MW00489386

ICD-10-CM Expert for Hospitals

The complete official code set

Codes valid from October 1, 2019
through September 30, 2020

2020

THE NEW WEBSITE HAS
LAUNCHED!
VISIT OPTUM360CODING.COM

Publisher's Notice

The *ICD-10-CM Expert for Hospitals: The Complete Official Code Set* is designed to be an accurate and authoritative source regarding coding and every reasonable effort has been made to ensure accuracy and completeness of the content. However, Optum360 makes no guarantee, warranty, or representation that this publication is accurate, complete or without errors. It is understood that Optum360 is not rendering any legal or other professional services or advice in this publication and that Optum360 bears no liability for any results or consequences that may arise from the use of this book.

Acknowledgments

Marianne Randall, CPC, *Product Manager*
Karen Schmidt, BSN, *Technical Director*
Anita Schmidt, BS, RHIA, AHIMA-approved ICD-10-CM/PCS
    Trainer, *Clinical Technical Editor*
Karen Krawzik, RHIT, CCS, AHIMA-approved ICD-10-CM/PCS
    Trainer, *Clinical Technical Editor*
Peggy Willard, CCS, AHIMA-approved ICD-10-CM/PCS
    Trainer, *Clinical Technical Editor*
Leanne Patterson, CPC, *Clinical Technical Editor*
LaJuana Green, RHIA, CCS, *Clinical Technical Editor*
Stacy Perry, *Manager, Desktop Publishing*
Lisa Singley, *Project Manager*
Tracy Betzler, *Senior Desktop Publishing Specialist*
Hope M. Dunn, *Senior Desktop Publishing Specialist*
Katie Russell, *Desktop Publishing Specialist*
Kate Holden, *Editor*

Our Commitment to Accuracy

Optum360 is committed to producing accurate and reliable materials.

To report corrections, please visit www.optum360coding.com/accuracy or email accuracy@optum.com. You can also reach customer service by calling 1.800.464.3649, option 1.

Copyright

Property of Optum360, LLC. Optum360 and the Optum360 logo are trademarks of Optum360, LLC. All other brand or product names are trademarks or registered trademarks of their respective owner.

© 2019 Optum360, LLC. All rights reserved.

Made in the USA
ISBN 978-1-62254-526-1

Anita Schmidt, BS, RHIA, AHIMA-approved ICD-10-CM/PCS Trainer

Ms. Schmidt has expertise in ICD-10-CM/PCS, DRG, and CPT with more than 15 years' experience in coding in multiple settings, including inpatient, observation, and same-day surgery. Her experience includes analysis of medical record documentation, assignment of ICD-10-CM and PCS codes, and DRG validation. She has conducted training for ICD-10-CM/PCS and electronic health record. She has also collaborated with clinical documentation specialists to identify documentation needs and potential areas for physician education. Most recently she has been developing content for resource and educational products related to ICD-10-CM, ICD-10-PCS, DRG, and CPT. Ms. Schmidt is an AHIMA-approved ICD-10-CM/PCS trainer and is an active member of the American Health Information Management Association (AHIMA) and the Minnesota Health Information Management Association.

Peggy Willard, CCS, AHIMA-approved ICD-10-CM/PCS Trainer

Ms. Willard has 18 years of experience in the healthcare field. Her expertise is in ICD-10-CM and ICD-10-PCS, including in-depth analysis of medical record documentation, ICD-10-CM/PCS code and DRG assignment, as well as clinical documentation improvement (CDI). In recent years Ms. Willard has been responsible for the creation and development of several products for Optum360 Coding Solutions that are designed to assist with appropriate application of the ICD-10-CM and ICD-10-PCS coding systems. She has several years of prior experience in Level I adult and pediatric trauma hospital and inpatient rehabilitation facility (IRF) coding, specializing in ICD-9-CM diagnosis and procedural coding, with emphasis in conducting coding audits, and conducting coding training for coding staff and clinical documentation specialists. Ms. Willard is an AHIMA-approved ICD-10 CM/PCS trainer and is an active member of the American Health Information Management Association (AHIMA) and the Minnesota Health Information Management Association (MHIMA).

2020 ICD-10-CM Official Guidelines for Coding and Reporting

Optum360 is pleased to provide you with this 2020 ICD-10-CM code book that INCLUDES the 2020 Official Guidelines for Coding and Reporting.

Contents

Preface

ICD-10-CM Official Preface

This FY 2020 update of the International Statistical Classification of Diseases and Related Health Problems, 10th revision, Clinical Modification (ICD-10-CM) is being published by the United States government in recognition of its responsibility to promulgate this classification throughout the United States for morbidity coding. The International Statistical Classification of Diseases and Related Health Problems, 10th Revision (ICD-10), published by the World Health Organization (WHO), is the foundation of ICD-10-CM. ICD-10 continues to be the classification used in cause-of-death coding in the United States. The ICD-10-CM is comparable with the ICD-10. The WHO Collaborating Center for the Family of International Classifications in North America, housed at the Centers for Disease Control and Prevention's National Center for Health Statistics (NCHS), has responsibility for the implementation of ICD and other WHO-FIC classifications and serves as a liaison with the WHO, fulfilling international obligations for comparable classifications and the national health data needs of the United States. The historical background of ICD and ICD-10 can be found in the Introduction to the International Classification of Diseases and Related Health Problems (ICD-10), 2010, World Health Organization, Geneva, Switzerland.

ICD-10-CM is the United States' clinical modification of the World Health Organization's ICD-10. The term "clinical" is used to emphasize the modification's intent: to serve as a useful tool in the area of classification of morbidity data for indexing of health records, medical care review, and ambulatory and other health care programs, as well as for basic health statistics. To describe the clinical picture of the patient the codes must be more precise than those needed only for statistical groupings and trend analysis.

Characteristics of ICD-10-CM

ICD-10-CM far exceeds its predecessors in the number of concepts and codes provided. The disease classification has been expanded to include health-related conditions and to provide greater specificity at the sixth and seventh character level. The sixth and seventh characters are not optional and are intended for use in recording the information documented in the clinical record.

ICD-10-CM extensions, interpretations, modifications, addenda, or errata other than those approved by the Centers for Disease Control and Prevention are not to be considered official and should not be utilized. Continuous maintenance of the ICD-10-CM is the responsibility of the aforementioned agencies. However, because the ICD-10-CM represents the best in contemporary thinking of clinicians, nosologists, epidemiologists, and statisticians from both public and private sectors, when future modifications are considered, advice will be sought from all stakeholders.

All official authorized addenda since the last complete update (October 1, 2019) have been included in this revision. For more detailed information please see the complete official authorized addenda to ICD-10-CM, including the "ICD-10-CM Official Guidelines for Coding and Reporting," and a description of the ICD-10-CM updating and maintenance process.

How to Use ICD-10-CM Expert for Hospitals 2020

Introduction

ICD-10-CM Expert for Hospitals: The Complete Official Code Set is your definitive coding resource, combining the work of the National Center for Health Statistics (NCHS), Centers for Medicare and Medicaid Services (CMS), American Hospital Association (AHA), and Optum360 experts to provide the information you need for coding accuracy.

The International Classification of Diseases, 10th Revision, Clinical Modification (ICD-10-CM), is an adaptation of ICD-10, copyrighted by the World Health Organization (WHO). The development and maintenance of this clinical modification (CM) is the responsibility of the NCHS as authorized by WHO. Any new concepts added to ICD-10-CM are based on an established update process through the collaboration of WHO's Update and Revision Committee and the ICD-10-CM Coordination and Maintenance Committee.

In addition to the ICD-10-CM classification, other official government source information has been included in this manual. Depending on the source, updates to information may be annual or quarterly. This manual provides the most current information that was available at the time of publication. For updates to the source documents that may have occurred after this manual was published, please refer to the following:

- **National Center for Health Statistics (NCHS), International Classification of Diseases, Tenth Revision, Clinical Modification (ICD-10-CM)**

  https://www.cdc.gov/nchs/icd/icd10cm.htm

  https://www.cms.gov/Medicare/Coding/ICD10/2020-ICD-10-CM.html

- **Centers for Medicare and Medicaid Services (CMS) Inpatient Prospective Payment System Proposed Rule, FY2020**

  https://www.cms.gov/Medicare/Medicare-Fee-for-Service-Payment/AcuteInpatientPPS/IPPS-Regulations-and-Notices.html

- **Centers for Medicare and Medicaid Services (CMS) Inpatient Prospective Payment Final Rule Data Files, FY2019 - Definition of Medicare Code Edits, version 36 and ICD-10 MS-DRG Definitions Manual, version 36R1**

  https://www.cms.gov/Medicare/Medicare-Fee-for-Service-Payment/AcuteInpatientPPS/MS-DRG-Classifications-and-Software.html

- **Centers for Medicare & Medicaid Services (CMS) Risk Adjustment Model, version 24**

  https://www.cms.gov/Medicare/Health-Plans/MedicareAdvtgSpecRateStats/Risk-Adjustors.html

- **Centers for Medicare & Medicaid Services (CMS) Long-term Care Hospital Prospective Payment System Final Rule and Data Files**

  https://www.cms.gov/Medicare/Medicare-Fee-for-Service-Payment/LongTermCareHospitalPPS/LTCHPPS-Regulations-and-Notices-Items/LTCH-PPS-CMS-1694-F.html

- **American Hospital Association (AHA) Coding Clinics**

  https://www.codingclinicadvisor.com/

The official NCHS ICD-10-CM classification includes three main sections: the guidelines, the indexes, and the tabular list, all of which make up the bulk of this coding manual. To complement the classification, Optum360's coding experts have incorporated Medicare-related coding edits and proprietary features, such as supplementary notations, coding tools, and appendixes, into a comprehensive and easy-to-use reference. This publication is organized as follows:

What's New for 2020

This section provides a high-level overview of the changes made to the ICD-10-CM official code set for fiscal 2020, identifying codes that have been added and deleted from the classification, codes that had validity changes as a result of these additions and deletions, as well as codes that had revisions to their descriptions. All changes are based on the 2020 official addendum, posted June 20, 2019, by the National Center for Health Statistics (NCHS), the agency charged with maintaining and updating ICD-10-CM. NCHS is part of the Centers for Disease Control and Prevention (CDC).

Conversion Table

The conversion table was developed by National Center for Healthcare Statistics (NCHS) to help facilitate data retrieval as new codes are added to the ICD-10-CM classification. This table provides a crosswalk from each FY 2020 new code to the equivalent code(s) assigned prior to October 1, 2019, for that particular diagnosis or condition. For the full conversion table, including code crosswalks before October 1, 2019, refer to the 2020 Conversion Table zip file at https://www.cms.gov/Medicare/Coding/ICD10/2020-ICD-10-CM.html.

10 Steps to Correct Coding

This step-by-step tutorial walks the coder through the process of finding the correct code — from locating the code in the official indexes to verifying the code in the tabular section — while following applicable conventions, guidelines, and instructional notes. Specific examples are provided with detailed explanations of each coding step along with advice for proper sequencing.

Official ICD-10-CM Guidelines for Coding and Reporting

This section provides the full official conventions and guidelines regulating the appropriate assignment and reporting of ICD-10-CM codes. These conventions and guidelines are published by the U.S. Department of Health and Human Services (DHHS) and approved by the cooperating parties (American Health Information Management Association [AHIMA], National Center for Health Statistics [NCHS], Centers for Disease Control and Prevention [CDC], and the American Hospital Association [AHA]).

Indexes

Index to Diseases and Injuries

The Index to Diseases and Injuries is arranged in alphabetic order by terms specific to a disease, condition, illness, injury, eponym, or abbreviation as well as terms that describe circumstances other than a disease or injury that may require attention from a health care professional.

Neoplasm Table

The Neoplasm Table is arranged in alphabetic order by anatomical site. Codes are then listed in individual columns based upon the histological behavior (malignant, in situ, benign, uncertain, or unspecified) of the neoplasm.

Table of Drugs and Chemicals

The Table of Drugs and Chemicals is arranged in alphabetic order by the specific drug or chemical name. Codes are listed in individual columns based upon the associated intent (poisoning, adverse effect, or underdosing).

External Causes Index

The External Causes Index is arranged in alphabetic order by main terms that describe the cause, the intent, the place of occurrence, the activity, and the status of the patient at the time the injury occurred or health condition arose.

Index Notations

With

The word "with" or "in" should be interpreted to mean "associated with" or "due to." The classification presumes a causal relationship between the two conditions linked by these terms in the index. These conditions should be coded as related even in the absence of provider documentation explicitly linking them unless the documentation clearly states the conditions are unrelated or when another guideline specifically requires a documented linkage between two conditions (e.g., the sepsis guideline for "acute organ dysfunction that is not clearly associated with the sepsis"). For conditions not specifically linked by these relational terms in the classification or when a guideline requires explicit documentation of a linkage between two conditions, provider documentation must link the conditions to code them as related.

The word "with" in the index is sequenced immediately following the main term, not in alphabetical order.

> **Dermatopolymyositis** M33.90
> with
>   myopathy M33.92
>   respiratory involvement M33.91
>   specified organ involvement NEC M33.99
> in neoplastic disease — *see also* Neoplasm D49.9 [M36.0]

See

When the instruction "see" follows a term in the index, it indicates that another term must be referenced to locate the correct code.

> **Hematoperitoneum** — *see* Hemoperitoneum

See Also

The instructional note "see also" simply provides alternative terms the coder may reference that may be useful in determining the correct code but are not necessary to follow if the main term supplies the appropriate code.

> **Hematinuria** — *see also* Hemaglobinuria
>   malarial B50.8

Default Codes

In the index, the default code is the code listed next to the main term and represents the condition most commonly associated with that main term. This code may be assigned when documentation does not support reporting a more specific code. Alternatively, it may provide an unspecified code for the condition.

> **Headache** R51
>   allergic NEC G44.89
>   associated with sexual activity G44.82
>   chronic daily R51

Parentheses

Parentheses in the indexes enclose nonessential modifiers, supplementary words that may be present or absent in the statement of a disease without affecting the code.

> **Pseudomeningocele** (cerebral) (infective) (post-traumatic) G96.19
>   postprocedural (spinal) G97.82

Brackets

ICD-10-CM has a coding convention addressing code assignment for manifestations that occur as a result of an underlying condition. This convention requires the underlying condition to be sequenced first, followed by the code or codes for the associated manifestation. In the index, italicized codes in brackets identify manifestation codes.

> **Polyneuropathy** (peripheral) G62.9
>   alcoholic G62.1
>   amyloid (Portuguese) E85.1 *[G63]*
>   transthyretin-related (ATTR) familial E85.1 *[G63]*

Shaded Guides

Exclusive vertical shaded guides in the Index to Diseases and Injuries and External Causes Index help the user easily follow the indent levels for the subentries under a main term. Sequencing rules may apply depending on the level of indent for separate subentries.

> **Hemicrania**
>   congenital malformation Q00.0
>   continua G44.51
>   meaning migraine — *see also* Migraine G43.909
>   paroxysmal G44.039
>   chronic G44.049
>   intractable G44.041
>   not intractable G44.049
>   episodic G44.039
>   intractable G44.031
>   not intractable G44.039
>   intractable G44.031
>   not intractable G44.039

Following References

The Index to Diseases and Injuries includes following references to assist in locating out-of-sequence codes in the tabular list. Out-of-sequence codes contain an alphabetic character (letter) in the third- or 4th-character position. These codes are placed according to the classification rules — according to condition — not according to alphabetic or numeric sequencing rules.

> **Carcinoma** (malignant) — *see also* Neoplasm, by site, malignant
>   neuroendocrine — *see also* Tumor, neuroendocrine
>   high grade, any site C7A.1 (*following* C75)
>   poorly differentiated, any site C7A.1 (*following* C75)

Additional Character Required

The Index to Diseases and Injuries, Neoplasm Table, and External Causes Index provide an icon after certain codes to signify to the user that additional characters are required to make the code valid. The tabular list should be consulted for appropriate character selection.

> **Fall, falling** (accidental) W19 ☑
>   building W20.1 ☑

Tabular List of Diseases

ICD-10-CM codes and descriptions are arranged numerically within the tabular list of diseases with 19 separate chapters providing codes associated with a particular body system or nature of injury or disease. There is also a chapter providing codes for external causes of an injury or health conditions and finally a chapter for codes that address encounters with healthcare facilities for circumstances other than a disease or injury.

Code and Code Descriptions

ICD-10-CM is an alphanumeric classification system that contains categories, subcategories, and valid codes. The first character is always a letter with any additional characters represented by either a letter or number. A three-character category without further subclassification is equivalent to a valid three-character code. Valid codes may be three, four, five, six, or seven characters in length, with each level of subdivision after a three-character category representing a subcategory. The final level of subdivision is a valid code.

Boldface

Boldface type is used for all codes and descriptions in the tabular list.

Italics

Italicized type is used to identify manifestation codes, those codes that should not be reported as first-listed diagnoses.

Deleted Text

Strikethrough on a code and code description indicates a deletion from the classification for the current year.

Key Word

Green font is used throughout the Tabular List of Diseases to differentiate the key words that appear in similar code descriptions in a given category or subcategory. The key word convention is used only in those categories in which there are multiple codes with very similar descriptions with only a few words that differentiate them.

For example, refer to the list of codes below from category H55:

> ✓4ᵗʰ **H55** **Nystagmus and other** irregular eye movements
> ✓5ᵗʰ **H55.Ø** **Nystagmus**
> **H55.ØØ** **Unspecified nystagmus**
> **H55.Ø1** **Congenital nystagmus**
> **H55.Ø2** **Latent nystagmus**
> **H55.Ø3** **Visual deprivation nystagmus**
> **H55.Ø4** **Dissociated nystagmus**
> **H55.Ø9** **Other forms of nystagmus**

The portion of the code description that appears in **green font** in the tabular list helps the coder quickly identify the key terms and the correct code. This convention is especially useful when the codes describe laterality, such as the following codes from subcategory H4Ø.22:

> ✓6ᵗʰ **H4Ø.22** **Chronic angle-closure glaucoma**
> Chronic primary angle-closure glaucoma
> ✓7ᵗʰ **H4Ø.221** **Chronic angle-closure glaucoma, right eye**
> ✓7ᵗʰ **H4Ø.222** **Chronic angle-closure glaucoma, left eye**
> ✓7ᵗʰ **H4Ø.223** **Chronic angle-closure glaucoma, bilateral**
> ✓7ᵗʰ **H4Ø.229** **Chronic angle-closure glaucoma, unspecified eye**

Tabular Notations

Official parenthetical notes as well as Optum360's supplementary notations are provided at the chapter, code block, category, subcategory, and individual code level to help the user assign proper codes. The information in the notation can apply to one or more codes depending on where the citation is placed.

Official Notations

Includes Notes

The word INCLUDES appears immediately under certain categories to further define, clarify, or give examples of the content of a code category.

Inclusion Terms

Lists of inclusion terms are included under certain codes. These terms indicate some of the conditions for which that code number may be used. Inclusion terms may be synonyms with the code title, or, in the case of "other specified" codes, the terms may also provide a list of various conditions included within a classification code. The inclusion terms are not exhaustive. The index may provide additional terms that may also be assigned to a given code.

Excludes Notes

ICD-10-CM has two types of excludes notes. Each note has a different definition for use. However, they are similar in that they both indicate that codes excluded from each other are independent of each other.

Excludes 1

An EXCLUDES 1 note is a "pure" excludes. It means "NOT CODED HERE!" An Excludes 1 note indicates mutually exclusive codes: two conditions that cannot be reported together. An Excludes1 note indicates that the code excluded should never be used at the same time as the code above the Excludes1 note. An Excludes1 is used when two conditions cannot occur together, such as a congenital form versus an acquired form of the same condition.

An exception to the Excludes 1 definition is when the two conditions are unrelated to each other. If it is not clear whether the two conditions involving an Excludes 1 note are related or not, query the provider. For example, code F45.8 Other somatoform disorders, has an Excludes 1 note for "sleep related teeth grinding (G47.63)" because "teeth grinding" is an inclusion term under F45.8. Only one of these two codes should be assigned for teeth grinding. However, psychogenic dysmenorrhea is also an inclusion term under F45.8, and a patient could have both this condition and sleep-related teeth grinding. In this case, the two conditions are clearly unrelated to each other, so it would be appropriate to report F45.8 and G47.63 together.

Excludes 2

An EXCLUDES 2 note means "NOT INCLUDED HERE." An Excludes 2 note indicates that although the excluded condition is not part of the condition it is excluded from, a patient may have both conditions at the same time. Therefore, when an Excludes 2 note appears under a code, it may be acceptable to use both the code and the excluded code together if supported by the medical documentation.

Note

The term "NOTE" appears as an icon and precedes the instructional information. These notes function as alerts to highlight coding instructions within the text.

Code First/Use additional code

These instructional notes provide sequencing instruction. They may appear independently of each other or to designate certain etiology/manifestation paired codes. These instructions signal the coder that an additional code should be reported to provide a more complete picture of that diagnosis.

In etiology/manifestation coding, ICD-10-CM requires the underlying condition to be sequenced first, followed by the manifestation. In these situations, codes with "In diseases classified elsewhere" in the code description are never permitted as a first-listed or principal diagnosis code and must be sequenced following the underlying condition code.

Code Also

A "code also" note alerts the coder that more than one code may be required to fully describe the condition. The sequencing depends on the circumstances of the encounter. Factors that may determine sequencing include severity and reason for the encounter.

Revised Text

The revised text ►◄ "bow ties" alert the user to changes in official notations for the current year. Revised text may include the following:

- A change in a current parenthetical description

- A change in the code(s) associated with a current parenthetical note

- A change in how a current parenthetical note is classified (e.g., an Excludes 1 note that changed to an Excludes 2 note)

- Addition of a new parenthetical note(s) to a code

Deleted Text
~~Strikethrough~~ on official notations indicate a deletion from the classification for the current year.

Optum360 Notations

AHA Coding Clinic Citations
Coding Clinics are official American Hospital Associated (AHA) publications that provide coding advice specific to ICD-10-CM and ICD-10-PCS.

These citations identify the year, quarter, and page number of one or more *Coding Clinic* publications that may have coding advice relevant to a particular code or group of codes. With the most current citation listed first, these notations are preceded by the symbol **AHA:** and appear in purple type.

> **I15.1** **Hypertension secondary to** other renal disorders
> **AHA:** 2016, 3Q, 22

Definitions
Definitions explain a specific term, condition, or disease process in layman's terms. These notations are preceded by the symbol **DEF:** and appear in purple type.

> ✓5ᵗʰ **M51.4 Schmorl's nodes**
> **DEF:** Irregular bone defect in the margin of the vertebral body that causes herniation into the end plate of the vertebral body.

Coding Tips
The tips in the tabular list offer coding advice that is not readily available within the ICD-10-CM classification. It may relate official coding guidelines, indexing nuances, or advice from *AHA's Coding Clinic for ICD-10-CM/PCS*. These notations are preceded by the symbol **TIP:** and appear in brown type.

> **P15.8 Other specified birth injuries**
> **TIP:** Use for any injury of newborn from scalpel.

CC Excludes Notations
The assignment of an MS-DRG or MS-LTC-DRG often depends on the presence or absence of a secondary diagnosis code that is designated as an MCC or CC. However, in some instances the MCC or CC designation for that secondary diagnosis code is negated due to its relationship with the principal diagnosis.

To save space in this coding manual and provide a more comprehensive reference for the user, the CC Exclusion notations have been restructured. Instead of the individual codes being listed in the reference, which can in many cases be extensive, only the principal diagnosis collection (PDX collection) number is provided. A PDX collection contains a specific list of ICD-10-CM codes and their official descriptions that when used as principal diagnosis would render the MCC/CC designation ineffective. Each PDX collection is provided in an easily searchable data file which can be accessed at the following:

https://www.optum360coding.com/ProductUpdates/
Title: "2020 ICD-10-CM for Hospitals CC Excludes Data File"
Password: OptumCCExcl20

Similar to the parenthetical notes, the CC Exclusion notations are provided at the category, subcategory, and/or code level. If a CC Exclusion notation is found at the category or subcategory level, all the CC and/or MCC codes

in that category or subcategory share the same PDX collection listed in that notation. For example:

> ✓5ᵗʰ **G43.6 Persistent migraine aura with cerebral infarction**
> Code also the type of cerebral infarction (I63.-)
> **CC Excl: For CC codes in subcategory G43.6, unless otherwise noted:** PDX collection 584

Often a CC exclusion reference is specific to laterality for CC/MCC codes in a category or subcategory. Where possible, a CC exclusion reference is placed at the category or subcategory level with the PDX collection identified for the right, left, or unspecified side. For example:

> ✓4ᵗʰ **S58 Traumatic amputation of elbow and forearm**
> An amputation not identified as partial or complete should be coded to complete.
> EXCLUDES 1 *traumatic amputation of wrist and hand (S68.-)*
>
> The appropriate 7th character is to be added to each code from category S58.
> A initial encounter
> D subsequent encounter
> S sequela
>
> **CC Excl: For CC codes in category S58:**
> **Right side:** PDX collection 1266
> **Left side:** PDX collection 1267
> **Unspecified side:** PDX collection 1268

Where possible a "see" reference may also be used, referring the user to a previously designated CC excludes notation. For example:

> ✓5ᵗʰ **S72.0 Fracture of head and neck of femur**
> EXCLUDES 2 *physeal fracture of upper end of femur (S79.0-)*
> **AHA:** 2016, 3Q, 16
> **CC Excl: For CC/MCC codes in subcategory S72.0:**
> **Right side:** See code S72.001
> **Left side:** See code S72.002
> **Unspecified side:** See code S72.009

Note: CC Excludes notations in chapters 13 and 19 apply to 7th character A, unless otherwise noted.

Certain codes may also have no principal diagnosis codes to which they would be excluded from functioning as a CC or MCC. These are identified as follows:

> **I16.1 Hypertensive emergency**   CC
> **CC Excl:** No Excl

Icons
Note: The following icons are placed to the left of the code.

- ● **New Code**
  Codes that have been added to the classification system for the current year.

- ▲ **Revised Code Title**
  Codes that have had a change to their description or validity change for the current year. For additional information on codes with validity changes, see the "What's New" section.

- ✓ **Additional Characters Required**
  ✓4ᵗʰ This symbol indicates that the code requires a 4th character.

  ✓5ᵗʰ This symbol indicates that the code requires a 5th character.

  ✓6ᵗʰ This symbol indicates that the code requires a 6th character.

  ✓7ᵗʰ This symbol indicates that the code requires a 7th character.

> ✓5ᵗʰ **H60.3 Other infective otitis externa**
> ✓6ᵗʰ **H60.31** Diffuse otitis externa
> **H60.311** Diffuse otitis externa, right ear
> **H60.312** Diffuse otitis externa, left ear
> **H60.313** Diffuse otitis externa, bilateral
> **H60.319** Diffuse otitis externa, unspecified ear

✓x7ᵗʰ Placeholder Alert

This symbol indicates that the code requires a 7th character following the placeholder "X". Codes with fewer than six characters that require a 7th character must contain placeholder "X" to fill in the empty character(s).

> **✓x7ᵗʰ T16.1** Foreign body in **right** ear

Optum360 has provided a searchable data file that includes each edit listed below and all ICD-10-CM codes associated with that edit. These comprehensive lists are based on FY 2020 IPPS final rule official files, effective October 1, 2019:

- Age
- Sex
- Hospital-acquired condition (HAC)
- CC
- MCC
- HIV
- Manifestation code
- Unacceptable diagnosis
- Questionable diagnosis

This data file can be accessed at the following:

https://www.optum360coding.com/ProductUpdates/
Title: "2020 ICD-10-CM for Hospital IPPS Data File"
Password: OptumIPPS20

Note: The following icons are placed to the right of the code description.

Age Edits

Codes intended for a specific age group based on CMS MCE designations, v36.

Ⓝ Newborn Age: 0

These diagnoses are intended for newborns and neonates and the patient's age must be 0 years.

> **N47.0** Adherent prepuce, newborn　　　　Ⓝ♂

Ⓟ Pediatric Age: 0-17

These diagnoses are intended for children and the patient's age must be between 0 and 17 years.

> **L21.1** Seborrheic infantile dermatitis　　　　Ⓟ

Ⓜ Maternity Age: 9-64

These diagnoses are intended for childbearing patients between the age of 9 and 64 years.

> **O02.9** Abnormal product of conception, unspecified　　Ⓜ♀

Ⓐ Adult Age: 15-124

These diagnoses are intended for patients between the age of 15 and 124 years.

> **R54** Age-related physical debility　　　　Ⓐ
> 　　　Frailty
> 　　　Old age
> 　　　Senescence
> 　　　Senile asthenia
> 　　　Senile debility
> 　　　**EXCLUDES 1** *age-related cognitive decline (R41.81)*
> 　　　　　*sarcopenia (M62.84)*
> 　　　　　*senile psychosis (F03)*
> 　　　　　*senility NOS (R41.81)*

Sex Edits

Codes intended for a specific sex based on CMS MCE designations, v36.

♂ Male diagnosis only

> **Q98.0** Klinefelter syndrome karyotype 47, XXY　　♂

♀ Female diagnosis only

> **N35.12** Postinfective urethral stricture, not elsewhere classified, **female**　　♀

H1 - H14 Hospital Acquired Condition (HAC)

These codes identify conditions that are high cost or high volume or both, are either a complication or comorbidity (CC) or major complication or comorbidity (MCC) that as a secondary diagnosis results in assignment of a case to a higher-paying MS-DRG. These conditions are reasonably preventable through the application of evidence-based guidelines. If the condition is not present on admission (meaning it developed during the hospital admission), the case will not group to the higher-paying MS-DRG based solely upon the reporting of the HAC code. Many of these HACs are conditional, and are based on reporting the specific diagnosis code(s) in combination with certain procedure codes, notated in footnotes.

Note: Hospital-acquired conditions do not impact MS-LTC-DRG assignment.

The comprehensive list of HAC tables that coincide with these icon numbers appears in appendix G of this book.

> **N15.1** Renal and perinephric abscess　　　MCC H6
> 　　　**CC Excl:** PDX collection 919

CC CC Condition

This symbol designates a complication or comorbidity diagnosis that may affect DRG assignment. A complication or comorbidity diagnosis, CC condition, is defined as a significant acute disease, a significant acute manifestation of a chronic disease, an advanced or end-stage chronic disease, or a chronic disease associated with systemic physiological decompensation and debility that have consistently greater impact on hospital resources.

A comprehensive list of ICD-10-CM codes considered a CC appears in appendix E of this book.

> **G90.59** Complex regional pain syndrome I of other specified site　　CC

MCC MCC Condition

This symbol designates a major complication or comorbidity diagnosis that may affect DRG assignment. An MCC condition meets the same criteria as a CC condition but is associated with a higher acuity level and hospital resource consumption is expected to be higher than that for a CC condition. There are fewer conditions that meet the criteria as an MCC than those for a CC condition.

A comprehensive list of ICD-10-CM codes considered an MCC appears in appendix D of this book.

> **✓7ᵗʰ S35.238** Other injury of inferior mesenteric artery　　MCC

HIV HIV-related Condition

This symbol indicates that the condition is considered a major HIV-related diagnosis. When the condition is coded in combination with a diagnosis of human immunodeficiency virus (HIV), code B20, the case will move from MS-DRG/MS-LTC-DRG 977 to MS-DRGs/MS-LTC-DRGs 974-976.

> **G96.9** Disorder of central nervous system, unspecified　　HIV

CMS-HCC Condition

Identify conditions that are considered a CMS-HCC (hierarchical condition category) diagnosis.

The HCC codes represented in this manual have been updated to reflect the 2020 Initial ICD-10-CM Mappings for CMS-HCC Model v24. Midyear final mappings were not available at the time this publication went to print; refer to the following CMS website for final mappings: https://www.cms.gov/Medicare/Health-Plans/MedicareAdvtgSpecRateStats/Risk-Adjustors.html.

> **Y62.2** **Failure of sterile precautions during kidney dialysis and other perfusion** `HCC`

Severe Wound Diagnosis

This symbol indicates that the condition is considered a severe wound diagnosis. Depending on the facility from which the patient is discharged, these conditions may not require that the payment rate for that admission be adjusted.

A comprehensive list of ICD-10-CM codes considered a severe wound diagnosis appears in appendix K of this book.

> **L89.014** **Pressure ulcer of right elbow, stage 4** `CC` `HCC` `SW`

Color Bars

Manifestation Code

Codes defined as manifestation codes appear in italic type, with a blue color bar over the code description. A manifestation cannot be reported as a first-listed code; it is sequenced as a secondary diagnosis with the underlying disease code listed first.

> *G32.89* *Other specified degenerative disorders of nervous system in diseases classified elsewhere*
>   Degenerative encephalopathy in diseases classified elsewhere

Unacceptable Principal Diagnoses

Unacceptable principal diagnoses will appear with a purple color bar over the code description. These codes do not describe a current illness or injury, but a circumstance which influences a patient's health status. They are considered an unacceptable principal diagnosis for *inpatient* admission.

> `✓7ᵗʰ` **T48.5X5** **Adverse effect of other anti-common-cold drugs**

Questionable Admission Diagnoses

Questionable admission diagnoses will appear with a yellow color bar over the code description. These codes, although not unacceptable as a PDx, may be considered a "questionable admission" when used as PDx in an acute care hospital.

> **E66.09** **Other obesity due to excess calories**

Wrong Procedure Performed Edit

An orange color bar over the code title indicates the Wrong Procedure Performed edit. This edit was created to identify cases in which wrong surgeries occurred. Any claim with a code from Y65.51–Y65.53 will be denied and returned to the provider. A surgical or other invasive procedure is considered to be a wrong procedure if one of the following is true:

- The procedure was performed on the wrong site.
- The procedure was performed on the wrong patient.
- The incorrect procedure was performed on a patient.

> **Y65.51** **Performance of wrong procedure (operation) on correct patient**
>   Wrong device implanted into correct surgical site
>   `EXCLUDES 1` *performance of correct procedure (operation) on wrong side or body part (Y65.53)*

Unspecified Diagnosis

Codes that appear with a gray color bar over the alphanumeric code identify unspecified diagnoses. These codes should be used in limited circumstances, when neither the diagnostic statement nor the documentation provides enough information to assign a more specific diagnosis code. The abbreviation NOS, "not otherwise specified," in the tabular list may be interpreted as "unspecified."

> **G03.9** **Meningitis, unspecified**
>   Arachnoiditis (spinal) NOS

Footnotes

Certain codes in the tabular section have a numerical superscript located to the upper left of the code. This numerical superscript corresponds to a specific footnote description.

For example:

> [1] **R57.1** **Hypovolemic shock** `MCC` `HCC`

For convenience, the footnote descriptions are provided on the front cover.

The following list also provides the footnote descriptions of all numerical superscripts found in the Tabular List of Diseases:

1. These codes are considered major complication/comorbidity (MCC) conditions only if the patient is discharged alive.
2. This condition is considered an MCC only when reported as an initial encounter for an open fracture (7th character B or C specific to category).
3. This condition is considered a CC only when reported as an initial encounter for a fracture (7th character A, B, or C specific to category) or a subsequent encounter for nonunion or malunion fracture (7th character K, M, N, P, Q, or R specific to category).
4. This condition is considered a CC only when reported as a subsequent encounter for a nonunion or malunion fracture (7th character K, M, N, P, Q, or R specific to category).
5. This condition is considered a CC only when reported as an initial encounter or subsequent encounter (7th character A or D).
6. This condition is considered an HCC when reported as initial encounter (7th character A, B, or C specific to category).
7. This condition is considered an HCC when reported as initial encounter (7th character A or B specific to category) or as a sequela.
8. This condition is considered an HCC when reported as a sequela.

Chapter-Level Notations

Chapter-Specific Guidelines with Coding Examples

Each chapter begins with the Official Guidelines for Coding and Reporting specific to that chapter, where provided. Coding examples specific to outpatient care settings have been provided to illustrate the coding and/or sequencing guidance in these guidelines.

Muscle and Tendon Table

ICD-10-CM categorizes certain muscles and tendons in the upper and lower extremities by their action (e.g., extension or flexion) as well as their anatomical location. The Muscle/Tendon table is provided at the beginning of chapter 13 and chapter 19 to help users when code selection depends on the action of the muscle and/or tendon.

Note: This table is not all-inclusive, and proper code assignment should be based on the provider's documentation.

Appendixes

The additional resources described below have been included as appendixes for the *ICD-10-CM Expert for Hospitals*. These resources further instruct the professional coder on the appropriate application of the ICD-10-CM code set.

Appendix A: Valid 3-character ICD-10-CM Codes

The user may consult this table to confirm that no further specificity, such as the use of 4th, 5th, 6th, or 7th characters or placeholders (X), is necessary. All ICD-10-CM codes that are valid at the three-character level are listed.

Appendix B: Pharmacology List 2020

This reference is a comprehensive but not all-inclusive list of pharmacological agents used to treat acute and/or chronic conditions. Drugs are listed in alphabetical order by their brand and/or generic names along with their drug action and indications for which they may commonly be prescribed. Some drugs have also been mapped to their appropriate long-term drug use Z code.

Appendix C: Z Codes for Long-Term Drug Use with Associated Drugs

This resource correlates Z codes that are used to identify current long-term drug use with a list of drugs that are typically categorized to that class of drug.

Note: These tables are not all-inclusive but list some of the more commonly used drugs.

Appendix D: Major Complication and Comorbidity (MCC) Code List

This is a full listing of conditions considered to be major complications and/or comorbidities that when present as a secondary diagnosis may affect DRG assignment under the Medicare Severity DRG (MS-DRG) system.

Appendix E: Complication and Comorbidity (CC) Code List

This is a full listing of conditions considered to be complications and/or comorbidities that when present as a secondary diagnosis may affect DRG assignment under the MS-DRG system.

Appendix F: Present on Admission (POA) Tutorial

This tutorial walks the coder through the process of assigning the appropriate present-on-admission (POA) indicator for inpatient codes based on the POA reporting guidelines. Detailed scenarios for a variety of situations are provided and discussed.

Appendix G: Hospital Acquired Conditions

This comprehensive table displays codes that identify conditions that are considered reasonably preventable when occurring during the hospital admission and may prevent the case from grouping to a higher-paying MS-DRG. Many of these HACs are conditional and are based on reporting the specific diagnosis code(s) in combination with certain procedure codes, which are also noted in this table.

Appendix H: Centers for Medicare & Medicaid Services (CMS) Hierarchical Condition Categories (HCC) (CMS-HCC)

This resource provides the framework behind CMS's Medicare Advantage (MA) program, a risk-adjustment model developed as a means of compensating health care plans with large numbers of Medicare Part C beneficiaries. It includes a brief synopsis of the evolution of the program from its inception; insight into the various elements needed to predict risk, including the principles used to develop the hierarchical condition categories (HCCs), one of the fundamental components of the risk adjustment model; and a description of the audit process used to ensure the accuracy of payments made to MA plans.

Appendix I: Long-term Care Hospital Prospective Payment System Overview

The long-term care hospital prospective payment system (LTCH PPS) provides payment rates for LTCH facilities certified by Medicare as LTCH with an average length of stay (LOS) of 25 days or longer. This resource summarizes the certification qualifications for LTCH facilities, payment methodology, and current fiscal year PPS updates.

Appendix J: Long-Term Care Hospital Quality Reporting Program

The LTCH QRP is a mandatory reporting component for LTCH facilities certified by Medicare as LTCH with an average LOS of 25 days or longer. Much of the current QRP for LTCH, like other post-acute care providers, is based upon the requirements of the 2014 IMPACT Act. This resource summarizes the current QRP requirements for facilities certified as LTCH under Medicare, including required data set items and market-basket payment impact.

Appendix K: Severe Wound Diagnosis Codes by Category

This resource includes a full listing of codes identified as severe wound diagnoses that may allow certain discharges from LTCHs a temporary exception from the site-neutral payment rate.

Illustrations

This section includes illustrations of normal anatomy with ICD-10-CM-specific terminology.

Official Updates

The official ICD-10-CM addendum was posted to the Centers for Medicare and Medicaid Services (CMS) website on June 20, 2019, identifying the changes to the ICD-10-CM code set for fiscal 2020, effective October 1, 2019, to September 30, 2020. These changes were made by the agency charged with maintaining and updating the ICD-10-CM code set, the National Center for Health Statistics (NCHS), a section of the Centers for Disease Control and Prevention (CDC). A summary of the changes is provided below:

15 Codes with a Change in Validity

Note: Validity changes are the result of codes being added to or deleted from the classification. Codes that change from valid to invalid allow the creation of a new subcategory to which new codes can be assigned that provide greater detail about the condition. Codes that change from invalid to valid are the result of codes being deleted from a subcategory in the classification, when the detail provided in those codes is no longer required.

Valid to Invalid

D81.3	I48.1	I48.2	Q66.0	Q66.1
Q66.21	Q66.22	Q66.3	Q66.4	Q66.7
Q66.9	Q79.6	Q87.1	R82.8	

Invalid to Valid

H81.4

7 Codes Deleted from the Classification

H81.41	Vertigo of central origin, right ear
H81.42	Vertigo of central origin, left ear
H81.43	Vertigo of central origin, bilateral
H81.49	Vertigo of central origin, unspecified ear
T67.0XXA	Heatstroke and sunstroke, initial encounter
T67.0XXD	Heatstroke and sunstroke, subsequent encounter
T67.0XXS	Heatstroke and sunstroke, sequela

273 New Codes Added to the Classification

D75.A	Glucose-6-phosphate dehydrogenase (G6PD) deficiency without anemia
D81.30	Adenosine deaminase deficiency, unspecified
D81.31	Severe combined immunodeficiency due to adenosine deaminase deficiency
D81.32	Adenosine deaminase 2 deficiency
D81.39	Other adenosine deaminase deficiency
I26.93	Single subsegmental pulmonary embolism without acute cor pulmonale
I26.94	Multiple subsegmental pulmonary emboli without acute cor pulmonale
I48.11	Longstanding persistent atrial fibrillation
I48.19	Other persistent atrial fibrillation
I48.20	Chronic atrial fibrillation, unspecified
I48.21	Permanent atrial fibrillation
I80.241	Phlebitis and thrombophlebitis of right peroneal vein
I80.242	Phlebitis and thrombophlebitis of left peroneal vein
I80.243	Phlebitis and thrombophlebitis of peroneal vein, bilateral
I80.249	Phlebitis and thrombophlebitis of unspecified peroneal vein
I80.251	Phlebitis and thrombophlebitis of right calf muscular vein
I80.252	Phlebitis and thrombophlebitis of left calf muscular vein
I80.253	Phlebitis and thrombophlebitis of calf muscular vein, bilateral
I80.259	Phlebitis and thrombophlebitis of unspecified calf muscular vein
I82.451	Acute embolism and thrombosis of right peroneal vein
I82.452	Acute embolism and thrombosis of left peroneal vein
I82.453	Acute embolism and thrombosis of peroneal vein, bilateral
I82.459	Acute embolism and thrombosis of unspecified peroneal vein
I82.461	Acute embolism and thrombosis of right calf muscular vein
I82.462	Acute embolism and thrombosis of left calf muscular vein
I82.463	Acute embolism and thrombosis of calf muscular vein, bilateral
I82.469	Acute embolism and thrombosis of unspecified calf muscular vein
I82.551	Chronic embolism and thrombosis of right peroneal vein
I82.552	Chronic embolism and thrombosis of left peroneal vein
I82.553	Chronic embolism and thrombosis of peroneal vein, bilateral
I82.559	Chronic embolism and thrombosis of unspecified peroneal vein
I82.561	Chronic embolism and thrombosis of right calf muscular vein
I82.562	Chronic embolism and thrombosis of left calf muscular vein
I82.563	Chronic embolism and thrombosis of calf muscular vein, bilateral
I82.569	Chronic embolism and thrombosis of unspecified calf muscular vein
L89.006	Pressure-induced deep tissue damage of unspecified elbow
L89.016	Pressure-induced deep tissue damage of right elbow
L89.026	Pressure-induced deep tissue damage of left elbow
L89.106	Pressure-induced deep tissue damage of unspecified part of back
L89.116	Pressure-induced deep tissue damage of right upper back
L89.126	Pressure-induced deep tissue damage of left upper back
L89.136	Pressure-induced deep tissue damage of right lower back
L89.146	Pressure-induced deep tissue damage of left lower back
L89.156	Pressure-induced deep tissue damage of sacral region
L89.206	Pressure-induced deep tissue damage of unspecified hip
L89.216	Pressure-induced deep tissue damage of right hip
L89.226	Pressure-induced deep tissue damage of left hip
L89.306	Pressure-induced deep tissue damage of unspecified buttock
L89.316	Pressure-induced deep tissue damage of right buttock
L89.326	Pressure-induced deep tissue damage of left buttock
L89.46	Pressure-induced deep tissue damage of contiguous site of back, buttock and hip
L89.506	Pressure-induced deep tissue damage of unspecified ankle
L89.516	Pressure-induced deep tissue damage of right ankle
L89.526	Pressure-induced deep tissue damage of left ankle
L89.606	Pressure-induced deep tissue damage of unspecified heel

L89.616	Pressure-induced deep tissue damage of right heel
L89.626	Pressure-induced deep tissue damage of left heel
L89.816	Pressure-induced deep tissue damage of head
L89.896	Pressure-induced deep tissue damage of other site
L89.96	Pressure-induced deep tissue damage of unspecified site
N63.15	Unspecified lump in the right breast, overlapping quadrants
N63.25	Unspecified lump in the left breast, overlapping quadrants
N99.85	Post endometrial ablation syndrome
Q66.00	Congenital talipes equinovarus, unspecified foot
Q66.01	Congenital talipes equinovarus, right foot
Q66.02	Congenital talipes equinovarus, left foot
Q66.10	Congenital talipes calcaneovarus, unspecified foot
Q66.11	Congenital talipes calcaneovarus, right foot
Q66.12	Congenital talipes calcaneovarus, left foot
Q66.211	Congenital metatarsus primus varus, right foot
Q66.212	Congenital metatarsus primus varus, left foot
Q66.219	Congenital metatarsus primus varus, unspecified foot
Q66.221	Congenital metatarsus adductus, right foot
Q66.222	Congenital metatarsus adductus, left foot
Q66.229	Congenital metatarsus adductus, unspecified foot
Q66.30	Other congenital varus deformities of feet, unspecified foot
Q66.31	Other congenital varus deformities of feet, right foot
Q66.32	Other congenital varus deformities of feet, left foot
Q66.40	Congenital talipes calcaneovalgus, unspecified foot
Q66.41	Congenital talipes calcaneovalgus, right foot
Q66.42	Congenital talipes calcaneovalgus, left foot
Q66.70	Congenital pes cavus, unspecified foot
Q66.71	Congenital pes cavus, right foot
Q66.72	Congenital pes cavus, left foot
Q66.90	Congenital deformity of feet, unspecified, unspecified foot
Q66.91	Congenital deformity of feet, unspecified, right foot
Q66.92	Congenital deformity of feet, unspecified, left foot
Q79.60	Ehlers-Danlos syndrome, unspecified
Q79.61	Classical Ehlers-Danlos syndrome
Q79.62	Hypermobile Ehlers-Danlos syndrome
Q79.63	Vascular Ehlers-Danlos syndrome
Q79.69	Other Ehlers-Danlos syndromes
Q87.11	Prader-Willi syndrome
Q87.19	Other congenital malformation syndromes predominantly associated with short stature
R11.15	Cyclical vomiting syndrome unrelated to migraine
R82.81	Pyuria
R82.89	Other abnormal findings on cytological and histological examination of urine
S02.121A	Fracture of orbital roof, right side, initial encounter for closed fracture
S02.121B	Fracture of orbital roof, right side, initial encounter for open fracture
S02.121D	Fracture of orbital roof, right side, subsequent encounter for fracture with routine healing
S02.121G	Fracture of orbital roof, right side, subsequent encounter for fracture with delayed healing
S02.121K	Fracture of orbital roof, right side, subsequent encounter for fracture with nonunion
S02.121S	Fracture of orbital roof, right side, sequela
S02.122A	Fracture of orbital roof, left side, initial encounter for closed fracture
S02.122B	Fracture of orbital roof, left side, initial encounter for open fracture
S02.122D	Fracture of orbital roof, left side, subsequent encounter for fracture with routine healing
S02.122G	Fracture of orbital roof, left side, subsequent encounter for fracture with delayed healing
S02.122K	Fracture of orbital roof, left side, subsequent encounter for fracture with nonunion
S02.122S	Fracture of orbital roof, left side, sequela
S02.129A	Fracture of orbital roof, unspecified side, initial encounter for closed fracture
S02.129B	Fracture of orbital roof, unspecified side, initial encounter for open fracture
S02.129D	Fracture of orbital roof, unspecified side, subsequent encounter for fracture with routine healing
S02.129G	Fracture of orbital roof, unspecified side, subsequent encounter for fracture with delayed healing
S02.129K	Fracture of orbital roof, unspecified side, subsequent encounter for fracture with nonunion
S02.129S	Fracture of orbital roof, unspecified side, sequela
S02.831A	Fracture of medial orbital wall, right side, initial encounter for closed fracture
S02.831B	Fracture of medial orbital wall, right side, initial encounter for open fracture
S02.831D	Fracture of medial orbital wall, right side, subsequent encounter for fracture with routine healing
S02.831G	Fracture of medial orbital wall, right side, subsequent encounter for fracture with delayed healing
S02.831K	Fracture of medial orbital wall, right side, subsequent encounter for fracture with nonunion
S02.831S	Fracture of medial orbital wall, right side, sequela
S02.832A	Fracture of medial orbital wall, left side, initial encounter for closed fracture
S02.832B	Fracture of medial orbital wall, left side, initial encounter for open fracture
S02.832D	Fracture of medial orbital wall, left side, subsequent encounter for fracture with routine healing
S02.832G	Fracture of medial orbital wall, left side, subsequent encounter for fracture with delayed healing
S02.832K	Fracture of medial orbital wall, left side, subsequent encounter for fracture with nonunion
S02.832S	Fracture of medial orbital wall, left side, sequela
S02.839A	Fracture of medial orbital wall, unspecified side, initial encounter for closed fracture
S02.839B	Fracture of medial orbital wall, unspecified side, initial encounter for open fracture
S02.839D	Fracture of medial orbital wall, unspecified side, subsequent encounter for fracture with routine healing
S02.839G	Fracture of medial orbital wall, unspecified side, subsequent encounter for fracture with delayed healing
S02.839K	Fracture of medial orbital wall, unspecified side, subsequent encounter for fracture with nonunion
S02.839S	Fracture of medial orbital wall, unspecified side, sequela

S02.841A	Fracture of lateral orbital wall, right side, initial encounter for closed fracture
S02.841B	Fracture of lateral orbital wall, right side, initial encounter for open fracture
S02.841D	Fracture of lateral orbital wall, right side, subsequent encounter for fracture with routine healing
S02.841G	Fracture of lateral orbital wall, right side, subsequent encounter for fracture with delayed healing
S02.841K	Fracture of lateral orbital wall, right side, subsequent encounter for fracture with nonunion
S02.841S	Fracture of lateral orbital wall, right side, sequela
S02.842A	Fracture of lateral orbital wall, left side, initial encounter for closed fracture
S02.842B	Fracture of lateral orbital wall, left side, initial encounter for open fracture
S02.842D	Fracture of lateral orbital wall, left side, subsequent encounter for fracture with routine healing
S02.842G	Fracture of lateral orbital wall, left side, subsequent encounter for fracture with delayed healing
S02.842K	Fracture of lateral orbital wall, left side, subsequent encounter for fracture with nonunion
S02.842S	Fracture of lateral orbital wall, left side, sequela
S02.849A	Fracture of lateral orbital wall, unspecified side, initial encounter for closed fracture
S02.849B	Fracture of lateral orbital wall, unspecified side, initial encounter for open fracture
S02.849D	Fracture of lateral orbital wall, unspecified side, subsequent encounter for fracture with routine healing
S02.849G	Fracture of lateral orbital wall, unspecified side, subsequent encounter for fracture with delayed healing
S02.849K	Fracture of lateral orbital wall, unspecified side, subsequent encounter for fracture with nonunion
S02.849S	Fracture of lateral orbital wall, unspecified side, sequela
S02.85XA	Fracture of orbit, unspecified, initial encounter for closed fracture
S02.85XB	Fracture of orbit, unspecified, initial encounter for open fracture
S02.85XD	Fracture of orbit, unspecified, subsequent encounter for fracture with routine healing
S02.85XG	Fracture of orbit, unspecified, subsequent encounter for fracture with delayed healing
S02.85XK	Fracture of orbit, unspecified, subsequent encounter for fracture with nonunion
S02.85XS	Fracture of orbit, unspecified, sequela
T50.911A	Poisoning by multiple unspecified drugs, medicaments and biological substances, accidental (unintentional), initial encounter
T50.911D	Poisoning by multiple unspecified drugs, medicaments and biological substances, accidental (unintentional), subsequent encounter
T50.911S	Poisoning by multiple unspecified drugs, medicaments and biological substances, accidental (unintentional), sequela
T50.912A	Poisoning by multiple unspecified drugs, medicaments and biological substances, intentional self-harm, initial encounter
T50.912D	Poisoning by multiple unspecified drugs, medicaments and biological substances, intentional self-harm, subsequent encounter
T50.912S	Poisoning by multiple unspecified drugs, medicaments and biological substances, intentional self-harm, sequela
T50.913A	Poisoning by multiple unspecified drugs, medicaments and biological substances, assault, initial encounter
T50.913D	Poisoning by multiple unspecified drugs, medicaments and biological substances, assault, subsequent encounter
T50.913S	Poisoning by multiple unspecified drugs, medicaments and biological substances, assault, sequela
T50.914A	Poisoning by multiple unspecified drugs, medicaments and biological substances, undetermined, initial encounter
T50.914D	Poisoning by multiple unspecified drugs, medicaments and biological substances, undetermined, subsequent encounter
T50.914S	Poisoning by multiple unspecified drugs, medicaments and biological substances, undetermined, sequela
T50.915A	Adverse effect of multiple unspecified drugs, medicaments and biological substances, initial encounter
T50.915D	Adverse effect of multiple unspecified drugs, medicaments and biological substances, subsequent encounter
T50.915S	Adverse effect of multiple unspecified drugs, medicaments and biological substances, sequela
T50.916A	Underdosing of multiple unspecified drugs, medicaments and biological substances, initial encounter
T50.916D	Underdosing of multiple unspecified drugs, medicaments and biological substances, subsequent encounter
T50.916S	Underdosing of multiple unspecified drugs, medicaments and biological substances, sequela
T67.01XA	Heatstroke and sunstroke, initial encounter
T67.01XD	Heatstroke and sunstroke, subsequent encounter
T67.01XS	Heatstroke and sunstroke, sequela
T67.02XA	Exertional heatstroke, initial encounter
T67.02XD	Exertional heatstroke, subsequent encounter
T67.02XS	Exertional heatstroke, sequela
T67.09XA	Other heatstroke and sunstroke, initial encounter
T67.09XD	Other heatstroke and sunstroke, subsequent encounter
T67.09XS	Other heatstroke and sunstroke, sequela
Y35.009A	Legal intervention involving unspecified firearm discharge, unspecified person injured, initial encounter
Y35.009D	Legal intervention involving unspecified firearm discharge, unspecified person injured, subsequent encounter
Y35.009S	Legal intervention involving unspecified firearm discharge, unspecified person injured, sequela
Y35.019A	Legal intervention involving injury by machine gun, unspecified person injured, initial encounter
Y35.019D	Legal intervention involving injury by machine gun, unspecified person injured, subsequent encounter
Y35.019S	Legal intervention involving injury by machine gun, unspecified person injured, sequela
Y35.029A	Legal intervention involving injury by handgun, unspecified person injured, initial encounter
Y35.029D	Legal intervention involving injury by handgun, unspecified person injured, subsequent encounter
Y35.029S	Legal intervention involving injury by handgun, unspecified person injured, sequela
Y35.039A	Legal intervention involving injury by rifle pellet, unspecified person injured, initial encounter
Y35.039D	Legal intervention involving injury by rifle pellet, unspecified person injured, subsequent encounter

Y35.039S Legal intervention involving injury by rifle pellet, unspecified person injured, sequela

Y35.049A Legal intervention involving injury by rubber bullet, unspecified person injured, initial encounter

Y35.049D Legal intervention involving injury by rubber bullet, unspecified person injured, subsequent encounter

Y35.049S Legal intervention involving injury by rubber bullet, unspecified person injured, sequela

Y35.099A Legal intervention involving other firearm discharge, unspecified person injured, initial encounter

Y35.099D Legal intervention involving other firearm discharge, unspecified person injured, subsequent encounter

Y35.099S Legal intervention involving other firearm discharge, unspecified person injured, sequela

Y35.109A Legal intervention involving unspecified explosives, unspecified person injured, initial encounter

Y35.109D Legal intervention involving unspecified explosives, unspecified person injured, subsequent encounter

Y35.109S Legal intervention involving unspecified explosives, unspecified person injured, sequela

Y35.119A Legal intervention involving injury by dynamite, unspecified person injured, initial encounter

Y35.119D Legal intervention involving injury by dynamite, unspecified person injured, subsequent encounter

Y35.119S Legal intervention involving injury by dynamite, unspecified person injured, sequela

Y35.129A Legal intervention involving injury by explosive shell, unspecified person injured, initial encounter

Y35.129D Legal intervention involving injury by explosive shell, unspecified person injured, subsequent encounter

Y35.129S Legal intervention involving injury by explosive shell, unspecified person injured, sequela

Y35.199A Legal intervention involving other explosives, unspecified person injured, initial encounter

Y35.199D Legal intervention involving other explosives, unspecified person injured, subsequent encounter

Y35.199S Legal intervention involving other explosives, unspecified person injured, sequela

Y35.209A Legal intervention involving unspecified gas, unspecified person injured, initial encounter

Y35.209D Legal intervention involving unspecified gas, unspecified person injured, subsequent encounter

Y35.209S Legal intervention involving unspecified gas, unspecified person injured, sequela

Y35.219A Legal intervention involving injury by tear gas, unspecified person injured, initial encounter

Y35.219D Legal intervention involving injury by tear gas, unspecified person injured, subsequent encounter

Y35.219S Legal intervention involving injury by tear gas, unspecified person injured, sequela

Y35.299A Legal intervention involving other gas, unspecified person injured, initial encounter

Y35.299D Legal intervention involving other gas, unspecified person injured, subsequent encounter

Y35.299S Legal intervention involving other gas, unspecified person injured, sequela

Y35.309A Legal intervention involving unspecified blunt objects, unspecified person injured, initial encounter

Y35.309D Legal intervention involving unspecified blunt objects, unspecified person injured, subsequent encounter

Y35.309S Legal intervention involving unspecified blunt objects, unspecified person injured, sequela

Y35.319A Legal intervention involving baton, unspecified person injured, initial encounter

Y35.319D Legal intervention involving baton, unspecified person injured, subsequent encounter

Y35.319S Legal intervention involving baton, unspecified person injured, sequela

Y35.399A Legal intervention involving other blunt objects, unspecified person injured, initial encounter

Y35.399D Legal intervention involving other blunt objects, unspecified person injured, subsequent encounter

Y35.399S Legal intervention involving other blunt objects, unspecified person injured, sequela

Y35.409A Legal intervention involving unspecified sharp objects, unspecified person injured, initial encounter

Y35.409D Legal intervention involving unspecified sharp objects, unspecified person injured, subsequent encounter

Y35.409S Legal intervention involving unspecified sharp objects, unspecified person injured, sequela

Y35.419A Legal intervention involving bayonet, unspecified person injured, initial encounter

Y35.419D Legal intervention involving bayonet, unspecified person injured, subsequent encounter

Y35.419S Legal intervention involving bayonet, unspecified person injured, sequela

Y35.499A Legal intervention involving other sharp objects, unspecified person injured, initial encounter

Y35.499D Legal intervention involving other sharp objects, unspecified person injured, subsequent encounter

Y35.499S Legal intervention involving other sharp objects, unspecified person injured, sequela

Y35.819A Legal intervention involving manhandling, unspecified person injured, initial encounter

Y35.819D Legal intervention involving manhandling, unspecified person injured, subsequent encounter

Y35.819S Legal intervention involving manhandling, unspecified person injured, sequela

Y35.831A Legal intervention involving a conducted energy device, law enforcement official injured, initial encounter

Y35.831D Legal intervention involving a conducted energy device, law enforcement official injured, subsequent encounter

Y35.831S Legal intervention involving a conducted energy device, law enforcement official injured, sequela

Y35.832A Legal intervention involving a conducted energy device, bystander injured, initial encounter

Y35.832D Legal intervention involving a conducted energy device, bystander injured, subsequent encounter

Y35.832S Legal intervention involving a conducted energy device, bystander injured, sequela

Y35.833A Legal intervention involving a conducted energy device, suspect injured, initial encounter

Y35.833D Legal intervention involving a conducted energy device, suspect injured, subsequent encounter

Y35.833S Legal intervention involving a conducted energy device, suspect injured, sequela

Y35.839A	Legal intervention involving a conducted energy device, unspecified person injured, initial encounter
Y35.839D	Legal intervention involving a conducted energy device, unspecified person injured, subsequent encounter
Y35.839S	Legal intervention involving a conducted energy device, unspecified person injured, sequela
Y35.99XA	Legal intervention, means unspecified, unspecified person injured, initial encounter
Y35.99XD	Legal intervention, means unspecified, unspecified person injured, subsequent encounter
Y35.99XS	Legal intervention, means unspecified, unspecified person injured, sequela
Z01.020	Encounter for examination of eyes and vision following failed vision screening without abnormal findings
Z01.021	Encounter for examination of eyes and vision following failed vision screening with abnormal findings
Z11.7	Encounter for testing for latent tuberculosis infection
Z22.7	Latent tuberculosis
Z71.84	Encounter for health counseling related to travel
Z86.002	Personal history of in-situ neoplasm of other and unspecified genital organs
Z86.003	Personal history of in-situ neoplasm of oral cavity, esophagus and stomach
Z86.004	Personal history of in-situ neoplasm of other and unspecified digestive organs
Z86.005	Personal history of in-situ neoplasm of middle ear and respiratory system
Z86.006	Personal history of melanoma in-situ
Z86.007	Personal history of in-situ neoplasm of skin
Z86.15	Personal history of latent tuberculosis infection
Z96.82	Presence of neurostimulator

30 Code Descriptions Revised

Note: Each code is listed with its revised description only. Please refer to the full FY 2020 official addenda code files at https://www.cms.gov/Medicare/Coding/ICD10/2020-ICD-10-CM.html for the specific changes made to the codes listed.

B96.21	Shiga toxin-producing Escherichia coli [E. coli] [STEC] O157 as the cause of diseases classified elsewhere
B96.22	Other specified Shiga toxin-producing Escherichia coli [E. coli] [STEC] as the cause of diseases classified elsewhere
B96.23	Unspecified Shiga toxin-producing Escherichia coli [E. coli] [STEC] as the cause of diseases classified elsewhere
G43.A0	Cyclical vomiting, in migraine, not intractable
G43.A1	Cyclical vomiting, in migraine, intractable
I70.238	Atherosclerosis of native arteries of right leg with ulceration of other part of lower leg
I70.248	Atherosclerosis of native arteries of left leg with ulceration of other part of lower leg
J44.0	Chronic obstructive pulmonary disease with (acute) lower respiratory infection
M50.120	Mid-cervical disc disorder, unspecified level
M66.88	Spontaneous rupture of other tendons, other sites

M67.839	Other specified disorders of synovium and tendon, unspecified wrist
M77.50	Other enthesopathy of unspecified foot and ankle
M77.51	Other enthesopathy of right foot and ankle
M77.52	Other enthesopathy of left foot and ankle
N35.814	Other anterior urethral stricture, male
R82.993	Hyperuricosuria
T40.906A	Underdosing of unspecified psychodysleptics [hallucinogens], initial encounter
T40.906D	Underdosing of unspecified psychodysleptics [hallucinogens], subsequent encounter
T40.906S	Underdosing of unspecified psychodysleptics [hallucinogens], sequela
T40.996A	Underdosing of other psychodysleptics [hallucinogens], initial encounter
T40.996D	Underdosing of other psychodysleptics [hallucinogens], subsequent encounter
T40.996S	Underdosing of other psychodysleptics [hallucinogens], sequela
T44.1X6A	Underdosing of other parasympathomimetics [cholinergics], initial encounter
T44.1X6D	Underdosing of other parasympathomimetics [cholinergics], subsequent encounter
T44.1X6S	Underdosing of other parasympathomimetics [cholinergics], sequela
V43.13XA	Car passenger injured in collision with pick-up truck in nontraffic accident, initial encounter
V43.13XD	Car passenger injured in collision with pick-up truck in nontraffic accident, subsequent encounter
V43.13XS	Car passenger injured in collision with pick-up truck in nontraffic accident, sequela
Z45.42	Encounter for adjustment and management of neurostimulator
Z68.43	Body mass index (BMI) 50.0-59.9, adult

Proprietary Updates

The following proprietary features have also been added:

- 40+ new definitions that describe, in lay terms, a specific condition or disease process

- 40+ new coding tips that provide coding advice beyond the code classification

- Updated *AHA Coding Clinic* references through second quarter 2019

Conversion Table of ICD-10-CM Codes

Code Assignment Beginning 10/1/2019	Previous Code(s) Assignment	Code Assignment Beginning 10/1/2019	Previous Code(s) Assignment	Code Assignment Beginning 10/1/2019	Previous Code(s) Assignment
D75.A	D55.0	L89.316	L89.310	S02.121A	S02.19A*
D81.30	D81.3	L89.326	L89.320	S02.121B	S02.19B*
D81.31	D81.3	L89.46	L89.45	S02.121D	S02.19D*
D81.32	D81.3	L89.506	L89.500	S02.121G	S02.19G*
D81.39	D81.3	L89.516	L89.510	S02.121K	S02.19K*
H81.4	H81.41–H81.43; H81.49	L89.526	L89.520	S02.121S	S02.19S*
I26.93	I26.99	L89.606	L89.600	S02.122A	S02.19A*
I26.94	I26.99	L89.616	L89.610	S02.122B	S02.19B*
I48.11	I48.1	L89.626	L89.620	S02.122D	S02.19D*
I48.19	I48.1	L89.816	L89.810	S02.122G	S02.19G*
I48.20	I48.2	L89.896	L89.890	S02.122K	S02.19K*
I48.21	I48.2	L89.96	L89.95	S02.122S	S02.19S*
I80.241	I80.291	N63.15	N63.11–N63.14	S02.129A	S02.19A*
I80.242	I80.292	N63.25	N63.21–N63.24	S02.129B	S02.19B*
I80.243	I80.293	N99.85	N99.89	S02.129D	S02.19D*
I80.249	I80.299	Q66.00	Q66.0	S02.129G	S02.19G*
I80.251	I80.291	Q66.01	Q66.0	S02.129K	S02.19K*
I80.252	I80.292	Q66.02	Q66.0	S02.129S	S02.19S*
I80.253	I80.293	Q66.10	Q66.1	S02.831A	S02.81XA
I80.259	I80.299	Q66.11	Q66.1	S02.831B	S02.81XB
I82.451	I80.491	Q66.12	Q66.1	S02.831D	S02.81XD
I82.452	I80.492	Q66.211	Q66.21	S02.831G	S02.81XG
I82.453	I80.493	Q66.212	Q66.21	S02.831K	S02.81XK
I82.459	I80.499	Q66.219	Q66.21	S02.831S	S02.81XS
I82.461	I80.491	Q66.221	Q66.22	S02.832A	S02.82XA
I82.462	I80.492	Q66.222	Q66.22	S02.832B	S02.82XB
I82.463	I80.493	Q66.229	Q66.22	S02.832D	S02.82XD
I82.469	I80.499	Q66.30	Q66.3	S02.832G	S02.82XG
I82.551	I80.591	Q66.31	Q66.3	S02.832K	S02.82XK
I82.552	I80.592	Q66.32	Q66.3	S02.832S	S02.82XS
I82.553	I80.593	Q66.40	Q66.4	S02.839A	S02.80XA
I82.559	I80.599	Q66.41	Q66.4	S02.839B	S02.80XB
I82.561	I80.591	Q66.42	Q66.4	S02.839D	S02.80XD
I82.562	I80.592	Q66.70	Q66.7	S02.839G	S02.80XG
I82.563	I80.593	Q66.71	Q66.7	S02.839K	S02.80XK
I82.569	I80.599	Q66.72	Q66.7	S02.839S	S02.80XS
L89.006	L89.000	Q66.90	Q66.9	S02.841A	S02.81XA
L89.016	L89.010	Q66.91	Q66.9	S02.841B	S02.81XB
L89.026	L89.020	Q66.92	Q66.9	S02.841D	S02.81XD
L89.106	L89.100	Q79.60	Q79.6	S02.841G	S02.81XG
L89.116	L89.110	Q79.61	Q79.6	S02.841K	S02.81XK
L89.126	L89.120	Q79.62	Q79.6	S02.841S	S02.81XS
L89.136	L89.130	Q79.63	Q79.6	S02.842A	S02.82XA
L89.146	L89.140	Q79.69	Q79.6	S02.842B	S02.82XB
L89.156	L89.150	Q87.11	Q87.1	S02.842D	S02.82XD
L89.206	L89.200	Q87.19	Q87.1	S02.842G	S02.82XG
L89.216	L89.210	R11.15	K31.89 and a code from R11-	S02.842K	S02.82XK
L89.226	L89.220			S02.842S	S02.82XS
L89.306	L89.300	R82.81	R82.8	S02.849A	S02.80XA
		R82.89	R82.8	S02.849B	S02.80XB

Code Assignment Beginning 10/1/2019	Previous Code(s) Assignment	Code Assignment Beginning 10/1/2019	Previous Code(s) Assignment	Code Assignment Beginning 10/1/2019	Previous Code(s) Assignment
S02.849D	S02.80XD	Y35.029A	None	Y35.409D	None
S02.849G	S02.80XG	Y35.029D	None	Y35.409S	None
S02.849K	S02.80XK	Y35.029S	None	Y35.419A	None
S02.849S	S02.80XS	Y35.039A	None	Y35.419D	None
S02.85XA	S02.80XA	Y35.039D	None	Y35.419S	None
S02.85XB	S02.80XB	Y35.039S	None	Y35.499A	None
S02.85XD	S02.80XD	Y35.049A	None	Y35.499D	None
S02.85XG	S02.80XG	Y35.049D	None	Y35.499S	None
S02.85XK	S02.80XK	Y35.049S	None	Y35.819A	None
S02.85XS	S02.80XS	Y35.099A	None	Y35.819D	None
T50.911A	T50.991A	Y35.099D	None	Y35.819S	None
T50.911D	T50.991D	Y35.099S	None	Y35.831A	Y35.891A
T50.911S	T50.991S	Y35.109A	None	Y35.831D	Y35.891D
T50.912A	T50.992A	Y35.109D	None	Y35.831S	Y35.891S
T50.912D	T50.992D	Y35.109S	None	Y35.832A	Y35.892A
T50.912S	T50.992S	Y35.119A	None	Y35.832D	Y35.892D
T50.913A	T50.993A	Y35.119D	None	Y35.832S	Y35.892S
T50.913D	T50.993D	Y35.119S	None	Y35.833A	Y35.893A
T50.913S	T50.993S	Y35.129A	None	Y35.833D	Y35.893D
T50.914A	T50.994A	Y35.129D	None	Y35.833S	Y35.893S
T50.914D	T50.994D	Y35.129S	None	Y35.839A	None
T50.914S	T50.994S	Y35.199A	None	Y35.839D	None
T50.915A	T50.995A	Y35.199D	None	Y35.839S	None
T50.915D	T50.995D	Y35.199S	None	Y35.99XA	None
T50.915S	T50.995S	Y35.209A	None	Y35.99XD	None
T50.916A	T50.996A	Y35.209D	None	Y35.99XS	None
T50.916D	T50.996D	Y35.209S	None	Z01.020	Z01.00
T50.916S	T50.996S	Y35.219A	None	Z01.021	Z01.01
T67.01XA	T67.0XXA	Y35.219D	None	Z11.7	Z11.1
T67.01XD	T67.0XXD	Y35.219S	None	Z22.7	R76.11
T67.01XS	T67.0XXS	Y35.299A	None	Z71.84	Z71.89
T67.02XA	T67.0XXA	Y35.299D	None	Z86.002	Z86.008
T67.02XD	T67.0XXD	Y35.299S	None	Z86.003	Z86.008
T67.02XS	T67.0XXS	Y35.309A	None	Z86.004	Z86.008
T67.09XA	T67.0XXA	Y35.309D	None	Z86.005	Z86.008
T67.09XD	T67.0XXD	Y35.309S	None	Z86.006	Z86.008
T67.09XS	T67.0XXS	Y35.319A	None	Z86.007	Z86.008
Y35.009A	None	Y35.319D	None	Z86.15	R76.11
Y35.009D	None	Y35.319S	None	Z96.82	Z96.89
Y35.009S	None	Y35.399A	None		
Y35.019A	None	Y35.399D	None		
Y35.019D	None	Y35.399S	None		
Y35.019S	None	Y35.409A	None		

* These codes are listed exactly as found in the official conversion table from the CDC.

10 Steps to Correct Coding

Follow the 10 steps below to correctly code encounters for health care services.

Step 1: Identify the reason for the visit or encounter (i.e., a sign, symptom, diagnosis and/or condition).

The medical record documentation should accurately reflect the patient's condition, using terminology that includes specific diagnoses and symptoms or clearly states the reasons for the encounter.

Choosing the main term that best describes the reason chiefly responsible for the service provided is the most important step in coding. If symptoms are present and documented but a definitive diagnosis has not yet been determined, code the symptoms. *For outpatient cases, do not code conditions that are referred to as "rule out," "suspected," "probable," or "questionable."* Diagnoses often are not established at the time of the initial encounter/visit and may require two or more visits to be established. Code only what is documented in the available outpatient records and only to the highest degree of certainty known at the time of the patient's visit. For inpatient medical records, uncertain diagnoses may be reported if documented at the time of discharge.

Step 2: After selecting the reason for the encounter, consult the alphabetic index.

The most critical rule is to begin code selection in the alphabetic index. Never turn first to the tabular list. The index provides cross-references, essential and nonessential modifiers, and other instructional notations that may not be found in the tabular list.

Step 3: Locate the main term entry.

The alphabetic index lists conditions, which may be expressed as nouns or eponyms, with critical use of adjectives. Some conditions known by several names have multiple main entries. Reasons for encounters may be located under general terms such as admission, encounter, and examination. Other general terms such as history, status (post), or presence (of) can be used to locate other factors influencing health.

Step 4: Scan subterm entries.

Scan the subterm entries, as appropriate, being sure to review continued lines and additional subterms that may appear in the next column or on the next page. Shaded vertical guidelines in the index indicate the indentation level for each subterm in relation to the main terms.

Step 5: Pay close attention to index instructions.

- Parentheses ( ) enclose nonessential modifiers, terms that are supplementary words or explanatory information that may or may not appear in the diagnostic statement and do not affect code selection.

- Brackets [ ] enclose manifestation codes that can be used only as secondary codes to the underlying condition code immediately preceding it. If used, manifestation codes must be reported with the appropriate etiology codes.

- Default codes are listed next to the main term and represent the condition most commonly associated with the main term or the unspecified code for the main term.

- "See" cross-references, identified by italicized type and "code by" cross-references indicate that another term *must be referenced* to locate the correct code.

- "See also" cross-references, identified by italicized type, provide alternative terms that may be useful to look up but *are not mandatory.*

- "Omit code" cross-references identify instances when a code is not applicable depending on the condition being coded.

- "With" subterms are listed out of alphabetic order and identify a presumed causal relationship between the two conditions they link.

- "Due to" subterms identify a relationship between the two conditions they link.

- "NEC," abbreviation for "not elsewhere classified," follows some main terms or subterms and indicates that there is no specific code for the condition even though the medical documentation may be very specific.

- "NOS," abbreviation for "not otherwise specified," follows some main terms or subterms and is the equivalent of unspecified; NOS signifies that the information in the medical record is insufficient for assigning a more specific code.

- *Following* references help coders locate alphanumeric codes that are out of sequence in the tabular section.

- Check-additional-character symbols flag codes that require additional characters to make the code valid; the characters available to complete the code should be verified in the tabular section.

Step 6: Choose a potential code and locate it in the tabular list.

To prevent coding errors, always use both the alphabetic index (to identify a code) and the tabular list (to verify a code), as the index does not include the important instructional notes found in the tabular list. An added benefit of using the tabular list, which groups like things together, is that while looking at one code in the list, a coder might see a more specific one that would have been missed had the coder relied solely on the alphabetic index. Additionally, many of the codes require a fourth, fifth, sixth, or seventh character to be valid, and many of these characters can be found only in the tabular list.

Step 7: Read all instructional material in the tabular section.

The coder must follow any Includes, Excludes 1 and Excludes 2 notes, and other instructional notes, such as "Code first" and "Use additional code," listed in the tabular list for the chapter, category, subcategory, and subclassification levels of code selection that direct the coder to use a different or additional code. Any codes in the tabular range A00.0- through T88.9- may be used to identify the diagnostic reason for the encounter. The tabular list encompasses many codes describing disease and injury classifications (e.g., infectious and parasitic diseases, neoplasms, symptoms, nervous and circulatory system etc.).

Codes that describe symptoms and signs, as opposed to definitive diagnoses, should be reported when an established diagnosis has not been made (confirmed) by the physician. Chapter 18 of the ICD-10-CM code book, "Symptoms, Signs, and Abnormal Clinical and Laboratory Findings, Not Elsewhere Classified" (codes R00.--R99), contains many, but not all, codes for symptoms.

ICD-10-CM classifies encounters with health care providers for circumstances other than a disease or injury in chapter 21, "Factors Influencing Health Status and Contact with Health Services" (codes Z00–Z99). Circumstances other than a disease or injury often are recorded as chiefly responsible for the encounter.

A code is invalid if it does not include the full number of characters (greatest level of specificity) required. Codes in ICD-10-CM can contain from three to seven alphanumeric characters. A three-character code is to be used only if the category is not further subdivided into four-, five-, six-, or seven-character codes. Placeholder character X is used as part of an alphanumeric code to allow for future expansion and as a placeholder for empty characters in a code that requires a seventh character but has no fourth, fifth, or sixth character. Note that certain categories require seventh characters that apply to all codes in that category. Always check the category level for applicable seventh characters for that category.

Step 8: Consult the official ICD-10-CM conventions and guidelines.

The *ICD-10-CM Official Guidelines for Coding and Reporting* govern the use of certain codes. These guidelines provide both general and chapter-specific coding guidance.

Step 9: Confirm and assign the code.

Having reviewed all relevant information concerning the possible code choices, assign the code that most completely describes the condition.

Repeat steps 1 through 9 for all additional documented conditions that meet the following criteria:

- They exist at the time of the visit *AND*
- They require or affect patient care, treatment, or management

Step 10: Sequence codes correctly.

Sequencing is the order in which the codes are listed on the claim. List first the ICD-10-CM code for the diagnosis, condition, problem, or other reason for the encounter/visit that is shown in the medical record to be chiefly responsible for the services provided. List additional codes that describe any coexisting conditions. Follow the official coding guidelines (see the guidelines, section II, "Selection of Principal Diagnosis"; section III, "Reporting Additional Diagnoses"; and section IV, "Diagnostic Coding and Reporting Guidelines for Outpatient Services") on proper sequencing of codes.

Coding Examples

Diagnosis: Anorexia

Step 1: The reason for the encounter was the condition, anorexia.

Step 2: Consult the alphabetic index.

Step 3: Locate the main term "Anorexia."

Step 4: Two possible subterms are available, "hysterical" and "nervosa." Neither is documented in this instance, however, so they cannot be used in code selection.

Step 5: The code listed next to the main term is called the default code selection. Because the two subentries (essential modifiers) do not apply in this instance, the default code (R63.Ø) should be used.

Step 6: Turn to code R63.Ø in the tabular list and read all instructional notes.

Step 7: The Excludes 1 note at code R63.Ø indicates that anorexia nervosa and loss of appetite determined to be of nonorganic origin should be reported with a code from chapter 5. The diagnostic statement does not describe the condition as anorexia nervosa, however, and does not indicate that the anorexia is of a nonorganic origin. There is no further division of the category past the fourth-character subcategory. Therefore, code R63.Ø is at the highest level of specificity.

Step 8: Review of official guideline I.C.18 indicates that a symptom code is appropriate when a more definitive diagnosis is not documented.

Step 9: The default code, R63.Ø Anorexia, is the correct code selection.

Repeat steps 1 through 9 for any concomitant diagnoses.

Step 10: Since anorexia is listed as the chief reason for the health care encounter, the first-listed, or principal, diagnosis is R63.Ø. Note that this is a chapter 18 symptom code but can be assigned for both inpatient and outpatient records since the provider did not establish a more definitive diagnosis, according to sections II.A and IV.D.

Diagnosis: Acute bronchitis

Step 1: The reason for the encounter was the condition, acute bronchitis.

Step 2: Consult the alphabetic index.

Step 3: Locate the main term "Bronchitis."

Step 4: There is a subterm for "acute or subacute." Additional subterms are not included in the diagnostic statement.

Step 5: Review the instructional notes. Nonessential modifiers (with bronchospasm or obstruction) are terms that do not affect code assignment. Since no other subterms indented under "acute" apply here, the code listed next to this subentry—in this case J20.9—should be chosen.

Step 6: Turn to code J20.9 in the tabular list and read all instructional notes.

Step 7: The Includes note under category J20 lists alternative terms for acute bronchitis. Note that the list is not exhaustive but is only a representative selection of diagnoses that are included in the subcategory. The Excludes 1 note refers to category J40 for bronchitis and tracheobronchitis NOS. There are several conditions in the Excludes 2 notes that, if applicable, can be coded in addition to this code.

Note that the codes included in J20 represent acute bronchitis due to various infectious organisms that could be selected if identified in the documentation. In this case, the organism was not identified and there is no further division of the category past the fourth character subcategory. Therefore, code J20.9 is at the highest level of specificity.

Step 8: Review of official guideline I.C.10 provides no additional information affecting the code selected.

Step 9: Assign code J20.9 Acute bronchitis, unspecified.

Repeat steps 1 through 9 for any concomitant diagnoses.

Step 10: In the absence of additional diagnoses that may affect sequencing, code J20.9 should be sequenced as the first-listed, or principal, diagnosis.

Diagnosis: Cerebellar ataxia in myxedema

Step 1: The reason for the encounter was the condition, cerebellar ataxia.

Step 2: Consult the alphabetic index.

Step 3: Locate the main term "Ataxia."

Step 4: Available subterms include "cerebellar (hereditary)," with additional indented subterms for "in" and "myxedema," all essential modifiers that are included in the diagnostic statement. Two codes are provided, E03.9 and G13.2, the latter of which is in brackets.

Step 5: Note the nonessential modifier (in parentheses) after the subterm cerebellar includes the term "hereditary." Because it is in parentheses, this term is not required in the diagnostic statement for this subentry to apply. The brackets around G13.2 identify this code as a manifestation of the condition described by code E03.9 and indicate that the two must be reported together and sequencing rules apply.

Step 6: Locate codes E03.9 and G13.2 in the tabular list, and read all instructional notes.

Step 7: For code E03.9, there are no instructional notes in the tabular list at the category E03 or code level that indicate that this condition should be coded elsewhere in the classification or that additional codes are required. Without further information from the diagnostic statement, myxedema, not otherwise specified (NOS), is appropriately reported with code E03.9 Hypothyroidism, unspecified, according to the inclusion term at this code.

Code G13.2 in the tabular list has an instructional note to "Code first underlying disease," which includes conditions found in category E03.-. Based on this note, codes E03.9 and G13.2 are to be coded together, with G13.2 listed only as a secondary diagnosis. This correlates with what the alphabetic index indicated. As there is no further division of codes in category G13 beyond the fourth character, G13.2 is at the highest level of specificity.

Step 8: Although there are some general conventions, such as how to interpret brackets in the alphabetic index, no chapter-specific guidelines apply to this coding scenario.

Step 9: Assign codes E03.9 Hypothyroidism, unspecified, and G13.2 Systemic atrophy primarily affecting the central nervous system in myxedema.

Repeat steps 1 through 9 for any concomitant diagnoses.

Step 10: Based on the alphabetic index and tabular instructional notations, code E03.9 should be sequenced as the first-listed, or principal, diagnosis followed by G13.2 as a secondary diagnosis.

Diagnosis: Decubitus ulcer of right elbow with skin loss and necrosis of subcutaneous tissue

Step 1: The reason for the encounter was the condition, decubitus ulcer.

Step 2: Consult the alphabetic index.

Step 3: Locate the main term "Ulcer."

Step 4: For the subterm "decubitus," there is no code provided or additional subterms indented, but a cross-reference is listed.

Step 5: The italicized cross-reference instructs the coder to "*see* Ulcer, pressure, by site."

Repeat steps 3 through 5 for the cross-reference.

Step 3: Locate the main term "Ulcer."

Step 4: Review the subentries for the subterm "pressure." The next level of indent lists either the site of the ulcer or the specific stage of the ulcer (stage 1–4, unstageable, and unspecified stages). The diagnostic statement provides the site, right elbow, and the extent of tissue damage (skin loss and necrosis of subcutaneous tissue) but does not specifically state that the ulcer is stage 1, stage 2, etc. Nonessential modifiers (in parentheses) at each stage include a description of the typical extent of damage at each stage. For example, stage 1 describes "pre-ulcer skin changes limited to persistent focal edema." Based on the documentation in the record, the coder can correlate the documentation to the nonessential modifiers and choose the specific stage from the index. The coder can also go directly to the body site, choosing the stage of the ulcer after reviewing the code options and instructional notations in the tabular list.

The diagnostic statement indicates that the extent of the damage to the elbow includes skin loss and necrosis of subcutaneous tissue, coinciding with the nonessential modifier next to the subentry "stage 3." The body site of elbow (L89.0-) is listed as another level of indent with other body sites.

Step 5: Note that code L89.0 is followed by a dash and an additional-character-required icon, which indicate that more characters are needed to complete the code. From here, the tabular listing for L89.0- can be consulted.

Step 6: Locate code L89.0- in the tabular list and read all instructional notes.

Step 7: The tabular listing at category L89 has an Includes note for "decubitus ulcer," which confirms that category L89 is the appropriate category to represent what is documented in the diagnostic statement.

Several Excludes 2 notes are also listed at the category level. Excludes 2 notes represent conditions that can occur concomitantly with the decubitus ulcer and can be coded in addition to code L89, if supported by the documentation.

The subcategory codes under L89.0 indicate that the fifth character describes laterality. Locate the right elbow at subcategory L89.01. See that an additional sixth character to specify the stage of the ulcer is now needed to complete the code. The stage can be determined either by the specific documentation of the stage (e.g., stage 1, stage 2) or, in this case, a description that matches one of the inclusion terms that follow

each stage code. For example, the diagnostic description in this case of "skin loss and necrosis of the subcutaneous tissue" matches the inclusion term under L89.013 Pressure ulcer of right elbow, stage 3. No additional characters are required because code L89.013 is at its highest level of specificity.

Step 8: The official guidelines contain quite a bit of information relating to pressure ulcers in chapter-specific guideline I.C.12 as well as information in general guideline I.B.14. These and any other pertinent guidelines should be reviewed to ensure appropriate code assignment.

Step 9: Assign code L89.013 Pressure ulcer of right elbow, stage 3.

Repeat steps 1 through 9 for any concomitant diagnoses.

Step 10: Since the decubitus ulcer is listed as the chief reason for the health care encounter, the first-listed, or principal, diagnosis is L89.013. However, according to the code first instructional note at the L89 category level, gangrene (I96) would be sequenced before the pressure ulcer if it were documented.

Diagnosis: Emergency department visit for bimalleolar fracture of the right ankle due to trauma

Step 1: The reason for the encounter was the condition, bimalleolar fracture.

Step 2: Consult the alphabetic index.

Step 3: Locate the main term "Fracture." Note that many main terms represent fractures: "Fracture, burst," "Fracture, chronic," "Fracture, insufficiency," "Fracture, nontraumatic NEC," "Fracture, pathological," and "Fracture, traumatic." Since the diagnostic statement specifically states that this fracture was the result of trauma, the main term "Fracture, traumatic" should be used.

Step 4: Subterms that should be referenced are "ankle" and "bimalleolar (displaced)," which lists code S82.84-.

Step 5: A nonessential modifier (in parentheses) next to the term bimalleolar for "displaced" indicates that S82.84- is the default category unless the fracture is specifically identified as "nondisplaced."

Note that code S82.84- is followed by a dash and an additional-character icon, both of which indicate that more characters are required. From here, the tabular list can be consulted.

Step 6: Locate code S82.84- in the tabular list and read all instructional notes.

Step: 7 The instructional notes at category S82 indicate that fractures not specified as displaced or nondisplaced default to displaced and that fractures not designated as open or closed default to closed. Additional instructional notes can be found at the category level but none pertain to the current scenario.

Read through the subcategory codes under S82.84, and note that the sixth character specifies displaced or nondisplaced and laterality. Based on the index nonessential modifier (displaced) and the code note at category S82, code selection should identify a displaced fracture of the right side. A displaced bimalleolar fracture of the right lower leg is coded to S82.841.

To complete the code, a seventh character must be assigned to identify the type of encounter (initial, subsequent, or sequela) and whether the fracture is open or closed. Most of the codes in category S82 require a seventh character represented in the list at the category level. However, it is important to note that some subcategories have their own specific set of seventh characters. In this instance, subcategory S82.84- does not have a unique set of seventh characters and the list provided at the category level should be used. Without documentation of the fracture being open, the tabular notation indicates that the default is closed. Character A, representing "initial encounter for closed fracture," listed in the box at the category level is the most appropriate option.

Step 8: Assign code S82.841A Displaced bimalleolar fracture of right lower leg, initial encounter for closed fracture.

Repeat steps 1 through 9 for any concomitant diagnoses.

Step 9: Review chapter-specific guideline I.C.19. and any other official conventions or guidelines to ensure appropriate code assignment.

Step 10: Additional codes can be applied to relate the specific cause of the injury, the place of occurrence, the activity of the patient at the time of the injury, and the patient's status, when this information is available in the record. However, coding this information is voluntary and reporting requirements depend on state mandates and/or facility-specific reporting requirements. If assigned, the external cause codes should be reported as secondary diagnoses only with the injury (fracture) sequenced first. Most codes in chapter 20, "External Causes of Morbidity," require a seventh character to identify the type of encounter. The seventh character assigned to an external cause code should match the seventh character of the code assigned for the associated injury or condition for the encounter.

2020 ICD-10-CM Official Guidelines for Coding and Reporting

Narrative changes appear in **bold** text

Items <u>underlined</u> have been moved within the guidelines since the FY 2019 version

Italics are used to indicate revisions to heading changes

The Centers for Medicare and Medicaid Services (CMS) and the National Center for Health Statistics (NCHS), two departments within the U.S. Federal Government's Department of Health and Human Services (DHHS) provide the following guidelines for coding and reporting using the International Classification of Diseases, 10th Revision, Clinical Modification (ICD-10-CM). These guidelines should be used as a companion document to the official version of the ICD-10-CM as published on the NCHS website. The ICD-10-CM is a morbidity classification published by the United States for classifying diagnoses and reason for visits in all health care settings. The ICD-10-CM is based on the ICD-10, the statistical classification of disease published by the World Health Organization (WHO).

These guidelines have been approved by the four organizations that make up the Cooperating Parties for the ICD-10-CM: the American Hospital Association (AHA), the American Health Information Management Association (AHIMA), CMS, and NCHS.

These guidelines are a set of rules that have been developed to accompany and complement the official conventions and instructions provided within the ICD-10-CM itself. The instructions and conventions of the classification take precedence over guidelines. These guidelines are based on the coding and sequencing instructions in the Tabular List and Alphabetic Index of ICD-10-CM, but provide additional instruction. Adherence to these guidelines when assigning ICD-10-CM diagnosis codes is required under the Health Insurance Portability and Accountability Act (HIPAA). The diagnosis codes (Tabular List and Alphabetic Index) have been adopted under HIPAA for all healthcare settings. A joint effort between the healthcare provider and the coder is essential to achieve complete and accurate documentation, code assignment, and reporting of diagnoses and procedures. These guidelines have been developed to assist both the healthcare provider and the coder in identifying those diagnoses that are to be reported. The importance of consistent, complete documentation in the medical record cannot be overemphasized. Without such documentation accurate coding cannot be achieved. The entire record should be reviewed to determine the specific reason for the encounter and the conditions treated.

The term encounter is used for all settings, including hospital admissions. In the context of these guidelines, the term provider is used throughout the guidelines to mean physician or any qualified health care practitioner who is legally accountable for establishing the patient's diagnosis. Only this set of guidelines, approved by the Cooperating Parties, is official.

The guidelines are organized into sections. Section I includes the structure and conventions of the classification and general guidelines that apply to the entire classification, and chapter-specific guidelines that correspond to the chapters as they are arranged in the classification. Section II includes guidelines for selection of principal diagnosis for non-outpatient settings. Section III includes guidelines for reporting additional diagnoses in non-outpatient settings. Section IV is for outpatient coding and reporting. It is necessary to review all sections of the guidelines to fully understand all of the rules and instructions needed to code properly.

2020 ICD-10-CM Official Guidelines for Coding and Reporting

Section I. Conventions, general coding guidelines and chapter specific guidelines

The conventions, general guidelines and chapter-specific guidelines are applicable to all health care settings unless otherwise indicated. The conventions and instructions of the classification take precedence over guidelines.

A. Conventions for the ICD-10-CM

The conventions for the ICD-10-CM are the general rules for use of the classification independent of the guidelines. These conventions are incorporated within the Alphabetic Index and Tabular List of the ICD-10-CM as instructional notes.

1. **The Alphabetic Index and Tabular List**
   The ICD-10-CM is divided into the Alphabetic Index, an alphabetical list of terms and their corresponding code, and the Tabular List, a structured list of codes divided into chapters based on body system or condition. The Alphabetic Index consists of the following parts: the Index of Diseases and Injury, the Index of External Causes of Injury, the Table of Neoplasms and the Table of Drugs and Chemicals.
   See Section I.C2. General guidelines
   See Section I.C.19. Adverse effects, poisoning, underdosing and toxic effects

2. **Format and Structure:**
   The ICD-10-CM Tabular List contains categories, subcategories and codes. Characters for categories, subcategories and codes may be either a letter or a number. All categories are 3 characters. A three-character category that has no further subdivision is equivalent to a code. Subcategories are either 4 or 5 characters. Codes may be 3, 4, 5, 6 or 7 characters. That is, each level of subdivision after a category is a subcategory. The final level of subdivision is a code. Codes that have applicable 7th characters are still referred to as codes, not subcategories. A code that has an applicable 7th character is considered invalid without the 7th character.
   The ICD-10-CM uses an indented format for ease in reference.

3. **Use of codes for reporting purposes**
   For reporting purposes only codes are permissible, not categories or subcategories, and any applicable 7th character is required.

4. **Placeholder character**
   The ICD-10-CM utilizes a placeholder character "X". The "X" is used as a placeholder at certain codes to allow for future expansion. An example of this is at the poisoning, adverse effect and underdosing codes, categories T36–T50.
   Where a placeholder exists, the X must be used in order for the code to be considered a valid code.

5. **7th Characters**
   Certain ICD-10-CM categories have applicable 7th characters. The applicable 7th character is required for all codes within the category, or as the notes in the Tabular List instruct. The 7th character must always be the 7th character in the data field. If a code that requires a 7th character is not 6 characters, a placeholder X must be used to fill in the empty characters.

6. **Abbreviations**
   a. **Alphabetic Index abbreviations**
   NEC "Not elsewhere classifiable" — *not in book* —9— .8—8—
   This abbreviation in the Alphabetic Index represents "other specified." When a specific code is not available for a condition, the Alphabetic Index directs the coder to the "other specified" code in the Tabular List.

   NOS "Not otherwise specified" — *Dr didnt specify*

This abbreviation is the equivalent of unspecified.

   b. **Tabular List abbreviations**
   NEC "Not elsewhere classifiable"
   This abbreviation in the Tabular List represents "other specified". When a specific code is not available for a condition, the Tabular List includes an NEC entry under a code to identify the code as the "other specified" code.

   NOS "Not otherwise specified"
   This abbreviation is the equivalent of unspecified.

7. **Punctuation**
   [ ] Brackets are used in the Tabular List to enclose synonyms, alternative wording or explanatory phrases. Brackets are used in the Alphabetic Index to identify manifestation codes.
   ( ) Parentheses are used in both the Alphabetic Index and Tabular List to enclose supplementary words that may be present or absent in the statement of a disease or procedure without affecting the code number to which it is assigned. The terms within the parentheses are referred to as nonessential modifiers. The nonessential modifiers in the Alphabetic Index to Diseases apply to subterms following a main term except when a nonessential modifier and a subentry are mutually exclusive, the subentry takes precedence. For example, in the ICD-10-CM Alphabetic Index under the main term Enteritis, "acute" is a nonessential modifier and "chronic" is a subentry. In this case, the nonessential modifier "acute" does not apply to the subentry "chronic".
   : Colons are used in the Tabular List after an incomplete term which needs one or more of the modifiers following the colon to make it assignable to a given category.

8. **Use of "and"**
   See Section I.A.14. Use of the term "And"

9. **Other and Unspecified codes**
   a. **"Other" codes** NOS .9
   Codes titled "other" or "other specified" are for use when the information in the medical record provides detail for which a specific code does not exist. Alphabetic Index entries with NEC in the line designate "other" codes in the Tabular List. These Alphabetic Index entries represent specific disease entities for which no specific code exists so the term is included under an "other" code.

   b. **"Unspecified" codes** NEC .8
   Codes titled "unspecified" are for use when the information in the medical record is insufficient to assign a more specific code. For those categories for which an unspecified code is not provided, the "other specified" code may represent both other and unspecified.
   See Section I.B.18 Use of Signs/Symptom/Unspecified Codes

10. **Includes Notes**
    This note appears immediately under a three character code title to further define, or give examples of, the content of the category.

11. **Inclusion terms**
    List of terms is included under some codes. These terms are the conditions for which that code is to be used. The terms may be synonyms of the code title, or, in the case of "other specified" codes, the terms are a list of the various conditions assigned to that code. The inclusion terms are not necessarily exhaustive. Additional terms found only in the Alphabetic Index may also be assigned to a code.

12. **Excludes Notes**
    The ICD-10-CM has two types of excludes notes. Each type of note has a different definition for use but they are all similar in that they indicate that codes excluded from each other are independent of each other.
    a. **Excludes1**
    A type 1 Excludes note is a pure excludes note. It means "NOT CODED HERE!" An Excludes1 note indicates that the code excluded should never be used at the same time as the code above the Excludes1 note. An Excludes1 is used when two conditions cannot occur together, such as a congenital form versus an acquired form of the same condition.

    An exception to the Excludes1 definition is the circumstance when the two conditions are unrelated to each other. If it is not clear whether the two conditions involving an Excludes1 note are related or not, query the provider. For example, code F45.8, Other somatoform disorders, has an Excludes1 note for "sleep related teeth grinding (G47.63)," because "teeth grinding" is an inclusion term under F45.8. Only one of these two codes should be assigned for teeth grinding. However psychogenic dysmenorrhea is also an inclusion term under F45.8, and a patient could have both this condition and sleep related

2020 ICD-10-CM Official Guidelines for Coding and Reporting

teeth grinding. In this case, the two conditions are clearly unrelated to each other, and so it would be appropriate to report F45.8 and G47.63 together.

b. Excludes2

A type 2 Excludes note represents "Not included here." An excludes2 note indicates that the condition excluded is not part of the condition represented by the code, but a patient may have both conditions at the same time. When an Excludes2 note appears under a code, it is acceptable to use both the code and the excluded code together, when appropriate.

13. Etiology/manifestation convention ("code first", "use additional code" and "in diseases classified elsewhere" notes)

Certain conditions have both an underlying etiology and multiple body system manifestations due to the underlying etiology. For such conditions, the ICD-10-CM has a coding convention that requires the underlying condition be sequenced first, if applicable, followed by the manifestation. Wherever such a combination exists, there is a "use additional code" note at the etiology code, and a "code first" note at the manifestation code. These instructional notes indicate the proper sequencing order of the codes, etiology followed by manifestation.

In most cases the manifestation codes will have in the code title, "in diseases classified elsewhere." Codes with this title are a component of the etiology/ manifestation convention. The code title indicates that it is a manifestation code. "In diseases classified elsewhere" codes are never permitted to be used as first-listed or principal diagnosis codes. They must be used in conjunction with an underlying condition code and they must be listed following the underlying condition. See category F02, Dementia in other diseases classified elsewhere, for an example of this convention.

There are manifestation codes that do not have "in diseases classified elsewhere" in the title. For such codes, there is a "use additional code" note at the etiology code and a "code first" note at the manifestation code, and the rules for sequencing apply.

In addition to the notes in the Tabular List, these conditions also have a specific Alphabetic Index entry structure. In the Alphabetic Index both conditions are listed together with the etiology code first followed by the manifestation codes in brackets. The code in brackets is always to be sequenced second.

An example of the etiology/manifestation convention is dementia in Parkinson's disease. In the Alphabetic Index, code G20 is listed first, followed by code F02.80 or F02.81 in brackets. Code G20 represents the underlying etiology, Parkinson's disease, and must be sequenced first, whereas code F02.80 and F02.81 represent the manifestation of dementia in diseases classified elsewhere, with or without behavioral disturbance.

"Code first" and "Use additional code" notes are also used as sequencing rules in the classification for certain codes that are not part of an etiology/ manifestation combination.

See Section I.B.7. Multiple coding for a single condition.

14. "And"

The word "and" should be interpreted to mean either "and" or "or" when it appears in a title.

For example, cases of "tuberculosis of bones", "tuberculosis of joints" and "tuberculosis of bones and joints" are classified to subcategory A18.0, Tuberculosis of bones and joints.

15. "With"

The word "with" or "in" should be interpreted to mean "associated with" or "due to" when it appears in a code title, the Alphabetic Index (either under a main term or subterm), or an instructional note in the Tabular List. The classification presumes a causal relationship between the two conditions linked by these terms in the Alphabetic Index or Tabular List. These conditions should be coded as related even in the absence of provider documentation explicitly linking them, unless the documentation clearly states the conditions are unrelated or when another guideline exists that specifically requires a documented linkage between two conditions (e.g., sepsis guideline for "acute organ dysfunction that is not clearly associated with the sepsis").

For conditions not specifically linked by these relational terms in the classification or when a guideline requires that a linkage between two conditions be explicitly documented, provider documentation must link the conditions in order to code them as related.

The word "with" in the Alphabetic Index is sequenced immediately following the main term **or subterm**, not in alphabetical order.

16. "See" and "See Also"

The "see" instruction following a main term in the Alphabetic Index indicates that another term should be referenced. It is necessary to go to the main term referenced with the "see" note to locate the correct code.

A "see also" instruction following a main term in the Alphabetic Index instructs that there is another main term that may also be referenced that may provide additional Alphabetic Index entries that may be useful. It is not necessary to follow the "see also" note when the original main term provides the necessary code.

17. "Code also" note

A "code also" note instructs that two codes may be required to fully describe a condition, but this note does not provide sequencing direction. The sequencing depends on the circumstances of the encounter.

18. Default codes

A code listed next to a main term in the ICD-10-CM Alphabetic Index is referred to as a default code. The default code represents that condition that is most commonly associated with the main term, or is the unspecified code for the condition. If a condition is documented in a medical record (for example, appendicitis) without any additional information, such as acute or chronic, the default code should be assigned.

19. Code assignment and Clinical Criteria

The assignment of a diagnosis code is based on the provider's diagnostic statement that the condition exists. The provider's statement that the patient has a particular condition is sufficient. Code assignment is not based on clinical criteria used by the provider to establish the diagnosis.

B. General Coding Guidelines

1. Locating a code in the ICD-10-CM

To select a code in the classification that corresponds to a diagnosis or reason for visit documented in a medical record, first locate the term in the Alphabetic Index, and then verify the code in the Tabular List. Read and be guided by instructional notations that appear in both the Alphabetic Index and the Tabular List.

It is essential to use both the Alphabetic Index and Tabular List when locating and assigning a code. The Alphabetic Index does not always provide the full code. Selection of the full code, including laterality and any applicable 7th character can only be done in the Tabular List. A dash (-) at the end of an Alphabetic Index entry indicates that additional characters are required. Even if a dash is not included at the Alphabetic Index entry, it is necessary to refer to the Tabular List to verify that no 7th character is required.

2. Level of Detail in Coding

Diagnosis codes are to be used and reported at their highest number of characters available.

ICD-10-CM diagnosis codes are composed of codes with 3, 4, 5, 6 or 7 characters. Codes with three characters are included in ICD-10-CM as the heading of a category of codes that may be further subdivided by the use of fourth and/or fifth characters and/or sixth characters, which provide greater detail.

A three-character code is to be used only if it is not further subdivided. A code is invalid if it has not been coded to the full number of characters required for that code, including the 7th character, if applicable.

3. Code or codes from A00.0 through T88.9, Z00-Z99.8

The appropriate code or codes from A00.0 through T88.9, Z00-Z99.8 must be used to identify diagnoses, symptoms, conditions, problems, complaints or other reason(s) for the encounter/visit.

4. Signs and symptoms

Codes that describe symptoms and signs, as opposed to diagnoses, are acceptable for reporting purposes when a related definitive diagnosis has not been established (confirmed) by the provider. Chapter 18 of ICD-10-CM, Symptoms, Signs, and Abnormal Clinical and Laboratory Findings, Not Elsewhere Classified (codes R00.0 - R99) contains many, but not all, codes for symptoms.

See Section I.B.18 Use of Signs/Symptom/Unspecified Codes

5. Conditions that are an integral part of a disease process

Signs and symptoms that are associated routinely with a disease process should not be assigned as additional codes, unless otherwise instructed by the classification.

6. Conditions that are not an integral part of a disease process

Additional signs and symptoms that may not be associated routinely with a disease process should be coded when present.

7. Multiple coding for a single condition

In addition to the etiology/manifestation convention that requires two codes to fully describe a single condition that affects multiple body systems, there are other single conditions that also require more than one code. "Use additional code" notes are found in the Tabular List at codes that are not part of an etiology/manifestation pair where a secondary code is useful to fully describe a condition. The sequencing rule is the same as the etiology/manifestation pair, "use additional code" indicates that a secondary code should be added, if known.

For example, for bacterial infections that are not included in chapter 1, a secondary code from category B95, Streptococcus, Staphylococcus, and Enterococcus, as the cause of diseases classified elsewhere, or B96, Other bacterial agents as the cause of diseases classified elsewhere, may be required to identify the bacterial organism causing the infection. A "use additional code" note will normally be found at the infectious disease code, indicating a need for the organism code to be added as a secondary code.

"Code first" notes are also under certain codes that are not specifically manifestation codes but may be due to an underlying cause. When there is a "code first" note and an underlying condition is present, the underlying condition should be sequenced first, if known.

"Code, if applicable, any causal condition first" notes indicate that this code may be assigned as a principal diagnosis when the causal condition is unknown or not applicable. If a causal condition is known, then the code for that condition should be sequenced as the principal or first-listed diagnosis.

Multiple codes may be needed for sequela, complication codes and obstetric codes to more fully describe a condition. See the specific guidelines for these conditions for further instruction.

8. Acute and Chronic Conditions

If the same condition is described as both acute (subacute) and chronic, and separate subentries exist in the Alphabetic Index at the same indentation level, code both and sequence the acute (subacute) code first.

9. Combination Code

A combination code is a single code used to classify:

> Two diagnoses, or
>
> A diagnosis with an associated secondary process (manifestation)
>
> A diagnosis with an associated complication

Combination codes are identified by referring to subterm entries in the Alphabetic Index and by reading the inclusion and exclusion notes in the Tabular List.

Assign only the combination code when that code fully identifies the diagnostic conditions involved or when the Alphabetic Index so directs. Multiple coding should not be used when the classification provides a combination code that clearly identifies all of the elements documented in the diagnosis. When the combination code lacks necessary specificity in describing the manifestation or complication, an additional code should be used as a secondary code.

10. Sequela (Late Effects)

A sequela is the residual effect (condition produced) after the acute phase of an illness or injury has terminated. There is no time limit on when a sequela code can be used. The residual may be apparent early, such as in cerebral infarction, or it may occur months or years later, such as that due to a previous injury. Examples of sequela include: scar formation resulting from a burn, deviated septum due to a nasal fracture, and infertility due to tubal occlusion from old tuberculosis. Coding of sequela generally requires two codes sequenced in the following order: the condition or nature of the sequela is sequenced first. The sequela code is sequenced second.

An exception to the above guidelines are those instances where the code for the sequela is followed by a manifestation code identified in the Tabular List and title, or the sequela code has been expanded (at the fourth, fifth or sixth character levels) to include the manifestation(s). The code for the acute phase of an illness or injury that led to the sequela is never used with a code for the late effect.

See Section I.C.9. Sequelae of cerebrovascular disease

See Section I.C.15. Sequelae of complication of pregnancy, childbirth and the puerperium

See Section I.C.19. Application of 7th characters for Chapter 19

11. Impending or Threatened Condition

Code any condition described at the time of discharge as "impending" or "threatened" as follows:

> If it did occur, code as confirmed diagnosis.

If it did not occur, reference the Alphabetic Index to determine if the condition has a subentry term for "impending" or "threatened" and also reference main term entries for "Impending" and for "Threatened."

If the subterms are listed, assign the given code.

If the subterms are not listed, code the existing underlying condition(s) and not the condition described as impending or threatened.

12. Reporting Same Diagnosis Code more than Once

Each unique ICD-10-CM diagnosis code may be reported only once for an encounter. This applies to bilateral conditions when there are no distinct codes identifying laterality or two different conditions classified to the same ICD-10-CM diagnosis code.

13. Laterality

Some ICD-10-CM codes indicate laterality, specifying whether the condition occurs on the left, right or is bilateral. If no bilateral code is provided and the condition is bilateral, assign separate codes for both the left and right side. If the side is not identified in the medical record, assign the code for the unspecified side.

When a patient has a bilateral condition and each side is treated during separate encounters, assign the "bilateral" code (as the condition still exists on both sides), including for the encounter to treat the first side. For the second encounter for treatment after one side has previously been treated and the condition no longer exists on that side, assign the appropriate unilateral code for the side where the condition still exists (e.g., cataract surgery performed on each eye in separate encounters). The bilateral code would not be assigned for the subsequent encounter, as the patient no longer has the condition in the previously-treated site. If the treatment on the first side did not completely resolve the condition, then the bilateral code would still be appropriate.

14. Documentation *by Clinicians Other than the Patient's Provider*

Code assignment is based on the documentation by patient's provider (i.e., physician or other qualified healthcare practitioner legally accountable for establishing the patient's diagnosis). There are a few exceptions, such as codes for the Body Mass Index (BMI), depth of non-pressure chronic ulcers, pressure ulcer stage, coma scale, and NIH stroke scale (NIHSS) codes, code assignment may be based on medical record documentation from clinicians who are not the patient's provider (i.e., physician or other qualified healthcare practitioner legally accountable for establishing the patient's diagnosis), since this information is typically documented by other clinicians involved in the care of the patient (e.g., a dietitian often documents the BMI, a nurse often documents the pressure ulcer stages, and an emergency medical technician often documents the coma scale). However, the associated diagnosis (such as overweight, obesity, acute stroke, or pressure ulcer) must be documented by the patient's provider. If there is conflicting medical record documentation, either from the same clinician or different clinicians, the patient's attending provider should be queried for clarification.

For social determinants of health, such as information found in categories Z55-Z65, Persons with potential health hazards related to socioeconomic and psychosocial circumstances, code assignment may be based on medical record documentation from clinicians involved in the care of the patient who are not the patient's provider since this information represents social information, rather than medical diagnoses.

The BMI, coma scale, NIHSS codes and categories Z55-Z65 should only be reported as secondary diagnoses.

15. Syndromes

Follow the Alphabetic Index guidance when coding syndromes. In the absence of Alphabetic Index guidance, assign codes for the documented manifestations of the syndrome. Additional codes for manifestations that are not an integral part of the disease process may also be assigned when the condition does not have a unique code.

16. Documentation of Complications of Care

Code assignment is based on the provider's documentation of the relationship between the condition and the care or procedure, unless otherwise instructed by the classification. The guideline extends to any complications of care, regardless of the chapter the code is located in. It is important to note that not all conditions that occur during or following medical care or surgery are classified as complications. There must be a cause-and-effect relationship between the care provided and the condition, and an indication in the documentation that it is a complication. Query the provider for clarification, if the complication is not clearly documented.

17. Borderline Diagnosis

If the provider documents a "borderline" diagnosis at the time of discharge, the diagnosis is coded as confirmed, unless the classification provides a specific entry (e.g., borderline diabetes). If a borderline condition has a specific index entry in ICD-10-CM, it should be coded as such. Since borderline conditions are not uncertain diagnoses, no distinction is made between the care setting (inpatient versus outpatient). Whenever the documentation is unclear regarding a borderline condition, coders are encouraged to query for clarification.

18. Use of Sign/Symptom/Unspecified Codes

Sign/symptom and "unspecified" codes have acceptable, even necessary, uses. While specific diagnosis codes should be reported when they are supported by the available medical record documentation and clinical knowledge of the patient's health condition, there are instances when signs/symptoms or unspecified codes are the best choices for accurately reflecting the healthcare encounter. Each healthcare encounter should be coded to the level of certainty known for that encounter.

If a definitive diagnosis has not been established by the end of the encounter, it is appropriate to report codes for sign(s) and/or symptom(s) in lieu of a definitive diagnosis. When sufficient clinical information isn't known or available about a particular health condition to assign a more specific code, it is acceptable to report the appropriate "unspecified" code (e.g., a diagnosis of pneumonia has been determined, but not the specific type). Unspecified codes should be reported when they are the codes that most accurately reflect what is known about the patient's condition at the time of that particular encounter. It would be inappropriate to select a specific code that is not supported by the medical record documentation or conduct medically unnecessary diagnostic testing in order to determine a more specific code.

19. Coding for Healthcare Encounters in Hurricane Aftermath

a. Use of External Cause of Morbidity Codes

An external cause of morbidity code should be assigned to identify the cause of the injury(ies) incurred as a result of the hurricane. The use of external cause of morbidity codes is supplemental to the application of ICD-10-CM codes. External cause of morbidity codes are never to be recorded as a principal diagnosis (first-listed in non-inpatient settings). The appropriate injury code should be sequenced before any external cause codes. The external cause of morbidity codes capture how the injury or health condition happened (cause), the intent (unintentional or accidental; or intentional, such as suicide or assault), the place where the event occurred, the activity of the patient at the time of the event, and the person's status (e.g., civilian, military). They should not be assigned for encounters to treat hurricane victims' medical conditions when no injury, adverse effect or poisoning is involved. External cause of morbidity codes should be assigned for each encounter for care and treatment of the injury. External cause of morbidity codes may be assigned in all health care settings. For the purpose of capturing complete and accurate ICD-10-CM data in the aftermath of the hurricane, a healthcare setting should be considered as any location where medical care is provided by licensed healthcare professionals.

b. Sequencing of External Causes of Morbidity Codes

Codes for cataclysmic events, such as a hurricane, take priority over all other external cause codes except child and adult abuse and terrorism and should be sequenced before other external cause of injury codes. Assign as many external cause of morbidity codes as necessary to fully explain each cause. For example, if an injury occurs as a result of a building collapse during the hurricane, external cause codes for both the hurricane and the building collapse should be assigned, with the external causes code for hurricane being sequenced as the first external cause code. For injuries incurred as a direct result of the hurricane, assign the appropriate code(s) for the injuries, followed by the code X37.0-, Hurricane (with the appropriate 7th character), and any other applicable external cause of injury codes. Code X37.0- also should be assigned when an injury is incurred as a result of flooding caused by a levee breaking related to the hurricane. Code X38.-, Flood (with the appropriate 7th character), should be assigned when an injury is from flooding resulting directly from the storm. Code X36.0.-, Collapse of dam or man-made structure, should not be assigned when the cause of the collapse is due to the hurricane. Use of code X36.0- is limited to collapses of man-made structures due to earth surface movements, not due to storm surges directly from a hurricane.

c. Other External Causes of Morbidity Code Issues

For injuries that are not a direct result of the hurricane, such as an evacuee that has incurred an injury as a result of a motor vehicle accident, assign the appropriate external cause of morbidity code(s) to

describe the cause of the injury, but do not assign code X37.0-, Hurricane. If it is not clear whether the injury was a direct result of the hurricane, assume the injury is due to the hurricane and assign code X37.0-, Hurricane, as well as any other applicable external cause of morbidity codes. In addition to code X37.0-, Hurricane, other possible applicable external cause of morbidity codes include:

> W54.0-, Bitten by dog
>
> X30-, Exposure to excessive natural heat
>
> X31-, Exposure to excessive natural cold
>
> X38-, Flood

d. Use of Z codes

Z codes (other reasons for healthcare encounters) may be assigned as appropriate to further explain the reasons for presenting for healthcare services, including transfers between healthcare facilities. The ICD-10-CM Official Guidelines for Coding and Reporting identify which codes maybe assigned as principal or first-listed diagnosis only, secondary diagnosis only, or principal/first-listed or secondary (depending on the circumstances). Possible applicable Z codes include:

> Z59.0, Homelessness
>
> Z59.1, Inadequate housing
>
> Z59.5, Extreme poverty
>
> Z75.1, Person awaiting admission to adequate facility elsewhere
>
> Z75.3, Unavailability and inaccessibility of health-care facilities
>
> Z75.4, Unavailability and inaccessibility of other helping agencies
>
> Z76.2, Encounter for health supervision and care of other healthy infant and child
>
> Z99.12, Encounter for respirator [ventilator] dependence during power failure

The external cause of morbidity codes and the Z codes listed above are not an all-inclusive list. Other codes may be applicable to the encounter based upon the documentation. Assign as many codes as necessary to fully explain each healthcare encounter. Since patient history information may be very limited, use any available documentation to assign the appropriate external cause of morbidity and Z codes.

C. Chapter-Specific Coding Guidelines

In addition to general coding guidelines, there are guidelines for specific diagnoses and/or conditions in the classification. Unless otherwise indicated, these guidelines apply to all health care settings. Please refer to Section II for guidelines on the selection of principal diagnosis.

1. Chapter 1: Certain Infectious and Parasitic Diseases (A00-B99)

a. Human Immunodeficiency Virus (HIV) Infections

1) Code only confirmed cases

Code only confirmed cases of HIV infection/illness. This is an exception to the hospital inpatient guideline Section II, H.

In this context, "confirmation" does not require documentation of positive serology or culture for HIV; the provider's diagnostic statement that the patient is HIV positive, or has an HIV-related illness is sufficient.

2) Selection and sequencing of HIV codes

(a) Patient admitted for HIV-related condition

If a patient is admitted for an HIV-related condition, the principal diagnosis should be B20, Human immunodeficiency virus [HIV] disease followed by additional diagnosis codes for all reported HIV-related conditions.

(b) Patient with HIV disease admitted for unrelated condition

If a patient with HIV disease is admitted for an unrelated condition (such as a traumatic injury), the code for the unrelated condition (e.g., the nature of injury code) should be the principal diagnosis. Other diagnoses would be B20 followed by additional diagnosis codes for all reported HIV-related conditions.

(c) Whether the patient is newly diagnosed

Whether the patient is newly diagnosed or has had previous admissions/encounters for HIV conditions is irrelevant to the sequencing decision.

(d) Asymptomatic human immunodeficiency virus

Z21, Asymptomatic human immunodeficiency virus [HIV] infection status, is to be applied when the patient without any documentation of symptoms is listed as being "HIV positive," "known HIV," "HIV test positive," or similar terminology. Do not use this code if the term "AIDS" is used or if the patient is treated for any HIV-related illness or is described as having any condition(s) resulting from his/her HIV positive status; use B20 in these cases.

(e) Patients with inconclusive HIV serology

Patients with inconclusive HIV serology, but no definitive diagnosis or manifestations of the illness, may be assigned code R75, Inconclusive laboratory evidence of human immunodeficiency virus [HIV].

(f) Previously diagnosed HIV-related illness

Patients with any known prior diagnosis of an HIV-related illness should be coded to B20. Once a patient has developed an HIV-related illness, the patient should always be assigned code B20 on every subsequent admission/encounter. Patients previously diagnosed with any HIV illness (B20) should never be assigned to R75 or Z21, Asymptomatic human immunodeficiency virus [HIV] infection status.

(g) HIV Infection in Pregnancy, Childbirth and the Puerperium

During pregnancy, childbirth or the puerperium, a patient admitted (or presenting for a health care encounter) because of an HIV-related illness should receive a principal diagnosis code of O98.7-, Human immunodeficiency [HIV] disease complicating pregnancy, childbirth and the puerperium, followed by B20 and the code(s) for the HIV-related illness(es). Codes from Chapter 15 always take sequencing priority.

Patients with asymptomatic HIV infection status admitted (or presenting for a health care encounter) during pregnancy, childbirth, or the puerperium should receive codes of O98.7- and Z21.

(h) Encounters for testing for HIV

If a patient is being seen to determine his/her HIV status, use code Z11.4, Encounter for screening for human immunodeficiency virus [HIV]. Use additional codes for any associated high risk behavior.

If a patient with signs or symptoms is being seen for HIV testing, code the signs and symptoms. An additional counseling code Z71.7, Human immunodeficiency virus [HIV] counseling, may be used if counseling is provided during the encounter for the test.

When a patient returns to be informed of his/her HIV test results and the test result is negative, use code Z71.7, Human immunodeficiency virus [HIV] counseling.

If the results are positive, see previous guidelines and assign codes as appropriate.

b. Infectious agents as the cause of diseases classified to other chapters

Certain infections are classified in chapters other than Chapter 1 and no organism is identified as part of the infection code. In these instances, it is necessary to use an additional code from Chapter 1 to identify the organism. A code from category B95, Streptococcus, Staphylococcus, and Enterococcus as the cause of diseases classified to other chapters, B96, Other bacterial agents as the cause of diseases classified to other chapters, or B97, Viral agents as the cause of diseases classified to other chapters, is to be used as an additional code to identify the organism. An instructional note will be found at the infection code advising that an additional organism code is required.

c. Infections resistant to antibiotics

Many bacterial infections are resistant to current antibiotics. It is necessary to identify all infections documented as antibiotic resistant. Assign a code from category Z16, Resistance to antimicrobial drugs, following the infection code only if the infection code does not identify drug resistance.

d. Sepsis, Severe Sepsis, and Septic Shock

1) Coding of Sepsis and Severe Sepsis

(a) Sepsis

For a diagnosis of sepsis, assign the appropriate code for the underlying systemic infection. If the type of infection or causal organism is not further specified, assign code A41.9, Sepsis, unspecified organism.

A code from subcategory R65.2, Severe sepsis, should not be assigned unless severe sepsis or an associated acute organ dysfunction is documented.

(i) Negative or inconclusive blood cultures and sepsis

Negative or inconclusive blood cultures do not preclude a diagnosis of sepsis in patients with clinical evidence of the condition; however, the provider should be queried.

(ii) Urosepsis

The term urosepsis is a nonspecific term. It is not to be considered synonymous with sepsis. It has no default code in the Alphabetic Index. Should a provider use this term, he/she must be queried for clarification.

(iii) Sepsis with organ dysfunction

If a patient has sepsis and associated acute organ dysfunction or multiple organ dysfunction (MOD), follow the instructions for coding severe sepsis.

(iv) Acute organ dysfunction that is not clearly associated with the sepsis

If a patient has sepsis and an acute organ dysfunction, but the medical record documentation indicates that the acute organ dysfunction is related to a medical condition other than the sepsis, do not assign a code from subcategory R65.2, Severe sepsis. An acute organ dysfunction must be associated with the sepsis in order to assign the severe sepsis code. If the documentation is not clear as to whether an acute organ dysfunction is related to the sepsis or another medical condition, query the provider.

(b) Severe sepsis

The coding of severe sepsis requires a minimum of 2 codes: first a code for the underlying systemic infection, followed by a code from subcategory R65.2, Severe sepsis. If the causal organism is not documented, assign code A41.9, Sepsis, unspecified organism, for the infection. Additional code(s) for the associated acute organ dysfunction are also required.

Due to the complex nature of severe sepsis, some cases may require querying the provider prior to assignment of the codes.

2) Septic shock

(a) Septic shock generally refers to circulatory failure associated with severe sepsis, and therefore, it represents a type of acute organ dysfunction.

For cases of septic shock, the code for the systemic infection should be sequenced first, followed by code R65.21, Severe sepsis with septic shock or code T81.12, Postprocedural septic shock. Any additional codes for the other acute organ dysfunctions should also be assigned. As noted in the sequencing instructions in the Tabular List, the code for septic shock cannot be assigned as a principal diagnosis.

3) Sequencing of severe sepsis

If severe sepsis is present on admission, and meets the definition of principal diagnosis, the underlying systemic infection should be assigned as principal diagnosis followed by the appropriate code from subcategory R65.2 as required by the sequencing rules in the Tabular List. A code from subcategory R65.2 can never be assigned as a principal diagnosis.

When severe sepsis develops during an encounter (it was not present on admission), the underlying systemic infection and the appropriate code from subcategory R65.2 should be assigned as secondary diagnoses.

Severe sepsis may be present on admission, but the diagnosis may not be confirmed until sometime after admission. If the documentation is not clear whether severe sepsis was present on admission, the provider should be queried.

4) Sepsis *or* severe sepsis with a localized infection

If the reason for admission is sepsis or severe sepsis and a localized infection, such as pneumonia or cellulitis, a code(s) for the underlying systemic infection should be assigned first and the code for the localized infection should be assigned as a secondary diagnosis. If the patient has severe sepsis, a code from subcategory R65.2 should also be assigned as a secondary diagnosis. If the patient is admitted with a localized infection, such as pneumonia, and sepsis/severe sepsis doesn't develop until after admission, the localized infection should be assigned first, followed by the appropriate sepsis/severe sepsis codes.

5) Sepsis due to a postprocedural infection

(a) Documentation of causal relationship

As with all postprocedural complications, code assignment is based on the provider's documentation of the relationship between the infection and the procedure.

(b) Sepsis due to a postprocedural infection

For infections following a procedure, a code from T81.40, to T81.43 Infection following a procedure, or a code from O86.00 to O86.03, Infection of obstetric surgical wound, that identifies the site of the infection should be coded first, if known. Assign an additional code for sepsis following a procedure (T81.44) or sepsis following an obstetrical procedure (O86.04). Use an additional code to identify the infectious agent. If the patient has severe sepsis, the appropriate code from subcategory R65.2 should also be assigned with the additional code(s) for any acute organ dysfunction.

For infections following infusion, transfusion, therapeutic injection, or immunization, a code from subcategory T80.2, Infections following infusion, transfusion, and therapeutic injection, or code T88.0-, Infection following immunization, should be coded first, followed by the code for the specific infection. If the patient has severe sepsis, the appropriate code from subcategory R65.2 should also be assigned, with the additional codes(s) for any acute organ dysfunction.

(c) Postprocedural infection and postprocedural septic shock

If a postprocedural infection has resulted in postprocedural septic shock, assign the codes indicated above for sepsis due to a postprocedural infection, followed by code T81.12-, Postprocedural septic shock. Do not assign code R65.21, Severe sepsis with septic shock. Additional code(s) should be assigned for any acute organ dysfunction.

6) Sepsis and severe sepsis associated with a noninfectious process (condition)

In some cases a noninfectious process (condition), such as trauma, may lead to an infection which can result in sepsis or severe sepsis. If sepsis or severe sepsis is documented as associated with a noninfectious condition, such as a burn or serious injury, and this condition meets the definition for principal diagnosis, the code for the noninfectious condition should be sequenced first, followed by the code for the resulting infection. If severe sepsis is present, a code from subcategory R65.2 should also be assigned with any associated organ dysfunction(s) codes. It is not necessary to assign a code from subcategory R65.1, Systemic inflammatory response syndrome (SIRS) of non-infectious origin, for these cases.

If the infection meets the definition of principal diagnosis, it should be sequenced before the non-infectious condition. When both the associated non-infectious condition and the infection meet the definition of principal diagnosis, either may be assigned as principal diagnosis.

Only one code from category R65, Symptoms and signs specifically associated with systemic inflammation and infection, should be assigned. Therefore, when a non-infectious condition leads to an infection resulting in severe sepsis, assign the appropriate code from subcategory R65.2, Severe sepsis. Do not additionally assign a code from subcategory R65.1, Systemic inflammatory response syndrome (SIRS) of non-infectious origin.

See Section I.C.18. SIRS due to non-infectious process

7) Sepsis and septic shock complicating abortion, pregnancy, childbirth, and the puerperium

See Section I.C.15. Sepsis and septic shock complicating abortion, pregnancy, childbirth and the puerperium

8) Newborn sepsis

See Section I.C.16. f. Bacterial sepsis of Newborn

e. Methicillin Resistant Staphylococcus aureus (MRSA) Conditions

1) Selection and sequencing of MRSA codes

(a) Combination codes for MRSA infection

When a patient is diagnosed with an infection that is due to methicillin resistant *Staphylococcus aureus* (MRSA), and that infection has a combination code that includes the causal organism (e.g., sepsis, pneumonia) assign the appropriate combination code for the condition (e.g., code A41.02, Sepsis due to Methicillin resistant Staphylococcus aureus or code J15.212, Pneumonia due to Methicillin resistant Staphylococcus aureus). Do not assign code B95.62, Methicillin resistant Staphylococcus aureus infection as the cause of diseases classified elsewhere, as an additional code, because the combination code includes the type of infection and the MRSA organism. Do not assign a code from subcategory Z16.11, Resistance to penicillins, as an additional diagnosis.

See Section C.1. for instructions on coding and sequencing of sepsis and severe sepsis.

(b) Other codes for MRSA infection

When there is documentation of a current infection (e.g., wound infection, stitch abscess, urinary tract infection) due to MRSA, and that infection does not have a combination code that includes the causal organism, assign the appropriate code to identify the condition along with code B95.62, Methicillin resistant Staphylococcus aureus infection as the cause of diseases classified elsewhere for the MRSA infection. Do not assign a code from subcategory Z16.11, Resistance to penicillins.

(c) Methicillin susceptible Staphylococcus aureus (MSSA) and MRSA colonization

The condition or state of being colonized or carrying MSSA or MRSA is called colonization or carriage, while an individual person is described as being colonized or being a carrier. Colonization means that MSSA or MSRA is present on or in the body without necessarily causing illness. A positive MRSA colonization test might be documented by the provider as "MRSA screen positive" or "MRSA nasal swab positive".

Assign code Z22.322, Carrier or suspected carrier of Methicillin resistant Staphylococcus aureus, for patients documented as having MRSA colonization. Assign code Z22.321, Carrier or suspected carrier of Methicillin susceptible Staphylococcus aureus, for patients documented as having MSSA colonization. Colonization is not necessarily indicative of a disease process or as the cause of a specific condition the patient may have unless documented as such by the provider.

(d) MRSA colonization and infection

If a patient is documented as having both MRSA colonization and infection during a hospital admission, code Z22.322, Carrier or suspected carrier of Methicillin resistant Staphylococcus aureus, and a code for the MRSA infection may both be assigned.

f. Zika virus infections

1) Code only confirmed cases

Code only a confirmed diagnosis of Zika virus (A92.5, Zika virus disease) as documented by the provider. This is an exception to the hospital inpatient guideline Section II, H. In this context, "confirmation" does not require documentation of the type of test performed; the **provider's** diagnostic statement that the condition is confirmed is sufficient. This code should be assigned regardless of the stated mode of transmission.

If the provider documents "suspected", "possible" or "probable" Zika, do not assign code A92.5. Assign a code(s) explaining the reason for encounter (such as fever, rash, or joint pain) or Z20.821, Contact with and (suspected) exposure to Zika virus.

2. Chapter 2: Neoplasms (C00-D49)
General guidelines

Chapter 2 of the ICD-10-CM contains the codes for most benign and all malignant neoplasms. Certain benign neoplasms, such as prostatic adenomas, may be found in the specific body system chapters. To properly code a neoplasm it is necessary to determine from the record if the neoplasm is benign, in-situ, malignant, or of uncertain histologic behavior. If malignant, any secondary (metastatic) sites should also be determined.

Primary malignant neoplasms overlapping site boundaries

A primary malignant neoplasm that overlaps two or more contiguous (next to each other) sites should be classified to the subcategory/code .8 ('overlapping lesion'), unless the combination is specifically indexed elsewhere. For multiple neoplasms of the same site that are not contiguous such as tumors in different quadrants of the same breast, codes for each site should be assigned.

Malignant neoplasm of ectopic tissue

Malignant neoplasms of ectopic tissue are to be coded to the site of origin mentioned, e.g., ectopic pancreatic malignant neoplasms involving the stomach are coded to malignant neoplasm of pancreas, unspecified (C25.9).

The neoplasm table in the Alphabetic Index should be referenced first. However, if the histological term is documented, that term should be referenced first, rather than going immediately to the Neoplasm Table, in order to determine which column in the Neoplasm Table is appropriate. For example, if the documentation indicates "adenoma," refer to the term in the Alphabetic Index to review the entries under this term and the instructional note to "see also neoplasm, by site, benign." The table provides the proper code based on the type of neoplasm and the site. It is important to select the proper column in the table that corresponds to the type of neoplasm. The Tabular List should then be referenced to verify that the correct code has been selected from the table and that a more specific site code does not exist.

See Section I.C.21. Factors influencing health status and contact with health services, Status, for information regarding Z15.0, codes for genetic susceptibility to cancer.

a. Treatment directed at the malignancy

If the treatment is directed at the malignancy, designate the malignancy as the principal diagnosis.

The only exception to this guideline is if a patient admission/encounter is solely for the administration of chemotherapy, immunotherapy or external beam radiation therapy, assign the appropriate Z51.-- code as the first-listed or principal diagnosis, and the diagnosis or problem for which the service is being performed as a secondary diagnosis.

b. Treatment of secondary site

When a patient is admitted because of a primary neoplasm with metastasis and treatment is directed toward the secondary site only, the secondary neoplasm is designated as the principal diagnosis even though the primary malignancy is still present.

c. Coding and sequencing of complications

Coding and sequencing of complications associated with the malignancies or with the therapy thereof are subject to the following guidelines:

1) Anemia associated with malignancy

When admission/encounter is for management of an anemia associated with the malignancy, and the treatment is only for anemia, the appropriate code for the malignancy is sequenced as the principal or first-listed diagnosis followed by the appropriate code for the anemia (such as code D63.0, Anemia in neoplastic disease).

2) Anemia associated with chemotherapy, immunotherapy and radiation therapy

When the admission/encounter is for management of an anemia associated with an adverse effect of the administration of chemotherapy or immunotherapy and the only treatment is for the anemia, the anemia code is sequenced first followed by the appropriate codes for the neoplasm and the adverse effect (T45.1X5-, Adverse effect of antineoplastic and immunosuppressive drugs).

When the admission/encounter is for management of an anemia associated with an adverse effect of radiotherapy, the anemia code should be sequenced first, followed by the appropriate neoplasm code and code Y84.2, Radiological procedure and radiotherapy as the cause of abnormal reaction of the patient, or of later complication, without mention of misadventure at the time of the procedure.

3) Management of dehydration due to the malignancy

When the admission/encounter is for management of dehydration due to the malignancy and only the dehydration is being treated (intravenous rehydration), the dehydration is sequenced first, followed by the code(s) for the malignancy.

4) Treatment of a complication resulting from a surgical procedure

When the admission/encounter is for treatment of a complication resulting from a surgical procedure, designate the complication as the principal or first-listed diagnosis if treatment is directed at resolving the complication.

d. Primary malignancy previously excised

When a primary malignancy has been previously excised or eradicated from its site and there is no further treatment directed to that site and there is no evidence of any existing primary malignancy at that site, a code from category Z85, Personal history of malignant neoplasm, should be used to indicate the former site of the malignancy. Any mention of extension, invasion, or metastasis to another site is coded as a secondary malignant neoplasm to that site. The secondary site may be the principal or first-listed **diagnosis** with the Z85 code used as a secondary code.

e. Admissions/Encounters involving chemotherapy, immunotherapy and radiation therapy

1) Episode of care involves surgical removal of neoplasm

When an episode of care involves the surgical removal of a neoplasm, primary or secondary site, followed by adjunct chemotherapy or radiation treatment during the same episode of care, the code for the neoplasm should be assigned as principal or first-listed diagnosis.

2) Patient admission/encounter solely for administration of chemotherapy, immunotherapy and radiation therapy

If a patient admission/encounter is solely for the administration of chemotherapy, immunotherapy or external beam radiation therapy assign code Z51.0, Encounter for antineoplastic radiation therapy, or Z51.11, Encounter for antineoplastic chemotherapy, or Z51.12, Encounter for antineoplastic immunotherapy as the first-listed or principal diagnosis. If a patient receives more than one of these therapies during the same admission more than one of these codes may be assigned, in any sequence.

The malignancy for which the therapy is being administered should be assigned as a secondary diagnosis.

If a patient admission/encounter is for the insertion or implantation of radioactive elements (e.g., brachytherapy) the appropriate code for the malignancy is sequenced as the principal or first-listed diagnosis. Code Z51.0 should not be assigned.

3) Patient admitted for radiation therapy, chemotherapy or immunotherapy and develops complications

When a patient is admitted for the purpose of external beam radiotherapy, immunotherapy or chemotherapy and develops complications such as uncontrolled nausea and vomiting or dehydration, the principal or first-listed diagnosis is Z51.0, Encounter for antineoplastic radiation therapy, or Z51.11, Encounter for antineoplastic chemotherapy, or Z51.12, Encounter for antineoplastic immunotherapy followed by any codes for the complications.

When a patient is admitted for the purpose of insertion or implantation of radioactive elements (e.g., brachytherapy) and develops complications such as uncontrolled nausea and vomiting or dehydration, the principal or first-listed diagnosis is the appropriate code for the malignancy followed by any codes for the complications.

f. Admission/encounter to determine extent of malignancy

When the reason for admission/encounter is to determine the extent of the malignancy, or for a procedure such as paracentesis or thoracentesis, the primary malignancy or appropriate metastatic site is designated as the principal or first-listed diagnosis, even though chemotherapy or radiotherapy is administered.

g. Symptoms, signs, and abnormal findings listed in Chapter 18 associated with neoplasms

Symptoms, signs, and ill-defined conditions listed in Chapter 18 characteristic of, or associated with, an existing primary or secondary site malignancy cannot be used to replace the malignancy as principal or first-listed diagnosis, regardless of the number of admissions or encounters for treatment and care of the neoplasm.

See section I.C.21. Factors influencing health status and contact with health services, Encounter for prophylactic organ removal.

h. Admission/encounter for pain control/management

See Section I.C.6. for information on coding admission/encounter for pain control/management.

i. **Malignancy in two or more noncontiguous sites**
A patient may have more than one malignant tumor in the same organ. These tumors may represent different primaries or metastatic disease, depending on the site. Should the documentation be unclear, the provider should be queried as to the status of each tumor so that the correct codes can be assigned.

j. **Disseminated malignant neoplasm, unspecified**
Code C80.0, Disseminated malignant neoplasm, unspecified, is for use only in those cases where the patient has advanced metastatic disease and no known primary or secondary sites are specified. It should not be used in place of assigning codes for the primary site and all known secondary sites.

k. **Malignant neoplasm without specification of site**
Code C80.1, Malignant (primary) neoplasm, unspecified, equates to Cancer, unspecified. This code should only be used when no determination can be made as to the primary site of a malignancy. This code should rarely be used in the inpatient setting.

l. **Sequencing of neoplasm codes**
1) **Encounter for treatment of primary malignancy**
If the reason for the encounter is for treatment of a primary malignancy, assign the malignancy as the principal/first-listed diagnosis. The primary site is to be sequenced first, followed by any metastatic sites.

2) **Encounter for treatment of secondary malignancy**
When an encounter is for a primary malignancy with metastasis and treatment is directed toward the metastatic (secondary) site(s) only, the metastatic site(s) is designated as the principal/first-listed diagnosis. The primary malignancy is coded as an additional code.

3) **Malignant neoplasm in a pregnant patient**
When a pregnant woman has a malignant neoplasm, a code from subcategory O9A.1-, Malignant neoplasm complicating pregnancy, childbirth, and the puerperium, should be sequenced first, followed by the appropriate code from Chapter 2 to indicate the type of neoplasm.

4) **Encounter for complication associated with a neoplasm**
When an encounter is for management of a complication associated with a neoplasm, such as dehydration, and the treatment is only for the complication, the complication is coded first, followed by the appropriate code(s) for the neoplasm.

The exception to this guideline is anemia. When the admission/encounter is for management of an anemia associated with the malignancy, and the treatment is only for anemia, the appropriate code for the malignancy is sequenced as the principal or first-listed diagnosis followed by code D63.0, Anemia in neoplastic disease.

5) **Complication from surgical procedure for treatment of a neoplasm**
When an encounter is for treatment of a complication resulting from a surgical procedure performed for the treatment of the neoplasm, designate the complication as the principal/first-listed diagnosis. See **the** guideline regarding the coding of a current malignancy versus personal history to determine if the code for the neoplasm should also be assigned.

6) **Pathologic fracture due to a neoplasm**
When an encounter is for a pathological fracture due to a neoplasm, and the focus of treatment is the fracture, a code from subcategory M84.5, Pathological fracture in neoplastic disease, should be sequenced first, followed by the code for the neoplasm.

If the focus of treatment is the neoplasm with an associated pathological fracture, the neoplasm code should be sequenced first, followed by a code from M84.5 for the pathological fracture.

m. **Current malignancy versus personal history of malignancy**
When a primary malignancy has been excised but further treatment, such as an additional surgery for the malignancy, radiation therapy or chemotherapy is directed to that site, the primary malignancy code should be used until treatment is completed.

When a primary malignancy has been previously excised or eradicated from its site, there is no further treatment (of the malignancy) directed to that site, and there is no evidence of any existing primary malignancy at that site, a code from category Z85, Personal history of malignant neoplasm, should be used to indicate the former site of the malignancy.

Subcategories Z85.0 – Z85.7 should only be assigned for the former site of a primary malignancy, not the site of a secondary malignancy. Codes from subcategory Z85.8-, may be assigned for the former site(s) of either a primary or secondary malignancy included in this subcategory.
See Section I.C.21. Factors influencing health status and contact with health services, History (of)

n. **Leukemia, Multiple Myeloma, and Malignant Plasma Cell Neoplasms in remission versus personal history**
The categories for leukemia, and category C90, Multiple myeloma and malignant plasma cell neoplasms, have codes indicating whether or not the leukemia has achieved remission. There are also codes Z85.6, Personal history of leukemia, and Z85.79, Personal history of other malignant neoplasms of lymphoid, hematopoietic and related tissues. If the documentation is unclear as to whether the leukemia has achieved remission, the provider should be queried.
See Section I.C.21. Factors influencing health status and contact with health services, History (of)

o. **Aftercare following surgery for neoplasm**
See Section I.C.21. Factors influencing health status and contact with health services, Aftercare

p. **Follow-up care for completed treatment of a malignancy**
See Section I.C.21. Factors influencing health status and contact with health services, Follow-up

q. **Prophylactic organ removal for prevention of malignancy**
See Section I.C. 21, Factors influencing health status and contact with health services, Prophylactic organ removal

r. **Malignant neoplasm associated with transplanted organ**
A malignant neoplasm of a transplanted organ should be coded as a transplant complication. Assign first the appropriate code from category T86.-, Complications of transplanted organs and tissue, followed by code C80.2, Malignant neoplasm associated with transplanted organ. Use an additional code for the specific malignancy.

3. **Chapter 3: Disease of the blood and blood-forming organs and certain disorders involving the immune mechanism (D50-D89)**
Reserved for future guideline expansion

4. **Chapter 4: Endocrine, Nutritional, and Metabolic Diseases (E00-E89)**
a. **Diabetes mellitus**
The diabetes mellitus codes are combination codes that include the type of diabetes mellitus, the body system affected, and the complications affecting that body system. As many codes within a particular category as are necessary to describe all of the complications of the disease may be used. They should be sequenced based on the reason for a particular encounter. Assign as many codes from categories E08 – E13 as needed to identify all of the associated conditions that the patient has.

1) **Type of diabetes**
The age of a patient is not the sole determining factor, though most type 1 diabetics develop the condition before reaching puberty. For this reason type 1 diabetes mellitus is also referred to as juvenile diabetes.

2) **Type of diabetes mellitus not documented**
If the type of diabetes mellitus is not documented in the medical record the default is E11.-, Type 2 diabetes mellitus.

3) **Diabetes mellitus and the use of insulin and oral hypoglycemics**
If the documentation in a medical record does not indicate the type of diabetes but does indicate that the patient uses insulin, code E11.-, Type 2 diabetes mellitus, should be assigned. An additional code should be assigned from category Z79 to identify the long-term (current) use of insulin or oral hypoglycemic drugs. If the patient is treated with both oral medications and insulin, only the code for long-term (current) use of insulin should be assigned. Code Z79.4 should not be assigned if insulin is given temporarily to bring a type 2 patient's blood sugar under control during an encounter.

4) **Diabetes mellitus in pregnancy and gestational diabetes**
See Section I.C.15. Diabetes mellitus in pregnancy.
See Section I.C.15. Gestational (pregnancy induced) diabetes

5) **Complications due to insulin pump malfunction**

(a) **Underdose of insulin due to insulin pump failure**

An underdose of insulin due to an insulin pump failure should be assigned to a code from subcategory T85.6, Mechanical complication of other specified internal and external prosthetic devices, implants and grafts, that specifies the type of pump malfunction, as the principal or first-listed code, followed by code T38.3X6-, Underdosing of insulin and oral hypoglycemic [antidiabetic] drugs. Additional codes for the type of diabetes mellitus and any associated complications due to the underdosing should also be assigned.

(b) **Overdose of insulin due to insulin pump failure**

The principal or first-listed code for an encounter due to an insulin pump malfunction resulting in an overdose of insulin, should also be T85.6-, Mechanical complication of other specified internal and external prosthetic devices, implants and grafts, followed by code T38.3X1-, Poisoning by insulin and oral hypoglycemic [antidiabetic] drugs, accidental (unintentional).

6) **Secondary diabetes mellitus**

Codes under categories E08, Diabetes mellitus due to underlying condition, E09, Drug or chemical induced diabetes mellitus, and E13, Other specified diabetes mellitus, identify complications/manifestations associated with secondary diabetes mellitus. Secondary diabetes is always caused by another condition or event (e.g., cystic fibrosis, malignant neoplasm of pancreas, pancreatectomy, adverse effect of drug, or poisoning).

(a) **Secondary diabetes mellitus and the use of insulin or oral hypoglycemic drugs**

For patients with secondary diabetes mellitus who routinely use insulin or oral hypoglycemic drugs, an additional code from category Z79 should be assigned to identify the long-term (current) use of insulin or oral hypoglycemic drugs. If the patient is treated with both oral medications and insulin, only the code for long-term (current) use of insulin should be assigned. Code Z79.4 should not be assigned if insulin is given temporarily to bring a secondary diabetic patient's blood sugar under control during an encounter.

(b) **Assigning and sequencing secondary diabetes codes and its causes**

The sequencing of the secondary diabetes codes in relationship to codes for the cause of the diabetes is based on the Tabular List instructions for categories E08, E09 and E13.

(i) **Secondary diabetes mellitus due to pancreatectomy**

For postpancreatectomy diabetes mellitus (lack of insulin due to the surgical removal of all or part of the pancreas), assign code E89.1, Postprocedural hypoinsulinemia. Assign a code from category E13 and a code from subcategory Z90.41, Acquired absence of pancreas, as additional codes.

(ii) **Secondary diabetes due to drugs**

Secondary diabetes may be caused by an adverse effect of correctly administered medications, poisoning or sequela of poisoning.

See section I.C.19.e for coding of adverse effects and poisoning, and section I.C.20 for external cause code reporting.

5. **Chapter 5: Mental, Behavioral and Neurodevelopmental disorders (F01–F99)**

a. **Pain disorders related to psychological factors**

Assign code F45.41, for pain that is exclusively related to psychological disorders. As indicated by the Excludes 1 note under category G89, a code from category G89 should not be assigned with code F45.41.

Code F45.42, Pain disorders with related psychological factors, should be used with a code from category G89, Pain, not elsewhere classified, if there is documentation of a psychological component for a patient with acute or chronic pain.

See Section I.C.6. Pain

b. **Mental and behavioral disorders due to psychoactive substance use**

1) **In Remission**

Selection of codes for "in remission" for categories F10-F19, Mental and behavioral disorders due to psychoactive substance use (categories F10-F19 with -.11, -.21) requires the provider's clinical judgment. The appropriate codes for "in remission" are assigned only on the basis of provider documentation (as defined in the Official Guidelines for Coding and Reporting), unless otherwise instructed by the classification.

Mild substance use disorders in early or sustained remission are classified to the appropriate codes for substance abuse in remission, and moderate or severe substance use disorders in early or sustained remission are classified to the appropriate codes for substance dependence in remission.

2) **Psychoactive Substance Use, Abuse and Dependence**

When the provider documentation refers to use, abuse and dependence of the same substance (e.g. alcohol, opioid, cannabis, etc.), only one code should be assigned to identify the pattern of use based on the following hierarchy:

- If both use and abuse are documented, assign only the code for abuse
- If both abuse and dependence are documented, assign only the code for dependence
- If use, abuse and dependence are all documented, assign only the code for dependence
- If both use and dependence are documented, assign only the code for dependence.

3) **Psychoactive Substance Use, Unspecified**

As with all other unspecified diagnoses, the codes for unspecified psychoactive substance use (F10.9-, F11.9-, F12.9-, F13.9-, F14.9-, F15.9-, F16.9-, F18.9-, F19.9-) should only be assigned based on provider documentation and when they meet the definition of a reportable diagnosis (see Section III, Reporting Additional Diagnoses). These codes are to be used only when the psychoactive substance use is associated with a physical, mental or behavioral disorder, and such a relationship is documented by the provider.

c. **Factitious Disorder**

Factitious disorder imposed on self or Munchausen's syndrome is a disorder in which a person falsely reports or causes his or her own physical or psychological signs or symptoms. For patients with documented factitious disorder on self or Munchausen's syndrome, assign the appropriate code from subcategory F68.1-, Factitious disorder imposed on self.

Munchausen's syndrome by proxy (MSBP) is a disorder in which a caregiver (perpetrator) falsely reports or causes an illness or injury in another person (victim) under his or her care, such as a child, an elderly adult, or a person who has a disability. The condition is also referred to as "factitious disorder imposed on another" or "factitious disorder by proxy." The perpetrator, not the victim, receives this diagnosis. Assign code F68.A, Factitious disorder imposed on another, to the perpetrator's record. For the victim of a patient suffering from MSBP, assign the appropriate code from categories T74, Adult and child abuse, neglect and other maltreatment, confirmed, or T76, Adult and child abuse, neglect and other maltreatment, suspected.

See Section I.C.19.f. Adult and child abuse, neglect and other maltreatment

6. **Chapter 6: Diseases of the Nervous System (G00-G99)**

a. **Dominant/nondominant side**

Codes from category G81, Hemiplegia and hemiparesis, and subcategories G83.1, Monoplegia of lower limb, G83.2, Monoplegia of upper limb, and G83.3, Monoplegia, unspecified, identify whether the dominant or nondominant side is affected. Should the affected side be documented, but not specified as dominant or nondominant, and the classification system does not indicate a default, code selection is as follows:

- For ambidextrous patients, the default should be dominant.
- If the left side is affected, the default is non-dominant.
- If the right side is affected, the default is dominant.

b. **Pain - Category G89**

1) **General coding information**

Codes in category G89, Pain, not elsewhere classified, may be used in conjunction with codes from other categories and chapters to provide more detail about acute or chronic pain and neoplasm-related pain, unless otherwise indicated below.

If the pain is not specified as acute or chronic, post-thoracotomy, postprocedural, or neoplasm-related, do not assign codes from category G89.

A code from category G89 should not be assigned if the underlying (definitive) diagnosis is known, unless the reason for the encounter is pain control/ management and not management of the underlying condition.

When an admission or encounter is for a procedure aimed at treating the underlying condition (e.g., spinal fusion, kyphoplasty), a code for the underlying condition (e.g., vertebral fracture, spinal stenosis) should be assigned as the principal diagnosis. No code from category G89 should be assigned.

(a) Category G89 Codes as Principal or First-Listed Diagnosis

Category G89 codes are acceptable as principal diagnosis or the first-listed code:

- When pain control or pain management is the reason for the admission/encounter (e.g., a patient with displaced intervertebral disc, nerve impingement and severe back pain presents for injection of steroid into the spinal canal). The underlying cause of the pain should be reported as an additional diagnosis, if known.

- When a patient is admitted for the insertion of a neurostimulator for pain control, assign the appropriate pain code as the principal or first-listed diagnosis. When an admission or encounter is for a procedure aimed at treating the underlying condition and a neurostimulator is inserted for pain control during the same admission/encounter, a code for the underlying condition should be assigned as the principal diagnosis and the appropriate pain code should be assigned as a secondary diagnosis.

(b) Use of Category G89 Codes in Conjunction with Site Specific Pain Codes

(i) Assigning Category G89 and Site-Specific Pain Codes

Codes from category G89 may be used in conjunction with codes that identify the site of pain (including codes from chapter 18) if the category G89 code provides additional information. For example, if the code describes the site of the pain, but does not fully describe whether the pain is acute or chronic, then both codes should be assigned.

(ii) Sequencing of Category G89 Codes with Site-Specific Pain Codes

The sequencing of category G89 codes with site-specific pain codes (including chapter 18 codes), is dependent on the circumstances of the encounter/admission as follows:

- If the encounter is for pain control or pain management, assign the code from category G89 followed by the code identifying the specific site of pain (e.g., encounter for pain management for acute neck pain from trauma is assigned code G89.11, Acute pain due to trauma, followed by code M54.2, Cervicalgia, to identify the site of pain).

- If the encounter is for any other reason except pain control or pain management, and a related definitive diagnosis has not been established (confirmed) by the provider, assign the code for the specific site of pain first, followed by the appropriate code from category G89.

2) Pain due to devices, implants and grafts

See Section I.C.19. Pain due to medical devices

3) Postoperative Pain

The provider's documentation should be used to guide the coding of postoperative pain, as well as *Section III. Reporting Additional Diagnoses and Section IV. Diagnostic Coding and Reporting in the Outpatient Setting.*

The default for post-thoracotomy and other postoperative pain not specified as acute or chronic is the code for the acute form.

Routine or expected postoperative pain immediately after surgery should not be coded.

(a) Postoperative pain not associated with specific postoperative complication

Postoperative pain not associated with a specific postoperative complication is assigned to the appropriate postoperative pain code in category G89.

(b) Postoperative pain associated with specific postoperative complication

Postoperative pain associated with a specific postoperative complication (such as painful wire sutures) is assigned to the appropriate code(s) found in Chapter 19, Injury, poisoning, and certain other consequences of external causes. If appropriate, use additional code(s) from category G89 to identify acute or chronic pain (G89.18 or G89.28).

4) Chronic pain

Chronic pain is classified to subcategory G89.2. There is no time frame defining when pain becomes chronic pain. The provider's documentation should be used to guide use of these codes.

5) Neoplasm Related Pain

Code G89.3 is assigned to pain documented as being related, associated or due to cancer, primary or secondary malignancy, or tumor. This code is assigned regardless of whether the pain is acute or chronic.

This code may be assigned as the principal or first-listed code when the stated reason for the admission/encounter is documented as pain control/pain management. The underlying neoplasm should be reported as an additional diagnosis.

When the reason for the admission/encounter is management of the neoplasm and the pain associated with the neoplasm is also documented, code G89.3 may be assigned as an additional diagnosis. It is not necessary to assign an additional code for the site of the pain.

See Section I.C.2 for instructions on the sequencing of neoplasms for all other stated reasons for the admission/encounter (except for pain control/pain management).

6) Chronic pain syndrome

Central pain syndrome (G89.0) and chronic pain syndrome (G89.4) are different than the term "chronic pain," and therefore codes should only be used when the provider has specifically documented this condition.

See Section I.C.5. Pain disorders related to psychological factors

7. Chapter 7: Diseases of the Eye and Adnexa (H00-H59)

a. Glaucoma

1) Assigning Glaucoma Codes

Assign as many codes from category H40, Glaucoma, as needed to identify the type of glaucoma, the affected eye, and the glaucoma stage.

2) Bilateral glaucoma with same type and stage

When a patient has bilateral glaucoma and both eyes are documented as being the same type and stage, and there is a code for bilateral glaucoma, report only the code for the type of glaucoma, bilateral, with the seventh character for the stage.

When a patient has bilateral glaucoma and both eyes are documented as being the same type and stage, and the classification does not provide a code for bilateral glaucoma (i.e. subcategories H40.10 and H40.20) report only one code for the type of glaucoma with the appropriate seventh character for the stage.

3) Bilateral glaucoma stage with different types or stages

When a patient has bilateral glaucoma and each eye is documented as having a different type or stage, and the classification distinguishes laterality, assign the appropriate code for each eye rather than the code for bilateral glaucoma.

When a patient has bilateral glaucoma and each eye is documented as having a different type, and the classification does not distinguish laterality (i.e. subcategories H40.10 and H40.20), assign one code for each type of glaucoma with the appropriate seventh character for the stage.

When a patient has bilateral glaucoma and each eye is documented as having the same type, but different stage, and the classification does not distinguish laterality (i.e. subcategories H40.10 and H40.20), assign a code for the type of glaucoma for each eye with the seventh character for the specific glaucoma stage documented for each eye.

4) Patient admitted with glaucoma and stage evolves during the admission

If a patient is admitted with glaucoma and the stage progresses during the admission, assign the code for highest stage documented.

5) Indeterminate stage glaucoma

Assignment of the seventh character "4" for "indeterminate stage" should be based on the clinical documentation. The seventh character "4" is used for glaucomas whose stage cannot be clinically determined. This seventh character should not be confused with the seventh character "0", unspecified, which should be assigned when there is no documentation regarding the stage of the glaucoma.

b. Blindness

If "blindness" or "low vision" of both eyes is documented but the visual impairment category is not documented, assign code H54.3, Unqualified visual loss, both eyes. If "blindness" or "low vision" in one eye is documented but the visual impairment category is not documented, assign a code from H54.6-, Unqualified visual loss, one eye. If "blindness" or "visual loss" is documented without any information about whether one or both eyes are affected, assign code H54.7, Unspecified visual loss.

8. Chapter 8: Diseases of the Ear and Mastoid Process (H60-H95)

Reserved for future guideline expansion

9. Chapter 9: Diseases of the Circulatory System (I00-I99)

a. Hypertension

The classification presumes a causal relationship between hypertension and heart involvement and between hypertension and kidney involvement, as the two conditions are linked by the term "with" in the Alphabetic Index. These conditions should be coded as related even in the absence of provider documentation explicitly linking them, unless the documentation clearly states the conditions are unrelated.

For hypertension and conditions not specifically linked by relational terms such as "with," "associated with" or "due to" in the classification, provider documentation must link the conditions in order to code them as related.

1) Hypertension with Heart Disease

Hypertension with heart conditions classified to I50.- or I51.4-I51.7, I51.89, I51.9, are assigned to a code from category I11, Hypertensive heart disease. Use additional code(s) from category I50, Heart failure, to identify the type(s) of heart failure in those patients with heart failure.

The same heart conditions (I50.-, I51.4-I51.7, I51.89, I51.9) with hypertension are coded separately if the provider has documented they are unrelated to the hypertension. Sequence according to the circumstances of the admission/encounter.

2) Hypertensive Chronic Kidney Disease

Assign codes from category I12, Hypertensive chronic kidney disease, when both hypertension and a condition classifiable to category N18, Chronic kidney disease (CKD), are present. CKD should not be coded as hypertensive if the provider indicates the CKD is not related to the hypertension.

The appropriate code from category N18 should be used as a secondary code with a code from category I12 to identify the stage of chronic kidney disease.

See Section I.C.14. Chronic kidney disease.

If a patient has hypertensive chronic kidney disease and acute renal failure, an additional code for the acute renal failure is required.

3) Hypertensive Heart and Chronic Kidney Disease

Assign codes from combination category I13, Hypertensive heart and chronic kidney disease, when there is hypertension with both heart and kidney involvement. If heart failure is present, assign an additional code from category I50 to identify the type of heart failure.

The appropriate code from category N18, Chronic kidney disease, should be used as a secondary code with a code from category I13 to identify the stage of chronic kidney disease.

See Section I.C.14. Chronic kidney disease.

The codes in category I13, Hypertensive heart and chronic kidney disease, are combination codes that include hypertension, heart

disease and chronic kidney disease. The Includes note at I13 specifies that the conditions included at I11 and I12 are included together in I13. If a patient has hypertension, heart disease and chronic kidney disease, then a code from I13 should be used, not individual codes for hypertension, heart disease and chronic kidney disease, or codes from I11 or I12.

For patients with both acute renal failure and chronic kidney disease, an additional code for acute renal failure is required.

4) Hypertensive Cerebrovascular Disease

For hypertensive cerebrovascular disease, first assign the appropriate code from categories I60-I69, followed by the appropriate hypertension code.

5) Hypertensive Retinopathy

Subcategory H35.0, Background retinopathy and retinal vascular changes, should be used with a code from category I10- I15, Hypertensive disease to include the systemic hypertension. The sequencing is based on the reason for the encounter.

6) Hypertension, Secondary

Secondary hypertension is due to an underlying condition. Two codes are required: one to identify the underlying etiology and one from category I15 to identify the hypertension. Sequencing of codes is determined by the reason for admission/encounter.

7) Hypertension, Transient

Assign code R03.0, Elevated blood pressure reading without diagnosis of hypertension, unless patient has an established diagnosis of hypertension. Assign code O13.-, Gestational [pregnancy-induced] hypertension without significant proteinuria, or O14.-, Pre-eclampsia, for transient hypertension of pregnancy.

8) Hypertension, Controlled

This diagnostic statement usually refers to an existing state of hypertension under control by therapy. Assign the appropriate code from categories I10-I15, Hypertensive diseases.

9) Hypertension, Uncontrolled

Uncontrolled hypertension may refer to untreated hypertension or hypertension not responding to current therapeutic regimen. In either case, assign the appropriate code from categories I10-I15, Hypertensive diseases.

10) Hypertensive Crisis

Assign a code from category I16, Hypertensive crisis, for documented hypertensive urgency, hypertensive emergency or unspecified hypertensive crisis. Code also any identified hypertensive disease (I10-I15). The sequencing is based on the reason for the encounter.

11) Pulmonary Hypertension

Pulmonary hypertension is classified to category I27, Other pulmonary heart diseases. For secondary pulmonary hypertension (I27.1, I27.2-), code also any associated conditions or adverse effects of drugs or toxins. The sequencing is based on the reason for the encounter, except for adverse effects of drugs (See Section I.C.19.e.).

b. Atherosclerotic Coronary Artery Disease and Angina

ICD-10-CM has combination codes for atherosclerotic heart disease with angina pectoris. The subcategories for these codes are I25.11, Atherosclerotic heart disease of native coronary artery with angina pectoris and I25.7, Atherosclerosis of coronary artery bypass graft(s) and coronary artery of transplanted heart with angina pectoris.

When using one of these combination codes it is not necessary to use an additional code for angina pectoris. A causal relationship can be assumed in a patient with both atherosclerosis and angina pectoris, unless the documentation indicates the angina is due to something other than the atherosclerosis.

If a patient with coronary artery disease is admitted due to an acute myocardial infarction (AMI), the AMI should be sequenced before the coronary artery disease.

See Section I.C.9. Acute myocardial infarction (AMI)

c. Intraoperative and Postprocedural Cerebrovascular Accident

Medical record documentation should clearly specify the cause-and-effect relationship between the medical intervention and the cerebrovascular accident in order to assign a code for intraoperative or postprocedural cerebrovascular accident.

Proper code assignment depends on whether it was an infarction or hemorrhage and whether it occurred intraoperatively or postoperatively. If it was a cerebral hemorrhage, code assignment depends on the type of procedure performed.

d. Sequelae of Cerebrovascular Disease

1) Category I69, Sequelae of Cerebrovascular disease

Category I69 is used to indicate conditions classifiable to categories I60-I67 as the causes of sequela (neurologic deficits), themselves classified elsewhere. These "late effects" include neurologic deficits that persist after initial onset of conditions classifiable to categories I60-I67. The neurologic deficits caused by cerebrovascular disease may be present from the onset or may arise at any time after the onset of the condition classifiable to categories I60-I67.

Codes from category I69, Sequelae of cerebrovascular disease, that specify hemiplegia, hemiparesis and monoplegia identify whether the dominant or nondominant side is affected. Should the affected side be documented, but not specified as dominant or nondominant, and the classification system does not indicate a default, code selection is as follows:

- For ambidextrous patients, the default should be dominant.
- If the left side is affected, the default is non-dominant.
- If the right side is affected, the default is dominant.

2) Codes from category I69 with codes from I60-I67

Codes from category I69 may be assigned on a health care record with codes from I60-I67, if the patient has a current cerebrovascular disease and deficits from an old cerebrovascular disease.

3) Codes from category I69 and Personal history of transient ischemic attack (TIA) and cerebral infarction (Z86.73)

Codes from category I69 should not be assigned if the patient does not have neurologic deficits.

See Section I.C.21. 4. History (of) for use of personal history codes

e. Acute myocardial infarction (AMI)

1) Type 1 ST elevation myocardial infarction (STEMI) and non-ST elevation myocardial infarction (NSTEMI)

The ICD-10-CMcodes for type 1 acute myocardial infarction (AMI) identify the site, such as anterolateral wall or true posterior wall. Subcategories I21.0-I21.2 and code I21.3 are used for type 1 ST elevation myocardial infarction (STEMI). Code I21.4, Non-ST elevation (NSTEMI) myocardial infarction, is used for type 1 non ST elevation myocardial infarction (NSTEMI) and nontransmural MIs.

If a type 1 NSTEMI evolves to STEMI, assign the STEMI code. If a type 1 STEMI converts to NSTEMI due to thrombolytic therapy, it is still coded as STEMI.

For encounters occurring while the myocardial infarction is equal to, or less than, four weeks old, including transfers to another acute setting or a postacute setting, and the myocardial infarction meets the definition for "other diagnoses" (see Section III, Reporting Additional Diagnoses), codes from category I21 may continue to be reported. For encounters after the 4 week time frame and the patient is still receiving care related to the myocardial infarction, the appropriate aftercare code should be assigned, rather than a code from category I21. For old or healed myocardial infarctions not requiring further care, code I25.2, Old myocardial infarction, may be assigned.

2) Acute myocardial infarction, unspecified

Code I21.9, Acute myocardial infarction, unspecified, is the default for unspecified acute myocardial infarction or unspecified type. If only type 1 STEMI or transmural MI without the site is documented, assign code I21.3, ST elevation (STEMI) myocardial infarction of unspecified site.

3) AMI documented as nontransmural or subendocardial but site provided

If an AMI is documented as nontransmural or subendocardial, but the site is provided, it is still coded as a subendocardial AMI.

See Section I.C.21.3 for information on coding status post administration of tPA in a different facility within the last 24 hours.

4) Subsequent acute myocardial infarction

A code from category I22, Subsequent ST elevation (STEMI) and non-ST elevation (NSTEMI) myocardial infarction, is to be used when a patient who has suffered a type 1 or unspecified AMI has a new AMI within the 4 week time frame of the initial AMI. A code from category I22 must be used in conjunction with a code from

category I21. The sequencing of the I22 and I21 codes depends on the circumstances of the encounter.

Do not assign code I22 for subsequent myocardial infarctions other than type 1 or unspecified. For subsequent type 2 AMI assign only code I21.A1. For subsequent type 4 or type 5 AMI, assign only code I21.A9.

If a subsequent myocardial infarction of one type occurs within 4 weeks of a myocardial infarction of a different type, assign the appropriate codes from category I21 to identify each type. Do not assign a code from I22. Codes from category I22 should only be assigned if both the initial and subsequent myocardial infarctions are type 1 or unspecified.

5) Other Types of Myocardial Infarction

The ICD-10-CM provides codes for different types of myocardial infarction. Type 1 myocardial infarctions are assigned to codes I21.0-I21.4.

Type 2 myocardial infarction (myocardial infarction due to demand ischemia or secondary to ischemic **im**balance), is assigned to code I21.A1, Myocardial infarction type 2 with the underlying cause **coded first**. Do not assign code I24.8, Other forms of acute ischemic heart disease, for the demand ischemia. **If** a type 2 AMI is described as NSTEMI or STEMI, only assign code I21.A1. Codes I21.01-I21.4 should only be assigned for type 1 AMIs.

Acute myocardial infarctions type 3, 4a, 4b, 4c and 5 are assigned to code I21.A9, Other myocardial infarction type.

The "Code also" and "Code first" notes should be followed related to complications, and for coding of postprocedural myocardial infarctions during or following cardiac surgery.

10. Chapter 10: Diseases of the Respiratory System (J00-J99)

a. Chronic Obstructive Pulmonary Disease [COPD] and Asthma

1) Acute exacerbation of chronic obstructive bronchitis and asthma

The codes in categories J44 and J45 distinguish between uncomplicated cases and those in acute exacerbation. An acute exacerbation is a worsening or a decompensation of a chronic condition. An acute exacerbation is not equivalent to an infection superimposed on a chronic condition, though an exacerbation may be triggered by an infection.

b. Acute Respiratory Failure

1) Acute respiratory failure as principal diagnosis

A code from subcategory J96.0, Acute respiratory failure, or subcategory J96.2, Acute and chronic respiratory failure, may be assigned as a principal diagnosis when it is the condition established after study to be chiefly responsible for occasioning the admission to the hospital, and the selection is supported by the Alphabetic Index and Tabular List. However, chapter-specific coding guidelines (such as obstetrics, poisoning, HIV, newborn) that provide sequencing direction take precedence.

2) Acute respiratory failure as secondary diagnosis

Respiratory failure may be listed as a secondary diagnosis if it occurs after admission, or if it is present on admission, but does not meet the definition of principal diagnosis.

3) Sequencing of acute respiratory failure and another acute condition

When a patient is admitted with respiratory failure and another acute condition, (e.g., myocardial infarction, cerebrovascular accident, aspiration pneumonia), the principal diagnosis will not be the same in every situation. This applies whether the other acute condition is a respiratory or nonrespiratory condition. Selection of the principal diagnosis will be dependent on the circumstances of admission. If both the respiratory failure and the other acute condition are equally responsible for occasioning the admission to the hospital, and there are no chapter-specific sequencing rules, the guideline regarding two or more diagnoses that equally meet the definition for principal diagnosis *(Section II, C.)* may be applied in these situations.

If the documentation is not clear as to whether acute respiratory failure and another condition are equally responsible for occasioning the admission, query the provider for clarification.

c. Influenza due to certain identified influenza viruses

Code only confirmed cases of influenza due to certain identified influenza viruses (category J09), and due to other identified influenza virus (category J10). This is an exception to the hospital inpatient guideline Section II, H. (Uncertain Diagnosis).

In this context, "confirmation" does not require documentation of positive laboratory testing specific for avian or other novel influenza A or other identified influenza virus. However, coding should be based on the provider's diagnostic statement that the patient has avian influenza, or other novel influenza A, for category J09, or has another particular identified strain of influenza, such as H1N1 or H3N2, but not identified as novel or variant, for category J10.

If the provider records "suspected" or "possible" or "probable" avian influenza, or novel influenza, or other identified influenza, then the appropriate influenza code from category J11, Influenza due to unidentified influenza virus, should be assigned. A code from category J09, Influenza due to certain identified influenza viruses, should not be assigned nor should a code from category J10, Influenza due to other identified influenza virus.

d. **Ventilator associated Pneumonia**
   1) **Documentation of Ventilator associated Pneumonia**
      As with all procedural or postprocedural complications, code assignment is based on the provider's documentation of the relationship between the condition and the procedure.

      Code J95.851, Ventilator associated pneumonia, should be assigned only when the provider has documented ventilator associated pneumonia (VAP). An additional code to identify the organism (e.g., Pseudomonas aeruginosa, code B96.5) should also be assigned. Do not assign an additional code from categories J12-J18 to identify the type of pneumonia.

      Code J95.851 should not be assigned for cases where the patient has pneumonia and is on a mechanical ventilator and the provider has not specifically stated that the pneumonia is ventilator-associated pneumonia. If the documentation is unclear as to whether the patient has a pneumonia that is a complication attributable to the mechanical ventilator, query the provider.

   2) **Ventilator associated Pneumonia Develops after Admission**
      A patient may be admitted with one type of pneumonia (e.g., code J13, Pneumonia due to Streptococcus pneumonia) and subsequently develop VAP. In this instance, the principal diagnosis would be the appropriate code from categories J12-J18 for the pneumonia diagnosed at the time of admission. Code J95.851, Ventilator associated pneumonia, would be assigned as an additional diagnosis when the provider has also documented the presence of ventilator associated pneumonia.

11. **Chapter 11: Diseases of the Digestive System (K00-K95)**
    Reserved for future guideline expansion

12. **Chapter 12: Diseases of the Skin and Subcutaneous Tissue (L00-L99)**
    a. **Pressure ulcer stage codes**
       1) **Pressure ulcer stages**
          Codes in category L89, Pressure ulcer, identify the site and stage of the pressure ulcer.

          The ICD-10-CM classifies pressure ulcer stages based on severity, which is designated by stages 1-4, **deep tissue pressure injury,** unspecified stage and unstageable.

          Assign as many codes from category L89 as needed to identify all the pressure ulcers the patient has, if applicable.

          See Section I.B.14 for pressure ulcer stage documentation by clinicians other than patient's provider

       2) **Unstageable pressure ulcers**
          Assignment of the code for unstageable pressure ulcer (L89.--0) should be based on the clinical documentation. These codes are used for pressure ulcers whose stage cannot be clinically determined (e.g., the ulcer is covered by eschar or has been treated with a skin or muscle graft). This code should not be confused with the codes for unspecified stage (L89.--9). When there is no documentation regarding the stage of the pressure ulcer, assign the appropriate code for unspecified stage (L89.--9).

       3) **Documented pressure ulcer stage**
          Assignment of the pressure ulcer stage code should be guided by clinical documentation of the stage or documentation of the terms found in the Alphabetic Index. For clinical terms describing the stage that are not found in the Alphabetic Index, and there is no documentation of the stage, the provider should be queried.

       4) **Patients admitted with pressure ulcers documented as healed**
          No code is assigned if the documentation states that the pressure ulcer is completely healed **at the time of admission.**

5) **Pressure ulcers documented as healing**
   Pressure ulcers described as healing should be assigned the appropriate pressure ulcer stage code based on the documentation in the medical record. If the documentation does not provide information about the stage of the healing pressure ulcer, assign the appropriate code for unspecified stage.

   If the documentation is unclear as to whether the patient has a current (new) pressure ulcer or if the patient is being treated for a healing pressure ulcer, query the provider.

   For ulcers that were present on admission but healed at the time of discharge, assign the code for the site and stage of the pressure ulcer at the time of admission.

6) **Patient admitted with pressure ulcer evolving into another stage during the admission**
   If a patient is admitted to an inpatient hospital with a pressure ulcer at one stage and it progresses to a higher stage, two separate codes should be assigned: one code for the site and stage of the ulcer on admission and a second code for the same ulcer site and the highest stage reported during the stay.

7) **Pressure-induced deep tissue damage**
   For pressure-induced deep tissue damage or deep tissue pressure injury, assign only the appropriate code for pressure-induced deep tissue damage (L89.--6).

b. **Non-Pressure Chronic Ulcers**
   1) **Patients admitted with non-pressure ulcers documented as healed**
      No code is assigned if the documentation states that the non-pressure ulcer is completely healed **at the time of admission.**

   2) **Non-pressure ulcers documented as healing**
      Non-pressure ulcers described as healing should be assigned the appropriate non-pressure ulcer code based on the documentation in the medical record. If the documentation does not provide information about the severity of the healing non-pressure ulcer, assign the appropriate code for unspecified severity.

      If the documentation is unclear as to whether the patient has a current (new) non-pressure ulcer or if the patient is being treated for a healing non-pressure ulcer, query the provider.

      For ulcers that were present on admission but healed at the time of discharge, assign the code for the site and severity of the non-pressure ulcer at the time of admission.

   3) **Patient admitted with non-pressure ulcer that progresses to another severity level during the admission**
      If a patient is admitted to an inpatient hospital with a non-pressure ulcer at one severity level and it progresses to a higher severity level, two separate codes should be assigned: one code for the site and severity level of the ulcer on admission and a second code for the same ulcer site and the highest severity level reported during the stay.

      See Section I.B.14 for pressure ulcer stage documentation by clinicians other than patient's provider

13. **Chapter 13: Diseases of the Musculoskeletal System and Connective Tissue (M00-M99)**
    a. **Site and laterality**
       Most of the codes within Chapter 13 have site and laterality designations. The site represents the bone, joint or the muscle involved. For some conditions where more than one bone, joint or muscle is usually involved, such as osteoarthritis, there is a "multiple sites" code available. For categories where no multiple site code is provided and more than one bone, joint or muscle is involved, multiple codes should be used to indicate the different sites involved.

       1) **Bone versus joint**
          For certain conditions, the bone may be affected at the upper or lower end, (e.g., avascular necrosis of bone, M87, Osteoporosis, M80, M81). Though the portion of the bone affected may be at the joint, the site designation will be the bone, not the joint.

    b. **Acute traumatic versus chronic or recurrent musculoskeletal conditions**
       Many musculoskeletal conditions are a result of previous injury or trauma to a site, or are recurrent conditions. Bone, joint or muscle conditions that are the result of a healed injury are usually found in chapter 13. Recurrent bone, joint or muscle conditions are also usually found in chapter 13. Any current, acute injury should be coded to the

appropriate injury code from chapter 19. Chronic or recurrent conditions should generally be coded with a code from chapter 13. If it is difficult to determine from the documentation in the record which code is best to describe a condition, query the provider.

c. Coding of Pathologic Fractures

7th character A is for use as long as the patient is receiving active treatment for the fracture. While the patient may be seen by a new or different provider over the course of treatment for a pathological fracture, assignment of the 7th character is based on whether the patient is undergoing active treatment and not whether the provider is seeing the patient for the first time.

7th character D is to be used for encounters after the patient has completed active treatment for the fracture and is receiving routine care for the fracture during the healing or recovery phase. The other 7th characters, listed under each subcategory in the Tabular List, are to be used for subsequent encounters for treatment of problems associated with the healing, such as malunions, nonunions, and sequelae.

Care for complications of surgical treatment for fracture repairs during the healing or recovery phase should be coded with the appropriate complication codes.

See Section I.C.19. Coding of traumatic fractures.

d. Osteoporosis

Osteoporosis is a systemic condition, meaning that all bones of the musculoskeletal system are affected. Therefore, site is not a component of the codes under category M81, Osteoporosis without current pathological fracture. The site codes under category M80, Osteoporosis with current pathological fracture, identify the site of the fracture, not the osteoporosis.

1) Osteoporosis without pathological fracture

Category M81, Osteoporosis without current pathological fracture, is for use for patients with osteoporosis who do not currently have a pathologic fracture due to the osteoporosis, even if they have had a fracture in the past. For patients with a history of osteoporosis fractures, status code Z87.310, Personal history of (healed) osteoporosis fracture, should follow the code from M81.

2) Osteoporosis with current pathological fracture

Category M80, Osteoporosis with current pathological fracture, is for patients who have a current pathologic fracture at the time of an encounter. The codes under M80 identify the site of the fracture. A code from category M80, not a traumatic fracture code, should be used for any patient with known osteoporosis who suffers a fracture, even if the patient had a minor fall or trauma, if that fall or trauma would not usually break a normal, healthy bone.

14. Chapter 14: Diseases of Genitourinary System (N00-N99)

a. Chronic kidney disease

1) Stages of chronic kidney disease (CKD)

The ICD-10-CM classifies CKD based on severity. The severity of CKD is designated by stages 1-5. Stage 2, code N18.2, equates to mild CKD; stage 3, code N18.3, equates to moderate CKD; and stage 4, code N18.4, equates to severe CKD. Code N18.6, End stage renal disease (ESRD), is assigned when the provider has documented end-stage-renal disease (ESRD).

If both a stage of CKD and ESRD are documented, assign code N18.6 only.

2) Chronic kidney disease and kidney transplant status

Patients who have undergone kidney transplant may still have some form of chronic kidney disease (CKD) because the kidney transplant may not fully restore kidney function. Therefore, the presence of CKD alone does not constitute a transplant complication. Assign the appropriate N18 code for the patient's stage of CKD and code Z94.0, Kidney transplant status. If a transplant complication such as failure or rejection or other transplant complication is documented, see section I.C.19.g for information on coding complications of a kidney transplant. If the documentation is unclear as to whether the patient has a complication of the transplant, query the provider.

3) Chronic kidney disease with other conditions

Patients with CKD may also suffer from other serious conditions, most commonly diabetes mellitus and hypertension. The sequencing of the CKD code in relationship to codes for other contributing conditions is based on the conventions in the Tabular List.

See I.C.9. Hypertensive chronic kidney disease.

See I.C.19. Chronic kidney disease and kidney transplant complications.

15. Chapter 15: Pregnancy, Childbirth, and the Puerperium (O00-O9A)

a. General Rules for Obstetric Cases

1) Codes from chapter 15 and sequencing priority

Obstetric cases require codes from chapter 15, codes in the range O00-O9A, Pregnancy, Childbirth, and the Puerperium. Chapter 15 codes have sequencing priority over codes from other chapters. Additional codes from other chapters may be used in conjunction with chapter 15 codes to further specify conditions. Should the provider document that the pregnancy is incidental to the encounter, then code Z33.1, Pregnant state, incidental, should be used in place of any chapter 15 codes. It is the provider's responsibility to state that the condition being treated is not affecting the pregnancy.

2) Chapter 15 codes used only on the maternal record

Chapter 15 codes are to be used only on the maternal record, never on the record of the newborn.

3) Final character for trimester

The majority of codes in Chapter 15 have a final character indicating the trimester of pregnancy. The timeframes for the trimesters are indicated at the beginning of the chapter. If trimester is not a component of a code, it is because the condition always occurs in a specific trimester, or the concept of trimester of pregnancy is not applicable. Certain codes have characters for only certain trimesters because the condition does not occur in all trimesters, but it may occur in more than just one.

Assignment of the final character for trimester should be based on the provider's documentation of the trimester (or number of weeks) for the current admission/encounter. This applies to the assignment of trimester for pre-existing conditions as well as those that develop during or are due to the pregnancy. The provider's documentation of the number of weeks may be used to assign the appropriate code identifying the trimester.

Whenever delivery occurs during the current admission, and there is an "in childbirth" option for the obstetric complication being coded, the "in childbirth" code should be assigned.

4) Selection of trimester for inpatient admissions that encompass more than one trimester

In instances when a patient is admitted to a hospital for complications of pregnancy during one trimester and remains in the hospital into a subsequent trimester, the trimester character for the antepartum complication code should be assigned on the basis of the trimester when the complication developed, not the trimester of the discharge. If the condition developed prior to the current admission/encounter or represents a pre-existing condition, the trimester character for the trimester at the time of the admission/encounter should be assigned.

5) Unspecified trimester

Each category that includes codes for trimester has a code for "unspecified trimester." The "unspecified trimester" code should rarely be used, such as when the documentation in the record is insufficient to determine the trimester and it is not possible to obtain clarification.

6) 7th character for Fetus Identification

Where applicable, a 7th character is to be assigned for certain categories (O31, O32, O33.3 - O33.6, O35, O36, O40, O41, O60.1, O60.2, O64, and O69) to identify the fetus for which the complication code applies.

Assign 7th character "0":

- For single gestations
- When the documentation in the record is insufficient to determine the fetus affected and it is not possible to obtain clarification.
- When it is not possible to clinically determine which fetus is affected.

b. Selection of OB Principal or First-listed Diagnosis

1) Routine outpatient prenatal visits

For routine outpatient prenatal visits when no complications are present, a code from category Z34, Encounter for supervision of normal pregnancy, should be used as the first-listed diagnosis. These codes should not be used in conjunction with chapter 15 codes.

2) Supervision of High-Risk Pregnancy

Codes from category O09, Supervision of high-risk pregnancy, are intended for use only during the prenatal period. For complications during the labor or delivery episode as a result of a high-risk pregnancy, assign the applicable complication codes from Chapter 15. If there are no complications during the labor or delivery episode, assign code O80, Encounter for full-term uncomplicated delivery.

For routine prenatal outpatient visits for patients with high-risk pregnancies, a code from category O09, Supervision of high-risk pregnancy, should be used as the first-listed diagnosis. Secondary chapter 15 codes may be used in conjunction with these codes if appropriate.

3) Episodes when no delivery occurs

In episodes when no delivery occurs, the principal diagnosis should correspond to the principal complication of the pregnancy which necessitated the encounter. Should more than one complication exist, all of which are treated or monitored, any of the complication codes may be sequenced first.

4) When a delivery occurs

When an obstetric patient is admitted and delivers during that admission, the condition that prompted the admission should be sequenced as the principal diagnosis. If multiple conditions prompted the admission, sequence the one most related to the delivery as the principal diagnosis. A code for any complication of the delivery should be assigned as an additional diagnosis. In cases of cesarean delivery, if the patient was admitted with a condition that resulted in the performance of a cesarean procedure, that condition should be selected as the principal diagnosis. If the reason for the admission was unrelated to the condition resulting in the cesarean delivery, the condition related to the reason for the admission should be selected as the principal diagnosis.

5) Outcome of delivery

A code from category Z37, Outcome of delivery, should be included on every maternal record when a delivery has occurred. These codes are not to be used on subsequent records or on the newborn record.

c. Pre-existing conditions versus conditions due to the pregnancy

Certain categories in Chapter 15 distinguish between conditions of the mother that existed prior to pregnancy (pre-existing) and those that are a direct result of pregnancy. When assigning codes from Chapter 15, it is important to assess if a condition was pre-existing prior to pregnancy or developed during or due to the pregnancy in order to assign the correct code.

Categories that do not distinguish between pre-existing and pregnancy-related conditions may be used for either. It is acceptable to use codes specifically for the puerperium with codes complicating pregnancy and childbirth if a condition arises postpartum during the delivery encounter.

d. Pre-existing hypertension in pregnancy

Category O10, Pre-existing hypertension complicating pregnancy, childbirth and the puerperium, includes codes for hypertensive heart and hypertensive chronic kidney disease. When assigning one of the O10 codes that includes hypertensive heart disease or hypertensive chronic kidney disease, it is necessary to add a secondary code from the appropriate hypertension category to specify the type of heart failure or chronic kidney disease.

See Section I.C.9. Hypertension.

e. Fetal Conditions Affecting the Management of the Mother

1) Codes from categories O35 and O36

Codes from categories O35, Maternal care for known or suspected fetal abnormality and damage, and O36, Maternal care for other fetal problems, are assigned only when the fetal condition is actually responsible for modifying the management of the mother, i.e., by requiring diagnostic studies, additional observation, special care, or termination of pregnancy. The fact that the fetal condition exists does not justify assigning a code from this series to the mother's record.

2) In utero surgery

In cases when surgery is performed on the fetus, a diagnosis code from category O35, Maternal care for known or suspected fetal abnormality and damage, should be assigned identifying the fetal condition. Assign the appropriate procedure code for the procedure performed.

No code from Chapter 16, the perinatal codes, should be used on the mother's record to identify fetal conditions. Surgery performed in utero on a fetus is still to be coded as an obstetric encounter.

f. HIV Infection in Pregnancy, Childbirth and the Puerperium

During pregnancy, childbirth or the puerperium, a patient admitted because of an HIV-related illness should receive a principal diagnosis from subcategory O98.7-, Human immunodeficiency [HIV] disease complicating pregnancy, childbirth and the puerperium, followed by the code(s) for the HIV-related illness(es).

Patients with asymptomatic HIV infection status admitted during pregnancy, childbirth, or the puerperium should receive codes of O98.7- and Z21, Asymptomatic human immunodeficiency virus [HIV] infection status.

g. Diabetes mellitus in pregnancy

Diabetes mellitus is a significant complicating factor in pregnancy. Pregnant women who are diabetic should be assigned a code from category O24, Diabetes mellitus in pregnancy, childbirth, and the puerperium, first, followed by the appropriate diabetes code(s) (E08-E13) from Chapter 4.

h. Long term use of insulin and oral hypoglycemics

See section I.C.4.a.3 for information on the long term use of insulin and oral hypoglycemic.

i. Gestational (pregnancy induced) diabetes

Gestational (pregnancy induced) diabetes can occur during the second and third trimester of pregnancy in women who were not diabetic prior to pregnancy. Gestational diabetes can cause complications in the pregnancy similar to those of pre-existing diabetes mellitus. It also puts the woman at greater risk of developing diabetes after the pregnancy. Codes for gestational diabetes are in subcategory O24.4, Gestational diabetes mellitus. No other code from category O24, Diabetes mellitus in pregnancy, childbirth, and the puerperium, should be used with a code from O24.4.

The codes under subcategory O24.4 include diet controlled, insulin controlled, and controlled by oral hypoglycemic drugs. If a patient with gestational diabetes is treated with both diet and insulin, only the code for insulin-controlled is required. If a patient with gestational diabetes is treated with both diet and oral hypoglycemic medications, only the code for "controlled by oral hypoglycemic drugs" is required. Code Z79.4, Long-term (current) use of insulin or code Z79.84, Long-term (current) use of oral hypoglycemic drugs, should not be assigned with codes from subcategory O24.4.

An abnormal glucose tolerance in pregnancy is assigned a code from subcategory O99.81, Abnormal glucose complicating pregnancy, childbirth, and the puerperium.

j. Sepsis and septic shock complicating abortion, pregnancy, childbirth and the puerperium

When assigning a chapter 15 code for sepsis complicating abortion, pregnancy, childbirth, and the puerperium, a code for the specific type of infection should be assigned as an additional diagnosis. If severe sepsis is present, a code from subcategory R65.2, Severe sepsis, and code(s) for associated organ dysfunction(s) should also be assigned as additional diagnoses.

k. Puerperal sepsis

Code O85, Puerperal sepsis, should be assigned with a secondary code to identify the causal organism (e.g., for a bacterial infection, assign a code from category B95-B96, Bacterial infections in conditions classified elsewhere). A code from category A40, Streptococcal sepsis, or A41, Other sepsis, should not be used for puerperal sepsis. If applicable, use additional codes to identify severe sepsis (R65.2-) and any associated acute organ dysfunction.

l. Alcohol, tobacco and drug use during pregnancy, childbirth and the puerperium

1) Alcohol use during pregnancy, childbirth and the puerperium

Codes under subcategory O99.31, Alcohol use complicating pregnancy, childbirth, and the puerperium, should be assigned for any pregnancy case when a mother uses alcohol during the pregnancy or postpartum. A secondary code from category F10, Alcohol related disorders, should also be assigned to identify manifestations of the alcohol use.

2) Tobacco use during pregnancy, childbirth and the puerperium

Codes under subcategory O99.33, Smoking (tobacco) complicating pregnancy, childbirth, and the puerperium, should be assigned for any pregnancy case when a mother uses any type of tobacco product during the pregnancy or postpartum. A secondary code from category F17, Nicotine dependence, should also be assigned to identify the type of nicotine dependence.

3) Drug use during pregnancy, childbirth and the puerperium
Codes under subcategory O99.32, Drug use complicating pregnancy, childbirth, and the puerperium, should be assigned for any pregnancy case when a mother uses drugs during the pregnancy or postpartum. This can involve illegal drugs, or inappropriate use or abuse of prescription drugs. Secondary code(s) from categories F11-F16 and F18-F19 should also be assigned to identify manifestations of the drug use.

m. Poisoning, toxic effects, adverse effects and underdosing in a pregnant patient
A code from subcategory O9A.2, Injury, poisoning and certain other consequences of external causes complicating pregnancy, childbirth, and the puerperium, should be sequenced first, followed by the appropriate injury, poisoning, toxic effect, adverse effect or underdosing code, and then the additional code(s) that specifies the condition caused by the poisoning, toxic effect, adverse effect or underdosing.
See Section I.C.19. Adverse effects, poisoning, underdosing and toxic effects.

n. Normal Delivery, Code O80

1) Encounter for full term uncomplicated delivery
Code O80 should be assigned when a woman is admitted for a full-term normal delivery and delivers a single, healthy infant without any complications antepartum, during the delivery, or postpartum during the delivery episode. Code O80 is always a principal diagnosis. It is not to be used if any other code from chapter 15 is needed to describe a current complication of the antenatal, delivery, or **postnatal** period. Additional codes from other chapters may be used with code O80 if they are not related to or are in any way complicating the pregnancy.

2) Uncomplicated delivery with resolved antepartum complication
Code O80 may be used if the patient had a complication at some point during the pregnancy, but the complication is not present at the time of the admission for delivery.

3) Outcome of delivery for O80
Z37.0, Single live birth, is the only outcome of delivery code appropriate for use with O80.

o. The Peripartum and Postpartum Periods

1) Peripartum and Postpartum periods
The postpartum period begins immediately after delivery and continues for six weeks following delivery. The peripartum period is defined as the last month of pregnancy to five months postpartum.

2) Peripartum and postpartum complication
A postpartum complication is any complication occurring within the six-week period.

3) Pregnancy-related complications after 6 week period
Chapter 15 codes may also be used to describe pregnancy-related complications after the peripartum or postpartum period if the provider documents that a condition is pregnancy related.

4) Admission for routine postpartum care following delivery outside hospital
When the mother delivers outside the hospital prior to admission and is admitted for routine postpartum care and no complications are noted, code Z39.0, Encounter for care and examination of mother immediately after delivery, should be assigned as the principal diagnosis.

5) Pregnancy associated cardiomyopathy
Pregnancy associated cardiomyopathy, code O90.3, is unique in that it may be diagnosed in the third trimester of pregnancy but may continue to progress months after delivery. For this reason, it is referred to as peripartum cardiomyopathy. Code O90.3 is only for use when the cardiomyopathy develops as a result of pregnancy in a woman who did not have pre-existing heart disease.

p. Code O94, Sequelae of complication of pregnancy, childbirth, and the puerperium

1) Code O94
Code O94, Sequelae of complication of pregnancy, childbirth, and the puerperium, is for use in those cases when an initial

complication of a pregnancy develops a sequelae requiring care or treatment at a future date.

2) After the initial postpartum period
This code may be used at any time after the initial postpartum period.

3) Sequencing of Code O94
This code, like all sequela codes, is to be sequenced following the code describing the sequelae of the complication.

q. Termination of Pregnancy and Spontaneous abortions

1) Abortion with Liveborn Fetus
When an attempted termination of pregnancy results in a liveborn fetus, assign code Z33.2, Encounter for elective termination of pregnancy and a code from category Z37, Outcome of Delivery.

2) Retained Products of Conception following an abortion
Subsequent encounters for retained products of conception following a spontaneous abortion or elective termination of pregnancy, without complications are assigned O03.4, Incomplete spontaneous abortion without complication, or code O07.4, Failed attempted termination of pregnancy without complication. This advice is appropriate even when the patient was discharged previously with a discharge diagnosis of complete abortion. If the patient has a specific complication associated with the spontaneous abortion or elective termination of pregnancy in addition to retained products of conception, assign the appropriate complication **code (e.g., O03.-, O04.-, O07.-)** instead of code O03.4 or O07.4

3) Complications leading to abortion
Codes from Chapter 15 may be used as additional codes to identify any documented complications of the pregnancy in conjunction with codes in categories in O04, O07 and O08.

r. Abuse in a pregnant patient
For suspected or confirmed cases of abuse of a pregnant patient, a code(s) from subcategories O9A.3, Physical abuse complicating pregnancy, childbirth, and the puerperium, O9A.4, Sexual abuse complicating pregnancy, childbirth, and the puerperium, and O9A.5, Psychological abuse complicating pregnancy, childbirth, and the puerperium, should be sequenced first, followed by the appropriate codes (if applicable) to identify any associated current injury due to physical abuse, sexual abuse, and the perpetrator of abuse.
See Section I.C.19. Adult and child abuse, neglect and other maltreatment.

16. Chapter 16: Certain Conditions Originating in the Perinatal Period (P00-P96)
For coding and reporting purposes the perinatal period is defined as before birth through the 28th day following birth. The following guidelines are provided for reporting purposes.

a. General Perinatal Rules

1) Use of Chapter 16 Codes
Codes in this chapter are <u>never</u> for use on the maternal record. Codes from Chapter 15, the obstetric chapter, are never permitted on the newborn record. Chapter 16 codes may be used throughout the life of the patient if the condition is still present.

2) Principal Diagnosis for Birth Record
When coding the birth episode in a newborn record, assign a code from category Z38, Liveborn infants according to place of birth and type of delivery, as the principal diagnosis. A code from category Z38 is assigned only once, to a newborn at the time of birth. If a newborn is transferred to another institution, a code from category Z38 should not be used at the receiving hospital.

A code from category Z38 is used only on the newborn record, not on the mother's record.

3) Use of Codes from other Chapters with Codes from Chapter 16
Codes from other chapters may be used with codes from chapter 16 if the codes from the other chapters provide more specific detail. Codes for signs and symptoms may be assigned when a definitive diagnosis has not been established. If the reason for the encounter is a perinatal condition, the code from chapter 16 should be sequenced first.

4) Use of Chapter 16 Codes after the Perinatal Period
Should a condition originate in the perinatal period, and continue throughout the life of the patient, the perinatal code should continue to be used regardless of the patient's age.

5) Birth process or community acquired conditions

If a newborn has a condition that may be either due to the birth process or community acquired and the documentation does not indicate which it is, the default is due to the birth process and the code from Chapter 16 should be used. If the condition is community-acquired, a code from Chapter 16 should not be assigned.

6) Code all clinically significant conditions

All clinically significant conditions noted on routine newborn examination should be coded. A condition is clinically significant if it requires:

- clinical evaluation; or
- therapeutic treatment; or
- diagnostic procedures; or
- extended length of hospital stay; or
- increased nursing care and/or monitoring; or
- has implications for future health care needs

Note: The perinatal guidelines listed above are the same as the general coding guidelines for "additional diagnoses," except for the final point regarding implications for future health care needs. Codes should be assigned for conditions that have been specified by the provider as having implications for future health care needs.

b. Observation and Evaluation of Newborns for Suspected Conditions not Found

1) Use of Z05 codes

Assign a code from category Z05, Observation and evaluation of newborns and infants for suspected conditions ruled out, to identify those instances when a healthy newborn is evaluated for a suspected condition that is determined after study not to be present. Do not use a code from category Z05 when the patient has identified signs or symptoms of a suspected problem; in such cases code the sign or symptom.

2) Z05 on other than the birth record

A code from category Z05 may also be assigned as a principal or first-listed code for readmissions or encounters when the code from category Z38 code no longer applies. Codes from category Z05 are for use only for healthy newborns and infants for which no condition after study is found to be present.

3) Z05 on a birth record

A code from category Z05 is to be used as a secondary code after the code from category Z38, Liveborn infants according to place of birth and type of delivery.

c. Coding Additional Perinatal Diagnoses

1) Assigning codes for conditions that require treatment

Assign codes for conditions that require treatment or further investigation, prolong the length of stay, or require resource utilization.

2) Codes for conditions specified as having implications for future health care needs

Assign codes for conditions that have been specified by the provider as having implications for future health care needs.

Note: This guideline should not be used for adult patients.

d. Prematurity and Fetal Growth Retardation

Providers utilize different criteria in determining prematurity. A code for prematurity should not be assigned unless it is documented. Assignment of codes in categories P05, Disorders of newborn related to slow fetal growth and fetal malnutrition, and P07, Disorders of newborn related to short gestation and low birth weight, not elsewhere classified, should be based on the recorded birth weight and estimated gestational age.

When both birth weight and gestational age are available, two codes from category P07 should be assigned, with the code for birth weight sequenced before the code for gestational age.

e. Low birth weight and immaturity status

Codes from category P07, Disorders of newborn related to short gestation and low birth weight, not elsewhere classified, are for use for a child or adult who was premature or had a low birth weight as a newborn and this is affecting the patient's current health status.

See Section I.C.21. Factors influencing health status and contact with health services, Status.

f. Bacterial Sepsis of Newborn

Category P36, Bacterial sepsis of newborn, includes congenital sepsis. If a perinate is documented as having sepsis without documentation

of congenital or community acquired, the default is congenital and a code from category P36 should be assigned. If the P36 code includes the causal organism, an additional code from category B95, Streptococcus, Staphylococcus, and Enterococcus as the cause of diseases classified elsewhere, or B96, Other bacterial agents as the cause of diseases classified elsewhere, should not be assigned. If the P36 code does not include the causal organism, assign an additional code from category B96. If applicable, use additional codes to identify severe sepsis (R65.2-) and any associated acute organ dysfunction.

g. Stillbirth

Code P95, Stillbirth, is only for use in institutions that maintain separate records for stillbirths. No other code should be used with P95. Code P95 should not be used on the mother's record.

17. Chapter 17: Congenital malformations, deformations, and chromosomal abnormalities (Q00-Q99)

Assign an appropriate code(s) from categories Q00-Q99, Congenital malformations, deformations, and chromosomal abnormalities when a malformation/deformation or chromosomal abnormality is documented. A malformation/deformation/or chromosomal abnormality may be the principal/first-listed diagnosis on a record or a secondary diagnosis.

When a malformation/deformation or chromosomal abnormality does not have a unique code assignment, assign additional code(s) for any manifestations that may be present.

When the code assignment specifically identifies the malformation/deformation or chromosomal abnormality, manifestations that are an inherent component of the anomaly should not be coded separately. Additional codes should be assigned for manifestations that are not an inherent component.

Codes from Chapter 17 may be used throughout the life of the patient. If a congenital malformation or deformity has been corrected, a personal history code should be used to identify the history of the malformation or deformity. Although present at birth, **a** malformation/deformation/or chromosomal abnormality may not be identified until later in life. Whenever the condition is diagnosed by the **provider**, it is appropriate to assign a code from codes Q00-Q99. For the birth admission, the appropriate code from category Z38, Liveborn infants, according to place of birth and type of delivery, should be sequenced as the principal diagnosis, followed by any congenital anomaly codes, Q00- Q99.

18. Chapter 18: Symptoms, signs, and abnormal clinical and laboratory findings, not elsewhere classified (R00-R99)

Chapter 18 includes symptoms, signs, abnormal results of clinical or other investigative procedures, and ill-defined conditions regarding which no diagnosis classifiable elsewhere is recorded. Signs and symptoms that point to a specific diagnosis have been assigned to a category in other chapters of the classification.

a. Use of symptom codes

Codes that describe symptoms and signs are acceptable for reporting purposes when a related definitive diagnosis has not been established (confirmed) by the provider.

b. Use of a symptom code with a definitive diagnosis code

Codes for signs and symptoms may be reported in addition to a related definitive diagnosis when the sign or symptom is not routinely associated with that diagnosis, such as the various signs and symptoms associated with complex syndromes. The definitive diagnosis code should be sequenced before the symptom code.

Signs or symptoms that are associated routinely with a disease process should not be assigned as additional codes, unless otherwise instructed by the classification.

c. Combination codes that include symptoms

ICD-10-CM contains a number of combination codes that identify both the definitive diagnosis and common symptoms of that diagnosis.

When using one of these combination codes, an additional code should not be assigned for the symptom.

d. Repeated falls

Code R29.6, Repeated falls, is for use for encounters when a patient has recently fallen and the reason for the fall is being investigated.

Code Z91.81, History of falling, is for use when a patient has fallen in the past and is at risk for future falls. When appropriate, both codes R29.6 and Z91.81 may be assigned together.

e. Coma scale

The coma scale codes (R40.2-) can be used in conjunction with traumatic brain injury codes, acute cerebrovascular disease or sequelae of cerebrovascular disease codes. These codes are primarily for use by trauma registries, but they may be used in any setting where this information is collected. The coma scale may also be used to assess the status of the central nervous system for other non-trauma conditions, such as monitoring patients in the intensive care unit regardless of medical condition. The coma scale codes should be sequenced after the diagnosis code(s).

These codes, one from each subcategory, are needed to complete the scale. The 7th character indicates when the scale was recorded. The 7th character should match for all three codes.

At a minimum, report the initial score documented on presentation at your facility. This may be a score from the emergency medicine technician (EMT) or in the emergency department. If desired, a facility may choose to capture multiple coma scale scores.

Assign code R40.24, Glasgow coma scale, total score, when only the total score is documented in the medical record and not the individual score(s).

Do not report codes for individual or total Glasgow coma scale scores for a patient with a medically induced coma or a sedated patient.

See Section I.B.14 for coma scale documentation by clinicians other than patient's provider

f. **Functional quadriplegia**
    GUIDELINE HAS BEEN DELETED EFFECTIVE OCTOBER 1, 2017

g. **SIRS due to Non-Infectious Process**
    The systemic inflammatory response syndrome (SIRS) can develop as a result of certain non-infectious disease processes, such as trauma, malignant neoplasm, or pancreatitis. When SIRS is documented with a noninfectious condition, and no subsequent infection is documented, the code for the underlying condition, such as an injury, should be assigned, followed by code R65.10, Systemic inflammatory response syndrome (SIRS) of non-infectious origin without acute organ dysfunction, or code R65.11, Systemic inflammatory response syndrome (SIRS) of non-infectious origin with acute organ dysfunction. If an associated acute organ dysfunction is documented, the appropriate code(s) for the specific type of organ dysfunction(s) should be assigned in addition to code R65.11. If acute organ dysfunction is documented, but it cannot be determined if the acute organ dysfunction is associated with SIRS or due to another condition (e.g., directly due to the trauma), the provider should be queried.

h. **Death NOS**
    Code R99, Ill-defined and unknown cause of mortality, is only for use in the very limited circumstance when a patient who has already died is brought into an emergency department or other healthcare facility and is pronounced dead upon arrival. It does not represent the discharge disposition of death.

i. **NIHSS Stroke Scale**
    The NIH stroke scale (NIHSS) codes (R29.7- -) can be used in conjunction with acute stroke codes (I63) to identify the patient's neurological status and the severity of the stroke. The stroke scale codes should be sequenced after the acute stroke diagnosis code(s).

    At a minimum, report the initial score documented. If desired, a facility may choose to capture multiple stroke scale scores.

    See Section I.B.14 for NIHSS stroke scale documentation by clinicians other than patient's provider

19. **Chapter 19: Injury, poisoning, and certain other consequences of external causes (S00-T88)**

a. **Application of 7th Characters in Chapter 19**
    Most categories in chapter 19 have a 7th character requirement for each applicable code. Most categories in this chapter have three 7th character values (with the exception of fractures): A, initial encounter, D, subsequent encounter and S, sequela. Categories for traumatic fractures have additional 7th character values. While the patient may be seen by a new or different provider over the course of treatment for an injury, assignment of the 7th character is based on whether the patient is undergoing active treatment and not whether the provider is seeing the patient for the first time.

    For complication codes, active treatment refers to treatment for the condition described by the code, even though it may be related to an earlier precipitating problem. For example, code T84.50XA, Infection and inflammatory reaction due to unspecified internal joint prosthesis, initial encounter, is used when active treatment is provided for the infection, even though the condition relates to the prosthetic device, implant or graft that was placed at a previous encounter.

    7th character "A", initial encounter is used for each encounter where the patient is receiving active treatment for the condition.

7th character "D" subsequent encounter is used for encounters after the patient has completed active treatment of the condition and is receiving routine care for the condition during the healing or recovery phase.

The aftercare Z codes should not be used for aftercare for conditions such as injuries or poisonings, where 7th characters are provided to identify subsequent care. For example, for aftercare of an injury, assign the acute injury code with the 7th character "D" (subsequent encounter).

7th character "S", sequela, is for use for complications or conditions that arise as a direct result of a condition, such as scar formation after a burn. The scars are sequelae of the burn. When using 7th character "S", it is necessary to use both the injury code that precipitated the sequela and the code for the sequela itself. The "S" is added only to the injury code, not the sequela code. The 7th character "S" identifies the injury responsible for the sequela. The specific type of sequela (e.g. scar) is sequenced first, followed by the injury code.

See Section I.B.10 Sequelae, (Late Effects)

b. **Coding of Injuries**
    When coding injuries, assign separate codes for each injury unless a combination code is provided, in which case the combination code is assigned. Codes from category T07, Unspecified multiple injuries should not be assigned in the inpatient setting unless information for a more specific code is not available. Traumatic injury codes (S00-T14.9) are not to be used for normal, healing surgical wounds or to identify complications of surgical wounds.

    The code for the most serious injury, as determined by the provider and the focus of treatment, is sequenced first.

    1) **Superficial injuries**
        Superficial injuries such as abrasions or contusions are not coded when associated with more severe injuries of the same site.

    2) **Primary injury with damage to nerves/blood vessels**
        When a primary injury results in minor damage to peripheral nerves or blood vessels, the primary injury is sequenced first with additional code(s) for injuries to nerves and spinal cord (such as category S04), and/or injury to blood vessels (such as category S15). When the primary injury is to the blood vessels or nerves, that injury should be sequenced first.

    3) **Iatrogenic injuries**
        Injury codes from Chapter 19 should not be assigned for injuries that occur during, or as a result of, a medical intervention. Assign the appropriate complication code(s).

c. **Coding of Traumatic Fractures**
    The principles of multiple coding of injuries should be followed in coding fractures. Fractures of specified sites are coded individually by site in accordance with both the provisions within categories S02, S12, S22, S32, S42, S49, S52, S59, S62, S72, S79, S82, S89, S92 and the level of detail furnished by medical record content.

    A fracture not indicated as open or closed should be coded to closed. A fracture not indicated whether displaced or not displaced should be coded to displaced.

    More specific guidelines are as follows:

    1) **Initial vs. subsequent encounter for fractures**
        Traumatic fractures are coded using the appropriate 7th character for initial encounter (A, B, C) for each encounter where the patient is receiving active treatment for the fracture. The appropriate 7th character for initial encounter should also be assigned for a patient who delayed seeking treatment for the fracture or nonunion.

        Fractures are coded using the appropriate 7th character for subsequent care for encounters after the patient has completed active treatment of the fracture and is receiving routine care for the fracture during the healing or recovery phase.

        Care for complications of surgical treatment for fracture repairs during the healing or recovery phase should be coded with the appropriate complication codes.

        Care of complications of fractures, such as malunion and nonunion, should be reported with the appropriate 7th character for subsequent care with nonunion (K, M, N,) or subsequent care with malunion (P, Q, R).

        Malunion/nonunion: The appropriate 7th character for initial encounter should also be assigned for a patient who delayed seeking treatment for the fracture or nonunion.

The open fracture designations in the assignment of the 7th character for fractures of the forearm, femur and lower leg, including ankle are based on the Gustilo open fracture classification. When the Gustilo classification type is not specified for an open fracture, the 7th character for open fracture type I or II should be assigned (B, E, H, M, Q).

A code from category M80, not a traumatic fracture code, should be used for any patient with known osteoporosis who suffers a fracture, even if the patient had a minor fall or trauma, if that fall or trauma would not usually break a normal, healthy bone.

See Section I.C.13. Osteoporosis.

The aftercare Z codes should not be used for aftercare for traumatic fractures. For aftercare of a traumatic fracture, assign the acute fracture code with the appropriate 7th character.

2) **Multiple fractures sequencing**
Multiple fractures are sequenced in accordance with the severity of the fracture.

3) **Physeal fractures**
For physeal fractures, assign only the code identifying the type of physeal fracture. Do not assign a separate code to identify the specific bone that is fractured.

d. **Coding of Burns and Corrosions**
The ICD-10-CM makes a distinction between burns and corrosions. The burn codes are for thermal burns, except sunburns, that come from a heat source, such as a fire or hot appliance. The burn codes are also for burns resulting from electricity and radiation. Corrosions are burns due to chemicals. The guidelines are the same for burns and corrosions.

Current burns (T20-T25) are classified by depth, extent and by agent (X code). Burns are classified by depth as first degree (erythema), second degree (blistering), and third degree (full-thickness involvement). Burns of the eye and internal organs (T26-T28) are classified by site, but not by degree.

1) **Sequencing of burn and related condition codes**
Sequence first the code that reflects the highest degree of burn when more than one burn is present.

   a.   When the reason for the admission or encounter is for treatment of external multiple burns, sequence first the code that reflects the burn of the highest degree.

   b.   When a patient has both internal and external burns, the circumstances of admission govern the selection of the principal diagnosis or first-listed diagnosis.

   c.   When a patient is admitted for burn injuries and other related conditions such as smoke inhalation and/or respiratory failure, the circumstances of admission govern the selection of the principal or first-listed diagnosis.

2) **Burns of the same anatomic site**
Classify burns of the same anatomic site and on the same side but of different degrees to the subcategory identifying the highest degree recorded in the diagnosis (e.g., for second and third degree burns of right thigh, assign only code T24.311-).

3) **Non-healing burns**
Non-healing burns are coded as acute burns.
Necrosis of burned skin should be coded as a non-healed burn.

4) **Infected *burn***
For any documented infected burn site, use an additional code for the infection.

5) **Assign separate codes for each burn site**
When coding burns, assign separate codes for each burn site. Category T30, Burn and corrosion, body region unspecified is extremely vague and should rarely be used.

Codes for burns of "multiple sites" should only be assigned when the medical record documentation does not specify the individual sites.

6) **Burns and corrosions classified according to extent of body surface involved**
Assign codes from category T31, Burns classified according to extent of body surface involved, or T32, Corrosions classified according to extent of body surface involved, when the site of the burn is not specified or when there is a need for additional data. It is advisable to use category T31 as additional coding when needed to provide data for evaluating burn mortality, such as that needed by burn units. It is also advisable to use category T31 as an additional code for reporting purposes when there is mention

of a third-degree burn involving 20 percent or more of the body surface.

Categories T31 and T32 are based on the classic "rule of nines" in estimating body surface involved: head and neck are assigned nine percent, each arm nine percent, each leg 18 percent, the anterior trunk 18 percent, posterior trunk 18 percent, and genitalia one percent. Providers may change these percentage assignments where necessary to accommodate infants and children who have proportionately larger heads than adults, and patients who have large buttocks, thighs, or abdomen that involve burns.

7) **Encounters for treatment of sequela of burns**
Encounters for the treatment of the late effects of burns or corrosions (i.e., scars or joint contractures) should be coded with a burn or corrosion code with the 7th character "S" for sequela.

8) **Sequelae with a late effect code and current burn**
When appropriate, both a code for a current burn or corrosion with 7th character "A" or "D" and a burn or corrosion code with 7th character "S" may be assigned on the same record (when both a current burn and sequelae of an old burn exist). Burns and corrosions do not heal at the same rate and a current healing wound may still exist with sequela of a healed burn or corrosion.

See Section I.B.10 Sequela (Late Effects)

9) **Use of an external cause code with burns and corrosions**
An external cause code should be used with burns and corrosions to identify the source and intent of the burn, as well as the place where it occurred.

e. **Adverse Effects, Poisoning, Underdosing and Toxic Effects**
Codes in categories T36-T65 are combination codes that include the substance that was taken as well as the intent. No additional external cause code is required for poisonings, toxic effects, adverse effects and underdosing codes.

1) **Do not code directly from the Table of Drugs**
Do not code directly funderdosinrom the Table of Drugs and Chemicals. Always refer back to the Tabular List.

2) **Use as many codes as necessary to describe**
Use as many codes as necessary to describe completely all drugs, medicinal or biological substances.

3) **If the same code would describe the causative agent**
If the same code would describe the causative agent for more than one adverse reaction, poisoning, toxic effect or underdosing, assign the code only once.

4) **If two or more drugs, medicinal or biological substances**
If two or more drugs, medicinal or biological substances are **taken**, code each individually unless a combination code is listed in the Table of Drugs and Chemicals.

If multiple unspecified drugs, medicinal or biological substances were taken, assign the appropriate code from subcategory T50.91, Poisoning by, adverse effect of and underdosing of multiple unspecified drugs, medicaments and biological substances.

5) **The occurrence of drug toxicity is classified in ICD-10-CM as follows:**

   (a) **Adverse Effect**
   When coding an adverse effect of a drug that has been correctly prescribed and properly administered, assign the appropriate code for the nature of the adverse effect followed by the appropriate code for the adverse effect of the drug (T36-T50). The code for the drug should have a 5th or 6th character "5" (for example T36.0X5-) Examples of the nature of an adverse effect are tachycardia, delirium, gastrointestinal hemorrhaging, vomiting, hypokalemia, hepatitis, renal failure, or respiratory failure.

   (b) **Poisoning**
   When coding a poisoning or reaction to the improper use of a medication (e.g., overdose, wrong substance given or taken in error, wrong route of administration), first assign the appropriate code from categories T36-T50. The poisoning codes have an associated intent as their 5th or 6th character (accidental, intentional self-harm, assault and undetermined. If the intent of the poisoning is unknown or unspecified, code the intent as accidental intent. The undetermined

intent is only for use if the documentation in the record specifies that the intent cannot be determined. Use additional code(s) for all manifestations of poisonings.

If there is also a diagnosis of abuse or dependence of the substance, the abuse or dependence is assigned as an additional code.

Examples of poisoning include:

(i) Error was made in drug prescription
Errors made in drug prescription or in the administration of the drug by provider, nurse, patient, or other person.

(ii) Overdose of a drug intentionally taken
If an overdose of a drug was intentionally taken or administered and resulted in drug toxicity, it would be coded as a poisoning.

(iii) Nonprescribed drug taken with correctly prescribed and properly administered drug
If a nonprescribed drug or medicinal agent was taken in combination with a correctly prescribed and properly administered drug, any drug toxicity or other reaction resulting from the interaction of the two drugs would be classified as a poisoning.

(iv) Interaction of drug(s) and alcohol
When a reaction results from the interaction of a drug(s) and alcohol, this would be classified as poisoning.

See Section I.C.4. if poisoning is the result of insulin pump malfunctions.

(c) Underdosing

Underdosing refers to taking less of a medication than is prescribed by a provider or a manufacturer's instruction. Discontinuing the use of a prescribed medication on the patient's own initiative (not directed by the patient's provider) is also classified as an underdosing. For underdosing, assign the code from categories T36-T50 (fifth or sixth character "6").

Codes for underdosing should never be assigned as principal or first-listed codes. If a patient has a relapse or exacerbation of the medical condition for which the drug is prescribed because of the reduction in dose, then the medical condition itself should be coded.

Noncompliance (Z91.12-, Z91.13- and Z91.14-) or complication of care (Y63.6-Y63.9) codes are to be used with an underdosing code to indicate intent, if known.

(d) Toxic Effects

When a harmful substance is ingested or comes in contact with a person, this is classified as a toxic effect. The toxic effect codes are in categories T51-T65.

Toxic effect codes have an associated intent: accidental, intentional self-harm, assault and undetermined.

f. Adult and child abuse, neglect and other maltreatment

Sequence first the appropriate code from categories T74, Adult and child abuse, neglect and other maltreatment, confirmed) or T76, Adult and child abuse, neglect and other maltreatment, suspected) for abuse, neglect and other maltreatment, followed by any accompanying mental health or injury code(s).

If the documentation in the medical record states abuse or neglect it is coded as confirmed (T74.-). It is coded as suspected if it is documented as suspected (T76.-).

For cases of confirmed abuse or neglect an external cause code from the assault section (X92-Y09) should be added to identify the cause of any physical injuries. A perpetrator code (Y07) should be added when the perpetrator of the abuse is known. For suspected cases of abuse or neglect, do not report external cause or perpetrator code.

If a suspected case of abuse, neglect or mistreatment is ruled out during an encounter code Z04.71, Encounter for examination and observation following alleged physical adult abuse, ruled out, or code Z04.72, Encounter for examination and observation following alleged child physical abuse, ruled out, should be used, not a code from T76.

If a suspected case of alleged rape or sexual abuse is ruled out during an encounter code Z04.41, Encounter for examination and observation following alleged adult rape or code Z04.42, Encounter for examination and observation following alleged child rape, should be used, not a code from T76.

If a suspected case of forced sexual exploitation or forced labor exploitation is ruled out during an encounter, code Z04.81, Encounter

for examination and observation of victim following forced sexual exploitation, or code Z04.82, Encounter for examination and observation of victim following forced labor exploitation, should be used, not a code from T76.

See Section I.C.15. Abuse in a pregnant patient.

g. Complications of care

1) General guidelines for complications of care

(a) Documentation of complications of care

See Section I.B.16. for information on documentation of complications of care.

2) Pain due to medical devices

Pain associated with devices, implants or grafts left in a surgical site (for example painful hip prosthesis) is assigned to the appropriate code(s) found in Chapter 19, Injury, poisoning, and certain other consequences of external causes. Specific codes for pain due to medical devices are found in the T code section of the ICD-10-CM. Use additional code(s) from category G89 to identify acute or chronic pain due to presence of the device, implant or graft (G89.18 or G89.28).

3) Transplant complications

(a) Transplant complications other than kidney

Codes under category T86, Complications of transplanted organs and tissues, are for use for both complications and rejection of transplanted organs. A transplant complication code is only assigned if the complication affects the function of the transplanted organ. Two codes are required to fully describe a transplant complication: the appropriate code from category T86 and a secondary code that identifies the complication.

Pre-existing conditions or conditions that develop after the transplant are not coded as complications unless they affect the function of the transplanted organs.

See I.C.21. for transplant organ removal status

See I.C.2. for malignant neoplasm associated with transplanted organ.

(b) Kidney transplant complications

Patients who have undergone kidney transplant may still have some form of chronic kidney disease (CKD) because the kidney transplant may not fully restore kidney function. Code T86.1- should be assigned for documented complications of a kidney transplant, such as transplant failure or rejection or other transplant complication. Code T86.1- should not be assigned for post kidney transplant patients who have chronic kidney (CKD) unless a transplant complication such as transplant failure or rejection is documented. If the documentation is unclear as to whether the patient has a complication of the transplant, query the provider.

Conditions that affect the function of the transplanted kidney, other than CKD, should be assigned a code from subcategory T86.1, Complications of transplanted organ, Kidney, and a secondary code that identifies the complication.

For patients with CKD following a kidney transplant, but who do not have a complication such as failure or rejection, *see section I.C.14. Chronic kidney disease and kidney transplant status.*

4) Complication codes that include the external cause

As with certain other T codes, some of the complications of care codes have the external cause included in the code. The code includes the nature of the complication as well as the type of procedure that caused the complication. No external cause code indicating the type of procedure is necessary for these codes.

5) Complications of care codes within the body system chapters

Intraoperative and postprocedural complication codes are found within the body system chapters with codes specific to the organs and structures of that body system. These codes should be sequenced first, followed by a code(s) for the specific complication, if applicable.

Complication codes from the body system chapters should be assigned for intraoperative and postprocedural complications (e.g., the appropriate complication code from chapter 9 would be assigned for a vascular intraoperative or postprocedural complication) unless the complication is specifically indexed to a T code in chapter 19.

20. Chapter 20: External Causes of Morbidity (VØØ-Y99)

The external causes of morbidity codes should never be sequenced as the first-listed or principal diagnosis.

External cause codes are intended to provide data for injury research and evaluation of injury prevention strategies. These codes capture how the injury or health condition happened (cause), the intent (unintentional or accidental; or intentional, such as suicide or assault), the place where the event occurred the activity of the patient at the time of the event, and the person's status (e.g., civilian, military).

There is no national requirement for mandatory ICD-10-CM external cause code reporting. Unless a provider is subject to a state-based external cause code reporting mandate or these codes are required by a particular payer, reporting of ICD-10-CM codes in Chapter 2Ø, External Causes of Morbidity, is not required. In the absence of a mandatory reporting requirement, providers are encouraged to voluntarily report external cause codes, as they provide valuable data for injury research and evaluation of injury prevention strategies.

a. General External Cause Coding Guidelines

1) Used with any code in the range of AØØ.Ø-T88.9 ZØØ-Z99

An external cause code may be used with any code in the range of AØØ.Ø-T88.9, ZØØ-Z99, classification that represents a health condition due to an external cause. Though they are most applicable to injuries, they are also valid for use with such things as infections or diseases due to an external source, and other health conditions, such as a heart attack that occurs during strenuous physical activity.

2) External cause code used for length of treatment

Assign the external cause code, with the appropriate 7th character (initial encounter, subsequent encounter or sequela) for each encounter for which the injury or condition is being treated.

Most categories in chapter 20 have a 7th character requirement for each applicable code. Most categories in this chapter have three 7th character values: A, initial encounter, D, subsequent encounter and S, sequela. While the patient may be seen by a new or different provider over the course of treatment for an injury or condition, assignment of the 7th character for external cause should match the 7th character of the code assigned for the associated injury or condition for the encounter.

3) Use the full range of external cause codes

Use the full range of external cause codes to completely describe the cause, the intent, the place of occurrence, and if applicable, the activity of the patient at the time of the event, and the patient's status, for all injuries, and other health conditions due to an external cause.

4) Assign as many external cause codes as necessary

Assign as many external cause codes as necessary to fully explain each cause. If only one external cause code can be recorded, assign the code most related to the principal diagnosis.

5) The selection of the appropriate external cause code

The selection of the appropriate external cause code is guided by the Alphabetic Index of External Causes and by Inclusion and Exclusion notes in the Tabular List.

6) External cause code can never be a principal diagnosis

An external cause code can never be a principal (first-listed) diagnosis.

7) Combination external cause codes

Certain of the external cause codes are combination codes that identify sequential events that result in an injury, such as a fall which results in striking against an object. The injury may be due to either event or both. The combination external cause code used should correspond to the sequence of events regardless of which caused the most serious injury.

8) No external cause code needed in certain circumstances

No external cause code from Chapter 20 is needed if the external cause and intent are included in a code from another chapter (e.g. T36.ØX1- Poisoning by penicillins, accidental (unintentional)).

b. Place of Occurrence Guideline

Codes from category Y92, Place of occurrence of the external cause, are secondary codes for use after other external cause codes to identify the location of the patient at the time of injury or other condition.

Generally, a place of occurrence code is assigned only once, at the initial encounter for treatment. However, in the rare instance that a new injury occurs during hospitalization, an additional place of occurrence code may be assigned. No 7th characters are used for Y92.

Do not use place of occurrence code Y92.9 if the place is not stated or is not applicable.

c. Activity Code

Assign a code from category Y93, Activity code, to describe the activity of the patient at the time the injury or other health condition occurred.

An activity code is used only once, at the initial encounter for treatment. Only one code from Y93 should be recorded on a medical record.

The activity codes are not applicable to poisonings, adverse effects, misadventures or sequela.

Do not assign Y93.9, Unspecified activity, if the activity is not stated.

A code from category Y93 is appropriate for use with external cause and intent codes if identifying the activity provides additional information about the event.

d. Place of Occurrence, Activity, and Status Codes Used with other External Cause Code

When applicable, place of occurrence, activity, and external cause status codes are sequenced after the main external cause code(s). Regardless of the number of external cause codes assigned, generally there should be only one place of occurrence code, one activity code, and one external cause status code assigned to an encounter. However, in the rare instance that a new injury occurs during hospitalization, an additional place of occurrence code may be assigned.

e. If the Reporting Format Limits the Number of External Cause Codes

If the reporting format limits the number of external cause codes that can be used in reporting clinical data, report the code for the cause/intent most related to the principal diagnosis. If the format permits capture of additional external cause codes, the cause/intent, including medical misadventures, of the additional events should be reported rather than the codes for place, activity, or external status.

f. Multiple External Cause Coding Guidelines

More than one external cause code is required to fully describe the external cause of an illness or injury. The assignment of external cause codes should be sequenced in the following priority:

If two or more events cause separate injuries, an external cause code should be assigned for each cause. The first-listed external cause code will be selected in the following order:

External codes for child and adult abuse take priority over all other external cause codes.

See Section I.C.19., Child and Adult abuse guidelines.

External cause codes for terrorism events take priority over all other external cause codes except child and adult abuse.

External cause codes for cataclysmic events take priority over all other external cause codes except child and adult abuse and terrorism.

External cause codes for transport accidents take priority over all other external cause codes except cataclysmic events, child and adult abuse and terrorism.

Activity and external cause status codes are assigned following all causal (intent) external cause codes.

The first-listed external cause code should correspond to the cause of the most serious diagnosis due to an assault, accident, or self-harm, following the order of hierarchy listed above.

g. Child and Adult Abuse Guideline

Adult and child abuse, neglect and maltreatment are classified as assault. Any of the assault codes may be used to indicate the external cause of any injury resulting from the confirmed abuse.

For confirmed cases of abuse, neglect and maltreatment, when the perpetrator is known, a code from YØ7, Perpetrator of maltreatment and neglect, should accompany any other assault codes.

See Section I.C.19. Adult and child abuse, neglect and other maltreatment

h. Unknown or Undetermined Intent Guideline

If the intent (accident, self-harm, assault) of the cause of an injury or other condition is unknown or unspecified, code the intent as accidental intent. All transport accident categories assume accidental intent.

1) Use of undetermined intent
External cause codes for events of undetermined intent are only for use if the documentation in the record specifies that the intent cannot be determined.

i. Sequelae (Late Effects) of External Cause Guidelines
1) Sequelae external cause codes
Sequela are reported using the external cause code with the 7th character "S" for sequela. These codes should be used with any report of a late effect or sequela resulting from a previous injury.
See Section I.B.10 Sequela (Late Effects)

2) Sequela external cause code with a related current injury
A sequela external cause code should never be used with a related current nature of injury code.

3) Use of sequela external cause codes for subsequent visits
Use a late effect external cause code for subsequent visits when a late effect of the initial injury is being treated. Do not use a late effect external cause code for subsequent visits for follow-up care (e.g., to assess healing, to receive rehabilitative therapy) of the injury when no late effect of the injury has been documented.

j. Terrorism Guidelines
1) Cause of injury identified by the Federal Government (FBI) as terrorism
When the cause of an injury is identified by the Federal Government (FBI) as terrorism, the first-listed external cause code should be a code from category Y38, Terrorism. The definition of terrorism employed by the FBI is found at the inclusion note at the beginning of category Y38. Use additional code for place of occurrence (Y92.-). More than one Y38 code may be assigned if the injury is the result of more than one mechanism of terrorism.

2) Cause of an injury is suspected to be the result of terrorism
When the cause of an injury is suspected to be the result of terrorism a code from category Y38 should not be assigned. Suspected cases should be classified as assault.

3) Code Y38.9, Terrorism, secondary effects
Assign code Y38.9, Terrorism, secondary effects, for conditions occurring subsequent to the terrorist event. This code should not be assigned for conditions that are due to the initial terrorist act.

It is acceptable to assign code Y38.9 with another code from Y38 if there is an injury due to the initial terrorist event and an injury that is a subsequent result of the terrorist event.

k. External Cause Status
A code from category Y99, External cause status, should be assigned whenever any other external cause code is assigned for an encounter, including an Activity code, except for the events noted below. Assign a code from category Y99, External cause status, to indicate the work status of the person at the time the event occurred. The status code indicates whether the event occurred during military activity, whether a non-military person was at work, whether an individual including a student or volunteer was involved in a non-work activity at the time of the causal event.

A code from Y99, External cause status, should be assigned, when applicable, with other external cause codes, such as transport accidents and falls. The external cause status codes are not applicable to poisonings, adverse effects, misadventures or late effects.

Do not assign a code from category Y99 if no other external cause codes (cause, activity) are applicable for the encounter.

An external cause status code is used only once, at the initial encounter for treatment. Only one code from Y99 should be recorded on a medical record.

Do not assign code Y99.9, Unspecified external cause status, if the status is not stated.

21. Chapter 21: Factors influencing health status and contact with health services (Z00-Z99)
Note: The chapter specific guidelines provide additional information about the use of Z codes for specified encounters.

a. Use of Z Codes in Any Healthcare Setting
Z codes are for use in any healthcare setting. Z codes may be used as either a first-listed (principal diagnosis code in the inpatient setting) or secondary code, depending on the circumstances of the encounter. Certain Z codes may only be used as first-listed or principal diagnosis.

b. Z Codes Indicate a Reason for an Encounter
Z codes are not procedure codes. A corresponding procedure code must accompany a Z code to describe any procedure performed.

c. Categories of Z Codes
1) Contact/Exposure
Category Z20 indicates contact with, and suspected exposure to, communicable diseases. These codes are for patients who do not show any sign or symptom of a disease but are suspected to have been exposed to it by close personal contact with an infected individual or are in an area where a disease is epidemic.

Category Z77, Other contact with and (suspected) exposures hazardous to health, indicates contact with and suspected exposures hazardous to health.

Contact/exposure codes may be used as a first-listed code to explain an encounter for testing, or, more commonly, as a secondary code to identify a potential risk.

2) Inoculations and vaccinations
Code Z23 is for encounters for inoculations and vaccinations. It indicates that a patient is being seen to receive a prophylactic inoculation against a disease. Procedure codes are required to identify the actual administration of the injection and the type(s) of immunizations given. Code Z23 may be used as a secondary code if the inoculation is given as a routine part of preventive health care, such as a well-baby visit.

3) Status
Status codes indicate that a patient is either a carrier of a disease or has the sequelae or residual of a past disease or condition. This includes such things as the presence of prosthetic or mechanical devices resulting from past treatment. A status code is informative, because the status may affect the course of treatment and its outcome. A status code is distinct from a history code. The history code indicates that the patient no longer has the condition.

A status code should not be used with a diagnosis code from one of the body system chapters, if the diagnosis code includes the information provided by the status code. For example, code Z94.1, Heart transplant status, should not be used with a code from subcategory T86.2, Complications of heart transplant. The status code does not provide additional information. The complication code indicates that the patient is a heart transplant patient.

For encounters for weaning from a mechanical ventilator, assign a code from subcategory J96.1, Chronic respiratory failure, followed by code Z99.11, Dependence on respirator [ventilator] status.

The status Z codes/categories are:

Z14   Genetic carrier

Genetic carrier status indicates that a person carries a gene, associated with a particular disease, which may be passed to offspring who may develop that disease. The person does not have the disease and is not at risk of developing the disease.

Z15   Genetic susceptibility to disease

Genetic susceptibility indicates that a person has a gene that increases the risk of that person developing the disease.

Codes from category Z15 should not be used as principal or first-listed codes. If the patient has the condition to which he/she is susceptible, and that condition is the reason for the encounter, the code for the current condition should be sequenced first. If the patient is being seen for follow-up after completed treatment for this condition, and the condition no longer exists, a follow-up code should be sequenced first, followed by the appropriate personal history and genetic susceptibility codes. If the purpose of the encounter is genetic counseling associated with procreative management, code Z31.5, Encounter for genetic counseling, should be assigned as the first-listed code, followed by a code from category Z15. Additional codes should be assigned for any applicable family or personal history.

Z16   Resistance to antimicrobial drugs

This code indicates that a patient has a condition that is resistant to antimicrobial drug treatment. Sequence the infection code first.

Z17   Estrogen receptor status

Z18   Retained foreign body fragments

Z19   Hormone sensitivity malignancy status

Z21   Asymptomatic HIV infection status

This code indicates that a patient has tested positive for HIV but has manifested no signs or symptoms of the disease.

Z22   Carrier of infectious disease

Carrier status indicates that a person harbors the specific organisms of a disease without manifest symptoms and is capable of transmitting the infection.

Z28.3   Underimmunization status

Z33.1   Pregnant state, incidental

This code is a secondary code only for use when the pregnancy is in no way complicating the reason for visit. Otherwise, a code from the obstetric chapter is required.

Z66   Do not resuscitate

This code may be used when it is documented by the provider that a patient is on do not resuscitate status at any time during the stay.

Z67   Blood type

Z68   Body mass index (BMI)

BMI codes should only be assigned when **there is an associated, reportable diagnosis (such as obesity).** Do not assign BMI codes during pregnancy.

See Section I.B.14 for BMI documentation by clinicians other than the patient's provider.

Z74.Ø1 Bed confinement status

Z76.82 Awaiting organ transplant status

Z78   Other specified health status

Code Z78.1, Physical restraint status, may be used when it is documented by the provider that a patient has been put in restraints during the current encounter. Please note that this code should not be reported when it is documented by the provider that a patient is temporarily restrained during a procedure.

Z79   Long-term (current) drug therapy

Codes from this category indicate a patient's continuous use of a prescribed drug (including such things as aspirin therapy) for the long-term treatment of a condition or for prophylactic use. It is not for use for patients who have addictions to drugs. This subcategory is not for use of medications for detoxification or maintenance programs to prevent withdrawal symptoms in patients with drug dependence (e.g., methadone maintenance for opiate dependence). Assign the appropriate code for the drug dependence instead.

Assign a code from Z79 if the patient is receiving a medication for an extended period as a prophylactic measure (such as for the prevention of deep vein thrombosis) or as treatment of a chronic condition (such as arthritis) or a disease requiring a lengthy course of treatment (such as cancer). Do not assign a code from category Z79 for medication being administered for a brief period of time to treat an acute illness or injury (such as a course of antibiotics to treat acute bronchitis).

Z88   Allergy status to drugs, medicaments and biological substances

Except: Z88.9, Allergy status to unspecified drugs, medicaments and biological substances status

Z89   Acquired absence of limb

Z9Ø   Acquired absence of organs, not elsewhere classified

Z91.Ø- Allergy status, other than to drugs and biological substances

Z92.82 Status post administration of tPA (rtPA) in a different facility within the last 24 hours prior to admission to a current facility

Assign code Z92.82, Status post administration of tPA (rtPA) in a different facility within the last 24 hours prior to admission to current facility, as a secondary diagnosis when a patient is received by transfer into a facility and documentation indicates they were administered tissue

plasminogen activator (tPA) within the last 24 hours prior to admission to the current facility.

This guideline applies even if the patient is still receiving the tPA at the time they are received into the current facility.

The appropriate code for the condition for which the tPA was administered (such as cerebrovascular disease or myocardial infarction) should be assigned first.

Code Z92.82 is only applicable to the receiving facility record and not to the transferring facility record.

Z93   Artificial opening status

Z94   Transplanted organ and tissue status

Z95   Presence of cardiac and vascular implants and grafts

Z96   Presence of other functional implants

Z97   Presence of other devices

Z98   Other postprocedural states

Assign code Z98.85, Transplanted organ removal status, to indicate that a transplanted organ has been previously removed. This code should not be assigned for the encounter in which the transplanted organ is removed. The complication necessitating removal of the transplant organ should be assigned for that encounter.

See section I.C19. for information on the coding of organ transplant complications.

Z99   Dependence on enabling machines and devices, not elsewhere classified

Note: Categories Z89-Z9Ø and Z93-Z99 are for use only if there are no complications or malfunctions of the organ or tissue replaced, the amputation site or the equipment on which the patient is dependent.

4) **History (of)**

There are two types of history Z codes, personal and family. Personal history codes explain a patient's past medical condition that no longer exists and is not receiving any treatment, but that has the potential for recurrence, and therefore may require continued monitoring.

Family history codes are for use when a patient has a family member(s) who has had a particular disease that causes the patient to be at higher risk of also contracting the disease.

Personal history codes may be used in conjunction with follow-up codes and family history codes may be used in conjunction with screening codes to explain the need for a test or procedure. History codes are also acceptable on any medical record regardless of the reason for visit. A history of an illness, even if no longer present, is important information that may alter the type of treatment ordered.

The history Z code categories are:

Z8Ø   Family history of primary malignant neoplasm

Z81   Family history of mental and behavioral disorders

Z82   Family history of certain disabilities and chronic diseases (leading to disablement)

Z83   Family history of other specific disorders

Z84   Family history of other conditions

Z85   Personal history of malignant neoplasm

Z86   Personal history of certain other diseases

Z87   Personal history of other diseases and conditions

Z91.4- Personal history of psychological trauma, not elsewhere classified

Z91.5   Personal history of self-harm

Z91.81 History of falling

Z91.82 Personal history of military deployment

Z92   Personal history of medical treatment

Except: Z92.Ø, Personal history of contraception

Except: Z92.82, Status post administration of tPA (rtPA) in a different facility within the last 24 hours prior to admission to a current facility

5) **Screening**

Screening is the testing for disease or disease precursors in seemingly well individuals so that early detection and treatment can be provided for those who test positive for the disease (e.g., screening mammogram).

The testing of a person to rule out or confirm a suspected diagnosis because the patient has some sign or symptom is a diagnostic examination, not a screening. In these cases, the sign or symptom is used to explain the reason for the test.

A screening code may be a first-listed code if the reason for the visit is specifically the screening exam. It may also be used as an additional code if the screening is done during an office visit for other health problems. A screening code is not necessary if the screening is inherent to a routine examination, such as a pap smear done during a routine pelvic examination.

Should a condition be discovered during the screening then the code for the condition may be assigned as an additional diagnosis.

The Z code indicates that a screening exam is planned. A procedure code is required to confirm that the screening was performed.

The screening Z codes/categories:

Z11	Encounter for screening for infectious and parasitic diseases
Z12	Encounter for screening for malignant neoplasms
Z13	Encounter for screening for other diseases and disorders
	Except: Z13.9, Encounter for screening, unspecified
Z36	Encounter for antenatal screening for mother

6) Observation

There are three observation Z code categories. They are for use in very limited circumstances when a person is being observed for a suspected condition that is ruled out. The observation codes are not for use if an injury or illness or any signs or symptoms related to the suspected condition are present. In such cases the diagnosis/symptom code is used with the corresponding external cause code.

The observation codes are to be used as principal diagnosis only. The only exception to this is when the principal diagnosis is required to be a code from category Z38, Liveborn infants according to place of birth and type of delivery. Then a code from category Z05, Encounter for observation and evaluation of newborn for suspected diseases and conditions ruled out, is sequenced after the Z38 code. Additional codes may be used in addition to the observation code, but only if they are unrelated to the suspected condition being observed.

Codes from subcategory Z03.7, Encounter for suspected maternal and fetal conditions ruled out, may either be used as a first-listed or as an additional code assignment depending on the case. They are for use in very limited circumstances on a maternal record when an encounter is for a suspected maternal or fetal condition that is ruled out during that encounter (for example, a maternal or fetal condition may be suspected due to an abnormal test result). These codes should not be used when the condition is confirmed. In those cases, the confirmed condition should be coded. In addition, these codes are not for use if an illness or any signs or symptoms related to the suspected condition or problem are present. In such cases the diagnosis/symptom code is used.

Additional codes may be used in addition to the code from subcategory Z03.7, but only if they are unrelated to the suspected condition being evaluated.

Codes from subcategory Z03.7 may not be used for encounters for antenatal screening of mother. See Section I.C.21. Screening.

For encounters for suspected fetal condition that are inconclusive following testing and evaluation, assign the appropriate code from category O35, O36, O40 or O41.

The observation Z code categories:

Z03	Encounter for medical observation for suspected diseases and conditions ruled out
Z04	Encounter for examination and observation for other reasons
	Except: Z04.9, Encounter for examination and observation for unspecified reason
Z05	Encounter for observation and evaluation of newborn for suspected diseases and conditions ruled out

7) Aftercare

Aftercare visit codes cover situations when the initial treatment of a disease has been performed and the patient requires continued care during the healing or recovery phase, or for the long-term consequences of the disease. The aftercare Z code should not be used if treatment is directed at a current, acute disease. The diagnosis code is to be used in these cases. Exceptions to this rule are codes Z51.0, Encounter for antineoplastic radiation therapy, and codes from subcategory Z51.1, Encounter for antineoplastic chemotherapy and immunotherapy. These codes are to be first-listed, followed by the diagnosis code when a patient's encounter is solely to receive radiation therapy, chemotherapy, or immunotherapy for the treatment of a neoplasm. If the reason for the encounter is more than one type of antineoplastic therapy, code Z51.0 and a code from subcategory Z51.1 may be assigned together, in which case one of these codes would be reported as a secondary diagnosis.

The aftercare Z codes should also not be used for aftercare for injuries. For aftercare of an injury, assign the acute injury code with the appropriate 7th character (for subsequent encounter).

The aftercare codes are generally first-listed to explain the specific reason for the encounter. An aftercare code may be used as an additional code when some type of aftercare is provided in addition to the reason for admission and no diagnosis code is applicable. An example of this would be the closure of a colostomy during an encounter for treatment of another condition.

Aftercare codes should be used in conjunction with other aftercare codes or diagnosis codes to provide better detail on the specifics of an aftercare encounter visit, unless otherwise directed by the classification. The sequencing of multiple aftercare codes depends on the circumstances of the encounter.

Certain aftercare Z code categories need a secondary diagnosis code to describe the resolving condition or sequelae. For others, the condition is included in the code title.

Additional Z code aftercare category terms include fitting and adjustment, and attention to artificial openings.

Status Z codes may be used with aftercare Z codes to indicate the nature of the aftercare. For example, code Z95.1, Presence of aortocoronary bypass graft, may be used with code Z48.812, Encounter for surgical aftercare following surgery on the circulatory system, to indicate the surgery for which the aftercare is being performed. A status code should not be used when the aftercare code indicates the type of status, such as using Z43.0, Encounter for attention to tracheostomy, with Z93.0, Tracheostomy status.

The aftercare Z category/codes:

Z42	Encounter for plastic and reconstructive surgery following medical procedure or healed injury
Z43	Encounter for attention to artificial openings
Z44	Encounter for fitting and adjustment of external prosthetic device
Z45	Encounter for adjustment and management of implanted device
Z46	Encounter for fitting and adjustment of other devices
Z47	Orthopedic aftercare
Z48	Encounter for other postprocedural aftercare
Z49	Encounter for care involving renal dialysis
Z51	Encounter for other aftercare and medical care

8) Follow-up

The follow-up codes are used to explain continuing surveillance following completed treatment of a disease, condition, or injury. They imply that the condition has been fully treated and no longer exists. They should not be confused with aftercare codes, or injury codes with a 7th character for subsequent encounter, that explain ongoing care of a healing condition or its sequelae. Follow-up codes may be used in conjunction with history codes to provide the full picture of the healed condition and its treatment. The follow-up code is sequenced first, followed by the history code.

A follow-up code may be used to explain multiple visits. Should a condition be found to have recurred on the follow-up visit, then the diagnosis code for the condition should be assigned in place of the follow-up code.

The follow-up Z code categories:

Z08   Encounter for follow-up examination after completed treatment for malignant neoplasm

Z09   Encounter for follow-up examination after completed treatment for conditions other than malignant neoplasm

Z39   Encounter for maternal postpartum care and examination

9) Donor
Codes in category Z52, Donors of organs and tissues, are used for living individuals who are donating blood or other body tissue. These codes are only for individuals donating for others, not for self-donations. They are not used to identify cadaveric donations.

10) Counseling
Counseling Z codes are used when a patient or family member receives assistance in the aftermath of an illness or injury, or when support is required in coping with family or social problems.

The counseling Z codes/categories:

Z30.0- Encounter for general counseling and advice on contraception

Z31.5   Encounter for procreative genetic counseling

Z31.6- Encounter for general counseling and advice on procreation

Z32.2   Encounter for childbirth instruction

Z32.3   Encounter for childcare instruction

Z69   Encounter for mental health services for victim and perpetrator of abuse

Z70   Counseling related to sexual attitude, behavior and orientation

Z71   Persons encountering health services for other counseling and medical advice, not elsewhere classified

Note: Code Z71.84, Encounter for health counseling related to travel, is to be used for health risk and safety counseling for future travel purposes.

Z76.81 Expectant mother prebirth pediatrician visit

11) Encounters for Obstetrical and Reproductive Services
See Section I.C.15. Pregnancy, Childbirth, and the Puerperium, for further instruction on the use of these codes.

Z codes for pregnancy are for use in those circumstances when none of the problems or complications included in the codes from the Obstetrics chapter exist (a routine prenatal visit or postpartum care). Codes in category Z34, Encounter for supervision of normal pregnancy, are always first-listed and are not to be used with any other code from the OB chapter.

Codes in category Z3A, Weeks of gestation, may be assigned to provide additional information about the pregnancy. Category Z3A codes should not be assigned for pregnancies with abortive outcomes (categories O00-O08), elective termination of pregnancy (code Z33.2), nor for postpartum conditions, as category Z3A is not applicable to these conditions. The date of the admission should be used to determine weeks of gestation for inpatient admissions that encompass more than one gestational week.

The outcome of delivery, category Z37, should be included on all maternal delivery records. It is always a secondary code. Codes in category Z37 should not be used on the newborn record.

Z codes for family planning (contraceptive) or procreative management and counseling should be included on an obstetric record either during the pregnancy or the postpartum stage, if applicable.

Z codes/categories for obstetrical and reproductive services:

Z30   Encounter for contraceptive management

Z31   Encounter for procreative management

Z32.2   Encounter for childbirth instruction

Z32.3   Encounter for childcare instruction

Z33   Pregnant state

Z34   Encounter for supervision of normal pregnancy

Z36   Encounter for antenatal screening of mother

Z3A   Weeks of gestation

Z37   Outcome of delivery

Z39   Encounter for maternal postpartum care and examination

Z76.81 Expectant mother prebirth pediatrician visit

12) Newborns and Infants
See Section I.C.16. Newborn (Perinatal) Guidelines, for further instruction on the use of these codes.

Newborn Z codes/categories:

Z76.1   Encounter for health supervision and care of foundling

Z00.1- Encounter for routine child health examination

Z38   Liveborn infants according to place of birth and type of delivery

13) Routine and Administrative Examinations
The Z codes allow for the description of encounters for routine examinations, such as, a general check-up, or, examinations for administrative purposes, such as, a pre-employment physical. The codes are not to be used if the examination is for diagnosis of a suspected condition or for treatment purposes. In such cases the diagnosis code is used. During a routine exam, should a diagnosis or condition be discovered, it should be coded as an additional code. Pre-existing and chronic conditions and history codes may also be included as additional codes as long as the examination is for administrative purposes and not focused on any particular condition.

Some of the codes for routine health examinations distinguish between "with" and "without" abnormal findings. Code assignment depends on the information that is known at the time the encounter is being coded. For example, if no abnormal findings were found during the examination, but the encounter is being coded before test results are back, it is acceptable to assign the code for "without abnormal findings." When assigning a code for "with abnormal findings," additional code(s) should be assigned to identify the specific abnormal finding(s).

Pre-operative examination and pre-procedural laboratory examination Z codes are for use only in those situations when a patient is being cleared for a procedure or surgery and no treatment is given.

The Z codes/categories for routine and administrative examinations:

Z00   Encounter for general examination without complaint, suspected or reported diagnosis

Z01   Encounter for other special examination without complaint, suspected or reported diagnosis

Z02   Encounter for administrative examination
       Except: Z02.9, Encounter for administrative examinations, unspecified

Z32.0- Encounter for pregnancy test

14) Miscellaneous Z *Codes*
The miscellaneous Z codes capture a number of other health care encounters that do not fall into one of the other categories. Certain of these codes identify the reason for the encounter; others are for use as additional codes that provide useful information on circumstances that may affect a patient's care and treatment.

Prophylactic Organ Removal
For encounters specifically for prophylactic removal of an organ (such as prophylactic removal of breasts due to a genetic susceptibility to cancer or a family history of cancer), the principal or first-listed code should be a code from category Z40, Encounter for prophylactic surgery, followed by the appropriate codes to identify the associated risk factor (such as genetic susceptibility or family history).

If the patient has a malignancy of one site and is having prophylactic removal at another site to prevent either a new primary malignancy or metastatic disease, a code for the malignancy should also be assigned in addition to a code from subcategory Z40.0, Encounter for prophylactic surgery for risk factors related to malignant neoplasms. A Z40.0 code should not be assigned if the patient is having organ removal for treatment of a malignancy, such as the removal of the testes for the treatment of prostate cancer.

Miscellaneous Z codes/categories:

Z28   Immunization not carried out

       Except: Z28.3, Underimmunization status

Z29   Encounter for other prophylactic measures

Z40   Encounter for prophylactic surgery

Z41   Encounter for procedures for purposes other than remedying health state

       Except: Z41.9, Encounter for procedure for purposes other than remedying health state, unspecified

Z53   Persons encountering health services for specific procedures and treatment, not carried out

Z55   Problems related to education and literacy

Z56   Problems related to employment and unemployment

Z57   Occupational exposure to risk factors

Z58   Problems related to physical environment

Z59   Problems related to housing and economic circumstances

Z60   Problems related to social environment

Z62   Problems related to upbringing

Z63   Other problems related to primary support group, including family circumstances

Z64   Problems related to certain psychosocial circumstances

Z65   Problems related to other psychosocial circumstances

Z72   Problems related to lifestyle

       Note: These codes should be assigned only when the documentation specifies that the patient has an associated problem

Z73   Problems related to life management difficulty

Z74   Problems related to care provider dependency

       Except: Z74.01, Bed confinement status

Z75   Problems related to medical facilities and other health care

Z76.0 Encounter for issue of repeat prescription

Z76.3 Healthy person accompanying sick person

Z76.4 Other boarder to healthcare facility

Z76.5 Malingerer [conscious simulation]

Z91.1- Patient's noncompliance with medical treatment and regimen

Z91.83 Wandering in diseases classified elsewhere

Z91.84- Oral health risk factors

Z91.89 Other specified personal risk factors, not elsewhere classified

See Section I.B.14 for Z55-Z65 Persons with potential health hazards related to socioeconomic and psychosocial circumstances, documentation by clinicians other than the patient's provider.

15) Nonspecific Z Codes

Certain Z codes are so non-specific, or potentially redundant with other codes in the classification, that there can be little justification for their use in the inpatient setting. Their use in the outpatient setting should be limited to those instances when there is no further documentation to permit more precise coding. Otherwise, any sign or symptom or any other reason for visit that is captured in another code should be used.

Nonspecific Z codes/categories:

Z02.9 Encounter for administrative examinations, unspecified

Z04.9 Encounter for examination and observation for unspecified reason

Z13.9 Encounter for screening, unspecified

Z41.9 Encounter for procedure for purposes other than remedying health state, unspecified

Z52.9 Donor of unspecified organ or tissue

Z86.59 Personal history of other mental and behavioral disorders

Z88.9 Allergy status to unspecified drugs, medicaments and biological substances status

Z92.0 Personal history of contraception

16) Z Codes That May Only be Principal/First-Listed Diagnosis

The following Z codes/categories may only be reported as the principal/first-listed diagnosis, except when there are multiple encounters on the same day and the medical records for the encounters are combined:

Z00   Encounter for general examination without complaint, suspected or reported diagnosis

       Except: Z00.6

Z01   Encounter for other special examination without complaint, suspected or reported diagnosis

Z02   Encounter for administrative examination

Z03   Encounter for medical observation for suspected diseases and conditions ruled out

Z04   Encounter for examination and observation for other reasons

Z33.2 Encounter for elective termination of pregnancy

Z31.81 Encounter for male factor infertility in female patient

Z31.83 Encounter for assisted reproductive fertility procedure cycle

Z31.84 Encounter for fertility preservation procedure

Z34   Encounter for supervision of normal pregnancy

Z39   Encounter for maternal postpartum care and examination

Z38   Liveborn infants according to place of birth and type of delivery

Z40   Encounter for prophylactic surgery

Z42   Encounter for plastic and reconstructive surgery following medical procedure or healed injury

Z51.0 Encounter for antineoplastic radiation therapy

Z51.1- Encounter for antineoplastic chemotherapy and immunotherapy

Z52   Donors of organs and tissues

       Except: Z52.9, Donor of unspecified organ or tissue

Z76.1 Encounter for health supervision and care of foundling

Z76.2 Encounter for health supervision and care of other healthy infant and child

Z99.12 Encounter for respirator [ventilator] dependence during power failure

Section II. Selection of Principal Diagnosis

The circumstances of inpatient admission always govern the selection of principal diagnosis. The principal diagnosis is defined in the Uniform Hospital Discharge Data Set (UHDDS) as "that condition established after study to be chiefly responsible for occasioning the admission of the patient to the hospital for care."

The UHDDS definitions are used by hospitals to report inpatient data elements in a standardized manner. These data elements and their definitions can be found in the July 31, 1985, Federal Register (Vol. 50, No, 147), pp. 31038-40.

Since that time the application of the UHDDS definitions has been expanded to include all non-outpatient settings (acute care, short term, long term care and psychiatric hospitals; home health agencies; rehab facilities; nursing homes, etc). The UHDDS definitions also apply to hospice services (all levels of care).

In determining principal diagnosis, coding conventions in the ICD-10-CM, the Tabular List and Alphabetic Index take precedence over these official coding guidelines.

(See Section I.A., Conventions for the ICD-10-CM)

The importance of consistent, complete documentation in the medical record cannot be overemphasized. Without such documentation the application of all coding guidelines is a difficult, if not impossible, task.

A. Codes for symptoms, signs, and ill-defined conditions

Codes for symptoms, signs, and ill-defined conditions from Chapter 18 are not to be used as principal diagnosis when a related definitive diagnosis has been established.

B. Two or more interrelated conditions, each potentially meeting the definition for principal diagnosis.

When there are two or more interrelated conditions (such as diseases in the same ICD-10-CM chapter or manifestations characteristically associated with a certain disease) potentially meeting the definition of principal diagnosis, either condition may be sequenced first, unless the circumstances of the admission, the therapy provided, the Tabular List, or the Alphabetic Index indicate otherwise.

C. Two or more diagnoses that equally meet the definition for principal diagnosis

In the unusual instance when two or more diagnoses equally meet the criteria for principal diagnosis as determined by the circumstances of admission, diagnostic workup and/or therapy provided, and the Alphabetic Index, Tabular List, or another coding guidelines does not provide sequencing direction, any one of the diagnoses may be sequenced first.

D. Two or more comparative or contrasting conditions

In those rare instances when two or more contrasting or comparative diagnoses are documented as "either/or" (or similar terminology), they are coded as if the diagnoses were confirmed and the diagnoses are sequenced according to the circumstances of the admission. If no further determination can be made as to which diagnosis should be principal, either diagnosis may be sequenced first.

E. A symptom(s) followed by contrasting/comparative diagnoses

GUIDELINE HAS BEEN DELETED EFFECTIVE OCTOBER 1, 2014

F. Original treatment plan not carried out

Sequence as the principal diagnosis the condition, which after study occasioned the admission to the hospital, even though treatment may not have been carried out due to unforeseen circumstances.

G. Complications of surgery and other medical care

When the admission is for treatment of a complication resulting from surgery or other medical care, the complication code is sequenced as the principal diagnosis. If the complication is classified to the T80-T88 series and the code lacks the necessary specificity in describing the complication, an additional code for the specific complication should be assigned.

H. Uncertain Diagnosis

If the diagnosis documented at the time of discharge is qualified as "probable," "suspected," "likely," "questionable," "possible," or "still to be ruled out," **"compatible with," "consistent with,"** or other similar terms indicating uncertainty, code the condition as if it existed or was established. The bases for these guidelines are the diagnostic workup, arrangements for further workup or observation, and initial therapeutic approach that correspond most closely with the established diagnosis.

Note: This guideline is applicable only to inpatient admissions to short-term, acute, long-term care and psychiatric hospitals.

I. Admission from Observation Unit

1. Admission Following Medical Observation

When a patient is admitted to an observation unit for a medical condition, which either worsens or does not improve, and is subsequently admitted as an inpatient of the same hospital for this same medical condition, the principal diagnosis would be the medical condition which led to the hospital admission.

2. Admission Following Post-Operative Observation

When a patient is admitted to an observation unit to monitor a condition (or complication) that develops following outpatient surgery, and then is subsequently admitted as an inpatient of the same hospital, hospitals should apply the Uniform Hospital Discharge Data Set (UHDDS) definition of principal diagnosis as "that condition established after study to be chiefly responsible for occasioning the admission of the patient to the hospital for care."

J. Admission from Outpatient Surgery

When a patient receives surgery in the hospital's outpatient surgery department and is subsequently admitted for continuing inpatient care at the same hospital, the following guidelines should be followed in selecting the principal diagnosis for the inpatient admission:

- If the reason for the inpatient admission is a complication, assign the complication as the principal diagnosis.
- If no complication, or other condition, is documented as the reason for the inpatient admission, assign the reason for the outpatient surgery as the principal diagnosis.
- If the reason for the inpatient admission is another condition unrelated to the surgery, assign the unrelated condition as the principal diagnosis.

K. Admissions/Encounters for Rehabilitation

When the purpose for the admission/encounter is rehabilitation, sequence first the code for the condition for which the service is being performed. For example, for an admission/encounter for rehabilitation for right-sided dominant hemiplegia following a cerebrovascular infarction, report code I69.351, Hemiplegia and hemiparesis following cerebral infarction affecting right dominant side, as the first-listed or principal diagnosis.

If the condition for which the rehabilitation service is being provided is no longer present, report the appropriate aftercare code as the first-listed or principal diagnosis, unless the rehabilitation service is being provided following an injury. For rehabilitation services following active treatment of an injury, assign the injury code with the appropriate seventh character for subsequent encounter as the first-listed or principal diagnosis. For example, if a patient with severe degenerative osteoarthritis of the hip, underwent hip replacement and the current encounter/admission is for rehabilitation, report code Z47.1, Aftercare following joint replacement surgery, as the first-listed or principal diagnosis. If the patient requires rehabilitation post hip replacement for right intertrochanteric femur fracture, report code S72.141D, Displaced intertrochanteric fracture of right femur, subsequent encounter for closed fracture with routine healing, as the first-listed or principal diagnosis.

See Section I.C.21.c.7, Factors influencing health states and contact with health services, Aftercare.

See Section I.C.19.a for additional information about the use of 7th characters for injury codes.

Section III. Reporting Additional Diagnoses

GENERAL RULES FOR OTHER (ADDITIONAL) DIAGNOSES

For reporting purposes the definition for "other diagnoses" is interpreted as additional conditions that affect patient care in terms of requiring:

clinical evaluation; or
therapeutic treatment; or
diagnostic procedures; or
extended length of hospital stay; or
increased nursing care and/or monitoring.

The UHDDS item #11-b defines Other Diagnoses as "all conditions that coexist at the time of admission, that develop subsequently, or that affect the treatment received and/or the length of stay. Diagnoses that relate to an earlier episode which have no bearing on the current hospital stay are to be excluded." UHDDS definitions apply to inpatients in acute care, short-term, long term care and psychiatric hospital setting. The UHDDS definitions are used by acute care short-term hospitals to report inpatient data elements in a standardized manner. These data elements and their definitions can be found in the July 31, 1985, Federal Register (Vol. 50, No, 147), pp. 31038-40.

Since that time the application of the UHDDS definitions has been expanded to include all non-outpatient settings (acute care, short term, long term care and psychiatric hospitals; home health agencies; rehab facilities; nursing homes, etc). The UHDDS definitions also apply to hospice services (all levels of care).

The following guidelines are to be applied in designating "other diagnoses" when neither the Alphabetic Index nor the Tabular List in ICD-10-CM provide direction. The listing of the diagnoses in the patient record is the responsibility of the attending provider.

A. Previous conditions

If the provider has included a diagnosis in the final diagnostic statement, such as the discharge summary or the face sheet, it should ordinarily be coded. Some providers include in the diagnostic statement resolved conditions or diagnoses and status-post procedures from previous admission that have no bearing on the current stay. Such conditions are not to be reported and are coded only if required by hospital policy.

However, history codes (categories Z80-Z87) may be used as secondary codes if the historical condition or family history has an impact on current care or influences treatment.

B. Abnormal findings

Abnormal findings (laboratory, x-ray, pathologic, and other diagnostic results) are not coded and reported unless the provider indicates their clinical significance. If the findings are outside the normal range and the attending provider has ordered other tests to evaluate the condition or prescribed treatment, it is appropriate to ask the provider whether the abnormal finding should be added.

Please note: This differs from the coding practices in the outpatient setting for coding encounters for diagnostic tests that have been interpreted by a provider.

C. Uncertain Diagnosis

If the diagnosis documented at the time of discharge is qualified as "probable," "suspected," "likely," "questionable," "possible," or "still to be ruled out," **"compatible with," "consistent with,"** or other similar terms indicating uncertainty, code the condition as if it existed or was

2020 ICD-10-CM Official Guidelines for Coding and Reporting

established. The bases for these guidelines are the diagnostic workup, arrangements for further workup or observation, and initial therapeutic approach that correspond most closely with the established diagnosis.

Note: This guideline is applicable only to inpatient admissions to short-term, acute, long-term care and psychiatric hospitals.

Section IV.Diagnostic Coding and Reporting Guidelines for Outpatient Services

These coding guidelines for outpatient diagnoses have been approved for use by hospitals/ providers in coding and reporting hospital-based outpatient services and provider-based office visits. Guidelines in Section I, Conventions, general coding guidelines and chapter-specific guidelines, should also be applied for outpatient services and office visits.

Information about the use of certain abbreviations, punctuation, symbols, and other conventions used in the ICD-10-CM Tabular List (code numbers and titles), can be found in Section IA of these guidelines, under "Conventions Used in the Tabular List." Section I.B. contains general guidelines that apply to the entire classification. Section I.C. contains chapter-specific guidelines that correspond to the chapters as they are arranged in the classification. Information about the correct sequence to use in finding a code is also described in Section I.

The terms encounter and visit are often used interchangeably in describing outpatient service contacts and, therefore, appear together in these guidelines without distinguishing one from the other.

Though the conventions and general guidelines apply to all settings, coding guidelines for outpatient and provider reporting of diagnoses will vary in a number of instances from those for inpatient diagnoses, recognizing that:

The Uniform Hospital Discharge Data Set (UHDDS) definition of principal diagnosis does not apply to hospital-based outpatient services and provider-based office visits.

Coding guidelines for inconclusive diagnoses (probable, suspected, rule out, etc.) were developed for inpatient reporting and do not apply to outpatients.

A. **Selection of first-listed condition**
   In the outpatient setting, the term first-listed diagnosis is used in lieu of principal diagnosis.

   In determining the first-listed diagnosis the coding conventions of ICD-10-CM, as well as the general and disease specific guidelines take precedence over the outpatient guidelines.

   Diagnoses often are not established at the time of the initial encounter/visit. It may take two or more visits before the diagnosis is confirmed.

   The most critical rule involves beginning the search for the correct code assignment through the Alphabetic Index. Never begin searching initially in the Tabular List as this will lead to coding errors.

   1. **Outpatient Surgery**
      When a patient presents for outpatient surgery (same day surgery), code the reason for the surgery as the first-listed diagnosis (reason for the encounter), even if the surgery is not performed due to a contraindication.

   2. **Observation Stay**
      When a patient is admitted for observation for a medical condition, assign a code for the medical condition as the first-listed diagnosis.

      When a patient presents for outpatient surgery and develops complications requiring admission to observation, code the reason for the surgery as the first reported diagnosis (reason for the encounter), followed by codes for the complications as secondary diagnoses.

B. **Codes from A00.0 through T88.9, Z00-Z99**
   The appropriate code(s) from A00.0 through T88.9, Z00-Z99 must be used to identify diagnoses, symptoms, conditions, problems, complaints, or other reason(s) for the encounter/visit.

C. **Accurate reporting of ICD-10-CM diagnosis codes**
   For accurate reporting of ICD-10-CM diagnosis codes, the documentation should describe the patient's condition, using terminology which includes specific diagnoses as well as symptoms, problems, or reasons for the encounter. There are ICD-10-CM codes to describe all of these.

D. **Codes that describe symptoms and signs**
   Codes that describe symptoms and signs, as opposed to diagnoses, are acceptable for reporting purposes when a diagnosis has not been established (confirmed) by the provider. Chapter 18 of ICD-10-CM, Symptoms, Signs, and Abnormal Clinical and Laboratory Findings Not Elsewhere Classified (codes R00-R99) contain many, but not all codes for symptoms.

E. **Encounters for circumstances other than a disease or injury**
   ICD-10-CM provides codes to deal with encounters for circumstances other than a disease or injury. The Factors Influencing Health Status and Contact with Health Services codes (Z00-Z99) are provided to deal with occasions when circumstances other than a disease or injury are recorded as diagnosis or problems.

   See Section I.C.21. Factors influencing health status and contact with health services.

F. **Level of Detail in Coding**
   1. **ICD-10-CM codes with 3, 4, 5, 6 or 7 characters**
      ICD-10-CM is composed of codes with 3, 4, 5, 6 or 7 characters. Codes with three characters are included in ICD-10-CM as the heading of a category of codes that may be further subdivided by the use of fourth, fifth, sixth or seventh characters to provide greater specificity.

   2. **Use of full number of characters required for a code**
      A three-character code is to be used only if it is not further subdivided. A code is invalid if it has not been coded to the full number of characters required for that code, including the 7th character, if applicable.

G. **ICD-10-CM code for the diagnosis, condition, problem, or other reason for encounter/visit**
   List first the ICD-10-CM code for the diagnosis, condition, problem, or other reason for encounter/visit shown in the medical record to be chiefly responsible for the services provided. List additional codes that describe any coexisting conditions. In some cases the first-listed diagnosis may be a symptom when a diagnosis has not been established (confirmed) by the **provider.**

H. **Uncertain diagnosis**
   Do not code diagnoses documented as "probable", "suspected," "questionable," "rule out," **"compatible with," "consistent with,"** or "working diagnosis" or other similar terms indicating uncertainty. Rather, code the condition(s) to the highest degree of certainty for that encounter/visit, such as symptoms, signs, abnormal test results, or other reason for the visit.

   Please note: This differs from the coding practices used by short-term, acute care, long-term care and psychiatric hospitals.

I. **Chronic diseases**
   Chronic diseases treated on an ongoing basis may be coded and reported as many times as the patient receives treatment and care for the condition(s)

J. **Code all documented conditions that coexist**
   Code all documented conditions that coexist at the time of the encounter/visit, and require or affect patient care treatment or management. Do not code conditions that were previously treated and no longer exist. However, history codes (categories Z80-Z87) may be used as secondary codes if the historical condition or family history has an impact on current care or influences treatment.

K. **Patients receiving diagnostic services only**
   For patients receiving diagnostic services only during an encounter/visit, sequence first the diagnosis, condition, problem, or other reason for encounter/visit shown in the medical record to be chiefly responsible for the outpatient services provided during the encounter/visit. Codes for other diagnoses (e.g., chronic conditions) may be sequenced as additional diagnoses.

   For encounters for routine laboratory/radiology testing in the absence of any signs, symptoms, or associated diagnosis, assign Z01.89, Encounter for other specified special examinations. If routine testing is performed during the same encounter as a test to evaluate a sign, symptom, or diagnosis, it is appropriate to assign both the Z code and the code describing the reason for the non-routine test.

   For outpatient encounters for diagnostic tests that have been interpreted by a physician, and the final report is available at the time of coding, code any confirmed or definitive diagnosis(es) documented in the interpretation. Do not code related signs and symptoms as additional diagnoses.

   Please note: This differs from the coding practice in the hospital inpatient setting regarding abnormal findings on test results.

L. **Patients receiving therapeutic services only**
   For patients receiving therapeutic services only during an encounter/visit, sequence first the diagnosis, condition, problem, or other reason for encounter/visit shown in the medical record to be chiefly responsible for the outpatient services provided during the encounter/visit. Codes for other diagnoses (e.g., chronic conditions) may be sequenced as additional diagnoses.

The only exception to this rule is that when the primary reason for the admission/encounter is chemotherapy or radiation therapy, the appropriate Z code for the service is listed first, and the diagnosis or problem for which the service is being performed listed second.

M. Patients receiving preoperative evaluations only

For patients receiving preoperative evaluations only, sequence first a code from subcategory Z01.81, Encounter for pre-procedural examinations, to describe the pre-op consultations. Assign a code for the condition to describe the reason for the surgery as an additional diagnosis. Code also any findings related to the pre-op evaluation.

N. Ambulatory surgery

For ambulatory surgery, code the diagnosis for which the surgery was performed. If the postoperative diagnosis is known to be different from the preoperative diagnosis at the time the diagnosis is confirmed, select the postoperative diagnosis for coding, since it is the most definitive.

O. Routine outpatient prenatal visits

See Section I.C.15. Routine outpatient prenatal visits.

P. Encounters for general medical examinations with abnormal findings

The subcategories for encounters for general medical examinations, Z00.0- and encounter for routine child health examination, Z00.12-, provide codes for with and without abnormal findings. Should a general medical examination result in an abnormal finding, the code for general medical examination with abnormal finding should be assigned as the first-listed diagnosis. An examination with abnormal findings refers to a condition/diagnosis that is newly identified or a change in severity of a chronic condition (such as uncontrolled hypertension, or an acute exacerbation of chronic obstructive pulmonary disease) during a routine physical examination. A secondary code for the abnormal finding should also be coded.

Q. Encounters for routine health screenings

See Section I.C.21. Factors influencing health status and contact with health services, Screening

Appendix I. Present on Admission Reporting Guidelines

Introduction

These guidelines are to be used as a supplement to the *ICD-10-CM Official Guidelines for Coding and Reporting* to facilitate the assignment of the Present on Admission (POA) indicator for each diagnosis and external cause of injury code reported on claim forms (UB-04 and 837 Institutional).

These guidelines are not intended to replace any guidelines in the main body of the *ICD-10-CM Official Guidelines for Coding and Reporting*. The POA guidelines are not intended to provide guidance on when a condition should be coded, but rather, how to apply the POA indicator to the final set of diagnosis codes that have been assigned in accordance with Sections I, II, and III of the official coding guidelines. Subsequent to the assignment of the ICD-10-CM codes, the POA indicator should then be assigned to those conditions that have been coded.

As stated in the Introduction to the *ICD-10-CM Official Guidelines for Coding and Reporting*, a joint effort between the healthcare provider and the coder is essential to achieve complete and accurate documentation, code assignment, and reporting of diagnoses and procedures. The importance of consistent, complete documentation in the medical record cannot be overemphasized. Medical record documentation from any provider involved in the care and treatment of the patient may be used to support the determination of whether a condition was present on admission or not. In the context of the official coding guidelines, the term "provider" means a physician or any qualified healthcare practitioner who is legally accountable for establishing the patient's diagnosis.

These guidelines are not a substitute for the provider's clinical judgment as to the determination of whether a condition was/was not present on admission. The provider should be queried regarding issues related to the linking of signs/symptoms, timing of test results, and the timing of findings.

Please see the CDC website for the detailed list of ICD-10-CM codes that do not require the use of a POA indicator (https://www.cdc.gov/nchs/icd/icd10cm.htm). The codes and categories on this exempt list are for circumstances regarding the healthcare encounter or factors influencing health status that do not represent a current disease or injury or that describe conditions that are always present on admission.

General Reporting Requirements

All claims involving inpatient admissions to general acute care hospitals or other facilities that are subject to a law or regulation mandating collection of present on admission information.

Present on admission is defined as present at the time the order for inpatient admission occurs -- conditions that develop during an outpatient encounter, including emergency department, observation, or outpatient surgery, are considered as present on admission.

POA indicator is assigned to principal and secondary diagnoses (as defined in Section II of the Official Guidelines for Coding and Reporting) and the external cause of injury codes.

Issues related to inconsistent, missing, conflicting or unclear documentation must still be resolved by the provider.

If a condition would not be coded and reported based on UHDDS definitions and current official coding guidelines, then the POA indicator would not be reported.

Reporting Options

Y - Yes

N - No

U - Unknown

W – Clinically undetermined

Unreported/Not used – (Exempt from POA reporting)

Reporting Definitions

Y = present at the time of inpatient admission

N = not present at the time of inpatient admission

U = documentation is insufficient to determine if condition is present on admission

W = provider is unable to clinically determine whether condition was present on admission or not

Timeframe for POA Identification and Documentation

There is no required timeframe as to when a provider (per the definition of "provider" used in these guidelines) must identify or document a condition to be present on admission. In some clinical situations, it may not be possible for a provider to make a definitive diagnosis (or a condition may not be recognized or reported by the patient) for a period of time after admission. In some cases it may be several days before the provider arrives at a definitive diagnosis. This does not mean that the condition was not present on admission. Determination of whether the condition was present on admission or not will be based on the applicable POA guideline as identified in this document, or on the provider's best clinical judgment.

If at the time of code assignment the documentation is unclear as to whether a condition was present on admission or not, it is appropriate to query the provider for clarification.

Assigning the POA Indicator

Condition is on the "Exempt from Reporting" list

Leave the "present on admission" field blank if the condition is on the list of ICD-10-CM codes for which this field is not applicable. This is the only circumstance in which the field may be left blank.

POA Explicitly Documented

Assign Y for any condition the provider explicitly documents as being present on admission.

Assign N for any condition the provider explicitly documents as not present at the time of admission.

Conditions diagnosed prior to inpatient admission

Assign "Y" for conditions that were diagnosed prior to admission (example: hypertension, diabetes mellitus, asthma)

Conditions diagnosed during the admission but clearly present before admission

Assign "Y" for conditions diagnosed during the admission that were clearly present but not diagnosed until after admission occurred.

Diagnoses subsequently confirmed after admission are considered present on admission if at the time of admission they are documented as suspected, possible, rule out, differential diagnosis, or constitute an underlying cause of a symptom that is present at the time of admission.

Condition develops during outpatient encounter prior to inpatient admission

Assign Y for any condition that develops during an outpatient encounter prior to a written order for inpatient admission.

Documentation does not indicate whether condition was present on admission

Assign "U" when the medical record documentation is unclear as to whether the condition was present on admission. "U" should not be routinely assigned and used only in very limited circumstances. Coders are encouraged to query the providers when the documentation is unclear.

Documentation states that it cannot be determined whether the condition was or was not present on admission

Assign "W" when the medical record documentation indicates that it cannot be clinically determined whether or not the condition was present on admission.

Chronic condition with acute exacerbation during the admission

If a single code identifies both the chronic condition and the acute exacerbation, see POA guidelines pertaining to codes that contain multiple clinical concepts.

If a single code only identifies the chronic condition and not the acute exacerbation (e.g., acute exacerbation of chronic leukemia), assign "Y."

Conditions documented as possible, probable, suspected, or rule out at the time of discharge

If the final diagnosis contains a possible, probable, suspected, or rule out diagnosis, and this diagnosis was based on signs, symptoms or clinical findings suspected at the time of inpatient admission, assign "Y."

If the final diagnosis contains a possible, probable, suspected, or rule out diagnosis, and this diagnosis was based on signs, symptoms or clinical findings that were not present on admission, assign "N".

Conditions documented as impending or threatened at the time of discharge

If the final diagnosis contains an impending or threatened diagnosis, and this diagnosis is based on symptoms or clinical findings that were present on admission, assign "Y".

If the final diagnosis contains an impending or threatened diagnosis, and this diagnosis is based on symptoms or clinical findings that were not present on admission, assign "N".

Acute and Chronic Conditions

Assign "Y" for acute conditions that are present at time of admission and N for acute conditions that are not present at time of admission.

Assign "Y" for chronic conditions, even though the condition may not be diagnosed until after admission.

If a single code identifies both an acute and chronic condition, see the POA guidelines for codes that contain multiple clinical concepts.

Codes That Contain Multiple Clinical Concepts

Assign "N" if at least one of the clinical concepts included in the code was not present on admission (e.g., COPD with acute exacerbation and the exacerbation was not present on admission; gastric ulcer that does not start bleeding until after admission; asthma patient develops status asthmaticus after admission).

Assign "Y" if all of the clinical concepts included in the code were present on admission (e.g., duodenal ulcer that perforates prior to admission).

For infection codes that include the causal organism, assign "Y" if the infection (or signs of the infection) were present on admission, even though the culture results may not be known until after admission (e.g., patient is admitted with pneumonia and the provider documents Pseudomonas as the causal organism a few days later).

Same Diagnosis Code for Two or More Conditions

When the same ICD-10-CM diagnosis code applies to two or more conditions during the same encounter (e.g. two separate conditions classified to the same ICD-10-CM diagnosis code):

Assign "Y" if all conditions represented by the single ICD-10-CM code were present on admission (e.g. bilateral unspecified age-related cataracts).

Assign "N" if any of the conditions represented by the single ICD-10-CM code was not present on admission (e.g. traumatic secondary and recurrent hemorrhage and seroma is assigned to a single code T79.2, but only one of the conditions was present on admission).

Obstetrical conditions

Whether or not the patient delivers during the current hospitalization does not affect assignment of the POA indicator. The determining factor for POA assignment is whether the pregnancy complication or obstetrical condition described by the code was present at the time of admission or not.

If the pregnancy complication or obstetrical condition was present on admission (e.g., patient admitted in preterm labor), assign "Y".

If the pregnancy complication or obstetrical condition was not present on admission (e.g., 2nd degree laceration during delivery, postpartum hemorrhage that occurred during current hospitalization, fetal distress develops after admission), assign "N".

If the obstetrical code includes more than one diagnosis and any of the diagnoses identified by the code were not present on admission assign "N". (e.g., Category O11, Pre-existing hypertension with pre-eclampsia)

Perinatal conditions

Newborns are not considered to be admitted until after birth. Therefore, any condition present at birth or that developed in utero is considered present at admission and should be assigned "Y". This includes conditions that occur during delivery (e.g., injury during delivery, meconium aspiration, exposure to streptococcus B in the vaginal canal).

Congenital conditions and anomalies

Assign "Y" for congenital conditions and anomalies except for categories Q00-Q99, Congenital anomalies, which are on the exempt list. Congenital conditions are always considered present on admission.

External cause of injury codes

Assign "Y" for any external cause code representing an external cause of morbidity that occurred prior to inpatient admission (e.g., patient fell out of bed at home, patient fell out of bed in emergency room prior to admission)

Assign "N" for any external cause code representing an external cause of morbidity that occurred during inpatient hospitalization (e.g., patient fell out of hospital bed during hospital stay, patient experienced an adverse reaction to a medication administered after inpatient admission).

A

Aarskog's syndrome Q87.19
Abandonment — *see* Maltreatment
Abasia (-astasia) (hysterical) F44.4
Abderhalden-Kaufmann-Lignac syndrome (cystinosis) E72.04
Abdomen, abdominal — *see also* condition
  muscle deficiency syndrome Q79.4
  angina K55.1
  acute R10.0
Abdominalgia — *see* Pain, abdominal
Abduction contracture, hip or other joint — *see* Contraction, joint
Aberrant (congenital) — *see also* Malposition, congenital
  hepatic duct Q44.5
  endocrine gland NEC Q89.2
  breast Q83.8
  artery (peripheral) Q27.8
    basilar NEC Q28.1
    cerebral Q28.3
    coronary Q24.5
    digestive system Q27.8
    eye Q15.8
    lower limb Q27.8
    precerebral Q28.1
    pulmonary Q25.79
    renal Q27.2
    retina Q14.1
    specified site NEC Q27.8
    subclavian Q27.8
    upper limb Q27.8
    vertebral Q28.1
  adrenal gland Q89.1
  pancreas Q45.3
  parathyroid gland Q89.2
  pituitary gland Q89.2
  sebaceous glands, mucous membrane, mouth, congenital Q38.6
  spleen Q89.09
  subclavian artery Q27.8
  thymus (gland) Q89.2
  thyroid gland Q89.2
  vein (peripheral) NEC Q27.8
    cerebral Q28.3
    digestive system Q27.8
    lower limb Q27.8
    precerebral Q28.1
    specified site NEC Q27.8
    upper limb Q27.8
Aberration
  distantial — *see* Disturbance, visual
  mental F99
Abetalipoproteinemia E78.6
Abiotrophy R68.89
Ablatio, ablation
  retinae — *see* Detachment, retina
Ablepharia, ablepharon Q10.3
Abnormal, abnormality, abnormalities — *see also* Anomaly
  acid-base balance (mixed) E87.4
  albumin R77.0
  alphafetoprotein R77.2
  alveolar ridge K08.9
  anatomical relationship Q89.9
  apertures, congenital, diaphragm Q79.1
  auditory perception H93.29- ✔
    diplacusis — *see* Diplacusis
    hyperacusis — *see* Hyperacusis
    recruitment — *see* Recruitment, auditory
    threshold shift — *see* Shift, auditory threshold
  autosomes Q99.9
    fragile site Q95.5
  basal metabolic rate R94.8
  biosynthesis, testicular androgen E29.1
  bleeding time R79.1
  blood level (of)
    cobalt R79.0
    copper R79.0
    iron R79.0
    lithium R78.89
    magnesium R79.0

Abnormal, abnormality, abnormalities — *continued*
  blood level — *continued*
    mineral NEC R79.0
    zinc R79.0
  blood pressure
    elevated R03.0
    low reading (nonspecific) R03.1
  blood sugar R73.09
  blood-gas level R79.81
  bowel sounds R19.15
    absent R19.11
    hyperactive R19.12
  brain scan R94.02
  breathing R06.9
  caloric test R94.138
  cerebrospinal fluid R83.9
    cytology R83.6
    drug level R83.2
    enzyme level R83.0
    hormones R83.1
    immunology R83.4
    microbiology R83.5
    nonmedicinal level R83.3
    specified type NEC R83.8
  chemistry, blood R79.9
    C-reactive protein R79.82
    drugs — *see* Findings, abnormal, in blood
    gas level R79.81
    minerals R79.0
    pancytopenia D61.818
    PTT R79.1
    specified NEC R79.89
    toxins — *see* Findings, abnormal, in blood
  chest sounds (friction) (rales) R09.89
  chromosome, chromosomal Q99.9
    with more than three X chromosomes, female Q97.1
    analysis result R89.8
      bronchial washings R84.8
      cerebrospinal fluid R83.8
      cervix uteri NEC R87.89
      nasal secretions R84.8
      nipple discharge R89.8
      peritoneal fluid R85.89
      pleural fluid R84.8
      prostatic secretions R86.8
      saliva R85.89
      seminal fluid R86.8
      sputum R84.8
      synovial fluid R89.8
      throat scrapings R84.8
      vagina R87.89
      vulva R87.89
      wound secretions R89.8
    dicentric replacement Q93.2
    ring replacement Q93.2
    sex Q99.8
      female phenotype Q97.9
        specified NEC Q97.8
      male phenotype Q98.9
        specified NEC Q98.8
      structural male Q98.6
    specified NEC Q99.8
  clinical findings NEC R68.89
  coagulation D68.9
    newborn, transient P61.6
    profile R79.1
    time R79.1
  communication — *see* Fistula
  conjunctiva, vascular H11.41- ✔
  coronary artery Q24.5
  cortisol-binding globulin E27.8
  course, eustachian tube Q17.8
  creatinine clearance R94.4
  cytology
    anus R85.619
      atypical squamous cells cannot exclude high grade squamous intraepithelial lesion (ASC-H) R85.611
      atypical squamous cells of undetermined significance (ASC-US) R85.610
      cytologic evidence of malignancy R85.614

Abnormal, abnormality, abnormalities — *continued*
  cytology — *continued*
    anus — *continued*
      high grade squamous intraepithelial lesion (HGSIL) R85.613
      human papillomavirus (HPV) DNA test
        high risk positive R85.81
        low risk postive R85.82
      inadequate smear R85.615
      low grade squamous intraepithelial lesion (LGSIL) R85.612
      satisfactory anal smear but lacking transformation zone R85.616
      specified NEC R85.618
      unsatisfactory smear R85.615
    female genital organs — *see* Abnormal, Papanicolaou (smear)
  dark adaptation curve H53.61
  dentofacial NEC — *see* Anomaly, dentofacial
  development, developmental Q89.9
    central nervous system Q07.9
  diagnostic imaging
    abdomen, abdominal region NEC R93.5
    biliary tract R93.2
    bladder R93.41
    breast R92.8
    central nervous system NEC R90.89
    cerebrovascular NEC R90.89
    coronary circulation R93.1
    digestive tract NEC R93.3
    gastrointestinal (tract) R93.3
    genitourinary organs R93.89
    head R93.0
    heart R93.1
    intrathoracic organ NEC R93.89
    kidney R93.42- ✔
    limbs R93.6
    liver R93.2
    lung (field) R91.8
    musculoskeletal system NEC R93.7
    renal pelvis R93.41
    retroperitoneum R93.5
    site specified NEC R93.89
    skin and subcutaneous tissue R93.89
    skull R93.0
    testis R93.81- ✔
    ureter R93.41
    urinary organs specified NEC R93.49
  direction, teeth, fully erupted M26.30
  ear ossicles, acquired NEC H74.39- ✔
    ankylosis — *see* Ankylosis, ear ossicles
    discontinuity — *see* Discontinuity, ossicles, ear
    partial loss — *see* Loss, ossicles, ear (partial)
  Ebstein Q22.5
  echocardiogram R93.1
  echoencephalogram R90.81
  echogram — *see* Abnormal, diagnostic imaging
  electrocardiogram [ECG] [EKG] R94.31
  electroencephalogram [EEG] R94.01
  electrolyte — *see* Imbalance, electrolyte
  electromyogram [EMG] R94.131
  electro-oculogram [EOG] R94.110
  electrophysiological intracardiac studies R94.39
  electroretinogram [ERG] R94.111
  erythrocytes
    congenital, with perinatal jaundice D58.9
  feces (color) (contents) (mucus) R19.5
  finding — *see* Findings, abnormal, without diagnosis
  fluid
    amniotic — *see* Abnormal, specimen, specified
    cerebrospinal — *see* Abnormal, cerebrospinal fluid
    peritoneal — *see* Abnormal, specimen, digestive organs
    pleural — *see* Abnormal, specimen, respiratory organs
    synovial — *see* Abnormal, specimen, specified
    thorax (bronchial washings) (pleural fluid) — *see* Abnormal, specimen, respiratory organs
    vaginal — *see* Abnormal, specimen, female genital organs
  form
    teeth K00.2

Abnormal, abnormality, abnormalities — continued
form — continued
  uterus — see Anomaly, uterus
  function studies
    auditory R94.120
    bladder R94.8
    brain R94.09
    cardiovascular R94.30
    ear R94.128
    endocrine NEC R94.7
    eye NEC R94.118
    kidney R94.4
    liver R94.5
    nervous system
      central NEC R94.09
      peripheral NEC R94.138
    pancreas R94.8
    placenta R94.8
    pulmonary R94.2
    special senses NEC R94.128
    spleen R94.8
    thyroid R94.6
    vestibular R94.121
  gait — see Gait
    hysterical F44.4
  gastrin secretion E16.4
  globulin R77.1
    cortisol-binding E27.8
    thyroid-binding E07.89
  glomerular, minor — see also N00-N07 with fourth
    character .0 N05.0
  glucagon secretion E16.3
  glucose tolerance (test) (non-fasting) R73.09
  gravitational (G) forces or states (effect of) T75.81 ☑
  hair (color) (shaft) L67.9
    specified NEC L67.8
  hard tissue formation in pulp (dental) K04.3
  head movement R25.0
  heart
    rate R00.9
      specified NEC R00.8
    shadow R93.1
    sounds NEC R01.2
  hemoglobin (disease) — see also Disease, hemoglobin
    D58.2
    trait — see Trait, hemoglobin, abnormal
  histology NEC R89.7
  immunological findings R89.4
    in serum R76.9
      specified NEC R76.8
  increase in appetite R63.2
  involuntary movement — see Abnormal, movement,
    involuntary
  jaw closure M26.51
  karyotype R89.8
  kidney function test R94.4
  knee jerk R29.2
  leukocyte (cell) (differential) NEC D72.9
  liver function test R94.5
  loss of
    height R29.890
    weight R63.4
  mammogram NEC R92.8
    calcification (calculus) R92.1
    microcalcification R92.0
  Mantoux test R76.11
  movement (disorder) — see also Disorder, movement
    head R25.0
    involuntary R25.9
      fasciculation R25.3
      of head R25.0
      spasm R25.2
      specified type NEC R25.8
      tremor R25.1
  myoglobin (Aberdeen) (Annapolis) R89.7
  neonatal screening P09
  oculomotor study R94.113
  palmar creases Q82.8
  Papanicolaou (smear)
    anus R85.619
      atypical squamous cells cannot exclude high
        grade squamous intraepithelial lesion
        (ASC-H) R85.611
      atypical squamous cells of undetermined signif-
        icance (ASC-US) R85.610
      cytologic evidence of malignancy R85.614

Abnormal, abnormality, abnormalities — continued
Papanicolaou — continued
  anus — continued
    high grade squamous intraepithelial lesion
      (HGSIL) R85.613
    human papillomavirus (HPV) DNA test
      high risk positive R85.81
      low risk postive R85.82
    inadequate smear R85.615
    low grade squamous intraepithelial lesion (LGSIL)
      R85.612
    satisfactory anal smear but lacking transforma-
      tion zone R85.616
    specified NEC R85.618
    unsatisfactory smear R85.615
  bronchial washings R84.6
  cerebrospinal fluid R83.6
  cervix R87.619
    atypical squamous cells cannot exclude high
      grade squamous intraepithelial lesion
      (ASC-H) R87.611
    atypical squamous cells of undetermined signif-
      icance (ASC-US) R87.610
    cytologic evidence of malignancy R87.614
    high grade squamous intraepithelial lesion
      (HGSIL) R87.613
    inadequate smear R87.615
    low grade squamous intraepithelial lesion (LGSIL)
      R87.612
    non-atypical endometrial cells R87.618
    satisfactory cervical smear but lacking transfor-
      mation zone R87.616
    specified NEC R87.618
    thin preparaton R87.619
    unsatisfactory smear R87.615
  nasal secretions R84.6
  nipple discharge R89.6
  peritoneal fluid R85.69
  pleural fluid R84.6
  prostatic secretions R86.6
  saliva R85.69
  seminal fluid R86.6
  sites NEC R89.6
  sputum R84.6
  synovial fluid R89.6
  throat scrapings R84.6
  vagina R87.629
    atypical squamous cells cannot exclude high
      grade squamous intraepithelial lesion
      (ASC-H) R87.621
    atypical squamous cells of undetermined signif-
      icance (ASC-US) R87.620
    cytologic evidence of malignancy R87.624
    high grade squamous intraepithelial lesion
      (HGSIL) R87.623
    inadequate smear R87.625
    low grade squamous intraepithelial lesion (LGSIL)
      R87.622
    specified NEC R87.628
    thin preparation R87.629
    unsatisfactory smear R87.625
  vulva R87.69
  wound secretions R89.6
partial thromboplastin time (PTT) R79.1
pelvis (bony) — see Deformity, pelvis
percussion, chest (tympany) R09.89
periods (grossly) — see Menstruation
phonocardiogram R94.39
plantar reflex R29.2
plasma
  protein R77.9
    specified NEC R77.8
  viscosity R70.1
pleural (folds) Q34.0
posture R29.3
product of conception O02.9
  specified type NEC O02.89
prothrombin time (PT) R79.1
pulmonary
  artery, congenital Q25.79
  function, newborn P28.89
  test results R94.2
pulsations in neck R00.2
pupillary H21.56- ☑
  function (reaction) (reflex) — see Anomaly, pupil,
    function
radiological examination — see Abnormal, diagnostic
  imaging

Abnormal, abnormality, abnormalities — continued
red blood cell(s) (morphology) (volume) R71.8
reflex — see Reflex
renal function test R94.4
response to nerve stimulation R94.130
retinal correspondence H53.31
retinal function study R94.111
rhythm, heart — see also Arrhythmia
saliva — see Abnormal, specimen, digestive organs
scan
  kidney R94.4
  liver R93.2
  thyroid R94.6
secretion
  gastrin E16.4
  glucagon E16.3
semen, seminal fluid — see Abnormal, specimen, male
  genital organs
serum level (of)
  acid phosphatase R74.8
  alkaline phosphatase R74.8
  amylase R74.8
  enzymes R74.9
    specified NEC R74.8
  lipase R74.8
  triacylglycerol lipase R74.8
shape
  gravid uterus — see Anomaly, uterus
sinus venosus Q21.1
size, tooth, teeth K00.2
spacing, tooth, teeth, fully erupted M26.30
specimen
  digestive organs (peritoneal fluid) (saliva) R85.9
    cytology R85.69
    drug level R85.2
    enzyme level R85.0
    histology R85.7
    hormones R85.1
    immunology R85.4
    microbiology R85.5
    nonmedicinal level R85.3
    specified type NEC R85.89
  female genital organs (secretions) (smears) R87.9
    cytology R87.69
      cervix R87.619
        human papillomavirus (HPV) DNA test
          high risk positive R87.810
          low risk positive R87.820
        inadequate (unsatisfactory) smear
          R87.615
        non-atypical endometrial cells R87.618
        specified NEC R87.618
      vagina R87.629
        human papillomavirus (HPV) DNA test
          high risk positive R87.811
          low risk positive R87.821
        inadequate (unsatisfactory) smear
          R87.625
      vulva R87.69
    drug level R87.2
    enzyme level R87.0
    histological R87.7
    hormones R87.1
    immunology R87.4
    microbiology R87.5
    nonmedicinal level R87.3
    specified type NEC R87.89
  male genital organs (prostatic secretions) (semen)
    R86.9
    cytology R86.6
    drug level R86.2
    enzyme level R86.0
    histological R86.7
    hormones R86.1
    immunology R86.4
    microbiology R86.5
    nonmedicinal level R86.3
    specified type NEC R86.8
  nipple discharge — see Abnormal, specimen, spec-
    ified
  respiratory organs (bronchial washings) (nasal secre-
    tions) (pleural fluid) (sputum) R84.9
    cytology R84.6
    drug level R84.2
    enzyme level R84.0
    histology R84.7
    hormones R84.1
    immunology R84.4

☑ Additional Character Required — Refer to the Tabular List for Character Selection

▽ Subterms under main terms may continue to next column or page

Abnormal, abnormality, abnormalities — *continued*
  specimen — *continued*
    respiratory organs — *continued*
      microbiology R84.5
      nonmedicinal level R84.3
      specified type NEC R84.8
    specified organ, system and tissue NOS R89.9
      cytology R89.6
      drug level R89.2
      enzyme level R89.0
      histology R89.7
      hormones R89.1
      immunology R89.4
      microbiology R89.5
      nonmedicinal level R89.3
      specified type NEC R89.8
    synovial fluid — *see* Abnormal, specimen, specified
    thorax (bronchial washings) (pleural fluids) — *see* Abnormal, specimen, respiratory organs
    vagina (secretion) (smear) R87.629
    vulva (secretion) (smear) R87.69
    wound secretion — *see* Abnormal, specimen, specified
  spermatozoa — *see* Abnormal, specimen, male genital organs
  sputum (amount) (color) (odor) R09.3
  stool (color) (contents) (mucus) R19.5
    bloody K92.1
    guaiac positive R19.5
  synchondrosis Q78.8
  thermography — *see also* Abnormal, diagnostic imaging R93.89
  thyroid-binding globulin E07.89
  tooth, teeth (form) (size) K00.2
  toxicology (findings) R78.9
  transport protein E88.09
  tumor marker NEC R97.8
  ultrasound results — *see* Abnormal, diagnostic imaging
  umbilical cord complicating delivery O69.9 ☑
  urination NEC R39.198
  urine (constituents) R82.90
    bile R82.2
    cytological examination R82.89
    drugs R82.5
    fat R82.0
    glucose R81
    heavy metals R82.6
    hemoglobin R82.3
    histological examination R82.89
    ketones R82.4
    microbiological examination (culture) R82.79
    myoglobin R82.1
    positive culture R82.79
    protein — *see* Proteinuria
    specified substance NEC R82.998
      chromoabnormality NEC R82.91
    substances nonmedical R82.6
  uterine hemorrhage — *see* Hemorrhage, uterus
  vectorcardiogram R94.39
  visually evoked potential (VEP) R94.112
  white blood cells D72.9
    specified NEC D72.89
  X-ray examination — *see* Abnormal, diagnostic imaging
Abnormity (any organ or part) — *see* Anomaly
Abocclusion M26.29
  hemolytic disease (newborn) P55.1
  incompatibility reaction ABO — *see* Complication(s), transfusion, incompatibility reaction, ABO
Abolition, language R48.8
Aborter, habitual or recurrent — *see* Loss (of), pregnancy, recurrent
Abortion (complete) (spontaneous) O03.9
  with
    retained products of conception — *see* Abortion, incomplete
  attempted (elective) (failed) O07.4
    complicated by O07.30
      afibrinogenemia O07.1
      cardiac arrest O07.36
      chemical damage of pelvic organ(s) O07.34
      circulatory collapse O07.31
      cystitis O07.38
      defibrination syndrome O07.1
      electrolyte imbalance O07.33
      embolism (air) (amniotic fluid) (blood clot) (fat) (pulmonary) (septic) (soap) O07.2
      endometritis O07.0

Abortion — *continued*
  attempted — *continued*
    complicated by — *continued*
      genital tract and pelvic infection O07.0
      hemolysis O07.1
      hemorrhage (delayed) (excessive) O07.1
      infection
        genital tract or pelvic O07.0
        urinary tract tract O07.38
      intravascular coagulation O07.1
      laceration of pelvic organ(s) O07.34
      metabolic disorder O07.33
      oliguria O07.32
      oophoritis O07.0
      parametritis O07.0
      pelvic peritonitis O07.0
      perforation of pelvic organ(s) O07.34
      renal failure or shutdown O07.32
      salpingitis or salpingo-oophoritis O07.0
      sepsis O07.37
      shock O07.31
      specified condition NEC O07.39
      tubular necrosis (renal) O07.32
      uremia O07.32
      urinary tract infection O07.38
      venous complication NEC O07.35
        embolism (air) (amniotic fluid) (blood clot) (fat) (pulmonary) (septic) (soap) O07.2
  complicated (by) (following) O03.80
    afibrinogenemia O03.6
    cardiac arrest O03.86
    chemical damage of pelvic organ(s) O03.84
    circulatory collapse O03.81
    cystitis O03.88
    defibrination syndrome O03.6
    electrolyte imbalance O03.83
    embolism (air) (amniotic fluid) (blood clot) (fat) (pulmonary) (septic) (soap) O03.7
    endometritis O03.5
    genital tract and pelvic infection O03.5
    hemolysis O03.6
    hemorrhage (delayed) (excessive) O03.6
    infection
      genital tract or pelvic O03.5
      urinary tract O03.88
    intravascular coagulation O03.6
    laceration of pelvic organ(s) O03.84
    metabolic disorder O03.83
    oliguria O03.82
    oophoritis O03.5
    parametritis O03.5
    pelvic peritonitis O03.5
    perforation of pelvic organ(s) O03.84
    renal failure or shutdown O03.82
    salpingitis or salpingo-oophoritis O03.5
    sepsis O03.87
    shock O03.81
    specified condition NEC O03.89
    tubular necrosis (renal) O03.82
    uremia O03.82
    urinary tract infection O03.88
    venous complication NEC O03.85
      embolism (air) (amniotic fluid) (blood clot) (fat) (pulmonary) (septic) (soap) O03.7
  failed — *see* Abortion, attempted
  habitual or recurrent N96
    with current abortion — *see* categories O03-O04
    without current pregnancy N96
    care in current pregnancy O26.2- ☑
  incomplete (spontaneous) O03.4
    complicated (by) (following) O03.30
      afibrinogenemia O03.1
      cardiac arrest O03.36
      chemical damage of pelvic organ(s) O03.34
      circulatory collapse O03.31
      cystitis O03.38
      defibrination syndrome O03.1
      electrolyte imbalance O03.33
      embolism (air) (amniotic fluid) (blood clot) (fat) (pulmonary) (septic) (soap) O03.2
      endometritis O03.0
      genital tract and pelvic infection O03.0
      hemolysis O03.1
      hemorrhage (delayed) (excessive) O03.1
      infection
        genital tract or pelvic O03.0
        urinary tract O03.38
      intravascular coagulation O03.1
      laceration of pelvic organ(s) O03.34

Abortion — *continued*
  incomplete — *continued*
    complicated — *continued*
      metabolic disorder O03.33
      oliguria O03.32
      oophoritis O03.0
      parametritis O03.0
      pelvic peritonitis O03.0
      perforation of pelvic organ(s) O03.34
      renal failure or shutdown O03.32
      salpingitis or salpingo-oophoritis O03.0
      sepsis O03.37
      shock O03.31
      specified condition NEC O03.39
      tubular necrosis (renal) O03.32
      uremia O03.32
      urinary infection O03.38
      venous complication NEC O03.35
        embolism (air) (amniotic fluid) (blood clot) (fat) (pulmonary) (septic) (soap) O03.2
  induced (encounter for) Z33.2
    complicated by O04.80
      afibrinogenemia O04.6
      cardiac arrest O04.86
      chemical damage of pelvic organ(s) O04.84
      circulatory collapse O04.81
      cystitis O04.88
      defibrination syndrome O04.6
      electrolyte imbalance O04.83
      embolism (air) (amniotic fluid) (blood clot) (fat) (pulmonary) (septic) (soap) O04.7
      endometritis O04.5
      genital tract and pelvic infection O04.5
      hemolysis O04.6
      hemorrhage (delayed) (excessive) O04.6
      infection
        genital tract or pelvic O04.5
        urinary tract O04.88
      intravascular coagulation O04.6
      laceration of pelvic organ(s) O04.84
      metabolic disorder O04.83
      oliguria O04.82
      oophoritis O04.5
      parametritis O04.5
      pelvic peritonitis O04.5
      perforation of pelvic organ(s) O04.84
      renal failure or shutdown O04.82
      salpingitis or salpingo-oophoritis O04.5
      sepsis O04.87
      shock O04.81
      specified condition NEC O04.89
      tubular necrosis (renal) O04.82
      uremia O04.82
      urinary tract infection O04.88
      venous complication NEC O04.85
        embolism (air) (amniotic fluid) (blood clot) (fat) (pulmonary) (septic) (soap) O04.7
  missed O02.1
  spontaneous — *see* Abortion (complete) (spontaneous)
    threatened O20.0
  threatened (spontaneous) O20.0
  tubal O00.10-
    with intrauterine pregnancy O00.11- ☑
Abortus fever A23.1
Aboulomania F60.7
Abrami's disease D59.8
Abramov-Fiedler myocarditis (acute isolated myocarditis) I40.1
Abrasion T14.8 ☑
  abdomen, abdominal (wall) S30.811 ☑
  alveolar process S00.512 ☑
  ankle S90.51- ☑
  antecubital space — *see* Abrasion, elbow
  anus S30.817 ☑
  arm (upper) S40.81- ☑
  auditory canal — *see* Abrasion, ear
  auricle — *see* Abrasion, ear
  axilla — *see* Abrasion, arm
  back, lower S30.810 ☑
  breast S20.11- ☑
  brow S00.81 ☑
  buttock S30.810 ☑
  calf — *see* Abrasion, leg
  canthus — *see* Abrasion, eyelid
  cheek S00.81 ☑
    internal S00.512 ☑
  chest wall — *see* Abrasion, thorax
  chin S00.81 ☑

Abrasion — *continued*
- clitoris S30.814 ☑
- cornea S05.0- ☑
- costal region — *see* Abrasion, thorax
- dental K03.1
- digit(s)
  - foot — *see* Abrasion, toe
  - hand — *see* Abrasion, finger
- ear S00.41- ☑
- elbow S50.31- ☑
- epididymis S30.813 ☑
- epigastric region S30.811 ☑
- epiglottis S10.11 ☑
- esophagus (thoracic) S27.818 ☑
  - cervical S10.11 ☑
- eyebrow — *see* Abrasion, eyelid
- eyelid S00.21- ☑
- face S00.81 ☑
- finger(s) S60.41- ☑
  - index S60.41- ☑
  - little S60.41- ☑
  - middle S60.41- ☑
  - ring S60.41- ☑
- flank S30.811 ☑
- foot (except toe(s) alone) S90.81- ☑
  - toe — *see* Abrasion, toe
- forearm S50.81- ☑
  - elbow only — *see* Abrasion, elbow
- forehead S00.81 ☑
- genital organs, external
  - female S30.816 ☑
  - male S30.815 ☑
- groin S30.811 ☑
- gum S00.512 ☑
- hand S60.51- ☑
- head S00.91 ☑
  - ear — *see* Abrasion, ear
  - eyelid — *see* Abrasion, eyelid
  - lip S00.511 ☑
  - nose S00.31 ☑
  - oral cavity S00.512 ☑
  - scalp S00.01 ☑
  - specified site NEC S00.81 ☑
- heel — *see* Abrasion, foot
- hip S70.21- ☑
- inguinal region S30.811 ☑
- interscapular region S20.419 ☑
- jaw S00.81 ☑
- knee S80.21- ☑
- labium (majus) (minus) S30.814 ☑
- larynx S10.11 ☑
- leg (lower) S80.81- ☑
  - knee — *see* Abrasion, knee
  - upper — *see* Abrasion, thigh
- lip S00.511 ☑
- lower back S30.810 ☑
- lumbar region S30.810 ☑
- malar region S00.81 ☑
- mammary — *see* Abrasion, breast
- mastoid region S00.81 ☑
- mouth S00.512 ☑
- nail
  - finger — *see* Abrasion, finger
  - toe — *see* Abrasion, toe
- nape S10.81 ☑
- nasal S00.31 ☑
- neck S10.91 ☑
  - specified site NEC S10.81 ☑
  - throat S10.11 ☑
- nose S00.31 ☑
- occipital region S00.01 ☑
- oral cavity S00.512 ☑
- orbital region — *see* Abrasion, eyelid
- palate S00.512 ☑
- palm — *see* Abrasion, hand
- parietal region S00.01 ☑
- pelvis S30.810 ☑
- penis S30.812 ☑
- perineum
  - female S30.814 ☑
  - male S30.810 ☑
- periocular area — *see* Abrasion, eyelid
- phalanges
  - finger — *see* Abrasion, finger
  - toe — *see* Abrasion, toe
- pharynx S10.11 ☑

Abrasion — *continued*
- pinna — *see* Abrasion, ear
- popliteal space — *see* Abrasion, knee
- prepuce S30.812 ☑
- pubic region S30.810 ☑
- pudendum
  - female S30.816 ☑
  - male S30.815 ☑
- sacral region S30.810 ☑
- scalp S00.01 ☑
- scapular region — *see* Abrasion, shoulder
- scrotum S30.813 ☑
- shin — *see* Abrasion, leg
- shoulder S40.21- ☑
- skin NEC T14.8 ☑
- sternal region S20.319 ☑
- submaxillary region S00.81 ☑
- submental region S00.81 ☑
- subungual
  - finger(s) — *see* Abrasion, finger
  - toe(s) — *see* Abrasion, toe
- supraclavicular fossa S10.81 ☑
- supraorbital S00.81 ☑
- temple S00.81 ☑
- temporal region S00.81 ☑
- testis S30.813 ☑
- thigh S70.31- ☑
- thorax, thoracic (wall) S20.91 ☑
  - back S20.41- ☑
  - front S20.31- ☑
- throat S10.11 ☑
- thumb S60.31- ☑
- toe(s) (lesser) S90.416 ☑
  - great S90.41- ☑
- tongue S00.512 ☑
- tooth, teeth (dentifrice) (habitual) (hard tissues) (occupational) (ritual) (traditional) K03.1
- trachea S10.11 ☑
- tunica vaginalis S30.813 ☑
- tympanum, tympanic membrane — *see* Abrasion, ear
- uvula S00.512 ☑
- vagina S30.814 ☑
- vocal cords S10.11 ☑
- vulva S30.814 ☑
- wrist S60.81- ☑

Abrism — *see* Poisoning, food, noxious, plant
Abruptio placentae O45.9- ☑
- with
  - afibrinogenemia O45.01- ☑
  - coagulation defect O45.00- ☑
    - specified NEC O45.09- ☑
  - disseminated intravascular coagulation O45.02- ☑
  - hypofibrinogenemia O45.01- ☑
- specified NEC O45.8- ☑
Abruption, placenta — *see* Abruptio placentae
Abscess (connective tissue) (embolic) (fistulous) (infective) (metastatic) (multiple) (pernicious) (pyogenic) (septic) L02.91
- with
  - diverticular disease (intestine) K57.80
    - with bleeding K57.81
    - large intestine K57.20
      - with
        - bleeding K57.21
        - small intestine K57.40
          - with bleeding K57.41
      - small intestine K57.00
        - with
          - bleeding K57.01
          - large intestine K57.40
            - with bleeding K57.41
  - lymphangitis — *code by* site under Abscess
- abdomen, abdominal
  - cavity K65.1
  - wall L02.211
- abdominopelvic K65.1
- accessory sinus — *see* Sinusitis
- adrenal (capsule) (gland) E27.8
- alveolar K04.7
  - with sinus K04.6
- amebic A06.4
  - brain (and liver or lung abscess) A06.6
  - genitourinary tract A06.82
  - liver (without mention of brain or lung abscess) A06.4
  - lung (and liver) (without mention of brain abscess) A06.5

Abscess — *continued*
- amebic — *continued*
  - specified site NEC A06.89
  - spleen A06.89
- anerobic A48.0
- ankle — *see* Abscess, lower limb
- anorectal K61.2
- antecubital space — *see* Abscess, upper limb
- antrum (chronic) (Highmore) — *see* Sinusitis, maxillary
- anus K61.0
- apical (tooth) K04.7
  - with sinus (alveolar) K04.6
- appendix K35.33
- areola (acute) (chronic) (nonpuerperal) N61.1
  - puerperal, postpartum or gestational — *see* Infection, nipple
- arm (any part) — *see* Abscess, upper limb
- artery (wall) I77.89
- atheromatous I77.2
- auricle, ear — *see* Abscess, ear, external
- axilla (region) L02.41- ☑
  - lymph gland or node L04.2
- back (any part, except buttock) L02.212
- Bartholin's gland N75.1
  - with
    - abortion — *see* Abortion, by type complicated by, sepsis
    - ectopic or molar pregnancy O08.0
  - following ectopic or molar pregnancy O08.0
- Bezold's — *see* Mastoiditis, acute
- bilharziasis B65.1
- bladder (wall) — *see* Cystitis, specified type NEC
- bone (subperiosteal) — *see also* Osteomyelitis, specified type NEC
  - accessory sinus (chronic) — *see* Sinusitis
  - chronic or old — *see* Osteomyelitis, chronic
  - jaw (lower) (upper) M27.2
  - mastoid — *see* Mastoiditis, acute, subperiosteal
  - petrous — *see* Petrositis
  - spinal (tuberculous) A18.01
    - nontuberculous — *see* Osteomyelitis, vertebra
- bowel K63.0
- brain (any part) (cystic) (otogenic) G06.0
  - amebic (with abscess of any other site) A06.6
  - gonococcal A54.82
  - pheomycotic (chromomycotic) B43.1
  - tuberculous A17.81
- breast (acute) (chronic) (nonpuerperal) N61.1
  - newborn P39.0
  - puerperal, postpartum, gestational — *see* Mastitis, obstetric, purulent
- broad ligament N73.2
  - acute N73.0
  - chronic N73.1
- Brodie's (localized) (chronic) M86.8X- ☑
- bronchi J98.09
- buccal cavity K12.2
- bulbourethral gland N34.0
- bursa M71.00
  - ankle M71.07- ☑
  - elbow M71.02- ☑
  - foot M71.07- ☑
  - hand M71.04- ☑
  - hip M71.05- ☑
  - knee M71.06- ☑
  - multiple sites M71.09
  - pharyngeal J39.1
  - shoulder M71.01- ☑
  - specified site NEC M71.08
  - wrist M71.03- ☑
- buttock L02.31
- canthus — *see* Blepharoconjunctivitis
- cartilage — *see* Disorder, cartilage, specified type NEC
- cecum K35.33
- cerebellum, cerebellar G06.0
  - sequelae G09
- cerebral (embolic) G06.0
  - sequelae G09
- cervical (meaning neck) L02.11
  - lymph gland or node L04.0
- cervix (stump) (uteri) — *see* Cervicitis
- cheek (external) L02.01
  - inner K12.2
- chest J86.9
  - with fistula J86.0
  - wall L02.213
- chin L02.01
- choroid — *see* Inflammation, chorioretinal

Abscess — *continued*
- circumtonsillar J36
- cold (lung) (tuberculous) — *see also* Tuberculosis, abscess, lung
  - articular — *see* Tuberculosis, joint
- colon (wall) K63.0
- colostomy K94.02
- conjunctiva — *see* Conjunctivitis, acute
- cornea H16.31- ☑
- corpus
  - cavernosum N48.21
  - luteum — *see* Oophoritis
- Cowper's gland N34.0
- cranium G06.0
- cul-de-sac (Douglas') (posterior) — *see* Peritonitis, pelvic, female
- cutaneous — *see* Abscess, by site
- dental K04.7
  - with sinus (alveolar) K04.6
- dentoalveolar K04.7
  - with sinus K04.6
- diaphragm, diaphragmatic K65.1
- Douglas' cul-de-sac or pouch — *see* Peritonitis, pelvic, female
- Dubois A50.59
- ear (middle) — *see also* Otitis, media, suppurative
  - acute — *see* Otitis, media, suppurative, acute
  - external H60.0- ☑
- entamebic — *see* Abscess, amebic
- enterostomy K94.12
- epididymis N45.4
- epidural G06.2
  - brain G06.0
  - spinal cord G06.1
- epiglottis J38.7
- epiploon, epiploic K65.1
- erysipelatous — *see* Erysipelas
- esophagus K20.8
- ethmoid (bone) (chronic) (sinus) J32.2
- external auditory canal — *see* Abscess, ear, external
- extradural G06.2
  - brain G06.0
    - sequelae G09
  - spinal cord G06.1
- extraperitoneal K68.19
- eye — *see* Endophthalmitis, purulent
- eyelid H00.03- ☑
- face (any part, except ear, eye and nose) L02.01
- fallopian tube — *see* Salpingitis
- fascia M72.8
- fauces J39.1
- fecal K63.0
- femoral (region) — *see* Abscess, lower limb
- filaria, filarial — *see* Infestation, filarial
- finger (any) — *see also* Abscess, hand
  - nail — *see* Cellulitis, finger
- foot L02.61- ☑
- forehead L02.01
- frontal sinus (chronic) J32.1
- gallbladder K81.0
- genital organ or tract
  - female (external) N76.4
  - male N49.9
    - multiple sites N49.8
    - specified NEC N49.8
- gestational mammary O91.11- ☑
- gestational subareolar O91.11- ☑
- gingival — *see* Periodontitis, localized
- gland, glandular (lymph) (acute) — *see* Lymphadenitis, acute
- gluteal (region) L02.31
- gonorrheal — *see* Gonococcus
- groin L02.214
- gum — *see* Periodontitis, localized
- hand L02.51- ☑
- head NEC L02.811
  - face (any part, except ear, eye and nose) L02.01
- heart — *see* Carditis
- heel — *see* Abscess, foot
- helminthic — *see* Infestation, helminth
- hepatic (cholangitic) (hematogenic) (lymphogenic) (pylephlebitic) K75.0
  - amebic A06.4
- hip (region) — *see* Abscess, lower limb
- horseshoe K61.31
- ileocecal K35.33
- ileostomy (bud) K94.12
- iliac (region) L02.214

Abscess — *continued*
- iliac — *continued*
  - fossa K35.33
- infraclavicular (fossa) — *see* Abscess, upper limb
- inguinal (region) L02.214
  - lymph gland or node L04.1
- intersphincteric K61.4
- intestine, intestinal NEC K63.0
  - rectal K61.1
- intra-abdominal — *see also* Abscess, peritoneum K65.1
  - following procedure T81.43 ☑
    - obstetrical O86.03
  - postprocedural T81.49 ☑
    - retroperitoneal K68.11
- intracranial G06.0
- intramammary — *see* Abscess, breast
- intramuscular, following procedure T81.42 ☑
  - obstetrical O86.02
- intraorbital — *see* Abscess, orbit
- intraperitoneal K65.1
- intrasphincteric (anus) K61.4
- intraspinal G06.1
- intratonsillar J36
- ischiorectal (fossa) (specified NEC) K61.39
- jaw (bone) (lower) (upper) M27.2
- joint — *see* Arthritis, pyogenic or pyemic
  - spine (tuberculous) A18.01
    - nontuberculous — *see* Spondylopathy, infective
- kidney N15.1
  - with calculus N20.0
    - with hydronephrosis N13.6
  - puerperal (postpartum) O86.21
- knee — *see also* Abscess, lower limb
  - joint M00.9
- labium (majus) (minus) N76.4
- lacrimal
  - caruncle — *see* Inflammation, lacrimal, passages, acute
  - gland — *see* Dacryoadenitis
  - passages (duct) (sac) — *see* Inflammation, lacrimal, passages, acute
- lacunar N34.0
- larynx J38.7
- lateral (alveolar) K04.7
  - with sinus K04.6
- leg (any part) — *see* Abscess, lower limb
- lens H27.8
- lingual K14.0
  - tonsil J36
- lip K13.0
- Littre's gland N34.0
- liver (cholangitic) (hematogenic) (lymphogenic) (pylephlebitic) (pyogenic) K75.0
  - amebic (due to Entamoeba histolytica) (dysenteric) (tropical) A06.4
    - with
      - brain abscess (and liver or lung abscess) A06.6
      - lung abscess A06.5
- loin (region) L02.211
- lower limb L02.41- ☑
- lumbar (tuberculous) A18.01
  - nontuberculous L02.212
- lung (miliary) (putrid) J85.2
  - with pneumonia J85.1
    - due to specified organism (see Pneumonia, in (due to))
  - amebic (with liver abscess) A06.5
    - with
      - brain abscess A06.6
      - pneumonia A06.5
- lymph, lymphatic, gland or node (acute) — *see also* Lymphadenitis, acute
  - mesentery I88.0
- malar M27.2
- mammary gland — *see* Abscess, breast
- marginal, anus K61.0
- mastoid — *see* Mastoiditis, acute
- maxilla, maxillary M27.2
  - molar (tooth) K04.7
    - with sinus K04.6
  - premolar K04.7
  - sinus (chronic) J32.0
- mediastinum J85.3
- meibomian gland — *see* Hordeolum
- meninges G06.2
- mesentery, mesenteric K65.1
- mesosalpinx — *see* Salpingitis
- mons pubis L02.215

Abscess — *continued*
- mouth (floor) K12.2
- muscle — *see* Myositis, infective
- myocardium I40.0
- nabothian (follicle) — *see* Cervicitis
- nasal J32.9
- nasopharyngeal J39.1
- navel L02.216
  - newborn P38.9
    - with mild hemorrhage P38.1
    - without hemorrhage P38.9
- neck (region) L02.11
  - lymph gland or node L04.0
- nephritic — *see* Abscess, kidney
- nipple N61.1
  - associated with
    - lactation — *see* Pregnancy, complicated by
    - pregnancy — *see* Pregnancy, complicated by
- nose (external) (fossa) (septum) J34.0
  - sinus (chronic) — *see* Sinusitis
- omentum K65.1
- operative wound T81.49 ☑
- orbit, orbital — *see* Cellulitis, orbit
- otogenic G06.0
- ovary, ovarian (corpus luteum) — *see* Oophoritis
- oviduct — *see* Oophoritis
- palate (soft) K12.2
  - hard M27.2
- palmar (space) — *see* Abscess, hand
- pancreas (duct) — *see* Pancreatitis, acute
- parafrenal N48.21
- parametric, parametrium N73.2
  - acute N73.0
  - chronic N73.1
- paranephric N15.1
- parapancreatic — *see* Pancreatitis, acute
- parapharyngeal J39.0
- pararectal K61.1
- parasinus — *see* Sinusitis
- parauterine — *see also* Disease, pelvis, inflammatory N73.2
- paravaginal — *see* Vaginitis
- parietal region (scalp) L02.811
- parodontal — *see* Periodontitis, aggressive, localized
- parotid (duct) (gland) K11.3
  - region K12.2
- pectoral (region) L02.213
- pelvis, pelvic
  - female — *see* Disease, pelvis, inflammatory
  - male, peritoneal K65.1
- penis N48.21
  - gonococcal (accessory gland) (periurethral) A54.1
- perianal K61.0
- periapical K04.7
  - with sinus (alveolar) K04.6
- periappendicular K35.33
- pericardial I30.1
- pericecal K35.33
- pericemental — *see* Periodontitis, aggressive, localized
- pericholecystic — *see* Cholecystitis, acute
- pericoronal — *see* Periodontitis, aggressive, localized
- peridental — *see* Periodontitis, aggressive, localized
- perimetric — *see also* Disease, pelvis, inflammatory N73.2
- perinephric, perinephritic — *see* Abscess, kidney
- perineum, perineal (superficial) L02.215
  - urethra N34.0
- periodontal (parietal) — *see* Periodontitis, aggressive, localized
  - apical K04.7
- periosteum, periosteal — *see also* Osteomyelitis, specified type NEC
  - with osteomyelitis — *see also* Osteomyelitis, specified type NEC
    - acute — *see* Osteomyelitis, acute
    - chronic — *see* Osteomyelitis, chronic
- peripharyngeal J39.0
- peripleuritic J86.9
  - with fistula J86.0
- periprostatic N41.2
- perirectal K61.1
- perirenal (tissue) — *see* Abscess, kidney
- perisinuous (nose) — *see* Sinusitis
- peritoneum, peritoneal (perforated) (ruptured) K65.1
  - with appendicitis — *see also* Appendicitis K35.33
  - pelvic
    - female — *see* Peritonitis, pelvic, female
    - male K65.1

Abscess — *continued*
  peritoneum, peritoneal — *continued*
    postoperative T81.49 ☑
    puerperal, postpartum, childbirth O85
    tuberculous A18.31
  peritonsillar J36
  perityphlic K35.33
  periureteral N28.89
  periurethral N34.0
    gonococcal (accessory gland) (periurethral) A54.1
  periuterine — *see also* Disease, pelvis, inflammatory N73.2
  perivesical — *see* Cystitis, specified type NEC
  petrous bone — *see* Petrositis
  phagedenic NOS L02.91
    chancroid A57
  pharynx, pharyngeal (lateral) J39.1
  pilonidal L05.01
  pituitary (gland) E23.6
  pleura J86.9
    with fistula J86.0
  popliteal — *see* Abscess, lower limb
  postcecal K35.33
  postlaryngeal J38.7
  postnasal J34.0
  postoperative (any site) — *see also* Infection, postoperative wound T81.49 ☑
    retroperitoneal K68.11
  postpharyngeal J39.0
  posttonsillar J36
  post-typhoid A01.09
  pouch of Douglas — *see* Peritonitis, pelvic, female
  premammary — *see* Abscess, breast
  prepatellar — *see* Abscess, lower limb
  prostate N41.2
    gonococcal (acute) (chronic) A54.22
  psoas muscle K68.12
  puerperal — *code by* site under Puerperal, abscess
  pulmonary — *see* Abscess, lung
  pulp, pulpal (dental) K04.01
    irreversible K04.02
    reversible K04.01
  rectovaginal septum K63.0
  rectovesical — *see* Cystitis, specified type NEC
  rectum K61.1
  renal — *see* Abscess, kidney
  retina — *see* Inflammation, chorioretinal
  retrobulbar — *see* Abscess, orbit
  retrocecal K65.1
  retrolaryngeal J38.7
  retromammary — *see* Abscess, breast
  retroperitoneal NEC K68.19
    postprocedural K68.11
  retropharyngeal J39.0
  retrouterine — *see* Peritonitis, pelvic, female
  retrovesical — *see* Cystitis, specified type NEC
  root, tooth K04.7
    with sinus (alveolar) K04.6
  round ligament — *see also* Disease, pelvis, inflammatory N73.2
  rupture (spontaneous) NOS L02.91
  sacrum (tuberculous) A18.01
    nontuberculous M46.28
  salivary (duct) (gland) K11.3
  scalp (any part) L02.811
  scapular — *see* Osteomyelitis, specified type NEC
  sclera — *see* Scleritis
  scrofulous (tuberculous) A18.2
  scrotum N49.2
  seminal vesicle N49.0
  septal, dental K04.7
    with sinus (alveolar) K04.6
  serous — *see* Periostitis
  shoulder (region) — *see* Abscess, upper limb
  sigmoid K63.0
  sinus (accessory) (chronic) (nasal) — *see also* Sinusitis
    intracranial venous (any) G06.0
  Skene's duct or gland N34.0
  skin — *see* Abscess, by site
  specified site NEC L02.818
  spermatic cord N49.1
  sphenoidal (sinus) (chronic) J32.3
  spinal cord (any part) (staphylococcal) G06.1
    tuberculous A17.81
  spine (column) (tuberculous) A18.01
    epidural G06.1
    nontuberculous — *see* Osteomyelitis, vertebra
  spleen D73.3

Abscess — *continued*
  spleen — *continued*
    amebic A06.89
  stitch T81.41
    following an obstetrical procedure O86.01
  subarachnoid G06.2
    brain G06.0
    spinal cord G06.1
  subareolar — *see* Abscess, breast
  subcecal K35.33
  subcutaneous — *see also* Abscess, by site
    following procedure T81.41 ☑
      obstetrical O86.01
    pheomycotic (chromomycotic) B43.2
  subdiaphragmatic K65.1
  subdural G06.2
    brain G06.0
      sequelae G09
    spinal cord G06.1
  sub-fascial, following an obstetrical procedure O86.02
  subgaleal L02.811
  subhepatic K65.1
  sublingual K12.2
    gland K11.3
  submammary — *see* Abscess, breast
  submandibular (region) (space) (triangle) K12.2
    gland K11.3
  submaxillary (region) L02.01
    gland K11.3
  submental L02.01
    gland K11.3
  subperiosteal — *see* Osteomyelitis, specified type NEC
  subphrenic K65.1
    following an obstetrical procedure O86.03
    postoperative T81.43 ☑
  suburethral N34.0
  sudoriparous L75.8
  supraclavicular (fossa) — *see* Abscess, upper limb
  supralevator K61.5
  suprapelvic, acute N73.0
  suprarenal (capsule) (gland) E27.8
  sweat gland L74.8
  tear duct — *see* Inflammation, lacrimal, passages, acute
  temple L02.01
  temporal region L02.01
  temporosphenoidal G06.0
  tendon (sheath) M65.00
    ankle M65.07- ☑
    foot M65.07- ☑
    forearm M65.03- ☑
    hand M65.04- ☑
    lower leg M65.06- ☑
    pelvic region M65.05- ☑
    shoulder region M65.01- ☑
    specified site NEC M65.08
    thigh M65.05- ☑
    upper arm M65.02- ☑
  testis N45.4
  thigh — *see* Abscess, lower limb
  thorax J86.9
    with fistula J86.0
  throat J39.1
  thumb — *see also* Abscess, hand
    nail — *see* Cellulitis, finger
  thymus (gland) E32.1
  thyroid (gland) E06.0
  toe (any) — *see also* Abscess, foot
    nail — *see* Cellulitis, toe
  tongue (staphylococcal) K14.0
  tonsil(s) (lingual) J36
  tonsillopharyngeal J36
  tooth, teeth (root) K04.7
    with sinus (alveolar) K04.6
    supporting structures NEC — *see* Periodontitis, aggressive, localized
  trachea J39.8
  trunk L02.219
    abdominal wall L02.211
    back L02.212
    chest wall L02.213
    groin L02.214
    perineum L02.215
    umbilicus L02.216
  tubal — *see* Salpingitis
  tuberculous — *see* Tuberculosis, abscess
  tubo-ovarian — *see* Salpingo-oophoritis
  tunica vaginalis N49.1
  umbilicus L02.216

Abscess — *continued*
  upper
    limb L02.41- ☑
    respiratory J39.8
  urethral (gland) N34.0
  urinary N34.0
  uterus, uterine (wall) — *see also* Endometritis
    ligament — *see also* Disease, pelvis, inflammatory N73.2
    neck — *see* Cervicitis
  uvula K12.2
  vagina (wall) — *see* Vaginitis
  vaginorectal — *see* Vaginitis
  vas deferens N49.1
  vermiform appendix K35.33
  vertebra (column) (tuberculous) A18.01
    nontuberculous — *see* Osteomyelitis, vertebra
  vesical — *see* Cystitis, specified type NEC
  vesico-uterine pouch — *see* Peritonitis, pelvic, female
  vitreous (humor) — *see* Endophthalmitis, purulent
  vocal cord J38.3
  von Bezold's — *see* Mastoiditis, acute
  vulva N76.4
  vulvovaginal gland N75.1
  web space — *see* Abscess, hand
  wound T81.49 ☑
  wrist — *see* Abscess, upper limb
Absence (of) (organ or part) (complete or partial)
  adrenal (gland) (congenital) Q89.1
    acquired E89.6
  albumin in blood E88.09
  alimentary tract (congenital) Q45.8
    upper Q40.8
  alveolar process (acquired) — *see* Anomaly, alveolar
  ankle (acquired) Z89.44- ☑
  anus (congenital) Q42.3
    with fistula Q42.2
  aorta (congenital) Q25.41
  appendix, congenital Q42.8
  arm (acquired) Z89.20- ☑
    above elbow Z89.22- ☑
      congenital (with hand present) — *see* Agenesis, arm, with hand present
      and hand — *see* Agenesis, forearm, and hand
    below elbow Z89.21- ☑
      congenital (with hand present) — *see* Agenesis, arm, with hand present
      and hand — *see* Agenesis, forearm, and hand
    congenital — *see* Defect, reduction, upper limb
    shoulder (following explanation of shoulder joint prosthesis) (joint) (with or without presence of antibiotic-impregnated cement spacer) Z89.23- ☑
      congenital (with hand present) — *see* Agenesis, arm, with hand present
  artery (congenital) (peripheral) Q27.8
    brain Q28.3
    coronary Q24.5
    pulmonary Q25.79
    specified NEC Q27.8
    umbilical Q27.0
  atrial septum (congenital) Q21.1
  auditory canal (congenital) (external) Q16.1
  auricle (ear), congenital Q16.0
  bile, biliary duct, congenital Q44.5
  bladder (acquired) Z90.6
    congenital Q64.5
  bowel sounds R19.11
  brain Q00.0
    part of Q04.3
  breast(s) (and nipple(s)) (acquired) Z90.1- ☑
    congenital Q83.8
  broad ligament Q50.6
  bronchus (congenital) Q32.4
  canaliculus lacrimalis, congenital Q10.4
  cerebellum (vermis) Q04.3
  cervix (acquired) (with uterus) Z90.710
    with remaining uterus Z90.712
    congenital Q51.5
  chin, congenital Q18.8
  cilia (congenital) Q10.3
    acquired — *see* Madarosis
  clitoris (congenital) Q52.6
  coccyx, congenital Q76.49
  cold sense R20.8
  congenital
    lumen — *see* Atresia
    organ or site NEC — *see* Agenesis

☑ **Additional Character Required** — Refer to the Tabular List for Character Selection   ▽ **Subterms under main terms may continue to next column or page**

Absence — *continued*
  congenital — *continued*
    septum — *see* Imperfect, closure
  corpus callosum Q04.0
  cricoid cartilage, congenital Q31.8
  diaphragm (with hernia), congenital Q79.1
  digestive organ(s) or tract, congenital Q45.8
    acquired NEC Z90.49
    upper Q40.8
  ductus arteriosus Q28.8
  duodenum (acquired) Z90.49
    congenital Q41.0
  ear, congenital Q16.9
    acquired H93.8- ☑
    auricle Q16.0
    external Q16.0
    inner Q16.5
    lobe, lobule Q17.8
    middle, except ossicles Q16.4
      ossicles Q16.3
    ossicles Q16.3
  ejaculatory duct (congenital) Q55.4
  endocrine gland (congenital) NEC Q89.2
    acquired E89.89
  epididymis (congenital) Q55.4
    acquired Z90.79
  epiglottis, congenital Q31.8
  esophagus (congenital) Q39.8
    acquired (partial) Z90.49
  eustachian tube (congenital) Q16.2
  extremity (acquired) Z89.9
    congenital Q73.0
    knee (following explantation of knee joint prosthe-
      sis) (joint) (with or without presence of antibi-
      otic-impregnated cement spacer) Z89.52- ☑
    lower (above knee) Z89.619
      below knee Z89.51- ☑
    upper — *see* Absence, arm
  eye (acquired) Z90.01
    congenital Q11.1
    muscle (congenital) Q10.3
  eyeball (acquired) Z90.01
  eyelid (fold) (congenital) Q10.3
    acquired Z90.01
  face, specified part NEC Q18.8
  fallopian tube(s) (acquired) Z90.79
    congenital Q50.6
  family member (causing problem in home) NEC — *see
    also* Disruption, family Z63.32
  femur, congenital — *see* Defect, reduction, lower limb,
    longitudinal, femur
  fibrinogen (congenital) D68.2
    acquired D65
  finger(s) (acquired) Z89.02- ☑
    congenital — *see* Agenesis, hand
  foot (acquired) Z89.43- ☑
    congenital — *see* Agenesis, foot
  forearm (acquired) — *see* Absence, arm, below elbow
  gallbladder (acquired) Z90.49
    congenital Q44.0
  gamma globulin in blood D80.1
    hereditary D80.0
  genital organs
    acquired (female) (male) Z90.79
    female, congenital Q52.8
      external Q52.71
      internal NEC Q52.8
    male, congenital Q55.8
  genitourinary organs, congenital NEC
    female Q52.8
    male Q55.8
  globe (acquired) Z90.01
    congenital Q11.1
  glottis, congenital Q31.8
  hand and wrist (acquired) Z89.11- ☑
    congenital — *see* Agenesis, hand
  head, part (acquired) NEC Z90.09
  heat sense R20.8
  hip (following explantation of hip joint prosthesis)
    (joint) (with or without presence of antibiotic-
    impregnated cement spacer) Z89.62- ☑
  hymen (congenital) Q52.4
  ileum (acquired) Z90.49
    congenital Q41.2
  immunoglobulin, isolated NEC D80.3
    IgA D80.2
    IgG D80.3
    IgM D80.4

Absence — *continued*
  incus (acquired) — *see* Loss, ossicles, ear
    congenital Q16.3
  inner ear, congenital Q16.5
  intestine (acquired) (small) Z90.49
    congenital Q41.9
      specified NEC Q41.8
    large Z90.49
      congenital Q42.9
        specified NEC Q42.8
  iris, congenital Q13.1
  jejunum (acquired) Z90.49
    congenital Q41.1
  joint
    acquired
      hip (following explantation of hip joint prosthe-
        sis) (with or without presence of antibiotic-
        impregnated cement spacer) Z89.62- ☑
      knee (following explantation of knee joint pros-
        thesis) (with or without presence of antibi-
        otic-impregnated cement spacer)
        Z89.52- ☑
      shoulder (following explantation of shoulder
        joint prosthesis) (with or without presence
        of antibiotic-impregnated cement spacer)
        Z89.23- ☑
    congenital NEC Q74.8
  kidney(s) (acquired) Z90.5
    congenital Q60.2
      bilateral Q60.1
      unilateral Q60.0
  knee (following explantation of knee joint prosthesis)
    (joint) (with or without presence of antibiotic-
    impregnated cement spacer) Z89.52- ☑
  labyrinth, membranous Q16.5
  larynx (congenital) Q31.8
    acquired Z90.02
  leg (acquired) (above knee) Z89.61- ☑
    below knee (acquired) Z89.51- ☑
    congenital — *see* Defect, reduction, lower limb
  lens (acquired) — *see also* Aphakia
    congenital Q12.3
    post cataract extraction Z98.4- ☑
  limb (acquired) — *see* Absence, extremity
  lip Q38.6
  liver (congenital) Q44.7
  lung (fissure) (lobe) (bilateral) (unilateral) (congenital)
    Q33.3
    acquired (any part) Z90.2
  menstruation — *see* Amenorrhea
  muscle (congenital) (pectoral) Q79.8
    ocular Q10.3
  neck, part Q18.8
  neutrophil — *see* Agranulocytosis
  nipple(s) (with breast(s)) (acquired) Z90.1- ☑
    congenital Q83.2
  nose (congenital) Q30.1
    acquired Z90.09
  organ
    of Corti, congenital Q16.5
    or site, congenital NEC Q89.8
      acquired NEC Z90.89
  osseous meatus (ear) Q16.4
  ovary (acquired)
    bilateral Z90.722
    congenital
      bilateral Q50.02
      unilateral Q50.01
    unilateral Z90.721
  oviduct (acquired)
    bilateral Z90.722
    congenital Q50.6
    unilateral Z90.721
  pancreas (congenital) Q45.0
    acquired Z90.410
      complete Z90.410
      partial Z90.411
      total Z90.410
  parathyroid gland (acquired) E89.2
    congenital Q89.2
  patella, congenital Q74.1
  penis (congenital) Q55.5
    acquired Z90.79
  pericardium (congenital) Q24.8
  pituitary gland (congenital) Q89.2
    acquired E89.3
  prostate (acquired) Z90.79
    congenital Q55.4

Absence — *continued*
  pulmonary valve Q22.0
  punctum lacrimale (congenital) Q10.4
  radius, congenital — *see* Defect, reduction, upper limb,
    longitudinal, radius
  rectum (congenital) Q42.1
    with fistula Q42.0
    acquired Z90.49
  respiratory organ NOS Q34.9
  rib (acquired) Z90.89
    congenital Q76.6
  sacrum, congenital Q76.49
  salivary gland(s), congenital Q38.4
  scrotum, congenital Q55.29
  seminal vesicles (congenital) Q55.4
    acquired Z90.79
  septum
    atrial (congenital) Q21.1
    between aorta and pulmonary artery Q21.4
    ventricular (congenital) Q20.4
  sex chromosome
    female phenotype Q97.8
    male phenotype Q98.8
  skull bone (congenital) Q75.8
    with
      anencephaly Q00.0
      encephalocele — *see* Encephalocele
      hydrocephalus Q03.9
        with spina bifida — *see* Spina bifida, by site,
          with hydrocephalus
      microcephaly Q02
  spermatic cord, congenital Q55.4
  spine, congenital Q76.49
  spleen (congenital) Q89.01
    acquired Z90.81
  sternum, congenital Q76.7
  stomach (acquired) (partial) Z90.3
    congenital Q40.2
  superior vena cava, congenital Q26.8
  teeth, tooth (congenital) K00.0
    acquired (complete) K08.109
      class I K08.101
      class II K08.102
      class III K08.103
      class IV K08.104
      due to
        caries K08.139
          class I K08.131
          class II K08.132
          class III K08.133
          class IV K08.134
        periodontal disease K08.129
          class I K08.121
          class II K08.122
          class III K08.123
          class IV K08.124
        specified NEC K08.199
          class I K08.191
          class II K08.192
          class III K08.193
          class IV K08.194
        trauma K08.119
          class I K08.111
          class II K08.112
          class III K08.113
          class IV K08.114
      partial K08.409
        class I K08.401
        class II K08.402
        class III K08.403
        class IV K08.404
        due to
          caries K08.439
            class I K08.431
            class II K08.432
            class III K08.433
            class IV K08.434
          periodontal disease K08.429
            class I K08.421
            class II K08.422
            class III K08.423
            class IV K08.424
          specified NEC K08.499
            class I K08.491
            class II K08.492
            class III K08.493
            class IV K08.494
          trauma K08.419
            class I K08.411

Absence — *continued*
  teeth, tooth — *continued*
    acquired — *continued*
      partial — *continued*
        due to — *continued*
          trauma — *continued*
            class II K08.412
            class III K08.413
            class IV K08.414
  tendon (congenital) Q79.8
  testis (congenital) Q55.0
    acquired Z90.79
  thumb (acquired) Z89.01- ☑
    congenital — *see* Agenesis, hand
  thymus gland Q89.2
  thyroid (gland) (acquired) E89.0
    cartilage, congenital Q31.8
    congenital E03.1
  toe(s) (acquired) Z89.42- ☑
    with foot — *see* Absence, foot and ankle
    congenital — *see* Agenesis, foot
    great Z89.41- ☑
  tongue, congenital Q38.3
  trachea (cartilage), congenital Q32.1
  transverse aortic arch, congenital Q25.49
  tricuspid valve Q22.4
  umbilical artery, congenital Q27.0
  upper arm and forearm with hand present, congenital
    — *see* Agenesis, arm, with hand present
  ureter (congenital) Q62.4
    acquired Z90.6
  urethra, congenital Q64.5
  uterus (acquired) Z90.710
    with cervix Z90.710
    with remaining cervical stump Z90.711
    congenital Q51.0
  uvula, congenital Q38.5
  vagina, congenital Q52.0
  vas deferens (congenital) Q55.4
    acquired Z90.79
  vein (peripheral) congenital NEC Q27.8
    cerebral Q28.3
    digestive system Q27.8
    great Q26.8
    lower limb Q27.8
    portal Q26.5
    precerebral Q28.1
    specified site NEC Q27.8
    upper limb Q27.8
  vena cava (inferior) (superior), congenital Q26.8
  ventricular septum Q20.4
  vertebra, congenital Q76.49
  vulva, congenital Q52.71
  wrist (acquired) Z89.12- ☑
Absorbent system disease I87.8
Absorption
  carbohydrate, disturbance K90.49
  chemical — *see* Table of Drugs and Chemicals
    through placenta (newborn) P04.9
      environmental substance P04.6
      nutritional substance P04.5
      obstetric anesthetic or analgesic drug P04.0
  drug NEC — *see* Table of Drugs and Chemicals
    addictive
      through placenta (newborn) — *see also* New-
        born, affected by, maternal, use of P04.40
        cocaine P04.41
        hallucinogens P04.42
        specified drug NEC P04.49
    medicinal
      through placenta (newborn) P04.19
    through placenta (newborn) P04.19
      obstetric anesthetic or analgesic drug P04.0
  fat, disturbance K90.49
    pancreatic K90.3
  noxious substance — *see* Table of Drugs and Chemicals
  protein, disturbance K90.49
  starch, disturbance K90.49
  toxic substance — *see* Table of Drugs and Chemicals
  uremic — *see* Uremia
Abstinence symptoms, syndrome
  alcohol F10.239
    with delirium F10.231
  cocaine F14.23
  neonatal P96.1
  nicotine — *see* Dependence, drug, nicotine, with,
    withdrawal
  opioid F11.93

Abstinence symptoms, syndrome — *continued*
  opioid — *continued*
    with dependence F11.23
  psychoactive NEC F19.939
    with
      delirium F19.931
      dependence F19.239
        with
          delirium F19.231
            perceptual disturbance F19.232
          uncomplicated F19.230
      perceptual disturbance F19.932
    uncomplicated F19.930
  sedative F13.939
    with
      delirium F13.931
      dependence F13.239
        with
          delirium F13.231
            perceptual disturbance F13.232
          uncomplicated F13.230
      perceptual disturbance F13.932
    uncomplicated F13.930
  stimulant NEC F15.93
    with dependence F15.23
Abulia R68.89
Abulomania F60.7
Abuse
  adult — *see* Maltreatment, adult
    as reason for
      couple seeking advice (including offender) Z63.0
  alcohol (non-dependent) F10.10
    with
      anxiety disorder F10.180
      intoxication F10.129
        with delirium F10.121
        uncomplicated F10.120
      mood disorder F10.14
      other specified disorder F10.188
      psychosis F10.159
        delusions F10.150
        hallucinations F10.151
      sexual dysfunction F10.181
      sleep disorder F10.182
      unspecified disorder F10.19
    counseling and surveillance Z71.41
    in remission (early) (sustained) F10.11
  amphetamine (or related substance) — *see also* Abuse,
    drug, stimulant NEC
    stimulant NEC F15.10
      with
        anxiety disorder F15.180
        intoxication F15.129
          with
            delirium F15.121
            perceptual disturbance F15.122
  analgesics (non-prescribed) (over the counter) F55.8
  antacids F55.0
  antidepressants — *see* Abuse, drug, psychoactive NEC
  anxiolytic — *see* Abuse, drug, sedative
  barbiturates — *see* Abuse, drug, sedative
  caffeine — *see* Abuse, drug, stimulant NEC
  cannabis, cannabinoids — *see* Abuse, drug, cannabis
  child — *see* Maltreatment, child
  cocaine — *see* Abuse, drug, cocaine
  drug NEC (non-dependent) F19.10
    with sleep disorder F19.182
    amphetamine type — *see* Abuse, drug, stimulant
      NEC
    analgesics (non-prescribed) (over the counter) F55.8
    antacids F55.0
    antidepressants — *see* Abuse, drug, psychoactive
      NEC
    anxiolytics — *see* Abuse, drug, sedative
    barbiturates — *see* Abuse, drug, sedative
    caffeine — *see* Abuse, drug, stimulant NEC
    cannabis F12.10
      with
        anxiety disorder F12.180
        intoxication F12.129
          with
            delirium F12.121
            perceptual disturbance F12.122
          uncomplicated F12.120
      other specified disorder F12.188
      psychosis F12.159
        delusions F12.150
        hallucinations F12.151

Abuse — *continued*
  drug — *continued*
    cannabis — *continued*
      with — *continued*
        unspecified disorder F12.19
      in remission (early) (sustained) F12.11
    cocaine F14.10
      with
        anxiety disorder F14.180
        intoxication F14.129
          with
            delirium F14.121
            perceptual disturbance F14.122
          uncomplicated F14.120
        mood disorder F14.14
        other specified disorder F14.188
        psychosis F14.159
          delusions F14.150
          hallucinations F14.151
        sexual dysfunction F14.181
        sleep disorder F14.182
        unspecified disorder F14.19
      in remission (early) (sustained) F14.11
    counseling and surveillance Z71.51
    hallucinogen F16.10
      with
        anxiety disorder F16.180
        flashbacks F16.183
        intoxication F16.129
          with
            delirium F16.121
            perceptual disturbance F16.122
          uncomplicated F16.120
        mood disorder F16.14
        other specified disorder F16.188
        perception disorder, persisting F16.183
        psychosis F16.159
          delusions F16.150
          hallucinations F16.151
        unspecified disorder F16.19
      in remission (early) (sustained) F16.11
    hashish — *see* Abuse, drug, cannabis
    herbal or folk remedies F55.1
    hormones F55.3
    hypnotics — *see* Abuse, drug, sedative
    in remission (early) (sustained) F19.11
    inhalant F18.10
      with
        anxiety disorder F18.180
        dementia, persisting F18.17
        intoxication F18.129
          with delirium F18.121
          uncomplicated F18.120
        mood disorder F18.14
        other specified disorder F18.188
        psychosis F18.159
          delusions F18.150
          hallucinations F18.151
        unspecified disorder F18.19
      in remission (early) (sustained) F18.11
    laxatives F55.2
    LSD — *see* Abuse, drug, hallucinogen
    marihuana — *see* Abuse, drug, cannabis
    morphine type (opioids) — *see* Abuse, drug, opioid
    opioid F11.10
      with
        intoxication F11.129
          with
            delirium F11.121
            perceptual disturbance F11.122
          uncomplicated F11.120
        mood disorder F11.14
        other specified disorder F11.188
        psychosis F11.159
          delusions F11.150
          hallucinations F11.151
        sexual dysfunction F11.181
        sleep disorder F11.182
        unspecified disorder F11.19
      in remission (early) (sustained) F11.11
    PCP (phencyclidine) (or related substance) — *see*
      Abuse, drug, hallucinogen
    psychoactive NEC F19.10
      with
        amnestic disorder F19.16
        anxiety disorder F19.180
        dementia F19.17
        intoxication F19.129

Abuse — *continued*
  drug — *continued*
    psychoactive — *continued*
      with — *continued*
        intoxication — *continued*
          with
            delirium F19.121
            perceptual disturbance F19.122
          uncomplicated F19.120
        mood disorder F19.14
        other specified disorder F19.188
        psychosis F19.159
          delusions F19.150
          hallucinations F19.151
        sexual dysfunction F19.181
        sleep disorder F19.182
        unspecified disorder F19.19
    sedative, hypnotic or anxiolytic F13.10
      with
        anxiety disorder F13.180
        intoxication F13.129
          with delirium F13.121
          uncomplicated F13.120
        mood disorder F13.14
        other specified disorder F13.188
        psychosis F13.159
          delusions F13.150
          hallucinations F13.151
        sexual dysfunction F13.181
        sleep disorder F13.182
        unspecified disorder F13.19
      in remission (early) (sustained) F13.11
    solvent — *see* Abuse, drug, inhalant
    steroids F55.3
    stimulant NEC F15.10
      with
        anxiety disorder F15.180
        intoxication F15.129
          with
            delirium F15.121
            perceptual disturbance F15.122
          uncomplicated F15.120
        mood disorder F15.14
        other specified disorder F15.188
        psychosis F15.159
          delusions F15.150
          hallucinations F15.151
        sexual dysfunction F15.181
        sleep disorder F15.182
        unspecified disorder F15.19
      in remission (early) (sustained) F15.11
    tranquilizers — *see* Abuse, drug, sedative
    vitamins F55.4
  hallucinogens — *see* Abuse, drug, hallucinogen
  hashish — *see* Abuse, drug, cannabis
  herbal or folk remedies F55.1
  hormones F55.3
  hypnotic — *see* Abuse, drug, sedative
  inhalant — *see* Abuse, drug, inhalant
  laxatives F55.2
  LSD — *see* Abuse, drug, hallucinogen
  marihuana — *see* Abuse, drug, cannabis
  morphine type (opioids) — *see* Abuse, drug, opioid
  non-psychoactive substance NEC F55.8
    antacids F55.0
    folk remedies F55.1
    herbal remedies F55.1
    hormones F55.3
    laxatives F55.2
    steroids F55.3
    vitamins F55.4
  opioids — *see* Abuse, drug, opioid
  PCP (phencyclidine) (or related substance) — *see* Abuse, drug, hallucinogen
  physical (adult) (child) — *see* Maltreatment
  psychoactive substance — *see* Abuse, drug, psychoactive NEC
  psychological (adult) (child) — *see* Maltreatment
  sedative — *see* Abuse, drug, sedative
  sexual — *see* Maltreatment
  solvent — *see* Abuse, drug, inhalant
  steroids F55.3
  vitamins F55.4
Acalculia R48.8
  developmental F81.2
Acanthamebiasis (with) B60.10
  conjunctiva B60.12
  keratoconjunctivitis B60.13

Acanthamebiasis — *continued*
  meningoencephalitis B60.11
  other specified B60.19
Acanthocephaliasis B83.8
Acanthocheilonemiasis B74.4
Acanthocytosis E78.6
Acantholysis L11.9
Acanthosis (acquired) (nigricans) L83
  benign Q82.8
  congenital Q82.8
  seborrheic L82.1
    inflamed L82.0
  tongue K14.3
Acapnia E87.3
Acarbia E87.2
Acardia, acardius Q89.8
Acardiacus amorphus Q89.8
Acardiotrophia I51.4
Acariasis B88.0
  scabies B86
Acarodermatitis (urticarioides) B88.0
Acarophobia F40.218
Acatalasemia, acatalasia E80.3
Acathisia (drug induced) G25.71
Accelerated atrioventricular conduction I45.6
Accentuation of personality traits (type A) Z73.1
Accessory (congenital)
  adrenal gland Q89.1
  anus Q43.4
  appendix Q43.4
  atrioventricular conduction I45.6
  auditory ossicles Q16.3
  auricle (ear) Q17.0
  biliary duct or passage Q44.5
  bladder Q64.79
  blood vessels NEC Q27.9
    coronary Q24.5
  bone NEC Q79.8
  breast tissue, axilla Q83.1
  carpal bones Q74.0
  cecum Q43.4
  chromosome(s) NEC (nonsex) Q92.9
    with complex rearrangements NEC Q92.5
      seen only at prometaphase Q92.8
    13 — *see* Trisomy, 13
    18 — *see* Trisomy, 18
    21 — *see* Trisomy, 21
    partial Q92.9
    sex
      female phenotype Q97.8
  coronary artery Q24.5
  cusp(s), heart valve NEC Q24.8
    pulmonary Q22.3
  cystic duct Q44.5
  digit(s) Q69.9
  ear (auricle) (lobe) Q17.0
  endocrine gland NEC Q89.2
  eye muscle Q10.3
  eyelid Q10.3
  face bone(s) Q75.8
  fallopian tube (fimbria) (ostium) Q50.6
  finger(s) Q69.0
  foreskin N47.8
  frontonasal process Q75.8
  gallbladder Q44.1
  genital organ(s)
    female Q52.8
      external Q52.79
      internal NEC Q52.8
    male Q55.8
  genitourinary organs NEC Q89.8
    female Q52.8
    male Q55.8
  hallux Q69.2
  heart Q24.8
    valve NEC Q24.8
      pulmonary Q22.3
  hepatic ducts Q44.5
  hymen Q52.4
  intestine (large) (small) Q43.4
  kidney Q63.0
  lacrimal canal Q10.6
  leaflet, heart valve NEC Q24.8
  ligament, broad Q50.6
  liver Q44.7
    duct Q44.5
  lobule (ear) Q17.0
  lung (lobe) Q33.1

Accessory — *continued*
  muscle Q79.8
  navicular of carpus Q74.0
  nervous system, part NEC Q07.8
  nipple Q83.3
  nose Q30.8
  organ or site not listed — *see* Anomaly, by site
  ovary Q50.31
  oviduct Q50.6
  pancreas Q45.3
  parathyroid gland Q89.2
  parotid gland (and duct) Q38.4
  pituitary gland Q89.2
  preauricular appendage Q17.0
  prepuce N47.8
  renal arteries (multiple) Q27.2
  rib Q76.6
    cervical Q76.5
  roots (teeth) K00.2
  salivary gland Q38.4
  sesamoid bones Q74.8
    foot Q74.2
    hand Q74.0
  skin tags Q82.8
  spleen Q89.09
  sternum Q76.7
  submaxillary gland Q38.4
  tarsal bones Q74.2
  teeth, tooth K00.1
  tendon Q79.8
  thumb Q69.1
  thymus gland Q89.2
  thyroid gland Q89.2
  toes Q69.2
  tongue Q38.3
  tooth, teeth K00.1
  tragus Q17.0
  ureter Q62.5
  urethra Q64.79
  urinary organ or tract NEC Q64.8
  uterus Q51.28
  vagina Q52.10
  valve, heart NEC Q24.8
    pulmonary Q22.3
  vertebra Q76.49
  vocal cords Q31.8
  vulva Q52.79
Accident
  birth — *see* Birth, injury
  cardiac — *see* Infarct, myocardium
  cerebral I63.9
  cerebrovascular (embolic) (ischemic) (thrombotic) I63.9
    aborted I63.9
    hemorrhage — *see* Hemorrhage, intracranial, intracerebral
    old (without sequelae) Z86.73
      with sequelae (of) — *see* Sequelae, infarction, cerebral
    coronary — *see* Infarct, myocardium
  craniovascular I63.9
  vascular, brain I63.9
Accidental — *see* condition
Accommodation (disorder) — *see also* condition
  hysterical paralysis of F44.89
  insufficiency of H52.4
  paresis — *see* Paresis, of accommodation
  spasm — *see* Spasm, of accommodation
Accouchement — *see* Delivery
Accreta placenta O43.21- ☑
Accretio cordis (nonrheumatic) I31.0
Accretions, tooth, teeth K03.6
Acculturation difficulty Z60.3
Accumulation secretion, prostate N42.89
Acephalia, acephalism, acephalus, acephaly Q00.0
Acephalobrachia monster Q89.8
Acephalochirus monster Q89.8
Acephalogaster Q89.8
Acephalostomus monster Q89.8
Acephalothorax Q89.8
Acerophobia F40.298
Acetonemia R79.89
  in Type 1 diabetes E10.10
    with coma E10.11
Acetonuria R82.4
Achalasia (cardia) (esophagus) K22.0
  congenital Q39.5
  pylorus Q40.0
  sphincteral NEC K59.8

Index

Abuse — Achalasia

Ache(s) — *see* Pain
Acheilia Q38.6
Achillobursitis — *see* Tendinitis, Achilles
Achillodynia — *see* Tendinitis, Achilles
Achlorhydria, achlorhydric (neurogenic) K31.83
   anemia D50.8
   diarrhea K31.83
   psychogenic F45.8
   secondary to vagotomy K91.1
Achluophobia F40.228
Acholia K82.8
Acholuric jaundice (familial) (splenomegalic) — *see also*
      Spherocytosis
   acquired D59.8
Achondrogenesis Q77.0
Achondroplasia (osteosclerosis congenita) Q77.4
Achroma, cutis L80
Achromat (ism), achromatopsia (acquired) (congenital)
      H53.51
Achromia, congenital — *see* Albinism
Achromia parasitica B36.0
Achylia gastrica K31.89
   psychogenic F45.8
Acid
   burn — *see* Corrosion
   deficiency
      amide nicotinic E52
      ascorbic E54
      folic E53.8
      nicotinic E52
      pantothenic E53.8
   intoxication E87.2
   peptic disease K30
   phosphatase deficiency E83.39
   stomach K30
      psychogenic F45.8
Acidemia E87.2
   argininosuccinic E72.22
   isovaleric E71.110
   metabolic (newborn) P19.9
      first noted before onset of labor P19.0
      first noted during labor P19.1
      noted at birth P19.2
   methylmalonic E71.120
   pipecolic E72.3
   propionic E71.121
Acidity, gastric (high) K30
   psychogenic F45.8
Acidocytopenia — *see* Agranulocytosis
Acidocytosis D72.1
Acidopenia — *see* Agranulocytosis
Acidosis (lactic) (respiratory) E87.2
   in Type 1 diabetes E10.10
      with coma E10.11
   kidney, tubular N25.89
   lactic E87.2
   metabolic NEC E87.2
      with respiratory acidosis E87.4
      hyperchloremic, of newborn P74.421
      late, of newborn P74.0
   mixed metabolic and respiratory, newborn P84
   newborn P84
   renal (hyperchloremic) (tubular) N25.89
   respiratory E87.2
      complicated by
         metabolic
            acidosis E87.4
            alkalosis E87.4
Aciduria
   4-hydroxybutyric E72.81
   argininosuccinic E72.22
   gamma-hydroxybutyric E72.81
   glutaric (type I) E72.3
      type II E71.313
      type III E71.5- ☑
   orotic (congenital) (hereditary) (pyrimidine deficiency)
      E79.8
      anemia D53.0
Acladiosis (skin) B36.0
Aclasis, diaphyseal Q78.6
Acleistocardia Q21.1
Aclusion — *see* Anomaly, dentofacial, malocclusion
Acne L70.9
   artificialis L70.8
   atrophica L70.2
   cachecticorum (Hebra) L70.8
   conglobata L70.1
   cystic L70.0

Acne — *continued*
   decalvans L66.2
   excoriée (des jeunes filles) L70.5
   frontalis L70.2
   indurata L70.0
   infantile L70.4
   keloid L73.0
   lupoid L70.2
   necrotic, necrotica (miliaris) L70.2
   neonatal L70.4
   nodular L70.0
   occupational L70.8
   picker's L70.5
   pustular L70.0
   rodens L70.2
   rosacea L71.9
   specified NEC L70.8
   tropica L70.3
   varioliformis L70.2
   vulgaris L70.0
Acnitis (primary) A18.4
Acosta's disease T70.29 ☑
Acoustic — *see* condition
Acousticophobia F40.298
Acquired — *see also* condition
   immunodeficiency syndrome (AIDS) B20
Acrania Q00.0
Acroangiodermatitis I78.9
Acroasphyxia, chronic I73.89
Acrobystitis N47.7
Acrocephalopolysyndactyly Q87.0
Acrocephalosyndactyly Q87.0
Acrocephaly Q75.0
Acrochondrohyperplasia — *see* Syndrome, Marfan's
Acrocyanosis I73.89
   newborn P28.2
      meaning transient blue hands and feet — *omit code*
Acrodermatitis L30.8
   atrophicans (chronica) L90.4
   continua (Hallopeau) L40.2
   enteropathica (hereditary) E83.2
   Hallopeau's L40.2
   infantile papular L44.4
   perstans L40.2
   pustulosa continua L40.2
   recalcitrant pustular L40.2
Acrodynia — *see* Poisoning, mercury
Acromegaly, acromegalia E22.0
Acromelalgia I73.81
Acromicria, acromikria Q79.8
Acronyx L60.0
Acropachy, thyroid — *see* Thyrotoxicosis
Acroparesthesia (simple) (vasomotor) I73.89
Acropathy, thyroid — *see* Thyrotoxicosis
Acrophobia F40.241
Acroposthitis N47.7
Acroscleriasis, acroscleroderma, acrosclerosis — *see*
      Sclerosis, systemic
Acrosphacelus I96
Acrospiroma, eccrine — *see* Neoplasm, skin, benign
Acrostealgia — *see* Osteochondropathy
Acrotrophodynia — *see* Immersion
ACTH ectopic syndrome E24.3
Actinic — *see* condition
Actinobacillosis, actinobacillus A28.8
   mallei A24.0
   muris A25.1
Actinomyces israelii (infection) — *see* Actinomycosis
Actinomycetoma (foot) B47.1
Actinomycosis, actinomycotic A42.9
   with pneumonia A42.0
   abdominal A42.1
   cervicofacial A42.2
   cutaneous A42.89
   gastrointestinal A42.1
   pulmonary A42.0
   sepsis A42.7
   specified site NEC A42.89
Actinoneuritis G62.82
Action, heart
   disorder I49.9
   irregular I49.9
      psychogenic F45.8
Activated protein C resistance D68.51
Activation
   mast cell (disorder) (syndrome) D89.40
      idiopathic D89.42

Activation — *continued*
   mast cell — *continued*
      monoclonal D89.41
      secondary D89.43
      specified type NEC D89.49
Active — *see* condition
Acute — *see also* condition
   abdomen R10.0
   gallbladder — *see* Cholecystitis, acute
Acyanotic heart disease (congenital) Q24.9
Acystia Q64.5
Adair-Dighton syndrome (brittle bones and blue sclera,
      deafness) Q78.0
Adamantinoblastoma — *see* Ameloblastoma
Adamantinoma — *see also* Cyst, calcifying odontogenic
   long bones C40.90
      lower limb C40.2- ☑
      upper limb C40.0- ☑
   malignant C41.1
      jaw (bone) (lower) C41.1
         upper C41.0
   tibial C40.2- ☑
Adamantoblastoma — *see* Ameloblastoma
Adams-Stokes (-Morgagni) disease or syndrome I45.9
Adaption reaction — *see* Disorder, adjustment
Addiction — *see also* Dependence F19.20
   alcohol, alcoholic (ethyl) (methyl) (wood) (without re-
      mission) F10.20
      with remission F10.21
   drug — *see* Dependence, drug
   ethyl alcohol (without remission) F10.20
      with remission F10.21
   heroin — *see* Dependence, drug, opioid
   methyl alcohol (without remission) F10.20
      with remission F10.21
   methylated spirit (without remission) F10.20
      with remission F10.21
   morphine (-like substances) — *see* Dependence, drug,
      opioid
   nicotine — *see* Dependence, drug, nicotine
   opium and opioids — *see* Dependence, drug, opioid
   tobacco — *see* Dependence, drug, nicotine
Addison-Biermer anemia (pernicious) D51.0
Addisonian crisis E27.2
Addison's
   anemia (pernicious) D51.0
   disease (bronze) or syndrome E27.1
      tuberculous A18.7
   keloid L94.0
Addison-Schilder complex E71.528
Additional — *see also* Accessory
   chromosome(s) Q99.8
      21 — *see* Trisomy, 21
      sex — *see* Abnormal, chromosome, sex
Adduction contracture, hip or other joint — *see*
      Contraction, joint
Adenitis — *see also* Lymphadenitis
   acute, unspecified site L04.9
   axillary I88.9
      acute L04.2
      chronic or subacute I88.1
   Bartholin's gland N75.8
   bulbourethral gland — *see* Urethritis
   cervical I88.9
      acute L04.0
      chronic or subacute I88.1
   chancroid (Hemophilus ducreyi) A57
   chronic, unspecified site I88.1
   Cowper's gland — *see* Urethritis
   due to Pasteurella multocida (P. septica) A28.0
   epidemic, acute B27.09
   gangrenous L04.9
   gonorrheal NEC A54.89
   groin I88.9
      acute L04.1
      chronic or subacute I88.1
   infectious (acute) (epidemic) B27.09
   inguinal I88.9
      acute L04.1
      chronic or subacute I88.1
   lymph gland or node, except mesenteric I88.9
      acute — *see* Lymphadenitis, acute
      chronic or subacute I88.1
   mesenteric (acute) (chronic) (nonspecific) (subacute)
      I88.0
   parotid gland (suppurative) — *see* Sialoadenitis
   salivary gland (any) (suppurative) — *see* Sialoadenitis
   scrofulous (tuberculous) A18.2

Adenitis — *continued*
  Skene's duct or gland — *see* Urethritis
  strumous, tuberculous A18.2
  subacute, unspecified site I88.1
  sublingual gland (suppurative) — *see* Sialoadenitis
  submandibular gland (suppurative) — *see* Sialoadenitis
  submaxillary gland (suppurative) — *see* Sialoadenitis
  tuberculous — *see* Tuberculosis, lymph gland
  urethral gland — *see* Urethritis
  Wharton's duct (suppurative) — *see* Sialoadenitis
Adenoacanthoma — *see* Neoplasm, malignant, by site
Adenoameloblastoma — *see* Cyst, calcifying odonto-genic
Adenocarcinoid (tumor) — *see* Neoplasm, malignant, by site
Adenocarcinoma — *see also* Neoplasm, malignant, by site
  acidophil
    specified site — *see* Neoplasm, malignant, by site
    unspecified site C75.1
  adrenal cortical C74.0- ☑
  alveolar — *see* Neoplasm, lung, malignant
  apocrine
    breast — *see* Neoplasm, breast, malignant
    in situ
      breast D05.8- ☑
      specified site NEC — *see* Neoplasm, skin, in situ
      unspecified site D04.9
    specified site NEC — *see* Neoplasm, skin, malignant
    unspecified site C44.99
  basal cell
    specified site — *see* Neoplasm, skin, malignant
    unspecified site C08.9
  basophil
    specified site — *see* Neoplasm, malignant, by site
    unspecified site C75.1
  bile duct type C22.1
    liver C22.1
    specified site NEC — *see* Neoplasm, malignant, by site
    unspecified site C22.1
  bronchiolar — *see* Neoplasm, lung, malignant
  bronchioloalveolar — *see* Neoplasm, lung, malignant
  ceruminous C44.29- ☑
  cervix, in situ — *see also* Carcinoma, cervix uteri, in situ D06.9
  chromophobe
    specified site — *see* Neoplasm, malignant, by site
    unspecified site C75.1
  diffuse type
    specified site — *see* Neoplasm, malignant, by site
    unspecified site C16.9
  duct
    infiltrating
      with Paget's disease — *see* Neoplasm, breast, malignant
      specified site — *see* Neoplasm, malignant, by site
      unspecified site (female) C50.91- ☑
        male C50.92- ☑
    specified site — *see* Neoplasm, malignant, by site
    unspecified site
      female C56.9
      male C61
  eosinophil
    specified site — *see* Neoplasm, malignant, by site
    unspecified site C75.1
  follicular
    with papillary C73
    moderately differentiated C73
    specified site — *see* Neoplasm, malignant, by site
    trabecular C73
    unspecified site C73
    well differentiated C73
  Hurthle cell C73
  in
    adenomatous
      polyposis coli C18.9
  infiltrating duct
    with Paget's disease — *see* Neoplasm, breast, ma-lignant
    specified site — *see* Neoplasm, by site, malignant
    unspecified site (female) C50.91- ☑
      male C50.92- ☑
  inflammatory
    specified site — *see* Neoplasm, by site, malignant
    unspecified site (female) C50.91- ☑

Adenocarcinoma — *continued*
  inflammatory — *continued*
    unspecified site — *continued*
      male C50.92- ☑
  intestinal type
    specified site — *see* Neoplasm, by site, malignant
    unspecified site C16.9
  intracystic papillary
  intraductal
    breast D05.1- ☑
    noninfiltrating
      breast D05.1- ☑
      papillary
        with invasion
          specified site — *see* Neoplasm, by site, malignant
          unspecified site (female) C50.91- ☑
            male C50.92- ☑
        breast D05.1- ☑
        specified site NEC — *see* Neoplasm, in situ, by site
        unspecified site D05.1- ☑
      specified site NEC — *see* Neoplasm, in situ, by site
      unspecified site D05.1- ☑
    papillary
      with invasion
        specified site — *see* Neoplasm, malignant, by site
        unspecified site (female) C50.91- ☑
          male C50.92- ☑
      breast D05.1- ☑
      specified site — *see* Neoplasm, in situ, by site
      unspecified site D05.1- ☑
    specified site NEC — *see* Neoplasm, in situ, by site
    unspecified site D05.1- ☑
  islet cell
    with exocrine, mixed
      specified site — *see* Neoplasm, malignant, by site
      unspecified site C25.9
    pancreas C25.4
    specified site NEC — *see* Neoplasm, malignant, by site
    unspecified site C25.4
  lobular
    in situ
      breast D05.0- ☑
      specified site NEC — *see* Neoplasm, in situ, by site
      unspecified site D05.0- ☑
    specified site — *see* Neoplasm, malignant, by site
    unspecified site (female) C50.91- ☑
      male C50.92- ☑
  mucoid — *see also* Neoplasm, malignant, by site
    cell
      specified site — *see* Neoplasm, malignant, by site
      unspecified site C75.1
  nonencapsulated sclerosing C73
  papillary
    with follicular C73
    follicular variant C73
    intraductal (noninfiltrating)
      with invasion
        specified site — *see* Neoplasm, malignant, by site
        unspecified site (female) C50.91- ☑
          male C50.92- ☑
      breast D05.1- ☑
      specified site NEC — *see* Neoplasm, in situ, by site
      unspecified site D05.1- ☑
    serous
      specified site — *see* Neoplasm, malignant, by site
      unspecified site C56.9
  papillocystic
    specified site — *see* Neoplasm, malignant, by site
    unspecified site C56.9
  pseudomucinous
    specified site — *see* Neoplasm, malignant, by site
    unspecified site C56.9
  renal cell C64- ☑
  sebaceous — *see* Neoplasm, skin, malignant
  serous — *see also* Neoplasm, malignant, by site

Adenocarcinoma — *continued*
  serous — *see also* Neoplasm, malignant, by site — *continued*
    papillary
      specified site — *see* Neoplasm, malignant, by site
      unspecified site C56.9
  sweat gland — *see* Neoplasm, skin, malignant
  water-clear cell C75.0
Adenocarcinoma-in-situ — *see also* Neoplasm, in situ, by site
  breast D05.9- ☑
Adenofibroma
  clear cell — *see* Neoplasm, benign, by site
  endometrioid D27.9
    borderline malignancy D39.10
    malignant C56- ☑
  mucinous
    specified site — *see* Neoplasm, benign, by site
    unspecified site D27.9
  papillary
    specified site — *see* Neoplasm, benign, by site
    unspecified site D27.9
  prostate — *see* Enlargement, enlarged, prostate
  serous
    specified site — *see* Neoplasm, benign, by site
    unspecified site D27.9
  specified site — *see* Neoplasm, benign, by site
  unspecified site D27.9
Adenofibrosis
  breast — *see* Fibroadenosis, breast
  endometrioid N80.0
Adenoiditis (chronic) J35.02
  with tonsillitis J35.03
  acute J03.90
    recurrent J03.91
    specified organism NEC J03.80
      recurrent J03.81
    staphylococcal J03.80
      recurrent J03.81
    streptococcal J03.00
      recurrent J03.01
Adenoids — *see* condition
Adenolipoma — *see* Neoplasm, benign, by site
Adenolipomatosis, Launois-Bensaude E88.89
Adenolymphoma
  specified site — *see* Neoplasm, benign, by site
  unspecified site D11.9
Adenoma — *see also* Neoplasm, benign, by site
  acidophil
    specified site — *see* Neoplasm, benign, by site
    unspecified site D35.2
  acidophil-basophil, mixed
    specified site — *see* Neoplasm, benign, by site
    unspecified site D35.2
  adrenal (cortical) D35.00
    clear cell D35.00
    compact cell D35.00
    glomerulosa cell D35.00
    heavily pigmented variant D35.00
    mixed cell D35.00
  alpha-cell
    pancreas D13.7
    specified site NEC — *see* Neoplasm, benign, by site
    unspecified site D13.7
  alveolar D14.30
  apocrine
    breast D24- ☑
    specified site NEC — *see* Neoplasm, skin, benign, by site
    unspecified site D23.9
  basal cell D11.9
  basophil
    specified site — *see* Neoplasm, benign, by site
    unspecified site D35.2
  basophil-acidophil, mixed
    specified site — *see* Neoplasm, benign, by site
    unspecified site D35.2
  beta-cell
    pancreas D13.7
    specified site NEC — *see* Neoplasm, benign, by site
    unspecified site D13.7
  bile duct D13.4
    common D13.5
    extrahepatic D13.5
    intrahepatic D13.4
    specified site NEC — *see* Neoplasm, benign, by site
    unspecified site D13.4

▽ Subterms under main terms may continue to next column or page   ☑ Additional Character Required — Refer to the Tabular List for Character Selection   11

Adenitis — Adenoma

Index

Adenoma — Adhesions, adhesive

Adenoma — *continued*
- black D35.00
- bronchial D38.1
  - cylindroid type — *see* Neoplasm, lung, malignant
- ceruminous D23.2- ☑
- chief cell D35.1
- chromophobe
  - specified site — *see* Neoplasm, benign, by site
  - unspecified site D35.2
- colloid
  - specified site — *see* Neoplasm, benign, by site
  - unspecified site D34
- duct
- eccrine, papillary — *see* Neoplasm, skin, benign
- endocrine, multiple
  - single specified site — *see* Neoplasm, uncertain behavior, by site
  - two or more specified sites D44- ☑
  - unspecified site D44.9
- endometrioid — *see also* Neoplasm, benign
  - borderline malignancy — *see* Neoplasm, uncertain behavior, by site
- eosinophil
  - specified site — *see* Neoplasm, benign, by site
  - unspecified site D35.2
- fetal
  - specified site — *see* Neoplasm, benign, by site
  - unspecified site D34
- follicular
  - specified site — *see* Neoplasm, benign, by site
  - unspecified site D34
- hepatocellular D13.4
- Hurthle cell D34
- islet cell
  - pancreas D13.7
  - specified site NEC — *see* Neoplasm, benign, by site
  - unspecified site D13.7
- liver cell D13.4
- macrofollicular
  - specified site — *see* Neoplasm, benign, by site
  - unspecified site D34
- malignant, malignum — *see* Neoplasm, malignant, by site
- microcystic
  - pancreas D13.6
  - specified site NEC — *see* Neoplasm, benign, by site
  - unspecified site D13.6
- microfollicular
  - specified site — *see* Neoplasm, benign, by site
  - unspecified site D34
- mucoid cell
  - specified site — *see* Neoplasm, benign, by site
  - unspecified site D35.2
- multiple endocrine
  - single specified site — *see* Neoplasm, uncertain behavior, by site
  - two or more specified sites D44- ☑
  - unspecified site D44.9
- nipple D24- ☑
- papillary — *see also* Neoplasm, benign, by site
  - eccrine — *see* Neoplasm, skin, benign
- Pick's tubular
  - specified site — *see* Neoplasm, benign, by site
  - unspecified site
    - female D27.9
    - male D29.20
- pleomorphic
  - carcinoma in — *see* Neoplasm, salivary gland, malignant
    - specified site — *see* Neoplasm, malignant, by site
    - unspecified site C08.9
- polypoid — *see also* Neoplasm, benign
  - adenocarcinoma in — *see* Neoplasm, malignant, by site
  - adenocarcinoma in situ — *see* Neoplasm, in situ, by site
- prostate — *see* Neoplasm, benign, prostate
- rete cell D29.20
- sebaceous — *see* Neoplasm, skin, benign
- Sertoli cell
  - specified site — *see* Neoplasm, benign, by site
  - unspecified site
    - female D27.9
    - male D29.20
- skin appendage — *see* Neoplasm, skin, benign
- sudoriferous gland — *see* Neoplasm, skin, benign
- sweat gland — *see* Neoplasm, skin, benign

Adenoma — *continued*
- testicular
  - specified site — *see* Neoplasm, benign, by site
  - unspecified site
    - female D27.9
    - male D29.20
- tubular — *see also* Neoplasm, benign, by site
  - adenocarcinoma in — *see* Neoplasm, malignant, by site
  - adenocarcinoma in situ — *see* Neoplasm, in situ, by site
  - Pick's
    - specified site — *see* Neoplasm, benign, by site
    - unspecified site
      - female D27.9
      - male D29.20
- tubulovillous — *see also* Neoplasm, benign, by site
  - adenocarcinoma in — *see* Neoplasm, malignant, by site
  - adenocarcinoma in situ — *see* Neoplasm, in situ, by site
- villous — *see* Neoplasm, uncertain behavior, by site
  - adenocarcinoma in — *see* Neoplasm, malignant, by site
  - adenocarcinoma in situ — *see* Neoplasm, in situ, by site
- water-clear cell D35.1

Adenomatosis
- endocrine (multiple) E31.20
  - single specified site — *see* Neoplasm, uncertain behavior, by site
- erosive of nipple D24- ☑
- pluriendocrine — *see* Adenomatosis, endocrine
- pulmonary D38.1
  - malignant — *see* Neoplasm, lung, malignant
- specified site — *see* Neoplasm, benign, by site
- unspecified site D12.6

Adenomatous
- goiter (nontoxic) E04.9
  - with hyperthyroidism — *see* Hyperthyroidism, with, goiter, nodular
  - toxic — *see* Hyperthyroidism, with, goiter, nodular

Adenomyoma — *see also* Neoplasm, benign, by site
- prostate — *see* Enlarged, prostate

Adenomyometritis N80.0

Adenomyosis N80.0

Adenopathy (lymph gland) R59.9
- generalized R59.1
- inguinal R59.0
- localized R59.0
- mediastinal R59.0
- mesentery R59.0
- syphilitic (secondary) A51.49
- tracheobronchial R59.0
  - tuberculous A15.4
    - primary (progressive) A15.7
- tuberculous — *see also* Tuberculosis, lymph gland
  - tracheobronchial A15.4
    - primary (progressive) A15.7

Adenosalpingitis — *see* Salpingitis

Adenosarcoma — *see* Neoplasm, malignant, by site

Adenosclerosis I88.8

Adenosis (sclerosing) breast — *see* Fibroadenosis, breast

Adenovirus, as cause of disease classified elsewhere B97.0

Adentia (complete) (partial) — *see* Absence, teeth

Adherent — *see also* Adhesions
- labia (minora) N90.89
- pericardium (nonrheumatic) I31.0
  - rheumatic I09.2
- placenta (with hemorrhage) O72.0
  - without hemorrhage O73.0
- prepuce, newborn N47.0
- scar (skin) L90.5
- tendon in scar L90.5

Adhesions, adhesive (postinfective) K66.0
- with intestinal obstruction K56.50
  - complete K56.52
  - incomplete K56.51
  - partial K56.51
- abdominal (wall) — *see* Adhesions, peritoneum
- appendix K38.8
- bile duct (common) (hepatic) K83.8
- bladder (sphincter) N32.89
- bowel — *see* Adhesions, peritoneum
- cardiac I31.0
  - rheumatic I09.2
- cecum — *see* Adhesions, peritoneum

Adhesions, adhesive — *continued*
- cervicovaginal N88.1
  - congenital Q52.8
  - postpartal O90.89
  - old N88.1
- cervix N88.1
- ciliary body NEC — *see* Adhesions, iris
- clitoris N90.89
- colon — *see* Adhesions, peritoneum
- common duct K83.8
- congenital — *see also* Anomaly, by site
  - fingers — *see* Syndactylism, complex, fingers
  - omental, anomalous Q43.3
  - peritoneal Q43.3
  - tongue (to gum or roof of mouth) Q38.3
- conjunctiva (acquired) H11.21- ☑
  - congenital Q15.8
- cystic duct K82.8
- diaphragm — *see* Adhesions, peritoneum
- due to foreign body — *see* Foreign body
- duodenum — *see* Adhesions, peritoneum
- ear
  - middle H74.1- ☑
- epididymis N50.89
- epidural — *see* Adhesions, meninges
- epiglottis J38.7
- eyelid H02.59
- female pelvis N73.6
- gallbladder K82.8
- globe H44.89
- heart I31.0
  - rheumatic I09.2
- ileocecal (coil) — *see* Adhesions, peritoneum
- ileum — *see* Adhesions, peritoneum
- intestine — *see also* Adhesions, peritoneum
  - with obstruction K56.50
    - complete K56.52
    - incomplete K56.51
    - partial K56.51
- intra-abdominal — *see* Adhesions, peritoneum
- iris H21.50- ☑
  - anterior H21.51- ☑
  - goniosynechiae H21.52- ☑
  - posterior H21.54- ☑
  - to corneal graft T85.898 ☑
- joint — *see* Ankylosis
  - knee M23.8X ☑
  - temporomandibular M26.61- ☑
- labium (majus) (minus), congenital Q52.5
- liver — *see* Adhesions, peritoneum
- lung J98.4
- mediastinum J98.59
- meninges (cerebral) (spinal) G96.12
  - congenital Q07.8
  - tuberculous (cerebral) (spinal) A17.0
- mesenteric — *see* Adhesions, peritoneum
- nasal (septum) (to turbinates) J34.89
- ocular muscle — *see* Strabismus, mechanical
- omentum — *see* Adhesions, peritoneum
- ovary N73.6
  - congenital (to cecum, kidney or omentum) Q50.39
- paraovarian N73.6
- pelvic (peritoneal)
  - female N73.6
    - postprocedural N99.4
  - male — *see* Adhesions, peritoneum
  - postpartal (old) N73.6
  - tuberculous A18.17
- penis to scrotum (congenital) Q55.8
- periappendiceal — *see also* Adhesions, peritoneum
- pericardium (nonrheumatic) I31.0
  - focal I31.8
  - rheumatic I09.2
  - tuberculous A18.84
- pericholecystic K82.8
- perigastric — *see* Adhesions, peritoneum
- periovarian N73.6
- periprostatic N42.89
- perirectal — *see* Adhesions, peritoneum
- perirenal N28.89
- peritoneum, peritoneal (postinfective) K66.0
  - with obstruction (intestinal) K56.50
    - complete K56.52
    - incomplete K56.51
    - partial K56.51
  - congenital Q43.3
  - pelvic, female N73.6
    - postprocedural N99.4

Adhesions, adhesive — *continued*
  peritoneum, peritoneal — *continued*
    postpartal, pelvic N73.6
    postprocedural K66.0
    to uterus N73.6
  peritubal N73.6
  periureteral N28.89
  periuterine N73.6
  perivesical N32.89
  perivesicular (seminal vesicle) N50.89
  pleura, pleuritic J94.8
    tuberculous NEC A15.6
  pleuropericardial J94.8
  postoperative (gastrointestinal tract) K66.0
    with obstruction — *see also* Obstruction, intestine, postoperative K91.30
    due to foreign body accidentally left in wound — *see* Foreign body, accidentally left during a procedure
    pelvic peritoneal N99.4
    urethra — *see* Stricture, urethra, postprocedural
    vagina N99.2
  postpartal, old (vulva or perineum) N90.89
  preputial, prepuce N47.5
  pulmonary J98.4
  pylorus — *see* Adhesions, peritoneum
  sciatic nerve — *see* Lesion, nerve, sciatic
  seminal vesicle N50.89
  shoulder (joint) — *see* Capsulitis, adhesive
  sigmoid flexure — *see* Adhesions, peritoneum
  spermatic cord (acquired) N50.89
    congenital Q55.4
  spinal canal G96.12
  stomach — *see* Adhesions, peritoneum
  subscapular — *see* Capsulitis, adhesive
  temporomandibular M26.61- ☑
  tendinitis (*see also* Tenosynovitis, specified type NEC)
    shoulder — *see* Capsulitis, adhesive
  testis N44.8
  tongue, congenital (to gum or roof of mouth) Q38.3
    acquired K14.8
  trachea J39.8
  tubo-ovarian N73.6
  tunica vaginalis N44.8
  uterus N73.6
    internal N85.6
    to abdominal wall N73.6
  vagina (chronic) N89.5
    postoperative N99.2
  vitreomacular H43.82- ☑
  vitreous H43.89
  vulva N90.89
Adiaspiromycosis B48.8
Adie (-Holmes) **pupil or syndrome** — *see* Anomaly, pupil, function, tonic pupil
Adiponecrosis neonatorum P83.88
Adiposis — *see also* Obesity
  cerebralis E23.6
  dolorosa E88.2
Adiposity — *see also* Obesity
  heart — *see* Degeneration, myocardial
  localized E65
Adiposogenital dystrophy E23.6
Adjustment
  disorder — *see* Disorder, adjustment
  implanted device — *see* Encounter (for), adjustment (of)
  prosthesis, external — *see* Fitting
  reaction — *see* Disorder, adjustment
Administration of tPA (rtPA) in a different facility within the last 24 hours prior to admission to current facility Z92.82
Admission (for) — *see also* Encounter (for)
  adjustment (of)
    artificial
      arm Z44.00- ☑
        complete Z44.01- ☑
        partial Z44.02- ☑
      eye Z44.2 ☑
      leg Z44.10- ☑
        complete Z44.11- ☑
        partial Z44.12- ☑
    brain neuropacemaker Z46.2
      implanted Z45.42
    breast
      implant Z45.81 ☑
      prosthesis (external) Z44.3 ☑

Admission — *continued*
  adjustment — *continued*
    colostomy belt Z46.89
    contact lenses Z46.0
    cystostomy device Z46.6
    dental prosthesis Z46.3
    device NEC
      abdominal Z46.89
      implanted Z45.89
        cardiac Z45.09
          defibrillator (with synchronous cardiac pacemaker) Z45.02
          pacemaker (cardiac resynchronization therapy (CRT-P)) Z45.018
          pulse generator Z45.010
          resynchronization therapy defibrillator (CRT-D) Z45.02
        hearing device Z45.328
          bone conduction Z45.320
          cochlear Z45.321
        infusion pump Z45.1
        nervous system Z45.49
          CSF drainage Z45.41
          hearing device — *see* Admission, adjustment, device, implanted, hearing device
          neuropacemaker Z45.42
          visual substitution Z45.31
        specified NEC Z45.89
        vascular access Z45.2
        visual substitution Z45.31
    nervous system Z46.2
      implanted — *see* Admission, adjustment, device, implanted, nervous system
    orthodontic Z46.4
    prosthetic Z44.9
      arm — *see* Admission, adjustment, artificial, arm
      breast Z44.3 ☑
      dental Z46.3
      eye Z44.2 ☑
      leg — *see* Admission, adjustment, artificial, leg
      specified type NEC Z44.8
    substitution
      auditory Z46.2
        implanted — *see* Admission, adjustment, device, implanted, hearing device
      nervous system Z46.2
        implanted — *see* Admission, adjustment, device, implanted, nervous system
      visual Z46.2
        implanted Z45.31
    urinary Z46.6
  hearing aid Z46.1
    implanted — *see* Admission, adjustment, device, implanted, hearing device
  ileostomy device Z46.89
  intestinal appliance or device NEC Z46.89
  neuropacemaker (brain) (peripheral nerve) (spinal cord) Z46.2
    implanted Z45.42
  orthodontic device Z46.4
  orthopedic (brace) (cast) (device) (shoes) Z46.89
  pacemaker (cardiac resynchronization therapy (CRT-P))
    cardiac Z45.018
      pulse generator Z45.010
    nervous system Z46.2
      implanted Z45.42
  portacath (port-a-cath) Z45.2
  prosthesis Z44.9
    arm — *see* Admission, adjustment, artificial, arm
    breast Z44.3 ☑
    dental Z46.3
    eye Z44.2 ☑
    leg — *see* Admission, adjustment, artificial, leg
    specified NEC Z44.8
  spectacles Z46.0
  aftercare — *see also* Aftercare Z51.89
    postpartum
      immediately after delivery Z39.0
      routine follow-up Z39.2
    radiation therapy (antineoplastic) Z51.0
  attention to artificial opening (of) Z43.9
    artificial vagina Z43.7
    colostomy Z43.3
    cystostomy Z43.5

Admission — *continued*
  attention to artificial opening — *continued*
    enterostomy Z43.4
    gastrostomy Z43.1
    ileostomy Z43.2
    jejunostomy Z43.4
    nephrostomy Z43.6
    specified site NEC Z43.8
      intestinal tract Z43.4
      urinary tract Z43.6
    tracheostomy Z43.0
    ureterostomy Z43.6
    urethrostomy Z43.6
  breast augmentation or reduction Z41.1
  breast reconstruction following mastectomy Z42.1
  change of
    dressing (nonsurgical) Z48.00
    neuropacemaker device (brain) (peripheral nerve) (spinal cord) Z46.2
      implanted Z45.42
    surgical dressing Z48.01
  circumcision, ritual or routine (in absence of diagnosis) Z41.2
  clinical research investigation (control) (normal comparison) (participant) Z00.6
  contraceptive management Z30.9
  cosmetic surgery NEC Z41.1
  counseling — *see also* Counseling
    dietary Z71.3
    gestational carrier Z31.7
    HIV Z71.7
    human immunodeficiency virus Z71.7
    nonattending third party Z71.0
    procreative management NEC Z31.69
  delivery, full-term, uncomplicated O80
    cesarean, without indication O82
  desensitization to allergens Z51.6
  dietary surveillance and counseling Z71.3
  ear piercing Z41.3
  examination at health care facility (adult) — *see also* Examination Z00.00
    with abnormal findings Z00.01
    clinical research investigation (control) (normal comparison) (participant) Z00.6
    dental Z01.20
      with abnormal findings Z01.21
    donor (potential) Z00.5
    ear Z01.10
      with abnormal findings NEC Z01.118
    eye Z01.00
      with abnormal findings Z01.01
      following failed vision screening Z01.020
        with abnormal findings Z01.021
    general, specified reason NEC Z00.8
    hearing Z01.10
      with abnormal findings NEC Z01.118
      infant or child (over 28 days old) Z00.129
        with abnormal findings Z00.121
    postpartum checkup Z39.2
    psychiatric (general) Z00.8
    requested by authority Z04.6
    vision Z01.00
      with abnormal findings Z01.01
      following failed vision screening Z01.020
        with abnormal findings Z01.021
      infant or child (over 28 days old) Z00.129
        with abnormal findings Z00.121
  fitting (of)
    artificial
      arm — *see* Admission, adjustment, artificial, arm
      eye Z44.2 ☑
      leg — *see* Admission, adjustment, artificial, leg
    brain neuropacemaker Z46.2
      implanted Z45.42
    breast prosthesis (external) Z44.3 ☑
    colostomy belt Z46.89
    contact lenses Z46.0
    cystostomy device Z46.6
    dental prosthesis Z46.3
    dentures Z46.3
    device NEC
      abdominal Z46.89
      nervous system Z46.2
        implanted — *see* Admission, adjustment, device, implanted, nervous system
      orthodontic Z46.4
      prosthetic Z44.9
        breast Z44.3 ☑

Admission — *continued*
  fitting — *continued*
    device — *continued*
      prosthetic — *continued*
        dental Z46.3
        eye Z44.2 ☑
      substitution
        auditory Z46.2
          implanted — *see* Admission, adjustment, device, implanted, hearing device
        nervous system Z46.2
          implanted — *see* Admission, adjustment, device, implanted, nervous system
        visual Z46.2
          implanted Z45.31
    hearing aid Z46.1
    ileostomy device Z46.89
    intestinal appliance or device NEC Z46.89
    neuropacemaker (brain) (peripheral nerve) (spinal cord) Z46.2
      implanted Z45.42
    orthodontic device Z46.4
    orthopedic device (brace) (cast) (shoes) Z46.89
    prosthesis Z44.9
      arm — *see* Admission, adjustment, artificial, arm
      breast Z44.3 ☑
      dental Z46.3
      eye Z44.2 ☑
      leg — *see* Admission, adjustment, artificial, leg
      specified type NEC Z44.8
    spectacles Z46.0
  follow-up examination Z09
  intrauterine device management Z30.431
    initial prescription Z30.014
  mental health evaluation Z00.8
    requested by authority Z04.6
  observation — *see* Observation
  Papanicolaou smear, cervix Z12.4
    for suspected malignant neoplasm Z12.4
  plastic and reconstructive surgery following medical procedure or healed injury NEC Z42.8
  plastic surgery, cosmetic NEC Z41.1
  postpartum observation
    immediately after delivery Z39.0
    routine follow-up Z39.2
  poststerilization (for restoration) Z31.0
    aftercare Z31.42
  procreative management Z31.9
  prophylactic (measure) — *see also* Encounter, prophylactic measures
    organ removal Z40.00
      breast Z40.01
      fallopian tube(s) Z40.03
        with ovary(s) Z40.02
      ovary(s) Z40.02
      specified organ NEC Z40.09
      testes Z40.09
    vaccination Z23
  psychiatric examination (general) Z00.8
    requested by authority Z04.6
  radiation therapy (antineoplastic) Z51.0
  reconstructive surgery following medical procedure or healed injury NEC Z42.8
  removal of
    cystostomy catheter Z43.5
    drains Z48.03
    dressing (nonsurgical) Z48.00
    implantable subdermal contraceptive Z30.46
    intrauterine contraceptive device Z30.432
    neuropacemaker (brain) (peripheral nerve) (spinal cord) Z46.2
      implanted Z45.42
    staples Z48.02
    surgical dressing Z48.01
    sutures Z48.02
    ureteral stent Z46.6
  respirator [ventilator] use during power failure Z99.12
  restoration of organ continuity (poststerilization) Z31.0
    aftercare Z31.42
  sensitivity test — *see also* Test, skin
    allergy NEC Z01.82
    Mantoux Z11.1
  tuboplasty following previous sterilization Z31.0
    aftercare Z31.42
  vasoplasty following previous sterilization Z31.0
    aftercare Z31.42
  vision examination Z01.00
    with abnormal findings Z01.01

Admission — *continued*
  vision examination — *continued*
    following failed vision screening Z01.020
      with abnormal findings Z01.021
    infant or child (over 28 days old) Z00.129
      with abnormal findings Z00.121
  waiting period for admission to other facility Z75.1
Adnexitis (suppurative) — *see* Salpingo-oophoritis
Adolescent X-linked adrenoleukodystrophy E71.521
Adrenal (gland) — *see* condition
Adrenalism, tuberculous A18.7
Adrenalitis, adrenitis E27.8
  autoimmune E27.1
  meningococcal, hemorrhagic A39.1
Adrenarche, premature E27.0
Adrenocortical syndrome — *see* Cushing's, syndrome
Adrenogenital syndrome E25.9
  acquired E25.8
  congenital E25.0
  salt loss E25.0
Adrenogenitalism, congenital E25.0
Adrenoleukodystrophy E71.529
  neonatal E71.511
  X-linked E71.529
    Addison only phenotype E71.528
    Addison-Schilder E71.528
    adolescent E71.521
    adrenomyeloneuropathy E71.522
    childhood cerebral E71.520
    other specified E71.528
Adrenomyeloneuropathy E71.522
Adventitious bursa — *see* Bursopathy, specified type NEC
Adverse effect — *see* Table of Drugs and Chemicals, categories T36-T50, with 6th character 5
Advice — *see* Counseling
Adynamia (episodica) (hereditary) (periodic) G72.3
Aeration lung imperfect, newborn — *see* Atelectasis
Aerobullosis T70.3 ☑
Aerocele — *see* Embolism, air
Aerodermectasia
  subcutaneous (traumatic) T79.7 ☑
Aerodontalgia T70.29 ☑
Aeroembolism T70.3 ☑
Aerogenes capsulatus infection A48.0
Aero-otitis media T70.0 ☑
Aerophagy, aerophagia (psychogenic) F45.8
Aerophobia F40.228
Aerosinusitis T70.1 ☑
Aerotitis T70.0 ☑
Affection — *see* Disease
Afibrinogenemia — *see also* Defect, coagulation D68.8
  acquired D65
  congenital D68.2
  following ectopic or molar pregnancy O08.1
  in abortion — *see* Abortion, by type, complicated by, afibrinogenemia
  puerperal O72.3
African
  sleeping sickness B56.9
  tick fever A68.1
  trypanosomiasis B56.9
    gambian B56.0
    rhodesian B56.1
Aftercare — *see also* Care Z51.89
  following surgery (for) (on)
    amputation Z47.81
    attention to
      drains Z48.03
      dressings (nonsurgical) Z48.00
        surgical Z48.01
      sutures Z48.02
    circulatory system Z48.812
    delayed (planned) wound closure Z48.1
    digestive system Z48.815
    explantation of joint prosthesis (staged procedure)
      hip Z47.32
      knee Z47.33
      shoulder Z47.31
    genitourinary system Z48.816
    joint replacement Z47.1
    neoplasm Z48.3
    nervous system Z48.811
    oral cavity Z48.814
    organ transplant
      bone marrow Z48.290
      heart Z48.21
      heart-lung Z48.280

Aftercare — *continued*
  following surgery — *continued*
    organ transplant — *continued*
      kidney Z48.22
      liver Z48.23
      lung Z48.24
      multiple organs NEC Z48.288
      specified NEC Z48.298
    orthopedic NEC Z47.89
    planned wound closure Z48.1
    removal of internal fixation device Z47.2
    respiratory system Z48.813
    scoliosis Z47.82
    sense organs Z48.810
    skin and subcutaneous tissue Z48.817
    specified body system
      circulatory Z48.812
      digestive Z48.815
      genitourinary Z48.816
      nervous Z48.811
      oral cavity Z48.814
      respiratory Z48.813
      sense organs Z48.810
      skin and subcutaneous tissue Z48.817
      teeth Z48.814
    specified NEC Z48.89
    spinal Z47.89
    teeth Z48.814
  fracture — *code to* fracture with seventh character D
  involving
    removal of
      drains Z48.03
      dressings (nonsurgical) Z48.00
      staples Z48.02
      surgical dressings Z48.01
      sutures Z48.02
  neuropacemaker (brain) (peripheral nerve) (spinal cord) Z46.2
    implanted Z45.42
  orthopedic NEC Z47.89
  postprocedural — *see* Aftercare, following surgery
After-cataract — *see* Cataract, secondary
Agalactia (primary) O92.3
  elective, secondary or therapeutic O92.5
Agammaglobulinemia (acquired (secondary)) (nonfamilial) D80.1
  with
    immunoglobulin-bearing B-lymphocytes D80.1
    lymphopenia D81.9
  autosomal recessive (Swiss type) D80.0
  Bruton's X-linked D80.0
  common variable (CVAgamma) D80.1
  congenital sex-linked D80.0
  hereditary D80.0
  lymphopenic D81.9
  Swiss type (autosomal recessive) D80.0
  X-linked (with growth hormone deficiency) (Bruton) D80.0
Aganglionosis (bowel) (colon) Q43.1
Age (old) — *see* Senility
Agenesis
  adrenal (gland) Q89.1
  alimentary tract (complete) (partial) NEC Q45.8
    upper Q40.8
  anus, anal (canal) Q42.3
    with fistula Q42.2
  aorta Q25.41
  appendix Q42.8
  arm (complete) Q71.0- ☑
    with hand present Q71.1- ☑
  artery (peripheral) Q27.9
    brain Q28.3
    coronary Q24.5
    pulmonary Q25.79
    specified NEC Q27.8
    umbilical Q27.0
  auditory (canal) (external) Q16.1
  auricle (ear) Q16.0
  bile duct or passage Q44.5
  bladder Q64.5
  bone Q79.9
  brain Q00.0
    part of Q04.3
  breast (with nipple present) Q83.8
    with absent nipple Q83.0
  bronchus Q32.4
  canaliculus lacrimalis Q10.4
  carpus — *see* Agenesis, hand

Agenesis — *continued*
cartilage Q79.9
cecum Q42.8
cerebellum Q04.3
cervix Q51.5
chin Q18.8
cilia Q10.3
circulatory system, part NOS Q28.9
clavicle Q74.0
clitoris Q52.6
coccyx Q76.49
colon Q42.9
  specified NEC Q42.8
corpus callosum Q04.0
cricoid cartilage Q31.8
diaphragm (with hernia) Q79.1
digestive organ(s) or tract (complete) (partial) NEC Q45.8
  upper Q40.8
ductus arteriosus Q28.8
duodenum Q41.0
ear Q16.9
  auricle Q16.0
  lobe Q17.8
ejaculatory duct Q55.4
endocrine (gland) NEC Q89.2
epiglottis Q31.8
esophagus Q39.8
eustachian tube Q16.2
eye Q11.1
  adnexa Q15.8
eyelid (fold) Q10.3
face
  bones NEC Q75.8
  specified part NEC Q18.8
fallopian tube Q50.6
femur — *see* Defect, reduction, lower limb, longitudinal, femur
fibula — *see* Defect, reduction, lower limb, longitudinal, fibula
finger (complete) (partial) — *see* Agenesis, hand
foot (and toes) (complete) (partial) Q72.3- ☑
forearm (with hand present) — *see* Agenesis, arm, with hand present
  and hand Q71.2- ☑
gallbladder Q44.0
gastric Q40.2
genitalia, genital (organ(s))
  female Q52.8
    external Q52.71
    internal NEC Q52.8
  male Q55.8
glottis Q31.8
hair Q84.0
hand (and fingers) (complete) (partial) Q71.3- ☑
heart Q24.8
  valve NEC Q24.8
    pulmonary Q22.0
hepatic Q44.7
humerus — *see* Defect, reduction, upper limb
hymen Q52.4
ileum Q41.2
incus Q16.3
intestine (small) Q41.9
  large Q42.9
    specified NEC Q42.8
iris (dilator fibers) Q13.1
jaw M26.09
jejunum Q41.1
kidney(s) (partial) Q60.2
  bilateral Q60.1
  unilateral Q60.0
labium (majus) (minus) Q52.71
labyrinth, membranous Q16.5
lacrimal apparatus Q10.4
larynx Q31.8
leg (complete) Q72.0- ☑
  with foot present Q72.1- ☑
  lower leg (with foot present) — *see* Agenesis, leg, with foot present
    and foot Q72.2- ☑
lens Q12.3
limb (complete) Q73.0
  lower — *see* Agenesis, leg
  upper — *see* Agenesis, arm
lip Q38.0
liver Q44.7
lung (fissure) (lobe) (bilateral) (unilateral) Q33.3

Agenesis — *continued*
mandible, maxilla M26.09
metacarpus — *see* Agenesis, hand
metatarsus — *see* Agenesis, foot
muscle Q79.8
  eyelid Q10.3
  ocular Q15.8
musculoskeletal system NEC Q79.8
nail(s) Q84.3
neck, part Q18.8
nerve Q07.8
nervous system, part NEC Q07.8
nipple Q83.2
nose Q30.1
nuclear Q07.8
organ
  of Corti Q16.5
  or site not listed — *see* Anomaly, by site
osseous meatus (ear) Q16.1
ovary
  bilateral Q50.02
  unilateral Q50.01
oviduct Q50.6
pancreas Q45.0
parathyroid (gland) Q89.2
parotid gland(s) Q38.4
patella Q74.1
pelvic girdle (complete) (partial) Q74.2
penis Q55.5
pericardium Q24.8
pituitary (gland) Q89.2
prostate Q55.4
punctum lacrimale Q10.4
radioulnar — *see* Defect, reduction, upper limb
radius — *see* Defect, reduction, upper limb, longitudinal, radius
rectum Q42.1
  with fistula Q42.0
renal Q60.2
  bilateral Q60.1
  unilateral Q60.0
respiratory organ NEC Q34.8
rib Q76.6
roof of orbit Q75.8
round ligament Q52.8
sacrum Q76.49
salivary gland Q38.4
scapula Q74.0
scrotum Q55.29
seminal vesicles Q55.4
septum
  atrial Q21.1
  between aorta and pulmonary artery Q21.4
  ventricular Q20.4
shoulder girdle (complete) (partial) Q74.0
skull (bone) Q75.8
  with
    anencephaly Q00.0
    encephalocele — *see* Encephalocele
    hydrocephalus Q03.9
      with spina bifida — *see* Spina bifida, by site, with hydrocephalus
    microcephaly Q02
spermatic cord Q55.4
spinal cord Q06.0
spine Q76.49
spleen Q89.01
sternum Q76.7
stomach Q40.2
submaxillary gland(s) (congenital) Q38.4
tarsus — *see* Agenesis, foot
tendon Q79.8
testicle Q55.0
thymus (gland) Q89.2
thyroid (gland) E03.1
  cartilage Q31.8
tibia — *see* Defect, reduction, lower limb, longitudinal, tibia
tibiofibular — *see* Defect, reduction, lower limb, specified type NEC
toe (and foot) (complete) (partial) — *see* Agenesis, foot
tongue Q38.3
trachea (cartilage) Q32.1
ulna — *see* Defect, reduction, upper limb, longitudinal, ulna
upper limb — *see* Agenesis, arm
ureter Q62.4
urethra Q64.5

Agenesis — *continued*
urinary tract NEC Q64.8
uterus Q51.0
uvula Q38.5
vagina Q52.0
vas deferens Q55.4
vein(s) (peripheral) Q27.9
  brain Q28.3
  great NEC Q26.8
  portal Q26.5
vena cava (inferior) (superior) Q26.8
vermis of cerebellum Q04.3
vertebra Q76.49
vulva Q52.71
Ageusia R43.2
Agitated — *see* condition
Agitation R45.1
Aglossia (congenital) Q38.3
Aglossia-adactylia syndrome Q87.0
Aglycogenosis E74.00
Agnosia (body image) (other senses) (tactile) R48.1
  developmental F88
  verbal R48.1
    auditory R48.1
      developmental F80.2
    developmental F80.2
  visual (object) R48.3
Agoraphobia F40.00
  with panic disorder F40.01
  without panic disorder F40.02
Agrammatism R48.8
Agranulocytopenia — *see* Agranulocytosis
Agranulocytosis (chronic) (cyclical) (genetic) (infantile) (periodic) (pernicious) — *see also* Neutropenia D70.9
  congenital D70.0
  cytoreductive cancer chemotherapy sequela D70.1
  drug-induced D70.2
    due to cytoreductive cancer chemotherapy D70.1
  due to infection D70.3
  secondary D70.4
    drug-induced D70.2
      due to cytoreductive cancer chemotherapy D70.1
Agraphia (absolute) R48.8
  with alexia R48.0
  developmental F81.81
Ague (dumb) — *see* Malaria
Agyria Q04.3
Ahumada-del Castillo syndrome E23.0
Aichomophobia F40.298
AIDS (related complex) B20
Ailment heart — *see* Disease, heart
Ailurophobia F40.218
AIN — *see* Neoplasia, intraepithelial, anal
Ainhum (disease) L94.6
AIPHI (acute idiopathic pulmonary hemorrhage in infants (over 28 days old)) R04.81
Air
  anterior mediastinum J98.2
  compressed, disease T70.3 ☑
  conditioner lung or pneumonitis J67.7
  embolism (artery) (cerebral) (any site) T79.0 ☑
    with ectopic or molar pregnancy O08.2
    due to implanted device NEC — *see* Complications, by site and type, specified NEC
    following
      abortion — *see* Abortion by type, complicated by, embolism
      ectopic or molar pregnancy O08.2
    infusion, therapeutic injection or transfusion T80.0 ☑
    in pregnancy, childbirth or puerperium — *see* Embolism, obstetric
    traumatic T79.0 ☑
  hunger, psychogenic F45.8
  rarefied, effects of — *see* Effect, adverse, high altitude
  sickness T75.3 ☑
Airplane sickness T75.3 ☑
Akathisia (drug-induced) (treatment-induced) G25.71
  neuroleptic induced (acute) G25.71
  tardive G25.71
Akinesia R29.898
Akinetic mutism R41.89
Akureyri's disease G93.3
Alactasia, congenital E73.0
Alagille's syndrome Q44.7
Alastrim B03

Index

Agenesis — Alastrim

Blood alch level Y90. (handwritten)

Albers-Schönberg syndrome Q78.2
Albert's syndrome — *see* Tendinitis, Achilles
Albinism, albino E70.30
  with hematologic abnormality E70.339
    Chédiak-Higashi syndrome E70.330
    Hermansky-Pudlak syndrome E70.331
    other specified E70.338
  I E70.320
  II E70.321
  ocular E70.319
    autosomal recessive E70.311
    other specified E70.318
    X-linked E70.310
  oculocutaneous E70.329
    other specified E70.328
    tyrosinase (ty) negative E70.320
    tyrosinase (ty) positive E70.321
  other specified E70.39
Albinismus E70.30
Albright (-McCune)(-Sternberg) syndrome Q78.1
Albuminous — *see* condition
Albuminuria, albuminuric (acute) (chronic) (subacute)
  — *see also* Proteinuria R80.9
  complicating pregnancy — *see* Proteinuria, gestational
    with
      gestational hypertension — *see* Pre-eclampsia
      pre-existing hypertension — *see* Hypertension,
        complicating pregnancy, pre-existing,
        with, pre-eclampsia
  gestational — *see* Proteinuria, gestational
    with
      gestational hypertension — *see* Pre-eclampsia
      pre-existing hypertension — *see* Hypertension,
        complicating pregnancy, pre-existing,
        with, pre-eclampsia
  orthostatic R80.2
  postural R80.2
  pre-eclamptic — *see* Pre-eclampsia
  scarlatinal A38.8
Albuminurophobia F40.298
Alcaptonuria E70.29
Alcohol, alcoholic, alcohol-induced
  addiction (without remission) F10.20
    with remission F10.21
  amnestic disorder, persisting F10.96
    with dependence F10.26
  anxiety disorder F10.980
  bipolar and related disorder F10.94
  brain syndrome, chronic F10.97
    with dependence F10.27
  cardiopathy I42.6
  counseling and surveillance Z71.41
    family member Z71.42
  delirium (acute) (tremens) (withdrawal) F10.231
    with intoxication F10.921
      in
        abuse F10.121
        dependence F10.221
  dementia F10.97
    with dependence F10.27
  depressive disorder F10.94
  deterioration F10.97
    with dependence F10.27
  hallucinosis (acute) F10.951
    in
      abuse F10.151
      dependence F10.251
  insanity F10.959
  intoxication (acute) (without dependence) F10.129
    with
      delirium F10.121
      dependence F10.229
        with delirium F10.221
        uncomplicated F10.220
      uncomplicated F10.120
  jealousy F10.988
  Korsakoff's, Korsakov's, Korsakow's F10.26
  liver K70.9
    acute — *see* Disease, liver, alcoholic, hepatitis
  major neurocognitive disorder, amnestic-confabulatory
    type F10.96
  major neurocognitive disorder, nonamnestic-confabu-
    latory type F10.97
  mania (acute) (chronic) F10.959
  mild neurocognitive disorder F10.988
  paranoia, paranoid (type) psychosis F10.950
  pellagra E52

Alcohol, alcoholic, alcohol-induced — *continued*
  poisoning, accidental (acute) NEC — *see* Table of Drugs
    and Chemicals, alcohol, poisoning
  psychosis — *see* Psychosis, alcoholic
  psychotic disorder F10.959
  sexual dysfunction F10.981
  sleep disorder F10.982
  withdrawal (without convulsions) F10.239
    with delirium F10.231
Alcoholism (chronic) (without remission) F10.20
  with
    psychosis — *see* Psychosis, alcoholic
    remission F10.21
  Korsakov's F10.96
    with dependence F10.26
Alder (-Reilly) **anomaly or syndrome** (leukocyte granulation) D72.0
Aldosteronism E26.9
  familial (type I) E26.02
  glucocorticoid-remediable E26.02
  primary (due to (bilateral) adrenal hyperplasia) E26.09
  primary NEC E26.09
  secondary E26.1
  specified NEC E26.89
Aldosteronoma D44.10
Aldrich (-Wiskott) **syndrome** (eczema-thrombocytopenia) D82.0
Alektorophobia F40.218
Aleppo boil B55.1
Aleukemic — *see* condition
Aleukia
  congenital D70.0
  hemorrhagica D61.9
    congenital D61.09
  splenica D73.1
Alexia R48.0
  developmental F81.0
  secondary to organic lesion R48.0
Algoneurodystrophy M89.00
  ankle M89.07- ☑
  foot M89.07- ☑
  forearm M89.03- ☑
  hand M89.04- ☑
  lower leg M89.06- ☑
  multiple sites M89.0- ☑
  shoulder M89.01- ☑
  specified site NEC M89.08
  thigh M89.05- ☑
  upper arm M89.02- ☑
Algophobia F40.298
Alienation, mental — *see* Psychosis
Alkalemia E87.3
Alkalosis E87.3
  metabolic E87.3
    with respiratory acidosis E87.4
    of newborn P74.41
  respiratory E87.3
Alkaptonuria E70.29
Allen-Masters syndrome N83.8
Allergy, allergic (reaction) (to) T78.40 ☑
  air-borne substance NEC (rhinitis) J30.89
  alveolitis (extrinsic) J67.9
    due to
      Aspergillus clavatus J67.4
      Cryptostroma corticale J67.6
      organisms (fungal, thermophilic actinomycete)
        growing in ventilation (air conditioning)
        systems J67.7
    specified type NEC J67.8
  anaphylactic reaction or shock T78.2 ☑
  angioneurotic edema T78.3 ☑
  animal (dander) (epidermal) (hair) (rhinitis) J30.81
  bee sting (anaphylactic shock) — *see* Toxicity, venom,
    arthropod, bee
  biological — *see* Allergy, drug
  colitis — *see also* Colitis, allergic K52.29
  dander (animal) (rhinitis) J30.81
  dandruff (rhinitis) J30.81
  dental restorative material (existing) K08.55
  dermatitis — *see* Dermatitis, contact, allergic
  diathesis — *see* History, allergy
  drug, medicament & biological (any) (external) (inter-
    nal) T78.40 ☑
    correct substance properly administered — *see* Ta-
      ble of Drugs and Chemicals, by drug, adverse
      effect

Allergy, allergic — *continued*
  drug, medicament & biological — *continued*
    wrong substance given or taken NEC (by accident)
      — *see* Table of Drugs and Chemicals, by drug,
      poisoning
  due to pollen J30.1
  dust (house) (stock) (rhinitis) J30.89
    with asthma — *see* Asthma, allergic extrinsic
  eczema — *see* Dermatitis, contact, allergic
  epidermal (animal) (rhinitis) J30.81
  feathers (rhinitis) J30.89
  food (any) (ingested) NEC T78.1 ☑
    anaphylactic shock — *see* Shock, anaphylactic, due
      to food
    dermatitis — *see* Dermatitis, due to, food
    dietary counseling and surveillance Z71.3
    in contact with skin L23.6
    rhinitis J30.5
    status (without reaction) Z91.018
      eggs Z91.012
      milk products Z91.011
      peanuts Z91.010
      seafood Z91.013
      specified NEC Z91.018
  gastrointestinal — *see also* specific type of allergic re-
    action
    meaning colitis — *see also* Colitis, allergic K52.29
    meaning gastroenteritis — *see also* Gastroenteritis,
      allergic K52.29
    meaning other adverse food reaction not elsewhere
      classified T78.1 ☑
  grain J30.1
  grass (hay fever) (pollen) J30.1
    asthma — *see* Asthma, allergic extrinsic
  hair (animal) (rhinitis) J30.81
  history (of) — *see* History, allergy
  horse serum — *see* Allergy, serum
  inhalant (rhinitis) J30.89
    pollen J30.1
  kapok (rhinitis) J30.89
  medicine — *see* Allergy, drug
  milk protein — *see also* Allergy, food Z91.011
    anaphylactic reaction T78.07 ☑
    dermatitis L27.2
    enterocolitis syndrome K52.21
    enteropathy K52.22
    gastroenteritis K52.29
    gastroesophageal reflux — *see also* Reaction, ad-
      verse, food K21.9
      with esophagitis K21.0
    proctocolitis K52.82
  nasal, seasonal due to pollen J30.1
  pneumonia J82
  pollen (any) (hay fever) J30.1
    asthma — *see* Asthma, allergic extrinsic
  primrose J30.1
  primula J30.1
  proctocolitis K52.82
  purpura D69.0
  ragweed (hay fever) (pollen) J30.1
    asthma — *see* Asthma, allergic extrinsic
  rose (pollen) J30.1
  seasonal NEC J30.2
  Senecio jacobae (pollen) J30.1
  serum — *see also* Reaction, serum T80.69 ☑
    anaphylactic shock T80.59 ☑
  shock (anaphylactic) T78.2 ☑
    due to
      administration of blood and blood products
        T80.51 ☑
      adverse effect of correct medicinal substance
        properly administered T88.6 ☑
      immunization T80.52 ☑
      serum NEC T80.59 ☑
      vaccination T80.52 ☑
  specific NEC T78.49 ☑
  tree (any) (hay fever) (pollen) J30.1
    asthma — *see* Asthma, allergic extrinsic
  upper respiratory J30.9
  urticaria L50.0
  vaccine — *see* Allergy, serum
  wheat — *see* Allergy, food
Allescheriasis B48.2
Alligator skin disease Q80.9
Allocheiria, allochiria R20.8
Almeida's disease — *see* Paracoccidioidomycosis
Alopecia (hereditaria) (seborrheica) L65.9

Alopecia — *continued*
  androgenic L64.9
    drug-induced L64.0
    specified NEC L64.8
  areata L63.9
    ophiasis L63.2
    specified NEC L63.8
    totalis L63.0
    universalis L63.1
  cicatricial L66.9
    specified NEC L66.8
  circumscripta L63.9
  congenital, congenitalis Q84.0
  due to cytotoxic drugs NEC L65.8
  mucinosa L65.2
  postinfective NEC L65.8
  postpartum L65.0
  premature L64.8
  specific (syphilitic) A51.32
  specified NEC L65.8
  syphilitic (secondary) A51.32
  totalis (capitis) L63.0
  universalis (entire body) L63.1
  X-ray L58.1
Alpers' disease G31.81
Alpine sickness T70.29 ☑
Alport syndrome Q87.81
ALTE (apparent life threatening event) **in newborn and infant** R68.13
Alteration (of), **Altered**
  awareness
    transient R40.4
    unintended under general anesthesia, during procedure T88.53 ☑
  mental status R41.82
  pattern of family relationships affecting child Z62.898
  sensation
    following
      cerebrovascular disease I69.998
        cerebral infarction I69.398
        intracerebral hemorrhage I69.198
        nontraumatic intracranial hemorrhage NEC I69.298
        specified disease NEC I69.898
        subarachnoid hemorrhage I69.098
Alternating — *see* condition
Altitude, high (effects) — *see* Effect, adverse, high altitude
Aluminosis (of lung) J63.0
Alveolitis
  allergic (extrinsic) — *see* Pneumonitis, hypersensitivity
  due to
    Aspergillus clavatus J67.4
    Cryptostroma corticale J67.6
  fibrosing (cryptogenic) (idiopathic) J84.112
  jaw M27.3
  sicca dolorosa M27.3
Alveolus, alveolar — *see* condition
Alymphocytosis D72.810
  thymic (with immunodeficiency) D82.1
Alymphoplasia, thymic D82.1
Alzheimer's disease or sclerosis — *see* Disease, Alzheimer's
Amastia (with nipple present) Q83.8
  with absent nipple Q83.0
Amathophobia F40.228
Amaurosis (acquired) (congenital) — *see also* Blindness
  fugax G45.3
  hysterical F44.6
  Leber's congenital H35.50
  uremic — *see* Uremia
Amaurotic idiocy (infantile) (juvenile) (late) E75.4
Amaxophobia F40.248
Ambiguous genitalia Q56.4
Amblyopia (congenital) (ex anopsia) (partial) (suppression) H53.00- ☑
  anisometropic — *see* Amblyopia, refractive
  deprivation H53.01- ☑
  hysterical F44.6
  nocturnal — *see also* Blindness, night
    vitamin A deficiency E50.5
  refractive H53.02- ☑
  strabismic H53.03- ☑
  suspect H53.04- ☑
  tobacco H53.8
  toxic NEC H53.8
  uremic — *see* Uremia
Ameba, amebic (histolytica) — *see also* Amebiasis

Ameba, amebic — *continued*
  abscess (liver) A06.4
Amebiasis A06.9
  with abscess — *see* Abscess, amebic
  acute A06.0
  chronic (intestine) A06.1
    with abscess — *see* Abscess, amebic
  cutaneous A06.7
  cutis A06.7
  cystitis A06.81
  genitourinary tract NEC A06.82
  hepatic — *see* Abscess, liver, amebic
  intestine A06.0
  nondysenteric colitis A06.2
  skin A06.7
  specified site NEC A06.89
Ameboma (of intestine) A06.3
Amelia Q73.0
  lower limb — *see* Agenesis, leg
  upper limb — *see* Agenesis, arm
Ameloblastoma — *see also* Cyst, calcifying odontogenic
  long bones C40.9- ☑
    lower limb C40.2- ☑
    upper limb C40.0- ☑
  malignant C41.1
    jaw (bone) (lower) C41.1
      upper C41.0
  tibial C40.2- ☑
Amelogenesis imperfecta K00.5
  nonhereditaria (segmentalis) K00.4
Amenorrhea N91.2
  hyperhormonal E28.8
  primary N91.0
  secondary N91.1
Amentia — *see* Disability, intellectual
  Meynert's (nonalcoholic) F04
American
  leishmaniasis B55.2
  mountain tick fever A93.2
Ametropia — *see* Disorder, refraction
AMH (asymptomatic microscopic hematuria) R31.21
Amianthosis J61
Amimia R48.8
Amino-acid disorder E72.9
  anemia D53.0
Aminoacidopathy E72.9
Aminoaciduria E72.9
Amnesia R41.3
  anterograde R41.1
  auditory R48.8
  dissociative F44.0
    with dissociative fugue F44.1
  hysterical F44.0
  postictal in epilepsy — *see* Epilepsy
  psychogenic F44.0
  retrograde R41.2
  transient global G45.4
Amnes(t)ic syndrome (post-traumatic) F04
  induced by
    alcohol F10.96
      with dependence F10.26
    psychoactive NEC F19.96
      with
        abuse F19.16
        dependence F19.26
    sedative F13.96
      with dependence F13.26
Amnion, amniotic — *see* condition
Amnionitis — *see* Pregnancy, complicated by
Amok F68.8
Amoral traits F60.89
Amphetamine (or other stimulant) **-induced**
  anxiety disorder F15.980
  bipolar and related disorder F15.94
  delirium F15.921
  depressive disorder F15.94
  obsessive-compulsive and related disorder F15.988
  psychotic disorder F15.959
  sexual dysfunction F15.981
  sleep disorder F15.982
  stimulant withdrawal F15.23
Ampulla
  lower esophagus K22.8
  phrenic K22.8
Amputation — *see also* Absence, by site, acquired
  neuroma (postoperative) (traumatic) — *see* Complications, amputation stump, neuroma

Amputation — *continued*
  stump (surgical)
    abnormal, painful, or with complication (late) — *see* Complications, amputation stump
    healed or old NOS Z89.9
  traumatic (complete) (partial)
    arm (upper) (complete) S48.91- ☑
      at
        elbow S58.01- ☑
          partial S58.02- ☑
        shoulder joint (complete) S48.01- ☑
          partial S48.02- ☑
      between
        elbow and wrist (complete) S58.11- ☑
          partial S58.12- ☑
        shoulder and elbow (complete) S48.11- ☑
          partial S48.12- ☑
      partial S48.92- ☑
    breast (complete) S28.21- ☑
      partial S28.22- ☑
    clitoris (complete) S38.211
      partial S38.212
    ear (complete) S08.11- ☑
      partial S08.12- ☑
    finger (complete) (metacarpophalangeal) S68.11- ☑
      index S68.11- ☑
      little S68.11- ☑
      middle S68.11- ☑
      partial S68.12- ☑
        index S68.12- ☑
        little S68.12- ☑
        middle S68.12- ☑
        ring S68.12- ☑
      ring S68.11- ☑
      thumb — *see* Amputation, traumatic, thumb
      transphalangeal (complete) S68.61- ☑
        index S68.61- ☑
        little S68.61- ☑
        middle S68.61- ☑
        partial S68.62- ☑
          index S68.62- ☑
          little S68.62- ☑
          middle S68.62- ☑
          ring S68.62- ☑
        ring S68.61- ☑
    foot (complete) S98.91- ☑
      at ankle level S98.01- ☑
        partial S98.02- ☑
      midfoot S98.31- ☑
        partial S98.32- ☑
      partial S98.92- ☑
    forearm (complete) S58.91- ☑
      at elbow level (complete) S58.01- ☑
        partial S58.02- ☑
      between elbow and wrist (complete) S58.11- ☑
        partial S58.12- ☑
      partial S58.92- ☑
    genital organ(s) (external)
      female (complete) S38.211
        partial S38.212
      male
        penis (complete) S38.221
          partial S38.222
        scrotum (complete) S38.231
          partial S38.232
        testes (complete) S38.231
          partial S38.232
    hand (complete) (wrist level) S68.41- ☑
      finger(s) alone — *see* Amputation, traumatic, finger
      partial S68.42- ☑
      thumb alone — *see* Amputation, traumatic, thumb
      transmetacarpal (complete) S68.71- ☑
        partial S68.72- ☑
    head
      ear — *see* Amputation, traumatic, ear
      nose (partial) S08.812
        complete S08.811
      part S08.89
        scalp S08.0 ☑
    hip (and thigh) (complete) S78.91- ☑
      at hip joint (complete) S78.01- ☑
        partial S78.02- ☑
      between hip and knee (complete) S78.11- ☑
        partial S78.12- ☑

▽ Subterms under main terms may continue to next column or page   ☑ **Additional Character Required** — **Refer to the Tabular List for Character Selection**   **17**

Alopecia — Amputation

Amputation — *continued*
  traumatic — *continued*
    hip — *continued*
      partial S78.92- ☑
    labium (majus) (minus) (complete) S38.21- ☑
      partial S38.21- ☑
    leg (lower) S88.91- ☑
      at knee level S88.01- ☑
        partial S88.02- ☑
      between knee and ankle S88.11- ☑
        partial S88.12- ☑
      partial S88.92- ☑
    nose (partial) S08.812 ☑
      complete S08.811 ☑
    penis (complete) S38.221 ☑
      partial S38.222 ☑
    scrotum (complete) S38.231 ☑
      partial S38.232 ☑
    shoulder — *see* Amputation, traumatic, arm
      at shoulder joint — *see* Amputation, traumatic, arm, at shoulder joint
    testes (complete) S38.231 ☑
      partial S38.232 ☑
    thigh — *see* Amputation, traumatic, hip
    thorax, part of S28.1 ☑
      breast — *see* Amputation, traumatic, breast
    thumb (complete) (metacarpophalangeal) S68.01- ☑
      partial S68.02- ☑
      transphalangeal (complete) S68.51- ☑
        partial S68.52- ☑
    toe (lesser) S98.13- ☑
      great S98.11- ☑
        partial S98.12- ☑
      more than one S98.21- ☑
        partial S98.22- ☑
      partial S98.14- ☑
    vulva (complete) S38.211 ☑
      partial S38.212 ☑
Amputee (bilateral) (old) Z89.9
Amsterdam dwarfism Q87.19
Amusia R48.8
  developmental F80.89
Amyelencephalus, amyelencephaly Q00.0
Amyelia Q06.0
Amygdalitis — *see* Tonsillitis
Amygdalolith J35.8
Amyloid heart (disease) E85.4 *[I43]*
Amyloidosis (generalized) (primary) E85.9
  with lung involvement E85.4 *[J99]*
  familial E85.2
  genetic E85.2
  heart E85.4 *[I43]*
  hemodialysis-associated E85.3
  light chain (AL) E85.81
  liver E85.4 *[K77]*
  localized E85.4
  neuropathic heredofamilial E85.1
  non-neuropathic heredofamilial E85.0
  organ limited E85.4
  Portuguese E85.1
  pulmonary E85.4 *[J99]*
  secondary systemic E85.3
  senile systemic (SSA) E85.82
  skin (lichen) (macular) E85.4 *[L99]*
  specified NEC E85.89
  subglottic E85.4 *[J99]*
  wild-type transthyretin-related (ATTR) E85.82
Amylopectinosis (brancher enzyme deficiency) E74.03
Amylophagia — *see* Pica
Amyoplasia congenita Q79.8
Amyotonia M62.89
  congenita G70.2
Amyotrophia, amyotrophy, amyotrophic G71.8
  congenita Q79.8
  diabetic — *see* Diabetes, amyotrophy
  lateral sclerosis G12.21
  neuralgic G54.5
  spinal progressive G12.25
Anacidity, gastric K31.83
  psychogenic F45.8
Anaerosis of newborn P28.89
Analbuminemia E88.09
Analgesia — *see* Anesthesia
Analphalipoproteinemia E78.6
Anaphylactic
  purpura D69.0

Anaphylactic — *continued*
  shock or reaction — *see* Shock, anaphylactic
Anaphylactoid shock or reaction — *see* Shock, anaphylactic
Anaphylactoid syndrome of pregnancy O88.01- ☑
Anaphylaxis — *see* Shock, anaphylactic
Anaplasia cervix — *see also* Dysplasia, cervix N87.9
Anaplasmosis, human A77.49
Anarthria R47.1
Anasarca R60.1
  cardiac — *see* Failure, heart, congestive
  lung J18.2
  newborn P83.2
  nutritional E43
  pulmonary J18.2
  renal N04.9
Anastomosis
  aneurysmal — *see* Aneurysm
  arteriovenous ruptured brain I60.8
    intracerebral I61.8
    intraparenchymal I61.8
    intraventricular I61.5
    subarachnoid I60.8
  intestinal K63.89
    complicated NEC K91.89
      involving urinary tract N99.89
  retinal and choroidal vessels (congenital) Q14.8
Anatomical narrow angle H40.03- ☑
Ancylostoma, ancylostomiasis (braziliense) (caninum) (ceylanicum) (duodenale) B76.0
  Necator americanus B76.1
Andersen's disease (glycogen storage) E74.09
Anderson-Fabry disease E75.21
Andes disease T70.29 ☑
Andrews' disease (bacterid) L08.89
Androblastoma
  benign
    specified site — *see* Neoplasm, benign, by site
    unspecified site
      female D27.9
      male D29.20
  malignant
    specified site — *see* Neoplasm, malignant, by site
    unspecified site
      female C56.9
      male C62.90
  specified site — *see* Neoplasm, uncertain behavior, by site
  tubular
    with lipid storage
      specified site — *see* Neoplasm, benign, by site
      unspecified site
        female D27.9
        male D29.20
    specified site — *see* Neoplasm, benign, by site
    unspecified site
      female D27.9
      male D29.20
  unspecified site
    female D39.10
    male D40.10
Androgen insensitivity syndrome — *see also* Syndrome, androgen insensitivity E34.50
Androgen resistance syndrome — *see also* Syndrome, androgen insensitivity E34.50
Android pelvis Q74.2
  with disproportion (fetopelvic) O33.3 ☑
    causing obstructed labor O65.3
Androphobia F40.290
Anectasis, pulmonary (newborn) — *see* Atelectasis
Anemia (essential) (general) (hemoglobin deficiency) (infantile) (primary) (profound) D64.9
  with (due to) (in)
    disorder of
      anaerobic glycolysis D55.2
      pentose phosphate pathway D55.1
    koilonychia D50.9
  achlorhydric D50.8
  achrestic D53.1
  Addison (-Biermer) (pernicious) D51.0
  agranulocytic — *see* Agranulocytosis
  amino-acid-deficiency D53.0
  aplastic D61.9
    congenital D61.09
    drug-induced D61.1
    due to
      drugs D61.1
      external agents NEC D61.2

Anemia — *continued*
  aplastic — *continued*
    due to — *continued*
      infection D61.2
      radiation D61.2
    idiopathic D61.3
    red cell (pure) D60.9
      chronic D60.0
      congenital D61.01
      specified type NEC D60.8
      transient D60.1
    specified type NEC D61.89
    toxic D61.2
  aregenerative
    congenital D61.09
  asiderotic D50.9
  atypical (primary) D64.9
  Baghdad spring D55.0
  Balantidium coli A07.0
  Biermer's (pernicious) D51.0
  blood loss (chronic) D50.0
    acute D62
  bothriocephalus B70.0 *[D63.8]*
  brickmaker's B76.9 *[D63.8]*
  cerebral I67.89
  childhood D58.9
  chlorotic D50.8
  chronic
    blood loss D50.0
    hemolytic D58.9
      idiopathic D59.9
    simple D53.9
  chronica congenita aregenerativa D61.09
  combined system disease NEC D51.0 *[G32.0]*
    due to dietary vitamin B12 deficiency D51.3 *[G32.0]*
  complicating pregnancy, childbirth or puerperium — *see* Pregnancy, complicated by (management affected by), anemia
  congenital P61.4
    aplastic D61.09
    due to isoimmunization NOS P55.9
    dyserythropoietic, dyshematopoietic D64.4
    following fetal blood loss P61.3
    Heinz body D58.2
    hereditary hemolytic NOS D58.9
    pernicious D51.0
    spherocytic D58.0
  Cooley's (erythroblastic) D56.1
  cytogenic D51.0
  deficiency D53.9
    2, 3 diphosphoglycurate mutase D55.2
    2, 3 PG D55.2
    6 phosphogluconate dehydrogenase D55.1
    6-PGD D55.1
    amino-acid D53.0
    combined B12 and folate D53.1
    enzyme D55.9
      drug-induced (hemolytic) D59.2
      glucose-6-phosphate dehydrogenase (G6PD) D55.0
      glycolytic D55.2
      nucleotide metabolism D55.3
      related to hexose monophosphate (HMP) shunt pathway NEC D55.1
      specified type NEC D55.8
    erythrocytic glutathione D55.1
    folate D52.9
      dietary D52.0
      drug-induced D52.1
    folic acid D52.9
      dietary D52.0
      drug-induced D52.1
    G SH D55.1
    G6PD D55.0
    GGS-R D55.1
    glucose-6-phosphate dehydrogenase D55.0
    glutathione reductase D55.1
    glyceraldehyde phosphate dehydrogenase D55.2
    hexokinase D55.2
    iron D50.9
      secondary to blood loss (chronic) D50.0
    nutritional D53.9
      with
        poor iron absorption D50.8
        specified deficiency NEC D53.8
    phosphofructo-aldolase D55.2
    phosphoglycerate kinase D55.2
    PK D55.2
    protein D53.0

☑ **Additional Character Required** — **Refer to the Tabular List for Character Selection**   ▽ **Subterms under main terms may continue to next column or page**

Anemia — *continued*
  deficiency — *continued*
    pyruvate kinase D55.2
    transcobalamin II D51.2
    triose-phosphate isomerase D55.2
    vitamin B12 NOS D51.9
      dietary D51.3
      due to
        intrinsic factor deficiency D51.0
        selective vitamin B12 malabsorption with
          proteinuria D51.1
      pernicious D51.0
      specified type NEC D51.8
  Diamond-Blackfan (congenital hypoplastic) D61.01
  dibothriocephalus B70.0 *[D63.8]*
  dimorphic D53.1
  diphasic D53.1
  Diphyllobothrium (Dibothriocephalus) B70.0 *[D63.8]*
  due to (in) (with)
    antineoplastic chemotherapy D64.81
    blood loss (chronic) D50.0
      acute D62
    chemotherapy, antineoplastic D64.81
    chronic disease classified elsewhere NEC D63.8
    chronic kidney disease D63.1
    deficiency
      amino-acid D53.0
      copper D53.8
      folate (folic acid) D52.9
        dietary D52.0
        drug-induced D52.1
      molybdenum D53.8
      protein D53.0
      zinc D53.8
    dietary vitamin B12 deficiency D51.3
    disorder of
      glutathione metabolism D55.1
      nucleotide metabolism D55.3
    drug — *see* Anemia, by type — *see also* Table of
      Drugs and Chemicals
    end stage renal disease D63.1
    enzyme disorder D55.9
    fetal blood loss P61.3
    fish tapeworm (D.latum) infestation B70.0 *[D63.8]*
    hemorrhage (chronic) D50.0
      acute D62
    impaired absorption D50.9
    loss of blood (chronic) D50.0
      acute D62
    myxedema E03.9 *[D63.8]*
    Necator americanus B76.1 *[D63.8]*
    prematurity P61.2
    selective vitamin B12 malabsorption with protein-
      uria D51.1
    transcobalamin II deficiency D51.2
  Dyke-Young type (secondary) (symptomatic) D59.1
  dyserythropoietic (congenital) D64.4
  dyshematopoietic (congenital) D64.4
  Egyptian B76.9 *[D63.8]*
  elliptocytosis — *see* Elliptocytosis
  enzyme-deficiency, drug-induced D59.2
  epidemic — *see also* Ancylostomiasis B76.9 *[D63.8]*
  erythroblastic
    familial D56.1
    newborn — *see also* Disease, hemolytic P55.9
    of childhood D56.1
  erythrocytic glutathione deficiency D55.1
  erythropoietin-resistant anemia (EPO resistant anemia)
    D63.1
  Faber's (achlorhydric anemia) D50.9
  factitious (self-induced blood letting) D50.0
  familial erythroblastic D56.1
  Fanconi's (congenital pancytopenia) D61.09
  favism D55.0
  fish tapeworm (D. latum) infestation B70.0 *[D63.8]*
  folate (folic acid) deficiency D52.9
  glucose-6-phosphate dehydrogenase (G6PD) deficiency
    D55.0
  glutathione-reductase deficiency D55.1
  goat's milk D52.0
  granulocytic — *see* Agranulocytosis
  Heinz body, congenital D58.2
  hemolytic D58.9
    acquired D59.9
      with hemoglobinuria NEC D59.6
      autoimmune NEC D59.1
      infectious D59.4
      specified type NEC D59.8

Anemia — *continued*
  hemolytic — *continued*
    acquired — *continued*
      toxic D59.4
    acute D59.9
      due to enzyme deficiency specified type NEC
        D55.8
      Lederer's D59.1
    autoimmune D59.1
      drug-induced D59.0
    chronic D58.9
      idiopathic D59.9
    cold type (secondary) (symptomatic) D59.1
    congenital (spherocytic) — *see* Spherocytosis
    due to
      cardiac conditions D59.4
      drugs (nonautoimmune) D59.2
        autoimmune D59.0
      enzyme disorder D55.9
        drug-induced D59.2
      presence of shunt or other internal prosthetic
        device D59.4
    familial D58.9
    hereditary D58.9
      due to enzyme disorder D55.9
        specified type NEC D55.8
      specified type NEC D58.8
    idiopathic (chronic) D59.9
    mechanical D59.4
    microangiopathic D59.4
    nonautoimmune D59.4
      drug-induced D59.2
    nonspherocytic
      congenital or hereditary NEC D55.8
        glucose-6-phosphate dehydrogenase deficien-
          cy D55.0
        pyruvate kinase deficiency D55.2
        type
          I D55.1
          II D55.2
      type
        I D55.1
        II D55.2
    secondary D59.4
      autoimmune D59.1
    specified (hereditary) type NEC D58.8
    Stransky-Regala type — *see also* Hemoglobinopathy
      D58.8
    symptomatic D59.4
      autoimmune D59.1
    toxic D59.4
    warm type (secondary) (symptomatic) D59.1
  hemorrhagic (chronic) D50.0
    acute D62
  Herrick's D57.1
  hexokinase deficiency D55.2
  hookworm B76.9 *[D63.8]*
  hypochromic (idiopathic) (microcytic) (normoblastic)
    D50.9
    due to blood loss (chronic) D50.0
      acute D62
    familial sex-linked D64.0
    pyridoxine-responsive D64.3
    sideroblastic, sex-linked D64.0
  hypoplasia, red blood cells D61.9
    congenital or familial D61.01
  hypoplastic (idiopathic) D61.9
    congenital or familial (of childhood) D61.01
  hypoproliferative (refractive) D61.9
  idiopathic D64.9
    aplastic D61.3
    hemolytic, chronic D59.9
  in (due to) (with)
    chronic kidney disease D63.1
    end stage renal disease D63.1
    failure, kidney (renal) D63.1
    neoplastic disease — *see also* Neoplasm D63.0
  intertropical — *see also* Ancylostomiasis D63.8
  iron deficiency D50.9
    secondary to blood loss (chronic) D50.0
      acute D62
    specified type NEC D50.8
  Joseph-Diamond-Blackfan (congenital hypoplastic)
    D61.01
  Lederer's (hemolytic) D59.1
  leukoerythroblastic D61.82
  macrocytic D53.9
    nutritional D52.0
    tropical D52.8

Anemia — *continued*
  malarial — *see also* Malaria B54 *[D63.8]*
  malignant (progressive) D51.0
  malnutrition D53.9
  marsh — *see also* Malaria B54 *[D63.8]*
  Mediterranean (with other hemoglobinopathy) D56.9
  megaloblastic D53.1
    combined B12 and folate deficiency D53.1
    hereditary D51.1
    nutritional D52.0
    orotic aciduria D53.0
    refractory D53.1
    specified type NEC D53.1
  megalocytic D53.1
  microcytic (hypochromic) D50.9
    due to blood loss (chronic) D50.0
      acute D62
    familial D56.8
  microdrepanocytosis D57.40
  microelliptopoikilocytic (Rietti-Greppi- Micheli) D56.9
  miner's B76.9 *[D63.8]*
  myelodysplastic D46.9
  myelofibrosis D75.81
  myelogenous D64.89
  myelopathic D64.89
  myelophthisic D61.82
  myeloproliferative D47.Z9 (*following* D47.4)
  newborn P61.4
    due to
      ABO (antibodies, isoimmunization, maternal/fetal
        incompatibility) P55.1
      Rh (antibodies, isoimmunization, maternal/fetal
        incompatibility) P55.0
    following fetal blood loss P61.3
    posthemorrhagic (fetal) P61.3
  nonspherocytic hemolytic — *see* Anemia, hemolytic,
    nonspherocytic
  normocytic (infectional) D64.9
    due to blood loss (chronic) D50.0
      acute D62
    myelophthisic D61.82
  nutritional (deficiency) D53.9
    with
      poor iron absorption D50.8
      specified deficiency NEC D53.8
    megaloblastic D52.0
  of prematurity P61.2
  orotaciduric (congenital) (hereditary) D53.0
  osteosclerotic D64.89
  ovalocytosis (hereditary) — *see* Elliptocytosis
  paludal — *see also* Malaria B54 *[D63.8]*
  pernicious (congenital) (malignant) (progressive) D51.0
  pleochromic D64.89
    of sprue D52.8
  posthemorrhagic (chronic) D50.0
    acute D62
    newborn P61.3
  postoperative (postprocedural)
    due to (acute) blood loss D62
      chronic blood loss D50.0
    specified NEC D64.9
  postpartum O90.81
  pressure D64.89
  progressive D64.9
    malignant D51.0
    pernicious D51.0
  protein-deficiency D53.0
  pseudoleukemica infantum D64.89
  pure red cell D60.9
    congenital D61.01
  pyridoxine-responsive D64.3
  pyruvate kinase deficiency D55.2
  refractory D46.4
    with
      excess of blasts D46.20
        1 (RAEB 1) D46.21
        2 (RAEB 2) D46.22
        in transformation (RAEB T) — *see* Leukemia,
          acute myeloblastic
      hemochromatosis D46.1
      sideroblasts (ring) (RARS) D46.1
    megaloblastic D53.1
    sideroblastic D46.1
    sideropenic D50.9
    without ring sideroblasts, so stated D46.0
    without sideroblasts without excess of blasts D46.0
  Rietti-Greppi-Micheli D56.9
  scorbutic D53.2

Anemia — *continued*
- secondary to
  - blood loss (chronic) D50.0
    - acute D62
  - hemorrhage (chronic) D50.0
    - acute D62
- semiplastic D61.89
- sickle-cell — *see* Disease, sickle-cell
- sideroblastic D64.3
  - hereditary D64.0
  - hypochromic, sex-linked D64.0
  - pyridoxine-responsive NEC D64.3
  - refractory D46.1
  - secondary (due to)
    - disease D64.1
    - drugs and toxins D64.2
  - specified type NEC D64.3
- sideropenic (refractory) D50.9
  - due to blood loss (chronic) D50.0
    - acute D62
- simple chronic D53.9
- specified type NEC D64.89
- spherocytic (hereditary) — *see* Spherocytosis
- splenic D64.89
- splenomegalic D64.89
- stomatocytosis D58.8
- syphilitic (acquired) (late) A52.79 *[D63.8]*
- target cell D64.89
- thalassemia D56.9
- thrombocytopenic — *see* Thrombocytopenia
- toxic D61.2
- tropical B76.9 *[D63.8]*
  - macrocytic D52.8
- tuberculous A18.89 *[D63.8]*
- vegan D51.3
- vitamin
  - B12 deficiency (dietary) pernicious D51.0
  - B6-responsive D64.3
- von Jaksch's D64.89
- Witts' (achlorhydric anemia) D50.8

Anemophobia F40.228

Anencephalus, anencephaly Q00.0

Anergasia — *see* Psychosis, organic

Anesthesia, anesthetic R20.0
- complication or reaction NEC — *see also* Complications, anesthesia T88.59 ☑
  - due to
    - correct substance properly administered — *see* Table of Drugs and Chemicals, by drug, adverse effect
    - overdose or wrong substance given — *see* Table of Drugs and Chemicals, by drug, poisoning
  - unintended awareness under general anesthesia during procedure T88.53 ☑
    - personal history of Z92.84
- cornea H18.81- ☑
- dissociative F44.6
- functional (hysterical) F44.6
- hyperesthetic, thalamic G89.0
- hysterical F44.6
- local skin lesion R20.0
- sexual (psychogenic) F52.1
- shock (due to) T88.2 ☑
- skin R20.0
- testicular N50.9

Anetoderma (maculosum) (of) L90.8
- Jadassohn-Pellizzari L90.2
- Schweniger-Buzzi L90.1

Aneurin deficiency E51.9

Aneurysm (anastomotic) (artery) (cirsoid) (diffuse) (false) (fusiform) (multiple) (saccular) I72.9
- abdominal (aorta) I71.4
  - ruptured I71.3
  - syphilitic A52.01
- aorta, aortic (nonsyphilitic) I71.9
  - abdominal I71.4
    - ruptured I71.3
  - arch I71.2
    - ruptured I71.1
  - arteriosclerotic I71.9
    - ruptured I71.8
  - ascending I71.2
    - ruptured I71.1
  - congenital Q25.43
  - descending I71.9
    - abdominal I71.4
      - ruptured I71.3

Aneurysm — *continued*
- aorta, aortic — *continued*
  - descending — *continued*
    - ruptured I71.8
    - thoracic I71.2
      - ruptured I71.1
  - root Q25.43
  - ruptured I71.8
  - sinus, congenital Q25.43
  - syphilitic A52.01
  - thoracic I71.2
    - ruptured I71.1
  - thoracoabdominal I71.6
    - ruptured I71.5
  - thorax, thoracic (arch) I71.2
    - ruptured I71.1
  - transverse I71.2
    - ruptured I71.1
  - valve (heart) — *see also* Endocarditis, aortic I35.8
- arteriosclerotic I72.9
  - cerebral I67.1
    - ruptured — *see* Hemorrhage, intracranial, sub-arachnoid
- arteriovenous (congenital) — *see also* Malformation, arteriovenous
  - acquired I77.0
    - brain I67.1
      - ruptured — *see* Aneurysm, arteriovenous, brain, ruptured
    - coronary I25.41
    - pulmonary I28.0
  - brain Q28.2
    - ruptured I60.8
      - intracerebral I61.8
      - intraparenchymal I61.8
      - intraventricular I61.5
      - subarachnoid I60.8
  - peripheral — *see* Malformation, arteriovenous, peripheral
  - precerebral vessels Q28.0
  - specified site NEC — *see also* Malformation, arteriovenous
    - acquired I77.0
- basal — *see* Aneurysm, brain
- basilar (trunk) I72.5
- berry (congenital) (nonruptured) I67.1
  - ruptured I60.7
- brain I67.1
  - arteriosclerotic I67.1
    - ruptured — *see* Hemorrhage, intracranial, sub-arachnoid
  - arteriovenous (congenital) (nonruptured) Q28.2
    - acquired I67.1
      - ruptured — *see* Aneurysm, arteriovenous, brain, ruptured I60.8
    - ruptured — *see* Aneurysm, arteriovenous, brain, ruptured I60.8
  - berry (congenital) (nonruptured) I67.1
    - ruptured — *see also* Hemorrhage, intracranial, subarachnoid I60.7
  - congenital Q28.3
    - ruptured I60.7
  - meninges I67.1
    - ruptured I60.8
  - miliary (congenital) (nonruptured) I67.1
    - ruptured — *see also* Hemorrhage, intracranial, subarachnoid I60.7
  - mycotic I33.0
  - ruptured — *see* Aneurysm, arteriovenous, brain, ruptured I60.8
  - syphilitic (hemorrhage) A52.05
- cardiac (false) — *see also* Aneurysm, heart I25.3
- carotid artery (common) (external) I72.0
  - internal (intracranial) I67.1
    - extracranial portion I72.0
    - ruptured into brain I60.0- ☑
  - syphilitic A52.09
    - intracranial A52.05
- cavernous sinus I67.1
  - arteriovenous (congenital) (nonruptured) Q28.3
    - ruptured I60.8
- celiac I72.8
- central nervous system, syphilitic A52.05
- cerebral — *see* Aneurysm, brain
- chest — *see* Aneurysm, thorax
- circle of Willis I67.1
  - congenital Q28.3
    - ruptured I60.6

Aneurysm — *continued*
- circle of Willis — *continued*
  - ruptured I60.6
- common iliac artery I72.3
- congenital (peripheral) Q27.8
  - aorta (root) (sinus) Q25.43
  - brain Q28.3
    - ruptured I60.7
  - coronary Q24.5
  - digestive system Q27.8
  - lower limb Q27.8
  - pulmonary Q25.79
  - retina Q14.1
  - specified site NEC Q27.8
  - upper limb Q27.8
- conjunctiva — *see* Abnormality, conjunctiva, vascular
- conus arteriosus — *see* Aneurysm, heart
- coronary (arteriosclerotic) (artery) I25.41
  - arteriovenous, congenital Q24.5
  - congenital Q24.5
  - ruptured — *see* Infarct, myocardium
  - syphilitic A52.06
  - vein I25.89
- cylindroid (aorta) I71.9
  - ruptured I71.8
  - syphilitic A52.01
- ductus arteriosus Q25.0
- endocardial, infective (any valve) I33.0
- femoral (artery) (ruptured) I72.4
- gastroduodenal I72.8
- gastroepiploic I72.8
- heart (wall) (chronic or with a stated duration of over 4 weeks) I25.3
  - valve — *see* Endocarditis
- hepatic I72.8
- iliac (common) (artery) (ruptured) I72.3
- infective I72.9
  - endocardial (any valve) I33.0
- innominate (nonsyphilitic) I72.8
  - syphilitic A52.09
- interauricular septum — *see* Aneurysm, heart
- interventricular septum — *see* Aneurysm, heart
- intrathoracic (nonsyphilitic) I71.2
  - ruptured I71.1
  - syphilitic A52.01
- lower limb I72.4
- lung (pulmonary artery) I28.1
- mediastinal (nonsyphilitic) I72.8
  - syphilitic A52.09
- miliary (congenital) I67.1
  - ruptured — *see* Hemorrhage, intracerebral, subarachnoid, intracranial
- mitral (heart) (valve) I34.8
- mural — *see* Aneurysm, heart
- mycotic I72.9
  - endocardial (any valve) I33.0
  - ruptured, brain — *see* Hemorrhage, intracerebral, subarachnoid
- myocardium — *see* Aneurysm, heart
- neck I72.0
- pancreaticoduodenal I72.8
- patent ductus arteriosus Q25.0
- peripheral NEC I72.8
  - congenital Q27.8
    - digestive system Q27.8
    - lower limb Q27.8
    - specified site NEC Q27.8
    - upper limb Q27.8
- popliteal (artery) (ruptured) I72.4
- precerebral
  - congenital (nonruptured) Q28.1
  - specified site, NEC I72.5
- pulmonary I28.1
  - arteriovenous Q25.72
    - acquired I28.0
  - syphilitic A52.09
  - valve (heart) — *see* Endocarditis, pulmonary
- racemose (peripheral) I72.9
  - congenital — *see* Aneurysm, congenital
- radial I72.1
- Rasmussen NEC A15.0
- renal (artery) I72.2
- retina — *see also* Disorder, retina, microaneurysms
  - congenital Q14.1
  - diabetic — *see* E08-E13 with .3-
- sinus of Valsalva Q25.49
- specified NEC I72.8
- spinal (cord) I72.8

☑ **Additional Character Required** — Refer to the Tabular List for Character Selection   ▽ **Subterms under main terms may continue to next column or page**

Aneurysm — continued
  spinal — continued
    syphilitic (hemorrhage) A52.09
  splenic I72.8
  subclavian (artery) (ruptured) I72.8
    syphilitic A52.09
  superior mesenteric I72.8
  syphilitic (aorta) A52.01
    central nervous system A52.05
    congenital (late) A50.54 [I79.0]
    spine, spinal A52.09
  thoracoabdominal (aorta) I71.6
    ruptured I71.5
    syphilitic A52.01
  thorax, thoracic (aorta) (arch) (nonsyphilitic) I71.2
    ruptured I71.1
    syphilitic A52.01
  traumatic (complication) (early), specified site — see Injury, blood vessel
  tricuspid (heart) (valve) I07.8
  ulnar I72.1
  upper limb (ruptured) I72.1
  valve, valvular — see Endocarditis
  venous — see also Varix I86.8
    congenital Q27.8
      digestive system Q27.8
      lower limb Q27.8
      specified site NEC Q27.8
      upper limb Q27.8
  ventricle — see Aneurysm, heart
  vertebral artery I72.6
  visceral NEC I72.8
Angelman syndrome Q93.51
Anger R45.4
Angiectasis, angiectopia I99.8
Angiitis I77.6
  allergic granulomatous M30.1
  hypersensitivity M31.0
  necrotizing M31.9
    specified NEC M31.8
  nervous system, granulomatous I67.7
Angina (attack) (cardiac) (chest) (heart) (pectoris) (syndrome) (vasomotor) I20.9
  with
    atherosclerotic heart disease — see Arteriosclerosis, coronary (artery),
    documented spasm I20.1
  abdominal K55.1
  accelerated — see Angina, unstable
  agranulocytic — see Agranulocytosis
  angiospastic — see Angina, with documented spasm
  aphthous B08.5
  crescendo — see Angina, unstable
  croupous J05.0
  cruris I73.9
  de novo effort — see Angina, unstable
  diphtheritic, membranous A36.0
  equivalent I20.8
  exudative, chronic J37.0
  following acute myocardial infarction I23.7
  gangrenous diphtheritic A36.0
  intestinal K55.1
  Ludovici K12.2
  Ludwig's K12.2
  malignant diphtheritic A36.0
  membranous J05.0
    diphtheritic A36.0
    Vincent's A69.1
  mesenteric K55.1
  monocytic — see Mononucleosis, infectious
  of effort — see Angina, specified NEC
  phlegmonous J36
    diphtheritic A36.0
  post-infarctional I23.7
  pre-infarctional — see Angina, unstable
  Prinzmetal — see Angina, with documented spasm
  progressive — see Angina, unstable
  pseudomembranous A69.1
  pultaceous, diphtheritic A36.0
  spasm-induced — see Angina, with documented spasm
  specified NEC I20.8
  stable I20.8
  stenocardia — see Angina, specified NEC
  stridulous, diphtheritic A36.2
  tonsil J36
  trachealis J05.0
  unstable I20.0
  variant — see Angina, with documented spasm

Angina — continued
  Vincent's A69.1
  worsening effort — see Angina, unstable
Angioblastoma — see Neoplasm, connective tissue, uncertain behavior
Angiocholecystitis — see Cholecystitis, acute
Angiocholitis — see also Cholecystitis, acute K83.09
Angiodysgenesis spinalis G95.19
Angiodysplasia (cecum) (colon) K55.20
  with bleeding K55.21
  duodenum (and stomach) K31.819
    with bleeding K31.811
  stomach (and duodenum) K31.819
    with bleeding K31.811
Angioedema (allergic) (any site) (with urticaria) T78.3 ☑
  hereditary D84.1
Angioendothelioma — see Neoplasm, uncertain behavior, by site
  benign D18.00
    intra-abdominal D18.03
    intracranial D18.02
    skin D18.01
    specified site NEC D18.09
  bone — see Neoplasm, bone, malignant
  Ewing's — see Neoplasm, bone, malignant
Angioendotheliomatosis C85.8- ☑
Angiofibroma — see also Neoplasm, benign, by site
  juvenile
    specified site — see Neoplasm, benign, by site
    unspecified site D10.6
Angiohemophilia (A) (B) D68.0
Angioid streaks (choroid) (macula) (retina) H35.33
Angiokeratoma — see Neoplasm, skin, benign
  corporis diffusum E75.21
Angioleiomyoma — see Neoplasm, connective tissue, benign
Angiolipoma — see also Lipoma
  infiltrating — see Lipoma
Angioma — see also Hemangioma, by site
  capillary I78.1
  hemorrhagicum hereditaria I78.0
  intra-abdominal D18.03
  intracranial D18.02
  malignant — see Neoplasm, connective tissue, malignant
  plexiform D18.00
    intra-abdominal D18.03
    intracranial D18.02
    skin D18.01
    specified site NEC D18.09
  senile I78.1
  serpiginosum L81.7
  skin D18.01
  specified site NEC D18.09
  spider I78.1
  stellate I78.1
  venous Q28.3
Angiomatosis Q82.8
  bacillary A79.89
  encephalotrigeminal Q85.8
  hemorrhagic familial I78.0
  hereditary familial I78.0
  liver K76.4
Angiomyolipoma — see Lipoma
Angiomyoliposarcoma — see Neoplasm, connective tissue, malignant
Angiomyoma — see Neoplasm, connective tissue, benign
Angiomyosarcoma — see Neoplasm, connective tissue, malignant
Angiomyxoma — see Neoplasm, connective tissue, uncertain behavior
Angioneurosis F45.8
Angioneurotic edema (allergic) (any site) (with urticaria) T78.3 ☑
  hereditary D84.1
Angiopathia, angiopathy I99.9
  cerebral I67.9
    amyloid E85.4 [I68.0]
  diabetic (peripheral) — see Diabetes, angiopathy
  peripheral I73.9
    diabetic — see Diabetes, angiopathy
    specified type NEC I73.89
  retinae syphilitica A52.05
  retinalis (juvenilis)
    diabetic — see Diabetes, retinopathy
    proliferative — see Retinopathy, proliferative
Angiosarcoma — see also Neoplasm, connective tissue, malignant

Angiosarcoma — continued
  liver C22.3
Angiosclerosis — see Arteriosclerosis
Angiospasm (peripheral) (traumatic) (vessel) I73.9
  brachial plexus G54.0
  cerebral G45.9
  cervical plexus G54.2
  nerve
    arm — see Mononeuropathy, upper limb
      axillary G54.0
      median — see Lesion, nerve, median
      ulnar — see Lesion, nerve, ulnar
    axillary G54.0
    leg — see Mononeuropathy, lower limb
    median — see Lesion, nerve, median
    plantar — see Lesion, nerve, plantar
    ulnar — see Lesion, nerve, ulnar
Angiospastic disease or edema I73.9
Angiostrongyliasis
  due to
    Parastrongylus
      cantonensis B83.2
      costaricensis B81.3
  intestinal B81.3
Anguillulosis — see Strongyloidiasis
Angulation
  cecum — see Obstruction, intestine
  coccyx (acquired) — see also subcategory M43.8 ☑
    congenital NEC Q76.49
  femur (acquired) — see also Deformity, limb, specified type NEC, thigh
    congenital Q74.2
  intestine (large) (small) — see Obstruction, intestine
  sacrum (acquired) — see also subcategory M43.8 ☑
    congenital NEC Q76.49
  sigmoid (flexure) — see Obstruction, intestine
  spine — see Dorsopathy, deforming, specified NEC
  tibia (acquired) — see also Deformity, limb, specified type NEC, lower leg
    congenital Q74.2
  ureter N13.5
    with infection N13.6
  wrist (acquired) — see also Deformity, limb, specified type NEC, forearm
    congenital Q74.0
Angulus infectiosus (lips) K13.0
Anhedonia R45.84
  sexual F52.0
Anhidrosis L74.4
Anhydration E86.0
Anhydremia E86.0
Anidrosis L74.4
Aniridia (congenital) Q13.1
Anisakiasis (infection) (infestation) B81.0
Anisakis larvae infestation B81.0
Aniseikonia H52.32
Anisocoria (pupil) H57.02
  congenital Q13.2
Anisocytosis R71.8
Anisometropia (congenital) H52.31
Ankle — see condition
Ankyloblepharon (eyelid) (acquired) — see also Blepharophimosis
  filiforme (adnatum) (congenital) Q10.3
  total Q10.3
Ankyloglossia Q38.1
Ankylosis (fibrous) (osseous) (joint) M24.60
  ankle M24.67- ☑
  arthrodesis status Z98.1
  cricoarytenoid (cartilage) (joint) (larynx) J38.7
  dental K03.5
  ear ossicles H74.31- ☑
  elbow M24.62- ☑
  foot M24.67- ☑
  hand M24.64- ☑
  hip M24.65- ☑
  incostapedial joint (infectional) — see Ankylosis, ear ossicles
  jaw (temporomandibular) M26.61- ☑
  knee M24.66- ☑
  lumbosacral (joint) M43.27
  postoperative (status) Z98.1
  produced by surgical fusion, status Z98.1
  sacro-iliac (joint) M43.28
  shoulder M24.61- ☑
  spine (joint) — see also Fusion, spine
    spondylitic — see Spondylitis, ankylosing

Ankylosis — continued
  surgical Z98.1
  temporomandibular M26.61- ☑
  tooth, teeth (hard tissues) K03.5
  wrist M24.63- ☑
Ankylostoma — see Ancylostoma
Ankylostomiasis — see Ancylostomiasis
Ankylurethria — see Stricture, urethra
Annular — see also condition
  detachment, cervix N88.8
  organ or site, congenital NEC — see Distortion
  pancreas (congenital) Q45.1
Anodontia (complete) (partial) (vera) K00.0
  acquired K08.10 ☑
Anomaly, anomalous (congenital) (unspecified type)
    Q89.9
  abdominal wall NEC Q79.59
  acoustic nerve Q07.8
  adrenal (gland) Q89.1
  Alder (-Reilly) (leukocyte granulation) D72.0
  alimentary tract Q45.9
    upper Q40.9
  alveolar M26.70
    hyperplasia M26.79
      mandibular M26.72
      maxillary M26.71
    hypoplasia M26.79
      mandibular M26.74
      maxillary M26.73
    ridge (process) M26.79
    specified NEC M26.79
  ankle (joint) Q74.2
  anus Q43.9
  aorta (arch) NEC Q25.40
    coarctation (preductal) (postductal) Q25.1
  aortic cusp or valve Q23.9
  appendix Q43.8
  apple peel syndrome Q41.1
  aqueduct of Sylvius Q03.0
    with spina bifida — see Spina bifida, with hydro-
        cephalus
  arm Q74.0
  arteriovenous NEC
    coronary Q24.5
    gastrointestinal Q27.33
      acquired — see Angiodysplasia
  artery (peripheral) Q27.9
    basilar NEC Q28.1
    cerebral Q28.3
    coronary Q24.5
    digestive system Q27.8
    eye Q15.8
    great Q25.9
      specified NEC Q25.8
    lower limb Q27.8
    peripheral Q27.9
      specified NEC Q27.8
    pulmonary NEC Q25.79
    renal Q27.2
    retina Q14.1
    specified site NEC Q27.8
    subclavian Q27.8
      origin Q25.48
    umbilical Q27.0
    upper limb Q27.8
    vertebral NEC Q28.1
  aryteno-epiglottic folds Q31.8
  atrial
    bands or folds Q20.8
    septa Q21.1
  atrioventricular
    excitation I45.6
    septum Q21.0
  auditory canal Q17.8
  auricle
    ear Q17.8
      causing impairment of hearing Q16.9
    heart Q20.8
  Axenfeld's Q15.0
  back Q89.9
  band
    atrial Q20.8
    heart Q24.8
    ventricular Q24.8
  Bartholin's duct Q38.4
  biliary duct or passage Q44.5
  bladder Q64.70
    absence Q64.5

Anomaly, anomalous — continued
  bladder — continued
    diverticulum Q64.6
    exstrophy Q64.10
      cloacal Q64.12
      extroversion Q64.19
      specified type NEC Q64.19
      supravesical fissure Q64.11
    neck obstruction Q64.31
    specified type NEC Q64.79
  bone Q79.9
    arm Q74.9
    face Q75.9
    leg Q74.2
    pelvic girdle Q74.2
    shoulder girdle Q74.0
    skull Q75.9
      with
        anencephaly Q00.0
        encephalocele — see Encephalocele
        hydrocephalus Q03.9
          with spina bifida — see Spina bifida, by
              site, with hydrocephalus
        microcephaly Q02
  brain (multiple) Q04.9
    vessel Q28.3
  breast Q83.9
  broad ligament Q50.6
  bronchus Q32.4
  bulbus cordis Q21.9
  bursa Q79.9
  canal of Nuck Q52.4
  canthus Q10.3
  capillary Q27.9
  cardiac Q24.9
    chambers Q20.9
      specified NEC Q20.8
    septal closure Q21.9
      specified NEC Q21.8
    valve NEC Q24.8
      pulmonary Q22.3
  cardiovascular system Q28.8
  carpus Q74.0
  caruncle, lacrimal Q10.6
  cascade stomach Q40.2
  cauda equina Q06.3
  cecum Q43.9
  cerebral Q04.9
    vessels Q28.3
  cervix Q51.9
  Chédiak-Higashi (-Steinbrinck) (congenital gigantism
      of peroxidase granules) E70.330
  cheek Q18.9
  chest wall Q67.8
    bones Q76.9
  chin Q18.9
  chordae tendineae Q24.8
  choroid Q14.3
    plexus Q07.8
  chromosomes, chromosomal Q99.9
    D (1) — see condition, chromosome 13
    E (3) — see condition, chromosome 18
    G — see condition, chromosome 21
    sex
      female phenotype Q97.8
      gonadal dysgenesis (pure) Q99.1
      Klinefelter's Q98.4
      male phenotype Q98.9
      Turner's Q96.9
      specified NEC Q99.8
  cilia Q10.3
  circulatory system Q28.9
  clavicle Q74.0
  clitoris Q52.6
  coccyx Q76.49
  colon Q43.9
  common duct Q44.5
  communication
    coronary artery Q24.5
    left ventricle with right atrium Q21.0
  concha (ear) Q17.3
  connection
    portal vein Q26.5
    pulmonary venous Q26.4
      partial Q26.3
      total Q26.2
    renal artery with kidney Q27.2
  cornea (shape) Q13.4
  coronary artery or vein Q24.5

Anomaly, anomalous — continued
  cranium — see Anomaly, skull
  cricoid cartilage Q31.8
  cystic duct Q44.5
  dental
    alveolar — see Anomaly, alveolar
    arch relationship M26.20
      specified NEC M26.29
  dentofacial M26.9
    alveolar — see Anomaly, alveolar
    dental arch relationship M26.20
      specified NEC M26.29
    functional M26.50
      specified NEC M26.59
    jaw size M26.00
      macrogenia M26.05
      mandibular
        hyperplasia M26.03
        hypoplasia M26.04
      maxillary
        hyperplasia M26.01
        hypoplasia M26.02
      microgenia M26.06
      specified type NEC M26.09
    jaw-cranial base relationship M26.10
      asymmetry M26.12
        maxillary M26.11
      specified type NEC M26.19
    malocclusion M26.4
      dental arch relationship NEC M26.29
      jaw size — see Anomaly, dentofacial, jaw size
      jaw-cranial base relationship — see Anomaly,
          dentofacial, jaw-cranial base relationship
    specified type NEC M26.89
    temporomandibular joint M26.60- ☑
      adhesions M26.61- ☑
      ankylosis M26.61- ☑
      arthralgia M26.62- ☑
      articular disc M26.63- ☑
      specified type NEC M26.69
    tooth position, fully erupted M26.30
      specified NEC M26.39
  dermatoglyphic Q82.8
  diaphragm (apertures) NEC Q79.1
  digestive organ(s) or tract Q45.9
    lower Q43.9
    upper Q40.9
  distance, interarch (excessive) (inadequate) M26.25
  distribution, coronary artery Q24.5
  ductus
    arteriosus Q25.0
    botalli Q25.0
  duodenum Q43.9
  dura (brain) Q04.9
    spinal cord Q06.9
  ear (external) Q17.9
    causing impairment of hearing Q16.9
    inner Q16.5
    middle (causing impairment of hearing) Q16.4
    ossicles Q16.3
  Ebstein's (heart) (tricuspid valve) Q22.5
  ectodermal Q82.9
  Eisenmenger's (ventricular septal defect) Q21.8
  ejaculatory duct Q55.4
  elbow Q74.0
  endocrine gland NEC Q89.2
  epididymis Q55.4
  epiglottis Q31.8
  esophagus Q39.9
  eustachian tube Q17.8
  eye Q15.9
    anterior segment Q13.9
      specified NEC Q13.89
    posterior segment Q14.9
      specified NEC Q14.8
    ptosis (eyelid) Q10.0
    specified NEC Q15.8
  eyebrow Q18.8
  eyelid Q10.3
    ptosis Q10.0
  face Q18.9
    bone(s) Q75.9
  fallopian tube Q50.6
  fascia Q79.9
  femur NEC Q74.2
  fibula NEC Q74.2
  finger Q74.0
  fixation, intestine Q43.3

☑ **Additional Character Required** — Refer to the Tabular List for Character Selection

▽ **Subterms under main terms may continue to next column or page**

Anomaly, anomalous — *continued*
- flexion (joint) NOS Q74.9
  - hip or thigh Q65.89
- foot NEC Q74.2
  - varus (congenital) Q66.3- ☑
- foramen
  - Botalli Q21.1
  - ovale Q21.1
- forearm Q74.0
- forehead Q75.8
- form, teeth K00.2
- fovea centralis Q14.1
- frontal bone — *see* Anomaly, skull
- gallbladder (position) (shape) (size) Q44.1
- Gartner's duct Q52.4
- gastrointestinal tract Q45.9
- genitalia, genital organ(s) or system
  - female Q52.9
    - external Q52.70
    - internal NOS Q52.9
  - male Q55.9
    - hydrocele P83.5
    - specified NEC Q55.8
- genitourinary NEC
  - female Q52.9
  - male Q55.9
- Gerbode Q21.0
- glottis Q31.8
- granulation or granulocyte, genetic (constitutional) (leukocyte) D72.0
- gum Q38.6
- gyri Q07.9
- hair Q84.2
- hand Q74.0
- hard tissue formation in pulp K04.3
- head — *see* Anomaly, skull
- heart Q24.9
  - auricle Q20.8
  - bands or folds Q24.8
  - fibroelastosis cordis I42.4
  - obstructive NEC Q24.6
  - patent ductus arteriosus (Botalli) Q25.0
  - septum Q21.9
    - auricular Q21.1
    - interatrial Q21.1
    - interventricular Q21.0
      - with pulmonary stenosis or atresia, dextraposition of aorta and hypertrophy of right ventricle Q21.3
    - specified NEC Q21.8
    - ventricular Q21.0
      - with pulmonary stenosis or atresia, dextraposition of aorta and hypertrophy of right ventricle Q21.3
  - tetralogy of Fallot Q21.3
  - valve NEC Q24.8
    - aortic
      - bicuspid valve Q23.1
      - insufficiency Q23.1
      - stenosis Q23.0
        - subaortic Q24.4
    - mitral
      - insufficiency Q23.3
      - stenosis Q23.2
    - pulmonary Q22.3
      - atresia Q22.0
      - insufficiency Q22.2
      - stenosis Q22.1
        - infundibular Q24.3
        - subvalvular Q24.3
    - tricuspid
      - atresia Q22.4
      - stenosis Q22.4
  - ventricle Q20.8
- heel NEC Q74.2
- Hegglin's D72.0
- hemianencephaly Q00.0
- hemicephaly Q00.0
- hemicrania Q00.0
- hepatic duct Q44.5
- hip NEC Q74.2
- hourglass stomach Q40.2
- humerus Q74.0
- hydatid of Morgagni
  - female Q50.5
  - male (epididymal) Q55.4
    - testicular Q55.29
- hymen Q52.4
- hypersegmentation of neutrophils, hereditary D72.0

Anomaly, anomalous — *continued*
- hypophyseal Q89.2
- ileocecal (coil) (valve) Q43.9
- ileum Q43.9
- ilium NEC Q74.2
- integument Q84.9
  - specified NEC Q84.8
- interarch distance (excessive) (inadequate) M26.25
- intervertebral cartilage or disc Q76.49
- intestine (large) (small) Q43.9
  - with anomalous adhesions, fixation or malrotation Q43.3
- iris Q13.2
- ischium NEC Q74.2
- jaw — *see* Anomaly, dentofacial
  - alveolar — *see* Anomaly, alveolar
  - jaw-cranial base relationship — *see* Anomaly, dentofacial, jaw-cranial base relationship
- jejunum Q43.8
- joint Q74.9
  - specified NEC Q74.8
- Jordan's D72.0
- kidney(s) (calyx) (pelvis) Q63.9
  - artery Q27.2
  - specified NEC Q63.8
- Klippel-Feil (brevicollis) Q76.1
- knee Q74.1
- labium (majus) (minus) Q52.70
- labyrinth, membranous Q16.5
- lacrimal apparatus or duct Q10.6
- larynx, laryngeal (muscle) Q31.9
  - web (bed) Q31.0
- lens Q12.9
- leukocytes, genetic D72.0
  - granulation (constitutional) D72.0
- lid (fold) Q10.3
- ligament Q79.9
  - broad Q50.6
  - round Q52.8
- limb Q74.9
  - lower NEC Q74.2
    - reduction deformity — *see* Defect, reduction, lower limb
  - upper Q74.0
- lip Q38.0
- liver Q44.7
  - duct Q44.5
- lower limb NEC Q74.2
- lumbosacral (joint) (region) Q76.49
  - kyphosis — *see* Kyphosis, congenital
  - lordosis — *see* Lordosis, congenital
- lung (fissure) (lobe) Q33.9
- mandible — *see* Anomaly, dentofacial
- maxilla — *see* Anomaly, dentofacial
- May (-Hegglin) D72.0
- meatus urinarius NEC Q64.79
- meningeal bands or folds Q07.9
  - constriction of Q07.8
  - spinal Q06.9
- meninges Q07.9
  - cerebral Q04.8
  - spinal Q06.9
- meningocele Q05.9
- mesentery Q45.9
- metacarpus Q74.0
- metatarsus NEC Q74.2
- middle ear Q16.4
  - ossicles Q16.3
- mitral (leaflets) (valve) Q23.9
  - insufficiency Q23.3
  - specified NEC Q23.8
  - stenosis Q23.2
- mouth Q38.6
- Müllerian — *see also* Anomaly, by site
  - uterus NEC Q51.818
- multiple NEC Q89.7
- muscle Q79.9
  - eyelid Q10.3
- musculoskeletal system, except limbs Q79.9
- myocardium Q24.8
- nail Q84.6
- narrowness, eyelid Q10.3
- nasal sinus (wall) Q30.8
- neck (any part) Q18.9
- nerve Q07.9
  - acoustic Q07.8
  - optic Q07.8
- nervous system (central) Q07.9

Anomaly, anomalous — *continued*
- nipple Q83.9
- nose, nasal (bones) (cartilage) (septum) (sinus) Q30.9
  - specified NEC Q30.8
- ocular muscle Q15.8
- omphalomesenteric duct Q43.0
- opening, pulmonary veins Q26.4
- optic
  - disc Q14.2
  - nerve Q07.8
- opticociliary vessels Q13.2
- orbit (eye) Q10.7
- organ Q89.9
  - of Corti Q16.5
- origin
  - artery
    - innominate Q25.8
    - pulmonary Q25.79
    - renal Q27.2
    - subclavian Q25.48
- osseous meatus (ear) Q16.1
- ovary Q50.39
- oviduct Q50.6
- palate (hard) (soft) NEC Q38.5
- pancreas or pancreatic duct Q45.3
- papillary muscles Q24.8
- parathyroid gland Q89.2
- paraurethral ducts Q64.79
- parotid (gland) Q38.4
- patella Q74.1
- Pelger-Huët (hereditary hyposegmentation) D72.0
- pelvic girdle NEC Q74.2
- pelvis (bony) NEC Q74.2
  - rachitic E64.3
- penis (glans) Q55.69
- pericardium Q24.8
- peripheral vascular system Q27.9
- Peter's Q13.4
- pharynx Q38.8
- pigmentation L81.9
  - congenital Q82.8
- pituitary (gland) Q89.2
- pleural (folds) Q34.0
- portal vein Q26.5
  - connection Q26.5
- position, tooth, teeth, fully erupted M26.30
  - specified NEC M26.39
- precerebral vessel Q28.1
- prepuce Q55.69
- prostate Q55.4
- pulmonary Q33.9
  - artery NEC Q25.79
  - valve Q22.3
    - atresia Q22.0
    - insufficiency Q22.2
    - specified type NEC Q22.3
    - stenosis Q22.1
      - infundibular Q24.3
      - subvalvular Q24.3
  - venous connection Q26.4
    - partial Q26.3
    - total Q26.2
- pupil Q13.2
  - function H57.00
    - anisocoria H57.02
    - Argyll Robertson pupil H57.01
    - miosis H57.03
    - mydriasis H57.04
    - specified type NEC H57.09
    - tonic pupil H57.05- ☑
- pylorus Q40.3
- radius Q74.0
- rectum Q43.9
- reduction (extremity) (limb)
  - femur (longitudinal) — *see* Defect, reduction, lower limb, longitudinal, femur
  - fibula (longitudinal) — *see* Defect, reduction, lower limb, longitudinal, fibula
  - lower limb — *see* Defect, reduction, lower limb
  - radius (longitudinal) — *see* Defect, reduction, upper limb, longitudinal, radius
  - tibia (longitudinal) — *see* Defect, reduction, lower limb, longitudinal, tibia
  - ulna (longitudinal) — *see* Defect, reduction, upper limb, longitudinal, ulna
  - upper limb — *see* Defect, reduction, upper limb
- refraction — *see* Disorder, refraction
- renal Q63.9

Index

Anomaly, anomalous — Anticoagulant, circulating

Anomaly, anomalous — *continued*
renal — *continued*
artery Q27.2
pelvis Q63.9
specified NEC Q63.8
respiratory system Q34.9
specified NEC Q34.8
retina Q14.1
rib Q76.6
cervical Q76.5
Rieger's Q13.81
rotation — *see* Malrotation
hip or thigh Q65.89
round ligament Q52.8
sacroiliac (joint) NEC Q74.2
sacrum NEC Q76.49
kyphosis — *see* Kyphosis, congenital
lordosis — *see* Lordosis, congenital
saddle nose, syphilitic A50.57
salivary duct or gland Q38.4
scapula Q74.0
scrotum — *see* Malformation, testis and scrotum
sebaceous gland Q82.9
seminal vesicles Q55.4
sense organs NEC Q07.8
sex chromosomes NEC — *see also* Anomaly, chromosomes
female phenotype Q97.8
male phenotype Q98.9
shoulder (girdle) (joint) Q74.0
sigmoid (flexure) Q43.9
simian crease Q82.8
sinus of Valsalva Q25.49
skeleton generalized Q78.9
skin (appendage) Q82.9
skull Q75.9
with
anencephaly Q00.0
encephalocele — *see* Encephalocele
hydrocephalus Q03.9
with spina bifida — *see* Spina bifida, by site, with hydrocephalus
microcephaly Q02
specified organ or site NEC Q89.8
spermatic cord Q55.4
spine, spinal NEC Q76.49
column NEC Q76.49
kyphosis — *see* Kyphosis, congenital
lordosis — *see* Lordosis, congenital
cord Q06.9
nerve root Q07.8
spleen Q89.09
agenesis Q89.01
stenonian duct Q38.4
sternum NEC Q76.7
stomach Q40.3
submaxillary gland Q38.4
tarsus NEC Q74.2
tendon Q79.9
testis — *see* Malformation, testis and scrotum
thigh NEC Q74.2
thorax (wall) Q67.8
bony Q76.9
throat Q38.8
thumb Q74.0
thymus gland Q89.2
thyroid (gland) Q89.2
cartilage Q31.8
tibia NEC Q74.2
saber A50.56
toe Q74.2
tongue Q38.3
tooth, teeth K00.9
eruption K00.6
position, fully erupted M26.30
spacing, fully erupted M26.30
trachea (cartilage) Q32.1
tragus Q17.9
tricuspid (leaflet) (valve) Q22.9
atresia or stenosis Q22.4
Ebstein's Q22.5
Uhl's (hypoplasia of myocardium, right ventricle) Q24.8
ulna Q74.0
umbilical artery Q27.0
union
cricoid cartilage and thyroid cartilage Q31.8
thyroid cartilage and hyoid bone Q31.8
trachea with larynx Q31.8

Anomaly, anomalous — *continued*
upper limb Q74.0
urachus Q64.4
ureter Q62.8
obstructive NEC Q62.39
cecoureterocele Q62.32
orthotopic ureterocele Q62.31
urethra Q64.70
absence Q64.5
double Q64.74
fistula to rectum Q64.73
obstructive Q64.39
stricture Q64.32
prolapse Q64.71
specified type NEC Q64.79
urinary tract Q64.9
uterus Q51.9
with only one functioning horn Q51.4
uvula Q38.5
vagina Q52.4
valleculae Q31.8
valve (heart) NEC Q24.8
coronary sinus Q24.5
inferior vena cava Q24.8
pulmonary Q22.3
sinus coronario Q24.5
venae cavae inferioris Q24.8
vas deferens Q55.4
vascular Q27.9
brain Q28.3
ring Q25.45
vein(s) (peripheral) Q27.9
brain Q28.3
cerebral Q28.3
coronary Q24.5
developmental Q28.3
great Q26.9
specified NEC Q26.8
vena cava (inferior) (superior) Q26.9
venous — *see* Anomaly, vein(s)
venous return Q26.8
ventricular
bands or folds Q24.8
septa Q21.0
vertebra Q76.49
kyphosis — *see* Kyphosis, congenital
lordosis — *see* Lordosis, congenital
vesicourethral orifice Q64.79
vessel(s) Q27.9
optic papilla Q14.2
precerebral Q28.1
vitelline duct Q43.0
vitreous body or humor Q14.0
vulva Q52.70
wrist (joint) Q74.0
Anomia R48.8
Anonychia (congenital) Q84.3
acquired L60.8
Anophthalmos, anophthalmus (congenital) (globe) Q11.1
acquired Z90.01
Anopia, anopsia H53.46- ☑
quadrant H53.46- ☑
Anorchia, anorchism, anorchidism Q55.0
Anorexia R63.0
hysterical F44.89
nervosa F50.00
atypical F50.9
binge-eating type F50.2
with purging F50.02
restricting type F50.01
Anorgasmy, psychogenic (female) F52.31
male F52.32
Anosmia R43.0
hysterical F44.6
postinfectional J39.8
Anosognosia R41.89
Anosteoplasia Q78.9
Anovulatory cycle N97.0
Anoxemia R09.02
newborn P84
Anoxia (pathological) R09.02
altitude T70.29 ☑
cerebral G93.1
complicating
anesthesia (general) (local) or other sedation T88.59 ☑
in labor and delivery O74.3

Anoxia — *continued*
cerebral — *continued*
complicating — *continued*
anesthesia or other sedation — *continued*
in pregnancy O29.21- ☑
postpartum, puerperal O89.2
delivery (cesarean) (instrumental) O75.4
during a procedure G97.81
newborn P84
resulting from a procedure G97.82
due to
drowning T75.1 ☑
high altitude T70.29 ☑
heart — *see* Insufficiency, coronary
intrauterine P84
myocardial — *see* Insufficiency, coronary
newborn P84
spinal cord G95.11
systemic (by suffocation) (low content in atmosphere) — *see* Asphyxia, traumatic
Anteflexion — *see* Anteversion
Antenatal
care (normal pregnancy) Z34.90
screening (encounter for) of mother — *see also* Encounter, antenatal screening Z36.9
Antepartum — *see* condition
Anterior — *see* condition
Antero-occlusion M26.220
Anteversion
cervix — *see* Anteversion, uterus
femur (neck), congenital Q65.89
uterus, uterine (cervix) (postinfectional) (postpartal, old) N85.4
congenital Q51.818
in pregnancy or childbirth — *see* Pregnancy, complicated by
Anthophobia F40.228
Anthracosilicosis J60
Anthracosis (lung) (occupational) J60
lingua K14.3
Anthrax A22.9
with pneumonia A22.1
cerebral A22.8
colitis A22.2
cutaneous A22.0
gastrointestinal A22.2
inhalation A22.1
intestinal A22.2
meningitis A22.8
pulmonary A22.1
respiratory A22.1
sepsis A22.7
specified manifestation NEC A22.8
Anthropoid pelvis Q74.2
with disproportion (fetopelvic) O33.0
Anthropophobia F40.10
generalized F40.11
Antibodies, maternal (blood group) — *see* Isoimmunization, affecting management of pregnancy
anti-D — *see* Isoimmunization, affecting management of pregnancy, Rh
newborn P55.0
Antibody
anticardiolipin R76.0
with
hemorrhagic disorder D68.312
hypercoagulable state D68.61
antiphosphatidylglycerol R76.0
with
hemorrhagic disorder D68.312
hypercoagulable state D68.61
antiphosphatidylinositol R76.0
with
hemorrhagic disorder D68.312
hypercoagulable state D68.61
antiphosphatidylserine R76.0
with
hemorrhagic disorder D68.312
hypercoagulable state D68.61
antiphospholipid R76.0
with
hemorrhagic disorder D68.312
hypercoagulable state D68.61
Anticardiolipin syndrome D68.61
Anticoagulant, circulating (intrinsic) — *see also* Disorder, hemorrhagic D68.318
drug-induced (extrinsic) — *see also* Disorder, hemorrhagic D68.32

☑ **Additional Character Required** — **Refer to the Tabular List for Character Selection**   ▽ **Subterms under main terms may continue to next column or page**

Anticoagulant, circulating — *continued*
  iatrogenic D68.32
Antidiuretic hormone syndrome E22.2
Antimonial cholera — *see* Poisoning, antimony
Antiphospholipid
  antibody
    with hemorrhagic disorder D68.312
    syndrome D68.61
Antisocial personality F60.2
Antithrombinemia — *see* Circulating anticoagulants
Antithromboplastinemia D68.318
Antithromboplastinogenemia D68.318
Antitoxin complication or reaction — *see* Complications, vaccination
Antlophobia F40.228
Antritis J32.0
  maxilla J32.0
    acute J01.00
      recurrent J01.01
  stomach K29.60
    with bleeding K29.61
Antrum, antral — *see* condition
Anuria R34
  calculous (impacted) (recurrent) — *see also* Calculus, urinary N20.9
  following
    abortion — *see* Abortion by type complicated by, renal failure
    ectopic or molar pregnancy O08.4
  newborn P96.0
  postprocedural N99.0
  postrenal N13.8
  traumatic (following crushing) T79.5 ☑
Anus, anal — *see* condition
Anusitis K62.89
Anxiety F41.9
  depression F41.8
  episodic paroxysmal F41.0
  generalized F41.1
  hysteria F41.8
  neurosis F41.1
  panic type F41.0
  reaction F41.1
  separation, abnormal (of childhood) F93.0
  specified NEC F41.8
  state F41.1
Aorta, aortic — *see* condition
Aortectasia — *see* Ectasia, aorta
  with aneurysm — *see* Aneurysm, aorta
Aortitis (nonsyphilitic) (calcific) I77.6
  arteriosclerotic I70.0
  Doehle-Heller A52.02
  luetic A52.02
  rheumatic — *see* Endocarditis, acute, rheumatic
  specific (syphilitic) A52.02
  syphilitic A52.02
    congenital A50.54 *[I79.1]*
Apathetic thyroid storm — *see* Thyrotoxicosis
Apathy R45.3
Apeirophobia F40.228
Apepsia K30
  psychogenic F45.8
Aperistalsis, esophagus K22.0
Apertognathia M26.29
Apert's syndrome Q87.0
Aphagia R13.0
  psychogenic F50.9
Aphakia (acquired) (postoperative) H27.0- ☑
  congenital Q12.3
Aphasia (amnestic) (global) (nominal) (semantic) (syntactic) R47.01
  acquired, with epilepsy (Landau-Kleffner syndrome) — *see* Epilepsy, specified NEC
  auditory (developmental) F80.2
  developmental (receptive type) F80.2
    expressive type F80.1
    Wernicke's F80.2
  following
    cerebrovascular disease I69.920
      cerebral infarction I69.320
      intracerebral hemorrhage I69.120
      nontraumatic intracranial hemorrhage NEC I69.220
      specified disease NEC I69.820
      subarachnoid hemorrhage I69.020
  primary progressive G31.01 *[F02.80]*
    with behavioral disturbance G31.01 *[F02.81]*
  progressive isolated G31.01 *[F02.80]*

Aphasia — *continued*
  progressive isolated — *continued*
    with behavioral disturbance G31.01 *[F02.81]*
  sensory F80.2
  syphilis, tertiary A52.19
  Wernicke's (developmental) F80.2
Aphonia (organic) R49.1
  hysterical F44.4
  psychogenic F44.4
Aphthae, aphthous — *see also* condition
  Bednar's K12.0
  cachectic K14.0
  epizootic B08.8
  fever B08.8
  oral (recurrent) K12.0
  stomatitis (major) (minor) K12.0
  thrush B37.0
  ulcer (oral) (recurrent) K12.0
    genital organ(s) NEC
      female N76.6
      male N50.89
    larynx J38.7
Apical — *see* condition
Apiphobia F40.218
Aplasia — *see also* Agenesis
  abdominal muscle syndrome Q79.4
  alveolar process (acquired) — *see* Anomaly, alveolar
    congenital Q38.6
  aorta (congenital) Q25.41
  axialis extracorticalis (congenita) E75.29
  bone marrow (myeloid) D61.9
    congenital D61.01
  brain Q00.0
    part of Q04.3
  bronchus Q32.4
  cementum K00.4
  cerebellum Q04.3
  cervix (congenital) Q51.5
  congenital pure red cell D61.01
  corpus callosum Q04.0
  cutis congenita Q84.8
  erythrocyte congenital D61.01
  extracortical axial E75.29
  eye Q11.1
  fovea centralis (congenital) Q14.1
  gallbladder, congenital Q44.0
  iris Q13.1
  labyrinth, membranous Q16.5
  limb (congenital) Q73.8
    lower — *see* Defect, reduction, lower limb
    upper — *see* Agenesis, arm
  lung, congenital (bilateral) (unilateral) Q33.3
  pancreas Q45.0
  parathyroid-thymic D82.1
  Pelizaeus-Merzbacher E75.29
  penis Q55.5
  prostate Q55.4
  red cell (with thymoma) D60.9
    acquired D60.9
      due to drugs D60.9
    adult D60.9
    chronic D60.0
    congenital D61.01
    constitutional D61.01
    due to drugs D60.9
    hereditary D61.01
    of infants D61.01
    primary D61.01
    pure D61.01
      due to drugs D60.9
    specified type NEC D60.8
    transient D60.1
  round ligament Q52.8
  skin Q84.8
  spermatic cord Q55.4
  spleen Q89.01
  testicle Q55.0
  thymic, with immunodeficiency D82.1
  thyroid (congenital) (with myxedema) E03.1
  uterus Q51.0
  ventral horn cell Q06.1
Apnea, apneic (of) (spells) R06.81
  newborn NEC P28.4
    obstructive P28.4
    sleep (central) (obstructive) (primary) P28.3
  prematurity P28.4
  sleep G47.30
    central (primary) G47.31

Apnea, apneic — *continued*
  sleep — *continued*
    central — *continued*
      idiopathic G47.31
      in conditions classified elsewhere G47.37
    obstructive (adult) (pediatric) G47.33
      hypopnea G47.33
    primary central G47.31
    specified NEC G47.39
Apneumatosis, newborn P28.0
Apocrine metaplasia (breast) — *see* Dysplasia, mammary, specified type NEC
Apophysitis (bone) — *see also* Osteochondropathy
  calcaneus M92.8
  juvenile M92.9
Apoplectiform convulsions (cerebral ischemia) I67.82
Apoplexia, apoplexy, apoplectic
  adrenal A39.1
  heart (auricle) (ventricle) — *see* Infarct, myocardium
  heat T67.01 ☑
  hemorrhagic (stroke) — *see* Hemorrhage, intracranial
  meninges, hemorrhagic — *see* Hemorrhage, intracranial, subarachnoid
  uremic N18.9 *[I68.8]*
Appearance
  bizarre R46.1
  specified NEC R46.89
  very low level of personal hygiene R46.0
Appendage
  epididymal (organ of Morgagni) Q55.4
  intestine (epiploic) Q43.8
  preauricular Q17.0
  testicular (organ of Morgagni) Q55.29
Appendicitis (pneumococcal) (retrocecal) K37
  with
    gangrene K35.891
    perforation NOS K35.32
    peritoneal abscess K35.33
    peritonitis NEC K35.33
      generalized (with perforation or rupture) K35.20
        with abscess K35.21
      localized K35.30
        with
          gangrene K35.31
          perforation K35.32
            and abscess K35.33
      rupture (with localized peritonitis) K35.32
  acute (catarrhal) (fulminating) (gangrenous) (obstructive) (retrocecal) (suppurative) K35.80
    with
      gangrene K35.891
      peritoneal abscess K35.33
      peritonitis NEC K35.33
        generalized (with perforation or rupture) K35.20
          with abscess K35.21
        localized K35.30
          with
            gangrene K35.31
            perforation K35.32
              and abscess K35.33
    specified NEC K35.890
      with gangrene K35.891
  amebic A06.89
  chronic (recurrent) K36
  exacerbation — *see* Appendicitis, acute
  gangrenous — *see* Appendicitis, acute
  healed (obliterative) K36
  interval K36
  neurogenic K36
  obstructive K36
  recurrent K36
  relapsing K36
  ruptured NOS (with localized peritonitis) K35.32
  subacute (adhesive) K36
  subsiding K36
  suppurative — *see* Appendicitis, acute
  tuberculous A18.32
Appendicopathia oxyurica B80
Appendix, appendicular — *see also* condition
  epididymis Q55.4
  Morgagni
    female Q50.5
    male (epididymal) Q55.4
      testicular Q55.29
  testis Q55.29
Appetite
  depraved — *see* Pica

(handwritten note: K90-postop intestinal obstruction)

Appetite — *continued*
excessive R63.2
lack or loss — *see also* Anorexia R63.0
nonorganic origin F50.89
psychogenic F50.89
perverted (hysterical) — *see* Pica
Apple peel syndrome Q41.1
Apprehension state F41.1
Apprehensiveness, abnormal F41.9
Approximal wear K03.0
Apraxia (classic) (ideational) (ideokinetic) (ideomotor)
(motor) (verbal) R48.2
following
cerebrovascular disease I69.990
cerebral infarction I69.390
intracerebral hemorrhage I69.190
nontraumatic intracranial hemorrhage NEC
I69.290
specified disease NEC I69.890
subarachnoid hemorrhage I69.090
oculomotor, congenital H51.8
Aptyalism K11.7
Apudoma — *see* Neoplasm, uncertain behavior, by site
Aqueous misdirection H40.83- ☑
Arabicum elephantiasis — *see* Infestation, filarial
Arachnitis — *see* Meningitis
Arachnodactyly — *see* Syndrome, Marfan's
Arachnoiditis (acute) (adhesive) (basal) (brain) (cere-
brospinal) — *see* Meningitis
Arachnophobia F40.210
Arboencephalitis, Australian A83.4
Arborization block (heart) I45.5
ARC (AIDS-related complex) B20
Arch
aortic Q25.49
bovine Q25.49
Arches — *see* condition
Arcuate uterus Q51.810
Arcuatus uterus Q51.810
Arcus (cornea) senilis — *see* Degeneration, cornea, senile
Arc-welder's lung J63.4
Areflexia R29.2
Areola — *see* condition
Argentaffinoma — *see also* Neoplasm, uncertain behav-
ior, by site
malignant — *see* Neoplasm, malignant, by site
syndrome E34.0
Argininemia E72.21
Arginosuccinic aciduria E72.22
Argyll Robertson phenomenon, pupil or syndrome
(syphilitic) A52.19
atypical H57.09
nonsyphilitic H57.09
Argyria, argyriasis
conjunctival H11.13- ☑
from drug or medicament — *see* Table of Drugs and
Chemicals, by substance
Argyrosis, conjunctival H11.13- ☑
Arhinencephaly Q04.1
Ariboflavinosis E53.0
Arm — *see* condition
Arnold-Chiari disease, obstruction or syndrome (type
II) Q07.00
with
hydrocephalus Q07.02
with spina bifida Q07.03
spina bifida Q07.01
with hydrocephalus Q07.03
type III — *see* Encephalocele
type IV Q04.8
Aromatic amino-acid metabolism disorder E70.9
specified NEC E70.8
Arousals, confusional G47.51
Arrest, arrested
cardiac I46.9
complicating
abortion — *see* Abortion, by type, complicated
by, cardiac arrest
anesthesia (general) (local) or other sedation —
see Table of Drugs and Chemicals, by drug
in labor and delivery O74.2
in pregnancy O29.11- ☑
postpartum, puerperal O89.1
delivery (cesarean) (instrumental) O75.4
due to
cardiac condition I46.2
specified condition NEC I46.8

Arrest, arrested — *continued*
cardiac — *continued*
intraoperative I97.71- ☑
newborn P29.81
personal history, successfully resuscitated Z86.74
postprocedural I97.12- ☑
obstetric procedure O75.4
cardiorespiratory — *see* Arrest, cardiac
circulatory — *see* Arrest, cardiac
deep transverse O64.0 ☑
development or growth
bone — *see* Disorder, bone, development or growth
child R62.50
tracheal rings Q32.1
epiphyseal
complete
femur M89.15- ☑
humerus M89.12- ☑
tibia M89.16- ☑
ulna M89.13- ☑
forearm M89.13- ☑
specified NEC M89.13- ☑
ulna — *see* Arrest, epiphyseal, by type, ulna
lower leg M89.16- ☑
specified NEC M89.168
tibia — *see* Arrest, epiphyseal, by type, tibia
partial
femur M89.15- ☑
humerus M89.12- ☑
tibia M89.16- ☑
ulna M89.13- ☑
specified NEC M89.18
granulopoiesis — *see* Agranulocytosis
growth plate — *see* Arrest, epiphyseal
heart — *see* Arrest, cardiac
legal, anxiety concerning Z65.3
physeal — *see* Arrest, epiphyseal
respiratory R09.2
newborn P28.81
sinus I45.5
spermatogenesis (complete) — *see* Azoospermia
incomplete — *see* Oligospermia
transverse (deep) O64.0 ☑
Arrhenoblastoma
benign
specified site — *see* Neoplasm, benign, by site
unspecified site
female D27.9
male D29.20
malignant
specified site — *see* Neoplasm, malignant, by site
unspecified site
female C56.9
male C62.90
specified site — *see* Neoplasm, uncertain behavior, by
site
unspecified site
female D39.10
male D40.10
Arrhythmia (auricle) (cardiac) (juvenile) (nodal) (reflex)
(sinus) (supraventricular) (transitory) (ventricle) I49.9
block I45.9
extrasystolic I49.49
newborn
bradycardia P29.12
occurring before birth P03.819
before onset of labor P03.810
during labor P03.811
tachycardia P29.11
psychogenic F45.8
specified NEC I49.8
vagal R55
ventricular re-entry I47.0
Arrillaga-Ayerza syndrome (pulmonary sclerosis with
pulmonary hypertension) I27.0
Arsenical pigmentation L81.8
from drug or medicament — *see* Table of Drugs and
Chemicals
Arsenism — *see* Poisoning, arsenic
Arterial — *see* condition
Arteriofibrosis — *see* Arteriosclerosis
Arteriolar sclerosis — *see* Arteriosclerosis
Arteriolith — *see* Arteriosclerosis
Arteriolitis I77.6
necrotizing, kidney I77.5
renal — *see* Hypertension, kidney
Arteriolosclerosis — *see* Arteriosclerosis

Arterionephrosclerosis — *see* Hypertension, kidney
Arteriopathy I77.9
cerebral autosomal dominant, with subcortical infarcts
and leukoencephalopathy (CADASIL) I67.850
Arteriosclerosis, arteriosclerotic (diffuse) (obliterans)
(of) (senile) (with calcification) I70.90
aorta I70.0
arteries of extremities — *see* Arteriosclerosis, extremities
brain I67.2
bypass graft
coronary — *see* Arteriosclerosis, coronary, bypass
graft
extremities — *see* Arteriosclerosis, extremities, bypass graft
cardiac — *see* Disease, heart, ischemic, atherosclerotic
cardiopathy — *see* Disease, heart, ischemic,
atherosclerotic
cardiorenal — *see* Hypertension, cardiorenal
cardiovascular — *see* Disease, heart, ischemic,
atherosclerotic
carotid — *see also* Occlusion, artery, carotid I65.2- ☑
central nervous system I67.2
cerebral I67.2
cerebrovascular I67.2
coronary (artery)
due to
calcified coronary lesion (severely) I25.84
lipid rich plaque I25.83
bypass graft I25.810
with
angina pectoris I25.709
with documented spasm I25.701
specified type NEC I25.708
unstable I25.700
ischemic chest pain I25.709
autologous artery I25.810
with
angina pectoris I25.729
with documented spasm I25.721
specified type I25.728
unstable I25.720
ischemic chest pain I25.729
autologous vein I25.810
with
angina pectoris I25.719
with documented spasm I25.711
specified type I25.718
unstable I25.710
ischemic chest pain I25.719
nonautologous biological I25.810
with
angina pectoris I25.739
with documented spasm I25.731
specified type I25.738
unstable I25.730
ischemic chest pain I25.739
specified type NEC I25.810
with
angina pectoris I25.799
with documented spasm I25.791
specified type I25.798
unstable I25.790
ischemic chest pain I25.799
native vessel
with
angina pectoris I25.119
with documented spasm I25.111
specified type NEC I25.118
unstable I25.110
ischemic chest pain I25.119
transplanted heart I25.811
bypass graft I25.812
with
angina pectoris I25.769
with documented spasm I25.761
specified type I25.768
unstable I25.760
ischemic chest pain I25.769
native coronary artery I25.811
with
angina pectoris I25.759
with documented spasm I25.751
specified type I25.758
unstable I25.750
ischemic chest pain I25.759
extremities (native arteries) I70.209
bypass graft I70.309

Arteriosclerosis, arteriosclerotic — *continued*
  extremities — *continued*
    bypass graft — *continued*
      autologous vein graft I70.409
        leg I70.409
          with
            gangrene (and intermittent claudication, rest pain and ulcer) I70.469
            intermittent claudication I70.419
            rest pain (and intermittent claudication) I70.429
          bilateral I70.403
            with
              gangrene (and intermittent claudication, rest pain and ulcer) I70.463
              intermittent claudication I70.463
              rest pain (and intermittent claudication) I70.423
            specified type NEC I70.493
          left I70.402
            with
              gangrene (and intermittent claudication, rest pain and ulcer) I70.462
              intermittent claudication I70.412
              rest pain (and intermittent claudication) I70.422
              ulceration (and intermittent claudication and rest pain) I70.449
                ankle I70.443
                calf I70.442
                foot site NEC I70.445
                heel I70.444
                lower leg NEC I70.448
                midfoot I70.444
                thigh I70.441
            specified type NEC I70.492
          right I70.401
            with
              gangrene (and intermittent claudication, rest pain and ulcer) I70.461
              intermittent claudication I70.411
              rest pain (and intermittent claudication) I70.421
              ulceration (and intermittent claudication and rest pain) I70.439
                ankle I70.433
                calf I70.432
                foot site NEC I70.435
                heel I70.434
                lower leg NEC I70.438
                midfoot I70.434
                thigh I70.431
            specified type NEC I70.491
        specified NEC I70.408
          with
            gangrene (and intermittent claudication, rest pain and ulcer) I70.468
            intermittent claudication I70.418
            rest pain (and intermittent claudication) I70.428
            ulceration (and intermittent claudication and rest pain) I70.45
          specified type NEC I70.498
      leg I70.309
        with
          gangrene (and intermittent claudication, rest pain and ulcer) I70.369
          intermittent claudication I70.319
          rest pain (and intermittent claudication) I70.329
        bilateral I70.303
          with
            gangrene (and intermittent claudication, rest pain and ulcer) I70.363
            intermittent claudication I70.313
            rest pain (and intermittent claudication) I70.323
          specified type NEC I70.393
        left I70.302
          with
            gangrene (and intermittent claudication, rest pain and ulcer) I70.362
            intermittent claudication I70.312
            rest pain (and intermittent claudication) I70.322

Arteriosclerosis, arteriosclerotic — *continued*
  extremities — *continued*
    bypass graft — *continued*
      leg — *continued*
        left — *continued*
          with — *continued*
            ulceration (and intermittent claudication and rest pain) I70.349
              ankle I70.343
              calf I70.342
              foot site NEC I70.345
              heel I70.344
              lower leg NEC I70.348
              midfoot I70.344
              thigh I70.341
          specified type NEC I70.392
        right I70.301
          with
            gangrene (and intermittent claudication, rest pain and ulcer) I70.361
            intermittent claudication I70.311
            rest pain (and intermittent claudication) I70.321
            ulceration (and intermittent claudication and rest pain) I70.339
              ankle I70.333
              calf I70.332
              foot site NEC I70.335
              heel I70.334
              lower leg NEC I70.338
              midfoot I70.334
              thigh I70.331
          specified type NEC I70.391
        specified type NEC I70.399
      nonautologous biological graft I70.509
        leg I70.509
          with
            gangrene (and intermittent claudication, rest pain and ulcer) I70.569
            intermittent claudication I70.519
            rest pain (and intermittent claudication) I70.529
          bilateral I70.503
            with
              gangrene (and intermittent claudication, rest pain and ulcer) I70.563
              intermittent claudication I70.513
              rest pain (and intermittent claudication) I70.523
            specified type NEC I70.593
          left I70.502
            with
              gangrene (and intermittent claudication, rest pain and ulcer) I70.562
              intermittent claudication I70.512
              rest pain (and intermittent claudication) I70.522
              ulceration (and intermittent claudication and rest pain) I70.549
                ankle I70.543
                calf I70.542
                foot site NEC I70.545
                heel I70.544
                lower leg NEC I70.548
                midfoot I70.544
                thigh I70.541
            specified type NEC I70.592
          right I70.501
            with
              gangrene (and intermittent claudication, rest pain and ulcer) I70.561
              intermittent claudication I70.511
              rest pain (and intermittent claudication) I70.521
              ulceration (and intermittent claudication and rest pain) I70.539
                ankle I70.533
                calf I70.532
                foot site NEC I70.535
                heel I70.534
                lower leg NEC I70.538
                midfoot I70.534
                thigh I70.531
            specified type NEC I70.591
          specified type NEC I70.599
        specified NEC I70.508

Arteriosclerosis, arteriosclerotic — *continued*
  extremities — *continued*
    bypass graft — *continued*
      nonautologous biological graft — *continued*
        specified — *continued*
          with
            gangrene (and intermittent claudication, rest pain and ulcer) I70.568
            intermittent claudication I70.518
            rest pain (and intermittent claudication) I70.528
            ulceration (and intermittent claudication and rest pain) I70.55
          specified type NEC I70.598
      nonbiological graft I70.609
        leg I70.609
          with
            gangrene (and intermittent claudication, rest pain and ulcer) I70.669
            intermittent claudication I70.619
            rest pain (and intermittent claudication) I70.629
          bilateral I70.603
            with
              gangrene (and intermittent claudication, rest pain and ulcer) I70.663
              intermittent claudication I70.613
              rest pain (and intermittent claudication) I70.623
            specified type NEC I70.693
          left I70.602
            with
              gangrene (and intermittent claudication, rest pain and ulcer) I70.662
              intermittent claudication I70.612
              rest pain (and intermittent claudication) I70.622
              ulceration (and intermittent claudication and rest pain) I70.649
                ankle I70.643
                calf I70.642
                foot site NEC I70.645
                heel I70.644
                lower leg NEC I70.648
                midfoot I70.644
                thigh I70.641
            specified type NEC I70.692
          right I70.601
            with
              gangrene (and intermittent claudication, rest pain and ulcer) I70.661
              intermittent claudication I70.611
              rest pain (and intermittent claudication) I70.621
              ulceration (and intermittent claudication and rest pain) I70.639
                ankle I70.633
                calf I70.632
                foot site NEC I70.635
                heel I70.634
                lower leg NEC I70.638
                midfoot I70.634
                thigh I70.631
            specified type NEC I70.691
          specified type NEC I70.699
        specified NEC I70.608
          with
            gangrene (and intermittent claudication, rest pain and ulcer) I70.668
            intermittent claudication I70.618
            rest pain (and intermittent claudication) I70.628
            ulceration (and intermittent claudication and rest pain) I70.65
          specified type NEC I70.698
      specified graft NEC I70.709
        leg I70.709
          with
            gangrene (and intermittent claudication, rest pain and ulcer) I70.769
            intermittent claudication I70.719
            rest pain (and intermittent claudication) I70.729
          bilateral I70.703

Arteriosclerosis, arteriosclerotic — Arthritis, arthritic

Arteriosclerosis, arteriosclerotic — *continued*
  extremities — *continued*
    bypass graft — *continued*
      specified graft — *continued*
        leg — *continued*
          bilateral — *continued*
            with
              gangrene (and intermittent claudication, rest pain and ulcer) I70.763
              intermittent claudication I70.713
              rest pain (and intermittent claudication) I70.723
              specified type NEC I70.793
          left I70.702
            with
              gangrene (and intermittent claudication, rest pain and ulcer) I70.762
              intermittent claudication I70.712
              rest pain (and intermittent claudication) I70.722
              ulceration (and intermittent claudication and rest pain) I70.749
                ankle I70.743
                calf I70.742
                foot site NEC I70.745
                heel I70.744
                lower leg NEC I70.748
                midfoot I70.744
                thigh I70.741
              specified type NEC I70.792
          right I70.701
            with
              gangrene (and intermittent claudication, rest pain and ulcer) I70.761
              intermittent claudication I70.711
              rest pain (and intermittent claudication) I70.721
              ulceration (and intermittent claudication and rest pain) I70.739
                ankle I70.733
                calf I70.732
                foot site NEC I70.735
                heel I70.734
                lower leg NEC I70.738
                midfoot I70.734
                thigh I70.731
              specified type NEC I70.791
          specified type NEC I70.799
      specified NEC I70.708
        with
          gangrene (and intermittent claudication, rest pain and ulcer) I70.768
          intermittent claudication I70.718
          rest pain (and intermittent claudication) I70.728
          ulceration (and intermittent claudication and rest pain) I70.75
          specified type NEC I70.798
    specified NEC I70.308
      with
        gangrene (and intermittent claudication, rest pain and ulcer) I70.368
        intermittent claudication I70.318
        rest pain (and intermittent claudication) I70.328
        ulceration (and intermittent claudication and rest pain) I70.35
        specifiec type NEC I70.398
    leg I70.209
      with
        gangrene (and intermittent claudication, rest pain and ulcer) I70.269
        intermittent claudication I70.219
        rest pain (and intermittent claudication) I70.229
      bilateral I70.203
        with
          gangrene (and intermittent claudication, rest pain and ulcer) I70.263
          intermittent claudication I70.213
          rest pain (and intermittent claudication) I70.223
          specified type NEC I70.293
      left I70.202

Arteriosclerosis, arteriosclerotic — *continued*
  extremities — *continued*
    leg — *continued*
      left — *continued*
        with
          gangrene (and intermittent claudication, rest pain and ulcer) I70.262
          intermittent claudication I70.212
          rest pain (and intermittent claudication) I70.222
          ulceration (and intermittent claudication and rest pain) I70.249
            ankle I70.243
            calf I70.242
            foot site NEC I70.245
            heel I70.244
            lower leg NEC I70.248
            midfoot I70.244
            thigh I70.241
        specified type NEC I70.292
      right I70.201
        with
          gangrene (and intermittent claudication, rest pain and ulcer) I70.261
          intermittent claudication I70.211
          rest pain (and intermittent claudication) I70.221
          ulceration (and intermittent claudication and rest pain) I70.239
            ankle I70.233
            calf I70.232
            foot site NEC I70.235
            heel I70.234
            lower leg NEC I70.238
            midfoot I70.234
            thigh I70.231
        specified type NEC I70.291
      specified type NEC I70.299
    specified site NEC I70.208
      with
        gangrene (and intermittent claudication, rest pain and ulcer) I70.268
        intermittent claudication I70.218
        rest pain (and intermittent claudication) I70.228
        ulceration (and intermittent claudication and rest pain) I70.25
        specified type NEC I70.298
  generalized I70.91
  heart (disease) — *see* Arteriosclerosis, coronary (artery),
  kidney — *see* Hypertension, kidney
  medial — *see* Arteriosclerosis, extremities
  mesenteric (artery) K55.1
  Mönckeberg's — *see* Arteriosclerosis, extremities
  myocarditis I51.4
  peripheral (of extremities) — *see* Arteriosclerosis, extremities
  pulmonary (idiopathic) I27.0
  renal (arterioles) — *see also* Hypertension, kidney
    artery I70.1
  retina (vascular) I70.8 *[H35.0-]* ☑
  specified artery NEC I70.8
  spinal (cord) G95.19
  vertebral (artery) I67.2
Arteriospasm I73.9
Arteriovenous — *see* condition
Arteritis I77.6
  allergic M31.0
  aorta (nonsyphilitic) I77.6
    syphilitic A52.02
  aortic arch M31.4
  brachiocephalic M31.4
  brain I67.7
    syphilitic A52.04
  cerebral I67.7
    in systemic lupus erythematosus M32.19
    listerial A32.89
    syphilitic A52.04
    tuberculous A18.89
  coronary (artery) I25.89
    rheumatic I01.8
      chronic I09.89
    syphilitic A52.06
  cranial (left) (right), giant cell M31.6
  deformans — *see* Arteriosclerosis
  giant cell NEC M31.6
    with polymyalgia rheumatica M31.5
  necrosing or necrotizing M31.9

Arteritis — *continued*
  necrosing or necrotizing — *continued*
    specified NEC M31.8
  nodosa M30.0
  obliterans — *see* Arteriosclerosis
  pulmonary I28.8
  rheumatic — *see* Fever, rheumatic
  senile — *see* Arteriosclerosis
  suppurative I77.2
  syphilitic (general) A52.09
    brain A52.04
    coronary A52.06
    spinal A52.09
  temporal, giant cell M31.6
  young female aortic arch syndrome M31.4
Artery, arterial — *see also* condition
  abscess I77.89
  single umbilical Q27.0
Arthralgia (allergic) — *see also* Pain, joint
  in caisson disease T70.3 ☑
  temporomandibular M26.62- ☑
Arthritis, arthritic (acute) (chronic) (nonpyogenic) (subacute) M19.90
  allergic — *see* Arthritis, specified form NEC
  ankylosing (crippling) (spine) — *see also* Spondylitis, ankylosing
    sites other than spine — *see* Arthritis, specified form NEC
  atrophic — *see* Osteoarthritis
    spine — *see* Spondylitis, ankylosing
  back — *see* Spondylopathy, inflammatory
  blennorrhagic (gonococcal) A54.42
  Charcot's — *see* Arthropathy, neuropathic
    diabetic — *see* Diabetes, arthropathy, neuropathic
    syringomyelic G95.0
  chylous (filarial) — *see also* category M01 B74.9
  climacteric (any site) NEC — *see* Arthritis, specified form NEC
  crystal (-induced) — *see* Arthritis, in, crystals
  deformans — *see* Osteoarthritis
  degenerative — *see* Osteoarthritis
  due to or associated with
    acromegaly E22.0
    brucellosis — *see* Brucellosis
    caisson disease T70.3 ☑
    diabetes — *see* Diabetes, arthropathy
    dracontiasis — *see also* category M01 B72
    enteritis NEC
      regional — *see* Enteritis, regional
    erysipelas — *see also* category M01 A46
    erythema
      epidemic A25.1
      nodosum L52
    filariasis NOS B74.9
    glanders A24.0
    helminthiasis — *see also* category M01 B83.9
    hemophilia D66 *[M36.2]*
    Henoch- (Schönlein) purpura D69.0 *[M36.4]*
    human parvovirus — *see also* category M01 B97.6
    infectious disease NEC M01 ☑
    leprosy (see also category M01) — *see also* Leprosy A30.9
    Lyme disease A69.23
    mycobacteria — *see also* category M01 A31.8
    parasitic disease NEC — *see also* category M01 B89
    paratyphoid fever (see also category M01) — *see also* Fever, paratyphoid A01.4
    rat bite fever — *see also* category M01 A25.1
    regional enteritis — *see* Enteritis, regional
    respiratory disorder NOS J98.9
    serum sickness — *see also* Reaction, serum T80.69 ☑
    syringomyelia G95.0
    typhoid fever A01.04
  epidemic erythema A25.1
  febrile — *see* Fever, rheumatic
  gonococcal A54.42
  gouty (acute) — *see* Gout
  in (due to)
    acromegaly — *see also* subcategory M14.8- E22.0
    amyloidosis — *see also* subcategory M14.8- E85.4
    bacterial disease — *see also* subcategory M01 A49.9
    Behçet's syndrome M35.2
    caisson disease — *see also* subcategory M14.8- T70.3 ☑
    coliform bacilli (Escherichia coli) — *see* Arthritis, in, pyogenic organism NEC

☑ **Additional Character Required** — Refer to the Tabular List for Character Selection   ▽ Subterms under main terms may continue to next column or page

Arthritis, arthritic — *continued*
  in — *continued*
    crystals M11.9
      dicalcium phosphate — *see* Arthritis, in, crystals, specified type NEC
      hydroxyapatite M11.0- ☑
      pyrophosphate — *see* Arthritis, in, crystals, specified type NEC
      specified type NEC M11.80
        ankle M11.87- ☑
        elbow M11.82- ☑
        foot joint M11.87- ☑
        hand joint M11.84- ☑
        hip M11.85- ☑
        knee M11.86- ☑
        multiple sites M11.8- ☑
        shoulder M11.81- ☑
        vertebrae M11.88
        wrist M11.83- ☑
    dermatoarthritis, lipoid E78.81
    dracontiasis (dracunculiasis) — *see also* category M01 B72
    endocrine disorder NEC — *see also* subcategory M14.8- E34.9
    enteritis, infectious NEC — *see also* category M01 A09
      specified organism NEC — *see also* category M01 A08.8
    erythema
      multiforme — *see also* subcategory M14.8- L51.9
      nodosum — *see also* subcategory M14.8- L52
    gout — *see* Gout
    helminthiasis NEC — *see also* category M01 B83.9
    hemochromatosis — *see also* subcategory M14.8- E83.118
    hemoglobinopathy NEC D58.2 *[M36.3]*
    hemophilia NEC D66 *[M36.2]*
    Hemophilus influenzae M00.8- ☑ *[B96.3]*
    Henoch (-Schönlein) purpura D69.0 *[M36.4]*
    hyperparathyroidism NEC — *see also* subcategory M14.8- E21.3
    hypersensitivity reaction NEC T78.49 ☑ *[M36.4]*
    hypogammaglobulinemia — *see also* subcategory M14.8- D80.1
    hypothyroidism NEC — *see also* subcategory M14.8- E03.9
    infection — *see* Arthritis, pyogenic or pyemic
      spine — *see* Spondylopathy, infective
    infectious disease NEC M01 ☑
    leprosy — *see also* category M01 A30.9
    leukemia NEC C95.9- ☑ *[M36.1]*
    lipoid dermatoarthritis E78.81
    Lyme disease A69.23
    Mediterranean fever, familial — *see also* subcategory M14.8- M04.1
    Meningococcus A39.83
    metabolic disorder NEC — *see also* subcategory M14.8- E88.9
    multiple myelomatosis C90.0- ☑ *[M36.1]*
    mumps B26.85
    mycosis NEC — *see also* category M01 B49
    myelomatosis (multiple) C90.0- ☑ *[M36.1]*
    neurological disorder NEC G98.0
    ochronosis — *see also* subcategory M14.8- E70.29
    O'nyong-nyong — *see also* category M01 A92.1
    parasitic disease NEC — *see also* category M01 B89
    paratyphoid fever — *see also* category M01 A01.4
    Pseudomonas — *see* Arthritis, pyogenic, bacterial NEC
    psoriasis L40.50
    pyogenic organism NEC — *see* Arthritis, pyogenic, bacterial NEC
    Reiter's disease — *see* Reiter's disease
    respiratory disorder NEC — *see also* subcategory M14.8- J98.9
    reticulosis, malignant — *see also* subcategory M14.8- C86.0
    rubella B06.82
    Salmonella (arizonae) (cholerae-suis) (enteritidis) (typhimurium) A02.23
    sarcoidosis D86.86
    specified bacteria NEC — *see* Arthritis, pyogenic, bacterial NEC
    sporotrichosis B42.82
    syringomyelia G95.0
    thalassemia NEC D56.9 *[M36.3]*
    tuberculosis — *see* Tuberculosis, arthritis

Arthritis, arthritic — *continued*
  in — *continued*
    typhoid fever A01.04
    urethritis, Reiter's — *see* Reiter's disease
    viral disease NEC — *see also* category M01 B34.9
  infectious or infective — *see also* Arthritis, pyogenic or pyemic
    spine — *see* Spondylopathy, infective
  juvenile M08.90
    with systemic onset — *see* Still's disease
    ankle M08.97- ☑
    elbow M08.92- ☑
    foot joint M08.97- ☑
    hand joint M08.94- ☑
    hip M08.95- ☑
    knee M08.96- ☑
    multiple site M08.99
    pauciarticular M08.40
      ankle M08.47- ☑
      elbow M08.42- ☑
      foot joint M08.47- ☑
      hand joint M08.44- ☑
      hip M08.45- ☑
      knee M08.46- ☑
      shoulder M08.41- ☑
      vertebrae M08.48
      wrist M08.43- ☑
    psoriatic L40.54
    rheumatoid — *see* Arthritis, rheumatoid, juvenile
    shoulder M08.91- ☑
    specified type NEC M08.80
      ankle M08.87- ☑
      elbow M08.82- ☑
      foot joint M08.87- ☑
      hand joint M08.84- ☑
      hip M08.85- ☑
      knee M08.86- ☑
      multiple site M08.89
      shoulder M08.81- ☑
      specified joint NEC M08.88
      vertebrae M08.88
      wrist M08.83- ☑
    wrist M08.93- ☑
  meaning osteoarthritis — *see* Osteoarthritis
  meningococcal A39.83
  menopausal (any site) NEC — *see* Arthritis, specified form NEC
  mutilans (psoriatic) L40.52
  mycotic NEC — *see also* category M01 B49
  neuropathic (Charcot) — *see* Arthropathy, neuropathic
    diabetic — *see* Diabetes, arthropathy, neuropathic
    nonsyphilitic NEC G98.0
    syringomyelic G95.0
  ochronotic — *see also* subcategory M14.8- E70.29
  palindromic (any site) — *see* Rheumatism, palindromic
  pneumococcal M00.10
    ankle M00.17- ☑
    elbow M00.12- ☑
    foot joint — *see* Arthritis, pneumococcal, ankle
    hand joint M00.14- ☑
    hip M00.15- ☑
    knee M00.16- ☑
    multiple site M00.19
    shoulder M00.11- ☑
    vertebra M00.18
    wrist M00.13- ☑
  postdysenteric — *see* Arthropathy, postdysenteric
  postmeningococcal A39.84
  postrheumatic, chronic — *see* Arthropathy, postrheumatic, chronic
  primary progressive — *see also* Arthritis, specified form NEC
    spine — *see* Spondylitis, ankylosing
  psoriatic L40.50
  purulent (any site except spine) — *see* Arthritis, pyogenic or pyemic
    spine — *see* Spondylopathy, infective
  pyogenic or pyemic (any site except spine) M00.9
    bacterial NEC M00.80
      ankle M00.87- ☑
      elbow M00.82- ☑
      foot joint — *see* Arthritis, pyogenic, bacterial NEC, ankle
      hand joint M00.84- ☑
      hip M00.85- ☑
      knee M00.86- ☑
      multiple site M00.89

Arthritis, arthritic — *continued*
  pyogenic or pyemic — *continued*
    bacterial — *continued*
      shoulder M00.81- ☑
      vertebra M00.88
      wrist M00.83- ☑
    pneumococcal — *see* Arthritis, pneumococcal
    spine — *see* Spondylopathy, infective
    staphylococcal — *see* Arthritis, staphylococcal
    streptococcal — *see* Arthritis, streptococcal NEC
      pneumococcal — *see* Arthritis, pneumococcal
  reactive — *see* Reiter's disease
  rheumatic — *see also* Arthritis, rheumatoid
    acute or subacute — *see* Fever, rheumatic
  rheumatoid M06.9
    with
      carditis — *see* Rheumatoid, carditis
      endocarditis — *see* Rheumatoid, carditis
      heart involvement NEC — *see* Rheumatoid, carditis
      lung involvement — *see* Rheumatoid, lung
      myocarditis — *see* Rheumatoid, carditis
      myopathy — *see* Rheumatoid, myopathy
      pericarditis — *see* Rheumatoid, carditis
      polyneuropathy — *see* Rheumatoid, polyneuropathy
      rheumatoid factor — *see* Arthritis, rheumatoid, seropositive
      splenoadenomegaly and leukopenia — *see* Felty's syndrome
      vasculitis — *see* Rheumatoid, vasculitis
      visceral involvement NEC — *see* Rheumatoid, arthritis, with involvement of organs NEC
    juvenile (with or without rheumatoid factor) M08.00
      ankle M08.07- ☑
      elbow M08.02- ☑
      foot joint M08.07- ☑
      hand joint M08.04- ☑
      hip M08.05- ☑
      knee M08.06- ☑
      multiple site M08.09
      shoulder M08.01- ☑
      vertebra M08.08
      wrist M08.03- ☑
    seronegative M06.00
      ankle M06.07- ☑
      elbow M06.02- ☑
      foot joint M06.07- ☑
      hand joint M06.04- ☑
      hip M06.05- ☑
      knee M06.06- ☑
      multiple site M06.09
      shoulder M06.01- ☑
      vertebra M06.08
      wrist M06.03- ☑
    seropositive M05.9
      specified NEC M05.80
        ankle M05.87- ☑
        elbow M05.82- ☑
        foot joint M05.87- ☑
        hand joint M05.84- ☑
        hip M05.85- ☑
        knee M05.86- ☑
        multiple sites M05.89
        shoulder M05.81- ☑
        vertebra — *see* Spondylitis, ankylosing
        wrist M05.83- ☑
      without organ involvement M05.70
        ankle M05.77- ☑
        elbow M05.72- ☑
        foot joint M05.77- ☑
        hand joint M05.74- ☑
        hip M05.75- ☑
        knee M05.76- ☑
        multiple sites M05.79
        shoulder M05.71- ☑
        vertebra — *see* Spondylitis, ankylosing
        wrist M05.73- ☑
    specified type NEC M06.80
      ankle M06.87- ☑
      elbow M06.82- ☑
      foot joint M06.87- ☑
      hand joint M06.84- ☑
      hip M06.85- ☑
      knee M06.86- ☑
      multiple site M06.89

Arthritis, arthritic — *continued*
  rheumatoid — *continued*
    specified type — *continued*
      shoulder M06.81- ☑
      vertebra M06.88
      wrist M06.83- ☑
    spine — *see* Spondylitis, ankylosing
  rubella B06.82
  scorbutic — *see also* subcategory M14.8- E54
  senile or senescent — *see* Osteoarthritis
  septic (any site except spine) — *see* Arthritis, pyogenic
    or pyemic
    spine — *see* Spondylopathy, infective
  serum (nontherapeutic) (therapeutic) — *see*
    Arthropathy, postimmunization
  specified form NEC M13.80
    ankle M13.87- ☑
    elbow M13.82- ☑
    foot joint M13.87- ☑
    hand joint M13.84- ☑
    hip M13.85- ☑
    knee M13.86- ☑
    multiple site M13.89
    shoulder M13.81- ☑
    specified joint NEC M13.88
    wrist M13.83- ☑
  spine — *see also* Spondylopathy, inflammatory
    infectious or infective NEC — *see* Spondylopathy,
      infective
    Marie-Strümpell — *see* Spondylitis, ankylosing
    pyogenic — *see* Spondylopathy, infective
    rheumatoid — *see* Spondylitis, ankylosing
    traumatic (old) — *see* Spondylopathy, traumatic
    tuberculous A18.01
  staphylococcal M00.00
    ankle M00.07- ☑
    elbow M00.02- ☑
    foot joint — *see* Arthritis, staphylococcal, ankle
    hand joint M00.04- ☑
    hip M00.05- ☑
    knee M00.06- ☑
    multiple site M00.09
    shoulder M00.01- ☑
    vertebra M00.08
    wrist M00.03- ☑
  streptococcal NEC M00.20
    ankle M00.27- ☑
    elbow M00.22- ☑
    foot joint — *see* Arthritis, streptococcal, ankle
    hand joint M00.24- ☑
    hip M00.25- ☑
    knee M00.26- ☑
    multiple site M00.29
    shoulder M00.21- ☑
    vertebra M00.28
    wrist M00.23- ☑
  suppurative — *see* Arthritis, pyogenic or pyemic
  syphilitic (late) A52.16
    congenital A50.55 *[M12.80]*
  syphilitica deformans (Charcot) A52.16
  temporomandibular M26.69
  toxic of menopause (any site) — *see* Arthritis, specified
    form NEC
  transient — *see* Arthropathy, specified form NEC
  traumatic (chronic) — *see* Arthropathy, traumatic
  tuberculous A18.02
    spine A18.01
  uratic — *see* Gout
  urethritica (Reiter's) — *see* Reiter's disease
  vertebral — *see* Spondylopathy, inflammatory
  villous (any site) — *see* Arthropathy, specified form
    NEC
Arthrocele — *see* Effusion, joint
Arthrodesis status Z98.1
Arthrodynia — *see also* Pain, joint
Arthrodysplasia Q74.9
Arthrofibrosis, joint — *see* Ankylosis
Arthrogryposis (congenital) Q68.8
  multiplex congenita Q74.3
Arthrokatadysis M24.7
Arthropathy — *see also* Arthritis M12.9
  Charcot's — *see* Arthropathy, neuropathic
    diabetic — *see* Diabetes, arthropathy, neuropathic
    syringomyelic G95.0
  cricoarytenoid J38.7
  crystal (-induced) — *see* Arthritis, in, crystals
  diabetic NEC — *see* Diabetes, arthropathy

Arthropathy — *continued*
  distal interphalangeal, psoriatic L40.51
  enteropathic M07.60
    ankle M07.67- ☑
    elbow M07.62- ☑
    foot joint M07.67- ☑
    hand joint M07.64- ☑
    hip M07.65- ☑
    knee M07.66- ☑
    multiple site M07.69
    shoulder M07.61- ☑
    vertebra M07.68
    wrist M07.63- ☑
  following intestinal bypass M02.00
    ankle M02.07- ☑
    elbow M02.02- ☑
    foot joint M02.07- ☑
    hand joint M02.04- ☑
    hip M02.05- ☑
    knee M02.06- ☑
    multiple site M02.09
    shoulder M02.01- ☑
    vertebra M02.08
    wrist M02.03- ☑
  gouty — *see also* Gout
    in (due to)
      Lesch-Nyhan syndrome E79.1 *[M14.8-]* ☑
      sickle-cell disorders D57- ☑ *[M14.8-]* ☑
  hemophilic NEC D66 *[M36.2]*
    in (due to)
      hyperparathyroidism NEC E21.3 *[M14.8-]* ☑
      metabolic disease NOS E88.9 *[M14.8-]* ☑
  in (due to)
    acromegaly E22.0 *[M14.8-]* ☑
    amyloidosis E85.4 *[M14.8-]* ☑
    blood disorder NOS D75.9 *[M36.3]*
    diabetes — *see* Diabetes, arthropathy
    endocrine disease NOS E34.9 *[M14.8-]* ☑
    erythema
      multiforme L51.9 *[M14.8-]* ☑
      nodosum L52 *[M14.8-]* ☑
    hemochromatosis E83.118 *[M14.8-]* ☑
    hemoglobinopathy NEC D58.2 *[M36.3]*
    hemophilia NEC D66 *[M36.2]*
    Henoch-Schönlein purpura D69.0 *[M36.4]*
    hyperthyroidism E05.90 *[M14.8-]* ☑
    hypothyroidism E03.9 *[M14.8-]* ☑
    infective endocarditis I33.0 *[M12.80]*
    leukemia NEC C95.9- ☑ *[M36.1]*
    malignant histiocytosis C96.A *[M36.1]*
    metabolic disease NOS E88.9 *[M14.8-]* ☑
    multiple myeloma C90.0- ☑ *[M36.1]*
    neoplastic disease NOS (*see also* Neoplasm)
      D49.9 *[M36.1]*
    nutritional deficiency — *see also* subcategory
      M14.8- E63.9
    psoriasis NOS L40.50
    sarcoidosis D86.86
    syphilis (late) A52.77
      congenital A50.55 *[M12.80]*
    thyrotoxicosis — *see also* subcategory M14.8-
      E05.90
    ulcerative colitis K51.90 *[M07.60]*
    viral hepatitis (postinfectious) NEC B19.9 *[M12.80]*
    Whipple's disease — *see also* subcategory M14.8-
      K90.81
  Jaccoud — *see* Arthropathy, postrheumatic, chronic
  juvenile — *see* Arthritis, juvenile
    psoriatic L40.54
  mutilans (psoriatic) L40.52
  neuropathic (Charcot) M14.60
    ankle M14.67- ☑
    diabetic — *see* Diabetes, arthropathy, neuropathic
    elbow M14.62- ☑
    foot joint M14.67- ☑
    hand joint M14.64- ☑
    hip M14.65- ☑
    knee M14.66- ☑
    multiple site M14.69
    nonsyphilitic NEC G98.0
    shoulder M14.61- ☑
    syringomyelic G95.0
    vertebra M14.68
    wrist M14.63- ☑
  osteopulmonary — *see* Osteoarthropathy, hyper-
    trophic, specified NEC

Arthropathy — *continued*
  postdysenteric M02.10
    ankle M02.17- ☑
    elbow M02.12- ☑
    foot joint M02.17- ☑
    hand joint M02.14- ☑
    hip M02.15- ☑
    knee M02.16- ☑
    multiple site M02.19
    shoulder M02.11- ☑
    vertebra M02.18
    wrist M02.13- ☑
  postimmunization M02.20
    ankle M02.27- ☑
    elbow M02.22- ☑
    foot joint M02.27- ☑
    hand joint M02.24- ☑
    hip M02.25- ☑
    knee M02.26- ☑
    multiple site M02.29
    shoulder M02.21- ☑
    vertebra M02.28
    wrist M02.23- ☑
  postinfectious NEC B99 ☑ *[M12.80]*
    in (due to)
      enteritis due to Yersinia enterocolitica
        A04.6 *[M12.80]*
      syphilis A52.77
      viral hepatitis NEC B19.9 *[M12.80]*
  postrheumatic, chronic (Jaccoud) M12.00
    ankle M12.07- ☑
    elbow M12.02- ☑
    foot joint M12.07- ☑
    hand joint M12.04- ☑
    hip M12.05- ☑
    knee M12.06- ☑
    multiple site M12.09
    shoulder M12.01- ☑
    specified joint NEC M12.08
    vertebrae M12.08
    wrist M12.03- ☑
  psoriatic NEC L40.59
    interphalangeal, distal L40.51
  reactive M02.9
    in (due to)
      infective endocarditis I33.0 *[M02.9]*
      specified type NEC M02.80
        ankle M02.87- ☑
        elbow M02.82- ☑
        foot joint M02.87- ☑
        hand joint M02.84- ☑
        hip M02.85- ☑
        knee M02.86- ☑
        multiple site M02.89
        shoulder M02.81- ☑
        vertebra M02.88
        wrist M02.83- ☑
  specified form NEC M12.80
    ankle M12.87- ☑
    elbow M12.82- ☑
    foot joint M12.87- ☑
    hand joint M12.84- ☑
    hip M12.85- ☑
    knee M12.86- ☑
    multiple site M12.89
    shoulder M12.81- ☑
    specified joint NEC M12.88
    vertebrae M12.88
    wrist M12.83- ☑
  syringomyelic G95.0
  tabes dorsalis A52.16
  tabetic A52.16
  transient — *see* Arthropathy, specified form NEC
  traumatic M12.50
    ankle M12.57- ☑
    elbow M12.52- ☑
    foot joint M12.57- ☑
    hand joint M12.54- ☑
    hip M12.55- ☑
    knee M12.56- ☑
    multiple site M12.59
    shoulder M12.51- ☑
    specified joint NEC M12.58
    vertebrae M12.58
    wrist M12.53- ☑
Arthropyosis — *see* Arthritis, pyogenic or pyemic

  ☑ **Additional Character Required** — Refer to the Tabular List for Character Selection   ▽ Subterms under main terms may continue to next column or page

Arthrosis (deformans) (degenerative) (localized) — *see also* Osteoarthritis M19.90
- spine — *see* Spondylosis

Arthus' phenomenon or reaction T78.41 ☑
- due to
  - drug — *see* Table of Drugs and Chemicals, by drug

Articular — *see* condition

Articulation, reverse (teeth) M26.24

Artificial
- insemination complication — *see* Complications, artificial, fertilization
- opening status (functioning) (without complication) Z93.9
  - anus (colostomy) Z93.3
  - colostomy Z93.3
  - cystostomy Z93.50
    - appendico-vesicostomy Z93.52
    - cutaneous Z93.51
    - specified NEC Z93.59
  - enterostomy Z93.4
  - gastrostomy Z93.1
  - ileostomy Z93.2
  - intestinal tract NEC Z93.4
  - jejunostomy Z93.4
  - nephrostomy Z93.6
  - specified site NEC Z93.8
  - tracheostomy Z93.0
  - ureterostomy Z93.6
  - urethrostomy Z93.6
  - urinary tract NEC Z93.6
  - vagina Z93.8
- vagina status Z93.8

Arytenoid — *see* condition

Asbestosis (occupational) J61

Ascariasis B77.9
- with
  - complications NEC B77.89
  - intestinal complications B77.0
  - pneumonia, pneumonitis B77.81

Ascaridosis, ascariadiasis — *see* Ascariasis

Ascaris (infection) (infestation) (lumbricoides) — *see* Ascariasis

Ascending — *see* condition

ASC-H (atypical squamous cells cannot exclude high grade squamous intraepithelial lesion on cytologic smear)
- anus R85.611
- cervix R87.611
- vagina R87.621

Aschoff's bodies — *see* Myocarditis, rheumatic

Ascites (abdominal) R18.8
- cardiac — *see also* Failure, heart, right I50.810
- chylous (nonfilarial) I89.8
  - filarial — *see* Infestation, filarial
- due to
  - cirrhosis, alcoholic K70.31
  - hepatitis
    - alcoholic K70.11
    - chronic active K71.51
  - S. japonicum B65.2
- heart — *see also* Failure, heart, right I50.810
- malignant R18.0
- pseudochylous R18.8
- syphilitic A52.74
- tuberculous A18.31

ASC-US (atypical squamous cells of undetermined significance on cytologic smear)
- anus R85.610
- cervix R87.610
- vagina R87.620

Aseptic — *see* condition

Asherman's syndrome N85.6

Asialia K11.7

Asiatic cholera — *see* Cholera

Asimultagnosia (simultanagnosia) R48.3

Askin's tumor — *see* Neoplasm, connective tissue, malignant

Asocial personality F60.2

Asomatognosia R41.4

Aspartylglucosaminuria E77.1

Asperger's disease or syndrome F84.5

Aspergilloma — *see* Aspergillosis

Aspergillosis (with pneumonia) B44.9
- bronchopulmonary, allergic B44.81
- disseminated B44.7
- generalized B44.7
- pulmonary NEC B44.1
  - allergic B44.81
  - invasive B44.0

Aspergillosis — *continued*
- specified NEC B44.89
- tonsillar B44.2

Aspergillus (flavus) (fumigatus) (infection) (terreus) — *see* Aspergillosis

Aspermatogenesis — *see* Azoospermia

Aspermia (testis) — *see* Azoospermia

Asphyxia, asphyxiation (by) R09.01
- antenatal P84
- birth P84
- bunny bag — *see* Asphyxia, due to, mechanical threat to breathing, trapped in bed clothes
- crushing S28.0 ☑
- drowning T75.1 ☑
- gas, fumes, or vapor — *see* Table of Drugs and Chemicals
- inhalation — *see* Inhalation
- intrauterine P84
- local I73.00
  - with gangrene I73.01
- mucus — *see also* Foreign body, respiratory tract, causing asphyxia
- newborn P84
- pathological R09.01
- postnatal P84
  - mechanical — *see* Asphyxia, due to, mechanical threat to breathing
- prenatal P84
- reticularis R23.1
- strangulation — *see* Asphyxia, due to, mechanical threat to breathing
- submersion T75.1 ☑
- traumatic T71.9 ☑
  - due to
    - crushed chest S28.0 ☑
    - foreign body (in) — *see* Foreign body, respiratory tract, causing asphyxia
    - low oxygen content of ambient air T71.20 ☑
      - due to
        - being trapped in
          - low oxygen environment T71.29 ☑
            - in car trunk T71.221 ☑
              - circumstances undetermined T71.224 ☑
              - done with intent to harm by
                - another person T71.223 ☑
                - self T71.222 ☑
            - in refrigerator T71.231 ☑
              - circumstances undetermined T71.234 ☑
              - done with intent to harm by
                - another person T71.233 ☑
                - self T71.232 ☑
        - cave-in T71.21 ☑
    - mechanical threat to breathing (accidental) T71.191 ☑
      - circumstances undetermined T71.194 ☑
      - done with intent to harm by
        - another person T71.193 ☑
        - self T71.192 ☑
      - hanging T71.161 ☑
        - circumstances undetermined T71.164 ☑
        - done with intent to harm by
          - another person T71.163 ☑
          - self T71.162 ☑
      - plastic bag T71.121 ☑
        - circumstances undetermined T71.124 ☑
        - done with intent to harm by
          - another person T71.123 ☑
          - self T71.122 ☑
      - smothering
        - in furniture T71.151 ☑
          - circumstances undetermined T71.154 ☑
          - done with intent to harm by
            - another person T71.153 ☑
            - self T71.152 ☑
        - under
          - another person's body T71.141 ☑
            - circumstances undetermined T71.144 ☑
            - done with intent to harm T71.143 ☑
          - pillow T71.111 ☑
            - circumstances undetermined T71.114 ☑
            - done with intent to harm by
              - another person T71.113 ☑

Asphyxia, asphyxiation — *continued*
- traumatic — *continued*
  - due to — *continued*
    - mechanical threat to breathing — *continued*
      - smothering — *continued*
        - under — *continued*
          - pillow — *continued*
            - done with intent to harm by — *continued*
              - self T71.112 ☑
          - trapped in bed clothes T71.131 ☑
            - circumstances undetermined T71.134 ☑
            - done with intent to harm by
              - another person T71.133 ☑
              - self T71.132 ☑
- vomiting, vomitus — *see* Foreign body, respiratory tract, causing asphyxia

Aspiration
- amniotic (clear) fluid (newborn) P24.10
  - with
    - pneumonia (pneumonitis) P24.11
    - respiratory symptoms P24.11
- blood
  - newborn (without respiratory symptoms) P24.20
    - with
      - pneumonia (pneumonitis) P24.21
      - respiratory symptoms P24.21
  - specified age NEC — *see* Foreign body, respiratory tract
- bronchitis J69.0
- food or foreign body (with asphyxiation) — *see* Asphyxia, food
- liquor (amnii) (newborn) P24.10
  - with
    - pneumonia (pneumonitis) P24.11
    - respiratory symptoms P24.11
- meconium (newborn) (without respiratory symptoms) P24.00
  - with
    - pneumonitis (pneumonitis) P24.01
    - respiratory symptoms P24.01
- milk (newborn) (without respiratory symptoms) P24.30
  - with
    - pneumonia (pneumonitis) P24.31
    - respiratory symptoms P24.31
  - specified age NEC — *see* Foreign body, respiratory tract
- mucus — *see also* Foreign body, by site, causing asphyxia
  - newborn P24.10
    - with
      - pneumonia (pneumonitis) P24.11
      - respiratory symptoms P24.11
- neonatal P24.9
  - specific NEC (without respiratory symptoms) P24.80
    - with
      - pneumonia (pneumonitis) P24.81
      - respiratory symptoms P24.81
- newborn P24.9
  - specific NEC (without respiratory symptoms) P24.80
    - with
      - pneumonia (pneumonitis) P24.81
      - respiratory symptoms P24.81
- pneumonia J69.0
- pneumonitis J69.0
- syndrome of newborn — *see* Aspiration, by substance, with pneumonia
- vernix caseosa (newborn) P24.80
  - with
    - pneumonia (pneumonitis) P24.81
    - respiratory symptoms P24.81
- vomitus — *see also* Foreign body, respiratory tract
  - newborn (without respiratory symptoms) P24.30
    - with
      - pneumonia (pneumonitis) P24.31
      - respiratory symptoms P24.31

Asplenia (congenital) Q89.01
- postsurgical Z90.81

Assam fever B55.0

Assault, sexual — *see* Maltreatment

Assmann's focus NEC A15.0

Astasia (-abasia) (hysterical) F44.4

Asteatosis cutis L85.3

Astereognosia, astereognosis R48.1

Asterixis R27.8
- in liver disease K71.3

Asteroid hyalitis — *see* Deposit, crystalline

Asthenia, asthenic R53.1

Asthenia, asthenic — *continued*
  cardiac — *see also* Failure, heart I50.9
    psychogenic F45.8
  cardiovascular — *see also* Failure, heart I50.9
    psychogenic F45.8
  heart — *see also* Failure, heart I50.9
    psychogenic F45.8
  hysterical F44.4
  myocardial — *see also* Failure, heart I50.9
    psychogenic F45.8
  nervous F48.8
  neurocirculatory F45.8
  neurotic F48.8
  psychogenic F48.8
  psychoneurotic F48.8
  psychophysiologic F48.8
  reaction (psychophysiologic) F48.8
  senile R54
Asthenopia — *see also* Discomfort, visual
  hysterical F44.6
  psychogenic F44.6
Asthenospermia — *see* Abnormal, specimen, male
    genital organs
Asthma, asthmatic (bronchial) (catarrh) (spasmodic)
    J45.909
  with
    chronic obstructive bronchitis J44.9
      with
        acute lower respiratory infection J44.0
        exacerbation (acute) J44.1
    chronic obstructive pulmonary disease J44.9
      with
        acute lower respiratory infection J44.0
        exacerbation (acute) J44.1
    exacerbation (acute) J45.901
    hay fever — *see* Asthma, allergic extrinsic
    rhinitis, allergic — *see* Asthma, allergic extrinsic
    status asthmaticus J45.902
  allergic extrinsic J45.909
    with
      exacerbation (acute) J45.901
      status asthmaticus J45.902
  atopic — *see* Asthma, allergic extrinsic
  cardiac — *see* Failure, ventricular, left
  cardiobronchial I50.1
  childhood J45.909
    with
      exacerbation (acute) J45.901
      status asthmaticus J45.902
  chronic obstructive J44.9
    with
      acute lower respiratory infection J44.0
      exacerbation (acute) J44.1
  collier's J60
  cough variant J45.991
  detergent J69.8
  due to
    detergent J69.8
    inhalation of fumes J68.3
  eosinophilic J82
  extrinsic, allergic — *see* Asthma, allergic extrinsic
  grinder's J62.8
  hay — *see* Asthma, allergic extrinsic
  heart I50.1
  idiosyncratic — *see* Asthma, nonallergic
  intermittent (mild) J45.20
    with
      exacerbation (acute) J45.21
      status asthmaticus J45.22
  intrinsic, nonallergic — *see* Asthma, nonallergic
  Kopp's E32.8
  late-onset J45.909
    with
      exacerbation (acute) J45.901
      status asthmaticus J45.902
  mild intermittent J45.20
    with
      exacerbation (acute) J45.21
      status asthmaticus J45.22
  mild persistent J45.30
    with
      exacerbation (acute) J45.31
      status asthmaticus J45.32
  Millar's (laryngismus stridulus) J38.5
  miner's J60
  mixed J45.909
    with
      exacerbation (acute) J45.901

Asthma, asthmatic — *continued*
  mixed — *continued*
    with — *continued*
      status asthmaticus J45.902
  moderate persistent J45.40
    with
      exacerbation (acute) J45.41
      status asthmaticus J45.42
  nervous — *see* Asthma, nonallergic
  nonallergic (intrinsic) J45.909
    with
      exacerbation (acute) J45.901
      status asthmaticus J45.902
  persistent
    mild J45.30
      with
        exacerbation (acute) J45.31
        status asthmaticus J45.32
    moderate J45.40
      with
        exacerbation (acute) J45.41
        status asthmaticus J45.42
    severe J45.50
      with
        exacerbation (acute) J45.51
        status asthmaticus J45.52
  platinum J45.998
  pneumoconiotic NEC J64
  potter's J62.8
  predominantly allergic J45.909
  psychogenic F54
  pulmonary eosinophilic J82
  red cedar J67.8
  Rostan's I50.1
  sandblaster's J62.8
  sequoiosis J67.8
  severe persistent J45.50
    with
      exacerbation (acute) J45.51
      status asthmaticus J45.52
  specified NEC J45.998
  stonemason's J62.8
  thymic E32.8
  tuberculous — *see* Tuberculosis, pulmonary
  Wichmann's (laryngismus stridulus) J38.5
  wood J67.8
Astigmatism (compound) (congenital) H52.20- ☑
  irregular H52.21- ☑
  regular H52.22- ☑
Astraphobia F40.220
Astroblastoma
  specified site — *see* Neoplasm, malignant, by site
  unspecified site C71.9
Astrocytoma (cystic)
  anaplastic
    specified site — *see* Neoplasm, malignant, by site
    unspecified site C71.9
  fibrillary
    specified site — *see* Neoplasm, malignant, by site
    unspecified site C71.9
  fibrous
    specified site — *see* Neoplasm, malignant, by site
    unspecified site C71.9
  gemistocytic
    specified site — *see* Neoplasm, malignant, by site
    unspecified site C71.9
  juvenile
    specified site — *see* Neoplasm, malignant, by site
    unspecified site C71.9
  pilocytic
    specified site — *see* Neoplasm, malignant, by site
    unspecified site C71.9
  piloid
    specified site — *see* Neoplasm, malignant, by site
    unspecified site C71.9
  protoplasmic
    specified site — *see* Neoplasm, malignant, by site
    unspecified site C71.9
  specified site NEC — *see* Neoplasm, malignant, by site
  subependymal D43.2
    giant cell
      specified site — *see* Neoplasm, uncertain behavior, by site
      unspecified site D43.2
  specified site — *see* Neoplasm, uncertain behavior, by site
  unspecified site C71.9

Astroglioma
  specified site — *see* Neoplasm, malignant, by site
  unspecified site C71.9
Asymbolia R48.8
Asymmetry — *see also* Distortion
  between native and reconstructed breast N65.1
  face Q67.0
  jaw (lower) — *see* Anomaly, dentofacial, jaw-cranial
    base relationship, asymmetry
Asynergia, asynergy R27.8
  ventricular I51.89
Asystole (heart) — *see* Arrest, cardiac
At risk
  for
    dental caries Z91.849
      high Z91.843
      low Z91.841
      moderate Z91.842
    falling Z91.81
Ataxia, ataxy, ataxic R27.0
  acute R27.8
  brain (hereditary) G11.9
  cerebellar (hereditary) G11.9
    with defective DNA repair G11.3
    alcoholic G31.2
    early-onset G11.1
    in
      alcoholism G31.2
      myxedema E03.9 *[G13.2]*
      neoplastic disease — *see also* Neoplasm
        D49.9 *[G32.81]*
      specified disease NEC G32.81
    late-onset (Marie's) G11.2
  cerebral (hereditary) G11.9
  congenital nonprogressive G11.0
  family, familial — *see* Ataxia, hereditary
  following
    cerebrovascular disease I69.993
      cerebral infarction I69.393
      intracerebral hemorrhage I69.193
      nontraumatic intracranial hemorrhage NEC
        I69.293
      specified disease NEC I69.893
      subarachnoid hemorrhage I69.093
  Friedreich's (heredofamilial) (cerebellar) (spinal) G11.1
  gait R26.0
    hysterical F44.4
  general R27.8
  gluten M35.9 *[G32.81]*
    with celiac disease K90.0 *[G32.81]*
  hereditary G11.9
    with neuropathy G60.2
    cerebellar — *see* Ataxia, cerebellar
    spastic G11.4
    specified NEC G11.8
    spinal (Friedreich's) G11.1
  heredofamilial — *see* Ataxia, hereditary
  Hunt's G11.1
  hysterical F44.4
  locomotor (progressive) (syphilitic) (partial) (spastic)
    A52.11
    diabetic — *see* Diabetes, ataxia
  Marie's (cerebellar) (heredofamilial) (late- onset) G11.2
  nonorganic origin F44.4
  nonprogressive, congenital G11.0
  psychogenic F44.4
  Roussy-Lévy G60.0
  Sanger-Brown's (hereditary) G11.2
  spastic hereditary G11.4
  spinal
    hereditary (Friedreich's) G11.1
    progressive (syphilitic) A52.11
  spinocerebellar, X-linked recessive G11.1
  telangiectasia (Louis-Bar) G11.3
Ataxia-telangiectasia (Louis-Bar) G11.3
Atelectasis (massive) (partial) (pressure) (pulmonary)
    J98.11
  newborn P28.10
    due to resorption P28.11
    partial P28.19
    primary P28.0
    secondary P28.19
  primary (newborn) P28.0
  tuberculous — *see* Tuberculosis, pulmonary
Atelocardia Q24.9
Atelomyelia Q06.1

☑ **Additional Character Required — Refer to the Tabular List for Character Selection**   � **Subterms under main terms may continue to next column or page**

Atheroembolism
  of
    extremities
      lower I75.02- ☑
      upper I75.01- ☑
    kidney I75.81
    specified NEC I75.89
Atheroma, atheromatous — *see also* Arteriosclerosis I70.90
  aorta, aortic I70.0
    valve — *see also* Endocarditis, aortic I35.8
  aorto-iliac I70.0
  artery — *see* Arteriosclerosis
  basilar (artery) I67.2
  carotid (artery) (common) (internal) I67.2
  cerebral (arteries) I67.2
  coronary (artery) I25.10
    with angina pectoris — *see* Arteriosclerosis, coronary (artery),
  degeneration — *see* Arteriosclerosis
  heart, cardiac — *see* Disease, heart, ischemic, atherosclerotic
  mitral (valve) I34.8
  myocardium, myocardial — *see* Disease, heart, ischemic, atherosclerotic
  pulmonary valve (heart) — *see also* Endocarditis, pulmonary I37.8
  tricuspid (heart) (valve) I36.8
  valve, valvular — *see* Endocarditis
  vertebral (artery) I67.2
Atheromatosis — *see* Arteriosclerosis
Atherosclerosis — *see also* Arteriosclerosis
  coronary
    artery I25.10
      with angina pectoris — *see* Arteriosclerosis, coronary (artery),
      due to
        calcified coronary lesion (severely) I25.84
        lipid rich plaque I25.83
    transplanted heart I25.811
      bypass graft I25.812
        with angina pectoris — *see* Arteriosclerosis, coronary (artery),
      native coronary artery I25.811
        with angina pectoris — *see* Arteriosclerosis, coronary (artery),
Athetosis (acquired) R25.8
  bilateral (congenital) G80.3
  congenital (bilateral) (double) G80.3
  double (congenital) G80.3
  unilateral R25.8
Athlete's
  foot B35.3
  heart I51.7
Athrepsia E41
Athyrea (acquired) — *see also* Hypothyroidism
  congenital E03.1
Atonia, atony, atonic
  bladder (sphincter) (neurogenic) N31.2
  capillary I78.8
  cecum K59.8
    psychogenic F45.8
  colon — *see* Atony, intestine
  congenital P94.2
  esophagus K22.8
  intestine K59.8
    psychogenic F45.8
  stomach K31.89
    neurotic or psychogenic F45.8
  uterus (during labor) O62.2
    with hemorrhage (postpartum) O72.1
    postpartum (with hemorrhage) O72.1
      without hemorrhage O75.89
Atopy — *see* History, allergy
Atransferrinemia, congenital E88.09
Atresia, atretic
  alimentary organ or tract NEC Q45.8
    upper Q40.8
  ani, anus, anal (canal) Q42.3
    with fistula Q42.2
  aorta (ring) Q25.29
  aortic (orifice) (valve) Q23.0
    arch Q25.21
      congenital with hypoplasia of ascending aorta and defective development of left ventricle (with mitral stenosis) Q23.4
    in hypoplastic left heart syndrome Q23.4
  aqueduct of Sylvius Q03.0

Atresia, atretic — *continued*
  aqueduct of Sylvius — *continued*
    with spina bifida — *see* Spina bifida, with hydrocephalus
  artery NEC Q27.8
    cerebral Q28.3
    coronary Q24.5
    digestive system Q27.8
    eye Q15.8
    lower limb Q27.8
    pulmonary Q25.5
    specified site NEC Q27.8
    umbilical Q27.0
    upper limb Q27.8
  auditory canal (external) Q16.1
  bile duct (common) (congenital) (hepatic) Q44.2
    acquired — *see* Obstruction, bile duct
  bladder (neck) Q64.39
    obstruction Q64.31
  bronchus Q32.4
  cecum Q42.8
  cervix (acquired) N88.2
    congenital Q51.828
    in pregnancy or childbirth — *see* Anomaly, cervix, in pregnancy or childbirth
      causing obstructed labor O65.5
  choana Q30.0
  colon Q42.9
    specified NEC Q42.8
  common duct Q44.2
  cricoid cartilage Q31.8
  cystic duct Q44.2
    acquired K82.8
      with obstruction K82.0
  digestive organs NEC Q45.8
  duodenum Q41.0
  ear canal Q16.1
  ejaculatory duct Q55.4
  epiglottis Q31.8
  esophagus Q39.0
    with tracheoesophageal fistula Q39.1
  eustachian tube Q17.8
  fallopian tube (congenital) Q50.6
    acquired N97.1
  follicular cyst N83.0- ☑
  foramen of
    Luschka Q03.1
      with spina bifida — *see* Spina bifida, with hydrocephalus
    Magendie Q03.1
      with spina bifida — *see* Spina bifida, with hydrocephalus
  gallbladder Q44.1
  genital organ
    external
      female Q52.79
      male Q55.8
    internal
      female Q52.8
      male Q55.8
  glottis Q31.8
  gullet Q39.0
    with tracheoesophageal fistula Q39.1
  heart valve NEC Q24.8
    pulmonary Q22.0
    tricuspid Q22.4
  hymen Q52.3
    acquired (postinfective) N89.6
  ileum Q41.2
  intestine (small) Q41.9
    large Q42.9
      specified NEC Q42.8
  iris, filtration angle Q15.0
  jejunum Q41.1
  lacrimal apparatus Q10.4
  larynx Q31.8
  meatus urinarius Q64.33
  mitral valve Q23.2
    in hypoplastic left heart syndrome Q23.4
  nares (anterior) (posterior) Q30.0
  nasopharynx Q34.8
  nose, nostril Q30.0
    acquired J34.89
  organ or site NEC Q89.8
  osseous meatus (ear) Q16.1
  oviduct (congenital) Q50.6
    acquired N97.1
  parotid duct Q38.4
    acquired K11.8

Atresia, atretic — *continued*
  pulmonary (artery) Q25.5
    valve Q22.0
  pulmonic Q22.0
  pupil Q13.2
  rectum Q42.1
    with fistula Q42.0
  salivary duct Q38.4
    acquired K11.8
  sublingual duct Q38.4
    acquired K11.8
  submandibular duct Q38.4
    acquired K11.8
  submaxillary duct Q38.4
    acquired K11.8
  thyroid cartilage Q31.8
  trachea Q32.1
  tricuspid valve Q22.4
  ureter Q62.10
    pelvic junction Q62.11
    vesical orifice Q62.12
  ureteropelvic junction Q62.11
  ureterovesical orifice Q62.12
  urethra (valvular) Q64.39
    stricture Q64.32
  urinary tract NEC Q64.8
  uterus Q51.818
    acquired N85.8
  vagina (congenital) Q52.4
    acquired (postinfectional) (senile) N89.5
  vas deferens Q55.3
  vascular NEC Q27.8
    cerebral Q28.3
    digestive system Q27.8
    lower limb Q27.8
    specified site NEC Q27.8
    upper limb Q27.8
  vein NEC Q27.8
    digestive system Q27.8
    great Q26.8
    lower limb Q27.8
    portal Q26.5
    pulmonary Q26.4
      partial Q26.3
      total Q26.2
    specified site NEC Q27.8
    upper limb Q27.8
  vena cava (inferior) (superior) Q26.8
  vesicourethral orifice Q64.31
  vulva Q52.79
    acquired N90.5
Atrichia, atrichosis — *see* Alopecia
Atrophia — *see also* Atrophy
  cutis senilis L90.8
    due to radiation L57.8
  gyrata of choroid and retina H31.23
  senilis R54
    dermatological L90.8
      due to radiation (nonionizing) (solar) L57.8
  unguium L60.3
    congenita Q84.6
Atrophie blanche (en plaque) (de Milian) L95.0
Atrophoderma, atrophodermia (of) L90.9
  diffusum (idiopathic) L90.4
  maculatum L90.8
    et striatum L90.8
      due to syphilis A52.79
    syphilitic A51.39
  neuriticum L90.8
  Pasini and Pierini L90.3
  pigmentosum Q82.1
  reticulatum symmetricum faciei L66.4
  senile L90.8
    due to radiation (nonionizing) (solar) L57.8
  vermiculata (cheeks) L66.4
Atrophy, atrophic (of)
  adrenal (capsule) (gland) E27.49
    primary (autoimmune) E27.1
  alveolar process or ridge (edentulous) K08.20
  anal sphincter (disuse) N81.84
  appendix K38.8
  arteriosclerotic — *see* Arteriosclerosis
  bile duct (common) (hepatic) K83.8
  bladder N32.89
    neurogenic N31.8
  blanche (en plaque) (of Milian) L95.0
  bone (senile) NEC — *see also* Disorder, bone, specified type NEC

Atrophy, atrophic — *continued*
- bone — *see also* Disorder, bone, specified type — *continued*
  - due to
    - tabes dorsalis (neurogenic) A52.11
- brain (cortex) (progressive) G31.9
  - frontotemporal circumscribed G31.01 *[F02.80]*
    - with behavioral disturbance G31.01 *[F02.81]*
  - senile NEC G31.1
- breast N64.2
  - obstetric — *see* Disorder, breast, specified type NEC
- buccal cavity K13.79
- cardiac — *see* Degeneration, myocardial
- cartilage (infectional) (joint) — *see* Disorder, cartilage, specified NEC
- cerebellar — *see* Atrophy, brain
- cerebral — *see* Atrophy, brain
- cervix (mucosa) (senile) (uteri) N88.8
  - menopausal N95.8
- Charcot-Marie-Tooth G60.0
- choroid (central) (macular) (myopic) (retina) H31.10- ☑
  - diffuse secondary H31.12- ☑
  - gyrate H31.23
  - senile H31.11- ☑
- ciliary body — *see* Atrophy, iris
- conjunctiva (senile) H11.89
- corpus cavernosum N48.89
- cortical — *see* Atrophy, brain
- cystic duct K82.8
- Déjérine-Thomas G23.8
- disuse NEC — *see* Atrophy, muscle
- Duchenne-Aran G12.21
- ear H93.8- ☑
- edentulous alveolar ridge K08.20
- endometrium (senile) N85.8
  - cervix N88.8
- enteric K63.89
- epididymis N50.89
- eyeball — *see* Disorder, globe, degenerated condition, atrophy
- eyelid (senile) — *see* Disorder, eyelid, degenerative
- facial (skin) L90.9
- fallopian tube (senile) N83.32- ☑
  - with ovary N83.33- ☑
- fascioscapulohumeral (Landouzy- Déjérine) G71.02
- fatty, thymus (gland) E32.8
- gallbladder K82.8
- gastric K29.40
  - with bleeding K29.41
- gastrointestinal K63.89
- glandular I89.8
- globe H44.52- ☑
- gum — *see* Recession, gingival
- hair L67.8
- heart (brown) — *see* Degeneration, myocardial
- hemifacial Q67.4
  - Romberg G51.8
- infantile E41
  - paralysis, acute — *see* Poliomyelitis, paralytic
- intestine K63.89
- iris (essential) (progressive) H21.26- ☑
  - specified NEC H21.29
- kidney (senile) (terminal) — *see also* Sclerosis, renal N26.1
  - congenital or infantile Q60.5
    - bilateral Q60.4
    - unilateral Q60.3
  - hydronephrotic — *see* Hydronephrosis
- lacrimal gland (primary) H04.14- ☑
  - secondary H04.15- ☑
- Landouzy-Déjérine G71.02
- laryngitis, infective J37.0
- larynx J38.7
- Leber's optic (hereditary) H47.22
- lip K13.0
- liver (yellow) K72.90
  - with coma K72.91
  - acute, subacute K72.00
    - with coma K72.01
  - chronic K72.10
    - with coma K72.11
- lung (senile) J98.4
- macular (dermatological) L90.8
  - syphilitic, skin A51.39
    - striated A52.79
- mandible (edentulous) K08.20
  - minimal K08.21
  - moderate K08.22

Atrophy, atrophic — *continued*
- mandible — *continued*
  - severe K08.23
- maxilla K08.20
  - minimal K08.24
  - moderate K08.25
  - severe K08.26
- muscle, muscular (diffuse) (general) (idiopathic) (primary) M62.50
  - ankle M62.57- ☑
  - Duchenne-Aran G12.21
  - foot M62.57- ☑
  - forearm M62.53- ☑
  - hand M62.54- ☑
  - infantile spinal G12.0
  - lower leg M62.56- ☑
  - multiple sites M62.59
  - myelopathic — *see* Atrophy, muscle, spinal
  - myotonic G71.11
  - neuritic G58.9
  - neuropathic (peroneal) (progressive) G60.0
  - pelvic (disuse) N81.84
  - peroneal G60.0
  - progressive (bulbar) G12.21
    - adult G12.1
    - infantile (spinal) G12.0
    - spinal G12.25
      - adult G12.1
      - infantile G12.0
  - pseudohypertrophic G71.02
  - shoulder region M62.51- ☑
  - specified site NEC M62.58
  - spinal G12.9
    - adult form G12.1
    - Aran-Duchenne G12.21
    - childhood form, type II G12.1
    - distal G12.1
    - hereditary NEC G12.1
    - infantile, type I (Werdnig-Hoffmann) G12.0
    - juvenile form, type III (Kugelberg- Welander) G12.1
    - progressive G12.25
    - scapuloperoneal form G12.1
    - specified NEC G12.8
  - syphilitic A52.78
  - thigh M62.55- ☑
  - upper arm M62.52- ☑
- myocardium — *see* Degeneration, myocardial
- myometrium (senile) N85.8
  - cervix N88.8
- myopathic NEC — *see* Atrophy, muscle
- myotonia G71.11
- nail L60.3
- nasopharynx J31.1
- nerve — *see also* Disorder, nerve
  - abducens — *see* Strabismus, paralytic, sixth nerve
  - accessory G52.8
  - acoustic or auditory H93.3 ☑
  - cranial G52.9
    - eighth (auditory) H93.3 ☑
    - eleventh (accessory) G52.8
    - fifth (trigeminal) G50.8
    - first (olfactory) G52.0
    - fourth (trochlear) — *see* Strabismus, paralytic, fourth nerve
    - second (optic) H47.20
    - sixth (abducens) — *see* Strabismus, paralytic, sixth nerve
    - tenth (pneumogastric) (vagus) G52.2
    - third (oculomotor) — *see* Strabismus, paralytic, third nerve
    - twelfth (hypoglossal) G52.3
  - hypoglossal G52.3
  - oculomotor — *see* Strabismus, paralytic, third nerve
  - olfactory G52.0
  - optic (papillomacular bundle)
    - syphilitic (late) A52.15
      - congenital A50.44
  - pneumogastric G52.2
  - trigeminal G50.8
  - trochlear — *see* Strabismus, paralytic, fourth nerve
  - vagus (pneumogastric) G52.2
- neurogenic, bone, tabetic A52.11
- nutritional E41
- old age R54
- olivopontocerebellar G23.8
- optic (nerve) H47.20
  - glaucomatous H47.23- ☑

Atrophy, atrophic — *continued*
- optic — *continued*
  - hereditary H47.22
  - primary H47.21- ☑
  - specified type NEC H47.29- ☑
  - syphilitic (late) A52.15
    - congenital A50.44
- orbit H05.31- ☑
- ovary (senile) N83.31- ☑
  - with fallopian tube N83.33- ☑
- oviduct (senile) — *see* Atrophy, fallopian tube
- palsy, diffuse (progressive) G12.22
- pancreas (duct) (senile) K86.89
- parotid gland K11.0
- pelvic muscle N81.84
- penis N48.89
- pharynx J39.2
- pluriglandular E31.8
  - autoimmune E31.0
- polyarthritis M15.9
- prostate N42.89
- pseudohypertrophic (muscle) G71.02
- renal — *see also* Sclerosis, renal N26.1
- retina, retinal (postinfectional) H35.89
- rhinitis J31.0
- salivary gland K11.0
- scar L90.5
- sclerosis, lobar (of brain) G31.09 *[F02.80]*
  - with behavioral disturbance G31.09 *[F02.81]*
- scrotum N50.89
- seminal vesicle N50.89
- senile R54
  - due to radiation (nonionizing) (solar) L57.8
- skin (patches) (spots) L90.9
  - degenerative (senile) L90.8
  - due to radiation (nonionizing) (solar) L57.8
  - senile L90.8
- spermatic cord N50.89
- spinal (acute) (cord) G95.89
  - muscular — *see* Atrophy, muscle, spinal
  - paralysis G12.20
    - acute — *see* Poliomyelitis, paralytic
    - meaning progressive muscular atrophy G12.25
- spine (column) — *see* Spondylopathy, specified NEC
- spleen (senile) D73.0
- stomach K29.40
  - with bleeding K29.41
- striate (skin) L90.6
  - syphilitic A52.79
- subcutaneous L90.9
- sublingual gland K11.0
- submandibular gland K11.0
- submaxillary gland K11.0
- Sudeck's — *see* Algoneurodystrophy
- suprarenal (capsule) (gland) E27.49
  - primary E27.1
- systemic affecting central nervous system in
  - myxedema E03.9 *[G13.2]*
  - neoplastic disease — *see also* Neoplasm D49.9 *[G13.1]*
  - specified disease NEC G13.8
- tarso-orbital fascia, congenital Q10.3
- testis N50.0
- thenar, partial — *see* Syndrome, carpal tunnel
- thymus (fatty) E32.8
- thyroid (gland) (acquired) E03.4
  - with cretinism E03.1
  - congenital (with myxedema) E03.1
- tongue (senile) K14.8
  - papillae K14.4
- trachea J39.8
- tunica vaginalis N50.89
- turbinate J34.89
- tympanic membrane (nonflaccid) H73.82- ☑
  - flaccid H73.81- ☑
- upper respiratory tract J39.8
- uterus, uterine (senile) N85.8
  - cervix N88.8
  - due to radiation (intended effect) N85.8
    - adverse effect or misadventure N99.89
- vagina (senile) N95.2
- vas deferens N50.89
- vascular I99.8
- vertebra (senile) — *see* Spondylopathy, specified NEC
- vulva (senile) N90.5
- Werdnig-Hoffmann G12.0
- yellow — *see* Failure, hepatic

Attack, attacks
  with alteration of consciousness (with automatisms) — *see* Epilepsy, localization-related, symptomatic, with complex partial seizures
  Adams-Stokes I45.9
  akinetic — *see* Epilepsy, generalized, specified NEC
  angina — *see* Angina
  atonic — *see* Epilepsy, generalized, specified NEC
  benign shuddering G25.83
  cataleptic — *see* Catalepsy
  coronary — *see* Infarct, myocardium
  cyanotic, newborn P28.2
  drop NEC R55
  epileptic — *see* Epilepsy
  heart — *see* infarct, myocardium
  hysterical F44.9
  jacksonian — *see* Epilepsy, localization-related, symptomatic, with simple partial seizures
  myocardium, myocardial — *see* Infarct, myocardium
  myoclonic — *see* Epilepsy, generalized, specified NEC
  panic F41.0
  psychomotor — *see* Epilepsy, localization-related, symptomatic, with complex partial seizures
  salaam — *see* Epilepsy, spasms
  schizophreniform, brief F23
  shuddering, benign G25.83
  Stokes-Adams I45.9
  syncope R55
  transient ischemic (TIA) G45.9
    specified NEC G45.8
  unconsciousness R55
    hysterical F44.89
  vasomotor R55
  vasovagal (paroxysmal) (idiopathic) R55
  without alteration of consciousness — *see* Epilepsy, localization-related, symptomatic, with simple partial seizures
Attention (to)
  artificial
    opening (of) Z43.9
      digestive tract NEC Z43.4
        colon Z43.3
        ilium Z43.2
        stomach Z43.1
      specified NEC Z43.8
      trachea Z43.0
      urinary tract NEC Z43.6
        cystostomy Z43.5
        nephrostomy Z43.6
        ureterostomy Z43.6
        urethrostomy Z43.6
    vagina Z43.7
  colostomy Z43.3
  cystostomy Z43.5
  deficit disorder or syndrome F98.8
    with hyperactivity — *see* Disorder, attention-deficit hyperactivity
  gastrostomy Z43.1
  ileostomy Z43.2
  jejunostomy Z43.4
  nephrostomy Z43.6
  surgical dressings Z48.01
  sutures Z48.02
  tracheostomy Z43.0
  ureterostomy Z43.6
  urethrostomy Z43.6
Attrition
  gum — *see* Recession, gingival
  tooth, teeth (excessive) (hard tissues) K03.0
Atypical, atypism — *see also* condition
  cells (on cytolgocial smear) (endocervical) (endometrial) (glandular)
    cervix R87.619
    vagina R87.629
  cervical N87.9
  endometrium N85.9
    hyperplasia N85.00
  parenting situation Z62.9
Auditory — *see* condition
Aujeszky's disease B33.8
Aurantiasis, cutis E67.1
Auricle, auricular — *see also* condition
  cervical Q18.2
Auriculotemporal syndrome G50.8
Austin Flint murmur (aortic insufficiency) I35.1
Australian
  Q fever A78
  X disease A83.4

Autism, autistic (childhood) (infantile) F84.0
  atypical F84.9
  spectrum disorder F84.0
Autodigestion R68.89
Autoerythrocyte sensitization (syndrome) D69.2
Autographism L50.3
Autoimmune
  disease (systemic) M35.9
  inhibitors to clotting factors D68.311
  lymphoproliferative syndrome [ALPS] D89.82
  thyroiditis E06.3
Autointoxication R68.89
Automatism G93.89
  with temporal sclerosis G93.81
  epileptic — *see* Epilepsy, localization-related, symptomatic, with complex partial seizures
  paroxysmal, idiopathic — *see* Epilepsy, localization-related, symptomatic, with complex partial seizures
Autonomic, autonomous
  bladder (neurogenic) N31.2
  hysteria seizure F44.5
Autosensitivity, erythrocyte D69.2
Autosensitization, cutaneous L30.2
Autosome — *see* condition by chromosome involved
Autotopagnosia R48.1
Autotoxemia R68.89
Autumn — *see* condition
Avellis' syndrome G46.8
Aversion
  oral R63.3
    newborn P92.- ☑
    nonorganic origin F98.2 ☑
  sexual F52.1
Aviator's
  disease or sickness — *see* Effect, adverse, high altitude
  ear T70.0 ☑
Avitaminosis (multiple) — *see also* Deficiency, vitamin E56.9
  B E53.9
    with
      beriberi E51.11
      pellagra E52
  B2 E53.0
  B6 E53.1
  B12 E53.8
  D E55.9
    with rickets E55.0
  G E53.0
  K E56.1
  nicotinic acid E52
AVNRT (atrioventricular nodal re-entrant tachycardia) I47.1
AVRT (atrioventricular nodal re-entrant tachycardia) I47.1
Avulsion (traumatic)
  blood vessel — *see* Injury, blood vessel
  bone — *see* Fracture, by site
  cartilage — *see also* Dislocation, by site
    symphyseal (inner), complicating delivery O71.6
  external site other than limb — *see* Wound, open, by site
  eye S05.7- ☑
  head (intracranial)
    external site NEC S08.89 ☑
    scalp S08.0 ☑
  internal organ or site — *see* Injury, by site
  joint — *see also* Dislocation, by site
    capsule — *see* Sprain, by site
  kidney S37.06- ☑
  ligament — *see* Sprain, by site
  limb — *see also* Amputation, traumatic, by site
    skin and subcutaneous tissue — *see* Wound, open, by site
  muscle — *see* Injury, muscle
  nerve (root) — *see* Injury, nerve
  scalp S08.0 ☑
  skin and subcutaneous tissue — *see* Wound, open, by site
  spleen S36.032 ☑
  symphyseal cartilage (inner), complicating delivery O71.6
  tendon — *see* Injury, muscle
  tooth S03.2 ☑
Awareness of heart beat R00.2
Axenfeld's
  anomaly or syndrome Q15.0
  degeneration (calcareous) Q13.4

Axilla, axillary — *see also* condition
  breast Q83.1
Axonotmesis — *see* Injury, nerve
Ayerza's disease or syndrome (pulmonary artery sclerosis with pulmonary hypertension) I27.0
Azoospermia (organic) N46.01
  due to
    drug therapy N46.021
    efferent duct obstruction N46.023
    infection N46.022
    radiation N46.024
    specified cause NEC N46.029
    systemic disease N46.025
Azotemia R79.89
  meaning uremia N19
Aztec ear Q17.3
Azygos
  continuation inferior vena cava Q26.8
  lobe (lung) Q33.1

B

Baastrup's disease — *see* Kissing spine
Babesiosis B60.0
Babington's disease (familial hemorrhagic telangiectasia) I78.0
Babinski's syndrome A52.79
Baby
  crying constantly R68.11
  floppy (syndrome) P94.2
Bacillary — *see* condition
Bacilluria R82.71
Bacillus — *see also* Infection, bacillus
  abortus infection A23.1
  anthracis infection A22.9
  coli infection — *see also* Escherichia coli B96.20
  Flexner's A03.1
  mallei infection A24.0
  Shiga's A03.0
  suipestifer infection — *see* Infection, salmonella
Back — *see* condition
Backache (postural) M54.9
  sacroiliac M53.3
  specified NEC M54.89
Backflow — *see* Reflux
Backward reading (dyslexia) F81.0
Bacteremia R78.81
  with sepsis — *see* Sepsis
Bactericholia — *see* Cholecystitis, acute
Bacterid, bacteride (pustular) L40.3
Bacterium, bacteria, bacterial
  agent NEC, as cause of disease classified elsewhere B96.89
  in blood — *see* Bacteremia
  in urine — *see* Bacteriuria
Bacteriuria, bacteruria R82.71
  asymptomatic R82.71
Bacteroides
  fragilis, as cause of disease classified elsewhere B96.6
Bad
  heart — *see* Disease, heart
  trip
    due to drug abuse — *see* Abuse, drug, hallucinogen
    due to drug dependence — *see* Dependence, drug, hallucinogen
Baelz's disease (cheilitis glandularis apostematosa) K13.0
Baerensprung's disease (eczema marginatum) B35.6
Bagasse disease or pneumonitis J67.1
Bagassosis J67.1
Baker's cyst — *see* Cyst, Baker's
Bakwin-Krida syndrome (metaphyseal dysplasia) Q78.5
Balancing side interference M26.56
Balanitis (circinata) (erosiva) (gangrenosa) (phagedenic) (vulgaris) N48.1
  amebic A06.82
  candidal B37.42
  due to Haemophilus ducreyi A57
  gonococcal (acute) (chronic) A54.23
  xerotica obliterans N48.0
Balanoposthitis N47.6
  gonococcal (acute) (chronic) A54.23
  ulcerative (specific) A63.8
Balanorrhagia — *see* Balanitis
Balantidiasis, balantidiosis A07.0
Bald tongue K14.4
Baldness — *see also* Alopecia
  male-pattern — *see* Alopecia, androgenic

Balkan grippe A78
Balloon disease — *see* Effect, adverse, high altitude
Balo's disease (concentric sclerosis) G37.5
Bamberger-Marie disease — *see* Osteoarthropathy, hypertrophic, specified type NEC
Bancroft's filariasis B74.0
Band(s)
  adhesive — *see* Adhesions, peritoneum
  anomalous or congenital — *see also* Anomaly, by site
    heart (atrial) (ventricular) Q24.8
    intestine Q43.3
    omentum Q43.3
  cervix N88.1
  constricting, congenital Q79.8
  gallbladder (congenital) Q44.1
  intestinal (adhesive) — *see* Adhesions, peritoneum
  obstructive
    intestine K56.50
      complete K56.52
      incomplete K56.51
      partial K56.51
    peritoneum K56.50
      complete K56.52
      incomplete K56.51
      partial K56.51
  periappendiceal, congenital Q43.3
  peritoneal (adhesive) — *see* Adhesions, peritoneum
  uterus N73.6
    internal N85.6
  vagina N89.5
Bandemia D72.825
Bandl's ring (contraction), complicating delivery O62.4
Bangkok hemorrhagic fever A91
Bang's disease (brucella abortus) A23.1
Bankruptcy, anxiety concerning Z59.8
Bannister's disease T78.3 ☑
  hereditary D84.1
Banti's disease or syndrome (with cirrhosis) (with portal hypertension) K76.6
Bar, median, prostate — *see* Enlargement, enlarged, prostate
Barcoo disease or rot — *see* Ulcer, skin
Barlow's disease E54
Barodontalgia T70.29 ☑
Baron Münchausen syndrome — *see* Disorder, factitious
Barosinusitis T70.1 ☑
Barotitis T70.0 ☑
Barotrauma T70.29 ☑
  odontalgia T70.29 ☑
  otitic T70.0 ☑
  sinus T70.1 ☑
Barraquer (-Simons) **disease or syndrome** (progressive lipodystrophy) E88.1
Barré-Guillain disease or syndrome G61.0
Barrel chest M95.4
Barré-Liéou syndrome (posterior cervical sympathetic) M53.0
Barrett's
  disease — *see* Barrett's, esophagus
  esophagus K22.70
    with dysplasia K22.719
      high grade K22.711
      low grade K22.710
    without dysplasia K22.70
  syndrome — *see* Barrett's, esophagus
  ulcer K22.10
    with bleeding K22.11
    without bleeding K22.10
Bársony (-Polgár) (-Teschendorf) **syndrome** (corkscrew esophagus) K22.4
Barth syndrome E78.71
Bartholinitis (suppurating) N75.8
  gonococcal (acute) (chronic) (with abscess) A54.1
Bartonellosis A44.9
  cutaneous A44.1
  mucocutaneous A44.1
  specified NEC A44.8
  systemic A44.0
Barton's fracture S52.56- ☑
Bartter's syndrome E26.81
Basal — *see* condition
Basan's (hidrotic) ectodermal dysplasia Q82.4
Baseball finger — *see* Dislocation, finger
Basedow's disease (exophthalmic goiter) — *see* Hyperthyroidism, with, goiter
Basic — *see* condition

Basilar — *see* condition
Bason's (hidrotic) ectodermal dysplasia Q82.4
Basopenia — *see* Agranulocytosis
Basophilia D72.824
Basophilism (cortico-adrenal) (Cushing's) (pituitary) E24.0
Bassen-Kornzweig disease or syndrome E78.6
Bat ear Q17.5
Bateman's
  disease B08.1
  purpura (senile) D69.2
Bathing cramp T75.1 ☑
Bathophobia F40.248
Batten (-Mayou) **disease** E75.4
  retina E75.4 *[H36]*
Batten-Steinert syndrome G71.11
Battered — *see* Maltreatment
Battey Mycobacterium infection A31.0
Battle exhaustion F43.0
Battledore placenta O43.19- ☑
Baumgarten-Cruveilhier cirrhosis, disease or syndrome K74.69
Bauxite fibrosis (of lung) J63.1
Bayle's disease (general paresis) A52.17
Bazin's disease (primary) (tuberculous) A18.4
Beach ear — *see* Swimmer's, ear
Beaded hair (congenital) Q84.1
Béal conjunctivitis or syndrome B30.2
Beard's disease (neurasthenia) F48.8
Beat(s)
  atrial, premature I49.1
  ectopic I49.49
  elbow — *see* Bursitis, elbow
  escaped, heart I49.49
  hand — *see* Bursitis, hand
  knee — *see* Bursitis, knee
  premature I49.40
    atrial I49.1
    auricular I49.1
    supraventricular I49.1
Beau's
  disease or syndrome — *see* Degeneration, myocardial
  lines (transverse furrows on fingernails) L60.4
Bechterev's syndrome — *see* Spondylitis, ankylosing
Becker's
  cardiomyopathy I42.8
  disease
    idiopathic mural endomyocardial disease I42.3
    myotonia congenita, recessive form G71.12
  dystrophy G71.01
  pigmented hairy nevus D22.5
Beck's syndrome (anterior spinal artery occlusion) I65.8
Beckwith-Wiedemann syndrome Q87.3
Bed confinement status Z74.01
Bed sore — *see* Ulcer, pressure, by site
Bedbug bite(s) — *see* Bite(s), by site, superficial, insect
Bedclothes, asphyxiation or suffocation by — *see* Asphyxia, traumatic, due to, mechanical, trapped
Bednar's
  aphthae K12.0
  tumor — *see* Neoplasm, malignant, by site
Bedridden Z74.01
Bedsore — *see* Ulcer, pressure, by site
Bedwetting — *see* Enuresis
Bee sting (with allergic or anaphylactic shock) — *see* Toxicity, venom, arthropod, bee
Beer drinker's heart (disease) I42.6
Begbie's disease (exophthalmic goiter) — *see* Hyperthyroidism, with, goiter
Behavior
  antisocial
    adult Z72.811
    child or adolescent Z72.810
  disorder, disturbance — *see* Disorder, conduct
  disruptive — *see* Disorder, conduct
  drug seeking Z76.5
  inexplicable R46.2
  marked evasiveness R46.5
  obsessive-compulsive R46.81
  overactivity R46.3
  poor responsiveness R46.4
  self-damaging (life-style) Z72.89
  sleep-incompatible Z72.821
  slowness R46.4
  specified NEC R46.89
  strange (and inexplicable) R46.2
  suspiciousness R46.5
  type A pattern Z73.1

Behavior — *continued*
  undue concern or preoccupation with stressful events R46.6
  verbosity and circumstantial detail obscuring reason for contact R46.7
Behçet's disease or syndrome M35.2
Behr's disease — *see* Degeneration, macula
Beigel's disease or morbus (white piedra) B36.2
Bejel A65
Bekhterev's syndrome — *see* Spondylitis, ankylosing
Belching — *see* Eructation
Bell's
  mania F30.8
  palsy, paralysis G51.0
    infant or newborn P11.3
  spasm G51.3- ☑
Bence Jones albuminuria or proteinuria NEC R80.3
Bends T70.3 ☑
Benedikt's paralysis or syndrome G46.3
Benign — *see also* condition
  prostatic hyperplasia — *see* Hyperplasia, prostate
Bennett's fracture (displaced) S62.21- ☑
Benson's disease — *see* Deposit, crystalline
Bent
  back (hysterical) F44.4
  nose M95.0
    congenital Q67.4
Bereavement (uncomplicated) Z63.4
Bergeron's disease (hysterical chorea) F44.4
Berger's disease — *see* Nephropathy, IgA
Beriberi (dry) E51.11
  heart (disease) E51.12
  polyneuropathy E51.11
  wet E51.12
  involving circulatory system E51.11
Berlin's disease or edema (traumatic) S05.8X- ☑
Berlock (berloque) **dermatitis** L56.2
Bernard-Horner syndrome G90.2
Bernard-Soulier disease or thrombopathia D69.1
Bernhardt (-Roth) **disease** — *see* Mononeuropathy, lower limb, meralgia paresthetica
Bernheim's syndrome — *see* Failure, heart, right
Bertielliasis B71.8
Berylliosis (lung) J63.2
Besnier-Boeck (-Schaumann) **disease** — *see* Sarcoidosis
Besnier's
  lupus pernio D86.3
  prurigo L20.0
Bestiality F65.89
Best's disease H35.50
Betalipoproteinemia, broad or floating E78.2
Beta-mercaptolactate-cysteine disulfiduria E72.09
Betting and gambling Z72.6
  pathological (compulsive) F63.0
Bezoar T18.9 ☑
  intestine T18.3 ☑
  stomach T18.2 ☑
Bezold's abscess — *see* Mastoiditis, acute
Bianchi's syndrome R48.8
Bicornate or bicornis uterus Q51.3
  in pregnancy or childbirth O34.00
    causing obstructed labor O65.5
Bicuspid aortic valve Q23.1
Biedl-Bardet syndrome Q87.89
Bielschowsky (-Jansky) disease E75.4
Biermer's (pernicious) anemia or disease D51.0
Biett's disease L93.0
Bifid (congenital)
  apex, heart Q24.8
  clitoris Q52.6
  kidney Q63.8
  nose Q30.2
  patella Q74.1
  scrotum Q55.29
  toe NEC Q74.2
  tongue Q38.3
  ureter Q62.8
  uterus Q51.3
  uvula Q35.7
Biforis uterus (suprasimplex) Q51.3
Bifurcation (congenital)
  gallbladder Q44.1
  kidney pelvis Q63.8
  renal pelvis Q63.8
  rib Q76.6
  tongue, congenital Q38.3
  trachea Q32.1

☑ **Additional Character Required** — Refer to the Tabular List for Character Selection   ▽ **Subterms under main terms may continue to next column or page**

Bifurcation — *continued*
ureter Q62.8
urethra Q64.74
vertebra Q76.49
Big spleen syndrome D73.1
Bigeminal pulse R00.8
Bilateral — *see* condition
Bile
duct — *see* condition
pigments in urine R82.2
Bilharziasis — *see also* Schistosomiasis
chyluria B65.0
cutaneous B65.3
galacturia B65.0
hematochyluria B65.0
intestinal B65.1
lipemia B65.9
lipuria B65.0
oriental B65.2
piarhemia B65.9
pulmonary NOS B65.9 *[J99]*
pneumonia B65.9 *[J17]*
tropical hematuria B65.0
vesical B65.0
Biliary — *see* condition
Bilirubin metabolism disorder E80.7
specified NEC E80.6
Bilirubinemia, familial nonhemolytic E80.4
Bilirubinuria R82.2
Biliuria R82.2
Bilocular stomach K31.2
Binswanger's disease I67.3
Biparta, bipartite
carpal scaphoid Q74.0
patella Q74.1
vagina Q52.10
Bird
face Q75.8
fancier's disease or lung J67.2
Birth
complications in mother — *see* Delivery, complicated
compression during NOS P15.9
defect — *see* Anomaly
immature (less than 37 completed weeks) — *see* Preterm, newborn
extremely (less than 28 completed weeks) — *see* Immaturity, extreme
inattention, at or after — *see* Maltreatment, child, neglect
injury NOS P15.9
basal ganglia P11.1
brachial plexus NEC P14.3
brain (compression) (pressure) P11.2
central nervous system NOS P11.9
cerebellum P11.1
cerebral hemorrhage P10.1
external genitalia P15.5
eye P15.3
face P15.4
fracture
bone P13.9
specified NEC P13.8
clavicle P13.4
femur P13.2
humerus P13.3
long bone, except femur P13.3
radius and ulna P13.3
skull P13.0
spine P11.5
tibia and fibula P13.3
intracranial P11.2
laceration or hemorrhage P10.9
specified NEC P10.8
intraventricular hemorrhage P10.2
laceration
brain P10.1
by scalpel P15.8
peripheral nerve P14.9
liver P15.0
meninges
brain P11.1
spinal cord P11.5
nerve
brachial plexus P14.3
cranial NEC (except facial) P11.4
facial P11.3
peripheral P14.9
phrenic (paralysis) P14.2

Birth — *continued*
injury — *continued*
paralysis
facial nerve P11.3
spinal P11.5
penis P15.5
rupture
spinal cord P11.5
scalp P12.9
scalpel wound P15.8
scrotum P15.5
skull NEC P13.1
fracture P13.0
specified type NEC P15.8
spinal cord P11.5
spine P11.5
spleen P15.1
sternomastoid (hematoma) P15.2
subarachnoid hemorrhage P10.3
subcutaneous fat necrosis P15.6
subdural hemorrhage P10.0
tentorial tear P10.4
testes P15.5
vulva P15.5
lack of care, at or after — *see* Maltreatment, child, neglect
neglect, at or after — *see* Maltreatment, child, neglect
palsy or paralysis, newborn, NOS (birth injury) P14.9
premature (infant) — *see* Preterm, newborn
shock, newborn P96.89
trauma — *see* Birth, injury
weight
low (2499 grams or less) — *see* Low, birthweight
extremely (999 grams or less) — *see* Low, birthweight, extreme
4000 grams to 4499 grams P08.1
4500 grams or more P08.0
Birthmark Q82.5
Birt-Hogg-Dube syndrome Q87.89
Bisalbuminemia E88.09
Biskra's button B55.1
Bite(s) (animal) (human)
abdomen, abdominal
wall S31.159 ☑
with penetration into peritoneal cavity S31.659 ☑
epigastric region S31.152 ☑
with penetration into peritoneal cavity S31.652 ☑
left
lower quadrant S31.154 ☑
with penetration into peritoneal cavity S31.654 ☑
upper quadrant S31.151 ☑
with penetration into peritoneal cavity S31.651 ☑
periumbilic region S31.155 ☑
with penetration into peritoneal cavity S31.655 ☑
right
lower quadrant S31.153 ☑
with penetration into peritoneal cavity S31.653 ☑
upper quadrant S31.150 ☑
with penetration into peritoneal cavity S31.650 ☑
superficial NEC S30.871 ☑
insect S30.861 ☑
alveolar (process) — *see* Bite, oral cavity
amphibian (venomous) — *see* Venom, bite, amphibian
animal — *see also* Bite, by site
venomous — *see* Venom
ankle S91.05- ☑
superficial NEC S90.57- ☑
insect S90.56- ☑
antecubital space — *see* Bite, elbow
anus S31.835 ☑
superficial NEC S30.877 ☑
insect S30.867 ☑
arm (upper) S41.15- ☑
lower — *see* Bite, forearm
superficial NEC S40.87- ☑
insect S40.86- ☑
arthropod NEC — *see* Venom, bite, arthropod
auditory canal (external) (meatus) — *see* Bite, ear
auricle, ear — *see* Bite, ear
axilla — *see* Bite, arm

Bite(s) — *continued*
back — *see also* Bite, thorax, back
lower S31.050 ☑
with penetration into retroperitoneal space S31.051 ☑
superficial NEC S30.870 ☑
insect S30.860 ☑
bedbug — *see* Bite(s), by site, superficial, insect
breast S21.05- ☑
superficial NEC S20.17- ☑
insect S20.16- ☑
brow — *see* Bite, head, specified site NEC
buttock S31.805 ☑
left S31.825 ☑
right S31.815 ☑
superficial NEC S30.870 ☑
insect S30.860 ☑
calf — *see* Bite, leg
canaliculus lacrimalis — *see* Bite, eyelid
canthus, eye — *see* Bite, eyelid
centipede — *see* Toxicity, venom, arthropod, centipede
cheek (external) S01.45- ☑
internal — *see* Bite, oral cavity
superficial NEC S00.87 ☑
insect S00.86 ☑
chest wall — *see* Bite, thorax
chigger B88.0
chin — *see* Bite, head, specified site NEC
clitoris — *see* Bite, vulva
costal region — *see* Bite, thorax
digit(s)
hand — *see* Bite, finger
toe — *see* Bite, toe
ear (canal) (external) S01.35- ☑
superficial NEC S00.47- ☑
insect S00.46- ☑
elbow S51.05- ☑
superficial NEC S50.37- ☑
insect S50.36- ☑
epididymis — *see* Bite, testis
epigastric region — *see* Bite, abdomen
epiglottis — *see* Bite, neck, specified site NEC
esophagus, cervical S11.25 ☑
superficial NEC S10.17 ☑
insect S10.16 ☑
eyebrow — *see* Bite, eyelid
eyelid S01.15- ☑
superficial NEC S00.27- ☑
insect S00.26- ☑
face NEC — *see* Bite, head, specified site NEC
finger(s) S61.259 ☑
with
damage to nail S61.359 ☑
index S61.258 ☑
with
damage to nail S61.358 ☑
left S61.251 ☑
with
damage to nail S61.351 ☑
right S61.250 ☑
with
damage to nail S61.350 ☑
superficial NEC S60.478 ☑
insect S60.46- ☑
little S61.25- ☑
with
damage to nail S61.35- ☑
superficial NEC S60.47- ☑
insect S60.46- ☑
middle S61.25- ☑
with
damage to nail S61.35- ☑
superficial NEC S60.47- ☑
insect S60.46- ☑
ring S61.25- ☑
with
damage to nail S61.35- ☑
superficial NEC S60.47- ☑
insect S60.46- ☑
superficial NEC S60.479 ☑
insect S60.469 ☑
thumb — *see* Bite, thumb
flank — *see* Bite, abdomen, wall
flea — *see* Bite, by site, superficial, insect
foot (except toe(s) alone) S91.35- ☑
superficial NEC S90.87- ☑

⚐ **Subterms under main terms may continue to next column or page**   ☑ **Additional Character Required** — Refer to the Tabular List for Character Selection   **37**

Bifurcation — Bite

Bite(s) — *continued*
- foot(s alone) — *continued*
  - superficial — *continued*
    - insect S90.86- ☑
    - toe — *see* Bite, toe
- forearm S51.85- ☑
  - elbow only — *see* Bite, elbow
  - superficial NEC S50.87- ☑
    - insect S50.86- ☑
- forehead — *see* Bite, head, specified site NEC
- genital organs, external
  - female S31.552 ☑
    - superficial NEC S30.876 ☑
      - insect S30.866 ☑
    - vagina and vulva — *see* Bite, vulva
  - male S31.551 ☑
    - penis — *see* Bite, penis
    - scrotum — *see* Bite, scrotum
    - superficial NEC S30.875 ☑
      - insect S30.865 ☑
    - testes — *see* Bite, testis
- groin — *see* Bite, abdomen, wall
- gum — *see* Bite, oral cavity
- hand S61.45- ☑
  - finger — *see* Bite, finger
  - superficial NEC S60.57- ☑
    - insect S60.56- ☑
  - thumb — *see* Bite, thumb
- head S01.95 ☑
  - cheek — *see* Bite, cheek
  - ear — *see* Bite, ear
  - eyelid — *see* Bite, eyelid
  - lip — *see* Bite, lip
  - nose — *see* Bite, nose
  - oral cavity — *see* Bite, oral cavity
  - scalp — *see* Bite, scalp
  - specified site NEC S01.85 ☑
    - superficial NEC S00.87 ☑
      - insect S00.86 ☑
  - superficial NEC S00.97 ☑
    - insect S00.96 ☑
  - temporomandibular area — *see* Bite, cheek
- heel — *see* Bite, foot
- hip S71.05- ☑
  - superficial NEC S70.27- ☑
    - insect S70.26- ☑
- hymen S31.45 ☑
- hypochondrium — *see* Bite, abdomen, wall
- hypogastric region — *see* Bite, abdomen, wall
- inguinal region — *see* Bite, abdomen, wall
- insect — *see* Bite, by site, superficial, insect
- instep — *see* Bite, foot
- interscapular region — *see* Bite, thorax, back
- jaw — *see* Bite, head, specified site NEC
- knee S81.05- ☑
  - superficial NEC S80.27- ☑
    - insect S80.26- ☑
- labium (majus) (minus) — *see* Bite, vulva
- lacrimal duct — *see* Bite, eyelid
- larynx S11.015 ☑
  - superficial NEC S10.17 ☑
    - insect S10.16 ☑
- leg (lower) S81.85- ☑
  - ankle — *see* Bite, ankle
  - foot — *see* Bite, foot
  - knee — *see* Bite, knee
  - superficial NEC S80.87- ☑
    - insect S80.86- ☑
  - toe — *see* Bite, toe
  - upper — *see* Bite, thigh
- lip S01.551 ☑
  - superficial NEC S00.571 ☑
    - insect S00.561 ☑
- lizard (venomous) — *see* Venom, bite, reptile
- loin — *see* Bite, abdomen, wall
- lower back — *see* Bite, back, lower
- lumbar region — *see* Bite, back, lower
- malar region — *see* Bite, head, specified site NEC
- mammary — *see* Bite, breast
- marine animals (venomous) — *see* Toxicity, venom, marine animal
- mastoid region — *see* Bite, head, specified site NEC
- mouth — *see* Bite, oral cavity
- nail
  - finger — *see* Bite, finger
  - toe — *see* Bite, toe

Bite(s) — *continued*
- nape — *see* Bite, neck, specified site NEC
- nasal (septum) (sinus) — *see* Bite, nose
- nasopharynx — *see* Bite, head, specified site NEC
- neck S11.95 ☑
  - involving
    - cervical esophagus — *see* Bite, esophagus, cervical
    - larynx — *see* Bite, larynx
    - pharynx — *see* Bite, pharynx
    - thyroid gland S11.15 ☑
    - trachea — *see* Bite, trachea
  - specified site NEC S11.85 ☑
    - superficial NEC S10.87 ☑
      - insect S10.86 ☑
  - superficial NEC S10.97 ☑
    - insect S10.96 ☑
  - throat S11.85 ☑
    - superficial NEC S10.17 ☑
      - insect S10.16 ☑
- nose (septum) (sinus) S01.25 ☑
  - superficial NEC S00.37 ☑
    - insect S00.36 ☑
- occipital region — *see* Bite, scalp
- oral cavity S01.552 ☑
  - superficial NEC S00.572 ☑
    - insect S00.562 ☑
- orbital region — *see* Bite, eyelid
- palate — *see* Bite, oral cavity
- palm — *see* Bite, hand
- parietal region — *see* Bite, scalp
- pelvis S31.050 ☑
  - with penetration into retroperitoneal space S31.051 ☑
  - superficial NEC S30.870 ☑
    - insect S30.860 ☑
- penis S31.25 ☑
  - superficial NEC S30.872 ☑
    - insect S30.862 ☑
- perineum
  - female — *see* Bite, vulva
  - male — *see* Bite, pelvis
- periocular area (with or without lacrimal passages) — *see* Bite, eyelid
- phalanges
  - finger — *see* Bite, finger
  - toe — *see* Bite, toe
- pharynx S11.25 ☑
  - superficial NEC S10.17 ☑
    - insect S10.16 ☑
- pinna — *see* Bite, ear
- poisonous — *see* Venom
- popliteal space — *see* Bite, knee
- prepuce — *see* Bite, penis
- pubic region — *see* Bite, abdomen, wall
- rectovaginal septum — *see* Bite, vulva
- red bug B88.0
- reptile NEC — *see also* Venom, bite, reptile
  - nonvenomous — *see* Bite, by site
  - snake — *see* Venom, bite, snake
- sacral region — *see* Bite, back, lower
- sacroiliac region — *see* Bite, back, lower
- salivary gland — *see* Bite, oral cavity
- scalp S01.05 ☑
  - superficial NEC S00.07 ☑
    - insect S00.06 ☑
- scapular region — *see* Bite, shoulder
- scrotum S31.35 ☑
  - superficial NEC S30.873 ☑
    - insect S30.863 ☑
- sea-snake (venomous) — *see* Toxicity, venom, snake, sea snake
- shin — *see* Bite, leg
- shoulder S41.05- ☑
  - superficial NEC S40.27- ☑
    - insect S40.26- ☑
- snake — *see also* Venom, bite, snake
  - nonvenomous — *see* Bite, by site
- spermatic cord — *see* Bite, testis
- spider (venomous) — *see* Toxicity, venom, spider
  - nonvenomous — *see* Bite, by site, superficial, insect
- sternal region — *see* Bite, thorax, front
- submaxillary region — *see* Bite, head, specified site NEC
- submental region — *see* Bite, head, specified site NEC

Bite(s) — *continued*
- subungual
  - finger(s) — *see* Bite, finger
  - toe — *see* Bite, toe
- superficial — *see* Bite, by site, superficial
- supraclavicular fossa S11.85 ☑
- supraorbital — *see* Bite, head, specified site NEC
- temple, temporal region — *see* Bite, head, specified site NEC
- temporomandibular area — *see* Bite, cheek
- testis S31.35 ☑
  - superficial NEC S30.873 ☑
    - insect S30.863 ☑
- thigh S71.15- ☑
  - superficial NEC S70.37- ☑
    - insect S70.36- ☑
- thorax, thoracic (wall) S21.95 ☑
  - back S21.25- ☑
    - with penetration into thoracic cavity S21.45- ☑
  - breast — *see* Bite, breast
  - front S21.15- ☑
    - with penetration into thoracic cavity S21.35- ☑
  - superficial NEC S20.97 ☑
    - back S20.47- ☑
    - front S20.37- ☑
    - insect S20.96 ☑
      - back S20.46- ☑
      - front S20.36- ☑
- throat — *see* Bite, neck, throat
- thumb S61.05- ☑
  - with
    - damage to nail S61.15- ☑
  - superficial NEC S60.37- ☑
    - insect S60.36- ☑
- thyroid S11.15 ☑
  - superficial NEC S10.87 ☑
    - insect S10.86 ☑
- toe(s) S91.15- ☑
  - with
    - damage to nail S91.25- ☑
  - great S91.15- ☑
    - with
      - damage to nail S91.25- ☑
  - lesser S91.15- ☑
    - with
      - damage to nail S91.25- ☑
  - superficial NEC S90.47- ☑
    - great S90.47- ☑
    - insect S90.46- ☑
      - great S90.46- ☑
- tongue S01.552 ☑
- trachea S11.025 ☑
  - superficial NEC S10.17 ☑
    - insect S10.16 ☑
- tunica vaginalis — *see* Bite, testis
- tympanum, tympanic membrane — *see* Bite, ear
- umbilical region S31.155 ☑
- uvula — *see* Bite, oral cavity
- vagina — *see* Bite, vulva
- venomous — *see* Venom
- vocal cords S11.035 ☑
  - superficial NEC S10.17 ☑
    - insect S10.16 ☑
- vulva S31.45 ☑
  - superficial NEC S30.874 ☑
    - insect S30.864 ☑
- wrist S61.55- ☑
  - superficial NEC S60.87- ☑
    - insect S60.86- ☑

Biting, cheek or lip K13.1
Biventricular failure (heart) I50.82
Björck (-Thorson) **syndrome** (malignant carcinoid) E34.0
Black
- death A20.9
- eye S00.1- ☑
- hairy tongue K14.3
- heel (foot) S90.3- ☑
- lung (disease) J60
- palm (hand) S60.22- ☑

Blackfan-Diamond anemia or syndrome (congenital hypoplastic anemia) D61.01
Blackhead L70.0
Blackout R55
Bladder — *see* condition
Blast (air) (hydraulic) (immersion) (underwater)
- blindness S05.8X- ☑

Blast — *continued*
  injury
    abdomen or thorax — *see* Injury, by site
    ear (acoustic nerve trauma) — *see* Injury, nerve,
      acoustic, specified type NEC
    syndrome NEC T70.8 ☑
Blastoma — *see* Neoplasm, malignant, by site
  pulmonary — *see* Neoplasm, lung, malignant
Blastomycosis, blastomycotic B40.9
  Brazilian — *see* Paracoccidioidomycosis
  cutaneous B40.3
  disseminated B40.7
  European — *see* Cryptococcosis
  generalized B40.7
  keloidal B48.0
  North American B40.9
  primary pulmonary B40.0
  pulmonary B40.2
    acute B40.0
    chronic B40.1
  skin B40.3
  South American — *see* Paracoccidioidomycosis
  specified NEC B40.89
Bleb(s) R23.8
  emphysematous (lung) (solitary) J43.9
  endophthalmitis H59.43
  filtering (vitreous), after glaucoma surgery Z98.83
  inflamed (infected), postprocedural H59.40
    stage 1 H59.41
    stage 2 H59.42
    stage 3 H59.43
  lung (ruptured) J43.9
    congenital — *see* Atelectasis
    newborn P25.8
  subpleural (emphysematous) J43.9
Blebitis, postprocedural H59.40
  stage 1 H59.41
  stage 2 H59.42
  stage 3 H59.43
Bleeder (familial) (hereditary) — *see* Hemophilia
Bleeding — *see also* Hemorrhage
  anal K62.5
  anovulatory N97.0
  atonic, following delivery O72.1
  capillary I78.8
    puerperal O72.2
  contact (postcoital) N93.0
  due to uterine subinvolution N85.3
  ear — *see* Otorrhagia
  excessive, associated with menopausal onset N92.4
  familial — *see* Defect, coagulation
  following intercourse N93.0
  gastrointestinal K92.2
  hemorrhoids — *see* Hemorrhoids
  intermenstrual (regular) N92.3
    irregular N92.1
  intraoperative — *see* Complication, intraoperative,
    hemorrhage
  irregular N92.6
  menopausal N92.4
  newborn, intraventricular — *see* Newborn, affected
    by, hemorrhage, intraventricular
  nipple N64.59
  nose R04.0
  ovulation N92.3
  perimenopausal N92.4
  postclimacteric N95.0
  postcoital N93.0
  postmenopausal N95.0
  postoperative — *see* Complication, postprocedural,
    hemorrhage
  preclimacteric N92.4
  pre-pubertal vaginal N93.1
  puberty (excessive, with onset of menstrual periods)
    N92.2
  rectum, rectal K62.5
    newborn P54.2
  tendencies — *see* Defect, coagulation
  throat R04.1
  tooth socket (post-extraction) K91.840
  umbilical stump P51.9
  uterus, uterine NEC N93.9
    climacteric N92.4
    dysfunctional or functional N93.8
    menopausal N92.4
    preclimacteric or premenopausal N92.4
    unrelated to menstrual cycle N93.9
  vagina, vaginal (abnormal) N93.9

Bleeding — *continued*
  vagina, vaginal — *continued*
    dysfunctional or functional N93.8
    newborn P54.6
    pre-pubertal N93.1
  vicarious N94.89
Blennorrhagia, blennorrhagic — *see* Gonorrhea
Blennorrhea (acute) (chronic) — *see also* Gonorrhea
  inclusion (neonatal) (newborn) P39.1
  lower genitourinary tract (gonococcal) A54.00
  neonatorum (gonococcal ophthalmia) A54.31
Blepharelosis — *see* Entropion
Blepharitis (angularis) (ciliaris) (eyelid) (marginal)
  (nonulcerative) H01.009
  herpes zoster B02.39
  left H01.006
    lower H01.005
    upper H01.004
    upper and lower H01.00B
  right H01.003
    lower H01.002
    upper H01.001
    upper and lower H01.00A
  squamous H01.029
    left H01.026
      lower H01.025
      upper H01.024
      upper and lower H01.02B
    right H01.023
      lower H01.022
      upper H01.021
      upper and lower H01.02A
  ulcerative H01.019
    left H01.016
      lower H01.015
      upper H01.014
      upper and lower H01.01B
    right H01.013
      lower H01.012
      upper H01.011
      upper and lower H01.01A
Blepharochalasis H02.30
  congenital Q10.0
  left H02.36
    lower H02.35
    upper H02.34
  right H02.33
    lower H02.32
    upper H02.31
Blepharoclonus H02.59
Blepharoconjunctivitis H10.50- ☑
  angular H10.52- ☑
  contact H10.53- ☑
  ligneous H10.51- ☑
Blepharophimosis (eyelid) H02.529
  congenital Q10.3
  left H02.526
    lower H02.525
    upper H02.524
  right H02.523
    lower H02.522
    upper H02.521
Blepharoptosis H02.40- ☑
  congenital Q10.0
  mechanical H02.41- ☑
  myogenic H02.42- ☑
  neurogenic H02.43- ☑
  paralytic H02.43- ☑
Blepharopyorrhea, gonococcal A54.39
Blepharospasm G24.5
  drug induced G24.01
Blighted ovum O02.0
Blind — *see also* Blindness
  bronchus (congenital) Q32.4
  loop syndrome K90.2
    congenital Q43.8
  sac, fallopian tube (congenital) Q50.6
  spot, enlarged — *see* Defect, visual field, localized,
    scotoma, blind spot area
  tract or tube, congenital NEC — *see* Atresia, by site
Blindness (acquired) (congenital) (both eyes) H54.0X- ☑
  blast S05.8X- ☑
  color — *see* Deficiency, color vision
  concussion S05.8X- ☑
  cortical H47.619
    left brain H47.612
    right brain H47.611
  day H53.11

Blindness — *continued*
  due to injury (current episode) S05.9- ☑
    sequelae — *code to* injury with seventh character
      S
  eclipse (total) — *see* Retinopathy, solar
  emotional (hysterical) F44.6
  face H53.16
  hysterical F44.6
  legal (both eyes) (USA definition) H54.8
  mind R48.8
  night H53.60
    abnormal dark adaptation curve H53.61
    acquired H53.62
    congenital H53.63
    specified type NEC H53.69
    vitamin A deficiency E50.5
  one eye (other eye normal) H54.40
    left (normal vision on right) H54.42- ☑
      low vision on right H54.12- ☑
    low vision, other eye H54.10
    right (normal vision on left) H54.41- ☑
      low vision on left H54.11- ☑
  psychic R48.8
  river B73.01
  snow — *see* Photokeratitis
  sun, solar — *see* Retinopathy, solar
  transient — *see* Disturbance, vision, subjective, loss,
    transient
  traumatic (current episode) S05.9- ☑
  word (developmental) F81.0
    acquired R48.0
    secondary to organic lesion R48.0
Blister (nonthermal)
  abdominal wall S30.821 ☑
  alveolar process S00.522 ☑
  ankle S90.52- ☑
  antecubital space — *see* Blister, elbow
  anus S30.827 ☑
  arm (upper) S40.82- ☑
  auditory canal — *see* Blister, ear
  auricle — *see* Blister, ear
  axilla — *see* Blister, arm
  back, lower S30.820 ☑
  beetle dermatitis L24.89
  breast S20.12- ☑
  brow S00.82 ☑
  calf — *see* Blister, leg
  canthus — *see* Blister, eyelid
  cheek S00.82 ☑
    internal S00.522 ☑
  chest wall — *see* Blister, thorax
  chin S00.82 ☑
  costal region — *see* Blister, thorax
  digit(s)
    foot — *see* Blister, toe
    hand — *see* Blister, finger
  due to burn — *see* Burn, by site, second degree
  ear S00.42- ☑
  elbow S50.32- ☑
  epiglottis S10.12 ☑
  esophagus, cervical S10.12 ☑
  eyebrow — *see* Blister, eyelid
  eyelid S00.22- ☑
  face S00.82 ☑
  fever B00.1
  finger(s) S60.429 ☑
    index S60.42- ☑
    little S60.42- ☑
    middle S60.42- ☑
    ring S60.42- ☑
  foot (except toe(s) alone) S90.82- ☑
    toe — *see* Blister, toe
  forearm S50.82- ☑
    elbow only — *see* Blister, elbow
  forehead S00.82 ☑
  fracture — *omit code*
  genital organ
    female S30.826 ☑
    male S30.825 ☑
  gum S00.522 ☑
  hand S60.52- ☑
  head S00.92 ☑
    ear — *see* Blister, ear
    eyelid — *see* Blister, eyelid
    lip S00.521 ☑
    nose S00.32 ☑

Blister — *continued*
- head — *continued*
  - oral cavity S00.522 ☑
  - scalp S00.02 ☑
  - specified site NEC S00.82 ☑
- heel — *see* Blister, foot
- hip S70.22- ☑
- interscapular region S20.429 ☑
- jaw S00.82 ☑
- knee S80.22- ☑
- larynx S10.12 ☑
- leg (lower) S80.82- ☑
  - knee — *see* Blister, knee
  - upper — *see* Blister, thigh
- lip S00.521 ☑
- malar region S00.82 ☑
- mammary — *see* Blister, breast
- mastoid region S00.82 ☑
- mouth S00.522 ☑
- multiple, skin, nontraumatic R23.8
- nail
  - finger — *see* Blister, finger
  - toe — *see* Blister, toe
- nasal S00.32 ☑
- neck S10.92 ☑
  - specified site NEC S10.82 ☑
  - throat S10.12 ☑
- nose S00.32 ☑
- occipital region S00.02 ☑
- oral cavity S00.522 ☑
- orbital region — *see* Blister, eyelid
- palate S00.522 ☑
- palm — *see* Blister, hand
- parietal region S00.02 ☑
- pelvis S30.820 ☑
- penis S30.822 ☑
- periocular area — *see* Blister, eyelid
- phalanges
  - finger — *see* Blister, finger
  - toe — *see* Blister, toe
- pharynx S10.12 ☑
- pinna — *see* Blister, ear
- popliteal space — *see* Blister, knee
- scalp S00.02 ☑
- scapular region — *see* Blister, shoulder
- scrotum S30.823 ☑
- shin — *see* Blister, leg
- shoulder S40.22- ☑
- sternal region S20.329 ☑
- submaxillary region S00.82 ☑
- submental region S00.82 ☑
- subungual
  - finger(s) — *see* Blister, finger
  - toe(s) — *see* Blister, toe
- supraclavicular fossa S10.82 ☑
- supraorbital S00.82 ☑
- temple S00.82 ☑
- temporal region S00.82 ☑
- testis S30.823 ☑
- thermal — *see* Burn, second degree, by site
- thigh S70.32- ☑
- thorax, thoracic (wall) S20.92 ☑
  - back S20.42- ☑
  - front S20.32- ☑
- throat S10.12 ☑
- thumb S60.32- ☑
- toe(s) S90.42- ☑
  - great S90.42- ☑
- tongue S00.522 ☑
- trachea S10.12 ☑
- tympanum, tympanic membrane — *see* Blister, ear
- upper arm — *see* Blister, arm (upper)
- uvula S00.522 ☑
- vagina S30.824 ☑
- vocal cords S10.12 ☑
- vulva S30.824 ☑
- wrist S60.82- ☑

Bloating R14.0
Bloch-Sulzberger disease or syndrome Q82.3
Block, blocked
- alveolocapillary J84.10
- arborization (heart) I45.5
- arrhythmic I45.9
- atrioventricular (incomplete) (partial) I44.30
  - with atrioventricular dissociation I44.2
    - complete I44.2

Block, blocked — *continued*
- atrioventricular — *continued*
  - complete — *continued*
    - congenital Q24.6
  - congenital Q24.6
  - first degree I44.0
  - second degree (types I and II) I44.1
  - specified NEC I44.39
  - third degree I44.2
  - types I and II I44.1
- auriculoventricular — *see* Block, atrioventricular
- bifascicular (cardiac) I45.2
- bundle-branch (complete) (false) (incomplete) I45.4
  - bilateral I45.2
  - left I44.7
    - with right bundle branch block I45.2
    - hemiblock I44.60
      - anterior I44.4
      - posterior I44.5
    - incomplete I44.7
      - with right bundle branch block I45.2
  - right I45.10
    - with
      - left bundle branch block I45.2
      - left fascicular block I45.2
    - specified NEC I45.19
  - Wilson's type I45.19
- cardiac I45.9
- conduction I45.9
  - complete I44.2
- fascicular (left) I44.60
  - anterior I44.4
  - posterior I44.5
  - right I45.0
  - specified NEC I44.69
- foramen Magendie (acquired) G91.1
  - congenital Q03.1
    - with spina bifida — *see* Spina bifida, by site, with hydrocephalus
- heart I45.9
  - bundle branch I45.4
    - bilateral I45.2
  - complete (atrioventricular) I44.2
  - congenital Q24.6
  - first degree (atrioventricular) I44.0
  - second degree (atrioventricular) I44.1
  - specified type NEC I45.5
  - third degree (atrioventricular) I44.2
- hepatic vein I82.0
- intraventricular (nonspecific) I45.4
  - bundle branch
    - bilateral I45.2
- kidney N28.9
  - postcystoscopic or postprocedural N99.0
- Mobitz (types I and II) I44.1
- myocardial — *see* Block, heart
- nodal I45.5
- organ or site, congenital NEC — *see* Atresia, by site
- portal (vein) I81
- second degree (types I and II) I44.1
- sinoatrial I45.5
- sinoauricular I45.5
- third degree I44.2
- trifascicular I45.3
- tubal N97.1
- vein NOS I82.90
- Wenckebach (types I and II) I44.1
Blockage — *see* Obstruction
Blocq's disease F44.4
Blood
- constituents, abnormal R78.9
- disease D75.9
- donor — *see* Donor, blood
- dyscrasia D75.9
  - with
    - abortion — *see* Abortion, by type, complicated by, hemorrhage
    - ectopic pregnancy O08.1
    - molar pregnancy O08.1
  - following ectopic or molar pregnancy O08.1
  - newborn P61.9
  - puerperal, postpartum O72.3
- flukes NEC — *see* Schistosomiasis
- in
  - feces K92.1
    - occult R19.5
  - urine — *see* Hematuria
- mole O02.0

Blood — *continued*
- occult in feces R19.5
- pressure
  - decreased, due to shock following injury T79.4 ☑
  - examination only Z01.30
  - fluctuating I99.8
  - high — *see* Hypertension
    - borderline R03.0
    - incidental reading, without diagnosis of hypertension R03.0
  - low — *see also* Hypotension
    - incidental reading, without diagnosis of hypotension R03.1
- spitting — *see* Hemoptysis
- staining cornea — *see* Pigmentation, cornea, stromal
- transfusion
  - reaction or complication — *see* Complications, transfusion
- type
  - A (Rh positive) Z67.10
    - Rh negative Z67.11
  - AB (Rh positive) Z67.30
    - Rh negative Z67.31
  - B (Rh positive) Z67.20
    - Rh negative Z67.21
  - O (Rh positive) Z67.40
    - Rh negative Z67.41
  - Rh (positive) Z67.90
    - negative Z67.91
- vessel rupture — *see* Hemorrhage
- vomiting — *see* Hematemesis
Blood-forming organs, disease D75.9
Bloodgood's disease — *see* Mastopathy, cystic
Bloom (-Machacek)(-Torre) **syndrome** Q82.8
Blount's disease or osteochondrosis — *see* Osteochondrosis, juvenile, tibia
Blue
- baby Q24.9
- diaper syndrome E72.09
- dome cyst (breast) — *see* Cyst, breast
- dot cataract Q12.0
- nevus D22.9
- sclera Q13.5
  - with fragility of bone and deafness Q78.0
- toe syndrome I75.02- ☑
Blueness — *see* Cyanosis
Blues, postpartal O90.6
- baby O90.6
Blurring, visual H53.8
Blushing (abnormal) (excessive) R23.2
BMI — *see* Body, mass index
Boarder, hospital NEC Z76.4
- accompanying sick person Z76.3
- healthy infant or child Z76.2
  - foundling Z76.1
Bockhart's impetigo L01.02
Bodechtel-Guttman disease (subacute sclerosing panencephalitis) A81.1
Boder-Sedgwick syndrome (ataxia-telangiectasia) G11.3
Body, bodies
- Aschoff's — *see* Myocarditis, rheumatic
- asteroid, vitreous — *see* Deposit, crystalline
- cytoid (retina) — *see* Occlusion, artery, retina
- drusen (degenerative) (macula) (retinal) — *see also* Degeneration, macula, drusen
  - optic disc — *see* Drusen, optic disc
- foreign — *see* Foreign body
- loose
  - joint, except knee — *see* Loose, body, joint
    - knee M23.4- ☑
  - sheath, tendon — *see* Disorder, tendon, specified type NEC
- mass index (BMI)
  - adult
    - 19.9 or less Z68.1
    - 20.0-20.9 Z68.20
    - 21.0-21.9 Z68.21
    - 22.0-22.9 Z68.22
    - 23.0-23.9 Z68.23
    - 24.0-24.9 Z68.24
    - 25.0-25.9 Z68.25
    - 26.0-26.9 Z68.26
    - 27.0-27.9 Z68.27
    - 28.0-28.9 Z68.28
    - 29.0-29.9 Z68.29
    - 30.0-30.9 Z68.30
    - 31.0-31.9 Z68.31
    - 32.0-32.9 Z68.32

Body, bodies — *continued*
  mass index — *continued*
    adult — *continued*
      33.0-33.9 Z68.33
      34.0-34.9 Z68.34
      35.0-35.9 Z68.35
      36.0-36.9 Z68.36
      37.0-37.9 Z68.37
      38.0-38.9 Z68.38
      39.0-39.9 Z68.39
      40.0-44.9 Z68.41
      45.0-49.9 Z68.42
      50.0-59.9 Z68.43
      60.0-69.9 Z68.44
      70 and over Z68.45
    pediatric
      5th percentile to less than 85th percentile for age Z68.52
      85th percentile to less than 95th percentile for age Z68.53
      greater than or equal to ninety-fifth percentile for age Z68.54
      less than fifth percentile for age Z68.51
  Mooser's A75.2
  rice — *see also* Loose, body, joint
    knee M23.4- ☑
  rocking F98.4
Boeck's
  disease or sarcoid — *see* Sarcoidosis
  lupoid (miliary) D86.3
Boerhaave's syndrome (spontaneous esophageal rupture) K22.3
Boggy
  cervix N88.8
  uterus N85.8
Boil — *see also* Furuncle, by site
  Aleppo B55.1
  Baghdad B55.1
  Delhi B55.1
  lacrimal
    gland — *see* Dacryoadenitis
    passages (duct) (sac) — *see* Inflammation, lacrimal, passages, acute
  Natal B55.1
  orbit, orbital — *see* Abscess, orbit
  tropical B55.1
Bold hives — *see* Urticaria
Bombé, iris — *see* Membrane, pupillary
Bone — *see* condition
Bonnevie-Ullrich syndrome — *see also* Turner's syndrome Q87.19
Bonnier's syndrome H81.8 ☑
Bonvale dam fever T73.3 ☑
Bony block of joint — *see* Ankylosis
BOOP (bronchiolitis obliterans organized pneumonia) J84.89
Borderline
  diabetes mellitus R73.03
  hypertension R03.0
  osteopenia M85.8- ☑
  pelvis, with obstruction during labor O65.1
  personality F60.3
Borna disease A83.9
Bornholm disease B33.0
Boston exanthem A88.0
Botalli, ductus (patent) (persistent) Q25.0
Bothriocephalus latus infestation B70.0
Botulism (foodborne intoxication) A05.1
  infant A48.51
  non-foodborne A48.52
  wound A48.52
Bouba — *see* Yaws
Bouchard's nodes (with arthropathy) M15.2
Bouffée délirante F23
Bouillaud's disease or syndrome (rheumatic heart disease) I01.9
Bourneville's disease Q85.1
Boutonniere deformity (finger) — *see* Deformity, finger, boutonniere
Bouveret (-Hoffmann) **syndrome** (paroxysmal tachycardia) I47.9
Bovine heart — *see* Hypertrophy, cardiac
Bowel — *see* condition
Bowen's
  dermatosis (precancerous) — *see* Neoplasm, skin, in situ
  disease — *see* Neoplasm, skin, in situ

Bowen's — *continued*
  epithelioma — *see* Neoplasm, skin, in situ
  type
    epidermoid carcinoma-in-situ — *see* Neoplasm, skin, in situ
    intraepidermal squamous cell carcinoma — *see* Neoplasm, skin, in situ
Bowing
  femur — *see also* Deformity, limb, specified type NEC, thigh
    congenital Q68.3
  fibula — *see also* Deformity, limb, specified type NEC, lower leg
    congenital Q68.4
  forearm — *see* Deformity, limb, specified type NEC, forearm
  leg(s), long bones, congenital Q68.5
  radius — *see* Deformity, limb, specified type NEC, forearm
  tibia — *see also* Deformity, limb, specified type NEC, lower leg
    congenital Q68.4
Bowleg(s) (acquired) M21.16- ☑
  congenital Q68.5
  rachitic E64.3
Boyd's dysentery A03.2
Brachial — *see* condition
Brachycardia R00.1
Brachycephaly Q75.0
Bradley's disease A08.19
Bradyarrhythmia, cardiac I49.8
Bradycardia (sinoatrial) (sinus) (vagal) R00.1
  neonatal P29.12
  reflex G90.09
  tachycardia syndrome I49.5
Bradykinesia R25.8
Bradypnea R06.89
Bradytachycardia I49.5
Brailsford's disease or osteochondrosis — *see* Osteochondrosis, juvenile, radius
Brain — *see also* condition
  death G93.82
  syndrome — *see* Syndrome, brain
Branched-chain amino-acid disorder E71.2
Branchial — *see* condition
  cartilage, congenital Q18.2
Branchiogenic remnant (in neck) Q18.0
Brandt's syndrome (acrodermatitis enteropathica) E83.2
Brash (water) R12
Bravais-jacksonian epilepsy — *see* Epilepsy, localization-related, symptomatic, with simple partial seizures
Braxton Hicks contractions — *see* False, labor
Brazilian leishmaniasis B55.2
BRBPR K62.5
Break, retina (without detachment) H33.30- ☑
  with retinal detachment — *see* Detachment, retina
  horseshoe tear H33.31- ☑
  multiple H33.33- ☑
  round hole H33.32- ☑
Breakdown
  device, graft or implant — *see also* Complications, by site and type, mechanical T85.618 ☑
    arterial graft NEC — *see* Complication, cardiovascular device, mechanical, vascular
    breast (implant) T85.41 ☑
    catheter NEC T85.618 ☑
      cystostomy T83.010 ☑
      dialysis (renal) T82.41 ☑
        intraperitoneal T85.611 ☑
      Hopkins T83.018 ☑
      ileostomy T83.018 ☑
      infusion NEC T82.514 ☑
        cranial T85.610- ☑
        epidural T85.610 ☑
        intrathecal T85.610 ☑
        spinal T85.610 ☑
        subarachnoid T85.610 ☑
        subdural T85.610 ☑
      nephrostomy T83.012 ☑
      urethral indwelling T83.011 ☑
      urinary NEC T83.018 ☑
      urostomy T83.018 ☑
    electronic (electrode) (pulse generator) (stimulator)
      bone T84.310 ☑
      cardiac T82.119 ☑
        electrode T82.110 ☑

Breakdown — *continued*
  device, graft or implant — *see also* Complications, by site and type, mechanical — *continued*
    electronic — *continued*
      cardiac — *continued*
        pulse generator T82.111 ☑
        specified type NEC T82.118 ☑
      nervous system — *see* Complication, prosthetic device, mechanical, electronic nervous system stimulator
      urinary — *see* Complication, genitourinary, device, urinary, mechanical
    fixation, internal (orthopedic) NEC — *see* Complication, fixation device, mechanical
    gastrointestinal — *see* Complications, prosthetic device, mechanical, gastrointestinal device
    genital NEC T83.418 ☑
      intrauterine contraceptive device T83.31 ☑
      penile prosthesis (cylinder) (implanted) (pump) (resevoir) T83.410 ☑
      testicular prosthesis T83.411 ☑
    heart NEC — *see* Complication, cardiovascular device, mechanical
    intrathecal infusion pump T85.615 ☑
    joint prosthesis — *see* Complications…, joint prosthesis,internal, mechanical, by site
    nervous system, specified device NEC T85.615 ☑
    ocular NEC — *see* Complications, prosthetic device, mechanical, ocular device
    orthopedic NEC — *see* Complication, orthopedic, device, mechanical
    specified NEC T85.618 ☑
    subcutaneous device pocket
      nervous system prosthetic device, implant, or graft T85.890 ☑
      other internal prosthetic device, implant, or graft T85.898 ☑
    sutures, permanent T85.612 ☑
      used in bone repair — *see* Complications, fixation device, internal (orthopedic), mechanical
    urinary NEC T83.118 ☑
      graft T83.21 ☑
      sphincter, implanted T83.111 ☑
      stent (ileal conduit) (nephroureteral) T83.113 ☑
        ureteral indwelling T83.112 ☑
    vascular NEC — *see* Complication, cardiovascular device, mechanical
    ventricular intracranial shunt T85.01 ☑
  nervous F48.8
  perineum O90.1
  respirator J95.850
    specified NEC J95.859
  ventilator J95.850
    specified NEC J95.859
Breast — *see also* condition
  buds E30.1
    in newborn P96.89
  dense R92.2
  nodule — *see also* Lump, breast N63.0
Breath
  foul R19.6
  holder, child R06.89
  holding spell R06.89
  shortness R06.02
Breathing
  labored — *see* Hyperventilation
  mouth R06.5
    causing malocclusion M26.5 ☑
  periodic R06.3
    high altitude G47.32
Breathlessness R06.81
Breda's disease — *see* Yaws
Breech presentation (mother) O32.1 ☑
  causing obstructed labor O64.1 ☑
  footling O32.8 ☑
    causing obstructed labor O64.8 ☑
  incomplete O32.8 ☑
    causing obstructed labor O64.8 ☑
Breisky's disease N90.4
Brennemann's syndrome I88.0
Brenner
  tumor (benign) D27.9
    borderline malignancy D39.1- ☑
    malignant C56 ☑
    proliferating D39.1- ☑
Bretonneau's disease or angina A36.0
Breus' mole O02.0

Brevicollis Q76.49
Brickmakers' anemia B76.9 *[D63.8]*
Bridge, myocardial Q24.5
Bright red blood per rectum (BRBPR) K62.5
Bright's disease — *see also* Nephritis
  arteriosclerotic — *see* Hypertension, kidney
Brill (-Zinsser) **disease** (recrudescent typhus) A75.1
Brill-Symmers' disease C82.90
Brion-Kayser disease — *see* Fever, parathyroid
Briquet's disorder or syndrome F45.0
Brissaud's
  infantilism or dwarfism E23.0
  motor-verbal tic F95.2
Brittle
  bones disease Q78.0
  nails L60.3
    congenital Q84.6
Broad — *see also* condition
  beta disease E78.2
  ligament laceration syndrome N83.8
Broad- or floating-betalipoproteinemia E78.2
Brock's syndrome (atelectasis due to enlarged lymph
    nodes) J98.19
Brocq-Duhring disease (dermatitis herpetiformis) L13.0
Brodie's abscess or disease M86.8X- ☑
Broken
  arches — *see also* Deformity, limb, flat foot
  arm (meaning upper limb) — *see* Fracture, arm
  back — *see* Fracture, vertebra
  bone — *see* Fracture
  implant or internal device — *see* Complications, by site
    and type, mechanical
  leg (meaning lower limb) — *see* Fracture, leg
  nose S02.2 ☑
  tooth, teeth — *see* Fracture, tooth
Bromhidrosis, bromidrosis L75.0
Bromidism, bromism G92
  due to
    correct substance properly administered — *see* Ta-
      ble of Drugs and Chemicals, by drug, adverse
      effect
    overdose or wrong substance given or taken — *see*
      Table of Drugs and Chemicals, by drug, poi-
      soning
  chronic (dependence) F13.20
Bromidrosiphobia F40.298
Bronchi, bronchial — *see* condition
Bronchiectasis (cylindrical) (diffuse) (fusiform) (localized)
    (saccular) J47.9
  with
    acute
      bronchitis J47.0
      lower respiratory infection J47.0
    exacerbation (acute) J47.1
  congenital Q33.4
  tuberculous NEC — *see* Tuberculosis, pulmonary
Bronchiolectasis — *see* Bronchiectasis
Bronchiolitis (acute) (infective) (subacute) J21.9
  with
    bronchospasm or obstruction J21.9
    influenza, flu or grippe — *see* Influenza, with, respi-
      ratory manifestations NEC
  chemical (chronic) J68.4
    acute J68.0
  chronic (fibrosing) (obliterative) J44.9
  due to
    external agent — *see* Bronchitis, acute, due to
    human metapneumovirus J21.1
    respiratory syncytial virus (RSV) J21.0
    specified organism NEC J21.8
  fibrosa obliterans J44.9
  influenzal — *see* Influenza, with, respiratory manifesta-
    tions NEC
  obliterans J42
    with organizing pneumonia (BOOP) J84.89
  obliterative (chronic) (subacute) J44.9
    due to fumes or vapors J68.4
    due to chemicals, gases, fumes or vapors (inhalation)
      J68.4
  respiratory, interstitial lung disease J84.115
Bronchitis (diffuse) (fibrinous) (hypostatic) (infective)
    (membranous) J40
  with
    influenza, flu or grippe — *see* Influenza, with, respi-
      ratory manifestations NEC
    obstruction (airway) (lung) J44.9
    tracheitis (15 years of age and above) J40

Bronchitis — *continued*
  with — *continued*
    tracheitis — *continued*
      acute or subacute J20.9
      chronic J42
      under 15 years of age J20.9
  acute or subacute (with bronchospasm or obstruction)
    J20.9
    with
      bronchiectasis J47.0
      chronic obstructive pulmonary disease J44.0
    chemical (due to gases, fumes or vapors) J68.0
    due to
      fumes or vapors J68.0
      Haemophilus influenzae J20.1
      Mycoplasma pneumoniae J20.0
      radiation J70.0
      specified organism NEC J20.8
      Streptococcus J20.2
      virus
        coxsackie J20.3
        echovirus J20.7
        parainfluenzae J20.4
        respiratory syncytial (RSV) J20.5
        rhinovirus J20.6
    viral NEC J20.8
  allergic (acute) J45.909
    with
      exacerbation (acute) J45.901
      status asthmaticus J45.902
  arachidic T17.528 ☑
  aspiration (due to fumes or vapors) J68.0
  asthmatic J45.9 ☑
    chronic J44.9
      with
        acute lower respiratory infection J44.0
        exacerbation (acute) J44.1
  capillary — *see* Pneumonia, broncho
  caseous (tuberculous) A15.5
  Castellani's A69.8
  catarrhal (15 years of age and above) J40
    acute — *see* Bronchitis, acute
    chronic J41.0
    under 15 years of age J20.9
  chemical (acute) (subacute) J68.0
    chronic J68.4
    due to fumes or vapors J68.0
      chronic J68.4
  chronic J42
    with
      airways obstruction J44.9
      tracheitis (chronic) J42
    asthmatic (obstructive) J44.9
    catarrhal J41.0
    chemical (due to fumes or vapors) J68.4
    due to
      chemicals, gases, fumes or vapors (inhalation)
        J68.4
      radiation J70.1
      tobacco smoking J41.0
    emphysematous J44.9
    mucopurulent J41.1
    non-obstructive J41.0
    obliterans J44.9
    obstructive J44.9
    purulent J41.1
    simple J41.0
  croupous — *see* Bronchitis, acute
  due to gases, fumes or vapors (chemical) J68.0
  emphysematous (obstructive) J44.9
  exudative — *see* Bronchitis, acute
  fetid J41.1
  grippal — *see* Influenza, with, respiratory manifesta-
    tions NEC
  in those under 15 years age — *see* Bronchitis, acute
    chronic — *see* Bronchitis, chronic
  influenzal — *see* Influenza, with, respiratory manifesta-
    tions NEC
  mixed simple and mucopurulent J41.8
  moulder's J62.8
  mucopurulent (chronic) (recurrent) J41.1
    acute or subacute J20.9
    simple (mixed) J41.8
  obliterans (chronic) J44.9
  obstructive (chronic) (diffuse) J44.9
  pituitous J41.1
  pneumococcal, acute or subacute J20.2

Bronchitis — *continued*
  pseudomembranous, acute or subacute — *see* Bronchi-
    tis, acute
  purulent (chronic) (recurrent) J41.1
    acute or subacute — *see* Bronchitis, acute
  putrid J41.1
  senile (chronic) J42
  simple and mucopurulent (mixed) J41.8
  smokers' J41.0
  spirochetal NEC A69.8
  subacute — *see* Bronchitis, acute
  suppurative (chronic) J41.1
    acute or subacute — *see* Bronchitis, acute
  tuberculous A15.5
  under 15 years of age — *see* Bronchitis, acute
    chronic — *see* Bronchitis, chronic
  viral NEC, acute or subacute — *see also* Bronchitis,
    acute J20.8
Bronchoalveolitis J18.0
Bronchoaspergillosis B44.1
Bronchocele meaning goiter E04.0
Broncholithiasis J98.09
  tuberculous NEC A15.5
Bronchomalacia J98.09
  congenital Q32.2
Bronchomycosis NOS B49 *[J99]*
  candidal B37.1
Bronchopleuropneumonia — *see* Pneumonia, broncho
Bronchopneumonia — *see* Pneumonia, broncho
Bronchopneumonitis — *see* Pneumonia, broncho
Bronchopulmonary — *see* condition
Bronchopulmonitis — *see* Pneumonia, broncho
Bronchorrhagia (see Hemoptysis)
Bronchorrhea J98.09
  acute J20.9
  chronic (infective) (purulent) J42
Bronchospasm (acute) J98.01
  with
    bronchiolitis, acute J21.9
    bronchitis, acute (conditions in J20) — *see* Bronchi-
      tis, acute
  due to external agent — *see* condition, respiratory,
    acute, due to
  exercise induced J45.990
Bronchospirochetosis A69.8
  Castellani A69.8
Bronchostenosis J98.09
Bronchus — *see* condition
Brontophobia F40.220
Bronze baby syndrome P83.88
Brooke's tumor — *see* Neoplasm, skin, benign
Brown enamel of teeth (hereditary) K00.5
Brown's sheath syndrome H50.61- ☑
Brown-Séquard disease, paralysis or syndrome
    G83.81
Bruce sepsis A23.0
Brucellosis (infection) A23.9
  abortus A23.1
  canis A23.3
  dermatitis A23.9
  melitensis A23.0
  mixed A23.8
  sepsis A23.9
    melitensis A23.0
    specified NEC A23.8
  suis A23.2
Bruck-de Lange disease Q87.19
Bruck's disease — *see* Deformity, limb
BRUE (brief resolved unexplained event) R68.13
Brugsch's syndrome Q82.8
Bruise (skin surface intact) — *see also* Contusion
  with
    open wound — *see* Wound, open
  internal organ — *see* Injury, by site
  newborn P54.5
  scalp, due to birth injury, newborn P12.3
  umbilical cord O69.5 ☑
Bruit (arterial) R09.89
  cardiac R01.1
Brush burn — *see* Abrasion, by site
Bruton's X-linked agammaglobulinemia D80.0
Bruxism
  psychogenic F45.8
  sleep related G47.63
Bubbly lung syndrome P27.0
Bubo I88.8
  blennorrhagic (gonococcal) A54.89

Bubo — *continued*
  chancroidal A57
  climatic A55
  due to Haemophilus ducreyi A57
  gonococcal A54.89
  indolent (nonspecific) I88.8
  inguinal (nonspecific) I88.8
    chancroidal A57
    climatic A55
    due to H. ducreyi A57
    infective I88.8
  scrofulous (tuberculous) A18.2
  soft chancre A57
  suppurating — *see* Lymphadenitis, acute
  syphilitic (primary) A51.0
    congenital A50.07
  tropical A55
  virulent (chancroidal) A57
Bubonic plague A20.0
Bubonocele — *see* Hernia, inguinal
Buccal — *see* condition
Buchanan's disease or osteochondrosis M91.0
Buchem's syndrome (hyperostosis corticalis) M85.2
Bucket-handle fracture or tear (semilunar cartilage) — *see* Tear, meniscus
Budd-Chiari syndrome (hepatic vein thrombosis) I82.0
Budgerigar fancier's disease or lung J67.2
Buds
  breast E30.1
    in newborn P96.89
Buerger's disease (thromboangiitis obliterans) I73.1
Bulbar — *see* condition
Bulbus cordis (left ventricle) (persistent) Q21.8
Bulimia (nervosa) F50.2
  atypical F50.9
  normal weight F50.9
Bulky
  stools R19.5
  uterus N85.2
Bulla (e) R23.8
  lung (emphysematous) (solitary) J43.9
    newborn P25.8
Bullet wound — *see also* Wound, open
  fracture — *code as* Fracture, by site
  internal organ — *see* Injury, by site
Bundle
  branch block (complete) (false) (incomplete) — *see* Block, bundle-branch
  of His — *see* condition
Bunion M21.61- ☑
  tailor's M21.62- ☑
Bunionette M21.62- ☑
Buphthalmia, buphthalmos (congenital) Q15.0
Burdwan fever B55.0
Bürger-Grütz disease or syndrome E78.3
Buried
  penis (congenital) Q55.64
    acquired N48.83
  roots K08.3
Burke's syndrome K86.89
Burkitt
  cell leukemia C91.0- ☑
  lymphoma (malignant) C83.7- ☑
    small noncleaved, diffuse C83.7- ☑
    spleen C83.77
    undifferentiated C83.7- ☑
  tumor C83.7- ☑
  type
    acute lymphoblastic leukemia C91.0- ☑
    undifferentiated C83.7- ☑
Burn (electricity) (flame) (hot gas, liquid or hot object) (radiation) (steam) (thermal) T30.0
  abdomen, abdominal (muscle) (wall) T21.02 ☑
    first degree T21.12 ☑
    second degree T21.22 ☑
    third degree T21.32 ☑
  above elbow T22.039 ☑
    first degree T22.139 ☑
    left T22.032 ☑
      first degree T22.132 ☑
      second degree T22.232 ☑
      third degree T22.332 ☑
    right T22.031 ☑
      first degree T22.131 ☑
      second degree T22.231 ☑
      third degree T22.331 ☑
    second degree T22.239 ☑

Burn — *continued*
  above elbow — *continued*
    third degree T22.339 ☑
  acid (caustic) (external) (internal) — *see* Corrosion, by site
  alimentary tract NEC T28.2 ☑
    esophagus T28.1 ☑
    mouth T28.0 ☑
    pharynx T28.0 ☑
  alkaline (caustic) (external) (internal) — *see* Corrosion, by site
  ankle T25.019 ☑
    first degree T25.119 ☑
    left T25.012 ☑
      first degree T25.112 ☑
      second degree T25.212 ☑
      third degree T25.312 ☑
    multiple with foot — *see* Burn, lower, limb, multiple, ankle and foot
    right T25.011 ☑
      first degree T25.111 ☑
      second degree T25.211 ☑
      third degree T25.311 ☑
    second degree T25.219 ☑
    third degree T25.319 ☑
  anus — *see* Burn, buttock
  arm (lower) (upper) — *see* Burn, upper, limb
  axilla T22.049 ☑
    first degree T22.149 ☑
    left T22.042 ☑
      first degree T22.142 ☑
      second degree T22.242 ☑
      third degree T22.342 ☑
    right T22.041 ☑
      first degree T22.141 ☑
      second degree T22.241 ☑
      third degree T22.341 ☑
    second degree T22.249 ☑
    third degree T22.349 ☑
  back (lower) T21.04 ☑
    first degree T21.14 ☑
    second degree T21.24 ☑
    third degree T21.34 ☑
    upper T21.03 ☑
      first degree T21.13 ☑
      second degree T21.23 ☑
      third degree T21.33 ☑
  blisters — *code as* Burn, second degree, by site
  breast(s) — *see* Burn, chest wall
  buttock(s) T21.05 ☑
    first degree T21.15 ☑
    second degree T21.25 ☑
    third degree T21.35 ☑
  calf T24.039 ☑
    first degree T24.139 ☑
    left T24.032 ☑
      first degree T24.132 ☑
      second degree T24.232 ☑
      third degree T24.332 ☑
    right T24.031 ☑
      first degree T24.131 ☑
      second degree T24.231 ☑
      third degree T24.331 ☑
    second degree T24.239 ☑
    third degree T24.339 ☑
  canthus (eye) — *see* Burn, eyelid
  caustic acid or alkaline — *see* Corrosion, by site
  cervix T28.3 ☑
  cheek T20.06 ☑
    first degree T20.16 ☑
    second degree T20.26 ☑
    third degree T20.36 ☑
  chemical (acids) (alkalines) (caustics) (external) (internal) — *see* Corrosion, by site
  chest wall T21.01 ☑
    first degree T21.11 ☑
    second degree T21.21 ☑
    third degree T21.31 ☑
  chin T20.03 ☑
    first degree T20.13 ☑
    second degree T20.23 ☑
    third degree T20.33 ☑
  colon T28.2 ☑
  conjunctiva (and cornea) — *see* Burn, cornea
  cornea (and conjunctiva) T26.1- ☑
    chemical — *see* Corrosion, cornea

Burn — *continued*
  corrosion (external) (internal) — *see* Corrosion, by site
  deep necrosis of underlying tissue — *code as* Burn, third degree, by site
  dorsum of hand T23.069 ☑
    first degree T23.169 ☑
    left T23.062 ☑
      first degree T23.162 ☑
      second degree T23.262 ☑
      third degree T23.362 ☑
    right T23.061 ☑
      first degree T23.161 ☑
      second degree T23.261 ☑
      third degree T23.361 ☑
    second degree T23.269 ☑
    third degree T23.369 ☑
  due to ingested chemical agent — *see* Corrosion, by site
  ear (auricle) (external) (canal) T20.01 ☑
    first degree T20.11 ☑
    second degree T20.21 ☑
    third degree T20.31 ☑
  elbow T22.029 ☑
    first degree T22.129 ☑
    left T22.022 ☑
      first degree T22.122 ☑
      second degree T22.222 ☑
      third degree T22.322 ☑
    right T22.021 ☑
      first degree T22.121 ☑
      second degree T22.221 ☑
      third degree T22.321 ☑
    second degree T22.229 ☑
    third degree T22.329 ☑
  epidermal loss — *code as* Burn, second degree, by site
  erythema, erythematous — *code as* Burn, first degree, by site
  esophagus T28.1 ☑
  extent (percentage of body surface)
    less than 10 percent T31.0
    10-19 percent T31.10
      with 0-9 percent third degree burns T31.10
      with 10-19 percent third degree burns T31.11
    20-29 percent T31.20
      with 0-9 percent third degree burns T31.20
      with 10-19 percent third degree burns T31.21
      with 20-29 percent third degree burns T31.22
    30-39 percent T31.30
      with 0-9 percent third degree burns T31.30
      with 10-19 percent third degree burns T31.31
      with 20-29 percent third degree burns T31.32
      with 30-39 percent third degree burns T31.33
    40-49 percent T31.40
      with 0-9 percent third degree burns T31.40
      with 10-19 percent third degree burns T31.41
      with 20-29 percent third degree burns T31.42
      with 30-39 percent third degree burns T31.43
      with 40-49 percent third degree burns T31.44
    50-59 percent T31.50
      with 0-9 percent third degree burns T31.50
      with 10-19 percent third degree burns T31.51
      with 20-29 percent third degree burns T31.52
      with 30-39 percent third degree burns T31.53
      with 40-49 percent third degree burns T31.54
      with 50-59 percent third degree burns T31.55
    60-69 percent T31.60
      with 0-9 percent third degree burns T31.60
      with 10-19 percent third degree burns T31.61
      with 20-29 percent third degree burns T31.62
      with 30-39 percent third degree burns T31.63
      with 40-49 percent third degree burns T31.64
      with 50-59 percent third degree burns T31.65
      with 60-69 percent third degree burns T31.66
    70-79 percent T31.70
      with 0-9 percent third degree burns T31.70
      with 10-19 percent third degree burns T31.71
      with 20-29 percent third degree burns T31.72
      with 30-39 percent third degree burns T31.73
      with 40-49 percent third degree burns T31.74
      with 50-59 percent third degree burns T31.75
      with 60-69 percent third degree burns T31.76
      with 70-79 percent third degree burns T31.77
    80-89 percent T31.80
      with 0-9 percent third degree burns T31.80
      with 10-19 percent third degree burns T31.81
      with 20-29 percent third degree burns T31.82
      with 30-39 percent third degree burns T31.83

Subterms under main terms may continue to next column or page   ☑ Additional Character Required — Refer to the Tabular List for Character Selection   43

Bubo — Burn

Burn — *continued*
  extent — *continued*
    80-89 percent — *continued*
      with 40-49 percent third degree burns T31.84
      with 50-59 percent third degree burns T31.85
      with 60-69 percent third degree burns T31.86
      with 70-79 percent third degree burns T31.87
      with 80-89 percent third degree burns T31.88
    90 percent or more T31.90
      with 0-9 percent third degree burns T31.90
      with 10-19 percent third degree burns T31.91
      with 20-29 percent third degree burns T31.92
      with 30-39 percent third degree burns T31.93
      with 40-49 percent third degree burns T31.94
      with 50-59 percent third degree burns T31.95
      with 60-69 percent third degree burns T31.96
      with 70-79 percent third degree burns T31.97
      with 80-89 percent third degree burns T31.98
      with 90 percent or more third degree burns
        T31.99
  extremity — *see* Burn, limb
  eye(s) and adnexa T26.4- ☑
    with resulting rupture and destruction of eyeball
      T26.2- ☑
    conjunctival sac — *see* Burn, cornea
    cornea — *see* Burn, cornea
    lid — *see* Burn, eyelid
    periocular area — *see* Burn, eyelid
    specified site NEC T26.3- ☑
  eyeball — *see* Burn, eye
  eyelid(s) T26.0- ☑
    chemical — *see* Corrosion, eyelid
  face — *see* Burn, head
  finger T23.029 ☑
    first degree T23.129 ☑
    left T23.022 ☑
      first degree T23.122 ☑
      second degree T23.222 ☑
      third degree T23.322 ☑
    multiple sites (without thumb) T23.039 ☑
      with thumb T23.049 ☑
        first degree T23.149 ☑
        left T23.042 ☑
          first degree T23.142 ☑
          second degree T23.242 ☑
          third degree T23.342 ☑
        right T23.041 ☑
          first degree T23.141 ☑
          second degree T23.241 ☑
          third degree T23.341 ☑
      second degree T23.249 ☑
      third degree T23.349 ☑
    first degree T23.139 ☑
    left T23.032 ☑
      first degree T23.132 ☑
      second degree T23.232 ☑
      third degree T23.332 ☑
    right T23.031 ☑
      first degree T23.131 ☑
      second degree T23.231 ☑
      third degree T23.331 ☑
    second degree T23.239 ☑
    third degree T23.339 ☑
    right T23.021 ☑
      first degree T23.121 ☑
      second degree T23.221 ☑
      third degree T23.321 ☑
    second degree T23.229 ☑
    third degree T23.329 ☑
  flank — *see* Burn, abdominal wall
  foot T25.029 ☑
    first degree T25.129 ☑
    left T25.022 ☑
      first degree T25.122 ☑
      second degree T25.222 ☑
      third degree T25.322 ☑
    multiple with ankle — *see* Burn, lower, limb, multi-
      ple, ankle and foot
    right T25.021 ☑
      first degree T25.121 ☑
      second degree T25.221 ☑
      third degree T25.321 ☑
    second degree T25.229 ☑
    third degree T25.329 ☑
  forearm T22.019 ☑
    first degree T22.119 ☑

Burn — *continued*
  forearm — *continued*
    left T22.012 ☑
      first degree T22.112 ☑
      second degree T22.212 ☑
      third degree T22.312 ☑
    right T22.011 ☑
      first degree T22.111 ☑
      second degree T22.211 ☑
      third degree T22.311 ☑
    second degree T22.219 ☑
    third degree T22.319 ☑
  forehead T20.06 ☑
    first degree T20.16 ☑
    second degree T20.26 ☑
    third degree T20.36 ☑
  fourth degree — *code as* Burn, third degree, by site
  friction — *see* Burn, by site
  from swallowing caustic or corrosive substance NEC
    — *see* Corrosion, by site
  full thickness skin loss — *code as* Burn, third degree,
    by site
  gastrointestinal tract NEC T28.2 ☑
    from swallowing caustic or corrosive substance
      T28.7 ☑
  genital organs
    external
      female T21.07 ☑
        first degree T21.17 ☑
        second degree T21.27 ☑
        third degree T21.37 ☑
      male T21.06 ☑
        first degree T21.16 ☑
        second degree T21.26 ☑
        third degree T21.36 ☑
    internal T28.3 ☑
      from caustic or corrosive substance T28.8 ☑
  groin — *see* Burn, abdominal wall
  hand(s) T23.009 ☑
    back — *see* Burn, dorsum of hand
    finger — *see* Burn, finger
    first degree T23.109 ☑
    left T23.002 ☑
      first degree T23.102 ☑
      second degree T23.202 ☑
      third degree T23.302 ☑
    multiple sites with wrist T23.099 ☑
      first degree T23.199 ☑
      left T23.092 ☑
        first degree T23.192 ☑
        second degree T23.292 ☑
        third degree T23.392 ☑
      right T23.091 ☑
        first degree T23.191 ☑
        second degree T23.291 ☑
        third degree T23.391 ☑
      second degree T23.299 ☑
      third degree T23.399 ☑
    palm — *see* Burn, palm
    right T23.001 ☑
      first degree T23.101 ☑
      second degree T23.201 ☑
      third degree T23.301 ☑
    second degree T23.209 ☑
    third degree T23.309 ☑
    thumb — *see* Burn, thumb
  head (and face) (and neck) T20.00 ☑
    cheek — *see* Burn, cheek
    chin — *see* Burn, chin
    ear — *see* Burn, ear
    eye(s) only — *see* Burn, eye
    first degree T20.10 ☑
    forehead — *see* Burn, forehead
    lip — *see* Burn, lip
    multiple sites T20.09 ☑
      first degree T20.19 ☑
      second degree T20.29 ☑
      third degree T20.39 ☑
    neck — *see* Burn, neck
    nose — *see* Burn, nose
    scalp — *see* Burn, scalp
    second degree T20.20 ☑
    third degree T20.30 ☑
  hip(s) — *see* Burn, thigh
  inhalation — *see* Burn, respiratory tract

Burn — *continued*
  inhalation — *see* Burn, respiratory tract — *contin-*
    ued
    caustic or corrosive substance (fumes) — *see* Corro-
      sion, respiratory tract
  internal organ(s) T28.40 ☑
    alimentary tract T28.2 ☑
      esophagus T28.1 ☑
    eardrum T28.41 ☑
    esophagus T28.1 ☑
    from caustic or corrosive substance (swallowing)
      NEC — *see* Corrosion, by site
    genitourinary T28.3 ☑
    mouth T28.0 ☑
    pharynx T28.0 ☑
    respiratory tract — *see* Burn, respiratory tract
    specified organ NEC T28.49 ☑
  interscapular region — *see* Burn, back, upper
  intestine (large) (small) T28.2 ☑
  knee T24.029 ☑
    first degree T24.129 ☑
    left T24.022 ☑
      first degree T24.122 ☑
      second degree T24.222 ☑
      third degree T24.322 ☑
    right T24.021 ☑
      first degree T24.121 ☑
      second degree T24.221 ☑
      third degree T24.321 ☑
    second degree T24.229 ☑
    third degree T24.329 ☑
  labium (majus) (minus) — *see* Burn, genital organs,
    external, female
  lacrimal apparatus, duct, gland or sac — *see* Burn, eye,
    specified site NEC
  larynx T27.0 ☑
    with lung T27.1 ☑
  leg(s) (lower) (upper) — *see* Burn, lower, limb
  lightning — *see* Burn, by site
  limb(s)
    lower (except ankle or foot alone) — *see* Burn,
      lower, limb
    upper — *see* Burn, upper limb
  lip(s) T20.02 ☑
    first degree T20.12 ☑
    second degree T20.22 ☑
    third degree T20.32 ☑
  lower
    back — *see* Burn, back
    limb T24.009 ☑
      ankle — *see* Burn, ankle
      calf — *see* Burn, calf
      first degree T24.109 ☑
      foot — *see* Burn, foot
      hip — *see* Burn, thigh
      knee — *see* Burn, knee
      left T24.002 ☑
        first degree T24.102 ☑
        second degree T24.202 ☑
        third degree T24.302 ☑
      multiple sites, except ankle and foot T24.099 ☑
        ankle and foot T25.099 ☑
          first degree T25.199 ☑
          left T25.092 ☑
            first degree T25.192 ☑
            second degree T25.292 ☑
            third degree T25.392 ☑
          right T25.091 ☑
            first degree T25.191 ☑
            second degree T25.291 ☑
            third degree T25.391 ☑
          second degree T25.299 ☑
          third degree T25.399 ☑
        first degree T24.199 ☑
        left T24.092 ☑
          first degree T24.192 ☑
          second degree T24.292 ☑
          third degree T24.392 ☑
        right T24.091 ☑
          first degree T24.191 ☑
          second degree T24.291 ☑
          third degree T24.391 ☑
        second degree T24.299 ☑
        third degree T24.399 ☑
      right T24.001 ☑
        first degree T24.101 ☑

☑ **Additional Character Required** — **Refer to the Tabular List for Character Selection**   ▽ **Subterms under main terms may continue to next column or page**

Burn — *continued*
 lower — *continued*
  limb — *continued*
   right — *continued*
    second degree T24.201 ☑
     third degree T24.301 ☑
   second degree T24.209 ☑
   thigh — *see* Burn, thigh
   third degree T24.309 ☑
   toe — *see* Burn, toe
 lung (with larynx and trachea) T27.1 ☑
 mouth T28.0 ☑
 neck T20.07 ☑
  first degree T20.17 ☑
  second degree T20.27 ☑
  third degree T20.37 ☑
 nose (septum) T20.04 ☑
  first degree T20.14 ☑
  second degree T20.24 ☑
  third degree T20.34 ☑
 ocular adnexa — *see* Burn, eye
 orbit region — *see* Burn, eyelid
 palm T23.059 ☑
  first degree T23.159 ☑
  left T23.052 ☑
   first degree T23.152 ☑
   second degree T23.252 ☑
   third degree T23.352 ☑
  right T23.051 ☑
   first degree T23.151 ☑
   second degree T23.251 ☑
   third degree T23.351 ☑
  second degree T23.259 ☑
  third degree T23.359 ☑
 partial thickness — *code as* Burn, degree, by site
 pelvis — *see* Burn, trunk
 penis — *see* Burn, genital organs, external, male
 perineum
  female — *see* Burn, genital organs, external, female
  male — *see* Burn, genital organs, external, male
 periocular area — *see* Burn, eyelid
 pharynx T28.0 ☑
 rectum T28.2 ☑
 respiratory tract T27.3 ☑
  larynx — *see* Burn, larynx
  specified part NEC T27.2 ☑
  trachea — *see* Burn, trachea
 sac, lacrimal — *see* Burn, eye, specified site NEC
 scalp T20.05 ☑
  first degree T20.15 ☑
  second degree T20.25 ☑
  third degree T20.35 ☑
 scapular region T22.069 ☑
  first degree T22.169 ☑
  left T22.062 ☑
   first degree T22.162 ☑
   second degree T22.262 ☑
   third degree T22.362 ☑
  right T22.061 ☑
   first degree T22.161 ☑
   second degree T22.261 ☑
   third degree T22.361 ☑
  second degree T22.269 ☑
  third degree T22.369 ☑
 sclera — *see* Burn, eye, specified site NEC
 scrotum — *see* Burn, genital organs, external, male
 shoulder T22.059 ☑
  first degree T22.159 ☑
  left T22.052 ☑
   first degree T22.152 ☑
   second degree T22.252 ☑
   third degree T22.352 ☑
  right T22.051 ☑
   first degree T22.151 ☑
   second degree T22.251 ☑
   third degree T22.351 ☑
  second degree T22.259 ☑
  third degree T22.359 ☑
 stomach T28.2 ☑
 temple — *see* Burn, head
 testis — *see* Burn, genital organs, external, male
 thigh T24.019 ☑
  first degree T24.119 ☑
  left T24.012 ☑
   first degree T24.112 ☑
   second degree T24.212 ☑

Burn — *continued*
 thigh — *continued*
  left — *continued*
   third degree T24.312 ☑
  right T24.011 ☑
   first degree T24.111 ☑
   second degree T24.211 ☑
   third degree T24.311 ☑
  second degree T24.219 ☑
  third degree T24.319 ☑
 thorax (external) — *see* Burn, trunk
 throat (meaning pharynx) T28.0 ☑
 thumb(s) T23.019 ☑
  first degree T23.119 ☑
  left T23.012 ☑
   first degree T23.112 ☑
   second degree T23.212 ☑
   third degree T23.312 ☑
  multiple sites with fingers T23.049 ☑
   first degree T23.149 ☑
   left T23.042 ☑
    first degree T23.142 ☑
    second degree T23.242 ☑
    third degree T23.342 ☑
   right T23.041 ☑
    first degree T23.141 ☑
    second degree T23.241 ☑
    third degree T23.341 ☑
   second degree T23.249 ☑
   third degree T23.349 ☑
  right T23.011 ☑
   first degree T23.111 ☑
   second degree T23.211 ☑
   third degree T23.311 ☑
  second degree T23.219 ☑
  third degree T23.319 ☑
 toe T25.039 ☑
  first degree T25.139 ☑
  left T25.032 ☑
   first degree T25.132 ☑
   second degree T25.232 ☑
   third degree T25.332 ☑
  right T25.031 ☑
   first degree T25.131 ☑
   second degree T25.231 ☑
   third degree T25.331 ☑
  second degree T25.239 ☑
  third degree T25.339 ☑
 tongue T28.0 ☑
 tonsil(s) T28.0 ☑
 trachea T27.0 ☑
  with lung T27.1 ☑
 trunk T21.00 ☑
  abdominal wall — *see* Burn, abdominal wall
  anus — *see* Burn, buttock
  axilla — *see* Burn, upper limb
  back — *see* Burn, back
  breast — *see* Burn, chest wall
  buttock — *see* Burn, buttock
  chest wall — *see* Burn, chest wall
  first degree T21.10 ☑
  flank — *see* Burn, abdominal wall
  genital
   female — *see* Burn, genital organs, external, female
   male — *see* Burn, genital organs, external, male
  groin — *see* Burn, abdominal wall
  interscapular region — *see* Burn, back, upper
  labia — *see* Burn, genital organs, external, female
  lower back — *see* Burn, back
  penis — *see* Burn, genital organs, external, male
  perineum
   female — *see* Burn, genital organs, external, female
   male — *see* Burn, genital organs, external, male
  scapula region — *see* Burn, scapular region
  scrotum — *see* Burn, genital organs, external, male
  second degree T21.20 ☑
  specified site NEC T21.09 ☑
   first degree T21.19 ☑
   second degree T21.29 ☑
   third degree T21.39 ☑
  testes — *see* Burn, genital organs, external, male
  third degree T21.30 ☑
  upper back — *see* Burn, back, upper
  vulva — *see* Burn, genital organs, external, female

Burn — *continued*
 unspecified site with extent of body surface involved specified
  less than 10 percent T31.0
  10-19 percent (0-9 percent third degree) T31.10
   with 10-19 percent third degree T31.11
  20-29 percent (0-9 percent third degree) T31.20
   with
    10-19 percent third degree T31.21
    20-29 percent third degree T31.22
  30-39 percent (0-9 percent third degree) T31.30
   with
    10-19 percent third degree T31.31
    20-29 percent third degree T31.32
    30-39 percent third degree T31.33
  40-49 percent (0-9 percent third degree) T31.40
   with
    10-19 percent third degree T31.41
    20-29 percent third degree T31.42
    30-39 percent third degree T31.43
    40-49 percent third degree T31.44
  50-59 percent (0-9 percent third degree) T31.50
   with
    10-19 percent third degree T31.51
    20-29 percent third degree T31.52
    30-39 percent third degree T31.53
    40-49 percent third degree T31.54
    50-59 percent third degree T31.55
  60-69 percent (0-9 percent third degree) T31.60
   with
    10-19 percent third degree T31.61
    20-29 percent third degree T31.62
    30-39 percent third degree T31.63
    40-49 percent third degree T31.64
    50-59 percent third degree T31.65
    60-69 percent third degree T31.66
  70-79 percent (0-9 percent third degree) T31.70
   with
    10-19 percent third degree T31.71
    20-29 percent third degree T31.72
    30-39 percent third degree T31.73
    40-49 percent third degree T31.74
    50-59 percent third degree T31.75
    60-69 percent third degree T31.76
    70-79 percent third degree T31.77
  80-89 percent (0-9 percent third degree) T31.80
   with
    10-19 percent third degree T31.81
    20-29 percent third degree T31.82
    30-39 percent third degree T31.83
    40-49 percent third degree T31.84
    50-59 percent third degree T31.85
    60-69 percent third degree T31.86
    70-79 percent third degree T31.87
    80-89 percent third degree T31.88
  90 percent or more (0-9 percent third degree) T31.90
   with
    10-19 percent third degree T31.91
    20-29 percent third degree T31.92
    30-39 percent third degree T31.93
    40-49 percent third degree T31.94
    50-59 percent third degree T31.95
    60-69 percent third degree T31.96
    70-79 percent third degree T31.97
    80-89 percent third degree T31.98
    90-99 percent third degree T31.99
 upper limb T22.00 ☑
  above elbow — *see* Burn, above elbow
  axilla — *see* Burn, axilla
  elbow — *see* Burn, elbow
  first degree T22.10 ☑
  forearm — *see* Burn, forearm
  hand — *see* Burn, hand
  interscapular region — *see* Burn, back, upper
  multiple sites T22.099 ☑
   first degree T22.199 ☑
   left T22.092 ☑
    first degree T22.192 ☑
    second degree T22.292 ☑
    third degree T22.392 ☑
   right T22.091 ☑
    first degree T22.191 ☑
    second degree T22.291 ☑
    third degree T22.391 ☑
   second degree T22.299 ☑
   third degree T22.399 ☑
  scapular region — *see* Burn, scapular region
  second degree T22.20 ☑

⛛ Subterms under main terms may continue to next column or page   ☑ Additional Character Required — Refer to the Tabular List for Character Selection   45

Burn — Burn

Burn — *continued*
upper limb — *continued*
shoulder — *see* Burn, shoulder
third degree T22.30 ☑
wrist — *see* Burn, wrist
uterus T28.3 ☑
vagina T28.3 ☑
vulva — *see* Burn, genital organs, external, female
wrist T23.079 ☑
first degree T23.179 ☑
left T23.072 ☑
first degree T23.172 ☑
second degree T23.272 ☑
third degree T23.372 ☑
multiple sites with hand T23.099 ☑
first degree T23.199 ☑
left T23.092 ☑
first degree T23.192 ☑
second degree T23.292 ☑
third degree T23.392 ☑
right T23.091 ☑
first degree T23.191 ☑
second degree T23.291 ☑
third degree T23.391 ☑
second degree T23.299 ☑
third degree T23.399 ☑
right T23.071 ☑
first degree T23.171 ☑
second degree T23.271 ☑
third degree T23.371 ☑
second degree T23.279 ☑
third degree T23.379 ☑
Burnett's syndrome E83.52
Burning
feet syndrome E53.9
sensation R20.8
tongue K14.6
Burn-out (state) Z73.0
Burns' disease or osteochondrosis — *see* Osteochondrosis, juvenile, ulna
Bursa — *see* condition
Bursitis M71.9
Achilles — *see* Tendinitis, Achilles
adhesive — *see* Bursitis, specified NEC
ankle — *see* Enthesopathy, lower limb, ankle, specified type NEC
calcaneal — *see* Enthesopathy, foot, specified type NEC
collateral ligament, tibial — *see* Bursitis, tibial collateral
due to use, overuse, pressure — *see also* Disorder, soft tissue, due to use, specified type NEC
specified NEC — *see* Disorder, soft tissue, due to use, specified NEC
Duplay's M75.0 ☑
elbow NEC M70.3- ☑
olecranon M70.2- ☑
finger — *see* Disorder, soft tissue, due to use, specified type NEC, hand
foot — *see* Enthesopathy, foot, specified type NEC
gonococcal A54.49
gouty — *see* Gout
hand M70.1- ☑
hip NEC M70.7- ☑
trochanteric M70.6- ☑
infective NEC M71.10
abscess — *see* Abscess, bursa
ankle M71.17- ☑
elbow M71.12- ☑
foot M71.17- ☑
hand M71.14- ☑
hip M71.15- ☑
knee M71.16- ☑
multiple sites M71.19
shoulder M71.11- ☑
specified site NEC M71.18
wrist M71.13- ☑
ischial — *see* Bursitis, hip
knee NEC M70.5- ☑
prepatellar M70.4- ☑
occupational NEC — *see also* Disorder, soft tissue, due to, use
olecranon — *see* Bursitis, elbow, olecranon
pharyngeal J39.1
popliteal — *see* Bursitis, knee
prepatellar M70.4- ☑
radiohumeral M77.8
rheumatoid M06.20

Bursitis — *continued*
rheumatoid — *continued*
ankle M06.27- ☑
elbow M06.22- ☑
foot joint M06.27- ☑
hand joint M06.24- ☑
hip M06.25- ☑
knee M06.26- ☑
multiple site M06.29
shoulder M06.21- ☑
vertebra M06.28
wrist M06.23- ☑
scapulohumeral — *see* Bursitis, shoulder
semimembranous muscle (knee) — *see* Bursitis, knee
shoulder M75.5- ☑
adhesive — *see* Capsulitis, adhesive
specified NEC M71.50
ankle M71.57- ☑
due to use, overuse or pressure — *see* Disorder, soft tissue, due to, use
elbow M71.52- ☑
foot M71.57- ☑
hand M71.54- ☑
hip M71.55- ☑
knee M71.56- ☑
shoulder — *see* Bursitis, shoulder
specified site NEC M71.58
tibial collateral M76.4- ☑
wrist M71.53- ☑
subacromial — *see* Bursitis, shoulder
subcoracoid — *see* Bursitis, shoulder
subdeltoid — *see* Bursitis, shoulder
syphilitic A52.78
Thornwaldt, Tornwaldt J39.2
tibial collateral M76.4- ☑
toe — *see* Enthesopathy, foot, specified type NEC
trochanteric (area) — *see* Bursitis, hip, trochanteric
wrist — *see* Bursitis, hand
Bursopathy M71.9
specified type NEC M71.80
ankle M71.87- ☑
elbow M71.82- ☑
foot M71.87- ☑
hand M71.84- ☑
hip M71.85- ☑
knee M71.86- ☑
multiple sites M71.89
shoulder M71.81- ☑
specified site NEC M71.88
wrist M71.83- ☑
Burst stitches or sutures (complication of surgery) T81.31 ☑
external operation wound T81.31 ☑
internal operation wound T81.32 ☑
Buruli ulcer A31.1
Bury's disease L95.1
Buschke's
disease B45.3
scleredema — *see* Sclerosis, systemic
Busse-Buschke disease B45.3
Buttock — *see* condition
Button
Biskra B55.1
Delhi B55.1
oriental B55.1
Buttonhole deformity (finger) — *see* Deformity, finger, boutonniere
Bwamba fever A92.8
Byssinosis J66.0
Bywaters' syndrome T79.5 ☑

C

Cachexia R64
cancerous R64
cardiac — *see* Disease, heart
dehydration E86.0
due to malnutrition R64
exophthalmic — *see* Hyperthyroidism
heart — *see* Disease, heart
hypophyseal E23.0
hypopituitary E23.0
lead — *see* Poisoning, lead
malignant R64
marsh — *see* Malaria
nervous F48.8

Cachexia — *continued*
old age R54
paludal — *see* Malaria
pituitary E23.0
renal N28.9
saturnine — *see* Poisoning, lead
senile R54
Simmonds' E23.0
splenica D73.0
strumipriva E03.4
tuberculous NEC — *see* Tuberculosis
CADASIL (cerebral autosomal dominant arteriopathy with subcortical infarcts and leukoencephalopathy) I67.850
Café, au lait spots L81.3
Caffeine-induced
anxiety disorder F15.980
sleep disorder F15.982
Caffey's syndrome Q78.8
Caisson disease T70.3 ☑
Cake kidney Q63.1
Caked breast (puerperal, postpartum) O92.79
Calabar swelling B74.3
Calcaneal spur — *see* Spur, bone, calcaneal
Calcaneo-apophysitis M92.8
Calcareous — *see* condition
Calcicosis J62.8
Calciferol (vitamin D) deficiency E55.9
with rickets E55.0
Calcification
adrenal (capsule) (gland) E27.49
tuberculous E35 [B90.8]
aorta I70.0
artery (annular) — *see* Arteriosclerosis
auricle (ear) — *see* Disorder, pinna, specified type NEC
basal ganglia G23.8
bladder N32.89
due to Schistosoma hematobium B65.0
brain (cortex) — *see* Calcification, cerebral
bronchus J98.09
bursa M71.40
ankle M71.47- ☑
elbow M71.42- ☑
foot M71.47- ☑
hand M71.44- ☑
hip M71.45- ☑
knee M71.46- ☑
multiple sites M71.49
shoulder M75.3- ☑
specified site NEC M71.48
wrist M71.43- ☑
cardiac — *see* Degeneration, myocardial
cerebral (cortex) G93.89
artery I67.2
cervix (uteri) N88.8
choroid plexus G93.89
conjunctiva — *see* Concretion, conjunctiva
corpora cavernosa (penis) N48.89
cortex (brain) — *see* Calcification, cerebral
dental pulp (nodular) K04.2
dentinal papilla K00.4
fallopian tube N83.8
falx cerebri G96.19
gallbladder K82.8
general E83.59
heart — *see also* Degeneration, myocardial
valve — *see* Endocarditis
idiopathic infantile arterial (IIAC) Q28.8
intervertebral cartilage or disc (postinfective) — *see* Disorder, disc, specified NEC
intracranial — *see* Calcification, cerebral
joint — *see* Disorder, joint, specified type NEC
kidney N28.89
tuberculous N29 [B90.1]
larynx (senile) J38.7
lens — *see* Cataract, specified NEC
lung (active) (postinfectional) J98.4
tuberculous B90.9
lymph gland or node (postinfectional) I89.8
tuberculous — *see also* Tuberculosis, lymph gland B90.8
mammographic R92.1
massive (paraplegic) — *see* Myositis, ossificans, in, quadriplegia
medial — *see* Arteriosclerosis, extremities
meninges (cerebral) (spinal) G96.19
metastatic E83.59

Calcification — *continued*
  Mönckeberg's — *see* Arteriosclerosis, extremities
  muscle M61.9
    due to burns — *see* Myositis, ossificans, in, burns
    paralytic — *see* Myositis, ossificans, in, quadriplegia
    specified type NEC M61.40
      ankle M61.47- ☑
      foot M61.47- ☑
      forearm M61.43- ☑
      hand M61.44- ☑
      lower leg M61.46- ☑
      multiple sites M61.49
      pelvic region M61.45- ☑
      shoulder region M61.41- ☑
      specified site NEC M61.48
      thigh M61.45- ☑
      upper arm M61.42- ☑
  myocardium, myocardial — *see* Degeneration, myocardial
  ovary N83.8
  pancreas K86.89
  penis N48.89
  periarticular — *see* Disorder, joint, specified type NEC
  pericardium — *see also* Pericarditis I31.1
  pineal gland E34.8
  pleura J94.8
    postinfectional J94.8
    tuberculous NEC B90.9
  pulpal (dental) (nodular) K04.2
  sclera H15.89
  spleen D73.89
  subcutaneous L94.2
  suprarenal (capsule) (gland) E27.49
  tendon (sheath) — *see also* Tenosynovitis, specified
      type NEC
    with bursitis, synovitis or tenosynovitis — *see* Tendinitis, calcific
  trachea J39.8
  ureter N28.89
  uterus N85.8
  vitreous — *see* Deposit, crystalline
Calcified — *see* Calcification
Calcinosis (interstitial) (tumoral) (universalis) E83.59
  with Raynaud's phenomenon, esophageal dysfunction,
      sclerodactyly, telangiectasia (CREST syndrome)
      M34.1
  circumscripta (skin) L94.2
  cutis L94.2
Calciphylaxis — *see also* Calcification, by site E83.59
Calcium
  deposits — *see* Calcification, by site
  metabolism disorder E83.50
  salts or soaps in vitreous — *see* Deposit, crystalline
Calciuria R82.994
Calculi — *see* Calculus
Calculosis, intrahepatic — *see* Calculus, bile duct
Calculus, calculi, calculous
  ampulla of Vater — *see* Calculus, bile duct
  anuria (impacted) (recurrent) — *see also* Calculus, urinary N20.9
  appendix K38.1
  bile duct (common) (hepatic) K80.50
    with
      calculus of gallbladder — *see* Calculus, gallbladder and bile duct
      cholangitis K80.30
        with
          cholecystitis — *see* Calculus, bile duct, with cholecystitis
          obstruction K80.31
        acute K80.32
          with
            chronic cholangitis K80.36
              with obstruction K80.37
            obstruction K80.33
        chronic K80.34
          with
            acute cholangitis K80.36
              with obstruction K80.37
            obstruction K80.35
      cholecystitis (with cholangitis) K80.40
        with obstruction K80.41
        acute K80.42
          with
            chronic cholecystitis K80.46
              with obstruction K80.47
            obstruction K80.43
        chronic K80.44

Calculus, calculi, calculous — *continued*
  bile duct — *continued*
    with — *continued*
      cholecystitis — *continued*
        chronic — *continued*
          with
            acute cholecystitis K80.46
              with obstruction K80.47
            obstruction K80.45
  biliary — *see also* Calculus, gallbladder
    specified NEC K80.80
      with obstruction K80.81
  bilirubin, multiple — *see* Calculus, gallbladder
  bladder (encysted) (impacted) (urinary) (diverticulum)
      N21.0
  bronchus J98.09
  calyx (kidney) (renal) — *see* Calculus, kidney
  cholesterol (pure) (solitary) — *see* Calculus, gallbladder
  common duct (bile) — *see* Calculus, bile duct
  conjunctiva — *see* Concretion, conjunctiva
  cystic N21.0
    duct — *see* Calculus, gallbladder
  dental (subgingival) (supragingival) K03.6
  diverticulum
    bladder N21.0
    kidney N20.0
  epididymis N50.89
  gallbladder K80.20
    with
      bile duct calculus — *see* Calculus, gallbladder
        and bile duct
      cholecystitis K80.10
        with obstruction K80.11
        acute K80.00
          with
            chronic cholecystitis K80.12
              with obstruction K80.13
            obstruction K80.01
        chronic K80.10
          with
            acute cholecystitis K80.12
              with obstruction K80.13
            obstruction K80.11
      specified NEC K80.18
        with obstruction K80.19
    obstruction K80.21
  gallbladder and bile duct K80.70
    with
      cholecystitis K80.60
        with obstruction K80.61
        acute K80.62
          with
            chronic cholecystitis K80.66
              with obstruction K80.67
            obstruction K80.63
        chronic K80.64
          with
            acute cholecystitis K80.66
              with obstruction K80.67
            obstruction K80.65
    obstruction K80.71
  hepatic (duct) — *see* Calculus, bile duct
  ileal conduit N21.8
  intestinal (impaction) (obstruction) K56.49
  kidney (impacted) (multiple) (pelvis) (recurrent)
      (staghorn) N20.0
    with calculus, ureter N20.2
    congenital Q63.8
  lacrimal passages — *see* Dacryolith
  liver (impacted) — *see* Calculus, bile duct
  lung J98.4
  mammographic R92.1
  nephritic (impacted) (recurrent) — *see* Calculus, kidney
  nose J34.89
  pancreas (duct) K86.89
  parotid duct or gland K11.5
  pelvis, encysted — *see* Calculus, kidney
  prostate N42.0
  pulmonary J98.4
  pyelitis (impacted) (recurrent) N20.0
    with hydronephrosis N13.6
  pyelonephritis (impacted) (recurrent) — *see* category
      N20 ☑
    with hydronephrosis N13.6
  renal (impacted) (recurrent) — *see* Calculus, kidney
  salivary (duct) (gland) K11.5
  seminal vesicle N50.89
  staghorn — *see* Calculus, kidney

Calculus, calculi, calculous — *continued*
  Stensen's duct K11.5
  stomach K31.89
  sublingual duct or gland K11.5
    congenital Q38.4
  submandibular duct, gland or region K11.5
  submaxillary duct, gland or region K11.5
  suburethral N21.8
  tonsil J35.8
  tooth, teeth (subgingival) (supragingival) K03.6
  tunica vaginalis N50.89
  ureter (impacted) (recurrent) N20.1
    with calculus, kidney N20.2
      with hydronephrosis N13.2
        with infection N13.6
  urethra (impacted) N21.1
  urinary (duct) (impacted) (passage) (tract) N20.9
    with hydronephrosis N13.2
      with infection N13.6
    in (due to)
      lower N21.9
        specified NEC N21.8
  vagina N89.8
  vesical (impacted) N21.0
  Wharton's duct K11.5
  xanthine E79.8 *[N22]*
Calicectasis N28.89
Caliectasis N28.89
California
  disease B38.9
  encephalitis A83.5
Caligo cornea — *see* Opacity, cornea, central
Callositas, callosity (infected) L84
Callus (infected) L84
  bone — *see* Osteophyte
    excessive, following fracture — *code as* Sequelae
      of fracture
CALME (childhood asymmetric labium majus enlargement) N90.61
Calorie deficiency or malnutrition — *see also* Malnutrition E46
Calvé-Perthes disease — *see* Legg-Calvé-Perthes disease
Calvé's disease — *see* Osteochondrosis, juvenile, spine
Calvities — *see* Alopecia, androgenic
Cameroon fever — *see* Malaria
Camptocormia (hysterical) F44.4
Camurati-Engelmann syndrome Q78.3
Canal — *see also* condition
  atrioventricular common Q21.2
Canaliculitis (lacrimal) (acute) (subacute) H04.33- ☑
  Actinomyces A42.89
  chronic H04.42- ☑
Canavan's disease E75.29
Canceled procedure (surgical) Z53.9
  because of
    contraindication Z53.09
      smoking Z53.01
    left against medical advice (AMA) Z53.29
    patient's decision Z53.20
      for reasons of belief or group pressure Z53.1
      specified reason NEC Z53.29
    specified reason NEC Z53.8
Cancer — *see also* Neoplasm, by site, malignant
  bile duct type liver C22.1
  blood — *see* Leukemia
  breast — *see also* Neoplasm, breast, malignant
      C50.91- ☑
  hepatocellular C22.0
  lung — *see also* Neoplasm, lung, malignant C34.90
  ovarian — *see also* Neoplasm ovary, malignant C56.9
  unspecified site (primary) C80.1
Cancer (o)**phobia** F45.29
Cancerous — *see* Neoplasm, malignant, by site
Cancrum oris A69.0
Candidiasis, candidal B37.9
  balanitis B37.42
  bronchitis B37.1
  cheilitis B37.83
  congenital P37.5
  cystitis B37.41
  disseminated B37.7
  endocarditis B37.6
  enteritis B37.82
  esophagitis B37.81
  intertrigo B37.2
  lung B37.1
  meningitis B37.5

Candidiasis, candidal — *continued*
- mouth B37.0
- nails B37.2
- neonatal P37.5
- onychia B37.2
- oral B37.0
- osteomyelitis B37.89
- otitis externa B37.84
- paronychia B37.2
- perionyxis B37.2
- pneumonia B37.1
- proctitis B37.82
- pulmonary B37.1
- pyelonephritis B37.49
- sepsis B37.7
- skin B37.2
- specified site NEC B37.89
- stomatitis B37.0
- systemic B37.7
- urethritis B37.41
- urogenital site NEC B37.49
- vagina B37.3
- vulva B37.3
- vulvovaginitis B37.3

Candidid L30.2
Candidosis — *see* Candidiasis
Candiru infection or infestation B88.8
Canities (premature) L67.1
- congenital Q84.2

Canker (mouth) (sore) K12.0
- rash A38.9

Cannabinosis J66.2
Cannabis induced
- anxiety disorder F12.980
- psychotic disorder F12.959
- sleep disorder F12.988

Canton fever A75.9
Cantrell's syndrome Q87.89
Capillariasis (intestinal) B81.1
- hepatic B83.8

Capillary — *see* condition
Caplan's syndrome — *see* Rheumatoid, lung
Capsule — *see* condition
Capsulitis (joint) — *see also* Enthesopathy
- adhesive (shoulder) M75.0- ☑
- hepatic K65.8
- labyrinthine — *see* Otosclerosis, specified NEC
- thyroid E06.9

Caput
- crepitus Q75.8
- medusae I86.8
- succedaneum P12.81

Car sickness T75.3 ☑
Carapata (disease) A68.0
Carate — *see* Pinta
Carbon lung J60
Carbuncle L02.93
- abdominal wall L02.231
- anus K61.0
- auditory canal, external — *see* Abscess, ear, external
- auricle ear — *see* Abscess, ear, external
- axilla L02.43- ☑
- back (any part) L02.232
- breast N61.1
- buttock L02.33
- cheek (external) L02.03
- chest wall L02.233
- chin L02.03
- corpus cavernosum N48.21
- ear (any part) (external) (middle) — *see* Abscess, ear, external
- external auditory canal — *see* Abscess, ear, external
- eyelid — *see* Abscess, eyelid
- face NEC L02.03
- femoral (region) — *see* Carbuncle, lower limb
- finger — *see* Carbuncle, hand
- flank L02.231
- foot L02.63- ☑
- forehead L02.03
- genital — *see* Abscess, genital
- gluteal (region) L02.33
- groin L02.234
- hand L02.53- ☑
- head NEC L02.831
- heel — *see* Carbuncle, foot
- hip — *see* Carbuncle, lower limb
- kidney — *see* Abscess, kidney

Carbuncle — *continued*
- knee — *see* Carbuncle, lower limb
- labium (majus) (minus) N76.4
- lacrimal
  - gland — *see* Dacryoadenitis
  - passages (duct) (sac) — *see* Inflammation, lacrimal, passages, acute
- leg — *see* Carbuncle, lower limb
- lower limb L02.43- ☑
- malignant A22.0
- navel L02.236
- neck L02.13
- nose (external) (septum) J34.0
- orbit, orbital — *see* Abscess, orbit
- palmar (space) — *see* Carbuncle, hand
- partes posteriores L02.33
- pectoral region L02.233
- penis N48.21
- perineum L02.235
- pinna — *see* Abscess, ear, external
- popliteal — *see* Carbuncle, lower limb
- scalp L02.831
- seminal vesicle N49.0
- shoulder — *see* Carbuncle, upper limb
- specified site NEC L02.838
- temple (region) L02.03
- thumb — *see* Carbuncle, hand
- toe — *see* Carbuncle, foot
- trunk L02.239
  - abdominal wall L02.231
  - back L02.232
  - chest wall L02.233
  - groin L02.234
  - perineum L02.235
  - umbilicus L02.236
- umbilicus L02.236
- upper limb L02.43- ☑
- urethra N34.0
- vulva N76.4

Carbunculus — *see* Carbuncle
Carcinoid (tumor) — *see* Tumor, carcinoid
Carcinoidosis E34.0
Carcinoma (malignant) — *see also* Neoplasm, by site, malignant
- acidophil
  - specified site — *see* Neoplasm, malignant, by site
  - unspecified site C75.1
- acidophil-basophil, mixed
  - specified site — *see* Neoplasm, malignant, by site
  - unspecified site C75.1
- adnexal (skin) — *see* Neoplasm, skin, malignant
- adrenal cortical C74.0- ☑
- alveolar — *see* Neoplasm, lung, malignant
  - cell — *see* Neoplasm, lung, malignant
- ameloblastic C41.1
  - upper jaw (bone) C41.0
- apocrine
  - breast — *see* Neoplasm, breast, malignant
  - specified site NEC — *see* Neoplasm, skin, malignant
  - unspecified site C44.99
- basal cell (pigmented) (*see also* Neoplasm, skin, malignant) C44.91
  - fibro-epithelial — *see* Neoplasm, skin, malignant
  - morphea — *see* Neoplasm, skin, malignant
  - multicentric — *see* Neoplasm, skin, malignant
- basaloid
- basal-squamous cell, mixed — *see* Neoplasm, skin, malignant
- basophil
  - specified site — *see* Neoplasm, malignant, by site
  - unspecified site C75.1
- basophil-acidophil, mixed
  - specified site — *see* Neoplasm, malignant, by site
  - unspecified site C75.1
- basosquamous — *see* Neoplasm, skin, malignant
- bile duct
  - with hepatocellular, mixed C22.0
  - liver C22.1
  - specified site NEC — *see* Neoplasm, malignant, by site
  - unspecified site C22.1
- branchial or branchiogenic C10.4
- bronchial or bronchogenic — *see* Neoplasm, lung, malignant
- bronchiolar — *see* Neoplasm, lung, malignant
- bronchioloalveolar — *see* Neoplasm, lung, malignant

Carcinoma — *continued*
- C cell
  - specified site — *see* Neoplasm, malignant, by site
  - unspecified site C73
- ceruminous C44.29- ☑
- cervix uteri
  - in situ D06.9
    - endocervix D06.0
    - exocervix D06.1
    - specified site NEC D06.7
- chorionic
  - specified site — *see* Neoplasm, malignant, by site
  - unspecified site
    - female C58
    - male C62.90
- chromophobe
  - specified site — *see* Neoplasm, malignant, by site
  - unspecified site C75.1
- cloacogenic
  - specified site — *see* Neoplasm, malignant, by site
  - unspecified site C21.2
- diffuse type
  - specified site — *see* Neoplasm, malignant, by site
  - unspecified site C16.9
- duct (cell)
  - with Paget's disease — *see* Neoplasm, breast, malignant
  - infiltrating
    - with lobular carcinoma (in situ)
      - specified site — *see* Neoplasm, malignant, by site
      - unspecified site (female) C50.91- ☑
        - male C50.92- ☑
    - specified site — *see* Neoplasm, malignant, by site
    - unspecified site (female) C50.91- ☑
      - male C50.92- ☑
- ductal
  - with lobular
    - specified site — *see* Neoplasm, malignant, by site
    - unspecified site (female) C50.91- ☑
      - male C50.92- ☑
- ductular, infiltrating
  - specified site — *see* Neoplasm, malignant, by site
  - unspecified site (female) C50.91- ☑
    - male C50.92- ☑
- embryonal
  - liver C22.7
- endometrioid
  - specified site — *see* Neoplasm, malignant, by site
  - unspecified site
    - female C56.9
    - male C61
- eosinophil
  - specified site — *see* Neoplasm, malignant, by site
  - unspecified site C75.1
- epidermoid — *see also* Neoplasm, skin, malignant
  - in situ, Bowen's type — *see* Neoplasm, skin, in situ
- fibroepithelial, basal cell — *see* Neoplasm, skin, malignant
- follicular
  - with papillary (mixed) C73
  - moderately differentiated C73
  - pure follicle C73
  - specified site — *see* Neoplasm, malignant, by site
  - trabecular C73
  - unspecified site C73
  - well differentiated C73
- generalized, with unspecified primary site C80.0
- glycogen-rich — *see* Neoplasm, breast, malignant
- granulosa cell C56- ☑
- hepatic cell C22.0
- hepatocellular C22.0
  - with bile duct, mixed C22.0
  - fibrolamellar C22.0
- hepatocholangiolitic C22.0
- Hurthle cell C73
- in
  - adenomatous
    - polyposis coli C18.9
  - pleomorphic adenoma — *see* Neoplasm, salivary glands, malignant
  - situ — *see* Carcinoma-in-situ

Carcinoma — *continued*
- infiltrating
  - duct
    - with lobular
      - specified site — *see* Neoplasm, malignant, by site
      - unspecified site (female) C50.91- ☑
        - male C50.92- ☑
    - with Paget's disease — *see* Neoplasm, breast, malignant
    - specified site — *see* Neoplasm, malignant
    - unspecified site (female) C50.91- ☑
      - male C50.92- ☑
  - ductular
    - specified site — *see* Neoplasm, malignant
    - unspecified site (female) C50.91- ☑
      - male C50.92- ☑
  - lobular
    - specified site — *see* Neoplasm, malignant
    - unspecified site (female) C50.91- ☑
      - male C50.92- ☑
- inflammatory
  - specified site — *see* Neoplasm, malignant
  - unspecified site (female) C50.91- ☑
    - male C50.92- ☑
- intestinal type
  - specified site — *see* Neoplasm, malignant, by site
  - unspecified site C16.9
- intracystic
  - noninfiltrating — *see* Neoplasm, in situ, by site
- intraductal (noninfiltrating)
  - with Paget's disease — *see* Neoplasm, breast, malignant
  - breast D05.1- ☑
  - papillary
    - with invasion
      - specified site — *see* Neoplasm, malignant, by site
      - unspecified site (female) C50.91- ☑
        - male C50.92- ☑
    - breast D05.1- ☑
    - specified site NEC — *see* Neoplasm, in situ, by site
    - unspecified site (female) D05.1- ☑
  - specified site NEC — *see* Neoplasm, in situ, by site
  - unspecified site (female) D05.1- ☑
- intraepidermal — *see* Neoplasm, in situ
  - squamous cell, Bowen's type — *see* Neoplasm, skin, in situ
- intraepithelial — *see* Neoplasm, in situ, by site
  - squamous cell — *see* Neoplasm, in situ, by site
- intraosseous C41.1
  - upper jaw (bone) C41.0
- islet cell
  - with exocrine, mixed
    - specified site — *see* Neoplasm, malignant, by site
    - unspecified site C25.9
  - pancreas C25.4
  - specified site NEC — *see* Neoplasm, malignant, by site
  - unspecified site C25.4
- juvenile, breast — *see* Neoplasm, breast, malignant
- large cell
  - small cell
    - specified site — *see* Neoplasm, malignant, by site
    - unspecified site C34.90
- Leydig cell (testis)
  - specified site — *see* Neoplasm, malignant, by site
  - unspecified site
    - female C56.9
    - male C62.90
- lipid-rich (female) C50.91- ☑
  - male C50.92- ☑
- liver cell C22.0
- liver NEC C22.7
- lobular (infiltrating)
  - with intraductal
    - specified site — *see* Neoplasm, malignant, by site
    - unspecified site (female) C50.91- ☑
      - male C50.92- ☑
  - noninfiltrating
    - breast D05.0- ☑
    - specified site NEC — *see* Neoplasm, in situ, by site

Carcinoma — *continued*
- lobular — *continued*
  - noninfiltrating — *continued*
    - unspecified site D05.0- ☑
  - specified site — *see* Neoplasm, malignant, by site
  - unspecified site (female) C50.91- ☑
    - male C50.92- ☑
- medullary
  - with
    - amyloid stroma
      - specified site — *see* Neoplasm, malignant, by site
      - unspecified site C73
    - lymphoid stroma
      - specified site — *see* Neoplasm, malignant, by site
      - unspecified site (female) C50.91- ☑
        - male C50.92- ☑
- Merkel cell C4A.9 (*following* C43)
  - anal margin C4A.51 (*following* C43)
  - anal skin C4A.51 (*following* C43)
  - canthus C4A.1- ☑ (*following* C43)
  - ear and external auricular canal C4A.2- ☑ (*following* C43)
  - external auricular canal C4A.2- ☑ (*following* C43)
  - eyelid, including canthus C4A.1- ☑ (*following* C43)
  - face C4A.30 (*following* C43)
    - specified NEC C4A.39 (*following* C43)
  - hip C4A.7- ☑ (*following* C43)
  - lip C4A.0 (*following* C43)
  - lower limb, including hip C4A.7- ☑ (*following* C43)
  - neck C4A.4 (*following* C43)
  - nodal presentation C7B.1 (*following* C75)
  - nose C4A.31 (*following* C43)
  - overlapping sites C4A.8 (*following* C43)
  - perianal skin C4A.51 (*following* C43)
  - scalp C4A.4 (*following* C43)
  - secondary C7B.1 (*following* C75)
  - shoulder C4A.6- ☑ (*following* C43)
  - skin of breast C4A.52 (*following* C43)
  - trunk NEC C4A.59 (*following* C43)
  - upper limb, including shoulder C4A.6- ☑ (*following* C43)
  - visceral metastatic C7B.1 (*following* C75)
- metastatic — *see* Neoplasm, secondary, by site
- metatypical — *see* Neoplasm, skin, malignant
- morphea, basal cell — *see* Neoplasm, skin, malignant
- mucoid
  - cell
    - specified site — *see* Neoplasm, malignant, by site
    - unspecified site C75.1
- neuroendocrine — *see also* Tumor, neuroendocrine
  - high grade, any site C7A.1 (*following* C75)
  - poorly differentiated, any site C7A.1 (*following* C75)
- nonencapsulated sclerosing C73
- noninfiltrating
  - intracystic — *see* Neoplasm, in situ, by site
  - intraductal
    - breast D05.1- ☑
    - papillary
      - breast D05.1- ☑
      - specified site NEC — *see* Neoplasm, in situ, by site
      - unspecified site D05.1- ☑
    - specified site — *see* Neoplasm, in situ, by site
    - unspecified site D05.1- ☑
  - lobular
    - breast D05.0- ☑
    - specified site NEC — *see* Neoplasm, in situ, by site
    - unspecified site (female) D05.0- ☑
- oat cell
  - specified site — *see* Neoplasm, malignant, by site
  - unspecified site C34.90
- odontogenic C41.1
  - upper jaw (bone) C41.0
- papillary
  - with follicular (mixed) C73
  - follicular variant C73
  - intraductal (noninfiltrating)
    - with invasion
      - specified site — *see* Neoplasm, malignant, by site
      - unspecified site (female) C50.91- ☑
        - male C50.92- ☑
    - breast D05.1- ☑

Carcinoma — *continued*
- papillary — *continued*
  - intraductal — *continued*
    - specified site NEC — *see* Neoplasm, in situ, by site
    - unspecified site D05.1- ☑
  - serous
    - specified site — *see* Neoplasm, malignant, by site
    - surface
      - specified site — *see* Neoplasm, malignant, by site
      - unspecified site C56.9
    - unspecified site C56.9
- papillocystic
  - specified site — *see* Neoplasm, malignant, by site
  - unspecified site C56.9
- parafollicular cell
  - specified site — *see* Neoplasm, malignant, by site
  - unspecified site C73
- pilomatrix — *see* Neoplasm, skin, malignant
- pseudomucinous
  - specified site — *see* Neoplasm, malignant, by site
  - unspecified site C56.9
- renal cell C64- ☑
- Schmincke — *see* Neoplasm, nasopharynx, malignant
- Schneiderian
  - specified site — *see* Neoplasm, malignant, by site
  - unspecified site C30.0
- sebaceous — *see* Neoplasm, skin, malignant
- secondary — *see also* Neoplasm, secondary, by site
  - Merkel cell C7B.1 (*following* C75)
- secretory, breast — *see* Neoplasm, breast, malignant
- serous
  - papillary
    - specified site — *see* Neoplasm, malignant, by site
    - unspecified site C56.9
  - surface, papillary
    - specified site — *see* Neoplasm, malignant, by site
    - unspecified site C56.9
- Sertoli cell
  - specified site — *see* Neoplasm, malignant, by site
  - unspecified site C62.90
    - female C56.9
    - male C62.90
- skin appendage — *see* Neoplasm, skin, malignant
- small cell
  - fusiform cell
    - specified site — *see* Neoplasm, malignant, by site
    - unspecified site C34.90
  - intermediate cell
    - specified site — *see* Neoplasm, malignant, by site
    - unspecified site C34.90
  - large cell
    - specified site — *see* Neoplasm, malignant, by site
    - unspecified site C34.90
- solid
  - with amyloid stroma
    - specified site — *see* Neoplasm, malignant, by site
    - unspecified site C73
  - microinvasive
    - specified site — *see* Neoplasm, malignant, by site
    - unspecified site C53.9
- sweat gland — *see* Neoplasm, skin, malignant
- theca cell C56.- ☑
- thymic C37
- unspecified site (primary) C80.1
- water-clear cell C75.0
Carcinoma-in-situ — *see also* Neoplasm, in situ, by site
- breast NOS D05.9- ☑
  - specified type NEC D05.8- ☑
- epidermoid — *see also* Neoplasm, in situ, by site
  - with questionable stromal invasion
    - cervix D06.9
    - specified site NEC — *see* Neoplasm, in situ, by site
    - unspecified site D06.9
  - Bowen's type — *see* Neoplasm, skin, in situ
- intraductal
  - breast D05.1- ☑
  - specified site NEC — *see* Neoplasm, in situ, by site

Carcinoma-in-situ — *continued*
  intraductal — *continued*
    unspecified site D05.1- ☑
  lobular
    with
      infiltrating duct
        breast (female) C50.91- ☑
          male C50.92- ☑
        specified site NEC — *see* Neoplasm, malignant
        unspecified site (female) C50.91- ☑
          male C50.92- ☑
      intraductal
        breast D05.8- ☑
        specified site NEC — *see* Neoplasm, in situ, by site
        unspecified site (female) D05.8- ☑
    breast D05.0- ☑
    specified site NEC — *see* Neoplasm, in situ, by site
    unspecified site D05.0- ☑
  squamous cell — *see also* Neoplasm, in situ, by site
    with questionable stromal invasion
      cervix D06.9
      specified site NEC — *see* Neoplasm, in situ, by site
      unspecified site D06.9
Carcinomaphobia F45.29
Carcinomatosis C80.0
  peritonei C78.6
  unspecified site (primary) (secondary) C80.0
Carcinosarcoma — *see* Neoplasm, malignant, by site
  embryonal — *see* Neoplasm, malignant, by site
Cardia, cardial — *see* condition
Cardiac — *see also* condition
  death, sudden — *see* Arrest, cardiac
  pacemaker
    in situ Z95.0
    management or adjustment Z45.018
  tamponade I31.4
Cardialgia — *see* Pain, precordial
Cardiectasis — *see* Hypertrophy, cardiac
Cardiochalasia K21.9
Cardiomalacia I51.5
Cardiomegalia glycogenica diffusa E74.02 *[I43]*
Cardiomegaly — *see also* Hypertrophy, cardiac
  congenital Q24.8
  glycogen E74.02 *[I43]*
  idiopathic I51.7
Cardiomyoliposis I51.5
Cardiomyopathy (familial) (idiopathic) I42.9
  alcoholic I42.6
  amyloid E85.4 *[I43]*
    transthyretin-related (ATTR) familial E85.4 *[I43]*
  arteriosclerotic — *see* Disease, heart, ischemic, atherosclerotic
  beriberi E51.12
  cobalt-beer I42.6
  congenital I42.4
  congestive I42.0
  constrictive NOS I42.5
  dilated I42.0
  due to
    alcohol I42.6
    beriberi E51.12
    cardiac glycogenosis E74.02 *[I43]*
    drugs I42.7
    external agents NEC I42.7
    Friedreich's ataxia G11.1
    myotonia atrophica G71.11 *[I43]*
    progressive muscular dystrophy G71.09 *[I43]*
  glycogen storage E74.02 *[I43]*
  hypertensive — *see* Hypertension, heart
  hypertrophic (nonobstructive) I42.2
    obstructive I42.1
      congenital Q24.8
  in
    Chagas' disease (chronic) B57.2
      acute B57.0
    sarcoidosis D86.85
  ischemic I25.5
  metabolic E88.9 *[I43]*
    thyrotoxic E05.90 *[I43]*
      with thyroid storm E05.91 *[I43]*
  newborn I42.8
    congenital I42.4
  non-ischemic — *see also* by cause I42.8
  nutritional E63.9 *[I43]*
    beriberi E51.12

Cardiomyopathy — *continued*
  obscure of Africa I42.8
  peripartum O90.3
  postpartum O90.3
  restrictive NEC I42.5
  rheumatic I09.0
  secondary I42.9
  specified NEC I42.8
  stress induced I51.81
  takotsubo I51.81
  thyrotoxic E05.90 *[I43]*
    with thyroid storm E05.91 *[I43]*
  toxic NEC I42.7
  transthyretin-related (ATTR) familial amyloid E85.4
  tuberculous A18.84
  viral B33.24
Cardionephritis — *see* Hypertension, cardiorenal
Cardionephropathy — *see* Hypertension, cardiorenal
Cardionephrosis — *see* Hypertension, cardiorenal
Cardiopathia nigra I27.0
Cardiopathy — *see also* Disease, heart I51.9
  idiopathic I42.9
  mucopolysaccharidosis E76.3 *[I52]*
Cardiopericarditis — *see* Pericarditis
Cardiophobia F45.29
Cardiorenal — *see* condition
Cardiorrhexis — *see* Infarct, myocardium
Cardiosclerosis — *see* Disease, heart, ischemic, atherosclerotic
Cardiosis — *see* Disease, heart
Cardiospasm (esophagus) (reflex) (stomach) K22.0
  congenital Q39.5
    with megaesophagus Q39.5
Cardiostenosis — *see* Disease, heart
Cardiosymphysis I31.0
Cardiovascular — *see* condition
Carditis (acute) (bacterial) (chronic) (subacute) I51.89
  meningococcal A39.50
  rheumatic — *see* Disease, heart, rheumatic
  rheumatoid — *see* Rheumatoid, carditis
  viral B33.20
Care (of) (for) (following)
  child (routine) Z76.2
  family member (handicapped) (sick)
    creating problem for family Z63.6
    provided away from home for holiday relief Z75.5
    unavailable, due to
      absence (person rendering care) (sufferer) Z74.2
      inability (any reason) of person rendering care Z74.2
  foundling Z76.1
  holiday relief Z75.5
  improper — *see* Maltreatment
  lack of (at or after birth) (infant) — *see* Maltreatment, child, neglect
  lactating mother Z39.1
  palliative Z51.5
  postpartum
    immediately after delivery Z39.0
    routine follow-up Z39.2
  respite Z75.5
  unavailable, due to
    absence of person rendering care Z74.2
    inability (any reason) of person rendering care Z74.2
  well-baby Z76.2
Caries
  bone NEC A18.03
  dental (dentino enamel junction) (early childhood) (of dentine) (pre-eruptive) (recurrent) (to the pulp) K02.9
    arrested (coronal) (root) K02.3
    chewing surface
      limited to enamel K02.51
      penetrating into dentin K02.52
      penetrating into pulp K02.53
    coronal surface
      chewing surface
        limited to enamel K02.51
        penetrating into dentin K02.52
        penetrating into pulp K02.53
      pit and fissure surface
        limited to enamel K02.51
        penetrating into dentin K02.52
        penetrating into pulp K02.53
      smooth surface
        limited to enamel K02.61
        penetrating into dentin K02.62
        penetrating into pulp K02.63

Caries — *continued*
  dental — *continued*
    pit and fissure surface
      limited to enamel K02.51
      penetrating into dentin K02.52
      penetrating into pulp K02.53
    primary, cervical origin K02.52
    root K02.7
    smooth surface
      limited to enamel K02.61
      penetrating into dentin K02.62
      penetrating into pulp K02.63
  external meatus — *see* Disorder, ear, external, specified type NEC
  hip (tuberculous) A18.02
  initial (tooth)
    chewing surface K02.51
    pit and fissure surface K02.51
    smooth surface K02.61
  knee (tuberculous) A18.02
  labyrinth H83.8 ☑
  limb NEC (tuberculous) A18.03
  mastoid process (chronic) — *see* Mastoiditis, chronic
    tuberculous A18.03
  middle ear H74.8 ☑
  nose (tuberculous) A18.03
  orbit (tuberculous) A18.03
  ossicles, ear — *see* Abnormal, ear ossicles
  petrous bone — *see* Petrositis
  root (dental) (tooth) K02.7
  sacrum (tuberculous) A18.01
  spine, spinal (column) (tuberculous) A18.01
  syphilitic A52.77
    congenital (early) A50.02 *[M90.80]*
  tooth, teeth — *see* Caries, dental
  tuberculous A18.03
  vertebra (column) (tuberculous) A18.01
Carious teeth — *see* Caries, dental
Carneous mole O02.0
Carnitine insufficiency E71.40
Carotenemia (dietary) E67.1
Carotenosis (cutis) (skin) E67.1
Carotid body or sinus syndrome G90.01
Carotidynia G90.01
Carpal tunnel syndrome — *see* Syndrome, carpal tunnel
Carpenter's syndrome Q87.0
Carpopedal spasm — *see* Tetany
Carr-Barr-Plunkett syndrome Q97.1
Carrier (suspected) of
  amebiasis Z22.1
  bacterial disease NEC Z22.39
    diphtheria Z22.2
    intestinal infectious NEC Z22.1
      typhoid Z22.0
    meningococcal Z22.31
    sexually transmitted Z22.4
    specified NEC Z22.39
    staphylococcal (Methicillin susceptible) Z22.321
      Methicillin resistant Z22.322
    streptococcal Z22.338
      group B Z22.330
        complicating pregnancy or delivery O99.82- ☑
    typhoid Z22.0
  cholera Z22.1
  diphtheria Z22.2
  gastrointestinal pathogens NEC Z22.1
  genetic Z14.8
    cystic fibrosis Z14.1
    hemophilia A (asymptomatic) Z14.01
      symptomatic Z14.02
  gestational, pregnant Z33.1
  gonorrhea Z22.4
  HAA (hepatitis Australian-antigen) B18.8
  HB (c)(s)-AG B18.1
  hepatitis (viral) B18.9
    Australia-antigen (HAA) B18.8
    B surface antigen (HBsAg) B18.1
      with acute delta- (super)infection B17.0
    C B18.2
    specified NEC B18.8
  human T-cell lymphotropic virus type-1 (HTLV-1) infection Z22.6
  infectious organism Z22.9
    specified NEC Z22.8
  meningococci Z22.31
  Salmonella typhosa Z22.0
  serum hepatitis — *see* Carrier, hepatitis

☑ Additional Character Required — *Refer to the Tabular List for Character Selection*
▼ Subterms under main terms may continue to next column or page

Carrier of — *continued*
staphylococci (Methicillin susceptible) Z22.321
Methicillin resistant Z22.322
streptococci Z22.338
group B Z22.330
complicating pregnancy or delivery O99.82- ☑
syphilis Z22.4
typhoid Z22.0
venereal disease NEC Z22.4
Carrion's disease A44.0
Carter's relapsing fever (Asiatic) A68.1
Cartilage — *see* condition
Caruncle (inflamed)
conjunctiva (acute) — *see* Conjunctivitis, acute
labium (majus) (minus) N90.89
lacrimal — *see* Inflammation, lacrimal, passages
myrtiform N89.8
urethral (benign) N36.2
Cascade stomach K31.2
Caseation lymphatic gland (tuberculous) A18.2
Cassidy (-Scholte) syndrome (malignant carcinoid) E34.0
Castellani's disease A69.8
Castration, traumatic, male S38.231 ☑
Casts in urine R82.998
Cat
cry syndrome Q93.4
ear Q17.3
eye syndrome Q92.8
Catabolism, senile R54
Catalepsy (hysterical) F44.2
schizophrenic F20.2
Cataplexy (idiopathic) — *see* Narcolepsy
Cataract (cortical) (immature) (incipient) H26.9
with
neovascularization — *see* Cataract, complicated
age-related — *see* Cataract, senile
anterior
and posterior axial embryonal Q12.0
pyramidal Q12.0
associated with
galactosemia E74.21 *[H28]*
myotonic disorders G71.19 *[H28]*
blue Q12.0
central Q12.0
cerulean Q12.0
complicated H26.20
with
neovascularization H26.21- ☑
ocular disorder H26.22- ☑
glaucomatous flecks H26.23- ☑
congenital Q12.0
coraliform Q12.0
coronary Q12.0
crystalline Q12.0
diabetic — *see* Diabetes, cataract
drug-induced H26.3- ☑
due to
ocular disorder — *see* Cataract, complicated
radiation H26.8
electric H26.8
extraction status Z98.4- ☑
glass-blower's H26.8
heat ray H26.8
heterochromic — *see* Cataract, complicated
hypermature — *see* Cataract, senile, morgagnian type
in (due to)
chronic iridocyclitis — *see* Cataract, complicated
diabetes — *see* Diabetes, cataract
endocrine disease E34.9 *[H28]*
eye disease — *see* Cataract, complicated
hypoparathyroidism E20.9 *[H28]*
malnutrition-dehydration E46 *[H28]*
metabolic disease E88.9 *[H28]*
myotonic disorders G71.19 *[H28]*
nutritional disease E63.9 *[H28]*
infantile — *see* Cataract, presenile
irradiational — *see* Cataract, specified NEC
juvenile — *see* Cataract, presenile
malnutrition-dehydration E46 *[H28]*
morgagnian — *see* Cataract, senile, morgagnian type
myotonic G71.19 *[H28]*
myxedema E03.9 *[H28]*
nuclear
embryonal Q12.0
sclerosis — *see* Cataract, senile, nuclear
presenile H26.00- ☑
combined forms H26.06- ☑

Cataract — *continued*
presenile — *continued*
cortical H26.01- ☑
lamellar — *see* Cataract, presenile, cortical
nuclear H26.03- ☑
specified NEC H26.09
subcapsular polar (anterior) H26.04- ☑
posterior H26.05- ☑
zonular — *see* Cataract, presenile, cortical
secondary H26.40
Soemmering's ring H26.41- ☑
specified NEC H26.49- ☑
to eye disease — *see* Cataract, complicated
senile H25.9
brunescens — *see* Cataract, senile, nuclear
combined forms H25.81- ☑
coronary — *see* Cataract, senile, incipient
cortical H25.01- ☑
hypermature — *see* Cataract, senile, morgagnian type
incipient (mature) (total) H25.09- ☑
cortical — *see* Cataract, senile, cortical
subcapsular — *see* Cataract, senile, subcapsular
morgagnian type (hypermature) H25.2- ☑
nuclear (sclerosis) H25.1- ☑
polar subcapsular (anterior) (posterior) — *see* Cataract, senile, incipient
punctate — *see* Cataract, senile, incipient
specified NEC H25.89
subcapsular polar (anterior) H25.03- ☑
posterior H25.04- ☑
snowflake — *see* Diabetes, cataract
specified NEC H26.8
toxic — *see* Cataract, drug-induced
traumatic H26.10- ☑
localized H26.11- ☑
partially resolved H26.12- ☑
total H26.13- ☑
zonular (perinuclear) Q12.0
Cataracta — *see also* Cataract
brunescens — *see* Cataract, senile, nuclear
centralis pulverulenta Q12.0
cerulea Q12.0
complicata — *see* Cataract, complicated
congenita Q12.0
coralliformis Q12.0
coronaria Q12.0
diabetic — *see* Diabetes, cataract
membranacea
accreta — *see* Cataract, secondary
congenita Q12.0
nigra — *see* Cataract, senile, nuclear
sunflower — *see* Cataract, complicated
Catarrh, catarrhal (acute) (febrile) (infectious) (inflammation) — *see also* condition J00
bronchial — *see* Bronchitis
chest — *see* Bronchitis
chronic J31.0
due to congenital syphilis A50.03
enteric — *see* Enteritis
eustachian H68.009
fauces — *see* Pharyngitis
gastrointestinal — *see* Enteritis
gingivitis K05.00
nonplaque induced K05.01
plaque induced K05.00
hay — *see* Fever, hay
intestinal — *see* Enteritis
larynx, chronic J37.0
liver B15.9
with hepatic coma B15.0
lung — *see* Bronchitis
middle ear, chronic — *see* Otitis, media, nonsuppurative, chronic, serous
mouth K12.1
nasal (chronic) — *see* Rhinitis
nasobronchial J31.1
nasopharyngeal (chronic) J31.1
acute J00
pulmonary — *see* Bronchitis
spring (eye) (vernal) — *see* Conjunctivitis, acute, atopic
summer (hay) — *see* Fever, hay
throat J31.2
tubotympanal — *see also* Otitis, media, nonsuppurative
chronic — *see* Otitis, media, nonsuppurative, chronic, serous
Catatonia (schizophrenic) F20.2

Catatonic
disorder due to known physiologic condition F06.1
schizophrenia F20.2
stupor R40.1
Cat-scratch — *see also* Abrasion
disease or fever A28.1
Cauda equina — *see* condition
Cauliflower ear M95.1- ☑
Causalgia (upper limb) G56.4- ☑
lower limb G57.7- ☑
Cause
external, general effects T75.89 ☑
Caustic burn — *see* Corrosion, by site
Cavare's disease (familial periodic paralysis) G72.3
Cave-in, injury
crushing (severe) — *see* Crush
suffocation — *see* Asphyxia, traumatic, due to low oxygen, due to cave-in
Cavernitis (penis) N48.29
Cavernositis N48.29
Cavernous — *see* condition
Cavitation of lung — *see also* Tuberculosis, pulmonary
nontuberculous J98.4
Cavities, dental — *see* Caries, dental
Cavity
lung — *see* Cavitation of lung
optic papilla Q14.2
pulmonary — *see* Cavitation of lung
Cavovarus foot, congenital Q66.1- ☑
Cavus foot (congenital) Q66.7- ☑
acquired — *see* Deformity, limb, foot, specified NEC
Cazenave's disease L10.2
Cecitis K52.9
with perforation, peritonitis, or rupture K65.8
Cecoureterocele Q62.32
Cecum — *see* condition
Celiac
artery compression syndrome I77.4
disease (with steatorrhea) K90.0
infantilism K90.0
Cell(s), cellular — *see also* condition
in urine R82.998
Cellulitis (diffuse) (phlegmonous) (septic) (suppurative) L03.90
abdominal wall L03.311
anaerobic A48.0
ankle — *see* Cellulitis, lower limb
anus K61.0
arm — *see* Cellulitis, upper limb
auricle (ear) — *see* Cellulitis, ear
axilla L03.11- ☑
back (any part) L03.312
breast (acute) (nonpuerperal) (subacute) N61.0
nipple N61.0
broad ligament
acute N73.0
buttock L03.317
cervical (meaning neck) L03.221
cervix (uteri) — *see* Cervicitis
cheek (external) L03.211
internal K12.2
chest wall L03.313
chronic L03.90
clostridial A48.0
corpus cavernosum N48.22
digit
finger — *see* Cellulitis, finger
toe — *see* Cellulitis, toe
Douglas' cul-de-sac or pouch
acute N73.0
drainage site (following operation) T81.49 ☑
ear (external) H60.1- ☑
eosinophilic (granulomatous) L98.3
erysipelatous — *see* Erysipelas
external auditory canal — *see* Cellulitis, ear
eyelid — *see* Abscess, eyelid
face NEC L03.211
finger (intrathecal) (periosteal) (subcutaneous) (subcuticular) L03.01- ☑
foot — *see* Cellulitis, lower limb
gangrenous — *see* Gangrene
genital organ NEC
female (external) N76.4
male N49.9
multiple sites N49.8
specified NEC N49.8
gluteal (region) L03.317

Cellulitis — *continued*
  gonococcal A54.89
  groin L03.314
  hand — *see* Cellulitis, upper limb
  head NEC L03.811
    face (any part, except ear, eye and nose) L03.211
  heel — *see* Cellulitis, lower limb
  hip — *see* Cellulitis, lower limb
  jaw (region) L03.211
  knee — *see* Cellulitis, lower limb
  labium (majus) (minus) — *see* Vulvitis
  lacrimal passages — *see* Inflammation, lacrimal, passages
  larynx J38.7
  leg — *see* Cellulitis, lower limb
  lip K13.0
  lower limb L03.11- ☑
    toe — *see* Cellulitis, toe
  mouth (floor) K12.2
  multiple sites, so stated L03.90
  nasopharynx J39.1
  navel L03.316
    newborn P38.9
      with mild hemorrhage P38.1
      without hemorrhage P38.9
  neck (region) L03.221
  nipple (acute) (nonpuerperal) (subacute) N61.0
  nose (septum) (external) J34.0
  orbit, orbital H05.01- ☑
  palate (soft) K12.2
  pectoral (region) L03.313
  pelvis, pelvic (chronic)
    female — *see also* Disease, pelvis, inflammatory N73.2
      acute N73.0
    following ectopic or molar pregnancy O08.0
    male K65.0
  penis N48.22
  perineal, perineum L03.315
  periorbital L03.213
  perirectal K61.1
  peritonsillar J36
  periurethral N34.0
  periuterine — *see also* Disease, pelvis, inflammatory N73.2
    acute N73.0
  pharynx J39.1
  preseptal L03.213
  rectum K61.1
  retroperitoneal K68.9
  round ligament
    acute N73.0
  scalp (any part) L03.811
  scrotum N49.2
  seminal vesicle N49.0
  shoulder — *see* Cellulitis, upper limb
  specified site NEC L03.818
  submandibular (region) (space) (triangle) K12.2
    gland K11.3
  submaxillary (region) K12.2
    gland K11.3
  thigh — *see* Cellulitis, lower limb
  thumb (intrathecal) (periosteal) (subcutaneous) (subcuticular) — *see* Cellulitis, finger
  toe (intrathecal) (periosteal) (subcutaneous) (subcuticular) L03.03- ☑
  tonsil J36
  trunk L03.319
    abdominal wall L03.311
    back (any part) L03.312
    buttock L03.317
    chest wall L03.313
    groin L03.314
    perineal, perineum L03.315
    umbilicus L03.316
  tuberculous (primary) A18.4
  umbilicus L03.316
  upper limb L03.11- ☑
    axilla — *see* Cellulitis, axilla
    finger — *see* Cellulitis, finger
    thumb — *see* Cellulitis, finger
  vaccinal T88.0 ☑
  vocal cord J38.3
  vulva — *see* Vulvitis
  wrist — *see* Cellulitis, upper limb
Cementoblastoma, benign — *see* Cyst, calcifying odontogenic
Cementoma — *see* Cyst, calcifying odontogenic

Cementoperiostitis — *see* Periodontitis
Cementosis K03.4
Central auditory processing disorder H93.25
Central pain syndrome G89.0
Cephalematocele, cephal (o)hematocele
  newborn P52.8
    birth injury P10.8
  traumatic — *see* Hematoma, brain
Cephalematoma, cephalhematoma (calcified)
  newborn (birth injury) P12.0
  traumatic — *see* Hematoma, brain
Cephalgia, cephalalgia — *see also* Headache
  histamine G44.009
    intractable G44.001
    not intractable G44.009
  trigeminal autonomic (TAC) NEC G44.099
    intractable G44.091
    not intractable G44.099
Cephalic — *see* condition
Cephalitis — *see* Encephalitis
Cephalocele — *see* Encephalocele
Cephalomenia N94.89
Cephalopelvic — *see* condition
Cerclage (with cervical incompetence) in pregnancy — *see* Incompetence, cervix, in pregnancy
Cerebellitis — *see* Encephalitis
Cerebellum, cerebellar — *see* condition
Cerebral — *see* condition
Cerebritis — *see* Encephalitis
Cerebro-hepato-renal syndrome Q87.89
Cerebromalacia — *see* Softening, brain
  sequelae of cerebrovascular disease I69.398
Cerebroside lipidosis E75.22
Cerebrospasticity (congenital) G80.1
Cerebrospinal — *see* condition
Cerebrum — *see* condition
Ceroid-lipofuscinosis, neuronal E75.4
Cerumen (accumulation) (impacted) H61.2- ☑
Cervical — *see also* condition
  auricle Q18.2
  dysplasia in pregnancy — *see* Abnormal, cervix, in pregnancy or childbirth
  erosion in pregnancy — *see* Abnormal, cervix, in pregnancy or childbirth
  fibrosis in pregnancy — *see* Abnormal, cervix, in pregnancy or childbirth
  fusion syndrome Q76.1
  rib Q76.5
  shortening (complicating pregnancy) O26.87- ☑
Cervicalgia M54.2
Cervicitis (acute) (chronic) (nonvenereal) (senile (atrophic)) (subacute) (with ulceration) N72
  with
    abortion — *see* Abortion, by type complicated by genital tract and pelvic infection
    ectopic pregnancy O08.0
    molar pregnancy O08.0
  chlamydial A56.09
  gonococcal A54.03
  herpesviral A60.03
  puerperal (postpartum) O86.11
  syphilitic A52.76
  trichomonal A59.09
  tuberculous A18.16
Cervicocolpitis (emphysematosa) — *see also* Cervicitis N72
Cervix — *see* condition
Cesarean delivery, previous, affecting management of pregnancy O34.219
  classical (vertical) scar O34.212
  low transverse scar O34.211
Céstan (-Chenais) paralysis or syndrome G46.3
Céstan-Raymond syndrome I65.8
Cestode infestation B71.9
  specified type NEC B71.8
Cestodiasis B71.9
Chabert's disease A22.9
Chacaleh E53.8
Chafing L30.4
Chagas' (-Mazza) disease (chronic) B57.2
  with
    cardiovascular involvement NEC B57.2
    digestive system involvement B57.30
      megacolon B57.32
      megaesophagus B57.31
      other specified B57.39
    megacolon B57.32

Chagas' disease — *continued*
  with — *continued*
    megaesophagus B57.31
    myocarditis B57.2
    nervous system involvement B57.40
      meningitis B57.41
      meningoencephalitis B57.42
      other specified B57.49
    specified organ involvement NEC B57.5
  acute (with) B57.1
    cardiovascular NEC B57.0
    myocarditis B57.0
Chagres fever B50.9
Chairridden Z74.09
Chalasia (cardiac sphincter) K21.9
Chalazion H00.19
  left H00.16
    lower H00.15
    upper H00.14
  right H00.13
    lower H00.12
    upper H00.11
Chalcosis — *see also* Disorder, globe, degenerative, chalcosis
  cornea — *see* Deposit, cornea
  crystalline lens — *see* Cataract, complicated
  retina H35.89
Chalicosis (pulmonum) J62.8
Chancre (any genital site) (hard) (hunterian) (mixed) (primary) (seronegative) (seropositive) (syphilitic) A51.0
  congenital A50.07
  conjunctiva NEC A51.2
  Ducrey's A57
  extragenital A51.2
  eyelid A51.2
  lip A51.2
  nipple A51.2
  Nisbet's A57
  of
    carate A67.0
    pinta A67.0
    yaws A66.0
  palate, soft A51.2
  phagedenic A57
  simple A57
  soft A57
    bubo A57
    palate A51.2
  urethra A51.0
  yaws A66.0
Chancroid (anus) (genital) (penis) (perineum) (rectum) (urethra) (vulva) A57
Chandler's disease (osteochondritis dissecans, hip) — *see* Osteochondritis, dissecans, hip
Change(s) (in) (of) — *see also* Removal
  arteriosclerotic — *see* Arteriosclerosis
  bone — *see also* Disorder, bone
    diabetic — *see* Diabetes, bone change
  bowel habit R19.4
  cardiorenal (vascular) — *see* Hypertension, cardiorenal
  cardiovascular — *see* Disease, cardiovascular
  circulatory I99.9
  cognitive (mild) (organic) R41.89
  color, tooth, teeth
    during formation K00.8
    posteruptive K03.7
  contraceptive device Z30.433
  corneal membrane H18.30
    Bowman's membrane fold or rupture H18.31- ☑
    Descemet's membrane
      fold H18.32- ☑
      rupture H18.33- ☑
  coronary — *see* Disease, heart, ischemic
  degenerative, spine or vertebra — *see* Spondylosis
  dental pulp, regressive K04.2
  dressing (nonsurgical) Z48.00
    surgical Z48.01
  heart — *see* Disease, heart
  hip joint — *see* Derangement, joint, hip
  hyperplastic larynx J38.7
  hypertrophic
    nasal sinus J34.89
    turbinate, nasal J34.3
    upper respiratory tract J39.8
  indwelling catheter Z46.6
  inflammatory — *see also* Inflammation
    sacroiliac M46.1

Change(s) — continued
job, anxiety concerning Z56.1
joint — see Derangement, joint
life — see Menopause
mental status R41.82
minimal (glomerular) — see also N00-N07 with fourth character .0 N05.0
myocardium, myocardial — see Degeneration, myocardial
of life — see Menopause
pacemaker Z45.018
pulse generator Z45.010
personality (enduring) F68.8
due to (secondary to)
general medical condition F07.0
secondary (nonspecific) F60.89
regressive, dental pulp K04.2
renal — see Disease, renal
retina H35.9
myopic — see also Myopia, degenerative H44.2- ☑
sacroiliac joint M53.3
senile — see also condition R54
sensory R20.8
skin R23.9
acute, due to ultraviolet radiation L56.9
specified NEC L56.8
chronic, due to nonionizing radiation L57.9
specified NEC L57.8
cyanosis R23.0
flushing R23.2
pallor R23.1
petechiae R23.3
specified change NEC R23.8
swelling — see Mass, localized
texture R23.4
trophic
arm — see Mononeuropathy, upper limb
leg — see Mononeuropathy, lower limb
vascular I99.9
vasomotor I73.9
voice R49.9
psychogenic F44.4
specified NEC R49.8
Changing sleep-work schedule, affecting sleep G47.26
Changuinola fever A93.1
Chapping skin T69.8 ☑
Charcot-Marie-Tooth disease, paralysis or syndrome G60.0
Charcot's
arthropathy — see Arthropathy, neuropathic
cirrhosis K74.3
disease (tabetic arthropathy) A52.16
joint (disease) (tabetic) A52.16
diabetic — see Diabetes, with, arthropathy
syringomyelic G95.0
syndrome (intermittent claudication) I73.9
CHARGE association Q89.8
Charley-horse (quadriceps) M62.831
traumatic (quadriceps) S76.11- ☑
Charlouis' disease — see Yaws
Cheadle's disease E54
Checking (of)
cardiac pacemaker (battery) (electrode(s)) Z45.018
pulse generator Z45.010
implantable subdermal contraceptive Z30.46
intrauterine contraceptive device Z30.431
wound Z48.0- ☑
due to injury — code to Injury, by site, using appropriate seventh character for subsequent encounter
Check-up — see Examination
Chédiak-Higashi (-Steinbrinck) **syndrome** (congenital gigantism of peroxidase granules) E70.330
Cheek — see condition
Cheese itch B88.0
Cheese-washer's lung J67.8
Cheese-worker's lung J67.8
Cheilitis (acute) (angular) (catarrhal) (chronic) (exfoliative) (gangrenous) (glandular) (infectional) (suppurative) (ulcerative) (vesicular) K13.0
actinic (due to sun) L56.8
other than from sun L59.8
candidal B37.83
Cheilodynia K13.0
Cheiloschisis — see Cleft, lip
Cheilosis (angular) K13.0
with pellagra E52

Cheilosis — continued
due to
vitamin B2 (riboflavin) deficiency E53.0
Cheiromegaly M79.89
Cheiropompholyx L30.1
Cheloid — see Keloid
Chemical burn — see Corrosion, by site
Chemodectoma — see Paraganglioma, nonchromaffin
Chemosis, conjunctiva — see Edema, conjunctiva
Chemotherapy (session) (for)
cancer Z51.11
neoplasm Z51.11
Cherubism M27.8
Chest — see condition
Cheyne-Stokes breathing (respiration) R06.3
Chiari's
disease or syndrome (hepatic vein thrombosis) I82.0
malformation
type I G93.5
type II — see Spina bifida
net Q24.8
Chicago disease B40.9
Chickenpox — see Varicella
Chiclero ulcer or sore B55.1
Chigger (infestation) B88.0
Chignon (disease) B36.8
newborn (from vacuum extraction) (birth injury) P12.1
Chilaiditi's syndrome (subphrenic displacement, colon) Q43.3
Chilblain(s) (lupus) T69.1 ☑
Child
custody dispute Z65.3
Childbirth — see Delivery
Childhood
cerebral X-linked adrenoleukodystrophy E71.520
period of rapid growth Z00.2
Chill(s) R68.83
with fever R50.9
congestive in malarial regions B54
without fever R68.83
Chilomastigiasis A07.8
Chimera 46,XX/46,XY Q99.0
Chin — see condition
Chinese dysentery A03.9
Chionophobia F40.228
Chitral fever A93.1
Chlamydia, chlamydial A74.9
cervicitis A56.09
conjunctivitis A74.0
cystitis A56.01
endometritis A56.11
epididymitis A56.19
female
pelvic inflammatory disease A56.11
pelviperitonitis A56.11
orchitis A56.19
peritonitis A74.81
pharyngitis A56.4
proctitis A56.3
psittaci (infection) A70
salpingitis A56.11
sexually-transmitted infection NEC A56.8
specified NEC A74.89
urethritis A56.01
vulvovaginitis A56.02
Chlamydiosis — see Chlamydia
Chloasma (skin) (idiopathic) (symptomatic) L81.1
eyelid H02.719
hyperthyroid E05.90 [H02.719]
with thyroid storm E05.91 [H02.719]
left H02.716
lower H02.715
upper H02.714
right H02.713
lower H02.712
upper H02.711
Chloroma C92.3- ☑
Chlorosis D50.9
Egyptian B76.9 [D63.8]
miner's B76.9 [D63.8]
Chlorotic anemia D50.8
Chocolate cyst (ovary) N80.1
Choked
disc or disk — see Papilledema
on food, phlegm, or vomitus NOS — see Foreign body, by site
while vomiting NOS — see Foreign body, by site

Chokes (resulting from bends) T70.3 ☑
Choking sensation R09.89
Cholangiectasis K83.8
Cholangiocarcinoma
with hepatocellular carcinoma, combined C22.0
liver C22.1
specified site NEC — see Neoplasm, malignant, by site
unspecified site C22.1
Cholangiohepatitis K83.8
due to fluke infestation B66.1
Cholangiohepatoma C22.0
Cholangiolitis (acute) (chronic) (extrahepatic) (gangrenous) (intrahepatic) K83.09
paratyphoidal — see Fever, paratyphoid
typhoidal A01.09
Cholangioma D13.4
malignant — see Cholangiocarcinoma
Cholangitis (ascending) (recurrent) (secondary) (stenosing) (suppurative) K83.09
with calculus, bile duct — see Calculus, bile duct, with cholangitis
chronic nonsuppurative destructive K74.3
primary K83.09
sclerosing K83.01
sclerosing K83.09
Cholecystectasia K82.8
Cholecystitis K81.9
with
calculus, stones in
bile duct (common) (hepatic) — see Calculus, bile duct, with cholecystitis
cystic duct — see Calculus, gallbladder, with cholecystitis
gallbladder — see Calculus, gallbladder, with cholecystitis
choledocholithiasis — see Calculus, bile duct, with cholecystitis
cholelithiasis — see Calculus, gallbladder, with cholecystitis
gangrene of gallbladder K82.A1
perforation of gallbladder K82.A2
acute (emphysematous) (gangrenous) (suppurative) K81.0
with
calculus, stones in
cystic duct — see Calculus, gallbladder, with cholecystitis, acute
gallbladder — see Calculus, gallbladder, with cholecystitis, acute
choledocholithiasis — see Calculus, bile duct, with cholecystitis, acute *K80.46*
cholelithiasis — see Calculus, gallbladder, with cholecystitis, acute *K80.00*
chronic cholecystitis K81.2
with gallbladder calculus K80.12
with obstruction K80.13
chronic K81.1
with acute cholecystitis K81.2
with gallbladder calculus K80.12
with obstruction K80.13
emphysematous (acute) — see Cholecystitis, acute
gangrenous — see Cholecystitis, acute
paratyphoidal, current A01.4
suppurative — see Cholecystitis, acute
typhoidal A01.09
Cholecystolithiasis — see Calculus, gallbladder
Choledochitis (suppurative) K83.09
Choledocholith — see Calculus, bile duct
Choledocholithiasis (common duct) (hepatic duct) — see Calculus, bile duct
cystic — see Calculus, gallbladder
typhoidal A01.09
Cholelithiasis (cystic duct) (gallbladder) (impacted) (multiple) — see Calculus, gallbladder
bile duct (common) (hepatic) — see Calculus, bile duct
hepatic duct — see Calculus, bile duct
specified NEC K80.80
with obstruction K80.81
Cholemia — see also Jaundice
familial (simple) (congenital) E80.4
Gilbert's E80.4
Choleperitoneum, choleperitonitis K65.3
Cholera (Asiatic) (epidemic) (malignant) A00.9
antimonial — see Poisoning, antimony
classical A00.0
due to Vibrio cholerae 01 A00.9
biovar cholerae A00.0

Cholera — *continued*
due to Vibrio cholerae 01 — *continued*
biovar eltor A00.1
el tor A00.1
el tor A00.1
Cholerine — *see* Cholera
Cholestasis NEC K83.1
with hepatocyte injury K71.0
due to total parenteral nutrition (TPN) K76.89
pure K71.0
Cholesteatoma (ear) (middle) (with reaction) H71.9- ☑
attic H71.0- ☑
external ear (canal) H60.4- ☑
mastoid H71.2- ☑
postmastoidectomy cavity (recurrent) — *see* Complications, postmastoidectomy, recurrent cholesteatoma
recurrent (postmastoidectomy) — *see* Complications, postmastoidectomy, recurrent cholesteatoma
tympanum H71.1- ☑
Cholesteatosis, diffuse H71.3- ☑
Cholesteremia E78.00
Cholesterin in vitreous — *see* Deposit, crystalline
Cholesterol
deposit
retina H35.89
vitreous — *see* Deposit, crystalline
elevated (high) E78.00
with elevated (high) triglycerides E78.2
screening for Z13.220
imbibition of gallbladder K82.4
Cholesterolemia (essential) (pure) E78.00
familial E78.01
hereditary E78.01
Cholesterolosis, cholesterosis (gallbladder) K82.4
cerebrotendinous E75.5
Cholocolic fistula K82.3
Choluria R82.2
Chondritis M94.8X9
aurical H61.03- ☑
costal (Tietze's) M94.0
external ear H61.03- ☑
patella, posttraumatic — *see* Chondromalacia, patella
pinna H61.03- ☑
purulent M94.8X- ☑
tuberculous NEC A18.02
intervertebral A18.01
Chondroblastoma — *see also* Neoplasm, bone, benign
malignant — *see* Neoplasm, bone, malignant
Chondrocalcinosis M11.20
ankle M11.27- ☑
elbow M11.22- ☑
familial M11.10
ankle M11.17- ☑
elbow M11.12- ☑
foot joint M11.17- ☑
hand joint M11.14- ☑
hip M11.15- ☑
knee M11.16- ☑
multiple site M11.19
shoulder M11.11- ☑
vertebrae M11.18
wrist M11.13- ☑
foot joint M11.27- ☑
hand joint M11.24- ☑
hip M11.25- ☑
knee M11.26- ☑
multiple site M11.29
shoulder M11.21- ☑
specified type NEC M11.20
ankle M11.27- ☑
elbow M11.22- ☑
foot joint M11.27- ☑
hand joint M11.24- ☑
hip M11.25- ☑
knee M11.26- ☑
multiple site M11.29
shoulder M11.21- ☑
vertebrae M11.28
wrist M11.23- ☑
vertebrae M11.28
wrist M11.23- ☑
Chondrodermatitis nodularis helicis or anthelicis — *see* Perichondritis, ear
Chondrodysplasia Q78.9
with hemangioma Q78.4
calcificans congenita Q77.3

Chondrodysplasia — *continued*
fetalis Q77.4
metaphyseal (Jansen's) (McKusick's) (Schmid's) Q78.8
punctata Q77.3
Chondrodystrophy, chondrodystrophia (familial) (fetalis) (hypoplastic) Q78.9
calcificans congenita Q77.3
myotonic (congenital) G71.13
punctata Q77.3
Chondroectodermal dysplasia Q77.6
Chondrogenesis imperfecta Q77.4
Chondrolysis M94.35-
Chondroma — *see also* Neoplasm, cartilage, benign
juxtacortical — *see* Neoplasm, bone, benign
periosteal — *see* Neoplasm, bone, benign
Chondromalacia (systemic) M94.20
acromioclavicular joint M94.21- ☑
ankle M94.27- ☑
elbow M94.22- ☑
foot joint M94.27- ☑
glenohumeral joint M94.21- ☑
hand joint M94.24- ☑
hip M94.25- ☑
knee M94.26- ☑
patella M22.4- ☑
multiple sites M94.29
patella M22.4- ☑
rib M94.28
sacroiliac joint M94.259
shoulder M94.21- ☑
sternoclavicular joint M94.21- ☑
vertebral joint M94.28
wrist M94.23- ☑
Chondromatosis — *see also* Neoplasm, cartilage, uncertain behavior
internal Q78.4
Chondromyxosarcoma — *see* Neoplasm, cartilage, malignant
Chondro-osteodysplasia (Morquio-Brailsford type) E76.219
Chondro-osteodystrophy E76.29
Chondro-osteoma — *see* Neoplasm, bone, benign
Chondropathia tuberosa M94.0
Chondrosarcoma — *see* Neoplasm, cartilage, malignant
juxtacortical — *see* Neoplasm, bone, malignant
mesenchymal — *see* Neoplasm, connective tissue, malignant
myxoid — *see* Neoplasm, cartilage, malignant
Chordee (nonvenereal) N48.89
congenital Q54.4
gonococcal A54.09
Chorditis (fibrinous) (nodosa) (tuberosa) J38.2
Chordoma — *see* Neoplasm, vertebral (column), malignant
Chorea (chronic) (gravis) (posthemiplegic) (senile) (spasmodic) G25.5
with
heart involvement I02.0
active or acute (conditions in I01-) I02.0
rheumatic I02.9
with valvular disorder I02.0
rheumatic heart disease (chronic) (inactive)(quiescent) — *code to* rheumatic heart condition involved
drug-induced G25.4
habit F95.8
hereditary G10
Huntington's G10
hysterical F44.4
minor I02.9
with heart involvement I02.0
progressive G25.5
hereditary G10
rheumatic (chronic) I02.9
with heart involvement I02.0
Sydenham's I02.9
with heart involvement — *see* Chorea, with rheumatic heart disease
nonrheumatic G25.5
Choreoathetosis (paroxysmal) G25.5
Chorioadenoma (destruens) D39.2
Chorioamnionitis O41.12- ☑
Chorioangioma D26.7
Choriocarcinoma — *see* Neoplasm, malignant, by site
combined with
embryonal carcinoma — *see* Neoplasm, malignant, by site

Choriocarcinoma — *continued*
combined with — *continued*
other germ cell elements — *see* Neoplasm, malignant, by site
teratoma — *see* Neoplasm, malignant, by site
specified site — *see* Neoplasm, malignant, by site
unspecified site
female C58
male C62.90
Chorioencephalitis (acute) (lymphocytic) (serous) A87.2
Chorioepithelioma — *see* Choriocarcinoma
Choriomeningitis (acute) (lymphocytic) (serous) A87.2
Chorionepithelioma — *see* Choriocarcinoma
Chorioretinitis — *see also* Inflammation, chorioretinal
disseminated — *see also* Inflammation, chorioretinal, disseminated
in neurosyphilis A52.19
Egyptian B76.9 *[D63.8]*
focal — *see also* Inflammation, chorioretinal, focal
histoplasmic B39.9 *[H32]*
in (due to)
histoplasmosis B39.9 *[H32]*
syphilis (secondary) A51.43
late A52.71
toxoplasmosis (acquired) B58.01
congenital (active) P37.1 *[H32]*
tuberculosis A18.53
juxtapapillary, juxtapapillaris — *see* Inflammation, chorioretinal, focal, juxtapapillary
leprous A30.9 *[H32]*
miner's B76.9 *[D63.8]*
progressive myopia (degeneration) — *see also* Myopia, degenerative H44.2- ☑
syphilitic (secondary) A51.43
congenital (early) A50.01 *[H32]*
late A50.32
late A52.71
tuberculous A18.53
Chorioretinopathy, central serous H35.71- ☑
Choroid — *see* condition
Choroideremia H31.21
Choroiditis — *see* Chorioretinitis
Choroidopathy — *see* Disorder, choroid
Choroidoretinitis — *see* Chorioretinitis
Choroidoretinopathy, central serous — *see* Chorioretinopathy, central serous
Christian-Weber disease M35.6
Christmas disease D67
Chromaffinoma — *see also* Neoplasm, benign, by site
malignant — *see* Neoplasm, malignant, by site
Chromatopsia — *see* Deficiency, color vision
Chromhidrosis, chromidrosis L75.1
Chromoblastomycosis — *see* Chromomycosis
Chromoconversion R82.91
Chromomycosis B43.9
brain abscess B43.1
cerebral B43.1
cutaneous B43.0
skin B43.0
specified NEC B43.8
subcutaneous abscess or cyst B43.2
Chromophytosis B36.0
Chromosome — *see* Anomaly, by chromosome involved
D (1) — *see* Anomaly, chromosome 13
E (3) — *see* Anomaly, chromosome 18
G — *see* Anomaly, chromosome 21
Chromotrichomycosis B36.8
Chronic — *see* condition
fracture — *see* Fracture, pathological
Churg-Strauss syndrome M30.1
Chyle cyst, mesentery I89.8
Chylocele (nonfilarial) I89.8
filarial — *see also* Infestation, filarial B74.9 *[N51]*
tunica vaginalis N50.89
filarial — *see also* Infestation, filarial B74.9 *[N51]*
Chylomicronemia (fasting) (with hyperprebetalipoproteinemia) E78.3
Chylopericardium I31.3
acute I30.9
Chylothorax (nonfilarial) I89.8
filarial — *see also* Infestation, filarial B74.9 *[J91.8]*
Chylous — *see* condition
Chyluria (nonfilarial) R82.0
due to
bilharziasis B65.0
Brugia (malayi) B74.1
timori B74.2

Chyluria — *continued*
  due to — *continued*
    schistosomiasis (bilharziasis) B65.0
      Wuchereria (bancrofti) B74.0
  filarial — *see* Infestation, filarial
Cicatricial (deformity) — *see* Cicatrix
Cicatrix (adherent) (contracted) (painful) (vicious) — *see also* Scar L90.5
  adenoid (and tonsil) J35.8
  alveolar process M26.79
  anus K62.89
  auricle — *see* Disorder, pinna, specified type NEC
  bile duct (common) (hepatic) K83.8
  bladder N32.89
  bone — *see* Disorder, bone, specified type NEC
  brain G93.89
  cervix (postoperative) (postpartal) N88.1
  common duct K83.8
  cornea H17.9
    tuberculous A18.59
  duodenum (bulb), obstructive K31.5
  esophagus K22.2
  eyelid — *see* Disorder, eyelid function
  hypopharynx J39.2
  lacrimal passages — *see* Obstruction, lacrimal
  larynx J38.7
  lung J98.4
  middle ear H74.8 ☑
  mouth K13.79
  muscle M62.89
    with contracture — *see* Contraction, muscle NEC
  nasopharynx J39.2
  palate (soft) K13.79
  penis N48.89
  pharynx J39.2
  prostate N42.89
  rectum K62.89
  retina — *see* Scar, chorioretinal
  semilunar cartilage — *see* Derangement, meniscus
  seminal vesicle N50.89
  skin L90.5
    infected L08.89
    postinfective L90.5
    tuberculous B90.8
  specified site NEC L90.5
  throat J39.2
  tongue K14.8
  tonsil (and adenoid) J35.8
  trachea J39.8
  tuberculous NEC B90.9
  urethra N36.8
  uterus N85.8
  vagina N89.8
    postoperative N99.2
  vocal cord J38.3
  wrist, constricting (annular) L90.5
CIDP (chronic inflammatory demyelinating polyneuropathy) G61.81
CIN — *see* Neoplasia, intraepithelial, cervix
CINCA (chronic infantile neurological, cutaneous and articular syndrome) M04.2
Cinchonism — *see* Deafness, ototoxic
  correct substance properly administered — *see* Table of Drugs and Chemicals, by drug, adverse effect
  overdose or wrong substance given or taken — *see* Table of Drugs and Chemicals, by drug, poisoning
Circle of Willis — *see* condition
Circular — *see* condition
Circulating anticoagulants — *see also* Disorder, hemorrhagic D68.318
  due to drugs — *see also* Disorder, hemorrhagic D68.32
  following childbirth O72.3
Circulation
  collateral, any site I99.8
  defective (lower extremity) I99.9
    congenital Q28.9
  embryonic Q28.9
  failure (peripheral) R57.9
    newborn P29.89
  fetal, persistent P29.38
  heart, incomplete Q28.9
Circulatory system — *see* condition
Circulus senilis (cornea) — *see* Degeneration, cornea, senile
Circumcision (in absence of medical indication) (ritual) (routine) Z41.2
Circumscribed — *see* condition
Circumvallate placenta O43.11- ☑

Cirrhosis, cirrhotic (hepatic) (liver) K74.60
  alcoholic K70.30
    with ascites K70.31
  atrophic — *see* Cirrhosis, liver
  Baumgarten-Cruveilhier K74.69
  biliary (cholangiolitic) (cholangitic) (hypertrophic) (obstructive) (pericholangiolitic) K74.5
    due to
      Clonorchiasis B66.1
      flukes B66.3
    primary K74.3
    secondary K74.4
  cardiac (of liver) K76.1
  Charcot's K74.3
  cholangiolitic, cholangitic, cholostatic (primary) K74.3
  congestive K76.1
  Cruveilhier-Baumgarten K74.69
  cryptogenic (liver) K74.69
  due to
    hepatolenticular degeneration E83.01
    Wilson's disease E83.01
    xanthomatosis E78.2
  fatty K76.0
    alcoholic K70.0
  Hanot's (hypertrophic) K74.3
  hepatic — *see* Cirrhosis, liver
  hypertrophic K74.3
  Indian childhood K74.69
  kidney — *see* Sclerosis, renal
  Laennec's K70.30
    with ascites K70.31
    alcoholic K70.30
      with ascites K70.31
    nonalcoholic K74.69
  liver K74.60
    alcoholic K70.30
      with ascites K70.31
    fatty K70.0
    congenital P78.81
    syphilitic A52.74
  lung (chronic) J84.10
  macronodular K74.69
    alcoholic K70.30
      with ascites K70.31
  micronodular K74.69
    alcoholic K70.30
      with ascites K70.31
  mixed type K74.69
  monolobular K74.3
  nephritis — *see* Sclerosis, renal
  nutritional K74.69
    alcoholic K70.30
      with ascites K70.31
  obstructive — *see* Cirrhosis, biliary
  ovarian N83.8
  pancreas (duct) K86.89
  pigmentary E83.110
  portal K74.69
    alcoholic K70.30
      with ascites K70.31
  postnecrotic K74.69
    alcoholic K70.30
      with ascites K70.31
  pulmonary J84.10
  renal — *see* Sclerosis, renal
  spleen D73.2
  stasis K76.1
  Todd's K74.3
  unilobar K74.3
  xanthomatous (biliary) K74.5
    due to xanthomatosis (familial) (metabolic) (primary) E78.2
Cistern, subarachnoid R93.0
Citrullinemia E72.23
Citrullinuria E72.23
Civatte's disease or poikiloderma L57.3
Clam digger's itch B65.3
Clammy skin R23.1
Clap — *see* Gonorrhea
Clarke-Hadfield syndrome (pancreatic infantilism) K86.89
Clark's paralysis G80.9
Clastothrix L67.8
Claude Bernard-Horner syndrome G90.2
  traumatic — *see* Injury, nerve, cervical sympathetic
Claude's disease or syndrome G46.3
Claudicatio venosa intermittens I87.8
Claudication (intermittent) I73.9

Claudication — *continued*
  cerebral (artery) G45.9
  spinal cord (arteriosclerotic) G95.19
    syphilitic A52.09
  venous (axillary) I87.8
Claustrophobia F40.240
Clavus (infected) L84
Clawfoot (congenital) Q66.89
  acquired — *see* Deformity, limb, clawfoot
Clawhand (acquired) — *see also* Deformity, limb, clawhand
  congenital Q68.1
Clawtoe (congenital) Q66.89
  acquired — *see* Deformity, toe, specified NEC
Clay eating — *see* Pica
Cleansing of artificial opening — *see* Attention to, artificial, opening
Cleft (congenital) — *see also* Imperfect, closure
  alveolar process M26.79
  branchial (persistent) Q18.2
    cyst Q18.0
      fistula Q18.0
      sinus Q18.0
  cricoid cartilage, posterior Q31.8
  cyst Q18.0
    fistula Q18.0
    sinus Q18.0
  foot Q72.7 ☑
  hand Q71.6 ☑
  lip (unilateral) Q36.9
    with cleft palate Q37.9
      hard Q37.1
        with soft Q37.5
      soft Q37.3
        with hard Q37.5
      bilateral Q36.0
        with cleft palate Q37.8
          hard Q37.0
            with soft Q37.4
          soft Q37.2
            with hard Q37.4
    median Q36.1
  nose Q30.2
  palate Q35.9
    with cleft lip (unilateral) Q37.9
      bilateral Q37.8
    hard Q35.1
      with
        cleft lip (unilateral) Q37.1
          bilateral Q37.0
        soft Q35.5
          with cleft lip (unilateral) Q37.5
            bilateral Q37.4
    medial Q35.5
    soft Q35.3
      with
        cleft lip (unilateral) Q37.3
          bilateral Q37.2
        hard Q35.5
          with cleft lip (unilateral) Q37.5
            bilateral Q37.4
  penis Q55.69
  scrotum Q55.29
  thyroid cartilage Q31.8
  uvula Q35.7
Cleidocranial dysostosis Q74.0
Cleptomania F63.2
Clicking hip (newborn) R29.4
Climacteric (female) — *see also* Menopause
  arthritis (any site) NEC — *see* Arthritis, specified form NEC
  depression (single episode) F32.89
    recurrent episode F33.8
  male (symptoms) (syndrome) NEC N50.89
  melancholia (single episode) F32.89
    recurrent episode F33.8
  paranoid state F22
  polyarthritis NEC — *see* Arthritis, specified form NEC
  symptoms (female) N95.1
Clinical research investigation (clinical trial) (control subject) (normal comparison) (participant) Z00.6
Clitoris — *see* condition
Cloaca (persistent) Q43.7
Clonorchiasis, clonorchis infection (liver) B66.1
Clonus R25.8
Closed bite M26.29
Clostridium (C.) perfringens, as cause of disease classified elsewhere B96.7

Closure
- congenital, nose Q30.0
- cranial sutures, premature Q75.0
- defective or imperfect NEC — *see* Imperfect, closure
- fistula, delayed — *see* Fistula
- foramen ovale, imperfect Q21.1
- hymen N89.6
- interauricular septum, defective Q21.1
- interventricular septum, defective Q21.0
- lacrimal duct — *see also* Stenosis, lacrimal, duct
  - congenital Q10.5
- nose (congenital) Q30.0
  - acquired M95.0
- of artificial opening — *see* Attention to, artificial, opening
- vagina N89.5
- valve — *see* Endocarditis
- vulva N90.5

Clot (blood) — *see also* Embolism
- artery (obstruction) (occlusion) — *see* Embolism
- bladder N32.89
- brain (intradural or extradural) — *see* Occlusion, artery, cerebral
- circulation I74.9
- heart — *see also* Infarct, myocardium
  - not resulting in infarction I51.3
- vein — *see* Thrombosis

Clouded state R40.1
- epileptic — *see* Epilepsy, specified NEC
- paroxysmal — *see* Epilepsy, specified NEC

Cloudy antrum, antra J32.0

Clouston's (hidrotic) **ectodermal dysplasia** Q82.4

Clubbed nail pachydermoperiostosis M89.40 *[L62]*

Clubbing of finger(s) (nails) R68.3

Clubfinger R68.3
- congenital Q68.1

Clubfoot (congenital) Q66.89
- acquired — *see* Deformity, limb, clubfoot
- equinovarus Q66.0- ☑
- paralytic — *see* Deformity, limb, clubfoot

Clubhand (congenital) (radial) Q71.4- ☑
- acquired — *see* Deformity, limb, clubhand

Clubnail R68.3
- congenital Q84.6

Clump, kidney Q63.1

Clumsiness, clumsy child syndrome F82

Cluttering F80.81

Clutton's joints A50.51 *[M12.80]*

Coagulation, intravascular (diffuse) (disseminated) — *see also* Defibrination syndrome
- complicating abortion — *see* Abortion, by type, complicated by, intravascular coagulation
- following ectopic or molar pregnancy O08.1

Coagulopathy — *see also* Defect, coagulation
- consumption D65
- intravascular D65
  - newborn P60

Coalition
- calcaneo-scaphoid Q66.89
- tarsal Q66.89

Coalminer's
- elbow — *see* Bursitis, elbow, olecranon
- lung or pneumoconiosis J60

Coalworker's lung or pneumoconiosis J60

Coarctation
- aorta (preductal) (postductal) Q25.1
- pulmonary artery Q25.71

Coated tongue K14.3

Coats' disease (exudative retinopathy) — *see* Retinopathy, exudative

Cocaine-induced
- anxiety disorder F14.980
- bipolar and related disorder F14.94
- depressive disorder F14.94
- obsessive-compulsive and related disorder F14.988
- psychotic disorder F14.959
- sexual dysfunction F14.981
- sleep disorder F14.982

Cocainism — *see* Disorder, cocaine use

Coccidioidomycosis B38.9
- cutaneous B38.3
- disseminated B38.7
- generalized B38.7
- meninges B38.4
- prostate B38.81
- pulmonary B38.2
  - acute B38.0

Coccidioidomycosis — *continued*
- pulmonary — *continued*
  - chronic B38.1
- skin B38.3
- specified NEC B38.89

Coccidioidosis — *see* Coccidioidomycosis

Coccidiosis (intestinal) A07.3

Coccydynia, coccygodynia M53.3

Coccyx — *see* condition

Cochin-China diarrhea K90.1

Cockayne's syndrome Q87.19

Cocked up toe — *see* Deformity, toe, specified NEC

Cock's peculiar tumor L72.3

Codman's tumor — *see* Neoplasm, bone, benign

Coenurosis B71.8

Coffee-worker's lung J67.8

Cogan's syndrome H16.32- ☑
- oculomotor apraxia H51.8

Coitus, painful (female) N94.10
- male N53.12
- psychogenic F52.6

Cold J00
- with influenza, flu, or grippe — *see* Influenza, with, respiratory manifestations NEC
- agglutinin disease or hemoglobinuria (chronic) D59.1
- bronchial — *see* Bronchitis
- chest — *see* Bronchitis
- common (head) J00
- effects of T69.9 ☑
  - specified effect NEC T69.8 ☑
- excessive, effects of T69.9 ☑
  - specified effect NEC T69.8 ☑
- exhaustion from T69.8 ☑
- exposure to T69.9 ☑
  - specified effect NEC T69.8 ☑
- head J00
- injury syndrome (newborn) P80.0
- on lung — *see* Bronchitis
- rose J30.1
- sensitivity, auto-immune D59.1
- symptoms J00
- virus J00

Coldsore B00.1

Colibacillosis A49.8
- as the cause of other disease — *see also* Escherichia coli B96.20
- generalized A41.50

Colic (bilious) (infantile) (intestinal) (recurrent) (spasmodic) R10.83
- abdomen R10.83
  - psychogenic F45.8
- appendix, appendicular K38.8
- bile duct — *see* Calculus, bile duct
- biliary — *see* Calculus, bile duct
- common duct — *see* Calculus, bile duct
- cystic duct — *see* Calculus, gallbladder
- Devonshire NEC — *see* Poisoning, lead
- gallbladder — *see* Calculus, gallbladder
- gallstone — *see* Calculus, gallbladder
  - gallbladder or cystic duct — *see* Calculus, gallbladder
- hepatic (duct) — *see* Calculus, bile duct
- hysterical F45.8
- kidney N23
- lead NEC — *see* Poisoning, lead
- mucous K58.9
  - with diarrhea K58.0
  - psychogenic F54
- nephritic N23
- painter's NEC — *see* Poisoning, lead
- pancreas K86.89
- psychogenic F45.8
- renal N23
- saturnine NEC — *see* Poisoning, lead
- ureter N23
- urethral N36.8
  - due to calculus N21.1
- uterus NEC N94.89
  - menstrual — *see* Dysmenorrhea
- worm NOS B83.9

Colicystitis — *see* Cystitis

Colitis (acute) (catarrhal) (chronic) (noninfective) (hemorrhagic) — *see also* Enteritis K52.9
- allergic K52.29
  - with
    - food protein-induced enterocolitis syndrome K52.21

Colitis — *continued*
- allergic — *continued*
  - with — *continued*
    - proctocolitis K52.82
- amebic (acute) — *see also* Amebiasis A06.0
  - nondysenteric A06.2
- anthrax A22.2
- bacillary — *see* Infection, Shigella
- balantidial A07.0
- Clostridium difficile
  - not specified as recurrent A04.72
  - recurrent A04.71
- coccidial A07.3
- collagenous K52.831
- cystica superficialis K52.89
- dietary counseling and surveillance (for) Z71.3
- dietetic — *see also* Colitis, allergic K52.29
- drug-induced K52.1
- due to radiation K52.0
- eosinophilic K52.82
- food hypersensitivity — *see also* Colitis, allergic K52.29
- giardial A07.1
- granulomatous — *see* Enteritis, regional, large intestine
- indeterminate, so stated K52.3
- infectious — *see* Enteritis, infectious
- ischemic K55.9
  - acute (subacute) — *see also* Ischemia, intestine, acute K55.039
  - chronic K55.1
  - due to mesenteric artery insufficiency K55.1
  - fulminant (acute) — *see also* Ischemia, intestine, acute K55.039
- left sided K51.50
  - with
    - abscess K51.514
    - complication K51.519
      - specified NEC K51.518
    - fistula K51.513
    - obstruction K51.512
    - rectal bleeding K51.511
- lymphocytic K52.832
- membranous
  - psychogenic F54
- microscopic K52.839
  - specified NEC K52.838
- mucous — *see* Syndrome, irritable, bowel
  - psychogenic F54
- noninfective K52.9
  - specified NEC K52.89
- polyposa — *see* Polyp, colon, inflammatory
- protozoal A07.9
- pseudomembranous
  - not specified as recurrent A04.72
  - recurrent A04.71
- pseudomucinous — *see* Syndrome, irritable, bowel
- regional — *see* Enteritis, regional, large intestine
  - infectious A09
- segmental — *see* Enteritis, regional, large intestine
- septic — *see* Enteritis, infectious
- spastic K58.9
  - with diarrhea K58.0
  - psychogenic F54
- staphylococcal A04.8
  - foodborne A05.0
- subacute ischemic — *see also* Ischemia, intestine, acute K55.039
- thromboulcerative — *see also* Ischemia, intestine, acute K55.039
- toxic NEC K52.1
  - due to Clostridium difficile
    - not specified as recurrent A04.72
    - recurrent A04.71
- transmural — *see* Enteritis, regional, large intestine
- trichomonal A07.8
- tuberculous (ulcerative) A18.32
- ulcerative (chronic) K51.90
  - with
    - complication K51.919
      - abscess K51.914
      - fistula K51.913
      - obstruction K51.912
      - rectal bleeding K51.911
      - specified complication NEC K51.918
  - enterocolitis — *see* Enterocolitis, ulcerative
  - ileocolitis — *see* Ileocolitis, ulcerative
  - mucosal proctocolitis — *see* Proctocolitis, mucosal
  - proctitis — *see* Proctitis, ulcerative
  - pseudopolyposis — *see* Polyp, colon, inflammatory

☑ **Additional Character Required — Refer to the Tabular List for Character Selection**

🔻 Subterms under main terms may continue to next column or page

Colitis — *continued*
  ulcerative — *continued*
    psychogenic F54
    rectosigmoiditis — *see* Rectosigmoiditis, ulcerative
    specified type NEC K51.80
      with
        complication K51.819
          abscess K51.814
          fistula K51.813
          obstruction K51.812
          rectal bleeding K51.811
          specified complication NEC K51.818
Collagenosis, collagen disease (nonvascular) (vascular)
  M35.9
  cardiovascular I42.8
  reactive perforating L87.1
  specified NEC M35.8
Collapse R55
  adrenal E27.2
  cardiorespiratory R57.0
  cardiovascular R57.0
    newborn P29.89
  circulatory (peripheral) R57.9
    during or after labor and delivery O75.1
    following ectopic or molar pregnancy O08.3
    newborn P29.89
  during or
    after labor and delivery O75.1
    resulting from a procedure, not elsewhere classified
      T81.10 ☑
  external ear canal — *see* Stenosis, external ear canal
  general R55
  heart — *see* Disease, heart
  heat T67.1 ☑
  hysterical F44.89
  labyrinth, membranous (congenital) Q16.5
  lung (massive) — *see also* Atelectasis J98.19
    pressure due to anesthesia (general) (local) or other
      sedation T88.2 ☑
      during labor and delivery O74.1
      in pregnancy O29.02- ☑
      postpartum, puerperal O89.09
  myocardial — *see* Disease, heart
  nervous F48.8
  neurocirculatory F45.8
  nose M95.0
  postoperative T81.10 ☑
  pulmonary — *see also* Atelectasis J98.19
    newborn — *see* Atelectasis
  trachea J39.8
  tracheobronchial J98.09
  valvular — *see* Endocarditis
  vascular (peripheral) R57.9
    during or after labor and delivery O75.1
    following ectopic or molar pregnancy O08.3
    newborn P29.89
  vertebra M48.50- ☑
    cervical region M48.52- ☑
    cervicothoracic region M48.53- ☑
    in (due to)
      metastasis — *see* Collapse, vertebra, in, specified
        disease NEC
      osteoporosis — *see also* Osteoporosis M80.88 ☑
        cervical region M80.88 ☑
        cervicothoracic region M80.88 ☑
        lumbar region M80.88 ☑
        lumbosacral region M80.88 ☑
        multiple sites M80.88 ☑
        occipito-atlanto-axial region M80.88 ☑
        sacrococcygeal region M80.88 ☑
        thoracic region M80.88 ☑
        thoracolumbar region M80.88 ☑
      specified disease NEC M48.50- ☑
        cervical region M48.52- ☑
        cervicothoracic region M48.53- ☑
        lumbar region M48.56- ☑
        lumbosacral region M48.57- ☑
        occipito-atlanto-axial region M48.51- ☑
        sacrococcygeal region M48.58- ☑
        thoracic region M48.54- ☑
        thoracolumbar region M48.55- ☑
    lumbar region M48.56- ☑
    lumbosacral region M48.57- ☑
    occipito-atlanto-axial region M48.51- ☑
    sacrococcygeal region M48.58- ☑
    thoracic region M48.54- ☑
    thoracolumbar region M48.55- ☑

Collateral — *see also* condition
  circulation (venous) I87.8
  dilation, veins I87.8
Colles' fracture S52.53- ☑
Collet (-Sicard) syndrome G52.7
Collier's asthma or lung J60
Collodion baby Q80.2
Colloid nodule (of thyroid) (cystic) E04.1
Coloboma (iris) Q13.0
  eyelid Q10.3
  fundus Q14.8
  lens Q12.2
  optic disc (congenital) Q14.2
    acquired H47.31- ☑
Coloenteritis — *see* Enteritis
Colon — *see* condition
Colonization
  MRSA (Methicillin resistant Staphylococcus aureus)
    Z22.322
  MSSA (Methicillin susceptible Staphylococcus aureus)
    Z22.321
  status — *see* Carrier (suspected) of
Coloptosis K63.4
Color blindness — *see* Deficiency, color vision
Colostomy
  attention to Z43.3
  fitting or adjustment Z46.89
  malfunctioning K94.03
  status Z93.3
Colpitis (acute) — *see* Vaginitis
Colpocele N81.5
Colpocystitis — *see* Vaginitis
Colpospasm N94.2
Column, spinal, vertebral — *see* condition
Coma R40.20
  with
    motor response (none) R40.231 ☑
      abnormal extensor posturing to pain or noxious
        stimuli (< 2 years of age) R40.232 ☑
      abnormal flexure posturing to pain or noxious
        stimuli (0-5 years of age) R40.233 ☑
      extensor posturing to pain or noxious stimuli (2-
        5 years of age) R40.232 ☑
      flexion/decorticate posturing (< 2 years of age)
        R40.233 ☑
      localizes pain (2-5 years of age) R40.235 ☑
      normal or spontaneous movement (< 2 years of
        age) R40.236 ☑
      obeys commands (2-5 years of age) R40.236 ☑
      score of
        1 R40.231 ☑
        2 R40.232 ☑
        3 R40.233 ☑
        4 R40.234 ☑
        5 R40.235 ☑
        6 R40.236 ☑
      withdraws from pain or noxious stimuli (0-5 years
        of age) R40.234 ☑
      withdraws to touch (< 2 years of age) R40.235 ☑
    opening of eyes (never) R40.211 ☑
      in response to
        pain R40.212 ☑
        sound R40.213 ☑
      score of
        1 R40.211 ☑
        2 R40.212 ☑
        3 R40.213 ☑
        4 R40.214 ☑
      spontaneous R40.214 ☑
    verbal response (none) R40.221 ☑
      confused conversation R40.224 ☑
      cooing or babbling or crying appropriately (<2
        years of age) R40.225 ☑
      inappropriate crying or screaming (< 2 years of
        age) R40.223 ☑
      inappropriate words (2-5 years of age)
        R40.224 ☑
      incomprehensible sounds (2-5 years of age)
        R40.222 ☑
      incomprehensible words R40.222 ☑
      irritable cries (< 2 years of age) R40.224 ☑
      moans/grunts to pain; restless (< 2 years old)
        R40.222 ☑
      oriented R40.225 ☑
      score of
        1 R40.221 ☑
        2 R40.222 ☑

Coma — *continued*
  with — *continued*
    verbal response — *continued*
      score of — *continued*
        3 R40.223 ☑
        4 R40.224 ☑
        5 R40.225 ☑
      screaming (2-5 years of age) R40.223 ☑
      uses appropriate words (2-5 years of age)
        R40.225 ☑
  eclamptic — *see* Eclampsia
  epileptic — *see* Epilepsy
  Glasgow, scale score — *see* Glasgow coma scale
  hepatic — *see* Failure, hepatic, by type, with coma
  hyperglycemic (diabetic) — *see* Diabetes, by type, with
    hyperosmolarity, with coma
  hyperosmolar (diabetic) — *see* Diabetes, by type, with
    hyperosmolarity, with coma
  hypoglycemic (diabetic) — *see* Diabetes, by type, with
    hypoglycemia, with coma
    nondiabetic E15
  in diabetes — *see* Diabetes, coma
  insulin-induced — *see* Coma, hypoglycemic
  ketoacidotic (diabetic) — *see* Diabetes, by type, with
    ketoacidosis, with coma
  myxedematous E03.5
  newborn P91.5
  persistent vegetative state R40.3
  specified NEC, without documented Glasgow coma
    scale score, or with partial Glasgow coma scale
    score reported R40.244 ☑
Comatose — *see* Coma
Combat fatigue F43.0
Combined — *see* condition
Comedo, comedones (giant) L70.0
Comedocarcinoma — *see also* Neoplasm, breast, malignant
  noninfiltrating
    breast D05.8- ☑
    specified site — *see* Neoplasm, in situ, by site
    unspecified site D05.8- ☑
Comedomastitis — *see* Ectasia, mammary duct
Comminuted fracture — *code as* Fracture, closed
Common
  arterial trunk Q20.0
  atrioventricular canal Q21.2
  atrium Q21.1
  cold (head) J00
  truncus (arteriosus) Q20.0
  variable immunodeficiency — *see* Immunodeficiency,
    common variable
  ventricle Q20.4
Commotio, commotion (current)
  brain — *see* Injury, intracranial, concussion
  cerebri — *see* Injury, intracranial, concussion
  retinae S05.8X- ☑
  spinal cord — *see* Injury, spinal cord, by region
  spinalis — *see* Injury, spinal cord, by region
Communication
  between
    base of aorta and pulmonary artery Q21.4
    left ventricle and right atrium Q20.5
    pericardial sac and pleural sac Q34.8
    pulmonary artery and pulmonary vein, congenital
      Q25.72
  congenital between uterus and digestive or urinary
    tract Q51.7
Compartment syndrome (deep) (posterior) (traumatic)
  T79.A0 ☑ (*following* T79.7)
  abdomen T79.A3 ☑ (*following* T79.7)
  lower extremity (hip, buttock, thigh, leg, foot, toes)
    T79.A2 ☑ (*following* T79.7)
  nontraumatic
    abdomen M79.A3 (*following* M79.7)
    lower extremity (hip, buttock, thigh, leg, foot, toes)
      M79.A2- ☑ (*following* M79.7)
    specified site NEC M79.A9 (*following* M79.7)
    upper extremity (shoulder, arm, forearm, wrist,
      hand, fingers) M79.A1- ☑ (*following* M79.7)
  specified site NEC T79.A9 ☑ (*following* T79.7)
  upper extremity (shoulder, arm, forearm, wrist, hand,
    fingers) T79.A1- ☑ (*following* T79.7)
Compensation
  failure — *see* Disease, heart
  neurosis, psychoneurosis — *see* Disorder, factitious
Complaint — *see also* Disease
  bowel, functional K59.9

Complaint — *continued*
  bowel, functional — *continued*
    psychogenic F45.8
    intestine, functional K59.9
      psychogenic F45.8
  kidney — *see* Disease, renal
  miners' J60
Complete — *see* condition
Complex
  Addison-Schilder E71.528
  cardiorenal — *see* Hypertension, cardiorenal
  Costen's M26.69
  disseminated mycobacterium avium- intracellulare
    (DMAC) A31.2
  Eisenmenger's (ventricular septal defect) I27.83
  hypersexual F52.8
  jumped process, spine — *see* Dislocation, vertebra
  primary, tuberculous A15.7
  Schilder-Addison E71.528
  subluxation (vertebral) M99.19
    abdomen M99.19
    acromioclavicular M99.17
    cervical region M99.11
    cervicothoracic M99.11
    costochondral M99.18
    costovertebral M99.18
    head region M99.10
    hip M99.15
    lower extremity M99.16
    lumbar region M99.13
    lumbosacral M99.13
    occipitocervical M99.10
    pelvic region M99.15
    pubic M99.15
    rib cage M99.18
    sacral region M99.14
    sacrococcygeal M99.14
    sacroiliac M99.14
    specified NEC M99.19
    sternochondral M99.18
    sternoclavicular M99.17
    thoracic region M99.12
    thoracolumbar M99.12
    upper extremity M99.17
  Taussig-Bing (transposition, aorta and overriding pulmonary artery) Q20.1
Complication(s) (from) (of)
  accidental puncture or laceration during a procedure (of) — *see* Complications, intraoperative (intraprocedural), puncture or laceration
  amputation stump (surgical) (late) NEC T87.9
    dehiscence T87.81
    infection or inflammation T87.40
      lower limb T87.4- ☑
      upper limb T87.4- ☑
    necrosis T87.50
      lower limb T87.5- ☑
      upper limb T87.5- ☑
    neuroma T87.30
      lower limb T87.3- ☑
      upper limb T87.3- ☑
    specified type NEC T87.89
  anastomosis (and bypass) — *see also* Complications, prosthetic device or implant
    intestinal (internal) NEC K91.89
      involving urinary tract N99.89
    urinary tract (involving intestinal tract) N99.89
    vascular — *see* Complications, cardiovascular device or implant
  anesthesia, anesthetic — *see also* Anesthesia, complication T88.59
    brain, postpartum, puerperal O89.2
    cardiac
      in
        labor and delivery O74.2
        pregnancy O29.19- ☑
      postpartum, puerperal O89.1
    central nervous system
      in
        labor and delivery O74.3
        pregnancy O29.29- ☑
      postpartum, puerperal O89.2
    difficult or failed intubation T88.4 ☑
      in pregnancy O29.6- ☑
    failed sedation (conscious) (moderate) during procedure T88.52 ☑
    general, unintended awareness during procedure T88.53 ☑

Complication(s) — *continued*
  anesthesia, anesthetic — *see also* Anesthesia, complication — *continued*
    hyperthermia, malignant T88.3 ☑
    hypothermia T88.51 ☑
    intubation failure T88.4 ☑
    malignant hyperthermia T88.3 ☑
    pulmonary
      in
        labor and delivery O74.1
        pregnancy NEC O29.09- ☑
      postpartum, puerperal O89.09
    shock T88.2 ☑
    spinal and epidural
      in
        labor and delivery NEC O74.6
          headache O74.5
        pregnancy NEC O29.5X- ☑
      postpartum, puerperal NEC O89.5
        headache O89.4
    unintended awareness under general anesthesia
      during procedure T88.53 ☑
  anti-reflux device — *see* Complications, esophageal anti-reflux device
  aortic (bifurcation) graft — *see* Complications, graft, vascular
  aortocoronary (bypass) graft — *see* Complications, coronary artery (bypass) graft
  aortofemoral (bypass) graft — *see* Complications, extremity artery (bypass) graft
  arteriovenous
    fistula, surgically created T82.9 ☑
      embolism T82.818 ☑
      fibrosis T82.828 ☑
      hemorrhage T82.838 ☑
      infection or inflammation T82.7 ☑
      mechanical
        breakdown T82.510 ☑
        displacement T82.520 ☑
        leakage T82.530 ☑
        malposition T82.520 ☑
        obstruction T82.590 ☑
        perforation T82.590 ☑
        protrusion T82.590 ☑
      pain T82.848 ☑
      specified type NEC T82.898 ☑
      stenosis T82.858 ☑
      thrombosis T82.868 ☑
    shunt, surgically created T82.9 ☑
      embolism T82.818 ☑
      fibrosis T82.828 ☑
      hemorrhage T82.838 ☑
      infection or inflammation T82.7 ☑
      mechanical
        breakdown T82.511 ☑
        displacement T82.521 ☑
        leakage T82.531 ☑
        malposition T82.521 ☑
        obstruction T82.591 ☑
        perforation T82.591 ☑
        protrusion T82.591 ☑
      pain T82.848 ☑
      specified type NEC T82.898 ☑
      stenosis T82.858 ☑
      thrombosis T82.868 ☑
  arthroplasty — *see* Complications, joint prosthesis
  artificial
    fertilization or insemination N98.9
      attempted introduction (of)
        embryo in embryo transfer N98.3
        ovum following in vitro fertilization N98.2
      hyperstimulation of ovaries N98.1
      infection N98.0
      specified NEC N98.8
    heart T82.9 ☑
      embolism T82.817 ☑
      fibrosis T82.827 ☑
      hemorrhage T82.837 ☑
      infection or inflammation T82.7 ☑
      mechanical
        breakdown T82.512 ☑
        displacement T82.522 ☑
        leakage T82.532 ☑
        malposition T82.522 ☑
        obstruction T82.592 ☑
        perforation T82.592 ☑

Complication(s) — *continued*
  artificial — *continued*
    heart — *continued*
      mechanical — *continued*
        protrusion T82.592 ☑
      pain T82.847 ☑
      specified type NEC T82.897 ☑
      stenosis T82.857 ☑
      thrombosis T82.867 ☑
    opening
      cecostomy — *see* Complications, colostomy
      colostomy — *see* Complications, colostomy
      cystostomy — *see* Complications, cystostomy
      enterostomy — *see* Complications, enterostomy
      gastrostomy — *see* Complications, gastrostomy
      ileostomy — *see* Complications, enterostomy
      jejunostomy — *see* Complications, enterostomy
      nephrostomy — *see* Complications, stoma, urinary tract
      tracheostomy — *see* Complications, tracheostomy
      ureterostomy — *see* Complications, stoma, urinary tract
      urethrostomy — *see* Complications, stoma, urinary tract
  balloon implant or device
    gastrointestinal T85.9 ☑
      embolism T85.818 ☑
      fibrosis T85.828 ☑
      hemorrhage T85.838 ☑
      infection and inflammation T85.79 ☑
      pain T85.848 ☑
      specified type NEC T85.898 ☑
      stenosis T85.858 ☑
      thrombosis T85.868 ☑
    vascular (counterpulsation) T82.9 ☑
      embolism T82.818 ☑
      fibrosis T82.828 ☑
      hemorrhage T82.838 ☑
      infection or inflammation T82.7 ☑
      mechanical
        breakdown T82.513 ☑
        displacement T82.523 ☑
        leakage T82.533 ☑
        malposition T82.523 ☑
        obstruction T82.593 ☑
        perforation T82.593 ☑
        protrusion T82.593 ☑
      pain T82.848 ☑
      specified type NEC T82.898 ☑
      stenosis T82.858 ☑
      thrombosis T82.868 ☑
  bariatric procedure
    gastric band procedure K95.09
      infection K95.01
    specified procedure NEC K95.89
      infection K95.81
  bile duct implant (prosthetic) T85.9 ☑
    embolism T85.818 ☑
    fibrosis T85.828 ☑
    hemorrhage T85.838 ☑
    infection and inflammation T85.79 ☑
    mechanical
      breakdown T85.510 ☑
      displacement T85.520 ☑
      malfunction T85.510 ☑
      malposition T85.520 ☑
      obstruction T85.590 ☑
      perforation T85.590 ☑
      protrusion T85.590 ☑
      specified NEC T85.590 ☑
    pain T85.848 ☑
    specified type NEC T85.898 ☑
    stenosis T85.858 ☑
    thrombosis T85.868 ☑
  bladder device (auxiliary) — *see* Complications, genitourinary, device or implant, urinary system
  bleeding (postoperative) — *see* Complication, postoperative, hemorrhage
    intraoperative — *see* Complication, intraoperative, hemorrhage
  blood vessel graft — *see* Complications, graft, vascular
  bone
    device NEC T84.9 ☑
      embolism T84.81 ☑
      fibrosis T84.82 ☑

Complication(s) — *continued*
- bone — *continued*
  - device — *continued*
    - hemorrhage T84.83 ☑
    - infection or inflammation T84.7 ☑
    - mechanical
      - breakdown T84.318 ☑
      - displacement T84.328 ☑
      - malposition T84.328 ☑
      - obstruction T84.398 ☑
      - perforation T84.398 ☑
      - protrusion T84.398 ☑
    - pain T84.84 ☑
    - specified type NEC T84.89 ☑
    - stenosis T84.85 ☑
    - thrombosis T84.86 ☑
  - graft — *see* Complications, graft, bone
  - growth stimulator (electrode) — *see* Complications, electronic stimulator device, bone
  - marrow transplant — *see* Complications, transplant, bone, marrow
- brain neurostimulator (electrode) — *see* Complications, electronic stimulator device, brain
- breast implant (prosthetic) T85.9 ☑
  - capsular contracture T85.44 ☑
  - embolism T85.818 ☑
  - fibrosis T85.828 ☑
  - hemorrhage T85.838 ☑
  - infection and inflammation T85.79 ☑
  - mechanical
    - breakdown T85.41 ☑
    - displacement T85.42 ☑
    - leakage T85.43 ☑
    - malposition T85.42 ☑
    - obstruction T85.49 ☑
    - perforation T85.49 ☑
    - protrusion T85.49 ☑
    - specified NEC T85.49 ☑
  - pain T85.848 ☑
  - specified type NEC T85.898 ☑
  - stenosis T85.858 ☑
  - thrombosis T85.868 ☑
- bypass — *see also* Complications, prosthetic device or implant
  - aortocoronary — *see* Complications, coronary artery (bypass) graft
  - arterial — *see also* Complications, graft, vascular
    - extremity — *see* Complications, extremity artery (bypass) graft
- cardiac — *see also* Disease, heart
  - device, implant or graft T82.9 ☑
    - embolism T82.817 ☑
    - fibrosis T82.827 ☑
    - hemorrhage T82.837 ☑
    - infection or inflammation T82.7 ☑
      - valve prosthesis T82.6 ☑
    - mechanical
      - breakdown T82.519 ☑
        - specified device NEC T82.518 ☑
      - displacement T82.529 ☑
        - specified device NEC T82.528 ☑
      - leakage T82.539 ☑
        - specified device NEC T82.538 ☑
      - malposition T82.529 ☑
        - specified device NEC T82.528 ☑
      - obstruction T82.599 ☑
        - specified device NEC T82.598 ☑
      - perforation T82.599 ☑
        - specified device NEC T82.598 ☑
      - protrusion T82.599 ☑
        - specified device NEC T82.598 ☑
    - pain T82.847 ☑
    - specified type NEC T82.897 ☑
    - stenosis T82.857 ☑
    - thrombosis T82.867 ☑
- cardiovascular device, graft or implant T82.9 ☑
  - aortic graft — *see* Complications, graft, vascular
  - arteriovenous
    - fistula, artificial — *see* Complication, arteriovenous, fistula, surgically created
    - shunt — *see* Complication, arteriovenous, shunt, surgically created
  - artificial heart — *see* Complication, artificial, heart
  - balloon (counterpulsation) device — *see* Complication, balloon implant, vascular

Complication(s) — *continued*
- cardiovascular device, graft or implant — *continued*
  - carotid artery graft — *see* Complications, graft, vascular
  - coronary bypass graft — *see* Complication, coronary artery (bypass) graft
  - dialysis catheter (vascular) — *see* Complication, catheter, dialysis
  - electronic T82.9 ☑
    - electrode T82.9 ☑
      - embolism T82.817 ☑
      - fibrosis T82.827 ☑
      - hemorrhage T82.837 ☑
      - infection T82.7 ☑
      - mechanical
        - breakdown T82.110 ☑
        - displacement T82.120 ☑
        - leakage T82.190 ☑
        - obstruction T82.190 ☑
        - perforation T82.190 ☑
        - protrusion T82.190 ☑
        - specified type NEC T82.190 ☑
      - pain T82.847 ☑
      - specified NEC T82.897 ☑
      - stenosis T82.857 ☑
      - thrombosis T82.867 ☑
    - embolism T82.817 ☑
    - fibrosis T82.827 ☑
    - hemorrhage T82.837 ☑
    - infection T82.7 ☑
    - mechanical
      - breakdown T82.119 ☑
      - displacement T82.129 ☑
      - leakage T82.199 ☑
      - obstruction T82.199 ☑
      - perforation T82.199 ☑
      - protrusion T82.199 ☑
      - specified type NEC T82.199 ☑
    - pain T82.847 ☑
    - pulse generator T82.9 ☑
      - embolism T82.817 ☑
      - fibrosis T82.827 ☑
      - hemorrhage T82.837 ☑
      - infection T82.7 ☑
      - mechanical
        - breakdown T82.111 ☑
        - displacement T82.121 ☑
        - leakage T82.191 ☑
        - obstruction T82.191 ☑
        - perforation T82.191 ☑
        - protrusion T82.191 ☑
        - specified type NEC T82.191 ☑
      - pain T82.847 ☑
      - specified NEC T82.897 ☑
      - stenosis T82.857 ☑
      - thrombosis T82.867 ☑
    - specified condition NEC T82.897 ☑
    - specified device NEC T82.9 ☑
      - embolism T82.817 ☑
      - fibrosis T82.827 ☑
      - hemorrhage T82.837 ☑
      - infection T82.7 ☑
      - mechanical
        - breakdown T82.118 ☑
        - displacement T82.128 ☑
        - leakage T82.198 ☑
        - obstruction T82.198 ☑
        - perforation T82.198 ☑
        - protrusion T82.198 ☑
        - specified type NEC T82.198 ☑
      - pain T82.847 ☑
      - specified NEC T82.897 ☑
      - stenosis T82.857 ☑
      - thrombosis T82.867 ☑
    - stenosis T82.857 ☑
    - thrombosis T82.867 ☑
  - extremity artery graft — *see* Complication, extremity artery (bypass) graft
  - femoral artery graft — *see* Complication, extremity artery (bypass) graft
  - heart
    - transplant — *see* Complication, transplant, heart
    - valve — *see* Complication, prosthetic device, heart valve
      - graft — *see* Complication, heart, valve, graft

Complication(s) — *continued*
- cardiovascular device, graft or implant — *continued*
  - heart-lung transplant — *see* Complication, transplant, heart, with lung
  - infection or inflammation T82.7 ☑
  - umbrella device — *see* Complication, umbrella device, vascular
  - vascular graft (or anastomosis) — *see* Complication, graft, vascular
- carotid artery (bypass) graft — *see* Complications, graft, vascular
- catheter (device) NEC — *see also* Complications, prosthetic device or implant
  - cranial infusion
    - infection and inflammation T85.735 ☑
    - mechanical
      - breakdown T85.610 ☑
      - displacement T85.620 ☑
      - leakage T85.630 ☑
      - malfunction T85.690 ☑
      - malposition T85.620 ☑
      - obstruction T85.690 ☑
      - perforation T85.690 ☑
      - protrusion T85.690 ☑
      - specified NEC T85.690 ☑
  - cystostomy T83.9 ☑
    - embolism T83.81 ☑
    - fibrosis T83.82 ☑
    - hemorrhage T83.83 ☑
    - infection and inflammation T83.510 ☑
    - mechanical
      - breakdown T83.010 ☑
      - displacement T83.020 ☑
      - leakage T83.030 ☑
      - malposition T83.020 ☑
      - obstruction T83.090 ☑
      - perforation T83.090 ☑
      - protrusion T83.090 ☑
      - specified NEC T83.090 ☑
    - pain T83.84 ☑
    - specified type NEC T83.89 ☑
    - stenosis T83.85 ☑
    - thrombosis T83.86 ☑
  - dialysis (vascular) T82.9 ☑
    - embolism T82.818 ☑
    - fibrosis T82.828 ☑
    - hemorrhage T82.838 ☑
    - infection and inflammation T82.7 ☑
    - intraperitoneal — *see* Complications, catheter, intraperitoneal
    - mechanical
      - breakdown T82.41 ☑
      - displacement T82.42 ☑
      - leakage T82.43 ☑
      - malposition T82.42 ☑
      - obstruction T82.49 ☑
      - perforation T82.49 ☑
      - protrusion T82.49 ☑
    - pain T82.848 ☑
    - specified type NEC T82.898 ☑
    - stenosis T82.858 ☑
    - thrombosis T82.868 ☑
  - epidural infusion T85.9 ☑
    - embolism T85.810 ☑
    - fibrosis T85.820 ☑
    - hemorrhage T85.830 ☑
    - infection and inflammation T85.735 ☑
    - mechanical
      - breakdown T85.610 ☑
      - displacement T85.620 ☑
      - leakage T85.630 ☑
      - malfunction T85.610 ☑
      - malposition T85.620 ☑
      - obstruction T85.690 ☑
      - perforation T85.690 ☑
      - protrusion T85.690 ☑
      - specified NEC T85.690 ☑
    - pain T85.840 ☑
    - specified type NEC T85.890 ☑
    - stenosis T85.850 ☑
    - thrombosis T85.860 ☑
  - intraperitoneal dialysis T85.9 ☑
    - embolism T85.818 ☑
    - fibrosis T85.828 ☑
    - hemorrhage T85.838 ☑
    - infection and inflammation T85.71 ☑

⬙ **Subterms under main terms may continue to next column or page**   ☑ **Additional Character Required — Refer to the Tabular List for Character Selection**   59

Complication — Complication

Complication(s) — *continued*
  catheter — *see also* Complications, prosthetic device or implant — *continued*
    intraperitoneal dialysis — *continued*
      mechanical
        breakdown T85.611 ☑
        displacement T85.621 ☑
        leakage T85.631 ☑
        malfunction T85.611 ☑
        malposition T85.621 ☑
        obstruction T85.691 ☑
        perforation T85.691 ☑
        protrusion T85.691 ☑
        specified NEC T85.691 ☑
      pain T85.848 ☑
      specified type NEC T85.898 ☑
      stenosis T85.858 ☑
      thrombosis T85.868 ☑
    intrathecal infusion
      infection and inflammation T85.735 ☑
      mechanical
        breakdown T85.610 ☑
        displacement T85.620 ☑
        leakage T85.630 ☑
        malfunction T85.690 ☑
        malposition T85.620 ☑
        obstruction T85.690 ☑
        perforation T85.690 ☑
        protrusion T85.690 ☑
        specified NEC T85.690 ☑
    intravenous infusion T82.9 ☑
      embolism T82.818 ☑
      fibrosis T82.828 ☑
      hemorrhage T82.838 ☑
      infection or inflammation T82.7 ☑
      mechanical
        breakdown T82.514 ☑
        displacement T82.524 ☑
        leakage T82.534 ☑
        malposition T82.524 ☑
        obstruction T82.594 ☑
        perforation T82.594 ☑
        protrusion T82.594 ☑
      pain T82.848 ☑
      specified type NEC T82.898 ☑
      stenosis T82.858 ☑
      thrombosis T82.868 ☑
    spinal infusion
      infection and inflammation T85.735 ☑
      mechanical
        breakdown T85.610 ☑
        displacement T85.620 ☑
        leakage T85.630 ☑
        malfunction T85.690 ☑
        malposition T85.620 ☑
        obstruction T85.690 ☑
        perforation T85.690 ☑
        protrusion T85.690 ☑
        specified NEC T85.690 ☑
    subarachnoid infusion
      infection and inflammation T85.735 ☑
      mechanical
        breakdown T85.610 ☑
        displacement T85.620 ☑
        leakage T85.630 ☑
        malfunction T85.690 ☑
        malposition T85.620 ☑
        obstruction T85.690 ☑
        perforation T85.690 ☑
        protrusion T85.690 ☑
        specified NEC T85.690 ☑
    subdural infusion T85.9 ☑
      embolism T85.810 ☑
      fibrosis T85.820 ☑
      hemorrhage T85.830 ☑
      infection and inflammation T85.735 ☑
      mechanical
        breakdown T85.610 ☑
        displacement T85.620 ☑
        leakage T85.630 ☑
        malfunction T85.610 ☑
        malposition T85.620 ☑
        obstruction T85.690 ☑
        perforation T85.690 ☑
        protrusion T85.690 ☑
        specified NEC T85.690 ☑

Complication(s) — *continued*
  catheter — *see also* Complications, prosthetic device or implant — *continued*
    subdural infusion — *continued*
      pain T85.840 ☑
      specified type NEC T85.890 ☑
      stenosis T85.850 ☑
      thrombosis T85.860 ☑
    urethral T83.9 ☑
      displacement T83.028 ☑
      embolism T83.81 ☑
      fibrosis T83.82 ☑
      hemorrhage T83.83 ☑
      indwelling
        breakdown T83.011 ☑
        displacement T83.021 ☑
        infection and inflammation T83.511 ☑
        leakage T83.031 ☑
        specified complication NEC T83.091 ☑
      infection and inflammation T83.511 ☑
      leakage T83.038 ☑
      malposition T83.028 ☑
      mechanical
        breakdown T83.011 ☑
      obstruction (mechanical) T83.091 ☑
      pain T83.84 ☑
      perforation T83.091 ☑
      protrusion T83.091 ☑
      specified type NEC T83.091 ☑
      stenosis T83.85 ☑
      thrombosis T83.86 ☑
    urinary NEC
      breakdown T83.018 ☑
      displacement T83.028 ☑
      infection and inflammation T83.518 ☑
      leakage T83.038 ☑
      specified complication NEC T83.098 ☑
  cecostomy (stoma) — *see* Complications, colostomy
  cesarean delivery wound NEC O90.89
    disruption O90.0
    hematoma O90.2
    infection (following delivery) O86.00
  chemotherapy (antineoplastic) NEC T88.7 ☑
  chin implant (prosthetic) — *see* Complication, prosthetic device or implant, specified NEC
  circulatory system I99.8
    intraoperative I97.88
    postprocedural I97.89
      following cardiac surgery — *see also* Infarct, myocardium, associated with revascularization procedure I97.19- ☑
        postcardiotomy syndrome I97.0
      hypertension I97.3
      lymphedema after mastectomy I97.2
      postcardiotomy syndrome I97.0
      specified NEC I97.89
  colostomy (stoma) K94.00
    hemorrhage K94.01
    infection K94.02
    malfunction K94.03
    mechanical K94.03
    specified complication NEC K94.09
  contraceptive device, intrauterine — *see* Complications, intrauterine, contraceptive device
  cord (umbilical) — *see* Complications, umbilical cord
  corneal graft — *see* Complications, graft, cornea
  coronary artery (bypass) graft T82.9 ☑
    atherosclerosis — *see* Arteriosclerosis, coronary (artery),
    embolism T82.818 ☑
    fibrosis T82.828 ☑
    hemorrhage T82.838 ☑
    infection and inflammation T82.7 ☑
    mechanical
      breakdown T82.211 ☑
      displacement T82.212 ☑
      leakage T82.213 ☑
      malposition T82.212 ☑
      obstruction T82.218 ☑
      perforation T82.218 ☑
      protrusion T82.218 ☑
      specified NEC T82.218 ☑
    pain T82.848 ☑
    specified type NEC T82.898 ☑
    stenosis T82.858 ☑
    thrombosis T82.868 ☑

Complication(s) — *continued*
  counterpulsation device (balloon), intra- aortic — *see* Complications, balloon implant, vascular
  cystostomy (stoma) N99.518
    catheter — *see* Complications, catheter, cystostomy
    hemorrhage N99.510
    infection N99.511
    malfunction N99.512
    specified type NEC N99.518
  delivery — *see also* Complications, obstetric O75.9
    procedure (instrumental) (manual) (surgical) O75.4
    specified NEC O75.89
  dialysis (peritoneal) (renal) — *see also* Complications, infusion
    catheter (vascular) — *see* Complication, catheter, dialysis
    peritoneal, intraperitoneal — *see* Complications, catheter, intraperitoneal
  dorsal column (spinal) neurostimulator — *see* Complications, electronic stimulator device, spinal cord
  drug NEC T88.7 ☑
  ear procedure — *see also* Disorder, ear
    intraoperative H95.88
      hematoma — *see* Complications, intraoperative, hemorrhage (hematoma) (of), ear
      hemorrhage — *see* Complications, intraoperative, hemorrhage (hematoma) (of), ear
      laceration — *see* Complications, intraoperative, puncture or laceration..., ear
      specified NEC H95.88
    postoperative H95.89
      external ear canal stenosis H95.81- ☑
      hematoma — *see* Complications, postprocedural, hematoma (of), ear
      hemorrhage — *see* Complications, postprocedural, hemorrhage (of), ear
      postmastoidectomy — *see* Complications, postmastoidectomy
      seroma — *see* Complications, postprocedural, seroma (of), mastoid process
      specified NEC H95.89
  ectopic pregnancy O08.9
    damage to pelvic organs O08.6
    embolism O08.2
    genital infection O08.0
    hemorrhage (delayed) (excessive) O08.1
    metabolic disorder O08.5
    renal failure O08.4
    shock O08.3
    specified type NEC O08.0
    venous complication NEC O08.7
  electronic stimulator device
    bladder (urinary) — *see* Complications, electronic stimulator device, urinary
    bone T84.9 ☑
      breakdown T84.310 ☑
      displacement T84.320 ☑
      embolism T84.81 ☑
      fibrosis T84.82 ☑
      hemorrhage T84.83 ☑
      infection or inflammation T84.7 ☑
      malfunction T84.310 ☑
      malposition T84.320 ☑
      mechanical NEC T84.390 ☑
      obstruction T84.390 ☑
      pain T84.84 ☑
      perforation T84.390 ☑
      protrusion T84.390 ☑
      specified type NEC T84.89 ☑
      stenosis T84.85 ☑
      thrombosis T84.86 ☑
    brain T85.9 ☑
      embolism T85.810 ☑
      fibrosis T85.820 ☑
      hemorrhage T85.830 ☑
      infection and inflammation T85.731 ☑
      mechanical
        breakdown T85.110 ☑
        displacement T85.120 ☑
        leakage T85.190 ☑
        malposition T85.120 ☑
        obstruction T85.190 ☑
        perforation T85.190 ☑
        protrusion T85.190 ☑
        specified NEC T85.190 ☑
      pain T85.840 ☑
      specified type NEC T85.890 ☑

☑ **Additional Character Required — Refer to the Tabular List for Character Selection**   ▽ **Subterms under main terms may continue to next column or page**

Complication — Complication

Complication(s) — *continued*
  electronic stimulator device — *continued*
    brain — *continued*
      stenosis T85.850 ☑
      thrombosis T85.860 ☑
    cardiac (defibrillator) (pacemaker) — *see* Complications, cardiovascular device or implant, electronic
    generator (brain) (gastric) (peripheral) (sacral) (spinal)
      breakdown T85.113 ☑
      displacement T85.123 ☑
      leakage T85.193 ☑
      malposition T85.123 ☑
      obstruction T85.193 ☑
      perforation T85.193 ☑
      protrusion T85.193 ☑
      specified type NEC T85.193 ☑
    muscle T84.9 ☑
      breakdown T84.418 ☑
      displacement T84.428 ☑
      embolism T84.81 ☑
      fibrosis T84.82 ☑
      hemorrhage T84.83 ☑
      infection or inflammation T84.7 ☑
      mechanical NEC T84.498 ☑
      pain T84.84 ☑
      specified type NEC T84.89 ☑
      stenosis T84.85 ☑
      thrombosis T84.86 ☑
    nervous system T85.9 ☑
      brain — *see* Complications, electronic stimulator device, brain
      cranial nerve — *see* Complications, electronic stimulator device, peripheral nerve
      embolism T85.810 ☑
      fibrosis T85.820 ☑
      gastric nerve — *see* Complications, electronic stimulator device, peripheral nerve
      hemorrhage T85.830 ☑
      infection and inflammation T85.738 ☑
      mechanical
        breakdown T85.118 ☑
        displacement T85.128 ☑
        leakage T85.199 ☑
        malposition T85.128 ☑
        obstruction T85.199 ☑
        perforation T85.199 ☑
        protrusion T85.199 ☑
        specified NEC T85.199 ☑
      pain T85.840 ☑
      peripheral nerve — *see* Complications, electronic stimulator device, peripheral nerve
      sacral nerve — *see* Complications, electronic stimulator device, peripheral nerve
      specified type NEC T85.890 ☑
      spinal cord — *see* Complications, electronic stimulator device, spinal cord
      stenosis T85.850 ☑
      thrombosis T85.860 ☑
      vagal nerve — *see* Complications, electronic stimulator device, peripheral nerve
    peripheral nerve T85.9 ☑
      embolism T85.810 ☑
      fibrosis T85.820 ☑
      hemorrhage T85.830 ☑
      infection and inflammation T85.732 ☑
      mechanical
        breakdown T85.111 ☑
        displacement T85.121 ☑
        leakage T85.191 ☑
        malposition T85.121 ☑
        obstruction T85.191 ☑
        perforation T85.191 ☑
        protrusion T85.191 ☑
        specified NEC T85.191 ☑
      pain T85.840 ☑
      specified type NEC T85.890 ☑
      stenosis T85.850 ☑
      thrombosis T85.860 ☑
    spinal cord T85.9 ☑
      embolism T85.810 ☑
      fibrosis T85.820 ☑
      hemorrhage T85.830 ☑
      infection and inflammation T85.733 ☑

Complication(s) — *continued*
  electronic stimulator device — *continued*
    spinal cord — *continued*
      mechanical
        breakdown T85.112 ☑
        displacement T85.122 ☑
        leakage T85.192 ☑
        malposition T85.122 ☑
        obstruction T85.192 ☑
        perforation T85.192 ☑
        protrusion T85.192 ☑
        specified NEC T85.192 ☑
      pain T85.840 ☑
      specified type NEC T85.890 ☑
      stenosis T85.850 ☑
      thrombosis T85.860 ☑
    urinary T83.9
      embolism T83.81 ☑
      fibrosis T83.82 ☑
      hemorrhage T83.83 ☑
      infection and inflammation T83.598 ☑
      mechanical
        breakdown T83.110 ☑
        displacement T83.120 ☑
        malposition T83.120 ☑
        perforation T83.190 ☑
        protrusion T83.190 ☑
        specified NEC T83.190 ☑
      pain T83.84 ☑
      specified type NEC T83.89 ☑
      stenosis T83.85 ☑
      thrombosis T83.86 ☑
  electroshock therapy T88.9 ☑
    specified NEC T88.8 ☑
  endocrine E34.9
    postprocedural
      adrenal hypofunction E89.6
      hypoinsulinemia E89.1
      hypoparathyroidism E89.2
      hypopituitarism E89.3
      hypothyroidism E89.0
      ovarian failure E89.40
        asymptomatic E89.40
        symptomatic E89.41
      specified NEC E89.89
      testicular hypofunction E89.5
  endodontic treatment NEC M27.59
  enterostomy (stoma) K94.10
    hemorrhage K94.11
    infection K94.12
    malfunction K94.13
    mechanical K94.13
    specified complication NEC K94.19
  episiotomy, disruption O90.1
  esophageal anti-reflux device T85.9 ☑
    embolism T85.818 ☑
    fibrosis T85.828 ☑
    hemorrhage T85.838 ☑
    infection and inflammation T85.79 ☑
    mechanical
      breakdown T85.511 ☑
      displacement T85.521 ☑
      malfunction T85.511 ☑
      malposition T85.521 ☑
      obstruction T85.591 ☑
      perforation T85.591 ☑
      protrusion T85.591 ☑
      specified NEC T85.591 ☑
    pain T85.848 ☑
    specified type NEC T85.898 ☑
    stenosis T85.858 ☑
    thrombosis T85.868 ☑
  esophagostomy K94.30
    hemorrhage K94.31
    infection K94.32
    malfunction K94.33
    mechanical K94.33
    specified complication NEC K94.39
  extracorporeal circulation T80.90 ☑
  extremity artery (bypass) graft T82.9 ☑
    arteriosclerosis — *see* Arteriosclerosis, extremities, bypass graft
    embolism T82.818 ☑
    fibrosis T82.828 ☑
    hemorrhage T82.838 ☑
    infection and inflammation T82.7 ☑

Complication(s) — *continued*
  extremity artery graft — *continued*
    mechanical
      breakdown T82.318 ☑
        femoral artery T82.312 ☑
      displacement T82.328 ☑
        femoral artery T82.322 ☑
      leakage T82.338 ☑
        femoral artery T82.332 ☑
      malposition T82.328 ☑
        femoral artery T82.322 ☑
      obstruction T82.398 ☑
        femoral artery T82.392 ☑
      perforation T82.398 ☑
        femoral artery T82.392 ☑
      protrusion T82.398 ☑
        femoral artery T82.392 ☑
    pain T82.848 ☑
    specified type NEC T82.898 ☑
    stenosis T82.858 ☑
    thrombosis T82.868 ☑
  eye H57.9
    corneal graft — *see* Complications, graft, cornea
    implant (prosthetic) T85.9 ☑
      embolism T85.818 ☑
      fibrosis T85.828 ☑
      hemorrhage T85.838 ☑
      infection and inflammation T85.79 ☑
      mechanical
        breakdown T85.318 ☑
        displacement T85.328 ☑
        leakage T85.398 ☑
        malposition T85.328 ☑
        obstruction T85.398 ☑
        perforation T85.398 ☑
        protrusion T85.398 ☑
        specified NEC T85.398 ☑
      pain T85.848 ☑
      specified type NEC T85.898 ☑
      stenosis T85.858 ☑
      thrombosis T85.868 ☑
    intraocular lens — *see* Complications, intraocular lens
    orbital prosthesis — *see* Complications, orbital prosthesis
  female genital N94.9
    device, implant or graft NEC — *see* Complications, genitourinary, device or implant, genital tract
  femoral artery (bypass) graft — *see* Complication, extremity artery (bypass) graft
  fixation device, internal (orthopedic) T84.9 ☑
    infection and inflammation T84.60 ☑
      arm T84.61- ☑
        humerus T84.61- ☑
        radius T84.61- ☑
        ulna T84.61- ☑
      leg T84.629 ☑
        femur T84.62- ☑
        fibula T84.62- ☑
        tibia T84.62- ☑
      specified site NEC T84.89 ☑
      spine T84.63 ☑
    mechanical
      breakdown
        limb T84.119 ☑
          carpal T84.210 ☑
          femur T84.11- ☑
          fibula T84.11- ☑
          humerus T84.11- ☑
          metacarpal T84.210 ☑
          metatarsal T84.213 ☑
          phalanx
            foot T84.213 ☑
            hand T84.210 ☑
          radius T84.11- ☑
          tarsal T84.213 ☑
          tibia T84.11- ☑
          ulna T84.11- ☑
        specified bone NEC T84.218 ☑
        spine T84.216 ☑
      displacement
        limb T84.129 ☑
          carpal T84.220 ☑
          femur T84.12- ☑
          fibula T84.12- ☑
          humerus T84.12- ☑

Complication(s) — *continued*
  fixation device, internal — *continued*
    mechanical — *continued*
      displacement — *continued*
        limb — *continued*
          metacarpal T84.220 ☑
          metatarsal T84.223 ☑
          phalanx
            foot T84.223 ☑
            hand T84.220 ☑
          radius T84.12-☑
          tarsal T84.223 ☑
          tibia T84.12-☑
          ulna T84.12-☑
        specified bone NEC T84.228 ☑
        spine T84.226 ☑
      malposition — *see* Complications, fixation device, internal, mechanical, displacement
      obstruction — *see* Complications, fixation device, internal, mechanical, specified type NEC
      perforation — *see* Complications, fixation device, internal, mechanical, specified type NEC
      protrusion — *see* Complications, fixation device, internal, mechanical, specified type NEC
      specified type NEC
        limb T84.199 ☑
          carpal T84.290 ☑
          femur T84.19-☑
          fibula T84.19-☑
          humerus T84.19-☑
          metacarpal T84.290 ☑
          metatarsal T84.293 ☑
          phalanx
            foot T84.293 ☑
            hand T84.290 ☑
          radius T84.19-☑
          tarsal T84.293 ☑
          tibia T84.19-☑
          ulna T84.19-☑
        specified bone NEC T84.298 ☑
        vertebra T84.296 ☑
    specified type NEC T84.89 ☑
      embolism T84.81 ☑
      fibrosis T84.82 ☑
      hemorrhage T84.83 ☑
      pain T84.84 ☑
      specified complication NEC T84.89 ☑
      stenosis T84.85 ☑
      thrombosis T84.86 ☑
  following
    acute myocardial infarction NEC I23.8
      aneurysm (false) (of cardiac wall) (of heart wall) (ruptured) I23.3
      angina I23.7
      atrial
        septal defect I23.1
        thrombosis I23.6
      cardiac wall rupture I23.3
      chordae tendinae rupture I23.4
      defect
        septal
          atrial (heart) I23.1
          ventricular (heart) I23.2
      hemopericardium I23.0
      papillary muscle rupture I23.5
      rupture
        cardiac wall I23.3
          with hemopericardium I23.0
        chordae tendineae I23.4
        papillary muscle I23.5
      specified NEC I23.8
      thrombosis
        atrium I23.6
        auricular appendage I23.6
        ventricle (heart) I23.6
      ventricular
        septal defect I23.2
        thrombosis I23.6
    ectopic or molar pregnancy O08.9
      cardiac arrest O08.81
      sepsis O08.82
      specified type NEC O08.89
      urinary tract infection O08.83
    termination of pregnancy — *see* Abortion
  gastrointestinal K92.9
    bile duct prosthesis — *see* Complications, bile duct implant

Complication(s) — *continued*
  gastrointestinal — *continued*
    esophageal anti-reflux device — *see* Complications, esophageal anti-reflux device
    postoperative
      colostomy — *see* Complications, colostomy
      dumping syndrome K91.1
      enterostomy — *see* Complications, enterostomy
      gastrostomy — *see* Complications, gastrostomy
      malabsorption NEC K91.2
      obstruction — *see also* Obstruction, intestine, postoperative K91.30
      postcholecystectomy syndrome K91.5
      specified NEC K91.89
      vomiting after GI surgery K91.0
    prosthetic device or implant
      bile duct prosthesis — *see* Complications, bile duct implant
      esophageal anti-reflux device — *see* Complications, esophageal anti-reflux device
      specified type NEC
        embolism T85.818 ☑
        fibrosis T85.828 ☑
        hemorrhage T85.838 ☑
        mechanical
          breakdown T85.518 ☑
          displacement T85.528 ☑
          malfunction T85.518 ☑
          malposition T85.528 ☑
          obstruction T85.598 ☑
          perforation T85.598 ☑
          protrusion T85.598 ☑
          specified NEC T85.598 ☑
        pain T85.848 ☑
        specified complication NEC T85.898 ☑
        stenosis T85.858 ☑
        thrombosis T85.868 ☑
  gastrostomy (stoma) K94.20
    hemorrhage K94.21
    infection K94.22
    malfunction K94.23
    mechanical K94.23
    specified complication NEC K94.29
  genitourinary
    device or implant T83.9 ☑
      genital tract T83.9 ☑
        infection or inflammation T83.69 ☑
        intrauterine contraceptive device — *see* Complications, intrauterine, contraceptive device
        mechanical — *see* Complications, by device, mechanical
        mesh — *see* Complications, prosthetic device or implant, mesh
        penile prosthesis — *see* Complications, prosthetic device, penile
        specified type NEC T83.89 ☑
          embolism T83.81 ☑
          fibrosis T83.82 ☑
          hemorrhage T83.83 ☑
          pain T83.84 ☑
          specified complication NEC T83.89 ☑
          stenosis T83.85 ☑
          thrombosis T83.86 ☑
        vaginal mesh — *see* Complications, prosthetic device or implant, mesh
      urinary system T83.9 ☑
        cystostomy catheter — *see* Complication, catheter, cystostomy
        electronic stimulator — *see* Complications, electronic stimulator device, urinary
        indwelling urethral catheter — *see* Complications, catheter, urethral, indwelling
        infection or inflammation T83.598 ☑
          indwelling urethral catheter T83.511 ☑
        kidney transplant — *see* Complication, transplant, kidney
        organ graft — *see* Complication, graft, urinary organ
        specified type NEC T83.89 ☑
          embolism T83.81 ☑
          fibrosis T83.82 ☑
          hemorrhage T83.83 ☑
          mechanical T83.198 ☑
            breakdown T83.118 ☑
            displacement T83.128 ☑
            malfunction T83.118 ☑

Complication(s) — *continued*
  genitourinary — *continued*
    device or implant — *continued*
      urinary system — *continued*
        specified type — *continued*
          mechanical — *continued*
            malposition T83.128 ☑
            obstruction T83.198 ☑
            perforation T83.198 ☑
            protrusion T83.198 ☑
            specified NEC T83.198 ☑
          sphincter implant — *see* Complications, implant, urinary sphincter
          sphincter, implanted T83.191 ☑
          stent (ileal conduit) (nephroureteral) T83.193 ☑
          pain T83.84 ☑
          specified complication NEC T83.89 ☑
          stenosis T83.85 ☑
          thrombosis T83.86 ☑
          ureteral indwelling T83.192 ☑
    postprocedural
      pelvic peritoneal adhesions N99.4
      renal failure N99.0
      specified NEC N99.89
      stoma — *see* Complications, stoma, urinary tract
      urethral stricture — *see* Stricture, urethra, postprocedural
      vaginal
        adhesions N99.2
        vault prolapse N99.3
  graft (bypass) (patch) — *see also* Complications, prosthetic device or implant
    aorta — *see* Complications, graft, vascular
    arterial — *see* Complication, graft, vascular
    bone T86.839
      failure T86.831
      infection T86.832
      mechanical T84.318 ☑
        breakdown T84.318 ☑
        displacement T84.328 ☑
        protrusion T84.398 ☑
        specified type NEC T84.398 ☑
      rejection T86.830
      specified type NEC T86.838
    carotid artery — *see* Complications, graft, vascular
    cornea T86.849
      failure T86.841
      infection T86.842
      mechanical T85.398 ☑
        breakdown T85.318 ☑
        displacement T85.328 ☑
        protrusion T85.398 ☑
        specified type NEC T85.398 ☑
      rejection T86.840
      retroprosthetic membrane T85.398 ☑
      specified type NEC T86.848
    femoral artery (bypass) — *see* Complication, extremity artery (bypass) graft
    genital organ or tract — *see* Complications, genitourinary, device or implant, genital tract
    muscle T84.9 ☑
      breakdown T84.410 ☑
      displacement T84.420 ☑
      embolism T84.81 ☑
      fibrosis T84.82 ☑
      hemorrhage T84.83 ☑
      infection and inflammation T84.7 ☑
      mechanical NEC T84.490 ☑
      pain T84.84 ☑
      specified type NEC T84.89 ☑
      stenosis T84.85 ☑
      thrombosis T84.86 ☑
    nerve — *see* Complication, prosthetic device or implant, specified NEC
    skin — *see* Complications, prosthetic device or implant, skin graft
    tendon T84.9 ☑
      breakdown T84.410 ☑
      displacement T84.420 ☑
      embolism T84.81 ☑
      fibrosis T84.82 ☑
      hemorrhage T84.83 ☑
      infection and inflammation T84.7 ☑
      mechanical NEC T84.490 ☑
      pain T84.84 ☑
      specified type NEC T84.89 ☑

☑ **Additional Character Required — Refer to the Tabular List for Character Selection** ▽ Subterms under main terms may continue to next column or page

Complication(s) — continued
graft — see also Complications, prosthetic device or implant — continued
  tendon — continued
    stenosis T84.85 ☑
    thrombosis T84.86 ☑
  urinary organ T83.9 ☑
    embolism T83.81 ☑
    fibrosis T83.82 ☑
    hemorrhage T83.83 ☑
    infection and inflammation T83.598 ☑
      indwelling urethral catheter T83.511 ☑
    mechanical
      breakdown T83.21 ☑
      displacement T83.22 ☑
      erosion T83.24 ☑
      exposure T83.25 ☑
      leakage T83.23 ☑
      malposition T83.22 ☑
      obstruction T83.29 ☑
      perforation T83.29 ☑
      protrusion T83.29 ☑
      specified NEC T83.29 ☑
    pain T83.84 ☑
    specified type NEC T83.89 ☑
    stenosis T83.85 ☑
    thrombosis T83.86 ☑
  vascular T82.9 ☑
    embolism T82.818 ☑
    femoral artery — see Complication, extremity artery (bypass) graft
    fibrosis T82.828 ☑
    hemorrhage T82.838 ☑
    mechanical
      breakdown T82.319 ☑
        aorta (bifurcation) T82.310 ☑
        carotid artery T82.311 ☑
        specified vessel NEC T82.318 ☑
      displacement T82.329 ☑
        aorta (bifurcation) T82.320 ☑
        carotid artery T82.321 ☑
        specified vessel NEC T82.328 ☑
      leakage T82.339 ☑
        aorta (bifurcation) T82.330 ☑
        carotid artery T82.331 ☑
        specified vessel NEC T82.338 ☑
      malposition T82.329 ☑
        aorta (bifurcation) T82.320 ☑
        carotid artery T82.321 ☑
        specified vessel NEC T82.328 ☑
      obstruction T82.399 ☑
        aorta (bifurcation) T82.390 ☑
        carotid artery T82.391 ☑
        specified vessel NEC T82.398 ☑
      perforation T82.399 ☑
        aorta (bifurcation) T82.390 ☑
        carotid artery T82.391 ☑
        specified vessel NEC T82.398 ☑
      protrusion T82.399 ☑
        aorta (bifurcation) T82.390 ☑
        carotid artery T82.391 ☑
        specified vessel NEC T82.398 ☑
    pain T82.848 ☑
    specified complication NEC T82.898 ☑
    stenosis T82.858 ☑
    thrombosis T82.868 ☑
heart I51.9
  assist device
    infection and inflammation T82.7 ☑
  following acute myocardial infarction — see Complications, following, acute myocardial infarction
  postoperative — see Complications, circulatory system
  transplant — see Complication, transplant, heart and lung(s) — see Complications, transplant, heart, with lung
  valve
    graft (biological) T82.9 ☑
      embolism T82.817 ☑
      fibrosis T82.827 ☑
      hemorrhage T82.837 ☑
      infection and inflammation T82.7 ☑
      mechanical T82.228 ☑
        breakdown T82.221 ☑
        displacement T82.222 ☑

Complication(s) — continued
heart — continued
  valve — continued
    graft — continued
      mechanical — continued
        leakage T82.223 ☑
        malposition T82.222 ☑
        obstruction T82.228 ☑
        perforation T82.228 ☑
        protrusion T82.228 ☑
      pain T82.847 ☑
      specified type NEC T82.897 ☑
      stenosis T82.857 ☑
      thrombosis T82.867 ☑
    prosthesis T82.9 ☑
      embolism T82.817 ☑
      fibrosis T82.827 ☑
      hemorrhage T82.837 ☑
      infection or inflammation T82.6 ☑
      mechanical T82.09 ☑
        breakdown T82.01 ☑
        displacement T82.02 ☑
        leakage T82.03 ☑
        malposition T82.02 ☑
        obstruction T82.09 ☑
        perforation T82.09 ☑
        protrusion T82.09 ☑
      pain T82.847 ☑
      specified type NEC T82.897 ☑
        mechanical T82.09 ☑
      stenosis T82.857 ☑
      thrombosis T82.867 ☑
hematoma
  intraoperative — see Complication, intraoperative, hemorrhage
  postprocedural — see Complication, postprocedural, hematoma
hemodialysis — see Complications, dialysis
hemorrhage
  intraoperative — see Complication, intraoperative, hemorrhage
  postprocedural — see Complication, postprocedural, hemorrhage
ileostomy (stoma) — see Complications, enterostomy
immunization (procedure) — see Complications, vaccination
implant — see also Complications, by site and type
  urinary sphincter T83.9 ☑
    embolism T83.81 ☑
    fibrosis T83.82 ☑
    hemorrhage T83.83 ☑
    infection and inflammation T83.591 ☑
    mechanical
      breakdown T83.111 ☑
      displacement T83.121 ☑
      leakage T83.191 ☑
      malposition T83.121 ☑
      obstruction T83.191 ☑
      perforation T83.191 ☑
      protrusion T83.191 ☑
      specified NEC T83.191 ☑
    pain T83.84 ☑
    specified type NEC T83.89 ☑
    stenosis T83.85 ☑
    thrombosis T83.86 ☑
infusion (procedure) T80.90 ☑
  air embolism T80.0 ☑
  blood — see Complications, transfusion
  catheter — see Complications, catheter
  infection T80.29 ☑
  pump — see Complications, cardiovascular, device or implant
  sepsis T80.29 ☑
  serum reaction — see also Reaction, serum T80.69 ☑
    anaphylactic shock — see also Shock, anaphylactic T80.59 ☑
  specified type NEC T80.89 ☑
inhalation therapy NEC T81.81 ☑
injection (procedure) T80.90 ☑
  drug reaction — see Reaction, drug
  infection T80.29 ☑
  sepsis T80.29 ☑
  serum (prophylactic) (therapeutic) — see Complications, vaccination
  specified type NEC T80.89 ☑

Complication(s) — continued
injection — continued
  vaccine (any) — see Complications, vaccination
inoculation (any) — see Complications, vaccination
insulin pump
  infection and inflammation T85.72 ☑
  mechanical
    breakdown T85.614 ☑
    displacement T85.624 ☑
    leakage T85.633 ☑
    malposition T85.624 ☑
    obstruction T85.694 ☑
    perforation T85.694 ☑
    protrusion T85.694 ☑
    specified NEC T85.694 ☑
intestinal pouch NEC K91.858
intraocular lens (prosthetic) T85.9 ☑
  embolism T85.818 ☑
  fibrosis T85.828 ☑
  hemorrhage T85.838 ☑
  infection and inflammation T85.79 ☑
  mechanical
    breakdown T85.21 ☑
    displacement T85.22 ☑
    malposition T85.22 ☑
    obstruction T85.29 ☑
    perforation T85.29 ☑
    protrusion T85.29 ☑
    specified NEC T85.29 ☑
  pain T85.848 ☑
  specified type NEC T85.898 ☑
  stenosis T85.858 ☑
  thrombosis T85.868 ☑
intraoperative (intraprocedural)
  cardiac arrest — see also Infarct, myocardium, associated with revascularization procedure
    during cardiac surgery I97.710
    during other surgery I97.711
  cardiac functional disturbance NEC — see also Infarct, myocardium, associated with revascularization procedure
    during cardiac surgery I97.790
    during other surgery I97.791
  hemorrhage (hematoma) (of)
    circulatory system organ or structure
      during cardiac bypass I97.411
      during cardiac catheterization I97.410
      during other circulatory system procedure I97.418
      during other procedure I97.42
    digestive system organ
      during procedure on digestive system K91.61
      during procedure on other organ K91.62
    ear
      during procedure on ear and mastoid process H95.21
      during procedure on other organ H95.22
    endocrine system organ or structure
      during procedure on endocrine system organ or structure E36.01
      during procedure on other organ E36.02
    eye and adnexa
      during ophthalmic procedure H59.11- ☑
      during other procedure H59.12- ☑
    genitourinary organ or structure
      during procedure on genitourinary organ or structure N99.61
      during procedure on other organ N99.62
    mastoid process
      during procedure on ear and mastoid process H95.21
      during procedure on other organ H95.22
    musculoskeletal structure
      during musculoskeletal surgery M96.810
      during non-orthopedic surgery M96.811
      during orthopedic surgery M96.810
    nervous system
      during a nervous system procedure G97.31
      during other procedure G97.32
    respiratory system
      during other procedure J95.62
      during procedure on respiratory system organ or structure J95.61
    skin and subcutaneous tissue
      during a dermatologic procedure L76.01
      during a procedure on other organ L76.02
    spleen
      during a procedure on other organ D78.02

Complication(s) — *continued*
  intraoperative — *continued*
    hemorrhage — *continued*
      spleen — *continued*
        during a procedure on the spleen D78.01
      puncture or laceration (accidental) (unintentional) (of)
        brain
          during a nervous system procedure G97.48
          during other procedure G97.49
        circulatory system organ or structure
          during circulatory system procedure I97.51
          during other procedure I97.52
        digestive system
          during procedure on digestive system K91.71
          during procedure on other organ K91.72
        ear
          during procedure on ear and mastoid process H95.31
          during procedure on other organ H95.32
        endocrine system organ or structure
          during procedure on endocrine system organ or structure E36.11
          during procedure on other organ E36.12
        eye and adnexa
          during ophthalmic procedure H59.21- ☑
          during other procedure H59.22- ☑
        genitourinary organ or structure
          during procedure on genitourinary organ or structure N99.71
          during procedure on other organ N99.72
        mastoid process
          during procedure on ear and mastoid process H95.31
          during procedure on other organ H95.32
        musculoskeletal structure
          during musculoskeletal surgery M96.820
          during non-orthopedic surgery M96.821
          during orthopedic surgery M96.820
        nervous system
          during a nervous system procedure G97.48
          during other procedure G97.49
        respiratory system
          during other procedure J95.72
          during procedure on respiratory system organ or structure J95.71
        skin and subcutaneous tissue
          during a dermatologic procedure L76.11
          during a procedure on other organ L76.12
        spleen
          during a procedure on other organ D78.12
          during a procedure on the spleen D78.11
    specified NEC
      circulatory system I97.88
      digestive system K91.81
      ear H95.88
      endocrine system E36.8
      eye and adnexa H59.88
      genitourinary system N99.81
      mastoid process H95.88
      musculoskeletal structure M96.89
      nervous system G97.81
      respiratory system J95.88
      skin and subcutaneous tissue L76.81
      spleen D78.81
  intraperitoneal catheter (dialysis) (infusion) — *see* Complications, catheter, intraperitoneal
  intrathecal infusion pump
    infection and inflammation T85.738 ☑
    mechanical
      breakdown T85.615 ☑
      displacement T85.625 ☑
      leakage T85.635 ☑
      malfunction T85.695 ☑
      malposition T85.625 ☑
      obstruction T85.695 ☑
      perforation T85.695 ☑
      protrusion T85.695 ☑
      specified NEC T85.695 ☑
  intrauterine
    contraceptive device
      embolism T83.81 ☑
      fibrosis T83.82 ☑
      hemorrhage T83.83 ☑
      infection and inflammation T83.69 ☑
      mechanical
        breakdown T83.31 ☑
        displacement T83.32 ☑

Complication(s) — *continued*
  intrauterine — *continued*
    contraceptive device — *continued*
      mechanical — *continued*
        malposition T83.32 ☑
        obstruction T83.39 ☑
        perforation T83.39 ☑
        protrusion T83.39 ☑
        specified NEC T83.39 ☑
      pain T83.84 ☑
      specified type NEC T83.89 ☑
      stenosis T83.85 ☑
      thrombosis T83.86 ☑
    procedure (fetal), to newborn P96.5
  jejunostomy (stoma) — *see* Complications, enterostomy
  joint prosthesis, internal T84.9 ☑
    breakage (fracture) T84.01- ☑
    dislocation T84.02- ☑
    fracture T84.01- ☑
    infection or inflammation T84.50 ☑
      hip T84.5- ☑
      knee T84.5- ☑
      specified joint NEC T84.59 ☑
    instability T84.02- ☑
    malposition — *see* Complications, joint prosthesis, mechanical, displacement
    mechanical
      breakage, broken T84.01- ☑
      dislocation T84.02- ☑
      fracture T84.01- ☑
      instability T84.02- ☑
      leakage — *see* Complications, joint prosthesis, mechanical, specified NEC
      loosening T84.039 ☑
        hip T84.03- ☑
        knee T84.03- ☑
        specified joint NEC T84.038 ☑
      obstruction — *see* Complications, joint prosthesis, mechanical, specified NEC
      perforation — *see* Complications, joint prosthesis, mechanical, specified NEC
      osteolysis T84.059 ☑
        hip T84.05- ☑
        knee T84.05- ☑
        other specified joint T84.058 ☑
      periprosthetic T84.059 ☑
      protrusion — *see* Complications, joint prosthesis, mechanical, specified NEC
      specified complication NEC T84.099 ☑
        hip T84.09- ☑
        knee T84.09- ☑
        other specified joint T84.098 ☑
      subluxation T84.02- ☑
      wear of articular bearing surface T84.069 ☑
        hip T84.06- ☑
        knee T84.06- ☑
        other specified joint T84.068 ☑
    specified joint NEC T84.89 ☑
      embolism T84.81 ☑
      fibrosis T84.82 ☑
      hemorrhage T84.83 ☑
      pain T84.84 ☑
      specified complication NEC T84.89 ☑
      stenosis T84.85 ☑
      thrombosis T84.86 ☑
    subluxation T84.02- ☑
  kidney transplant — *see* Complications, transplant, kidney
  labor O75.9
    specified NEC O75.89
  liver transplant (immune or nonimmune) — *see* Complications, transplant, liver
  lumbar puncture G97.1
    cerebrospinal fluid leak G97.0
    headache or reaction G97.1
  lung transplant — *see* Complications, transplant, lung
    and heart — *see* Complications, transplant, lung, with heart
  male genital N50.9
    device, implant or graft — *see* Complications, genitourinary, device or implant, genital tract
    postprocedural or postoperative — *see* Complications, genitourinary, postprocedural
    specified NEC N99.89

Complication(s) — *continued*
  mastoid (process) procedure
    intraoperative H95.88
      hematoma — *see* Complications, intraoperative, hemorrhage (hematoma) (of), mastoid process
      hemorrhage — *see* Complications, intraoperative, hemorrhage (hematoma) (of), mastoid process
      laceration — *see* Complications, intraoperative, puncture or laceration, mastoid process
      specified NEC H95.88
    postmastoidectomy — *see* Complications, postmastoidectomy
    postoperative H95.89
      external ear canal stenosis H95.81 ☑
      hematoma — *see* Complications, postprocedural, hematoma (of), mastoid process
      hemorrhage — *see* Complications, postprocedural, hemorrhage (of), mastoid process
      postmastoidectomy — *see* Complications, postmastoidectomy
      seroma — *see* Complications, postprocedural, seroma (of), mastoid process
      specified NEC H95.89
  mastoidectomy cavity — *see* Complications, postmastoidectomy
  mechanical — *see* Complications, by site and type, mechanical
  medical procedures — *see also* Complication(s), intraoperative T88.9 ☑
  metabolic E88.9
    postoperative E89.89
    specified NEC E89.89
  molar pregnancy NOS O08.9
    damage to pelvic organs O08.6
    embolism O08.2
    genital infection O08.0
    hemorrhage (delayed) (excessive) O08.1
    metabolic disorder O08.5
    renal failure O08.4
    shock O08.3
    specified type NEC O08.0
    venous complication NEC O08.7
  musculoskeletal system — *see also* Complication, intraoperative (intraprocedural), by site
    device, implant or graft NEC — *see* Complications, orthopedic, device or implant
    internal fixation (nail) (plate) (rod) — *see* Complications, fixation device, internal
    joint prosthesis — *see* Complications, joint prosthesis
    post radiation M96.89
      kyphosis M96.2
      scoliosis M96.5
      specified complication NEC M96.89
    postoperative (postprocedural) M96.89
      with osteoporosis — *see* Osteoporosis
      fracture following insertion of device — *see* Fracture, following insertion of orthopedic implant, joint prosthesis or bone plate
      joint instability after prosthesis removal M96.89
      lordosis M96.4
      postlaminectomy syndrome NEC M96.1
        kyphosis M96.3
      pseudarthrosis M96.0
      specified complication NEC M96.89
  nephrostomy (stoma) — *see* Complications, stoma, urinary tract, external NEC
  nervous system G98.8
    central G96.9
    device, implant or graft — *see also* Complication, prosthetic device or implant, specified NEC
      electronic stimulator (electrode(s)) — *see* Complications, electronic stimulator device
      specified NEC
        infection and inflammation T85.738 ☑
        mechanical T85.695 ☑
          breakdown T85.615 ☑
          displacement T85.625 ☑
          leakage T85.635 ☑
          malfunction T85.695 ☑
          malposition T85.625 ☑
          obstruction T85.695 ☑
          perforation T85.695 ☑
          protrusion T85.695 ☑
          specified NEC T85.695 ☑

Complication(s) — *continued*
  nervous system — *continued*
    device, implant or graft — *see also* Complication, prosthetic device or implant, specified — *continued*
      ventricular shunt — *see* Complications, ventricular shunt
      electronic stimulator (electrode(s)) — *see* Complications, electronic stimulator device
      postprocedural G97.82
        intracranial hypotension G97.2
        specified NEC G97.82
        spinal fluid leak G97.0
  newborn, due to intrauterine (fetal) procedure P96.5
  nonabsorbable (permanent) sutures — *see* Complication, sutures, permanent
  obstetric O75.9
    procedure (instrumental) (manual) (surgical) specified NEC O75.4
    specified NEC O75.89
    surgical wound NEC O90.89
      hematoma O90.2
      infection O86.00
  ocular lens implant — *see* Complications, intraocular lens
  ophthalmologic
    postprocedural bleb — *see* Blebitis
  orbital prosthesis T85.9 ☑
    embolism T85.818 ☑
    fibrosis T85.828 ☑
    hemorrhage T85.838 ☑
    infection and inflammation T85.79 ☑
    mechanical
      breakdown T85.31- ☑
      displacement T85.32- ☑
      malposition T85.32- ☑
      obstruction T85.39- ☑
      perforation T85.39- ☑
      protrusion T85.39- ☑
      specified NEC T85.39- ☑
    pain T85.848 ☑
    specified type NEC T85.898 ☑
    stenosis T85.858 ☑
    thrombosis T85.868 ☑
  organ or tissue transplant (partial) (total) — *see* Complications, transplant
  orthopedic — *see also* Disorder, soft tissue
    device or implant T84.9 ☑
      bone
        device or implant — *see* Complication, bone, device NEC
        graft — *see* Complication, graft, bone
      breakdown T84.418 ☑
      displacement T84.428 ☑
      electronic bone stimulator — *see* Complications, electronic stimulator device, bone
      embolism T84.81 ☑
      fibrosis T84.82 ☑
      fixation device — *see* Complication, fixation device, internal
      hemorrhage T84.83 ☑
      infection or inflammation T84.7 ☑
      joint prosthesis — *see* Complication, joint prosthesis, internal
      malfunction T84.418 ☑
      malposition T84.428 ☑
      mechanical NEC T84.498 ☑
      muscle graft — *see* Complications, graft, muscle
      obstruction T84.498 ☑
      pain T84.84 ☑
      perforation T84.498 ☑
      protrusion T84.498 ☑
      specified complication NEC T84.89 ☑
      stenosis T84.85 ☑
      tendon graft — *see* Complications, graft, tendon
      thrombosis T84.86 ☑
    fracture (following insertion of device) — *see* Fracture, following insertion of orthopedic implant, joint prosthesis or bone plate
    postprocedural M96.89
      fracture — *see* Fracture, following insertion of orthopedic implant, joint prosthesis or bone plate
      postlaminectomy syndrome NEC M96.1
        kyphosis M96.3
        lordosis M96.4

Complication(s) — *continued*
  orthopedic — *see also* Disorder, soft tissue — *continued*
    postprocedural — *continued*
      postradiation
        kyphosis M96.2
        scoliosis M96.5
      pseudarthrosis post-fusion M96.0
      specified type NEC M96.89
  pacemaker (cardiac) — *see* Complications, cardiovascular device or implant, electronic
  pancreas transplant — *see* Complications, transplant, pancreas
  penile prosthesis (implant) — *see* Complications, prosthetic device, penile
  perfusion NEC T80.90 ☑
  perineal repair (obstetrical) NEC O90.89
    disruption O90.1
    hematoma O90.2
    infection (following delivery) O86.09
  phototherapy T88.9 ☑
    specified NEC T88.8 ☑
  postmastoidectomy NEC H95.19- ☑
    cyst, mucosal H95.13- ☑
    granulation H95.12- ☑
    inflammation, chronic H95.11- ☑
    recurrent cholesteatoma H95.0- ☑
  postoperative — *see* Complications, postprocedural
    circulatory — *see* Complications, circulatory system
    ear — *see* Complications, ear
    endocrine — *see* Complications, endocrine
    eye — *see* Complications, eye
    lumbar puncture G97.1
      cerebrospinal fluid leak G97.0
    nervous system (central) (peripheral) — *see* Complications, nervous system
    respiratory system — *see* Complications, respiratory system
  postprocedural — *see also* Complications, surgical procedure
    cardiac arrest — *see also* Infarct, myocardium, associated with revascularization procedure
      following cardiac surgery I97.120
      following other surgery I97.121
    cardiac functional disturbance NEC — *see also* Infarct, myocardium, associated with revascularization procedure
      following cardiac surgery I97.190
      following other surgery I97.191
    cardiac insufficiency
      following cardiac surgery I97.110
      following other surgery I97.111
    chorioretinal scars following retinal surgery H59.81- ☑
    following cataract surgery
      cataract (lens) fragments H59.02- ☑
      cystoid macular edema H59.03- ☑
      specified NEC H59.09- ☑
      vitreous (touch) syndrome H59.01- ☑
    heart failure
      following cardiac surgery I97.130
      following other surgery I97.131
    hematoma (of)
      circulatory system organ or structure
        following cardiac bypass I97.631
        following cardiac catheterization I97.630
        following other circulatory system procedure I97.638
        following other procedure I97.621
      digestive system
        following procedure on digestive system K91.870
        following procedure on other organ K91.871
      ear
        following other procedure H95.52
        following procedure on ear and mastoid process H95.51
      endocrine system
        following endocrine system procedure E89.820
        following other procedure E89.821
      eye and adnexa
        following ophthalmic procedure H59.33- ☑
        following other procedure H59.34- ☑
      genitourinary organ or structure
        following procedure on genitourinary organ or structure N99.840
        following procedure on other organ N99.841

Complication(s) — *continued*
  postprocedural — *see also* Complications, surgical procedure — *continued*
    hematoma — *continued*
      mastoid process
        following other procedure H95.52
        following procedure on ear and mastoid process H95.51
      musculoskeletal structure
        following musculoskeletal surgery M96.840
        following non-orthopedic surgery M96.841
        following orthopedic surgery M96.840
      nervous system
        following nervous system procedure G97.61
        following other procedure G97.62
      respiratory system
        following other procedure J95.861
        following procedure on respiratory system organ or structure J95.860
      skin and subcutaneous tissue
        following dermatologic procedure L76.31
        following procedure on other organ L76.32
      spleen
        following procedure on other organ D78.32
        following procedure on the spleen D78.31
    hemorrhage (of)
      circulatory system organ or structure
        following cardiac bypass I97.611
        following cardiac catheterization I97.610
        following other circulatory system procedure I97.618
        following other procedure I97.620
      digestive system
        following procedure on digestive system K91.840
        following procedure on other organ K91.841
      ear
        following other procedure H95.42
        following procedure on ear and mastoid process H95.41
      endocrine system
        following endocrine system procedure E89.810
        following other procedure E89.811
      eye and adnexa
        following ophthalmic procedure H59.31- ☑
        following other procedure H59.32- ☑
      genitourinary organ or structure
        following procedure on genitourinary organ or structure N99.820
        following procedure on other organ N99.821
      mastoid process
        following other procedure H95.42
        following procedure on ear and mastoid process H95.41
      musculoskeletal structure
        following musculoskeletal surgery M96.830
        following non-orthopedic surgery M96.831
        following orthopedic surgery M96.830
      nervous system
        following nervous system procedure G97.51
        following other procedure G97.52
      respiratory system
        following a respiratory system procedure J95.830
        following other procedure J95.831
      skin and subcutaneous tissue
        following a procedure on other organ L76.22
        following dermatologic procedure L76.21
      spleen
        following procedure on other organ D78.22
        following procedure on the spleen D78.21
    seroma (of)
      circulatory system organ or structure
        following cardiac bypass I97.641
        following cardiac catheterization I97.640
        following other circulatory system procedure I97.648
        following other procedure I97.622
      digestive system
        following procedure on digestive system K91.872
        following procedure on other organ K91.873
      ear
        following other procedure H95.54
        following procedure on ear and mastoid process H95.53

Complication — Complication

Complication(s) — *continued*
postprocedural — *see also* Complications, surgical
procedure — *continued*
seroma — *continued*
endocrine system
following endocrine system procedure
E89.822
following other procedure E89.823
eye and adnexa
following ophthalmic procedure H59.35- ☑
following other procedure H59.36- ☑
genitourinary organ or structure
following procedure on genitourinary organ
or structure N99.842
following procedure on other organ N99.843
mastoid process
following other procedure H95.54
following procedure on ear and mastoid process H95.53
musculoskeletal structure
following musculoskeletal surgery M96.842
following non-orthopedic surgery M96.843
following orthopedic surgery M96.842
nervous system
following nervous system procedure G97.63
following other procedure G97.64
respiratory system
following other procedure J95.863
following procedure on respiratory system
organ or structure J95.862
skin and subcutaneous tissue
following dermatologic procedure L76.33
following procedure on other organ L76.34
spleen
following procedure on other organ D78.34
following procedure on the spleen D78.33
specified NEC
circulatory system I97.89
digestive K91.89
ear H95.89
endocrine E89.89
eye and adnexa H59.89
genitourinary N99.89
mastoid process H95.89
metabolic E89.89
musculoskeletal structure M96.89
nervous system G97.82
respiratory system J95.89
skin and subcutaneous tissue L76.82
spleen D78.89
pregnancy NEC — *see* Pregnancy, complicated by
prosthetic device or implant T85.9 ☑
bile duct — *see* Complications, bile duct implant
breast — *see* Complications, breast implant
bulking agent
ureteral
erosion T83.714 ☑
exposure T83.724 ☑
urethral
erosion T83.713 ☑
exposure T83.723 ☑
cardiac and vascular NEC — *see* Complications,
cardiovascular device or implant
corneal transplant — *see* Complications, graft,
cornea
electronic nervous system stimulator — *see* Complications, electronic stimulator device
epidural infusion catheter — *see* Complications,
catheter, epidural
esophageal anti-reflux device — *see* Complications,
esophageal anti-reflux device
genital organ or tract — *see* Complications, genitourinary, device or implant, genital tract
specified NEC T83.79- ☑
heart valve — *see* Complications, heart, valve,
prosthesis
infection or inflammation T85.79 ☑
intestine transplant T86.892
liver transplant T86.43
lung transplant T86.812
pancreas transplant T86.892
skin graft T86.822
intraocular lens — *see* Complications, intraocular
lens
intraperitoneal (dialysis) catheter — *see* Complications, catheter, intraperitoneal
joint — *see* Complications, joint prosthesis, internal
mechanical NEC T85.698 ☑

Complication(s) — *continued*
prosthetic device or implant — *continued*
mechanical — *continued*
dialysis catheter (vascular) — *see also* Complication, catheter, dialysis, mechanical
peritoneal — *see* Complication, catheter, intraperitoneal, mechanical
gastrointestinal device T85.598 ☑
ocular device T85.398 ☑
subdural (infusion) catheter T85.690 ☑
suture, permanent T85.692 ☑
that for bone repair — *see* Complications,
fixation device, internal (orthopedic),
mechanical
ventricular shunt
breakdown T85.01 ☑
displacement T85.02 ☑
leakage T85.03 ☑
malposition T85.02 ☑
obstruction T85.09 ☑
perforation T85.09 ☑
protrusion T85.09 ☑
specified NEC T85.09 ☑
mesh
erosion (to surrounding organ or tissue)
T83.718 ☑
urethral (into pelvic floor muscles) T83.712 ☑
vaginal (into pelvic floor muscles) T83.711 ☑
exposure (into surrounding organ or tissue)
T83.728 ☑
urethral (through urethral wall) T83.722 ☑
vaginal (into vagina) (through vaginal wall)
T83.721 ☑
orbital — *see* Complications, orbital prosthesis
penile T83.9 ☑
embolism T83.81 ☑
fibrosis T83.82 ☑
hemorrhage T83.83 ☑
infection and inflammation T83.61 ☑
mechanical
breakdown T83.410 ☑
displacement T83.420 ☑
leakage T83.490 ☑
malposition T83.420 ☑
obstruction T83.490 ☑
perforation T83.490 ☑
protrusion T83.490 ☑
specified NEC T83.490 ☑
pain T83.84 ☑
specified type NEC T83.89 ☑
stenosis T83.85 ☑
thrombosis T83.86 ☑
prosthetic materials NEC
erosion (to surrounding organ or tissue)
T83.718 ☑
exposure (into surrounding organ or tissue)
T83.728 ☑
skin graft T86.829
artificial skin or decellularized allodermis
embolism T85.818 ☑
fibrosis T85.828 ☑
hemorrhage T85.838 ☑
infection and inflammation T85.79 ☑
mechanical
breakdown T85.613 ☑
displacement T85.623 ☑
malfunction T85.613 ☑
malposition T85.623 ☑
obstruction T85.693 ☑
perforation T85.693 ☑
protrusion T85.693 ☑
specified NEC T85.693 ☑
pain T85.848 ☑
specified type NEC T85.898 ☑
stenosis T85.858 ☑
thrombosis T85.868 ☑
failure T86.821
infection T86.822
rejection T86.820
specified NEC T86.828
sling
urethral (female) (male)
erosion T83.712 ☑
exposure T83.722 ☑
specified NEC T85.9 ☑
embolism T85.818 ☑

Complication(s) — *continued*
prosthetic device or implant — *continued*
specified — *continued*
fibrosis T85.828 ☑
hemorrhage T85.838 ☑
infection and inflammation T85.79 ☑
mechanical
breakdown T85.618 ☑
displacement T85.628 ☑
leakage T85.638 ☑
malfunction T85.618 ☑
malposition T85.628 ☑
obstruction T85.698 ☑
perforation T85.698 ☑
protrusion T85.698 ☑
specified NEC T85.698 ☑
pain T85.848 ☑
specified type NEC T85.898 ☑
stenosis T85.858 ☑
thrombosis T85.868 ☑
subdural infusion catheter — *see* Complications,
catheter, subdural
sutures — *see* Complications, sutures
urinary organ or tract NEC — *see* Complications,
genitourinary, device or implant, urinary system
vascular — *see* Complications, cardiovascular device
or implant
ventricular shunt — *see* Complications, ventricular
shunt (device)
puerperium — *see* Puerperal
puncture, spinal G97.1
cerebrospinal fluid leak G97.0
headache or reaction G97.1
pyelogram N99.89
radiation
kyphosis M96.2
scoliosis M96.5
reattached
extremity (infection) (rejection)
lower T87.1X- ☑
upper T87.0X- ☑
specified body part NEC T87.2
reconstructed breast
asymmetry between native and reconstructed
breast N65.1
deformity N65.0
disproportion between native and reconstructed
breast N65.1
excess tissue N65.0
misshappen N65.0
reimplant NEC — *see also* Complications, prosthetic
device or implant
limb (infection) (rejection) — *see* Complications,
reattached, extremity
organ (partial) (total) — *see* Complications, transplant
prosthetic device NEC — *see* Complications, prosthetic device
renal N28.9
allograft — *see* Complications, transplant, kidney
dialysis — *see* Complications, dialysis
respirator
mechanical J95.850
specified NEC J95.859
respiratory system J98.9
device, implant or graft — *see* Complication, prosthetic device or implant, specified NEC
lung transplant — *see* Complications, prosthetic
device or implant, lung transplant
postoperative J95.89
air leak J95.812
Mendelson's syndrome (chemical pneumonitis)
J95.4
pneumothorax J95.811
pulmonary insufficiency (acute) (after nonthoracic surgery) J95.2
chronic J95.3
following thoracic surgery J95.1
respiratory failure (acute) J95.821
acute and chronic J95.822
specified NEC J95.89
subglottic stenosis J95.5
tracheostomy complication — *see* Complications, tracheostomy
therapy T81.89 ☑
sedation during labor and delivery O74.9

☑ **Additional Character Required** — **Refer to the Tabular List for Character Selection**   ▽ **Subterms under main terms may continue to next column or page**

Complication(s) — *continued*

sedation during labor and delivery — *continued*
- cardiac O74.2
- central nervous system O74.3
- pulmonary NEC O74.1

shunt — *see also* Complications, prosthetic device or implant
- arteriovenous — *see* Complications, arteriovenous, shunt
- ventricular (communicating) — *see* Complications, ventricular shunt

skin
- graft T86.829
  - failure T86.821
  - infection T86.822
  - rejection T86.820
  - specified type NEC T86.828

spinal
- anesthesia — *see* Complications, anesthesia, spinal
- catheter (epidural) (subdural) — *see* Complications, catheter
- puncture or tap G97.1
  - cerebrospinal fluid leak G97.0
  - headache or reaction G97.1

stent
- bile duct — *see* Complications, bile duct prosthesis
- ureteral indwelling
  - breakdown T83.112 ☑
  - displacement T83.122 ☑
  - leakage T83.192 ☑
  - malposition T83.122 ☑
  - obstruction T83.192 ☑
  - perforation T83.192 ☑
  - protrusion T83.192 ☑
  - specified NEC T83.192 ☑
- urinary NEC (ileal conduit) (nephroureteral) T83.193 ☑
  - embolism T83.81 ☑
  - fibrosis T83.82 ☑
  - hemorrhage T83.83 ☑
  - infection and inflammation T83.593 ☑
  - mechanical
    - breakdown T83.113 ☑
    - displacement T83.123 ☑
    - leakage T83.193 ☑
    - malposition T83.123 ☑
    - obstruction T83.193 ☑
    - perforation T83.193 ☑
    - protrusion T83.193 ☑
    - specified NEC T83.193 ☑
  - pain T83.84 ☑
  - specified type NEC T83.89 ☑
  - stenosis T83.85 ☑
  - thrombosis T83.86 ☑
- vascular
  - end stent stenosis — *see* Restenosis, stent
  - in stent stenosis — *see* Restenosis, stent

stoma
- digestive tract
  - colostomy — *see* Complications, colostomy
  - enterostomy — *see* Complications, enterostomy
  - esophagostomy — *see* Complications, esophagostomy
  - gastrostomy — *see* Complications, gastrostomy
- urinary tract N99.528
  - continent N99.538
    - hemorrhage N99.530
    - herniation N99.533
    - infection N99.531
    - malfunction N99.532
    - specified type NEC N99.538
    - stenosis N99.534
  - cystostomy — *see* Complications, cystostomy
  - external NOS N99.528
  - hemorrhage N99.520
  - herniation N99.523
  - incontinent N99.528
    - hemorrhage N99.520
    - herniation N99.523
    - infection N99.521
    - malfunction N99.522
    - specified type NEC N99.528
    - stenosis N99.524
  - infection N99.521
  - malfunction N99.522
  - specified type NEC N99.528
  - stenosis N99.524

Complication(s) — *continued*

stomach banding — *see* Complications, bariatric procedure
stomach stapling — *see* Complications, bariatric procedure
surgical material, nonabsorbable — *see* Complication, suture, permanent
surgical procedure (on) T81.9 ☑
- amputation stump (late) — *see* Complications, amputation stump
- cardiac — *see* Complications, circulatory system
- cholesteatoma, recurrent — *see* Complications, postmastoidectomy, recurrent cholesteatoma
- circulatory (early) — *see* Complications, circulatory system
- digestive system — *see* Complications, gastrointestinal
- dumping syndrome (postgastrectomy) K91.1
- ear — *see* Complications, ear
- elephantiasis or lymphedema I97.89
  - postmastectomy I97.2
- emphysema (surgical) T81.82 ☑
- endocrine — *see* Complications, endocrine
- eye — *see* Complications, eye
- fistula (persistent postoperative) T81.83 ☑
- foreign body inadvertently left in wound (sponge) (suture) (swab) — *see* Foreign body, accidentally left during a procedure
- gastrointestinal — *see* Complications, gastrointestinal
- genitourinary NEC N99.89
- hematoma
  - intraoperative — *see* Complication, intraoperative, hemorrhage
  - postprocedural — *see* Complication, postprocedural, hematoma
- hemorrhage
  - intraoperative — *see* Complication, intraoperative, hemorrhage
  - postprocedural — *see* Complication, postprocedural, hemorrhage
- hepatic failure K91.82
- hyperglycemia (postpancreatectomy) E89.1
- hypoinsulinemia (postpancreatectomy) E89.1
- hypoparathyroidism (postparathyroidectomy) E89.2
- hypopituitarism (posthypophysectomy) E89.3
- hypothyroidism (post-thyroidectomy) E89.0
- intestinal obstruction — *see also* Obstruction, intestine, postoperative K91.30
- intracranial hypotension following ventricular shunting (ventriculostomy) G97.2
- lymphedema I97.89
  - postmastectomy I97.2
- malabsorption (postsurgical) NEC K91.2
  - osteoporosis — *see* Osteoporosis, postsurgical malabsorption
- mastoidectomy cavity NEC — *see* Complications, postmastoidectomy
- metabolic E89.89
  - specified NEC E89.89
- musculoskeletal — *see* Complications, musculoskeletal system
- nervous system (central) (peripheral) — *see* Complications, nervous system
- ovarian failure E89.40
  - asymptomatic E89.40
  - symptomatic E89.41
- peripheral vascular — *see* Complications, surgical procedure, vascular
- postcardiotomy syndrome I97.0
- postcholecystectomy syndrome K91.5
- postcommissurotomy syndrome I97.0
- postgastrectomy dumping syndrome K91.1
- postlaminectomy syndrome NEC M96.1
  - kyphosis M96.3
- postmastectomy lymphedema syndrome I97.2
- postmastoidectomy cholesteatoma — *see* Complications, postmastoidectomy, recurrent cholesteatoma
- postvagotomy syndrome K91.1
- postvalvulotomy syndrome I97.0
- pulmonary insufficiency (acute) J95.2
  - chronic J95.3
  - following thoracic surgery J95.1
- reattached body part — *see* Complications, reattached
- respiratory — *see* Complications, respiratory system
- shock (hypovolemic) T81.19 ☑

Complication(s) — *continued*

surgical procedure — *continued*
- spleen (postoperative) D78.89
  - intraoperative D78.81
- stitch abscess T81.41 ☑
- subglottic stenosis (postsurgical) J95.5
- testicular hypofunction E89.5
- transplant — *see* Complications, organ or tissue transplant
- urinary NEC N99.89
- vaginal vault prolapse (posthysterectomy) N99.3
- vascular (peripheral)
  - artery T81.719 ☑
    - mesenteric T81.710 ☑
    - renal T81.711 ☑
    - specified NEC T81.718 ☑
  - vein T81.72 ☑
- wound infection T81.49 ☑

suture, permanent (wire) NEC T85.9 ☑
- with repair of bone — *see* Complications, fixation device, internal
- embolism T85.818 ☑
- fibrosis T85.828 ☑
- hemorrhage T85.838 ☑
- infection and inflammation T85.79 ☑
- mechanical
  - breakdown T85.612 ☑
  - displacement T85.622 ☑
  - malfunction T85.612 ☑
  - malposition T85.622 ☑
  - obstruction T85.692 ☑
  - perforation T85.692 ☑
  - protrusion T85.692 ☑
  - specified NEC T85.692 ☑
- pain T85.848 ☑
- specified type NEC T85.898 ☑
- stenosis T85.858 ☑
- thrombosis T85.868 ☑

tracheostomy J95.00
- granuloma J95.09
- hemorrhage J95.01
- infection J95.02
- malfunction J95.03
- mechanical J95.03
- obstruction J95.03
- specified type NEC J95.09
- tracheo-esophageal fistula J95.04

transfusion (blood) (lymphocytes) (plasma) T80.92 ☑
- air embolism T80.0 ☑
- circulatory overload E87.71
- febrile nonhemolytic transfusion reaction R50.84
- hemochromatosis E83.111
- hemolysis T80.89 ☑
- hemolytic reaction (antigen unspecified) T80.919 ☑
- incompatibility reaction (antigen unspecified) T80.919 ☑
  - ABO T80.30 ☑
    - delayed serologic (DSTR) T80.39 ☑
    - hemolytic transfusion reaction (HTR) (unspecified time after transfusion) T80.319 ☑
      - acute (AHTR) (less than 24 hours after transfusion) T80.310 ☑
      - delayed (DHTR) (24 hours or more after transfusion) T80.311 ☑
    - specified NEC T80.39 ☑
  - acute (antigen unspecified) T80.910 ☑
  - delayed (antigen unspecified) T80.911 ☑
  - delayed serologic (DSTR) T80.89 ☑
  - non-ABO (minor antigens (Duffy) (K) (Kell) (Kidd) (Lewis) (M) (N) (P) (S)) T80.A0 ☑ (*following* T80.4)
    - delayed serologic (DSTR) T80.A9 ☑ (*following* T80.4)
    - hemolytic transfusion reaction (HTR) (unspecified time after transfusion) T80.A19 ☑ (*following* T80.4)
      - acute (AHTR) (less than 24 hours after transfusion) T80.A10 ☑ (*following* T80.4)
      - delayed (DHTR) (24 hours or more after transfusion) T80.A11 ☑ (*following* T80.4)
    - specified NEC T80.A9 ☑ (*following* T80.4)
  - Rh (antigens (C) (c) (D) (E) (e)) (factor) T80.40 ☑
    - delayed serologic (DSTR) T80.49 ☑
    - hemolytic transfusion reaction (HTR) (unspecified time after transfusion) T80.419 ☑

Complication(s) — *continued*
  transfusion — *continued*
    incompatibility reaction — *continued*
      Rh — *continued*
        hemolytic transfusion reaction — *continued*
          acute (AHTR) (less than 24 hours after transfusion) T80.410 ☑
          delayed (DHTR) (24 hours or more after transfusion) T80.411 ☑
          specified NEC T80.49 ☑
    infection T80.29 ☑
      acute T80.22- ☑
    reaction NEC T80.89 ☑
    sepsis T80.29 ☑
    shock T80.89 ☑
  transplant T86.90
    bone T86.839
      failure T86.831
      infection T86.832
      rejection T86.830
      specified type NEC T86.838
    bone marrow T86.00
      failure T86.02
      infection T86.03
      rejection T86.01
      specified type NEC T86.09
    cornea T86.849
      failure T86.841
      infection T86.842
      rejection T86.840
      specified type NEC T86.848
    failure T86.92
    heart T86.20
      with lung T86.30
      cardiac allograft vasculopathy T86.290
        failure T86.32
        infection T86.33
        rejection T86.31
        specified type NEC T86.39
      failure T86.22
      infection T86.23
      rejection T86.21
      specified type NEC T86.298
    infection T86.93
    intestine T86.859
      failure T86.851
      infection T86.852
      rejection T86.850
      specified type NEC T86.858
    kidney T86.10
      failure T86.12
      infection T86.13
      rejection T86.11
      specified type NEC T86.19
    liver T86.40
      failure T86.42
      infection T86.43
      rejection T86.41
      specified type NEC T86.49
    lung T86.819
      with heart T86.30
        failure T86.32
        infection T86.33
        rejection T86.31
        specified type NEC T86.39
      failure T86.811
      infection T86.812
      rejection T86.810
      specified type NEC T86.818
    malignant neoplasm C80.2
    pancreas T86.899
      failure T86.891
      infection T86.892
      rejection T86.890
      specified type NEC T86.898
    peripheral blood stem cells T86.5
    post-transplant lymphoproliferative disorder (PTLD) D47.Z1 (*following* D47.4)
    rejection T86.91
    skin T86.829
      failure T86.821
      infection T86.822
      rejection T86.820
      specified type NEC T86.828
    specified
      tissue T86.899
        failure T86.891

Complication(s) — *continued*
  transplant — *continued*
    specified — *continued*
      tissue — *continued*
        infection T86.892
        rejection T86.890
        specified type NEC T86.898
      type NEC T86.99
    stem cell (from peripheral blood) (from umbilical cord) T86.5
    umbilical cord stem cells T86.5
  trauma (early) T79.9 ☑
    specified NEC T79.8 ☑
  ultrasound therapy NEC T88.9 ☑
  umbilical cord NEC
    complicating delivery O69.9 ☑
      specified NEC O69.89 ☑
  umbrella device, vascular T82.9 ☑
    embolism T82.818 ☑
    fibrosis T82.828 ☑
    hemorrhage T82.838 ☑
    infection or inflammation T82.7 ☑
    mechanical
      breakdown T82.515 ☑
      displacement T82.525 ☑
      leakage T82.535 ☑
      malposition T82.525 ☑
      obstruction T82.595 ☑
      perforation T82.595 ☑
      protrusion T82.595 ☑
    pain T82.848 ☑
    specified type NEC T82.898 ☑
    stenosis T82.858 ☑
    thrombosis T82.868 ☑
  urethral catheter — *see* Complications, catheter, urethral, indwelling
  vaccination T88.1 ☑
    anaphylaxis NEC T80.52 ☑
    arthropathy — *see* Arthropathy, postimmunization
    cellulitis T88.0 ☑
    encephalitis or encephalomyelitis G04.02
    infection (general) (local) NEC T88.0 ☑
    meningitis G03.8
    myelitis G04.02
    protein sickness T80.62 ☑
    rash T88.1 ☑
    reaction (allergic) T88.1 ☑
      serum T80.62 ☑
    sepsis T88.0 ☑
    serum intoxication, sickness, rash, or other serum reaction NEC T80.62 ☑
    anaphylactic shock T80.52 ☑
    shock (allergic) (anaphylactic) T80.52 ☑
    vaccinia (generalized) (localized) T88.1 ☑
  vas deferens device or implant — *see* Complications, genitourinary, device or implant, genital tract
  vascular I99.9
    device or implant T82.9 ☑
      embolism T82.818 ☑
      fibrosis T82.828 ☑
      hemorrhage T82.838 ☑
      infection or inflammation T82.7 ☑
      mechanical
        breakdown T82.519 ☑
          specified device NEC T82.518 ☑
        displacement T82.529 ☑
          specified device NEC T82.528 ☑
        leakage T82.539 ☑
          specified device NEC T82.538 ☑
        malposition T82.529 ☑
          specified device NEC T82.528 ☑
        obstruction T82.599 ☑
          specified device NEC T82.598 ☑
        perforation T82.599 ☑
          specified device NEC T82.598 ☑
        protrusion T82.599 ☑
          specified device NEC T82.598 ☑
      pain T82.848 ☑
      specified type NEC T82.898 ☑
      stenosis T82.858 ☑
      thrombosis T82.868 ☑
    dialysis catheter — *see* Complication, catheter, dialysis
    following infusion, therapeutic injection or transfusion T80.1 ☑
    graft T82.9 ☑

Complication(s) — *continued*
  vascular — *continued*
    graft — *continued*
      embolism T82.818 ☑
      fibrosis T82.828 ☑
      hemorrhage T82.838 ☑
      mechanical
        breakdown T82.319 ☑
          aorta (bifurcation) T82.310 ☑
          carotid artery T82.311 ☑
          specified vessel NEC T82.318 ☑
        displacement T82.329 ☑
          aorta (bifurcation) T82.320 ☑
          carotid artery T82.321 ☑
          specified vessel NEC T82.328 ☑
        leakage T82.339 ☑
          aorta (bifurcation) T82.330 ☑
          carotid artery T82.331 ☑
          specified vessel NEC T82.338 ☑
        malposition T82.329 ☑
          aorta (bifurcation) T82.320 ☑
          carotid artery T82.321 ☑
          specified vessel NEC T82.328 ☑
        obstruction T82.399 ☑
          aorta (bifurcation) T82.390 ☑
          carotid artery T82.391 ☑
          specified vessel NEC T82.398 ☑
        perforation T82.399 ☑
          aorta (bifurcation) T82.390 ☑
          carotid artery T82.391 ☑
          specified vessel NEC T82.398 ☑
        protrusion T82.399 ☑
          aorta (bifurcation) T82.390 ☑
          carotid artery T82.391 ☑
          specified vessel NEC T82.398 ☑
      pain T82.848 ☑
      specified complication NEC T82.898 ☑
      stenosis T82.858 ☑
      thrombosis T82.868 ☑
    postoperative — *see* Complications, postoperative, circulatory
  vena cava device (filter) (sieve) (umbrella) — *see* Complications, umbrella device, vascular
  ventilation therapy NEC T81.81 ☑
  ventilator
    mechanical J95.850
      specified NEC J95.859
  ventricular (communicating) shunt (device) T85.9 ☑
    embolism T85.810 ☑
    fibrosis T85.820 ☑
    hemorrhage T85.830 ☑
    infection and inflammation T85.730 ☑
    mechanical
      breakdown T85.01 ☑
      displacement T85.02 ☑
      leakage T85.03 ☑
      malposition T85.02 ☑
      obstruction T85.09 ☑
      perforation T85.09 ☑
      protrusion T85.09 ☑
      specified NEC T85.09 ☑
    pain T85.840 ☑
    specified type NEC T85.890 ☑
    stenosis T85.850 ☑
    thrombosis T85.860 ☑
  wire suture, permanent (implanted) — *see* Complications, suture, permanent

Compressed air disease T70.3 ☑
Compression
  with injury — *code by* Nature of injury
  artery I77.1
    celiac, syndrome I77.4
  brachial plexus G54.0
  brain (stem) G93.5
    due to
      contusion (diffuse) — *see* Injury, intracranial, diffuse
        focal — *see* Injury, intracranial, focal
      injury NEC — *see* Injury, intracranial, diffuse
      traumatic — *see* Injury, intracranial, diffuse
  bronchus J98.09
  cauda equina G83.4
  celiac (artery) (axis) I77.4
  cerebral — *see* Compression, brain
  cervical plexus G54.2

Compression — *continued*
  cord
    spinal — *see* Compression, spinal
    umbilical — *see* Compression, umbilical cord
  cranial nerve G52.9
    eighth H93.3 ☑
    eleventh G52.8
    fifth G50.8
    first G52.0
    fourth — *see* Strabismus, paralytic, fourth nerve
    ninth G52.1
    second — *see* Disorder, nerve, optic
    seventh G51.8
    sixth — *see* Strabismus, paralytic, sixth nerve
    tenth G52.2
    third — *see* Strabismus, paralytic, third nerve
    twelfth G52.3
  diver's squeeze T70.3 ☑
  during birth (newborn) P15.9
  esophagus K22.2
  eustachian tube — *see* Obstruction, eustachian tube, cartilaginous
  facies Q67.1
  fracture
    nontraumatic NOS — *see* Collapse, vertebra
    pathological — *see* Fracture, pathological
    traumatic — *see* Fracture, traumatic
  heart — *see* Disease, heart
  intestine — *see* Obstruction, intestine
  laryngeal nerve, recurrent G52.2
    with paralysis of vocal cords and larynx J38.00
      bilateral J38.02
      unilateral J38.01
  lumbosacral plexus G54.1
  lung J98.4
  lymphatic vessel I89.0
  medulla — *see* Compression, brain
  nerve — *see also* Disorder, nerve G58.9
    arm NEC — *see* Mononeuropathy, upper limb
    axillary G54.0
    cranial — *see* Compression, cranial nerve
    leg NEC — *see* Mononeuropathy, lower limb
    median (in carpal tunnel) — *see* Syndrome, carpal tunnel
    optic — *see* Disorder, nerve, optic
    plantar — *see* Lesion, nerve, plantar
    posterior tibial (in tarsal tunnel) — *see* Syndrome, tarsal tunnel
    root or plexus NOS (in) G54.9
      intervertebral disc disorder NEC — *see* Disorder, disc, with, radiculopathy
      with myelopathy — *see* Disorder, disc, with, myelopathy
      neoplastic disease — *see also* Neoplasm D49.9 *[G55]*
      spondylosis — *see* Spondylosis, with radiculopathy
    sciatic (acute) — *see* Lesion, nerve, sciatic
    sympathetic G90.8
    traumatic — *see* Injury, nerve
    ulnar — *see* Lesion, nerve, ulnar
    upper extremity NEC — *see* Mononeuropathy, upper limb
  spinal (cord) G95.20
    by displacement of intervertebral disc NEC — *see also* Disorder, disc, with, myelopathy
    nerve root NOS G54.9
      due to displacement of intervertebral disc NEC — *see* Disorder, disc, with, radiculopathy
      with myelopathy — *see* Disorder, disc, with, myelopathy
    specified NEC G95.29
    spondylogenic (cervical) (lumbar, lumbosacral) (thoracic) — *see* Spondylosis, with myelopathy NEC
    anterior — *see* Syndrome, anterior, spinal artery, compression
    traumatic — *see* Injury, spinal cord, by region
  subcostal nerve (syndrome) — *see* Mononeuropathy, upper limb, specified NEC
  sympathetic nerve NEC G90.8
  syndrome T79.5 ☑
  trachea J39.8
  ulnar nerve (by scar tissue) — *see* Lesion, nerve, ulnar
  umbilical cord
    complicating delivery O69.2 ☑
      cord around neck O69.1 ☑

Compression — *continued*
  umbilical cord — *continued*
    complicating delivery — *continued*
      prolapse O69.0 ☑
      specified NEC O69.2 ☑
  ureter N13.5
  vein I87.1
  vena cava (inferior) (superior) I87.1
Compulsion, compulsive
  gambling F63.0
  neurosis F42.8
  personality F60.5
  states F42.8
  swearing F42.8
    in Gilles de la Tourette's syndrome F95.2
  tics and spasms F95.9
Concato's disease (pericardial polyserositis) A19.9
  nontubercular I31.1
  pleural — *see* Pleurisy, with effusion
Concavity chest wall M95.4
Concealed penis Q55.64
Concern (normal) **about sick person in family** Z63.6
Concrescence (teeth) K00.2
Concretio cordis I31.1
  rheumatic I09.2
Concretion — *see also* Calculus
  appendicular K38.1
  canaliculus — *see* Dacryolith
  clitoris N90.89
  conjunctiva H11.12- ☑
  eyelid — *see* Disorder, eyelid, specified type NEC
  lacrimal passages — *see* Dacryolith
  prepuce (male) N47.8
  salivary gland (any) K11.5
  seminal vesicle N50.89
  tonsil J35.8
Concussion (brain) (cerebral) (current) S06.0X9 ☑
  with
    loss of consciousness of 30 minutes or less S06.0X1 ☑
    loss of consciousness of unspecified duration S06.0X9 ☑
  blast (air) (hydraulic) (immersion) (underwater)
    abdomen or thorax — *see* Injury, blast, by site
    ear with acoustic nerve injury — *see* Injury, nerve, acoustic, specified type NEC
  cauda equina S34.3 ☑
  conus medullaris S34.02 ☑
  ocular S05.8X- ☑
  spinal (cord)
    cervical S14.0 ☑
    lumbar S34.01 ☑
    sacral S34.02 ☑
    thoracic S24.0 ☑
  syndrome F07.81
  without loss of consciousness S06.0X0 ☑
Condition — *see* Disease
Conditions arising in the perinatal period — *see* Newborn, affected by
Conduct disorder — *see* Disorder, conduct
Condyloma A63.0
  acuminatum A63.0
  gonorrheal A54.09
  latum A51.31
  syphilitic A51.31
    congenital A50.07
  venereal, syphilitic A51.31
Conflagration — *see also* Burn
  asphyxia (by inhalation of gases, fumes or vapors) — *see also* Table of Drugs and Chemicals T59.9- ☑
Conflict (with) — *see also* Discord
  family Z73.9
  marital Z63.0
    involving divorce or estrangement Z63.5
  parent-child Z62.820
    parent-adopted child Z62.821
    parent-biological child Z62.820
    parent-foster child Z62.822
  social role NEC Z73.5
Confluent — *see* condition
Confusion, confused R41.0
  epileptic F05
  mental state (psychogenic) F44.89
  psychogenic F44.89
  reactive (from emotional stress, psychological trauma) F44.89
Confusional arousals G47.51

Congelation T69.9 ☑
Congenital — *see also* condition
  aortic septum Q25.49
  intrinsic factor deficiency D51.0
  malformation — *see* Anomaly
Congestion, congestive
  bladder N32.89
  bowel K63.89
  brain G93.89
  breast N64.59
  bronchial J98.09
  catarrhal J31.0
  chest R09.89
  chill, malarial — *see* Malaria
  circulatory NEC I99.8
  duodenum K31.89
  eye — *see* Hyperemia, conjunctiva
  facial, due to birth injury P15.4
  general R68.89
  glottis J37.0
  heart — *see* Failure, heart, congestive
  hepatic K76.1
  hypostatic (lung) — *see* Edema, lung
  intestine K63.89
  kidney N28.89
  labyrinth H83.8 ☑
  larynx J37.0
  liver K76.1
  lung R09.89
    active or acute — *see* Pneumonia
  malaria, malarial — *see* Malaria
  nasal R09.81
  nose R09.81
  orbit, orbital — *see also* Exophthalmos
    inflammatory (chronic) — *see* Inflammation, orbit
  ovary N83.8
  pancreas K86.89
  pelvic, female N94.89
  pleural J94.8
  prostate (active) N42.1
  pulmonary — *see* Congestion, lung
  renal N28.89
  retina H35.81
  seminal vesicle N50.1
  spinal cord G95.19
  spleen (chronic) D73.2
  stomach K31.89
  trachea — *see* Tracheitis
  urethra N36.8
  uterus N85.8
    with subinvolution N85.3
  venous (passive) I87.8
  viscera R68.89
Congestive — *see* Congestion
Conical
  cervix (hypertrophic elongation) N88.4
  cornea — *see* Keratoconus
  teeth K00.2
Conjoined twins Q89.4
Conjugal maladjustment Z63.0
  involving divorce or estrangement Z63.5
Conjunctiva — *see* condition
Conjunctivitis (staphylococcal) (streptococcal) NOS H10.9
  Acanthamoeba B60.12
  acute H10.3- ☑
    atopic H10.1- ☑
    chemical — *see also* Corrosion, cornea H10.21- ☑
    mucopurulent H10.02- ☑
      follicular H10.01- ☑
    pseudomembranous H10.22- ☑
    serous except viral H10.23- ☑
      viral — *see* Conjunctivitis, viral
    toxic H10.21- ☑
  adenoviral (acute) (follicular) B30.1
  allergic (acute) — *see* Conjunctivitis, acute, atopic
    chronic H10.45
      vernal H10.44
  anaphylactic — *see* Conjunctivitis, acute, atopic
  Apollo B30.3
  atopic (acute) — *see* Conjunctivitis, acute, atopic
  Béal's B30.2
  blennorrhagic (gonococcal) (neonatorum) A54.31
  chemical (acute) — *see also* Corrosion, cornea H10.21- ☑
  chlamydial A74.0
    due to trachoma A71.1
    neonatal P39.1

▽ **Subterms under main terms may continue to next column or page**   ☑ **Additional Character Required — Refer to the Tabular List for Character Selection**   **69**

Compression — Conjunctivitis

   ☑ **Additional Character Required** — **Refer to the Tabular List for Character Selection**   ▽ **Subterms under main terms may continue to next column or page**

Constrictive — *see* condition
Consultation
  medical — *see* Counseling, medical
  religious Z71.81
  specified reason NEC Z71.89
  spiritual Z71.81
  without complaint or sickness Z71.9
    feared complaint unfounded Z71.1
    specified reason NEC Z71.89
Consumption — *see* Tuberculosis
Contact (with) — *see also* Exposure (to)
  acariasis Z20.7
  AIDS virus Z20.6
  air pollution Z77.110
  algae and algae toxins Z77.121
  algae bloom Z77.121
  anthrax Z20.810
  aromatic amines Z77.020
  aromatic (hazardous) compounds NEC Z77.028
  aromatic dyes NOS Z77.028
  arsenic Z77.010
  asbestos Z77.090
  bacterial disease NEC Z20.818
  benzene Z77.021
  blue-green algae bloom Z77.121
  body fluids (potentially hazardous) Z77.21
  brown tide Z77.121
  chemicals (chiefly nonmedicinal) (hazardous) NEC
      Z77.098
  cholera Z20.09
  chromium compounds Z77.018
  communicable disease Z20.9
    bacterial NEC Z20.818
    specified NEC Z20.89
    viral NEC Z20.828
    Zika virus Z20.821
  cyanobacteria bloom Z77.121
  dyes Z77.098
  Escherichia coli (E. coli) Z20.01
  fiberglass — *see* Table of Drugs and Chemicals, fiber-
      glass
  German measles Z20.4
  gonorrhea Z20.2
  hazardous metals NEC Z77.018
  hazardous substances NEC Z77.29
  hazards in the physical environment NEC Z77.128
  hazards to health NEC Z77.9
  HIV Z20.6
  HTLV-III/LAV Z20.6
  human immunodeficiency virus (HIV) Z20.6
  infection Z20.9
    specified NEC Z20.89
  infestation (parasitic) NEC Z20.7
  intestinal infectious disease NEC Z20.09
    Escherichia coli (E. coli) Z20.01
  lead Z77.011
  meningococcus Z20.811
  mold (toxic) Z77.120
  nickel dust Z77.018
  noise Z77.122
  parasitic disease Z20.7
  pediculosis Z20.7
  pfiesteria piscicida Z77.121
  poliomyelitis Z20.89
  pollution
    air Z77.110
    environmental NEC Z77.118
    soil Z77.112
    water Z77.111
  polycyclic aromatic hydrocarbons Z77.028
  rabies Z20.3
  radiation, naturally occurring NEC Z77.123
  radon Z77.123
  red tide (Florida) Z77.121
  rubella Z20.4
  sexually-transmitted disease Z20.2
  smallpox (laboratory) Z20.89
  syphilis Z20.2
  tuberculosis Z20.1
  uranium Z77.012
  varicella Z20.820
  venereal disease Z20.2
  viral disease NEC Z20.828
  viral hepatitis Z20.5
  water pollution Z77.111
  Zika virus Z20.821
Contamination, food — *see* Intoxication, foodborne

Contraception, contraceptive
  advice Z30.09
  counseling Z30.09
  device (intrauterine) (in situ) Z97.5
    causing menorrhagia T83.83 ☑
    checking Z30.431
    complications — *see* Complications, intrauterine,
        contraceptive device
    in place Z97.5
    initial prescription Z30.014
    reinsertion Z30.433
    removal Z30.432
    replacement Z30.433
  emergency (postcoital) Z30.012
  initial prescription Z30.019
    barrier Z30.018
    diaphragm Z30.018
    injectable Z30.013
    intrauterine device Z30.014
    pills Z30.011
    postcoital (emergency) Z30.012
    specified type NEC Z30.018
    subdermal implantable Z30.017
    transdermal patch hormonal Z30.016
    vaginal ring hormonal Z30.015
  maintenance Z30.40
    barrier Z30.49
    diaphragm Z30.49
    examination Z30.8
    injectable Z30.42
    intrauterine device Z30.431
    pills Z30.41
    specified type NEC Z30.49
    subdermal implantable Z30.46
    transdermal patch hormonal Z30.45
    vaginal ring hormonal Z30.44
  management Z30.9
    specified NEC Z30.8
  postcoital (emergency) Z30.012
  prescription Z30.019
    repeat Z30.40
  sterilization Z30.2
  surveillance (drug) — *see* Contraception, maintenance
Contraction(s), contracture, contracted
  Achilles tendon — *see also* Short, tendon, Achilles
    congenital Q66.89
  amputation stump (surgical) (flexion) (late) (next
      proximal joint) T87.89
  anus K59.8
  bile duct (common) (hepatic) K83.8
  bladder N32.89
    neck or sphincter N32.0
  bowel, cecum, colon or intestine, any part — *see* Ob-
      struction, intestine
  Braxton Hicks — *see* False, labor
  breast implant, capsular T85.44 ☑
  bronchial J98.09
  burn (old) — *see* Cicatrix
  cervix — *see* Stricture, cervix
  cicatricial — *see* Cicatrix
  conjunctiva, trachomatous, active A71.1
    sequelae (late effect) B94.0
  Dupuytren's M72.0
  eyelid — *see* Disorder, eyelid function
  fascia (lata) (postural) M72.8
    Dupuytren's M72.0
    palmar M72.0
    plantar M72.2
  finger NEC — *see also* Deformity, finger
    congenital Q68.1
    joint — *see* Contraction, joint, hand
  flaccid — *see* Contraction, paralytic
  gallbladder K82.0
  heart valve — *see* Endocarditis
  hip — *see* Contraction, joint, hip
  hourglass
    bladder N32.89
      congenital Q64.79
    gallbladder K82.0
      congenital Q44.1
    stomach K31.89
      congenital Q40.2
      psychogenic F45.8
    uterus (complicating delivery) O62.4
  hysterical F44.4
  internal os — *see* Stricture, cervix
  joint (abduction) (acquired) (adduction) (flexion) (rota-
      tion) M24.50

Contraction(s), contracture, contracted —
    continued
  joint — *continued*
    ankle M24.57- ☑
    congenital NEC Q68.8
      hip Q65.89
    elbow M24.52- ☑
    foot joint M24.57- ☑
    hand joint M24.54- ☑
    hip M24.55- ☑
      congenital Q65.89
    hysterical F44.4
    knee M24.56- ☑
    shoulder M24.51- ☑
    wrist M24.53- ☑
  kidney (granular) (secondary) N26.9
    congenital Q63.8
    hydronephritic — *see* Hydronephrosis
    Page N26.2
    pyelonephritic — *see* Pyelitis, chronic
    tuberculous A18.11
  ligament — *see also* Disorder, ligament
    congenital Q79.8
  muscle (postinfective) (postural) NEC M62.40
    with contracture of joint — *see* Contraction, joint
    ankle M62.47- ☑
    congenital Q79.8
      sternocleidomastoid Q68.0
    extraocular — *see* Strabismus
    eye (extrinsic) — *see* Strabismus
    foot M62.47- ☑
    forearm M62.43- ☑
    hand M62.44- ☑
    hysterical F44.4
    ischemic (Volkmann's) T79.6 ☑
    lower leg M62.46- ☑
    multiple sites M62.49
    pelvic region M62.45- ☑
    posttraumatic — *see* Strabismus, paralytic
    psychogenic F45.8
      conversion reaction F44.4
    shoulder region M62.41- ☑
    specified site NEC M62.48
    thigh M62.45- ☑
    upper arm M62.42- ☑
  neck — *see* Torticollis
  ocular muscle — *see* Strabismus
  organ or site, congenital NEC — *see* Atresia, by site
  outlet (pelvis) — *see* Contraction, pelvis
  palmar fascia M72.0
  paralytic
    joint — *see* Contraction, joint
    muscle — *see also* Contraction, muscle NEC
      ocular — *see* Strabismus, paralytic
  pelvis (acquired) (general) M95.5
    with disproportion (fetopelvic) O33.1
      causing obstructed labor O65.1
    inlet O33.2
    mid-cavity O33.3 ☑
    outlet O33.3 ☑
  plantar fascia M72.2
  premature
    atrium I49.1
    auriculoventricular I49.49
    heart I49.49
    junctional I49.2
    supraventricular I49.1
    ventricular I49.3
  prostate N42.89
  pylorus NEC — *see also* Pylorospasm
    psychogenic F45.8
  rectum, rectal (sphincter) K59.8
  ring (Bandl's) (complicating delivery) O62.4
  scar — *see* Cicatrix
  spine — *see* Dorsopathy, deforming
  sternocleidomastoid (muscle), congenital Q68.0
  stomach K31.89
    hourglass K31.89
      congenital Q40.2
      psychogenic F45.8
    psychogenic F45.8
  tendon (sheath) M62.40
    with contracture of joint — *see* Contraction, joint
    Achilles — *see* Short, tendon, Achilles
    ankle M62.47- ☑
      Achilles — *see* Short, tendon, Achilles
    foot M62.47- ☑

Contraction(s), contracture, contracted — *continued*
- tendon — *continued*
  - forearm M62.43- ☑
  - hand M62.44- ☑
  - lower leg M62.46- ☑
  - multiple sites M62.49
  - neck M62.48
  - pelvic region M62.45- ☑
  - shoulder region M62.41- ☑
  - specified site NEC M62.48
  - thigh M62.45- ☑
  - thorax M62.48
  - trunk M62.48
  - upper arm M62.42- ☑
- toe — *see* Deformity, toe, specified NEC
- ureterovesical orifice (postinfectional) N13.5
  - with infection N13.6
- urethra — *see also* Stricture, urethra
  - orifice N32.0
- uterus N85.8
  - abnormal NEC O62.9
  - clonic (complicating delivery) O62.4
  - dyscoordinate (complicating delivery) O62.4
  - hourglass (complicating delivery) O62.4
  - hypertonic O62.4
  - hypotonic NEC O62.2
  - inadequate
    - primary O62.0
    - secondary O62.1
  - incoordinate (complicating delivery) O62.4
  - poor O62.2
  - tetanic (complicating delivery) O62.4
- vagina (outlet) N89.5
- vesical N32.89
  - neck or urethral orifice N32.0
- visual field — *see* Defect, visual field, generalized
- Volkmann's (ischemic) T79.6

Contusion (skin surface intact) T14.8 ☑
- abdomen, abdominal (muscle) (wall) S30.1 ☑
- adnexa, eye NEC S05.8X- ☑
- adrenal gland S37.812 ☑
- alveolar process S00.532 ☑
- ankle S90.0- ☑
- antecubital space — *see* Contusion, forearm
- anus S30.3 ☑
- arm (upper) S40.02- ☑
  - lower (with elbow) — *see* Contusion, forearm
- auditory canal — *see* Contusion, ear
- auricle — *see* Contusion, ear
- axilla — *see* Contusion, arm, upper
- back — *see also* Contusion, thorax, back
  - lower S30.0 ☑
- bile duct S36.13 ☑
- bladder S37.22 ☑
- bone NEC T14.8 ☑
- brain (diffuse) — *see* Injury, intracranial, diffuse
  - focal — *see* Injury, intracranial, focal
- brainstem S06.38- ☑
- breast S20.0- ☑
- broad ligament S37.892 ☑
- brow S00.83 ☑
- buttock S30.0 ☑
- canthus, eye S00.1- ☑
- cauda equina S34.3 ☑
- cerebellar, traumatic S06.37- ☑
- cerebral S06.33- ☑
  - left side S06.32- ☑
  - right side S06.31- ☑
- cheek S00.83 ☑
  - internal S00.532 ☑
- chest (wall) — *see* Contusion, thorax
- chin S00.83 ☑
- clitoris S30.23 ☑
- colon — *see* Injury, intestine, large, contusion
- common bile duct S36.13 ☑
- conjunctiva S05.1- ☑
  - with foreign body (in conjunctival sac) — *see* Foreign body, conjunctival sac
- conus medullaris (spine) S34.139 ☑
- cornea — *see* Contusion, eyeball
  - with foreign body — *see* Foreign body, cornea
- corpus cavernosum S30.21 ☑
- cortex (brain) (cerebral) — *see* Injury, intracranial, diffuse
  - focal — *see* Injury, intracranial, focal
- costal region — *see* Contusion, thorax

Contusion — *continued*
- cystic duct S36.13 ☑
- diaphragm S27.802 ☑
- duodenum S36.420 ☑
- ear S00.43- ☑
- elbow S50.0- ☑
  - with forearm — *see* Contusion, forearm
- epididymis S30.22 ☑
- epigastric region S30.1 ☑
- epiglottis S10.0 ☑
- esophagus (thoracic) S27.812 ☑
  - cervical S10.0 ☑
- eyeball S05.1- ☑
- eyebrow S00.1- ☑
- eyelid (and periocular area) S00.1- ☑
- face NEC S00.83 ☑
- fallopian tube S37.529 ☑
  - bilateral S37.522 ☑
  - unilateral S37.521 ☑
- femoral triangle S30.1 ☑
- finger(s) S60.00 ☑
  - with damage to nail (matrix) S60.10 ☑
  - index S60.02- ☑
    - with damage to nail S60.12- ☑
  - little S60.05- ☑
    - with damage to nail S60.15- ☑
  - middle S60.03- ☑
    - with damage to nail S60.13- ☑
  - ring S60.04- ☑
    - with damage to nail S60.14- ☑
  - thumb — *see* Contusion, thumb
- flank S30.1 ☑
- foot (except toe(s) alone) S90.3- ☑
  - toe — *see* Contusion, toe
- forearm S50.1- ☑
  - elbow only — *see* Contusion, elbow
- forehead S00.83 ☑
- gallbladder S36.122 ☑
- genital organs, external
  - female S30.202 ☑
  - male S30.201 ☑
- globe (eye) — *see* Contusion, eyeball
- groin S30.1 ☑
- gum S00.532 ☑
- hand S60.22- ☑
  - finger(s) — *see* Contusion, finger
  - wrist — *see* Contusion, wrist
- head S00.93 ☑
  - ear — *see* Contusion, ear
  - eyelid — *see* Contusion, eyelid
  - lip S00.531 ☑
  - nose S00.33 ☑
  - oral cavity S00.532 ☑
  - scalp S00.03 ☑
  - specified part NEC S00.83 ☑
- heart — *see also* Injury, heart S26.91 ☑
- heel — *see* Contusion, foot
- hepatic duct S36.13 ☑
- hip S70.0- ☑
- ileum S36.428 ☑
- iliac region S30.1 ☑
- inguinal region S30.1 ☑
- interscapular region S20.229 ☑
- intra-abdominal organ S36.92 ☑
  - colon — *see* Injury, intestine, large, contusion
  - liver S36.112 ☑
  - pancreas — *see* Contusion, pancreas
  - rectum S36.62 ☑
  - small intestine — *see* Injury, intestine, small, contusion
  - specified organ NEC S36.892 ☑
  - spleen — *see* Contusion, spleen
  - stomach S36.32 ☑
- iris (eye) — *see* Contusion, eyeball
- jaw S00.83 ☑
- jejunum S36.428 ☑
- kidney S37.01- ☑
  - major (greater than 2 cm) S37.02- ☑
  - minor (less than 2 cm) S37.01- ☑
- knee S80.0- ☑
- labium (majus) (minus) S30.23 ☑
- lacrimal apparatus, gland or sac S05.8X- ☑
- larynx S10.0 ☑
- leg (lower) S80.1- ☑
  - knee — *see* Contusion, knee
- lens — *see* Contusion, eyeball

Contusion — *continued*
- lip S00.531 ☑
- liver S36.112 ☑
- lower back S30.0 ☑
- lumbar region S30.0 ☑
- lung S27.329 ☑
  - bilateral S27.322 ☑
  - unilateral S27.321 ☑
- malar region S00.83 ☑
- mastoid region S00.83 ☑
- membrane, brain — *see* Injury, intracranial, diffuse
  - focal — *see* Injury, intracranial, focal
- mesentery S36.892 ☑
- mesosalpinx S37.892 ☑
- mouth S00.532 ☑
- muscle — *see* Contusion, by site
- nail
  - finger — *see* Contusion, finger, with damage to nail
  - toe — *see* Contusion, toe, with damage to nail
- nasal S00.33 ☑
- neck S10.93 ☑
  - specified site NEC S10.83 ☑
  - throat S10.0 ☑
- nerve — *see* Injury, nerve
- newborn P54.5
- nose S00.33 ☑
- occipital
  - lobe (brain) — *see* Injury, intracranial, diffuse
    - focal — *see* Injury, intracranial, focal
  - region (scalp) S00.03 ☑
- orbit (region) (tissues) S05.1- ☑
- ovary S37.429 ☑
  - bilateral S37.422 ☑
  - unilateral S37.421 ☑
- palate S00.532 ☑
- pancreas S36.229 ☑
  - body S36.221 ☑
  - head S36.220 ☑
  - tail S36.222 ☑
- parietal
  - lobe (brain) — *see* Injury, intracranial, diffuse
    - focal — *see* Injury, intracranial, focal
  - region (scalp) S00.03 ☑
- pelvic organ S37.92 ☑
  - adrenal gland S37.812 ☑
  - bladder S37.22 ☑
  - fallopian tube — *see* Contusion, fallopian tube
  - kidney — *see* Contusion, kidney
  - ovary — *see* Contusion, ovary
  - prostate S37.822 ☑
  - specified organ NEC S37.892 ☑
  - ureter S37.12 ☑
  - urethra S37.32 ☑
  - uterus S37.62 ☑
- pelvis S30.0 ☑
- penis S30.21 ☑
- perineum
  - female S30.23 ☑
  - male S30.0 ☑
- periocular area S00.1- ☑
- peritoneum S36.81 ☑
- periurethral tissue — *see* Contusion, urethra
- pharynx S10.0 ☑
- pinna — *see* Contusion, ear
- popliteal space — *see* Contusion, knee
- prepuce S30.21 ☑
- prostate S37.822 ☑
- pubic region S30.1 ☑
- pudendum
  - female S30.202 ☑
  - male S30.201 ☑
- quadriceps femoris — *see* Contusion, thigh
- rectum S36.62 ☑
- retroperitoneum S36.892 ☑
- round ligament S37.892 ☑
- sacral region S30.0 ☑
- scalp S00.03 ☑
  - due to birth injury P12.3
- scapular region — *see* Contusion, shoulder
- sclera — *see* Contusion, eyeball
- scrotum S30.22 ☑
- seminal vesicle S37.892 ☑
- shoulder S40.01- ☑
- skin NEC T14.8 ☑
- small intestine — *see* Injury, intestine, small, contusion
- spermatic cord S30.22 ☑

Contusion — *continued*
- spinal cord — *see* Injury, spinal cord, by region
  - cauda equina S34.3 ☑
  - conus medullaris S34.139 ☑
- spleen S36.029 ☑
  - major S36.021 ☑
  - minor S36.020 ☑
- sternal region S20.219 ☑
- stomach S36.32 ☑
- subconjunctival S05.1- ☑
- subcutaneous NEC T14.8 ☑
- submaxillary region S00.83 ☑
- submental region S00.83 ☑
- subperiosteal NEC T14.8 ☑
- subungual
  - finger — *see* Contusion, finger, with damage to nail
  - toe — *see* Contusion, toe, with damage to nail
- supraclavicular fossa S10.83 ☑
- supraorbital S00.83 ☑
- suprarenal gland S37.812 ☑
- temple (region) S00.83 ☑
- temporal
  - lobe (brain) — *see* Injury, intracranial, diffuse
  - focal — *see* Injury, intracranial, focal
  - region S00.83 ☑
- testis S30.22 ☑
- thigh S70.1- ☑
- thorax (wall) S20.20 ☑
  - back S20.22- ☑
  - front S20.21- ☑
- throat S10.0 ☑
- thumb S60.01- ☑
  - with damage to nail S60.11- ☑
- toe(s) (lesser) S90.12- ☑
  - with damage to nail S90.22- ☑
  - great S90.11- ☑
    - with damage to nail S90.21- ☑
- tongue S00.532 ☑
- trachea (cervical) S10.0 ☑
  - thoracic S27.52 ☑
- tunica vaginalis S30.22 ☑
- tympanum, tympanic membrane — *see* Contusion, ear
- ureter S37.12 ☑
- urethra S37.32 ☑
- urinary organ NEC S37.892 ☑
- uterus S37.62 ☑
- uvula S00.532 ☑
- vagina S30.23 ☑
- vas deferens S37.892 ☑
- vesical S37.22 ☑
- vocal cord(s) S10.0 ☑
- vulva S30.23 ☑
- wrist S60.21- ☑

Conus (congenital) (any type) Q14.8
- cornea — *see* Keratoconus
- medullaris syndrome G95.81

Conversion hysteria, neurosis or reaction F44.9
Converter, tuberculosis (test reaction) R76.11
Conviction (legal), **anxiety concerning** Z65.0
- with imprisonment Z65.1
Convulsions (idiopathic) — *see also* Seizure(s) R56.9
- apoplectiform (cerebral ischemia) I67.82
- dissociative F44.5
- epileptic — *see* Epilepsy
- epileptiform, epileptoid — *see* Seizure, epileptiform
- ether (anesthetic) — *see* Table of Drugs and Chemicals, by drug
- febrile R56.00
  - with status epilepticus G40.901
  - complex R56.01
    - with status epilepticus G40.901
  - simple R56.00
- hysterical F44.5
- infantile P90
  - epilepsy — *see* Epilepsy
- jacksonian — *see* Epilepsy, localization-related, symptomatic, with simple partial seizures
- myoclonic G25.3
- newborn P90
- obstetrical (nephritic) (uremic) — *see* Eclampsia
- paretic A52.17
- post traumatic R56.1
- psychomotor — *see* Epilepsy, localization-related, symptomatic, with complex partial seizures
- recurrent R56.9

Convulsions — *continued*
- reflex R25.8
- scarlatinal A38.8
- tetanus, tetanic — *see* Tetanus
- thymic E32.8
Convulsive — *see also* Convulsions
Cooley's anemia D56.1
Coolie itch B76.9
Cooper's
- disease — *see* Mastopathy, cystic
- hernia — *see* Hernia, abdomen, specified site NEC
Copra itch B88.0
Coprophagy F50.89
Coprophobia F40.298
Coproporphyria, hereditary E80.29
Cor
- biloculare Q20.8
- bovis, bovinum — *see* Hypertrophy, cardiac
- pulmonale (chronic) I27.81
  - acute I26.09
- triatriatum, triatrium Q24.2
- triloculare Q20.8
  - biatrium Q20.4
  - biventriculare Q21.1
Corbus' disease (gangrenous balanitis) N48.1
Cord — *see also* condition
- around neck
  - complicating delivery O69.81 ☑
    - with compression O69.1 ☑
- bladder G95.89
  - tabetic A52.19
Cordis ectopia Q24.8
Corditis (spermatic) N49.1
Corectopia Q13.2
Cori's disease (glycogen storage) E74.03
Corkhandler's disease or lung J67.3
Corkscrew esophagus K22.4
Corkworker's disease or lung J67.3
Corn (infected) L84
Cornea — *see also* condition
- donor Z52.5
- plana Q13.4
Cornelia de Lange syndrome Q87.19
Cornu cutaneum L85.8
Cornual gestation or pregnancy O00.80
- with intrauterine pregnancy O00.81
Coronary (artery) — *see* condition
Coronavirus, as cause of disease classified elsewhere B97.29
- SARS-associated B97.21
Corpora — *see also* condition
- amylacea, prostate N42.89
- cavernosa — *see* condition
Corpulence — *see* Obesity
Corpus — *see* condition
Corrected transposition Q20.5
Corrosion (injury) (acid) (caustic) (chemical) (lime) (external) (internal) T30.4
- abdomen, abdominal (muscle) (wall) T21.42 ☑
  - first degree T21.52 ☑
  - second degree T21.62 ☑
  - third degree T21.72 ☑
- above elbow T22.439 ☑
  - first degree T22.539 ☑
  - left T22.432 ☑
    - first degree T22.532 ☑
    - second degree T22.632 ☑
    - third degree T22.732 ☑
  - right T22.431 ☑
    - first degree T22.531 ☑
    - second degree T22.631 ☑
    - third degree T22.731 ☑
  - second degree T22.639 ☑
  - third degree T22.739 ☑
- alimentary tract NEC T28.7 ☑
- ankle T25.419 ☑
  - first degree T25.519 ☑
  - left T25.412 ☑
    - first degree T25.512 ☑
    - second degree T25.612 ☑
    - third degree T25.712 ☑
  - multiple with foot — *see* Corrosion, lower, limb, multiple, ankle and foot
  - right T25.411 ☑
    - first degree T25.511 ☑
    - second degree T25.611 ☑

Corrosion — *continued*
- ankle — *continued*
  - right — *continued*
    - third degree T25.711 ☑
  - second degree T25.619 ☑
  - third degree T25.719 ☑
- anus — *see* Corrosion, buttock
- arm(s) (meaning upper limb(s)) — *see* Corrosion, upper limb
- axilla T22.449 ☑
  - first degree T22.549 ☑
  - left T22.442 ☑
    - first degree T22.542 ☑
    - second degree T22.642 ☑
    - third degree T22.742 ☑
  - right T22.441 ☑
    - first degree T22.541 ☑
    - second degree T22.641 ☑
    - third degree T22.741 ☑
  - second degree T22.649 ☑
  - third degree T22.749 ☑
- back (lower) T21.44 ☑
  - first degree T21.54 ☑
  - second degree T21.64 ☑
  - third degree T21.74 ☑
  - upper T21.43 ☑
    - first degree T21.53 ☑
    - second degree T21.63 ☑
    - third degree T21.73 ☑
- blisters — *code as* Corrosion, second degree, by site
- breast(s) — *see* Corrosion, chest wall
- buttock(s) T21.45 ☑
  - first degree T21.55 ☑
  - second degree T21.65 ☑
  - third degree T21.75 ☑
- calf T24.439 ☑
  - first degree T24.539 ☑
  - left T24.432 ☑
    - first degree T24.532 ☑
    - second degree T24.632 ☑
    - third degree T24.732 ☑
  - right T24.431 ☑
    - first degree T24.531 ☑
    - second degree T24.631 ☑
    - third degree T24.731 ☑
  - second degree T24.639 ☑
  - third degree T24.739 ☑
- canthus (eye) — *see* Corrosion, eyelid
- cervix T28.8 ☑
- cheek T20.46 ☑
  - first degree T20.56 ☑
  - second degree T20.66 ☑
  - third degree T20.76 ☑
- chest wall T21.41 ☑
  - first degree T21.51 ☑
  - second degree T21.61 ☑
  - third degree T21.71 ☑
- chin T20.43 ☑
  - first degree T20.53 ☑
  - second degree T20.63 ☑
  - third degree T20.73 ☑
- colon T28.7 ☑
- conjunctiva (and cornea) — *see* Corrosion, cornea
- cornea (and conjunctiva) T26.6- ☑
- deep necrosis of underlying tissue — *code as* Corrosion, third degree, by site
- dorsum of hand T23.469 ☑
  - first degree T23.569 ☑
  - left T23.462 ☑
    - first degree T23.562 ☑
    - second degree T23.662 ☑
    - third degree T23.762 ☑
  - right T23.461 ☑
    - first degree T23.561 ☑
    - second degree T23.661 ☑
    - third degree T23.761 ☑
  - second degree T23.669 ☑
  - third degree T23.769 ☑
- ear (auricle) (external) (canal) T20.41 ☑
  - drum T28.91 ☑
  - first degree T20.51 ☑
  - second degree T20.61 ☑
  - third degree T20.71 ☑
- elbow T22.429 ☑
  - first degree T22.529 ☑
  - left T22.422 ☑

Corrosion — *continued*
  elbow — *continued*
    left — *continued*
      first degree T22.522 ☑
      second degree T22.622 ☑
      third degree T22.722 ☑
    right T22.421 ☑
      first degree T22.521 ☑
      second degree T22.621 ☑
      third degree T22.721 ☑
    second degree T22.629 ☑
    third degree T22.729 ☑
  entire body — *see* Corrosion, multiple body regions
  epidermal loss — *code as* Corrosion, second degree, by site
  epiglottis T27.4 ☑
  erythema, erythematous — *code as* Corrosion, first degree, by site
  esophagus T28.6 ☑
  extent (percentage of body surface)
    less than 10 percent T32.0
    10-19 percent (0-9 percent third degree) T32.10
      with 10-19 percent third degree T32.11
    20-29 percent (0-9 percent third degree) T32.20
      with
        10-19 percent third degree T32.21
        20-29 percent third degree T32.22
    30-39 percent (0-9 percent third degree) T32.30
      with
        10-19 percent third degree T32.31
        20-29 percent third degree T32.32
        30-39 percent third degree T32.33
    40-49 percent (0-9 percent third degree) T32.40
      with
        10-19 percent third degree T32.41
        20-29 percent third degree T32.42
        30-39 percent third degree T32.43
        40-49 percent third degree T32.44
    50-59 percent (0-9 percent third degree) T32.50
      with
        10-19 percent third degree T32.51
        20-29 percent third degree T32.52
        30-39 percent third degree T32.53
        40-49 percent third degree T32.54
        50-59 percent third degree T32.55
    60-69 percent (0-9 percent third degree) T32.60
      with
        10-19 percent third degree T32.61
        20-29 percent third degree T32.62
        30-39 percent third degree T32.63
        40-49 percent third degree T32.64
        50-59 percent third degree T32.65
        60-69 percent third degree T32.66
    70-79 percent (0-9 percent third degree) T32.70
      with
        10-19 percent third degree T32.71
        20-29 percent third degree T32.72
        30-39 percent third degree T32.73
        40-49 percent third degree T32.74
        50-59 percent third degree T32.75
        60-69 percent third degree T32.76
        70-79 percent third degree T32.77
    80-89 percent (0-9 percent third degree) T32.80
      with
        10-19 percent third degree T32.81
        20-29 percent third degree T32.82
        30-39 percent third degree T32.83
        40-49 percent third degree T32.84
        50-59 percent third degree T32.85
        60-69 percent third degree T32.86
        70-79 percent third degree T32.87
        80-89 percent third degree T32.88
    90 percent or more (0-9 percent third degree) T32.90
      with
        10-19 percent third degree T32.91
        20-29 percent third degree T32.92
        30-39 percent third degree T32.93
        40-49 percent third degree T32.94
        50-59 percent third degree T32.95
        60-69 percent third degree T32.96
        70-79 percent third degree T32.97
        80-89 percent third degree T32.98
        90-99 percent third degree T32.99
  extremity — *see* Corrosion, limb
  eye(s) and adnexa T26.9-
    with resulting rupture and destruction of eyeball T26.7-
    conjunctival sac — *see* Corrosion, cornea

Corrosion — *continued*
  eye(s) and adnexa — *continued*
    cornea — *see* Corrosion, cornea
    lid — *see* Corrosion, eyelid
    periocular area — *see* Corrosion eyelid
    specified site NEC T26.8- ☑
  eyeball — *see* Corrosion, eye
  eyelid(s) T26.5-
  face — *see* Corrosion, head
  finger T23.429 ☑
    first degree T23.529 ☑
    left T23.422 ☑
      first degree T23.522 ☑
      second degree T23.622 ☑
      third degree T23.722 ☑
    multiple sites (without thumb) T23.439 ☑
      with thumb T23.449 ☑
        first degree T23.549 ☑
        left T23.442 ☑
          first degree T23.542 ☑
          second degree T23.642 ☑
          third degree T23.742 ☑
        right T23.441 ☑
          first degree T23.541 ☑
          second degree T23.641 ☑
          third degree T23.741 ☑
        second degree T23.649 ☑
        third degree T23.749 ☑
      first degree T23.539 ☑
      left T23.432 ☑
        first degree T23.532 ☑
        second degree T23.632 ☑
        third degree T23.732 ☑
      right T23.431 ☑
        first degree T23.531 ☑
        second degree T23.631 ☑
        third degree T23.731 ☑
      second degree T23.639 ☑
      third degree T23.739 ☑
    right T23.421 ☑
      first degree T23.521 ☑
      second degree T23.621 ☑
      third degree T23.721 ☑
    second degree T23.629 ☑
    third degree T23.729 ☑
  flank — *see* Corrosion, abdomen
  foot T25.429 ☑
    first degree T25.529 ☑
    left T25.422 ☑
      first degree T25.522 ☑
      second degree T25.622 ☑
      third degree T25.722 ☑
    multiple with ankle — *see* Corrosion, lower, limb, multiple, ankle and foot
    right T25.421 ☑
      first degree T25.521 ☑
      second degree T25.621 ☑
      third degree T25.721 ☑
    second degree T25.629 ☑
    third degree T25.729 ☑
  forearm T22.419 ☑
    first degree T22.519 ☑
    left T22.412 ☑
      first degree T22.512 ☑
      second degree T22.612 ☑
      third degree T22.712 ☑
    right T22.411 ☑
      first degree T22.511 ☑
      second degree T22.611 ☑
      third degree T22.711 ☑
    second degree T22.619 ☑
    third degree T22.719 ☑
  forehead T20.46 ☑
    first degree T20.56 ☑
    second degree T20.66 ☑
    third degree T20.76 ☑
  fourth degree — *code as* Corrosion, third degree, by site
  full thickness skin loss — *code as* Corrosion, third degree, by site
  gastrointestinal tract NEC T28.7 ☑
  genital organs
    external
      female T21.47 ☑
        first degree T21.57 ☑
        second degree T21.67 ☑

Corrosion — *continued*
  genital organs — *continued*
    external — *continued*
      female — *continued*
        third degree T21.77 ☑
      male T21.46 ☑
        first degree T21.56 ☑
        second degree T21.66 ☑
        third degree T21.76 ☑
    internal T28.8 ☑
  groin — *see* Corrosion, abdominal wall
  hand(s) T23.409 ☑
    back — *see* Corrosion, dorsum of hand
    finger — *see* Corrosion, finger
    first degree T23.509 ☑
    left T23.402 ☑
      first degree T23.502 ☑
      second degree T23.602 ☑
      third degree T23.702 ☑
    multiple sites with wrist T23.499 ☑
      first degree T23.599 ☑
      left T23.492 ☑
        first degree T23.592 ☑
        second degree T23.692 ☑
        third degree T23.792 ☑
      right T23.491 ☑
        first degree T23.591 ☑
        second degree T23.691 ☑
        third degree T23.791 ☑
      second degree T23.699 ☑
      third degree T23.799 ☑
    palm — *see* Corrosion, palm
    right T23.401 ☑
      first degree T23.501 ☑
      second degree T23.601 ☑
      third degree T23.701 ☑
    second degree T23.609 ☑
    third degree T23.709 ☑
    thumb — *see* Corrosion, thumb
  head (and face) (and neck) T20.40 ☑
    cheek — *see* Corrosion, cheek
    chin — *see* Corrosion, chin
    ear — *see* Corrosion, ear
    eye(s) only — *see* Corrosion, eye
    first degree T20.50 ☑
    forehead — *see* Corrosion, forehead
    lip — *see* Corrosion, lip
    multiple sites T20.49 ☑
      first degree T20.59 ☑
      second degree T20.69 ☑
      third degree T20.79 ☑
    neck — *see* Corrosion, neck
    nose — *see* Corrosion, nose
    scalp — *see* Corrosion, scalp
    second degree T20.60 ☑
    third degree T20.70 ☑
  hip(s) — *see* Corrosion, lower, limb
  inhalation — *see* Corrosion, respiratory tract
  internal organ(s) — *see also* Corrosion, by site T28.90 ☑
    alimentary tract T28.7 ☑
      esophagus T28.6 ☑
    esophagus T28.6 ☑
    genitourinary T28.8 ☑
    mouth T28.5 ☑
    pharynx T28.5 ☑
    specified organ NEC T28.99 ☑
  interscapular region — *see* Corrosion, back, upper
  intestine (large) (small) T28.7 ☑
  knee T24.429 ☑
    first degree T24.529 ☑
    left T24.422 ☑
      first degree T24.522 ☑
      second degree T24.622 ☑
      third degree T24.722 ☑
    right T24.421 ☑
      first degree T24.521 ☑
      second degree T24.621 ☑
      third degree T24.721 ☑
    second degree T24.629 ☑
    third degree T24.729 ☑
  labium (majus) (minus) — *see* Corrosion, genital organs, external, female
  lacrimal apparatus, duct, gland or sac — *see* Corrosion, eye, specified site NEC
  larynx T27.4 ☑

Corrosion — continued
  larynx — continued
    with lung T27.5 ☑
  leg(s) (meaning lower limb(s)) — see Corrosion, lower limb
  limb(s)
    lower — see Corrosion, lower limb
    upper — see Corrosion, upper limb
  lip(s) T20.42 ☑
    first degree T20.52 ☑
    second degree T20.62 ☑
    third degree T20.72 ☑
  lower
    back — see Corrosion, back
    limb T24.409 ☑
      ankle — see Corrosion, ankle
      calf — see Corrosion, calf
      first degree T24.509 ☑
      foot — see Corrosion, foot
      knee — see Corrosion, knee
      left T24.402 ☑
        first degree T24.502 ☑
        second degree T24.602 ☑
        third degree T24.702 ☑
      multiple sites, except ankle and foot T24.499 ☑
        ankle and foot T25.499 ☑
          first degree T25.599 ☑
          left T25.492 ☑
            first degree T25.592 ☑
            second degree T25.692 ☑
            third degree T25.792 ☑
          right T25.491 ☑
            first degree T25.591 ☑
            second degree T25.691 ☑
            third degree T25.791 ☑
          second degree T25.699 ☑
          third degree T25.799 ☑
        first degree T24.599 ☑
        left T24.492 ☑
          first degree T24.592 ☑
          second degree T24.692 ☑
          third degree T24.792 ☑
        right T24.491 ☑
          first degree T24.591 ☑
          second degree T24.691 ☑
          third degree T24.791 ☑
        second degree T24.699 ☑
        third degree T24.799 ☑
      right T24.401 ☑
        first degree T24.501 ☑
        second degree T24.601 ☑
        third degree T24.701 ☑
      second degree T24.609 ☑
      thigh — see Corrosion, thigh
      third degree T24.709 ☑
  lung (with larynx and trachea) T27.5 ☑
  mouth T28.5 ☑
  neck T20.47 ☑
    first degree T20.57 ☑
    second degree T20.67 ☑
    third degree T20.77 ☑
  nose (septum) T20.44 ☑
    first degree T20.54 ☑
    second degree T20.64 ☑
    third degree T20.74 ☑
  ocular adnexa — see Corrosion, eye
  orbit region — see Corrosion, eyelid
  palm T23.459 ☑
    first degree T23.559 ☑
    left T23.452 ☑
      first degree T23.552 ☑
      second degree T23.652 ☑
      third degree T23.752 ☑
    right T23.451 ☑
      first degree T23.551 ☑
      second degree T23.651 ☑
      third degree T23.751 ☑
    second degree T23.659 ☑
    third degree T23.759 ☑
  partial thickness — code as Corrosion, unspecified degree, by site
  pelvis — see Corrosion, trunk
  penis — see Corrosion, genital organs, external, male
  perineum
    female — see Corrosion, genital organs, external, female

Corrosion — continued
  perineum — continued
    male — see Corrosion, genital organs, external, male
  periocular area — see Corrosion, eyelid
  pharynx T28.5 ☑
  rectum T28.7 ☑
  respiratory tract T27.7 ☑
    larynx — see Corrosion, larynx
    specified part NEC T27.6 ☑
    trachea — see Corrosion, larynx
  sac, lacrimal — see Corrosion, eye, specified site NEC
  scalp T20.45 ☑
    first degree T20.55 ☑
    second degree T20.65 ☑
    third degree T20.75 ☑
  scapular region T22.469 ☑
    first degree T22.569 ☑
    left T22.462 ☑
      first degree T22.562 ☑
      second degree T22.662 ☑
      third degree T22.762 ☑
    right T22.461 ☑
      first degree T22.561 ☑
      second degree T22.661 ☑
      third degree T22.761 ☑
    second degree T22.669 ☑
    third degree T22.769 ☑
  sclera — see Corrosion, eye, specified site NEC
  scrotum — see Corrosion, genital organs, external, male
  shoulder T22.459 ☑
    first degree T22.559 ☑
    left T22.452 ☑
      first degree T22.552 ☑
      second degree T22.652 ☑
      third degree T22.752 ☑
    right T22.451 ☑
      first degree T22.551 ☑
      second degree T22.651 ☑
      third degree T22.751 ☑
    second degree T22.659 ☑
    third degree T22.759 ☑
  stomach T28.7 ☑
  temple — see Corrosion, head
  testis — see Corrosion, genital organs, external, male
  thigh T24.419 ☑
    first degree T24.519 ☑
    left T24.412 ☑
      first degree T24.512 ☑
      second degree T24.612 ☑
      third degree T24.712 ☑
    right T24.411 ☑
      first degree T24.511 ☑
      second degree T24.611 ☑
      third degree T24.711 ☑
    second degree T24.619 ☑
    third degree T24.719 ☑
  thorax (external) — see Corrosion, trunk
  throat (meaning pharynx) T28.5 ☑
  thumb(s) T23.419 ☑
    first degree T23.519 ☑
    left T23.412 ☑
      first degree T23.512 ☑
      second degree T23.612 ☑
      third degree T23.712 ☑
    multiple sites with fingers T23.449 ☑
      first degree T23.549 ☑
      left T23.442 ☑
        first degree T23.542 ☑
        second degree T23.642 ☑
        third degree T23.742 ☑
      right T23.441 ☑
        first degree T23.541 ☑
        second degree T23.641 ☑
        third degree T23.741 ☑
      second degree T23.649 ☑
      third degree T23.749 ☑
    right T23.411 ☑
      first degree T23.511 ☑
      second degree T23.611 ☑
      third degree T23.711 ☑
    second degree T23.619 ☑
    third degree T23.719 ☑
  toe T25.439 ☑
    first degree T25.539 ☑
    left T25.432 ☑

Corrosion — continued
  toe — continued
    left — continued
      first degree T25.532 ☑
      second degree T25.632 ☑
      third degree T25.732 ☑
    right T25.431 ☑
      first degree T25.531 ☑
      second degree T25.631 ☑
      third degree T25.731 ☑
    second degree T25.639 ☑
    third degree T25.739 ☑
  tongue T28.5 ☑
  tonsil(s) T28.5 ☑
  total body — see Corrosion, multiple body regions
  trachea T27.4 ☑
    with lung T27.5 ☑
  trunk T21.40 ☑
    abdominal wall — see Corrosion, abdominal wall
    anus — see Corrosion, buttock
    axilla — see Corrosion, upper limb
    back — see Corrosion, back
    breast — see Corrosion, chest wall
    buttock — see Corrosion, buttock
    chest wall — see Corrosion, chest wall
    first degree T21.50 ☑
    flank — see Corrosion, abdominal wall
    genital
      female — see Corrosion, genital organs, external, female
      male — see Corrosion, genital organs, external, male
    groin — see Corrosion, abdominal wall
    interscapular region — see Corrosion, back, upper
    labia — see Corrosion, genital organs, external, female
    lower back — see Corrosion, back
    penis — see Corrosion, genital organs, external, male
    perineum
      female — see Corrosion, genital organs, external, female
      male — see Corrosion, genital organs, external, male
    scapular region — see Corrosion, upper limb
    scrotum — see Corrosion, genital organs, external, male
    second degree T21.60 ☑
    shoulder — see Corrosion, upper limb
    specified site NEC T21.49 ☑
      first degree T21.59 ☑
      second degree T21.69 ☑
      third degree T21.79 ☑
    testes — see Corrosion, genital organs, external, male
    third degree T21.70 ☑
    upper back — see Corrosion, back, upper
    vagina T28.8 ☑
    vulva — see Corrosion, genital organs, external, female
  unspecified site with extent of body surface involved specified
    less than 10 percent T32.0
    10-19 percent (0-9 percent third degree) T32.10
      with 10-19 percent third degree T32.11
    20-29 percent (0-9 percent third degree) T32.20
      with
        10-19 percent third degree T32.21
        20-29 percent third degree T32.22
    30-39 percent (0-9 percent third degree) T32.30
      with
        10-19 percent third degree T32.31
        20-29 percent third degree T32.32
        30-39 percent third degree T32.33
    40-49 percent (0-9 percent third degree) T32.40
      with
        10-19 percent third degree T32.41
        20-29 percent third degree T32.42
        30-39 percent third degree T32.43
        40-49 percent third degree T32.44
    50-59 percent (0-9 percent third degree) T32.50
      with
        10-19 percent third degree T32.51
        20-29 percent third degree T32.52
        30-39 percent third degree T32.53
        40-49 percent third degree T32.54
        50-59 percent third degree T32.55

Corrosion — *continued*
unspecified site with extent of body surface involved
specified — *continued*
60-69 percent (0-9 percent third degree) T32.60
with
10-19 percent third degree T32.61
20-29 percent third degree T32.62
30-39 percent third degree T32.63
40-49 percent third degree T32.64
50-59 percent third degree T32.65
60-69 percent third degree T32.66
70-79 percent (0-9 percent third degree) T32.70
with
10-19 percent third degree T32.71
20-29 percent third degree T32.72
30-39 percent third degree T32.73
40-49 percent third degree T32.74
50-59 percent third degree T32.75
60-69 percent third degree T32.76
70-79 percent third degree T32.77
80-89 percent (0-9 percent third degree) T32.80
with
10-19 percent third degree T32.81
20-29 percent third degree T32.82
30-39 percent third degree T32.83
40-49 percent third degree T32.84
50-59 percent third degree T32.85
60-69 percent third degree T32.86
70-79 percent third degree T32.87
80-89 percent third degree T32.88
90 percent or more (0-9 percent third degree) T32.90
with
10-19 percent third degree T32.91
20-29 percent third degree T32.92
30-39 percent third degree T32.93
40-49 percent third degree T32.94
50-59 percent third degree T32.95
60-69 percent third degree T32.96
70-79 percent third degree T32.97
80-89 percent third degree T32.98
90-99 percent third degree T32.99
upper limb (axilla) (scapular region) T22.40 ☑
above elbow — *see* Corrosion, above elbow
axilla — *see* Corrosion, axilla
elbow — *see* Corrosion, elbow
first degree T22.50 ☑
forearm — *see* Corrosion, forearm
hand — *see* Corrosion, hand
interscapular region — *see* Corrosion, back, upper
multiple sites T22.499 ☑
first degree T22.599 ☑
left T22.492 ☑
first degree T22.592 ☑
second degree T22.692 ☑
third degree T22.792 ☑
right T22.491 ☑
first degree T22.591 ☑
second degree T22.691 ☑
third degree T22.791 ☑
second degree T22.699 ☑
third degree T22.799 ☑
scapular region — *see* Corrosion, scapular region
second degree T22.60 ☑
shoulder — *see* Corrosion, shoulder
third degree T22.70 ☑
wrist — *see* Corrosion, hand
uterus T28.8 ☑
vagina T28.8 ☑
vulva — *see* Corrosion, genital organs, external, female
wrist T23.479 ☑
first degree T23.579 ☑
left T23.472 ☑
first degree T23.572 ☑
second degree T23.672 ☑
third degree T23.772 ☑
multiple sites with hand T23.499 ☑
first degree T23.599 ☑
left T23.492 ☑
first degree T23.592 ☑
second degree T23.692 ☑
third degree T23.792 ☑
right T23.491 ☑
first degree T23.591 ☑
second degree T23.691 ☑
third degree T23.791 ☑
second degree T23.699 ☑
third degree T23.799 ☑

Corrosion — *continued*
wrist — *continued*
right T23.471 ☑
first degree T23.571 ☑
second degree T23.671 ☑
third degree T23.771 ☑
second degree T23.679 ☑
third degree T23.779 ☑
Corrosive burn — *see* Corrosion
Corsican fever — *see* Malaria
Cortical — *see* condition
Cortico-adrenal — *see* condition
Coryza (acute) J00
with grippe or influenza — *see* Influenza, with, respiratory manifestations NEC
syphilitic
congenital (chronic) A50.05
Costen's syndrome or complex M26.69
Costiveness — *see* Constipation
Costochondritis M94.0
Cot death R99
Cotard's syndrome F22
Cotia virus B08.8
Cotton wool spots (retinal) H35.81
Cotungo's disease — *see* Sciatica
Cough (affected) (chronic) (epidemic) (nervous) R05
with hemorrhage — *see* Hemoptysis
bronchial R05
with grippe or influenza — *see* Influenza, with, respiratory manifestations NEC
functional F45.8
hysterical F45.8
laryngeal, spasmodic R05
psychogenic F45.8
smokers' J41.0
tea taster's B49
Counseling (for) Z71.9
abuse NEC
perpetrator Z69.82
victim Z69.81
alcohol abuser Z71.41
family Z71.42
child abuse
nonparental
perpetrator Z69.021
victim Z69.020
parental
perpetrator Z69.011
victim Z69.010
consanguinity Z71.89
contraceptive Z30.09
dietary Z71.3
drug abuser Z71.51
family member Z71.52
exercise Z71.82
family Z71.89
fertility preservation (prior to cancer therapy) (prior to removal of gonads) Z31.62
for non-attending third party Z71.0
related to sexual behavior or orientation Z70.2
genetic
nonprocreative Z71.83
procreative NEC Z31.5
gestational carrier Z31.7
health (advice) (education) (instruction) — *see* Counseling, medical
risk for travel (international) Z71.84
human immunodeficiency virus (HIV) Z71.7
impotence Z70.1
insulin pump use Z46.81
medical (for) Z71.9
boarding school resident Z59.3
consanguinity Z71.89
feared complaint and no disease found Z71.1
human immunodeficiency virus (HIV) Z71.7
institutional resident Z59.3
on behalf of another Z71.0
related to sexual behavior or orientation Z70.2
person living alone Z60.2
specified reason NEC Z71.89
natural family planning
procreative Z31.61
to avoid pregnancy Z30.02
perpetrator (of)
abuse NEC Z69.82
child abuse
non-parental Z69.021
parental Z69.011

Counseling — *continued*
perpetrator — *continued*
rape NEC Z69.82
spousal abuse Z69.12
procreative NEC Z31.69
fertility preservation (prior to cancer therapy) (prior to removal of gonads) Z31.62
using natural family planning Z31.61
promiscuity Z70.1
rape victim Z69.81
religious Z71.81
safety for travel (international) Z71.84
sex, sexual (related to) Z70.9
attitude(s) Z70.0
behavior or orientation Z70.1
combined concerns Z70.3
non-responsiveness Z70.1
on behalf of third party Z70.2
specified reason NEC Z70.8
specified reason NEC Z71.89
spiritual Z71.81
spousal abuse (perpetrator) Z69.12
victim Z69.11
substance abuse Z71.89
alcohol Z71.41
drug Z71.51
tobacco Z71.6
tobacco use Z71.6
travel (international) Z71.84
use (of)
insulin pump Z46.81
victim (of)
abuse Z69.81
child abuse
by parent Z69.010
non-parental Z69.020
rape NEC Z69.81
Coupled rhythm R00.8
Couvelaire syndrome or uterus (complicating delivery) O45.8X- ☑
Cowperitis — *see* Urethritis
Cowper's gland — *see* condition
Cowpox B08.010
due to vaccination T88.1 ☑
Coxa
magna M91.4-
plana M91.2- ☑
valga (acquired) — *see also* Deformity, limb, specified type NEC, thigh
congenital Q65.81
sequelae (late effect) of rickets E64.3
vara (acquired) — *see also* Deformity, limb, specified type NEC, thigh
congenital Q65.82
sequelae (late effect) of rickets E64.3
Coxalgia, coxalgic (nontuberculous) — *see also* Pain, joint, hip
tuberculous A18.02
Coxitis — *see* Monoarthritis, hip
Coxsackie (virus) (infection) B34.1
as cause of disease classified elsewhere B97.11
carditis B33.20
central nervous system NEC A88.8
endocarditis B33.21
enteritis A08.39
meningitis (aseptic) A87.0
myocarditis B33.22
pericarditis B33.23
pharyngitis B08.5
pleurodynia B33.0
specific disease NEC B33.8
Crabs, meaning pubic lice B85.3
Crack baby P04.41
Cracked nipple N64.0
associated with
lactation O92.13
pregnancy O92.11- ☑
puerperium O92.12
Cracked tooth K03.81
Cradle cap L21.0
Craft neurosis F48.8
Cramp(s) R25.2
abdominal — *see* Pain, abdominal
bathing T75.1 ☑
colic R10.83
psychogenic F45.8
due to immersion T75.1 ☑
fireman T67.2 ☑

Cramp(s) — *continued*
  heat T67.2 ☑
  immersion T75.1 ☑
  intestinal — *see* Pain, abdominal
    psychogenic F45.8
  leg, sleep related G47.62
  limb (lower) (upper) NEC R25.2
    sleep related G47.62
  linotypist's F48.8
    organic G25.89
  muscle (limb) (general) R25.2
    due to immersion T75.1 ☑
    psychogenic F45.8
  occupational (hand) F48.8
    organic G25.89
  salt-depletion E87.1
  sleep related, leg G47.62
  stoker's T67.2 ☑
  swimmer's T75.1 ☑
  telegrapher's F48.8
    organic G25.89
  typist's F48.8
    organic G25.89
  uterus N94.89
    menstrual — *see* Dysmenorrhea
  writer's F48.8
    organic G25.89
Cranial — *see* condition
Craniocleidodysostosis Q74.0
Craniofenestria (skull) Q75.8
Craniolacunia (skull) Q75.8
Craniopagus Q89.4
Craniopathy, metabolic M85.2
Craniopharyngeal — *see* condition
Craniopharyngioma D44.4
Craniorachischisis (totalis) Q00.1
Cranioschisis Q75.8
Craniostenosis Q75.0
Craniosynostosis Q75.0
Craniotabes (cause unknown) M83.8
  neonatal P96.3
  rachitic E64.3
  syphilitic A50.56
Cranium — *see* condition
Craw-craw — *see* Onchocerciasis
Creaking joint — *see* Derangement, joint, specified type NEC
Creeping
  eruption B76.9
  palsy or paralysis G12.22
Crenated tongue K14.8
Creotoxism A05.9
Crepitus
  caput Q75.8
  joint — *see* Derangement, joint, specified type NEC
Crescent or conus choroid, congenital Q14.3
CREST syndrome M34.1
Cretin, cretinism (congenital) (endemic) (nongoitrous) (sporadic) E00.9
  pelvis
    with disproportion (fetopelvic) O33.0
      causing obstructed labor O65.0
  type
    hypothyroid E00.1
    mixed E00.2
    myxedematous E00.1
    neurological E00.0
Creutzfeldt-Jakob disease or syndrome (with dementia) A81.00
  familial A81.09
  iatrogenic A81.09
  specified NEC A81.09
  sporadic A81.09
  variant (vCJD) A81.01
Crib death R99
Cribriform hymen Q52.3
Cri-du-chat syndrome Q93.4
Crigler-Najjar disease or syndrome E80.5
Crime, victim of Z65.4
Crimean hemorrhagic fever A98.0
Criminalism F60.2
Crisis
  abdomen R10.0
  acute reaction F43.0
  addisonian E27.2
  adrenal (cortical) E27.2
  celiac K90.0

Crisis — *continued*
  Dietl's N13.8
  emotional — *see also* Disorder, adjustment
    acute reaction to stress F43.0
    specific to childhood and adolescence F93.8
  glaucomatocyclitic — *see* Glaucoma, secondary, inflammation
  heart — *see* Failure, heart
  nitritoid I95.2
    correct substance properly administered — *see* Table of Drugs and Chemicals, by drug, adverse effect
    overdose or wrong substance given or taken — *see* Table of Drugs and Chemicals, by drug, poisoning
  oculogyric H51.8
    psychogenic F45.8
  Pel's (tabetic) A52.11
  psychosexual identity F64.2
  renal N28.0
  sickle-cell D57.00
    with
      acute chest syndrome D57.01
      splenic sequestration D57.02
  state (acute reaction) F43.0
  tabetic A52.11
  thyroid — *see* Thyrotoxicosis with thyroid storm
  thyrotoxic — *see* Thyrotoxicosis with thyroid storm
Crocq's disease (acrocyanosis) I73.89
Crohn's disease — *see* Enteritis, regional
Crooked septum, nasal J34.2
Cross syndrome E70.328
Crossbite (anterior) (posterior) M26.24
Cross-eye — *see* Strabismus, convergent concomitant
Croup, croupous (catarrhal) (infectious) (inflammatory) (nondiphtheritic) J05.0
  bronchial J20.9
  diphtheritic A36.2
  false J38.5
  spasmodic J38.5
    diphtheritic A36.2
  stridulous J38.5
    diphtheritic A36.2
Crouzon's disease Q75.1
Crowding, tooth, teeth, fully erupted M26.31
CRST syndrome M34.1
Cruchet's disease A85.8
Cruelty in children — *see also* Disorder, conduct
Crural ulcer — *see* Ulcer, lower limb
Crush, crushed, crushing T14.8 ☑
  abdomen S38.1 ☑
  ankle S97.0- ☑
  arm (upper) (and shoulder) S47.- ☑
  axilla — *see* Crush, arm
  back, lower S38.1 ☑
  buttock S38.1 ☑
  cheek S07.0 ☑
  chest S28.0 ☑
  cranium S07.1 ☑
  ear S07.0 ☑
  elbow S57.0- ☑
  extremity
    lower
      ankle — *see* Crush, ankle
      below knee — *see* Crush, leg
      foot — *see* Crush, foot
      hip — *see* Crush, hip
      knee — *see* Crush, knee
      thigh — *see* Crush, thigh
      toe — *see* Crush, toe
    upper
      below elbow S67.9- ☑
      elbow — *see* Crush, elbow
      finger — *see* Crush, finger
      forearm — *see* Crush, forearm
      hand — *see* Crush, hand
      thumb — *see* Crush, thumb
      upper arm — *see* Crush, arm
      wrist — *see* Crush, wrist
  face S07.0 ☑
  finger(s) S67.1- ☑
    with hand (and wrist) — *see* Crush, hand, specified site NEC
    index S67.19- ☑
    little S67.19- ☑
    middle S67.19- ☑
    ring S67.19- ☑

Crush, crushed, crushing — *continued*
  finger(s) — *continued*
    thumb — *see* Crush, thumb
  foot S97.8- ☑
    toe — *see* Crush, toe
  forearm S57.8- ☑
  genitalia, external
    female S38.002 ☑
      vagina S38.03 ☑
      vulva S38.03 ☑
    male S38.001 ☑
      penis S38.01 ☑
      scrotum S38.02 ☑
      testis S38.02 ☑
  hand (except fingers alone) S67.2- ☑
    with wrist S67.4- ☑
  head S07.9 ☑
    specified NEC S07.8 ☑
  heel — *see* Crush, foot
  hip S77.0- ☑
    with thigh S77.2- ☑
  internal organ (abdomen, chest, or pelvis) NEC T14.8 ☑
  knee S87.0- ☑
  labium (majus) (minus) S38.03 ☑
  larynx S17.0 ☑
  leg (lower) S87.8- ☑
    knee — *see* Crush, knee
  lip S07.0 ☑
  lower
    back S38.1 ☑
    leg — *see* Crush, leg
  neck S17.9 ☑
  nerve — *see* Injury, nerve
  nose S07.0 ☑
  pelvis S38.1 ☑
  penis S38.01 ☑
  scalp S07.8 ☑
  scapular region — *see* Crush, arm
  scrotum S38.02 ☑
  severe, unspecified site T14.8 ☑
  shoulder (and upper arm) — *see* Crush, arm
  skull S07.1 ☑
  syndrome (complication of trauma) T79.5 ☑
  testis S38.02 ☑
  thigh S77.1- ☑
    with hip S77.2- ☑
  throat S17.8 ☑
  thumb S67.0- ☑
    with hand (and wrist) — *see* Crush, hand, specified site NEC
  toe(s) S97.10- ☑
    great S97.11- ☑
    lesser S97.12- ☑
  trachea S17.0 ☑
  vagina S38.03 ☑
  vulva S38.03 ☑
  wrist S67.3- ☑
    with hand S67.4- ☑
Crusta lactea L21.0
Crusts R23.4
Crutch paralysis — *see* Injury, brachial plexus
Cruveilhier-Baumgarten cirrhosis, disease or syndrome K74.69
Cruveilhier's atrophy or disease G12.8
Crying (constant) (continuous) (excessive)
  child, adolescent, or adult R45.83
  infant (baby) (newborn) R68.11
Cryofibrinogenemia D89.2
Cryoglobulinemia (essential) (idiopathic) (mixed) (primary) (purpura) (secondary) (vasculitis) D89.1
  with lung involvement D89.1 [J99]
Cryptitis (anal) (rectal) K62.89
Cryptococcosis, cryptococcus (infection) (neoformans) B45.9
  bone B45.3
  cerebral B45.1
  cutaneous B45.2
  disseminated B45.7
  generalized B45.7
  meningitis B45.1
  meningocerebralis B45.1
  osseous B45.3
  pulmonary B45.0
  skin B45.2
  specified NEC B45.8
Cryptopapillitis (anus) K62.89

Cryptophthalmos Q11.2
 syndrome Q87.0
Cryptorchid, cryptorchism, cryptorchidism Q53.9
 bilateral Q53.20
  abdominal Q53.211
  perineal Q53.22
 unilateral Q53.10
  abdominal Q53.111
  perineal Q53.12
Cryptosporidiosis A07.2
 hepatobiliary B88.8
 respiratory B88.8
Cryptostromosis J67.6
Crystalluria R82.998
Cubitus
 congenital Q68.8
 valgus (acquired) M21.0- ☑
  congenital Q68.8
  sequelae (late effect) of rickets E64.3
 varus (acquired) M21.1- ☑
  congenital Q68.8
  sequelae (late effect) of rickets E64.3
Cultural deprivation or shock Z60.3
Curling esophagus K22.4
Curling's ulcer — *see* Ulcer, peptic, acute
Curschmann (-Batten) (-Steinert) **disease or syndrome**
  G71.11
Curse, Ondine's — *see* Apnea, sleep
Curvature
 organ or site, congenital NEC — *see* Distortion
 penis (lateral) Q55.61
 Pott's (spinal) A18.01
 radius, idiopathic, progressive (congenital) Q74.0
 spine (acquired) (angular) (idiopathic) (incorrect)
   (postural) — *see* Dorsopathy, deforming
  congenital Q67.5
  due to or associated with
   Charcot-Marie-Tooth disease — *see also* subcat-
     egory M49.8 G60.0
   osteitis
    deformans M88.88
    fibrosa cystica — *see also* subcategory M49.8
      E21.0
   tuberculosis (Pott's curvature) A18.01
  sequelae (late effect) of rickets E64.3
  tuberculous A18.01
Cushingoid due to steroid therapy E24.2
 correct substance properly administered — *see* Table
   of Drugs and Chemicals, by drug, adverse effect
 overdose or wrong substance given or taken — *see*
   Table of Drugs and Chemicals, by drug, poisoning
Cushing's
 syndrome or disease E24.9
  drug-induced E24.2
  iatrogenic E24.2
  pituitary-dependent E24.0
  specified NEC E24.8
 ulcer — *see* Ulcer, peptic, acute
Cusp, Carabelli — *omit code*
Cut (external) — *see also* Laceration
 muscle — *see* Injury, muscle
Cutaneous — *see also* condition
 hemorrhage R23.3
 larva migrans B76.9
Cutis — *see also* condition
 hyperelastica Q82.8
  acquired L57.4
 laxa (hyperelastica) — *see* Dermatolysis
 marmorata R23.8
 osteosis L94.2
 pendula — *see* Dermatolysis
 rhomboidalis nuchae L57.2
 verticis gyrata Q82.8
  acquired L91.8
Cyanosis R23.0
 due to
  patent foramen botalli Q21.1
  persistent foramen ovale Q21.1
 enterogenous D74.8
 paroxysmal digital — *see* Raynaud's disease
  with gangrene I73.01
 retina, retinal H35.89
Cyanotic heart disease I24.9
 congenital Q24.9
Cycle
 anovulatory N97.0
 menstrual, irregular N92.6
Cyclencephaly Q04.9

Cyclical vomiting, in migraine — *see also* Vomiting,
 cyclical G43.A0 (*following* G43.7)
 psychogenic F50.89
Cyclitis — *see also* Iridocyclitis H20.9
 chronic — *see* Iridocyclitis, chronic
 Fuchs' heterochromic H20.81- ☑
 granulomatous — *see* Iridocyclitis, chronic
 lens-induced — *see* Iridocyclitis, lens-induced
 posterior H30.2- ☑
Cycloid personality F34.0
Cyclophoria H50.54
Cyclopia, cyclops Q87.0
Cyclopism Q87.0
Cyclosporiasis A07.4
Cyclothymia F34.0
Cyclothymic personality F34.0
Cyclotropia H50.41- ☑
Cylindroma — *see also* Neoplasm, malignant, by site
 eccrine dermal — *see* Neoplasm, skin, benign
 skin — *see* Neoplasm, skin, benign
Cylindruria R82.998
Cynanche
 diphtheritic A36.2
 tonsillaris J36
Cynophobia F40.218
Cynorexia R63.2
Cyphosis — *see* Kyphosis
Cyprus fever — *see* Brucellosis
Cyst (colloid) (mucous) (simple) (retention)
 adenoid (infected) J35.8
 adrenal gland E27.8
  congenital Q89.1
 air, lung J98.4
 allantoic Q64.4
 alveolar process (jaw bone) M27.40
 amnion, amniotic O41.8X- ☑
 aneurysmal M27.49
 anterior
  chamber (eye) — *see* Cyst, iris
  nasopalatine K09.1
 antrum J34.1
 anus K62.89
 apical (tooth) (periodontal) K04.8
 appendix K38.8
 arachnoid, brain (acquired) G93.0
  congenital Q04.6
 arytenoid J38.7
 Baker's M71.2- ☑
  ruptured M66.0
  tuberculous A18.02
 Bartholin's gland N75.0
 bile duct (common) (hepatic) K83.5
 bladder (multiple) (trigone) N32.89
 blue dome (breast) — *see* Cyst, breast
 bone (local) NEC M85.60
  aneurysmal M85.50
   ankle M85.57- ☑
   foot M85.57- ☑
   forearm M85.53- ☑
   hand M85.54- ☑
   jaw M27.49
   lower leg M85.56- ☑
   multiple site M85.59
   neck M85.58
   rib M85.58
   shoulder M85.51- ☑
   skull M85.58
   specified site NEC M85.58
   thigh M85.55- ☑
   toe M85.57- ☑
   upper arm M85.52- ☑
   vertebra M85.58
  solitary M85.40
   ankle M85.47- ☑
   fibula M85.46- ☑
   foot M85.47- ☑
   hand M85.44- ☑
   humerus M85.42- ☑
   jaw M27.49
   neck M85.48
   pelvis M85.45- ☑
   radius M85.43- ☑
   rib M85.48
   shoulder M85.41- ☑
   skull M85.48
   specified site NEC M85.48
   tibia M85.46- ☑

Cyst — *continued*
 bone — *continued*
  solitary — *continued*
   toe M85.47- ☑
   ulna M85.43- ☑
   vertebra M85.48
  specified type NEC M85.60
   ankle M85.67- ☑
   foot M85.67- ☑
   forearm M85.63- ☑
   hand M85.64- ☑
   jaw M27.40
    developmental (nonodontogenic) K09.1
     odontogenic K09.0
    latent M27.0
   lower leg M85.66- ☑
   multiple site M85.69
   neck M85.68
   rib M85.68
   shoulder M85.61- ☑
   skull M85.68
   specified site NEC M85.68
   thigh M85.65- ☑
   toe M85.67- ☑
   upper arm M85.62- ☑
   vertebra M85.68
 brain (acquired) G93.0
  congenital Q04.6
  hydatid B67.99 *[G94]*
  third ventricle (colloid), congenital Q04.6
 branchial (cleft) Q18.0
 branchiogenic Q18.0
 breast (benign) (blue dome) (pedunculated) (solitary)
   N60.0- ☑
  involution — *see* Dysplasia, mammary, specified
    type NEC
  sebaceous — *see* Dysplasia, mammary, specified
    type NEC
 broad ligament (benign) N83.8
 bronchogenic (mediastinal) (sequestration) J98.4
  congenital Q33.0
 buccal K09.8
 bulbourethral gland N36.8
 bursa, bursal NEC M71.30
  with rupture — *see* Rupture, synovium
  ankle M71.37- ☑
  elbow M71.32- ☑
  foot M71.37- ☑
  hand M71.34- ☑
  hip M71.35- ☑
  multiple sites M71.39
  pharyngeal J39.2
  popliteal space — *see* Cyst, Baker's
  shoulder M71.31- ☑
  specified site NEC M71.38
  wrist M71.33- ☑
 calcifying odontogenic D16.5
  upper jaw (bone) (maxilla) D16.4
 canal of Nuck (female) N94.89
  congenital Q52.4
 canthus — *see* Cyst, conjunctiva
 carcinomatous — *see* Neoplasm, malignant, by site
 cauda equina G95.89
 cavum septi pellucidi — *see* Cyst, brain
 celomic (pericardium) Q24.8
 cerebellopontine (angle) — *see* Cyst, brain
 cerebellum — *see* Cyst, brain
 cerebral — *see* Cyst, brain
 cervical lateral Q18.0
 cervix NEC N88.8
  embryonic Q51.6
  nabothian N88.8
 chiasmal optic NEC — *see* Disorder, optic, chiasm
 chocolate (ovary) N80.1
 choledochus, congenital Q44.4
 chorion O41.8X- ☑
 choroid plexus G93.0
  congenital Q04.6
 ciliary body — *see* Cyst, iris
 clitoris N90.7
 colon K63.89
 common (bile) duct K83.5
 congenital NEC Q89.8
  adrenal gland Q89.1
  epiglottis Q31.8
  esophagus Q39.8
  fallopian tube Q50.4
  kidney Q61.00

78 ☑ **Additional Character Required — Refer to the Tabular List for Character Selection** ▽ **Subterms under main terms may continue to next column or page**

Cryptophthalmos — Cyst

Cyst — *continued*
  congenital — *continued*
    kidney — *continued*
      more than one (multiple) Q61.02
        specified as polycystic Q61.3
          adult type Q61.2
          infantile type NEC Q61.19
            collecting duct dilation Q61.11
      solitary Q61.01
    larynx Q31.8
    liver Q44.6
    lung Q33.0
    mediastinum Q34.1
    ovary Q50.1
    oviduct Q50.4
    periurethral (tissue) Q64.79
    prepuce Q55.69
    salivary gland (any) Q38.4
    sublingual Q38.6
    submaxillary gland Q38.6
    thymus (gland) Q89.2
    tongue Q38.3
    ureterovesical orifice Q62.8
    vulva Q52.79
  conjunctiva H11.44- ☑
  cornea H18.89- ☑
  corpora quadrigemina G93.0
  corpus
    albicans N83.29- ☑
    luteum (hemorrhagic) (ruptured) N83.1- ☑
  Cowper's gland (benign) (infected) N36.8
  cranial meninges G93.0
  craniobuccal pouch E23.6
  craniopharyngeal pouch E23.6
  cystic duct K82.8
  Cysticercus — *see* Cysticercosis
  Dandy-Walker Q03.1
    with spina bifida — *see* Spina bifida
  dental (root) K04.8
    developmental K09.0
    eruption K09.0
    primordial K09.0
  dentigerous (mandible) (maxilla) K09.0
  dermoid — *see* Neoplasm, benign, by site
    with malignant transformation C56.- ☑
    implantation
      external area or site (skin) NEC L72.0
      iris — *see* Cyst, iris, implantation
      vagina N89.8
      vulva N90.7
    mouth K09.8
    oral soft tissue K09.8
    sacrococcygeal — *see* Cyst, pilonidal
  developmental K09.1
    odontogenic K09.0
    oral region (nonodontogenic) K09.1
    ovary, ovarian Q50.1
  dura (cerebral) G93.0
    spinal G96.19
  ear (external) Q18.1
  echinococcal — *see* Echinococcus
  embryonic
    cervix uteri Q51.6
    fallopian tube Q50.4
    vagina Q52.4
  endometrium, endometrial (uterus) N85.8
    ectopic — *see* Endometriosis
  enterogenous Q43.8
  epidermal, epidermoid (inclusion) (*see also* Cyst, skin) L72.0
    mouth K09.8
    oral soft tissue K09.8
  epididymis N50.3
  epiglottis J38.7
  epiphysis cerebri E34.8
  epithelial (inclusion) L72.0
  epoophoron Q50.5
  eruption K09.0
  esophagus K22.8
  ethmoid sinus J34.1
  external female genital organs NEC N90.7
  eyelid (sebaceous) H02.829
    infected — *see* Hordeolum
    left H02.826
      lower H02.825
      upper H02.824
    right H02.823
      lower H02.822

Cyst — *continued*
  eyelid — *continued*
    right — *continued*
      upper H02.821
  eye NEC H57.89
    congenital Q15.8
  fallopian tube N83.8
    congenital Q50.4
  fimbrial (twisted) Q50.4
  fissural (oral region) K09.1
  follicle (graafian) (hemorrhagic) N83.0- ☑
    nabothian N88.8
  follicular (atretic) (hemorrhagic) (ovarian) N83.0- ☑
    dentigerous K09.0
    odontogenic K09.0
    skin L72.9
      specified NEC L72.8
  frontal sinus J34.1
  gallbladder K82.8
  ganglion — *see* Ganglion
  Gartner's duct Q52.4
  gingiva K09.0
  gland of Moll — *see* Cyst, eyelid
  globulomaxillary K09.1
  graafian follicle (hemorrhagic) N83.0- ☑
  granulosal lutein (hemorrhagic) N83.1- ☑
  hemangiomatous D18.00
    intra-abdominal D18.03
    intracranial D18.02
    skin D18.01
    specified site NEC D18.09
  hemorrhagic M27.49
  hydatid — *see also* Echinococcus B67.90
    brain B67.99 *[G94]*
    liver — *see also* Cyst, liver, hydatid B67.8
    lung NEC B67.99 *[J99]*
    Morgagni
      female Q50.5
      male (epididymal) Q55.4
        testicular Q55.29
    specified site NEC B67.99
  hymen N89.8
    embryonic Q52.4
  hypopharynx J39.2
  hypophysis, hypophyseal (duct) (recurrent) E23.6
    cerebri E23.6
  implantation (dermoid)
    external area or site (skin) NEC L72.0
    iris — *see* Cyst, iris, implantation
    vagina N89.8
    vulva N90.7
  incisive canal K09.1
  inclusion (epidermal) (epithelial) (epidermoid) (squamous) L72.0
    not of skin — *code under* Cyst, by site
  intestine (large) (small) K63.89
  intracranial — *see* Cyst, brain
  intraligamentous — *see also* Disorder, ligament
    knee — *see* Derangement, knee
  intrasellar E23.6
  iris H21.309
    exudative H21.31- ☑
    idiopathic H21.30- ☑
    implantation H21.32- ☑
    parasitic H21.33- ☑
    pars plana (primary) H21.34- ☑
      exudative H21.35- ☑
  jaw (bone) M27.40
    aneurysmal M27.49
    developmental (odontogenic) K09.0
    fissural K09.1
    hemorrhagic M27.49
    traumatic M27.49
  joint NEC — *see* Disorder, joint, specified type NEC
  kidney (acquired) N28.1
    calyceal — *see* Hydronephrosis
    congenital Q61.00
    more than one (multiple) Q61.02
      specified as polycystic Q61.3
        adult type (autosomal dominant) Q61.2
        infantile type (autosomal recessive) NEC Q61.19
          collecting duct dilation Q61.11
    pyelogenic — *see* Hydronephrosis
    simple N28.1
    solitary (single) Q61.01
      acquired N28.1
  labium (majus) (minus) N90.7

Cyst — *continued*
  labium — *continued*
    sebaceous N90.7
  lacrimal — *see also* Disorder, lacrimal system, specified NEC
    gland H04.13- ☑
    passages or sac — *see* Disorder, lacrimal system, specified NEC
  larynx J38.7
  lateral periodontal K09.0
  lens H27.8
    congenital Q12.8
  lip (gland) K13.0
  liver (idiopathic) (simple) K76.89
    congenital Q44.6
    hydatid B67.8
      granulosus B67.0
      multilocularis B67.5
  lung J98.4
    congenital Q33.0
    giant bullous J43.9
  lutein N83.1- ☑
  lymphangiomatous D18.1
  lymphoepithelial, oral soft tissue K09.8
  macula — *see* Degeneration, macula, hole
  malignant — *see* Neoplasm, malignant, by site
  mammary gland — *see* Cyst, breast
  mandible M27.40
    dentigerous K09.0
    radicular K04.8
  maxilla M27.40
    dentigerous K09.0
    radicular K04.8
  medial, face and neck Q18.8
  median
    anterior maxillary K09.1
    palatal K09.1
  mediastinum, congenital Q34.1
  meibomian (gland) — *see* Chalazion
    infected — *see* Hordeolum
  membrane, brain G93.0
  meninges (cerebral) G93.0
    spinal G96.19
  meniscus, knee — *see* Derangement, knee, meniscus, cystic
  mesentery, mesenteric K66.8
    chyle I89.8
  mesonephric duct
    female Q50.5
    male Q55.4
  milk N64.89
  Morgagni (hydatid)
    female Q50.5
    male (epididymal) Q55.4
      testicular Q55.29
  mouth K09.8
  Müllerian duct Q50.4
    appendix testis Q55.29
    cervix Q51.6
    fallopian tube Q50.4
    female Q50.4
    male Q55.29
    prostatic utricle Q55.4
    vagina (embryonal) Q52.4
  multilocular (ovary) D39.10
    benign — *see* Neoplasm, benign, by site
  myometrium N85.8
  nabothian (follicle) (ruptured) N88.8
  nasoalveolar K09.1
  nasolabial K09.1
  nasopalatine (anterior) (duct) K09.1
  nasopharynx J39.2
  neoplastic — *see* Neoplasm, uncertain behavior, by site
    benign — *see* Neoplasm, benign, by site
  nervous system NEC G96.8
  neuroenteric (congenital) Q06.8
  nipple — *see* Cyst, breast
  nose (turbinates) J34.1
    sinus J34.1
  odontogenic, developmental K09.0
  omentum (lesser) K66.8
    congenital Q45.8
  ora serrata — *see* Cyst, retina, ora serrata
  oral
    region K09.9
      developmental (nonodontogenic) K09.1
      specified NEC K09.8

Index

Cyst — Cyst

Cyst — *continued*
  oral — *continued*
    soft tissue K09.9
      specified NEC K09.8
  orbit H05.81- ☑
  ovary, ovarian (twisted) N83.20- ☑
    adherent N83.20- ☑
    chocolate N80.1
    corpus
      albicans N83.29- ☑
      luteum (hemorrhagic) N83.1- ☑
    dermoid D27.9
    developmental Q50.1
    due to failure of involution NEC N83.20- ☑
    endometrial N80.1
    follicular (graafian) (hemorrhagic) N83.0- ☑
    hemorrhagic N83.20- ☑
    in pregnancy or childbirth O34.8- ☑
      with obstructed labor O65.5
    multilocular D39.10
    pseudomucinous D27.9
    retention N83.29- ☑
    serous N83.20- ☑
    specified NEC N83.29- ☑
    theca lutein (hemorrhagic) N83.1- ☑
    tuberculous A18.18
  oviduct N83.8
  palate (median) (fissural) K09.1
  palatine papilla (jaw) K09.1
  pancreas, pancreatic (hemorrhagic) (true) K86.2
    congenital Q45.2
    false K86.3
  paralabral
    hip M24.85- ☑
    shoulder S43.43- ☑
  paramesonephric duct Q50.4
    female Q50.4
    male Q55.29
  paranephric N28.1
  paraphysis, cerebri, congenital Q04.6
  parasitic B89
  parathyroid (gland) E21.4
  paratubal N83.8
  paraurethral duct N36.8
  paroophoron Q50.5
  parotid gland K11.6
  parovarian Q50.5
  pelvis, female N94.89
    in pregnancy or childbirth O34.8- ☑
      causing obstructed labor O65.5
  penis (sebaceous) N48.89
  periapical K04.8
  pericardial (congenital) Q24.8
    acquired (secondary) I31.8
  pericoronal K09.0
  periodontal K04.8
    lateral K09.0
  peripelvic (lymphatic) N28.1
  peritoneum K66.8
    chylous I89.8
  periventricular, acquired, newborn P91.1
  pharynx (wall) J39.2
  pilar L72.11
  pilonidal (infected) (rectum) L05.91
    with abscess L05.01
    malignant C44.59- ☑
  pituitary (duct) (gland) E23.6
  placenta O43.19- ☑
  pleura J94.8
  popliteal — *see* Cyst, Baker's
  porencephalic Q04.6
    acquired G93.0
  postanal (infected) — *see* Cyst, pilonidal
  postmastoidectomy cavity (mucosal) — *see* Complications, postmastoidectomy, cyst
  preauricular Q18.1
  prepuce N47.4
    congenital Q55.69
  primordial (jaw) K09.0
  prostate N42.83
  pseudomucinous (ovary) D27.9
  pupillary, miotic H21.27- ☑
  radicular (residual) K04.8
  radiculodental K04.8
  ranular K11.8
  Rathke's pouch E23.6
  rectum (epithelium) (mucous) K62.89
  renal — *see* Cyst, kidney

Cyst — *continued*
  residual (radicular) K04.8
  retention (ovary) N83.29- ☑
    salivary gland K11.6
  retina H33.19- ☑
    ora serrata H33.11- ☑
    parasitic H33.12- ☑
  retroperitoneal K68.9
  sacrococcygeal (dermoid) — *see* Cyst, pilonidal
  salivary gland or duct (mucous extravasation or retention) K11.6
  Sampson's N80.1
  sclera H15.89
  scrotum L72.9
    sebaceous L72.3
  sebaceous (duct) (gland) L72.3
    breast — *see* Dysplasia, mammary, specified type NEC
    eyelid — *see* Cyst, eyelid
    genital organ NEC
      female N94.89
      male N50.89
    scrotum L72.3
  semilunar cartilage (knee) (multiple) — *see* Derangement, knee, meniscus, cystic
  seminal vesicle N50.89
  serous (ovary) N83.20- ☑
  sinus (accessory) (nasal) J34.1
  Skene's gland N36.8
  skin L72.9
    breast — *see* Dysplasia, mammary, specified type NEC
    epidermal, epidermoid L72.0
    epithelial L72.0
    eyelid — *see* Cyst, eyelid
    genital organ NEC
      female N90.7
      male N50.89
    inclusion L72.0
    scrotum L72.9
    sebaceous L72.3
    sweat gland or duct L74.8
  solitary
    bone — *see* Cyst, bone, solitary
    jaw M27.40
    kidney N28.1
  spermatic cord N50.89
  sphenoid sinus J34.1
  spinal meninges G96.19
  spleen NEC D73.4
    congenital Q89.09
    hydatid — *see also* Echinococcus B67.99 *[D77]*
  Stafne's M27.0
  subarachnoid intrasellar R93.0
  subcutaneous, pheomycotic (chromomycotic) B43.2
  subdural (cerebral) G93.0
    spinal cord G96.19
  sublingual gland K11.6
  submandibular gland K11.6
  submaxillary gland K11.6
  suburethral N36.8
  suprarenal gland E27.8
  suprasellar — *see* Cyst, brain
  sweat gland or duct L74.8
  synovial — *see also* Cyst, bursa
    ruptured — *see* Rupture, synovium
  tarsal — *see* Chalazion
  tendon (sheath) — *see* Disorder, tendon, specified type NEC
  testis N44.2
    tunica albuginea N44.1
  theca lutein (ovary) N83.1- ☑
  Thornwaldt's J39.2
  thymus (gland) E32.8
  thyroglossal duct (infected) (persistent) Q89.2
  thyroid (gland) E04.1
  thyrolingual duct (infected) (persistent) Q89.2
  tongue K14.8
  tonsil J35.8
  tooth — *see* Cyst, dental
  Tornwaldt's J39.2
  trichilemmal (proliferating) L72.12
  trichodermal L72.12
  tubal (fallopian) N83.8
    inflammatory — *see* Salpingitis, chronic
  tubo-ovarian N83.8
    inflammatory N70.13

Cyst — *continued*
  tunica
    albuginea testis N44.1
    vaginalis N50.89
  turbinate (nose) J34.1
  Tyson's gland N48.89
  urachus, congenital Q64.4
  ureter N28.89
  ureterovesical orifice N28.89
  urethra, urethral (gland) N36.8
  uterine ligament N83.8
  uterus (body) (corpus) (recurrent) N85.8
    embryonic Q51.818
      cervix Q51.6
  vagina, vaginal (implantation) (inclusion) (squamous cell) (wall) N89.8
    embryonic Q52.4
  vallecula, vallecular (epiglottis) J38.7
  vesical (orifice) N32.89
  vitreous body H43.89
  vulva (implantation) (inclusion) N90.7
    congenital Q52.79
    sebaceous gland N90.7
  vulvovaginal gland N90.7
  wolffian
    female Q50.5
    male Q55.4
Cystadenocarcinoma — *see* Neoplasm, malignant, by site
  bile duct C22.1
  endometrioid — *see* Neoplasm, malignant, by site
    specified site — *see* Neoplasm, malignant, by site
    unspecified site
      female C56.9
      male C61
  mucinous
    papillary
      specified site — *see* Neoplasm, malignant, by site
      unspecified site C56.9
    specified site — *see* Neoplasm, malignant, by site
    unspecified site C56.9
  papillary
    mucinous
      specified site — *see* Neoplasm, malignant, by site
      unspecified site C56.9
    pseudomucinous
      specified site — *see* Neoplasm, malignant, by site
      unspecified site C56.9
    serous
      specified site — *see* Neoplasm, malignant, by site
      unspecified site C56.9
    specified site — *see* Neoplasm, malignant, by site
    unspecified site C56.9
  pseudomucinous
    papillary
      specified site — *see* Neoplasm, malignant, by site
      unspecified site C56.9
    specified site — *see* Neoplasm, malignant, by site
    unspecified site C56.9
  serous
    papillary
      specified site — *see* Neoplasm, malignant, by site
      unspecified site C56.9
    specified site — *see* Neoplasm, malignant, by site
    unspecified site C56.9
Cystadenofibroma
  clear cell — *see* Neoplasm, benign, by site
  endometrioid D27.9
    borderline malignancy D39.1- ☑
    malignant C56.- ☑
  mucinous
    specified site — *see* Neoplasm, benign, by site
    unspecified site D27.9
  serous
    specified site — *see* Neoplasm, benign, by site
    unspecified site D27.9
  specified site — *see* Neoplasm, benign, by site
  unspecified site D27.9
Cystadenoma — *see also* Neoplasm, benign, by site
  bile duct D13.4
  endometrioid — *see* Neoplasm, benign, by site

☑ **Additional Character Required — Refer to the Tabular List for Character Selection**   ▽ **Subterms under main terms may continue to next column or page**

Cystadenoma — *continued*
  endometrioid — *see* Neoplasm, benign, by site — *continued*
    borderline malignancy — *see* Neoplasm, uncertain behavior, by site
  malignant — *see* Neoplasm, malignant, by site
  mucinous
    borderline malignancy
      ovary C56.- ☑
      specified site NEC — *see* Neoplasm, uncertain behavior, by site
      unspecified site C56.9
    papillary
      borderline malignancy
        ovary C56.- ☑
        specified site NEC — *see* Neoplasm, uncertain behavior, by site
        unspecified site C56.9
      specified site — *see* Neoplasm, benign, by site
      unspecified site D27.9
    specified site — *see* Neoplasm, benign, by site
    unspecified site D27.9
  papillary
    borderline malignancy
      ovary C56.- ☑
      specified site NEC — *see* Neoplasm, uncertain behavior, by site
      unspecified site C56.9
    lymphomatosum
      specified site — *see* Neoplasm, benign, by site
      unspecified site D11.9
    mucinous
      borderline malignancy
        ovary C56.- ☑
        specified site NEC — *see* Neoplasm, uncertain behavior, by site
        unspecified site C56.9
      specified site — *see* Neoplasm, benign, by site
      unspecified site D27.9
    pseudomucinous
      borderline malignancy
        ovary C56.- ☑
        specified site NEC — *see* Neoplasm, uncertain behavior, by site
        unspecified site C56.9
      specified site — *see* Neoplasm, benign, by site
      unspecified site D27.9
    serous
      borderline malignancy
        ovary C56.- ☑
        specified site NEC — *see* Neoplasm, uncertain behavior, by site
        unspecified site C56.9
      specified site — *see* Neoplasm, benign, by site
      unspecified site D27.9
  pseudomucinous
    borderline malignancy
      ovary C56.- ☑
      specified site NEC — *see* Neoplasm, uncertain behavior, by site
      unspecified site C56.9
    papillary
      borderline malignancy
        ovary C56.- ☑
        specified site NEC — *see* Neoplasm, uncertain behavior, by site
        unspecified site C56.9
      specified site — *see* Neoplasm, benign, by site
      unspecified site D27.9
    specified site — *see* Neoplasm, benign, by site
    unspecified site D27.9
  serous
    borderline malignancy
      ovary C56.- ☑
      specified site NEC — *see* Neoplasm, uncertain behavior, by site
      unspecified site C56.9

Cystadenoma — *continued*
  serous — *continued*
    papillary
      borderline malignancy
        ovary C56.- ☑
        specified site NEC — *see* Neoplasm, uncertain behavior, by site
        unspecified site C56.9
      specified site — *see* Neoplasm, benign, by site
      unspecified site D27.9
    specified site — *see* Neoplasm, benign, by site
    unspecified site D27.9
Cystathionine synthase deficiency E72.11
Cystathioninemia E72.19
Cystathioninuria E72.19
Cystic — *see also* condition
  breast (chronic) — *see* Mastopathy, cystic
  corpora lutea (hemorrhagic) N83.1-
  duct — *see* condition
  eyeball (congenital) Q11.0
  fibrosis — *see* Fibrosis, cystic
  kidney (congenital) Q61.9
    adult type Q61.2
    infantile type NEC Q61.19
      collecting duct dilatation Q61.11
    medullary Q61.5
  liver, congenital Q44.6
  lung disease J98.4
    congenital Q33.0
  mastitis, chronic — *see* Mastopathy, cystic
  medullary, kidney Q61.5
  meniscus — *see* Derangement, knee, meniscus, cystic
  ovary N83.20- ☑
Cysticercosis, cysticerciasis B69.9
  with
    epileptiform fits B69.0
    myositis B69.81
  brain B69.0
  central nervous system B69.0
  cerebral B69.0
  ocular B69.1
  specified NEC B69.89
Cysticercus cellulose infestation — *see* Cysticercosis
Cystinosis (malignant) E72.04
Cystinuria E72.01
Cystitis (exudative) (hemorrhagic) (septic) (suppurative) N30.90
  with
    fibrosis — *see* Cystitis, chronic, interstitial
    hematuria N30.91
    leukoplakia — *see* Cystitis, chronic, interstitial
    malakoplakia — *see* Cystitis, chronic, interstitial
    metaplasia — *see* Cystitis, chronic, interstitial
    prostatitis N41.3
  acute N30.00
    with hematuria N30.01
    of trigone N30.30
      with hematuria N30.31
  allergic — *see* Cystitis, specified type NEC
  amebic A06.81
  bilharzial B65.9 *[N33]*
  blennorrhagic (gonococcal) A54.01
  bullous — *see* Cystitis, specified type NEC
  calculous N21.0
  chlamydial A56.01
  chronic N30.20
    with hematuria N30.21
    interstitial N30.10
      with hematuria N30.11
    of trigone N30.30
      with hematuria N30.31
    specified NEC N30.20
      with hematuria N30.21
  cystic (a) — *see* Cystitis, specified type NEC
  diphtheritic A36.85
  echinococcal
    granulosus B67.39
    multilocularis B67.69
  emphysematous — *see* Cystitis, specified type NEC
  encysted — *see* Cystitis, specified type NEC

Cystitis — *conti...*
  eosinophili...
  follicular...
  gang...
  gla...

  irritat...
  malignan...
  of trigone ...
    with hema...
  panmural — se...
  polyposa — *see* Cy...
  prostatic N41.3
  puerperal (postpartum)...
  radiation — *see* Cystitis, irr...
  specified type NEC N30.80
    with hematuria N30.81
  subacute — *see* Cystitis, chronic
  submucous — *see* Cystitis, chronic, int...
  syphilitic (late) A52.76
  trichomonal A59.03
  tuberculous A18.12
  ulcerative — *see* Cystitis, chronic, interstitial
Cystocele (-urethrocele)
  female N81.10
    with prolapse of uterus — *see* Prolapse, uterus
    lateral N81.12
    midline N81.11
    paravaginal N81.12
  in pregnancy or childbirth O34.8- ☑
    causing obstructed labor O65.5
  male N32.89
Cystolithiasis N21.0
Cystoma — *see also* Neoplasm, benign, by site
  endometrial, ovary N80.1
  mucinous
    specified site — *see* Neoplasm, benign, by site
    unspecified site D27.9
  serous
    specified site — *see* Neoplasm, benign, by site
    unspecified site D27.9
  simple (ovary) N83.29- ☑
Cystoplegia N31.2
Cystoptosis N32.89
Cystopyelitis — *see* Pyelonephritis
Cystorrhagia N32.89
Cystosarcoma phyllodes D48.6- ☑
  benign D24- ☑
  malignant — *see* Neoplasm, breast, malignant
Cystostomy
  attention to Z43.5
  complication — *see* Complications, cystostomy
  status Z93.50
    appendico-vesicostomy Z93.52
    cutaneous Z93.51
    specified NEC Z93.59
Cystourethritis — *see* Urethritis
Cystourethrocele — *see also* Cystocele
  female N81.10
    with uterine prolapse — *see* Prolapse, uterus
    lateral N81.12
    midline N81.11
    paravaginal N81.12
  male N32.89
Cytomegalic inclusion disease
  congenital P35.1
Cytomegalovirus infection B25.9
Cytomycosis (reticuloendothelial) B39.4
Cytopenia D75.9
  refractory
    with multilineage dysplasia D46.A (*following* D46.2)
    and ring sideroblasts (RCMD RS) D46.B (*following* D46.2)
Czerny's disease (periodic hydrarthrosis of the knee) — *see* Effusion, joint, knee

(Side tab, rotated) **Da Costa's syndrome** — Index
Da Costa's syndrome
Daae (-Finsen) disease B3...
Dabney's grip B33...
Dacryoadenitis H04.01-...
  acute H04...
  chronic H04...
Dacryocystitis...
Dacryocystitis...
  acute H04...
  chronic H...
  neonata...
  phlegm...
  syphili...
tra...
Da...
D...

(Vertical tab, right edge) **Cystadenoma — Czerny's disease**

D

Da Costa's syndrome — Defect, defective

e F45.8
ase (epidemic pleurodynia) B33.0
...0
dacryadenitis H04.00- ☑
☑
02- ☑
s H04.30- ☑
32- ☑
04.41- ☑
P39.1
onous H04.31- ☑
ic A52.71
ongenital (early) A50.01
nomatous, active A71.1
sequelae (late effect) B94.0
ryocystoblenorrhea — see Inflammation, lacrimal, passages, chronic
acryocystocele — see Disorder, lacrimal system, changes

Dacryolith, dacryolithiasis H04.51- ☑
Dacryoma — see Disorder, lacrimal system, changes
Dacryopericystitis — see Dacryocystitis
Dacryops H04.11- ☑
Dacryostenosis — see also Stenosis, lacrimal
  congenital Q10.5
Dactylitis
  bone — see Osteomyelitis
  sickle-cell D57.00
    Hb C D57.219
    Hb SS D57.00
    specified NEC D57.819
  skin L08.9
  syphilitic A52.77
  tuberculous A18.03
Dactylolysis spontanea (ainhum) L94.6
Dactylosymphysis Q70.9
  fingers — see Syndactylism, complex, fingers
  toes — see Syndactylism, complex, toes
Damage
  arteriosclerotic — see Arteriosclerosis
  brain (nontraumatic) G93.9
    anoxic, hypoxic G93.1
      resulting from a procedure G97.82
    child NEC G80.9
    due to birth injury P11.2
  cardiorenal (vascular) — see Hypertension, cardiorenal
  cerebral NEC — see Damage, brain
  coccyx, complicating delivery O71.6
  coronary — see Disease, heart, ischemic
  deep tissue, pressure-induced — see also L89 with final character .6
  eye, birth injury P15.3
  liver (nontraumatic) K76.9
    alcoholic K70.9
    due to drugs — see Disease, liver, toxic
    toxic — see Disease, liver, toxic
  medication T88.7 ☑
  pelvic
    joint or ligament, during delivery O71.6
    organ NEC
      during delivery O71.5
      following ectopic or molar pregnancy O08.6
  renal — see Disease, renal
  subendocardium, subendocardial — see Degeneration, myocardial
  vascular I99.9
Dana-Putnam syndrome (subacute combined sclerosis with pernicious anemia) — see Degeneration, combined
Danbolt (-Cross) syndrome (acrodermatitis enteropathica) E83.2
Dandruff L21.0
Dandy-Walker syndrome Q03.1
  with spina bifida — see Spina bifida
Danlos' syndrome — see also Syndrome, Ehlers-Danlos Q79.60
Darier (-White) disease (congenital) Q82.8
  meaning erythema annulare centrifugum L53.1
Darier-Roussy sarcoid D86.3
Darling's disease or histoplasmosis B39.4
Darwin's tubercle Q17.8
Dawson's (inclusion body) **encephalitis** A81.1
De Beurmann (-Gougerot) **disease** B42.1
De la Tourette's syndrome F95.2

De Lange's syndrome Q87.19
De Morgan's spots (senile angiomas) I78.1
De Quervain's
  disease (tendon sheath) M65.4
  syndrome E34.51
  thyroiditis (subacute granulomatous thyroiditis) E06.1
De Toni-Fanconi (-Debré) **syndrome** E72.09
  with cystinosis E72.04
Dead
  fetus, retained (mother) O36.4 ☑
    early pregnancy O02.1
  labyrinth H83.2 ☑
  ovum, retained O02.0
Deaf nonspeaking NEC H91.3
Deafmutism (acquired) (congenital) NEC H91.3
  hysterical F44.6
  syphilitic, congenital — see also subcategory H94.8 A50.09
Deafness (acquired) (complete) (hereditary) (partial) H91.9- ☑
  with blue sclera and fragility of bone Q78.0
  auditory fatigue — see Deafness, specified type NEC
  aviation T70.0 ☑
    nerve injury — see Injury, nerve, acoustic, specified type NEC
  boilermaker's H83.3 ☑
  central — see Deafness, sensorineural
  conductive H90.2
    and sensorineural
      mixed H90.8
        bilateral H90.6
    bilateral H90.0
    unilateral H90.1- ☑
      with restricted hearing on the contralateral side H90.A- ☑
  congenital H90.5
    with blue sclera and fragility of bone Q78.0
  due to toxic agents — see Deafness, ototoxic
  emotional (hysterical) F44.6
  functional (hysterical) F44.6
  high frequency H91.9- ☑
  hysterical F44.6
  low frequency H91.9- ☑
  mental R48.8
  mixed conductive and sensorineural H90.8
    bilateral H90.6
    unilateral H90.7- ☑
  nerve — see Deafness, sensorineural
  neural — see Deafness, sensorineural
  noise-induced — see also subcategory H83.3 ☑
    nerve injury — see Injury, nerve, acoustic, specified type NEC
  nonspeaking H91.3
  ototoxic H91.0 ☑
  perceptive — see Deafness, sensorineural
  psychogenic (hysterical) F44.6
  sensorineural H90.5
    and conductive
      bilateral H90.6
      mixed H90.8
        bilateral H90.6
    bilateral H90.3
    unilateral H90.4- ☑
      with restricted hearing on the contralateral side H90.A- ☑
  sensory — see Deafness, sensorineural
  specified type NEC H91.8 ☑
  sudden (idiopathic) H91.2- ☑
  syphilitic A52.15
  transient ischemic H93.01- ☑
  traumatic — see Injury, nerve, acoustic, specified type NEC
  word (developmental) H93.25
Death (cause unknown) (of) (unexplained) (unspecified cause) R99
  brain G93.82
  cardiac (sudden) (with successful resuscitation) — code to underlying disease
    family history of Z82.41
    personal history of Z86.74
  family member (assumed) Z63.4
Debility (chronic) (general) (nervous) R53.81
  congenital or neonatal NOS P96.9
  nervous R53.81
  old age R54
  senile R54
Débove's disease (splenomegaly) R16.1

Decalcification
  bone — see Osteoporosis
  teeth K03.89
Decapsulation, kidney N28.89
Decay
  dental — see Caries, dental
  senile R54
  tooth, teeth — see Caries, dental
Deciduitis (acute)
  following ectopic or molar pregnancy O08.0
Decline (general) — see Debility
  cognitive, age-associated R41.81
Decompensation
  cardiac (acute) (chronic) — see Disease, heart
  cardiovascular — see Disease, cardiovascular
  heart — see Disease, heart
  hepatic — see Failure, hepatic
  myocardial (acute) (chronic) — see Disease, heart
  respiratory J98.8
Decompression sickness T70.3 ☑
Decrease (d)
  absolute neutrophil count — see Neutropenia
  blood
    platelets — see Thrombocytopenia
    pressure R03.1
      due to shock following
        injury T79.4 ☑
        operation T81.19 ☑
  estrogen E28.39
    postablative E89.40
      asymptomatic E89.40
      symptomatic E89.41
  fragility of erythrocytes D58.8
  function
    lipase (pancreatic) K90.3
    ovary in hypopituitarism E23.0
    parenchyma of pancreas K86.89
    pituitary (gland) (anterior) (lobe) E23.0
      posterior (lobe) E23.0
  functional activity R68.89
  glucose R73.09
  hematocrit R71.0
  hemoglobin R71.0
  leukocytes D72.819
    specified NEC D72.818
  libido R68.82
  lymphocytes D72.810
  platelets D69.6
  respiration, due to shock following injury T79.4 ☑
  sexual desire R68.82
  tear secretion NEC — see Syndrome, dry eye
  tolerance
    fat K90.49
    glucose R73.09
    pancreatic K90.3
    salt and water E87.8
  vision NEC H54.7
  white blood cell count D72.819
    specified NEC D72.818
Decubitus (ulcer) — see Ulcer, pressure, by site
  cervix N86
Deepening acetabulum — see Derangement, joint, specified type NEC, hip
Defect, defective Q89.9
  3-beta-hydroxysteroid dehydrogenase E25.0
  11-hydroxylase E25.0
  21-hydroxylase E25.0
  abdominal wall, congenital Q79.59
  antibody immunodeficiency D80.9
  aorticopulmonary septum Q21.4
  atrial septal (ostium secundum type) Q21.1
    following acute myocardial infarction (current complication) I23.1
    ostium primum type Q21.2
  atrioventricular
    canal Q21.2
    septum Q21.2
  auricular septal Q21.1
  bilirubin excretion NEC E80.6
  biosynthesis, androgen (testicular) E29.1
  bulbar septum Q21.0
  catalase E80.3
  cell membrane receptor complex (CR3) D71
  circulation I99.9
    congenital Q28.9
    newborn Q28.9
  coagulation (factor) — see also Deficiency, factor D68.9

Defect, defective — *continued*
- coagulation — *see also* Deficiency, factor — *continued*
  - with
    - ectopic pregnancy O08.1
    - molar pregnancy O08.1
  - acquired D68.4
  - antepartum with hemorrhage — *see* Hemorrhage, antepartum, with coagulation defect
  - due to
    - liver disease D68.4
    - vitamin K deficiency D68.4
  - hereditary NEC D68.2
  - intrapartum O67.0
  - newborn, transient P61.6
  - postpartum O99.13
    - with hemorrhage O72.3
  - specified type NEC D68.8
- complement system D84.1
- conduction (heart) I45.9
  - bone — *see* Deafness, conductive
- congenital, organ or site not listed — *see* Anomaly, by site
- coronary sinus Q21.1
- cushion, endocardial Q21.2
- degradation, glycoprotein E77.1
- dental bridge, crown, fillings — *see* Defect, dental restoration
- dental restoration K08.50
  - specified NEC K08.59
- dentin (hereditary) K00.5
- Descemet's membrane, congenital Q13.89
- developmental — *see also* Anomaly
  - cauda equina Q06.3
- diaphragm
  - with elevation, eventration or hernia — *see* Hernia, diaphragm
  - congenital Q79.1
    - with hernia Q79.0
    - gross (with hernia) Q79.0
- ectodermal, congenital Q82.9
- Eisenmenger's Q21.8
- enzyme
  - catalase E80.3
  - peroxidase E80.3
- esophagus, congenital Q39.9
- extensor retinaculum M62.89
- fibrin polymerization D68.2
- filling
  - bladder R93.41
  - kidney R93.42- ☑
  - renal pelvis R93.41
  - stomach R93.3
  - ureter R93.41
  - urinary organs, specified NEC R93.49
- GABA (gamma aminobutyric acid) metabolic E72.81
- Gerbode Q21.0
- glycoprotein degradation E77.1
- Hageman (factor) D68.2
- hearing — *see* Deafness
- high grade F70
- interatrial septal Q21.1
- interauricular septal Q21.1
- interventricular septal Q21.0
  - with dextroposition of aorta, pulmonary stenosis and hypertrophy of right ventricle Q21.3
  - in tetralogy of Fallot Q21.3
- learning (specific) — *see* Disorder, learning
- lymphocyte function antigen-1 (LFA-1) D84.0
- lysosomal enzyme, post-translational modification E77.0
- major osseous M89.70
  - ankle M89.77- ☑
  - carpus M89.74- ☑
  - clavicle M89.71- ☑
  - femur M89.75- ☑
  - fibula M89.76- ☑
  - fingers M89.74- ☑
  - foot M89.77- ☑
  - forearm M89.73- ☑
  - hand M89.74- ☑
  - humerus M89.72- ☑
  - lower leg M89.76- ☑
  - metacarpus M89.74- ☑
  - metatarsus M89.77- ☑
  - multiple sites M89.79
  - pelvic region M89.75- ☑
  - pelvis M89.75- ☑

Defect, defective — *continued*
- major osseous — *continued*
  - radius M89.73- ☑
  - scapula M89.71- ☑
  - shoulder region M89.71- ☑
  - specified NEC M89.78
  - tarsus M89.77- ☑
  - thigh M89.75- ☑
  - tibia M89.76- ☑
  - toes M89.77- ☑
  - ulna M89.73- ☑
- mental — *see* Disability, intellectual
- modification, lysosomal enzymes, post-translational E77.0
- obstructive, congenital
  - renal pelvis Q62.39
  - ureter Q62.39
    - atresia — *see* Atresia, ureter
    - cecoureterocele Q62.32
    - megaureter Q62.2
    - orthotopic ureterocele Q62.31
- osseous, major M89.70
  - ankle M89.77- ☑
  - carpus M89.74- ☑
  - clavicle M89.71- ☑
  - femur M89.75- ☑
  - fibula M89.76- ☑
  - fingers M89.74- ☑
  - foot M89.77- ☑
  - forearm M89.73- ☑
  - hand M89.74- ☑
  - humerus M89.72- ☑
  - lower leg M89.76- ☑
  - metacarpus M89.74- ☑
  - metatarsus M89.77- ☑
  - multiple sites M89.9
  - pelvic region M89.75- ☑
  - pelvis M89.75- ☑
  - radius M89.73- ☑
  - scapula M89.71- ☑
  - shoulder region M89.71- ☑
  - specified NEC M89.78
  - tarsus M89.77- ☑
  - thigh M89.75- ☑
  - tibia M89.76- ☑
  - toes M89.77- ☑
  - ulna M89.73- ☑
- osteochondral NEC — *see also* Deformity M95.8
- ostium
  - primum Q21.2
  - secundum Q21.1
- peroxidase E80.3
- placental blood supply — *see* Insufficiency, placental
- platelets, qualitative D69.1
  - constitutional D68.0
- postural NEC, spine — *see* Dorsopathy, deforming
- reduction
  - limb Q73.8
    - lower Q72.9- ☑
      - absence — *see* Agenesis, leg
        - foot — *see* Agenesis, foot
      - longitudinal
        - femur Q72.4- ☑
        - fibula Q72.6- ☑
        - tibia Q72.5- ☑
      - specified type NEC Q72.89- ☑
      - split foot Q72.7- ☑
    - specified type NEC Q73.8
    - upper Q71.9- ☑
      - absence — *see* Agenesis, arm
        - forearm — *see* Agenesis, forearm
        - hand — *see* Agenesis, hand
      - lobster-claw hand Q71.6- ☑
      - longitudinal
        - radius Q71.4- ☑
        - ulna Q71.5- ☑
      - specified type NEC Q71.89- ☑
- renal pelvis Q63.8
  - obstructive Q62.39
- respiratory system, congenital Q34.9
- restoration, dental K08.50
  - specified NEC K08.59
- retinal nerve bundle fibers H35.89
- septal (heart) NOS Q21.9
  - acquired (atrial) (auricular) (ventricular) (old) I51.0
  - atrial Q21.1

Defect, defective — *continued*
- septal — *continued*
  - atrial — *continued*
    - concurrent with acute myocardial infarction — *see* Infarct, myocardium
    - following acute myocardial infarction (current complication) I23.1
    - ventricular — *see also* Defect, ventricular septal Q21.0
  - sinus venosus Q21.1
- speech R47.9
  - developmental F80.9
  - specified NEC R47.89
- Taussig-Bing (aortic transposition and overriding pulmonary artery) Q20.1
- teeth, wedge K03.1
- vascular (local) I99.9
  - congenital Q27.9
- ventricular septal Q21.0
  - concurrent with acute myocardial infarction — *see* Infarct, myocardium
  - following acute myocardial infarction (current complication) I23.2
  - in tetralogy of Fallot Q21.3
- vision NEC H54.7
- visual field H53.40
  - bilateral
    - heteronymous H53.47
    - homonymous H53.46- ☑
  - generalized contraction H53.48- ☑
  - localized
    - arcuate H53.43- ☑
    - scotoma (central area) H53.41- ☑
      - blind spot area H53.42- ☑
    - sector H53.43- ☑
  - specified type NEC H53.45- ☑
- voice R49.9
  - specified NEC R49.8
- wedge, tooth, teeth (abrasion) K03.1

Deferentitis N49.1
- gonorrheal (acute) (chronic) A54.23

Defibrination (syndrome) D65
- antepartum — *see* Hemorrhage, antepartum, with coagulation defect, disseminated intravascular coagulation
- following ectopic or molar pregnancy O08.1
- intrapartum O67.0
- newborn P60
- postpartum O72.3

Deficiency, deficient
- 3-beta hydroxysteroid dehydrogenase E25.0
- 5-alpha reductase (with male pseudohermaphroditism) E29.1
- 11-hydroxylase E25.0
- 21-hydroxylase E25.0
- abdominal muscle syndrome Q79.4
- AC globulin (congenital) (hereditary) D68.2
  - acquired D68.4
- accelerator globulin (Ac G) (blood) D68.2
- acid phosphatase E83.39
- activating factor (blood) D68.2
- ADA2 (adenosine deaminase 2) D81.32
- adenosine deaminase (ADA) D81.30
  - with severe combined immunodeficiency (SCID) D81.31
  - partial (type 1) D81.39
  - specified NEC D81.39
  - type 1 (without SCID) (without severe combined immunodeficiency) D81.39
  - type 2 D81.32
- aldolase (hereditary) E74.19
- alpha-1-antitrypsin E88.01
- amino-acids E72.9
- anemia — *see* Anemia
- aneurin E51.9
- antibody with
  - hyperimmunoglobulinemia D80.6
  - near-normal immunoglobins D80.6
- antidiuretic hormone E23.2
- anti-hemophilic
  - factor (A) D66
    - B D67
    - C D68.1
  - globulin (AHG) NEC D66
- antithrombin (antithrombin III) D68.59
- ascorbic acid E54
- attention (disorder) (syndrome) F98.8

Deficiency, deficient — *continued*
attention — *continued*
  with hyperactivity — *see* Disorder, attention-deficit hyperactivity
autoprothrombin
  C D68.2
  I D68.2
  II D67
beta-glucuronidase E76.29
biotin E53.8
biotin-dependent carboxylase D81.819
biotinidase D81.810
brancher enzyme (amylopectinosis) E74.03
C1 esterase inhibitor (C1-INH) D84.1
calciferol E55.9
  with
    adult osteomalacia M83.8
    rickets — *see* Rickets
calcium (dietary) E58
calorie, severe E43
  with marasmus E41
    and kwashiorkor E42
cardiac — *see* Insufficiency, myocardial
carnitine E71.40
  due to
    hemodialysis E71.43
    inborn errors of metabolism E71.42
    Valproic acid therapy E71.43
  iatrogenic E71.43
  muscle palmityltransferase E71.314
  primary E71.41
  secondary E71.448
carotene E50.9
central nervous system G96.8
ceruloplasmin (Wilson) E83.01
choline E53.8
Christmas factor D67
chromium E61.4
clotting (blood) — *see also* Deficiency, coagulation factor D68.9
clotting factor NEC (hereditary) — *see also* Deficiency, factor D68.2
coagulation NOS D68.9
  with
    ectopic pregnancy O08.1
    molar pregnancy O08.1
  acquired (any) D68.4
  antepartum hemorrhage — *see* Hemorrhage, antepartum, with coagulation defect
  clotting factor NEC — *see also* Deficiency, factor D68.2
  due to
    hyperprothrombinemia D68.4
    liver disease D68.4
    vitamin K deficiency D68.4
  newborn, transient P61.6
  postpartum O72.3
  specified NEC D68.8
cognitive F09
color vision H53.50
  achromatopsia H53.51
  acquired H53.52
  deuteranomaly H53.53
  protanomaly H53.54
  specified type NEC H53.59
  tritanomaly H53.55
combined glucocorticoid and mineralocorticoid E27.49
contact factor D68.2
copper (nutritional) E61.0
corticoadrenal E27.40
  primary E27.1
craniofacial axis Q75.0
cyanocobalamin E53.8
debrancher enzyme (limit dextrinosis) E74.03
dehydrogenase
  long chain/very long chain acyl CoA E71.310
  medium chain acyl CoA E71.311
  short chain acyl CoA E71.312
diet E63.9
dihydropyrimidine dehydrogenase (DPD) E88.89
disaccharidase E73.9
edema — *see* Malnutrition, severe
endocrine E34.9
energy-supply — *see* Malnutrition
enzymes, circulating NEC E88.09
ergosterol E55.9
  with
    adult osteomalacia M83.8

Deficiency, deficient — *continued*
ergosterol — *continued*
  with — *continued*
    rickets — *see* Rickets
essential fatty acid (EFA) E63.0
factor — *see also* Deficiency, coagulation
  Hageman D68.2
  I (congenital) (hereditary) D68.2
  II (congenital) (hereditary) D68.2
  IX (congenital) (functional) (hereditary) (with functional defect) D67
  multiple (congenital) D68.8
    acquired D68.4
  V (congenital) (hereditary) D68.2
  VII (congenital) (hereditary) D68.2
  VIII (congenital) (functional) (hereditary) (with functional defect) D66
    with vascular defect D68.0
  X (congenital) (hereditary) D68.2
  XI (congenital) (hereditary) D68.1
  XII (congenital) (hereditary) D68.2
  XIII (congenital) (hereditary) D68.2
femoral, proximal focal (congenital) — *see* Defect, reduction, lower limb, longitudinal, femur
fibrinase D68.2
fibrinogen (congenital) (hereditary) D68.2
  acquired D65
fibrin-stabilizing factor (congenital) (hereditary) D68.2
  acquired D68.4
folate E53.8
folic acid E53.8
foreskin N47.3
fructokinase E74.11
fructose 1,6-diphosphatase E74.19
fructose-1-phosphate aldolase E74.19
GABA (gamma aminobutyric acid) transaminase E72.81
GABA-T (gamma aminobutyric acid transaminase)-T E72.81
galactokinase E74.29
galactose-1-phosphate uridyl transferase E74.29
gammaglobulin in blood D80.1
  hereditary D80.0
glass factor D68.2
glucocorticoid E27.49
  mineralocorticoid E27.49
glucose-6-phosphatase E74.01
glucose-6-phosphate dehydrogenase
  anemia D55.0
  without anemia D75.A
glucuronyl transferase E80.5
glycogen synthetase E74.09
gonadotropin (isolated) E23.0
growth hormone (idiopathic) (isolated) E23.0
Hageman factor D68.2
hemoglobin D64.9
hepatophosphorylase E74.09
homogentisate 1,2-dioxygenase E70.29
hormone
  anterior pituitary (partial) NEC E23.0
    growth E23.0
  growth (isolated) E23.0
  pituitary E23.0
  testicular E29.1
hypoxanthine- (guanine)-phosphoribosyltransferase (HG- PRT) (total H-PRT) E79.1
immunity D84.9
  cell-mediated D84.8
    with thrombocytopenia and eczema D82.0
  combined D81.9
  humoral D80.9
  IgA (secretory) D80.2
  IgG D80.3
  IgM D80.4
immuno — *see* Immunodeficiency
immunoglobulin, selective
  A (IgA) D80.2
  G (IgG) (subclasses) D80.3
  M (IgM) D80.4
inositol (B complex) E53.8
intrinsic
  factor (congenital) D51.0
  sphincter N36.42
    with urethral hypermobility N36.43
iodine E61.8
  congenital syndrome — *see* Syndrome, iodine-deficiency, congenital
iron E61.1
  anemia D50.9
kalium E87.6

Deficiency, deficient — *continued*
kappa-light chain D80.8
labile factor (congenital) (hereditary) D68.2
  acquired D68.4
lacrimal fluid (acquired) — *see also* Syndrome, dry eye
  congenital Q10.6
lactase
  congenital E73.0
  secondary E73.1
Laki-Lorand factor D68.2
lecithin cholesterol acyltransferase E78.6
lipocaic K86.89
lipoprotein (familial) (high density) E78.6
liver phosphorylase E74.09
lysosomal alpha-1, 4 glucosidase E74.02
magnesium E61.2
major histocompatibility complex
  class I D81.6
  class II D81.7
manganese E61.3
menadione (vitamin K) E56.1
  newborn P53
mental (familial) (hereditary) — *see* Disability, intellectual
methylenetetrahydrofolate reductase (MTHFR) E72.12
mevalonate kinase M04.1
mineralocorticoid E27.49
  with glucocorticoid E27.49
mineral NEC E61.8
molybdenum (nutritional) E61.5
moral F60.2
multiple nutrient elements E61.7
multiple sulfatase (MSD) E75.26
muscle
  carnitine (palmityltransferase) E71.314
  phosphofructokinase E74.09
myoadenylate deaminase E79.2
myocardial — *see* Insufficiency, myocardial
myophosphorylase E74.04
NADH diaphorase or reductase (congenital) D74.0
NADH-methemoglobin reductase (congenital) D74.0
natrium E87.1
niacin (amide) (-tryptophan) E52
nicotinamide E52
nicotinic acid E52
number of teeth — *see* Anodontia
nutrient element E61.9
  multiple E61.7
  specified NEC E61.8
nutrition, nutritional E63.9
  sequelae — *see* Sequelae, nutritional deficiency
  specified NEC E63.8
of interleukin 1 receptor antagonist [DIRA] M04.8
ornithine transcarbamylase E72.4
ovarian E28.39
oxygen — *see* Anoxia
pantothenic acid E53.8
parathyroid (gland) E20.9
perineum (female) N81.89
phenylalanine hydroxylase E70.1
phosphoenolpyruvate carboxykinase E74.4
phosphofructokinase E74.19
phosphomannomutase E74.8
phosphomannose isomerase E74.8
phosphomannosyl mutase E74.8
phosphorylase kinase, liver E74.09
pituitary hormone (isolated) E23.0
plasma thromboplastin
  antecedent (PTA) D68.1
  component (PTC) D67
plasminogen (type 1) (type 2) E88.02
platelet NEC D69.1
  constitutional D68.0
polyglandular E31.8
  autoimmune E31.0
potassium (K) E87.6
prepuce N47.3
proaccelerin (congenital) (hereditary) D68.2
  acquired D68.4
proconvertin factor (congenital) (hereditary) D68.2
  acquired D68.4
protein — *see also* Malnutrition E46
  anemia D53.0
  C D68.59
  S D68.59
prothrombin (congenital) (hereditary) D68.2
  acquired D68.4
Prower factor D68.2

☑ Additional Character Required — Refer to the Tabular List for Character Selection   ▽ Subterms under main terms may continue to next column or page

Deficiency, deficient — *continued*
pseudocholinesterase E88.09
PTA (plasma thromboplastin antecedent) D68.1
PTC (plasma thromboplastin component) D67
purine nucleoside phosphorylase (PNP) D81.5
pyracin (alpha) (beta) E53.1
pyridoxal E53.1
pyridoxamine E53.1
pyridoxine (derivatives) E53.1
pyruvate
  carboxylase E74.4
  dehydrogenase E74.4
riboflavin (vitamin B2) E53.0
salt E87.1
secretion
  ovary E28.39
  salivary gland (any) K11.7
  urine R34
selenium (dietary) E59
serum antitrypsin, familial E88.01
short stature homeobox gene (SHOX)
  with
    dyschondrosteosis Q78.8
    short stature (idiopathic) E34.3
    Turner's syndrome Q96.9
sodium (Na) E87.1
SPCA (factor VII) D68.2
sphincter, intrinsic N36.42
  with urethral hypermobility N36.43
stable factor (congenital) (hereditary) D68.2
  acquired D68.4
Stuart-Prower (factor X) D68.2
succinic semialdehyde dehydrogenase E72.81
sucrase E74.39
sulfatase E75.26
sulfite oxidase E72.19
thiamin, thiaminic (chloride) E51.9
  beriberi (dry) E51.11
    wet E51.12
thrombokinase D68.2
  newborn P53
thyroid (gland) — *see* Hypothyroidism
tocopherol E56.0
tooth bud K00.0
transcobalamine II (anemia) D51.2
vanadium E61.6
vascular I99.9
vasopressin E23.2
vertical ridge K06.8
viosterol — *see* Deficiency, calciferol
vitamin (multiple) NOS E56.9
  A E50.9
    with
      Bitot's spot (corneal) E50.1
      follicular keratosis E50.8
      keratomalacia E50.4
      manifestations NEC E50.8
      night blindness E50.5
      scar of cornea, xerophthalmic E50.6
      xeroderma E50.8
      xerophthalmia E50.7
      xerosis
        conjunctival E50.0
          and Bitot's spot E50.1
        cornea E50.2
          and ulceration E50.3
    sequelae E64.1
  B (complex) NOS E53.9
    with
      beriberi (dry) E51.11
        wet E51.12
      pellagra E52
  B1 NOS E51.9
    beriberi (dry) E51.11
      with circulatory system manifestations E51.11
      wet E51.12
  B12 E53.8
  B2 (riboflavin) E53.0
  B6 E53.1
  C E54
    sequelae E64.2
  D E55.9
    with
      adult osteomalacia M83.8
      rickets — *see* Rickets
    25-hydroxylase E83.32
  E E56.0
  folic acid E53.8
  G E53.0

Deficiency, deficient — *continued*
vitamin — *continued*
  group B E53.9
    specified NEC E53.8
  H (biotin) E53.8
  K E56.1
    of newborn P53
  nicotinic E52
  P E56.8
  PP (pellagra-preventing) E52
  specified NEC E56.8
  thiamin E51.9
    beriberi — *see* Beriberi
zinc, dietary E60
Deficit — *see also* Deficiency
attention and concentration R41.840
  disorder — *see* Attention, deficit
  following
    cerebral infarction I69.310
    cerebrovascular disease I69.910
      specified disease NEC I69.810
    nontraumatic
      intracerebral hemorrhage I69.110
      specified intracranial hemorrhage NEC I69.210
      subarachnoid hemorrhage I69.010
cognitive
  communication R41.841
  emotional
    following
      cerebral infarction I69.315
      cerebrovascular disease I69.915
        specified disease NEC I69.815
      nontraumatic
        intracerebral hemorrhage I69.115
        specified intracranial hemorrhage NEC I69.215
        subarachnoid hemorrhage I69.015
  following
    cerebral infarction I69.319
    cerebrovascular disease I69.919
      specified disease NEC I69.819
    nontraumatic
      intracerebral hemorrhage I69.119
      specified intracranial hemorrhage NEC I69.219
      subarachnoid hemorrhage I69.019
  social
    following
      cerebral infarction I69.315
      cerebrovascular disease I69.915
        specified disease NEC I69.815
      nontraumatic
        intracerebral hemorrhage I69.115
        specified intracranial hemorrhage NEC I69.215
        subarachnoid hemorrhage I69.015
cognitive NEC R41.89
  following
    cerebral infarction I69.318
    cerebrovascular disease I69.918
      specified disease NEC I69.818
    nontraumatic
      intracerebral hemorrhage I69.118
      specified intracranial hemorrhage NEC I69.218
      subarachnoid hemorrhage I69.018
concentration R41.840
executive function R41.844
  following
    cerebral infarction I69.314
    cerebrovascular disease I69.914
      specified disease NEC I69.814
    nontraumatic
      intracerebral hemorrhage I69.114
      specified intracranial hemorrhage NEC I69.214
      subarachnoid hemorrhage I69.014
frontal lobe R41.844
  following
    cerebral infarction I69.314
    cerebrovascular disease I69.914
      specified disease NEC I69.814
    nontraumatic
      intracerebral hemorrhage I69.114
      specified intracranial hemorrhage NEC I69.214
      subarachnoid hemorrhage I69.014
memory
  following
    cerebral infarction I69.311
    cerebrovascular disease I69.911
      specified disease NEC I69.811

Deficit — *continued*
memory — *continued*
  following — *continued*
    nontraumatic
      intracerebral hemorrhage I69.111
      specified intracranial hemorrhage NEC I69.211
      subarachnoid hemorrhage I69.011
neurologic NEC R29.818
  ischemic
    reversible (RIND) I63.9
      prolonged (PRIND) I63.9
oxygen R09.02
prolonged reversible ischemic neurologic (PRIND) I63.9
psychomotor R41.843
  following
    cerebral infarction I69.313
    cerebrovascular disease I69.913
      specified disease NEC I69.813
    nontraumatic
      intracerebral hemorrhage I69.113
      specified intracranial hemorrhage NEC I69.213
      subarachnoid hemorrhage I69.013
visuospatial R41.842
  following
    cerebral infarction I69.312
    cerebrovascular disease I69.912
      specified disease NEC I69.812
    nontraumatic
      intracerebral hemorrhage I69.112
      specified intracranial hemorrhage NEC I69.212
      subarachnoid hemorrhage I69.012
Deflection
radius — *see* Deformity, limb, specified type NEC, forearm
septum (acquired) (nasal) (nose) J34.2
spine — *see* Curvature, spine
turbinate (nose) J34.2
Defluvium
capillorum — *see* Alopecia
ciliorum — *see* Madarosis
unguium L60.8
Deformity Q89.9
abdomen, congenital Q89.9
abdominal wall
  acquired M95.8
  congenital Q79.59
acquired (unspecified site) M95.9
adrenal gland Q89.1
alimentary tract, congenital Q45.9
  upper Q40.9
ankle (joint) (acquired) — *see also* Deformity, limb, lower leg
  abduction — *see* Contraction, joint, ankle
  congenital Q68.8
  contraction — *see* Contraction, joint, ankle
  specified type NEC — *see* Deformity, limb, foot, specified NEC
anus (acquired) K62.89
  congenital Q43.9
aorta (arch) (congenital) Q25.40
  acquired I77.89
aortic
  arch, acquired I77.89
  cusp or valve (congenital) Q23.8
    acquired — *see also* Endocarditis, aortic I35.8
arm (acquired) (upper) — *see also* Deformity, limb, upper arm
  congenital Q68.8
  forearm — *see* Deformity, limb, forearm
artery (congenital) (peripheral) NOS Q27.9
  acquired I77.89
  coronary (acquired) I25.9
    congenital Q24.5
  umbilical Q27.0
atrial septal Q21.1
auditory canal (external) (congenital) — *see also* Malformation, ear, external
  acquired — *see* Disorder, ear, external, specified type NEC
auricle
  ear (congenital) — *see also* Malformation, ear, external
    acquired — *see* Disorder, pinna, deformity
back — *see* Dorsopathy, deforming
bile duct (common) (congenital) (hepatic) Q44.5
  acquired K83.8
biliary duct or passage (congenital) Q44.5
  acquired K83.8

▽ Subterms under main terms may continue to next column or page   ☑ Additional Character Required — Refer to the Tabular List for Character Selection   85

Deficiency, deficient — Deformity

Deformity — *continued*
- bladder (neck) (trigone) (sphincter) (acquired) N32.89
  - congenital Q64.79
- bone (acquired) NOS M95.9
  - congenital Q79.9
  - turbinate M95.0
- brain (congenital) Q04.9
  - acquired G93.89
  - reduction Q04.3
- breast (acquired) N64.89
  - congenital Q83.9
  - reconstructed N65.0
- bronchus (congenital) Q32.4
  - acquired NEC J98.09
- bursa, congenital Q79.9
- canaliculi (lacrimalis) (acquired) — *see also* Disorder, lacrimal system, changes
  - congenital Q10.6
- canthus, acquired — *see* Disorder, eyelid, specified type NEC
- capillary (acquired) I78.8
- cardiovascular system, congenital Q28.9
- caruncle, lacrimal (acquired) — *see also* Disorder, lacrimal system, changes
  - congenital Q10.6
- cascade, stomach K31.2
- cecum (congenital) Q43.9
  - acquired K63.89
- cerebral, acquired G93.89
  - congenital Q04.9
- cervix (uterus) (acquired) NEC N88.8
  - congenital Q51.9
- cheek (acquired) M95.2
  - congenital Q18.9
- chest (acquired) (wall) M95.4
  - congenital Q67.8
  - sequelae (late effect) of rickets E64.3
- chin (acquired) M95.2
  - congenital Q18.9
- choroid (congenital) Q14.3
  - acquired H31.8
  - plexus Q07.8
    - acquired G96.19
- cicatricial — *see* Cicatrix
- cilia, acquired — *see* Disorder, eyelid, specified type NEC
- clavicle (acquired) M95.8
  - congenital Q68.8
- clitoris (congenital) Q52.6
  - acquired N90.89
- clubfoot — *see* Clubfoot
- coccyx (acquired) — *see* subcategory M43.8 ☑
- colon (congenital) Q43.9
  - acquired K63.89
- concha (ear), congenital — *see also* Malformation, ear, external
  - acquired — *see* Disorder, pinna, deformity
- cornea (acquired) H18.70
  - congenital Q13.4
  - descemetocele — *see* Descemetocele
  - ectasia — *see* Ectasia, cornea
  - specified NEC H18.79- ☑
  - staphyloma — *see* Staphyloma, cornea
- coronary artery (acquired) I25.9
  - congenital Q24.5
- cranium (acquired) — *see* Deformity, skull
- cricoid cartilage (congenital) Q31.8
  - acquired J38.7
- cystic duct (congenital) Q44.5
  - acquired K82.8
- Dandy-Walker Q03.1
  - with spina bifida — *see* Spina bifida
- diaphragm (congenital) Q79.1
  - acquired J98.6
- digestive organ NOS Q45.9
- ductus arteriosus Q25.0
- duodenal bulb K31.89
- duodenum (congenital) Q43.9
  - acquired K31.89
- dura — *see* Deformity, meninges
- ear (acquired) — *see also* Disorder, pinna, deformity
  - congenital (external) Q17.9
    - internal Q16.5
    - middle Q16.4
      - ossicles Q16.3
    - ossicles Q16.3
- ectodermal (congenital) NEC Q84.9
- ejaculatory duct (congenital) Q55.4

Deformity — *continued*
- ejaculatory duct — *continued*
  - acquired N50.89
- elbow (joint) (acquired) — *see also* Deformity, limb, upper arm
  - congenital Q68.8
  - contraction — *see* Contraction, joint, elbow
- endocrine gland NEC Q89.2
- epididymis (congenital) Q55.4
  - acquired N50.89
- epiglottis (congenital) Q31.8
  - acquired J38.7
- esophagus (congenital) Q39.9
  - acquired K22.8
- eustachian tube (congenital) NEC Q17.8
- eye, congenital Q15.9
- eyebrow (congenital) Q18.8
- eyelid (acquired) — *see also* Disorder, eyelid, specified type NEC
  - congenital Q10.3
- face (acquired) M95.2
  - congenital Q18.9
- fallopian tube, acquired N83.8
- femur (acquired) — *see* Deformity, limb, specified type NEC, thigh
- fetal
  - with fetopelvic disproportion O33.7 ☑
  - causing obstructed labor O66.3
- finger (acquired) M20.00- ☑
  - boutonniere M20.02- ☑
  - congenital Q68.1
  - flexion contracture — *see* Contraction, joint, hand
  - mallet finger M20.01- ☑
  - specified NEC M20.09- ☑
  - swan-neck M20.03- ☑
- flexion (joint) (acquired) — *see also* Deformity, limb, flexion M21.20
  - congenital NOS Q74.9
    - hip Q65.89
- foot (acquired) — *see also* Deformity, limb, lower leg
  - cavovarus (congenital) Q66.1- ☑
  - congenital NOS Q66.9- ☑
    - specified type NEC Q66.89
  - specified type NEC — *see* Deformity, limb, foot, specified NEC
  - valgus (congenital) Q66.6
    - acquired — *see* Deformity, valgus, ankle
  - varus (congenital) NEC Q66.3- ☑
    - acquired — *see* Deformity, varus, ankle
- forearm (acquired) — *see also* Deformity, limb, forearm
  - congenital Q68.8
- forehead (acquired) M95.2
  - congenital Q75.8
- frontal bone (acquired) M95.2
  - congenital Q75.8
- gallbladder (congenital) Q44.1
  - acquired K82.8
- gastrointestinal tract (congenital) NOS Q45.9
  - acquired K63.89
- genitalia, genital organ(s) or system NEC
  - female (congenital) Q52.9
    - acquired N94.89
    - external Q52.70
  - male (congenital) Q55.9
    - acquired N50.89
- globe (eye) (congenital) Q15.8
  - acquired H44.89
- gum, acquired NEC K06.8
- hand (acquired) — *see* Deformity, limb, hand
  - congenital Q68.1
- head (acquired) M95.2
  - congenital Q75.8
- heart (congenital) Q24.9
  - septum Q21.9
    - auricular Q21.1
    - ventricular Q21.0
  - valve (congenital) NEC Q24.8
    - acquired — *see* Endocarditis
- heel (acquired) — *see* Deformity, foot
- hepatic duct (congenital) Q44.5
  - acquired K83.8
- hip (joint) (acquired) (*see also* Deformity, limb, thigh)
  - congenital Q65.9
  - due to (previous) juvenile osteochondrosis — *see* Coxa, plana
  - flexion — *see* Contraction, joint, hip
- hourglass — *see* Contraction, hourglass
- humerus (acquired) M21.82- ☑

Deformity — *continued*
- humerus — *continued*
  - congenital Q74.0
- hypophyseal (congenital) Q89.2
- ileocecal (coil) (valve) (acquired) K63.89
  - congenital Q43.9
- ileum (congenital) Q43.9
  - acquired K63.89
- ilium (acquired) M95.5
  - congenital Q74.2
- integument (congenital) Q84.9
- intervertebral cartilage or disc (acquired) — *see* Disorder, disc, specified NEC
- intestine (large) (small) (congenital) NOS Q43.9
  - acquired K63.89
- intrinsic minus or plus (hand) — *see* Deformity, limb, specified type NEC, forearm
- iris (acquired) H21.89
  - congenital Q13.2
- ischium (acquired) M95.5
  - congenital Q74.2
- jaw (acquired) (congenital) M26.9
- joint (acquired) NEC M21.90
  - congenital Q68.8
  - elbow M21.92- ☑
  - hand M21.94- ☑
  - hip M21.95- ☑
  - knee M21.96- ☑
  - shoulder M21.92- ☑
  - wrist M21.93- ☑
- kidney(s) (calyx) (pelvis) (congenital) Q63.9
  - acquired N28.89
  - artery (congenital) Q27.2
    - acquired I77.89
- Klippel-Feil (brevicollis) Q76.1
- knee (acquired) NEC — *see* Deformity, limb, lower leg
  - congenital Q68.2
- labium (majus) (minus) (congenital) Q52.79
  - acquired N90.89
- lacrimal passages or duct (congenital) NEC Q10.6
  - acquired — *see* Disorder, lacrimal system, changes
- larynx (muscle) (congenital) Q31.8
  - acquired J38.7
  - web (glottic) Q31.0
- leg (upper) (acquired) NEC — *see* Deformity, limb, thigh
  - congenital Q68.8
  - lower leg — *see* Deformity, limb, lower leg
- lens (acquired) H27.8
  - congenital Q12.9
- lid (fold) (acquired) — *see also* Disorder, eyelid, specified type NEC
  - congenital Q10.3
- ligament (acquired) — *see* Disorder, ligament
  - congenital Q79.9
- limb (acquired) M21.90
  - clawfoot M21.53- ☑
  - clawhand M21.51- ☑
  - clubfoot M21.54- ☑
  - clubhand M21.52- ☑
  - congenital, except reduction deformity Q74.9
  - flat foot M21.4- ☑
  - flexion M21.20
    - ankle M21.27- ☑
    - elbow M21.22- ☑
    - finger M21.24- ☑
    - hip M21.25- ☑
    - knee M21.26- ☑
    - shoulder M21.21- ☑
    - toe M21.27- ☑
    - wrist M21.23- ☑
  - foot
    - claw — *see* Deformity, limb, clawfoot
    - club — *see* Deformity, limb, clubfoot
    - drop M21.37- ☑
    - flat — *see* Deformity, limb, flat foot
    - specified NEC M21.6X- ☑
  - forearm M21.93- ☑
  - hand M21.94- ☑
  - lower leg M21.96- ☑
  - specified type NEC M21.80
    - forearm M21.83- ☑
    - lower leg M21.86- ☑
    - thigh M21.85- ☑
    - upper arm M21.82- ☑
  - thigh M21.95- ☑

Deformity — *continued*
  limb — *continued*
    unequal length M21.70
      short site is
        femur M21.75- ☑
        fibula M21.76- ☑
        humerus M21.72- ☑
        radius M21.73- ☑
        tibia M21.76- ☑
        ulna M21.73- ☑
      upper arm M21.92- ☑
      valgus — *see* Deformity, valgus
      varus — *see* Deformity, varus
      wrist drop M21.33- ☑
  lip (acquired) NEC K13.0
    congenital Q38.0
  liver (congenital) Q44.7
    acquired K76.89
  lumbosacral (congenital) (joint) (region) Q76.49
    acquired — *see* subcategory M43.8 ☑
    kyphosis — *see* Kyphosis, congenital
    lordosis — *see* Lordosis, congenital
  lung (congenital) Q33.9
    acquired J98.4
  lymphatic system, congenital Q89.9
  Madelung's (radius) Q74.0
  mandible (acquired) (congenital) M26.9
  maxilla (acquired) (congenital) M26.9
  meninges or membrane (congenital) Q07.9
    cerebral Q04.8
      acquired G96.19
    spinal cord (congenital) G96.19
      acquired G96.19
  metacarpus (acquired) — *see* Deformity, limb, forearm
    congenital Q74.0
  metatarsus (acquired) — *see* Deformity, foot
    congenital Q66.9- ☑
  middle ear (congenital) Q16.4
    ossicles Q16.3
  mitral (leaflets) (valve) I05.8
    parachute Q23.2
    stenosis, congenital Q23.2
  mouth (acquired) K13.79
    congenital Q38.6
  multiple, congenital NEC Q89.7
  muscle (acquired) M62.89
    congenital Q79.9
      sternocleidomastoid Q68.0
  musculoskeletal system (acquired) M95.9
    congenital Q79.9
    specified NEC M95.8
  nail (acquired) L60.8
    congenital Q84.6
  nasal — *see* Deformity, nose
  neck (acquired) M95.3
    congenital Q18.9
      sternocleidomastoid Q68.0
  nervous system (congenital) Q07.9
  nipple (congenital) Q83.9
    acquired N64.89
  nose (acquired) (cartilage) M95.0
    bone (turbinate) M95.0
    congenital Q30.9
      bent or squashed Q67.4
    saddle M95.0
      syphilitic A50.57
    septum (acquired) J34.2
      congenital Q30.8
    sinus (wall) (congenital) Q30.8
      acquired M95.0
    syphilitic (congenital) A50.57
      late A52.73
  ocular muscle (congenital) Q10.3
    acquired — *see* Strabismus, mechanical
  opticociliary vessels (congenital) Q13.2
  orbit (eye) (acquired) H05.30
    atrophy — *see* Atrophy, orbit
    congenital Q10.7
    due to
      bone disease NEC H05.32- ☑
      trauma or surgery H05.33- ☑
    enlargement — *see* Enlargement, orbit
    exostosis — *see* Exostosis, orbit
  organ of Corti (congenital) Q16.5
  ovary (congenital) Q50.39
    acquired N83.8
  oviduct, acquired N83.8
  palate (congenital) Q38.5

Deformity — *continued*
  palate — *continued*
    acquired M27.8
    cleft (congenital) — *see* Cleft, palate
  pancreas (congenital) Q45.3
    acquired K86.89
  parathyroid (gland) Q89.2
  parotid (gland) (congenital) Q38.4
    acquired K11.8
  patella (acquired) — *see* Disorder, patella, specified NEC
  pelvis, pelvic (acquired) (bony) M95.5
    with disproportion (fetopelvic) O33.0
      causing obstructed labor O65.0
    congenital Q74.2
    rachitic sequelae (late effect) E64.3
  penis (glans) (congenital) Q55.69
    acquired N48.89
  pericardium (congenital) Q24.8
    acquired — *see* Pericarditis
  pharynx (congenital) Q38.8
    acquired J39.2
  pinna, acquired — *see also* Disorder, pinna, deformity
    congenital Q17.9
  pituitary (congenital) Q89.2
  posture — *see* Dorsopathy, deforming
  prepuce (congenital) Q55.69
    acquired N47.8
  prostate (congenital) Q55.4
    acquired N42.89
  pupil (congenital) Q13.2
    acquired — *see* Abnormality, pupillary
  pylorus (congenital) Q40.3
    acquired K31.89
  rachitic (acquired), old or healed E64.3
  radius (acquired) — *see also* Deformity, limb, forearm
    congenital Q68.8
  rectum (congenital) Q43.9
    acquired K62.89
  reduction (extremity) (limb), congenital — *see also* condition and site Q73.8
    brain Q04.3
    lower — *see* Defect, reduction, lower limb
    upper — *see* Defect, reduction, upper limb
  renal — *see* Deformity, kidney
  respiratory system (congenital) Q34.9
  rib (acquired) M95.4
    congenital Q76.6
    cervical Q76.5
  rotation (joint) (acquired) — *see* Deformity, limb, specified site NEC
    congenital Q74.9
    hip — *see* Deformity, limb, specified type NEC, thigh
      congenital Q65.89
  sacroiliac joint (congenital) — *see* subcategory Q74.2
    acquired — *see* subcategory M43.8 ☑
  sacrum (acquired) — *see* subcategory M43.8 ☑
  saddle
    back — *see* Lordosis
    nose M95.0
      syphilitic A50.57
  salivary gland or duct (congenital) Q38.4
    acquired K11.8
  scapula (acquired) M95.8
    congenital Q68.8
  scrotum (congenital) — *see also* Malformation, testis and scrotum
    acquired N50.8
  seminal vesicles (congenital) Q55.4
    acquired N50.89
  septum, nasal (acquired) J34.2
  shoulder (joint) (acquired) — *see* Deformity, limb, upper arm
    congenital Q74.0
    contraction — *see* Contraction, joint, shoulder
  sigmoid (flexure) (congenital) Q43.9
    acquired K63.89
  skin (congenital) Q82.9
  skull (acquired) M95.2
    congenital Q75.8
      with
        anencephaly Q00.0
        encephalocele — *see* Encephalocele
        hydrocephalus Q03.9
          with spina bifida — *see* Spina bifida, by site, with hydrocephalus
        microcephaly Q02

Deformity — *continued*
  soft parts, organs or tissues (of pelvis)
    in pregnancy or childbirth NEC O34.8- ☑
      causing obstructed labor O65.5
  spermatic cord (congenital) Q55.4
    acquired N50.89
    torsion — *see* Torsion, spermatic cord
  spinal — *see* Dorsopathy, deforming
    column (acquired) — *see* Dorsopathy, deforming
    congenital Q67.5
    cord (congenital) Q06.9
      acquired G95.89
    nerve root (congenital) Q07.9
  spine (acquired) — *see also* Dorsopathy, deforming
    congenital Q67.5
    rachitic E64.3
    specified NEC — *see* Dorsopathy, deforming, specified NEC
  spleen
    acquired D73.89
    congenital Q89.09
  Sprengel's (congenital) Q74.0
  sternocleidomastoid (muscle), congenital Q68.0
  sternum (acquired) M95.4
    congenital NEC Q76.7
  stomach (congenital) Q40.3
    acquired K31.89
  submandibular gland (congenital) Q38.4
  submaxillary gland (congenital) Q38.4
    acquired K11.8
  talipes — *see* Talipes
  testis (congenital) — *see also* Malformation, testis and scrotum
    acquired N44.8
    torsion — *see* Torsion, testis
  thigh (acquired) — *see also* Deformity, limb, thigh
    congenital NEC Q68.8
  thorax (acquired) (wall) M95.4
    congenital Q67.8
    sequelae of rickets E64.3
  thumb (acquired) — *see also* Deformity, finger
    congenital NEC Q68.1
  thymus (tissue) (congenital) Q89.2
  thyroid (gland) (congenital) Q89.2
    cartilage Q31.8
      acquired J38.7
  tibia (acquired) — *see also* Deformity, limb, specified type NEC, lower leg
    congenital NEC Q68.8
    saber (syphilitic) A50.56
  toe (acquired) M20.6- ☑
    congenital Q66.9- ☑
    hallux rigidus M20.2- ☑
    hallux valgus M20.1- ☑
    hallux varus M20.3- ☑
    hammer toe M20.4- ☑
    specified NEC M20.5X- ☑
  tongue (congenital) Q38.3
    acquired K14.8
  tooth, teeth K00.2
  trachea (rings) (congenital) Q32.1
    acquired J39.8
  transverse aortic arch (congenital) Q25.49
  tricuspid (leaflets) (valve) I07.8
    atresia or stenosis Q22.4
    Ebstein's Q22.5
  trunk (acquired) M95.8
    congenital Q89.9
  ulna (acquired) — *see also* Deformity, limb, forearm
    congenital NEC Q68.8
  urachus, congenital Q64.4
  ureter (opening) (congenital) Q62.8
    acquired N28.89
  urethra (congenital) Q64.79
    acquired N36.8
  urinary tract (congenital) Q64.9
    urachus Q64.4
  uterus (congenital) Q51.9
    acquired N85.8
  uvula (congenital) Q38.5
  vagina (acquired) N89.8
    congenital Q52.4
  valgus NEC M21.00
    ankle M21.07- ☑
    elbow M21.02- ☑
    hip M21.05- ☑
    knee M21.06- ☑
  valve, valvular (congenital) (heart) Q24.8

Deformity — *continued*
  valve, valvular — *continued*
    acquired — *see* Endocarditis
  varus NEC M21.1Ø
    ankle M21.17- ☑
    elbow M21.12- ☑
    hip M21.15 ☑
    knee M21.16- ☑
    tibia — *see* Osteochondrosis, juvenile, tibia
  vas deferens (congenital) Q55.4
    acquired N5Ø.89
  vein (congenital) Q27.9
    great Q26.9
  vertebra — *see* Dorsopathy, deforming
  vertical talus (congenital) Q66.8Ø
    left foot Q66.82
    right foot Q66.81
  vesicourethral orifice (acquired) N32.89
    congenital NEC Q64.79
  vessels of optic papilla (congenital) Q14.2
  visual field (contraction) — *see* Defect, visual field
  vitreous body, acquired H43.89
  vulva (congenital) Q52.79
    acquired N9Ø.89
  wrist (joint) (acquired) — *see also* Deformity, limb,
      forearm
    congenital Q68.8
    contraction — *see* Contraction, joint, wrist

Degeneration, degenerative
  adrenal (capsule) (fatty) (gland) (hyaline) (infectional)
      E27.8
  amyloid — *see also* Amyloidosis E85.9
  anterior cornua, spinal cord G12.29
  anterior labral S43.49- ☑
  aorta, aortic I7Ø.Ø
    fatty I77.89
  aortic valve (heart) — *see* Endocarditis, aortic
  arteriovascular — *see* Arteriosclerosis
  artery, arterial (atheromatous) (calcareous) — *see also*
      Arteriosclerosis
    cerebral, amyloid E85.4 [I68.Ø]
    medial — *see* Arteriosclerosis, extremities
  articular cartilage NEC — *see* Derangement, joint, artic-
      ular cartilage, by site
  atheromatous — *see* Arteriosclerosis
  basal nuclei or ganglia G23.9
    specified NEC G23.8
  bone NEC — *see* Disorder, bone, specified type NEC
  brachial plexus G54.Ø
  brain (cortical) (progressive) G31.9
    alcoholic G31.2
    arteriosclerotic I67.2
    childhood G31.9
      specified NEC G31.89
    cystic G31.89
      congenital QØ4.6
    in
      alcoholism G31.2
      beriberi E51.2
      cerebrovascular disease I67.9
      congenital hydrocephalus QØ3.9
        with spina bifida — *see also* Spina bifida
      Fabry-Anderson disease E75.21
      Gaucher's disease E75.22
      Hunter's syndrome E76.1
      lipidosis
        cerebral E75.4
        generalized E75.6
      mucopolysaccharidosis — *see* Mucopolysaccha-
          ridosis
      myxedema EØ3.9 [G32.89]
      neoplastic disease — *see also* Neoplasm
          D49.6 [G32.89]
      Niemann-Pick disease E75.249 [G32.89]
      sphingolipidosis E75.3 [G32.89]
      vitamin B12 deficiency E53.8 [G32.89]
    senile NEC G31.1
  breast N64.89
  Bruch's membrane — *see* Degeneration, choroid
  capillaries (fatty) I78.8
    amyloid E85.89 [I79.8]
  cardiac — *see also* Degeneration, myocardial
    valve, valvular — *see* Endocarditis
  cardiorenal — *see* Hypertension, cardiorenal
  cardiovascular — *see also* Disease, cardiovascular
    renal — *see* Hypertension, cardiorenal
  cerebellar NOS G31.9
    alcoholic G31.2

Degeneration, degenerative — *continued*
  cerebellar — *continued*
    primary (hereditary) (sporadic) G11.9
  cerebral — *see* Degeneration, brain
  cerebrovascular I67.9
    due to hypertension I67.4
  cervical plexus G54.2
  cervix N88.8
    due to radiation (intended effect) N88.8
      adverse effect or misadventure N99.89
  chamber angle H21.21- ☑
  changes, spine or vertebra — *see* Spondylosis
  chorioretinal — *see also* Degeneration, choroid
    hereditary H31.2Ø
  choroid (colloid) (drusen) H31.1Ø- ☑
    atrophy — *see* Atrophy, choroidal
    hereditary — *see* Dystrophy, choroidal, hereditary
  ciliary body H21.22- ☑
  cochlear — *see* subcategory H83.8 ☑
  combined (spinal cord) (subacute) E53.8 [G32.Ø]
    with anemia (pernicious) D51.Ø [G32.Ø]
      due to dietary vitamin B12 deficiency
          D51.3 [G32.Ø]
    in (due to)
      vitamin B12 deficiency E53.8 [G32.Ø]
        anemia D51.9 [G32.Ø]
  conjunctiva H11.1Ø
    concretions — *see* Concretion, conjunctiva
    deposits — *see* Deposit, conjunctiva
    pigmentations — *see* Pigmentation, conjunctiva
    pinguecula — *see* Pinguecula
    xerosis — *see* Xerosis, conjunctiva
  cornea H18.4Ø
    calcerous H18.43
      band keratopathy H18.42- ☑
    familial, hereditary — *see* Dystrophy, cornea
    hyaline (of old scars) H18.49
    keratomalacia — *see* Keratomalacia
    nodular H18.45- ☑
    peripheral H18.46- ☑
    senile H18.41- ☑
    specified type NEC H18.49
  cortical (cerebellar) (parenchymatous) G31.89
    alcoholic G31.2
    diffuse, due to arteriopathy I67.2
  corticobasal G31.85
  cutis L98.8
    amyloid E85.4 [L99]
  dental pulp KØ4.2
  disc disease — *see* Degeneration, intervertebral disc
      NEC
  dorsolateral (spinal cord) — *see* Degeneration, com-
      bined
  extrapyramidal G25.9
  eye, macular — *see also* Degeneration, macula
    congenital or hereditary — *see* Dystrophy, retina
  facet joints — *see* Spondylosis
  fatty
    liver NEC K76.Ø
      alcoholic K7Ø.Ø
  grey matter (brain) (Alpers') G31.81
  heart — *see also* Degeneration, myocardial
    amyloid E85.4 [I43]
    atheromatous — *see* Disease, heart, ischemic,
        atherosclerotic
    ischemic — *see* Disease, heart, ischemic
  hepatolenticular (Wilson's) E83.Ø1
  hepatorenal K76.7
  hyaline (diffuse) (generalized)
    localized — *see* Degeneration, by site
  infrapatellar fat pad M79.4
  intervertebral disc NOS
    with
      myelopathy — *see* Disorder, disc, with,
          myelopathy
      radiculitis or radiculopathy — *see* Disorder, disc,
          with, radiculopathy
    cervical, cervicothoracic — *see* Disorder, disc, cervi-
        cal, degeneration
      with
        myelopathy — *see* Disorder, disc, cervical,
            with myelopathy
        neuritis, radiculitis or radiculopathy — *see*
            Disorder, disc, cervical, with neuritis
    lumbar region M51.36
      with
        myelopathy M51.Ø6

Degeneration, degenerative — *continued*
  intervertebral disc — *continued*
    lumbar region — *continued*
      with — *continued*
        neuritis, radiculitis, radiculopathy or sciatica
            M51.16
    lumbosacral region M51.37
      with
        neuritis, radiculitis, radiculopathy or sciatica
            M51.17
    sacrococcygeal region M53.3
    thoracic region M51.34
      with
        myelopathy M51.Ø4
        neuritis, radiculitis, radiculopathy M51.14
    thoracolumbar region M51.35
      with
        myelopathy M51.Ø5
        neuritis, radiculitis, radiculopathy M51.15
  intestine, amyloid E85.4
  iris (pigmentary) H21.23- ☑
  ischemic — *see* Ischemia
  joint disease — *see* Osteoarthritis
  kidney N28.89
    amyloid E85.4 [N29]
    cystic, congenital Q61.9
    fatty N28.89
    polycystic Q61.3
      adult type (autosomal dominant) Q61.2
      infantile type (autosomal recessive) NEC Q61.19
        collecting duct dilatation Q61.11
  Kuhnt-Junius — *see also* Degeneration, macula
      H35.32- ☑
  lens — *see* Cataract
  lenticular (familial) (progressive) (Wilson's) (with cirrho-
      sis of liver) E83.Ø1
  liver (diffuse) NEC K76.89
    amyloid E85.4 [K77]
    cystic K76.89
      congenital Q44.6
    fatty NEC K76.Ø
      alcoholic K7Ø.Ø
    hypertrophic K76.89
    parenchymatous, acute or subacute K72.ØØ
      with coma K72.Ø1
    pigmentary K76.89
    toxic (acute) K71.9
  lung J98.4
  lymph gland I89.8
    hyaline I89.8
  macula, macular (acquired) (age-related) (senile)
      H35.3Ø
    angioid streaks H35.33
    atrophic age-related H35.31- ☑
    congenital or hereditary — *see* Dystrophy, retina
    cystoid H35.35- ☑
    drusen H35.36- ☑
    dry age-related H35.31- ☑
    exudative H35.32- ☑
    hole H35.34- ☑
    nonexudative H35.31- ☑
    puckering H35.37- ☑
    toxic H35.38- ☑
    wet age-related H35.32- ☑
  membranous labyrinth, congenital (causing impair-
      ment of hearing) Q16.5
  meniscus — *see* Derangement, meniscus
  mitral — *see* Insufficiency, mitral
  Mönckeberg's — *see* Arteriosclerosis, extremities
  motor centers, senile G31.1
  multi-system G90.3
  mural — *see* Degeneration, myocardial
  muscle (fatty) (fibrous) (hyaline) (progressive) M62.89
    heart — *see* Degeneration, myocardial
  myelin, central nervous system G37.9
  myocardial, myocardium (fatty) (hyaline) (senile) I51.5
    with rheumatic fever (conditions in IØØ) IØ9.Ø
      active, acute or subacute IØ1.2
        with chorea IØ2.Ø
      inactive or quiescent (with chorea) IØ9.Ø
    hypertensive — *see* Hypertension, heart
    rheumatic — *see* Degeneration, myocardial, with
        rheumatic fever
    syphilitic A52.Ø6
  nasal sinus (mucosa) J32.9
    frontal J32.1
    maxillary J32.Ø
  nerve — *see* Disorder, nerve

Degeneration, degenerative — continued
nervous system G31.9
  alcoholic G31.2
  amyloid E85.4 *[G99.8]*
  autonomic G90.9
  fatty G31.89
  specified NEC G31.89
nipple N64.89
olivopontocerebellar (hereditary) (familial) G23.8
osseous labyrinth — *see* subcategory H83.8 ☑
ovary N83.8
  cystic N83.20- ☑
  microcystic N83.20- ☑
pallidal pigmentary (progressive) G23.0
pancreas K86.89
  tuberculous A18.83
penis N48.89
pigmentary (diffuse) (general)
  localized — *see* Degeneration, by site
  pallidal (progressive) G23.0
pineal gland E34.8
pituitary (gland) E23.6
popliteal fat pad M79.4
posterolateral (spinal cord) — *see* Degeneration, combined
pulmonary valve (heart) I37.8
pulp (tooth) K04.2
pupillary margin H21.24- ☑
renal — *see* Degeneration, kidney
retina H35.9
  hereditary (cerebroretinal) (congenital) (juvenile) (macula) (peripheral) (pigmentary) — *see* Dystrophy, retina
  Kuhnt-Junius — *see also* Degeneration, macula H35.32- ☑
  macula (cystic) (exudative) (hole) (nonexudative) (pseudohole) (senile) (toxic) — *see* Degeneration, macula
  peripheral H35.40
    lattice H35.41- ☑
    microcystoid H35.42- ☑
    paving stone H35.43- ☑
    secondary
      pigmentary H35.45- ☑
      vitreoretinal H35.46- ☑
    senile reticular H35.44- ☑
  pigmentary (primary) — *see also* Dystrophy, retina
    secondary — *see* Degeneration, retina, peripheral, secondary
  posterior pole — *see* Degeneration, macula
saccule, congenital (causing impairment of hearing) Q16.5
senile R54
  brain G31.1
  cardiac, heart or myocardium — *see* Degeneration, myocardial
  motor centers G31.1
  vascular — *see* Arteriosclerosis
sinus (cystic) — *see also* Sinusitis
  polypoid J33.1
skin L98.8
  amyloid E85.4 *[L99]*
  colloid L98.8
spinal (cord) G31.89
  amyloid E85.4 *[G32.89]*
  combined (subacute) — *see* Degeneration, combined
  dorsolateral — *see* Degeneration, combined
  familial NEC G31.89
  fatty G31.89
  funicular — *see* Degeneration, combined
  posterolateral — *see* Degeneration, combined
  subacute combined — *see* Degeneration, combined
  tuberculous A17.81
spleen D73.0
  amyloid E85.4 *[D77]*
stomach K31.89
striatonigral G23.2
suprarenal (capsule) (gland) E27.8
synovial membrane (pulpy) — *see* Disorder, synovium, specified type NEC
tapetoretinal — *see* Dystrophy, retina
thymus (gland) E32.8
  fatty E32.8
thyroid (gland) E07.89
tricuspid (heart) (valve) I07.9
tuberculous NEC — *see* Tuberculosis
turbinate J34.89

Degeneration, degenerative — continued
uterus (cystic) N85.8
vascular (senile) — *see* Arteriosclerosis
  hypertensive — *see* Hypertension
vitreoretinal, secondary — *see* Degeneration, retina, peripheral, secondary, vitreoretinal
vitreous (body) H43.81- ☑
Wallerian — *see* Disorder, nerve
Wilson's hepatolenticular E83.01
Deglutition
paralysis R13.0
  hysterical F44.4
pneumonia J69.0
Degos' disease I77.89
Dehiscence (of)
amputation stump T87.81
cesarean wound O90.0
closure of
  cornea T81.31 ☑
  craniotomy T81.32 ☑
  fascia (muscular) (superficial) T81.32 ☑
  internal organ or tissue T81.32 ☑
  laceration (external) (internal) T81.33 ☑
  ligament T81.32 ☑
  mucosa T81.31 ☑
  muscle or muscle flap T81.32 ☑
  ribs or rib cage T81.32 ☑
  skin and subcutaneous tissue (full-thickness) (superficial) T81.31 ☑
  skull T81.32 ☑
  sternum (sternotomy) T81.32 ☑
  tendon T81.32 ☑
  traumatic laceration (external) (internal) T81.33 ☑
episiotomy O90.1
operation wound NEC T81.31 ☑
  external operation wound (superficial) T81.31 ☑
  internal operation wound (deep) T81.32 ☑
perineal wound (postpartum) O90.1
traumatic injury wound repair T81.33 ☑
wound T81.30 ☑
  traumatic repair T81.33 ☑
Dehydration E86.0
newborn P74.1
Déjérine-Roussy syndrome G89.0
Déjérine-Sottas disease or neuropathy (hypertrophic) G60.0
Déjérine-Thomas atrophy G23.8
Delay, delayed
any plane in pelvis
  complicating delivery O66.9
birth or delivery NOS O63.9
closure, ductus arteriosus (Botalli) P29.38
coagulation — *see* Defect, coagulation
conduction (cardiac) (ventricular) I45.9
delivery, second twin, triplet, etc O63.2
development R62.50
  global F88
  intellectual (specific) F81.9
  language F80.9
    due to hearing loss F80.4
  learning F81.9
  pervasive F84.9
  physiological R62.50
    specified stage NEC R62.0
  reading F81.0
  sexual E30.0
  speech F80.9
    due to hearing loss F80.4
  spelling F81.81
ejaculation F52.32
gastric emptying K30
menarche E30.0
menstruation (cause unknown) N91.0
milestone R62.0
passage of meconium (newborn) P76.0
primary respiration P28.9
puberty (constitutional) E30.0
separation of umbilical cord P96.82
sexual maturation, female E30.0
sleep phase syndrome G47.21
union, fracture — *see* Fracture, by site
vaccination Z28.9
Deletion(s)
autosome Q93.9
  identified by fluorescence in situ hybridization (FISH) Q93.89
  identified by in situ hybridization (ISH) Q93.89

Deletion(s) — continued
chromosome
  with complex rearrangements NEC Q93.7
  part of NEC Q93.59
  seen only at prometaphase Q93.89
  short arm
    22q11.2 Q93.81
    4 Q93.3
    5p Q93.4
  specified NEC Q93.89
  long arm chromosome 18 or 21 Q93.89
    with complex rearrangements NEC Q93.7
  microdeletions NEC Q93.88
Delhi boil or button B55.1
Delinquency (juvenile) (neurotic) F91.8
group Z72.810
Delinquent immunization status Z28.3
Delirium, delirious (acute or subacute) (not alcohol- or drug-induced) (with dementia) R41.0
alcoholic (acute) (tremens) (withdrawal) F10.921
  with intoxication F10.921
    in
      abuse F10.121
      dependence F10.221
due to (secondary to)
  alcohol
    intoxication F10.921
      in
        abuse F10.121
        dependence F10.221
    withdrawal F10.231
  amphetamine intoxication F15.921
    in
      abuse F15.121
      dependence F15.221
  anxiolytic
    intoxication F13.921
      in
        abuse F13.121
        dependence F13.221
    withdrawal F13.231
  cannabis intoxication (acute) F12.921
    in
      abuse F12.121
      dependence F12.221
  cocaine intoxication (acute) F14.921
    in
      abuse F14.121
      dependence F14.221
  general medical condition F05
  hallucinogen intoxication F16.921
    in
      abuse F16.121
      dependence F16.221
  hypnotic
    intoxication F13.921
      in
        abuse F13.121
        dependence F13.221
    withdrawal F13.231
  inhalant intoxication (acute) F18.921
    in
      abuse F18.121
      dependence F18.221
  multiple etiologies F05
  opioid intoxication (acute) F11.921
    in
      abuse F11.121
      dependence F11.221
  other (or unknown) substance F19.921
  phencyclidine intoxication (acute) F16.921
    in
      abuse F16.121
      dependence F16.221
  psychoactive substance NEC intoxication (acute) F19.921
    in
      abuse F19.121
      dependence F19.221
  sedative
    intoxication F13.921
      in
        abuse F13.121
        dependence F13.221
    withdrawal F13.231
  unknown etiology R41.0
exhaustion F43.0
hysterical F44.89
postprocedural (postoperative) F05

(handwritten annotations: "resulting from physiological condition F05", "code condition first")

Delirium, delirious — *continued*
puerperal F05
thyroid — *see* Thyrotoxicosis with thyroid storm
traumatic — *see* Injury, intracranial
tremens (alcohol-induced) F10.231
sedative-induced F13.231
Delivery (childbirth) (labor)
arrested active phase O62.1
cesarean (for)
abnormal
pelvis (bony) (deformity) (major) NEC with disproportion (fetopelvic) O33.0
with obstructed labor O65.0
presentation or position O32.9 ☑
abruptio placentae — *see also* Abruptio placentae
O45.9- ☑
acromion presentation O32.2 ☑
atony, uterus O62.2
breech presentation O32.1 ☑
incomplete O32.8 ☑
brow presentation O32.3 ☑
cephalopelvic disproportion O33.9
cerclage O34.3- ☑
chin presentation O32.3 ☑
cicatrix of cervix O34.4- ☑
contracted pelvis (general)
inlet O33.2
outlet O33.3 ☑
cord presentation or prolapse O69.0 ☑
cystocele O34.8- ☑
deformity (acquired) (congenital)
pelvic organs or tissues NEC O34.8- ☑
pelvis (bony) NEC O33.0
disproportion NOS O33.9
eclampsia — *see* Eclampsia
face presentation O32.3 ☑
failed
forceps O66.5
induction of labor O61.9
instrumental O61.1
mechanical O61.1
medical O61.0
specified NEC O61.8
surgical O61.1
trial of labor NOS O66.40
following previous cesarean delivery O66.41
vacuum extraction O66.5
ventouse O66.5
fetal-maternal hemorrhage O43.01- ☑
hemorrhage (intrapartum) O67.9
with coagulation defect O67.0
specified cause NEC O67.8
high head at term O32.4 ☑
hydrocephalic fetus O33.6 ☑
incarceration of uterus O34.51- ☑
incoordinate uterine action O62.4
increased size, fetus O33.5 ☑
inertia, uterus O62.2
primary O62.0
secondary O62.1
lateroversion, uterus O34.59- ☑
mal lie O32.9 ☑
malposition
fetus O32.9 ☑
pelvic organs or tissues NEC O34.8- ☑
uterus NEC O34.59- ☑
malpresentation NOS O32.9 ☑
oblique presentation O32.2 ☑
occurring after 37 completed weeks of gestation
but before 39 completed weeks gestation due
to (spontaneous) onset of labor O75.82
oversize fetus O33.5 ☑
pelvic tumor NEC O34.8- ☑
placenta previa O44.0- ☑
complete O44.0- ☑
with hemorrhage O44.1- ☑
placental insufficiency O36.51- ☑
planned, occurring after 37 completed weeks of
gestation but before 39 completed weeks
gestation due to (spontaneous) onset of labor
O75.82
polyp, cervix O34.4- ☑
causing obstructed labor O65.5
poor dilatation, cervix O62.0
pre-eclampsia O14.94
mild O14.04
moderate O14.04

Delivery — *continued*
cesarean — *continued*
pre-eclampsia — *continued*
severe O14.14
with hemolysis, elevated liver enzymes and
low platelet count (HELLP) O14.24
previous
cesarean delivery O34.219
classical (vertical) scar O34.212
low transverse scar O34.211
surgery (to)
cervix O34.4- ☑
gynecological NEC O34.8- ☑
rectum O34.7- ☑
uterus O34.29
vagina O34.6- ☑
prolapse
arm or hand O32.2 ☑
uterus O34.52- ☑
prolonged labor NOS O63.9
rectocele O34.8- ☑
retroversion
uterus O34.53- ☑
rigid
cervix O34.4- ☑
pelvic floor O34.8- ☑
perineum O34.7- ☑
vagina O34.6- ☑
vulva O34.7- ☑
sacculation, pregnant uterus O34.59- ☑
scar(s)
cervix O34.4- ☑
cesarean delivery O34.219
classical (vertical) O34.212
low transverse O34.211
transmural uterine O34.29
uterus O34.29
Shirodkar suture in situ O34.3- ☑
shoulder presentation O32.2 ☑
stenosis or stricture, cervix O34.4- ☑
streptococcus group B (GBS) carrier state O99.824
transmural uterine scar O34.29
transverse presentation or lie O32.2 ☑
tumor, pelvic organs or tissues NEC O34.8- ☑
cervix O34.4- ☑
umbilical cord presentation or prolapse O69.0 ☑
without indication O82
completely normal case O80
complicated O75.9
by
abnormal, abnormality (of)
forces of labor O62.9
specified type NEC O62.8
glucose O99.814
uterine contractions NOS O62.9
abruptio placentae — *see also* Abruptio placentae O45.9- ☑
abuse
physical O9A.32 (*following* O99)
psychological O9A.52 (*following* O99)
sexual O9A.42 (*following* O99)
adherent placenta O72.0
without hemorrhage O73.0
alcohol use O99.314
anemia (pre-existing) O99.02
anesthetic death O74.8
annular detachment of cervix O71.3
atony, uterus O62.2
attempted vacuum extraction and forceps O66.5
Bandl's ring O62.4
bariatric surgery status O99.844
biliary tract disorder O26.62
bleeding — *see* Delivery, complicated by, hemorrhage
blood disorder NEC O99.12
cervical dystocia (hypotonic) O62.2
primary O62.0
secondary O62.1
circulatory system disorder O99.42
compression of cord (umbilical) NEC O69.2 ☑
condition NEC O99.89
contraction, contracted ring O62.4
cord (umbilical)
around neck
with compression O69.1 ☑
without compression O69.81 ☑
bruising O69.5 ☑
complication O69.9 ☑

Delivery — *continued*
complicated — *continued*
by — *continued*
cord — *continued*
complication — *continued*
specified NEC O69.89 ☑
compression NEC O69.2 ☑
entanglement O69.2 ☑
without compression O69.82 ☑
hematoma O69.5 ☑
presentation O69.0 ☑
prolapse O69.0 ☑
short O69.3 ☑
thrombosis (vessels) O69.5 ☑
vascular lesion O69.5 ☑
Couvelaire uterus O45.8X- ☑
damage to (injury to) NEC
perineum O71.82
periurethral tissue O71.82
vulva O71.82
delay following rupture of membranes (spontaneous) — *see* Pregnancy, complicated by,
premature rupture of membranes
depressed fetal heart tones O76
diabetes O24.92
gestational O24.429
diet controlled O24.420
insulin controlled O24.424
oral drug controlled (antidiabetic) (hypoglycemic) O24.425
pre-existing O24.32
specified NEC O24.82
type 1 O24.02
type 2 O24.12
diastasis recti (abdominis) O71.89
dilatation
bladder O66.8
cervix incomplete, poor or slow O62.0
disease NEC O99.89
disruptio uteri — *see* Delivery, complicated by,
rupture, uterus
drug use O99.324
dysfunction, uterus NOS O62.9
hypertonic O62.4
hypotonic O62.2
primary O62.0
secondary O62.1
incoordinate O62.4
eclampsia O15.1
embolism (pulmonary) — *see* Embolism, obstetric
endocrine, nutritional or metabolic disease NEC
O99.284
failed
attempted vaginal birth after previous cesarean delivery O66.41
induction of labor O61.9
instrumental O61.1
mechanical O61.1
medical O61.0
specified NEC O61.8
surgical O61.1
trial of labor O66.40
female genital mutilation O65.5
fetal
abnormal acid-base balance O68
acidemia O68
acidosis O68
alkalosis O68
death, early O02.1
deformity O66.3
heart rate or rhythm (abnormal) (non-reassuring) O76
hypoxia O77.8
stress O77.9
due to drug administration O77.1
electrocardiographic evidence of O77.8
specified NEC O77.8
ultrasound evidence of O77.8
fever during labor O75.2
gastric banding status O99.844
gastric bypass status O99.844
gastrointestinal disease NEC O99.62
gestational
diabetes O24.429
diet controlled O24.420
insulin (and diet) controlled O24.424

Delivery — *continued*
  complicated — *continued*
    by — *continued*
      gestational — *continued*
        diabetes — *continued*
          oral drug controlled (antidiabetic) (hypo-glycemic) O24.425
        edema O12.04
          with proteinuria O12.24
        proteinuria O12.14
      gonorrhea O98.22
      hematoma O71.7
        ischial spine O71.7
        pelvic O71.7
        vagina O71.7
        vulva or perineum O71.7
      hemorrhage (uterine) O67.9
        associated with
          afibrinogenemia O67.0
          coagulation defect O67.0
          hyperfibrinolysis O67.0
          hypofibrinogenemia O67.0
        due to
          low implantation of placenta O44.5- ☑
          low-lying placenta O44.5- ☑
          placenta previa O44.1- ☑
            marginal O44.3- ☑
            partial O44.3- ☑
          premature separation of placenta (normal-ly implanted) — *see also* Abruptio placentae O45.9- ☑
          retained placenta O72.0
          uterine leiomyoma O67.8
        placenta NEC O67.8
        postpartum NEC (atonic) (immediate) O72.1
          with retained or trapped placenta O72.0
          delayed O72.2
          secondary O72.2
          third stage O72.0
      hourglass contraction, uterus O62.4
      hypertension, hypertensive (pre-existing) — *see* Hypertension, complicated by, childbirth (labor)
      hypotension O26.5- ☑
      incomplete dilatation (cervix) O62.0
      incoordinate uterus contractions O62.4
      inertia, uterus O62.2
        during latent phase of labor O62.0
        primary O62.0
        secondary O62.1
      infection (maternal) O98.92
        carrier state NEC O99.834
        gonorrhea O98.22
        human immunodeficiency virus (HIV) O98.72
        sexually transmitted NEC O98.32
        specified NEC O98.82
        syphilis O98.12
        tuberculosis O98.02
        viral hepatitis O98.42
        viral NEC O98.52
      injury (to mother) — *see also* Delivery, complicat-ed, by, damage to O71.9
        nonobstetric O9A.22 (*following* O99)
          caused by abuse — *see* Delivery, compli-cated by, abuse
      intrauterine fetal death, early O02.1
      inversion, uterus O71.2
      laceration (perineal) O70.9
        anus (sphincter) O70.4
          with third degree laceration — *see also* Delivery, complicated, by, lacera-tion, perineum, third degree O70.20
            with mucosa O70.3
          without third degree laceration O70.2 ☑
        bladder (urinary) O71.5
        bowel O71.5
        cervix (uteri) O71.3
        fourchette O70.0
        hymen O70.0
        labia O70.0
        pelvic
          floor O70.1
          organ NEC O71.5
        perineum, perineal O70.9
          first degree O70.0
          fourth degree O70.3
          muscles O70.1

Delivery — *continued*
  complicated — *continued*
    by — *continued*
      laceration — *continued*
        perineum, perineal — *continued*
          second degree O70.1
          skin O70.0
          slight O70.0
          third degree O70.20
            with
              both external anal sphincter (EAS) and internal anal sphincter (IAS) torn (IIIc) O70.23
              less than 50% of external anal sphincter (EAS) thickness torn (IIIa) O70.21
              more than 50% external anal sphincter (EAS) thickness torn (IIIb) O70.22
            IIIa O70.21
            IIIb O70.22
            IIIc O70.23
        peritoneum (pelvic) O71.5
        rectovaginal (septum) (without perineal lacer-ation) O71.4
          with perineum — *see also* Delivery, complicated, by, laceration, per-ineum, third degree O70.20
            with anal or rectal mucosa O70.3
        specified NEC O71.89
        sphincter ani — *see* Delivery, complicated, by, laceration, anus (sphincter)
        urethra O71.5
        uterus O71.81
          before labor O71.81
        vagina, vaginal (deep) (high) (without per-ineal laceration) O71.4
          with perineum O70.0
          muscles, with perineum O70.1
        vulva O70.0
      liver disorder O26.62
      malignancy O9A.12 (*following* O99)
      malnutrition O25.2
      malposition, malpresentation
        uterus or cervix O65.5
        placenta O44.0- ☑
          with hemorrhage O44.1- ☑
        without obstruction — *see also* Delivery, complicated, by, obstruction O32.9 ☑
          breech O32.1 ☑
          compound O32.6 ☑
          face (brow) (chin) O32.3 ☑
          footling O32.8 ☑
          high head O32.4 ☑
          oblique O32.2 ☑
          specified NEC O32.8 ☑
          transverse O32.2 ☑
          unstable lie O32.0 ☑
      meconium in amniotic fluid O77.0
      mental disorder NEC O99.344
      metrorrhexis — *see* Delivery, complicated by, rupture, uterus
      nervous system disorder O99.354
      obesity (pre-existing) O99.214
      obesity surgery status O99.844
      obstetric trauma O71.9
        specified NEC O71.89
      obstructed labor
        due to
          breech (complete) (frank) presentation O64.1 ☑
            incomplete O64.8 ☑
          brow presentation O64.3 ☑
          buttock presentation O64.1 ☑
          chin presentation O64.2 ☑
          compound presentation O64.5 ☑
          contracted pelvis O65.1
          deep transverse arrest O64.0 ☑
          deformed pelvis O65.0
          dystocia (fetal) O66.9
            due to
              conjoined twins O66.3
              fetal
                abnormality NEC O66.3
                ascites O66.3
                hydrops O66.3
                meningomyelocele O66.3
                sacral teratoma O66.3

Delivery — *continued*
  complicated — *continued*
    by — *continued*
      obstructed labor — *continued*
        due to — *continued*
          dystocia — *continued*
            due to — *continued*
              fetal — *continued*
                tumor O66.3
              hydrocephalic fetus O66.3
              shoulder O66.0
          face presentation O64.2 ☑
          fetopelvic disproportion O65.4
          footling presentation O64.8 ☑
          impacted shoulders O66.0
          incomplete rotation of fetal head O64.0 ☑
          large fetus O66.2
          locked twins O66.1
          malposition O64.9 ☑
            specified NEC O64.8 ☑
          malpresentation O64.9 ☑
            specified NEC O64.8 ☑
          multiple fetuses NEC O66.6
          pelvic
            abnormality (maternal) O65.9
              organ O65.5
              specified NEC O65.8
            contraction
              inlet O65.2
              mid-cavity O65.3
              outlet O65.3
          persistent (position)
            occipitoiliac O64.0 ☑
            occipitoposterior O64.0 ☑
            occipitosacral O64.0 ☑
            occipitotransverse O64.0 ☑
          prolapsed arm O64.4 ☑
          shoulder presentation O64.4 ☑
          specified NEC O66.8
      pathological retraction ring, uterus O62.4
      penetration, pregnant uterus by instrument O71.1
      perforation — *see* Delivery, complicated by, lac-eration
      placenta, placental
        ablatio — *see also* Abruptio placentae O45.9- ☑
        abnormality O43.9- ☑
          specified NEC O43.89- ☑
        abruptio — *see also* Abruptio placentae O45.9- ☑
        accreta O43.21- ☑
        adherent (with hemorrhage) O72.0
          without hemorrhage O73.0
        detachment (premature) — *see also* Abruptio placentae O45.9- ☑
        disorder O43.9- ☑
          specified NEC O43.89- ☑
        hemorrhage NEC O67.8
        increta O43.22- ☑
        low (implantation) (lying) O44.4- ☑
          with hemorrhage O44.5- ☑
        malformation O43.10- ☑
        malposition O44.0- ☑
          without hemorrhage O44.1- ☑
        percreta O43.23- ☑
        previa (central) (complete) (lateral) (total) O44.0- ☑
          with hemorrhage O44.1- ☑
          marginal O44.2- ☑
            with hemorrhage O44.3- ☑
          partial O44.2- ☑
            with hemorrhage O44.3- ☑
        retained (with hemorrhage) O72.0
          without hemorrhage O73.0
        separation (premature) O45.9- ☑
          specified NEC O45.8X- ☑
        vicious insertion O44.1- ☑
      precipitate labor O62.3
      premature rupture, membranes — *see also* Pregnancy, complicated by, premature rupture of membranes O42.90
      prolapse
        arm or hand O32.2 ☑
        cord (umbilical) O69.0 ☑
        foot or leg O32.8 ☑

⚇ Subterms under main terms may continue to next column or page   ☑ Additional Character Required — Refer to the Tabular List for Character Selection   91

Delivery — Delivery

Delivery — *continued*
  complicated — *continued*
    by — *continued*
      prolapse — *continued*
        uterus O34.52- ☑
      prolonged labor O63.9
        first stage O63.0
        second stage O63.1
      protozoal disease (maternal) O98.62
      respiratory disease NEC O99.52
      retained membranes or portions of placenta O72.2
        without hemorrhage O73.1
      retarded birth O63.9
      retention of secundines (with hemorrhage) O72.0
        without hemorrhage O73.0
        partial O72.2
          without hemorrhage O73.1
      rupture
        bladder (urinary) O71.5
        cervix O71.3
        pelvic organ NEC O71.5
        urethra O71.5
        uterus (during or after labor) O71.1
          before labor O71.0- ☑
      separation, pubic bone (symphysis pubis) O71.6
      shock O75.1
      shoulder presentation O64.4 ☑
      skin disorder NEC O99.72
      spasm, cervix O62.4
      stenosis or stricture, cervix O65.5
      streptococcus group B (GBS) carrier state O99.824
      subluxation of symphysis (pubis) O26.72
      syphilis (maternal) O98.12
      tear — *see* Delivery, complicated by, laceration
      tetanic uterus O62.4
      trauma (obstetrical) — *see also* Delivery, complicated, by, damage to O71.9
        non-obstetric O9A.22 (*following* O99)
        periurethral O71.82
        specified NEC O71.89
      tuberculosis (maternal) O98.02
      tumor, pelvic organs or tissues NEC O65.5
      umbilical cord around neck
        with compression O69.1 ☑
        without compression O69.81 ☑
      uterine inertia O62.2
        during latent phase of labor O62.0
        primary O62.0
        secondary O62.1
      vasa previa O69.4 ☑
      velamentous insertion of cord O43.12- ☑
    specified complication NEC O75.89
  delayed NOS O63.9
    following rupture of membranes
      artificial O75.5
    second twin, triplet, etc. O63.2
  forceps, low following failed vacuum extraction O66.5
  missed (at or near term) O36.4 ☑
  normal O80
  obstructed — *see* Delivery, complicated by, obstructed labor
  precipitate O62.3
  preterm — *see also* Pregnancy, complicated by, preterm labor O60.10 ☑
  spontaneous O80
  term pregnancy NOS O80
  uncomplicated O80
  vaginal, following previous cesarean delivery O34.219
    classical (vertical) scar O34.212
    low transverse scar O34.211
Delusions (paranoid) — *see* Disorder, delusional
Dementia (degenerative (primary)) (old age) (persisting) F03.90
  with
    aggressive behavior F03.91
    behavioral disturbance F03.91
    combative behavior F03.91
    Lewy bodies G31.83 *[F02.80]*
      with behavioral disturbance G31.83 *[F02.81]*
    Parkinsonism G31.83 *[F02.80]*
      with behavioral disturbance G31.83 *[F02.81]*
    Parkinson's disease G20 *[F02.80]*
      with behavioral disturbance G20 *[F02.81]*
    violent behavior F03.91
  alcoholic F10.97
    with dependence F10.27
  Alzheimer's type — *see* Disease, Alzheimer's

Dementia — *continued*
  arteriosclerotic — *see* Dementia, vascular
  atypical, Alzheimer's type — *see* Disease, Alzheimer's, specified NEC
  congenital — *see* Disability, intellectual
  frontal (lobe) G31.09 *[F02.80]*
    with behavioral disturbance G31.09 *[F02.81]*
  frontotemporal G31.09 *[F02.80]*
    with behavioral disturbance G31.09 *[F02.81]*
    specified NEC G31.09 *[F02.80]*
      with behavioral disturbance G31.09 *[F02.81]*
  Huntington's disease or chorea G10
    with dementia G10 *[F02.80]*
  in (due to)
    with behavioral disturbance G31.83 *[F02.81]*
    alcohol F10.97
      with dependence F10.27
    Alzheimer's disease — *see* Disease, Alzheimer's
    arteriosclerotic brain disease — *see* Dementia, vascular
    cerebral lipidoses E75.- *[F02.80]*
      with behavioral disturbance E75.- ☑ *[F02.81]*
    Creutzfeldt-Jakob disease — *see also* Creutzfeldt-Jakob disease or syndrome (with dementia) A81.00
    epilepsy G40.- ☑ *[F02.80]*
      with behavioral disturbance G40.- ☑ *[F02.81]*
    hepatolenticular degeneration E83.01 *[F02.80]*
      with behavioral disturbance E83.01 *[F02.81]*
    human immunodeficiency virus (HIV) disease B20 *[F02.80]*
      with behavioral disturbance B20 *[F02.81]*
    Huntington's disease or chorea G10 *[F02.80]*
      with behavioral disturbance G10 *[F02.81]*
    hypercalcemia E83.52 *[F02.80]*
      with behavioral disturbance E83.52 *[F02.81]*
    hypothyroidism, acquired E03.9 *[F02.80]*
      with behavioral disturbance E03.9 *[F02.81]*
      due to iodine deficiency E01.8 *[F02.80]*
        with behavioral disturbance E01.8 *[F02.81]*
    inhalants F18.97
      with dependence F18.27
    multiple
      etiologies F03 ☑
      sclerosis G35 *[F02.80]*
        with behavioral disturbance G35 *[F02.81]*
    neurosyphilis A52.17 *[F02.80]*
      with behavioral disturbance A52.17 *[F02.81]*
      juvenile A50.49 *[F02.80]*
        with behavioral disturbance A50.49 *[F02.81]*
    niacin deficiency E52 *[F02.80]*
      with behavioral disturbance E52 *[F02.81]*
    paralysis agitans G20 *[F02.80]*
      with behavioral disturbance G20 *[F02.81]*
    Parkinson's disease G20 *[F02.80]*
    pellagra E52 *[F02.80]*
      with behavioral disturbance E52 *[F02.81]*
    Pick's G31.01 *[F02.80]*
      with behavioral disturbance G31.01 *[F02.81]*
    polyarteritis nodosa M30.0 *[F02.80]*
      with behavioral disturbance M30.0 *[F02.81]*
    psychoactive drug F19.97
      with dependence F19.27
      inhalants F18.97
        with dependence F18.27
      sedatives, hypnotics or anxiolytics F13.97
        with dependence F13.27
    sedatives, hypnotics or anxiolytics F13.97
      with dependence F13.27
    systemic lupus erythematosus M32.- ☑ *[F02.80]*
      with behavioral disturbance M32.- ☑ *[F02.81]*
    trypanosomiasis
      African B56.9 *[F02.80]*
        with behavioral disturbance B56.9 *[F02.81]*
    unknown etiology F03 ☑
    vitamin B12 deficiency E53.8 *[F02.80]*
      with behavioral disturbance E53.8 *[F02.81]*
    volatile solvents F18.97
      with dependence F18.27
  infantile, infantilis F84.3
  Lewy body G31.83 *[F02.80]*
    with behavioral disturbance G31.83 *[F02.81]*
  multi-infarct — *see* Dementia, vascular
  paralytica, paralytic (syphilitic) A52.17 *[F02.80]*
    with behavioral disturbance A52.17 *[F02.81]*
    juvenilis A50.45
  paretic A52.17

Dementia — *continued*
  praecox — *see* Schizophrenia
  presenile F03 ☑
    Alzheimer's type — *see* Disease, Alzheimer's, early onset
  primary degenerative F03 ☑
  progressive, syphilitic A52.17
  senile F03 ☑
    with acute confusional state F05
    Alzheimer's type — *see* Disease, Alzheimer's, late onset
    depressed or paranoid type F03 ☑
  vascular (acute onset) (mixed) (multi-infarct) (subcortical) F01.50
    with behavioral disturbance F01.51
Demineralization, bone — *see* Osteoporosis
Demodex folliculorum (infestation) B88.0
Demophobia F40.248
Demoralization R45.3
Demyelination, demyelinization
  central nervous system G37.9
    specified NEC G37.8
  corpus callosum (central) G37.1
  disseminated, acute G36.9
    specified NEC G36.8
  global G35
  in optic neuritis G36.0
Dengue (classical) (fever) A90
  hemorrhagic A91
  sandfly A93.1
Dennie-Marfan syphilitic syndrome A50.45
Dens evaginatus, in dente or invaginatus K00.2
Dense breasts R92.2
Density
  increased, bone (disseminated) (generalized) (spotted) — *see* Disorder, bone, density and structure, specified type NEC
  lung (nodular) J98.4
Dental — *see also* condition
  examination Z01.20
    with abnormal findings Z01.21
  restoration
    aesthetically inadequate or displeasing K08.56
    defective K08.50
      specified NEC K08.59
    failure of marginal integrity K08.51
    failure of periodontal anatomical integrity K08.54
Dentia praecox K00.6
Denticles (pulp) K04.2
Dentigerous cyst K09.0
Dentin
  irregular (in pulp) K04.3
  opalescent K00.5
  secondary (in pulp) K04.3
  sensitive K03.89
Dentinogenesis imperfecta K00.5
Dentinoma — *see* Cyst, calcifying odontogenic
Dentition (syndrome) K00.7
  delayed K00.6
  difficult K00.7
  precocious K00.6
  premature K00.6
  retarded K00.6
Dependence (on) (syndrome) F19.20
  with remission F19.21
  alcohol (ethyl) (methyl) (without remission) F10.20
    with
      amnestic disorder, persisting F10.26
      anxiety disorder F10.280
      dementia, persisting F10.27
      intoxication F10.229
        with delirium F10.221
        uncomplicated F10.220
      mood disorder F10.24
      psychotic disorder F10.259
        with
          delusions F10.250
          hallucinations F10.251
      remission F10.21
      sexual dysfunction F10.281
      sleep disorder F10.282
      specified disorder NEC F10.288
      withdrawal F10.239
        with
          delirium F10.231
          perceptual disturbance F10.232
        uncomplicated F10.230
    counseling and surveillance Z71.41

☑ Additional Character Required — Refer to the Tabular List for Character Selection   ▽ Subterms under main terms may continue to next column or page

Dependence — *continued*
amobarbital — *see* Dependence, drug, sedative
amphetamine(s) (type) — *see* Dependence, drug, stimulant NEC
amytal (sodium) — *see* Dependence, drug, sedative
analgesic NEC F55.8
anesthetic (agent) (gas) (general) (local) NEC — *see* Dependence, drug, psychoactive NEC
anxiolytic NEC — *see* Dependence, drug, sedative
barbital(s) — *see* Dependence, drug, sedative
barbiturate(s) (compounds) (drugs classifiable to T42) — *see* Dependence, drug, sedative
benzedrine — *see* Dependence, drug, stimulant NEC
bhang — *see* Dependence, drug, cannabis
bromide(s) NEC — *see* Dependence, drug, sedative
caffeine — *see* Dependence, drug, stimulant NEC
cannabis (sativa) (indica) (resin) (derivatives) (type) — *see* Dependence, drug, cannabis
chloral (betaine) (hydrate) — *see* Dependence, drug, sedative
chlordiazepoxide — *see* Dependence, drug, sedative
coca (leaf) (derivatives) — *see* Dependence, drug, cocaine
cocaine — *see* Dependence, drug, cocaine
codeine — *see* Dependence, drug, opioid
combinations of drugs F19.20
dagga — *see* Dependence, drug, cannabis
demerol — *see* Dependence, drug, opioid
dexamphetamine — *see* Dependence, drug, stimulant NEC
dexedrine — *see* Dependence, drug, stimulant NEC
dextromethorphan — *see* Dependence, drug, opioid
dextromoramide — *see* Dependence, drug, opioid
dextro-nor-pseudo-ephedrine — *see* Dependence, drug, stimulant NEC
dextrorphan — *see* Dependence, drug, opioid
diazepam — *see* Dependence, drug, sedative
dilaudid — *see* Dependence, drug, opioid
D-lysergic acid diethylamide — *see* Dependence, drug, hallucinogen
drug NEC F19.20
  with sleep disorder F19.282
  cannabis F12.20
    with
      anxiety disorder F12.280
      intoxication F12.229
        with
          delirium F12.221
          perceptual disturbance F12.222
        uncomplicated F12.220
      other specified disorder F12.288
      psychosis F12.259
        delusions F12.250
        hallucinations F12.251
      unspecified disorder F12.29
      withdrawal F12.23
    in remission F12.21
  cocaine F14.20
    with
      anxiety disorder F14.280
      intoxication F14.229
        with
          delirium F14.221
          perceptual disturbance F14.222
        uncomplicated F14.220
      mood disorder F14.24
      other specified disorder F14.288
      psychosis F14.259
        delusions F14.250
        hallucinations F14.251
      sexual dysfunction F14.281
      sleep disorder F14.282
      unspecified disorder F14.29
      withdrawal F14.23
    in remission F14.21
    withdrawal symptoms in newborn P96.1
  counseling and surveillance Z71.51
  hallucinogen F16.20
    with
      anxiety disorder F16.280
      flashbacks F16.283
      intoxication F16.229
        with delirium F16.221
        uncomplicated F16.220
      mood disorder F16.24
      other specified disorder F16.288
      perception disorder, persisting F16.283
      psychosis F16.259

Dependence — *continued*
drug — *continued*
  hallucinogen — *continued*
    with — *continued*
      psychosis — *continued*
        delusions F16.250
        hallucinations F16.251
      unspecified disorder F16.29
    in remission F16.21
  in remission F19.21
  inhalant F18.20
    with
      anxiety disorder F18.280
      dementia, persisting F18.27
      intoxication F18.229
        with delirium F18.221
        uncomplicated F18.220
      mood disorder F18.24
      other specified disorder F18.288
      psychosis F18.259
        delusions F18.250
        hallucinations F18.251
      unspecified disorder F18.29
    in remission F18.21
  nicotine F17.200
    with disorder F17.209
      in remission F17.201
      specified disorder NEC F17.208
      withdrawal F17.203
    chewing tobacco F17.220
      with disorder F17.229
        in remission F17.221
        specified disorder NEC F17.228
        withdrawal F17.223
    cigarettes F17.210
      with disorder F17.219
        in remission F17.211
        specified disorder NEC F17.218
        withdrawal F17.213
    specified product NEC F17.290
      with disorder F17.299
        remission F17.291
        specified disorder NEC F17.298
        withdrawal F17.293
  opioid F11.20
    with
      intoxication F11.229
        with
          delirium F11.221
          perceptual disturbance F11.222
        uncomplicated F11.220
      mood disorder F11.24
      other specified disorder F11.288
      psychosis F11.259
        delusions F11.250
        hallucinations F11.251
      sexual dysfunction F11.281
      sleep disorder F11.282
      unspecified disorder F11.29
      withdrawal F11.23
    in remission F11.21
  psychoactive NEC F19.20
    with
      amnestic disorder F19.26
      anxiety disorder F19.280
      dementia F19.27
      intoxication F19.229
        with
          delirium F19.221
          perceptual disturbance F19.222
        uncomplicated F19.220
      mood disorder F19.24
      other specified disorder F19.288
      psychosis F19.259
        delusions F19.250
        hallucinations F19.251
      sexual dysfunction F19.281
      sleep disorder F19.282
      unspecified disorder F19.29
      withdrawal F19.239
        with
          delirium F19.231
          perceptual disturbance F19.232
        uncomplicated F19.230
  sedative, hypnotic or anxiolytic F13.20
    with
      amnestic disorder F13.26
      anxiety disorder F13.280
      dementia, persisting F13.27

Dependence — *continued*
drug — *continued*
  sedative, hypnotic or anxiolytic — *continued*
    with — *continued*
      intoxication F13.229
        with delirium F13.221
        uncomplicated F13.220
      mood disorder F13.24
      other specified disorder F13.288
      psychosis F13.259
        delusions F13.250
        hallucinations F13.251
      sexual dysfunction F13.281
      sleep disorder F13.282
      unspecified disorder F13.29
      withdrawal F13.239
        with
          delirium F13.231
          perceptual disturbance F13.232
        uncomplicated F13.230
    in remission F13.21
  stimulant NEC F15.20
    with
      anxiety disorder F15.280
      intoxication F15.229
        with
          delirium F15.221
          perceptual disturbance F15.222
        uncomplicated F15.220
      mood disorder F15.24
      other specified disorder F15.288
      psychosis F15.259
        delusions F15.250
        hallucinations F15.251
      sexual dysfunction F15.281
      sleep disorder F15.282
      unspecified disorder F15.29
      withdrawal F15.23
    in remission F15.21
  ethyl
    alcohol (without remission) F10.20
      with remission F10.21
    bromide — *see* Dependence, drug, sedative
    carbamate F19.20
    chloride F19.20
    morphine — *see* Dependence, drug, opioid
  ganja — *see* Dependence, drug, cannabis
  glue (airplane) (sniffing) — *see* Dependence, drug, inhalant
  glutethimide — *see* Dependence, drug, sedative
  hallucinogenics — *see* Dependence, drug, hallucinogen
  hashish — *see* Dependence, drug, cannabis
  hemp — *see* Dependence, drug, cannabis
  heroin (salt) (any) — *see* Dependence, drug, opioid
  hypnotic NEC — *see* Dependence, drug, sedative
  Indian hemp — *see* Dependence, drug, cannabis
  inhalants — *see* Dependence, drug, inhalant
  khat — *see* Dependence, drug, stimulant NEC
  laudanum — *see* Dependence, drug, opioid
  LSD (-25) (derivatives) — *see* Dependence, drug, hallucinogen
  luminal — *see* Dependence, drug, sedative
  lysergic acid — *see* Dependence, drug, hallucinogen
  maconha — *see* Dependence, drug, cannabis
  marihuana — *see* Dependence, drug, cannabis
  meprobamate — *see* Dependence, drug, sedative
  mescaline — *see* Dependence, drug, hallucinogen
  methadone — *see* Dependence, drug, opioid
  methamphetamine(s) — *see* Dependence, drug, stimulant NEC
  methaqualone — *see* Dependence, drug, sedative
  methyl
    alcohol (without remission) F10.20
      with remission F10.21
    bromide — *see* Dependence, drug, sedative
    morphine — *see* Dependence, drug, opioid
    phenidate — *see* Dependence, drug, stimulant NEC
    sulfonal — *see* Dependence, drug, sedative
  morphine (sulfate) (sulfite) (type) — *see* Dependence, drug, opioid
  narcotic (drug) NEC — *see* Dependence, drug, opioid
  nembutal — *see* Dependence, drug, sedative
  neraval — *see* Dependence, drug, sedative
  neravan — *see* Dependence, drug, sedative
  neurobarb — *see* Dependence, drug, sedative
  nicotine — *see* Dependence, drug, nicotine
  nitrous oxide F19.20

[handwritten annotation at top:] derangement of knee due to injury is dislocation → under S83.104, S83.105   S83.2

Dependence — *continued*
nonbarbiturate sedatives and tranquilizers with similar
    effect — *see* Dependence, drug, sedative
on
    artificial heart (fully implantable) (mechanical)
        Z95.812
    aspirator Z99.0
    care provider (because of) Z74.9
        impaired mobility Z74.09
        need for
            assistance with personal care Z74.1
            continuous supervision Z74.3
        no other household member able to render care
            Z74.2
        specified reason NEC Z74.8
    machine Z99.89
        enabling NEC Z99.89
        specified type NEC Z99.89
    renal dialysis (hemodialysis) (peritoneal) Z99.2
    respirator Z99.11
    ventilator Z99.11
    wheelchair Z99.3
opiate — *see* Dependence, drug, opioid
opioids — *see* Dependence, drug, opioid
opium (alkaloids) (derivatives) (tincture) — *see* Dependence, drug, opioid
oxygen (long-term) (supplemental) Z99.81
paraldehyde — *see* Dependence, drug, sedative
paregoric — *see* Dependence, drug, opioid
PCP (phencyclidine) (or related substance) — *see* Dependence, drug, hallucinogen
pentobarbital — *see* Dependence, drug, sedative
pentobarbitone (sodium) — *see* Dependence, drug, sedative
pentothal — *see* Dependence, drug, sedative
peyote — *see* Dependence, drug, hallucinogen
phencyclidine (PCP) (or related substance) — *see* Dependence, drug, hallucinogen
phenmetrazine — *see* Dependence, drug, stimulant NEC
phenobarbital — *see* Dependence, drug, sedative
polysubstance F19.20
psilocibin, psilocin, psilocyn, psilocyline — *see* Dependence, drug, hallucinogen
psychostimulant NEC — *see* Dependence, drug, stimulant NEC
secobarbital — *see* Dependence, drug, sedative
seconal — *see* Dependence, drug, sedative
sedative NEC — *see* Dependence, drug, sedative
specified drug NEC — *see* Dependence, drug
stimulant NEC — *see* Dependence, drug, stimulant NEC
substance NEC — *see* Dependence, drug
supplemental oxygen Z99.81
tobacco — *see* Dependence, drug, nicotine
    counseling and surveillance Z71.6
tranquilizer NEC — *see* Dependence, drug, sedative
vitamin B6 E53.1
volatile solvents — *see* Dependence, drug, inhalant

Dependency
care-provider Z74.9
passive F60.7
reactions (persistent) F60.7

Depersonalization (in neurotic state) (neurotic) (syndrome) F48.1

Depletion
extracellular fluid E86.9
plasma E86.1
potassium E87.6
    nephropathy N25.89
salt or sodium E87.1
    causing heat exhaustion or prostration T67.4 ☑
    nephropathy N28.9
volume NOS E86.9

Deployment (current) (military) status Z56.82
in theater or in support of military war, peacekeeping
    and humanitarian operations Z56.82
personal history of Z91.82
    military war, peacekeeping and humanitarian deployment (current or past conflict) Z91.82
returned from Z91.82

Depolarization, premature I49.40
atrial I49.1
junctional I49.2
specified NEC I49.49
ventricular I49.3

Deposit
bone in Boeck's sarcoid D86.89
calcareous, calcium — *see* Calcification

Deposit — *continued*
cholesterol
    retina H35.89
    vitreous (body) (humor) — *see* Deposit, crystalline
conjunctiva H11.11- ☑
cornea H18.00- ☑
    argentous H18.02- ☑
    due to metabolic disorder H18.03- ☑
    Kayser-Fleischer ring H18.04- ☑
    pigmentation — *see* Pigmentation, cornea
crystalline, vitreous (body) (humor) H43.2- ☑
hemosiderin in old scars of cornea — *see* Pigmentation, cornea, stromal
metallic in lens — *see* Cataract, specified NEC
skin R23.8
tooth, teeth (betel) (black) (green) (materia alba) (orange) (tobacco) K03.6
urate, kidney — *see* Calculus, kidney

Depraved appetite — *see* Pica

Depressed
HDL cholesterol E78.6

Depression (acute) (mental) F32.9
agitated (single episode) F32.2
anaclitic — *see* Disorder, adjustment
anxiety F41.8
    persistent F34.1
arches — *see also* Deformity, limb, flat foot
atypical (single episode) F32.89
    recurrent episode F33.8
basal metabolic rate R94.8
bone marrow D75.89
central nervous system R09.2
cerebral R29.818
    newborn P91.4
cerebrovascular I67.9
chest wall M95.4
climacteric (single episode) F32.89
    recurrent episode F33.8
endogenous (without psychotic symptoms) F33.2
    with psychotic symptoms F33.3
functional activity R68.89
hysterical F44.89
involutional (single episode) F32.89
    recurrent episode F33.8
major F32.9
    with psychotic symptoms F32.3
    recurrent — *see* Disorder, depressive, recurrent
manic-depressive — *see* Disorder, depressive, recurrent
masked (single episode) F32.89
medullary G93.89
menopausal (single episode) F32.89
    recurrent episode F33.8
metatarsus — *see* Depression, arches
monopolar F33.9
nervous F34.1
neurotic F34.1
nose M95.0
postnatal (NOS) F53.0
postpartum (NOS) F53.0
post-psychotic of schizophrenia F32.89
post-schizophrenic F32.89
psychogenic (reactive) (single episode) F32.9
psychoneurotic F34.1
psychotic (single episode) F32.3
    recurrent F33.3
reactive (psychogenic) (single episode) F32.9
    psychotic (single episode) F32.3
recurrent — *see* Disorder, depressive, recurrent
respiratory center G93.89
seasonal — *see* Disorder, depressive, recurrent
senile F03 ☑
severe, single episode F32.2
situational F43.21
skull Q67.4
specified NEC (single episode) F32.89
sternum M95.4
visual field — *see* Defect, visual field
vital (recurrent) (without psychotic symptoms) F33.2
    with psychotic symptoms F33.3
    single episode F32.2

Deprivation
cultural Z60.3
effects NOS T73.9 ☑
    specified NEC T73.8 ☑
emotional NEC Z65.8
    affecting infant or child — *see* Maltreatment, child, psychological
food T73.0 ☑

Deprivation — *continued*
protein — *see* Malnutrition
sleep Z72.820
social Z60.4
    affecting infant or child — *see* Maltreatment, child, psychological
specified NEC T73.8 ☑
vitamins — *see* Deficiency, vitamin
water T73.1 ☑

Derangement
ankle (internal) — *see* Derangement, joint, ankle
cartilage (articular) NEC — *see* Derangement, joint, articular cartilage, by site
    recurrent — *see* Dislocation, recurrent
cruciate ligament, anterior, current injury — *see* Sprain, knee, cruciate, anterior
elbow (internal) — *see* Derangement, joint, elbow
hip (joint) (internal) (old) — *see* Derangement, joint, hip
joint (internal) M24.9
    ankylosis — *see* Ankylosis
    articular cartilage M24.10
        ankle M24.17- ☑
        elbow M24.12- ☑
        foot M24.17- ☑
        hand M24.14- ☑
        hip M24.15- ☑
        knee NEC M23.9- ☑
        loose body — *see* Loose, body
        shoulder M24.11- ☑
        wrist M24.13- ☑
    contracture — *see* Contraction, joint
    current injury — *see also* Dislocation
        knee, meniscus or cartilage — *see* Tear, meniscus
    dislocation
        pathological — *see* Dislocation, pathological
        recurrent — *see* Dislocation, recurrent
    knee — *see* Derangement, knee
    ligament — *see* Disorder, ligament
    loose body — *see* Loose, body
    recurrent — *see* Dislocation, recurrent
    specified type NEC M24.80
        ankle M24.87- ☑
        elbow M24.82- ☑
        foot joint M24.87- ☑
        hand joint M24.84- ☑
        hip M24.85- ☑
        shoulder M24.81- ☑
        wrist M24.83- ☑
    temporomandibular M26.69
knee (recurrent) M23.9- ☑
    ligament disruption, spontaneous M23.60- ☑
        anterior cruciate M23.61- ☑
        capsular M23.67- ☑
        instability, chronic M23.5- ☑
        lateral collateral M23.64- ☑
        medial collateral M23.63- ☑
        posterior cruciate M23.62- ☑
    loose body M23.4- ☑
    meniscus M23.30- ☑
        cystic M23.00- ☑
            lateral M23.002
                anterior horn M23.04- ☑
                posterior horn M23.05- ☑
                specified NEC M23.06- ☑
            medial M23.005
                anterior horn M23.01- ☑
                posterior horn M23.02- ☑
                specified NEC M23.03- ☑
        degenerate — *see* Derangement, knee, meniscus, specified NEC
        detached — *see* Derangement, knee, meniscus, specified NEC
        due to old tear or injury M23.20- ☑
            lateral M23.20- ☑
                anterior horn M23.24- ☑
                posterior horn M23.25- ☑
                specified NEC M23.26- ☑
            medial M23.20- ☑
                anterior horn M23.21- ☑
                posterior horn M23.22- ☑
                specified NEC M23.23- ☑
        retained — *see* Derangement, knee, meniscus, specified NEC
        specified NEC M23.30- ☑
            lateral M23.30- ☑

Derangement — *continued*
  knee — *continued*
    meniscus — *continued*
      specified — *continued*
        lateral — *continued*
          anterior horn M23.34- ☑
          posterior horn M23.35- ☑
          specified NEC M23.36- ☑
        medial M23.30- ☑
          anterior horn M23.31- ☑
          posterior horn M23.32- ☑
          specified NEC M23.33- ☑
    old M23.8X- ☑
    specified NEC — *see* subcategory M23.8 ☑
  low back NEC — *see* Dorsopathy, specified NEC
  meniscus — *see* Derangement, knee, meniscus
  mental — *see* Psychosis
  patella, specified NEC — *see* Disorder, patella, derangement NEC
  semilunar cartilage (knee) — *see* Derangement, knee, meniscus, specified NEC
  shoulder (internal) — *see* Derangement, joint, shoulder
Dercum's disease E88.2
Derealization (neurotic) F48.1
Dermal — *see* condition
Dermaphytid — *see* Dermatophytosis
Dermatitis (eczematous) L30.9
  ab igne L59.0
  acarine B88.0
  actinic (due to sun) L57.8
    other than from sun L59.8
  allergic — *see* Dermatitis, contact, allergic
  ambustionis, due to burn or scald — *see* Burn
  amebic A06.7
  ammonia L22
  arsenical (ingested) L27.8
  artefacta L98.1
    psychogenic F54
  atopic L20.9
    psychogenic F54
    specified NEC L20.89
  autoimmune progesterone L30.8
  berlock, berloque L56.2
  blastomycotic B40.3
  blister beetle L24.89
  bullous, bullosa L13.9
    mucosynechial, atrophic L12.1
    seasonal L30.8
    specified NEC L13.8
  calorica L59.0
    due to burn or scald — *see* Burn
  caterpillar L24.89
  cercarial B65.3
  combustionis L59.0
    due to burn or scald — *see* Burn
  congelationis T69.1 ☑
  contact (occupational) L25.9
    allergic L23.9
      due to
        adhesives L23.1
        cement L23.5
        chemical products NEC L23.5
        chromium L23.0
        cosmetics L23.2
        dander (cat) (dog) L23.81
        drugs in contact with skin L23.3
        dyes L23.4
        food in contact with skin L23.6
        hair (cat) (dog) L23.81
        insecticide L23.5
        metals L23.0
        nickel L23.0
        plants, non-food L23.7
        plastic L23.5
        rubber L23.5
        specified agent NEC L23.89
    due to
      cement L25.3
      chemical products NEC L25.3
      cosmetics L25.0
      dander (cat) (dog) L23.81
      drugs in contact with skin L25.1
      dyes L25.2
      food in contact with skin L25.4
      hair (cat) (dog) L23.81
      plants, non-food L25.5
      specified agent NEC L25.8
    irritant L24.9

Dermatitis — *continued*
  contact — *continued*
    irritant — *continued*
      due to
        cement L24.5
        chemical products NEC L24.5
        cosmetics L24.3
        detergents L24.0
        drugs in contact with skin L24.4
        food in contact with skin L24.6
        oils and greases L24.1
        plants, non-food L24.7
        solvents L24.2
        specified agent NEC L24.89
  contusiformis L52
  diabetic — *see* E08-E13 with .620
  diaper L22
  diphtheritica A36.3
  dry skin L85.3
  due to
    acetone (contact) (irritant) L24.2
    acids (contact) (irritant) L24.5
    adhesive(s) (allergic) (contact) (plaster) L23.1
      irritant L24.5
    alcohol (irritant) (skin contact) (substances in category T51) L24.2
      taken internally L27.8
    alkalis (contact) (irritant) L24.5
    arsenic (ingested) L27.8
    carbon disulfide (contact) (irritant) L24.2
    caustics (contact) (irritant) L24.5
    cement L25.3
    cereal (ingested) L27.2
    chemical(s) NEC L25.3
      taken internally L27.8
    chlorocompounds L24.2
    chromium (contact) (irritant) L24.81
    coffee (ingested) L27.2
    cold weather L30.8
    cosmetics (contact) L25.0
      allergic L23.2
      irritant L24.3
    cyclohexanes L24.2
    dander (cat) (dog) L23.81
    Demodex species B88.0
    Dermanyssus gallinae B88.0
    detergents (contact) (irritant) L24.0
    dichromate L24.81
    drugs and medicaments (generalized) (internal use) L27.0
      external — *see* Dermatitis, due to, drugs, in contact with skin
      in contact with skin L25.1
        allergic L23.3
        irritant L24.4
      localized skin eruption L27.1
      specified substance — *see* Table of Drugs and Chemicals
    dyes (contact) L25.2
      allergic L23.4
      irritant L24.89
    epidermophytosis — *see* Dermatophytosis
    esters L24.2
    external irritant NEC L24.9
    fish (ingested) L27.2
    flour (ingested) L27.2
    food (ingested) L27.2
      in contact with skin L25.4
    fruit (ingested) L27.2
    furs (allergic) (contact) L23.81
    glues — *see* Dermatitis, due to, adhesives
    glycols L24.2
    greases NEC (contact) (irritant) L24.1
    hair (cat) (dog) L23.81
    hot
      objects and materials — *see* Burn
      weather or places L59.0
    hydrocarbons L24.2
    infrared rays L59.8
    ingestion, ingested substance L27.9
      chemical NEC L27.8
      drugs and medicaments — *see* Dermatitis, due to, drugs
      food L27.2
      specified NEC L27.8
    insecticide in contact with skin L24.5
    internal agent L27.9

Dermatitis — *continued*
  due to — *continued*
    internal agent — *continued*
      drugs and medicaments (generalized) — *see* Dermatitis, due to, drugs
      food L27.2
    irradiation — *see* Dermatitis, due to, radioactive substance
    ketones L24.2
    lacquer tree (allergic) (contact) L23.7
    light (sun) NEC L57.8
      acute L56.8
      other L59.8
    Liponyssoides sanguineus B88.0
    low temperature L30.8
    meat (ingested) L27.2
    metals, metal salts (contact) (irritant) L24.81
    milk (ingested) L27.2
    nickel (contact) (irritant) L24.81
    nylon (contact) (irritant) L24.5
    oils NEC (contact) (irritant) L24.1
    paint solvent (contact) (irritant) L24.2
    petroleum products (contact) (irritant) (substances in T52.0) L24.2
    plants NEC (contact) L25.5
      allergic L23.7
      irritant L24.7
    plasters (adhesive) (any) (allergic) (contact) L23.1
      irritant L24.5
    plastic (contact) L25.3
    preservatives (contact) — *see* Dermatitis, due to, chemical, in contact with skin
    primrose (allergic) (contact) L23.7
    primula (allergic) (contact) L23.7
    radiation L59.8
      nonionizing (chronic exposure) L57.8
      sun NEC L57.8
        acute L56.8
    radioactive substance L58.9
      acute L58.0
      chronic L58.1
    radium L58.9
      acute L58.0
      chronic L58.1
    ragweed (allergic) (contact) L23.7
    Rhus (allergic) (contact) (diversiloba) (radicans) (toxicodendron) (venenata) (verniciflua) L23.7
    rubber (contact) L24.5
    Senecio jacobaea (allergic) (contact) L23.7
    solvents (contact) (irritant) (substances in category T52) L24.2
    specified agent NEC (contact) L25.8
      allergic L23.89
      irritant L24.89
    sunshine NEC L57.8
      acute L56.8
    tetrachlorethylene (contact) (irritant) L24.2
    toluene (contact) (irritant) L24.2
    turpentine (contact) L24.2
    ultraviolet rays (sun NEC) (chronic exposure) L57.8
      acute L56.8
    vaccine or vaccination L27.0
      specified substance — *see* Table of Drugs and Chemicals
    varicose veins — *see* Varix, leg, with, inflammation
    X-rays L58.9
      acute L58.0
      chronic L58.1
  dyshydrotic L30.1
  dysmenorrheica N94.6
  escharotica — *see* Burn
  exfoliative, exfoliativa (generalized) L26
    neonatorum L00
  eyelid — *see also* Dermatosis, eyelid
    allergic H01.119
      left H01.116
        lower H01.115
        upper H01.114
      right H01.113
        lower H01.112
        upper H01.111
    contact — *see* Dermatitis, eyelid, allergic
    due to
      Demodex species B88.0
      herpes (zoster) B02.39
        simplex B00.59
    eczematous H01.139
      left H01.136

☁ Subterms under main terms may continue to next column or page   ☑ Additional Character Required — Refer to the Tabular List for Character Selection   **95**

Derangement — Dermatitis

Index

Dermatitis — continued
  eyelid — see also Dermatosis, eyelid — continued
    eczematous — continued
      left — continued
        lower H01.135
        upper H01.134
      right H01.133
        lower H01.132
        upper H01.131
  facta, factitia, factitial L98.1
    psychogenic F54
  flexural NEC L20.82
  friction L30.4
  fungus B36.9
    specified type NEC B36.8
  gangrenosa, gangrenous infantum L08.0
  harvest mite B88.0
  heat L59.0
  herpesviral, vesicular (ear) (lip) B00.1
  herpetiformis (bullous) (erythematous) (pustular)
      (vesicular) L13.0
    juvenile L12.2
    senile L12.0
  hiemalis L30.8
  hypostatic, hypostatica — see Varix, leg, with, inflam-
      mation
  infectious eczematoid L30.3
  infective L30.3
  irritant — see Dermatitis, contact, irritant
  Jacquet's (diaper dermatitis) L22
  Leptus B88.0
  lichenified NEC L28.0
  medicamentosa (generalized) (internal use) — see
      Dermatitis, due to drugs
  mite B88.0
  multiformis L13.0
    juvenile L12.2
  napkin L22
  neurotica L13.0
  nummular L30.0
  papillaris capillitii L73.0
  pellagrous E52
  perioral L71.0
  photocontact L56.2
  polymorpha dolorosa L13.0
  pruriginosa L13.0
  pruritic NEC L30.8
  psychogenic F54
  purulent L08.0
  pustular
    contagious B08.02
    subcorneal L13.1
  pyococcal L08.0
  pyogenica L08.0
  repens L40.2
  Ritter's (exfoliativa) L00
  Schamberg's L81.7
  schistosome B65.3
  seasonal bullous L30.8
  seborrheic L21.9
    infantile L21.1
    specified NEC L21.8
  sensitization NOS L23.9
  septic L08.0
  solare L57.8
  specified NEC L30.8
  stasis I87.2
    with
      varicose ulcer — see Varix, leg, with ulcer, with
          inflammation
      varicose veins — see Varix, leg, with, inflamma-
          tion
    due to postthrombotic syndrome — see Syndrome,
        postthrombotic
  suppurative L08.0
  traumatic NEC L30.4
  trophoneurotica L13.0
  ultraviolet (sun) (chronic exposure) L57.8
    acute L56.8
  varicose — see Varix, leg, with, inflammation
  vegetans L10.1
  verrucosa B43.0
  vesicular, herpesviral B00.1
Dermatoarthritis, lipoid E78.81
Dermatochalasis, eyelid H02.839
  left H02.836
    lower H02.835
    upper H02.834

Dermatochalasis, eyelid — continued
  right H02.833
    lower H02.832
    upper H02.831
Dermatofibroma (lenticulare) — see Neoplasm, skin,
    benign
  protuberans — see Neoplasm, skin, uncertain behavior
Dermatofibrosarcoma (pigmented) (protuberans) —
    see Neoplasm, skin, malignant
Dermatographia L50.3
Dermatolysis (exfoliativa) (congenital) Q82.8
  acquired L57.4
  eyelids — see Blepharochalasis
  palpebrarum — see Blepharochalasis
  senile L57.4
Dermatomegaly NEC Q82.8
Dermatomucosomyositis M33.10
  with
    myopathy M33.12
    respiratory involvement M33.11
    specified organ involvement NEC M33.19
Dermatomycosis B36.9
  furfuracea B36.0
  specified type NEC B36.8
Dermatomyositis (acute) (chronic) — see also Der-
    matopolymyositis
  adult — see also Dermatomyositis, specified NEC
      M33.10
  in (due to) neoplastic disease — see also Neoplasm
      D49.9 [M36.0]
  juvenile M33.00
    with
      myopathy M33.02
      respiratory involvement M33.01
      specified organ involvement NEC M33.09
    without myopathy M33.03
  specified NEC M33.10
    with
      myopathy M33.12
      respiratory involvement M33.11
      specified organ involvement NEC M33.19
    without myopathy M33.13
Dermatoneuritis of children — see Poisoning, mercury
Dermatophilosis A48.8
Dermatophytid L30.2
Dermatophytide — see Dermatophytosis
Dermatophytosis (epidermophyton) (infection) (Mi-
    crosporum) (tinea) (Trichophyton) B35.9
  beard B35.0
  body B35.4
  capitis B35.0
  corporis B35.4
  deep-seated B35.8
  disseminated B35.8
  foot B35.3
  granulomatous B35.8
  groin B35.6
  hand B35.2
  nail B35.1
  perianal (area) B35.6
  scalp B35.0
  specified NEC B35.8
Dermatopolymyositis M33.90
  with
    myopathy M33.92
    respiratory involvement M33.91
    specified organ involvement NEC M33.99
  in neoplastic disease — see also Neoplasm
      D49.9 [M36.0]
  juvenile M33.00
    with
      myopathy M33.02
      respiratory involvement M33.01
      specified organ involvement NEC M33.09
  specified NEC M33.10
    myopathy M33.12
    respiratory involvement M33.11
    specified organ involvement NEC M33.19
  without myopathy M33.93
Dermatopolyneuritis — see Poisoning, mercury
Dermatorrhexis — see also Syndrome, Ehlers-Danlos
    Q79.60
  acquired L57.4
Dermatosclerosis — see also Scleroderma
  localized L94.0
Dermatosis L98.9
  Andrews' L08.89
  Bowen's — see Neoplasm, skin, in situ

Dermatosis — continued
  bullous L13.9
    specified NEC L13.8
  exfoliativa L26
  eyelid (noninfectious)
    dermatitis — see Dermatitis, eyelid
    discoid lupus erythematosus — see Lupus, erythe-
        matosus, eyelid
    xeroderma — see Xeroderma, acquired, eyelid
  factitial L98.1
  febrile neutrophilic L98.2
  gonococcal A54.89
  herpetiformis L13.0
    juvenile L12.2
  linear IgA L13.8
  menstrual NEC L98.8
  neutrophilic, febrile L98.2
  occupational — see Dermatitis, contact
  papulosa nigra L82.1
  pigmentary L81.9
    progressive L81.7
    Schamberg's L81.7
  psychogenic F54
  purpuric, pigmented L81.7
  pustular, subcorneal L13.1
  transient acantholytic L11.1
Dermographia, dermographism L50.3
Dermoid (cyst) — see also Neoplasm, benign, by site
  with malignant transformation C56- ☑
  due to radiation (nonionizing) L57.8
Dermopathy
  infiltrative with thyrotoxicosis — see Thyrotoxicosis
  nephrogenic fibrosing L90.8
Dermophytosis — see Dermatophytosis
Descemetocele H18.73- ☑
Descemet's membrane — see condition
Descending — see condition
Descensus uteri — see Prolapse, uterus
Desert
  rheumatism B38.0
  sore — see Ulcer, skin
Desertion (newborn) — see Maltreatment
Desmoid (extra-abdominal) (tumor) — see Neoplasm,
    connective tissue, uncertain behavior
  abdominal D48.1
Despondency F32.9
Desquamation, skin R23.4
Destruction, destructive — see also Damage
  articular facet — see also Derangement, joint, specified
      type NEC
    knee M23.8X- ☑
    vertebra — see Spondylosis
  bone — see also Disorder, bone, specified type NEC
    syphilitic A52.77
  joint — see also Derangement, joint, specified type
      NEC
    sacroiliac M53.3
  rectal sphincter K62.89
  septum (nasal) J34.89
  tuberculous NEC — see Tuberculosis
  tympanum, tympanic membrane (nontraumatic) —
      see Disorder, tympanic membrane, specified NEC
  vertebral disc — see Degeneration, intervertebral disc
Destructiveness — see also Disorder, conduct
  adjustment reaction — see Disorder, adjustment
Desultory labor O62.2
Detachment
  cartilage — see Sprain
  cervix, annular N88.8
    complicating delivery O71.3
  choroid (old) (postinfectional) (simple) (spontaneous)
      H31.40- ☑
    hemorrhagic H31.41- ☑
    serous H31.42- ☑
  ligament — see Sprain
  meniscus (knee) — see also Derangement, knee,
      meniscus, specified NEC
    current injury — see Tear, meniscus
    due to old tear or injury — see Derangement, knee,
        meniscus, due to old tear
  retina (without retinal break) (serous) H33.2- ☑
    with retinal:
      break H33.00- ☑
        giant H33.03- ☑
        multiple H33.02- ☑
        single H33.01- ☑
      dialysis H33.04- ☑

☑ **Additional Character Required** — Refer to the Tabular List for Character Selection — Subterms under main terms may continue to next column or page

Dermatitis — Detachment

Detachment — *continued*
  retina — *continued*
    pigment epithelium — *see* Degeneration, retina, separation of layers, pigment epithelium detachment
    rhegmatogenous — *see* Detachment, retina, with retinal, break
    specified NEC H33.8
    total H33.05- ☑
    traction H33.4- ☑
  vitreous (body) H43.81 ☑
Detergent asthma J69.8
Deterioration
  epileptic F06.8
  general physical R53.81
  heart, cardiac — *see* Degeneration, myocardial
  mental — *see* Psychosis
  myocardial, myocardium — *see* Degeneration, myocardial
  senile (simple) R54
Deuteranomaly (anomalous trichromat) H53.53
Deuteranopia (complete) (incomplete) H53.53
Development
  abnormal, bone Q79.9
  arrested R62.50
    bone — *see* Arrest, development or growth, bone
    child R62.50
    due to malnutrition E45
  defective, congenital — *see also* Anomaly, by site
    cauda equina Q06.3
    left ventricle Q24.8
      in hypoplastic left heart syndrome Q23.4
    valve Q24.8
      pulmonary Q22.3
  delayed — *see also* Delay, development R62.50
    arithmetical skills F81.2
    language (skills) (expressive) F80.1
    learning skill F81.9
    mixed skills F88
    motor coordination F82
    reading F81.0
    specified learning skill NEC F81.89
    speech F80.9
    spelling F81.81
    written expression F81.81
  imperfect, congenital — *see also* Anomaly, by site
    heart Q24.9
    lungs Q33.6
  incomplete
    bronchial tree Q32.4
    organ or site not listed — *see* Hypoplasia, by site
    respiratory system Q34.9
  sexual, precocious NEC E30.1
  tardy, mental — *see also* Disability, intellectual F79
Developmental — *see* condition
  testing, infant or child — *see* Examination, child
Devergie's disease (pityriasis rubra pilaris) L44.0
Deviation (in)
  conjugate palsy (eye) (spastic) H51.0
  esophagus (acquired) K22.8
  eye, skew H51.8
  midline (jaw) (teeth) (dental arch) M26.29
    specified site NEC — *see* Malposition
  nasal septum J34.2
    congenital Q67.4
  opening and closing of the mandible M26.53
  organ or site, congenital NEC — *see* Malposition, congenital
  septum (nasal) (acquired) J34.2
    congenital Q67.4
  sexual F65.9
    bestiality F65.89
    erotomania F52.8
    exhibitionism F65.2
    fetishism, fetishistic F65.0
      transvestism F65.1
    frotteurism F65.81
    masochism F65.51
    multiple F65.89
    necrophilia F65.89
    nymphomania F52.8
    pederosis F65.4
    pedophilia F65.4
    sadism, sadomasochism F65.52
    satyriasis F52.8
    specified type NEC F65.89
    transvestism F64.1
    voyeurism F65.3

Deviation — *continued*
  teeth, midline M26.29
  trachea J39.8
  ureter, congenital Q62.61
Device
  cerebral ventricle (communicating) in situ Z98.2
  contraceptive — *see* Contraceptive, device
  drainage, cerebrospinal fluid, in situ Z98.2
Devic's disease G36.0
Devil's
  grip B33.0
  pinches (purpura simplex) D69.2
Devitalized tooth K04.99
Devonshire colic — *see* Poisoning, lead
Dextraposition, aorta Q20.3
  in tetralogy of Fallot Q21.3
Dextrinosis, limit (debrancher enzyme deficiency) E74.03
Dextrocardia (true) Q24.0
  with
    complete transposition of viscera Q89.3
    situs inversus Q89.3
Dextrotransposition, aorta Q20.3
d-glycericacidemia E72.59
Dhat syndrome F48.8
Dhobi itch B35.6
Di George's syndrome D82.1
Di Guglielmo's disease C94.0- ☑
Diabetes, diabetic (mellitus) (sugar) E11.9
  with
    amyotrophy E11.44
    arthropathy NEC E11.618
    autonomic (poly)neuropathy E11.43
    cataract E11.36
    Charcot's joints E11.610
    chronic kidney disease E11.22
    circulatory complication NEC E11.59
    complication E11.8
      specified NEC E11.69
    dermatitis E11.620
    foot ulcer E11.621
    gangrene E11.52
    gastroparalysis E11.43
    gastroparesis E11.43
    glomerulonephrosis, intracapillary E11.21
    glomerulosclerosis, intercapillary E11.21
    hyperglycemia E11.65
    hyperosmolarity E11.00
      with coma E11.01
    hypoglycemia E11.649
      with coma E11.641
    ketoacidosis E11.10
      with coma E11.11
    kidney complications NEC E11.29
    Kimmelstiel-Wilson disease E11.21
    loss of protective sensation (LOPS) — *see* Diabetes, by type, with neuropathy
    mononeuropathy E11.41
    myasthenia E11.44
    necrobiosis lipoidica E11.620
    nephropathy E11.21
    neuralgia E11.42
    neurologic complication NEC E11.49
    neuropathic arthropathy E11.610
    neuropathy E11.40
    ophthalmic complication NEC E11.39
    oral complication NEC E11.638
    osteomyelitis E11.69
    periodontal disease E11.630
    peripheral angiopathy E11.51
      with gangrene E11.52
    polyneuropathy E11.42
    renal complication NEC E11.29
    renal tubular degeneration E11.29
    retinopathy E11.319
      with macular edema E11.311
        resolved following treatment E11.37- ☑
      nonproliferative E11.329 ☑
        with macular edema E11.321 ☑
        mild E11.329 ☑
          with macular edema E11.321 ☑
        moderate E11.339 ☑
          with macular edema E11.331 ☑
        severe E11.349 ☑
          with macular edema E11.341 ☑
      proliferative E11.359 ☑

Diabetes, diabetic — *continued*
  with — *continued*
    retinopathy — *continued*
      proliferative — *continued*
        with
          combined traction retinal detachment and rhegmatogenous retinal detachment E11.354 ☑
          macular edema E11.351 ☑
          stable proliferative diabetic retinopathy E11.355 ☑
          traction retinal detachment involving the macula E11.352 ☑
          traction retinal detachment not involving the macula E11.353 ☑
      resolved following treatment E09.37 ☑
    skin complication NEC E11.628
    skin ulcer NEC E11.622
  brittle — *see* Diabetes, type 1
  bronzed E83.110
  complicating pregnancy — *see* Pregnancy, complicated by, diabetes
  dietary counseling and surveillance Z71.3
  due to
    autoimmune process — *see* Diabetes, type 1
    immune mediated pancreatic islet beta-cell destruction — *see* Diabetes, type 1
  due to drug or chemical E09.9
    with
      amyotrophy E09.44
      arthropathy NEC E09.618
      autonomic (poly)neuropathy E09.43
      cataract E09.36
      Charcot's joints E09.610
      chronic kidney disease E09.22
      circulatory complication NEC E09.59
      complication E09.8
        specified NEC E09.69
      dermatitis E09.620
      foot ulcer E09.621
      gangrene E09.52
      gastroparalysis E09.43
      gastroparesis E09.43
      glomerulonephrosis, intracapillary E09.21
      glomerulosclerosis, intercapillary E09.21
      hyperglycemia E09.65
      hyperosmolarity E09.00
        with coma E09.01
      hypoglycemia E09.649
        with coma E09.641
      ketoacidosis E09.10
        with coma E09.11
      kidney complications NEC E09.29
      Kimmelstiel-Wilson disease E09.21
      mononeuropathy E09.41
      myasthenia E09.44
      necrobiosis lipoidica E09.620
      nephropathy E09.21
      neuralgia E09.42
      neurologic complication NEC E09.49
      neuropathic arthropathy E09.610
      neuropathy E09.40
      ophthalmic complication NEC E09.39
      oral complication NEC E09.638
      periodontal disease E09.630
      peripheral angiopathy E09.51
        with gangrene E09.52
      polyneuropathy E09.42
      renal complication NEC E09.29
      renal tubular degeneration E09.29
      retinopathy E09.319
        with macular edema E09.311
        resolved following treatment E09.37 ☑
        nonproliferative E09.329 ☑
          with macular edema E09.321 ☑
          mild E09.329 ☑
            with macular edema E09.321 ☑
          moderate E09.339 ☑
            with macular edema E09.331 ☑
          severe E09.349 ☑
            with macular edema E09.341 ☑
        proliferative E09.359 ☑
          with
            combined traction retinal detachment and rhegmatogenous retinal detachment E09.354 ☑
            macular edema E09.351 ☑

Detachment — Diabetes, diabetic

▼ Subterms under main terms may continue to next column or page   ☑ Additional Character Required — Refer to the Tabular List for Character Selection   97

Diabetes, diabetic — *continued*
  due to drug or chemical — *continued*
    with — *continued*
      retinopathy — *continued*
        proliferative — *continued*
          with — *continued*
            stable proliferative diabetic retinopathy E09.355 ☑
            traction retinal detachment involving the macula E09.352 ☑
            traction retinal detachment not involving the macula E09.353 ☑
      skin complication NEC E09.628
      skin ulcer NEC E09.622
  due to underlying condition E08.9
    with
      amyotrophy E08.44
      arthropathy NEC E08.618
      autonomic (poly)neuropathy E08.43
      cataract E08.36
      Charcot's joints E08.610
      chronic kidney disease E08.22
      circulatory complication NEC E08.59
      complication E08.8
        specified NEC E08.69
      dermatitis E08.620
      foot ulcer E08.621
      gangrene E08.52
      gastroparalysis E08.43
      gastroparesis E08.43
      glomerulonephrosis, intracapillary E08.21
      glomerulosclerosis, intercapillary E08.21
      hyperglycemia E08.65
      hyperosmolarity E08.00
        with coma E08.01
      hypoglycemia E08.649
        with coma E08.641
      ketoacidosis E08.10
        with coma E08.11
      kidney complications NEC E08.29
      Kimmelsteil-Wilson disease E08.21
      mononeuropathy E08.41
      myasthenia E08.44
      necrobiosis lipoidica E08.620
      nephropathy E08.21
      neuralgia E08.42
      neurologic complication NEC E08.49
      neuropathic arthropathy E08.610
      neuropathy E08.40
      ophthalmic complication NEC E08.39
      oral complication NEC E08.638
      periodontal disease E08.630
      peripheral angiopathy E08.51
        with gangrene E08.52
      polyneuropathy E08.42
      renal complication NEC E08.29
      renal tubular degeneration E08.29
      retinopathy E08.319
        with macular edema E08.311
        resolved following treatment E08.37 ☑
        nonproliferative E08.329 ☑
          with macular edema E08.321 ☑
          mild E08.329 ☑
            with macular edema E08.321 ☑
          moderate E08.339 ☑
            with macular edema E08.331 ☑
          severe E08.349 ☑
            with macular edema E08.341 ☑
        proliferative E08.359 ☑
          with
            combined traction retinal detachment and rhegmatogenous retinal detachment E08.354 ☑
            macular edema E08.351 ☑
            stable proliferative diabetic retinopathy E08.355 ☑
            traction retinal detachment involving the macula E08.352 ☑
            traction retinal detachment not involving the macula E08.353 ☑
      skin complication NEC E08.628
      skin ulcer NEC E08.622
  gestational (in pregnancy) O24.419
    affecting newborn P70.0
    diet controlled O24.410
    in childbirth O24.429
      diet controlled O24.420
      insulin (and diet) controlled O24.424

Diabetes, diabetic — *continued*
  gestational — *continued*
    in childbirth — *continued*
      oral drug controlled (antidiabetic) (hypoglycemic) O24.425
    insulin (and diet) controlled O24.414
    oral drug controlled (antidiabetic) (hypoglycemic) O24.415
    puerperal O24.439
      diet controlled O24.430
      insulin (and diet) controlled O24.434
      oral drug controlled (antidiabetic) (hypoglycemic) O24.435
  hepatogenous E13.9
  idiopathic — *see* Diabetes, type 1
  inadequately controlled — *code to* Diabetes, by type, with hyperglycemia
  insipidus E23.2
    nephrogenic N25.1
    pituitary E23.2
    vasopressin resistant N25.1
  insulin dependent — *code to* type of diabetes
  juvenile-onset — *see* Diabetes, type 1
  ketosis-prone — *see* Diabetes, type 1
  latent R73.03
  neonatal (transient) P70.2
  non-insulin dependent — *code to* type of diabetes
  out of control — *code to* Diabetes, by type, with hyperglycemia
  phosphate E83.39
  poorly controlled — *code to* Diabetes, by type, with hyperglycemia
  postpancreatectomy — *see* Diabetes, specified type NEC
  postprocedural — *see* Diabetes, specified type NEC
  secondary diabetes mellitus NEC — *see* Diabetes, specified type NEC
  specified type NEC E13.9
    with
      amyotrophy E13.44
      arthropathy NEC E13.618
      autonomic (poly)neuropathy E13.43
      cataract E13.36
      Charcot's joints E13.610
      chronic kidney disease E13.22
      circulatory complication NEC E13.59
      complication E13.8
        specified NEC E13.69
      dermatitis E13.620
      foot ulcer E13.621
      gangrene E13.52
      gastroparalysis E13.43
      gastroparesis E13.43
      glomerulonephrosis, intracapillary E13.21
      glomerulosclerosis, intercapillary E13.21
      hyperglycemia E13.65
      hyperosmolarity E13.00
        with coma E13.01
      hypoglycemia E13.649
        with coma E13.641
      ketoacidosis E13.10
        with coma E13.11
      kidney complications NEC E13.29
      Kimmelsteil-Wilson disease E13.21
      mononeuropathy E13.41
      myasthenia E13.44
      necrobiosis lipoidica E13.620
      nephropathy E13.21
      neuralgia E13.42
      neurologic complication NEC E13.49
      neuropathic arthropathy E13.610
      neuropathy E13.40
      ophthalmic complication NEC E13.39
      oral complication NEC E13.638
      periodontal disease E13.630
      peripheral angiopathy E13.51
        with gangrene E13.52
      polyneuropathy E13.42
      renal complication NEC E13.29
      renal tubular degeneration E13.29
      retinopathy E13.319
        with macular edema E13.311
        resolved following treatment E13.37 ☑
        nonproliferative E13.329 ☑
          with macular edema E13.321 ☑
          mild E13.329 ☑
            with macular edema E13.321 ☑
          moderate E13.339 ☑

Diabetes, diabetic — *continued*
  specified type — *continued*
    with — *continued*
      retinopathy — *continued*
        nonproliferative — *continued*
          moderate — *continued*
            with macular edema E13.331 ☑
          severe E13.349 ☑
            with macular edema E13.341 ☑
        proliferative E13.359 ☑
          with
            combined traction retinal detachment and rhegmatogenous retinal detachment E13.354 ☑
            macular edema E13.351 ☑
            stable proliferative diabetic retinopathy E13.355 ☑
            traction retinal detachment involving the macula E13.352 ☑
            traction retinal detachment not involving the macula E13.353 ☑
      skin complication NEC E13.628
      skin ulcer NEC E13.622
  steroid-induced — *see* Diabetes, due to, drug or chemical
  type 1 E10.9
    with
      amyotrophy E10.44
      arthropathy NEC E10.618
      autonomic (poly)neuropathy E10.43
      cataract E10.36
      Charcot's joints E10.610
      chronic kidney disease E10.22
      circulatory complication NEC E10.59
      complication E10.8
        specified NEC E10.69
      dermatitis E10.620
      foot ulcer E10.621
      gangrene E10.52
      gastroparalysis E10.43
      gastroparesis E10.43
      glomerulonephrosis, intracapillary E10.21
      glomerulosclerosis, intercapillary E10.21
      hyperglycemia E10.65
      hypoglycemia E10.649
        with coma E10.641
      ketoacidosis E10.10
        with coma E10.11
      kidney complications NEC E10.29
      Kimmelsteil-Wilson disease E10.21
      mononeuropathy E10.41
      myasthenia E10.44
      necrobiosis lipoidica E10.620
      nephropathy E10.21
      neuralgia E10.42
      neurologic complication NEC E10.49
      neuropathic arthropathy E10.610
      neuropathy E10.40
      ophthalmic complication NEC E10.39
      oral complication NEC E10.638
      osteomyelitis E10.69
      periodontal disease E10.630
      peripheral angiopathy E10.51
        with gangrene E10.52
      polyneuropathy E10.42
      renal complication NEC E10.29
      renal tubular degeneration E10.29
      retinopathy E10.319
        with macular edema E10.311
        resolved following treatment E10.37 ☑
        nonproliferative E10.329 ☑
          with macular edema E10.321 ☑
          mild E10.329 ☑
            with macular edema E10.321 ☑
          moderate E10.339 ☑
            with macular edema E10.331 ☑
          severe E10.349 ☑
            with macular edema E10.341 ☑
        proliferative E10.359 ☑
          with
            combined traction retinal detachment and rhegmatogenous retinal detachment E10.354 ☑
            macular edema E10.351 ☑
            stable proliferative diabetic retinopathy E10.355 ☑
            traction retinal detachment involving the macula E10.352 ☑

Diabetes, diabetic — *continued*
  type 1 — *continued*
    with — *continued*
      retinopathy — *continued*
        proliferative — *continued*
          with — *continued*
            traction retinal detachment not involving the macula E10.353 ☑
      skin complication NEC E10.628
      skin ulcer NEC E10.622
  type 2 E11.9
    with
      amyotrophy E11.44
      arthropathy NEC E11.618
      autonomic (poly)neuropathy E11.43
      cataract E11.36
      Charcot's joints E11.610
      chronic kidney disease E11.22
      circulatory complication NEC E11.59
      complication E11.8
        specified NEC E11.69
      dermatitis E11.620
      foot ulcer E11.621
      gangrene E11.52
      gastroparalysis E11.43
      gastroparesis E11.43
      glomerulonephrosis, intracapillary E11.21
      glomerulosclerosis, intercapillary E11.21
      hyperglycemia E11.65
      hyperosmolarity E11.00
        with coma E11.01
      hypoglycemia E11.649
        with coma E11.641
      ketoacidosis E11.10
        with coma E11.11
      kidney complications NEC E11.29
      Kimmelstiel-Wilson disease E11.21
      mononeuropathy E11.41
      myasthenia E11.44
      necrobiosis lipoidica E11.620
      nephropathy E11.21
      neuralgia E11.42
      neurologic complication NEC E11.49
      neuropathic arthropathy E11.610
      neuropathy E11.40
      ophthalmic complication NEC E11.39
      oral complication NEC E11.638
      osteomyelitis E11.69
      periodontal disease E11.630
      peripheral angiopathy E11.51
        with gangrene E11.52
      polyneuropathy E11.42
      renal complication NEC E11.29
      renal tubular degeneration E11.29
      retinopathy E11.319
        with macular edema E11.311
        resolved following treatment E11.37 ☑
        nonproliferative E11.329 ☑
          with macular edema E11.321 ☑
          mild E11.329 ☑
            with macular edema E11.321 ☑
          moderate E11.339 ☑
            with macular edema E11.331 ☑
          severe E11.349 ☑
            with macular edema E11.341 ☑
        proliferative E11.359 ☑
          with
            combined traction retinal detachment and rhegmatogenous retinal detachment E11.354 ☑
            macular edema E11.351 ☑
            stable proliferative diabetic retinopathy E11.355 ☑
            traction retinal detachment involving the macula E11.352 ☑
            traction retinal detachment not involving the macula E11.353 ☑
      skin complication NEC E11.628
      skin ulcer NEC E11.622
  uncontrolled
    meaning
      hyperglycemia — *see* Diabetes, by type, with, hyperglycemia
      hypoglycemia — *see* Diabetes, by type, with, hypoglycemia
Diacyclothrombopathia D69.1
Diagnosis deferred R69

Dialysis (intermittent) (treatment)
  noncompliance (with) Z91.15
  renal (hemodialysis) (peritoneal), status Z99.2
  retina, retinal — *see* Detachment, retina, with retinal, dialysis
Diamond-Blackfan anemia (congenital hypoplastic) D61.01
Diamond-Gardener syndrome (autoerythrocyte sensitization) D69.2
Diaper rash L22
Diaphoresis (excessive) R61
Diaphragm — *see* condition
Diaphragmalgia R07.1
Diaphragmatitis, diaphragmitis J98.6
Diaphysial aclasis Q78.6
Diaphysitis — *see* Osteomyelitis, specified type NEC
Diarrhea, diarrheal (disease) (infantile) (inflammatory) R19.7
  achlorhydric K31.83
  allergic K52.29
    due to
      colitis — *see* Colitis, allergic
      enteritis — *see* Enteritis, allergic
  amebic — *see also* Amebiasis A06.0
    with abscess — *see* Abscess, amebic
    acute A06.0
    chronic A06.1
    nondysenteric A06.2
  bacillary — *see* Dysentery, bacillary
  balantidial A07.0
  cachectic NEC K52.89
  Chilomastix A07.8
  choleriformis A00.1
  chronic (noninfectious) K52.9
  coccidial A07.3
  Cochin-China K90.1
    strongyloidiasis B78.0
  Dientamoeba A07.8
  dietetic — *see also* Diarrhea, allergic K52.29
  drug-induced K52.1
  due to
    bacteria A04.9
      specified NEC A04.8
    Campylobacter A04.5
    Capillaria philippinensis B81.1
    Clostridium difficile
      not specified as recurrent A04.72
      recurrent A04.71
    Clostridium perfringens (C) (F) A04.8
    Cryptosporidium A07.2
    drugs K52.1
    Escherichia coli A04.4
      enteroaggregative A04.4
      enterohemorrhagic A04.3
      enteroinvasive A04.2
      enteropathogenic A04.0
      enterotoxigenic A04.1
      specified NEC A04.4
    food hypersensitivity — *see also* Diarrhea, allergic K52.29
    Necator americanus B76.1
    S. japonicum B65.2
    specified organism NEC A08.8
      bacterial A04.8
      viral A08.39
    Staphylococcus A04.8
    Trichuris trichiuria B79
    virus — *see* Enteritis, viral
    Yersinia enterocolitica A04.6
  dysenteric A09
  endemic A09
  epidemic A09
  flagellate A07.9
  Flexner's (ulcerative) A03.1
  functional K59.1
    following gastrointestinal surgery K91.89
    psychogenic F45.8
  Giardia lamblia A07.1
  giardial A07.1
  hill K90.1
  infectious A09
  malarial — *see* Malaria
  mite B88.0
  mycotic NEC B49
  neonatal (noninfectious) P78.3
  nervous F45.8
  neurogenic K59.1
  noninfectious K52.9

Diarrhea, diarrheal — *continued*
  postgastrectomy K91.1
  postvagotomy K91.1
  protozoal A07.9
    specified NEC A07.8
  psychogenic F45.8
  specified
    bacterium NEC A04.8
    virus NEC A08.39
  strongyloidiasis B78.0
  toxic K52.1
  trichomonal A07.8
  tropical K90.1
  tuberculous A18.32
  viral — *see* Enteritis, viral
Diastasis
  cranial bones M84.88
    congenital NEC Q75.8
  joint (traumatic) — *see* Dislocation
  muscle M62.00
    ankle M62.07- ☑
    congenital Q79.8
    foot M62.07- ☑
    forearm M62.03- ☑
    hand M62.04- ☑
    lower leg M62.06- ☑
    pelvic region M62.05- ☑
    shoulder region M62.01- ☑
    specified site NEC M62.08
    thigh M62.05- ☑
    upper arm M62.02- ☑
  recti (abdomen)
    complicating delivery O71.89
    congenital Q79.59
Diastema, tooth, teeth, fully erupted M26.32
Diastematomyelia Q06.2
Diataxia, cerebral G80.4
Diathesis
  allergic — *see* History, allergy
  bleeding (familial) D69.9
  cystine (familial) E72.00
  gouty — *see* Gout
  hemorrhagic (familial) D69.9
    newborn NEC P53
  spasmophilic R29.0
Diaz's disease or osteochondrosis (juvenile) (talus) — *see* Osteochondrosis, juvenile, tarsus
Dibothriocephalus, dibothriocephaliasis (latus) (infection) (infestation) B70.0
  larval B70.1
Dicephalus, dicephaly Q89.4
Dichotomy, teeth K00.2
Dichromat, dichromatopsia (congenital) — *see* Deficiency, color vision
Dichuchwa A65
Dicroceliasis B66.2
Didelphia, didelphys — *see* Double uterus
Didymytis N45.1
  with orchitis N45.3
Dietary
  inadequacy or deficiency E63.9
  surveillance and counseling Z71.3
Dietl's crisis N13.8
Dieulafoy lesion (hemorrhagic)
  duodenum K31.82
  esophagus K22.8
  intestine (colon) K63.81
  stomach K31.82
Difficult, difficulty (in)
  acculturation Z60.3
  feeding R63.3
    newborn P92.9
      breast P92.5
      specified NEC P92.8
    nonorganic (infant or child) F98.29
  intubation, in anesthesia T88.4 ☑
  mechanical, gastroduodenal stoma K91.89
    causing obstruction — *see also* Obstruction, intestine, postoperative K91.30
  micturition
    need to immediately re-void R39.191
    position dependent R39.192
    specified NEC R39.198
  reading (developmental) F81.0
    secondary to emotional disorders F93.9
  spelling (specific) F81.81
    with reading disorder F81.89
    due to inadequate teaching Z55.8

▽ **Subterms under main terms may continue to next column or page**   ☑ **Additional Character Required — Refer to the Tabular List for Character Selection**   **99**

Diabetes, diabetic — Difficult, difficulty

Difficult, difficulty — *continued*
swallowing — *see* Dysphagia
walking R26.2
work
conditions NEC Z56.5
schedule Z56.3
Diffuse — *see* condition
Digestive — *see* condition
Dihydropyrimidine dehydrogenase disease (DPD) E88.89
Diktyoma — *see* Neoplasm, malignant, by site
Dilaceration, tooth K00.4
Dilatation
anus K59.8
venule — *see* Hemorrhoids
aorta (focal) (general) — *see* Ectasia, aorta
with aneuysm — *see* Aneurysm, aorta
congenital Q25.44
artery — *see* Aneurysm
bladder (sphincter) N32.89
congenital Q64.79
blood vessel I99.8
bronchial J47.9
with
exacerbation (acute) J47.1
lower respiratory infection J47.0
calyx (due to obstruction) — *see* Hydronephrosis
capillaries I78.8
cardiac (acute) (chronic) — *see also* Hypertrophy, cardiac
congenital Q24.8
valve NEC Q24.8
pulmonary Q22.3
valve — *see* Endocarditis
cavum septi pellucidi Q06.8
cervix (uteri) — *see also* Incompetency, cervix
incomplete, poor, slow complicating delivery O62.0
colon K59.39
congenital Q43.1
psychogenic F45.8
toxic K59.31
common duct (acquired) K83.8
congenital Q44.5
cystic duct (acquired) K82.8
congenital Q44.5
duct, mammary — *see* Ectasia, mammary duct
duodenum K59.8
esophagus K22.8
congenital Q39.5
due to achalasia K22.0
eustachian tube, congenital Q17.8
gallbladder K82.8
gastric — *see* Dilatation, stomach
heart (acute) (chronic) — *see also* Hypertrophy, cardiac
congenital Q24.8
valve — *see* Endocarditis
ileum K59.8
psychogenic F45.8
jejunum K59.8
psychogenic F45.8
kidney (calyx) (collecting structures) (cystic) (parenchyma) (pelvis) (idiopathic) N28.89
lacrimal passages or duct — *see* Disorder, lacrimal system, changes
lymphatic vessel I89.0
mammary duct — *see* Ectasia, mammary duct
Meckel's diverticulum (congenital) Q43.0
malignant — *see* Table of Neoplasms, small intestine, malignant
myocardium (acute) (chronic) — *see* Hypertrophy, cardiac
organ or site, congenital NEC — *see* Distortion
pancreatic duct K86.89
pericardium — *see* Pericarditis
pharynx J39.2
prostate N42.89
pulmonary
artery (idiopathic) I28.8
valve, congenital Q22.3
pupil H57.04
rectum K59.39
saccule, congenital Q16.5
salivary gland (duct) K11.8
sphincter ani K62.89
stomach K31.89
acute K31.0
psychogenic F45.8
submaxillary duct K11.8

Dilatation — *continued*
trachea, congenital Q32.1
ureter (idiopathic) N28.82
congenital Q62.2
due to obstruction N13.4
urethra (acquired) N36.8
vasomotor I73.9
vein I86.8
ventricular, ventricle (acute) (chronic) — *see also* Hypertrophy, cardiac
cerebral, congenital Q04.8
venule NEC I86.8
vesical orifice N32.89
Dilated, dilation — *see* Dilatation
Diminished, diminution
hearing (acuity) — *see* Deafness
sense or sensation (cold) (heat) (tactile) (vibratory) R20.8
vision NEC H54.7
vital capacity R94.2
Diminuta taenia B71.0
Dimitri-Sturge-Weber disease Q85.8
Dimple
congenital sacral Q82.6
parasacral Q82.6
pilonidal or postanal — *see* Cyst, pilonidal
Dioctophyme renalis (infection) (infestation) B83.8
Dipetalonemiasis B74.4
Diphallus Q55.69
Diphtheria, diphtheritic (gangrenous) (hemorrhagic) A36.9
carrier (suspected) Z22.2
cutaneous A36.3
faucial A36.0
infection of wound A36.3
laryngeal A36.2
myocarditis A36.81
nasal, anterior A36.89
nasopharyngeal A36.1
neurological complication A36.89
pharyngeal A36.0
specified site NEC A36.89
tonsillar A36.0
Diphyllobothriasis (intestine) B70.0
larval B70.1
Diplacusis H93.22- ✓
Diplegia (upper limbs) G83.0
congenital (cerebral) G80.8
facial G51.0
lower limbs G82.20
spastic G80.1
Diplococcus, diplococcal — *see* condition
Diplopia H53.2
Dipsomania F10.20
with
psychosis — *see* Psychosis, alcoholic
remission F10.21
Dipylidiasis B71.1
DIRA (deficiency of interleukin 1 receptor antagonist) M04.8
Direction, teeth, abnormal, fully erupted M26.30
Dirofilariasis B74.8
Dirt-eating child F98.3
Disability, disabilities
heart — *see* Disease, heart
intellectual F79
with
autistic features F84.9
mild (I.Q. 50-69) F70
moderate (I.Q. 35-49) F71
profound (I.Q. under 20) F73
severe (I.Q. 20-34) F72
specified level NEC F78
knowledge acquisition F81.9
learning F81.9
limiting activities Z73.6
spelling, specific F81.81
Disappearance of family member Z63.4
Disarticulation — *see* Amputation
meaning traumatic amputation — *see* Amputation, traumatic
Discharge (from)
abnormal finding in — *see* Abnormal, specimen
breast (female) (male) N64.52
diencephalic autonomic idiopathic — *see* Epilepsy, specified NEC
ear — *see also* Otorrhea
blood — *see* Otorrhagia

Discharge — *continued*
excessive urine R35.8
nipple N64.52
penile R36.9
postnasal R09.82
prison, anxiety concerning Z65.2
urethral R36.9
without blood R36.0
hematospermia R36.1
vaginal N89.8
Discitis, diskitis M46.40
cervical region M46.42
cervicothoracic region M46.43
lumbar region M46.46
lumbosacral region M46.47
multiple sites M46.49
occipito-atlanto-axial region M46.41
pyogenic — *see* Infection, intervertebral disc, pyogenic
sacrococcygeal region M46.48
thoracic region M46.44
thoracolumbar region M46.45
Discoid
meniscus (congenital) Q68.6
semilunar cartilage (congenital) — *see* Derangement, knee, meniscus, specified NEC
Discoloration
nails L60.8
teeth (posteruptive) K03.7
during formation K00.8
Discomfort
chest R07.89
visual H53.14- ✓
Discontinuity, ossicles, ear H74.2- ✓
Discord (with)
boss Z56.4
classmates Z55.4
counselor Z64.4
employer Z56.4
family Z63.8
fellow employees Z56.4
in-laws Z63.1
landlord Z59.2
lodgers Z59.2
neighbors Z59.2
probation officer Z64.4
social worker Z64.4
teachers Z55.4
workmates Z56.4
Discordant connection
atrioventricular (congenital) Q20.5
ventriculoarterial Q20.3
Discrepancy
centric occlusion maximum intercuspation M26.55
leg length (acquired) — *see* Deformity, limb, unequal length
congenital — *see* Defect, reduction, lower limb
uterine size date O26.84- ✓
Discrimination
ethnic Z60.5
political Z60.5
racial Z60.5
religious Z60.5
sex Z60.5
Disease, diseased — *see also* Syndrome
absorbent system I87.8
acid-peptic K30
Acosta's T70.29 ✓
Adams-Stokes (-Morgagni) (syncope with heart block) I45.9
Addison's anemia (pernicious) D51.0
adenoids (and tonsils) J35.9
adrenal (capsule) (cortex) (gland) (medullary) E27.9
hyperfunction E27.0
specified NEC E27.8
ainhum L94.6
airway
obstructive, chronic J44.9
due to
cotton dust J66.0
specific organic dusts NEC J66.8
reactive — *see* Asthma
akamushi (scrub typhus) A75.3
Albers-Schönberg (marble bones) Q78.2
Albert's — *see* Tendinitis, Achilles
alimentary canal K63.9
alligator-skin Q80.9
acquired L85.0
alpha heavy chain C88.3

Disease, diseased — continued
- alpine T70.29 ☑
- altitude T70.20 ☑
- alveolar ridge
  - edentulous K06.9
    - specified NEC K06.8
- alveoli, teeth K08.9
- Alzheimer's G30.9 *[F02.80]*
  - with behavioral disturbance G30.9 *[F02.81]*
  - early onset G30.0 *[F02.80]*
    - with behavioral disturbance G30.0 *[F02.81]*
  - late onset G30.1 *[F02.80]*
    - with behavioral disturbance G30.1 *[F02.81]*
  - specified NEC G30.8 *[F02.80]*
    - with behavioral disturbance G30.8 *[F02.81]*
- amyloid — see Amyloidosis
- Andersen's (glycogenosis IV) E74.09
- Andes T70.29 ☑
- Andrews' (bacterid) L08.89
- angiospastic I73.9
  - cerebral G45.9
  - vein I87.8
- anterior
  - chamber H21.9
  - horn cell G12.29
- antiglomerular basement membrane (anti- GBM) antibody M31.0
  - tubulo-interstitial nephritis N12
- antral — see Sinusitis, maxillary
- anus K62.9
  - specified NEC K62.89
- aorta (nonsyphilitic) I77.9
  - syphilitic NEC A52.02
- aortic (heart) (valve) I35.9
  - rheumatic I06.9
- Apollo B30.3
- aponeuroses — see Enthesopathy
- appendix K38.9
  - specified NEC K38.8
- aqueous (chamber) H21.9
- Arnold-Chiari — see Arnold-Chiari disease
- arterial I77.9
  - occlusive — see Occlusion, by site
    - due to stricture or stenosis I77.1
  - peripheral I73.9
- arteriocardiorenal — see Hypertension, cardiorenal
- arteriolar (generalized) (obliterative) I77.9
- arteriorenal — see Hypertension, kidney
- arteriosclerotic — see also Arteriosclerosis
  - cardiovascular — see Disease, heart, ischemic, atherosclerotic
  - coronary (artery) — see Disease, heart, ischemic, atherosclerotic
  - heart — see Disease, heart, ischemic, atherosclerotic
- artery I77.9
  - cerebral I67.9
  - coronary I25.10
    - with angina pectoris — see Arteriosclerosis, coronary (artery)
  - peripheral I73.9
- arthropod-borne NOS (viral) A94
  - specified type NEC A93.8
- atticoantral, chronic H66.20
  - left H66.22
    - with right H66.23
  - right H66.21
    - with left H66.23
- auditory canal — see Disorder, ear, external
- auricle, ear NEC — see Disorder, pinna
- Australian X A83.4
- autoimmune (systemic) NOS M35.9
  - hemolytic (cold type) (warm type) D59.1
    - drug-induced D59.0
  - thyroid E06.3
- autoinflammatory M04.9
  - NOD2-associated M04.8
  - specified type NEC M04.8
- aviator's — see Effect, adverse, high altitude
- Ayerza's (pulmonary artery sclerosis with pulmonary hypertension) I27.0
- Babington's (familial hemorrhagic telangiectasia) I78.0
- bacterial A49.9
  - specified NEC A48.8
  - zoonotic A28.9
    - specified type NEC A28.8
- Baelz's (cheilitis glandularis apostematosa) K13.0
- bagasse J67.1
- balloon — see Effect, adverse, high altitude

Disease, diseased — continued
- Bang's (brucella abortus) A23.1
- Bannister's T78.3
- barometer makers' — see Poisoning, mercury
- Barraquer (-Simons') (progressive lipodystrophy) E88.1
- Barrett's — see Barrett's, esophagus
- Bartholin's gland N75.9
- basal ganglia G25.9
  - degenerative G23.9
    - specified NEC G23.8
  - specified NEC G25.89
- Basedow's (exophthalmic goiter) — see Hyperthyroidism, with, goiter (diffuse)
- Bateman's B08.1
- Batten-Steinert G71.11
- Battey A31.0
- Beard's (neurasthenia) F48.8
- Becker
  - idiopathic mural endomyocardial I42.3
  - myotonia congenita G71.12
- Begbie's (exophthalmic goiter) — see Hyperthyroidism, with, goiter (diffuse)
- behavioral, organic F07.9
- Beigel's (white piedra) B36.2
- Benson's — see Deposit, crystalline
- Bernard-Soulier (thrombopathy) D69.1
- Bernhardt (-Roth) — see Mononeuropathy, lower limb, meralgia paresthetica
- Biermer's (pernicious anemia) D51.0
- bile duct (common) (hepatic) K83.9
  - with calculus, stones — see Calculus, bile duct
  - specified NEC K83.8
- biliary (tract) K83.9
  - specified NEC K83.8
- Billroth's — see Spina bifida
- bird fancier's J67.2
- black lung J60
- bladder N32.9
  - in (due to)
    - schistosomiasis (bilharziasis) B65.0 *[N33]*
  - specified NEC N32.89
- bleeder's D66
- blood D75.9
  - forming organs D75.9
  - vessel I99.9
- Bloodgood's — see Mastopathy, cystic
- Bodechtel-Guttmann (subacute sclerosing panencephalitis) A81.1
- bone — see also Disorder, bone
  - aluminum M83.4
  - fibrocystic NEC
    - jaw M27.49
- bone-marrow D75.9
- Borna A83.9
- Bornholm (epidemic pleurodynia) B33.0
- Bouchard's (myopathic dilatation of the stomach) K31.0
- Bouillaud's (rheumatic heart disease) I01.9
- Bourneville (-Brissaud) (tuberous sclerosis) Q85.1
- Bouveret (-Hoffmann) (paroxysmal tachycardia) I47.9
- bowel K63.9
  - functional K59.9
    - psychogenic F45.8
- brain G93.9
  - arterial, artery I67.9
  - arteriosclerotic I67.2
  - congenital Q04.9
  - degenerative — see Degeneration, brain
  - inflammatory — see Encephalitis
  - organic G93.9
    - arteriosclerotic I67.2
  - parasitic NEC B71.9 *[G94]*
  - senile NEC G31.1
  - specified NEC G93.89
- breast — see also Disorder, breast N64.9
  - cystic (chronic) — see Mastopathy, cystic
  - fibrocystic — see Mastopathy, cystic
  - Paget's
    - female, unspecified side C50.91- ☑
    - male, unspecified side C50.92- ☑
  - specified NEC N64.89
- Breda's — see Yaws
- Bretonneau's (diphtheritic malignant angina) A36.0
- Bright's — see Nephritis
  - arteriosclerotic — see Hypertension, kidney
- Brill's (recrudescent typhus) A75.1
- Brill-Zinsser (recrudescent typhus) A75.1
- Brion-Kayser — see Fever, paratyphoid

Disease, diseased — continued
- broad
  - beta E78.2
  - ligament (noninflammatory) N83.9
    - inflammatory — see Disease, pelvis, inflammatory
    - specified NEC N83.8
- Brocq-Duhring (dermatitis herpetiformis) L13.0
- Brocq's
  - meaning
    - dermatitis herpetiformis L13.0
    - prurigo L28.2
- bronchopulmonary J98.4
- bronchus NEC J98.09
- bronze Addison's E27.1
  - tuberculous A18.7
- budgerigar fancier's J67.2
- Buerger's (thromboangiitis obliterans) I73.1
- bullous L13.9
  - chronic of childhood L12.2
  - specified NEC L13.8
- Bürger-Grütz (essential familial hyperlipemia) E78.3
- bursa — see Bursopathy
- caisson T70.3 ☑
- California — see Coccidioidomycosis
- capillaries I78.9
  - specified NEC I78.8
- Carapata A68.0
- cardiac — see Disease, heart
- cardiopulmonary, chronic I27.9
- cardiorenal (hepatic) (hypertensive) (vascular) — see Hypertension, cardiorenal
- cardiovascular (atherosclerotic) I25.10
  - with angina pectoris — see Arteriosclerosis, coronary (artery),
  - congenital Q28.9
  - hypertensive — see Hypertension, heart
  - newborn P29.9
    - specified NEC P29.89
  - renal (hypertensive) — see Hypertension, cardiorenal
  - syphilitic (asymptomatic) A52.00
- cartilage — see Disorder, cartilage
- Castellani's A69.8
- Castleman (unicentric) (multicentric) D47.Z2
  - HHV-8-associated — see also Herpesvirus, human, 8 D47.Z2
- cat-scratch A28.1
- Cavare's (familial periodic paralysis) G72.3
- cecum K63.9
- celiac (adult) (infantile) (with steatorrhea) K90.0
- cellular tissue L98.9
- central core G71.2
- cerebellar, cerebellum — see Disease, brain
- cerebral — see also Disease, brain
  - degenerative — see Degeneration, brain
- cerebrospinal G96.9
- cerebrovascular I67.9
  - acute I67.89
    - embolic I63.4- ☑
    - thrombotic I63.3- ☑
  - arteriosclerotic I67.2
  - hereditary NEC I67.858
  - specified NEC I67.89
- cervix (uteri) (noninflammatory) N88.9
  - inflammatory — see Cervicitis
  - specified NEC N88.8
- Chabert's A22.9
- Chandler's (osteochondritis dissecans, hip) — see Osteochondritis, dissecans, hip
- Charlouis — see Yaws
- Chédiak-Steinbrinck (-Higashi) (congenital gigantism of peroxidase granules) E70.330
- chest J98.9
- Chiari's (hepatic vein thrombosis) I82.0
- Chicago B40.9
- Chignon B36.8
- chigo, chigoe B88.1
- childhood granulomatous D71
- Chinese liver fluke B66.1
- chlamydial A74.9
  - specified NEC A74.89
- cholecystic K82.9
- choroid H31.9
  - specified NEC H31.8
- Christmas D67
- chronic bullous of childhood L12.2
- chylomicron retention E78.3

Disease, diseased — *continued*
- ciliary body H21.9
  - specified NEC H21.89
- circulatory (system) NEC I99.8
  - newborn P29.9
  - syphilitic A52.00
    - congenital A50.54
- coagulation factor deficiency (congenital) — *see* Defect, coagulation
- coccidioidal — *see* Coccidioidomycosis
- cold
  - agglutinin or hemoglobinuria D59.1
    - paroxysmal D59.6
  - hemagglutinin (chronic) D59.1
- collagen NOS (nonvascular) (vascular) M35.9
  - specified NEC M35.8
- colon K63.9
  - functional K59.9
    - congenital Q43.2
  - ischemic — *see also* Ischemia, intestine, acute K55.039
- colonic inflammatory bowel, unclassified (IBDU) K52.3
- combined system — *see* Degeneration, combined
- compressed air T70.3 ☑
- Concato's (pericardial polyserositis) A19.9
  - nontubercular I31.1
  - pleural — *see* Pleurisy, with effusion
- conjunctiva H11.9
  - chlamydial A74.0
  - specified NEC H11.89
  - viral B30.9
    - specified NEC B30.8
- connective tissue, systemic (diffuse) M35.9
  - in (due to)
    - hypogammaglobulinemia D80.1 *[M36.8]*
    - ochronosis E70.29 *[M36.8]*
  - specified NEC M35.8
- Conor and Bruch's (boutonneuse fever) A77.1
- Cooper's — *see* Mastopathy, cystic
- Cori's (glycogenosis III) E74.03
- corkhandler's or corkworker's J67.3
- cornea H18.9
  - specified NEC H18.89- ☑
- coronary (artery) — *see* Disease, heart, ischemic, atherosclerotic
  - congenital Q24.5
  - ostial, syphilitic (aortic) (mitral) (pulmonary) A52.03
- corpus cavernosum N48.9
  - specified NEC N48.89
- Cotugno's — *see* Sciatica
- coxsackie (virus) NEC B34.1
- cranial nerve NOS G52.9
- Creutzfeldt-Jakob — *see* Creutzfeldt-Jakob disease or syndrome
- Crocq's (acrocyanosis) I73.89
- Crohn's — *see* Enteritis, regional
- Curschmann G71.11
- cystic
  - breast (chronic) — *see* Mastopathy, cystic
  - kidney, congenital Q61.9
  - liver, congenital Q44.6
  - lung J98.4
    - congenital Q33.0
- cytomegalic inclusion (generalized) B25.9
  - with pneumonia B25.0
  - congenital P35.1
- cytomegaloviral B25.9
  - specified NEC B25.8
- Czerny's (periodic hydrarthrosis of the knee) — *see* Effusion, joint, knee
- Daae (-Finsen) (epidemic pleurodynia) B33.0
- Darling's — *see* Histoplasmosis capsulati
- de Quervain's (tendon sheath) M65.4
  - thyroid (subacute granulomatous thyroiditis) E06.1
- Débove's (splenomegaly) R16.1
- deer fly — *see* Tularemia
- Degos' I77.89
- demyelinating, demyelinizating (nervous system) G37.9
  - multiple sclerosis G35
  - specified NEC G37.8
- dense deposit — *see also* N00-N07 with fourth character .6 N05.6
- deposition, hydroxyapatite — *see* Disease, hydroxyapatite deposition
- Devergie's (pityriasis rubra pilaris) L44.0
- Devic's G36.0
- diaphorase deficiency D74.0
- diaphragm J98.6

Disease, diseased — *continued*
- diarrheal, infectious NEC A09
- digestive system K92.9
  - specified NEC K92.89
- disc, degenerative — *see* Degeneration, intervertebral disc
- discogenic — *see also* Displacement, intervertebral disc NEC
  - with myelopathy — *see* Disorder, disc, with, myelopathy
- diverticular — *see* Diverticula
- Dubois (thymus) A50.59 *[E35]*
- Duchenne-Griesinger G71.01
- Duchenne's
  - muscular dystrophy G71.01
  - pseudohypertrophy, muscles G71.01
- ductless glands E34.9
- Duhring's (dermatitis herpetiformis) L13.0
- duodenum K31.9
  - specified NEC K31.89
- Dupré's (meningism) R29.1
- Dupuytren's (muscle contracture) M72.0
- Durand-Nicholas-Favre (climatic bubo) A55
- Duroziez's (congenital mitral stenosis) Q23.2
- ear — *see* Disorder, ear
- Eberth's — *see* Fever, typhoid
- Ebola (virus) A98.4
- Ebstein's heart Q22.5
- Echinococcus — *see* Echinococcus
- echovirus NEC B34.1
- Eddowes' (brittle bones and blue sclera) Q78.0
- edentulous (alveolar) ridge K06.9
  - specified NEC K06.8
- Edsall's T67.2 ☑
- Eichstedt's (pityriasis versicolor) B36.0
- Eisenmenger's (irreversible) I27.83
- Ellis-van Creveld (chondroectodermal dysplasia) Q77.6
- end stage renal (ESRD) N18.6
  - due to hypertension I12.0
- endocrine glands or system NEC E34.9
- endomyocardial (eosinophilic) I42.3
- English (rickets) E55.0
- enteroviral, enterovirus NEC B34.1
  - central nervous system NEC A88.8
- epidemic B99.9
  - specified NEC B99.8
- epididymis N50.9
- epidural — *see* Erb (-Landouzy) G71.02
- Erb (-Landouzy) G71.02
- Erdheim-Chester (ECD) E88.89
- esophagus K22.9
  - functional K22.4
  - psychogenic F45.8
  - specified NEC K22.8
- Eulenburg's (congenital paramyotonia) G71.19
- eustachian tube — *see* Disorder, eustachian tube
- external
  - auditory canal — *see* Disorder, ear, external
  - ear — *see* Disorder, ear, external
- extrapyramidal G25.9
  - specified NEC G25.89
- eye H57.9
  - anterior chamber H21.9
  - inflammatory NEC H57.89
  - muscle (external) — *see* Strabismus
  - specified NEC H57.89
  - syphilitic — *see* Oculopathy, syphilitic
- eyeball H44.9
  - specified NEC H44.89
- eyelid — *see* Disorder, eyelid
  - specified NEC — *see* Disorder, eyelid, specified type NEC
- eyeworm of Africa B74.3
- facial nerve (seventh) G51.9
  - newborn (birth injury) P11.3
- Fahr (of brain) G23.8
- Fahr Volhard (of kidney) I12.- ☑
- fallopian tube (noninflammatory) N83.9
  - inflammatory — *see* Salpingo-oophoritis
  - specified NEC N83.8
- familial periodic paralysis G72.3
- Fanconi's (congenital pancytopenia) D61.09
- fascia NEC — *see also* Disorder, muscle
  - inflammatory — *see* Myositis
  - specified NEC M62.89
- Fauchard's (periodontitis) — *see* Periodontitis
- Favre-Durand-Nicolas (climatic bubo) A55
- Fede's K14.0
- Feer's — *see* Poisoning, mercury

Disease, diseased — *continued*
- female pelvic inflammatory — *see also* Disease, pelvis, inflammatory N73.9
  - syphilitic (secondary) A51.42
  - tuberculous A18.17
- Fernels' (aortic aneurysm) I71.9
- fibrocaseous of lung — *see* Tuberculosis, pulmonary
- fibrocystic — *see* Fibrocystic disease
- Fiedler's (leptospiral jaundice) A27.0
- fifth B08.3
- file-cutter's — *see* Poisoning, lead
- fish-skin Q80.9
  - acquired L85.0
- Flajani (-Basedow) (exophthalmic goiter) — *see* Hyperthyroidism, with, goiter (diffuse)
- flax-dresser's J66.1
- fluke — *see* Infestation, fluke
- foot and mouth B08.8
- foot process N04.9
- Forbes' (glycogenosis III) E74.03
- Fordyce-Fox (apocrine miliaria) L75.2
- Fordyce's (ectopic sebaceous glands) (mouth) Q38.6
- Forestier's (rhizomelic pseudopolyarthritis) M35.3
  - meaning ankylosing hyperostosis — *see* Hyperostosis, ankylosing
- Fothergill's
  - neuralgia — *see* Neuralgia, trigeminal
  - scarlatina anginosa A38.9
- Fournier (gangrene) N49.3
  - female N76.89
- fourth B08.8
- Fox (-Fordyce) (apocrine miliaria) L75.2
- Francis' — *see* Tularemia
- Franklin C88.2
- Frei's (climatic bubo) A55
- Friedreich's
  - combined systemic or ataxia G11.1
  - myoclonia G25.3
- frontal sinus — *see* Sinusitis, frontal
- fungus NEC B49
- Gaisböck's (polycythemia hypertonica) D75.1
- gallbladder K82.9
  - calculus — *see* Calculus, gallbladder
  - cholecystitis — *see* Cholecystitis
  - cholesterolosis K82.4
  - fistula — *see* Fistula, gallbladder
  - hydrops K82.1
  - obstruction — *see* Obstruction, gallbladder
  - perforation K82.2
  - specified NEC K82.8
- gamma heavy chain C88.2
- Gamna's (siderotic splenomegaly) D73.2
- Gamstorp's (adynamia episodica hereditaria) G72.3
- Gandy-Nanta (siderotic splenomegaly) D73.2
- ganister J62.8
- gastric — *see* Disease, stomach
- gastroesophageal reflux (GERD) K21.9
  - with esophagitis K21.0
- gastrointestinal (tract) K92.9
  - amyloid E85.4
  - functional K59.9
    - psychogenic F45.8
  - specified NEC K92.89
- Gee (-Herter) (-Heubner) (-Thaysen) (nontropical sprue) K90.0
- genital organs
  - female N94.9
  - male N50.9
- Gerhardt's (erythromelalgia) I73.81
- Gibert's (pityriasis rosea) L42
- Gierke's (glycogenosis I) E74.01
- Gilles de la Tourette's (motor-verbal tic) F95.2
- gingiva K06.9
  - plaque induced K05.00
  - specified NEC K06.8
- gland (lymph) I89.9
- Glanzmann's (hereditary hemorrhagic thrombasthenia) D69.1
- glass-blower's (cataract) — *see* Cataract, specified NEC
  - salivary gland hypertrophy K11.1
- Glisson's — *see* Rickets
- globe H44.9
  - specified NEC H44.89
- glomerular — *see also* Glomerulonephritis
  - with edema — *see* Nephrosis
  - acute — *see* Nephritis, acute
  - chronic — *see* Nephritis, chronic
  - minimal change N05.0

Disease, diseased — *continued*

glomerular — *see also* Glomerulonephritis — *continued*
  rapidly progressive N01.9
glycogen storage E74.00
  Andersen's E74.09
  Cori's E74.03
  Forbes' E74.03
  generalized E74.00
  glucose-6-phosphatase deficiency E74.01
  heart E74.02 *[143]*
  hepatorenal E74.09
  Hers' E74.09
  liver and kidney E74.09
  McArdle's E74.04
  muscle phosphofructokinase E74.09
  myocardium E74.02 *[143]*
  Pompe's E74.02
  Tauri's E74.09
  type 0 E74.09
  type I E74.01
  type II E74.02
  type III E74.03
  type IV E74.09
  type V E74.04
  type VI-XI E74.09
  Von Gierke's E74.01
Goldstein's (familial hemorrhagic telangiectasia) I78.0
gonococcal NOS A54.9
graft-versus-host (GVH) D89.813
  acute D89.810
  acute on chronic D89.812
  chronic D89.811
grainhandler's J67.8
granulomatous (childhood) (chronic) D71
Graves' (exophthalmic goiter) — *see* Hyperthyroidism, with, goiter (diffuse)
Griesinger's — *see* Ancylostomiasis
Grisel's M43.6
Gruby's (tinea tonsurans) B35.0
Guillain-Barré G61.0
Guinon's (motor-verbal tic) F95.2
gum K06.9
gynecological N94.9
H (Hartnup's) E72.02
Haff — *see* Poisoning, mercury
Hageman (congenital factor XII deficiency) D68.2
hair (color) (shaft) L67.9
  follicles L73.9
    specified NEC L73.8
Hamman's (spontaneous mediastinal emphysema) J98.2
hand, foot and mouth B08.4
Hansen's — *see* Leprosy
Hantavirus, with pulmonary manifestations B33.4
  with renal manifestations A98.5
Harada's H30.81- ☑
Hartnup (pellagra-cerebellar ataxia-renal aminoaciduria) E72.02
Hart's (pellagra-cerebellar ataxia-renal aminoaciduria) E72.02
Hashimoto's (struma lymphomatosa) E06.3
Hb — *see* Disease, hemoglobin
heart (organic) I51.9
  with
    pulmonary edema (acute) — *see also* Failure, ventricular, left I50.1
    rheumatic fever (conditions in I00)
      active I01.9
        with chorea I02.0
        specified NEC I01.8
      inactive or quiescent (with chorea) I09.9
        specified NEC I09.89
  amyloid E85.4 *[143]*
  aortic (valve) I35.9
  arteriosclerotic or sclerotic (senile) — *see* Disease, heart, ischemic, atherosclerotic
  artery, arterial — *see* Disease, heart, ischemic, atherosclerotic
  beer drinkers' I42.6
  beriberi (wet) E51.12
  black I27.0
  congenital Q24.9
    cyanotic Q24.9
    specified NEC Q24.8
  coronary — *see* Disease, heart, ischemic
  cryptogenic I51.9
  fibroid — *see* Myocarditis

Disease, diseased — *continued*

heart — *continued*
  functional I51.89
    psychogenic F45.8
  glycogen storage E74.02 *[143]*
  gonococcal A54.83
  hypertensive — *see* Hypertension, heart
  hyperthyroid — *see also* Hyperthyroidism E05.90 *[143]*
    with thyroid storm E05.91 *[143]*
  ischemic (chronic or with a stated duration of over 4 weeks) I25.9
    atherosclerotic (of) I25.10
      with angina pectoris — *see* Arteriosclerosis, coronary (artery)
      coronary artery bypass graft — *see* Arteriosclerosis, coronary (artery),
    cardiomyopathy I25.5
    diagnosed on ECG or other special investigation, but currently presenting no symptoms I25.6
    silent I25.6
    specified form NEC I25.89
  kyphoscoliotic I27.1
  meningococcal A39.50
    endocarditis A39.51
    myocarditis A39.52
    pericarditis A39.53
  mitral I05.9
    specified NEC I05.8
  muscular — *see* Degeneration, myocardial
  psychogenic (functional) F45.8
  pulmonary (chronic) I27.9
    in schistosomiasis B65.9 *[152]*
    specified NEC I27.89
  rheumatic (chronic) (inactive) (old) (quiescent) (with chorea) I09.9
    active or acute I01.9
      with chorea (acute) (rheumatic) (Sydenham's) I02.0
    specified NEC I09.89
  senile — *see* Myocarditis
  syphilitic A52.06
    aortic A52.03
      aneurysm A52.01
    congenital A50.54 *[152]*
  thyrotoxic — *see also* Thyrotoxicosis E05.90 *[143]*
    with thyroid storm E05.91 *[143]*
  valve, valvular (obstructive) (regurgitant) — *see also* Endocarditis
    congenital NEC Q24.8
      pulmonary Q22.3
  vascular — *see* Disease, cardiovascular
heavy chain NEC C88.2
  alpha C88.3
  gamma C88.2
  mu C88.2
Hebra's
  pityriasis
    maculata et circinata L42
    rubra pilaris L44.0
  prurigo L28.2
hematopoietic organs D75.9
hemoglobin or Hb
  abnormal (mixed) NEC D58.2
    with thalassemia D56.9
  AS genotype D57.3
  Bart's D56.0
  C (Hb-C) D58.2
    with other abnormal hemoglobin NEC D58.2
    elliptocytosis D58.1
    Hb-S D57.2- ☑
    sickle-cell D57.2- ☑
    thalassemia D56.8
  Constant Spring D58.2
  D (Hb-D) D58.2
  E (Hb-E) D58.2
  E-beta thalassemia D56.5
  elliptocytosis D58.1
  H (Hb-H) (thalassemia) D56.0
    with other abnormal hemoglobin NEC D56.9
    Constant Spring D56.0
  I thalassemia D56.9
  M D74.0
  S or SS D57.1
  SC D57.2- ☑
  SD D57.8- ☑
  SE D57.8- ☑

Disease, diseased — *continued*

hemoglobin or Hb — *continued*
  spherocytosis D58.0
  unstable, hemolytic D58.2
  hemolytic (newborn) P55.9
    autoimmune (cold type) (warm type) D59.1
    drug-induced D59.0
    due to or with
      incompatibility
        ABO (blood group) P55.1
        blood (group) (Duffy) (K) (Kell) (Kidd) (Lewis) (M) (S) NEC P55.8
        Rh (blood group) (factor) P55.0
        Rh negative mother P55.0
    specified type NEC P55.8
    unstable hemoglobin D58.2
hemorrhagic D69.9
  newborn P53
Henoch (-Schönlein) (purpura nervosa) D69.0
hepatic — *see* Disease, liver
hepatolenticular E83.01
heredodegenerative NEC
  spinal cord G95.89
herpesviral, disseminated B00.7
Hers' (glycogenosis VI) E74.09
Herter (-Gee) (-Heubner) (nontropical sprue) K90.0
Heubner-Herter (nontropical sprue) K90.0
high fetal gene or hemoglobin thalassemia D56.9
Hildenbrand's — *see* Typhus
hip (joint) M25.9
  congenital Q65.89
  suppurative M00.9
  tuberculous A18.02
His (-Werner) (trench fever) A79.0
Hodgson's I71.2
  ruptured I71.1
Holla — *see* Spherocytosis
hookworm B76.9
  specified NEC B76.8
host-versus-graft D89.813
  acute D89.810
  acute on chronic D89.812
  chronic D89.811
human immunodeficiency virus (HIV) B20
Huntington's G10
  with dementia G10 *[F02.80]*
Hutchinson's (cheiropompholyx) — *see* Hutchinson's disease
hyaline (diffuse) (generalized)
  membrane (lung) (newborn) P22.0
    adult J80
hydatid — *see* Echinococcus
hydroxyapatite deposition M11.00
  ankle M11.07- ☑
  elbow M11.02- ☑
  foot joint M11.07- ☑
  hand joint M11.04- ☑
  hip M11.05- ☑
  knee M11.06- ☑
  multiple site M11.09
  shoulder M11.01- ☑
  vertebra M11.08
  wrist M11.03- ☑
hyperkinetic — *see* Hyperkinesia
hypertensive — *see* Hypertension
hypophysis E23.7
Iceland G93.3
I-cell E77.0
immune D89.9
immunoproliferative (malignant) C88.9
  small intestinal C88.3
  specified NEC C88.8
inclusion B25.9
  salivary gland B25.9
infectious, infective B99.9
  congenital P37.9
    specified NEC P37.8
    viral P35.9
      specified type NEC P35.8
  specified NEC B99.8
inflammatory
  penis N48.29
    abscess N48.21
    cellulitis N48.22
  prepuce N47.7
    balanoposthitis N47.6
  tubo-ovarian — *see* Salpingo-oophoritis
intervertebral disc — *see also* Disorder, disc

▽ Subterms under main terms may continue to next column or page   ☑ Additional Character Required — Refer to the Tabular List for Character Selection   103

Disease, diseased — Disease, diseased

Disease, diseased — *continued*
  intervertebral disc — *see also* Disorder, disc — *continued*
    with myelopathy — *see* Disorder, disc, with, myelopathy
    cervical, cervicothoracic — *see* Disorder, disc, cervical
      with
        myelopathy — *see* Disorder, disc, cervical, with myelopathy
        neuritis, radiculitis or radiculopathy — *see* Disorder, disc, cervical, with neuritis
        specified NEC — *see* Disorder, disc, cervical, specified type NEC
    lumbar (with)
      myelopathy M51.06
      neuritis, radiculitis, radiculopathy or sciatica M51.16
      specified NEC M51.86
    lumbosacral (with)
      neuritis, radiculitis, radiculopathy or sciatica M51.17
      specified NEC M51.87
    specified NEC — *see* Disorder, disc, specified NEC
    thoracic (with)
      myelopathy M51.04
      neuritis, radiculitis or radiculopathy M51.14
      specified NEC M51.84
    thoracolumbar (with)
      myelopathy M51.05
      neuritis, radiculitis or radiculopathy M51.15
      specified NEC M51.85
  intestine K63.9
    functional K59.9
      psychogenic F45.8
      specified NEC K59.8
    organic K63.9
    protozoal A07.9
    specified NEC K63.89
  iris H21.9
    specified NEC H21.89
  iron metabolism or storage E83.10
  island (scrub typhus) A75.3
  itai-itai — *see* Poisoning, cadmium
  Jakob-Creutzfeldt — *see* Creutzfeldt-Jakob disease or syndrome
  jaw M27.9
    fibrocystic M27.49
    specified NEC M27.8
  jigger B88.1
  joint — *see also* Disorder, joint
    Charcot's — *see* Arthropathy, neuropathic (Charcot)
    degenerative — *see* Osteoarthritis
      multiple M15.9
      spine — *see* Spondylosis
    hypertrophic — *see* Osteoarthritis
    sacroiliac M53.3
    specified NEC — *see* Disorder, joint, specified type NEC
    spine NEC — *see* Dorsopathy
    suppurative — *see* Arthritis, pyogenic or pyemic
  Jourdain's (acute gingivitis) K05.00
    nonplaque induced K05.01
    plaque induced K05.00
  Kaschin-Beck (endemic polyarthritis) M12.10
    ankle M12.17- ☑
    elbow M12.12- ☑
    foot joint M12.17- ☑
    hand joint M12.14- ☑
    hip M12.15- ☑
    knee M12.16- ☑
    multiple site M12.19
    shoulder M12.11- ☑
    vertebra M12.18
    wrist M12.13- ☑
  Katayama B65.2
  Kedani (scrub typhus) A75.3
  Keshan E59
  kidney (functional) (pelvis) N28.9
    chronic N18.9
      hypertensive — *see* Hypertension, kidney
      stage 1 N18.1
      stage 2 (mild) N18.2
      stage 3 (moderate) N18.3
      stage 4 (severe) N18.4
      stage 5 N18.5
    complicating pregnancy — *see* Pregnancy, complicated by, renal disease

Disease, diseased — *continued*
  kidney — *continued*
    cystic (congenital) Q61.9
    fibrocystic (congenital) Q61.8
    hypertensive — *see* Hypertension, kidney
    in (due to)
      schistosomiasis (bilharziasis) B65.9 *[N29]*
    multicystic Q61.4
    polycystic Q61.3
      adult type Q61.2
      childhood type NEC Q61.19
        collecting duct dilatation Q61.11
  Kimmelstiel (-Wilson) (intercapillary polycystic (congenital) glomerulosclerosis) — *see* E08-E13 with .21
  Kinnier Wilson's (hepatolenticular degeneration) E83.01
  kissing — *see* Mononucleosis, infectious
  Klebs' — *see also* Glomerulonephritis N05- ☑
  Klippel-Feil (brevicollis) Q76.1
  Köhler-Pellegrini-Stieda (calcification, knee joint) — *see* Bursitis, tibial collateral
  Kok Q89.8
  König's (osteochondritis dissecans) — *see* Osteochondritis, dissecans
  Korsakoff's (nonalcoholic) F04
    alcoholic F10.96
      with dependence F10.26
  Kostmann's (infantile genetic agranulocytosis) D70.0
  kuru A81.81
  Kyasanur Forest A98.2
  labyrinth, ear — *see* Disorder, ear, inner
  lacrimal system — *see* Disorder, lacrimal system
  Lafora's — *see* Epilepsy, generalized, idiopathic
  Lancereaux-Mathieu (leptospiral jaundice) A27.0
  Landry's G61.0
  Larrey-Weil (leptospiral jaundice) A27.0
  larynx J38.7
  legionnaires' A48.1
    nonpneumonic A48.2
  Lenegre's I44.2
  lens H27.9
    specified NEC H27.8
  Lev's (acquired complete heart block) I44.2
  Lewy body (dementia) G31.83 *[F02.80]*
    with behavioral disturbance G31.83 *[F02.81]*
  Lichtheim's (subacute combined sclerosis with pernicious anemia) D51.0
  Lightwood's (renal tubular acidosis) N25.89
  Lignac's (cystinosis) E72.04
  lip K13.0
  lipid-storage E75.6
    specified NEC E75.5
  Lipschütz's N76.6
  liver (chronic) (organic) K76.9
    alcoholic (chronic) K70.9
      acute — *see* Disease, liver, alcoholic, hepatitis
      cirrhosis K70.30
        with ascites K70.31
      failure K70.40
        with coma K70.41
      fatty liver K70.0
      fibrosis K70.2
      hepatitis K70.10
        with ascites K70.11
      sclerosis K70.2
    cystic, congenital Q44.6
    drug-induced (idiosyncratic) (toxic) (predictable) (unpredictable) — *see* Disease, liver, toxic
    end stage K72.90
      due to hepatitis — *see* Hepatitis
    fatty, nonalcoholic (NAFLD) K76.0
      alcoholic K70.0
    fibrocystic (congenital) Q44.6
    fluke
      Chinese B66.1
      oriental B66.1
      sheep B66.3
    gestational alloimmune (GALD) P78.84
    glycogen storage E74.09 *[K77]*
    in (due to)
      schistosomiasis (bilharziasis) B65.9 *[K77]*
    inflammatory K75.9
      alcoholic K70.1 ☑
      specified NEC K75.89
    polycystic (congenital) Q44.6
    toxic K71.9
      with
        cholestasis K71.0
        cirrhosis (liver) K71.7

Disease, diseased — *continued*
  liver — *continued*
    toxic — *continued*
      with — *continued*
        fibrosis (liver) K71.7
        focal nodular hyperplasia K71.8
        hepatic granuloma K71.8
        hepatic necrosis K71.10
          with coma K71.11
        hepatitis NEC K71.6
          acute K71.2
          chronic
            active K71.50
              with ascites K71.51
            lobular K71.4
            persistent K71.3
          lupoid K71.50
            with ascites K71.51
        peliosis hepatis K71.8
        veno-occlusive disease (VOD) of liver K71.8
      veno-occlusive K76.5
  Lobo's (keloid blastomycosis) B48.0
  Lobstein's (brittle bones and blue sclera) Q78.0
  Ludwig's (submaxillary cellulitis) K12.2
  lumbosacral region M53.87
  lung J98.4
    black J60
    congenital Q33.9
    cystic J98.4
      congenital Q33.0
    fibroid (chronic) — *see* Fibrosis, lung
    fluke B66.4
      oriental B66.4
    in
      amyloidosis E85.4 *[J99]*
      sarcoidosis D86.0
      Sjögren's syndrome M35.02
      systemic
        lupus erythematosus M32.13
        sclerosis M34.81
    interstitial J84.9
      of childhood, specified NEC J84.848
      respiratory bronchiolitis J84.115
      specified NEC J84.89
    obstructive (chronic) J43.9
      with
        acute
          bronchitis J44.0
          exacerbation NEC J44.1
          lower respiratory infection J44.0
        alveolitis, allergic J67.9
        asthma J44.9
        bronchiectasis J47.9
          with
            exacerbation (acute) J47.1
            lower respiratory infection J47.0
        bronchitis J44.9
          with
            exacerbation (acute) J44.1
            lower respiratory infection J44.0
        emphysema J43.9
        hypersensitivity pneumonitis J67.9
      decompensated J44.1
        with
          exacerbation (acute) J44.1
    polycystic J98.4
      congenital Q33.0
    rheumatoid (diffuse) (interstitial) — *see* Rheumatoid, lung
  Lutembacher's (atrial septal defect with mitral stenosis) Q21.1
  Lyme A69.20
  lymphatic (gland) (system) (channel) (vessel) I89.9
  lymphoproliferative D47.9
    specified NEC D47.Z9 *(following D47.4)*
    T-gamma D47.Z9 *(following D47.4)*
    X-linked D82.3
  Magitot's M27.2
  malarial — *see* Malaria
  malignant — *see also* Neoplasm, malignant, by site
  Manson's B65.1
  maple bark J67.6
  maple-syrup-urine E71.0
  Marburg (virus) A98.3
  Marion's (bladder neck obstruction) N32.0
  Marsh's (exophthalmic goiter) — *see* Hyperthyroidism, with, goiter (diffuse)
  mastoid (process) — *see* Disorder, ear, middle
  Mathieu's (leptospiral jaundice) A27.0

☑ **Additional Character Required** — Refer to the Tabular List for Character Selection   ▽ **Subterms under main terms may continue to next column or page**

Disease, diseased — *continued*
- Maxcy's A75.2
- McArdle (-Schmid-Pearson) (glycogenosis V) E74.04
- mediastinum J98.59
- medullary center (idiopathic) (respiratory) G93.89
- Meige's (chronic hereditary edema) Q82.0
- meningococcal — *see* Infection, meningococcal
- mental F99
  - organic F09
- mesenchymal M35.9
- mesenteric embolic — *see also* Ischemia, intestine, acute K55.039
- metabolic, metabolism E88.9
  - bilirubin E80.7
- metal-polisher's J62.8
- metastatic — *see also* Neoplasm, secondary, by site C79.9
- microvascular - code to condition
- microvillus
  - atrophy Q43.8
  - inclusion (MVD) Q43.8
- middle ear — *see* Disorder, ear, middle
- Mikulicz' (dryness of mouth, absent or decreased lacrimation) K11.8
- Milroy's (chronic hereditary edema) Q82.0
- Minamata — *see* Poisoning, mercury
- minicore G71.2
- Minor's G95.19
- Minot's (hemorrhagic disease, newborn) P53
- Minot-von Willebrand-Jürgens (angiohemophilia) D68.0
- Mitchell's (erythromelalgia) I73.81
- mitral (valve) I05.9
  - nonrheumatic I34.9
- mixed connective tissue M35.1
- moldy hay J67.0
- Monge's T70.29 ☑
- Morgagni-Adams-Stokes (syncope with heart block) I45.9
- Morgagni's (syndrome) (hyperostosis frontalis interna) M85.2
- Morton's (with metatarsalgia) — *see* Lesion, nerve, plantar
- Morvan's G60.8
- motor neuron (bulbar) (mixed type) (spinal) G12.20
  - amyotrophic lateral sclerosis G12.21
  - familial G12.24
  - progressive bulbar palsy G12.22
  - specified NEC G12.29
- moyamoya I67.5
- mu heavy chain disease C88.2
- multicore G71.2
- muscle — *see also* Disorder, muscle
  - inflammatory — *see* Myositis
  - ocular (external) — *see* Strabismus
- musculoskeletal system, soft tissue — *see also* Disorder, soft tissue
  - specified NEC — *see* Disorder, soft tissue, specified type NEC
- mushroom workers' J67.5
- mycotic B49
- myelodysplastic, not classified C94.6
- myeloproliferative, not classified C94.6
  - chronic D47.1
- myocardium, myocardial — *see also* Degeneration, myocardial I51.5
  - primary (idiopathic) I42.9
- myoneural G70.9
- Naegeli's D69.1
- nails L60.9
  - specified NEC L60.8
- Nairobi (sheep virus) A93.8
- nasal J34.9
- nemaline body G71.2
- nerve — *see* Disorder, nerve
- nervous system G98.8
  - autonomic G90.9
  - central G96.9
    - specified NEC G96.8
  - congenital Q07.9
  - parasympathetic G90.9
  - specified NEC G98.8
  - sympathetic G90.9
  - vegetative G90.9
- neuromuscular system G70.9
- Newcastle B30.8
- Nicolas (-Durand)-Favre (climatic bubo) A55
- nipple N64.9
  - Paget's C50.01- ☑

Disease, diseased — *continued*
- nipple — *continued*
  - Paget's — *continued*
    - female C50.01- ☑
    - male C50.02- ☑
- Nishimoto (-Takeuchi) I67.5
- nonarthropod-borne NOS (viral) B34.9
  - enterovirus NEC B34.1
- nonautoimmune hemolytic D59.4
  - drug-induced D59.2
- Nonne-Milroy-Meige (chronic hereditary edema) Q82.0
- nose J34.9
- nucleus pulposus — *see* Disorder, disc
- nutritional E63.9
- oast-house-urine E72.19
  - ocular
    - herpesviral B00.50
    - zoster B02.30
- obliterative vascular I77.1
- Ohara's — *see* Tularemia
- Opitz's (congestive splenomegaly) D73.2
- Oppenheim-Urbach (necrobiosis lipoidica diabetico-rum) — *see* E08-E13 with .620
- optic nerve NEC — *see* Disorder, nerve, optic
- orbit — *see* Disorder, orbit
- Oriental liver fluke B66.1
- Oriental lung fluke B66.4
- Ormond's N13.5
- Oropouche virus A93.0
- Osler-Rendu (familial hemorrhagic telangiectasia) I78.0
- osteofibrocystic E21.0
- Otto's M24.7
- outer ear — *see* Disorder, ear, external
- ovary (noninflammatory) N83.9
  - cystic N83.20- ☑
  - inflammatory — *see* Salpingo-oophoritis
  - polycystic E28.2
  - specified NEC N83.8
- Owren's (congenital) — *see* Defect, coagulation
- pancreas K86.9
  - cystic K86.2
  - fibrocystic E84.9
  - specified NEC K86.89
- panvalvular I08.9
  - specified NEC I08.8
- parametrium (noninflammatory) N83.9
- parasitic B89
  - cerebral NEC B71.9 *[G94]*
  - intestinal NOS B82.9
  - mouth B37.0
  - skin NOS B88.9
  - specified type — *see* Infestation
  - tongue B37.0
- parathyroid (gland) E21.5
  - specified NEC E21.4
- Parkinson's G20
- parodontal K05.6
- Parrot's (syphilitic osteochondritis) A50.02
- Parry's (exophthalmic goiter) — *see* Hyperthyroidism, with, goiter (diffuse)
- Parson's (exophthalmic goiter) — *see* Hyperthyroidism, with, goiter (diffuse)
- Paxton's (white piedra) B36.2
- pearl-worker's — *see* Osteomyelitis, specified type NEC
- Pellegrini-Stieda (calcification, knee joint) — *see* Bursitis, tibial collateral
- pelvis, pelvic
  - female NOS N94.9
    - specified NEC N94.89
  - gonococcal (acute) (chronic) A54.24
  - inflammatory (female) N73.9
    - acute N73.0
    - chlamydial A56.11
    - chronic N73.1
    - specified NEC N73.8
    - syphilitic (secondary) A51.42
      - late A52.76
    - tuberculous A18.17
  - organ, female N94.9
  - peritoneum, female NEC N94.89
- penis N48.9
  - inflammatory N48.29
    - abscess N48.21
    - cellulitis N48.22
  - specified NEC N48.89
- periapical tissues NOS K04.90
- periodontal K05.6
  - specified NEC K05.5

Disease, diseased — *continued*
- periosteum — *see* Disorder, bone, specified type NEC
- peripheral
  - arterial I73.9
  - autonomic nervous system G90.9
  - nerves — *see* Polyneuropathy
  - vascular NOS I73.9
- peritoneum K66.9
  - pelvic, female NEC N94.89
  - specified NEC K66.8
- persistent mucosal (middle ear) H66.20
  - left H66.22
    - with right H66.23
  - right H66.21
    - with left H66.23
- Petit's — *see* Hernia, abdomen, specified site NEC
- pharynx J39.2
  - specified NEC J39.2
- Phocas' — *see* Mastopathy, cystic
- photochromogenic (acid-fast bacilli) (pulmonary) A31.0
  - nonpulmonary A31.9
- Pick's G31.01 *[F02.80]*
  - with behavioral disturbance G31.01 *[F02.81]*
  - brain G31.01 *[F02.80]*
    - with behavioral disturbance G31.01 *[F02.81]*
  - of pericardium (pericardial pseudocirrhosis of liver) I31.1
- pigeon fancier's J67.2
- pineal gland E34.8
- pink — *see* Poisoning, mercury
- Pinkus' (lichen nitidus) L44.1
- pinworm B80
- Piry virus A93.8
- pituitary (gland) E23.7
- pituitary-snuff-taker's J67.8
- pleura (cavity) J94.9
  - specified NEC J94.8
- pneumatic drill (hammer) T75.21 ☑
- Pollitzer's (hidradenitis suppurativa) L73.2
- polycystic
  - kidney or renal Q61.3
    - adult type Q61.2
    - childhood type NEC Q61.19
      - collecting duct dilatation Q61.11
  - liver or hepatic Q44.6
  - lung or pulmonary J98.4
    - congenital Q33.0
  - ovary, ovaries E28.2
  - spleen Q89.09
- polyethylene T84.05- ☑
- Pompe's (glycogenosis II) E74.02
- Posadas-Wernicke B38.9
- Potain's (pulmonary edema) — *see* Edema, lung
- prepuce N47.8
  - inflammatory N47.7
    - balanoposthitis N47.6
- Pringle's (tuberous sclerosis) Q85.1
- prion, central nervous system A81.9
  - specified NEC A81.89
- prostate N42.9
  - specified NEC N42.89
- protozoal B64
  - acanthamebiasis — *see* Acanthamebiasis
  - African trypanosomiasis — *see* African trypanosomiasis
  - babesiosis B60.0
  - Chagas disease — *see* Chagas disease
  - intestine, intestinal A07.9
  - leishmaniasis — *see* Leishmaniasis
  - malaria — *see* Malaria
  - naegleriasis B60.2
  - pneumocystosis B59
  - specified organism NEC B60.8
  - toxoplasmosis — *see* Toxoplasmosis
- pseudo-Hurler's E77.0
- psychiatric F99
- psychotic — *see* Psychosis
- Puente's (simple glandular cheilitis) K13.0
- puerperal — *see also* Puerperal O90.89
- pulmonary — *see also* Disease, lung
  - artery I28.9
  - chronic obstructive J44.9
    - with
      - acute bronchitis J44.0
      - exacerbation (acute) J44.1
      - lower respiratory infection (acute) J44.0
    - decompensated J44.1

Disease, diseased — *continued*
  pulmonary — *see also* Disease, lung — *continued*
    chronic obstructive — *continued*
      decompensated — *continued*
        with
          exacerbation (acute) J44.1
    heart I27.9
      specified NEC I27.89
    hypertensive (vascular) — *see also* Hypertension, pulmonary I27.20
      NEC I27.2 ☑
      primary (idiopathic) I27.0
    valve I37.9
      rheumatic I09.89
  pulp (dental) NOS K04.90
  pulseless M31.4
  Putnam's (subacute combined sclerosis with pernicious anemia) D51.0
  Pyle (-Cohn) (metaphyseal dysplasia) Q78.5
  ragpicker's or ragsorter's A22.1
  Raynaud's — *see* Raynaud's disease
  reactive airway — *see* Asthma
  Reclus' (cystic) — *see* Mastopathy, cystic
  rectum K62.9
    specified NEC K62.89
  Refsum's (heredopathia atactica polyneuritiformis) G60.1
  renal (functional) (pelvis) — *see also* Disease, kidney N28.9
    with
      edema — *see* Nephrosis
      glomerular lesion — *see* Glomerulonephritis
        with edema — *see* Nephrosis
      interstitial nephritis N12
    acute N28.9
    chronic — *see also* Disease, kidney, chronic N18.9
    cystic, congenital Q61.9
    diabetic — *see* E08-E13 with .22
    end-stage (failure) N18.6
      due to hypertension I12.0
    fibrocystic (congenital) Q61.8
    hypertensive — *see* Hypertension, kidney
    lupus M32.14
    phosphate-losing (tubular) N25.0
    polycystic (congenital) Q61.3
      adult type Q61.2
      childhood type NEC Q61.19
        collecting duct dilatation Q61.11
    rapidly progressive N01.9
    subacute N01.9
  Rendu-Osler-Weber (familial hemorrhagic telangiectasia) I78.0
  renovascular (arteriosclerotic) — *see* Hypertension, kidney
  respiratory (tract) J98.9
    acute or subacute NOS J06.9
      due to
        chemicals, gases, fumes or vapors (inhalation) J68.3
        external agent J70.9
          specified NEC J70.8
        radiation J70.0
        smoke inhalation J70.5
      noninfectious J39.8
    chronic NOS J98.9
      due to
        chemicals, gases, fumes or vapors J68.4
        external agent J70.9
          specified NEC J70.8
        radiation J70.1
      newborn P27.9
        specified NEC P27.8
    due to
      chemicals, gases, fumes or vapors J68.9
        acute or subacute NEC J68.3
        chronic J68.4
      external agent J70.9
        specified NEC J70.8
    newborn P28.9
      specified type NEC P28.89
    upper J39.9
      acute or subacute J06.9
      noninfectious NEC J39.8
      specified NEC J39.8
      streptococcal J06.9
  retina, retinal H35.9
    Batten's or Batten-Mayou E75.4 *[H36]*
    specified NEC H35.89

Disease, diseased — *continued*
  rheumatoid — *see* Arthritis, rheumatoid
  rickettsial NOS A79.9
    specified type NEC A79.89
  Riga (-Fede) (cachectic aphthae) K14.0
  Riggs' (compound periodontitis) — *see* Periodontitis
  Ritter's L00
  Rivalta's (cervicofacial actinomycosis) A42.2
  Robles' (onchocerciasis) B73.01
  Roger's (congenital interventricular septal defect) Q21.0
  Rosenthal's (factor XI deficiency) D68.1
  Ross River B33.1
  Rossbach's (hyperchlorhydria) K31.89
    psychogenic F45.8
  Rotes Quérol — *see* Hyperostosis, ankylosing
  Roth (-Bernhardt) — *see* Mononeuropathy, lower limb, meralgia paresthetica
  Runeberg's (progressive pernicious anemia) D51.0
  sacroiliac NEC M53.3
  salivary gland or duct K11.9
    inclusion B25.9
    specified NEC K11.8
    virus B25.9
  sandworm B76.9
  Schimmelbusch's — *see* Mastopathy, cystic
  Schmorl's — *see* Schmorl's disease or nodes
  Schönlein (-Henoch) (purpura rheumatica) D69.0
  Schottmüller's — *see* Fever, paratyphoid
  Schultz's (agranulocytosis) — *see* Agranulocytosis
  Schwalbe-Ziehen-Oppenheim G24.1
  Schwartz-Jampel G71.13
  sclera H15.9
    specified NEC H15.89
  scrofulous (tuberculous) A18.2
  scrotum N50.9
  sebaceous glands L73.9
  semilunar cartilage, cystic — *see also* Derangement, knee, meniscus, cystic
  seminal vesicle N50.9
  serum NEC — *see also* Reaction, serum T80.69 ☑
  sexually transmitted A64
    anogenital
      herpesviral infection — *see* Herpes, anogenital
      warts A63.0
    chancroid A57
    chlamydial infection — *see* Chlamydia
    gonorrhea — *see* Gonorrhea
    granuloma inguinale A58
    specified organism NEC A63.8
    syphilis — *see* Syphilis
    trichomoniasis — *see* Trichomoniasis
  Sézary C84.1- ☑
  shimamushi (scrub typhus) A75.3
  shipyard B30.0
  sickle-cell D57.1
    with crisis (vasoocclusive pain) D57.00
      with
        acute chest syndrome D57.01
        splenic sequestration D57.02
    elliptocytosis D57.8- ☑
    Hb-C D57.20
      with crisis (vasoocclusive pain) D57.219
        with
          acute chest syndrome D57.211
          splenic sequestration D57.212
      without crisis D57.20
    Hb-SD D57.80
      with crisis D57.819
        with
          acute chest syndrome D57.811
          splenic sequestration D57.812
    Hb-SE D57.80
      with crisis D57.819
        with
          acute chest syndrome D57.811
          splenic sequestration D57.812
    specified NEC D57.80
      with crisis D57.819
        with
          acute chest syndrome D57.811
          splenic sequestration D57.812
    spherocytosis D57.80
      with crisis D57.819
        with
          acute chest syndrome D57.811
          splenic sequestration D57.812
    thalassemia D57.40
      with crisis (vasoocclusive pain) D57.419

Disease, diseased — *continued*
  sickle-cell — *continued*
    thalassemia — *continued*
      with crisis — *continued*
        with
          acute chest syndrome D57.411
          splenic sequestration D57.412
      without crisis D57.40
  silo-filler's J68.8
    bronchitis J68.0
    pneumonitis J68.0
    pulmonary edema J68.1
  simian B B00.4
  Simons' (progressive lipodystrophy) E88.1
  sin nombre virus B33.4
  sinus — *see* Sinusitis
  Sirkari's B55.0
  sixth B08.20
    due to human herpesvirus 6 B08.21
    due to human herpesvirus 7 B08.22
  skin L98.9
    due to metabolic disorder NEC E88.9 *[L99]*
    specified NEC L98.8
  slim (HIV) B20
  small vessel I73.9
  Sneddon-Wilkinson (subcorneal pustular dermatosis) L13.1
  South African creeping B88.0
  spinal (cord) G95.9
    congenital Q06.9
    specified NEC G95.89
  spine — *see also* Spondylopathy
    joint — *see* Dorsopathy
    tuberculous A18.01
  spinocerebellar (hereditary) G11.9
    specified NEC G11.8
  spleen D73.9
    amyloid E85.4 *[D77]*
    organic D73.9
    polycystic Q89.09
    postinfectional D73.89
  sponge-diver's — *see* Toxicity, venom, marine animal, sea anemone
  Startle Q89.8
  Steinert's G71.11
  Sticker's (erythema infectiosum) B08.3
  Stieda's (calcification, knee joint) — *see* Bursitis, tibial collateral
  Stokes' (exophthalmic goiter) — *see* Hyperthyroidism, with, goiter (diffuse)
  Stokes-Adams (syncope with heart block) I45.9
  stomach K31.9
    functional, psychogenic F45.8
    specified NEC K31.89
  stonemason's J62.8
  storage
    glycogen — *see* Disease, glycogen storage
    mucopolysaccharide — *see* Mucopolysaccharidosis
  striatopallidal system NEC G25.89
  Stuart-Prower (congenital factor X deficiency) D68.2
  Stuart's (congenital factor X deficiency) D68.2
  subcutaneous tissue — *see* Disease, skin
  supporting structures of teeth K08.9
    specified NEC K08.89
  suprarenal (capsule) (gland) E27.9
    hyperfunction E27.0
    specified NEC E27.8
  sweat glands L74.9
    specified NEC L74.8
  Sweeley-Klionsky E75.21
  Swift (-Feer) — *see* Poisoning, mercury
  swimming-pool granuloma A31.1
  Sylvest's (epidemic pleurodynia) B33.0
  sympathetic nervous system G90.9
  synovium — *see* Disorder, synovium
  syphilitic — *see* Syphilis
  systemic tissue mast cell D47.02
  tanapox (virus) B08.71
  Tangier E78.6
  Tarral-Besnier (pityriasis rubra pilaris) L44.0
  Tauri's E74.09
  tear duct — *see* Disorder, lacrimal system
  tendon, tendinous — *see also* Disorder, tendon
    nodular — *see* Trigger finger
  terminal vessel I73.9
  testis N50.9
  thalassemia Hb-S — *see* Disease, sickle-cell, thalassemia
  Thaysen-Gee (nontropical sprue) K90.0

Disease, diseased — *continued*
Thomsen G71.12
throat J39.2
  septic J02.0
thromboembolic — *see* Embolism
thymus (gland) E32.9
  specified NEC E32.8
thyroid (gland) E07.9
  heart — *see also* Hyperthyroidism E05.90 *[I43]*
    with thyroid storm E05.91 *[I43]*
  specified NEC E07.89
Tietze's M94.0
tongue K14.9
  specified NEC K14.8
tonsils, tonsillar (and adenoids) J35.9
tooth, teeth K08.9
  hard tissues K03.9
    specified NEC K03.89
  pulp NEC K04.99
  specified NEC K08.89
Tourette's F95.2
trachea NEC J39.8
tricuspid I07.9
  nonrheumatic I36.9
triglyceride-storage E75.5
trophoblastic — *see* Mole, hydatidiform
tsutsugamushi A75.3
tube (fallopian) (noninflammatory) N83.9
  inflammatory — *see* Salpingitis
  specified NEC N83.8
tuberculous NEC — *see* Tuberculosis
tubo-ovarian (noninflammatory) N83.9
  inflammatory — *see* Salpingo-oophoritis
  specified NEC N83.8
tubotympanic, chronic — *see* Otitis, media, suppurative, chronic, tubotympanic
tubulo-interstitial N15.9
  specified NEC N15.8
tympanum — *see* Disorder, tympanic membrane
Uhl's Q24.8
Underwood's (sclerema neonatorum) P83.0
Unverricht (-Lundborg) — *see* Epilepsy, generalized, idiopathic
Urbach-Oppenheim (necrobiosis lipoidica diabeticorum) — *see* E08-E13 with .620
ureter N28.9
  in (due to)
    schistosomiasis (bilharziasis) B65.0 *[N29]*
urethra N36.9
  specified NEC N36.8
urinary (tract) N39.9
  bladder N32.9
    specified NEC N32.89
  specified NEC N39.8
uterus (noninflammatory) N85.9
  infective — *see* Endometritis
  inflammatory — *see* Endometritis
  specified NEC N85.8
uveal tract (anterior) H21.9
  posterior H31.9
vagabond's B85.1
vagina, vaginal (noninflammatory) N89.9
  inflammatory NEC N76.89
  specified NEC N89.8
valve, valvular I38
  multiple I08.9
    specified NEC I08.8
van Creveld-von Gierke (glycogenosis I) E74.01
vas deferens N50.9
vascular I99.9
  arteriosclerotic — *see* Arteriosclerosis
  ciliary body NEC — *see* Disorder, iris, vascular
  hypertensive — *see* Hypertension
  iris NEC — *see* Disorder, iris, vascular
  obliterative I77.1
    peripheral I73.9
  occlusive I99.8
  peripheral (occlusive) I73.9
    in diabetes mellitus — *see* E08-E13 with .51
vasomotor I73.9
vasospastic I73.9
vein I87.9
venereal — *see also* Disease, sexually transmitted A64
  chlamydial NEC A56.8
    anus A56.3
    genitourinary NOS A56.2
    pharynx A56.4
    rectum A56.3

Disease, diseased — *continued*
venereal — *see also* Disease, sexually transmitted — *continued*
  fifth A55
  sixth A55
  specified nature or type NEC A63.8
vertebra, vertebral — *see also* Spondylopathy
  disc — *see* Disorder, disc
vibration — *see* Vibration, adverse effects
viral, virus — *see also* Disease, by type of virus B34.9
  arbovirus NOS A94
  arthropod-borne NOS A94
  congenital P35.9
    specified NEC P35.8
  Hanta (with renal manifestations) (Dobrava) (Puumala) (Seoul) A98.5
    with pulmonary manifestations (Andes) (Bayou) (Bermejo) (Black Creek Canal) (Choclo) (Juquitiba) (Laguna negra) (Lechiguanas) (New York) (Oran) (Sin nombre) B33.4
  Hantaan (Korean hemorrhagic fever) A98.5
  human immunodeficiency (HIV) B20
  Kunjin A83.4
  nonarthropod-borne NOS B34.9
  Powassan A84.8
  Rocio (encephalitis) A83.6
  Sin nombre (Hantavirus) (cardio)-pulmonary syndrome) B33.4
  Tahyna B33.8
  vesicular stomatitis A93.8
vitreous H43.9
  specified NEC H43.89
vocal cord J38.3
Volkmann's, acquired T79.6 ☑
von Eulenburg's (congenital paramyotonia) G71.19
von Gierke's (glycogenosis I) E74.01
von Graefe's — *see* Strabismus, paralytic, ophthalmoplegia, progressive
von Willebrand (-Jürgens) (angiohemophilia) D68.0
Vrolik's (osteogenesis imperfecta) Q78.0
vulva (noninflammatory) N90.9
  inflammatory NEC N76.89
  specified NEC N90.89
Wallgren's (obstruction of splenic vein with collateral circulation) I87.8
Wassilieff's (leptospiral jaundice) A27.0
wasting NEC R64
  due to malnutrition E41
Waterhouse-Friderichsen A39.1
Wegner's (syphilitic osteochondritis) A50.02
Weil's (leptospiral jaundice of lung) A27.0
Weir Mitchell's (erythromelalgia) I73.81
Werdnig-Hoffmann G12.0
Wermer's E31.21
Werner-His (trench fever) A79.0
Werner-Schultz (neutropenic splenomegaly) D73.81
Wernicke-Posadas B38.9
whipworm B79
white blood cells D72.9
  specified NEC D72.89
white matter R90.82
white-spot, meaning lichen sclerosus et atrophicus L90.0
  penis N48.0
  vulva N90.4
Wilkie's K55.1
Wilkinson-Sneddon (subcorneal pustular dermatosis) L13.1
Willis' — *see* Diabetes
Wilson's (hepatolenticular degeneration) E83.01
woolsorter's A22.1
yaba monkey tumor B08.72
yaba pox (virus) B08.72
Zika virus A92.5
  congenital P35.4
zoonotic, bacterial A28.9
  specified type NEC A28.8
Disfigurement (due to scar) L90.5
Disgerminoma — *see* Dysgerminoma
DISH (diffuse idiopathic skeletal hyperostosis) — *see* Hyperostosis, ankylosing
Disinsertion, retina — *see* Detachment, retina
Dislocatable hip, congenital Q65.6
Dislocation (articular)
with fracture — *see* Fracture
acromioclavicular (joint) S43.10- ☑
  with displacement
    100%-200% S43.12- ☑

Dislocation — *continued*
acromioclavicular — *continued*
  with displacement — *continued*
    more than 200% S43.13- ☑
    inferior S43.14- ☑
    posterior S43.15- ☑
ankle S93.0- ☑
astragalus — *see* Dislocation, ankle
atlantoaxial S13.121 ☑
atlantooccipital S13.111 ☑
atloidooccipital S13.111 ☑
breast bone S23.29 ☑
capsule, joint — *code by* site under Dislocation
carpal (bone) — *see* Dislocation, wrist
carpometacarpal (joint) NEC S63.05- ☑
  thumb S63.04- ☑
cartilage (joint) — *code by* site under Dislocation
cervical spine (vertebra) — *see* Dislocation, vertebra, cervical
chronic — *see* Dislocation, recurrent
clavicle — *see* Dislocation, acromioclavicular joint
coccyx S33.2 ☑
congenital NEC Q68.8
coracoid — *see* Dislocation, shoulder
costal cartilage S23.29 ☑
costochondral S23.29 ☑
cricoarytenoid articulation S13.29 ☑
cricothyroid articulation S13.29 ☑
dorsal vertebra — *see* Dislocation, vertebra, thoracic
ear ossicle — *see* Discontinuity, ossicles, ear
elbow S53.10- ☑
  congenital Q68.8
  pathological — *see* Dislocation, pathological NEC, elbow
  radial head alone — *see* Dislocation, radial head
  recurrent — *see* Dislocation, recurrent, elbow
  traumatic S53.10- ☑
    anterior S53.11- ☑
    lateral S53.14- ☑
    medial S53.13- ☑
    posterior S53.12- ☑
    specified type NEC S53.19- ☑
eye, nontraumatic — *see* Luxation, globe
eyeball, nontraumatic — *see* Luxation, globe
femur
  distal end — *see* Dislocation, knee
  proximal end — *see* Dislocation, hip
fibula
  distal end — *see* Dislocation, ankle
  proximal end — *see* Dislocation, knee
finger S63.25- ☑
  index S63.25- ☑
  interphalangeal S63.27- ☑
    distal S63.29- ☑
      index S63.29- ☑
      little S63.29- ☑
      middle S63.29- ☑
      ring S63.29- ☑
    index S63.27- ☑
    little S63.27- ☑
    middle S63.27- ☑
    proximal S63.28- ☑
      index S63.28- ☑
      little S63.28- ☑
      middle S63.28- ☑
      ring S63.28- ☑
    ring S63.27- ☑
  little S63.25- ☑
  metacarpophalangeal S63.26- ☑
    index S63.26- ☑
    little S63.26- ☑
    middle S63.26- ☑
    ring S63.26- ☑
  middle S63.25- ☑
  recurrent — *see* Dislocation, recurrent, finger
  ring S63.25- ☑
  thumb — *see* Dislocation, thumb
foot S93.30- ☑
  recurrent — *see* Dislocation, recurrent, foot
  specified site NEC S93.33- ☑
  tarsal joint S93.31- ☑
  tarsometatarsal joint S93.32- ☑
  toe — *see* Dislocation, toe
fracture — *see* Fracture
glenohumeral (joint) — *see* Dislocation, shoulder
glenoid — *see* Dislocation, shoulder

Dislocation — *continued*
  habitual — *see* Dislocation, recurrent
  hip S73.00- ☑
    anterior S73.03- ☑
      obturator S73.02- ☑
    central S73.04- ☑
    congenital (total) Q65.2
      bilateral Q65.1
      partial Q65.5
        bilateral Q65.4
        unilateral Q65.3-
      unilateral Q65.0-
    developmental M24.85- ☑
    pathological — *see* Dislocation, pathological NEC, hip
    posterior S73.01- ☑
    recurrent — *see* Dislocation, recurrent, hip
  humerus, proximal end — *see* Dislocation, shoulder
  incomplete — *see* Subluxation, by site
  incus — *see* Discontinuity, ossicles, ear
  infracoracoid — *see* Dislocation, shoulder
  innominate (pubic junction) (sacral junction) S33.39 ☑
    acetabulum — *see* Dislocation, hip
  interphalangeal (joint(s))
    finger S63.279 ☑
      distal S63.29- ☑
        index S63.29- ☑
        little S63.29- ☑
        middle S63.29- ☑
        ring S63.29- ☑
      index S63.27- ☑
      little S63.27- ☑
      middle S63.27- ☑
      proximal S63.28- ☑
        index S63.28- ☑
        little S63.28- ☑
        middle S63.28- ☑
        ring S63.28- ☑
      ring S63.27- ☑
    foot or toe — *see* Dislocation, toe
    thumb S63.12- ☑
  jaw (cartilage) (meniscus) S03.0- ☑
  joint prosthesis — *see* Complications, joint prosthesis, mechanical, displacement, by site
  knee S83.106 ☑
    cap — *see* Dislocation, patella
    congenital Q68.2
    old M23.8X- ☑
    patella — *see* Dislocation, patella
    pathological — *see* Dislocation, pathological NEC, knee
    proximal tibia
      anteriorly S83.11- ☑
      laterally S83.14- ☑
      medially S83.13- ☑
      posteriorly S83.12- ☑
    recurrent — *see also* Derangement, knee, specified NEC
    specified type NEC S83.19- ☑
  lacrimal gland H04.16- ☑
  lens (complete) H27.10
    anterior H27.12- ☑
    congenital Q12.1
    ocular implant — *see* Complications, intraocular lens
    partial H27.11- ☑
    posterior H27.13- ☑
    traumatic S05.8X- ☑
  ligament — *code by* site under Dislocation
  lumbar (vertebra) — *see* Dislocation, vertebra, lumbar
  lumbosacral (vertebra) — *see also* Dislocation, vertebra, lumbar
    congenital Q76.49
  mandible S03.0- ☑
  meniscus (knee) — *see* Tear, meniscus
    other sites - code by site under Dislocation
  metacarpal (bone)
    distal end — *see* Dislocation, finger
    proximal end S63.06- ☑
  metacarpophalangeal (joint)
    finger S63.26- ☑
      index S63.26- ☑
      little S63.26- ☑
      middle S63.26- ☑
      ring S63.26- ☑
    thumb S63.11- ☑

Dislocation — *continued*
  metatarsal (bone) — *see* Dislocation, foot
  metatarsophalangeal (joint(s)) — *see* Dislocation, toe
  midcarpal (joint) S63.03- ☑
  midtarsal (joint) — *see* Dislocation, foot
  neck S13.20 ☑
    specified site NEC S13.29 ☑
    vertebra — *see* Dislocation, vertebra, cervical
  nose (septal cartilage) S03.1 ☑
  occipitoatloid S13.111 ☑
  old — *see* Derangement, joint, specified type NEC
  ossicles, ear — *see* Discontinuity, ossicles, ear
  partial — *see* Subluxation, by site
  patella S83.006 ☑
    congenital Q74.1
    lateral S83.01- ☑
    recurrent (nontraumatic) M22.0- ☑
      incomplete M22.1- ☑
    specified type NEC S83.09- ☑
  pathological NEC M24.30 ☑
    ankle M24.37- ☑
    elbow M24.32- ☑
    foot joint M24.37- ☑
    hand joint M24.34- ☑
    hip M24.35- ☑
    knee M24.36- ☑
    lumbosacral joint — *see* subcategory M53.2 ☑
    pelvic region — *see* Dislocation, pathological, hip
    sacroiliac — *see* subcategory M53.2 ☑
    shoulder M24.31- ☑
    wrist M24.33- ☑
  pelvis NEC S33.30 ☑
    specified NEC S33.39 ☑
  phalanx
    finger or hand — *see* Dislocation, finger
    foot or toe — *see* Dislocation, toe
  prosthesis, internal — *see* Complications, prosthetic device, by site, mechanical
  radial head S53.006 ☑
    anterior S53.01- ☑
    posterior S53.02- ☑
    specified type NEC S53.09- ☑
  radiocarpal (joint) S63.02- ☑
  radiohumeral (joint) — *see* Dislocation, radial head
  radioulnar (joint)
    distal S63.01- ☑
    proximal — *see* Dislocation, elbow
  radius
    distal end — *see* Dislocation, wrist
    proximal end — *see* Dislocation, radial head
  recurrent M24.40 ☑
    ankle M24.47- ☑
    elbow M24.42- ☑
    finger M24.44- ☑
    foot joint M24.47- ☑
    hand joint M24.44- ☑
    hip M24.45- ☑
    knee M24.46- ☑
      patella — *see* Dislocation, patella, recurrent
    patella — *see* Dislocation, patella, recurrent
    sacroiliac — *see* subcategory M53.2 ☑
    shoulder M24.41- ☑
    toe M24.47- ☑
    vertebra — *see also* subcategory M43.5 ☑
      atlantoaxial M43.4
        with myelopathy M43.3
    wrist M24.43- ☑
  rib (cartilage) S23.29 ☑
  sacrococcygeal S33.2 ☑
  sacroiliac (joint) (ligament) S33.2 ☑
    congenital Q74.2
    recurrent — *see* subcategory M53.2 ☑
  sacrum S33.2 ☑
  scaphoid (bone) (hand) (wrist) — *see* Dislocation, wrist
    foot — *see* Dislocation, foot
  scapula — *see* Dislocation, shoulder, girdle, scapula
  semilunar cartilage, knee — *see* Tear, meniscus
  septal cartilage (nose) S03.1 ☑
  septum (nasal) (old) J34.2
  sesamoid bone — *code by* site under Dislocation
  shoulder (blade) (ligament) (joint) (traumatic) S43.006 ☑
    acromioclavicular — *see* Dislocation, acromioclavicular
    chronic — *see* Dislocation, recurrent, shoulder
    congenital Q68.8

Dislocation — *continued*
  shoulder — *continued*
    girdle S43.30- ☑
      scapula S43.31- ☑
      specified site NEC S43.39- ☑
    humerus S43.00- ☑
      anterior S43.01- ☑
      inferior S43.03- ☑
      posterior S43.02- ☑
    pathological — *see* Dislocation, pathological NEC, shoulder
    recurrent — *see* Dislocation, recurrent, shoulder
    specified type NEC S43.08- ☑
  spine
    cervical — *see* Dislocation, vertebra, cervical
    congenital Q76.49
    due to birth trauma P11.5
    lumbar — *see* Dislocation, vertebra, lumbar
    thoracic — *see* Dislocation, vertebra, thoracic
  spontaneous — *see* Dislocation, pathological
  sternoclavicular (joint) S43.206 ☑
    anterior S43.21- ☑
    posterior S43.22- ☑
  sternum S23.29 ☑
  subglenoid — *see* Dislocation, shoulder
  symphysis pubis S33.4 ☑
  talus — *see* Dislocation, ankle
  tarsal (bone(s)) (joint(s)) — *see* Dislocation, foot
  tarsometatarsal (joint(s)) — *see* Dislocation, foot
  temporomandibular (joint) S03.0- ☑
  thigh, proximal end — *see* Dislocation, hip
  thorax S23.20 ☑
    specified site NEC S23.29 ☑
    vertebra — *see* Dislocation, vertebra
  thumb S63.10- ☑
    interphalangeal joint — *see* Dislocation, interphalangeal (joint), thumb
    metacarpophalangeal joint — *see* Dislocation, metacarpophalangeal (joint), thumb
  thyroid cartilage S13.29 ☑
  tibia
    distal end — *see* Dislocation, ankle
    proximal end — *see* Dislocation, knee
  tibiofibular (joint)
    distal — *see* Dislocation, ankle
    superior — *see* Dislocation, knee
  toe(s) S93.106 ☑
    great S93.10- ☑
      interphalangeal joint S93.11- ☑
      metatarsophalangeal joint S93.12- ☑
    interphalangeal joint S93.119 ☑
    lesser S93.106 ☑
      interphalangeal joint S93.11- ☑
      metatarsophalangeal joint S93.12- ☑
    metatarsophalangeal joint S93.12- ☑
  tooth S03.2 ☑
  trachea S23.29 ☑
  ulna
    distal end S63.07- ☑
    proximal end — *see* Dislocation, elbow
  ulnohumeral (joint) — *see* Dislocation, elbow
  vertebra (articular process) (body) (traumatic)
    cervical S13.101 ☑
      atlantoaxial joint S13.121 ☑
      atlantooccipital joint S13.111 ☑
      atloidooccipital joint S13.111 ☑
      joint between
        C0 and C1 S13.111 ☑
        C1 and C2 S13.121 ☑
        C2 and C3 S13.131 ☑
        C3 and C4 S13.141 ☑
        C4 and C5 S13.151 ☑
        C5 and C6 S13.161 ☑
        C6 and C7 S13.171 ☑
        C7 and T1 S13.181 ☑
      occipitoatloid joint S13.111 ☑
    congenital Q76.49
    lumbar S33.101 ☑
      joint between
        L1 and L2 S33.111 ☑
        L2 and L3 S33.121 ☑
        L3 and L4 S33.131 ☑
        L4 and L5 S33.141 ☑
    nontraumatic — *see* Displacement, intervertebral disc
    partial — *see* Subluxation, by site

☑ **Additional Character Required — Refer to the Tabular List for Character Selection**   ▽ **Subterms under main terms may continue to next column or page**

Dislocation — *continued*
  vertebra — *continued*
    recurrent NEC — *see* subcategory M43.5 ☑
    thoracic S23.101 ☑
      joint between
        T1 and T2 S23.111 ☑
        T2 and T3 S23.121 ☑
        T3 and T4 S23.123 ☑
        T4 and T5 S23.131 ☑
        T5 and T6 S23.133 ☑
        T6 and T7 S23.141 ☑
        T7 and T8 S23.143 ☑
        T8 and T9 S23.151 ☑
        T9 and T10 S23.153 ☑
        T10 and T11 S23.161 ☑
        T11 and T12 S23.163 ☑
        T12 and L1 S23.171 ☑
  wrist (carpal bone) S63.006 ☑
    carpometacarpal joint — *see* Dislocation, carpometacarpal (joint)
    distal radioulnar joint — *see* Dislocation, radioulnar (joint), distal
    metacarpal bone, proximal — *see* Dislocation, metacarpal (bone), proximal end
    midcarpal — *see* Dislocation, midcarpal (joint)
    radiocarpal joint — *see* Dislocation, radiocarpal (joint)
    recurrent — *see* Dislocation, recurrent, wrist
    specified site NEC S63.09- ☑
    ulna — *see* Dislocation, ulna, distal end
  xiphoid cartilage S23.29 ☑

Disorder (of) — *see also* Disease
  acantholytic L11.9
    specified NEC L11.8
  acute
    psychotic — *see* Psychosis, acute
    stress F43.0
  adjustment (grief) F43.20
    with
      anxiety F43.22
        with depressed mood F43.23
      conduct disturbance F43.24
        with emotional disturbance F43.25
      depressed mood F43.21
        with anxiety F43.23
      other specified symptom F43.29
  adrenal (capsule) (gland) (medullary) E27.9
    specified NEC E27.8
  adrenogenital E25.9
    drug-induced E25.8
    iatrogenic E25.8
    idiopathic E25.8
  adult personality (and behavior) F69
    specified NEC F68.8
  affective (mood) — *see* Disorder, mood
  aggressive, unsocialized F91.1
  alcohol use
    mild F10.10
      with
        alcohol intoxication F10.129
          delirium F10.121
        alcohol-induced
          anxiety disorder F10.180
          bipolar and related disorder F10.14
          depressive disorder F10.14
          psychotic disorder F10.159
          sexual dysfunction F10.181
          sleep disorder F10.182
      in remission (early) (sustained) F10.11
    moderate or severe F10.20
      with
        alcohol intoxication F10.229
          delirium F10.221
        alcohol-induced
          anxiety disorder F10.280
          bipolar and related disorder F10.24
          depressive disorder F10.24
          major neurocognitive disorder, amnestic-confabulatory type F10.26
          major neurocognitive disorder, non-amnestic-confabulatory type F10.27
          mild neurocognitive disorder F10.288
          psychotic disorder F10.259
          sexual dysfunction F10.281
          sleep disorder F10.282
      in remission (early) (sustained) F10.21
  alcohol-related F10.99

Disorder — *continued*
  alcohol-related — *continued*
    with
      amnestic disorder, persisting F10.96
      anxiety disorder F10.980
      dementia, persisting F10.97
      intoxication F10.929
        with delirium F10.921
        uncomplicated F10.920
      mood disorder F10.94
      other specified F10.988
      psychotic disorder F10.959
        with
          delusions F10.950
          hallucinations F10.951
      sexual dysfunction F10.981
      sleep disorder F10.982
  allergic — *see* Allergy
  alveolar NEC J84.09
  amino-acid
    cystathioninuria E72.19
    cystinosis E72.04
    cystinuria E72.01
    glycinuria E72.09
    homocystinuria E72.11
    metabolism — *see* Disturbance, metabolism, amino-acid
    specified NEC E72.89
    neonatal, transitory P74.8
    renal transport NEC E72.09
    transport NEC E72.09
  amnesic, amnestic
    alcohol-induced F10.96
      with dependence F10.26
    due to (secondary to) general medical condition F04
    psychoactive NEC-induced F19.96
      with
        abuse F19.16
        dependence F19.26
    sedative, hypnotic or anxiolytic-induced F13.96
      with dependence F13.26
  amphetamine (or other stimulant) use
    mild
      with
        amphetamine, cocaine, or other stimulant intoxication
          with perceptual disturbances F15.122
          without perceptual disturbances F15.129
        amphetamine (or other stimulant) -induced
          anxiety disorder F15.180
          bipolar and related disorder F15.14
          depressive disorder F15.14
          obsessive-compulsive and related disorder F15.188
          psychotic disorder F15.159
          sexual dysfunction F15.181
        intoxication delirium F15.121
    moderate or severe
      with
        amphetamine, cocaine, or other stimulant intoxication
          with perceptual disturbances F15.222
          without perceptual disturbances F15.229
        amphetamine (or other stimulant) -induced
          anxiety disorder F15.280
          bipolar and related disorder F15.24
          depressive disorder F15.24
          obsessive-compulsive and related disorder F15.288
          psychotic disorder F15.259
          sexual dysfunction F15.281
        intoxication delirium F15.221
  amphetamine-type substance use
    mild F15.10
      in remission (early) (sustained) F15.11
    moderate F15.20
      in remission (early) (sustained) F15.21
    severe F15.20
      in remission (early) (sustained) F15.21
  anaerobic glycolysis with anemia D55.2
  anxiety F41.9
    due to (secondary to)
      alcohol F10.980
        in
          abuse F10.180
          dependence F10.280
      amphetamine F15.980
        in
          abuse F15.180

Disorder — *continued*
  anxiety — *continued*
    due to — *continued*
      amphetamine — *continued*
        in — *continued*
          dependence F15.280
      anxiolytic F13.980
        in
          abuse F13.180
          dependence F13.280
      caffeine F15.980
        in
          abuse F15.180
          dependence F15.280
      cannabis F12.980
        in
          abuse F12.180
          dependence F12.280
      cocaine F14.980
        in
          abuse F14.180
          dependence F14.180
      general medical condition F06.4
      hallucinogen F16.980
        in
          abuse F16.180
          dependence F16.280
      hypnotic F13.980
        in
          abuse F13.180
          dependence F13.280
      inhalant F18.980
        in
          abuse F18.180
          dependence F18.280
      phencyclidine F16.980
        in
          abuse F16.180
          dependence F16.280
      psychoactive substance NEC F19.980
        in
          abuse F19.180
          dependence F19.280
      sedative F13.980
        in
          abuse F13.180
          dependence F13.280
      volatile solvents F18.980
        in
          abuse F18.180
          dependence F18.280
    generalized F41.1
    illness F45.21
    mixed
      with depression (mild) F41.8
      specified NEC F41.3
    organic F06.4
    phobic F40.9
      of childhood F40.8
    specified NEC F41.8
  aortic valve — *see* Endocarditis, aortic
  aromatic amino-acid metabolism E70.9
    specified NEC E70.8
  arteriole NEC I77.89
  artery NEC I77.89
  articulation — *see* Disorder, joint
  attachment (childhood)
    disinhibited F94.2
    reactive F94.1
  attention-deficit hyperactivity (adolescent) (adult) (child) F90.9
    combined
      presentation F90.2
      type F90.2
    hyperactive
      impulsive presentation F90.1
      type F90.1
    inattentive
      presentation F90.0
      type F90.0
    specified type NEC F90.8
  attention-deficit without hyperactivity (adolescent) (adult) (child) F98.8
  auditory processing (central) H93.25
  autism spectrum F84.0
  autistic F84.0
  autoimmune D89.89
  autonomic nervous system G90.9
    specified NEC G90.8

Disorder — *continued*
avoidant
  child or adolescent F40.10
  restrictive food intake F50.82
balance
  acid-base E87.8
    mixed E87.4
  electrolyte E87.8
  fluid NEC E87.8
behavioral (disruptive) — *see* Disorder, conduct
beta-amino-acid metabolism E72.89
bile acid and cholesterol metabolism E78.70
  Barth syndrome E78.71
  other specified E78.79
  Smith-Lemli-Opitz syndrome E78.72
bilirubin excretion E80.6
binge eating F50.81
binocular
  movement H51.9
    convergence
      excess H51.12
      insufficiency H51.11
    internuclear ophthalmoplegia — *see* Ophthalmo-
      plegia, internuclear
    palsy of conjugate gaze H51.0
    specified type NEC H51.8
  vision NEC — *see* Disorder, vision, binocular
bipolar (I) (type I) F31.9
  and related due to a known physiological condition
    with
      manic features F06.33
      manic- or hypomanic-like episodes F06.33
      mixed features F06.34
  current (or most recent) episode
    depressed F31.9
      with psychotic features F31.5
      without psychotic features F31.30
        mild F31.31
        moderate F31.32
        severe (without psychotic features) F31.4
          with psychotic features F31.5
    hypomanic F31.0
    manic F31.9
      with psychotic features F31.2
      without psychotic features F31.10
        mild F31.11
        moderate F31.12
        severe (without psychotic features)
          F31.13
          with psychotic features F31.2
    mixed F31.60
      mild F31.61
      moderate F31.62
      severe (without psychotic features) F31.63
        with psychotic features F31.64
    severe depression (without psychotic features)
      F31.4
      with psychotic features F31.5
  in remission (currently) F31.70
    in full remission
      most recent episode
        depressed F31.76
        hypomanic F31.72
        manic F31.74
        mixed F31.78
    in partial remission
      most recent episode
        depressed F31.75
        hypomanic F31.71
        manic F31.73
        mixed F31.77
  organic F06.30
  single manic episode F30.9
    mild F30.11
    moderate F30.12
    severe (without psychotic symptoms) F30.13
      with psychotic symptoms F30.2
  specified type NEC F31.89
bipolar II (type 2) F31.81
bladder N32.9
  functional NEC N31.9
  in schistosomiasis B65.0 *[N33]*
  specified NEC N32.89
bleeding D68.9
blood D75.9
  in congenital early syphilis A50.09 *[D77]*
body dysmorphic F45.22
bone M89.9
  continuity M84.9

Disorder — *continued*
bone — *continued*
  continuity — *continued*
    specified type NEC M84.80
      ankle M84.87- ☑
      fibula M84.86- ☑
      foot M84.87- ☑
      hand M84.84- ☑
      humerus M84.82- ☑
      neck M84.88
      pelvis M84.859
      radius M84.83- ☑
      rib M84.88
      shoulder M84.81- ☑
      skull M84.88
      thigh M84.85- ☑
      tibia M84.86- ☑
      ulna M84.83- ☑
      vertebra M84.88
  density and structure M85.9
    cyst — *see also* Cyst, bone, specified type NEC
      aneurysmal — *see* Cyst, bone, aneurysmal
      solitary — *see* Cyst, bone, solitary
    diffuse idiopathic skeletal hyperostosis — *see*
      Hyperostosis, ankylosing
    fibrous dysplasia (monostotic) — *see* Dysplasia,
      fibrous, bone
    fluorosis — *see* Fluorosis, skeletal
    hyperostosis of skull M85.2
    osteitis condensans — *see* Osteitis, condensans
    specified type NEC M85.8- ☑
      ankle M85.87- ☑
      foot M85.87- ☑
      forearm M85.83- ☑
      hand M85.84- ☑
      lower leg M85.86- ☑
      multiple sites M85.89
      neck M85.88
      rib M85.88
      shoulder M85.81- ☑
      skull M85.88
      thigh M85.85- ☑
      upper arm M85.82- ☑
      vertebra M85.88
  development and growth NEC M89.20
    carpus M89.24- ☑
    clavicle M89.21- ☑
    femur M89.25- ☑
    fibula M89.26- ☑
    finger M89.24- ☑
    humerus M89.22- ☑
    ilium M89.259
    ischium M89.259
    metacarpus M89.24- ☑
    metatarsus M89.27- ☑
    multiple sites M89.29
    neck M89.28
    radius M89.23- ☑
    rib M89.28
    scapula M89.21- ☑
    skull M89.28
    tarsus M89.27- ☑
    tibia M89.26- ☑
    toe M89.27- ☑
    ulna M89.23- ☑
    vertebra M89.28
    specified type NEC M89.8X- ☑
brachial plexus G54.0
branched-chain amino-acid metabolism E71.2
  specified NEC E71.19
breast N64.9
  agalactia — *see* Agalactia
  associated with
    lactation O92.70
      specified NEC O92.79
    pregnancy O92.20
      specified NEC O92.29
    puerperium O92.20
      specified NEC O92.29
  cracked nipple — *see* Cracked nipple
  galactorrhea — *see* Galactorrhea
  hypogalactia O92.4
  lactation disorder NEC O92.79
  mastitis — *see* Mastitis
  nipple infection — *see* Infection, nipple
  retracted nipple — *see* Retraction, nipple
  specified type NEC N64.89

Disorder — *continued*
Briquet's F45.0
bullous, in diseases classified elsewhere L14
caffeine use
  mild
    with
      caffeine-induced
        anxiety disorder F15.180
        sleep disorder F15.182
  moderate or severe
    with
      caffeine-induced
        anxiety disorder F15.280
        sleep disorder F15.282
cannabis use
  mild F12.10
    with
      cannabis intoxication delirium F12.121
        with perceptual disturbances F12.122
        without perceptual disturbances F12.129
      cannabis-induced
        anxiety disorder F12.180
        psychotic disorder F12.159
        sleep disorder F12.188
    in remission (early) (sustained) F12.11
  moderate or severe F12.20
    with
      cannabis intoxication
        with perceptual disturbances F12.222
        without perceptual disturbances F12.229
      cannabis-induced
        anxiety disorder F12.280
        psychotic disorder F12.259
        sleep disorder F12.288
      delirium F12.221
    in remission (early) (sustained) F12.21
carbohydrate
  absorption, intestinal NEC E74.39
  metabolism (congenital) E74.9
    specified NEC E74.8
cardiac, functional I51.89
carnitine metabolism E71.40
cartilage M94.9
  articular NEC — *see* Derangement, joint, articular
    cartilage
  chondrocalcinosis — *see* Chondrocalcinosis
  specified type NEC M94.8X- ☑
    articular — *see* Derangement, joint, articular
      cartilage
    multiple sites M94.8X0
catatonia (due to known physiological condition) (with
  another mental disorder) F06.1
catatonic
  due to (secondary to) known physiological condition
    F06.1
  organic F06.1
central auditory processing H93.25
cervical
  region NEC M53.82
  root (nerve) NEC G54.2
character NOS F60.9
childhood disintegrative NEC F84.3
cholesterol and bile acid metabolism E78.70
  Barth syndrome E78.71
  other specified E78.79
  Smith-Lemli-Opitz syndrome E78.72
choroid H31.9
  atrophy — *see* Atrophy, choroid
  degeneration — *see* Degeneration, choroid
  detachment — *see* Detachment, choroid
  dystrophy — *see* Dystrophy, choroid
  hemorrhage — *see* Hemorrhage, choroid
  rupture — *see* Rupture, choroid
  scar — *see* Scar, chorioretinal
  solar retinopathy — *see* Retinopathy, solar
  specified type NEC H31.8
ciliary body — *see* Disorder, iris
  degeneration — *see* Degeneration, ciliary body
coagulation (factor) — *see also* Defect, coagulation
  D68.9
  newborn, transient P61.6
cocaine use
  mild F14.10
    with
      amphetamine, cocaine, or other stimulant
        intoxication
        with perceptual disturbances F14.122
        without perceptual disturbances F14.129

☑ Additional Character Required — Refer to the Tabular List for Character Selection
▽ Subterms under main terms may continue to next column or page

Disorder — *continued*
  cocaine use — *continued*
    mild — *continued*
      with — *continued*
        cocaine intoxication delirium F14.121
        cocaine-induced
          anxiety disorder F14.180
          bipolar and related disorder F14.14
          depressive disorder F14.14
          obsessive-compulsive and related disorder F14.188
          psychotic disorder F14.159
          sexual dysfunction F14.181
          sleep disorder F14.182
      in remission (early) (sustained) F14.11
    moderate or severe F14.20
      with
        amphetamine, cocaine, or other stimulant intoxication
          with perceptual disturbances F14.222
          without perceptual disturbances F14.229
        cocaine intoxication delirium F14.221
        cocaine-induced
          anxiety disorder F14.280
          bipolar and related disorder F14.24
          depressive disorder F14.24
          obsessive-compulsive and related disorder F14.288
          psychotic disorder F14.259
          sexual dysfunction F14.281
          sleep disorder F14.282
      in remission (early) (sustained) F14.21
  coccyx NEC M53.3
  cognitive F09
    due to (secondary to) general medical condition F09
    persisting R41.89
      due to
        alcohol F10.97
          with dependence F10.27
        anxiolytics F13.97
          with dependence F13.27
        hypnotics F13.97
          with dependence F13.27
        sedatives F13.97
          with dependence F13.27
        specified substance NEC F19.97
          with
            abuse F19.17
            dependence F19.27
  communication F80.9
    social pragmatic F80.82
  conduct (childhood) F91.9
    adjustment reaction — *see* Disorder, adjustment
    adolescent onset type F91.2
    childhood onset type F91.1
    compulsive F63.9
    confined to family context F91.0
    depressive F91.8
    group type F91.2
    hyperkinetic — *see* Disorder, attention-deficit hyperactivity
    oppositional defiance F91.3
    socialized F91.2
    solitary aggressive type F91.1
    specified NEC F91.8
    unsocialized (aggressive) F91.1
  conduction, heart I45.9
  congenital glycosylation (CDG) E74.8
  conjunctiva H11.9
    infection — *see* Conjunctivitis
  connective tissue, localized L94.9
    specified NEC L94.8
  conversion (functional neurological symptom disorder)
    with
      abnormal movement F44.4
      anesthesia or sensory loss F44.6
      attacks or seizures F44.5
      mixed symptoms F44.7
      special sensory symptoms F44.6
      speech symptoms F44.4
      swallowing symptoms F44.4
      weakness or paralysis F44.4
  convulsive (secondary) — *see* Convulsions
  cornea H18.9
    deformity — *see* Deformity, cornea
    degeneration — *see* Degeneration, cornea
    deposits — *see* Deposit, cornea
    due to contact lens H18.82- ☑

Disorder — *continued*
  cornea — *continued*
    due to contact lens — *continued*
      specified as edema — *see* Edema, cornea
    edema — *see* Edema, cornea
    keratitis — *see* Keratitis
    keratoconjunctivitis — *see* Keratoconjunctivitis
    membrane change — *see* Change, corneal membrane
    neovascularization — *see* Neovascularization, cornea
    scar — *see* Opacity, cornea
    specified type NEC H18.89- ☑
    ulcer — *see* Ulcer, cornea
  corpus cavernosum N48.9
  cranial nerve — *see* Disorder, nerve, cranial
  cyclothymic F34.0
  defiant oppositional F91.3
  delusional (persistent) (systematized) F22
    induced F24
  depersonalization F48.1
  depressive F32.9
    due to known physiological condition
      with
        depressive features F06.31
        major depressive-like episode F06.32
        mixed features F06.34
    major F32.9
      with psychotic symptoms F32.3
      in remission (full) F32.5
        partial F32.4
      recurrent F33.9
        with psychotic features F33.3
      single episode F32.9
        mild F32.0
        moderate F32.1
        severe (without psychotic symptoms) F32.2
          with psychotic symptoms F32.3
    organic F06.31
    persistent F34.1
    recurrent F33.9
      current episode
        mild F33.0
        moderate F33.1
        severe (without psychotic symptoms) F33.2
          with psychotic symptoms F33.3
      in remission F33.40
        full F33.42
        partial F33.41
      specified NEC F33.8
    single episode — *see* Episode, depressive
    specified NEC F32.89
  developmental F89
    arithmetical skills F81.2
    coordination (motor) F82
    expressive writing F81.81
    language F80.9
      expressive F80.1
      mixed receptive and expressive F80.2
      receptive type F80.2
      specified NEC F80.89
    learning F81.9
      arithmetical F81.2
      reading F81.0
    mixed F88
    motor coordination or function F82
    pervasive F84.9
      specified NEC F84.8
    phonological F80.0
    reading F81.0
    scholastic skills — *see also* Disorder, learning
      mixed F81.89
    specified NEC F88
    speech F80.9
      articulation F80.0
      specified NEC F80.89
    written expression F81.81
  diaphragm J98.6
  digestive (system) K92.9
    newborn P78.9
      specified NEC P78.89
    postprocedural — *see* Complication, gastrointestinal
    psychogenic F45.8
  disc (intervertebral) M51.9
    with
      myelopathy
        cervical region M50.00
        cervicothoracic region M50.03

Disorder — *continued*
  disc — *continued*
    with — *continued*
      myelopathy — *continued*
        high cervical region M50.01
        lumbar region M51.06
        mid-cervical region M50.020
        sacrococcygeal region M53.3
        thoracic region M51.04
        thoracolumbar region M51.05
      radiculopathy
        cervical region M50.10
        cervicothoracic region M50.13
        high cervical region M50.11
        lumbar region M51.16
        lumbosacral region M51.17
        mid-cervical region M50.120
        sacrococcygeal region M53.3
        thoracic region M51.14
        thoracolumbar region M51.15
    cervical M50.90
      with
        myelopathy M50.00
          C2-C3 M50.01
          C3-C4 M50.01
          C4-C5 M50.021
          C5-C6 M50.022
          C6-C7 M50.023
          C7-T1 M50.03
          cervicothoracic region M50.03
          high cervical region M50.01
          mid-cervical region M50.020
        neuritis, radiculitis or radiculopathy M50.10
          C2-C3 M50.11
          C3-C4 M50.11
          C4-C5 M50.121
          C5-C6 M50.122
          C6-C7 M50.123
          C7-T1 M50.13
          cervicothoracic region M50.13
          high cervical region M50.11
          mid-cervical region M50.120
        C2-C3 M50.91
        C3-C4 M50.91
        C4-C5 M50.921
        C5-C6 M50.922
        C6-C7 M50.923
        C7-T1 M50.93
        cervicothoracic region M50.93
        degeneration M50.30
          C2-C3 M50.31
          C3-C4 M50.31
          C4-C5 M50.321
          C5-C6 M50.322
          C6-C7 M50.323
          C7-T1 M50.33
          cervicothoracic region M50.33
          high cervical region M50.31
          mid-cervical region M50.320
        displacement M50.20
          C2-C3 M50.21
          C3-C4 M50.21
          C4-C5 M50.221
          C5-C6 M50.222
          C6-C7 M50.223
          C7-T1 M50.23
          cervicothoracic region M50.23
          high cervical region M50.21
          mid-cervical region M50.220
        high cervical region M50.91
        mid-cervical region M50.920
        specified type NEC M50.80
          C2-C3 M50.81
          C3-C4 M50.81
          C4-C5 M50.821
          C5-C6 M50.822
          C6-C7 M50.823
          C7-T1 M50.83
          cervicothoracic region M50.83
          high cervical region M50.81
          mid-cervical region M50.820
    specified NEC
      lumbar region M51.86
      lumbosacral region M51.87
      sacrococcygeal region M53.3
      thoracic region M51.84
      thoracolumbar region M51.85
  disinhibited attachment (childhood) F94.2
  disintegrative, childhood NEC F84.3

Disorder — continued
- disruptive F91.9
  - mood dysregulation F34.81
  - specified NEC F91.8
- disruptive behavior — *see* Disorder, conduct
- dissocial personality F60.2
- dissociative F44.9
  - affecting
    - motor function F44.4
      - and sensation F44.7
    - sensation F44.6
      - and motor function F44.7
  - brief reactive F43.0
  - due to (secondary to) general medical condition F06.8
  - mixed F44.7
  - organic F06.8
  - other specified NEC F44.89
- double heterozygous sickling — *see* Disease, sickle-cell
- dream anxiety F51.5
- drug induced hemorrhagic D68.32
- drug related F19.99
  - abuse — *see* Abuse, drug
  - dependence — *see* Dependence, drug
- dysmorphic body F45.22
- dysthymic F34.1
- ear H93.9- ☑
  - bleeding — *see* Otorrhagia
  - deafness — *see* Deafness
  - degenerative H93.09- ☑
  - discharge — *see* Otorrhea
  - external H61.9- ☑
    - auditory canal stenosis — *see* Stenosis, external ear canal
    - exostosis — *see* Exostosis, external ear canal
    - impacted cerumen — *see* Impaction, cerumen
    - otitis — *see* Otitis, externa
    - perichondritis — *see* Perichondritis, ear
    - pinna — *see* Disorder, pinna
    - specified type NEC H61.89- ☑
  - inner H83.9- ☑
    - vestibular dysfunction — *see* Disorder, vestibular function
  - middle H74.9- ☑
    - adhesive H74.1- ☑
    - ossicle — *see* Abnormal, ear ossicles
    - polyp — *see* Polyp, ear (middle)
    - specified NEC, in diseases classified elsewhere H75.8- ☑
  - postprocedural — *see* Complications, ear, procedure
  - specified NEC, in diseases classified elsewhere H94.8- ☑
- eating (adult) (psychogenic) F50.9
  - anorexia — *see* Anorexia
  - binge F50.81
  - bulimia F50.2
  - child F98.29
    - pica F98.3
    - rumination disorder F98.21
  - pica F50.89
    - childhood F98.3
- electrolyte (balance) NEC E87.8
  - with
    - abortion — *see* Abortion by type complicated by specified condition NEC
    - ectopic pregnancy O08.5
    - molar pregnancy O08.5
  - acidosis (metabolic) (respiratory) E87.2
  - alkalosis (metabolic) (respiratory) E87.3
- elimination, transepidermal L87.9
  - specified NEC L87.8
- emotional (persistent) F34.9
  - of childhood F93.9
    - specified NEC F93.8
- endocrine E34.9
  - postprocedural E89.89
  - specified NEC E89.89
- erectile (male) (organic) — *see also* Dysfunction, sexual, male, erectile N52.9
  - nonorganic F52.21
- erythematous — *see* Erythema
- esophagus K22.9
  - functional K22.4
  - psychogenic F45.8
- eustachian tube H69.9- ☑
  - infection — *see* Salpingitis, eustachian
  - obstruction — *see* Obstruction, eustachian tube
  - patulous — *see* Patulous, eustachian tube

Disorder — continued
- eustachian tube — *continued*
  - specified NEC H69.8- ☑
- exhibitionistic F65.2
- extrapyramidal G25.9
  - in deseases classified elsewhere — *see* category G26
  - specified type NEC G25.89
- eye H57.9
  - postprocedural — *see* Complication, postprocedural, eye
- eyelid H02.9
  - cyst — *see* Cyst, eyelid
  - degenerative H02.70
    - chloasma — *see* Chloasma, eyelid
    - madarosis — *see* Madarosis
    - specified type NEC H02.79
    - vitiligo — *see* Vitiligo, eyelid
    - xanthelasma — *see* Xanthelasma
  - dermatochalasis — *see* Dermatochalasis
  - edema — *see* Edema, eyelid
  - elephantiasis — *see* Elephantiasis, eyelid
  - foreign body, retained — *see* Foreign body, retained, eyelid
  - function H02.59
    - abnormal innervation syndrome — *see* Syndrome, abnormal innervation
    - blepharochalasis — *see* Blepharochalasis
    - blepharoclonus — *see* Blepharoclonus
    - blepharophimosis — *see* Blepharophimosis
    - blepharoptosis — *see* Blepharoptosis
    - lagophthalmos — *see* Lagophthalmos
    - lid retraction — *see* Retraction, lid
  - hypertrichosis — *see* Hypertrichosis, eyelid
  - specified type NEC H02.89
  - vascular H02.879
    - left H02.876
      - lower H02.875
      - upper H02.874
    - right H02.873
      - lower H02.872
      - upper H02.871
- factitious
  - by proxy F68.A
  - imposed on another F68.A
  - imposed on self F68.10
    - with predominantly
      - psychological symptoms F68.11
        - with physical symptoms F68.13
      - physical symptoms F68.12
        - with psychological symptoms F68.13
- factor, coagulation — *see* Defect, coagulation
- fatty acid
  - metabolism E71.30
    - specified NEC E71.39
  - oxidation
    - LCAD E71.310
    - MCAD E71.311
    - SCAD E71.312
    - specified deficiency NEC E71.318
- feeding (infant or child) — *see also* Disorder, eating R63.3
  - or eating disorder F50.9
  - specified NEC F50.9
- feigned (with obvious motivation) Z76.5
  - without obvious motivation — *see* Disorder, factitious
- female
  - hypoactive sexual desire F52.0
  - orgasmic F52.31
  - sexual interest/arousal F52.22
- fetishistic F65.0
- fibroblastic M72.9
  - specified NEC M72.8
- fluency
  - adult onset F98.5
  - childhood onset F80.81
  - following
    - cerebral infarction I69.323
    - cerebrovascular disease I69.923
      - specified disease NEC I69.823
    - intracerebral hemorrhage I69.123
    - nontraumatic intracranial hemorrhage NEC I69.223
    - subarachnoid hemorrhage I69.023
  - in conditions classified elsewhere R47.82
- fluid balance E87.8
- follicular (skin) L73.9

Disorder — continued
- follicular — *continued*
  - specified NEC L73.8
- frotteuristic F65.81
- fructose metabolism E74.10
  - essential fructosuria E74.11
  - fructokinase deficiency E74.11
  - fructose-1, 6-diphosphatase deficiency E74.19
  - hereditary fructose intolerance E74.12
  - other specified E74.19
- functional polymorphonuclear neutrophils D71
- gallbladder, biliary tract and pancreas in diseases classified elsewhere K87
- gambling F63.0
- gamma aminobutyric acid (GABA) metabolism E72.81
- gamma-glutamyl cycle E72.89
- gastric (functional) K31.9
  - motility K30
  - psychogenic F45.8
  - secretion K30
- gastrointestinal (functional) NOS K92.9
  - newborn P78.9
  - psychogenic F45.8
- gender-identity or -role F64.9
  - childhood F64.2
  - effect on relationship F66
  - of adolescence or adulthood F64.0
    - nontranssexual F64.8
  - specified NEC F64.8
  - uncertainty F66
- genito-pelvic pain penetration F52.6
- genitourinary system
  - female N94.9
  - male N50.9
  - psychogenic F45.8
- globe H44.9
  - degenerated condition H44.50
    - absolute glaucoma H44.51- ☑
    - atrophy H44.52- ☑
    - leucocoria H44.53- ☑
  - degenerative H44.30
    - chalcosis H44.31- ☑
    - myopia — *see also* Myopia, degenerative H44.2- ☑
    - siderosis H44.32- ☑
    - specified type NEC H44.39- ☑
  - endophthalmitis — *see* Endophthalmitis
  - foreign body, retained — *see* Foreign body, intraocular, old, retained
  - hemophthalmos — *see* Hemophthalmos
  - hypotony H44.40
    - due to
      - ocular fistula H44.42- ☑
      - specified disorder NEC H44.43- ☑
    - flat anterior chamber H44.41- ☑
    - primary H44.44- ☑
  - luxation — *see* Luxation, globe
  - specified type NEC H44.89
- glomerular (in) N05.9
  - amyloidosis E85.4 *[N08]*
  - cryoglobulinemia D89.1 *[N08]*
  - disseminated intravascular coagulation D65 *[N08]*
  - Fabry's disease E75.21 *[N08]*
  - familial lecithin cholesterol acyltransferase deficiency E78.6 *[N08]*
  - Goodpasture's syndrome M31.0
  - hemolytic-uremic syndrome D59.3
  - Henoch (-Schönlein) purpura D69.0 *[N08]*
  - malariae malaria B52.0
  - microscopic polyangiitis M31.7 *[N08]*
  - multiple myeloma C90.0- ☑ *[N08]*
  - mumps B26.83
  - schistosomiasis B65.9 *[N08]*
  - sepsis NEC A41.- ☑ *[N08]*
    - streptococcal A40.- ☑ *[N08]*
  - sickle-cell disorders D57.- ☑ *[N08]*
  - strongyloidiasis B78.9 *[N08]*
  - subacute bacterial endocarditis I33.0 *[N08]*
  - syphilis A52.75
  - systemic lupus erythematosus M32.14
  - thrombotic thrombocytopenic purpura M31.1 *[N08]*
  - Waldenström macroglobulinemia C88.0 *[N08]*
  - Wegener's granulomatosis M31.31
- gluconeogenesis E74.4
- glucosaminoglycan metabolism — *see* Disorder, metabolism, glucosaminoglycan
- glycine metabolism E72.50
  - d-glycericacidemia E72.59

☑ Additional Character Required — Refer to the Tabular List for Character Selection   ▽ Subterms under main terms may continue to next column or page

Disorder — *continued*
glycine metabolism — *continued*
  hyperhydroxyprolinemia E72.59
  hyperoxaluria R82.992
    primary E72.53
  hyperprolinemia E72.59
  non-ketotic hyperglycinemia E72.51
  oxalosis E72.53
  oxaluria E72.53
  sarcosinemia E72.59
  trimethylaminuria E72.52
glycoprotein metabolism E77.9
  specified NEC E77.8
habit (and impulse) F63.9
  involving sexual behavior NEC F65.9
  specified NEC F63.89
hallucinogen use
  mild F16.10
    with
      hallucinogen intoxication delirium F16.121
      hallucinogen-induced
        anxiety disorder F16.180
        bipolar and related disorder F16.14
        depressive disorder F16.14
        psychotic disorder F16.159
      other hallucinogen intoxication F16.129
    in remission (early) (sustained) F16.11
  moderate or severe F16.20
    with
      hallucinogen intoxication delirium F16.221
      hallucinogen-induced
        anxiety disorder F16.280
        bipolar and related disorder F16.24
        depressive disorder F16.24
        psychotic disorder F16.259
      other hallucinogen intoxication F16.229
    in remission (early) (sustained) F16.21
heart action I49.9
hematological D75.9
  newborn (transient) P61.9
    specified NEC P61.8
hematopoietic organs D75.9
hemorrhagic NEC D69.9
  drug-induced D68.32
  due to
    extrinsic circulating anticoagulants D68.32
    increase in
      anti-IIa D68.32
      anti-Xa D68.32
    intrinsic
      circulating anticoagulants D68.318
      increase in
        anti-IXa D68.318
        antithrombin D68.318
        anti-VIIIa D68.318
        anti-XIa D68.318
  following childbirth O72.3
hemostasis — *see* Defect, coagulation
histidine metabolism E70.40
  histidinemia E70.41
  other specified E70.49
hoarding F42.3
hyperkinetic — *see* Disorder, attention-deficit hyperactivity
hyperleucine-isoleucinemia E71.19
hypervalinemia E71.19
hypoactive sexual desire F52.0
hypochondriacal F45.20
  body dysmorphic F45.22
  neurosis F45.21
  other specified F45.29
identity
  dissociative F44.81
  illness anxiety F45.21
  of childhood F93.8
immune mechanism (immunity) D89.9
  specified type NEC D89.89
impaired renal tubular function N25.9
  specified NEC N25.89
impulse (control) F63.9
inflammatory
  pelvic, in diseases classified elsewhere — *see* category N74
  penis N48.29
    abscess N48.21
    cellulitis N48.22
inhalant use
  mild F18.10

Disorder — *continued*
inhalant use — *continued*
  mild — *continued*
    with
      inhalant intoxication F18.129
      inhalant intoxication delirium F18.121
      inhalant-induced
        anxiety disorder F18.180
        depressive disorder F18.14
        major neurocognitive disorder F18.17
        mild neurocognitive disorder F18.188
        psychotic disorder F18.159
    in remission (early) (sustained) F18.11
  moderate or severe F18.20
    with
      inhalant intoxication F18.229
      inhalant intoxication delirium F18.221
      inhalant-induced
        anxiety disorder F18.280
        depressive disorder F18.24
        major neurocognitive disorder F18.27
        mild neurocognitive disorder F18.288
        psychotic disorder F18.259
    in remission (early) (sustained) F18.21
integument, newborn P83.9
  specified NEC P83.88
intermittent explosive F63.81
internal secretion pancreas — *see* Increased, secretion, pancreas, endocrine
intestine, intestinal
  carbohydrate absorption NEC E74.39
    postoperative K91.2
  functional NEC K59.9
    postoperative K91.89
  psychogenic F45.8
  vascular K55.9
    chronic K55.1
    specified NEC K55.8
intraoperative (intraprocedural) — *see* Complications, intraoperative
involuntary emotional expression (IEED) F07.89
iris H21.9
  adhesions — *see* Adhesions, iris
  atrophy — *see* Atrophy, iris
  chamber angle recession — *see* Recession, chamber angle
  cyst — *see* Cyst, iris
  degeneration — *see* Degeneration, iris
  in diseases classified elsewhere H22
  iridodialysis — *see* Iridodialysis
  iridoschisis — *see* Iridoschisis
  miotic pupillary cyst — *see* Cyst, pupillary
  pupillary
    abnormality — *see* Abnormality, pupillary
    membrane — *see* Membrane, pupillary
  specified type NEC H21.89
  vascular NEC H21.1X- ☑
iron metabolism E83.10
  specified NEC E83.19
isovaleric acidemia E71.110
jaw, developmental M27.0
  temporomandibular — *see also* Anomaly, dentofacial, temporomandibular joint M26.60- ☑
joint M25.9
  derangement — *see* Derangement, joint
  effusion — *see* Effusion, joint
  fistula — *see* Fistula, joint
  hemarthrosis — *see* Hemarthrosis
  instability — *see* Instability, joint
  osteophyte — *see* Osteophyte
  pain — *see* Pain, joint
  psychogenic F45.8
  specified type NEC M25.80
    ankle M25.87- ☑
    elbow M25.82- ☑
    foot joint M25.87- ☑
    hand joint M25.84- ☑
    hip M25.85- ☑
    knee M25.86- ☑
    shoulder M25.81- ☑
    wrist M25.83- ☑
  stiffness — *see* Stiffness, joint
ketone metabolism E71.32
kidney N28.9
  functional (tubular) N25.9
  in
    schistosomiasis B65.9 *[N29]*
  tubular function N25.9

Disorder — *continued*
kidney — *continued*
  tubular function — *continued*
    specified NEC N25.89
lacrimal system H04.9
  changes H04.69
    fistula — *see* Fistula, lacrimal
  gland H04.19
    atrophy — *see* Atrophy, lacrimal gland
    cyst — *see* Cyst, lacrimal, gland
    dacryops — *see* Dacryops
    dislocation — *see* Dislocation, lacrimal gland
    dry eye syndrome — *see* Syndrome, dry eye
    infection — *see* Dacryoadenitis
  granuloma — *see* Granuloma, lacrimal
  inflammation — *see* Inflammation, lacrimal
  obstruction — *see* Obstruction, lacrimal
  specified NEC H04.89
lactation NEC O92.79
language (developmental) F80.9
  expressive F80.1
  mixed receptive and expressive F80.2
  receptive F80.2
late luteal phase dysphoric N94.89
learning (specific) F81.9
  acalculia R48.8
  alexia R48.0
  mathematics F81.2
  reading F81.0
  specified
    with impairment in
      mathematics F81.2
      reading F81.0
      written expression F81.81
  specified NEC F81.89
  spelling F81.81
  written expression F81.81
lens H27.9
  aphakia — *see* Aphakia
  cataract — *see* Cataract
  dislocation — *see* Dislocation, lens
  specified type NEC H27.8
ligament M24.20
  ankle M24.27- ☑
  attachment, spine — *see* Enthesopathy, spinal
  elbow M24.22- ☑
  foot joint M24.27- ☑
  hand joint M24.24- ☑
  hip M24.25- ☑
  knee — *see* Derangement, knee, specified NEC
  shoulder M24.21- ☑
  vertebra M24.28
  wrist M24.23- ☑
ligamentous attachments — *see also* Enthesopathy
  spine — *see* Enthesopathy, spinal
lipid
  metabolism, congenital E78.9
  storage E75.6
    specified NEC E75.5
lipoprotein
  deficiency (familial) E78.6
  metabolism E78.9
    specified NEC E78.89
liver K76.9
  malarial B54 *[K77]*
low back — *see also* Dorsopathy, specified NEC
lumbosacral
  plexus G54.1
  root (nerve) NEC G54.4
lung, interstitial, drug-induced J70.4
  acute J70.2
  chronic J70.3
lymphoproliferative, post-transplant (PTLD) D47.Z1
  (*following* D47.4)
lysine and hydroxylysine metabolism E72.3
major neurocognitive — *see* Dementia, in (due to)
male
  erectile (organic) — *see also* Dysfunction, sexual, male, erectile N52.9
    nonorganic F52.21
  hypoactive sexual desire F52.0
  orgasmic F52.32
manic F30.9
  organic F06.33
mast cell activation — *see* Activation, mast cell
mastoid — *see also* Disorder, ear, middle
  postprocedural — *see* Complications, ear, procedure
meniscus — *see* Derangement, knee, meniscus

Disorder — *continued*
- menopausal N95.9
  - specified NEC N95.8
- menstrual N92.6
  - psychogenic F45.8
  - specified NEC N92.5
- mental (or behavioral) (nonpsychotic) F99
  - due to (secondary to)
    - amphetamine
      - due to drug abuse — *see* Abuse, drug, stimulant
      - due to drug dependence — *see* Dependence, drug, stimulant
    - brain disease, damage and dysfunction F09
    - caffeine use
      - due to drug abuse — *see* Abuse, drug, stimulant
      - due to drug dependence — *see* Dependence, drug, stimulant
    - cannabis use
      - due to drug abuse — *see* Abuse, drug, cannabis
      - due to drug dependence — *see* Dependence, drug, cannabis
    - general medical condition F09
    - sedative or hypnotic use
      - due to drug abuse — *see* Abuse, drug, sedative
      - due to drug dependence — *see* Dependence, drug, sedative
    - tobacco (nicotine) use — *see* Dependence, drug, nicotine
  - following organic brain damage F07.9
    - frontal lobe syndrome F07.0
    - personality change F07.0
    - postconcussional syndrome F07.81
    - specified NEC F07.89
  - infancy, childhood or adolescence F98.9
  - neurotic — *see* Neurosis
  - organic or symptomatic F09
  - presenile, psychotic F03 ☑
  - problem NEC
  - psychoneurotic — *see* Neurosis
  - psychotic — *see* Psychosis
  - puerperal F53.0
  - senile, psychotic NEC F03 ☑
- metabolic, amino acid, transitory, newborn P74.8
- metabolism NOS E88.9
  - amino-acid E72.9
    - aromatic E70.9
      - albinism — *see* Albinism
      - histidine E70.40
        - histidinemia E70.41
        - other specified E70.49
      - hyperphenylalaninemia E70.1
        - classical phenylketonuria E70.0
      - other specified E70.8
      - tryptophan E70.5
      - tyrosine E70.20
        - hypertyrosinemia E70.21
        - other specified E70.29
    - branched chain E71.2
      - 3-methylglutaconic aciduria E71.111
      - hyperleucine-isoleucinemia E71.19
      - hypervalinemia E71.19
      - isovaleric acidemia E71.110
      - maple syrup urine disease E71.0
      - methylmalonic acidemia E71.120
      - organic aciduria NEC E71.118
      - other specified E71.19
      - proprionate NEC E71.128
      - proprionic acidemia E71.121
    - glycine E72.50
      - d-glycericacidemia E72.59
      - hyperhydroxyprolinemia E72.59
      - hyperoxaluria R82.992
        - primary E72.53
      - hyperprolinemia E72.59
      - non-ketotic hyperglycinemia E72.51
      - other specified E72.59
      - sarcosinemia E72.59
      - trimethylaminuria E72.52
    - hydroxylysine E72.3
    - lysine E72.3
    - ornithine E72.4
    - other specified E72.89
      - beta-amino acid E72.89
      - gamma-glutamyl cycle E72.89

Disorder — *continued*
- metabolism — *continued*
  - amino-acid — *continued*
    - straight-chain E72.89
    - sulfur-bearing E72.10
      - homocystinuria E72.11
      - methylenetetrahydrofolate reductase deficiency E72.12
      - other specified E72.19
  - bile acid and cholesterol metabolism E78.70
  - bilirubin E80.7
    - specified NEC E80.6
  - calcium E83.50
    - hypercalcemia E83.52
    - hypocalcemia E83.51
    - other specified E83.59
  - carbohydrate E74.9
    - specified NEC E74.8
  - cholesterol and bile acid metabolism E78.70
  - congenital E88.9
  - copper E83.00
    - specified type NEC E83.09
    - Wilson's disease E83.01
  - cystinuria E72.01
  - fructose E74.10
  - galactose E74.20
  - glucosaminoglycan E76.9
    - mucopolysaccharidosis — *see* Mucopolysaccharidosis
    - specified NEC E76.8
  - glutamine E72.89
  - glycine E72.50
  - glycogen storage (hepatorenal) E74.09
  - glycoprotein E77.9
    - specified NEC E77.8
  - glycosaminoglycan E76.9
    - specified NEC E76.8
  - in labor and delivery O75.89
  - iron E83.10
  - isoleucine E71.19
  - leucine E71.19
  - lipoid E78.9
  - lipoprotein E78.9
    - specified NEC E78.89
  - magnesium E83.40
    - hypermagnesemia E83.41
    - hypomagnesemia E83.42
    - other specified E83.49
  - mineral E83.9
    - specified NEC E83.89
  - mitochondrial E88.40
    - MELAS syndrome E88.41
    - MERRF syndrome (myoclonic epilepsy associated with ragged-red fibers) E88.42
    - other specified E88.49
  - ornithine E72.4
  - phosphatases E83.30
  - phosphorus E83.30
    - acid phosphatase deficiency E83.39
    - hypophosphatasia E83.39
    - hypophosphatemia E83.39
      - familial E83.31
    - other specified E83.39
    - pseudovitamin D deficiency E83.32
  - plasma protein NEC E88.09
  - porphyrin — *see* Porphyria
  - postprocedural E89.89
    - specified NEC E89.89
  - purine E79.9
    - specified NEC E79.8
  - pyrimidine E79.9
    - specified NEC E79.8
  - pyruvate E74.4
  - serine E72.89
  - sodium E87.8
  - specified NEC E88.89
  - threonine E72.89
  - valine E71.19
  - zinc E83.2
- methylmalonic acidemia E71.120
- micturition NEC — *see also* Difficulty, micturition R39.198
  - feeling of incomplete emptying R39.14
  - hesitancy R39.11
  - poor stream R39.12
  - psychogenic F45.8
  - split stream R39.13
  - straining R39.16
  - urgency R39.15

Disorder — *continued*
- mild neurocognitive G31.84
- mitochondrial metabolism E88.40
- mitral (valve) — *see* Endocarditis, mitral
- mixed
  - anxiety and depressive F41.8
  - of scholastic skills (developmental) F81.89
  - receptive expressive language F80.2
- mood F39
  - bipolar — *see* Disorder, bipolar
  - depressive — *see* Disorder, depressive
  - due to (secondary to)
    - alcohol F10.94
    - amphetamine F15.94
      - in
        - abuse F15.14
        - dependence F15.24
    - anxiolytic F13.94
      - in
        - abuse F13.14
        - dependence F13.24
    - cocaine F14.94
      - in
        - abuse F14.14
        - dependence F14.24
    - general medical condition F06.30
    - hallucinogen F16.94
      - in
        - abuse F16.14
        - dependence F16.24
    - hypnotic F13.94
      - in
        - abuse F13.14
        - dependence F13.24
    - inhalant F18.94
      - in
        - abuse F18.14
        - dependence F18.24
    - opioid F11.94
      - in
        - abuse F11.14
        - dependence F11.24
    - phencyclidine (PCP) F16.94
      - in
        - abuse F16.14
        - dependence F16.24
    - physiological condition F06.30
      - with
        - depressive features F06.31
        - major depressive-like episode F06.32
        - manic features F06.33
        - mixed features F06.34
    - psychoactive substance NEC F19.94
      - in
        - abuse F19.14
        - dependence F19.24
    - sedative F13.94
      - in
        - abuse F13.14
        - dependence F13.24
    - volatile solvents F18.94
      - in
        - abuse F18.14
        - dependence F18.24
  - manic episode F30.9
    - with psychotic symptoms F30.2
    - in remission (full) F30.4
      - partial F30.3
    - specified type NEC F30.8
    - without psychotic symptoms F30.10
      - mild F30.11
      - moderate F30.12
      - severe F30.13
  - organic F06.30
    - right hemisphere F07.89
  - persistent F34.9
    - cyclothymia F34.0
    - dysthymia F34.1
    - specified type NEC F34.89
  - recurrent F39
  - right hemisphere organic F07.89
- movement G25.9
  - drug-induced G25.70
    - akathisia G25.71
    - specified NEC G25.79
  - hysterical F44.4
  - in diseases classified elsewhere — *see* category G26
  - periodic limb G47.61
    - sleep related G47.61

Disorder — *continued*
- movement — *continued*
  - sleep related NEC G47.69
  - specified NEC G25.89
  - stereotyped F98.4
  - treatment-induced G25.9
- multiple personality F44.81
- muscle M62.9
  - attachment, spine — *see* Enthesopathy, spinal
  - in trichinellosis — *see* Trichinellosis, with muscle disorder
  - psychogenic F45.8
  - specified type NEC M62.89
  - tone, newborn P94.9
    - specified NEC P94.8
- muscular
  - attachments — *see also* Enthesopathy
    - spine — *see* Enthesopathy, spinal
  - urethra N36.44
- musculoskeletal system, soft tissue — *see* Disorder, soft tissue
  - postprocedural M96.89
  - psychogenic F45.8
- myoneural G70.9
  - due to lead G70.1
  - specified NEC G70.89
  - toxic G70.1
- myotonic NEC G71.19
- nail, in diseases classified elsewhere L62
- neck region NEC — *see* Dorsopathy, specified NEC
- neonatal onset multisystemic inflammatory (NOMID) M04.2
- nerve G58.9
  - abducent NEC — *see* Strabismus, paralytic, sixth nerve
  - accessory G52.8
  - acoustic — *see* subcategory H93.3 ☑
  - auditory — *see* subcategory H93.3 ☑
  - auriculotemporal G50.8
  - axillary G54.0
  - cerebral — *see* Disorder, nerve, cranial
  - cranial G52.9
    - eighth — *see* subcategory H93.3 ☑
    - eleventh G52.8
    - fifth G50.9
    - first G52.0
    - fourth NEC — *see* Strabismus, paralytic, fourth nerve
    - multiple G52.7
    - ninth G52.1
    - second NEC — *see* Disorder, nerve, optic
    - seventh NEC G51.8
    - sixth NEC — *see* Strabismus, paralytic, sixth nerve
    - specified NEC G52.8
    - tenth G52.2
    - third NEC — *see* Strabismus, paralytic, third nerve
    - twelfth G52.3
  - entrapment — *see* Neuropathy, entrapment
  - facial G51.9
    - specified NEC G51.8
  - femoral — *see* Lesion, nerve, femoral
  - glossopharyngeal NEC G52.1
  - hypoglossal G52.3
  - intercostal G58.0
  - lateral
    - cutaneous of thigh — *see* Mononeuropathy, lower limb, meralgia paresthetica
    - popliteal — *see* Lesion, nerve, popliteal
  - lower limb — *see* Mononeuropathy, lower limb
  - medial popliteal — *see* Lesion, nerve, popliteal, medial
  - median NEC — *see* Lesion, nerve, median
  - multiple G58.7
  - oculomotor NEC — *see* Strabismus, paralytic, third nerve
  - olfactory G52.0
  - optic NEC H47.09- ☑
    - hemorrhage into sheath — *see* Hemorrhage, optic nerve
    - ischemic H47.01- ☑
  - peroneal — *see* Lesion, nerve, popliteal
  - phrenic G58.8
  - plantar — *see* Lesion, nerve, plantar
  - pneumogastric G52.2
  - posterior tibial — *see* Syndrome, tarsal tunnel
  - radial — *see* Lesion, nerve, radial
  - recurrent laryngeal G52.2
  - root G54.9

Disorder — *continued*
- nerve — *continued*
  - root — *continued*
    - cervical G54.2
    - lumbosacral G54.1
    - specified NEC G54.8
    - thoracic G54.3
  - sciatic NEC — *see* Lesion, nerve, sciatic
  - specified NEC G58.8
    - lower limb — *see* Mononeuropathy, lower limb, specified NEC
    - upper limb — *see* Mononeuropathy, upper limb, specified NEC
  - sympathetic G90.9
  - tibial — *see* Lesion, nerve, popliteal, medial
  - trigeminal G50.9
    - specified NEC G50.8
  - trochlear NEC — *see* Strabismus, paralytic, fourth nerve
  - ulnar — *see* Lesion, nerve, ulnar
  - upper limb — *see* Mononeuropathy, upper limb
  - vagus G52.2
- nervous system G98.8
  - autonomic (peripheral) G90.9
    - specified NEC G90.8
  - central G96.9
    - specified NEC G96.8
  - parasympathetic G90.9
  - specified NEC G98.8
  - sympathetic G90.9
  - vegetative G90.9
- neurocognitive R41.9
  - major
    - with
      - aggressive behavior F01.51
      - combative behavior F01.51
      - violent behavior F01.51
    - due to vascular disease, with behavioral disturbance F01.51
    - in (due to) (other diseases classified elsewhere) — *see also* Dementia, in (due to) F02.80
      - with
        - aggressive behavior F02.81
        - combative behavior F02.81
        - violent behavior F02.81
      - without behavioral disturbance F01.50
  - mild G31.84
- neurodevelopmental F89
  - specified NEC F88
- neurohypophysis NEC E23.3
- neurological NEC R29.818
- neuromuscular G70.9
  - hereditary NEC G71.9
  - specified NEC G70.89
  - toxic G70.1
- neurotic F48.9
  - specified NEC F48.8
- neutrophil, polymorphonuclear D71
- nicotine use — *see* Dependence, drug, nicotine
- nightmare F51.5
- non-rapid eye movement sleep arousal
  - sleep terror type F51.4
  - sleepwalking type F51.3
- nose J34.9
  - specified NEC J34.89
- obsessive-compulsive F42.9
  - and related disorder due to a known physiological condition F06.8
- odontogenesis NOS K00.9
- opioid use
  - with
    - opioid-induced psychotic disorder F11.959
      - with
        - delusions F11.950
        - hallucinations F11.951
    - due to drug abuse — *see* Abuse, drug, opioid
    - due to drug dependence — *see* Dependence, drug, opioid
  - mild F11.10
    - with
      - opioid-induced
        - anxiety disorder F11.188
        - depressive disorder F11.14
        - sexual dysfunction F11.181
      - opioid intoxication
        - with perceptual disturbances F11.122
        - delirium F11.121
        - without perceptual disturbances F11.129

Disorder — *continued*
- opioid use — *continued*
  - mild — *continued*
    - in remission (early) (sustained) F11.11
  - moderate or severe F11.20
    - with
      - opioid-induced
        - anxiety disorder F11.288
        - anxiety disorder F11.988
        - depressive disorder F11.24
        - depressive disorder F11.94
        - sexual dysfunction F11.281
        - sexual dysfunction F11.981
      - opioid intoxication
        - with perceptual disturbances F11.222
        - delirium F11.221
        - without perceptual disturbances F11.229
    - in remission (early) (sustained) F11.21
- oppositional defiant F91.3
- optic
  - chiasm H47.49
    - due to
      - inflammatory disorder H47.41
      - neoplasm H47.42
      - vascular disorder H47.43
  - disc H47.39- ☑
    - coloboma — *see* Coloboma, optic disc
    - drusen — *see* Drusen, optic disc
    - pseudopapilledema — *see* Pseudopapilledema
  - radiations — *see* Disorder, visual, pathway
  - tracts — *see* Disorder, visual, pathway
- orbit H05.9
  - cyst — *see* Cyst, orbit
  - deformity — *see* Deformity, orbit
  - edema — *see* Edema, orbit
  - enophthalmos — *see* Enophthalmos
  - exophthalmos — *see* Exophthalmos
  - hemorrhage — *see* Hemorrhage, orbit
  - inflammation — *see* Inflammation, orbit
  - myopathy — *see* Myopathy, extraocular muscles
  - retained foreign body — *see* Foreign body, orbit, old
  - specified type NEC H05.89
- organic
  - anxiety F06.4
  - catatonic F06.1
  - delusional F06.2
  - dissociative F06.8
  - emotionally labile (asthenic) F06.8
  - mood (affective) F06.30
  - schizophrenia-like F06.2
- orgasmic (female) F52.31
  - male F52.32
- ornithine metabolism E72.4
- overanxious F41.1
  - of childhood F93.8
- pain
  - with related psychological factors F45.42
  - exclusively related to psychological factors F45.41
  - genito-pelvic penetration disorder F52.6
- pancreatic internal secretion E16.9
  - specified NEC E16.8
- panic F41.0
  - with agoraphobia F40.01
- papulosquamous L44.9
  - in diseases classified elsewhere L45
  - specified NEC L44.8
- paranoid F22
  - induced F24
  - shared F24
- paraphilic F65.9
  - specified NEC F65.89
- parathyroid (gland) E21.5
  - specified NEC E21.4
- parietoalveolar NEC J84.09
- paroxysmal, mixed R56.9
- patella M22.9- ☑
  - chondromalacia — *see* Chondromalacia, patella
  - derangement NEC M22.3X- ☑
  - recurrent
    - dislocation — *see* Dislocation, patella, recurrent
    - subluxation — *see* Dislocation, patella, recurrent, incomplete
  - specified NEC M22.8X- ☑
- patellofemoral M22.2X- ☑
- pedophilic F65.4
- pentose phosphate pathway with anemia D55.1
- perception, due to hallucinogens F16.983

Disorder — *continued*
  perception, due to hallucinogens — *continued*
    in
      abuse F16.183
      dependence F16.283
  peripheral nervous system NEC G64
  peroxisomal E71.50
    biogenesis
      neonatal adrenoleukodystrophy E71.511
      specified disorder NEC E71.518
      Zellweger syndrome E71.510
    rhizomelic chondrodysplasia punctata E71.540
    specified form NEC E71.548
      group 1 E71.518
      group 2 E71.53
      group 3 E71.542
    X-linked adrenoleukodystrophy E71.529
      adolescent E71.521
      adrenomyeloneuropathy E71.522
      childhood E71.520
      specified form NEC E71.528
    Zellweger-like syndrome E71.541
  persistent
    (somatoform) pain F45.41
    affective (mood) F34.9
  personality — *see also* Personality F60.9
    affective F34.0
    aggressive F60.3
    amoral F60.2
    anankastic F60.5
    antisocial F60.2
    anxious F60.6
    asocial F60.2
    asthenic F60.7
    avoidant F60.6
    borderline F60.3
    change (secondary) due to general medical condition F07.0
    compulsive F60.5
    cyclothymic F34.0
    dependent (passive) F60.7
    depressive F34.1
    dissocial F60.2
    emotional instability F60.3
    expansive paranoid F60.0
    explosive F60.3
    following organic brain damage F07.9
    histrionic F60.4
    hyperthymic F34.0
    hypothymic F34.1
    hysterical F60.4
    immature F60.89
    inadequate F60.7
    labile F60.3
    mixed (nonspecific) F60.89
    moral deficiency F60.2
    narcissistic F60.81
    negativistic F60.89
    obsessional F60.5
    obsessive (-compulsive) F60.5
    organic F07.9
    overconscientious F60.5
    paranoid F60.0
    passive (-dependent) F60.7
    passive-aggressive F60.89
    pathological NEC F60.9
    pseudosocial F60.2
    psychopathic F60.2
    schizoid F60.1
    schizotypal F21
    self-defeating F60.7
    specified NEC F60.89
    type A F60.5
    unstable (emotional) F60.3
  pervasive, developmental F84.9
  phencyclidine use
    mild F16.10
      with
        phencyclidine intoxication F16.129
        phencyclidine intoxication delirium F16.121
        phencyclidine-induced
          anxiety disorder F16.180
          bipolar and related disorder F16.14
          depressive disorder F16.14
          psychotic disorder F16.159
      in remission (early) (sustained) F16.11
    moderate or severe F16.20
      with
        phencyclidine intoxication F16.229

Disorder — *continued*
  phencyclidine use — *continued*
    moderate or severe — *continued*
      with — *continued*
        phencyclidine intoxication delirium F16.221
        phencyclidine-induced
          anxiety disorder F16.280
          bipolar and related disorder F16.14
          depressive disorder F16.24
          psychotic disorder F16.259
      in remission (early) (sustained) F16.21
  phobic anxiety, childhood F40.8
  phosphate-losing tubular N25.0
  pigmentation L81.9
    choroid, congenital Q14.3
    diminished melanin formation L81.6
    iron L81.8
    specified NEC L81.8
  pinna (noninfective) H61.10- ☑
    deformity, acquired H61.11- ☑
    hematoma H61.12- ☑
    perichondritis — *see* Perichondritis, ear
    specified type NEC H61.19- ☑
  pituitary gland E23.7
    iatrogenic (postprocedural) E89.3
    specified NEC E23.6
  platelets D69.1
  plexus G54.9
    specified NEC G54.8
  polymorphonuclear neutrophils D71
  porphyrin metabolism — *see* Porphyria
  postconcussional F07.81
  posthallucinogen perception F16.983
    in
      abuse F16.183
      dependence F16.283
  postmenopausal N95.9
    specified NEC N95.8
  postprocedural (postoperative) — *see* Complications, postprocedural
  post-transplant lymphoproliferative D47.Z1 (*following* D47.4)
  post-traumatic stress (PTSD) F43.10
    acute F43.11
    chronic F43.12
  premenstrual dysphoric (PMDD) F32.81
  prepuce N47.8
  propionic acidemia E71.121
  prostate N42.9
    specified NEC N42.89
  psychogenic NOS — *see also* condition F45.9
    anxiety F41.8
    appetite F50.9
    asthenic F48.8
    cardiovascular (system) F45.8
    compulsive F42.8
    cutaneous F54
    depressive F32.9
    digestive (system) F45.8
    dysmenorrheic F45.8
    dyspneic F45.8
    endocrine (system) F54
    eye NEC F45.8
    feeding — *see* Disorder, eating
    functional NEC F45.8
    gastric F45.8
    gastrointestinal (system) F45.8
    genitourinary (system) F45.8
    heart (function) (rhythm) F45.8
    hyperventilatory F45.8
    hypochondriacal — *see* Disorder, hypochondriacal
    intestinal F45.8
    joint F45.8
    learning F81.9
    limb F45.8
    lymphatic (system) F45.8
    menstrual F45.8
    micturition F45.8
    monoplegic NEC F44.4
    motor F44.4
    muscle F45.8
    musculoskeletal F45.8
    neurocirculatory F45.8
    obsessive F42.8
    occupational F48.8
    organ or part of body NEC F45.8
    paralytic NEC F44.4
    phobic F40.9

Disorder — *continued*
  psychogenic — *see also* condition — *continued*
    physical NEC F45.8
    rectal F45.8
    respiratory (system) F45.8
    rheumatic F45.8
    sexual (function) F52.9
    skin (allergic) (eczematous) F54
    sleep F51.9
    specified part of body NEC F45.8
    stomach F45.8
  psychological F99
    associated with
      disease classified elsewhere F54
      sexual
        development F66
        relationship F66
      uncertainty about gender identity F64.9
  psychomotor NEC F44.4
    hysterical F44.4
  psychoneurotic — *see also* Neurosis
    mixed NEC F48.8
  psychophysiologic — *see* Disorder, somatoform
  psychosexual F65.9
    development F66
    identity of childhood F64.2
  psychosomatic NOS — *see* Disorder, somatoform
    multiple F45.0
    undifferentiated F45.1
  psychotic — *see* Psychosis
    transient (acute) F23
  puberty E30.9
    specified NEC E30.8
  pulmonary (valve) — *see* Endocarditis, pulmonary
  purine metabolism E79.9
  pyrimidine metabolism E79.9
  pyruvate metabolism E74.4
  reactive attachment (childhood) F94.1
  reading R48.0
    developmental (specific) F81.0
  receptive language F80.2
  receptor, hormonal, peripheral — *see also* Syndrome, androgen insensitivity E34.50
  recurrent brief depressive F33.8
  reflex R29.2
  refraction H52.7
    aniseikonia H52.32
    anisometropia H52.31
    astigmatism — *see* Astigmatism
    hypermetropia — *see* Hypermetropia
    myopia — *see* Myopia
    presbyopia H52.4
    specified NEC H52.6
  relationship F68.8
    due to sexual orientation F66
  REM sleep behavior G47.52
  renal function, impaired (tubular) N25.9
  resonance R49.9
    specified NEC R49.8
  respiratory function, impaired — *see also* Failure, respiration
    postprocedural — *see* Complication, postoperative, respiratory system
    psychogenic F45.8
  retina H35.9
    angioid streaks H35.33
    changes in vascular appearance H35.01- ☑
    degeneration — *see* Degeneration, retina
    dystrophy (hereditary) — *see* Dystrophy, retina
    edema H35.81
    hemorrhage — *see* Hemorrhage, retina
    ischemia H35.82
    macular degeneration — *see* Degeneration, macula
    microaneurysms H35.04- ☑
    microvascular abnormality NEC H35.09
    neovascularization — *see* Neovascularization, retina
    retinopathy — *see* Retinopathy
    separation of layers H35.70
      central serous chorioretinopathy H35.71- ☑
      pigment epithelium detachment (serous) H35.72- ☑
        hemorrhagic H35.73- ☑
    specified type NEC H35.89
    telangiectasis — *see* Telangiectasis, retina
    vasculitis — *see* Vasculitis, retina
  retroperitoneal K68.9
  right hemisphere organic affective F07.89
  rumination (infant or child) F98.21

Disorder — *continued*
  sacrum, sacrococcygeal NEC M53.3
  schizoaffective F25.9
    bipolar type F25.0
    depressive type F25.1
    manic type F25.0
    mixed type F25.0
    specified NEC F25.8
  schizoid of childhood F84.5
  schizophrenia spectrum and other psychotic disorder F29
    specified NEC F28
  schizophreniform F20.81
    brief F23
  schizotypal (personality) F21
  secretion, thyrocalcitonin E07.0
  sedative, hypnotic, or anxiolytic use
    mild F13.10
      with
        sedative, hypnotic, or anxiolytic intoxication F13.129
        sedative, hypnotic, or anxiolytic intoxication delirium F13.121
        sedative, hypnotic, or anxiolytic-induced
          anxiety disorder F13.180
          bipolar and related disorder F13.14
          depressive disorder F13.14
          psychotic disorder F13.159
          sexual dysfunction F13.181
      in remission (early) (sustained) F13.11
    moderate or severe F13.20
      with
        sedative, hypnotic, or anxiolytic intoxication F13.229
        sedative, hypnotic, or anxiolytic intoxication delirium F13.221
        sedative, hypnotic, or anxiolytic-induced
          anxiety disorder F13.280
          bipolar and related disorder F13.24
          depressive disorder F13.24
          major neurocognitive disorder F13.27
          mild neurocognitive disorder F13.288
          psychotic disorder F13.259
          sexual dysfunction F13.281
      in remission (early) (sustained) F13.21
  seizure — *see also* Epilepsy G40.909
    intractable G40.919
      with status epilepticus G40.911
  semantic pragmatic F80.89
    with autism F84.0
  sense of smell R43.1
    psychogenic F45.8
  separation anxiety, of childhood F93.0
  sexual
    aversion F52.1
    function, psychogenic F52.9
    interest/arousal, female F52.22
    masochism F65.51
    maturation F66
    nonorganic F52.9
    preference — *see also* Deviation, sexual F65.9
      fetishistic transvestism F65.1
    relationship F66
    sadism F65.52
  shyness, of childhood and adolescence F40.10
  sibling rivalry F93.8
  sickle-cell (sickling) (homozygous) — *see* Disease, sickle-cell
    heterozygous D57.3
    specified type NEC D57.8- ☑
    trait D57.3
  sinus (nasal) J34.9
    specified NEC J34.89
  skin L98.9
    atrophic L90.9
      specified NEC L90.8
    granulomatous L92.9
      specified NEC L92.8
    hypertrophic L91.9
      specified NEC L91.8
    infiltrative NEC L98.6
    newborn P83.9
      specified NEC P83.88
    picking F42.4
    psychogenic (allergic) (eczematous) F54
  sleep G47.9
    breathing-related — *see* Apnea, sleep
    circadian rhythm G47.20
      advance sleep phase type G47.22

Disorder — *continued*
  sleep — *continued*
    circadian rhythm — *continued*
      delayed sleep phase type G47.21
      due to
        alcohol
          abuse F10.182
          dependence F10.282
          use F10.982
        amphetamines
          abuse F15.182
          dependence F15.282
          use F15.982
        caffeine
          abuse F15.182
          dependence F15.282
          use F15.982
        cocaine
          abuse F14.182
          dependence F14.282
          use F14.982
        drug NEC
          abuse F19.182
          dependence F19.282
          use F19.982
        opioid
          abuse F11.182
          dependence F11.282
          use F11.982
        psychoactive substance NEC
          abuse F19.182
          dependence F19.282
          use F19.982
        sedative, hypnotic, or anxiolytic
          abuse F13.182
          dependence F13.282
          use F13.982
        stimulant NEC
          abuse F15.182
          dependence F15.282
          use F15.982
      free running type G47.24
      in conditions classified elsewhere G47.27
      irregular sleep wake type G47.23
      jet lag type G47.25
      non-24-hour sleep-wake type G47.24
      shift work type G47.26
      specified NEC G47.29
    due to
      alcohol
        abuse F10.182
        dependence F10.282
        use F10.982
      amphetamine
        abuse F15.182
        dependence F15.282
        use F15.982
      anxiolytic
        abuse F13.182
        dependence F13.282
        use F13.982
      caffeine
        abuse F15.182
        dependence F15.282
        use F15.982
      cocaine
        abuse F14.182
        dependence F14.282
        use F14.982
      drug NEC
        abuse F19.182
        dependence F19.282
        use F19.982
      hypnotic
        abuse F13.182
        dependence F13.282
        use F13.982
      opioid
        abuse F11.182
        dependence F11.282
        use F11.982
      psychoactive substance NEC
        abuse F19.182
        dependence F19.282
        use F19.982
      sedative
        abuse F13.182
        dependence F13.282
        use F13.982

Disorder — *continued*
  sleep — *continued*
    due to — *continued*
      stimulant NEC
        abuse F15.182
        dependence F15.282
        use F15.982
    emotional F51.9
    excessive somnolence — *see* Hypersomnia
    hypersomnia type — *see* Hypersomnia
    initiating or maintaining — *see* Insomnia
    nightmares F51.5
    nonorganic F51.9
      specified NEC F51.8
    parasomnia type G47.50
    specified NEC G47.8
    terrors F51.4
    walking F51.3
  sleep-wake pattern or schedule — *see also* Disorder, sleep, circadian rhythm G47.9
    specified NEC G47.8
  social
    anxiety (of childhood) F40.10
      generalized F40.11
    functioning in childhood F94.9
      specified NEC F94.8
    pragmatic F80.82
  soft tissue M79.9
    ankle M79.9
    due to use, overuse and pressure M70.90
      ankle M70.97- ☑
      bursitis — *see* Bursitis
      foot M70.97- ☑
      forearm M70.93- ☑
      hand M70.94- ☑
      lower leg M70.96- ☑
      multiple sites M70.99
      pelvic region M70.95- ☑
      shoulder region M70.91- ☑
      specified site NEC M70.98
      specified type NEC M70.80
        ankle M70.87- ☑
        foot M70.87- ☑
        forearm M70.83- ☑
        hand M70.84- ☑
        lower leg M70.86- ☑
        multiple sites M70.89
        pelvic region M70.85- ☑
        shoulder region M70.81- ☑
        specified site NEC M70.88
        thigh M70.85- ☑
        upper arm M70.82- ☑
      thigh M70.95- ☑
      upper arm M70.92- ☑
    foot M79.9
    forearm M79.9
    hand M79.9
    lower leg M79.9
    multiple sites M79.9
    occupational — *see* Disorder, soft tissue, due to use, overuse and pressure
    pelvic region M79.9
    shoulder region M79.9
    specified type NEC M79.89
    thigh M79.9
    upper arm M79.9
  somatic symptom F45.1
  somatization F45.0
  somatoform F45.9
    pain (persistent) F45.41
    somatization (multiple) (long-lasting) F45.0
    specified NEC F45.8
    undifferentiated F45.1
  somnolence, excessive — *see* Hypersomnia
  specific
    arithmetical F81.2
    developmental, of motor F82
    reading F81.0
    speech and language F80.9
    spelling F81.81
    written expression F81.81
  speech R47.9
    articulation (functional) (specific) F80.0
    developmental F80.9
    specified NEC R47.89
  speech-sound F80.0
  spelling (specific) F81.81
  spine — *see also* Dorsopathy

⬇ **Subterms under main terms may continue to next column or page**   ☑ **Additional Character Required — Refer to the Tabular List for Character Selection**   **117**

Disorder — Disorder

Disorder — continued

spine — see also Dorsopathy — continued
 ligamentous or muscular attachments, peripheral — see Enthesopathy, spinal
 specified NEC — see Dorsopathy, specified NEC
stereotyped, habit or movement F98.4
stimulant use (other) (unspecified)
 mild F15.10
 in remission (early) (sustained) F15.11
 moderate or severe F15.20
 in remission (early) (sustained) F15.21
stomach (functional) — see Disorder, gastric
stress F43.9
 acute F43.0
 post-traumatic F43.10
 acute F43.11
 chronic F43.12
substance use (other) (unknown)
 mild F19.10
 with substance-induced
 anxiety disorder F19.180
 bipolar and related disorder F19.14
 depressive disorder F19.14
 major neurocognitive disorder F19.17
 mild neurocognitive disorder F19.188
 obsessive-compulsive and related disorder F19.188
 sexual dysfunction F19.181
 substance intoxication F19.129
 substance intoxication delirium F19.121
 moderate or severe F19.20
 with substance-induced
 anxiety disorder F19.280
 bipolar and related disorder F19.24
 depressive disorder F19.24
 major neurocognitive disorder F19.27
 mild neurocognitive disorder F19.288
 obsessive-compulsive and related disorder F19.288
 sexual dysfunction F19.281
 in remission (early) (sustained) F19.21
 substance intoxication F19.229
 substance intoxication delirium F19.221
sulfur-bearing amino-acid metabolism E72.10
sweat gland (eccrine) L74.9
 apocrine L75.9
 specified NEC L75.8
 specified NEC L74.8
synovium M67.90
 acromioclavicular M67.91- ☑
 ankle M67.97- ☑
 elbow M67.92- ☑
 foot M67.97- ☑
 forearm M67.93- ☑
 hand M67.94- ☑
 hip M67.95- ☑
 knee M67.96- ☑
 multiple sites M67.99
 rupture — see Rupture, synovium
 shoulder M67.91- ☑
 specified type NEC M67.80
 acromioclavicular M67.81- ☑
 ankle M67.87- ☑
 elbow M67.82- ☑
 foot M67.87- ☑
 hand M67.84- ☑
 hip M67.85- ☑
 knee M67.86- ☑
 multiple sites M67.89
 wrist M67.83- ☑
 synovitis — see Synovitis
 upper arm M67.92- ☑
 wrist M67.93- ☑
temperature regulation, newborn P81.9
 specified NEC P81.8
temporomandibular joint M26.60- ☑
tendon M67.90
 acromioclavicular M67.91- ☑
 ankle M67.97- ☑
 contracture — see Contracture, tendon
 elbow M67.92- ☑
 foot M67.97- ☑
 forearm M67.93- ☑
 hand M67.94- ☑
 hip M67.95- ☑
 knee M67.96- ☑
 multiple sites M67.99

Disorder — continued

tendon — continued
 rupture — see Rupture, tendon
 shoulder M67.91- ☑
 specified type NEC M67.80
 acromioclavicular M67.81- ☑
 ankle M67.87- ☑
 elbow M67.82- ☑
 foot M67.87- ☑
 hand M67.84- ☑
 hip M67.85- ☑
 knee M67.86- ☑
 multiple sites M67.89
 trunk M67.88
 wrist M67.83- ☑
 synovitis — see Synovitis
 tendinitis — see Tendinitis
 tenosynovitis — see Tenosynovitis
 trunk M67.98
 upper arm M67.92- ☑
 wrist M67.93- ☑
thoracic root (nerve) NEC G54.3
thyrocalcitonin hypersecretion E07.0
thyroid (gland) E07.9
 function NEC, neonatal, transitory P72.2
 iodine-deficiency related E01.8
 specified NEC E07.89
tic — see Tic
tobacco use
 chewing tobacco (mild) (moderate) (severe)
 in remission (early) (sustained) F17.221
 cigarettes (mild) (moderate) (severe)
 in remission (early) (sustained) F17.211
 mild F17.200
 in remission (early) (sustained) F17.201
 moderate F17.200
 in remission (early) (sustained) F17.201
 severe F17.200
 in remission (early) (sustained) F17.201
 specified product NEC (mild) (moderate) (severe)
 in remission (early) (sustained) F17.291
tooth K08.9
 development K00.9
 specified NEC K00.8
 eruption K00.6
Tourette's F95.2
trance and possession F44.89
transvestic F65.1
trauma and stressor-related F43.9
 other specified F43.8
tricuspid (valve) — see Endocarditis, tricuspid
tryptophan metabolism E70.5
tubular, phosphate-losing N25.0
tubulo-interstitial (in)
 brucellosis A23.9 [N16]
 cystinosis E72.04
 diphtheria A36.84
 glycogen storage disease E74.00 [N16]
 leukemia NEC C95.9- ☑ [N16]
 lymphoma NEC C85.9- ☑ [N16]
 mixed cryoglobulinemia D89.1 [N16]
 multiple myeloma C90.0- ☑ [N16]
 Salmonella infection A02.25
 sarcoidosis D86.84
 sepsis A41.9 [N16]
 streptococcal A40.9 [N16]
 systemic lupus erythematosus M32.15
 toxoplasmosis B58.83
 transplant rejection T86.91 [N16]
 Wilson's disease E83.01 [N16]
tubulo-renal function, impaired N25.9
 specified NEC N25.89
tympanic membrane H73.9- ☑
 atrophy — see Atrophy, tympanic membrane
 infection — see Myringitis
 perforation — see Perforation, tympanum
 specified NEC H73.89- ☑
unsocialized aggressive F91.1
urea cycle metabolism E72.20
 argininemia E72.21
 arginosuccinic aciduria E72.22
 citrullinemia E72.23
 ornithine transcarbamylase deficiency E72.4
 other specified E72.29
ureter (in) N28.9
 schistosomiasis B65.0 [N29]
 tuberculosis A18.11
urethra N36.9

Disorder — continued

urethra — continued
 specified NEC N36.8
urinary system N39.9
 specified NEC N39.8
valve, heart
 aortic — see Endocarditis, aortic
 mitral — see Endocarditis, mitral
 pulmonary — see Endocarditis, pulmonary
 rheumatic
 aortic — see Endocarditis, aortic, rheumatic
 mitral — see Endocarditis, mitral
 pulmonary — see Endocarditis, pulmonary, rheumatic
 tricuspid — see Endocarditis, tricuspid
 tricuspid — see Endocarditis, tricuspid
vestibular function H81.9- ☑
 specified NEC — see subcategory H81.8 ☑
 in diseases classified elsewhere H82.- ☑
 vertigo — see Vertigo
vision, binocular H53.30
 abnormal retinal correspondence H53.31
 diplopia H53.2
 fusion with defective stereopsis H53.32
 simultaneous perception H53.33
 suppression H53.34
visual
 cortex
 blindness H47.619
 left brain H47.612
 right brain H47.611
 due to
 inflammatory disorder H47.629
 left brain H47.622
 right brain H47.621
 neoplasm H47.639
 left brain H47.632
 right brain H47.631
 vascular disorder H47.649
 left brain H47.642
 right brain H47.641
 pathway H47.9
 due to
 inflammatory disorder H47.51- ☑
 neoplasm H47.52- ☑
 vascular disorder H47.53- ☑
 optic chiasm — see Disorder, optic, chiasm
vitreous body H43.9
 crystalline deposits — see Deposit, crystalline
 degeneration — see Degeneration, vitreous
 hemorrhage — see Hemorrhage, vitreous
 opacities — see Opacity, vitreous
 prolapse — see Prolapse, vitreous
 specified type NEC H43.89
voice R49.9
 specified type NEC R49.8
volatile solvent use
 due to drug abuse — see Abuse, drug, inhalant
 due to drug dependence — see Dependence, drug, inhalant
voyeuristic F65.3
white blood cells D72.9
 specified NEC D72.89
withdrawing, child or adolescent F40.10
Disorientation R41.0
Displacement, displaced
 acquired traumatic of bone, cartilage, joint, tendon NEC — see Dislocation
 adrenal gland (congenital) Q89.1
 appendix, retrocecal (congenital) Q43.8
 auricle (congenital) Q17.4
 bladder (acquired) N32.89
 congenital Q64.19
 brachial plexus (congenital) Q07.8
 brain stem, caudal (congenital) Q04.8
 canaliculus (lacrimalis), congenital Q10.6
 cardia through esophageal hiatus (congenital) Q40.1
 cerebellum, caudal (congenital) Q04.8
 cervix — see Malposition, uterus
 colon (congenital) Q43.3
 device, implant or graft — see also Complications, by site and type, mechanical T85.628 ☑
 arterial graft NEC — see Complication, cardiovascular device, mechanical, vascular
 breast (implant) T85.42 ☑
 catheter NEC T85.628 ☑
 dialysis (renal) T82.42 ☑
 intraperitoneal T85.621 ☑

☑ Additional Character Required — Refer to the Tabular List for Character Selection   ▽ Subterms under main terms may continue to next column or page

Displacement, displaced — *continued*
device, implant or graft — *see also* Complications, by
    site and type, mechanical — *continued*
    catheter — *continued*
      infusion NEC T82.524 ☑
        spinal (epidural) (subdural) T85.620 ☑
      urinary
        cystostomy T83.020 ☑
        Hopkins T83.028 ☑
        ileostomy T83.028 ☑
        indwelling T83.021 ☑
        nephrostomy T83.022 ☑
        specified NEC T83.028 ☑
        urostomy T83.028 ☑
    electronic (electrode) (pulse generator) (stimulator)
      — *see* Complication, electronic stimulator
    fixation, internal (orthopedic) NEC — *see* Complica-
      tion, fixation device, mechanical
    gastrointestinal — *see* Complications, prosthetic
      device, mechanical, gastrointestinal device
    genital NEC T83.428 ☑
      intrauterine contraceptive device (string)
        T83.32 ☑
      penile prosthesis (cylinder) (implanted) (pump)
        (reservoir) T83.420 ☑
      testicular prosthesis T83.421 ☑
    heart NEC — *see* Complication, cardiovascular de-
      vice, mechanical
    joint prosthesis — *see* Complications, joint prosthe-
      sis, mechanical
    ocular — *see* Complications, prosthetic device,
      mechanical, ocular device
    orthopedic NEC — *see* Complication, orthopedic,
      device or graft, mechanical
    specified NEC T85.628 ☑
    urinary NEC T83.128 ☑
      graft T83.22 ☑
      sphincter, implanted T83.121 ☑
      stent (ileal conduit) (nephroureteral) T83.123 ☑
      ureteral indwelling T83.122 ☑
    vascular NEC — *see* Complication, cardiovascular
      device, mechanical
    ventricular intracranial shunt T85.02 ☑
electronic stimulator
    bone T84.320 ☑
    cardiac — *see* Complications, cardiac device, elec-
      tronic
    nervous system — *see* Complication, prosthetic
      device, mechanical, electronic nervous system
      stimulator
    urinary — *see* Complications, electronic stimulator,
      urinary
esophageal mucosa into cardia of stomach, congenital
    Q39.8
esophagus (acquired) K22.8
    congenital Q39.8
eyeball (acquired) (lateral) (old) — *see* Displacement,
    globe
    congenital Q15.8
    current — *see* Avulsion, eye
fallopian tube (acquired) N83.4- ☑
    congenital Q50.6
    opening (congenital) Q50.6
gallbladder (congenital) Q44.1
gastric mucosa (congenital) Q40.2
globe (acquired) (old) (lateral) H05.21- ☑
    current — *see* Avulsion, eye
heart (congenital) Q24.8
    acquired I51.89
hymen (upward) (congenital) Q52.4
intervertebral disc NEC
    with myelopathy — *see* Disorder, disc, with,
      myelopathy
    cervical, cervicothoracic (with) M50.20
      myelopathy — *see* Disorder, disc, cervical, with
        myelopathy
      neuritis, radiculitis or radiculopathy — *see* Disor-
        der, disc, cervical, with neuritis
    due to trauma — *see* Dislocation, vertebra
    lumbar region M51.26
      with
        myelopathy M51.06
        neuritis, radiculitis, radiculopathy or sciatica
          M51.16
    lumbosacral region M51.27

Displacement, displaced — *continued*
intervertebral disc — *continued*
    lumbosacral region — *continued*
      with
        neuritis, radiculitis, radiculopathy or sciatica
          M51.17
    sacrococcygeal region M53.3
    thoracic region M51.24
      with
        myelopathy M51.04
        neuritis, radiculitis, radiculopathy M51.14
    thoracolumbar region M51.25
      with
        myelopathy M51.05
        neuritis, radiculitis, radiculopathy M51.15
intrauterine device (string) T83.32 ☑
kidney (acquired) N28.83
    congenital Q63.2
lachrymal, lacrimal apparatus or duct (congenital) Q10.6
lens, congenital Q12.1
macula (congenital) Q14.1
Meckel's diverticulum Q43.0
    malignant — *see* Table of Neoplasms, small intes-
      tine, malignant
nail (congenital) Q84.6
    acquired L60.8
opening of Wharton's duct in mouth Q38.4
organ or site, congenital NEC — *see* Malposition, con-
    genital
ovary (acquired) N83.4- ☑
    congenital Q50.39
    free in peritoneal cavity (congenital) Q50.39
    into hernial sac N83.4- ☑
oviduct (acquired) N83.4- ☑
    congenital Q50.6
parathyroid (gland) E21.4
parotid gland (congenital) Q38.4
punctum lacrimale (congenital) Q10.6
sacro-iliac (joint) (congenital) Q74.2
    current injury S33.2 ☑
    old — *see* subcategory M53.2 ☑
salivary gland (any) (congenital) Q38.4
spleen (congenital) Q89.09
stomach, congenital Q40.2
sublingual duct Q38.4
tongue (downward) (congenital) Q38.3
tooth, teeth, fully erupted M26.30
    horizontal M26.33
    vertical M26.34
trachea (congenital) Q32.1
ureter or ureteric opening or orifice (congenital) Q62.62
uterine opening of oviducts or fallopian tubes Q50.6
uterus, uterine — *see* Malposition, uterus
ventricular septum Q21.0
    with rudimentary ventricle Q20.4

Disproportion
between native and reconstructed breast N65.1
fiber-type G71.2
Disruptio uteri — *see* Rupture, uterus
Disruption (of)
ciliary body NEC H21.89
closure of
    cornea T81.31 ☑
    craniotomy T81.32 ☑
    fascia (muscular) (superficial) T81.32 ☑
    internal organ or tissue T81.32 ☑
    laceration (external) (internal) T81.33 ☑
    ligament T81.32 ☑
    mucosa T81.31 ☑
    muscle or muscle flap T81.32 ☑
    ribs or rib cage T81.32 ☑
    skin and subcutaneous tissue (full-thickness) (super-
      ficial) T81.31 ☑
    skull T81.32 ☑
    sternum (sternotomy) T81.32 ☑
    tendon T81.32 ☑
    traumatic laceration (external) (internal) T81.33 ☑
family Z63.8
    due to
      absence of family member due to military deploy-
        ment Z63.31
      absence of family member NEC Z63.32
      alcoholism and drug addiction in family Z63.72
      bereavement Z63.4
      death (assumed) or disappearance of family
        member Z63.4
      divorce or separation Z63.5
      drug addiction in family Z63.72

Disruption — *continued*
family — *continued*
    due to — *continued*
      return of family member from military deploy-
        ment (current or past conflict) Z63.71
      stressful life events NEC Z63.79
iris NEC H21.89
ligament(s) — *see also* Sprain
    knee
      current injury — *see* Dislocation, knee
      old (chronic) — *see* Derangement, knee, instabil-
        ity
      spontaneous NEC — *see* Derangement, knee,
        disruption ligament
ossicular chain — *see* Discontinuity, ossicles, ear
pelvic ring (stable) S32.810 ☑
    unstable S32.811 ☑
traumatic injury wound repair T81.33 ☑
wound T81.30 ☑
    episiotomy O90.1
    operation T81.31 ☑
      cesarean O90.0
      external operation wound (superficial) T81.31 ☑
      internal operation wound (deep) T81.32 ☑
    perineal (obstetric) O90.1
    traumatic injury repair T81.33 ☑
Dissatisfaction with
employment Z56.9
school environment Z55.4
Dissecting — *see* condition
Dissection
aorta I71.00
    abdominal I71.02
    thoracic I71.01
    thoracoabdominal I71.03
artery I77.70
    basilar (trunk) I77.75
    carotid I77.71
    cerebral (nonruptured) I67.0
      ruptured — *see* Hemorrhage, intracranial, sub-
        arachnoid
    coronary I25.42
    extremity
      lower I77.77
      upper I77.76
    iliac I77.72
    precerebral
      congenital (nonruptured) Q28.1
      specified site NEC I77.75
    renal I77.73
    specified NEC I77.79
    vertebral I77.74
precerebral artery, congenital (nonruptured) Q28.1
    Heartland A93.8
traumatic — *see* Wound, open, by site
vascular I99.8
wound — *see* Wound, open
Disseminated — *see* condition
Dissociation
auriculoventricular or atrioventricular (AV) (any degree)
    (isorhythmic) I45.89
    with heart block I44.2
interference I45.89
Dissociative reaction, state F44.9
Dissolution, vertebra — *see* Osteoporosis
Distension, distention
abdomen R14.0
bladder N32.89
cecum K63.89
colon K63.89
gallbladder K82.8
intestine K63.89
kidney N28.89
liver K76.89
seminal vesicle N50.89
stomach K31.89
    acute K31.0
    psychogenic F45.8
ureter — *see* Dilatation, ureter
uterus N85.8
Distoma hepaticum infestation B66.3
Distomiasis B66.9
bile passages B66.3
hemic B65.9
hepatic B66.3
    due to Clonorchis sinensis B66.1
intestinal B66.5
liver B66.3

Distomiasis — continued
  liver — continued
    due to Clonorchis sinensis B66.1
  lung B66.4
  pulmonary B66.4
Distomolar (fourth molar) K00.1
Disto-occlusion (Division I) (Division II) M26.212
Distortion(s) (congenital)
  adrenal (gland) Q89.1
  arm NEC Q68.8
  bile duct or passage Q44.5
  bladder Q64.79
  brain Q04.9
  cervix (uteri) Q51.9
  chest (wall) Q67.8
    bones Q76.8
  clavicle Q74.0
  clitoris Q52.6
  coccyx Q76.49
  common duct Q44.5
  coronary Q24.5
  cystic duct Q44.5
  ear (auricle) (external) Q17.3
    inner Q16.5
    middle Q16.4
      ossicles Q16.3
  endocrine NEC Q89.2
  eustachian tube Q17.8
  eye (adnexa) Q15.8
  face bone(s) NEC Q75.8
  fallopian tube Q50.6
  femur NEC Q68.8
  fibula NEC Q68.8
  finger(s) Q68.1
  foot Q66.9- ☑
  genitalia, genital organ(s)
    female Q52.8
      external Q52.79
      internal NEC Q52.8
  gyri Q04.8
  hand bone(s) Q68.1
  heart (auricle) (ventricle) Q24.8
    valve (cusp) Q24.8
  hepatic duct Q44.5
  humerus NEC Q68.8
  hymen Q52.4
  intrafamilial communications Z63.8
  jaw NEC M26.89
  labium (majus) (minus) Q52.79
  leg NEC Q68.8
  lens Q12.8
  liver Q44.7
  lumbar spine Q76.49
    with disproportion O33.8
      causing obstructed labor O65.0
  lumbosacral (joint) (region) Q76.49
    kyphosis — see Kyphosis, congenital
    lordosis — see Lordosis, congenital
  nerve Q07.8
  nose Q30.8
  organ
    of Corti Q16.5
    or site not listed — see Anomaly, by site
  ossicles, ear Q16.3
  oviduct Q50.6
  pancreas Q45.3
  parathyroid (gland) Q89.2
  pituitary (gland) Q89.2
  radius NEC Q68.8
  sacroiliac joint Q74.2
  sacrum Q76.49
  scapula Q74.0
  shoulder girdle Q74.0
  skull bone(s) NEC Q75.8
    with
      anencephalus Q00.0
      encephalocele — see Encephalocele
      hydrocephalus Q03.9
        with spina bifida — see Spina bifida, with
          hydrocephalus
      microcephaly Q02
  spinal cord Q06.8
  spine Q76.49
    kyphosis — see Kyphosis, congenital
    lordosis — see Lordosis, congenital
  spleen Q89.09
  sternum NEC Q76.7
  thorax (wall) Q67.8

Distortion(s) — continued
  thorax — continued
    bony Q76.8
  thymus (gland) Q89.2
  thyroid (gland) Q89.2
  tibia NEC Q68.8
  toe(s) Q66.9- ☑
  tongue Q38.3
  trachea (cartilage) Q32.1
  ulna NEC Q68.8
  ureter Q62.8
  urethra Q64.79
    causing obstruction Q64.39
  uterus Q51.9
  vagina Q52.4
  vertebra Q76.49
    kyphosis — see Kyphosis, congenital
    lordosis — see Lordosis, congenital
  visual — see also Disturbance, vision
    shape and size H53.15
  vulva Q52.79
  wrist (bones) (joint) Q68.8
Distress
  abdomen — see Pain, abdominal
  acute respiratory R06.03
    syndrome (adult) (child) J80
  epigastric R10.13
  fetal P84
    complicating pregnancy — see Stress, fetal
  gastrointestinal (functional) K30
    psychogenic F45.8
  intestinal (functional) NOS K59.9
    psychogenic F45.8
  maternal, during labor and delivery O75.0
  relationship, with spouse or intimate partner Z63.0
  respiratory (adult) (child) R06.03
    newborn P22.9
      specified NEC P22.8
    orthopnea R06.01
    psychogenic F45.8
    shortness of breath R06.02
    specified type NEC R06.09
Distribution vessel, atypical Q27.9
  coronary artery Q24.5
  precerebral Q28.1
Districhiasis L68.8
Disturbance(s) — see also Disease
  absorption K90.9
    calcium E58
    carbohydrate K90.49
    fat K90.49
      pancreatic K90.3
    protein K90.49
    starch K90.49
    vitamin — see Deficiency, vitamin
  acid-base equilibrium E87.8
    mixed E87.4
  activity and attention (with hyperkinesis) — see Disor-
    der, attention-deficit hyperactivity
  amino acid transport E72.00
  assimilation, food K90.9
  auditory nerve, except deafness — see subcategory
    H93.3 ☑
  behavior — see Disorder, conduct
  blood clotting (mechanism) — see also Defect, coagu-
    lation D68.9
  cerebral
    nerve — see Disorder, nerve, cranial
    status, newborn P91.9
      specified NEC P91.88
  circulatory I99.9
  conduct — see also Disorder, conduct F91.9
    adjustment reaction — see Disorder, adjustment
    compulsive F63.9
    disruptive F91.9
    hyperkinetic — see Disorder, attention-deficit hy-
      peractivity
    socialized F91.2
    specified NEC F91.8
    unsocialized F91.1
  coordination R27.8
  cranial nerve — see Disorder, nerve, cranial
  deep sensibility — see Disturbance, sensation
  digestive K30
    psychogenic F45.8
  electrolyte — see also Imbalance, electrolyte
    newborn, transitory P74.49
      hyperammonemia P74.6

Disturbance(s) — continued
  electrolyte — see also Imbalance, electrolyte — contin-
    ued
    newborn, transitory — continued
      hyperchloremia P74.421
      hyperchloremic metabolic acidosis P74.421
      hypochloremia P74.422
      potassium balance
        hyperkalemia P74.31
        hypokalemia P74.32
      sodium balance
        hypernatremia P74.21
        hyponatremia P74.22
      specified type NEC P74.49
  emotions specific to childhood and adolescence F93.9
    with
      anxiety and fearfulness NEC F93.8
      elective mutism F94.0
      oppositional disorder F91.3
      sensitivity (withdrawal) F40.10
      shyness F40.10
      social withdrawal F40.10
    involving relationship problems F93.8
    mixed F93.8
    specified NEC F93.8
  endocrine (gland) E34.9
    neonatal, transitory P72.9
      specified NEC P72.8
  equilibrium R42
  fructose metabolism E74.10
  gait — see Gait
    hysterical F44.4
    psychogenic F44.4
  gastrointestinal (functional) K30
    psychogenic F45.8
  habit, child F98.9
  hearing, except deafness and tinnitus — see Abnormal,
    auditory perception
  heart, functional (conditions in I44-I50)
    due to presence of (cardiac) prosthesis I97.19- ☑
    postoperative I97.89
      cardiac surgery — see also Infarct, myocardium,
        associated with revascularization proce-
        dure I97.19- ☑
  hormones E34.9
  innervation uterus (parasympathetic) (sympathetic)
    N85.8
  keratinization NEC
    gingiva K05.10
      nonplaque induced K05.11
      plaque induced K05.10
    lip K13.0
    oral (mucosa) (soft tissue) K13.29
    tongue K13.29
  learning (specific) — see Disorder, learning
  memory — see Amnesia
    mild, following organic brain damage F06.8
  mental F99
    associated with diseases classified elsewhere F54
  metabolism E88.9
    with
      abortion — see Abortion, by type with other
        specified complication
      ectopic pregnancy O08.5
      molar pregnancy O08.5
    amino-acid E72.9
      aromatic E70.9
      branched-chain E71.2
      straight-chain E72.89
      sulfur-bearing E72.10
    ammonia E72.20
    arginine E72.21
    arginosuccinic acid E72.22
    carbohydrate E74.9
    cholesterol E78.9
    citrulline E72.23
    cystathionine E72.19
    general E88.9
    glutamine E72.89
    histidine E70.40
    homocystine E72.19
    hydroxylysine E72.3
    in labor or delivery O75.89
    iron E83.10
    lipoid E78.9
    lysine E72.3
    methionine E72.19
    neonatal, transitory P74.9

Disturbance(s) — *continued*
metabolism — *continued*
neonatal, transitory — *continued*
calcium and magnesium P71.9
specified type NEC P71.8
carbohydrate metabolism P70.9
specified type NEC P70.8
specified NEC P74.8
ornithine E72.4
phosphate E83.39
sodium NEC E87.8
threonine E72.89
tryptophan E70.5
tyrosine E70.20
urea cycle E72.20
motor R29.2
nervous, functional R45.0
neuromuscular mechanism (eye), due to syphilis A52.15
nutritional E63.9
nail L60.3
ocular motion H51.9
psychogenic F45.8
oculogyric H51.8
psychogenic F45.8
oculomotor H51.9
psychogenic F45.8
olfactory nerve R43.1
optic nerve NEC — *see* Disorder, nerve, optic
oral epithelium, including tongue NEC K13.29
perceptual due to
alcohol withdrawal F10.232
amphetamine intoxication F15.922
in
abuse F15.122
dependence F15.222
anxiolytic withdrawal F13.232
cannabis intoxication (acute) F12.922
in
abuse F12.122
dependence F12.222
cocaine intoxication (acute) F14.922
in
abuse F14.122
dependence F14.222
hypnotic withdrawal F13.232
opioid intoxication (acute) F11.922
in
abuse F11.122
dependence F11.222
phencyclidine intoxication (acute) F16.122
sedative withdrawal F13.232
personality (pattern) (trait) — *see also* Disorder, personality F60.9
following organic brain damage F07.9
polyglandular E31.9
specified NEC E31.8
potassium balance, newborn
hyperkalemia P74.31
hypokalemia P74.32
psychogenic F45.9
psychomotor F44.4
psychophysical visual H53.16
pupillary — *see* Anomaly, pupil, function
reflex R29.2
rhythm, heart I49.9
salivary secretion K11.7
sensation (cold) (heat) (localization) (tactile discrimination) (texture) (vibratory) NEC R20.9
hysterical F44.6
skin R20.9
anesthesia R20.0
hyperesthesia R20.3
hypoesthesia R20.1
paresthesia R20.2
specified type NEC R20.8
smell R43.9
and taste (mixed) R43.8
anosmia R43.0
parosmia R43.1
specified NEC R43.8
taste R43.9
and smell (mixed) R43.8
parageusia R43.2
specified NEC R43.8
sensory — *see* Disturbance, sensation
situational (transient) — *see also* Disorder, adjustment
acute F43.0
sleep G47.9
nonorganic origin F51.9

Disturbance(s) — *continued*
smell — *see* Disturbance, sensation, smell
sociopathic F60.2
sodium balance, newborn
hypernatremia P74.21
hyponatremia P74.22
speech R47.9
developmental F80.9
specified NEC R47.89
stomach (functional) K31.9
sympathetic (nerve) G90.9
taste — *see* Disturbance, sensation, taste
temperature
regulation, newborn P81.9
specified NEC P81.8
sense R20.8
hysterical F44.6
tooth
eruption K00.6
formation K00.4
structure, hereditary NEC K00.5
touch — *see* Disturbance, sensation
vascular I99.9
arteriosclerotic — *see* Arteriosclerosis
vasomotor I73.9
vasospastic I73.9
vision, visual H53.9
following
cerebral infarction I69.398
cerebrovascular disease I69.998
specified NEC I69.898
intracerebral hemorrhage I69.198
nontraumatic intracranial hemorrhage NEC I69.298
specified disease NEC I69.898
subarachnoid hemorrhage I69.098
psychophysical H53.16
specified NEC H53.8
subjective H53.10
day blindness H53.11
discomfort H53.14- ☑
distortions of shape and size H53.15
loss
sudden H53.13- ☑
transient H53.12- ☑
specified type NEC H53.19
voice R49.9
psychogenic F44.4
specified NEC R49.8
Diuresis R35.8
Diver's palsy, paralysis or squeeze T70.3 ☑
Diverticulitis (acute) K57.92
bladder — *see* Cystitis
ileum — *see* Diverticulitis, intestine, small
intestine K57.92
with
abscess, perforation or peritonitis K57.80
with bleeding K57.81
bleeding K57.93
congenital Q43.8
large K57.32
with
abscess, perforation or peritonitis K57.20
with bleeding K57.21
bleeding K57.33
small intestine K57.52
with
abscess, perforation or peritonitis K57.40
with bleeding K57.41
bleeding K57.53
small K57.12
with
abscess, perforation or peritonitis K57.00
with bleeding K57.01
bleeding K57.13
large intestine K57.52
with
abscess, perforation or peritonitis K57.40
with bleeding K57.41
bleeding K57.53
Diverticulosis K57.90
with bleeding K57.91
large intestine K57.30
with
bleeding K57.31
small intestine K57.50

Diverticulosis — *continued*
large intestine — *continued*
with — *continued*
small intestine — *continued*
with bleeding K57.51
small intestine K57.10
with
bleeding K57.11
large intestine K57.50
with bleeding K57.51
Diverticulum, diverticula (multiple) K57.90
appendix (noninflammatory) K38.2
bladder (sphincter) N32.3
congenital Q64.6
bronchus (congenital) Q32.4
acquired J98.09
calyx, calyceal (kidney) N28.89
cardia (stomach) K31.4
cecum — *see* Diverticulosis, intestine, large
congenital Q43.8
colon — *see* Diverticulosis, intestine, large
congenital Q43.8
duodenum — *see* Diverticulosis, intestine, small
congenital Q43.8
epiphrenic (esophagus) K22.5
esophagus (congenital) Q39.6
acquired (epiphrenic) (pulsion) (traction) K22.5
eustachian tube — *see* Disorder, eustachian tube, specified NEC
fallopian tube N83.8
gastric K31.4
heart (congenital) Q24.8
ileum — *see* Diverticulosis, intestine, small
jejunum — *see* Diverticulosis, intestine, small
kidney (pelvis) (calyces) N28.89
with calculus — *see* Calculus, kidney
Meckel's (displaced) (hypertrophic) Q43.0
malignant — *see* Table of Neoplasms, small intestine, malignant
midthoracic K22.5
organ or site, congenital NEC — *see* Distortion
pericardium (congenital) (cyst) Q24.8
acquired I31.8
pharyngoesophageal (congenital) Q39.6
acquired K22.5
pharynx (congenital) Q38.7
rectosigmoid — *see* Diverticulosis, intestine, large
congenital Q43.8
rectum — *see* Diverticulosis, intestine, large
Rokitansky's K22.5
seminal vesicle N50.89
sigmoid — *see* Diverticulosis, intestine, large
congenital Q43.8
stomach (acquired) K31.4
congenital Q40.2
trachea (acquired) J39.8
ureter (acquired) N28.89
congenital Q62.8
ureterovesical orifice N28.89
urethra (acquired) N36.1
congenital Q64.79
ventricle, left (congenital) Q24.8
vesical N32.3
congenital Q64.6
Zenker's (esophagus) K22.5
Division
cervix uteri (acquired) N88.8
glans penis Q55.69
labia minora (congenital) Q52.79
ligament (partial or complete) (current) — *see also* Sprain
with open wound — *see* Wound, open
muscle (partial or complete) (current) — *see also* Injury, muscle
with open wound — *see* Wound, open
nerve (traumatic) — *see* Injury, nerve
spinal cord — *see* Injury, spinal cord, by region
vein I87.8
Divorce, causing family disruption Z63.5
Dix-Hallpike neurolabyrinthitis — *see* Neuronitis, vestibular
Dizziness R42
hysterical F44.89
psychogenic F45.8
DMAC (disseminated mycobacterium avium-intracellulare complex) A31.2
DNR (do not resuscitate) Z66

Doan-Wiseman syndrome (primary splenic neutropenia) — *see* Agranulocytosis
Doehle-Heller aortitis A52.02
Dog bite — *see* Bite
Dohle body panmyelopathic syndrome D72.0
Dolichocephaly Q67.2
Dolichocolon Q43.8
Dolichostenomelia — *see* Syndrome, Marfan's
Donohue's syndrome E34.8
Donor (organ or tissue) Z52.9
  blood (whole) Z52.000
    autologous Z52.010
    specified component (lymphocytes) (platelets) NEC Z52.008
      autologous Z52.018
      specified donor NEC Z52.098
    specified donor NEC Z52.090
    stem cells Z52.001
      autologous Z52.011
      specified donor NEC Z52.091
  bone Z52.20
    autologous Z52.21
    marrow Z52.3
    specified type NEC Z52.29
  cornea Z52.5
  egg (Oocyte) Z52.819
    age 35 and over Z52.812
      anonymous recipient Z52.812
      designated recipient Z52.813
    under age 35 Z52.810
      anonymous recipient Z52.810
      designated recipient Z52.811
  kidney Z52.4
  liver Z52.6
  lung Z52.89
  lymphocyte — *see* Donor, blood, specified components NEC
  Oocyte — *see* Donor, egg
  platelets Z52.008
  potential, examination of Z00.5
  semen Z52.89
  skin Z52.10
    autologous Z52.11
    specified type NEC Z52.19
  specified organ or tissue NEC Z52.89
  sperm Z52.89
Donovanosis A58
Dorsalgia M54.9
  psychogenic F45.41
  specified NEC M54.89
Dorsopathy M53.9
  deforming M43.9
    specified NEC — *see* subcategory M43.8 ☑
  specified NEC M53.80
    cervical region M53.82
    cervicothoracic region M53.83
    lumbar region M53.86
    lumbosacral region M53.87
    occipito-atlanto-axial region M53.81
    sacrococcygeal region M53.88
    thoracic region M53.84
    thoracolumbar region M53.85
Double
  albumin E88.09
  aortic arch Q25.45
  auditory canal Q17.8
  auricle (heart) Q20.8
  bladder Q64.79
  cervix Q51.820
    with doubling of uterus (and vagina) Q51.10
      with obstruction Q51.11
  inlet ventricle Q20.4
  kidney with double pelvis (renal) Q63.0
  meatus urinarius Q64.75
  monster Q89.4
  outlet
    left ventricle Q20.2
    right ventricle Q20.1
  pelvis (renal) with double ureter Q62.5
  tongue Q38.3
  ureter (one or both sides) Q62.5
    with double pelvis (renal) Q62.5
  urethra Q64.74
  urinary meatus Q64.75
  uterus Q51.20
    with
      doubling of cervix (and vagina) Q51.10
        with obstruction Q51.11

Double — *continued*
  uterus — *continued*
    complete Q51.21
    in pregnancy or childbirth O34.0- ☑
      causing obstructed labor O65.5
    partial Q51.22
    specified NEC Q51.28
  vagina Q52.10
    with doubling of uterus (and cervix) Q51.10
      with obstruction Q51.11
  vision H53.2
  vulva Q52.79
Douglas' pouch, cul-de-sac — *see* condition
Down syndrome Q90.9
  meiotic nondisjunction Q90.0
  mitotic nondisjunction Q90.1
  mosaicism Q90.1
  translocation Q90.2
DPD (dihydropyrimidine dehydrogenase deficiency) E88.89
Dracontiasis B72
Dracunculiasis, dracunculosis B72
Dream state, hysterical F44.89
Drepanocytic anemia — *see* Disease, sickle-cell
Dresbach's syndrome (elliptocytosis) D58.1
Dreschlera (hawaiiensis) (infection) B43.8
Dressler's syndrome I24.1
Drift, ulnar — *see* Deformity, limb, specified type NEC, forearm
Drinking (alcohol)
  excessive, to excess NEC (without dependence) F10.10
    habitual (continual) (without remission) F10.20
      with remission F10.21
Drip, postnasal (chronic) R09.82
  due to
    allergic rhinitis — *see* Rhinitis, allergic
    common cold J00
    gastroesophageal reflux — *see* Reflux, gastroesophageal
    nasopharyngitis — *see* Nasopharyngitis
    other known condition — *code to* condition
    sinusitis — *see* Sinusitis
Droop
  facial R29.810
    cerebrovascular disease I69.992
      cerebral infarction I69.392
      intracerebral hemorrhage I69.192
      nontraumatic intracranial hemorrhage NEC I69.292
      specified disease NEC I69.892
      subarachnoid hemorrhage I69.092
Drop (in)
  attack NEC R55
  finger — *see* Deformity, finger
  foot — *see* Deformity, limb, foot, drop
  hematocrit (precipitous) R71.0
  hemoglobin R71.0
  toe — *see* Deformity, toe, specified NEC
  wrist — *see* Deformity, limb, wrist drop
Dropped heart beats I45.9
Dropsy, dropsical — *see also* Hydrops
  abdomen R18.8
  brain — *see* Hydrocephalus
  cardiac, heart — *see* Failure, heart, congestive
  gangrenous — *see* Gangrene
  heart — *see* Failure, heart, congestive
  kidney — *see* Nephrosis
  lung — *see* Edema, lung
  newborn due to isoimmunization P56.0
  pericardium — *see* Pericarditis
Drowned, drowning (near) T75.1 ☑
Drowsiness R40.0
Drug
  abuse counseling and surveillance Z71.51
  addiction — *see* Dependence
  dependence — *see* Dependence
  habit — *see* Dependence
  harmful use — *see* Abuse, drug
  induced fever R50.2
  overdose — *see* Table of Drugs and Chemicals, by drug, poisoning
  poisoning — *see* Table of Drugs and Chemicals, by drug, poisoning
  resistant organism infection — *see also* Resistant, organism, to, drug Z16.30

Drug — *continued*
  therapy
    long term (current) (prophylactic) — *see* Therapy, drug long-term (current) (prophylactic)
    short term — *omit code*
  wrong substance given or taken in error — *see* Table of Drugs and Chemicals, by drug, poisoning
Drunkenness (without dependence) F10.129
  acute in alcoholism F10.229
  chronic (without remission) F10.20
    with remission F10.21
  pathological (without dependence) F10.129
    with dependence F10.229
  sleep F51.9
Drusen
  macula (degenerative) (retina) — *see* Degeneration, macula, drusen
  optic disc H47.32- ☑
Dry, dryness — *see also* condition
  larynx J38.7
  mouth R68.2
    due to dehydration E86.0
  nose J34.89
  socket (teeth) M27.3
  throat J39.2
DSAP L56.5
Duane's syndrome H50.81- ☑
Dubin-Johnson disease or syndrome E80.6
Dubois' disease (thymus gland) A50.59 *[E35]*
Dubowitz' syndrome Q87.19
Duchenne-Aran muscular atrophy G12.21
Duchenne-Griesinger disease G71.01
Duchenne's
  disease or syndrome
    motor neuron disease G12.22
    muscular dystrophy G71.01
  locomotor ataxia (syphilitic) A52.11
  paralysis
    birth injury P14.0
    due to or associated with
      motor neuron disease G12.22
      muscular dystrophy G71.01
Ducrey's chancre A57
Duct, ductus — *see* condition
Duhring's disease (dermatitis herpetiformis) L13.0
Dullness, cardiac (decreased) (increased) R01.2
Dumb ague — *see* Malaria
Dumbness — *see* Aphasia
Dumdum fever B55.0
Dumping syndrome (postgastrectomy) K91.1
Duodenitis (nonspecific) (peptic) K29.80
  with bleeding K29.81
Duodenocholangitis — *see* Cholangitis
Duodenum, duodenal — *see* condition
Duplay's bursitis or periarthritis — *see* Tendinitis, calcific, shoulder
Duplication, duplex — *see also* Accessory
  alimentary tract Q45.8
  anus Q43.4
  appendix (and cecum) Q43.4
  biliary duct (any) Q44.5
  bladder Q64.79
  cecum (and appendix) Q43.4
  cervix Q51.820
  chromosome NEC
    with complex rearrangements NEC Q92.5
    seen only at prometaphase Q92.8
  cystic duct Q44.5
  digestive organs Q45.8
  esophagus Q39.8
  frontonasal process Q75.8
  intestine (large) (small) Q43.4
  kidney Q63.0
  liver Q44.7
  pancreas Q45.3
  penis Q55.69
  respiratory organs NEC Q34.8
  salivary duct Q38.4
  spinal cord (incomplete) Q06.2
  stomach Q40.2
Dupré's disease (meningism) R29.1
Dupuytren's contraction or disease M72.0
Durand-Nicolas-Favre disease A55
Durotomy (inadvertent) (incidental) G97.41
Duroziez's disease (congenital mitral stenosis) Q23.2
Dutton's relapsing fever (West African) A68.1
Dwarfism E34.3
  achondroplastic Q77.4

☑ **Additional Character Required** — Refer to the Tabular List for Character Selection   ▽ Subterms under main terms may continue to next column or page

Dwarfism — *continued*
congenital E34.3
constitutional E34.3
hypochondroplastic Q77.4
hypophyseal E23.0
infantile E34.3
Laron-type E34.3
Lorain (-Levi) type E23.0
metatropic Q77.8
nephrotic-glycosuric (with hypophosphatemic rickets) E72.09
nutritional E45
pancreatic K86.89
pituitary E23.0
renal N25.0
thanatophoric Q77.1
Dyke-Young anemia (secondary) (symptomatic) D59.1
Dysacusis — *see* Abnormal, auditory perception
Dysadrenocortism E27.9
hyperfunction E27.0
Dysarthria R47.1
following
cerebral infarction I69.322
cerebrovascular disease I69.922
specified disease NEC I69.822
intracerebral hemorrhage I69.122
nontraumatic intracranial hemorrhage NEC I69.222
subarachnoid hemorrhage I69.022
Dysautonomia (familial) G90.1
Dysbarism T70.3 ☑
Dysbasia R26.2
angiosclerotica intermittens I73.9
hysterical F44.4
lordotica (progressiva) G24.1
nonorganic origin F44.4
psychogenic F44.4
Dysbetalipoproteinemia (familial) E78.2
Dyscalculia R48.8
developmental F81.2
Dyschezia K59.00
Dyschondroplasia (with hemangiomata) Q78.4
Dyschromia (skin) L81.9
Dyscollagenosis M35.9
Dyscranio-pygo-phalangy Q87.0
Dyscrasia
blood (with) D75.9
antepartum hemorrhage — *see* Hemorrhage, antepartum, with coagulation defect
intrapartum hemorrhage O67.0
newborn P61.9
specified type NEC P61.8
puerperal, postpartum O72.3
polyglandular, pluriglandular E31.9
Dysendocrinism E34.9
Dysentery, dysenteric (catarrhal) (diarrhea) (epidemic) (hemorrhagic) (infectious) (sporadic) (tropical) A09
abscess, liver A06.4
amebic — *see also* Amebiasis A06.0
with abscess — *see* Abscess, amebic
acute A06.0
chronic A06.1
arthritis — *see also* category M01 A09
bacillary (*see also* category M01) A03.9
bacillary A03.9
arthritis — *see also* category M01 A03.9
Boyd A03.2
Flexner A03.1
Schmitz (-Stutzer) A03.0
Shiga (-Kruse) A03.0
Shigella A03.9
boydii A03.2
dysenteriae A03.0
flexneri A03.1
group A A03.0
group B A03.1
group C A03.2
group D A03.3
sonnei A03.3
specified type NEC A03.8
Sonne A03.3
specified type NEC A03.8
balantidial A07.0
Balantidium coli A07.0
Boyd's A03.2
candidal B37.82
Chilomastix A07.8
Chinese A03.9
coccidial A07.3

Dysentery, dysenteric — *continued*
Dientamoeba (fragilis) A07.8
Embadomonas A07.8
Entamoeba, entambic — *see* Dysentery, amebic
Flexner-Boyd A03.2
Flexner's A03.1
Giardia lamblia A07.1
Hiss-Russell A03.1
Lamblia A07.1
leishmanial B55.0
malarial — *see* Malaria
metazoal B82.0
monilial B37.82
protozoal A07.9
Salmonella A02.0
schistosomal B65.1
Schmitz (-Stutzer) A03.0
Shiga (-Kruse) A03.0
Shigella NOS — *see* Dysentery, bacillary
Sonne A03.3
strongyloidiasis B78.0
trichomonal A07.8
viral — *see also* Enteritis, viral A08.4
Dysequilibrium R42
Dysesthesia R20.8
hysterical F44.6
Dysfibrinogenemia (congenital) D68.2
Dysfunction
adrenal E27.9
hyperfunction E27.0
autonomic
due to alcohol G31.2
somatoform F45.8
bladder N31.9
neurogenic NOS — *see* Dysfunction, bladder, neuromuscular
neuromuscular NOS N31.9
atonic (motor) (sensory) N31.2
autonomous N31.2
flaccid N31.2
nonreflex N31.2
reflex N31.1
specified NEC N31.8
uninhibited N31.0
bleeding, uterus N93.8
cerebral G93.89
colon K59.9
psychogenic F45.8
colostomy K94.03
cystic duct K82.8
cystostomy (stoma) — *see* Complications, cystostomy
ejaculatory N53.19
anejaculatory orgasm N53.13
painful N53.12
premature F52.4
retarded N53.11
endocrine NOS E34.9
endometrium N85.8
enterostomy K94.13
erectile — *see* Dysfunction, sexual, male, erectile
gallbladder K82.8
gastrostomy (stoma) K94.23
gland, glandular NOS E34.9
meibomian, of eyelid — *see* Dysfunction, meibomian gland
heart I51.89
hemoglobin D75.89
hepatic K76.89
hypophysis E23.7
hypothalamic NEC E23.3
ileostomy (stoma) K94.13
jejunostomy (stoma) K94.13
kidney — *see* Disease, renal
labyrinthine — *see* subcategory H83.2 ☑
left ventricular, following sudden emotional stress I51.81
liver K76.89
male — *see* Dysfunction, sexual, male
meibomian gland, of eyelid H02.889
left H02.886
lower H02.885
upper H02.884
upper and lower eyelids H02.88B
right H02.883
lower H02.882
upper H02.881
upper and lower eyelids H02.88A
orgasmic (female) F52.31

Dysfunction — *continued*
orgasmic — *continued*
male F52.32
ovary E28.9
specified NEC E28.8
papillary muscle I51.89
parathyroid E21.4
physiological NEC R68.89
psychogenic F59
pineal gland E34.8
pituitary (gland) E23.3
platelets D69.1
polyglandular E31.9
specified NEC E31.8
psychophysiologic F59
psychosexual F52.9
with
dyspareunia F52.6
premature ejaculation F52.4
vaginismus F52.5
pylorus K31.9
rectum K59.9
psychogenic F45.8
reflex (sympathetic) — *see* Syndrome, pain, complex regional I
segmental — *see* Dysfunction, somatic
senile R54
sexual (due to) R37
alcohol F10.981
amphetamine F15.981
in
abuse F15.181
dependence F15.281
anxiolytic F13.981
in
abuse F13.181
dependence F13.281
cocaine F14.981
in
abuse F14.181
dependence F14.281
excessive sexual drive F52.8
failure of genital response (male) F52.21
female F52.22
female N94.9
aversion F52.1
dyspareunia N94.10
psychogenic F52.6
frigidity F52.22
nymphomania F52.8
orgasmic F52.31
psychogenic F52.9
aversion F52.1
dyspareunia F52.6
frigidity F52.22
nymphomania F52.8
orgasmic F52.31
vaginismus F52.5
vaginismus N94.2
psychogenic F52.5
hypnotic F13.981
in
abuse F13.181
dependence F13.281
inhibited orgasm (female) F52.31
male F52.32
lack
of sexual enjoyment F52.1
or loss of sexual desire F52.0
male N53.9
anejaculatory orgasm N53.13
ejaculatory N53.19
painful N53.12
premature F52.4
retarded N53.11
erectile N52.9
drug induced N52.2
due to
disease classified elsewhere N52.1
drug N52.2
postoperative (postprocedural) N52.39
following
cryotherapy N52.37
interstitial seed therapy N52.36
prostate ablative therapy N52.37
prostatectomy N52.34
radical N52.31
radiation therapy N52.35
radical cystectomy N52.32

Dysfunction — *continued*
  sexual — *continued*
    male — *continued*
      erectile — *continued*
        postoperative — *continued*
          following — *continued*
            ultrasound ablative therapy N52.37
            urethral surgery N52.33
        psychogenic F52.21
        specified cause NEC N52.8
        vasculogenic
          arterial insufficiency N52.01
            with corporo-venous occlusive N52.03
          corporo-venous occlusive N52.02
            with arterial insufficiency N52.03
      impotence — *see* Dysfunction, sexual, male, erectile
    psychogenic F52.9
      aversion F52.1
      erectile F52.21
      orgasmic F52.32
      premature ejaculation F52.4
      satyriasis F52.8
      specified type NEC F52.8
    specified type NEC N53.8
  nonorganic F52.9
    specified NEC F52.8
  opioid F11.981
    in
      abuse F11.181
      dependence F11.281
  orgasmic dysfunction (female) F52.31
    male F52.32
  premature ejaculation F52.4
  psychoactive substances NEC F19.981
    in
      abuse F19.181
      dependence F19.281
  psychogenic F52.9
  sedative F13.981
    in
      abuse F13.181
      dependence F13.281
  sexual aversion F52.1
  vaginismus (nonorganic) (psychogenic) F52.5
  sinoatrial node I49.5
  somatic M99.09
    abdomen M99.09
    acromioclavicular M99.07
    cervical region M99.01
    cervicothoracic M99.01
    costochondral M99.08
    costovertebral M99.08
    head region M99.00
    hip M99.05
    lower extremity M99.06
    lumbar region M99.03
    lumbosacral M99.03
    occipitocervical M99.00
    pelvic region M99.05
    pubic M99.05
    rib cage M99.08
    sacral region M99.04
    sacrococcygeal M99.04
    sacroiliac M99.04
    specified NEC M99.09
    sternochondral M99.08
    sternoclavicular M99.07
    thoracic region M99.02
    thoracolumbar M99.02
    upper extremity M99.07
  somatoform autonomic F45.8
  stomach K31.89
    psychogenic F45.8
  suprarenal E27.9
    hyperfunction E27.0
  symbolic R48.9
    specified type NEC R48.8
  temporomandibular (joint) M26.69
    joint-pain syndrome M26.62- ☑
  testicular (endocrine) E29.9
    specified NEC E29.8
  thymus E32.9
  thyroid E07.9
  ureterostomy (stoma) — *see* Complications, stoma, urinary tract
  urethrostomy (stoma) — *see* Complications, stoma, urinary tract
  uterus, complicating delivery O62.9

Dysfunction — *continued*
  uterus, complicating delivery — *continued*
    hypertonic O62.4
    hypotonic O62.2
      primary O62.0
      secondary O62.1
  ventricular I51.9
    with congestive heart failure — *see also* Failure, heart I50.9
    left, reversible, following sudden emotional stress I51.81

Dysgenesis
  gonadal (due to chromosomal anomaly) Q96.9
    pure Q99.1
  renal Q60.5
    bilateral Q60.4
    unilateral Q60.3
  reticular D72.0
  tidal platelet D69.3

Dysgerminoma
  specified site — *see* Neoplasm, malignant, by site
  unspecified site
    female C56.9
    male C62.90

Dysgeusia R43.2
Dysgraphia R27.8
Dyshidrosis, dysidrosis L30.1
Dyskaryotic cervical smear R87.619
Dyskeratosis L85.8
  cervix — *see* Dysplasia, cervix
  congenital Q82.8
  uterus NEC N85.8
Dyskinesia G24.9
  biliary (cystic duct or gallbladder) K82.8
  drug induced
    orofacial G24.01
  esophagus K22.4
  hysterical F44.4
  intestinal K59.8
  nonorganic origin F44.4
  orofacial (idiopathic) G24.4
    drug induced G24.01
  psychogenic F44.4
  subacute, drug induced G24.01
  tardive G24.01
    neuroleptic induced G24.01
  trachea J39.8
  tracheobronchial J98.09
Dyslalia (developmental) F80.0
Dyslexia R48.0
  developmental F81.0
Dyslipidemia E78.5
  depressed HDL cholesterol E78.6
  elevated fasting triglycerides E78.1
Dysmaturity — *see also* Light for dates
  pulmonary (newborn) (Wilson-Mikity) P27.0
Dysmenorrhea (essential) (exfoliative) N94.6
  congestive (syndrome) N94.6
  primary N94.4
  psychogenic F45.8
  secondary N94.5
Dysmetabolic syndrome X E88.81
Dysmetria R27.8
Dysmorphism (due to)
  alcohol Q86.0
  exogenous cause NEC Q86.8
  hydantoin Q86.1
  warfarin Q86.2
Dysmorphophobia (nondelusional) F45.22
  delusional F22
Dysnomia R47.01
Dysorexia R63.0
  psychogenic F50.89
Dysostosis
  cleidocranial, cleidocranialis Q74.0
  craniofacial Q75.1
  Fairbank's (idiopathic familial generalized osteophytosis) Q78.9
  mandibulofacial (incomplete) Q75.4
  multiplex E76.01
  oculomandibular Q75.5
Dyspareunia (female) N94.10
  deep N94.12
  male N53.12
  nonorganic F52.6
  psychogenic F52.6
  secondary N94.19
  specified NEC N94.19

Dyspareunia — *continued*
  superficial (introital) N94.11
Dyspepsia R10.13
  atonic K30
  functional (allergic) (congenital) (gastrointestinal) (occupational) (reflex) K30
  intestinal K59.8
  nervous F45.8
  neurotic F45.8
  psychogenic F45.8
Dysphagia R13.10
  cervical R13.19
  following
    cerebral infarction I69.391
    cerebrovascular disease I69.991
      specified NEC I69.891
    intracerebral hemorrhage I69.191
    nontraumatic intracranial hemorrhage NEC I69.291
    specified disease NEC I69.891
    subarachnoid hemorrhage I69.091
  functional (hysterical) F45.8
  hysterical F45.8
  nervous (hysterical) F45.8
  neurogenic R13.19
  oral phase R13.11
  oropharyngeal phase R13.12
  pharyngeal phase R13.13
  pharyngoesophageal phase R13.14
  psychogenic F45.8
  sideropenic D50.1
  spastica K22.4
  specified NEC R13.19
Dysphagocytosis, congenital D71
Dysphasia R47.02
  developmental
    expressive type F80.1
    receptive type F80.2
  following
    cerebrovascular disease I69.921
      cerebral infarction I69.321
      intracerebral hemorrhage I69.121
      nontraumatic intracranial hemorrhage NEC I69.221
      specified disease NEC I69.821
      subarachnoid hemorrhage I69.021
Dysphonia R49.0
  functional F44.4
  hysterical F44.4
  psychogenic F44.4
  spastica J38.3
Dysphoria
  gender F64.9
    in
      adolescence and adulthood F64.0
      children F64.2
    specified NEC F64.8
  postpartal O90.6
Dyspituitarism E23.3
Dysplasia — *see also* Anomaly
  acetabular, congenital Q65.89
  alveolar capillary, with vein misalignment J84.843
  anus (histologically confirmed) (mild) (moderate) K62.82
    severe D01.3
  arrhythmogenic right ventricular I42.8
  arterial, fibromuscular I77.3
  asphyxiating thoracic (congenital) Q77.2
  brain Q07.9
  bronchopulmonary, perinatal P27.1
  cervix (uteri) N87.9
    mild N87.0
    moderate N87.1
    severe D06.9
  chondroectodermal Q77.6
  colon D12.6
  craniometaphyseal Q78.8
  dentinal K00.5
  diaphyseal, progressive Q78.3
  dystrophic Q77.5
  ectodermal (anhidrotic) (congenital) (hereditary) Q82.4
    hydrotic Q82.8
  epithelial, uterine cervix — *see* Dysplasia, cervix
  eye (congenital) Q11.2
  fibrous
    bone NEC (monostotic) M85.00
      ankle M85.07- ☑
      foot M85.07- ☑
      forearm M85.03- ☑

Dysplasia — *continued*
  fibrous — *continued*
    bone — *continued*
      hand M85.04- ☑
      lower leg M85.06- ☑
      multiple site M85.09
      neck M85.08
      rib M85.08
      shoulder M85.01- ☑
      skull M85.08
      specified site NEC M85.08
      thigh M85.05- ☑
      toe M85.07- ☑
      upper arm M85.02- ☑
      vertebra M85.08
    diaphyseal, progressive Q78.3
    jaw M27.8
    polyostotic Q78.1
  florid osseous — *see also* Cyst, calcifying odontogenic
  high grade, focal D12.6
  hip, congenital Q65.89
  joint, congenital Q74.8
  kidney Q61.4
    multicystic Q61.4
  leg Q74.2
  lung, congenital (not associated with short gestation) Q33.6
  mammary (gland) (benign) N60.9- ☑
    cyst (solitary) — *see* Cyst, breast
    cystic — *see* Mastopathy, cystic
    duct ectasia — *see* Ectasia, mammary duct
    fibroadenosis — *see* Fibroadenosis, breast
    fibrosclerosis — *see* Fibrosclerosis, breast
    specified type NEC N60.8- ☑
  metaphyseal Q78.5
  muscle Q79.8
  oculodentodigital Q87.0
  periapical (cemental) (cemento-osseous) — *see* Cyst, calcifying odontogenic
  periosteum — *see* Disorder, bone, specified type NEC
  polyostotic fibrous Q78.1
  prostate — *see also* Neoplasia, intraepithelial, prostate N42.30
    severe D07.5
    specified NEC N42.39
  renal Q61.4
    multicystic Q61.4
  retinal, congenital Q14.1
  right ventricular, arrhythmogenic I42.8
  septo-optic Q04.4
  skin L98.8
  spinal cord Q06.1
  spondyloepiphyseal Q77.7
  thymic, with immunodeficiency D82.1
  vagina N89.3
    mild N89.0
    moderate N89.1
    severe NEC D07.2
  vulva N90.3
    mild N90.0
    moderate N90.1
    severe NEC D07.1
Dysplasminogenemia E88.02
Dyspnea (nocturnal) (paroxysmal) R06.00
  asthmatic (bronchial) J45.909
    with
      bronchitis J45.909
        with
          exacerbation (acute) J45.901
          status asthmaticus J45.902
        chronic J44.9
      exacerbation (acute) J45.901
      status asthmaticus J45.902
    cardiac — *see* Failure, ventricular, left
  cardiac — *see* Failure, ventricular, left
  functional F45.8
  hyperventilation R06.4
  hysterical F45.8
  newborn P28.89
  orthopnea R06.01
  psychogenic F45.8
  shortness of breath R06.02
  specified type NEC R06.09
Dyspraxia R27.8
  developmental (syndrome) F82
Dysproteinemia E88.09
Dysreflexia, autonomic G90.4

Dysrhythmia
  cardiac I49.9
    newborn
      bradycardia P29.12
      occurring before birth P03.819
        before onset of labor P03.810
        during labor P03.811
      tachycardia P29.11
    postoperative I97.89
  cerebral or cortical — *see* Epilepsy
Dyssomnia — *see* Disorder, sleep
Dyssynergia
  biliary K83.8
  bladder sphincter N36.44
  cerebellaris myoclonica (Hunt's ataxia) G11.1
Dysthymia F34.1
Dysthyroidism E07.9
Dystocia O66.9
  affecting newborn P03.1
  cervical (hypotonic) O62.2
    affecting newborn P03.6
    primary O62.0
    secondary O62.1
  contraction ring O62.4
  fetal O66.9
    abnormality NEC O66.3
    conjoined twins O66.3
    oversize O66.2
  maternal O66.9
  positional O64.9 ☑
  shoulder (girdle) O66.0
    causing obstructed labor O66.0
  uterine NEC O62.4
Dystonia G24.9
  cervical G24.3
  deformans progressiva G24.1
  drug induced NEC G24.09
    acute G24.02
    specified NEC G24.09
  familial G24.1
  idiopathic G24.1
    familial G24.1
    nonfamilial G24.2
    orofacial G24.4
  lenticularis G24.8
  musculorum deformans G24.1
  neuroleptic induced (acute) G24.02
  orofacial (idiopathic) G24.4
  oromandibular G24.4
    due to drug G24.01
  specified NEC G24.8
  torsion (familial) (idiopathic) G24.1
    acquired G24.8
    genetic G24.1
    symptomatic (nonfamilial) G24.2
Dystonic movements R25.8
Dystrophy, dystrophia
  adiposogenital E23.6
  autosomal recessive, childhood type, muscular dystrophy resembling Duchenne or Becker G71.01
  Becker's type G71.01
  cervical sympathetic G90.2
  choroid (hereditary) H31.20
    central areolar H31.22
    choroideremia H31.21
    gyrate atrophy H31.23
    specified type NEC H31.29
  cornea (hereditary) H18.50
    endothelial H18.51
    epithelial H18.52
    granular H18.53
    lattice H18.54
    macular H18.55
    specified type NEC H18.59
  Duchenne's type G71.01
  due to malnutrition E45
  Erb's G71.02
  Fuchs' H18.51
  Gower's muscular G71.01
  hair L67.8
  infantile neuraxonal G31.89
  Landouzy-Déjérine G71.02
  Leyden-Möbius G71.09
  muscular G71.00
    autosomal recessive, childhood type, muscular dystrophy resembling Duchenne or Becker G71.01
    benign (Becker type) G71.01

Dystrophy, dystrophia — *continued*
  muscular — *continued*
    benign — *continued*
      scapuloperoneal with early contractures [Emery-Dreifuss] G71.09
    congenital (hereditary) (progressive) (with specific morphological abnormalities of the muscle fiber) G71.09
      myotonic G71.11
    distal G71.09
    Duchenne type G71.01
    Emery-Dreifuss G71.09
    Erb type G71.02
    facioscapulohumeral G71.02
    Gower's G71.01
    hereditary (progressive) G71.09
    Landouzy-Déjérine type G71.02
    limb-girdle G71.09
    myotonic G71.11
    progressive (hereditary) G71.09
      Charcot-Marie (-Tooth) type G60.0
    pseudohypertrophic (infantile) G71.01
    scapulohumeral G71.02
    scapuloperoneal G71.09
    severe (Duchenne type) G71.01
    specified type NEC G71.09
  myocardium, myocardial — *see* Degeneration, myocardial
  nail L60.3
    congenital Q84.6
  nutritional E45
  ocular G71.09
  oculocerebrorenal E72.03
  oculopharyngeal G71.09
  ovarian N83.8
  polyglandular E31.8
  reflex (neuromuscular) (sympathetic) — *see* Syndrome, pain, complex regional I
  retinal (hereditary) H35.50
    in
      lipid storage disorders E75.6 [H36]
      systemic lipidoses E75.6 [H36]
    involving
      pigment epithelium H35.54
      sensory area H35.53
    pigmentary H35.52
    vitreoretinal H35.51
  Salzmann's nodular — *see* Degeneration, cornea, nodular
  scapuloperoneal G71.09
  skin NEC L98.8
  sympathetic (reflex) — *see* Syndrome, pain, complex regional I
    cervical G90.2
  tapetoretinal H35.54
  thoracic, asphyxiating Q77.2
  unguium L60.3
    congenital Q84.6
  vitreoretinal H35.51
  vulva N90.4
  yellow (liver) — *see* Failure, hepatic
Dysuria R30.0
  psychogenic F45.8

E

Eales' disease H35.06- ☑
Ear — *see also* condition
  piercing Z41.3
  tropical NEC B36.9 [H62.40]
    in
      aspergillosis B44.89
      candidiasis B37.84
      moniliasis B37.84
  wax (impacted) H61.20
    left H61.22
      with right H61.23
    right H61.21
      with left H61.23
Earache — *see* subcategory H92.0 ☑
Early satiety R68.81
Eaton-Lambert syndrome — *see* Syndrome, Lambert-Eaton
Eberth's disease (typhoid fever) A01.00
Ebola virus disease A98.4
Ebstein's anomaly or syndrome (heart) Q22.5
Eccentro-osteochondrodysplasia E76.29
Ecchondroma — *see* Neoplasm, bone, benign

Ecchondrosis D48.0
Ecchymosis R58
  conjunctiva — *see* Hemorrhage, conjunctiva
  eye (traumatic) — *see* Contusion, eyeball
  eyelid (traumatic) — *see* Contusion, eyelid
  newborn P54.5
  spontaneous R23.3
  traumatic — *see* Contusion
Echinococciasis — *see* Echinococcus
Echinococcosis — *see* Echinococcus
Echinococcus (infection) B67.90
  granulosus B67.4
    bone B67.2
    liver B67.0
    lung B67.1
    multiple sites B67.32
    specified site NEC B67.39
    thyroid B67.31
  liver NOS B67.8
    granulosus B67.0
    multilocularis B67.5
  lung NEC B67.99
    granulosus B67.1
    multilocularis B67.69
  multilocularis B67.7
    liver B67.5
    multiple sites B67.61
    specified site NEC B67.69
  specified site NEC B67.99
    granulosus B67.39
    multilocularis B67.69
  thyroid NEC B67.99
    granulosus B67.31
    multilocularis B67.69 *[E35]*
Echinorhynchiasis B83.8
Echinostomiasis B66.8
Echolalia R48.8
Echovirus, as cause of disease classified elsewhere B97.12
Eclampsia, eclamptic (coma) (convulsions) (delirium) (with hypertension) NEC O15.9
  complicating
    labor and delivery O15.1
    postpartum O15.2
    pregnancy O15.0- ☑
    puerperium O15.2
Economic circumstances affecting care Z59.9
Economo's disease A85.8
Ectasia, ectasis
  annuloaortic I35.8
  aorta I77.819
    with aneurysm — *see* Aneurysm, aorta
    abdominal I77.811
    thoracic I77.810
    thoracoabdominal I77.812
  breast — *see* Ectasia, mammary duct
  capillary I78.8
  cornea H18.71- ☑
  gastric antral vascular (GAVE) K31.819
    with hemorrhage K31.811
    without hemorrhage K31.819
  mammary duct N60.4- ☑
  salivary gland (duct) K11.8
  sclera — *see* Sclerectasia
Ecthyma L08.0
  contagiosum B08.02
  gangrenosum L08.0
  infectiosum B08.02
Ectocardia Q24.8
Ectodermal dysplasia (anhidrotic) Q82.4
Ectodermosis erosiva pluriorificialis L51.1
Ectopic, ectopia (congenital)
  abdominal viscera Q45.8
    due to defect in anterior abdominal wall Q79.59
  ACTH syndrome E24.3
  adrenal gland Q89.1
  anus Q43.5
  atrial beats I49.1
  beats I49.49
    atrial I49.1
    ventricular I49.3
  bladder Q64.10
  bone and cartilage in lung Q33.5
  brain Q04.8
  breast tissue Q83.8
  cardiac Q24.8
  cerebral Q04.8
  cordis Q24.8

Ectopic, ectopia — *continued*
  endometrium — *see* Endometriosis
  gastric mucosa Q40.2
  gestation — *see* Pregnancy, by site
  heart Q24.8
  hormone secretion NEC E34.2
  kidney (crossed) (pelvis) Q63.2
  lens, lentis Q12.1
  mole — *see* Pregnancy, by site
  organ or site NEC — *see* Malposition, congenital
  pancreas Q45.3
  pregnancy — *see* Pregnancy, ectopic
  pupil — *see* Abnormality, pupillary
  renal Q63.2
  sebaceous glands of mouth Q38.6
  spleen Q89.09
  testis Q53.00
    bilateral Q53.02
    unilateral Q53.01
  thyroid Q89.2
  tissue in lung Q33.5
  ureter Q62.63
  ventricular beats I49.3
  vesicae Q64.10
Ectromelia Q73.8
  lower limb — *see* Defect, reduction, limb, lower, specified type NEC
  upper limb — *see* Defect, reduction, limb, upper, specified type NEC
Ectropion H02.109
  cervix N86
    with cervicitis N72
  congenital Q10.1
  eyelid H02.109
    cicatricial H02.119
      left H02.116
        lower H02.115
        upper H02.114
      right H02.113
        lower H02.112
        upper H02.111
    congenital Q10.1
    left H02.106
      lower H02.105
      upper H02.104
    mechanical H02.129
      left H02.126
        lower H02.125
        upper H02.124
      right H02.123
        lower H02.122
        upper H02.121
    paralytic H02.159
      left H02.156
        lower H02.155
        upper H02.154
      right H02.153
        lower H02.152
        upper H02.151
    right H02.103
      lower H02.102
      upper H02.101
    senile H02.139
      left H02.136
        lower H02.135
        upper H02.134
      right H02.133
        lower H02.132
        upper H02.131
    spastic H02.149
      left H02.146
        lower H02.145
        upper H02.144
      right H02.143
        lower H02.142
        upper H02.141
  iris H21.89
  lip (acquired) K13.0
    congenital Q38.0
  urethra N36.8
  uvea H21.89
Eczema (acute) (chronic) (erythematous) (fissum) (rubrum) (squamous) — *see also* Dermatitis L30.9
  contact — *see* Dermatitis, contact
  dyshidrotic L30.1
  external ear — *see* Otitis, externa, acute, eczematoid
  flexural L20.82
  herpeticum B00.0

Eczema — *continued*
  hypertrophicum L28.0
  hypostatic — *see* Varix, leg, with, inflammation
  impetiginous L01.1
  infantile (due to any substance) L20.83
    intertriginous L21.1
    seborrheic L21.1
  intertriginous NEC L30.4
    infantile L21.1
  intrinsic (allergic) L20.84
  lichenified NEC L28.0
  marginatum (hebrae) B35.6
  pustular L30.3
  stasis I87.2
    with varicose veins — *see* Varix, leg, with, inflammation
  vaccination, vaccinatum T88.1 ☑
  varicose — *see* Varix, leg, with, inflammation
Eczematid L30.2
Eddowes (-Spurway) **syndrome** Q78.0
Edema, edematous (infectious) (pitting) (toxic) R60.9
  with nephritis — *see* Nephrosis
  allergic T78.3 ☑
  amputation stump (surgical) (sequelae (late effect)) T87.89
  angioneurotic (allergic) (any site) (with urticaria) T78.3 ☑
    hereditary D84.1
  angiospastic I73.9
  Berlin's (traumatic) S05.8X- ☑
  brain (cytotoxic) (vasogenic) G93.6
    due to birth injury P11.0
    newborn (anoxia or hypoxia) P52.4
      birth injury P11.0
    traumatic — *see* Injury, intracranial, cerebral edema
  cardiac — *see* Failure, heart, congestive
  cardiovascular — *see* Failure, heart, congestive
  cerebral — *see* Edema, brain
  cerebrospinal — *see* Edema, brain
  cervix (uteri) (acute) N88.8
    puerperal, postpartum O90.89
  chronic hereditary Q82.0
  circumscribed, acute T78.3 ☑
    hereditary D84.1
  conjunctiva H11.42- ☑
  cornea H18.2- ☑
    idiopathic H18.22- ☑
    secondary H18.23- ☑
      due to contact lens H18.21- ☑
  due to
    lymphatic obstruction I89.0
    salt retention E87.0
  epiglottis — *see* Edema, glottis
  essential, acute T78.3 ☑
    hereditary D84.1
  extremities, lower — *see* Edema, legs
  eyelid NEC H02.849
    left H02.846
      lower H02.845
      upper H02.844
    right H02.843
      lower H02.842
      upper H02.841
  familial, hereditary Q82.0
  famine — *see* Malnutrition, severe
  generalized R60.1
  glottis, glottic, glottidis (obstructive) (passive) J38.4
    allergic T78.3 ☑
      hereditary D84.1
  heart — *see* Failure, heart, congestive
  heat T67.7 ☑
  hereditary Q82.0
  inanition — *see* Malnutrition, severe
  intracranial G93.6
  iris H21.89
  joint — *see* Effusion, joint
  larynx — *see* Edema, glottis
  legs R60.0
    due to venous obstruction I87.1
    hereditary Q82.0
  localized R60.0
    due to venous obstruction I87.1
  lower limbs — *see* Edema, legs
  lung J81.1
    with heart condition or failure — *see* Failure, ventricular, left
    acute J81.0
    chemical (acute) J68.1

Edema, edematous — *continued*
- lung — *continued*
  - chemical — *continued*
    - chronic J68.1
    - chronic J81.1
      - due to
        - chemicals, gases, fumes or vapors (inhalation) J68.1
        - external agent J70.9
          - specified NEC J70.8
        - radiation J70.1
  - due to
    - chemicals, fumes or vapors (inhalation) J68.1
    - external agent J70.9
      - specified NEC J70.8
    - high altitude T70.29 ☑
    - near drowning T75.1 ☑
    - radiation J70.0
  - meaning failure, left ventricle I50.1
- lymphatic I89.0
  - due to mastectomy I97.2
- macula H35.81
  - cystoid, following cataract surgery — *see* Complications, postprocedural, following cataract surgery
  - diabetic — *see* Diabetes, by type, with, retinopathy, with macular edema
- malignant — *see* Gangrene, gas
- Milroy's Q82.0
- nasopharynx J39.2
- newborn P83.30
  - hydrops fetalis — *see* Hydrops, fetalis
  - specified NEC P83.39
- nutritional — *see also* Malnutrition, severe
  - with dyspigmentation, skin and hair E40
- optic disc or nerve — *see* Papilledema
- orbit H05.22- ☑
- pancreas K86.89
- papilla, optic — *see* Papilledema
- penis N48.89
- periodic T78.3 ☑
  - hereditary D84.1
- pharynx J39.2
- pulmonary — *see* Edema, lung
- Quincke's T78.3 ☑
  - hereditary D84.1
- renal — *see* Nephrosis
- retina H35.81
  - diabetic — *see* Diabetes, by type, with, retinopathy, with macular edema
- salt E87.0
- scrotum N50.89
- seminal vesicle N50.89
- spermatic cord N50.89
- spinal (cord) (vascular) (nontraumatic) G95.19
- starvation — *see* Malnutrition, severe
- stasis — *see* Hypertension, venous, (chronic)
- subglottic — *see* Edema, glottis
- supraglottic — *see* Edema, glottis
- testis N44.8
- tunica vaginalis N50.89
- vas deferens N50.89
- vulva (acute) N90.89

Edentulism — *see* Absence, teeth, acquired
Edsall's disease T67.2 ☑
Educational handicap Z55.9
- specified NEC Z55.8
Edward's syndrome — *see* Trisomy, 18
Effect(s) (of) (from) — *see* Effect, adverse NEC
Effect, adverse
- abnormal gravitational (G) forces or states T75.81 ☑
- abuse — *see* Maltreatment
- air pressure T70.9 ☑
  - specified NEC T70.8 ☑
- altitude (high) — *see* Effect, adverse, high altitude
- anesthesia — *see also* Anesthesia T88.59 ☑
  - in labor and delivery O74.9
  - local, toxic
    - in labor and delivery O74.4
    - in pregnancy NEC O29.3- ☑
    - postpartum, puerperal O89.3
  - postpartum, puerperal O89.9
  - specified NEC T88.59 ☑
    - in labor and delivery O74.8
    - postpartum, puerperal O89.8
  - spinal and epidural T88.59 ☑
    - headache T88.59 ☑

Effect, adverse — *continued*
- anesthesia — *see also* Anesthesia — *continued*
  - spinal and epidural — *continued*
    - headache — *continued*
      - in labor and delivery O74.5
      - postpartum, puerperal O89.4
    - specified NEC
      - in labor and delivery O74.6
      - postpartum, puerperal O89.5
- antitoxin — *see* Complications, vaccination
- atmospheric pressure T70.9 ☑
  - due to explosion T70.8 ☑
  - high T70.3 ☑
  - low — *see* Effect, adverse, high altitude
  - specified effect NEC T70.8 ☑
- biological, correct substance properly administered — *see* Effect, adverse, drug
- blood (derivatives) (serum) (transfusion) — *see* Complications, transfusion
- chemical substance — *see* Table of Drugs and Chemicals
- cold (temperature) (weather) T69.9 ☑
  - chilblains T69.1 ☑
  - frostbite — *see* Frostbite
  - specified effect NEC T69.8 ☑
- drugs and medicaments T88.7 ☑
  - specified drug — *see* Table of Drugs and Chemicals, by drug, adverse effect
  - specified effect — *code to* condition
- electric current, electricity (shock) T75.4 ☑
  - burn — *see* Burn
- exertion (excessive) T73.3 ☑
- exposure — *see* Exposure
- external cause NEC T75.89 ☑
- foodstuffs T78.1 ☑
  - allergic reaction — *see* Allergy, food
    - causing anaphylaxis — *see* Shock, anaphylactic, due to food
  - noxious — *see* Poisoning, food, noxious
- gases, fumes, or vapors T59.9- ☑
  - specified agent — *see* Table of Drugs and Chemicals
- glue (airplane) sniffing
  - due to drug abuse — *see* Abuse, drug, inhalant
  - due to drug dependence — *see* Dependence, drug, inhalant
- heat — *see* Heat
- high altitude NEC T70.29 ☑
  - anoxia T70.29 ☑
  - on
    - ears T70.0 ☑
    - sinuses T70.1 ☑
  - polycythemia D75.1
- high pressure fluids T70.4 ☑
- hot weather — *see* Heat
- hunger T73.0 ☑
- immersion, foot — *see* Immersion
- immunization — *see* Complications, vaccination
- immunological agents — *see* Complications, vaccination
- infrared (radiation) (rays) NOS T66 ☑
  - dermatitis or eczema L59.8
- infusion — *see* Complications, infusion
- lack of care of infants — *see* Maltreatment, child
- lightning — *see* Lightning
- medical care T88.9 ☑
  - specified NEC T88.8 ☑
- medicinal substance, correct, properly administered — *see* Effect, adverse, drug
- motion T75.3 ☑
- noise, on inner ear — *see* subcategory H83.3 ☑
- overheated places — *see* Heat
- psychosocial, of work environment Z56.5
- radiation (diagnostic) (infrared) (natural source) (therapeutic) (ultraviolet) (X-ray) NOS T66 ☑
  - dermatitis or eczema — *see* Dermatitis, due to, radiation
  - fibrosis of lung J70.1
  - pneumonitis J70.0
  - pulmonary manifestations
    - acute J70.0
    - chronic J70.1
  - skin L59.9
- radioactive substance NOS
  - dermatitis or eczema — *see* Radiodermatitis
- reduced temperature T69.9 ☑
  - immersion foot or hand — *see* Immersion
  - specified effect NEC T69.8 ☑

Effect, adverse — *continued*
- serum NEC — *see also* Reaction, serum T80.69 ☑
- specified NEC T78.8 ☑
  - external cause NEC T75.89 ☑
- strangulation — *see* Asphyxia, traumatic
- submersion T75.1 ☑
- thirst T73.1 ☑
- toxic — *see* Toxicity
- transfusion — *see* Complications, transfusion
- ultraviolet (radiation) (rays) NOS T66 ☑
  - burn — *see* Burn
  - dermatitis or eczema — *see* Dermatitis, due to, ultraviolet rays
    - acute L56.8
- vaccine (any) — *see* Complications, vaccination
- vibration — *see* Vibration, adverse effects
- water pressure NEC T70.9 ☑
  - specified NEC T70.8 ☑
- weightlessness T75.82 ☑
- whole blood — *see* Complications, transfusion
- work environment Z56.5

Effects, late — *see* Sequelae
Effluvium
- anagen L65.1
- telogen L65.0
Effort syndrome (psychogenic) F45.8
Effusion
- amniotic fluid — *see* Pregnancy, complicated by, prematue rupture of membranes
- brain (serous) G93.6
- bronchial — *see* Bronchitis
- cerebral G93.6
- cerebrospinal — *see also* Meningitis
  - vessel G93.6
- chest — *see* Effusion, pleura
- chylous, chyliform (pleura) J94.0
- intracranial G93.6
- joint M25.40
  - ankle M25.47- ☑
  - elbow M25.42- ☑
  - foot joint M25.47- ☑
  - hand joint M25.44- ☑
  - hip M25.45- ☑
  - knee M25.46- ☑
  - shoulder M25.41- ☑
  - specified joint NEC M25.48
  - wrist M25.43- ☑
- malignant pleural J91.0
- meninges — *see* Meningitis
- pericardium, pericardial (noninflammatory) I31.3
  - acute — *see* Pericarditis, acute
- peritoneal (chronic) R18.8
- pleura, pleurisy, pleuritic, pleuropericardial J90
  - chylous, chyliform J94.0
  - due to systemic lupus erythematosis M32.13
  - in conditions classified elsewhere J91.8
  - influenzal — *see* Influenza, with, respiratory manifestations NEC
  - malignant J91.0
  - newborn P28.89
  - tuberculous NEC A15.6
    - primary (progressive) A15.7
- spinal — *see* Meningitis
- thorax, thoracic — *see* Effusion, pleura
Egg shell nails L60.3
- congenital Q84.6
Egyptian splenomegaly B65.1
Ehlers-Danlos syndrome — *see also* Syndrome, Ehlers-Danlos Q79.60
Ehrlichiosis A77.40
- due to
  - E. chafeensis A77.41
  - E. sennetsu A79.81
  - specified organism NEC A77.49
Eichstedt's disease B36.0
Eisenmenger's
- complex or syndrome I27.83
- defect Q21.8
Ejaculation
- delayed F52.32
- painful N53.12
- premature F52.4
- retarded N53.11
- retrograde N53.14
- semen, painful N53.12
  - psychogenic F52.6
Ekbom's syndrome (restless legs) G25.81

Ekman's syndrome (brittle bones and blue sclera) Q78.0
Elastic skin Q82.8
acquired L57.4
Elastofibroma — *see* Neoplasm, connective tissue, benign
Elastoma (juvenile) Q82.8
Miescher's L87.2
Elastomyofibrosis I42.4
Elastosis
actinic, solar L57.8
atrophicans (senile) L57.4
perforans serpiginosa L87.2
senilis L57.4
Elbow — *see* condition
Electric current, electricity, effects (concussion) (fatal) (nonfatal) (shock) T75.4 ☑
burn — *see* Burn
Electric feet syndrome E53.8
Electrocution T75.4 ☑
from electroshock gun (taser) T75.4 ☑
Electrolyte imbalance E87.8
with
abortion — *see* Abortion by type, complicated by, electrolyte imbalance
ectopic pregnancy O08.5
molar pregnancy O08.5
Elephantiasis (nonfilarial) I89.0
arabicum — *see* Infestation, filarial
bancroftian B74.0
congenital (any site) (hereditary) Q82.0
due to
Brugia (malayi) B74.1
timori B74.2
mastectomy I97.2
Wuchereria (bancrofti) B74.0
eyelid H02.859
left H02.856
lower H02.855
upper H02.854
right H02.853
lower H02.852
upper H02.851
filarial, filariensis — *see* Infestation, filarial
glandular I89.0
graecorum A30.9
lymphangiectatic I89.0
lymphatic vessel I89.0
due to mastectomy I97.2
scrotum (nonfilarial) I89.0
streptococcal I89.0
surgical I97.89
postmastectomy I97.2
telangiectodes I89.0
vulva (nonfilarial) N90.89
Elevated, elevation
antibody titer R76.0
basal metabolic rate R94.8
blood pressure — *see also* Hypertension
reading (incidental) (isolated) (nonspecific), no diagnosis of hypertension R03.0
blood sugar R73.9
body temperature (of unknown origin) R50.9
cancer antigen 125 [CA 125] R97.1
carcinoembryonic antigen [CEA] R97.0
cholesterol E78.00
with high triglycerides E78.2
conjugate, eye H51.0
C-reactive protein (CRP) R79.82
diaphragm, congenital Q79.1
erythrocyte sedimentation rate R70.0
fasting glucose R73.01
fasting triglycerides E78.1
finding on laboratory examination — *see* Findings, abnormal, inconclusive, without diagnosis, by type of exam
GFR (glomerular filtration rate) — *see* Findings, abnormal, inconclusive, without diagnosis, by type of exam
glucose tolerance (oral) R73.02
immunoglobulin level R76.8
indoleacetic acid R82.5
lactic acid dehydrogenase (LDH) level R74.0
leukocytes D72.829
lipoprotein a (Lp(a)) level E78.41
liver function
study R94.5
test R79.89
alkaline phosphatase R74.8

Elevated, elevation — *continued*
liver function — *continued*
test — *continued*
aminotransferase R74.0
bilirubin R17
hepatic enzyme R74.8
lactate dehydrogenase R74.0
Lp(a) (lipoprotein(a)) E78.41
lymphocytes D72.820
prostate specific antigen [PSA] R97.20
Rh titer — *see* Complication(s), transfusion, incompatibility reaction, Rh (factor)
scapula, congenital Q74.0
sedimentation rate R70.0
SGOT R74.0
SGPT R74.0
transaminase level R74.0
triglycerides E78.1
with high cholesterol E78.2
tumor associated antigens [TAA] NEC R97.8
tumor specific antigens [TSA] NEC R97.8
urine level of
17-ketosteroids R82.5
catecholamine R82.5
indoleacetic acid R82.5
steroids R82.5
vanillylmandelic acid (VMA) R82.5
venous pressure I87.8
white blood cell count D72.829
specified NEC D72.828
Elliptocytosis (congenital) (hereditary) D58.1
Hb C (disease) D58.1
hemoglobin disease D58.1
sickle-cell (disease) D57.8- ☑
trait D57.3
Ellison-Zollinger syndrome E16.4
Ellis-van Creveld syndrome (chondroectodermal dysplasia) Q77.6
Elongated, elongation (congenital) — *see also* Distortion
bone Q79.9
cervix (uteri) Q51.828
acquired N88.4
hypertrophic N88.4
colon Q43.8
common bile duct Q44.5
cystic duct Q44.5
frenulum, penis Q55.69
labia minora (acquired) N90.69
ligamentum patellae Q74.1
petiolus (epiglottidis) Q31.8
tooth, teeth K00.2
uvula Q38.6
Eltor cholera A00.1
Emaciation (due to malnutrition) E41
Embadomoniasis A07.8
Embedded tooth, teeth K01.0
root only K08.3
Embolic — *see* condition
Embolism (multiple) (paradoxical) I74.9
air (any site) (traumatic) T79.0 ☑
following
abortion — *see* Abortion by type complicated by embolism
ectopic pregnancy O08.2
infusion, therapeutic injection or transfusion T80.0 ☑
molar pregnancy O08.2
procedure NEC
artery T81.719 ☑
mesenteric T81.710 ☑
renal T81.711 ☑
specified NEC T81.718 ☑
vein T81.72 ☑
in pregnancy, childbirth or puerperium — *see* Embolism, obstetric
amniotic fluid (pulmonary) — *see also* Embolism, obstetric
following
abortion — *see* Abortion by type complicated by embolism
ectopic pregnancy O08.2
molar pregnancy O08.2
aorta, aortic I74.10
abdominal I74.09
saddle I74.01
bifurcation I74.09
saddle I74.01

Embolism — *continued*
aorta, aortic — *continued*
thoracic I74.11
artery I74.9
auditory, internal I65.8
basilar — *see* Occlusion, artery, basilar
carotid (common) (internal) — *see* Occlusion, artery, carotid
cerebellar (anterior inferior) (posterior inferior) (superior) I66.3
cerebral — *see* Occlusion, artery, cerebral
choroidal (anterior) I65.8
communicating posterior I65.8
coronary — *see also* Infarct, myocardium
not resulting in infarction I24.0
extremity I74.4
lower I74.3
upper I74.2
hypophyseal I65.8
iliac I74.5
limb I74.4
lower I74.3
upper I74.2
mesenteric (with gangrene) — *see also* Ischemia, intestine, acute K55.059
ophthalmic — *see* Occlusion, artery, retina
peripheral I74.4
pontine I65.8
precerebral — *see* Occlusion, artery, precerebral
pulmonary — *see* Embolism, pulmonary
renal N28.0
retinal — *see* Occlusion, artery, retina
septic I76
specified NEC I74.8
vertebral — *see* Occlusion, artery, vertebral
basilar (artery) I65.1
blood clot
following
abortion — *see* Abortion by type complicated by embolism
ectopic or molar pregnancy O08.2
in pregnancy, childbirth or puerperium — *see* Embolism, obstetric
brain — *see also* Occlusion, artery, cerebral
following
abortion — *see* Abortion by type complicated by embolism
ectopic or molar pregnancy O08.2
puerperal, postpartum, childbirth — *see* Embolism, obstetric
capillary I78.8
cardiac — *see also* Infarct, myocardium
not resulting in infarction I51.3
carotid (artery) (common) (internal) — *see* Occlusion, artery, carotid
cavernous sinus (venous) — *see* Embolism, intracranial venous sinus
cerebral — *see* Occlusion, artery, cerebral
cholesterol — *see* Atheroembolism
coronary (artery or vein) (systemic) — *see* Occlusion, coronary
due to device, implant or graft — *see also* Complications, by site and type, specified NEC
arterial graft NEC T82.818 ☑
breast (implant) T85.818 ☑
catheter NEC T85.818 ☑
dialysis (renal) T82.818 ☑
intraperitoneal T85.818 ☑
infusion NEC T82.818 ☑
spinal (epidural) (subdural) T85.810 ☑
urinary (indwelling) T83.81 ☑
electronic (electrode) (pulse generator) (stimulator)
bone T84.81 ☑
cardiac T82.817 ☑
nervous system (brain) (peripheral nerve) (spinal) T85.810 ☑
urinary T83.81 ☑
fixation, internal (orthopedic) NEC T84.81 ☑
gastrointestinal (bile duct) (esophagus) T85.818 ☑
genital NEC T83.81 ☑
heart (graft) (valve) T82.817 ☑
joint prosthesis T84.81 ☑
ocular (corneal graft) (orbital implant) T85.818 ☑
orthopedic (bone graft) NEC T86.838
specified NEC T85.818 ☑
urinary (graft) NEC T83.81 ☑
vascular NEC T82.818 ☑

☑ Additional Character Required — Refer to the Tabular List for Character Selection   ᵂ Subterms under main terms may continue to next column or page

Embolism — *continued*
  due to device, implant or graft — *see also* Complications, by site and type, specified — *continued*
    ventricular intracranial shunt T85.810 ☑
  extremities
    lower — *see* Embolism, vein, lower extremity
      arterial I74.3
    upper I74.2
  eye H34.9
  fat (cerebral) (pulmonary) (systemic) T79.1 ☑
    complicating delivery — *see* Embolism, obstetric
    following
      abortion — *see* Abortion by type complicated by embolism
      ectopic or molar pregnancy O08.2
  following
    abortion — *see* Abortion by type complicated by embolism
    ectopic or molar pregnancy O08.2
    infusion, therapeutic injection or transfusion air T80.0 ☑
  heart (fatty) — *see also* Infarct, myocardium
    not resulting in infarction I51.3
  hepatic (vein) I82.0
  in pregnancy, childbirth or puerperium — *see* Embolism, obstetric
  intestine (artery) (vein) (with gangrene) — *see also* Ischemia, intestine, acute K55.039
  intracranial — *see also* Occlusion, artery, cerebral
    venous sinus (any) G08
      nonpyogenic I67.6
  intraspinal venous sinuses or veins G08
    nonpyogenic G95.19
  kidney (artery) N28.0
  lateral sinus (venous) — *see* Embolism, intracranial, venous sinus
  leg — *see* Embolism, vein, lower extremity
    arterial I74.3
  longitudinal sinus (venous) — *see* Embolism, intracranial, venous sinus
  lung (massive) — *see* Embolism, pulmonary
  meninges I66.8
  mesenteric (artery) (vein) (with gangrene) — *see also* Ischemia, intestine, acute K55.059
  obstetric (in) (pulmonary)
    childbirth O88.22
      air O88.02
      amniotic fluid O88.12
      blood clot O88.22
      fat O88.82
      pyemic O88.32
      septic O88.32
      specified type NEC O88.82
    pregnancy O88.21- ☑
      air O88.01- ☑
      amniotic fluid O88.11- ☑
      blood clot O88.21- ☑
      fat O88.81- ☑
      pyemic O88.31- ☑
      septic O88.31- ☑
      specified type NEC O88.81- ☑
    puerperal O88.23
      air O88.03
      amniotic fluid O88.13
      blood clot O88.23
      fat O88.83
      pyemic O88.33
      septic O88.33
      specified type NEC O88.83
  ophthalmic — *see* Occlusion, artery, retina
  penis N48.81
  peripheral artery NOS I74.4
  pituitary E23.6
  popliteal (artery) I74.3
  portal (vein) I81
  postoperative, postprocedural
    artery T81.719 ☑
      mesenteric T81.710 ☑
      renal T81.711 ☑
      specified NEC T81.718 ☑
    vein T81.72 ☑
  precerebral artery — *see* Occlusion, artery, precerebral
  puerperal — *see* Embolism, obstetric
  pulmonary (acute) (artery) (vein) I26.99
    with acute cor pulmonale I26.09
    chronic I27.82

Embolism — *continued*
  pulmonary — *continued*
    following
      abortion — *see* Abortion by type complicated by embolism
      ectopic or molar pregnancy O08.2
    healed or old Z86.711
    in pregnancy, childbirth or puerperium — *see* Embolism, obstetric
    multiple subsegmental without acute cor pulmonale I26.94
    personal history of Z86.711
    saddle I26.92
      with acute cor pulmonale I26.02
    septic I26.90
      with acute cor pulmonale I26.01
    single subsegmental without acute cor pulmonale I26.93
    subsegmental NOS I26.93
  pyemic (multiple) I76
    following
      abortion — *see* Abortion by type complicated by embolism
      ectopic or molar pregnancy O08.2
    Hemophilus influenzae A41.3
    pneumococcal A40.3
      with pneumonia J13
    puerperal, postpartum, childbirth (any organism) — *see* Embolism, obstetric
    specified organism NEC A41.89
    staphylococcal A41.2
    streptococcal A40.9
  renal (artery) N28.0
    vein I82.3
  retina, retinal — *see* Occlusion, artery, retina
  saddle
    abdominal aorta I74.01
    pulmonary artery I26.92
      with acute cor pulmonale I26.02
  septic (arterial) I76
    complicating abortion — *see* Abortion, by type, complicated by, embolism
  sinus — *see* Embolism, intracranial, venous sinus
  soap complicating abortion — *see* Abortion, by type, complicated by, embolism
  spinal cord G95.19
    pyogenic origin G06.1
  spleen, splenic (artery) I74.8
  upper extremity I74.2
  vein (acute) I82.90
    antecubital I82.61- ☑
      chronic I82.71- ☑
    axillary I82.A1- ☑ (*following* I82.7)
      chronic I82.A2- ☑ (*following* I82.7)
    basilic I82.61- ☑
      chronic I82.71- ☑
    brachial I82.62- ☑
      chronic I82.72- ☑
    brachiocephalic (innominate) I82.290
      chronic I82.291
    cephalic I82.61- ☑
      chronic I82.71- ☑
    chronic I82.91
    deep (DVT) I82.40- ☑
      calf I82.4Z- ☑
        chronic I82.5Z- ☑
      lower leg I82.4Z- ☑
        chronic I82.5Z- ☑
      thigh I82.4Y- ☑
        chronic I82.5Y- ☑
      upper leg I82.4Y ☑
        chronic I82.5Y-
    femoral I82.41- ☑
      chronic I82.51- ☑
    iliac (iliofemoral) I82.42- ☑
      chronic I82.52- ☑
    innominate I82.290
      chronic I82.291
    internal jugular I82.C1- ☑ (*following* I82.7)
      chronic I82.C2- ☑ (*following* I82.7)
    lower extremity
      deep I82.40- ☑
        chronic I82.50- ☑
        specified NEC I82.49- ☑
          chronic NEC I82.59- ☑
      distal
        deep I82.4Z- ☑

Embolism — *continued*
  vein — *continued*
    lower extremity — *continued*
      proximal
        deep I82.4Y- ☑
          chronic I82.5Y- ☑
        superficial I82.81- ☑
    popliteal I82.43- ☑
      chronic I82.53- ☑
    radial I82.62- ☑
      chronic I82.72- ☑
    renal I82.3
    saphenous (greater) (lesser) I82.81- ☑
    specified NEC I82.890
      chronic NEC I82.891
    subclavian I82.B1- ☑ (*following* I82.7)
      chronic I82.B2- ☑ (*following* I82.7)
    thoracic NEC I82.290
      chronic I82.291
    tibial I82.44- ☑
      chronic I82.54- ☑
    ulnar I82.62- ☑
      chronic I82.72- ☑
    upper extremity I82.60- ☑
      chronic I82.70- ☑
      deep I82.62- ☑
        chronic I82.72- ☑
      superficial I82.61- ☑
        chronic I82.71- ☑
  vena cava
    inferior (acute) I82.220
      chronic I82.221
    superior (acute) I82.210
      chronic I82.211
  venous sinus G08
  vessels of brain — *see* Occlusion, artery, cerebral
Embolus — *see* Embolism
Embryoma — *see also* Neoplasm, uncertain behavior, by site
  benign — *see* Neoplasm, benign, by site
  kidney C64.- ☑
  liver C22.0
  malignant — *see also* Neoplasm, malignant, by site
    kidney C64.- ☑
    liver C22.0
    testis C62.9- ☑
      descended (scrotal) C62.1- ☑
      undescended C62.0- ☑
  testis C62.9- ☑
    descended (scrotal) C62.1- ☑
    undescended C62.0- ☑
Embryonic
  circulation Q28.9
  heart Q28.9
  vas deferens Q55.4
Embryopathia NOS Q89.9
Embryotoxon Q13.4
Emesis — *see* Vomiting
Emotional lability R45.86
Emotionality, pathological F60.3
Emotogenic disease — *see* Disorder, psychogenic
Emphysema (atrophic) (bullous) (chronic) (interlobular) (lung) (obstructive) (pulmonary) (senile) (vesicular) J43.9
  cellular tissue (traumatic) T79.7 ☑
    surgical T81.82 ☑
  centrilobular J43.2
  compensatory J98.3
  congenital (interstitial) P25.0
  conjunctiva H11.89
  connective tissue (traumatic) T79.7 ☑
    surgical T81.82 ☑
  due to chemicals, gases, fumes or vapors J68.4
  eyelid(s) — *see* Disorder, eyelid, specified type NEC
    surgical T81.82 ☑
    traumatic T79.7 ☑
  interstitial J98.2
    congenital P25.0
    perinatal period P25.0
  laminated tissue T79.7 ☑
    surgical T81.82 ☑
  mediastinal J98.2
    newborn P25.2
  orbit, orbital — *see* Disorder, orbit, specified type NEC
  panacinar J43.1
  panlobular J43.1
  specified NEC J43.8

▽ Subterms under main terms may continue to next column or page   ☑ Additional Character Required — Refer to the Tabular List for Character Selection   129

Embolism — Emphysema

Emphysema — continued
  subcutaneous (traumatic) T79.7 ☑
    nontraumatic J98.2
    postprocedural T81.82 ☑
    surgical T81.82 ☑
  surgical T81.82 ☑
  thymus (gland) (congenital) E32.8
  traumatic (subcutaneous) T79.7 ☑
  unilateral J43.0
Empty nest syndrome Z60.0
Empyema (acute) (chest) (double) (pleura) (supradiaphragmatic) (thorax) J86.9
  with fistula J86.0
  accessory sinus (chronic) — see Sinusitis
  antrum (chronic) — see Sinusitis, maxillary
  brain (any part) — see Abscess, brain
  ethmoidal (chronic) (sinus) — see Sinusitis, ethmoidal
  extradural — see Abscess, extradural
  frontal (chronic) (sinus) — see Sinusitis, frontal
  gallbladder K81.0
  mastoid (process) (acute) — see Mastoiditis, acute
  maxilla, maxillary M27.2
    sinus (chronic) — see Sinusitis, maxillary
  nasal sinus (chronic) — see Sinusitis
  sinus (accessory) (chronic) (nasal) — see Sinusitis
  sphenoidal (sinus) (chronic) — see Sinusitis, sphenoidal
  subarachnoid — see Abscess, extradural
  subdural — see Abscess, subdural
  tuberculous A15.6
  ureter — see Ureteritis
  ventricular — see Abscess, brain
En coup de sabre lesion L94.1
Enamel pearls K00.2
Enameloma K00.2
Enanthema, viral B09
Encephalitis (chronic) (hemorrhagic) (idiopathic) (nonepidemic) (spurious) (subacute) G04.90
  acute — see also Encephalitis, viral A86
    disseminated G04.00
      infectious G04.01
      noninfectious G04.81
      postimmunization (postvaccination) G04.02
      postinfectious G04.01
    inclusion body A85.8
    necrotizing hemorrhagic G04.30
      postimmunization G04.32
      postinfectious G04.31
      specified NEC G04.39
  arboviral, arbovirus NEC A85.2
  arthropod-borne NEC (viral) A85.2
  Australian A83.4
  California (virus) A83.5
  Central European (tick-borne) A84.1
  Czechoslovakian A84.1
  Dawson's (inclusion body) A81.1
  diffuse sclerosing A81.1
  disseminated, acute G04.00
  due to
    cat scratch disease A28.1
    human immunodeficiency virus (HIV) disease B20 [G05.3]
    malaria — see Malaria
    rickettsiosis — see Rickettsiosis
    smallpox inoculation G04.02
    typhus — see Typhus
  Eastern equine A83.2
  endemic (viral) A86
  epidemic NEC (viral) A86
  equine (acute) (infectious) (viral) A83.9
    Eastern A83.2
    Venezuelan A92.2
    Western A83.1
  Far Eastern (tick-borne) A84.0
  following vaccination or other immunization procedure G04.02
  herpes zoster B02.0
  herpesviral B00.4
    due to herpesvirus 6 B10.01
    due to herpesvirus 7 B10.09
    specified NEC B10.09
  Ilheus (virus) A83.8
  in (due to)
    actinomycosis A42.82
    adenovirus A85.1
    African trypanosomiasis B56.9 [G05.3]
    Chagas' disease (chronic) B57.42
    cytomegalovirus B25.8
    enterovirus A85.0

Encephalitis — continued
  in — continued
    herpes (simplex) virus B00.4
      due to herpesvirus 6 B10.01
      due to herpesvirus 7 B10.09
      specified NEC B10.09
    infectious disease NEC B99 ☑ [G05.3]
    influenza — see Influenza, with, encephalopathy
    listeriosis A32.12
    measles B05.0
    mumps B26.2
    naegleriasis B60.2
    parasitic disease NEC B89 [G05.3]
    poliovirus A80.9 [G05.3]
    rubella B06.01
    syphilis
      congenital A50.42
      late A52.14
    systemic lupus erythematosus M32.19
    toxoplasmosis (acquired) B58.2
      congenital P37.1
    tuberculosis A17.82
    zoster B02.0
  inclusion body A81.1
  infectious (acute) (virus) NEC A86
  Japanese (B type) A83.0
  La Crosse A83.5
  lead — see Poisoning, lead
  lethargica (acute) (infectious) A85.8
  louping ill A84.8
  lupus erythematosus, systemic M32.19
  lymphatica A87.2
  Mengo A85.8
  meningococcal A39.81
  Murray Valley A83.4
  otitic NEC H66.40 [G05.3]
  parasitic NOS B71.9
  periaxial G37.0
  periaxialis (concentrica) (diffuse) G37.5
  postchickenpox B01.11
  postexanthematous NEC B09
  postimmunization G04.02
  postinfectious NEC G04.01
  postmeasles B05.0
  postvaccinal G04.02
  postvaricella B01.11
  postviral NEC A86
  Powassan A84.8
  Rasmussen G04.81
  Rio Bravo A85.8
  Russian
    autumnal A83.0
    spring-summer (taiga) A84.0
  saturnine — see Poisoning, lead
  specified NEC G04.81
  St. Louis A83.3
  subacute sclerosing A81.1
  summer A83.0
  suppurative G04.81
  tick-borne A84.9
  Torula, torular (cryptococcal) B45.1
  toxic NEC G92
  trichinosis B75 [G05.3]
  type
    B A83.0
    C A83.3
  van Bogaert's A81.1
  Venezuelan equine A92.2
  Vienna A85.8
  viral, virus A86
    arthropod-borne NEC A85.2
      mosquito-borne A83.9
        Australian X disease A83.4
        California virus A83.5
        Eastern equine A83.2
        Japanese (B type) A83.0
        Murray Valley A83.4
        specified NEC A83.8
        St. Louis A83.3
        type B A83.0
        type C A83.3
        Western equine A83.1
      tick-borne A84.9
        biundulant A84.1
        central European A84.1
        Czechoslovakian A84.1
        diphasic meningoencephalitis A84.1
        Far Eastern A84.0

Encephalitis — continued
  viral, virus — continued
    arthropod-borne — continued
      tick-borne — continued
        Russian spring-summer (taiga) A84.0
        specified NEC A84.8
      specified type NEC A85.8
    Western equine A83.1
Encephalocele Q01.9
  frontal Q01.0
  nasofrontal Q01.1
  occipital Q01.2
  specified NEC Q01.8
Encephalocystocele — see Encephalocele
Encephaloduroarteriomyosynangiosis (EDAMS) I67.5
Encephalomalacia (brain) (cerebellar) (cerebral) — see Softening, brain
Encephalomeningitis — see Meningoencephalitis
Encephalomeningocele — see Encephalocele
Encephalomeningomyelitis — see Meningoencephalitis
Encephalomyelitis — see also Encephalitis G04.90
  acute disseminated G04.00
    infectious G04.01
    noninfectious G04.81
    postimmunization G04.02
    postinfection G04.01
  acute necrotizing hemorrhagic G04.30
    postimmunization G04.32
    postinfectious G04.31
    specified NEC G04.39
  benign myalgic G93.3
  equine A83.9
    Eastern A83.2
    Venezuelan A92.2
    Western A83.1
  in diseases classified elsewhere G05.3
  myalgic, benign G93.3
  postchickenpox B01.11
  postinfectious NEC G04.01
  postmeasles B05.0
  postvaccinal G04.02
  postvaricella B01.11
  rubella B06.01
  specified NEC G04.81
  Venezuelan equine A92.2
Encephalomyelocele — see Encephalocele
Encephalomyelomeningitis — see Meningoencephalitis
Encephalomyelopathy G96.9
Encephalomyeloradiculitis (acute) G61.0
Encephalomyeloradiculoneuritis (acute) (Guillain-Barré) G61.0
Encephalomyeloradiculopathy G96.9
Encephalopathia hyperbilirubinemica, newborn P57.9
  due to isoimmunization (conditions in P55) P57.0
Encephalopathy (acute) G93.40
  acute necrotizing hemorrhagic G04.30
    postimmunization G04.32
    postinfectious G04.31
    specified NEC G04.39
  alcoholic G31.2
  anoxic — see Damage, brain, anoxic
  arteriosclerotic I67.2
  centrolobar progressive (Schilder) G37.0
  congenital Q07.9
  degenerative, in specified disease NEC G32.89
  demyelinating callosal G37.1
  due to
    drugs — see also Table of Drugs and Chemicals G92
  hepatic — see Failure, hepatic
  hyperbilirubinemic, newborn P57.9
    due to isoimmunization (conditions in P55) P57.0
  hypertensive I67.4
  hypoglycemic E16.2
  hypoxic — see Damage, brain, anoxic
  hypoxic ischemic P91.60
    mild P91.61
    moderate P91.62
    severe P91.63
  in (due to) (with)
    birth injury P11.1
    hyperinsulinism E16.1 [G94]
    influenza — see Influenza, with, encephalopathy
    lack of vitamin — see also Deficiency, vitamin E56.9 [G32.89]
    neoplastic disease — see also Neoplasm D49.9 [G13.1]
    serum — see also Reaction, serum T80.69 ☑

☑ Additional Character Required — Refer to the Tabular List for Character Selection   ▽ Subterms under main terms may continue to next column or page

Encephalopathy — continued
- in — continued
  - syphilis A52.17
  - trauma (postconcussional) F07.81
    - current injury — see Injury, intracranial
  - vaccination G04.02
- lead — see Poisoning, lead
- metabolic G93.41
  - drug induced G92
  - toxic G92
- myoclonic, early, symptomatic — see Epilepsy, generalized, specified NEC
- necrotizing, subacute (Leigh) G31.82
- neonatal P91.819
  - in diseases classified elsewhere P91.811
- pellagrous E52 [G32.89]
- portosystemic — see Failure, hepatic
- postcontusional F07.81
  - current injury — see Injury, intracranial, diffuse
- posthypoglycemic (coma) E16.1 [G94]
- postradiation G93.89
- saturnine — see Poisoning, lead
- septic G93.41
- specified NEC G93.49
- spongioform, subacute (viral) A81.09
- toxic G92
  - metabolic G92
- traumatic (postconcussional) F07.81
  - current injury — see Injury, intracranial
- vitamin B deficiency NEC E53.9 [G32.89]
  - vitamin B1 E51.2
  - Wernicke's E51.2

Encephalorrhagia — see Hemorrhage, intracranial, intracerebral

Encephalosis, posttraumatic F07.81

Enchondroma — see also Neoplasm, bone, benign

Enchondromatosis (cartilaginous) (multiple) Q78.4

Encopresis R15.9
- functional F98.1
- nonorganic origin F98.1
- psychogenic F98.1

Encounter (with health service) (for) Z76.89
- adjustment and management (of)
  - breast implant Z45.81 ☑
  - implanted device NEC Z45.89
  - myringotomy device (stent) (tube) Z45.82
  - neurostimulator (brain) (gastric) (peripheral nerve) (sacral nerve) (spinal cord) (vagus nerve) Z45.42
- administrative purpose only Z02.9
  - examination for
    - adoption Z02.82
    - armed forces Z02.3
    - disability determination Z02.71
    - driving license Z02.4
    - employment Z02.1
    - insurance Z02.6
    - medical certificate NEC Z02.79
    - paternity testing Z02.81
    - residential institution admission Z02.2
    - school admission Z02.0
    - sports Z02.5
    - specified reason NEC Z02.89
- aftercare — see Aftercare
- antenatal screening Z36.9
  - cervical length Z36.86
  - chromosomal anomalies Z36.0
  - congenital cardiac abnormalities Z36.83
  - elevated maternal serum alphafetoprotein Z36.1
  - fetal growth retardation Z36.4
  - fetal lung maturity Z36.84
  - fetal macrosomia Z36.88
  - hydrops fetalis Z36.81
  - intrauterine growth restriction (IUGR) /small-for-dates Z36.4
  - isoimmunization Z36.5
  - large-for-dates Z36.88
  - malformations Z36.3
  - non-visualized anatomy on a previous scan Z36.2
  - nuchal translucency Z36.82
  - raised alphafetoprotein level Z36.1
  - risk of pre-term labor Z36.86
  - specified follow-up NEC Z36.2
  - specified genetic defects NEC Z36.8A
  - specified type NEC Z36.89
  - Streptococcus B Z36.85
  - suspected anomaly Z36.3
  - uncertain dates Z36.87

Encounter — continued
- assisted reproductive fertility procedure cycle Z31.83
- blood typing Z01.83
  - Rh typing Z01.83
- breast augmentation or reduction Z41.1
- breast implant exchange (different material) (different size) Z45.81 ☑
- breast reconstruction following mastectomy Z42.1
- check-up — see Examination
- chemotherapy for neoplasm Z51.11
- colonoscopy, screening Z12.11
- counseling — see Counseling
- delivery, full-term, uncomplicated O80
  - cesarean, without indication O82
- desensitization to allergens Z51.6
- ear piercing Z41.3
- examination — see Examination
- expectant parent(s) (adoptive) pre-birth pediatrician visit Z76.81
- fertility preservation procedure (prior to cancer therapy) (prior to removal of gonads) Z31.84
- fitting (of) — see Fitting (and adjustment) (of)
- genetic
  - counseling
    - nonprocreative Z71.83
    - procreative Z31.5
  - testing — see Test, genetic
- hearing conservation and treatment Z01.12
- immunotherapy for neoplasm Z51.12
- in vitro fertilization cycle Z31.83
- instruction (in)
  - child care (postpartal) (prenatal) Z32.3
  - childbirth Z32.2
  - natural family planning
    - procreative Z31.61
    - to avoid pregnancy Z30.02
- insulin pump titration Z46.81
- joint prosthesis insertion following prior explantation of joint prosthesis (staged procedure)
  - hip Z47.32
  - knee Z47.33
  - shoulder Z47.31
- laboratory (as part of a general medical examination) Z00.00
  - with abnormal findings Z00.01
- mental health services (for)
  - abuse NEC
    - perpetrator Z69.82
    - victim Z69.81
  - child abuse
    - nonparental
      - perpetrator Z69.021
      - victim Z69.020
    - parental
      - perpetrator Z69.011
      - victim Z69.010
  - child neglect
    - nonparental
      - perpetrator Z69.021
      - victim Z69.020
    - parental
      - perpetrator Z69.011
      - victim Z69.010
  - child psychological abuse
    - nonparental
      - perpetrator Z69.021
      - victim Z69.020
    - parental
      - perpetrator Z69.011
      - victim Z69.010
  - child sexual abuse
    - nonparental
      - perpetrator Z69.021
      - victim Z69.020
    - parental
      - perpetrator Z69.011
      - victim Z69.010
  - non-spousal adult abuse
    - perpetrator Z69.82
    - victim Z69.81
  - spousal or partner
    - abuse
      - perpetrator Z69.12
      - victim Z69.11
    - neglect
      - perpetrator Z69.12
      - victim Z69.11
    - psychological abuse
      - perpetrator Z69.12

Encounter — continued
- mental health services — continued
  - spousal or partner — continued
    - psychological abuse — continued
      - victim Z69.11
    - violence
      - perpetrator (physical) (sexual) Z69.12
      - victim (physical) Z69.11
      - sexual Z69.81
- observation (for) (ruled out)
  - exposure to (suspected)
    - anthrax Z03.810
    - biological agent NEC Z03.818
- pediatrician visit, by expectant parent(s) (adoptive) Z76.81
- placental sample (taken vaginally) — see also Encounter, antenatal screening Z36.9
- plastic and reconstructive surgery following medical procedure or healed injury NEC Z42.8
- pregnancy
  - supervision of — see Pregnancy, supervision of
  - test Z32.00
    - result negative Z32.02
    - result positive Z32.01
- procreative management and counseling for gestational carrier Z31.7
- prophylactic measures Z29.9
  - antivenin Z29.12
  - fluoride administration Z29.3
  - immunotherapy for respiratory syncytial virus (RSV) Z29.11
  - rabies immune globin Z29.14
  - Rho (D) immune globulin Z29.13
  - specified NEC Z29.8
- radiation therapy (antineoplastic) Z51.0
- radiological (as part of a general medical examination) Z00.00
  - with abnormal findings Z00.01
- reconstructive surgery following medical procedure or healed injury NEC Z42.8
- removal (of) — see also Removal
  - artificial
    - arm Z44.00- ☑
      - complete Z44.01- ☑
      - partial Z44.02- ☑
    - eye Z44.2- ☑
    - leg Z44.10- ☑
      - complete Z44.11- ☑
      - partial Z44.12- ☑
  - breast implant Z45.81 ☑
    - tissue expander (with or without synchronous insertion of permanent implant) Z45.81 ☑
  - device Z46.9
    - specified NEC Z46.89
  - external
    - fixation device — code to fracture with seventh character D
    - prosthesis, prosthetic device Z44.9
      - breast Z44.3- ☑
      - specified NEC Z44.8
  - implanted device NEC Z45.89
  - insulin pump Z46.81
  - internal fixation device Z47.2
  - myringotomy device (stent) (tube) Z45.82
  - nervous system device NEC Z46.2
    - brain neuropacemaker Z46.2
    - visual substitution device Z46.2
      - implanted Z45.31
  - non-vascular catheter Z46.82
  - orthodontic device Z46.4
  - stent
    - ureteral Z46.6
  - urinary device Z46.6
- repeat cervical smear to confirm findings of recent normal smear following initial abnormal smear Z01.42
- respirator [ventilator] use during power failure Z99.12
- Rh typing Z01.83
- screening — see Screening
- specified NEC Z76.89
- sterilization Z30.2
- suspected condition, ruled out
  - amniotic cavity and membrane Z03.71
  - cervical shortening Z03.75
  - fetal anomaly Z03.73
  - fetal growth Z03.74
  - maternal and fetal conditions NEC Z03.79
  - oligohydramnios Z03.71

Index

Encephalopathy — Encounter

Encounter — *continued*
  suspected condition, ruled out — *continued*
    placental problem Z03.72
    polyhydramnios Z03.71
  suspected exposure (to), ruled out
    anthrax Z03.810
    biological agents NEC Z03.818
  termination of pregnancy, elective Z33.2
  testing — *see* Test
  therapeutic drug level monitoring Z51.81
  titration, insulin pump Z46.81
  to determine fetal viability of pregnancy O36.80 ☑
  training
    insulin pump Z46.81
  X-ray of chest (as part of a general medical examination) Z00.00
    with abnormal findings Z00.01
Encystment — *see* Cyst
Endarteritis (bacterial, subacute) (infective) I77.6
  brain I67.7
  cerebral or cerebrospinal I67.7
  deformans — *see* Arteriosclerosis
  embolic — *see* Embolism
  obliterans — *see also* Arteriosclerosis
    pulmonary I28.8
  pulmonary I28.8
  retina — *see* Vasculitis, retina
  senile — *see* Arteriosclerosis
  syphilitic A52.09
    brain or cerebral A52.04
    congenital A50.54 [I79.8]
  tuberculous A18.89
Endemic — *see* condition
Endocarditis (chronic) (marantic) (nonbacterial) (thrombotic) (valvular) I38
  with rheumatic fever (conditions in I00)
    active — *see* Endocarditis, acute, rheumatic
    inactive or quiescent (with chorea) I09.1
  acute or subacute I33.9
    infective I33.0
    rheumatic (aortic) (mitral) (pulmonary) (tricuspid) I01.1
      with chorea (acute) (rheumatic) (Sydenham's) I02.0
  aortic (heart) (nonrheumatic) (valve) I35.8
    with
      mitral disease I08.0
        with tricuspid (valve) disease I08.3
          active or acute I01.1
            with chorea (acute) (rheumatic) (Sydenham's) I02.0
        rheumatic fever (conditions in I00)
          active — *see* Endocarditis, acute, rheumatic
          inactive or quiescent (with chorea) I06.9
      tricuspid (valve) disease I08.2
        with mitral (valve) disease I08.3
    acute or subacute I33.9
    arteriosclerotic I35.8
    rheumatic I06.9
      with mitral disease I08.0
        with tricuspid (valve) disease I08.3
          active or acute I01.1
            with chorea (acute) (rheumatic) (Sydenham's) I02.0
      active or acute I01.1
        with chorea (acute) (rheumatic) (Sydenham's) I02.0
    specified NEC I06.8
    specified cause NEC I35.8
    syphilitic A52.03
  arteriosclerotic I38
  atypical verrucous (Libman-Sacks) M32.11
  bacterial (acute) (any valve) (subacute) I33.0
  candidal B37.6
  congenital Q24.8
  constrictive I33.0
  Coxiella burnetii A78 [I39]
  Coxsackie B33.21
  due to
    prosthetic cardiac valve T82.6 ☑
    Q fever A78 [I39]
    Serratia marcescens I33.0
    typhoid (fever) A01.02
  gonococcal A54.83
  infectious or infective (acute) (any valve) (subacute) I33.0
  lenta (acute) (any valve) (subacute) I33.0
  Libman-Sacks M32.11

Endocarditis — *continued*
  listerial A32.82
  Löffler's I42.3
  malignant (acute) (any valve) (subacute) I33.0
  meningococcal A39.51
  mitral (chronic) (double) (fibroid) (heart) (inactive) (valve) (with chorea) I05.9
    with
      aortic (valve) disease I08.0
        with tricuspid (valve) disease I08.3
          active or acute I01.1
            with chorea (acute) (rheumatic) (Sydenham's) I02.0
      rheumatic fever (conditions in I00)
        active — *see* Endocarditis, acute, rheumatic
        inactive or quiescent (with chorea) I05.9
      tricuspid (valve) disease I08.1
        with aortic (valve) disease I08.3
    active or acute I01.1
      with chorea (acute) (rheumatic) (Sydenham's) I02.0
    bacterial I33.0
    arteriosclerotic I34.8
    nonrheumatic I34.8
      acute or subacute I33.9
    specified NEC I05.8
  monilial B37.6
  multiple valves I08.9
    specified disorders I08.8
  mycotic (acute) (any valve) (subacute) I33.0
  pneumococcal (acute) (any valve) (subacute) I33.0
  pulmonary (chronic) (heart) (valve) I37.8
    with rheumatic fever (conditions in I00)
      active — *see* Endocarditis, acute, rheumatic
      inactive or quiescent (with chorea) I09.89
        with aortic, mitral or tricuspid disease I08.8
    acute or subacute I33.9
      rheumatic I01.1
        with chorea (acute) (rheumatic) (Sydenham's) I02.0
    arteriosclerotic I37.8
    congenital Q22.2
    rheumatic (chronic) (inactive) (with chorea) I09.89
      active or acute I01.1
        with chorea (acute) (rheumatic) (Sydenham's) I02.0
    syphilitic A52.03
  purulent (acute) (any valve) (subacute) I33.0
  Q fever A78 [I39]
  rheumatic (chronic) (inactive) (with chorea) I09.1
    active or acute (aortic) (mitral) (pulmonary) (tricuspid) I01.1
      with chorea (acute) (rheumatic) (Sydenham's) I02.0
  rheumatoid — *see* Rheumatoid, carditis
  septic (acute) (any valve) (subacute) I33.0
  streptococcal (acute) (any valve) (subacute) I33.0
  subacute — *see* Endocarditis, acute
  suppurative (acute) (any valve) (subacute) I33.0
  syphilitic A52.03
  toxic I33.9
  tricuspid (chronic) (heart) (inactive) (rheumatic) (valve) (with chorea) I07.9
    with
      aortic (valve) disease I08.2
        mitral (valve) disease I08.3
      mitral (valve) disease I08.1
        aortic (valve) disease I08.3
      rheumatic fever (conditions in I00)
        active — *see* Endocarditis, acute, rheumatic
        inactive or quiescent (with chorea) I07.8
    active or acute I01.1
      with chorea (acute) (rheumatic) (Sydenham's) I02.0
    arteriosclerotic I36.8
    nonrheumatic I36.8
      acute or subacute I33.9
    specified cause, except rheumatic I36.8
  tuberculous — *see* Tuberculosis, endocarditis
  typhoid A01.02
  ulcerative (acute) (any valve) (subacute) I33.0
  vegetative (acute) (any valve) (subacute) I33.0
  verrucous (atypical) (nonbacterial) (nonrheumatic) M32.11
Endocardium, endocardial — *see also* condition
  cushion defect Q21.2
Endocervicitis — *see also* Cervicitis
  due to intrauterine (contraceptive) device T83.69 ☑

Endocervicitis — *continued*
  hyperplastic N72
Endocrine — *see* condition
Endocrinopathy, pluriglandular E31.9
Endodontic
  overfill M27.52
  underfill M27.53
Endodontitis K04.01
  irreversible K04.02
  reversible K04.01
Endomastoiditis — *see* Mastoiditis
Endometrioma N80.9
Endometriosis N80.9
  appendix N80.5
  bladder N80.8
  bowel N80.5
  broad ligament N80.3
  cervix N80.0
  colon N80.5
  cul-de-sac (Douglas') N80.3
  exocervix N80.0
  fallopian tube N80.2
  female genital organ NEC N80.8
  gallbladder N80.8
  in scar of skin N80.6
  internal N80.0
  intestine N80.5
  lung N80.8
  myometrium N80.0
  ovary N80.1
  parametrium N80.3
  pelvic peritoneum N80.3
  peritoneal (pelvic) N80.3
  rectovaginal septum N80.4
  rectum N80.5
  round ligament N80.3
  skin (scar) N80.6
  specified site NEC N80.8
  stromal D39.0
  thorax N80.8
  umbilicus N80.8
  uterus (internal) N80.0
  vagina N80.4
  vulva N80.8
Endometritis (decidual) (nonspecific) (purulent) (senile) (atrophic) (suppurative) N71.9
  with ectopic pregnancy O08.0
  acute N71.0
  blenorrhagic (gonococcal) (acute) (chronic) A54.24
  cervix, cervical (with erosion or ectropion) — *see also* Cervicitis
    hyperplastic N72
  chlamydial A56.11
  chronic N71.1
  following
    abortion — *see* Abortion by type complicated by genital infection
    ectopic or molar pregnancy O08.0
  gonococcal, gonorrheal (acute) (chronic) A54.24
  hyperplastic — *see also* Hyperplasia, endometrial N85.00
    cervix N72
  puerperal, postpartum, childbirth O86.12
  subacute N71.0
  tuberculous A18.17
Endometrium — *see* condition
Endomyocardiopathy, South African I42.3
Endomyocarditis — *see* Endocarditis
Endomyofibrosis I42.3
Endomyometritis — *see* Endometritis
Endopericarditis — *see* Endocarditis
Endoperineuritis — *see* Disorder, nerve
Endophlebitis — *see* Phlebitis
Endophthalmia — *see* Endophthalmitis, purulent
Endophthalmitis (acute) (infective) (metastatic) (subacute) H44.009
  bleb associated — *see also* Bleb, inflamed (infected), postprocedural H59.4 ☑
  gonorrheal A54.39
  in (due to)
    cysticercosis B69.1
    onchocerciasis B73.01
    toxocariasis B83.0
  panuveitis — *see* Panuveitis
  parasitic H44.12- ☑
  purulent H44.00- ☑
    panophthalmitis — *see* Panophthalmitis
    vitreous abscess H44.02- ☑

Endophthalmitis — *continued*
- specified NEC H44.19
- sympathetic — *see* Uveitis, sympathetic

Endosalpingioma D28.2

Endosalpingiosis N94.89

Endosteitis — *see* Osteomyelitis

Endothelioma, bone — *see* Neoplasm, bone, malignant

Endotheliosis (hemorrhagic infectional) D69.8

Endotoxemia — code to condition

Endotrachelitis — *see* Cervicitis

Engelmann (-Camurati) **syndrome** Q78.3

English disease — *see* Rickets

Engman's disease L30.3

Engorgement
- breast N64.59
  - newborn P83.4
  - puerperal, postpartum O92.79
- lung (passive) — *see* Edema, lung
- pulmonary (passive) — *see* Edema, lung
- stomach K31.89
- venous, retina — *see* Occlusion, retina, vein, engorgement

Enlargement, enlarged — *see also* Hypertrophy
- adenoids J35.2
  - with tonsils J35.3
- alveolar ridge K08.89
  - congenital — *see* Anomaly, alveolar
- apertures of diaphragm (congenital) Q79.1
- gingival K06.1
- heart, cardiac — *see* Hypertrophy, cardiac
- labium majus, childhood asymmetric (CALME) N90.61
- lacrimal gland, chronic H04.03- ☑
- liver — *see* Hypertrophy, liver
- lymph gland or node R59.9
  - generalized R59.1
  - localized R59.0
- orbit H05.34- ☑
- organ or site, congenital NEC — *see* Anomaly, by site
- parathyroid (gland) E21.0
- pituitary fossa R93.0
- prostate N40.0
  - with lower urinary tract symptoms (LUTS) N40.1
  - without lower urinary tract symtpoms (LUTS) N40.0
- sella turcica R93.0
- spleen — *see* Splenomegaly
- thymus (gland) (congenital) E32.0
- thyroid (gland) — *see* Goiter
- tongue K14.8
- tonsils J35.1
  - with adenoids J35.3
- uterus N85.2
- vestibular aqueduct Q16.5

Enophthalmos H05.40- ☑
- due to
  - orbital tissue atrophy H05.41- ☑
  - trauma or surgery H05.42- ☑

Enostosis M27.8

Entamebic, entamebiasis — *see* Amebiasis

Entanglement
- umbilical cord(s) O69.82 ☑
  - with compression O69.2 ☑
  - around neck (with compression) O69.81 ☑
    - with compression O69.1 ☑
    - without compression O69.81 ☑
  - of twins in monoamniotic sac O69.2 ☑
  - without compression O69.82 ☑

Enteralgia — *see* Pain, abdominal

Enteric — *see* condition

Enteritis (acute) (diarrheal) (hemorrhagic) (noninfective) K52.9
- adenovirus A08.2
- aertrycke infection A02.0
- allergic K52.29
  - with
    - eosinophilic gastritis or gastroenteritis K52.81
    - food protein-induced enterocolitis syndrome K52.21
    - food protein-induced enteropathy K52.22
    - FPIES K52.21
- amebic (acute) A06.0
  - with abscess — *see* Abscess, amebic
  - chronic A06.1
    - with abscess — *see* Abscess, amebic
    - nondysenteric A06.2
  - nondysenteric A06.2
- astrovirus A08.32
- bacillary NOS A03.9

Enteritis — *continued*
- bacterial A04.9
  - specified NEC A04.8
- calicivirus A08.31
- candidal B37.82
- Chilomastix A07.8
- choleriformis A00.1
- chronic (noninfectious) K52.9
  - ulcerative — *see* Colitis, ulcerative
- cicatrizing (chronic) — *see* Enteritis, regional, small intestine
- Clostridium
  - botulinum (food poisoning) A05.1
  - difficile
    - not specified as recurrent A04.72
    - recurrent A04.71
- coccidial A07.3
- coxsackie virus A08.39
- dietetic — *see also* Enteritis, allergic K52.29
- drug-induced K52.1
- due to
  - astrovirus A08.32
  - calicivirus A08.31
  - coxsackie virus A08.39
  - drugs K52.1
  - echovirus A08.39
  - enterovirus NEC A08.39
  - food hypersensitivity — *see also* Enteritis, allergic K52.29
  - infectious organism (bacterial) (viral) — *see* Enteritis, infectious
  - torovirus A08.39
  - Yersinia enterocolitica A04.6
- echovirus A08.39
- eltor A00.1
- enterovirus NEC A08.39
- eosinophilic K52.81
- epidemic (infectious) A09
- fulminant — *see also* Ischemia, intestine, acute K55.019
- gangrenous — *see* Enteritis, infectious
- giardial A07.1
- infectious NOS A09
  - due to
    - adenovirus A08.2
    - Aerobacter aerogenes A04.8
    - Arizona (bacillus) A02.0
    - bacteria NOS A04.9
      - specified NEC A04.8
    - Campylobacter A04.5
    - Clostridium difficile
      - not specified as recurrent A04.72
      - recurrent A04.71
    - Clostridium perfringens A04.8
    - Enterobacter aerogenes A04.8
    - enterovirus A08.39
    - Escherichia coli A04.4
      - enteroaggregative A04.4
      - enterohemorrhagic A04.3
      - enteroinvasive A04.2
      - enteropathogenic A04.0
      - enterotoxigenic A04.1
      - specified NEC A04.4
    - specified
      - bacteria NEC A04.8
      - virus NEC A08.39
    - Staphylococcus A04.8
    - virus NEC A08.4
      - specified type NEC A08.39
    - Yersinia enterocolitica A04.6
  - specified organism NEC A08.8
- influenzal — *see* Influenza, with, digestive manifestations
- ischemic K55.9
  - acute — *see also* Ischemia, intestine, acute K55.019
  - chronic K55.1
- microsporidial A07.8
- mucomembranous, myxomembranous — *see* Syndrome, irritable bowel
- mucous — *see* Syndrome, irritable bowel
- necroticans A05.2
- necrotizing of newborn — *see* Enterocolitis, necrotizing, in newborn
- neurogenic — *see* Syndrome, irritable bowel
- newborn necrotizing — *see* Enterocolitis, necrotizing, in newborn
- noninfectious K52.9
- norovirus A08.11
- parasitic NEC B82.9

Enteritis — *continued*
- paratyphoid (fever) — *see* Fever, paratyphoid
- protozoal A07.9
  - specified NEC A07.8
- radiation K52.0
- regional (of) K50.90
  - with
    - complication K50.919
      - abscess K50.914
      - fistula K50.913
      - intestinal obstruction K50.912
      - rectal bleeding K50.911
      - specified complication NEC K50.918
  - colon — *see* Enteritis, regional, large intestine
  - duodenum — *see* Enteritis, regional, small intestine
  - ileum — *see* Enteritis, regional, small intestine
  - jejunum — *see* Enteritis, regional, small intestine
  - large bowel — *see* Enteritis, regional, large intestine
  - large intestine (colon) (rectum) K50.10
    - with
      - complication K50.119
        - abscess K50.114
        - fistula K50.113
        - intestinal obstruction K50.112
        - rectal bleeding K50.111
        - small intestine (duodenum) (ileum) (jejunum) involvement K50.80
          - with
            - complication K50.819
              - abscess K50.814
              - fistula K50.813
              - intestinal obstruction K50.812
              - rectal bleeding K50.811
              - specified complication NEC K50.818
        - specified complication NEC K50.118
  - rectum — *see* Enteritis, regional, large intestine
  - small intestine (duodenum) (ileum) (jejunum) K50.00
    - with
      - complication K50.019
        - abscess K50.014
        - fistula K50.013
        - intestinal obstruction K50.012
        - large intestine (colon) (rectum) involvement K50.80
          - with
            - complication K50.819
              - abscess K50.814
              - fistula K50.813
              - intestinal obstruction K50.812
              - rectal bleeding K50.811
              - specified complication NEC K50.818
        - rectal bleeding K50.011
        - specified complication NEC K50.018
- rotaviral A08.0
- Salmonella, salmonellosis (arizonae) (cholerae-suis) (enteritidis) (typhimurium) A02.0
- segmental — *see* Enteritis, regional
- septic A09
- Shigella — *see* Infection, Shigella
- small round structured NEC A08.19
- spasmodic, spastic — *see* Syndrome, irritable bowel
- staphylococcal A04.8
  - due to food A05.0
- torovirus A08.39
- toxic NEC K52.1
  - due to Clostridium difficile
    - not specified as recurrent A04.72
    - recurrent A04.71
- trichomonal A07.8
- tuberculous A18.32
- typhosa A01.00
- ulcerative (chronic) — *see* Colitis, ulcerative
- viral A08.4
  - adenovirus A08.2
  - enterovirus A08.39
  - Rotavirus A08.0
  - small round structured NEC A08.19
  - specified NEC A08.39
  - virus specified NEC A08.39

Enterobiasis B80

Enterobius vermicularis (infection) (infestation) B80

Enterocele — *see also* Hernia, abdomen
- pelvic, pelvis (acquired) (congenital) N81.5
- vagina, vaginal (acquired) (congenital) NEC N81.5

Enterocolitis — *see also* Enteritis K52.9

Enterocolitis — continued
  due to Clostridium difficile
    not specified as recurrent A04.72
    recurrent A04.71
  fulminant ischemic — see also Ischemia, intestine,
    acute K55.059
  granulomatous — see Enteritis, regional
  hemorrhagic (acute) — see also Ischemia, intestine,
    acute K55.059
    chronic K55.1
  infectious NEC A09
  ischemic K55.9
  necrotizing K55.30
    with
      perforation K55.33
      pneumatosis K55.32
        and perforation K55.33
    due to Clostridium difficile
      not specified as recurrent A04.72
      recurrent A04.71
    in non-newborn K55.30
      stage 1 (without pneumatosis, without perfora-
        tion) K55.31
      stage 2 (with pneumatosis, without perforation)
        K55.32
      stage 3 (with pneumatosis, with perforation)
        K55.33
    in newborn P77.9
      stage 1 (without pneumatosis, without perfora-
        tion) P77.1
      stage 2 (with pneumatosis, without perforation)
        P77.2
      stage 3 (with pneumatosis, with perforation)
        P77.3
    without pneumatosis or perforation K55.31
  noninfectious K52.9
    newborn — see Enterocolitis, necrotizing, in new-
      born
  pseudomembranous (newborn)
    not specified as recurrent A04.72
    recurrent A04.71
  radiation K52.0
    newborn — see Enterocolitis, necrotizing, in new-
      born
  ulcerative (chronic) — see Pancolitis, ulcerative
    (chronic)
Enterogastritis — see Enteritis
Enteropathy K63.9
  celiac-gluten-sensitive K90.0
    non-celiac K90.41
  food protein-induced K52.22
  hemorrhagic, terminal — see also Ischemia, intestine,
    acute K55.059
  protein-losing K90.49
Enteroperitonitis — see Peritonitis
Enteroptosis K63.4
Enterorrhagia K92.2
Enterospasm — see also Syndrome, irritable, bowel
  psychogenic F45.8
Enterostenosis — see also Obstruction, intestine, specified NEC K56.699
Enterostomy
  complication — see Complication, enterostomy
  status Z93.4
Enterovirus, as cause of disease classified elsewhere
    B97.10
  coxsackievirus B97.11
  echovirus B97.12
  other specified B97.19
Enthesopathy (peripheral) M77.9
  Achilles tendinitis — see Tendinitis, Achilles
  ankle and tarsus M77.5- ☑
    specified type NEC — see Enthesopathy, foot,
      specified type NEC
  anterior tibial syndrome M76.81- ☑
  calcaneal spur — see Spur, bone, calcaneal
  elbow region M77.8
    lateral epicondylitis — see Epicondylitis, lateral
    medial epicondylitis — see Epicondylitis, medial
  foot NEC M77.9
    metatarsalgia — see Metatarsalgia
    specified type NEC M77.5- ☑
  forearm M77.9
  gluteal tendinitis — see Tendinitis, gluteal
  hand M77.9
  hip — see Enthesopathy, lower limb, specified type
    NEC
  iliac crest spur — see Spur, bone, iliac crest

Enthesopathy — continued
  iliotibial band syndrome — see Syndrome, iliotibial
    band
  knee — see Enthesopathy, lower limb, lower leg,
    specified type NEC
  lateral epicondylitis — see Epicondylitis, lateral
  lower limb (excluding foot) M76.9
    Achilles tendinitis — see Tendinitis, Achilles
    ankle and tarsus M77.5- ☑
      specified type NEC — see Enthesopathy, foot,
        specified type NEC
    anterior tibial syndrome M76.81- ☑
    gluteal tendinitis — see Tendinitis, gluteal
    iliac crest spur — see Spur, bone, iliac crest
    iliotibial band syndrome — see Syndrome, iliotibial
      band
    patellar tendinitis — see Tendinitis, patellar
    pelvic region — see Enthesopathy, lower limb,
      specified type NEC
    peroneal tendinitis — see Tendinitis, peroneal
    posterior tibial syndrome M76.82- ☑
    psoas tendinitis — see Tendinitis, psoas
    specified type NEC M76.89- ☑
    tibial collateral bursitis — see Bursitis, tibial collater-
      al
  medial epicondylitis — see Epicondylitis, medial
  metatarsalgia — see Metatarsalgia
  multiple sites M77.9
  patellar tendinitis — see Tendinitis, patellar
  pelvis M77.9
  periarthritis of wrist — see Periarthritis, wrist
  peroneal tendinitis — see Tendinitis, peroneal
  posterior tibial syndrome M76.82- ☑
  psoas tendinitis — see Tendinitis, psoas
  shoulder M77.9
  shoulder region — see Lesion, shoulder
  specified site NEC M77.9
  specified type NEC M77.8
  spinal M46.00
    cervical region M46.02
    cervicothoracic region M46.03
    lumbar region M46.06
    lumbosacral region M46.07
    multiple sites M46.09
    occipito-atlanto-axial region M46.01
    sacrococcygeal region M46.08
    thoracic region M46.04
    thoracolumbar region M46.05
  tibial collateral bursitis — see Bursitis, tibial collateral
  upper arm M77.9
  wrist and carpus NEC M77.8
    calcaneal spur — see Spur, bone, calcaneal
    periarthritis of wrist — see Periarthritis, wrist
Entomophobia F40.218
Entomophthoromycosis B46.8
Entrance, air into vein — see Embolism, air
Entrapment, nerve — see Neuropathy, entrapment
Entropion (eyelid) (paralytic) H02.009
  cicatricial H02.019
    left H02.016
      lower H02.015
      upper H02.014
    right H02.013
      lower H02.012
      upper H02.011
  congenital Q10.2
  left H02.006
    lower H02.005
    upper H02.004
  mechanical H02.029
    left H02.026
      lower H02.025
      upper H02.024
    right H02.023
      lower H02.022
      upper H02.021
  right H02.003
    lower H02.002
    upper H02.001
  senile H02.039
    left H02.036
      lower H02.035
      upper H02.034
    right H02.033
      lower H02.032
      upper H02.031
  spastic H02.049
    left H02.046

Entropion — continued
  spastic — continued
    left — continued
      lower H02.045
      upper H02.044
    right H02.043
      lower H02.042
      upper H02.041
Enucleated eye (traumatic, current) S05.7- ☑
Enuresis R32
  functional F98.0
  habit disturbance F98.0
  nocturnal N39.44
    psychogenic F98.0
  nonorganic origin F98.0
  psychogenic F98.0
Eosinopenia — see Agranulocytosis
Eosinophilia (allergic) (hereditary) (idiopathic) (secondary) D72.1
  with
    angiolymphoid hyperplasia (ALHE) D18.01
  infiltrative J82
  Löffler's J82
  peritoneal — see Peritonitis, eosinophilic
  pulmonary NEC J82
  tropical (pulmonary) J82
Eosinophilia-myalgia syndrome M35.8
Ependymitis (acute) (cerebral) (chronic) (granular) —
  see Encephalomyelitis
Ependymoblastoma
  specified site — see Neoplasm, malignant, by site
  unspecified site C71.9
Ependymoma (epithelial) (malignant)
  anaplastic
    specified site — see Neoplasm, malignant, by site
    unspecified site C71.9
  benign
    specified site — see Neoplasm, benign, by site
    unspecified site D33.2
  myxopapillary D43.2
    specified site — see Neoplasm, uncertain behavior,
      by site
    unspecified site D43.2
  papillary D43.2
    specified site — see Neoplasm, uncertain behavior,
      by site
    unspecified site D43.2
  specified site — see Neoplasm, malignant, by site
  unspecified site C71.9
Ependymopathy G93.89
Ephelis, ephelides L81.2
Epiblepharon (congenital) Q10.3
Epicanthus, epicanthic fold (eyelid) (congenital) Q10.3
Epicondylitis (elbow)
  lateral M77.1- ☑
  medial M77.0- ☑
Epicystitis — see Cystitis
Epidemic — see condition
Epidermidalization, cervix — see Dysplasia, cervix
Epidermis, epidermal — see condition
Epidermodysplasia verruciformis B07.8
Epidermolysis
  bullosa (congenital) Q81.9
    acquired L12.30
      drug-induced L12.31
      specified cause NEC L12.35
    dystrophica Q81.2
    letalis Q81.1
    simplex Q81.0
    specified NEC Q81.8
  necroticans combustiformis L51.2
    due to drug — see Table of Drugs and Chemicals,
      by drug
Epidermophytid — see Dermatophytosis
Epidermophytosis (infected) — see Dermatophytosis
Epididymis — see condition
Epididymitis (acute) (nonvenereal) (recurrent) (residual)
  N45.1
  with orchitis N45.3
  blennorrhagic (gonococcal) A54.23
  caseous (tuberculous) A18.15
  chlamydial A56.19
  filarial — see also Infestation, filarial B74.9 [N51]
  gonococcal A54.23
  syphilitic A52.76
  tuberculous A18.15
Epididymo-orchitis — see also Epididymitis N45.3
Epidural — see condition

Epigastrium, epigastric — *see* condition
Epigastrocele — *see* Hernia, ventral
Epiglottis — *see* condition
Epiglottitis, epiglottiditis (acute) J05.10
  with obstruction J05.11
  chronic J37.0
Epignathus Q89.4
Epilepsia partialis continua — *see also* Kozhevnikof's
  epilepsy G40.1- ☑
Epilepsy, epileptic, epilepsia (attack) (cerebral) (convulsion) (fit) (seizure) G40.909

> Note: the following terms are to be considered equivalent to intractable: pharmacoresistant (pharmacologically resistant), treatment resistant, refractory (medically) and poorly controlled

with
  complex partial seizures — *see* Epilepsy, localization-related, symptomatic, with complex partial seizures
  grand mal seizures on awakening — *see* Epilepsy, generalized, specified NEC
  myoclonic absences — *see* Epilepsy, generalized, specified NEC
  myoclonic-astatic seizures — *see* Epilepsy, generalized, specified NEC
  simple partial seizures — *see* Epilepsy, localization-related, symptomatic, with simple partial seizures
akinetic — *see* Epilepsy, generalized, specified NEC
benign childhood with centrotemporal EEG spikes — *see* Epilepsy, localization-related, idiopathic
benign myoclonic in infancy G40.80- ☑
Bravais-jacksonian — *see* Epilepsy, localization-related, symptomatic, with simple partial seizures
childhood
  with occipital EEG paroxysms — *see* Epilepsy, localization-related, idiopathic
  absence G40.A09 (*following* G40.3)
    intractable G40.A19 (*following* G40.3)
      with status epilepticus G40.A11 (*following* G40.3)
      without status epilepticus G40.A19 (*following* G40.3)
    not intractable G40.A09 (*following* G40.3)
      with status epilepticus G40.A01 (*following* G40.3)
      without status epilepticus G40.A09 (*following* G40.3)
climacteric — *see* Epilepsy, specified NEC
cysticercosis B69.0
deterioration (mental) F06.8
due to syphilis A52.19
focal — *see* Epilepsy, localization-related, symptomatic, with simple partial seizures
generalized
  idiopathic G40.309
    intractable G40.319
      with status epilepticus G40.311
      without status epilepticus G40.319
    not intractable G40.309
      with status epilepticus G40.301
      without status epilepticus G40.309
  specified NEC G40.409
    intractable G40.419
      with status epilepticus G40.411
      without status epilepticus G40.419
    not intractable G40.409
      with status epilepticus G40.401
      without status epilepticus G40.409
impulsive petit mal — *see* Epilepsy, juvenile myoclonic
intractable G40.919
  with status epilepticus G40.911
  without status epilepticus G40.919
juvenile absence G40.A09 (*following* G40.3)
  intractable G40.A19 (*following* G40.3)
    with status epilepticus G40.A11 (*following* G40.3)
    without status epilepticus G40.A19 (*following* G40.3)
  not intractable G40.A09 (*following* G40.3)
    with status epilepticus G40.A01 (*following* G40.3)
    without status epilepticus G40.A09 (*following* G40.3)
juvenile myoclonic G40.B09 (*following* G40.3)
  intractable G40.B19 (*following* G40.3)
    with status epilepticus G40.B11 (*following* G40.3)
    without status epilepticus G40.B19 (*following* G40.3)

Epilepsy, epileptic, epilepsia — *continued*
juvenile myoclonic — *continued*
  not intractable G40.B09 (*following* G40.3)
    with status epilepticus G40.B01 (*following* G40.3)
    without status epilepticus G40.B09 (*following* G40.3)
localization-related (focal) (partial)
  idiopathic G40.009
    with seizures of localized onset G40.009
      intractable G40.019
        with status epilepticus G40.011
        without status epilepticus G40.019
      not intractable G40.009
        with status epilepticus G40.001
        without status epilepticus G40.009
  symptomatic
    with complex partial seizures G40.209
      intractable G40.219
        with status epilepticus G40.211
        without status epilepticus G40.219
      not intractable G40.209
        with status epilepticus G40.201
        without status epilepticus G40.209
    with simple partial seizures G40.109
      intractable G40.119
        with status epilepticus G40.111
        without status epilepticus G40.119
      not intractable G40.109
        with status epilepticus G40.101
        without status epilepticus G40.109
myoclonus, myoclonic — *see* Epilepsy, generalized, specified NEC
progressive — *see* Epilepsy, generalized, idiopathic
not intractable G40.909
  with status epilepticus G40.901
  without status epilepticus G40.909
on awakening — *see* Epilepsy, generalized, specified NEC
parasitic NOS B71.9 *[G94]*
partialis continua — *see also* Kozhevnikof's epilepsy G40.1- ☑
peripheral — *see* Epilepsy, specified NEC
procursiva — *see* Epilepsy, localization-related, symptomatic, with simple partial seizures
progressive (familial) myoclonic — *see* Epilepsy, generalized, idiopathic
reflex — *see* Epilepsy, specified NEC
related to
  alcohol G40.509
    not intractable G40.509
      with status epilepticus G40.501
      without status epliepticus G40.509
  drugs G40.509
    not intractable G40.509
      with status epilepticus G40.501
      without status epliepticus G40.509
  external causes G40.509
    not intractable G40.509
      with status epilepticus G40.501
      without status epliepticus G40.509
  hormonal changes G40.509
    not intractable G40.509
      with status epilepticus G40.501
      without status epliepticus G40.509
  sleep deprivation G40.509
    not intractable G40.509
      with status epilepticus G40.501
      without status epliepticus G40.509
  stress G40.509
    not intractable G40.509
      with status epilepticus G40.501
      without status epliepticus G40.509
somatomotor — *see* Epilepsy, localization-related, symptomatic, with simple partial seizures
somatosensory — *see* Epilepsy, localization-related, symptomatic, with simple partial seizures
spasms G40.822
  intractable G40.824
    with status epilepticus G40.823
    without status epilepticus G40.824
  not intractable G40.822
    with status epilepticus G40.821
    without status epilepticus G40.822
specified NEC G40.802
  intractable G40.804
    with status epilepticus G40.803
    without status epilepticus G40.804
  not intractable G40.802

Epilepsy, epileptic, epilepsia — *continued*
specified — *continued*
  not intractable — *continued*
    with status epilepticus G40.801
    without status epilepticus G40.802
syndromes
  generalized
    idiopathic G40.309
      intractable G40.319
        with status epilepticus G40.311
        without status epilepticus G40.319
      not intractable G40.309
        with status epilepticus G40.301
        without status epilepticus G40.309
    specified NEC G40.409
      intractable G40.419
        with status epilepticus G40.411
        without status epilepticus G40.419
      not intractable G40.409
        with status epilepticus G40.401
        without status epilepticus G40.409
  localization-related (focal) (partial)
    idiopathic G40.009
      with seizures of localized onset G40.009
        intractable G40.019
          with status epilepticus G40.011
          without status epilepticus G40.019
        not intractable G40.009
          with status epilepticus G40.001
          without status epilepticus G40.009
    symptomatic
      with complex partial seizures G40.209
        intractable G40.219
          with status epilepticus G40.211
          without status epilepticus G40.219
        not intractable G40.209
          with status epilepticus G40.201
          without status epilepticus G40.209
      with simple partial seizures G40.109
        intractable G40.119
          with status epilepticus G40.111
          without status epilepticus G40.119
        not intractable G40.109
          with status epilepticus G40.101
          without status epilepticus G40.109
  specified NEC G40.802
    intractable G40.804
      with status epilepticus G40.803
      without status epilepticus G40.804
    not intractable G40.802
      with status epilepticus G40.801
      without status epilepticus G40.802
tonic (-clonic) — *see* Epilepsy, generalized, specified NEC
twilight F05
uncinate (gyrus) — *see* Epilepsy, localization-related, symptomatic, with complex partial seizures
Unverricht (-Lundborg) (familial myoclonic) — *see* Epilepsy, generalized, idiopathic
visceral — *see* Epilepsy, specified NEC
visual — *see* Epilepsy, specified NEC
Epiloia Q85.1
Epimenorrhea N92.0
Epipharyngitis — *see* Nasopharyngitis
Epiphora H04.20- ☑
  due to
    excess lacrimation H04.21- ☑
    insufficient drainage H04.22- ☑
Epiphyseal arrest — *see* Arrest, epiphyseal
Epiphyseolysis, epiphysiolysis — *see* Osteochondropathy
Epiphysitis — *see also* Osteochondropathy
  juvenile M92.9
  syphilitic (congenital) A50.02
Epiplocele — *see* Hernia, abdomen
Epiploitis — *see* Peritonitis
Epiplosarcomphalocele — *see* Hernia, umbilicus
Episcleritis (suppurative) H15.10- ☑
  in (due to)
    syphilis A52.71
    tuberculosis A18.51
  nodular H15.12- ☑
  periodica fugax H15.11- ☑
    angioneurotic — *see* Edema, angioneurotic
  syphilitic (late) A52.71
  tuberculous A18.51
Episode
  affective, mixed F39

Episode — continued
depersonalization (in neurotic state) F48.1
depressive F32.9
major F32.9
mild F32.0
moderate F32.1
severe (without psychotic symptoms) F32.2
with psychotic symptoms F32.3
recurrent F33.9
brief F33.8
specified NEC F32.89
hypomanic F30.8
manic F30.9
with
psychotic symptoms F30.2
remission (full) F30.4
partial F30.3
other specified F30.8
recurrent F31.89
without psychotic symptoms F30.10
mild F30.11
moderate F30.12
severe (without psychotic symptoms) F30.13
with psychotic symptoms F30.2
psychotic F23
organic F06.8
schizophrenic (acute) NEC, brief F23
Epispadias (female) (male) Q64.0
Episplenitis D73.89
Epistaxis (multiple) R04.0
hereditary I78.0
vicarious menstruation N94.89
Epithelioma (malignant) — see also Neoplasm, malignant, by site
adenoides cysticum — see Neoplasm, skin, benign
basal cell — see Neoplasm, skin, malignant
benign — see Neoplasm, benign, by site
Bowen's — see Neoplasm, skin, in situ
calcifying, of Malherbe — see Neoplasm, skin, benign
external site — see Neoplasm, skin, malignant
intraepidermal, Jadassohn — see Neoplasm, skin, benign
squamous cell — see Neoplasm, malignant, by site
Epitheliomatosis pigmented Q82.1
Epitheliopathy, multifocal placoid pigment
H30.14- ☑
Epithelium, epithelial — see condition
Epituberculosis (with atelectasis) (allergic) A15.7
Eponychia Q84.6
Epstein's
nephrosis or syndrome — see Nephrosis
pearl K09.8
Epulis (gingiva) (fibrous) (giant cell) K06.8
Equinia A24.0
Equinovarus (congenital) (talipes) Q66.0- ☑
acquired — see Deformity, limb, clubfoot
Equivalent
convulsive (abdominal) — see Epilepsy, specified NEC
epileptic (psychic) — see Epilepsy, localization-related, symptomatic, with complex partial seizures
Erb (-Duchenne) **paralysis** (birth injury) (newborn) P14.0
Erb-Goldflam disease or syndrome G70.00
with exacerbation (acute) G70.01
in crisis G70.01
Erb's
disease G71.02
palsy, paralysis (brachial) (birth) (newborn) P14.0
spinal (spastic) syphilitic A52.17
pseudohypertrophic muscular dystrophy G71.02
Erdheim's syndrome (acromegalic macrospondylitis)
E22.0
Erection, painful (persistent) — see Priapism
Ergosterol deficiency (vitamin D) E55.9
with
adult osteomalacia M83.8
rickets — see Rickets
Ergotism — see also Poisoning, food, noxious, plant
from ergot used as drug (migraine therapy) — see Table of Drugs and Chemicals
Erosio interdigitalis blastomycetica B37.2
Erosion
artery I77.2
without rupture I77.89
bone — see Disorder, bone, density and structure, specified NEC
bronchus J98.09

Erosion — continued
cartilage (joint) — see Disorder, cartilage, specified type NEC
cervix (uteri) (acquired) (chronic) (congenital) N86
with cervicitis N72
cornea (nontraumatic) — see Ulcer, cornea
recurrent H18.83- ☑
traumatic — see Abrasion, cornea
dental (idiopathic) (occupational) (due to diet, drugs or vomiting) K03.2
duodenum, postpyloric — see Ulcer, duodenum
esophagus K22.10
with bleeding K22.11
gastric — see Ulcer, stomach
gastrojejunal — see Ulcer, gastrojejunal
implanted mesh — see Complications, prosthetic device or implant, mesh
intestine K63.3
lymphatic vessel I89.8
pylorus, pyloric (ulcer) — see Ulcer, stomach
spine, aneurysmal A52.09
stomach — see Ulcer, stomach
subcutaneous device pocket
nervous system prosthetic device, implant, or graft T85.890 ☑
other internal prosthetic device, implant, or graft T85.898 ☑
teeth (idiopathic) (occupational) (due to diet, drugs or vomiting) K03.2
urethra N36.8
uterus N85.8
Erotomania F52.8
Error
metabolism, inborn — see Disorder, metabolism
refractive — see Disorder, refraction
Eructation R14.2
nervous or psychogenic F45.8
Eruption
creeping B76.9
drug (generalized) (taken internally) L27.0
fixed L27.1
in contact with skin — see Dermatitis, due to drugs
localized L27.1
Hutchinson, summer L56.4
Kaposi's varicelliform B00.0
napkin L22
polymorphous light (sun) L56.4
recalcitrant pustular L13.8
ringed R23.8
skin (nonspecific) R21
creeping (meaning hookworm) B76.9
due to inoculation/vaccination (generalized) — see also Dermatitis, due to, vaccine L27.0
localized L27.1
erysipeloid A26.0
feigned L98.1
Kaposi's varicelliform B00.0
lichenoid L28.0
meaning dermatitis — see Dermatitis
toxic NEC L53.0
tooth, teeth, abnormal (incomplete) (late) (premature) (sequence) K00.6
vesicular R23.8
Erysipelas (gangrenous) (infantile) (newborn) (phlegmonous) (suppurative) A46
external ear A46 [H62.40]
puerperal, postpartum O86.89
Erysipeloid A26.9
cutaneous (Rosenbach's) A26.0
disseminated A26.8
sepsis A26.7
specified NEC A26.8
Erythema, erythematous (infectional) (inflammation)
L53.9
ab igne L59.0
annulare (centrifugum) (rheumaticum) L53.1
arthriticum epidemicum A25.1
brucellum — see Brucellosis
chronic figurate NEC L53.3
chronicum migrans (Borrelia burgdorferi) A69.20
diaper L22
due to
chemical NEC L53.0
in contact with skin L24.5
drug (internal use) — see Dermatitis, due to, drugs
elevatum diutinum L95.1
endemic E52
epidemic, arthritic A25.1

Erythema, erythematous — continued
figuratum perstans L53.3
gluteal L22
heat — code by site under Burn, first degree
ichthyosiforme congenitum bullous Q80.3
in diseases classified elsewhere L54
induratum (nontuberculous) L52
tuberculous A18.4
infectiosum B08.3
intertrigo L30.4
iris L51.9
marginatum L53.2
in (due to) acute rheumatic fever I00
medicamentosum — see Dermatitis, due to, drugs
migrans A26.0
chronicum A69.20
tongue K14.1
multiforme (major) (minor) L51.9
bullous, bullosum L51.1
conjunctiva L51.1
nonbullous L51.0
pemphigoides L12.0
specified NEC L51.8
napkin L22
neonatorum P83.88
toxic P83.1
nodosum L52
tuberculous A18.4
palmar L53.8
pernio T69.1 ☑
rash, newborn P83.88
scarlatiniform (recurrent) (exfoliative) L53.8
solare L55.0
specified NEC L53.8
toxic, toxicum NEC L53.0
newborn P83.1
tuberculous (primary) A18.4
Erythematous, erythematosus — see condition
Erythermalgia (primary) I73.81
Erythralgia I73.81
Erythrasma L08.1
Erythredema (polyneuropathy) — see Poisoning, mercury
Erythremia (acute) C94.0- ☑
chronic D45
secondary D75.1
Erythroblastopenia — see also Aplasia, red cell D60.9
congenital D61.01
Erythroblastophthisis D61.09
Erythroblastosis (fetalis) (newborn) P55.9
due to
ABO (antibodies) (incompatibility) (isoimmunization) P55.1
Rh (antibodies) (incompatibility) (isoimmunization) P55.0
Erythrocyanosis (crurum) I73.89
Erythrocythemia — see Erythremia
Erythrocytosis (megalosplenic) (secondary) D75.1
familial D75.0
oval, hereditary — see Elliptocytosis
secondary D75.1
stress D75.1
Erythroderma (secondary) — see also Erythema L53.9
bullous ichthyosiform, congenital Q80.3
desquamativum L21.1
ichthyosiform, congenital (bullous) Q80.3
neonatorum P83.88
psoriaticum L40.8
Erythrodysesthesia, palmar plantar (PPE) L27.1
Erythrogenesis imperfecta D61.09
Erythroleukemia C94.0- ☑
Erythromelalgia I73.81
Erythrophagocytosis D75.89
Erythrophobia F40.298
Erythroplakia, oral epithelium, and tongue K13.29
Erythroplasia (Queyrat) D07.4
specified site — see Neoplasm, skin, in situ
unspecified site D07.4
Escherichia coli (E. coli), **as cause of disease classified elsewhere** B96.20
non-O157 Shiga toxin-producing (with known O group) B96.22
non-Shiga toxin-producing B96.29
O157 with confirmation of Shiga toxin when H antigen is unknown, or is not H7 B96.21
O157:H- (nonmotile) with confirmation of Shiga toxin B96.21

☑ **Additional Character Required — Refer to the Tabular List for Character Selection**   ▽ Subterms under main terms may continue to next column or page

Escherichia coli (E. coli), **as cause of disease classified elsewhere** — *continued*
  O157:H7 with or without confirmation of Shiga toxin-production B96.21
    specified NEC B96.22-
  Shiga toxin-producing (with unspecified O group) (STEC) B96.23
  O157 B96.21
  specified NEC B96.29
Esophagismus K22.4
Esophagitis (acute) (alkaline) (chemical) (chronic) (infectional) (necrotic) (peptic) (postoperative) K20.9
  candidal B37.81
  due to gastrointestinal reflux disease K21.0
  eosinophilic K20.0
  reflux K21.0
  specified NEC K20.8
  tuberculous A18.83
  ulcerative K22.10
    with bleeding K22.11
Esophagocele K22.5
Esophagomalacia K22.8
Esophagospasm K22.4
Esophagostenosis K22.2
Esophagostomiasis B81.8
Esophagotracheal — *see* condition
Esophagus — *see* condition
Esophoria H50.51
  convergence, excess H51.12
  divergence, insufficiency H51.8
Esotropia — *see* Strabismus, convergent concomitant
Espundia B55.2
Essential — *see* condition
Esthesioneuroblastoma C30.0
Esthesioneurocytoma C30.0
Esthesioneuroepithelioma C30.0
Esthiomene A55
Estivo-autumnal malaria (fever) B50.9
Estrangement (marital) Z63.5
  parent-child NEC Z62.890
Estriasis — *see* Myiasis
Ethanolism — *see* Alcoholism
Etherism — *see* Dependence, drug, inhalant
Ethmoid, ethmoidal — *see* condition
Ethmoiditis (chronic) (nonpurulent) (purulent) — *see also* Sinusitis, ethmoidal
  influenzal — *see* Influenza, with, respiratory manifestations NEC
  Woakes' J33.1
Ethylism — *see* Alcoholism
Eulenburg's disease (congenital paramyotonia) G71.19
Eumycetoma B47.0
Eunuchoidism E29.1
  hypogonadotropic E23.0
European blastomycosis — *see* Cryptococcosis
Eustachian — *see* condition
Evaluation (for) (of)
  development state
    adolescent Z00.3
    period of
      delayed growth in childhood Z00.70
        with abnormal findings Z00.71
      rapid growth in childhood Z00.2
      puberty Z00.3
  growth and developmental state (period of rapid growth) Z00.2
    delayed growth Z00.70
      with abnormal findings Z00.71
  mental health (status) Z00.8
    requested by authority Z04.6
  period of
    delayed growth in childhood Z00.70
      with abnormal findings Z00.71
    rapid growth in childhood Z00.2
  suspected condition — *see* Observation
Evans syndrome D69.41
Event
  apparent life threatening in newborn and infant (ALTE) R68.13
  brief resolved unexplained event (BRUE) R68.13
Eventration — *see also* Hernia, ventral
  colon into chest — *see* Hernia, diaphragm
  diaphragm (congenital) Q79.1
Eversion
  bladder N32.89
  cervix (uteri) N86
    with cervicitis N72

Eversion — *continued*
  foot NEC — *see also* Deformity, valgus, ankle
    congenital Q66.6
  punctum lacrimale (postinfectional) (senile) H04.52- ☑
  ureter (meatus) N28.89
  urethra (meatus) N36.8
  uterus N81.4
Evidence
  cytologic
    of malignancy on anal smear R85.614
    of malignancy on cervical smear R87.614
    of malignancy on vaginal smear R87.624
Evisceration
  birth injury P15.8
  traumatic NEC
    eye — *see* Enucleated eye
Evulsion — *see* Avulsion
Ewing's sarcoma or tumor — *see* Neoplasm, bone, malignant
Examination (for) (following) (general) (of) (routine) Z00.00
  with abnormal findings Z00.01
  abuse, physical (alleged), ruled out
    adult Z04.71
    child Z04.72
  adolescent (development state) Z00.3
  alleged rape or sexual assault (victim), ruled out
    adult Z04.41
    child Z04.42
  allergy Z01.82
  annual (adult) (periodic) (physical) Z00.00
    with abnormal findings Z00.01
    gynecological Z01.419
      with abnormal findings Z01.411
  antibody response Z01.84
  blood — *see* Examination, laboratory
  blood pressure Z01.30
    with abnormal findings Z01.31
  cancer staging — *see* Neoplasm, malignant, by site
  cervical Papanicolaou smear Z12.4
    as part of routine gynecological examination Z01.419
      with abnormal findings Z01.411
  child (over 28 days old) Z00.129
    with abnormal findings Z00.121
    under 28 days old — *see* Newborn, examination
  clinical research control or normal comparison (control) (participant) Z00.6
  contraceptive (drug) maintenance (routine) Z30.8
    device (intrauterine) Z30.431
  dental Z01.20
    with abnormal findings Z01.21
  developmental — *see* Examination, child
  donor (potential) Z00.5
  ear Z01.10
    with abnormal findings NEC Z01.118
  eye Z01.00
    with abnormal findings Z01.01
    following failed vision screening Z01.020
      with abnormal findings Z01.021
  follow-up (routine) (following) Z09
    chemotherapy NEC Z09
      malignant neoplasm Z08
    fracture Z09
    malignant neoplasm Z08
    postpartum Z39.2
    psychotherapy Z09
    radiotherapy NEC Z09
      malignant neoplasm Z08
    surgery NEC Z09
      malignant neoplasm Z08
  following
    accident NEC Z04.3
      transport Z04.1
      work Z04.2
    assault, alleged, ruled out
      adult Z04.71
      child Z04.72
    motor vehicle accident Z04.1
    treatment (for) Z09
      combined NEC Z09
        fracture Z09
        malignant neoplasm Z08
      malignant neoplasm Z08
      mental disorder Z09
      specified condition NEC Z09
  forced sexual exploitation Z04.81
  forced labor exploitation Z04.82

Examination — *continued*
  gynecological Z01.419
    with abnormal findings Z01.411
    for contraceptive maintenance Z30.8
  health — *see* Examination, medical
  hearing Z01.10
    with abnormal findings NEC Z01.118
    following failed hearing screening Z01.110
    infant or child (over 28 days old) Z00.129
      with abnormal findings Z00.121
  immunity status testing Z01.84
  laboratory (as part of a general medical examination) Z00.00
    with abnormal findings Z00.01
    preprocedural Z01.812
  lactating mother Z39.1
  medical (adult) (for) (of) Z00.00
    with abnormal findings Z00.01
    administrative purpose only Z02.9
      specified NEC Z02.89
    admission to
      armed forces Z02.3
      old age home Z02.2
      prison Z02.89
      residential institution Z02.2
      school Z02.0
        following illness or medical treatment Z02.0
      summer camp Z02.89
    adoption Z02.82
    blood alcohol or drug level Z02.83
    camp (summer) Z02.89
    clinical research, normal subject (control) (participant) Z00.6
    control subject in clinical research (normal comparison) (participant) Z00.6
    donor (potential) Z00.5
    driving license Z02.4
    general (adult) Z00.00
      with abnormal findings Z00.01
    immigration Z02.89
    insurance purposes Z02.6
    marriage Z02.89
    medicolegal reasons NEC Z04.89
    naturalization Z02.89
    participation in sport Z02.5
    paternity testing Z02.81
    population survey Z00.8
    pre-employment Z02.1
    pre-operative — *see* Examination, pre-procedural
    pre-procedural
      cardiovascular Z01.810
      respiratory Z01.811
      specified NEC Z01.818
    preschool children
      for admission to school Z02.0
    prisoners
      for entrance into prison Z02.89
    recruitment for armed forces Z02.3
    specified NEC Z00.8
    sport competition Z02.5
  medicolegal reason NEC Z04.89
    following
      forced sexual exploitation Z04.81
      forced labor exploitation Z04.82
  newborn — *see* Newborn, examination
  pelvic (annual) (periodic) Z01.419
    with abnormal findings Z01.411
  period of rapid growth in childhood Z00.2
  periodic (adult) (annual) (routine) Z00.00
    with abnormal findings Z00.01
  physical (adult) — *see also* Examination, medical Z00.00
    sports Z02.5
  postpartum
    immediately after delivery Z39.0
    routine follow-up Z39.2
  pre-chemotherapy (antineoplastic) Z01.818
  prenatal (normal pregnancy) — *see also* Pregnancy, normal Z34.9- ☑
  pre-procedural (pre-operative)
    cardiovascular Z01.810
    laboratory Z01.812
    respiratory Z01.811
    specified NEC Z01.818
  prior to chemotherapy (antineoplastic) Z01.818
  psychiatric NEC Z00.8
    follow-up not needing further care Z09
    requested by authority Z04.6
  radiological (as part of a general medical examination) Z00.00

▽ Subterms under main terms may continue to next column or page   ☑ Additional Character Required — Refer to the Tabular List for Character Selection   137

Escherichia coli — Examination

Examination — *continued*
  radiological — *continued*
    with abnormal findings Z00.01
    repeat cervical smear to confirm findings of recent
        normal smear following initial abnormal smear
        Z01.42
  skin (hypersensitivity) Z01.82
  special — *see also* Examination, by type Z01.89
    specified type NEC Z01.89
  specified type or reason NEC Z04.89
  teeth Z01.20
    with abnormal findings Z01.21
  urine — *see* Examination, laboratory
  vision Z01.00
    with abnormal findings Z01.01
    following failed vision screening Z01.020
      with abnormal findings Z01.021
    infant or child (over 28 days old) Z00.129
      with abnormal findings Z00.121
Exanthem, exanthema — *see also* Rash
  with enteroviral vesicular stomatitis B08.4
  Boston A88.0
  epidemic with meningitis A88.0 *[G02]*
  subitum B08.20
    due to human herpesvirus 6 B08.21
    due to human herpesvirus 7 B08.22
  viral, virus B09
    specified type NEC B08.8
Excess, excessive, excessively
  alcohol level in blood R78.0
  androgen (ovarian) E28.1
  attrition, tooth, teeth K03.0
  carotene, carotin (dietary) E67.1
  cold, effects of T69.9 ☑
    specified effect NEC T69.8 ☑
  convergence H51.12
  crying
    in child, adolescent, or adult R45.83
    in infant R68.11
  development, breast N62
  divergence H51.8
  drinking (alcohol) NEC (without dependence) F10.10
    habitual (continual) (without remission) F10.20
  eating R63.2
  estrogen E28.0
  fat — *see also* Obesity
    in heart — *see* Degeneration, myocardial
    localized E65
  foreskin N47.8
  gas R14.0
  glucagon E16.3
  heat — *see* Heat
  intermaxillary vertical dimension of fully erupted teeth
      M26.37
  interocclusal distance of fully erupted teeth M26.37
  kalium E87.5
  large
    colon K59.39
      congenital Q43.8
    infant P08.0
    organ or site, congenital NEC — *see* Anomaly, by
        site
  long
    organ or site, congenital NEC — *see* Anomaly, by
        site
  menstruation (with regular cycle) N92.0
    with irregular cycle N92.1
  napping Z72.821
  natrium E87.0
  number of teeth K00.1
  nutrient (dietary) NEC R63.2
  potassium (K) E87.5
  salivation K11.7
  secretion — *see also* Hypersecretion
    milk O92.6
    sputum R09.3
    sweat R61
  sexual drive F52.8
  short
    organ or site, congenital NEC — *see* Anomaly, by
        site
    umbilical cord in labor or delivery O69.3 ☑
  skin L98.7
    and subcutaneous tissue L98.7
    eyelid (acquired) — *see* Blepharochalasis
      congenital Q10.3
  sodium (Na) E87.0
  spacing of fully erupted teeth M26.32

Excess, excessive, excessively — *continued*
  sputum R09.3
  sweating R61
  thirst R63.1
    due to deprivation of water T73.1 ☑
  tuberosity of jaw M26.07
  vitamin
    A (dietary) E67.0
      administered as drug (prolonged intake) — *see*
          Table of Drugs and Chemicals, vitamins,
          adverse effect
      overdose or wrong substance given or taken —
          see Table of Drugs and Chemicals, vita-
          mins, poisoning
    D (dietary) E67.3
      administered as drug (prolonged intake) — *see*
          Table of Drugs and Chemicals, vitamins,
          adverse effect
      overdose or wrong substance given or taken —
          see Table of Drugs and Chemicals, vita-
          mins, poisoning
  weight
    gain R63.5
    loss R63.4
Excitability, abnormal, under minor stress (personal-
    ity disorder) F60.3
Excitation
  anomalous atrioventricular I45.6
  psychogenic F30.8
  reactive (from emotional stress, psychological trauma)
      F30.8
Excitement
  hypomanic F30.8
  manic F30.9
  mental, reactive (from emotional stress, psychological
      trauma) F30.8
  state, reactive (from emotional stress, psychological
      trauma) F30.8
Excoriation (traumatic) — *see also* Abrasion
  neurotic L98.1
  skin picking disorder F42.4
Exfoliation
  due to erythematous conditions according to extent
      of body surface involved L49.0
    10-19 percent of body surface L49.1
    20-29 percent of body surface L49.2
    30-39 percent of body surface L49.3
    40-49 percent of body surface L49.4
    50-59 percent of body surface L49.5
    60-69 percent of body surface L49.6
    70-79 percent of body surface L49.7
    80-89 percent of body surface L49.8
    90-99 percent of body surface L49.9
    less than 10 percent of body surface L49.0
  teeth, due to systemic causes K08.0
Exfoliative — *see* condition
Exhaustion, exhaustive (physical NEC) R53.83
  battle F43.0
  cardiac — *see* Failure, heart
  delirium F43.0
  due to
    cold T69.8 ☑
    excessive exertion T73.3 ☑
    exposure T73.2 ☑
    neurasthenia F48.8
  heart — *see* Failure, heart
  heat — *see also* Heat, exhaustion T67.5 ☑
    due to
      salt depletion T67.4 ☑
      water depletion T67.3 ☑
  maternal, complicating delivery O75.81
  mental F48.8
  myocardium, myocardial — *see* Failure, heart
  nervous F48.8
  old age R54
  psychogenic F48.8
  psychosis F43.0
  senile R54
  vital NEC Z73.0
Exhibitionism F65.2
Exocervicitis — *see* Cervicitis
Exomphalos Q79.2
  meaning hernia — *see* Hernia, umbilicus
Exophoria H50.52
  convergence, insufficiency H51.11
  divergence, excess H51.8
Exophthalmos H05.2- ☑
  congenital Q15.8

Exophthalmos — *continued*
  constant NEC H05.24- ☑
  displacement, globe — *see* Displacement, globe
  due to thyrotoxicosis (hyperthyroidism) — *see* Hyper-
      thyroidism, with, goiter (diffuse)
  dysthyroid — *see* Hyperthyroidism, with, goiter (dif-
      fuse)
  goiter — *see* Hyperthyroidism, with, goiter (diffuse)
  intermittent NEC H05.25- ☑
  malignant — *see* Hyperthyroidism, with, goiter (diffuse)
  orbital
    edema — *see* Edema, orbit
    hemorrhage — *see* Hemorrhage, orbit
  pulsating NEC H05.26- ☑
  thyrotoxic, thyrotropic — *see* Hyperthyroidism, with,
      goiter (diffuse)
Exostosis — *see also* Disorder, bone
  cartilaginous — *see* Neoplasm, bone, benign
  congenital (multiple) Q78.6
  external ear canal H61.81- ☑
  gonococcal A54.49
  jaw (bone) M27.8
  multiple, congenital Q78.6
  orbit H05.35- ☑
  osteocartilaginous — *see* Neoplasm, bone, benign
  syphilitic A52.77
Exotropia — *see* Strabismus, divergent concomitant
Explanation of
  investigation finding Z71.2
  medication Z71.89
Exposure (to) — *see also* Contact, with T75.89 ☑
  acariasis Z20.7
  AIDS virus Z20.6
  air pollution Z77.110
  algae and algae toxins Z77.121
  algae bloom Z77.121
  anthrax Z20.810
  aromatic amines Z77.020
  aromatic (hazardous) compounds NEC Z77.028
  aromatic dyes NOS Z77.028
  arsenic Z77.010
  asbestos Z77.090
  bacterial disease NEC Z20.818
  benzene Z77.021
  blue-green algae bloom Z77.121
  body fluids (potentially hazardous) Z77.21
  brown tide Z77.121
  chemicals (chiefly nonmedicinal) (hazardous) NEC
      Z77.098
  cholera Z20.09
  chromium compounds Z77.018
  cold, effects of T69.9 ☑
    specified effect NEC T69.8 ☑
  communicable disease Z20.9
    bacterial NEC Z20.818
    specified NEC Z20.89
    viral NEC Z20.828
    Zika virus Z20.821
  cyanobacteria bloom Z77.121
  disaster Z65.5
  discrimination Z60.5
  dyes Z77.098
  effects of T73.9 ☑
  environmental tobacco smoke (acute) (chronic) Z77.22
  Escherichia coli (E. coli) Z20.01
  exhaustion due to T73.2 ☑
  fiberglass — *see* Table of Drugs and Chemicals, fiber-
      glass
  German measles Z20.4
  gonorrhea Z20.2
  hazardous metals NEC Z77.018
  hazardous substances NEC Z77.29
  hazards in the physical environment NEC Z77.128
  hazards to health NEC Z77.9
  human immunodeficiency virus (HIV) Z20.6
  human T-lymphotropic virus type-1 (HTLV-1) Z20.89
  implanted
    mesh — *see* Complications, prosthetic devise or
        implant, mesh
    prosthetic materials NEC — *see* Complications,
        prosthetic materials NEC
  infestation (parasitic) NEC Z20.7
  intestinal infectious disease NEC Z20.09
    Escherichia coli (E. coli) Z20.01
  lead Z77.011
  meningococcus Z20.811
  mold (toxic) Z77.120
  nickel dust Z77.018

☑ **Additional Character Required** — **Refer to the Tabular List for Character Selection**   ⬝ Subterms under main terms may continue to next column or page

Exposure — *continued*
  noise Z77.122
  occupational
    air contaminants NEC Z57.39
    dust Z57.2
    environmental tobacco smoke Z57.31
    extreme temperature Z57.6
    noise Z57.0
    radiation Z57.1
    risk factors Z57.9
      specified NEC Z57.8
    toxic agents (gases) (liquids) (solids) (vapors) in
      agriculture Z57.4
    toxic agents (gases) (liquids) (solids) (vapors) in in-
      dustry NEC Z57.5
    vibration Z57.7
  parasitic disease NEC Z20.7
  pediculosis Z20.7
  persecution Z60.5
  pfiesteria piscicida Z77.121
  poliomyelitis Z20.89
  pollution
    air Z77.110
    environmental NEC Z77.118
    soil Z77.112
    water Z77.111
  polycyclic aromatic hydrocarbons Z77.028
  prenatal (drugs) (toxic chemicals) — *see* Newborn, af-
    fected by, noxious substances transmitted via
    placenta or breast milk
  rabies Z20.3
  radiation, naturally occurring NEC Z77.123
  radon Z77.123
  red tide (Florida) Z77.121
  rubella Z20.4
  second hand tobacco smoke (acute) (chronic) Z77.22
    in the perinatal period P96.81
  sexually-transmitted disease Z20.2
  smallpox (laboratory) Z20.89
  syphilis Z20.2
  terrorism Z65.4
  torture Z65.4
  tuberculosis Z20.1
  uranium Z77.012
  varicella Z20.820
  venereal disease Z20.2
  viral disease NEC Z20.828
  war Z65.5
  water pollution Z77.111
  Zika virus Z20.821
Exsanguination — *see* Hemorrhage
Exstrophy
  abdominal contents Q45.8
  bladder Q64.10
    cloacal Q64.12
    specified type NEC Q64.19
    supravesical fissure Q64.11
Extensive — *see* condition
Extra — *see also* Accessory
  marker chromosomes (normal individual) Q92.61
    in abnormal individual Q92.62
  rib Q76.6
    cervical Q76.5
Extrasystoles (supraventricular) I49.49
  atrial I49.1
  auricular I49.1
  junctional I49.2
  ventricular I49.3
Extrauterine gestation or pregnancy — *see* Pregnancy,
  by site
Extravasation
  blood R58
  chyle into mesentery I89.8
  pelvicalyceal N13.8
  pyelosinus N13.8
  urine (from ureter) R39.0
  vesicant agent
    antineoplastic chemotherapy T80.810 ☑
    other agent NEC T80.818 ☑
Extremity — *see* condition, limb
Extrophy — *see* Exstrophy
Extroversion
  bladder Q64.19
  uterus N81.4
    complicating delivery O71.2
    postpartal (old) N81.4
Extruded tooth (teeth) M26.34

Extrusion
  breast implant (prosthetic) T85.42 ☑
  eye implant (globe) (ball) T85.328 ☑
  intervertebral disc — *see* Displacement, intervertebral
    disc
  ocular lens implant (prosthetic) — *see* Complications,
    intraocular lens
  vitreous — *see* Prolapse, vitreous
Exudate
  pleural — *see* Effusion, pleura
  retina H35.89
Exudative — *see* condition
Eye, eyeball, eyelid — *see* condition
Eyestrain — *see* Disturbance, vision, subjective
Eyeworm disease of Africa B74.3

F

Faber's syndrome (achlorhydric anemia) D50.9
Fabry (-Anderson) **disease** E75.21
Faciocephalalgia, autonomic — *see also* Neuropathy,
  peripheral, autonomic G90.09
Factor(s)
  psychic, associated with diseases classified elsewhere
    F54
  psychological
    affecting physical conditions F54
    or behavioral
      affecting general medical condition F54
      associated with disorders or diseases classified
        elsewhere F54
Fahr disease (of brain) G23.8
Fahr Volhard disease (of kidney) I12.- ☑
Failure, failed
  abortion — *see* Abortion, attempted
  aortic (valve) I35.8
    rheumatic I06.8
  attempted abortion — *see* Abortion, attempted
  biventricular I50.82
    due to left heart failure I50.814
  bone marrow — *see* Anemia, aplastic
  cardiac — *see* Failure, heart
  cardiorenal (chronic) — *see also* Failure, renal, and
    Failure, heart I50.9
    hypertensive I13.2
  cardiorespiratory — *see also* Failure, heart R09.2
  cardiovascular (chronic) — *see* Failure, heart
  cerebrovascular I67.9
  cervical dilatation in labor O62.0
  circulation, circulatory (peripheral) R57.9
    newborn P29.89
  compensation — *see* Disease, heart
  compliance with medical treatment or regimen — *see*
    Noncompliance
  congestive — *see* Failure, heart, congestive
  dental implant (endosseous) M27.69
    due to
      failure of dental prosthesis M27.63
      lack of attached gingiva M27.62
      occlusal trauma (poor prosthetic design) M27.62
      parafunctional habits M27.62
      periodontal infection (peri-implantitis) M27.62
      poor oral hygiene M27.62
    osseointegration M27.61
      due to
        complications of systemic disease M27.61
        poor bone quality M27.61
      iatrogenic M27.61
    post-osseointegration
      biological M27.62
      due to complications of systemic disease M27.62
      iatrogenic M27.62
      mechanical M27.63
    pre-integration M27.61
    pre-osseointegration M27.61
    specified NEC M27.69
  descent of head (at term) of pregnancy (mother)
    O32.4 ☑
  endosseous dental implant — *see* Failure, dental im-
    plant
  engagement of head (term of pregnancy) (mother)
    O32.4 ☑
  erection (penile) — *see also* Dysfunction, sexual, male,
    erectile N52.9
    nonorganic F52.21
  examination(s), anxiety concerning Z55.2

Failure, failed — *continued*
  expansion terminal respiratory units (newborn) (prima-
    ry) P28.0
  forceps NOS (with subsequent cesarean delivery) O66.5
  gain weight (child over 28 days old) R62.51
    adult R62.7
    newborn P92.6
  genital response (male) F52.21
    female F52.22
  heart (acute) (senile) (sudden) I50.9
    with
      acute pulmonary edema — *see* Failure, ventricu-
        lar, left
      decompensation — *see also* Failure, heart, by
        type as diastolic or systolic, acute and
        chronic I50.9
      dilatation — *see* Disease, heart
      hypertension — *see* Hypertension, heart
      normal ejection fraction — *see* Failure, heart,
        diastolic
      preserved ejection fraction — *see* Failure, heart,
        diastolic
      reduced ejection fraction — *see* Failure, heart,
        systolic
    arteriosclerotic I70.90
    biventricular I50.82
      due to left heart failure I50.814
    combined left-right sided I50.82
      due to left heart failure I50.814
    compensated — *see also* Failure, heart, by type as
      diastolic or systolic, chronic I50.9
    complicating
      anesthesia (general) (local) or other sedation
        in labor and delivery O74.2
        in pregnancy O29.12- ☑
        postpartum, puerperal O89.1
      delivery (cesarean) (instrumental) O75.4
    congestive I50.9
      with rheumatic fever (conditions in I00)
        active I01.8
        inactive or quiescent (with chorea) I09.81
      newborn P29.0
      rheumatic (chronic) (inactive) (with chorea)
        I09.81
        active or acute I01.8
          with chorea I02.0
    decompensated — *see also* Failure, heart, by type
      as diastolic or systolic, acute and chronic I50.9
    degenerative — *see* Degeneration, myocardial
    diastolic (congestive) (left ventricular) I50.30
      acute (congestive) I50.31
        and (on) chronic (congestive) I50.33
      chronic (congestive) I50.32
        and (on) acute (congestive) I50.33
      combined with systolic (congestive) I50.40
        acute (congestive) I50.41
          and (on) chronic (congestive) I50.43
        chronic (congestive) I50.42
          and (on) acute (congestive) I50.43
    due to presence of cardiac prosthesis I97.13- ☑
    end stage — *see also* Failure, heart, by type as dias-
      tolic or systolic, chronic I50.84
    following cardiac surgery I97.13- ☑
    high output NOS I50.83
    hypertensive — *see* Hypertension, heart
    left (ventricular) — *see also* Failure, ventricular, left
      combined diastolic and systolic — *see* Failure,
        heart, diastolic, combined with systolic
      diastolic — *see* Failure, heart, diastolic
      systolic — *see* Failure, heart, systolic
    low output (syndrome) NOS I50.9
    newborn P29.0
    organic — *see* Disease, heart
    peripartum O90.3
    postprocedural I97.13- ☑
    rheumatic (chronic) (inactive) I09.9
    right (isolated) (ventricular) I50.810
      acute I50.811
        and (on) chronic I50.813
      chronic I50.812
        and acute I50.813
      secondary to left heart failure I50.814

Failure, failed — *continued*
  heart — *continued*
    specified NEC I50.89

> *Note: heart failure stages A, B, C, and D are based on the American College of Cardiology and American Heart Association stages of heart failure, which complement and should not be confused with the New York Heart Association Classification of Heart Failure, into Class I, Class II, Class III, and Class IV*

    stage A Z91.89
    stage B — *see also* Failure, heart, by type as diastolic or systolic I50.9
    stage C — *see also* Failure, heart, by type as diastolic or systolic I50.9
    stage D — *see also* Failure, heart, by type as diastolic or systolic, chronic I50.84
    systolic (congestive) (left ventricular) I50.20
      acute (congestive) I50.21
        and (on) chronic (congestive) I50.23
      chronic (congestive) I50.22
        and (on) acute (congestive) I50.23
      combined with diastolic (congestive) I50.40
        acute (congestive) I50.41
          and (on) chronic (congestive) I50.43
        chronic (congestive) I50.42
          and (on) acute (congestive) I50.43
    thyrotoxic — *see also* Thyrotoxicosis E05.90 *[I43]*
      with
        high output — *see also* Thyrotoxicosis I50.83
        thyroid storm E05.91 *[I43]*
          high output — *see also* Thyrotoxicosis I50.83
    valvular — *see* Endocarditis
  hepatic K72.90
    with coma K72.91
    acute or subacute K72.00
      with coma K72.01
      due to drugs K71.10
        with coma K71.11
    alcoholic (acute) (chronic) (subacute) K70.40
      with coma K70.41
    chronic K72.10
      with coma K72.11
      due to drugs (acute) (subacute) (chronic) K71.10
        with coma K71.11
    due to drugs (acute) (subacute) (chronic) K71.10
      with coma K71.11
    postprocedural K91.82
  hepatorenal K76.7
  induction (of labor) O61.9
    abortion — *see* Abortion, attempted
    by
      oxytocic drugs O61.0
      prostaglandins O61.0
    instrumental O61.1
    mechanical O61.1
    medical O61.0
    specified NEC O61.8
    surgical O61.1
  intubation during anesthesia T88.4 ☑
    in pregnancy O29.6- ☑
    labor and delivery O74.7
    postpartum, puerperal O89.6
  involution, thymus (gland) E32.0
  kidney — *see also* Disease, kidney, chronic N19
    acute — *see also* Failure, renal, acute N17.9
  lactation (complete) O92.3
    partial O92.4
  Leydig's cell, adult E29.1
  liver — *see* Failure, hepatic
  menstruation at puberty N91.0
  mitral I05.8
  myocardial, myocardium — *see also* Failure, heart I50.9
    chronic — *see also* Failure, heart, congestive I50.9
    congestive — *see also* Failure, heart, congestive I50.9
  orgasm (female) (psychogenic) F52.31
    male F52.32
  ovarian (primary) E28.39
    iatrogenic E89.40
      asymptomatic E89.40
      symptomatic E89.41
    postprocedural (postablative) (postirradiation) (postsurgical) E89.40
      asymptomatic E89.40
      symptomatic E89.41
  ovulation causing infertility N97.0

Failure, failed — *continued*
  polyglandular, autoimmune E31.0
  prosthetic joint implant — *see* Complications, joint prosthesis, mechanical, breakdown, by site
  renal N19
    with
      tubular necrosis (acute) N17.0
    acute N17.9
      with
        cortical necrosis N17.1
        medullary necrosis N17.2
        tubular necrosis N17.0
      specified NEC N17.8
    chronic N18.9
      hypertensive — *see* Hypertension, kidney
    congenital P96.0
    end stage (chronic) N18.6
      due to hypertension I12.0
    following
      abortion — *see* Abortion by type complicated by specified condition NEC
      crushing T79.5 ☑
      ectopic or molar pregnancy O08.4
      labor and delivery (acute) O90.4
    hypertensive — *see* Hypertension, kidney
    postprocedural N99.0
  respiration, respiratory J96.90
    with
      hypercapnia J96.92
      hypercarbia J96.92
      hypoxia J96.91
    acute J96.00
      with
        hypercapnia J96.02
        hypercarbia J96.02
        hypoxia J96.01
    center G93.89
    acute and (on) chronic J96.20
      with
        hypercapnia J96.22
        hypercarbia J96.22
        hypoxia J96.21
    chronic J96.10
      with
        hypercapnia J96.12
        hypercarbia J96.12
        hypoxia J96.11
    newborn P28.5
    postprocedural (acute) J95.821
      acute and chronic J95.822
  rotation
    cecum Q43.3
    colon Q43.3
    intestine Q43.3
    kidney Q63.2
  sedation (conscious) (moderate) during procedure T88.52 ☑
    history of Z92.83
  segmentation — *see also* Fusion
    fingers — *see* Syndactylism, complex, fingers
    vertebra Q76.49
      with scoliosis Q76.3
  seminiferous tubule, adult E29.1
  senile (general) R54
  sexual arousal (male) F52.21
    female F52.22
  testicular endocrine function E29.1
  to thrive (child over 28 days old) R62.51
    adult R62.7
    newborn P92.6
  transplant T86.92
    bone T86.831
      marrow T86.02
    cornea T86.841
    heart T86.22
      with lung(s) T86.32
    intestine T86.851
    kidney T86.12
    liver T86.42
    lung(s) T86.811
      with heart T86.32
    pancreas T86.891
    skin (allograft) (autograft) T86.821
    specified organ or tissue NEC T86.891
    stem cell (peripheral blood) (umbilical cord) T86.5
  trial of labor (with subsequent cesarean delivery) O66.40
    following previous cesarean delivery O66.41

Failure, failed — *continued*
  tubal ligation N99.89
  urinary — *see* Disease, kidney, chronic
  vacuum extraction NOS (with subsequent cesarean delivery) O66.5
  vasectomy N99.89
  ventouse NOS (with subsequent cesarean delivery) O66.5
  ventricular — *see also* Failure, heart I50.9
    left — *see also* Failure, heart, left I50.1
      with rheumatic fever (conditions in I00)
        active I01.8
          with chorea I02.0
        inactive or quiescent (with chorea) I09.81
      rheumatic (chronic) (inactive) (with chorea) I09.81
        active or acute I01.8
          with chorea I02.0
    right — *see* Failure, heart, right
  vital centers, newborn P91.88
Fainting (fit) R55
Fallen arches — *see* Deformity, limb, flat foot
Falling, falls (repeated) R29.6
  any organ or part — *see* Prolapse
Fallopian
  insufflation Z31.41
  tube — *see* condition
Fallot's
  pentalogy Q21.8
  tetrad or tetralogy Q21.3
  triad or trilogy Q22.3
False — *see also* condition
  croup J38.5
  joint — *see* Nonunion, fracture
  labor (pains) O47.9
    at or after 37 completed weeks of gestation O47.1
    before 37 completed weeks of gestation O47.0- ☑
  passage, urethra (prostatic) N36.5
  pregnancy F45.8
Family, familial — *see also* condition
  disruption Z63.8
    involving divorce or separation Z63.5
  Li-Fraumeni (syndrome) Z15.01
  planning advice Z30.09
  problem Z63.9
    specified NEC Z63.8
  retinoblastoma C69.2- ☑
Famine (effects of) T73.0 ☑
  edema — *see* Malnutrition, severe
Fanconi (-de Toni)(-Debré) **syndrome** E72.09
  with cystinosis E72.04
Fanconi's anemia (congenital pancytopenia) D61.09
Farber's disease or syndrome E75.29
Farcy A24.0
Farmer's
  lung J67.0
  skin L57.8
Farsightedness — *see* Hypermetropia
Fascia — *see* condition
Fasciculation R25.3
Fasciitis M72.9
  diffuse (eosinophilic) M35.4
  infective M72.8
    necrotizing M72.6
  necrotizing M72.6
  nodular M72.4
  perirenal (with ureteral obstruction) N13.5
    with infection N13.6
  plantar M72.2
  specified NEC M72.8
  traumatic (old) M72.8
    current — *code by* site under Sprain
Fascioliasis B66.3
Fasciolopsis, fasciolopsiasis (intestinal) B66.5
Fascioscapulohumeral myopathy G71.02
Fast pulse R00.0
Fat
  embolism — *see* Embolism, fat
  excessive — *see also* Obesity
    in heart — *see* Degeneration, myocardial
  in stool R19.5
  localized (pad) E65
    heart — *see* Degeneration, myocardial
    knee M79.4
    retropatellar M79.4
  necrosis
    breast N64.1
    mesentery K65.4

Fat — *continued*
  necrosis — *continued*
    omentum K65.4
    pad E65
      knee M79.4
Fatigue R53.83
  auditory deafness — *see* Deafness
  chronic R53.82
  combat F43.0
  general R53.83
    psychogenic F48.8
  heat (transient) T67.6 ☑
  muscle M62.89
  myocardium — *see* Failure, heart
  neoplasm-related R53.0
  nervous, neurosis F48.8
  operational F48.8
  psychogenic (general) F48.8
  senile R54
  voice R49.8
Fatness — *see* Obesity
Fatty — *see also* condition
  apron E65
  degeneration — *see* Degeneration, fatty
  heart (enlarged) — *see* Degeneration, myocardial
  liver NEC K76.0
    alcoholic K70.0
    nonalcoholic K76.0
  necrosis — *see* Degeneration, fatty
Fauces — *see* condition
Fauchard's disease (periodontitis) — *see* Periodontitis
Faucitis J02.9
Favism (anemia) D55.0
Favus — *see* Dermatophytosis
Fazio-Londe disease or syndrome G12.1
Fear complex or reaction F40.9
Fear of — *see* Phobia
Feared complaint unfounded Z71.1
Febris, febrile — *see also* Fever
  flava — *see also* Fever, yellow A95.9
  melitensis A23.0
  pestis — *see* Plague
  recurrens — *see* Fever, relapsing
  rubra A38.9
Fecal
  incontinence R15.9
  smearing R15.1
  soiling R15.1
  urgency R15.2
Fecalith (impaction) K56.41
  appendix K38.1
  congenital P76.8
Fede's disease K14.0
Feeble rapid pulse due to shock following injury
  T79.4 ☑
Feeble-minded F70
Feeding
  difficulties R63.3
  problem R63.3
    newborn P92.9
      specified NEC P92.8
    nonorganic (adult) — *see* Disorder, eating
Feeling (of)
  foreign body in throat R09.89
Feer's disease — *see* Poisoning, mercury
Feet — *see* condition
Feigned illness Z76.5
Feil-Klippel syndrome (brevicollis) Q76.1
Feinmesser's (hidrotic) **ectodermal dysplasia** Q82.4
Felinophobia F40.218
Felon — *see also* Cellulitis, digit
  with lymphangitis — *see* Lymphangitis, acute, digit
Felty's syndrome M05.00
  ankle M05.07- ☑
  elbow M05.02- ☑
  foot joint M05.07- ☑
  hand joint M05.04- ☑
  hip M05.05- ☑
  knee M05.06- ☑
  multiple site M05.09
  shoulder M05.01- ☑
  vertebra — *see* Spondylitis, ankylosing
  wrist M05.03- ☑
Female genital cutting status — *see* Female genital
  mutilation status (FGM)
Female genital mutilation status (FGM) N90.810
  specified NEC N90.818

Female genital mutilation status — *continued*
  type I (clitorectomy status) N90.811
  type II (clitorectomy with excision of labia minora status) N90.812
  type III (infibulation status) N90.813
  type IV N90.818
Femur, femoral — *see* condition
Fenestration, fenestrated — *see also* Imperfect, closure
  aortico-pulmonary Q21.4
  cusps, heart valve NEC Q24.8
    pulmonary Q22.3
  pulmonic cusps Q22.3
Fernell's disease (aortic aneurysm) I71.9
Fertile eunuch syndrome E23.0
Fetid
  breath R19.6
  sweat L75.0
Fetishism F65.0
  transvestic F65.1
Fetus, fetal — *see also* condition
  alcohol syndrome (dysmorphic) Q86.0
  compressus O31.0- ☑
  hydantoin syndrome Q86.1
  lung tissue P28.0
  papyraceous O31.0- ☑
Fever (inanition) (of unknown origin) (persistent) (with chills) (with rigor) R50.9
  abortus A23.1
  Aden (dengue) A90
  African tick-borne A68.1
  American
    mountain (tick) A93.2
    spotted A77.0
  aphthous B08.8
  arbovirus, arboviral A94
    hemorrhagic A94
    specified NEC A93.8
  Argentinian hemorrhagic A96.0
  Assam B55.0
  Australian Q A78
  Bangkok hemorrhagic A91
  Barmah forest A92.8
  Bartonella A44.0
  bilious, hemoglobinuric B50.8
  blackwater B50.8
  blister B00.1
  Bolivian hemorrhagic A96.1
  Bonvale dam T73.3 ☑
  boutonneuse A77.1
  brain — *see* Encephalitis
  Brazilian purpuric A48.4
  breakbone A90
  Bullis A77.0
  Bunyamwera A92.8
  Burdwan B55.0
  Bwamba A92.8
  Cameroon — *see* Malaria
  Canton A75.9
  catarrhal (acute) J00
    chronic J31.0
  cat-scratch A28.1
  Central Asian hemorrhagic A98.0
  cerebral — *see* Encephalitis
  cerebrospinal meningococcal A39.0
  Chagres B50.9
  Chandipura A92.8
  Changuinola A93.1
  Charcot's (biliary) (hepatic) (intermittent) — *see* Calculus, bile duct
  Chikungunya (viral) (hemorrhagic) A92.0
  Chitral A93.1
  Colombo — *see* Fever, paratyphoid
  Colorado tick (virus) A93.2
  congestive (remittent) — *see* Malaria
  Congo virus A98.0
  continued malarial B50.9
  Corsican — *see* Malaria
  Crimean-Congo hemorrhagic A98.0
  Cyprus — *see* Brucellosis
  dandy A90
  deer fly — *see* Tularemia
  dengue (virus) A90
    hemorrhagic A91
    sandfly A93.1
  desert B38.0
  drug induced R50.2
  due to
    conditions classified elsewhere R50.81

Fever — *continued*
  due to — *continued*
    heat T67.01 ☑
  enteric A01.00
  enteroviral exanthematous (Boston exanthem) A88.0
  ephemeral (of unknown origin) R50.9
  epidemic hemorrhagic A98.5
  erysipelatous — *see* Erysipelas
  estivo-autumnal (malarial) B50.9
  famine A75.0
  five day A79.0
  following delivery O86.4
  Fort Bragg A27.89
  gastroenteric A01.00
  gastromalarial — *see* Malaria
  Gibraltar — *see* Brucellosis
  glandular — *see* Mononucleosis, infectious
  Guama (viral) A92.8
  Haverhill A25.1
  hay (allergic) J30.1
    with asthma (bronchial) J45.909
      with
        exacerbation (acute) J45.901
        status asthmaticus J45.902
    due to
      allergen other than pollen J30.89
      pollen, any plant or tree J30.1
  heat (effects) T67.01 ☑
  hematuric, bilious B50.8
  hemoglobinuric (malarial) (bilious) B50.8
  hemorrhagic (arthropod-borne) NOS A94
    with renal syndrome A98.5
    arenaviral A96.9
      specified NEC A96.8
    Argentinian A96.0
    Bangkok A91
    Bolivian A96.1
    Central Asian A98.0
    Chikungunya A92.0
    Crimean-Congo A98.0
    dengue (virus) A91
    epidemic A98.5
    Junin (virus) A96.0
    Korean A98.5
    Kyasanur forest A98.2
    Machupo (virus) A96.1
    mite-borne A93.8
    mosquito-borne A92.8
    Omsk A98.1
    Philippine A91
    Russian A98.5
    Singapore A91
    Southeast Asia A91
    Thailand A91
    tick-borne NEC A93.8
    viral A99
      specified NEC A98.8
  hepatic — *see* Cholecystitis
  herpetic — *see* Herpes
  icterohemorrhagic A27.0
  Indiana A93.8
  infective B99.9
    specified NEC B99.8
  intermittent (bilious) — *see also* Malaria
    of unknown origin R50.9
    pernicious B50.9
  iodide R50.2
  Japanese river A75.3
  jungle — *see also* Malaria
    yellow A95.0
  Junin (virus) hemorrhagic A96.0
  Katayama B65.2
  kedani A75.3
  Kenya (tick) A77.1
  Kew Garden A79.1
  Korean hemorrhagic A98.5
  Lassa A96.2
  Lone Star A77.0
  Machupo (virus) hemorrhagic A96.1
  malaria, malarial — *see* Malaria
  Malta A23.9
  Marseilles A77.1
  marsh — *see* Malaria
  Mayaro (viral) A92.8
  Mediterranean — *see also* Brucellosis A23.9
    familial M04.1
    tick A77.1
  meningeal — *see* Meningitis

Subterms under main terms may continue to next column or page   ☑ Additional Character Required — Refer to the Tabular List for Character Selection   141

Fat — Fever

Fever — *continued*
Meuse A79.0
Mexican A75.2
mianeh A68.1
miasmatic — *see* Malaria
mosquito-borne (viral) A92.9
  hemorrhagic A92.8
mountain — *see also* Brucellosis
  meaning Rocky Mountain spotted fever A77.0
  tick (American) (Colorado) (viral) A93.2
Mucambo (viral) A92.8
mud A27.9
Neapolitan — *see* Brucellosis
neutropenic D70.9
newborn P81.9
  environmental P81.0
Nine-Mile A78
non-exanthematous tick A93.2
North Asian tick-borne A77.2
Omsk hemorrhagic A98.1
O'nyong-nyong (viral) A92.1
Oropouche (viral) A93.0
Oroya A44.0
paludal — *see* Malaria
Panama (malarial) B50.9
Pappataci A93.1
paratyphoid A01.4
  A A01.1
  B A01.2
  C A01.3
parrot A70
periodic (Mediterranean) M04.1
persistent (of unknown origin) R50.9
petechial A39.0
pharyngoconjunctival B30.2
Philippine hemorrhagic A91
phlebotomus A93.1
Piry (virus) A93.8
Pixuna (viral) A92.8
Plasmodium ovale B53.0
polioviral (nonparalytic) A80.4
Pontiac A48.2
postimmunization R50.83
postoperative R50.82
  due to infection T81.40 ☑
posttransfusion R50.84
postvaccination R50.83
presenting with conditions classified elsewhere R50.81
pretibial A27.89
puerperal O86.4
Q A78
quadrilateral A78
quartan (malaria) B52.9
Queensland (coastal) (tick) A77.3
quintan A79.0
rabbit — *see* Tularemia
rat-bite A25.9
  due to
    Spirillum A25.0
    Streptobacillus moniliformis A25.1
recurrent — *see* Fever, relapsing
relapsing (Borrelia) A68.9
  Carter's (Asiatic) A68.1
  Dutton's (West African) A68.1
  Koch's A68.9
  louse-borne A68.0
  Novy's
    louse-borne A68.0
    tick-borne A68.1
  Obermeyer's (European) A68.0
  tick-borne A68.1
remittent (bilious) (congestive) (gastric) — *see* Malaria
rheumatic (active) (acute) (chronic) (subacute) I00
  with central nervous system involvement I02.9
  active with heart involvement — *see* category I01 ☑
  inactive or quiescent with
    cardiac hypertrophy I09.89
    carditis I09.9
    endocarditis I09.1
      aortic (valve) I06.9
        with mitral (valve) disease I08.0
      mitral (valve) I05.9
        with aortic (valve) disease I08.0
      pulmonary (valve) I09.89
      tricuspid (valve) I07.8
    heart disease NEC I09.89
    heart failure (congestive) (conditions in category
      I50.) I09.81

Fever — *continued*
  rheumatic — *continued*
    inactive or quiescent with — *continued*
      left ventricular failure (conditions in I50.1- I50.4-)
        I09.81
      myocarditis, myocardial degeneration (condi-
        tions in I51.4) I09.0
      pancarditis I09.9
      pericarditis I09.2
Rift Valley (viral) A92.4
Rocky Mountain spotted A77.0
rose J30.1
Ross River B33.1
Russian hemorrhagic A98.5
San Joaquin (Valley) B38.0
sandfly A93.1
Sao Paulo A77.0
scarlet A38.9
seven day (leptospirosis) (autumnal) (Japanese) A27.89
  dengue A90
shin-bone A79.0
Singapore hemorrhagic A91
solar A90
Songo A98.5
sore B00.1
South African tick-bite A68.1
Southeast Asia hemorrhagic A91
spinal — *see* Meningitis
spirillary A25.0
splenic — *see* Anthrax
spotted A77.9
  American A77.0
  Brazilian A77.0
  cerebrospinal meningitis A39.0
  Colombian A77.0
  due to Rickettsia
    australis A77.3
    conorii A77.1
    rickettsii A77.0
    sibirica A77.2
    specified type NEC A77.8
  Ehrlichiosis A77.40
    due to
      E. chafeensis A77.41
      specified organism NEC A77.49
  Rocky Mountain A77.0
steroid R50.2
streptobacillary A25.1
subtertian B50.9
Sumatran mite A75.3
sun A90
swamp A27.9
swine A02.8
sylvatic, yellow A95.0
Tahyna B33.8
tertian — *see* Malaria, tertian
Thailand hemorrhagic A91
thermic T67.01 ☑
three-day A93.1
tick
  American mountain A93.2
  Colorado A93.2
  Kemerovo A93.8
  Mediterranean A77.1
  mountain A93.2
  nonexanthematous A93.2
  Quaranfil A93.8
tick-bite NEC A93.8
tick-borne (hemorrhagic) NEC A93.8
trench A79.0
tsutsugamushi A75.3
typhogastric A01.00
typhoid (abortive) (hemorrhagic) (intermittent) (malig-
    nant) A01.00
  complicated by
    arthritis A01.04
    heart involvement A01.02
    meningitis A01.01
    osteomyelitis A01.05
    pneumonia A01.03
    specified NEC A01.09
typhomalarial — *see* Malaria
typhus — *see* Typhus (fever)
undulant — *see* Brucellosis
unknown origin R50.9
uveoparotid D86.89
valley B38.0
Venezuelan equine A92.2

Fever — *continued*
  vesicular stomatitis A93.8
  viral hemorrhagic — *see* Fever, hemorrhagic, by type
    of virus
  Volhynian A79.0
  Wesselsbron (viral) A92.8
  West
    African B50.8
    Nile (viral) A92.30
      with
        complications NEC A92.39
        cranial nerve disorders A92.32
        encephalitis A92.31
        encephalomyelitis A92.31
        neurologic manifestation NEC A92.32
        optic neuritis A92.32
        polyradiculitis A92.32
  Whitmore's — *see* Melioidosis
  Wolhynian A79.0
  worm B83.9
  yellow A95.9
    jungle A95.0
    sylvatic A95.0
    urban A95.1
  Zika virus A92.5
Fibrillation
  atrial or auricular (established) I48.91
    chronic I48.20
      persistent I48.19
    paroxysmal I48.0
    permanent I48.21
    persistent (chronic) (NOS) (other) I48.19
      longstanding I48.11
  cardiac I49.8
  heart I49.8
  muscular M62.89
  ventricular I49.01
Fibrin
  ball or bodies, pleural (sac) J94.1
  chamber, anterior (eye) (gelatinous exudate) — *see*
    Iridocyclitis, acute
Fibrinogenolysis — *see* Fibrinolysis
Fibrinogenopenia D68.8
  acquired D65
  congenital D68.2
Fibrinolysis (hemorrhagic) (acquired) D65
  antepartum hemorrhage — *see* Hemorrhage, antepar-
    tum, with coagulation defect
  following
    abortion — *see* Abortion by type complicated by
      hemorrhage
    ectopic or molar pregnancy O08.1
  intrapartum O67.0
  newborn, transient P60
  postpartum O72.3
Fibrinopenia (hereditary) D68.2
  acquired D68.4
Fibrinopurulent — *see* condition
Fibrinous — *see* condition
Fibroadenoma
  cellular intracanalicular D24- ☑
  giant D24- ☑
  intracanalicular
    cellular D24- ☑
    giant D24- ☑
    specified site — *see* Neoplasm, benign, by site
    unspecified site D24- ☑
  juvenile D24- ☑
  pericanalicular
    specified site — *see* Neoplasm, benign, by site
    unspecified site D24- ☑
  phyllodes D24- ☑
  prostate D29.1
  specified site NEC — *see* Neoplasm, benign, by site
  unspecified site D24- ☑
Fibroadenosis, breast (chronic) (cystic) (diffuse) (period-
    ic) (segmental) N60.2- ☑
Fibroangioma — *see also* Neoplasm, benign, by site
  juvenile
    specified site — *see* Neoplasm, benign, by site
    unspecified site D10.6
Fibrochondrosarcoma — *see* Neoplasm, cartilage, ma-
    lignant
Fibrocystic
  disease — *see also* Fibrosis, cystic
    breast — *see* Mastopathy, cystic
    jaw M27.49
    kidney (congenital) Q61.8

Fibrocystic — *continued*
  disease — *see also* Fibrosis, cystic — *continued*
    liver Q44.6
    pancreas E84.9
    kidney (congenital) Q61.8
Fibrodysplasia ossificans progressiva — *see* Myositis, ossificans, progressiva
Fibroelastosis (cordis) (endocardial) (endomyocardial) I42.4
Fibroid (tumor) — *see also* Neoplasm, connective tissue, benign
  disease, lung (chronic) — *see* Fibrosis, lung
  heart (disease) — *see* Myocarditis
  in pregnancy or childbirth O34.1- ☑
    causing obstructed labor O65.5
  induration, lung (chronic) — *see* Fibrosis, lung
  lung — *see* Fibrosis, lung
  pneumonia (chronic) — *see* Fibrosis, lung
  uterus — *see also* Leiomyoma, uterus D25.9
Fibrolipoma — *see* Lipoma
Fibroliposarcoma — *see* Neoplasm, connective tissue, malignant
Fibroma — *see also* Neoplasm, connective tissue, benign
  ameloblastic — *see* Cyst, calcifying odontogenic
  bone (nonossifying) — *see* Disorder, bone, specified type NEC
    ossifying — *see* Neoplasm, bone, benign
  cementifying — *see* Neoplasm, bone, benign
  chondromyxoid — *see* Neoplasm, bone, benign
  desmoplastic — *see* Neoplasm, connective tissue, uncertain behavior
  durum — *see* Neoplasm, connective tissue, benign
  fascial — *see* Neoplasm, connective tissue, benign
  invasive — *see* Neoplasm, connective tissue, uncertain behavior
  molle — *see* Lipoma
  myxoid — *see* Neoplasm, connective tissue, benign
  nasopharynx, nasopharyngeal (juvenile) D10.6
  nonosteogenic (nonossifying) — *see* Dysplasia, fibrous
  odontogenic (central) — *see* Cyst, calcifying odontogenic
  ossifying — *see* Neoplasm, bone, benign
  periosteal — *see* Neoplasm, bone, benign
  soft — *see* Lipoma
Fibromatosis M72.9
  abdominal — *see* Neoplasm, connective tissue, uncertain behavior
  aggressive — *see* Neoplasm, connective tissue, uncertain behavior
  congenital generalized — *see* Neoplasm, connective tissue, uncertain behavior
  Dupuytren's M72.0
  gingival K06.1
  palmar (fascial) M72.0
  plantar (fascial) M72.2
  pseudosarcomatous (proliferative) (subcutaneous) M72.4
  retroperitoneal D48.3
  specified NEC M72.8
Fibromyalgia M79.7
Fibromyoma — *see also* Neoplasm, connective tissue, benign
  uterus (corpus) — *see also* Leiomyoma, uterus
    in pregnancy or childbirth — *see* Fibroid, in pregnancy or childbirth
    causing obstructed labor O65.5
Fibromyositis M79.7
Fibromyxolipoma D17.9
Fibromyxoma — *see* Neoplasm, connective tissue, benign
Fibromyxosarcoma — *see* Neoplasm, connective tissue, malignant
Fibro-odontoma, ameloblastic — *see* Cyst, calcifying odontogenic
Fibro-osteoma — *see* Neoplasm, bone, benign
Fibroplasia, retrolental H35.17- ☑
Fibropurulent — *see* condition
Fibrosarcoma — *see also* Neoplasm, connective tissue, malignant
  ameloblastic C41.1
    upper jaw (bone) C41.0
  congenital — *see* Neoplasm, connective tissue, malignant
  fascial — *see* Neoplasm, connective tissue, malignant
  infantile — *see* Neoplasm, connective tissue, malignant
  odontogenic C41.1
    upper jaw (bone) C41.0

Fibrosarcoma — *continued*
  periosteal — *see* Neoplasm, bone, malignant
Fibrosclerosis
  breast N60.3- ☑
  multifocal M35.5
  penis (corpora cavernosa) N48.6
Fibrosis, fibrotic
  adrenal (gland) E27.8
  amnion O41.8X- ☑
  anal papillae K62.89
  arteriocapillary — *see* Arteriosclerosis
  bladder N32.89
    interstitial — *see* Cystitis, chronic, interstitial
    localized submucosal — *see* Cystitis, chronic, interstitial
    panmural — *see* Cystitis, chronic, interstitial
  breast — *see* Fibrosclerosis, breast
  capillary — *see also* Arteriosclerosis I70.90
    lung (chronic) — *see* Fibrosis, lung
  cardiac — *see* Myocarditis
  cervix N88.8
  chorion O41.8X- ☑
  corpus cavernosum (sclerosing) N48.6
  cystic (of pancreas) E84.9
    with
      distal intestinal obstruction syndrome E84.19
      fecal impaction E84.19
      intestinal manifestations NEC E84.19
      pulmonary manifestations E84.0
      specified manifestations NEC E84.8
  due to device, implant or graft — *see also* Complications, by site and type, specified NEC T85.828 ☑
    arterial graft NEC T82.828 ☑
    breast (implant) T85.828 ☑
    catheter NEC T85.828 ☑
      dialysis (renal) T82.828 ☑
        intraperitoneal T85.828 ☑
      infusion NEC T82.828 ☑
        spinal (epidural) (subdural) T85.820 ☑
      urinary (indwelling) T83.82 ☑
    electronic (electrode) (pulse generator) (stimulator)
      bone T84.82 ☑
      cardiac T82.827 ☑
      nervous system (brain) (peripheral nerve) (spinal) T85.820 ☑
      urinary T83.82 ☑
    fixation, internal (orthopedic) NEC T84.82 ☑
    gastrointestinal (bile duct) (esophagus) T85.828 ☑
    genital NEC T83.82 ☑
    heart NEC T82.827 ☑
    joint prosthesis T84.82 ☑
    ocular (corneal graft) (orbital implant) NEC T85.828 ☑
    orthopedic NEC T84.82 ☑
    specified NEC T85.828 ☑
    urinary NEC T83.82 ☑
    vascular NEC T82.828 ☑
    ventricular intracranial shunt T85.820 ☑
  ejaculatory duct N50.89
  endocardium — *see* Endocarditis
  endomyocardial (tropical) I42.3
  epididymis N50.89
  eye muscle — *see* Strabismus, mechanical
  heart — *see* Myocarditis
  hepatic — *see* Fibrosis, liver
  hepatolienal (portal hypertension) K76.6
  hepatosplenic (portal hypertension) K76.6
  infrapatellar fat pad M79.4
  intrascrotal N50.89
  kidney N26.9
  liver K74.0
    with sclerosis K74.2
    alcoholic K70.2
  lung (atrophic) (chronic) (confluent) (massive) (perialveolar) (peribronchial) J84.10
    with
      anthracosilicosis J60
      anthracosis J60
      asbestosis J61
      bagassosis J67.1
      bauxite J63.1
      berylliosis J63.2
      byssinosis J66.0
      calcicosis J62.8
      chalicosis J62.8
      dust reticulation J64
      farmer's lung J67.0

Fibrosis, fibrotic — *continued*
  lung — *continued*
    with — *continued*
      ganister disease J62.8
      graphite J63.3
      pneumoconiosis NOS J64
      siderosis J63.4
      silicosis J62.8
    capillary J84.10
    congenital P27.8
    diffuse (idiopathic) J84.10
      chemicals, gases, fumes or vapors (inhalation) J68.4
      interstitial J84.10
        acute J84.114
      talc J62.0
    following radiation J70.1
    idiopathic J84.112
    postinflammatory J84.10
    silicotic J62.8
    tuberculous — *see* Tuberculosis, pulmonary
  lymphatic gland I89.8
  median bar — *see* Hyperplasia, prostate
  mediastinum (idiopathic) J98.59
  meninges G96.19
  myocardium, myocardial — *see* Myocarditis
  ovary N83.8
  oviduct N83.8
  pancreas K86.89
  penis NEC N48.6
  pericardium I31.0
  perineum, in pregnancy or childbirth O34.7- ☑
    causing obstructed labor O65.5
  pleura J94.1
  popliteal fat pad M79.4
  prostate (chronic) — *see* Hyperplasia, prostate
  pulmonary — *see also* Fibrosis, lung J84.10
    congenital P27.8
    idiopathic J84.112
  rectal sphincter K62.89
  retroperitoneal, idiopathic (with ureteral obstruction) N13.5
    with infection N13.6
  sclerosing mesenteric (idiopathic) K65.4
  scrotum N50.89
  seminal vesicle N50.89
  senile R54
  skin L90.5
  spermatic cord N50.89
  spleen D73.89
    in schistosomiasis (bilharziasis) B65.9 *[D77]*
  subepidermal nodular — *see* Neoplasm, skin, benign
  submucous (oral) (tongue) K13.5
  testis N44.8
    chronic, due to syphilis A52.76
  thymus (gland) E32.8
  tongue, submucous K13.5
  tunica vaginalis N50.89
  uterus (non-neoplastic) N85.8
  vagina N89.8
  valve, heart — *see* Endocarditis
  vas deferens N50.89
  vein I87.8
Fibrositis (periarticular) M79.7
  nodular, chronic (Jaccoud's) (rheumatoid) — *see* Arthropathy, postrheumatic, chronic
Fibrothorax J94.1
Fibrotic — *see* Fibrosis
Fibrous — *see* condition
Fibroxanthoma — *see also* Neoplasm, connective tissue, benign
  atypical — *see* Neoplasm, connective tissue, uncertain behavior
  malignant — *see* Neoplasm, connective tissue, malignant
Fibroxanthosarcoma — *see* Neoplasm, connective tissue, malignant
Fiedler's
  disease (icterohemorrhagic leptospirosis) A27.0
  myocarditis (acute) I40.1
Fifth disease B08.3
  venereal A55
Filaria, filarial, filariasis — *see* Infestation, filarial
Filatov's disease — *see* Mononucleosis, infectious
File-cutter's disease — *see* Poisoning, lead
Filling defect
  biliary tract R93.2
  bladder R93.41

Filling defect — *continued*
duodenum R93.3
gallbladder R93.2
gastrointestinal tract R93.3
intestine R93.3
kidney R93.42- ☑
stomach R93.3
ureter R93.41
urinary organs, specified NEC R93.49
Fimbrial cyst Q50.4
Financial problem affecting care NOS Z59.9
bankruptcy Z59.8
foreclosure on loan Z59.8
Findings, abnormal, inconclusive, without diagnosis
— *see also* Abnormal
17-ketosteroids, elevated R82.5
acetonuria R82.4
alcohol in blood R78.0
anisocytosis R71.8
antenatal screening of mother O28.9
biochemical O28.1
chromosomal O28.5
cytological O28.2
genetic O28.5
hematological O28.0
radiological O28.4
specified NEC O28.8
ultrasonic O28.3
antibody titer, elevated R76.0
anticardiolipin antibody R76.0
antiphosphatidylglycerol antibody R76.0
antiphosphatidylinositol antibody R76.0
antiphosphatidylserine antibody R76.0
antiphospholipid antibody R76.0
bacteriuria R82.71
bicarbonate E87.8
bile in urine R82.2
blood sugar R73.09
high R73.9
low (transient) E16.2
body fluid or substance, specified NEC R88.8
casts, urine R82.998
catecholamines R82.5
cells, urine R82.998
chloride E87.8
cholesterol E78.9
high E78.00
with high triglycerides E78.2
chyluria R82.0
cloudy
dialysis effluent R88.0
urine R82.90
creatinine clearance R94.4
crystals, urine R82.998
culture
blood R78.81
positive — *see* Positive, culture
echocardiogram R93.1
electrolyte level, urinary R82.998
function study NEC R94.8
bladder R94.8
endocrine NEC R94.7
thyroid R94.6
kidney R94.4
liver R94.5
pancreas R94.8
placenta R94.8
pulmonary R94.2
spleen R94.8
gallbladder, nonvisualization R93.2
glucose (tolerance test) (non-fasting) R73.09
glycosuria R81
heart
shadow R93.1
sounds R01.2
hematinuria R82.3
hematocrit drop (precipitous) R71.0
hemoglobinuria R82.3
human papillomavirus (HPV) DNA test positive
cervix
high risk R87.810
low risk R87.820
vagina
high risk R87.811
low risk R87.821
in blood (of substance not normally found in blood)
R78.9
addictive drug NEC R78.4
alcohol (excessive level) R78.0

Findings, abnormal, inconclusive, without diagnosis
— *continued*
in blood — *continued*
cocaine R78.2
hallucinogen R78.3
heavy metals (abnormal level) R78.79
lead R78.71
lithium (abnormal level) R78.89
opiate drug R78.1
psychotropic drug R78.5
specified substance NEC R78.89
steroid agent R78.6
indoleacetic acid, elevated R82.5
ketonuria R82.4
lactic acid dehydrogenase (LDH) R74.0
liver function test R79.89
mammogram NEC R92.8
calcification (calculus) R92.1
inconclusive result (due to dense breasts) R92.2
microcalcification R92.0
mediastinal shift R93.89
melanin, urine R82.998
myoglobinuria R82.1
neonatal screening P09
nonvisualization of gallbladder R93.2
odor of urine NOS R82.90
Papanicolaou cervix R87.619
non-atypical endometrial cells R87.618
pneumoencephalogram R93.0
poikilocytosis R71.8
potassium (deficiency) E87.6
excess E87.5
PPD R76.11
radiologic (X-ray) R93.89
abdomen R93.5
biliary tract R93.2
breast R92.8
gastrointestinal tract R93.3
genitourinary organs R93.89
head R93.0
inconclusive due to excess body fat of patient R93.9
intrathoracic organs NEC R93.1
musculoskeletal
limbs R93.6
other than limb R93.7
placenta R93.89
retroperitoneum R93.5
skin R93.89
skull R93.0
subcutaneous tissue R93.89
testis R93.81- ☑
red blood cell (count) (morphology) (sickling) (volume)
R71.8
scan NEC R94.8
bladder R94.8
bone R94.8
kidney R94.4
liver R93.2
lung R94.2
pancreas R94.8
placental R94.8
spleen R94.8
thyroid R94.6
sedimentation rate, elevated R70.0
SGOT R74.0
SGPT R74.0
sodium (deficiency) E87.1
excess E87.0
specified body fluid NEC R88.8
stress test R94.39
testis R93.81- ☑
thyroid (function) (metabolic rate) (scan) (uptake) R94.6
transaminase (level) R74.0
triglycerides E78.9
high E78.1
with high cholesterol E78.2
tuberculin skin test (without active tuberculosis) R76.11
urine R82.90
acetone R82.4
bacteria R82.71
bile R82.2
casts or cells R82.998
chyle R82.0
culture positive R82.79
glucose R81
hemoglobin R82.3
ketone R82.4
sugar R81
vanillylmandelic acid (VMA), elevated R82.5

Findings, abnormal, inconclusive, without diagnosis
— *continued*
vectorcardiogram (VCG) R94.39
ventriculogram R93.0
white blood cell (count) (differential) (morphology)
D72.9
xerography R92.8
Finger — *see* condition
Fire, Saint Anthony's — *see* Erysipelas
Fire-setting
pathological (compulsive) F63.1
Fish hook stomach K31.89
Fishmeal-worker's lung J67.8
Fissure, fissured
anus, anal K60.2
acute K60.0
chronic K60.1
congenital Q43.8
ear, lobule, congenital Q17.8
epiglottis (congenital) Q31.8
larynx J38.7
congenital Q31.8
lip K13.0
congenital — *see* Cleft, lip
nipple N64.0
associated with
lactation O92.13
pregnancy O92.11- ☑
puerperium O92.12
nose Q30.2
palate (congenital) — *see* Cleft, palate
skin R23.4
spine (congenital) — *see also* Spina bifida
with hydrocephalus — *see* Spina bifida, by site, with
hydrocephalus
tongue (acquired) K14.5
congenital Q38.3
Fistula (cutaneous) L98.8
abdomen (wall) K63.2
bladder N32.2
intestine NEC K63.2
ureter N28.89
uterus N82.5
abdominorectal K63.2
abdominosigmoidal K63.2
abdominothoracic J86.0
abdominouterine N82.5
congenital Q51.7
abdominovesical N32.2
accessory sinuses — *see* Sinusitis
actinomycotic — *see* Actinomycosis
alveolar antrum — *see* Sinusitis, maxillary
alveolar process K04.6
anorectal K60.5
antrobuccal — *see* Sinusitis, maxillary
antrum — *see* Sinusitis, maxillary
anus, anal (recurrent) (infectional) K60.3
congenital Q43.6
with absence, atresia and stenosis Q42.2
tuberculous A18.32
aorta-duodenal I77.2
appendix, appendicular K38.3
arteriovenous (acquired) (nonruptured) I77.0
brain I67.1
congenital Q28.2
ruptured — *see* Fistula, arteriovenous, brain,
ruptured
ruptured I60.8
intracerebral I61.8
intraparenchymal I61.8
intraventricular I61.5
subarachnoid I60.8
cerebral — *see* Fistula, arteriovenous, brain
congenital (peripheral) — *see also* Malformation,
arteriovenous
brain Q28.2
ruptured — *see* Fistula, arteriovenous, brain,
ruptured
coronary Q24.5
pulmonary Q25.72
coronary I25.41
congenital Q24.5
pulmonary I28.0
congenital Q25.72
surgically created (for dialysis) Z99.2
complication — *see* Complication, arteriovenous,
fistula, surgically created
traumatic — *see* Injury, blood vessel

☑ **Additional Character Required** — Refer to the Tabular List for Character Selection   ☜ Subterms under main terms may continue to next column or page

Fistula — *continued*
artery I77.2
aural (mastoid) — *see* Mastoiditis, chronic
auricle — *see also* Disorder, pinna, specified type NEC
    congenital Q18.1
Bartholin's gland N82.8
bile duct (common) (hepatic) K83.3
    with calculus, stones — *see* Calculus, bile duct
biliary (tract) — *see* Fistula, bile duct
bladder (sphincter) NEC — *see also* Fistula, vesico-
    N32.2
    into seminal vesicle N32.2
bone — *see also* Disorder, bone, specified type NEC
    with osteomyelitis, chronic — *see* Osteomyelitis,
        chronic, with draining sinus
brain G93.89
    arteriovenous (acquired) — *see also* Fistula, arteri-
        ovenous, brain I67.1
    congenital Q28.2
branchial (cleft) Q18.0
branchiogenous Q18.0
breast N61.0
    puerperal, postpartum or gestational, due to mastitis
        (purulent) — *see* Mastitis, obstetric, purulent
bronchial J86.0
bronchocutaneous, bronchomediastinal, bronchopleu-
    ral, bronchopleuromediastinal (infective) J86.0
    tuberculous NEC A15.5
bronchoesophageal J86.0
    congenital Q39.2
        with atresia of esophagus Q39.1
bronchovisceral J86.0
buccal cavity (infective) K12.2
cecosigmoidal K63.2
cecum K63.2
cerebrospinal (fluid) G96.0
cervical, lateral Q18.1
cervicoaural Q18.1
cervicosigmoidal N82.4
cervicovesical N82.1
cervix N82.8
chest (wall) J86.0
cholecystenteric — *see* Fistula, gallbladder
cholecystocolic — *see* Fistula, gallbladder
cholecystocolonic — *see* Fistula, gallbladder
cholecystoduodenal — *see* Fistula, gallbladder
cholecystogastric — *see* Fistula, gallbladder
cholecystointestinal — *see* Fistula, gallbladder
choledochoduodenal — *see* Fistula, bile duct
cholocolic K82.3
coccyx — *see* Sinus, pilonidal
colon K63.2
colostomy K94.09
colovesical N32.1
common duct — *see* Fistula, bile duct
congenital, site not listed — *see* Anomaly, by site
coronary, arteriovenous I25.41
    congenital Q24.5
costal region J86.0
cul-de-sac, Douglas' N82.8
cystic duct — *see also* Fistula, gallbladder
    congenital Q44.5
dental K04.6
diaphragm J86.0
duodenum K31.6
ear (external) (canal) — *see* Disorder, ear, external,
    specified type NEC
enterocolic K63.2
enterocutaneous K63.2
enterouterine N82.4
    congenital Q51.7
enterovaginal N82.4
    congenital Q52.2
    large intestine N82.3
    small intestine N82.2
enterovesical N32.1
epididymis N50.89
    tuberculous A18.15
esophagobronchial J86.0
    congenital Q39.2
        with atresia of esophagus Q39.1
esophagocutaneous K22.8
esophagopleural-cutaneous J86.0
esophagotracheal J86.0
    congenital Q39.2
        with atresia of esophagus Q39.1
esophagus K22.8
    congenital Q39.2

Fistula — *continued*
esophagus — *continued*
    congenital — *continued*
        with atresia of esophagus Q39.1
ethmoid — *see* Sinusitis, ethmoidal
eyeball (cornea) (sclera) — *see* Disorder, globe, hy-
    potony
eyelid H01.8
fallopian tube, external N82.5
fecal K63.2
    congenital Q43.6
from periapical abscess K04.6
frontal sinus — *see* Sinusitis, frontal
gallbladder K82.3
    with calculus, cholelithiasis, stones — *see* Calculus,
        gallbladder
gastric K31.6
gastrocolic K31.6
    congenital Q40.2
    tuberculous A18.32
gastroenterocolic K31.6
gastroesophageal K31.6
gastrojejunal K31.6
gastrojejunocolic K31.6
genital tract (female) N82.9
    specified NEC N82.8
    to intestine NEC N82.4
    to skin N82.5
hepatic artery-portal vein, congenital Q26.6
hepatopleural J86.0
hepatopulmonary J86.0
ileorectal or ileosigmoidal K63.2
ileovaginal N82.2
ileovesical N32.1
ileum K63.2
in ano K60.3
    tuberculous A18.32
inner ear (labyrinth) — *see* subcategory H83.1 ☑
intestine NEC K63.2
intestinocolonic (abdominal) K63.2
intestinoureteral N28.89
intestinouterine N82.4
intestinovaginal N82.4
    large intestine N82.3
    small intestine N82.2
intestinovesical N32.1
ischiorectal (fossa) K61.39
jejunum K63.2
joint M25.10
    ankle M25.17- ☑
    elbow M25.12- ☑
    foot joint M25.17- ☑
    hand joint M25.14- ☑
    hip M25.15- ☑
    knee M25.16- ☑
    shoulder M25.11- ☑
    specified joint NEC M25.18
    tuberculous — *see* Tuberculosis, joint
    vertebrae M25.18
    wrist M25.13- ☑
kidney N28.89
labium (majus) (minus) N82.8
labyrinth — *see* subcategory H83.1 ☑
lacrimal (gland) (sac) H04.61- ☑
lacrimonasal duct — *see* Fistula, lacrimal
laryngotracheal, congenital Q34.8
larynx J38.7
lip K13.0
    congenital Q38.0
lumbar, tuberculous A18.01
lung J86.0
lymphatic I89.8
mammary (gland) N61.0
mastoid (process) (region) — *see* Mastoiditis, chronic
maxillary J32.0
medial, face and neck Q18.8
mediastinal J86.0
mediastinobronchial J86.0
mediastinocutaneous J86.0
middle ear — *see* subcategory H74.8 ☑
mouth K12.2
nasal J34.89
    sinus — *see* Sinusitis
nasopharynx J39.2
nipple N64.0
nose J34.89
oral (cutaneous) K12.2
    maxillary J32.0

Fistula — *continued*
oral — *continued*
    nasal (with cleft palate) — *see* Cleft, palate
orbit, orbital — *see* Disorder, orbit, specified type NEC
oroantral J32.0
oviduct, external N82.5
palate (hard) M27.8
pancreatic K86.89
pancreaticoduodenal K86.89
parotid (gland) K11.4
    region K12.2
penis N48.89
perianal K60.3
pericardium (pleura) (sac) — *see* Pericarditis
pericecal K63.2
perineorectal K60.4
perineosigmoidal K63.2
perineum, perineal (with urethral involvement) NEC
    N36.0
    tuberculous A18.13
    ureter N28.89
perirectal K60.4
    tuberculous A18.32
peritoneum K65.9
pharyngoesophageal J39.2
pharynx J39.2
    branchial cleft (congenital) Q18.0
pilonidal (infected) (rectum) — *see* Sinus, pilonidal
pleura, pleural, pleurocutaneous, pleuroperitoneal
    J86.0
    tuberculous NEC A15.6
pleuropericardial I31.8
portal vein-hepatic artery, congenital Q26.6
postauricular H70.81- ☑
postoperative, persistent T81.83 ☑
    specified site — *see* Fistula, by site
preauricular (congenital) Q18.1
prostate N42.89
pulmonary J86.0
    arteriovenous I28.0
        congenital Q25.72
    tuberculous — *see* Tuberculosis, pulmonary
pulmonoperitoneal J86.0
rectolabial N82.4
rectosigmoid (intercommunicating) K63.2
rectoureteral N28.89
rectourethral N36.0
    congenital Q64.73
rectouterine N82.4
    congenital Q51.7
rectovaginal N82.3
    congenital Q52.2
    tuberculous A18.18
rectovesical N32.1
    congenital Q64.79
rectovesicovaginal N82.3
rectovulval N82.4
    congenital Q52.79
rectum (to skin) K60.4
    congenital Q43.6
        with absence, atresia and stenosis Q42.0
    tuberculous A18.32
renal N28.89
retroauricular — *see* Fistula, postauricular
salivary duct or gland (any) K11.4
    congenital Q38.4
scrotum (urinary) N50.89
    tuberculous A18.15
semicircular canals — *see* subcategory H83.1 ☑
sigmoid K63.2
    to bladder N32.1
sinus — *see* Sinusitis
skin L98.8
    to genital tract (female) N82.5
splenocolic D73.89
stercoral K63.2
stomach K31.6
sublingual gland K11.4
submandibular gland K11.4
submaxillary (gland) K11.4
    region K12.2
thoracic J86.0
    duct I89.8
thoracoabdominal J86.0
thoracogastric J86.0
thoracointestinal J86.0
thorax J86.0
thyroglossal duct Q89.2

Fistula — *continued*
 thyroid E07.89
 trachea, congenital (external) (internal) Q32.1
 tracheoesophageal J86.0
  congenital Q39.2
   with atresia of esophagus Q39.1
  following tracheostomy J95.04
 traumatic arteriovenous — *see* Injury, blood vessel, by
   site
 tuberculous — *code by* site under Tuberculosis
 typhoid A01.09
 umbilicourinary Q64.8
 urachus, congenital Q64.4
 ureter (persistent) N28.89
 ureteroabdominal N28.89
 ureterorectal N28.89
 ureterosigmoido-abdominal N28.89
 ureterovaginal N82.1
 ureterovesical N32.2
 urethra N36.0
  congenital Q64.79
  tuberculous A18.13
 urethroperineal N36.0
 urethroperineovesical N32.2
 urethrorectal N36.0
  congenital Q64.73
 urethroscrotal N50.89
 urethrovaginal N82.1
 urethrovesical N32.2
 urinary (tract) (persistent) (recurrent) N36.0
 uteroabdominal N82.5
  congenital Q51.7
 uteroenteric, uterointestinal N82.4
  congenital Q51.7
 uterorectal N82.4
  congenital Q51.7
 uteroureteric N82.1
 uterourethral Q51.7
 uterovaginal N82.8
 uterovesical N82.1
  congenital Q51.7
 uterus N82.8
 vagina (postpartal) (wall) N82.8
 vaginocutaneous (postpartal) N82.5
 vaginointestinal NEC N82.4
  large intestine N82.3
  small intestine N82.2
 vaginoperineal N82.5
 vasocutaneous, congenital Q55.7
 vesical NEC N32.2
 vesicoabdominal N32.2
 vesicocervicovaginal N82.1
 vesicocolic N32.1
 vesicocutaneous N32.2
 vesicoenteric N32.1
 vesicointestinal N32.1
 vesicometrorectal N82.4
 vesicoperineal N32.2
 vesicorectal N32.1
  congenital Q64.79
 vesicosigmoidal N32.1
 vesicosigmoidovaginal N82.3
 vesicoureteral N32.2
 vesicoureterovaginal N82.1
 vesicourethral N32.2
 vesicourethrorectal N32.1
 vesicouterine N82.1
  congenital Q51.7
 vesicovaginal N82.0
 vulvorectal N82.4
  congenital Q52.79
Fit R56.9
 epileptic — *see* Epilepsy
 fainting R55
 hysterical F44.5
 newborn P90
Fitting (and adjustment) (of)
 artificial
  arm — *see* Admission, adjustment, artificial, arm
  breast Z44.3 ☑
  eye Z44.2 ☑
  leg — *see* Admission, adjustment, artificial, leg
 automatic implantable cardiac defibrillator (with synchronous cardiac pacemaker) Z45.02
 brain neuropacemaker Z46.2
  implanted Z45.42
 cardiac defibrillator — *see* Fitting (and adjustment)
   (of), automatic implantable cardiac defibrillator

Fitting — *continued*
 catheter, non-vascular Z46.82
 colostomy belt Z46.89
 contact lenses Z46.0
 CRT-D (resynchronization therapy defibrillator) Z45.02
 CRT-P (cardiac resynchronization therapy pacemaker)
   Z45.018
  pulse generator Z45.010
 cystostomy device Z46.6
 defibrillator, cardiac — *see* Fitting (and adjustment)
   (of), automatic implantable cardiac defibrillator
 dentures Z46.3
 device NOS Z46.9
  abdominal Z46.89
  gastrointestinal NEC Z46.59
  implanted NEC Z45.89
  nervous system Z46.2
   implanted — *see* Admission, adjustment, device,
     implanted, nervous system
  orthodontic Z46.4
  orthoptic Z46.0
  orthotic Z46.89
  prosthetic (external) Z44.9
   breast Z44.3 ☑
   dental Z46.3
   eye Z44.2 ☑
   specified NEC Z44.8
  specified NEC Z46.89
  substitution
   auditory Z46.2
    implanted — *see* Admission, adjustment,
      device, implanted, hearing device
   nervous system Z46.2
    implanted — *see* Admission, adjustment,
      device, implanted, nervous system
   visual Z46.2
    implanted Z45.31
  urinary Z46.6
 gastric lap band Z46.51
 gastrointestinal appliance NEC Z46.59
 glasses (reading) Z46.0
 hearing aid Z46.1
 ileostomy device Z46.89
 insulin pump Z46.81
 intestinal appliance NEC Z46.89
 myringotomy device (stent) (tube) Z45.82
 neuropacemaker Z46.2
  implanted Z45.42
 non-vascular catheter Z46.82
 orthodontic device Z46.4
 orthopedic device (brace) (cast) (corset) (shoes) Z46.89
 pacemaker (cardiac) (cardiac resynchronization therapy
   (CRT-P)) Z45.018
  nervous system (brain) (peripheral nerve) (spinal
    cord) Z46.2
   implanted Z45.42
  pulse generator Z45.010
 portacath (port-a-cath) Z45.2
 prosthesis (external) Z44.9
  arm — *see* Admission, adjustment, artificial, arm
  breast Z44.3 ☑
  dental Z46.3
  eye Z44.2 ☑
  leg — *see* Admission, adjustment, artificial, leg
  specified NEC Z44.8
 spectacles Z46.0
 wheelchair Z46.89
Fitzhugh-Curtis syndrome
 due to
  Chlamydia trachomatis A74.81
  Neisseria gonorrhorea (gonococcal peritonitis)
    A54.85
Fitz's syndrome (acute hemorrhagic pancreatitis) — *see
 also* Pancreatitis, acute K85.80
Fixation
 joint — *see* Ankylosis
 larynx J38.7
 stapes — *see* Ankylosis, ear ossicles
  deafness — *see* Deafness, conductive
 uterus (acquired) — *see* Malposition, uterus
 vocal cord J38.3
Flabby ridge K06.8
Flaccid — *see also* condition
 palate, congenital Q38.5
Flail
 chest S22.5 ☑
  newborn (birth injury) P13.8
 joint (paralytic) M25.20

Flail — *continued*
 joint — *continued*
  ankle M25.27- ☑
  elbow M25.22- ☑
  foot joint M25.27- ☑
  hand joint M25.24- ☑
  hip M25.25- ☑
  knee M25.26- ☑
  shoulder M25.21- ☑
  specified joint NEC M25.28
  wrist M25.23- ☑
Flajani's disease — *see* Hyperthyroidism, with, goiter
 (diffuse)
Flap, liver K71.3
Flashbacks (residual to hallucinogen use) F16.283
Flat
 chamber (eye) — *see* Disorder, globe, hypotony, flat
   anterior chamber
 chest, congenital Q67.8
 foot (acquired) (fixed type) (painful) (postural) — *see
   also* Deformity, limb, flat foot
  congenital (rigid) (spastic (everted)) Q66.5- ☑
  rachitic sequelae (late effect) E64.3
 organ or site, congenital NEC — *see* Anomaly, by site
 pelvis M95.5
  with disproportion (fetopelvic) O33.0
   causing obstructed labor O65.0
  congenital Q74.2
Flatau-Schilder disease G37.0
Flatback syndrome M40.30
 lumbar region M40.36
 lumbosacral region M40.37
 thoracolumbar region M40.35
Flattening
 head, femur M89.8X5
 hip — *see* Coxa, plana
 lip (congenital) Q18.8
 nose (congenital) Q67.4
  acquired M95.0
Flatulence R14.3
 psychogenic F45.8
Flatus R14.3
 vaginalis N89.8
Flax-dresser's disease J66.1
Flea bite — *see* Injury, bite, by site, superficial, insect
Flecks, glaucomatous (subcapsular) — *see* Cataract,
 complicated
Fleischer (-Kayser) **ring** (cornea) H18.04- ☑
Fleshy mole O02.0
Flexibilitas cerea — *see* Catalepsy
Flexion
 amputation stump (surgical) T87.89
 cervix — *see* Malposition, uterus
 contracture, joint — *see* Contraction, joint
 deformity, joint — *see also* Deformity, limb, flexion
   M21.20
  hip, congenital Q65.89
 uterus — *see also* Malposition, uterus
  lateral — *see* Lateroversion, uterus
Flexner-Boyd dysentery A03.2
Flexner's dysentery A03.1
Flexure — *see* Flexion
Flint murmur (aortic insufficiency) I35.1
Floater, vitreous — *see* Opacity, vitreous
Floating
 cartilage (joint) — *see also* Loose, body, joint
  knee — *see* Derangement, knee, loose body
 gallbladder, congenital Q44.1
 kidney N28.89
  congenital Q63.8
 spleen D73.89
Flooding N92.0
Floor — *see* condition
Floppy
 baby syndrome (nonspecific) P94.2
 iris syndrome (intraoperative) (IFIS) H21.81
 nonrheumatic mitral valve syndrome I34.1
Flu — *see also* Influenza
 avian — *see also* Influenza, due to, identified novel influenza A virus J09.X2
 bird — *see also* Influenza, due to, identified novel influenza A virus J09.X2
 intestinal NEC A08.4
 swine (viruses that normally cause infections in pigs)
   — *see also* Influenza, due to, identified novel
   influenza A virus J09.X2
Fluctuating blood pressure I99.8

Fluid
abdomen R18.8
chest J94.8
heart — *see* Failure, heart, congestive
joint — *see* Effusion, joint
loss (acute) E86.9
lung — *see* Edema, lung
overload E87.70
  specified NEC E87.79
peritoneal cavity R18.8
pleural cavity J94.8
retention R60.9
Flukes NEC — *see also* Infestation, fluke
blood NEC — *see* Schistosomiasis
liver B66.3
Fluor (vaginalis) N89.8
trichomonal or due to Trichomonas (vaginalis) A59.00
Fluorosis
dental K00.3
skeletal M85.10
  ankle M85.17-☑
  foot M85.17-☑
  forearm M85.13-☑
  hand M85.14-☑
  lower leg M85.16-☑
  multiple site M85.19
  neck M85.18
  rib M85.18
  shoulder M85.11-☑
  skull M85.18
  specified site NEC M85.18
  thigh M85.15-☑
  toe M85.17-☑
  upper arm M85.12-☑
  vertebra M85.18
Flush syndrome E34.0
Flushing R23.2
menopausal N95.1
Flutter
atrial or auricular I48.92
  atypical I48.4
  type I I48.3
  type II I48.4
  typical I48.3
heart I49.8
  atrial or auricular I48.92
    atypical I48.4
    type I I48.3
    type II I48.4
    typical I48.3
  ventricular I49.02
ventricular I49.02
FNHTR (febrile nonhemolytic transfusion reaction) R50.84
Fochier's abscess — *code by* site under Abscess
Focus, Assmann's — *see* Tuberculosis, pulmonary
Fogo selvagem L10.3
Foix-Alajouanine syndrome G95.19
Fold, folds (anomalous) — *see also* Anomaly, by site
Descemet's membrane — *see* Change, corneal membrane, Descemet's, fold
epicanthic Q10.3
heart Q24.8
Folie à deux F24
Follicle
cervix (nabothian) (ruptured) N88.8
graafian, ruptured, with hemorrhage N83.0-☑
nabothian N88.8
Follicular — *see* condition
Folliculitis (superficial) L73.9
abscedens et suffodiens L66.3
cyst N83.0-☑
decalvans L66.2
deep — *see* Furuncle, by site
gonococcal (acute) (chronic) A54.01
keloid, keloidalis L73.0
pustular L01.02
ulerythematosa reticulata L66.4
Folliculome lipidique
specified site — *see* Neoplasm, benign, by site
unspecified site
  female D27.9
  male D29.20
Følling's disease E70.0
Follow-up — *see* Examination, follow-up
Fong's syndrome (hereditary osteo-onychodysplasia) Q87.2

Food
allergy L27.2
asphyxia (from aspiration or inhalation) — *see* Foreign body, by site
choked on — *see* Foreign body, by site
deprivation T73.0☑
  specified kind of food NEC E63.8
intoxication — *see* Poisoning, food
lack of T73.0☑
poisoning — *see* Poisoning, food
rejection NEC — *see* Disorder, eating
strangulation or suffocation — *see* Foreign body, by site
toxemia — *see* Poisoning, food
Foot — *see* condition
Foramen ovale (nonclosure) (patent) (persistent) Q21.1
Forbes' glycogen storage disease E74.03
Fordyce-Fox disease L75.2
Fordyce's disease (mouth) Q38.6
Forearm — *see* condition
Foreign body
with
  laceration — *see* Laceration, by site, with foreign body
  puncture wound — *see* Puncture, by site, with foreign body
accidentally left following a procedure T81.509☑
  aspiration T81.506☑
    resulting in
      adhesions T81.516☑
      obstruction T81.526☑
      perforation T81.536☑
      specified complication NEC T81.596☑
  cardiac catheterization T81.505☑
    resulting in
      acute reaction T81.60☑
        aseptic peritonitis T81.61☑
          specified NEC T81.69☑
      adhesions T81.515☑
      obstruction T81.525☑
      perforation T81.535☑
      specified complication NEC T81.595☑
  causing
    acute reaction T81.60☑
      aseptic peritonitis T81.61☑
        specified complication NEC T81.69☑
    adhesions T81.519☑
    aseptic peritonitis T81.61☑
    obstruction T81.529☑
    perforation T81.539☑
    specified complication NEC T81.599☑
  endoscopy T81.504☑
    resulting in
      adhesions T81.514☑
      obstruction T81.524☑
      perforation T81.534☑
      specified complication NEC T81.594☑
  immunization T81.503☑
    resulting in
      adhesions T81.513☑
      obstruction T81.523☑
      perforation T81.533☑
      specified complication NEC T81.593☑
  infusion T81.501☑
    resulting in
      adhesions T81.511☑
      obstruction T81.521☑
      perforation T81.531☑
      specified complication NEC T81.591☑
  injection T81.503☑
    resulting in
      adhesions T81.513☑
      obstruction T81.523☑
      perforation T81.533☑
      specified complication NEC T81.593☑
  kidney dialysis T81.502☑
    resulting in
      adhesions T81.512☑
      obstruction T81.522☑
      perforation T81.532☑
      specified complication NEC T81.592☑
  packing removal T81.507☑
    resulting in
      acute reaction T81.60☑
        aseptic peritonitis T81.61☑
          specified NEC T81.69☑

Foreign body — *continued*
accidentally left following a procedure — *continued*
  packing removal — *continued*
    resulting in — *continued*
      adhesions T81.517☑
      obstruction T81.527☑
      perforation T81.537☑
      specified complication NEC T81.597☑
  puncture T81.506☑
    resulting in
      adhesions T81.516☑
      obstruction T81.526☑
      perforation T81.536☑
      specified complication NEC T81.596☑
  specified procedure NEC T81.508☑
    resulting in
      acute reaction T81.60☑
        aseptic peritonitis T81.61☑
          specified NEC T81.69☑
      adhesions T81.518☑
      obstruction T81.528☑
      perforation T81.538☑
      specified complication NEC T81.598☑
  surgical operation T81.500☑
    resulting in
      acute reaction T81.60☑
        aseptic peritonitis T81.61☑
          specified NEC T81.69☑
      adhesions T81.510☑
      obstruction T81.520☑
      perforation T81.530☑
      specified complication NEC T81.590☑
  transfusion T81.501☑
    resulting in
      adhesions T81.511☑
      obstruction T81.521☑
      perforation T81.531☑
      specified complication NEC T81.591☑
alimentary tract T18.9☑
  anus T18.5☑
  colon T18.4☑
  esophagus — *see* Foreign body, esophagus
  mouth T18.0☑
  multiple sites T18.8☑
  rectosigmoid (junction) T18.5☑
  rectum T18.5☑
  small intestine T18.3☑
  specified site NEC T18.8☑
  stomach T18.2☑
anterior chamber (eye) S05.5-☑
auditory canal — *see* Foreign body, entering through orifice, ear
bronchus T17.508☑
  causing
    asphyxiation T17.500☑
      food (bone) (seed) T17.520☑
      gastric contents (vomitus) T17.510☑
      specified type NEC T17.590☑
    injury NEC T17.508☑
      food (bone) (seed) T17.528☑
      gastric contents (vomitus) T17.518☑
      specified type NEC T17.598☑
canthus — *see* Foreign body, conjunctival sac
ciliary body (eye) S05.5-☑
conjunctival sac T15.1-☑
cornea T15.0-☑
entering through orifice
  accessory sinus T17.0☑
  alimentary canal T18.9☑
    multiple parts T18.8☑
    specified part NEC T18.8☑
  alveolar process T18.0☑
  antrum (Highmore's) T17.0☑
  anus T18.5☑
  appendix T18.4☑
  auditory canal — *see* Foreign body, entering through orifice, ear
  auricle — *see* Foreign body, entering through orifice, ear
  bladder T19.1☑
  bronchioles — *see* Foreign body, respiratory tract, specified site NEC
  bronchus (main) — *see* Foreign body, bronchus
  buccal cavity T18.0☑
  canthus (inner) — *see* Foreign body, conjunctival sac

▽ Subterms under main terms may continue to next column or page ☑ Additional Character Required — Refer to the Tabular List for Character Selection 147

Fluid — Foreign body

☑ **Additional Character Required — Refer to the Tabular List for Character Selection**   ▽ **Subterms under main terms may continue to next column or page**

Foreign body — *continued*
retina S05.5- ☑
superficial, without open wound
  abdomen, abdominal (wall) S30.851 ☑
  alveolar process S00.552 ☑
  ankle S90.55- ☑
  antecubital space — *see* Foreign body, superficial, forearm
  anus S30.857 ☑
  arm (upper) S40.85- ☑
  auditory canal — *see* Foreign body, superficial, ear
  auricle — *see* Foreign body, superficial, ear
  axilla — *see* Foreign body, superficial, arm
  back, lower S30.850 ☑
  breast S20.15- ☑
  brow S00.85 ☑
  buttock S30.850 ☑
  calf — *see* Foreign body, superficial, leg
  canthus — *see* Foreign body, superficial, eyelid
  cheek S00.85 ☑
    internal S00.552 ☑
  chest wall — *see* Foreign body, superficial, thorax
  chin S00.85 ☑
  clitoris S30.854 ☑
  costal region — *see* Foreign body, superficial, thorax
  digit(s)
    foot — *see* Foreign body, superficial, toe
    hand — *see* Foreign body, superficial, finger
  ear S00.45- ☑
  elbow S50.35- ☑
  epididymis S30.853 ☑
  epigastric region S30.851 ☑
  epiglottis S10.15 ☑
  esophagus, cervical S10.15 ☑
  eyebrow — *see* Foreign body, superficial, eyelid
  eyelid S00.25- ☑
  face S00.85 ☑
  finger(s) S60.459 ☑
    index S60.45- ☑
    little S60.45- ☑
    middle S60.45- ☑
    ring S60.45- ☑
  flank S30.851 ☑
  foot (except toe(s) alone) S90.85- ☑
    toe — *see* Foreign body, superficial, toe
  forearm S50.85- ☑
    elbow only — *see* Foreign body, superficial, elbow
  forehead S00.85 ☑
  genital organs, external
    female S30.856 ☑
    male S30.855 ☑
  groin S30.851 ☑
  gum S00.552 ☑
  hand S60.55- ☑
  head S00.95 ☑
    ear — *see* Foreign body, superficial, ear
    eyelid — *see* Foreign body, superficial, eyelid
    lip S00.551 ☑
    nose S00.35 ☑
    oral cavity S00.552 ☑
    scalp S00.05 ☑
    specified site NEC S00.85 ☑
  heel — *see* Foreign body, superficial, foot
  hip S70.25- ☑
  inguinal region S30.851 ☑
  interscapular region S20.459 ☑
  jaw S00.85 ☑
  knee S80.25- ☑
  labium (majus) (minus) S30.854 ☑
  larynx S10.15 ☑
  leg (lower) S80.85- ☑
    knee — *see* Foreign body, superficial, knee
    upper — *see* Foreign body, superficial, thigh
  lip S00.551 ☑
  lower back S30.850 ☑
  lumbar region S30.850 ☑
  malar region S00.85 ☑
  mammary — *see* Foreign body, superficial, breast
  mastoid region S00.85 ☑
  mouth S00.552 ☑
  nail
    finger — *see* Foreign body, superficial, finger
    toe — *see* Foreign body, superficial, toe
  nape S10.85 ☑
  nasal S00.35 ☑

Foreign body — *continued*
superficial, without open wound — *continued*
  neck S10.95 ☑
    specified site NEC S10.85 ☑
    throat S10.15 ☑
  nose S00.35 ☑
  occipital region S00.05 ☑
  oral cavity S00.552 ☑
  orbital region — *see* Foreign body, superficial, eyelid
  palate S00.552 ☑
  palm — *see* Foreign body, superficial, hand
  parietal region S00.05 ☑
  pelvis S30.850 ☑
  penis S30.852 ☑
  perineum
    female S30.854 ☑
    male S30.850 ☑
  periocular area — *see* Foreign body, superficial, eyelid
  phalanges
    finger — *see* Foreign body, superficial, finger
    toe — *see* Foreign body, superficial, toe
  pharynx S10.15 ☑
  pinna — *see* Foreign body, superficial, ear
  popliteal space — *see* Foreign body, superficial, knee
  prepuce S30.852 ☑
  pubic region S30.850 ☑
  pudendum
    female S30.856 ☑
    male S30.855 ☑
  sacral region S30.850 ☑
  scalp S00.05 ☑
  scapular region — *see* Foreign body, superficial, shoulder
  scrotum S30.853 ☑
  shin — *see* Foreign body, superficial, leg
  shoulder S40.25- ☑
  sternal region S20.359 ☑
  submaxillary region S00.85 ☑
  submental region S00.85 ☑
  subungual
    finger(s) — *see* Foreign body, superficial, finger
    toe(s) — *see* Foreign body, superficial, toe
  supraclavicular fossa S10.85 ☑
  supraorbital S00.85 ☑
  temple S00.85 ☑
  temporal region S00.85 ☑
  testis S70.35- ☑
  thigh S70.35- ☑
  thorax, thoracic (wall) S20.95 ☑
    back S20.45- ☑
    front S20.35- ☑
  throat S10.15 ☑
  thumb S60.35- ☑
  toe(s) (lesser) S90.456 ☑
    great S90.45- ☑
  tongue S00.552 ☑
  trachea S10.15 ☑
  tunica vaginalis S30.853 ☑
  tympanum, tympanic membrane — *see* Foreign body, superficial, ear
  uvula S00.552 ☑
  vagina S30.854 ☑
  vocal cords S10.15 ☑
  vulva S30.854 ☑
  wrist S60.85- ☑
swallowed T18.9 ☑
trachea T17.408 ☑
  causing
    asphyxiation T17.400 ☑
      food (bone) (seed) T17.420 ☑
      gastric contents (vomitus) T17.410 ☑
      specified type NEC T17.490 ☑
    injury NEC T17.408 ☑
      food (bone) (seed) T17.428 ☑
      gastric contents (vomitus) T17.418 ☑
      specified type NEC T17.498 ☑
type of fragment — *see* Retained, foreign body fragments (type of)
vitreous (humor) S05.5- ☑
Forestier's disease (rhizomelic pseudopolyarthritis) M35.3
meaning ankylosing hyperostosis — *see* Hyperostosis, ankylosing

Formation
hyalin in cornea — *see* Degeneration, cornea
sequestrum in bone (due to infection) — *see* Osteomyelitis, chronic
valve
  colon, congenital Q43.8
  ureter (congenital) Q62.39
Formication R20.2
Fort Bragg fever A27.89
Fossa — *see also* condition
pyriform — *see* condition
Foster-Kennedy syndrome H47.14- ☑
Fothergill's
disease (trigeminal neuralgia) — *see also* Neuralgia, trigeminal
scarlatina anginosa A38.9
Foul breath R19.6
Foundling Z76.1
Fournier disease or gangrene N49.3
female N76.89
Fourth
cranial nerve — *see* condition
molar K00.1
Foville's (peduncular) **disease or syndrome** G46.3
Fox (-Fordyce) disease (apocrine miliaria) L75.2
FPIES (food protein-induced enterocolitis syndrome) K52.21
Fracture, burst — *see* Fracture, traumatic, by site
Fracture, chronic — *see* Fracture, pathological, by site
Fracture, insufficiency — *see* Fracture, pathological, by site
Fracture, nontraumatic, NEC
atypical
  femur M84.750- ☑
    complete
      oblique M84.759 ☑
        left side M84.758 ☑
        right side M84.757 ☑
      transverse M84.756 ☑
        left side M84.755 ☑
        right side M84.754 ☑
    incomplete M84.753 ☑
      left side M84.752 ☑
      right side M84.751 ☑
Fracture, pathological (pathologic) — *see also* Fracture, traumatic M84.40 ☑
ankle M84.47- ☑
carpus M84.44- ☑
clavicle M84.41- ☑
compression (not due to trauma) — *see also* Collapse, vertebra M48.50- ☑
dental implant M27.63
dental restorative material K08.539
  with loss of material K08.531
  without loss of material K08.530
due to
  neoplastic disease NEC — *see also* Neoplasm M84.50 ☑
    ankle M84.57- ☑
    carpus M84.54- ☑
    clavicle M84.51- ☑
    femur M84.55- ☑
    fibula M84.56- ☑
    finger M84.54- ☑
    hip M84.559 ☑
    humerus M84.52- ☑
    ilium M84.550 ☑
    ischium M84.550 ☑
    metacarpus M84.54- ☑
    metatarsus M84.57- ☑
    neck M84.58 ☑
    pelvis M84.550 ☑
    radius M84.53- ☑
    rib M84.58 ☑
    scapula M84.51- ☑
    skull M84.58 ☑
    specified site NEC M84.58 ☑
    tarsus M84.57- ☑
    tibia M84.56- ☑
    toe M84.57- ☑
    ulna M84.53- ☑
    vertebra M84.58 ☑
  osteoporosis M80.00 ☑
    disuse — *see* Osteoporosis, specified type NEC, with pathological fracture

Fracture, pathological — continued
  due to — continued
    osteoporosis — continued
      drug-induced — see Osteoporosis, drug induced, with pathological fracture
      idiopathic — see Osteoporosis, specified type NEC, with pathological fracture
      postmenopausal — see Osteoporosis, post-menopausal, with pathological fracture
      postoophorectomy — see Osteoporosis, pos-toophorectomy, with pathological fracture
      postsurgical malabsorption — see Osteoporosis, specified type NEC, with pathological fracture
      specified cause NEC — see Osteoporosis, speci-fied type NEC, with pathological fracture
    specified disease NEC M84.60 ☑
      ankle M84.67- ☑
      carpus M84.64- ☑
      clavicle M84.61- ☑
      femur M84.65- ☑
      fibula M84.66- ☑
      finger M84.64- ☑
      hip M84.65- ☑
      humerus M84.62- ☑
      ilium M84.650 ☑
      ischium M84.650 ☑
      metacarpus M84.64- ☑
      metatarsus M84.67- ☑
      neck M84.68 ☑
      radius M84.63- ☑
      rib M84.68 ☑
      scapula M84.61- ☑
      skull M84.68 ☑
      tarsus M84.67- ☑
      tibia M84.66- ☑
      toe M84.67- ☑
      ulna M84.63- ☑
      vertebra M84.68 ☑
  femur M84.45- ☑
  fibula M84.46- ☑
  finger M84.44- ☑
  hip M84.459 ☑
  humerus M84.42- ☑
  ilium M84.454 ☑
  ischium M84.454 ☑
  joint prosthesis — see Complications, joint prosthesis, mechanical, breakdown, by site
  periprosthetic — see Fracture, pathological, periprosthetic
  metacarpus M84.44- ☑
  metatarsus M84.47- ☑
  neck M84.48 ☑
  pelvis M84.454 ☑
  periprosthetic M97.9 ☑
    ankle M97.2- ☑
    elbow M97.4- ☑
    finger M97.8 ☑
    hip M97.0- ☑
    knee M97.1- ☑
    other specified joint M97.8 ☑
    shoulder M97.3- ☑
    spinal joint M97.8 ☑
    toe joint M97.8 ☑
    wrist joint M97.8 ☑
  radius M84.43- ☑
  restorative material (dental) K08.539
    with loss of material K08.531
    without loss of material K08.530
  rib M84.48 ☑
  scapula M84.41- ☑
  skull M84.48 ☑
  tarsus M84.47- ☑
  tibia M84.46- ☑
  toe M84.47- ☑
  ulna M84.43- ☑
  vertebra M84.48 ☑

Fracture, traumatic (abduction) (adduction) (separation) — see also Fracture, pathological T14.8 ☑
  acetabulum S32.40- ☑
    column
      anterior (displaced) (iliopubic) S32.43- ☑
        nondisplaced S32.436 ☑
      posterior (displaced) (ilioischial) S32.443 ☑
        nondisplaced S32.44- ☑
    dome (displaced) S32.48- ☑

Fracture, traumatic — continued
  acetabulum — continued
    dome — continued
      nondisplaced S32.48 ☑
    specified NEC S32.49- ☑
    transverse (displaced) S32.45- ☑
      with associated posterior wall fracture (displaced) S32.46- ☑
      nondisplaced S32.46- ☑
      nondisplaced S32.45- ☑
    wall
      anterior (displaced) S32.41- ☑
        nondisplaced S32.41- ☑
      medial (displaced) S32.47- ☑
        nondisplaced S32.47- ☑
      posterior (displaced) S32.42- ☑
        with associated transverse fracture (displaced) S32.46- ☑
        nondisplaced S32.46- ☑
        nondisplaced S32.42- ☑
  acromion — see Fracture, scapula, acromial process
  ankle S82.899 ☑
    bimalleolar (displaced) S82.84- ☑
      nondisplaced S82.84- ☑
    lateral malleolus only (displaced) S82.6- ☑
      nondisplaced S82.6- ☑
    medial malleolus (displaced) S82.5- ☑
      associated with Maisonneuve's fracture — see Fracture, Maisonneuve's
      nondisplaced S82.5- ☑
    talus — see Fracture, tarsal, talus
    trimalleolar (displaced) S82.85- ☑
      nondisplaced S82.85- ☑
  arm (upper) — see also Fracture, humerus, shaft
    humerus — see Fracture, humerus
    radius — see Fracture, radius
    ulna — see Fracture, ulna
  astragalus — see Fracture, tarsal, talus
  atlas — see Fracture, neck, cervical vertebra, first
  axis — see Fracture, neck, cervical vertebra, second
  back — see Fracture, vertebra
  Barton's — see Barton's fracture
  base of skull — see Fracture, skull, base
  basicervical (basal) (femoral) S72.0 ☑
  Bennett's — see Bennett's fracture
  bimalleolar — see Fracture, ankle, bimalleolar
  blow-out S02.3- ☑
  bone NEC T14.8 ☑
    birth injury P13.9
    following insertion of orthopedic implant, joint prosthesis or bone plate — see Fracture, fol-lowing insertion of orthopedic implant, joint prosthesis or bone plate
    in (due to) neoplastic disease NEC — see Fracture, pathological, due to, neoplastic disease
    pathological (cause unknown) — see Fracture, pathological
  breast bone — see Fracture, sternum
  bucket handle (semilunar cartilage) — see Tear, meniscus
  burst — see Fracture, traumatic, by site
  calcaneus — see Fracture, tarsal, calcaneus
  carpal bone(s) S62.10- ☑
    capitate (displaced) S62.13- ☑
      nondisplaced S62.13- ☑
    cuneiform — see Fracture, carpal bone, triquetrum
    hamate (body) (displaced) S62.143 ☑
      hook process (displaced) S62.15- ☑
        nondisplaced S62.15- ☑
      nondisplaced S62.14- ☑
    larger multangular — see Fracture, carpal bones, trapezium
    lunate (displaced) S62.12- ☑
      nondisplaced S62.12- ☑
    navicular S62.00- ☑
      distal pole (displaced) S62.01- ☑
        nondisplaced S62.01- ☑
      middle third (displaced) S62.02- ☑
        nondisplaced S62.02- ☑
      proximal third (displaced) S62.03- ☑
        nondisplaced S62.03- ☑
      volar tuberosity — see Fracture, carpal bones, navicular, distal pole
    os magnum — see Fracture, carpal bones, capitate
    pisiform (displaced) S62.16- ☑
      nondisplaced S62.16- ☑

Fracture, traumatic — continued
  carpal bone(s) — continued
    semilunar — see Fracture, carpal bones, lunate
    smaller multangular — see Fracture, carpal bones, trapezoid
    trapezium (displaced) S62.17- ☑
      nondisplaced S62.17- ☑
    trapezoid (displaced) S62.18- ☑
      nondisplaced S62.18- ☑
    triquetrum (displaced) S62.11- ☑
      nondisplaced S62.11- ☑
    unciform — see Fracture, carpal bones, hamate
  cervical — see Fracture, vertebra, cervical
  clavicle S42.00- ☑
    acromial end (displaced) S42.03- ☑
      nondisplaced S42.03- ☑
    birth injury P13.4
    lateral end — see Fracture, clavicle, acromial end
    shaft (displaced) S42.02- ☑
      nondisplaced S42.02- ☑
    sternal end (anterior) (displaced) S42.01- ☑
      nondisplaced S42.01- ☑
      posterior S42.01- ☑
  coccyx S32.2 ☑
  collapsed — see Collapse, vertebra
  collar bone — see Fracture, clavicle
  Colles' — see Colles' fracture
  coronoid process — see Fracture, ulna, upper end, coronoid process
  corpus cavernosum penis S39.840 ☑
  costochondral cartilage S23.41 ☑
  costochondral, costosternal junction — see Fracture, rib
  cranium — see Fracture, skull
  cricoid cartilage S12.8 ☑
  cuboid (ankle) — see Fracture, tarsal, cuboid
  cuneiform
    foot — see Fracture, tarsal, cuneiform
    wrist — see Fracture, carpal, triquetrum
  delayed union — see Delay, union, fracture
  dental restorative material K08.539
    with loss of material K08.531
    without loss of material K08.530
  due to
    birth injury — see Birth, injury, fracture
    osteoporosis — see Osteoporosis, with fracture
  Dupuytren's — see Fracture, ankle, lateral malleolus
  elbow S42.40- ☑
  ethmoid (bone) (sinus) — see Fracture, skull, base
  face bone S02.92 ☑
  fatigue — see also Fracture, stress
    vertebra M48.40 ☑
      cervical region M48.42 ☑
      cervicothoracic region M48.43 ☑
      lumbar region M48.46 ☑
      lumbosacral region M48.47 ☑
      occipito-atlanto-axial region M48.41 ☑
      sacrococcygeal region M48.48 ☑
      thoracic region M48.44 ☑
      thoracolumbar region M48.45 ☑
  femur, femoral S72.9- ☑
    basicervical (basal) S72.0 ☑
    birth injury P13.2
    capital epiphyseal S79.01- ☑
    condyles, epicondyles — see Fracture, femur, lower end
    distal end — see Fracture, femur, lower end
    epiphysis
      head — see Fracture, femur, upper end, epiphysis
      lower — see Fracture, femur, lower end, epiph-ysis
      upper — see Fracture, femur, upper end, epiph-ysis
    following insertion of implant, prosthesis or plate M96.66- ☑
    head — see Fracture, femur, upper end, head
    intertrochanteric — see Fracture, femur, trochanteric
    intratrochanteric — see Fracture, femur, trochanteric
    lower end S72.40- ☑
      condyle (displaced) S72.41- ☑
        lateral (displaced) S72.42- ☑
          nondisplaced S72.42- ☑
        medial (displaced) S72.43- ☑
          nondisplaced S72.43- ☑

Index

Fracture, traumatic — *continued*
  femur, femoral — *continued*
    lower end — *continued*
      condyle — *continued*
        nondisplaced S72.41- ☑
      epiphysis (displaced) S72.44- ☑
        nondisplaced S72.44- ☑
      physeal S79.10- ☑
        Salter-Harris
          Type I S79.11- ☑
          Type II S79.12- ☑
          Type III S79.13- ☑
          Type IV S79.14- ☑
        specified NEC S79.19- ☑
      specified NEC S72.49- ☑
      supracondylar (displaced) S72.45- ☑
        with intracondylar extension (displaced) S72.46- ☑
          nondisplaced S72.46- ☑
        nondisplaced S72.45- ☑
      torus S72.47- ☑
    neck — *see* Fracture, femur, upper end, neck
    pertrochanteric — *see* Fracture, femur, trochanteric
    shaft (lower third) (middle third) (upper third) S72.30- ☑
      comminuted (displaced) S72.35- ☑
        nondisplaced S72.35- ☑
      oblique (displaced) S72.33- ☑
        nondisplaced S72.33- ☑
      segmental (displaced) S72.36- ☑
        nondisplaced S72.36- ☑
      specified NEC S72.39- ☑
      spiral (displaced) S72.34- ☑
        nondisplaced S72.34- ☑
      transverse (displaced) S72.32- ☑
        nondisplaced S72.32- ☑
    specified site NEC — *see* subcategory S72.8 ☑
    subcapital (displaced) S72.01- ☑
    subtrochanteric (region) (section) (displaced) S72.2- ☑
      nondisplaced S72.2- ☑
    transcervical — *see* Fracture, femur, midcervical
    transtrochanteric — *see* Fracture, femur, trochanteric
    trochanteric S72.10- ☑
      apophyseal (displaced) S72.13- ☑
        nondisplaced S72.13- ☑
      greater trochanter (displaced) S72.11- ☑
        nondisplaced S72.11- ☑
      intertrochanteric (displaced) S72.14- ☑
        nondisplaced S72.14- ☑
      lesser trochanter (displaced) S72.12- ☑
        nondisplaced S72.12- ☑
    upper end S72.00- ☑
      apophyseal (displaced) S72.13- ☑
        nondisplaced S72.13- ☑
      cervicotrochanteric — *see* Fracture, femur, upper end, neck, base
      epiphysis (displaced) S72.02- ☑
        nondisplaced S72.02- ☑
      head S72.05- ☑
        articular (displaced) S72.06- ☑
          nondisplaced S72.06- ☑
        specified NEC S72.09- ☑
      intertrochanteric (displaced) S72.14- ☑
        nondisplaced S72.14- ☑
      intracapsular S72.01- ☑
      midcervical (displaced) S72.03- ☑
        nondisplaced S72.03- ☑
      neck S72.00- ☑
        base (displaced) S72.04- ☑
          nondisplaced S72.04- ☑
        specified NEC S72.09- ☑
      pertrochanteric — *see* Fracture, femur, upper end, trochanteric
      physeal S79.00- ☑
        Salter-Harris type I S79.01- ☑
        specified NEC S79.09- ☑
      subcapital (displaced) S72.01- ☑
      subtrochanteric (displaced) S72.2- ☑
        nondisplaced S72.2- ☑
      transcervical — *see* Fracture, femur, upper end, midcervical
      trochanteric S72.10- ☑
        greater (displaced) S72.11- ☑
          nondisplaced S72.11- ☑

Fracture, traumatic — *continued*
  femur, femoral — *continued*
    upper end — *continued*
      trochanteric — *continued*
        lesser (displaced) S72.12- ☑
          nondisplaced S72.12- ☑
  fibula (shaft) (styloid) S82.40- ☑
    comminuted (displaced) S82.45- ☑
      nondisplaced S82.45- ☑
    following insertion of implant, prosthesis or plate M96.67- ☑
    involving ankle or malleolus — *see* Fracture, fibula, lateral malleolus
    lateral malleolus (displaced) S82.6- ☑
      nondisplaced S82.6- ☑
    lower end
      physeal S89.30- ☑
        Salter-Harris
          Type I S89.31- ☑
          Type II S89.32- ☑
        specified NEC S89.39- ☑
      specified NEC S82.83- ☑
      torus S82.82- ☑
    oblique (displaced) S82.43- ☑
      nondisplaced S82.43- ☑
    segmental (displaced) S82.46- ☑
      nondisplaced S82.46- ☑
    specified NEC S82.49- ☑
    spiral (displaced) S82.44- ☑
      nondisplaced S82.44- ☑
    transverse (displaced) S82.42- ☑
      nondisplaced S82.42- ☑
    upper end
      physeal S89.20- ☑
        Salter-Harris
          Type I S89.21- ☑
          Type II S89.22- ☑
        specified NEC S89.29- ☑
      specified NEC S82.83- ☑
      torus S82.81- ☑
  finger (except thumb) S62.60- ☑
    distal phalanx (displaced) S62.63- ☑
      nondisplaced S62.66- ☑
    index S62.60- ☑
      distal phalanx (displaced) S62.63- ☑
        nondisplaced S62.66- ☑
      middle phalanx (displaced) S62.62- ☑
        nondisplaced S62.65- ☑
      proximal phalanx (displaced) S62.61- ☑
        nondisplaced S62.64- ☑
    little S62.60- ☑
      distal phalanx (displaced) S62.63- ☑
        nondisplaced S62.66- ☑
      middle phalanx (displaced) S62.62- ☑
        nondisplaced S62.65- ☑
      proximal phalanx (displaced) S62.61- ☑
        nondisplaced S62.64- ☑
    middle S62.60- ☑
      distal phalanx (displaced) S62.63- ☑
        nondisplaced S62.66- ☑
      middle phalanx (displaced) S62.62- ☑
        nondisplaced S62.65- ☑
      proximal phalanx (displaced) S62.61- ☑
        nondisplaced S62.64- ☑
    middle phalanx (displaced) S62.62- ☑
      nondisplaced S62.65- ☑
    proximal phalanx (displaced) S62.61- ☑
      nondisplaced S62.64- ☑
    ring S62.60- ☑
      distal phalanx (displaced) S62.63- ☑
        nondisplaced S62.66- ☑
      middle phalanx (displaced) S62.62- ☑
        nondisplaced S62.65- ☑
      proximal phalanx (displaced) S62.61- ☑
        nondisplaced S62.64- ☑
    thumb — *see* Fracture, thumb
  following insertion (intraoperative) (postoperative) of orthopedic implant, joint prosthesis or bone plate M96.69
    femur M96.66- ☑
    fibula M96.67- ☑
    humerus M96.62- ☑
    pelvis M96.65
    radius M96.63- ☑
    specified bone NEC M96.69
    tibia M96.67- ☑

Fracture, traumatic — *continued*
  following insertion of orthopedic implant, joint prosthesis or bone plate — *continued*
    ulna M96.63- ☑
  foot S92.90- ☑
    astragalus — *see* Fracture, tarsal, talus
    calcaneus — *see* Fracture, tarsal, calcaneus
    cuboid — *see* Fracture, tarsal, cuboid
    cuneiform — *see* Fracture, tarsal, cuneiform
    metatarsal — *see* Fracture, metatarsal
    navicular — *see* Fracture, tarsal, navicular
    sesamoid S92.81- ☑
    specified NEC S92.81- ☑
    talus — *see* Fracture, tarsal, talus
    tarsal — *see* Fracture, tarsal
    toe — *see* Fracture, toe
  forearm S52.9- ☑
    radius — *see* Fracture, radius
    ulna — *see* Fracture, ulna
  fossa (anterior) (middle) (posterior) S02.19 ☑
  fragility — *see* Fracture, pathological, due to osteoporosis
  frontal (bone) (skull) S02.0 ☑
    sinus S02.19 ☑
  glenoid (cavity) (scapula) — *see* Fracture, scapula, glenoid cavity
  greenstick — *see* Fracture, by site
  hallux — *see* Fracture, toe, great
  hand S62.9- ☑
    carpal — *see* Fracture, carpal bone
    finger (except thumb) — *see* Fracture, finger
    metacarpal — *see* Fracture, metacarpal
    navicular (scaphoid) (hand) — *see* Fracture, carpal bone, navicular
    thumb — *see* Fracture, thumb
  healed or old
    with complications — *code by* Nature of the complication
  heel bone — *see* Fracture, tarsal, calcaneus
  Hill-Sachs S42.29- ☑
  hip — *see* Fracture, femur, neck
  humerus S42.30- ☑
    anatomical neck — *see* Fracture, humerus, upper end
    articular process — *see* Fracture, humerus, lower end
    capitellum — *see* Fracture, humerus, lower end, condyle, lateral
    distal end — *see* Fracture, humerus, lower end
    epiphysis
      lower — *see* Fracture, humerus, lower end, physeal
      upper — *see* Fracture, humerus, upper end, physeal
    external condyle — *see* Fracture, humerus, lower end, condyle, lateral
    following insertion of implant, prosthesis or plate M96.62- ☑
    great tuberosity — *see* Fracture, humerus, upper end, greater tuberosity
    intercondylar — *see* Fracture, humerus, lower end
    internal epicondyle — *see* Fracture, humerus, lower end, epicondyle, medial
    lesser tuberosity — *see* Fracture, humerus, upper end, lesser tuberosity
    lower end S42.40- ☑
      condyle
        lateral (displaced) S42.45- ☑
          nondisplaced S42.45- ☑
        medial (displaced) S42.46- ☑
          nondisplaced S42.46- ☑
      epicondyle
        lateral (displaced) S42.43- ☑
          nondisplaced S42.43- ☑
        medial (displaced) S42.44- ☑
          incarcerated S42.44- ☑
          nondisplaced S42.44- ☑
      physeal S49.10- ☑
        Salter-Harris
          Type I S49.11- ☑
          Type II S49.12- ☑
          Type III S49.13- ☑
          Type IV S49.14- ☑
        specified NEC S49.19- ☑
      specified NEC (displaced) S42.49- ☑
        nondisplaced S42.49- ☑

Fracture, traumatic — Fracture, traumatic

Fracture, traumatic — *continued*
  humerus — *continued*
    lower end — *continued*
      supracondylar (simple) (displaced) S42.41- ☑
        with intercondylar fracture — *see* Fracture, humerus, lower end
        comminuted (displaced) S42.42- ☑
          nondisplaced S42.42- ☑
        nondisplaced S42.41- ☑
      torus S42.48- ☑
      transcondylar (displaced) S42.47- ☑
        nondisplaced S42.47- ☑
    proximal end — *see* Fracture, humerus, upper end
    shaft S42.30- ☑
      comminuted (displaced) S42.35- ☑
        nondisplaced S42.35- ☑
      greenstick S42.31- ☑
      oblique (displaced) S42.33- ☑
        nondisplaced S42.33- ☑
      segmental (displaced) S42.36- ☑
        nondisplaced S42.36- ☑
      specified NEC S42.39- ☑
      spiral (displaced) S42.34- ☑
        nondisplaced S42.34- ☑
      transverse (displaced) S42.32- ☑
        nondisplaced S42.32- ☑
    supracondylar — *see* Fracture, humerus, lower end
    surgical neck — *see* Fracture, humerus, upper end, surgical neck
    trochlea — *see* Fracture, humerus, lower end, condyle, medial
    tuberosity — *see* Fracture, humerus, upper end
    upper end S42.20- ☑
      anatomical neck — *see* Fracture, humerus, upper end, specified NEC
      articular head — *see* Fracture, humerus, upper end, specified NEC
      epiphysis — *see* Fracture, humerus, upper end, physeal
      greater tuberosity (displaced) S42.25- ☑
        nondisplaced S42.25- ☑
      lesser tuberosity (displaced) S42.26- ☑
        nondisplaced S42.26- ☑
      physeal S49.00- ☑
        Salter-Harris
          Type I S49.01- ☑
          Type II S49.02- ☑
          Type III S49.03- ☑
          Type IV S49.04- ☑
        specified NEC S49.09- ☑
      specified NEC (displaced) S42.29- ☑
        nondisplaced S42.29- ☑
      surgical neck (displaced) S42.21- ☑
        four-part S42.24- ☑
        nondisplaced S42.21- ☑
        three-part S42.23- ☑
        two-part (displaced) S42.22- ☑
          nondisplaced S42.22- ☑
      torus S42.27- ☑
      transepiphyseal — *see* Fracture, humerus, upper end, physeal
  hyoid bone S12.8 ☑
  ilium S32.30- ☑
    with disruption of pelvic ring — *see* Disruption, pelvic ring
    avulsion (displaced) S32.31- ☑
      nondisplaced S32.31- ☑
    specified NEC S32.39- ☑
  impaction, impacted — *code as* Fracture, by site
  innominate bone — *see* Fracture, ilium
  instep — *see* Fracture, foot
  ischium S32.60- ☑
    with disruption of pelvic ring — *see* Disruption, pelvic ring
    avulsion (displaced) S32.61- ☑
      nondisplaced S32.61- ☑
    specified NEC S32.69- ☑
  jaw (bone) (lower) — *see* Fracture, mandible
    upper — *see* Fracture, maxilla
  joint prosthesis — *see* Complications, joint prosthesis, mechanical, breakdown, by site
    periprosthetic — *see* Fracture, traumatic, periprosthetic
  knee cap — *see* Fracture, patella
  larynx S12.8 ☑
  late effects — *see* Sequelae, fracture

  leg (lower) S82.9-
    ankle — *see* Fracture, ankle
    femur — *see* Fracture, femur
    fibula — *see* Fracture, fibula
    malleolus — *see* Fracture, ankle
    patella — *see* Fracture, patella
    specified site NEC S82.89-
    tibia — *see* Fracture, tibia
  lumbar spine — *see* Fracture, vertebra, lumbar
  lumbosacral spine S32.9
  Maisonneuve's (displaced) S82.86- ☑
    nondisplaced S82.86- ☑
  malar bone — *see also* Fracture, maxilla S02.400 ☑
    left side S02.40B ☑
    right side S02.40A ☑
  malleolus — *see* Fracture, ankle
  malunion — *see* Fracture, by site
  mandible (lower jaw (bone)) S02.609 ☑
    alveolus S02.67- ☑
    angle (of jaw) S02.65- ☑
    body, unspecified S02.600 ☑
      left side S02.602 ☑
      right side S02.601 ☑
    condylar process S02.61- ☑
    coronoid process S02.63- ☑
    ramus, unspecified S02.64- ☑
    specified site NEC S02.69 ☑
    subcondylar process S02.62- ☑
    symphysis S02.66 ☑
  manubrium (sterni) S22.21 ☑
    dissociation from sternum S22.23 ☑
  march — *see* Fracture, traumatic, stress, by site
  maxilla, maxillary (bone) (sinus) (superior) (upper jaw) S02.401 ☑
    alveolus S02.42 ☑
    inferior — *see* Fracture, mandible
    LeFort I S02.411 ☑
    LeFort II S02.412 ☑
    LeFort III S02.413 ☑
    left side S02.40D ☑
    right side S02.40C ☑
  metacarpal S62.309 ☑
    base (displaced) S62.319 ☑
      nondisplaced S62.349 ☑
    fifth S62.30- ☑
      base (displaced) S62.31- ☑
        nondisplaced S62.34- ☑
      neck (displaced) S62.33- ☑
        nondisplaced S62.36- ☑
      shaft (displaced) S62.32- ☑
        nondisplaced S62.35- ☑
      specified NEC S62.398 ☑
    first S62.20- ☑
      base NEC (displaced) S62.23- ☑
        nondisplaced S62.23- ☑
      Bennett's — *see* Bennett's fracture
      neck (displaced) S62.25- ☑
        nondisplaced S62.25- ☑
      shaft (displaced) S62.24- ☑
        nondisplaced S62.24- ☑
      specified NEC S62.29- ☑
    fourth S62.30- ☑
      base (displaced) S62.31- ☑
        nondisplaced S62.34- ☑
      neck (displaced) S62.33- ☑
        nondisplaced S62.36- ☑
      shaft (displaced) S62.32- ☑
        nondisplaced S62.35- ☑
      specified NEC S62.39- ☑
    neck (displaced) S62.33- ☑
      nondisplaced S62.36- ☑
    Rolando's — *see* Rolando's fracture
    second S62.30- ☑
      base (displaced) S62.31- ☑
        nondisplaced S62.34- ☑
      neck (displaced) S62.33- ☑
        nondisplaced S62.36- ☑
      shaft (displaced) S62.32- ☑
        nondisplaced S62.35- ☑
      specified NEC S62.39- ☑
    shaft (displaced) S62.32- ☑
      nondisplaced S62.35- ☑
    specified NEC S62.399 ☑
    third S62.30- ☑
      base (displaced) S62.31- ☑

  metacarpal — *continued*
    third — *continued*
      base — *continued*
        nondisplaced S62.34- ☑
      neck (displaced) S62.33- ☑
        nondisplaced S62.36- ☑
      shaft (displaced) S62.32- ☑
        nondisplaced S62.35- ☑
      specified NEC S62.39- ☑
  metastatic — *see* Fracture, pathological, due to, neoplastic disease — *see also* Neoplasm
  metatarsal bone S92.30- ☑
    fifth (displaced) S92.35- ☑
      nondisplaced S92.35- ☑
    first (displaced) S92.31- ☑
      nondisplaced S92.31- ☑
    fourth (displaced) S92.34- ☑
      nondisplaced S92.34- ☑
    physeal S99.10- ☑
      Salter-Harris
        Type I S99.11- ☑
        Type II S99.12- ☑
        Type III S99.13- ☑
        Type IV S99.14- ☑
      specified NEC S99.19- ☑
    second (displaced) S92.32- ☑
      nondisplaced S92.32- ☑
    third (displaced) S92.33- ☑
      nondisplaced S92.33- ☑
  Monteggia's — *see* Monteggia's fracture
  multiple
    hand (and wrist) NEC — *see* Fracture, by site
    ribs — *see* Fracture, rib, multiple
  nasal (bone(s)) S02.2
  navicular (scaphoid) (foot) — *see also* Fracture, tarsal, navicular
    hand — *see* Fracture, carpal, navicular
  neck S12.9 ☑
    cervical vertebra S12.9 ☑
      fifth (displaced) S12.400 ☑
        nondisplaced S12.401 ☑
        specified type NEC (displaced) S12.490 ☑
          nondisplaced S12.491 ☑
      first (displaced) S12.000 ☑
        burst (stable) S12.01 ☑
          unstable S12.02 ☑
        lateral mass (displaced) S12.040 ☑
          nondisplaced S12.041 ☑
        nondisplaced S12.001 ☑
        posterior arch (displaced) S12.030 ☑
          nondisplaced S12.031 ☑
        specified type NEC (displaced) S12.090 ☑
          nondisplaced S12.091 ☑
      fourth (displaced) S12.300 ☑
        nondisplaced S12.301 ☑
        specified type NEC (displaced) S12.390 ☑
          nondisplaced S12.391 ☑
      second (displaced) S12.100 ☑
        dens (anterior) (displaced) (type II) S12.110 ☑
          nondisplaced S12.112 ☑
          posterior S12.111 ☑
          specified type NEC (displaced) S12.120 ☑
            nondisplaced S12.121 ☑
        nondisplaced S12.101 ☑
        specified type NEC (displaced) S12.190 ☑
          nondisplaced S12.191 ☑
      seventh (displaced) S12.600 ☑
        nondisplaced S12.601 ☑
        specified type NEC (displaced) S12.690 ☑
          nondisplaced S12.691 ☑
      sixth (displaced) S12.500 ☑
        nondisplaced S12.501 ☑
        specified type NEC (displaced) S12.590 ☑
          nondisplaced S12.591 ☑
      third (displaced) S12.200 ☑
        nondisplaced S12.201 ☑
        specified type NEC (displaced) S12.290 ☑
          nondisplaced S12.291 ☑
    hyoid bone S12.8 ☑
    larynx S12.8 ☑
    specified site NEC S12.8 ☑
    thyroid cartilage S12.8 ☑
    trachea S12.8 ☑
  neoplastic NEC — *see* Fracture, pathological, due to, neoplastic disease

☑ **Additional Character Required — Refer to the Tabular List for Character Selection**   ▽ Subterms under main terms may continue to next column or page

Fracture, traumatic — *continued*
neural arch — *see* Fracture, vertebra
newborn — *see* Birth, injury, fracture
nontraumatic — *see* Fracture, pathological
nonunion — *see* Nonunion, fracture
nose, nasal (bone) (septum) S02.2 ☑
occiput — *see* Fracture, skull, base, occiput
odontoid process — *see* Fracture, neck, cervical vertebra, second
olecranon (process) (ulna) — *see* Fracture, ulna, upper end, olecranon process
orbit, orbital (bone) (region) S02.85 ☑
   floor (blow-out) S02.3- ☑
   roof S02.12- ☑
   wall S02.85 ☑
      lateral S02.84- ☑
      medial S02.83- ☑
os
   calcis — *see* Fracture, tarsal, calcaneus
   magnum — *see* Fracture, carpal, capitate
   pubis — *see* Fracture, pubis
palate S02.8- ☑
parietal bone (skull) S02.0 ☑
patella S82.00- ☑
   comminuted (displaced) S82.04- ☑
      nondisplaced S82.04- ☑
   longitudinal (displaced) S82.02- ☑
      nondisplaced S82.02- ☑
   osteochondral (displaced) S82.01- ☑
      nondisplaced S82.01- ☑
   specified NEC S82.09- ☑
   transverse (displaced) S82.03- ☑
      nondisplaced S82.03- ☑
pedicle (of vertebral arch) — *see* Fracture, vertebra
pelvis, pelvic (bone) S32.9 ☑
   acetabulum — *see* Fracture, acetabulum
   circle — *see* Disruption, pelvic ring
   following insertion of implant, prosthesis or plate M96.65
   ilium — *see* Fracture, ilium
   ischium — *see* Fracture, ischium
   multiple
      with disruption of pelvic ring (circle) — *see* Disruption, pelvic ring
      without disruption of pelvic ring (circle) S32.82 ☑
   pubis — *see* Fracture, pubis
   sacrum — *see* Fracture, sacrum
   specified site NEC S32.89 ☑
periprosthetic, around internal prosthetic joint M97.9 ☑
   ankle M97.2- ☑
   elbow M97.4- ☑
   finger M97.8 ☑
   hip M97.0- ☑
   knee M97.1- ☑
   shoulder M97.3- ☑
   specified joint NEC M97.8 ☑
   spine M97.8 ☑
   toe M97.8 ☑
   wrist M97.8 ☑
phalanx
   foot — *see* Fracture, toe
   hand — *see* Fracture, finger
pisiform — *see* Fracture, carpal, pisiform
pond — *see* Fracture, skull
prosthetic device, internal — *see* Complications, prosthetic device, by site, mechanical
pubis S32.50- ☑
   with disruption of pelvic ring — *see* Disruption, pelvic ring
   specified site NEC S32.59- ☑
   superior rim S32.51- ☑
radius S52.9- ☑
   distal end — *see* Fracture, radius, lower end
   following insertion of implant, prosthesis or plate M96.63- ☑
   head — *see* Fracture, radius, upper end, head
   lower end S52.50- ☑
      Barton's — *see* Barton's fracture
      Colles' — *see* Colles' fracture
      extraarticular NEC S52.55- ☑
      intraarticular NEC S52.57- ☑
      physeal S59.20- ☑
         Salter-Harris
            Type I S59.21- ☑

radius — *continued*
   lower end — *continued*
      physeal — *continued*
         Salter-Harris — *continued*
            Type II S59.22- ☑
            Type III S59.23- ☑
            Type IV S59.24- ☑
         specified NEC S59.29- ☑
      Smith's — *see* Smith's fracture
      specified NEC S52.59- ☑
      styloid process (displaced) S52.51- ☑
         nondisplaced S52.51- ☑
      torus S52.52- ☑
   neck — *see* Fracture, radius, upper end
   proximal end — *see* Fracture, radius, upper end
   shaft S52.30- ☑
      bent bone S52.38- ☑
      comminuted (displaced) S52.35- ☑
         nondisplaced S52.35- ☑
      Galeazzi's — *see* Galeazzi's fracture
      greenstick S52.31- ☑
      oblique (displaced) S52.33- ☑
         nondisplaced S52.33- ☑
      segmental (displaced) S52.36- ☑
         nondisplaced S52.36- ☑
      specified NEC S52.39- ☑
      spiral (displaced) S52.34- ☑
         nondisplaced S52.34- ☑
      transverse (displaced) S52.32- ☑
         nondisplaced S52.32- ☑
   upper end S52.10- ☑
      head (displaced) S52.12- ☑
         nondisplaced S52.12- ☑
      neck (displaced) S52.13- ☑
         nondisplaced S52.13- ☑
      physeal S59.10- ☑
         Salter-Harris
            Type I S59.11- ☑
            Type II S59.12- ☑
            Type III S59.13- ☑
            Type IV S59.14- ☑
         specified NEC S59.19- ☑
      specified NEC S52.18- ☑
      torus S52.11- ☑
ramus
   inferior or superior, pubis — *see* Fracture, pubis
   mandible — *see* Fracture, mandible
restorative material (dental) K08.539
   with loss of material K08.531
   without loss of material K08.530
rib S22.3- ☑
   with flail chest — *see* Flail, chest
   multiple S22.4- ☑
      with flail chest — *see* Flail, chest
root, tooth — *see* Fracture, tooth
sacrum S32.10 ☑
   specified NEC S32.19 ☑
   Type
      1 S32.14 ☑
      2 S32.15 ☑
      3 S32.16 ☑
      4 S32.17 ☑
   Zone
      I S32.119 ☑
         displaced (minimally) S32.111 ☑
            severely S32.112 ☑
         nondisplaced S32.110 ☑
      II S32.129 ☑
         displaced (minimally) S32.121 ☑
            severely S32.122 ☑
         nondisplaced S32.120 ☑
      III S32.139 ☑
         displaced (minimally) S32.131 ☑
            severely S32.132 ☑
         nondisplaced S32.130 ☑
scaphoid (hand) — *see also* Fracture, carpal, navicular
   foot — *see* Fracture, tarsal, navicular
scapula S42.10- ☑
   acromial process (displaced) S42.12- ☑
      nondisplaced S42.12- ☑
   body (displaced) S42.11- ☑
      nondisplaced S42.11- ☑
   coracoid process (displaced) S42.13- ☑
      nondisplaced S42.13- ☑
   glenoid cavity (displaced) S42.14- ☑

scapula — *continued*
   glenoid cavity — *continued*
      nondisplaced S42.14- ☑
   neck (displaced) S42.15- ☑
      nondisplaced S42.15- ☑
   specified NEC S42.19- ☑
semilunar bone, wrist — *see* Fracture, carpal, lunate
sequelae — *see* Sequelae, fracture
sesamoid bone
   foot S92.81- ☑
   hand — *see* Fracture, carpal
   other — *see* Fracture, traumatic, by site
shepherd's — *see* Fracture, tarsal, talus
shoulder (girdle) S42.9- ☑
   blade — *see* Fracture, scapula
sinus (ethmoid) (frontal) S02.19 ☑
skull S02.91 ☑
   base S02.10- ☑
      occiput S02.119 ☑
         condyle S02.113 ☑
         specified NEC S02.118 ☑
            left side S02.11H ☑
            right side S02.11G ☑
         type I S02.110 ☑
            left side S02.11B ☑
            right side S02.11A ☑
         type II S02.111 ☑
            left side S02.11D ☑
            right side S02.11C ☑
         type III S02.112 ☑
            left side S02.11F ☑
            right side S02.11E ☑
         specified NEC S02.19 ☑
   birth injury P13.0
   frontal bone S02.0 ☑
   parietal bone S02.0 ☑
   specified site NEC S02.8- ☑
   temporal bone S02.19 ☑
   vault S02.0 ☑
Smith's — *see* Smith's fracture
sphenoid (bone) (sinus) S02.19 ☑
spine — *see* Fracture, vertebra
spinous process — *see* Fracture, vertebra
spontaneous (cause unknown) — *see* Fracture, pathological
stave (of thumb) — *see* Fracture, metacarpal, first
sternum S22.20 ☑
   with flail chest — *see* Flail, chest
   body S22.22 ☑
   manubrium S22.21 ☑
   xiphoid (process) S22.24 ☑
stress M84.30 ☑
   ankle M84.37- ☑
   carpus M84.34- ☑
   clavicle M84.31- ☑
   femoral neck M84.359 ☑
   femur M84.35- ☑
   fibula M84.36- ☑
   finger M84.34- ☑
   hip M84.359 ☑
   humerus M84.32- ☑
   ilium M84.350 ☑
   ischium M84.350 ☑
   metacarpus M84.34- ☑
   metatarsus M84.37- ☑
   neck — *see* Fracture, fatigue, vertebra
   pelvis M84.350 ☑
   radius M84.33- ☑
   rib M84.38 ☑
   scapula M84.31- ☑
   skull M84.38 ☑
   tarsus M84.37- ☑
   tibia M84.36- ☑
   toe M84.37- ☑
   ulna M84.33- ☑
   vertebra — *see* Fracture, fatigue, vertebra
supracondylar, elbow — *see* Fracture, humerus, lower end, supracondylar
symphysis pubis — *see* Fracture, pubis
talus (ankle bone) — *see* Fracture, tarsal, talus
tarsal bone(s) S92.20- ☑
   astragalus — *see* Fracture, tarsal, talus
   calcaneus S92.00- ☑
      anterior process (displaced) S92.02- ☑
         nondisplaced S92.02- ☑

Fracture, traumatic — *continued*
  tarsal bone(s) — *continued*
    calcaneus — *continued*
      body (displaced) S92.01- ✓
        nondisplaced S92.01- ✓
      extraarticular NEC (displaced) S92.05- ✓
        nondisplaced S92.05- ✓
      intraarticular (displaced) S92.06- ✓
        nondisplaced S92.06- ✓
      physeal S99.00- ✓
        Salter-Harris
          Type I S99.01- ✓
          Type II S99.02- ✓
          Type III S99.03- ✓
          Type IV S99.04- ✓
        specified NEC S99.09- ✓
      tuberosity (displaced) S92.04- ✓
        avulsion (displaced) S92.03- ✓
          nondisplaced S92.03- ✓
        nondisplaced S92.04- ✓
    cuboid (displaced) S92.21- ✓
      nondisplaced S92.21- ✓
    cuneiform
      intermediate (displaced) S92.23- ✓
        nondisplaced S92.23- ✓
      lateral (displaced) S92.22- ✓
        nondisplaced S92.22- ✓
      medial (displaced) S92.24- ✓
        nondisplaced S92.24- ✓
    navicular (displaced) S92.25- ✓
      nondisplaced S92.25- ✓
    scaphoid — *see* Fracture, tarsal, navicular
    talus S92.10- ✓
      avulsion (displaced) S92.15- ✓
        nondisplaced S92.15- ✓
      body (displaced) S92.12- ✓
        nondisplaced S92.12- ✓
      dome (displaced) S92.14- ✓
        nondisplaced S92.14- ✓
      head (displaced) S92.12- ✓
        nondisplaced S92.12- ✓
      lateral process (displaced) S92.14- ✓
        nondisplaced S92.14- ✓
      neck (displaced) S92.11- ✓
        nondisplaced S92.11- ✓
      posterior process (displaced) S92.13- ✓
        nondisplaced S92.13- ✓
      specified NEC S92.19- ✓
  temporal bone (styloid) S02.19 ✓
  thorax (bony) S22.9 ✓
    with flail chest — *see* Flail, chest
    rib S22.3- ✓
      multiple S22.4- ✓
        with flail chest — *see* Flail, chest
    sternum S22.20 ✓
      body S22.22 ✓
      manubrium S22.21 ✓
      xiphoid process S22.24 ✓
    vertebra (displaced) S22.009 ✓
      burst (stable) S22.001 ✓
        unstable S22.002 ✓
      eighth S22.069 ✓
        burst (stable) S22.061 ✓
          unstable S22.062 ✓
        specified type NEC S22.068 ✓
        wedge compression S22.060 ✓
      eleventh S22.089 ✓
        burst (stable) S22.081 ✓
          unstable S22.082 ✓
        specified type NEC S22.088 ✓
        wedge compression S22.080 ✓
      fifth S22.059 ✓
        burst (stable) S22.051 ✓
          unstable S22.052 ✓
        specified type NEC S22.058 ✓
        wedge compression S22.050 ✓
      first S22.019 ✓
        burst (stable) S22.011 ✓
          unstable S22.012 ✓
        specified type NEC S22.018 ✓
        wedge compression S22.010 ✓
      fourth S22.049 ✓
        burst (stable) S22.041 ✓
          unstable S22.042 ✓
        specified type NEC S22.048 ✓
        wedge compression S22.040 ✓

Fracture, traumatic — *continued*
  thorax — *continued*
    vertebra — *continued*
      ninth S22.079 ✓
        burst (stable) S22.071 ✓
          unstable S22.072 ✓
        specified type NEC S22.078 ✓
        wedge compression S22.070 ✓
      nondisplaced S22.001 ✓
      second S22.029 ✓
        burst (stable) S22.021 ✓
          unstable S22.022 ✓
        specified type NEC S22.028 ✓
        wedge compression S22.020 ✓
      seventh S22.069 ✓
        burst (stable) S22.061 ✓
          unstable S22.062 ✓
        specified type NEC S22.068 ✓
        wedge compression S22.060 ✓
      sixth S22.059 ✓
        burst (stable) S22.051 ✓
          unstable S22.052 ✓
        specified type NEC S22.058 ✓
        wedge compression S22.050 ✓
      specified type NEC S22.008 ✓
      tenth S22.079 ✓
        burst (stable) S22.071 ✓
          unstable S22.072 ✓
        specified type NEC S22.078 ✓
        wedge compression S22.070 ✓
      third S22.039 ✓
        burst (stable) S22.031 ✓
          unstable S22.032 ✓
        specified type NEC S22.038 ✓
        wedge compression S22.030 ✓
      twelfth S22.089 ✓
        burst (stable) S22.081 ✓
          unstable S22.082 ✓
        specified type NEC S22.088 ✓
        wedge compression S22.080 ✓
      wedge compression S22.000 ✓
  thumb S62.50- ✓
    distal phalanx (displaced) S62.52- ✓
      nondisplaced S62.52- ✓
    proximal phalanx (displaced) S62.51- ✓
      nondisplaced S62.51- ✓
  thyroid cartilage S12.8 ✓
  tibia (shaft) S82.20- ✓
    comminuted (displaced) S82.25- ✓
      nondisplaced S82.25- ✓
    condyles — *see* Fracture, tibia, upper end
    distal end — *see* Fracture, tibia, lower end
    epiphysis
      lower — *see* Fracture, tibia, lower end
      upper — *see* Fracture, tibia, upper end
    following insertion of implant, prosthesis or plate
      M96.67- ✓
    head (involving knee joint) — *see* Fracture, tibia, upper end
    intercondyloid eminence — *see* Fracture, tibia, upper end
    involving ankle or malleolus — *see* Fracture, ankle, medial malleolus
    lower end S82.30- ✓
      physeal S89.10- ✓
        Salter-Harris
          Type I S89.11- ✓
          Type II S89.12- ✓
          Type III S89.13- ✓
          Type IV S89.14- ✓
        specified NEC S89.19- ✓
      pilon (displaced) S82.87- ✓
        nondisplaced S82.87- ✓
      specified NEC S82.39- ✓
      torus S82.31- ✓
    malleolus — *see* Fracture, ankle, medial malleolus
    oblique (displaced) S82.23- ✓
      nondisplaced S82.23- ✓
    pilon — *see* Fracture, tibia, lower end, pilon
    proximal end — *see* Fracture, tibia, upper end
    segmental (displaced) S82.26- ✓
      nondisplaced S82.26- ✓
    specified NEC S82.29- ✓
    spine — *see* Fracture, tibia, upper end, spine
    spiral (displaced) S82.24- ✓
      nondisplaced S82.24- ✓

Fracture, traumatic — *continued*
  tibia — *continued*
    transverse (displaced) S82.22- ✓
      nondisplaced S82.22- ✓
    tuberosity — *see* Fracture, tibia, upper end, tuberosity
    upper end S82.10- ✓
      bicondylar (displaced) S82.14- ✓
        nondisplaced S82.14- ✓
      lateral condyle (displaced) S82.12- ✓
        nondisplaced S82.12- ✓
      medial condyle (displaced) S82.13- ✓
        nondisplaced S82.13- ✓
      physeal S89.00- ✓
        Salter-Harris
          Type I S89.01- ✓
          Type II S89.02- ✓
          Type III S89.03- ✓
          Type IV S89.04- ✓
        specified NEC S89.09- ✓
      plateau — *see* Fracture, tibia, upper end, bicondylar
      specified NEC S82.19- ✓
      spine (displaced) S82.11- ✓
        nondisplaced S82.11- ✓
      torus S82.16- ✓
      tuberosity (displaced) S82.15- ✓
        nondisplaced S82.15- ✓
  toe S92.91- ✓
    great (displaced) S92.40- ✓
      distal phalanx (displaced) S92.42- ✓
        nondisplaced S92.42- ✓
      nondisplaced S92.40- ✓
      proximal phalanx (displaced) S92.41- ✓
        nondisplaced S92.41- ✓
      specified NEC S92.49- ✓
    lesser (displaced) S92.50- ✓
      distal phalanx (displaced) S92.53- ✓
        nondisplaced S92.53- ✓
      middle phalanx (displaced) S92.52- ✓
        nondisplaced S92.52- ✓
      nondisplaced S92.50- ✓
      proximal phalanx (displaced) S92.51- ✓
        nondisplaced S92.51- ✓
      specified NEC S92.59- ✓
    physeal
      phalanx S99.20- ✓
        Salter-Harris
          Type I S99.21- ✓
          Type II S99.22- ✓
          Type III S99.23- ✓
          Type IV S99.24- ✓
        specified NEC S99.29- ✓
  tooth (root) S02.5 ✓
  trachea (cartilage) S12.8 ✓
  transverse process — *see* Fracture, vertebra
  trapezium or trapezoid bone — *see* Fracture, carpal
  trimalleolar — *see* Fracture, ankle, trimalleolar
  triquetrum (cuneiform of carpus) — *see* Fracture, carpal, triquetrum
  trochanter — *see* Fracture, femur, trochanteric
  tuberosity (external) — *see* Fracture, traumatic, by site
  ulna (shaft) S52.20- ✓
    bent bone S52.28- ✓
    coronoid process — *see* Fracture, ulna, upper end, coronoid process
    distal end — *see* Fracture, ulna, lower end
    following insertion of implant, prosthesis or plate M96.63- ✓
    head S52.60- ✓
    lower end S52.60- ✓
      physeal S59.00- ✓
        Salter-Harris
          Type I S59.01- ✓
          Type II S59.02- ✓
          Type III S59.03- ✓
          Type IV S59.04- ✓
        specified NEC S59.09- ✓
      specified NEC S52.69- ✓
      styloid process (displaced) S52.61- ✓
        nondisplaced S52.61- ✓
      torus S52.62- ✓
    proximal end — *see* Fracture, ulna, upper end
    shaft S52.20- ✓
      comminuted (displaced) S52.25- ✓
        nondisplaced S52.25- ✓

Fracture, traumatic — *continued*
  ulna — *continued*
    shaft — *continued*
      greenstick S52.21- ☑
      Monteggia's — *see* Monteggia's fracture
      oblique (displaced) S52.23- ☑
        nondisplaced S52.23- ☑
      segmental (displaced) S52.26- ☑
        nondisplaced S52.26- ☑
      specified NEC S52.29- ☑
      spiral (displaced) S52.24- ☑
        nondisplaced S52.24- ☑
      transverse (displaced) S52.22- ☑
        nondisplaced S52.22- ☑
    upper end S52.00- ☑
      coronoid process (displaced) S52.04- ☑
        nondisplaced S52.04- ☑
      olecranon process (displaced) S52.02- ☑
        with intraarticular extension S52.03- ☑
        nondisplaced S52.02- ☑
          with intraarticular extension S52.03- ☑
      specified NEC S52.09- ☑
      torus S52.01- ☑
  unciform — *see* Fracture, carpal, hamate
  vault of skull S02.0 ☑
  vertebra, vertebral (arch) (body) (column) (neural arch) (pedicle) (spinous process) (transverse process)
    atlas — *see* Fracture, neck, cervical vertebra, first
    axis — *see* Fracture, neck, cervical vertebra, second
    cervical (teardrop) S12.9 ☑
      axis — *see* Fracture, neck, cervical vertebra, second
      first (atlas) — *see* Fracture, neck, cervical vertebra, first
      second (axis) — *see* Fracture, neck, cervical vertebra, second
    chronic M84.48 ☑
    coccyx S32.2 ☑
    dorsal — *see* Fracture, thorax, vertebra
    lumbar S32.009 ☑
      burst (stable) S32.001 ☑
        unstable S32.002 ☑
      fifth S32.059 ☑
        burst (stable) S32.051 ☑
          unstable S32.052 ☑
        specified type NEC S32.058 ☑
        wedge compression S32.050 ☑
      first S32.019 ☑
        burst (stable) S32.011 ☑
          unstable S32.012 ☑
        specified type NEC S32.018 ☑
        wedge compression S32.010 ☑
      fourth S32.049 ☑
        burst (stable) S32.041 ☑
          unstable S32.042 ☑
        specified type NEC S32.048 ☑
        wedge compression S32.040 ☑
      second S32.029 ☑
        burst (stable) S32.021 ☑
          unstable S32.022 ☑
        specified type NEC S32.028 ☑
        wedge compression S32.020 ☑
      specified type NEC S32.008 ☑
      third S32.039 ☑
        burst (stable) S32.031 ☑
          unstable S32.032 ☑
        specified type NEC S32.038 ☑
        wedge compression S32.030 ☑
      wedge compression S32.000 ☑
    metastatic — *see* Collapse, vertebra, in, specified disease NEC — *see also* Neoplasm
    newborn (birth injury) P11.5
    sacrum S32.10 ☑
      specified NEC S32.19 ☑
      Type
        1 S32.14 ☑
        2 S32.15 ☑
        3 S32.16 ☑
        4 S32.17 ☑
      Zone
        I S32.119 ☑
          displaced (minimally) S32.111 ☑
            severely S32.112 ☑
          nondisplaced S32.110 ☑
        II S32.129 ☑
          displaced (minimally) S32.121 ☑

Fracture, traumatic — *continued*
  vertebra, vertebral — *continued*
    sacrum — *continued*
      Zone — *continued*
        II — *continued*
          displaced — *continued*
            severely S32.122 ☑
          nondisplaced S32.120 ☑
        III S32.139 ☑
          displaced (minimally) S32.131 ☑
            severely S32.132 ☑
          nondisplaced S32.130 ☑
    thoracic — *see* Fracture, thorax, vertebra
  vertex S02.0 ☑
  vomer (bone) S02.2 ☑
  wrist S62.10- ☑
    carpal — *see* Fracture, carpal bone
    navicular (scaphoid) (hand) — *see* Fracture, carpal, navicular
  xiphisternum, xiphoid (process) S22.24 ☑
  zygoma S02.402 ☑
    left side S02.40F ☑
    right side S02.40E ☑
Fragile, fragility
  autosomal site Q95.5
  bone, congenital (with blue sclera) Q78.0
  capillary (hereditary) D69.8
  hair L67.8
  nails L60.3
  non-sex chromosome site Q95.5
  X chromosome Q99.2
Fragilitas
  crinium L67.8
  ossium (with blue sclerae) (hereditary) Q78.0
  unguium L60.3
    congenital Q84.6
Fragments, cataract (lens), **following cataract surgery** H59.02- ☑
  retained foreign body — *see* Retained, foreign body fragments (type of)
Frailty (frail) R54
  mental R41.81
Frambesia, frambesial (tropica) — *see also* Yaws
  initial lesion or ulcer A66.0
  primary A66.0
Frambeside
  gummatous A66.4
  of early yaws A66.2
Frambesioma A66.1
Franceschetti-Klein (-Wildervanck) **disease or syndrome** Q75.4
Francis' disease — *see* Tularemia
Franklin disease C88.2
Frank's essential thrombocytopenia D69.3
Fraser's syndrome Q87.0
Freckle(s) L81.2
  malignant melanoma in — *see* Melanoma
  melanotic (Hutchinson's) — *see* Melanoma, in situ
  retinal D49.81
Frederickson's hyperlipoproteinemia, type
  I and V E78.3
  IIA E78.00
  IIB and III E78.2
  IV E78.1
Freeman Sheldon syndrome Q87.0
Freezing — *see also* Effect, adverse, cold T69.9 ☑
Freiberg's disease (infraction of metatarsal head or osteochondrosis) — *see* Osteochondrosis, juvenile, metatarsus
Frei's disease A55
Fremitus, friction, cardiac R01.2
Frenum, frenulum
  external os Q51.828
  tongue (shortening) (congenital) Q38.1
Frequency micturition (nocturnal) R35.0
  psychogenic F45.8
Frey's syndrome
  auriculotemporal G50.8
  hyperhidrosis L74.52
Friction
  burn — *see* Burn, by site
  fremitus, cardiac R01.2
  precordial R01.2
  sounds, chest R09.89
Friderichsen-Waterhouse syndrome or disease A39.1
Friedländer's B (bacillus) **NEC** — *see also* condition A49.8

Friedreich's
  ataxia G11.1
  combined systemic disease G11.1
  facial hemihypertrophy Q67.4
  sclerosis (cerebellum) (spinal cord) G11.1
Frigidity F52.22
Fröhlich's syndrome E23.6
Frontal — *see also* condition
  lobe syndrome F07.0
Frostbite (superficial) T33.90 ☑
  with
    partial thickness skin loss — *see* Frostbite (superficial), by site
    tissue necrosis T34.90 ☑
  abdominal wall T33.3 ☑
    with tissue necrosis T34.3 ☑
  ankle T33.81- ☑
    with tissue necrosis T34.81- ☑
  arm T33.4- ☑
    with tissue necrosis T34.4- ☑
    finger(s) — *see* Frostbite, finger
    hand — *see* Frostbite, hand
    wrist — *see* Frostbite, wrist
  ear T33.01- ☑
    with tissue necrosis T34.01- ☑
  face T33.09 ☑
    with tissue necrosis T34.09 ☑
  finger T33.53- ☑
    with tissue necrosis T34.53- ☑
  foot T33.82- ☑
    with tissue necrosis T34.82- ☑
  hand T33.52- ☑
    with tissue necrosis T34.52- ☑
  head T33.09 ☑
    with tissue necrosis T34.09 ☑
    ear — *see* Frostbite, ear
    nose — *see* Frostbite, nose
  hip (and thigh) T33.6- ☑
    with tissue necrosis T34.6- ☑
  knee T33.7- ☑
    with tissue necrosis T34.7- ☑
  leg T33.9- ☑
    with tissue necrosis T34.9- ☑
    ankle — *see* Frostbite, ankle
    foot — *see* Frostbite, foot
    knee — *see* Frostbite, knee
    lower T33.7- ☑
      with tissue necrosis T34.7- ☑
    thigh — *see* Frostbite, hip
    toe — *see* Frostbite, toe
  limb
    lower T33.99 ☑
      with tissue necrosis T34.99 ☑
    upper — *see* Frostbite, arm
  neck T33.1 ☑
    with tissue necrosis T34.1 ☑
  nose T33.02 ☑
    with tissue necrosis T34.02 ☑
  pelvis T33.3 ☑
    with tissue necrosis T34.3 ☑
  specified site NEC T33.99 ☑
    with tissue necrosis T34.99 ☑
  thigh — *see* Frostbite, hip
  thorax T33.2 ☑
    with tissue necrosis T34.2 ☑
  toes T33.83- ☑
    with tissue necrosis T34.83- ☑
  trunk T33.99 ☑
    with tissue necrosis T34.99 ☑
  wrist T33.51- ☑
    with tissue necrosis T34.51- ☑
Frotteurism F65.81
Frozen — *see also* Effect, adverse, cold T69.9 ☑
  pelvis (female) N94.89
    male K66.8
  shoulder — *see* Capsulitis, adhesive
Fructokinase deficiency E74.11
Fructose 1,6 diphosphatase deficiency E74.19
Fructosemia (benign) (essential) E74.12
Fructosuria (benign) (essential) E74.11
Fuchs'
  black spot (myopic) — *see also* Myopia, degenerative H44.2- ☑
  dystrophy (corneal endothelium) H18.51
  heterochromic cyclitis — *see* Cyclitis, Fuchs' heterochromic

Fucosidosis E77.1
Fugue R68.89
  dissociative F44.1
  hysterical (dissociative) F44.1
  postictal in epilepsy — *see* Epilepsy
  reaction to exceptional stress (transient) F43.0
Fulminant, fulminating — *see* condition
Functional — *see also* condition
  bleeding (uterus) N93.8
Functioning, intellectual, borderline R41.83
Fundus — *see* condition
Fungemia NOS B49
Fungus, fungous
  cerebral G93.89
  disease NOS B49
  infection — *see* Infection, fungus
Funiculitis (acute) (chronic) (endemic) N49.1
  gonococcal (acute) (chronic) A54.23
  tuberculous A18.15
Funnel
  breast (acquired) M95.4
    congenital Q67.6
    sequelae (late effect) of rickets E64.3
  chest (acquired) M95.4
    congenital Q67.6
    sequelae (late effect) of rickets E64.3
  pelvis (acquired) M95.5
    with disproportion (fetopelvic) O33.3 ☑
      causing obstructed labor O65.3
    congenital Q74.2
FUO (fever of unknown origin) R50.9
Furfur L21.0
  microsporon B36.0
Furrier's lung J67.8
Furrowed K14.5
  nail(s) (transverse) L60.4
    congenital Q84.6
  tongue K14.5
    congenital Q38.3
Furuncle L02.92
  abdominal wall L02.221
  ankle — *see* Furuncle, lower limb
  antecubital space — *see* Furuncle, upper limb
  anus K61.0
  arm — *see* Furuncle, upper limb
  auditory canal, external — *see* Abscess, ear, external
  auricle (ear) — *see* Abscess, ear, external
  axilla (region) L02.42- ☑
  back (any part) L02.222
  breast N61.1
  buttock L02.32
  cheek (external) L02.02
  chest wall L02.223
  chin L02.02
  corpus cavernosum N48.21
  ear, external — *see* Abscess, ear, external
  external auditory canal — *see* Abscess, ear, external
  eyelid — *see* Abscess, eyelid
  face L02.02
  femoral (region) — *see* Furuncle, lower limb

Furuncle — *continued*
  finger — *see* Furuncle, hand
  flank L02.221
  foot L02.62- ☑
  forehead L02.02
  gluteal (region) L02.32
  groin L02.224
  hand L02.52- ☑
  head L02.821
    face L02.02
  hip — *see* Furuncle, lower limb
  kidney — *see* Abscess, kidney
  knee — *see* Furuncle, lower limb
  labium (majus) (minus) N76.4
  lacrimal
    gland — *See* Dacryoadenitis
    passages (duct) (sac) — *see* Inflammation, lacrimal,
      passages, acute
  leg (any part) — *see* Furuncle, lower limb
  lower limb L02.42- ☑
  malignant A22.0
  mouth K12.2
  navel L02.226
  neck L02.12
  nose J34.0
  orbit, orbital — *see* Abscess, orbit
  palmar (space) — *see* Furuncle, hand
  partes posteriores L02.32
  pectoral region L02.223
  penis N48.21
  perineum L02.225
  pinna — *see* Abscess, ear, external
  popliteal — *see* Furuncle, lower limb
  prepatellar — *see* Furuncle, lower limb
  scalp L02.821
  seminal vesicle N49.0
  shoulder — *see* Furuncle, upper limb
  specified site NEC L02.828
  submandibular K12.2
  temple (region) L02.02
  thumb — *see* Furuncle, hand
  toe — *see* Furuncle, foot
  trunk L02.229
    abdominal wall L02.221
    back L02.222
    chest wall L02.223
    groin L02.224
    perineum L02.225
    umbilicus L02.226
  umbilicus L02.226
  upper limb L02.42- ☑
  vulva N76.4
Furunculosis — *see* Furuncle
Fused — *see* Fusion, fused
Fusion, fused (congenital)
  astragaloscaphoid Q74.2
  atria Q21.1
  auditory canal Q16.1
  auricles, heart Q21.1
  binocular with defective stereopsis H53.32

Fusion, fused — *continued*
  bone Q79.8
  cervical spine M43.22
  choanal Q30.0
  commissure, mitral valve Q23.2
  cusps, heart valve NEC Q24.8
    mitral Q23.2
    pulmonary Q22.1
    tricuspid Q22.4
  ear ossicles Q16.3
  fingers Q70.0 ☑
  hymen Q52.3
  joint (acquired) — *see also* Ankylosis
    congenital Q74.8
  kidneys (incomplete) Q63.1
  labium (majus) (minus) Q52.5
  larynx and trachea Q34.8
  limb, congenital Q74.8
    lower Q74.2
    upper Q74.0
  lobes, lung Q33.8
  lumbosacral (acquired) M43.27
    arthrodesis status Z98.1
    congenital Q76.49
    postprocedural status Z98.1
  nares, nose, nasal, nostril(s) Q30.0
  organ or site not listed — *see* Anomaly, by site
  ossicles Q79.9
    auditory Q16.3
  pulmonic cusps Q22.1
  ribs Q76.6
  sacroiliac (joint) (acquired) M43.28
    arthrodesis status Z98.1
    congenital Q74.2
    postprocedural status Z98.1
  spine (acquired) NEC M43.20
    arthrodesis status Z98.1
    cervical region M43.22
    cervicothoracic region M43.23
    congenital Q76.49
    lumbar M43.26
    lumbosacral region M43.27
    occipito-atlanto-axial region M43.21
    postoperative status Z98.1
    sacrococcygeal region M43.28
    thoracic region M43.24
    thoracolumbar region M43.25
  sublingual duct with submaxillary duct at opening in
    mouth Q38.4
  testes Q55.1
  toes Q70.2- ☑
  tooth, teeth K00.2
  trachea and esophagus Q39.8
  twins Q89.4
  vagina Q52.4
  ventricles, heart Q21.0
  vertebra (arch) — *see* Fusion, spine
  vulva Q52.5
Fusospirillosis (mouth) (tongue) (tonsil) A69.1
Fussy baby R68.12

☑ **Additional Character Required — Refer to the Tabular List for Character Selection**   🔻 **Subterms under main terms may continue to next column or page**

G

Gain in weight (abnormal) (excessive) — see also Weight, gain
Gaisböck's disease (polycythemia hypertonica) D75.1
Gait abnormality R26.9
  ataxic R26.0
  falling R29.6
  hysterical (ataxic) (staggering) F44.4
  paralytic R26.1
  spastic R26.1
  specified type NEC R26.89
  staggering R26.0
  unsteadiness R26.81
  walking difficulty NEC R26.2
Galactocele (breast) N64.89
  puerperal, postpartum O92.79
Galactokinase deficiency E74.29
Galactophoritis N61.0
  gestational, puerperal, postpartum O91.2- ☑
Galactorrhea O92.6
  not associated with childbirth N64.3
Galactosemia (classic) (congenital) E74.21
Galactosuria E74.29
Galacturia R82.0
  schistosomiasis (bilharziasis) B65.0
GALD (gestational alloimmune liver disease) P78.84
Galeazzi's fracture S52.37- ☑
Galen's vein — see condition
Galeophobia F40.218
Gall duct — see condition
Gallbladder — see also condition
  acute K81.0
Gallop rhythm R00.8
Gallstone (colic) (cystic duct) (gallbladder) (impacted) (multiple) — see also Calculus, gallbladder
  with
    cholecystitis — see Calculus, gallbladder, with cholecystitis
  bile duct (common) (hepatic) — see Calculus, bile duct
  causing intestinal obstruction K56.3
  specified NEC K80.80
    with obstruction K80.81
Gambling Z72.6
  pathological (compulsive) F63.0
Gammopathy (of undetermined significance [MGUS]) D47.2
  associated with lymphoplasmacytic dyscrasia D47.2
  monoclonal D47.2
  polyclonal D89.0
Gamna's disease (siderotic splenomegaly) D73.1
Gamophobia F40.298
Gampsodactylia (congenital) Q66.7- ☑
Gamstorp's disease (adynamia episodica hereditaria) G72.3
Gandy-Nanta disease (siderotic splenomegaly) D73.1
Gang
  membership offenses Z72.810
Gangliocytoma D36.10
Ganglioglioma — see Neoplasm, uncertain behavior, by site
Ganglion (compound) (diffuse) (joint) (tendon (sheath)) M67.40
  ankle M67.47- ☑
  foot M67.47- ☑
  forearm M67.43- ☑
  hand M67.44- ☑
  lower leg M67.46- ☑
  multiple sites M67.49
  of yaws (early) (late) A66.6
  pelvic region M67.45- ☑
  periosteal — see Periostitis
  shoulder region M67.41- ☑
  specified site NEC M67.48
  thigh region M67.45- ☑
  tuberculous A18.09
  upper arm M67.42- ☑
  wrist M67.43- ☑
Ganglioneuroblastoma — see Neoplasm, nerve, malignant
Ganglioneuroma D36.10
  malignant — see Neoplasm, nerve, malignant
Ganglioneuromatosis D36.10
Ganglionitis
  fifth nerve — see Neuralgia, trigeminal
  gasserian (postherpetic) (postzoster) B02.21

Ganglionitis — continued
  geniculate G51.1
    newborn (birth injury) P11.3
    postherpetic, postzoster B02.21
  herpes zoster B02.21
  postherpetic geniculate B02.21
Gangliosidosis E75.10
  GM1 E75.19
  GM2 E75.00
    other specified E75.09
    Sandhoff disease E75.01
    Tay-Sachs disease E75.02
  GM3 E75.19
  mucolipidosis IV E75.11
Gangosa A66.5
Gangrene, gangrenous (connective tissue) (dropsical) (dry) (moist) (skin) (ulcer) — see also Necrosis I96
  with diabetes (mellitus) — see Diabetes, gangrene
  abdomen (wall) I96
  alveolar M27.3
  appendix K35.80
    with
      peritonitis, localized — see also Appendicitis K35.31
  arteriosclerotic (general) (senile) — see Arteriosclerosis, extremities, with, gangrene
  auricle I96
  Bacillus welchii A48.0
  bladder (infectious) — see Cystitis, specified type NEC
  bowel, cecum, or colon — see Gangrene, intestine
  Clostridium perfringens or welchii A48.0
  cornea H18.89- ☑
  corpora cavernosa N48.29
    noninfective N48.89
  cutaneous, spreading I96
  decubital — see Ulcer, pressure, by site
  diabetic (any site) — see Diabetes, gangrene
  emphysematous — see Gangrene, gas
  epidemic — see Poisoning, food, noxious, plant
  epididymis (infectional) N45.1
  erysipelas — see Erysipelas
  extremity (lower) (upper) I96
  Fournier N49.3
    female N76.89
  fusospirochetal A69.0
  gallbladder — see Cholecystitis, acute
  gas (bacillus) A48.0
    following
      abortion — see Abortion by type complicated by infection
      ectopic or molar pregnancy O08.0
  glossitis K14.0
  hernia — see Hernia, by site, with gangrene
  intestine, intestinal (hemorrhagic) (massive) — see also Infarct, intestine K55.069
    with
      mesenteric embolism — see also Infarct, intestine K55.069
      obstruction — see Obstruction, intestine
  laryngitis J04.0
  limb (lower) (upper) I96
  lung J85.0
    spirochetal A69.8
  lymphangitis I89.1
  Meleney's (synergistic) — see Ulcer, skin
  mesentery — see also Infarct, intestine K55.069
    with
      embolism — see also Infarct, intestine K55.069
      intestinal obstruction — see Obstruction, intestine
  mouth A69.0
  ovary — see Oophoritis
  pancreas — see Pancreatitis, acute
  penis N48.29
    noninfective N48.89
  perineum I96
  pharynx — see also Pharyngitis
    Vincent's A69.1
  presenile I73.1
  progressive synergistic — see Ulcer, skin
  pulmonary J85.0
  pulpal (dental) K04.1
  quinsy J36
  Raynaud's (symmetric gangrene) I73.01
  retropharyngeal J39.2
  scrotum N49.3
    noninfective N50.89

Gangrene, gangrenous — continued
  senile (atherosclerotic) — see Arteriosclerosis, extremities, with, gangrene
  spermatic cord N49.1
    noninfective N50.89
  spine I96
  spirochetal NEC A69.8
  spreading cutaneous I96
  stomatitis A69.0
  symmetrical I73.01
  testis (infectional) N45.2
    noninfective N44.8
  throat — see also Pharyngitis
    diphtheritic A36.0
    Vincent's A69.1
  thyroid (gland) E07.89
  tooth (pulp) K04.1
  tuberculous NEC — see Tuberculosis
  tunica vaginalis N49.1
    noninfective N50.89
  umbilicus I96
  uterus — see Endometritis
  uvulitis K12.2
  vas deferens N49.1
    noninfective N50.89
  vulva N76.89
Ganister disease J62.8
Ganser's syndrome (hysterical) F44.89
Gardner-Diamond syndrome (autoerythrocyte sensitization) D69.2
Gargoylism E76.01
Garré's disease, osteitis (sclerosing), osteomyelitis — see Osteomyelitis, specified type NEC
Garrod's pad, knuckle M72.1
Gartner's duct
  cyst Q52.4
  persistent Q50.6
Gas R14.3
  asphyxiation, inhalation, poisoning, suffocation NEC — see Table of Drugs and Chemicals
  excessive R14.0
  gangrene A48.0
    following
      abortion — see Abortion by type complicated by infection
      ectopic or molar pregnancy O08.0
  on stomach R14.0
  pains R14.1
Gastralgia — see also Pain, abdominal
Gastrectasis K31.0
  psychogenic F45.8
Gastric — see condition
Gastrinoma
  malignant
    pancreas C25.4
    specified site NEC — see Neoplasm, malignant, by site
    unspecified site C25.4
  specified site — see Neoplasm, uncertain behavior
  unspecified site D37.9
Gastritis (simple) K29.70
  with bleeding K29.71
  acute (erosive) K29.00
    with bleeding K29.01
  alcoholic K29.20
    with bleeding K29.21
  allergic K29.60
    with bleeding K29.61
  atrophic (chronic) K29.40
    with bleeding K29.41
  chronic (antral) (fundal) K29.50
    with bleeding K29.51
    atrophic K29.40
      with bleeding K29.41
    superficial K29.30
      with bleeding K29.31
  dietary counseling and surveillance Z71.3
  due to diet deficiency E63.9
  eosinophilic K52.81
  giant hypertrophic K29.60
    with bleeding K29.61
  granulomatous K29.60
    with bleeding K29.61
  hypertrophic (mucosa) K29.60
    with bleeding K29.61
  nervous F54
  spastic K29.60
    with bleeding K29.61

⬇ Subterms under main terms may continue to next column or page   ☑ Additional Character Required — Refer to the Tabular List for Character Selection   157

Gain in weight — Gastritis

Gastritis — *continued*
  specified NEC K29.60
    with bleeding K29.61
  superficial chronic K29.30
    with bleeding K29.31
  tuberculous A18.83
  viral NEC A08.4
Gastrocarcinoma — *see* Neoplasm, malignant, stomach
Gastrocolic — *see* condition
Gastrodisciasis, gastrodiscoidiasis B66.8
Gastroduodenitis K29.90
  with bleeding K29.91
  virus, viral A08.4
    specified type NEC A08.39
Gastrodynia — *see* Pain, abdominal
Gastroenteritis (acute) (chronic) (noninfectious) — *see also* Enteritis K52.9
  allergic K52.29
    with
      eosinophilic gastritis or gastroenteritis K52.81
      food protein-induced enterocolitis syndrome K52.21
      food protein-induced enteropathy K52.22
  dietetic — *see also* Gastroenteritis, allergic K52.29
  drug-induced K52.1
  due to
    Cryptosporidium A07.2
    drugs K52.1
    food poisoning — *see* Intoxication, foodborne
    radiation K52.0
  eosinophilic K52.81
  epidemic (infectious) A09
  food hypersensitivity — *see also* Gastroenteritis, allergic K52.29
  infectious — *see* Enteritis, infectious
  influenzal — *see* Influenza, with gastroenteritis
  noninfectious K52.9
    specified NEC K52.89
  rotaviral A08.0
  Salmonella A02.0
  toxic K52.1
  viral NEC A08.4
    acute infectious A08.39
      type Norwalk A08.11
    infantile (acute) A08.39
    Norwalk agent A08.11
    rotaviral A08.0
    severe of infants A08.39
    specified type NEC A08.39
Gastroenteropathy — *see also* Gastroenteritis K52.9
  acute, due to Norovirus A08.11
  acute, due to Norwalk agent A08.11
  infectious A09
Gastroenteroptosis K63.4
Gastroesophageal laceration- hemorrhage syndrome K22.6
Gastrointestinal — *see* condition
Gastrojejunal — *see* condition
Gastrojejunitis — *see also* Enteritis K52.9
Gastrojejunocolic — *see* condition
Gastroliths K31.89
Gastromalacia K31.89
Gastroparalysis K31.84
  diabetic — *see* Diabetes, gastroparalysis
Gastroparesis K31.84
  diabetic — *see* Diabetes, by type, with gastroparesis
Gastropathy K31.9
  congestive portal K31.89
  erythematous K29.70
  exudative K90.89
  portal hypertensive K31.89
Gastroptosis K31.89
Gastrorrhagia K92.2
  psychogenic F45.8
Gastroschisis (congenital) Q79.3
Gastrospasm (neurogenic) (reflex) K31.89
  neurotic F45.8
  psychogenic F45.8
Gastrostaxis — *see* Gastritis, with bleeding
Gastrostenosis K31.89
Gastrostomy
  attention to Z43.1
  status Z93.1
Gastrosuccorrhea (continuous) (intermittent) K31.89
  neurotic F45.8
  psychogenic F45.8
Gatophobia F40.218

Gaucher's disease or splenomegaly (adult) (infantile) E75.22
Gee (-Herter)(-Thaysen) **disease** (nontropical sprue) K90.0
Gélineau's syndrome G47.419
  with cataplexy G47.411
Gemination, tooth, teeth K00.2
Gemistocytoma
  specified site — *see* Neoplasm, malignant, by site
  unspecified site C71.9
General, generalized — *see* condition
Genetic
  carrier (status)
    cystic fibrosis Z14.1
    hemophilia A (asymptomatic) Z14.01
      symptomatic Z14.02
    specified NEC Z14.8
  susceptibility to disease NEC Z15.89
    malignant neoplasm Z15.09
      breast Z15.01
      endometrium Z15.04
      ovary Z15.02
      prostate Z15.03
      specified NEC Z15.09
    multiple endocrine neoplasia Z15.81
Genital — *see* condition
Genito-anorectal syndrome A55
Genitourinary system — *see* condition
Genu
  congenital Q74.1
  extrorsum (acquired) — *see also* Deformity, varus, knee
    congenital Q74.1
    sequelae (late effect) of rickets E64.3
  introrsum (acquired) — *see also* Deformity, valgus, knee
    congenital Q74.1
    sequelae (late effect) of rickets E64.3
  rachitic (old) E64.3
  recurvatum (acquired) — *see also* Deformity, limb, specified type NEC, lower leg
    congenital Q68.2
    sequelae (late effect) of rickets E64.3
  valgum (acquired) (knock-knee) M21.06- ☑
    congenital Q74.1
    sequelae (late effect) of rickets E64.3
  varum (acquired) (bowleg) M21.16- ☑
    congenital Q74.1
    sequelae (late effect) of rickets E64.3
Geographic tongue K14.1
Geophagia — *see* Pica
Geotrichosis B48.3
  stomatitis B48.3
Gephyrophobia F40.242
Gerbode defect Q21.0
GERD (gastroesophageal reflux disease) K21.9
Gerhardt's
  disease (erythromelalgia) I73.81
  syndrome (vocal cord paralysis) J38.00
    bilateral J38.02
    unilateral J38.01
German measles — *see also* Rubella
  exposure to Z20.4
Germinoblastoma (diffuse) C85.9- ☑
  follicular C82.9- ☑
Germinoma — *see* Neoplasm, malignant, by site
Gerontoxon — *see* Degeneration, cornea, senile
Gerstmann's syndrome R48.8
  developmental F81.2
Gerstmann-Sträussler-Scheinker syndrome (GSS) A81.82
Gestation (period) — *see also* Pregnancy
  ectopic — *see* Pregnancy, by site
  multiple O30.9- ☑
    greater than quadruplets — *see* Pregnancy, multiple (gestation), specified NEC
    specified NEC — *see* Pregnancy, multiple (gestation), specified NEC
Gestational
  mammary abscess O91.11- ☑
  purulent mastitis O91.11- ☑
  subareolar abscess O91.11- ☑
Ghon tubercle, primary infection A15.7
Ghost
  teeth K00.4
  vessels (cornea) H16.41- ☑
Ghoul hand A66.3
Gianotti-Crosti disease L44.4

Giant
  cell
    epulis K06.8
    peripheral granuloma K06.8
  esophagus, congenital Q39.5
  kidney, congenital Q63.3
  urticaria T78.3 ☑
    hereditary D84.1
Giardiasis A07.1
Gibert's disease or pityriasis L42
Giddiness R42
  hysterical F44.89
  psychogenic F45.8
Gierke's disease (glycogenosis I) E74.01
Gigantism (cerebral) (hypophyseal) (pituitary) E22.0
  constitutional E34.4
Gilbert's disease or syndrome E80.4
Gilchrist's disease B40.9
Gilford-Hutchinson disease E34.8
Gilles de la Tourette's disease or syndrome (motor-verbal tic) F95.2
Gingivitis K05.10
  acute (catarrhal) K05.00
    necrotizing A69.1
    nonplaque induced K05.01
    plaque induced K05.00
  chronic (desquamative) (hyperplastic) (simple marginal) (pregnancy associated) (ulcerative) K05.10
    nonplaque induced K05.11
    plaque induced K05.10
  expulsiva — *see* Periodontitis
  necrotizing ulcerative (acute) A69.1
  pellagrous E52
    acute necrotizing A69.1
  Vincent's A69.1
Gingivoglossitis K14.0
Gingivopericementitis — *see* Periodontitis
Gingivosis — *see* Gingivitis, chronic
Gingivostomatitis K05.10
  herpesviral B00.2
  necrotizing ulcerative (acute) A69.1
Gland, glandular — *see* condition
Glanders A24.0
Glanzmann (-Naegeli) **disease or thrombasthenia** D69.1
Glasgow coma scale
  total score
    13-15 R40.241 ☑
    3-8 R40.243 ☑
    9-12 R40.242 ☑
Glass-blower's disease (cataract) — *see* Cataract, specified NEC
Glaucoma H40.9
  with
    increased episcleral venous pressure H40.81- ☑
    pseudoexfoliation of lens — *see* Glaucoma, open angle, primary, capsular
  absolute H44.51- ☑
  angle-closure (primary) H40.20- ☑
    acute (attack) (crisis) H40.21- ☑
    chronic H40.22- ☑
    intermittent H40.23- ☑
    residual stage H40.24- ☑
  borderline H40.00- ☑
  capsular (with pseudoexfoliation of lens) — *see* Glaucoma, open angle, primary, capsular
  childhood Q15.0
  closed angle — *see* Glaucoma, angle-closure
  congenital Q15.0
  corticosteroid-induced — *see* Glaucoma, secondary, drugs
  hypersecretion H40.82- ☑
  in (due to)
    amyloidosis E85.4 *[H42]*
    aniridia Q13.1 *[H42]*
    concussion of globe — *see* Glaucoma, secondary, trauma
    dislocation of lens — *see* Glaucoma, secondary
    disorder of lens NEC — *see* Glaucoma, secondary
    drugs — *see* Glaucoma, secondary, drugs
    endocrine disease NOS E34.9 *[H42]*
    eye
      inflammation — *see* Glaucoma, secondary, inflammation
      trauma — *see* Glaucoma, secondary, trauma
    hypermature cataract — *see* Glaucoma, secondary

☑ **Additional Character Required — Refer to the Tabular List for Character Selection**   ⌐ **Subterms under main terms may continue to next column or page**

Glaucoma — *continued*
  in — *continued*
    iridocyclitis — *see* Glaucoma, secondary, inflammation
    lens disorder — *see* Glaucoma, secondary
    Lowe's syndrome E72.03 *[H42]*
    metabolic disease NOS E88.9 *[H42]*
    ocular disorders NEC — *see* Glaucoma, secondary
    onchocerciasis B73.02
    pupillary block — *see* Glaucoma, secondary
    retinal vein occlusion — *see* Glaucoma, secondary
    Rieger's anomaly Q13.81 *[H42]*
    rubeosis of iris — *see* Glaucoma, secondary
    tumor of globe — *see* Glaucoma, secondary
  infantile Q15.0
  low tension — *see* Glaucoma, open angle, primary, low-tension
  malignant H40.83- ☑
  narrow angle — *see* Glaucoma, angle-closure
  newborn Q15.0
  noncongestive (chronic) — *see* Glaucoma, open angle
  nonobstructive — *see* Glaucoma, open angle
  obstructive — *see also* Glaucoma, angle-closure
    due to lens changes — *see* Glaucoma, secondary
  open angle H40.10- ☑
    primary H40.11- ☑
      capsular (with pseudoexfoliation of lens) H40.14- ☑
      low-tension H40.12- ☑
      pigmentary H40.13- ☑
      residual stage H40.15- ☑
  phacolytic — *see* Glaucoma, secondary
  pigmentary — *see* Glaucoma, open angle, primary, pigmentary
  postinfectious — *see* Glaucoma, secondary, inflammation
  secondary (to) H40.5- ☑
    drugs H40.6- ☑
    inflammation H40.4- ☑
    trauma H40.3- ☑
  simple (chronic) H40.11- ☑
  simplex H40.11- ☑
  specified type NEC H40.89
  suspect H40.00- ☑
  syphilitic A52.71
  traumatic — *see also* Glaucoma, secondary, trauma
    newborn (birth injury) P15.3
  tuberculous A18.59
Glaucomatous flecks (subcapsular) — *see* Cataract, complicated
Glazed tongue K14.4
Gleet (gonococcal) A54.01
Glénard's disease K63.4
Glioblastoma (multiforme)
  with sarcomatous component
    specified site — *see* Neoplasm, malignant, by site
    unspecified site C71.9
  giant cell
    specified site — *see* Neoplasm, malignant, by site
    unspecified site C71.9
  specified site — *see* Neoplasm, malignant, by site
  unspecified site C71.9
Glioma (malignant)
  astrocytic
    specified site — *see* Neoplasm, malignant, by site
    unspecified site C71.9
  mixed
    specified site — *see* Neoplasm, malignant, by site
    unspecified site C71.9
  nose Q30.8
  specified site NEC — *see* Neoplasm, malignant, by site
  subependymal D43.2
    specified site — *see* Neoplasm, uncertain behavior, by site
    unspecified site D43.2
  unspecified site C71.9
Gliomatosis cerebri C71.0
Glioneuroma — *see* Neoplasm, uncertain behavior, by site
Gliosarcoma
  specified site — *see* Neoplasm, malignant, by site
  unspecified site C71.9
Gliosis (cerebral) G93.89
  spinal G95.89
Glisson's disease — *see* Rickets
Globinuria R82.3
Globus (hystericus) F45.8

Glomangioma D18.00
  intra-abdominal D18.03
  intracranial D18.02
  skin D18.01
  specified site NEC D18.09
Glomangiomyoma D18.00
  intra-abdominal D18.03
  intracranial D18.02
  skin D18.01
  specified site NEC D18.09
Glomangiosarcoma — *see* Neoplasm, connective tissue, malignant
Glomerular
  disease in syphilis A52.75
  nephritis — *see* Glomerulonephritis
Glomerulitis — *see* Glomerulonephritis
Glomerulonephritis — *see also* Nephritis N05.9
  with
    edema — *see* Nephrosis
    minimal change N05.0
    minor glomerular abnormality N05.0
  acute N00.9
  chronic N03.9
  crescentic (diffuse) NEC — *see also* N00-N07 with fourth character .7 N05.7
  dense deposit — *see also* N00-N07 with fourth character .6 N05.6
  diffuse
    crescentic — *see also* N00-N07 with fourth character .7 N05.7
    endocapillary proliferative — *see also* N00-N07 with fourth character .4 N05.4
    membranous — *see also* N00-N07 with fourth character .2 N05.2
    mesangial proliferative — *see also* N00-N07 with fourth character .3 N05.3
    mesangiocapillary — *see also* N00-N07 with fourth character .5 N05.5
    sclerosing N18.9
  endocapillary proliferative (diffuse) NEC — *see also* N00-N07 with fourth character .4 N05.4
  extracapillary NEC — *see also* N00-N07 with fourth character .7 N05.7
  focal (and segmental) — *see also* N00-N07 with fourth character .1 N05.1
  hypocomplementemic — *see* Glomerulonephritis, membranoproliferative
  IgA — *see* Nephropathy, IgA
  immune complex (circulating) NEC N05.8
  in (due to)
    amyloidosis E85.4 *[N08]*
    bilharziasis B65.9 *[N08]*
    cryoglobulinemia D89.1 *[N08]*
    defibrination syndrome D65 *[N08]*
    diabetes mellitus — *see* Diabetes, glomerulosclerosis
    disseminated intravascular coagulation D65 *[N08]*
    Fabry (-Anderson) disease E75.21 *[N08]*
    Goodpasture's syndrome M31.0
    hemolytic-uremic syndrome D59.3
    Henoch (-Schönlein) purpura D69.0 *[N08]*
    lecithin cholesterol acyltransferase deficiency E78.6 *[N08]*
    microscopic polyangiitis M31.7 *[N08]*
    multiple myeloma C90.0- ☑ *[N08]*
    Plasmodium malariae B52.0
    schistosomiasis B65.9 *[N08]*
    sepsis A41.9 *[N08]*
      streptococcal A40- ☑ *[N08]*
    sickle-cell disorders D57.- ☑ *[N08]*
    strongyloidiasis B78.9 *[N08]*
    subacute bacterial endocarditis I33.0 *[N08]*
    syphilis (late) congenital A50.59 *[N08]*
    systemic lupus erythematosus M32.14
    thrombotic thrombocytopenic purpura M31.1 *[N08]*
    typhoid fever A01.09
    Waldenström macroglobulinemia C88.0 *[N08]*
    Wegener's granulomatosis M31.31
  latent or quiescent N03.9
  lobular, lobulonodular — *see* Glomerulonephritis, membranoproliferative
  membranoproliferative (diffuse)(type 1 or 3) — *see also* N00-N07 with fourth character .5 N05.5
    dense deposit (type 2) NEC — *see also* N00-N07 with fourth character .6 N05.6
  membranous (diffuse) NEC — *see also* N00-N07 with fourth character .2 N05.2

Glomerulonephritis — *continued*
  mesangial
    IgA/IgG — *see* Nephropathy, IgA
    proliferative (diffuse) NEC — *see also* N00-N07 with fourth character .3 N05.3
  mesangiocapillary (diffuse) NEC — *see also* N00-N07 with fourth character .5 N05.5
  necrotic, necrotizing NEC — *see also* N00- N07 with fourth character .8 N05.8
  nodular — *see* Glomerulonephritis, membranoproliferative
  poststreptococcal NEC N05.9
    acute N00.9
    chronic N03.9
    rapidly progressive N01.9
  proliferative (diffuse) NEC — *see also* N00-N07 with fourth character .8 N05.8
    diffuse (lupus) M32.14
  rapidly progressive N01.9
  sclerosing, diffuse N18.9
  specified pathology NEC — *see also* N00- N07 with fourth character .8 N05.8
  subacute N01.9
Glomerulopathy — *see* Glomerulonephritis
Glomerulosclerosis — *see also* Sclerosis, renal
  intercapillary (nodular) (with diabetes) — *see* Diabetes, glomerulosclerosis
  intracapillary — *see* Diabetes, glomerulosclerosis
Glossagra K14.6
Glossalgia K14.6
Glossitis (chronic superficial) (gangrenous) (Moeller's) K14.0
  areata exfoliativa K14.1
  atrophic K14.4
  benign migratory K14.1
  cortical superficial, sclerotic K14.0
  Hunter's D51.0
  interstitial, sclerous K14.0
  median rhomboid K14.2
  pellagrous E52
  superficial, chronic K14.0
Glossocele K14.8
Glossodynia K14.6
  exfoliativa K14.4
Glossoncus K14.8
Glossopathy K14.9
Glossophytia K14.3
Glossoplegia K14.8
Glossoptosis K14.8
Glossopyrosis K14.6
Glossotrichia K14.3
Glossy skin L90.8
Glottis — *see* condition
Glottitis — *see also* Laryngitis J04.0
Glucagonoma
  pancreas
    benign D13.7
    malignant C25.4
    uncertain behavior D37.8
  specified site NEC
    benign — *see* Neoplasm, benign, by site
    malignant — *see* Neoplasm, malignant, by site
    uncertain behavior — *see* Neoplasm, uncertain behavior, by site
  unspecified site
    benign D13.7
    malignant C25.4
    uncertain behavior D37.8
Glucoglycinuria E72.51
Glucose-galactose malabsorption E74.39
Glue
  ear — *see* Otitis, media, nonsuppurative, chronic, mucoid
  sniffing (airplane) — *see* Abuse, drug, inhalant
    dependence — *see* Dependence, drug, inhalant
Glutaric aciduria E72.3
Glycinemia E72.51
Glycinuria (renal) (with ketosis) E72.09
Glycogen
  infiltration — *see* Disease, glycogen storage
  storage disease — *see* Disease, glycogen storage
Glycogenosis (diffuse) (generalized) — *see also* Disease, glycogen storage
  cardiac E74.02 *[I43]*
  diabetic, secondary — *see* Diabetes, glycogenosis, secondary
  pulmonary interstitial J84.842

Index

Glaucoma — Glycogenosis

Glycopenia E16.2
Glycosuria R81
  renal E74.8
Gnathostoma spinigerum (infection) (infestation), **gnathostomiasis** (wandering swelling) B83.1
Goiter (plunging) (substernal) E04.9
  with
    hyperthyroidism (recurrent) — *see* Hyperthyroidism, with, goiter
    thyrotoxicosis — *see* Hyperthyroidism, with, goiter
  adenomatous — *see* Goiter, nodular
  cancerous C73
  congenital (nontoxic) E03.0
    diffuse E03.0
    parenchymatous E03.0
    transitory, with normal functioning P72.0
  cystic E04.2
    due to iodine-deficiency E01.1
  due to
    enzyme defect in synthesis of thyroid hormone E07.1
    iodine-deficiency (endemic) E01.2
  dyshormonogenetic (familial) E07.1
  endemic (iodine-deficiency) E01.2
    diffuse E01.0
    multinodular E01.1
  exophthalmic — *see* Hyperthyroidism, with, goiter
  iodine-deficiency (endemic) E01.2
    diffuse E01.0
    multinodular E01.1
    nodular E01.1
  lingual Q89.2
  lymphadenoid E06.3
  malignant C73
  multinodular (cystic) (nontoxic) E04.2
    toxic or with hyperthyroidism E05.20
      with thyroid storm E05.21
  neonatal NEC P72.0
  nodular (nontoxic) (due to) E04.9
    with
      hyperthyroidism E05.20
        with thyroid storm E05.21
      thyrotoxicosis E05.20
        with thyroid storm E05.21
    endemic E01.1
    iodine-deficiency E01.1
    sporadic E04.9
    toxic E05.20
      with thyroid storm E05.21
  nontoxic E04.9
    diffuse (colloid) E04.0
    multinodular E04.2
    simple E04.0
    specified NEC E04.8
    uninodular E04.1
  simple E04.0
  toxic — *see* Hyperthyroidism, with, goiter
  uninodular (nontoxic) E04.1
    toxic or with hyperthyroidism E05.10
      with thyroid storm E05.11
Goiter-deafness syndrome E07.1
Goldberg syndrome Q89.8
Goldberg-Maxwell syndrome E34.51
Goldblatt's hypertension or kidney I70.1
Goldenhar (-Gorlin) **syndrome** Q87.0
Goldflam-Erb disease or syndrome G70.00
  with exacerbation (acute) G70.01
  in crisis G70.01
Goldscheider's disease Q81.8
Goldstein's disease (familial hemorrhagic telangiectasia) I78.0
Golfer's elbow — *see* Epicondylitis, medial
Gonadoblastoma
  specified site — *see* Neoplasm, uncertain behavior, by site
  unspecified site
    female D39.10
    male D40.10
Gonecystitis — *see* Vesiculitis
Gongylonemiasis B83.8
Goniosynechiae — *see* Adhesions, iris, goniosynechiae
Gonococcemia A54.86
Gonococcus, gonococcal (disease) (infection) — *see also* condition A54.9
  anus A54.6
  bursa, bursitis A54.49
  conjunctiva, conjunctivitis (neonatorum) A54.31
  endocardium A54.83

Gonococcus, gonococcal — *continued*
  eye A54.30
    conjunctivitis A54.31
    iridocyclitis A54.32
    keratitis A54.33
    newborn A54.31
    other specified A54.39
  fallopian tubes (acute) (chronic) A54.24
  genitourinary (organ) (system) (tract) (acute)
    lower A54.00
      with abscess (accessory gland) (periurethral) A54.1
    upper — *see also* condition A54.29
  heart A54.83
  iridocyclitis A54.32
  joint A54.42
  lymphatic (gland) (node) A54.89
  meninges, meningitis A54.81
  musculoskeletal A54.40
    arthritis A54.42
    osteomyelitis A54.43
    other specified A54.49
    spondylopathy A54.41
  pelviperitonitis A54.24
  pelvis (acute) (chronic) A54.24
  pharynx A54.5
  proctitis A54.6
  pyosalpinx (acute) (chronic) A54.24
  rectum A54.6
  skin A54.89
  specified site NEC A54.89
  tendon sheath A54.49
  throat A54.5
  urethra (acute) (chronic) A54.01
    with abscess (accessory gland) (periurethral) A54.1
  vulva (acute) (chronic) A54.02
Gonocytoma
  specified site — *see* Neoplasm, uncertain behavior, by site
  unspecified site
    female D39.10
    male D40.10
Gonorrhea (acute) (chronic) A54.9
  Bartholin's gland (acute) (chronic) (purulent) A54.02
    with abscess (accessory gland) (periurethral) A54.1
  bladder A54.01
  cervix A54.03
  conjunctiva, conjunctivitis (neonatorum) A54.31
  contact Z20.2
  Cowper's gland (with abscess) A54.1
  exposure to Z20.2
  fallopian tube (acute) (chronic) A54.24
  kidney (acute) (chronic) A54.21
  lower genitourinary tract A54.00
    with abscess (accessory gland) (periurethral) A54.1
  ovary (acute) (chronic) A54.24
  pelvis (acute) (chronic) A54.24
    female pelvic inflammatory disease A54.24
  penis A54.09
  prostate (acute) (chronic) A54.22
  seminal vesicle (acute) (chronic) A54.23
  specified site not listed — *see also* Gonococcus A54.89
  spermatic cord (acute) (chronic) A54.23
  urethra A54.01
    with abscess (accessory gland) (periurethral) A54.1
  vagina A54.02
  vas deferens (acute) (chronic) A54.23
  vulva A54.02
Goodall's disease A08.19
Goodpasture's syndrome M31.0
Gopalan's syndrome (burning feet) E53.0
Gorlin-Chaudry-Moss syndrome Q87.0
Gottron's papules L94.4
Gougerot-Blum syndrome (pigmented purpuric lichenoid dermatitis) L81.7
Gougerot-Carteaud disease or syndrome (confluent reticulate papillomatosis) L83
Gougerot's syndrome (trisymptomatic) L81.7
Gouley's syndrome (constrictive pericarditis) I31.1
Goundou A66.6
Gout, chronic — *see also* Gout, gouty M1A.9 ☑ (*following* M08)
  drug-induced M1A.20 ☑ (*following* M08)
    ankle M1A.27- ☑ (*following* M08)
    elbow M1A.22- ☑ (*following* M08)
    foot joint M1A.27- ☑ (*following* M08)
    hand joint M1A.24- ☑ (*following* M08)
    hip M1A.25- ☑ (*following* M08)

Gout, chronic — *continued*
  drug-induced — *continued*
    knee M1A.26- ☑ (*following* M08)
    multiple site M1A.29- ☑ (*following* M08)
    shoulder M1A.21- ☑ (*following* M08)
    vertebrae M1A.28 ☑ (*following* M08)
    wrist M1A.23- ☑ (*following* M08)
  idiopathic M1A.00 ☑ (*following* M08)
    ankle M1A.07- ☑ (*following* M08)
    elbow M1A.02- ☑ (*following* M08)
    foot joint M1A.07- ☑ (*following* M08)
    hand joint M1A.04- ☑ (*following* M08)
    hip M1A.05- ☑ (*following* M08)
    knee M1A.06- ☑ (*following* M08)
    multiple site M1A.09 ☑ (*following* M08)
    shoulder M1A.01- ☑ (*following* M08)
    vertebrae M1A.08 ☑ (*following* M08)
    wrist M1A.03- ☑ (*following* M08)
  in (due to) renal impairment M1A.30 ☑ (*following* M08)
    ankle M1A.37- ☑ (*following* M08)
    elbow M1A.32- ☑ (*following* M08)
    foot joint M1A.37- ☑ (*following* M08)
    hand joint M1A.34- ☑ (*following* M08)
    hip M1A.35- ☑ (*following* M08)
    knee M1A.36- ☑ (*following* M08)
    multiple site M1A.39 ☑ (*following* M08)
    shoulder M1A.31- ☑ (*following* M08)
    vertebrae M1A.38 ☑ (*following* M08)
    wrist M1A.33- ☑ (*following* M08)
  lead-induced M1A.10 ☑ (*following* M08)
    ankle M1A.17- ☑ (*following* M08)
    elbow M1A.12- ☑ (*following* M08)
    foot joint M1A.17- ☑ (*following* M08)
    hand joint M1A.14- ☑ (*following* M08)
    hip M1A.15- ☑ (*following* M08)
    knee M1A.16- ☑ (*following* M08)
    multiple site M1A.19 ☑ (*following* M08)
    shoulder M1A.11- ☑ (*following* M08)
    vertebrae M1A.18 ☑ (*following* M08)
    wrist M1A.13- ☑ (*following* M08)
  primary — *see* Gout, chronic, idiopathic
  saturnine — *see* Gout, chronic, lead-induced
  secondary NEC M1A.40 ☑ (*following* M08)
    ankle M1A.47- ☑ (*following* M08)
    elbow M1A.42- ☑ (*following* M08)
    foot joint M1A.47- ☑ (*following* M08)
    hand joint M1A.44- ☑ (*following* M08)
    hip M1A.45- ☑ (*following* M08)
    knee M1A.46- ☑ (*following* M08)
    multiple site M1A.49 ☑ (*following* M08)
    shoulder M1A.41- ☑ (*following* M08)
    vertebrae M1A.48 ☑ (*following* M08)
    wrist M1A.43- ☑ (*following* M08)
  syphilitic — *see also* subcategory M14.8- A52.77
  tophi M1A.9 ☑ (*following* M08)
Gout, gouty (acute) (attack) (flare) — *see also* Gout, chronic M10.9
  drug-induced M10.20
    ankle M10.27- ☑
    elbow M10.22- ☑
    foot joint M10.27- ☑
    hand joint M10.24- ☑
    hip M10.25- ☑
    knee M10.26- ☑
    multiple site M10.29
    shoulder M10.21- ☑
    vertebrae M10.28
    wrist M10.23- ☑
  idiopathic M10.00
    ankle M10.07- ☑
    elbow M10.02- ☑
    foot joint M10.07- ☑
    hand joint M10.04- ☑
    hip M10.05- ☑
    knee M10.06- ☑
    multiple site M10.09
    shoulder M10.01- ☑
    vertebrae M10.08
    wrist M10.03- ☑
  in (due to) renal impairment M10.30
    ankle M10.37- ☑
    elbow M10.32- ☑
    foot joint M10.37- ☑
    hand joint M10.34- ☑
    hip M10.35- ☑
    knee M10.36- ☑

Gout, gouty — continued
  in renal impairment — continued
    multiple site M10.39
    shoulder M10.31- ☑
    vertebrae M10.38
    wrist M10.33- ☑
  lead-induced M10.10
    ankle M10.17- ☑
    elbow M10.12- ☑
    foot joint M10.17- ☑
    hand joint M10.14- ☑
    hip M10.15- ☑
    knee M10.16- ☑
    multiple site M10.19
    shoulder M10.11- ☑
    vertebrae M10.18
    wrist M10.13- ☑
  primary — see Gout, idiopathic
  saturnine — see Gout, lead-induced
  secondary NEC M10.40
    ankle M10.47- ☑
    elbow M10.42- ☑
    foot joint M10.47- ☑
    hand joint M10.44- ☑
    hip M10.45- ☑
    knee M10.46- ☑
    multiple site M10.49
    shoulder M10.41- ☑
    vertebrae M10.48
    wrist M10.43- ☑
  syphilitic — see also subcategory M14.8- A52.77
  tophi — see Gout, chronic
Gower's
  muscular dystrophy G71.01
  syndrome (vasovagal attack) R55
Gradenigo's syndrome — see Otitis, media, suppurative, acute
Graefe's disease — see Strabismus, paralytic, ophthalmoplegia, progressive
Graft-versus-host disease D89.813
  acute D89.810
  acute on chronic D89.812
  chronic D89.811
Grain mite (itch) B88.0
Grainhandler's disease or lung J67.8
Grand mal — see Epilepsy, generalized, specified NEC
Grand multipara status only (not pregnant) Z64.1
  pregnant — see Pregnancy, complicated by, grand multiparity
Granite worker's lung J62.8
Granular — see also condition
  inflammation, pharynx J31.2
  kidney (contracting) — see Sclerosis, renal
  liver K74.69
Granulation tissue (abnormal) (excessive) L92.9
  postmastoidectomy cavity — see Complications, postmastoidectomy, granulation
Granulocytopenia (primary) (malignant) — see Agranulocytosis
Granuloma L92.9
  abdomen K66.8
    from residual foreign body L92.3
    pyogenicum L98.0
  actinic L57.5
  annulare (perforating) L92.0
  apical K04.5
  aural — see Otitis, externa, specified NEC
  beryllium (skin) L92.3
  bone
    eosinophilic C96.6
    from residual foreign body — see Osteomyelitis, specified type NEC
    lung C96.6
  brain (any site) G06.0
    schistosomiasis B65.9 [G07]
  canaliculus lacrimalis — see Granuloma, lacrimal
  candidal (cutaneous) B37.2
  cerebral (any site) G06.0
  coccidioidal (primary) (progressive) B38.7
    lung B38.1
    meninges B38.4
  colon K63.89
  conjunctiva H11.22- ☑
  dental K04.5
  ear, middle — see Cholesteatoma
  eosinophilic C96.6
    bone C96.6

Granuloma — continued
  eosinophilic — continued
    lung C96.6
    oral mucosa K13.4
    skin L92.2
  eyelid H01.8
  facial (e) L92.2
  foreign body (in soft tissue) NEC M60.20
    ankle M60.27- ☑
    foot M60.27- ☑
    forearm M60.23- ☑
    hand M60.24- ☑
    in operation wound — see Foreign body, accidentally left during a procedure
    lower leg M60.26- ☑
    pelvic region M60.25- ☑
    shoulder region M60.21- ☑
    skin L92.3
    specified site NEC M60.28
    subcutaneous tissue L92.3
    thigh M60.25- ☑
    upper arm M60.22- ☑
  gangraenescens M31.2
  genito-inguinale A58
  giant cell (central) (reparative) (jaw) M27.1
    gingiva (peripheral) K06.8
  gland (lymph) I88.8
  hepatic NEC K75.3
    in (due to)
      berylliosis J63.2 [K77]
      sarcoidosis D86.89
  Hodgkin C81.9
  ileum K63.89
  infectious B99.9
    specified NEC B99.8
  inguinale (Donovan) (venereal) A58
  intestine NEC K63.89
  intracranial (any site) G06.0
  intraspinal (any part) G06.1
  iridocyclitis — see Iridocyclitis, chronic
  jaw (bone) (central) M27.1
    reparative giant cell M27.1
  kidney — see also Infection, kidney N15.8
  lacrimal H04.81- ☑
  larynx J38.7
  lethal midline (faciale(e)) M31.2
  liver NEC — see Granuloma, hepatic
  lung (infectious) — see also Fibrosis, lung
    coccidioidal B38.1
    eosinophilic C96.6
  Majocchi's B35.8
  malignant (facial(e)) M31.2
  mandible (central) M27.1
  midline (lethal) M31.2
  monilial (cutaneous) B37.2
  nasal sinus — see Sinusitis
  operation wound T81.89 ☑
    foreign body — see Foreign body, accidentally left during a procedure
    stitch T81.89 ☑
    talc — see Foreign body, accidentally left during a procedure
  oral mucosa K13.4
  orbit, orbital H05.11- ☑
  paracoccidioidal B41.8
  penis, venereal A58
  periapical K04.5
  peritoneum K66.8
    due to ova of helminths NOS — see also Helminthiasis B83.9 [K67]
  postmastoidectomy cavity — see Complications, postmastoidectomy, recurrent cholesteatoma
  prostate N42.89
  pudendi (ulcerating) A58
  pulp, internal (tooth) K03.3
  pyogenic, pyogenicum (of) (skin) L98.0
    gingiva K06.8
    maxillary alveolar ridge K04.5
    oral mucosa K13.4
  rectum K62.89
  reticulohistiocytic D76.3
  rubrum nasi L74.8
  Schistosoma — see Schistosomiasis
  septic (skin) L98.0
  silica (skin) L92.3
  sinus (accessory) (infective) (nasal) — see Sinusitis
  skin L92.9
    from residual foreign body L92.3

Granuloma — continued
  skin — continued
    pyogenicum L98.0
  spine
    syphilitic (epidural) A52.19
    tuberculous A18.01
  stitch (postoperative) T81.89 ☑
  suppurative (skin) L98.0
  swimming pool A31.1
  talc — see also Granuloma, foreign body
    in operation wound — see Foreign body, accidentally left during a procedure
  telangiectaticum (skin) L98.0
  tracheostomy J95.09
  trichophyticum B35.8
  tropicum A66.4
  umbilical P83.81
  umbilicus P83.81
  urethra N36.8
  uveitis — see Iridocyclitis, chronic
  vagina A58
  venereum A58
  vocal cord J38.3
Granulomatosis L92.9
  lymphoid C83.8- ☑
  miliary (listerial) A32.89
  necrotizing, respiratory M31.30
  progressive septic D71
  specified NEC L92.8
  Wegener's M31.30
    with renal involvement M31.31
Granulomatous tissue (abnormal) (excessive) L92.9
Granulosis rubra nasi L74.8
Graphite fibrosis (of lung) J63.3
Graphospasm F48.8
  organic G25.89
Grating scapula M89.8X1
Gravel (urinary) — see Calculus, urinary
Graves' disease — see Hyperthyroidism, with, goiter
Gravis — see condition
Grawitz tumor C64.- ☑
Gray syndrome (newborn) P93.0
Grayness, hair (premature) L67.1
  congenital Q84.2
Green sickness D50.8
Greenfield's disease
  meaning
    concentric sclerosis (encephalitis periaxialis concentrica) G37.5
    metachromatic leukodystrophy E75.25
Greenstick fracture — code as Fracture, by site
Grey syndrome (newborn) P93.0
Grief F43.21
  prolonged F43.29
  reaction — see also Disorder, adjustment F43.20
Griesinger's disease B76.0
Grinder's lung or pneumoconiosis J62.8
Grinding, teeth
  psychogenic F45.8
  sleep related G47.63
Grip
  Dabney's B33.0
  devil's B33.0
Grippe, grippal — see also Influenza
  Balkan A78
  summer, of Italy A93.1
Grisel's disease M43.6
Groin — see condition
Grooved tongue K14.5
Ground itch B76.9
Grover's disease or syndrome L11.1
Growing pains, children R29.898
Growth (fungoid) (neoplastic) (new) — see also Neoplasm
  adenoid (vegetative) J35.8
  benign — see Neoplasm, benign, by site
  malignant — see Neoplasm, malignant, by site
  rapid, childhood Z00.2
  secondary — see Neoplasm, secondary, by site
Gruby's disease B35.0
Gubler-Millard paralysis or syndrome G46.3
Guerin-Stern syndrome Q74.3
Guidance, insufficient anterior (occlusal) M26.54
Guillain-Barré disease or syndrome G61.0
  sequelae G65.0
Guinea worms (infection) (infestation) B72
Guinon's disease (motor-verbal tic) F95.2
Gull's disease E03.4

Gum — *see* condition
Gumboil K04.7
  with sinus K04.6
Gumma (syphilitic) A52.79
  artery A52.09
    cerebral A52.04
  bone A52.77
    of yaws (late) A66.6
  brain A52.19
  cauda equina A52.19
  central nervous system A52.3
  ciliary body A52.71
  congenital A50.59
  eyelid A52.71
  heart A52.06
  intracranial A52.19
  iris A52.71
  kidney A52.75
  larynx A52.73
  leptomeninges A52.19
  liver A52.74
  meninges A52.19
  myocardium A52.06
  nasopharynx A52.73
  neurosyphilitic A52.3
  nose A52.73
  orbit A52.71
  palate (soft) A52.79
  penis A52.76
  pericardium A52.06
  pharynx A52.73
  pituitary A52.79
  scrofulous (tuberculous) A18.4
  skin A52.79
  specified site NEC A52.79
  spinal cord A52.19
  tongue A52.79
  tonsil A52.73
  trachea A52.73
  tuberculous A18.4
  ulcerative due to yaws A66.4
  ureter A52.75
  yaws A66.4
    bone A66.6
Gunn's syndrome Q07.8
Gunshot wound — *see also* Wound, open
  fracture — *code as* Fracture, by site
  internal organs — *see* Injury, by site
Gynandrism Q56.0
Gynandroblastoma
  specified site — *see* Neoplasm, uncertain behavior, by site
  unspecified site
    female D39.10
    male D40.10
Gynecological examination (periodic) (routine) Z01.419
  with abnormal findings Z01.411
Gynecomastia N62
Gynephobia F40.291
Gyrate scalp Q82.8

H

H (Hartnup's) **disease** E72.02
Haas' disease or osteochondrosis (juvenile) (head of humerus) — *see* Osteochondrosis, juvenile, humerus
Habit, habituation
  bad sleep Z72.821
  chorea F95.8
  disturbance, child F98.9
  drug — *see* Dependence, drug
  irregular sleep Z72.821
  laxative F55.2
  spasm — *see* Tic
  tic — *see* Tic
Haemophilus (H.) **influenzae, as cause of disease classified elsewhere** B96.3
Haff disease — *see* Poisoning, mercury
Hageman's factor defect, deficiency or disease D68.2
Haglund's disease or osteochondrosis (juvenile) (os tibiale externum) — *see* Osteochondrosis, juvenile, tarsus
Hailey-Hailey disease Q82.8
Hair — *see also* condition
  plucking F63.3
    in stereotyped movement disorder F98.4
  tourniquet syndrome — *see also* Constriction, external, by site

Hair — *continued*
  tourniquet syndrome — *see also* Constriction, external, by site — *continued*
    finger S60.44- ☑
    penis S30.842 ☑
    thumb S60.34- ☑
    toe S90.44- ☑
Hairball in stomach T18.2 ☑
Hair-pulling, pathological (compulsive) F63.3
Hairy black tongue K14.3
Half vertebra Q76.49
Halitosis R19.6
Hallerman-Streiff syndrome Q87.0
Hallervorden-Spatz disease G23.0
Hallopeau's acrodermatitis or disease L40.2
Hallucination R44.3
  auditory R44.0
  gustatory R44.2
  olfactory R44.2
  specified NEC R44.2
  tactile R44.2
  visual R44.1
Hallucinosis (chronic) F28
  alcoholic (acute) F10.951
    in
      abuse F10.151
      dependence F10.251
  drug-induced F19.951
    cannabis F12.951
    cocaine F14.951
    hallucinogen F16.151
    in
      abuse F19.151
        cannabis F12.151
        cocaine F14.151
        hallucinogen F16.151
        inhalant F18.151
        opioid F11.151
        sedative, anxiolytic or hypnotic F13.151
        stimulant NEC F15.151
      dependence F19.251
        cannabis F12.251
        cocaine F14.251
        hallucinogen F16.251
        inhalant F18.251
        opioid F11.251
        sedative, anxiolytic or hypnotic F13.251
        stimulant NEC F15.251
    inhalant F18.951
    opioid F11.951
    sedative, anxiolytic or hypnotic F13.951
    stimulant NEC F15.951
  organic F06.0
Hallux
  deformity (acquired) NEC M20.5X- ☑
  limitus M20.5X- ☑
  malleus (acquired) NEC M20.3- ☑
  rigidus (acquired) M20.2- ☑
    congenital Q74.2
    sequelae (late effect) of rickets E64.3
  valgus (acquired) M20.1- ☑
    congenital Q66.6
  varus (acquired) M20.3- ☑
    congenital Q66.3- ☑
Halo, visual H53.19
Hamartoma, hamartoblastoma Q85.9
  epithelial (gingival), odontogenic, central or peripheral — *see* Cyst, calcifying odontogenic
Hamartosis Q85.9
Hamman-Rich syndrome J84.114
Hammer toe (acquired) NEC — *see also* Deformity, toe, hammer toe
  congenital Q66.89
  sequelae (late effect) of rickets E64.3
Hand — *see* condition
Hand-foot syndrome L27.1
Handicap, handicapped
  educational Z55.9
    specified NEC Z55.8
Hand-Schüller-Christian disease or syndrome C96.5
Hanging (asphyxia) (strangulation) (suffocation) — *see* Asphyxia, traumatic, due to mechanical threat
Hangnail — *see also* Cellulitis, digit
  with lymphangitis — *see* Lymphangitis, acute, digit
Hangover (alcohol) F10.129
Hanhart's syndrome Q87.0
Hanot-Chauffard (-Troisier) **syndrome** E83.19

Hanot's cirrhosis or disease K74.3
Hansen's disease — *see* Leprosy
Hantaan virus disease (Korean hemorrhagic fever) A98.5
Hantavirus disease (with renal manifestations) (Dobrava) (Puumala) (Seoul) A98.5
  with pulmonary manifestations (Andes) (Bayou) (Bermejo) (Black Creek Canal) (Choclo) (Juquitiba) (Laguna negra) (Lechiguanas) (New York) (Oran) (Sin nombre) B33.4
Happy puppet syndrome Q93.51
Harada's disease or syndrome H30.81- ☑
Hardening
  artery — *see* Arteriosclerosis
  brain G93.89
Harelip (complete) (incomplete) — *see* Cleft, lip
Harlequin (newborn) Q80.4
Harley's disease D59.6
Harmful use (of)
  alcohol F10.10
  anxiolytics — *see* Abuse, drug, sedative
  cannabinoids — *see* Abuse, drug, cannabis
  cocaine — *see* Abuse, drug, cocaine
  drug — *see* Abuse, drug
  hallucinogens — *see* Abuse, drug, hallucinogen
  hypnotics — *see* Abuse, drug, sedative
  opioids — *see* Abuse, drug, opioid
  PCP (phencyclidine) — *see* Abuse, drug, hallucinogen
  sedatives — *see* Abuse, drug, sedative
  stimulants NEC — *see* Abuse, drug, stimulant
Harris' lines — *see* Arrest, epiphyseal
Hartnup's disease E72.02
Harvester's lung J67.0
Harvesting ovum for in vitro fertilization Z31.83
Hashimoto's disease or thyroiditis E06.3
Hashitoxicosis (transient) E06.3
Hassal-Henle bodies or warts (cornea) H18.49
Haut mal — *see* Epilepsy, generalized, specified NEC
Haverhill fever A25.1
Hay fever — *see also* Fever, hay J30.1
Hayem-Widal syndrome D59.8
Haygarth's nodes M15.8
Haymaker's lung J67.0
Hb (abnormal)
  Bart's disease D56.0
  disease — *see* Disease, hemoglobin
  trait — *see* Trait
Head — *see* condition
Headache R51
  allergic NEC G44.89
  associated with sexual activity G44.82
  chronic daily R51
  cluster G44.009
    chronic G44.029
      intractable G44.021
      not intractable G44.029
    episodic G44.019
      intractable G44.011
      not intractable G44.019
    intractable G44.001
    not intractable G44.009
  cough (primary) G44.83
  daily chronic R51
  drug-induced NEC G44.40
    intractable G44.41
    not intractable G44.40
  exertional (primary) G44.84
  histamine G44.009
    intractable G44.001
    not intractable G44.009
  hypnic G44.81
  lumbar puncture G97.1
  medication overuse G44.40
    intractable G44.41
    not intractable G44.40
  menstrual — *see* Migraine, menstrual
  migraine (type) — *see also* Migraine G43.909
  nasal septum R51
  neuralgiform, short lasting unilateral, with conjunctival injection and tearing (SUNCT) G44.059
    intractable G44.051
    not intractable G44.059
  new daily persistent (NDPH) G44.52
  orgasmic G44.82
  periodic syndromes in adults and children G43.C0 (*following* G43.7)
    with refractory migraine G43.C1 (*following* G43.7)
    intractable G43.C1 (*following* G43.7)

☑ **Additional Character Required** — **Refer to the Tabular List for Character Selection**   � **Subterms under main terms may continue to next column or page**

Headache — *continued*
  periodic syndromes in adults and children — *continued*
    not intractable G43.CØ (*following* G43.7)
    without refractory migraine G43.CØ (*following* G43.7)
  postspinal puncture G97.1
  post-traumatic G44.3Ø9
    acute G44.319
      intractable G44.311
      not intractable G44.319
    chronic G44.329
      intractable G44.321
      not intractable G44.329
    intractable G44.3Ø1
    not intractable G44.3Ø9
  pre-menstrual — *see* Migraine, menstrual
  preorgasmic G44.82
  primary
    cough G44.83
    exertional G44.84
    stabbing G44.85
    thunderclap G44.53
  rebound G44.4Ø
    intractable G44.41
    not intractable G44.4Ø
  short lasting unilateral neuralgiform, with conjunctival injection and tearing (SUNCT) G44.Ø59
    intractable G44.Ø51
    not intractable G44.Ø59
  specified syndrome NEC G44.89
  spinal and epidural anesthesia - induced T88.59 ☑
    in labor and delivery O74.5
    in pregnancy O29.4- ☑
    postpartum, puerperal O89.4
  spinal fluid loss (from puncture) G97.1
  stabbing (primary) G44.85
  tension (-type) G44.2Ø9
    chronic G44.229
      intractable G44.221
      not intractable G44.229
    episodic G44.219
      intractable G44.211
      not intractable G44.219
    intractable G44.2Ø1
    not intractable G44.2Ø9
  thunderclap (primary) G44.53
  vascular NEC G44.1
Healthy
  infant
    accompanying sick mother Z76.3
    receiving care Z76.2
  person accompanying sick person Z76.3
Hearing examination ZØ1.1Ø
  with abnormal findings NEC ZØ1.118
  following failed hearing screening ZØ1.11Ø
  for hearing conservation and treatment ZØ1.12
  infant or child (over 28 days old) ZØØ.129
    with abnormal findings ZØØ.121
Heart — *see* condition
Heart beat
  abnormality RØØ.9
    specified NEC RØØ.8
  awareness RØØ.2
  rapid RØØ.Ø
  slow RØØ.1
Heartburn R12
  psychogenic F45.8
Heartland virus disease A93.8
Heat (effects) T67.9 ☑
  apoplexy T67.Ø1 ☑
  burn — *see also* Burn L55.9
  collapse T67.1 ☑
  cramps T67.2 ☑
  dermatitis or eczema L59.Ø
  edema T67.7 ☑
  erythema — *code by site under* Burn, first degree
  excessive T67.9 ☑
    specified effect NEC T67.8 ☑
  exhaustion T67.5 ☑
    anhydrotic T67.3 ☑
    due to
      salt (and water) depletion T67.4 ☑
      water depletion T67.3 ☑
        with salt depletion T67.4 ☑
  fatigue (transient) T67.6 ☑
  fever T67.Ø1 ☑
  hyperpyrexia T67.Ø1 ☑
  prickly L74.Ø

Heat — *continued*
  prostration — *see* Heat, exhaustion
  pyrexia T67.Ø1 ☑
  rash L74.Ø
  specified effect NEC T67.8 ☑
  stroke T67.Ø1 ☑
    exertional T67.Ø2 ☑
    specified NEC T67.Ø9 ☑
  sunburn — *see* Sunburn
  syncope T67.1 ☑
Heavy-for-dates NEC (infant) (4ØØØg to 4499g) PØ8.1
  exceptionally (45ØØg or more) PØ8.Ø
Hebephrenia, hebephrenic (schizophrenia) F2Ø.1
Heberden's disease or nodes (with arthropathy) M15.1
Hebra's
  pityriasis L26
  prurigo L28.2
Heel — *see* condition
Heerfordt's disease D86.89
Hegglin's anomaly or syndrome D72.Ø
Heilmeyer-Schoner disease D45
Heine-Medin disease A8Ø.9
Heinz body anemia, congenital D58.2
Heliophobia F4Ø.228
Heller's disease or syndrome F84.3
HELLP syndrome (hemolysis, elevated liver enzymes and low platelet count) O14.2- ☑
  complicating
    childbirth O14.24
    puerperium O14.25
Helminthiasis — *see also* Infestation, helminth
  Ancylostoma B76.Ø
  intestinal B82.Ø
    mixed types (types classifiable to more than one of the titles B65.Ø-B81.3 and B81.8) B81.4
    specified type NEC B81.8
  mixed types (intestinal) (types classifiable to more than one of the titles B65.Ø-B81.3 and B81.8) B81.4
  Necator (americanus) B76.1
  specified type NEC B83.8
Heloma L84
Hemangioblastoma — *see* Neoplasm, connective tissue, uncertain behavior
  malignant — *see* Neoplasm, connective tissue, malignant
Hemangioendothelioma — *see also* Neoplasm, uncertain behavior, by site
  benign D18.ØØ
    intra-abdominal D18.Ø3
    intracranial D18.Ø2
    skin D18.Ø1
    specified site NEC D18.Ø9
  bone (diffuse) — *see* Neoplasm, bone, malignant
  epithelioid — *see also* Neoplasm, uncertain behavior, by site
    malignant — *see* Neoplasm, malignant, by site
  malignant — *see* Neoplasm, connective tissue, malignant
Hemangiofibroma — *see* Neoplasm, benign, by site
Hemangiolipoma — *see* Lipoma
Hemangioma D18.ØØ
  arteriovenous D18.ØØ
    intra-abdominal D18.Ø3
    intracranial D18.Ø2
    skin D18.Ø1
    specified site NEC D18.Ø9
  capillary I78.1
    intra-abdominal D18.Ø3
    intracranial D18.Ø2
    skin D18.Ø1
    specified site NEC D18.Ø9
  cavernous D18.ØØ
    intra-abdominal D18.Ø3
    intracranial D18.Ø2
    skin D18.Ø1
    specified site NEC D18.Ø9
  epithelioid D18.ØØ
    intra-abdominal D18.Ø3
    intracranial D18.Ø2
    skin D18.Ø1
    specified site NEC D18.Ø9
  histiocytoid D18.ØØ
    intra-abdominal D18.Ø3
    intracranial D18.Ø2
    skin D18.Ø1
    specified site NEC D18.Ø9
  infantile D18.ØØ
    intra-abdominal D18.Ø3

Hemangioma — *continued*
  infantile — *continued*
    intracranial D18.Ø2
    skin D18.Ø1
    specified site NEC D18.Ø9
  intra-abdominal D18.Ø3
  intracranial D18.Ø2
  intramuscular D18.ØØ
    intra-abdominal D18.Ø3
    intracranial D18.Ø2
    skin D18.Ø1
    specified site NEC D18.Ø9
  intrathoracic structures D18.Ø9
  juvenile D18.ØØ
  malignant — *see* Neoplasm, connective tissue, malignant
  plexiform D18.ØØ
    intra-abdominal D18.Ø3
    intracranial D18.Ø2
    skin D18.Ø1
    specified site NEC D18.Ø9
  racemose D18.ØØ
    intra-abdominal D18.Ø3
    intracranial D18.Ø2
    skin D18.Ø1
    specified site NEC D18.Ø9
  sclerosing — *see* Neoplasm, skin, benign
  simplex D18.ØØ
    intra-abdominal D18.Ø3
    intracranial D18.Ø2
    skin D18.Ø1
    specified site NEC D18.Ø9
  skin D18.Ø1
  specified site NEC D18.Ø9
  venous D18.ØØ
    intra-abdominal D18.Ø3
    intracranial D18.Ø2
    skin D18.Ø1
    specified site NEC D18.Ø9
  verrucous keratotic D18.ØØ
    intra-abdominal D18.Ø3
    intracranial D18.Ø2
    skin D18.Ø1
    specified site NEC D18.Ø9
Hemangiomatosis (systemic) I78.8
  involving single site — *see* Hemangioma
Hemangiopericytoma — *see also* Neoplasm, connective tissue, uncertain behavior
  benign — *see* Neoplasm, connective tissue, benign
  malignant — *see* Neoplasm, connective tissue, malignant
Hemangiosarcoma — *see* Neoplasm, connective tissue, malignant
Hemarthrosis (nontraumatic) M25.ØØ
  ankle M25.Ø7- ☑
  elbow M25.Ø2- ☑
  foot joint M25.Ø7- ☑
  hand joint M25.Ø4- ☑
  hip M25.Ø5- ☑
  in hemophilic arthropathy — *see* Arthropathy, hemophilic
  knee M25.Ø6- ☑
  shoulder M25.Ø1- ☑
  specified joint NEC M25.Ø8
  traumatic — *see* Sprain, by site
  vertebrae M25.Ø8
  wrist M25.Ø3- ☑
Hematemesis K92.Ø
  with ulcer — *code by site under* Ulcer, with hemorrhage K27.4
  newborn, neonatal P54.Ø
    due to swallowed maternal blood P78.2
Hematidrosis L74.8
Hematinuria — *see also* Hemoglobinuria
  malarial B5Ø.8
Hematobilia K83.8
Hematocele
  female NEC N94.89
    with ectopic pregnancy OØØ.9Ø
      with intrauterine pregnancy OØØ.91
    ovary N83.8
  male N5Ø.1
Hematochezia — *see also* Melena K92.1
Hematochyluria — *see also* Infestation, filarial
  schistosomiasis (bilharziasis) B65.Ø
Hematocolpos (with hematometra or hematosalpinx) N89.7
Hematocornea — *see* Pigmentation, cornea, stromal

Hematogenous — *see* condition
Hematoma (traumatic) (skin surface intact) — *see also*
    Contusion
  with
    injury of internal organs — *see* Injury, by site
    open wound — *see* Wound, open
  amputation stump (surgical) (late) T87.89
  aorta, dissecting I71.00
    abdominal I71.02
    thoracic I71.01
    thoracoabdominal I71.03
  aortic intramural — *see* Dissection, aorta
  arterial (complicating trauma) — *see* Injury, blood
    vessel, by site
  auricle — *see* Contusion, ear
    nontraumatic — *see* Disorder, pinna, hematoma
  birth injury NEC P15.8
  brain (traumatic)
    with
      cerebral laceration or contusion (diffuse) — *see*
        Injury, intracranial, diffuse
        focal — *see* Injury, intracranial, focal
    cerebellar, traumatic S06.37- ☑
    intracerebral, traumatic — *see* Injury, intracranial,
      intracerebral hemorrhage
    newborn NEC P52.4
      birth injury P10.1
    nontraumatic — *see* Hemorrhage, intracranial
    subarachnoid, arachnoid, traumatic — *see* Injury,
      intracranial, subarachnoid hemorrhage
    subdural, traumatic — *see* Injury, intracranial, sub-
      dural hemorrhage
  breast (nontraumatic) N64.89
  broad ligament (nontraumatic) N83.7
    traumatic S37.892 ☑
  cerebellar, traumatic S06.37- ☑
  cerebral — *see* Hematoma, brain
  cerebrum S06.36- ☑
    left S06.35- ☑
    right S06.34- ☑
  cesarean delivery wound O90.2
  complicating delivery (perineal) (pelvic) (vagina) (vulva)
    O71.7
  corpus cavernosum (nontraumatic) N48.89
  epididymis (nontraumatic) N50.1
  epidural (traumatic) — *see* Injury, intracranial, epidural
    hemorrhage
    spinal — *see* Injury, spinal cord, by region
  episiotomy O90.2
  face, birth injury P15.4
  genital organ NEC (nontraumatic)
    female (nonobstetric) N94.89
      traumatic S30.202 ☑
    male N50.1
      traumatic S30.201 ☑
  internal organs — *see* Injury, by site
  intracerebral, traumatic — *see* Injury, intracranial, in-
    tracerebral hemorrhage
  intraoperative — *see* Complications, intraoperative,
    hemorrhage
  labia (nontraumatic) (nonobstetric) N90.89
  liver (subcapsular) (nontraumatic) K76.89
    birth injury P15.0
  mediastinum — *see* Injury, intrathoracic
  mesosalpinx (nontraumatic) N83.7
    traumatic S37.898 ☑
  muscle — code by site under Contusion
  nontraumatic
    muscle M79.81
    soft tissue M79.81
  obstetrical surgical wound O90.2
  orbit, orbital (nontraumatic) — *see also* Hemorrhage,
    orbit
    traumatic — *see* Contusion, orbit
  pelvis (female) (nontraumatic) (nonobstetric) N94.89
    obstetric O71.7
    traumatic — *see* Injury, by site
  penis (nontraumatic) N48.89
    birth injury P15.5
  perianal (nontraumatic) K64.5
  perineal S30.23 ☑
    complicating delivery O71.7
  perirenal — *see* Injury, kidney
  pinna — *see* Contusion, ear
    nontraumatic — *see* Disorder, pinna, hematoma
  placenta O43.89- ☑

Hematoma — *continued*
  postoperative (postprocedural) — *see* Complication,
    postprocedural, hematoma
  retroperitoneal (nontraumatic) K66.1
    traumatic S36.892 ☑
  scrotum, superficial S30.22 ☑
    birth injury P15.5
  seminal vesicle (nontraumatic) N50.1
    traumatic S37.892 ☑
  spermatic cord (traumatic) S37.892 ☑
    nontraumatic N50.1
  spinal (cord) (meninges) — *see also* Injury, spinal cord,
    by region
    newborn (birth injury) P11.5
  spleen D73.5
    intraoperative — *see* Complications, intraoperative,
      hemorrhage, spleen
    postprocedural (postoperative) — *see* Complica-
      tions, postprocedural, hemorrhage, spleen
  sternocleidomastoid, birth injury P15.2
  sternomastoid, birth injury P15.2
  subarachnoid (traumatic) — *see* Injury, intracranial,
    subarachnoid hemorrhage
    newborn (nontraumatic) P52.5
      due to birth injury P10.3
    nontraumatic — *see* Hemorrhage, intracranial,
      subarachnoid
  subdural (traumatic) — *see* Injury, intracranial, subdural
    hemorrhage
    newborn (localized) P52.8
      birth injury P10.0
    nontraumatic — *see* Hemorrhage, intracranial,
      subdural
  superficial, newborn P54.5
  testis (nontraumatic) N50.1
    birth injury P15.5
  tunica vaginalis (nontraumatic) N50.1
  umbilical cord, complicating delivery O69.5 ☑
  uterine ligament (broad) (nontraumatic) N83.7
    traumatic S37.892 ☑
  vagina (ruptured) (nontraumatic) N89.8
    complicating delivery O71.7
  vas deferens (nontraumatic) N50.1
    traumatic S37.892 ☑
  vitreous — *see* Hemorrhage, vitreous
  vulva (nontraumatic) (nonobstetric) N90.89
    complicating delivery O71.7
    newborn (birth injury) P15.5
Hematometra N85.7
  with hematocolpos N89.7
Hematomyelia (central) G95.19
  newborn (birth injury) P11.5
    traumatic T14.8 ☑
Hematomyelitis G04.90
Hematoperitoneum — *see* Hemoperitoneum
Hematophobia F40.230
Hematopneumothorax (see Hemothorax)
Hematopoiesis, cyclic D70.4
Hematoporphyria — *see* Porphyria
Hematorachis, hematorrhachis G95.19
  newborn (birth injury) P11.5
Hematosalpinx N83.6
  with
    hematocolpos N89.7
    hematometra N85.7
      with hematocolpos N89.7
  infectional — *see* Salpingitis
Hematospermia R36.1
Hematothorax (see Hemothorax)
Hematuria R31.9
  benign (familial) (of childhood) — *see also* Hematuria,
    idiopathic
    essential microscopic R31.1
  due to sulphonamide, sulfonamide — *see* Table of
    Drugs and Chemicals, by drug
  endemic — *see also* Schistosomiasis B65.0
  gross R31.0
  idiopathic N02.9
    with glomerular lesion
      crescentic (diffuse) glomerulonephritis N02.7
      dense deposit disease N02.6
      endocapillary proliferative glomerulonephritis
        N02.4
      focal and segmental hyalinosis or sclerosis N02.1
      membranoproliferative (diffuse) N02.5
      membranous (diffuse) N02.2
      mesangial proliferative (diffuse) N02.3
      mesangiocapillary (diffuse) N02.5

Hematuria — *continued*
  idiopathic — *continued*
    with glomerular lesion — *continued*
      minor abnormality N02.0
      proliferative NEC N02.8
      specified pathology NEC N02.8
  intermittent — *see* Hematuria, idiopathic
  malarial B50.8
  microscopic NEC (with symptoms) R31.29
    asymptomatic R31.21
    benign essential R31.1
  paroxysmal — *see also* Hematuria, idiopathic
    nocturnal D59.5
  persistent — *see* Hematuria, idiopathic
  recurrent — *see* Hematuria, idiopathic
  tropical — *see also* Schistosomiasis B65.0
  tuberculous A18.13
Hemeralopia (day blindness) H53.11
  vitamin A deficiency E50.5
Hemi-akinesia R41.4
Hemianalgesia R20.0
Hemianencephaly Q00.0
Hemianesthesia R20.0
Hemianopia, hemianopsia (heteronymous) H53.47
  homonymous H53.46- ☑
  syphilitic A52.71
Hemiathetosis R25.8
Hemiatrophy R68.89
  cerebellar G31.9
  face, facial, progressive (Romberg) G51.8
  tongue K14.8
Hemiballism (us) G25.5
Hemicardia Q24.8
Hemicephalus, hemicephaly Q00.0
Hemichorea G25.5
Hemicolitis, left — *see* Colitis, left sided
Hemicrania
  congenital malformation Q00.0
  continua G44.51
  meaning migraine — *see also* Migraine G43.909
  paroxysmal G44.039
    chronic G44.049
      intractable G44.041
      not intractable G44.049
    episodic G44.039
      intractable G44.031
      not intractable G44.039
    intractable G44.031
    not intractable G44.039
Hemidystrophy — *see* Hemiatrophy
Hemiectromelia Q73.8
Hemihypalgesia R20.8
Hemihypesthesia R20.1
Hemi-inattention R41.4
Hemimelia Q73.8
  lower limb — *see* Defect, reduction, lower limb, speci-
    fied type NEC
  upper limb — *see* Defect, reduction, upper limb, spec-
    ified type NEC
Hemiparalysis — *see* Hemiplegia
Hemiparesis — *see* Hemiplegia
Hemiparesthesia R20.2
Hemiparkinsonism G20
Hemiplegia G81.9- ☑
  alternans facialis G83.89
  ascending NEC G81.90
    spinal G95.89
  congenital (cerebral) G80.8
    spastic G80.2
  embolic (current episode) I63.4- ☑
  flaccid G81.0- ☑
  following
    cerebrovascular disease I69.959
      cerebral infarction I69.35- ☑
      intracerebral hemorrhage I69.15- ☑
      nontraumatic intracranial hemorrhage NEC
        I69.25- ☑
      specified disease NEC I69.85- ☑
      stroke NOS I69.35- ☑
      subarachnoid hemorrhage I69.05- ☑
  hysterical F44.4
  newborn NEC P91.88
    birth injury P11.9
  spastic G81.1- ☑
    congenital G80.2
  thrombotic (current episode) I63.3- ☑

☑ **Additional Character Required — Refer to the Tabular List for Character Selection**   ▽ **Subterms under main terms may continue to next column or page**

Hemisection, spinal cord — see Injury, spinal cord, by region
Hemispasm (facial) R25.2
Hemisporosis B48.8
Hemitremor R25.1
Hemivertebra Q76.49
  failure of segmentation with scoliosis Q76.3
  fusion with scoliosis Q76.3
Hemochromatosis E83.119
  with refractory anemia D46.1
  due to repeated red blood cell transfusion E83.111
  hereditary (primary) E83.110
  neonatal P78.84
  primary E83.110
  specified NEC E83.118
Hemoglobin — see also condition
  abnormal (disease) — see Disease, hemoglobin
  AS genotype D57.3
  Constant Spring D58.2
  E-beta thalassemia D56.5
  fetal, hereditary persistence (HPFH) D56.4
  H Constant Spring D56.0
  low NOS D64.9
  S (Hb S), heterozygous D57.3
Hemoglobinemia D59.9
  due to blood transfusion T80.89 ☑
  paroxysmal D59.6
    nocturnal D59.5
Hemoglobinopathy (mixed) D58.2
  with thalassemia D56.8
  sickle-cell D57.1
    with thalassemia D57.40
      with crisis (vasoocclusive pain) D57.419
        with
          acute chest syndrome D57.411
          splenic sequestration D57.412
      without crisis D57.40
Hemoglobinuria R82.3
  with anemia, hemolytic, acquired (chronic) NEC D59.6
  cold (agglutinin) (paroxysmal) (with Raynaud's syndrome) D59.6
  due to exertion or hemolysis NEC D59.6
  intermittent D59.6
  malarial B50.8
  march D59.6
  nocturnal (paroxysmal) D59.5
  paroxysmal (cold) D59.6
    nocturnal D59.5
Hemolymphangioma D18.1
Hemolysis
  intravascular
    with
      abortion — see Abortion, by type, complicated by, hemorrhage
      ectopic or molar pregnancy O08.1
      hemorrhage
        antepartum — see Hemorrhage, antepartum, with coagulation defect
        intrapartum — see also Hemorrhage, complicating, delivery O67.0
      postpartum O72.3
  neonatal (excessive) P58.9
    specified NEC P58.8
Hemolytic — see condition
Hemopericardium I31.2
  following acute myocardial infarction (current complication) I23.0
  newborn P54.8
  traumatic — see Injury, heart, with hemopericardium
Hemoperitoneum K66.1
  infectional K65.9
  traumatic S36.899 ☑
    with open wound — see Wound, open, with penetration into peritoneal cavity
Hemophilia (classical) (familial) (hereditary) D66
  A D66
  acquired D68.311
  autoimmune D68.311
  B D67
  C D68.1
  calcipriva — see also Defect, coagulation D68.4
  nonfamilial — see also Defect, coagulation D68.4
  secondary D68.311
  vascular D68.0
Hemophthalmos H44.81- ☑
Hemopneumothorax — see also Hemothorax
  traumatic S27.2 ☑
Hemoptysis R04.2

Hemoptysis — continued
  newborn P26.9
  tuberculous — see Tuberculosis, pulmonary
Hemorrhage, hemorrhagic (concealed) R58
  abdomen R58
  accidental antepartum — see Hemorrhage, antepartum
  acute idiopathic pulmonary, in infants R04.81
  adenoid J35.8
  adrenal (capsule) (gland) E27.49
    medulla E27.8
    newborn P54.4
  after delivery — see Hemorrhage, postpartum
  alveolar
    lung, newborn P26.8
    process K08.89
  alveolus K08.89
  amputation stump (surgical) T87.89
  anemia (chronic) D50.0
    acute D62
  antepartum (with) O46.90
    with coagulation defect O46.00- ☑
      afibrinogenemia O46.01- ☑
      disseminated intravascular coagulation O46.02- ☑
      hypofibrinogenemia O46.01- ☑
      specified defect NEC O46.09- ☑
    before 20 weeks gestation O20.9
      specified type NEC O20.8
      threatened abortion O20.0
    due to
      abruptio placenta — see also Abruptio placentae O45.9- ☑
      leiomyoma, uterus — see Hemorrhage, antepartum, specified cause NEC
      placenta previa O44.1- ☑
    specified cause NEC — see subcategory O46.8X- ☑
  anus (sphincter) K62.5
  apoplexy (stroke) — see Hemorrhage, intracranial, intracerebral
  arachnoid — see Hemorrhage, intracranial, subarachnoid
  artery R58
    brain — see Hemorrhage, intracranial, intracerebral
  basilar (ganglion) I61.0
  bladder N32.89
  bowel K92.2
    newborn P54.3
  brain (miliary) (nontraumatic) — see Hemorrhage, intracranial, intracerebral
    due to
      birth injury P10.1
      syphilis A52.05
    epidural or extradural (traumatic) — see Injury, intracranial, epidural hemorrhage
    newborn P52.4
      birth injury P10.1
    subarachnoid — see Hemorrhage, intracranial, subarachnoid
    subdural — see Hemorrhage, intracranial, subdural
  brainstem (nontraumatic) I61.3
    traumatic S06.38- ☑
  breast N64.59
  bronchial tube — see Hemorrhage, lung
  bronchopulmonary — see Hemorrhage, lung
  bronchus — see Hemorrhage, lung
  bulbar I61.5
  capillary I78.8
    primary D69.8
  cecum K92.2
  cerebellar, cerebellum (nontraumatic) I61.4
    newborn P52.6
    traumatic S06.37- ☑
  cerebral, cerebrum — see also Hemorrhage, intracranial, intracerebral
    lobe I61.1
    newborn (anoxic) P52.4
      birth injury P10.1
  cerebromeningeal I61.8
  cerebrospinal — see Hemorrhage, intracranial, intracerebral
  cervix (uteri) (stump) NEC N88.8
  chamber, anterior (eye) — see Hyphema
  childbirth — see Hemorrhage, complicating, delivery
  choroid H31.30- ☑
    expulsive H31.31- ☑
  ciliary body — see Hyphema
  cochlea — see subcategory H83.8 ☑
  colon K92.2

Hemorrhage, hemorrhagic — continued
  complicating
    abortion — see Abortion, by type, complicated by, hemorrhage
    delivery O67.9
      associated with coagulation defect (afibrinogenemia) (DIC) (hyperfibrinolysis) O67.0
      specified cause NEC O67.8
    surgical procedure — see Hemorrhage, intraoperative
  conjunctiva H11.3- ☑
    newborn P54.8
  cord, newborn (stump) P51.9
  corpus luteum (ruptured) cyst N83.1- ☑
  cortical (brain) I61.1
  cranial — see Hemorrhage, intracranial
  cutaneous R23.3
    due to autosensitivity, erythrocyte D69.2
    newborn P54.5
  delayed
    following ectopic or molar pregnancy O08.1
    postpartum O72.2
  diathesis (familial) D69.9
  disease D69.9
    newborn P53
    specified type NEC D69.8
  due to or associated with
    afibrinogenemia or other coagulation defect (conditions in categories D65- D69)
      antepartum — see Hemorrhage, antepartum, with coagulation defect
      intrapartum O67.0
    dental implant M27.61
    device, implant or graft — see also Complications, by site and type, specified NEC T85.838 ☑
      arterial graft NEC T82.838 ☑
      breast T85.838 ☑
      catheter NEC T85.838 ☑
        dialysis (renal) T82.838 ☑
          intraperitoneal T85.838 ☑
        infusion NEC T82.838 ☑
          spinal (epidural) (subdural) T85.830 ☑
        urinary (indwelling) T83.83 ☑
      electronic (electrode) (pulse generator) (stimulator)
        bone T84.83 ☑
        cardiac T82.837 ☑
        nervous system (brain) (peripheral nerve) (spinal) T85.830 ☑
        urinary T83.83 ☑
      fixation, internal (orthopedic) NEC T84.83 ☑
      gastrointestinal (bile duct) (esophagus) T85.838 ☑
      genital NEC T83.83 ☑
      heart NEC T82.837 ☑
      joint prosthesis T84.83 ☑
      ocular (corneal graft) (orbital implant) NEC T85.838 ☑
      orthopedic NEC T84.83 ☑
        bone graft T86.838
      specified NEC T85.838 ☑
      urinary NEC T83.83 ☑
      vascular NEC T82.838 ☑
      ventricular intracranial shunt T85.830 ☑
  duodenum, duodenal K92.2
    ulcer — see Ulcer, duodenum, with hemorrhage
  dura mater — see Hemorrhage, intracranial, subdural
  endotracheal — see Hemorrhage, lung
  epicranial subaponeurotic (massive), birth injury P12.2
  epidural (traumatic) — see also Injury, intracranial, epidural hemorrhage
    nontraumatic I62.1
  esophagus K22.8
    varix I85.01
      secondary I85.11
  excessive, following ectopic gestation (subsequent episode) O08.1
  extradural (traumatic) — see Injury, intracranial, epidural hemorrhage
    birth injury P10.8
    newborn (anoxic) (nontraumatic) P52.8
    nontraumatic I62.1
  eye NEC H57.89
    fundus — see Hemorrhage, retina
    lid — see Disorder, eyelid, specified type NEC
  fallopian tube N83.6
  fibrinogenolysis — see Fibrinolysis

Hemorrhage, hemorrhagic — *continued*
fibrinolytic (acquired) — *see* Fibrinolysis
from
  ear (nontraumatic) — *see* Otorrhagia
  tracheostomy stoma J95.01
fundus, eye — *see* Hemorrhage, retina
funis — *see* Hemorrhage, umbilicus, cord
gastric — *see* Hemorrhage, stomach
gastroenteric K92.2
  newborn P54.3
gastrointestinal (tract) K92.2
  newborn P54.3
genital organ, male N50.1
genitourinary (tract) NOS R31.9
gingiva K06.8
globe (eye) — *see* Hemophthalmos
graafian follicle cyst (ruptured) N83.0- ☑
gum K06.8
heart I51.89
hypopharyngeal (throat) R04.1
intermenstrual (regular) N92.3
  irregular N92.1
internal (organs) NEC R58
  capsule I61.0
  ear — *see* subcategory H83.8 ☑
  newborn P54.8
intestine K92.2
  newborn P54.3
intra-abdominal R58
intra-alveolar (lung), newborn P26.8
intracerebral (nontraumatic) — *see* Hemorrhage, intracranial, intracerebral
intracranial (nontraumatic) I62.9
  birth injury P10.9
  epidural, nontraumatic I62.1
  extradural, nontraumatic I62.1
  intracerebral (nontraumatic) (in) I61.9
    brain stem I61.3
    cerebellum I61.4
    hemisphere I61.2
      cortical (superficial) I61.1
      subcortical (deep) I61.0
    intraoperative
      during a nervous system procedure G97.31
      during other procedure G97.32
    intraventricular I61.5
    multiple localized I61.6
    newborn P52.4
      birth injury P10.1
    postprocedural
      following a nervous system procedure G97.51
      following other procedure G97.52
    specified NEC I61.8
    superficial I61.1
    traumatic (diffuse) — *see* Injury, intracranial, diffuse
      focal — *see* Injury, intracranial, focal
  newborn P52.9
    specified NEC P52.8
  subarachnoid (nontraumatic) (from) I60.9
    intracranial (cerebral) artery I60.7
      anterior communicating I60.2
      basilar I60.4
      carotid siphon and bifurcation I60.0- ☑
      communicating I60.7
        anterior I60.2
        posterior I60.3- ☑
      middle cerebral I60.1- ☑
      posterior communicating I60.3- ☑
      specified artery NEC I60.6
      vertebral I60.5- ☑
    newborn P52.5
      birth injury P10.3
    specified NEC I60.8
    traumatic S06.6X- ☑
  subdural (nontraumatic) I62.00
    acute I62.01
    birth injury P10.0
    chronic I62.03
    newborn (anoxic) (hypoxic) P52.8
      birth injury P10.0
    spinal G95.19
    subacute I62.02
    traumatic — *see* Injury, intracranial, subdural hemorrhage
  traumatic — *see* Injury, intracranial, focal brain injury
intramedullary NEC G95.19

Hemorrhage, hemorrhagic — *continued*
intraocular — *see* Hemophthalmos
intraoperative, intraprocedural — *see* Complication, hemorrhage (hematoma), intraoperative (intraprocedural), by site
intrapartum — *see* Hemorrhage, complicating, delivery
intrapelvic
  female N94.89
  male K66.1
intraperitoneal K66.1
intrapontine I61.3
intraprocedural — *see* Complication, hemorrhage (hematoma), intraoperative (intraprocedural), by site
intrauterine N85.7
  complicating delivery — *see also* Hemorrhage, complicating, delivery O67.9
  postpartum — *see* Hemorrhage, postpartum
intraventricular I61.5
  newborn (nontraumatic) — *see also* Newborn, affected by, hemorrhage P52.3
    due to birth injury P10.2
    grade
      1 P52.0
      2 P52.1
      3 P52.21
      4 P52.22
intravesical N32.89
iris (postinfectional) (postinflammatory) (toxic) — *see* Hyphema
joint (nontraumatic) — *see* Hemarthrosis
kidney N28.89
knee (joint) (nontraumatic) — *see* Hemarthrosis, knee
labyrinth — *see* subcategory H83.8 ☑
lenticular striate artery I61.0
ligature, vessel — *see* Hemorrhage, postoperative
liver K76.89
lung R04.89
  newborn P26.9
    massive P26.1
    specified NEC P26.8
  tuberculous — *see* Tuberculosis, pulmonary
massive umbilical, newborn P51.0
mediastinum — *see* Hemorrhage, lung
medulla I61.3
membrane (brain) I60.8
  spinal cord — *see* Hemorrhage, spinal cord
meninges, meningeal (brain) (middle) I60.8
  spinal cord — *see* Hemorrhage, spinal cord
mesentery K66.1
metritis — *see* Endometritis
mouth K13.79
mucous membrane NEC R58
  newborn P54.8
muscle M62.89
nail (subungual) L60.8
nasal turbinate R04.0
  newborn P54.8
navel, newborn P51.9
newborn P54.9
  specified NEC P54.8
nipple N64.59
nose R04.0
  newborn P54.8
omentum K66.1
optic nerve (sheath) H47.02- ☑
orbit, orbital H05.23- ☑
ovary NEC N83.8
oviduct N83.6
pancreas K86.89
parathyroid (gland) (spontaneous) E21.4
parturition — *see* Hemorrhage, complicating, delivery
penis N48.89
pericardium, pericarditis I31.2
peritoneum, peritoneal K66.1
peritonsillar tissue J35.8
  due to infection J36
petechial R23.3
  due to autosensitivity, erythrocyte D69.2
pituitary (gland) E23.6
pleura — *see* Hemorrhage, lung
polioencephalitis, superior E51.2
polymyositis — *see* Polymyositis
pons, pontine I61.3
posterior fossa (nontraumatic) I61.8
  newborn P52.6
postmenopausal N95.0
postnasal R04.0

Hemorrhage, hemorrhagic — *continued*
postoperative — *see* Complications, postprocedural, hemorrhage, by site
postpartum NEC (following delivery of placenta) O72.1
  delayed or secondary O72.2
  retained placenta O72.0
  third stage O72.0
pregnancy — *see* Hemorrhage, antepartum
preretinal — *see* Hemorrhage, retina
prostate N42.1
puerperal — *see* Hemorrhage, postpartum
  delayed or secondary O72.2
pulmonary R04.89
  newborn P26.9
    massive P26.1
    specified NEC P26.8
  tuberculous — *see* Tuberculosis, pulmonary
purpura (primary) D69.3
rectum (sphincter) K62.5
  newborn P54.2
recurring, following initial hemorrhage at time of injury T79.2 ☑
renal N28.89
respiratory passage or tract R04.9
  specified NEC R04.89
retina, retinal (vessels) H35.6- ☑
  diabetic — *see* Diabetes, retinal, hemorrhage
retroperitoneal R58
scalp R58
scrotum N50.1
secondary (nontraumatic) R58
  following initial hemorrhage at time of injury T79.2 ☑
seminal vesicle N50.1
skin R23.3
  newborn P54.5
slipped umbilical ligature P51.8
spermatic cord N50.1
spinal (cord) G95.19
  newborn (birth injury) P11.5
spleen D73.5
  intraoperative — *see* Complications, intraoperative, hemorrhage, spleen
  postprocedural — *see* Complications, postprocedural, hemorrhage, spleen
stomach K92.2
  newborn P54.3
  ulcer — *see* Ulcer, stomach, with hemorrhage
subarachnoid (nontraumatic) — *see* Hemorrhage, intracranial, subarachnoid
subconjunctival — *see also* Hemorrhage, conjunctiva
  birth injury P15.3
subcortical (brain) I61.0
subcutaneous R23.3
subdiaphragmatic R58
subdural (acute) (nontraumatic) — *see* Hemorrhage, intracranial, subdural
subependymal
  newborn P52.0
    with intraventricular extension P52.1
      and intracerebral extension P52.22
subgaleal P12.2
subhyaloid — *see* Hemorrhage, retina
subperiosteal — *see* Disorder, bone, specified type NEC
subretinal — *see* Hemorrhage, retina
subtentorial — *see* Hemorrhage, intracranial, subdural
subungual L60.8
suprarenal (capsule) (gland) E27.49
  newborn P54.4
tentorium (traumatic) NEC — *see* Hemorrhage, brain
  newborn (birth injury) P10.4
testis N50.1
third stage (postpartum) O72.0
thorax — *see* Hemorrhage, lung
throat R04.1
thymus (gland) E32.8
thyroid (cyst) (gland) E07.89
tongue K14.8
tonsil J35.8
trachea — *see* Hemorrhage, lung
tracheobronchial R04.89
  newborn P26.0
traumatic — *code to* specific injury
  cerebellar — *see* Hemorrhage, brain
  intracranial — *see* Hemorrhage, brain
  recurring or secondary (following initial hemorrhage at time of injury) T79.2 ☑

☑ **Additional Character Required — Refer to the Tabular List for Character Selection**   ▽ **Subterms under main terms may continue to next column or page**

Hemorrhage, hemorrhagic — *continued*
  tuberculous NEC — *see also* Tuberculosis, pulmonary A15.Ø
  tunica vaginalis N5Ø.1
  ulcer — *code by* site under Ulcer, with hemorrhage K27.4
  umbilicus, umbilical
    cord
      after birth, newborn P51.9
      complicating delivery O69.5 ☑
    newborn P51.9
      massive P51.Ø
      slipped ligature P51.8
    stump P51.9
  urethra (idiopathic) N36.8
  uterus, uterine (abnormal) N93.9
    climacteric N92.4
    complicating delivery — *see* Hemorrhage, complicating, delivery
    dysfunctional or functional N93.8
    intermenstrual (regular) N92.3
      irregular N92.1
    postmenopausal N95.Ø
    postpartum — *see* Hemorrhage, postpartum
    preclimacteric or premenopausal N92.4
    prepubertal N93.8
    pubertal N92.2
  vagina (abnormal) N93.9
    newborn P54.6
  vas deferens N5Ø.1
  vasa previa O69.4 ☑
  ventricular I61.5
  vesical N32.89
  viscera NEC R58
    newborn P54.8
  vitreous (humor) (intraocular) H43.1- ☑
  vulva N9Ø.89
Hemorrhoids (bleeding) (without mention of degree) K64.9
  1st degree (grade/stage I) (without prolapse outside of anal canal) K64.Ø
  2nd degree (grade/stage II) (that prolapse with straining but retract spontaneously) K64.1
  3rd degree (grade/stage III) (that prolapse with straining and require manual replacement back inside anal canal) K64.2
  4th degree (grade/stage IV) (with prolapsed tissue that cannot be manually replaced) K64.3
  complicating
    pregnancy O22.4 ☑
    puerperium O87.2
  external K64.4
    with
      thrombosis K64.5
  internal (without mention of degree) K64.8
  prolapsed K64.8
  skin tags
    anus K64.4
    residual K64.4
  specified NEC K64.8
  strangulated — *see also* Hemorrhoids, by degree K64.8
  thrombosed — *see also* Hemorrhoids, by degree K64.5
  ulcerated — *see also* Hemorrhoids, by degree K64.8
Hemosalpinx N83.6
  with
    hematocolpos N89.7
    hematometra N85.7
      with hematocolpos N89.7
Hemosiderosis (dietary) E83.19
  pulmonary, idiopathic E83.1- ☑ *[J84.Ø3]*
  transfusion T8Ø.89 ☑
Hemothorax (bacterial) (nontuberculous) J94.2
  newborn P54.8
  traumatic S27.1 ☑
    with pneumothorax S27.2 ☑
  tuberculous NEC A15.6
Henoch (-Schönlein) **disease or syndrome** (purpura) D69.Ø
Henpue, henpuye A66.6
Hepar lobatum (syphilitic) A52.74
Hepatalgia K76.89
Hepatitis K75.9
  acute B17.9
    with coma K72.Ø1
    with hepatic failure — *see* Failure, hepatic
    alcoholic — *see* Hepatitis, alcoholic
    infectious B17.9
    non-viral K72.Ø ☑

Hepatitis — *continued*
  acute — *continued*
    viral B17.9
  alcoholic (acute) (chronic) K7Ø.1Ø
    with ascites K7Ø.11
  amebic — *see* Abscess, liver, amebic
  anicteric, (viral) — *see* Hepatitis, viral
  antigen-associated (HAA) — *see* Hepatitis, B
  Australia-antigen (positive) — *see* Hepatitis, B
  autoimmune K75.4
  B B19.1Ø
    with hepatic coma B19.11
    acute B16.9
      with
        delta-agent (coinfection) (without hepatic coma) B16.1
          with hepatic coma B16.Ø
        hepatic coma (without delta-agent coinfection) B16.2
    chronic B18.1
      with delta-agent B18.Ø
  bacterial NEC K75.89
  C (viral) B19.2Ø
    with hepatic coma B19.21
    acute B17.1Ø
      with hepatic coma B17.11
    chronic B18.2
  catarrhal (acute) B15.9
    with hepatic coma B15.Ø
  cholangiolitic K75.89
  cholestatic K75.89
  chronic K73.9
    active NEC K73.2
    lobular NEC K73.1
    persistent NEC K73.Ø
    specified NEC K73.8
  cytomegaloviral B25.1
  due to ethanol (acute) (chronic) — *see* Hepatitis, alcoholic
  epidemic B15.9
    with hepatic coma B15.Ø
  fulminant NEC (viral) — *see* Hepatitis, viral
  granulomatous NEC K75.3
  herpesviral BØØ.81
  history of
    B Z86.19
    C Z86.19
  homologous serum — *see* Hepatitis, viral, type B
  in (due to)
    mumps B26.81
    toxoplasmosis (acquired) B58.1
      congenital (active) P37.1 *[K77]*
  infectious, infective B15.9
    acute (subacute) B17.9
    chronic B18.9
  inoculation — *see* Hepatitis, viral, type B
  interstitial (chronic) K74.69
  lupoid NEC K75.4
  malignant NEC (with hepatic failure) K72.9Ø
    with coma K72.91
  neonatal (idiopathic) (toxic) P59.29
  neonatal giant cell P59.29
  newborn P59.29
  non-viral K72.Ø ☑
  postimmunization — *see* Hepatitis, viral, type B
  post-transfusion — *see* Hepatitis, viral, type B
  reactive, nonspecific K75.2
  serum — *see* Hepatitis, viral, type B
  specified type NEC
    with hepatic failure — *see* Failure, hepatic
  syphilitic (late) A52.74
    congenital (early) A5Ø.Ø8 *[K77]*
      late A5Ø.59 *[K77]*
    secondary A51.45
  toxic — *see also* Disease, liver, toxic K71.6
  tuberculous A18.83
  viral, virus B19.9
    with hepatic coma B19.Ø
    acute B17.9
    chronic B18.9
      specified NEC B18.8
    type
      B B18.1
        with delta-agent B18.Ø
      C B18.2
    congenital P35.3
    coxsackie B33.8 *[K77]*
    cytomegalic inclusion B25.1

Hepatitis — *continued*
  viral, virus — *continued*
    in remission, any type — *code to* Hepatitis, chronic, by type
    non-A, non-B B17.8
    specified type NEC (with or without coma) B17.8
    type
      A B15.9
        with hepatic coma B15.Ø
      B B19.1Ø
        with hepatic coma B19.11
        acute B16.9
          with
            delta-agent (coinfection) (without hepatic coma) B16.1
              with hepatic coma B16.Ø
            hepatic coma (without delta-agent coinfection) B16.2
        chronic B18.1
          with delta-agent B18.Ø
      C B19.2Ø
        with hepatic coma B19.21
        acute B17.1Ø
          with hepatic coma B17.11
        chronic B18.2
      E B17.2
      non-A, non-B B17.8
Hepatization lung (acute) — *see* Pneumonia, lobar
Hepatoblastoma C22.2
Hepatocarcinoma C22.Ø
Hepatocholangiocarcinoma C22.Ø
Hepatocholangioma, benign D13.4
Hepatocholangitis K75.89
Hepatolenticular degeneration E83.Ø1
Hepatoma (malignant) C22.Ø
  benign D13.4
  embryonal C22.Ø
Hepatomegaly — *see also* Hypertrophy, liver
  with splenomegaly R16.2
  congenital Q44.7
  in mononucleosis
    gammaherpesviral B27.Ø9
    infectious specified NEC B27.89
Hepatoptosis K76.89
Hepatorenal syndrome following labor and delivery O90.4
Hepatosis K76.89
Hepatosplenomegaly R16.2
  hyperlipemic (Bürger-Grütz type) E78.3 *[K77]*
Hereditary — *see* condition
Heredodegeneration, macular — *see* Dystrophy, retina
Heredopathia atactica polyneuritiformis G6Ø.1
Heredosyphilis — *see* Syphilis, congenital
Herlitz' syndrome Q81.1
Hermansky-Pudlak syndrome E7Ø.331
Hermaphrodite, hermaphroditism (true) Q56.Ø
  46,XX with streak gonads Q99.1
  46,XX/46,XY Q99.Ø
  46,XY with streak gonads Q99.1
  chimera 46,XX/46,XY Q99.Ø
Hernia, hernial (acquired) (recurrent) K46.9
  with
    gangrene — *see* Hernia, by site, with, gangrene
    incarceration — *see* Hernia, by site, with, obstruction
    irreducible — *see* Hernia, by site, with, obstruction
    obstruction — *see* Hernia, by site, with, obstruction
    strangulation — *see* Hernia, by site, with, obstruction
  abdomen, abdominal K46.9
    with
      gangrene (and obstruction) K46.1
      obstruction K46.Ø
    femoral — *see* Hernia, femoral
    incisional — *see* Hernia, incisional
    inguinal — *see* Hernia, inguinal
    specified site NEC K45.8
      with
        gangrene (and obstruction) K45.1
        obstruction K45.Ø
    umbilical — *see* Hernia, umbilical
    wall — *see* Hernia, ventral
  appendix — *see* Hernia, abdomen
  bladder (mucosa) (sphincter)
    congenital (female) (male) Q79.51
    female — *see* Cystocele
    male N32.89
  brain, congenital — *see* Encephalocele

Index

Hernia, hernial — Herpes, herpesvirus, herpetic

Hernia, hernial — *continued*
cartilage, vertebra — *see* Displacement, intervertebral disc
cerebral, congenital — *see also* Encephalocele
   endaural Q01.8
ciliary body (traumatic) S05.2- ☑
colon — *see* Hernia, abdomen
Cooper's — *see* Hernia, abdomen, specified site NEC
crural — *see* Hernia, femoral
diaphragm, diaphragmatic K44.9
   with
      gangrene (and obstruction) K44.1
      obstruction K44.0
   congenital Q79.0
direct (inguinal) — *see* Hernia, inguinal
diverticulum, intestine — *see* Hernia, abdomen
double (inguinal) — *see* Hernia, inguinal, bilateral
due to adhesions (with obstruction) K56.50
epigastric — *see also* Hernia, ventral K43.9
esophageal hiatus — *see* Hernia, hiatal
external (inguinal) — *see* Hernia, inguinal
fallopian tube N83.4- ☑
fascia M62.89
femoral K41.90
   with
      gangrene (and obstruction) K41.40
         not specified as recurrent K41.40
         recurrent K41.41
      obstruction K41.30
         not specified as recurrent K41.30
         recurrent K41.31
   not specified as recurrent K41.90
   recurrent K41.91
   bilateral K41.20
      with
         gangrene (and obstruction) K41.10
            not specified as recurrent K41.10
            recurrent K41.11
         obstruction K41.00
            not specified as recurrent K41.00
            recurrent K41.01
      not specified as recurrent K41.20
      recurrent K41.21
   unilateral K41.90
      with
         gangrene (and obstruction) K41.40
            not specified as recurrent K41.40
            recurrent K41.41
         obstruction K41.30
            not specified as recurrent K41.30
            recurrent K41.31
      not specified as recurrent K41.90
      recurrent K41.91
foramen magnum G93.5
   congenital Q01.8
funicular (umbilical) — *see also* Hernia, umbilicus
   spermatic (cord) — *see* Hernia, inguinal
gastrointestinal tract — *see* Hernia, abdomen
Hesselbach's — *see* Hernia, femoral, specified site NEC
hiatal (esophageal) (sliding) K44.9
   with
      gangrene (and obstruction) K44.1
      obstruction K44.0
   congenital Q40.1
hypogastric — *see* Hernia, ventral
incarcerated — *see also* Hernia, by site, with obstruction
   with gangrene — *see* Hernia, by site, with gangrene
incisional K43.2
   with
      gangrene (and obstruction) K43.1
      obstruction K43.0
indirect (inguinal) — *see* Hernia, inguinal
inguinal (direct) (external) (funicular) (indirect) (internal) (oblique) (scrotal) (sliding) K40.90
   with
      gangrene (and obstruction) K40.40
         not specified as recurrent K40.40
         recurrent K40.41
      obstruction K40.30
         not specified as recurrent K40.30
         recurrent K40.31
   not specified as recurrent K40.90
   recurrent K40.91
   bilateral K40.20
      with
         gangrene (and obstruction) K40.10
            not specified as recurrent K40.10

Hernia, hernial — *continued*
inguinal — *continued*
   bilateral — *continued*
      with — *continued*
         gangrene — *continued*
            recurrent K40.11
         obstruction K40.00
            not specified as recurrent K40.00
            recurrent K40.01
      not specified as recurrent K40.20
      recurrent K40.21
   unilateral K40.90
      with
         gangrene (and obstruction) K40.40
            not specified as recurrent K40.40
            recurrent K40.41
         obstruction K40.30
            not specified as recurrent K40.30
            recurrent K40.31
      not specified as recurrent K40.90
      recurrent K40.91
internal — *see also* Hernia, abdomen
   inguinal — *see* Hernia, inguinal
interstitial — *see* Hernia, abdomen
intervertebral cartilage or disc — *see* Displacement, intervertebral disc
intestine, intestinal — *see* Hernia, by site
intra-abdominal — *see* Hernia, abdomen
iris (traumatic) S05.2- ☑
irreducible — *see also* Hernia, by site, with obstruction
   with gangrene — *see* Hernia, by site, with gangrene
ischiatic — *see* Hernia, abdomen, specified site NEC
ischiorectal — *see* Hernia, abdomen, specified site NEC
lens (traumatic) S05.2- ☑
linea (alba) (semilunaris) — *see* Hernia, ventral
Littre's — *see* Hernia, abdomen
lumbar — *see* Hernia, abdomen, specified site NEC
lung (subcutaneous) J98.4
mediastinum J98.59
mesenteric (internal) — *see* Hernia, abdomen
midline — *see* Hernia, ventral
muscle (sheath) M62.89
nucleus pulposus — *see* Displacement, intervertebral disc
oblique (inguinal) — *see* Hernia, inguinal
obstructive — *see also* Hernia, by site, with obstruction
   with gangrene — *see* Hernia, by site, with gangrene
obturator — *see* Hernia, abdomen, specified site NEC
omental — *see* Hernia, abdomen
ovary N83.4- ☑
oviduct N83.4- ☑
paraesophageal — *see also* Hernia, diaphragm
   congenital Q40.1
parastomal K43.5
   with
      gangrene (and obstruction) K43.4
      obstruction K43.3
paraumbilical — *see* Hernia, umbilicus
perineal — *see* Hernia, abdomen, specified site NEC
Petit's — *see* Hernia, abdomen, specified site NEC
postoperative — *see* Hernia, incisional
pregnant uterus — *see* Abnormal, uterus in pregnancy or childbirth
prevesical N32.89
properitoneal — *see* Hernia, abdomen, specified site NEC
pudendal — *see* Hernia, abdomen, specified site NEC
rectovaginal N81.6
retroperitoneal — *see* Hernia, abdomen, specified site NEC
Richter's — *see* Hernia, abdomen, with obstruction
Rieux's, Riex's — *see* Hernia, abdomen, specified site NEC
sac condition (adhesion) (dropsy) (inflammation) (laceration) (suppuration) — *code by site under* Hernia
sciatic — *see* Hernia, abdomen, specified site NEC
scrotum, scrotal — *see* Hernia, inguinal
sliding (inguinal) — *see also* Hernia, inguinal
   hiatus — *see* Hernia, hiatal
spigelian — *see* Hernia, ventral
spinal — *see* Spina bifida
strangulated — *see also* Hernia, by site, with obstruction
   with gangrene — *see* Hernia, by site, with gangrene
subxiphoid — *see* Hernia, ventral
supra-umbilicus — *see* Hernia, ventral

Hernia, hernial — *continued*
tendon — *see* Disorder, tendon, specified type NEC
Treitz's (fossa) — *see* Hernia, abdomen, specified site NEC
tunica vaginalis Q55.29
umbilicus, umbilical K42.9
   with
      gangrene (and obstruction) K42.1
      obstruction K42.0
ureter N28.89
urethra, congenital Q64.79
urinary meatus, congenital Q64.79
uterus N81.4
   pregnant — *see* Abnormal, uterus in pregnancy or childbirth
vaginal (anterior) (wall) — *see* Cystocele
Velpeau's — *see* Hernia, femoral
ventral K43.9
   with
      gangrene (and obstruction) K43.7
      obstruction K43.6
   incisional K43.2
      with
         gangrene (and obstruction) K43.1
         obstruction K43.0
      recurrent — *see* Hernia, incisional
   specified NEC K43.9
      with
         gangrene (and obstruction) K43.7
         obstruction K43.6
vesical
   congenital (female) (male) Q79.51
   female — *see* Cystocele
   male N32.89
vitreous (into wound) S05.2- ☑
   into anterior chamber — *see* Prolapse, vitreous
Herniation — *see also* Hernia
brain (stem) G93.5
cerebral G93.5
mediastinum J98.59
nucleus pulposus — *see* Displacement, intervertebral disc
Herpangina B08.5
Herpes, herpesvirus, herpetic B00.9
anogenital A60.9
   perianal skin A60.1
   rectum A60.1
   urogenital tract A60.00
      cervix A60.03
      male genital organ NEC A60.02
      penis A60.01
      specified site NEC A60.09
      vagina A60.04
      vulva A60.04
blepharitis (zoster) B02.39
   simplex B00.59
circinatus B35.4
   bullosus L12.0
conjunctivitis (simplex) B00.53
   zoster B02.31
cornea B02.33
encephalitis B00.4
   due to herpesvirus 6 B10.01
   due to herpesvirus 7 B10.09
   specified NEC B10.09
eye (zoster) B02.30
   simplex B00.50
eyelid (zoster) B02.39
   simplex B00.59
facialis B00.1
febrilis B00.1
geniculate ganglionitis B02.21
genital, genitalis A60.00
   female A60.09
   male A60.02
gestational, gestationis O26.4- ☑
gingivostomatitis B00.2
human B00.9
   1 — *see* Herpes, simplex
   2 — *see* Herpes, simplex
   3 — *see* Varicella
   4 — *see* Mononucleosis, Epstein-Barr (virus)
   5 — *see* Disease, cytomegalic inclusion (generalized)
   6
      encephalitis B10.01
      specified NEC B10.81
   7
      encephalitis B10.09

☑ **Additional Character Required** — Refer to the Tabular List for Character Selection   ▽ **Subterms under main terms may continue to next column or page**

Herpes, herpesvirus, herpetic — *continued*
  human — *continued*
    7 — *continued*
      specified NEC B10.82
    8 B10.89
    infection NEC B10.89
      Kaposi's sarcoma associated B10.89
    iridocyclitis (simplex) B00.51
      zoster B02.32
    iris (vesicular erythema multiforme) L51.9
    iritis (simplex) B00.51
    Kaposi's sarcoma associated B10.89
    keratitis (simplex) (dendritic) (disciform) (interstitial) B00.52
      zoster (interstitial) B02.33
    keratoconjunctivitis (simplex) B00.52
      zoster B02.33
    labialis B00.1
    lip B00.1
    meningitis (simplex) B00.3
      zoster B02.1
    ophthalmicus (zoster) NEC B02.30
      simplex B00.50
    penis A60.01
    perianal skin A60.1
    pharyngitis, pharyngotonsillitis B00.2
    rectum A60.1
    scrotum A60.02
    sepsis B00.7
    simplex B00.9
      complicated NEC B00.89
      congenital P35.2
      conjunctivitis B00.53
      external ear B00.1
      eyelid B00.59
      hepatitis B00.81
      keratitis (interstitial) B00.52
      myeltis B00.82
      specified complication NEC B00.89
      visceral B00.89
    stomatitis B00.2
    tonsurans B35.0
    visceral B00.89
    vulva A60.04
    whitlow B00.89
    zoster — *see also* condition B02.9
      auricularis B02.21
      complicated NEC B02.8
      conjunctivitis B02.31
      disseminated B02.7
      encephalitis B02.0
      eye (lid) B02.39
      geniculate ganglionitis B02.21
      keratitis (interstitial) B02.33
      meningitis B02.1
      myelitis B02.24
      neuritis, neuralgia B02.29
      ophthalmicus NEC B02.30
      oticus B02.21
      polyneuropathy B02.23
      specified complication NEC B02.8
      trigeminal neuralgia B02.22
Herpesvirus (human) — *see* Herpes
Herpetophobia F40.218
Herrick's anemia — *see* Disease, sickle-cell
Hers' disease E74.09
Herter-Gee syndrome K90.0
Herxheimer's reaction R68.89
Hesitancy
  of micturition R39.11
  urinary R39.11
Hesselbach's hernia — *see* Hernia, femoral, specified site NEC
Heterochromia (congenital) Q13.2
  cataract — *see* Cataract, complicated
  cyclitis (Fuchs) — *see* Cyclitis, Fuchs' heterochromic
  hair L67.1
  iritis — *see* Cyclitis, Fuchs' heterochromic
  retained metallic foreign body (nonmagnetic) — *see* Foreign body, intraocular, old, retained
    magnetic — *see* Foreign body, intraocular, old, retained, magnetic
  uveitis — *see* Cyclitis, Fuchs' heterochromic
Heterophoria — *see* Strabismus, heterophoria
Heterophyes, heterophyiasis (small intestine) B66.8
Heterotopia, heterotopic — *see also* Malposition, congenital
  cerebralis Q04.8

Heterotropia — *see* Strabismus
Heubner-Herter disease K90.0
Hexadactylism Q69.9
HGSIL (cytology finding) (high grade squamous intraepithelial lesion on cytologic smear) (Pap smear finding)
  anus R85.613
  cervix R87.613
    biopsy (histology) finding — *see* Neoplasia, intraepithelial, cervix, grade II or grade III
  vagina R87.623
    biopsy (histology) finding — *see* Neoplasia, intraepithelial, cervix, grade II or grade III
Hibernoma — *see* Lipoma
Hiccup, hiccough R06.6
  epidemic B33.0
  psychogenic F45.8
Hidden penis (congenital) Q55.64
  acquired N48.83
Hidradenitis (axillaris) (suppurative) L73.2
Hidradenoma (nodular) — *see also* Neoplasm, skin, benign
  clear cell — *see* Neoplasm, skin, benign
  papillary — *see* Neoplasm, skin, benign
Hidrocystoma — *see* Neoplasm, skin, benign
High
  altitude effects T70.20 ☑
    anoxia T70.29 ☑
    on
      ears T70.0 ☑
      sinuses T70.1 ☑
    polycythemia D75.1
  arch
    foot Q66.7- ☑
    palate, congenital Q38.5
  arterial tension — *see* Hypertension
  basal metabolic rate R94.8
  blood pressure — *see also* Hypertension
    borderline R03.0
    reading (incidental) (isolated) (nonspecific), without diagnosis of hypertension R03.0
  cholesterol E78.00
    with high triglycerides E78.2
  diaphragm (congenital) Q79.1
  expressed emotional level within family Z63.8
  head at term O32.4 ☑
  palate, congenital Q38.5
  risk
    infant NEC Z76.2
    sexual behavior (heterosexual) Z72.51
      bisexual Z72.53
      homosexual Z72.52
  scrotal testis, testes
    bilateral Q53.23
    unilateral Q53.13
  temperature (of unknown origin) R50.9
  thoracic rib Q76.6
  triglycerides E78.1
    with high cholesterol E78.2
Hildenbrand's disease A75.0
Hilum — *see* condition
Hip — *see* condition
Hippel's disease Q85.8
Hippophobia F40.218
Hippus H57.09
Hirschsprung's disease or megacolon Q43.1
Hirsutism, hirsuties L68.0
Hirudiniasis
  external B88.3
  internal B83.4
Hiss-Russell dysentery A03.1
Histidinemia, histidinuria E70.41
Histiocytoma — *see also* Neoplasm, skin, benign
  fibrous — *see also* Neoplasm, skin, benign
    atypical — *see* Neoplasm, connective tissue, uncertain behavior
    malignant — *see* Neoplasm, connective tissue, malignant
Histiocytosis D76.3
  acute differentiated progressive C96.0
  Langerhans' cell NEC C96.6
    multifocal X
      multisystemic (disseminated) C96.0
      unisystemic C96.5
    pulmonary, adult (adult PLCH) J84.82
    unifocal (X) C96.6
  lipid, lipoid D76.3

Histiocytosis — *continued*
  lipid, lipoid — *continued*
    essential E75.29
  malignant C96.A (*following* C96.6)
  mononuclear phagocytes NEC D76.1
    Langerhans' cells C96.6
  non-Langerhans cell D76.3
  polyostotic sclerosing D76.3
  sinus, with massive lymphadenopathy D76.3
  syndrome NEC D76.3
  X NEC C96.6
    acute (progressive) C96.0
    chronic C96.6
    multifocal C96.5
    multisystemic C96.0
    unifocal C96.6
Histoplasmosis B39.9
  with pneumonia NEC B39.2
  African B39.5
  American — *see* Histoplasmosis, capsulati
  capsulati B39.4
    disseminated B39.3
    generalized B39.3
    pulmonary B39.2
      acute B39.0
      chronic B39.1
  Darling's B39.4
  duboisii B39.5
  lung NEC B39.2
History
  family (of) — *see also* History, personal (of)
    alcohol abuse Z81.1
    allergy NEC Z84.89
    anemia Z83.2
    arthritis Z82.61
    asthma Z82.5
    blindness Z82.1
    cardiac death (sudden) Z82.41
    carrier of genetic disease Z84.81
    chromosomal anomaly Z82.79
    chronic
      disabling disease NEC Z82.8
      lower respiratory disease Z82.5
    colonic polyps Z83.71
    congenital malformations and deformations Z82.79
      polycystic kidney Z82.71
    consanguinity Z84.3
    deafness Z82.2
    diabetes mellitus Z83.3
    disability NEC Z82.8
    disease or disorder (of)
      allergic NEC Z84.89
      behavioral NEC Z81.8
      blood and blood-forming organs Z83.2
      cardiovascular NEC Z82.49
      chronic disabling NEC Z82.8
      digestive Z83.79
      ear NEC Z83.52
      elevated lipoprotein (a) (Lp(a)) Z83.430
      endocrine NEC Z83.49
      eye NEC Z83.518
        glaucoma Z83.511
      familial hypercholesterolemia Z83.42
      genitourinary NEC Z84.2
      glaucoma Z83.511
      hematological Z83.2
      immune mechanism Z83.2
      infectious NEC Z83.1
      ischemic heart Z82.49
      kidney Z84.1
      lipoprotein metabolism Z83.438
      mental NEC Z81.8
      metabolic Z83.49
      musculoskeletal NEC Z82.69
      neurological NEC Z82.0
      nutritional Z83.49
      parasitic NEC Z83.1
      psychiatric NEC Z81.8
      respiratory NEC Z83.6
      skin and subcutaneous tissue NEC Z84.0
      specified NEC Z84.89
    drug abuse NEC Z81.3
    elevated lipoprotein (a) (Lp(a)) Z83.430
    epilepsy Z82.0
    familial hypercholesterolemia Z83.42
    genetic disease carrier Z84.81
    glaucoma Z83.511
    hearing loss Z82.2
    human immunodeficiency virus (HIV) infection Z83.0

History — continued

family — see also History, personal — continued
    Huntington's chorea Z82.0
    hyperlipidemia, familial combined Z83.438
    intellectual disability Z81.0
    leukemia Z80.6
    lipidemia NEC Z83.438
    malignant neoplasm (of) NOS Z80.9
      bladder Z80.52
      breast Z80.3
      bronchus Z80.1
      digestive organ Z80.0
      gastrointestinal tract Z80.0
      genital organ Z80.49
        ovary Z80.41
        prostate Z80.42
        specified organ NEC Z80.49
        testis Z80.43
      hematopoietic NEC Z80.7
      intrathoracic organ NEC Z80.2
      kidney Z80.51
      lung Z80.1
      lymphatic NEC Z80.7
      ovary Z80.41
      prostate Z80.42
      respiratory organ NEC Z80.2
      specified site NEC Z80.8
      testis Z80.43
      trachea Z80.1
      urinary organ or tract Z80.59
        bladder Z80.52
        kidney Z80.51
    mental
      disorder NEC Z81.8
    multiple endocrine neoplasia (MEN) syndrome Z83.41
    osteoporosis Z82.62
    polycystic kidney Z82.71
    polyps (colon) Z83.71
    psychiatric disorder Z81.8
    psychoactive substance abuse NEC Z81.3
    respiratory condition NEC Z83.6
      asthma and other lower respiratory conditions Z82.5
    self-harmful behavior Z81.8
    SIDS (sudden infant death syndrome) Z84.82
    skin condition Z84.0
    specified condition NEC Z84.89
    stroke (cerebrovascular) Z82.3
    substance abuse NEC Z81.4
      alcohol Z81.1
      drug NEC Z81.3
      psychoactive NEC Z81.3
      tobacco Z81.2
    sudden
      cardiac death Z82.41
      infant death syndrome (SIDS) Z84.82
    tobacco abuse Z81.2
    violence, violent behavior Z81.8
    visual loss Z82.1

personal (of) — see also History, family (of)
    abuse
      adult Z91.419
        forced labor or sexual exploitation Z91.42
        physical and sexual Z91.410
        psychological Z91.411
      childhood Z62.819
        forced labor or sexual exploitation in childhood Z62.813
        physical Z62.810
        psychological Z62.811
        sexual Z62.810
    alcohol dependence F10.21
    allergy (to) Z88.9
      analgesic agent NEC Z88.6
      anesthetic Z88.4
      antibiotic agent NEC Z88.1
      anti-infective agent NEC Z88.3
      contrast media Z91.041
      drugs, medicaments and biological substances Z88.9
        specified NEC Z88.8
      food Z91.018
        additives Z91.02
        eggs Z91.012
        milk products Z91.011
        peanuts Z91.010
        seafood Z91.013
        specified food NEC Z91.018

History — continued

personal — see also History, family — continued
    allergy — continued
      insect Z91.038
        bee Z91.030
      latex Z91.040
      medicinal agents Z88.9
        specified NEC Z88.8
      narcotic agent NEC Z88.5
      nonmedicinal agents Z91.048
      penicillin Z88.0
      serum Z88.7
      specified NEC Z91.09
      sulfonamides Z88.2
      vaccine Z88.7
    anaphylactic shock Z87.892
    anaphylaxis Z87.892
    behavioral disorders Z86.59
    benign carcinoid tumor Z86.012
    benign neoplasm Z86.018
      brain Z86.011
      carcinoid Z86.012
      colonic polyps Z86.010
    brain injury (traumatic) Z87.820
    breast implant removal Z98.86
    calculi, renal Z87.442
    cancer — see History, personal (of), malignant neoplasm (of)
    cardiac arrest (death), successfully resuscitated Z86.74
    cerebral infarction without residual deficit Z86.73
    cervical dysplasia Z87.410
    chemotherapy for neoplastic condition Z92.21
    childhood abuse — see History, personal (of), abuse
    cleft lip (corrected) Z87.730
    cleft palate (corrected) Z87.730
    collapsed vertebra (healed) Z87.311
      due to osteoporosis Z87.310
    combat and operational stress reaction Z86.51
    congenital malformation (corrected) Z87.798
      circulatory system (corrected) Z87.74
      digestive system (corrected) NEC Z87.738
      ear (corrected) Z87.721
      eye (corrected) Z87.720
      face and neck (corrected) Z87.790
      genitourinary system (corrected) NEC Z87.718
      heart (corrected) Z87.74
      integument (corrected) Z87.76
      limb(s) (corrected) Z87.76
      musculoskeletal system (corrected) Z87.76
      neck (corrected) Z87.790
      nervous system (corrected) NEC Z87.728
      respiratory system (corrected) Z87.75
      sense organs (corrected) NEC Z87.728
      specified NEC Z87.798
    contraception Z92.0
    deployment (military) Z91.82
    diabetic foot ulcer Z86.31
    disease or disorder (of) Z87.898
      anaphylaxis Z87.892
      blood and blood-forming organs Z86.2
      circulatory system Z86.79
        specified condition NEC Z86.79
      connective tissue Z87.39
      digestive system Z87.19
        colonic polyp Z86.010
        peptic ulcer disease Z87.11
        specified condition NEC Z87.19
      ear Z86.69
      endocrine Z86.39
        diabetic foot ulcer Z86.31
        gestational diabetes Z86.32
        specified type NEC Z86.39
      eye Z86.69
      genital (track) system NEC
        female Z87.42
        male Z87.438
      hematological Z86.2
      Hodgkin Z85.71
      immune mechanism Z86.2
      infectious Z86.19
        malaria Z86.13
        Methicillin resistant Staphylococcus aureus (MRSA) Z86.14
        poliomyelitis Z86.12
        specified NEC Z86.19
        tuberculosis Z86.11
      mental NEC Z86.59
      metabolic Z86.39

History — continued

personal — see also History, family — continued
    disease or disorder — continued
      metabolic — continued
        diabetic foot ulcer Z86.31
        gestational diabetes Z86.32
        specified type NEC Z86.39
      musculoskeletal NEC Z87.39
      nervous system Z86.69
      nutritional Z86.39
      parasitic Z86.19
      respiratory system NEC Z87.09
      sense organs Z86.69
      skin Z87.2
      specified site or type NEC Z87.898
      subcutaneous tissue Z87.2
      trophoblastic Z87.59
      urinary system NEC Z87.448
    drug dependence — see Dependence, drug, by type, in remission
    drug therapy
      antineoplastic chemotherapy Z92.21
      estrogen Z92.23
      immunosupression Z92.25
      inhaled steroids Z92.240
      monoclonal drug Z92.22
      specified NEC Z92.29
      steroid Z92.241
      systemic steroids Z92.241
    dysplasia
      cervical (mild) (moderate) Z87.410
        severe (grade III) Z86.001
      prostatic Z87.430
      vaginal (mild) (moderate) Z87.411
        severe (grade III) Z86.002
      vulvar (mild) (moderate) Z87.412
        severe (grade III) Z86.002
    embolism (venous) Z86.718
      pulmonary Z86.711
    encephalitis Z86.61
    estrogen therapy Z92.23
    extracorporeal membrane oxygenation (ECMO) Z92.81
    failed conscious sedation Z92.83
    failed moderate sedation Z92.83
    fall, falling Z91.81
    forced labor or sexual exploitation Z91.42
      in childhood Z62.813
    fracture (healed)
      fatigue Z87.312
      fragility Z87.310
      osteoporosis Z87.310
      pathological NEC Z87.311
      stress Z87.312
      traumatic Z87.81
    gestational diabetes Z86.32
    hepatitis
      B Z86.19
      C Z86.19
    Hodgkin disease Z85.71
    hyperthermia, malignant Z88.4
    hypospadias (corrected) Z87.710
    hysterectomy Z90.710
    immunosupression therapy Z92.25
    in situ neoplasm
      breast Z86.000
      cervix uteri Z86.001
      digestive organs, specified NEC Z86.004
      esophagus Z86.003
      genital organs, specified NEC Z86.002
      melanoma Z86.006
      middle ear Z86.005
      oral cavity Z86.003
      respiratory system Z86.005
      skin Z86.007
      specified NEC Z86.008
      stomach Z86.003
    in utero procedure during pregnancy Z98.870
    in utero procedure while a fetus Z98.871
    infection NEC Z86.19
      central nervous system Z86.61
      latent tuberculosis Z86.15
      Methicillin resistant Staphylococcus aureus (MRSA) Z86.14
      urinary (recurrent) (tract) Z87.440
    injury NEC Z87.828
    irradiation Z92.3
    kidney stones Z87.442
    latent tuberculosis infection Z86.15

History — *continued*
  personal — *see also* History, family — *continued*
    leukemia Z85.6
    lymphoma (non-Hodgkin) Z85.72
    malignant melanoma (skin) Z85.820
    malignant neoplasm (of) Z85.9
      accessory sinuses Z85.22
      anus NEC Z85.048
        carcinoid Z85.040
      bladder Z85.51
      bone Z85.830
      brain Z85.841
      breast Z85.3
      bronchus NEC Z85.118
        carcinoid Z85.110
      carcinoid — *see* History, personal (of), malignant
        neoplasm, by site, carcinioid
      cervix Z85.41
      colon NEC Z85.038
        carcinoid Z85.030
      digestive organ Z85.00
        specified NEC Z85.09
      endocrine gland NEC Z85.858
      epididymis Z85.48
      esophagus Z85.01
      eye Z85.840
      gastrointestinal tract — *see* History, malignant
        neoplasm, digestive organ
      genital organ
        female Z85.40
          specified NEC Z85.44
        male Z85.45
          specified NEC Z85.49
      hematopoietic NEC Z85.79
      intrathoracic organ Z85.20
      kidney NEC Z85.528
        carcinoid Z85.520
      large intestine NEC Z85.038
        carcinoid Z85.030
      larynx Z85.21
      liver Z85.05
      lung NEC Z85.118
        carcinoid Z85.110
      mediastinum Z85.29
      Merkel cell Z85.821
      middle ear Z85.22
      nasal cavities Z85.22
      nervous system NEC Z85.848
      oral cavity Z85.819
        specified site NEC Z85.818
      ovary Z85.43
      pancreas Z85.07
      pelvis Z85.53
      pharynx Z85.819
        specified site NEC Z85.818
      pleura Z85.29
      prostate Z85.46
      rectosigmoid junction NEC Z85.048
        carcinoid Z85.040
      rectum NEC Z85.048
        carcinoid Z85.040
      respiratory organ Z85.20
      sinuses, accessory Z85.22
      skin NEC Z85.828
        melanoma Z85.820
        Merkel cell Z85.821
      small intestine NEC Z85.068
        carcinoid Z85.060
      soft tissue Z85.831
      specified site NEC Z85.89
      stomach NEC Z85.028
        carcinoid Z85.020
      testis Z85.47
      thymus NEC Z85.238
        carcinoid Z85.230
      thyroid Z85.850
      tongue Z85.810
      trachea Z85.12
      urinary organ or tract Z85.50
        specified NEC Z85.59
      uterus Z85.42
    maltreatment Z91.89
    medical treatment NEC Z92.89
    melanoma Z85.820
      in situ Z86.006
      malignant (skin) Z85.820
    meningitis Z86.61
    mental disorder Z86.59
    Merkel cell carcinoma (skin) Z85.821

History — *continued*
  personal — *see also* History, family — *continued*
    Methicillin resistant Staphylococcus aureus (MRSA)
      Z86.14
    military deployment Z91.82
    military war, peacekeeping and humanitarian de-
      ployment (current or past conflict) Z91.82
    myocardial infarction (old) I25.2
    neglect (in)
      adult Z91.412
      childhood Z62.812
    neoplasia
      anal intraepithelial, III [AIN III] Z86.004
      high-grade prostatic intraepithelial, III [HGPIN
        III] Z86.002
      vaginal intraepithelial, III [VAIN III] Z86.002
      vulvar intraepithelial, III [VIN III] Z86.002
    neoplasm
      benign Z86.018
        brain Z86.011
        colon polyp Z86.010
      in situ
        breast Z86.000
        cervix uteri Z86.001
        digestive organs, specified NEC Z86.004
        esophagus Z86.003
        genital organs, specified NEC Z86.002
        melanoma Z86.006
        middle ear Z86.005
        oral cavity Z86.003
        respiratory system Z86.005
        skin Z86.007
        specified NEC Z86.008
        stomach Z86.003
      malignant — *see* History of, malignant neoplasm
      uncertain behavior Z86.03
    nephrotic syndrome Z87.441
    nicotine dependence Z87.891
    noncompliance with medical treatment or regimen
        — *see* Noncompliance
    nutritional deficiency Z86.39
    obstetric complications Z87.59
      childbirth Z87.59
      pregnancy Z87.59
      pre-term labor Z87.51
      puerperium Z87.59
    osteoporosis fractures Z87.31 ☑
    parasuicide (attempt) Z91.5
    physical trauma NEC Z87.828
      self-harm or suicide attempt Z91.5
    pneumonia (recurrent) Z87.01
    poisoning NEC Z91.89
      self-harm or suicide attempt Z91.5
    poor personal hygiene Z91.89
    preterm labor Z87.51
    procedure during pregnancy Z98.870
    procedure while a fetus Z98.871
    prolonged reversible ischemic neurologic deficit
      (PRIND) Z86.73
    prostatic dysplasia Z87.430
    psychological
      abuse
        adult Z91.411
        child Z62.811
      trauma, specified NEC Z91.49
    radiation therapy Z92.3
    removal
      implant
        breast Z98.86
      renal calculi Z87.442
    respiratory condition NEC Z87.09
    retained foreign body fully removed Z87.821
    risk factors NEC Z91.89
    self-harm Z91.5
    self-poisoning attempt Z91.5
    sex reassignment Z87.890
    sleep-wake cycle problem Z72.821
    specified NEC Z87.898
    steroid therapy (systemic) Z92.241
      inhaled Z92.240
    stroke without residual deficits Z86.73
    substance abuse NEC F10-F19
    sudden cardiac arrest Z86.74
    sudden cardiac death successfully resuscitated
      Z86.74
    suicide attempt Z91.5
    surgery NEC Z98.890
      with uterine scar Z98.891
      sex reassignment Z87.890

History — *continued*
  personal — *see also* History, family — *continued*
    surgery — *continued*
      transplant — *see* Transplant
    thrombophlebitis Z86.72
    thrombosis (venous) Z86.718
      pulmonary Z86.711
    tobacco dependence Z87.891
    transient ischemic attack (TIA) without residual
      deficits Z86.73
    trauma (physical) NEC Z87.828
      psychological NEC Z91.49
      self-harm Z91.5
    traumatic brain injury Z87.820
    tuberculosis, latent infection Z86.15
    unhealthy sleep-wake cycle Z72.821
    unintended awareness under general anesthesia
      Z92.84
    urinary calculi Z87.442
    urinary (recurrent) (tract) infection(s) Z87.440
    uterine scar from previous surgery Z98.891
    vaginal dysplasia Z87.411
    venous thrombosis or embolism Z86.718
      pulmonary Z86.711
    vulvar dysplasia Z87.412
His-Werner disease A79.0
HIV — *see also* Human, immunodeficiency virus B20
  laboratory evidence (nonconclusive) R75
  nonconclusive test (in infants) R75
  positive, seropositive Z21
Hives (bold) — *see* Urticaria
Hoarseness R49.0
Hobo Z59.0
Hodgkin disease — *see* Lymphoma, Hodgkin
Hodgson's disease I71.2
  ruptured I71.1
Hoffa-Kastert disease E88.89
Hoffa's disease E88.89
Hoffmann-Bouveret syndrome I47.9
Hoffmann's syndrome E03.9 *[G73.7]*
Hole (round)
  macula H35.34- ☑
  retina (without detachment) — *see* Break, retina, round
    hole
    with detachment — *see* Detachment, retina, with
      retinal, break
Holiday relief care Z75.5
Hollenhorst's plaque — *see* Occlusion, artery, retina
Hollow foot (congenital) Q66.7- ☑
  acquired — *see* Deformity, limb, foot, specified NEC
Holoprosencephaly Q04.2
Holt-Oram syndrome Q87.2
Homelessness Z59.0
Homesickness — *see* Disorder, adjustment
Homocystinemia, homocystinuria E72.11
Homogentisate 1,2-dioxygenase deficiency E70.29
Homologous serum hepatitis (prophylactic) (therapeu-
  tic) — *see* Hepatitis, viral, type B
Honeycomb lung J98.4
  congenital Q33.0
Hooded
  clitoris Q52.6
  penis Q55.69
Hookworm (disease) (infection) (infestation) B76.9
  with anemia B76.9 *[D63.8]*
  specified NEC B76.8
Hordeolum (eyelid) (externum) (recurrent) H00.019
  internum H00.029
    left H00.026
      lower H00.025
      upper H00.024
    right H00.023
      lower H00.022
      upper H00.021
  left H00.016
    lower H00.015
    upper H00.014
  right H00.013
    lower H00.012
    upper H00.011
Horn
  cutaneous L85.8
  nail L60.2
    congenital Q84.6
Horner (-Claude Bernard) **syndrome** G90.2
  traumatic — *see* Injury, nerve, cervical sympathetic
Horseshoe kidney (congenital) Q63.1

Horton's headache or neuralgia G44.099
  intractable G44.091
  not intractable G44.099
Hospital hopper syndrome — *see* Disorder, factitious
Hospitalism in children — *see* Disorder, adjustment
Hostility R45.5
  towards child Z62.3
Hot flashes
  menopausal N95.1
Hourglass (contracture) — *see also* Contraction, hourglass
  stomach K31.89
    congenital Q40.2
    stricture K31.2
Household, housing circumstance affecting care Z59.9
  specified NEC Z59.8
Housemaid's knee — *see* Bursitis, prepatellar
Hudson (-Stähli) **line** (cornea) — *see* Pigmentation, cornea, anterior
Human
  bite (open wound) — *see also* Bite
    intact skin surface — *see* Bite, superficial
  herpesvirus — *see* Herpes
  immunodeficiency virus (HIV) disease (infection) B20
    asymptomatic status Z21
    contact Z20.6
    counseling Z71.7
    dementia B20 [F02.80]
      with behavioral disturbance B20 [F02.81]
    exposure to Z20.6
    laboratory evidence R75
    type-2 (HIV 2) as cause of disease classified elsewhere B97.35
  papillomavirus (HPV)
    DNA test positive
      high risk
        cervix R87.810
        vagina R87.811
      low risk
        cervix R87.820
        vagina R87.821
    screening for Z11.51
  T-cell lymphotropic virus
    type-1 (HTLV-I) infection B33.3
      as cause of disease classified elsewhere B97.33
      carrier Z22.6
    type-2 (HTLV-II) as cause of disease classified elsewhere B97.34
Humidifier lung or pneumonitis J67.7
Humiliation (experience) **in childhood** Z62.898
Humpback (acquired) — *see* Kyphosis
Hunchback (acquired) — *see* Kyphosis
Hunger T73.0 ☑
  air, psychogenic F45.8
Hungry bone syndrome E83.81
Hunner's ulcer — *see* Cystitis, chronic, interstitial
Hunter's
  glossitis D51.0
  syndrome E76.1
Huntington's disease or chorea G10
  with dementia G10 [F02.80]
    with behavioral disturbance G10 [F02.81]
Hunt's
  disease or syndrome (herpetic geniculate ganglionitis) B02.21
    dyssynergia cerebellaris myoclonica G11.1
  neuralgia B02.21
Hurler (-Scheie) **disease or syndrome** E76.02
Hurst's disease G36.1
Hurthle cell
  adenocarcinoma C73
  adenoma D34
  carcinoma C73
  tumor D34
Hutchinson-Boeck disease or syndrome — *see* Sarcoidosis
Hutchinson-Gilford disease or syndrome E34.8
Hutchinson's
  disease, meaning
    angioma serpiginosum L81.7
    pompholyx (cheiropompholyx) L30.1
    prurigo estivalis L56.4
    summer eruption or summer prurigo L56.4
  melanotic freckle — *see* Melanoma, in situ
    malignant melanoma in — *see* Melanoma
  teeth or incisors (congenital syphilis) A50.52
  triad (congenital syphilis) A50.53

Hyalin plaque, sclera, senile H15.89
Hyaline membrane (disease) (lung) (pulmonary) (newborn) P22.0
Hyalinosis
  cutis (et mucosae) E78.89
  focal and segmental (glomerular) — *see also* N00-N07
    with fourth character .1 N05.1
Hyalitis, hyalosis, asteroid — *see also* Deposit, crystalline
  syphilitic (late) A52.71
Hydatid
  cyst or tumor — *see* Echinococcus
  mole — *see* Hydatidiform mole
  Morgagni
    female Q50.5
    male (epididymal) Q55.4
      testicular Q55.29
Hydatidiform mole (benign) (complicating pregnancy) (delivered) (undelivered) O01.9
  classical O01.0
  complete O01.0
  incomplete O01.1
  invasive D39.2
  malignant D39.2
  partial O01.1
Hydatidosis — *see* Echinococcus
Hydradenitis (axillaris) (suppurative) L73.2
Hydradenoma — *see* Hidradenoma
Hydramnios O40.-
Hydrancephaly, hydranencephaly Q04.3
  with spina bifida — *see* Spina bifida, with hydrocephalus
Hydrargyrism NEC — *see* Poisoning, mercury
Hydrarthrosis — *see also* Effusion, joint
  gonococcal A54.42
  intermittent M12.40
    ankle M12.47- ☑
    elbow M12.42- ☑
    foot joint M12.47- ☑
    hand joint M12.44- ☑
    hip M12.45- ☑
    knee M12.46- ☑
    multiple site M12.49
    shoulder M12.41- ☑
    specified joint NEC M12.48
    wrist M12.43- ☑
  of yaws (early) (late) — *see also* subcategory M14.8- A66.6
  syphilitic (late) A52.77
    congenital A50.55 [M12.80]
Hydremia D64.89
Hydrencephalocele (congenital) — *see* Encephalocele
Hydrencephalomeningocele (congenital) — *see* Encephalocele
Hydroa R23.8
  aestivale L56.4
  vacciniforme L56.4
Hydroadenitis (axillaris) (suppurative) L73.2
Hydrocalycosis — *see* Hydronephrosis
Hydrocele (spermatic cord) (testis) (tunica vaginalis) N43.3
  canal of Nuck N94.89
  communicating N43.2
    congenital P83.5
  congenital P83.5
  encysted N43.0
  female NEC N94.89
  infected N43.1
  newborn P83.5
  round ligament N94.89
  specified NEC N43.2
  spinalis — *see* Spina bifida
  vulva N90.89
Hydrocephalus (acquired) (external) (internal) (malignant) (recurrent) G91.9
  aqueduct Sylvius stricture Q03.0
  causing disproportion O33.6 ☑
    with obstructed labor O66.3
  communicating G91.0
  congenital (external) (internal) Q03.9
    with spina bifida Q05.4
      cervical Q05.0
      dorsal Q05.1
      lumbar Q05.2
      lumbosacral Q05.2
      sacral Q05.3
      thoracic Q05.1

Hydrocephalus — *continued*
  congenital — *continued*
    with spina bifida — *continued*
      thoracolumbar Q05.1
    specified NEC Q03.8
  due to toxoplasmosis (congenital) P37.1
  foramen Magendie block (acquired) G91.1
    congenital — *see also* Hydrocephalus, congenital Q03.1
  in (due to)
    infectious disease NEC B89 [G91.4]
    neoplastic disease NEC — *see also* Neoplasm G91.4
    parasitic disease B89 [G91.4]
  newborn Q03.9
    with spina bifida — *see* Spina bifida, with hydrocephalus
  noncommunicating G91.1
  normal pressure G91.2
    secondary G91.0
  obstructive G91.1
  otitic G93.2
  post-traumatic NEC G91.3
  secondary G91.4
    post-traumatic G91.3
  specified NEC G91.8
  syphilitic, congenital A50.49
Hydrocolpos (congenital) N89.8
Hydrocystoma — *see* Neoplasm, skin, benign
Hydroencephalocele (congenital) — *see* Encephalocele
Hydroencephalomeningocele (congenital) — *see* Encephalocele
Hydrohematopneumothorax — *see* Hemothorax
Hydromeningitis — *see* Meningitis
Hydromeningocele (spinal) — *see also* Spina bifida
  cranial — *see* Encephalocele
Hydrometra N85.8
Hydrometrocolpos N89.8
Hydromicrocephaly Q02
Hydromphalos (since birth) Q45.8
Hydromyelia Q06.4
Hydromyelocele — *see* Spina bifida
Hydronephrosis (atrophic) (early) (functionless) (intermittent) (primary) (secondary) NEC N13.30
  with
    infection N13.6
    obstruction (by) (of)
      renal calculus N13.2
        with infection N13.6
      ureteral NEC N13.1
        with infection N13.6
        calculus N13.2
          with infection N13.6
      ureteropelvic junction (congenital) Q62.11
        acquired N13.0
          with infection N13.6
    ureteral stricture NEC N13.1
      with infection N13.6
  congenital Q62.0
    due to acquired occlusion of ureteropelvic junction N13.0
  specified type NEC N13.39
  tuberculous A18.11
Hydropericarditis — *see* Pericarditis
Hydropericardium — *see* Pericarditis
Hydroperitoneum R18.8
Hydrophobia — *see* Rabies
Hydrophthalmos Q15.0
Hydropneumohemothorax — *see* Hemothorax
Hydropneumopericarditis — *see* Pericarditis
Hydropneumopericardium — *see* Pericarditis
Hydropneumothorax J94.8
  traumatic — *see* Injury, intrathoracic, lung
  tuberculous NEC A15.6
Hydrops R60.9
  abdominis R18.8
  articulorum intermittens — *see* Hydrarthrosis, intermittent
  cardiac — *see* Failure, heart, congestive
  causing obstructed labor (mother) O66.3
  endolymphatic H81.0- ☑
  fetal — *see* Pregnancy, complicated by, hydrops, fetalis
  fetalis P83.2
    due to
      ABO isoimmunization P56.0
      alpha thalassemia D56.0
      hemolytic disease P56.90
        specified NEC P56.99
      isoimmunization (ABO) (Rh) P56.0

☑ **Additional Character Required** — Refer to the Tabular List for Character Selection
▽ **Subterms under main terms may continue to next column or page**

Hydrops — *continued*
  fetalis — *continued*
    due to — *continued*
      other specified nonhemolytic disease NEC P83.2
      Rh incompatibility P56.0
    during pregnancy — *see* Pregnancy, complicated
      by, hydrops, fetalis
  gallbladder K82.1
  joint — *see* Effusion, joint
  labyrinth H81.0- ✓
  newborn (idiopathic) P83.2
    due to
      ABO isoimmunization P56.0
      alpha thalassemia D56.0
      hemolytic disease P56.90
        specified NEC P56.99
      isoimmunization (ABO) (Rh) P56.0
      Rh incompatibility P56.0
  nutritional — *see* Malnutrition, severe
  pericardium — *see* Pericarditis
  pleura — *see* Hydrothorax
  spermatic cord — *see* Hydrocele
Hydropyonephrosis N13.6
Hydrorachis Q06.4
Hydrorrhea (nasal) J34.89
  pregnancy — *see* Rupture, membranes, premature
Hydrosadenitis (axillaris) (suppurative) L73.2
Hydrosalpinx (fallopian tube) (follicularis) N70.11
Hydrothorax (double) (pleura) J94.8
  chylous (nonfilarial) I89.8
    filarial — *see also* Infestation, filarial B74.9 *[J91.8]*
  traumatic — *see* Injury, intrathoracic
  tuberculous NEC (non primary) A15.6
Hydroureter — *see also* Hydronephrosis N13.4
  with infection N13.6
  congenital Q62.39
Hydroureteronephrosis — *see* Hydronephrosis
Hydrourethra N36.8
Hydroxykynureninuria E70.8
Hydroxylysinemia E72.3
Hydroxyprolinemia E72.59
Hygiene, sleep
  abuse Z72.821
  inadequate Z72.821
  poor Z72.821
Hygroma (congenital) (cystic) D18.1
  praepatellare, prepatellar — *see* Bursitis, prepatellar
Hymen — *see* condition
Hymenolepis, hymenolepiasis (diminuta) (infection)
  (infestation) (nana) B71.0
Hypalgesia R20.8
Hyperacidity (gastric) K31.89
  psychogenic F45.8
Hyperactive, hyperactivity F90.9
  basal cell, uterine cervix — *see* Dysplasia, cervix
  bowel sounds R19.12
  cervix epithelial (basal) — *see* Dysplasia, cervix
  child F90.9
    attention deficit — *see* Disorder, attention-deficit
      hyperactivity
  detrusor muscle N32.81
  gastrointestinal K31.89
    psychogenic F45.8
  nasal mucous membrane J34.3
  stomach K31.89
  thyroid (gland) — *see* Hyperthyroidism
Hyperacusis H93.23- ✓
Hyperadrenalism E27.5
Hyperadrenocorticism E24.9
  congenital E25.0
  iatrogenic E24.2
    correct substance properly administered — *see* Table of Drugs and Chemicals, by drug, adverse effect
    overdose or wrong substance given or taken — *see* Table of Drugs and Chemicals, by drug, poisoning
  not associated with Cushing's syndrome E27.0
  pituitary-dependent E24.0
Hyperaldosteronism E26.9
  familial (type I) E26.02
  glucocorticoid-remediable E26.02
  primary (due to (bilateral) adrenal hyperplasia) E26.09
  primary NEC E26.09
  secondary E26.1
  specified NEC E26.89
Hyperalgesia R20.8

Hyperalimentation R63.2
  carotene, carotin E67.1
  specified NEC E67.8
  vitamin
    A E67.0
    D E67.3
Hyperaminoaciduria
  arginine E72.21
  cystine E72.01
  lysine E72.3
  ornithine E72.4
Hyperammonemia (congenital) E72.20
Hyperazotemia — *see* Uremia
Hyperbetalipoproteinemia (familial) E78.00
  with prebetalipoproteinemia E78.2
Hyperbicarbonatemia P74.41
Hyperbilirubinemia
  constitutional E80.6
  familial conjugated E80.6
  neonatal (transient) — *see* Jaundice, newborn
Hypercalcemia, hypocalciuric, familial E83.52
Hypercalciuria, idiopathic R82.994
Hypercapnia R06.89
  newborn P84
Hypercarotenemia (dietary) E67.1
Hypercementosis K03.4
Hyperchloremia E87.8
Hyperchlorhydria K31.89
  neurotic F45.8
  psychogenic F45.8
Hypercholesterinemia — *see* Hypercholesterolemia
Hypercholesterolemia (essential) (primary) (pure) E78.00
  with hyperglyceridemia, endogenous E78.2
  dietary counseling and surveillance Z71.3
  familial E78.01
  hereditary E78.01
Hyperchylia gastrica, psychogenic F45.8
Hyperchylomicronemia (familial) (primary) E78.3
  with hyperbetalipoproteinemia E78.3
Hypercoagulable (state) D68.59
  activated protein C resistance D68.51
  antithrombin (III) deficiency D68.59
  factor V Leiden mutation D68.51
  primary NEC D68.59
  protein C deficiency D68.59
  protein S deficiency D68.59
  prothrombin gene mutation D68.52
  secondary D68.69
  specified NEC D68.69
Hypercoagulation (state) D68.59
Hypercorticalism, pituitary-dependent E24.0
Hypercorticosolism — *see* Cushing's, syndrome
Hypercorticosteronism E24.2
  correct substance properly administered — *see* Table of Drugs and Chemicals, by drug, adverse effect
  overdose or wrong substance given or taken — *see* Table of Drugs and Chemicals, by drug, poisoning
Hypercortisonism E24.2
  correct substance properly administered — *see* Table of Drugs and Chemicals, by drug, adverse effect
  overdose or wrong substance given or taken — *see* Table of Drugs and Chemicals, by drug, poisoning
Hyperekplexia Q89.8
Hyperelectrolytemia E87.8
Hyperemesis R11.10
  with nausea R11.2
  gravidarum (mild) O21.0
    with
      carbohydrate depletion O21.1
      dehydration O21.1
      electrolyte imbalance O21.1
      metabolic disturbance O21.1
    severe (with metabolic disturbance) O21.1
  projectile R11.12
  psychogenic F45.8
Hyperemia (acute) (passive) R68.89
  anal mucosa K62.89
  bladder N32.89
  cerebral I67.89
  conjunctiva H11.43- ✓
  ear internal, acute — *see* subcategory H83.0 ✓
  enteric K59.8
  eye — *see* Hyperemia, conjunctiva
  eyelid (active) (passive) — *see* Disorder, eyelid, specified type NEC
  intestine K59.8
  iris — *see* Disorder, iris, vascular
  kidney N28.89

Hyperemia — *continued*
  labyrinth — *see* subcategory H83.0 ✓
  liver (active) K76.89
  lung (passive) — *see* Edema, lung
  pulmonary (passive) — *see* Edema, lung
  renal N28.89
  retina H35.89
  stomach K31.89
Hyperesthesia (body surface) R20.3
  larynx (reflex) J38.7
    hysterical F44.89
  pharynx (reflex) J39.2
    hysterical F44.89
Hyperestrogenism (drug-induced) (iatrogenic) E28.0
Hyperexplexia Q89.8
Hyperfibrinolysis — *see* Fibrinolysis
Hyperfructosemia E74.19
Hyperfunction
  adrenal cortex, not associated with Cushing's syndrome E27.0
    medulla E27.5
      adrenomedullary E27.5
    virilism E25.9
      congenital E25.0
  ovarian E28.8
  pancreas K86.89
  parathyroid (gland) E21.3
  pituitary (gland) (anterior) E22.9
    specified NEC E22.8
  polyglandular E31.1
  testicular E29.0
Hypergammaglobulinemia D89.2
  polyclonal D89.0
  Waldenström D89.0
Hypergastrinemia E16.4
Hyperglobulinemia R77.1
Hyperglycemia, hyperglycemic (transient) R73.9
  coma — *see* Diabetes, by type, with coma
  postpancreatectomy E89.1
Hyperglyceridemia (endogenous) (essential) (familial) (hereditary) (pure) E78.1
  mixed E78.3
Hyperglycinemia (non-ketotic) E72.51
Hypergonadism
  ovarian E28.8
  testicular (primary) (infantile) E29.0
Hyperheparinemia D68.32
Hyperhidrosis, hyperidrosis R61
  focal
    primary L74.519
      axilla L74.510
      face L74.511
      palms L74.512
      soles L74.513
    secondary L74.52
  generalized R61
  localized
    primary L74.519
      axilla L74.510
      face L74.511
      palms L74.512
      soles L74.513
    secondary L74.52
  psychogenic F45.8
  secondary R61
    focal L74.52
Hyperhistidinemia E70.41
Hyperhomocysteinemia E72.11
Hyperhydroxyprolinemia E72.59
Hyperinsulinism (functional) E16.1
  with
    coma (hypoglycemic) E15
    encephalopathy E16.1 *[G94]*
  ectopic E16.1
  therapeutic misadventure (from administration of insulin) — *see* subcategory T38.3 ✓
Hyperkalemia E87.5
Hyperkeratosis — *see also* Keratosis L85.9
  cervix N88.0
  due to yaws (early) (late) (palmar or plantar) A66.3
  follicularis Q82.8
    penetrans (in cutem) L87.0
  palmoplantaris climacterica L85.1
  pinta A67.1
  senile (with pruritus) L57.0
  universalis congenita Q80.8
  vocal cord J38.3
  vulva N90.4

Index

Hydrops — Hyperkeratosis

Index

Hyperkinesia, hyperkinetic — Hypersegmentation, leukocytic, hereditary

Hyperkinesia, hyperkinetic (disease) (reaction) (syndrome) (childhood) (adolescence) — *see also* Disorder, attention-deficit hyperactivity
  heart I51.89
Hyperleucine-isoleucinemia E71.19
Hyperlipemia, hyperlipidemia E78.5
  combined E78.2
    familial E78.49
  group
    A E78.00
    B E78.1
    C E78.2
    D E78.3
  mixed E78.2
  specified NEC E78.49
Hyperlipidosis E75.6
  hereditary NEC E75.5
Hyperlipoproteinemia E78.5
  Fredrickson's type
    I E78.3
    IIa E78.00
    IIb E78.2
    III E78.2
    IV E78.1
    V E78.3
  low-density-lipoprotein-type (LDL) E78.00
  very-low-density-lipoprotein-type (VLDL) E78.1
Hyperlucent lung, unilateral J43.0
Hyperlysinemia E72.3
Hypermagnesemia E83.41
  neonatal P71.8
Hypermenorrhea N92.0
Hypermethioninemia E72.19
Hypermetropia (congenital) H52.0- ☑
Hypermobility, hypermotility
  cecum — *see* Syndrome, irritable bowel
  coccyx — *see* subcategory M53.2 ☑
  colon — *see* Syndrome, irritable bowel
    psychogenic F45.8
  ileum K58.9
  intestine — *see also* Syndrome, irritable bowel K58.9
    psychogenic F45.8
  meniscus (knee) — *see* Derangement, knee, meniscus
  scapula — *see* Instability, joint, shoulder
  stomach K31.89
    psychogenic F45.8
  syndrome M35.7
  urethra N36.41
    with intrinsic sphincter deficiency N36.43
Hypernasality R49.21
Hypernatremia E87.0
Hypernephroma C64.- ☑
Hyperopia — *see* Hypermetropia
Hyperorexia nervosa F50.2
Hyperornithinemia E72.4
Hyperosmia R43.1
Hyperosmolality E87.0
Hyperostosis (monomelic) — *see also* Disorder, bone, density and structure, specified NEC
  ankylosing (spine) M48.10
    cervical region M48.12
    cervicothoracic region M48.13
    lumbar region M48.16
    lumbosacral region M48.17
    multiple sites M48.19
    occipito-atlanto-axial region M48.11
    sacrococcygeal region M48.18
    thoracic region M48.14
    thoracolumbar region M48.15
  cortical (skull) M85.2
    infantile M89.8X- ☑
  frontal, internal of skull M85.2
  interna frontalis M85.2
  skeletal, diffuse idiopathic — *see* Hyperostosis, ankylosing
  skull M85.2
    congenital Q75.8
  vertebral, ankylosing — *see* Hyperostosis, ankylosing
Hyperovarism E28.8
Hyperoxaluria R82.992
  primary E72.53
Hyperparathyroidism E21.3
  primary E21.0
  secondary (renal) N25.81
    non-renal E21.1
  specified NEC E21.2
  tertiary E21.2
Hyperpathia R20.8

Hyperperistalsis R19.2
  psychogenic F45.8
Hyperpermeability, capillary I78.8
Hyperphagia R63.2
Hyperphenylalaninemia NEC E70.1
Hyperphoria (alternating) H50.53
Hyperphosphatemia E83.39
Hyperpiesis, hyperpiesia — *see* Hypertension
Hyperpigmentation — *see also* Pigmentation
  melanin NEC L81.4
  postinflammatory L81.0
Hyperpinealism E34.8
Hyperpituitarism E22.9
Hyperplasia, hyperplastic
  adenoids J35.2
  adrenal (capsule) (cortex) (gland) E27.8
    with
      sexual precocity (male) E25.9
        congenital E25.0
      virilism, adrenal E25.9
        congenital E25.0
      virilization (female) E25.9
        congenital E25.0
    congenital E25.0
    salt-losing E25.0
  adrenomedullary E27.5
  angiolymphoid, eosinophilia (ALHE) D18.01
  appendix (lymphoid) K38.0
  artery, fibromuscular I77.3
  bone — *see also* Hypertrophy, bone
    marrow D75.89
  breast — *see also* Hypertrophy, breast
    atypical, atypia N60.9- ☑
      ductal N60.9- ☑
      lobular N60.9- ☑
  C-cell, thyroid E07.0
  cementation (tooth) (teeth) K03.4
  cervical gland R59.0
  cervix (uteri) (basal cell) (endometrium) (polypoid) — *see also* Dysplasia, cervix
    congenital Q51.828
  clitoris, congenital Q52.6
  denture K06.2
  endocervicitis N72
  endometrium, endometrial (adenomatous) (cystic) (glandular) (glandular-cystic) (polypoid) N85.00
    with atypia N85.02
    benign N85.01
    cervix — *see* Dysplasia, cervix
    complex (without atypia) N85.01
    simple (without atypia) N85.01
  epithelial L85.9
    focal, oral, including tongue K13.29
    nipple N62
    skin L85.9
    tongue K13.29
    vaginal wall N89.3
  erythroid D75.89
  fibromuscular of artery (carotid) (renal) I77.3
  genital
    female NEC N94.89
    male N50.89
  gingiva K06.1
  glandularis cystica uteri (interstitialis) — *see also* Hyperplasia, endometrial N85.00
  gum K06.1
  hymen, congenital Q52.4
  irritative, edentulous (alveolar) K06.2
  jaw M26.09
    alveolar M26.79
    lower M26.03
      alveolar M26.72
    upper M26.01
      alveolar M26.71
  kidney (congenital) Q63.3
  labia N90.69
    epithelial N90.3
  liver (congenital) Q44.7
    nodular, focal K76.89
  lymph gland or node R59.9
  mandible, mandibular M26.03
    alveolar M26.72
    unilateral condylar M27.8
  maxilla, maxillary M26.01
    alveolar M26.71
  myometrium, myometrial N85.2
  neuroendocrine cell, of infancy J84.841

Hyperplasia, hyperplastic — *continued*
  nose
    lymphoid J34.89
    polypoid J33.9
  oral mucosa (irritative) K13.6
  organ or site, congenital NEC — *see* Anomaly, by site
  ovary N83.8
  palate, papillary (irritative) K13.6
  pancreatic islet cells E16.9
    alpha E16.8
      with excess
        gastrin E16.4
        glucagon E16.3
    beta E16.1
  parathyroid (gland) E21.0
  pharynx (lymphoid) J39.2
  prostate (adenofibromatous) (nodular) N40.0
    with lower urinary tract symptoms (LUTS) N40.1
    without lower urinary tract symtpoms (LUTS) N40.0
  renal artery I77.89
  reticulo-endothelial (cell) D75.89
  salivary gland (any) K11.1
  Schimmelbusch's — *see* Mastopathy, cystic
  suprarenal capsule (gland) E27.8
  thymus (gland) (persistent) E32.0
  thyroid (gland) — *see* Goiter
  tonsils (faucial) (infective) (lingual) (lymphoid) J35.1
    with adenoids J35.3
  unilateral condylar M27.8
  uterus, uterine N85.2
    endometrium (glandular) — *see also* Hyperplasia, endometrial N85.00
  vulva N90.69
    epithelial N90.3
Hyperpnea — *see* Hyperventilation
Hyperpotassemia E87.5
Hyperprebetalipoproteinemia (familial) E78.1
Hyperprolactinemia E22.1
Hyperprolinemia (type I) (type II) E72.59
Hyperproteinemia E88.09
Hyperprothrombinemia, causing coagulation factor deficiency D68.4
Hyperpyrexia R50.9
  heat (effects) T67.01 ☑
  malignant, due to anesthetic T88.3 ☑
  rheumatic — *see* Fever, rheumatic
  unknown origin R50.9
Hyper-reflexia R29.2
Hypersalivation K11.7
Hypersecretion
  ACTH (not associated with Cushing's syndrome) E27.0
    pituitary E24.0
  adrenaline E27.5
  adrenomedullary E27.5
  androgen (testicular) E29.0
    ovarian (drug-induced) (iatrogenic) E28.1
  calcitonin E07.0
  catecholamine E27.5
  corticoadrenal E24.9
  cortisol E24.9
  epinephrine E27.5
  estrogen E28.0
  gastric K31.89
    psychogenic F45.8
  gastrin E16.4
  glucagon E16.3
  hormone(s)
    ACTH (not associated with Cushing's syndrome) E27.0
      pituitary E24.0
    antidiuretic E22.2
    growth E22.0
    intestinal NEC E34.1
    ovarian androgen E28.1
    pituitary E22.9
    testicular E29.0
    thyroid stimulating E05.80
      with thyroid storm E05.81
  insulin — *see* Hyperinsulinism
  lacrimal glands — *see* Epiphora
  medulloadrenal E27.5
  milk O92.6
  ovarian androgens E28.1
  salivary gland (any) K11.7
  thyrocalcitonin E07.0
  upper respiratory J39.8
Hypersegmentation, leukocytic, hereditary D72.0

☑ **Additional Character Required** — Refer to the Tabular List for Character Selection   ▽ **Subterms under main terms may continue to next column or page**

Hypersensitive, hypersensitiveness, hypersensitivity
— *see also* Allergy
  carotid sinus G90.01
  colon — *see* Irritable, colon
  drug T88.7 ☑
  gastrointestinal K52.29
    immediate K52.29
    psychogenic F45.8
  labyrinth — *see* subcategory H83.2 ☑
  pain R20.8
  pneumonitis — *see* Pneumonitis, allergic
  reaction T78.40 ☑
    upper respiratory tract NEC J39.3
Hypersomnia (organic) G47.10
  due to
    alcohol
      abuse F10.182
      dependence F10.282
      use F10.982
    amphetamines
      abuse F15.182
      dependence F15.282
      use F15.982
    caffeine
      abuse F15.182
      dependence F15.282
      use F15.982
    cocaine
      abuse F14.182
      dependence F14.282
      use F14.982
    drug NEC
      abuse F19.182
      dependence F19.282
      use F19.982
    medical condition G47.14
    mental disorder F51.13
    opioid
      abuse F11.182
      dependence F11.282
      use F11.982
    psychoactive substance NEC
      abuse F19.182
      dependence F19.282
      use F19.982
    sedative, hypnotic, or anxiolytic
      abuse F13.182
      dependence F13.282
      use F13.982
    stimulant NEC
      abuse F15.182
      dependence F15.282
      use F15.982
  idiopathic G47.11
    with long sleep time G47.11
    without long sleep time G47.12
  menstrual related G47.13
  nonorganic origin F51.11
    specified NEC F51.19
  not due to a substance or known physiological condition F51.11
    specified NEC F51.19
  primary F51.11
  recurrent G47.13
  specified NEC G47.19
Hypersplenia, hypersplenism D73.1
Hyperstimulation, ovaries (associated with induced ovulation) N98.1
Hypersusceptibility — *see* Allergy
Hypertelorism (ocular) (orbital) Q75.2
Hypertension, hypertensive (accelerated) (benign) (essential) (idiopathic) (malignant) (systemic) I10
  with
    heart failure (congestive) I11.0
    heart involvement (conditions in I50.-, I51.4- I51.9 due to hypertension) — *see* Hypertension, heart
    kidney involvement — *see* Hypertension, kidney
  benign, intracranial G93.2
  borderline R03.0
  cardiorenal (disease) I13.10
    with heart failure I13.0
      with stage 1 through stage 4 chronic kidney disease I13.0
      with stage 5 or end stage renal disease I13.2
    without heart failure I13.10
      with stage 1 through stage 4 chronic kidney disease I13.10

Hypertension, hypertensive — *continued*
  cardiorenal — *continued*
    without heart failure — *continued*
      with stage 5 or end stage renal disease I13.11
  cardiovascular
    disease (arteriosclerotic) (sclerotic) — *see* Hypertension, heart
    renal (disease) — *see* Hypertension, cardiorenal
  chronic venous — *see* Hypertension, venous (chronic)
  complicating
    childbirth (labor) O16.4
      pre-existing O10.92
        with
          heart disease O10.12
            with renal disease O10.32
          pre-eclampsia O11.4
          renal disease O10.22
            with heart disease O10.32
        essential O10.02
      secondary O10.42
    pregnancy O16.- ☑
      with edema — *see also* Pre-eclampsia O14.9- ☑
      gestational (pregnancy induced) (without proteinuria) O13.- ☑
        with proteinuria O14.9- ☑
          mild pre-eclampsia O14.0- ☑
          moderate pre-eclampsia O14.0- ☑
          severe pre-eclampsia O14.1- ☑
            with hemolysis, elevated liver enzymes and low platelet count (HELLP) O14.2- ☑
      pre-existing O10.91- ☑
        with
          heart disease O10.11- ☑
            with renal disease O10.31- ☑
          pre-eclampsia — *see* category O11
          renal disease O10.21- ☑
            with heart disease O10.31- ☑
        essential O10.01- ☑
        secondary O10.41- ☑
      transient O13- ☑
    puerperium, pre-existing O16.5
      pre-existing
        with
          heart disease O10.13
            with renal disease O10.33
          pre-eclampsia O11.5
          renal disease O10.23
            with heart disease O10.33
        essential O10.03
      pregnancy-induced O13.9
      secondary O10.43
  crisis I16.9
  due to
    endocrine disorders I15.2
    pheochromocytoma I15.2
    renal disorders NEC I15.1
      arterial I15.0
    renovascular disorders I15.0
    specified disease NEC I15.8
  emergency I16.1
  encephalopathy I67.4
  gestational (without significant proteinuria) (pregnancy-induced) (transient) O13.- ☑
    with significant proteinuria — *see* Pre-eclampsia
    complicating
      delivery O13.4
      puerperium O13.5
  Goldblatt's I70.1
  heart (disease) (conditions in I51.4-I51.9 due to hypertension) I11.9
    with
      heart failure (congestive) I11.0
      kidney disease (chronic) — *see* Hypertension, cardiorenal
  intracranial (benign) G93.2
  kidney I12.9
    with
      heart disease — *see* Hypertension, cardiorenal
      stage 1 through stage 4 chronic kidney disease I12.9
      stage 5 chronic kidney disease (CKD) or end stage renal disease (ESRD) I12.0
  lesser circulation I27.0
  maternal O16- ☑
  newborn P29.2
    pulmonary (persistent) P29.30
  ocular H40.05- ☑

Hypertension, hypertensive — *continued*
  pancreatic duct — *code to* underlying condition
    with chronic pancreatitis K86.1
  portal (due to chronic liver disease) (idiopathic) K76.6
    gastropathy K31.89
    in (due to) schistosomiasis (bilharziasis) B65.9 *[K77]*
  postoperative I97.3
  psychogenic F45.8
  pulmonary I27.20
    with
      cor pulmonale (chronic) I27.29
        acute I26.09
      right heart ventricular strain/failure I27.29
        acute I26.09
      right to left shunt related to congenital heart disease I27.83
      unclear multifactorial mechanisms I27.29
    arterial (associated) (drug-induced) (toxin-induced) I27.21
    chronic thromboembolic I27.24
    due to
      hematologic disorders I27.29
      left heart disease I27.22
      lung diseases and hypoxia I27.23
      metabolic disorders I27.29
      specified systemic disorders I27.29
    group 1 (associated) (drug-induced) (toxin-induced) I27.21
    group 2 I27.22
    group 3 I27.23
    group 4 I27.24
    group 5 I27.29
    of newborn (persistent) P29.30
    primary (idiopathic) I27.0
    secondary
      arterial I27.21
      specified NEC I27.29
  renal — *see* Hypertension, kidney
  renovascular I15.0
  secondary NEC I15.9
    due to
      endocrine disorders I15.2
      pheochromocytoma I15.2
      renal disorders NEC I15.1
        arterial I15.0
      renovascular disorders I15.0
    specified NEC I15.8
  transient R03.0
    of pregnancy O13.- ☑
  urgency I16.0
  venous (chronic)
    due to
      deep vein thrombosis — *see* Syndrome, post-thrombotic
    idiopathic I87.309
      with
        inflammation I87.32- ☑
          with ulcer I87.33- ☑
        specified complication NEC I87.39- ☑
        ulcer I87.31- ☑
          with inflammation I87.33- ☑
      asymptomatic I87.30- ☑
Hypertensive urgency — *see* Hypertension
Hyperthecosis ovary E28.8
Hyperthermia (of unknown origin) — *see also* Hyperpyrexia
  malignant, due to anesthesia T88.3 ☑
  newborn P81.9
    environmental P81.0
Hyperthyroid (recurrent) — *see* Hyperthyroidism
Hyperthyroidism (latent) (pre-adult) (recurrent) E05.90
  with
    goiter (diffuse) E05.00
      with thyroid storm E05.01
      nodular (multinodular) E05.20
        with thyroid storm E05.21
        uninodular E05.10
          with thyroid storm E05.11
    storm E05.91
  due to ectopic thyroid tissue E05.30
    with thyroid storm E05.31
  neonatal, transitory P72.1
  specified NEC E05.80
    with thyroid storm E05.81
Hypertony, hypertonia, hypertonicity
  bladder N31.8
  congenital P94.1
  stomach K31.89

Hypertony, hypertonia, hypertonicity — continued
  stomach — continued
    psychogenic F45.8
  uterus, uterine (contractions) (complicating delivery) O62.4
Hypertrichosis L68.9
  congenital Q84.2
  eyelid H02.869
    left H02.866
      lower H02.865
      upper H02.864
    right H02.863
      lower H02.862
      upper H02.861
  lanuginosa Q84.2
    acquired L68.1
  localized L68.2
  specified NEC L68.8
Hypertriglyceridemia, essential E78.1
Hypertrophy, hypertrophic
  adenofibromatous, prostate — see Enlargement, enlarged, prostate
  adenoids (infective) J35.2
    with tonsils J35.3
  adrenal cortex E27.8
  alveolar process or ridge — see Anomaly, alveolar
  anal papillae K62.89
  artery I77.89
    congenital NEC Q27.8
      digestive system Q27.8
      lower limb Q27.8
      specified site NEC Q27.8
      upper limb Q27.8
  auricular — see Hypertrophy, cardiac
  Bartholin's gland N75.8
  bile duct (common) (hepatic) K83.8
  bladder (sphincter) (trigone) N32.89
  bone M89.30
    carpus M89.34- ☑
    clavicle M89.31- ☑
    femur M89.35- ☑
    fibula M89.36- ☑
    finger M89.34- ☑
    humerus M89.32- ☑
    ilium M89.359
    ischium M89.359
    metacarpus M89.34- ☑
    metatarsus M89.37- ☑
    multiple sites M89.39
    neck M89.38
    radius M89.33- ☑
    rib M89.38
    scapula M89.31- ☑
    skull M89.38
    tarsus M89.37- ☑
    tibia M89.36- ☑
    toe M89.37- ☑
    ulna M89.33- ☑
    vertebra M89.38
  brain G93.89
  breast N62
    cystic — see Mastopathy, cystic
    newborn P83.4
    pubertal, massive N62
    puerperal, postpartum — see Disorder, breast, specified type NEC
    senile (parenchymatous) N62
  cardiac (chronic) (idiopathic) I51.7
    with rheumatic fever (conditions in I00)
      active I01.8
      inactive or quiescent (with chorea) I09.89
    congenital NEC Q24.8
    fatty — see Degeneration, myocardial
    hypertensive — see Hypertension, heart
    rheumatic (with chorea) I09.89
      active or acute I01.8
        with chorea I02.0
    valve — see Endocarditis
  cartilage — see Disorder, cartilage, specified type NEC
  cecum — see Megacolon
  cervix (uteri) N88.8
    congenital Q51.828
    elongation N88.4
  clitoris (cirrhotic) N90.89
    congenital Q52.6
  colon — see also Megacolon
    congenital Q43.2

Hypertrophy, hypertrophic — continued
  conjunctiva, lymphoid H11.89
  corpora cavernosa N48.89
  cystic duct K82.8
  duodenum K31.89
  endometrium (glandular) — see also Hyperplasia, endometrial N85.00
    cervix N88.8
  epididymis N50.89
  esophageal hiatus (congenital) Q79.1
    with hernia — see Hernia, hiatal
  eyelid — see Disorder, eyelid, specified type NEC
  fat pad E65
    knee (infrapatellar) (popliteal) (prepatellar) (retropatellar) M79.4
  foot (congenital) Q74.2
  frenulum, frenum (tongue) K14.8
    lip K13.0
  gallbladder K82.8
  gastric mucosa K29.60
    with bleeding K29.61
  gland, glandular R59.9
    generalized R59.1
    localized R59.0
  gum (mucous membrane) K06.1
  heart (idiopathic) — see also Hypertrophy, cardiac
    valve — see also Endocarditis I38
  hemifacial Q67.4
  hepatic — see Hypertrophy, liver
  hiatus (esophageal) Q79.1
  hilus gland R59.0
  hymen, congenital Q52.4
  ileum K63.89
  intestine NEC K63.89
  jejunum K63.89
  kidney (compensatory) N28.81
    congenital Q63.3
  labium (majus) (minus) N90.60
  ligament — see Disorder, ligament
  lingual tonsil (infective) J35.1
    with adenoids J35.3
  lip K13.0
    congenital Q18.6
  liver R16.0
    acute K76.89
    cirrhotic — see Cirrhosis, liver
    congenital Q44.7
    fatty — see Fatty, liver
  lymph, lymphatic gland R59.9
    generalized R59.1
    localized R59.0
    tuberculous — see Tuberculosis, lymph gland
  mammary gland — see Hypertrophy, breast
  Meckel's diverticulum (congenital) Q43.0
    malignant — see Table of Neoplasms, small intestine, malignant
  median bar — see Hyperplasia, prostate
  meibomian gland — see Chalazion
  meniscus, knee, congenital Q74.1
  metatarsal head — see Hypertrophy, bone, metatarsus
  metatarsus — see Hypertrophy, bone, metatarsus
  mucous membrane
    alveolar ridge K06.2
    gum K06.1
    nose (turbinate) J34.3
  muscle M62.89
  muscular coat, artery I77.89
  myocardium — see also Hypertrophy, cardiac
    idiopathic I42.2
  myometrium N85.2
  nail L60.2
    congenital Q84.5
  nasal J34.89
    alae J34.89
    bone J34.89
    cartilage J34.89
    mucous membrane (septum) J34.3
    sinus J34.89
    turbinate J34.3
  nasopharynx, lymphoid (infectional) (tissue) (wall) J35.2
  nipple N62
  organ or site, congenital NEC — see Anomaly, by site
  ovary N83.8
  palate (hard) M27.8
    soft K13.79
  pancreas, congenital Q45.3
  parathyroid (gland) E21.0
  parotid gland K11.1

Hypertrophy, hypertrophic — continued
  penis N48.89
  pharyngeal tonsil J35.2
  pharynx J39.2
    lymphoid (infectional) (tissue) (wall) J35.2
  pituitary (anterior) (fossa) (gland) E23.6
  prepuce (congenital) N47.8
    female N90.89
  prostate — see Enlargement, enlarged, prostate
    congenital Q55.4
  pseudomuscular G71.09
  pylorus (adult) (muscle) (sphincter) K31.1
    congenital or infantile Q40.0
  rectal, rectum (sphincter) K62.89
  rhinitis (turbinate) J31.0
  salivary gland (any) K11.1
    congenital Q38.4
  scaphoid (tarsal) — see Hypertrophy, bone, tarsus
  scar L91.0
  scrotum N50.89
  seminal vesicle N50.89
  sigmoid — see Megacolon
  skin L91.9
    specified NEC L91.8
  spermatic cord N50.89
  spleen — see Splenomegaly
  spondylitis — see Spondylosis
  stomach K31.89
  sublingual gland K11.1
  submandibular gland K11.1
  suprarenal cortex (gland) E27.8
  synovial NEC M67.20
    acromioclavicular M67.21- ☑
    ankle M67.27- ☑
    elbow M67.22- ☑
    foot M67.27- ☑
    hand M67.24- ☑
    hip M67.25- ☑
    knee M67.26- ☑
    multiple sites M67.29
    specified site NEC M67.28
    wrist M67.23- ☑
  tendon — see Disorder, tendon, specified type NEC
  testis N44.8
    congenital Q55.29
  thymic, thymus (gland) (congenital) E32.0
  thyroid (gland) — see Goiter
  toe (congenital) Q74.2
    acquired — see also Deformity, toe, specified NEC
  tongue K14.8
    congenital Q38.2
    papillae (foliate) K14.3
  tonsils (faucial) (infective) (lingual) (lymphoid) J35.1
    with adenoids J35.3
  tunica vaginalis N50.89
  ureter N28.89
  urethra N36.8
  uterus N85.2
    neck (with elongation) N88.4
    puerperal O90.89
  uvula K13.79
  vagina N89.8
  vas deferens N50.89
  vein I87.8
  ventricle, ventricular (heart) — see also Hypertrophy, cardiac
    congenital Q24.8
    in tetralogy of Fallot Q21.3
  verumontanum N36.8
  vocal cord J38.3
  vulva N90.60
    stasis (nonfilarial) N90.69
Hypertropia H50.2- ☑
Hypertyrosinemia E70.21
Hyperuricemia (asymptomatic) E79.0
Hyperuricosuria R82.993
Hypervalinemia E71.19
Hyperventilation (tetany) R06.4
  hysterical F45.8
  psychogenic F45.8
  syndrome F45.8
Hypervitaminosis (dietary) NEC E67.8
  A E67.0
    administered as drug (prolonged intake) — see Table of Drugs and Chemicals, vitamins, adverse effect

Hypervitaminosis — *continued*
  A — *continued*
    overdose or wrong substance given or taken — *see* Table of Drugs and Chemicals, vitamins, poisoning
  B6 E67.2
  D E67.3
    administered as drug (prolonged intake) — *see* Table of Drugs and Chemicals, vitamins, adverse effect
    overdose or wrong substance given or taken — *see* Table of Drugs and Chemicals, vitamins, poisoning
  K E67.8
    administered as drug (prolonged intake) — *see* Table of Drugs and Chemicals, vitamins, adverse effect
    overdose or wrong substance given or taken — *see* Table of Drugs and Chemicals, vitamins, poisoning
Hypervolemia E87.70
  specified NEC E87.79
Hypesthesia R20.1
  cornea — *see* Anesthesia, cornea
Hyphema H21.0- ☑
  traumatic S05.1- ☑
Hypoacidity, gastric K31.89
  psychogenic F45.8
Hypoadrenalism, hypoadrenia E27.40
  primary E27.1
  tuberculous A18.7
Hypoadrenocorticism E27.40
  pituitary E23.0
  primary E27.1
Hypoalbuminemia E88.09
Hypoaldosteronism E27.40
Hypoalphalipoproteinemia E78.6
Hypobarism T70.29 ☑
Hypobaropathy T70.29 ☑
Hypobetalipoproteinemia (familial) E78.6
Hypocalcemia E83.51
  dietary E58
  neonatal P71.1
    due to cow's milk P71.0
  phosphate-loading (newborn) P71.1
Hypochloremia E87.8
Hypochlorhydria K31.89
  neurotic F45.8
  psychogenic F45.8
Hypochondria, hypochondriac, hypochondriasis (reaction) F45.21
  sleep F51.03
Hypochondrogenesis Q77.0
Hypochondroplasia Q77.4
Hypochromasia, blood cells D50.8
Hypocitraturia R82.991
Hypodontia — *see* Anodontia
Hypoeosinophilia D72.89
Hypoesthesia R20.1
Hypofibrinogenemia D68.8
  acquired D65
  congenital (hereditary) D68.2
Hypofunction
  adrenocortical E27.40
    drug-induced E27.3
    postprocedural E89.6
    primary E27.1
  adrenomedullary, postprocedural E89.6
  cerebral R29.818
  corticoadrenal NEC E27.40
  intestinal K59.8
  labyrinth — *see* subcategory H83.2 ☑
  ovary E28.39
  pituitary (gland) (anterior) E23.0
  testicular E29.1
    postprocedural (postsurgical) (postirradiation) (iatrogenic) E89.5
Hypogalactia O92.4
Hypogammaglobulinemia — *see also* Agammaglobulinemia D80.1
  hereditary D80.0
  nonfamilial D80.1
  transient, of infancy D80.7
Hypogenitalism (congenital) — *see* Hypogonadism
Hypoglossia Q38.3
Hypoglycemia (spontaneous) E16.2
  coma E15

Hypoglycemia — *continued*
  coma — *continued*
    diabetic — *see* Diabetes, by type, with hypoglycemia, with coma
  diabetic — *see* Diabetes, hypoglycemia
  dietary counseling and surveillance Z71.3
  drug-induced E16.0
    with coma (nondiabetic) E15
  due to insulin E16.0
    with coma (nondiabetic) E15
    therapeutic misadventure — *see* subcategory T38.3 ☑
  functional, nonhyperinsulinemic E16.1
  iatrogenic E16.0
    with coma (nondiabetic) E15
  in infant of diabetic mother P70.1
    gestational diabetes P70.0
  infantile E16.1
  leucine-induced E71.19
  neonatal (transitory) P70.4
    iatrogenic P70.3
  reactive (not drug-induced) E16.1
  transitory neonatal P70.4
Hypogonadism
  female E28.39
  hypogonadotropic E23.0
  male E29.1
  ovarian (primary) E28.39
  pituitary E23.0
  testicular (primary) E29.1
Hypohidrosis, hypoidrosis L74.4
Hypoinsulinemia, postprocedural E89.1
Hypokalemia E87.6
Hypoleukocytosis — *see* Agranulocytosis
Hypolipoproteinemia (alpha) (beta) E78.6
Hypomagnesemia E83.42
  neonatal P71.2
Hypomania, hypomanic reaction F30.8
Hypomenorrhea — *see* Oligomenorrhea
Hypometabolism R63.8
Hypomotility
  gastrointestinal (tract) K31.89
    psychogenic F45.8
  intestine K59.8
    psychogenic F45.8
  stomach K31.89
    psychogenic F45.8
Hyponasality R49.22
Hyponatremia E87.1
Hypo-osmolality E87.1
Hypo-ovarianism, hypo-ovarism E28.39
Hypoparathyroidism E20.9
  familial E20.8
  idiopathic E20.0
  neonatal, transitory P71.4
  postprocedural E89.2
  specified NEC E20.8
Hypoperfusion (in)
  newborn P96.89
Hypopharyngitis — *see* Laryngopharyngitis
Hypophoria H50.53
Hypophosphatemia, hypophosphatasia (acquired) (congenital) (renal) E83.39
  familial E83.31
Hypophyseal, hypophysis — *see also* condition
  dwarfism E23.0
  gigantism E22.0
Hypopiesis — *see* Hypotension
Hypopinealism E34.8
Hypopituitarism (juvenile) E23.0
  drug-induced E23.1
  due to
    hypophysectomy E89.3
    radiotherapy E89.3
  iatrogenic NEC E23.1
  postirradiation E89.3
  postpartum O99.285
  postprocedural E89.3
Hypoplasia, hypoplastic
  adrenal (gland), congenital Q89.1
  alimentary tract, congenital Q45.8
    upper Q40.8
  anus, anal (canal) Q42.3
    with fistula Q42.2
  aorta, aortic Q25.42
    ascending, in hypoplastic left heart syndrome Q23.4
    valve Q23.1
      in hypoplastic left heart syndrome Q23.4

Hypoplasia, hypoplastic — *continued*
  areola, congenital Q83.8
  arm (congenital) — *see* Defect, reduction, upper limb
  artery (peripheral) Q27.8
    brain (congenital) Q28.3
    coronary Q24.5
    digestive system Q27.8
    lower limb Q27.8
    pulmonary Q25.79
      functional, unilateral J43.0
    retinal (congenital) Q14.1
    specified site NEC Q27.8
    umbilical Q27.0
    upper limb Q27.8
  auditory canal Q17.8
    causing impairment of hearing Q16.9
  biliary duct or passage Q44.5
  bone NOS Q79.9
    face Q75.8
    marrow D61.9
      megakaryocytic D69.49
    skull — *see* Hypoplasia, skull
  brain Q02
    gyri Q04.3
    part of Q04.3
  breast (areola) N64.82
  bronchus Q32.4
  cardiac Q24.8
  carpus — *see* Defect, reduction, upper limb, specified type NEC
  cartilage hair Q78.8
  cecum Q42.8
  cementum K00.4
  cephalic Q02
  cerebellum Q04.3
  cervix (uteri), congenital Q51.821
  clavicle (congenital) Q74.0
  coccyx Q76.49
  colon Q42.9
    specified NEC Q42.8
  corpus callosum Q04.0
  cricoid cartilage Q31.2
  digestive organ(s) or tract NEC Q45.8
    upper (congenital) Q40.8
  ear (auricle) (lobe) Q17.2
    middle Q16.4
  enamel of teeth (neonatal) (postnatal) (prenatal) K00.4
  endocrine (gland) NEC Q89.2
  endometrium N85.8
  epididymis (congenital) Q55.4
  epiglottis Q31.2
  erythroid, congenital D61.01
  esophagus (congenital) Q39.8
  eustachian tube Q17.8
  eye Q11.2
  eyelid (congenital) Q10.3
  face Q18.8
    bone(s) Q75.8
  femur (congenital) — *see* Defect, reduction, lower limb, specified type NEC
  fibula (congenital) — *see* Defect, reduction, lower limb, specified type NEC
  finger (congenital) — *see* Defect, reduction, upper limb, specified type NEC
  focal dermal Q82.8
  foot — *see* Defect, reduction, lower limb, specified type NEC
  gallbladder Q44.0
  genitalia, genital organ(s)
    female, congenital Q52.8
      external Q52.79
      internal NEC Q52.8
    in adiposogenital dystrophy E23.6
  glottis Q31.2
  hair Q84.2
  hand (congenital) — *see* Defect, reduction, upper limb, specified type NEC
  heart Q24.8
  humerus (congenital) — *see* Defect, reduction, upper limb, specified type NEC
  intestine (small) Q41.9
    large Q42.9
      specified NEC Q42.8
  jaw M26.09
    alveolar M26.79
    lower M26.04
      alveolar M26.74
    upper M26.02

Hypoplasia, hypoplastic — continued
jaw — continued
  upper — continued
    alveolar M26.73
  kidney(s) Q60.5
    bilateral Q60.4
    unilateral Q60.3
  labium (majus) (minus), congenital Q52.79
  larynx Q31.2
  left heart syndrome Q23.4
  leg (congenital) — see Defect, reduction, lower limb
  limb Q73.8
    lower (congenital) — see Defect, reduction, lower limb
    upper (congenital) — see Defect, reduction, upper limb
  liver Q44.7
  lung (lobe) (not associated with short gestation) Q33.6
    associated with immaturity, low birth weight, prematurity, or short gestation P28.0
  mammary (areola), congenital Q83.8
  mandible, mandibular M26.04
    alveolar M26.74
    unilateral condylar M27.8
  maxillary M26.02
    alveolar M26.73
  medullary D61.9
  megakaryocytic D69.49
  metacarpus — see Defect, reduction, upper limb, specified type NEC
  metatarsus — see Defect, reduction, lower limb, specified type NEC
  muscle Q79.8
  nail(s) Q84.6
  nose, nasal Q30.1
  optic nerve H47.03- ☑
  osseous meatus (ear) Q17.8
  ovary, congenital Q50.39
  pancreas Q45.0
  parathyroid (gland) Q89.2
  parotid gland Q38.4
  patella Q74.1
  pelvis, pelvic girdle Q74.2
  penis (congenital) Q55.62
  peripheral vascular system Q27.8
    digestive system Q27.8
    lower limb Q27.8
    specified site NEC Q27.8
    upper limb Q27.8
  pituitary (gland) (congenital) Q89.2
  pulmonary (not associated with short gestation) Q33.6
    artery, functional J43.0
    associated with short gestation P28.0
  radioulnar — see Defect, reduction, upper limb, specified type NEC
  radius — see Defect, reduction, upper limb
  rectum Q42.1
    with fistula Q42.0
  respiratory system NEC Q34.8
  rib Q76.6
  right heart syndrome Q22.6
  sacrum Q76.49
  scapula Q74.0
  scrotum Q55.1
  shoulder girdle Q74.0
  skin Q82.8
  skull (bone) Q75.8
    with
      anencephaly Q00.0
      encephalocele — see Encephalocele
      hydrocephalus Q03.9
        with spina bifida — see Spina bifida, by site, with hydrocephalus
      microcephaly Q02
  spinal (cord) (ventral horn cell) Q06.1
  spine Q76.49
  sternum Q76.7
  tarsus — see Defect, reduction, lower limb, specified type NEC
  testis Q55.1
  thymic, with immunodeficiency D82.1
  thymus (gland) Q89.2
    with immunodeficiency D82.1
  thyroid (gland) E03.1
    cartilage Q31.2
  tibiofibular (congenital) — see Defect, reduction, lower limb, specified type NEC

Hypoplasia, hypoplastic — continued
toe — see Defect, reduction, lower limb, specified type NEC
tongue Q38.3
Turner's Q00.4
ulna (congenital) — see Defect, reduction, upper limb
umbilical artery Q27.0
unilateral condylar M27.8
ureter Q62.8
uterus, congenital Q51.811
vagina Q52.4
vascular NEC peripheral Q27.8
  brain Q28.3
  digestive system Q27.8
  lower limb Q27.8
  specified site NEC Q27.8
  upper limb Q27.8
vein(s) (peripheral) Q27.8
  brain Q28.3
  digestive system Q27.8
  great Q26.8
  lower limb Q27.8
  specified site NEC Q27.8
  upper limb Q27.8
vena cava (inferior) (superior) Q26.8
vertebra Q76.49
vulva, congenital Q52.79
zonule (ciliary) Q12.8
Hypoplasminogenemia E88.02
Hypopnea, obstructive sleep apnea G47.33
Hypopotassemia E87.6
Hypoproconvertinemia, congenital (hereditary) D68.2
Hypoproteinemia E77.8
Hypoprothrombinemia (congenital) (hereditary) (idiopathic) D68.2
  acquired D68.4
  newborn, transient P61.6
Hypoptyalism K11.7
Hypopyon (eye) (anterior chamber) — see Iridocyclitis, acute, hypopyon
Hypopyrexia R68.0
Hyporeflexia R29.2
Hyposecretion
  ACTH E23.0
  antidiuretic hormone E23.2
  ovary E28.39
  salivary gland (any) K11.7
  vasopressin E23.2
Hyposegmentation, leukocytic, hereditary D72.0
Hyposiderinemia D50.9
Hypospadias Q54.9
  balanic Q54.0
  coronal Q54.0
  glandular Q54.0
  penile Q54.1
  penoscrotal Q54.2
  perineal Q54.3
  specified NEC Q54.8
Hypospermatogenesis — see Oligospermia
Hyposplenism D73.0
Hypostasis pulmonary, passive — see Edema, lung
Hypostatic — see condition
Hyposthenuria N28.89
Hypotension (arterial) (constitutional) I95.9
  chronic I95.89
  due to (of) hemodialysis I95.3
  drug-induced I95.2
  iatrogenic I95.89
  idiopathic (permanent) I95.0
  intracranial, following ventricular shunting (ventriculostomy) G97.2
  intra-dialytic I95.3
  maternal, syndrome (following labor and delivery) O26.5- ☑
  neurogenic, orthostatic G90.3
  orthostatic (chronic) I95.1
    due to drugs I95.2
    neurogenic G90.3
  postoperative I95.81
  postural I95.1
  specified NEC I95.89
Hypothermia (accidental) T68 ☑
  due to anesthesia, anesthetic T88.51 ☑
  low environmental temperature T68 ☑
  neonatal P80.9
    environmental (mild) NEC P80.8
    mild P80.8
    severe (chronic) (cold injury syndrome) P80.0

Hypothermia — continued
  neonatal — continued
    specified NEC P80.8
  not associated with low environmental temperature R68.0
Hypothyroidism (acquired) E03.9
  autoimmune — see Thyroiditis, autoimmune
  congenital (without goiter) E03.1
    with goiter (diffuse) E03.0
  due to
    exogenous substance NEC E03.2
    iodine-deficiency, acquired E01.8
      subclinical E02
    irradiation therapy E89.0
    medicament NEC E03.2
    P-aminosalicylic acid (PAS) E03.2
    phenylbutazone E03.2
    resorcinol E03.2
    sulfonamide E03.2
    surgery E89.0
    thiourea group drugs E03.2
  iatrogenic NEC E03.2
  iodine-deficiency (acquired) E01.8
    congenital — see Syndrome, iodine- deficiency, congenital
    subclinical E02
  neonatal, transitory P72.2
  postinfectious E03.3
  postirradiation E89.0
  postprocedural E89.0
  postsurgical E89.0
  specified NEC E03.8
  subclinical, iodine-deficiency related E02
Hypotonia, hypotonicity, hypotony
  bladder N31.2
  congenital (benign) P94.2
  eye — see Disorder, globe, hypotony
Hypotrichosis — see Alopecia
Hypotropia H50.2- ☑
Hypoventilation R06.89
  congenital central alveolar G47.35
  sleep related
    idiopathic nonobstructive alveolar G47.34
    in conditions classified elsewhere G47.36
Hypovitaminosis — see Deficiency, vitamin
Hypovolemia E86.1
  surgical shock T81.19 ☑
  traumatic (shock) T79.4 ☑
Hypoxemia R09.02
  newborn P84
  sleep related, in conditions classified elsewhere G47.36
Hypoxia — see also Anoxia R09.02
  cerebral, during a procedure NEC G97.81
    postprocedural NEC G97.82
  intrauterine P84
  myocardial — see Insufficiency, coronary
  newborn P84
  sleep-related G47.34
Hypsarrhythmia — see Epilepsy, generalized, specified NEC
Hysteralgia, pregnant uterus O26.89- ☑
Hysteria, hysterical (conversion) (dissociative state) F44.9
  anxiety F41.8
  convulsions F44.5
  psychosis, acute F44.9
Hysteroepilepsy F44.5

I

IBDU (colonic inflammatory bowel dissease unclassified) K52.3
Ichthyoparasitism due to Vandellia cirrhosa B88.8
Ichthyosis (congenital) Q80.9
  acquired L85.0
  fetalis Q80.4
  hystrix Q80.8
  lamellar Q80.2
  lingual K13.29
  palmaris and plantaris Q82.8
  simplex Q80.0
  vera Q80.8
  vulgaris Q80.0
  X-linked Q80.1
Ichthyotoxism — see Poisoning, fish
  bacterial — see Intoxication, foodborne
Icteroanemia, hemolytic (acquired) D59.9
  congenital — see Spherocytosis

Icterus — *see also* Jaundice
  conjunctiva R17
  gravis, newborn P55.0
  hematogenous (acquired) D59.9
  hemolytic (acquired) D59.9
    congenital — *see* Spherocytosis
  hemorrhagic (acute) (leptospiral) (spirochetal) A27.0
    newborn P53
  infectious B15.9
    with hepatic coma B15.0
    leptospiral A27.0
    spirochetal A27.0
  neonatorum — *see* Jaundice, newborn
  newborn P59.9
  spirochetal A27.0
Ictus solaris, solis T67.01 ☑
Id reaction (due to bacteria) L30.2
Ideation
  homicidal R45.850
  suicidal R45.851
Identity disorder (child) F64.9
  gender role F64.2
  psychosexual F64.2
Idioglossia F80.0
Idiopathic — *see* condition
Idiot, idiocy (congenital) F73
  amaurotic (Bielschowsky(-Jansky)) (family) (infantile
    (late)) (juvenile (late)) (Vogt-Spielmeyer) E75.4
  microcephalic Q02
IgE asthma J45.909
IIAC (idiopathic infantile arterial calcification) Q28.8
Ileitis (chronic) (noninfectious) — *see also* Enteritis K52.9
  backwash — *see* Pancolitis, ulcerative (chronic)
  infectious A09
  regional (ulcerative) — *see* Enteritis, regional, small
    intestine
  segmental — *see* Enteritis, regional
  terminal (ulcerative) — *see* Enteritis, regional, small
    intestine
Ileocolitis — *see also* Enteritis K52.9
  infectious A09
  regional — *see* Enteritis, regional
  ulcerative K51.0- ☑
Ileostomy
  attention to Z43.2
  malfunctioning K94.13
  status Z93.2
    with complication — *see* Complications, enterosto-
      my
Ileotyphus — *see* Typhoid
Ileum — *see* condition
Ileus (bowel) (colon) (inhibitory) (intestine) K56.7
  adynamic K56.0
  due to gallstone (in intestine) K56.3
  duodenal (chronic) K31.5
  gallstone K56.3
  mechanical NEC — *see also* Obstruction, intestine,
    specified NEC K56.699
  meconium P76.0
    in cystic fibrosis E84.11
    meaning meconium plug (without cystic fibrosis)
      P76.0
  myxedema K59.8
  neurogenic K56.0
    Hirschsprung's disease or megacolon Q43.1
  newborn
    due to meconium P76.0
      in cystic fibrosis E84.11
      meaning meconium plug (without cystic fibrosis)
        P76.0
    transitory P76.1
  obstructive — *see also* Obstruction, intestine, specified
    NEC K56.699
  paralytic K56.0
  postoperative K91.89
Iliac — *see* condition
Iliotibial band syndrome M76.3- ☑
Illiteracy Z55.0
Illness — *see also* Disease R69
  manic-depressive — *see* Disorder, bipolar
Imbalance R26.89
  autonomic G90.8
  constituents of food intake E63.1
  electrolyte E87.8
    with
      abortion — *see* Abortion by type, complicated
        by, electrolyte imbalance
      molar pregnancy O08.5

Imbalance — *continued*
  electrolyte — *continued*
    due to hyperemesis gravidarum O21.1
    following ectopic or molar pregnancy O08.5
    neonatal, transitory NEC P74.49
      potassium
        hyperkalemia P74.31
        hypokalemia P74.32
      sodium
        hypernatremia P74.21
        hyponatremia P74.22
  endocrine E34.9
  eye muscle NOS H50.9
  hormone E34.9
  hysterical F44.4
  labyrinth — *see* subcategory H83.2 ☑
  posture R29.3
  protein-energy — *see* Malnutrition
  sympathetic G90.8
Imbecile, imbecility (I.Q. 35-49) F71
Imbedding, intrauterine device T83.39 ☑
Imbibition, cholesterol (gallbladder) K82.4
Imbrication, teeth,, fully erupted M26.30
Imerslund (-Gräsbeck) **syndrome** D51.1
Immature — *see also* Immaturity
  birth (less than 37 completed weeks) — *see* Preterm,
    newborn
    extremely (less than 28 completed weeks) — *see*
      Immaturity, extreme
  personality F60.89
Immaturity (less than 37 completed weeks) — *see also*
    Preterm, newborn
  extreme of newborn (less than 28 completed weeks of
    gestation) (less than 196 completed days of
    gestation) (unspecified weeks of gestation)
    P07.20
    gestational age
      23 completed weeks (23 weeks, 0 days through
        23 weeks, 6 days) P07.22
      24 completed weeks (24 weeks, 0 days through
        24 weeks, 6 days) P07.23
      25 completed weeks (25 weeks, 0 days through
        25 weeks, 6 days) P07.24
      26 completed weeks (26 weeks, 0 days through
        26 weeks, 6 days) P07.25
      27 completed weeks (27 weeks, 0 days through
        27 weeks, 6 days) P07.26
      less than 23 completed weeks P07.21
  fetus or infant light-for-dates — *see* Light-for-dates
  lung, newborn P28.0
  organ or site NEC — *see* Hypoplasia
  pulmonary, newborn P28.0
  reaction F60.89
  sexual (female) (male), after puberty E30.0
Immersion T75.1 ☑
  foot T69.02- ☑
  hand T69.01- ☑
Immobile, immobility
  complete, due to severe physical disability or frailty
    R53.2
  intestine K59.8
  syndrome (paraplegic) M62.3
Immune reconstitution (inflammatory) syndrome [IRIS]
    D89.3
Immunization — *see also* Vaccination
  ABO — *see* Incompatibility, ABO
    in newborn P55.1
  appropriate for age
    child (over 28 days old) Z00.129
      with abnormal findings Z00.121
  complication — *see* Complications, vaccination
  encounter for Z23
  not done (not carried out) Z28.9
    because (of)
      acute illness of patient Z28.01
      allergy to vaccine (or component) Z28.04
      caregiver refusal Z28.82
      chronic illness of patient Z28.02
      contraindication NEC Z28.09
      delay in delivery of vaccine Z28.83
      group pressure Z28.1
      guardian refusal Z28.82
      immune compromised state of patient Z28.03
      lack of availability of vaccine Z28.83
      manufacturer delay of vaccine Z28.83
      parent refusal Z28.82
      patient had disease being vaccinated against
        Z28.81

Immunization — *continued*
  not done — *continued*
    because — *continued*
      patient refusal Z28.21
      patient's belief Z28.1
      religious beliefs of patient Z28.1
      specified reason NEC Z28.89
        of patient Z28.29
      unavailability of vaccine Z28.83
      unspecified patient reason Z28.20
    Rh factor
      affecting management of pregnancy NEC O36.09- ☑
        anti-D antibody O36.01- ☑
      from transfusion — *see* Complication(s), transfusion,
        incompatibility reaction, Rh (factor)
Immunocytoma C83.0-
Immunodeficiency D84.9
  with
    adenosine-deaminase deficiency — *see also* Defi-
      ciency, adenosine deaminase D81.30
    antibody defects D80.9
      specified type NEC D80.8
    hyperimmunoglobulinemia D80.6
    increased immunoglobulin M (IgM) D80.5
    major defect D82.9
      specified type NEC D82.8
    partial albinism D82.8
    short-limbed stature D82.2
    thrombocytopenia and eczema D82.0
  antibody with
    hyperimmunoglobulinemia D80.6
    near-normal immunoglobulins D80.6
  autosomal recessive, Swiss type D80.0
  combined D81.9
    biotin-dependent carboxylase D81.819
      biotinidase D81.810
      holocarboxylase synthetase D81.818
      specified type NEC D81.818
    severe (SCID) D81.9
      with
        low or normal B-cell numbers D81.2
        low T- and B-cell numbers D81.1
        reticular dysgenesis D81.0
      specified type NEC D81.89
  common variable D83.9
    with
      abnormalities of B-cell numbers and function
        D83.0
      autoantibodies to B- or T-cells D83.2
      immunoregulatory T-cell disorders D83.1
    specified type NEC D83.8
  following hereditary defective response to Epstein-Barr
    virus (EBV) D82.3
  selective, immunoglobulin
    A (IgA) D80.2
    G (IgG) (subclasses) D80.3
    M (IgM) D80.4
  severe combined (SCID) D81.9
    due to adenosine deaminase deficiency D81.31
  specified type NEC D84.8
  X-linked, with increased IgM D80.5
Immunotherapy (encounter for)
  antineoplastic Z51.12
Impaction, impacted
  bowel, colon, rectum — *see also* Impaction, fecal
    K56.49
    by gallstone K56.3
  calculus — *see* Calculus
  cerumen (ear) (external) H61.2- ☑
  cuspid — *see* Impaction, tooth
  dental (same or adjacent tooth) K01.1
  fecal, feces K56.41
  fracture — *see* Fracture, by site
  gallbladder — *see* Calculus, gallbladder
  gallstone(s) — *see* Calculus, gallbladder
    bile duct (common) (hepatic) — *see* Calculus, bile
      duct
    cystic duct — *see* Calculus, gallbladder
    in intestine, with obstruction (any part) K56.3
  intestine (calculous) NEC — *see also* Impaction, fecal
    K56.49
    gallstone, with ileus K56.3
  intrauterine device (IUD) T83.39 ☑
  molar — *see* Impaction, tooth
  shoulder, causing obstructed labor O66.0
  tooth, teeth K01.1
  turbinate J34.89

Index

Impaired, impairment —Inappropriate

Impaired, impairment (function)
auditory discrimination — see Abnormal, auditory perception
cognitive, mild, so stated G31.84
dual sensory Z73.82
fasting glucose R73.01
glucose tolerance (oral) R73.02
hearing — see Deafness
heart — see Disease, heart
kidney N28.9
  disorder resulting from N25.9
    specified NEC N25.89
liver K72.90
  with coma K72.91
mastication K08.89
mild cognitive, so stated G31.84
mobility
  ear ossicles — see Ankylosis, ear ossicles
  requiring care provider Z74.09
myocardium, myocardial — see Insufficiency, myocardial
rectal sphincter R19.8
renal (acute) (chronic) N28.9
  disorder resulting from N25.9
    specified NEC N25.89
vision NEC H54.7
  both eyes H54.3
Impediment, speech R47.9
psychogenic (childhood) F98.8
slurring R47.81
specified NEC R47.89
Impending
coronary syndrome I20.0
delirium tremens F10.239
myocardial infarction I20.0
Imperception auditory (acquired) — see also Deafness
congenital H93.25
Imperfect
aeration, lung (newborn) NEC — see Atelectasis
closure (congenital)
  alimentary tract NEC Q45.8
    lower Q43.8
    upper Q40.8
  atrioventricular ostium Q21.2
  atrium (secundum) Q21.1
  branchial cleft NOS Q18.2
    cyst Q18.0
    fistula Q18.0
    sinus Q18.0
  choroid Q14.3
  cricoid cartilage Q31.8
  cusps, heart valve NEC Q24.8
    pulmonary Q22.3
  ductus
    arteriosus Q25.0
    Botalli Q25.0
  ear drum (causing impairment of hearing) Q16.4
  esophagus with communication to bronchus or trachea Q39.1
  eyelid Q10.3
  foramen
    botalli Q21.1
    ovale Q21.1
  genitalia, genital organ(s) or system
    female Q52.8
      external Q52.79
      internal NEC Q52.8
    male Q55.8
  glottis Q31.8
  interatrial ostium or septum Q21.1
  interauricular ostium or septum Q21.1
  interventricular ostium or septum Q21.0
  larynx Q31.8
  lip — see Cleft, lip
  nasal septum Q30.3
  nose Q30.2
  omphalomesenteric duct Q43.0
  optic nerve entry Q14.2
  organ or site not listed — see Anomaly, by site
  ostium
    interatrial Q21.1
    interauricular Q21.1
    interventricular Q21.0
  palate — see Cleft, palate
  preauricular sinus Q18.1
  retina Q14.1
  roof of orbit Q75.8
  sclera Q13.5

Imperfect — continued
closure — continued
  septum
    aorticopulmonary Q21.4
    atrial (secundum) Q21.1
    between aorta and pulmonary artery Q21.4
    heart Q21.9
    interatrial (secundum) Q21.1
    interauricular (secundum) Q21.1
    interventricular Q21.0
      in tetralogy of Fallot Q21.3
    nasal Q30.3
    ventricular Q21.0
      with pulmonary stenosis or atresia, dextraposition of aorta, and hypertrophy of right ventricle Q21.3
      in tetralogy of Fallot Q21.3
  skull Q75.0
    with
      anencephaly Q00.0
      encephalocele — see Encephalocele
      hydrocephalus Q03.9
        with spina bifida — see Spina bifida, by site, with hydrocephalus
      microcephaly Q02
  spine (with meningocele) — see Spina bifida
  trachea Q32.1
  tympanic membrane (causing impairment of hearing) Q16.4
  uterus Q51.818
  vitelline duct Q43.0
erection — see Dysfunction, sexual, male, erectile
fusion — see Imperfect, closure
inflation, lung (newborn) — see Atelectasis
posture R29.3
rotation, intestine Q43.3
septum, ventricular Q21.0
Imperfectly descended testis — see Cryptorchid
Imperforate (congenital) — see also Atresia
anus Q42.3
  with fistula Q42.2
cervix (uteri) Q51.828
esophagus Q39.0
  with tracheoesophageal fistula Q39.1
hymen Q52.3
jejunum Q41.1
pharynx Q38.8
rectum Q42.1
  with fistula Q42.0
urethra Q64.39
vagina Q52.4
Impervious (congenital) — see also Atresia
anus Q42.3
  with fistula Q42.2
bile duct Q44.2
esophagus Q39.0
  with tracheoesophageal fistula Q39.1
intestine (small) Q41.9
  large Q42.9
    specified NEC Q42.8
rectum Q42.1
  with fistula Q42.0
ureter — see Atresia, ureter
urethra Q64.39
Impetiginization of dermatoses L01.1
Impetigo (any organism) (any site) (circinate) (contagiosa) (simplex) (vulgaris) L01.00
Bockhart's L01.02
bullous, bullosa L01.03
external ear L01.00 [H62.40]
follicularis L01.02
furfuracea L30.5
herpetiformis L40.1
  nonobstetrical L40.1
neonatorum L01.03
nonbullous L01.01
specified type NEC L01.09
ulcerative L01.09
Impingement (on teeth)
joint — see Disorder, joint, specified type NEC
soft tissue
  anterior M26.81
  posterior M26.82
Implant, endometrial N80.9
Implantation
anomalous — see Anomaly, by site
  ureter Q62.63

Implantation — continued
cyst
  external area or site (skin) NEC L72.0
  iris — see Cyst, iris, implantation
  vagina N89.8
  vulva N90.7
dermoid (cyst) — see Implantation, cyst
Impotence (sexual) N52.9
counseling Z70.1
organic origin — see also Dysfunction, sexual, male, erectile N52.9
psychogenic F52.21
Impression, basilar Q75.8
Imprisonment, anxiety concerning Z65.1
Improper care (child) (newborn) — see Maltreatment
Improperly tied umbilical cord (causing hemorrhage) P51.8
Impulsiveness (impulsive) R45.87
Inability to swallow — see Aphagia
Inaccessible, inaccessibility
health care NEC Z75.3
  due to
    waiting period Z75.2
      for admission to facility elsewhere Z75.1
  other helping agencies Z75.4
Inactive — see condition
Inadequate, inadequacy
aesthetics of dental restoration K08.56
biologic, constitutional, functional, or social F60.7
development
  child R62.50
  genitalia
    after puberty NEC E30.0
    congenital
      female Q52.8
        external Q52.79
        internal Q52.8
      male Q55.8
  lungs Q33.6
    associated with short gestation P28.0
  organ or site not listed — see Anomaly, by site
diet (causing nutritional deficiency) E63.9
eating habits Z72.4
environment, household Z59.1
family support Z63.8
food (supply) NEC Z59.4
  hunger effects T73.0 ☑
functional F60.7
household care, due to
  family member
    handicapped or ill Z74.2
    on vacation Z75.5
    temporarily away from home Z74.2
  technical defects in home Z59.1
  temporary absence from home of person rendering care Z74.2
housing (heating) (space) Z59.1
income (financial) Z59.6
intrafamilial communication Z63.8
material resources Z59.9
mental — see Disability, intellectual
parental supervision or control of child Z62.0
personality F60.7
pulmonary
  function R06.89
    newborn P28.5
  ventilation, newborn P28.5
sample of cytologic smear
  anus R85.615
  cervix R87.615
  vagina R87.625
social F60.7
  insurance Z59.7
  skills NEC Z73.4
supervision of child by parent Z62.0
teaching affecting education Z55.8
welfare support Z59.7
Inanition R64
with edema — see Malnutrition, severe
due to
  deprivation of food T73.0 ☑
  malnutrition — see Malnutrition
fever R50.9
Inappropriate
change in quantitative human chorionic gonadotropin (hCG) in early pregnancy O02.81
diet or eating habits Z72.4

☑ Additional Character Required — Refer to the Tabular List for Character Selection   ▽ Subterms under main terms may continue to next column or page

Inappropriate — *continued*
 level of quantitative human chorionic gonadotropin (hCG) for gestational age in early pregnancy O02.81
 secretion
  antidiuretic hormone (ADH) (excessive) E22.2
   deficiency E23.2
  pituitary (posterior) E22.2
Inattention at or after birth — *see* Neglect
Incarceration, incarcerated
 enterocele K46.0
  gangrenous K46.1
 epiplocele K46.0
  gangrenous K46.1
 exomphalos K42.0
  gangrenous K42.1
 hernia — *see also* Hernia, by site, with obstruction
  with gangrene — *see* Hernia, by site, with gangrene
 iris, in wound — *see* Injury, eye, laceration, with prolapse
 lens, in wound — *see* Injury, eye, laceration, with prolapse
 omphalocele K42.0
 prison, anxiety concerning Z65.1
 rupture — *see* Hernia, by site
 sarcoepiplocele K46.0
  gangrenous K46.1
 sarcoepiplomphalocele K42.0
  with gangrene K42.1
 uterus N85.8
  gravid O34.51- ☑
   causing obstructed labor O65.5
Incised wound
 external — *see* Laceration
 internal organs — *see* Injury, by site
Incision, incisional
 hernia K43.2
  with
   gangrene (and obstruction) K43.1
   obstruction K43.0
  surgical, complication — *see* Complications, surgical procedure
  traumatic
   external — *see* Laceration
   internal organs — *see* Injury, by site
Inclusion
 azurophilic leukocytic D72.0
 blennorrhea (neonatal) (newborn) P39.1
 gallbladder in liver (congenital) Q44.1
Incompatibility
 ABO
  affecting management of pregnancy O36.11- ☑
   anti-A sensitization O36.11- ☑
   anti-B sensitization O36.19- ☑
   specified NEC O36.19- ☑
  infusion or transfusion reaction — *see* Complication(s), transfusion, incompatibility reaction, ABO
  newborn P55.1
 blood (group) (Duffy) (K) (Kell) (Kidd) (Lewis) (M) (S) NEC
  affecting management of pregnancy O36.11- ☑
   anti-A sensitization O36.11- ☑
   anti-B sensitization O36.19- ☑
  infusion or transfusion reaction T80.89 ☑
  newborn P55.8
 divorce or estrangement Z63.5
 Rh (blood group) (factor) Z31.82
  affecting management of pregnancy NEC O36.09- ☑
   anti-D antibody O36.01- ☑
  infusion or transfusion reaction — *see* Complication(s), transfusion, incompatibility reaction, Rh (factor)
  newborn P55.0
 rhesus — *see* Incompatibility, Rh
Incompetency, incompetent, incompetence
 annular
  aortic (valve) — *see* Insufficiency, aortic
  mitral (valve) I34.0
  pulmonary valve (heart) I37.1
 aortic (valve) — *see* Insufficiency, aortic
 cardiac valve — *see* Endocarditis
 cervix, cervical (os) N88.3
  in pregnancy O34.3- ☑
 chronotropic I45.89
  with
   autonomic dysfunction G90.8
   ischemic heart disease I25.89

Incompetency, incompetent, incompetence — *continued*
 chronotropic — *continued*
  with — *continued*
   left ventricular dysfunction I51.89
   sinus node dysfunction I49.8
 esophagogastric (junction) (sphincter) K22.0
 mitral (valve) — *see* Insufficiency, mitral
 pelvic fundus N81.89
 pubocervical tissue N81.82
 pulmonary valve (heart) I37.1
  congenital Q22.3
 rectovaginal tissue N81.83
 tricuspid (annular) (valve) — *see* Insufficiency, tricuspid
 valvular — *see* Endocarditis
  congenital Q24.8
 vein, venous (saphenous) (varicose) — *see* Varix, leg
Incomplete — *see also* condition
 bladder, emptying R33.9
 defecation R15.0
 expansion lungs (newborn) NEC — *see* Atelectasis
 rotation, intestine Q43.3
Inconclusive
 diagnostic imaging due to excess body fat of patient R93.9
 findings on diagnostic imaging of breast NEC R92.8
 mammogram (due to dense breasts) R92.2
Incontinence R32
 anal sphincter R15.9
 coital N39.491
 feces R15.9
  nonorganic origin F98.1
 insensible (urinary) N39.42
 overflow N39.490
 postural (urinary) N39.492
 psychogenic F45.8
 rectal R15.9
 reflex N39.498
 stress (female) (male) N39.3
  and urge N39.46
 urethral sphincter R32
 urge N39.41
  and stress (female) (male) N39.46
 urine (urinary) R32
  continuous N39.45
  due to cognitive impairment, or severe physical disability or immobility R39.81
  functional R39.81
  insensible N39.42
  mixed (stress and urge) N39.46
  nocturnal N39.44
  nonorganic origin F98.0
  overflow N39.490
  post dribbling N39.43
  postural N39.492
  reflex N39.498
  specified NEC N39.498
  stress (female) (male) N39.3
   and urge N39.46
  total N39.498
  unaware N39.42
  urge N39.41
   and stress (female) (male) N39.46
Incontinentia pigmenti Q82.3
Incoordinate, incoordination
 esophageal-pharyngeal (newborn) — *see* Dysphagia
 muscular R27.8
 uterus (action) (contractions) (complicating delivery) O62.4
Increase, increased
 abnormal, in development R63.8
 androgens (ovarian) E28.1
 anticoagulants (antithrombin) (anti-VIIIa) (anti-IXa) (anti-Xa) (anti-XIa) — *see* Circulating anticoagulants
 cold sense R20.8
 estrogen E28.0
 function
  adrenal
   cortex — *see* Cushing's, syndrome
   medulla E27.5
  pituitary (gland) (anterior) (lobe) E22.9
   posterior E22.2
 heat sense R20.8
 intracranial pressure (benign) G93.2
 permeability, capillaries I78.8
 pressure, intracranial G93.2

Increase, increased — *continued*
 secretion
  gastrin E16.4
  glucagon E16.3
  pancreas, endocrine E16.9
   growth hormone-releasing hormone E16.8
   pancreatic polypeptide E16.8
   somatostatin E16.8
   vasoactive-intestinal polypeptide E16.8
  sphericity, lens Q12.4
  splenic activity D73.1
  venous pressure I87.8
   portal K76.6
Increta placenta O43.22- ☑
Incrustation, cornea, foreign body (lead)(zinc) — *see* Foreign body, cornea
Incyclophoria H50.54
Incyclotropia — *see* Cyclotropia
Indeterminate sex Q56.4
India rubber skin Q82.8
Indigestion (acid) (bilious) (functional) K30
 catarrhal K31.89
 due to decomposed food NOS A05.9
 nervous F45.8
 psychogenic F45.8
Indirect — *see* condition
Induratio penis plastica N48.6
Induration, indurated
 brain G93.89
 breast (fibrous) N64.51
  puerperal, postpartum O92.29
 broad ligament N83.8
 chancre
  anus A51.1
  congenital A50.07
  extragenital NEC A51.2
 corpora cavernosa (penis) (plastic) N48.6
 liver (chronic) K76.89
 lung (black) (chronic) (fibroid) — *see also* Fibrosis, lung J84.10
  essential brown J84.03
 penile (plastic) N48.6
 phlebitic — *see* Phlebitis
 skin R23.4
Inebriety (without dependence) — *see* Alcohol, intoxication
Inefficiency, kidney N28.9
Inelasticity, skin R23.4
Inequality, leg (length) (acquired) — *see also* Deformity, limb, unequal length
 congenital — *see* Defect, reduction, lower limb
 lower leg — *see* Deformity, limb, unequal length
Inertia
 bladder (neurogenic) N31.2
 stomach K31.89
  psychogenic F45.8
 uterus, uterine during labor O62.2
  during latent phase of labor O62.0
  primary O62.0
  secondary O62.1
 vesical (neurogenic) N31.2
Infancy, infantile, infantilism — *see also* condition
 celiac K90.0
 genitalia, genitals (after puberty) E30.0
 Herter's (nontropical sprue) K90.0
 intestinal K90.0
 Lorain E23.0
 pancreatic K86.89
 pelvis M95.5
  with disproportion (fetopelvic) O33.1
   causing obstructed labor O65.1
 pituitary E23.0
 renal N25.0
 uterus — *see* Infantile, genitalia
Infant(s) — *see also* Infancy
 excessive crying R68.11
 irritable child R68.12
 lack of care — *see* Neglect
 liveborn (singleton) Z38.2
  born in hospital Z38.00
   by cesarean Z38.01
  born outside hospital Z38.1
  multiple NEC Z38.8
   born in hospital Z38.68
    by cesarean Z38.69
   born outside hospital Z38.7
  quadruplet Z38.8
   born in hospital Z38.63

Index

Infant — Infection, infected, infective

Infant(s) — continued
  liveborn — continued
    quadruplet — continued
      born in hospital — continued
        by cesarean Z38.64
      born outside hospital Z38.7
    quintuplet Z38.8
      born in hospital Z38.65
        by cesarean Z38.66
      born outside hospital Z38.7
    triplet Z38.8
      born in hospital Z38.61
        by cesarean Z38.62
      born outside hospital Z38.7
    twin Z38.5
      born in hospital Z38.30
        by cesarean Z38.31
      born outside hospital Z38.4
  of diabetic mother (syndrome of) P70.1
    gestational diabetes P70.0
Infantile — see also condition
  genitalia, genitals E30.0
  os, uterine E30.0
  penis E30.0
  testis E29.1
  uterus E30.0
Infantilism — see Infancy
Infarct, infarction
  adrenal (capsule) (gland) E27.49
  appendices epiploicae — see also Infarct, intestine K55.069
  bowel — see also Infarct, intestine K55.069
  brain (stem) — see Infarct, cerebral
  breast N64.89
  brewer's (kidney) N28.0
  cardiac — see Infarct, myocardium
  cerebellar — see Infarct, cerebral
  cerebral (acute) (chronic) — see also Occlusion, artery cerebral or precerebral, with infarction I63.9
    aborted I63.9
    cortical I63.9
    due to
      cerebral venous thrombosis, nonpyogenic I63.6
      embolism
        cerebral arteries I63.4- ☑
        precerebral arteries I63.1- ☑
      occlusion NEC
        cerebral arteries I63.5- ☑
        precerebral arteries I63.2- ☑
        small artery I63.81
      stenosis NEC
        cerebral arteries I63.5- ☑
        precerebral arteries I63.2- ☑
        small artery I63.81
      thrombosis
        cerebral artery I63.3- ☑
        precerebral artery I63.0- ☑
    intraoperative
      during cardiac surgery I97.810
      during other surgery I97.811
    postprocedural
      following cardiac surgery I97.820
      following other surgery I97.821
    specified NEC I63.89
  colon (acute) (agnogenic) (embolic) (hemorrhagic) (nonocclusive) (nonthrombotic) (occlusive) (segmental) (thrombotic) (with gangrene) — see also Infarct, intestine K55.069
  coronary artery — see Infarct, myocardium
  embolic — see Embolism
  fallopian tube N83.8
  gallbladder K82.8
  heart — see Infarct, myocardium
  hepatic K76.3
  hypophysis (anterior lobe) E23.6
  impending (myocardium) I20.0
  intestine (acute) (agnogenic) (embolic) (hemorrhagic) (nonocclusive) (nonthrombotic) (occlusive) (thrombotic) (with gangrene) K55.069
    diffuse K55.062
    focal K55.061
    large K55.049
      diffuse K55.042
      focal K55.041
    small K55.029
      diffuse K55.022
      focal K55.021
  kidney N28.0

Infarct, infarction — continued
  lacunar I63.81
  liver K76.3
  lung (embolic) (thrombotic) — see Embolism, pulmonary
  lymph node I89.8
  mesentery, mesenteric (embolic) (thrombotic) (with gangrene) — see also Infarct, intestine K55.069
  muscle (ischemic) M62.20
    ankle M62.27- ☑
    foot M62.27- ☑
    forearm M62.23- ☑
    hand M62.24- ☑
    lower leg M62.26- ☑
    pelvic region M62.25- ☑
    shoulder region M62.21- ☑
    specified site NEC M62.28
    thigh M62.25- ☑
    upper arm M62.22- ☑
  myocardium, myocardial (acute) (with stated duration of 4 weeks or less) I21.9
    associated with revascularization procedure I21.A9
    diagnosed on ECG, but presenting no symptoms I25.2
    due to
      demand ischemia I21.A1
      ischemic imbalance I21.A1
    healed or old I25.2
    intraoperative — see also Infarct, myocardium, associated with revascularization procedure
      during cardiac surgery I97.790
      during other surgery I97.791
    non-Q wave I21.4
    non-ST elevation (NSTEMI) I21.4
      subsequent I22.2
    nontransmural I21.4
    past (diagnosed on ECG or other investigation, but currently presenting no symptoms) I25.2
    postprocedural — see also Infarct, myocardium, associated with revascularization procedure
      following cardiac surgery — see also Infarct, myocardium, type 4 or type 5 I97.190
      following other surgery I97.191
    Q wave (see also Infarct, myocardium, by site) I21.3
    secondary to
      demand ischemia I21.A1
      ischemic imbalance I21.A1
    ST elevation (STEMI) I21.3
      anterior (anteroapical) (anterolateral) (anteroseptal) (Q wave) (wall) I21.09
        subsequent I22.0
      inferior (diaphragmatic) (inferolateral) (inferoposterior) (wall) NEC I21.19
        subsequent I22.1
      inferoposterior transmural (Q wave) I21.11
      involving
        coronary artery of anterior wall NEC I21.09
        coronary artery of inferior wall NEC I21.19
        diagonal coronary artery I21.02
        left anterior descending coronary artery I21.02
        left circumflex coronary artery I21.21
        left main coronary artery I21.01
        oblique marginal coronary artery I21.21
        right coronary artery I21.11
      lateral (apical-lateral) (basal-lateral) (high) I21.29
        subsequent I22.8
      posterior (posterobasal) (posterolateral) (posteroseptal) (true) I21.29
        subsequent I22.8
      septal I21.29
        subsequent I22.8
      specified NEC I21.29
        subsequent I22.8
      subsequent I22.9
    subsequent (recurrent) (reinfarction) I22.9
      anterior (anteroapical) (anterolateral) (anteroseptal) (wall) I22.0
      diaphragmatic (wall) I22.1
      inferior (diaphragmatic) (inferolateral) (inferoposterior) (wall) I22.1
      lateral (apical-lateral) (basal-lateral) (high) I22.8
      non-ST elevation (NSTEMI) I22.2
      posterior (posterobasal) (posterolateral) (posteroseptal) (true) I22.8
      septal I22.8
      specified NEC I22.8
      ST elevation I22.9

Infarct, infarction — continued
  myocardium, myocardial — continued
    subsequent — continued
      ST elevation — continued
        anterior (anteroapical) (anterolateral) (anteroseptal) (wall) I22.0
        inferior (diaphragmatic) (inferolateral) (inferoposterior) (wall) I22.1
        specified NEC I22.8
      subendocardial I22.2
      transmural I22.9
        anterior (anteroapical) (anterolateral) (anteroseptal) (wall) I22.0
        diaphragmatic (wall) I22.1
        inferior (diaphragmatic) (inferolateral) (inferoposterior) (wall) I22.1
        lateral (apical-lateral) (basal-lateral) (high) I22.8
        posterior (posterobasal) (posterolateral) (posteroseptal) (true) I22.8
        specified NEC I22.8
      type 1 — see also Infarction, myocardial, subsequent, by site, or by ST elevation or non-ST elevation I22.9
      type 2 I21.A1
      type 3 I21.A9
      type 4 I21.A9
      type 5 I21.A9
    syphilitic A52.06
    transmural I21.9
      anterior (anteroapical) (anterolateral) (anteroseptal) (Q wave) (wall) NEC I21.09
      inferior (diaphragmatic) (inferolateral) (inferoposterior) (Q wave) (wall) NEC I21.19
      inferoposterior (Q wave) I21.11
      lateral (apical-lateral) (basal-lateral) (high) NEC I21.29
      posterior (posterobasal) (posterolateral) (posteroseptal) (true) NEC I21.29
      septal NEC I21.29
      specified NEC I21.29
      type 1 — see also Infarction, myocardial, by site, or by ST elevation or non-ST elevation I21.9
      type 2 I21.A1
      type 3 I21.A9
      type 4 (a) (b) (c) I21.A9
      type 5 I21.A9
  nontransmural I21.4
  omentum — see also Infarct, intestine K55.069
  ovary N83.8
  pancreas K86.89
  papillary muscle — see Infarct, myocardium
  parathyroid gland E21.4
  pituitary (gland) E23.6
  placenta O43.81- ☑
  prostate N42.89
  pulmonary (artery) (vein) (hemorrhagic) — see Embolism, pulmonary
  renal (embolic) (thrombotic) N28.0
  retina, retinal (artery) — see Occlusion, artery, retina
  spinal (cord) (acute) (embolic) (nonembolic) G95.11
  spleen D73.5
    embolic or thrombotic I74.8
  subendocardial (acute) (nontransmural) I21.4
  suprarenal (capsule) (gland) E27.49
  testis N50.1
  thrombotic — see also Thrombosis
    artery, arterial — see Embolism
  thyroid (gland) E07.89
  ventricle (heart) — see Infarct, myocardium
Infecting — see condition
Infection, infected, infective (opportunistic) B99.9
  with
    drug resistant organism — see Resistance (to), drug — see also specific organism
    lymphangitis — see Lymphangitis
    organ dysfunction (acute) R65.20
      with septic shock R65.21
  abscess (skin) — code by site under Abscess
  Absidia — see Mucormycosis
  Acanthamoeba — see Acanthamebiasis
  Acanthocheilonema (perstans) (streptocerca) B74.4
  accessory sinus (chronic) — see Sinusitis
  achorion — see Dermatophytosis
  Acremonium falciforme B47.0
  acromioclavicular M00.9
  Actinobacillus (actinomycetem-comitans) A28.8
    mallei A24.0

Infection, infected, infective — *continued*

Actinobacillus — *continued*
  muris A25.1
Actinomadura B47.1
Actinomyces (israelii) — *see also* Actinomycosis A42.9
Actinomycetales — *see* Actinomycosis
actinomycotic NOS — *see* Actinomycosis
adenoid (and tonsil) J03.90
  chronic J35.02
adenovirus NEC
  as cause of disease classified elsewhere B97.0
  unspecified nature or site B34.0
aerogenes capsulatus A48.0
aertrycke — *see* Infection, salmonella
alimentary canal NOS — *see* Enteritis, infectious
Allescheria boydii B48.2
Alternaria B48.8
alveolus, alveolar (process) K04.7
Ameba, amebic (histolytica) — *see* Amebiasis
amniotic fluid, sac or cavity O41.10- ☑
  chorioamnionitis O41.12- ☑
  placentitis O41.14- ☑
amputation stump (surgical) — *see* Complication, amputation stump, infection
Ancylostoma (duodenalis) B76.0
Anisakiasis, Anisakis larvae B81.0
anthrax — *see* Anthrax
antrum (chronic) — *see* Sinusitis, maxillary
anus, anal (papillae) (sphincter) K62.89
arbovirus (arbor virus) A94
  specified type NEC A93.8
artificial insemination N98.0
Ascaris lumbricoides — *see* Ascariasis
Ascomycetes B47.0
Aspergillus (flavus) (fumigatus) (terreus) — *see* Aspergillosis
atypical
  acid-fast (bacilli) — *see* Mycobacterium, atypical
  mycobacteria — *see* Mycobacterium, atypical
  virus A81.9
    specified type NEC A81.89
auditory meatus (external) — *see* Otitis, externa, infective
auricle (ear) — *see* Otitis, externa, infective
axillary gland (lymph) L04.2
Bacillus A49.9
  abortus A23.1
  anthracis — *see* Anthrax
  Ducrey's (any location) A57
  Flexner's A03.1
  Friedländer's NEC A49.8
  gas (gangrene) A48.0
  mallei A24.0
  melitensis A23.0
  paratyphoid, paratyphosus A01.4
    A A01.1
    B A01.2
    C A01.3
  Shiga (-Kruse) A03.0
  suipestifer — *see* Infection, salmonella
  swimming pool A31.1
  typhosa A01.00
  welchii — *see* Gangrene, gas
bacterial NOS A49.9
  as cause of disease classified elsewhere B96.89
    Bacteroides fragilis [B. fragilis] B96.6
    Clostridium perfringens [C. perfringens] B96.7
    Enterobacter sakazakii B96.89
    Enterococcus B95.2
    Escherichia coli [E. coli] — *see also* Escherichia coli B96.20
    Helicobacter pylori [H.pylori] B96.81
    Hemophilus influenzae [H. influenzae] B96.3
    Klebsiella pneumoniae [K. pneumoniae] B96.1
    Mycoplasma pneumoniae [M. pneumoniae] B96.0
    Proteus (mirabilis) (morganii) B96.4
    Pseudomonas (aeruginosa) (mallei) (pseudomallei) B96.5
    Staphylococcus B95.8
      aureus (methicillin susceptible) (MSSA) B95.61
        methicillin resistant (MRSA) B95.62
      specified NEC B95.7
    Streptococcus B95.5
      group A B95.0
      group B B95.1
      pneumoniae B95.3
      specified NEC B95.4

Infection, infected, infective — *continued*

bacterial — *continued*
  as cause of disease classified elsewhere — *continued*
    Vibrio vulnificus B96.82
    specified NEC A48.8
Bacterium
  paratyphosum A01.4
    A A01.1
    B A01.2
    C A01.3
  typhosum A01.00
Bacteroides NEC A49.8
  fragilis, as cause of disease classified elsewhere B96.6
Balantidium coli A07.0
Bartholin's gland N75.8
Basidiobolus B46.8
bile duct (common) (hepatic) — *see* Cholangitis
bladder — *see* Cystitis
Blastomyces, blastomycotic — *see also* Blastomycosis
  brasiliensis — *see* Paracoccidioidomycosis
  dermatitidis — *see* Blastomycosis
  European — *see* Cryptococcosis
  Loboi B48.0
  North American B40.9
  South American — *see* Paracoccidioidomycosis
bleb, postprocedure — *see* Blebitis
bone — *see* Osteomyelitis
Bordetella — *see* Whooping cough
Borrelia bergdorfi A69.20
brain — *see also* Encephalitis G04.90
  membranes — *see* Meningitis
  septic G06.0
    meninges — *see* Meningitis, bacterial
branchial cyst Q18.0
breast — *see* Mastitis
bronchus — *see* Bronchitis
Brucella A23.9
  abortus A23.1
  canis A23.3
  melitensis A23.0
  mixed A23.8
  specified NEC A23.8
  suis A23.2
Brugia (malayi) B74.1
  timori B74.2
bursa — *see* Bursitis, infective
buttocks (skin) L08.9
Campylobacter, intestinal A04.5
  as cause of disease classified elsewhere B96.81
Candida (albicans) (tropicalis) — *see* Candidiasis
candiru B88.8
Capillaria (intestinal) B81.1
  hepatica B83.8
  philippinensis B81.1
cartilage — *see* Disorder, cartilage, specified type NEC
cat liver fluke B66.0
catheter-related bloodstream (CRBSI) T80.211 ☑
cellulitis — *code by* site under Cellulitis
central line-associated T80.219 ☑
  bloodstream (CLABSI) T80.211 ☑
  specified NEC T80.218 ☑
Cephalosporium falciforme B47.0
cerebrospinal — *see* Meningitis
cervical gland (lymph) L04.0
cervix — *see* Cervicitis
cesarean delivery wound (puerperal) O86.00
cestodes — *see* Infestation, cestodes
chest J22
Chilomastix (intestinal) A07.8
Chlamydia, chlamydial A74.9
  anus A56.3
  genitourinary tract A56.2
    lower A56.00
    specified NEC A56.19
  lymphogranuloma A55
  pharynx A56.4
  psittaci A70
  rectum A56.3
  sexually transmitted NEC A56.8
cholera — *see* Cholera
Cladosporium
  bantianum (brain abscess) B43.1
  carrionii B43.0
  castellanii B36.1
  trichoides (brain abscess) B43.1
  werneckii B36.1

Infection, infected, infective — *continued*

Clonorchis (sinensis) (liver) B66.1
Clostridium NEC
  bifermentans A48.0
  botulinum (food poisoning) A05.1
    infant A48.51
    wound A48.52
  difficile
    as cause of disease classified elsewhere B96.89
    foodborne (disease)
      not specified as recurrent A04.72
      recurrent A04.71
    gas gangrene A48.0
    necrotizing enterocolitis
      not specified as recurrent A04.72
      recurrent A04.71
    sepsis A41.4
  gas-forming NEC A48.0
  histolyticum A48.0
  novyi, causing gas gangrene A48.0
  oedematiens A48.0
  perfringens
    as cause of disease classified elsewhere B96.7
    due to food A05.2
    foodborne (disease) A05.2
    gas gangrene A48.0
    sepsis A41.4
  septicum, causing gas gangrene A48.0
  sordellii, causing gas gangrene A48.0
  welchii
    as cause of disease classified elsewhere B96.7
    foodborne (disease) A05.2
    gas gangrene A48.0
    necrotizing enteritis A05.2
    sepsis A41.4
Coccidioides (immitis) — *see* Coccidioidomycosis
colon — *see* Enteritis, infectious
colostomy K94.02
common duct — *see* Cholangitis
congenital P39.9
  Candida (albicans) P37.5
  cytomegalovirus P35.1
  hepatitis, viral P35.3
  herpes simplex P35.2
  infectious or parasitic disease P37.9
    specified NEC P37.8
  listeriosis (disseminated) P37.2
  malaria NEC P37.4
    falciparum P37.3
  Plasmodium falciparum P37.3
  poliomyelitis P35.8
  rubella P35.0
  skin P39.4
  toxoplasmosis (acute) (subacute) (chronic) P37.1
  tuberculosis P37.0
  urinary (tract) P39.3
  vaccinia P35.8
  virus P35.9
    specified type NEC P35.8
Conidiobolus B46.8
coronavirus NEC B34.2
  as cause of disease classified elsewhere B97.29
  severe acute respiratory syndrome (SARS associated) B97.21
corpus luteum — *see* Salpingo-oophoritis
Corynebacterium diphtheriae — *see* Diphtheria
cotia virus B08.8
Coxiella burnetii A78
coxsackie — *see* Coxsackie
Cryptococcus neoformans — *see* Cryptococcosis
Cryptosporidium A07.2
Cunninghamella — *see* Mucormycosis
cyst — *see* Cyst
cystic duct — *see also* Cholecystitis K81.9
Cysticercus cellulosae — *see* Cysticercosis
cytomegalovirus, cytomegaloviral B25.9
  congenital P35.1
  maternal, maternal care for (suspected) damage to fetus O35.3 ☑
  mononucleosis B27.10
    with
      complication NEC B27.19
      meningitis B27.12
      polyneuropathy B27.11
delta-agent (acute), in hepatitis B carrier B17.0
dental (pulpal origin) K04.7
Deuteromycetes B47.0
Dicrocoelium dendriticum B66.2

Infection, infected, infective — *continued*
- Dipetalonema (perstans) (streptocerca) B74.4
- diphtherial — *see* Diphtheria
- Diphyllobothrium (adult) (latum) (pacificum) B70.0
  - larval B70.1
- Diplogonoporus (grandis) B71.8
- Dipylidium caninum B67.4
- Dirofilaria B74.8
- Dracunculus medinensis B72
- Drechslera (hawaiiensis) B43.8
- Ducrey Haemophilus (any location) A57
- due to or resulting from
  - artificial insemination N98.0
  - central venous catheter T80.219 ☑
    - bloodstream T80.211 ☑
    - exit or insertion site T80.212 ☑
    - localized T80.212 ☑
    - port or reservoir T80.212 ☑
    - specified NEC T80.218 ☑
    - tunnel T80.212 ☑
  - device, implant or graft — *see also* Complications, by site and type, infection or inflammation T85.79 ☑
    - arterial graft NEC T82.7 ☑
    - breast (implant) T85.79 ☑
    - catheter NEC T85.79 ☑
      - dialysis (renal) T82.7 ☑
        - intraperitoneal T85.71 ☑
      - infusion NEC T82.7 ☑
        - cranial T85.735 ☑
        - intrathecal T85.735 ☑
        - spinal (epidural) (subdural) T85.735 ☑
        - subarachnoid T85.735 ☑
      - urinary T83.518 ☑
        - cystostomy T83.510 ☑
        - Hopkins T83.518 ☑
        - ileostomy T83.518 ☑
        - nephrostomy T83.512 ☑
        - specified NEC T83.518 ☑
        - urethral indwelling T83.511 ☑
        - urostomy T83.518 ☑
    - electronic (electrode) (pulse generator) (stimulator)
      - bone T84.7 ☑
      - cardiac T82.7 ☑
      - nervous system T85.738 ☑
        - brain T85.731 ☑
        - cranial nerve T85.732 ☑
        - gastric nerve T85.732 ☑
        - generator pocket T85.734 ☑
        - neurostimulator generator T85.734 ☑
        - peripheral nerve T85.732 ☑
        - sacral nerve T85.732 ☑
        - spinal cord T85.733 ☑
        - vagal nerve T85.732 ☑
      - urinary (indwelling) T83.51 ☑
    - fixation, internal (orthopedic) NEC — *see* Complication, fixation device, infection
    - gastrointestinal (bile duct) (esophagus) T85.79 ☑
      - neurostimulator electrode (lead) T85.732 ☑
    - genital NEC T83.69 ☑
    - heart NEC T82.7 ☑
      - valve (prosthesis) T82.6 ☑
        - graft T82.7 ☑
    - joint prosthesis — *see* Complication, joint prosthesis, infection
    - ocular (corneal graft) (orbital implant) NEC T85.79 ☑
    - orthopedic NEC T84.7 ☑
    - penile (cylinder) (pump) (resevoir) T83.61 ☑
    - specified NEC T85.79 ☑
    - testicular T83.62 ☑
    - urinary NEC T83.598 ☑
      - ileal conduit stent T83.593 ☑
      - implanted neurostimulation T83.590 ☑
      - implanted sphincter T83.591 ☑
      - indwelling ureteral stent T83.592 ☑
      - nephroureteral stent T83.593 ☑
      - specified stent NEC T83.593 ☑
    - vascular NEC T82.7 ☑
    - ventricular intracranial (communicating) shunt T85.730 ☑
  - Hickman catheter T80.219 ☑
    - bloodstream T80.211 ☑
    - localized T80.212 ☑
    - specified NEC T80.218 ☑

Infection, infected, infective — *continued*
- due to or resulting from — *continued*
  - immunization or vaccination T88.0 ☑
  - infusion, injection or transfusion NEC T80.29 ☑
  - injury NEC — *code by* site under Wound, open
  - peripherally inserted central catheter (PICC) T80.219 ☑
    - bloodstream T80.211 ☑
    - localized T80.212 ☑
    - specified NEC T80.218 ☑
  - portacath (port-a-cath) T80.219 ☑
    - bloodstream T80.211 ☑
    - localized T80.212 ☑
    - specified NEC T80.218 ☑
  - pulmonary artery catheter — *see* Infection, due to or resulting from, central venous catheter
  - surgery T81.40 ☑
  - Swan Ganz catheter — *see* Infection, due to or resulting from, central venous catheter
  - triple lumen catheter T80.219 ☑
    - bloodstream T80.211 ☑
    - localized T80.212 ☑
    - specified NEC T80.218 ☑
  - umbilical venous catheter T80.219 ☑
    - bloodstream T80.211 ☑
    - localized T80.212 ☑
    - specified NEC T80.218 ☑
- during labor NEC O75.3
- ear (middle) — *see also* Otitis media
  - external — *see* Otitis, externa, infective
  - inner — *see* subcategory H83.0 ☑
- Eberthella typhosa A01.00
- Echinococcus — *see* Echinococcus
- echovirus
  - as cause of disease classified elsewhere B97.12
  - unspecified nature or site B34.1
- endocardium I33.0
- endocervix — *see* Cervicitis
- Entamoeba — *see* Amebiasis
- enteric — *see* Enteritis, infectious
- Enterobacter sakazakii B96.89
- Enterobius vermicularis B80
- enterostomy K94.12
- enterovirus B34.1
  - as cause of disease classified elsewhere B97.10
    - coxsackievirus B97.11
    - echovirus B97.12
    - specified NEC B97.19
- Entomophthora B46.8
- Epidermophyton — *see* Dermatophytosis
- epididymis — *see* Epididymitis
- episiotomy (puerperal) O86.09
- Erysipelothrix (insidiosa) (rhusiopathiae) — *see* Erysipeloid
- erythema infectiosum B08.3
- Escherichia (E.) coli NEC A49.8
  - as cause of disease classified elsewhere — *see also* Escherichia coli B96.20
  - congenital P39.8
    - sepsis P36.4
  - generalized A41.51
  - intestinal — *see* Enteritis, infectious, due to, Escherichia coli
- ethmoidal (chronic) (sinus) — *see* Sinusitis, ethmoidal
- eustachian tube (ear) — *see* Salpingitis, eustachian
- external auditory canal (meatus) NEC — *see* Otitis, externa, infective
- eye (purulent) — *see* Endophthalmitis, purulent
- eyelid — *see* Inflammation, eyelid
- fallopian tube — *see* Salpingo-oophoritis
- Fasciola (gigantica) (hepatica) (indica) B66.3
- Fasciolopsis (buski) B66.5
- filarial — *see* Infestation, filarial
- finger (skin) L08.9
  - nail L03.01- ☑
    - fungus B35.1
- fish tapeworm B70.0
  - larval B70.1
- flagellate, intestinal A07.9
- fluke — *see* Infestation, fluke
- focal
  - teeth (pulpal origin) K04.7
  - tonsils J35.01
- Fonsecaea (compactum) (pedrosoi) B43.0
- food — *see* Intoxication, foodborne
- foot (skin) L08.9
  - dermatophytic fungus B35.3

Infection, infected, infective — *continued*
- Francisella tularensis — *see* Tularemia
- frontal (sinus) (chronic) — *see* Sinusitis, frontal
- fungus NOS B49
  - beard B35.0
  - dermatophytic — *see* Dermatophytosis
  - foot B35.3
  - groin B35.6
  - hand B35.2
  - nail B35.1
  - pathogenic to compromised host only B48.8
  - perianal (area) B35.6
  - scalp B35.0
  - skin B36.9
    - foot B35.3
    - hand B35.2
    - toenails B35.1
- Fusarium B48.8
- gallbladder — *see* Cholecystitis
- gas bacillus — *see* Gangrene, gas
- gastrointestinal — *see* Enteritis, infectious
- generalized NEC — *see* Sepsis
- generator pocket, implanted electronic neurostimulator T85.734 ☑
- genital organ or tract
  - female — *see* Disease, pelvis, inflammatory
  - male N49.9
    - multiple sites N49.8
    - specified NEC N49.8
- Ghon tubercle, primary A15.7
- Giardia lamblia A07.1
- gingiva (chronic) K05.10
  - acute K05.00
    - nonplaque induced K05.01
    - plaque induced K05.00
  - nonplaque induced K05.11
  - plaque induced K05.10
- glanders A24.0
- glenosporopsis B48.0
- Gnathostoma (spinigerum) B83.1
- Gongylonema B83.8
- gonococcal — *see* Gonococcus
- gram-negative bacilli NOS A49.9
- guinea worm B72
- gum (chronic) K05.10
  - acute K05.00
    - nonplaque induced K05.01
    - plaque induced K05.00
  - nonplaque induced K05.11
  - plaque induced K05.10
- Haemophilus — *see* Infection, Hemophilus
- heart — *see* Carditis
- Helicobacter pylori A04.8
  - as cause of disease classified elsewhere B96.81
- helminths B83.9
  - intestinal B82.0
    - mixed (types classifiable to more than one of the titles B65.0-B81.3 and B81.8) B81.4
    - specified type NEC B81.8
  - specified type NEC B83.8
- Hemophilus
  - aegyptius, systemic A48.4
  - ducrey (any location) A57
  - generalized A41.3
  - influenzae NEC A49.2
    - as cause of disease classified elsewhere B96.3
- herpes (simplex) — *see also* Herpes
  - congenital P35.2
  - disseminated B00.7
  - zoster B02.9
- herpesvirus, herpesviral — *see* Herpes
- Heterophyes (heterophyes) B66.8
- hip (joint) NEC M00.9
  - due to internal joint prosthesis
    - left T84.52 ☑
    - right T84.51 ☑
  - skin NEC L08.9
- Histoplasma — *see* Histoplasmosis
  - American B39.4
  - capsulatum B39.4
- hookworm B76.9
- human
  - papilloma virus A63.0
  - T-cell lymphotropic virus type-1 (HTLV-1) B33.3
- hydrocele N43.0
- Hymenolepis B71.0
- hypopharynx — *see* Pharyngitis
- inguinal (lymph) glands L04.1

Infection, infected, infective — *continued*
inguinal glands — *continued*
due to soft chancre A57
intervertebral disc, pyogenic M46.30
cervical region M46.32
cervicothoracic region M46.33
lumbar region M46.36
lumbosacral region M46.37
multiple sites M46.39
occipito-atlanto-axial region M46.31
sacrococcygeal region M46.38
thoracic region M46.34
thoracolumbar region M46.35
intestine, intestinal — *see* Enteritis, infectious
specified NEC A08.8
intra-amniotic affecting newborn NEC P39.2
Isospora belli or hominis A07.3
Japanese B encephalitis A83.0
jaw (bone) (lower) (upper) M27.2
joint NEC M00.9
due to internal joint prosthesis T84.50 ☑
kidney (cortex) (hematogenous) N15.9
with calculus N20.0
with hydronephrosis N13.6
following ectopic gestation O08.83
pelvis and ureter (cystic) N28.85
puerperal (postpartum) O86.21
specified NEC N15.8
Klebsiella (K.) pneumoniae NEC A49.8
as cause of disease classified elsewhere B96.1
knee (joint) NEC M00.9
joint M00.9
due to internal joint prosthesis
left T84.54 ☑
right T84.53 ☑
skin L08.9
Koch's — *see* Tuberculosis
labia (majora) (minora) (acute) — *see* Vulvitis
lacrimal
gland — *see* Dacryoadenitis
passages (duct) (sac) — *see* Inflammation, lacrimal, passages
lancet fluke B66.2
larynx NEC J38.7
leg (skin) NOS L08.9
Legionella pneumophila A48.1
nonpneumonic A48.2
Leishmania — *see also* Leishmaniasis
aethiopica B55.1
braziliensis B55.2
chagasi B55.0
donovani B55.0
infantum B55.0
major B55.1
mexicana B55.1
tropica B55.1
lentivirus, as cause of disease classified elsewhere B97.31
Leptosphaeria senegalensis B47.0
Leptospira interrogans A27.9
autumnalis A27.89
canicola A27.89
hebdomadis A27.89
icterohaemorrhagiae A27.0
pomona A27.89
specified type NEC A27.89
leptospirochetal NEC — *see* Leptospirosis
Listeria monocytogenes — *see also* Listeriosis
congenital P37.2
Loa loa B74.3
with conjunctival infestation B74.3
eyelid B74.3
Loboa loboi B48.0
local, skin (staphylococcal) (streptococcal) L08.9
abscess — *code by* site under Abscess
cellulitis — *code by* site under Cellulitis
specified NEC L08.89
ulcer — *see* Ulcer, skin
Loefflerella mallei A24.0
lung — *see also* Pneumonia J18.9
atypical Mycobacterium A31.0
spirochetal A69.8
tuberculous — *see* Tuberculosis, pulmonary
virus — *see* Pneumonia, viral
lymph gland — *see also* Lymphadenitis, acute
mesenteric I88.0
lymphoid tissue, base of tongue or posterior pharynx, NEC (chronic) J35.03

Infection, infected, infective — *continued*
Madurella (grisea) (mycetomii) B47.0
major
following ectopic or molar pregnancy O08.0
puerperal, postpartum, childbirth O85
Malassezia furfur B36.0
Malleomyces
mallei A24.0
pseudomallei (whitmori) — *see* Melioidosis
mammary gland N61.0
Mansonella (ozzardi) (perstans) (streptocerca) B74.4
mastoid — *see* Mastoiditis
maxilla, maxillary M27.2
sinus (chronic) — *see* Sinusitis, maxillary
mediastinum J98.51
Medina (worm) B72
meibomian cyst or gland — *see* Hordeolum
meninges — *see* Meningitis, bacterial
meningococcal — *see also* condition A39.9
adrenals A39.1
brain A39.81
cerebrospinal A39.0
conjunctiva A39.89
endocardium A39.51
heart A39.50
endocardium A39.51
myocardium A39.52
pericardium A39.53
joint A39.83
meninges A39.0
meningococcemia A39.4
acute A39.2
chronic A39.3
myocardium A39.52
pericardium A39.53
retrobulbar neuritis A39.82
specified site NEC A39.89
mesenteric lymph nodes or glands NEC I88.0
Metagonimus B66.8
metatarsophalangeal M00.9
methicillin
resistant Staphylococcus aureus (MRSA) A49.02
susceptible Staphylococcus aureus (MSSA) A49.01
Microsporum, microsporic — *see* Dermatophytosis
mixed flora (bacterial) NEC A49.8
Monilia — *see* Candidiasis
Monosporium apiospermum B48.2
mouth, parasitic B37.0
Mucor — *see* Mucormycosis
muscle NEC — *see* Myositis, infective
mycelium NOS B49
mycetoma B47.9
actinomycotic NEC B47.1
mycotic NEC B47.0
Mycobacterium, mycobacterial — *see* Mycobacterium
Mycoplasma NEC A49.3
pneumoniae, as cause of disease classified elsewhere B96.0
mycotic NOS B49
pathogenic to compromised host only B48.8
skin NOS B36.9
myocardium NEC I40.0
nail (chronic)
with lymphangitis — *see* Lymphangitis, acute, digit
finger L03.01- ☑
fungus B35.1
ingrowing L60.0
toe L03.03- ☑
fungus B35.1
nasal sinus (chronic) — *see* Sinusitis
nasopharynx — *see* Nasopharyngitis
navel L08.82
Necator americanus B76.1
Neisseria — *see* Gonococcus
Neotestudina rosatii B47.0
newborn P39.9
intra-amniotic NEC P39.2
skin P39.4
specified type NEC P39.8
nipple N61.0
associated with
lactation O91.03
pregnancy O91.01- ☑
puerperium O91.02
Nocardia — *see* Nocardiosis
obstetrical surgical wound (puerperal) O86.00
incisional site
deep O86.02

Infection, infected, infective — *continued*
obstetrical surgical wound — *continued*
incisional site — *continued*
superficial O86.01
organ and space site O86.03
surgical site specified NEC O86.09
Oesophagostomum (apiostomum) B81.8
Oestrus ovis — *see* Myiasis
Oidium albicans B37.9
Onchocerca (volvulus) — *see* Onchocerciasis
oncovirus, as cause of disease classified elsewhere B97.32
operation wound T81.49 ☑
Opisthorchis (felineus) (viverrini) B66.0
orbit, orbital — *see* Inflammation, orbit
orthopoxvirus NEC B08.09
ovary — *see* Salpingo-oophoritis
Oxyuris vermicularis B80
pancreas (acute) — *see* Pancreatitis, acute
abscess — *see* Pancreatitis, acute
specified NEC — *see also* Pancreatitis, acute K85.80
papillomavirus, as cause of disease classified elsewhere B97.7
papovavirus NEC B34.4
Paracoccidioides brasiliensis — *see* Paracoccidioidomy- cosis
Paragonimus (westermani) B66.4
parainfluenza virus B34.8
parameningococcus NOS A39.9
parapoxvirus B08.60
specified NEC B08.69
parasitic B89
Parastrongylus
cantonensis B83.2
costaricensis B81.3
paratyphoid A01.4
Type A A01.1
Type B A01.2
Type C A01.3
paraurethral ducts N34.2
parotid gland — *see* Sialoadenitis
parvovirus NEC B34.3
as cause of disease classified elsewhere B97.6
Pasteurella NEC A28.0
multocida A28.0
pestis — *see* Plague
pseudotuberculosis A28.0
septica (cat bite) (dog bite) A28.0
tularensis — *see* Tularemia
pelvic, female — *see* Disease, pelvis, inflammatory
Penicillium (marneffei) B48.4
penis (glans) (retention) NEC N48.29
periapical K04.5
peridental, periodontal K05.20
generalized — *see* Periodontitis, aggressive, gener- alized
localized — *see* Periodontitis, aggressive, localized
perinatal period P39.9
specified type NEC P39.8
perineal repair (puerperal) O86.09
periorbital — *see* Inflammation, orbit
perirectal K62.89
perirenal — *see* Infection, kidney
peritoneal — *see* Peritonitis
periureteral N28.89
Petriellidium boydii B48.2
pharynx — *see also* Pharyngitis
coxsackievirus B08.5
posterior, lymphoid (chronic) J35.03
Phialophora
gougerotii (subcutaneous abscess or cyst) B43.2
jeanselmei (subcutaneous abscess or cyst) B43.2
verrucosa (skin) B43.0
Piedraia hortae B36.3
pinta A67.9
intermediate A67.1
late A67.2
mixed A67.3
primary A67.0
pinworm B80
pityrosporum furfur B36.0
pleuro-pneumonia-like organism (PPLO) NEC A49.3
as cause of disease classified elsewhere B96.0
pneumococcus, pneumococcal NEC A49.1
as cause of disease classified elsewhere B95.3
generalized (purulent) A40.3
with pneumonia J13
Pneumocystis carinii (pneumonia) B59

Infection, infected, infective — *continued*
Pneumocystis jiroveci (pneumonia) B59
port or reservoir T80.212 ☑
postoperative T81.40 ☑
postoperative wound T81.49 ☑
 surgical site
  deep incisional T81.42 ☑
  organ and space T81.43 ☑
  specified NEC T81.49 ☑
  superficial incisional T81.41 ☑
postprocedural T81.40 ☑
postvaccinal T88.0 ☑
prepuce NEC N47.7
 with penile inflammation N47.6
prion — *see* Disease, prion, central nervous system
prostate (capsule) — *see* Prostatitis
Proteus (mirabilis) (morganii) (vulgaris) NEC A49.8
 as cause of disease classified elsewhere B96.4
protozoal NEC B64
 intestinal A07.9
  specified NEC A07.8
 specified NEC B60.8
Pseudoallescheria boydii B48.2
Pseudomonas NEC A49.8
 as cause of disease classified elsewhere B96.5
 mallei A24.0
 pneumonia J15.1
 pseudomallei — *see* Melioidosis
puerperal O86.4
 genitourinary tract NEC O86.89
 major or generalized O85
 minor O86.4
 specified NEC O86.89
pulmonary — *see* Infection, lung
purulent — *see* Abscess
Pyrenochaeta romeroi B47.0
Q fever A78
rectum (sphincter) K62.89
renal — *see also* Infection, kidney
 pelvis and ureter (cystic) N28.85
reovirus, as cause of disease classified elsewhere B97.5
respiratory (tract) NEC J98.8
 acute J22
 chronic J98.8
 influenzal (upper) (acute) — *see* Influenza, with,
  respiratory manifestations NEC
 lower (acute) J22
  chronic — *see* Bronchitis, chronic
 rhinovirus J00
 syncytial virus (RSV) — *see* Infection, virus, respiratory syncytial (RSV)
 upper (acute) NOS J06.9
  chronic J39.8
  streptococcal J06.9
  viral NOS J06.9
   due to respiratory syncytial virus (RSV)
    J06.9 [B97.4]
resulting from
 presence of internal prosthesis, implant, graft —
  see Complications, by site and type, infection
retortamoniasis A07.8
retroperitoneal NEC K68.9
retrovirus B33.3
 as cause of disease classified elsewhere B97.30 ☑
  human
   immunodeficiency, type 2 (HIV 2) B97.35
   T-cell lymphotropic
    type I (HTLV-I) B97.33
    type II (HTLV-II) B97.34
  lentivirus B97.31
  oncovirus B97.32
  specified NEC B97.39
Rhinosporidium (seeberi) B48.1
rhinovirus
 as cause of disease classified elsewhere B97.89
 unspecified nature or site B34.8
Rhizopus — *see* Mucormycosis
rickettsial NOS A79.9
roundworm (large) NEC B82.0
 Ascariasis — *see also* Ascariasis B77.9
rubella — *see* Rubella
Saccharomyces — *see* Candidiasis
salivary duct or gland (any) — *see* Sialoadenitis
Salmonella (aertrycke) (arizonae) (callinarum) (cholerae-
  suis) (enteritidis) (suipestifer) (typhimurium)
  A02.9
 with
  (gastro)enteritis A02.0

Infection, infected, infective — *continued*
Salmonella — *continued*
 with — *continued*
  sepsis A02.1
  specified manifestation NEC A02.8
 due to food (poisoning) A02.9
 hirschfeldii A01.3
 localized A02.20
  arthritis A02.23
  meningitis A02.21
  osteomyelitis A02.24
  pneumonia A02.22
  pyelonephritis A02.25
  specified NEC A02.29
 paratyphi A01.4
  A A01.1
  B A01.2
  C A01.3
 schottmuelleri A01.2
 typhi, typhosa — *see* Typhoid
Sarcocystis A07.8
scabies B86
Schistosoma — *see* Infestation, Schistosoma
scrotum (acute) NEC N49.2
seminal vesicle — *see* Vesiculitis
septic
 localized, skin — *see* Abscess
sheep liver fluke B66.3
Shigella A03.9
 boydii A03.2
 dysenteriae A03.0
 flexneri A03.1
 group
  A A03.0
  B A03.1
  C A03.2
  D A03.3
 Schmitz (-Stutzer) A03.0
 schmitzii A03.0
 shigae A03.0
 sonnei A03.3
 specified NEC A03.8
shoulder (joint) NEC M00.9
 due to internal joint prosthesis T84.59 ☑
 skin NEC L08.9
sinus (accessory) (chronic) (nasal) — *see also* Sinusitis
 pilonidal — *see* Sinus, pilonidal
 skin NEC L08.89
Skene's duct or gland — *see* Urethritis
skin (local) (staphylococcal) (streptococcal) L08.9
 abscess — *code by* site under Abscess
 cellulitis — *code by* site under Cellulitis
 due to fungus B36.9
  specified type NEC B36.8
 mycotic B36.9
  specified type NEC B36.8
 newborn P39.4
 ulcer — *see* Ulcer, skin
slow virus A81.9
 specified NEC A81.89
Sparganum (mansoni) (proliferum) (baxteri) B70.1
specific — *see also* Syphilis
 to perinatal period — *see* Infection, congenital
specified NEC B99.8
spermatic cord NEC N49.1
sphenoidal (sinus) — *see* Sinusitis, sphenoidal
spinal cord NOS — *see also* Myelitis G04.91
 abscess G06.1
 meninges — *see* Meningitis
 streptococcal G04.89
Spirillum A25.0
spirochetal NOS A69.9
 lung A69.8
 specified NEC A69.8
Spirometra larvae B70.1
spleen D73.89
Sporotrichum, Sporothrix (schenckii) — *see* Sporotrichosis
staphylococcal, unspecified site
 as cause of disease classified elsewhere B95.8
  aureus (methicillin susceptible) (MSSA) B95.61
   methicillin resistant (MRSA) B95.62
  specified NEC B95.7
 aureus (methicillin susceptible) (MSSA) A49.01
  methicillin resistant (MRSA) A49.02
 food poisoning A05.0
 generalized (purulent) A41.2
 pneumonia — *see* Pneumonia, staphylococcal

Infection, infected, infective — *continued*
Stellantchasmus falcatus B66.8
streptobacillus moniliformis A25.1
streptococcal NEC A49.1
 as cause of disease classified elsewhere B95.5
 B genitourinary complicating
  childbirth O98.82
  pregnancy O98.81- ☑
  puerperium O98.83
 congenital
  sepsis P36.10
   group B P36.0
   specified NEC P36.19
 generalized (purulent) A40.9
Streptomyces B47.1
Strongyloides (stercoralis) — *see* Strongyloidiasis
stump (amputation) (surgical) — *see* Complication,
  amputation stump, infection
subcutaneous tissue, local L08.9
suipestifer — *see* Infection, salmonella
swimming pool bacillus A31.1
Taenia — *see* Infestation, Taenia
Taeniarhynchus saginatus B68.1
tapeworm — *see* Infestation, tapeworm
tendon (sheath) — *see* Tenosynovitis, infective NEC
Ternidens diminutus B81.8
testis — *see* Orchitis
threadworm B80
throat — *see* Pharyngitis
thyroglossal duct K14.8
toe (skin) L08.9
 cellulitis L03.03- ☑
  fungus B35.1
 nail L03.03- ☑
  fungus B35.1
tongue NEC K14.0
 parasitic B37.0
tonsil (and adenoid) (faucial) (lingual) (pharyngeal) —
  see Tonsillitis
tooth, teeth K04.7
 periapical K04.7
 peridental, periodontal K05.20
  generalized — *see* Periodontitis, aggressive,
   generalized
  localized — *see* Periodontitis, aggressive, localized
 pulp K04.01
  irreversible K04.02
  reversible K04.01
 socket M27.3
TORCH — *see* Infection, congenital
 without active infection P00.2
Torula histolytica — *see* Cryptococcosis
Toxocara (canis) (cati) (felis) B83.0
Toxoplasma gondii — *see* Toxoplasma
trachea, chronic J42
trematode NEC — *see* Infestation, fluke
trench fever A79.0
Treponema pallidum — *see* Syphilis
Trichinella (spiralis) B75
Trichomonas A59.9
 cervix A59.09
 intestine A07.8
 prostate A59.02
 specified site NEC A59.8
 urethra A59.03
 urogenitalis A59.00
 vagina A59.01
 vulva A59.01
Trichophyton, trichophytic — *see* Dermatophytosis
Trichosporon (beigelii) cutaneum B36.2
Trichostrongylus B81.2
Trichuris (trichiura) B79
Trombicula (irritans) B88.0
Trypanosoma
 brucei
  gambiense B56.0
  rhodesiense B56.1
 cruzi — *see* Chagas' disease
tubal — *see* Salpingo-oophoritis
tuberculous
 latent (LTBI) Z22.7
 NEC — *see* Tuberculosis
tubo-ovarian — *see* Salpingo-oophoritis
tunica vaginalis N49.1
tunnel T80.212 ☑
tympanic membrane NEC — *see* Myringitis
typhoid (abortive) (ambulant) (bacillus) — *see* Typhoid

Infection, infected, infective — *continued*
- typhus A75.9
  - flea-borne A75.2
  - mite-borne A75.3
  - recrudescent A75.1
  - tick-borne A77.9
    - African A77.1
    - North Asian A77.2
- umbilicus L08.82
- ureter — *see* Ureteritis
- urethra — *see* Urethritis
- urinary (tract) N39.0
  - bladder — *see* Cystitis
  - complicating
    - pregnancy O23.4- ☑
      - specified type NEC O23.3- ☑
  - kidney — *see* Infection, kidney
  - newborn P39.3
  - puerperal (postpartum) O86.20
  - tuberculous A18.13
  - urethra — *see* Urethritis
- uterus, uterine — *see* Endometritis
- vaccination T88.0 ☑
- vaccinia not from vaccination B08.011
- vagina (acute) — *see* Vaginitis
- varicella B01.9
- varicose veins — *see* Varix
- vas deferens NEC N49.1
- vesical — *see* Cystitis
- Vibrio
  - cholerae A00.0
    - El Tor A00.1
  - parahaemolyticus (food poisoning) A05.3
  - vulnificus
    - as cause of disease classified elsewhere B96.82
    - foodborne intoxication A05.5
- Vincent's (gum) (mouth) (tonsil) A69.1
- virus, viral NOS B34.9
  - adenovirus
    - as cause of disease classified elsewhere B97.0
    - unspecified nature or site B34.0
  - arborvirus, arbovirus arthropod-borne A94
  - as cause of disease classified elsewhere B97.89
    - adenovirus B97.0
    - coronavirus B97.29
      - SARS-associated B97.21
    - coxsackievirus B97.11
    - echovirus B97.12
    - enterovirus B97.10
      - coxsackievirus B97.11
      - echovirus B97.12
      - specified NEC B97.19
    - human
      - immunodeficiency, type 2 (HIV 2) B97.35
      - metapneumovirus B97.81
      - T-cell lymphotropic,
        - type I (HTLV-I) B97.33
        - type II (HTLV-II) B97.34
    - papillomavirus B97.7
    - parvovirus B97.6
    - reovirus B97.5
    - respiratory syncytial (RSV) — *see* Infection, virus, respiratory syncytial (RSV)
    - retrovirus B97.30
      - human
        - immunodeficiency, type 2 (HIV 2) B97.35
        - T-cell lymphotropic,
          - type I (HTLV-I) B97.33
          - type II (HTLV-II) B97.34
      - lentivirus B97.31
      - oncovirus B97.32
      - specified NEC B97.39
    - specified NEC B97.89
  - central nervous system A89
    - atypical A81.9
      - specified NEC A81.89
    - enterovirus NEC A88.8
      - meningitis A87.0
    - slow virus A81.9
      - specified NEC A81.89
    - specified NEC A88.8
  - chest J98.8
  - cotia B08.8
  - coxsackie — *see also* Infection, coxsackie B34.1
    - as cause of disease classified elsewhere B97.11
  - ECHO
    - as cause of disease classified elsewhere B97.12
    - unspecified nature or site B34.1

Infection, infected, infective — *continued*
- virus, viral — *continued*
  - encephalitis, tick-borne A84.9
  - enterovirus, as cause of disease classified elsewhere B97.10
    - coxsackievirus B97.11
    - echovirus B97.12
    - specified NEC B97.19
  - exanthem NOS B09
  - human metapneumovirus as cause of disease classified elsewhere B97.81
  - human papilloma as cause of disease classified elsewhere B97.7
  - intestine — *see* Enteritis, viral
  - respiratory syncytial (RSV)
    - as cause of disease classified elsewhere B97.4
    - bronchiolitis J21.0
    - bronchitis J20.5
    - bronchopneumonia J12.1
    - otitis media H65- ☑ *[B97.4]*
    - pneumonia J12.1
    - upper respiratory infection J06.9 *[B97.4]*
  - rhinovirus
    - as cause of disease classified elsewhere B97.89
    - unspecified nature or site B34.8
  - slow A81.9
    - specified NEC A81.89
  - specified type NEC B33.8
    - as cause of disease classified elsewhere B97.89
    - unspecified nature or site B34.8
  - unspecified nature or site B34.9
  - West Nile — *see* Virus, West Nile
- vulva (acute) — *see* Vulvitis
- West Nile — *see* Virus, West Nile
- whipworm B79
- worms B83.9
  - specified type NEC B83.8
- Wuchereria (bancrofti) B74.0
  - malayi B74.1
- yatapoxvirus B08.70
  - specified NEC B08.79
- yeast — *see also* Candidiasis B37.9
- yellow fever — *see* Fever, yellow
- Yersinia
  - enterocolitica (intestinal) A04.6
  - pestis — *see* Plague
  - pseudotuberculosis A28.2
- Zeis' gland — *see* Hordeolum
- Zika virus A92.5
  - congenital P35.4
- zoonotic bacterial NOS A28.9
- Zopfia senegalensis B47.0

Infective, infectious — *see* condition
Infertility
- female N97.9
  - age-related N97.8
  - associated with
    - anovulation N97.0
    - cervical (mucus) disease or anomaly N88.3
    - congenital anomaly
      - cervix N88.3
      - fallopian tube N97.1
      - uterus N97.2
      - vagina N97.8
    - dysmucorrhea N88.3
    - fallopian tube disease or anomaly N97.1
    - pituitary-hypothalamic origin E23.0
    - specified origin NEC N97.8
    - Stein-Leventhal syndrome E28.2
    - uterine disease or anomaly N97.2
    - vaginal disease or anomaly N97.8
  - due to
    - cervical anomaly N88.3
    - fallopian tube anomaly N97.1
    - ovarian failure E28.39
    - Stein-Leventhal syndrome E28.2
    - uterine anomaly N97.2
    - vaginal anomaly N97.8
  - nonimplantation N97.2
  - origin
    - cervical N88.3
    - tubal (block) (occlusion) (stenosis) N97.1
    - uterine N97.2
    - vaginal N97.8
- male N46.9
  - azoospermia N46.01
    - extratesticular cause N46.029
      - drug therapy N46.021

Infertility — *continued*
- male — *continued*
  - azoospermia — *continued*
    - extratesticular cause — *continued*
      - efferent duct obstruction N46.023
      - infection N46.022
      - radiation N46.024
      - specified cause NEC N46.029
      - systemic disease N46.025
  - oligospermia N46.11
    - extratesticular cause N46.129
      - drug therapy N46.121
      - efferent duct obstruction N46.123
      - infection N46.122
      - radiation N46.124
      - specified cause NEC N46.129
      - systemic disease N46.125
  - specified type NEC N46.8

Infestation B88.9
- Acanthocheilonema (perstans) (streptocerca) B74.4
- Acariasis B88.0
  - demodex folliculorum B88.0
  - sarcoptes scabiei B86
  - trombiculae B88.0
- Agamofilaria streptocerca B74.4
- Ancylostoma, ankylostoma (braziliense) (caninum) (ceylanicum) (duodenale) B76.0
  - americanum B76.1
  - new world B76.1
- Anisakis larvae, anisakiasis B81.0
- arthropod NEC B88.2
- Ascaris lumbricoides — *see* Ascariasis
- Balantidium coli A07.0
- beef tapeworm B68.1
- Bothriocephalus (latus) B70.0
  - larval B70.1
- broad tapeworm B70.0
  - larval B70.1
- Brugia (malayi) B74.1
  - timori B74.2
- candiru B88.8
- Capillaria
  - hepatica B83.8
  - philippinensis B81.1
- cat liver fluke B66.0
- cestodes B71.9
  - diphyllobothrium — *see* Infestation, diphyllobothrium
  - dipylidiasis B71.1
  - hymenolepiasis B71.0
  - specified type NEC B71.8
- chigger B88.0
- chigo, chigoe B88.1
- Clonorchis (sinensis) (liver) B66.1
- coccidial A07.3
- crab-lice B85.3
- Cysticercus cellulosae — *see* Cysticercosis
- Demodex (folliculorum) B88.0
- Dermanyssus gallinae B88.0
- Dermatobia (hominis) — *see* Myiasis
- Dibothriocephalus (latus) B70.0
  - larval B70.1
- Dicrocoelium dendriticum B66.2
- Diphyllobothrium (adult) (latum) (intestinal) (pacificum) B70.0
  - larval B70.1
- Diplogonoporus (grandis) B71.8
- Dipylidium caninum B67.4
- Distoma hepaticum B66.3
- dog tapeworm B67.4
- Dracunculus medinensis B72
- dragon worm B72
- dwarf tapeworm B71.0
- Echinococcus — *see* Echinococcus
- Echinostomum ilocanum B66.8
- Entamoeba (histolytica) — *see* Infection, Ameba
- Enterobius vermicularis B80
- eyelid
  - in (due to)
    - leishmaniasis B55.1
    - loiasis B74.3
    - onchocerciasis B73.09
    - phthiriasis B85.3
  - parasitic NOS B89
- eyeworm B74.3
- Fasciola (gigantica) (hepatica) (indica) B66.3
- Fasciolopsis (buski) (intestine) B66.5
- filarial B74.9

Infestation — *continued*
  filarial — *continued*
    bancroftian B74.0
    conjunctiva B74.9
    due to
      Acanthocheilonema (perstans) (streptocerca) B74.4
      Brugia (malayi) B74.1
        timori B74.2
      Dracunculus medinensis B72
      guinea worm B72
      loa loa B74.3
      Mansonella (ozzardi) (perstans) (streptocerca) B74.4
      Onchocerca volvulus B73.00
        eye B73.00
        eyelid B73.09
      Wuchereria (bancrofti) B74.0
    Malayan B74.1
    ozzardi B74.4
    specified type NEC B74.8
  fish tapeworm B70.0
    larval B70.1
  fluke B66.9
    blood NOS — *see* Schistosomiasis
    cat liver B66.0
    intestinal B66.5
    lancet B66.2
    liver (sheep) B66.3
      cat B66.0
      Chinese B66.1
      due to clonorchiasis B66.1
      oriental B66.1
    lung (oriental) B66.4
    sheep liver B66.3
    specified type NEC B66.8
  fly larvae — *see* Myiasis
  Gasterophilus (intestinalis) — *see* Myiasis
  Gastrodiscoides hominis B66.8
  Giardia lamblia A07.1
  Gnathostoma (spinigerum) B83.1
  Gongylonema B83.8
  guinea worm B72
  helminth B83.9
    angiostrongyliasis B83.2
      intestinal B81.3
    gnathostomiasis B83.1
    hirudiniasis, internal B83.4
    intestinal B82.0
      angiostrongyliasis B81.3
      anisakiasis B81.0
      ascariasis — *see* Ascariasis
      capillariasis B81.1
      cysticercosis — *see* Cysticercosis
      diphyllobothriasis — *see* Infestation, diphyllobothriasis
      dracunculiasis B72
      echinococcus — *see* Echinococcosis
      enterobiasis B80
      filariasis — *see* Infestation, filarial
      fluke — *see* Infestation, fluke
      hookworm — *see* Infestation, hookworm
      mixed (types classifiable to more than one of the titles B65.0-B81.3 and B81.8) B81.4
      onchocerciasis — *see* Onchocerciasis
      schistosomiasis — *see* Infestation, schistosoma
      specified
        cestode NEC — *see* Infestation, cestode type NEC B81.8
      strongyloidiasis — *see* Strongyloidiasis
      taenia — *see* Infestation, taenia
      trichinellosis B75
      trichostrongyliasis B81.2
      trichuriasis B79
    specified type NEC B83.8
    syngamiasis B83.3
    visceral larva migrans B83.0
  Heterophyes (heterophyes) B66.8
  hookworm B76.9
    ancylostomiasis B76.0
    necatoriasis B76.1
    specified type NEC B76.8
  Hymenolepis (diminuta) (nana) B71.0
  intestinal NEC B82.9
  leeches (aquatic) (land) — *see* Hirudiniasis
  Leishmania — *see* Leishmaniasis
  lice, louse — *see* Infestation, Pediculus
  Linguatula B88.8

Liponyssoides sanguineus B88.0
Loa loa B74.3
  conjunctival B74.3
  eyelid B74.3
louse — *see* Infestation, Pediculus
maggots — *see* Myiasis
Mansonella (ozzardi) (perstans) (streptocerca) B74.4
Medina (worm) B72
Metagonimus (yokogawai) B66.8
microfilaria streptocerca — *see* Onchocerciasis
  eye B73.00
  eyelid B73.09
mites B88.9
  scabic B86
Monilia (albicans) — *see* Candidiasis
mouth B37.0
Necator americanus B76.1
nematode NEC (intestinal) B82.0
  Ancylostoma B76.0
  conjunctiva NEC B83.9
  Enterobius vermicularis B80
  Gnathostoma spinigerum B83.1
  physaloptera B80
  specified NEC B81.8
  trichostrongylus B81.2
  trichuris (trichuria) B79
Oesophagostomum (apiostomum) B81.8
Oestrus ovis — *see also* Myiasis B87.9
Onchocerca (volvulus) — *see* Onchocerciasis
Opisthorchis (felineus) (viverrini) B66.0
orbit, parasitic NOS B89
Oxyuris vermicularis B80
Paragonimus (westermani) B66.4
parasite, parasitic B89
  eyelid B89
  intestinal NOS B82.9
  mouth B37.0
  skin B88.9
  tongue B37.0
Parastrongylus
  cantonensis B83.2
  costaricensis B81.3
Pediculus B85.2
  body B85.1
  capitis (humanus) (any site) B85.0
  corporis (humanus) (any site) B85.1
  head B85.0
  mixed (classifiable to more than one of the titles B85.0 - B85.3) B85.4
  pubis (any site) B85.3
Pentastoma B88.8
Phthirus (pubis) (any site) B85.3
  with any infestation classifiable to B85.0 - B85.2 B85.4
pinworm B80
pork tapeworm (adult) B68.0
protozoal NEC B64
  intestinal A07.9
    specified NEC A07.8
  specified NEC B60.8
pubic, louse B85.3
rat tapeworm B71.0
red bug B88.0
roundworm (large) NEC B82.0
  Ascariasis — *see also* Ascariasis B77.9
sandflea B88.1
Sarcoptes scabiei B86
scabies B86
Schistosoma B65.9
  bovis B65.8
  cercariae B65.3
  haematobium B65.0
  intercalatum B65.8
  japonicum B65.2
  mansoni B65.1
  mattheei B65.8
  mekongi B65.8
  specified type NEC B65.8
  spindale B65.8
screw worms — *see* Myiasis
skin NOS B88.9
Sparganum (mansoni) (proliferum) (baxteri) B70.1
  larval B70.1
specified type NEC B88.8
Spirometra larvae B70.1
Stellantchasmus falcatus B66.8
Strongyloides stercoralis — *see* Strongyloidiasis

Taenia B68.9
  diminuta B71.0
  echinococcus — *see* Echinococcus
  mediocanellata B68.1
  nana B71.0
  saginata B68.1
  solium (intestinal form) B68.0
    larval form — *see* Cysticercosis
Taeniarhynchus saginatus B68.1
tapeworm B71.9
  beef B68.1
  broad B70.0
    larval B70.1
  dog B67.4
  dwarf B71.0
  fish B70.0
    larval B70.1
  pork B68.0
  rat B71.0
Ternidens diminutus B81.8
Tetranychus molestissimus B88.0
threadworm B80
tongue B37.0
Toxocara (canis) (cati) (felis) B83.0
trematode(s) NEC — *see* Infestation, fluke
Trichinella (spiralis) B75
Trichocephalus B79
Trichomonas — *see* Trichomoniasis
Trichostrongylus B81.2
Trichuris (trichiura) B79
Trombicula (irritans) B88.0
Tunga penetrans B88.1
Uncinaria americana B76.1
Vandellia cirrhosa B88.8
whipworm B79
worms B83.9
  intestinal B82.0
Wuchereria (bancrofti) B74.0
Infiltrate, infiltration
  amyloid (generalized) (localized) — *see* Amyloidosis
  calcareous NEC R89.7
    localized — *see* Degeneration, by site
  calcium salt R89.7
  cardiac
    fatty — *see* Degeneration, myocardial
    glycogenic E74.02 *[I43]*
  corneal — *see* Edema, cornea
  eyelid — *see* Inflammation, eyelid
  glycogen, glycogenic — *see* Disease, glycogen storage
  heart, cardiac
    fatty — *see* Degeneration, myocardial
    glycogenic E74.02 *[I43]*
  inflammatory in vitreous H43.89
  kidney N28.89
  leukemic — *see* Leukemia
  liver K76.89
    fatty — *see* Fatty, liver NEC
    glycogen — *see also* Disease, glycogen storage E74.03 *[K77]*
  lung R91.8
    eosinophilic J82
  lymphatic — *see also* Leukemia, lymphatic C91.9- ☑
    gland I88.9
  muscle, fatty M62.89
  myocardium, myocardial
    fatty — *see* Degeneration, myocardial
    glycogenic E74.02 *[I43]*
  on chest x-ray R91.8
  pulmonary R91.8
    with eosinophilia J82
  skin (lymphocytic) L98.6
  thymus (gland) (fatty) E32.8
  urine R39.0
  vesicant agent
    antineoplastic chemotherapy T80.810 ☑
    other agent NEC T80.818 ☑
  vitreous body H43.89
Infirmity R68.89
  senile R54
Inflammation, inflamed, inflammatory (with exudation)
  abducent (nerve) — *see* Strabismus, paralytic, sixth nerve
  accessory sinus (chronic) — *see* Sinusitis
  adrenal (gland) E27.8
  alveoli, teeth M27.3
    scorbutic E54

Inflammation, inflamed, inflammatory — *continued*
- anal canal, anus K62.89
- antrum (chronic) — *see* Sinusitis, maxillary
- appendix — *see* Appendicitis
- arachnoid — *see* Meningitis
- areola N61.0
  - puerperal, postpartum or gestational — *see* Infection, nipple
- areolar tissue NOS L08.9
- artery — *see* Arteritis
- auditory meatus (external) — *see* Otitis, externa
- Bartholin's gland N75.8
- bile duct (common) (hepatic) or passage — *see* Cholangitis
- bladder — *see* Cystitis
- bone — *see* Osteomyelitis
- brain — *see also* Encephalitis
  - membrane — *see* Meningitis
- breast N61.0
  - puerperal, postpartum, gestational — *see* Mastitis, obstetric
- broad ligament — *see* Disease, pelvis, inflammatory
- bronchi — *see* Bronchitis
- catarrhal J00
- cecum — *see* Appendicitis
- cerebral — *see also* Encephalitis
  - membrane — *see* Meningitis
- cerebrospinal
  - meningococcal A39.0
- cervix (uteri) — *see* Cervicitis
- chest J98.8
- chorioretinal H30.9- ☑
  - cyclitis — *see* Cyclitis
  - disseminated H30.10- ☑
    - generalized H30.13- ☑
    - peripheral H30.12- ☑
    - posterior pole H30.11- ☑
  - epitheliopathy — *see* Epitheliopathy
  - focal H30.00- ☑
    - juxtapapillary H30.01- ☑
    - macular H30.04- ☑
    - paramacular — *see* Inflammation, chorioretinal, focal, macular
    - peripheral H30.03- ☑
    - posterior pole H30.02- ☑
  - specified type NEC H30.89- ☑
- choroid — *see* Inflammation, chorioretinal
- chronic, postmastoidectomy cavity — *see* Complications, postmastoidectomy, inflammation
- colon — *see* Enteritis
- connective tissue (diffuse) NEC — *see* Disorder, soft tissue, specified type NEC
- cornea — *see* Keratitis
- corpora cavernosa N48.29
- cranial nerve — *see* Disorder, nerve, cranial
- Douglas' cul-de-sac or pouch (chronic) N73.0
- due to device, implant or graft — *see also* Complications, by site and type, infection or inflammation
  - arterial graft T82.7 ☑
  - breast (implant) T85.79 ☑
  - catheter T85.79 ☑
    - dialysis (renal) T82.7 ☑
      - intraperitoneal T85.71 ☑
    - infusion T82.7 ☑
      - cranial T85.735 ☑
      - intrathecal T85.735 ☑
      - spinal (epidural) (subdural) T85.735 ☑
      - subarachnoid T85.735 ☑
    - urinary T83.518 ☑
      - cystostomy T83.510 ☑
      - Hopkins T83.518 ☑
      - ileostomy T83.518 ☑
      - nephrostomy T83.512 ☑
      - specified NEC T83.518 ☑
      - urethral indwelling T83.511 ☑
      - urostomy T83.518 ☑
  - electronic (electrode) (pulse generator) (stimulator)
    - bone T84.7 ☑
    - cardiac T82.7 ☑
    - nervous system T85.738 ☑
      - brain T85.731 ☑
      - cranial nerve T85.732 ☑
      - gastric nerve T85.732 ☑
      - neurostimulator generator T85.734 ☑
      - peripheral nerve T85.732 ☑

Inflammation, inflamed, inflammatory — *continued*
- due to device, implant or graft — *see also* Complications, by site and type, infection or inflammation — *continued*
  - electronic — *continued*
    - nervous system — *continued*
      - sacral nerve T85.732 ☑
      - spinal cord T85.733 ☑
      - vagal nerve T85.732 ☑
    - urinary T83.590 ☑
  - fixation, internal (orthopedic) NEC — *see* Complication, fixation device, infection
  - gastrointestinal (bile duct) (esophagus) T85.79 ☑
    - neurostimulator electrode (lead) T85.732 ☑
  - genital NEC T83.69 ☑
  - heart NEC T82.7 ☑
    - valve (prosthesis) T82.6 ☑
      - graft T82.7 ☑
  - joint prosthesis — *see* Complication, joint prosthesis, infection
  - ocular (corneal graft) (orbital implant) NEC T85.79 ☑
  - orthopedic NEC T84.7 ☑
  - penile (cylinder) (pump) (resevoir) T83.61 ☑
  - specified NEC T85.79 ☑
  - testicular T83.62 ☑
  - urinary NEC T83.598 ☑
    - ileal conduit stent T83.593 ☑
    - implanted neurostimulation T83.590 ☑
    - implanted sphincter T83.591 ☑
    - indwelling ureteral stent T83.592 ☑
    - nephroureteral stent T83.593 ☑
    - specified stent NEC T83.593 ☑
  - vascular NEC T82.7 ☑
  - ventricular intracranial (communicating) shunt T85.730 ☑
- duodenum K29.80
  - with bleeding K29.81
- dura mater — *see* Meningitis
- ear (middle) — *see also* Otitis, media
  - external — *see* Otitis, externa
  - inner — *see* subcategory H83.0 ☑
- epididymis — *see* Epididymitis
- esophagus K20.9
- ethmoidal (sinus) (chronic) — *see* Sinusitis, ethmoidal
- eustachian tube (catarrhal) — *see* Salpingitis, eustachian
- eyelid H01.9
  - abscess — *see* Abscess, eyelid
  - blepharitis — *see* Blepharitis
  - chalazion — *see* Chalazion
  - dermatosis (noninfectious) — *see* Dermatosis, eyelid
  - hordeolum — *see* Hordeolum
  - specified NEC H01.8
- fallopian tube — *see* Salpingo-oophoritis
- fascia — *see* Myositis
- follicular, pharynx J31.2
- frontal (sinus) (chronic) — *see* Sinusitis, frontal
- gallbladder — *see* Cholecystitis
- gastric — *see* Gastritis
- gastrointestinal — *see* Enteritis
- genital organ (internal) (diffuse)
  - female — *see* Disease, pelvis, inflammatory
  - male N49.9
    - multiple sites N49.8
    - specified NEC N49.8
- gland (lymph) — *see* Lymphadenitis
- glottis — *see* Laryngitis
- granular, pharynx J31.2
- gum K05.10
  - nonplaque induced K05.11
  - plaque induced K05.10
- heart — *see* Carditis
- hepatic duct — *see* Cholangitis
- ileoanal (internal) pouch K91.850
- ileum — *see also* Enteritis
  - regional or terminal — *see* Enteritis, regional
- intestinal pouch K91.850
- intestine (any part) — *see* Enteritis
- jaw (acute) (bone) (chronic) (lower) (suppurative) (upper) M27.2
- joint NEC — *see* Arthritis
  - sacroiliac M46.1
- kidney — *see* Nephritis
- knee (joint) M13.169
  - tuberculous A18.02
- labium (majus) (minus) — *see* Vulvitis

Inflammation, inflamed, inflammatory — *continued*
- lacrimal
  - gland — *see* Dacryoadenitis
  - passages (duct) (sac) — *see also* Dacryocystitis
    - canaliculitis — *see* Canaliculitis, lacrimal
- larynx — *see* Laryngitis
- leg NOS L08.9
- lip K13.0
- liver (capsule) — *see also* Hepatitis
  - chronic K73.9
  - suppurative K75.0
- lung (acute) — *see also* Pneumonia
  - chronic J98.4
- lymph gland or node — *see* Lymphadenitis
- lymphatic vessel — *see* Lymphangitis
- maxilla, maxillary M27.2
  - sinus (chronic) — *see* Sinusitis, maxillary
- membranes of brain or spinal cord — *see* Meningitis
- meninges — *see* Meningitis
- mouth K12.1
- muscle — *see* Myositis
- myocardium — *see* Myocarditis
- nasal sinus (chronic) — *see* Sinusitis
- nasopharynx — *see* Nasopharyngitis
- navel L08.82
- nerve NEC — *see* Neuralgia
- nipple N61.0
  - puerperal, postpartum or gestational — *see* Infection, nipple
- nose — *see* Rhinitis
- oculomotor (nerve) — *see* Strabismus, paralytic, third nerve
- optic nerve — *see* Neuritis, optic
- orbit (chronic) H05.10
  - acute H05.00
    - abscess — *see* Abscess, orbit
    - cellulitis — *see* Cellulitis, orbit
    - osteomyelitis — *see* Osteomyelitis, orbit
    - periostitis — *see* Periostitis, orbital
    - tenonitis — *see* Tenonitis, eye
  - granuloma — *see* Granuloma, orbit
  - myositis — *see* Myositis, orbital
- ovary — *see* Salpingo-oophoritis
- oviduct — *see* Salpingo-oophoritis
- pancreas (acute) — *see* Pancreatitis
- parametrium N73.0
- parotid region L08.9
- pelvis, female — *see* Disease, pelvis, inflammatory
- penis (corpora cavernosa) N48.29
- perianal K62.89
- pericardium — *see* Pericarditis
- perineum (female) (male) L08.9
- perirectal K62.89
- peritoneum — *see* Peritonitis
- periuterine — *see* Disease, pelvis, inflammatory
- perivesical — *see* Cystitis
- petrous bone (acute) (chronic) — *see* Petrositis
- pharynx (acute) — *see* Pharyngitis
- pia mater — *see* Meningitis
- pleura — *see* Pleurisy
- polyp, colon — *see also* Polyp, colon, inflammatory K51.40
- prostate — *see also* Prostatitis
  - specified type NEC N41.8
- rectosigmoid — *see* Rectosigmoiditis
- rectum — *see also* Proctitis K62.89
- respiratory, upper — *see also* Infection, respiratory, upper J06.9
  - acute, due to radiation J70.0
  - chronic, due to external agent — *see* condition, respiratory, chronic, due to
  - due to
    - chemicals, gases, fumes or vapors (inhalation) J68.2
    - radiation J70.1
- retina — *see* Chorioretinitis
- retrocecal — *see* Appendicitis
- retroperitoneal — *see* Peritonitis
- salivary duct or gland (any) (suppurative) — *see* Sialoadenitis
- scorbutic, alveoli, teeth E54
- scrotum N49.2
- seminal vesicle — *see* Vesiculitis
- sigmoid — *see* Enteritis
- sinus — *see* Sinusitis
- Skene's duct or gland — *see* Urethritis

Inflammation, inflamed, inflammatory — *continued*
skin L08.9
spermatic cord N49.1
sphenoidal (sinus) — *see* Sinusitis, sphenoidal
spinal
  cord — *see* Encephalitis
  membrane — *see* Meningitis
  nerve — *see* Disorder, nerve
spine — *see* Spondylopathy, inflammatory
spleen (capsule) D73.89
stomach — *see* Gastritis
subcutaneous tissue L08.9
suprarenal (gland) E27.8
synovial — *see* Tenosynovitis
tendon (sheath) NEC — *see* Tenosynovitis
testis — *see* Orchitis
throat (acute) — *see* Pharyngitis
thymus (gland) E32.8
thyroid (gland) — *see* Thyroiditis
tongue K14.0
tonsil — *see* Tonsillitis
trachea — *see* Tracheitis
trochlear (nerve) — *see* Strabismus, paralytic, fourth
  nerve
tubal — *see* Salpingo-oophoritis
tuberculous NEC — *see* Tuberculosis
tubo-ovarian — *see* Salpingo-oophoritis
tunica vaginalis N49.1
tympanic membrane — *see* Tympanitis
umbilicus, umbilical L08.82
uterine ligament — *see* Disease, pelvis, inflammatory
uterus (catarrhal) — *see* Endometritis
uveal tract (anterior) NOS — *see also* Iridocyclitis
  posterior — *see* Chorioretinitis
vagina — *see* Vaginitis
vas deferens N49.1
vein — *see also* Phlebitis
  intracranial or intraspinal (septic) G08
  thrombotic I80.9
    leg — *see* Phlebitis, leg
    lower extremity — *see* Phlebitis, leg
vocal cord J38.3
vulva — *see* Vulvitis
Wharton's duct (suppurative) — *see* Sialoadenitis
Inflation, lung, imperfect (newborn) — *see* Atelectasis
Influenza (bronchial) (epidemic) (respiratory (upper))
  (unidentified influenza virus) J11.1
  with
    digestive manifestations J11.2
    encephalopathy J11.81
    enteritis J11.2
    gastroenteritis J11.2
    gastrointestinal manifestations J11.2
    laryngitis J11.1
    myocarditis J11.82
    otitis media J11.83
    pharyngitis J11.1
    pneumonia J11.00
      specified type J11.08
    respiratory manifestations NEC J11.1
    specified manifestation NEC J11.89
  A/H5N1 — *see also* Influenza, due to, identified novel
    influenza A virus J09.X2
  avian — *see also* Influenza, due to, identified novel in-
    fluenza A virus J09.X2
  bird — *see also* Influenza, due to, identified novel in-
    fluenza A virus J09.X2
  novel (2009) H1N1 influenza — *see also* Influenza, due
    to, identified influenza virus NEC J10.1
  novel influenza A/H1N1 — *see also* Influenza, due to,
    identified influenza virus NEC J10.1
  due to
    avian — *see also* Influenza, due to, identified novel
      influenza A virus J09.X2
    identified influenza virus NEC J10.1
      with
        digestive manifestations J10.2
        encephalopathy J10.81
        enteritis J10.2
        gastroenteritis J10.2
        gastrointestinal manifestations J10.2
        laryngitis J10.1
        myocarditis J10.82
        otitis media J10.83
        pharyngitis J10.1
        pneumonia (unspecified type) J10.00

Influenza — *continued*
due to — *continued*
  identified influenza virus — *continued*
    with — *continued*
      pneumonia — *continued*
        with same identified influenza virus
          J10.01
        specified type NEC J10.08
      respiratory manifestations NEC J10.1
      specified manifestation NEC J10.89
  identified novel influenza A virus J09.X2
    with
      digestive manifestations J09.X3
      encephalopathy J09.X9
      enteritis J09.X3
      gastroenteritis J09.X3
      gastrointestinal manifestations J09.X3
      laryngitis J09.X2
      myocarditis J09.X9
      otitis media J09.X9
      pharyngitis J09.X2
      pneumonia J09.X1
      respiratory manifestations NEC J09.X2
      specified manifestation NEC J09.X9
      upper respiratory symptoms J09.X2
  of other animal origin, not bird or swine — *see also*
    Influenza, due to, identified novel influenza A
    virus J09.X2
  swine (viruses that normally cause infections in pigs)
    — *see also* Influenza, due to, identified novel
    influenza A virus J09.X2
Influenzal — *see* Influenza
Influenza-like disease — *see* Influenza
Infraction, Freiberg's (metatarsal head) — *see* Osteochondrosis, juvenile, metatarsus
Infraeruption of tooth (teeth) M26.34
Infusion complication, misadventure, or reaction —
  see Complications, infusion
Ingestion
chemical — *see* Table of Drugs and Chemicals, by
  substance, poisoning
drug or medicament
  correct substance properly administered — *see* Ta-
    ble of Drugs and Chemicals, by drug, adverse
    effect
  overdose or wrong substance given or taken — *see*
    Table of Drugs and Chemicals, by drug, poi-
    soning
foreign body — *see* Foreign body, alimentary tract
multiple drug — *see* Table of Drugs and Chemicals,
  multiple
tularemia A21.3
Ingrowing
hair (beard) L73.1
nail (finger) (toe) L60.0
Inguinal — *see also* condition
testicle Q53.9
  bilateral Q53.212
  unilateral Q53.112
Inhalant-induced
anxiety disorder F18.980
depressive disorder F18.94
major neurocognitive disorder F18.97
mild neurocognitive disorder F18.988
psychotic disorder F18.959
Inhalation
anthrax A22.1
flame T27.3 ☑
food or foreign body — *see* Foreign body, by site
gases, fumes, or vapors NEC T59.9- ☑
  specified agent — *see* Table of Drugs and Chemicals,
    by substance
liquid or vomitus — *see* Asphyxia
meconium (newborn) P24.00
  with
    with respiratory symptoms P24.01
    pneumonia (pneumonitis) P24.01
mucus — *see* Asphyxia, mucus
oil or gasoline (causing suffocation) — *see* Foreign
  body, by site
smoke J70.5
  due to chemicals, gases, fumes and vapors J68.9
steam — *see* Toxicity, vapors
stomach contents or secretions — *see* Foreign body,
  by site
  due to anesthesia (general) (local) or other sedation
    T88.59 ☑
    in labor and delivery O74.0

Inhalation — *continued*
stomach contents or secretions — *see* Foreign body,
  by site — *continued*
  due to anesthesia or other sedation — *continued*
    in pregnancy O29.01- ☑
    postpartum, puerperal O89.01
Inhibition, orgasm
female F52.31
male F52.32
Inhibitor, systemic lupus erythematosus (presence
  of) D68.62
Iniencephalus, iniencephaly Q00.2
Injection, traumatic jet (air) (industrial) (water) (paint
  or dye) T70.4 ☑
Injury — *see also* specified injury type T14.90 ☑
abdomen, abdominal S39.91 ☑
  blood vessel — *see* Injury, blood vessel, abdomen
  cavity — *see* Injury, intra-abdominal
  contusion S30.1 ☑
  internal — *see* Injury, intra-abdominal
  intra-abdominal organ — *see* Injury, intra-abdomi-
    nal
  nerve — *see* Injury, nerve, abdomen
  open — *see* Wound, open, abdomen
  specified NEC S39.81 ☑
  superficial — *see* Injury, superficial, abdomen
Achilles tendon S86.00- ☑
  laceration S86.02- ☑
  specified type NEC S86.09- ☑
  strain S86.01- ☑
acoustic, resulting in deafness — *see* Injury, nerve,
  acoustic
adrenal (gland) S37.819 ☑
  contusion S37.812 ☑
  laceration S37.813 ☑
  specified type NEC S37.818 ☑
alveolar (process) S09.93 ☑
ankle S99.91- ☑
  contusion — *see* Contusion, ankle
  dislocation — *see* Dislocation, ankle
  fracture — *see* Fracture, ankle
  nerve — *see* Injury, nerve, ankle
  open — *see* Wound, open, ankle
  specified type NEC S99.81- ☑
  sprain — *see* Sprain, ankle
  superficial — *see* Injury, superficial, ankle
anterior chamber, eye — *see* Injury, eye, specified site
  NEC
anus — *see* Injury, abdomen
aorta (thoracic) S25.00 ☑
  abdominal S35.00 ☑
    laceration (minor) (superficial) S35.01 ☑
      major S35.02 ☑
    specified type NEC S35.09 ☑
  laceration (minor) (superficial) S25.01 ☑
    major S25.02 ☑
  specified type NEC S25.09 ☑
arm (upper) S49.9- ☑
  blood vessel — *see* Injury, blood vessel, arm
  contusion — *see* Contusion, arm, upper
  fracture — *see* Fracture, humerus
  lower — *see* Injury, forearm
  muscle — *see* Injury, muscle, shoulder
  nerve — *see* Injury, nerve, arm
  open — *see* Wound, open, arm
  specified type NEC S49.8- ☑
  superficial — *see* Injury, superficial, arm
artery (complicating trauma) — *see also* Injury, blood
  vessel, by site
  cerebral or meningeal — *see* Injury, intracranial
auditory canal (external) (meatus) S09.91 ☑
auricle, auris, ear S09.91 ☑
axilla — *see* Injury, shoulder
back — *see* Injury, back, lower
bile duct S36.13 ☑
birth — *see also* Birth, injury P15.9
bladder (sphincter) S37.20 ☑
  at delivery O71.5
  contusion S37.22 ☑
  laceration S37.23 ☑
  obstetrical trauma O71.5
  specified type NEC S37.29 ☑
blast (air) (hydraulic) (immersion) (underwater) NEC
  T14.8 ☑
  acoustic nerve trauma — *see* Injury, nerve, acoustic
  bladder — *see* Injury, bladder

☑ Additional Character Required — Refer to the Tabular List for Character Selection   ▽ Subterms under main terms may continue to next column or page

Injury — continued
  blast — continued
    brain — see Concussion
    colon — see Injury, intestine, large
    ear (primary) S09.31- ☑
      secondary S09.39- ☑
    generalized T70.8 ☑
    lung — see Injury, intrathoracic, lung
    multiple body organs T70.8 ☑
    peritoneum S36.81 ☑
    rectum S36.61 ☑
    retroperitoneum S36.898 ☑
    small intestine S36.419 ☑
      duodenum S36.410 ☑
      specified site NEC S36.418 ☑
    specified
      intra-abdominal organ NEC S36.898 ☑
      pelvic organ NEC S37.899 ☑
  blood vessel NEC T14.8 ☑
    abdomen S35.9 ☑
      aorta — see Injury, aorta, abdominal
      celiac artery — see Injury, blood vessel, celiac
        artery
      iliac vessel — see Injury, blood vessel, iliac
      laceration S35.91
      mesenteric vessel — see Injury, mesenteric
      portal vein — see Injury, blood vessel, portal vein
      renal vessel — see Injury, blood vessel, renal
      specified vessel NEC S35.8X-
      splenic vessel — see Injury, blood vessel, splenic
      vena cava — see Injury, vena cava, inferior
    ankle — see Injury, blood vessel, foot
    aorta (abdominal) (thoracic) — see Injury, aorta
    arm (upper) NEC S45.90- ☑
      forearm — see Injury, blood vessel, forearm
      laceration S45.91- ☑
      specified
        site NEC S45.80- ☑
          laceration S45.81- ☑
          specified type NEC S45.89- ☑
        type NEC S45.99- ☑
      superficial vein S45.30- ☑
        laceration S45.31- ☑
        specified type NEC S45.39- ☑
    axillary
      artery S45.00- ☑
        laceration S45.01- ☑
        specified type NEC S45.09- ☑
      vein S45.20- ☑
        laceration S45.21- ☑
        specified type NEC S45.29- ☑
    azygos vein — see Injury, blood vessel, thoracic,
      specified site NEC
    brachial
      artery S45.10- ☑
        laceration S45.11- ☑
        specified type NEC S45.19- ☑
      vein S45.20- ☑
        laceration S45.219 ☑
        specified type NEC S45.29- ☑
    carotid artery (common) (external) (internal, extracra-
      nial) S15.00- ☑
      internal, intracranial S06.8- ☑
      laceration (minor) (superficial) S15.01- ☑
        major S15.02- ☑
      specified type NEC S15.09- ☑
    celiac artery S35.219 ☑
      branch S35.299 ☑
        laceration (minor) (superficial) S35.291 ☑
          major S35.292 ☑
        specified NEC S35.298 ☑
      laceration (minor) (superficial) S35.211 ☑
        major S35.212 ☑
      specified type NEC S35.218 ☑
    cerebral — see Injury, intracranial
    deep plantar — see Injury, blood vessel, plantar
      artery
    digital (hand) — see Injury, blood vessel, finger
    dorsal
      artery (foot) S95.00- ☑
        laceration S95.01- ☑
        specified type NEC S95.09- ☑
      vein (foot) S95.20- ☑
        laceration S95.21- ☑
        specified type NEC S95.29- ☑

Injury — continued
  blood vessel — continued
    due to accidental laceration during procedure —
      see Laceration, accidental complicating
      surgery
    extremity — see Injury, blood vessel, limb
    femoral
      artery (common) (superficial) S75.00- ☑
        laceration (minor) (superficial) S75.01- ☑
          major S75.02- ☑
        specified type NEC S75.09- ☑
      vein (hip level) (thigh level) S75.10- ☑
        laceration (minor) (superficial) S75.11- ☑
          major S75.12- ☑
        specified type NEC S75.19- ☑
    finger S65.50- ☑
      index S65.50- ☑
        laceration S65.51- ☑
        specified type NEC S65.59- ☑
      laceration S65.51- ☑
      little S65.50- ☑
        laceration S65.51- ☑
        specified type NEC S65.59- ☑
      middle S65.50- ☑
        laceration S65.51- ☑
        specified type NEC S65.59- ☑
      specified type NEC S65.59- ☑
      thumb — see Injury, blood vessel, thumb
    foot S95.90- ☑
      dorsal
        artery — see Injury, blood vessel, dorsal,
          artery
        vein — see Injury, blood vessel, dorsal, vein
      laceration S95.91- ☑
      plantar artery — see Injury, blood vessel, plantar
        artery
      specified
        site NEC S95.80- ☑
          laceration S95.81- ☑
          specified type NEC S95.89- ☑
        specified type NEC S95.99- ☑
    forearm S55.90- ☑
      laceration S55.91- ☑
      radial artery — see Injury, blood vessel, radial
        artery
      specified
        site NEC S55.80- ☑
          laceration S55.81- ☑
          specified type NEC S55.89- ☑
        type NEC S55.99- ☑
      ulnar artery — see Injury, blood vessel, ulnar
        artery
      vein S55.20- ☑
        laceration S55.21- ☑
        specified type NEC S55.29- ☑
    gastric
      artery — see Injury, mesenteric, artery, branch
      vein — see Injury, blood vessel, abdomen
    gastroduodenal artery — see Injury, mesenteric,
      artery, branch
    greater saphenous vein (lower leg level) S85.30- ☑
      hip (and thigh) level S75.20- ☑
        laceration (minor) (superficial) S75.21- ☑
          major S75.22- ☑
        specified type NEC S75.29- ☑
      laceration S85.31- ☑
      specified type NEC S85.39- ☑
    hand (level) S65.90- ☑
      finger — see Injury, blood vessel, finger
      laceration S65.91- ☑
      palmar arch — see Injury, blood vessel, palmar
        arch
      radial artery — see Injury, blood vessel, radial
        artery, hand
      specified
        site NEC S65.80- ☑
          laceration S65.81- ☑
          specified type NEC S65.89- ☑
        type NEC S65.99- ☑
      thumb — see Injury, blood vessel, thumb
      ulnar artery — see Injury, blood vessel, ulnar
        artery, hand
    head S09.0 ☑
      intracranial — see Injury, intracranial
      multiple S09.0 ☑

Injury — continued
  blood vessel — continued
    hepatic
      artery — see Injury, mesenteric, artery
      vein — see Injury, vena cava, inferior
    hip S75.90- ☑
      femoral artery — see Injury, blood vessel,
        femoral, artery
      femoral vein — see Injury, blood vessel, femoral,
        vein
      greater saphenous vein — see Injury, blood ves-
        sel, greater saphenous, hip level
      laceration S75.91- ☑
      specified
        site NEC S75.80- ☑
          laceration S75.81- ☑
          specified type NEC S75.89- ☑
        type NEC S75.99- ☑
    hypogastric (artery) (vein) — see Injury, blood ves-
      sel, iliac
    iliac S35.5- ☑
      artery S35.51- ☑
      specified vessel NEC S35.5- ☑
      uterine vessel — see Injury, blood vessel, uterine
      vein S35.51- ☑
    innominate — see Injury, blood vessel, thoracic, in-
      nominate
    intercostal (artery) (vein) — see Injury, blood vessel,
      thoracic, intercostal
    jugular vein (external) S15.20- ☑
      internal S15.30- ☑
        laceration (minor) (superficial) S15.31- ☑
          major S15.32- ☑
        specified type NEC S15.39- ☑
      laceration (minor) (superficial) S15.21- ☑
        major S15.22- ☑
      specified type NEC S15.29- ☑
    leg (level) (lower) S85.90- ☑
      greater saphenous — see Injury, blood vessel,
        greater saphenous
      laceration S85.91- ☑
      lesser saphenous — see Injury, blood vessel,
        lesser saphenous
      peroneal artery — see Injury, blood vessel, per-
        oneal artery
      popliteal
        artery — see Injury, blood vessel, popliteal,
          artery
        vein — see Injury, blood vessel, popliteal, vein
      specified
        site NEC S85.80- ☑
          laceration S85.81- ☑
          specified type NEC S85.89- ☑
        type NEC S85.99- ☑
      thigh — see Injury, blood vessel, hip
      tibial artery — see Injury, blood vessel, tibial
        artery
    lesser saphenous vein (lower leg level) S85.40- ☑
      laceration S85.41- ☑
      specified type NEC S85.49- ☑
    limb
      lower — see Injury, blood vessel, leg
      upper — see Injury, blood vessel, arm
    lower back — see Injury, blood vessel, abdomen
      specified NEC — see Injury, blood vessel, ab-
        domen, specified, site NEC
    mammary (artery) (vein) — see Injury, blood vessel,
      thoracic, specified site NEC
    mesenteric (inferior) (superior)
      artery — see Injury, mesenteric, artery
      vein — see Injury, blood vessel, mesenteric, vein
    neck S15.9 ☑
      specified site NEC S15.8 ☑
    ovarian (artery) (vein) — see subcategory S35.8 ☑
    palmar arch (superficial) S65.20- ☑
      deep S65.30- ☑
        laceration S65.31- ☑
        specified type NEC S65.39- ☑
      laceration S65.21- ☑
      specified type NEC S65.29- ☑
    pelvis — see Injury, blood vessel, abdomen
      specified NEC — see Injury, blood vessel, ab-
        domen, specified, site NEC
    peroneal artery S85.20- ☑
      laceration S85.21- ☑
      specified type NEC S85.29- ☑

▽ **Subterms under main terms may continue to next column or page**   ☑ **Additional Character Required — Refer to the Tabular List for Character Selection**   **191**

Injury — Injury

Injury — *continued*
　blood vessel — *continued*
　　plantar artery (deep) (foot) S95.10- ☑
　　　laceration S95.11- ☑
　　　specified type NEC S95.19- ☑
　　popliteal
　　　artery S85.00- ☑
　　　　laceration S85.01- ☑
　　　　specified type NEC S85.09- ☑
　　　vein S85.50- ☑
　　　　laceration S85.51- ☑
　　　　specified type NEC S85.59- ☑
　　portal vein S35.319 ☑
　　　laceration S35.311 ☑
　　　specified type NEC S35.318 ☑
　　precerebral — *see* Injury, blood vessel, neck
　　pulmonary (artery) (vein) — *see* Injury, blood vessel, thoracic, pulmonary
　　radial artery (forearm level) S55.10- ☑
　　　hand and wrist (level) S65.10- ☑
　　　　laceration S65.11- ☑
　　　　specified type NEC S65.19- ☑
　　　laceration S55.11- ☑
　　　specified type NEC S55.19- ☑
　　renal
　　　artery S35.40- ☑
　　　　laceration S35.41- ☑
　　　　specified NEC S35.49- ☑
　　　vein S35.40- ☑
　　　　laceration S35.41- ☑
　　　　specified NEC S35.49- ☑
　　saphenous vein (greater) (lower leg level) — *see* Injury, blood vessel, greater saphenous
　　　hip and thigh level — *see* Injury, blood vessel, greater saphenous, hip level
　　　lesser — *see* Injury, blood vessel, lesser saphenous
　　shoulder
　　　specified NEC — *see* Injury, blood vessel, arm, specified site NEC
　　　superficial vein — *see* Injury, blood vessel, arm, superficial vein
　　specified NEC T14.8 ☑
　　splenic
　　　artery — *see* Injury, blood vessel, celiac artery, branch
　　　vein S35.329 ☑
　　　　laceration S35.321 ☑
　　　　specified NEC S35.328 ☑
　　subclavian — *see* Injury, blood vessel, thoracic, innominate
　　thigh — *see* Injury, blood vessel, hip
　　thoracic S25.90 ☑
　　　aorta S25.00 ☑
　　　　laceration (minor) (superficial) S25.01 ☑
　　　　　major S25.02 ☑
　　　　specified type NEC S25.09 ☑
　　　azygos vein — *see* Injury, blood vessel, thoracic, specified, site NEC
　　　innominate
　　　　artery S25.10- ☑
　　　　　laceration (minor) (superficial) S25.11- ☑
　　　　　　major S25.12- ☑
　　　　　specified type NEC S25.19- ☑
　　　　vein S25.30- ☑
　　　　　laceration (minor) (superficial) S25.31- ☑
　　　　　　major S25.32- ☑
　　　　　specified type NEC S25.39- ☑
　　　intercostal S25.50- ☑
　　　　laceration S25.51- ☑
　　　　specified type NEC S25.59- ☑
　　　laceration S25.91 ☑
　　　mammary vessel — *see* Injury, blood vessel, thoracic, specified, site NEC
　　　pulmonary S25.40- ☑
　　　　laceration (minor) (superficial) S25.41- ☑
　　　　　major S25.42- ☑
　　　　specified type NEC S25.49- ☑
　　　specified
　　　　site NEC S25.80- ☑
　　　　　laceration S25.81 ☑
　　　　　specified type NEC S25.89 ☑
　　　　type NEC S25.99 ☑
　　　subclavian — *see* Injury, blood vessel, thoracic, innominate
　　　vena cava (superior) S25.20 ☑

Injury — *continued*
　blood vessel — *continued*
　　thoracic — *continued*
　　　vena cava — *continued*
　　　　laceration (minor) (superficial) S25.21 ☑
　　　　　major S25.22 ☑
　　　　specified type NEC S25.29 ☑
　　thumb S65.40- ☑
　　　laceration S65.41- ☑
　　　specified type NEC S65.49- ☑
　　tibial artery S85.10- ☑
　　　anterior S85.13- ☑
　　　　laceration S85.14- ☑
　　　　specified injury NEC S85.15- ☑
　　　laceration S85.11- ☑
　　　posterior S85.16- ☑
　　　　laceration S85.17- ☑
　　　　specified injury NEC S85.18- ☑
　　　specified injury NEC S85.12- ☑
　　ulnar artery (forearm level) S55.00- ☑
　　　hand and wrist (level) S65.00- ☑
　　　　laceration S65.01- ☑
　　　　specified type NEC S65.09- ☑
　　　laceration S55.01- ☑
　　　specified type NEC S55.09- ☑
　　upper arm (level) — *see* Injury, blood vessel, arm
　　　superficial vein — *see* Injury, blood vessel, arm, superficial vein
　　uterine S35.5- ☑
　　　artery S35.53- ☑
　　　vein S35.53- ☑
　　vena cava — *see* Injury, vena cava
　　vertebral artery S15.10- ☑
　　　laceration (minor) (superficial) S15.11- ☑
　　　　major S15.12- ☑
　　　specified type NEC S15.19- ☑
　　wrist (level) — *see* Injury, blood vessel, hand
　brachial plexus S14.3 ☑
　　newborn P14.3
　brain (traumatic) S06.9- ☑
　　diffuse (axonal) S06.2X- ☑
　　focal S06.30- ☑
　brainstem S06.38- ☑
　breast NOS S29.9 ☑
　broad ligament — *see* Injury, pelvic organ, specified site NEC
　bronchus, bronchi — *see* Injury, intrathoracic, bronchus
　brow S09.90 ☑
　buttock S39.92 ☑
　canthus, eye S05.90 ☑
　cardiac plexus — *see* Injury, nerve, thorax, sympathetic
　cauda equina S34.3 ☑
　cavernous sinus — *see* Injury, intracranial
　cecum — *see* Injury, colon
　celiac ganglion or plexus — *see* Injury, nerve, lumbosacral, sympathetic
　cerebellum — *see* Injury, intracranial
　cerebral — *see* Injury, intracranial
　cervix (uteri) — *see* Injury, uterus
　cheek (wall) S09.93 ☑
　chest — *see* Injury, thorax
　childbirth (newborn) — *see also* Birth, injury
　　maternal NEC O71.9
　chin S09.93 ☑
　choroid (eye) — *see* Injury, eye, specified site NEC
　clitoris S39.94 ☑
　coccyx — *see also* Injury, back, lower
　　complicating delivery O71.6
　colon — *see* Injury, intestine, large
　common bile duct — *see* Injury, liver
　conjunctiva (superficial) — *see* Injury, eye, conjunctiva
　conus medullaris — *see* Injury, spinal, sacral
　cord
　　spermatic (pelvic region) S37.898 ☑
　　　scrotal region S39.848 ☑
　　spinal — *see* Injury, spinal cord, by region
　cornea — *see* Injury, eye, specified site NEC
　　abrasion — *see* Injury, eye, cornea, abrasion
　cortex (cerebral) — *see also* Injury, intracranial
　　visual — *see* Injury, nerve, optic
　costal region NEC S29.9 ☑
　costochondral NEC S29.9 ☑
　cranial
　　cavity — *see* Injury, intracranial
　　nerve — *see* Injury, nerve, cranial
　crushing — *see* Crush

Injury — *continued*
　cutaneous sensory nerve
　cystic duct — *see* Injury, liver
　deep tissue — *see* Contusion, by site
　　meaning pressure ulcer — *see* Ulcer, pressure, unstageable, by site
　delivery (newborn) P15.9
　　maternal NEC O71.9
　Descemet's membrane — *see* Injury, eyeball, penetrating
　diaphragm — *see* Injury, intrathoracic, diaphragm
　duodenum — *see* Injury, intestine, small, duodenum
　ear (auricle) (external) (canal) S09.91 ☑
　　abrasion — *see* Abrasion, ear
　　bite — *see* Bite, ear
　　blister — *see* Blister, ear
　　bruise — *see* Contusion, ear
　　contusion — *see* Contusion, ear
　　external constriction — *see* Constriction, external, ear
　　hematoma — *see* Hematoma, ear
　　inner — *see* Injury, ear, middle
　　laceration — *see* Laceration, ear
　　middle S09.30- ☑
　　　blast — *see* Injury, blast, ear
　　　specified NEC S09.39- ☑
　　puncture — *see* Puncture, ear
　　superficial — *see* Injury, superficial, ear
　eighth cranial nerve (acoustic or auditory) — *see* Injury, nerve, acoustic
　elbow S59.90- ☑
　　contusion — *see* Contusion, elbow
　　dislocation — *see* Dislocation, elbow
　　fracture — *see* Fracture, ulna, upper end
　　open — *see* Wound, open, elbow
　　specified NEC S59.80- ☑
　　sprain — *see* Sprain, elbow
　　superficial — *see* Injury, superficial, elbow
　eleventh cranial nerve (accessory) — *see* Injury, nerve, accessory
　epididymis S39.94 ☑
　epigastric region S39.91 ☑
　epiglottis NEC S19.89 ☑
　esophageal plexus — *see* Injury, nerve, thorax, sympathetic
　esophagus (thoracic part) — *see also* Injury, intrathoracic, esophagus
　　cervical NEC S19.85 ☑
　eustachian tube S09.30 ☑
　eye S05.9- ☑
　　avulsion S05.7- ☑
　　ball — *see* Injury, eyeball
　　conjunctiva S05.0- ☑
　　cornea
　　　abrasion S05.0- ☑
　　　laceration S05.3- ☑
　　　　with prolapse S05.2- ☑
　　lacrimal apparatus S05.8X- ☑
　　orbit penetration S05.4- ☑
　　specified site NEC S05.8X- ☑
　eyeball S05.8X- ☑
　　contusion S05.1- ☑
　　penetrating S05.6- ☑
　　　with
　　　　foreign body S05.5- ☑
　　　　prolapse or loss of intraocular tissue S05.2- ☑
　　　　without prolapse or loss of intraocular tissue S05.3- ☑
　　　specified type NEC S05.8- ☑
　eyebrow S09.93 ☑
　eyelid S09.93 ☑
　　abrasion — *see* Abrasion, eyelid
　　contusion — *see* Contusion, eyelid
　　open — *see* Wound, open, eyelid
　face S09.93 ☑
　fallopian tube S37.509 ☑
　　bilateral S37.502 ☑
　　　blast injury S37.512 ☑
　　　contusion S37.522 ☑
　　　laceration S37.532 ☑
　　　specified type NEC S37.592 ☑
　　blast injury (primary) S37.519 ☑
　　　bilateral S37.512 ☑
　　　secondary — *see* Injury, fallopian tube, specified type NEC
　　　unilateral S37.511 ☑

Injury — *continued*
- fallopian tube — *continued*
  - contusion S37.529 ☑
    - bilateral S37.522 ☑
    - unilateral S37.521 ☑
  - laceration S37.539 ☑
    - bilateral S37.532 ☑
    - unilateral S37.531 ☑
  - specified type NEC S37.599 ☑
    - bilateral S37.592 ☑
    - unilateral S37.591 ☑
  - unilateral S37.501 ☑
    - blast injury S37.511 ☑
    - contusion S37.521 ☑
    - laceration S37.531 ☑
    - specified type NEC S37.591 ☑
- fascia — *see* Injury, muscle
- fifth cranial nerve (trigeminal) — *see* Injury, nerve, trigeminal
- finger (nail) S69.9- ☑
  - blood vessel — *see* Injury, blood vessel, finger
  - contusion — *see* Contusion, finger
  - dislocation — *see* Dislocation, finger
  - fracture — *see* Fracture, finger
  - muscle — *see* Injury, muscle, finger
  - nerve — *see* Injury, nerve, digital, finger
  - open — *see* Wound, open, finger
  - specified NEC S69.8- ☑
  - sprain — *see* Sprain, finger
  - superficial — *see* Injury, superficial, finger
- first cranial nerve (olfactory) — *see* Injury, nerve, olfactory
- flank — *see* Injury, abdomen
- foot S99.92- ☑
  - blood vessel — *see* Injury, blood vessel, foot
  - contusion — *see* Contusion, foot
  - dislocation — *see* Dislocation, foot
  - fracture — *see* Fracture, foot
  - muscle — *see* Injury, muscle, foot
  - open — *see* Wound, open, foot
  - specified type NEC S99.82- ☑
  - sprain — *see* Sprain, foot
  - superficial — *see* Injury, superficial, foot
- forceps NOS P15.9
- forearm S59.91- ☑
  - blood vessel — *see* Injury, blood vessel, forearm
  - contusion — *see* Contusion, forearm
  - fracture — *see* Fracture, forearm
  - muscle — *see* Injury, muscle, forearm
  - nerve — *see* Injury, nerve, forearm
  - open — *see* Wound, open, forearm
  - specified NEC S59.81- ☑
  - superficial — *see* Injury, superficial, forearm
- forehead S09.90 ☑
- fourth cranial nerve (trochlear) — *see* Injury, nerve, trochlear
- gallbladder S36.129 ☑
  - contusion S36.122 ☑
  - laceration S36.123 ☑
  - specified NEC S36.128 ☑
- ganglion
  - celiac, coeliac — *see* Injury, nerve, lumbosacral, sympathetic
  - gasserian — *see* Injury, nerve, trigeminal
  - stellate — *see* Injury, nerve, thorax, sympathetic
  - thoracic sympathetic — *see* Injury, nerve, thorax, sympathetic
- gasserian ganglion — *see* Injury, nerve, trigeminal
- gastric artery — *see* Injury, blood vessel, celiac artery, branch
- gastroduodenal artery — *see* Injury, blood vessel, celiac artery, branch
- gastrointestinal tract — *see* Injury, intra-abdominal
  - with open wound into abdominal cavity — *see* Wound, open, with penetration into peritoneal cavity
  - colon — *see* Injury, intestine, large
  - rectum — *see* Injury, intestine, large, rectum
    - with open wound into abdominal cavity S36.61 ☑
  - small intestine — *see* Injury, intestine, small
  - specified site NEC — *see* Injury, intra-abdominal, specified, site NEC
  - stomach — *see* Injury, stomach
- genital organ(s)
  - external S39.94 ☑

Injury — *continued*
- genital organ(s) — *continued*
  - external — *continued*
    - specified NEC S39.848 ☑
  - internal S37.90 ☑
    - fallopian tube — *see* Injury, fallopian tube
    - ovary — *see* Injury, ovary
    - prostate — *see* Injury, prostate
    - seminal vesicle — *see* Injury, pelvis, organ, specified site NEC
    - uterus — *see* Injury, uterus
    - vas deferens — *see* Injury, pelvis, organ, specified site NEC
  - obstetrical trauma O71.9
- gland
  - lacrimal laceration — *see* Injury, eye, specified site NEC
  - salivary S09.93 ☑
  - thyroid NEC S19.84 ☑
- globe (eye) S05.90 ☑
  - specified NEC S05.8X- ☑
- groin — *see* Injury, abdomen
- gum S09.90 ☑
- hand S69.9- ☑
  - blood vessel — *see* Injury, blood vessel, hand
  - contusion — *see* Contusion, hand
  - fracture — *see* Fracture, hand
  - muscle — *see* Injury, muscle, hand
  - nerve — *see* Injury, nerve, hand
  - open — *see* Wound, open, hand
  - specified NEC S69.8- ☑
  - sprain — *see* Sprain, hand
  - superficial — *see* Injury, superficial, hand
- head S09.90 ☑
  - with loss of consciousness S06.9- ☑
  - specified NEC S09.8 ☑
- heart S26.90 ☑
  - with hemopericardium S26.00 ☑
    - contusion S26.01 ☑
    - laceration (mild) S26.020 ☑
      - major S26.022 ☑
      - moderate S26.021 ☑
    - specified type NEC S26.09 ☑
  - contusion S26.91 ☑
  - laceration S26.92 ☑
  - specified type NEC S26.99 ☑
  - without hemopericardium S26.10 ☑
    - contusion S26.11 ☑
    - laceration S26.12 ☑
    - specified type NEC S26.19 ☑
- heel — *see* Injury, foot
- hepatic
  - artery — *see* Injury, blood vessel, celiac artery, branch
  - duct — *see* Injury, liver
  - vein — *see* Injury, vena cava, inferior
- hip S79.91- ☑
  - blood vessel — *see* Injury, blood vessel, hip
  - contusion — *see* Contusion, hip
  - dislocation — *see* Dislocation, hip
  - fracture — *see* Fracture, femur, neck
  - muscle — *see* Injury, muscle, hip
  - nerve — *see* Injury, nerve, hip
  - open — *see* Wound, open, hip
  - specified NEC S79.81- ☑
  - sprain — *see* Sprain, hip
  - superficial — *see* Injury, superficial, hip
- hymen S39.94 ☑
- hypogastric
  - blood vessel — *see* Injury, blood vessel, iliac
  - plexus — *see* Injury, nerve, lumbosacral, sympathetic
- ileum — *see* Injury, intestine, small
- iliac region S39.91 ☑
- instrumental (during surgery) — *see* Laceration, accidental complicating surgery
  - birth injury — *see* Birth, injury
  - nonsurgical — *see* Injury, by site
- obstetrical O71.9
  - bladder O71.5
  - cervix O71.3
  - high vaginal O71.4
  - perineal NOS O70.9
  - urethra O71.5
  - uterus O71.5
    - with rupture or perforation O71.1

Injury — *continued*
- internal T14.8 ☑
  - aorta — *see* Injury, aorta
  - bladder (sphincter) — *see* Injury, bladder
    - with
      - ectopic or molar pregnancy O08.6
      - following ectopic or molar pregnancy O08.6
      - obstetrical trauma O71.5
  - bronchus, bronchi — *see* Injury, intrathoracic, bronchus
  - cecum — *see* Injury, intestine, large
  - cervix (uteri) — *see also* Injury, uterus
    - with ectopic or molar pregnancy O08.6
    - following ectopic or molar pregnancy O08.6
    - obstetrical trauma O71.3
  - chest — *see* Injury, intrathoracic
  - gastrointestinal tract — *see* Injury, intra-abdominal
  - heart — *see* Injury, heart
  - intestine NEC — *see* Injury, intestine
  - intrauterine — *see* Injury, uterus
  - mesentery — *see* Injury, intra-abdominal, specified, site NEC
  - pelvis, pelvic (organ) S37.90 ☑
    - following ectopic or molar pregnancy (subsequent episode) O08.6
    - obstetrical trauma NEC O71.5
      - rupture or perforation O71.1
    - specified NEC S39.83 ☑
  - rectum — *see* Injury, intestine, large, rectum
  - stomach — *see* Injury, stomach
  - ureter — *see* Injury, ureter
  - urethra (sphincter) following ectopic or molar pregnancy O08.6
  - uterus — *see* Injury, uterus
- interscapular area — *see* Injury, thorax
- intestine
  - large S36.509 ☑
    - ascending (right) S36.500 ☑
      - blast injury (primary) S36.510 ☑
        - secondary S36.590 ☑
      - contusion S36.520 ☑
      - laceration S36.530 ☑
      - specified type NEC S36.590 ☑
    - blast injury (primary) S36.519 ☑
      - ascending (right) S36.510 ☑
      - descending (left) S36.512 ☑
      - rectum S36.61 ☑
      - sigmoid S36.513 ☑
      - specified site NEC S36.518 ☑
      - transverse S36.511 ☑
    - contusion S36.529 ☑
      - ascending (right) S36.520 ☑
      - descending (left) S36.522 ☑
      - rectum S36.62 ☑
      - sigmoid S36.523 ☑
      - specified site NEC S36.528 ☑
      - transverse S36.521 ☑
    - descending (left) S36.502 ☑
      - blast injury (primary) S36.512 ☑
        - secondary S36.592 ☑
      - contusion S36.522 ☑
      - laceration S36.532 ☑
      - specified type NEC S36.592 ☑
    - laceration S36.539 ☑
      - ascending (right) S36.530 ☑
      - descending (left) S36.532 ☑
      - rectum S36.63 ☑
      - sigmoid S36.533 ☑
      - specified site NEC S36.538 ☑
      - transverse S36.531 ☑
    - rectum S36.60 ☑
      - blast injury (primary) S36.61 ☑
        - secondary S36.69 ☑
      - contusion S36.62 ☑
      - laceration S36.63 ☑
      - specified type NEC S36.69 ☑
    - sigmoid S36.503 ☑
      - blast injury (primary) S36.513 ☑
        - secondary S36.593 ☑
      - contusion S36.523 ☑
      - laceration S36.533 ☑
      - specified type NEC S36.593 ☑
    - specified
      - site NEC S36.508 ☑
        - blast injury (primary) S36.518 ☑
          - secondary S36.598 ☑

▽ Subterms under main terms may continue to next column or page   ☑ Additional Character Required — Refer to the Tabular List for Character Selection   193

Injury — Injury

Injury — *continued*
  intestine — *continued*
    large — *continued*
      specified — *continued*
        site — *continued*
          contusion S36.528 ☑
          laceration S36.538 ☑
          specified type NEC S36.598 ☑
        type NEC S36.599 ☑
          ascending (right) S36.590 ☑
          descending (left) S36.592 ☑
          rectum S36.69 ☑
          sigmoid S36.593 ☑
          specified site NEC S36.598 ☑
          transverse S36.591 ☑
      transverse S36.501 ☑
        blast injury (primary) S36.511 ☑
          secondary S36.591 ☑
        contusion S36.521 ☑
        laceration S36.531 ☑
        specified type NEC S36.591 ☑
    small S36.409 ☑
      blast injury (primary) S36.419 ☑
        duodenum S36.410 ☑
        secondary S36.499 ☑
          duodenum S36.490 ☑
          specified site NEC S36.498 ☑
        specified site NEC S36.418 ☑
      contusion S36.429 ☑
        duodenum S36.420 ☑
        specified site NEC S36.428 ☑
      duodenum S36.400 ☑
        blast injury (primary) S36.410 ☑
          secondary S36.490 ☑
        contusion S36.420 ☑
        laceration S36.430 ☑
        specified NEC S36.490 ☑
      laceration S36.439 ☑
        duodenum S36.430 ☑
        specified site NEC S36.438 ☑
      specified
        site NEC S36.408 ☑
        type NEC S36.499 ☑
          duodenum S36.490 ☑
          specified site NEC S36.498 ☑
  intra-abdominal S36.90 ☑
    adrenal gland — *see* Injury, adrenal gland
    bladder — *see* Injury, bladder
    colon — *see* Injury, intestine, large
    contusion S36.92 ☑
    fallopian tube — *see* Injury, fallopian tube
    gallbladder — *see* Injury, gallbladder
    intestine — *see* Injury, intestine
    kidney — *see* Injury, kidney
    laceration S36.93 ☑
    liver — *see* Injury, liver
    ovary — *see* Injury, ovary
    pancreas — *see* Injury, pancreas
    pelvic NOS S37.90 ☑
    peritoneum — *see* Injury, intra-abdominal, specified, site NEC
    prostate — *see* Injury, prostate
    rectum — *see* Injury, intestine, large, rectum
    retroperitoneum — *see* Injury, intra-abdominal, specified, site NEC
    seminal vesicle — *see* Injury, pelvis, organ, specified site NEC
    small intestine — *see* Injury, intestine, small
    specified
      pelvic S37.90 ☑
        specified
          site NEC S37.899 ☑
            specified type NEC S37.898 ☑
          type NEC S37.99 ☑
      site NEC S36.899 ☑
        contusion S36.892 ☑
        laceration S36.893 ☑
        specified type NEC S36.898 ☑
      type NEC S36.99 ☑
    spleen — *see* Injury, spleen
    stomach — *see* Injury, stomach
    ureter — *see* Injury, ureter
    urethra — *see* Injury, urethra
    uterus — *see* Injury, uterus
    vas deferens — *see* Injury, pelvis, organ, specified site NEC

Injury — *continued*
  intracranial (traumatic) S06.9- ☑
    cerebellar hemorrhage, traumatic — *see* Injury, intracranial, focal
    cerebral edema, traumatic S06.1X- ☑
      diffuse S06.1X- ☑
      focal S06.1X- ☑
    diffuse (axonal) S06.2X- ☑
    epidural hemorrhage (traumatic) S06.4X- ☑
    focal brain injury S06.30- ☑
      contusion — *see* Contusion, cerebral
      laceration — *see* Laceration, cerebral
      intracerebral hemorrhage, traumatic S06.36- ☑
        left side S06.35- ☑
        right side S06.34- ☑
    subarachnoid hemorrhage, traumatic S06.6X- ☑
    subdural hemorrhage, traumatic S06.5X- ☑
  intraocular — *see* Injury, eyeball, penetrating
  intrathoracic S27.9 ☑
    bronchus S27.409 ☑
      bilateral S27.402 ☑
      blast injury (primary) S27.419 ☑
        bilateral S27.412 ☑
        secondary — *see* Injury, intrathoracic, bronchus, specified type NEC
        unilateral S27.411 ☑
      contusion S27.429 ☑
        bilateral S27.422 ☑
        unilateral S27.421 ☑
      laceration S27.439 ☑
        bilateral S27.432 ☑
        unilateral S27.431 ☑
      specified type NEC S27.499 ☑
        bilateral S27.492 ☑
        unilateral S27.491 ☑
      unilateral S27.401 ☑
    diaphragm S27.809 ☑
      contusion S27.802 ☑
      laceration S27.803 ☑
      specified type NEC S27.808 ☑
    esophagus (thoracic) S27.819 ☑
      contusion S27.812 ☑
      laceration S27.813 ☑
      specified type NEC S27.818 ☑
    heart — *see* Injury, heart
    hemopneumothorax S27.2 ☑
    hemothorax S27.1 ☑
    lung S27.309 ☑
      aspiration J69.0
      bilateral S27.302 ☑
      blast injury (primary) S27.319 ☑
        bilateral S27.312 ☑
        secondary — *see* Injury, intrathoracic, lung, specified type NEC
        unilateral S27.311 ☑
      contusion S27.329 ☑
        bilateral S27.322 ☑
        unilateral S27.321 ☑
      laceration S27.339 ☑
        bilateral S27.332 ☑
        unilateral S27.331 ☑
      specified type NEC S27.399 ☑
        bilateral S27.392 ☑
        unilateral S27.391 ☑
      unilateral S27.301 ☑
    pleura S27.60 ☑
      laceration S27.63 ☑
      specified type NEC S27.69 ☑
    pneumothorax S27.0 ☑
    specified organ NEC S27.899 ☑
      contusion S27.892 ☑
      laceration S27.893 ☑
      specified type NEC S27.898 ☑
    thoracic duct — *see* Injury, intrathoracic, specified organ NEC
    thymus gland — *see* Injury, intrathoracic, specified organ NEC
    trachea, thoracic S27.50 ☑
      blast (primary) S27.51 ☑
      contusion S27.52 ☑
      laceration S27.53 ☑
      specified type NEC S27.59 ☑
  iris — *see* Injury, eye, specified site NEC
    penetrating — *see* Injury, eyeball, penetrating
  jaw S09.93 ☑
  jejunum — *see* Injury, intestine, small

Injury — *continued*
  joint NOS T14.8 ☑
    old or residual — *see* Disorder, joint, specified type NEC
  kidney S37.00- ☑
    acute (nontraumatic) N17.9
    contusion — *see* Contusion, kidney
    laceration — *see* Laceration, kidney
    specified NEC S37.09- ☑
  knee S89.9- ☑
    contusion — *see* Contusion, knee
    dislocation — *see* Dislocation, knee
    meniscus (lateral) (medial) — *see* Sprain, knee, specified site NEC
      old injury or tear — *see* Derangement, knee, meniscus, due to old injury
    open — *see* Wound, open, knee
    specified NEC S89.8- ☑
    sprain — *see* Sprain, knee
    superficial — *see* Injury, superficial, knee
  labium (majus) (minus) S39.94 ☑
  labyrinth, ear S09.30- ☑
  lacrimal apparatus, duct, gland, or sac — *see* Injury, eye, specified site NEC
  larynx NEC S19.81 ☑
  leg (lower) S89.9- ☑
    blood vessel — *see* Injury, blood vessel, leg
    contusion — *see* Contusion, leg
    fracture — *see* Fracture, leg
    muscle — *see* Injury, muscle, leg
    nerve — *see* Injury, nerve, leg
    open — *see* Wound, open, leg
    specified NEC S89.8- ☑
    superficial — *see* Injury, superficial, leg
  lens, eye — *see* Injury, eye, specified site NEC
    penetrating — *see* Injury, eyeball, penetrating
  limb NEC T14.8 ☑
  lip S09.93 ☑
  liver S36.119 ☑
    contusion S36.112 ☑
    laceration S36.113 ☑
      major (stellate) S36.116 ☑
      minor S36.114 ☑
      moderate S36.115 ☑
    specified NEC S36.118 ☑
  lower back S39.92 ☑
    specified NEC S39.82 ☑
  lumbar, lumbosacral (region) S39.92 ☑
    plexus — *see* Injury, lumbosacral plexus
  lumbosacral plexus S34.4 ☑
  lung — *see also* Injury, intrathoracic, lung
    aspiration J69.0
    transfusion-related (TRALI) J95.84
  lymphatic thoracic duct — *see* Injury, intrathoracic, specified organ NEC
  malar region S09.93 ☑
  mastoid region S09.90 ☑
  maxilla S09.93 ☑
  mediastinum — *see* Injury, intrathoracic, specified organ NEC
  membrane, brain — *see* Injury, intracranial
  meningeal artery — *see* Injury, intracranial, subdural hemorrhage
  meninges (cerebral) — *see* Injury, intracranial
  mesenteric
    artery
      branch S35.299 ☑
        laceration (minor) (superficial) S35.291 ☑
          major S35.292 ☑
        specified NEC S35.298 ☑
      inferior S35.239 ☑
        laceration (minor) (superficial) S35.231 ☑
          major S35.232 ☑
        specified NEC S35.238 ☑
      superior S35.229 ☑
        laceration (minor) (superficial) S35.221 ☑
          major S35.222 ☑
        specified NEC S35.228 ☑
    plexus (inferior) (superior) — *see* Injury, nerve, lumbosacral, sympathetic
    vein
      inferior S35.349 ☑
        laceration S35.341 ☑
        specified NEC S35.348 ☑
      superior S35.339 ☑
        laceration S35.331 ☑

☑ **Additional Character Required** — Refer to the Tabular List for Character Selection   ▽ Subterms under main terms may continue to next column or page

Injury — *continued*
  mesenteric — *continued*
    vein — *continued*
      superior — *continued*
        specified NEC S35.338 ☑
  mesentery — *see* Injury, intra-abdominal, specified site
      NEC
  mesosalpinx — *see* Injury, pelvic organ, specified site
      NEC
  middle ear S09.30- ☑
  midthoracic region NOS S29.9 ☑
  mouth S09.93 ☑
  multiple NOS T07 ☑
  muscle (and fascia) (and tendon)
    abdomen S39.001 ☑
      laceration S39.021 ☑
      specified type NEC S39.091 ☑
      strain S39.011 ☑
    abductor
      thumb, forearm level — *see* Injury, muscle,
        thumb, abductor
    adductor
      thigh S76.20- ☑
        laceration S76.22- ☑
        specified type NEC S76.29- ☑
        strain S76.21- ☑
    ankle — *see* Injury, muscle, foot
    anterior muscle group, at leg level (lower) S86.20- ☑
      laceration S86.22- ☑
      specified type NEC S86.29- ☑
      strain S86.21- ☑
    arm (upper) — *see* Injury, muscle, shoulder
    biceps (parts NEC) S46.20- ☑
      laceration S46.22- ☑
      long head S46.10- ☑
        laceration S46.12- ☑
        specified type NEC S46.19- ☑
        strain S46.11- ☑
      specified type NEC S46.29- ☑
      strain S46.21- ☑
    extensor
      finger(s) (other than thumb) — *see* Injury, mus-
        cle, finger by site, extensor
      forearm level, specified NEC — *see* Injury, muscle,
        forearm, extensor
      thumb — *see* Injury, muscle, thumb, extensor
      toe (large) (ankle level) (foot level) — *see* Injury,
        muscle, toe, extensor
    finger
      extensor (forearm level) S56.40- ☑
        hand level S66.309 ☑
          laceration S66.329 ☑
          specified type NEC S66.399 ☑
          strain S66.319 ☑
        laceration S56.429 ☑
        specified type NEC S56.499 ☑
        strain S56.419 ☑
      flexor (forearm level) S56.10- ☑
        hand level S66.109 ☑
          laceration S66.129 ☑
          specified type NEC S66.199 ☑
          strain S66.119 ☑
        laceration S56.129 ☑
        specified type NEC S56.199 ☑
        strain S56.119 ☑
      index
        extensor (forearm level)
          hand level S66.308 ☑
            laceration S66.32- ☑
            specified type NEC S66.39- ☑
            strain S66.31- ☑
          specified type NEC S56.492- ☑
        flexor (forearm level)
          hand level S66.108 ☑
            laceration S66.12- ☑
            specified type NEC S66.19- ☑
            strain S66.11- ☑
          specified type NEC S56.19- ☑
          strain S56.11- ☑
        intrinsic S66.50- ☑
          laceration S66.52- ☑
          specified type NEC S66.59- ☑
          strain S66.51- ☑
        intrinsic S66.509 ☑
          laceration S66.529 ☑
          specified type NEC S66.599 ☑

Injury — *continued*
  muscle — *continued*
    finger — *continued*
      intrinsic — *continued*
        strain S66.519 ☑
      little
        extensor (forearm level)
          hand level S66.30- ☑
            laceration S66.32- ☑
            specified type NEC S66.39- ☑
            strain S66.31- ☑
          laceration S56.42- ☑
          specified type NEC S56.49- ☑
          strain S56.41- ☑
        flexor (forearm level)
          hand level S66.10- ☑
            laceration S66.12- ☑
            specified type NEC S66.19- ☑
            strain S66.11- ☑
          laceration S56.12- ☑
          specified type NEC S56.19- ☑
          strain S56.11- ☑
        intrinsic S66.50- ☑
          laceration S66.52- ☑
          specified type NEC S66.59- ☑
          strain S66.51- ☑
      middle
        extensor (forearm level)
          hand level S66.30- ☑
            laceration S66.32- ☑
            specified type NEC S66.39- ☑
            strain S66.31- ☑
          laceration S56.42- ☑
          specified type NEC S56.49- ☑
          strain S56.41- ☑
        flexor (forearm level)
          hand level S66.10- ☑
            laceration S66.12- ☑
            specified type NEC S66.19- ☑
            strain S66.11- ☑
          laceration S56.12- ☑
          specified type NEC S56.19- ☑
          strain S56.11- ☑
        intrinsic S66.50- ☑
          laceration S66.52- ☑
          specified type NEC S66.59- ☑
          strain S66.51- ☑
      ring
        extensor (forearm level)
          hand level S66.30- ☑
            laceration S66.32- ☑
            specified type NEC S66.39- ☑
            strain S66.31- ☑
          laceration S56.42- ☑
          specified type NEC S56.49- ☑
          strain S56.41- ☑
        flexor (forearm level)
          hand level S66.10- ☑
            laceration S66.12- ☑
            specified type NEC S66.19- ☑
            strain S66.11- ☑
          laceration S56.12- ☑
          specified type NEC S56.19- ☑
          strain S56.11- ☑
        intrinsic S66.50- ☑
          laceration S66.52- ☑
          specified type NEC S66.59- ☑
          strain S66.51- ☑
    flexor
      finger(s) (other than thumb) — *see* Injury, mus-
        cle, finger
      forearm level, specified NEC — *see* Injury, muscle,
        forearm, flexor
      thumb — *see* Injury, muscle, thumb, flexor
      toe (long) (ankle level) (foot level) — *see* Injury,
        muscle, toe, flexor
    foot S96.90- ☑
      intrinsic S96.20- ☑
        laceration S96.22- ☑
        specified type NEC S96.29- ☑
        strain S96.21- ☑
      laceration S96.92- ☑
      long extensor, toe — *see* Injury, muscle, toe, ex-
        tensor
      long flexor, toe — *see* Injury, muscle, toe, flexor

Injury — *continued*
  muscle — *continued*
    foot — *continued*
      specified
        site NEC S96.80- ☑
          laceration S96.82- ☑
          specified type NEC S96.89- ☑
          strain S96.81- ☑
        type S96.99- ☑
      strain S96.91- ☑
    forearm (level) S56.90- ☑
      extensor S56.50- ☑
        laceration S56.52- ☑
        specified type NEC S56.59- ☑
        strain S56.51- ☑
      flexor S56.20- ☑
        laceration S56.22- ☑
        specified type NEC S56.29- ☑
        strain S56.21- ☑
      laceration S56.92- ☑
      specified S56.99- ☑
        site NEC S56.80- ☑
          laceration S56.82- ☑
          strain S56.81- ☑
          type NEC S56.89- ☑
      strain S56.91- ☑
    hand (level) S66.90- ☑
      laceration S66.92- ☑
      specified
        site NEC S66.80- ☑
          laceration S66.82- ☑
          specified type NEC S66.89- ☑
          strain S66.81- ☑
        type NEC S66.99- ☑
      strain S66.91- ☑
    head S09.10 ☑
      laceration S09.12 ☑
      specified type NEC S09.19 ☑
      strain S09.11 ☑
    hip NEC S76.00- ☑
      laceration S76.02- ☑
      specified type NEC S76.09- ☑
      strain S76.01- ☑
    intrinsic
      ankle and foot level — *see* Injury, muscle, foot,
        intrinsic
      finger (other than thumb) — *see* Injury, muscle,
        finger by site, intrinsic
      foot (level) — *see* Injury, muscle, foot, intrinsic
      thumb — *see* Injury, muscle, thumb, intrinsic
    leg (level) (lower) S86.90- ☑
      Achilles tendon — *see* Injury, Achilles tendon
      anterior muscle group — *see* Injury, muscle, an-
        terior muscle group
      laceration S86.92- ☑
      peroneal muscle group — *see* Injury, muscle,
        peroneal muscle group
      posterior muscle group — *see* Injury, muscle,
        posterior muscle group, leg level
      specified
        site NEC S86.80- ☑
          laceration S86.82- ☑
          specified type NEC S86.89- ☑
          strain S86.81- ☑
        type NEC S86.99- ☑
      strain S86.91- ☑
    long
      extensor toe, at ankle and foot level — *see* Injury,
        muscle, toe, extensor
      flexor, toe, at ankle and foot level — *see* Injury,
        muscle, toe, flexor
      head, biceps — *see* Injury, muscle, biceps, long
        head
    lower back S39.002 ☑
      laceration S39.022 ☑
      specified type NEC S39.092 ☑
      strain S39.012 ☑
    neck (level) S16.9 ☑
      laceration S16.2 ☑
      specified type NEC S16.8 ☑
      strain S16.1 ☑
    pelvis S39.003 ☑
      laceration S39.023 ☑
      specified type NEC S39.093 ☑
      strain S39.013 ☑

Injury — *continued*
  muscle — *continued*
    peroneal muscle group, at leg level (lower)
      S86.30- ☑
      laceration S86.32- ☑
      specified type NEC S86.39- ☑
      strain S86.31- ☑
    posterior muscle (group)
      leg level (lower) S86.10- ☑
        laceration S86.12- ☑
        specified type NEC S86.19- ☑
        strain S86.11- ☑
      thigh level S76.30- ☑
        laceration S76.32- ☑
        specified type NEC S76.39- ☑
        strain S76.31- ☑
    quadriceps (thigh) S76.10- ☑
      laceration S76.12- ☑
      specified type NEC S76.19- ☑
      strain S76.11- ☑
    shoulder S46.90- ☑
      laceration S46.92- ☑
      rotator cuff — *see* Injury, rotator cuff
      specified site NEC S46.80- ☑
        laceration S46.82- ☑
        specified type NEC S46.89- ☑
        strain S46.81- ☑
      specified type NEC S46.99- ☑
      strain S46.91- ☑
    thigh NEC (level) S76.90- ☑
      adductor — *see* Injury, muscle, adductor, thigh
      laceration S76.92- ☑
      posterior muscle (group) — *see* Injury, muscle,
        posterior muscle, thigh level
      quadriceps — *see* Injury, muscle, quadriceps
      specified
        site NEC S76.80- ☑
          laceration S76.82- ☑
          specified type NEC S76.89- ☑
          strain S76.81- ☑
        type NEC S76.99- ☑
      strain S76.91- ☑
    thorax (level) S29.009 ☑
      back wall S29.002 ☑
      front wall S29.001 ☑
      laceration S29.029 ☑
        back wall S29.022 ☑
        front wall S29.021 ☑
      specified type NEC S29.099 ☑
        back wall S29.092 ☑
        front wall S29.091 ☑
      strain S29.019 ☑
        back wall S29.012 ☑
        front wall S29.011 ☑
    thumb
      abductor (forearm level) S56.30- ☑
        laceration S56.32- ☑
        specified type NEC S56.39- ☑
        strain S56.31- ☑
      extensor (forearm level) S56.30- ☑
        hand level S66.20- ☑
          laceration S66.22- ☑
          specified type NEC S66.29- ☑
          strain S66.21- ☑
        laceration S56.32- ☑
        specified type NEC S56.39- ☑
        strain S56.31- ☑
      flexor (forearm level) S56.00- ☑
        hand level S66.00- ☑
          laceration S66.02- ☑
          specified type NEC S66.09- ☑
          strain S66.01- ☑
        laceration S56.02- ☑
        specified type NEC S56.09- ☑
        strain S56.01- ☑
        wrist level — *see* Injury, muscle, thumb, flex-
          or, hand level
      intrinsic S66.40- ☑
        laceration S66.42- ☑
        specified type NEC S66.49- ☑
        strain S66.41- ☑
    toe — *see also* Injury, muscle, foot
      extensor, long S96.10- ☑
        laceration S96.12- ☑
        specified type NEC S96.19- ☑
        strain S96.11- ☑

Injury — *continued*
  muscle — *continued*
    toe — *see also* Injury, muscle, foot — *continued*
      flexor, long S96.00- ☑
        laceration S96.02- ☑
        specified type NEC S96.09- ☑
        strain S96.01- ☑
      triceps S46.30- ☑
        laceration S46.32- ☑
        specified type NEC S46.39- ☑
        strain S46.31- ☑
    wrist (and hand) level — *see* Injury, muscle, hand
  musculocutaneous nerve — *see* Injury, nerve, muscu-
    locutaneous
  myocardium — *see* Injury, heart
  nape — *see* Injury, neck
  nasal (septum) (sinus) S09.92 ☑
  nasopharynx S09.92 ☑
  neck S19.9
    specified NEC S19.80 ☑
      specified site NEC S19.89 ☑
  nerve NEC T14.8 ☑
    abdomen S34.9 ☑
      peripheral S34.6 ☑
      specified site NEC S34.8 ☑
    abducens S04.4- ☑
      contusion S04.4- ☑
      laceration S04.4- ☑
      specified type NEC S04.4- ☑
    abducent — *see* Injury, nerve, abducens
    accessory S04.7- ☑
      contusion S04.7- ☑
      laceration S04.7- ☑
      specified type NEC S04.7- ☑
    acoustic S04.6- ☑
      contusion S04.6- ☑
      laceration S04.6- ☑
      specified type NEC S04.6- ☑
    ankle S94.9- ☑
      cutaneous sensory S94.3- ☑
      specified site NEC — *see* subcategory S94.8 ☑
    anterior crural, femoral — *see* Injury, nerve, femoral
    arm (upper) S44.9- ☑
      axillary — *see* Injury, nerve, axillary
      cutaneous — *see* Injury, nerve, cutaneous, arm
      median — *see* Injury, nerve, median, upper arm
      musculocutaneous — *see* Injury, nerve, muscu-
        locutaneous
      radial — *see* Injury, nerve, radial, upper arm
      specified site NEC — *see* subcategory S44.8 ☑
      ulnar — *see* Injury, nerve, ulnar, arm
    auditory — *see* Injury, nerve, acoustic
    axillary S44.3- ☑
    brachial plexus — *see* Injury, brachial plexus
    cervical sympathetic S14.5 ☑
    cranial S04.9
      contusion S04.9 ☑
      eighth (acoustic or auditory) — *see* Injury, nerve,
        acoustic
      eleventh (accessory) — *see* Injury, nerve, acces-
        sory
      fifth (trigeminal) — *see* Injury, nerve, trigeminal
      first (olfactory) — *see* Injury, nerve, olfactory
      fourth (trochlear) — *see* Injury, nerve, trochlear
      laceration S04.9 ☑
      ninth (glossopharyngeal) — *see* Injury, nerve,
        glossopharyngeal
      second (optic) — *see* Injury, nerve, optic
      seventh (facial) — *see* Injury, nerve, facial
      sixth (abducent) — *see* Injury, nerve, abducens
      specified
        nerve NEC S04.89- ☑
          contusion S04.89- ☑
          laceration S04.89- ☑
          specified type NEC S04.89- ☑
        type NEC S04.9 ☑
      tenth (pneumogastric or vagus) — *see* Injury,
        nerve, vagus
      third (oculomotor) — *see* Injury, nerve, oculomo-
        tor
      twelfth (hypoglossal) — *see* Injury, nerve, hy-
        poglossal
    cutaneous sensory
      ankle (level) S94.3- ☑
      arm (upper) (level) S44.5- ☑

Injury — *continued*
  nerve — *continued*
    cutaneous sensory — *continued*
      foot (level) — *see* Injury, nerve, cutaneous senso-
        ry, ankle
      forearm (level) S54.3- ☑
      hip (level) S74.2- ☑
      leg (lower level) S84.2- ☑
      shoulder (level) — *see* Injury, nerve, cutaneous
        sensory, arm
      thigh (level) — *see* Injury, nerve, cutaneous
        sensory, hip
    deep peroneal — *see* Injury, nerve, peroneal, foot
    digital
      finger S64.4- ☑
        index S64.49- ☑
        little S64.49- ☑
        middle S64.49- ☑
        ring S64.49- ☑
      thumb S64.3- ☑
      toe — *see* Injury, nerve, ankle, specified site NEC
    eighth cranial (acoustic or auditory) — *see* Injury,
      nerve, acoustic
    eleventh cranial (accessory) — *see* Injury, nerve,
      accessory
    facial S04.5- ☑
      contusion S04.5- ☑
      laceration S04.5- ☑
      newborn P11.3
      specified type NEC S04.5- ☑
    femoral (hip level) (thigh level) S74.1- ☑
    fifth cranial (trigeminal) — *see* Injury, nerve,
      trigeminal
    finger (digital) — *see* Injury, nerve, digital, finger
    first cranial (olfactory) — *see* Injury, nerve, olfactory
    foot S94.9- ☑
      cutaneous sensory S94.3- ☑
      deep peroneal S94.2- ☑
      lateral plantar S94.0- ☑
      medial plantar S94.1- ☑
      specified site NEC — *see* subcategory S94.8 ☑
    forearm (level) S54.9- ☑
      cutaneous sensory — *see* Injury, nerve, cuta-
        neous sensory, forearm
      median — *see* Injury, nerve, median
      radial — *see* Injury, nerve, radial
      specified site NEC — *see* subcategory S54.8 ☑
      ulnar — *see* Injury, nerve, ulnar
    fourth cranial (trochlear) — *see* Injury, nerve,
      trochlear
    glossopharyngeal S04.89- ☑
      specified type NEC S04.89- ☑
    hand S64.9- ☑
      median — *see* Injury, nerve, median, hand
      radial — *see* Injury, nerve, radial, hand
      specified NEC — *see* subcategory S64.8 ☑
      ulnar — *see* Injury, nerve, ulnar, hand
    hip (level) S74.9- ☑
      cutaneous sensory — *see* Injury, nerve, cuta-
        neous sensory, hip
      femoral — *see* Injury, nerve, femoral
      sciatic — *see* Injury, nerve, sciatic
      specified site NEC — *see* subcategory S74.8 ☑
    hypoglossal S04.89- ☑
      specified type NEC S04.89- ☑
    lateral plantar S94.0- ☑
    leg (lower) S84.9- ☑
      cutaneous sensory — *see* Injury, nerve, cuta-
        neous sensory, leg
      peroneal — *see* Injury, nerve, peroneal
      specified site NEC — *see* subcategory S84.8 ☑
      tibial — *see* Injury, nerve, tibial
      upper — *see* Injury, nerve, thigh
    lower
      back — *see* Injury, nerve, abdomen, specified
        site NEC
        peripheral — *see* Injury, nerve, abdomen,
          peripheral
      limb — *see* Injury, nerve, leg
    lumbar plexus — *see* Injury, nerve, lumbosacral,
      sympathetic
    lumbar spinal — *see* Injury, nerve, spinal, lumbar
    lumbosacral
      plexus — *see* Injury, nerve, lumbosacral, sympa-
        thetic
      sympathetic S34.5 ☑

196

☑ Additional Character Required — Refer to the Tabular List for Character Selection   ▽ Subterms under main terms may continue to next column or page

Injury — *continued*
  nerve — *continued*
    medial plantar S94.1- ☑
    median (forearm level) S54.1- ☑
      hand (level) S64.1- ☑
      upper arm (level) S44.1- ☑
      wrist (level) — *see* Injury, nerve, median, hand
    musculocutaneous S44.4- ☑
    musculospiral (upper arm level) — *see* Injury, nerve, radial, upper arm
    neck S14.9 ☑
      peripheral S14.4 ☑
      specified site NEC S14.8 ☑
      sympathetic S14.5 ☑
    ninth cranial (glossopharyngeal) — *see* Injury, nerve, glossopharyngeal
    oculomotor S04.1- ☑
      contusion S04.1- ☑
      laceration S04.1- ☑
      specified type NEC S04.1- ☑
    olfactory S04.81- ☑
      specified type NEC S04.81- ☑
    optic S04.01- ☑
      contusion S04.01- ☑
      laceration S04.01- ☑
      specified type NEC S04.01- ☑
    pelvic girdle — *see* Injury, nerve, hip
    pelvis — *see* Injury, nerve, abdomen, specified site NEC
      peripheral — *see* Injury, nerve, abdomen, peripheral
    peripheral NEC T14.8 ☑
      abdomen — *see* Injury, nerve, abdomen, peripheral
      lower back — *see* Injury, nerve, abdomen, peripheral
      neck — *see* Injury, nerve, neck, peripheral
      pelvis — *see* Injury, nerve, abdomen, peripheral
      specified NEC T14.8 ☑
    peroneal (lower leg level) S84.1- ☑
      foot S94.2- ☑
    plexus
      brachial — *see* Injury, brachial plexus
      celiac, coeliac — *see* Injury, nerve, lumbosacral, sympathetic
      mesenteric, inferior — *see* Injury, nerve, lumbosacral, sympathetic
      sacral — *see* Injury, lumbosacral plexus
      spinal
        brachial — *see* Injury, brachial plexus
        lumbosacral — *see* Injury, lumbosacral plexus
    pneumogastric — *see* Injury, nerve, vagus
    radial (forearm level) S54.2- ☑
      hand (level) S64.2- ☑
      upper arm (level) S44.2- ☑
      wrist (level) — *see* Injury, nerve, radial, hand
    root — *see* Injury, nerve, spinal, root
    sacral plexus — *see* Injury, lumbosacral plexus
    sacral spinal — *see* Injury, nerve, spinal, sacral
    sciatic (hip level) (thigh level) S74.0- ☑
    second cranial (optic) — *see* Injury, nerve, optic
    seventh cranial (facial) — *see* Injury, nerve, facial
    shoulder — *see* Injury, nerve, arm
    sixth cranial (abducent) — *see* Injury, nerve, abducens
    spinal
      plexus — *see* Injury, nerve, plexus, spinal
      root
        cervical S14.2 ☑
        dorsal S24.2 ☑
        lumbar S34.21 ☑
        sacral S34.22 ☑
        thoracic — *see* Injury, nerve, spinal, root, dorsal
    splanchnic — *see* Injury, nerve, lumbosacral, sympathetic
    sympathetic NEC — *see* Injury, nerve, lumbosacral, sympathetic
      cervical — *see* Injury, nerve, cervical sympathetic
    tenth cranial (pneumogastric or vagus) — *see* Injury, nerve, vagus
    thigh (level) — *see* Injury, nerve, hip
      cutaneous sensory — *see* Injury, nerve, cutaneous sensory, hip
      femoral — *see* Injury, nerve, femoral
      sciatic — *see* Injury, nerve, sciatic

Injury — *continued*
  nerve — *continued*
    thigh — *see* Injury, nerve, hip — *continued*
      specified NEC — *see* Injury, nerve, hip
    third cranial (oculomotor) — *see* Injury, nerve, oculomotor
    thorax S24.9 ☑
      peripheral S24.3 ☑
      specified site NEC S24.8 ☑
      sympathetic S24.4 ☑
    thumb, digital — *see* Injury, nerve, digital, thumb
    tibial (lower leg level) (posterior) S84.0- ☑
    toe — *see* Injury, nerve, ankle
    trigeminal S04.3- ☑
      contusion S04.3- ☑
      laceration S04.3- ☑
      specified type NEC S04.3- ☑
    trochlear S04.2- ☑
      contusion S04.2- ☑
      laceration S04.2- ☑
      specified type NEC S04.2- ☑
    twelfth cranial (hypoglossal) — *see* Injury, nerve, hypoglossal
    ulnar (forearm level) S54.0- ☑
      arm (upper) (level) S44.0- ☑
      hand (level) S64.0- ☑
      wrist (level) — *see* Injury, nerve, ulnar, hand
    vagus S04.89- ☑
      specified type NEC S04.89- ☑
    wrist (level) — *see* Injury, nerve, hand
  ninth cranial nerve (glossopharyngeal) — *see* Injury, nerve, glossopharyngeal
  nose (septum) S09.92 ☑
  obstetrical O71.9
    specified NEC O71.89
  occipital (region) (scalp) S09.90 ☑
    lobe — *see* Injury, intracranial
  optic chiasm S04.02 ☑
  optic radiation S04.03- ☑
  optic tract and pathways S04.03- ☑
  orbit, orbital (region) — *see* Injury, eye
    penetrating (with foreign body) — *see* Injury, eye, orbit, penetrating
    specified NEC — *see* Injury, eye, specified site NEC
  ovary, ovarian S37.409 ☑
    bilateral S37.402 ☑
      contusion S37.422 ☑
      laceration S37.432 ☑
      specified type NEC S37.492 ☑
    blood vessel — *see* Injury, blood vessel, ovarian
    contusion S37.429 ☑
      bilateral S37.422 ☑
      unilateral S37.421 ☑
    laceration S37.439 ☑
      bilateral S37.432 ☑
      unilateral S37.431 ☑
    specified type NEC S37.499 ☑
      bilateral S37.492 ☑
      unilateral S37.491 ☑
    unilateral S37.401 ☑
      contusion S37.421 ☑
      laceration S37.431 ☑
      specified type NEC S37.491 ☑
  palate (hard) (soft) S09.93 ☑
  pancreas S36.209 ☑
    body S36.201 ☑
      contusion S36.221 ☑
      laceration S36.231 ☑
        major S36.261 ☑
        minor S36.241 ☑
        moderate S36.251 ☑
      specified type NEC S36.291 ☑
    contusion S36.229 ☑
    head S36.200 ☑
      contusion S36.220 ☑
      laceration S36.230 ☑
        major S36.260 ☑
        minor S36.240 ☑
        moderate S36.250 ☑
      specified type NEC S36.290 ☑
    laceration S36.239 ☑
      major S36.269 ☑
      minor S36.249 ☑
      moderate S36.259 ☑
    specified type NEC S36.299 ☑
    tail S36.202 ☑

Injury — *continued*
  pancreas — *continued*
    tail — *continued*
      contusion S36.222 ☑
      laceration S36.232 ☑
        major S36.262 ☑
        minor S36.242 ☑
        moderate S36.252 ☑
      specified type NEC S36.292 ☑
  parietal (region) (scalp) S09.90 ☑
    lobe — *see* Injury, intracranial
  patellar ligament (tendon) S76.10- ☑
    laceration S76.12- ☑
    specified NEC S76.19- ☑
    strain S76.11- ☑
  pelvis, pelvic (floor) S39.93 ☑
    complicating delivery O70.1
    joint or ligament, complicating delivery O71.6
    organ S37.90 ☑
      with ectopic or molar pregnancy O08.6
      complication of abortion — *see* Abortion
      contusion S37.92 ☑
      following ectopic or molar pregnancy O08.6
      laceration S37.93 ☑
      obstetrical trauma NEC O71.5
      specified
        site NEC S37.899 ☑
          contusion S37.892 ☑
          laceration S37.893 ☑
          specified type NEC S37.898 ☑
        type NEC S37.99 ☑
    specified NEC S39.83 ☑
  penis S39.94 ☑
  perineum S39.94 ☑
  peritoneum S36.81 ☑
    laceration S36.893 ☑
  periurethral tissue — *see* Injury, urethra
    complicating delivery O71.82
  phalanges
    foot — *see* Injury, foot
    hand — *see* Injury, hand
  pharynx NEC S19.85 ☑
  pleura — *see* Injury, intrathoracic, pleura
  plexus
    brachial — *see* Injury, brachial plexus
    cardiac — *see* Injury, nerve, thorax, sympathetic
    celiac, coeliac — *see* Injury, nerve, lumbosacral, sympathetic
    esophageal — *see* Injury, nerve, thorax, sympathetic
    hypogastric — *see* Injury, nerve, lumbosacral, sympathetic
    lumbar, lumbosacral — *see* Injury, lumbosacral plexus
    mesenteric — *see* Injury, nerve, lumbosacral, sympathetic
    pulmonary — *see* Injury, nerve, thorax, sympathetic
  postcardiac surgery (syndrome) I97.0
  prepuce S39.94 ☑
  pressure
    injury — *see* Ulcer, pressure, by site
  prostate S37.829 ☑
    contusion S37.822 ☑
    laceration S37.823 ☑
    specified type NEC S37.828 ☑
  pubic region S39.94 ☑
  pudendum S39.94 ☑
  pulmonary plexus — *see* Injury, nerve, thorax, sympathetic
  rectovaginal septum NEC S39.83 ☑
  rectum — *see* Injury, intestine, large, rectum
  retina — *see* Injury, eye, specified site NEC
    penetrating — *see* Injury, eyeball, penetrating
  retroperitoneal — *see* Injury, intra-abdominal, specified site NEC
  rotator cuff (muscle(s)) (tendon(s)) S46.00- ☑
    laceration S46.02- ☑
    specified type NEC S46.09- ☑
    strain S46.01- ☑
  round ligament — *see* Injury, pelvic organ, specified site NEC
  sacral plexus — *see* Injury, lumbosacral plexus
  salivary duct or gland S09.93 ☑
  scalp S09.90 ☑
    newborn (birth injury) P12.9
      due to monitoring (electrode) (sampling incision) P12.4

▽ Subterms under main terms may continue to next column or page   ☑ Additional Character Required — Refer to the Tabular List for Character Selection   197

Injury — Injury

Injury — *continued*
　superficial — *continued*
　　canthus, eye — *see* Injury, superficial, periocular area
　　cheek (external) — *see* Injury, superficial, head, specified NEC
　　　internal — *see* Injury, superficial, oral cavity
　　chest wall — *see* Injury, superficial, thorax
　　chin — *see* Injury, superficial, head NEC
　　clitoris S30.95 ☑
　　conjunctiva — *see* Injury, eye, conjunctiva
　　　with foreign body (in conjunctival sac) — *see* Foreign body, conjunctival sac
　　contusion — *see* Contusion, by site
　　costal region — *see* Injury, superficial, thorax
　　digit(s)
　　　hand — *see* Injury, superficial, finger
　　ear (auricle) (canal) (external) S00.40- ☑
　　　abrasion — *see* Abrasion, ear
　　　bite — *see* Bite, superficial, ear
　　　contusion — *see* Contusion, ear
　　　external constriction — *see* Constriction, external, ear
　　　foreign body — *see* Foreign body, superficial, ear
　　elbow S50.90- ☑
　　　abrasion — *see* Abrasion, elbow
　　　bite — *see* Bite, superficial, elbow
　　　blister — *see* Blister, elbow
　　　contusion — *see* Contusion, elbow
　　　external constriction — *see* Constriction, external, elbow
　　　foreign body — *see* Foreign body, superficial, elbow
　　epididymis S30.94 ☑
　　epigastric region S30.92 ☑
　　epiglottis — *see* Injury, superficial, throat
　　esophagus
　　　cervical — *see* Injury, superficial, throat
　　external constriction — *see* Constriction, external, by site
　　extremity NEC T14.8 ☑
　　eyeball NEC — *see* Injury, eye, specified site NEC
　　eyebrow — *see* Injury, superficial, periocular area
　　eyelid S00.20- ☑
　　　abrasion — *see* Abrasion, eyelid
　　　bite — *see* Bite, superficial, eyelid
　　　contusion — *see* Contusion, eyelid
　　　external constriction — *see* Constriction, external, eyelid
　　　foreign body — *see* Foreign body, superficial, eyelid
　　face NEC — *see* Injury, superficial, head, specified NEC
　　finger(s) S60.949 ☑
　　　abrasion — *see* Abrasion, finger
　　　bite — *see* Bite, superficial, finger
　　　blister — *see* Blister, finger
　　　contusion — *see* Contusion, finger
　　　external constriction — *see* Constriction, external, finger
　　　foreign body — *see* Foreign body, superficial, finger
　　　index S60.94- ☑
　　　insect bite — *see* Bite, by site, superficial, insect
　　　little S60.94- ☑
　　　middle S60.94- ☑
　　　ring S60.94- ☑
　　flank S30.92 ☑
　　foot S90.92- ☑
　　　abrasion — *see* Abrasion, foot
　　　bite — *see* Bite, foot
　　　blister — *see* Blister, foot
　　　contusion — *see* Contusion, foot
　　　external constriction — *see* Constriction, external, foot
　　　foreign body — *see* Foreign body, superficial, foot
　　forearm S50.91- ☑
　　　abrasion — *see* Abrasion, forearm
　　　bite — *see* Bite, forearm, superficial
　　　blister — *see* Blister, forearm
　　　contusion — *see* Contusion, forearm
　　　elbow only — *see* Injury, superficial, elbow
　　　external constriction — *see* Constriction, external, forearm

Injury — *continued*
　superficial — *continued*
　　forearm — *continued*
　　　foreign body — *see* Foreign body, superficial, forearm
　　forehead — *see* Injury, superficial, head NEC
　　foreign body — *see* Foreign body, superficial
　　genital organs, external
　　　female S30.97 ☑
　　　male S30.96 ☑
　　globe (eye) — *see* Injury, eye, specified site NEC
　　groin S30.92 ☑
　　gum — *see* Injury, superficial, oral cavity
　　hand S60.92- ☑
　　　abrasion — *see* Abrasion, hand
　　　bite — *see* Bite, superficial, hand
　　　contusion — *see* Contusion, hand
　　　external constriction — *see* Constriction, external, hand
　　　foreign body — *see* Foreign body, superficial, hand
　　head S00.90 ☑
　　　ear — *see* Injury, superficial, ear
　　　eyelid — *see* Injury, superficial, eyelid
　　　nose S00.30 ☑
　　　oral cavity S00.502 ☑
　　　scalp S00.00 ☑
　　　specified site NEC S00.80 ☑
　　heel — *see* Injury, superficial, foot
　　hip S70.91- ☑
　　　abrasion — *see* Abrasion, hip
　　　bite — *see* Bite, superficial, hip
　　　blister — *see* Blister, hip
　　　contusion — *see* Contusion, hip
　　　external constriction — *see* Constriction, external, hip
　　　foreign body — *see* Foreign body, superficial, hip
　　iliac region — *see* Injury, superficial, abdomen
　　inguinal region — *see* Injury, superficial, abdomen
　　insect bite — *see* Bite, by site, superficial, insect
　　interscapular region — *see* Injury, superficial, thorax, back
　　jaw — *see* Injury, superficial, head, specified NEC
　　knee S80.91- ☑
　　　abrasion — *see* Abrasion, knee
　　　bite — *see* Bite, superficial, knee
　　　blister — *see* Blister, knee
　　　contusion — *see* Contusion, knee
　　　external constriction — *see* Constriction, external, knee
　　　foreign body — *see* Foreign body, superficial, knee
　　labium (majus) (minus) S30.95 ☑
　　lacrimal (apparatus) (gland) (sac) — *see* Injury, eye, specified site NEC
　　larynx — *see* Injury, superficial, throat
　　leg (lower) S80.92- ☑
　　　abrasion — *see* Abrasion, leg
　　　bite — *see* Bite, superficial, leg
　　　contusion — *see* Contusion, leg
　　　external constriction — *see* Constriction, external, leg
　　　foreign body — *see* Foreign body, superficial, leg
　　　knee — *see* Injury, superficial, knee
　　limb NEC T14.8 ☑
　　lip S00.501 ☑
　　lower back S30.91 ☑
　　lumbar region S30.91 ☑
　　malar region — *see* Injury, superficial, head, specified NEC
　　mammary — *see* Injury, superficial, breast
　　mastoid region — *see* Injury, superficial, head, specified NEC
　　mouth — *see* Injury, superficial, oral cavity
　　muscle NEC T14.8 ☑
　　nail NEC T14.8 ☑
　　　finger — *see* Injury, superficial, finger
　　　toe — *see* Injury, superficial, toe
　　nasal (septum) — *see* Injury, superficial, nose
　　neck S10.90 ☑
　　　specified site NEC S10.80 ☑
　　nose (septum) S00.30 ☑
　　occipital region — *see* Injury, superficial, scalp
　　oral cavity S00.502 ☑

Injury — *continued*
　superficial — *continued*
　　orbital region — *see* Injury, superficial, periocular area
　　palate — *see* Injury, superficial, oral cavity
　　palm — *see* Injury, superficial, hand
　　parietal region — *see* Injury, superficial, scalp
　　pelvis S30.91 ☑
　　　girdle — *see* Injury, superficial, hip
　　penis S30.93 ☑
　　perineum
　　　female S30.95 ☑
　　　male S30.91 ☑
　　periocular area S00.20- ☑
　　　abrasion — *see* Abrasion, eyelid
　　　bite — *see* Bite, superficial, eyelid
　　　contusion — *see* Contusion, eyelid
　　　external constriction — *see* Constriction, external, eyelid
　　　foreign body — *see* Foreign body, superficial, eyelid
　　phalanges
　　　finger — *see* Injury, superficial, finger
　　　toe — *see* Injury, superficial, toe
　　pharynx — *see* Injury, superficial, throat
　　pinna — *see* Injury, superficial, ear
　　popliteal space — *see* Injury, superficial, knee
　　prepuce S30.93 ☑
　　pubic region S30.91 ☑
　　pudendum
　　　female S30.97 ☑
　　　male S30.96 ☑
　　sacral region S30.91 ☑
　　scalp S00.00 ☑
　　scapular region — *see* Injury, superficial, shoulder
　　sclera — *see* Injury, eye, specified site NEC
　　scrotum S30.94 ☑
　　shin — *see* Injury, superficial, leg
　　shoulder S40.91- ☑
　　　abrasion — *see* Abrasion, shoulder
　　　bite — *see* Bite, superficial, shoulder
　　　blister — *see* Blister, shoulder
　　　contusion — *see* Contusion, shoulder
　　　external constriction — *see* Constriction, external, shoulder
　　　foreign body — *see* Foreign body, superficial, shoulder
　　skin NEC T14.8 ☑
　　sternal region — *see* Injury, superficial, thorax, front
　　subconjunctival — *see* Injury, eye, specified site NEC
　　subcutaneous NEC T14.8 ☑
　　submaxillary region — *see* Injury, superficial, head, specified NEC
　　submental region — *see* Injury, superficial, head, specified NEC
　　subungual
　　　finger(s) — *see* Injury, superficial, finger
　　　toe(s) — *see* Injury, superficial, toe
　　supraclavicular fossa — *see* Injury, superficial, neck
　　supraorbital — *see* Injury, superficial, head, specified NEC
　　temple — *see* Injury, superficial, head, specified NEC
　　temporal region — *see* Injury, superficial, head, specified NEC
　　testis S30.94 ☑
　　thigh S70.92- ☑
　　　abrasion — *see* Abrasion, thigh
　　　bite — *see* Bite, superficial, thigh
　　　blister — *see* Blister, thigh
　　　contusion — *see* Contusion, thigh
　　　external constriction — *see* Constriction, external, thigh
　　　foreign body — *see* Foreign body, superficial, thigh
　　thorax, thoracic (wall) S20.90 ☑
　　　abrasion — *see* Abrasion, thorax
　　　back S20.40- ☑
　　　bite — *see* Bite, thorax, superficial
　　　blister — *see* Blister, thorax
　　　contusion — *see* Contusion, thorax
　　　external constriction — *see* Constriction, external, thorax
　　　foreign body — *see* Foreign body, superficial, thorax
　　　front S20.30- ☑
　　throat S10.10 ☑

Injury — *continued*
  superficial — *continued*
    throat — *continued*
      abrasion S10.11 ☑
      bite S10.17 ☑
        insect S10.16 ☑
      blister S10.12 ☑
      contusion S10.0 ☑
      external constriction S10.14 ☑
      foreign body S10.15 ☑
    thumb S60.93- ☑
      abrasion — *see* Abrasion, thumb
      bite — *see* Bite, superficial, thumb
      blister — *see* Blister, thumb
      contusion — *see* Contusion, thumb
      external constriction — *see* Constriction, external, thumb
      foreign body — *see* Foreign body, superficial, thumb
      insect bite — *see* Bite, by site, superficial, insect
      specified type NEC S60.39 ☑
    toe(s) S90.93- ☑
      abrasion — *see* Abrasion, toe
      bite — *see* Bite, toe
      blister — *see* Blister, toe
      contusion — *see* Contusion, toe
      external constriction — *see* Constriction, external, toe
      foreign body — *see* Foreign body, superficial, toe
      great S90.93- ☑
    tongue — *see* Injury, superficial, oral cavity
    tooth, teeth — *see* Injury, superficial, oral cavity
    trachea S10.10 ☑
    tunica vaginalis S30.94 ☑
    tympanum, tympanic membrane — *see* Injury, superficial, ear
    uvula — *see* Injury, superficial, oral cavity
    vagina S30.95 ☑
    vocal cords — *see* Injury, superficial, throat
    vulva S30.95 ☑
    wrist S60.91- ☑
  supraclavicular region — *see* Injury, neck
  supraorbital S09.93 ☑
  suprarenal gland (multiple) — *see* Injury, adrenal
  surgical complication (external or internal site) — *see* Laceration, accidental complicating surgery
  temple S09.90 ☑
  temporal region S09.90 ☑
  tendon — *see also* Injury, muscle, by site
    abdomen — *see* Injury, muscle, abdomen
    Achilles — *see* Injury, Achilles tendon
    lower back — *see* Injury, muscle, lower back
    pelvic organs — *see* Injury, muscle, pelvis
  tenth cranial nerve (pneumogastric or vagus) — *see* Injury, nerve, vagus
  testis S39.94 ☑
  thigh S79.92- ☑
    blood vessel — *see* Injury, blood vessel, hip
    contusion — *see* Contusion, thigh
    fracture — *see* Fracture, femur
    muscle — *see* Injury, muscle, thigh
    nerve — *see* Injury, nerve, thigh
    open — *see* Wound, open, thigh
    specified NEC S79.82- ☑
    superficial — *see* Injury, superficial, thigh
  third cranial nerve (oculomotor) — *see* Injury, nerve, oculomotor
  thorax, thoracic S29.9 ☑
    blood vessel — *see* Injury, blood vessel, thorax
    cavity — *see* Injury, intrathoracic
    dislocation — *see* Dislocation, thorax
    external (wall) S29.9 ☑
      contusion — *see* Contusion, thorax
      nerve — *see* Injury, nerve, thorax
      open — *see* Wound, open, thorax
      specified NEC S29.8 ☑
      sprain — *see* Sprain, thorax
      superficial — *see* Injury, superficial, thorax
    fracture — *see* Fracture, thorax
    internal — *see* Injury, intrathoracic
    intrathoracic organ — *see* Injury, intrathoracic
    sympathetic ganglion — *see* Injury, nerve, thorax, sympathetic
  throat — *see also* Injury, neck S19.9 ☑
  thumb S69.9- ☑

Injury — *continued*
  thumb — *continued*
    blood vessel — *see* Injury, blood vessel, thumb
    contusion — *see* Contusion, thumb
    dislocation — *see* Dislocation, thumb
    fracture — *see* Fracture, thumb
    muscle — *see* Injury, muscle, thumb
    nerve — *see* Injury, nerve, digital, thumb
    open — *see* Wound, open, thumb
    specified NEC S69.8- ☑
    sprain — *see* Sprain, thumb
    superficial — *see* Injury, superficial, thumb
  thymus (gland) — *see* Injury, intrathoracic, specified organ NEC
  thyroid (gland) NEC S19.84 ☑
  toe S99.92- ☑
    contusion — *see* Contusion, toe
    dislocation — *see* Dislocation, toe
    fracture — *see* Fracture, toe
    muscle — *see* Injury, muscle, toe
    open — *see* Wound, open, toe
    specified type NEC S99.82- ☑
    sprain — *see* Sprain, toe
    superficial — *see* Injury, superficial, toe
  tongue S09.93 ☑
  tonsil S09.93 ☑
  tooth S09.93 ☑
  trachea (cervical) NEC S19.82 ☑
    thoracic — *see* Injury, intrathoracic, trachea, thoracic
  transfusion-related acute lung (TRALI) J95.84
  tunica vaginalis S39.94 ☑
  twelfth cranial nerve (hypoglossal) — *see* Injury, nerve, hypoglossal
  ureter S37.10 ☑
    contusion S37.12 ☑
    laceration S37.13 ☑
    specified type NEC S37.19 ☑
  urethra (sphincter) S37.30 ☑
    at delivery O71.5
    contusion S37.32 ☑
    laceration S37.33 ☑
    specified type NEC S37.39 ☑
  urinary organ S37.90 ☑
    contusion S37.92 ☑
    laceration S37.93 ☑
    specified
      site NEC S37.899 ☑
        contusion S37.892 ☑
        laceration S37.893 ☑
        specified type NEC S37.898 ☑
      type NEC S37.99 ☑
  uterus, uterine S37.60 ☑
    with ectopic or molar pregnancy O08.6
    blood vessel — *see* Injury, blood vessel, iliac
    contusion S37.62 ☑
    laceration S37.63 ☑
      cervix at delivery O71.3
    rupture associated with obstetrics — *see* Rupture, uterus
    specified type NEC S37.69 ☑
  uvula S09.93 ☑
  vagina S39.93 ☑
    abrasion S30.814 ☑
    bite S31.45 ☑
      insect S30.864 ☑
      superficial NEC S30.874 ☑
    contusion S30.23 ☑
    crush S38.03 ☑
    during delivery — *see* Laceration, vagina, during delivery
    external constriction S30.844 ☑
    insect bite S30.864 ☑
    laceration S31.41 ☑
      with foreign body S31.42 ☑
    open wound S31.40 ☑
    puncture S31.43 ☑
      with foreign body S31.44 ☑
    superficial S30.95 ☑
      foreign body S30.854 ☑
  vas deferens — *see* Injury, pelvic organ, specified site NEC
  vascular NEC T14.8 ☑
  vein — *see* Injury, blood vessel
  vena cava (superior) S25.20 ☑
    inferior S35.10 ☑
      laceration (minor) (superficial) S35.11 ☑

Injury — *continued*
  vena cava — *continued*
    inferior — *continued*
      laceration — *continued*
        major S35.12 ☑
        specified type NEC S35.19 ☑
    laceration (minor) (superficial) S25.21 ☑
      major S25.22 ☑
    specified type NEC S25.29 ☑
  vesical (sphincter) — *see* Injury, bladder
  visual cortex S04.04- ☑
  vitreous (humor) S05.90 ☑
    specified NEC S05.8X- ☑
  vocal cord NEC S19.83 ☑
  vulva S39.94 ☑
    abrasion S30.814 ☑
    bite S31.45 ☑
      insect S30.864 ☑
      superficial NEC S30.874 ☑
    contusion S30.23 ☑
    crush S38.03 ☑
    during delivery — *see* Laceration, perineum, female, during delivery
    external constriction S30.844 ☑
    insect bite S30.864 ☑
    laceration S31.41 ☑
      with foreign body S31.42 ☑
    open wound S31.40 ☑
    puncture S31.43 ☑
      with foreign body S31.44 ☑
    superficial S30.95 ☑
      foreign body S30.854 ☑
  whiplash (cervical spine) S13.4 ☑
  wrist S69.9- ☑
    blood vessel — *see* Injury, blood vessel, hand
    contusion — *see* Contusion, wrist
    dislocation — *see* Dislocation, wrist
    fracture — *see* Fracture, wrist
    muscle — *see* Injury, muscle, hand
    nerve — *see* Injury, nerve, hand
    open — *see* Wound, open, wrist
    specified NEC S69.8- ☑
    sprain — *see* Sprain, wrist
    superficial — *see* Injury, superficial, wrist
Inoculation — *see also* Vaccination
  complication or reaction — *see* Complications, vaccination
Insanity, insane — *see also* Psychosis
  adolescent — *see* Schizophrenia
  confusional F28
    acute or subacute F05
  delusional F22
  senile F03 ☑
Insect
  bite — *see* Bite, by site, superficial, insect
  venomous, poisoning NEC (by) — *see* Venom, arthropod
Insensitivity
  adrenocorticotropin hormone (ACTH) E27.49
  androgen E34.50
    complete E34.51
    partial E34.52
Insertion
  cord (umbilical) lateral or velamentous O43.12- ☑
  intrauterine contraceptive device (encounter for) — *see* Intrauterine contraceptive device
Insolation (sunstroke) T67.01 ☑
Insomnia (organic) G47.00
  adjustment F51.02
  adjustment disorder F51.02
  behavioral, of childhood Z73.819
    combined type Z73.812
    limit setting type Z73.811
    sleep-onset association type Z73.810
  childhood Z73.819
  chronic F51.04
    somatized tension F51.04
  conditioned F51.04
  due to
    alcohol
      abuse F10.182
      dependence F10.282
      use F10.982
    amphetamines
      abuse F15.182
      dependence F15.282
      use F15.982

Insomnia — *continued*
  due to — *continued*
    anxiety disorder F51.05
    caffeine
      abuse F15.182
      dependence F15.282
      use F15.982
    cocaine
      abuse F14.182
      dependence F14.282
      use F14.982
    depression F51.05
    drug NEC
      abuse F19.182
      dependence F19.282
      use F19.982
    medical condition G47.01
    mental disorder NEC F51.05
    opioid
      abuse F11.182
      dependence F11.282
      use F11.982
    psychoactive substance NEC
      abuse F19.182
      dependence F19.182
      use F19.982
    sedative, hypnotic, or anxiolytic
      abuse F13.182
      dependence F13.282
      use F13.982
    stimulant NEC
      abuse F15.182
      dependence F15.282
      use F15.982
  fatal familial (FFI) A81.83
  idiopathic F51.01
  learned F51.3
  nonorganic origin F51.01
  not due to a substance or known physiological condition F51.01
    specified NEC F51.09
  paradoxical F51.03
  primary F51.01
  psychiatric F51.05
  psychophysiologic F51.04
  related to psychopathology F51.05
  short-term F51.02
  specified NEC G47.09
  stress-related F51.02
  transient F51.02
  without objective findings F51.02
Inspiration
  food or foreign body — *see* Foreign body, by site
  mucus — *see* Asphyxia, mucus
Inspissated bile syndrome (newborn) P59.1
Instability
  emotional (excessive) F60.3
  joint (post-traumatic) M25.30
    ankle M25.37- ☑
    due to old ligament injury — *see* Disorder, ligament
    elbow M25.32- ☑
    flail — *see* Flail, joint
    foot M25.37- ☑
    hand M25.34- ☑
    hip M25.35- ☑
    knee M25.36- ☑
    lumbosacral — *see* subcategory M53.2 ☑
    prosthesis — *see* Complications, joint prosthesis, mechanical, displacement, by site
    sacroiliac — *see* subcategory M53.2 ☑
    secondary to
      old ligament injury — *see* Disorder, ligament
      removal of joint prosthesis M96.89
    shoulder (region) M25.31- ☑
    spine — *see* subcategory M53.2 ☑
    wrist M25.33- ☑
  knee (chronic) M23.5- ☑
  lumbosacral — *see* subcategory M53.2 ☑
  nervous F48.8
  personality (emotional) F60.3
  spine — *see* Instability, joint, spine
  vasomotor R55
Institutional syndrome (childhood) F94.2
Institutionalization, affecting child Z62.22
  disinhibited attachment F94.2
Insufficiency, insufficient
  accommodation, old age H52.4
  adrenal (gland) E27.40

Insufficiency, insufficient — *continued*
  adrenal — *continued*
    primary E27.1
  adrenocortical E27.40
    drug-induced E27.3
    iatrogenic E27.3
    primary E27.1
  anatomic crown height K08.89
  anterior (occlusal) guidance M26.54
  anus K62.89
  aortic (valve) I35.1
    with
      mitral (valve) disease I08.0
        with tricuspid (valve) disease I08.3
      stenosis I35.2
      tricuspid (valve) disease I08.2
        with mitral (valve) disease I08.3
    congenital Q23.1
    rheumatic I06.1
      with
        mitral (valve) disease I08.0
          with tricuspid (valve) disease I08.3
        stenosis I06.2
          with mitral (valve) disease I08.0
            with tricuspid (valve) disease I08.3
        tricuspid (valve) disease I08.2
          with mitral (valve) disease I08.3
    specified cause NEC I35.1
    syphilitic A52.03
  arterial I77.1
    basilar G45.0
    carotid (hemispheric) G45.1
    cerebral I67.81
    coronary (acute or subacute) I24.8
    mesenteric K55.1
    peripheral I73.9
    precerebral (multiple) (bilateral) G45.2
    vertebral G45.0
  arteriovenous I99.8
  biliary K83.8
  cardiac — *see also* Insufficiency, myocardial
    due to presence of (cardiac) prosthesis I97.11- ☑
    postprocedural I97.11- ☑
  cardiorenal, hypertensive I13.2
  cardiovascular — *see* Disease, cardiovascular
  cerebrovascular (acute) I67.81
    with transient focal neurological signs and symptoms G45.8
  circulatory NEC I99.8
    newborn P29.89
  clinical crown length K08.89
  convergence H51.11
  coronary (acute or subacute) I24.8
    chronic or with a stated duration of over 4 weeks I25.89
  corticoadrenal E27.40
    primary E27.1
  dietary E63.9
  divergence H51.8
  food T73.0 ☑
  gastroesophageal K22.8
  gonadal
    ovary E28.39
    testis E29.1
  heart — *see also* Insufficiency, myocardial
    newborn P29.0
    valve — *see* Endocarditis
  hepatic — *see* Failure, hepatic
  idiopathic autonomic G90.09
  interocclusal distance of fully erupted teeth (ridge) M26.36
  kidney N28.9
    acute N28.9
    chronic N18.9
  lacrimal (secretion) H04.12- ☑
    passages — *see* Stenosis, lacrimal
  liver — *see* Failure, hepatic
  lung — *see* Insufficiency, pulmonary
  mental (congenital) — *see* Disability, intellectual
  mesenteric K55.1
  mitral (valve) I34.0
    with
      aortic valve disease I08.0
        with tricuspid (valve) disease I08.3
      obstruction or stenosis I05.2
        with aortic valve disease I08.0
      tricuspid (valve) disease I08.1
        with aortic (valve) disease I08.3

Insufficiency, insufficient — *continued*
  mitral — *continued*
    congenital Q23.3
    rheumatic I05.1
      with
        aortic valve disease I08.0
          with tricuspid (valve) disease I08.3
        obstruction or stenosis I05.2
          with aortic valve disease I08.0
            with tricuspid (valve) disease I08.3
        tricuspid (valve) disease I08.1
          with aortic (valve) disease I08.3
      active or acute I01.1
        with chorea, rheumatic (Sydenham's) I02.0
    specified cause, except rheumatic I34.0
  muscle — *see also* Disease, muscle
    heart — *see* Insufficiency, myocardial
    ocular NEC H50.9
  myocardial, myocardium (with arteriosclerosis) — *see also* Failure, heart I50.9
    with
      rheumatic fever (conditions in I00) I09.0
        active, acute or subacute I01.2
          with chorea I02.0
        inactive or quiescent (with chorea) I09.0
    congenital Q24.8
    hypertensive — *see* Hypertension, heart
    newborn P29.0
    rheumatic I09.0
      active, acute, or subacute I01.2
    syphilitic A52.06
  nourishment T73.0 ☑
  pancreatic K86.89
    exocrine K86.81
  parathyroid (gland) E20.9
  peripheral vascular (arterial) I73.9
  pituitary E23.0
  placental (mother) O36.51- ☑
  platelets D69.6
  prenatal care affecting management of pregnancy O09.3- ☑
  progressive pluriglandular E31.0
  pulmonary J98.4
    acute, following surgery (nonthoracic) J95.2
      thoracic J95.1
    chronic, following surgery J95.3
    following
      shock J98.4
      trauma J98.4
    newborn P28.89
    valve I37.1
      with stenosis I37.2
      congenital Q22.2
      rheumatic I09.89
        with aortic, mitral or tricuspid (valve) disease I08.8
  pyloric K31.89
  renal (acute) N28.9
    chronic N18.9
  respiratory R06.89
    newborn P28.5
  rotation — *see* Malrotation
  sleep syndrome F51.12
  social insurance Z59.7
  suprarenal E27.40
    primary E27.1
  tarso-orbital fascia, congenital Q10.3
  testis E29.1
  thyroid (gland) (acquired) E03.9
    congenital E03.1
  tricuspid (valve) (rheumatic) I07.1
    with
      aortic (valve) disease I08.2
        with mitral (valve) disease I08.3
      mitral (valve) disease I08.1
        with aortic (valve) disease I08.3
      obstruction or stenosis I07.2
        with aortic (valve) disease I08.2
          with mitral (valve) disease I08.3
    congenital Q22.8
    nonrheumatic I36.1
      with stenosis I36.2
  urethral sphincter R32
  valve, valvular (heart) I38
    aortic — *see* Insufficiency, aortic (valve)
    congenital Q24.8
    mitral — *see* Insufficiency, mitral (valve)
    pulmonary — *see* Insufficiency, pulmonary, valve

Insufficiency, insufficient — *continued*
  valve, valvular — *continued*
    tricuspid — *see* Insufficiency, tricuspid (valve)
  vascular I99.8
    intestine K55.9
      acute — *see also* Ischemia, intestine, acute K55.059
    mesenteric K55.1
    peripheral I73.9
    renal — *see* Hypertension, kidney
  velopharyngeal
    acquired K13.79
    congenital Q38.8
  venous (chronic) (peripheral) I87.2
  ventricular — *see* Insufficiency, myocardial
  welfare support Z59.7
Insufflation, fallopian Z31.41
Insular — *see* condition
Insulinoma
  pancreas
    benign D13.7
    malignant C25.4
    uncertain behavior D37.8
  specified site
    benign — *see* Neoplasm, by site, benign
    malignant — *see* Neoplasm, by site, malignant
    uncertain behavior — *see* Neoplasm, by site, uncertain behavior
  unspecified site
    benign D13.7
    malignant C25.4
    uncertain behavior D37.8
Insuloma — *see* Insulinoma
Interference
  balancing side M26.56
  non-working side M26.56
Intermenstrual — *see* condition
Intermittent — *see* condition
Internal — *see* condition
Interrogation
  cardiac defibrillator (automatic) (implantable) Z45.02
  cardiac pacemaker Z45.018
  cardiac (event) (loop) recorder Z45.09
  infusion pump (implanted) (intrathecal) Z45.1
  neurostimulator Z46.2
Interruption
  aortic arch Q25.21
  bundle of His I44.30
  phase-shift, sleep cycle — *see* Disorder, sleep, circadian rhythm
  sleep phase-shift, or 24 hour sleep-wake cycle — *see* Disorder, sleep, circadian rhythm
Interstitial — *see* condition
Intertrigo L30.4
  labialis K13.0
Intervertebral disc — *see* condition
Intestine, intestinal — *see* condition
Intolerance
  carbohydrate K90.49
  disaccharide, hereditary E73.0
  fat NEC K90.49
    pancreatic K90.3
  food K90.49
    dietary counseling and surveillance Z71.3
  fructose E74.10
    hereditary E74.12
  glucose (-galactose) E74.39
  gluten K90.41
  lactose E73.9
    specified NEC E73.8
  lysine E72.3
  milk NEC K90.49
    lactose E73.9
  protein K90.49
  starch NEC K90.49
  sucrose (-isomaltose) E74.31
Intoxicated NEC (without dependence) — *see* Alcohol, intoxication
Intoxication
  acid E87.2
  alcoholic (acute) (without dependence) — *see* Alcohol, intoxication
  alimentary canal K52.1
  amphetamine (without dependence) — *see also* Abuse, drug, stimulant, with intoxication
    with dependence — *see* Dependence, drug, stimulant, with intoxication
    stimulant NEC F15.10

Intoxication — *continued*
  amphetamine — *see also* Abuse, drug, stimulant, with intoxication — *continued*
    stimulant — *continued*
      with
        anxiety disorder F15.180
        intoxication F15.129
          with
            delirium F15.121
            perceptual disturbance F15.122
  anxiolytic (acute) (without dependence) — *see* Abuse, drug, sedative, with intoxication
    with dependence — *see* Dependence, drug, sedative, with intoxication
  caffeine F15.929
    with dependence — *see* Dependence, drug, stimulant, with intoxication
  cannabinoids (acute) (without dependence) — *see* Use, cannabis, with intoxication
    with
      abuse — *see* Abuse, drug, cannabis, with intoxication
      dependence — *see* Dependence, drug, cannabis, with intoxication
  chemical — *see* Table of Drugs and Chemicals
    via placenta or breast milk — *see* - Absorption, chemical, through placenta
  cocaine (acute) (without dependence) — *see* Abuse, drug, cocaine, with intoxication
    with dependence — *see* Dependence, drug, cocaine, with intoxication
  drug
    acute (without dependence) — *see* Abuse, drug, by type with intoxication
      with dependence — *see* Dependence, drug, by type with intoxication
    addictive
      via placenta or breast milk — *see* Absorption, drug, addictive, through placenta
    newborn P93.8
      gray baby syndrome P93.0
    overdose or wrong substance given or taken — *see* Table of Drugs and Chemicals, by drug, poisoning
  enteric K52.1
  foodborne A05.9
    bacterial A05.9
    classical (Clostridium botulinum) A05.1
    due to
      Bacillus cereus A05.4
      bacterium A05.9
        specified NEC A05.8
      Clostridium
        botulinum A05.1
        perfringens A05.2
        welchii A05.2
      Salmonella A02.9
        with
          (gastro)enteritis A02.0
          localized infection(s) A02.20
            arthritis A02.23
            meningitis A02.21
            osteomyelitis A02.24
            pneumonia A02.22
            pyelonephritis A02.25
            specified NEC A02.29
          sepsis A02.1
          specified manifestation NEC A02.8
      Staphylococcus A05.0
      Vibrio
        parahaemolyticus A05.3
        vulnificus A05.5
    enterotoxin, staphylococcal A05.0
    noxious — *see* Poisoning, food, noxious
  gastrointestinal K52.1
  hallucinogenic (without dependence) — *see* Abuse, drug, hallucinogen, with intoxication
    with dependence — *see* Dependence, drug, hallucinogen, with intoxication
  hypnotic (acute) (without dependence) — *see* Abuse, drug, sedative, with intoxication
    with dependence — *see* Dependence, drug, sedative, with intoxication
  inhalant (acute) (without dependence) — *see* Abuse, drug, inhalant, with intoxication
    with dependence — *see* Dependence, drug, inhalant, with intoxication

Intoxication — *continued*
  meaning
    inebriation — *see* category F10 ☑
    poisoning — *see* Table of Drugs and Chemicals
  methyl alcohol (acute) (without dependence) — *see* Alcohol, intoxication
  opioid (acute) (without dependence) — *see* Abuse, drug, opioid, with intoxication
    with dependence — *see* Dependence, drug, opioid, with intoxication
  pathologic NEC (without dependence) — *see* Alcohol, intoxication
  phencyclidine (without dependence) — *see* Abuse, drug, hallucinogen, with intoxication
    with dependence — *see* Dependence, drug, hallucinogen, with intoxication
  potassium (K) E87.5
  psychoactive substance NEC (without dependence) — *see* Abuse, drug, psychoactive NEC, with intoxication
    with dependence — *see* Dependence, drug, psychoactive NEC, with intoxication
  sedative (acute) (without dependence) — *see* Abuse, drug, sedative, with intoxication
    with dependence — *see* Dependence, drug, sedative, with intoxication
  serum — *see also* Reaction, serum T80.69 ☑
  uremic — *see* Uremia
  volatile solvents (acute) (without dependence) — *see* Abuse, drug, inhalant, with intoxication
    with dependence — *see* Dependence, drug, inhalant, with intoxication
  water E87.79
Intraabdominal testis, testes
  bilateral Q53.211
  unilateral Q53.111
Intracranial — *see* condition
Intrahepatic gallbladder Q44.1
Intraligamentous — *see* condition
Intrathoracic — *see also* condition
  kidney Q63.2
Intrauterine contraceptive device
  checking Z30.431
  in situ Z97.5
  insertion Z30.430
    immediately following removal Z30.433
  management Z30.431
  reinsertion Z30.433
  removal Z30.432
  replacement Z30.433
  retention in pregnancy O26.3- ☑
Intraventricular — *see* condition
Intrinsic deformity — *see* Deformity
Intubation, difficult or failed T88.4 ☑
Intumescence, lens (eye) (cataract) — *see* Cataract
Intussusception (bowel) (colon) (enteric) (ileocecal) (ileocolic) (intestine) (rectum) K56.1
  appendix K38.8
  congenital Q43.8
  ureter (with obstruction) N13.5
Invagination (bowel, colon, intestine or rectum) K56.1
Inversion
  albumin-globulin (A-G) ratio E88.09
  bladder N32.89
  cecum — *see* Intussusception
  cervix N88.8
  chromosome in normal individual Q95.1
  circadian rhythm — *see* Disorder, sleep, circadian rhythm
  nipple N64.59
    congenital Q83.8
    gestational — *see* Retraction, nipple
    puerperal, postpartum — *see* Retraction, nipple
  nyctohemeral rhythm — *see* Disorder, sleep, circadian rhythm
  optic papilla Q14.2
  organ or site, congenital NEC — *see* Anomaly, by site
  sleep rhythm — *see* Disorder, sleep, circadian rhythm
  testis (congenital) Q55.29
  uterus (chronic) (postinfectional) (postpartal, old) N85.5
    postpartum O71.2
  vagina (posthysterectomy) N99.3
  ventricular Q20.5
Investigation — *see also* Examination Z04.9
  clinical research subject (control) (normal comparison) (participant) Z00.6
Involuntary movement, abnormal R25.9

Involution, involutional — see also condition
    breast, cystic — see Dysplasia, mammary, specified
        type NEC
    depression (single episode) F32.89
        recurrent episode F33.9
    melancholia (single episode) F32.89
        recurrent episode F33.8
    ovary, senile — see Atrophy, ovary
    thymus failure E32.8
I.Q.
    20-34 F72
    35-49 F71
    50-69 F70
    under 20 F73
IRDS (type I) P22.0
    type II P22.1
Irideremia Q13.1
Iridis rubeosis — see Disorder, iris, vascular
Iridochoroiditis (panuveitis) — see Panuveitis
Iridocyclitis H20.9
    acute H20.0- ☑
        hypopyon H20.05- ☑
        primary H20.01- ☑
        recurrent H20.02- ☑
        secondary (noninfectious) H20.04- ☑
            infectious H20.03- ☑
    chronic H20.1- ☑
    due to allergy — see Iridocyclitis, acute, secondary
    endogenous — see Iridocyclitis, acute, primary
    Fuchs' — see Cyclitis, Fuchs' heterochromic
    gonococcal A54.32
    granulomatous — see Iridocyclitis, chronic
    herpes, herpetic (simplex) B00.51
        zoster B02.32
    hypopyon — see Iridocyclitis, acute, hypopyon
    in (due to)
        ankylosing spondylitis M45.9
        gonococcal infection A54.32
        herpes (simplex) virus B00.51
            zoster B02.32
        infectious disease NOS B99 ☑
        parasitic disease NOS B89 [H22]
        sarcoidosis D86.83
        syphilis A51.43
        tuberculosis A18.54
        zoster B02.32
    lens-induced H20.2- ☑
    nongranulomatous — see Iridocyclitis, acute
    recurrent — see Iridocyclitis, acute, recurrent
    rheumatic — see Iridocyclitis, chronic
    subacute — see Iridocyclitis, acute
    sympathetic — see Uveitis, sympathetic
    syphilitic (secondary) A51.43
    tuberculous (chronic) A18.54
    Vogt-Koyanagi H20.82- ☑
Iridocyclochoroiditis (panuveitis) — see Panuveitis
Iridodialysis H21.53- ☑
Iridodonesis H21.89
Iridoplegia (complete) (partial) (reflex) H57.09
Iridoschisis H21.25- ☑
Iris — see also condition
    bombé — see Membrane, pupillary
Iritis — see also Iridocyclitis
    chronic — see Iridocyclitis, chronic
    diabetic — see E08-E13 with .39
    due to
        herpes simplex B00.51
        leprosy A30.9 [H22]
    gonococcal A54.32
    gouty — see also Gout, by type M10.9 [H22]
    granulomatous — see Iridocyclitis, chronic
    lens induced — see Iridocyclitis, lens-induced
    papulosa (syphilitic) A52.71
    rheumatic — see Iridocyclitis, chronic
    syphilitic (secondary) A51.43
        congenital (early) A50.01
        late A52.71
    tuberculous A18.54
Iron — see condition
Iron-miner's lung J63.4
Irradiated enamel (tooth, teeth) K03.89
Irradiation effects, adverse T66 ☑
Irreducible, irreducibility — see condition
Irregular, irregularity
    action, heart I49.9
    alveolar process K08.89
    bleeding N92.6

Irregular, irregularity — continued
    breathing R06.89
    contour of cornea (acquired) — see Deformity, cornea
        congenital Q13.4
    contour, reconstructed breast N65.0
    dentin (in pulp) K04.3
    eye movements H55.89
        nystagmus — see Nystagmus
        saccadic H55.81
    labor O62.2
    menstruation (cause unknown) N92.6
    periods N92.6
    prostate N42.9
    pupil — see Abnormality, pupillary
    reconstructed breast N65.0
    respiratory R06.89
    septum (nasal) J34.2
    shape, organ or site, congenital NEC — see Distortion
    sleep-wake pattern (rhythm) G47.23
Irritable, irritability R45.4
    bladder N32.89
    bowel (syndrome) K58.9
        with
            constipation K58.1
            diarrhea K58.0
        mixed K58.2
        psychogenic F45.8
        specified NEC K58.8
    bronchial — see Bronchitis
    cerebral, in newborn P91.3
    colon — see also Irritable, bowel K58.9
        with diarrhea K58.0
        psychogenic F45.8
    duodenum K59.8
    heart (psychogenic) F45.8
    hip — see Derangement, joint, specified type NEC, hip
    ileum K59.8
    infant R68.12
    jejunum K59.8
    rectum K59.8
    stomach K31.89
        psychogenic F45.8
    sympathetic G90.8
    urethra N36.8
Irritation
    anus K62.89
    axillary nerve G54.0
    bladder N32.89
    brachial plexus G54.0
    bronchial — see Bronchitis
    cervical plexus G54.2
    cervix — see Cervicitis
    choroid, sympathetic — see Endophthalmitis
    cranial nerve — see Disorder, nerve, cranial
    gastric K31.89
        psychogenic F45.8
    globe, sympathetic — see Uveitis, sympathetic
    labyrinth — see subcategory H83.2 ☑
    lumbosacral plexus G54.1
    meninges (traumatic) — see Injury, intracranial
        nontraumatic — see Meningismus
    nerve — see Disorder, nerve
    nervous R45.0
    penis N48.89
    perineum NEC L29.3
    peripheral autonomic nervous system G90.8
    peritoneum — see Peritonitis
    pharynx J39.2
    plantar nerve — see Lesion, nerve, plantar
    spinal (cord) (traumatic) — see also Injury, spinal cord,
        by region
        nerve G58.9
            root NEC — see Radiculopathy
        nontraumatic — see Myelopathy
    stomach K31.89
        psychogenic F45.8
    sympathetic nerve NEC G90.8
    ulnar nerve — see Lesion, nerve, ulnar
    vagina N89.8
Ischemia, ischemic I99.8
    bowel (transient)
        acute — see also Ischemia, intestine, acute K55.059
        chronic K55.1
        due to mesenteric artery insufficiency K55.1
    brain — see Ischemia, cerebral
    cardiac (see Disease, heart, ischemic)
    cardiomyopathy I25.5
    cerebral (chronic) (generalized) I67.82

Ischemia, ischemic — continued
    cerebral — continued
        arteriosclerotic I67.2
        intermittent G45.9
        newborn P91.0
        recurrent focal G45.8
        transient G45.9
    colon chronic (due to mesenteric artery insufficiency)
        K55.1
    coronary — see Disease, heart, ischemic
    demand (coronary) — see also Angina I24.8
        with myocardial infarction I21.A1
        resulting in myocardial infarction I21.A1
    heart (chronic or with a stated duration of over 4 weeks)
        I25.9
        acute or with a stated duration of 4 weeks or less
            I24.9
        subacute I24.9
    infarction, muscle — see Infarct, muscle
    intestine (large) (small) (transient) K55.9
        acute K55.059
            diffuse K55.052
            focal K55.051
            large K55.039
                diffuse K55.032
                focal K55.031
            small K55.019
                diffuse K55.012
                focal K55.011
        chronic K55.1
        due to mesenteric artery insufficiency K55.1
    kidney N28.0
    mesenteric, acute — see also Ischemia, intestine, acute
        K55.059
    muscle, traumatic T79.6 ☑
    myocardium, myocardial (chronic or with a stated du-
        ration of over 4 weeks) I25.9
        acute, without myocardial infarction I51.3
        silent (asymptomatic) I25.6
        transient of newborn P29.4
    renal N28.0
    retina, retinal — see Occlusion, artery, retina
    small bowel
        acute K55.019
            diffuse K55.012
            focal K55.011
        chronic K55.1
        due to mesenteric artery insufficiency K55.1
    spinal cord G95.11
    subendocardial — see Insufficiency, coronary
    supply (coronary) — see also Angina I25.9
        due to vasospasm I20.1
Ischial spine — see condition
Ischialgia — see Sciatica
Ischiopagus Q89.4
Ischium, ischial — see condition
Ischuria R34
Iselin's disease or osteochondrosis — see Osteochon-
    drosis, juvenile, metatarsus
Islands of
    parotid tissue in
        lymph nodes Q38.6
        neck structures Q38.6
    submaxillary glands in
        fascia Q38.6
        lymph nodes Q38.6
        neck muscles Q38.6
Islet cell tumor, pancreas D13.7
Isoimmunization NEC — see also Incompatibility
    affecting management of pregnancy (ABO) (with hy-
        drops fetalis) O36.11- ☑
        anti-A sensitization O36.11- ☑
        anti-B sensitization O36.19- ☑
        anti-c sensitization O36.09- ☑
        anti-C sensitization O36.09- ☑
        anti-e sensitization O36.09- ☑
        anti-E sensitization O36.09- ☑
        Rh NEC O36.09- ☑
            anti-D antibody O36.01- ☑
        specified NEC O36.19- ☑
    newborn P55.9
        with
            hydrops fetalis P56.0
            kernicterus P57.0
        ABO (blood groups) P55.1
        Rhesus (Rh) factor P55.0
        specified type NEC P55.8

Index

Isolation, isolated
- dwelling Z59.8
- family Z63.79
- social Z60.4

Isoleucinosis E71.19
Isomerism atrial appendages (with asplenia or polysplenia) Q20.6
Isosporiasis, isosporosis A07.3
Isovaleric acidemia E71.110
Issue of
- medical certificate Z02.79
  - for disability determination Z02.71
- repeat prescription (appliance) (glasses) (medicinal substance, medicament, medicine) Z76.0
- contraception — see Contraception

Itch, itching — see also Pruritus
- baker's L23.6
- barber's B35.0
- bricklayer's L24.5
- cheese B88.0
- clam digger's B65.3
- coolie B76.9
- copra B88.0
- dew B76.9
- dhobi B35.6
- filarial — see Infestation, filarial
- grain B88.0
- grocer's B88.0
- ground B76.9
- harvest B88.0
- jock B35.6
- Malabar B35.5
  - beard B35.0
  - foot B35.3
  - scalp B35.0
- meaning scabies B86
- Norwegian B86
- perianal L29.0
- poultrymen's B88.0
- sarcoptic B86
- scabies B86
- scrub B88.0
- straw B88.0
- swimmer's B65.3
- water B76.9
- winter L29.8

Ivemark's syndrome (asplenia with congenital heart disease) Q89.01
Ivory bones Q78.2
Ixodiasis NEC B88.8

J

Jaccoud's syndrome — see Arthropathy, postrheumatic, chronic
Jackson's
- membrane Q43.3
- paralysis or syndrome G83.89
- veil Q43.3

Jacquet's dermatitis (diaper dermatitis) L22
Jadassohn-Pellizari's disease or anetoderma L90.2
Jadassohn's
- blue nevus — see Nevus
- intraepidermal epithelioma — see Neoplasm, skin, benign

Jaffe-Lichtenstein (-Uehlinger) **syndrome** — see Dysplasia, fibrous, bone NEC
Jakob-Creutzfeldt disease or syndrome — see Creutzfeldt-Jakob disease or syndrome
Jaksch-Luzet disease D64.89
Jamaican
- neuropathy G92
- paraplegic tropical ataxic-spastic syndrome G92

Janet's disease F48.8
Janiceps Q89.4
Jansky-Bielschowsky amaurotic idiocy E75.4
Japanese
- B-type encephalitis A83.0
- river fever A75.3

Jaundice (yellow) R17
- acholuric (familial) (splenomegalic) — see also Spherocytosis
  - acquired D59.8
- breast-milk (inhibitor) P59.3
- catarrhal (acute) B15.9
  - with hepatic coma B15.0
- cholestatic (benign) R17

Jaundice — continued
- due to or associated with
  - delayed conjugation P59.8
    - associated with (due to) preterm delivery P59.0
  - preterm delivery P59.0
- epidemic (catarrhal) B15.9
  - with hepatic coma B15.0
  - leptospiral A27.0
  - spirochetal A27.0
- familial nonhemolytic (congenital) (Gilbert) E80.4
  - Crigler-Najjar E80.5
- febrile (acute) B15.9
  - with hepatic coma B15.0
  - leptospiral A27.0
  - spirochetal A27.0
- hematogenous D59.9
- hemolytic (acquired) D59.9
  - congenital — see Spherocytosis
- hemorrhagic (acute) (leptospiral) (spirochetal) A27.0
- infectious (acute) (subacute) B15.9
  - with hepatic coma B15.0
  - leptospiral A27.0
  - spirochetal A27.0
- leptospiral (hemorrhagic) A27.0
- malignant (without coma) K72.90
  - with coma K72.91
- neonatal — see Jaundice, newborn
- newborn P59.9
  - due to or associated with
    - ABO
      - antibodies P55.1
      - incompatibility, maternal/fetal P55.1
      - isoimmunization P55.1
    - absence or deficiency of enzyme system for bilirubin conjugation (congenital) P59.8
    - bleeding P58.1
    - breast milk inhibitors to conjugation P59.3
      - associated with preterm delivery P59.0
    - bruising P58.0
    - Crigler-Najjar syndrome E80.5
    - delayed conjugation P59.8
      - associated with preterm delivery P59.0
    - drugs or toxins
      - given to newborn P58.42
      - transmitted from mother P58.41
    - excessive hemolysis P58.9
      - due to
        - bleeding P58.1
        - bruising P58.0
        - drugs or toxins
          - given to newborn P58.42
          - transmitted from mother P58.41
        - infection P58.2
        - polycythemia P58.3
        - swallowed maternal blood P58.5
      - specified type NEC P58.8
    - galactosemia E74.21
    - Gilbert syndrome E80.4
    - hemolytic disease P55.9
      - ABO isoimmunization P55.1
      - Rh isoimmunization P55.0
      - specified NEC P55.8
    - hepatocellular damage P59.20
      - specified NEC P59.29
    - hereditary hemolytic anemia P58.8
    - hypothyroidism, congenital E03.1
    - incompatibility, maternal/fetal NOS P55.9
    - infection P58.2
    - inspissated bile syndrome P59.1
    - isoimmunization NOS P55.9
    - mucoviscidosis E84.9
    - polycythemia P58.3
    - preterm delivery P59.0
    - Rh
      - antibodies P55.0
      - incompatibility, maternal/fetal P55.0
      - isoimmunization P55.0
    - specified cause NEC P59.8
    - swallowed maternal blood P58.5
  - spherocytosis (congenital) D58.0
- nonhemolytic congenital familial (Gilbert) E80.4
- nuclear, newborn — see also Kernicterus of newborn P57.9
- obstructive — see also Obstruction, bile duct K83.1
- post-immunization — see Hepatitis, viral, type, B
- post-transfusion — see Hepatitis, viral, type, B
- regurgitation — see also Obstruction, bile duct K83.1

Jaundice — continued
- serum (homologous) (prophylactic) (therapeutic) — see Hepatitis, viral, type, B
- spirochetal (hemorrhagic) A27.0
- symptomatic R17
  - newborn P59.9

Jaw — see condition
Jaw-winking phenomenon or syndrome Q07.8
Jealousy
- alcoholic F10.988
- childhood F93.8
- sibling F93.8

Jejunitis — see Enteritis
Jejunostomy status Z93.4
Jejunum, jejunal — see condition
Jensen's disease — see Inflammation, chorioretinal, focal, juxtapapillary
Jerks, myoclonic G25.3
Jervell-Lange-Nielsen syndrome I45.81
Jeune's disease Q77.2
Jigger disease B88.1
Job's syndrome (chronic granulomatous disease) D71
Joint — see also condition
- mice — see Loose, body, joint
  - knee M23.4- ☑

Jordan's anomaly or syndrome D72.0
Joseph-Diamond-Blackfan anemia (congenital hypoplastic) D61.01
Jungle yellow fever A95.0
Jüngling's disease — see Sarcoidosis
Juvenile — see condition

K

Kahler's disease C90.0- ☑
Kakke E51.11
Kala-azar B55.0
Kallmann's syndrome E23.0
Kanner's syndrome (autism) — see Psychosis, childhood
Kaposi's
- dermatosis (xeroderma pigmentosum) Q82.1
- lichen ruber L44.0
  - acuminatus L44.0
- sarcoma
  - colon C46.4
  - connective tissue C46.1
  - gastrointestinal organ C46.4
  - lung C46.5- ☑
  - lymph node (multiple) C46.3
  - palate (hard) (soft) C46.2
  - rectum C46.4
  - skin (multiple sites) C46.0
  - specified site NEC C46.7
  - stomach C46.4
  - unspecified site C46.9
- varicelliform eruption B00.0
  - vaccinia T88.1 ☑

Kartagener's syndrome or triad (sinusitis, bronchiectasis, situs inversus) Q89.3
Karyotype
- with abnormality except iso (Xq) Q96.2
- 45,X Q96.0
- 46,X
  - iso (Xq) Q96.1
- 46,XX Q98.3
  - with streak gonads Q50.32
  - hermaphrodite (true) Q99.1
  - male Q98.3
- 46,XY
  - with streak gonads Q56.1
  - female Q97.3
  - hermaphrodite (true) Q99.1
- 47,XXX Q97.0
- 47,XXY Q98.0
- 47,XYY Q98.5

Kaschin-Beck disease — see Disease, Kaschin-Beck
Katayama's disease or fever B65.2
Kawasaki's syndrome M30.3
Kayser-Fleischer ring (cornea) (pseudosclerosis) H18.04- ☑
Kaznelson's syndrome (congenital hypoplastic anemia) D61.01
Kearns-Sayre syndrome H49.81- ☑
Kedani fever A75.3
Kelis L91.0
Kelly (-Patterson) **syndrome** (sideropenic dysphagia) D50.1

☑ Additional Character Required — Refer to the Tabular List for Character Selection ▽ Subterms under main terms may continue to next column or page

Isolation, isolated — Kelly

Keloid, cheloid L91.0
  acne L73.0
  Addison's L94.0
  cornea — see Opacity, cornea
  Hawkin's L91.0
  scar L91.0
Keloma L91.0
Kenya fever A77.1
Keratectasia — see also Ectasia, cornea
  congenital Q13.4
Keratinization of alveolar ridge mucosa
  excessive K13.23
  minimal K13.22
Keratinized residual ridge mucosa
  excessive K13.23
  minimal K13.22
Keratitis (nodular) (nonulcerative) (simple) (zonular)
    H16.9
  with ulceration (central) (marginal) (perforated) (ring)
    — see Ulcer, cornea
  actinic — see Photokeratitis
  arborescens (herpes simplex) B00.52
  areolar H16.11- ☑
  bullosa H16.8
  deep H16.309
    specified type NEC H16.399
  dendritic (a) (herpes simplex) B00.52
  disciform (is) (herpes simplex) B00.52
    varicella B01.81
  filamentary H16.12- ☑
  gonococcal (congenital or prenatal) A54.33
  herpes, herpetic (simplex) B00.52
    zoster B02.33
  in (due to)
    acanthamebiasis B60.13
    adenovirus B30.0
    exanthema — see also Exanthem B09
    herpes (simplex) virus B00.52
    measles B05.81
    syphilis A50.31
    tuberculosis A18.52
    zoster B02.33
  interstitial (nonsyphilitic) H16.30- ☑
    diffuse H16.32- ☑
    herpes, herpetic (simplex) B00.52
      zoster B02.33
    sclerosing H16.33- ☑
    specified type NEC H16.39- ☑
    syphilitic (congenital) (late) A50.31
    tuberculous A18.52
  macular H16.11-
  nummular H16.11- ☑
  oyster shuckers' H16.8
  parenchymatous — see Keratitis, interstitial
  petrificans H16.8
  postmeasles B05.81
  punctata
    leprosa A30.9 [H16.14-] ☑
    syphilitic (profunda) A50.31
  punctate H16.14- ☑
  purulent H16.8
  rosacea L71.8
  sclerosing H16.33- ☑
  specified type NEC H16.8
  stellate H16.11- ☑
  striate H16.11- ☑
  superficial H16.10- ☑
    with conjunctivitis — see Keratoconjunctivitis
    due to light — see Photokeratitis
  suppurative H16.8
  syphilitic (congenital) (prenatal) A50.31
  trachomatous A71.1
    sequelae B94.0
  tuberculous A18.52
  vesicular H16.8
  xerotic — see also Keratomalacia H16.8
    vitamin A deficiency E50.4
Keratoacanthoma L85.8
Keratocele — see Descemetocele
Keratoconjunctivitis H16.20- ☑
  Acanthamoeba B60.13
  adenoviral B30.0
  epidemic B30.0
  exposure H16.21- ☑
  herpes, herpetic (simplex) B00.52
    zoster B02.33
  in exanthema — see also Exanthem B09
  infectious B30.0

Keratoconjunctivitis — continued
  lagophthalmic — see Keratoconjunctivitis, specified
    type NEC
  neurotrophic H16.23- ☑
  phlyctenular H16.25- ☑
  postmeasles B05.81
  shipyard B30.0
  sicca (Sjogren's) M35.0- ☑
    not Sjogren's H16.22- ☑
  specified type NEC H16.29- ☑
  tuberculous (phlyctenular) A18.52
  vernal H16.26- ☑
Keratoconus H18.60- ☑
  congenital Q13.4
  stable H18.61- ☑
  unstable H18.62- ☑
Keratocyst (dental) (odontogenic) — see Cyst, calcifying
    odontogenic
Keratoderma, keratodermia (congenital) (palmaris et
    plantaris) (symmetrical) Q82.8
  acquired L85.1
    in diseases classified elsewhere L86
  climactericum L85.1
  gonococcal A54.89
  gonorrheal A54.89
  punctata L85.2
  Reiter's — see Reiter's disease
Keratodermatocele — see Descemetocele
Keratoglobus H18.79 ☑
  congenital Q15.8
    with glaucoma Q15.0
Keratohemia — see Pigmentation, cornea, stromal
Keratoiritis — see also Iridocyclitis
  syphilitic A50.39
  tuberculous A18.54
Keratoma L57.0
  palmaris and plantaris hereditarium Q82.8
  senile L57.0
Keratomalacia H18.44- ☑
  vitamin A deficiency E50.4
Keratomegaly Q13.4
Keratomycosis B49
  nigrans, nigricans (palmaris) B36.1
Keratopathy H18.9
  band H18.42- ☑
  bullous (aphakic), following cataract surgery H59.01- ☑
  bullous H18.1- ☑
Keratoscleritis, tuberculous A18.52
Keratosis L57.0
  actinic L57.0
  arsenical L85.8
  congenital, specified NEC Q80.8
  female genital NEC N94.89
  follicularis Q82.8
    acquired L11.0
    congenita Q82.8
    et parafollicularis in cutem penetrans L87.0
    spinulosa (decalvans) Q82.8
    vitamin A deficiency E50.8
  gonococcal A54.89
  male genital (external) N50.89
  nigricans L83
  obturans, external ear (canal) — see Cholesteatoma,
    external ear
  palmaris et plantaris (inherited) (symmetrical) Q82.8
    acquired L85.1
  penile N48.89
  pharynx J39.2
  pilaris, acquired L85.8
  punctata (palmaris et plantaris) L85.2
  scrotal N50.89
  seborrheic L82.1
    inflamed L82.0
  senile L57.0
  solar L57.0
  tonsillaris J35.8
  vagina N89.4
  vegetans Q82.8
  vitamin A deficiency E50.8
  vocal cord J38.3
Kerato-uveitis — see Iridocyclitis
Kerion (celsi) B35.0
Kernicterus of newborn (not due to isoimmunization)
    P57.9
  due to isoimmunization (conditions in P55.0-P55.9)
    P57.0
  specified type NEC P57.8
Kerunoparalysis T75.09 ☑

Keshan disease E59
Ketoacidosis E87.2
  diabetic — see Diabetes, by type, with ketoacidosis
Ketonuria R82.4
Ketosis NEC E88.89
  diabetic — see Diabetes, by type, with ketoacidosis
Kew Garden fever A79.1
Kidney — see condition
Kienböck's disease — see also Osteochondrosis, juvenile,
    hand, carpal lunate
  adult M93.1
Kimmelstiel (-Wilson) disease — see Diabetes, Kimmel-
    stiel (-Wilson) disease
Kink, kinking
  artery I77.1
  hair (acquired) L67.8
  ileum or intestine — see Obstruction, intestine
  Lane's — see Obstruction, intestine
  organ or site, congenital NEC — see Anomaly, by site
  ureter (pelvic junction) N13.5
    with
      hydronephrosis N13.1
        with infection N13.6
      pyelonephritis (chronic) N11.1
    congenital Q62.39
  vein(s) I87.8
    caval I87.1
    peripheral I87.1
Kinnier Wilson's disease (hepatolenticular degenera-
    tion) E83.01
Kissing spine M48.20
  cervical region M48.22
  cervicothoracic region M48.23
  lumbar region M48.26
  lumbosacral region M48.27
  occipito-atlanto-axial region M48.21
  thoracic region M48.24
  thoracolumbar region M48.25
Klatskin's tumor C22.1
Klauder's disease A26.8
Klebs' disease — see also Glomerulonephritis N05- ☑
**Klebsiella (K.) pneumoniae, as cause of disease clas-
    sified elsewhere** B96.1
Klein (e)-Levin syndrome G47.13
Kleptomania F63.2
Klinefelter's syndrome Q98.4
  karyotype 47,XXY Q98.0
  male with more than two X chromosomes Q98.1
Klippel-Feil deficiency, disease, or syndrome (brevi-
    collis) Q76.1
Klippel's disease I67.2
Klippel-Trenaunay (-Weber) syndrome Q87.2
Klumpke (-Déjerine) palsy, paralysis (birth) (newborn)
    P14.1
Knee — see condition
Knock knee (acquired) M21.06- ☑
  congenital Q74.1
Knot(s)
  intestinal, syndrome (volvulus) K56.2
  surfer S89.8- ☑
  umbilical cord (true) O69.2 ☑
Knotting (of)
  hair L67.8
  intestine K56.2
Knuckle pad (Garrod's) M72.1
Koch's
  infection — see Tuberculosis
  relapsing fever A68.9
Koch-Weeks' conjunctivitis — see Conjunctivitis, acute,
    mucopurulent
Köebner's syndrome Q81.8
Köenig's disease (osteochondritis dissecans) — see Os-
    teochondritis, dissecans
Köhler-Pellegrini-Steida disease or syndrome (calci-
    fication, knee joint) — see Bursitis, tibial collateral
Köhler's disease
  patellar — see Osteochondrosis, juvenile, patella
  tarsal navicular — see Osteochondrosis, juvenile, tarsus
Koilonychia L60.3
  congenital Q84.6
Kojevnikov's, epilepsy — see Kozhevnikof's epilepsy
Koplik's spots B05.9
Kopp's asthma E32.8
**Korsakoff's (Wernicke) disease, psychosis or syn-
    drome** (alcoholic) F10.96
  with dependence F10.26

Korsakoff's (Wernicke) **disease, psychosis or syndrome** — *continued*
drug-induced
due to drug abuse — *see* Abuse, drug, by type, with amnestic disorder
due to drug dependence — *see* Dependence, drug, by type, with amnestic disorder
nonalcoholic F04
Korsakov's disease, psychosis or syndrome — *see* Korsakoff's disease
Korsakow's disease, psychosis or syndrome — *see* Korsakoff's disease
Kostmann's disease or syndrome (infantile genetic agranulocytosis) — *see* Agranulocytosis
Kozhevnikof's epilepsy G40.109
intractable G40.119
with status epilepticus G40.111
without status epilepticus G40.119
not intractable G40.109
with status epilepticus G40.101
without status epilepticus G40.109
Krabbe's
disease E75.23
syndrome, congenital muscle hypoplasia Q79.8
Kraepelin-Morel disease — *see* Schizophrenia
Kraft-Weber-Dimitri disease Q85.8
Kraurosis
ani K62.89
penis N48.0
vagina N89.8
vulva N90.4
Kreotoxism A05.9
Krukenberg's
spindle — *see* Pigmentation, cornea, posterior
tumor C79.6- ☑
Kufs' disease E75.4
Kugelberg-Welander disease G12.1
Kuhnt-Junius degeneration — *see also* Degeneration, macula H35.32-
Kümmell's disease or spondylitis — *see* Spondylopathy, traumatic
Kupffer cell sarcoma C22.3
Kuru A81.81
Kussmaul's
disease M30.0
respiration E87.2
in diabetic acidosis — *see* Diabetes, by type, with ketoacidosis
Kwashiorkor E40
marasmic, marasmus type E42
Kyasanur Forest disease A98.2
Kyphoscoliosis, kyphoscoliotic (acquired) — *see also* Scoliosis M41.9
congenital Q67.5
heart (disease) I27.1
sequelae of rickets E64.3
tuberculous A18.01
Kyphosis, kyphotic (acquired) M40.209
cervical region M40.202
cervicothoracic region M40.203
congenital Q76.419
cervical region Q76.412
cervicothoracic region Q76.413
occipito-atlanto-axial region Q76.411
thoracic region Q76.414
thoracolumbar region Q76.415
Morquio-Brailsford type (spinal) — *see also* subcategory M49.8 E76.219
postlaminectomy M96.3
postradiation therapy M96.2
postural (adolescent) M40.00
cervicothoracic region M40.03
thoracic region M40.04
thoracolumbar region M40.05
secondary NEC M40.10
cervical region M40.12
cervicothoracic region M40.13
thoracic region M40.14
thoracolumbar region M40.15
sequelae of rickets E64.3
specified type NEC M40.299
cervical region M40.292
cervicothoracic region M40.293
thoracic region M40.294
thoracolumbar region M40.295
syphilitic, congenital A50.56
thoracic region M40.204
thoracolumbar region M40.205

Kyphosis, kyphotic — *continued*
tuberculous A18.01
Kyrle disease L87.0

L

Labia, labium — *see* condition
Labile
blood pressure R09.89
vasomotor system I73.9
Labioglossal paralysis G12.29
Labium leporinum — *see* Cleft, lip
Labor — *see* Delivery
Labored breathing — *see* Hyperventilation
Labyrinthitis (circumscribed) (destructive) (diffuse) (inner ear) (latent) (purulent) (suppurative) — *see also* subcategory H83.0 ☑
syphilitic A52.79
Laceration
with abortion — *see* Abortion, by type, complicated by laceration of pelvic organs
abdomen, abdominal
wall S31.119 ☑
with
foreign body S31.129 ☑
penetration into peritoneal cavity S31.619 ☑
with foreign body S31.629 ☑
epigastric region S31.112 ☑
with
foreign body S31.122 ☑
penetration into peritoneal cavity S31.612 ☑
with foreign body S31.622 ☑
left
lower quadrant S31.114 ☑
with
foreign body S31.124 ☑
penetration into peritoneal cavity S31.614 ☑
with foreign body S31.624 ☑
upper quadrant S31.111 ☑
with
foreign body S31.121 ☑
penetration into peritoneal cavity S31.611 ☑
with foreign body S31.621 ☑
periumbilic region S31.115 ☑
with
foreign body S31.125 ☑
penetration into peritoneal cavity S31.615 ☑
with foreign body S31.625 ☑
right
lower quadrant S31.113 ☑
with
foreign body S31.123 ☑
penetration into peritoneal cavity S31.613 ☑
with foreign body S31.623 ☑
upper quadrant S31.110 ☑
with
foreign body S31.120 ☑
penetration into peritoneal cavity S31.610 ☑
with foreign body S31.620 ☑
accidental, complicating surgery — *see* Complications, surgical, accidental puncture or laceration
Achilles tendon S86.02- ☑
adrenal gland S37.813 ☑
alveolar (process) — *see* Laceration, oral cavity
ankle S91.01- ☑
with
foreign body S91.02- ☑
antecubital space — *see* Laceration, elbow
anus (sphincter) S31.831 ☑
with
ectopic or molar pregnancy O08.6
foreign body S31.832 ☑
complicating delivery — *see* Delivery, complicated, by, laceration, anus (sphincter)
following ectopic or molar pregnancy O08.6
nontraumatic, nonpuerperal — *see* Fissure, anus
arm (upper) S41.11- ☑
with foreign body S41.12- ☑
lower — *see* Laceration, forearm

Laceration — *continued*
auditory canal (external) (meatus) — *see* Laceration, ear
auricle, ear — *see* Laceration, ear
axilla — *see* Laceration, arm
back — *see also* Laceration, thorax, back
lower S31.010 ☑
with
foreign body S31.020 ☑
with penetration into retroperitoneal space S31.021 ☑
penetration into retroperitoneal space S31.011 ☑
bile duct S36.13 ☑
bladder S37.23 ☑
with ectopic or molar pregnancy O08.6
following ectopic or molar pregnancy O08.6
obstetrical trauma O71.5
blood vessel — *see* Injury, blood vessel
bowel — *see also* Laceration, intestine
with ectopic or molar pregnancy O08.6
complicating abortion — *see* Abortion, by type, complicated by, specified condition NEC
following ectopic or molar pregnancy O08.6
obstetrical trauma O71.5
brain (any part) (cortex) (diffuse) (membrane) — *see also* Injury, intracranial, diffuse
during birth P10.8
with hemorrhage P10.1
focal — *see* Injury, intracranial, focal brain injury
brainstem S06.38- ☑
breast S21.01- ☑
with foreign body S21.02- ☑
broad ligament S37.893 ☑
with ectopic or molar pregnancy O08.6
following ectopic or molar pregnancy O08.6
laceration syndrome N83.8
obstetrical trauma O71.6
syndrome (laceration) N83.8
buttock S31.801 ☑
with foreign body S31.802 ☑
left S31.821 ☑
with foreign body S31.822 ☑
right S31.811 ☑
with foreign body S31.812 ☑
calf — *see* Laceration, leg
canaliculus lacrimalis — *see* Laceration, eyelid
canthus, eye — *see* Laceration, eyelid
capsule, joint — *see* Sprain
causing eversion of cervix uteri (old) N86
central (perineal), complicating delivery O70.9
cerebellum, traumatic S06.37- ☑
cerebral S06.33- ☑
during birth P10.8
with hemorrhage P10.1
left side S06.32- ☑
right side S06.31- ☑
cervix (uteri)
with ectopic or molar pregnancy O08.6
following ectopic or molar pregnancy O08.6
nonpuerperal, nontraumatic N88.1
obstetrical trauma (current) O71.3
old (postpartal) N88.1
traumatic S37.63 ☑
cheek (external) S01.41- ☑
with foreign body S01.42- ☑
internal — *see* Laceration, oral cavity
chest wall — *see* Laceration, thorax
chin — *see* Laceration, head, specified site NEC
chordae tendinae NEC I51.1
concurrent with acute myocardial infarction — *see* Infarct, myocardium
following acute myocardial infarction (current complication) I23.4
clitoris — *see* Laceration, vulva
colon — *see* Laceration, intestine, large, colon
common bile duct S36.13 ☑
cortex (cerebral) — *see* Injury, intracranial, diffuse
costal region — *see* Laceration, thorax
cystic duct S36.13 ☑
diaphragm S27.803 ☑
digit(s)
foot — *see* Laceration, toe
hand — *see* Laceration, finger
duodenum S36.430 ☑
ear (canal) (external) S01.31- ☑
with foreign body S01.32- ☑

Laceration — continued
  ear — continued
    drum S09.2- ☑
  elbow S51.01- ☑
    with
      foreign body S51.02- ☑
  epididymis — see Laceration, testis
  epigastric region — see Laceration, abdomen, wall,
    epigastric region
  esophagus K22.8
    traumatic
      cervical S11.21
        with foreign body S11.22 ☑
      thoracic S27.813 ☑
  eye (ball) S05.3- ☑
    with prolapse or loss of intraocular tissue S05.2- ☑
    penetrating S05.6- ☑
  eyebrow — see Laceration, eyelid
  eyelid S01.11- ☑
    with foreign body S01.12- ☑
  face NEC — see Laceration, head, specified site NEC
  fallopian tube S37.539 ☑
    bilateral S37.532 ☑
    unilateral S37.531 ☑
  finger(s) S61.219 ☑
    with
      damage to nail S61.319 ☑
        with
          foreign body S61.329 ☑
      foreign body S61.229 ☑
    index S61.218 ☑
      with
        damage to nail S61.318 ☑
          with
            foreign body S61.328 ☑
        foreign body S61.228 ☑
      left S61.211 ☑
        with
          damage to nail S61.311 ☑
            with
              foreign body S61.321 ☑
          foreign body S61.221 ☑
      right S61.210 ☑
        with
          damage to nail S61.310 ☑
            with
              foreign body S61.320 ☑
          foreign body S61.220 ☑
    little S61.218 ☑
      with
        damage to nail S61.318 ☑
          with
            foreign body S61.328 ☑
        foreign body S61.228 ☑
      left S61.217 ☑
        with
          damage to nail S61.317 ☑
            with
              foreign body S61.327 ☑
          foreign body S61.227 ☑
      right S61.216 ☑
        with
          damage to nail S61.316 ☑
            with
              foreign body S61.326 ☑
          foreign body S61.226 ☑
    middle S61.218 ☑
      with
        damage to nail S61.318 ☑
          with
            foreign body S61.328 ☑
        foreign body S61.228 ☑
      left S61.213 ☑
        with
          damage to nail S61.313 ☑
            with
              foreign body S61.323 ☑
          foreign body S61.223 ☑
      right S61.212 ☑
        with
          damage to nail S61.312 ☑
            with
              foreign body S61.322 ☑
          foreign body S61.222 ☑
    ring S61.218 ☑

Laceration — continued
  finger(s) — continued
    ring — continued
      with
        damage to nail S61.318 ☑
          with
            foreign body S61.328 ☑
        foreign body S61.228 ☑
      left S61.215 ☑
        with
          damage to nail S61.315 ☑
            with
              foreign body S61.325 ☑
          foreign body S61.225 ☑
      right S61.214 ☑
        with
          damage to nail S61.314 ☑
            with
              foreign body S61.324 ☑
          foreign body S61.224 ☑
  flank S31.119 ☑
    with foreign body S31.129 ☑
  foot (except toe(s) alone) S91.319 ☑
    with foreign body S91.329 ☑
    left S91.312 ☑
      with foreign body S91.322 ☑
    right S91.311 ☑
      with foreign body S91.321 ☑
    toe — see Laceration, toe
  forearm S51.819 ☑
    with
      foreign body S51.829 ☑
    elbow only — see Laceration, elbow
    left S51.812 ☑
      with
        foreign body S51.822 ☑
    right S51.811 ☑
      with
        foreign body S51.821 ☑
  forehead S01.81 ☑
    with foreign body S01.82 ☑
  fourchette O70.0
    with ectopic or molar pregnancy O08.6
    complicating delivery O70.0
    following ectopic or molar pregnancy O08.6
  gallbladder S36.123 ☑
  genital organs, external
    female S31.512 ☑
      with foreign body S31.522 ☑
      vagina — see Laceration, vagina
      vulva — see Laceration, vulva
    male S31.511 ☑
      with foreign body S31.521 ☑
      penis — see Laceration, penis
      scrotum — see Laceration, scrotum
      testis — see Laceration, testis
  groin — see Laceration, abdomen, wall
  gum — see Laceration, oral cavity
  hand S61.419 ☑
    with
      foreign body S61.429 ☑
    finger — see Laceration, finger
    left S61.412 ☑
      with
        foreign body S61.422 ☑
    right S61.411 ☑
      with
        foreign body S61.421 ☑
    thumb — see Laceration, thumb
  head S01.91 ☑
    with foreign body S01.92 ☑
    cheek — see Laceration, cheek
    ear — see Laceration, ear
    eyelid — see Laceration, eyelid
    lip — see Laceration, lip
    nose — see Laceration, nose
    oral cavity — see Laceration, oral cavity
    scalp S01.01 ☑
      with foreign body S01.02 ☑
    specified site NEC S01.81 ☑
      with foreign body S01.82 ☑
    temporomandibular area — see Laceration, cheek
  heart — see Injury, heart, laceration
  heel — see Laceration, foot
  hepatic duct S36.13 ☑
  hip S71.019 ☑

Laceration — continued
  hip — continued
    with foreign body S71.029 ☑
    left S71.012 ☑
      with foreign body S71.022 ☑
    right S71.011 ☑
      with foreign body S71.021 ☑
  hymen — see Laceration, vagina
  hypochondrium — see Laceration, abdomen, wall
  hypogastric region — see Laceration, abdomen, wall
  ileum S36.438 ☑
  inguinal region — see Laceration, abdomen, wall
  instep — see Laceration, foot
  internal organ — see Injury, by site
  interscapular region — see Laceration, thorax, back
  intestine
    large
      colon S36.539 ☑
        ascending S36.530 ☑
        descending S36.532 ☑
        sigmoid S36.533 ☑
        specified site NEC S36.538 ☑
      rectum S36.63 ☑
        transverse S36.531 ☑
    small S36.439 ☑
      duodenum S36.430 ☑
      specified site NEC S36.438 ☑
  intra-abdominal organ S36.93 ☑
    intestine — see Laceration, intestine
    liver — see Laceration, liver
    pancreas — see Laceration, pancreas
    peritoneum S36.81 ☑
    specified site NEC S36.893 ☑
    spleen — see Laceration, spleen
    stomach — see Laceration, stomach
  intracranial NEC — see also Injury, intracranial, diffuse
    birth injury P10.9
  jaw — see Laceration, head, specified site NEC
  jejunum S36.438 ☑
  joint capsule — see Sprain, by site
  kidney S37.03- ☑
    major (greater than 3 cm) (massive) (stellate)
      S37.06- ☑
    minor (less than 1 cm) S37.04- ☑
    moderate (1 to 3 cm) S37.05- ☑
    multiple S37.06- ☑
  knee S81.01- ☑
    with foreign body S81.02- ☑
  labium (majus) (minus) — see Laceration, vulva
  lacrimal duct — see Laceration, eyelid
  large intestine — see Laceration, intestine, large
  larynx S11.011 ☑
    with foreign body S11.012 ☑
  leg (lower) S81.819 ☑
    with foreign body S81.829 ☑
    foot — see Laceration, foot
    knee — see Laceration, knee
    left S81.812 ☑
      with foreign body S81.822 ☑
    right S81.811 ☑
      with foreign body S81.821 ☑
    upper — see Laceration, thigh
  ligament — see Sprain
  lip S01.511 ☑
    with foreign body S01.521 ☑
  liver S36.113 ☑
    major (stellate) S36.116 ☑
    minor S36.114 ☑
    moderate S36.115 ☑
  loin — see Laceration, abdomen, wall
  lower back — see Laceration, back, lower
  lumbar region — see Laceration, back, lower
  lung S27.339 ☑
    bilateral S27.332 ☑
    unilateral S27.331 ☑
  malar region — see Laceration, head, specified site NEC
  mammary — see Laceration, breast
  mastoid region — see Laceration, head, specified site
    NEC
  meninges — see Injury, intracranial, diffuse
  meniscus — see Tear, meniscus
  mesentery S36.893 ☑
  mesosalpinx S37.893 ☑
  mouth — see Laceration, oral cavity
  muscle — see Injury, muscle, by site, laceration

Laceration — *continued*
- nail
  - finger — *see* Laceration, finger, with damage to nail
  - toe — *see* Laceration, toe, with damage to nail
- nasal (septum) (sinus) — *see* Laceration, nose
- nasopharynx — *see* Laceration, head, specified site NEC
- neck S11.91 ☑
  - with foreign body S11.92 ☑
  - involving
    - cervical esophagus S11.21 ☑
      - with foreign body S11.22 ☑
    - larynx — *see* Laceration, larynx
    - pharynx — *see* Laceration, pharynx
    - thyroid gland — *see* Laceration, thyroid gland
    - trachea — *see* Laceration, trachea
  - specified site NEC S11.81 ☑
    - with foreign body S11.82 ☑
- nerve — *see* Injury, nerve
- nose (septum) (sinus) S01.21 ☑
  - with foreign body S01.22 ☑
- ocular NOS S05.3-
  - adnexa NOS S01.11- ☑
- oral cavity S01.512 ☑
  - with foreign body S01.522 ☑
- orbit (eye) — *see* Wound, open, ocular, orbit
- ovary S37.439 ☑
  - bilateral S37.432 ☑
  - unilateral S37.431 ☑
- palate — *see* Laceration, oral cavity
- palm — *see* Laceration, hand
- pancreas S36.239 ☑
- pelvic S31.010 ☑
  - with
    - foreign body S31.020 ☑
      - penetration into retroperitoneal cavity S31.021 ☑
    - penetration into retroperitoneal cavity S31.011 ☑
  - floor — *see also* Laceration, back, lower
    - with ectopic or molar pregnancy O08.6
    - complicating delivery O70.1
    - following ectopic or molar pregnancy O08.6
    - old (postpartal) N81.89
  - organ S37.93 ☑
- penis S31.21 ☑
  - with foreign body S31.22 ☑
- perineum
  - female S31.41 ☑
    - with
      - ectopic or molar pregnancy O08.6
      - foreign body S31.42 ☑
    - during delivery O70.9
      - first degree O70.0
      - fourth degree O70.3
      - second degree O70.1
      - third degree — *see also* Delivery, complicated, by, laceration, perineum, third degree O70.20
    - old (postpartal) N81.89
    - postpartal N81.89
    - secondary (postpartal) O90.1
  - male S31.119 ☑
    - with foreign body S31.129 ☑
- periocular area (with or without lacrimal passages) — *see* Laceration, eyelid
- peritoneum S36.893 ☑
- periumbilic region — *see* Laceration, abdomen, wall, periumbilic
- periurethral tissue — *see* Laceration, urethra
- phalanges
  - finger — *see* Laceration, finger
  - toe — *see* Laceration, toe
- pharynx S11.21 ☑
  - with foreign body S11.22 ☑
- pinna — *see* Laceration, ear
- popliteal space — *see* Laceration, knee
- prepuce — *see* Laceration, penis
- prostate S37.823 ☑
- pubic region S31.119 ☑
  - with foreign body S31.129 ☑
- pudendum — *see* Laceration, genital organs, external
- rectovaginal septum — *see* Laceration, vagina
- rectum S36.63 ☑
- retroperitoneum S36.893 ☑
- round ligament S37.893 ☑
- sacral region — *see* Laceration, back, lower

Laceration — *continued*
- sacroiliac region — *see* Laceration, back, lower
- salivary gland — *see* Laceration, oral cavity
- scalp S01.01 ☑
  - with foreign body S01.02 ☑
- scapular region — *see* Laceration, shoulder
- scrotum S31.31 ☑
  - with foreign body S31.32 ☑
- seminal vesicle S37.893 ☑
- shin — *see* Laceration, leg
- shoulder S41.019 ☑
  - with foreign body S41.029 ☑
  - left S41.012 ☑
    - with foreign body S41.022 ☑
  - right S41.011 ☑
    - with foreign body S41.021 ☑
- small intestine — *see* Laceration, intestine, small
- spermatic cord — *see* Laceration, testis
- spinal cord (meninges) — *see also* Injury, spinal cord, by region
  - due to injury at birth P11.5
  - newborn (birth injury) P11.5
- spleen S36.039 ☑
  - major (massive) (stellate) S36.032 ☑
  - moderate S36.031 ☑
  - superficial (minor) S36.030 ☑
- sternal region — *see* Laceration, thorax, front
- stomach S36.33 ☑
- submaxillary region — *see* Laceration, head, specified site NEC
- submental region — *see* Laceration, head, specified site NEC
- subungual
  - finger(s) — *see* Laceration, finger, with damage to nail
  - toe(s) — *see* Laceration, toe, with damage to nail
- suprarenal gland — *see* Laceration, adrenal gland
- temple, temporal region — *see* Laceration, head, specified site NEC
- temporomandibular area — *see* Laceration, cheek
- tendon — *see* Injury, muscle, by site, laceration
  - Achilles S86.02- ☑
- tentorium cerebelli — *see* Injury, intracranial, diffuse
- testis S31.31 ☑
  - with foreign body S31.32 ☑
- thigh S71.11- ☑
  - with foreign body S71.12- ☑
- thorax, thoracic (wall) S21.91 ☑
  - with foreign body S21.92 ☑
    - back S21.22- ☑
      - with penetration into thoracic cavity S21.42- ☑
    - front S21.12- ☑
      - with penetration into thoracic cavity S21.32- ☑
  - back S21.21- ☑
    - with
      - foreign body S21.22- ☑
        - with penetration into thoracic cavity S21.42- ☑
      - penetration into thoracic cavity S21.41- ☑
  - breast — *see* Laceration, breast
  - front S21.11- ☑
    - with
      - foreign body S21.12- ☑
        - with penetration into thoracic cavity S21.32- ☑
      - penetration into thoracic cavity S21.31- ☑
- thumb S61.019 ☑
  - with
    - damage to nail S61.119 ☑
      - with
        - foreign body S61.129 ☑
    - foreign body S61.029 ☑
  - left S61.012 ☑
    - with
      - damage to nail S61.112 ☑
        - with
          - foreign body S61.122 ☑
      - foreign body S61.022 ☑
  - right S61.011 ☑
    - with
      - damage to nail S61.111 ☑
        - with
          - foreign body S61.121 ☑
      - foreign body S61.021 ☑

Laceration — *continued*
- thyroid gland S11.11 ☑
  - with foreign body S11.12 ☑
- toe(s) S91.119 ☑
  - with
    - damage to nail S91.219 ☑
      - with
        - foreign body S91.229 ☑
    - foreign body S91.129 ☑
  - great S91.113 ☑
    - with
      - damage to nail S91.213 ☑
        - with
          - foreign body S91.223 ☑
      - foreign body S91.123 ☑
    - left S91.112 ☑
      - with
        - damage to nail S91.212 ☑
          - with
            - foreign body S91.222 ☑
        - foreign body S91.122 ☑
    - right S91.111 ☑
      - with
        - damage to nail S91.211 ☑
          - with
            - foreign body S91.221 ☑
        - foreign body S91.121 ☑
  - lesser S91.116 ☑
    - with
      - damage to nail S91.216 ☑
        - with
          - foreign body S91.226 ☑
      - foreign body S91.126 ☑
    - left S91.115 ☑
      - with
        - damage to nail S91.215 ☑
          - with
            - foreign body S91.225 ☑
        - foreign body S91.125 ☑
    - right S91.114 ☑
      - with
        - damage to nail S91.214 ☑
          - with
            - foreign body S91.224 ☑
        - foreign body S91.124 ☑
- tongue — *see* Laceration, oral cavity
- trachea S11.021 ☑
  - with foreign body S11.022 ☑
- tunica vaginalis — *see* Laceration, testis
- tympanum, tympanic membrane — *see* Laceration, ear, drum
- umbilical region S31.115 ☑
  - with foreign body S31.125 ☑
- ureter S37.13 ☑
- urethra S37.33 ☑
  - with or following ectopic or molar pregnancy O08.6
  - obstetrical trauma O71.5
- urinary organ NEC S37.893 ☑
- uterus S37.63 ☑
  - with ectopic or molar pregnancy O08.6
  - following ectopic or molar pregnancy O08.6
  - nonpuerperal, nontraumatic N85.8
  - obstetrical trauma NEC O71.81
  - old (postpartal) N85.8
- uvula — *see* Laceration, oral cavity
- vagina S31.41 ☑
  - with
    - ectopic or molar pregnancy O08.6
    - foreign body S31.42 ☑
  - during delivery O71.4
    - with perineal laceration — *see* Laceration, perineum, female, during delivery
  - following ectopic or molar pregnancy O08.6
  - nonpuerperal, nontraumatic N89.8
  - old (postpartal) N89.8
- vas deferens S37.893 ☑
- vesical — *see* Laceration, bladder
- vocal cords S11.031 ☑
  - with foreign body S11.032 ☑
- vulva S31.41 ☑
  - with
    - ectopic or molar pregnancy O08.6
    - foreign body S31.42 ☑
  - complicating delivery O70.0
  - following ectopic or molar pregnancy O08.6
  - nonpuerperal, nontraumatic N90.89
  - old (postpartal) N90.89

☑ **Additional Character Required — Refer to the Tabular List for Character Selection**   ▽ **Subterms under main terms may continue to next column or page**

Index

Laceration — *continued*
- wrist S61.519 ☑
  - with
    - foreign body S61.529 ☑
  - left S61.512 ☑
    - with
      - foreign body S61.522 ☑
  - right S61.511 ☑
    - with
      - foreign body S61.521 ☑

Lack of
- achievement in school Z55.3
- adequate
  - food Z59.4
  - intermaxillary vertical dimension of fully erupted teeth M26.36
  - sleep Z72.820
- appetite (see Anorexia) R63.0
- awareness R41.9
- care
  - in home Z74.2
  - of infant (at or after birth) T76.02 ☑
    - confirmed T74.02 ☑
- cognitive functions R41.9
- coordination R27.9
  - ataxia R27.0
  - specified type NEC R27.8
- development (physiological) R62.50
  - failure to thrive (child over 28 days old) R62.51
    - adult R62.7
    - newborn P92.6
  - short stature R62.52
  - specified type NEC R62.59
- energy R53.83
- financial resources Z59.6
- food T73.0 ☑
- growth R62.52
- heating Z59.1
- housing (permanent) (temporary) Z59.0
  - adequate Z59.1
- learning experiences in childhood Z62.898
- leisure time (affecting life-style) Z73.2
- material resources Z59.9
- memory — *see also* Amnesia
  - mild, following organic brain damage F06.8
- ovulation N97.0
- parental supervision or control of child Z62.0
- person able to render necessary care Z74.2
- physical exercise Z72.3
- play experience in childhood Z62.898
- posterior occlusal support M26.57
- relaxation (affecting life-style) Z73.2
- sexual
  - desire F52.0
  - enjoyment F52.1
- shelter Z59.0
- sleep (adequate) Z72.820
- supervision of child by parent Z62.0
- support, posterior occlusal M26.57
- water T73.1 ☑

Lacrimal — *see* condition
Lacrimation, abnormal — *see* Epiphora
Lacrimonasal duct — *see* condition
Lactation, lactating (breast) (puerperal, postpartum)
- associated
  - cracked nipple O92.13
  - retracted nipple O92.03
- defective O92.4
- disorder NEC O92.79
- excessive O92.6
- failed (complete) O92.3
  - partial O92.4
- mastitis NEC — *see* Mastitis, obstetric
- mother (care and/or examination) Z39.1
- nonpuerperal N64.3

Lacticemia, excessive E87.2
Lacunar skull Q75.8
Laennec's cirrhosis K70.30
- with ascites K70.31
- nonalcoholic K74.69

Lafora's disease — *see* Epilepsy, generalized, idiopathic
Lag, lid (nervous) — *see* Retraction, lid
Lagophthalmos (eyelid) (nervous) H02.209
- bilateral, upper and lower eyelids H02.20C
- cicatricial H02.219
  - bilateral, upper and lower eyelids H02.21C
  - left H02.216
    - lower H02.215

Lagophthalmos — *continued*
- cicatricial — *continued*
  - left — *continued*
    - upper H02.214
    - upper and lower eyelids H02.21B
  - right H02.213
    - lower H02.212
    - upper H02.211
    - upper and lower eyelids H02.21A
- keratoconjunctivitis — *see* Keratoconjunctivitis
- left H02.206
  - lower H02.205
  - upper H02.204
  - upper and lower eyelids H02.20B
- mechanical H02.229
  - bilateral, upper and lower eyelids H02.22C
  - left H02.226
    - lower H02.225
    - upper H02.224
    - upper and lower eyelids H02.22B
  - right H02.223
    - lower H02.222
    - upper H02.221
    - upper and lower eyelids H02.22A
- paralytic H02.239
  - bilateral, upper and lower eyelids H02.23C
  - left H02.236
    - lower H02.235
    - upper H02.234
    - upper and lower eyelids H02.23B
  - right H02.233
    - lower H02.232
    - upper H02.231
    - upper and lower eyelids H02.23A
- right H02.203
  - lower H02.202
  - upper H02.201
  - upper and lower eyelids H02.20A

Laki-Lorand factor deficiency — *see* Defect, coagulation, specified type NEC
Lalling F80.0
Lambert-Eaton syndrome — *see* Syndrome, Lambert-Eaton
Lambliasis, lambliosis A07.1
Landau-Kleffner syndrome — *see* Epilepsy, specified NEC
Landouzy-Déjérine dystrophy or facioscapulohumeral atrophy G71.02
Landouzy's disease (icterohemorrhagic leptospirosis) A27.0
Landry-Guillain-Barré, syndrome or paralysis G61.0
Landry's disease or paralysis G61.0
Lane's
- band Q43.3
- kink — *see* Obstruction, intestine
- syndrome K90.2

Langdon Down syndrome — *see* Trisomy, 21
Lapsed immunization schedule status Z28.3
Large
- baby (regardless of gestational age) (4000g to 4499g) P08.1
- ear, congenital Q17.1
- physiological cup Q14.2
- stature R68.89

Large-for-dates NEC (infant) (4000g to 4499g) P08.1
- affecting management of pregnancy O36.6- ☑
- exceptionally (4500g or more) P08.0

Larsen-Johansson disease orosteochondrosis — *see* Osteochondrosis, juvenile, patella
Larsen's syndrome (flattened facies and multiple congenital dislocations) Q74.8
Larva migrans
- cutaneous B76.9
  - Ancylostoma B76.0
- visceral B83.0

Laryngeal — *see* condition
Laryngismus (stridulus) J38.5
- congenital P28.89
- diphtheritic A36.2

Laryngitis (acute) (edematous) (fibrinous) (infective) (infiltrative) (malignant) (membranous) (phlegmonous) (pneumococcal) (pseudomembranous) (septic) (subglottic) (suppurative) (ulcerative) J04.0
- with
  - influenza, flu, or grippe — *see* Influenza, with, laryngitis
  - tracheitis (acute) — *see* Laryngotracheitis
- atrophic J37.0

Laryngitis — *continued*
- catarrhal J37.0
- chronic J37.0
  - with tracheitis (chronic) J37.1
- diphtheritic A36.2
- due to external agent — *see* Inflammation, respiratory, upper, due to
- H. influenzae J04.0
- Hemophilus influenzae J04.0
- hypertrophic J37.0
- influenzal — *see* Influenza, with, respiratory manifestations NEC
- obstructive J05.0
- sicca J37.0
- spasmodic J05.0
  - acute J04.0
- streptococcal J04.0
- stridulous J05.0
- syphilitic (late) A52.73
  - congenital A50.59 *[J99]*
  - early A50.03 *[J99]*
- tuberculous A15.5
- Vincent's A69.1

Laryngocele (congenital) (ventricular) Q31.3
Laryngofissure J38.7
- congenital Q31.8
Laryngomalacia (congenital) Q31.5
Laryngopharyngitis (acute) J06.0
- chronic J37.0
- due to external agent — *see* Inflammation, respiratory, upper, due to
Laryngoplegia J38.00
- bilateral J38.02
- unilateral J38.01
Laryngoptosis J38.7
Laryngospasm J38.5
Laryngostenosis J38.6
Laryngotracheitis (acute) (Infectional) (infective) (viral) J04.2
- atrophic J37.1
- catarrhal J37.1
- chronic J37.1
- diphtheritic A36.2
- due to external agent — *see* Inflammation, respiratory, upper, due to
- Hemophilus influenzae J04.2
- hypertrophic J37.1
- influenzal — *see* Influenza, with, respiratory manifestations NEC
- pachydermic J38.7
- sicca J37.1
- spasmodic J38.5
  - acute J05.0
- streptococcal J04.2
- stridulous J38.5
- syphilitic (late) A52.73
  - congenital A50.59 *[J99]*
  - early A50.03 *[J99]*
- tuberculous A15.5
- Vincent's A69.1

Laryngotracheobronchitis — *see* Bronchitis
Larynx, laryngeal — *see* condition
Lassa fever A96.2
Lassitude — *see* Weakness
Late
- talker R62.0
- walker R62.0
Late effect(s) — *see* Sequelae
Latent — *see* condition
Laterocession — *see* Lateroversion
Lateroflexion — *see* Lateroversion
Lateroversion
- cervix — *see* Lateroversion, uterus
- uterus, uterine (cervix) (postinfectional) (postpartal, old) N85.4
  - congenital Q51.818
  - in pregnancy or childbirth O34.59- ☑
Lathyrism — *see* Poisoning, food, noxious, plant
Launois' syndrome (pituitary gigantism) E22.0
Launois-Bensaude adenolipomatosis E88.89
Laurence-Moon (-Bardet)-**Biedl syndrome** Q87.89
Lax, laxity — *see also* Relaxation
- ligament (ous) — *see also* Disorder, ligament
  - familial M35.7
  - knee — *see* Derangement, knee
- skin (acquired) L57.4
  - congenital Q82.8
Laxative habit F55.2

Laceration — Laxative habit

Lazy leukocyte syndrome D70.8
Lead miner's lung J63.6
Leak, leakage
  air NEC J93.82
    postprocedural J95.812
  amniotic fluid — see Rupture, membranes, premature
  blood (microscopic), fetal, into maternal circulation
    affecting management of pregnancy — see
    Pregnancy, complicated by
  cerebrospinal fluid G96.0
    from spinal (lumbar) puncture G97.0
  device, implant or graft — see also Complications, by
    site and type, mechanical
    arterial graft NEC — see Complication, cardiovascu-
      lar device, mechanical, vascular
    breast (implant) T85.43 ☑
    catheter NEC T85.638 ☑
      dialysis (renal) T82.43 ☑
        intraperitoneal T85.631 ☑
      infusion NEC T82.534 ☑
        spinal (epidural) (subdural) T85.630 ☑
      urinary T83.038 ☑
        cystostomy T83.030 ☑
        Hopkins T83.038 ☑
        ileostomy T83.038 ☑
        indwelling T83.031 ☑
        nephrostomy T83.032 ☑
        specified T83.038 ☑
        urostomy T83.038 ☑
    gastrointestinal — see Complications, prosthetic
      device, mechanical, gastrointestinal device
    genital NEC T83.498 ☑
      penile prosthesis (cylinder) (implanted) (pump)
        (reservoir) T83.490 ☑
      testicular prosthesis T83.491 ☑
    heart NEC — see Complication, cardiovascular de-
      vice, mechanical
    joint prosthesis — see Complications, joint prosthe-
      sis, mechanical, specified NEC, by site
    ocular NEC — see Complications, prosthetic device,
      mechanical, ocular device
    orthopedic NEC — see Complication, orthopedic,
      device, mechanical
    persistent air J93.82
    specified NEC T85.638 ☑
    urinary NEC — see also Complication, genitourinary,
      device, urinary, mechanical
      graft T83.23 ☑
    vascular NEC — see Complication, cardiovascular
      device, mechanical
    ventricular intracranial shunt T85.03 ☑
  urine — see Incontinence
Leaky heart — see Endocarditis
Learning defect (specific) F81.9
Leather bottle stomach C16.9
Leber's
  congenital amaurosis H35.50
  optic atrophy (hereditary) H47.22
Lederer's anemia D59.1
Leeches (external) — see Hirudiniasis
Leg — see condition
Legg (-Calvé)-**Perthes disease, syndrome or osteo-
  chondrosis** M91.1- ☑
Legionellosis A48.1
  nonpneumonic A48.2
Legionnaires'
  disease A48.1
    nonpneumonic A48.2
    pneumonia A48.1
Leigh's disease G31.82
Leiner's disease L21.1
Leiofibromyoma — see Leiomyoma
Leiomyoblastoma — see Neoplasm, connective tissue,
  benign
Leiomyofibroma — see also Neoplasm, connective tissue, benign
  uterus (cervix) (corpus) D25.9
Leiomyoma — see also Neoplasm, connective tissue,
  benign
  bizarre — see Neoplasm, connective tissue, benign
  cellular — see Neoplasm, connective tissue, benign
  epithelioid — see Neoplasm, connective tissue, benign
  uterus (cervix) (corpus) D25.9
    intramural D25.1
    submucous D25.0
    subserosal D25.2
  vascular — see Neoplasm, connective tissue, benign

Leiomyoma, leiomyomatosis (intravascular) — see
  Neoplasm, connective tissue, uncertain behavior
Leiomyosarcoma — see also Neoplasm, connective tissue, malignant
  epithelioid — see Neoplasm, connective tissue, malig-
    nant
  myxoid — see Neoplasm, connective tissue, malignant
Leishmaniasis B55.9
  American (mucocutaneous) B55.2
    cutaneous B55.1
  Asian Desert B55.1
  Brazilian B55.2
  cutaneous (any type) B55.1
  dermal — see also Leishmaniasis, cutaneous
    post-kala-azar B55.0
  eyelid B55.1
  infantile B55.0
  Mediterranean B55.0
  mucocutaneous (American) (New World) B55.2
  naso-oral B55.2
  nasopharyngeal B55.2
  old world B55.1
  tegumentaria diffusa B55.1
  visceral B55.0
Leishmanoid, dermal — see also Leishmaniasis, cutaneous
  post-kala-azar B55.0
Lenegre's disease I44.2
Lengthening, leg — see Deformity, limb, unequal length
Lennert's lymphoma — see Lymphoma, Lennert's
Lennox-Gastaut syndrome G40.812
  intractable G40.814
    with status epilepticus G40.813
    without status epilepticus G40.814
  not intractable G40.812
    with status epilepticus G40.811
    without status epilepticus G40.812
Lens — see condition
Lenticonus (anterior) (posterior) (congenital) Q12.8
Lenticular degeneration, progressive E83.01
Lentiglobus (posterior) (congenital) Q12.8
Lentigo (congenital) L81.4
  maligna — see also Melanoma, in situ
    melanoma — see Melanoma
Lentivirus, as cause of disease classified elsewhere
  B97.31
Leontiasis
  ossium M85.2
  syphilitic (late) A52.78
    congenital A50.59
Lepothrix A48.8
Lepra — see Leprosy
Leprechaunism E34.8
Leprosy A30.- ☑
  with muscle disorder A30.9 *[M63.80]*
    ankle A30.9 *[M63.87-]* ☑
    foot A30.9 *[M63.87-]* ☑
    forearm A30.9 *[M63.83-]* ☑
    hand A30.9 *[M63.84-]* ☑
    lower leg A30.9 *[M63.86-]* ☑
    multiple sites A30.9 *[M63.89]*
    pelvic region A30.9 *[M63.85-]* ☑
    shoulder region A30.9 *[M63.81-]* ☑
    specified site NEC A30.9 *[M63.88]*
    thigh A30.9 *[M63.85-]* ☑
    upper arm A30.9 *[M63.82-]* ☑
  anesthetic A30.9
  BB A30.3
  BL A30.4
  borderline (infiltrated) (neuritic) A30.3
    lepromatous A30.4
    tuberculoid A30.2
  BT A30.2
  dimorphous (infiltrated) (neuritic) A30.3
  I A30.0
  indeterminate (macular) (neuritic) A30.0
  lepromatous (diffuse) (infiltrated) (macular) (neuritic)
    (nodular) A30.5
  LL A30.5
  macular (early) (neuritic) (simple) A30.9
  maculoanesthetic A30.9
  mixed A30.3
  neural A30.9
  nodular A30.5
  primary neuritic A30.3
  specified type NEC A30.8
  TT A30.1

Leprosy — continued
  tuberculoid (major) (minor) A30.1
Leptocytosis, hereditary D56.9
Leptomeningitis (chronic) (circumscribed) (hemorrhagic)
  (nonsuppurative) — see Meningitis
Leptomeningopathy G96.19
Leptospiral — see condition
Leptospirochetal — see condition
Leptospirosis A27.9
  canicola A27.89
  due to Leptospira interrogans serovar icterohaemorrha-
    giae A27.0
  icterohemorrhagica A27.0
  pomona A27.89
  Weil's disease A27.0
Leptus dermatitis B88.0
Leriche's syndrome (aortic bifurcation occlusion) I74.09
Leri's pleonosteosis Q78.8
Leri-Weill syndrome Q77.8
Lermoyez' syndrome — see Vertigo, peripheral NEC
Lesch-Nyhan syndrome E79.1
Leser-Trélat disease L82.1
  inflamed L82.0
Lesion(s) (nontraumatic)
  abducens nerve — see Strabismus, paralytic, sixth nerve
  alveolar process K08.9
  angiocentric immunoproliferative D47.Z9 (following
    D47.4)
  anorectal K62.9
  aortic (valve) I35.9
  auditory nerve — see subcategory H93.3 ☑
  basal ganglion G25.9
  bile duct — see Disease, bile duct
  biomechanical M99.9
    specified type NEC M99.89
      abdomen M99.89
      acromioclavicular M99.87
      cervical region M99.81
      cervicothoracic M99.81
      costochondral M99.88
      costovertebral M99.88
      head region M99.80
      hip M99.85
      lower extremity M99.86
      lumbar region M99.83
      lumbosacral M99.83
      occipitocervical M99.80
      pelvic region M99.85
      pubic M99.85
      rib cage M99.88
      sacral region M99.84
      sacrococcygeal M99.84
      sacroiliac M99.84
      specified NEC M99.89
      sternochondral M99.88
      sternoclavicular M99.87
      thoracic region M99.82
      thoracolumbar M99.82
      upper extremity M99.87
  bladder N32.9
  bone — see Disorder, bone
  brachial plexus G54.0
  brain G93.9
    congenital Q04.9
    vascular I67.9
      degenerative I67.9
      hypertensive I67.4
  buccal cavity K13.79
  calcified — see Calcification
  canthus — see Disorder, eyelid
  carate — see Pinta, lesions
  cardia K31.9
  cardiac — see also Disease, heart I51.9
    congenital Q24.9
    valvular — see Endocarditis
  cauda equina G83.4
  cecum K63.9
  cerebral — see Lesion, brain
  cerebrovascular I67.9
    degenerative I67.9
    hypertensive I67.4
  cervical (nerve) root NEC G54.2
  chiasmal — see Disorder, optic, chiasm
  chorda tympani G51.8
  coin, lung R91.1
  colon K63.9
  combined periodontic - endodontic K05.5
  congenital — see Anomaly, by site

☑ **Additional Character Required** — Refer to the Tabular List for Character Selection   ▽ **Subterms under main terms may continue to next column or page**

Lesion(s) — *continued*
conjunctiva H11.9
conus medullaris — *see* Injury, conus medullaris
coronary artery — *see* Ischemia, heart
cranial nerve G52.9
  eighth — *see* Disorder, ear
  eleventh G52.9
  fifth G50.9
  first G52.0
  fourth — *see* Strabismus, paralytic, fourth nerve
  seventh G51.9
  sixth — *see* Strabismus, paralytic, sixth nerve
  tenth G52.2
  twelfth G52.3
cystic — *see* Cyst
degenerative — *see* Degeneration
duodenum K31.9
edentulous (alveolar) ridge, associated with trauma,
    due to traumatic occlusion K06.2
en coup de sabre L94.1
eyelid — *see* Disorder, eyelid
gasserian ganglion G50.8
gastric K31.9
gastroduodenal K31.9
gastrointestinal K63.9
gingiva, associated with trauma K06.2
glomerular
  focal and segmental — *see also* N00-N07 with fourth
    character .1 N05.1
  minimal change — *see also* N00-N07 with fourth
    character .0 N05.0
heart (organic) — *see* Disease, heart
hyperchromic, due to pinta (carate) A67.1
hyperkeratotic — *see* Hyperkeratosis
hypothalamic E23.7
ileocecal K63.9
ileum K63.9
iliohypogastric nerve G57.8- ☑
inflammatory — *see* Inflammation
intestine K63.9
intracerebral — *see* Lesion, brain
intrachiasmal (optic) — *see* Disorder, optic, chiasm
intracranial, space-occupying R90.0
joint — *see* Disorder, joint
  sacroiliac (old) M53.3
keratotic — *see* Keratosis
kidney — *see* Disease, renal
laryngeal nerve (recurrent) G52.2
lip K13.0
liver K76.9
lumbosacral
  plexus G54.1
  root (nerve) NEC G54.4
lung (coin) R91.1
maxillary sinus J32.0
mitral I05.9
Morel-Lavallée — *see* Hematoma, by site
motor cortex NEC G93.89
mouth K13.79
nerve G58.9
  femoral G57.2- ☑
  median G56.1- ☑
    carpal tunnel syndrome — *see* Syndrome, carpal
      tunnel
  plantar G57.6- ☑
  popliteal (lateral) G57.3- ☑
    medial G57.4- ☑
  radial G56.3- ☑
  sciatic G57.0- ☑
  spinal — *see* Injury, nerve, spinal
  ulnar G56.2- ☑
nervous system, congenital Q07.9
nonallopathic — *see* Lesion, biomechanical
nose (internal) J34.89
obstructive — *see* Obstruction
obturator nerve G57.8- ☑
oral mucosa K13.70
organ or site NEC — *see* Disease, by site
osteolytic — *see* Osteolysis
peptic K27.9
periodontal, due to traumatic occlusion K05.5
pharynx J39.2
pigment, pigmented (skin) L81.9
pinta — *see* Pinta, lesions
polypoid — *see* Polyp
prechiasmal (optic) — *see* Disorder, optic, chiasm
primary — *see also* Syphilis, primary A51.0

Lesion(s) — *continued*
primary — *see also* Syphilis, primary — *continued*
  carate A67.0
  pinta A67.0
  yaws A66.0
pulmonary J98.4
  valve I37.9
pylorus K31.9
rectosigmoid K63.9
retina, retinal H35.9
sacroiliac (joint) (old) M53.3
salivary gland K11.9
  benign lymphoepithelial K11.8
saphenous nerve G57.8- ☑
sciatic nerve G57.0- ☑
secondary — *see* Syphilis, secondary
shoulder (region) M75.9-
  specified NEC M75.8- ☑
sigmoid K63.9
sinus (accessory) (nasal) J34.89
skin L98.9
  suppurative L08.0
SLAP S43.43- ☑
spinal cord G95.9
  congenital Q06.9
spleen D73.89
stomach K31.9
superior glenoid labrum S43.43- ☑
syphilitic — *see* Syphilis
tertiary — *see* Syphilis, tertiary
thoracic root (nerve) NEC G54.3
tonsillar fossa J35.9
tooth, teeth K08.9
  white spot
    chewing surface K02.51
    pit and fissure surface K02.51
    smooth surface K02.61
traumatic — *see* specific type of injury by site
tricuspid (valve) I07.9
  nonrheumatic I36.9
trigeminal nerve G50.9
ulcerated or ulcerative — *see* Ulcer, skin
uterus N85.9
vagina N89.8
vagus nerve G52.2
valvular — *see* Endocarditis
vascular I99.9
  affecting central nervous system I67.9
  following trauma NEC T14.8 ☑
  umbilical cord, complicating delivery O69.5 ☑
vulva N90.89
warty — *see* Verruca
white spot (tooth)
  chewing surface K02.51
  pit and fissure surface K02.51
  smooth surface K02.61
Lethargic — *see* condition
Lethargy R53.83
Letterer-Siwe's disease C96.0
Leukemia, leukemic C95.9- ☑
acute basophilic C94.8- ☑
acute bilineal C95.0- ☑
acute erythroid C94.0- ☑
acute lymphoblastic C91.0- ☑
acute megakaryoblastic C94.2- ☑
acute megakaryocytic C94.2- ☑
acute mixed lineage C95.0- ☑
acute monoblastic (monoblastic/monocytic) C93.0- ☑
acute monocytic (monoblastic/monocytic) C93.0- ☑
acute myeloblastic (minimal differentiation) (with
    maturation) C92.0- ☑
acute myeloid, NOS C92.0- ☑
  with
    11q23-abnormality C92.6- ☑
    dysplasia of remaining hematopoesis and/or
      myelodysplastic disease in its history
      C92.A- ☑ (*following* C92.6)
    multilineage dysplasia C92.A- ☑ (*following*
      C92.6)
    variation of MLL-gene C92.6- ☑
  M6 (a)(b) C94.0- ☑
  M7 C94.2- ☑
acute myelomonocytic C92.5- ☑
acute promyelocytic C92.4- ☑
adult T-cell (HTLV-1-associated) (acute variant)
    (chronic variant) (lymphomatoid variant)
    (smouldering variant) C91.5- ☑

Leukemia, leukemic — *continued*
aggressive NK-cell C94.8- ☑
AML (1/ETO) (M0) (M1) (M2) (without a FAB classifica-
    tion) C92.0- ☑
AML M3 C92.4- ☑
AML M4 (Eo with inv(16) or t(16;16)) C92.5- ☑
AML M5 C93.0- ☑
AML M5a C93.0- ☑
AML M5b C93.0- ☑
AML Me with t (15;17) and variants C92.4- ☑
atypical chronic myeloid, BCR/ABL-negative C92.2- ☑
biphenotypic acute C95.0- ☑
blast cell C95.0- ☑
Burkitt-type, mature B-cell C91.A- ☑ (*following* C91.6)
chronic lymphocytic, of B-cell type C91.1- ☑
chronic monocytic C93.1- ☑
chronic myelogenous (Philadelphia chromosome (Ph1)
    positive) (t(9;22)) (q34;q11) (with crisis of blast
    cells) C92.1- ☑
chronic myeloid, BCR/ABL-positive C92.1- ☑
  atypical, BCR/ABL-negative C92.2- ☑
chronic myelomonocytic C93.1- ☑
chronic neutrophilic D47.1
CMML (-1) (-2) (with eosinophilia) C93.1- ☑
granulocytic — *see also* Category C92 C92.9- ☑
hairy cell C91.4- ☑
juvenile myelomonocytic C93.3- ☑
lymphoid C91.9- ☑
  specified NEC C91.Z- ☑ (*following* C91.6)
mast cell C94.3- ☑
mature B-cell, Burkitt-type C91.A- ☑ (*following* C91.6)
monocytic (subacute) C93.9- ☑
  specified NEC C93.Z- ☑ (*following* C93.3)
myelogenous — *see also* Category C92 C92.9- ☑
myeloid C92.9- ☑
  specified NEC C92.Z- ☑ (*following* C92.6)
plasma cell C90.1- ☑
plasmacytic C90.1- ☑
prolymphocytic
  of B-cell type C91.3- ☑
  of T-cell type C91.6- ☑
specified NEC C94.8- ☑
stem cell, of unclear lineage C95.0- ☑
subacute lymphocytic C91.9- ☑
T-cell large granular lymphocytic C91.Z- ☑ (*following*
    C91.6)
unspecified cell type C95.9- ☑
  acute C95.0- ☑
  chronic C95.1- ☑
Leukemoid reaction — *see also* Reaction, leukemoid
  D72.823
Leukoaraiosis (hypertensive) I67.81
Leukoariosis — *see* Leukoaraiosis
Leukocoria — *see* Disorder, globe, degenerated condition, leucocoria
Leukocytopenia D72.819
Leukocytosis D72.829
  eosinophilic D72.1
Leukoderma, leukodermia NEC L81.5
  syphilitic A51.39
    late A52.79
Leukodystrophy E75.29
Leukoedema, oral epithelium K13.29
Leukoencephalitis G04.81
  acute (subacute) hemorrhagic G36.1
    postimmunization or postvaccinal G04.02
  postinfectious G04.01
  subacute sclerosing A81.1
  van Bogaert's (sclerosing) A81.1
Leukoencephalopathy — *see also* Encephalopathy
  G93.49
  Binswanger's I67.3
  heroin vapor G92
  metachromatic E75.25
  multifocal (progressive) A81.2
  postimmunization and postvaccinal G04.02
  progressive multifocal A81.2
  reversible, posterior G93.6
  van Bogaert's (sclerosing) A81.1
  vascular, progressive I67.3
Leukoerythroblastosis D75.9
Leukokeratosis — *see also* Leukoplakia
  mouth K13.21
  nicotina palati K13.24
  oral mucosa K13.21
  tongue K13.21
  vocal cord J38.3

Leukokraurosis vulva (e) N90.4
Leukoma (cornea) — *see also* Opacity, cornea
  adherent H17.0- ☑
  interfering with central vision — *see* Opacity, cornea, central
Leukomalacia, cerebral, newborn P91.2
  periventricular P91.2
Leukomelanopathy, hereditary D72.0
Leukonychia (punctata) (striata) L60.8
  congenital Q84.4
Leukopathia unguium L60.8
  congenital Q84.4
Leukopenia D72.819
  basophilic D72.818
  chemotherapy (cancer) induced D70.1
  congenital D70.0
  cyclic D70.0
  drug induced NEC D70.2
    due to cytoreductive cancer chemotherapy D70.1
  eosinophilic D72.818
  familial D70.0
  infantile genetic D70.0
  malignant D70.9
  periodic D70.0
  transitory neonatal P61.5
Leukopenic — *see* condition
Leukoplakia
  anus K62.89
  bladder (postinfectional) N32.89
  buccal K13.21
  cervix (uteri) N88.0
  esophagus K22.8
  gingiva K13.21
  hairy (oral mucosa) (tongue) K13.3
  kidney (pelvis) N28.89
  larynx J38.7
  lip K13.21
  mouth K13.21
  oral epithelium, including tongue (mucosa) K13.21
  palate K13.21
  pelvis (kidney) N28.89
  penis (infectional) N48.0
  rectum K62.89
  syphilitic (late) A52.79
  tongue K13.21
  ureter (postinfectional) N28.89
  urethra (postinfectional) N36.8
  uterus N85.8
  vagina N89.4
  vocal cord J38.3
  vulva N90.4
Leukorrhea N89.8
  due to Trichomonas (vaginalis) A59.00
  trichomonal A59.00
Leukosarcoma C85.9- ☑
Levocardia (isolated) Q24.1
  with situs inversus Q89.3
Levotransposition Q20.5
Lev's disease or syndrome (acquired complete heart block) I44.2
Levulosuria — *see* Fructosuria
Levurid L30.2
Lewy body (ies) (dementia) (disease) G31.83
Leyden-Moebius dystrophy G71.09
Leydig cell
  carcinoma
    specified site — *see* Neoplasm, malignant, by site
    unspecified site
      female C56.9
      male C62.9- ☑
  tumor
    benign
      specified site — *see* Neoplasm, benign, by site
      unspecified site
        female D27.- ☑
        male D29.2- ☑
    malignant
      specified site — *see* Neoplasm, malignant, by site
      unspecified site
        female C56.- ☑
        male C62.9- ☑
    specified site — *see* Neoplasm, uncertain behavior, by site
    unspecified site
      female D39.1- ☑
      male D40.1- ☑

Leydig-Sertoli cell tumor
  specified site — *see* Neoplasm, benign, by site
  unspecified site
    female D27.- ☑
    male D29.2- ☑
LGSIL (Low grade squamous intraepithelial lesion on cytologic smear of)
  anus R85.612
  cervix R87.612
  vagina R87.622
Liar, pathologic F60.2
Libido
  decreased R68.82
Libman-Sacks disease M32.11
Lice (infestation) B85.2
  body (Pediculus corporis) B85.1
  crab B85.3
  head (Pediculus capitis) B85.0
  mixed (classifiable to more than one of the titles B85.0-B85.3) B85.4
  pubic (Phthirus pubis) B85.3
Lichen L28.0
  albus L90.0
    penis N48.0
    vulva N90.4
  amyloidosis E85.4 *[L99]*
  atrophicus L90.0
    penis N48.0
    vulva N90.4
  congenital Q82.8
  myxedematosus L98.5
  nitidus L44.1
  pilaris Q82.8
    acquired L85.8
  planopilaris L66.1
  planus (chronicus) L43.9
    annularis L43.8
    bullous L43.1
    follicular L66.1
    hypertrophic L43.0
    moniliformis L44.3
    of Wilson L43.9
    specified NEC L43.8
    subacute (active) L43.3
    tropicus L43.3
  ruber
    acuminatus L44.0
    moniliformis L44.3
    planus L43.9
  sclerosus (et atrophicus) L90.0
    penis N48.0
    vulva N90.4
  scrofulosus (primary) (tuberculous) A18.4
  simplex (chronicus) (circumscriptus) L28.0
  striatus L44.2
  urticatus L28.2
Lichenification L28.0
Lichenoides tuberculosis (primary) A18.4
Lichtheim's disease or syndrome D51.0
Lien migrans D73.89
Ligament — *see* condition
Light
  for gestational age — *see* Light for dates
  headedness R42
Light-for-dates (infant) P05.00
  with weight of
    499 grams or less P05.01
    500-749 grams P05.02
    750-999 grams P05.03
    1000-1249 grams P05.04
    1250-1499 grams P05.05
    1500-1749 grams P05.06
    1750-1999 grams P05.07
    2000-2499 grams P05.08
    2500 grams and over P05.09
  affecting management of pregnancy O36.59- ☑
  and small-for-dates — *see* Small for dates
  specified NEC P05.09
Lightning (effects) (stroke) (struck by) T75.00 ☑
  burn — *see* Burn
  foot E53.8
  shock T75.01 ☑
  specified effect NEC T75.09 ☑
Lightwood-Albright syndrome N25.89
Lightwood's disease or syndrome (renal tubular acidosis) N25.89
Lignac (-de Toni) (-Fanconi) (-Debré) **disease or syndrome** E72.09

Lignac (-de Toni) (-Fanconi) (-Debré) **disease or syndrome** — *continued*
  with cystinosis E72.04
Ligneous thyroiditis E06.5
Likoff's syndrome I20.8
Limb — *see* condition
Limbic epilepsy personality syndrome F07.0
Limitation, limited
  activities due to disability Z73.6
  cardiac reserve — *see* Disease, heart
  eye muscle duction, traumatic — *see* Strabismus, mechanical
  mandibular range of motion M26.52
Lindau (-von Hippel) **disease** Q85.8
Line(s)
  Beau's L60.4
  Harris' — *see* Arrest, epiphyseal
  Hudson's (cornea) — *see* Pigmentation, cornea, anterior
  Stähli's (cornea) — *see* Pigmentation, cornea, anterior
Linea corneae senilis — *see* Change, cornea, senile
Lingua
  geographica K14.1
  nigra (villosa) K14.3
  plicata K14.5
  tylosis K13.29
Lingual — *see* condition
Linguatulosis B88.8
Linitis (gastric) **plastica** C16.9
Lip — *see* condition
Lipedema — *see* Edema
Lipemia — *see also* Hyperlipidemia
  retina, retinalis E78.3
Lipidosis E75.6
  cerebral (infantile) (juvenile) (late) E75.4
  cerebroretinal E75.4
  cerebroside E75.22
  cholesterol (cerebral) E75.5
  glycolipid E75.21
  hepatosplenomegalic E78.3
  sphingomyelin — *see* Niemann-Pick disease or syndrome
  sulfatide E75.29
Lipoadenoma — *see* Neoplasm, benign, by site
Lipoblastoma — *see* Lipoma
Lipoblastomatosis — *see* Lipoma
Lipochondrodystrophy E76.01
Lipochrome histiocytosis (familial) D71
Lipodermatosclerosis — *see* Varix, leg, with, inflammation
  ulcerated — *see* Varix, leg, with, ulcer, with inflammation by site
Lipodystrophia progressiva E88.1
Lipodystrophy (progressive) E88.1
  insulin E88.1
  intestinal K90.81
  mesenteric K65.4
Lipofibroma — *see* Lipoma
Lipofuscinosis, neuronal (with ceroidosis) E75.4
Lipogranuloma, sclerosing L92.8
Lipogranulomatosis E78.89
Lipoid — *see also* condition
  histiocytosis D76.3
    essential E75.29
  nephrosis N04.9
  proteinosis of Urbach E78.89
Lipoidemia — *see* Hyperlipidemia
Lipoidosis — *see* Lipidosis
Lipoma D17.9
  fetal D17.9
    fat cell D17.9
  infiltrating D17.9
  intramuscular D17.9
  pleomorphic D17.9
  site classification
    arms (skin) (subcutaneous) D17.2- ☑
    connective tissue D17.30
      intra-abdominal D17.5
      intrathoracic D17.4
      peritoneum D17.79
      retroperitoneum D17.79
      specified site NEC D17.39
      spermatic cord D17.6
    face (skin) (subcutaneous) D17.0
    genitourinary organ NEC D17.72
    head (skin) (subcutaneous) D17.0
    intra-abdominal D17.5
    intrathoracic D17.4

212

☑ Additional Character Required — Refer to the Tabular List for Character Selection   ▽ Subterms under main terms may continue to next column or page

Lipoma — *continued*
  site classification — *continued*
    kidney D17.71
    legs (skin) (subcutaneous) D17.2- ☑
    neck (skin) (subcutaneous) D17.Ø
    peritoneum D17.79
    retroperitoneum D17.79
    skin D17.3Ø
      specified site NEC D17.39
    specified site NEC D17.79
    spermatic cord D17.6
    subcutaneous D17.3Ø
      specified site NEC D17.39
    trunk (skin) (subcutaneous) D17.1
    unspecified D17.9
  spindle cell D17.9
Lipomatosis E88.2
  dolorosa (Dercum) E88.2
  fetal — *see* Lipoma
  Launois-Bensaude E88.89
Lipomyoma — *see* Lipoma
Lipomyxoma — *see* Lipoma
Lipomyxosarcoma — *see* Neoplasm, connective tissue, malignant
Lipoprotein metabolism disorder E78.9
Lipoproteinemia E78.5
  broad-beta E78.2
  floating-beta E78.2
  hyper-pre-beta E78.1
Liposarcoma — *see also* Neoplasm, connective tissue, malignant
  dedifferentiated — *see* Neoplasm, connective tissue, malignant
  differentiated type — *see* Neoplasm, connective tissue, malignant
  embryonal — *see* Neoplasm, connective tissue, malignant
  mixed type — *see* Neoplasm, connective tissue, malignant
  myxoid — *see* Neoplasm, connective tissue, malignant
  pleomorphic — *see* Neoplasm, connective tissue, malignant
  round cell — *see* Neoplasm, connective tissue, malignant
  well differentiated type — *see* Neoplasm, connective tissue, malignant
Liposynovitis prepatellaris E88.89
Lipping, cervix N86
Lipschütz disease or ulcer N76.6
Lipuria R82.Ø
  schistosomiasis (bilharziasis) B65.Ø
Lisping F8Ø.Ø
Lissauer's paralysis A52.17
Lissencephalia, lissencephaly QØ4.3
Listeriosis, listerellosis A32.9
  congenital (disseminated) P37.2
  cutaneous A32.Ø
  neonatal, newborn (disseminated) P37.2
  oculoglandular A32.81
  specified NEC A32.89
Lithemia E79.Ø
Lithiasis — *see* Calculus
Lithosis J62.8
Lithuria R82.998
Litigation, anxiety concerning Z65.3
Little leaguer's elbow — *see* Epicondylitis, medial
Little's disease G8Ø.9
Littre's
  gland — *see* condition
  hernia — *see* Hernia, abdomen
Littritis — *see* Urethritis
Livedo (annularis) (racemosa) (reticularis) R23.1
Liver — *see* condition
Living alone (problems with) Z6Ø.2
  with handicapped person Z74.2
Lloyd's syndrome — *see* Adenomatosis, endocrine
Loa loa, loaiasis, loasis B74.3
Lobar — *see* condition
Lobomycosis B48.Ø
Lobo's disease B48.Ø
Lobotomy syndrome FØ7.Ø
Lobstein (-Ekman) **disease or syndrome** Q78.Ø
Lobster-claw hand Q71.6- ☑
Lobulation (congenital) — *see also* Anomaly, by site
  kidney, Q63.1
  liver, abnormal Q44.7
  spleen Q89.Ø9

Lobule, lobular — *see* condition
Local, localized — *see* condition
Locked twins causing obstructed labor O66.1
Locked-in state G83.5
Locking
  joint — *see* Derangement, joint, specified type NEC
    knee — *see* Derangement, knee
Lockjaw — *see* Tetanus
Löffler's
  endocarditis I42.3
  eosinophilia J82
  pneumonia J82
  syndrome (eosinophilic pneumonitis) J82
Loiasis (with conjunctival infestation) (eyelid) B74.3
Lone Star fever A77.Ø
Long
  labor O63.9
    first stage O63.Ø
    second stage O63.1
  QT syndrome I45.81
Longitudinal stripes or grooves, nails L6Ø.8
  congenital Q84.6
Long-term (current) (prophylactic) **drug therapy** (use of)
  agents affecting estrogen receptors and estrogen levels NEC Z79.818
  anastrozole (Arimidex) Z79.811
  antibiotics Z79.2
    short-term use — *omit code*
  anticoagulants Z79.Ø1
  anti-inflammatory, non-steroidal (NSAID) Z79.1
  antiplatelet Z79.Ø2
  antithrombotics Z79.Ø2
  aromatase inhibitors Z79.811
  aspirin Z79.82
  birth control pill or patch Z79.3
  bisphosphonates Z79.83
  contraceptive, oral Z79.3
  drug, specified NEC Z79.899
  estrogen receptor downregulators Z79.818
  Evista Z79.81Ø
  exemestane (Aromasin) Z79.811
  Fareston Z79.81Ø
  fulvestrant (Faslodex) Z79.818
  gonadotropin-releasing hormone (GnRH) agonist Z79.818
  goserelin acetate (Zoladex) Z79.818
  hormone replacement Z79.89Ø
  insulin Z79.4
  letrozole (Femara) Z79.811
  leuprolide acetate (leuprorelin) (Lupron) Z79.818
  megestrol acetate (Megace) Z79.818
  methadone for pain management Z79.891
  Nolvadex Z79.81Ø
  non-steroidal anti-inflammatories (NSAID) Z79.1
  opiate analgesic Z79.891
  oral
    antidiabetic Z79.84
    contraceptive Z79.3
    hypoglycemic Z79.84
  raloxifene (Evista) Z79.81Ø
  selective estrogen receptor modulators (SERMs) Z79.81Ø
  steroids
    inhaled Z79.51
    systemic Z79.52
  tamoxifen (Nolvadex) Z79.81Ø
  toremifene (Fareston) Z79.81Ø
Loop
  intestine — *see* Volvulus
  vascular on papilla (optic) Q14.2
Loose — *see also* condition
  body
    joint M24.ØØ
      ankle M24.Ø7- ☑
      elbow M24.Ø2- ☑
      hand M24.Ø4- ☑
      hip M24.Ø5- ☑
      knee M23.4- ☑
      shoulder (region) M24.Ø1- ☑
      specified site NEC M24.Ø8
      toe M24.Ø7- ☑
      vertebra M24.Ø8
      wrist M24.Ø3- ☑
    knee M23.4- ☑
  sheath, tendon — *see* Disorder, tendon, specified type NEC
  cartilage — *see* Loose, body, joint

Loose — *continued*
  skin and subcutaneous tissue (following bariatric surgery weight loss) (following dietary weight loss) L98.7
  tooth, teeth KØ8.89
Loosening
  aseptic
    joint prosthesis — *see* Complications, joint prosthesis, mechanical, loosening, by site
    epiphysis — *see* Osteochondropathy
  mechanical
    joint prosthesis — *see* Complications, joint prosthesis, mechanical, loosening, by site
Looser-Milkman (-Debray) **syndrome** M83.8
Lop ear (deformity) Q17.3
Lorain (-Levi) **short stature syndrome** E23.Ø
Lordosis M4Ø.5Ø
  acquired — *see* Lordosis, specified type NEC
  congenital Q76.429
    lumbar region Q76.426
    lumbosacral region Q76.427
    sacral region Q76.428
    sacrococcygeal region Q76.428
    thoracolumbar region Q76.425
  lumbar region M4Ø.56
  lumbosacral region M4Ø.57
  postsurgical M96.4
  postural — *see* Lordosis, specified type NEC
  rachitic (late effect) (sequelae) E64.3
  sequelae of rickets E64.3
  specified type NEC M4Ø.4Ø
    lumbar region M4Ø.46
    lumbosacral region M4Ø.47
    thoracolumbar region M4Ø.45
  thoracolumbar region M4Ø.55
  tuberculous A18.Ø1
Loss (of)
  appetite — *see also* Anorexia R63.Ø
    hysterical F5Ø.89
    nonorganic origin F5Ø.89
    psychogenic F5Ø.89
  blood — *see* Hemorrhage
  bone — *see* Loss, substance of, bone
  consciousness, transient R55
    traumatic — *see* Injury, intracranial
  control, sphincter, rectum R15.9
    nonorganic origin F98.1
  elasticity, skin R23.4
  family (member) in childhood Z62.898
  fluid (acute) E86.9
  function of labyrinth — *see* subcategory H83.2 ☑
  hair, nonscarring — *see* Alopecia
  hearing — *see also* Deafness
    central NOS H9Ø.5
    conductive H9Ø.2
      bilateral H9Ø.Ø
      unilateral
        with
          restricted hearing on the contralateral side H9Ø.A1- ☑
          unrestricted hearing on the contralateral side H9Ø.1- ☑
    mixed conductive and sensorineural hearing loss H9Ø.8
      bilateral H9Ø.6
      unilateral
        with
          restricted hearing on the contralateral side H9Ø.A3- ☑
          unrestricted hearing on the contralateral side H9Ø.7- ☑
    neural NOS H9Ø.5
    perceptive NOS H9Ø.5
    sensorineural NOS H9Ø.5
      bilateral H9Ø.3
      unilateral
        with
          restricted hearing onthe contralateral side H9Ø.A2- ☑
          unrestricted hearing on the contralateral side H9Ø.4- ☑
    sensory NOS H9Ø.5
  height R29.89Ø
  limb or member, traumatic, current — *see* Amputation, traumatic
  love relationship in childhood Z62.898
  memory — *see also* Amnesia
    mild, following organic brain damage FØ6.8

▽ Subterms under main terms may continue to next column or page   ☑ Additional Character Required — Refer to the Tabular List for Character Selection

Loss — *continued*
  mind — *see* Psychosis
  occlusal vertical dimension of fully erupted teeth
    M26.37
  organ or part — *see* Absence, by site, acquired
  ossicles, ear (partial) H74.32- ☑
  parent in childhood Z63.4
  pregnancy, recurrent N96
    care in current pregnancy O26.2- ☑
    without current pregnancy N96
  recurrent pregnancy — *see* Loss, pregnancy, recurrent
  self-esteem, in childhood Z62.898
  sense of
    smell — *see* Disturbance, sensation, smell
    taste — *see* Disturbance, sensation, taste
    touch R20.8
  sensory R44.9
    dissociative F44.6
  sexual desire F52.0
  sight (acquired) (complete) (congenital) — *see* Blindness
  substance of
    bone — *see* Disorder, bone, density and structure, specified NEC
      horizontal alveolar K06.3
    cartilage — *see* Disorder, cartilage, specified type NEC
      auricle (ear) — *see* Disorder, pinna, specified type NEC
    vitreous (humor) H15.89
  tooth, teeth — *see* Absence, teeth, acquired
  vision, visual H54.7
    both eyes H54.3
    one eye H54.60
      left (normal vision on right) H54.62
      right (normal vision on left) H54.61
    specified as blindness — *see* Blindness
    subjective
      sudden H53.13- ☑
      transient H53.12- ☑
  vitreous — *see* Prolapse, vitreous
  voice — *see* Aphonia
  weight (abnormal) (cause unknown) R63.4
Louis-Bar syndrome (ataxia-telangiectasia) G11.3
Louping ill (encephalitis) A84.8
Louse, lousiness — *see* Lice
Low
  achiever, school Z55.3
  back syndrome M54.5
  basal metabolic rate R94.8
  birthweight (2499 grams or less) P07.10
    with weight of
      1000-1249 grams P07.14
      1250-1499 grams P07.15
      1500-1749 grams P07.16
      1750-1999 grams P07.17
      2000-2499 grams P07.18
    extreme (999 grams or less) P07.00
      with weight of
        499 grams or less P07.01
        500-749 grams P07.02
        750-999 grams P07.03
    for gestational age — *see* Light for dates
  blood pressure — *see also* Hypotension
    reading (incidental) (isolated) (nonspecific) R03.1
  cardiac reserve — *see* Disease, heart
  function — *see also* Hypofunction
    kidney N28.9
  hematocrit D64.9
  hemoglobin D64.9
  income Z59.6
  level of literacy Z55.0
  lying
    kidney N28.89
    organ or site, congenital — *see* Malposition, congenital
  output syndrome (cardiac) — *see* Failure, heart
  platelets (blood) — *see* Thrombocytopenia
  reserve, kidney N28.89
  salt syndrome E87.1
  self esteem R45.81
  set ears Q17.4
  vision H54.2X- ☑
    one eye (other eye normal) H54.50
      left (normal vision on right) H54.52A- ☑
      other eye blind — *see* Blindness
      right (normal vision on left) H54.511- ☑

Low-density-lipoprotein-type (LDL) **hyperlipoproteinemia** E78.00
Lowe's syndrome E72.03
Lown-Ganong-Levine syndrome I45.6
LSD reaction (acute) (without dependence) F16.90
  with dependence F16.20
L-shaped kidney Q63.8
LTBI (latent tuberculosis infection) Z22.7
Ludwig's angina or disease K12.2
Lues (venerea), **luetic** — *see* Syphilis
Luetscher's syndrome (dehydration) E86.0
Lumbago, lumbalgia M54.5
  with sciatica M54.4- ☑
    due to intervertebral disc disorder M51.17
  due to displacement, intervertebral disc M51.27
    with sciatica M51.17
Lumbar — *see* condition
Lumbarization, vertebra, congenital Q76.49
Lumbermen's itch B88.0
Lump — *see also* Mass
  breast N63.0
    axillary tail
      left N63.32
      right N63.31
    left
      lower inner quadrant N63.24
      lower outer quadrant N63.23
      overlapping quadrants N63.25
      unspecified quadrant N63.20
      upper inner quadrant N63.22
      upper outer quadrant N63.21
    right
      lower inner quadrant N63.14
      lower outer quadrant N63.13
      overlapping quadrants N63.15
      unspecified quadrant N63.10
      upper inner quadrant N63.12
      upper outer quadrant N63.11
    subareolar
      left N63.42
      right N63.41
Lunacy — *see* Psychosis
Lung — *see* condition
Lupoid (miliary) **of Boeck** D86.3
Lupus
  anticoagulant D68.62
    with
      hemorrhagic disorder D68.312
      hypercoagulable state D68.62
    finding without diagnosis R76.0
  discoid (local) L93.0
  erythematosus (discoid) (local) L93.0
    disseminated — *see* Lupus, erythematosus, systemic
    eyelid H01.129
      left H01.126
        lower H01.125
        upper H01.124
      right H01.123
        lower H01.122
        upper H01.121
    profundus L93.2
    specified NEC L93.2
    subacute cutaneous L93.1
    systemic M32.9
      with organ or system involvement M32.10
        endocarditis M32.11
        lung M32.13
        pericarditis M32.12
        renal (glomerular) M32.14
          tubulo-interstitial M32.15
        specified organ or system NEC M32.19
      drug-induced M32.0
      inhibitor (presence of) D68.62
        with
          hemorrhagic disorder D68.312
          hypercoagulable state D68.62
        finding without diagnosis R76.0
      specified NEC M32.8
  exedens A18.4
  hydralazine M32.0
    correct substance properly administered — *see* Table of Drugs and Chemicals, by drug, adverse effect
    overdose or wrong substance given or taken — *see* Table of Drugs and Chemicals, by drug, poisoning
  nephritis (chronic) M32.14
  nontuberculous, not disseminated L93.0

Lupus — *continued*
  panniculitis L93.2
  pernio (Besnier) D86.3
  systemic — *see* Lupus, erythematosus, systemic
  tuberculous A18.4
    eyelid A18.4
  vulgaris A18.4
    eyelid A18.4
Luteinoma D27.- ☑
Lutembacher's disease or syndrome (atrial septal defect with mitral stenosis) Q21.1
Luteoma D27.- ☑
Lutz (-Splendore-de Almeida) **disease** — *see* Paracoccidioidomycosis
Luxation — *see also* Dislocation
  eyeball (nontraumatic) — *see* Luxation, globe
    birth injury P15.3
  globe, nontraumatic H44.82- ☑
  lacrimal gland — *see* Dislocation, lacrimal gland
  lens (old) (partial) (spontaneous)
    congenital Q12.1
    syphilitic A50.39
Lycanthropy F22
Lyell's syndrome L51.2
  due to drug L51.2
    correct substance properly administered — *see* Table of Drugs and Chemicals, by drug, adverse effect
    overdose or wrong substance given or taken — *see* Table of Drugs and Chemicals, by drug, poisoning
Lyme disease A69.20
Lymph
  gland or node — *see* condition
  scrotum — *see* Infestation, filarial
Lymphadenitis I88.9
  with ectopic or molar pregnancy O08.0
  acute L04.9
    axilla L04.2
    face L04.0
    head L04.0
    hip L04.3
    limb
      lower L04.3
      upper L04.2
    neck L04.0
    shoulder L04.2
    specified site NEC L04.8
    trunk L04.1
  anthracosis (occupational) J60
  any site, except mesenteric I88.9
    chronic I88.1
    subacute I88.1
  breast
    gestational — *see* Mastitis, obstetric
    puerperal, postpartum (nonpurulent) O91.22
  chancroidal (congenital) A57
  chronic I88.1
    mesenteric I88.0
  due to
    Brugia (malayi) B74.1
      timori B74.2
    chlamydial lymphogranuloma A55
    diphtheria (toxin) A36.89
    lymphogranuloma venereum A55
    Wuchereria bancrofti B74.0
  following ectopic or molar pregnancy O08.0
  gonorrheal A54.89
  infective — *see* Lymphadenitis, acute
  mesenteric (acute) (chronic) (nonspecific) (subacute) I88.0
    due to Salmonella typhi A01.09
    tuberculous A18.39
  mycobacterial A31.8
  purulent — *see* Lymphadenitis, acute
  pyogenic — *see* Lymphadenitis, acute
  regional, nonbacterial I88.8
  septic — *see* Lymphadenitis, acute
  subacute, unspecified site I88.1
  suppurative — *see* Lymphadenitis, acute
  syphilitic (early) (secondary) A51.49
    late A52.79
  tuberculous — *see* Tuberculosis, lymph gland
  venereal (chlamydial) A55
Lymphadenoid goiter E06.3
Lymphadenopathy (generalized) R59.1
  angioimmunoblastic, with dysproteinemia (AILD) C86.5
  due to toxoplasmosis (acquired) B58.89

Lymphadenopathy — *continued*
　due to toxoplasmosis — *continued*
　　congenital (acute) (subacute) (chronic) P37.1
　localized R59.0
　syphilitic (early) (secondary) A51.49
Lymphadenosis R59.1
Lymphangiectasis I89.0
　conjunctiva H11.89
　postinfectional I89.0
　scrotum I89.0
Lymphangiectatic elephantiasis, nonfilarial I89.0
Lymphangioendothelioma D18.1
　malignant — *see* Neoplasm, connective tissue, malignant
Lymphangioleiomyomatosis J84.81
Lymphangioma D18.1
　capillary D18.1
　cavernous D18.1
　cystic D18.1
　malignant — *see* Neoplasm, connective tissue, malignant
Lymphangiomyoma D18.1
Lymphangiomyomatosis J84.81
Lymphangiosarcoma — *see* Neoplasm, connective tissue, malignant
Lymphangitis I89.1
　with
　　abscess — *code by* site under Abscess
　　cellulitis — *code by* site under Cellulitis
　　ectopic or molar pregnancy O08.0
　acute L03.91
　　abdominal wall L03.321
　　ankle — *see* Lymphangitis, acute, lower limb
　　arm — *see* Lymphangitis, acute, upper limb
　　auricle (ear) — *see* Lymphangitis, acute, ear
　　axilla L03.12- ☑
　　back (any part) L03.322
　　buttock L03.327
　　cervical (meaning neck) L03.222
　　cheek (external) L03.212
　　chest wall L03.323
　　digit
　　　finger — *see* Lymphangitis, acute, finger
　　　toe — *see* Lymphangitis, acute, toe
　　ear (external) H60.1- ☑
　　external auditory canal — *see* Lymphangitis, acute, ear
　　eyelid — *see* Abscess, eyelid
　　face NEC L03.212
　　finger (intrathecal) (periosteal) (subcutaneous) (subcuticular) L03.02- ☑
　　foot — *see* Lymphangitis, acute, lower limb
　　gluteal (region) L03.327
　　groin L03.324
　　hand — *see* Lymphangitis, acute, upper limb
　　head NEC L03.891
　　　face (any part, except ear, eye and nose) L03.212
　　heel — *see* Lymphangitis, acute, lower limb
　　hip — *see* Lymphangitis, acute, lower limb
　　jaw (region) L03.212
　　knee — *see* Lymphangitis, acute, lower limb
　　leg — *see* Lymphangitis, acute, lower limb
　　lower limb L03.12- ☑
　　　toe — *see* Lymphangitis, acute, toe
　　navel L03.326
　　neck (region) L03.222
　　orbit, orbital — *see* Cellulitis, orbit
　　pectoral (region) L03.323
　　perineal, perineum L03.325
　　scalp (any part) L03.891
　　shoulder — *see* Lymphangitis, acute, upper limb
　　specified site NEC L03.898
　　thigh — *see* Lymphangitis, acute, lower limb
　　thumb (intrathecal) (periosteal) (subcutaneous) (subcuticular) — *see* Lymphangitis, acute, finger
　　toe (intrathecal) (periosteal) (subcutaneous) (subcuticular) L03.04- ☑
　　trunk L03.329
　　　abdominal wall L03.321
　　　back (any part) L03.322
　　　buttock L03.327
　　　chest wall L03.323
　　　groin L03.324
　　　perineal, perineum L03.325
　　　umbilicus L03.326
　　umbilicus L03.326

Lymphangitis — *continued*
　acute — *continued*
　　upper limb L03.12- ☑
　　　axilla — *see* Lymphangitis, acute, axilla
　　　finger — *see* Lymphangitis, acute, finger
　　　thumb — *see* Lymphangitis, acute, finger
　　　wrist — *see* Lymphangitis, acute, upper limb
　breast
　　gestational — *see* Mastitis, obstetric
　chancroidal A57
　chronic (any site) I89.1
　due to
　　Brugia (malayi) B74.1
　　　timori B74.2
　　Wuchereria bancrofti B74.0
　following ectopic or molar pregnancy O08.89
　penis
　　acute N48.29
　　gonococcal (acute) (chronic) A54.09
　puerperal, postpartum, childbirth O86.89
　strumous, tuberculous A18.2
　subacute (any site) I89.1
　tuberculous — *see* Tuberculosis, lymph gland
Lymphatic (vessel) — *see* condition
Lymphatism E32.8
Lymphectasia I89.0
Lymphedema (acquired) — *see also* Elephantiasis
　congenital Q82.0
　hereditary (chronic) (idiopathic) Q82.0
　postmastectomy I97.2
　praecox I89.0
　secondary I89.0
　surgical NEC I97.89
　　postmastectomy (syndrome) I97.2
Lymphoblastic — *see* condition
Lymphoblastoma (diffuse) — *see* Lymphoma, lymphoblastic (diffuse)
　giant follicular — *see* Lymphoma, lymphoblastic (diffuse)
　macrofollicular — *see* Lymphoma, lymphoblastic (diffuse)
Lymphocele I89.8
Lymphocytic
　chorioencephalitis (acute) (serous) A87.2
　choriomeningitis (acute) (serous) A87.2
　meningoencephalitis A87.2
Lymphocytoma, benign cutis L98.8
Lymphocytopenia D72.810
Lymphocytosis (symptomatic) D72.820
　infectious (acute) B33.8
Lymphoepithelioma — *see* Neoplasm, malignant, by site
Lymphogranuloma (malignant) — *see also* Lymphoma, Hodgkin
　chlamydial A55
　inguinale A55
　venereum (any site) (chlamydial) (with stricture of rectum) A55
Lymphogranulomatosis (malignant) — *see also* Lymphoma, Hodgkin
　benign (Boeck's sarcoid) (Schaumann's) D86.1
Lymphohistiocytosis, hemophagocytic (familial) D76.1
Lymphoid — *see* condition
Lymphoma (of) (malignant) C85.90
　adult T-cell (HTLV-1-associated) (acute variant) (chronic variant) (lymphomatoid variant) (smouldering variant) C91.5- ☑
　anaplastic large cell
　　ALK-negative C84.7- ☑
　　ALK-positive C84.6- ☑
　　CD30-positive C84.6- ☑
　　primary cutaneous C86.6
　angioimmunoblastic T-cell C86.5
　BALT C88.4
　B-cell C85.1- ☑
　blastic NK-cell C86.4
　blastic plasmacytoid dendritic cell neoplasm (BPDCN) C86.4
　B-precursor C83.5- ☑
　bronchial-associated lymphoid tissue [BALT-lymphoma] C88.4
　Burkitt (atypical) C83.7- ☑
　Burkitt-like C83.7- ☑
　centrocytic C83.1- ☑
　cutaneous follicle center C82.6- ☑
　cutaneous T-cell C84.A- ☑ (*following* C84.7)
　diffuse follicle center C82.5- ☑

Lymphoma — *continued*
　diffuse large cell C83.3- ☑
　　anaplastic C83.3- ☑
　　B-cell C83.3- ☑
　　CD30-positive C83.3- ☑
　　centroblastic C83.3- ☑
　　immunoblastic C83.3- ☑
　　plasmablastic C83.3- ☑
　　subtype not specified C83.3- ☑
　　T-cell rich C83.3- ☑
　enteropathy-type (associated) (intestinal) T-cell C86.2
　extranodal marginal zone B-cell lymphoma of mucosa-associated lymphoid tissue [MALT-lymphoma] C88.4
　extranodal NK/T-cell, nasal type C86.0
　follicular C82.9- ☑
　　grade
　　　I C82.0- ☑
　　　II C82.1- ☑
　　　III C82.2- ☑
　　　IIIa C82.3- ☑
　　　IIIb C82.4- ☑
　　specified NEC C82.8- ☑
　hepatosplenic T-cell (alpha-beta) (gamma-delta) C86.1
　histiocytic C85.9- ☑
　　true C96.A (*following* C96.6)
　Hodgkin C81.9 ☑
　　lymphocyte depleted (classical) C81.3- ☑
　　lymphocyte-rich (classical) C81.4- ☑
　　mixed cellularity (classical) C81.2- ☑
　　nodular
　　　lymphocyte predominant C81.0- ☑
　　　sclerosis (classical) C81.1- ☑
　　nodular sclerosis (classical) C81.1- ☑
　　specified NEC (classical) C81.7- ☑
　intravascular large B-cell C83.8- ☑
　Lennert's C84.4- ☑
　lymphoblastic (diffuse) C83.5- ☑
　lymphoblastic B-cell C83.5- ☑
　lymphoblastic T-cell C83.5- ☑
　lymphoepithelioid C84.4- ☑
　lymphoplasmacytic C83.0- ☑
　　with IgM-production C88.0
　MALT C88.4
　mantle cell C83.1- ☑
　mature T-cell NEC C84.4- ☑
　mature T/NK-cell C84.9- ☑
　　specified NEC C84.Z- ☑ (*following* C84.7)
　mediastinal (thymic) large B-cell C85.2- ☑
　Mediterranean C88.3
　mucosa-associated lymphoid tissue [MALT-lymphoma] C88.4
　NK/T cell C84.9- ☑
　nodal marginal zone C83.0- ☑
　non-follicular (diffuse) C83.9- ☑
　　specified NEC C83.8- ☑
　non-Hodgkin — *see also* Lymphoma, by type C85.9- ☑
　　specified NEC C85.8- ☑
　non-leukemic variant of B-CLL C83.0- ☑
　peripheral T-cell, not classified C84.4- ☑
　primary cutaneous
　　anaplastic large cell C86.6
　　CD30-positive large T-cell C86.6
　primary effusion B-cell C83.8- ☑
　SALT C88.4
　skin-associated lymphoid tissue [SALT-lymphoma] C88.4
　small cell B-cell C83.0- ☑
　splenic marginal zone C83.0- ☑
　subcutaneous panniculitis-like T-cell C86.3
　T-precursor C83.5- ☑
　true histiocytic C96.A (*following* C96.6)
Lymphomatosis — *see* Lymphoma
Lymphopathia venereum, veneris A55
Lymphopenia D72.810
Lymphoplasmacytic leukemia — *see* Leukemia, chronic lymphocytic, B-cell type
Lymphoproliferation, X-linked disease D82.3
Lymphoreticulosis, benign (of inoculation) A28.1
Lymphorrhea I89.8
Lymphosarcoma (diffuse) — *see also* Lymphoma C85.9- ☑
Lymphostasis I89.8
Lypemania — *see* Melancholia
Lysine and hydroxylysine metabolism disorder E72.3
Lyssa — *see* Rabies

M

Macacus ear Q17.3
Maceration, wet feet, tropical (syndrome) T69.02- ☑
MacLeod's syndrome J43.0
Macrocephalia, macrocephaly Q75.3
Macrocheilia, macrochilia (congenital) Q18.6
Macrocolon — *see also* Megacolon Q43.1
Macrocornea Q15.8
  with glaucoma Q15.0
Macrocytic — *see* condition
Macrocytosis D75.89
Macrodactylia, macrodactylism (fingers) (thumbs) Q74.0
  toes Q74.2
Macrodontia K00.2
Macrogenia M26.05
Macrogenitosomia (adrenal) (male) (praecox) E25.9
  congenital E25.0
Macroglobulinemia (idiopathic) (primary) C88.0
  monoclonal (essential) D47.2
  Waldenström C88.0
Macroglossia (congenital) Q38.2
  acquired K14.8
Macrognathia, macrognathism (congenital) (mandibular) (maxillary) M26.09
Macrogyria (congenital) Q04.8
Macrohydrocephalus — *see* Hydrocephalus
Macromastia — *see* Hypertrophy, breast
Macrophthalmos Q11.3
  in congenital glaucoma Q15.0
Macropsia H53.15
Macrosigmoid K59.39
  congenital Q43.2
Macrospondylitis , acromegalic E22.0
Macrostomia (congenital) Q18.4
Macrotia (external ear) (congenital) Q17.1
Macula
  cornea, corneal — *see* Opacity, cornea
  degeneration (atrophic) (exudative) (senile) — *see also* Degeneration, macula
    hereditary — *see* Dystrophy, retina
Maculae ceruleae B85.1
Maculopathy, toxic — *see* Degeneration, macula, toxic
Madarosis (eyelid) H02.729
  left H02.726
    lower H02.725
    upper H02.724
  right H02.723
    lower H02.722
    upper H02.721
Madelung's
  deformity (radius) Q74.0
  disease
    radial deformity Q74.0
    symmetrical lipomas, neck E88.89
Madness — *see* Psychosis
Madura
  foot B47.9
    actinomycotic B47.1
    mycotic B47.0
Maduromycosis B47.0
Maffucci's syndrome Q78.4
Magnesium metabolism disorder — *see* Disorder, metabolism, magnesium
Main en griffe (acquired) — *see also* Deformity, limb, clawhand
  congenital Q74.0
Maintenance (encounter for)
  antineoplastic chemotherapy Z51.11
  antineoplastic radiation therapy Z51.0
  methadone F11.20
Majocchi's
  disease L81.7
  granuloma B35.8
Major — *see* condition
Mal de los pintos — *see* Pinta
Mal de mer T75.3 ☑
Malabar itch (any site) B35.5
Malabsorption K90.9
  calcium K90.89
  carbohydrate K90.49
  disaccharide E73.9
  fat K90.49
  galactose E74.20
  glucose (-galactose) E74.39

Malabsorption — *continued*
  intestinal K90.9
    specified NEC K90.89
  isomaltose E74.31
  lactose E73.9
  methionine E72.19
  monosaccharide E74.39
  postgastrectomy K91.2
  postsurgical K91.2
  protein K90.49
  starch K90.49
  sucrose E74.39
  syndrome K90.9
    postsurgical K91.2
Malacia, bone (adult) M83.9
  juvenile — *see* Rickets
Malacoplakia
  bladder N32.89
  pelvis (kidney) N28.89
  ureter N28.89
  urethra N36.8
Malacosteon, juvenile — *see* Rickets
Maladaptation — *see* Maladjustment
Maladie de Roger Q21.0
Maladjustment
  conjugal Z63.0
    involving divorce or estrangement Z63.5
  educational Z55.4
  family Z63.9
  marital Z63.0
    involving divorce or estrangement Z63.5
  occupational NEC Z56.89
  simple, adult — *see* Disorder, adjustment
  situational — *see* Disorder, adjustment
  social Z60.9
    due to
      acculturation difficulty Z60.3
      discrimination and persecution (perceived) Z60.5
      exclusion and isolation Z60.4
      life-cycle (phase of life) transition Z60.0
      rejection Z60.4
      specified reason NEC Z60.8
Malaise R53.81
Malakoplakia — *see* Malacoplakia
Malaria, malarial (fever) B54
  with
    blackwater fever B50.8
      hemoglobinuric (bilious) B50.8
    hemoglobinuria B50.8
  accidentally induced (therapeutically) — *code by* type under Malaria
  algid B50.9
  cerebral B50.0 *[G94]*
  clinically diagnosed (without parasitological confirmation) B54
  congenital NEC P37.4
    falciparum P37.3
  congestion, congestive B54
  continued (fever) B50.9
  estivo-autumnal B50.9
  falciparum B50.9
    with complications NEC B50.8
      cerebral B50.0 *[G94]*
      severe B50.8
  hemorrhagic B54
  malariae B52.9
    with
      complications NEC B52.8
      glomerular disorder B52.0
  malignant (tertian) — *see* Malaria, falciparum
  mixed infections — *code to* first listed type in B50-B53
  ovale B53.0
  parasitologically confirmed NEC B53.8
  pernicious, acute — *see* Malaria, falciparum
  Plasmodium (P.)
    falciparum NEC — *see* Malaria, falciparum
    malariae NEC B52.9
      with Plasmodium
        falciparum (and or vivax) — *see* Malaria, falciparum
        vivax — *see also* Malaria, vivax
          and falciparum — *see* Malaria, falciparum
    ovale B53.0
      with Plasmodium malariae — *see also* Malaria, malariae
      and vivax — *see also* Malaria, vivax
        and falciparum — *see* Malaria, falciparum
    simian B53.1

Malaria, malarial — *continued*
  Plasmodium — *continued*
    simian — *continued*
      with Plasmodium malariae — *see also* Malaria, malariae
      and vivax — *see also* Malaria, vivax
        and falciparum — *see* Malaria, falciparum
    vivax NEC B51.9
      with Plasmodium falciparum — *see* Malaria, falciparum
  quartan — *see* Malaria, malariae
  quotidian — *see* Malaria, falciparum
  recurrent B54
  remittent B54
  specified type NEC (parasitologically confirmed) B53.8
  spleen B54
  subtertian (fever) — *see* Malaria, falciparum
  tertian (benign) — *see also* Malaria, vivax
    malignant B50.9
  tropical B50.9
  typhoid B54
  vivax B51.9
    with
      complications NEC B51.8
      ruptured spleen B51.0
Malassez's disease (cystic) N50.89
Malassimilation K90.9
Maldescent, testis Q53.9
  bilateral Q53.20
    abdominal Q53.211
    perineal Q53.22
  unilateral Q53.10
    abdominal Q53.111
    perineal Q53.12
Maldevelopment — *see also* Anomaly
  brain Q07.9
  colon Q43.9
  hip Q74.2
    congenital dislocation Q65.2
      bilateral Q65.1
      unilateral Q65.0- ☑
  mastoid process Q75.8
  middle ear Q16.4
    except ossicles Q16.4
    ossicles Q16.3
  ossicles Q16.3
  spine Q76.49
  toe Q74.2
Male type pelvis Q74.2
  with disproportion (fetopelvic) O33.3 ☑
    causing obstructed labor O65.3
Malformation (congenital) — *see also* Anomaly
  adrenal gland Q89.1
  affecting multiple systems with skeletal changes NEC Q87.5
  alimentary tract Q45.9
    specified type NEC Q45.8
    upper Q40.9
      specified type NEC Q40.8
  aorta Q25.40
    absence Q25.41
    aneurysm, congenital Q25.43
    aplasia Q25.41
    atresia Q25.29
      aortic arch Q25.21
    coarctation (preductal) (postductal) Q25.1
    dilatation, congenital Q25.44
    hypoplasia Q25.42
    patent ductus arteriosus Q25.0
    specified type NEC Q25.49
    stenosis Q25.1
      supravalvular Q25.3
  aortic valve Q23.9
    specified NEC Q23.8
  arteriovenous, aneurysmatic (congenital) Q27.30
    brain Q28.2
      ruptured I60.8
        intracerebral I61.8
        intraparenchymal I61.8
        intraventricular I61.5
        subarachnoid I60.8
    cerebral — *see also* Malformation, arteriovenous, brain Q28.2
    peripheral Q27.30
      digestive system — *see* Angiodysplasia
        congenital Q27.33
      lower limb Q27.32
      other specified site Q27.39

☑ **Additional Character Required** — Refer to the Tabular List for Character Selection   ▽ Subterms under main terms may continue to next column or page

Malformation — *continued*
  arteriovenous, aneurysmatic — *continued*
    peripheral — *continued*
      renal vessel Q27.34
      upper limb Q27.31
    precerebral vessels (nonruptured) Q28.0
  auricle
    ear (congenital) Q17.3
      acquired H61.119
        left H61.112
          with right H61.113
        right H61.111
          with left H61.113
  bile duct Q44.5
  bladder Q64.79
    aplasia Q64.5
    diverticulum Q64.6
    exstrophy — *see* Exstrophy, bladder
    neck obstruction Q64.31
  bone Q79.9
    face Q75.9
      specified type NEC Q75.8
    skull Q75.9
      specified type NEC Q75.8
  brain (multiple) Q04.9
    arteriovenous Q28.2
    specified type NEC Q04.8
  branchial cleft Q18.2
  breast Q83.9
    specified type NEC Q83.8
  broad ligament Q50.6
  bronchus Q32.4
  bursa Q79.9
  cardiac
    chambers Q20.9
      specified type NEC Q20.8
    septum Q21.9
      specified type NEC Q21.8
  cerebral Q04.9
    vessels Q28.3
  cervix uteri Q51.9
    specified type NEC Q51.828
  Chiari
    Type I G93.5
    Type II Q07.01
  choroid (congenital) Q14.3
    plexus Q07.8
  circulatory system Q28.9
  cochlea Q16.5
  cornea Q13.4
  coronary vessels Q24.5
  corpus callosum (congenital) Q04.0
  diaphragm Q79.1
  digestive system NEC, specified type NEC Q45.8
  dura Q07.9
    brain Q04.9
    spinal Q06.9
  ear Q17.9
    causing impairment of hearing Q16.9
    external Q17.9
      accessory auricle Q17.0
      causing impairment of hearing Q16.9
        absence of
          auditory canal Q16.1
          auricle Q16.0
      macrotia Q17.1
      microtia Q17.2
      misplacement Q17.4
      misshapen NEC Q17.3
      prominence Q17.5
      specified type NEC Q17.8
    inner Q16.5
    middle Q16.4
      absence of eustachian tube Q16.2
      ossicles (fusion) Q16.3
    ossicles Q16.3
    specified type NEC Q17.8
  epididymis Q55.4
  esophagus Q39.9
    specified type NEC Q39.8
  eye Q15.9
    lid Q10.3
    specified NEC Q15.8
  fallopian tube Q50.6
  genital organ — *see* Anomaly, genitalia
  great
    artery Q25.9
      aorta — *see* Malformation, aorta

Malformation — *continued*
  great — *continued*
    artery — *continued*
      pulmonary artery — *see* Malformation, pul-
        monary, artery
      specified type NEC Q25.8
    vein Q26.9
      anomalous
        portal venous connection Q26.5
        pulmonary venous connection Q26.4
          partial Q26.3
          total Q26.2
      persistent left superior vena cava Q26.1
      portal vein-hepatic artery fistula Q26.6
      specified type NEC Q26.8
      vena cava stenosis, congenital Q26.0
  gum Q38.6
  hair Q84.2
  heart Q24.9
    specified type NEC Q24.8
  integument Q84.9
    specified type NEC Q84.8
  internal ear Q16.5
  intestine Q43.9
    specified type NEC Q43.8
  iris Q13.2
  joint Q74.9
    ankle Q74.2
    lumbosacral Q76.49
    sacroiliac Q74.2
    specified type NEC Q74.8
  kidney Q63.9
    accessory Q63.0
    giant Q63.3
    horseshoe Q63.1
    hydronephrosis Q62.0
    malposition Q63.2
    specified type NEC Q63.8
  lacrimal apparatus Q10.6
  lingual Q38.3
  lip Q38.0
  liver Q44.7
  lung Q33.9
  meninges or membrane (congenital) Q07.9
    cerebral Q04.8
    spinal (cord) Q06.9
  middle ear Q16.4
    ossicles Q16.3
  mitral valve Q23.9
    specified NEC Q23.8
  Mondini's (congenital) (malformation, cochlea) Q16.5
  mouth (congenital) Q38.6
  multiple types NEC Q89.7
  musculoskeletal system Q79.9
  myocardium Q24.8
  nail Q84.6
  nervous system (central) Q07.9
  nose Q30.9
    specified type NEC Q30.8
  optic disc Q14.2
  orbit Q10.7
  ovary Q50.39
  palate Q38.5
  parathyroid gland Q89.2
  pelvic organs or tissues NEC
    in pregnancy or childbirth O34.8- ☑
      causing obstructed labor O65.5
  penis Q55.69
    aplasia Q55.5
    curvature (lateral) Q55.61
    hypoplasia Q55.62
  pericardium Q24.8
  peripheral vascular system Q27.9
    specified type NEC Q27.8
  pharynx Q38.8
  precerebral vessels Q28.1
  prostate Q55.4
  pulmonary
    arteriovenous Q25.72
    artery Q25.9
      atresia Q25.5
      specified type NEC Q25.79
      stenosis Q25.6
    valve Q22.3
  renal artery Q27.2
  respiratory system Q34.9
  retina Q14.1
  scrotum — *see* Malformation, testis and scrotum
  seminal vesicles Q55.4

Malformation — *continued*
  sense organs NEC Q07.9
  skin Q82.9
  specified NEC Q89.8
  spinal
    cord Q06.9
    nerve root Q07.8
  spine Q76.49
    kyphosis — *see* Kyphosis, congenital
    lordosis — *see* Lordosis, congenital
  spleen Q89.09
  stomach Q40.3
    specified type NEC Q40.2
  teeth, tooth K00.9
  tendon Q79.9
  testis and scrotum Q55.20
    aplasia Q55.0
    hypoplasia Q55.1
    polyorchism Q55.21
    retractile testis Q55.22
    scrotal transposition Q55.23
    specified NEC Q55.29
  thorax, bony Q76.9
  throat Q38.8
  thyroid gland Q89.2
  tongue (congenital) Q38.3
    hypertrophy Q38.2
    tie Q38.1
  trachea Q32.1
  tricuspid valve Q22.9
    specified type NEC Q22.8
  umbilical cord NEC (complicating delivery) O69.89 ☑
  umbilicus Q89.9
  ureter Q62.8
    agenesis Q62.4
    duplication Q62.5
    malposition — *see* Malposition, congenital, ureter
    obstructive defect — *see* Defect, obstructive, ureter
    vesico-uretero-renal reflux Q62.7
  urethra Q64.79
    aplasia Q64.5
    duplication Q64.74
    posterior valves Q64.2
    prolapse Q64.71
    stricture Q64.32
  urinary system Q64.9
  uterus Q51.9
    specified type NEC Q51.818
  vagina Q52.4
  vas deferens Q55.4
    atresia Q55.3
  vascular system, peripheral Q27.9
  venous — *see* Anomaly, vein(s)
  vulva Q52.70
Malfunction — *see also* Dysfunction
  cardiac electronic device T82.119 ☑
    electrode T82.110 ☑
    pulse generator T82.111 ☑
    specified type NEC T82.118 ☑
  catheter device NEC T85.618 ☑
    cystostomy T83.010 ☑
    dialysis (renal) (vascular) T82.41 ☑
      intraperitoneal T85.611 ☑
    infusion NEC T82.514 ☑
      cranial T85.610 ☑
      epidural T85.610 ☑
      intrathecal T85.610 ☑
      spinal T85.610 ☑
      subarachnoid T85.610 ☑
      subdural T85.610 ☑
    urinary — *see also* Breakdown, device, catheter
      T83.018 ☑
  colostomy K94.03
    valve K94.03
  cystostomy (stoma) N99.512
    catheter T83.010 ☑
  enteric stoma K94.13
  enterostomy K94.13
  esophagostomy K94.33
  gastroenteric K31.89
  gastrostomy K94.23
  ileostomy K94.13
    valve K94.13
  intrathecal infusion pump T85.615 ☑
  jejunostomy K94.13
  nervous system device, implant or graft, specified NEC
    T85.615 ☑

Malfunction — continued
  pacemaker — see Malfunction, cardiac electronic device
  prosthetic device, internal — see Complications, prosthetic device, by site, mechanical
  tracheostomy J95.03
  urinary device NEC — see Complication, genitourinary, device, urinary, mechanical
  valve
    colostomy K94.03
    heart T82.09 ☑
    ileostomy K94.13
  vascular graft or shunt NEC — see Complication, cardiovascular device, mechanical, vascular
  ventricular (communicating shunt) T85.01 ☑
Malherbe's tumor — see Neoplasm, skin, benign
Malibu disease L98.8
Malignancy — see also Neoplasm, malignant, by site
  unspecified site (primary) C80.1
Malignant — see condition
Malingerer, malingering Z76.5
Mallet finger (acquired) — see Deformity, finger, mallet finger
  congenital Q74.0
  sequelae of rickets E64.3
Malleus A24.0
Mallory's bodies R89.7
Mallory-Weiss syndrome K22.6
Malnutrition E46
  degree
    · first E44.1
    mild (protein) E44.1
    moderate (protein) E44.0
    second E44.0
    severe (protein-energy) E43
      intermediate form E42
        with
          kwashiorkor (and marasmus) E42
          marasmus E41
    third E43
  following gastrointestinal surgery K91.2
  intrauterine
    light-for-dates — see Light for dates
    small-for-dates — see Small for dates
  lack of care, or neglect (child) (infant) T76.02 ☑
    confirmed T74.02 ☑
  malignant E40
  protein E46
    calorie E46
      mild E44.1
      moderate E44.0
      severe E43
        intermediate form E42
          with
            kwashiorkor (and marasmus) E42
            marasmus E41
    energy E46
      mild E44.1
      moderate E44.0
      severe E43
        intermediate form E42
          with
            kwashiorkor (and marasmus) E42
            marasmus E41
    severe (protein-energy) E43
      with
        kwashiorkor (and marasmus) E42
        marasmus E41
Malocclusion (teeth) M26.4
  Angle's M26.219
    class I M26.211
    class II M26.212
    class III M26.213
  due to
    abnormal swallowing M26.59
    mouth breathing M26.59
    tongue, lip or finger habits M26.59
  temporomandibular (joint) M26.69
Malposition
  cervix — see Malposition, uterus
  congenital
    adrenal (gland) Q89.1
    alimentary tract Q45.8
      lower Q43.8
      upper Q40.8
    aorta Q25.49
    appendix Q43.8
    arterial trunk Q20.0

Malposition — continued
  congenital — continued
    artery (peripheral) Q27.8
      coronary Q24.5
      digestive system Q27.8
      lower limb Q27.8
      pulmonary Q25.79
      specified site NEC Q27.8
      upper limb Q27.8
    auditory canal Q17.8
      causing impairment of hearing Q16.9
    auricle (ear) Q17.4
      causing impairment of hearing Q16.9
      cervical Q18.2
    biliary duct or passage Q44.5
    bladder (mucosa) — see Exstrophy, bladder
    brachial plexus Q07.8
    brain tissue Q04.8
    breast Q83.8
    bronchus Q32.4
    cecum Q43.8
    clavicle Q74.0
    colon Q43.8
    digestive organ or tract NEC Q45.8
      lower Q43.8
      upper Q40.8
    ear (auricle) (external) Q17.4
      ossicles Q16.3
    endocrine (gland) NEC Q89.2
    epiglottis Q31.8
    eustachian tube Q17.8
    eye Q15.8
    facial features Q18.8
    fallopian tube Q50.6
    finger(s) Q68.1
      supernumerary Q69.0
    foot Q66.9- ☑
    gallbladder Q44.1
    gastrointestinal tract Q45.8
    genitalia, genital organ(s) or tract
      female Q52.8
        external Q52.79
        internal NEC Q52.8
      male Q55.8
    glottis Q31.8
    hand Q68.1
    heart Q24.8
      dextrocardia Q24.0
        with complete transposition of viscera Q89.3
    hepatic duct Q44.5
    hip (joint) Q65.89
    intestine (large) (small) Q43.8
      with anomalous adhesions, fixation or malrotation Q43.3
    joint NEC Q68.8
    kidney Q63.2
    larynx Q31.8
    limb Q68.8
      lower Q68.8
      upper Q68.8
    liver Q44.7
    lung (lobe) Q33.8
    nail(s) Q84.6
    nerve Q07.8
    nervous system NEC Q07.8
    nose, nasal (septum) Q30.8
    organ or site not listed — see Anomaly, by site
    ovary Q50.39
    pancreas Q45.3
    parathyroid (gland) Q89.2
    patella Q74.1
    peripheral vascular system Q27.8
    pituitary (gland) Q89.2
    respiratory organ or system NEC Q34.8
    rib (cage) Q76.6
      supernumerary in cervical region Q76.5
    scapula Q74.0
    shoulder Q74.0
    spinal cord Q06.8
    spleen Q89.09
    sternum NEC Q76.7
    stomach Q40.2
    symphysis pubis Q74.2
    thymus (gland) Q89.2
    thyroid (gland) (tissue) Q89.2
      cartilage Q31.8
    toe(s) Q66.9- ☑
      supernumerary Q69.2
    tongue Q38.3

Malposition — continued
  congenital — continued
    trachea Q32.1
    ureter Q62.60
      deviation Q62.61
      displacement Q62.62
      ectopia Q62.63
      specified type NEC Q62.69
    uterus Q51.818
    vein(s) (peripheral) Q27.8
      great Q26.8
    vena cava (inferior) (superior) Q26.8
  device, implant or graft — see also Complications, by site and type, mechanical T85.628 ☑
    arterial graft NEC — see Complication, cardiovascular device, mechanical, vascular
    breast (implant) T85.42 ☑
    catheter NEC T85.628 ☑
      cystostomy T83.020 ☑
      dialysis (renal) T82.42 ☑
        intraperitoneal T85.621 ☑
      infusion NEC T82.524 ☑
        spinal (epidural) (subdural) T85.620 ☑
      urinary — see also Displacement, device, catheter, urinary T83.028 ☑
    electronic (electrode) (pulse generator) (stimulator)
      bone T84.320 ☑
      cardiac T82.129 ☑
        electrode T82.120 ☑
        pulse generator T82.121 ☑
        specified type NEC T82.128 ☑
      nervous system — see Complication, prosthetic device, mechanical, electronic nervous system stimulator
      urinary — see Complication, genitourinary, device, urinary, mechanical
    fixation, internal (orthopedic) NEC — see Complication, fixation device, mechanical
    gastrointestinal — see Complications, prosthetic device, mechanical, gastrointestinal device
    genital NEC T83.428 ☑
      intrauterine contraceptive device (string) T83.32 ☑
      penile prosthesis (cylinder) (implanted) (pump) (reservoir) T83.420 ☑
      testicular prosthesis T83.421 ☑
    heart NEC — see Complication, cardiovascular device, mechanical
    joint prosthesis — see Complication, joint prosthesis, mechanical
    ocular NEC — see Complications, prosthetic device, mechanical, ocular device
    orthopedic NEC — see Complication, orthopedic, device, mechanical
    specified NEC T85.628 ☑
    urinary NEC — see also Complication, genitourinary, device, urinary, mechanical
      graft T83.22 ☑
    vascular NEC — see Complication, cardiovascular device, mechanical
    ventricular intracranial shunt T85.02 ☑
  fetus — see Pregnancy, complicated by (management affected by), presentation, fetal
  gallbladder K82.8
  gastrointestinal tract, congenital Q45.8
  heart, congenital NEC Q24.8
  joint prosthesis — see Complications, joint prosthesis, mechanical, displacement, by site
  stomach K31.89
    congenital Q40.2
  tooth, teeth, fully erupted M26.30
  uterus (acute) (acquired) (adherent) (asymptomatic) (postinfectional) (postpartal, old) N85.4
    anteflexion or anteversion N85.4
      congenital Q51.818
    flexion N85.4
      lateral — see Lateroversion, uterus
    inversion N85.5
    lateral (flexion) (version) — see Lateroversion, uterus
      in pregnancy or childbirth — see subcategory O34.5
    retroflexion or retroversion — see Retroversion, uterus
Malposture R29.3
Malrotation
  cecum Q43.3
  colon Q43.3

☑ **Additional Character Required** — Refer to the Tabular List for Character Selection   ▽ **Subterms under main terms may continue to next column or page**

Malrotation — *continued*
  intestine Q43.3
  kidney Q63.2
Malta fever — *see* Brucellosis
Maltreatment
  adult
    abandonment
      confirmed T74.01 ☑
      suspected T76.01 ☑
    bullying
      confirmed T74.31 ☑
      suspected T76.31 ☑
    confirmed T74.91 ☑
    history of Z91.419
    intimidation (through social media)
      confirmed T74.31 ☑
      suspected T76.31 ☑
    neglect
      confirmed T74.01 ☑
      suspected T76.01 ☑
    physical abuse
      confirmed T74.11 ☑
      suspected T76.11 ☑
    psychological abuse
      confirmed T74.31 ☑
      history of Z91.411
      suspected T76.31 ☑
    sexual abuse
      confirmed T74.21 ☑
      suspected T76.21 ☑
    suspected T76.91 ☑
  child
    abandonment
      confirmed T74.02 ☑
      suspected T76.02 ☑
    bullying
      confirmed T74.32 ☑
      suspected T76.32 ☑
    confirmed T74.92 ☑
    history of — *see* History, personal (of), abuse
    intimidation (through social media)
      confirmed T74.32 ☑
      suspected T76.32 ☑
    neglect
      confirmed T74.02 ☑
      history of — *see* History, personal (of), abuse
      suspected T76.02 ☑
    physical abuse
      confirmed T74.12 ☑
      history of — *see* History, personal (of), abuse
      suspected T76.12 ☑
    psychological abuse
      confirmed T74.32 ☑
      history of — *see* History, personal (of), abuse
      suspected T76.32 ☑
    sexual abuse
      confirmed T74.22 ☑
      history of — *see* History, personal (of), abuse
      suspected T76.22 ☑
    suspected T76.92 ☑
    personal history of Z91.89
Maltworker's lung J67.4
Malunion, fracture — *see* Fracture, by site
Mammillitis N61.0
  puerperal, postpartum O91.02
Mammitis — *see* Mastitis
Mammogram (examination) Z12.39
  routine Z12.31
Mammoplasia N62
Management (of)
  bone conduction hearing device (implanted) Z45.320
  cardiac pacemaker NEC Z45.018
  cerebrospinal fluid drainage device Z45.41
  cochlear device (implanted) Z45.321
  contraceptive Z30.9
    specified NEC Z30.8
  implanted device Z45.9
    specified NEC Z45.89
  infusion pump Z45.1
  procreative Z31.9
    male factor infertility in female Z31.81
    specified NEC Z31.89
  prosthesis (external) — *see also* Fitting Z44.9
    implanted Z45.9
      specified NEC Z45.89
  renal dialysis catheter Z49.01
  vascular access device Z45.2

Mangled — *see* specified injury by site
Mania (monopolar) — *see also* Disorder, mood, manic
  episode
  with psychotic symptoms F30.2
  without psychotic symptoms F30.10
    mild F30.11
    moderate F30.12
    severe F30.13
  Bell's F30.8
  chronic (recurrent) F31.89
  hysterical F44.89
  puerperal F30.8
  recurrent F31.89
Manic depression F31.9
Manic-depressive insanity, psychosis, or syndrome
  — *see* Disorder, bipolar
Mannosidosis E77.1
Mansonelliasis, mansonellosis B74.4
Manson's
  disease B65.1
  schistosomiasis B65.1
Manual — *see* condition
Maple-bark-stripper's lung (disease) J67.6
Maple-syrup-urine disease E71.0
Marable's syndrome (celiac artery compression) I77.4
Marasmus E41
  due to malnutrition E41
  intestinal E41
  nutritional E41
  senile R54
  tuberculous NEC — *see* Tuberculosis
Marble
  bones Q78.2
  skin R23.8
Marburg virus disease A98.3
March
  fracture — *see* Fracture, traumatic, stress, by site
  hemoglobinuria D59.6
Marchesani (-Weill) **syndrome** Q87.0
Marchiafava (-Bignami) **syndrome or disease** G37.1
Marchiafava-Micheli syndrome D59.5
Marcus Gunn's syndrome Q07.8
Marfan's syndrome — *see* Syndrome, Marfan's
Marie-Bamberger disease — *see* Osteoarthropathy,
  hypertrophic, specified NEC
Marie-Charcot-Tooth neuropathic muscular atrophy
  G60.0
Marie's
  cerebellar ataxia (late-onset) G11.2
  disease or syndrome (acromegaly) E22.0
Marie-Strümpell arthritis, disease or spondylitis —
  see Spondylitis, ankylosing
Marion's disease (bladder neck obstruction) N32.0
Marital conflict Z63.0
Mark
  port wine Q82.5
  raspberry Q82.5
  strawberry Q82.5
  stretch L90.6
  tattoo L81.8
Marker heterochromatin — *see* Extra, marker chromo-
  somes
Maroteaux-Lamy syndrome (mild) (severe) E76.29
Marrow (bone)
  arrest D61.9
  poor function D75.89
Marseilles fever A77.1
Marsh fever — *see* Malaria
Marshall's (hidrotic) **ectodermal dysplasia** Q82.4
Marsh's disease (exophthalmic goiter) E05.00
  with storm E05.01
Masculinization (female) **with adrenal hyperplasia**
  E25.9
  congenital E25.0
Masculinovoblastoma D27.- ☑
Masochism (sexual) F65.51
Mason's lung J62.8
Mass
  abdominal R19.00
    epigastric R19.06
    generalized R19.07
    left lower quadrant R19.04
    left upper quadrant R19.02
    periumbilic R19.05
    right lower quadrant R19.03
    right upper quadrant R19.01
    specified site NEC R19.09

Mass — *continued*
  breast — *see also* Lump, breast N63.0
  chest R22.2
  cystic — *see* Cyst
  ear H93.8- ☑
  head R22.0
  intra-abdominal (diffuse) (generalized) — *see* Mass,
    abdominal
  kidney N28.89
  liver R16.0
  localized (skin) R22.9
    chest R22.2
    head R22.0
    limb
      lower R22.4- ☑
      upper R22.3- ☑
    neck R22.1
    trunk R22.2
  lung R91.8
  malignant — *see* Neoplasm, malignant, by site
  neck R22.1
  pelvic (diffuse) (generalized) — *see* Mass, abdominal
  specified organ NEC — *see* Disease, by site
  splenic R16.1
  substernal thyroid — *see* Goiter
  superficial (localized) R22.9
  umbilical (diffuse) (generalized) R19.09
Massive — *see* condition
Mast cell
  disease, systemic tissue D47.02
  leukemia C94.3- ☑
  neoplasm
    malignant C96.20
      specified type NEC C96.29
    of uncertain behavior NEC D47.09
  sarcoma C96.22
  tumor D47.09
Mastalgia N64.4
Masters-Allen syndrome N83.8
Mastitis (acute) (diffuse) (nonpuerperal) (subacute) N61.0
  with abscess N61.1
  chronic (cystic) — *see* Mastopathy, cystic
  cystic (Schimmelbusch's type) — *see* Mastopathy, cystic
  fibrocystic — *see* Mastopathy, cystic
  infective N61.0
    newborn P39.0
  interstitial, gestational or puerperal — *see* Mastitis,
    obstetric
  neonatal (noninfective) P83.4
    infective P39.0
  obstetric (interstitial) (nonpurulent)
    associated with
      lactation O91.23
      pregnancy O91.21- ☑
      puerperium O91.22
    purulent
      associated with
        lactation O91.13
        pregnancy O91.11- ☑
        puerperium O91.12
  periductal — *see* Ectasia, mammary duct
  phlegmonous — *see* Mastopathy, cystic
  plasma cell — *see* Ectasia, mammary duct
  without abscess N61.0
Mastocytoma (extracutaneous) D47.09
  malignant C96.29
  solitary D47.01
Mastocytosis D47.09
  aggressive systemic C96.21
  cutaneous (diffuse) (maculopapular) D47.01
    congenital Q82.2
    of neonatal onset Q82.2
    of newborn onset Q82.2
  indolent systemic D47.02
  isolated bone marrow D47.02
  malignant C96.29
  systemic (indolent) (smoldering)
    with an associated hematological non-mast cell
      lineage disease (SM-AHNMD) D47.02
Mastodynia N64.4
Mastoid — *see* condition
Mastoidalgia — *see* subcategory H92.0 ☑
Mastoiditis (coalescent) (hemorrhagic) (suppurative)
  H70.9- ☑
  acute, subacute H70.00- ☑
    complicated NEC H70.09- ☑
    subperiosteal H70.01- ☑

Mastoiditis — *continued*
  chronic (necrotic) (recurrent) H70.1- ☑
  in (due to)
    infectious disease NEC B99 ☑ *[H75.0-]* ☑
    parasitic disease NEC B89 *[H75.0-]* ☑
    tuberculosis A18.03
  petrositis — *see* Petrositis
  postauricular fistula — *see* Fistula, postauricular
  specified NEC H70.89- ☑
  tuberculous A18.03
Mastopathy, mastopathia N64.9
  chronica cystica — *see* Mastopathy, cystic
  cystic (chronic) (diffuse) N60.1- ☑
    with epithelial proliferation N60.3- ☑
  diffuse cystic — *see* Mastopathy, cystic
  estrogenic, oestrogenica N64.89
  ovarian origin N64.89
Mastoplasia, mastoplastia N62
Masturbation (excessive) F98.8
Maternal care (for) — *see* Pregnancy (complicated by) (management affected by)
Matheiu's disease (leptospiral jaundice) A27.0
Mauclaire's disease or osteochondrosis — *see* Osteochondrosis, juvenile, hand, metacarpal
Maxcy's disease A75.2
Maxilla, maxillary — *see* condition
May (-Hegglin) **anomaly or syndrome** D72.0
McArdle (-Schmid)(-Pearson) **disease** (glycogen storage) E74.04
McCune-Albright syndrome Q78.1
McQuarrie's syndrome (idiopathic familial hypoglycemia) E16.2
Meadow's syndrome Q86.1
Measles (black) (hemorrhagic) (suppressed) B05.9
  with
    complications NEC B05.89
    encephalitis B05.0
    intestinal complications B05.4
    keratitis (keratoconjunctivitis) B05.81
    meningitis B05.1
    otitis media B05.3
    pneumonia B05.2
  French — *see* Rubella
  German — *see* Rubella
  Liberty — *see* Rubella
Meatitis, urethral — *see* Urethritis
Meatus, meatal — *see* condition
Meat-wrappers' asthma J68.9
Meckel-Gruber syndrome Q61.9
Meckel's diverticulitis, diverticulum (displaced) (hypertrophic) Q43.0
  malignant — *see* Table of Neoplasms, small intestine, malignant
Meconium
  ileus, newborn P76.0
    in cystic fibrosis E84.11
    meaning meconium plug (without cystic fibrosis) P76.0
  obstruction, newborn P76.0
    due to fecaliths P76.0
    in mucoviscidosis E84.11
  peritonitis P78.0
  plug syndrome (newborn) NEC P76.0
Median — *see also* condition
  arcuate ligament syndrome I77.4
  bar (prostate) (vesical orifice) — *see* Hyperplasia, prostate
  rhomboid glossitis K14.2
Mediastinal shift R93.89
Mediastinitis (acute) (chronic) J98.51
  syphilitic A52.73
  tuberculous A15.8
Mediastinopericarditis — *see also* Pericarditis
  acute I30.9
  adhesive I31.0
  chronic I31.8
    rheumatic I09.2
Mediastinum, mediastinal — *see* condition
Medicine poisoning — *see* Table of Drugs and Chemicals, by drug, poisoning
Mediterranean
  fever — *see* Brucellosis
    familial M04.1
    tick A77.1
  kala-azar B55.0
  leishmaniasis B55.0
  tick fever A77.1

Medulla — *see* condition
Medullary cystic kidney Q61.5
Medullated fibers
  optic (nerve) Q14.8
  retina Q14.1
Medulloblastoma
  desmoplastic C71.6
  specified site — *see* Neoplasm, malignant, by site
  unspecified site C71.6
Medulloepithelioma — *see also* Neoplasm, malignant, by site
  teratoid — *see* Neoplasm, malignant, by site
Medullomyoblastoma
  specified site — *see* Neoplasm, malignant, by site
  unspecified site C71.6
Meekeren-Ehlers-Danlos syndrome — *see also* Syndrome, Ehlers-Danlos Q79.69
Megacolon (acquired) (functional) (not Hirschsprung's disease) (in) K59.39
  Chagas' disease B57.32
  congenital, congenitum (aganglionic) Q43.1
  Hirschsprung's (disease) Q43.1
  toxic NEC K59.31
    due to Clostridium difficile
      not specified as recurrent A04.72
      recurrent A04.71
Megaesophagus (functional) K22.0
  congenital Q39.5
  in (due to) Chagas' disease B57.31
Megalencephaly Q04.5
Megalerythema (epidemic) B08.3
Megaloappendix Q43.8
Megalocephalus, megalocephaly NEC Q75.3
Megalocornea Q15.8
  with glaucoma Q15.0
Megalocytic anemia D53.1
Megalodactylia (fingers) (thumbs) (congenital) Q74.0
  toes Q74.2
Megaloduodenum Q43.8
Megaloesophagus (functional) K22.0
  congenital Q39.5
Megalogastria (acquired) K31.89
  congenital Q40.2
Megalophthalmos Q11.3
Megalopsia H53.15
Megalosplenia — *see* Splenomegaly
Megaloureter N28.82
  congenital Q62.2
Megarectum K62.89
Megasigmoid K59.39
  congenital Q43.2
Megaureter N28.82
  congenital Q62.2
Megavitamin-B6 syndrome E67.2
Megrim — *see* Migraine
Meibomian
  cyst, infected — *see* Hordeolum
  gland — *see* condition
  sty, stye — *see* Hordeolum
Meibomitis — *see* Hordeolum
Meige-Milroy disease (chronic hereditary edema) Q82.0
Meige's syndrome Q82.0
Melalgia, nutritional E53.8
Melancholia F32.9
  climacteric (single episode) F32.89
    recurrent episode F33.8
  hypochondriac F45.29
  intermittent (single episode) F32.89
    recurrent episode F33.8
  involutional (single episode) F32.89
    recurrent episode F33.8
  menopausal (single episode) F32.89
    recurrent episode F33.8
  puerperal F32.89
  reactive (emotional stress or trauma) F32.3
  recurrent F33.9
  senile F03 ☑
  stuporous (single episode) F32.89
    recurrent episode F33.8
Melanemia R79.89
Melanoameloblastoma — *see* Neoplasm, bone, benign
Melanoblastoma — *see* Melanoma
Melanocarcinoma — *see* Melanoma
Melanocytoma, eyeball D31.9-
Melanocytosis, neurocutaneous Q82.8
Melanoderma, melanodermia L81.4
Melanodontia, infantile K03.89

Melanodontoclasia K03.89
Melanoepithelioma — *see* Melanoma
Melanoma (malignant) C43.9
  acral lentiginous, malignant — *see* Melanoma, skin, by site
  amelanotic — *see* Melanoma, skin, by site
  balloon cell — *see* Melanoma, skin, by site
  benign — *see* Nevus
  desmoplastic, malignant — *see* Melanoma, skin, by site
  epithelioid cell — *see* Melanoma, skin, by site
    with spindle cell, mixed — *see* Melanoma, skin, by site
  in
    giant pigmented nevus — *see* Melanoma, skin, by site
    Hutchinson's melanotic freckle — *see* Melanoma, skin, by site
    junctional nevus — *see* Melanoma, skin, by site
    precancerous melanosis — *see* Melanoma, skin, by site
  in situ D03.9
    abdominal wall D03.59
    ala nasi D03.39
    ankle D03.7- ☑
    anus, anal (margin) (skin) D03.51
    arm D03.6- ☑
    auditory canal D03.2- ☑
    auricle (ear) D03.2- ☑
    auricular canal (external) D03.2- ☑
    axilla, axillary fold D03.59
    back D03.59
    breast D03.52
    brow D03.39
    buttock D03.59
    canthus (eye) D03.1- ☑
    cheek (external) D03.39
    chest wall D03.59
    chin D03.39
    choroid D03.8
    conjunctiva D03.8
    ear (external) D03.2- ☑
    external meatus (ear) D03.2- ☑
    eye D03.8
    eyebrow D03.39
    eyelid (lower) (upper) D03.1- ☑
    face D03.30
      specified NEC D03.39
    female genital organ (external) NEC D03.8
    finger D03.6- ☑
    flank D03.59
    foot D03.7- ☑
    forearm D03.6- ☑
    forehead D03.39
    foreskin D03.8
    gluteal region D03.59
    groin D03.59
    hand D03.6- ☑
    heel D03.7- ☑
    helix D03.2- ☑
    hip D03.7- ☑
    interscapular region D03.59
    iris D03.8
    jaw D03.39
    knee D03.7- ☑
    labium (majus) (minus) D03.8
    lacrimal gland D03.8
    leg D03.7- ☑
    lip (lower) (upper) D03.0
    lower limb NEC D03.7- ☑
    male genital organ (external) NEC D03.8
    nail D03.9
      finger D03.6- ☑
      toe D03.7- ☑
    neck D03.4
    nose (external) D03.39
    orbit D03.8
    penis D03.8
    perianal skin D03.51
    perineum D03.51
    pinna D03.2- ☑
    popliteal fossa or space D03.7- ☑
    prepuce D03.8
    pudendum D03.8
    retina D03.8
    retrobulbar D03.8
    scalp D03.4

☑ Additional Character Required — Refer to the Tabular List for Character Selection   ▽ Subterms under main terms may continue to next column or page

Melanoma — *continued*
  in situ — *continued*
    scrotum D03.8
    shoulder D03.6- ☑
    specified site NEC D03.8
    submammary fold D03.52
    temple D03.39
    thigh D03.7- ☑
    toe D03.7- ☑
    trunk NEC D03.59
    umbilicus D03.59
    upper limb NEC D03.6- ☑
    vulva D03.8
  juvenile — *see* Nevus
  malignant, of soft parts except skin — *see* Neoplasm, connective tissue, malignant
  metastatic
    breast C79.81
    genital organ C79.82
    specified site NEC C79.89
  neurotropic, malignant — *see* Melanoma, skin, by site
  nodular — *see* Melanoma, skin, by site
  regressing, malignant — *see* Melanoma, skin, by site
  skin C43.9
    abdominal wall C43.59
    ala nasi C43.31
    ankle C43.7- ☑
    anus, anal (skin) C43.51
    arm C43.6- ☑
    auditory canal (external) C43.2- ☑
    auricle (ear) C43.2- ☑
    auricular canal (external) C43.2- ☑
    axilla, axillary fold C43.59
    back C43.59
    breast (female) (male) C43.52
    brow C43.39
    buttock C43.59
    canthus (eye) C43.1- ☑
    cheek (external) C43.39
    chest wall C43.59
    chin C43.39
    ear (external) C43.2- ☑
    elbow C43.6- ☑
    external meatus (ear) C43.2- ☑
    eyebrow C43.39
    eyelid (lower) (upper) C43.1- ☑
    face C43.30
      specified NEC C43.39
    female genital organ (external) NEC C51.9
    finger C43.6- ☑
    flank C43.59
    foot C43.7- ☑
    forearm C43.6- ☑
    forehead C43.39
    foreskin C60.0
    glabella C43.39
    gluteal region C43.59
    groin C43.59
    hand C43.6- ☑
    heel C43.7- ☑
    helix C43.2- ☑
    hip C43.7- ☑
    interscapular region C43.59
    jaw (external) C43.39
    knee C43.7- ☑
    labium C51.9
      majus C51.0
      minus C51.1
    leg C43.7- ☑
    lip (lower) (upper) C43.0
    lower limb NEC C43.7- ☑
    male genital organ (external) NEC C63.9
    nail
      finger C43.6- ☑
      toe C43.7- ☑
    nasolabial groove C43.39
    nates C43.59
    neck C43.4
    nose (external) C43.31
    overlapping site C43.8
    palpebra C43.1- ☑
    penis C60.9
    perianal skin C43.51
    perineum C43.51
    pinna C43.2- ☑
    popliteal fossa or space C43.7- ☑
    prepuce C60.0

Melanoma — *continued*
  skin — *continued*
    pudendum C51.9
    scalp C43.4
    scrotum C63.2
    shoulder C43.6- ☑
    skin NEC C43.9
    submammary fold C43.52
    temple C43.39
    thigh C43.7- ☑
    toe C43.7- ☑
    trunk NEC C43.59
    umbilicus C43.59
    upper limb NEC C43.6- ☑
    vulva C51.9
      overlapping sites C51.8
  spindle cell
    with epithelioid, mixed — *see* Melanoma, skin, by site
    type A C69.4- ☑
    type B C69.4- ☑
  superficial spreading — *see* Melanoma, skin, by site
Melanosarcoma — *see also* Melanoma
  epithelioid cell — *see* Melanoma
Melanosis L81.4
  addisonian E27.1
    tuberculous A18.7
  adrenal E27.1
  colon K63.89
  conjunctiva — *see* Pigmentation, conjunctiva
    congenital Q13.89
  cornea (presenile) (senile) — *see also* Pigmentation, cornea
    congenital Q13.4
  eye NEC H57.89
    congenital Q15.8
  lenticularis progressiva Q82.1
  liver K76.89
  precancerous — *see also* Melanoma, in situ
    malignant melanoma in — *see* Melanoma
  Riehl's L81.4
  sclera H15.89
    congenital Q13.89
  suprarenal E27.1
  tar L81.4
  toxic L81.4
Melanuria R82.998
MELAS syndrome E88.41
Melasma L81.1
  adrenal (gland) E27.1
  suprarenal (gland) E27.1
Melena K92.1
  with ulcer — *code by* site under Ulcer, with hemorrhage K27.4
  due to swallowed maternal blood P78.2
  newborn, neonatal P54.1
    due to swallowed maternal blood P78.2
Meleney's
  gangrene (cutaneous) — *see* Ulcer, skin
  ulcer (chronic undermining) — *see* Ulcer, skin
Melioidosis A24.9
  acute A24.1
  chronic A24.2
  fulminating A24.1
  pneumonia A24.1
  pulmonary (chronic) A24.2
    acute A24.1
    subacute A24.2
  sepsis A24.1
  specified NEC A24.3
  subacute A24.2
Melitensis, febris A23.0
Melkersson (-Rosenthal) **syndrome** G51.2
Mellitus, diabetes — *see* Diabetes
Melorheostosis (bone) — *see* Disorder, bone, density and structure, specified NEC
Meloschisis Q18.4
Melotia Q17.4
Membrana
  capsularis lentis posterior Q13.89
  epipapillaris Q14.2
Membranacea placenta O43.19- ☑
Membranaceous uterus N85.8
Membrane(s), membranous — *see also* condition
  cyclitic — *see* Membrane, pupillary
  folds, congenital — *see* Web
  Jackson's Q43.3
  over face of newborn P28.9

Membrane(s), membranous — *continued*
  premature rupture — *see* Rupture, membranes, premature
  pupillary H21.4- ☑
    persistent Q13.89
  retained (with hemorrhage) (complicating delivery) O72.2
    without hemorrhage O73.1
  secondary cataract — *see* Cataract, secondary
  unruptured (causing asphyxia) — *see* Asphyxia, newborn
  vitreous — *see* Opacity, vitreous, membranes and strands
Membranitis — *see* Chorioamnionitis
Memory disturbance, lack or loss — *see also* Amnesia
  mild, following organic brain damage F06.8
Menadione deficiency E56.1
Menarche
  delayed E30.0
  precocious E30.1
Mendacity, pathologic F60.2
Mendelson's syndrome (due to anesthesia) J95.4
  in labor and delivery O74.0
  in pregnancy O29.01- ☑
  obstetric O74.0
  postpartum, puerperal O89.01
Ménétrier's disease or syndrome K29.60
  with bleeding K29.61
Ménière's disease, syndrome or vertigo H81.0- ☑
Meninges, meningeal — *see* condition
Meningioma — *see also* Neoplasm, meninges, benign
  angioblastic — *see* Neoplasm, meninges, benign
  angiomatous — *see* Neoplasm, meninges, benign
  endotheliomatous — *see* Neoplasm, meninges, benign
  fibroblastic — *see* Neoplasm, meninges, benign
  fibrous — *see* Neoplasm, meninges, benign
  hemangioblastic — *see* Neoplasm, meninges, benign
  hemangiopericytic — *see* Neoplasm, meninges, benign
  malignant — *see* Neoplasm, meninges, malignant
  meningiothelial — *see* Neoplasm, meninges, benign
  meningotheliomatous — *see* Neoplasm, meninges, benign
  mixed — *see* Neoplasm, meninges, benign
  multiple — *see* Neoplasm, meninges, uncertain behavior
  papillary — *see* Neoplasm, meninges, uncertain behavior
  psammomatous — *see* Neoplasm, meninges, benign
  syncytial — *see* Neoplasm, meninges, benign
  transitional — *see* Neoplasm, meninges, benign
Meningiomatosis (diffuse) — *see* Neoplasm, meninges, uncertain behavior
Meningism — *see* Meningismus
Meningismus (infectional) (pneumococcal) R29.1
  due to serum or vaccine R29.1
  influenzal — *see* Influenza, with, manifestations NEC
Meningitis (basal) (basic) (brain) (cerebral) (cervical) (congestive) (diffuse) (hemorrhagic) (infantile) (membranous) (metastatic) (nonspecific) (pontine) (progressive) (simple) (spinal) (subacute) (sympathetic) (toxic) G03.9
  abacterial G03.0
  actinomycotic A42.81
  adenoviral A87.1
  arbovirus A87.8
  aseptic (acute) G03.0
  bacterial G00.9
    Escherichia coli (E. coli) G00.8
    Friedländer (bacillus) G00.8
    gram-negative G00.9
    H. influenzae G00.0
    Klebsiella G00.8
    pneumococcal G00.1
    specified organism NEC G00.8
    staphylococcal G00.3
    streptococcal (acute) G00.2
  benign recurrent (Mollaret) G03.2
  candidal B37.5
  caseous (tuberculous) A17.0
  cerebrospinal A39.0
  chronic NEC G03.1
  clear cerebrospinal fluid NEC G03.0
  coxsackievirus A87.0
  cryptococcal B45.1
  diplococcal (gram positive) A39.0
  echovirus A87.0
  enteroviral A87.0
  eosinophilic B83.2

▽ **Subterms under main terms may continue to next column or page**   ☑ **Additional Character Required** — Refer to the Tabular List for Character Selection   **221**

Melanoma — Meningitis

Meningitis — continued
epidemic NEC A39.0
Escherichia coli (E. coli) G00.8
fibrinopurulent G00.9
specified organism NEC G00.8
Friedländer (bacillus) G00.8
gonococcal A54.81
gram-negative cocci G00.9
gram-positive cocci G00.9
H. influenzae G00.0
Haemophilus (influenzae) G00.0
in (due to)
adenovirus A87.1
African trypanosomiasis B56.9 *[G02]*
anthrax A22.8
bacterial disease NEC A48.8 *[G01]*
Chagas' disease (chronic) B57.41
chickenpox B01.0
coccidioidomycosis B38.4
Diplococcus pneumoniae G00.1
enterovirus A87.0
herpes (simplex) virus B00.3
zoster B02.1
infectious mononucleosis B27.92
leptospirosis A27.81
Listeria monocytogenes A32.11
Lyme disease A69.21
measles B05.1
mumps (virus) B26.1
neurosyphilis (late) A52.13
parasitic disease NEC B89 *[G02]*
poliovirus A80.9 *[G02]*
preventive immunization, inoculation or vaccination G03.8
rubella B06.02
Salmonella infection A02.21
specified cause NEC G03.8
Streptococcal pneumoniae G00.1
typhoid fever A01.01
varicella B01.0
viral disease NEC A87.8
whooping cough A37.90
zoster B02.1
infectious G00.9
influenzal (H. influenzae) G00.0
Klebsiella G00.8
leptospiral (aseptic) A27.81
lymphocytic (acute) (benign) (serous) A87.2
meningococcal A39.0
Mima polymorpha G00.8
Mollaret (benign recurrent) G03.2
monilial B37.5
mycotic NEC B49 *[G02]*
Neisseria A39.0
nonbacterial G03.0
nonpyogenic NEC G03.0
ossificans G96.19
pneumococcal streptococcus pneumoniae G00.1
poliovirus A80.9 *[G02]*
postmeasles B05.1
purulent G00.9
specified organism NEC G00.8
pyogenic G00.9
specified organism NEC G00.8
Salmonella (arizonae) (Cholerae-Suis) (enteritidis) (typhimurium) A02.21
septic G00.9
specified organism NEC G00.8
serosa circumscripta NEC G03.0
serous NEC G93.2
specified organism NEC G00.8
sporotrichosis B42.81
staphylococcal G00.3
sterile G03.0
Streptococcal (acute) G00.2
pneumoniae G00.1
suppurative G00.9
specified organism NEC G00.8
syphilitic (late) (tertiary) A52.13
acute A51.41
congenital A50.41
secondary A51.41
Torula histolytica (cryptococcal) B45.1
traumatic (complication of injury) T79.8 ☑
tuberculous A17.0
typhoid A01.01
viral NEC A87.9
Yersinia pestis A20.3

Meningocele (spinal) — see also Spina bifida
with hydrocephalus — see Spina bifida, by site, with hydrocephalus
acquired (traumatic) G96.19
cerebral — see Encephalocele
Meningocerebritis — see Meningoencephalitis
Meningococcemia A39.4
acute A39.2
chronic A39.3
Meningococcus, meningococcal — see also condition A39.9
adrenalitis, hemorrhagic A39.1
carrier (suspected) of Z22.31
meningitis (cerebrospinal) A39.0
Meningoencephalitis — see also Encephalitis G04.90
acute NEC — see also Encephalitis, viral A86
bacterial NEC G04.2
California A83.5
diphasic A84.1
eosinophilic B83.2
epidemic A39.81
herpesviral, herpetic B00.4
due to herpesvirus 6 B10.01
due to herpesvirus 7 B10.09
specified NEC B10.09
in (due to)
blastomycosis NEC B40.81
diseases classified elsewhere G05.3
free-living amebae B60.2
H. influenzae G00.0
Hemophilus influenzae (H .influenzae) G00.0
herpes B00.4
due to herpesvirus 6 B10.01
due to herpesvirus 7 B10.09
specified NEC B10.09
Lyme disease A69.22
mercury — see subcategory T56.1 ☑
mumps B26.2
Naegleria (amebae) (organisms) (fowleri) B60.2
Parastrongylus cantonensis B83.2
toxoplasmosis (acquired) B58.2
congenital P37.1
infectious (acute) (viral) A86
influenzal (H. influenzae) G00.0
Listeria monocytogenes A32.12
lymphocytic (serous) A87.2
mumps B26.2
parasitic NEC B89 *[G05.3]*
pneumococcal G04.2
primary amebic B60.2
specific (syphilitic) A52.14
specified organism NEC G04.81
staphylococcal G04.2
streptococcal G04.2
syphilitic A52.14
toxic NEC G92
due to mercury — see subcategory T56.1 ☑
tuberculous A17.82
virus NEC A86
Meningoencephalocele — see also Encephalocele
syphilitic A52.19
congenital A50.49
Meningoencephalomyelitis — see also Meningoencephalitis
acute NEC (viral) A86
disseminated G04.00
postimmunization or postvaccination G04.02
postinfectious G04.01
due to
actinomycosis A42.82
Torula B45.1
Toxoplasma or toxoplasmosis (acquired) B58.2
congenital P37.1
postimmunization or postvaccination G04.02
Meningoencephalomyelopathy G96.9
Meningoencephalopathy G96.9
Meningomyelitis — see also Meningoencephalitis
bacterial NEC G04.2
blastomycotic NEC B40.81
cryptococcal B45.1
in diseases classified elsewhere G05.4
meningococcal A39.81
syphilitic A52.14
tuberculous A17.82
Meningomyelocele — see also Spina bifida
syphilitic A52.19
Meningomyeloneuritis — see Meningoencephalitis
Meningoradiculitis — see Meningitis

Meningovascular — see condition
Menkes' disease or syndrome E83.09
meaning maple-syrup-urine disease E71.0
Menometrorrhagia N92.1
Menopause, menopausal (asymptomatic) (state) Z78.0
arthritis (any site) NEC — see Arthritis, specified form NEC
bleeding N92.4
depression (single episode) F32.89
agitated (single episode) F32.2
recurrent episode F33.9
psychotic (single episode) F32.89
recurrent episode F33.9
recurrent episode F33.8
melancholia (single episode) F32.89
recurrent episode F33.8
paranoid state F22
premature E28.319
asymptomatic E28.319
postirradiation E89.40
postsurgical E89.40
symptomatic E28.310
postirradiation E89.41
postsurgical E89.41
psychosis NEC F28
symptomatic N95.1
toxic polyarthritis NEC — see Arthritis, specified form NEC
Menorrhagia (primary) N92.0
climacteric N92.4
menopausal N92.4
menopausal N92.4
perimenopausal N92.4
postclimacteric N95.0
postmenopausal N95.0
preclimacteric or premenopausal N92.4
pubertal (menses retained) N92.2
Menostaxis N92.0
Menses, retention N94.89
Menstrual — see Menstruation
Menstruation
absent — see Amenorrhea
anovulatory N97.0
cycle, irregular N92.6
delayed N91.0
disorder N93.9
psychogenic F45.8
during pregnancy O20.8
excessive (with regular cycle) N92.0
with irregular cycle N92.1
at puberty N92.2
frequent N92.0
infrequent — see Oligomenorrhea
irregular N92.6
specified NEC N92.5
latent N92.5
membranous N92.5
painful — see also Dysmenorrhea N94.6
primary N94.4
psychogenic F45.8
secondary N94.5
passage of clots N92.0
precocious E30.1
protracted N92.5
rare — see Oligomenorrhea
retained N94.89
retrograde N92.5
scanty — see Oligomenorrhea
suppression N94.89
vicarious (nasal) N94.89
Mental — see also condition
deficiency — see Disability, intellectual
deterioration — see Psychosis
disorder — see Disorder, mental
exhaustion F48.8
insufficiency (congenital) — see Disability, intellectual
observation without need for further medical care Z03.89
retardation — see Disability, intellectual
subnormality — see Disability, intellectuall
upset — see Disorder, mental
Meralgia paresthetica G57.1- ☑
Mercurial — see condition
Mercurialism — see subcategory T56.1 ☑
Merkel cell tumor — see Carcinoma, Merkel cell
Merocele — see Hernia, femoral
Meromelia
lower limb — see Defect, reduction, lower limb

222

☑ **Additional Character Required** — Refer to the Tabular List for Character Selection   ▽ **Subterms under main terms may continue to next column or page**

Meromelia — *continued*
  lower limb — *see* Defect, reduction, lower limb — *continued*
    intercalary
      femur — *see* Defect, reduction, lower limb, specified type NEC
        tibiofibular (complete) (incomplete) — *see* Defect, reduction, lower limb
  upper limb — *see* Defect, reduction, upper limb
    intercalary, humeral, radioulnar — *see* Agenesis, arm, with hand present
MERRF syndrome (myoclonic epilepsy associated with ragged-red fiber) E88.42
Merzbacher-Pelizaeus disease E75.29
Mesaortitis — *see* Aortitis
Mesarteritis — *see* Arteritis
Mesencephalitis — *see* Encephalitis
Mesenchymoma — *see also* Neoplasm, connective tissue, uncertain behavior
  benign — *see* Neoplasm, connective tissue, benign
  malignant — *see* Neoplasm, connective tissue, malignant
Mesenteritis
  retractile K65.4
  sclerosing K65.4
Mesentery, mesenteric — *see* condition
Mesiodens, mesiodentes K00.1
Mesio-occlusion M26.213
Mesocolon — *see* condition
Mesonephroma (malignant) — *see* Neoplasm, malignant, by site
  benign — *see* Neoplasm, benign, by site
Mesophlebitis — *see* Phlebitis
Mesostromal dysgenesia Q13.89
Mesothelioma (malignant) C45.9
  benign
    mesentery D19.1
    mesocolon D19.1
    omentum D19.1
    peritoneum D19.1
    pleura D19.0
    specified site NEC D19.7
    unspecified site D19.9
  biphasic C45.9
    benign
      mesentery D19.1
      mesocolon D19.1
      omentum D19.1
      peritoneum D19.1
      pleura D19.0
      specified site NEC D19.7
      unspecified site D19.9
  cystic D48.4
  epithelioid C45.9
    benign
      mesentery D19.1
      mesocolon D19.1
      omentum D19.1
      peritoneum D19.1
      pleura D19.0
      specified site NEC D19.7
      unspecified site D19.9
  fibrous C45.9
    benign
      mesentery D19.1
      mesocolon D19.1
      omentum D19.1
      peritoneum D19.1
      pleura D19.0
      specified site NEC D19.7
      unspecified site D19.9
  site classification
    liver C45.7
    lung C45.7
    mediastinum C45.7
    mesentery C45.1
    mesocolon C45.1
    omentum C45.1
    pericardium C45.2
    peritoneum C45.1
    pleura C45.0
      parietal C45.0
    retroperitoneum C45.7
    specified site NEC C45.7
    unspecified C45.9
Metabolic syndrome E88.81
Metagonimiasis B66.8
Metagonimus infestation (intestine) B66.8

Metal
  pigmentation L81.8
  polisher's disease J62.8
Metamorphopsia H53.15
Metaplasia
  apocrine (breast) — *see* Dysplasia, mammary, specified type NEC
  cervix (squamous) — *see* Dysplasia, cervix
  endometrium (squamous) (uterus) N85.8
  esophagus K22.7- ☑
  kidney (pelvis) (squamous) N28.89
  myelogenous D73.1
  myeloid (agnogenic) (megakaryocytic) D73.1
  spleen D73.1
  squamous cell, bladder N32.89
Metastasis, metastatic
  abscess — *see* Abscess
  calcification E83.59
  cancer
    from specified site — *see* Neoplasm, malignant, by site
    to specified site — *see* Neoplasm, secondary, by site
  deposits (in) — *see* Neoplasm, secondary, by site
  disease — *see also* Neoplasm, secondary, by site C79.9
  spread (to) — *see* Neoplasm, secondary, by site
Metastrongyliasis B83.8
Metatarsalgia M77.4- ☑
  anterior G57.6- ☑
  Morton's G57.6- ☑
Metatarsus, metatarsal — *see also* condition
  adductus, congenital Q66.22- ☑
  valgus (abductus), congenital Q66.6
  varus (congenital) Q66.22- ☑
    primus Q66.21- ☑
Methadone use — *see* Use, opioid
Methemoglobinemia D74.9
  acquired (with sulfhemoglobinemia) D74.8
  congenital D74.0
    enzymatic (congenital) D74.0
  Hb M disease D74.0
  hereditary D74.0
  toxic D74.8
Methemoglobinuria — *see* Hemoglobinuria
Methioninemia E72.19
Methylmalonic acidemia E71.120
Metritis (catarrhal) (hemorrhagic) (septic) (suppurative) — *see also* Endometritis
  cervical — *see* Cervicitis
Metropathia hemorrhagica N93.8
Metroperitonitis — *see* Peritonitis, pelvic, female
Metrorrhagia N92.1
  climacteric N92.4
  menopausal N92.4
  perimenopausal N92.4
  postpartum NEC (atonic) (following delivery of placenta) O72.1
    delayed or secondary O72.2
  preclimacteric or premenopausal N92.4
  psychogenic F45.8
Metrorrhexis — *see* Rupture, uterus
Metrosalpingitis N70.91
Metrostaxis N93.8
Metrovaginitis — *see* Endometritis
Meyer-Schwickerath and Weyers syndrome Q87.0
Meynert's amentia (nonalcoholic) F04
  alcoholic F10.96
    with dependence F10.26
Mibelli's disease (porokeratosis) Q82.8
Mice, joint — *see* Loose, body, joint
  knee M23.4- ☑
Micrencephalon, micrencephaly Q02
Microalbuminuria R80.9
Microaneurysm, retinal — *see also* Disorder, retina, microaneurysms
  diabetic — *see* E08-E13 with .31
Microangiopathy (peripheral) I73.9
  thrombotic M31.1
Microcalcifications, breast R92.0
Microcephalus, microcephalic, microcephaly Q02
  due to toxoplasmosis (congenital) P37.1
Microcheilia Q18.7
Microcolon (congenital) Q43.8
Microcornea (congenital) Q13.4
Microcytic — *see* condition
Microdeletions NEC Q93.88
Microdontia K00.2
Microdrepanocytosis D57.40

Microdrepanocytosis — *continued*
  with crisis (vasoocclusive pain) D57.419
    with
      acute chest syndrome D57.411
      splenic sequestration D57.412
Microembolism
  atherothrombotic — *see* Atheroembolism
  retinal — *see* Occlusion, artery, retina
Microencephalon Q02
Microfilaria streptocerca infestation — *see* Onchocerciasis
Microgastria (congenital) Q40.2
Microgenia M26.06
Microgenitalia, congenital
  female Q52.8
  male Q55.8
Microglioma — *see* Lymphoma, non-Hodgkin, specified NEC
Microglossia (congenital) Q38.3
Micrognathia, micrognathism (congenital) (mandibular) (maxillary) M26.09
Microgyria (congenital) Q04.3
Microinfarct of heart — *see* Insufficiency, coronary
Microlentia (congenital) Q12.8
Microlithiasis, alveolar, pulmonary J84.02
Micromastia N64.82
Micromyelia (congenital) Q06.8
Micropenis Q55.62
Microphakia (congenital) Q12.8
Microphthalmos, microphthalmia (congenital) Q11.2
  due to toxoplasmosis P37.1
Micropsia H53.15
Microscopic polyangiitis (polyarteritis) M31.7
Microsporidiosis B60.8
  intestinal A07.8
Microsporon furfur infestation B36.0
Microsporosis — *see also* Dermatophytosis
  nigra B36.1
Microstomia (congenital) Q18.5
Microtia (congenital) (external ear) Q17.2
Microtropia H50.40
Microvillus inclusion disease (MVD) (MVID) Q43.8
Micturition
  disorder NEC — *see also* Difficulty, micturition R39.198
    psychogenic F45.8
  frequency R35.0
    psychogenic F45.8
  hesitancy R39.11
  incomplete emptying R39.14
  nocturnal R35.1
  painful R30.9
    dysuria R30.0
    psychogenic F45.8
    tenesmus R30.1
  poor stream R39.12
  position dependent R39.192
  split stream R39.13
  straining R39.16
  urgency R39.15
Mid plane — *see* condition
Middle
  ear — *see* condition
  lobe (right) syndrome J98.19
Miescher's elastoma L87.2
Mietens' syndrome Q87.2
Migraine (idiopathic) G43.909
  with refractory migraine G43.919
    with status migrainosus G43.911
    without status migrainosus G43.919
  with aura (acute-onset) (prolonged) (typical) (without headache) G43.109
    with refractory migraine G43.119
      with status migrainosus G43.111
      without status migrainosus G43.119
    intractable G43.119
      with status migrainosus G43.111
      without status migrainosus G43.119
    not intractable G43.109
      with status migrainosus G43.101
      without status migrainosus G43.109
    persistent G43.509
      with cerebral infarction G43.609
        with refractory migraine G43.619
          with status migrainosus G43.611
          without status migrainosus G43.619
        intractable G43.619
          with status migrainosus G43.611
          without status migrainosus G43.619

Migraine — *continued*
 with aura — *continued*
  persistent — *continued*
   with cerebral infarction — *continued*
    not intractable G43.609
     with status migrainosus G43.601
     without status migrainosus G43.609
    without refractory migraine G43.609
     with status migrainosus G43.601
     without status migrainosus G43.609
   without cerebral infarction G43.509
    with refractory migraine G43.519
     with status migrainosus G43.511
     without status migrainosus G43.519
    intractable G43.519
     with status migrainosus G43.511
     without status migrainosus G43.519
    not intractable G43.509
     with status migrainosus G43.501
     without status migrainosus G43.509
    without refractory migraine G43.509
     with status migrainosus G43.501
     without status migrainosus G43.509
   without mention of refractory migraine G43.109
    with status migrainosus G43.101
    without status migrainosus G43.109
 abdominal G43.D0 (*following* G43.7)
  with refractory migraine G43.D1 (*following* G43.7)
  intractable G43.D1 (*following* G43.7)
  not intractable G43.D0 (*following* G43.7)
  without refractory migraine G43.D0 (*following* G43.7)
 basilar — *see* Migraine, with aura
 classical — *see* Migraine, with aura
 common — *see* Migraine, without aura
 complicated G43.109
 equivalents — *see* Migraine, with aura
 familial — *see* Migraine, hemiplegic
 hemiplegic G43.409
  with refractory migraine G43.419
   with status migrainosus G43.411
   without status migrainosus G43.419
  intractable G43.419
   with status migrainosus G43.411
   without status migrainosus G43.419
  not intractable G43.409
   with status migrainosus G43.401
   without status migrainosus G43.409
  without refractory migraine G43.409
   with status migrainosus G43.401
   without status migrainosus G43.409
 intractable G43.919
  with status migrainosus G43.911
  without status migrainosus G43.919
 menstrual G43.829
  with refractory migraine G43.839
   with status migrainosus G43.831
   without status migrainosus G43.839
  intractable G43.839
   with status migrainosus G43.831
   without status migrainosus G43.839
  not intractable 4G43.829
   with status migrainosus G43.821
   without status migrainosus G43.829
  without refractory migraine G43.829
   with status migrainosus G43.821
   without status migrainosus G43.829
 menstrually related — *see* Migraine, menstrual
 not intractable G43.909
  with status migrainosus G43.901
  without status migrainosus G43.919
 ophthalmoplegic G43.B0 (*following* G43.7)
  with refractory migraine G43.B1 (*following* G43.7)
  intractable G43.B1 (*following* G43.7)
  not intractable G43.B0 (*following* G43.7)
  without refractory migraine G43.B0 (*following* G43.7)
 persistent aura (with, without) cerebral infarction —
  see Migraine, with aura, persistent
 preceded or accompanied by transient focal neurological phenomena — *see* Migraine, with aura
 pre-menstrual — *see* Migraine, menstrual
 pure menstrual — *see* Migraine, menstrual
 retinal — *see* Migraine, with aura
 specified NEC G43.809
  intractable G43.819
   with status migrainosus G43.811
   without status migrainosus G43.819
  not intractable G43.809
   with status migrainosus G43.801

Migraine — *continued*
 specified — *continued*
  not intractable — *continued*
   without status migrainosus G43.809
 sporadic — *see* Migraine, hemiplegic
 transformed — *see* Migraine, without aura, chronic
 triggered seizures — *see* Migraine, with aura
 without aura G43.009
  with refractory migraine G43.019
   with status migrainosus G43.011
   without status migrainosus G43.019
  chronic G43.709
   with refractory migraine G43.719
    with status migrainosus G43.711
    without status migrainosus G43.719
   intractable
    with status migrainosus G43.711
    without status migrainosus G43.719
   not intractable
    with status migrainosus G43.701
    without status migrainosus G43.709
   without refractory migraine G43.709
    with status migrainosus G43.701
    without status migrainosus G43.709
  intractable
   with status migrainosus G43.011
   without status migrainosus G43.019
  not intractable
   with status migrainosus G43.001
   without status migrainosus G43.009
  without mention of refractory migraine G43.009
   with status migrainosus G43.001
   without status migrainosus G43.009
 without refractory migraine G43.909
  with status migrainosus G43.901
  without status migrainosus G43.919
Migrant, social Z59.0
Migration, anxiety concerning Z60.3
Migratory, migrating — *see also* condition
 person Z59.0
 testis Q55.29
Mikity-Wilson disease or syndrome P27.0
Mikulicz' disease or syndrome K11.8
Miliaria L74.3
 alba L74.1
 apocrine L75.2
 crystallina L74.1
 profunda L74.2
 rubra L74.0
 tropicalis L74.2
Miliary — *see* condition
Milium L72.0
 colloid L57.8
Milk
 crust L21.0
 excessive secretion O92.6
 poisoning — *see* Poisoning, food, noxious
 retention O92.79
 sickness — *see* Poisoning, food, noxious
 spots I31.0
Milk-alkali disease or syndrome E83.52
Milk-leg (deep vessels) (nonpuerperal) — *see* Embolism,
  vein, lower extremity
 complicating pregnancy O22.3- ☑
 puerperal, postpartum, childbirth O87.1
Milkman's disease or syndrome M83.8
Milky urine — *see* Chyluria
Millard-Gubler (-Foville) **paralysis or syndrome** G46.3
Millar's asthma J38.5
Miller Fisher syndrome G61.0
Mills' disease — *see* Hemiplegia
Millstone maker's pneumoconiosis J62.8
Milroy's disease (chronic hereditary edema) Q82.0
Minamata disease T56.1 ☑
Miners' asthma or lung J60
Minkowski-Chauffard syndrome — *see* Spherocytosis
Minor — *see* condition
Minor's disease (hematomyelia) G95.19
Minot's disease (hemorrhagic disease), newborn P53
Minot-von Willebrand-Jurgens disease or syndrome
  (angiohemophilia) D68.0
Minus (and plus) **hand** (intrinsic) — *see* Deformity, limb,
  specified type NEC, forearm
Miosis (pupil) H57.03
Mirizzi's syndrome (hepatic duct stenosis) K83.1
Mirror writing F81.0

Misadventure (of) (prophylactic) (therapeutic) — *see
  also* Complications T88.9 ☑
 administration of insulin (by accident) — *see* subcategory T38.3 ☑
 infusion — *see* Complications, infusion
 local applications (of fomentations, plasters, etc.)
  T88.9 ☑
  burn or scald — *see* Burn
  specified NEC T88.8 ☑
 medical care (early) (late) T88.9 ☑
  adverse effect of drugs or chemicals — *see* Table of
   Drugs and Chemicals
  burn or scald — *see* Burn
  specified NEC T88.8 ☑
 specified NEC T88.8 ☑
 surgical procedure (early) (late) — *see* Complications,
  surgical procedure
 transfusion — *see* Complications, transfusion
 vaccination or other immunological procedure — *see*
  Complications, vaccination
Miscarriage O03.9
Misdirection, aqueous H40.83- ☑
Misperception, sleep state F51.02
Misplaced, misplacement
 ear Q17.4
 kidney (acquired) N28.89
  congenital Q63.2
 organ or site, congenital NEC — *see* Malposition, congenital
Missed
 abortion O02.1
 delivery O36.4 ☑
Missing — *see also* Absence
 string of intrauterine contraceptive device T83.32- ☑
Misuse of drugs F19.99
Mitchell's disease (erythromelalgia) I73.81
Mite(s) (infestation) B88.9
 diarrhea B88.0
 grain (itch) B88.0
 hair follicle (itch) B88.0
 in sputum B88.0
Mitral — *see* condition
Mittelschmerz N94.0
Mixed — *see* condition
MMN (multifocal motor neuropathy) G61.82
MNGIE (Mitochondrial Neurogastrointestinal Encephalopathy) **syndrome** E88.49
Mobile, mobility
 cecum Q43.3
 excessive — *see* Hypermobility
 gallbladder, congenital Q44.1
 kidney N28.89
 organ or site, congenital NEC — *see* Malposition, congenital
Mobitz heart block (atrioventricular) I44.1
Moebius, Möbius
 disease (ophthalmoplegic migraine) — *see* Migraine,
  ophthalmoplegic
 syndrome Q87.0
  congenital oculofacial paralysis (with other anomalies) Q87.0
  ophthalmoplegic migraine — *see* Migraine, ophthalmoplegic
Moeller's glossitis K14.0
Mohr's syndrome (Types I and II) Q87.0
Mola destruens D39.2
Molar pregnancy O02.0
Molarization of premolars K00.2
Molding, head (during birth) — *omit code*
Mole (pigmented) — *see also* Nevus
 blood O02.0
 Breus' O02.0
 cancerous — *see* Melanoma
 carneous O02.0
 destructive D39.2
 fleshy O02.0
 hydatid, hydatidiform (benign) (complicating pregnancy) (delivered) (undelivered) O01.9
  classical O01.0
  complete O01.0
  incomplete O01.1
  invasive D39.2
  malignant D39.2
  partial O01.1
 intrauterine O02.0
 invasive (hydatidiform) D39.2

Mole — *continued*
  malignant
    meaning
      malignant hydatidiform mole D39.2
      melanoma — *see* Melanoma
    nonhydatidiform O02.0
    nonpigmented — *see* Nevus
    pregnancy NEC O02.0
    skin — *see* Nevus
    tubal O00.10- ☑
      with intrauterine pregnancy O00.11- ☑
  vesicular — *see* Mole, hydatidiform
Molimen, molimina (menstrual) N94.3
Molluscum contagiosum (epitheliale) B08.1
Mönckeberg's arteriosclerosis, disease, or sclerosis
  — *see* Arteriosclerosis, extremities
Mondini's malformation (cochlea) Q16.5
Mondor's disease I80.8
Monge's disease T70.29 ☑
Monilethrix (congenital) Q84.1
Moniliasis — *see also* Candidiasis B37.9
  neonatal P37.5
Monitoring (encounter for)
  therapeutic drug level Z51.81
Monkey malaria B53.1
Monkeypox B04
Monoarthritis M13.10
  ankle M13.17- ☑
  elbow M13.12- ☑
  foot joint M13.17- ☑
  hand joint M13.14- ☑
  hip M13.15- ☑
  knee M13.16- ☑
  shoulder M13.11- ☑
  wrist M13.13- ☑
Monoblastic — *see* condition
Monochromat (ism), monochromatopsia (acquired)
  (congenital) H53.51
Monocytic — *see* condition
Monocytopenia D72.818
Monocytosis (symptomatic) D72.821
Monomania — *see* Psychosis
Mononeuritis G58.9
  cranial nerve — *see* Disorder, nerve, cranial
  femoral nerve G57.2- ☑
  lateral
    cutaneous nerve of thigh G57.1- ☑
    popliteal nerve G57.3- ☑
  lower limb G57.9- ☑
    specified nerve NEC G57.8- ☑
  medial popliteal nerve G57.4- ☑
  median nerve G56.1- ☑
  multiplex G58.7
  plantar nerve G57.6- ☑
  posterior tibial nerve G57.5- ☑
  radial nerve G56.3- ☑
  sciatic nerve G57.0- ☑
  specified NEC G58.8
  tibial nerve G57.4- ☑
  ulnar nerve G56.2- ☑
  upper limb G56.9- ☑
    specified nerve NEC G56.8- ☑
  vestibular — *see* subcategory H93.3 ☑
Mononeuropathy G58.9
  carpal tunnel syndrome — *see* Syndrome, carpal tunnel
  diabetic NEC — *see* E08-E13 with .41
  femoral nerve — *see* Lesion, nerve, femoral
  ilioinguinal nerve G57.8- ☑
  in diseases classified elsewhere — *see* category G59
  intercostal G58.0
  lower limb G57.9- ☑
    causalgia — *see* Causalgia, lower limb
    femoral nerve — *see* Lesion, nerve, femoral
    meralgia paresthetica G57.1- ☑
    plantar nerve — *see* Lesion, nerve, plantar
    popliteal nerve — *see* Lesion, nerve, popliteal
    sciatic nerve — *see* Lesion, nerve, sciatic
    specified NEC G57.8- ☑
    tarsal tunnel syndrome — *see* Syndrome, tarsal
      tunnel
  median nerve — *see* Lesion, nerve, median
  multiplex G58.7
  obturator nerve G57.8- ☑
  popliteal nerve — *see* Lesion, nerve, popliteal
  radial nerve — *see* Lesion, nerve, radial
  saphenous nerve G57.8- ☑

Mononeuropathy — *continued*
  specified NEC G58.8
  tarsal tunnel syndrome — *see* Syndrome, tarsal tunnel
  tuberculous A17.83
  ulnar nerve — *see* Lesion, nerve, ulnar
  upper limb G56.9- ☑
    carpal tunnel syndrome — *see* Syndrome, carpal
      tunnel
    causalgia — *see* Causalgia
    median nerve — *see* Lesion, nerve, median
    radial nerve — *see* Lesion, nerve, radial
    specified site NEC G56.8- ☑
    ulnar nerve — *see* Lesion, nerve, ulnar
Mononucleosis, infectious B27.90
  with
    complication NEC B27.99
    meningitis B27.92
    polyneuropathy B27.91
  cytomegaloviral B27.10
    with
      complication NEC B27.19
      meningitis B27.12
      polyneuropathy B27.11
  Epstein-Barr (virus) B27.00
    with
      complication NEC B27.09
      meningitis B27.02
      polyneuropathy B27.01
  gammaherpesviral B27.00
    with
      complication NEC B27.09
      meningitis B27.02
      polyneuropathy B27.01
  specified NEC B27.80
    with
      complication NEC B27.89
      meningitis B27.82
      polyneuropathy B27.81
Monoplegia G83.3- ☑
  congenital (cerebral) G80.8
    spastic G80.1
  embolic (current episode) I63.4- ☑
  following
    cerebrovascular disease
      cerebral infarction
        lower limb I69.34- ☑
        upper limb I69.33- ☑
      intracerebral hemorrhage
        lower limb I69.14- ☑
        upper limb I69.13- ☑
      lower limb I69.94- ☑
      nontraumatic intracranial hemorrhage NEC
        lower limb I69.24- ☑
        upper limb I69.23- ☑
      specified disease NEC
        lower limb I69.84- ☑
        upper limb I69.83- ☑
      stroke NOS
        lower limb I69.34- ☑
        upper limb I69.33- ☑
      subarachnoid hemorrhage
        lower limb I69.04- ☑
        upper limb I69.03- ☑
      upper limb I69.93- ☑
  hysterical (transient) F44.4
  lower limb G83.1- ☑
  psychogenic (conversion reaction) F44.4
  thrombotic (current episode) I63.3- ☑
  transient R29.818
  upper limb G83.2- ☑
Monorchism, monorchidism Q55.0
Monosomy — *see also* Deletion, chromosome Q93.9
  specified NEC Q93.89
  whole chromosome
    meiotic nondisjunction Q93.0
    mitotic nondisjunction Q93.1
    mosaicism Q93.1
  X Q96.9
Monster, monstrosity (single) Q89.7
  acephalic Q00.0
  twin Q89.4
Monteggia's fracture (-dislocation) S52.27- ☑
Mooren's ulcer (cornea) — *see* Ulcer, cornea, Mooren's
Moore's syndrome — *see* Epilepsy, specified NEC
Mooser-Neill reaction A75.2
Mooser's bodies A75.2
Morbidity not stated or unknown R69

Morbilli — *see* Measles
Morbus — *see also* Disease
  angelicus, anglorum E55.0
  Beigel B36.2
  caducus — *see* Epilepsy
  celiacus K90.0
  comitialis — *see* Epilepsy
  cordis — *see also* Disease, heart I51.9
    valvulorum — *see* Endocarditis
  coxae senilis M16.9
    tuberculous A18.02
  hemorrhagicus neonatorum P53
  maculosus neonatorum P54.5
Morel (-Stewart)(-Morgagni) **syndrome** M85.2
Morel-Kraepelin disease — *see* Schizophrenia
Morel-Moore syndrome M85.2
Morgagni's
  cyst, organ, hydatid, or appendage
    female Q50.5
    male (epididymal) Q55.4
      testicular Q55.29
  syndrome M85.2
Morgagni-Stewart-Morel syndrome M85.2
Morgagni-Stokes-Adams syndrome I45.9
Morgagni-Turner (-Albright) **syndrome** Q96.9
Moria F07.0
Moron (I.Q. 50-69) F70
Morphea L94.0
Morphinism (without remission) F11.20
  with remission F11.21
Morphinomania (without remission) F11.20
  with remission F11.21
Morquio (-Ullrich)(-Brailsford) **disease or syndrome** —
  see Mucopolysaccharidosis
Mortification (dry) (moist) — *see* Gangrene
Morton's metatarsalgia (neuralgia)(neuroma) (syn-
  drome) G57.6- ☑
Morvan's disease or syndrome G60.8
Mosaicism, mosaic (autosomal) (chromosomal)
  45,X/46,XX Q96.3
  45,X/other cell lines NEC with abnormal sex chromo-
    some Q96.4
  sex chromosome
    female Q97.8
    lines with various numbers of X chromosomes Q97.2
    male Q98.7
  XY Q96.3
Moschowitz' disease M31.1
Mother yaw A66.0
Motion sickness (from travel, any vehicle) (from round-
  abouts or swings) T75.3 ☑
Mottled, mottling, teeth (enamel) (endemic) (nonen-
  demic) K00.3
Mounier-Kuhn syndrome Q32.4
  with bronchiectasis J47.9
    exacerbation (acute) J47.1
    lower respiratory infection J47.0
  acquired J98.09
    with bronchiectasis J47.9
      with
        exacerbation (acute) J47.1
        lower respiratory infection J47.0
Mountain
  sickness T70.29 ☑
    with polycythemia , acquired (acute) D75.1
  tick fever A93.2
Mouse, joint — *see* Loose, body, joint
  knee M23.4- ☑
Mouth — *see* condition
Movable
  coccyx — *see* subcategory M53.2 ☑
  kidney N28.89
    congenital Q63.8
  spleen D73.89
Movements, dystonic R25.8
Moyamoya disease I67.5
MRSA (Methicillin resistant Staphylococcus aureus)
  infection A49.02
    as the cause of diseases classified elsewhere B95.62
  sepsis A41.02
MSD (multiple sulfatase deficiency) E75.26
MSSA (Methicillin susceptible Staphylococcus aureus)
  infection A49.01
    as the cause of diseases classified elsewhere B95.61
  sepsis A41.01
Mucha-Habermann disease L41.0
Mucinosis (cutaneous) (focal) (papular) (skin) L98.5

Mucinosis — *continued*
  oral K13.79
Mucocele
  appendix K38.8
  buccal cavity K13.79
  gallbladder K82.1
  lacrimal sac, chronic H04.43- ☑
  nasal sinus J34.1
  nose J34.1
  salivary gland (any) K11.6
  sinus (accessory) (nasal) J34.1
  turbinate (bone) (middle) (nasal) J34.1
  uterus N85.8
Mucolipidosis
  I E77.1
  II, III E77.0
  IV E75.11
Mucopolysaccharidosis E76.3
  beta-gluduronidase deficiency E76.29
  cardiopathy E76.3 *[I52]*
  Hunter's syndrome E76.1
  Hurler's syndrome E76.01
  Hurler-Scheie syndrome E76.02
  Maroteaux-Lamy syndrome E76.29
  Morquio syndrome E76.219
    A E76.210
    B E76.211
    classic E76.210
  Sanfilippo syndrome E76.22
  Scheie's syndrome E76.03
  specified NEC E76.29
  type
    I
      Hurler's syndrome E76.01
      Hurler-Scheie syndrome E76.02
      Scheie's syndrome E76.03
    II E76.1
    III E76.22
    IV E76.219
    IVA E76.210
    IVB E76.211
    VI E76.29
    VII E76.29
Mucormycosis B46.5
  cutaneous B46.3
  disseminated B46.4
  gastrointestinal B46.2
  generalized B46.4
  pulmonary B46.0
  rhinocerebral B46.1
  skin B46.3
  subcutaneous B46.3
Mucositis (ulcerative) K12.30
  due to drugs NEC K12.32
  gastrointestinal K92.81
  mouth (oral) (oropharyngeal) K12.30
    due to antineoplastic therapy K12.31
    due to drugs NEC K12.32
    due to radiation K12.33
    specified NEC K12.39
    viral K12.39
  nasal J34.81
  oral cavity — *see* Mucositis, mouth
  oral soft tissues — *see* Mucositis, mouth
  vagina and vulva N76.81
Mucositis necroticans agranulocytica — *see* Agranulocytosis
Mucous — *see also* condition
  patches (syphilitic) A51.39
    congenital A50.07
Mucoviscidosis E84.9
  with meconium obstruction E84.11
Mucus
  asphyxia or suffocation — *see* Asphyxia, mucus
  in stool R19.5
  plug — *see* Asphyxia, mucus
Muguet B37.0
Mulberry molars (congenital syphilis) A50.52
Müllerian mixed tumor
  specified site — *see* Neoplasm, malignant, by site
  unspecified site C54.9
Multicystic kidney (development) Q61.4
Multiparity (grand) Z64.1
  affecting management of pregnancy, labor and delivery
    (supervision only) O09.4- ☑
  requiring contraceptive management — *see* Contraception
Multipartita placenta O43.19- ☑

Multiple, multiplex — *see also* condition
  digits (congenital) Q69.9
  endocrine neoplasia — *see* Neoplasia, endocrine, multiple (MEN)
  personality F44.81
Mumps B26.9
  arthritis B26.85
  complication NEC B26.89
  encephalitis B26.2
  hepatitis B26.81
  meningitis (aseptic) B26.1
  meningoencephalitis B26.2
  myocarditis B26.82
  oophoritis B26.89
  orchitis B26.0
  pancreatitis B26.3
  polyneuropathy B26.84
Mumu — *see also* Infestation, filarial B74.9 *[N51]*
Münchhausen's syndrome — *see* Disorder, factitious
Münchmeyer's syndrome — *see* Myositis, ossificans, progressiva
Mural — *see* condition
Murmur (cardiac) (heart) (organic) R01.1
  abdominal R19.15
  aortic (valve) — *see* Endocarditis, aortic
  benign R01.0
  diastolic — *see* Endocarditis
  Flint I35.1
  functional R01.0
  Graham Steell I37.1
  innocent R01.0
  mitral (valve) — *see* Insufficiency, mitral
  nonorganic R01.0
  presystolic, mitral — *see* Insufficiency, mitral
  pulmonic (valve) I37.8
  systolic R01.1
  tricuspid (valve) I07.9
  valvular — *see* Endocarditis
Murri's disease (intermittent hemoglobinuria) D59.6
Muscle, muscular — *see also* condition
  carnitine (palmityltransferase) deficiency E71.314
Musculoneuralgia — *see* Neuralgia
Mushrooming hip — *see* Derangement, joint, specified NEC, hip
Mushroom-workers' (pickers') **disease or lung** J67.5
Mutation(s)
  factor V Leiden D68.51
  prothrombin gene D68.52
  surfactant, of lung J84.83
Mutism — *see also* Aphasia
  deaf (acquired) (congenital) NEC H91.3
  elective (adjustment reaction) (childhood) F94.0
  hysterical F44.4
  selective (childhood) F94.0
MVD (microvillus inclusion disease) Q43.8
MVID (microvillus inclusion disease) Q43.8
Myalgia M79.10
  auxiliary muscles, head and neck M79.12
  epidemic (cervical) B33.0
  mastication muscle M79.11
  site specified NEC M79.18
  traumatic NEC T14.8 ☑
Myasthenia G70.9
  congenital G70.2
  cordis — *see* Failure, heart
  developmental G70.2
  gravis G70.00
    with exacerbation (acute) G70.01
    in crisis G70.01
    neonatal, transient P94.0
    pseudoparalytica G70.00
      with exacerbation (acute) G70.01
      in crisis G70.01
  stomach, psychogenic F45.8
  syndrome
    in
      diabetes mellitus — *see* E08-E13 with .44
      neoplastic disease — *see also* Neoplasm D49.9 *[G73.3]*
      pernicious anemia D51.0 *[G73.3]*
      thyrotoxicosis E05.90 *[G73.3]*
        with thyroid storm E05.91 *[G73.3]*
Myasthenic M62.81
Mycelium infection B49
Mycetismus — *see* Poisoning, food, noxious, mushroom
Mycetoma B47.9
  actinomycotic B47.1
  bone (mycotic) B47.9 *[M90.80]*

Mycetoma — *continued*
  eumycotic B47.0
  foot B47.9
    actinomycotic B47.1
    mycotic B47.0
  madurae NEC B47.9
    mycotic B47.0
  maduromycotic B47.0
  mycotic B47.0
  nocardial B47.1
Mycobacteriosis — *see* Mycobacterium
Mycobacterium, mycobacterial (infection) A31.9
  anonymous A31.9
  atypical A31.9
    cutaneous A31.1
    pulmonary A31.0
      tuberculous — *see* Tuberculosis, pulmonary
    specified site NEC A31.8
  avium (intracellulare complex) A31.0
  balnei A31.1
  Battey A31.0
  chelonei A31.8
  cutaneous A31.1
  extrapulmonary systemic A31.8
  fortuitum A31.8
  intracellulare (Battey bacillus) A31.0
  kakaferifu A31.8
  kansasii (yellow bacillus) A31.0
  kasongo A31.8
  leprae — *see also* Leprosy A30.9
  luciflavum A31.1
  marinum (M. balnei) A31.1
  nonspecific — *see* Mycobacterium, atypical
  pulmonary (atypical) A31.0
    tuberculous — *see* Tuberculosis, pulmonary
  scrofulaceum A31.8
  simiae A31.8
  systemic, extrapulmonary A31.8
  szulgai A31.8
  terrae A31.8
  triviale A31.8
  tuberculosis (human, bovine) — *see* Tuberculosis
  ulcerans A31.1
  xenopi A31.8
Mycoplasma (M.) **pneumoniae, as cause of disease classified elsewhere** B96.0
Mycosis, mycotic B49
  cutaneous NEC B36.9
  ear B36.9
    in
      aspergillosis B44.89
      candidiasis B37.84
      moniliasis B37.84
  fungoides (extranodal) (solid organ) C84.0- ☑
  mouth B37.0
  nails B35.1
  opportunistic B48.8
  skin NEC B36.9
  specified NEC B48.8
  stomatitis B37.0
  vagina, vaginitis (candidal) B37.3
Mydriasis (pupil) H57.04
Myelatelia Q06.1
Myelinolysis, pontine, central G37.2
Myelitis (acute) (ascending) (childhood) (chronic) (descending) (diffuse) (disseminated) (idiopathic) (pressure) (progressive) (spinal cord) (subacute) — *see also* Encephalitis G04.91
  herpes simplex B00.82
  herpes zoster B02.24
  in diseases classified elsewhere G05.4
  necrotizing, subacute G37.4
  optic neuritis in G36.0
  postchickenpox B01.12
  postherpetic B02.24
  postimmunization G04.02
  postinfectious NEC G04.89
  postvaccinal G04.02
  specified NEC G04.89
  syphilitic (transverse) A52.14
  toxic G92
  transverse (in demyelinating diseases of central nervous system) G37.3
  tuberculous A17.82
  varicella B01.12
Myeloblastic — *see* condition
Myeloblastoma
  granular cell — *see also* Neoplasm, connective tissue

Myeloblastoma — *continued*
  granular cell — *see also* Neoplasm, connective tissue
      — *continued*
    malignant — *see* Neoplasm, connective tissue, malignant
    tongue D10.1
Myelocele — *see* Spina bifida
Myelocystocele — *see* Spina bifida
Myelocytic — *see* condition
Myelodysplasia D46.9
  specified NEC D46.Z (*following* D46.4)
  spinal cord (congenital) Q06.1
Myelodysplastic syndrome D46.9
  with
    5q deletion D46.C (*following* D46.2)
    isolated del (5q) chromosomal abnormality D46.C
        (*following* D46.2)
  specified NEC D46.Z (*following* D46.4)
Myeloencephalitis — *see* Encephalitis
Myelofibrosis D75.81
  with myeloid metaplasia D47.4
  acute C94.4- ☑
  idiopathic (chronic) D47.4
  primary D47.1
  secondary D75.81
    in myeloproliferative disease D47.4
Myelogenous — *see* condition
Myeloid — *see* condition
Myelokathexis D70.9
Myeloleukodystrophy E75.29
Myelolipoma — *see* Lipoma
Myeloma (multiple) C90.0- ☑
  monostotic C90.3 ☑
    plasma cell C90.0- ☑
  plasma cell C90.0- ☑
  solitary — *see also* Plasmacytoma, solitary C90.3- ☑
Myelomalacia G95.89
Myelomatosis C90.0- ☑
Myelomeningitis — *see* Meningoencephalitis
Myelomeningocele (spinal cord) — *see* Spina bifida
Myelo-osteo-musculodysplasia hereditaria Q79.8
Myelopathic
  anemia D64.89
  muscle atrophy — *see* Atrophy, muscle, spinal
  pain syndrome G89.0
Myelopathy (spinal cord) G95.9
  drug-induced G95.89
  in (due to)
    degeneration or displacement, intervertebral disc
        NEC — *see* Disorder, disc, with, myelopathy
    infection — *see* Encephalitis
    intervertebral disc disorder — *see also* Disorder,
        disc, with, myelopathy
    mercury — *see* subcategory T56.1 ☑
    neoplastic disease — *see also* Neoplasm
        D49.9 *[G99.2]*
    pernicious anemia D51.0 *[G99.2]*
    spondylosis — *see* Spondylosis, with myelopathy
        NEC
  necrotic (subacute) (vascular) G95.19
  radiation-induced G95.89
  spondylogenic NEC — *see* Spondylosis, with
        myelopathy NEC
  toxic G95.89
  transverse, acute G37.3
  vascular G95.19
  vitamin B12 E53.8 *[G32.0]*
Myelophthisis D61.82
Myeloradiculitis G04.91
Myeloradiculodysplasia (spinal) Q06.1
Myelosarcoma C92.3- ☑
Myelosclerosis D75.89
  with myeloid metaplasia D47.4
  disseminated, of nervous system G35
  megakaryocytic D47.4
    with myeloid metaplasia D47.4
Myelosis
  acute C92.0- ☑
  aleukemic C92.9- ☑
  chronic D47.1
  erythremic (acute) C94.0- ☑
  megakaryocytic C94.2- ☑
  nonleukemic D72.828
  subacute C92.9- ☑
Myiasis (cavernous) B87.9
  aural B87.4
  creeping B87.0

Myiasis — *continued*
  cutaneous B87.0
  dermal B87.0
  ear (external) (middle) B87.4
  eye B87.2
  genitourinary B87.81
  intestinal B87.82
  laryngeal B87.3
  nasopharyngeal B87.3
  ocular B87.2
  orbit B87.2
  skin B87.0
  specified site NEC B87.89
  traumatic B87.1
  wound B87.1
Myoadenoma, prostate — *see* Hyperplasia, prostate
Myoblastoma
  granular cell — *see also* Neoplasm, connective tissue,
      benign
    malignant — *see* Neoplasm, connective tissue, malignant
  tongue D10.1
Myocardial — *see* condition
Myocardiopathy (congestive) (constrictive) (familial)
      (hypertrophic nonobstructive) (idiopathic) (infiltrative) (obstructive) (primary) (restrictive) (sporadic)
      — *see also* Cardiomyopathy I42.9
  alcoholic I42.6
  cobalt-beer I42.6
  glycogen storage E74.02 *[I43]*
  hypertrophic obstructive I42.1
  in (due to)
    beriberi E51.12
    cardiac glycogenosis E74.02 *[I43]*
    Friedreich's ataxia G11.1 *[I43]*
    myotonia atrophica G71.11 *[I43]*
    progressive muscular dystrophy G71.09 *[I43]*
  obscure (African) I42.8
  secondary I42.9
  thyrotoxic E05.90 *[I43]*
    with storm E05.91 *[I43]*
  toxic NEC I42.7
Myocarditis (with arteriosclerosis)(chronic)(fibroid) (interstitial) (old) (progressive) (senile) I51.4
  with
    rheumatic fever (conditions in I00) I09.0
      active — *see* Myocarditis, acute, rheumatic
      inactive or quiescent (with chorea) I09.0
  active I40.9
    rheumatic I01.2
      with chorea (acute) (rheumatic) (Sydenham's)
          I02.0
  acute or subacute (interstitial) I40.9
    due to
      streptococcus (beta-hemolytic) I01.2
    idiopathic I40.1
    rheumatic I01.2
      with chorea (acute) (rheumatic) (Sydenham's)
          I02.0
    specified NEC I40.8
  aseptic of newborn B33.22
  bacterial (acute) I40.0
  Coxsackie (virus) B33.22
  diphtheritic A36.81
  eosinophilic I40.1
  epidemic of newborn (Coxsackie) B33.22
  Fiedler's (acute) (isolated) I40.1
  giant cell (acute) (subacute) I40.1
  gonococcal A54.83
  granulomatous (idiopathic) (isolated) (nonspecific) I40.1
  hypertensive — *see* Hypertension, heart
  idiopathic (granulomatous) I40.1
  in (due to)
    diphtheria A36.81
    epidemic louse-borne typhus A75.0 *[I41]*
    Lyme disease A69.29
    sarcoidosis D86.85
    scarlet fever A38.1
    toxoplasmosis (acquired) B58.81
    typhoid A01.02
    typhus NEC A75.9 *[I41]*
  infective I40.0
  influenzal — *see* Influenza, with, myocarditis
  isolated (acute) I40.1
  meningococcal A39.52
  mumps B26.82
  nonrheumatic, active I40.9
  parenchymatous I40.9

Myocarditis — *continued*
  pneumococcal I40.0
  rheumatic (chronic) (inactive) (with chorea) I09.0
    active or acute I01.2
      with chorea (acute) (rheumatic) (Sydenham's)
          I02.0
  rheumatoid — *see* Rheumatoid, carditis
  septic I40.0
  staphylococcal I40.0
  suppurative I40.0
  syphilitic (chronic) A52.06
  toxic I40.8
    rheumatic — *see* Myocarditis, acute, rheumatic
  tuberculous A18.84
  typhoid A01.02
  valvular — *see* Endocarditis
  virus, viral I40.0
    of newborn (Coxsackie) B33.22
Myocardium, myocardial — *see* condition
Myocardosis — *see* Cardiomyopathy
Myoclonus, myoclonic, myoclonia (familial) (essential)
      (multifocal) (simplex) G25.3
  drug-induced G25.3
  epilepsy — *see also* Epilepsy, generalized, specified
      NEC G40.4- ☑
    familial (progressive) G25.3
  epileptica G40.409
    with status epilepticus G40.401
  facial G51.3- ☑
  familial progressive G25.3
  Friedreich's G25.3
  jerks G25.3
  massive G25.3
  palatal G25.3
  pharyngeal G25.3
Myocytolysis I51.5
Myodiastasis — *see* Diastasis, muscle
Myoendocarditis — *see* Endocarditis
Myoepithelioma — *see* Neoplasm, benign, by site
Myofasciitis (acute) — *see* Myositis
Myofibroma — *see also* Neoplasm, connective tissue,
      benign
  uterus (cervix) (corpus) — *see* Leiomyoma
Myofibromatosis D48.1
  infantile Q89.8
Myofibrosis M62.89
  heart — *see* Myocarditis
  scapulohumeral — *see* Lesion, shoulder, specified NEC
Myofibrositis M79.7
  scapulohumeral — *see* Lesion, shoulder, specified NEC
Myoglobulinuria, myoglobinuria (primary) R82.1
Myokymia, facial G51.4
Myolipoma — *see* Lipoma
Myoma — *see also* Neoplasm, connective tissue, benign
  malignant — *see* Neoplasm, connective tissue, malignant
  prostate D29.1
  uterus (cervix) (corpus) — *see* Leiomyoma
Myomalacia M62.89
Myometritis — *see* Endometritis
Myometrium — *see* condition
Myonecrosis, clostridial A48.0
Myopathy G72.9
  acute
    necrotizing G72.81
    quadriplegic G72.81
  alcoholic G72.1
  benign congenital G71.2
  central core G71.2
  centronuclear G71.2
  congenital (benign) G71.2
  critical illness G72.81
  distal G71.09
  drug-induced G72.0
  endocrine NEC E34.9 *[G73.7]*
  extraocular muscles H05.82- ☑
  facioscapulohumeral G71.02
  hereditary G71.9
    specified NEC G71.8
  immune NEC G72.49
  in (due to)
    Addison's disease E27.1 *[G73.7]*
    alcohol G72.1
    amyloidosis E85.0 *[G73.7]*
    cretinism E00.9 *[G73.7]*
    Cushing's syndrome E24.9 *[G73.7]*
    drugs G72.0

Myopathy — continued
  in — continued
    endocrine disease NEC E34.9 [G73.7]
    giant cell arteritis M31.6 [G73.7]
    glycogen storage disease E74.00 [G73.7]
    hyperadrenocorticism E24.9 [G73.7]
    hyperparathyroidism NEC E21.3 [G73.7]
    hypoparathyroidism E20.9 [G73.7]
    hypopituitarism E23.0 [G73.7]
    hypothyroidism E03.9 [G73.7]
    infectious disease NEC B99 ☑ [G73.7]
    lipid storage disease E75.6 [G73.7]
    metabolic disease NEC E88.9 [G73.7]
    myxedema E03.9 [G73.7]
    parasitic disease NEC B89 [G73.7]
    polyarteritis nodosa M30.0 [G73.7]
    rheumatoid arthritis — see Rheumatoid, myopathy
    sarcoidosis D86.87
    scleroderma M34.82
    sicca syndrome M35.03
    Sjögren's syndrome M35.03
    systemic lupus erythematosus M32.19
    thyrotoxicosis (hyperthyroidism) E05.90 [G73.7]
      with thyroid storm E05.91 [G73.7]
    toxic agent NEC G72.2
  inflammatory NEC G72.49
  intensive care (ICU) G72.81
  limb-girdle G71.09
  mitochondrial NEC G71.3
  myotubular G71.2
  mytonic, proximal (PROMM) G71.11
  nemaline G71.2
  ocular G71.09
  oculopharyngeal G71.09
  of critical illness G72.81
  primary G71.9
    specified NEC G71.8
  progressive NEC G72.89
  proximal myotonic (PROMM) G71.11
  rod G71.2
  scapulohumeral G71.02
  specified NEC G72.89
  toxic G72.2
Myopericarditis — see also Pericarditis
  chronic rheumatic I09.2
Myopia (axial) (congenital) H52.1- ☑
  degenerative (malignant) H44.20
    with
      choroidal neovascularization H44.2A- ☑
      foveoschisis H44.2D- ☑
      macular hole H44.2B- ☑
      retinal detachment H44.2C- ☑
      specified maculopathy NEC H44.2E- ☑
    bilateral H44.23
    left eye H44.22
    right eye H44.21
  malignant — see also Myopia, degenerative H44.2- ☑
  pernicious — see also Myopia, degenerative H44.2- ☑
  progressive high (degenerative) — see also Myopia, degenerative H44.2- ☑
Myosarcoma — see Neoplasm, connective tissue, malignant
Myosis (pupil) H57.03
  stromal (endolymphatic) D39.0
Myositis M60.9
  clostridial A48.0
  due to posture — see Myositis, specified type NEC
  epidemic B33.0
  fibrosa or fibrous (chronic), Volkmann's T79.6 ☑
  foreign body granuloma — see Granuloma, foreign body
  in (due to)
    bilharziasis B65.9 [M63.8-] ☑
    cysticercosis B69.81
    leprosy A30.9 [M63.8-] ☑
    mycosis B49 [M63.8-] ☑
    sarcoidosis D86.87
    schistosomiasis B65.9 [M63.8-] ☑
    syphilis
      late A52.78
      secondary A51.49
    toxoplasmosis (acquired) B58.82

Myositis — continued
  in — continued
    trichinellosis B75 [M63.8-] ☑
    tuberculosis A18.09
  inclusion body [IBM] G72.41
  infective M60.009
    arm M60.002
      left M60.001
      right M60.000
    leg M60.005
      left M60.004
      right M60.003
    lower limb M60.005
      ankle M60.07- ☑
      foot M60.07- ☑
      lower leg M60.06- ☑
      thigh M60.05- ☑
      toe M60.07- ☑
    multiple sites M60.09
    specified site NEC M60.08
    upper limb M60.002
      finger M60.04- ☑
      forearm M60.03- ☑
      hand M60.04- ☑
      shoulder region M60.01- ☑
      upper arm M60.02- ☑
  interstitial M60.10
    ankle M60.17- ☑
    foot M60.17- ☑
    forearm M60.13- ☑
    hand M60.14- ☑
    lower leg M60.16- ☑
    multiple sites M60.19
    shoulder region M60.11- ☑
    specified site NEC M60.18
    thigh M60.15- ☑
    upper arm M60.12- ☑
  mycotic B49 [M63.8-] ☑
  orbital, chronic H05.12- ☑
  ossificans or ossifying (circumscripta) — see also Ossification, muscle, specified NEC
    in (due to)
      burns M61.30
        ankle M61.37- ☑
        foot M61.37- ☑
        forearm M61.33- ☑
        hand M61.34- ☑
        lower leg M61.36- ☑
        multiple sites M61.39
        pelvic region M61.35- ☑
        shoulder region M61.31- ☑
        specified site NEC M61.38
        thigh M61.35- ☑
        upper arm M61.32- ☑
      quadriplegia or paraplegia M61.20
        ankle M61.27- ☑
        foot M61.27- ☑
        forearm M61.23- ☑
        hand M61.24- ☑
        lower leg M61.26- ☑
        multiple sites M61.29
        pelvic region M61.25- ☑
        shoulder region M61.21- ☑
        specified site NEC M61.28
        thigh M61.25- ☑
        upper arm M61.22- ☑
    progressiva M61.10
      ankle M61.17- ☑
      finger M61.14- ☑
      foot M61.17- ☑
      forearm M61.13- ☑
      hand M61.14- ☑
      lower leg M61.16- ☑
      multiple sites M61.19
      pelvic region M61.15- ☑
      shoulder region M61.11- ☑
      specified site NEC M61.18
      thigh M61.15- ☑
      toe M61.17- ☑
      upper arm M61.12- ☑
    traumatica M61.00

Myositis — continued
  ossificans or ossifying — see also Ossification, muscle, specified — continued
    traumatica — continued
      ankle M61.07- ☑
      foot M61.07- ☑
      forearm M61.03- ☑
      hand M61.04- ☑
      lower leg M61.06- ☑
      multiple sites M61.09
      pelvic region M61.05- ☑
      shoulder region M61.01- ☑
      specified site NEC M61.08
      thigh M61.05- ☑
      upper arm M61.02- ☑
  purulent — see Myositis, infective
  specified type NEC M60.80
    ankle M60.87- ☑
    foot M60.87- ☑
    forearm M60.83- ☑
    hand M60.84- ☑
    lower leg M60.86- ☑
    multiple sites M60.89
    pelvic region M60.85- ☑
    shoulder region M60.81- ☑
    specified site NEC M60.88
    thigh M60.85- ☑
    upper arm M60.82- ☑
  suppurative — see Myositis, infective
  traumatic (old) — see Myositis, specified type NEC
Myospasia impulsiva F95.2
Myotonia (acquisita) (intermittens) M62.89
  atrophica G71.11
  chondrodystrophic G71.13
  congenita (acetazolamide responsive) (dominant) (recessive) G71.12
  drug-induced G71.14
  dystrophica G71.11
  fluctuans G71.19
  levior G71.12
  permanens G71.19
  symptomatic G71.19
Myotonic pupil — see Anomaly, pupil, function, tonic pupil
Myriapodiasis B88.2
Myringitis H73.2- ☑
  with otitis media — see Otitis, media
  acute H73.00- ☑
    bullous H73.01- ☑
    specified NEC H73.09- ☑
  bullous — see Myringitis, acute, bullous
  chronic H73.1- ☑
Mysophobia F40.228
Mytilotoxism — see Poisoning, fish
Myxadenitis labialis K13.0
Myxedema (adult) (idiocy) (infantile) (juvenile) — see also Hypothyroidism E03.9
  circumscribed E05.90
    with storm E05.91
  coma E03.5
  congenital E00.1
  cutis L98.5
  localized (pretibial) E05.90
    with storm E05.91
  papular L98.5
Myxochondrosarcoma — see Neoplasm, cartilage, malignant
Myxofibroma — see Neoplasm, connective tissue, benign
  odontogenic — see Cyst, calcifying odontogenic
Myxofibrosarcoma — see Neoplasm, connective tissue, malignant
Myxolipoma D17.9
Myxoliposarcoma — see Neoplasm, connective tissue, malignant
Myxoma — see also Neoplasm, connective tissue, benign
  nerve sheath — see Neoplasm, nerve, benign
  odontogenic — see Cyst, calcifying odontogenic
Myxosarcoma — see Neoplasm, connective tissue, malignant

☑ Additional Character Required — Refer to the Tabular List for Character Selection   ▽ Subterms under main terms may continue to next column or page

Myopathy — Myxosarcoma

N

Naegeli's
  disease Q82.8
  leukemia, monocytic C93.1- ☑
Naegleriasis (with meningoencephalitis) B60.2
Naffziger's syndrome G54.0
Naga sore — see Ulcer, skin
Nägele's pelvis M95.5
  with disproportion (fetopelvic) O33.0
    causing obstructed labor O65.0
Nail — see also condition
  biting F98.8
  patella syndrome Q87.2
Nanism, nanosomia — see Dwarfism
Nanophyetiasis B66.8
Nanukayami A27.89
Napkin rash L22
Narcolepsy G47.419
  with cataplexy G47.411
  in conditions classified elsewhere G47.429
    with cataplexy G47.421
Narcosis R06.89
Narcotism — see Dependence
NARP (Neuropathy, Ataxia and Retinitis pigmentosa)
  syndrome E88.49
Narrow
  anterior chamber angle H40.03- ☑
  gingival width (of periodontal soft tissue) K05.5
  pelvis — see Contraction, pelvis
Narrowing — see also Stenosis
  artery I77.1
    auditory, internal I65.8
    basilar — see Occlusion, artery, basilar
    carotid — see Occlusion, artery, carotid
    cerebellar — see Occlusion, artery, cerebellar
    cerebral — see Occlusion artery, cerebral
    choroidal — see Occlusion, artery, precerebral,
      specified NEC
    communicating posterior — see Occlusion, artery,
      precerebral, specified NEC
    coronary — see also Disease, heart, ischemic,
      atherosclerotic
      congenital Q24.5
        syphilitic A50.54 [I52]
      due to syphilis NEC A52.06
    hypophyseal — see Occlusion, artery, precerebral,
      specified NEC
    pontine — see Occlusion, artery, precerebral, spec-
      ified NEC
    precerebral — see Occlusion, artery, precerebral
    vertebral — see Occlusion, artery, vertebral
    auditory canal (external) — see Stenosis, external ear
      canal
  eustachian tube — see Obstruction, eustachian tube
  eyelid — see Disorder, eyelid function
  larynx J38.6
  mesenteric artery — see also Ischemia, intestine, acute
    K55.059
  palate M26.89
  palpebral fissure — see Disorder, eyelid function
  ureter N13.5
    with infection N13.6
  urethra — see Stricture, urethra
Narrowness, abnormal, eyelid Q10.3
Nasal — see condition
Nasolachrymal, nasolacrimal — see condition
Nasopharyngeal — see also condition
  pituitary gland Q89.2
  torticollis M43.6
Nasopharyngitis (acute) (infective) (streptococcal)
  (subacute) J00
  chronic (suppurative) (ulcerative) J31.1
Nasopharynx, nasopharyngeal — see condition
Natal tooth, teeth K00.6
Nausea (without vomiting) R11.0
  with vomiting R11.2
  gravidarum — see Hyperemesis, gravidarum
  marina T75.3 ☑
  navalis T75.3 ☑
Navel — see condition
Neapolitan fever — see Brucellosis
Near drowning T75.1 ☑
Nearsightedness — see Myopia
Near-syncope R55
Nebula, cornea — see Opacity, cornea

Necator americanus infestation B76.1
Necatoriasis B76.1
Neck — see condition
Necrobiosis R68.89
  lipoidica NEC L92.1
    with diabetes — see E08-E13 with .620
Necrolysis, toxic epidermal L51.2
  due to drug
    correct substance properly administered — see Ta-
      ble of Drugs and Chemicals, by drug, adverse
      effect
    overdose or wrong substance given or taken — see
      Table of Drugs and Chemicals, by drug, poi-
      soning
Necrophilia F65.89
Necrosis, necrotic (ischemic) — see also Gangrene
  adrenal (capsule) (gland) E27.49
  amputation stump (surgical) (late) T87.50
    arm T87.5- ☑
    leg T87.5- ☑
  antrum J32.0
  aorta (hyaline) — see also Aneurysm, aorta
    cystic medial — see Dissection, aorta
  artery I77.5
  bladder (aseptic) (sphincter) N32.89
  bone — see also Osteonecrosis M87.9
    aseptic or avascular — see Osteonecrosis
      idiopathic M87.00
    ethmoid J32.2
    jaw M27.2
    tuberculous — see Tuberculosis, bone
  brain I67.89
  breast (aseptic) (fat) (segmental) N64.1
  bronchus J98.09
  central nervous system NEC I67.89
  cerebellar I67.89
  cerebral I67.89
  colon — see also Infarct, intestine K55.049
  cornea H18.89- ☑
  cortical (acute) (renal) N17.1
  cystic medial (aorta) — see Dissection, aorta
  dental pulp K04.1
  esophagus K22.8
  ethmoid (bone) J32.2
  eyelid — see Disorder, eyelid, degenerative
  fat, fatty (generalized) — see also Disorder, soft tissue,
    specified type NEC)
    abdominal wall K65.4
    breast (aseptic) (segmental) N64.1
    localized — see Degeneration, by site, fatty
    mesentery K65.4
    omentum K65.4
    pancreas K86.89
    peritoneum K65.4
    skin (subcutaneous), newborn P83.0
    subcutaneous, due to birth injury P15.6
  gallbladder — see Cholecystitis, acute
  heart — see Infarct, myocardium
  hip, aseptic or avascular — see Osteonecrosis, by type,
    femur
  intestine (acute) (hemorrhagic) (massive) — see also
    Infarct, intestine K55.069
  jaw M27.2
  kidney (bilateral) N28.0
    acute N17.9
    cortical (acute) (bilateral) N17.1
      with ectopic or molar pregnancy O08.4
    medullary (bilateral) (in acute renal failure) (papil-
      lary) N17.2
    papillary (bilateral) (in acute renal failure) N17.2
    tubular N17.0
      with ectopic or molar pregnancy O08.4
      complicating
        abortion — see Abortion, by type, complicat-
          ed by, tubular necrosis
        ectopic or molar pregnancy O08.4
        pregnancy — see Pregnancy, complicated by,
          diseases of, specified type or system
          NEC
      following ectopic or molar pregnancy O08.4
      traumatic T79.5 ☑
  larynx J38.7
  liver (with hepatic failure) (cell) — see Failure, hepatic
    hemorrhagic, central K76.2
  lung J85.0
  lymphatic gland — see Lymphadenitis, acute
  mammary gland (fat) (segmental) N64.1
  mastoid (chronic) — see Mastoiditis, chronic

Necrosis, necrotic — continued
  medullary (acute) (renal) N17.2
  mesentery — see also Infarct, intestine K55.069
    fat K65.4
  mitral valve — see Insufficiency, mitral
  myocardium, myocardial — see Infarct, myocardium
  nose J34.0
  omentum (with mesenteric infarction) — see also In-
    farct, intestine K55.069
    fat K65.4
  orbit, orbital — see Osteomyelitis, orbit
  ossicles, ear — see Abnormal, ear ossicles
  ovary N70.92
  pancreas (aseptic) (duct) (fat) K86.89
    acute (infective) — see Pancreatitis, acute
    infective — see Pancreatitis, acute
  papillary (acute) (renal) N17.2
  perineum N90.89
  peritoneum (with mesenteric infarction) — see also
    Infarct, intestine K55.069
    fat K65.4
  pharynx J02.9
    in granulocytopenia — see Neutropenia
    Vincent's A69.1
  phosphorus — see subcategory T54.2 ☑
  pituitary (gland) E23.0
    postpartum O99.285
    Sheehan O99.285
  pressure — see Ulcer, pressure, by site
  pulmonary J85.0
  pulp (dental) K04.1
  radiation — see Necrosis, by site
  radium — see Necrosis, by site
  renal — see Necrosis, kidney
  sclera H15.89
  scrotum N50.89
  skin or subcutaneous tissue NEC I96
  spine, spinal (column) — see also Osteonecrosis, by
    type, vertebra
    cord G95.19
  spleen D73.5
  stomach K31.89
  stomatitis (ulcerative) A69.0
  subcutaneous fat, newborn P83.88
  subendocardial (acute) I21.4
    chronic I25.89
  suprarenal (capsule) (gland) E27.49
  testis N50.89
  thymus (gland) E32.8
  tonsil J35.8
  trachea J39.8
  tuberculous NEC — see Tuberculosis
  tubular (acute) (anoxic) (renal) (toxic) N17.0
    postprocedural N99.0
  vagina N89.8
  vertebra — see also Osteonecrosis, by type, vertebra
    tuberculous A18.01
  vulva N90.89
  X-ray — see Necrosis, by site
Necrospermia — see Infertility, male
Need (for)
  care provider because (of)
    assistance with personal care Z74.1
    continuous supervision required Z74.3
    impaired mobility Z74.09
    no other household member able to render care
      Z74.2
    specified reason NEC Z74.8
  immunization — see Vaccination
  vaccination — see Vaccination
Neglect
  adult
    confirmed T74.01 ☑
    history of Z91.412
    suspected T76.01 ☑
  child (childhood)
    confirmed T74.02 ☑
    history of Z62.812
    suspected T76.02 ☑
  emotional, in childhood Z62.898
  hemispatial R41.4
  left-sided R41.4
  sensory R41.4
  visuospatial R41.4
Neisserian infection NEC — see Gonococcus
Nelaton's syndrome G60.8
Nelson's syndrome E24.1
Nematodiasis (intestinal) B82.0

Nematodiasis — *continued*
Ancylostoma B76.0
Neonatal — *see also* Newborn
acne L70.4
bradycardia P29.12
screening, abnormal findings on P09
tachycardia P29.11
tooth, teeth K00.6
Neonatorum — *see* condition
Neoplasia
endocrine, multiple (MEN) E31.20
type I E31.21
type IIA E31.22
type IIB E31.23
intraepithelial (histologically confirmed)
anal (AIN) (histologically confirmed) K62.82
grade I K62.82
grade II K62.82
severe D01.3
cervical glandular (histologically confirmed) D06.9
cervix (uteri) (CIN) (histologically confirmed) N87.9
glandular D06.9
grade I N87.0
grade II N87.1
grade III (severe dysplasia) — *see also* Carcinoma, cervix uteri, in situ D06.9
prostate (histologically confirmed) (PIN) N42.31
grade I N42.31
grade II N42.31
grade III (severe dysplasia) D07.5
vagina (histologically confirmed) (VAIN) N89.3
grade I N89.0
grade II N89.1
grade III (severe dysplasia) D07.2
vulva (histologically confirmed) (VIN) N90.3
grade I N90.0
grade II N90.1
grade III (severe dysplasia) D07.1
Neoplasm, neoplastic — *see also* Table of Neoplasms
lipomatous, benign — *see* Lipoma
malignant mast cell C96.20
specified type NEC C96.29
mast cell, of uncertain behavior NEC D47.09
Neovascularization
ciliary body — *see* Disorder, iris, vascular
cornea H16.40- ☑
deep H16.44- ☑
ghost vessels — *see* Ghost, vessels
localized H16.43- ☑
pannus — *see* Pannus
iris — *see* Disorder, iris, vascular
retina H35.05- ☑
Nephralgia N23
Nephritis, nephritic (albuminuric) (azotemic) (congenital) (disseminated) (epithelial) (familial) (focal) (granulomatous) (hemorrhagic) (infantile) (nonsuppurative, excretory) (uremic) N05.9
with
dense deposit disease N05.6
diffuse
crescentic glomerulonephritis N05.7
endocapillary proliferative glomerulonephritis N05.4
membranous glomerulonephritis N05.2
mesangial proliferative glomerulonephritis N05.3
mesangiocapillary glomerulonephritis N05.5
edema — *see* Nephrosis
focal and segmental glomerular lesions N05.1
foot process disease N04.9
glomerular lesion
diffuse sclerosing N05.8
hypocomplementemic — *see* Nephritis, membranoproliferative
IgA — *see* Nephropathy, IgA
lobular, lobulonodular — *see* Nephritis, membranoproliferative
nodular — *see* Nephritis, membranoproliferative
lesion of
glomerulonephritis, proliferative N05.8
renal necrosis N05.9
minor glomerular abnormality N05.0
specified morphological changes NEC N05.8
acute N00.9
with
dense deposit disease N00.6
diffuse
crescentic glomerulonephritis N00.7

Nephritis, nephritic — *continued*
acute — *continued*
with — *continued*
diffuse — *continued*
endocapillary proliferative glomerulonephritis N00.4
membranous glomerulonephritis N00.2
mesangial proliferative glomerulonephritis N00.3
mesangiocapillary glomerulonephritis N00.5
focal and segmental glomerular lesions N00.1
minor glomerular abnormality N00.0
specified morphological changes NEC N00.8
amyloid E85.4 *[N08]*
antiglomerular basement membrane (anti-GBM) antibody NEC
in Goodpasture's syndrome M31.0
antitubular basement membrane (tubulo-interstitial) NEC N12
toxic — *see* Nephropathy, toxic
arteriolar — *see* Hypertension, kidney
arteriosclerotic — *see* Hypertension, kidney
ascending — *see* Nephritis, tubulo-interstitial
atrophic N03.9
Balkan (endemic) N15.0
calculous, calculus — *see* Calculus, kidney
cardiac — *see* Hypertension, kidney
cardiovascular — *see* Hypertension, kidney
chronic N03.9
with
dense deposit disease N03.6
diffuse
crescentic glomerulonephritis N03.7
endocapillary proliferative glomerulonephritis N03.4
membranous glomerulonephritis N03.2
mesangial proliferative glomerulonephritis N03.3
mesangiocapillary glomerulonephritis N03.5
focal and segmental glomerular lesions N03.1
minor glomerular abnormality N03.0
specified morphological changes NEC N03.8
arteriosclerotic — *see* Hypertension, kidney
cirrhotic N26.9
complicating pregnancy O26.83- ☑
croupous N00.9
degenerative — *see* Nephrosis
diffuse sclerosing N05.8
due to
diabetes mellitus — *see* E08-E13 with .21
subacute bacterial endocarditis I33.0
systemic lupus erythematosus (chronic) M32.14
typhoid fever A01.09
gonococcal (acute) (chronic) A54.21
hypocomplementemic — *see* Nephritis, membranoproliferative
IgA — *see* Nephropathy, IgA
immune complex (circulating) NEC N05.8
infective — *see* Nephritis, tubulo-interstitial
interstitial — *see* Nephritis, tubulo-interstitial
lead N14.3
membranoproliferative (diffuse) (type 1 or 3) — *see also* N00-N07 with fourth character .5 N05.5
type 2 — *see also* N00-N07 with fourth character .6 N05.6
minimal change N05.0
necrotic, necrotizing NEC — *see also* N00-N07 with fourth character .8 N05.8
nephrotic — *see* Nephrosis
nodular — *see* Nephritis, membranoproliferative
polycystic Q61.3
adult type Q61.2
autosomal
dominant Q61.2
recessive NEC Q61.19
childhood type NEC Q61.19
infantile type NEC Q61.19
poststreptococcal N05.9
acute N00.9
chronic N03.9
rapidly progressive N01.9
proliferative NEC — *see also* N00-N07 with fourth character .8 N05.8
purulent — *see* Nephritis, tubulo-interstitial
rapidly progressive N01.9
with
dense deposit disease N01.6

Nephritis, nephritic — *continued*
rapidly progressive — *continued*
with — *continued*
diffuse
crescentic glomerulonephritis N01.7
endocapillary proliferative glomerulonephritis N01.4
membranous glomerulonephritis N01.2
mesangial proliferative glomerulonephritis N01.3
mesangiocapillary glomerulonephritis N01.5
focal and segmental glomerular lesions N01.1
minor glomerular abnormality N01.0
specified morphological changes NEC N01.8
salt losing or wasting NEC N28.89
saturnine N14.3
sclerosing, diffuse N05.8
septic — *see* Nephritis, tubulo-interstitial
specified pathology NEC — *see also* N00-N07 with fourth character .8 N05.8
subacute N01.9
suppurative — *see* Nephritis, tubulo-interstitial
syphilitic (late) A52.75
congenital A50.59 *[N08]*
early (secondary) A51.44
toxic — *see* Nephropathy, toxic
tubal, tubular — *see* Nephritis, tubulo-interstitial
tuberculous A18.11
tubulo-interstitial (in) N12
acute (infectious) N10
chronic (infectious) N11.9
nonobstructive N11.8
reflux-associated N11.0
obstructive N11.1
specified NEC N11.8
due to
brucellosis A23.9 *[N16]*
cryoglobulinemia D89.1 *[N16]*
glycogen storage disease E74.00 *[N16]*
Sjögren's syndrome M35.04
vascular — *see* Hypertension, kidney
war N00.9
Nephroblastoma (epithelial) (mesenchymal) C64- ☑
Nephrocalcinosis E83.59 *[N29]*
Nephrocystitis, pustular — *see* Nephritis, tubulo-interstitial
Nephrolithiasis (congenital) (pelvis) (recurrent) — *see also* Calculus, kidney
Nephroma C64- ☑
mesoblastic D41.0- ☑
Nephronephritis — *see* Nephrosis
Nephronophthisis Q61.5
Nephropathia epidemica A98.5
Nephropathy — *see also* Nephritis N28.9
with
edema — *see* Nephrosis
glomerular lesion — *see* Glomerulonephritis
amyloid, hereditary E85.0
analgesic N14.0
with medullary necrosis, acute N17.2
Balkan (endemic) N15.0
chemical — *see* Nephropathy, toxic
diabetic — *see* E08-E13 with .21
drug-induced N14.2
specified NEC N14.1
focal and segmental hyalinosis or sclerosis N02.1
heavy metal-induced N14.3
hereditary NEC N07.9
with
dense deposit disease N07.6
diffuse
crescentic glomerulonephritis N07.7
endocapillary proliferative glomerulonephritis N07.4
membranous glomerulonephritis N07.2
mesangial proliferative glomerulonephritis N07.3
mesangiocapillary glomerulonephritis N07.5
focal and segmental glomerular lesions N07.1
minor glomerular abnormality N07.0
specified morphological changes NEC N07.8
hypercalcemic N25.89
hypertensive — *see* Hypertension, kidney
hypokalemic (vacuolar) N25.89
IgA N02.8
with glomerular lesion N02.9
focal and segmental hyalinosis or sclerosis N02.1
membranoproliferative (diffuse) N02.5

Nephropathy — continued
  IgA — continued
    with glomerular lesion — continued
      membranous (diffuse) N02.2
      mesangial proliferative (diffuse) N02.3
      mesangiocapillary (diffuse) N02.5
      proliferative NEC N02.8
      specified pathology NEC N02.8
  lead N14.3
  membranoproliferative (diffuse) N02.5
  membranous (diffuse) N02.2
  mesangial (IgA/IgG) — see Nephropathy, IgA
    proliferative (diffuse) N02.3
  mesangiocapillary (diffuse) N02.5
  obstructive N13.8
  phenacetin N17.2
  phosphate-losing N25.0
  potassium depletion N25.89
  pregnancy-related O26.83- ☑
  proliferative NEC — see also N00-N07 with fourth
    character .8 N05.8
  protein-losing N25.89
  saturnine N14.3
  sickle-cell D57.- ☑ [N08]
  toxic NEC N14.4
    due to
      drugs N14.2
        analgesic N14.0
        specified NEC N14.1
      heavy metals N14.3
  vasomotor N17.0
  water-losing N25.89
Nephroptosis N28.83
Nephropyosis — see Abscess, kidney
Nephrorrhagia N28.89
Nephrosclerosis (arteriolar)(arteriosclerotic) (chronic)
  (hyaline) — see also Hypertension, kidney
  hyperplastic — see Hypertension, kidney
  senile N26.9
Nephrosis, nephrotic (Epstein's) (syndrome) (congenital)
  N04.9
  with
    foot process disease N04.9
    glomerular lesion N04.1
    hypocomplementemic N04.5
  acute N04.9
  anoxic — see Nephrosis, tubular
  chemical — see Nephrosis, tubular
  cholemic K76.7
  diabetic — see E08-E13 with .21
  Finnish type (congenital) Q89.8
  hemoglobin N10
  hemoglobinuric — see Nephrosis, tubular
  in
    amyloidosis E85.4 [N08]
    diabetes mellitus — see E08-E13 with .21
    epidemic hemorrhagic fever A98.5
    malaria (malariae) B52.0
  ischemic — see Nephrosis, tubular
  lipoid N04.9
  lower nephron — see Nephrosis, tubular
  malarial (malariae) B52.0
  minimal change N04.0
  myoglobin N10
  necrotizing — see Nephrosis, tubular
  osmotic (sucrose) N25.89
  radiation N04.9
  syphilitic (late) A52.75
  toxic — see Nephrosis, tubular
  tubular (acute) N17.0
    postprocedural N99.0
    radiation N04.9
Nephrosonephritis, hemorrhagic (endemic) A98.5
Nephrostomy
  attention to Z43.6
  status Z93.6
Nerve — see also condition
  injury — see Injury, nerve, by body site
Nerves R45.0
Nervous — see also condition R45.0
  heart F45.8
  stomach F45.8
  tension R45.0
Nervousness R45.0
Nesidioblastoma
  pancreas D13.7
  specified site NEC — see Neoplasm, benign, by site
  unspecified site D13.7

Nettleship's syndrome — see Urticaria pigmentosa
Neumann's disease or syndrome L10.1
Neuralgia, neuralgic (acute) M79.2
  accessory (nerve) G52.8
  acoustic (nerve) — see subcategory H93.3 ☑
  auditory (nerve) — see subcategory H93.3 ☑
  ciliary G44.009
    intractable G44.001
    not intractable G44.009
  cranial
    nerve — see also Disorder, nerve, cranial
      fifth or trigeminal — see Neuralgia, trigeminal
    postherpetic, postzoster B02.29
  ear — see subcategory H92.0 ☑
  facialis vera G51.1
  Fothergill's — see Neuralgia, trigeminal
  glossopharyngeal (nerve) G52.1
  Horton's G44.009
    intractable G44.091
    not intractable G44.099
  Hunt's B02.21
  hypoglossal (nerve) G52.3
  infraorbital — see Neuralgia, trigeminal
  malarial — see Malaria
  migrainous G44.009
    intractable G44.001
    not intractable G44.009
  Morton's G57.6- ☑
  nerve, cranial — see Disorder, nerve, cranial
  nose G52.0
  occipital M54.81
  olfactory G52.0
  penis N48.9
  perineum R10.2
  postherpetic NEC B02.29
    trigeminal B02.22
  pubic region R10.2
  scrotum R10.2
  Sluder's G44.89
  specified nerve NEC G58.8
  spermatic cord R10.2
  sphenopalatine (ganglion) G90.09
  trifacial — see Neuralgia, trigeminal
  trigeminal G50.0
    postherpetic, postzoster B02.22
  vagus (nerve) G52.2
  writer's F48.8
    organic G25.89
Neurapraxia — see Injury, nerve
Neurasthenia F48.8
  cardiac F45.8
  gastric F45.8
  heart F45.8
Neurilemmoma — see also Neoplasm, nerve, benign
  acoustic (nerve) D33.3
  malignant — see also Neoplasm, nerve, malignant
    acoustic (nerve) C72.4- ☑
Neurilemmosarcoma — see Neoplasm, nerve, malignant
Neurinoma — see Neoplasm, nerve, benign
Neurinomatosis — see Neoplasm, nerve, uncertain behavior
Neuritis (rheumatoid) M79.2
  abducens (nerve) — see Strabismus, paralytic, sixth
    nerve
  accessory (nerve) G52.8
  acoustic (nerve) — see also subcategory H93.3 ☑
    in (due to)
      infectious disease NEC B99 ☑ [H94.0-] ☑
      parasitic disease NEC B89 [H94.0-] ☑
      syphilitic A52.15
  alcoholic G62.1
    with psychosis — see Psychosis, alcoholic
  amyloid, any site E85.4 [G63]
  auditory (nerve) — see subcategory H93.3 ☑
  brachial — see Radiculopathy
    due to displacement, intervertebral disc — see Dis-
      order, disc, cervical, with neuritis
  cranial nerve
    due to Lyme disease A69.22
    eighth or acoustic or auditory — see subcategory
      H93.3 ☑
    eleventh or accessory G52.8
    fifth or trigeminal G51.0
    first or olfactory G52.0
    fourth or trochlear — see Strabismus, paralytic,
      fourth nerve
    second or optic — see Neuritis, optic

Neuritis — continued
  cranial nerve — continued
    seventh or facial G51.8
      newborn (birth injury) P11.3
    sixth or abducent — see Strabismus, paralytic, sixth
      nerve
    tenth or vagus G52.2
    third or oculomotor — see Strabismus, paralytic,
      third nerve
    twelfth or hypoglossal G52.3
  Déjérine-Sottas G60.0
  diabetic (mononeuropathy) — see E08-E13 with .41
    polyneuropathy — see E08-E13 with .42
  due to
    beriberi E51.11
    displacement, prolapse or rupture, intervertebral
      disc — see Disorder, disc, with, radiculopathy
    herniation, nucleus pulposus M51.9 [G55]
  endemic E51.11
  facial G51.8
    newborn (birth injury) P11.3
  general — see Polyneuropathy
  geniculate ganglion G51.1
    due to herpes (zoster) B02.21
  gouty — see also Gout, by type M10.9 [G63]
  hypoglossal (nerve) G52.3
  ilioinguinal (nerve) G57.9- ☑
  infectious (multiple) NEC G61.0
  interstitial hypertrophic progressive G60.0
  lumbar M54.16
  lumbosacral M54.17
  multiple — see also Polyneuropathy
    endemic E51.11
    infective, acute G61.0
  multiplex endemica E51.11
  nerve root — see Radiculopathy
  oculomotor (nerve) — see Strabismus, paralytic, third
    nerve
  olfactory nerve G52.0
  optic (nerve) (hereditary) (sympathetic) H46.9
    with demyelination G36.0
    in myelitis G36.0
    nutritional H46.2
    papillitis — see Papillitis, optic
    retrobulbar H46.1- ☑
    specified type NEC H46.8
    toxic H46.3
  peripheral (nerve) G62.9
    multiple — see Polyneuropathy
    single — see Mononeuritis
  pneumogastric (nerve) G52.2
  postherpetic, postzoster B02.29
  progressive hypertrophic interstitial G60.0
  retrobulbar — see also Neuritis, optic, retrobulbar
    in (due to)
      late syphilis A52.15
      meningococcal infection A39.82
    meningococcal A39.82
    syphilitic A52.15
  sciatic (nerve) — see also Sciatica
    due to displacement of intervertebral disc — see
      Disorder, disc, with, radiculopathy
  serum — see also Reaction, serum T80.69 ☑
  shoulder-girdle G54.5
  specified nerve NEC G58.8
  spinal (nerve) root — see Radiculopathy
  syphilitic A52.15
  thenar (median) G56.1- ☑
  thoracic M54.14
  toxic NEC G62.2
  trochlear (nerve) — see Strabismus, paralytic, fourth
    nerve
  vagus (nerve) G52.2
Neuroastrocytoma — see Neoplasm, uncertain behavior,
  by site
Neuroavitaminosis E56.9 [G99.8]
Neuroblastoma
  olfactory C30.0
  specified site — see Neoplasm, malignant, by site
  unspecified site C74.90
Neurochorioretinitis — see Chorioretinitis
Neurocirculatory asthenia F45.8
Neurocysticercosis B69.0
Neurocytoma — see Neoplasm, benign, by site
Neurodermatitis (circumscribed) (circumscripta) (local)
  L28.0
  atopic L20.81
  diffuse (Brocq) L20.81

Subterms under main terms may continue to next column or page   ☑ Additional Character Required — Refer to the Tabular List for Character Selection   231

Nephropathy — Neurodermatitis

Neurodermatitis — *continued*
  disseminated L20.81
Neuroencephalomyelopathy, optic G36.0
Neuroepithelioma — *see also* Neoplasm, malignant, by
    site
  olfactory C30.0
Neurofibroma — *see also* Neoplasm, nerve, benign
  melanotic — *see* Neoplasm, nerve, benign
  multiple — *see* Neurofibromatosis
  plexiform — *see* Neoplasm, nerve, benign
Neurofibromatosis (multiple) (nonmalignant) Q85.00
  acoustic Q85.02
  malignant — *see* Neoplasm, nerve, malignant
  specified NEC Q85.09
  type 1 (von Recklinghausen) Q85.01
  type 2 Q85.02
Neurofibrosarcoma — *see* Neoplasm, nerve, malignant
Neurogenic — *see also* condition
  bladder — *see also* Dysfunction, bladder, neuromuscu-
      lar N31.9
    cauda equina syndrome G83.4
  bowel NEC K59.2
  heart F45.8
Neuroglioma — *see* Neoplasm, uncertain behavior, by
    site
Neurolabyrinthitis (of Dix and Hallpike) — *see* Neuroni-
    tis, vestibular
Neurolathyrism — *see* Poisoning, food, noxious, plant
Neuroleprosy A30.9
Neuroma — *see also* Neoplasm, nerve, benign
  acoustic (nerve) D33.3
  amputation (stump) (traumatic) (surgical complication)
        (late) T87.3- ☑
      arm T87.3- ☑
      leg T87.3- ☑
  digital (toe) G57.6- ☑
  interdigital G58.8
    lower limb (toe) G57.8- ☑
    upper limb G56.8- ☑
  intermetatarsal G57.8- ☑
  Morton's G57.6- ☑
  nonneoplastic
    arm G56.9- ☑
    leg G57.9- ☑
    lower extremity G57.9- ☑
    upper extremity G56.9- ☑
  optic (nerve) D33.3
  plantar G57.6- ☑
  plexiform — *see* Neoplasm, nerve, benign
  surgical (nonneoplastic)
    arm G56.9- ☑
    leg G57.9- ☑
    lower extremity G57.9- ☑
    upper extremity G56.9- ☑
Neuromyalgia — *see* Neuralgia
Neuromyasthenia (epidemic) (postinfectious) G93.3
Neuromyelitis G36.9
  ascending G61.0
  optica G36.0
Neuromyopathy G70.9
  paraneoplastic D49.9 *[G13.0]*
Neuromyotonia (Isaacs) G71.19
Neuronevus — *see* Nevus
Neuronitis G58.9
  ascending (acute) G57.2- ☑
  vestibular H81.2- ☑
Neuroparalytic — *see* condition
Neuropathy, neuropathic G62.9
  acute motor G62.81
  alcoholic G62.1
    with psychosis — *see* Psychosis, alcoholic
  arm G56.9- ☑
  autonomic, peripheral — *see* Neuropathy, peripheral,
      autonomic
  axillary G56.9- ☑
  bladder N31.9
    atonic (motor) (sensory) N31.2
    autonomous N31.2
    flaccid N31.2
    nonreflex N31.2
    reflex N31.1
    uninhibited N31.0
  brachial plexus G54.0
  cervical plexus G54.2
  chronic
    progressive segmentally demyelinating G62.89
    relapsing demyelinating G62.89

Neuropathy, neuropathic — *continued*
  Déjérine-Sottas G60.0
  diabetic — *see* E08-E13 with .40
    mononeuropathy — *see* E08-E13 with .41
    polyneuropathy — *see* E08-E13 with .42
  entrapment G58.9
    iliohypogastric nerve G57.8- ☑
    ilioinguinal nerve G57.8- ☑
    lateral cutaneous nerve of thigh G57.1- ☑
    median nerve G56.0- ☑
    obturator nerve G57.8- ☑
    peroneal nerve G57.3- ☑
    posterior tibial nerve G57.5- ☑
    saphenous nerve G57.8- ☑
    ulnar nerve G56.2- ☑
  facial nerve G51.9
  hereditary G60.9
    motor and sensory (types I-IV) G60.0
    sensory G60.8
    specified NEC G60.8
  hypertrophic G60.0
    Charcot-Marie-Tooth G60.0
    Déjérine-Sottas G60.0
    interstitial progressive G60.0
    of infancy G60.0
    Refsum G60.1
  idiopathic G60.9
    progressive G60.3
    specified NEC G60.8
  in association with hereditary ataxia G60.2
  intercostal G58.0
  ischemic — *see* Disorder, nerve
  Jamaica (ginger) G62.2
  leg NEC G57.9- ☑
  lower extremity G57.9- ☑
  lumbar plexus G54.1
  median nerve G56.1- ☑
  motor and sensory — *see also* Polyneuropathy
    hereditary (types I-IV) G60.0
  multifocal motor (MMN) G61.82
  multiple (acute) (chronic) — *see* Polyneuropathy
  optic (nerve) — *see also* Neuritis, optic
    ischemic H47.01- ☑
  paraneoplastic (sensorial) (Denny Brown) D49.9 *[G13.0]*
  peripheral (nerve) — *see also* Polyneuropathy G62.9
    autonomic G90.9
      idiopathic G90.09
      in (due to)
        amyloidosis E85.4 *[G99.0]*
        diabetes mellitus — *see* E08-E13 with .43
        endocrine disease NEC E34.9 *[G99.0]*
        gout M10.00 *[G99.0]*
        hyperthyroidism E05.90 *[G99.0]*
          with thyroid storm E05.91 *[G99.0]*
        metabolic disease NEC E88.9 *[G99.0]*
    idiopathic G60.9
      progressive G60.3
    in (due to)
      antitetanus serum G62.0
      arsenic G62.2
      drugs NEC G62.0
      lead G62.2
      organophosphate compounds G62.2
      toxic agent NEC G62.2
  plantar nerves G57.6- ☑
  progressive
    hypertrophic interstitial G60.0
    inflammatory G62.81
  radicular NEC — *see* Radiculopathy
  sacral plexus G54.1
  sciatic G57.0- ☑
  serum G61.1
  toxic NEC G62.2
  trigeminal sensory G50.8
  ulnar nerve G56.2- ☑
  uremic N18.9 *[G63]*
  vitamin B12 E53.8 *[G63]*
    with anemia (pernicious) D51.0 *[G63]*
      due to dietary deficiency D51.3 *[G63]*
Neurophthisis — *see also* Disorder, nerve
  peripheral, diabetic — *see* E08-E13 with .42
Neuroretinitis — *see* Chorioretinitis
Neuroretinopathy, hereditary optic H47.22
Neurosarcoma — *see* Neoplasm, nerve, malignant
Neurosclerosis — *see* Disorder, nerve
Neurosis, neurotic F48.9
  anankastic F42.8

Neurosis, neurotic — *continued*
  anxiety (state) F41.1
    panic type F41.0
  asthenic F48.8
  bladder F45.8
  cardiac (reflex) F45.8
  cardiovascular F45.8
  character F60.9
  colon F45.8
  compensation F68.10
  compulsive, compulsion F42.8
  conversion F44.9
  craft F48.8
  cutaneous F45.8
  depersonalization F48.1
  depressive (reaction) (type) F34.1
  environmental F48.8
  excoriation L98.1
  fatigue F48.8
  functional — *see* Disorder, somatoform
  gastric F45.8
  gastrointestinal F45.8
  heart F45.8
  hypochondriacal F45.21
  hysterical F44.9
  incoordination F45.8
    larynx F45.8
    vocal cord F45.8
  intestine F45.8
  larynx (sensory) F45.8
    hysterical F44.4
  mixed NEC F48.8
  musculoskeletal F45.8
  obsessional F42.8
  obsessive-compulsive F42.8
  occupational F48.8
  ocular NEC F45.8
  organ — *see* Disorder, somatoform
  pharynx F45.8
  phobic F40.9
  posttraumatic (situational) F43.10
    acute F43.11
    chronic F43.12
  psychasthenic (type) F48.8
  railroad F48.8
  rectum F45.8
  respiratory F45.8
  rumination F45.8
  sexual F65.9
  situational F48.8
  social F40.10
    generalized F40.11
  specified type NEC F48.8
  state F48.9
    with depersonalization episode F48.1
  stomach F45.8
  traumatic F43.10
    acute F43.11
    chronic F43.12
  vasomotor F45.8
  visceral F45.8
  war F48.8
Neurospongioblastosis diffusa Q85.1
Neurosyphilis (arrested) (early) (gumma) (late) (latent)
    (recurrent) (relapse) A52.3
  with ataxia (cerebellar) (locomotor) (spastic) (spinal)
      A52.19
  aneurysm (cerebral) A52.05
  arachnoid (adhesive) A52.13
  arteritis (any artery) (cerebral) A52.04
  asymptomatic A52.2
  congenital A50.40
  dura (mater) A52.13
  general paresis A52.17
  hemorrhagic A52.05
  juvenile (asymptomatic) (meningeal) A50.40
  leptomeninges (aseptic) A52.13
  meningeal, meninges (adhesive) A52.13
  meningitis A52.13
  meningovascular (diffuse) A52.13
  optic atrophy A52.15
  parenchymatous (degenerative) A52.19
  paresis, paretic A52.17
    juvenile A50.45
  remission in (sustained) A52.3
  serological (without symptoms) A52.2
  specified nature or site NEC A52.19
  tabes, tabetic (dorsalis) A52.11
    juvenile A50.45

☑ **Additional Character Required** — **Refer to the Tabular List for Character Selection**   ▽ **Subterms under main terms may continue to next column or page**

Neurosyphilis — *continued*
  taboparesis A52.17
    juvenile A50.45
  thrombosis (cerebral) A52.05
  vascular (cerebral) NEC A52.05
Neurothekeoma — *see* Neoplasm, nerve, benign
Neurotic — *see* Neurosis
Neurotoxemia — *see* Toxemia
Neutroclusion M26.211
Neutropenia, neutropenic (chronic) (genetic) (idiopathic) (immune) (infantile) (malignant) (pernicious) (splenic) D70.9
  congenital (primary) D70.0
  cyclic D70.4
  cytoreductive cancer chemotherapy sequela D70.1
  drug-induced D70.2
    due to cytoreductive cancer chemotherapy D70.1
  due to infection D70.3
  fever D70.9
  neonatal, transitory (isoimmune) (maternal transfer) P61.5
  periodic D70.4
  secondary (cyclic) (periodic) (splenic) D70.4
    drug-induced D70.2
      due to cytoreductive cancer chemotherapy D70.1
  toxic D70.8
Neutrophilia, hereditary giant D72.0
Nevocarcinoma — *see* Melanoma
Nevus D22.9
  achromic — *see* Neoplasm, skin, benign
  amelanotic — *see* Neoplasm, skin, benign
  angiomatous D18.00
    intra-abdominal D18.03
    intracranial D18.02
    skin D18.01
    specified site NEC D18.09
  araneus I78.1
  balloon cell — *see* Neoplasm, skin, benign
  bathing trunk D48.5
  blue — *see* Neoplasm, skin, benign
    cellular — *see* Neoplasm, skin, benign
    giant — *see* Neoplasm, skin, benign
    Jadassohn's — *see* Neoplasm, skin, benign
    malignant — *see* Melanoma
  capillary D18.00
    intra-abdominal D18.03
    intracranial D18.02
    skin D18.01
    specified site NEC D18.09
  cavernous D18.00
    intra-abdominal D18.03
    intracranial D18.02
    skin D18.01
    specified site NEC D18.09
  cellular — *see* Neoplasm, skin, benign
    blue — *see* Neoplasm, skin, benign
  choroid D31.3- ☑
  comedonicus Q82.5
  conjunctiva D31.0- ☑
  dermal — *see* Neoplasm, skin, benign
    with epidermal nevus — *see* Neoplasm, skin, benign
  dysplastic — *see* Neoplasm, skin, benign
  eye D31.9- ☑
  flammeus Q82.5
  hemangiomatous D18.00
    intra-abdominal D18.03
    intracranial D18.02
    skin D18.01
    specified site NEC D18.09
  iris D31.4- ☑
  lacrimal gland D31.5- ☑
  lymphatic D18.1
  magnocellular
    specified site — *see* Neoplasm, benign, by site
    unspecified site D31.40
  malignant — *see* Melanoma
  meaning hemangioma D18.00
    intra-abdominal D18.03
    intracranial D18.02
    skin D18.01
    specified site NEC D18.09
  mouth (mucosa) D10.30
    specified site NEC D10.39
    white sponge Q38.6
  multiplex Q85.1
  non-neoplastic I78.1
  oral mucosa D10.30
    specified site NEC D10.39

Nevus — *continued*
  oral mucosa — *continued*
    white sponge Q38.6
  orbit D31.6- ☑
  pigmented
    giant — *see also* Neoplasm, skin, uncertain behavior D48.5
    malignant melanoma in — *see* Melanoma
  portwine Q82.5
  retina D31.2- ☑
  retrobulbar D31.6- ☑
  sanguineous Q82.5
  senile I78.1
  skin D22.9
    abdominal wall D22.5
    ala nasi D22.39
    ankle D22.7- ☑
    anus, anal D22.5
    arm D22.6- ☑
    auditory canal (external) D22.2- ☑
    auricle (ear) D22.2- ☑
    auricular canal (external) D22.2- ☑
    axilla, axillary fold D22.5
    back D22.5
    breast D22.5
    brow D22.39
    buttock D22.5
    canthus (eye) D22.1- ☑
    cheek (external) D22.39
    chest wall D22.5
    chin D22.39
    ear (external) D22.2- ☑
    external meatus (ear) D22.2- ☑
    eyebrow D22.39
    eyelid (lower) (upper) D22.1- ☑
    face D22.30
      specified NEC D22.39
    female genital organ (external) NEC D28.0
    finger D22.6- ☑
    flank D22.5
    foot D22.7- ☑
    forearm D22.6- ☑
    forehead D22.39
    foreskin D29.0
    genital organ (external) NEC
      female D28.0
      male D29.9
    gluteal region D22.5
    groin D22.5
    hand D22.6- ☑
    heel D22.7- ☑
    helix D22.2- ☑
    hip D22.7- ☑
    interscapular region D22.5
    jaw D22.39
    knee D22.7- ☑
    labium (majus) (minus) D28.0
    leg D22.7- ☑
    lip (lower) (upper) D22.0
    lower limb D22.7- ☑
    male genital organ (external) D29.9
    nail D22.9
      finger D22.6- ☑
      toe D22.7- ☑
    nasolabial groove D22.39
    nates D22.5
    neck D22.4
    nose (external) D22.39
    palpebra D22.1- ☑
    penis D29.0
    perianal skin D22.5
    perineum D22.5
    pinna D22.2- ☑
    popliteal fossa or space D22.7- ☑
    prepuce D29.0
    pudendum D28.0
    scalp D22.4
    scrotum D29.4
    shoulder D22.6- ☑
    submammary fold D22.5
    temple D22.39
    thigh D22.7- ☑
    toe D22.7- ☑
    trunk NEC D22.5
    umbilicus D22.5
    upper limb D22.6- ☑
    vulva D28.0

Nevus — *continued*
  specified site NEC — *see* Neoplasm, by site, benign
  spider I78.1
  stellar I78.1
  strawberry Q82.5
  Sutton's benign D22.9
  unius lateris Q82.5
  Unna's Q82.5
  vascular Q82.5
  verrucous Q82.5
Newborn (infant) (liveborn) (singleton) Z38.2
  abstinence syndrome P96.1
  acne L70.4
  affected by
    abnormalities of membranes P02.9
      specified NEC P02.8
    abruptio placenta P02.1
    amino-acid metabolic disorder, transitory P74.8
    amniocentesis (while in utero) P00.6
    amnionitis P02.78
    apparent life threatening event (ALTE) R68.13
    bleeding (into)
      cerebral cortex P52.22
      germinal matrix P52.0
      ventricles P52.1
    breech delivery P03.0
    cardiac arrest P29.81
    cardiomyopathy I42.8
      congenital I42.4
    cerebral ischemia P91.0
    Cesarean delivery P03.4
    chemotherapy agents P04.11
    chorioamnionitis P02.78
    cocaine (crack) P04.41
    complications of labor and delivery P03.9
      specified NEC P03.89
    compression of umbilical cord NEC P02.5
    contracted pelvis P03.1
    cyanosis P28.2
    delivery P03.9
      Cesarean P03.4
      forceps P03.2
      vacuum extractor P03.3
    drugs of addiction P04.40
      cocaine P04.41
      hallucinogens P04.42
      specified drug NEC P04.49
    entanglement (knot) in umbilical cord P02.5
    environmental chemicals P04.6
    fetal (intrauterine)
      growth retardation P05.9
      inflammatory response syndrome (FIRS) P02.70
      malnutrition not light or small for gestational age P05.2
    FIRS (fetal inflammatory response syndrome) P02.70
    forceps delivery P03.2
    heart rate abnormalities
      bradycardia P29.12
      intrauterine P03.819
        before onset of labor P03.810
        during labor P03.811
      tachycardia P29.11
    hemorrhage (antepartum) P02.1
      cerebellar (nontraumatic) P52.6
      intracerebral (nontraumatic) P52.4
      intracranial (nontraumatic) P52.9
        specified NEC P52.8
      intraventricular (nontraumatic) P52.3
        grade 1 P52.0
        grade 2 P52.1
        grade 3 P52.21
        grade 4 P52.22
      posterior fossa (nontraumatic) P52.6
      subarachnoid (nontraumatic) P52.5
      subependymal P52.0
        with intracerebral extension P52.22
        with intraventricular extension P52.1
          with enlargment of ventricles P52.21
        without intraventricular extension P52.0
    hypoxic ischemic encephalopathy [HIE] P91.60
      mild P91.61
      moderate P91.62
      severe P91.63
    induction of labor P03.89
    intestinal perforation P78.0
    intrauterine (fetal) blood loss P50.9
      due to (from)
        cut end of co-twin cord P50.5

Newborn — *continued*
  affected by — *continued*
    intrauterine blood loss — *continued*
      due to — *continued*
        hemorrhage into
          co-twin P50.3
            maternal circulation P50.4
          placenta P50.2
          ruptured cord blood P50.1
          vasa previa P50.0
        specified NEC P50.8
    intrauterine (fetal) hemorrhage P50.9
    intrauterine (in utero) procedure P96.5
    malpresentation (malposition) NEC P03.1
    maternal (complication of) (use of)
      alcohol P04.3
      amphetamines P04.16
      analgesia (maternal) P04.0
      anesthesia (maternal) P04.0
      anticonvulsants P04.13
      antidepressants P04.15
      antineoplastic chemotherapy P04.11
      anxiolytics P04.1A
      blood loss P02.1
      cannabis P04.81
      circulatory disease P00.3
      condition P00.9
        specified NEC P00.89
      cytotoxic drugs P04.12
      delivery P03.9
        Cesarean P03.4
        forceps P03.2
        vacuum extractor P03.3
      diabetes mellitus (pre-existing) P70.1
      disorder P00.9
        specified NEC P00.89
      drugs (addictive) (illegal) NEC P04.49
      ectopic pregnancy P01.4
      gestational diabetes P70.0
      hemorrhage P02.1
      hypertensive disorder P00.0
      incompetent cervix P01.0
      infectious disease P00.2
      injury P00.5
      labor and delivery P03.9
      malpresentation before labor P01.7
      maternal death P01.6
      medical procedure P00.7
      medication P04.19
        specified type NEC P04.18
      multiple pregnancy P01.5
      nutritional disorder P00.4
      oligohydramnios P01.2
      opiates P04.14
        administered for procedures during pregnan-
          cy or labor and delivery P04.0
      parasitic disease P00.2
      periodontal disease P00.81
      placenta previa P02.0
      polyhydramnios P01.3
      precipitate delivery P03.5
      pregnancy P01.9
        specified P01.8
      premature rupture of membranes P01.1
      renal disease P00.1
      respiratory disease P00.3
      sedative-hypnotics P04.17
      surgical procedure P00.6
      tranquilizers administered for procedures during
        pregnancy or labor and delivery P04.0
      urinary tract disease P00.1
      uterine contraction (abnormal) P03.6
    meconium peritonitis P78.0
    medication (legal) (maternal use) (prescribed)
      P04.19
    membrane abnormalities P02.9
      specified NEC P02.8
    membranitis P02.78
    methamphetamine(s) P04.49
    mixed metabolic and respiratory acidosis P84
    neonatal abstinence syndrome P96.1
    noxious substances transmitted via placenta or
      breast milk P04.9
      cannabis P04.81
      specified NEC P04.89
    nutritional supplements P04.5
    placenta previa P02.0
    placental
      abnormality (functional) (morphological) P02.20

Newborn — *continued*
  affected by — *continued*
    placental — *continued*
      abnormality — *continued*
        specified NEC P02.29
      dysfunction P02.29
      infarction P02.29
      insufficiency P02.29
      separation NEC P02.1
      transfusion syndromes P02.3
    placentitis P02.78
    precipitate delivery P03.5
    prolapsed cord P02.4
    respiratory arrest P28.81
    slow intrauterine growth P05.9
    tobacco P04.2
    twin to twin transplacental transfusion P02.3
    umbilical cord (tightly) around neck P02.5
    umbilical cord condition P02.60
      short cord P02.69
      specified NEC P02.69
    uterine contractions (abnormal) P03.6
    vasa previa P02.69
      from intrauterine blood loss P50.0
  apnea P28.4
    obstructive P28.4
    primary P28.3
    sleep (central) (obstructive) (primary) P28.3
  born in hospital Z38.00
    by cesarean Z38.01
  born outside hospital Z38.1
  breast buds P96.89
  breast engorgement P83.4
  check-up — *see* Newborn, examination
  convulsion P90
  dehydration P74.1
  examination
    8 to 28 days old Z00.111
    under 8 days old Z00.110
  fever P81.9
    environmentally-induced P81.0
  hyperbilirubinemia P59.9
    of prematurity P59.0
  hypernatremia P74.21
  hyponatremia P74.22
  infection P39.9
    candidal P37.5
    specified NEC P39.8
    urinary tract P39.3
  jaundice P59.9
    due to
      breast milk inhibitor P59.3
      hepatocellular damage P59.20
        specified NEC P59.29
      preterm delivery P59.0
    of prematurity P59.0
    specified NEC P59.8
  late metabolic acidosis P74.0
  mastitis P39.0
    infective P39.0
    noninfective P83.4
  multiple born NEC Z38.8
    born in hospital Z38.68
      by cesarean Z38.69
    born outside hospital Z38.7
  omphalitis P38.9
    with mild hemorrhage P38.1
    without hemorrhage P38.9
  post-term P08.21
  prolonged gestation (over 42 completed weeks) P08.22
  quadruplet Z38.8
    born in hospital Z38.63
      by cesarean Z38.64
    born outside hospital Z38.7
  quintuplet Z38.8
    born in hospital Z38.65
      by cesarean Z38.66
    born outside hospital Z38.7
  seizure P90
  sepsis (congenital) P36.9
    due to
      anaerobes NEC P36.5
      Escherichia coli P36.4
      Staphylococcus P36.30
        aureus P36.2
        specified NEC P36.39
      Streptococcus P36.10
        group B P36.0
        specified NEC P36.19

Newborn — *continued*
  sepsis — *continued*
    specified NEC P36.8
  triplet Z38.8
    born in hospital Z38.61
      by cesarean Z38.62
    born outside hospital Z38.7
  twin Z38.5
    born in hospital Z38.30
      by cesarean Z38.31
    born outside hospital Z38.4
  vomiting P92.09
    bilious P92.01
  weight check Z00.111
Newcastle conjunctivitis or disease B30.8
Nezelof's syndrome (pure alymphocytosis) D81.4
Niacin (amide) **deficiency** E52
Nicolas (-Durand)-**Favre disease** A55
Nicotine — *see* Tobacco
Nicotinic acid deficiency E52
Niemann-Pick disease or syndrome E75.249
  specified NEC E75.248
  type
    A E75.240
    B E75.241
    C E75.242
    D E75.243
Night
  blindness — *see* Blindness, night
  sweats R61
  terrors (child) F51.4
Nightmares (REM sleep type) F51.5
NIHSS (National Institutes of Health Stroke Scale) **score**
  R29.7- ☑
Nipple — *see* condition
Nisbet's chancre A57
Nishimoto (-Takeuchi) **disease** I67.5
Nitritoid crisis or reaction — *see* Crisis, nitritoid
Nitrosohemoglobinemia D74.8
Njovera A65
Nocardiosis, nocardiasis A43.9
  cutaneous A43.1
  lung A43.0
  pneumonia A43.0
  pulmonary A43.0
  specified site NEC A43.8
Nocturia R35.1
  psychogenic F45.8
Nocturnal — *see* condition
Nodal rhythm I49.8
Node(s) — *see also* Nodule
  Bouchard's (with arthropathy) M15.2
  Haygarth's M15.8
  Heberden's (with arthropathy) M15.1
  larynx J38.7
  lymph — *see* condition
  milker's B08.03
  Osler's I33.0
  Schmorl's — *see* Schmorl's disease
  singer's J38.2
  teacher's J38.2
  tuberculous — *see* Tuberculosis, lymph gland
  vocal cord J38.2
Nodule(s), **nodular**
  actinomycotic — *see* Actinomycosis
  breast NEC — *see also* Lump, breast N63.0
  colloid (cystic), thyroid E04.1
  cutaneous — *see* Swelling, localized
  endometrial (stromal) D26.1
  Haygarth's M15.8
  inflammatory — *see* Inflammation
  juxta-articular
    syphilitic A52.77
    yaws A66.7
  larynx J38.7
  lung, solitary (subsegmental branch of the bronchial
    tree) R91.1
    multiple R91.8
  milker's B08.03
  prostate N40.2
    with lower urinary tract symptoms (LUTS) N40.3
    without lower urinary tract symtpoms (LUTS) N40.2
  pulmonary, solitary (subsegmental branch of the
    bronchial tree) R91.1
  retrocardiac R09.89
  rheumatoid M06.30
    ankle M06.37- ☑
    elbow M06.32- ☑

☑ Additional Character Required — Refer to the Tabular List for Character Selection   ▽ Subterms under main terms may continue to next column or page

Nodule(s), **nodular** — *continued*
  rheumatoid — *continued*
    foot joint M06.37- ☑
    hand joint M06.34- ☑
    hip M06.35- ☑
    knee M06.36- ☑
    multiple site M06.39
    shoulder M06.31- ☑
    vertebra M06.38
    wrist M06.33- ☑
  scrotum (inflammatory) N49.2
  singer's J38.2
  solitary, lung (subsegmental branch of the bronchial tree) R91.1
    multiple R91.8
  subcutaneous — *see* Swelling, localized
  teacher's J38.2
  thyroid (cold) (gland) (nontoxic) E04.1
    with thyrotoxicosis E05.20
      with thyroid storm E05.21
    toxic or with hyperthyroidism E05.20
      with thyroid storm E05.21
  vocal cord J38.2
Noma (gangrenous) (hospital) (infective) A69.0
  auricle I96
  mouth A69.0
  pudendi N76.89
  vulvae N76.89
Nomad, nomadism Z59.0
NOMID (neonatal onset multisystemic inflammatory disorder) M04.2
Nonadherence to medical treatment Z91.19
Nonautoimmune hemolytic anemia D59.4
  drug-induced D59.2
Nonclosure — *see also* Imperfect, closure
  ductus arteriosus (Botallo's) Q25.0
  foramen
    botalli Q21.1
    ovale Q21.1
Noncompliance Z91.19
  with
    dialysis Z91.15
    dietary regimen Z91.11
    medical treatment Z91.19
    medication regimen NEC Z91.14
      underdosing — *see also* Table of Drugs and Chemicals, categories T36-T50, with final character 6 Z91.14
        intentional NEC Z91.128
          due to financial hardship of patient Z91.120
        unintentional NEC Z91.138
          due to patient's age related debility Z91.130
    renal dialysis Z91.15
Nondescent (congenital) — *see also* Malposition, congenital
  cecum Q43.3
  colon Q43.3
  testicle Q53.9
    bilateral Q53.20
      abdominal Q53.211
      perineal Q53.22
    unilateral Q53.10
      abdominal Q53.111
      perineal Q53.12
Nondevelopment
  brain Q02
    part of Q04.3
  heart Q24.8
  organ or site, congenital NEC — *see* Hypoplasia
Nonengagement
  head NEC O32.4 ☑
    in labor, causing obstructed labor O64.8 ☑
Nonexanthematous tick fever A93.2
Nonexpansion, lung (newborn) P28.0
Nonfunctioning
  cystic duct — *see also* Disease, gallbladder K82.8
  gallbladder — *see also* Disease, gallbladder K82.8
  kidney N28.9
  labyrinth — *see* subcategory H83.2 ☑
Non-Hodgkin lymphoma NEC — *see* Lymphoma, non-Hodgkin
Nonimplantation, ovum N97.2
Noninsufflation, fallopian tube N97.1
Non-ketotic hyperglycinemia E72.51
Nonne-Milroy syndrome Q82.0
Nonovulation N97.0

Non-palpable testicle(s)
  bilateral R39.84
  unilateral R39.83
Nonpatent fallopian tube N97.1
Nonpneumatization, lung NEC P28.0
Nonrotation — *see* Malrotation
Nonsecretion, urine — *see* Anuria
Nonunion
  fracture — *see* Fracture, by site
  joint, following fusion or arthrodesis M96.0
  organ or site, congenital NEC — *see* Imperfect, closure
  symphysis pubis, congenital Q74.2
Nonvisualization, gallbladder R93.2
Nonvital, nonvitalized tooth K04.99
Non-working side interference M26.56
Noonan's syndrome Q87.19
Normocytic anemia (infectional) due to blood loss (chronic) D50.0
  acute D62
Norrie's disease (congenital) Q15.8
North American blastomycosis B40.9
Norwegian itch B86
Nose, nasal — *see* condition
Nosebleed R04.0
Nose-picking F98.8
Nosomania F45.21
Nosophobia F45.22
Nostalgia F43.20
Notch of iris Q13.2
Notching nose, congenital (tip) Q30.2
Nothnagel's
  syndrome — *see* Strabismus, paralytic, third nerve
  vasomotor acroparesthesia I73.89
Novy's relapsing fever A68.9
  louse-borne A68.0
  tick-borne A68.1
Noxious
  foodstuffs, poisoning by — *see* Poisoning, food, noxious, plant
  substances transmitted through placenta or breast milk P04.9
Nucleus pulposus — *see* condition
Numbness R20.0
Nuns' knee — *see* Bursitis, prepatellar
Nursemaid's elbow S53.03- ☑
Nutcracker esophagus K22.4
Nutmeg liver K76.1
Nutrient element deficiency E61.9
  specified NEC E61.8
Nutrition deficient or insufficient — *see also* Malnutrition E46
  due to
    insufficient food T73.0 ☑
    lack of
      care (child) T76.02 ☑
        adult T76.01 ☑
      food T73.0 ☑
Nutritional stunting E45
Nyctalopia (night blindness) — *see* Blindness, night
Nycturia R35.1
  psychogenic F45.8
Nymphomania F52.8
Nystagmus H55.00
  benign paroxysmal — *see* Vertigo, benign paroxysmal
  central positional H81.4
  congenital H55.01
  dissociated H55.04
  latent H55.02
  miners' H55.09
  positional
    benign paroxysmal H81.4
    central H81.4
  specified form NEC H55.09
  visual deprivation H55.03

O

Obermeyer's relapsing fever (European) A68.0
Obesity E66.9
  with alveolar hypoventilation E66.2
  adrenal E27.8
  complicating
    childbirth O99.214
    pregnancy O99.21- ☑
    puerperium O99.215
  constitutional E66.8
  dietary counseling and surveillance Z71.3

Obesity — *continued*
  drug-induced E66.1
  due to
    drug E66.1
    excess calories E66.09
      morbid E66.01
      severe E66.01
  endocrine E66.8
  endogenous E66.8
  exogenous E66.09
  familial E66.8
  glandular E66.8
  hypothyroid — *see* Hypothyroidism
  hypoventilation syndrome (OHS) E66.2
  morbid E66.01
    with
      alveolar hypoventilation E66.2
      obesity hypoventilation syndrome (OHS) E66.2
    due to excess calories E66.01
  nutritional E66.09
  pituitary E23.6
  severe E66.01
  specified type NEC E66.8
Oblique — *see* condition
Obliteration
  appendix (lumen) K38.8
  artery I77.1
  bile duct (noncalculous) K83.1
  common duct (noncalculus) K83.1
  cystic duct — *see* Obstruction, gallbladder
  disease, arteriolar I77.1
  endometrium N85.8
  eye, anterior chamber — *see* Disorder, globe, hypotony
  fallopian tube N97.1
  lymphatic vessel I89.0
    due to mastectomy I97.2
  organ or site, congenital NEC — *see* Atresia, by site
  ureter N13.5
    with infection N13.6
  urethra — *see* Stricture, urethra
  vein I87.8
  vestibule (oral) K08.89
Observation (following) (for) (without need for further medical care) Z04.9
  accident NEC Z04.3
    at work Z04.2
    transport Z04.1
  adverse effect of drug Z03.6
  alleged rape or sexual assault (victim), ruled out
    adult Z04.41
    child Z04.42
  criminal assault Z04.89
  development state
    adolescent Z00.3
    period of rapid growth in childhood Z00.2
    puberty Z00.3
  disease, specified NEC Z03.89
  following work accident Z04.2
  forced sexual exploitation Z04.81
  forced labor exploitation Z04.82
  growth and development state — *see* Observation, development state
  injuries (accidental) NEC — *see also* Observation, accident
  newborn (for)
    suspected condition, related to exposure from the mother or birth process — *see* Newborn, affected by, maternal
    ruled out Z05.9
      cardiac Z05.0
      connective tissue Z05.73
      gastrointestinal Z05.5
      genetic Z05.41
      genitourinary Z05.6
      immunologic Z05.43
      infectious Z05.1
      metabolic Z05.42
      musculoskeletal Z05.72
      neurological Z05.2
      respiratory Z05.3
      skin and subcutaneous tissue Z05.71
      specified condition NEC Z05.8
  postpartum
    immediately after delivery Z39.0
    routine follow-up Z39.2
  pregnancy (normal) (without complication) Z34.9- ☑
    high risk O09.9- ☑
  suicide attempt, alleged NEC Z03.89

Observation — *continued*
  suicide attempt, alleged — *continued*
    self-poisoning Z03.6
  suspected, ruled out — *see also* Suspected condition, ruled out
    abuse, physical
      adult Z04.71
      child Z04.72
    accident at work Z04.2
    adult battering victim Z04.71
    child battering victim Z04.72
    condition NEC Z03.89
      newborn — *see also* Observation, newborn (for), suspected condition, ruled out Z05.9
    drug poisoning or adverse effect Z03.6
    exposure (to)
      anthrax Z03.810
      biological agent NEC Z03.818
    inflicted injury NEC Z04.89
    suicide attempt, alleged Z03.89
      self-poisoning Z03.6
    toxic effects from ingested substance (drug) (poison) Z03.6
  toxic effects from ingested substance (drug) (poison) Z03.6
Obsession, obsessional state F42.8
  mixed thoughts and acts F42.2
Obsessive-compulsive neurosis or reaction F42.8
Obstetric embolism, septic — *see* Embolism, obstetric, septic
Obstetrical trauma (complicating delivery) O71.9
  with or following ectopic or molar pregnancy O08.6
  specified type NEC O71.89
Obstipation — *see* Constipation
Obstruction, obstructed, obstructive
  airway J98.8
    with
      allergic alveolitis J67.9
      asthma J45.909
        with
          exacerbation (acute) J45.901
          status asthmaticus J45.902
      bronchiectasis J47.9
        with
          exacerbation (acute) J47.1
          lower respiratory infection J47.0
      bronchitis (chronic) J44.9
      emphysema J43.9
    chronic J44.9
      with
        allergic alveolitis — *see* Pneumonitis, hypersensitivity
        bronchiectasis J47.9
          with
            exacerbation (acute) J47.1
            lower respiratory infection J47.0
    due to
      foreign body — *see* Foreign body, by site, causing asphyxia
      inhalation of fumes or vapors J68.9
      laryngospasm J38.5
  ampulla of Vater K83.1
  aortic (heart) (valve) — *see* Stenosis, aortic
  aortoiliac I74.09
  aqueduct of Sylvius G91.1
    congenital Q03.0
      with spina bifida — *see* Spina bifida, by site, with hydrocephalus
  Arnold-Chiari — *see* Arnold-Chiari disease
  artery — *see also* Atherosclerosis, artery I70.9 ☑
    basilar (complete) (partial) — *see* Occlusion, artery, basilar
    carotid (complete) (partial) — *see* Occlusion, artery, carotid
    cerebellar — *see* Occlusion, artery, cerebellar
    cerebral (anterior) (middle) (posterior) — *see* Occlusion, artery, cerebral
    precerebral — *see* Occlusion, artery, precerebral
    renal N28.0
    retinal NEC — *see* Occlusion, artery, retina
    stent — *see* Restenosis, stent
    vertebral (complete) (partial) — *see* Occlusion, artery, vertebral
  band (intestinal) — *see also* Obstruction, intestine, specified NEC K56.699
  bile duct or passage (common) (hepatic) (noncalculous) K83.1
    with calculus K80.51

Obstruction, obstructed, obstructive — *continued*
  bile duct or passage — *continued*
    congenital (causing jaundice) Q44.3
    biliary (duct) (tract) K83.1
      gallbladder K82.0
  bladder-neck (acquired) N32.0
    congenital Q64.31
    due to hyperplasia (hypertrophy) of prostate — *see* Hyperplasia, prostate
  bowel — *see* Obstruction, intestine
  bronchus J98.09
  canal, ear — *see* Stenosis, external ear canal
  cardia K22.2
  caval veins (inferior) (superior) I87.1
  cecum — *see* Obstruction, intestine
  circulatory I99.8
  colon — *see* Obstruction, intestine
  common duct (noncalculous) K83.1
  coronary (artery) — *see* Occlusion, coronary
  cystic duct — *see also* Obstruction, gallbladder
    with calculus K80.21
  device, implant or graft — *see also* Complications, by site and type, mechanical T85.698 ☑
    arterial graft NEC — *see* Complication, cardiovascular device, mechanical, vascular
    catheter NEC T85.628 ☑
      cystostomy T83.090 ☑
      dialysis (renal) T82.49 ☑
        intraperitoneal T85.691 ☑
      Hopkins T83.098 ☑
      ileostomy T83.098 ☑
      infusion NEC T82.594 ☑
        spinal (epidural) (subdural) T85.690 ☑
      nephrostomy T83.092 ☑
      urethral indwelling T83.091 ☑
      urinary T83.098 ☑
      urostomy T83.098 ☑
    due to infection T85.79 ☑
    gastrointestinal — *see* Complications, prosthetic device, mechanical, gastrointestinal device
    genital NEC T83.498 ☑
      intrauterine contraceptive device T83.39 ☑
      penile prosthesis (cylinder) (implanted) (pump) (resevoir) T83.490 ☑
      testicular prosthesis T83.491 ☑
    heart NEC — *see* Complication, cardiovascular device, mechanical
    joint prosthesis — *see* Complications, joint prosthesis, mechanical, specified NEC, by site
    orthopedic NEC — *see* Complication, orthopedic, device, mechanical
    specified NEC T85.628 ☑
    urinary NEC — *see also* Complication, genitourinary, device, urinary, mechanical
      graft T83.29 ☑
    vascular NEC — *see* Complication, cardiovascular device, mechanical
    ventricular intracranial shunt T85.09 ☑
  due to foreign body accidentally left in operative wound T81.529 ☑
  duodenum K31.5
  ejaculatory duct N50.89
  esophagus K22.2
  eustachian tube (complete) (partial) H68.10- ☑
    cartilagenous (extrinsic) H68.13- ☑
      intrinsic H68.12- ☑
    osseous H68.11- ☑
  fallopian tube (bilateral) N97.1
  fecal K56.41
    with hernia — *see* Hernia, by site, with obstruction
  foramen of Monro (congenital) Q03.8
    with spina bifida — *see* Spina bifida, by site, with hydrocephalus
  foreign body — *see* Foreign body
  gallbladder K82.0
    with calculus, stones K80.21
    congenital Q44.1
  gastric outlet K31.1
  gastrointestinal — *see* Obstruction, intestine
  hepatic K76.89
    duct (noncalculous) K83.1
  ileum — *see* Obstruction, intestine
  iliofemoral (artery) I74.5
  intestine K56.609
    with
      adhesions (intestinal) (peritoneal) K56.50
        complete K56.52

Obstruction, obstructed, obstructive — *continued*
  intestine — *continued*
    with — *continued*
      adhesions — *continued*
        incomplete K56.51
        partial K56.51
    adynamic K56.0
    by gallstone K56.3
    complete K56.601
    congenital (small) Q41.9
      large Q42.9
        specified part NEC Q42.8
    incomplete K56.600
    neurogenic K56.0
      Hirschsprung's disease or megacolon Q43.1
    newborn P76.9
      due to
        fecaliths P76.8
        inspissated milk P76.2
        meconium (plug) P76.0
          in mucoviscidosis E84.11
      specified NEC P76.8
    partial K56.600
    postoperative K91.30
      complete K91.32
      incomplete K91.31
      partial K91.31
    reflex K56.0
    specified NEC K56.699
      complete K56.691
      incomplete K56.690
      partial K56.690
    volvulus K56.2
  intracardiac ball valve prosthesis T82.09 ☑
  jejunum — *see* Obstruction, intestine
  joint prosthesis — *see* Complications, joint prosthesis, mechanical, specified NEC, by site
  kidney (calices) N28.89
  labor — *see* Delivery
  lacrimal (passages) (duct)
    by
      dacryolith — *see* Dacryolith
      stenosis — *see* Stenosis, lacrimal
    congenital Q10.5
    neonatal H04.53- ☑
  lacrimonasal duct — *see* Obstruction, lacrimal
  lacteal, with steatorrhea K90.2
  laryngitis — *see* Laryngitis
  larynx NEC J38.6
    congenital Q31.8
  lung J98.4
    disease, chronic J44.9
  lymphatic I89.0
  meconium (plug)
    newborn P76.0
      due to fecaliths P76.0
      in mucoviscidosis E84.11
  mitral — *see* Stenosis, mitral
  nasal J34.89
  nasolacrimal duct — *see also* Obstruction, lacrimal
    congenital Q10.5
  nasopharynx J39.2
  nose J34.89
  organ or site, congenital NEC — *see* Atresia, by site
  pancreatic duct K86.89
  parotid duct or gland K11.8
  pelviureteral junction N13.5
    with hydronephrosis N13.0
    congenital Q62.39
  pharynx J39.2
  portal (circulation) (vein) I81
  prostate — *see also* Hyperplasia, prostate
    valve (urinary) N32.0
  pulmonary valve (heart) I37.0
  pyelonephritis (chronic) N11.1
  pylorus
    adult K31.1
    congenital or infantile Q40.0
  rectosigmoid — *see* Obstruction, intestine
  rectum K62.4
  renal N28.89
    outflow N13.8
    pelvis, congenital Q62.39
  respiratory J98.8
    chronic J44.9
  retinal (vessels) H34.9
  salivary duct (any) K11.8
    with calculus K11.5

236

☑ Additional Character Required — Refer to the Tabular List for Character Selection   ⁖ Subterms under main terms may continue to next column or page

Obstruction, obstructed, obstructive — *continued*
- sigmoid — *see* Obstruction, intestine
- sinus (accessory) (nasal) J34.89
- Stensen's duct K11.8
- stomach NEC K31.89
  - acute K31.0
  - congenital Q40.2
  - due to pylorospasm K31.3
- submandibular duct K11.8
- submaxillary gland K11.8
  - with calculus K11.5
- thoracic duct I89.0
- thrombotic — *see* Thrombosis
- trachea J39.8
- tracheostomy airway J95.03
- tricuspid (valve) — *see* Stenosis, tricuspid
- upper respiratory, congenital Q34.8
- ureter (functional) (pelvic junction) NEC N13.5
  - with
    - hydronephrosis N13.1
      - with infection N13.6
    - pyelonephritis (chronic) N11.1
  - congenital Q62.39
  - due to calculus — *see* Calculus, ureter
- urethra NEC N36.8
  - congenital Q64.39
- urinary (moderate) N13.9
  - due to hyperplasia (hypertrophy) of prostate — *see* Hyperplasia, prostate
  - organ or tract (lower) N13.9
  - prostatic valve N32.0
  - specified NEC N13.8
- uropathy N13.9
- uterus N85.8
- vagina N89.5
- valvular — *see* Endocarditis
- vein, venous I87.1
  - caval (inferior) (superior) I87.1
  - thrombotic — *see* Thrombosis
- vena cava (inferior) (superior) I87.1
- vesical NEC N32.0
- vesicourethral orifice N32.0
  - congenital Q64.31
- vessel NEC I99.8
  - stent — *see* Restenosis, stent

Obturator — *see* condition
Occlusal wear, teeth K03.0
Occlusio pupillae — *see* Membrane, pupillary
Occlusion, occluded
- anus K62.4
  - congenital Q42.3
    - with fistula Q42.2
- aortoiliac (chronic) I74.09
- aqueduct of Sylvius G91.1
  - congenital Q03.0
    - with spina bifida — *see* Spina bifida, by site, with hydrocephalus
- artery — *see also* Atherosclerosis, artery I70.9 ☑
  - auditory, internal I65.8
  - basilar I65.1
    - with
      - infarction I63.22
        - due to
          - embolism I63.12
          - thrombosis I63.02
  - brain or cerebral I66.9
    - with infarction (due to) I63.5- ☑
      - embolism I63.4- ☑
      - thrombosis I63.3- ☑
  - carotid I65.2- ☑
    - with
      - infarction I63.23- ☑
        - due to
          - embolism I63.13- ☑
          - thrombosis I63.03- ☑
  - cerebellar (anterior inferior) (posterior inferior) (superior) I66.3
    - with infarction I63.54- ☑
      - due to
        - embolism I63.44- ☑
        - thrombosis I63.34- ☑
  - cerebral I66.9
    - with infarction I63.50
      - due to
        - embolism I63.40
          - specified NEC I63.49
        - thrombosis I63.30
          - specified NEC I63.39

Occlusion, occluded — *continued*
- artery — *see also* Atherosclerosis, artery — *continued*
  - cerebral — *continued*
    - anterior I66.1- ☑
      - with infarction I63.52- ☑
        - due to
          - embolism I63.42- ☑
          - thrombosis I63.32- ☑
    - middle I66.0- ☑
      - with infarction I63.51- ☑
        - due to
          - embolism I63.41- ☑
          - thrombosis I63.31- ☑
    - posterior I66.2- ☑
      - with infarction I63.53- ☑
        - due to
          - embolism I63.43- ☑
          - thrombosis I63.33- ☑
    - specified NEC I66.8
      - with infarction I63.59
        - due to
          - embolism I63.4- ☑
          - thrombosis I63.3- ☑
  - choroidal (anterior) — *see* Occlusion, artery, precerebral, specified NEC
  - communicating posterior — *see* Occlusion, artery, precerebral, specified NEC
  - complete
    - coronary I25.82
    - extremities I70.92
  - coronary (acute) (thrombotic) (without myocardial infarction) I24.0
    - with myocardial infarction — *see* Infarction, myocardium
    - chronic total I25.82
    - complete I25.82
    - healed or old I25.2
    - total (chronic) I25.82
  - hypophyseal — *see* Occlusion, artery, precerebral, specified NEC
  - iliac I74.5
  - lower extremities due to stenosis or stricture I77.1
  - mesenteric (embolic) (thrombotic) — *see also* Infarct, intestine K55.069
  - perforating — *see* Occlusion, artery, cerebral, specified NEC
  - peripheral I77.9
    - thrombotic or embolic I74.4
  - pontine — *see* Occlusion, artery, precerebral, specified NEC
  - precerebral I65.9
    - with infarction I63.20
      - specified NEC I63.29
        - due to
          - embolism I63.10
            - specified NEC I63.19
          - thrombosis I63.00
            - specified NEC I63.09
    - basilar — *see* Occlusion, artery, basilar
    - carotid — *see* Occlusion, artery, carotid
    - puerperal O88.23
    - specified NEC I65.8
      - with infarction I63.29
        - due to
          - embolism I63.19
          - thrombosis I63.09
    - vertebral — *see* Occlusion, artery, vertebral
  - renal N28.0
  - retinal
    - branch H34.23- ☑
    - central H34.1- ☑
    - partial H34.21- ☑
    - transient H34.0- ☑
  - spinal — *see* Occlusion, artery, precerebral, vertebral
  - total (chronic)
    - coronary I25.82
    - extremities I70.92
  - vertebral I65.0- ☑
    - with
      - infarction I63.21- ☑
        - due to
          - embolism I63.11- ☑
          - thrombosis I63.01- ☑
- basilar artery — *see* Occlusion, artery, basilar
- bile duct (common) (hepatic) (noncalculous) K83.1
- bowel — *see* Obstruction, intestine

Occlusion, occluded — *continued*
- carotid (artery) (common) (internal) — *see* Occlusion, artery, carotid
- centric (of teeth) M26.59
  - maximum intercuspation discrepancy M26.55
- cerebellar (artery) — *see* Occlusion, artery, cerebellar
- cerebral (artery) — *see* Occlusion, artery, cerebral
- cerebrovascular — *see also* Occlusion, artery, cerebral
  - with infarction I63.5-
- cervical canal — *see* Stricture, cervix
- cervix (uteri) — *see* Stricture, cervix
- choanal Q30.0
- choroidal (artery) — *see* Occlusion, artery, precerebral, specified NEC
- colon — *see* Obstruction, intestine
- communicating posterior artery — *see* Occlusion, artery, precerebral, specified NEC
- coronary (artery) (vein) (thrombotic) — *see also* Infarct, myocardium
  - chronic total I25.82
  - healed or old I25.2
  - not resulting in infarction I24.0
  - total (chronic) I25.82
- cystic duct — *see* Obstruction, gallbladder
- embolic — *see* Embolism
- fallopian tube N97.1
  - congenital Q50.6
- gallbladder — *see also* Obstruction, gallbladder
  - congenital (causing jaundice) Q44.1
- gingiva, traumatic K06.2
- hymen N89.6
  - congenital Q52.3
- hypophyseal (artery) — *see* Occlusion, artery, precerebral, specified NEC
- iliac artery I74.5
- intestine — *see* Obstruction, intestine
- lacrimal passages — *see* Obstruction, lacrimal
- lung J98.4
- lymph or lymphatic channel I89.0
- mammary duct N64.89
- mesenteric artery (embolic) (thrombotic) — *see also* Infarct, intestine K55.069
- nose J34.89
  - congenital Q30.0
- organ or site, congenital NEC — *see* Atresia, by site
- oviduct N97.1
  - congenital Q50.6
- peripheral arteries
  - due to stricture or stenosis I77.1
  - upper extremity I74.2
- pontine (artery) — *see* Occlusion, artery, precerebral, specified NEC
- posterior lingual, of mandibular teeth M26.29
- precerebral artery — *see* Occlusion, artery, precerebral
- punctum lacrimale — *see* Obstruction, lacrimal
- pupil — *see* Membrane, pupillary
- pylorus, adult — *see also* Stricture, pylorus K31.1
- renal artery N28.0
- retina, retinal
  - artery — *see* Occlusion, artery, retinal
  - vein (central) H34.81- ☑
    - engorgement H34.82- ☑
    - tributary H34.83- ☑
  - vessels H34.9
- spinal artery — *see* Occlusion, artery, precerebral, vertebral
- teeth (mandibular) (posterior lingual) M26.29
- thoracic duct I89.0
- thrombotic — *see* Thrombosis, artery
- traumatic
  - edentulous (alveolar) ridge K06.2
  - gingiva K06.2
  - periodontal K05.5
- tubal N97.1
- ureter (complete) (partial) N13.5
  - congenital Q62.10
- ureteropelvic junction N13.5
  - congenital Q62.11
- ureterovesical orifice N13.5
  - congenital Q62.12
- urethra — *see* Stricture, urethra
- uterus N85.8
- vagina N89.5
- vascular NEC I99.8
- vein — *see* Thrombosis
  - retinal — *see* Occlusion, retinal, vein
- vena cava (inferior) (superior) — *see* Embolism, vena cava

Occlusion, occluded — *continued*
  ventricle (brain) NEC G91.1
  vertebral (artery) — *see* Occlusion, artery, vertebral
  vessel (blood) I99.8
  vulva N90.5
Occult
  blood in feces (stools) R19.5
Occupational
  problems NEC Z56.89
Ochlophobia — *see* Agoraphobia
Ochronosis (endogenous) E70.29
Ocular muscle — *see* condition
Oculogyric crisis or disturbance H51.8
  psychogenic F45.8
Oculomotor syndrome H51.9
Oculopathy
  syphilitic NEC A52.71
    congenital
      early A50.01
      late A50.30
    early (secondary) A51.43
    late A52.71
Oddi's sphincter spasm K83.4
Odontalgia K08.89
Odontoameloblastoma — *see* Cyst, calcifying odontogenic
Odontoclasia K03.89
Odontodysplasia, regional K00.4
Odontogenesis imperfecta K00.5
Odontoma (ameloblastic) (complex) (compound) (fibroameloblastic) — *see* Cyst, calcifying odontogenic
Odontomyelitis (closed) (open) K04.01
  irreversible K04.02
  reversible K04.01
Odontorrhagia K08.89
Odontosarcoma, ameloblastic C41.1
  upper jaw (bone) C41.0
Oestriasis — *see* Myiasis
Oguchi's disease H53.63
Ohara's disease — *see* Tularemia
OHS (obesity hypoventilation syndrome) E66.2
Oidiomycosis — *see* Candidiasis
Oidium albicans infection — *see* Candidiasis
Old age (without mention of debility) R54
  dementia F03 ☑
Old (previous) **myocardial infarction** I25.2
Olfactory — *see* condition
Oligemia — *see* Anemia
Oligoastrocytoma
  specified site — *see* Neoplasm, malignant, by site
  unspecified site C71.9
Oligocythemia D64.9
Oligodendroblastoma
  specified site — *see* Neoplasm, malignant, by site
  unspecified site C71.9
Oligodendroglioma
  anaplastic type
    specified site — *see* Neoplasm, malignant, by site
    unspecified site C71.9
  specified site — *see* Neoplasm, malignant, by site
  unspecified site C71.9
Oligodontia — *see* Anodontia
Oligoencephalon Q02
Oligohidrosis L74.4
Oligohydramnios O41.0- ☑
Oligohydrosis L74.4
Oligomenorrhea N91.5
  primary N91.3
  secondary N91.4
Oligophrenia — *see also* Disability, intellectual
  phenylpyruvic E70.0
Oligospermia N46.11
  due to
    drug therapy N46.121
    efferent duct obstruction N46.123
    infection N46.122
    radiation N46.124
    specified cause NEC N46.129
    systemic disease N46.125
Oligotrichia — *see* Alopecia
Oliguria R34
  with, complicating or following ectopic or molar pregnancy O08.4
  postprocedural N99.0
Ollier's disease Q78.4
Omenotocele — *see* Hernia, abdomen, specified site NEC
Omentitis — *see* Peritonitis

Omentum, omental — *see* condition
Omphalitis (congenital) (newborn) P38.9
  with mild hemorrhage P38.1
  without hemorrhage P38.9
  not of newborn L08.82
  tetanus A33
Omphalocele Q79.2
Omphalomesenteric duct, persistent Q43.0
Omphalorrhagia, newborn P51.9
Omsk hemorrhagic fever A98.1
Onanism (excessive) F98.8
Onchocerciasis, onchocercosis B73.1
  with
    eye disease B73.00
      endophthalmitis B73.01
      eyelid B73.09
      glaucoma B73.02
      specified NEC B73.09
    eyelid B73.09
    eye NEC B73.00
Oncocytoma — *see* Neoplasm, benign, by site
Oncovirus, as cause of disease classified elsewhere B97.32
Ondine's curse — *see* Apnea, sleep
Oneirophrenia F23
Onychauxis L60.2
  congenital Q84.5
Onychia — *see also* Cellulitis, digit
  with lymphangitis — *see* Lymphangitis, acute, digit
  candidal B37.2
  dermatophytic B35.1
Onychitis — *see also* Cellulitis, digit
  with lymphangitis — *see* Lymphangitis, acute, digit
Onychocryptosis L60.0
Onychodystrophy L60.3
  congenital Q84.6
Onychogryphosis, onychogryposis L60.2
Onycholysis L60.1
Onychomadesis L60.8
Onychomalacia L60.3
Onychomycosis (finger) (toe) B35.1
Onycho-osteodysplasia Q87.2
Onychophagia F98.8
Onychophosis L60.8
Onychoptosis L60.8
Onychorrhexis L60.3
  congenital Q84.6
Onychoschizia L60.3
Onyxis (finger) (toe) L60.0
Onyxitis — *see also* Cellulitis, digit
  with lymphangitis — *see* Lymphangitis, acute, digit
Oophoritis (cystic) (infectional) (interstitial) N70.92
  with salpingitis N70.93
  acute N70.02
    with salpingitis N70.03
  chronic N70.12
    with salpingitis N70.13
  complicating abortion — *see* Abortion, by type, complicated by, oophoritis
Oophorocele N83.4- ☑
Opacity, opacities
  cornea H17.- ☑
    central H17.1- ☑
    congenital Q13.3
    degenerative — *see* Degeneration, cornea
    hereditary — *see* Dystrophy, cornea
    inflammatory — *see* Keratitis
    minor H17.81- ☑
    peripheral H17.82- ☑
    sequelae of trachoma (healed) B94.0
    specified NEC H17.89
  enamel (teeth) (fluoride) (nonfluoride) K00.3
  lens — *see* Cataract
  snowball — *see* Deposit, crystalline
  vitreous (humor) NEC H43.39- ☑
    congenital Q14.0
    membranes and strands H43.31- ☑
Opalescent dentin (hereditary) K00.5
Open, opening
  abnormal, organ or site, congenital — *see* Imperfect, closure
  angle with
    borderline
      findings
        high risk H40.02- ☑
        low risk H40.01- ☑
      intraocular pressure H40.00- ☑

Open, opening — *continued*
  angle with — *continued*
    cupping of discs H40.01- ☑
    glaucoma (primary) — *see* Glaucoma, open angle
  bite
    anterior M26.220
    posterior M26.221
  false — *see* Imperfect, closure
  margin on tooth restoration K08.51
  restoration margins of tooth K08.51
  wound — *see* Wound, open
Operational fatigue F48.8
Operative — *see* condition
Operculitis — *see* Periodontitis
Operculum — *see* Break, retina
Ophiasis L63.2
Ophthalmia — *see also* Conjunctivitis H10.9
  actinic rays — *see* Photokeratitis
  allergic (acute) — *see* Conjunctivitis, acute, atopic
  blennorrhagic (gonococcal) (neonatorum) A54.31
  diphtheritic A36.86
  Egyptian A71.1
  electrica — *see* Photokeratitis
  gonococcal (neonatorum) A54.31
  metastatic — *see* Endophthalmitis, purulent
  migraine — *see* Migraine, ophthalmoplegic
  neonatorum, newborn P39.1
    gonococcal A54.31
  nodosa H16.24- ☑
  purulent — *see* Conjunctivitis, acute, mucopurulent
  spring — *see* Conjunctivitis, acute, atopic
  sympathetic — *see* Uveitis, sympathetic
Ophthalmitis — *see* Ophthalmia
Ophthalmocele (congenital) Q15.8
Ophthalmoneuromyelitis G36.0
Ophthalmoplegia — *see also* Strabismus, paralytic
  anterior internuclear — *see* Ophthalmoplegia, internuclear
  ataxia-areflexia G61.0
  diabetic — *see* E08-E13 with .39
  exophthalmic E05.00
    with thyroid storm E05.01
  external H49.88- ☑
    progressive H49.4- ☑
      with pigmentary retinopathy — *see* Kearns-Sayre syndrome
    total H49.3- ☑
  internal (complete) (total) H52.51- ☑
  internuclear H51.2- ☑
  migraine — *see* Migraine, ophthalmoplegic
  Parinaud's H49.88- ☑
  progressive external — *see* Ophthalmoplegia, external, progressive
  supranuclear, progressive G23.1
  total (external) — *see* Ophthalmoplegia, external, total
Opioid(s)
  abuse — *see* Abuse, drug, opioids
  dependence — *see* Dependence, drug, opioids
  induced, without use disorder
    anxiety disorder F11.988
    delirium F11.921
    depressive disorder F11.94
    sexual dysfunction F11.981
    sleep disorder F11.982
Opisthognathism M26.09
Opisthorchiasis (felineus) (viverrini) B66.0
Opitz' disease D73.2
Opiumism — *see* Dependence, drug, opioid
Oppenheim's disease G70.2
Oppenheim-Urbach disease (necrobiosis lipoidica diabeticorum) — *see* E08-E13 with .620
Optic nerve — *see* condition
Orbit — *see* condition
Orchioblastoma C62.9- ☑
Orchitis (gangrenous) (nonspecific) (septic) (suppurative) N45.2
  blennorrhagic (gonococcal) (acute) (chronic) A54.23
  chlamydial A56.19
  filarial — *see also* Infestation, filarial B74.9 *[N51]*
  gonococcal (acute) (chronic) A54.23
  mumps B26.0
  syphilitic A52.76
  tuberculous A18.15
Orf (virus disease) B08.02
Organic — *see also* condition
  brain syndrome F09
  heart — *see* Disease, heart

☑ **Additional Character Required** — Refer to the Tabular List for Character Selection ⬙ Subterms under main terms may continue to next column or page

Organic — *continued*
   mental disorder F09
   psychosis F09
Orgasm
   anejaculatory N53.13
Oriental
   bilharziasis B65.2
   schistosomiasis B65.2
Orifice — *see* condition
Origin of both great vessels from right ventricle
   Q20.1
Ormond's disease (with ureteral obstruction) N13.5
   with infection N13.6
Ornithine metabolism disorder E72.4
Ornithinemia (Type I) (Type II) E72.4
Ornithosis A70
Orotaciduria, oroticaciduria (congenital) (hereditary)
   (pyrimidine deficiency) E79.8
   anemia D53.0
Orthodontics
   adjustment Z46.4
   fitting Z46.4
Orthopnea R06.01
Orthopoxvirus B08.09
Os, uterus — *see* condition
Osgood-Schlatter disease or osteochondrosis — *see*
   Osteochondrosis, juvenile, tibia
Osler (-Weber)-**Rendu disease** I78.0
Osler's nodes I33.0
Osmidrosis L75.0
Osseous — *see* condition
Ossification
   artery — *see* Arteriosclerosis
   auricle (ear) — *see* Disorder, pinna, specified type NEC
   bronchial J98.09
   cardiac — *see* Degeneration, myocardial
   cartilage (senile) — *see* Disorder, cartilage, specified
     type NEC
   coronary (artery) — *see* Disease, heart, ischemic,
     atherosclerotic
   diaphragm J98.6
   ear, middle — *see* Otosclerosis
   falx cerebri G96.19
   fontanel, premature Q75.0
   heart — *see also* Degeneration, myocardial
     valve — *see* Endocarditis
   larynx J38.7
   ligament — *see* Disorder, tendon, specified type NEC
     posterior longitudinal — *see* Spondylopathy, spec-
      ified NEC
   meninges (cerebral) (spinal) G96.19
   multiple, eccentric centers — *see* Disorder, bone, de-
     velopment or growth
   muscle — *see also* Calcification, muscle
     due to burns — *see* Myositis, ossificans, in, burns
     paralytic — *see* Myositis, ossificans, in, quadriplegia
     progressive — *see* Myositis, ossificans, progressiva
     specified NEC M61.50
      ankle M61.57- ☑
      foot M61.57- ☑
      forearm M61.53- ☑
      hand M61.54- ☑
      lower leg M61.56- ☑
      multiple sites M61.59
      pelvic region M61.55- ☑
      shoulder region M61.51- ☑
      specified site NEC M61.58
      thigh M61.55- ☑
      upper arm M61.52- ☑
     traumatic — *see* Myositis, ossificans, traumatica
   myocardium, myocardial — *see* Degeneration, myocar-
     dial
   penis N48.89
   periarticular — *see* Disorder, joint, specified type NEC
   pinna — *see* Disorder, pinna, specified type NEC
   rider's bone — *see* Ossification, muscle, specified NEC
   sclera H15.89
   subperiosteal, post-traumatic M89.8X- ☑
   tendon — *see* Disorder, tendon, specified type NEC
   trachea J39.8
   tympanic membrane — *see* Disorder, tympanic mem-
     brane, specified NEC
   vitreous (humor) — *see* Deposit, crystalline
Osteitis — *see also* Osteomyelitis
   alveolar M27.3
   condensans M85.30
     ankle M85.37- ☑

Osteitis — *continued*
   condensans — *continued*
     foot M85.37- ☑
     forearm M85.33- ☑
     hand M85.34- ☑
     lower leg M85.36- ☑
     multiple site M85.39
     neck M85.38
     rib M85.38
     shoulder M85.31- ☑
     skull M85.38
     specified site NEC M85.38
     thigh M85.35- ☑
     toe M85.37- ☑
     upper arm M85.32- ☑
     vertebra M85.38
   deformans M88.9
     in (due to)
      malignant neoplasm of bone C41.9 *[M90.60]*
      neoplastic disease — *see also* Neoplasm
       D49.9 *[M90.60]*
       carpus D49.9 *[M90.64-]* ☑
       clavicle D49.9 *[M90.61-]* ☑
       femur D49.9 *[M90.65-]* ☑
       fibula D49.9 *[M90.66-]* ☑
       finger D49.9 *[M90.64-]* ☑
       humerus D49.9 *[M90.62-]* ☑
       ilium D49.9 *[M90.65-]* ☑
       ischium D49.9 *[M90.65-]* ☑
       metacarpus D49.9 *[M90.64-]* ☑
       metatarsus D49.9 *[M90.67-]* ☑
       multiple sites D49.9 *[M90.69]*
       neck D49.9 *[M90.68]*
       radius D49.9 *[M90.63-]* ☑
       rib D49.9 *[M90.68]*
       scapula D49.9 *[M90.61-]* ☑
       skull D49.9 *[M90.68]*
       tarsus D49.9 *[M90.67-]* ☑
       tibia D49.9 *[M90.66-]* ☑
       toe D49.9 *[M90.67-]* ☑
       ulna D49.9 *[M90.63-]* ☑
       vertebra D49.9 *[M90.68]*
     skull M88.0
     specified NEC — *see* Paget's disease, bone, by site
     vertebra M88.1
   due to yaws A66.6
   fibrosa NEC — *see* Cyst, bone, by site
     circumscripta — *see* Dysplasia, fibrous, bone NEC
     cystica (generalisata) E21.0
     disseminata Q78.1
     osteoplastica E21.0
   fragilitans Q78.0
   Garr's (sclerosing) — *see* Osteomyelitis, specified type
     NEC
   jaw (acute) (chronic) (lower) (suppurative) (upper)
     M27.2
   parathyroid E21.0
   petrous bone (acute) (chronic) — *see* Petrositis
   sclerotic, nonsuppurative — *see* Osteomyelitis, speci-
     fied type NEC
   tuberculosa A18.09
     cystica D86.89
     multiplex cystoides D86.89
Osteoarthritis M19.90
   ankle M19.07- ☑
   elbow M19.02- ☑
   foot joint M19.07- ☑
   generalized M15.9
     erosive M15.4
     primary M15.0
     specified NEC M15.8
   hand joint M19.04- ☑
     first carpometacarpal joint M18.9
   hip M16.1- ☑
     bilateral M16.0
     due to hip dysplasia (unilateral) M16.3- ☑
      bilateral M16.2
   interphalangeal
     distal (Heberden) M15.1
     proximal (Bouchard) M15.2
   knee M17.1- ☑
     bilateral M17.0
   post-traumatic NEC M19.92
     ankle M19.17- ☑
     elbow M19.12- ☑
     foot joint M19.17- ☑
     hand joint M19.14- ☑

Osteoarthritis — *continued*
   post-traumatic — *continued*
     hand joint — *continued*
      first carpometacarpal joint M18.3- ☑
       bilateral M18.2
     hip M16.5- ☑
      bilateral M16.4
     knee M17.3- ☑
      bilateral M17.2
     shoulder M19.11- ☑
     wrist M19.13- ☑
   primary M19.91
     ankle M19.07- ☑
     elbow M19.02- ☑
     foot joint M19.07- ☑
     hand joint M19.04- ☑
      first carpometacarpal joint M18.1- ☑
       bilateral M18.0
     hip M16.1- ☑
      bilateral M16.0
     knee M17.1- ☑
      bilateral M17.0
     multiple sites M89.49
     shoulder M19.01- ☑
     spine — *see* Spondylosis
     wrist M19.03- ☑
   secondary M19.93
     ankle M19.27- ☑
     elbow M19.22- ☑
     foot joint M19.27- ☑
     hand joint M19.24- ☑
      first carpometacarpal joint M18.5- ☑
       bilateral M18.4
     hip M16.7
      bilateral M16.6
     knee M17.5
      bilateral M17.4
     multiple M15.3
     shoulder M19.21- ☑
     spine — *see* Spondylosis
     wrist M19.23- ☑
   shoulder M19.01- ☑
   spine — *see* Spondylosis
   wrist M19.03- ☑
Osteoarthropathy (hypertrophic) M19.90
   ankle — *see* Osteoarthritis, primary, ankle
   elbow — *see* Osteoarthritis, primary, elbow
   foot joint — *see* Osteoarthritis, primary, foot
   hand joint — *see* Osteoarthritis, primary, hand joint
   knee joint — *see* Osteoarthritis, primary, knee
   multiple site — *see* Osteoarthritis, primary, multiple
     joint
   pulmonary — *see also* Osteoarthropathy, specified
     type NEC
     hypertrophic — *see* Osteoarthropathy, hypertrophic,
      specified type NEC
   secondary — *see* Osteoarthropathy, specified type NEC
   secondary hypertrophic — *see* Osteoarthropathy,
     specified type NEC
   shoulder — *see* Osteoarthritis, primary, shoulder
   specified joint NEC — *see* Osteoarthritis, primary,
     specified joint NEC
   specified type NEC M89.40
     carpus M89.44- ☑
     clavicle M89.41- ☑
     femur M89.45- ☑
     fibula M89.46- ☑
     finger M89.44- ☑
     humerus M89.42- ☑
     ilium M89.459
     ischium M89.459
     metacarpus M89.44- ☑
     metatarsus M89.47- ☑
     multiple sites M89.49
     neck M89.48
     radius M89.43- ☑
     rib M89.48
     scapula M89.41- ☑
     skull M89.48
     tarsus M89.47- ☑
     tibia M89.46- ☑
     toe M89.47- ☑
     ulna M89.43- ☑
     vertebra M89.48
   spine — *see* Spondylosis
   wrist — *see* Osteoarthritis, primary, wrist

Organic — Osteoarthropathy

Index

Osteoarthrosis (degenerative) (hypertrophic) (joint) — *see also* Osteoarthritis
  deformans alkaptonurica E70.29 *[M36.8]*
  erosive M15.4
  generalized M15.9
    primary M15.0
  polyarticular M15.9
  spine — *see* Spondylosis
Osteoblastoma — *see* Neoplasm, bone, benign
  aggressive — *see* Neoplasm, bone, uncertain behavior
Osteochondritis — *see also* Osteochondropathy, by site
  Brailsford's — *see* Osteochondrosis, juvenile, radius
  dissecans M93.20
    ankle M93.27- ☑
    elbow M93.22- ☑
    foot M93.27- ☑
    hand M93.24- ☑
    hip M93.25- ☑
    knee M93.26- ☑
    multiple sites M93.29
    shoulder joint M93.21- ☑
    specified site NEC M93.28
    wrist M93.23- ☑
  juvenile M92.9
    patellar — *see* Osteochondrosis, juvenile, patella
  syphilitic (congenital) (early) A50.02 *[M90.80]*
    ankle A50.02 *[M90.87-]* ☑
    elbow A50.02 *[M90.82-]* ☑
    foot A50.02 *[M90.87-]* ☑
    forearm A50.02 *[M90.83-]* ☑
    hand A50.02 *[M90.84-]* ☑
    hip A50.02 *[M90.85-]* ☑
    knee A50.02 *[M90.86-]* ☑
    multiple sites A50.02 *[M90.89]*
    shoulder joint A50.02 *[M90.81-]* ☑
    specified site NEC A50.02 *[M90.88]*
Osteochondroarthrosis deformans endemica — *see* Disease, Kaschin-Beck
Osteochondrodysplasia Q78.9
  with defects of growth of tubular bones and spine Q77.9
    specified NEC Q77.8
  specified NEC Q78.8
Osteochondrodystrophy E78.9
Osteochondrolysis — *see* Osteochondritis, dissecans
Osteochondroma — *see* Neoplasm, bone, benign
Osteochondromatosis D48.0
  syndrome Q78.4
Osteochondromyxosarcoma — *see* Neoplasm, bone, malignant
Osteochondropathy M93.90
  ankle M93.97- ☑
  elbow M93.92- ☑
  foot M93.97- ☑
  hand M93.94- ☑
  hip M93.95- ☑
  Kienböck's disease of adults M93.1
  knee M93.96- ☑
  multiple joints M93.99
  osteochondritis dissecans — *see* Osteochondritis, dissecans
  osteochondrosis — *see* Osteochondrosis
  shoulder region M93.91- ☑
  slipped upper femoral epiphysis — *see* Slipped, epiphysis, upper femoral
  specified joint NEC M93.98
  specified type NEC M93.80
    ankle M93.87- ☑
    elbow M93.82- ☑
    foot M93.87- ☑
    hand M93.84- ☑
    hip M93.85- ☑
    knee M93.86- ☑
    multiple joints M93.89
    shoulder region M93.81- ☑
    specified joint NEC M93.88
    wrist M93.83- ☑
  syphilitic, congenital
    early A50.02 *[M90.80]*
    late A50.56 *[M90.80]*
  wrist M93.93- ☑
Osteochondrosarcoma — *see* Neoplasm, bone, malignant
Osteochondrosis — *see also* Osteochondropathy, by site
  acetabulum (juvenile) M91.0

Osteochondrosis — *continued*
  adult — *see* Osteochondropathy, specified type NEC, by site
  astragalus (juvenile) — *see* Osteochondrosis, juvenile, tarsus
  Blount's — *see* Osteochondrosis, juvenile, tibia
  Buchanan's M91.0
  Burns' — *see* Osteochondrosis, juvenile, ulna
  calcaneus (juvenile) — *see* Osteochondrosis, juvenile, tarsus
  capitular epiphysis (femur) (juvenile) — *see* Legg-Calvé-Perthes disease
  carpal (juvenile) (lunate) (scaphoid) — *see* Osteochondrosis, juvenile, hand, carpal lunate
    adult M93.1
  coxae juvenilis — *see* Legg-Calvé-Perthes disease
  deformans juvenilis, coxae — *see* Legg-Calvé-Perthes disease
  Diaz's — *see* Osteochondrosis, juvenile, tarsus
  dissecans (knee) (shoulder) — *see* Osteochondritis, dissecans
  femoral capital epiphysis (juvenile) — *see* Legg-Calvé-Perthes disease
  femur (head), juvenile — *see* Legg-Calvé-Perthes disease
  fibula (juvenile) — *see* Osteochondrosis, juvenile, fibula
  foot NEC (juvenile) M92.8
  Freiberg's — *see* Osteochondrosis, juvenile, metatarsus
  Haas' (juvenile) — *see* Osteochondrosis, juvenile, humerus
  Haglund's — *see* Osteochondrosis, juvenile, tarsus
  hip (juvenile) — *see* Legg-Calvé-Perthes disease
  humerus (capitulum) (head) (juvenile) — *see* Osteochondrosis, juvenile, humerus
  ilium, iliac crest (juvenile) M91.0
  ischiopubic synchondrosis M91.0
  Iselin's — *see* Osteochondrosis, juvenile, metatarsus
  juvenile, juvenilis M92.9
    after congenital dislocation of hip reduction — *see* Osteochondrosis, juvenile, hip, specified NEC
    arm — *see* Osteochondrosis, juvenile, upper limb NEC
    capitular epiphysis (femur) — *see* Legg-Calvé-Perthes disease
    clavicle, sternal epiphysis — *see* Osteochondrosis, juvenile, upper limb NEC
    coxae — *see* Legg-Calvé-Perthes disease
    deformans M92.9
    fibula M92.5- ☑
    foot NEC M92.8
    hand M92.20- ☑
      carpal lunate M92.21- ☑
      metacarpal head M92.22- ☑
      specified site NEC M92.29- ☑
    head of femur — *see* Legg-Calvé-Perthes disease
    hip and pelvis M91.9-
      coxa plana — *see* Coxa, plana
      femoral head — *see* Legg-Calvé-Perthes disease
      pelvis M91.0
      pseudocoxalgia — *see* Pseudocoxalgia
      specified NEC M91.8- ☑
    humerus M92.0- ☑
    limb
      lower NEC M92.8
      upper NEC — *see* Osteochondrosis, juvenile, upper limb NEC
    medial cuneiform bone — *see* Osteochondrosis, juvenile, tarsus
    metatarsus M92.7- ☑
    patella M92.4- ☑
    radius M92.1- ☑
    specified site NEC M92.8
    spine M42.00
      cervical region M42.02
      cervicothoracic region M42.03
      lumbar region M42.06
      lumbosacral region M42.07
      multiple sites M42.09
      occipito-atlanto-axial region M42.01
      sacrococcygeal region M42.08
      thoracic region M42.04
      thoracolumbar region M42.05
    tarsus M92.6- ☑
    tibia M92.5- ☑
    ulna M92.1- ☑
    upper limb NEC M92.3- ☑

Osteochondrosis — *continued*
  juvenile, juvenilis — *continued*
    vertebra (body) (epiphyseal plates) (Calvé's) (Scheuermann's) — *see* Osteochondrosis, juvenile, spine
  Kienböck's — *see* Osteochondrosis, juvenile, hand, carpal lunate
    adult M93.1
  Köhler's
    patellar — *see* Osteochondrosis, juvenile, patella
    tarsal navicular — *see* Osteochondrosis, juvenile, tarsus
  Legg-Perthes (-Calvé)(-Waldenström) — *see* Legg-Calvé-Perthes disease
  limb
    lower NEC (juvenile) M92.8
    upper NEC (juvenile) — *see* Osteochondrosis, juvenile, upper limb NEC
  lunate bone (carpal) (juvenile) — *see also* Osteochondrosis, juvenile, hand, carpal lunate
    adult M93.1
  Mauclaire's — *see* Osteochondrosis, juvenile, hand, metacarpal
  metacarpal (head) (juvenile) — *see* Osteochondrosis, juvenile, hand, metacarpal
  metatarsus (fifth) (head) (juvenile) (second) — *see* Osteochondrosis, juvenile, metatarsus
  navicular (juvenile) — *see* Osteochondrosis, juvenile, tarsus
  os
    calcis (juvenile) — *see* Osteochondrosis, juvenile, tarsus
    tibiale externum (juvenile) — *see* Osteochondrosis, juvenile, tarsus
  Osgood-Schlatter — *see* Osteochondrosis, juvenile, tibia
  Panner's — *see* Osteochondrosis, juvenile, humerus
  patellar center (juvenile) (primary) (secondary) — *see* Osteochondrosis, juvenile, patella
  pelvis (juvenile) M91.0
  Pierson's M91.0
  radius (head) (juvenile) — *see* Osteochondrosis, juvenile, radius
  Scheuermann's — *see* Osteochondrosis, juvenile, spine
  Sever's — *see* Osteochondrosis, juvenile, tarsus
  Sinding-Larsen — *see* Osteochondrosis, juvenile, patella
  spine M42.9
    adult M42.10
      cervical region M42.12
      cervicothoracic region M42.13
      lumbar region M42.16
      lumbosacral region M42.17
      multiple sites M42.19
      occipito-atlanto-axial region M42.11
      sacrococcygeal region M42.18
      thoracic region M42.14
      thoracolumbar region M42.15
    juvenile — *see* Osteochondrosis, juvenile, spine
  symphysis pubis (juvenile) M91.0
  syphilitic (congenital) A50.02
  talus (juvenile) — *see* Osteochondrosis, juvenile, tarsus
  tarsus (navicular) (juvenile) — *see* Osteochondrosis, juvenile, tarsus
  tibia (proximal) (tubercle) (juvenile) — *see* Osteochondrosis, juvenile, tibia
  tuberculous — *see* Tuberculosis, bone
  ulna (lower) (juvenile) — *see* Osteochondrosis, juvenile, ulna
  van Neck's M91.0
  vertebral — *see* Osteochondrosis, spine
Osteoclastoma D48.0
  malignant — *see* Neoplasm, bone, malignant
Osteodynia — *see* Disorder, bone, specified type NEC
Osteodystrophy Q78.9
  azotemic N25.0
  congenital Q78.9
  parathyroid, secondary E21.1
  renal N25.0
Osteofibroma — *see* Neoplasm, bone, benign
Osteofibrosarcoma — *see* Neoplasm, bone, malignant
Osteogenesis imperfecta Q78.0
Osteogenic — *see* condition
Osteolysis M89.50
  carpus M89.54- ☑
  clavicle M89.51- ☑
  femur M89.55- ☑

Osteoarthrosis — Osteolysis

Osteolysis — *continued*
  fibula M89.56- ☑
  finger M89.54- ☑
  humerus M89.52- ☑
  ilium M89.559
  ischium M89.559
  joint prosthesis (periprosthetic) — *see* Complications,
     joint prosthesis, mechanical, periprosthetic, oste-
     olysis, by site
  metacarpus M89.54- ☑
  metatarsus M89.57- ☑
  multiple sites M89.59
  neck M89.58
  periprosthetic — *see* Complications, joint prosthesis,
     mechanical, periprosthetic, osteolysis, by site
  radius M89.53- ☑
  rib M89.58
  scapula M89.51- ☑
  skull M89.58
  tarsus M89.57- ☑
  tibia M89.56- ☑
  toe M89.57- ☑
  ulna M89.53- ☑
  vertebra M89.58
Osteoma — *see also* Neoplasm, bone, benign
  osteoid — *see also* Neoplasm, bone, benign
    giant — *see* Neoplasm, bone, benign
Osteomalacia M83.9
  adult M83.9
    drug-induced NEC M83.5
    due to
      malabsorption (postsurgical) M83.2
      malnutrition M83.3
    specified NEC M83.8
  aluminium-induced M83.4
  infantile — *see* Rickets
  juvenile — *see* Rickets
  oncogenic E83.89
  pelvis M83.8
  puerperal M83.0
  senile M83.1
  vitamin-D-resistant in adults E83.31 *[M90.8-]* ☑
    carpus E83.31 *[M90.84-]* ☑
    clavicle E83.31 *[M90.81-]* ☑
    femur E83.31 *[M90.85-]* ☑
    fibula E83.31 *[M90.86-]* ☑
    finger E83.31 *[M90.84-]* ☑
    humerus E83.31 *[M90.82-]* ☑
    ilium E83.31 *[M90.859]*
    ischium E83.31 *[M90.859]*
    metacarpus E83.31 *[M90.84-]* ☑
    metatarsus E83.31 *[M90.87-]* ☑
    multiple sites E83.31 *[M90.89]*
    neck E83.31 *[M90.88]*
    radius E83.31 *[M90.83-]* ☑
    rib E83.31 *[M90.88]*
    scapula E83.31 *[M90.819]*
    skull E83.31 *[M90.88]*
    tarsus E83.31 *[M90.879]*
    tibia E83.31 *[M90.869]*
    toe E83.31 *[M90.879]*
    ulna E83.31 *[M90.839]*
    vertebra E83.31 *[M90.88]*
Osteomyelitis (general) (infective) (localized) (neonatal)
    (purulent) (septic) (staphylococcal) (streptococcal)
    (suppurative) (with periostitis) M86.9
  acute M86.10
    carpus M86.14- ☑
    clavicle M86.11- ☑
    femur M86.15- ☑
    fibula M86.16- ☑
    finger M86.14- ☑
    hematogenous M86.00
      carpus M86.04- ☑
      clavicle M86.01- ☑
      femur M86.05- ☑
      fibula M86.06- ☑
      finger M86.04- ☑
      humerus M86.02- ☑
      ilium M86.059
      ischium M86.059
      mandible M27.2
      metacarpus M86.04- ☑
      metatarsus M86.07- ☑
      multiple sites M86.09
      neck M86.08
      orbit H05.02- ☑

Osteomyelitis — *continued*
  acute — *continued*
    hematogenous — *continued*
      petrous bone — *see* Petrositis
      radius M86.03- ☑
      rib M86.08
      scapula M86.01- ☑
      skull M86.08
      tarsus M86.07- ☑
      tibia M86.06- ☑
      toe M86.07- ☑
      ulna M86.03- ☑
      vertebra — *see* Osteomyelitis, vertebra
    humerus M86.12- ☑
    ilium M86.18
    ischium M86.18
    mandible M27.2
    metacarpus M86.14- ☑
    metatarsus M86.17- ☑
    multiple sites M86.19
    neck M86.18
    orbit H05.02- ☑
    petrous bone — *see* Petrositis
    radius M86.13- ☑
    rib M86.18
    scapula M86.11- ☑
    skull M86.18
    tarsus M86.17- ☑
    tibia M86.16- ☑
    toe M86.17- ☑
    ulna M86.13- ☑
    vertebra — *see* Osteomyelitis, vertebra
  chronic (or old) M86.60
    with draining sinus M86.40
      carpus M86.44- ☑
      clavicle M86.41- ☑
      femur M86.45- ☑
      fibula M86.46- ☑
      finger M86.44- ☑
      humerus M86.42- ☑
      ilium M86.459
      ischium M86.459
      mandible M27.2
      metacarpus M86.44- ☑
      metatarsus M86.47- ☑
      multiple sites M86.49
      neck M86.48
      orbit H05.02- ☑
      petrous bone — *see* Petrositis
      radius M86.43- ☑
      rib M86.48
      scapula M86.41- ☑
      skull M86.48
      tarsus M86.47- ☑
      tibia M86.46- ☑
      toe M86.47- ☑
      ulna M86.43- ☑
      vertebra — *see* Osteomyelitis, vertebra
    carpus M86.64- ☑
    clavicle M86.61- ☑
    femur M86.65- ☑
    fibula M86.66- ☑
    finger M86.64- ☑
    hematogenous NEC M86.50
      carpus M86.54- ☑
      clavicle M86.51- ☑
      femur M86.55- ☑
      fibula M86.56- ☑
      finger M86.54- ☑
      humerus M86.52- ☑
      ilium M86.559
      ischium M86.559
      mandible M27.2
      metacarpus M86.54- ☑
      metatarsus M86.57- ☑
      multifocal M86.30
        carpus M86.34- ☑
        clavicle M86.31- ☑
        femur M86.35- ☑
        fibula M86.36- ☑
        finger M86.34- ☑
        humerus M86.32- ☑
        ilium M86.359
        ischium M86.359
        metacarpus M86.34- ☑
        metatarsus M86.37- ☑

Osteomyelitis — *continued*
  chronic — *continued*
    hematogenous — *continued*
      multifocal — *continued*
        multiple sites M86.39
        neck M86.38
        radius M86.33- ☑
        rib M86.38
        scapula M86.31- ☑
        skull M86.38
        tarsus M86.37- ☑
        tibia M86.36- ☑
        toe M86.37- ☑
        ulna M86.33- ☑
        vertebra — *see* Osteomyelitis, vertebra
      multiple sites M86.59
      neck M86.58
      orbit H05.02- ☑
      petrous bone — *see* Petrositis
      radius M86.53- ☑
      rib M86.58
      scapula M86.51- ☑
      skull M86.58
      tarsus M86.57- ☑
      tibia M86.56- ☑
      toe M86.57- ☑
      ulna M86.53- ☑
      vertebra — *see* Osteomyelitis, vertebra
    humerus M86.62- ☑
    ilium M86.659
    ischium M86.659
    mandible M27.2
    metacarpus M86.64- ☑
    metatarsus M86.67- ☑
    multifocal — *see* Osteomyelitis, chronic,
      hematogenous, multifocal
    multiple sites M86.69
    neck M86.68
    orbit H05.02- ☑
    petrous bone — *see* Petrositis
    radius M86.63- ☑
    rib M86.68
    scapula M86.61- ☑
    skull M86.68
    tarsus M86.67- ☑
    tibia M86.66- ☑
    toe M86.67- ☑
    ulna M86.63- ☑
    vertebra — *see* Osteomyelitis, vertebra
  echinococcal B67.2
  Garr's — *see* Osteomyelitis, specified type NEC
  in diabetes mellitus — *see* E08-E13 with .69
  jaw (acute) (chronic) (lower) (neonatal) (suppurative)
    (upper) M27.2
  nonsuppurating — *see* Osteomyelitis, specified type
    NEC
  orbit H05.02- ☑
  petrous bone — *see* Petrositis
  Salmonella (arizonae) (cholerae-suis) (enteritidis) (ty-
    phimurium) A02.24
  sclerosing, nonsuppurative — *see* Osteomyelitis,
    specified type NEC
  specified type NEC — *see also* subcategory M86.8X- ☑
    mandible M27.2
    orbit H05.02- ☑
    petrous bone — *see* Petrositis
    vertebra — *see* Osteomyelitis, vertebra
  subacute M86.20
    carpus M86.24- ☑
    clavicle M86.21- ☑
    femur M86.25- ☑
    fibula M86.26- ☑
    finger M86.24- ☑
    humerus M86.22- ☑
    mandible M27.2
    metacarpus M86.24- ☑
    metatarsus M86.27- ☑
    multiple sites M86.29
    neck M86.28
    orbit H05.02- ☑
    petrous bone — *see* Petrositis
    radius M86.23- ☑
    rib M86.28
    scapula M86.21- ☑
    skull M86.28
    tarsus M86.27- ☑
    tibia M86.26- ☑

Osteomyelitis — *continued*
  subacute — *continued*
    toe M86.27- ☑
    ulna M86.23- ☑
    vertebra — *see* Osteomyelitis, vertebra
  syphilitic A52.77
    congenital (early) A50.02 *[M90.80]*
  tuberculous — *see* Tuberculosis, bone
  typhoid A01.05
  vertebra M46.20
    cervical region M46.22
    cervicothoracic region M46.23
    lumbar region M46.26
    lumbosacral region M46.27
    occipito-atlanto-axial region M46.21
    sacrococcygeal region M46.28
    thoracic region M46.24
    thoracolumbar region M46.25
Osteomyelofibrosis D47.4
Osteomyelosclerosis D75.89
Osteonecrosis M87.9
  due to
    drugs — *see* Osteonecrosis, secondary, due to, drugs
    trauma — *see* Osteonecrosis, secondary, due to, trauma
  idiopathic aseptic M87.00
    ankle M87.07- ☑
    carpus M87.03- ☑
    clavicle M87.01- ☑
    femur M87.05- ☑
    fibula M87.06- ☑
    finger M87.04- ☑
    humerus M87.02- ☑
    ilium M87.050
    ischium M87.050
    metacarpus M87.04- ☑
    metatarsus M87.07- ☑
    multiple sites M87.09
    neck M87.08
    pelvis M87.050
    radius M87.03- ☑
    rib M87.08
    scapula M87.01- ☑
    skull M87.08
    tarsus M87.07- ☑
    tibia M87.06- ☑
    toe M87.07- ☑
    ulna M87.03- ☑
    vertebra M87.08
  secondary NEC M87.30
    carpus M87.33- ☑
    clavicle M87.31- ☑
    due to
      drugs M87.10
        carpus M87.13- ☑
        clavicle M87.11- ☑
        femur M87.15- ☑
        fibula M87.16- ☑
        finger M87.14- ☑
        humerus M87.12- ☑
        ilium M87.159
        ischium M87.159
        jaw M87.180
        metacarpus M87.14- ☑
        metatarsus M87.17- ☑
        multiple sites M87.19
        neck M87.18
        radius M87.13- ☑
        rib M87.18
        scapula M87.11- ☑
        skull M87.18
        tarsus M87.17- ☑
        tibia M87.16- ☑
        toe M87.17- ☑
        ulna M87.13- ☑
        vertebra M87.18
      hemoglobinopathy NEC D58.2 *[M90.50]*
        carpus D58.2 *[M90.54-]* ☑
        clavicle D58.2 *[M90.51-]* ☑
        femur D58.2 *[M90.55-]* ☑
        fibula D58.2 *[M90.56-]* ☑
        finger D58.2 *[M90.54-]* ☑
        humerus D58.2 *[M90.52-]* ☑
        ilium D58.2 *[M90.55-]* ☑
        ischium D58.2 *[M90.55-]* ☑
        metacarpus D58.2 *[M90.54-]* ☑
        metatarsus D58.2 *[M90.57-]* ☑

Osteonecrosis — *continued*
  secondary — *continued*
    due to — *continued*
      hemoglobinopathy — *continued*
        multiple sites D58.2 *[M90.58]*
        neck D58.2 *[M90.58]*
        radius D58.2 *[M90.53-]* ☑
        rib D58.2 *[M90.58]*
        scapula D58.2 *[M90.51-]* ☑
        skull D58.2 *[M90.58]*
        tarsus D58.2 *[M90.57-]* ☑
        tibia D58.2 *[M90.56-]* ☑
        toe D58.2 *[M90.57-]* ☑
        ulna D58.2 *[M90.53-]* ☑
        vertebra D58.2 *[M90.58]*
      trauma (previous) M87.20
        carpus M87.23- ☑
        clavicle M87.21- ☑
        femur M87.25- ☑
        fibula M87.26- ☑
        finger M87.24- ☑
        humerus M87.22- ☑
        ilium M87.25- ☑
        ischium M87.25- ☑
        metacarpus M87.24- ☑
        metatarsus M87.27- ☑
        multiple sites M87.29
        neck M87.28
        radius M87.23- ☑
        rib M87.28
        scapula M87.21- ☑
        skull M87.28
        tarsus M87.27- ☑
        tibia M87.26- ☑
        toe M87.27- ☑
        ulna M87.23- ☑
        vertebra M87.28
    femur M87.35- ☑
    fibula M87.36- ☑
    finger M87.34- ☑
    humerus M87.32- ☑
    ilium M87.350
    in
      caisson disease T70.3 ☑ *[M90.50]*
        carpus T70.3 ☑ *[M90.54-]* ☑
        clavicle T70.3 ☑ *[M90.51-]* ☑
        femur T70.3 ☑ *[M90.55-]* ☑
        fibula T70.3 ☑ *[M90.56-]* ☑
        finger T70.3 ☑ *[M90.54-]* ☑
        humerus T70.3 ☑ *[M90.52-]* ☑
        ilium T70.3 ☑ *[M90.55-]* ☑
        ischium T70.3 ☑ *[M90.55-]* ☑
        metacarpus T70.3 ☑ *[M90.54-]* ☑
        metatarsus T70.3 ☑ *[M90.57-]* ☑
        multiple sites T70.3 ☑ *[M90.59]*
        neck T70.3 ☑ *[M90.58]*
        radius T70.3 ☑ *[M90.53-]* ☑
        rib T70.3 ☑ *[M90.58]*
        scapula T70.3 ☑ *[M90.51-]* ☑
        skull T70.3 ☑ *[M90.58]*
        tarsus T70.3 ☑ *[M90.57-]* ☑
        tibia T70.3 ☑ *[M90.56-]* ☑
        toe T70.3 ☑ *[M90.57-]* ☑
        ulna T70.3 ☑ *[M90.53-]* ☑
        vertebra T70.3 ☑ *[M90.58]*
    ischium M87.350
    metacarpus M87.34- ☑
    metatarsus M87.37- ☑
    multiple site M87.39
    neck M87.38
    radius M87.33- ☑
    rib M87.38
    scapula M87.319
    skull M87.38
    tarsus M87.379
    tibia M87.366
    toe M87.379
    ulna M87.33- ☑
    vertebra M87.38
  specified type NEC M87.80
    carpus M87.83- ☑
    clavicle M87.81- ☑
    femur M87.85- ☑
    fibula M87.86- ☑
    finger M87.84- ☑
    humerus M87.82- ☑

Osteonecrosis — *continued*
  specified type — *continued*
    ilium M87.85- ☑
    ischium M87.85- ☑
    metacarpus M87.84- ☑
    metatarsus M87.87- ☑
    multiple sites M87.89
    neck M87.88
    radius M87.83- ☑
    rib M87.88
    scapula M87.81- ☑
    skull M87.88
    tarsus M87.87- ☑
    tibia M87.86- ☑
    toe M87.87- ☑
    ulna M87.83- ☑
    vertebra M87.88
Osteo-onycho-arthro-dysplasia Q87.2
Osteo-onychodysplasia, hereditary Q87.2
Osteopathia condensans disseminata Q78.8
Osteopathy — *see also* Osteomyelitis, Osteonecrosis, Osteoporosis
  after poliomyelitis M89.60
    carpus M89.64- ☑
    clavicle M89.61- ☑
    femur M89.65- ☑
    fibula M89.66- ☑
    finger M89.64- ☑
    humerus M89.62- ☑
    ilium M89.659
    ischium M89.659
    metacarpus M89.64- ☑
    metatarsus M89.67- ☑
    multiple sites M89.69
    neck M89.68
    radius M89.63- ☑
    rib M89.68
    scapula M89.61- ☑
    skull M89.68
    tarsus M89.67- ☑
    tibia M89.66- ☑
    toe M89.67- ☑
    ulna M89.63- ☑
    vertebra M89.68
  in (due to)
    renal osteodystrophy N25.0
    specified diseases classified elsewhere — *see* sub-category M90.8 ☑
Osteopenia M85.8- ☑
  borderline M85.8- ☑
Osteoperiostitis — *see* Osteomyelitis, specified type NEC
Osteopetrosis (familial) Q78.2
Osteophyte M25.70
  ankle M25.77- ☑
  elbow M25.72- ☑
  foot joint M25.77- ☑
  hand joint M25.74- ☑
  hip M25.75- ☑
  knee M25.76- ☑
  shoulder M25.71- ☑
  spine M25.78
  vertebrae M25.78
  wrist M25.73- ☑
Osteopoikilosis Q78.8
Osteoporosis (female) (male) M81.0
  with current pathological fracture M80.00 ☑
  age-related M81.0
    with current pathologic fracture M80.00 ☑
      carpus M80.04- ☑
      clavicle M80.01- ☑
      fibula M80.06- ☑
      finger M80.04- ☑
      humerus M80.02- ☑
      ilium M80.05- ☑
      ischium M80.05- ☑
      metacarpus M80.04- ☑
      metatarsus M80.07- ☑
      pelvis M80.05- ☑
      radius M80.03- ☑
      scapula M80.01- ☑
      tarsus M80.07- ☑
      tibia M80.06- ☑
      toe M80.07- ☑
      ulna M80.03- ☑
      vertebra M80.08 ☑

☑ **Additional Character Required** — Refer to the Tabular List for Character Selection   ▽ **Subterms under main terms may continue to next column or page**

Osteoporosis — continued
  disuse M81.8
    with current pathological fracture M80.80 ☑
      carpus M80.84- ☑
      clavicle M80.81- ☑
      fibula M80.86- ☑
      finger M80.84- ☑
      humerus M80.82- ☑
      ilium M80.85- ☑
      ischium M80.85- ☑
      metacarpus M80.84- ☑
      metatarsus M80.87- ☑
      pelvis M80.85- ☑
      radius M80.83- ☑
      scapula M80.81- ☑
      tarsus M80.87- ☑
      tibia M80.86- ☑
      toe M80.87- ☑
      ulna M80.83- ☑
      vertebra M80.88 ☑
  drug-induced — see Osteoporosis, specified type NEC
  idiopathic — see Osteoporosis, specified type NEC
  involutional — see Osteoporosis, age-related
  Lequesne M81.6
  localized M81.6
  postmenopausal M81.0
    with pathological fracture M80.00 ☑
      carpus M80.04- ☑
      clavicle M80.01- ☑
      fibula M80.06- ☑
      finger M80.04- ☑
      humerus M80.02- ☑
      ilium M80.05- ☑
      ischium M80.05- ☑
      metacarpus M80.04- ☑
      metatarsus M80.07- ☑
      pelvis M80.05- ☑
      radius M80.03- ☑
      scapula M80.01- ☑
      tarsus M80.07- ☑
      tibia M80.06- ☑
      toe M80.07- ☑
      ulna M80.03- ☑
      vertebra M80.08 ☑
  postoophorectomy — see Osteoporosis, specified type NEC
  postsurgical malabsorption — see Osteoporosis, specified type NEC
  post-traumatic — see Osteoporosis, specified type NEC
  senile — see Osteoporosis, age-related
  specified type NEC M81.8
    with pathological fracture M80.80 ☑
      carpus M80.84- ☑
      clavicle M80.81- ☑
      fibula M80.86- ☑
      finger M80.84- ☑
      humerus M80.82- ☑
      ilium M80.85- ☑
      ischium M80.85- ☑
      metacarpus M80.84- ☑
      metatarsus M80.87- ☑
      pelvis M80.85- ☑
      radius M80.83- ☑
      scapula M80.81- ☑
      tarsus M80.87- ☑
      tibia M80.86- ☑
      toe M80.87- ☑
      ulna M80.83- ☑
      vertebra M80.88 ☑

Osteopsathyrosis (idiopathica) Q78.0
Osteoradionecrosis, jaw (acute) (chronic) (lower) (suppurative) (upper) M27.2
Osteosarcoma (any form) — see Neoplasm, bone, malignant
Osteosclerosis Q78.2
  acquired M85.8- ☑
  congenita Q77.4
  fragilitas (generalisata) Q78.2
  myelofibrosis D75.81
Osteosclerotic anemia D64.89
Osteosis
  cutis L94.2
  renal fibrocystic N25.0
Österreicher-Turner syndrome Q87.2
Ostium
  atrioventriculare commune Q21.2

Ostium — continued
  primum (arteriosum) (defect) (persistent) Q21.2
  secundum (arteriosum) (defect) (patent) (persistent) Q21.1
Ostrum-Furst syndrome Q75.8
Otalgia H92.0 ☑
Otitis (acute) H66.90
  with effusion — see also Otitis, media, nonsuppurative
    purulent — see Otitis, media, suppurative
  adhesive — see subcategory H74.1 ☑
  chronic — see also Otitis, media, chronic
    with effusion — see also Otitis, media, nonsuppurative, chronic
  externa H60.9- ☑
    abscess — see Abscess, ear, external
    acute (noninfective) H60.50- ☑
      actinic H60.51- ☑
      chemical H60.52- ☑
      contact H60.53- ☑
      eczematoid H60.54- ☑
      infective — see Otitis, externa, infective
      reactive H60.55- ☑
      specified NEC H60.59- ☑
    cellulitis — see Cellulitis, ear
    chronic H60.6- ☑
    diffuse — see Otitis, externa, infective, diffuse
    hemorrhagic — see Otitis, externa, infective, hemorrhagic
    in (due to)
      aspergillosis B44.89
      candidiasis B37.84
      erysipelas A46 [H62.40]
      herpes (simplex) virus infection B00.1
        zoster B02.8
      impetigo L01.00 [H62.40]
      infectious disease NEC B99 ☑ [H62.4-]
      mycosis NEC B36.9 [H62.40]
      parasitic disease NEC B89 [H62.40]
      viral disease NEC B34.9 [H62.40]
      zoster B02.8
    infective NEC H60.39- ☑
      abscess — see Abscess, ear, external
      cellulitis — see Cellulitis, ear
      diffuse H60.31- ☑
      hemorrhagic H60.32- ☑
      swimmer's ear — see Swimmer's, ear
    malignant H60.2- ☑
    mycotic NEC B36.9 [H62.40]
      in
        aspergillosis B44.89
        candidiasis B37.84
        moniliasis B37.84
    necrotizing — see Otitis, externa, malignant
    Pseudomonas aeruginosa — see Otitis, externa, malignant
    reactive — see Otitis, externa, acute, reactive
    specified NEC — see subcategory H60.8 ☑
    tropical NEC B36.9 [H62.40]
      in
        aspergillosis B44.89
        candidiasis B37.84
        moniliasis B37.84
  insidiosa — see Otosclerosis
  interna H83.0 ☑
  media (hemorrhagic) (staphylococcal) (streptococcal) H66.9- ☑
    with effusion (nonpurulent) — see Otitis, media, nonsuppurative
    acute, subacute H66.90
      allergic — see Otitis, media, nonsuppurative, acute, allergic
      exudative — see Otitis, media, nonsuppurative, acute
      mucoid — see Otitis, media, nonsuppurative, acute
      necrotizing — see also Otitis, media, suppurative, acute
        in
          measles B05.3
          scarlet fever A38.0
      nonsuppurative NEC — see Otitis, media, nonsuppurative, acute
      purulent — see Otitis, media, suppurative, acute
      sanguinous — see Otitis, media, nonsuppurative, acute
      secretory — see Otitis, media, nonsuppurative, acute, serous

Otitis — continued
  media — continued
    acute, subacute — continued
      seromucinous — see Otitis, media, nonsuppurative, acute
      serous — see Otitis, media, nonsuppurative, acute, serous
      suppurative — see Otitis, media, suppurative, acute
    allergic — see Otitis, media, nonsuppurative
    catarrhal — see Otitis, media, nonsuppurative
    chronic H66.90
      with effusion (nonpurulent) — see Otitis, media, nonsuppurative, chronic
      allergic — see Otitis, media, nonsuppurative, chronic, allergic
      benign suppurative — see Otitis, media, suppurative, chronic, tubotympanic
      catarrhal — see Otitis, media, nonsuppurative, chronic, serous
      exudative — see Otitis, media, nonsuppurative, chronic
      mucinous — see Otitis, media, nonsuppurative, chronic, mucoid
      mucoid — see Otitis, media, nonsuppurative, chronic, mucoid
      nonsuppurative NEC — see Otitis, media, nonsuppurative, chronic
      purulent — see Otitis, media, suppurative, chronic
      secretory — see Otitis, media, nonsuppurative, chronic, mucoid
      seromucinous — see Otitis, media, nonsuppurative, chronic
      serous — see Otitis, media, nonsuppurative, chronic, serous
      suppurative — see Otitis, media, suppurative, chronic
      transudative — see Otitis, media, nonsuppurative, chronic, mucoid
    exudative — see Otitis, media, suppurative
    in (due to) (with)
      influenza — see Influenza, with, otitis media
      measles B05.3
      scarlet fever A38.0
      tuberculosis A18.6
      viral disease NEC B34.- ☑ [H67.-] ☑
    mucoid — see Otitis, media, nonsuppurative
    nonsuppurative H65.9- ☑
      acute or subacute NEC H65.19- ☑
        allergic H65.11- ☑
          recurrent H65.11- ☑
        recurrent H65.19- ☑
        secretory — see Otitis, media, nonsuppurative, serous
        serous H65.0- ☑
          recurrent H65.0- ☑
      chronic H65.49- ☑
        allergic H65.41- ☑
        mucoid H65.3- ☑
        serous H65.2- ☑
    postmeasles B05.3
    purulent — see Otitis, media, suppurative
    secretory — see Otitis, media, nonsuppurative
    seromucinous — see Otitis, media, nonsuppurative
    serous — see Otitis, media, nonsuppurative
    suppurative H66.4- ☑
      acute H66.00- ☑
        with rupture of ear drum H66.01- ☑
        recurrent H66.00- ☑
          with rupture of ear drum H66.01- ☑
      chronic — see also subcategory H66.3 ☑
        atticoantral H66.2- ☑
        benign — see Otitis, media, suppurative, chronic, tubotympanic
        tubotympanic H66.1- ☑
    transudative — see Otitis, media, nonsuppurative
    tuberculous A18.6
Otocephaly Q18.2
Otolith syndrome — see subcategory H81.8 ☑
Otomycosis (diffuse) NEC B36.9 [H62.40]
  in
    aspergillosis B44.89
    candidiasis B37.84
    moniliasis B37.84
Otoporosis — see Otosclerosis
Otorrhagia (nontraumatic) H92.2- ☑

Otorrhagia — *continued*
  traumatic — *code by* Type of injury
Otorrhea H92.1- ☑
  cerebrospinal G96.0
Otosclerosis (general) H80.9- ☑
  cochlear (endosteal) H80.2- ☑
  involving
    otic capsule — *see* Otosclerosis, cochlear
    oval window
      nonobliterative H80.0- ☑
      obliterative H80.1- ☑
    round window — *see* Otosclerosis, cochlear
  nonobliterative — *see* Otosclerosis, involving, oval window, nonobliterative
  obliterative — *see* Otosclerosis, involving, oval window, obliterative
  specified NEC H80.8- ☑
Otospongiosis — *see* Otosclerosis
Otto's disease or pelvis M24.7
Outcome of delivery Z37.9
  multiple births Z37.9
    all liveborn Z37.50
      quadruplets Z37.52
      quintuplets Z37.53
      sextuplets Z37.54
      specified number NEC Z37.59
      triplets Z37.51
    all stillborn Z37.7
    some liveborn Z37.60
      quadruplets Z37.62
      quintuplets Z37.63
      sextuplets Z37.64
      specified number NEC Z37.69
      triplets Z37.61
  single NEC Z37.9
    liveborn Z37.0
    stillborn Z37.1
  twins NEC Z37.9
    both liveborn Z37.2
    both stillborn Z37.4
    one liveborn, one stillborn Z37.3
Outlet — *see* condition
Ovalocytosis (congenital) (hereditary) — *see* Elliptocytosis
Ovarian — *see* Condition
Ovariocele N83.4- ☑
Ovaritis (cystic) — *see* Oophoritis
Ovary, ovarian — *see also* condition
  resistant syndrome E28.39
  vein syndrome N13.8
Overactive — *see also* Hyperfunction
  adrenal cortex NEC E27.0
  bladder N32.81
  hypothalamus E23.3
  thyroid — *see* Hyperthyroidism
Overactivity R46.3
  child — *see* Disorder, attention-deficit hyperactivity
Overbite (deep) (excessive) (horizontal) (vertical) M26.29
Overbreathing — *see* Hyperventilation
Overconscientious personality F60.5
Overdevelopment — *see* Hypertrophy
Overdistension — *see* Distension
Overdose, overdosage (drug) — *see* Table of Drugs and Chemicals, by drug, poisoning
Overeating R63.2
  nonorganic origin F50.89
  psychogenic F50.89
Overexertion (effects) (exhaustion) T73.3 ☑
Overexposure (effects) T73.9 ☑
  exhaustion T73.2 ☑
Overfeeding — *see* Overeating
  newborn P92.4
Overfill, endodontic M27.52
Overgrowth, bone — *see* Hypertrophy, bone
Overhanging of dental restorative material (unrepairable) K08.52
Overheated (places) (effects) — *see* Heat
Overjet (excessive horizontal) M26.23
Overlaid, overlying (suffocation) — *see* Asphyxia, traumatic, due to mechanical threat
Overlap, excessive horizontal (teeth) M26.23
Overlapping toe (acquired) — *see also* Deformity, toe, specified NEC
  congenital (fifth toe) Q66.89
Overload
  circulatory, due to transfusion (blood) (blood components) (TACO) E87.71

Overload — *continued*
  fluid E87.70
    due to transfusion (blood) (blood components) E87.71
    specified NEC E87.79
  iron, due to repeated red blood cell transfusions E83.111
  potassium (K) E87.5
  sodium (Na) E87.0
Overnutrition — *see* Hyperalimentation
Overproduction — *see also* Hypersecretion
  ACTH E27.0
  catecholamine E27.5
  growth hormone E22.0
Overprotection, child by parent Z62.1
Overriding
  aorta Q25.49
  finger (acquired) — *see* Deformity, finger
    congenital Q68.1
  toe (acquired) — *see also* Deformity, toe, specified NEC
    congenital Q66.89
Overstrained R53.83
  heart — *see* Hypertrophy, cardiac
Overuse, muscle NEC M70.8- ☑
Overweight E66.3
Overworked R53.83
Oviduct — *see* condition
Ovotestis Q56.0
Ovulation (cycle)
  failure or lack of N97.0
  pain N94.0
Ovum — *see* condition
Owren's disease or syndrome (parahemophilia) D68.2
Ox heart — *see* Hypertrophy, cardiac
Oxalosis E72.53
Oxaluria E72.53
Oxycephaly, oxycephalic Q75.0
  syphilitic, congenital A50.02
Oxyuriasis B80
Oxyuris vermicularis (infestation) B80
Ozena J31.0

P

Pachyderma, pachydermia L85.9
  larynx (verrucosa) J38.7
Pachydermatocele (congenital) Q82.8
Pachydermoperiostosis — *see also* Osteoarthropathy, hypertrophic, specified type NEC
  clubbed nail M89.40 [L62]
Pachygyria Q04.3
Pachymeningitis (adhesive) (basal) (brain) (cervical) (chronic)(circumscribed) (external) (fibrous) (hemorrhagic) (hypertrophic) (internal) (purulent) (spinal) (suppurative) — *see* Meningitis
Pachyonychia (congenital) Q84.5
Pacinian tumor — *see* Neoplasm, skin, benign
Pad, knuckle or Garrod's M72.1
Paget's disease
  with infiltrating duct carcinoma — *see* Neoplasm, breast, malignant
  bone M88.9
    carpus M88.84- ☑
    clavicle M88.81- ☑
    femur M88.85- ☑
    fibula M88.86- ☑
    finger M88.84- ☑
    humerus M88.82- ☑
    ilium M88.85- ☑
    in neoplastic disease — *see* Osteitis, deformans, in neoplastic disease
    ischium M88.85- ☑
    metacarpus M88.84- ☑
    metatarsus M88.87- ☑
    multiple sites M88.89
    neck M88.88
    radius M88.83- ☑
    rib M88.88
    scapula M88.81- ☑
    skull M88.0
    specified NEC M88.88
    tarsus M88.87- ☑
    tibia M88.86- ☑
    toe M88.87- ☑
    ulna M88.83- ☑
    vertebra M88.1
  breast (female) C50.01- ☑

Paget's disease — *continued*
  breast — *continued*
    male C50.02- ☑
  extramammary — *see also* Neoplasm, skin, malignant
    anus C21.0
      margin C44.590
      skin C44.590
  intraductal carcinoma — *see* Neoplasm, breast, malignant
  malignant — *see* Neoplasm, skin, malignant
    breast (female) C50.01- ☑
      male C50.02- ☑
    unspecified site (female) C50.01- ☑
      male C50.02- ☑
  mammary — *see* Paget's disease, breast
  nipple — *see* Paget's disease, breast
  osteitis deformans — *see* Paget's disease, bone
Paget-Schroetter syndrome I82.890
Pain(s) — *see also* Painful R52
  abdominal R10.9
    colic R10.83
    generalized R10.84
      with acute abdomen R10.0
    lower R10.30
      left quadrant R10.32
      pelvic or perineal R10.2
      periumbilical R10.33
      right quadrant R10.31
    rebound — *see* Tenderness, abdominal, rebound
    severe with abdominal rigidity R10.0
    tenderness — *see* Tenderness, abdominal
    upper R10.10
      epigastric R10.13
      left quadrant R10.12
      right quadrant R10.11
  acute R52
    due to trauma G89.11
    neoplasm related G89.3
    postprocedural NEC G89.18
    post-thoracotomy G89.12
    specified by site — *code to* Pain, by site
  adnexa (uteri) R10.2
  anginoid — *see* Pain, precordial
  anus K62.89
  arm — *see* Pain, limb, upper
  axillary (axilla) M79.62- ☑
  back (postural) M54.9
  bladder R39.89
    associated with micturition — *see* Micturition, painful
    chronic R39.82
  bone — *see* Disorder, bone, specified type NEC
  breast N64.4
  broad ligament R10.2
  cancer associated (acute) (chronic) G89.3
  cecum — *see* Pain, abdominal
  cervicobrachial M53.1
  chest (central) R07.9
    anterior wall R07.89
    atypical R07.89
    ischemic I20.9
    musculoskeletal R07.89
    non-cardiac R07.89
    on breathing R07.1
    pleurodynia R07.81
    precordial R07.2
    wall (anterior) R07.89
  chronic G89.29
    associated with significant psychosocial dysfunction G89.4
    due to trauma G89.21
    neoplasm related G89.3
    postoperative NEC G89.28
    postprocedural NEC G89.28
    post-thoracotomy G89.22
    specified NEC G89.29
  coccyx M53.3
  colon — *see* Pain, abdominal
  coronary — *see* Angina
  costochondral R07.1
  diaphragm R07.1
  due to cancer G89.3
  due to device, implant or graft — *see also* Complications, by site and type, specified NEC T85.848 ☑
    arterial graft NEC T82.848 ☑
    breast (implant) T85.848 ☑
    catheter NEC T85.848 ☑
      dialysis (renal) T82.848 ☑

Pain(s) — *continued*
- due to device, implant or graft — *see also* Complications, by site and type, specified — *continued*
  - catheter — *continued*
    - dialysis — *continued*
      - intraperitoneal T85.848 ☑
    - infusion NEC T82.848 ☑
      - spinal (epidural) (subdural) T85.840 ☑
    - urinary (indwelling) T83.84 ☑
  - electronic (electrode) (pulse generator) (stimulator)
    - bone T85.840 ☑
    - cardiac T82.847 ☑
    - nervous system (brain) (peripheral nerve) (spinal) T85.84 ☑
    - urinary T83.84 ☑
  - fixation, internal (orthopedic) NEC T84.84 ☑
  - gastrointestinal (bile duct) (esophagus) T85.848 ☑
  - genital NEC T83.84 ☑
  - heart NEC T82.847 ☑
  - infusion NEC T85.848 ☑
  - joint prosthesis T84.84 ☑
  - ocular (corneal graft) (orbital implant) NEC T85.848 ☑
  - orthopedic NEC T84.84 ☑
  - specified NEC T85.848 ☑
  - urinary NEC T83.84 ☑
  - vascular NEC T82.848 ☑
  - ventricular intracranial shunt T85.840 ☑
- due to malignancy (primary) (secondary) G89.3
- ear — *see* subcategory H92.0 ☑
- epigastric, epigastrium R10.13
- eye — *see* Pain, ocular
- face, facial R51
  - atypical G50.1
- female genital organs NEC N94.89
- finger — *see* Pain, limb, upper
- flank — *see* Pain, abdominal
- foot — *see* Pain, limb, lower
- gallbladder K82.9
- gas (intestinal) R14.1
- gastric — *see* Pain, abdominal
- generalized NOS R52
- genital organ
  - female N94.89
  - male N50.89
- groin — *see* Pain, abdominal, lower
- hand — *see* Pain, limb, upper
- head — *see* Headache
- heart — *see* Pain, precordial
- infra-orbital — *see* Neuralgia, trigeminal
- intercostal R07.82
- intermenstrual N94.0
- jaw R68.84
- joint M25.50
  - ankle M25.57- ☑
  - elbow M25.52- ☑
  - finger M25.54- ☑
  - foot M25.57- ☑
  - hand M25.54- ☑
  - hip M25.55- ☑
  - knee M25.56- ☑
  - shoulder M25.51- ☑
  - toe M25.57- ☑
  - wrist M25.53- ☑
- kidney N23
- laryngeal R07.0
- leg — *see* Pain, limb, lower
- limb M79.609
  - lower M79.60- ☑
    - foot M79.67- ☑
    - lower leg M79.66- ☑
    - thigh M79.65- ☑
    - toe M79.67- ☑
  - upper M79.60- ☑
    - axilla M79.62- ☑
    - finger M79.64- ☑
    - forearm M79.63- ☑
    - hand M79.64- ☑
    - upper arm M79.62- ☑
- loin M54.5
- low back M54.5
- lumbar region M54.5
- mandibular R68.84
- mastoid — *see* subcategory H92.0 ☑
- maxilla R68.84
- menstrual — *see also* Dysmenorrhea N94.6
- metacarpophalangeal (joint) — *see* Pain, joint, hand

Pain(s) — *continued*
- metatarsophalangeal (joint) — *see* Pain, joint, foot
- mouth K13.79
- muscle — *see* Myalgia
- musculoskeletal — *see also* Pain, by site M79.18
- myofascial M79.18
- nasal J34.89
- nasopharynx J39.2
- neck NEC M54.2
- nerve NEC — *see* Neuralgia
- neuromuscular — *see* Neuralgia
- nose J34.89
- ocular H57.1- ☑
- ophthalmic — *see* Pain, ocular
- orbital region — *see* Pain, ocular
- ovary N94.89
- over heart — *see* Pain, precordial
- ovulation N94.0
- pelvic (female) R10.2
- penis N48.89
- pericardial — *see* Pain, precordial
- perineal, perineum R10.2
- pharynx J39.2
- pleura, pleural, pleuritic R07.81
- postoperative NOS G89.18
- postprocedural NOS G89.18
- post-thoracotomy G89.12
- precordial (region) R07.2
- premenstrual N94.3
- psychogenic (persistent) (any site) F45.41
- radicular (spinal) — *see* Radiculopathy
- rectum K62.89
- respiration R07.1
- retrosternal R07.2
- rheumatoid, muscular — *see* Myalgia
- rib R07.81
- root (spinal) — *see* Radiculopathy
- round ligament (stretch) R10.2
- sacroiliac M53.3
- sciatic — *see* Sciatica
- scrotum N50.82
- seminal vesicle N50.89
- shoulder M25.51- ☑
- spermatic cord N50.89
- spinal root — *see* Radiculopathy
- spine M54.9
  - cervical M54.2
  - low back M54.5
    - with sciatica M54.4- ☑
  - thoracic M54.6
- stomach — *see* Pain, abdominal
- substernal R07.2
- temporomandibular (joint) M26.62- ☑
- testis N50.81- ☑
- thoracic spine M54.6
  - with radicular and visceral pain M54.14
- throat R07.0
- tibia — *see* Pain, limb, lower
- toe — *see* Pain, limb, lower
- tongue K14.6
- tooth K08.89
- trigeminal — *see* Neuralgia, trigeminal
- tumor associated G89.3
- ureter N23
- urinary (organ) (system) N23
- uterus NEC N94.89
- vagina R10.2
- vertebrogenic (syndrome) M54.89
- vesical R39.89
  - associated with micturition — *see* Micturition, painful
- vulva R10.2

Painful — *see also* Pain
- coitus
  - female N94.10
  - male N53.12
  - psychogenic F52.6
- ejaculation (semen) N53.12
  - psychogenic F52.6
- erection — *see* Priapism
- feet syndrome E53.8
- joint replacement (hip) (knee) T84.84 ☑
- menstruation — *see* Dysmenorrhea
  - psychogenic F45.8
- micturition — *see* Micturition, painful
- respiration R07.1
- scar NEC L90.5
- wire sutures T81.89 ☑

Painter's colic — *see* subcategory T56.0 ☑
Palate — *see* condition
Palatoplegia K13.79
Palatoschisis — *see* Cleft, palate
Palilalia R48.8
Palliative care Z51.5
Pallor R23.1
- optic disc, temporal — *see* Atrophy, optic
Palmar — *see also* condition
- fascia — *see* condition
Palpable
- cecum K63.89
- kidney N28.89
- ovary N83.8
- prostate N42.9
- spleen — *see* Splenomegaly
Palpitations (heart) R00.2
- psychogenic F45.8
Palsy — *see also* Paralysis G83.9
- atrophic diffuse (progressive) G12.22
- Bell's — *see also* Palsy, facial
  - newborn P11.3
- brachial plexus NEC G54.0
  - newborn (birth injury) P14.3
- brain — *see* Palsy, cerebral
- bulbar (progressive) (chronic) G12.22
  - of childhood (Fazio-Londe) G12.1
  - pseudo NEC G12.29
  - supranuclear (progressive) G23.1
- cerebral (congenital) G80.9
  - ataxic G80.4
  - athetoid G80.3
  - choreathetoid G80.3
  - diplegic G80.8
    - spastic G80.1
  - dyskinetic G80.3
    - athetoid G80.3
    - choreathetoid G80.3
    - distonic G80.3
  - dystonic G80.3
  - hemiplegic G80.8
    - spastic G80.2
  - mixed G80.8
  - monoplegic G80.8
    - spastic G80.1
  - paraplegic G80.8
    - spastic G80.1
  - quadriplegic G80.8
    - spastic G80.0
  - spastic G80.1
    - diplegic G80.1
    - hemiplegic G80.2
    - monoplegic G80.1
    - quadriplegic G80.0
    - specified NEC G80.1
    - tetrapelgic G80.0
  - specified NEC G80.8
  - syphilitic A52.12
    - congenital A50.49
  - tetraplegic G80.8
    - spastic G80.0
- cranial nerve — *see also* Disorder, nerve, cranial
  - multiple G52.7
  - in
    - infectious disease B99 ☑ *[G53]*
    - neoplastic disease — *see also* Neoplasm D49.9 *[G53]*
    - parasitic disease B89 *[G53]*
    - sarcoidosis D86.82
- creeping G12.22
- diver's T70.3 ☑
- Erb's P14.0
- facial G51.0
  - newborn (birth injury) P11.3
- glossopharyngeal G52.1
- Klumpke (-Déjérine) P14.1
- lead — *see* subcategory T56.0 ☑
- median nerve (tardy) G56.1- ☑
- nerve G58.9
  - specified NEC G58.8
- peroneal nerve (acute) (tardy) G57.3- ☑
- progressive supranuclear G23.1
- pseudobulbar NEC G12.29
- radial nerve (acute) G56.3- ☑
- seventh nerve — *see also* Palsy, facial
  - newborn P11.3
- shaking — *see* Parkinsonism
- spastic (cerebral) (spinal) G80.1

Palsy — *continued*
   ulnar nerve (tardy) G56.2- ☑
   wasting G12.29
Paludism — *see* Malaria
Panangiitis M30.0
Panaris, panaritium — *see also* Cellulitis, digit
   with lymphangitis — *see* Lymphangitis, acute, digit
Panarteritis nodosa M30.0
   brain or cerebral I67.7
Pancake heart R93.1
   with cor pulmonale (chronic) I27.81
Pancarditis (acute) (chronic) I51.89
   rheumatic I09.89
    active or acute I01.8
Pancoast's syndrome or tumor C34.1- ☑
Pancolitis, ulcerative (chronic) K51.00
   with
    abscess K51.014
    complication K51.019
    fistula K51.013
    obstruction K51.012
    rectal bleeding K51.011
    specified complication NEC K51.018
Pancreas, pancreatic — *see* condition
Pancreatitis (annular) (apoplectic) (calcareous) (edematous) (hemorrhagic) (malignant) (recurrent) (subacute) (suppurative) K85.90
   with necrosis (uninfected) K85.91
    infected K85.92
   acute (without necrosis or infection) K85.90
    with necrosis (uninfected) K85.91
     infected K85.92
    alcohol induced (without necrosis or infection) K85.20
     with necrosis (uninfected) K85.21
      infected K85.22
    biliary (without necrosis or infection) K85.10
     with necrosis (uninfected) K85.11
      infected K85.12
    drug induced (without necrosis or infection) K85.30
     with necrosis (uninfected) K85.31
      infected K85.32
    gallstone (without necrosis or infection) K85.10
     with necrosis (uninfected) K85.11
      infected K85.12
    idiopathic (without necrosis or infection) K85.00
     with necrosis (uninfected) K85.01
      infected K85.02
    specified NEC (without necrosis or infection) K85.80
     with necrosis (uninfected) K85.81
      infected K85.82
   chronic (infectious) K86.1
    alcohol-induced K86.0
    recurrent K86.1
    relapsing K86.1
   cystic (chronic) K86.1
   cytomegaloviral B25.2
   fibrous (chronic) K86.1
   gallstone (without necrosis or infection) K85.10
    with necrosis (uninfected) K85.11
     infected K85.12
   gangrenous — *see* Pancreatitis, acute
   interstitial (chronic) K86.1
    acute — *see also* Pancreatitis, acute K85.80
   mumps B26.3
   recurrent (chronic) K86.1
   relapsing, chronic K86.1
   syphilitic A52.74
Pancreatoblastoma — *see* Neoplasm, pancreas, malignant
Pancreolithiasis K86.89
Pancytolysis D75.89
Pancytopenia (acquired) D61.818
   with
    malformations D61.09
    myelodysplastic syndrome — *see* Syndrome, myelodysplastic
   antineoplastic chemotherapy induced D61.810
   congenital D61.09
   drug-induced NEC D61.811
PANDAS (pediatric autoimmune neuropsychiatric disorders associated with streptococcal infections syndrome) D89.89
Panencephalitis, subacute, sclerosing A81.1
Panhematopenia D61.9
   congenital D61.09
   constitutional D61.09
   splenic, primary D73.1

Panhemocytopenia D61.9
   congenital D61.09
   constitutional D61.09
Panhypogonadism E29.1
Panhypopituitarism E23.0
   prepubertal E23.0
Panic (attack) (state) F41.0
   reaction to exceptional stress (transient) F43.0
Panmyelopathy, familial, constitutional D61.09
Panmyelophthisis D61.82
   congenital D61.09
Panmyelosis (acute) (with myelofibrosis) C94.4- ☑
Panner's disease — *see* Osteochondrosis, juvenile, humerus
Panneuritis endemica E51.11
Panniculitis (nodular) (nonsuppurative) M79.3
   back M54.00
    cervical region M54.02
    cervicothoracic region M54.03
    lumbar region M54.06
    lumbosacral region M54.07
    multiple sites M54.09
    occipito-atlanto-axial region M54.01
    sacrococcygeal region M54.08
    thoracic region M54.04
    thoracolumbar region M54.05
   lupus L93.2
   mesenteric K65.4
   neck M54.02
    cervicothoracic region M54.03
    occipito-atlanto-axial region M54.01
   relapsing M35.6
Panniculus adiposus (abdominal) E65
Pannus (allergic) (cornea) (degenerativus) (keratic) H16.42- ☑
   abdominal (symptomatic) E65
   trachomatosus, trachomatous (active) A71.1
Panophthalmitis H44.01- ☑
Pansinusitis (chronic) (hyperplastic) (nonpurulent) (purulent) J32.4
   acute J01.40
    recurrent J01.41
   tuberculous A15.8
Panuveitis (sympathetic) H44.11- ☑
Panvalvular disease I08.9
   specified NEC I08.8
PAPA (pyogenic arthritis, pyoderma gangrenosum, and acne syndrome) M04.8
Papanicolaou smear, cervix Z12.4
   as part of routine gynecological examination Z01.419
    with abnormal findings Z01.411
   for suspected neoplasm Z12.4
   nonspecific abnormal finding R87.619
   routine Z01.419
    with abnormal findings Z01.411
Papilledema (choked disc) H47.10
   associated with
    decreased ocular pressure H47.12
    increased intracranial pressure H47.11
    retinal disorder H47.13
   Foster-Kennedy syndrome H47.14- ☑
Papillitis H46.00
   anus K62.89
   chronic lingual K14.4
   necrotizing, kidney N17.2
   optic H46.0- ☑
   rectum K62.89
   renal, necrotizing N17.2
   tongue K14.0
Papilloma — *see also* Neoplasm, benign, by site
   acuminatum (female) (male) (anogenital) A63.0
   basal cell L82.1
    inflamed L82.0
   benign pinta (primary) A67.0
   bladder (urinary) (transitional cell) D41.4
   choroid plexus (lateral ventricle) (third ventricle) D33.0
    anaplastic C71.5
    fourth ventricle D33.1
    malignant C71.5
   renal pelvis (transitional cell) D41.1- ☑
    benign D30.1- ☑
   Schneiderian
    specified site — *see* Neoplasm, benign, by site
    unspecified site D14.0
   serous surface
    borderline malignancy
     specified site — *see* Neoplasm, uncertain behavior, by site

Papilloma — *continued*
   serous surface — *continued*
    borderline malignancy — *continued*
     unspecified site D39.10
    specified site — *see* Neoplasm, benign, by site
    unspecified site D27.9
   transitional (cell)
    bladder (urinary) D41.4
    inverted type — *see* Neoplasm, uncertain behavior, by site
    renal pelvis D41.1- ☑
    ureter D41.2- ☑
   ureter (transitional cell) D41.2- ☑
    benign D30.2- ☑
   urothelial — *see* Neoplasm, uncertain behavior, by site
   villous — *see* Neoplasm, uncertain behavior, by site
    adenocarcinoma in — *see* Neoplasm, malignant, by site
    in situ — *see* Neoplasm, in situ
   yaws, plantar or palmar A66.1
Papillomata, multiple, of yaws A66.1
Papillomatosis — *see also* Neoplasm, benign, by site
   confluent and reticulated L83
   cystic, breast — *see* Mastopathy, cystic
   ductal, breast — *see* Mastopathy, cystic
   intraductal (diffuse) — *see* Neoplasm, benign, by site
   subareolar duct D24- ☑
Papillomavirus, as cause of disease classified elsewhere B97.7
Papillon-Léage and Psaume syndrome Q87.0
Papule(s) R23.8
   carate (primary) A67.0
   fibrous, of nose D22.39
   Gottron's L94.4
   pinta (primary) A67.0
Papulosis
   lymphomatoid C86.6
   malignant I77.89
Papyraceous fetus O31.0- ☑
Para-albuminemia E88.09
Paracephalus Q89.7
Parachute mitral valve Q23.2
Paracoccidioidomycosis B41.9
   disseminated B41.7
   generalized B41.7
   mucocutaneous-lymphangitic B41.8
   pulmonary B41.0
   specified NEC B41.8
   visceral B41.8
Paradentosis K05.4
Paraffinoma T88.8 ☑
Paraganglioma D44.7
   adrenal D35.0- ☑
    malignant C74.1- ☑
   aortic body D44.7
    malignant C75.5
   carotid body D44.6
    malignant C75.4
   chromaffin — *see also* Neoplasm, benign, by site
    malignant — *see* Neoplasm, malignant, by site
   extra-adrenal D44.7
    malignant C75.5
     specified site — *see* Neoplasm, malignant, by site
     unspecified site C75.5
    specified site — *see* Neoplasm, uncertain behavior, by site
    unspecified site D44.7
   gangliocytic D13.2
    specified site — *see* Neoplasm, benign, by site
    unspecified site D13.2
   glomus jugulare D44.7
    malignant C75.5
   jugular D44.7
   malignant C75.5
    specified site — *see* Neoplasm, malignant, by site
    unspecified site C75.5
   nonchromaffin D44.7
    malignant C75.5
     specified site — *see* Neoplasm, malignant, by site
     unspecified site C75.5
    specified site — *see* Neoplasm, uncertain behavior, by site
    unspecified site D44.7
   parasympathetic D44.7

☑ Additional Character Required — Refer to the Tabular List for Character Selection   ▽ Subterms under main terms may continue to next column or page

Paraganglioma — *continued*
  parasympathetic — *continued*
    specified site — *see* Neoplasm, uncertain behavior, by site
    unspecified site D44.7
  specified site — *see* Neoplasm, uncertain behavior, by site
  sympathetic D44.7
    specified site — *see* Neoplasm, uncertain behavior, by site
    unspecified site D44.7
  unspecified site D44.7
Parageusia R43.2
  psychogenic F45.8
Paragonimiasis B66.4
Paragranuloma, Hodgkin — *see* Lymphoma, Hodgkin, specified NEC
Parahemophilia — *see also* Defect, coagulation D68.2
Parakeratosis R23.4
  variegata L41.0
Paralysis, paralytic (complete) (incomplete) G83.9
  with
    syphilis A52.17
  abducens, abducent (nerve) — *see* Strabismus, paralytic, sixth nerve
  abductor, lower extremity G57.9- ☑
  accessory nerve G52.8
  accommodation — *see also* Paresis, of accommodation
    hysterical F44.89
  acoustic nerve (except Deafness) H93.3 ☑
  agitans — *see also* Parkinsonism G20
    arteriosclerotic G21.4
  alternating (oculomotor) G83.89
  amyotrophic G12.21
  ankle G57.9- ☑
  anus (sphincter) K62.89
  arm — *see* Monoplegia, upper limb
  ascending (spinal), acute G61.0
  association G12.29
  asthenic bulbar G70.00
    with exacerbation (acute) G70.01
    in crisis G70.01
  ataxic (hereditary) G11.9
    general (syphilitic) A52.17
  atrophic G58.9
    infantile, acute — *see* Poliomyelitis, paralytic
    progressive G12.22
    spinal (acute) — *see* Poliomyelitis, paralytic
  axillary G54.0
  Babinski-Nageotte's G83.89
  Bell's G51.0
    newborn P11.3
  Benedikt's G46.3
  birth injury P14.9
    spinal cord P11.5
  bladder (neurogenic) (sphincter) N31.2
  bowel, colon or intestine K56.0
  brachial plexus G54.0
    birth injury P14.3
    newborn (birth injury) P14.3
  brain G83.9
    diplegia G83.0
    triplegia G83.89
  bronchial J98.09
  Brown-Séquard G83.81
  bulbar (chronic) (progressive) G12.22
    infantile — *see* Poliomyelitis, paralytic
    poliomyelitic — *see* Poliomyelitis, paralytic
    pseudo G12.29
  bulbospinal G70.00
    with exacerbation (acute) G70.01
    in crisis G70.01
  cardiac — *see also* Failure, heart I50.9
  cerebrocerebellar, diplegic G80.1
  cervical
    plexus G54.2
    sympathetic G90.09
  Céstan-Chenais G46.3
  Charcot-Marie-Tooth type G60.0
  Clark's G80.9
  colon K56.0
  compressed air T70.3 ☑
  compression
    arm G56.9- ☑
    leg G57.9- ☑
    lower extremity G57.9- ☑
    upper extremity G56.9- ☑
  congenital (cerebral) — *see* Palsy, cerebral

Paralysis, paralytic — *continued*
  conjugate movement (gaze) (of eye) H51.0
    cortical (nuclear) (supranuclear) H51.0
  cordis — *see* Failure, heart
  cranial or cerebral nerve G52.9
  creeping G12.22
  crossed leg G83.89
  crutch — *see* Injury, brachial plexus
  deglutition R13.0
    hysterical F44.4
  dementia A52.17
  descending (spinal) NEC G12.29
  diaphragm (flaccid) J98.6
    due to accidental dissection of phrenic nerve during procedure — *see* Puncture, accidental complicating surgery
  digestive organs NEC K59.8
  diplegic — *see* Diplegia
  divergence (nuclear) H51.8
  diver's T70.3 ☑
  Duchenne's
    birth injury P14.0
    due to or associated with
      motor neuron disease G12.22
      muscular dystrophy G71.01
  due to intracranial or spinal birth injury — *see* Palsy, cerebral
  embolic (current episode) I63.4- ☑
  Erb (-Duchenne) (birth) (newborn) P14.0
  Erb's syphilitic spastic spinal A52.17
  esophagus K22.8
  eye muscle (extrinsic) H49.9
    intrinsic — *see also* Paresis, of accommodation
  facial (nerve) G51.0
    birth injury P11.3
    congenital P11.3
    following operation NEC — *see* Puncture, accidental complicating surgery
    newborn (birth injury) P11.3
  familial (recurrent) (periodic) G72.3
    spastic G11.4
  fauces J39.2
  finger G56.9- ☑
  gait R26.1
  gastric nerve (nondiabetic) G52.2
  gaze, conjugate H51.0
  general (progressive) (syphilitic) A52.17
    juvenile A50.45
  glottis J38.00
    bilateral J38.02
    unilateral J38.01
  gluteal G54.1
  Gubler (-Millard) G46.3
  hand — *see* Monoplegia, upper limb
  heart — *see* Arrest, cardiac
  hemiplegic — *see* Hemiplegia
  hyperkalemic periodic (familial) G72.3
  hypoglossal (nerve) G52.3
  hypokalemic periodic G72.3
  hysterical F44.4
  ileus K56.0
  infantile — *see also* Poliomyelitis, paralytic A80.30
    bulbar — *see* Poliomyelitis, paralytic
    cerebral — *see* Palsy, cerebral
    spastic — *see* Palsy, cerebral, spastic
  infective — *see* Poliomyelitis, paralytic
  inferior nuclear G83.9
  internuclear — *see* Ophthalmoplegia, internuclear
  intestine K56.0
  iris H57.09
    due to diphtheria (toxin) A36.89
  ischemic, Volkmann's (complicating trauma) T79.6 ☑
  Jackson's G83.89
  jake — *see* Poisoning, food, noxious, plant
  Jamaica ginger (jake) G62.2
  juvenile general A50.45
  Klumpke (-Déjérine) (birth) (newborn) P14.1
  labioglossal (laryngeal) (pharyngeal) G12.29
  Landry's G61.0
  laryngeal nerve (recurrent) (superior) (unilateral) J38.00
    bilateral J38.02
    unilateral J38.01
  larynx J38.00
    bilateral J38.02
    due to diphtheria (toxin) A36.2
    unilateral J38.01
  lateral G12.23
  lead T56.0 ☑

Paralysis, paralytic — *continued*
  left side — *see* Hemiplegia
  leg G83.1- ☑
    both — *see* Paraplegia
    crossed G83.89
    hysterical F44.4
    psychogenic F44.4
    transient or transitory R29.818
      traumatic NEC — *see* Injury, nerve, leg
  levator palpebrae superioris — *see* Blepharoptosis, paralytic
  limb — *see* Monoplegia
  lip K13.0
  Lissauer's A52.17
  lower limb — *see* Monoplegia, lower limb
    both — *see* Paraplegia
  lung J98.4
  median nerve G56.1- ☑
  medullary (tegmental) G83.89
  mesencephalic NEC G83.89
    tegmental G83.89
  middle alternating G83.89
  Millard-Gubler-Foville G46.3
  monoplegic — *see* Monoplegia
  motor G83.9
  muscle, muscular NEC G72.89
    due to nerve lesion G58.9
    eye (extrinsic) H49.9
      intrinsic — *see* Paresis, of accommodation
      oblique — *see* Strabismus, paralytic, fourth nerve
    iris sphincter H21.9
    ischemic (Volkmann's) (complicating trauma) T79.6 ☑
    progressive G12.21
    progressive, spinal G12.25
    pseudohypertrophic G71.02
    spinal progressive G12.25
  musculocutaneous nerve G56.9- ☑
  musculospiral G56.9- ☑
  nerve — *see also* Disorder, nerve
    abducent — *see* Strabismus, paralytic, sixth nerve
    accessory G52.8
    auditory (except Deafness) H93.3 ☑
    birth injury P14.9
    cranial or cerebral G52.9
    facial G51.0
      birth injury P11.3
      congenital P11.3
      newborn (birth injury) P11.3
    fourth or trochlear — *see* Strabismus, paralytic, fourth nerve
    newborn (birth injury) P14.9
    oculomotor — *see* Strabismus, paralytic, third nerve
    phrenic (birth injury) P14.2
    radial G56.3- ☑
    seventh or facial G51.0
      newborn (birth injury) P11.3
    sixth or abducent — *see* Strabismus, paralytic, sixth nerve
    syphilitic A52.15
    third or oculomotor — *see* Strabismus, paralytic, third nerve
    trigeminal G50.9
    trochlear — *see* Strabismus, paralytic, fourth nerve
    ulnar G56.2- ☑
  normokalemic periodic G72.3
  ocular H49.9
    alternating G83.89
  oculofacial, congenital (Moebius) Q87.0
  oculomotor (external bilateral) (nerve) — *see* Strabismus, paralytic, third nerve
  palate (soft) K13.79
  paratrigeminal G50.9
  periodic (familial) (hyperkalemic) (hypokalemic) (myotonic) (normokalemic) (potassium sensitive) (secondary) G72.3
  peripheral autonomic nervous system — *see* Neuropathy, peripheral, autonomic
  peroneal (nerve) G57.3- ☑
  pharynx J39.2
  phrenic nerve G56.8- ☑
  plantar nerve(s) G57.6- ☑
  pneumogastric nerve G52.2
  poliomyelitis (current) — *see* Poliomyelitis, paralytic
  popliteal nerve G57.3- ☑
  postepileptic transitory G83.84
  progressive (atrophic) (bulbar) (spinal) G12.22
    general A52.17

Paralysis, paralytic — *continued*
  progressive — *continued*
    infantile acute — *see* Poliomyelitis, paralytic
    supranuclear G23.1
  pseudobulbar G12.29
  pseudohypertrophic (muscle) G71.09
  psychogenic F44.4
  quadriceps G57.9- ☑
  quadriplegic — *see* Tetraplegia
  radial nerve G56.3- ☑
  rectus muscle (eye) H49.9
  recurrent isolated sleep G47.53
  respiratory (muscle) (system) (tract) R06.81
    center NEC G93.89
    congenital P28.89
    newborn P28.89
  right side — *see* Hemiplegia
  saturnine T56.0 ☑
  sciatic nerve G57.0- ☑
  senile G83.9
  shaking — *see* Parkinsonism
  shoulder G56.9- ☑
  sleep, recurrent isolated G47.53
  spastic G83.9
    cerebral — *see* Palsy, cerebral, spastic
    congenital (cerebral) — *see* Palsy, cerebral, spastic
    familial G11.4
    hereditary G11.4
    quadriplegic G80.0
    syphilitic (spinal) A52.17
  sphincter, bladder — *see* Paralysis, bladder
  spinal (cord) G83.9
    accessory nerve G52.8
    acute — *see* Poliomyelitis, paralytic
    ascending acute G61.0
    atrophic (acute) — *see also* Poliomyelitis, paralytic
      spastic, syphilitic A52.17
    congenital NEC — *see* Palsy, cerebral
    hereditary G95.89
    infantile — *see* Poliomyelitis, paralytic
    progressive G12.21
      muscle G12.25
    sequelae NEC G83.89
  sternomastoid G52.8
  stomach K31.84
    diabetic — *see* Diabetes, by type, with gastroparesis
    nerve G52.2
      diabetic — *see* Diabetes, by type, with gastro-paresis
  stroke — *see* Infarct, brain
  subcapsularis G56.8- ☑
  supranuclear (progressive) G23.1
  sympathetic G90.8
    cervical G90.09
    nervous system — *see* Neuropathy, peripheral, autonomic
  syndrome G83.9
    specified NEC G83.89
  syphilitic spastic spinal (Erb's) A52.17
  thigh G57.9- ☑
  throat J39.2
    diphtheritic A36.0
    muscle J39.2
  thrombotic (current episode) I63.3- ☑
  thumb G56.9- ☑
  tick — *see* Toxicity, venom, arthropod, specified NEC
  Todd's (postepileptic transitory paralysis) G83.84
  toe G57.6- ☑
  tongue K14.8
  transient R29.5
    arm or leg NEC R29.818
    traumatic NEC — *see* Injury, nerve
  trapezius G52.8
  traumatic, transient NEC — *see* Injury, nerve
  trembling — *see* Parkinsonism
  triceps brachii G56.9- ☑
  trigeminal nerve G50.9
  trochlear (nerve) — *see* Strabismus, paralytic, fourth nerve
  ulnar nerve G56.2- ☑
  upper limb — *see* Monoplegia, upper limb
  uremic N18.9 *[G99.8]*
  uveoparotitic D86.89
  uvula K13.79
    postdiphtheritic A36.0
  vagus nerve G52.2
  vasomotor NEC G90.8
  velum palati K13.79

Paralysis, paralytic — *continued*
  vesical — *see* Paralysis, bladder
  vestibular nerve (except Vertigo) H93.3 ☑
  vocal cords J38.00
    bilateral J38.02
    unilateral J38.01
  Volkmann's (complicating trauma) T79.6 ☑
  wasting G12.29
  Weber's G46.3
  wrist G56.9- ☑
Paramedial urethrovesical orifice Q64.79
Paramenia N92.6
Parametritis — *see also* Disease, pelvis, inflammatory N73.2
  acute N73.0
  complicating abortion — *see* Abortion, by type, complicated by, parametritis
Parametrium, parametric — *see* condition
Paramnesia — *see* Amnesia
Paramolar K00.1
Paramyloidosis E85.89
Paramyoclonus multiplex G25.3
Paramyotonia (congenita) G71.19
Parangi — *see* Yaws
Paranoia (querulans) F22
  senile F03 ☑
Paranoid
  dementia (senile) F03 ☑
    praecox — *see* Schizophrenia
  personality F60.0
  psychosis (climacteric) (involutional) (menopausal) F22
    psychogenic (acute) F23
    senile F03 ☑
  reaction (acute) F23
    chronic F22
  schizophrenia F20.0
  state (climacteric) (involutional) (menopausal) (simple) F22
    senile F03 ☑
  tendencies F60.0
  traits F60.0
  trends F60.0
  type, psychopathic personality F60.0
Paraparesis — *see* Paraplegia
Paraphasia R47.02
Paraphilia F65.9
Paraphimosis (congenital) N47.2
  chancroidal A57
Paraphrenia, paraphrenic (late) F22
  schizophrenia F20.0
Paraplegia (lower) G82.20
  ataxic — *see* Degeneration, combined, spinal cord
  complete G82.21
  congenital (cerebral) G80.8
    spastic G80.1
  familial spastic G11.4
  functional (hysterical) F44.4
  hereditary, spastic G11.4
  hysterical F44.4
  incomplete G82.22
  Pott's A18.01
  psychogenic F44.4
  spastic
    Erb's spinal, syphilitic A52.17
    hereditary G11.4
    tropical G04.1
  syphilitic (spastic) A52.17
  traumatic
    current injury — code to injury with seventh character A
    sequela of previous injury — code to injury with seventh character S
  tropical spastic G04.1
Parapoxvirus B08.60
  specified NEC B08.69
Paraproteinemia D89.2
  benign (familial) D89.2
  monoclonal D47.2
  secondary to malignant disease D47.2
Parapsoriasis L41.9
  en plaques L41.4
  guttata L41.1
  large plaque L41.4
  retiform, retiformis L41.5
  small plaque L41.3
  specified NEC L41.8
  varioliformis (acuta) L41.0
Parasitic — *see also* condition

Parasitic — *continued*
  disease NEC B89
  stomatitis B37.0
  sycosis (beard) (scalp) B35.0
  twin Q89.4
Parasitism B89
  intestinal B82.9
  skin B88.9
  specified — *see* Infestation
Parasitophobia F40.218
Parasomnia G47.50
  due to
    alcohol
      abuse F10.182
      dependence F10.282
      use F10.982
    amphetamines
      abuse F15.182
      dependence F15.282
      use F15.982
    caffeine
      abuse F15.182
      dependence F15.282
      use F15.982
    cocaine
      abuse F14.182
      dependence F14.282
      use F14.982
    drug NEC
      abuse F19.182
      dependence F19.282
      use F19.982
    opioid
      abuse F11.182
      dependence F11.282
      use F11.982
    psychoactive substance NEC
      abuse F19.182
      dependence F19.282
      use F19.982
    sedative, hypnotic, or anxiolytic
      abuse F13.182
      dependence F13.282
      use F13.982
    stimulant NEC
      abuse F15.182
      dependence F15.282
      use F15.982
  in conditions classified elsewhere G47.54
  nonorganic origin F51.8
  organic G47.50
  specified NEC G47.59
Paraspadias Q54.9
Paraspasmus facialis G51.8
Parasuicide (attempt)
  history of (personal) Z91.5
    in family Z81.8
Parathyroid gland — *see* condition
Parathyroid tetany E20.9
Paratrachoma A74.0
Paratyphilitis — *see* Appendicitis
Paratyphoid (fever) — *see* Fever, paratyphoid
Paratyphus — *see* Fever, paratyphoid
Paraurethral duct Q64.79
Paraurethritis — *see also* Urethritis
  gonococcal (acute) (chronic) (with abscess) A54.1
Paravaccinia NEC B08.04
Paravaginitis — *see* Vaginitis
Parencephalitis — *see also* Encephalitis
  sequelae G09
Parent-child conflict — *see* Conflict, parent-child
  estrangement NEC Z62.890
Paresis — *see also* Paralysis
  accommodation — *see* Paresis, of accommodation
  Bernhardt's G57.1- ☑
  bladder (sphincter) — *see also* Paralysis, bladder
    tabetic A52.17
  bowel, colon or intestine K56.0
  extrinsic muscle, eye H49.9
  general (progressive) (syphilitic) A52.17
    juvenile A50.45
  heart — *see* Failure, heart
  insane (syphilitic) A52.17
  juvenile (general) A50.45
  of accommodation H52.52- ☑
  peripheral progressive (idiopathic) G60.3
  pseudohypertrophic G71.09
  senile G83.9

☑ **Additional Character Required** — Refer to the Tabular List for Character Selection
▽ **Subterms under main terms may continue to next column or page**

Paresis — *continued*
  syphilitic (general) A52.17
    congenital A50.45
  vesical NEC N31.2
Paresthesia — *see also* Disturbance, sensation, skin R20.2
  Bernhardt G57.1- ☑
Paretic — *see* condition
Parinaud's
  conjunctivitis H10.89
  oculoglandular syndrome H10.89
  ophthalmoplegia H49.88- ☑
Parkinsonism (idiopathic) (primary) G20
  with neurogenic orthostatic hypotension (symptomatic) G90.3
  arteriosclerotic G21.4
  dementia G31.83 *[F02.80]*
    with behavioral disturbance G31.83 *[F02.81]*
  due to
    drugs NEC G21.19
      neuroleptic G21.11
  medication-induced NEC G21.19
  neuroleptic induced G21.11
  postencephalitic G21.3
  secondary G21.9
    due to
      arteriosclerosis G21.4
      drugs NEC G21.19
        neuroleptic G21.11
      encephalitis G21.3
      external agents NEC G21.2
      syphilis A52.19
    specified NEC G21.8
  syphilitic A52.19
  treatment-induced NEC G21.19
  vascular G21.4
Parkinson's disease, syndrome or tremor — *see* Parkinsonism
Parodontitis — *see* Periodontitis
Parodontosis K05.4
Paronychia — *see also* Cellulitis, digit
  with lymphangitis — *see* Lymphangitis, acute, digit
  candidal (chronic) B37.2
  tuberculous (primary) A18.4
Parorexia (psychogenic) F50.89
Parosmia R43.1
  psychogenic F45.8
Parotid gland — *see* condition
Parotitis, parotiditis (allergic)(nonspecific toxic) (purulent) (septic) (suppurative) — *see also* Sialoadenitis
  epidemic — *see* Mumps
  infectious — *see* Mumps
  postoperative K91.89
  surgical K91.89
Parrot fever A70
Parrot's disease (early congenital syphilitic pseudoparalysis) A50.02
Parry-Romberg syndrome G51.8
Parry's disease or syndrome E05.00
  with thyroid storm E05.01
Pars planitis — *see* Cyclitis
Parsonage (-Aldren)-**Turner syndrome** G54.5
Parson's disease (exophthalmic goiter) E05.00
  with thyroid storm E05.01
Particolored infant Q82.8
Parturition — *see* Delivery
Parulis K04.7
  with sinus K04.6
Parvovirus, as cause of disease classified elsewhere B97.6
Pasini and Pierini's atrophoderma L90.3
Passage
  false, urethra N36.5
  meconium (newborn) during delivery P03.82
  of sounds or bougies — *see* Attention to, artificial, opening
Passive — *see* condition
  smoking Z77.22
Pasteurella septica A28.0
Pasteurellosis — *see* Infection, Pasteurella
PAT (paroxysmal atrial tachycardia) I47.1
Patau's syndrome — *see* Trisomy, 13
Patches
  mucous (syphilitic) A51.39
    congenital A50.07
  smokers' (mouth) K13.24
Patellar — *see* condition
Patent — *see also* Imperfect, closure

Patent — *continued*
  canal of Nuck Q52.4
  cervix N88.3
  ductus arteriosus or Botallo's Q25.0
  foramen
    botalli Q21.1
    ovale Q21.1
  interauricular septum Q21.1
  interventricular septum Q21.0
  omphalomesenteric duct Q43.0
  os (uteri) — *see* Patent, cervix
  ostium secundum Q21.1
  urachus Q64.4
  vitelline duct Q43.0
Paterson (-Brown)(-Kelly) **syndrome or web** D50.1
Pathologic, pathological — *see also* condition
  asphyxia R09.01
  fire-setting F63.1
  gambling F63.0
  ovum O02.0
  resorption, tooth K03.3
  stealing F63.2
Pathology (of) — *see* Disease
  periradicular, associated with previous endodontic treatment NEC M27.59
Pattern, sleep-wake, irregular G47.23
Patulous — *see also* Imperfect, closure (congenital)
  alimentary tract Q45.8
    lower Q43.8
    upper Q40.8
  eustachian tube H69.0- ☑
Pause, sinoatrial I49.5
Paxton's disease B36.2
Pearl(s)
  enamel K00.2
  Epstein's K09.8
Pearl-worker's disease — *see* Osteomyelitis, specified type NEC
Pectenosis K62.4
Pectoral — *see* condition
Pectus
  carinatum (congenital) Q67.7
    acquired M95.4
    rachitic sequelae (late effect) E64.3
  excavatum (congenital) Q67.6
    acquired M95.4
    rachitic sequelae (late effect) E64.3
  recurvatum (congenital) Q67.6
Pedatrophia E41
Pederosis F65.4
Pediculosis (infestation) B85.2
  capitis (head-louse) (any site) B85.0
  corporis (body-louse) (any site) B85.1
  eyelid B85.0
  mixed (classifiable to more than one of the titles B85.0-B85.3) B85.4
  pubis (pubic louse) (any site) B85.3
  vestimenti B85.1
  vulvae B85.3
Pediculus (infestation) — *see* Pediculosis
Pedophilia F65.4
Peg-shaped teeth K00.2
Pelade — *see* Alopecia, areata
Pelger-Huët anomaly or syndrome D72.0
Peliosis (rheumatica) D69.0
  hepatis K76.4
    with toxic liver disease K71.8
Pelizaeus-Merzbacher disease E75.29
Pellagra (alcoholic) (with polyneuropathy) E52
Pellagra-cerebellar-ataxia-renal aminoaciduria syndrome E72.02
Pellegrini (-Stieda) **disease or syndrome** — *see* Bursitis, tibial collateral
Pellizzi's syndrome E34.8
Pel's crisis A52.11
Pelvic — *see also* condition
  examination (periodic) (routine) Z01.419
    with abnormal findings Z01.411
  kidney, congenital Q63.2
Pelviolithiasis — *see* Calculus, kidney
Pelviperitonitis — *see also* Peritonitis, pelvic
  gonococcal A54.24
  puerperal O85
Pelvis — *see* condition or type
Pemphigoid L12.9
  benign, mucous membrane L12.1
  bullous L12.0
  cicatrical L12.1

Pemphigoid — *continued*
  juvenile L12.2
  ocular L12.1
  specified NEC L12.8
Pemphigus L10.9
  benign familial (chronic) Q82.8
  Brazilian L10.3
  circinatus L13.0
  conjunctiva L12.1
  drug-induced L10.5
  erythematosus L10.4
  foliaceous L10.2
  gangrenous — *see* Gangrene
  neonatorum L01.03
  ocular L12.1
  paraneoplastic L10.81
  specified NEC L10.89
  syphilitic (congenital) A50.06
  vegetans L10.1
  vulgaris L10.0
  wildfire L10.3
Pendred's syndrome E07.1
Pendulous
  abdomen, in pregnancy — *see* Pregnancy, complicated by, abnormal, pelvic organs or tissues NEC
  breast N64.89
Penetrating wound — *see also* Puncture
  with internal injury — *see* Injury, by site
  eyeball — *see* Puncture, eyeball
  orbit (with or without foreign body) — *see* Puncture, orbit
  uterus by instrument with or following ectopic or molar pregnancy O08.6
Penicillosis B48.4
Penis — *see* condition
Penitis N48.29
Pentalogy of Fallot Q21.8
Pentasomy X syndrome Q97.1
Pentosuria (essential) E74.8
Percreta placenta - O43.23 ☑
Peregrinating patient — *see* Disorder, factitious
Perforation, perforated (nontraumatic) (of)
  accidental during procedure (blood vessel) (nerve) (organ) — *see* Complication, accidental puncture or laceration
  antrum — *see* Sinusitis, maxillary
  appendix K35.32
    with localized peritonitis K35.32
  atrial septum, multiple Q21.1
  attic, ear — *see* Perforation, tympanum, attic
  bile duct (common) (hepatic) K83.2
    cystic K82.2
  bladder (urinary)
    with or following ectopic or molar pregnancy O08.6
    obstetrical trauma O71.5
    traumatic S37.29 ☑
      at delivery O71.5
  bowel K63.1
    with or following ectopic or molar pregnancy O08.6
    newborn P78.0
    obstetrical trauma O71.5
    traumatic — *see* Laceration, intestine
  broad ligament N83.8
    with or following ectopic or molar pregnancy O08.6
    obstetrical trauma O71.6
  by
    device, implant or graft — *see also* Complications, by site and type, mechanical T85.628 ☑
      arterial graft NEC — *see* Complication, cardiovascular device, mechanical, vascular
      breast (implant) T85.49 ☑
      catheter NEC T85.698 ☑
        cystostomy T83.090 ☑
        dialysis (renal) T82.49 ☑
          intraperitoneal T85.691 ☑
        infusion NEC T82.594 ☑
          spinal (epidural) (subdural) T85.690 ☑
        urinary — *see also* Complications, catheter, urinary T83.098 ☑
      electronic (electrode) (pulse generator) (stimulator)
        bone T84.390 ☑
        cardiac T82.199 ☑
          electrode T82.190 ☑
          pulse generator T82.191 ☑
          specified type NEC T82.198 ☑

Index

Perforation, perforated — Pericementitis

Perforation, perforated — *continued*
  by — *continued*
    device, implant or graft — *see also* Complications,
      by site and type, mechanical — *continued*
      electronic — *continued*
        nervous system — *see* Complication, prosthet-
          ic device, mechanical, electronic ner-
          vous system stimulator
        urinary — *see* Complication, genitourinary,
          device, urinary, mechanical
      fixation, internal (orthopedic) NEC — *see* Compli-
        cation, fixation device, mechanical
      gastrointestinal — *see* Complications, prosthetic
        device, mechanical, gastrointestinal device
      genital NEC T83.498 ☑
        intrauterine contraceptive device T83.39 ☑
        penile prosthesis T83.490 ☑
      heart NEC — *see* Complication, cardiovascular
        device, mechanical
      joint prosthesis — *see* Complications, joint
        prosthesis, mechanical, specified NEC, by
        site
      ocular NEC — *see* Complications, prosthetic de-
        vice, mechanical, ocular device
      orthopedic NEC — *see* Complication, orthopedic,
        device, mechanical
      specified NEC T85.628 ☑
      urinary NEC — *see also* Complication, genitouri-
        nary, device, urinary, mechanical
        graft T83.29 ☑
      vascular NEC — *see* Complication, cardiovascular
        device, mechanical
      ventricular intracranial shunt T85.09 ☑
      foreign body left accidentally in operative wound
        T81.539 ☑
      instrument (any) during a procedure, accidental —
        see Puncture, accidental complicating surgery
  cecum K35.32
    with localized peritonitis K35.32
  cervix (uteri) N88.8
    with or following ectopic or molar pregnancy O08.6
    obstetrical trauma O71.3
  colon K63.1
    newborn P78.0
    obstetrical trauma O71.5
    traumatic — *see* Laceration, intestine, large
  common duct (bile) K83.2
  cornea (due to ulceration) — *see* Ulcer, cornea, perfo-
    rated
  cystic duct K82.2
  diverticulum (intestine) K57.80
    with bleeding K57.81
    large intestine K57.20
      with
        bleeding K57.21
        small intestine K57.40
          with bleeding K57.41
      small intestine K57.00
      with
        bleeding K57.01
        large intestine K57.40
          with bleeding K57.41
  ear drum — *see* Perforation, tympanum
  esophagus K22.3
  ethmoidal sinus — *see* Sinusitis, ethmoidal
  frontal sinus — *see* Sinusitis, frontal
  gallbladder K82.2
  heart valve — *see* Endocarditis
  ileum K63.1
    newborn P78.0
    obstetrical trauma O71.5
    traumatic — *see* Laceration, intestine, small
  instrumental, surgical (accidental) (blood vessel) (nerve)
    (organ) — *see* Puncture, accidental complicating
    surgery
  intestine NEC K63.1
    with ectopic or molar pregnancy O08.6
    newborn P78.0
    obstetrical trauma O71.5
    traumatic — *see* Laceration, intestine
    ulcerative NEC K63.1
      newborn P78.0
  jejunum, jejunal K63.1
    obstetrical trauma O71.5
    traumatic — *see* Laceration, intestine, small
    ulcer — *see* Ulcer, gastrojejunal, with perforation
  joint prosthesis — *see* Complications, joint prosthesis,
    mechanical, specified NEC, by site

Perforation, perforated — *continued*
  mastoid (antrum) (cell) — *see* Disorder, mastoid,
    specified NEC
  maxillary sinus — *see* Sinusitis, maxillary
  membrana tympani — *see* Perforation, tympanum
  nasal
    septum J34.89
      congenital Q30.3
      syphilitic A52.73
    sinus J34.89
      congenital Q30.8
      due to sinusitis — *see* Sinusitis
  palate — *see also* Cleft, palate Q35.9
    syphilitic A52.79
  palatine vault — *see also* Cleft, palate, hard Q35.1
    syphilitic A52.79
    congenital A50.59
  pars flaccida (ear drum) — *see* Perforation, tympanum,
    attic
  pelvic
    floor S31.030 ☑
      with
        ectopic or molar pregnancy O08.6
        penetration into retroperitoneal space
          S31.031 ☑
        retained foreign body S31.040 ☑
          with penetration into retroperitoneal
            space S31.041 ☑
      following ectopic or molar pregnancy O08.6
      obstetrical trauma O70.1
    organ S37.99 ☑
      adrenal gland S37.818 ☑
      bladder — *see* Perforation, bladder
      fallopian tube S37.599 ☑
        bilateral S37.592 ☑
        unilateral S37.591 ☑
      kidney S37.09- ☑
      obstetrical trauma O71.5
      ovary S37.499 ☑
        bilateral S37.492 ☑
        unilateral S37.491 ☑
      prostate S37.828 ☑
      specified organ NEC S37.898 ☑
      ureter — *see* Perforation, ureter
      urethra — *see* Perforation, urethra
      uterus — *see* Perforation, uterus
  perineum — *see* Laceration, perineum
  pharynx J39.2
  rectum K63.1
    newborn P78.0
    obstetrical trauma O71.5
    traumatic S36.63 ☑
  root canal space due to endodontic treatment M27.51
  sigmoid K63.1
    newborn P78.0
    obstetrical trauma O71.5
    traumatic S36.533 ☑
  sinus (accessory) (chronic) (nasal) J34.89
  sphenoidal sinus — *see* Sinusitis, sphenoidal
  surgical (accidental) (by instrument) (blood vessel)
    (nerve) (organ) — *see* Puncture, accidental
    complicating surgery
  traumatic
    external — *see* Puncture
    eye — *see* Puncture, eyeball
    internal organ — *see* Injury, by site
  tympanum, tympanic (membrane) (persistent post-
    traumatic) (postinflammatory) H72.9- ☑
    attic H72.1- ☑
      multiple — *see* Perforation, tympanum, multiple
      total — *see* Perforation, tympanum, total
    central H72.0- ☑
      multiple — *see* Perforation, tympanum, multiple
      total — *see* Perforation, tympanum, total
    marginal NEC — *see* subcategory H72.2 ☑
    multiple H72.81- ☑
    pars flaccida — *see* Perforation, tympanum, attic
    total H72.82- ☑
    traumatic, current episode S09.2- ☑
  typhoid, gastrointestinal — *see* Typhoid
  ulcer — *see* Ulcer, by site, with perforation
  ureter N28.89
    traumatic S37.19 ☑
  urethra N36.8
    with ectopic or molar pregnancy O08.6
    following ectopic or molar pregnancy O08.6
    obstetrical trauma O71.5

Perforation, perforated — *continued*
  urethra — *continued*
    traumatic S37.39 ☑
      at delivery O71.5
  uterus
    with ectopic or molar pregnancy O08.6
    by intrauterine contraceptive device T83.39 ☑
    following ectopic or molar pregnancy O08.6
    obstetrical trauma O71.1
    traumatic S37.69 ☑
      obstetric O71.1
  uvula K13.79
    syphilitic A52.79
  vagina O71.4
    obstetrical trauma O71.4
    other trauma — *see* Puncture, vagina
Periadenitis mucosa necrotica recurrens K12.0
Periappendicitis (acute) — *see* Appendicitis
Periarteritis nodosa (disseminated) (infectious) (necrotizing) M30.0
Periarthritis (joint) — *see also* Enthesopathy
  Duplay's M75.0- ☑
  gonococcal A54.42
  humeroscapularis — *see* Capsulitis, adhesive
  scapulohumeral — *see* Capsulitis, adhesive
  shoulder — *see* Capsulitis, adhesive
  wrist M77.2- ☑
Periarthrosis (angioneural) — *see* Enthesopathy
Pericapsulitis, adhesive (shoulder) — *see* Capsulitis,
  adhesive
Pericarditis (with decompensation) (with effusion) I31.9
  with rheumatic fever (conditions in I00)
    active — *see* Pericarditis, rheumatic
    inactive or quiescent I09.2
  acute (hemorrhagic) (nonrheumatic) (Sicca) I30.9
    with chorea (acute) (rheumatic) (Sydenham's) I02.0
    benign I30.8
    nonspecific I30.0
    rheumatic I01.0
      with chorea (acute) (Sydenham's) I02.0
  adhesive or adherent (chronic) (external) (internal) I31.0
    acute — *see* Pericarditis, acute
    rheumatic I09.2
  bacterial (acute) (subacute) (with serous or seropuru-
    lent effusion) I30.1
  calcareous I31.1
  cholesterol (chronic) I31.8
    acute I30.9
  chronic (nonrheumatic) I31.9
    rheumatic I09.2
  constrictive (chronic) I31.1
  coxsackie B33.23
  fibrinocaseous (tuberculous) A18.84
  fibrinopurulent I30.1
  fibrinous I30.8
  fibrous I31.0
  gonococcal A54.83
  idiopathic I30.0
  in systemic lupus erythematosus M32.12
  infective I30.1
  meningococcal A39.53
  neoplastic (chronic) I31.8
    acute I30.9
  obliterans, obliterating I31.0
  plastic I31.0
  pneumococcal I30.1
  postinfarction I24.1
  purulent I30.1
  rheumatic (active) (acute) (with effusion) (with pneu-
    monia) I01.0
    with chorea (acute) (rheumatic) (Sydenham's) I02.0
    chronic or inactive (with chorea) I09.2
  rheumatoid — *see* Rheumatoid, carditis
  septic I30.1
  serofibrinous I30.8
  staphylococcal I30.1
  streptococcal I30.1
  suppurative I30.1
  syphilitic A52.06
  tuberculous A18.84
  uremic N18.9 *[I32]*
  viral I30.1
Pericardium, pericardial — *see* condition
Pericellulitis — *see* Cellulitis
Pericementitis (chronic) (suppurative) — *see also* Periodontitis
  acute K05.20

☑ **Additional Character Required** — Refer to the Tabular List for Character Selection ▽ **Subterms under main terms may continue to next column or page**

Pericementitis — *continued*
  acute — *continued*
    generalized — *see* Periodontitis, aggressive, generalized
    localized — *see* Periodontitis, aggressive, localized
Perichondritis
  auricle — *see* Perichondritis, ear
  bronchus J98.09
  ear (external) H61.00- ☑
    acute H61.01- ☑
    chronic H61.02- ☑
  external auditory canal — *see* Perichondritis, ear
  larynx J38.7
    syphilitic A52.73
    typhoid A01.09
  nose J34.89
  pinna — *see* Perichondritis, ear
  trachea J39.8
Periclasia K05.4
Pericoronitis — *see* Periodontitis
Pericystitis N30.90
  with hematuria N30.91
Peridiverticulitis (intestine) K57.92
  cecum — *see* Diverticulitis, intestine, large
  colon — *see* Diverticulitis, intestine, large
  duodenum — *see* Diverticulitis, intestine, small
  intestine — *see* Diverticulitis, intestine
  jejunum — *see* Diverticulitis, intestine, small
  rectosigmoid — *see* Diverticulitis, intestine, large
  rectum — *see* Diverticulitis, intestine, large
  sigmoid — *see* Diverticulitis, intestine, large
Periendocarditis — *see* Endocarditis
Periepididymitis N45.1
Perifolliculitis L01.02
  abscedens, caput, scalp L66.3
  capitis, abscedens (et suffodiens) L66.3
  superficial pustular L01.02
Perihepatitis K65.8
Perilabyrinthitis (acute) — *see* subcategory H83.0 ☑
Perimeningitis — *see* Meningitis
Perimetritis — *see* Endometritis
Perimetrosalpingitis — *see* Salpingo-oophoritis
Perineocele N81.81
Perinephric, perinephritic — *see* condition
Perinephritis — *see also* Infection, kidney
  purulent — *see* Abscess, kidney
Perineum, perineal — *see* condition
Perineuritis NEC — *see* Neuralgia
Periodic — *see* condition
Periodontitis (chronic) (complex) (compound) (local)
      (simplex) K05.30
    acute K05.20
      generalized K05.229
        moderate K05.222
        severe K05.223
        slight K05.221
      localized K05.219
        moderate K05.212
        severe K05.213
        slight K05.211
    apical K04.5
      acute (pulpal origin) K04.4
    generalized K05.329
      moderate K05.322
      severe K05.323
      slight K05.321
    localized K05.319
      moderate K05.312
      severe K05.313
      slight K05.311
Periodontoclasia K05.4
Periodontosis (juvenile) K05.4
Periods — *see also* Menstruation
  heavy N92.0
  irregular N92.6
  shortened intervals (irregular) N92.1
Perionychia — *see also* Cellulitis, digit
  with lymphangitis — *see* Lymphangitis, acute, digit
Perioophoritis — *see* Salpingo-oophoritis
Periorchitis N45.2
Periosteum, periosteal — *see* condition
Periostitis (albuminosa) (circumscribed) (diffuse) (infective) (monomelic) — *see also* Osteomyelitis
  alveolar M27.3
  alveolodental M27.3
  dental M27.3
  gonorrheal A54.43

Periostitis — *continued*
  jaw (lower) (upper) M27.2
  orbit H05.03- ☑
  syphilitic A52.77
    congenital (early) A50.02 *[M90.80]*
    secondary A51.46
  tuberculous — *see* Tuberculosis, bone
  yaws (hypertrophic) (early) (late) A66.6 *[M90.80]*
Periostosis (hyperplastic) — *see also* Disorder, bone, specified type NEC
  with osteomyelitis — *see* Osteomyelitis, specified type NEC
Peripartum
  cardiomyopathy O90.3
Periphlebitis — *see* Phlebitis
Periproctitis K62.89
Periprostatitis — *see* Prostatitis
Perirectal — *see* condition
Perirenal — *see* condition
Perisalpingitis — *see* Salpingo-oophoritis
Perisplenitis (infectional) D73.89
Peristalsis, visible or reversed R19.2
Peritendinitis — *see* Enthesopathy
Peritoneum, peritoneal — *see* condition
Peritonitis (adhesive) (bacterial) (fibrinous) (hemorrhagic)
      (idiopathic) (localized) (perforative) (primary) (with
      adhesions) (with effusion) K65.9
    with or following
      abscess K65.1
      appendicitis
        with perforation or rupture K35.32
        generalized — *see also* Appendicitis K35.20
        localized — *see also* Appendicitis K35.30
      diverticular disease (intestine) K57.80
        with bleeding K57.81
        ectopic or molar pregnancy O08.0
        large intestine K57.20
          with
            bleeding K57.21
            small intestine K57.40
              with bleeding K57.41
        small intestine K57.00
          with
            bleeding K57.01
            large intestine K57.40
              with bleeding K57.41
    acute (generalized) K65.0
    aseptic T81.61 ☑
    bile, biliary K65.3
    chemical T81.61 ☑
    chlamydial A74.81
    chronic proliferative K65.8
    complicating abortion — *see* Abortion, by type, complicated by, pelvic peritonitis
    congenital P78.1
    diaphragmatic K65.0
    diffuse K65.0
    diphtheritic A36.89
    disseminated K65.0
    due to
      bile K65.3
      foreign
        body or object accidentally left during a procedure (instrument) (sponge) (swab) T81.599 ☑
        substance accidentally left during a procedure (chemical) (powder) (talc) T81.61 ☑
      talc T81.61 ☑
      urine K65.8
    eosinophilic K65.8
      acute K65.0
    fibrocaseous (tuberculous) A18.31
    fibropurulent K65.0
    following ectopic or molar pregnancy O08.0
    general (ized) K65.0
    gonococcal A54.85
    meconium (newborn) P78.0
    neonatal P78.1
      meconium P78.0
    pancreatic K65.0
    paroxysmal, familial E85.0
      benign E85.0
    pelvic
      female N73.5
        acute N73.3
        chronic N73.4
          with adhesions N73.6
      male K65.0

Peritonitis — *continued*
  periodic, familial E85.0
  proliferative, chronic K65.8
  puerperal, postpartum, childbirth O85
  purulent K65.0
  septic K65.0
  specified NEC K65.8
  spontaneous bacterial K65.2
  subdiaphragmatic K65.0
  subphrenic K65.0
  suppurative K65.0
  syphilitic A52.74
    congenital (early) A50.08 *[K67]*
  talc T81.61 ☑
  tuberculous A18.31
  urine K65.8
Peritonsillar — *see* condition
Peritonsillitis J36
Perityphlitis K37
Periureteritis N28.89
Periurethral — *see* condition
Periurethritis (gangrenous) — *see* Urethritis
Periuterine — *see* condition
Perivaginitis — *see* Vaginitis
Perivasculitis, retinal H35.06- ☑
Perivasitis (chronic) N49.1
Perivesiculitis (seminal) — *see* Vesiculitis
Perlèche NEC K13.0
  due to
    candidiasis B37.83
    moniliasis B37.83
    riboflavin deficiency E53.0
    vitamin B2 (riboflavin) deficiency E53.0
Pernicious — *see* condition
Pernio, perniosis T69.1 ☑
Perpetrator (of abuse) — *see* Index to External Causes of Injury, Perpetrator
Persecution
  delusion F22
  social Z60.5
Perseveration (tonic) R48.8
Persistence, persistent (congenital)
  anal membrane Q42.3
    with fistula Q42.2
  arteria stapedia Q16.3
  atrioventricular canal Q21.2
  branchial cleft NOS Q18.2
    cyst Q18.0
    fistula Q18.0
    sinus Q18.0
  bulbus cordis in left ventricle Q21.8
  canal of Cloquet Q14.0
  capsule (opaque) Q12.8
  cilioretinal artery or vein Q14.8
  cloaca Q43.7
  communication — *see* Fistula, congenital
  convolutions
    aortic arch Q25.46
    fallopian tube Q50.6
    oviduct Q50.6
    uterine tube Q50.6
  double aortic arch Q25.45
  ductus arteriosus (Botalli) Q25.0
  fetal
    circulation P29.38
    form of cervix (uteri) Q51.828
    hemoglobin, hereditary (HPFH) D56.4
  foramen
    Botalli Q21.1
    ovale Q21.1
  Gartner's duct Q52.4
  hemoglobin, fetal (hereditary) (HPFH) D56.4
  hyaloid
    artery (generally incomplete) Q14.0
    system Q14.8
  hymen, in pregnancy or childbirth — *see* Pregnancy, complicated by, abnormal, vulva
  lanugo Q84.2
  left
    posterior cardinal vein Q26.8
    root with right arch of aorta Q25.49
    superior vena cava Q26.1
  Meckel's diverticulum Q43.0
    malignant — *see* Table of Neoplasms, small intestine, malignant
  mucosal disease (middle ear) — *see* Otitis, media, suppurative, chronic, tubotympanic
  nail(s), anomalous Q84.6

Persistence, persistent — *continued*
- omphalomesenteric duct Q43.0
- organ or site not listed — *see* Anomaly, by site
- ostium
  - atrioventriculare commune Q21.2
  - primum Q21.2
  - secundum Q21.1
- ovarian rests in fallopian tube Q50.6
- pancreatic tissue in intestinal tract Q43.8
- primary (deciduous)
  - teeth K00.6
  - vitreous hyperplasia Q14.0
- pupillary membrane Q13.89
- rhesus (Rh) titer — *see* Complication(s), transfusion, incompatibility reaction, Rh (factor)
- right aortic arch Q25.47
- sinus
  - urogenitalis
    - female Q52.8
    - male Q55.8
  - venosus with imperfect incorporation in right auricle Q26.8
- thymus (gland) (hyperplasia) E32.0
- thyroglossal duct Q89.2
- thyrolingual duct Q89.2
- truncus arteriosus or communis Q20.0
- tunica vasculosa lentis Q12.2
- umbilical sinus Q64.4
- urachus Q64.4
- vitelline duct Q43.0

Person (with)
- admitted for clinical research, as a control subject (normal comparison) (participant) Z00.6
- awaiting admission to adequate facility elsewhere Z75.1
- concern (normal) about sick person in family Z63.6
- consulting on behalf of another Z71.0
- feigning illness Z76.5
- living (in)
  - alone Z60.2
  - boarding school Z59.3
  - residential institution Z59.3
  - without
    - adequate housing (heating) (space) Z59.1
    - housing (permanent) (temporary) Z59.0
    - person able to render necessary care Z74.2
    - shelter Z59.0
- on waiting list Z75.1
- sick or handicapped in family Z63.6

Personality (disorder) F60.9
- accentuation of traits (type A pattern) Z73.1
- affective F34.0
- aggressive F60.3
- amoral F60.2
- anacastic, anankastic F60.5
- antisocial F60.2
- anxious F60.6
- asocial F60.2
- asthenic F60.7
- avoidant F60.6
- borderline F60.3
- change due to organic condition (enduring) F07.0
- compulsive F60.5
- cycloid F34.0
- cyclothymic F34.0
- dependent F60.7
- depressive F34.1
- dissocial F60.2
- dual F44.81
- eccentric F60.89
- emotionally unstable F60.3
- expansive paranoid F60.0
- explosive F60.3
- fanatic F60.0
- haltlose type F60.89
- histrionic F60.4
- hyperthymic F34.0
- hypothymic F34.1
- hysterical F60.4
- immature F60.89
- inadequate F60.7
- labile (emotional) F60.3
- mixed (nonspecific) F60.89
- morally defective F60.2
- multiple F44.81
- narcissistic F60.81
- obsessional F60.5
- obsessive (-compulsive) F60.5
- organic F07.0

Personality — *continued*
- overconscientious F60.5
- paranoid F60.0
- passive (-dependent) F60.7
- passive-aggressive F60.89
- pathologic F60.9
- pattern defect or disturbance F60.9
- pseudopsychopathic (organic) F07.0
- pseudoretarded (organic) F07.0
- psychoinfantile F60.4
- psychoneurotic NEC F60.89
- psychopathic F60.2
- querulant F60.0
- sadistic F60.89
- schizoid F60.1
- self-defeating F60.89
- sensitive paranoid F60.0
- sociopathic (amoral) (antisocial) (asocial) (dissocial) F60.2
- specified NEC F60.89
- type A Z73.1
- unstable (emotional) F60.3

Perthes' disease — *see* Legg-Calvé-Perthes disease
Pertussis — *see also* Whooping cough A37.90
Perversion, perverted
- appetite F50.89
  - psychogenic F50.89
- function
  - pituitary gland E23.2
    - posterior lobe E22.2
- sense of smell and taste R43.8
  - psychogenic F45.8
- sexual — *see* Deviation, sexual

Pervious, congenital — *see also* Imperfect, closure
- ductus arteriosus Q25.0

Pes (congenital) — *see also* Talipes
- acquired — *see also* Deformity, limb, foot, specified NEC
  - planus — *see* Deformity, limb, flat foot
- adductus Q66.89
- cavus Q66.7- ☑
- deformity NEC, acquired — *see* Deformity, limb, foot, specified NEC
- planus (acquired) (any degree) — *see also* Deformity, limb, flat foot
  - rachitic sequelae (late effect) E64.3
- valgus Q66.6

Pest, pestis — *see* Plague
Petechia, petechiae R23.3
- newborn P54.5
Petechial typhus A75.9
Peter's anomaly Q13.4
Petit mal seizure — *see* Epilepsy, childhood, absence
Petit's hernia — *see* Hernia, abdomen, specified site NEC
Petrellidosis B48.2
Petrositis H70.20- ☑
- acute H70.21- ☑
- chronic H70.22- ☑
Peutz-Jeghers disease or syndrome Q85.8
Peyronie's disease N48.6
PFAPA (periodic fever, aphthous stomatitis, pharyngitis, and adenopathy syndrome) M04.8
Pfeiffer's disease — *see* Mononucleosis, infectious
Phagedena (dry) (moist) (sloughing) — *see also* Gangrene
- geometric L88
- penis N48.29
- tropical — *see* Ulcer, skin
- vulva N76.6
Phagedenic — *see* condition
Phakoma H35.89
Phakomatosis — *see also* specific eponymous syndromes Q85.9
- Bourneville's Q85.1
- specified NEC Q85.8
Phantom limb syndrome (without pain) G54.7
- with pain G54.6
Pharyngeal pouch syndrome D82.1
Pharyngitis (acute) (catarrhal) (gangrenous) (infective) (malignant) (membranous) (phlegmonous) (pseudomembranous) (simple) (subacute) (suppurative) (ulcerative) (viral) J02.9
- with influenza, flu, or grippe — *see* Influenza, with, pharyngitis
- aphthous B08.5
- atrophic J31.2
- chlamydial A56.4
- chronic (atrophic) (granular) (hypertrophic) J31.2

Pharyngitis — *continued*
- coxsackievirus B08.5
- diphtheritic A36.0
- enteroviral vesicular B08.5
- follicular (chronic) J31.2
- fusospirochetal A69.1
- gonococcal A54.5
- granular (chronic) J31.2
- herpesviral B00.2
- hypertrophic J31.2
- infectional, chronic J31.2
- influenzal — *see* Influenza, with, respiratory manifestations NEC
- lymphonodular, acute (enteroviral) B08.8
- pneumococcal J02.8
- purulent J02.9
- putrid J02.9
- septic J02.0
- sicca J31.2
- specified organism NEC J02.8
- staphylococcal J02.8
- streptococcal J02.0
- syphilitic, congenital (early) A50.03
- tuberculous A15.8
- vesicular, enteroviral B08.5
- viral NEC J02.8
Pharyngoconjunctivitis, viral B30.2
Pharyngolaryngitis (acute) J06.0
- chronic J37.0
Pharyngoplegia J39.2
Pharyngotonsillitis, herpesviral B00.2
Pharyngotracheitis, chronic J42
Pharynx, pharyngeal — *see* condition
Phencyclidine-induced
- anxiety disorder F16.980
- bipolar and related disorder F16.94
- depressive disorder F16.94
- psychotic disorder F16.959
Phenomenon
- Arthus' — *see* Arthus' phenomenon
- jaw-winking Q07.8
- lupus erythematosus (LE) cell M32.9
- Raynaud's (secondary) I73.00
  - with gangrene I73.01
- vasomotor R55
- vasospastic I73.9
- vasovagal R55
- Wenckebach's I44.1
Phenylketonuria E70.1
- classical E70.0
- maternal E70.1
Pheochromoblastoma
- specified site — *see* Neoplasm, malignant, by site
- unspecified site C74.10
Pheochromocytoma
- malignant
  - specified site — *see* Neoplasm, malignant, by site
  - unspecified site C74.10
- specified site — *see* Neoplasm, benign, by site
- unspecified site D35.00
Pheohyphomycosis — *see* Chromomycosis
Pheomycosis — *see* Chromomycosis
Phimosis (congenital) (due to infection) N47.1
- chancroidal A57
Phlebectasia — *see also* Varix
- congenital Q27.4
Phlebitis (infective) (pyemic) (septic) (suppurative) I80.9
- antepartum — *see* Thrombophlebitis, antepartum
- blue — *see* Phlebitis, leg, deep
- breast, superficial I80.8
- calf muscular vein (NOS) I80.25- ☑
- cavernous (venous) sinus — *see* Phlebitis, intracranial (venous) sinus
- cerebral (venous) sinus — *see* Phlebitis, intracranial (venous) sinus
- chest wall, superficial I80.8
- cranial (venous) sinus — *see* Phlebitis, intracranial (venous) sinus
- deep (vessels) — *see* Phlebitis, leg, deep
- due to implanted device — *see* Complications, by site and type, specified NEC
- during or resulting from a procedure T81.72 ☑
- femoral vein (superficial) I80.1- ☑
- femoropopliteal vein I80.0- ☑
- gastrocnemial vein I80.25- ☑
- gestational — *see* Phlebopathy, gestational
- hepatic veins I80.8
- iliac vein (common) (external) (internal) I80.21- ☑

Index

Phlebitis — *Pityriasis*

Phlebitis — *continued*
iliofemoral — *see* Phlebitis, femoral vein
intracranial (venous) sinus (any) G08
nonpyogenic I67.6
intraspinal venous sinuses and veins G08
nonpyogenic G95.19
lateral (venous) sinus — *see* Phlebitis, intracranial (venous) sinus
leg I80.3
antepartum — *see* Thrombophlebitis, antepartum
deep (vessels) NEC I80.20- ☑
iliac I80.21- ☑
popliteal vein I80.22- ☑
specified vessel NEC I80.29- ☑
tibial vein (anterior) (posterior) I80.23- ☑
femoral vein (superficial) I80.1- ☑
superficial (vessels) I80.0- ☑
longitudinal sinus — *see* Phlebitis, intracranial (venous) sinus
lower limb — *see* Phlebitis, leg
migrans, migrating (superficial) I82.1
pelvic
with ectopic or molar pregnancy O08.0
following ectopic or molar pregnancy O08.0
puerperal, postpartum O87.1
peroneal vein I80.24- ☑
popliteal vein — *see* Phlebitis, leg, deep, popliteal
portal (vein) K75.1
postoperative T81.72 ☑
pregnancy — *see* Thrombophlebitis, antepartum
puerperal, postpartum, childbirth O87.0
deep O87.1
pelvic O87.1
superficial O87.0
retina — *see* Vasculitis, retina
saphenous (accessory) (great) (long) (small) — *see* Phlebitis, leg, superficial
sinus (meninges) — *see* Phlebitis, intracranial (venous) sinus
soleal vein I80.25- ☑
specified site NEC I80.8
syphilitic A52.09
tibial vein — *see* Phlebitis, leg, deep, tibial
ulcerative I80.9
leg — *see* Phlebitis, leg
umbilicus I80.8
uterus (septic) — *see* Endometritis
varicose (leg) (lower limb) — *see* Varix, leg, with, inflammation
Phlebofibrosis I87.8
Phleboliths I87.8
Phlebopathy,
gestational O22.9- ☑
puerperal O87.9
Phlebosclerosis I87.8
Phlebothrombosis — *see also* Thrombosis
antepartum — *see* Thrombophlebitis, antepartum
pregnancy — *see* Thrombophlebitis, antepartum
puerperal — *see* Thrombophlebitis, puerperal
Phlebotomus fever A93.1
Phlegmasia
alba dolens O87.1
nonpuerperal — *see* Phlebitis, femoral vein
cerulea dolens — *see* Phlebitis, leg, deep
Phlegmon — *see* Abscess
Phlegmonous — *see* condition
Phlyctenulosis (allergic) (keratoconjunctivitis) (nontuberculous) — *see also* Keratoconjunctivitis
cornea — *see* Keratoconjunctivitis
tuberculous A18.52
Phobia, phobic F40.9
animal F40.218
spiders F40.210
examination F40.298
reaction F40.9
simple F40.298
social F40.10
generalized F40.11
specific (isolated) F40.298
animal F40.218
spiders F40.210
blood F40.230
injection F40.231
injury F40.233
men F40.290
natural environment F40.228
thunderstorms F40.220

Phobia, phobic — *continued*
specific — *continued*
situational F40.248
bridges F40.242
closed in spaces F40.240
flying F40.243
heights F40.241
specified focus NEC F40.298
transfusion F40.231
women F40.291
specified NEC F40.8
medical care NEC F40.232
state F40.9
Phocas' disease — *see* Mastopathy, cystic
Phocomelia Q73.1
lower limb — *see* Agenesis, leg, with foot present
upper limb — *see* Agenesis, arm, with hand present
Phoria H50.50
Phosphate-losing tubular disorder N25.0
Phosphatemia E83.39
Phosphaturia E83.39
Photodermatitis (sun) L56.8
chronic L57.8
due to drug L56.8
light other than sun L59.8
Photokeratitis H16.13- ☑
Photophobia H53.14- ☑
Photophthalmia — *see* Photokeratitis
Photopsia H53.19
Photoretinitis — *see* Retinopathy, solar
Photosensitivity, photosensitization (sun) skin L56.8
light other than sun L59.8
Phrenitis — *see* Encephalitis
Phrynoderma (vitamin A deficiency) E50.8
Phthiriasis (pubis) B85.3
with any infestation classifiable to B85.0-B85.2 B85.4
Phthirus infestation — *see* Phthiriasis
Phthisis — *see also* Tuberculosis
bulbi (infectional) — *see* Disorder, globe, degenerated condition, atrophy
eyeball (due to infection) — *see* Disorder, globe, degenerated condition, atrophy
Phycomycosis — *see* Zygomycosis
Physalopteriasis B81.8
Physical restraint status Z78.1
Phytobezoar T18.9 ☑
intestine T18.3 ☑
stomach T18.2 ☑
Pian — *see* Yaws
Pianoma A66.1
Pica F50.89
in adults F50.89
infant or child F98.3
Picking, nose F98.8
Pick-Niemann disease — *see* Niemann-Pick disease or syndrome
Pick's
cerebral atrophy G31.01 *[F02.80]*
with behavioral disturbance G31.01 *[F02.81]*
disease or syndrome (brain) G31.01 *[F02.80]*
with behavioral disturbance G31.01 *[F02.81]*
brain G31.01 *[F02.80]*
with behavioral disturbance G31.01 *[F02.81]*
pericardium (pericardial pseudocirrhosis of liver) I31.1
syndrome
brain G31.01 *[F02.80]*
with behavioral disturbance G31.01 *[F02.81]*
of heart (pericardial pseudocirrhosis of liver) I31.1
Pickwickian syndrome E66.2
Piebaldism E70.39
Piedra (beard) (scalp) B36.8
black B36.3
white B36.2
Pierre Robin deformity or syndrome Q87.0
Pierson's disease or osteochondrosis M91.0
Pig-bel A05.2
Pigeon
breast or chest (acquired) M95.4
congenital Q67.7
rachitic sequelae (late effect) E64.3
breeder's disease or lung J67.2
fancier's disease or lung J67.2
toe — *see* Deformity, toe, specified NEC
Pigmentation (abnormal) (anomaly) L81.9
conjunctiva H11.13- ☑
cornea (anterior) H18.01- ☑

Pigmentation — *continued*
cornea — *continued*
posterior H18.05- ☑
stromal H18.06- ☑
diminished melanin formation NEC L81.6
iron L81.8
lids, congenital Q82.8
limbus corneae — *see* Pigmentation, cornea
metals L81.8
optic papilla, congenital Q14.2
retina, congenital (grouped) (nevoid) Q14.1
scrotum, congenital Q82.8
tattoo L81.8
Piles — *see also* Hemorrhoids K64.9
Pili
annulati or torti (congenital) Q84.1
incarnati L73.1
Pill roller hand (intrinsic) — *see* Parkinsonism
Pilomatrixoma — *see* Neoplasm, skin, benign
malignant — *see* Neoplasm, skin, malignant
Pilonidal — *see* condition
Pimple R23.8
PIN — *see* Neoplasia, intraepithelial, prostate
Pinched nerve — *see* Neuropathy, entrapment
Pindborg tumor — *see* Cyst, calcifying odontogenic
Pineal body or gland — *see* condition
Pinealoblastoma C75.3
Pinealoma D44.5
malignant C75.3
Pineoblastoma C75.3
Pineocytoma D44.5
Pinguecula H11.15- ☑
Pingueculitis H10.81- ☑
Pinhole meatus — *see also* Stricture, urethra N35.919
Pink
disease — *see* subcategory T56.1 ☑
eye — *see* Conjunctivitis, acute, mucopurulent
Pinkus' disease (lichen nitidus) L44.1
Pinpoint
meatus — *see* Stricture, urethra
os (uteri) — *see* Stricture, cervix
Pins and needles R20.2
Pinta A67.9
cardiovascular lesions A67.2
chancre (primary) A67.0
erythematous plaques A67.1
hyperchromic lesions A67.1
hyperkeratosis A67.1
lesions A67.9
cardiovascular A67.2
hyperchromic A67.1
intermediate A67.1
late A67.2
mixed A67.3
primary A67.0
skin (achromic) (cicatricial) (dyschromic) A67.2
hyperchromic A67.1
mixed (achromic and hyperchromic) A67.3
papule (primary) A67.0
skin lesions (achromic) (cicatricial) (dyschromic) A67.2
hyperchromic A67.1
mixed (achromic and hyperchromic) A67.3
vitiligo A67.2
Pintids A67.1
Pinworm (disease) (infection) (infestation) B80
Piroplasmosis B60.0
Pistol wound — *see* Gunshot wound
Pitchers' elbow — *see* Derangement, joint, specified type NEC, elbow
Pithecoid pelvis Q74.2
with disproportion (fetopelvic) O33.0
causing obstructed labor O65.0
Pithiatism F48.8
Pitted — *see* Pitting
Pitting — *see also* Edema R60.9
lip R60.0
nail L60.8
teeth K00.4
Pituitary gland — *see* condition
Pituitary-snuff-taker's disease J67.8
Pityriasis (capitis) L21.0
alba L30.5
circinata (et maculata) L42
furfuracea L21.0
Hebra's L26
lichenoides L41.0
chronica L41.1

Pityriasis — *continued*
  lichenoides — *continued*
    et varioliformis (acuta) L41.0
  maculata (et circinata) L30.5
  nigra B36.1
  pilaris, Hebra's L44.0
  rosea L42
  rotunda L44.8
  rubra (Hebra) pilaris L44.0
  simplex L30.5
  specified type NEC L30.5
  streptogenes L30.5
  versicolor (scrotal) B36.0
Placenta, placental — *see* Pregnancy, complicated by (care of) (management affected by), specified condition
Placentitis O41.14- ☑
Plagiocephaly Q67.3
Plague A20.9
  abortive A20.8
  ambulatory A20.8
  asymptomatic A20.8
  bubonic A20.0
  cellulocutaneous A20.1
  cutaneobubonic A20.1
  lymphatic gland A20.0
  meningitis A20.3
  pharyngeal A20.8
  pneumonic (primary) (secondary) A20.2
  pulmonary, pulmonic A20.2
  septicemic A20.7
  tonsillar A20.8
    septicemic A20.7
Planning, family
  contraception Z30.9
  procreation Z31.69
Plaque(s)
  artery, arterial — *see* Arteriosclerosis
  calcareous — *see* Calcification
  coronary, lipid rich I25.83
  epicardial I31.8
  erythematous, of pinta A67.1
  Hollenhorst's — *see* Occlusion, artery, retina
  lipid rich, coronary I25.83
  pleural (without asbestos) J92.9
    with asbestos J92.0
  tongue K13.29
Plasmacytoma C90.3- ☑
  extramedullary C90.2- ☑
  medullary C90.0- ☑
  solitary C90.3- ☑
Plasmacytopenia D72.818
Plasmacytosis D72.822
Plaster ulcer — *see* Ulcer, pressure, by site
Plateau iris syndrome (post-iridectomy) (postprocedural) (without glaucoma) H21.82
  with glaucoma H40.22- ☑
Platybasia Q75.8
Platyonychia (congenital) Q84.6
  acquired L60.8
Platypelloid pelvis M95.5
  with disproportion (fetopelvic) O33.0
    causing obstructed labor O65.0
  congenital Q74.2
Platyspondylisis Q76.49
Plaut (-Vincent) **disease** — *see also* Vincent's A69.1
Plethora R23.2
  newborn P61.1
Pleura, pleural — *see* condition
Pleuralgia R07.81
Pleurisy (acute) (adhesive) (chronic) (costal) (diaphragmatic) (double) (dry) (fibrinous) (fibrous) (interlobar) (latent) (plastic) (primary) (residual) (sicca) (sterile) (subacute) (unresolved) R09.1
  with
    adherent pleura J86.0
    effusion J90
      chylous, chyliform J94.0
      tuberculous (non primary) A15.6
        primary (progressive) A15.7
    tuberculosis — *see* Pleurisy, tuberculous (non primary)
  encysted — *see* Pleurisy, with effusion
  exudative — *see* Pleurisy, with effusion
  fibrinopurulent, fibropurulent — *see* Pyothorax
  hemorrhagic — *see* Hemothorax
  pneumococcal J90
  purulent — *see* Pyothorax

Pleurisy — *continued*
  septic — *see* Pyothorax
  serofibrinous — *see* Pleurisy, with effusion
  seropurulent — *see* Pyothorax
  serous — *see* Pleurisy, with effusion
  staphylococcal J86.9
  streptococcal J90
  suppurative — *see* Pyothorax
  traumatic (post) (current) — *see* Injury, intrathoracic, pleura
  tuberculous (with effusion) (non primary) A15.6
    primary (progressive) A15.7
Pleuritis sicca — *see* Pleurisy
Pleurobronchopneumonia — *see* Pneumonia, broncho-
Pleurodynia R07.81
  epidemic B33.0
  viral B33.0
Pleuropericarditis — *see also* Pericarditis
  acute I30.9
Pleuropneumonia (acute) (bilateral) (double) (septic) — *see also* Pneumonia J18.8
  chronic — *see* Fibrosis, lung
Pleuro-pneumonia-like-organism (PPLO), as cause of disease classified elsewhere B96.0
Pleurorrhea — *see* Pleurisy, with effusion
Plexitis, brachial G54.0
Plica
  polonica B85.0
  syndrome, knee M67.5- ☑
  tonsil J35.8
Plicated tongue K14.5
Plug
  bronchus NEC J98.09
  meconium (newborn) NEC syndrome P76.0
  mucus — *see* Asphyxia, mucus
Plumbism — *see* subcategory T56.0 ☑
Plummer's disease E05.20
  with thyroid storm E05.21
Plummer-Vinson syndrome D50.1
Pluricarential syndrome of infancy E40
Plus (and minus) **hand** (intrinsic) — *see* Deformity, limb, specified type NEC, forearm
Pneumathemia — *see* Air, embolism
Pneumatic hammer (drill) syndrome T75.21 ☑
Pneumatocele (lung) J98.4
  intracranial G93.89
  tension J44.9
Pneumatosis
  cystoides intestinalis K63.89
  intestinalis K63.89
  peritonei K66.8
Pneumaturia R39.89
Pneumoblastoma — *see* Neoplasm, lung, malignant
Pneumocephalus G93.89
Pneumococcemia A40.3
Pneumococcus, pneumococcal — *see* condition
Pneumoconiosis (due to) (inhalation of) J64
  with tuberculosis (any type in A15) J65
  aluminum J63.0
  asbestos J61
  bagasse, bagassosis J67.1
  bauxite J63.1
  beryllium J63.2
  coal miners' (simple) J60
  coalworkers' (simple) J60
  collier's J60
  cotton dust J66.0
  diatomite (diatomaceous earth) J62.8
  dust
    inorganic NEC J63.6
    lime J62.8
    marble J62.8
    organic NEC J66.8
  fumes or vapors (from silo) J68.9
  graphite J63.3
  grinder's J62.8
  kaolin J62.8
  mica J62.8
  millstone maker's J62.8
  mineral fibers NEC J61
  miner's J60
  moldy hay J67.0
  potter's J62.8
  rheumatoid — *see* Rheumatoid, lung
  sandblaster's J62.8
  silica, silicate NEC J62.8
    with carbon J60
  stonemason's J62.8

Pneumoconiosis — *continued*
  talc (dust) J62.0
Pneumocystis carinii pneumonia B59
Pneumocystis jiroveci (pneumonia) B59
Pneumocystosis (with pneumonia) B59
Pneumohemopericardium I31.2
Pneumohemothorax J94.2
  traumatic S27.2 ☑
Pneumohydropericardium — *see* Pericarditis
Pneumohydrothorax — *see* Hydrothorax
Pneumomediastinum J98.2
  congenital or perinatal P25.2
Pneumomycosis B49 *[J99]*
Pneumonia (acute) (double) (migratory) (purulent) (septic) (unresolved) J18.9
  with
    influenza — *see* Influenza, with, pneumonia
    lung abscess J85.1
      due to specified organism — *see* Pneumonia, in (due to)
  adenoviral J12.0
  adynamic J18.2
  alba A50.04
  allergic (eosinophilic) J82
  alveolar — *see* Pneumonia, lobar
  anaerobes J15.8
  anthrax A22.1
  apex, apical — *see* Pneumonia, lobar
  Ascaris B77.81
  aspiration J69.0
    due to
      aspiration of microorganisms
        bacterial J15.9
        viral J12.9
      food (regurgitated) J69.0
      gastric secretions J69.0
      milk (regurgitated) J69.0
      oils, essences J69.1
      solids, liquids NEC J69.8
      vomitus J69.0
    newborn P24.81
      amniotic fluid (clear) P24.11
      blood P24.21
      food (regurgitated) P24.31
      liquor (amnii) P24.11
      meconium P24.01
      milk P24.31
      mucus P24.11
      specified NEC P24.81
      stomach contents P24.31
    postprocedural J95.4
  atypical NEC J18.9
  bacillus J15.9
    specified NEC J15.8
  bacterial J15.9
    specified NEC J15.8
  Bacteroides (fragilis) (oralis) (melaninogenicus) J15.8
  basal, basic, basilar — *see* Pneumonia, by type
  bronchiolitis obliterans organized (BOOP) J84.89
  broncho-, bronchial (confluent) (croupous) (diffuse) (disseminated) (hemorrhagic) (involving lobes) (lobar) (terminal) J18.0
    allergic (eosinophilic) J82
    aspiration — *see* Pneumonia, aspiration
    bacterial J15.9
      specified NEC J15.8
    chronic — *see* Fibrosis, lung
    diplococcal J13
    Eaton's agent J15.7
    Escherichia coli (E. coli) J15.5
    Friedländer's bacillus J15.0
    Hemophilus influenzae J14
    hypostatic J18.2
    inhalation — *see also* Pneumonia, aspiration
      due to fumes or vapors (chemical) J68.0
      of oils or essences J69.1
    Klebsiella (pneumoniae) J15.0
    lipid, lipoid J69.1
      endogenous J84.89
    Mycoplasma (pneumoniae) J15.7
    pleuro-pneumonia-like-organisms (PPLO) J15.7
    pneumococcal J13
    Proteus J15.6
    Pseudomonas J15.1
    Serratia marcescens J15.6
    specified organism NEC J16.8
    staphylococcal — *see* Pneumonia, staphylococcal
    streptococcal NEC J15.4

☑ **Additional Character Required** — Refer to the Tabular List for Character Selection   ▽ **Subterms under main terms may continue to next column or page**

Pneumonia — *continued*
  broncho-, bronchial — *continued*
    streptococcal — *continued*
      group B J15.3
      pneumoniae J13
    viral, virus — *see* Pneumonia, viral
  Butyrivibrio (fibriosolvens) J15.8
  Candida B37.1
  caseous — *see* Tuberculosis, pulmonary
  catarrhal — *see* Pneumonia, broncho
  chlamydial J16.0
    congenital P23.1
  cholesterol J84.89
  cirrhotic (chronic) — *see* Fibrosis, lung
  Clostridium (haemolyticum) (novyi) J15.8
  confluent — *see* Pneumonia, broncho
  congenital (infective) P23.9
    due to
      bacterium NEC P23.6
      Chlamydia P23.1
      Escherichia coli P23.4
      Haemophilus influenzae P23.6
      infective organism NEC P23.8
      Klebsiella pneumoniae P23.6
      Mycoplasma P23.6
      Pseudomonas P23.5
      Staphylococcus P23.2
      Streptococcus (except group B) P23.6
        group B P23.3
      viral agent P23.0
    specified NEC P23.8
  croupous — *see* Pneumonia, lobar
  cryptogenic organizing J84.116
  cytomegalic inclusion B25.0
  cytomegaloviral B25.0
  deglutition — *see* Pneumonia, aspiration
  desquamative interstitial J84.117
  diffuse — *see* Pneumonia, broncho
  diplococcal, diplococcus (broncho-) (lobar) J13
  disseminated (focal) — *see* Pneumonia, broncho
  Eaton's agent J15.7
  embolic, embolism — *see* Embolism, pulmonary
  Enterobacter J15.6
  eosinophilic J82
  Escherichia coli (E. coli) J15.5
  Eubacterium J15.8
  fibrinous — *see* Pneumonia, lobar
  fibroid, fibrous (chronic) — *see* Fibrosis, lung
  Friedländer's bacillus J15.0
  Fusobacterium (nucleatum) J15.8
  gangrenous J85.0
  giant cell (measles) B05.2
  gonococcal A54.84
  gram-negative bacteria NEC J15.6
    anaerobic J15.8
  Hemophilus influenzae (broncho) (lobar) J14
  human metapneumovirus J12.3
  hypostatic (broncho) (lobar) J18.2
  in (due to)
    actinomycosis A42.0
    adenovirus J12.0
    anthrax A22.1
    ascariasis B77.81
    aspergillosis B44.9
    Bacillus anthracis A22.1
    Bacterium anitratum J15.6
    candidiasis B37.1
    chickenpox B01.2
    Chlamydia J16.0
      neonatal P23.1
    coccidioidomycosis B38.2
      acute B38.0
      chronic B38.1
    cytomegalovirus disease B25.0
    Diplococcus (pneumoniae) J13
    Eaton's agent J15.7
    Enterobacter J15.6
    Escherichia coli (E. coli) J15.5
    Friedländer's bacillus J15.0
    fumes and vapors (chemical) (inhalation) J68.0
    gonorrhea A54.84
    Hemophilus influenzae (H. influenzae) J14
    Herellea J15.6
    histoplasmosis B39.2
      acute B39.0
      chronic B39.1
    human metapneumovirus J12.3
    Klebsiella (pneumoniae) J15.0

Pneumonia — *continued*
  in — *continued*
    measles B05.2
    Mycoplasma (pneumoniae) J15.7
    nocardiosis, nocardiasis A43.0
    ornithosis A70
    parainfluenza virus J12.2
    pleuro-pneumonia-like-organism (PPLO) J15.7
    pneumococcus J13
    pneumocystosis (Pneumocystis carinii) (Pneumocys-
      tis jiroveci) B59
    Proteus J15.6
    Pseudomonas NEC J15.1
      pseudomallei A24.1
    psittacosis A70
    Q fever A78
    respiratory syncytial virus (RSV) J12.1
    rheumatic fever I00 *[J17]*
    rubella B06.81
    Salmonella (infection) A02.22
      typhi A01.03
    schistosomiasis B65.9 *[J17]*
    Serratia marcescens J15.6
    specified
      bacterium NEC J15.8
      organism NEC J16.8
    spirochetal NEC A69.8
    Staphylococcus J15.20
      aureus (methicillin susceptible) (MSSA) J15.211
        methicillin resistant (MRSA) J15.212
      specified NEC J15.29
    Streptococcus J15.4
      group B J15.3
      pneumoniae J13
      specified NEC J15.4
    toxoplasmosis B58.3
    tularemia A21.2
    typhoid (fever) A01.03
    varicella B01.2
    virus — *see* Pneumonia, viral
    whooping cough A37.91
      due to
        Bordetella parapertussis A37.11
        Bordetella pertussis A37.01
        specified NEC A37.81
    Yersinia pestis A20.2
  inhalation of food or vomit — *see* Pneumonia, aspira-
    tion
  interstitial J84.9
    chronic J84.111
    desquamative J84.117
    due to
      collagen vascular disease J84.17
      known underlying cause J84.17
    idiopathic NOS J84.111
    in disease classified elsewhere J84.17
    lymphocytic (due to collagen vascular disease) (in
      diseases classified elsewhere) J84.17
    lymphoid J84.2
    non-specific J84.89
      due to
        collagen vascular disease J84.17
        known underlying cause J84.17
      idiopathic J84.113
      in diseases classified elsewhere J84.17
    plasma cell B59
    pseudomonas J15.1
    usual J84.112
      due to collagen vascular disease J84.17
      idiopathic J84.112
      in diseases classified elsewhere J84.17
  Klebsiella (pneumoniae) J15.0
  lipid, lipoid (exogenous) J69.1
    endogenous J84.89
  lobar (disseminated) (double) (interstitial) J18.1
    bacterial J15.9
      specified NEC J15.8
    chronic — *see* Fibrosis, lung
    Escherichia coli (E. coli) J15.5
    Friedländer's bacillus J15.0
    Hemophilus influenzae J14
    hypostatic J18.2
    Klebsiella (pneumoniae) J15.0
    pneumococcal J13
    Proteus J15.6
    Pseudomonas J15.1
    specified organism NEC J16.8
    staphylococcal — *see* Pneumonia, staphylococcal
    streptococcal NEC J15.4

Pneumonia — *continued*
  lobar — *continued*
    Streptococcus pneumoniae J13
    viral, virus — *see* Pneumonia, viral
  lobular — *see* Pneumonia, broncho
  Löffler's J82
  lymphoid interstitial J84.2
  massive — *see* Pneumonia, lobar
  meconium P24.01
  MRSA (methicillin resistant Staphylococcus aureus)
    J15.212
  MSSA (methicillin susceptible Staphylococcus aureus)
    J15.211
  multilobar — *see* Pneumonia, by type
  Mycoplasma (pneumoniae) J15.7
  necrotic J85.0
  neonatal P23.9
    aspiration — *see* Aspiration, by substance, with
      pneumonia
  nitrogen dioxide J68.0
  organizing J84.89
    due to
      collagen vascular disease J84.17
      known underlying cause J84.17
    in diseases classified elsewhere J84.17
  orthostatic J18.2
  parainfluenza virus J12.2
  parenchymatous — *see* Fibrosis, lung
  passive J18.2
  patchy — *see* Pneumonia, broncho
  Peptococcus J15.8
  Peptostreptococcus J15.8
  plasma cell (of infants) B59
  pleurolobar — *see* Pneumonia, lobar
  pleuro-pneumonia-like organism (PPLO) J15.7
  pneumococcal (broncho) (lobar) J13
  Pneumocystis (carinii) (jiroveci) B59
  postinfectional NEC B99 ☑ *[J17]*
  postmeasles B05.2
  Proteus J15.6
  Pseudomonas J15.1
  psittacosis A70
  radiation J70.0
  respiratory syncytial virus (RSV) J12.1
  resulting from a procedure J95.89
  rheumatic I00 *[J17]*
  Salmonella (arizonae) (cholerae-suis) (enteritidis) (ty-
    phimurium) A02.22
    typhi A01.03
    typhoid fever A01.03
  SARS-associated coronavirus J12.81
  segmented, segmental — *see* Pneumonia, broncho-
  Serratia marcescens J15.6
  specified NEC J18.8
    bacterium NEC J15.8
    organism NEC J16.8
    virus NEC J12.89
  spirochetal NEC A69.8
  staphylococcal (broncho) (lobar) J15.20
    aureus (methicillin susceptible) (MSSA) J15.211
      methicillin resistant (MRSA) J15.212
    specified NEC J15.29
  static, stasis J18.2
  streptococcal NEC (broncho) (lobar) J15.4
    group
      A J15.4
      B J15.3
    specified NEC J15.4
  Streptococcus pneumoniae J13
  syphilitic, congenital (early) A50.04
  traumatic (complication) (early) (secondary) T79.8 ☑
  tuberculous (any) — *see* Tuberculosis, pulmonary
  tularemic A21.2
  varicella B01.2
  Veillonella J15.8
  ventilator associated J95.851
  viral, virus (broncho) (interstitial) (lobar) J12.9
    adenoviral J12.0
    congenital P23.0
    human metapneumovirus J12.3
    parainfluenza J12.2
    respiratory syncytial (RSV) J12.1
    SARS-associated coronavirus J12.81
    specified NEC J12.89
  white (congenital) A50.04
Pneumonic — *see* condition
Pneumonitis (acute) (primary) — *see also* Pneumonia
  air-conditioner J67.7

Pneumonitis — continued
  allergic (due to) J67.9
    organic dust NEC J67.8
    red cedar dust J67.8
    sequoiosis J67.8
    wood dust J67.8
  aspiration J69.0
    due to
      anesthesia J95.4
        during
          labor and delivery O74.0
            pregnancy O29.01- ☑
            puerperium O89.01
      fumes or gases J68.0
    obstetric O74.0
  chemical (due to gases, fumes or vapors) (inhalation) J68.0
    due to anesthesia J95.4
  cholesterol J84.89
  chronic — see Fibrosis, lung
  congenital rubella P35.0
  crack (cocaine) J68.0
  due to
    beryllium J68.0
    cadmium J68.0
    crack (cocaine) J68.0
    detergent J69.8
    fluorocarbon-polymer J68.0
    food, vomit (aspiration) J69.0
    fumes or vapors J68.0
    gases, fumes or vapors (inhalation) J68.0
    inhalation
      blood J69.8
      essences J69.1
      food (regurgitated), milk, vomit J69.0
      oils, essences J69.1
      saliva J69.0
      solids, liquids NEC J69.8
    manganese J68.0
    nitrogen dioxide J68.0
    oils, essences J69.1
    solids, liquids NEC J69.8
    toxoplasmosis (acquired) B58.3
      congenital P37.1
    vanadium J68.0
    ventilator J95.851
  eosinophilic J82
  hypersensitivity J67.9
    air conditioner lung J67.7
    bagassosis J67.1
    bird fancier's lung J67.2
    farmer's lung J67.0
    maltworker's lung J67.4
    maple bark-stripper's lung J67.6
    mushroom worker's lung J67.5
    specified organic dust NEC J67.8
    suberosis J67.3
  interstitial (chronic) J84.89
    acute J84.114
    lymphoid J84.2
    non-specific J84.89
      idiopathic J84.113
  lymphoid, interstitial J84.2
  meconium P24.01
  postanesthetic J95.4
    correct substance properly administered — see Table of Drugs and Chemicals, by drug, adverse effect
    in labor and delivery O74.0
    in pregnancy O29.01- ☑
    obstetric O74.0
    overdose or wrong substance given or taken (by accident) — see Table of Drugs and Chemicals, by drug, poisoning
    postpartum, puerperal O89.01
  postoperative J95.4
    obstetric O74.0
  radiation J70.0
  rubella, congenital P35.0
  ventilation (air-conditioning) J67.7
  ventilator associated J95.851
  wood-dust J67.8
Pneumonoconiosis — see Pneumoconiosis
Pneumoparotid K11.8
Pneumopathy NEC J98.4
  alveolar J84.09
  due to organic dust NEC J66.8
  parietoalveolar J84.09

Pneumopericarditis — see also Pericarditis
  acute I30.9
Pneumopericardium — see also Pericarditis
  congenital P25.3
  newborn P25.3
  traumatic (post) — see Injury, heart
Pneumophagia (psychogenic) F45.8
Pneumopleurisy, pneumopleuritis — see also Pneumonia J18.8
Pneumopyopericardium I30.1
Pneumopyothorax — see Pyopneumothorax
  with fistula J86.0
Pneumorrhagia — see also Hemorrhage, lung
  tuberculous — see Tuberculosis, pulmonary
Pneumothorax NOS J93.9
  acute J93.83
  chronic J93.81
  congenital P25.1
  perinatal period P25.1
  postprocedural J95.811
  specified NEC J93.83
  spontaneous NOS J93.83
    newborn P25.1
    primary J93.11
    secondary J93.12
    tension J93.0
  tense valvular, infectional J93.0
  tension (spontaneous) J93.0
  traumatic S27.0 ☑
    with hemothorax S27.2 ☑
  tuberculous — see Tuberculosis, pulmonary
Podagra — see also Gout M10.9
Podencephalus Q01.9
Poikilocytosis R71.8
Poikiloderma L81.6
  Civatte's L57.3
  congenital Q82.8
  vasculare atrophicans L94.5
Poikilodermatomyositis M33.10
  with
    myopathy M33.12
    respiratory involvement M33.11
    specified organ involvement NEC M33.19
Pointed ear (congenital) Q17.3
Poison ivy, oak, sumac or other plant dermatitis (allergic) (contact) L23.7
Poisoning (acute) — see also Table of Drugs and Chemicals
  algae and toxins T65.82- ☑
  Bacillus B (aertrycke) (cholerae (suis)) (paratyphosus) (suipestifer) A02.9
    botulinus A05.1
  bacterial toxins A05.9
  berries, noxious — see Poisoning, food, noxious, berries
  botulism A05.1
  ciguatera fish T61.0- ☑
  Clostridium botulinum A05.1
  death-cap (Amanita phalloides) (Amanita verna) — see Poisoning, food, noxious, mushrooms
  drug — see Table of Drugs and Chemicals, by drug, poisoning
  epidemic, fish (noxious) — see Poisoning, seafood
    bacterial A05.9
  fava bean D55.0
  fish (noxious) T61.9- ☑
    bacterial — see Intoxication, foodborne, by agent
    ciguatera fish — see Poisoning, ciguatera fish
    scombroid fish — see Poisoning, scombroid fish
    specified type NEC T61.77- ☑
  food NEC A05.9
    bacterial — see Intoxication, foodborne, by agent
    due to
      Bacillus (aertrycke) (choleraesuis) (paratyphosus) (suipestifer) A02.9
        botulinus A05.1
      Clostridium (perfringens) (Welchii) A05.2
      salmonella (aertrycke) (callinarum) (choleraesuis) (enteritidis) (paratyphi) (suipestifer) A02.9
        with
          gastroenteritis A02.0
          sepsis A02.1
      staphylococcus A05.0
      Vibrio
        parahaemolyticus A05.3
        vulnificus A05.5
    noxious or naturally toxic T62.9- ☑
      berries — see subcategory T62.1 ☑
      fish — see Poisoning, seafood

Poisoning — continued
  food — continued
    noxious or naturally toxic — continued
      mushrooms — see subcategory T62.0X ☑
      plants NEC — see subcategory T62.2X ☑
      seafood — see Poisoning, seafood
      specified NEC — see subcategory T62.8X ☑
  ichthyotoxism — see Poisoning, seafood
  kreotoxism, food A05.9
  latex T65.81- ☑
  lead T56.0- ☑
  mushroom — see Poisoning, food, noxious, mushroom
  mussels — see also Poisoning, shellfish
    bacterial — see Intoxication, foodborne, by agent
  nicotine (tobacco) T65.2- ☑
  noxious foodstuffs — see Poisoning, food, noxious
  plants, noxious — see Poisoning, food, noxious, plants NEC
  ptomaine — see Poisoning, food
  radiation J70.0
  Salmonella (arizonae) (cholerae-suis) (enteritidis) (typhimurium) A02.9
  scombroid fish T61.1- ☑
  seafood (noxious) T61.9- ☑
    bacterial — see Intoxication, foodborne, by agent
    fish — see Poisoning, fish
    shellfish — see Poisoning, shellfish
    specified NEC — see subcategory T61.8X ☑
  shellfish (amnesic) (azaspiracid) (diarrheic) (neurotoxic) (noxious) (paralytic) T61.78- ☑
    bacterial — see Intoxication, foodborne, by agent
    ciguatera mollusk — see Poisoning, ciguatera fish
  specified substance NEC T65.891 ☑
  Staphylococcus, food A05.0
  tobacco (nicotine) T65.2- ☑
  water E87.79
Poker spine — see Spondylitis, ankylosing
Poland syndrome Q79.8
Polioencephalitis (acute) (bulbar) A80.9
  inferior G12.22
  influenzal — see Influenza, with, encephalopathy
  superior hemorrhagic (acute) (Wernicke's) E51.2
  Wernicke's E51.2
Polioencephalomyelitis (acute) (anterior) A80.9
  with beriberi E51.2
Polioencephalopathy, superior hemorrhagic E51.2
  with
    beriberi E51.11
    pellagra E52
Poliomeningoencephalitis — see Meningoencephalitis
Poliomyelitis (acute) (anterior) (epidemic) A80.9
  with paralysis (bulbar) — see Poliomyelitis, paralytic
  abortive A80.4
  ascending (progressive) — see Poliomyelitis, paralytic
  bulbar (paralytic) — see Poliomyelitis, paralytic
  congenital P35.8
  nonepidemic A80.9
  nonparalytic A80.4
  paralytic A80.30
    specified NEC A80.39
    vaccine-associated A80.0
    wild virus
      imported A80.1
      indigenous A80.2
  spinal, acute A80.9
Poliosis (eyebrow) (eyelashes) L67.1
  circumscripta, acquired L67.1
Pollakiuria R35.0
  psychogenic F45.8
Pollinosis J30.1
Pollitzer's disease L73.2
Polyadenitis — see also Lymphadenitis
  malignant A20.0
Polyalgia M79.89
Polyangiitis M30.0
  microscopic M31.7
  overlap syndrome M30.8
Polyarteritis
  microscopic M31.7
  nodosa M30.0
    with lung involvement M30.1
    juvenile M30.2
    related condition NEC M30.8
Polyarthralgia — see Pain, joint
Polyarthritis, polyarthropathy — see also Arthritis M13.0

Polyarthritis, polyarthropathy — *continued*
  due to or associated with other specified conditions — *see* Arthritis
  epidemic (Australian) (with exanthema) B33.1
  infective — *see* Arthritis, pyogenic or pyemic
  inflammatory M06.4
  juvenile (chronic) (seronegative) M08.3
  migratory M13.8- ☑
  rheumatic, acute — *see* Fever, rheumatic
Polyarthrosis M15.9
  post-traumatic M15.3
  primary M15.0
  specified NEC M15.8
Polycarential syndrome of infancy E40
Polychondritis (atrophic) (chronic) — *see also* Disorder, cartilage, specified type NEC
  relapsing M94.1
Polycoria Q13.2
Polycystic (disease)
  degeneration, kidney Q61.3
    autosomal dominant (adult type) Q61.2
    autosomal recessive (infantile type) NEC Q61.19
  kidney Q61.3
    autosomal
      dominant Q61.2
      recessive NEC Q61.19
    autosomal dominant (adult type) Q61.2
    autosomal recessive (childhood type) NEC Q61.19
    infantile type NEC Q61.19
  liver Q44.6
  lung J98.4
    congenital Q33.0
  ovary, ovaries E28.2
  spleen Q89.09
Polycythemia (secondary) D75.1
  acquired D75.1
  benign (familial) D75.0
  due to
    donor twin P61.1
    erythropoietin D75.1
    fall in plasma volume D75.1
    high altitude D75.1
    maternal-fetal transfusion P61.1
    stress D75.1
  emotional D75.1
  erythropoietin D75.1
  familial (benign) D75.0
  Gaisböck's (hypertonica) D75.1
  high altitude D75.1
  hypertonica D75.1
  hypoxemic D75.1
  neonatorum P61.1
  nephrogenous D75.1
  relative D75.1
  secondary D75.1
  spurious D75.1
  stress D75.1
  vera D45
Polycytosis cryptogenica D75.1
Polydactylism, polydactyly Q69.9 — *extra digits — look up in Alpha*
  toes Q69.2
Polydipsia R63.1
Polydystrophy, pseudo-Hurler E77.0
Polyembryoma — *see* Neoplasm, malignant, by site
Polyglandular
  deficiency E31.0
  dyscrasia E31.9
  dysfunction E31.9
  syndrome E31.8
Polyhydramnios O40.- ☑
Polymastia Q83.1
Polymenorrhea N92.0
Polymyalgia M35.3
  arteritica, giant cell M31.5
  rheumatica M35.3
    with giant cell arteritis M31.5
Polymyositis (acute) (chronic) (hemorrhagic) M33.20
  with
    myopathy M33.22
    respiratory involvement M33.21
    skin involvement — *see* Dermatopolymyositis
    specified organ involvement NEC M33.29
  ossificans (generalisata) (progressiva) — *see* Myositis, ossificans, progressiva
Polyneuritis, polyneuritic — *see also* Polyneuropathy
  acute (post-)infective G61.0
  alcoholic G62.1
  cranialis G52.7

Polyneuritis, polyneuritic — *continued*
  demyelinating, chronic inflammatory (CIDP) G61.81
  diabetic — *see* Diabetes, polyneuropathy
  diphtheritic A36.83
  due to lack of vitamin NEC E56.9 *[G63]*
  endemic E51.11
  erythredema — *see* subcategory T56.1 ☑
  febrile, acute G61.0
  hereditary ataxic G60.1
  idiopathic, acute G61.0
  infective (acute) G61.0
  inflammatory, chronic demyelinating (CIDP) G61.81
  nutritional E63.9 *[G63]*
  postinfective (acute) G61.0
  specified NEC G62.89
Polyneuropathy (peripheral) G62.9
  alcoholic G62.1
  amyloid (Portuguese) E85.1 *[G63]*
    transthyretin-related (ATTR) familial E85.1 *[G63]*
  arsenical G62.2
  critical illness G62.81
  demyelinating, chronic inflammatory (CIDP) G61.81
  diabetic — *see* Diabetes, polyneuropathy
  drug-induced G62.0
  hereditary G60.9
    specified NEC G60.8
  idiopathic G60.9
    progressive G60.3
  in (due to)
    alcohol G62.1
      sequelae G65.2
    amyloidosis, familial (Portuguese) E85.1 *[G63]*
    antitetanus serum G61.1
    arsenic G62.2
      sequelae G65.2
    avitaminosis NEC E56.9 *[G63]*
    beriberi E51.11
    collagen vascular disease NEC M35.9 *[G63]*
    deficiency (of)
      B (-complex) vitamins E53.9 *[G63]*
      vitamin B6 E53.1 *[G63]*
    diabetes — *see* Diabetes, polyneuropathy
    diphtheria A36.83
    drug or medicament G62.0
      correct substance properly administered — *see* Table of Drugs and Chemicals, by drug, adverse effect
      overdose or wrong substance given or taken — *see* Table of Drugs and Chemicals, by drug, poisoning
    endocrine disease NEC E34.9 *[G63]*
    herpes zoster B02.23
    hypoglycemia E16.2 *[G63]*
    infectious
      disease NEC B99 ☑ *[G63]*
      mononucleosis B27.91
    lack of vitamin NEC E56.9 *[G63]*
    lead G62.2
      sequelae G65.2
    leprosy A30.9 *[G63]*
    Lyme disease A69.22
    metabolic disease NEC E88.9 *[G63]*
    microscopic polyangiitis M31.7 *[G63]*
    mumps B26.84
    neoplastic disease — *see also* Neoplasm D49.9 *[G63]*
    nutritional deficiency NEC E63.9 *[G63]*
    organophosphate compounds G62.2
      sequelae G65.2
    parasitic disease NEC B89 *[G63]*
    pellagra E52 *[G63]*
    polyarteritis nodosa M30.0
    porphyria E80.20 *[G63]*
    radiation G62.82
    rheumatoid arthritis — *see* Rheumatoid, polyneuropathy
    sarcoidosis D86.89
    serum G61.1
    syphilis (late) A52.15
      congenital A50.43
    systemic
      connective tissue disorder M35.9 *[G63]*
      lupus erythematosus M32.19
    toxic agent NEC G62.2
      sequelae G65.2
  inflammatory G61.9
    chronic demyelinating (CIDP) G61.81
    sequelae G65.1
    specified NEC G61.89

Polyneuropathy — *continued*
  lead G62.2
    sequelae G65.2
  nutritional NEC E63.9 *[G63]*
  postherpetic (zoster) B02.23
  progressive G60.3
  radiation-induced G62.82
  sensory (hereditary) (idiopathic) G60.8
  specified NEC G62.89
  syphilitic (late) A52.15
    congenital A50.43
  transthyretin-related (ATTR) familial amyloid E85.1
    triorthocresyl phosphate G62.2
      sequelae G65.2
    tuberculosis A17.89
    uremia N18.9 *[G63]*
    vitamin B12 deficiency E53.8 *[G63]*
      with anemia (pernicious) D51.0 *[G63]*
        due to dietary deficiency D51.3 *[G63]*
    zoster B02.23
Polyopia H53.8
Polyorchism, polyorchidism Q55.21
Polyosteoarthritis — *see also* Osteoarthritis, generalized M15.9
  post-traumatic M15.3
  specified NEC M15.8
Polyostotic fibrous dysplasia Q78.1
Polyotia Q17.0
Polyp, polypus
  accessory sinus J33.8
  adenocarcinoma in — *see* Neoplasm, malignant, by site
  adenocarcinoma in situ in — *see* Neoplasm, in situ, by site
  adenoid tissue J33.0
  adenomatous — *see also* Neoplasm, benign, by site
    adenocarcinoma in — *see* Neoplasm, malignant, by site
    adenocarcinoma in situ in — *see* Neoplasm, in situ, by site
    carcinoma in — *see* Neoplasm, malignant, by site
    carcinoma in situ in — *see* Neoplasm, in situ, by site
    multiple — *see* Neoplasm, benign, by site
      adenocarcinoma in — *see* Neoplasm, malignant, by site
      adenocarcinoma in situ in — *see* Neoplasm, in situ, by site
  antrum J33.8
  anus, anal (canal) K62.0
  Bartholin's gland N84.3
  bladder D41.4
  carcinoma in — *see* Neoplasm, malignant, by site
  carcinoma in situ in — *see* Neoplasm, in situ, by site
  cecum D12.0
  cervix (uteri) N84.1
    in pregnancy or childbirth — *see* Pregnancy, complicated by, abnormal, cervix
    mucous N84.1
    nonneoplastic N84.1
  choanal J33.0
  cholesterol K82.4
  clitoris N84.3
  colon K63.5
    adenomatous D12.6
    ascending D12.2
    cecum D12.0
    descending D12.4
    hyperplastic, (any site) K63.5
    inflammatory K51.40
      with
        abscess K51.414
        complication K51.419
          specified NEC K51.418
        fistula K51.413
        intestinal obstruction K51.412
        rectal bleeding K51.411
    sigmoid D12.5
    transverse D12.3
  corpus uteri N84.0
  dental K04.01
    irreversible K04.02
    reversible K04.01
  duodenum K31.7
  ear (middle) H74.4- ☑
  endometrium N84.0
  ethmoidal (sinus) J33.8
  fallopian tube N84.8
  female genital tract N84.9

▽ Subterms under main terms may continue to next column or page   ☑ Additional Character Required — Refer to the Tabular List for Character Selection   **257**

Polyarthritis, polyarthropathy — Polyp, polypus

Polyp, polypus — *continued*
  female genital tract — *continued*
    specified NEC N84.8
  frontal (sinus) J33.8
  gallbladder K82.4
  gingiva, gum K06.8
  labia, labium (majus) (minus) N84.3
  larynx (mucous) J38.1
    adenomatous D14.1
  malignant — *see* Neoplasm, malignant, by site
  maxillary (sinus) J33.8
  middle ear — *see* Polyp, ear (middle)
  myometrium N84.0
  nares
    anterior J33.9
    posterior J33.0
  nasal (mucous) J33.9
    cavity J33.0
    septum J33.0
  nasopharyngeal J33.0
  nose (mucous) J33.9
  oviduct N84.8
  pharynx J39.2
  placenta O90.89
  prostate — *see* Enlargement, enlarged, prostate
  pudenda, pudendum N84.3
  pulpal (dental) K04.01
    irreversible K04.02
    reversible K04.01
  rectum (nonadenomatous) K62.1
    adenomatous — *see* Polyp, adenomatous
  septum (nasal) J33.0
  sinus (accessory) (ethmoidal) (frontal) (maxillary)
    (sphenoidal) J33.8
  sphenoidal (sinus) J33.8
  stomach K31.7
    adenomatous D13.1
  tube, fallopian N84.8
  turbinate, mucous membrane J33.8
  umbilical, newborn P83.6
  ureter N28.89
  urethra N36.2
  uterus (body) (corpus) (mucous) N84.0
    cervix N84.1
    in pregnancy or childbirth — *see* Pregnancy, com-
      plicated by, tumor, uterus
  vagina N84.2
  vocal cord (mucous) J38.1
  vulva N84.3
Polyphagia R63.2
Polyploidy Q92.7
Polypoid — *see* condition
Polyposis — *see also* Polyp
  coli (adenomatous) D12.6
    adenocarcinoma in C18.9
    adenocarcinoma in situ in — *see* Neoplasm, in situ,
      by site
    carcinoma in C18.9
  colon (adenomatous) D12.6
  familial D12.6
    adenocarcinoma in situ in — *see* Neoplasm, in situ,
      by site
  intestinal (adenomatous) D12.6
  malignant lymphomatous C83.1- ☑
  multiple, adenomatous — *see also* Neoplasm, benign
    D36.9
Polyradiculitis — *see* Polyneuropathy
Polyradiculoneuropathy (acute) (postinfective) (seg-
  mentally demyelinating) G61.0
Polyserositis
  due to pericarditis I31.1
  pericardial I31.1
  periodic, familial E85.0
  tuberculous A19.9
    acute A19.1
    chronic A19.8
Polysplenia syndrome Q89.09
Polysyndactyly — *see also* Syndactylism, syndactyly
  Q70.4
Polytrichia L68.3
Polyunguia Q84.6
Polyuria R35.8
  nocturnal R35.1
  psychogenic F45.8
Pompe's disease (glycogen storage) E74.02
Pompholyx L30.1
Poncet's disease (tuberculous rheumatism) A18.09
Pond fracture — *see* Fracture, skull

Ponos B55.0
Pons, pontine — *see* condition
Poor
  aesthetic of existing restoration of tooth K08.56
  contractions, labor O62.2
  gingival margin to tooth restoration K08.51
  personal hygiene R46.0
  prenatal care, affecting management of pregnancy —
    see Pregnancy, complicated by, insufficient,
    prenatal care
  sucking reflex (newborn) R29.2
  urinary stream R39.12
  vision NEC H54.7
Poradenitis, nostras inguinalis or venerea A55
Porencephaly (congenital) (developmental) (true) Q04.6
  acquired G93.0
  nondevelopmental G93.0
  traumatic (post) F07.89
Porocephaliasis B88.8
Porokeratosis Q82.8
Poroma, eccrine — *see* Neoplasm, skin, benign
Porphyria (South African) E80.20
  acquired E80.20
  acute intermittent (hepatic) (Swedish) E80.21
  cutanea tarda (hereditary) (symptomatic) E80.1
  due to drugs E80.20
    correct substance properly administered — *see* Ta-
      ble of Drugs and Chemicals, by drug, adverse
      effect
    overdose or wrong substance given or taken — *see*
      Table of Drugs and Chemicals, by drug, poi-
      soning
  erythropoietic (congenital) (hereditary) E80.0
  hepatocutaneous type E80.1
  secondary E80.20
  toxic NEC E80.20
  variegata E80.20
Porphyrinuria — *see* Porphyria
Porphyruria — *see* Porphyria
Port wine nevus, mark, or stain Q82.5
Portal — *see* condition
Posadas-Wernicke disease B38.9
Positive
  culture (nonspecific)
    blood R78.81
    bronchial washings R84.5
    cerebrospinal fluid R83.5
    cervix uteri R87.5
    nasal secretions R84.5
    nipple discharge R89.5
    nose R84.5
      staphylococcus (Methicillin susceptible) Z22.321
        Methicillin resistant Z22.322
    peritoneal fluid R85.5
    pleural fluid R84.5
    prostatic secretions R86.5
    saliva R85.5
    seminal fluid R86.5
    sputum R84.5
    synovial fluid R89.5
    throat scrapings R84.5
    urine R82.79
    vagina R87.5
    vulva R87.5
    wound secretions R89.5
  PPD (skin test) R76.11
  serology for syphilis A53.0
    false R76.8
    with signs or symptoms — *code as* Syphilis, by site
      and stage
  skin test, tuberculin (without active tuberculosis) R76.11
  test, human immunodeficiency virus (HIV) R75
  VDRL A53.0
    with signs or symptoms — *code by* site and stage
      under Syphilis A53.9
  Wassermann reaction A53.0
Postcardiotomy syndrome I97.0
Postcaval ureter Q62.62
Postcholecystectomy syndrome K91.5
Postclimacteric bleeding N95.0
Postcommissurotomy syndrome I97.0
Postconcussional syndrome F07.81
Postcontusional syndrome F07.81
Postcricoid region — *see* condition
Post-dates (40-42 weeks) (pregnancy) (mother) O48.0
  more than 42 weeks gestation O48.1
Postencephalitic syndrome F07.89
Posterior — *see* condition

Posterolateral sclerosis (spinal cord) — *see* Degenera-
  tion, combined
Postexanthematous — *see* condition
Postfebrile — *see* condition
Postgastrectomy dumping syndrome K91.1
Posthemiplegic chorea — *see* Monoplegia
Posthemorrhagic anemia (chronic) D50.0
  acute D62
  newborn P61.3
Postherpetic neuralgia (zoster) B02.29
  trigeminal B02.22
Posthitis N47.7
Postimmunization complication or reaction — *see*
  Complications, vaccination
Postinfectious — *see* condition
Postlaminectomy syndrome NEC M96.1
Postleukotomy syndrome F07.0
Postmastectomy lymphedema (syndrome) I97.2
Postmaturity, postmature (over 42 weeks)
  maternal (over 42 weeks gestation) O48.1
  newborn P08.22
Postmeasles complication NEC — *see also* condition
  B05.89
Postmenopausal
  endometrium (atrophic) N95.8
    suppurative — *see also* Endometritis N71.9
  osteoporosis — *see* Osteoporosis, postmenopausal
Postnasal drip R09.82
  due to
    allergic rhinitis — *see* Rhinitis, allergic
    common cold J00
    gastroesophageal reflux — *see* Reflux, gastroe-
      sophageal
    nasopharyngitis — *see* Nasopharyngitis
    other known condition — *code to* condition
    sinusitis — *see* Sinusitis
Postnatal — *see* condition
Postoperative (postprocedural) — *see* Complication,
  postoperative
  pneumothorax, therapeutic Z98.3
  state NEC Z98.890
Postpancreatectomy hyperglycemia E89.1
Postpartum — *see* Puerperal
Postphlebitic syndrome — *see* Syndrome, postthrom-
  botic
Postpolio (myelitic) **syndrome** G14
Postpoliomyelitic — *see also* condition
  osteopathy — *see* Osteopathy, after poliomyelitis
Postprocedural — *see also* Postoperative
  hypoinsulinemia E89.1
Postschizophrenic depression F32.89
Postsurgery status — *see also* Status (post)
  pneumothorax, therapeutic Z98.3
Post-term (40-42 weeks) (pregnancy) (mother) O48.0
  infant P08.21
  more than 42 weeks gestation (mother) O48.1
Post-traumatic brain syndrome, nonpsychotic F07.81
Post-typhoid abscess A01.09
Postures, hysterical F44.2
Postvaccinal reaction or complication — *see* Complications, vaccination
Postvalvulotomy syndrome I97.0
Potain's
  disease (pulmonary edema) — *see* Edema, lung
  syndrome (gastrectasis with dyspepsia) K31.0
Potter's
  asthma J62.8
  facies Q60.6
  lung J62.8
  syndrome (with renal agenesis) Q60.6
Pott's
  curvature (spinal) A18.01
  disease or paraplegia A18.01
  spinal curvature A18.01
  tumor, puffy — *see* Osteomyelitis, specified type NEC
Pouch
  bronchus Q32.4
  Douglas' — *see* condition
  esophagus, esophageal, congenital Q39.6
    acquired K22.5
  gastric K31.4
  Hartmann's K82.8
  pharynx, pharyngeal (congenital) Q38.7
Pouchitis K91.850
Poultrymen's itch B88.0
Poverty NEC Z59.6
  extreme Z59.5

Poxvirus NEC B08.8
Prader-Willi syndrome Q87.11
Prader-Willi-like syndrome Q87.19
Preauricular appendage or tag Q17.0
Prebetalipoproteinemia (acquired) (essential) (familial) (hereditary) (primary) (secondary) E78.1
   with chylomicronemia E78.3
Precipitate labor or delivery O62.3
Preclimacteric bleeding (menorrhagia) N92.4
Precocious
   adrenarche E30.1
   menarche E30.1
   menstruation E30.1
   pubarche E30.1
   puberty E30.1
     central E22.8
   sexual development NEC E30.1
   thelarche E30.8
Precocity, sexual (constitutional) (cryptogenic) (female) (idiopathic) (male) E30.1
   with adrenal hyperplasia E25.9
     congenital E25.0
Precordial pain R07.2
Predeciduous teeth K00.2
Prediabetes, prediabetic R73.03
   complicating
     pregnancy — see Pregnancy, complicated by, diseases of, specified type or system NEC
     puerperium O99.89
Predislocation status of hip at birth Q65.6
Pre-eclampsia O14.9- ☑
   with pre-existing hypertension — see Hypertension, complicating pregnancy, pre-existing, with, pre-eclampsia
   complicating
     childbirth O14.94
     puerperium O14.95
   mild O14.0- ☑
     complicating
       childbirth O14.04
       puerperium O14.05
   moderate O14.0- ☑
     complicating
       childbirth O14.04
       puerperium O14.05
   severe O14.1- ☑
     with hemolysis, elevated liver enzymes and low platelet count (HELLP) O14.2- ☑
       complicating
         childbirth O14.24
         puerperium O14.25
     complicating
       childbirth O14.14
       puerperium O14.15
Pre-eruptive color change, teeth, tooth K00.8
Pre-excitation atrioventricular conduction I45.6
Preglaucoma H40.00- ☑
Pregnancy (single) (uterine) — see also Delivery and Puerperal

> Note: The Tabular must be reviewed for assignment of appropriate seventh character for multiple gestation codes in Chapter 15

> Note: The Tabular must be reviewed for assignment of the appropriate character indicating the trimester of the pregnancy

   abdominal (ectopic) O00.00
     with intrauterine pregnancy O00.01
     with viable fetus O36.7- ☑
   ampullar O00.10- ☑
     with intrauterine pregnancy O00.11- ☑
   biochemical O02.81
   broad ligament O00.80
     with intrauterine pregnancy O00.81
   cervical O00.8
     with intrauterine pregnancy O00.81
   chemical O02.81
   complicated by (care of) (management affected by)
     abnormal, abnormality
       cervix O34.4- ☑
         causing obstructed labor O65.5
       cord (umbilical) O69.9 ☑
       fetal heart rate or rhythm O36.83- ☑
       findings on antenatal screening of mother O28.9
         biochemical O28.1
         chromosomal O28.5

Pregnancy — continued
   complicated by — continued
     abnormal, abnormality — continued
       findings on antenatal screening of mother — continued
         cytological O28.2
         genetic O28.5
         hematological O28.0
         radiological O28.4
         specified NEC O28.8
         ultrasonic O28.3
       glucose (tolerance) NEC O99.810
       pelvic organs O34.9-
         specified NEC O34.8- ☑
           causing obstructed labor O65.5
       pelvis (bony) (major) NEC O33.0
       perineum O34.7- ☑
       position
         placenta O44.0- ☑
           with hemorrhage O44.1- ☑
         uterus O34.59- ☑
       uterus O34.59- ☑
         causing obstructed labor O65.5
         congenital O34.0- ☑
       vagina O34.6-
         causing obstructed labor O65.5
       vulva O34.7-
         causing obstructed labor O65.5
     abruptio placentae — see Abruptio placentae
     abscess or cellulitis
       bladder O23.1-
       breast O91.11- ☑
       genital organ or tract O23.9-
     abuse
       physical O9A.31 ☑ (following O99)
       psychological O9A.51 ☑ (following O99)
       sexual O9A.41 ☑ (following O99)
     adverse effect anesthesia O29.9-
       aspiration pneumonitis O29.01- ☑
       cardiac arrest O29.11- ☑
       cardiac complication NEC O29.19- ☑
       cardiac failure O29.12- ☑
       central nervous system complication NEC O29.29-
       cerebral anoxia O29.21- ☑
       failed or difficult intubation O29.6- ☑
       inhalation of stomach contents or secretions NOS O29.01-
       local, toxic reaction O29.3X ☑
       Mendelson's syndrome O29.01- ☑
       pressure collapse of lung O29.02- ☑
       pulmonary complications NEC O29.09- ☑
       specified NEC O29.8X- ☑
       spinal and epidural type NEC O29.5X ☑
         induced headache O29.4- ☑
     albuminuria — see also Proteinuria, gestational O12.1- ☑
     alcohol use O99.31- ☑
     amnionitis O41.12- ☑
     anaphylactoid syndrome of pregnancy O88.01- ☑
     anemia (conditions in D50-D64) (pre-existing) O99.01- ☑
       complicating the puerperium O99.03
     antepartum hemorrhage O46.9- ☑
       with coagulation defect — see Hemorrhage, antepartum, with coagulation defect
       specified NEC O46.8X- ☑
     appendicitis O99.61- ☑
     atrophy (yellow) (acute) liver (subacute) O26.61- ☑
     bariatric surgery status O99.84- ☑
     bicornis or bicornuate uterus O34.0- ☑
     biliary tract problems O26.61- ☑
     breech presentation O32.1 ☑
     cardiovascular diseases (conditions in I00-I09, I20-I52, I70-I99) O99.41- ☑
     cerebrovascular disorders (conditions in I60-I69) O99.41- ☑
     cervical shortening O26.87- ☑
     cervicitis O23.51- ☑
     chloasma (gravidarum) O26.89- ☑
     cholecystitis O99.61- ☑
     cholestasis (intrahepatic) O26.61- ☑
     chorioamnionitis O41.12- ☑
     circulatory system disorder (conditions in I00-I09, I20-I99, O99.41-)
     compound presentation O32.6 ☑

Pregnancy — continued
   complicated by — continued
     conjoined twins O30.02- ☑
     connective system disorders (conditions in M00-M99) O99.89
     contracted pelvis (general) O33.1
       inlet O33.2
       outlet O33.3 ☑
     convulsions (eclamptic) (uremic) — see also Eclampsia O15.9
     cracked nipple O92.11- ☑
     cystitis O23.1- ☑
     cystocele O34.8- ☑
     death of fetus (near term) O36.4 ☑
       early pregnancy O02.1
       of one fetus or more in multiple gestation O31.2- ☑
     deciduitis O41.14- ☑
     decreased fetal movement O36.81- ☑
     dental problems O99.61- ☑
     diabetes (mellitus) O24.91- ☑
       gestational (pregnancy induced) — see Diabetes, gestational
       pre-existing O24.31- ☑
         specified NEC O24.81- ☑
         type 1 O24.01- ☑
         type 2 O24.11- ☑
     digestive system disorders (conditions in K00-K93) O99.61- ☑
     diseases of — see Pregnancy, complicated by, specified body system disease
       biliary tract O26.61- ☑
       blood NEC (conditions in D65-D77) O99.11- ☑
       liver O26.61- ☑
       specified NEC O99.89
     disorders of — see Pregnancy, complicated by, specified body system disorder
       amniotic fluid and membranes O41.9- ☑
         specified NEC O41.8X- ☑
       biliary tract O26.61- ☑
       ear and mastoid process (conditions in H60-H95) O99.89
       eye and adnexa (conditions in H00-H59) O99.89
       liver O26.61- ☑
       skin (conditions in L00-L99) O99.71- ☑
       specified NEC O99.89
     displacement, uterus NEC O34.59- ☑
       causing obstructed labor O65.5
     disproportion (due to) O33.9
       fetal (ascites) (hydrops) (meningomyelocele) (sacral teratoma) (tumor) deformities NEC O33.7
       generally contracted pelvis O33.1
       hydrocephalic fetus O33.6 ☑
       inlet contraction of pelvis O33.2
       mixed maternal and fetal origin O33.4 ☑
       specified NEC O33.8
     double uterus O34.0- ☑
       causing obstructed labor O65.5
     drug use (conditions in F11-F19) O99.32- ☑
     eclampsia, eclamptic (coma) (convulsions) (delirium) (nephritis) (uremia) — see also Eclampsia O15.- ☑
     ectopic pregnancy — see Pregnancy, ectopic
     edema O12.0- ☑
       with
         gestational hypertension, mild — see also Pre-eclampsia O14.0- ☑
         proteinuria O12.2- ☑
     effusion, amniotic fluid — see Pregnancy, complicated by, premature rupture of membranes
     elderly
       multigravida O09.52- ☑
       primigravida O09.51- ☑
     embolism — see also Embolism, obstetric, pregnancy O88.- ☑
     endocrine diseases NEC O99.28- ☑
     endometritis O86.12
     excessive weight gain O26.0- ☑
     exhaustion O26.81- ☑
       during labor and delivery O75.81
     face presentation O32.3 ☑
     failed induction of labor O61.9
       instrumental O61.1
       mechanical O61.1
       medical O61.0
       specified NEC O61.8

▽ Subterms under main terms may continue to next column or page   ☑ Additional Character Required — Refer to the Tabular List for Character Selection   259

Poxvirus NEC — Pregnancy

Pregnancy — *continued*
  complicated by — *continued*
    failed induction of labor — *continued*
      surgical O61.1
    failed or difficult intubation for anesthesia O29.6- ☑
    false labor (pains) O47.9
      at or after 37 completed weeks of pregnancy O47.1
      before 37 completed weeks of pregnancy O47.0- ☑
    fatigue O26.81- ☑
      during labor and delivery O75.81
    fatty metamorphosis of liver O26.61- ☑
    female genital mutilation O34.8- ☑ *[N90.81-]* ☑
    fetal (maternal care for)
      abnormality or damage O35.9 ☑
        acid-base balance O68
        specified type NEC O35.8 ☑
      acidemia O68
      acidosis O68
      alkalosis O68
      anemia and thrombocytopenia O36.82- ☑
      anencephaly O35.0 ☑
      bradycardia O36.83- ☑
      chromosomal abnormality (conditions in Q90-Q99) O35.1 ☑
      conjoined twins O30.02- ☑
      damage from
        amniocentesis O35.7 ☑
        biopsy procedures O35.7 ☑
        drug addiction O35.5 ☑
        hematological investigation O35.7 ☑
        intrauterine contraceptive device O35.7 ☑
        maternal
          alcohol addiction O35.4 ☑
          cytomegalovirus infection O35.3 ☑
          disease NEC O35.8 ☑
          drug addiction O35.5 ☑
          listeriosis O35.8 ☑
          rubella O35.3 ☑
          toxoplasmosis O35.8 ☑
          viral infection O35.3 ☑
        medical procedure NEC O35.7 ☑
        radiation O35.6 ☑
      death (near term) O36.4 ☑
        early pregnancy O02.1
      decreased movement O36.81- ☑
      depressed heart rate tones O36.83- ☑
      disproportion due to deformity (fetal) O33.7 ☑
      excessive growth (large for dates) O36.6- ☑
      growth retardation O36.59- ☑
        light for dates O36.59- ☑
        small for dates O36.59- ☑
      heart rate irregularity (abnormal variability) (bradycardia) (decelerations) (tachycardia) O36.83- ☑
      hereditary disease O35.2 ☑
      hydrocephalus O35.0 ☑
      intrauterine death O36.4 ☑
      non-reassuring heart rate or rhythm O36.83- ☑
      poor growth O36.59- ☑
        light for dates O36.59- ☑
        small for dates O36.59- ☑
      problem O36.9- ☑
        specified NEC O36.89- ☑
      reduction (elective) O31.3- ☑
      selective termination O31.3- ☑
      spina bifida O35.0 ☑
      thrombocytopenia O36.82- ☑
    fibroid (tumor) (uterus) O34.1- ☑
    fissure of nipple O92.11- ☑
    gallstones O99.61- ☑
    gastric banding status O99.84- ☑
    gastric bypass status O99.84- ☑
    genital herpes (asymptomatic) (history of) (inactive) O98.3- ☑
    genital tract infection O23.9- ☑
    glomerular diseases (conditions in N00-N07) O26.83- ☑
      with hypertension, pre-existing — *see* Hypertension, complicating, pregnancy, pre-existing, with, renal disease
    gonorrhea O98.21- ☑
    grand multiparity O09.4 ☑
    habitual aborter — *see* Pregnancy, complicated by, recurrent pregnancy loss

Pregnancy — *continued*
  complicated by — *continued*
    HELLP syndrome (hemolysis, elevated liver enzymes and low platelet count) O14.2- ☑
    hemorrhage
      antepartum — *see* Hemorrhage, antepartum
      before 20 completed weeks gestation O20.9
        specified NEC O20.8
      due to premature separation, placenta — *see also* Abruptio placentae O45.9- ☑
      early O20.9
        specified NEC O20.8
      threatened abortion O20.0
    hemorrhoids O22.4- ☑
    hepatitis (viral) O98.41- ☑
    herniation of uterus O34.59- ☑
    high
      head at term O32.4 ☑
      risk — *see* Supervision (of) (for), high-risk
    history of in utero procedure during previous pregnancy O09.82- ☑
    HIV O98.71- ☑
    human immunodeficiency virus (HIV) disease O98.71- ☑
    hydatidiform mole — *see also* Mole, hydatidiform O01.9
    hydramnios O40.- ☑
    hydrocephalic fetus (disproportion) O33.6 ☑
    hydrops
      amnii O40.- ☑
      fetalis O36.2- ☑
        associated with isoimmunization — *see also* Pregnancy, complicated by, isoimmunization O36.11- ☑
    hydrorrhea O42.90
    hyperemesis (gravidarum) (mild) — *see also* Hyperemesis, gravidarum O21.0
    hypertension — *see* Hypertension, complicating pregnancy
    hypertensive
      heart and renal disease, pre-existing — *see* Hypertension, complicating, pregnancy, pre-existing, with, heart disease, with renal disease
      heart disease, pre-existing — *see* Hypertension, complicating, pregnancy, pre-existing, with, heart disease
      renal disease, pre-existing — *see* Hypertension, complicating, pregnancy, pre-existing, with, renal disease
    hypotension O26.5- ☑
    immune disorders NEC (conditions in D80-D89) O99.11- ☑
    incarceration, uterus O34.51- ☑
    incompetent cervix O34.3- ☑
    inconclusive fetal viability O36.80 ☑
    infection(s) O98.91- ☑
      amniotic fluid or sac O41.10- ☑
      bladder O23.1- ☑
      carrier state NEC O99.830
        streptococcus B O99.820
      genital organ or tract O23.9- ☑
        specified NEC O23.59- ☑
      genitourinary tract O23.9- ☑
      gonorrhea O98.21- ☑
      hepatitis (viral) O98.41- ☑
      HIV O98.71- ☑
      human immunodeficiency virus (HIV) O98.71- ☑
      kidney O23.0- ☑
      nipple O91.01- ☑
      parasitic disease O98.91- ☑
        specified NEC O98.81- ☑
      protozoal disease O98.61- ☑
      sexually transmitted NEC O98.31- ☑
      specified type NEC O98.81- ☑
      syphilis O98.11- ☑
      tuberculosis O98.01- ☑
      urethra O23.2- ☑
      urinary (tract) O23.4- ☑
        specified NEC O23.3- ☑
      viral disease O98.51- ☑
    injury or poisoning (conditions in S00-T88) O9A.21- ☑ *(following O99)*
      due to abuse
        physical O9A.31- ☑ *(following O99)*
        psychological O9A.51- ☑ *(following O99)*
        sexual O9A.41- ☑ *(following O99)*

Pregnancy — *continued*
  complicated by — *continued*
    insufficient
      prenatal care O09.3- ☑
      weight gain O26.1- ☑
    insulin resistance O26.89 ☑
    intrauterine fetal death (near term) O36.4 ☑
      early pregnancy O02.1
      multiple gestation (one fetus or more) O31.2- ☑
    isoimmunization O36.11- ☑
      anti-A sensitization O36.11- ☑
      anti-B sensitization O36.19- ☑
      Rh O36.09- ☑
        anti-D antibody O36.01- ☑
      specified NEC O36.19- ☑
    laceration of uterus NEC O71.81
    malformation
      placenta, placental (vessel) O43.10- ☑
        specified NEC O43.19- ☑
      uterus (congenital) O34.0- ☑
    malnutrition (conditions in E40-E46) O25.1- ☑
    maternal hypotension syndrome O26.5- ☑
    mental disorders (conditions in F01-F09, F20-F99) O99.34- ☑
      alcohol use O99.31- ☑
      drug use O99.32- ☑
      smoking O99.33- ☑
    mentum presentation O32.3 ☑
    metabolic disorders O99.28- ☑
    missed
      abortion O02.1
      delivery O36.4 ☑
    multiple gestations O30.9- ☑
      conjoined twins O30.02- ☑
      quadruplet — *see* Pregnancy, quadruplet
      specified complication NEC O31.8X- ☑
      specified number of multiples NEC — *see* Pregnancy, multiple (gestation), specified NEC
      triplet — *see* Pregnancy, triplet
      twin — *see* Pregnancy, twin
    musculoskeletal condition (conditions is M00-M99) O99.89
    necrosis, liver (conditions in K72) O26.61- ☑
    neoplasm
      benign
        cervix O34.4- ☑
        corpus uteri O34.1- ☑
        uterus O34.1- ☑
      malignant O9A.11- ☑ *(following O99)*
    nephropathy NEC O26.83- ☑
    nervous system condition (conditions in G00-G99) O99.35- ☑
    nutritional diseases NEC O99.28- ☑
    obesity (pre-existing) O99.21- ☑
    obesity surgery status O99.84- ☑
    oblique lie or presentation O32.2 ☑
    older mother — *see* Pregnancy, complicated by, elderly
    oligohydramnios O41.0- ☑
      with premature rupture of membranes — *see also* Pregnancy, complicated by, premature rupture of membranes O42.- ☑
    onset (spontaneous) of labor after 37 completed weeks of gestation but before 39 completed weeks gestation, with delivery by (planned) cesarean section O75.82
    oophoritis O23.52- ☑
    overdose, drug — *see also* Table of Drugs and Chemicals, by drug, poisoning O9A.21- ☑ *(following O99)*
    oversize fetus O33.5 ☑
    papyraceous fetus O31.0- ☑
    pelvic inflammatory disease O99.89
    periodontal disease O99.61- ☑
    peripheral neuritis O26.82- ☑
    peritoneal (pelvic) adhesions O99.89
    phlebitis O22.9- ☑
    phlebopathy O22.9- ☑
    phlebothrombosis (superficial) O22.2- ☑
      deep O22.3- ☑
    placenta accreta O43.21- ☑
    placenta increta O43.22- ☑
    placenta percreta O43.23- ☑
    placenta previa O44.0- ☑
      complete O44.0- ☑
        with hemorrhage O44.1- ☑

☑ Additional Character Required — Refer to the Tabular List for Character Selection   ▽ Subterms under main terms may continue to next column or page

Pregnancy — Pregnancy

Pregnancy — *continued*
  complicated by — *continued*
    placenta previa — *continued*
      marginal O44.2- ☑
        with hemorrhage O44.3- ☑
      partial O44.2- ☑
        with hemorrhage O44.3- ☑
    placental disorder O43.9- ☑
      specified NEC O43.89- ☑
    placental dysfunction O43.89- ☑
    placental infarction O43.81- ☑
    placental insufficiency O36.51- ☑
    placental transfusion syndromes
      fetomaternal O43.01- ☑
      fetus to fetus O43.02- ☑
      maternofetal O43.01- ☑
    placentitis O41.14- ☑
    pneumonia O99.51- ☑
    poisoning — *see also* Table of Drugs and Chemicals O9A.21 ☑ (*following* O99)
    polyhydramnios O40- ☑
    polymorphic eruption of pregnancy O26.86
    poor obstetric history NEC O09.29- ☑
    postmaturity (post-term) (40 to 42 weeks) O48.0
      more than 42 completed weeks gestation (prolonged) O48.1
    pre-eclampsia O14.9- ☑
      mild O14.0- ☑
      moderate O14.0- ☑
      severe O14.1- ☑
        with hemolysis, elevated liver enzymes and low platelet count (HELLP) O14.2- ☑
    premature labor — *see* Pregnancy, complicated by, preterm labor
    premature rupture of membranes O42.90
      with onset of labor
        within 24 hours O42.00
          at or after 37 weeks gestation, onset of labor within 24 hours of rupture O42.02
          pre-term (before 37 completed weeks of gestation) O42.01- ☑
        after 24 hours O42.10
          at or after 37 weeks gestation, onset of labor more than 24 hours following rupture O42.12
          pre-term (before 37 completed weeks of gestation) O42.11- ☑
      at or after 37 weeks gestation, unspecified as to length of time between rupture and onset of labor O42.92
      full-term, unspecified as to length of time between rupture and onset of labor O42.92
      pre-term (before 37 completed weeks of gestation) O42.91- ☑
    premature separation of placenta — *see also* Abruptio placentae O45.9- ☑
    presentation, fetal — *see* Delivery, complicated by, malposition
    preterm delivery O60.10 ☑
    preterm labor
      with delivery O60.10 ☑
        preterm O60.10 ☑
        term O60.20 ☑
      second trimester
        with term delivery O60.22 ☑
        without delivery O60.02 ☑
        with preterm delivery
          second trimester O60.12 ☑
          third trimester O60.13 ☑
      third trimester
        with term delivery O60.23 ☑
        without delivery O60.03
        with third trimester preterm delivery O60.14 ☑
      without delivery O60.00
        second trimester O60.02
        third trimester O60.03
    previous history of — *see* Pregnancy, supervision of, high-risk
    prolapse, uterus O34.52- ☑
    proteinuria (gestational) — *see also* Proteinuria, gestational O12.1- ☑
      with edema O12.2- ☑
    pruritic urticarial papules and plaques of pregnancy (PUPPP) O26.86
    pruritus (neurogenic) O26.89- ☑

Pregnancy — *continued*
  complicated by — *continued*
    psychosis or psychoneurosis (puerperal) F53.1
    ptyalism O26.89- ☑
    PUPPP (pruritic urticarial papules and plaques of pregnancy) O26.86
    pyelitis O23.0- ☑
    recurrent pregnancy loss O26.2- ☑
    renal disease or failure NEC O26.83- ☑
      with secondary hypertension, pre-existing — *see* Hypertension, complicating, pregnancy, pre-existing, secondary
      hypertensive, pre-existing — *see* Hypertension, complicating, pregnancy, pre-existing, with, renal disease
    respiratory condition (conditions in J00-J99) O99.51- ☑
    retained, retention
      dead ovum O02.0
      intrauterine contraceptive device O26.3- ☑
    retroversion, uterus O34.53- ☑
    Rh immunization, incompatibility or sensitization NEC O36.09- ☑
      anti-D antibody O36.01- ☑
    rupture
      amnion (premature) — *see also* Pregnancy, complicated by, premature rupture of membranes O42- ☑
      membranes (premature) — *see also* Pregnancy, complicated by, premature rupture of membranes O42- ☑
      uterus (during labor) O71.1
        before onset of labor O71.0- ☑
    salivation (excessive) O26.89- ☑
    salpingitis O23.52- ☑
    salpingo-oophoritis O23.52- ☑
    sepsis (conditions in A40, A41) O98.81- ☑
    size date discrepancy (uterine) O26.84- ☑
    skin condition (conditions in L00-L99) O99.71- ☑
    smoking (tobacco) O99.33- ☑
    social problem O09.7- ☑
    specified condition NEC O26.89- ☑
    spotting O26.85- ☑
    streptococcus group B (GBS) carrier state O99.820
    subluxation of symphysis (pubis) O26.71- ☑
    syphilis (conditions in A50-A53) O98.11- ☑
    threatened
      abortion O20.0
      labor O47.9
        at or after 37 completed weeks of gestation O47.1
        before 37 completed weeks of gestation O47.0- ☑
    thrombophlebitis (superficial) O22.2- ☑
    thrombosis O22.9- ☑
      cerebral venous O22.5- ☑
      cerebrovenous sinus O22.5- ☑
      deep O22.3- ☑
    tobacco use disorder (smoking) O99.33- ☑
    torsion of uterus O34.59- ☑
    toxemia O14.9- ☑
    transverse lie or presentation O32.2 ☑
    tuberculosis (conditions in A15-A19) O98.01- ☑
    tumor (benign)
      cervix O34.4- ☑
      malignant O9A.11- ☑ (*following* O99)
      uterus O34.1- ☑
    unstable lie O32.0 ☑
    upper respiratory infection O99.51- ☑
    urethritis O23.2- ☑
    uterine size date discrepancy O26.84- ☑
    vaginitis or vulvitis O23.59- ☑
    varicose veins (lower extremities) O22.0- ☑
      genitals O22.1- ☑
      legs O22.0- ☑
      perineal O22.1- ☑
      vaginal or vulval O22.1- ☑
    venereal disease NEC (conditions in A63.8) O98.31- ☑
    venous disorders O22.9- ☑
      specified NEC O22.8X- ☑
    very young mother — *see* Pregnancy, complicated by, young mother
    viral diseases (conditions in A80-B09, B25-B34) O98.51- ☑
    vomiting O21.9
      due to diseases classified elsewhere O21.8

Pregnancy — *continued*
  complicated by — *continued*
    vomiting — *continued*
      hyperemesis gravidarum (mild) — *see also* Hyperemesis, gravidarum O21.0
      late (occurring after 20 weeks of gestation) O21.2
    young mother
      multigravida O09.62- ☑
      primigravida O09.61- ☑
  complicated NOS O26.9- ☑
  concealed O09.3- ☑
  continuing following
    elective fetal reduction of one or more fetus O31.3- ☑
    intrauterine death of one or more fetus O31.2- ☑
    spontaneous abortion of one or more fetus O31.1- ☑
  cornual O00.80
    with intrauterine pregnancy O00.81
  ectopic (ruptured) O00.90
    with intrauterine pregnancy O00.91
    abdominal O00.00
      with
        intrauterine pregnancy O00.01
        viable fetus O36.7- ☑
    cervical O00.80
      with intrauterine pregnancy O00.81
    complicated (by) O08.9
      afibrinogenemia O08.1
      cardiac arrest O08.81
      chemical damage of pelvic organ(s) O08.6
      circulatory collapse O08.3
      defibrination syndrome O08.1
      electrolyte imbalance O08.5
      embolism (amniotic fluid) (blood clot) (pulmonary) (septic) O08.2
      endometritis O08.0
      genital tract and pelvic infection O08.0
      hemorrhage (delayed) (excessive) O08.1
      infection
        genital tract or pelvic O08.0
        kidney O08.83
        urinary tract O08.3
      intravascular coagulation O08.1
      laceration of pelvic organ(s) O08.6
      metabolic disorder O08.5
      oliguria O08.4
      oophoritis O08.0
      parametritis O08.0
      pelvic peritonitis O08.0
      perforation of pelvic organ(s) O08.6
      renal failure or shutdown O08.4
      salpingitis or salpingo-oophoritis O08.0
      sepsis O08.82
      shock O08.83
        septic O08.82
      specified condition NEC O08.89
      tubular necrosis (renal) O08.4
      uremia O08.4
      urinary infection O08.83
      venous complication NEC O08.7
        embolism O08.2
    cornual O00.80
      with intrauterine pregnancy O00.81
    intraligamentous O00.80
      with intrauterine pregnancy O00.81
    mural O00.80
      with intrauterine pregnancy O00.81
    ovarian O00.20- ☑
      with intrauterine pregnancy O00.21- ☑
    specified site NEC O00.80
      with intrauterine pregnancy O00.81
    tubal (ruptured) O00.10- ☑
      with intrauterine pregnancy O00.11- ☑
  examination (normal) Z34.9- ☑
    first Z34.0- ☑
    high-risk — *see* Pregnancy, supervision of, high-risk
    specified Z34.8- ☑
  extrauterine — *see* Pregnancy, ectopic
  fallopian O00.10- ☑
    with intrauterine pregnancy O00.11- ☑
  false F45.8
  gestational carrier Z33.3
  heptachorionic, hepta-amniotic (septuplets) O30.83- ☑
  hexachorionic, hexa-amniotic (sextuplets) O30.83- ☑
  hidden O09.3- ☑
  high-risk — *see* Pregnancy, supervision of, high-risk
  incidental finding Z33.1

Pregnancy — *continued*
- interstitial O00.80
  - with intrauterine pregnancy O00.81
- intraligamentous O00.80
  - with intrauterine pregnancy O00.81
- intramural O00.80
  - with intrauterine pregnancy O00.81
- intraperitoneal O00.00
  - with intrauterine pregnancy O00.01
- isthmian O00.10- ☑
  - with intrauterine pregnancy O00.11- ☑
- mesometric (mural) O00.80
  - with intrauterine pregnancy O00.81
- molar NEC O02.0
  - complicated (by) O08.9
    - afibrinogenemia O08.1
    - cardiac arrest O08.81
    - chemical damage of pelvic organ(s) O08.6
    - circulatory collapse O08.3
    - defibrination syndrome O08.1
    - electrolyte imbalance O08.5
    - embolism (amniotic fluid) (blood clot) (pulmonary) (septic) O08.2
    - endometritis O08.0
    - genital tract and pelvic infection O08.0
    - hemorrhage (delayed) (excessive) O08.1
    - infection
      - genital tract or pelvic O08.0
      - kidney O08.83
      - urinary tract O08.83
    - intravascular coagulation O08.1
    - laceration of pelvic organ(s) O08.6
    - metabolic disorder O08.5
    - oliguria O08.4
    - oophoritis O08.0
    - parametritis O08.0
    - pelvic peritonitis O08.0
    - perforation of pelvic organ(s) O08.6
    - renal failure or shutdown O08.4
    - salpingitis or salpingo-oophoritis O08.0
    - sepsis O08.82
    - shock O08.3
      - septic O08.82
    - specified condition NEC O08.89
    - tubular necrosis (renal) O08.4
    - uremia O08.4
    - urinary infection O08.83
    - venous complication NEC O08.7
      - embolism O08.2
  - hydatidiform — *see also* Mole, hydatidiform O01.9
- multiple (gestation) O30.9- ☑
  - greater than quadruplets — *see* Pregnancy, multiple (gestation), specified NEC
  - specified NEC O30.80- ☑
    - with
      - two or more monoamniotic fetuses O30.82- ☑
      - two or more monochorionic fetuses O30.81- ☑
      - number of chorions and amnions are both equal to the number of fetuses O30.83- ☑
      - two or more monoamniotic fetuses O30.82- ☑
      - two or more monochorionic fetuses O30.81- ☑
      - unable to determine number of placenta and number of amniotic sacs O30.89- ☑
      - unspecified number of placenta and unspecified number of amniotic sacs O30.80- ☑
  - mural O00.80
    - with intrauterine pregnancy O00.81
  - normal (supervision of) Z34.9- ☑
    - first Z34.0- ☑
    - high-risk — *see* Pregnancy, supervision of, high-risk
    - specified Z34.8- ☑
  - ovarian O00.20- ☑
    - with intrauterine pregnancy O00.21- ☑
  - pentachorionic, penta-amniotic (quintuplets) O30.83- ☑
  - postmature (40 to 42 weeks) O48.0
    - more than 42 weeks gestation O48.1
  - post-term (40 to 42 weeks) O48.0
  - prenatal care only Z34.9- ☑
    - first Z34.0- ☑
    - high-risk — *see* Pregnancy, supervision of, high-risk
    - specified Z34.8- ☑
  - prolonged (more than 42 weeks gestation) O48.1
  - quadruplet O30.20- ☑
    - with
      - two or more monoamniotic fetuses O30.22- ☑

Pregnancy — *continued*
- quadruplet — *continued*
  - with — *continued*
    - two or more monochorionic fetuses O30.21- ☑
    - quadrachorionic/quadra-amniotic O30.23- ☑
    - two or more monoamniotic fetuses O30.22- ☑
    - two or more monochorionic fetuses O30.21- ☑
    - unable to determine number of placenta and number of amniotic sacs O30.29- ☑
    - unspecified number of placenta and unspecified number of amniotic sacs O30.20- ☑
  - quintuplet — *see* Pregnancy, multiple (gestation), specified NEC
  - sextuplet — *see* Pregnancy, multiple (gestation), specified NEC
  - supervision of
    - concealed pregnancy O09.3- ☑
    - elderly mother
      - multigravida O09.52- ☑
      - primigravida O09.51- ☑
    - hidden pregnancy O09.3- ☑
    - high-risk O09.9- ☑
      - due to (history of)
        - ectopic pregnancy O09.1- ☑
        - elderly — *see* Pregnancy, supervision, elderly mother
        - grand multiparity O09.4 ☑
        - in utero procedure during previous pregnancy O09.82- ☑
        - in vitro fertilization O09.81- ☑
        - infertility O09.0- ☑
        - insufficient prenatal care O09.3- ☑
        - molar pregnancy O09.A- ☑
        - multiple previous pregnancies O09.4- ☑
        - older mother — *see* Pregnancy, supervision of, elderly mother
        - poor reproductive or obstetric history NEC O09.29- ☑
        - pre-term labor O09.21- ☑
        - previous
          - neonatal death O09.29- ☑
        - social problems O09.7- ☑
        - specified NEC O09.89- ☑
        - very young mother — *see* Pregnancy, supervision, young mother
      - resulting from in vitro fertilization O09.81- ☑
    - normal Z34.9- ☑
      - first Z34.0- ☑
      - specified NEC Z34.8- ☑
    - young mother
      - multigravida O09.62- ☑
      - primigravida O09.61- ☑
  - triplet O30.10- ☑
    - with
      - two or more monoamniotic fetuses O30.12- ☑
      - two or more monochorionic fetuses O30.11- ☑
    - trichorionic/triamniotic O30.13- ☑
    - two or more monoamniotic fetuses O30.12- ☑
    - two or more monochorionic fetuses O30.11- ☑
    - unable to determine number of placenta and number of amniotic sacs O30.19- ☑
    - unspecified number of placenta and unspecified number of amniotic sacs O30.10- ☑
  - tubal (with abortion) (with rupture) O00.10- ☑
    - with intrauterine pregnancy O00.11- ☑
  - twin O30.00- ☑
    - conjoined O30.02- ☑
    - dichorionic/diamniotic (two placenta, two amniotic sacs) O30.04- ☑
    - monochorionic/diamniotic (one placenta, two amniotic sacs) O30.03- ☑
    - monochorionic/monoamniotic (one placenta, one amniotic sac) O30.01- ☑
    - unable to determine number of placenta and number of amniotic sacs O30.09- ☑
    - unspecified number of placenta and unspecified number of amniotic sacs O30.00- ☑
  - unwanted Z64.0
  - weeks of gestation
    - 8 weeks Z3A.08 (*following* Z36)
    - 9 weeks Z3A.09 (*following* Z36)
    - 10 weeks Z3A.10 (*following* Z36)
    - 11 weeks Z3A.11 (*following* Z36)
    - 12 weeks Z3A.12 (*following* Z36)
    - 13 weeks Z3A.13 (*following* Z36)
    - 14 weeks Z3A.14 (*following* Z36)
    - 15 weeks Z3A.15 (*following* Z36)

Pregnancy — *continued*
- weeks of gestation — *continued*
  - 16 weeks Z3A.16 (*following* Z36)
  - 17 weeks Z3A.17 (*following* Z36)
  - 18 weeks Z3A.18 (*following* Z36)
  - 19 weeks Z3A.19 (*following* Z36)
  - 20 weeks Z3A.20 (*following* Z36)
  - 21 weeks Z3A.21 (*following* Z36)
  - 22 weeks Z3A.22 (*following* Z36)
  - 23 weeks Z3A.23 (*following* Z36)
  - 24 weeks Z3A.24 (*following* Z36)
  - 25 weeks Z3A.25 (*following* Z36)
  - 26 weeks Z3A.26 (*following* Z36)
  - 27 weeks Z3A.27 (*following* Z36)
  - 28 weeks Z3A.28 (*following* Z36)
  - 29 weeks Z3A.29 (*following* Z36)
  - 30 weeks Z3A.30 (*following* Z36)
  - 31 weeks Z3A.31 (*following* Z36)
  - 32 weeks Z3A.32 (*following* Z36)
  - 33 weeks Z3A.33 (*following* Z36)
  - 34 weeks Z3A.34 (*following* Z36)
  - 35 weeks Z3A.35 (*following* Z36)
  - 36 weeks Z3A.36 (*following* Z36)
  - 37 weeks Z3A.37 (*following* Z36)
  - 38 weeks Z3A.38 (*following* Z36)
  - 39 weeks Z3A.39 (*following* Z36)
  - 40 weeks Z3A.40 (*following* Z36)
  - 41 weeks Z3A.41 (*following* Z36)
  - 42 weeks Z3A.42 (*following* Z36)
  - greater than 42 weeks Z3A.49 (*following* Z36)
  - less than 8 weeks Z3A.01 (*following* Z36)
  - not specified Z3A.00 (*following* Z36)
- **Preiser's disease** — *see* Osteonecrosis, secondary, due to, trauma, metacarpus
- **Pre-kwashiorkor** — *see* Malnutrition, severe
- **Preleukemia** (syndrome) D46.9
- **Preluxation, hip, congenital** Q65.6
- **Premature** — *see also* condition
  - adrenarche E27.0
  - aging E34.8
  - beats I49.40
    - atrial I49.1
    - auricular I49.1
    - supraventricular I49.1
  - birth NEC — *see* Preterm, newborn
  - closure, foramen ovale Q21.8
  - contraction
    - atrial I49.1
    - atrioventricular I49.2
    - auricular I49.1
    - auriculoventricular I49.49
    - heart (extrasystole) I49.49
    - junctional I49.2
    - ventricular I49.3
  - delivery — *see also* Pregnancy, complicated by, preterm labor O60.10 ☑
  - ejaculation F52.4
  - infant NEC — *see* Preterm, newborn
    - light-for-dates — *see* Light for dates
  - labor — *see* Pregnancy, complicated by, preterm labor
  - lungs P28.0
  - menopause E28.319
    - asymptomatic E28.319
    - symptomatic E28.310
  - newborn
    - extreme (less than 28 completed weeks) — *see* Immaturity, extreme
    - less than 37 completed weeks — *see* Preterm, newborn
  - puberty E30.1
  - rupture membranes or amnion — *see* Pregnancy, complicated by, premature rupture of membranes
  - senility E34.8
  - thelarche E30.8
  - ventricular systole I49.3
- **Prematurity NEC** (less than 37 completed weeks) — *see* Preterm, newborn
  - extreme (less than 28 completed weeks) — *see* Immaturity, extreme
- **Premenstrual**
  - dysphoric disorder (PMDD) F32.81
  - tension (syndrome) N94.3
- **Premolarization, cuspids** K00.2
- **Prenatal**
  - care, normal pregnancy — *see* Pregnancy, normal
  - screening of mother — *see also* Encounter, antenatal screening Z36.9

☑ **Additional Character Required — Refer to the Tabular List for Character Selection**　　　▽ **Subterms under main terms may continue to next column or page**

Prenatal — *continued*
teeth K00.6
Preparatory care for subsequent treatment NEC
for dialysis Z49.01
peritoneal Z49.02
Prepartum — *see* condition
Preponderance, left or right ventricular I51.7
Prepuce — *see* condition
PRES (posterior reversible encephalopathy syndrome)
I67.83
Presbycardia R54
Presbycusis, presbyacusia H91.1- ☑
Presbyesophagus K22.8
Presbyophrenia F03 ☑
Presbyopia H52.4
Prescription of contraceptives (initial) Z30.019
barrier Z30.018
diaphragm Z30.018
emergency (postcoital) Z30.012
implantable subdermal Z30.017
injectable Z30.013
intrauterine contraceptive device Z30.014
pills Z30.011
postcoital (emergency) Z30.012
repeat Z30.40
barrier Z30.49
diaphragm Z30.49
implantable subdermal Z30.46
injectable Z30.42
pills Z30.41
specified type NEC Z30.49
transdermal patch hormonal Z30.45
vaginal ring hormonal Z30.44
specified type NEC Z30.018
transdermal patch hormonal Z30.016
vaginal ring hormonal Z30.015
Presence (of)
ankle-joint implant (functional) (prosthesis) Z96.66- ☑
aortocoronary (bypass) graft Z95.1
arterial-venous shunt (dialysis) Z99.2
artificial
eye (globe) Z97.0
heart (fully implantable) (mechanical) Z95.812
valve Z95.2
larynx Z96.3
lens (intraocular) Z96.1
limb (complete) (partial) Z97.1- ☑
arm Z97.1- ☑
bilateral Z97.15
leg Z97.1- ☑
bilateral Z97.16
audiological implant (functional) Z96.29
bladder implant (functional) Z96.0
bone
conduction hearing device Z96.29
implant (functional) NEC Z96.7
joint (prosthesis) — *see* Presence, joint implant
cardiac
defibrillator (functional) (with synchronous cardiac
pacemaker) Z95.810
implant or graft Z95.9
specified type NEC Z95.818
pacemaker Z95.0
resynchronization therapy
defibrillator Z95.810
pacemaker Z95.0
cardioverter-defibrillator (ICD) Z95.810
cerebrospinal fluid drainage device Z98.2
cochlear implant (functional) Z96.21
contact lens (es) Z97.3
coronary artery graft or prosthesis Z95.5
CRT-D (cardiac resynchronization therapy defibrillator)
Z95.810
CRT-P (cardiac resynchronization therapy pacemaker)
Z95.0
CSF shunt Z98.2
dental prosthesis device Z97.2
dentures Z97.2
device (external) NEC Z97.8
cardiac NEC Z95.818
heart assist Z95.811
implanted (functional) Z96.9
specified NEC Z96.89
prosthetic Z97.8
ear implant Z96.20
cochlear implant Z96.21
myringotomy tube Z96.22
specified type NEC Z96.29

Presence — *continued*
elbow-joint implant (functional) (prosthesis) Z96.62- ☑
endocrine implant (functional) NEC Z96.49
eustachian tube stent or device (functional) Z96.29
external hearing-aid or device Z97.4
finger-joint implant (functional) (prosthetic) Z96.69- ☑
functional implant Z96.9
specified NEC Z96.89
graft
cardiac NEC Z95.818
vascular NEC Z95.828
hearing-aid or device (external) Z97.4
implant (bone) (cochlear) (functional) Z96.21
heart assist device Z95.811
heart valve implant (functional) Z95.2
prosthetic Z95.2
specified type NEC Z95.4
xenogenic Z95.3
hip-joint implant (functional) (prosthesis) Z96.64- ☑
ICD (cardioverter-defibrillator) Z95.810
implanted device (artificial) (functional) (prosthetic)
Z96.9
automatic cardiac defibrillator (with synchronous
cardiac pacemaker) Z95.810
cardiac pacemaker Z95.0
cochlear Z96.21
dental Z96.5
heart Z95.812
heart valve Z95.2
prosthetic Z95.2
specified NEC Z95.4
xenogenic Z95.3
insulin pump Z96.41
intraocular lens Z96.1
joint Z96.60
ankle Z96.66- ☑
elbow Z96.62- ☑
finger Z96.69- ☑
hip Z96.64- ☑
knee Z96.65- ☑
shoulder Z96.61- ☑
specified NEC Z96.698
wrist Z96.63- ☑
larynx Z96.3
myringotomy tube Z96.22
otological Z96.20
cochlear Z96.21
eustachian stent Z96.29
myringotomy Z96.22
specified NEC Z96.29
stapes Z96.29
skin Z96.81
skull plate Z96.7
specified NEC Z96.89
urogenital Z96.0
insulin pump (functional) Z96.41
intestinal bypass or anastomosis Z98.0
intraocular lens (functional) Z96.1
intrauterine contraceptive device (IUD) Z97.5
intravascular implant (functional) (prosthetic) NEC
Z95.9
coronary artery Z95.5
defibrillator (with synchronous cardiac pacemaker)
Z95.810
peripheral vessel (with angioplasty) Z95.820
joint implant (prosthetic) (any) Z96.60
ankle — *see* Presence, ankle joint implant
elbow — *see* Presence, elbow joint implant
finger — *see* Presence, finger joint implant
hip — *see* Presence, hip joint implant
knee — *see* Presence, knee joint implant
shoulder — *see* Presence, shoulder joint implant
specified joint NEC Z96.698
wrist — *see* Presence, wrist joint implant
knee-joint implant (functional) (prosthesis) Z96.65- ☑
laryngeal implant (functional) Z96.3
mandibular implant (dental) Z96.5
myringotomy tube(s) Z96.22
neurostimulator (brain) (gastric) (peripheral nerve)
(sacral nerve) (spinal cord) (vagus nerve) Z96.82
orthopedic-joint implant (prosthetic) (any) — *see*
Presence, joint implant
otological implant (functional) Z96.29
shoulder-joint implant (functional) (prosthesis)
Z96.61- ☑
skull-plate implant Z96.7
spectacles Z97.3
stapes implant (functional) Z96.29

Presence — *continued*
systemic lupus erythematosus [SLE] inhibitor D68.62
tendon implant (functional) (graft) Z96.7
tooth root(s) implant Z96.5
ureteral stent Z96.0
urethral stent Z96.0
urogenital implant (functional) Z96.0
vascular implant or device Z95.9
access port device Z95.828
specified type NEC Z95.828
wrist-joint implant (functional) (prosthesis) Z96.63- ☑
Presenile — *see also* condition
dementia F03 ☑
premature aging E34.8
Presentation, fetal — *see* Delivery, complicated by,
malposition
Prespondylolisthesis (congenital) Q76.2
Pressure
area, skin — *see* Ulcer, pressure, by site
brachial plexus G54.0
brain G93.5
injury at birth NEC P11.1
cerebral — *see* Pressure, brain
chest R07.89
cone, tentorial G93.5
hyposystolic — *see also* Hypotension
incidental reading, without diagnosis of hypotension R03.1
increased
intracranial (benign) G93.2
injury at birth P11.0
intraocular H40.05- ☑
injury — *see* Ulcer, pressure, by site
lumbosacral plexus G54.1
mediastinum J98.59
necrosis (chronic) — *see* Ulcer, pressure, by site
parental, inappropriate (excessive) Z62.6
sore (chronic) — *see* Ulcer, pressure, by site
spinal cord G95.20
ulcer (chronic) — *see* Ulcer, pressure, by site
venous, increased I87.8
Pre-syncope R55
Preterm
delivery — *see also* Pregnancy, complicated by,
preterm labor O60.10 ☑
labor — *see* Pregnancy, complicated by, preterm labor
newborn (infant) P07.30
gestational age
28 completed weeks (28 weeks, 0 days through
28 weeks, 6 days) P07.31
29 completed weeks (29 weeks, 0 days through
29 weeks, 6 days) P07.32
30 completed weeks (30 weeks, 0 days through
30 weeks, 6 days) P07.33
31 completed weeks (31 weeks, 0 days through
31 weeks, 6 days) P07.34
32 completed weeks (32 weeks, 0 days through
32 weeks, 6 days) P07.35
33 completed weeks (33 weeks, 0 days through
33 weeks, 6 days) P07.36
34 completed weeks (34 weeks, 0 days through
34 weeks, 6 days) P07.37
35 completed weeks (35 weeks, 0 days through
35 weeks, 6 days) P07.38
36 completed weeks (36 weeks, 0 days through
36 weeks, 6 days) P07.39
Previa
placenta (total) (without hemorrhage) O44.0- ☑
with hemorrhage O44.1- ☑
complete O44.0- ☑
with hemorrhage O44.1- ☑
low — *see also* Delivery, complicated, by, placenta,
low O44.4- ☑
with hemorrhage O44.5- ☑
marginal O44.2- ☑
with hemorrhage O44.3- ☑
partial O44.2- ☑
with hemorrhage O44.3- ☑
vasa O69.4 ☑
Priapism N48.30
due to
disease classified elsewhere N48.32
drug N48.33
specified cause NEC N48.39
trauma N48.31
Prickling sensation (skin) R20.2
Prickly heat L74.0

⚐ Subterms under main terms may continue to next column or page   ☑ Additional Character Required — Refer to the Tabular List for Character Selection   263

Prenatal — Prickly heat

Primary — *see* condition

Primigravida

elderly, affecting management of pregnancy, labor and delivery (supervision only) — *see* Pregnancy, complicated by, elderly, primigravida

older, affecting management of pregnancy, labor and delivery (supervision only) — *see* Pregnancy, complicated by, elderly, primigravida

very young, affecting management of pregnancy, labor and delivery (supervision only) — *see* Pregnancy, complicated by, young mother, primigravida

Primipara

elderly, affecting management of pregnancy, labor and delivery (supervision only) — *see* Pregnancy, complicated by, elderly, primigravida

older, affecting management of pregnancy, labor and delivery (supervision only) — *see* Pregnancy, complicated by, elderly, primigravida

very young, affecting management of pregnancy, labor and delivery (supervision only) — *see* Pregnancy, complicated by, young mother, primigravida

Primus varus Q66.21- ☑

PRIND (Prolonged reversible ischemic neurologic deficit) I63.9

Pringle's disease (tuberous sclerosis) Q85.1

Prinzmetal angina I20.1

Prizefighter ear — *see* Cauliflower ear

Problem (with) (related to)

academic Z55.8

acculturation Z60.3

adjustment (to)

change of job Z56.1

life-cycle transition Z60.0

pension Z60.0

retirement Z60.0

adopted child Z62.821

alcoholism in family Z63.72

atypical parenting situation Z62.9

bankruptcy Z59.8

behavioral (adult) F69

drug seeking Z76.5

birth of sibling affecting child Z62.898

care (of)

provider dependency Z74.9

specified NEC Z74.8

sick or handicapped person in family or household Z63.6

child

abuse (affecting the child) — *see* Maltreatment, child

custody or support proceedings Z65.3

in care of non-parental family member Z62.21

in foster care Z62.21

in welfare custody Z62.21

living in orphanage or group home Z62.22

child-rearing Z62.9

specified NEC Z62.898

communication (developmental) F80.9

conflict or discord (with)

boss Z56.4

classmates Z55.4

counselor Z64.4

employer Z56.4

family Z63.9

specified NEC Z63.8

probation officer Z64.4

social worker Z64.4

teachers Z55.4

workmates Z56.4

conviction in legal proceedings Z65.0

with imprisonment Z65.1

counselor Z64.4

creditors Z59.8

digestive K92.9

drug addict in family Z63.72

ear — *see* Disorder, ear

economic Z59.9

affecting care Z59.9

specified NEC Z59.8

education Z55.9

specified NEC Z55.8

employment Z56.9

change of job Z56.1

discord Z56.4

environment Z56.5

sexual harassment Z56.81

specified NEC Z56.89

stressful schedule Z56.3

Problem — *continued*

employment — *continued*

stress NEC Z56.6

threat of job loss Z56.2

unemployment Z56.0

enuresis, child F98.0

eye H57.9

failed examinations (school) Z55.2

falling Z91.81

family — *see also* Disruption, family Z63.9

specified NEC Z63.8

feeding (elderly) (infant) R63.3

newborn P92.9

breast P92.5

overfeeding P92.4

slow P92.2

specified NEC P92.8

underfeeding P92.3

nonorganic F50.89

finance Z59.9

specified NEC Z59.8

foreclosure on loan Z59.8

foster child Z62.822

frightening experience(s) in childhood Z62.898

genital NEC

female N94.9

male N50.9

health care Z75.9

specified NEC Z75.8

hearing — *see* Deafness

homelessness Z59.0

housing Z59.9

inadequate Z59.1

isolated Z59.8

specified NEC Z59.8

identity (of childhood) F93.8

illegitimate pregnancy (unwanted) Z64.0

illiteracy Z55.0

impaired mobility Z74.09

imprisonment or incarceration Z65.1

inadequate teaching affecting education Z55.8

inappropriate (excessive) parental pressure Z62.6

influencing health status NEC Z78.9

in-law Z63.1

institutionalization, affecting child Z62.22

intrafamilial communication Z63.8

jealousy, child F93.8

landlord Z59.2

language (developmental) F80.9

learning (developmental) F81.9

legal Z65.3

conviction without imprisonment Z65.0

imprisonment Z65.1

release from prison Z65.2

life-management Z73.9

specified NEC Z73.89

life-style Z72.9

gambling Z72.6

high-risk sexual behavior (heterosexual) Z72.51

bisexual Z72.53

homosexual Z72.52

inappropriate eating habits Z72.4

self-damaging behavior NEC Z72.89

specified NEC Z72.89

tobacco use Z72.0

literacy Z55.9

low level Z55.0

specified NEC Z55.8

living alone Z60.2

lodgers Z59.2

loss of love relationship in childhood Z62.898

marital Z63.0

involving

divorce Z63.5

estrangement Z63.5

gender identity F66

mastication K08.89

medical

care, within family Z63.6

facilities Z75.9

specified NEC Z75.8

mental F48.9

multiparity Z64.1

negative life events in childhood Z62.9

altered pattern of family relationships Z62.898

frightening experience Z62.898

loss of

love relationship Z62.898

self-esteem Z62.898

Problem — *continued*

negative life events in childhood — *continued*

physical abuse (alleged) — *see* Maltreatment, child

removal from home Z62.29

specified event NEC Z62.898

neighbor Z59.2

neurological NEC R29.818

new step-parent affecting child Z62.898

none (feared complaint unfounded) Z71.1

occupational NEC Z56.89

parent-child — *see* Conflict, parent-child

personal hygiene Z91.89

personality F69

phase-of-life transition, adjustment Z60.0

presence of sick or disabled person in family or household Z63.79

needing care Z63.6

primary support group (family) Z63.9

specified NEC Z63.8

probation officer Z64.4

psychiatric F99

psychosexual (development) F66

psychosocial Z65.9

religious or spiritual Z65.8

specified NEC Z65.8

relationship Z63.9

childhood F93.8

release from prison Z65.2

religious or spiritual Z65.8

removal from home affecting child Z62.29

seeking and accepting known hazardous and harmful

behavioral or psychological interventions Z65.8

chemical, nutritional or physical interventions Z65.8

sexual function (nonorganic) F52.9

sight H54.7

sleep disorder, child F51.9

smell — *see* Disturbance, sensation, smell

social

environment Z60.9

specified NEC Z60.8

exclusion and rejection Z60.4

worker Z64.4

speech R47.9

developmental F80.9

specified NEC R47.89

swallowing — *see* Dysphagia

taste — *see* Disturbance, sensation, taste

tic, child F95.0

underachievement in school Z55.3

unemployment Z56.0

threatened Z56.2

unwanted pregnancy Z64.0

upbringing Z62.9

specified NEC Z62.898

urinary N39.9

voice production R47.89

work schedule (stressful) Z56.3

Procedure (surgical)

converted

arthroscopic to open Z53.33

laparoscopic to open Z53.31

specified procedure NEC to open Z53.39

thoracoscopic to open Z53.32

for purpose other than remedying health state Z41.9

specified NEC Z41.8

not done Z53.9

because of

administrative reasons Z53.8

contraindication Z53.09

smoking Z53.01

patient's decision Z53.20

for reasons of belief or group pressure Z53.1

left against medical advice (AMA) Z53.21

specified reason NEC Z53.29

specified reason NEC Z53.8

Procidentia (uteri) N81.3

Proctalgia K62.89

fugax K59.4

spasmodic K59.4

Proctitis K62.89

amebic (acute) A06.0

chlamydial A56.3

gonococcal A54.6

granulomatous — *see* Enteritis, regional, large intestine

herpetic A60.1

radiation K62.7

tuberculous A18.32

ulcerative (chronic) K51.20

☑ **Additional Character Required** — Refer to the Tabular List for Character Selection   ▽ **Subterms under main terms may continue to next column or page**

Proctitis — *continued*
  ulcerative — *continued*
    with
      complication K51.219
        abscess K51.214
        fistula K51.213
        obstruction K51.212
        rectal bleeding K51.211
        specified NEC K51.218
Proctocele
  female (without uterine prolapse) N81.6
    with uterine prolapse N81.2
      complete N81.3
  male K62.3
Proctocolitis
  food protein-induced K52.82
  food-induced eosinophilic K52.82
  milk protein-induced K52.82
  mucosal — *see* Rectosigmoiditis, ulcerative
Proctoptosis K62.3
Proctorrhagia K62.5
Proctosigmoiditis K63.89
  ulcerative (chronic) — *see* Rectosigmoiditis, ulcerative
Proctospasm K59.4
  psychogenic F45.8
Profichet's disease — *see* Disorder, soft tissue, specified
  type NEC
Progeria E34.8
Prognathism (mandibular) (maxillary) M26.19
Progonoma (melanotic) — *see* Neoplasm, benign, by
  site
Progressive — *see* condition
Prolactinoma
  specified site — *see* Neoplasm, benign, by site
  unspecified site D35.2
Prolapse, prolapsed
  anus, anal (canal) (sphincter) K62.2
  arm or hand O32.2 ☑
    causing obstructed labor O64.4 ☑
  bladder (mucosa) (sphincter) (acquired)
    congenital Q79.4
    female — *see* Cystocele
    male N32.89
  breast implant (prosthetic) T85.49 ☑
  cecostomy K94.09
  cecum K63.4
  cervix, cervical (hypertrophied) N81.2
    anterior lip, obstructing labor O65.5
    congenital Q51.828
    postpartal, old N81.2
    stump N81.85
  ciliary body (traumatic) — *see* Laceration, eye(ball),
    with prolapse or loss of interocular tissue
  colon (pedunculated) K63.4
  colostomy K94.09
  disc (intervertebral) — *see* Displacement, intervertebral
    disc
  eye implant (orbital) T85.398 ☑
    lens (ocular) — *see* Complications, intraocular lens
  fallopian tube N83.4- ☑
  gastric (mucosa) K31.89
  genital, female N81.9
    specified NEC N81.89
  globe, nontraumatic — *see* Luxation, globe
  ileostomy bud K94.19
  intervertebral disc — *see* Displacement, intervertebral
    disc
  intestine (small) K63.4
  iris (traumatic) — *see* Laceration, eye(ball), with pro-
    lapse or loss of interocular tissue
    nontraumatic H21.89
  kidney N28.83
    congenital Q63.2
  laryngeal muscles or ventricle J38.7
  liver K76.89
  meatus urinarius N36.8
  mitral (valve) I34.1
  ocular lens implant — *see* Complications, intraocular
    lens
  organ or site, congenital NEC — *see* Malposition, con-
    genital
  ovary N83.4- ☑
  pelvic floor, female N81.89
  perineum, female N81.89
  rectum (mucosa) (sphincter) K62.3
    due to trichuris trichiuria B79
  spleen D73.89
  stomach K31.89

Prolapse, prolapsed — *continued*
  umbilical cord
    complicating delivery O69.0 ☑
  urachus, congenital Q64.4
  ureter N28.89
    with obstruction N13.5
      with infection N13.6
  ureterovesical orifice N28.89
  urethra (acquired) (infected) (mucosa) N36.8
    congenital Q64.71
  urinary meatus N36.8
    congenital Q64.72
  uterovaginal N81.4
    complete N81.3
    incomplete N81.2
  uterus (with prolapse of vagina) N81.4
    complete N81.3
    congenital Q51.818
    first degree N81.2
    in pregnancy or childbirth — *see* Pregnancy, com-
      plicated by, abnormal, uterus
    incomplete N81.2
    postpartal (old) N81.4
    second degree N81.2
    third degree N81.3
  uveal (traumatic) — *see* Laceration, eye(ball), with
    prolapse or loss of interocular tissue
  vagina (anterior) (wall) — *see* Cystocele
    with prolapse of uterus N81.4
      complete N81.3
      incomplete N81.2
    posterior wall N81.6
    posthysterectomy N99.3
  vitreous (humor) H43.0- ☑
    in wound — *see* Laceration, eye(ball), with prolapse
      or loss of interocular tissue
  womb — *see* Prolapse, uterus
Prolapsus, female N81.9
  specified NEC N81.89
Proliferation(s)
  primary cutaneous CD30-positive large T-cell C86.6
  prostate, atypical small acinar N42.32
Proliferative — *see* condition
Prolonged, prolongation (of)
  bleeding (time) (idiopathic) R79.1
  coagulation (time) R79.1
  gestation (over 42 completed weeks)
    mother O48.1
    newborn P08.22
  interval I44.0
  labor O63.9
    first stage O63.0
    second stage O63.1
  partial thromboplastin time (PTT) R79.1
  pregnancy (more than 42 weeks gestation) O48.1
  prothrombin time R79.1
  QT interval R94.31
  uterine contractions in labor O62.4
Prominence, prominent
  auricle (congenital) (ear) Q17.5
  ischial spine or sacral promontory with disproportion
    (fetopelvic)
    with disproportion (fetopelvic) O33.0
      causing obstructed labor O65.0-
  nose (congenital) acquired M95.0
Promiscuity — *see* High, risk, sexual behavior
Pronation
  ankle — *see* Deformity, limb, foot, specified NEC
  foot — *see also* Deformity, limb, foot, specified NEC
    congenital Q74.2
Prophylactic
  administration of
    antibiotics, long-term Z79.2
      short-term use — *omit code*
    drug — *see also* Long-term (current) drug therapy
      (use of) Z79.899
  medication Z79.899
  organ removal (for neoplasia management) Z40.00
    breast Z40.01
    fallopian tube(s) Z40.03
      with ovary(s) Z40.02
    ovary(s) Z40.02
    specified site NEC Z40.09
  surgery Z40.9
    for risk factors related to malignant neoplasm —
      see Prophylactic, organ removal
    specified NEC Z40.8
  vaccination Z23

Propionic acidemia E71.121
Proptosis (ocular) — *see also* Exophthalmos
  thyroid — *see* Hyperthyroidism, with goiter
Prosecution, anxiety concerning Z65.3
Prosopagnosia R48.3
Prostadynia N42.81
Prostate, prostatic — *see* condition
Prostatism — *see* Hyperplasia, prostate
Prostatitis (congestive) (suppurative) (with cystitis) N41.9
  acute N41.0
  cavitary N41.8
  chronic N41.1
  diverticular N41.8
  due to Trichomonas (vaginalis) A59.02
  fibrous N41.1
  gonococcal (acute) (chronic) A54.22
  granulomatous N41.4
  hypertrophic N41.1
  subacute N41.1
  trichomonal A59.02
  tuberculous A18.14
Prostatocystitis N41.3
Prostatorrhea N42.89
Prostatosis N42.82
Prostration R53.83
  heat — *see also* Heat, exhaustion
    anhydrotic T67.3 ☑
    due to
      salt (and water) depletion T67.4 ☑
      water depletion T67.3 ☑
  nervous F48.8
  senile R54
Protanomaly (anomalous trichromat) H53.54
Protanopia (complete) (incomplete) H53.54
Protection (against) (from) — *see* Prophylactic
Protein
  deficiency NEC — *see* Malnutrition
  malnutrition — *see* Malnutrition
  sickness — *see also* Reaction, serum T80.69 ☑
Proteinemia R77.9
Proteinosis
  alveolar (pulmonary) J84.01
  lipid or lipoid (of Urbach) E78.89
Proteinuria R80.9
  Bence Jones R80.3
  complicating pregnancy — *see* Proteinuria, gestational
  gestational
    complicating
      childbirth O12.14
      pregnancy O12.1- ☑
        with edema O12.2- ☑
      puerperium O12.15
  idiopathic R80.0
  isolated R80.0
    with glomerular lesion N06.9
      dense deposit disease N06.6
      diffuse
        crescentic glomerulonephritis N06.7
        endocapillary proliferative glomerulonephritis
          N06.4
        mesangiocapillary glomerulonephritis N06.5
      focal and segmental hyalinosis or sclerosis N06.1
      membranous (diffuse) N06.2
      mesangial proliferative (diffuse) N06.3
      minimal change N06.0
      specified pathology NEC N06.8
  orthostatic R80.2
    with glomerular lesion — *see* Proteinuria, isolated,
      with glomerular lesion
  persistent R80.1
    with glomerular lesion — *see* Proteinuria, isolated,
      with glomerular lesion
  postural R80.2
    with glomerular lesion — *see* Proteinuria, isolated,
      with glomerular lesion
  pre-eclamptic — *see* Pre-eclampsia
  puerperal O12.15
  specified type NEC R80.8
Proteolysis, pathologic D65
Proteus (mirabilis) (morganii), **as cause of disease**
  classified elsewhere B96.4
Prothrombin gene mutation D68.52
Protoporphyria, erythropoietic E80.0
Protozoal — *see also* condition
  disease B64
    specified NEC B60.8

▽ Subterms under main terms may continue to next column or page   ☑ Additional Character Required — Refer to the Tabular List for Character Selection   265

Proctitis — Protozoal

Protrusion, protrusio
acetabuli M24.7
acetabulum (into pelvis) M24.7
device, implant or graft — see also Complications, by site and type, mechanical T85.698 ☑
  arterial graft NEC — see Complication, cardiovascular device, mechanical, vascular
  breast (implant) T85.49 ☑
  catheter NEC T85.698 ☑
    cystostomy T83.090 ☑
    dialysis (renal) T82.49 ☑
      intraperitoneal T85.691 ☑
    infusion NEC T82.594 ☑
      spinal (epidural) (subdural) T85.690 ☑
    urinary — see also Complications, catheter, urinary T83.098 ☑
  electronic (electrode) (pulse generator) (stimulator)
    bone T84.390 ☑
    nervous system — see Complication, prosthetic device, mechanical, electronic nervous system stimulator
  fixation, internal (orthopedic) NEC — see Complication, fixation device, mechanical
  gastrointestinal — see Complications, prosthetic device, mechanical, gastrointestinal device
  genital NEC T83.498 ☑
    intrauterine contraceptive device T83.39 ☑
    penile prosthesis (cylinder) (implanted) (pump) (resevoir) T83.490 ☑
    testicular prosthesis T83.491 ☑
  heart NEC — see Complication, cardiovascular device, mechanical
  joint prosthesis — see Complications, joint prosthesis, mechanical, specified NEC, by site
  ocular NEC — see Complications, prosthetic device, mechanical, ocular device
  orthopedic NEC — see Complication, orthopedic, device, mechanical
  specified NEC T85.628 ☑
  urinary NEC — see also Complication, genitourinary, device, urinary, mechanical
    graft T83.29 ☑
  vascular NEC — see Complication, cardiovascular device, mechanical
  ventricular intracranial shunt T85.09 ☑
intervertebral disc — see Displacement, intervertebral disc
joint prosthesis — see Complications, joint prosthesis, mechanical, specified NEC, by site
nucleus pulposus — see Displacement, intervertebral disc
Prune belly (syndrome) Q79.4
Prurigo (ferox) (gravis) (Hebrae) (Hebra's) (mitis) (simplex) L28.2
  Besnier's L20.0
  estivalis L56.4
  nodularis L28.1
  psychogenic F45.8
Pruritus, pruritic (essential) L29.9
  ani, anus L29.0
    psychogenic F45.8
  anogenital L29.3
    psychogenic F45.8
  due to onchocerca volvulus B73.1
  gravidarum — see Pregnancy, complicated by, specified pregnancy-related condition NEC
  hiemalis L29.8
  neurogenic (any site) F45.8
  perianal L29.0
  psychogenic (any site) F45.8
  scroti, scrotum L29.1
    psychogenic F45.8
  senile, senilis L29.8
  specified NEC L29.8
    psychogenic F45.8
  Trichomonas A59.9
  vulva, vulvae L29.2
    psychogenic F45.8
Pseudarthrosis, pseudoarthrosis (bone) — see Nonunion, fracture
  clavicle, congenital Q74.0
  joint, following fusion or arthrodesis M96.0
Pseudoaneurysm — see Aneurysm
Pseudoangina (pectoris) — see Angina
Pseudoangioma I81
Pseudoarteriosus Q28.8
Pseudoarthrosis — see Pseudarthrosis

Pseudobulbar affect (PBA) F48.2
Pseudochromhidrosis L67.8
Pseudocirrhosis, liver, pericardial I31.1
Pseudocowpox B08.03
Pseudocoxalgia M91.3- ☑
Pseudocroup J38.5
Pseudo-Cushing's syndrome, alcohol-induced E24.4
Pseudocyesis F45.8
Pseudocyst
  lung J98.4
  pancreas K86.3
  retina — see Cyst, retina
Pseudoelephantiasis neuroarthritica Q82.0
Pseudoexfoliation, capsule (lens) — see Cataract, specified NEC
Pseudofolliculitis barbae L73.1
Pseudoglioma H44.89
Pseudohemophilia (Bernuth's) (hereditary) (type B) D68.0
  Type A D69.8
  vascular D69.8
Pseudohermaphroditism Q56.3
  adrenal E25.8
  female Q56.2
    with adrenocortical disorder E25.8
    without adrenocortical disorder Q56.2
    adrenal (congenital) E25.0
    unspecified E25.9
  male Q56.1
    with
      5-alpha-reductase deficiency E29.1
      adrenocortical disorder E25.8
      androgen resistance E34.51
      cleft scrotum Q56.1
      feminizing testis E34.51
    without gonadal disorder Q56.1
    adrenal E25.8
    unspecified E25.9
Pseudo-Hurler's polydystrophy E77.0
Pseudohydrocephalus G93.2
Pseudohypertrophic muscular dystrophy (Erb's) G71.02
Pseudohypertrophy, muscle G71.09
Pseudohypoparathyroidism E20.1
Pseudoinsomnia F51.03
Pseudoleukemia, infantile D64.89
Pseudomembranous — see condition
Pseudomeningocele (cerebral) (infective) (post-traumatic) G96.19
  postprocedural (spinal) G97.82
Pseudomenses (newborn) P54.6
Pseudomenstruation (newborn) P54.6
Pseudomonas
  aeruginosa, as cause of disease classified elsewhere B96.5
  mallei infection A24.0
    as cause of disease classified elsewhere B96.5
  pseudomallei, as cause of disease classified elsewhere B96.5
Pseudomyotonia G71.19
Pseudomyxoma peritonei C78.6
Pseudoneuritis, optic (nerve) (disc) (papilla), **congenital** Q14.2
Pseudo-obstruction intestine (acute) (chronic) (idiopathic) (intermittent secondary) (primary) K59.8
Pseudopapilledema H47.33- ☑
  congenital Q14.2
Pseudoparalysis
  arm or leg R29.818
  atonic, congenital P94.2
Pseudopelade L66.0
Pseudophakia Z96.1
Pseudopolyarthritis, rhizomelic M35.3
Pseudopolycythemia D75.1
Pseudopseudohypoparathyroidism E20.1
Pseudopterygium H11.81- ☑
Pseudoptosis (eyelid) — see Blepharochalasis
Pseudopuberty, precocious
  female heterosexual E25.8
  male isosexual E25.8
Pseudorickets (renal) N25.0
Pseudorubella B08.20
Pseudosclerema, newborn P83.88
Pseudosclerosis (brain)
  Jakob's — see Creutzfeldt-Jakob disease or syndrome
  of Westphal (Strümpell) E83.01
  spastic — see Creutzfeldt-Jakob disease or syndrome

Pseudotetanus — see Convulsions
Pseudotetany R29.0
  hysterical F44.5
Pseudotruncus arteriosus Q25.49
Pseudotuberculosis A28.2
  enterocolitis A04.8
  pasteurella (infection) A28.0
Pseudotumor
  cerebri G93.2
  orbital H05.11 ☑
Pseudoxanthoma elasticum Q82.8
Psilosis (sprue) (tropical) K90.1
  nontropical K90.0
Psittacosis A70
Psoitis M60.88
Psoriasis L40.9
  arthropathic L40.50
    arthritis mutilans L40.52
    distal interphalangeal L40.51
    juvenile L40.54
    other specified L40.59
    spondylitis L40.53
  buccal K13.29
  flexural L40.8
  guttate L40.4
  mouth K13.29
  nummular L40.0
  plaque L40.0
  psychogenic F54
  pustular (generalized) L40.1
    palmaris et plantaris L40.3
  specified NEC L40.8
  vulgaris L40.0
Psychasthenia F48.8
Psychiatric disorder or problem F99
Psychogenic — see also condition
  factors associated with physical conditions F54
Psychological and behavioral factors affecting medical condition F59
Psychoneurosis, psychoneurotic — see also Neurosis
  anxiety (state) F41.1
  depersonalization F48.1
  hypochondriacal F45.21
  hysteria F44.9
  neurasthenic F48.8
  personality NEC F60.89
Psychopathy, psychopathic
  affectionless F94.2
  autistic F84.5
  constitution, post-traumatic F07.81
  personality — see Disorder, personality
  sexual — see Deviation, sexual
  state F60.2
Psychosexual identity disorder of childhood F64.2
Psychosis, psychotic F29
  acute (transient) F23
    hysterical F44.9
  affective — see Disorder, mood
  alcoholic F10.959
    with
      abuse F10.159
      anxiety disorder F10.980
        with
          abuse F10.180
          dependence F10.280
      delirium tremens F10.231
      delusions F10.950
        with
          abuse F10.150
          dependence F10.250
      dementia F10.97
        with dependence F10.27
      dependence F10.259
      hallucinosis F10.951
        with
          abuse F10.151
          dependence F10.251
      mood disorder F10.94
        with
          abuse F10.14
          dependence F10.24
      paranoia F10.950
        with
          abuse F10.150
          dependence F10.250
      persisting amnesia F10.96
        with dependence F10.26
    amnestic confabulatory F10.96

☑ **Additional Character Required** — Refer to the Tabular List for Character Selection   ▽ Subterms under main terms may continue to next column or page

Psychosis, psychotic — *continued*
alcoholic — *continued*
amnestic confabulatory — *continued*
with dependence F10.26
delirium tremens F10.231
Korsakoff's, Korsakov's, Korsakow's F10.26
paranoid type F10.950
with
abuse F10.150
dependence F10.250
anergastic — *see* Psychosis, organic
arteriosclerotic (simple type) (uncomplicated) F01.50
with behavioral disturbance F01.51
childhood F84.0
atypical F84.8
climacteric — *see* Psychosis, involutional
confusional F29
acute or subacute F05
reactive F23
cycloid F23
depressive — *see* Disorder, depressive
disintegrative (childhood) F84.3
drug-induced — *see* F11-F19 with .X59
paranoid and hallucinatory states — *see* F11-F19
with .X50 or .X51
due to or associated with
addiction, drug — *see* F11-F19 with .X59
dependence
alcohol F10.259
drug — *see* F11-F19 with .X59
epilepsy F06.8
Huntington's chorea F06.8
ischemia, cerebrovascular (generalized) F06.8
multiple sclerosis F06.8
physical disease F06.8
presenile dementia F03 ☑
senile dementia F03 ☑
vascular disease (arteriosclerotic) (cerebral) F01.50
with behavioral disturbance F01.51
epileptic F06.8
episode F23
due to or associated with physical condition F06.8
exhaustive F43.0
hallucinatory, chronic F28
hypomanic F30.8
hysterical (acute) F44.9
induced F24
infantile F84.0
atypical F84.8
infective (acute) (subacute) F05
involutional F28
depressive — *see* Disorder, depressive
melancholic — *see* Disorder, depressive
paranoid (state) F22
Korsakoff's, Korsakov's, Korsakow's (nonalcoholic) F04
alcoholic F10.96
in dependence F10.26
induced by other psychoactive substance — *see*
categories F11-F19 with .X5X
mania, manic (single episode) F30.2
recurrent type F31.89
manic-depressive — *see* Disorder, bipolar
menopausal — *see* Psychosis, involutional
mixed schizophrenic and affective F25.8
multi-infarct (cerebrovascular) F01.50
with behavioral disturbance F01.51
nonorganic F29
specified NEC F28
organic F09
due to or associated with
arteriosclerosis (cerebral) — *see* Psychosis, arteriosclerotic
cerebrovascular disease, arteriosclerotic — *see*
Psychosis, arteriosclerotic
childbirth — *see* Psychosis, puerperal
Creutzfeldt-Jakob disease or syndrome — *see*
Creutzfeldt-Jakob disease or syndrome
dependence, alcohol F10.259
disease
alcoholic liver F10.259
brain, arteriosclerotic — *see* Psychosis, arteriosclerotic
cerebrovascular F01.50
with behavioral disturbance F01.51
Creutzfeldt-Jakob — *see* Creutzfeldt-Jakob
disease or syndrome
endocrine or metabolic F06.8
acute or subacute F05

Psychosis, psychotic — *continued*
organic — *continued*
due to or associated with — *continued*
disease — *continued*
liver, alcoholic F10.259
epilepsy transient (acute) F05
infection
brain (intracranial) F06.8
acute or subacute F05
intoxication
alcoholic (acute) F10.259
drug F11-F19 with .x59
ischemia, cerebrovascular (generalized) — *see*
Psychosis, arteriosclerotic
puerperium — *see* Psychosis, puerperal
trauma, brain (birth) (from electric current) (surgical) F06.8
acute or subacute F05
infective F06.8
acute or subacute F05
post-traumatic F06.8
acute or subacute F05
paranoiac F22
paranoid (climacteric) (involutional) (menopausal) F22
psychogenic (acute) F23
schizophrenic F20.0
senile F03 ☑
postpartum (NOS) F53.1
presbyophrenic (type) F03 ☑
presenile F03 ☑
psychogenic (paranoid) F23
depressive F32.3
puerperal (NOS) F53.1
specified type — *see* Psychosis, by type
reactive (brief) (transient) (emotional stress) (psychological trauma) F23
depressive F32.3
recurrent F33.3
excitative type F30.8
schizoaffective F25.9
depressive type F25.1
manic type F25.0
schizophrenia, schizophrenic — *see* Schizophrenia
schizophrenia-like, in epilepsy F06.2
schizophreniform F20.81
affective type F25.9
brief F23
confusional type F23
mixed type F25.0
senile NEC F03 ☑
depressed or paranoid type F03 ☑
simple deterioration F03 ☑
specified type — *code to* condition
shared F24
situational (reactive) F23
symbiotic (childhood) F84.3
symptomatic F09
Psychosomatic — *see* Disorder, psychosomatic
Psychosyndrome, organic F07.9
**Psychotic episode due to or associated with physical
condition** F06.8
Pterygium (eye) H11.00- ☑
amyloid H11.01- ☑
central H11.02- ☑
colli Q18.3
double H11.03- ☑
peripheral
progressive H11.05- ☑
stationary H11.04- ☑
recurrent H11.06- ☑
Ptilosis (eyelid) — *see* Madarosis
Ptomaine (poisoning) — *see* Poisoning, food
Ptosis — *see also* Blepharoptosis
adiposa (false) — *see* Blepharoptosis
breast N64.81-
brow H57.81- ☑
cecum K63.4
colon K63.4
congenital (eyelid) Q10.0
specified site NEC — *see* Anomaly, by site
eyebrow H57.81- ☑
eyelid — *see* Blepharoptosis
congenital Q10.0
gastric K31.89
intestine K63.4
kidney N28.83
liver K76.89
renal N28.83

Ptosis — *continued*
splanchnic K63.4
spleen D73.89
stomach K31.89
viscera K63.4
PTP D69.51
Ptyalism (periodic) K11.7
hysterical F45.8
pregnancy — *see* Pregnancy, complicated by, specified
pregnancy-related condition NEC
psychogenic F45.8
Ptyalolithiasis K11.5
Pubarche, precocious E30.1
Pubertas praecox E30.1
Puberty (development state) Z00.3
bleeding (excessive) N92.2
delayed E30.0
precocious (constitutional) (cryptogenic) (idiopathic)
E30.1
central E22.8
due to
ovarian hyperfunction E28.1
estrogen E28.0
testicular hyperfunction E29.0
premature E30.1
due to
adrenal cortical hyperfunction E25.8
pineal tumor E34.8
pituitary (anterior) hyperfunction E22.8
Puckering, macula — *see* Degeneration, macula, puckering
Pudenda, pudendum — *see* condition
Puente's disease (simple glandular cheilitis) K13.0
Puerperal, puerperium (complicated by, complications)
abnormal glucose (tolerance test) O99.815
abscess
areola O91.02
associated with lactation O91.03
Bartholin's gland O86.19
breast O91.12
associated with lactation O91.13
cervix (uteri) O86.11
genital organ NEC O86.19
kidney O86.21
mammary O91.12
associated with lactation O91.13
nipple O91.02
associated with lactation O91.03
peritoneum O85
subareolar O91.12
associated with lactation O91.13
urinary tract — *see* Puerperal, infection, urinary
uterus O86.12
vagina (wall) O86.13
vaginorectal O86.13
vulvovaginal gland O86.13
adnexitis O86.19
afibrinogenemia, or other coagulation defect O72.3
albuminuria (acute) (subacute) — *see* Proteinuria,
gestational
alcohol use O99.315
anemia O90.81
pre-existing (pre-pregnancy) O99.03
anesthetic death O89.8
apoplexy O99.43
bariatric surgery status O99.845
blood disorder NEC O99.13
blood dyscrasia O72.3
cardiomyopathy O90.3
cerebrovascular disorder (conditions in I60-I69) O99.43
cervicitis O86.11
circulatory system disorder O99.43
coagulopathy (any) O99.13
with hemorrhage O72.3
complications O90.9
specified NEC O90.89
convulsions — *see* Eclampsia
cystitis O86.22
cystopyelitis O86.29
delirium NEC F05
diabetes O24.93
gestational — *see* Puerperal, gestational diabetes
pre-existing O24.33
specified NEC O24.83
type 1 O24.03
type 2 O24.13
digestive system disorder O99.63
disease O90.9

Puerperal, puerperium — *continued*
  disease — *continued*
    breast NEC O92.29
    cerebrovascular (acute) O99.43
      nonobstetric NEC O99.89
    tubo-ovarian O86.19
    Valsuani's O99.03
  disorder O90.9
    biliary tract O26.63
    lactation O92.70
    liver O26.63
    nonobstetric NEC O99.89
  disruption
    cesarean wound O90.0
    episiotomy wound O90.1
    perineal laceration wound O90.1
  drug use O99.325
  eclampsia (with pre-existing hypertension) O15.2
  embolism (pulmonary) (blood clot) — *see* Embolism, obstetric, puerperal
  endocrine, nutritional or metabolic disease NEC O99.285
  endophlebitis — *see* Puerperal, phlebitis
  endotrachelitis O86.11
  failure
    lactation (complete) O92.3
      partial O92.4
    renal, acute O90.4
  fever (of unknown origin) O86.4
    septic O85
  fissure, nipple O92.12
    associated with lactation O92.13
  fistula
    breast (due to mastitis) O91.12
      associated with lactation O91.13
    nipple O91.02
      associated with lactation O91.03
  galactophoritis O91.22
    associated with lactation O91.23
  galactorrhea O92.6
  gastric banding status O99.845
  gastric bypass status O99.845
  gastrointestinal disease NEC O99.63
  gestational
    diabetes O24.439
      diet controlled O24.430
      insulin (and diet) controlled O24.434
      oral drug controlled (antidiabetic) (hypoglycemic) O24.435
    edema O12.05
      with proteinuria O12.25
    proteinuria O12.15
  gonorrhea O98.23
  hematoma, subdural O99.43
  hemiplegia, cerebral O99.355
    due to cerbrovascular disorder O99.43
  hemorrhage O72.1
    brain O99.43
    bulbar O99.43
    cerebellar O99.43
    cerebral O99.43
    cortical O99.43
    delayed or secondary O72.2
    extradural O99.43
    internal capsule O99.43
    intracranial O99.43
    intrapontine O99.43
    meningeal O99.43
    pontine O99.43
    retained placenta O72.0
    subarachnoid O99.43
    subcortical O99.43
    subdural O99.43
    third stage O72.0
    uterine, delayed O72.2
    ventricular O99.43
  hemorrhoids O87.2
  hepatorenal syndrome O90.4
  hypertension — *see* Hypertension, complicating, puerperium
  hypertrophy, breast O92.29
  induration breast (fibrous) O92.29
  infection O86.4
    cervix O86.11
    generalized O85
    genital tract NEC O86.19
      obstetric surgical wound O86.09
    kidney (bacillus coli) O86.21
    maternal O98.93

Puerperal, puerperium — *continued*
  infection — *continued*
    maternal — *continued*
      carrier state NEC O99.835
      gonorrhea O98.23
      human immunodeficiency virus (HIV) O98.73
      protozoal O98.63
      sexually transmitted NEC O98.33
      specified NEC O98.83
      streptococcus group B (GBS) carrier state O99.825
      syphilis O98.13
      tuberculosis O98.03
      viral hepatitis O98.43
      viral NEC O98.53
    nipple O91.02
      associated with lactation O91.03
    peritoneum O85
    renal O86.21
    specified NEC O86.89
    urinary (asymptomatic) (tract) NEC O86.20
      bladder O86.22
      kidney O86.21
      specified site NEC O86.29
      urethra O86.22
    vagina O86.13
    vein — *see* Puerperal, phlebitis
  ischemia, cerebral O99.43
  lymphangitis O86.89
    breast O91.22
      associated with lactation O91.23
  malignancy O9A.13 (*following* O99)
  malnutrition O25.3
  mammillitis O91.02
    associated with lactation O91.03
  mammitis O91.22
    associated with lactation O91.23
  mania F30.8
  mastitis O91.22
    associated with lactation O91.23
    purulent O91.12
      associated with lactation O91.13
  melancholia — *see* Disorder, depressive
  mental disorder NEC O99.345
  metroperitonitis O85
  metrorrhagia — *see* Hemorrhage, postpartum
  metrosalpingitis O86.19
  metrovaginitis O86.13
  milk leg O87.1
  monoplegia, cerebral O99.43
  mood disturbance O90.6
  necrosis, liver (acute) (subacute) (conditions in subcategory K72.0) O26.63
    with renal failure O90.4
  nervous system disorder O99.355
  obesity (pre-existing prior to pregnancy) O99.215
  obesity surgery status O99.845
  occlusion, precerebral artery O99.43
  paralysis
    bladder (sphincter) O90.89
    cerebral O99.43
  paralytic stroke O99.43
  parametritis O85
  paravaginitis O86.13
  pelviperitonitis O85
  perimetritis O86.12
  perimetrosalpingitis O86.19
  perinephritis O86.21
  periphlebitis — *see* Puerperal phlebitis
  peritoneal infection O85
  peritonitis (pelvic) O85
  perivaginitis O86.13
  phlebitis O87.0
    deep O87.1
    pelvic O87.1
    superficial O87.0
  phlebothrombosis, deep O87.1
  phlegmasia alba dolens O87.1
  placental polyp O90.89
  pneumonia, embolic — *see* Embolism, obstetric, puerperal
  pre-eclampsia — *see* Pre-eclampsia
  psychosis (NOS) F53.1
  pyelitis O86.21
  pyelocystitis O86.29
  pyelonephritis O86.21
  pyelonephrosis O86.21
  pyemia O85
  pyocystitis O86.29
  pyohemia O85

Puerperal, puerperium — *continued*
  pyometra O86.12
  pyonephritis O86.21
  pyosalpingitis O86.19
  pyrexia (of unknown origin) O86.4
  renal
    disease NEC O90.89
    failure O90.4
  respiratory disease NEC O99.53
  retention
    decidua — *see* Retention, decidua
    placenta O72.0
    secundines — *see* Retention, secundines
  retrated nipple O92.02
  salpingo-ovaritis O86.19
  salpingoperitonitis O85
  secondary perineal tear O90.1
  sepsis (pelvic) O85
  sepsis O85
  septic thrombophlebitis O86.81
  skin disorder NEC O99.73
  specified condition NEC O99.89
  stroke O99.43
  subinvolution (uterus) O90.89
  subluxation of symphysis (pubis) O26.73
  suppuration — *see* Puerperal, abscess
  tetanus A34
  thelitis O91.02
    associated with lactation O91.03
  thrombocytopenia O72.3
  thrombophlebitis (superficial) O87.0
    deep O87.1
    pelvic O87.1
    septic O86.81
  thrombosis (venous) — *see* Thrombosis, puerperal
  thyroiditis O90.5
  toxemia (eclamptic) (pre-eclamptic) (with convulsions) O15.2
  trauma, non-obstetric O9A.23 (*following* O99)
    caused by abuse (physical) (suspected) O9A.33 (*following* O99)
      confirmed O9A.33 (*following* O99)
      psychological (suspected) O9A.53 (*following* O99)
        confirmed O9A.53 (*following* O99)
      sexual (suspected) O9A.43 (*following* O99)
        confirmed O9A.43 (*following* O99)
  uremia (due to renal failure) O90.4
  urethritis O86.22
  vaginitis O86.13
  varicose veins (legs) O87.4
    vulva or perineum O87.8
  venous O87.9
  vulvitis O86.19
  vulvovaginitis O86.13
  white leg O87.1
Puerperium — *see* Puerperal
Pulmolithiasis J98.4
Pulmonary — *see* condition
Pulpitis (acute) (anachoretic) (chronic) (hyperplastic) (putrescent) (suppurative) (ulcerative) K04.01
  irreversible K04.02
  reversible K04.01
Pulpless tooth K04.99
Pulse
  alternating R00.8
  bigeminal R00.8
  fast R00.0
  feeble, rapid due to shock following injury T79.4 ☑
  rapid R00.0
  weak R09.89
Pulsus alternans or trigeminus R00.8
Punch drunk F07.81
Punctum lacrimale occlusion — *see* Obstruction, lacrimal
Puncture
  abdomen, abdominal
    wall S31.139 ☑
      with
        foreign body S31.149 ☑
        penetration into peritoneal cavity S31.639 ☑
          with foreign body S31.649 ☑
      epigastric region S31.132 ☑
        with
          foreign body S31.142 ☑
          penetration into peritoneal cavity S31.632 ☑
            with foreign body S31.642 ☑

☑ Additional Character Required — Refer to the Tabular List for Character Selection ▽ Subterms under main terms may continue to next column or page

Puncture — *continued*
  abdomen, abdominal — *continued*
    wall — *continued*
      left
        lower quadrant S31.134 ☑
          with
            foreign body S31.144 ☑
            penetration into peritoneal cavity
              S31.634 ☑
              with foreign body S31.644 ☑
        upper quadrant S31.131 ☑
          with
            foreign body S31.141 ☑
            penetration into peritoneal cavity
              S31.631 ☑
              with foreign body S31.641 ☑
      periumbilic region S31.135 ☑
        with
          foreign body S31.145 ☑
          penetration into peritoneal cavity
            S31.635 ☑
            with foreign body S31.645 ☑
      right
        lower quadrant S31.133 ☑
          with
            foreign body S31.143 ☑
            penetration into peritoneal cavity
              S31.633 ☑
              with foreign body S31.643 ☑
        upper quadrant S31.130 ☑
          with
            foreign body S31.140 ☑
            penetration into peritoneal cavity
              S31.630 ☑
              with foreign body S31.640 ☑
  accidental, complicating surgery — *see* Complication, accidental puncture or laceration
  alveolar (process) — *see* Puncture, oral cavity
  ankle S91.039 ☑
    with
      foreign body S91.049 ☑
    left S91.032 ☑
      with
        foreign body S91.042 ☑
    right S91.031 ☑
      with
        foreign body S91.041 ☑
  anus S31.833 ☑
    with foreign body S31.834 ☑
  arm (upper) S41.139 ☑
    with foreign body S41.149 ☑
    left S41.132 ☑
      with foreign body S41.142 ☑
    lower — *see* Puncture, forearm
    right S41.131 ☑
      with foreign body S41.141 ☑
  auditory canal (external) (meatus) — *see* Puncture, ear
  auricle, ear — *see* Puncture, ear
  axilla — *see* Puncture, arm
  back — *see also* Puncture, thorax, back
    lower S31.030 ☑
      with
        foreign body S31.040 ☑
          with penetration into retroperitoneal space S31.041 ☑
        penetration into retroperitoneal space S31.031 ☑
  bladder (traumatic) S37.29 ☑
    nontraumatic N32.89
  breast S21.039 ☑
    with foreign body S21.049 ☑
    left S21.032 ☑
      with foreign body S21.042 ☑
    right S21.031 ☑
      with foreign body S21.041 ☑
  buttock S31.803 ☑
    with foreign body S31.804 ☑
    left S31.823 ☑
      with foreign body S31.824 ☑
    right S31.813 ☑
      with foreign body S31.814 ☑
  by
    device, implant or graft — *see* Complications, by site and type, mechanical
    foreign body left accidentally in operative wound T81.539 ☑

Puncture — *continued*
  by — *continued*
    instrument (any) during a procedure, accidental — *see* Puncture, accidental complicating surgery
  calf — *see* Puncture, leg
  canaliculus lacrimalis — *see* Puncture, eyelid
  canthus, eye — *see* Puncture, eyelid
  cervical esophagus S11.23 ☑
    with foreign body S11.24 ☑
  cheek (external) S01.439 ☑
    with foreign body S01.449 ☑
    internal — *see* Puncture, oral cavity
    left S01.432 ☑
      with foreign body S01.442 ☑
    right S01.431 ☑
      with foreign body S01.441 ☑
  chest wall — *see* Puncture, thorax
  chin — *see* Puncture, head, specified site NEC
  clitoris — *see* Puncture, vulva
  costal region — *see* Puncture, thorax
  digit(s)
    foot — *see* Puncture, toe
    hand — *see* Puncture, finger
  ear (canal) (external) S01.339 ☑
    with foreign body S01.349 ☑
    drum S09.2- ☑
    left S01.332 ☑
      with foreign body S01.342 ☑
    right S01.331 ☑
      with foreign body S01.341 ☑
  elbow S51.039 ☑
    with
      foreign body S51.049 ☑
    left S51.032 ☑
      with
        foreign body S51.042 ☑
    right S51.031 ☑
      with
        foreign body S51.041 ☑
  epididymis — *see* Puncture, testis
  epigastric region — *see* Puncture, abdomen, wall, epigastric
  epiglottis S11.83 ☑
    with foreign body S11.84 ☑
  esophagus
    cervical S11.23 ☑
      with foreign body S11.24 ☑
    thoracic S27.818 ☑
  eyeball S05.6- ☑
    with foreign body S05.5- ☑
  eyebrow — *see* Puncture, eyelid
  eyelid S01.13- ☑
    with foreign body S01.14- ☑
    left S01.132 ☑
      with foreign body S01.142 ☑
    right S01.131 ☑
      with foreign body S01.141 ☑
  face NEC — *see* Puncture, head, specified site NEC
  finger(s) S61.239 ☑
    with
      damage to nail S61.339 ☑
        with
          foreign body S61.349 ☑
      foreign body S61.249 ☑
    index S61.238 ☑
      with
        damage to nail S61.338 ☑
          with
            foreign body S61.348 ☑
        foreign body S61.248 ☑
      left S61.231 ☑
        with
          damage to nail S61.331 ☑
            with
              foreign body S61.341 ☑
          foreign body S61.241 ☑
      right S61.230 ☑
        with
          damage to nail S61.330 ☑
            with
              foreign body S61.340 ☑
          foreign body S61.240 ☑
    little S61.238 ☑
      with
        damage to nail S61.338 ☑

Puncture — *continued*
  finger(s) — *continued*
    little — *continued*
      with — *continued*
        damage to nail — *continued*
          with
            foreign body S61.348 ☑
        foreign body S61.248 ☑
      left S61.237 ☑
        with
          damage to nail S61.337 ☑
            with
              foreign body S61.347 ☑
          foreign body S61.247 ☑
      right S61.236 ☑
        with
          damage to nail S61.336 ☑
            with
              foreign body S61.346 ☑
          foreign body S61.246 ☑
    middle S61.238 ☑
      with
        damage to nail S61.338 ☑
          with
            foreign body S61.348 ☑
        foreign body S61.248 ☑
      left S61.233 ☑
        with
          damage to nail S61.333 ☑
            with
              foreign body S61.343 ☑
          foreign body S61.243 ☑
      right S61.232 ☑
        with
          damage to nail S61.332 ☑
            with
              foreign body S61.342 ☑
          foreign body S61.242 ☑
    ring S61.238 ☑
      with
        damage to nail S61.338 ☑
          with
            foreign body S61.348 ☑
        foreign body S61.248 ☑
      left S61.235 ☑
        with
          damage to nail S61.335 ☑
            with
              foreign body S61.345 ☑
          foreign body S61.245 ☑
      right S61.234 ☑
        with
          damage to nail S61.334 ☑
            with
              foreign body S61.344 ☑
          foreign body S61.244 ☑
  flank S31.139 ☑
    with foreign body S31.149 ☑
  foot (except toe(s) alone) S91.339 ☑
    with foreign body S91.349 ☑
    left S91.332 ☑
      with foreign body S91.342 ☑
    right S91.331 ☑
      with foreign body S91.341 ☑
    toe — *see* Puncture, toe
  forearm S51.839 ☑
    with
      foreign body S51.849 ☑
    elbow only — *see* Puncture, elbow
    left S51.832 ☑
      with
        foreign body S51.842 ☑
    right S51.831 ☑
      with
        foreign body S51.841 ☑
  forehead — *see* Puncture, head, specified site NEC
  genital organs, external
    female S31.532 ☑
      with foreign body S31.542 ☑
      vagina — *see* Puncture, vagina
      vulva — *see* Puncture, vulva
    male S31.531 ☑
      with foreign body S31.541 ☑
      penis — *see* Puncture, penis
      scrotum — *see* Puncture, scrotum
      testis — *see* Puncture, testis

▽ Subterms under main terms may continue to next column or page   ☑ Additional Character Required — Refer to the Tabular List for Character Selection   269

Puncture — Puncture

Puncture — *continued*

  groin — *see* Puncture, abdomen, wall
  gum — *see* Puncture, oral cavity
  hand S61.439 ☑
    with
      foreign body S61.449 ☑
    finger — *see* Puncture, finger
    left S61.432 ☑
      with
        foreign body S61.442 ☑
    right S61.431 ☑
      with
        foreign body S61.441 ☑
    thumb — *see* Puncture, thumb
  head S01.93 ☑
    with foreign body S01.94 ☑
    cheek — *see* Puncture, cheek
    ear — *see* Puncture, ear
    eyelid — *see* Puncture, eyelid
    lip — *see* Puncture, oral cavity
    nose — *see* Puncture, nose
    oral cavity — *see* Puncture, oral cavity
    scalp S01.03 ☑
      with foreign body S01.04 ☑
    specified site NEC S01.83 ☑
      with foreign body S01.84 ☑
    temporomandibular area — *see* Puncture, cheek
  heart S26.99 ☑
    with hemopericardium S26.09 ☑
    without hemopericardium S26.19 ☑
  heel — *see* Puncture, foot
  hip S71.039 ☑
    with foreign body S71.049 ☑
    left S71.032 ☑
      with foreign body S71.042 ☑
    right S71.031 ☑
      with foreign body S71.041 ☑
  hymen — *see* Puncture, vagina
  hypochondrium — *see* Puncture, abdomen, wall
  hypogastric region — *see* Puncture, abdomen, wall
  inguinal region — *see* Puncture, abdomen, wall
  instep — *see* Puncture, foot
  internal organs — *see* Injury, by site
  interscapular region — *see* Puncture, thorax, back
  intestine
    large
      colon S36.599 ☑
        ascending S36.590 ☑
        descending S36.592 ☑
        sigmoid S36.593 ☑
        specified site NEC S36.598 ☑
        transverse S36.591 ☑
      rectum S36.69 ☑
    small S36.499 ☑
      duodenum S36.490 ☑
      specified site NEC S36.498 ☑
  intra-abdominal organ S36.99 ☑
    gallbladder S36.128 ☑
    intestine — *see* Puncture, intestine
    liver S36.118 ☑
    pancreas — *see* Puncture, pancreas
    peritoneum S36.81 ☑
    specified site NEC S36.898 ☑
    spleen S36.09 ☑
    stomach S36.39 ☑
  jaw — *see* Puncture, head, specified site NEC
  knee S81.039 ☑
    with foreign body S81.049 ☑
    left S81.032 ☑
      with foreign body S81.042 ☑
    right S81.031 ☑
      with foreign body S81.041 ☑
  labium (majus) (minus) — *see* Puncture, vulva
  lacrimal duct — *see* Puncture, eyelid
  larynx S11.013 ☑
    with foreign body S11.014 ☑
  leg (lower) S81.839 ☑
    with foreign body S81.849 ☑
    foot — *see* Puncture, foot
    knee — *see* Puncture, knee
    left S81.832 ☑
      with foreign body S81.842 ☑
    right S81.831 ☑
      with foreign body S81.841 ☑
    upper — *see* Puncture, thigh
  lip S01.531 ☑

Puncture — *continued*

  lip — *continued*
    with foreign body S01.541 ☑
  loin — *see* Puncture, abdomen, wall
  lower back — *see* Puncture, back, lower
  lumbar region — *see* Puncture, back, lower
  malar region — *see* Puncture, head, specified site NEC
  mammary — *see* Puncture, breast
  mastoid region — *see* Puncture, head, specified site NEC
  mouth — *see* Puncture, oral cavity
  nail
    finger — *see* Puncture, finger, with damage to nail
    toe — *see* Puncture, toe, with damage to nail
  nasal (septum) (sinus) — *see* Puncture, nose
  nasopharynx — *see* Puncture, head, specified site NEC
  neck S11.93 ☑
    with foreign body S11.94 ☑
    involving
      cervical esophagus — *see* Puncture, cervical esophagus
      larynx — *see* Puncture, larynx
      pharynx — *see* Puncture, pharynx
      thyroid gland — *see* Puncture, thyroid gland
      trachea — *see* Puncture, trachea
    specified site NEC S11.83 ☑
      with foreign body S11.84 ☑
  nose (septum) (sinus) S01.23 ☑
    with foreign body S01.24 ☑
  ocular — *see* Puncture, eyeball
  oral cavity S01.532 ☑
    with foreign body S01.542 ☑
  orbit S05.4- ☑
  palate — *see* Puncture, oral cavity
  palm — *see* Puncture, hand
  pancreas S36.299 ☑
    body S36.291 ☑
    head S36.290 ☑
    tail S36.292 ☑
  pelvis — *see* Puncture, back, lower
  penis S31.23 ☑
    with foreign body S31.24 ☑
  perineum
    female S31.43 ☑
      with foreign body S31.44 ☑
    male S31.139 ☑
      with foreign body S31.149 ☑
  periocular area (with or without lacrimal passages) — *see* Puncture, eyelid
  phalanges
    finger — *see* Puncture, finger
    toe — *see* Puncture, toe
  pharynx S11.23 ☑
    with foreign body S11.24 ☑
  pinna — *see* Puncture, ear
  popliteal space — *see* Puncture, knee
  prepuce — *see* Puncture, penis
  pubic region S31.139 ☑
    with foreign body S31.149 ☑
  pudendum — *see* Puncture, genital organs, external
  rectovaginal septum — *see* Puncture, vagina
  sacral region — *see* Puncture, back, lower
  sacroiliac region — *see* Puncture, back, lower
  salivary gland — *see* Puncture, oral cavity
  scalp S01.03 ☑
    with foreign body S01.04 ☑
  scapular region — *see* Puncture, shoulder
  scrotum S31.33 ☑
    with foreign body S31.34 ☑
  shin — *see* Puncture, leg
  shoulder S41.039 ☑
    with foreign body S41.049 ☑
    left S41.032 ☑
      with foreign body S41.042 ☑
    right S41.031 ☑
      with foreign body S41.041 ☑
  spermatic cord — *see* Puncture, testis
  sternal region — *see* Puncture, thorax, front
  submaxillary region — *see* Puncture, head, specified site NEC
  submental region — *see* Puncture, head, specified site NEC
  subungual
    finger(s) — *see* Puncture, finger, with damage to nail
    toe — *see* Puncture, toe, with damage to nail

Puncture — *continued*

  supraclavicular fossa — *see* Puncture, neck, specified site NEC
  temple, temporal region — *see* Puncture, head, specified site NEC
  temporomandibular area — *see* Puncture, cheek
  testis S31.33 ☑
    with foreign body S31.34 ☑
  thigh S71.139 ☑
    with foreign body S71.149 ☑
    left S71.132 ☑
      with foreign body S71.142 ☑
    right S71.131 ☑
      with foreign body S71.141 ☑
  thorax, thoracic (wall) S21.93 ☑
    with foreign body S21.94 ☑
    back S21.23- ☑
      with
        foreign body S21.24- ☑
          with penetration S21.44 ☑
        penetration S21.43 ☑
    breast — *see* Puncture, breast
    front S21.13- ☑
      with
        foreign body S21.14- ☑
          with penetration S21.34 ☑
        penetration S21.33 ☑
  throat — *see* Puncture, neck
  thumb S61.039 ☑
    with
      damage to nail S61.139 ☑
        with
          foreign body S61.149 ☑
      foreign body S61.049 ☑
    left S61.032 ☑
      with
        damage to nail S61.132 ☑
          with
            foreign body S61.142 ☑
        foreign body S61.042 ☑
    right S61.031 ☑
      with
        damage to nail S61.131 ☑
          with
            foreign body S61.141 ☑
        foreign body S61.041 ☑
  thyroid gland S11.13 ☑
    with foreign body S11.14 ☑
  toe(s) S91.139 ☑
    with
      damage to nail S91.239 ☑
        with
          foreign body S91.249 ☑
      foreign body S91.149 ☑
    great S91.133 ☑
      with
        damage to nail S91.233 ☑
          with
            foreign body S91.243 ☑
        foreign body S91.143 ☑
      left S91.132 ☑
        with
          damage to nail S91.232 ☑
            with
              foreign body S91.242 ☑
          foreign body S91.142 ☑
      right S91.131 ☑
        with
          damage to nail S91.231 ☑
            with
              foreign body S91.241 ☑
          foreign body S91.141 ☑
    lesser S91.136 ☑
      with
        damage to nail S91.236 ☑
          with
            foreign body S91.246 ☑
        foreign body S91.146 ☑
      left S91.135 ☑
        with
          damage to nail S91.235 ☑
            with
              foreign body S91.245 ☑
          foreign body S91.145 ☑
      right S91.134 ☑

Index

Puncture — *continued*
　toe(s) — *continued*
　　lesser — *continued*
　　　right — *continued*
　　　　with
　　　　　damage to nail S91.234 ☑
　　　　　　with
　　　　　　　foreign body S91.244 ☑
　　　　　　foreign body S91.144 ☑
　tongue — *see* Puncture, oral cavity
　trachea S11.023 ☑
　　with foreign body S11.024 ☑
　tunica vaginalis — *see* Puncture, testis
　tympanum, tympanic membrane S09.2- ☑
　umbilical region S31.135 ☑
　　with foreign body S31.145 ☑
　uvula — *see* Puncture, oral cavity
　vagina S31.43 ☑
　　with foreign body S31.44 ☑
　vocal cords S11.033 ☑
　　with foreign body S11.034 ☑
　vulva S31.43 ☑
　　with foreign body S31.44 ☑
　wrist S61.539 ☑
　　with
　　　foreign body S61.549 ☑
　　left S61.532 ☑
　　　with
　　　　foreign body S61.542 ☑
　　right S61.531 ☑
　　　with
　　　　foreign body S61.541 ☑
PUO (pyrexia of unknown origin) R50.9
Pupillary membrane (persistent) Q13.89
Pupillotonia — *see* Anomaly, pupil, function, tonic pupil
Purpura D69.2
　abdominal D69.0
　allergic D69.0
　anaphylactoid D69.0
　annularis telangiectodes L81.7
　arthritic D69.0
　autoerythrocyte sensitization D69.2
　autoimmune D69.0
　bacterial D69.0
　Bateman's (senile) D69.2
　capillary fragility (hereditary) (idiopathic) D69.8
　cryoglobulinemic D89.1
　Devil's pinches D69.2
　fibrinolytic — *see* Fibrinolysis
　fulminans, fulminous D65
　gangrenous D65
　hemorrhagic, hemorrhagica D69.3
　　not due to thrombocytopenia D69.0
　Henoch (-Schönlein) (allergic) D69.0
　hypergammaglobulinemic (benign) (Waldenström) D89.0
　idiopathic (thrombocytopenic) D69.3
　　nonthrombocytopenic D69.0
　immune thrombocytopenic D69.3
　infectious D69.0
　malignant D69.0
　neonatorum P54.5
　nervosa D69.0
　newborn P54.5
　nonthrombocytopenic D69.2
　　hemorrhagic D69.0
　　idiopathic D69.0
　nonthrombopenic D69.2
　peliosis rheumatica D69.0
　posttransfusion (post-transfusion) (from (fresh) whole blood or blood products) D69.51
　primary D69.49
　red cell membrane sensitivity D69.2
　rheumatica D69.0
　Schönlein (-Henoch) (allergic) D69.0
　scorbutic E54 [D77]
　senile D69.2
　simplex D69.2
　symptomatica D69.0
　telangiectasia annularis L81.7
　thrombocytopenic D69.49
　　congenital D69.42
　　hemorrhagic D69.3
　　hereditary D69.42
　　idiopathic D69.3
　　immune D69.3
　　neonatal, transitory P61.0
　　thrombotic M31.1

Purpura — *continued*
　thrombohemolytic — *see* Fibrinolysis
　thrombolytic — *see* Fibrinolysis
　thrombopenic D69.49
　thrombotic, thrombocytopenic M31.1
　toxic D69.0
　vascular D69.0
　visceral symptoms D69.0
Purpuric spots R23.3
Purulent — *see* condition
Pus
　in
　　stool R19.5
　　urine N39.0
　tube (rupture) — *see* Salpingo-oophoritis
Pustular rash L08.0
Pustule (nonmalignant) L08.9
　malignant A22.0
Pustulosis palmaris et plantaris L40.3
Putnam (-Dana) **disease or syndrome** — *see* Degeneration, combined
Putrescent pulp (dental) K04.1
Pyarthritis, pyarthrosis — *see* Arthritis, pyogenic or pyemic
　tuberculous — *see* Tuberculosis, joint
Pyelectasis — *see* Hydronephrosis
Pyelitis (congenital) (uremic) — *see also* Pyelonephritis
　with
　　calculus — *see* category N20 ☑
　　　with hydronephrosis N13.6
　　contracted kidney N11.9
　acute N10
　chronic N11.9
　　with calculus — *see* category N20 ☑
　　　with hydronephrosis N13.6
　cystica N28.84
　puerperal (postpartum) O86.21
　tuberculous A18.11
Pyelocystitis — *see* Pyelonephritis
Pyelonephritis — *see also* Nephritis, tubulo-interstitial
　with
　　calculus — *see* category N20 ☑
　　　with hydronephrosis N13.6
　　contracted kidney N11.9
　acute N10
　calculous — *see* category N20 ☑
　　with hydronephrosis N13.6
　chronic N11.9
　　with calculus — *see* category N20 ☑
　　　with hydronephrosis N13.6
　　associated with ureteral obstruction or stricture N11.1
　　nonobstructive N11.8
　　　with reflux (vesicoureteral) N11.0
　　obstructive N11.1
　　specified NEC N11.8
　in (due to)
　　brucellosis A23.9 [N16]
　　cryoglobulinemia (mixed) D89.1 [N16]
　　cystinosis E72.04
　　diphtheria A36.84
　　glycogen storage disease E74.09 [N16]
　　leukemia NEC C95.9- ☑ [N16]
　　lymphoma NEC C85.90 [N16]
　　multiple myeloma C90.0- ☑ [N16]
　　obstruction N11.1
　　Salmonella infection A02.25
　　sarcoidosis D86.84
　　sepsis A41.9 [N16]
　　Sjögren's disease M35.04
　　toxoplasmosis B58.83
　　transplant rejection T86.91 [N16]
　　Wilson's disease E83.01 [N16]
　nonobstructive N12
　　with reflux (vesicoureteral) N11.0
　　chronic N11.8
　syphilitic A52.75
Pyelonephrosis (obstructive) N11.1
　chronic N11.9
Pyelophlebitis I80.8
Pyeloureteritis cystica N28.85
Pyemia, pyemic (fever) (infection) (purulent) — *see also* Sepsis
　joint — *see* Arthritis, pyogenic or pyemic
　liver K75.1
　pneumococcal A40.3
　portal K75.1

Pyemia, pyemic — *continued*
　postvaccinal T88.0 ☑
　puerperal, postpartum, childbirth O85
　specified organism NEC A41.89
　tuberculous — *see* Tuberculosis, miliary
Pygopagus Q89.4
Pyknoepilepsy (idiopathic) — *see* Pyknolepsy
Pyknolepsy G40.A09 (*following* G40.3)
　intractable G40.A19 (*following* G40.3)
　　with status epilepticus G40.A11 (*following* G40.3)
　　without status epilepticus G40.A19 (*following* G40.3)
　not intractable G40.A09 (*following* G40.3)
　　with status epilepticus G40.A01 (*following* G40.3)
　　without status epilepticus G40.A09 (*following* G40.3)
Pylephlebitis K75.1
Pyle's syndrome Q78.5
Pylethrombophlebitis K75.1
Pylethrombosis K75.1
Pyloritis K29.90
　with bleeding K29.91
Pylorospasm (reflex) **NEC** K31.3
　congenital or infantile Q40.0
　neurotic F45.8
　newborn Q40.0
　psychogenic F45.8
Pylorus, pyloric — *see* condition
Pyoarthrosis — *see* Arthritis, pyogenic or pyemic
Pyocele
　mastoid — *see* Mastoiditis, acute
　sinus (accessory) — *see* Sinusitis
　turbinate (bone) J32.9
　urethra — *see also* Urethritis N34.0
Pyocolpos — *see* Vaginitis
Pyocystitis N30.80
　with hematuria N30.81
Pyoderma, pyodermia L08.0
　gangrenosum L88
　newborn P39.4
　phagedenic L88
　vegetans L08.81
Pyodermatitis L08.0
　vegetans L08.81
Pyogenic — *see* condition
Pyohydronephrosis N13.6
Pyometra, pyometrium, pyometritis — *see* Endometritis
Pyomyositis (tropical) — *see* Myositis, infective
Pyonephritis N12
Pyonephrosis N13.6
　tuberculous A18.11
Pyo-oophoritis — *see* Salpingo-oophoritis
Pyo-ovarium — *see* Salpingo-oophoritis
Pyopericarditis, pyopericardium I30.1
Pyophlebitis — *see* Phlebitis
Pyopneumopericardium I30.1
Pyopneumothorax (infective) J86.9
　with fistula J86.0
　tuberculous NEC A15.6
Pyosalpinx, pyosalpingitis — *see also* Salpingo-oophoritis
Pyothorax J86.9
　with fistula J86.0
　tuberculous NEC A15.6
Pyoureter N28.89
　tuberculous A18.11
Pyramidopallidonigral syndrome G20
Pyrexia (of unknown origin) R50.9
　atmospheric T67.01 ☑
　during labor NEC O75.2
　heat T67.01 ☑
　newborn P81.9
　　environmentally-induced P81.0
　persistent R50.9
　puerperal O86.4
Pyroglobulinemia NEC E88.09
Pyromania F63.1
Pyrosis R12
Pyuria (bacterial) (sterile) R82.81

Q

Q fever A78
　with pneumonia A78
Quadricuspid aortic valve Q23.8
Quadrilateral fever A78
Quadriparesis — *see* Quadriplegia
　meaning muscle weakness M62.81

Puncture — Quadriparesis

Quadriplegia G82.50
  complete
    C1-C4 level G82.51
    C5-C7 level G82.53
  congenital (cerebral) (spinal) G80.8
    spastic G80.0
  embolic (current episode) I63.4- ☑
  functional R53.2
  incomplete
    C1-C4 level G82.52
    C5-C7 level G82.54
  thrombotic (current episode) I63.3- ☑
  traumatic — *code to* injury with seventh character S
    current episode — *see* Injury, spinal (cord), cervical
Quadruplet, pregnancy — *see* Pregnancy, quadruplet
Quarrelsomeness F60.3
Queensland fever A77.3
Quervain's disease M65.4
  thyroid E06.1
Queyrat's erythroplasia D07.4
  penis D07.4
  specified site — *see* Neoplasm, skin, in situ
  unspecified site D07.4
Quincke's disease or edema T78.3 ☑
  hereditary D84.1
Quinsy (gangrenous) J36
Quintan fever A79.0
Quintuplet, pregnancy — *see* Pregnancy, quintuplet

R

Rabbit fever — *see* Tularemia
Rabies A82.9
  contact Z20.3
  exposure to Z20.3
  inoculation reaction — *see* Complications, vaccination
  sylvatic A82.0
  urban A82.1
Rachischisis — *see* Spina bifida
Rachitic — *see also* condition
  deformities of spine (late effect) (sequelae) E64.3
  pelvis (late effect) (sequelae) E64.3
    with disproportion (fetopelvic) O33.0
      causing obstructed labor O65.0
Rachitis, rachitism (acute) (tarda) — *see also* Rickets
  renalis N25.0
  sequelae E64.3
Radial nerve — *see* condition
Radiation
  burn — *see* Burn
  effects NOS T66 ☑
  sickness NOS T66 ☑
  therapy, encounter for Z51.0
Radiculitis (pressure) (vertebrogenic) — *see* Radiculopathy
Radiculomyelitis — *see also* Encephalitis
  toxic, due to
    Clostridium tetani A35
    Corynebacterium diphtheriae A36.82
Radiculopathy M54.10
  cervical region M54.12
  cervicothoracic region M54.13
  due to
    disc disorder
      C3 M50.11
      C4 M50.11
      C5 M50.121
      C6 M50.122
      C7 M50.123
    displacement of intervertebral disc — *see* Disorder, disc, with, radiculopathy
  leg M54.1- ☑
  lumbar region M54.16
  lumbosacral region M54.17
  occipito-atlanto-axial region M54.11
  postherpetic B02.29
  sacrococcygeal region M54.18
  syphilitic A52.11
  thoracic region (with visceral pain) M54.14
  thoracolumbar region M54.15
Radiodermal burns (acute, chronic, or occupational) — *see* Burn
Radiodermatitis L58.9
  acute L58.0
  chronic L58.1
Radiotherapy session Z51.0
RAEB (refractory anemia with excess blasts) D46.2- ☑

Rage, meaning rabies — *see* Rabies
Ragpicker's disease A22.1
Ragsorter's disease A22.1
Raillietiniasis B71.8
Railroad neurosis F48.8
Railway spine F48.8
Raised — *see also* Elevated
  antibody titer R76.0
Rake teeth, tooth M26.39
Rales R09.89
Ramifying renal pelvis Q63.8
Ramsay-Hunt disease or syndrome — *see also* Hunt's disease B02.21
  meaning dyssynergia cerebellaris myoclonica G11.1
Ranula K11.6
  congenital Q38.4
Rape
  adult
    confirmed T74.21 ☑
    suspected T76.21 ☑
  alleged, observation or examination, ruled out
    adult Z04.41
    child Z04.42
  child
    confirmed T74.22 ☑
    suspected T76.22 ☑
Rapid
  feeble pulse, due to shock, following injury T79.4 ☑
  heart (beat) R00.0
    psychogenic F45.8
  second stage (delivery) O62.3
  time-zone change syndrome G47.25
Rarefaction, bone — *see* Disorder, bone, density and structure, specified NEC
Rash (toxic) R21
  canker A38.9
  diaper L22
  drug (internal use) L27.0
    contact — *see also* Dermatitis, due to, drugs, external L25.1
  following immunization T88.1 ☑
  food — *see* Dermatitis, due to, food
  heat L74.0
  napkin (psoriasiform) L22
  nettle — *see* Urticaria
  pustular L08.0
  rose R21
    epidemic B06.9
  scarlet A38.9
  serum — *see also* Reaction, serum T80.69 ☑
  wandering tongue K14.1
Rasmussen aneurysm — *see* Tuberculosis, pulmonary
Rasmussen encephalitis G04.81
Rat-bite fever A25.9
  due to Streptobacillus moniliformis A25.1
  spirochetal (morsus muris) A25.0
Rathke's pouch tumor D44.3
Raymond (-Céstan) **syndrome** I65.8
Raynaud's disease, phenomenon or syndrome (secondary) I73.00
  with gangrene (symmetric) I73.01
RDS (newborn) (type I) P22.0
  type II P22.1
Reaction — *see also* Disorder
  withdrawing, child or adolescent F93.8
  adaptation — *see* Disorder, adjustment
  adjustment (anxiety) (conduct disorder) (depressiveness) (distress) — *see* Disorder, adjustment
    with
      mutism, elective (child) (adolescent) F94.0
  adverse
    food (any) (ingested) NEC T78.1 ☑
      anaphylactic — *see* Shock, anaphylactic, due to food
  affective — *see* Disorder, mood
  allergic — *see* Allergy
  anaphylactic — *see* Shock, anaphylactic
  anaphylactoid — *see* Shock, anaphylactic
  anesthesia — *see* Anesthesia, complication
  antitoxin (prophylactic) (therapeutic) — *see* Complications, vaccination
  anxiety F41.1
  Arthus — *see* Arthus' phenomenon
  asthenic F48.8
  combat and operational stress F43.0
  compulsive F42.8
  conversion F44.9

Reaction — *continued*
  crisis, acute F43.0
  deoxyribonuclease (DNA) (DNase) hypersensitivity D69.2
  depressive (single episode) F32.9
    affective (single episode) F31.4
      recurrent episode F33.9
    neurotic F34.1
    psychoneurotic F34.1
    psychotic F32.3
    recurrent — *see* Disorder, depressive, recurrent
  dissociative F44.9
  drug NEC T88.7 ☑
    addictive — *see* Dependence, drug
      transmitted via placenta or breast milk — *see* Absorption, drug, addictive, through placenta
    allergic — *see* Allergy, drug
    lichenoid L43.2
    newborn P93.8
      gray baby syndrome P93.0
    overdose or poisoning (by accident) — *see* Table of Drugs and Chemicals, by drug, poisoning
    photoallergic L56.1
    phototoxic L56.0
    withdrawal — *see* Dependence, by drug, with, withdrawal
      infant of dependent mother P96.1
      newborn P96.1
    wrong substance given or taken (by accident) — *see* Table of Drugs and Chemicals, by drug, poisoning
  fear F40.9
    child (abnormal) F93.8
  febrile nonhemolytic transfusion (FNHTR) R50.84
  fluid loss, cerebrospinal G97.1
  foreign
    body NEC — *see* Granuloma, foreign body
      in operative wound (inadvertently left) — *see* Foreign body, accidentally left during a procedure
    substance accidentally left during a procedure (chemical) (powder) (talc) T81.60 ☑
      aseptic peritonitis T81.61 ☑
      body or object (instrument) (sponge) (swab) — *see* Foreign body, accidentally left during a procedure
      specified reaction NEC T81.69 ☑
  grief — *see* Disorder, adjustment
  Herxheimer's R68.89
  hyperkinetic — *see* Hyperkinesia
  hypochondriacal F45.20
  hypoglycemic, due to insulin E16.0
    with coma (diabetic) — *see* Diabetes, coma
    nondiabetic E15
    therapeutic misadventure — *see* subcategory T38.3 ☑
  hypomanic F30.8
  hysterical F44.9
  immunization — *see* Complications, vaccination
  incompatibility
    ABO blood group (infusion) (transfusion) — *see* Complication(s), transfusion, incompatibility reaction, ABO
      delayed serologic T80.39 ☑
    minor blood group (Duffy) (E) (K) (Kell) (Kidd) (Lewis) (M) (N) (P) (S) T80.89 ☑
    Rh (factor) (infusion) (transfusion) — *see* Complication(s), transfusion, incompatibility reaction, Rh (factor)
  inflammatory — *see* Infection
  infusion — *see* Complications, infusion
  inoculation (immune serum) — *see* Complications, vaccination
  insulin T38.3- ☑
  involutional psychotic — *see* Disorder, depressive
  leukemoid D72.823
    basophilic D72.823
    lymphocytic D72.823
    monocytic D72.823
    myelocytic D72.823
    neutrophilic D72.823
  LSD (acute)
    due to drug abuse — *see* Abuse, drug, hallucinogen
    due to drug dependence — *see* Dependence, drug, hallucinogen
  lumbar puncture G97.1
  manic-depressive — *see* Disorder, bipolar

☑ **Additional Character Required** — **Refer to the Tabular List for Character Selection**   ▽ **Subterms under main terms may continue to next column or page**

Reaction — *continued*
neurasthenic F48.8
neurogenic — *see* Neurosis
neurotic F48.9
neurotic-depressive F34.1
nitritoid — *see* Crisis, nitritoid
nonspecific
  to
    cell mediated immunity measurement of gamma
      interferon antigen response without active
      tuberculosis R76.12
    QuantiFERON-TB test (QFT) without active tuber-
      culosis R76.12
    tuberculin test — *see also* Reaction, tuberculin
      skin test R76.11
obsessive-compulsive F42.8
organic, acute or subacute — *see* Delirium
paranoid (acute) F23
  chronic F22
  senile F03 ☑
passive dependency F60.7
phobic F40.9
post-traumatic stress, uncomplicated Z73.3
psychogenic F99
psychoneurotic — *see also* Neurosis
  compulsive F42.8
  depersonalization F48.1
  depressive F34.1
  hypochondriacal F45.20
  neurasthenic F48.8
  obsessive F42.8
psychophysiologic — *see* Disorder, somatoform
psychosomatic — *see* Disorder, somatoform
psychotic — *see* Psychosis
scarlet fever toxin — *see* Complications, vaccination
schizophrenic F23
  acute (brief) (undifferentiated) F23
  latent F21
  undifferentiated (acute) (brief) F23
serological for syphilis — *see* Serology for syphilis
serum T80.69 ☑
  anaphylactic (immediate) — *see also* Shock, anaphy-
    lactic T80.59 ☑
  specified reaction NEC
    due to
      administration of blood and blood products
        T80.61 ☑
      immunization T80.62 ☑
      serum specified NEC T80.69 ☑
      vaccination T80.62 ☑
situational — *see* Disorder, adjustment
somatization — *see* Disorder, somatoform
spinal puncture G97.1
stress (severe) F43.9
  acute (agitation) ("daze") (disorientation) (distur-
    bance of consciousness) (flight reaction)
    (fugue) F43.0
  specified NEC F43.8
surgical procedure — *see* Complications, surgical procedure
tetanus antitoxin — *see* Complications, vaccination
toxic, to local anesthesia T88.59 ☑
  in labor and delivery O74.4
  in pregnancy O29.3X- ☑
  postpartum, puerperal O89.3
toxin-antitoxin — *see* Complications, vaccination
transfusion (blood) (bone marrow) (lymphocytes) (allergic) — *see* Complications, transfusion
tuberculin skin test, abnormal R76.11
vaccination (any) — *see* Complications, vaccination
Reactive airway disease — *see* Asthma
Reactive depression — *see* Reaction, depressive
Rearrangement
chromosomal
  balanced (in) Q95.9
    abnormal individual (autosomal) Q95.2
      non-sex (autosomal) chromosomes Q95.2
      sex/non-sex chromosomes Q95.3
    specified NEC Q95.8
Recalcitrant patient — *see* Noncompliance
Recanalization, thrombus — *see* Thrombosis
Recession, receding
chamber angle (eye) H21.55- ☑
chin M26.09
gingival (postinfective) (postoperative)
  generalized K06.020
    minimal K06.021
    moderate K06.022

Recession, receding — *continued*
gingival — *continued*
  generalized — *continued*
    severe K06.023
  localized K06.010
    minimal K06.011
    moderate K06.012
    severe K06.013
Recklinghausen disease Q85.01
bones E21.0
Reclus' disease (cystic) — *see* Mastopathy, cystic
Recrudescent typhus (fever) A75.1
Recruitment, auditory H93.21- ☑
Rectalgia K62.89
Rectitis K62.89
Rectocele
female (without uterine prolapse) N81.6
  with uterine prolapse N81.4
    incomplete N81.2
in pregnancy — *see* Pregnancy, complicated by, abnor-
  mal, pelvic organs or tissues NEC
male K62.3
Rectosigmoid junction — *see* condition
Rectosigmoiditis K63.89
ulcerative (chronic) K51.30
  with
    complication K51.319
      abscess K51.314
      fistula K51.313
      obstruction K51.312
      rectal bleeding K51.311
      specified NEC K51.318
Rectourethral — *see* condition
Rectovaginal — *see* condition
Rectovesical — *see* condition
Rectum, rectal — *see* condition
Recurrent — *see* condition
pregnancy loss — *see* Loss (of), pregnancy, recurrent
Red bugs B88.0
Red tide — *see also* Table of Drugs and Chemicals
  T65.82- ☑
Red-cedar lung or pneumonitis J67.8
Reduced
mobility Z74.09
ventilatory or vital capacity R94.2
Redundant, redundancy
anus (congenital) Q43.8
clitoris N90.89
colon (congenital) Q43.8
foreskin (congenital) N47.8
intestine (congenital) Q43.8
labia N90.69
organ or site, congenital NEC — *see* Accessory
panniculus (abdominal) E65
prepuce (congenital) N47.8
pylorus K31.89
rectum (congenital) Q43.8
scrotum N50.89
sigmoid (congenital) Q43.8
skin L98.7
  and subcutaneous tissue L98.7
  of face L57.4
    eyelids — *see* Blepharochalasis
stomach K31.89
Reduplication — *see* Duplication
Reflex R29.2
hyperactive gag J39.2
pupillary, abnormal — *see* Anomaly, pupil, function
vasoconstriction I73.9
vasovagal R55
Reflux K21.9
acid K21.9
esophageal K21.9
  with esophagitis K21.0
  newborn P78.83
gastroesophageal K21.9
  with esophagitis K21.0
mitral — *see* Insufficiency, mitral
ureteral — *see* Reflux, vesicoureteral
vesicoureteral (with scarring) N13.70
  with
    nephropathy N13.729
      with hydroureter N13.739
        bilateral N13.732
        unilateral N13.731
      bilateral N13.722
      unilateral N13.721
      without hydroureter N13.729

Reflux — *continued*
vesicoureteral — *continued*
  with — *continued*
    nephropathy — *continued*
      without hydroureter — *continued*
        bilateral N13.722
        unilateral N13.721
    pyelonephritis (chronic) N11.0
  congenital Q62.7
  without nephropathy N13.71
Reforming, artificial openings — *see* Attention to, artificial, opening
Refractive error — *see* Disorder, refraction
Refsum's disease or syndrome G60.1
Refusal of
food, psychogenic F50.89
treatment (because of) Z53.20
  left against medical advice (AMA) Z53.21
  patient's decision NEC Z53.29
  reasons of belief or group pressure Z53.1
Regional — *see* condition
Regurgitation R11.10
aortic (valve) — *see* Insufficiency, aortic
food — *see also* Vomiting
  with reswallowing — *see* Rumination
  newborn P92.1
gastric contents — *see* Vomiting
heart — *see* Endocarditis
mitral (valve) — *see* Insufficiency, mitral
  congenital Q23.3
myocardial — *see* Endocarditis
pulmonary (valve) (heart) I37.1
  congenital Q22.2
  syphilitic A52.03
tricuspid — *see* Insufficiency, tricuspid
valve, valvular — *see* Endocarditis
  congenital Q24.8
vesicoureteral — *see* Reflux, vesicoureteral
Reichmann's disease or syndrome K31.89
Reifenstein syndrome E34.52
Reinsertion
implantable subdermal contraceptive Z30.46
intrauterine contraceptive device Z30.433
Reiter's disease, syndrome, or urethritis M02.30
ankle M02.37- ☑
elbow M02.32- ☑
foot joint M02.37- ☑
hand joint M02.34- ☑
hip M02.35- ☑
knee M02.36- ☑
multiple site M02.39
shoulder M02.31- ☑
vertebra M02.38
wrist M02.33- ☑
Rejection
food, psychogenic F50.89
transplant T86.91
  bone T86.830
    marrow T86.01
  cornea T86.840
  heart T86.21
    with lung(s) T86.31
  intestine T86.850
  kidney T86.11
  liver T86.41
  lung(s) T86.810
    with heart T86.31
  organ (immune or nonimmune cause) T86.91
  pancreas T86.890
  skin (allograft) (autograft) T86.820
  specified NEC T86.890
  stem cell (peripheral blood) (umbilical cord) T86.5
Relapsing fever A68.9
Carter's (Asiatic) A68.1
Dutton's (West African) A68.1
Koch's A68.9
louse-borne (epidemic) A68.0
Novy's (American) A68.1
Obermeyers's (European) A68.0
Spirillum A68.9
tick-borne (endemic) A68.1
Relationship
occlusal
  open anterior M26.220
  open posterior M26.221
Relaxation
anus (sphincter) K62.89
  psychogenic F45.8

Relaxation — *continued*
  arch (foot) — *see also* Deformity, limb, flat foot
  back ligaments — *see* Instability, joint, spine
  bladder (sphincter) N31.2
  cardioesophageal K21.9
  cervix — *see* Incompetency, cervix
  diaphragm J98.6
  joint (capsule) (ligament) (paralytic) — *see* Flail, joint
    congenital NEC Q74.8
  lumbosacral (joint) — *see* subcategory M53.2 ☑
  pelvic floor N81.89
  perineum N81.89
  posture R29.3
  rectum (sphincter) K62.89
  sacroiliac (joint) — *see* subcategory M53.2 ☑
  scrotum N50.89
  urethra (sphincter) N36.44
  vesical N31.2
Release from prison, anxiety concerning Z65.2
Remains
  canal of Cloquet Q14.0
  capsule (opaque) Q14.8
Remittent fever (malarial) B54
Remnant
  canal of Cloquet Q14.0
  capsule (opaque) Q14.8
  cervix, cervical stump (acquired) (postoperative) N88.8
  cystic duct, postcholecystectomy K91.5
  fingernail L60.8
    congenital Q84.6
  meniscus, knee — *see* Derangement, knee, meniscus, specified NEC
  thyroglossal duct Q89.2
  tonsil J35.8
    infected (chronic) J35.01
  urachus Q64.4
Removal (from) (of)
  artificial
    arm Z44.00- ☑
      complete Z44.01- ☑
      partial Z44.02- ☑
    eye Z44.2- ☑
    leg Z44.10- ☑
      complete Z44.11- ☑
      partial Z44.12- ☑
  breast implant Z45.81 ☑
  cardiac pulse generator (battery) (end-of-life) Z45.010
  catheter (urinary) (indwelling) Z46.6
    from artificial opening — *see* Attention to, artificial, opening
    non-vascular Z46.82
    vascular NEC Z45.2
  device Z46.9
    contraceptive Z30.432
      implantable subdermal Z30.46
    implanted NEC Z45.89
    specified NEC Z46.89
  drains Z48.03
  dressing (nonsurgical) Z48.00
    surgical Z48.01
  external
    fixation device — *code to* fracture with seventh character D
    prosthesis, prosthetic device Z44.9
      breast Z44.3- ☑
      specified NEC Z44.8
  home in childhood (to foster home or institution) Z62.29
  ileostomy Z43.2
  insulin pump Z46.81
  myringotomy device (stent) (tube) Z45.82
  nervous system device NEC Z46.2
    brain neuropacemaker Z46.2
    visual substitution device Z46.2
      implanted Z45.31
  non-vascular catheter Z46.82
  organ, prophylactic (for neoplasia management) — *see* Prophylactic, organ removal
  orthodontic device Z46.4
  staples Z48.02
  stent
    ureteral Z46.6
  suture Z48.02
  urinary device Z46.6
  vascular access device or catheter Z45.2
Ren
  arcuatus Q63.1
  mobile, mobilis N28.89

Ren — *continued*
  mobile, mobilis — *continued*
    congenital Q63.8
  unguliformis Q63.1
Renal — *see* condition
Rendu-Osler-Weber disease or syndrome I78.0
Reninoma D41.0- ☑
Renon-Delille syndrome E23.3
Reovirus, as cause of disease classified elsewhere B97.5
Repeated falls NEC R29.6
Replaced chromosome by dicentric ring Q93.2
Replacement by artificial or mechanical device or prosthesis of
  bladder Z96.0
  blood vessel NEC Z95.828
  bone NEC Z96.7
  cochlea Z96.21
  coronary artery Z95.5
  eustachian tube Z96.29
  eye globe Z97.0
  heart Z95.812
    valve Z95.2
      prosthetic Z95.2
      specified NEC Z95.4
      xenogenic Z95.3
  intestine Z96.89
  joint Z96.60
    hip — *see* Presence, hip joint implant
    knee — *see* Presence, knee joint implant
    specified site NEC Z96.698
  larynx Z96.3
  lens Z96.1
  limb(s) — *see* Presence, artificial, limb
  mandible NEC (for tooth root implant(s)) Z96.5
  organ NEC Z96.89
  peripheral vessel NEC Z95.828
  stapes Z96.29
  teeth Z97.2
  tendon Z96.7
  tissue NEC Z96.89
  tooth root(s) Z96.5
  vessel NEC Z95.828
    coronary (artery) Z95.5
Request for expert evidence Z04.89
Reserve, decreased or low
  cardiac — *see* Disease, heart
  kidney N28.89
Residual — *see also* condition
  ovary syndrome N99.83
  state, schizophrenic F20.5
  urine R39.198
Resistance, resistant (to)
  activated protein C D68.51
  complicating pregnancy O26.89 ☑
  insulin E88.81
  organism(s)
    to
      drug Z16.30
        aminoglycosides Z16.29
        amoxicillin Z16.11
        ampicillin Z16.11
        antibiotic(s) Z16.20
          multiple Z16.24
          specified NEC Z16.29
        antifungal Z16.32
        antimicrobial (single) Z16.30
          multiple Z16.35
          specified NEC Z16.39
        antimycobacterial (single) Z16.341
          multiple Z16.342
        antiparasitic Z16.31
        antiviral Z16.33
        beta lactam antibiotics Z16.10
          specified NEC Z16.19
        cephalosporins Z16.19
        extended beta lactamase (ESBL) Z16.12
        fluoroquinolones Z16.23
        macrolides Z16.29
        methicillin — *see* MRSA
        multiple drugs (MDRO)
          antibiotics Z16.24
          antimicrobial Z16.35
          antimycobacterials Z16.342
        penicillins Z16.11
        quinine (and related compounds) Z16.31
        quinolones Z16.23
        sulfonamides Z16.29

Resistance, resistant — *continued*
  organism(s) — *continued*
    to — *continued*
      drug — *continued*
        tetracyclines Z16.29
        tuberculostatics (single) Z16.341
          multiple Z16.342
        vancomycin Z16.21
          related antibiotics Z16.22
  thyroid hormone E07.89
Resorption
  dental (roots) K03.3
    alveoli M26.79
  teeth (external) (internal) (pathological) (roots) K03.3
Respiration
  Cheyne-Stokes R06.3
  decreased due to shock, following injury T79.4 ☑
  disorder of, psychogenic F45.8
  insufficient, or poor R06.89
    newborn P28.5
  painful R07.1
  sighing, psychogenic F45.8
Respiratory — *see also* condition
  distress syndrome (newborn) (type I) P22.0
    type II P22.1
  syncytial virus, as cause of disease classified elsewhere — *see also* Virus, respiratory syncytial (RSV) B97.4
Respite care Z75.5
Response (drug)
  photoallergic L56.1
  phototoxic L56.0
Restenosis
  stent
    vascular
      end stent
        adjacent to stent — *see* Arteriosclerosis
        within the stent
          coronary T82.855 ☑
          peripheral T82.856 ☑
      in stent
        coronary vessel T82.855 ☑
        peripheral vessel T82.856 ☑
Restless legs (syndrome) G25.81
Restlessness R45.1
Restoration (of)
  dental
    aesthetically inadequate or displeasing K08.56
    defective K08.50
      specified NEC K08.59
    failure of marginal integrity K08.51
    failure of periodontal anatomical intergrity K08.54
  organ continuity from previous sterilization (tuboplasty) (vasoplasty) Z31.0
    aftercare Z31.42
  tooth (existing)
    contours biologically incompatible with oral health K08.54
    open margins K08.51
    overhanging K08.52
    poor aesthetic K08.56
    poor gingival margins K08.51
  unsatisfactory, of tooth K08.50
    specified NEC K08.59
Restorative material (dental)
  allergy to K08.55
  fractured K08.539
    with loss of material K08.531
    without loss of material K08.530
  unrepairable overhanging of K08.52
Restriction of housing space Z59.1
Rests, ovarian, in fallopian tube Q50.6
Restzustand (schizophrenic) F20.5
Retained — *see also* Retention
  cholelithiasis following cholecystectomy K91.86
  foreign body fragments (type of) Z18.9
    acrylics Z18.2
    animal quill(s) or spines Z18.31
    cement Z18.83
    concrete Z18.83
    crystalline Z18.83
    depleted isotope Z18.09
    depleted uranium Z18.01
    diethylhexyl phthalates Z18.2
    glass Z18.81
    isocyanate Z18.2
    magnetic metal Z18.11
    metal Z18.10
    nonmagnectic metal Z18.12

Retained — continued
  foreign body fragments — continued
    nontherapeutic radioactive Z18.09
    organic NEC Z18.39
    plastic Z18.2
    quill(s) (animal) Z18.31
    radioactive (nontherapeutic) NEC Z18.09
    specified NEC Z18.89
    spine(s) (animal) Z18.31
    stone Z18.83
    tooth (teeth) Z18.32
    wood Z18.33
  fragments (type of) Z18.9
    acrylics Z18.2
    animal quill(s) or spines Z18.31
    cement Z18.83
    concrete Z18.83
    crystalline Z18.83
    depleted isotope Z18.09
    depleted uranium Z18.01
    diethylhexyl phthalates Z18.2
    glass Z18.81
    isocyanate Z18.2
    magnetic metal Z18.11
    metal Z18.10
    nonmagnectic metal Z18.12
    nontherapeutic radioactive Z18.09
    organic NEC Z18.39
    plastic Z18.2
    quill(s) (animal) Z18.31
    radioactive (nontherapeutic) NEC Z18.09
    specified NEC Z18.89
    spine(s) (animal) Z18.31
    stone Z18.83
    tooth (teeth) Z18.32
    wood Z18.33
  gallstones, following cholecystectomy K91.86
Retardation
  development, developmental, specific — see Disorder, developmental
  endochondral bone growth — see Disorder, bone, development or growth
  growth R62.50
    due to malnutrition E45
  mental — see Disability, intellectual
  motor function, specific F82
  physical (child) R62.52
    due to malnutrition E45
  reading (specific) F81.0
  spelling (specific) (without reading disorder) F81.81
Retching — see Vomiting
Retention — see also Retained
  bladder — see Retention, urine
  carbon dioxide E87.2
  cholelithiasis following cholecystectomy K91.86
  cyst — see Cyst
  dead
    fetus (at or near term) (mother) O36.4 ☑
      early fetal death O02.1
    ovum O02.0
  decidua (fragments) (following delivery) (with hemorrhage) O72.2
    without hemorrhage O73.1
  deciduous tooth K00.6
  dental root K08.3
  fecal — see Constipation
  fetus
    dead O36.4 ☑
      early O02.1
  fluid R60.9
  foreign body — see also Foreign body, retained
    current trauma — code as Foreign body, by site or type
  gallstones, following cholecystectomy K91.86
  gastric K31.89
  intrauterine contraceptive device, in pregnancy — see Pregnancy, complicated by, retention, intrauterine device
  membranes (complicating delivery) (with hemorrhage) O72.2
    with abortion — see Abortion, by type
    without hemorrhage O73.1
  meniscus — see Derangement, meniscus
  menses N94.89
  milk (puerperal, postpartum) O92.79
  nitrogen, extrarenal R39.2
  ovary syndrome N99.83
  placenta (total) (with hemorrhage) O72.0

Retention — continued
  placenta — continued
    without hemorrhage O73.0
    portions or fragments (with hemorrhage) O72.2
      without hemorrhage O73.1
  products of conception
    early pregnancy (dead fetus) O02.1
    following
      delivery (with hemorrhage) O72.2
        without hemorrhage O73.1
  secundines (following delivery) (with hemorrhage) O72.0
    without hemorrhage O73.0
    complicating puerperium (delayed hemorrhage) O72.2
    partial O72.2
      without hemorrhage O73.1
  smegma, clitoris N90.89
  urine R33.9
    due to hyperplasia (hypertrophy) of prostate — see Hyperplasia, prostate
    drug-induced R33.0
    organic R33.8
      drug-induced R33.0
    psychogenic F45.8
    specified NEC R33.8
  water (in tissues) — see Edema
Reticulation, dust — see Pneumoconiosis
Reticulocytosis R70.1
Reticuloendotheliosis
  acute infantile C96.0
  leukemic C91.4- ☑
  nonlipid C96.0
Reticulohistiocytoma (giant-cell) D76.3
Reticuloid, actinic L57.1
Reticulosis (skin)
  acute of infancy C96.0
  hemophagocytic, familial D76.1
  histiocytic medullary C96.A (following C96.6)
  lipomelanotic I89.8
  malignant (midline) C86.0
  polymorphic C83.8- ☑
  Sézary — see Sézary disease
Retina, retinal — see also condition
  dark area D49.81
Retinitis — see also Inflammation, chorioretinal
  albuminurica N18.9 [H32]
  diabetic — see Diabetes, retinitis
  disciformis — see Degeneration, macula
  focal — see Inflammation, chorioretinal, focal
  gravidarum — see Pregnancy, complicated by, specified pregnancy-related condition NEC
  juxtapapillaris — see Inflammation, chorioretinal, focal, juxtapapillary
  luetic — see Retinitis, syphilitic
  pigmentosa H35.52
  proliferans — see Disorder, globe, degenerative, specified type NEC
  proliferating — see Disorder, globe, degenerative, specified type NEC
  renal N18.9 [H32]
  syphilitic (early) (secondary) A51.43
    central, recurrent A52.71
    congenital (early) A50.01 [H32]
    late A52.71
  tuberculous A18.53
Retinoblastoma C69.2- ☑
  differentiated C69.2- ☑
  undifferentiated C69.2- ☑
Retinochoroiditis — see also Inflammation, chorioretinal
  disseminated — see Inflammation, chorioretinal, disseminated
    syphilitic A52.71
  focal — see Inflammation, chorioretinal
  juxtapapillaris — see Inflammation, chorioretinal, focal, juxtapapillary
Retinopathy (background) H35.00
  arteriosclerotic I70.8 [H35.0-] ☑
  atherosclerotic I70.8 [H35.0-] ☑
  central serous — see Chorioretinopathy, central serous
  Coats H35.02- ☑
  diabetic — see Diabetes, retinopathy
  exudative H35.02- ☑
  hypertensive H35.03- ☑
  in (due to)
    diabetes — see Diabetes, retinopathy
    sickle-cell disorders D57.- ☑ [H36]

Retinopathy — continued
  of prematurity H35.10- ☑
    stage 0 H35.11- ☑
    stage 1 H35.12- ☑
    stage 2 H35.13- ☑
    stage 3 H35.14- ☑
    stage 4 H35.15- ☑
    stage 5 H35.16- ☑
  pigmentary, congenital — see Dystrophy, retina
  proliferative NEC H35.2- ☑
    diabetic — see Diabetes, retinopathy, proliferative
    sickle-cell D57.- ☑ [H36]
  solar H31.02- ☑
Retinoschisis H33.10- ☑
  congenital Q14.1
  specified type NEC H33.19- ☑
Retortamoniasis A07.8
Retractile testis Q55.22
Retraction
  cervix — see Retroversion, uterus
  drum (membrane) — see Disorder, tympanic membrane, specified NEC
  finger — see Deformity, finger
  lid H02.539
    left H02.536
      lower H02.535
      upper H02.534
    right H02.533
      lower H02.532
      upper H02.531
  lung J98.4
  mediastinum J98.59
  nipple N64.53
    associated with
      lactation O92.03
      pregnancy O92.01- ☑
      puerperium O92.02
    congenital Q83.8
  palmar fascia M72.0
  pleura — see Pleurisy
  ring, uterus (Bandl's) (pathological) O62.4
  sternum (congenital) Q76.7
    acquired M95.4
  uterus — see Retroversion, uterus
  valve (heart) — see Endocarditis
Retrobulbar — see condition
Retrocecal — see condition
Retrocession — see Retroversion
Retrodisplacement — see Retroversion
Retroflection, retroflexion — see Retroversion
Retrognathia, retrognathism (mandibular) (maxillary) M26.19
Retrograde menstruation N92.5
Retroperineal — see condition
Retroperitoneal — see condition
Retroperitonitis K68.9
Retropharyngeal — see condition
Retroplacental — see condition
Retroposition — see Retroversion
Retroprosthetic membrane T85.398 ☑
Retrosternal thyroid (congenital) Q89.2
Retroversion, retroverted
  cervix — see Retroversion, uterus
  female NEC — see Retroversion, uterus
  iris H21.89
  testis (congenital) Q55.29
  uterus (acquired) (acute) (any degree) (asymptomatic) (cervix) (postinfectional) (postpartal, old) N85.4
    congenital Q51.818
    in pregnancy O34.53- ☑
Retrovirus, as cause of disease classified elsewhere B97.30
  human
    immunodeficiency, type 2 (HIV 2) B97.35
    T-cell lymphotropic
      type I (HTLV-I) B97.33
      type II (HTLV-II) B97.34
  lentivirus B97.31
  oncovirus B97.32
  specified NEC B97.39
Retrusion, premaxilla (developmental) M26.09
Rett's disease or syndrome F84.2
Reverse peristalsis R19.2
Reye's syndrome G93.7
Rh (factor)
  hemolytic disease (newborn) P55.0

Index

Retained — Rh

Rh — *continued*
  incompatibility, immunization or sensitization
    affecting management of pregnancy NEC O36.09- ☑
      anti-D antibody O36.01- ☑
    newborn P55.0
    transfusion reaction — *see* Complication(s), transfusion, incompatibility reaction, Rh (factor)
    negative mother affecting newborn P55.0
    titer elevated — *see* Complication(s), transfusion, incompatibility reaction, Rh (factor)
    transfusion reaction — *see* Complication(s), transfusion, incompatibility reaction, Rh (factor)
Rhabdomyolysis (idiopathic) NEC M62.82
  traumatic T79.6
Rhabdomyoma — *see also* Neoplasm, connective tissue, benign
  adult — *see* Neoplasm, connective tissue, benign
  fetal — *see* Neoplasm, connective tissue, benign
  glycogenic — *see* Neoplasm, connective tissue, benign
Rhabdomyosarcoma (any type) — *see* Neoplasm, connective tissue, malignant
Rhabdosarcoma — *see* Rhabdomyosarcoma
Rhesus (factor) **incompatibility** — *see* Rh, incompatibility
Rheumatic (acute) (subacute)
  adherent pericardium I09.2
  chronic I09.89
  coronary arteritis I01.8
  degeneration, myocardium I09.0
  fever (acute) — *see* Fever, rheumatic
  heart — *see* Disease, heart, rheumatic
  myocardial degeneration — *see* Degeneration, myocardium
  myocarditis (chronic) (inactive) (with chorea) I09.0
    active or acute I01.2
    with chorea (acute) (rheumatic) (Sydenham's) I02.0
  pancarditis, acute I01.8
    with chorea (acute) (rheumatic) Sydenham's) I02.0
  pericarditis (active) (acute) (with effusion) (with pneumonia) I01.0
    with chorea (acute) (rheumatic) (Sydenham's) I02.0
    chronic or inactive I09.2
  pneumonia I00 *[J17]*
  torticollis M43.6
  typhoid fever A01.09
Rheumatism (articular) (neuralgic) (nonarticular) M79.0
  gout — *see* Arthritis, rheumatoid
  intercostal, meaning Tietze's disease M94.0
  palindromic (any site) M12.30
    ankle M12.37- ☑
    elbow M12.32- ☑
    foot joint M12.37- ☑
    hand joint M12.34- ☑
    hip M12.35- ☑
    knee M12.36- ☑
    multiple site M12.39
    shoulder M12.31- ☑
    specified joint NEC M12.38
    vertebrae M12.38
    wrist M12.33- ☑
  sciatic M54.4- ☑
Rheumatoid — *see also* condition
  arthritis — *see also* Arthritis, rheumatoid
    with involvement of organs NEC M05.60
      ankle M05.67- ☑
      elbow M05.62- ☑
      foot joint M05.67- ☑
      hand joint M05.64- ☑
      hip M05.65- ☑
      knee M05.66- ☑
      multiple site M05.69
      shoulder M05.61- ☑
      vertebra — *see* Spondylitis, ankylosing
      wrist M05.63- ☑
    seronegative — *see* Arthritis, rheumatoid, seronegative
    seropositive — *see* Arthritis, rheumatoid, seropositive
  carditis M05.30
    ankle M05.37- ☑
    elbow M05.32- ☑
    foot joint M05.37- ☑
    hand joint M05.34- ☑
    hip M05.35- ☑
    knee M05.36- ☑
    multiple site M05.39
    shoulder M05.31- ☑

Rheumatoid — *continued*
  carditis — *continued*
    vertebra — *see* Spondylitis, ankylosing
    wrist M05.33- ☑
  endocarditis — *see* Rheumatoid, carditis
  lung (disease) M05.10
    ankle M05.17- ☑
    elbow M05.12- ☑
    foot joint M05.17- ☑
    hand joint M05.14- ☑
    hip M05.15- ☑
    knee M05.16- ☑
    multiple site M05.19
    shoulder M05.11- ☑
    vertebra — *see* Spondylitis, ankylosing
    wrist M05.13- ☑
  myocarditis — *see* Rheumatoid, carditis
  myopathy M05.40
    ankle M05.47- ☑
    elbow M05.42- ☑
    foot joint M05.47- ☑
    hand joint M05.44- ☑
    hip M05.45- ☑
    knee M05.46- ☑
    multiple site M05.49
    shoulder M05.41- ☑
    vertebra — *see* Spondylitis, ankylosing
    wrist M05.43- ☑
  pericarditis — *see* Rheumatoid, carditis
  polyarthritis — *see* Arthritis, rheumatoid
  polyneuropathy M05.50
    ankle M05.57- ☑
    elbow M05.52- ☑
    foot joint M05.57- ☑
    hand joint M05.54- ☑
    hip M05.55- ☑
    knee M05.56- ☑
    multiple site M05.59
    shoulder M05.51- ☑
    vertebra — *see* Spondylitis, ankylosing
    wrist M05.53- ☑
  vasculitis M05.20
    ankle M05.27- ☑
    elbow M05.22- ☑
    foot joint M05.27- ☑
    hand joint M05.24- ☑
    hip M05.25- ☑
    knee M05.26- ☑
    multiple site M05.29
    shoulder M05.21- ☑
    vertebra — *see* Spondylitis, ankylosing
    wrist M05.23- ☑
Rhinitis (atrophic) (catarrhal) (chronic) (croupous) (fibrinous) (granulomatous) (hyperplastic) (hypertrophic) (membranous) (obstructive) (purulent) (suppurative) (ulcerative) J31.0
  with
    sore throat — *see* Nasopharyngitis
  acute J00
  allergic J30.9
    with asthma J45.909
      with
        exacerbation (acute) J45.901
        status asthmaticus J45.902
    due to
      food J30.5
      pollen J30.1
    nonseasonal J30.89
    perennial J30.89
    seasonal NEC J30.2
    specified NEC J30.89
  infective J00
  pneumococcal J00
  syphilitic A52.73
    congenital A50.05 *[J99]*
  tuberculous A15.8
  vasomotor J30.0
Rhinoantritis (chronic) — *see* Sinusitis, maxillary
Rhinodacryolith — *see* Dacryolith
Rhinolith (nasal sinus) J34.89
Rhinomegaly J34.89
Rhinopharyngitis (acute) (subacute) — *see also* Nasopharyngitis
  chronic J31.1
  destructive ulcerating A66.5
  mutilans A66.5
Rhinophyma L71.1

Rhinorrhea J34.89
  cerebrospinal (fluid) G96.0
  paroxysmal — *see* Rhinitis, allergic
  spasmodic — *see* Rhinitis, allergic
Rhinosalpingitis — *see* Salpingitis, eustachian
Rhinoscleroma A48.8
Rhinosporidiosis B48.1
Rhinovirus infection NEC B34.8
Rhizomelic chondrodysplasia punctata E71.540
Rhythm
  atrioventricular nodal I49.8
  disorder I49.9
    coronary sinus I49.8
    ectopic I49.8
    nodal I49.8
  escape I49.9
  heart, abnormal I49.9
  idioventricular I44.2
  nodal I49.8
  sleep, inversion G47.2- ☑
    nonorganic origin — *see* Disorder, sleep, circadian rhythm, psychogenic
Rhytidosis facialis L98.8
Rib — *see also* condition
  cervical Q76.5
Riboflavin deficiency E53.0
Rice bodies — *see also* Loose, body, joint
  knee M23.4- ☑
Richter syndrome — *see* Leukemia, chronic lymphocytic, B-cell type
Richter's hernia — *see* Hernia, abdomen, with obstruction
Ricinism — *see* Poisoning, food, noxious, plant
Rickets (active) (acute) (adolescent) (chest wall) (congenital) (current) (infantile) (intestinal) E55.0
  adult — *see* Osteomalacia
  celiac K90.0
  hypophosphatemic with nephrotic-glycosuric dwarfism E72.09
  inactive E64.3
  kidney N25.0
  renal N25.0
  sequelae, any E64.3
  vitamin-D-resistant E83.31 *[M90.80]*
Rickettsial disease A79.9
  specified type NEC A79.89
Rickettsialpox (Rickettsia akari) A79.1
Rickettsiosis A79.9
  due to
    Ehrlichia sennetsu A79.81
    Rickettsia akari (rickettsialpox) A79.1
  specified type NEC A79.89
  tick-borne A77.9
  vesicular A79.1
Rider's bone — *see* Ossification, muscle, specified NEC
Ridge, alveolus — *see also* condition
  flabby K06.8
Ridged ear, congenital Q17.3
Riedel's
  lobe, liver Q44.7
  struma, thyroiditis or disease E06.5
Rieger's anomaly or syndrome Q13.81
Riehl's melanosis L81.4
Rietti-Greppi-Micheli anemia D56.9
Rieux's hernia — *see* Hernia, abdomen, specified site NEC
Riga (-Fede) **disease** K14.0
Riggs' disease — *see* Periodontitis
Right aortic arch Q25.47
Right middle lobe syndrome J98.11
Rigid, rigidity — *see also* condition
  abdominal R19.30
    with severe abdominal pain R10.0
    epigastric R19.36
    generalized R19.37
    left lower quadrant R19.34
    left upper quadrant R19.32
    periumbilic R19.35
    right lower quadrant R19.33
    right upper quadrant R19.31
  articular, multiple, congenital Q68.8
  cervix (uteri) in pregnancy — *see* Pregnancy, complicated by, abnormal, cervix
  hymen (acquired) (congenital) N89.6
  nuchal R29.1
  pelvic floor in pregnancy — *see* Pregnancy, complicated by, abnormal, pelvic organs or tissues NEC

Rigid, rigidity — *continued*
　perineum or vulva in pregnancy — *see* Pregnancy,
　　complicated by, abnormal, vulva
　spine — *see* Dorsopathy, specified NEC
　vagina in pregnancy — *see* Pregnancy, complicated
　　by, abnormal, vagina
Rigors R68.89
　with fever R50.9
Riley-Day syndrome G90.1
RIND (reversible ischemic neurologic deficit) I63.9
Ring(s)
　aorta (vascular) Q25.45
　Bandl's O62.4
　contraction, complicating delivery O62.4
　esophageal, lower (muscular) K22.2
　Fleischer's (cornea) H18.04- ☑
　hymenal, tight (acquired) (congenital) N89.6
　Kayser-Fleischer (cornea) H18.04- ☑
　retraction, uterus, pathological O62.4
　Schatzki's (esophagus) (lower) K22.2
　　congenital Q39.3
　Soemmerring's — *see* Cataract, secondary
　vascular (congenital) Q25.8
　　aorta Q25.45
Ringed hair (congenital) Q84.1
Ringworm B35.9
　beard B35.0
　black dot B35.0
　body B35.4
　Burmese B35.5
　corporeal B35.4
　foot B35.3
　groin B35.6
　hand B35.2
　honeycomb B35.0
　nails B35.1
　perianal (area) B35.6
　scalp B35.0
　specified NEC B35.8
　Tokelau B35.5
Rise, venous pressure I87.8
Rising, PSA following treatment for malignant neo-
　　plasm of prostate R97.21
Risk
　for
　　dental caries Z91.849
　　　high Z91.843
　　　low Z91.841
　　　moderate Z91.842
　suicidal
　　meaning personal history of attempted suicide Z91.5
　　meaning suicidal ideation — *see* Ideation, suicidal
Ritter's disease L00
Rivalry, sibling Z62.891
Rivalta's disease A42.2
River blindness B73.01
Robert's pelvis Q74.2
　with disproportion (fetopelvic) O33.0
　　causing obstructed labor O65.0
Robin (-Pierre) **syndrome** Q87.0
Robinow-Silvermann-Smith syndrome Q87.19
Robinson's (hidrotic) **ectodermal dysplasia or syn-**
　　drome Q82.4
Robles' disease B73.01
Rocky Mountain (spotted) **fever** A77.0
Roetheln — *see* Rubella
Roger's disease Q21.0
Rokitansky-Aschoff sinuses (gallbladder) K82.8
Rolando's fracture (displaced) S62.22- ☑
　nondisplaced S62.22- ☑
Romano-Ward (prolonged QT interval) **syndrome** I45.81
Romberg's disease or syndrome G51.8
Roof, mouth — *see* condition
Rosacea L71.9
　acne L71.9
　keratitis L71.8
　specified NEC L71.8
Rosary, rachitic E55.0
Rose
　cold J30.1
　fever J30.1
　rash R21
　　epidemic B06.9
Rosenbach's erysipeloid A26.0
Rosenthal's disease or syndrome D68.1
Roseola B09
　infantum B08.20

Roseola — *continued*
　infantum — *continued*
　　due to human herpesvirus 6 B08.21
　　due to human herpesvirus 7 B08.22
Ross River disease or fever B33.1
Rossbach's disease K31.89
　psychogenic F45.8
Rostan's asthma (cardiac) — *see* Failure, ventricular, left
Rotation
　anomalous, incomplete or insufficient, intestine Q43.3
　cecum (congenital) Q43.3
　colon (congenital) Q43.3
　spine, incomplete or insufficient — *see* Dorsopathy,
　　deforming, specified NEC
　tooth, teeth, fully erupted M26.35
　vertebra, incomplete or insufficient — *see* Dorsopathy,
　　deforming, specified NEC
Rotes Quérol disease or syndrome — *see* Hyperostosis,
　　ankylosing
Roth (-Bernhardt) **disease or syndrome** — *see* Meralgia
　　paraesthetica
Rothmund (-Thomson) **syndrome** Q82.8
Rotor's disease or syndrome E80.6
Round
　back (with wedging of vertebrae) — *see* Kyphosis
　　sequelae (late effect) of rickets E64.3
　worms (large) (infestation) NEC B82.0
　　Ascariasis — *see also* Ascariasis B77.9
Roussy-Lévy syndrome G60.0
Rubella (German measles) B06.9
　complication NEC B06.09
　　neurological B06.00
　congenital P35.0
　contact Z20.4
　exposure to Z20.4
　maternal
　　care for (suspected) damage to fetus O35.3 ☑
　　　manifest rubella in infant P35.0
　　suspected damage to fetus affecting management
　　　of pregnancy O35.3 ☑
　specified complications NEC B06.89
Rubeola (meaning measles) — *see* Measles
　meaning rubella — *see* Rubella
Rubeosis, iris — *see* Disorder, iris, vascular
Rubinstein-Taybi syndrome Q87.2
Rudimentary (congenital) — *see also* Agenesis
　arm — *see* Defect, reduction, upper limb
　bone Q79.9
　cervix uteri Q51.828
　eye Q11.2
　lobule of ear Q17.3
　patella Q74.1
　respiratory organs in thoracopagus Q89.4
　tracheal bronchus Q32.4
　uterus Q51.818
　　in male Q56.1
　vagina Q52.0
Ruled out condition — *see* Observation, suspected
Rumination R11.10
　with nausea R11.2
　disorder of infancy F98.21
　neurotic F42.8
　newborn P92.1
　obsessional F42.8
　psychogenic F42.8
Runeberg's disease D51.0
Runny nose R09.89
Rupia (syphilitic) A51.39
　congenital A50.06
　tertiary A52.79
Rupture, ruptured
　abscess (spontaneous) — *code by* site under Abscess
　aneurysm — *see* Aneurysm
　anus (sphincter) — *see* Laceration, anus
　aorta, aortic I71.8
　　abdominal I71.3
　　arch I71.1
　　ascending I71.1
　　descending I71.8
　　　abdominal I71.3
　　　thoracic I71.1
　　syphilitic A52.01
　　thoracoabdominal I71.5
　　thorax, thoracic I71.1
　　transverse I71.1
　　traumatic — *see* Injury, aorta, laceration, major, by site
　　valve or cusp — *see also* Endocarditis, aortic I35.8

Rupture, ruptured — *continued*
　appendix (with peritonitis) — *see also* Appendicitis
　　K35.32
　　with localized peritonitis — *see also* Appendicitis
　　　K35.32
　arteriovenous fistula, brain — *see* Fistula, arteriove-
　　nous, brain, ruptured
　artery I77.2
　　brain — *see* Hemorrhage, intracranial, intracerebral
　　coronary — *see* Infarct, myocardium
　　heart — *see* Infarct, myocardium
　　pulmonary I28.8
　　traumatic (complication) — *see* Injury, blood vessel
　bile duct (common) (hepatic) K83.2
　　cystic K82.2
　bladder (sphincter) (nontraumatic) (spontaneous)
　　N32.89
　　following ectopic or molar pregnancy O08.6
　　obstetrical trauma O71.5
　　traumatic S37.29 ☑
　blood vessel — *see also* Hemorrhage
　　brain — *see* Hemorrhage, intracranial, intracerebral
　　heart — *see* Infarct, myocardium
　　traumatic (complication) — *see* Injury, blood vessel,
　　　laceration, major, by site
　bone — *see* Fracture
　bowel (nontraumatic) K63.1
　brain
　　aneurysm (congenital) — *see also* Hemorrhage, in-
　　　tracranial, subarachnoid
　　　syphilitic A52.05
　　hemorrhagic — *see* Hemorrhage, intracranial, intrac-
　　　erebral
　capillaries I78.8
　cardiac (auricle) (ventricle) (wall) I23.3
　　with hemopericardium I23.0
　　infectional I40.9
　　traumatic — *see* Injury, heart
　cartilage (articular) (current) — *see also* Sprain
　　knee S83.3- ☑
　　semilunar — *see* Tear, meniscus
　cecum (with peritonitis) K65.0
　　with peritoneal abscess K35.33
　　traumatic S36.598 ☑
　celiac artery, traumatic — *see* Injury, blood vessel,
　　celiac artery, laceration, major
　cerebral aneurysm (congenital) (see Hemorrhage, in-
　　tracranial, subarachnoid)
　cervix (uteri)
　　with ectopic or molar pregnancy O08.6
　　following ectopic or molar pregnancy O08.6
　　obstetrical trauma O71.3
　　traumatic S37.69 ☑
　chordae tendineae NEC I51.1
　　concurrent with acute myocardial infarction — *see*
　　　Infarct, myocardium
　　following acute myocardial infarction (current
　　　complication) I23.4
　choroid (direct) (indirect) (traumatic) H31.32- ☑
　circle of Willis I60.6
　colon (nontraumatic) K63.1
　　traumatic — *see* Injury, intestine, large
　cornea (traumatic) — *see* Injury, eye, laceration
　coronary (artery) (thrombotic) — *see* Infarct, myocardi-
　　um
　corpus luteum (infected) (ovary) N83.1- ☑
　cyst — *see* Cyst
　cystic duct K82.2
　Descemet's membrane — *see* Change, corneal mem-
　　brane, Descemet's; rupture
　　traumatic — *see* Injury, eye, laceration
　diaphragm, traumatic — *see* Injury, intrathoracic, di-
　　aphragm
　disc — *see* Rupture, intervertebral disc
　diverticulum (intestine) K57.80
　　with bleeding K57.81
　　bladder N32.3
　　large intestine K57.20
　　　with
　　　　bleeding K57.21
　　　　small intestine K57.40
　　　　　with bleeding K57.41
　　small intestine K57.00
　　　with
　　　　bleeding K57.01
　　　　large intestine K57.40
　　　　　with bleeding K57.41
　duodenal stump K31.89

Rupture, ruptured — *continued*

  ear drum (nontraumatic) — *see also* Perforation, tympanum
    traumatic S09.2- ☑
      due to blast injury — *see* Injury, blast, ear
  esophagus K22.3
  eye (without prolapse or loss of intraocular tissue) — *see* Injury, eye, laceration
  fallopian tube NEC (nonobstetric) (nontraumatic) N83.8
    due to pregnancy O00.10- ☑
      with intrauterine pregnancy O00.11- ☑
  fontanel P13.1
  gallbladder K82.2
    traumatic S36.128 ☑
  gastric — *see also* Rupture, stomach
    vessel K92.2
  globe (eye) (traumatic) — *see* Injury, eye, laceration
  graafian follicle (hematoma) N83.0- ☑
  heart — *see* Rupture, cardiac
  hymen (nontraumatic) (nonintentional) N89.8
  internal organ, traumatic — *see* Injury, by site
  intervertebral disc — *see* Displacement, intervertebral disc
    traumatic — *see* Rupture, traumatic, intervertebral disc
  intestine NEC (nontraumatic) K63.1
    traumatic — *see* Injury, intestine
  iris — *see also* Abnormality, pupillary
    traumatic — *see* Injury, eye, laceration
  joint capsule, traumatic — *see* Sprain
  kidney (traumatic) S37.06- ☑
    birth injury P15.8
    nontraumatic N28.89
  lacrimal duct (traumatic) — *see* Injury, eye, specified site NEC
  lens (cataract) (traumatic) — *see* Cataract, traumatic
  ligament, traumatic — *see* Rupture, traumatic, ligament, by site
  liver S36.116 ☑
    birth injury P15.0
  lymphatic vessel I89.8
  marginal sinus (placental) (with hemorrhage) — *see* Hemorrhage, antepartum, specified cause NEC
  membrana tympani (nontraumatic) — *see* Perforation, tympanum
  membranes (spontaneous)
    artificial
      delayed delivery following O75.5
    delayed delivery following — *see* Pregnancy, complicated by, premature rupture of membranes
  meningeal artery I60.8
  meniscus (knee) — *see also* Tear, meniscus
    old — *see* Derangement, meniscus
    site other than knee — *code as* Sprain
  mesenteric artery, traumatic — *see* Injury, mesenteric, artery, laceration, major
  mesentery (nontraumatic) K66.8
    traumatic — *see* Injury, intra-abdominal, specified, site NEC
  mitral (valve) I34.8
  muscle (traumatic) — *see also* Strain
    diastasis — *see* Diastasis, muscle
    nontraumatic M62.10
      ankle M62.17- ☑
      foot M62.17- ☑
      forearm M62.13- ☑
      hand M62.14- ☑
      lower leg M62.16- ☑
      pelvic region M62.15- ☑
      shoulder region M62.11- ☑
      specified site NEC M62.18
      thigh M62.15- ☑
      upper arm M62.12- ☑
    traumatic — *see* Strain, by site
  musculotendinous junction NEC, nontraumatic — *see* Rupture, tendon, spontaneous
  mycotic aneurysm causing cerebral hemorrhage — *see* Hemorrhage, intracranial, subarachnoid
  myocardium, myocardial — *see* Rupture, cardiac
    traumatic — *see* Injury, heart
  nontraumatic, meaning hernia — *see* Hernia
  obstructed — *see* Hernia, by site, obstructed
  operation wound — *see* Disruption, wound, operation
  ovary, ovarian N83.8
    corpus luteum cyst N83.1- ☑
    follicle (graafian) N83.0- ☑
  oviduct (nonobstetric) (nontraumatic) N83.8

Rupture, ruptured — *continued*

  oviduct — *continued*
    due to pregnancy O00.10- ☑
      with intrauterine pregnancy O00.11- ☑
  pancreas (nontraumatic) K86.89
    traumatic S36.299 ☑
  papillary muscle NEC I51.2
    following acute myocardial infarction (current complication) I23.5
  pelvic
    floor, complicating delivery O70.1
    organ NEC, obstetrical trauma O71.5
  perineum (nonobstetric) (nontraumatic) N90.89
    complicating delivery — *see* Delivery, complicated, by, laceration, anus (sphincter)
  postoperative wound — *see* Disruption, wound, operation
  prostate (traumatic) S37.828 ☑
  pulmonary
    artery I28.8
    valve (heart) I37.8
    vein I28.8
    vessel I28.8
  pus tube — *see* Salpingitis
  pyosalpinx — *see* Salpingitis
  rectum (nontraumatic) K63.1
    traumatic S36.69 ☑
  retina, retinal (traumatic) (without detachment) — *see also* Break, retina
    with detachment — *see* Detachment, retina, with retinal, break
  rotator cuff (nontraumatic) M75.10- ☑
    complete M75.12- ☑
    incomplete M75.11- ☑
  sclera — *see* Injury, eye, laceration
  sigmoid (nontraumatic) K63.1
    traumatic S36.593 ☑
  spinal cord — *see also* Injury, spinal cord, by region
    due to injury at birth P11.5
    newborn (birth injury) P11.5
  spleen (traumatic) S36.09 ☑
    birth injury P15.1
    congenital (birth injury) P15.1
    due to P. vivax malaria B51.0
    nontraumatic D73.5
    spontaneous D73.5
  splenic vein R58
    traumatic — *see* Injury, blood vessel, splenic vein
  stomach (nontraumatic) (spontaneous) K31.89
    traumatic S36.39 ☑
  supraspinatus (complete) (incomplete) (nontraumatic) — *see* Tear, rotator cuff
  symphysis pubis
    obstetric O71.6
    traumatic S33.4 ☑
  synovium (cyst) M66.10
    ankle M66.17- ☑
    elbow M66.12- ☑
    finger M66.14- ☑
    foot M66.17- ☑
    forearm M66.13- ☑
    hand M66.14- ☑
    pelvic region M66.15- ☑
    shoulder region M66.11- ☑
    specified site NEC M66.18
    thigh M66.15- ☑
    toe M66.17- ☑
    upper arm M66.12- ☑
    wrist M66.13- ☑
  tendon (traumatic) — *see* Strain
    nontraumatic (spontaneous) M66.9
      ankle M66.87- ☑
      extensor M66.20
        ankle M66.27- ☑
        foot M66.27- ☑
        forearm M66.23- ☑
        hand M66.24- ☑
        lower leg M66.26- ☑
        multiple sites M66.29
        pelvic region M66.25- ☑
        shoulder region M66.21- ☑
        specified site NEC M66.28
        thigh M66.25- ☑
        upper arm M66.22- ☑
      flexor M66.30
        ankle M66.37- ☑
        foot M66.37- ☑

Rupture, ruptured — *continued*

  tendon — *see* Strain — *continued*
    nontraumatic — *continued*
      flexor — *continued*
        forearm M66.33- ☑
        hand M66.34- ☑
        lower leg M66.36- ☑
        multiple sites M66.39
        pelvic region M66.35- ☑
        shoulder region M66.31- ☑
        specified site NEC M66.38
        thigh M66.35- ☑
        upper arm M66.32- ☑
      foot M66.87- ☑
      forearm M66.83- ☑
      hand M66.84- ☑
      lower leg M66.86- ☑
      multiple sites M66.89
      pelvic region M66.85- ☑
      shoulder region M66.81- ☑
      specified
        site NEC M66.88
        tendon M66.80
      thigh M66.85- ☑
      upper arm M66.82- ☑
  thoracic duct I89.8
  tonsil J35.8
  traumatic
    aorta — *see* Injury, aorta, laceration, major
    diaphragm — *see* Injury, intrathoracic, diaphragm
    external site — *see* Wound, open, by site
    eye — *see* Injury, eye, laceration
    internal organ — *see* Injury, by site
    intervertebral disc
      cervical S13.0 ☑
      lumbar S33.0 ☑
      thoracic S23.0 ☑
    kidney S37.06- ☑
    ligament — *see also* Sprain
      ankle — *see* Sprain, ankle
      carpus — *see* Rupture, traumatic, ligament, wrist
      collateral (hand) — *see* Rupture, traumatic, ligament, finger, collateral
      finger (metacarpophalangeal) (interphalangeal) S63.40- ☑
        collateral S63.41- ☑
          index S63.41- ☑
          little S63.41- ☑
          middle S63.41- ☑
          ring S63.41- ☑
        index S63.40- ☑
        little S63.40- ☑
        middle S63.40- ☑
        palmar S63.42- ☑
          index S63.42- ☑
          little S63.42- ☑
          middle S63.42- ☑
          ring S63.42- ☑
        ring S63.40- ☑
        specified site NEC S63.499 ☑
          index S63.49- ☑
          little S63.49- ☑
          middle S63.49- ☑
          ring S63.49- ☑
        volar plate S63.43- ☑
          index S63.43- ☑
          little S63.43- ☑
          middle S63.43- ☑
          ring S63.43- ☑
      foot — *see* Sprain, foot
      radial collateral S53.2- ☑
      radiocarpal — *see* Rupture, traumatic, ligament, wrist, radiocarpal
      ulnar collateral S53.3- ☑
      ulnocarpal — *see* Rupture, traumatic, ligament, wrist, ulnocarpal
      wrist S63.30- ☑
        collateral S63.31- ☑
        radiocarpal S63.32- ☑
        specified site NEC S63.39- ☑
        ulnocarpal (palmar) S63.33- ☑
    liver S36.116 ☑
    membrana tympani — *see* Rupture, ear drum, traumatic
    muscle or tendon — *see* Strain
    myocardium — *see* Injury, heart

   ☑ **Additional Character Required** — Refer to the Tabular List for Character Selection   ⍦ **Subterms under main terms may continue to next column or page**

Rupture, ruptured — *continued*
  traumatic — *continued*
    pancreas S36.299 ☑
    rectum S36.69 ☑
    sigmoid S36.593 ☑
    spleen S36.09 ☑
    stomach S36.39 ☑
    symphysis pubis S33.4 ☑
    tympanum, tympanic (membrane) — *see* Rupture, ear drum, traumatic
    ureter S37.19 ☑
    uterus S37.69 ☑
    vagina — *see* Injury, vagina
    vena cava — *see* Injury, vena cava, laceration, major
  tricuspid (heart) (valve) I07.8
  tube, tubal (nonobstetric) (nontraumatic) N83.8
    abscess — *see* Salpingitis
    due to pregnancy O00.10- ☑
      with intrauterine pregnancy O00.11- ☑
    tympanum, tympanic (membrane) (nontraumatic) —
      see also Perforation, tympanic membrane
      H72.9- ☑
      traumatic — *see* Rupture, ear drum, traumatic
  umbilical cord, complicating delivery O69.89 ☑
  ureter (traumatic) S37.19 ☑
    nontraumatic N28.89
  urethra (nontraumatic) N36.8
    with ectopic or molar pregnancy O08.6
    following ectopic or molar pregnancy O08.6
    obstetrical trauma O71.5
    traumatic S37.39 ☑
  uterosacral ligament (nonobstetric) (nontraumatic)
      N83.8
  uterus (traumatic) S37.69 ☑
    before labor O71.0- ☑
    during or after labor O71.1
    nonpuerperal, nontraumatic N85.8
    pregnant (during labor) O71.1
      before labor O71.0- ☑
  vagina — *see* Injury, vagina
  valve, valvular (heart) — *see* Endocarditis
  varicose vein — *see* Varix
  varix — *see* Varix
  vena cava R58
    traumatic — *see* Injury, vena cava, laceration, major
  vesical (urinary) N32.89
  vessel (blood) R58
    pulmonary I28.8
    traumatic — *see* Injury, blood vessel
  viscus R19.8
  vulva complicating delivery O70.0
Russell-Silver syndrome Q87.19
Russian spring-summer type encephalitis A84.0
Rust's disease (tuberculous cervical spondylitis) A18.01
Ruvalcaba-Myhre-Smith syndrome E71.440
Rytand-Lipsitch syndrome I44.2

S

Saber, sabre shin or tibia (syphilitic) A50.56 *[M90.8-]* ☑
Sac lacrimal — *see* condition
Saccharomyces infection B37.9
Saccharopinuria E72.3
Saccular — *see* condition
Sacculation
  aorta (nonsyphilitic) — *see* Aneurysm, aorta
  bladder N32.3
  intralaryngeal (congenital) (ventricular) Q31.3
  larynx (congenital) (ventricular) Q31.3
  organ or site, congenital — *see* Distortion
  pregnant uterus — *see* Pregnancy, complicated by, abnormal, uterus
  ureter N28.89
  urethra N36.1
  vesical N32.3
Sachs' amaurotic familial idiocy or disease E75.02
Sachs-Tay disease E75.02
Sacks-Libman disease M32.11
Sacralgia M53.3
Sacralization Q76.49
Sacrodynia M53.3
Sacroiliac joint — *see* condition
Sacroiliitis NEC M46.1
Sacrum — *see* condition
Saddle
  back — *see* Lordosis

Saddle — *continued*
  embolus
    abdominal aorta I74.01
    pulmonary artery I26.92
      with acute cor pulmonale I26.02
    injury — *code to* condition
    nose M95.0
      due to syphilis A50.57
Sadism (sexual) F65.52
Sadness, postpartal O90.6
Sadomasochism F65.50
Saemisch's ulcer (cornea) — *see* Ulcer, cornea, central
Sagging
  skin and subcutaneous tissue (following bariatric surgery weight loss) (following dietary weight loss) L98.7
Sahib disease B55.0
Sailors' skin L57.8
Saint
  Anthony's fire — *see* Erysipelas
  triad — *see* Hernia, diaphragm
  Vitus' dance — *see* Chorea, Sydenham's
Salaam
  attack(s) — *see* Epilepsy, spasms
  tic R25.8
Salicylism
  abuse F55.8
  overdose or wrong substance given — *see* Table of Drugs and Chemicals, by drug, poisoning
Salivary duct or gland — *see* condition
Salivation, excessive K11.7
Salmonella — *see* Infection, Salmonella
Salmonellosis A02.0
Salpingitis (catarrhal) (fallopian tube) (nodular) (pseud-ofollicular) (purulent) (septic) N70.91
  with oophoritis N70.93
  acute N70.01
    with oophoritis N70.03
  chlamydial A56.11
  chronic N70.11
    with oophoritis N70.13
  complicating abortion — *see* Abortion, by type, complicated by, salpingitis
  ear — *see* Salpingitis, eustachian
  eustachian (tube) H68.00- ☑
    acute H68.01- ☑
    chronic H68.02- ☑
  follicularis N70.11
    with oophoritis N70.13
  gonococcal (acute) (chronic) A54.24
  interstitial, chronic N70.11
    with oophoritis N70.13
  isthmica nodosa N70.11
    with oophoritis N70.13
  specific (gonococcal) (acute) (chronic) A54.24
  tuberculous (acute) (chronic) A18.17
  venereal (gonococcal) (acute) (chronic) A54.24
Salpingocele N83.4- ☑
Salpingo-oophoritis (catarrhal) (purulent) (ruptured) (septic) (suppurative) N70.93
  acute N70.03
    with ectopic or molar pregnancy O08.0
    following ectopic or molar pregnancy O08.0
    gonococcal A54.24
  chronic N70.13
  following ectopic or molar pregnancy O08.0
  gonococcal (acute) (chronic) A54.24
  puerperal O86.19
  specific (gonococcal) (acute) (chronic) A54.24
  subacute N70.03
  tuberculous (acute) (chronic) A18.17
  venereal (gonococcal) (acute) (chronic) A54.24
Salpingo-ovaritis — *see* Salpingo-oophoritis
Salpingoperitonitis — *see* Salpingo-oophoritis
Salzmann's nodular dystrophy — *see* Degeneration, cornea, nodular
Sampson's cyst or tumor N80.1
San Joaquin (Valley) **fever** B38.0
Sandblaster's asthma, lung or pneumoconiosis J62.8
Sander's disease (paranoia) F22
Sandfly fever A93.1
Sandhoff's disease E75.01
Sanfilippo (Type B) (Type C) (Type D) **syndrome** E76.22
Sanger-Brown ataxia G11.2
Sao Paulo fever or typhus A77.0
Saponification, mesenteric K65.8

Sarcocele (benign)
  syphilitic A52.76
    congenital A50.59
Sarcocystosis A07.8
Sarcoepiplocele — *see* Hernia
Sarcoepiplomphalocele Q79.2
Sarcoid — *see also* Sarcoidosis
  arthropathy D86.86
  Boeck's D86.9
  Darier-Roussy D86.3
  iridocyclitis D86.83
  meningitis D86.81
  myocarditis D86.85
  myositis D86.87
  pyelonephritis D86.84
  Spiegler-Fendt L08.89
Sarcoidosis D86.9
  with
    cranial nerve palsies D86.82
    hepatic granuloma D86.89
    polyarthritis D86.86
    tubulo-interstitial nephropathy D86.84
  combined sites NEC D86.89
  lung D86.0
    and lymph nodes D86.2
  lymph nodes D86.1
    and lung D86.2
  meninges D86.81
  skin D86.3
  specified type NEC D86.89
Sarcoma (of) — *see also* Neoplasm, connective tissue, malignant
  alveolar soft part — *see* Neoplasm, connective tissue, malignant
  ameloblastic C41.1
    upper jaw (bone) C41.0
  botryoid — *see* Neoplasm, connective tissue, malignant
  botryoides — *see* Neoplasm, connective tissue, malignant
  cerebellar C71.6
    circumscribed (arachnoidal) C71.6
  circumscribed (arachnoidal) cerebellar C71.6
  clear cell — *see also* Neoplasm, connective tissue, malignant
    kidney C64.- ☑
  dendritic cells (accessory cells) C96.4
  embryonal — *see* Neoplasm, connective tissue, malignant
  endometrial (stromal) C54.1
    isthmus C54.0
  epithelioid (cell) — *see* Neoplasm, connective tissue, malignant
  Ewing's — *see* Neoplasm, bone, malignant
  follicular dendritic cell C96.4
  germinoblastic (diffuse) — *see* Lymphoma, diffuse large cell
    follicular — *see* Lymphoma, follicular, specified NEC
  giant cell (except of bone) — *see also* Neoplasm, connective tissue, malignant
    bone — *see* Neoplasm, bone, malignant
  glomoid — *see* Neoplasm, connective tissue, malignant
  granulocytic C92.3- ☑
  hemangioendothelial — *see* Neoplasm, connective tissue, malignant
  hemorrhagic, multiple — *see* Sarcoma, Kaposi's
  histiocytic C96.A (*following* C96.6)
  Hodgkin — *see* Lymphoma, Hodgkin
  immunoblastic (diffuse) — *see* Lymphoma, diffuse large cell
  interdigitating dendritic cell C96.4
  Kaposi's
    colon C46.4
    connective tissue C46.1
    gastrointestinal organ C46.4
    lung C46.5- ☑
    lymph node(s) C46.3
    palate (hard) (soft) C46.2
    rectum C46.4
    skin C46.0
    specified site NEC C46.7
    stomach C46.4
    unspecified site C46.9
  Kupffer cell C22.3
  Langerhans cell C96.4
  leptomeningeal — *see* Neoplasm, meninges, malignant
  liver NEC C22.4
  lymphangioendothelial — *see* Neoplasm, connective tissue, malignant

Sarcoma — *continued*
  lymphoblastic — *see* Lymphoma, lymphoblastic (diffuse)
  lymphocytic — *see* Lymphoma, small cell B-cell
  mast cell C96.22
  melanotic — *see* Melanoma
  meningeal — *see* Neoplasm, meninges, malignant
  meningothelial — *see* Neoplasm, meninges, malignant
  mesenchymal — *see also* Neoplasm, connective tissue, malignant
    mixed — *see* Neoplasm, connective tissue, malignant
  mesothelial — *see* Mesothelioma
  monstrocellular
    specified site — *see* Neoplasm, malignant, by site
    unspecified site C71.9
  myeloid C92.3- ☑
  neurogenic — *see* Neoplasm, nerve, malignant
  odontogenic C41.1
    upper jaw (bone) C41.0
  osteoblastic — *see* Neoplasm, bone, malignant
  osteogenic — *see also* Neoplasm, bone, malignant
    juxtacortical — *see* Neoplasm, bone, malignant
    periosteal — *see* Neoplasm, bone, malignant
  periosteal — *see also* Neoplasm, bone, malignant
    osteogenic — *see* Neoplasm, bone, malignant
  pleomorphic cell — *see* Neoplasm, connective tissue, malignant
  reticulum cell (diffuse) — *see* Lymphoma, diffuse large cell
    nodular — *see* Lymphoma, follicular
    pleomorphic cell type — *see* Lymphoma, diffuse large cell
  rhabdoid — *see* Neoplasm, malignant, by site
  round cell — *see* Neoplasm, connective tissue, malignant
  small cell — *see* Neoplasm, connective tissue, malignant
  soft tissue — *see* Neoplasm, connective tissue, malignant
  spindle cell — *see* Neoplasm, connective tissue, malignant
  stromal (endometrial) C54.1
    isthmus C54.0
  synovial — *see also* Neoplasm, connective tissue, malignant
    biphasic — *see* Neoplasm, connective tissue, malignant
    epithelioid cell — *see* Neoplasm, connective tissue, malignant
    spindle cell — *see* Neoplasm, connective tissue, malignant
Sarcomatosis
  meningeal — *see* Neoplasm, meninges, malignant
  specified site NEC — *see* Neoplasm, connective tissue, malignant
  unspecified site C80.1
Sarcopenia (age-related) M62.84
Sarcosinemia E72.59
Sarcosporidiosis (intestinal) A07.8
Satiety, early R68.81
Saturnine — *see* condition
Saturnism
  overdose or wrong substance given or taken — *see* Table of Drugs and Chemicals, by drug, poisoning
Satyriasis F52.8
Sauriasis — *see* Ichthyosis
SBE (subacute bacterial endocarditis) I33.0
Scabies (any site) B86
Scabs R23.4
Scaglietti-Dagnini syndrome E22.0
Scald — *see* Burn
Scalenus anticus (anterior) **syndrome** G54.0
Scales R23.4
Scaling, skin R23.4
Scalp — *see* condition
Scapegoating affecting child Z62.3
Scaphocephaly Q75.0
Scapulalgia M89.8X1
Scapulohumeral myopathy G71.02
Scar, scarring — *see also* Cicatrix L90.5
  adherent L90.5
  atrophic L90.5
  cervix
    in pregnancy or childbirth — *see* Pregnancy, complicated by, abnormal cervix
  cheloid L91.0

Scar, scarring — *continued*
  chorioretinal H31.00- ☑
    posterior pole macula H31.01- ☑
    postsurgical H59.81- ☑
    solar retinopathy H31.02- ☑
    specified type NEC H31.09- ☑
  choroid — *see* Scar, chorioretinal
  conjunctiva H11.24- ☑
  cornea H17.9
    xerophthalmic — *see also* Opacity, cornea
      vitamin A deficiency E50.6
  duodenum, obstructive K31.5
  hypertrophic L91.0
  keloid L91.0
  labia N90.89
  lung (base) J98.4
  macula — *see* Scar, chorioretinal, posterior pole
  muscle M62.89
  myocardium, myocardial I25.2
  painful L90.5
  posterior pole (eye) — *see* Scar, chorioretinal, posterior pole
  retina — *see* Scar, chorioretinal
  trachea J39.8
  transmural uterine, in pregnancy O34.29
  uterus N85.8
    in pregnancy O34.29
  vagina N89.8
    postoperative N99.2
  vulva N90.89
Scarabiasis B88.2
Scarlatina (anginosa) (maligna) A38.9
  myocarditis (acute) A38.1
    old — *see* Myocarditis
  otitis media A38.0
  ulcerosa A38.8
Scarlet fever (albuminuria) (angina) A38.9
Schamberg's disease (progressive pigmentary dermatosis) L81.7
Schatzki's ring (acquired) (esophagus) (lower) K22.2
  congenital Q39.3
Schaufenster krankheit I20.8
Schaumann's
  benign lymphogranulomatosis D86.1
  disease or syndrome — *see* Sarcoidosis
Scheie's syndrome E76.03
Schenck's disease B42.1
Scheuermann's disease or osteochondrosis — *see* Osteochondrosis, juvenile, spine
Schilder (-Flatau) **disease** G37.0
Schilling-type monocytic leukemia C93.0- ☑
Schimmelbusch's disease, cystic mastitis, or hyperplasia — *see* Mastopathy, cystic
Schistosoma infestation — *see* Infestation, Schistosoma
Schistosomiasis B65.9
  with muscle disorder B65.9 *[M63.80]*
    ankle B65.9 *[M63.87-]* ☑
    foot B65.9 *[M63.87-]* ☑
    forearm B65.9 *[M63.83-]* ☑
    hand B65.9 *[M63.84-]* ☑
    lower leg B65.9 *[M63.86-]* ☑
    multiple sites B65.9 *[M63.89]*
    pelvic region B65.9 *[M63.85-]* ☑
    shoulder region B65.9 *[M63.81-]* ☑
    specified site NEC B65.9 *[M63.88]*
    thigh B65.9 *[M63.85-]* ☑
    upper arm B65.9 *[M63.82-]* ☑
  Asiatic B65.2
  bladder B65.0
  chestermani B65.8
  colon B65.1
  cutaneous B65.3
  due to
    S. haematobium B65.0
    S. japonicum B65.2
    S. mansoni B65.1
    S. mattheii B65.8
  Eastern B65.2
  genitourinary tract B65.0
  intestinal B65.1
  lung NEC B65.9 *[J99]*
    pneumonia B65.9 *[J17]*
  Manson's (intestinal) B65.1
  oriental B65.2
  pulmonary NEC B65.9 *[J99]*
    pneumonia B65.9

Schistosomiasis — *continued*
  Schistosoma
    haematobium B65.0
    japonicum B65.2
    mansoni B65.1
  specified type NEC B65.8
  urinary B65.0
  vesical B65.0
Schizencephaly Q04.6
Schizoaffective psychosis F25.9
Schizodontia K00.2
Schizoid personality F60.1
Schizophrenia, schizophrenic F20.9
  acute (brief) (undifferentiated) F23
  atypical (form) F20.3
  borderline F21
  catalepsy F20.2
  catatonic (type) (excited) (withdrawn) F20.2
  cenesthopathic, cenesthesiopathic F20.89
  childhood type F84.5
  chronic undifferentiated F20.5
  cyclic F25.0
  disorganized (type) F20.1
  flexibilitas cerea F20.2
  hebephrenic (type) F20.1
  incipient F21
  latent F21
  negative type F20.5
  paranoid (type) F20.0
  paraphrenic F20.0
  post-psychotic depression F32.89
  prepsychotic F21
  prodromal F21
  pseudoneurotic F21
  pseudopsychopathic F21
  reaction F23
  residual (state) (type) F20.5
  restzustand F20.5
  schizoaffective (type) — *see* Psychosis, schizoaffective
  simple (type) F20.89
  simplex F20.89
  specified type NEC F20.89
  spectrum and other psychotic disorder F29
    specified NEC F28
  stupor F20.2
  syndrome of childhood F84.5
  undifferentiated (type) F20.3
    chronic F20.5
Schizothymia (persistent) F60.1
Schlatter-Osgood disease or osteochondrosis — *see* Osteochondrosis, juvenile, tibia
Schlatter's tibia — *see* Osteochondrosis, juvenile, tibia
Schmidt's syndrome (polyglandular, autoimmune) E31.0
Schmincke's carcinoma or tumor — *see* Neoplasm, nasopharynx, malignant
Schmitz (-Stutzer) **dysentery** A03.0
Schmorl's disease or nodes
  lumbar region M51.46
  lumbosacral region M51.47
  sacrococcygeal region M53.3
  thoracic region M51.44
  thoracolumbar region M51.45
Schneiderian
  papilloma — *see* Neoplasm, nasopharynx, benign
    specified site — *see* Neoplasm, benign, by site
    unspecified site D14.0
  specified site — *see* Neoplasm, malignant, by site
    unspecified site C30.0
Scholte's syndrome (malignant carcinoid) E34.0
Scholz (-Bielchowsky-Henneberg) **disease or syndrome** E75.25
Schönlein (-Henoch) disease or purpura (primary) (rheumatic) D69.0
Schottmuller's disease A01.4
Schroeder's syndrome (endocrine hypertensive) E27.0
Schüller-Christian disease or syndrome C96.5
Schultze's type acroparesthesia, simple I73.89
Schultz's disease or syndrome — *see* Agranulocytosis
Schwalbe-Ziehen-Oppenheim disease G24.1
Schwannoma — *see also* Neoplasm, nerve, benign
  malignant — *see also* Neoplasm, nerve, malignant
    with rhabdomyoblastic differentiation — *see* Neoplasm, nerve, malignant
  melanocytic — *see* Neoplasm, nerve, benign
  pigmented — *see* Neoplasm, nerve, benign
Schwannomatosis Q85.03
Schwartz (-Jampel) **syndrome** G71.13
Schwartz-Bartter syndrome E22.2

Schweniger-Buzzi anetoderma L90.1
Sciatic — *see* condition
Sciatica (infective)
  with lumbago M54.4- ☑
    due to intervertebral disc disorder — *see* Disorder,
      disc, with, radiculopathy
    due to displacement of intervertebral disc (with lumba-
      go) — *see* Disorder, disc, with, radiculopathy
  wallet M54.3- ☑
Scimitar syndrome Q26.8
Sclera — *see* condition
Sclerectasia H15.84- ☑
Scleredema
  adultorum — *see* Sclerosis, systemic
  Buschke's — *see* Sclerosis, systemic
  newborn P83.0
Sclerema (adiposum) (edematosum) (neonatorum)
    (newborn) P83.0
  adultorum — *see* Sclerosis, systemic
Scleriasis — *see* Scleroderma
Scleritis H15.00- ☑
  with corneal involvement H15.04- ☑
  anterior H15.01- ☑
  brawny H15.02- ☑
  in (due to) zoster B02.34
  posterior H15.03- ☑
  specified type NEC H15.09- ☑
  syphilitic A52.71
  tuberculous (nodular) A18.51
Sclerochoroiditis H31.8
Scleroconjunctivitis — *see* Scleritis
Sclerocystic ovary syndrome E28.2
Sclerodactyly, sclerodactylia L94.3
Scleroderma, sclerodermia (acrosclerotic) (diffuse)
    (generalized) (progressive) (pulmonary) — *see also*
    Sclerosis, systemic M34.9
  circumscribed L94.0
  linear L94.1
  localized L94.0
  newborn P83.88
  systemic M34.9
Sclerokeratitis H16.8
  tuberculous A18.52
Scleroma nasi A48.8
Scleromalacia (perforans) H15.05- ☑
Scleromyxedema L98.5
Sclérose en plaques G35
Sclerosis, sclerotic
  adrenal (gland) E27.8
  Alzheimer's — *see* Disease, Alzheimer's
  amyotrophic (lateral) G12.21
  aorta, aortic I70.0
    valve — *see* Endocarditis, aortic
  artery, arterial, arteriolar, arteriovascular — *see* Arte-
    riosclerosis
  ascending multiple G35
  brain (generalized) (lobular) G37.9
    artery, arterial I67.2
    diffuse G37.0
    disseminated G35
    insular G35
    Krabbe's E75.23
    miliary G35
    multiple G35
    presenile (Alzheimer's) — *see* Disease, Alzheimer's,
      early onset
    senile (arteriosclerotic) I67.2
    stem, multiple G35
    tuberous Q85.1
  bulbar, multiple G35
  bundle of His I44.39
  cardiac — *see* Disease, heart, ischemic, atherosclerotic
  cardiorenal — *see* Hypertension, cardiorenal
  cardiovascular — *see also* Disease, cardiovascular
    renal — *see* Hypertension, cardiorenal
  cerebellar — *see* Sclerosis, brain
  cerebral — *see* Sclerosis, brain
  cerebrospinal (disseminated) (multiple) G35
  cerebrovascular I67.2
  choroid — *see* Degeneration, choroid
  combined (spinal cord) — *see also* Degeneration,
    combined
    multiple G35
  concentric (Balo) G37.5
  cornea — *see* Opacity, cornea
  coronary (artery) I25.10

Sclerosis, sclerotic — *continued*
  coronary — *continued*
    with angina pectoris — *see* Arteriosclerosis, coro-
      nary (artery),
  corpus cavernosum
    female N90.89
    male N48.6
  diffuse (brain) (spinal cord) G37.0
  disseminated G35
  dorsal G35
  dorsolateral (spinal cord) — *see* Degeneration, com-
    bined
  endometrium N85.5
  extrapyramidal G25.9
  eye, nuclear (senile) — *see* Cataract, senile, nuclear
  focal and segmental (glomerular) — *see also* N00-N07
    with fourth character .1 N05.1
  Friedreich's (spinal cord) G11.1
  funicular (spermatic cord) N50.89
  general (vascular) — *see* Arteriosclerosis
  gland (lymphatic) I89.8
  hepatic K74.1
    alcoholic K70.2
  hereditary
    cerebellar G11.9
    spinal (Friedreich's ataxia) G11.1
  hippocampal G93.81
  insular G35
  kidney — *see* Sclerosis, renal
  larynx J38.7
  lateral (amyotrophic) (descending) (spinal) G12.21
    primary G12.23
  lens, senile nuclear — *see* Cataract, senile, nuclear
  liver K74.1
    with fibrosis K74.2
      alcoholic K70.2
    alcoholic K70.2
    cardiac K76.1
  lung — *see* Fibrosis, lung
  mastoid — *see* Mastoiditis, chronic
  mesial temporal G93.81
  mitral I05.8
  Mönckeberg's (medial) — *see* Arteriosclerosis, extrem-
    ities
  multiple (brain stem) (cerebral) (generalized) (spinal
    cord) G35
  myocardium, myocardial — *see* Disease, heart, is-
    chemic, atherosclerotic
  nuclear (senile), eye — *see* Cataract, senile, nuclear
  ovary N83.8
  pancreas K86.89
  penis N48.6
  peripheral arteries — *see* Arteriosclerosis, extremities
  plaques G35
  pluriglandular E31.8
  polyglandular E31.8
  posterolateral (spinal cord) — *see* Degeneration,
    combined
  presenile (Alzheimer's) — *see* Disease, Alzheimer's,
    early onset
  primary, lateral G12.23
  progressive, systemic M34.0
  pulmonary — *see* Fibrosis, lung
    artery I27.0
    valve (heart) — *see* Endocarditis, pulmonary
  renal N26.9
    with
      cystine storage disease E72.09
      hypertensive heart disease (conditions in I11) —
        see Hypertension, cardiorenal
    arteriolar (hyaline) (hyperplastic) — *see* Hyperten-
      sion, kidney
  retina (senile) (vascular) H35.00
  senile (vascular) — *see* Arteriosclerosis
  spinal (cord) (progressive) G95.89
    ascending G61.0
    combined — *see also* Degeneration, combined
      multiple G35
      syphilitic A52.11
    disseminated G35
    dorsolateral — *see* Degeneration, combined
    hereditary (Friedreich's) (mixed form) G11.1
    lateral (amyotrophic) G12.21
      progressive G12.23
    multiple G35
    posterior (syphilitic) A52.11
  stomach K31.89
  subendocardial, congenital I42.4

Sclerosis, sclerotic — *continued*
  systemic M34.9
    with
      lung involvement M34.81
      myopathy M34.82
      polyneuropathy M34.83
    drug-induced M34.2
    due to chemicals NEC M34.2
    progressive M34.0
    specified NEC M34.89
  temporal (mesial) G93.81
  tricuspid (heart) (valve) I07.8
  tuberous (brain) Q85.1
  tympanic membrane — *see* Disorder, tympanic mem-
    brane, specified NEC
  valve, valvular (heart) — *see* Endocarditis
  vascular — *see* Arteriosclerosis
  vein I87.8
Scoliosis (acquired) (postural) M41.9
  adolescent (idiopathic) — *see* Scoliosis, idiopathic,
    adolescent
  congenital Q67.5
    due to bony malformation Q76.3
    failure of segmentation (hemivertebra) Q76.3
    hemivertebra fusion Q76.3
    postural Q67.5
  idiopathic M41.20
    adolescent M41.129
      cervical region M41.122
      cervicothoracic region M41.123
      lumbar region M41.126
      lumbosacral region M41.127
      thoracic region M41.124
      thoracolumbar region M41.125
    cervical region M41.22
    cervicothoracic region M41.23
    infantile M41.00
      cervical region M41.02
      cervicothoracic region M41.03
      lumbar region M41.06
      lumbosacral region M41.07
      sacrococcygeal region M41.08
      thoracic region M41.04
      thoracolumbar region M41.05
    juvenile M41.119
      cervical region M41.112
      cervicothoracic region M41.113
      lumbar region M41.116
      lumbosacral region M41.117
      thoracic region M41.114
      thoracolumbar region M41.115
    lumbar region M41.26
    lumbosacral region M41.27
    thoracic region M41.24
    thoracolumbar region M41.25
  infantile — *see* Scoliosis, idiopathic, infantile
  neuromuscular M41.40
    cervical region M41.42
    cervicothoracic region M41.43
    lumbar region M41.46
    lumbosacral region M41.47
    occipito-atlanto-axial region M41.41
    thoracic region M41.44
    thoracolumbar region M41.45
  paralytic — *see* Scoliosis, neuromuscular
  postradiation therapy M96.5
  rachitic (late effect or sequelae) E64.3 *[M49.80]*
    cervical region E64.3 *[M49.82]*
    cervicothoracic region E64.3 *[M49.83]*
    lumbar region E64.3 *[M49.86]*
    lumbosacral region E64.3 *[M49.87]*
    multiple sites E64.3 *[M49.89]*
    occipito-atlanto-axial region E64.3 *[M49.81]*
    sacrococcygeal region E64.3 *[M49.88]*
    thoracic region E64.3 *[M49.84]*
    thoracolumbar region E64.3 *[M49.85]*
  sciatic M54.4- ☑
  secondary (to) NEC M41.50
    cerebral palsy, Friedreich's ataxia, poliomyelitis,
      neuromuscular disorders — *see* Scoliosis,
      neuromuscular
    cervical region M41.52
    cervicothoracic region M41.53
    lumbar region M41.56
    lumbosacral region M41.57
    thoracic region M41.54
    thoracolumbar region M41.55
  specified form NEC M41.80

Scoliosis — continued
- specified form — continued
  - cervical region M41.82
  - cervicothoracic region M41.83
  - lumbar region M41.86
  - lumbosacral region M41.87
  - thoracic region M41.84
  - thoracolumbar region M41.85
  - thoracogenic M41.30
    - thoracic region M41.34
    - thoracolumbar region M41.35
  - tuberculous A18.01
Scoliotic pelvis
- with disproportion (fetopelvic) O33.0
  - causing obstructed labor O65.0
Scorbutus, scorbutic — see also Scurvy
- anemia D53.2
Score, NIHSS (National Institutes of Health Stroke Scale) R29.7- ☑
Scotoma (arcuate) (Bjerrum) (central) (ring) — see also Defect, visual field, localized, scotoma
- scintillating H53.19
Scratch — see Abrasion
Scratchy throat R09.89
Screening (for) Z13.9
- alcoholism Z13.39
- anemia Z13.0
- anomaly, congenital Z13.89
- antenatal, of mother — see also Encounter, antenatal screening Z36.9
- arterial hypertension Z13.6
- arthropod-borne viral disease NEC Z11.59
- autism Z13.41
- bacteriuria, asymptomatic Z13.89
- behavioral disorder Z13.30
  - specified NEC Z13.39
- brain injury, traumatic Z13.850
- bronchitis, chronic Z13.83
- brucellosis Z11.2
- cardiovascular disorder Z13.6
- cataract Z13.5
- chlamydial diseases Z11.8
- cholera Z11.0
- chromosomal abnormalities (nonprocreative) NEC Z13.79
- colonoscopy Z12.11
- congenital
  - dislocation of hip Z13.89
  - eye disorder Z13.5
  - malformation or deformation Z13.89
- contamination NEC Z13.88
- cystic fibrosis Z13.228
- dengue fever Z11.59
- dental disorder Z13.84
- depression (adult) (adolescent) (child) Z13.31
  - maternal Z13.32
  - perinatal Z13.32
- developmental
  - delays Z13.40
    - global (milestones) Z13.42
    - specified NEC Z13.49
  - handicap Z13.42
    - in early childhood Z13.42
- diabetes mellitus Z13.1
- diphtheria Z11.2
- disability, intellectual Z13.39
- disease or disorder Z13.9
  - bacterial NEC Z11.2
    - intestinal infectious Z11.0
    - respiratory tuberculosis Z11.1
  - behavioral Z13.30
    - specified NEC Z13.39
  - blood or blood-forming organ Z13.0
  - cardiovascular Z13.6
  - Chagas' Z11.6
  - chlamydial Z11.8
  - dental Z13.89
  - developmental delays Z13.40
    - global (milestones) Z13.42
    - specified NEC Z13.49
  - digestive tract NEC Z13.818
    - lower GI Z13.811
    - upper GI Z13.810
  - ear Z13.5
  - endocrine Z13.29
  - eye Z13.5
  - genitourinary Z13.89
  - heart Z13.6

Screening — continued
- disease or disorder — continued
  - human immunodeficiency virus (HIV) infection Z11.4
  - immunity Z13.0
  - infection
    - intestinal Z11.0
      - specified NEC Z11.6
    - infectious Z11.9
  - mental health and behavioral Z13.30
    - specified NEC Z13.39
  - metabolic Z13.228
  - neurological Z13.89
  - nutritional Z13.21
    - metabolic Z13.228
      - lipoid disorders Z13.220
  - protozoal Z11.6
    - intestinal Z11.0
  - respiratory Z13.83
  - rheumatic Z13.828
  - rickettsial Z11.8
  - sexually-transmitted NEC Z11.3
    - human immunodeficiency virus (HIV) Z11.4
  - sickle-cell (trait) Z13.0
  - skin Z13.89
  - specified NEC Z13.89
  - spirochetal Z11.8
  - thyroid Z13.29
  - vascular Z13.6
  - venereal Z11.3
  - viral NEC Z11.59
    - human immunodeficiency virus (HIV) Z11.4
    - intestinal Z11.0
- elevated titer Z13.89
- emphysema Z13.83
- encephalitis, viral (mosquito- or tick-borne) Z11.59
- exposure to contaminants (toxic) Z13.88
- fever
  - dengue Z11.59
  - hemorrhagic Z11.59
  - yellow Z11.59
- filariasis Z11.6
- galactosemia Z13.228
- gastrointestinal condition Z13.818
- genetic (nonprocreative) - for procreative management — see Testing, genetic, for procreative management
  - disease carrier status (nonprocreative) Z13.71
  - specified NEC (nonprocreative) Z13.79
- genitourinary condition Z13.89
- glaucoma Z13.5
- gonorrhea Z11.3
- gout Z13.89
- helminthiasis (intestinal) Z11.6
- hematopoietic malignancy Z12.89
- hemoglobinopathies NEC Z13.0
- hemorrhagic fever Z11.59
- Hodgkin disease Z12.89
- human immunodeficiency virus (HIV) Z11.4
- human papillomavirus Z11.51
- hypertension Z13.6
- immunity disorders Z13.0
- infant or child (over 28 days old) Z00.129
  - with abnormal findings Z00.121
- infection
  - mycotic Z11.8
  - parasitic Z11.8
- ingestion of radioactive substance Z13.88
- intellectual disability Z13.39
- intestinal
  - helminthiasis Z11.6
  - infectious disease Z11.0
- leishmaniasis Z11.6
- leprosy Z11.2
- leptospirosis Z11.8
- leukemia Z12.89
- lymphoma Z12.89
- malaria Z11.6
- malnutrition Z13.29
  - metabolic Z13.228
  - nutritional Z13.21
- measles Z11.59
- mental health disorder Z13.30
  - specified NEC Z13.39
- metabolic errors, inborn Z13.228
- multiphasic Z13.89
- musculoskeletal disorder Z13.828
  - osteoporosis Z13.820
- mycoses Z11.8
- myocardial infarction (acute) Z13.6

Screening — continued
- neoplasm (malignant) (of) Z12.9
  - bladder Z12.6
  - blood Z12.89
  - breast Z12.39
    - routine mammogram Z12.31
  - cervix Z12.4
  - colon Z12.11
  - genitourinary organs NEC Z12.79
    - bladder Z12.6
    - cervix Z12.4
    - ovary Z12.73
    - prostate Z12.5
    - testis Z12.71
    - vagina Z12.72
  - hematopoietic system Z12.89
  - intestinal tract Z12.10
    - colon Z12.11
    - rectum Z12.12
    - small intestine Z12.13
  - lung Z12.2
  - lymph (glands) Z12.89
  - nervous system Z12.82
  - oral cavity Z12.81
  - prostate Z12.5
  - rectum Z12.12
  - respiratory organs Z12.2
  - skin Z12.83
  - small intestine Z12.13
  - specified site NEC Z12.89
  - stomach Z12.0
- nephropathy Z13.89
- nervous system disorders NEC Z13.858
- neurological condition Z13.89
- osteoporosis Z13.820
- parasitic infestation Z11.9
  - specified NEC Z11.8
- phenylketonuria Z13.228
- plague Z11.2
- poisoning (chemical) (heavy metal) Z13.88
- poliomyelitis Z11.59
- postnatal, chromosomal abnormalities Z13.89
- prenatal, of mother — see also Encounter, antenatal screening Z36.9
- protozoal disease Z11.6
  - intestinal Z11.0
- pulmonary tuberculosis Z11.1
- radiation exposure Z13.88
- respiratory condition Z13.83
- respiratory tuberculosis Z11.1
- rheumatoid arthritis Z13.828
- rubella Z11.59
- schistosomiasis Z11.6
- sexually-transmitted disease NEC Z11.3
  - human immunodeficiency virus (HIV) Z11.4
- sickle-cell disease or trait Z13.0
- skin condition Z13.89
- sleeping sickness Z11.6
- special Z13.9
  - specified NEC Z13.89
- syphilis Z11.3
- tetanus Z11.2
- trachoma Z11.8
- traumatic brain injury Z13.850
- trypanosomiasis Z11.6
- tuberculosis, respiratory Z11.1
  - active Z11.1
  - latent Z11.7
- venereal disease Z11.3
- viral encephalitis (mosquito- or tick-borne) Z11.59
- whooping cough Z11.2
- worms, intestinal Z11.6
- yaws Z11.8
- yellow fever Z11.59
Scrofula, scrofulosis (tuberculosis of cervical lymph glands) A18.2
Scrofulide (primary) (tuberculous) A18.4
Scrofuloderma, scrofulodermia (any site) (primary) A18.4
Scrofulosus lichen (primary) (tuberculous) A18.4
Scrofulous — see condition
Scrotal tongue K14.5
Scrotum — see condition
Scurvy, scorbutic E54
- anemia D53.2
- gum E54
- infantile E54
- rickets E55.0 [M90.80]

Sealpox B08.62
Seasickness T75.3 ☑
Seatworm (infection) (infestation) B80
Sebaceous — *see also* condition
  cyst — *see* Cyst, sebaceous
Seborrhea, seborrheic L21.9
  capillitii R23.8
  capitis L21.0
  dermatitis L21.9
    infantile L21.1
  eczema L21.9
    infantile L21.1
  sicca L21.0
Seckel's syndrome Q87.19
Seclusion, pupil — *see* Membrane, pupillary
Second hand tobacco smoke exposure (acute)
  (chronic) Z77.22
  in the perinatal period P96.81
Secondary
  dentin (in pulp) K04.3
  neoplasm, secondaries — *see* Table of Neoplasms,
    secondary
Secretion
  antidiuretic hormone, inappropriate E22.2
  catecholamine, by pheochromocytoma E27.5
  hormone
    antidiuretic, inappropriate (syndrome) E22.2
    by
      carcinoid tumor E34.0
      pheochromocytoma E27.5
    ectopic NEC E34.2
  urinary
    excessive R35.8
    suppression R34
Section
  nerve, traumatic — *see* Injury, nerve
Sedative, hypnotic, or anxiolytic-induced
  anxiety disorder F13.980
  bipolar and related disorder F13.94
  delirium F13.921
  depressive disorder F13.94
  major neurocognitive disorder F13.97
  mild neurocognitive disorder F13.988
  psychotic disorder F13.959
  sexual dysfunction F13.981
  sleep disorder F13.982
Segmentation, incomplete (congenital) — *see also*
  Fusion
  bone NEC Q78.8
  lumbosacral (joint) (vertebra) Q76.49
Seitelberger's syndrome (infantile neuraxonal dystrophy) G31.89
Seizure(s) — *see also* Convulsions R56.9
  absence G40.A- ☑ (*following* G40.3)
  akinetic — *see* Epilepsy, generalized, specified NEC
  atonic — *see* Epilepsy, generalized, specified NEC
  autonomic (hysterical) F44.5
  convulsive — *see* Convulsions
  cortical (focal) (motor) — *see* Epilepsy, localization-re-
    lated, symptomatic, with simple partial seizures
  disorder — *see also* Epilepsy G40.909
  due to stroke — *see* Sequelae (of), disease, cerebrovas-
    cular, by type, specified NEC
  epileptic — *see* Epilepsy
  febrile (simple) R56.00
    with status epilepticus G40.901
    complex (atypical) (complicated) R56.01
      with status epilepticus G40.901
  grand mal G40.409
    intractable G40.419
      with status epilepticus G40.411
      without status epilepticus G40.419
    not intractable G40.409
      with status epilepticus G40.401
      without status epilepticus G40.409
  heart — *see* Disease, heart
  hysterical F44.5
  intractable G40.919
    with status epilepticus G40.911
  Jacksonian (focal) (motor type) (sensory type) — *see*
    Epilepsy, localization-related, symptomatic, with
    simple partial seizures
  newborn P90
  nonspecific epileptic
    atonic — *see* Epilepsy, generalized, specified NEC
    clonic — *see* Epilepsy, generalized, specified NEC
    myoclonic — *see* Epilepsy, generalized, specified
      NEC

Seizure(s) — *continued*
  nonspecific epileptic — *continued*
    tonic — *see* Epilepsy, generalized, specified NEC
    tonic-clonic — *see* Epilepsy, generalized, specified
      NEC
  partial, developing into secondarily generalized
    seizures
    complex — *see* Epilepsy, localization-related,
      symptomatic, with complex partial seizures
    simple — *see* Epilepsy, localization-related, symp-
      tomatic, with simple partial seizures
  petit mal G40.A- ☑ (*following* G40.3)
    intractable G40.419
      with status epilepticus G40.411
      without status epilepticus G40.419
    not intractable G40.409
      with status epilepticus G40.401
      without status epilepticus G40.409
  post traumatic R56.1
  recurrent G40.909
  specified NEC G40.89
  uncinate — *see* Epilepsy, localization-related, symp-
    tomatic, with complex partial seizures
Selenium deficiency, dietary E59
Self-damaging behavior (life-style) Z72.89
Self-harm (attempted)
  history (personal) Z91.5
    in family Z81.8
Self-mutilation (attempted)
  history (personal) Z91.5
    in family Z81.8
Self-poisoning
  history (personal) Z91.5
    in family Z81.8
  observation following (alleged) attempt Z03.6
Semicoma R40.1
Seminal vesiculitis N49.0
Seminoma C62.9- ☑
  specified site — *see* Neoplasm, malignant, by site
Senear-Usher disease or syndrome L10.4
Senectus R54
Senescence (without mention of psychosis) R54
Senile, senility — *see also* condition R41.81
  with
    acute confusional state F05
    mental changes NOS F03 ☑
    psychosis NEC — *see* Psychosis, senile
  asthenia R54
  cervix (atrophic) N88.8
  debility R54
  endometrium (atrophic) N85.8
  fallopian tube (atrophic) — *see* Atrophy, fallopian tube
  heart (failure) R54
  ovary (atrophic) — *see* Atrophy, ovary
  premature E34.8
  vagina, vaginitis (atrophic) N95.2
  wart L82.1
Sensation
  burning (skin) R20.8
    tongue K14.6
  loss of R20.8
  prickling (skin) R20.2
  tingling (skin) R20.2
Sense loss
  smell — *see* Disturbance, sensation, smell
  taste — *see* Disturbance, sensation, taste
  touch R20.8
Sensibility disturbance (cortical) (deep) (vibratory) R20.9
Sensitive, sensitivity — *see also* Allergy
  carotid sinus G90.01
  child (excessive) F93.8
  cold, autoimmune D59.1
  dentin K03.89
  gluten (non-celiac) K90.41
  latex Z91.040
  methemoglobin D74.8
  tuberculin, without clinical or radiological symptoms
    R76.11
  visual
    glare H53.71
    impaired contrast H53.72
Sensitiver Beziehungswahn F22
Sensitization, auto-erythrocytic D69.2
Separation
  anxiety, abnormal (of childhood) F93.0
  apophysis, traumatic — *code as* Fracture, by site
  choroid — *see* Detachment, choroid

Separation — *continued*
  epiphysis, epiphyseal
    nontraumatic — *see also* Osteochondropathy,
      specified type NEC
      upper femoral — *see* Slipped, epiphysis, upper
        femoral
    traumatic — *code as* Fracture, by site
  fracture — *see* Fracture
  infundibulum cardiac from right ventricle by a partition
    Q24.3
  joint (traumatic) (current) — *code by* site under Dislo-
    cation
  muscle (nontraumatic) — *see* Diastasis, muscle
  pubic bone, obstetrical trauma O71.6
  retina, retinal — *see* Detachment, retina
  symphysis pubis, obstetrical trauma O71.6
  tracheal ring, incomplete, congenital Q32.1
Sepsis (generalized) (unspecified organism) A41.9
  with
    organ dysfunction (acute) (multiple) R65.20
      with septic shock R65.21
  actinomycotic A42.7
  adrenal hemorrhage syndrome (meningococcal) A39.1
  anaerobic A41.4
  Bacillus anthracis A22.7
  Brucella — *see also* Brucellosis A23.9
  candidal B37.7
  cryptogenic A41.9
  due to device, implant or graft T85.79 ☑
    arterial graft NEC T82.7 ☑
    breast (implant) T85.79 ☑
    catheter NEC T85.79 ☑
      dialysis (renal) T82.7 ☑
        intraperitoneal T85.71 ☑
      infusion NEC T82.7 ☑
        spinal (cranial) (epidural) (intrathecal) (spinal)
          (subarachnoid) (subdural) T85.735 ☑
      urethral indwelling T83.511 ☑
      urinary T83.518 ☑
    ectopic or molar pregnancy O08.82
    electronic (electrode) (pulse generator) (stimulator)
      bone T84.7 ☑
      cardiac T82.7 ☑
      nervous system T85.738 ☑
        brain T85.731 ☑
        neurostimulator generator T85.734 ☑
        peripheral nerve T85.732 ☑
        spinal cord T85.733 ☑
      urinary T83.590 ☑
    fixation, internal (orthopedic) — *see* Complication,
      fixation device, infection
    gastrointestinal (bile duct) (esophagus) T85.79 ☑
      neurostimulator electrode (lead) T85.732 ☑
    genital T83.69 ☑
    heart NEC T82.7 ☑
      valve (prosthesis) T82.6 ☑
        graft T82.7 ☑
    joint prosthesis — *see* Complication, joint prosthe-
      sis, infection
    ocular (corneal graft) (orbital implant) T85.79 ☑
    orthopedic NEC T84.7 ☑
      fixation device, internal — *see* Complication,
        fixation device, infection
    specified NEC T85.79 ☑
    vascular T82.7 ☑
    ventricular intracranial (communicating) shunt
      T85.730 ☑
  during labor O75.3
  Enterococcus A41.81
  Erysipelothrix (rhusiopathiae) (erysipeloid) A26.7
  Escherichia coli (E. coli) A41.5 ☑
  extraintestinal yersiniosis A28.2
  following
    abortion (subsequent episode) O08.0
      current episode — *see* Abortion
    ectopic or molar pregnancy O08.82
    immunization T88.0 ☑
    infusion, therapeutic injection or transfusion NEC
      T80.29 ☑
    obstetrical procedure O86.04
  gangrenous A41.9
  gonococcal A54.86
  Gram-negative (organism) A41.5 ☑
    anaerobic A41.4
  Haemophilus influenzae A41.3
  herpesviral B00.7
  intra-abdominal K65.1

Sepsis — *continued*
- intraocular — *see* Endophthalmitis, purulent
- Listeria monocytogenes A32.7
- localized — *code to* specific localized infection
  - in operation wound T81.49 ☑
  - skin — *see* Abscess
- malleus A24.0
- melioidosis A24.1
- meningeal — *see* Meningitis
- meningococcal A39.4
  - acute A39.2
  - chronic A39.3
- MSSA (Methicillin susceptible Staphylococcus aureus) A41.01
- newborn P36.9
  - due to
    - anaerobes NEC P36.5
    - Escherichia coli P36.4
    - Staphylococcus P36.30
      - aureus P36.2
      - specified NEC P36.39
    - Streptococcus P36.10
      - group B P36.0
      - specified NEC P36.19
  - specified NEC P36.8
- Pasteurella multocida A28.0
- pelvic, puerperal, postpartum, childbirth O85
- pneumococcal A40.3 ☑
- postprocedural T81.44 ☑
- puerperal, postpartum, childbirth (pelvic) O85
- Salmonella (arizonae) (cholerae-suis) (enteritidis) (typhimurium) A02.1
- severe R65.20
  - with septic shock R65.21
- Shigella — *see also* Dysentery, bacillary A03.9
- skin, localized — *see* Abscess
- specified organism NEC A41.89
- Staphylococcus, staphylococcal A41.2
  - aureus (methicillin susceptible) (MSSA) A41.01
    - methicillin resistant (MRSA) A41.02
  - coagulase-negative A41.1
  - specified NEC A41.1
- Streptococcus, streptococcal A40.9
  - agalactiae A40.1
  - group
    - A A40.0
    - B A40.1
    - D A41.81
  - neonatal P36.10
    - group B P36.0
    - specified NEC P36.19
  - pneumoniae A40.3
  - pyogenes A40.0
  - specified NEC A40.8
- tracheostomy stoma J95.02
- tularemic A21.7
- umbilical, umbilical cord (newborn) — *see* Sepsis, newborn
- Yersinia pestis A20.7

Septate — *see* Septum
Septic — *see* condition
- arm — *see* Cellulitis, upper limb
  - with lymphangitis — *see* Lymphangitis, acute, upper limb
- embolus — *see* Embolism
- finger — *see* Cellulitis, digit
  - with lymphangitis — *see* Lymphangitis, acute, digit
- foot — *see* Cellulitis, lower limb
  - with lymphangitis — *see* Lymphangitis, acute, lower limb
- gallbladder (acute) K81.0
- hand — *see* Cellulitis, upper limb
  - with lymphangitis — *see* Lymphangitis, acute, upper limb
- joint — *see* Arthritis, pyogenic or pyemic
- leg — *see* Cellulitis, lower limb
  - with lymphangitis — *see* Lymphangitis, acute, lower limb
- nail — *see also* Cellulitis, digit
  - with lymphangitis — *see* Lymphangitis, acute, digit
- sore — *see also* Abscess
  - throat J02.0
    - streptococcal J02.0
- spleen (acute) D73.89
- teeth, tooth (pulpal origin) K04.4
- throat — *see* Pharyngitis
- thrombus — *see* Thrombosis
- toe — *see* Cellulitis, digit

Septic — *continued*
- toe — *see* Cellulitis, digit — *continued*
  - with lymphangitis — *see* Lymphangitis, acute, digit
- tonsils, chronic J35.01
  - with adenoiditis J35.03
- uterus — *see* Endometritis

Septicemia A41.9
- meaning sepsis — *see* Sepsis

Septum, septate (congenital) — *see also* Anomaly, by site
- anal Q42.3
  - with fistula Q42.2
- aqueduct of Sylvius Q03.0
  - with spina bifida — *see* Spina bifida, by site, with hydrocephalus
- uterus Q51.20
  - complete Q51.21
  - partial Q51.22
  - specified NEC Q51.28
- vagina Q52.10
  - in pregnancy — *see* Pregnancy, complicated by, abnormal vagina
    - causing obstructed labor O65.5
  - longitudinal Q52.129
    - microperforate
      - left side Q52.124
      - right side Q52.123
    - nonobstruction Q52.120
    - obstructing Q52.129
      - left side Q52.122
      - right side Q52.121
  - transverse Q52.11

Sequelae (of) — *see also* condition
- abscess, intracranial or intraspinal (conditions in G06) G09
- amputation — *code to* injury with seventh character S
- burn and corrosion — *code to* injury with seventh character S
- calcium deficiency E64.8
- cerebrovascular disease — *see* Sequelae, disease, cerebrovascular
- childbirth O94
- contusion — *code to* injury with seventh character S
- corrosion — *see* Sequelae, burn and corrosion
- crushing injury — *code to* injury with seventh character S
- disease
  - cerebrovascular I69.90
    - alteration of sensation I69.998
    - aphasia I69.920
    - apraxia I69.990
    - ataxia I69.993
    - cognitive deficits I69.91 ☑
    - disturbance of vision I69.998
    - dysarthria I69.922
    - dysphagia I69.991
    - dysphasia I69.921
    - facial droop I69.992
    - facial weakness I69.992
    - fluency disorder I69.923
    - hemiplegia I69.95- ☑
    - hemorrhage
      - intracerebral — *see* Sequelae, hemorrhage, intracerebral
      - intracranial, nontraumatic NEC — *see* Sequelae, hemorrhage, intracranial, nontraumatic
      - subarachnoid — *see* Sequelae, hemorrhage, subarachnoid
    - language deficit I69.928
    - monoplegia
      - lower limb I69.94- ☑
      - upper limb I69.93- ☑
    - paralytic syndrome I69.96- ☑
    - specified effect NEC I69.998
    - specified type NEC I69.80
      - alteration of sensation I69.898
      - aphasia I69.820
      - apraxia I69.890
      - ataxia I69.893
      - cognitive deficits I69.81 ☑
      - disturbance of vision I69.898
      - dysarthria I69.822
      - dysphagia I69.891
      - dysphasia I69.821
      - facial droop I69.892
      - facial weakness I69.892

Sequelae — *continued*
- disease — *continued*
  - cerebrovascular — *continued*
    - specified type — *continued*
      - fluency disorder I69.823
      - hemiplegia I69.85- ☑
      - language deficit I69.828
      - monoplegia
        - lower limb I69.84- ☑
        - upper limb I69.83- ☑
      - paralytic syndrome I69.86- ☑
      - specified effect NEC I69.898
    - speech deficit I69.928
      - speech deficit I69.828
    - stroke NOS — *see* Sequelae, stroke NOS
- dislocation — *code to* injury with seventh character S
- encephalitis or encephalomyelitis (conditions in G04) G09
  - in infectious disease NEC B94.8
  - viral B94.1
- external cause — *code to* injury with seventh character S
- foreign body entering natural orifice — *code to* injury with seventh character S
- fracture — *code to* injury with seventh character S
- frostbite — *code to* injury with seventh character S
- Hansen's disease B92
- hemorrhage
  - intracerebral I69.10
    - alteration of sensation I69.198
    - aphasia I69.120
    - apraxia I69.190
    - ataxia I69.193
    - cognitive deficits I69.11 ☑
    - disturbance of vision I69.198
    - dysarthria I69.122
    - dysphagia I69.191
    - dysphasia I69.121
    - facial droop I69.192
    - facial weakness I69.192
    - fluency disorder I69.123
    - hemiplegia I69.15- ☑
    - language deficit NEC I69.128
    - monoplegia
      - lower limb I69.14- ☑
      - upper limb I69.13- ☑
    - paralytic syndrome I69.16- ☑
    - specified effect NEC I69.198
    - speech deficit NEC I69.128
  - intracranial, nontraumatic NEC I69.20
    - alteration of sensation I69.298
    - aphasia I69.220
    - apraxia I69.290
    - ataxia I69.293
    - cognitive deficits I69.21 ☑
    - disturbance of vision I69.298
    - dysarthria I69.222
    - dysphagia I69.291
    - dysphasia I69.221
    - facial droop I69.292
    - facial weakness I69.292
    - fluency disorder I69.223
    - hemiplegia I69.25- ☑
    - language deficit NEC I69.228
    - monoplegia
      - lower limb I69.24- ☑
      - upper limb I69.23- ☑
    - paralytic syndrome I69.26- ☑
    - specified effect NEC I69.298
    - speech deficit NEC I69.228
  - subarachnoid I69.00
    - alteration of sensation I69.098
    - aphasia I69.020
    - apraxia I69.090
    - ataxia I69.093
    - cognitive deficits — *see* subcategory I69.01- ☑
    - disturbance of vision I69.098
    - dysarthria I69.022
    - dysphagia I69.091
    - dysphasia I69.021
    - facial droop I69.092
    - facial weakness I69.092
    - fluency disorder I69.023
    - hemiplegia I69.05- ☑
    - language deficit NEC I69.028
    - monoplegia
      - lower limb I69.04- ☑
      - upper limb I69.03- ☑

Sequelae — *continued*
  hemorrhage — *continued*
    subarachnoid — *continued*
      paralytic syndrome I69.06- ☑
      specified effect NEC I69.098
      speech deficit NEC I69.028
  hepatitis, viral B94.2
  hyperalimentation E68
  infarction
    cerebral I69.30
      alteration of sensation I69.398
      aphasia I69.320
      apraxia I69.390
      ataxia I69.393
      cognitive deficits I69.31 ☑
      disturbance of vision I69.398
      dysarthria I69.322
      dysphagia I69.391
      dysphasia I69.321
      facial droop I69.392
      facial weakness I69.392
      fluency disorder I69.323
      hemiplegia I69.35- ☑
      language deficit NEC I69.328
      monoplegia
        lower limb I69.34- ☑
        upper limb I69.33- ☑
      paralytic syndrome I69.36- ☑
      specified effect NEC I69.398
      speech deficit NEC I69.328
  infection, pyogenic, intracranial or intraspinal G09
  infectious disease B94.9
    specified NEC B94.8
  injury — *code to* injury with seventh character S
  leprosy B92
  meningitis
    bacterial (conditions in G00) G09
    other or unspecified cause (conditions in G03) G09
  muscle (and tendon) injury — *code to* injury with seventh character S
  myelitis — *see* Sequelae, encephalitis
  niacin deficiency E64.8
  nutritional deficiency E64.9
    specified NEC E64.8
  obstetrical condition O94
  parasitic disease B94.9
  phlebitis or thrombophlebitis of intracranial or intraspinal venous sinuses and veins (conditions in G08) G09
  poisoning — *code to* poisoning with seventh character S
    nonmedicinal substance — *see* Sequelae, toxic effect, nonmedicinal substance
  poliomyelitis (acute) B91
  pregnancy O94
  protein-energy malnutrition E64.0
  puerperium O94
  rickets E64.3
  selenium deficiency E64.8
  sprain and strain — *code to* injury with seventh character S
  stroke NOS I69.30
    alteration in sensation I69.398
    aphasia I69.320
    apraxia I69.390
    ataxia I69.393
    cognitive deficits I69.31 ☑
    disturbance of vision I69.398
    dysarthria I69.322
    dysphagia I69.391
    dysphasia I69.321
    facial droop I69.392
    facial weakness I69.392
    hemiplegia I69.35- ☑
    language deficit NEC I69.328
    monoplegia
      lower limb I69.34- ☑
      upper limb I69.33- ☑
    paralytic syndrome I69.36- ☑
    specified effect NEC I69.398
    speech deficit NEC I69.328
  tendon and muscle injury — *code to* injury with seventh character S
  thiamine deficiency E64.8
  trachoma B94.0
  tuberculosis B90.9
    bones and joints B90.2
    central nervous system B90.0

Sequelae — *continued*
  tuberculosis — *continued*
    genitourinary B90.1
    pulmonary (respiratory) B90.9
    specified organs NEC B90.8
  viral
    encephalitis B94.1
    hepatitis B94.2
  vitamin deficiency NEC E64.8
    A E64.1
    B E64.8
    C E64.2
  wound, open — *code to* injury with seventh character S
Sequestration — *see also* Sequestrum
  disk — *see* Displacement, intervertebral disk
  lung, congenital Q33.2
Sequestrum
  bone — *see* Osteomyelitis, chronic
  dental M27.2
  jaw bone M27.2
  orbit — *see* Osteomyelitis, orbit
  sinus (accessory) (nasal) — *see* Sinusitis
Sequoiosis lung or pneumonitis J67.8
Serology for syphilis
  doubtful
    with signs or symptoms — *code by* site and stage under Syphilis
    follow-up of latent syphilis — *see* Syphilis, latent
  negative, with signs or symptoms — *code by* site and stage under Syphilis
  positive A53.0
    with signs or symptoms — *code by* site and stage under Syphilis
  reactivated A53.0
Seroma — *see also* Hematoma
  postprocedural — *see* Complication, postprocedural, seroma
  traumatic, secondary and recurrent T79.2 ☑
Seropurulent — *see* condition
Serositis, multiple K65.8
  pericardial I31.1
  peritoneal K65.8
Serous — *see* condition
Sertoli cell
  adenoma
    specified site — *see* Neoplasm, benign, by site
    unspecified site
      female D27.9
      male D29.20
  carcinoma
    specified site — *see* Neoplasm, malignant, by site
    unspecified site (male) C62.9- ☑
      female C56.9
  tumor
    with lipid storage
      specified site — *see* Neoplasm, benign, by site
      unspecified site
        female D27.9
        male D29.20
    specified site — *see* Neoplasm, benign, by site
    unspecified site
      female D27.9
      male D29.20
Sertoli-Leydig cell tumor — *see* Neoplasm, benign, by site
  specified site — *see* Neoplasm, benign, by site
  unspecified site
    female D27.9
    male D29.20
Serum
  allergy, allergic reaction — *see also* Reaction, serum T80.69 ☑
    shock — *see also* Shock, anaphylactic T80.59 ☑
  arthritis — *see also* Reaction, serum T80.69 ☑
  complication or reaction NEC — *see also* Reaction, serum T80.69 ☑
  disease NEC — *see also* Reaction, serum T80.69 ☑
  hepatitis — *see* Hepatitis, viral, type B
    carrier (suspected) of B18.1
  intoxication — *see also* Reaction, serum T80.69 ☑
  neuritis — *see also* Reaction, serum T80.69 ☑
  neuropathy G61.1
  poisoning NEC — *see also* Reaction, serum T80.69 ☑
  rash NEC — *see also* Reaction, serum T80.69 ☑
  reaction NEC — *see also* Reaction, serum T80.69 ☑
  sickness NEC — *see also* Reaction, serum T80.69 ☑

Serum — *continued*
  urticaria — *see also* Reaction, serum T80.69 ☑
Sesamoiditis M25.8- ☑
Severe sepsis R65.20
  with septic shock R65.21
Sever's disease or osteochondrosis — *see* Osteochondrosis, juvenile, tarsus
Sex
  chromosome mosaics Q97.8
    lines with various numbers of X chromosomes Q97.2
  education Z70.8
  reassignment surgery status Z87.890
Sextuplet pregnancy — *see* Pregnancy, sextuplet
Sexual
  function, disorder of (psychogenic) F52.9
  immaturity (female) (male) E30.0
  impotence (psychogenic) organic origin NEC — *see* Dysfunction, sexual, male
  precocity (constitutional) (cryptogenic)(female) (idiopathic) (male) E30.1
Sexuality, pathologic — *see* Deviation, sexual
Sézary disease C84.1- ☑
Shadow, lung R91.8
Shaking palsy or paralysis — *see* Parkinsonism
Shallowness, acetabulum — *see* Derangement, joint, specified type NEC, hip
Shaver's disease J63.1
Sheath (tendon) — *see* condition
Sheathing, retinal vessels H35.01- ☑
Shedding
  nail L60.8
  premature, primary (deciduous) teeth K00.6
Sheehan's disease or syndrome E23.0
Shelf, rectal K62.89
Shell teeth K00.5
Shellshock (current) F43.0
  lasting state — *see* Disorder, post-traumatic stress
Shield kidney Q63.1
Shift
  auditory threshold (temporary) H93.24- ☑
  mediastinal R93.89
Shifting sleep-work schedule (affecting sleep) G47.26
Shiga (-Kruse) **dysentery** A03.0
Shiga's bacillus A03.0
Shigella (dysentery) — *see* Dysentery, bacillary
Shigellosis A03.9
  Group A A03.0
  Group B A03.1
  Group C A03.2
  Group D A03.3
Shin splints S86.89- ☑
Shingles — *see* Herpes, zoster
Shipyard disease or eye B30.0
Shirodkar suture, in pregnancy — *see* Pregnancy, complicated by, incompetent cervix
Shock R57.9
  with ectopic or molar pregnancy O08.3
  adrenal (cortical) (Addisonian) E27.2
  adverse food reaction (anaphylactic) — *see* Shock, anaphylactic, due to food
  allergic — *see* Shock, anaphylactic
  anaphylactic T78.2 ☑
    chemical — *see* Table of Drugs and Chemicals
    due to drug or medicinal substance
      correct substance properly administered T88.6 ☑
      overdose or wrong substance given or taken (by accident) — *see* Table of Drugs and Chemicals, by drug, poisoning
    due to food (nonpoisonous) T78.00 ☑
      additives T78.06 ☑
      dairy products T78.07 ☑
      eggs T78.08 ☑
      fish T78.03 ☑
        shellfish T78.02 ☑
      fruit T78.04 ☑
      milk T78.07 ☑
      nuts T78.05 ☑
        multiple types T78.05 ☑
        peanuts T78.01 ☑
      peanuts T78.01 ☑
      seeds T78.05 ☑
      specified type NEC T78.09 ☑
      vegetable T78.04 ☑
    following sting(s) — *see* Venom
    immunization T80.52 ☑
    serum T80.59 ☑
      blood and blood products T80.51 ☑

▽ Subterms under main terms may continue to next column or page   ☑ Additional Character Required — Refer to the Tabular List for Character Selection   285

Sequelae — Shock

Shock — *continued*
- anaphylactic — *continued*
  - serum — *continued*
    - immunization T80.52 ☑
    - specified NEC T80.59 ☑
    - vaccination T80.52 ☑
- anaphylactoid — *see* Shock, anaphylactic
- anesthetic
  - correct substance properly administered T88.2 ☑
  - overdose or wrong substance given or taken — *see* Table of Drugs and Chemicals, by drug, poisoning
  - specified anesthetic — *see* Table of Drugs and Chemicals, by drug, poisoning
- cardiogenic R57.0
- chemical substance — *see* Table of Drugs and Chemicals
- complicating ectopic or molar pregnancy O08.3
- culture — *see* Disorder, adjustment
- drug
  - due to correct substance properly administered T88.6 ☑
  - overdose or wrong substance given or taken (by accident) — *see* Table of Drugs and Chemicals, by drug, poisoning
- during or after labor and delivery O75.1
- electric T75.4 ☑
  - (taser) T75.4 ☑
- endotoxic R65.21
  - postprocedural (resulting from a procedure, not elsewhere classified) T81.12 ☑
- following
  - ectopic or molar pregnancy O08.3
  - injury (immediate) (delayed) T79.4 ☑
  - labor and delivery O75.1
- food (anaphylactic) — *see* Shock, anaphylactic, due to food
- from electroshock gun (taser) T75.4 ☑
- gram-negative R65.21
  - postprocedural (resulting from a procedure, not elsewhere classified) T81.12 ☑
- hematologic R57.8
- hemorrhagic R57.8
  - surgery (intraoperative) (postoperative) T81.19 ☑
  - trauma T79.4 ☑
- hypovolemic R57.1
  - surgical T81.19 ☑
  - traumatic T79.4 ☑
- insulin E15
  - therapeutic misadventure — *see* subcategory T38.3 ☑
- kidney N17.0
  - traumatic (following crushing) T79.5 ☑
- lightning T75.01 ☑
- liver K72.00
- lung J80
- obstetric O75.1
  - with ectopic or molar pregnancy O08.3
  - following ectopic or molar pregnancy O08.3
- pleural (surgical) T81.19 ☑
  - due to trauma T79.4 ☑
- postprocedural (postoperative) T81.10 ☑
  - with ectopic or molar pregnancy O08.3
  - cardiogenic T81.11 ☑
  - endotoxic T81.12 ☑
  - following ectopic or molar pregnancy O08.3
  - gram-negative T81.12 ☑
  - hypovolemic T81.19 ☑
  - septic T81.12 ☑
  - specified type NEC T81.19 ☑
- psychic F43.0
- septic (due to severe sepsis) R65.21
- specified NEC R57.8
- surgical T81.10 ☑
- taser gun (taser) T75.4 ☑
- therapeutic misadventure NEC T81.10 ☑
- thyroxin
  - overdose or wrong substance given or taken — *see* Table of Drugs and Chemicals, by drug, poisoning
- toxic, syndrome A48.3
- transfusion — *see* Complications, transfusion
- traumatic (immediate) (delayed) T79.4 ☑

Shoemaker's chest M95.4

Short, shortening, shortness
- arm (acquired) — *see also* Deformity, limb, unequal length

Short, shortening, shortness — *continued*
- arm — *see also* Deformity, limb, unequal length — *continued*
  - congenital Q71.81- ☑
  - forearm — *see* Deformity, limb, unequal length
- bowel syndrome K91.2
- breath R06.02
- cervical (complicating pregnancy) O26.87- ☑
  - non-gravid uterus N88.3
- common bile duct, congenital Q44.5
- cord (umbilical), complicating delivery O69.3 ☑
- cystic duct, congenital Q44.5
- esophagus (congenital) Q39.8
- femur (acquired) — *see* Deformity, limb, unequal length, femur
  - congenital — *see* Defect, reduction, lower limb, longitudinal, femur
- frenum, frenulum, linguae (congenital) Q38.1
- hip (acquired) — *see also* Deformity, limb, unequal length
  - congenital Q65.89
- leg (acquired) — *see also* Deformity, limb, unequal length
  - congenital Q72.81- ☑
  - lower leg — *see also* Deformity, limb, unequal length
- limbed stature, with immunodeficiency D82.2
- lower limb (acquired) — *see also* Deformity, limb, unequal length
  - congenital Q72.81- ☑
- organ or site, congenital NEC — *see* Distortion
- palate, congenital Q38.5
- radius (acquired) — *see also* Deformity, limb, unequal length
  - congenital — *see* Defect, reduction, upper limb, longitudinal, radius
- rib syndrome Q77.2
- stature (child) (hereditary) (idiopathic) NEC R62.52
  - constitutional E34.3
  - due to endocrine disorder E34.3
  - Laron-type E34.3
- tendon — *see also* Contraction, tendon
  - with contracture of joint — *see* Contraction, joint
  - Achilles (acquired) M67.0- ☑
    - congenital Q66.89
  - congenital Q79.8
- thigh (acquired) — *see also* Deformity, limb, unequal length, femur
  - congenital — *see* Defect, reduction, lower limb, longitudinal, femur
- tibialis anterior (tendon) — *see* Contraction, tendon
- umbilical cord
  - complicating delivery O69.3 ☑
- upper limb, congenital — *see* Defect, reduction, upper limb, specified type NEC
- urethra N36.8
- uvula, congenital Q38.5
- vagina (congenital) Q52.4

Shortsightedness — *see* Myopia

Shoshin (acute fulminating beriberi) E51.11

Shoulder — *see* condition

Shovel-shaped incisors K00.2

Shower, thromboembolic — *see* Embolism

Shunt
- arterial-venous (dialysis) Z99.2
- arteriovenous, pulmonary (acquired) I28.0
  - congenital Q25.72
- cerebral ventricle (communicating) in situ Z98.2
- surgical, prosthetic, with complications — *see* Complications, cardiovascular, device or implant

Shutdown, renal N28.9

Shy-Drager syndrome G90.3

Sialadenitis, sialadenosis (any gland) (chronic) (periodic) (suppurative) — *see* Sialoadenitis

Sialectasia K11.8

Sialidosis E77.1

Sialitis, silitis (any gland) (chronic) (suppurative) — *see* Sialoadenitis

Sialoadenitis (any gland) (periodic) (suppurative) K11.20
- acute K11.21
  - recurrent K11.22
- chronic K11.23

Sialoadenopathy K11.9

Sialoangitis — *see* Sialoadenitis

Sialodochitis (fibrinosa) — *see* Sialoadenitis

Sialodocholithiasis K11.5

Sialolithiasis K11.5

Sialometaplasia, necrotizing K11.8

Sialorrhea — *see also* Ptyalism
- periodic — *see* Sialoadenitis

Sialosis K11.7

Siamese twin Q89.4

Sibling rivalry Z62.891

Sicard's syndrome G52.7

Sicca syndrome M35.00
- with
  - keratoconjunctivitis M35.01
  - lung involvement M35.02
  - myopathy M35.03
  - renal tubulo-interstitial disorders M35.04
- specified organ involvement NEC M35.09

Sick R69
- or handicapped person in family Z63.79
  - needing care at home Z63.6
- sinus (syndrome) I49.5

Sick-euthyroid syndrome E07.81

Sickle-cell
- anemia — *see* Disease, sickle-cell
- trait D57.3

Sicklemia — *see also* Disease, sickle-cell
- trait D57.3

Sickness
- air (travel) T75.3 ☑
- airplane T75.3 ☑
- alpine T70.29 ☑
- altitude T70.20 ☑
- Andes T70.29 ☑
- aviator's T70.29 ☑
- balloon T70.29 ☑
- car T75.3 ☑
- compressed air T70.3 ☑
- decompression T70.3 ☑
- green D50.8
- milk — *see* Poisoning, food, noxious
- motion T75.3 ☑
- mountain T70.29 ☑
  - acute D75.1
- protein — *see also* Reaction, serum T80.69 ☑
- radiation T66 ☑
- roundabout (motion) T75.3 ☑
- sea T75.3 ☑
- serum NEC — *see also* Reaction, serum T80.69 ☑
- sleeping (African) B56.9
  - by Trypanosoma B56.9
    - brucei
      - gambiense B56.0
      - rhodesiense B56.1
    - East African B56.1
    - Gambian B56.0
    - Rhodesian B56.1
    - West African B56.0
- swing (motion) T75.3 ☑
- train (railway) (travel) T75.3 ☑
- travel (any vehicle) T75.3 ☑

Sideropenia — *see* Anemia, iron deficiency

Siderosilicosis J62.8

Siderosis (lung) J63.4
- eye (globe) — *see* Disorder, globe, degenerative, siderosis

Siemens' syndrome (ectodermal dysplasia) Q82.8

Sighing R06.89
- psychogenic F45.8

Sigmoid — *see also* condition
- flexure — *see* condition
- kidney Q63.1

Sigmoiditis — *see also* Enteritis K52.9
- infectious A09
- noninfectious K52.9

Silfversköld's syndrome Q78.9

Silicosiderosis J62.8

Silicosis, silicotic (simple) (complicated) J62.8
- with tuberculosis J65

Silicotuberculosis J65

Silo-fillers' disease J68.8
- bronchitis J68.0
- pneumonitis J68.0
- pulmonary edema J68.1

Silver's syndrome Q87.19

Simian malaria B53.1

Simmonds' cachexia or disease E23.0

Simons' disease or syndrome (progressive lipodystrophy) E88.1

Simple, simplex — *see* condition

Simulation, conscious (of illness) Z76.5

286

☑ **Additional Character Required** — Refer to the Tabular List for Character Selection   ▽ **Subterms under main terms may continue to next column or page**

Simultanagnosia (asimultagnosia) R48.3
Sin Nombre virus disease (Hantavirus) (cardio)-pulmonary syndrome) B33.4
Sinding-Larsen disease or osteochondrosis — *see* Osteochondrosis, juvenile, patella
Singapore hemorrhagic fever A91
Singer's node or nodule J38.2
Single
  atrium Q21.2
  coronary artery Q24.5
  umbilical artery Q27.0
  ventricle Q20.4
Singultus R06.6
  epidemicus B33.0
Sinus — *see also* Fistula
  abdominal K63.89
  arrest I45.5
  arrhythmia I49.8
  bradycardia R00.1
  branchial cleft (internal) (external) Q18.0
  coccygeal — *see* Sinus, pilonidal
  dental K04.6
  dermal (congenital) Q06.8
    with abscess Q06.8
    coccygeal, pilonidal — *see* Sinus, coccygeal
  infected, skin NEC L08.89
  marginal, ruptured or bleeding — *see* Hemorrhage, antepartum, specified cause NEC
  medial, face and neck Q18.8
  pause I45.5
  pericranii Q01.9
  pilonidal (infected) (rectum) L05.92
    with abscess L05.02
  preauricular Q18.1
  rectovaginal N82.3
  Rokitansky-Aschoff (gallbladder) K82.8
  sacrococcygeal (dermoid) (infected) — *see* Sinus, pilonidal
  tachycardia R00.0
    paroxysmal I47.1
  tarsi syndrome M25.57- ☑
  testis N50.89
  tract (postinfective) — *see* Fistula
  urachus Q64.4
Sinusitis (accessory) (chronic) (hyperplastic) (nasal) (nonpurulent) (purulent) J32.9
  acute J01.90
    ethmoidal J01.20
      recurrent J01.21
    frontal J01.10
      recurrent J01.11
    involving more than one sinus, other than pansinusitis J01.80
      recurrent J01.81
    maxillary J01.00
      recurrent J01.01
    pansinusitis J01.40
      recurrent J01.41
    recurrent J01.91
    specified NEC J01.80
      recurrent J01.81
    sphenoidal J01.30
      recurrent J01.31
  allergic — *see* Rhinitis, allergic
  due to high altitude T70.1 ☑
  ethmoidal J32.2
    acute J01.20
      recurrent J01.21
  frontal J32.1
    acute J01.10
      recurrent J01.11
  influenzal — *see* Influenza, with, respiratory manifestations NEC
  involving more than one sinus but not pansinusitis J32.8
    acute J01.80
      recurrent J01.81
  maxillary J32.0
    acute J01.00
      recurrent J01.01
  sphenoidal J32.3
    acute J01.30
      recurrent J01.31
  tuberculous, any sinus A15.8
Sinusitis-bronchiectasis-situs inversus (syndrome) (triad) Q89.3
Sipple's syndrome E31.22
Sirenomelia (syndrome) Q87.2

Siriasis T67.01 ☑
Sirkari's disease B55.0
Siti A65
Situation, psychiatric F99
Situational
  disturbance (transient) — *see* Disorder, adjustment
    acute F43.0
  maladjustment — *see* Disorder, adjustment
  reaction — *see* Disorder, adjustment
    acute F43.0
Situs inversus or transversus (abdominalis) (thoracis) Q89.3
Sixth disease B08.20
  due to human herpesvirus 6 B08.21
  due to human herpesvirus 7 B08.22
Sjögren-Larsson syndrome Q87.19
Sjögren's syndrome or disease — *see* Sicca syndrome
Skeletal — *see* condition
Skene's gland — *see* condition
Skenitis — *see* Urethritis
Skerljevo A65
Skevas-Zerfus disease — *see* Toxicity, venom, marine animal, sea anemone
Skin — *see also* condition
  clammy R23.1
  donor — *see* Donor, skin
  hidebound M35.9
Slate-dressers' or slate-miners' lung J62.8
Sleep
  apnea — *see* Apnea, sleep
  deprivation Z72.820
  disorder or disturbance G47.9
    child F51.9
    nonorganic origin F51.9
    specified NEC G47.8
  disturbance G47.9
    nonorganic origin F51.9
  drunkenness F51.9
  rhythm inversion G47.2- ☑
  terrors F51.4
  walking F51.3
    hysterical F44.89
Sleep hygiene
  abuse Z72.821
  inadequate Z72.821
  poor Z72.821
Sleeping sickness — *see* Sickness, sleeping
Sleeplessness — *see* Insomnia
  menopausal N95.1
Sleep-wake schedule disorder G47.20
Slim disease (in HIV infection) B20
Slipped, slipping
  epiphysis (traumatic) — *see also* Osteochondropathy, specified type NEC
    capital femoral (traumatic)
      acute (on chronic) S79.01- ☑
    current traumatic — *code as* Fracture, by site
    upper femoral (nontraumatic) M93.00- ☑
      acute M93.01- ☑
        on chronic M93.03- ☑
      chronic M93.02- ☑
  intervertebral disc — *see* Displacement, intervertebral disc
  ligature, umbilical P51.8
  patella — *see* Disorder, patella, derangement NEC
  rib M89.8X8
  sacroiliac joint — *see* subcategory M53.2 ☑
  tendon — *see* Disorder, tendon
  ulnar nerve, nontraumatic — *see* Lesion, nerve, ulnar
  vertebra NEC — *see* Spondylolisthesis
Slocumb's syndrome E27.0
Sloughing (multiple) (phagedena) (skin) — *see also* Gangrene
  abscess — *see* Abscess
  appendix K38.8
  fascia — *see* Disorder, soft tissue, specified type NEC
  scrotum N50.89
  tendon — *see* Disorder, tendon
  transplanted organ — *see* Rejection, transplant
  ulcer — *see* Ulcer, skin
Slow
  feeding, newborn P92.2
  flow syndrome, coronary I20.8
  heart (beat) R00.1
Slowing, urinary stream R39.198
Sluder's neuralgia (syndrome) G44.89
Slurred, slurring speech R47.81

Small (ness)
  for gestational age — *see* Small for dates
  introitus, vagina N89.6
  kidney (unknown cause) N27.9
    bilateral N27.1
    unilateral N27.0
  ovary (congenital) Q50.39
  pelvis
    with disproportion (fetopelvic) O33.1
      causing obstructed labor O65.1
  uterus N85.8
  white kidney N03.9
Small-and-light-for-dates — *see* Small for dates
Small-for-dates (infant) P05.10
  with weight of
    499 grams or less P05.11
    500-749 grams P05.12
    750-999 grams P05.13
    1000-1249 grams P05.14
    1250-1499 grams P05.15
    1500-1749 grams P05.16
    1750-1999 grams P05.17
    2000-2499 grams P05.18
    2500 grams and over P05.19
  specified NEC P05.19
Smallpox B03
Smearing, fecal R15.1
Smith-Lemli-Opitz syndrome E78.72
Smith's fracture S52.54- ☑
Smoker — *see* Dependence, drug, nicotine
Smoker's
  bronchitis J41.0
  cough J41.0
  palate K13.24
  throat J31.2
  tongue K13.24
Smoking
  passive Z77.22
Smothering spells R06.81
Snaggle teeth, tooth M26.39
Snapping
  finger — *see* Trigger finger
  hip — *see* Derangement, joint, specified type NEC, hip
    involving the iliotiblial band M76.3- ☑
  knee — *see* Derangement, knee
    involving the iliotiblial band M76.3- ☑
Sneddon-Wilkinson disease or syndrome (sub-corneal pustular dermatosis) L13.1
Sneezing (intractable) R06.7
Sniffing
  cocaine
    abuse — *see* Abuse, drug, cocaine
    dependence — *see* Dependence, drug, cocaine
  gasoline
    abuse — *see* Abuse, drug, inhalant
    dependence — *see* Dependence, drug, inhalant
  glue (airplane)
    abuse — *see* Abuse, drug, inhalant
    drug dependence — *see* Dependence, drug, inhalant
Sniffles
  newborn P28.89
Snoring R06.83
Snow blindness — *see* Photokeratitis
Snuffles (non-syphilitic) R06.5
  newborn P28.89
  syphilitic (infant) A50.05 *[J99]*
Social
  exclusion Z60.4
    due to discrimination or persecution (perceived) Z60.5
  migrant Z59.0
    acculturation difficulty Z60.3
  rejection Z60.4
    due to discrimination or persecution Z60.5
  role conflict NEC Z73.5
  skills inadequacy NEC Z73.4
  transplantation Z60.3
Sodoku A25.0
Soemmerring's ring — *see* Cataract, secondary
Soft — *see also* condition
  nails L60.3
Softening
  bone — *see* Osteomalacia
  brain (necrotic) (progressive) G93.89
    congenital Q04.8
    embolic I63.4- ☑

Softening — *continued*
  brain — *continued*
    hemorrhagic — *see* Hemorrhage, intracranial, intracerebral
    occlusive I63.5- ☑
    thrombotic I63.3- ☑
    cartilage M94.2- ☑
      patella M22.4- ☑
    cerebellar — *see* Softening, brain
    cerebral — *see* Softening, brain
    cerebrospinal — *see* Softening, brain
    myocardial, heart — *see* Degeneration, myocardial
    spinal cord G95.89
    stomach K31.89
Soldier's
  heart F45.8
  patches I31.0
Solitary
  cyst, kidney N28.1
  kidney, congenital Q60.0
Solvent abuse — *see* Abuse, drug, inhalant
  dependence — *see* Dependence, drug, inhalant
Somatization reaction, somatic reaction — *see* Disorder, somatoform
Somnambulism F51.3
  hysterical F44.89
Somnolence R40.0
  nonorganic origin F51.11
Sonne dysentery A03.3
Soor B37.0
Sore
  bed — *see* Ulcer, pressure, by site
  chiclero B55.1
  Delhi B55.1
  desert — *see* Ulcer, skin
  eye H57.1- ☑
  Lahore B55.1
  mouth K13.79
    canker K12.0
  muscle M79.10
  Naga — *see* Ulcer, skin
  of skin — *see* Ulcer, skin
  oriental B55.1
  pressure — *see* Ulcer, pressure, by site
  skin L98.9
  soft A57
  throat (acute) — *see also* Pharyngitis
    with influenza, flu, or grippe — *see* Influenza, with, respiratory manifestations NEC
    chronic J31.2
    coxsackie (virus) B08.5
    diphtheritic A36.0
    herpesviral B00.2
    influenzal — *see* Influenza, with, respiratory manifestations NEC
    septic J02.0
    streptococcal (ulcerative) J02.0
    viral NEC J02.8
      coxsackie B08.5
  tropical — *see* Ulcer, skin
  veldt — *see* Ulcer, skin
Soto's syndrome (cerebral gigantism) Q87.3
South African cardiomyopathy syndrome I42.8
Southeast Asian hemorrhagic fever A91
Spacing
  abnormal, tooth, teeth, fully erupted M26.30
  excessive, tooth, fully erupted M26.32
Spade-like hand (congenital) Q68.1
Spading nail L60.8
  congenital Q84.6
Spanish collar N47.1
Sparganosis B70.1
Spasm(s), spastic, spasticity — *see also* condition R25.2
  accommodation — *see* Spasm, of accommodation
  ampulla of Vater K83.4
  anus, ani (sphincter) (reflex) K59.4
    psychogenic F45.8
  artery I73.9
    cerebral G45.9
  Bell's G51.3- ☑
  bladder (sphincter, external or internal) N32.89
    psychogenic F45.8
  bronchus, bronchiole J98.01
  cardia K22.0
  cardiac I20.1
  carpopedal — *see* Tetany
  cerebral (arteries) (vascular) G45.9

Spasm(s), spastic, spasticity — *continued*
  cervix, complicating delivery O62.4
  ciliary body (of accommodation) — *see* Spasm, of accommodation
  colon — *see also* Irritable, bowel K58.9
    with diarrhea K58.0
    psychogenic F45.8
  common duct K83.8
  compulsive — *see* Tic
  conjugate H51.8
  coronary (artery) I20.1
  diaphragm (reflex) R06.6
    epidemic B33.0
    psychogenic F45.8
  duodenum K59.8
  epidemic diaphragmatic (transient) B33.0
  esophagus (diffuse) K22.4
    psychogenic F45.8
  facial G51.3- ☑
  fallopian tube N83.8
  gastrointestinal (tract) K31.89
    psychogenic F45.8
  glottis J38.5
    hysterical F44.4
    psychogenic F45.8
      conversion reaction F44.4
    reflex through recurrent laryngeal nerve J38.5
  habit — *see* Tic
  heart I20.1
  hemifacial (clonic) G51.3- ☑
  hourglass — *see* Contraction, hourglass
  hysterical F44.4
  infantile — *see* Epilepsy, spasms
  inferior oblique, eye H51.8
  intestinal — *see also* Syndrome, irritable bowel K58.9
    psychogenic F45.8
  larynx, laryngeal J38.5
    hysterical F44.4
    psychogenic F45.8
      conversion reaction F44.4
  levator palpebrae superioris — *see* Disorder, eyelid function
  muscle NEC M62.838
    back M62.830
  nerve, trigeminal G51.0
  nervous F45.8
  nodding F98.4
  occupational F48.8
  oculogyric H51.8
    psychogenic F45.8
  of accommodation H52.53- ☑
  ophthalmic artery — *see* Occlusion, artery, retina
  perineal, female N94.89
  peroneo-extensor — *see also* Deformity, limb, flat foot
  pharynx (reflex) J39.2
    hysterical F45.8
    psychogenic F45.8
  psychogenic F45.8
  pylorus NEC K31.3
    adult hypertrophic K31.89
    congenital or infantile Q40.0
    psychogenic F45.8
  rectum (sphincter) K59.4
    psychogenic F45.8
  retinal (artery) — *see* Occlusion, artery, retina
  sigmoid — *see also* Syndrome, irritable bowel K58.9
    psychogenic F45.8
  sphincter of Oddi K83.4
  stomach K31.89
    neurotic F45.8
  throat J39.2
    hysterical F45.8
    psychogenic F45.8
  tic F95.9
    chronic F95.1
    transient of childhood F95.0
  tongue K14.8
  torsion (progressive) G24.1
  trigeminal nerve — *see* Neuralgia, trigeminal
  ureter N13.5
  urethra (sphincter) N35.919
  uterus N85.8
    complicating labor O62.4
  vagina N94.2
    psychogenic F52.5
  vascular I73.9
  vasomotor I73.9
  vein NEC I87.8

Spasm(s), spastic, spasticity — *continued*
  viscera — *see* Pain, abdominal
Spasmodic — *see* condition
Spasmophilia — *see* Tetany
Spasmus nutans F98.4
Spastic, spasticity — *see also* Spasm
  child (cerebral) (congenital) (paralysis) G80.1
Speaker's throat R49.8
Specific, specified — *see* condition
Speech
  defect, disorder, disturbance, impediment R47.9
    psychogenic, in childhood and adolescence F98.8
    slurring R47.81
    specified NEC R47.89
Spencer's disease A08.19
Spens' syndrome (syncope with heart block) I45.9
Sperm counts (fertility testing) Z31.41
  postvasectomy Z30.8
    reversal Z31.42
Spermatic cord — *see* condition
Spermatocele N43.40
  congenital Q55.4
  multiple N43.42
  single N43.41
Spermatocystitis N49.0
Spermatocytoma C62.9- ☑
  specified site — *see* Neoplasm, malignant, by site
Spermatorrhea N50.89
Sphacelus — *see* Gangrene
Sphenoidal — *see* condition
Sphenoiditis (chronic) — *see* Sinusitis, sphenoidal
Sphenopalatine ganglion neuralgia G90.09
Sphericity, increased, lens (congenital) Q12.4
Spherocytosis (congenital) (familial) (hereditary) D58.0
  hemoglobin disease D58.0
  sickle-cell (disease) D57.8- ☑
Spherophakia Q12.4
Sphincter — *see* condition
Sphincteritis, sphincter of Oddi — *see* Cholangitis
Sphingolipidosis E75.3
  specified NEC E75.29
Sphingomyelinosis E75.3
Spicule tooth K00.2
Spider
  bite — *see* Toxicity, venom, spider
  fingers — *see* Syndrome, Marfan's
  nevus I78.1
  toes — *see* Syndrome, Marfan's
  vascular I78.1
Spiegler-Fendt
  benign lymphocytoma L98.8
  sarcoid L08.89
Spielmeyer-Vogt disease E75.4
Spina bifida (aperta) Q05.9
  with hydrocephalus NEC Q05.4
  cervical Q05.5
    with hydrocephalus Q05.0
  dorsal Q05.6
    with hydrocephalus Q05.1
  lumbar Q05.7
    with hydrocephalus Q05.2
  lumbosacral Q05.7
    with hydrocephalus Q05.2
  occulta Q76.0
  sacral Q05.8
    with hydrocephalus Q05.3
  thoracic Q05.6
    with hydrocephalus Q05.1
  thoracolumbar Q05.6
    with hydrocephalus Q05.1
Spindle, Krukenberg's — *see* Pigmentation, cornea, posterior
Spine, spinal — *see* condition
Spiradenoma (eccrine) — *see* Neoplasm, skin, benign
Spirillosis A25.0
Spirillum
  minus A25.0
  obermeieri infection A68.0
Spirochetal — *see* condition
Spirochetosis A69.9
  arthritic, arthritica A69.9
  bronchopulmonary A69.8
  icterohemorrhagic A27.0
  lung A69.8
Spirometrosis B70.1
Spitting blood — *see* Hemoptysis
Splanchnoptosis K63.4

Spleen, splenic — *see* condition
Splenectasis — *see* Splenomegaly
Splenitis (interstitial) (malignant) (nonspecific) D73.89
  malarial — *see also* Malaria B54 *[D77]*
  tuberculous A18.85
Splenocele D73.89
Splenomegaly, splenomegalia (Bengal) (cryptogenic)
    (idiopathic) (tropical) R16.1
  with hepatomegaly R16.2
  cirrhotic D73.2
  congenital Q89.09
  congestive, chronic D73.2
  Egyptian B65.1
  Gaucher's E75.22
  malarial — *see also* Malaria B54 *[D77]*
  neutropenic D73.81
  Niemann-Pick — *see* Niemann-Pick disease or syn-
      drome
  siderotic D73.2
  syphilitic A52.79
    congenital (early) A50.08 *[D77]*
Splenopathy D73.9
Splenoptosis D73.89
Splenosis D73.89
Splinter — *see* Foreign body, superficial, by site
Split, splitting
  foot Q72.7- ☑
  hand Q71.6 ☑
  heart sounds R01.2
  lip, congenital — *see* Cleft, lip
  nails L60.3
  urinary stream R39.13
Spondylarthrosis — *see* Spondylosis
Spondylitis (chronic) — *see also* Spondylopathy, inflam-
    matory
  ankylopoietica — *see* Spondylitis, ankylosing
  ankylosing (chronic) M45.9
    with lung involvement M45.9 *[J99]*
    cervical region M45.2
    cervicothoracic region M45.3
    juvenile M08.1
    lumbar region M45.6
    lumbosacral region M45.7
    multiple sites M45.0
    occipito-atlanto-axial region M45.1
    sacrococcygeal region M45.8
    thoracic region M45.4
    thoracolumbar region M45.5
  atrophic (ligamentous) — *see* Spondylitis, ankylosing
  deformans (chronic) — *see* Spondylosis
  gonococcal A54.41
  gouty — *see also* Gout, by type, vertebrae M10.08
  in (due to)
    brucellosis A23.9 *[M49.80]*
      cervical region A23.9 *[M49.82]*
      cervicothoracic region A23.9 *[M49.83]*
      lumbar region A23.9 *[M49.86]*
      lumbosacral region A23.9 *[M49.87]*
      multiple sites A23.9 *[M49.89]*
      occipito-atlanto-axial region A23.9 *[M49.81]*
      sacrococcygeal region A23.9 *[M49.88]*
      thoracic region A23.9 *[M49.84]*
      thoracolumbar region A23.9 *[M49.85]*
    enterobacteria — *see also* subcategory M49.8 A04.9
    tuberculosis A18.01
  infectious NEC — *see* Spondylopathy, infective
  juvenile ankylosing (chronic) M08.1
  Kümmell's — *see* Spondylopathy, traumatic
  Marie-Strümpell — *see* Spondylitis, ankylosing
  muscularis — *see* Spondylopathy, specified NEC
  psoriatic L40.53
  rheumatoid — *see* Spondylitis, ankylosing
  rhizomelica — *see* Spondylitis, ankylosing
  sacroiliac NEC M46.1
  senescent, senile — *see* Spondylosis
  traumatic (chronic) or post-traumatic — *see* Spondy-
      lopathy, traumatic
  tuberculous A18.01
  typhosa A01.05
Spondylolisthesis (acquired) (degenerative) M43.10
  with disproportion (fetopelvic) O33.0
    causing obstructed labor O65.0
  cervical region M43.12
  cervicothoracic region M43.13
  congenital Q76.2
  lumbar region M43.16
  lumbosacral region M43.17

Spondylolisthesis — *continued*
  multiple sites M43.19
  occipito-atlanto-axial region M43.11
  sacrococcygeal region M43.18
  thoracic region M43.14
  thoracolumbar region M43.15
  traumatic (old) M43.10
    acute
      fifth cervical (displaced) S12.430 ☑
        nondisplaced S12.431 ☑
        specified type NEC (displaced) S12.450 ☑
          nondisplaced S12.451 ☑
        type III S12.44 ☑
      fourth cervical (displaced) S12.330 ☑
        nondisplaced S12.331 ☑
        specified type NEC (displaced) S12.350 ☑
          nondisplaced S12.351 ☑
        type III S12.34 ☑
      second cervical (displaced) S12.130 ☑
        nondisplaced S12.131 ☑
        specified type NEC (displaced) S12.150 ☑
          nondisplaced S12.151 ☑
        type III S12.14 ☑
      seventh cervical (displaced) S12.630 ☑
        nondisplaced S12.631 ☑
        specified type NEC (displaced) S12.650 ☑
          nondisplaced S12.651 ☑
        type III S12.64 ☑
      sixth cervical (displaced) S12.530 ☑
        nondisplaced S12.531 ☑
        specified type NEC (displaced) S12.550 ☑
          nondisplaced S12.551 ☑
        type III S12.54 ☑
      third cervical (displaced) S12.230 ☑
        nondisplaced S12.231 ☑
        specified type NEC (displaced) S12.250 ☑
          nondisplaced S12.251 ☑
        type III S12.24 ☑
Spondylolysis (acquired) M43.00
  cervical region M43.02
  cervicothoracic region M43.03
  congenital Q76.2
  lumbar region M43.06
  lumbosacral region M43.07
    with disproportion (fetopelvic) O33.0
      causing obstructed labor O65.8
  multiple sites M43.09
  occipito-atlanto-axial region M43.01
  sacrococcygeal region M43.08
  thoracic region M43.04
  thoracolumbar region M43.05
Spondylopathy M48.9
  infective NEC M46.50
    cervical region M46.52
    cervicothoracic region M46.53
    lumbar region M46.56
    lumbosacral region M46.57
    multiple sites M46.59
    occipito-atlanto-axial region M46.51
    sacrococcygeal region M46.58
    thoracic region M46.54
    thoracolumbar region M46.55
  inflammatory M46.90
    cervical region M46.92
    cervicothoracic region M46.93
    lumbar region M46.96
    lumbosacral region M46.97
    multiple sites M46.99
    occipito-atlanto-axial region M46.91
    sacrococcygeal region M46.98
    specified type NEC M46.80
      cervical region M46.82
      cervicothoracic region M46.83
      lumbar region M46.86
      lumbosacral region M46.87
      multiple sites M46.89
      occipito-atlanto-axial region M46.81
      sacrococcygeal region M46.88
      thoracic region M46.84
      thoracolumbar region M46.85
    thoracic region M46.94
    thoracolumbar region M46.95
  neuropathic, in
    syringomyelia and syringobulbia G95.0
    tabes dorsalis A52.11
  specified NEC — *see* subcategory M48.8 ☑
  traumatic M48.30

Spondylopathy — *continued*
  traumatic — *continued*
    cervical region M48.32
    cervicothoracic region M48.33
    lumbar region M48.36
    lumbosacral region M48.37
    occipito-atlanto-axial region M48.31
    sacrococcygeal region M48.38
    thoracic region M48.34
    thoracolumbar region M48.35
Spondylosis M47.9
  with
    disproportion (fetopelvic) O33.0
      causing obstructed labor O65.0
    myelopathy NEC M47.10
      cervical region M47.12
      cervicothoracic region M47.13
      lumbar region M47.16
      occipito-atlanto-axial region M47.11
      thoracic region M47.14
      thoracolumbar region M47.15
    radiculopathy M47.20
      cervical region M47.22
      cervicothoracic region M47.23
      lumbar region M47.26
      lumbosacral region M47.27
      occipito-atlanto-axial region M47.21
      sacrococcygeal region M47.28
      thoracic region M47.24
      thoracolumbar region M47.25
  specified NEC M47.899
    cervical region M47.892
    cervicothoracic region M47.893
    lumbar region M47.896
    lumbosacral region M47.897
    occipito-atlanto-axial region M47.891
    sacrococcygeal region M47.898
    thoracic region M47.894
    thoracolumbar region M47.895
  traumatic — *see* Spondylopathy, traumatic
  without myelopathy or radiculopathy M47.819
    cervical region M47.812
    cervicothoracic region M47.813
    lumbar region M47.816
    lumbosacral region M47.817
    occipito-atlanto-axial region M47.811
    sacrococcygeal region M47.818
    thoracic region M47.814
    thoracolumbar region M47.815
Sponge
  inadvertently left in operation wound — *see* Foreign
      body, accidentally left during a procedure
  kidney (medullary) Q61.5
Sponge-diver's disease — *see* Toxicity, venom, marine
    animal, sea anemone
Spongioblastoma (any type) — *see* Neoplasm, malig-
    nant, by site
  specified site — *see* Neoplasm, malignant, by site
  unspecified site C71.9
Spongioneuroblastoma — *see* Neoplasm, malignant,
    by site
Spontaneous — *see also* condition
  fracture (cause unknown) — *see* Fracture, pathological
Spoon nail L60.3
  congenital Q84.6
Sporadic — *see* condition
Sporothrix schenckii infection — *see* Sporotrichosis
Sporotrichosis B42.9
  arthritis B42.82
  disseminated B42.7
  generalized B42.7
  lymphocutaneous (fixed) (progressive) B42.1
  pulmonary B42.0
  specified NEC B42.89
Spots, spotting (in) (of)
  Bitot's — *see also* Pigmentation, conjunctiva
    in the young child E50.1
      vitamin A deficiency E50.1
  café, au lait L81.3
  Cayenne pepper I78.1
  cotton wool, retina — *see* Occlusion, artery, retina
  de Morgan's (senile angiomas) I78.1
  Fuchs' black (myopic) — *see also* Myopia, degenerative
      H44.2- ☑
  intermenstrual (regular) N92.0
    irregular N92.1
  Koplik's B05.9
  liver L81.4

Spots, spotting — continued
    pregnancy O26.85- ☑
    purpuric R23.3
    ruby I78.1
Spotted fever — see Fever, spotted N92.3
Sprain (joint) (ligament)
    acromioclavicular joint or ligament S43.5- ☑
    ankle S93.40- ☑
        calcaneofibular ligament S93.41- ☑
        deltoid ligament S93.42- ☑
        internal collateral ligament — see Sprain, ankle,
            specified ligament NEC
        specified ligament NEC S93.49- ☑
        talofibular ligament — see Sprain, ankle, specified
            ligament NEC
        tibiofibular ligament S93.43- ☑
    anterior longitudinal, cervical S13.4 ☑
    atlas, atlanto-axial, atlanto-occipital S13.4 ☑
    breast bone — see Sprain, sternum
    calcaneofibular — see Sprain, ankle
    carpal — see Sprain, wrist
    carpometacarpal — see Sprain, hand, specified site
        NEC
    cartilage
        costal S23.41 ☑
        semilunar (knee) — see Sprain, knee, specified site
            NEC
            with current tear — see Tear, meniscus
        thyroid region S13.5 ☑
        xiphoid — see Sprain, sternum
    cervical, cervicodorsal, cervicothoracic S13.4 ☑
    chondrosternal S23.421 ☑
    coracoclavicular S43.8- ☑
    coracohumeral S43.41- ☑
    coronary, knee — see Sprain, knee, specified site NEC
    costal cartilage S23.41 ☑
    cricoarytenoid articulation or ligament S13.5 ☑
    cricothyroid articulation S13.5 ☑
    cruciate, knee — see Sprain, knee, cruciate
    deltoid, ankle — see Sprain, ankle
    dorsal (spine) S23.3 ☑
    elbow S53.40- ☑
        radial collateral ligament S53.43- ☑
        radiohumeral S53.41- ☑
        rupture
            radial collateral ligament — see Rupture, trau-
                matic, ligament, radial collateral
            ulnar collateral ligament — see Rupture, traumat-
                ic, ligament, ulnar collateral
        specified type NEC S53.49- ☑
        ulnar collateral ligament S53.44- ☑
        ulnohumeral S53.42- ☑
    femur, head — see Sprain, hip
    fibular collateral, knee — see Sprain, knee, collateral
    fibulocalcaneal — see Sprain, ankle
    finger(s) S63.61- ☑
        index S63.61- ☑
        interphalangeal (joint) S63.63- ☑
            index S63.63- ☑
            little S63.63- ☑
            middle S63.63- ☑
            ring S63.63- ☑
        little S63.61- ☑
        metacarpophalangeal (joint) S63.65- ☑
        middle S63.61- ☑
        ring S63.61- ☑
        specified site NEC S63.69- ☑
            index S63.69- ☑
            little S63.69- ☑
            middle S63.69- ☑
            ring S63.69- ☑
    foot S93.60- ☑
        specified ligament NEC S93.69- ☑
        tarsal ligament S93.61- ☑
        tarsometatarsal ligament S93.62- ☑
        toe — see Sprain, toe
    hand S63.9- ☑
        finger — see Sprain, finger
        specified site NEC — see subcategory S63.8 ☑
        thumb — see Sprain, thumb
    head S03.9 ☑
    hip S73.10- ☑
        iliofemoral ligament S73.11- ☑
        ischiocapsular (ligament) S73.12- ☑
        specified NEC S73.19- ☑
    iliofemoral — see Sprain, hip

Sprain — continued
    innominate
        acetabulum — see Sprain, hip
        sacral junction S33.6 ☑
    internal
        collateral, ankle — see Sprain, ankle
        semilunar cartilage — see Sprain, knee, specified
            site NEC
    interphalangeal
        finger — see Sprain, finger, interphalangeal (joint)
        toe — see Sprain, toe, interphalangeal joint
    ischiocapsular — see Sprain, hip
    ischiofemoral — see Sprain, hip
    jaw (articular disc) (cartilage) (meniscus) S03.4- ☑
        old M26.69
    knee S83.9- ☑
        collateral ligament S83.40- ☑
            lateral (fibular) S83.42- ☑
            medial (tibial) S83.41- ☑
        cruciate ligament S83.50- ☑
            anterior S83.51- ☑
            posterior S83.52- ☑
        lateral (fibular) collateral ligament S83.42- ☑
        medial (tibial) collateral ligament S83.41- ☑
        patellar ligament S76.11- ☑
        specified site NEC S83.8X- ☑
        superior tibiofibular joint (ligament) S83.6- ☑
    lateral collateral, knee — see Sprain, knee, collateral
    lumbar (spine) S33.5 ☑
    lumbosacral S33.9 ☑
    mandible (articular disc) S03.4- ☑
        old M26.69
    medial collateral, knee — see Sprain, knee, collateral
    meniscus
        jaw S03.4- ☑
            old M26.69
        knee — see Sprain, knee, specified site NEC
            with current tear — see Tear, meniscus
                old — see Derangement, knee, meniscus, due
                    to old tear
        mandible S03.4- ☑
            old M26.69
    metacarpal (distal) (proximal) — see Sprain, hand,
        specified site NEC
    metacarpophalangeal — see Sprain, finger, metacar-
        pophalangeal (joint)
    metatarsophalangeal — see Sprain, toe, metatarsopha-
        langeal joint
    midcarpal — see Sprain, hand, specified site NEC
    midtarsal — see Sprain, foot, specified site NEC
    neck S13.9 ☑
        anterior longitudinal cervical ligament S13.4 ☑
        atlanto-axial joint S13.4 ☑
        atlanto-occipital joint S13.4 ☑
        cervical spine S13.4 ☑
        cricoarytenoid ligament S13.5 ☑
        cricothyroid ligament S13.5 ☑
        specified site NEC S13.8 ☑
        thyroid region (cartilage) S13.5 ☑
    nose S03.8 ☑
    orbicular, hip — see Sprain, hip
    patella — see Sprain, knee, specified site NEC
    patellar ligament S76.11- ☑
    pelvis NEC S33.8 ☑
    phalanx
        finger — see Sprain, finger
        toe — see Sprain, toe
    pubofemoral — see Sprain, hip
    radiocarpal — see Sprain, wrist
    radiohumeral — see Sprain, elbow
    radius, collateral — see Rupture, traumatic, ligament,
        radial collateral
    rib (cage) S23.41 ☑
    rotator cuff (capsule) S43.42- ☑
    sacroiliac (region)
        chronic or old — see subcategory M53.2 ☑
        joint S33.6 ☑
    scaphoid (hand) — see Sprain, hand, specified site NEC
    scapula (r) — see Sprain, shoulder girdle, specified site
        NEC
    semilunar cartilage (knee) — see Sprain, knee, specified
        site NEC
        with current tear — see Tear, meniscus
            old — see Derangement, knee, meniscus, due to
                old tear
    shoulder joint S43.40- ☑

Sprain — continued
    shoulder joint — continued
        acromioclavicular joint (ligament) — see Sprain,
            acromioclavicular joint
        blade — see Sprain, shoulder, girdle, specified site
            NEC
        coracoclavicular joint (ligament) — see Sprain,
            coracoclavicular joint
        coracohumeral ligament — see Sprain, coracohumer-
            al joint
        girdle S43.9- ☑
            specified site NEC S43.8- ☑
        rotator cuff — see Sprain, rotator cuff
        specified site NEC S43.49- ☑
        sternoclavicular joint (ligament) — see Sprain,
            sternoclavicular joint
    spine
        cervical S13.4 ☑
        lumbar S33.5 ☑
        thoracic S23.3 ☑
    sternoclavicular joint S43.6- ☑
    sternum S23.429 ☑
        chondrosternal joint S23.421 ☑
        specified site NEC S23.428 ☑
        sternoclavicular (joint) (ligament) S23.420 ☑
    symphysis
        jaw S03.4- ☑
            old M26.69
        mandibular S03.4- ☑
            old M26.69
    talofibular — see Sprain, ankle
    tarsal — see Sprain, foot, specified site NEC
    tarsometatarsal — see Sprain, foot, specified site NEC
    temporomandibular S03.4- ☑
        old M26.69
    thorax S23.9 ☑
        ribs S23.41 ☑
        specified site NEC S23.8 ☑
        spine S23.3 ☑
        sternum — see Sprain, sternum
    thumb S63.60- ☑
        interphalangeal (joint) S63.62- ☑
        metacarpophalangeal (joint) S63.64- ☑
        specified site NEC S63.68- ☑
    thyroid cartilage or region S13.5 ☑
    tibia (proximal end) — see Sprain, knee, specified site
        NEC
    tibial collateral, knee — see Sprain, knee, collateral
    tibiofibular
        distal — see Sprain, ankle
        superior — see Sprain, knee, specified site NEC
    toe(s) S93.50- ☑
        great S93.50- ☑
        interphalangeal joint S93.51- ☑
            great S93.51- ☑
            lesser S93.51- ☑
        lesser S93.50- ☑
        metatarsophalangeal joint S93.52- ☑
            great S93.52- ☑
            lesser S93.52- ☑
    ulna, collateral — see Rupture, traumatic, ligament,
        ulnar collateral
    ulnohumeral — see Sprain, elbow
    wrist S63.50- ☑
        carpal S63.51- ☑
        radiocarpal S63.52- ☑
        specified site NEC S63.59- ☑
    xiphoid cartilage — see Sprain, sternum
Sprengel's deformity (congenital) Q74.0
Sprue (tropical) K90.1
    celiac K90.0
    idiopathic K90.49
    meaning thrush B37.0
    nontropical K90.0
Spur, bone — see also Enthesopathy
    calcaneal M77.3- ☑
    iliac crest M76.2- ☑
    nose (septum) J34.89
Spurway's syndrome Q78.0
Sputum
    abnormal (amount) (color) (odor) (purulent) R09.3
    blood-stained R04.2
    excessive (cause unknown) R09.3
Squamous — see also condition
    epithelium in
        cervical canal (congenital) Q51.828

290

☑ **Additional Character Required** — Refer to the Tabular List for Character Selection   ▼ **Subterms under main terms may continue to next column or page**

Squamous — *continued*
  epithelium in — *continued*
    uterine mucosa (congenital) Q51.818
Squashed nose M95.0
  congenital Q67.4
Squeeze, diver's T70.3 ☑
Squint — *see also* Strabismus
  accommodative — *see* Strabismus, convergent concomitant
SSADHD (succinic semialdehyde dehydrogenase deficiency) E72.81
St. Hubert's disease A82.9
Stab — *see also* Laceration
  internal organs — *see* Injury, by site
Stafne's cyst or cavity M27.0
Staggering gait R26.0
  hysterical F44.4
Staghorn calculus — *see* Calculus, kidney
Stähli's line (cornea) (pigment) — *see* Pigmentation, cornea, anterior
Stain, staining
  meconium (newborn) P96.83
  port wine Q82.5
  tooth, teeth (hard tissues) (extrinsic) K03.6
    due to
      accretions K03.6
      deposits (betel) (black) (green) (materia alba) (orange) (soft) (tobacco) K03.6
      metals (copper) (silver) K03.7
      nicotine K03.6
      pulpal bleeding K03.7
      tobacco K03.6
    intrinsic K00.8
Stammering — *see also* Disorder, fluency F80.81
Standstill
  auricular I45.5
  cardiac — *see* Arrest, cardiac
  sinoatrial I45.5
  ventricular — *see* Arrest, cardiac
Stannosis J63.5
Stanton's disease — *see* Melioidosis
Staphylitis (acute) (catarrhal) (chronic) (gangrenous) (membranous) (suppurative) (ulcerative) K12.2
Staphylococcal scalded skin syndrome L00
Staphylococcemia A41.2
Staphylococcus, staphylococcal — *see also* condition
  as cause of disease classified elsewhere B95.8
    aureus (methicillin susceptible) (MSSA) B95.61
      methicillin resistant (MRSA) B95.62
  specified NEC, as cause of disease classified elsewhere B95.7
Staphyloma (sclera)
  cornea H18.72- ☑
  equatorial H15.81- ☑
  localized (anterior) H15.82- ☑
  posticum H15.83- ☑
  ring H15.85- ☑
Stargardt's disease — *see* Dystrophy, retina
Starvation (inanition) (due to lack of food) T73.0 ☑
  edema — *see* Malnutrition, severe
Stasis
  bile (noncalculous) K83.1
  bronchus J98.09
    with infection — *see* Bronchitis
  cardiac — *see* Failure, heart, congestive
  cecum K59.8
  colon K59.8
  dermatitis I87.2
    with
      varicose ulcer — *see* Varix, leg, with ulcer, with inflammation
      varicose veins — *see* Varix, leg, with, inflammation
    due to postthrombotic syndrome — *see* Syndrome, postthrombotic
  duodenal K31.5
  eczema — *see* Varix, leg, with, inflammation
  edema — *see* Hypertension, venous (chronic), idiopathic
  foot T69.0- ☑
  ileocecal coil K59.8
  ileum K59.8
  intestinal K59.8
  jejunum K59.8
  kidney N19
  liver (cirrhotic) K76.1
  lymphatic I89.8

Stasis — *continued*
  pneumonia J18.2
  pulmonary — *see* Edema, lung
  rectal K59.8
  renal N19
    tubular N17.0
  ulcer — *see* Varix, leg, with, ulcer
    without varicose veins I87.2
  urine — *see* Retention, urine
  venous I87.8
State (of)
  affective and paranoid, mixed, organic psychotic F06.8
  agitated R45.1
    acute reaction to stress F43.0
  anxiety (neurotic) F41.1
  apprehension F41.1
  burn-out Z73.0
  climacteric, female Z78.0
    symptomatic N95.1
  compulsive F42.8
    mixed with obsessional thoughts F42.2
  confusional (psychogenic) F44.89
    acute — *see also* Delirium
      with
        arteriosclerotic dementia F01.50
          with behavioral disturbance F01.51
        senility or dementia F05
      alcoholic F10.231
    epileptic F05
    reactive (from emotional stress, psychological trauma) F44.89
    subacute — *see* Delirium
  convulsive — *see* Convulsions
  crisis F43.0
  depressive F32.9
    neurotic F34.1
  dissociative F44.9
  emotional shock (stress) R45.7
  hypercoagulation — *see* Hypercoagulable
  locked-in G83.5
  menopausal Z78.0
    symptomatic N95.1
  neurotic F48.9
    with depersonalization F48.1
  obsessional F42.8
  oneiroid (schizophrenia-like) F23
  organic
    hallucinatory (nonalcoholic) F06.0
    paranoid (-hallucinatory) F06.2
  panic F41.0
  paranoid F22
    climacteric F22
    involutional F22
    menopausal F22
    organic F06.2
    senile F03
    simple F22
  persistent vegetative R40.3
  phobic F40.9
  postleukotomy F07.0
  pregnant
    gestational carrier Z33.3
    incidental Z33.1
  psychogenic, twilight F44.89
  psychopathic (constitutional) F60.2
  psychotic, organic — *see also* Psychosis, organic
    mixed paranoid and affective F06.8
    senile or presenile F03 ☑
    transient NEC F06.8
      with
        depression F06.31
        hallucinations F06.0
  residual schizophrenic F20.5
  restlessness R45.1
  stress (emotional) R45.7
  tension (mental) F48.9
    specified NEC F48.8
  transient organic psychotic NEC F06.8
    depressive type F06.31
    hallucinatory type F06.0
  twilight
    epileptic F05
    psychogenic F44.89
  vegetative, persistent R40.3
  vital exhaustion Z73.0
  withdrawal, — *see* Withdrawal, state
Status (post) — *see also* Presence (of)

Status — *continued*
  absence, epileptic — *see* Epilepsy, by type, with status epilepticus
  administration of tPA (rtPA) in a different facility within the last 24 hours prior to admission to current facility Z92.82
  adrenalectomy (unilateral) (bilateral) E89.6
  anastomosis Z98.0
  anginosus I20.9
  angioplasty (peripheral) Z98.62
    with implant Z95.820
    coronary artery Z98.61
      with implant Z95.5
  aortocoronary bypass Z95.1
  arthrodesis Z98.1
  artificial opening (of) Z93.9
    gastrointestinal tract Z93.4
    specified NEC Z93.8
    urinary tract Z93.6
    vagina Z93.8
  asthmaticus — *see* Asthma, by type, with status asthmaticus
  awaiting organ transplant Z76.82
  bariatric surgery Z98.84
  bed confinement Z74.01
  bleb, filtering (vitreous), after glaucoma surgery Z98.83
  breast implant Z98.82
    removal Z98.86
  cataract extraction Z98.4- ☑
  cholecystectomy Z90.49
  clitorectomy N90.811
    with excision of labia minora N90.812
  colectomy (complete) (partial) Z90.49
  colonization — *see* Carrier (suspected) of
  colostomy Z93.3
  convulsivus idiopathicus — *see* Epilepsy, by type, with status epilepticus
  coronary artery angioplasty — *see* Status, angioplasty, coronary artery
  coronary artery bypass graft Z95.1
  cystectomy (urinary bladder) Z90.6
  cystostomy Z93.50
    appendico-vesicostomy Z93.52
    cutaneous Z93.51
    specified NEC Z93.59
  delinquent immunization Z28.3
  dental Z98.818
    crown Z98.811
    fillings Z98.811
    restoration Z98.811
    sealant Z98.810
    specified NEC Z98.818
  deployment (current) (military) Z56.82
  dialysis (hemodialysis) (peritoneal) Z99.2
  do not resuscitate (DNR) Z66
  donor — *see* Donor
  embedded fragments — *see* Retained, foreign body fragments (type of)
  embedded splinter — *see* Retained, foreign body fragments (type of)
  enterostomy Z93.4
  epileptic, epilepticus — *see also* Epilepsy, by type, with status epilepticus G40.901
  estrogen receptor
    negative Z17.1
    positive Z17.0
  female genital cutting — *see* Female genital mutilation status
  female genital mutilation — *see* Female genital mutilation status
  filtering (vitreous) bleb after glaucoma surgery Z98.83
  gastrectomy (complete) (partial) Z90.3
  gastric banding Z98.84
  gastric bypass for obesity Z98.84
  gastrostomy Z93.1
  human immunodeficiency virus (HIV) infection, asymptomatic Z21
  hysterectomy (complete) (total) Z90.710
    partial (with remaining cervial stump) Z90.711
  ileostomy Z93.2
  implant
    breast Z98.82
  infibulation N90.813
  intestinal bypass Z98.0
  jejunostomy Z93.4
  lapsed immunization schedule Z28.3
  laryngectomy Z90.02
  lymphaticus E32.8

Status — continued
  malignancy
    castrate resistant prostate Z19.2
    hormone resistant Z19.2
    hormone sensitive Z19.1
  marmoratus G80.3
  mastectomy (unilateral) (bilateral) Z90.1- ☑
  military deployment status (current) Z56.82
    in theater or in support of military war, peacekeeping and humanitarian operations Z56.82
  nephrectomy (unilateral) (bilateral) Z90.5
  nephrostomy Z93.6
  obesity surgery Z98.84
  oophorectomy
    bilateral Z90.722
    unilateral Z90.721
  organ replacement
    by artificial or mechanical device or prosthesis of
      artery Z95.828
      bladder Z96.0
      blood vessel Z95.828
      breast Z97.8
      eye globe Z97.0
      heart Z95.812
        valve Z95.2
      intestine Z97.8
      joint Z96.60
        hip — see Presence, hip joint implant
        knee — see Presence, knee joint implant
        specified site NEC Z96.698
      kidney Z97.8
      larynx Z96.3
      lens Z96.1
      limbs — see Presence, artificial, limb
      liver Z97.8
      lung Z97.8
      pancreas Z97.8
    by organ transplant (heterologous)(homologous) — see Transplant
  pacemaker
    brain Z96.89
    cardiac Z95.0
    specified NEC Z96.89
  pancreatectomy Z90.410
    complete Z90.410
    partial Z90.411
    total Z90.410
  physical restraint Z78.1
  pneumonectomy (complete) (partial) Z90.2
  pneumothorax, therapeutic Z98.3
  postcommotio cerebri F07.81
  postoperative (postprocedural) NEC Z98.890
    breast implant Z98.82
    dental Z98.818
      crown Z98.811
      fillings Z98.811
      restoration Z98.811
      sealant Z98.810
      specified NEC Z98.818
    pneumothorax, therapeutic Z98.3
    uterine scar Z98.891
  postpartum (routine follow-up) Z39.2
    care immediately after delivery Z39.0
  postsurgical (postprocedural) NEC Z98.890
    pneumothorax, therapeutic Z98.3
  pregnancy, incidental Z33.1
  prosthesis coronary angioplasty Z95.5
  pseudophakia Z96.1
  renal dialysis (hemodialysis) (peritoneal) Z99.2
  retained foreign body — see Retained, foreign body fragments (type of)
  reversed jejunal transposition (for bypass) Z98.0
  salpingo-oophorectomy
    bilateral Z90.722
    unilateral Z90.721
  sex reassignment surgery status Z87.890
  shunt
    arteriovenous (for dialysis) Z99.2
    cerebrospinal fluid Z98.2
    ventricular (communicating) (for drainage) Z98.2
  splenectomy Z90.81
  thymicolymphaticus E32.8
  thymicus E32.8
  thymolymphaticus E32.8
  thyroidectomy (hypothyroidism) E89.0
  tooth (teeth) extraction — see also Absence, teeth, acquired K08.409

Status — continued
  tPA (rtPA) administration in a different facility within the last 24 hours prior to admission to current facility Z92.82
  tracheostomy Z93.0
  transplant — see Transplant
    organ removed Z98.85
  tubal ligation Z98.51
  underimmunization Z28.3
  ureterostomy Z93.6
  urethrostomy Z93.6
  vagina, artificial Z93.8
  vasectomy Z98.52
  wheelchair confinement Z99.3
Stealing
  child problem F91.8
  in company with others Z72.810
  pathological (compulsive) F63.2
Steam burn — see Burn
Steatocystoma multiplex L72.2
Steatohepatitis (nonalcoholic) (NASH) K75.81
Steatoma L72.3
  eyelid (cystic) — see Dermatosis, eyelid
    infected — see Hordeolum
Steatorrhea (chronic) K90.9
  with lacteal obstruction K90.2
  idiopathic (adult) (infantile) K90.9
  pancreatic K90.3
  primary K90.0
  tropical K90.1
Steatosis E88.89
  heart — see Degeneration, myocardial
  kidney N28.89
  liver NEC K76.0
Steele-Richardson-Olszewski disease or syndrome G23.1
Steinbrocker's syndrome G90.8
Steinert's disease G71.11
Stein-Leventhal syndrome E28.2
Stein's syndrome E28.2
STEMI — see also Infarct, myocardium, ST elevation I21.3
Stenocardia I20.8
Stenocephaly Q75.8
Stenosis, stenotic (cicatricial) — see also Stricture
  ampulla of Vater K83.1
  anus, anal (canal) (sphincter) K62.4
    and rectum K62.4
    congenital Q42.3
      with fistula Q42.2
  aorta (ascending) (supraventricular) (congenital) Q25.1
    arteriosclerotic I70.0
    calcified I70.0
    supravalvular Q25.3
  aortic (valve) I35.0
    with insufficiency I35.2
    congenital Q23.0
    rheumatic I06.0
      with
        incompetency, insufficiency or regurgitation I06.2
          with mitral (valve) disease I08.0
            with tricuspid (valve) disease I08.3
        mitral (valve) disease I08.0
          with tricuspid (valve) disease I08.3
        tricuspid (valve) disease I08.2
          with mitral (valve) disease I08.3
    specified cause NEC I35.0
    syphilitic A52.03
  aqueduct of Sylvius (congenital) Q03.0
    with spina bifida — see Spina bifida, by site, with hydrocephalus
    acquired G91.1
  artery NEC — see also Arteriosclerosis I77.1
    celiac I77.4
    cerebral — see Occlusion, artery, cerebral
    extremities — see Arteriosclerosis, extremities
    precerebral — see Occlusion, artery, precerebral
    pulmonary (congenital) Q25.6
      acquired I28.8
    renal I70.1
    stent
      coronary T82.855 ☑
      peripheral T82.856 ☑
  bile duct (common) (hepatic) K83.1
    congenital Q44.3
  bladder-neck (acquired) N32.0
    congenital Q64.31
  brain G93.89

Stenosis, stenotic — continued
  bronchus J98.09
    congenital Q32.3
    syphilitic A52.72
  cardia (stomach) K22.2
    congenital Q39.3
  cardiovascular — see Disease, cardiovascular
  caudal
  cervix, cervical (canal) N88.2
    congenital Q51.828
    in pregnancy or childbirth — see Pregnancy, complicated by, abnormal cervix
  colon — see also Obstruction, intestine
    congenital Q42.9
      specified NEC Q42.8
  colostomy K94.03
  common (bile) duct K83.1
    congenital Q44.3
  coronary (artery) — see Disease, heart, ischemic, atherosclerotic
  cystic duct — see also Obstruction, gallbladder
  due to presence of device, implant or graft — see also Complications, by site and type, specified NEC T85.858 ☑
    arterial graft NEC T82.858 ☑
    breast (implant) T85.858 ☑
    catheter T85.858 ☑
      dialysis (renal) T82.858 ☑
        intraperitoneal T85.858 ☑
      infusion NEC T82.858 ☑
        spinal (epidural) (subdural) T85.850 ☑
      urinary (indwelling) T83.85 ☑
    fixation, internal (orthopedic) NEC T84.85 ☑
    gastrointestinal (bile duct) (esophagus) T85.858 ☑
    genital NEC T83.85 ☑
    heart NEC T82.857 ☑
    joint prosthesis T84.85 ☑
    ocular (corneal graft) (orbital implant) NEC T85.858 ☑
    orthopedic NEC T84.85 ☑
    specified NEC T85.858 ☑
    urinary NEC T83.85 ☑
    vascular NEC T82.858 ☑
    ventricular intracranial shunt T85.850 ☑
  duodenum K31.5
    congenital Q41.0
  ejaculatory duct NEC N50.89
    stent
      vascular
        end stent
          adjacent to stent — see Arteriosclerosis
          within the stent
            coronary T82.855 ☑
            peripheral T82.856 ☑
        in stent
          coronary vessel T82.855 ☑
          peripheral vessel T82.856 ☑
  endocervical os — see Stenosis, cervix
  enterostomy K94.13
  esophagus K22.2
    congenital Q39.3
    syphilitic A52.79
      congenital A50.59 [K23]
  eustachian tube — see Obstruction, eustachian tube
  external ear canal (acquired) H61.30- ☑
    congenital Q16.1
    due to
      inflammation H61.32- ☑
      trauma H61.31- ☑
    postprocedural H95.81- ☑
    specified cause NEC H61.39- ☑
  gallbladder — see Obstruction, gallbladder
  glottis J38.6
  heart valve (congenital) Q24.8
    aortic Q23.0
    mitral Q23.2
    pulmonary Q22.1
    tricuspid Q22.4
  hepatic duct K83.1
  hymen N89.6
  hypertrophic subaortic (idiopathic) I42.1
  ileum — see also Obstruction, intestine, specified NEC K56.699
    congenital Q41.2
  infundibulum cardia Q24.3
  intervertebral foramina — see also Lesion, biomechanical, specified NEC

☑ **Additional Character Required** — Refer to the Tabular List for Character Selection   ▽ **Subterms under main terms may continue to next column or page**

Stenosis, stenotic — *continued*
  intervertebral foramina — *see also* Lesion, biomechan-
    ical, specified — *continued*
    connective tissue M99.79
      abdomen M99.79
      cervical region M99.71
      cervicothoracic M99.71
      head region M99.70
      lumbar region M99.73
      lumbosacral M99.73
      occipitocervical M99.70
      sacral region M99.74
      sacrococcygeal M99.74
      sacroiliac M99.74
      specified NEC M99.79
      thoracic region M99.72
      thoracolumbar M99.72
    disc M99.79
      abdomen M99.79
      cervical region M99.71
      cervicothoracic M99.71
      head region M99.70
      lower extremity M99.76
      lumbar region M99.73
      lumbosacral M99.73
      occipitocervical M99.70
      pelvic M99.75
      rib cage M99.78
      sacral region M99.74
      sacrococcygeal M99.74
      sacroiliac M99.74
      specified NEC M99.79
      thoracic region M99.72
      thoracolumbar M99.72
      upper extremity M99.77
    osseous M99.69
      abdomen M99.69
      cervical region M99.61
      cervicothoracic M99.61
      head region M99.60
      lower extremity M99.66
      lumbar region M99.63
      lumbosacral M99.63
      occipitocervical M99.60
      pelvic M99.65
      rib cage M99.68
      sacral region M99.64
      sacrococcygeal M99.64
      sacroiliac M99.64
      specified NEC M99.69
      thoracic region M99.62
      thoracolumbar M99.62
      upper extremity M99.67
    subluxation — *see* Stenosis, intervertebral foramina,
      osseous
  intestine — *see also* Obstruction, intestine
    congenital (small) Q41.9
      large Q42.9
        specified NEC Q42.8
      specified NEC Q41.8
  jejunum — *see also* Obstruction, intestine, specified
    NEC K56.699
    congenital Q41.1
  lacrimal (passage)
    canaliculi H04.54- ☑
    congenital Q10.5
    duct H04.55- ☑
    punctum H04.56- ☑
    sac H04.57- ☑
  lacrimonasal duct — *see* Stenosis, lacrimal, duct
    congenital Q10.5
  larynx J38.6
    congenital NEC Q31.8
      subglottic Q31.1
    syphilitic A52.73
      congenital A50.59 *[J99]*
  mitral (chronic) (inactive) (valve) I05.0
    with
      aortic valve disease I08.0
      incompetency, insufficiency or regurgitation
        I05.2
    active or acute I01.1
      with rheumatic or Sydenham's chorea I02.0
    congenital Q23.2
    specified cause, except rheumatic I34.2
    syphilitic A52.03
  myocardium, myocardial — *see also* Degeneration,
    myocardial

Stenosis, stenotic — *continued*
  myocardium, myocardial — *see also* Degeneration,
    myocardial — *continued*
    hypertrophic subaortic (idiopathic) I42.1
  nares (anterior) (posterior) J34.89
    congenital Q30.0
  nasal duct — *see also* Stenosis, lacrimal, duct
    congenital Q10.5
  nasolacrimal duct — *see also* Stenosis, lacrimal, duct
    congenital Q10.5
  neural canal — *see also* Lesion, biomechanical, speci-
    fied NEC
    connective tissue M99.49
      abdomen M99.49
      cervical region M99.41
      cervicothoracic M99.41
      head region M99.40
      lower extremity M99.46
      lumbar region M99.43
      lumbosacral M99.43
      occipitocervical M99.40
      pelvic M99.45
      rib cage M99.48
      sacral region M99.44
      sacrococcygeal M99.44
      sacroiliac M99.44
      specified NEC M99.49
      thoracic region M99.42
      thoracolumbar M99.42
      upper extremity M99.47
    intervertebral disc M99.59
      abdomen M99.59
      cervical region M99.51
      cervicothoracic M99.51
      head region M99.50
      lower extremity M99.56
      lumbar region M99.53
      lumbosacral M99.53
      occipitocervical M99.50
      pelvic M99.55
      rib cage M99.58
      sacral region M99.54
      sacrococcygeal M99.54
      sacroiliac M99.54
      specified NEC M99.59
      thoracic region M99.52
      thoracolumbar M99.52
      upper extremity M99.57
    osseous M99.39
      abdomen M99.39
      cervical region M99.31
      cervicothoracic M99.31
      head region M99.30
      lower extremity M99.36
      lumbar region M99.33
      lumbosacral M99.33
      occipitocervical M99.30
      pelvic M99.35
      rib cage M99.38
      sacral region M99.34
      sacrococcygeal M99.34
      sacroiliac M99.34
      specified NEC M99.39
      thoracic region M99.32
      thoracolumbar M99.32
      upper extremity M99.37
    subluxation M99.29
      cervical region M99.21
      cervicothoracic M99.21
      head region M99.20
      lower extremity M99.26
      lumbar region M99.23
      lumbosacral M99.23
      occipitocervical M99.20
      pelvic M99.25
      rib cage M99.28
      sacral region M99.24
      sacrococcygeal M99.24
      sacroiliac M99.24
      specified NEC M99.29
      thoracic region M99.22
      thoracolumbar M99.22
      upper extremity M99.27
  organ or site, congenital NEC — *see* Atresia, by site
  papilla of Vater K83.1
  pulmonary (artery) (congenital) Q25.6
    with ventricular septal defect, transposition of aorta,
      and hypertrophy of right ventricle Q21.3
    acquired I28.8

Stenosis, stenotic — *continued*
  pulmonary — *continued*
    in tetralogy of Fallot Q21.3
    infundibular Q24.3
    subvalvular Q24.3
    supravalvular Q25.6
    valve I37.0
      with insufficiency I37.2
      congenital Q22.1
      rheumatic I09.89
        with aortic, mitral or tricuspid (valve) disease
          I08.8
    vein, acquired I28.8
    vessel NEC I28.8
  pulmonic (congenital) Q22.1
    infundibular Q24.3
    subvalvular Q24.3
  pylorus (hypertrophic) (acquired) K31.1
    adult K31.1
    congenital Q40.0
    infantile Q40.0
  rectum (sphincter) — *see* Stricture, rectum
  renal artery I70.1
    congenital Q27.1
  salivary duct (any) K11.8
  sphincter of Oddi K83.1
  spinal M48.00
    cervical region M48.02
    cervicothoracic region M48.03
    lumbar region (NOS) (without neurogenic claudica-
      tion) M48.061
      with neurogenic claudication M48.062
    lumbosacral region M48.07
    occipito-atlanto-axial region M48.01
    sacrococcygeal region M48.08
    thoracic region M48.04
    thoracolumbar region M48.05
  stomach, hourglass K31.2
  subaortic (congenital) Q24.4
    hypertrophic (idiopathic) I42.1
  subglottic J38.6
    congenital Q31.1
    postprocedural J95.5
  trachea J39.8
    congenital Q32.1
    syphilitic A52.73
    tuberculous NEC A15.5
  tracheostomy J95.03
  tricuspid (valve) I07.0
    with
      aortic (valve) disease I08.2
      incompetency, insufficiency or regurgitation
        I07.2
        with aortic (valve) disease I08.2
          with mitral (valve) disease I08.3
        mitral (valve) disease I08.1
        with aortic (valve) disease I08.3
    congenital Q22.4
    nonrheumatic I36.0
      with insufficiency I36.2
  tubal N97.1
  ureter — *see* Atresia, ureter
  ureteropelvic junction, congenital Q62.11
  ureterovesical orifice, congenital Q62.12
  urethra (valve) *see also* Stricture, urethra
    congenital Q64.32
  urinary meatus, congenital Q64.33
  vagina N89.5
    congenital Q52.4
    in pregnancy — *see* Pregnancy, complicated by,
      abnormal vagina
    causing obstructed labor O65.5
  valve (cardiac) (heart) — *see also* Endocarditis I38
    congenital Q24.8
      aortic Q23.0
      mitral Q23.2
      pulmonary Q22.1
      tricuspid Q22.4
  vena cava (inferior) (superior) I87.1
    congenital Q26.0
  vesicourethral orifice Q64.31
  vulva N90.5
Stent jail T82.897 ☑
Stercolith (impaction) K56.41
  appendix K38.1
Stercoraceous, stercoral ulcer K63.3
  anus or rectum K62.6
Stereotypies NEC F98.4

Sterility — *see* Infertility
Sterilization — *see* Encounter (for), sterilization
Sternalgia — *see* Angina
Sternopagus Q89.4
Sternum bifidum Q76.7
Steroid
  effects (adverse) (adrenocortical) (iatrogenic)
    cushingoid E24.2
      correct substance properly administered — *see*
        Table of Drugs and Chemicals, by drug,
        adverse effect
      overdose or wrong substance given or taken —
        see Table of Drugs and Chemicals, by drug,
        poisoning
    diabetes — *see* subcategory E09 ☑
      correct substance properly administered — *see*
        Table of Drugs and Chemicals, by drug,
        adverse effect
      overdose or wrong substance given or taken —
        see Table of Drugs and Chemicals, by drug,
        poisoning
    fever R50.2
    insufficiency E27.3
      correct substance properly administered — *see*
        Table of Drugs and Chemicals, by drug,
        adverse effect
      overdose or wrong substance given or taken —
        see Table of Drugs and Chemicals, by drug,
        poisoning
  responder H40.04- ☑
Stevens-Johnson disease or syndrome L51.1
  toxic epidermal necrolysis overlap L51.3
Stewart-Morel syndrome M85.2
Sticker's disease B08.3
Sticky eye — *see* Conjunctivitis, acute, mucopurulent
Stieda's disease — *see* Bursitis, tibial collateral
Stiff neck — *see* Torticollis
Stiff-man syndrome G25.82
Stiffness, joint NEC M25.60
  ankle M25.67- ☑
  ankylosis — *see* Ankylosis, joint
  contracture — *see* Contraction, joint
  elbow M25.62- ☑
  foot M25.67- ☑
  hand M25.64- ☑
  hip M25.65- ☑
  knee M25.66- ☑
  shoulder M25.61- ☑
  wrist M25.63- ☑
Stigmata congenital syphilis A50.59
Stillbirth P95
Still-Felty syndrome — *see* Felty's syndrome
Still's disease or syndrome (juvenile) M08.20
  adult-onset M06.1
  ankle M08.27- ☑
  elbow M08.22- ☑
  foot joint M08.27- ☑
  hand joint M08.24- ☑
  hip M08.25- ☑
  knee M08.26- ☑
  multiple site M08.29
  shoulder M08.21- ☑
  vertebra M08.28
  wrist M08.23- ☑
Stimulation, ovary E28.1
Sting (venomous) (with allergic or anaphylactic shock)
    — *see* Table of Drugs and Chemicals, by animal or
    substance, poisoning
Stippled epiphyses Q78.8
Stitch
  abscess T81.41 ☑
  burst (in operation wound) — *see* Disruption, wound,
    operation
Stokes' disease E05.00
  with thyroid storm E05.01
Stokes-Adams disease or syndrome I45.9
Stokvis (-Talma) **disease** D74.8
Stoma malfunction
  colostomy K94.03
  enterostomy K94.13
  gastrostomy K94.23
  ileostomy K94.13
  tracheostomy J95.03
Stomach — *see* condition
Stomatitis (denture) (ulcerative) K12.1
  angular K13.0
    due to dietary or vitamin deficiency E53.0

Stomatitis — *continued*
  aphthous K12.0
  bovine B08.61
  candidal B37.0
  catarrhal K12.1
  diphtheritic A36.89
  due to
    dietary deficiency E53.0
    thrush B37.0
    vitamin deficiency
      B group NEC E53.9
      B2 (riboflavin) E53.0
  epidemic B08.8
  epizootic B08.8
  follicular K12.1
  gangrenous A69.0
  Geotrichum B48.3
  herpesviral, herpetic B00.2
  herpetiformis K12.0
  malignant K12.1
  membranous acute K12.1
  monilial B37.0
  mycotic B37.0
  necrotizing ulcerative A69.0
  parasitic B37.0
  septic K12.1
  spirochetal A69.1
  suppurative (acute) K12.2
  ulceromembranous A69.1
  vesicular K12.1
    with exanthem (enteroviral) B08.4
    virus disease A93.8
  Vincent's A69.1
Stomatocytosis D58.8
Stomatomycosis B37.0
Stomatorrhagia K13.79
Stone(s) — *see also* Calculus
  bladder (diverticulum) N21.0
  cystine E72.09
  heart syndrome I50.1
  kidney N20.0
  prostate N42.0
  pulpal (dental) K04.2
  renal N20.0
  salivary gland or duct (any) K11.5
  urethra (impacted) N21.1
  urinary (duct) (impacted) (passage) N20.9
    bladder (diverticulum) N21.0
    lower tract N21.9
    specified NEC N21.8
  xanthine E79.8 *[N22]*
Stonecutter's lung J62.8
**Stonemason's asthma, disease, lung or pneumoco-
  niosis** J62.8
Stoppage
  heart — *see* Arrest, cardiac
  urine — *see* Retention, urine
Storm, thyroid — *see* Thyrotoxicosis
Strabismus (congenital) (nonparalytic) H50.9
  concomitant H50.40
    convergent — *see* Strabismus, convergent concomi-
      tant
    divergent — *see* Strabismus, divergent concomitant
  convergent concomitant H50.00
    accommodative component H50.43
    alternating H50.05
      with
        A pattern H50.06
        specified nonconcomitances NEC H50.08
        V pattern H50.07
    monocular H50.01- ☑
      with
        A pattern H50.02- ☑
        specified nonconcomitances NEC H50.04- ☑
        V pattern H50.03- ☑
      intermittent H50.31- ☑
        alternating H50.32
  cyclotropia H50.41
  divergent concomitant H50.10
    alternating H50.15
      with
        A pattern H50.16
        specified nonconcomitances NEC H50.18
        V pattern H50.17
    monocular H50.11- ☑
      with
        A pattern H50.12- ☑
        specified nonconcomitances NEC H50.14- ☑

Strabismus — *continued*
  divergent concomitant — *continued*
    monocular — *continued*
      with — *continued*
        V pattern H50.13- ☑
      intermittent H50.33 ☑
        alternating H50.34
  Duane's syndrome H50.81- ☑
  due to adhesions, scars H50.69
  heterophoria H50.50
    alternating H50.55
    cyclophoria H50.54
    esophoria H50.51
    exophoria H50.52
    vertical H50.53
  heterotropia H50.40
    intermittent H50.30
  hypertropia H50.2- ☑
  hypotropia — *see* Hypertropia
  latent H50.50
  mechanical H50.60
    Brown's sheath syndrome H50.61- ☑
    specified type NEC H50.69
  monofixation syndrome H50.42
  paralytic H49.9
    abducens nerve H49.2- ☑
    fourth nerve H49.1- ☑
    Kearns-Sayre syndrome H49.81- ☑
    ophthalmoplegia (external)
      progressive H49.4- ☑
        with pigmentary retinopathy H49.81- ☑
      total H49.3- ☑
    sixth nerve H49.2- ☑
    specified type NEC H49.88- ☑
    third nerve H49.0- ☑
    trochlear nerve H49.1- ☑
  specified type NEC H50.89
  vertical H50.2- ☑
Strain
  back S39.012 ☑
  cervical S16.1 ☑
  eye NEC — *see* Disturbance, vision, subjective
  heart — *see* Disease, heart
  low back S39.012 ☑
  mental NOS Z73.3
    work-related Z56.6
  muscle (tendon) — *see* Injury, muscle, by site, strain
  neck S16.1 ☑
  physical NOS Z73.3
    work-related Z56.6
  postural — *see also* Disorder, soft tissue, due to use
  psychological NEC Z73.3
  tendon — *see* Injury, muscle, by site, strain
Straining, on urination R39.16
Strand, vitreous — *see* Opacity, vitreous, membranes
  and strands
Strangulation, strangulated — *see also* Asphyxia,
  traumatic
  appendix K38.8
  bladder-neck N32.0
  bowel or colon K56.2
  food or foreign body — *see* Foreign body, by site
  hemorrhoids — *see* Hemorrhoids, with complication
  hernia — *see also* Hernia, by site, with obstruction
    with gangrene — *see* Hernia, by site, with gangrene
  intestine (large) (small) K56.2
    with hernia — *see also* Hernia, by site, with obstruc-
      tion
      with gangrene — *see* Hernia, by site, with gan-
        grene
  mesentery K56.2
  mucus — *see* Asphyxia, mucus
  omentum K56.2
  organ or site, congenital NEC — *see* Atresia, by site
  ovary — *see* Torsion, ovary
  penis N48.89
    foreign body T19.4 ☑
  rupture — *see* Hernia, by site, with obstruction
  stomach due to hernia — *see also* Hernia, by site, with
    obstruction
    with gangrene — *see* Hernia, by site, with gangrene
  vesicourethral orifice N32.0
Strangury R30.0
Straw itch B88.0
Strawberry
  gallbladder K82.4
  mark Q82.5

Strawberry — *continued*
 tongue (red) (white) K14.3
Streak(s)
 macula, angioid H35.33
 ovarian Q50.32
Strephosymbolia F81.0
 secondary to organic lesion R48.8
Streptobacillary fever A25.1
Streptobacillosis A25.1
Streptobacillus moniliformis A25.1
Streptococcus, streptococcal — *see also* condition
 as cause of disease classified elsewhere B95.5
 group
  A, as cause of disease classified elsewhere B95.0
  B, as cause of disease classified elsewhere B95.1
  D, as cause of disease classified elsewhere B95.2
 pneumoniae, as cause of disease classified elsewhere
  B95.3
 specified NEC, as cause of disease classified elsewhere
  B95.4
Streptomycosis B47.1
Streptotrichosis A48.8
Stress F43.9
 family — *see* Disruption, family
 fetal P84
  complicating pregnancy O77.9
   due to drug administration O77.1
 mental NEC Z73.3
  work-related Z56.6
 physical NEC Z73.3
  work-related Z56.6
 polycythemia D75.1
 reaction — *see also* Reaction, stress F43.9
 work schedule Z56.3
Stretching, nerve — *see* Injury, nerve
Striae albicantes, atrophicae or distensae (cutis) L90.6
Stricture — *see also* Stenosis
 ampulla of Vater K83.1
 anus (sphincter) K62.4
  congenital Q42.3
   with fistula Q42.2
  infantile Q42.3
   with fistula Q42.2
 aorta (ascending) (congenital) Q25.1
  arteriosclerotic I70.0
  calcified I70.0
  supravalvular, congenital Q25.3
 aortic (valve) — *see* Stenosis, aortic
 aqueduct of Sylvius (congenital) Q03.0
  with spina bifida — *see* Spina bifida, by site, with
   hydrocephalus
  acquired G91.1
 artery I77.1
  basilar — *see* Occlusion, artery, basilar
  carotid — *see* Occlusion, artery, carotid
  celiac I77.4
  congenital (peripheral) Q27.8
   cerebral Q28.3
   coronary Q24.5
   digestive system Q27.8
   lower limb Q27.8
   retinal Q14.1
   specified site NEC Q27.8
   umbilical Q27.0
   upper limb Q27.8
  coronary — *see* Disease, heart, ischemic,
   atherosclerotic
   congenital Q24.5
  precerebral — *see* Occlusion, artery, precerebral
  pulmonary (congenital) Q25.6
   acquired I28.8
  renal I70.1
  vertebral — *see* Occlusion, artery, vertebral
 auditory canal (external) (congenital)
  acquired — *see* Stenosis, external ear canal
 bile duct (common) (hepatic) K83.1
  congenital Q44.3
  postoperative K91.89
 bladder N32.89
  neck N32.0
 bowel — *see* Obstruction, intestine
 brain G93.89
 bronchus J98.09
  congenital Q32.3
  syphilitic A52.72
 cardia (stomach) K22.2
  congenital Q39.3
 cardiac — *see also* Disease, heart

Stricture — *continued*
 cardiac — *see also* Disease, heart — *continued*
  orifice (stomach) K22.2
 cecum — *see* Obstruction, intestine
 cervix, cervical (canal) N88.2
  congenital Q51.828
  in pregnancy — *see* Pregnancy, complicated by,
   abnormal cervix
   causing obstructed labor O65.5
 colon — *see also* Obstruction, intestine
  congenital Q42.9
  specified NEC Q42.8
 colostomy K94.03
 common (bile) duct K83.1
 coronary (artery) — *see* Disease, heart, ischemic,
  atherosclerotic
 cystic duct — *see* Obstruction, gallbladder
 digestive organs NEC, congenital Q45.8
 duodenum K31.5
  congenital Q41.0
 ear canal (external) (congenital) Q16.1
  acquired — *see* Stricture, auditory canal, acquired
 ejaculatory duct N50.89
 enterostomy K94.13
 esophagus K22.2
  congenital Q39.3
  syphilitic A52.79
   congenital A50.59 *[K23]*
 eustachian tube — *see also* Obstruction, eustachian
  tube
  congenital Q17.8
 fallopian tube N97.1
  gonococcal A54.24
  tuberculous A18.17
 gallbladder — *see* Obstruction, gallbladder
 glottis J38.6
 heart — *see also* Disease, heart
  valve — *see also* Endocarditis I38
   aortic Q23.0
   mitral Q23.2
   pulmonary Q22.1
   tricuspid Q22.4
 hepatic duct K83.1
 hourglass, of stomach K31.2
 hymen N89.6
 hypopharynx J39.2
 ileum — *see also* Obstruction, intestine, specified NEC
  K56.699
  congenital Q41.2
 intestine — *see also* Obstruction, intestine
  congenital (small) Q41.9
   large Q42.9
    specified NEC Q42.8
   specified NEC Q41.8
  ischemic K55.1
 jejunum — *see also* Obstruction, intestine, specified
  NEC K56.699
  congenital Q41.1
 lacrimal passages — *see also* Stenosis, lacrimal
  congenital Q10.5
 larynx J38.6
  congenital NEC Q31.8
   subglottic Q31.1
  syphilitic A52.73
   congenital A50.59 *[J99]*
 meatus
  ear (congenital) Q16.1
   acquired — *see* Stricture, auditory canal, ac-
    quired
   osseous (ear) (congenital) Q16.1
    acquired — *see* Stricture, auditory canal, ac-
     quired
  urinarius — *see also* Stricture, urethra
   congenital Q64.33
 mitral (valve) — *see* Stenosis, mitral
 myocardium, myocardial I51.5
  hypertrophic subaortic (idiopathic) I42.1
 nares (anterior) (posterior) J34.89
  congenital Q30.0
 nasal duct — *see also* Stenosis, lacrimal, duct
  congenital Q10.5
 nasolacrimal duct — *see also* Stenosis, lacrimal, duct
  congenital Q10.5
 nasopharynx J39.2
  syphilitic A52.73
 nose J34.89
  congenital Q30.0
 nostril (anterior) (posterior) J34.89

Stricture — *continued*
 nostril — *continued*
  congenital Q30.0
  syphilitic A52.73
   congenital A50.59 *[J99]*
 organ or site, congenital NEC — *see* Atresia, by site
 os uteri — *see* Stricture, cervix
 osseous meatus (ear) (congenital) Q16.1
  acquired — *see* Stricture, auditory canal, acquired
 oviduct — *see* Stricture, fallopian tube
 pelviureteric junction (congenital) Q62.11
  acquired, with hydronephrosis N13.0
 penis, by foreign body T19.4 ☑
 pharynx J39.2
 prostate N42.89
 pulmonary, pulmonic
  artery (congenital) Q25.6
   acquired I28.8
   noncongenital I28.8
  infundibulum (congenital) Q24.3
  valve I37.0
   congenital Q22.1
  vein, acquired I28.8
  vessel NEC I28.8
 punctum lacrimale — *see also* Stenosis, lacrimal,
  punctum
  congenital Q10.5
 pylorus (hypertrophic) K31.1
  adult K31.1
  congenital Q40.0
  infantile Q40.0
 rectosigmoid — *see also* Obstruction, intestine, specified NEC K56.699
 rectum (sphincter) K62.4
  congenital Q42.1
   with fistula Q42.0
  due to
   chlamydial lymphogranuloma A55
   irradiation K91.89
   lymphogranuloma venereum A55
  gonococcal A54.6
  inflammatory (chlamydial) A55
  syphilitic A52.74
  tuberculous A18.32
 renal artery I70.1
  congenital Q27.1
 salivary duct or gland (any) K11.8
 sigmoid (flexure) — *see* Obstruction, intestine
 spermatic cord N50.89
 stoma (following) (of)
  colostomy K94.03
  enterostomy K94.13
  gastrostomy K94.23
  ileostomy K94.13
  tracheostomy J95.03
 stomach K31.89
  congenital Q40.2
  hourglass K31.2
 subaortic Q24.4
  hypertrophic (acquired) (idiopathic) I42.1
 subglottic J38.6
 syphilitic NEC A52.79
 trachea J39.8
  congenital Q32.1
  syphilitic A52.73
  tuberculous NEC A15.5
 tracheostomy J95.03
 tricuspid (valve) — *see* Stenosis, tricuspid
 tunica vaginalis N50.89
 ureter (postoperative) N13.5
  with
   hydronephrosis N13.1
    with infection N13.6
   pyelonephritis (chronic) N11.1
  congenital — *see* Atresia, ureter
  tuberculous A18.11
 ureteropelvic junction (congenital) Q62.11
  acquired, with hydronephrosis N13.0
 ureterovesical orifice N13.5
  with infection N13.6
 urethra (organic) (spasmodic) — *see also* Stricture,
  urethra, male N35.919
  associated with schistosomiasis B65.0 *[N37]*
  congenital Q64.39
   valvular (posterior) Q64.2
  due to
   infection — *see* Stricture, urethra, postinfective
   trauma — *see* Stricture, urethra, post-traumatic

▽ Subterms under main terms may continue to next column or page   ☑ Additional Character Required — Refer to the Tabular List for Character Selection   **295**

Strawberry — Stricture

Stricture — *continued*

urethra — *see also* Stricture, urethra, male — *continued*

female N35.92

gonococcal, gonorrheal A54.01

infective NEC — *see* Stricture, urethra, postinfective

late effect (sequelae) of injury — *see* Stricture, urethra, post-traumatic

male N35.919

anterior urethra N35.914

bulbous urethra N35.912

meatal N35.911

membranous urethra N35.913

overlapping sites N35.916

postcatheterization — *see* Stricture, urethra, postprocedural

postinfective NEC

female N35.12

male N35.119

anterior urethra N35.114

bulbous urethra N35.112

meatal N35.111

membranous urethra N35.113

overlapping sites N35.116

postobstetric N35.021

postoperative — *see* Stricture, urethra, postprocedural

postprocedural

female N99.12

male N99.114

anterior bulbous urethra N99.113

bulbous urethra N99.111

fossa navicularis N99.115

meatal N99.110

membranous urethra N99.112

overlapping sites N99.116

post-traumatic

female N35.028

due to childbirth N35.021

male N35.014

anterior urethra N35.013

bulbous urethra N35.011

meatal N35.010

membranous urethra N35.012

overlapping sites N35.016

sequela (late effect) of

childbirth N35.021

injury — *see* Stricture, urethra, post-traumatic

specified cause NEC

female N35.82

male N35.819

anterior urethra N35.814

bulbous urethra N35.812

meatal N35.811

membranous urethra N35.813

overlapping sites N35.816

syphilitic A52.76

traumatic — *see* Stricture, urethra, post-traumatic

valvular (posterior), congenital Q64.2

urinary meatus — *see* Stricture, urethra

uterus, uterine (synechiae) N85.6

os (external) (internal) — *see* Stricture, cervix

vagina (outlet) — *see* Stenosis, vagina

valve (cardiac) (heart) — *see also* Endocarditis

congenital

aortic Q23.0

mitral Q23.2

pulmonary Q22.1

tricuspid Q22.4

vas deferens N50.89

congenital Q55.4

vein I87.1

vena cava (inferior) (superior) NEC I87.1

congenital Q26.0

vesicourethral orifice N32.0

congenital Q64.31

vulva (acquired) N90.5

Stridor R06.1

congenital (larynx) P28.89

Stridulous — *see* condition

Stroke (apoplectic) (brain) (embolic) (ischemic) (paralytic) (thrombotic) I63.9

cryptogenic — *see also* infarction, cerebral I63.9

epileptic — *see* Epilepsy

heat T67.01 ☑

exertional T67.02 ☑

specified NEC T67.09 ☑

in evolution I63.9

Stroke — *continued*

intraoperative

during cardiac surgery I97.810

during other surgery I97.811

lightning — *see* Lightning

meaning

cerebral hemorrhage — *code to* Hemorrhage, intracranial

cerebral infarction — *code to* Infarction, cerebral

postprocedural

following cardiac surgery I97.820

following other surgery I97.821

sun T67.01 ☑

specified NEC T67.09 ☑

unspecified (NOS) I63.9

Stromatosis, endometrial D39.0

Strongyloidiasis, strongyloidosis B78.9

cutaneous B78.1

disseminated B78.7

intestinal B78.0

Strophulus pruriginosus L28.2

Struck by lightning — *see* Lightning

Struma — *see also* Goiter

Hashimoto E06.3

lymphomatosa E06.3

nodosa (simplex) E04.9

endemic E01.2

multinodular E01.1

multinodular E04.2

iodine-deficiency related E01.1

toxic or with hyperthyroidism E05.20

with thyroid storm E05.21

multinodular E05.20

with thyroid storm E05.21

uninodular E05.10

with thyroid storm E05.11

toxicosa E05.20

with thyroid storm E05.21

multinodular E05.20

with thyroid storm E05.21

uninodular E05.10

with thyroid storm E05.11

uninodular E04.1

ovarii D27.- ☑

Riedel's E06.5

Strumipriva cachexia E03.4

Strümpell-Marie spine — *see* Spondylitis, ankylosing

Strümpell-Westphal pseudosclerosis E83.01

Stuart deficiency disease (factor X) D68.2

Stuart-Prower factor deficiency (factor X) D68.2

Student's elbow — *see* Bursitis, elbow, olecranon

Stump — *see* Amputation

Stunting, nutritional E45

Stupor (catatonic) R40.1

depressive (single episode) F32.89

recurrent episode F33.8

dissociative F44.2

manic F30.2

manic-depressive F31.89

psychogenic (anergic) F44.2

reaction to exceptional stress (transient) F43.0

Sturge (-Weber) (-Dimitri) (-Kalischer) **disease or syndrome** Q85.8

Stuttering F80.81

adult onset F98.5

childhood onset F80.81

following cerebrovascular disease — *see* Disorder, fluency, following cerebrovascular disease

in conditions classified elsewhere R47.82

Sty, stye (external) (internal) (meibomian) (zeisian) — *see* Hordeolum

Subacidity, gastric K31.89

psychogenic F45.8

Subacute — *see* condition

Subarachnoid — *see* condition

Subcortical — *see* condition

Subcostal syndrome, nerve compression — *see* Mononeuropathy, upper limb, specified site NEC

Subcutaneous, subcuticular — *see* condition

Subdural — *see* condition

Subendocardium — *see* condition

Subependymoma

specified site — *see* Neoplasm, uncertain behavior, by site

unspecified site D43.2

Suberosis J67.3

Subglossitis — *see* Glossitis

Subhemophilia D66

Subinvolution

breast (postlactational) (postpuerperal) N64.89

puerperal O90.89

uterus (chronic) (nonpuerperal) N85.3

puerperal O90.89

Sublingual — *see* condition

Sublinguitis — *see* Sialoadenitis

Subluxatable hip Q65.6

Subluxation — *see also* Dislocation

acromioclavicular S43.11- ☑

ankle S93.0- ☑

atlantoaxial, recurrent M43.4

with myelopathy M43.3

carpometacarpal (joint) NEC S63.05- ☑

thumb S63.04- ☑

complex, vertebral — *see* Complex, subluxation

congenital — *see also* Malposition, congenital

hip — *See* Dislocation, hip, congenital, partial

joint (excluding hip)

lower limb Q68.8

shoulder Q68.8

upper limb Q68.8

elbow (traumatic) S53.10- ☑

anterior S53.11- ☑

lateral S53.14- ☑

medial S53.13- ☑

posterior S53.12- ☑

specified type NEC S53.19- ☑

finger S63.20- ☑

index S63.20- ☑

interphalangeal S63.22- ☑

distal S63.24- ☑

index S63.24- ☑

little S63.24- ☑

middle S63.24- ☑

ring S63.24- ☑

index S63.22- ☑

little S63.22- ☑

middle S63.22- ☑

proximal S63.23- ☑

index S63.23- ☑

little S63.23- ☑

middle S63.23- ☑

ring S63.23- ☑

ring S63.22- ☑

little S63.20- ☑

metacarpophalangeal S63.21- ☑

index S63.21- ☑

little S63.21- ☑

middle S63.21- ☑

ring S63.21- ☑

middle S63.20- ☑

ring S63.20- ☑

foot S93.30- ☑

specified site NEC S93.33- ☑

tarsal joint S93.31- ☑

tarsometatarsal joint S93.32- ☑

toe — *see* Subluxation, toe

hip S73.00- ☑

anterior S73.03- ☑

obturator S73.02- ☑

central S73.04- ☑

posterior S73.01- ☑

interphalangeal (joint)

finger S63.22- ☑

distal joint S63.24- ☑

index S63.24- ☑

little S63.24- ☑

middle S63.24- ☑

ring S63.24- ☑

index S63.22- ☑

little S63.22- ☑

middle S63.22- ☑

proximal joint S63.23- ☑

index S63.23- ☑

little S63.23- ☑

middle S63.23- ☑

ring S63.23- ☑

ring S63.22- ☑

thumb S63.12- ☑

toe S93.13- ☑

great S93.13- ☑

lesser S93.13- ☑

joint prosthesis — *see* Complications, joint prosthesis, mechanical, displacement, by site

☑ **Additional Character Required** — Refer to the Tabular List for Character Selection

▽ **Subterms under main terms may continue to next column or page**

Subluxation — *continued*
 knee S83.10- ☑
  cap — *see* Subluxation, patella
  patella — *see* Subluxation, patella
  proximal tibia
   anteriorly S83.11- ☑
   laterally S83.14- ☑
   medially S83.13- ☑
   posteriorly S83.12- ☑
  specified type NEC S83.19- ☑
 lens — *see* Dislocation, lens, partial
 ligament, traumatic — *see* Sprain, by site
 metacarpal (bone)
  proximal end S63.06- ☑
 metacarpophalangeal (joint)
  finger S63.21- ☑
   index S63.21- ☑
   little S63.21- ☑
   middle S63.21- ☑
   ring S63.21- ☑
  thumb S63.11- ☑
 metatarsophalangeal joint S93.14- ☑
  great toe S93.14- ☑
  lesser toe S93.14- ☑
 midcarpal (joint) S63.03- ☑
 patella S83.00- ☑
  lateral S83.01- ☑
  recurrent (nontraumatic) — *see* Dislocation, patella, recurrent, incomplete
  specified type NEC S83.09- ☑
 pathological — *see* Dislocation, pathological
 radial head S53.00- ☑
  anterior S53.01- ☑
  nursemaid's elbow S53.03- ☑
  posterior S53.02- ☑
  specified type NEC S53.09- ☑
 radiocarpal (joint) S63.02- ☑
 radioulnar (joint)
  distal S63.01- ☑
  proximal — *see* Subluxation, elbow
 shoulder
  congenital Q68.8
  girdle S43.30- ☑
   scapula S43.31- ☑
   specified site NEC S43.39- ☑
  traumatic S43.00- ☑
   anterior S43.01- ☑
   inferior S43.03- ☑
   posterior S43.02- ☑
   specified type NEC S43.08- ☑
 sternoclavicular (joint) S43.20- ☑
  anterior S43.21- ☑
  posterior S43.22- ☑
 symphysis (pubis)
 thumb S63.103 ☑
  interphalangeal joint — *see* Subluxation, interphalangeal (joint), thumb
  metacarpophalangeal joint — *see* Subluxation, metacarpophalangeal (joint), thumb
 toe(s) S93.10- ☑
  great S93.10- ☑
   interphalangeal joint S93.13- ☑
   metatarsophalangeal joint S93.14- ☑
  interphalangeal joint S93.13- ☑
  lesser S93.10- ☑
   interphalangeal joint S93.13- ☑
   metatarsophalangeal joint S93.14- ☑
  metatarsophalangeal joint S93.149 ☑
 ulna
  distal end S63.07- ☑
  proximal end — *see* Subluxation, elbow
 ulnohumeral joint — *see* Subluxation, elbow
 vertebral
  recurrent NEC — *see* subcategory M43.5 ☑
  traumatic
   cervical S13.100 ☑
    atlantoaxial joint S13.120 ☑
    atlantooccipital joint S13.110 ☑
    atloidooccipital joint S13.110 ☑
    joint between
     C0 and C1 S13.110 ☑
     C1 and C2 S13.120 ☑
     C2 and C3 S13.130 ☑
     C3 and C4 S13.140 ☑
     C4 and C5 S13.150 ☑
     C5 and C6 S13.160 ☑

Subluxation — *continued*
 vertebral — *continued*
  traumatic — *continued*
   cervical — *continued*
    joint between — *continued*
     C6 and C7 S13.170 ☑
     C7 and T1 S13.180 ☑
    occipitoatloid joint S13.110 ☑
   lumbar S33.100 ☑
    joint between
     L1 and L2 S33.110 ☑
     L2 and L3 S33.120 ☑
     L3 and L4 S33.130 ☑
     L4 and L5 S33.140 ☑
   thoracic S23.100 ☑
    joint between
     T1 and T2 S23.110 ☑
     T2 and T3 S23.120 ☑
     T3 and T4 S23.122 ☑
     T4 and T5 S23.130 ☑
     T5 and T6 S23.132 ☑
     T6 and T7 S23.140 ☑
     T7 and T8 S23.142 ☑
     T8 and T9 S23.150 ☑
     T9 and T10 S23.152 ☑
     T10 and T11 S23.160 ☑
     T11 and T12 S23.162 ☑
     T12 and L1 S23.170 ☑
  wrist (carpal bone) S63.00- ☑
   carpometacarpal joint — *see* Subluxation, carpometacarpal (joint)
   distal radioulnar joint — *see* Subluxation, radioulnar (joint), distal
   metacarpal bone, proximal — *see* Subluxation, metacarpal (bone), proximal end
   midcarpal — *see* Subluxation, midcarpal (joint)
   radiocarpal joint — *see* Subluxation, radiocarpal (joint)
   recurrent — *see* Dislocation, recurrent, wrist
   specified site NEC S63.09- ☑
   ulna — *see* Subluxation, ulna, distal end
Submaxillary — *see* condition
Submersion (fatal) (nonfatal) T75.1 ☑
Submucous — *see* condition
Subnormal, subnormality
 accommodation (old age) H52.4
 mental — *see* Disability, intellectual
 temperature (accidental) T68 ☑
Subphrenic — *see* condition
Subscapular nerve — *see* condition
Subseptus uterus Q51.28
Subsiding appendicitis K36
Substance (other psychoactive) **-induced**
 anxiety disorder F19.980
 bipolar and related disorder F19.94
 delirium F19.921
 depressive disorder F19.94
 major neurocognitive disorder F19.97
 mild neurocognitive disorder F19.988
 obsessive-compulsive and related disorder F19.988
 psychotic disorder F19.959
 sexual dysfunction F19.981
 sleep disorder F19.982
Substernal thyroid E04.9
 congenital Q89.2
Substitution disorder F44.9
Subtentorial — *see* condition
Subthyroidism (acquired) — *see also* Hypothyroidism
 congenital E03.1
Succenturiate placenta O43.19- ☑
Sucking thumb, child (excessive) F98.8
Sudamen, sudamina L74.1
Sudanese kala-azar B55.0
Sudden
 hearing loss — *see* Deafness, sudden
 heart failure — *see* Failure, heart
Sudeck's atrophy, disease, or syndrome — *see* Algoneurodystrophy
Suffocation — *see* Asphyxia, traumatic
Sugar
 blood
  high (transient) R73.9
  low (transient) E16.2
 in urine R81
Suicide, suicidal (attempted) T14.91 ☑
 by poisoning — *see* Table of Drugs and Chemicals
 history of (personal) Z91.5

Suicide, suicidal — *continued*
 history of — *continued*
  in family Z81.8
 ideation — *see* Ideation, suicidal
 risk
  meaning personal history of attempted suicide Z91.5
  meaning suicidal ideation — *see* Ideation, suicidal
 tendencies
  meaning personal history of attempted suicide Z91.5
  meaning suicidal ideation — *see* Ideation, suicidal
 trauma — *see* nature of injury by site
Suipestifer infection — *see* Infection, salmonella
Sulfhemoglobinemia, sulphemoglobinemia (acquired) (with methemoglobinemia) D74.8
Sumatran mite fever A75.3
Summer — *see* condition
Sunburn L55.9
 due to
  tanning bed (acute) L56.8
   chronic L57.8
  ultraviolet radiation (acute) L56.8
   chronic L57.8
 first degree L55.0
 second degree L55.1
 third degree L55.2
SUNCT (short lasting unilateral neuralgiform headache with conjunctival injection and tearing) G44.059
 intractable G44.051
 not intractable G44.059
Sundowning F05
Sunken acetabulum — *see* Derangement, joint, specified type NEC, hip
Sunstroke T67.01 ☑
 specified NEC T67.09 ☑
Superfecundation — *see* Pregnancy, multiple
Superfetation — *see* Pregnancy, multiple
Superinvolution (uterus) N85.8
Supernumerary (congenital)
 aortic cusps Q23.8
 auditory ossicles Q16.3
 bone Q79.8
 breast Q83.1
 carpal bones Q74.0
 cusps, heart valve NEC Q24.8
  aortic Q23.8
  mitral Q23.2
  pulmonary Q22.3
 digit(s) Q69.9
 ear (lobule) Q17.0
 fallopian tube Q50.6
 finger Q69.0
 hymen Q52.4
 kidney Q63.0
 lacrimonasal duct Q10.6
 lobule (ear) Q17.0
 mitral cusps Q23.2
 muscle Q79.8
 nipple(s) Q83.3
 organ or site not listed — *see* Accessory
 ossicles, auditory Q16.3
 ovary Q50.31
 oviduct Q50.6
 pulmonary, pulmonic cusps Q22.3
 rib Q76.6
  cervical or first (syndrome) Q76.5
 roots (of teeth) K00.2
 spleen Q89.09
 tarsal bones Q74.2
 teeth K00.1
 testis Q55.29
 thumb Q69.1
 toe Q69.2
 uterus Q51.28
 vagina Q52.1 ☑
 vertebra Q76.49
Supervision (of)
 contraceptive — *see* Prescription, contraceptives
 dietary (for) Z71.3
  allergy (food) Z71.3
  colitis Z71.3
  diabetes mellitus Z71.3
  food allergy or intolerance Z71.3
  gastritis Z71.3
  hypercholesterolemia Z71.3
  hypoglycemia Z71.3
  intolerance (food) Z71.3
  obesity Z71.3
  specified NEC Z71.3

Supervision — continued
healthy infant or child Z76.2
foundling Z76.1
high-risk pregnancy — see Pregnancy, complicated by, high, risk
lactation Z39.1
pregnancy — see Pregnancy, supervision of
Supplemental teeth K00.1
Suppression
binocular vision H53.34
lactation O92.5
menstruation N94.89
ovarian secretion E28.39
renal N28.9
urine, urinary secretion R34
Suppuration, suppurative — see also condition
accessory sinus (chronic) — see Sinusitis
adrenal gland
antrum (chronic) — see Sinusitis, maxillary
bladder — see Cystitis
brain G06.0
sequelae G09
breast N61.1
puerperal, postpartum or gestational — see Mastitis, obstetric, purulent
dental periosteum M27.3
ear (middle) — see also Otitis, media
external NEC — see Otitis, externa, infective
internal — see subcategory H83.0 ☑
ethmoidal (chronic) (sinus) — see Sinusitis, ethmoidal
fallopian tube — see Salpingo-oophoritis
frontal (chronic) (sinus) — see Sinusitis, frontal
gallbladder (acute) K81.0
gum K05.20
generalized — see Periodontitis, aggressive, generalized
localized — see Periodontitis, aggressive, localized
intracranial G06.0
joint — see Arthritis, pyogenic or pyemic
labyrinthine — see subcategory H83.0 ☑
lung — see Abscess, lung
mammary gland N61.1
puerperal, postpartum O91.12
associated with lactation O91.13
maxilla, maxillary M27.2
sinus (chronic) — see Sinusitis, maxillary
muscle — see Myositis, infective
nasal sinus (chronic) — see Sinusitis
pancreas, acute — see also Pancreatitis, acute K85.80
parotid gland — see Sialoadenitis
pelvis, pelvic
female — see Disease, pelvis, inflammatory
male K65.0
pericranial — see Osteomyelitis
salivary duct or gland (any) — see Sialoadenitis
sinus (accessory) (chronic) (nasal) — see Sinusitis
sphenoidal sinus (chronic) — see Sinusitis, sphenoidal
thymus (gland) E32.1
thyroid (gland) E06.0
tonsil — see Tonsillitis
uterus — see Endometritis
Supraeruption of tooth (teeth) M26.34
Supraglottitis J04.30
with obstruction J04.31
Suprarenal (gland) — see condition
Suprascapular nerve — see condition
Suprasellar — see condition
Surfer's knots or nodules S89.8- ☑
Surgical
emphysema T81.82 ☑
procedures, complication or misadventure — see Complications, surgical procedures
shock T81.10 ☑
Surveillance (of) (for) — see also Observation
alcohol abuse Z71.41
contraceptive — see Prescription, contraceptives
dietary Z71.3
drug abuse Z71.51
Susceptibility to disease, genetic Z15.89
malignant neoplasm Z15.09
breast Z15.01
endometrium Z15.04
ovary Z15.02
prostate Z15.03
specified NEC Z15.09
multiple endocrine neoplasia Z15.81

Suspected condition, ruled out — see also Observation, suspected
amniotic cavity and membrane Z03.71
cervical shortening Z03.75
fetal anomaly Z03.73
fetal growth Z03.74
maternal and fetal conditions NEC Z03.79
newborn — see also Observation, newborn, suspected condition ruled out Z05.9
oligohydramnios Z03.71
placental problem Z03.72
polyhydramnios Z03.71
Suspended uterus
in pregnancy or childbirth — see Pregnancy, complicated by, abnormal uterus
Sutton's nevus D22.9
Suture
burst (in operation wound) T81.31 ☑
external operation wound T81.31 ☑
internal operation wound T81.32 ☑
inadvertently left in operation wound — see Foreign body, accidentally left during a procedure
removal Z48.02
Swab inadvertently left in operation wound — see Foreign body, accidentally left during a procedure
Swallowed, swallowing
difficulty — see Dysphagia
foreign body — see Foreign body, alimentary tract
Swan-neck deformity (finger) — see Deformity, finger, swan-neck
Swearing, compulsive F42.8
in Gilles de la Tourette's syndrome F95.2
Sweat, sweats
fetid L75.0
night R61
Sweating, excessive R61
Sweeley-Klionsky disease E75.21
Sweet's disease or dermatosis L98.2
Swelling (of) R60.9
abdomen, abdominal (not referable to any particular organ) — see Mass, abdominal
ankle — see Effusion, joint, ankle
arm M79.89
forearm M79.89
breast — see also Lump, breast N63.0
Calabar B74.3
cervical gland R59.0
chest, localized R22.2
ear H93.8- ☑
extremity (lower) (upper) — see Disorder, soft tissue, specified type NEC
finger M79.89
foot M79.89
glands R59.9
generalized R59.1
localized R59.0
hand M79.89
head (localized) R22.0
inflammatory — see Inflammation
intra-abdominal — see Mass, abdominal
joint — see Effusion, joint
leg M79.89
lower M79.89
limb — see Disorder, soft tissue, specified type NEC
localized (skin) R22.9
chest R22.2
head R22.0
limb
lower — see Mass, localized, limb, lower
upper — see Mass, localized, limb, upper
neck R22.1
trunk R22.2
neck (localized) R22.1
pelvic — see Mass, abdominal
scrotum N50.89
splenic — see Splenomegaly
testis N50.89
toe M79.89
umbilical R19.09
wandering, due to Gnathostoma (spinigerum) B83.1
white — see Tuberculosis, arthritis
Swift (-Feer) **disease**
overdose or wrong substance given or taken — see Table of Drugs and Chemicals, by drug, poisoning
Swimmer's
cramp T75.1 ☑
ear H60.33- ☑

Swimmer's — continued
itch B65.3
Swimming in the head R42
Swollen — see Swelling
Swyer syndrome Q99.1
Sycosis L73.8
barbae (not parasitic) L73.8
contagiosa (mycotic) B35.0
lupoides L73.8
mycotic B35.0
parasitic B35.0
vulgaris L73.8
Sydenham's chorea — see Chorea, Sydenham's
Sylvatic yellow fever A95.0
Sylvest's disease B33.0
Symblepharon H11.23- ☑
congenital Q10.3
Symond's syndrome G93.2
Sympathetic — see condition
Sympatheticotonia G90.8
Sympathicoblastoma
specified site — see Neoplasm, malignant, by site
unspecified site C74.90
Sympathogonioma — see Sympathicoblastoma
Symphalangy (fingers) (toes) Q70.9
Symptoms NEC R68.89
breast NEC N64.59
cold J00
development NEC R63.8
factitious, self-induced — see Disorder, factitious
genital organs, female R10.2
involving
abdomen NEC R19.8
appearance NEC R46.89
awareness R41.9
altered mental status R41.82
amnesia — see Amnesia
borderline intellectual functioning R41.83
coma — see Coma
disorientation R41.0
neurologic neglect syndrome R41.4
senile cognitive decline R41.81
specified symptom NEC R41.89
behavior NEC R46.89
cardiovascular system NEC R09.89
chest NEC R09.89
circulatory system NEC R09.89
cognitive functions R41.9
altered mental status R41.82
amnesia — see Amnesia
borderline intellectual functioning R41.83
coma — see Coma
disorientation R41.0
neurologic neglect syndrome R41.4
senile cognitive decline R41.81
specified symptom NEC R41.89
development NEC R62.50
digestive system NEC R19.8
emotional state NEC R45.89
emotional lability R45.86
food and fluid intake R63.8
general perceptions and sensations R44.9
specified NEC R44.8
musculoskeletal system R29.91
specified NEC R29.898
nervous system R29.90
specified NEC R29.818
pelvis NEC R19.8
respiratory system NEC R09.89
skin and integument R23.9
urinary system R39.9
menopausal N95.1
metabolism NEC R63.8
neurotic F48.8
of infancy R68.19
pelvis NEC, female R10.2
skin and integument NEC R23.9
subcutaneous tissue NEC R23.9
viral cold J00
Sympus Q74.2
Syncephalus Q89.4
Synchondrosis
abnormal (congenital) Q78.8
ischiopubic M91.0
Synchysis (scintillans) (senile) (vitreous body) H43.89
Syncope (near) (pre-) R55
anginosa I20.8
bradycardia R00.1

Syncope — *continued*
cardiac R55
carotid sinus G90.01
due to spinal (lumbar) puncture G97.1
heart R55
heat T67.1 ☑
laryngeal R05
psychogenic F48.8
tussive R05
vasoconstriction R55
vasodepressor R55
vasomotor R55
vasovagal R55
Syndactylism, syndactyly Q70.9
complex (with synostosis)
    fingers Q70.0- ☑
    toes Q70.2- ☑
simple (without synostosis)
    fingers Q70.1- ☑
    toes Q70.3- ☑
Syndrome — *see also* Disease
5q minus NOS D46.C (*following* D46.2)
48,XXXX Q97.1
49,XXXXX Q97.1
abdominal
  acute R10.0
  muscle deficiency Q79.4
abnormal innervation H02.519
  left H02.516
    lower H02.515
    upper H02.514
  right H02.513
    lower H02.512
    upper H02.511
abstinence, neonatal P96.1
acid pulmonary aspiration, obstetric O74.0
acquired immunodeficiency — *see* Human, immunod-
    eficiency virus (HIV) disease
acute abdominal R10.0
acute respiratory distress (adult) (child) J80
  idiopathic J84.114
Adair-Dighton Q78.0
Adams-Stokes (-Morgagni) I45.9
adiposogenital E23.6
adrenal
  hemorrhage (meningococcal) A39.1
  meningococcic A39.1
adrenocortical — *see* Cushing's, syndrome
adrenogenital E25.9
  congenital, associated with enzyme deficiency E25.0
afferent loop NEC K91.89
Alagille's Q44.7
alcohol withdrawal (without convulsions) — *see* De-
    pendence, alcohol, with, withdrawal
Alder's D72.0
Aldrich (-Wiskott) D82.0
alien hand R41.4
Alport Q87.81
alveolar hypoventilation E66.2
alveolocapillary block J84.10
amnesic, amnestic (confabulatory) (due to) — *see* Dis-
    order, amnesic
amyostatic (Wilson's disease) E83.01
androgen insensitivity E34.50
  complete E34.51
  partial E34.52
androgen resistance — *see also* Syndrome, androgen
    insensitivity E34.50
Angelman Q93.51
anginal — *see* Angina
ankyloglossia superior Q38.1
anterior
  chest wall R07.89
  cord G83.82
  spinal artery G95.19
    compression M47.019
      cervical region M47.012
      cervicothoracic region M47.013
      lumbar region M47.016
      occipito-atlanto-axial region M47.011
      thoracic region M47.014
      thoracolumbar region M47.015
  tibial M76.81- ☑
antibody deficiency D80.9
  agammaglobulinemic D80.1
    hereditary D80.0
  congenital D80.0
  hypogammaglobulinemic D80.1

Syndrome — *continued*
antibody deficiency — *continued*
  hypogammaglobulinemic — *continued*
    hereditary D80.0
anticardiolipin (-antibody) D68.61
antidepressant discontinuation T43.205 ☑
antiphospholipid (-antibody) D68.61
aortic
  arch M31.4
  bifurcation I74.09
aortomesenteric duodenum occlusion K31.5
apical ballooning (transient left ventricular) I51.81
arcuate ligament I77.4
argentaffin, argintaffinoma E34.0
Arnold-Chiari — *see* Arnold-Chiari disease
Arrillaga-Ayerza I27.0
arterial tortuosity Q87.82
arteriovenous steal T82.898- ☑
Asherman's N85.6
aspiration, of newborn — *see* Aspiration, by substance,
    with pneumonia
  meconium P24.01
ataxia-telangiectasia G11.3
auriculotemporal G50.8
autoerythrocyte sensitization (Gardner-Diamond) D69.2
autoimmune lymphoproliferative [ALPS] D89.82
autoimmune polyglandular E31.0
autoinflammatory M04.9
  specified type NEC M04.8
autosomal — *see* Abnormal, autosomes
Avellis' G46.8
Ayerza (-Arrillaga) I27.0
Babinski-Nageotte G83.89
Bakwin-Krida Q78.5
bare lymphocyte D81.6
Barré-Guillain G61.0
Barré-Liéou M53.0
Barrett's — *see* Barrett's, esophagus
Barsony-Polgar K22.4
Bársony-Teschendorf K22.4
Barth E78.71
Bartter's E26.81
basal cell nevus Q87.89
Basedow's E05.00
  with thyroid storm E05.01
basilar artery G45.0
Batten-Steinert G71.11
battered
  baby or child — *see* Maltreatment, child, physical
    abuse
  spouse — *see* Maltreatment, adult, physical abuse
Beals Q87.40
Beau's I51.5
Beck's I65.8
Benedikt's G46.3
Béquez César (-Steinbrinck-Chédiak-Higashi) E70.330
Bernhardt-Roth — *see* Meralgia paresthetica
Bernhein's — *see* Failure, heart, right
big spleen D73.1
Bing-Horton's — *see* Horton's headache
Birt-Hogg-Dube syndrome Q87.89
Björck (-Thorsen) E34.0
black
  lung J60
  widow spider bite — *see* Toxicity, venom, spider,
    black widow
Blackfan-Diamond D61.01
Blau M04.8
blind loop K90.2
  congenital Q43.8
  postsurgical K91.2
blue sclera Q78.0
blue toe I75.02- ☑
Boder-Sedgewick G11.3
Boerhaave's K22.3
Borjeson Forssman Lehmann Q89.8
Bouillaud's I01.9
Bourneville (-Pringle) Q85.1
Bouveret (-Hoffman) I47.9
brachial plexus G54.0
bradycardia-tachycardia I49.5
brain (nonpsychotic) F09
  with psychosis, psychotic reaction F09
    acute or subacute — *see* Delirium
  congenital — *see* Disability, intellectual
  organic F09
    post-traumatic (nonpsychotic) F07.81

Syndrome — *continued*
brain — *continued*
  organic — *continued*
    post-traumatic — *continued*
      psychotic F09
    personality change F07.0
    postcontusional F07.81
    post-traumatic, nonpsychotic F07.81
    psycho-organic F09
    psychotic F06.8
brain stem stroke G46.3
Brandt's (acrodermatitis enteropathica) E83.2
broad ligament laceration N83.8
Brock's J98.11
bronze baby P83.88
Brown-Sequard G83.81
Brugada I49.8
bubbly lung P27.0
Buchem's M85.2
Budd-Chiari I82.0
bulbar (progressive) G12.22
Bürger-Grütz E78.3
Burke's K86.89
Burnett's (milk-alkali) E83.52
burning feet E53.9
Bywaters' T79.5 ☑
Call-Fleming I67.841
carbohydrate-deficient glycoprotein (CDGS) E77.8
carcinogenic thrombophlebitis I82.1
carcinoid E34.0
cardiac asthma I50.1
cardiacos negros I27.0
cardiofaciocutaneous Q87.89
cardiopulmonary-obesity E66.2
cardiorenal — *see* Hypertension, cardiorenal
cardiorespiratory distress (idiopathic), newborn P22.0
cardiovascular renal — *see* Hypertension, cardiorenal
carotid
  artery (hemispheric) (internal) G45.1
  body G90.01
  sinus G90.01
carpal tunnel G56.0- ☑
Cassidy (-Scholte) E34.0
cat cry Q93.4
cat eye Q92.8
cauda equina G83.4
causalgia — *see* Causalgia
celiac K90.0
  artery compression I77.4
  axis I77.4
central pain G89.0
cerebellar
  hereditary G11.9
  stroke G46.4
cerebellomedullary malformation — *see* Spina bifida
cerebral
  artery
    anterior G46.1
    middle G46.0
    posterior G46.2
  gigantism E22.0
cervical (root) M53.1
  disc — *see* Disorder, disc, cervical, with neuritis
  fusion Q76.1
  posterior, sympathicus M53.0
  rib Q76.5
  sympathetic paralysis G90.2
cervicobrachial (diffuse) M53.1
cervicocranial M53.0
cervicodorsal outlet G54.2
cervicothoracic outlet G54.0
Céstan (-Raymond) I65.8
Charcot's (angina cruris) (intermittent claudication)
    I73.9
Charcot-Weiss-Baker G90.09
CHARGE Q89.8
Chédiak-Higashi (-Steinbrinck) E70.330
chest wall R07.1
Chiari's (hepatic vein thrombosis) I82.0
Chilaiditi's Q43.3
child maltreatment — *see* Maltreatment, child
chondrocostal junction M94.0
chondroectodermal dysplasia Q77.6
chromosome 4 short arm deletion Q93.3
chromosome 5 short arm deletion Q93.4
chronic
  infantile neurological, cutaneous and articular
    (CINCA) M04.2

Syndrome — *continued*
chronic — *continued*
　　pain G89.4
　　　personality F68.8
Churg-Strauss M30.1
Clarke-Hadfield K86.89
Clerambault's automatism G93.89
Clouston's (hidrotic ectodermal dysplasia) Q82.4
clumsiness, clumsy child F82
cluster headache G44.009
　　intractable G44.001
　　not intractable G44.009
Coffin-Lowry Q89.8
cold injury (newborn) P80.0
combined immunity deficiency D81.9
compartment (deep) (posterior) (traumatic) T79.A0 ☑
　　(*following* T79.7)
　　abdomen T79.A3 ☑ (*following* T79.7)
　　lower extremity (hip, buttock, thigh, leg, foot, toes)
　　　T79.A2 ☑ (*following* T79.7)
　　nontraumatic
　　　abdomen M79.A3 (*following* M79.7)
　　　lower extremity (hip, buttock, thigh, leg, foot,
　　　　toes) M79.A2- ☑ (*following* M79.7)
　　　specified site NEC M79.A9 (*following* M79.7)
　　　upper extremity (shoulder, arm, forearm, wrist,
　　　　hand, fingers) M79.A1- ☑ (*following*
　　　　M79.7)
　　postprocedural — *see* Syndrome, compartment,
　　　nontraumatic
　　specified site NEC T79.A9 ☑ (*following* T79.7)
　　upper extremity (shoulder, arm, forearm, wrist,
　　　hand, fingers) T79.A1 ☑ (*following* T79.7)
complex regional pain — *see* Syndrome, pain, complex
　　regional
compression T79.5 ☑
　　anterior spinal — *see* Syndrome, anterior, spinal
　　　artery, compression
　　cauda equina G83.4
　　celiac artery I77.4
　　vertebral artery M47.029
　　　cervical region M47.022
　　　occipito-atlanto-axial region M47.021
concussion F07.81
congenital
　　affecting multiple systems NEC Q87.89
　　central alveolar hypoventilation G47.35
　　facial diplegia Q87.0
　　muscular hypertrophy-cerebral Q87.89
　　oculo-auriculovertebral Q87.0
　　oculofacial diplegia (Moebius) Q87.0
　　rubella (manifest) P35.0
congestion-fibrosis (pelvic), female N94.89
congestive dysmenorrhea N94.6
connective tissue M35.9
　　overlap NEC M35.1
Conn's E26.01
conus medullaris G95.81
cord
　　anterior G83.82
　　posterior G83.83
coronary
　　acute NEC I24.9
　　insufficiency or intermediate I20.0
　　slow flow I20.8
Costen's (complex) M26.69
costochondral junction M94.0
costoclavicular G54.0
costovertebral E22.0
Cowden Q85.8
craniovertebral M53.9
Creutzfeldt-Jakob — *see* Creutzfeldt-Jakob disease or
　　syndrome
crib death R99
cricopharyngeal — *see* Dysphagia
cri-du-chat Q93.4
croup J05.0
CRPS I — *see* Syndrome, pain, complex regional I
crush T79.5 ☑
cryopyrin-associated perodic M04.2
cryptophthalmos Q87.0
cubital tunnel — *see* Lesion, nerve, ulnar
Curschmann (-Batten) (-Steinert) G71.11
Cushing's E24.9
　　alcohol-induced E24.4
　　due to
　　　alcohol
　　　drugs E24.2

Syndrome — *continued*
Cushing's — *continued*
　　due to — *continued*
　　　ectopic ACTH E24.3
　　　overproduction of pituitary ACTH E24.0
　　drug-induced E24.2
　　overdose or wrong substance given or taken — *see*
　　　Table of Drugs and Chemicals, by drug, poi-
　　　soning
　　pituitary-dependent E24.0
　　specified type NEC E24.8
cystic duct stump K91.5
Dana-Putnam D51.0
Danbolt (-Cross) (acrodermatitis enteropathica) E83.2
Dandy-Walker Q03.1
　　with spina bifida Q07.01
Danlos' — *see also* Syndrome, Ehlers-Danlos Q79.60
De Quervain E34.51
de Toni-Fanconi (-Debré) E72.09
　　with cystinosis E72.04
defibrination — *see also* Fibrinolysis
　　with
　　　antepartum hemorrhage — *see* Hemorrhage,
　　　　antepartum, with coagulation defect
　　　intrapartum hemorrhage — *see* Hemorrhage,
　　　　complicating, delivery
　　newborn P60
　　postpartum O72.3
Degos' I77.89
Déjérine-Roussy G89.0
delayed sleep phase G47.21
demyelinating G37.9
dependence — *see* F10-F19 with fourth character .2
depersonalization (-derealization) F48.1
di George's D82.1
diabetes mellitus in newborn infant P70.2
diabetes mellitus-hypertension-nephrosis — *see* Dia-
　　betes, nephrosis
diabetes-nephrosis — *see* Diabetes, nephrosis
diabetic amyotrophy — *see* Diabetes, amyotrophy
dialysis associated steal T82.898- ☑
Diamond-Blackfan D61.01
Diamond-Gardener D69.2
DIC (diffuse or disseminated intravascular coagulopa-
　　thy) D65
Dighton's Q78.0
disequilibrium E87.8
Döhle body-panmyelopathic D72.0
dorsolateral medullary G46.4
double athetosis G80.3
Down — *see also* Down syndrome Q90.9
Dresbach's (elliptocytosis) D58.1
Dressler's (postmyocardial infarction) I24.1
　　postcardiotomy I97.0
drug withdrawal, infant of dependent mother P96.1
dry eye H04.12- ☑
due to abnormality
　　chromosomal Q99.9
　　　sex
　　　　female phenotype Q97.9
　　　　male phenotype Q98.9
　　　　specified NEC Q99.8
dumping (postgastrectomy) K91.1
　　nonsurgical K31.89
Dupré's (meningism) R29.1
dysmetabolic X E88.81
dyspraxia, developmental F82
Eagle-Barrett Q79.4
Eaton-Lambert — *see* Syndrome, Lambert-Eaton
Ebstein's Q22.5
ectopic ACTH E24.3
eczema-thrombocytopenia D82.0
Eddowes' Q78.0
effort (psychogenic) F45.8
Ehlers-Danlos Q79.60
　　classical (cEDS) (classical EDS) Q79.61
　　hypermobile (hEDS) (hypermobile EDS) Q79.62
　　specified NEC Q79.69
　　vascular (vascular EDS) (vEDS) Q79.63
Eisenmenger's I27.83
Ekman's Q78.0
electric feet E53.8
Ellis-van Creveld Q77.6
empty nest Z60.0
endocrine-hypertensive E27.0
entrapment — *see* Neuropathy, entrapment
eosinophilia-myalgia M35.8
epileptic — *see also* Epilepsy, by type

Syndrome — *continued*
epileptic — *see also* Epilepsy, by type — *continued*
　　absence G40.A09 (*following* G40.3)
　　　intractable G40.A19 (*following* G40.3)
　　　　with status epilepticus G40.A11 (*following*
　　　　　G40.3)
　　　　without status epilepticus G40.A19 (*following*
　　　　　G40.3)
　　　not intractable G40.A09 (*following* G40.3)
　　　　with status epilepticus G40.A01 (*following*
　　　　　G40.3)
　　　　without status epilepticus G40.A09 (*following*
　　　　　G40.3)
Erdheim-Chester (ECD) E88.89
Erdheim's E22.0
erythrocyte fragmentation D59.4
Evans D69.41
exhaustion F48.8
extrapyramidal G25.9
　　specified NEC G25.89
eye retraction — *see* Strabismus
eyelid-malar-mandible Q87.0
Faber's D50.9
facial pain, paroxysmal G50.0
Fallot's Q21.3
familial cold autoinflammatory M04.2
familial eczema-thrombocytopenia (Wiskott-Aldrich)
　　D82.0
Fanconi (-de Toni) (-Debré) E72.09
　　with cystinosis E72.04
Fanconi's (anemia) (congenital pancytopenia) D61.09
fatigue
　　chronic R53.82
　　psychogenic F48.8
faulty bowel habit K59.39
Feil-Klippel (brevicollis) Q76.1
Felty's — *see* Felty's syndrome
fertile eunuch E23.0
fetal
　　alcohol (dysmorphic) Q86.0
　　hydantoin Q86.1
Fiedler's I40.1
first arch Q87.0
fish odor E72.89
Fisher's G61.0
Fitzhugh-Curtis
　　due to
　　　Chlamydia trachomatis A74.81
　　　Neisseria gonorrhorea (gonococcal peritonitis)
　　　　A54.85
Fitz's — *see also* Pancreatitis, acute K85.80
Flajani (-Basedow) E05.00
　　with thyroid storm E05.01
flatback — *see* Flatback syndrome
floppy
　　baby P94.2
　　iris (intraoeprative) (IFIS) H21.81
　　mitral valve I34.1
flush E34.0
Foix-Alajouanine G95.19
Fong's Q87.2
food protein-induced enterocolitis (FPIES) K52.21
foramen magnum G93.5
Foster-Kennedy H47.14- ☑
Foville's (peduncular) G46.3
fragile X Q99.2
Franceschetti Q75.4
Frey's
　　auriculotemporal G50.8
　　hyperhidrosis L74.52
Friderichsen-Waterhouse A39.1
Froin's G95.89
frontal lobe F07.0
Fukuhara E88.49
functional
　　bowel K59.9
　　prepubertal castrate E29.1
Gaisböck's D75.1
ganglion (basal ganglia brain) G25.9
　　geniculi G51.1
Gardner-Diamond D69.2
gastroesophageal
　　junction K22.0
　　laceration-hemorrhage K22.6
gastrojejunal loop obstruction K91.89
Gee-Herter-Heubner K90.0
Gelineau's G47.419
　　with cataplexy G47.411
genito-anorectal A55

Syndrome — *continued*
  Gerstmann-Sträussler-Scheinker (GSS) A81.82
  Gianotti-Crosti L44.4
  giant platelet (Bernard-Soulier) D69.1
  Gilles de la Tourette's F95.2
  Glass Q87.89
  goiter-deafness E07.1
  Goldberg Q89.8
  Goldberg-Maxwell E34.51
  Good's D83.8
  Gopalan' (burning feet) E53.8
  Gorlin's Q87.89
  Gougerot-Blum L81.7
  Gouley's I31.1
  Gower's R55
  gray or grey (newborn) P93.0
    platelet D69.1
  Gubler-Millard G46.3
  Guillain-Barré (-Strohl) G61.0
  gustatory sweating G50.8
  Hadfield-Clarke K86.89
  hair tourniquet — *see* Constriction, external, by site
  Hamman's J98.19
  hand-foot L27.1
  hand-shoulder G90.8
  hantavirus (cardio)-pulmonary (HPS) (HCPS) B33.4
  happy puppet Q93.51
  Harada's H30.81- ☑
  Hayem-Faber D50.9
  headache NEC G44.89
    complicated NEC G44.59
  Heberden's I20.8
  Hedinger's E34.0
  Hegglin's D72.0
  HELLP (hemolysis, elevated liver enzymes and low
      platelet count) O14.2- ☑
    complicating
      childbirth O14.24
      puerperium O14.25
  hemolytic-uremic D59.3
  hemophagocytic, infection-associated D76.2
  Henoch-Schönlein D69.0
  hepatic flexure K59.8
  hepatopulmonary K76.81
  hepatorenal K76.7
    following delivery O90.4
    postoperative or postprocedural K91.83
    postpartum, puerperal O90.4
  hepatourologic K76.7
  Herter (-Gee) (nontropical sprue) K90.0
  Heubner-Herter K90.0
  Heyd's K76.7
  Hilger's G90.09
  histamine-like (fish poisoning) — *see* Poisoning, fish
  histiocytic D76.3
  histiocytosis NEC D76.3
  HIV infection, acute B20
  Hoffmann-Werdnig G12.0
  Hollander-Simons E88.1
  Hoppe-Goldflam G70.00
    with exacerbation (acute) G70.01
    in crisis G70.01
  Horner's G90.2
  hungry bone E83.81
  hunterian glossitis D51.0
  Hutchinson's triad A50.53
  hyperabduction G54.0
  hyperammonemia-hyperornithinemia-homocitrulline-
      mia E72.4
  hypereosinophilic (idiopathic) D72.1
  hyperimmunoglobulin D M04.1
  hyperimmunoglobulin E (IgE) D82.4
  hyperkalemic E87.5
  hyperkinetic — *see* Hyperkinesia
  hypermobility M35.7
  hypernatremia E87.0
  hyperosmolarity E87.0
  hyperperfusion G97.82
  hypersplenic D73.1
  hypertransfusion, newborn P61.1
  hyperventilation F45.8
  hyperviscosity (of serum)
    polycythemic D75.1
    sclerothymic D58.8
  hypoglycemic (familial) (neonatal) E16.2
  hypokalemic E87.6
  hyponatremic E87.1
  hypopituitarism E23.0
  hypoplastic left-heart Q23.4

Syndrome — *continued*
  hypopotassemia E87.6
  hyposmolality E87.1
  hypotension, maternal O26.5- ☑
  hypothenar hammer I73.89
  hypoventilation, obesity (OHS) E66.2
  ICF (intravascular coagulation-fibrinolysis) D65
  idiopathic
    cardiorespiratory distress, newborn P22.0
    nephrotic (infantile) N04.9
  iliotibial band M76.3- ☑
  immobility, immobilization (paraplegic) M62.3
  immune reconstitution D89.3
  immune reconstitution inflammatory [IRIS] D89.3
  immunity deficiency, combined D81.9
  immunodeficiency
    acquired — *see* Human, immunodeficiency virus
        (HIV) disease
    combined D81.9
  impending coronary I20.0
  impingement, shoulder M75.4- ☑
  inappropriate secretion of antidiuretic hormone E22.2
  infant
    gestational diabetes P70.0
    of diabetic mother P70.1
  infantilism (pituitary) E23.0
  inferior vena cava I87.1
  inspissated bile (newborn) P59.1
  institutional (childhood) F94.2
  insufficient sleep F51.12
  intermediate coronary (artery) I20.0
  interspinous ligament — *see* Spondylopathy, specified
      NEC
  intestinal
    carcinoid E34.0
    knot K56.2
  intravascular coagulation-fibrinolysis (ICF) D65
  iodine-deficiency, congenital E00.9
    type
      mixed E00.2
      myxedematous E00.1
      neurological E00.0
  IRDS (idiopathic respiratory distress, newborn) P22.0
  irritable
    bowel K58.9
      with
        constipation K58.1
        diarrhea K58.0
      mixed K58.2
      psychogenic F45.8
      specified NEC K58.8
    heart (psychogenic) F45.8
    weakness F48.8
  ischemic
    bowel (transient) K55.9
      chronic K55.1
      due to mesenteric artery insufficiency K55.1
    steal T82.898 ☑
  IVC (intravascular coagulopathy) D65
  Ivemark's Q89.01
  Jaccoud's — *see* Arthropathy, postrheumatic, chronic
  Jackson's G83.89
  Jakob-Creutzfeldt — *see* Creutzfeldt-Jakob disease or
      syndrome
  jaw-winking Q07.8
  Jervell-Lange-Nielsen I45.81
  jet lag G47.25
  Job's D71
  Joseph-Diamond-Blackfan D61.01
  jugular foramen G52.7
  Kabuki Q89.8
  Kanner's (autism) F84.0
  Kartagener's Q89.3
  Kelly's D50.1
  Kimmelstiel-Wilson — *see* Diabetes, specified type,
      with Kimmelstiel-Wilson disease
  Klein (e)-Levine G47.13
  Klippel-Feil (brevicollis) Q76.1
  Köhler-Pellegrini-Steida — *see* Bursitis, tibial collateral
  König's K59.8
  Korsakoff (-Wernicke) (nonalcoholic) F04
    alcoholic F10.26
  Kostmann's D70.0
  Krabbe's congenital muscle hypoplasia Q79.8
  labyrinthine — *see* subcategory H83.2 ☑
  lacunar NEC G46.7
  Lambert-Eaton G70.80

Syndrome — *continued*
  Lambert-Eaton — *continued*
    in
      neoplastic disease G73.1
      specified disease NEC G70.81
  Landau-Kleffner — *see* Epilepsy, specified NEC
  Larsen's Q74.8
  lateral
    cutaneous nerve of thigh G57.1- ☑
    medullary G46.4
  Launois' E22.0
  lazy
    leukocyte D70.8
    posture M62.3
  Lemiere I80.8
  Lennox-Gastaut G40.812
    intractable G40.814
      with status epilepticus G40.813
      without status epilepticus G40.814
    not intractable G40.812
      with status epilepticus G40.811
      without status epilepticus G40.812
  lenticular, progressive E83.01
  Leopold-Levi's E05.90
  Lev's I44.2
  Lichtheim's D51.0
  Li-Fraumeni Z15.01
  Lightwood's N25.89
  Lignac (de Toni) (-Fanconi) (-Debré) E72.09
    with cystinosis E72.04
  Likoff's I20.8
  limbic epilepsy personality F07.0
  liver-kidney K76.7
  lobotomy F07.0
  Loffler's J82
  long arm 18 or 21 deletion Q93.89
  long QT I45.81
  Louis-Barré G11.3
  low
    atmospheric pressure T70.29 ☑
    back M54.5
    output (cardiac) I50.9
  lower radicular, newborn (birth injury) P14.8
  Luetscher's (dehydration) E86.0
  Lupus anticoagulant D68.62
  Lutembacher's Q21.1
  macrophage activation D76.1
    due to infection D76.2
  magnesium-deficiency R29.0
  Majeed M04.8
  Mal de Debarquement R42
  malabsorption K90.9
    postsurgical K91.2
  malformation, congenital, due to
    alcohol Q86.0
    exogenous cause NEC Q86.8
    hydantoin Q86.1
    warfarin Q86.2
  malignant
    carcinoid E34.0
    neuroleptic G21.0
  Mallory-Weiss K22.6
  mandibulofacial dysostosis Q75.4
  manic-depressive — *see* Disorder, bipolar
  maple-syrup-urine E71.0
  Marable's I77.4
  Marfan's Q87.40
    with
      cardiovascular manifestations Q87.418
        aortic dilation Q87.410
      ocular manifestations Q87.42
      skeletal manifestations Q87.43
  Marie's (acromegaly) E22.0
  mast cell activation — *see* Activation, mast cell
  maternal hypotension — *see* Syndrome, hypotension,
      maternal
  May (-Hegglin) D72.0
  McArdle (-Schmidt) (-Pearson) E74.04
  McQuarrie's E16.2
  meconium plug (newborn) P76.0
  median arcuate ligament I77.4
  Meekeren-Ehlers-Danlos Q79.6 ☑
  megavitamin-B6 E67.2
  Meige G24.4
  MELAS E88.41
  Mendelson's O74.0
  MERRF (myoclonic epilepsy associated with ragged-
      red fibers) E88.42

Syndrome — *continued*
  mesenteric
    artery (superior) K55.1
    vascular insufficiency K55.1
  metabolic E88.81
  metastatic carcinoid E34.0
  micrognathia-glossoptosis Q87.0
  midbrain NEC G93.89
  middle lobe (lung) J98.19
  middle radicular G54.0
  migraine — *see also* Migraine G43.909
  Mikulicz' K11.8
  milk-alkali E83.52
  Millard-Gubler G46.3
  Miller-Dieker Q93.88
  Miller-Fisher G61.0
  Minkowski-Chauffard D58.0
  Mirizzi's K83.1
  MNGIE (Mitochondrial Neurogastrointestinal Encephalopathy) E88.49
  Möbius, ophthalmoplegic migraine — *see* Migraine, ophthalmoplegic
  monofixation H50.42
  Morel-Moore M85.2
  Morel-Morgagni M85.2
  Morgagni (-Morel) (-Stewart) M85.2
  Morgagni-Adams-Stokes I45.9
  Mounier-Kuhn Q32.4
    with bronchiectasis J47.9
      with
        exacerbation (acute) J47.1
        lower respiratory infection J47.0
    acquired J98.09
      with bronchiectasis J47.9
        with
          exacerbation (acute) J47.1
          lower respiratory infection J47.0
  Muckle-Wells M04.2
  mucocutaneous lymph node (acute febrile) (MCLS) M30.3
  multiple endocrine neoplasia (MEN) — *see* Neoplasia, endocrine, multiple (MEN)
  multiple operations — *see* Disorder, factitious
  myasthenic G70.9
    in
      diabetes mellitus — *see* Diabetes, amyotrophy
      endocrine disease NEC E34.9 *[G73.3]*
      neoplastic disease — *see also* Neoplasm D49.9 *[G73.3]*
      thyrotoxicosis (hyperthyroidism) E05.90 *[G73.3]*
        with thyroid storm E05.91 *[G73.3]*
  myelodysplastic D46.9
    with
      5q deletion D46.C (*following* D46.2)
      isolated del (5q) chromosomal abnormality D46.C (*following* D46.2)
    lesions, low grade D46.20
    specified NEC D46.Z (*following* D46.4)
  myelopathic pain G89.0
  myeloproliferative (chronic) D47.1
  myofascial pain M79.18
  Naffziger's G54.0
  nail patella Q87.2
  NARP (Neuropathy, Ataxia and Retinitis pigmentosa) E88.49
  neonatal abstinence P96.1
  nephritic — *see also* Nephritis
    with edema — *see* Nephrosis
    acute N00.9
    chronic N03.9
    rapidly progressive N01.9
  nephrotic (congenital) — *see also* Nephrosis N04.9
    with
      dense deposit disease N04.6
      diffuse
        crescentic glomerulonephritis N04.7
        endocapillary proliferative glomerulonephritis N04.4
        membranous glomerulonephritis N04.2
        mesangial proliferative glomerulonephritis N04.3
        mesangiocapillary glomerulonephritis N04.5
      focal and segmental glomerular lesions N04.1
      minor glomerular abnormality N04.0
      specified morphological changes NEC N04.8
    diabetic — *see* Diabetes, nephrosis
  neurologic neglect R41.4
  Nezelof's D81.4

Syndrome — *continued*
  Nonne-Milroy-Meige Q82.0
  Nothnagel's vasomotor acroparesthesia I73.89
  obesity hypoventilation (OHS) E66.2
  oculomotor H51.9
  ophthalmoplegia-cerebellar ataxia — *see* Strabismus, paralytic, third nerve
  oral allergy T78.1 ☑
  oral-facial-digital Q87.0
  organic
    affective F06.30
    amnesic (not alcohol- or drug-induced) F04
    brain F09
    depressive F06.31
    hallucinosis F06.0
    personality F07.0
  Ormond's N13.5
  oro-facial-digital Q87.0
  os trigonum Q68.8
  Osler-Weber-Rendu I78.0
  osteoporosis-osteomalacia M83.8
  Österreicher-Turner Q87.2
  otolith — *see* subcategory H81.8 ☑
  oto-palatal-digital Q87.0
  outlet (thoracic) G54.0
  ovary
    polycystic E28.2
    resistant E28.39
    sclerocystic E28.2
  Owren's D68.2
  Paget-Schroetter I82.890
  pain — *see also* Pain
    complex regional I G90.50
      lower limb G90.52- ☑
      specified site NEC G90.59
      upper limb G90.51- ☑
    complex regional II — *see* Causalgia
  painful
    bruising D69.2
    feet E53.8
    prostate N42.81
  paralysis agitans — *see* Parkinsonism
  paralytic G83.9
    specified NEC G83.89
  Parinaud's H51.0
  parkinsonian — *see* Parkinsonism
  Parkinson's — *see* Parkinsonism
  paroxysmal facial pain G50.0
  Parry's E05.00
    with thyroid storm E05.01
  Parsonage (-Aldren)-Turner G54.5
  patella clunk M25.86- ☑
  Paterson (-Brown) (-Kelly) D50.1
  pectoral girdle I77.89
  pectoralis minor I77.89
  pediatric autoimmune neuropsychiatric disorders associated with streptococcal infections (PANDAS) D89.89
  Pelger-Huet D72.0
  pellagra-cerebellar ataxia-renal aminoaciduria E72.02
  pellagroid E52
  Pellegrini-Stieda — *see* Bursitis, tibial collateral
  pelvic congestion-fibrosis, female N94.89
  penta X Q97.1
  peptic ulcer — *see* Ulcer, peptic
  perabduction I77.89
  periodic fever M04.1
  periodic fever, aphthous stomatitis, pharyngitis, and adenopathy [PFAPA] M04.8
  periodic headache, in adults and children — *see* Headache, periodic syndromes in adults and children
  periurethral fibrosis N13.5
  phantom limb (without pain) G54.7
    with pain G54.6
  pharyngeal pouch D82.1
  Pick's — *see* Disease, Pick's
  Pickwickian E66.2
  PIE (pulmonary infiltration with eosinophilia) J82
  pigmentary pallidal degeneration (progressive) G23.0
  pineal E34.8
  pituitary E22.0
  placental transfusion — *see* Pregnancy, complicated by, placental transfusion syndromes
  plantar fascia M72.2
  plateau iris (post-iridectomy) (postprocedural) H21.82
  Plummer-Vinson D50.1
  pluricarential of infancy E40

Syndrome — *continued*
  plurideficiency E40
  pluriglandular (compensatory) E31.8
    autoimmune E31.0
  pneumatic hammer T75.21 ☑
  polyangiitis overlap M30.8
  polycarential of infancy E40
  polyglandular E31.8
    autoimmune E31.0
  polysplenia Q89.09
  pontine NEC G93.89
  popliteal
    artery entrapment I77.89
    post endometrial ablation N99.85
    web Q87.89
  post chemoembolization — *code to* associated conditions
  postcardiac injury
    postcardiotomy I97.0
    postmyocardial infarction I24.1
  postcardiotomy I97.0
  postcholecystectomy K91.5
  postcommissurotomy I97.0
  postconcussional F07.81
  postcontusional F07.81
  postencephalitic F07.89
  posterior
    cervical sympathetic M53.0
    cord G83.83
    fossa compression G93.5
    reversible encephalopathy (PRES) I67.83
  postgastrectomy (dumping) K91.1
  postgastric surgery K91.1
  postinfarction I24.1
  postlaminectomy NEC M96.1
  postleukotomy F07.0
  postmastectomy lymphedema I97.2
  postmyocardial infarction I24.1
  postoperative NEC T81.9 ☑
    blind loop K90.2
  postpartum panhypopituitary (Sheehan) E23.0
  postpolio (myelitic) G14
  postthrombotic I87.009
    with
      inflammation I87.02- ☑
        with ulcer I87.03- ☑
      specified complication NEC I87.09- ☑
      ulcer I87.01- ☑
        with inflammation I87.03- ☑
    asymptomatic I87.00- ☑
  postvagotomy K91.1
  postvalvulotomy I97.0
  postviral NEC G93.3
    fatigue G93.3
  Potain's K31.0
  potassium intoxication E87.5
  Prader-Willi Q87.11
  Prader-Willi-like Q87.19
  precerebral artery (multiple) (bilateral) G45.2
  preinfarction I20.0
  preleukemic D46.9
  premature senility E34.8
  premenstrual dysphoric F32.81
  premenstrual tension N94.3
  Prinzmetal-Massumi R07.1
  prune belly Q79.4
  pseudo -Turner's Q87.19
  pseudocarpal tunnel (sublimis) — *see* Syndrome, carpal tunnel
  pseudoparalytica G70.00
    with exacerbation (acute) G70.01
    in crisis G70.01
  psycho-organic (nonpsychotic severity) F07.9
    acute or subacute F05
    depressive type F06.31
    hallucinatory type F06.0
    nonpsychotic severity F07.0
    specified NEC F07.89
  pulmonary
    arteriosclerosis I27.0
    dysmaturity (Wilson-Mikity) P27.0
    hypoperfusion (idiopathic) P22.0
    renal (hemorrhagic) (Goodpasture's) M31.0
  pure
    motor lacunar G46.5
    sensory lacunar G46.6
  Putnam-Dana D51.0

☑ **Additional Character Required — Refer to the Tabular List for Character Selection**   ▽ **Subterms under main terms may continue to next column or page**

Syndrome — *continued*

pyogenic arthritis, pyoderma gangrenosum, and acne [PAPA] M04.8
pyramidopallidonigral G20
pyriformis — *see* Lesion, nerve, sciatic
QT interval prolongation I45.81
radicular NEC — *see* Radiculopathy
    upper limbs, newborn (birth injury) P14.3
rapid time-zone change G47.25
Rasmussen G04.81
Raymond (-Céstan) I65.8
Raynaud's I73.00
    with gangrene I73.01
RDS (respiratory distress syndrome, newborn) P22.0
reactive airways dysfunction J68.3
Refsum's G60.1
Reifenstein E34.52
renal glomerulohyalinosis-diabetic — *see* Diabetes, nephrosis
Rendu-Osler-Weber I78.0
residual ovary N99.83
resistant ovary E28.39
respiratory
    distress
        acute J80
            adult J80
            child J80
            idiopathic J84.114
        newborn (idiopathic) (type I) P22.0
            type II P22.1
restless legs G25.81
retinoblastoma (familial) C69.9 ☑
retroperitoneal fibrosis N13.5
retroviral seroconversion (acute) Z21
Reye's G93.7
Richter — *see* Leukemia, chronic lymphocytic, B-cell type
Ridley's I50.1
right
    heart, hypoplastic Q22.6
    ventricular obstruction — *see* Failure, heart, right
Romano-Ward (prolonged QT interval) I45.81
rotator cuff, shoulder — *see also* Tear, rotator cuff M75.10- ☑
Rotes Quérol — *see* Hyperostosis, ankylosing
Roth — *see* Meralgia paresthetica
rubella (congenital) P35.0
Ruvalcaba-Myhre-Smith E71.440
Rytand-Lipsitch I44.2
salt
    depletion E87.1
        due to heat NEC T67.8 ☑
            causing heat exhaustion or prostration T67.4 ☑
    low E87.1
salt-losing N28.89
SATB2-associated Q87.89
Scaglietti-Dagnini E22.0
scalenus anticus (anterior) G54.0
scapulocostal — *see* Mononeuropathy, upper limb, specified site NEC
scapuloperoneal G71.09
schizophrenic, of childhood NEC F84.5
Schnitzler D47.2
Scholte's E34.0
Schroeder's E27.0
Schüller-Christian C96.5
Schwachman's — *see* Syndrome, Shwachman's
Schwartz (-Jampel) G71.13
Schwartz-Bartter E22.2
scimitar Q26.8
sclerocystic ovary E28.2
Seitelberger's G31.89
septicemic adrenal hemorrhage A39.1
seroconversion, retroviral (acute) Z21
serous meningitis G93.2
severe acute respiratory (SARS) J12.81
shaken infant T74.4 ☑
shock (traumatic) T79.4 ☑
    kidney N17.0
        following crush injury T79.5 ☑
    toxic A48.3
shock-lung J80
Shone's — *code to* specific anomalies
short
    bowel K91.2
    rib Q77.2
shoulder-hand — *see* Algoneurodystrophy

Syndrome — *continued*

Shwachman's D70.4
sicca — *see* Sicca syndrome
sick
    cell E87.1
    sinus I49.5
sick-euthyroid E07.81
sideropenic D50.1
Siemens' ectodermal dysplasia Q82.4
Silfversköld's Q78.9
Simons' E88.1
sinus tarsi M25.57- ☑
sinusitis-bronchiectasis-situs inversus Q89.3
Sipple's E31.22
sirenomelia Q87.2
Slocumb's E27.0
slow flow, coronary I20.8
Sluder's G44.89
Smith-Magenis Q93.88
Sneddon-Wilkinson L13.1
Sotos' Q87.3
South African cardiomyopathy I42.8
spasmodic
    upward movement, eyes H51.8
    winking F95.8
Spen's I45.9
splenic
    agenesis Q89.01
    flexure K59.8
    neutropenia D73.81
Spurway's Q78.0
staphylococcal scalded skin L00
steal
    arteriovenous T82.898- ☑
    ischemic T82.898- ☑
    subclavian G45.8
Stein-Leventhal E28.2
Stein's E28.2
Stevens-Johnson syndrome L51.1
    toxic epidermal necrolysis overlap L51.3
Stewart-Morel M85.2
Stickler Q89.8
stiff baby Q89.8
stiff man G25.82
Still-Felty — *see* Felty's syndrome
Stokes (-Adams) I45.9
stone heart I50.1
straight back, congenital Q76.49
subclavian steal G45.8
subcoracoid-pectoralis minor G54.0
subcostal nerve compression I77.89
subphrenic interposition Q43.3
superior
    cerebellar artery I63.89
    mesenteric artery K55.1
    semi-circular canal dehiscence H83.8X- ☑
    vena cava I87.1
supine hypotensive (maternal) — *see* Syndrome, hypotension, maternal
suprarenal cortical E27.0
supraspinatus — *see also* Tear, rotator cuff M75.10- ☑
Susac G93.49
swallowed blood P78.2
sweat retention L74.0
Swyer Q99.1
Symond's G93.2
sympathetic
    cervical paralysis G90.2
    pelvic, female N94.89
systemic inflammatory response (SIRS), of non-infectious origin (without organ dysfunction) R65.10
    with acute organ dysfunction R65.11
tachycardia-bradycardia I49.5
takotsubo I51.81
TAR (thrombocytopenia with absent radius) Q87.2
tarsal tunnel G57.5- ☑
teething K00.7
tegmental G93.89
telangiectasic-pigmentation-cataract Q82.8
temporal pyramidal apex — *see* Otitis, media, suppurative, acute
temporomandibular joint-pain-dysfunction M26.62- ☑
Terry's — *see also* Myopia, degenerative H44.2- ☑
testicular feminization — *see also* Syndrome, androgen insensitivity E34.51
thalamic pain (hyperesthetic) G89.0
thoracic outlet (compression) G54.0
Thorson-Björck E34.0

Syndrome — *continued*

thrombocytopenia with absent radius (TAR) Q87.2
thyroid-adrenocortical insufficiency E31.0
tibial
    anterior M76.81- ☑
    posterior M76.82- ☑
Tietze's M94.0
time-zone (rapid) G47.25
Toni-Fanconi E72.09
    with cystinosis E72.04
Touraine's Q79.8
tourniquet — *see* Constriction, external, by site
toxic shock A48.3
transient left ventricular apical ballooning I51.81
traumatic vasospastic T75.22 ☑
Treacher Collins Q75.4
triple X, female Q97.0
trisomy Q92.9
    13 Q91.7
        meiotic nondisjunction Q91.4
        mitotic nondisjunction Q91.5
        mosaicism Q91.5
        translocation Q91.6
    18 Q91.3
        meiotic nondisjunction Q91.0
        mitotic nondisjunction Q91.1
        mosaicism Q91.1
        translocation Q91.2
    20 (q)(p) Q92.8
    21 Q90.9
        meiotic nondisjunction Q90.0
        mitotic nondisjunction Q90.1
        mosaicism Q90.1
        translocation Q90.2
    22 Q92.8
tropical wet feet T69.0- ☑
Trousseau's I82.1
tumor lysis (following antineoplastic chemotherapy) (spontaneous) NEC E88.3
tumor necrosis factor receptor associated periodic (TRAPS) M04.1
Twiddler's (due to)
    automatic implantable defibrillator T82.198 ☑
    cardiac pacemaker T82.198 ☑
Unverricht (-Lundborg) — *see* Epilepsy, generalized, idiopathic
upward gaze H51.8
uremia, chronic — *see also* Disease, kidney, chronic N18.9
urethral N34.3
urethro-oculo-articular — *see* Reiter's disease
urohepatic K76.7
vago-hypoglossal G52.7
van Buchem's M85.2
van der Hoeve's Q78.0
vascular NEC in cerebrovascular disease G46.8
vasoconstriction, reversible cerebrovascular I67.841
vasomotor I73.9
vasospastic (traumatic) T75.22 ☑
vasovagal R55
VATER Q87.2
velo-cardio-facial Q93.81
vena cava (inferior) (superior) (obstruction) I87.1
vertebral
    artery G45.0
        compression — *see* Syndrome, anterior, spinal artery, compression
    steal G45.0
vertebro-basilar artery G45.0
vertebrogenic (pain) M54.89
vertiginous — *see* Disorder, vestibular function
Vinson-Plummer D50.1
virus B34.9
visceral larva migrans B83.0
visual disorientation H53.8
vitamin B6 deficiency E53.1
vitreal corneal H59.01- ☑
vitreous (touch) H59.01- ☑
Vogt-Koyanagi H20.82- ☑
Volkmann's T79.6
von Schroetter's I82.890
von Willebrand (-Jürgen) D68.0
Waldenström-Kjellberg D50.1
Wallenberg's G46.3
water retention E87.79
Waterhouse (-Friderichsen) A39.1
Weber-Gubler G46.3
Weber-Leyden G46.3

Syndrome — *continued*
Weber's G46.3
Wegener's M31.30
with
kidney involvement M31.31
lung involvement M31.30
with kidney involvement M31.31
Weingarten's (tropical eosinophilia) J82
Weiss-Baker G90.09
Werdnig-Hoffman G12.0
Wermer's E31.21
Werner's E34.8
Wernicke-Korsakoff (nonalcoholic) F04
alcoholic F10.26
Westphal-Strümpell E83.01
West's — *see* Epilepsy, spasms
wet
feet (maceration) (tropical) T69.0- ☑
lung, newborn P22.1
whiplash S13.4 ☑
whistling face Q87.0
Wilkie's K55.1
Wilkinson-Sneddon L13.1
Willebrand (-Jürgens) D68.0
Williams Q93.82
Wilson's (hepatolenticular degeneration) E83.01
Wiskott-Aldrich D82.0
withdrawal — *see* Withdrawal, state
drug
infant of dependent mother P96.1
therapeutic use, newborn P96.2
Woakes' (ethmoiditis) J33.1
Wright's (hyperabduction) G54.0
X I20.9
XXXX Q97.1
XXXXX Q97.1
XXXXY Q98.1
XXY Q98.0
Yao M04.8
yellow nail L60.5
Zahorsky's B08.5
Zellweger syndrome E71.510
Zellweger-like syndrome E71.541
Synechia (anterior) (iris) (posterior) (pupil) — *see also* Adhesions, iris
intra-uterine (traumatic) N85.6
Synesthesia R20.8
Syngamiasis, syngamosis B83.3
Synodontia K00.2
Synorchidism, synorchism Q55.1
Synostosis (congenital) Q78.8
astragalo-scaphoid Q74.2
radioulnar Q74.0
Synovial sarcoma — *see* Neoplasm, connective tissue, malignant
Synovioma (malignant) — *see also* Neoplasm, connective tissue, malignant
benign — *see* Neoplasm, connective tissue, benign
Synoviosarcoma — *see* Neoplasm, connective tissue, malignant
Synovitis — *see also* Tenosynovitis M65.9
crepitant
hand M70.0- ☑
wrist M70.03- ☑
gonococcal A54.49
gouty — *see* Gout
in (due to)
crystals M65.8- ☑
gonorrhea A54.49
syphilis (late) A52.78
use, overuse, pressure — *see* Disorder, soft tissue, due to use
infective NEC — *see* Tenosynovitis, infective NEC
specified NEC — *see* Tenosynovitis, specified type NEC
syphilitic A52.78
congenital (early) A50.02
toxic — *see* Synovitis, transient
transient M67.3- ☑
ankle M67.37- ☑
elbow M67.32- ☑
foot joint M67.37- ☑
hand joint M67.34- ☑
hip M67.35- ☑
knee M67.36- ☑
multiple site M67.39
pelvic region M67.35- ☑
shoulder M67.31- ☑
specified joint NEC M67.38

Synovitis — *continued*
transient — *continued*
wrist M67.33- ☑
traumatic, current — *see* Sprain
tuberculous — *see* Tuberculosis, synovitis
villonodular (pigmented) M12.2- ☑
ankle M12.27- ☑
elbow M12.22- ☑
foot joint M12.27- ☑
hand joint M12.24- ☑
hip M12.25- ☑
knee M12.26- ☑
multiple site M12.29
pelvic region M12.25- ☑
shoulder M12.21- ☑
specified joint NEC M12.28
vertebrae M12.28
wrist M12.23- ☑
Syphilid A51.39
congenital A50.06
newborn A50.06
tubercular (late) A52.79
Syphilis, syphilitic (acquired) A53.9
abdomen (late) A52.79
acoustic nerve A52.15
adenopathy (secondary) A51.49
adrenal (gland) (with cortical hypofunction) A52.79
age under 2 years NOS — *see also* Syphilis, congenital, early
acquired A51.9
alopecia (secondary) A51.32
anemia (late) A52.79 *[D63.8]*
aneurysm (aorta) (ruptured) A52.01
central nervous system A52.05
congenital A50.54 *[I79.0]*
anus (late) A52.74
primary A51.1
secondary A51.39
aorta (arch) (abdominal) (thoracic) A52.02
aneurysm A52.01
aortic (insufficiency) (regurgitation) (stenosis) A52.03
aneurysm A52.01
arachnoid (adhesive) (cerebral) (spinal) A52.13
asymptomatic — *see* Syphilis, latent
ataxia (locomotor) A52.11
atrophoderma maculatum A51.39
auricular fibrillation A52.06
bladder (late) A52.76
bone A52.77
secondary A51.46
brain A52.17
breast (late) A52.79
bronchus (late) A52.72
bubo (primary) A51.0
bulbar palsy A52.19
bursa (late) A52.78
cardiac decompensation A52.06
cardiovascular A52.00
central nervous system (late) (recurrent) (relapse) (tertiary) A52.3
with
ataxia A52.11
general paralysis A52.17
juvenile A50.45
paresis (general) A52.17
juvenile A50.45
tabes (dorsalis) A52.11
juvenile A50.45
taboparesis A52.17
juvenile A50.45
aneurysm A52.05
congenital A50.40
juvenile A50.40
remission in (sustained) A52.3
serology doubtful, negative, or positive A52.3
specified nature or site NEC A52.19
vascular A52.05
cerebral A52.17
meningovascular A52.13
nerves (multiple palsies) A52.15
sclerosis A52.17
thrombosis A52.05
cerebrospinal (tabetic type) A52.12
cerebrovascular A52.05
cervix (late) A52.76
chancre (multiple) A51.0
extragenital A51.2
Rollet's A51.0

Syphilis, syphilitic — *continued*
Charcot's joint A52.16
chorioretinitis A51.43
congenital A50.01
late A52.71
prenatal A50.01
choroiditis — *see* Syphilitic chorioretinitis
choroidoretinitis — *see* Syphilitic chorioretinitis
ciliary body (secondary) A51.43
late A52.71
colon (late) A52.74
combined spinal sclerosis A52.11
condyloma (latum) A51.31
congenital A50.9
with
paresis (general) A50.45
tabes (dorsalis) A50.45
taboparesis A50.45
chorioretinitis, choroiditis A50.01 *[H32]*
early, or less than 2 years after birth NEC A50.2
with manifestations — *see* Syphilis, congenital, early, symptomatic
latent (without manifestations) A50.1
negative spinal fluid test A50.1
serology positive A50.1
symptomatic A50.09
cutaneous A50.06
mucocutaneous A50.07
oculopathy A50.01
osteochondropathy A50.02
pharyngitis A50.03
pneumonia A50.04
rhinitis A50.05
visceral A50.08
interstitial keratitis A50.31
juvenile neurosyphilis A50.45
late, or 2 years or more after birth NEC A50.7
chorioretinitis, choroiditis A50.32
interstitial keratitis A50.31
juvenile neurosyphilis A50.45
latent (without manifestations) A50.6
negative spinal fluid test A50.6
serology positive A50.6
symptomatic or with manifestations NEC A50.59
arthropathy A50.55
cardiovascular A50.54
Clutton's joints A50.51
Hutchinson's teeth A50.52
Hutchinson's triad A50.53
osteochondropathy A50.56
saddle nose A50.57
conjugal A53.9
tabes A52.11
conjunctiva (late) A52.71
contact Z20.2
cord bladder A52.19
cornea, late A52.71
coronary (artery) (sclerosis) A52.06
coryza, congenital A50.05
cranial nerve A52.15
multiple palsies A52.15
cutaneous — *see* Syphilis, skin
dacryocystitis (late) A52.71
degeneration, spinal cord A52.12
dementia paralytica A52.17
juvenilis A50.45
destruction of bone A52.77
dilatation, aorta A52.01
due to blood transfusion A53.9
dura mater A52.13
ear A52.79
inner A52.79
nerve (eighth) A52.15
neurorecurrence A52.15
early A51.9
cardiovascular A52.00
central nervous system A52.3
latent (without manifestations) (less than 2 years after infection) A51.5
negative spinal fluid test A51.5
serological relapse after treatment A51.5
serology positive A51.5
relapse (treated, untreated) A51.9
skin A51.39
symptomatic A51.9
extragenital chancre A51.2
primary, except extragenital chancre A51.0
secondary — *see also* Syphilis, secondary A51.39
relapse (treated, untreated) A51.49

Syphilis, syphilitic — *continued*
early — *continued*
ulcer A51.39
eighth nerve (neuritis) A52.15
endemic A65
endocarditis A52.03
aortic A52.03
pulmonary A52.03
epididymis (late) A52.76
epiglottis (late) A52.73
epiphysitis (congenital) (early) A50.02
episcleritis (late) A52.71
esophagus A52.79
eustachian tube A52.73
exposure to Z20.2
eye A52.71
eyelid (late) (with gumma) A52.71
fallopian tube (late) A52.76
fracture A52.77
gallbladder (late) A52.74
gastric (polyposis) (late) A52.74
general A53.9
paralysis A52.17
juvenile A50.45
genital (primary) A51.0
glaucoma A52.71
gumma NEC A52.79
cardiovascular system A52.00
central nervous system A52.3
congenital A50.59
heart (block) (decompensation) (disease) (failure) A52.06 *[I52]*
valve NEC A52.03
hemianesthesia A52.19
hemianopsia A52.71
hemiparesis A52.17
hemiplegia A52.17
hepatic artery A52.09
hepatis A52.74
hepatomegaly, congenital A50.08
hereditaria tarda — *see* Syphilis, congenital, late
hereditary — *see* Syphilis, congenital
Hutchinson's teeth A50.52
hyalitis A52.71
inactive — *see* Syphilis, latent
infantum — *see* Syphilis, congenital
inherited — *see* Syphilis, congenital
internal ear A52.79
intestine (late) A52.74
iris, iritis (secondary) A51.43
late A52.71
joint (late) A52.77
keratitis (congenital) (interstitial) (late) A50.31
kidney (late) A52.75
lacrimal passages (late) A52.71
larynx (late) A52.73
late A52.9
cardiovascular A52.00
central nervous system A52.3
kidney A52.75
latent or 2 years or more after infection (without manifestations) A52.8
negative spinal fluid test A52.8
serology positive A52.8
paresis A52.17
specified site NEC A52.79
symptomatic or with manifestations A52.79
tabes A52.11
latent A53.0
with signs or symptoms — *code by* site and stage under Syphilis
central nervous system A52.2
date of infection unspecified A53.0
early, or less than 2 years after infection A51.5
follow-up of latent syphilis A53.0
date of infection unspecified A53.0
late, or 2 years or more after infection A52.8
late, or 2 years or more after infection A52.8
positive serology (only finding) A53.0
date of infection unspecified A53.0
early, or less than 2 years after infection A51.5
late, or 2 years or more after infection A52.8
lens (late) A52.71
leukoderma A51.39
late A52.79
lienitis A52.79
lip A51.39
chancre (primary) A51.2

Syphilis, syphilitic — *continued*
lip — *continued*
late A52.79
Lissauer's paralysis A52.17
liver A52.74
locomotor ataxia A52.11
lung A52.72
lymph gland (early) (secondary) A51.49
late A52.79
lymphadenitis (secondary) A51.49
macular atrophy of skin A51.39
striated A52.79
mediastinum (late) A52.73
meninges (adhesive) (brain) (spinal cord) A52.13
meningitis A52.13
acute (secondary) A51.41
congenital A50.41
meningoencephalitis A52.14
meningovascular A52.13
congenital A50.41
mesarteritis A52.09
brain A52.04
middle ear A52.77
mitral stenosis A52.03
monoplegia A52.17
mouth (secondary) A51.39
late A52.79
mucocutaneous (secondary) A51.39
late A52.79
mucous
membrane (secondary) A51.39
late A52.79
patches A51.39
congenital A50.07
mulberry molars A50.52
muscle A52.78
myocardium A52.06
nasal sinus (late) A52.73
neonatorum — *see* Syphilis, congenital
nephrotic syndrome (secondary) A51.44
nerve palsy (any cranial nerve) A52.15
multiple A52.15
nervous system, central A52.3
neuritis A52.15
acoustic A52.15
neurorecidive of retina A52.19
neuroretinitis A52.19
newborn — *see* Syphilis, congenital
nodular superficial (late) A52.79
nonvenereal A65
nose (late) A52.73
saddle back deformity A50.57
occlusive arterial disease A52.09
oculopathy A52.71
ophthalmic (late) A52.71
optic nerve (atrophy) (neuritis) (papilla) A52.15
orbit (late) A52.71
organic A53.9
osseous (late) A52.77
osteochondritis (congenital) (early) A50.02 *[M90.80]*
osteoporosis A52.77
ovary (late) A52.76
oviduct (late) A52.76
palate (late) A52.79
pancreas (late) A52.74
paralysis A52.17
general A52.17
juvenile A50.45
paresis (general) A52.17
juvenile A50.45
paresthesia A52.19
Parkinson's disease or syndrome A52.19
paroxysmal tachycardia A52.06
pemphigus (congenital) A50.06
penis (chancre) A51.0
late A52.76
pericardium A52.06
perichondritis, larynx (late) A52.73
periosteum (late) A52.77
congenital (early) A50.02 *[M90.80]*
early (secondary) A51.46
peripheral nerve A52.79
petrous bone (late) A52.77
pharynx (late) A52.73
secondary A51.39
pituitary (gland) A52.79
pleura (late) A52.73
pneumonia, white A50.04
pontine lesion A52.17

Syphilis, syphilitic — *continued*
portal vein A52.09
primary A51.0
anal A51.1
and secondary — *see* Syphilis, secondary
central nervous system A52.3
extragenital chancre NEC A51.2
fingers A51.2
genital A51.0
lip A51.2
specified site NEC A51.2
tonsils A51.2
prostate (late) A52.76
ptosis (eyelid) A52.71
pulmonary (late) A52.72
artery A52.09
pyelonephritis (late) A52.75
recently acquired, symptomatic A51.9
rectum (late) A52.74
respiratory tract (late) A52.73
retina, late A52.71
retrobulbar neuritis A52.15
salpingitis A52.76
sclera (late) A52.71
sclerosis
cerebral A52.17
coronary A52.06
multiple A52.11
scotoma (central) A52.71
scrotum (late) A52.76
secondary (and primary) A51.49
adenopathy A51.49
anus A51.39
bone A51.46
chorioretinitis, choroiditis A51.43
hepatitis A51.45
liver A51.45
lymphadenitis A51.49
meningitis (acute) A51.41
mouth A51.39
mucous membranes A51.39
periosteum, periostitis A51.46
pharynx A51.39
relapse (treated, untreated) A51.49
skin A51.39
specified form NEC A51.49
tonsil A51.39
ulcer A51.39
viscera NEC A51.49
vulva A51.39
seminal vesicle (late) A52.76
seronegative with signs or symptoms — *code by* site and stage under Syphilis
seropositive
with signs or symptoms — *code by* site and stage under Syphilis
follow-up of latent syphilis — *see* Syphilis, latent
only finding — *see* Syphilis, latent
seventh nerve (paralysis) A52.15
sinus, sinusitis (late) A52.73
skeletal system A52.77
skin (with ulceration) (early) (secondary) A51.39
late or tertiary A52.79
small intestine A52.74
spastic spinal paralysis A52.17
spermatic cord (late) A52.76
spinal (cord) A52.12
spleen A52.79
splenomegaly A52.79
spondylitis A52.77
staphyloma A52.71
stigmata (congenital) A50.59
stomach A52.74
synovium A52.78
tabes dorsalis (late) A52.11
juvenile A50.45
tabetic type A52.11
juvenile A50.45
taboparesis A52.17
juvenile A50.45
tachycardia A52.06
tendon (late) A52.78
tertiary A52.9
with symptoms NEC A52.79
cardiovascular A52.00
central nervous system A52.3
multiple NEC A52.79
specified site NEC A52.79
testis A52.76

Index

Syphilis, syphilitic — System, systemic

Syphilis, syphilitic — *continued*
  thorax A52.73
  throat A52.73
  thymus (gland) (late) A52.79
  thyroid (late) A52.79
  tongue (late) A52.79
  tonsil (lingual) (late) A52.73
    primary A51.2
    secondary A51.39
  trachea (late) A52.73
  tunica vaginalis (late) A52.76
  ulcer (any site) (early) (secondary) A51.39
    late A52.79
    perforating A52.79
      foot A52.11
  urethra (late) A52.76
  urogenital (late) A52.76
  uterus (late) A52.76
  uveal tract (secondary) A51.43
    late A52.71
  uveitis (secondary) A51.43
    late A52.71

Syphilis, syphilitic — *continued*
  uvula (late) (perforated) A52.79
  vagina A51.0
    late A52.76
  valvulitis NEC A52.03
  vascular A52.00
    brain (cerebral) A52.05
  ventriculi A52.74
  vesicae urinariae (late) A52.76
  viscera (abdominal) (late) A52.74
    secondary A51.49
  vitreous (opacities) (late) A52.71
    hemorrhage A52.71
  vulva A51.0
    late A52.76
    secondary A51.39
Syphiloma A52.79
  cardiovascular system A52.00
  central nervous system A52.3
  circulatory system A52.00
  congenital A50.59
Syphilophobia F45.29

Syringadenoma — *see also* Neoplasm, skin, benign
  papillary — *see* Neoplasm, skin, benign
Syringobulbia G95.0
Syringocystadenoma — *see* Neoplasm, skin, benign
  papillary — *see* Neoplasm, skin, benign
Syringoma — *see also* Neoplasm, skin, benign
  chondroid — *see* Neoplasm, skin, benign
Syringomyelia G95.0
Syringomyelitis — *see* Encephalitis
Syringomyelocele — *see* Spina bifida
Syringopontia G95.0
System, systemic — *see also* condition
  disease, combined — *see* Degeneration, combined
  inflammatory response syndrome (SIRS) of non-infectious origin (without organ dysfunction) R65.10
    with acute organ dysfunction R65.11
  lupus erythematosus M32.9
    inhibitor present D68.62

☑ **Additional Character Required — Refer to the Tabular List for Character Selection**   ▽ **Subterms under main terms may continue to next column or page**

T

Tabacism, tabacosis, tabagism — *see also* Poisoning,
  tobacco
  meaning dependence (without remission) F17.200
    with
      disorder F17.299
        in remission F17.211
        specified disorder NEC F17.298
        withdrawal F17.203
Tabardillo A75.9
  flea-borne A75.2
  louse-borne A75.0
Tabes, tabetic A52.10
  with
    central nervous system syphilis A52.10
    Charcot's joint A52.16
    cord bladder A52.19
    crisis, viscera (any) A52.19
    paralysis, general A52.17
    paresis (general) A52.17
    perforating ulcer (foot) A52.19
  arthropathy (Charcot) A52.16
  bladder A52.19
  bone A52.11
  cerebrospinal A52.12
  congenital A50.45
  conjugal A52.10
  dorsalis A52.11
    juvenile A50.49
  juvenile A50.49
  latent A52.19
  mesenterica A18.39
  paralysis, insane, general A52.17
  spasmodic A52.17
  syphilis (cerebrospinal) A52.12
Taboparalysis A52.17
Taboparesis (remission) A52.17
  juvenile A50.45
TAC (trigeminal autonomic cephalgia) **NEC** G44.099
  intractable G44.091
  not intractable G44.099
Tache noir S60.22-☑
Tachyalimentation K91.2
Tachyarrhythmia, tachyrhythmia — *see* Tachycardia
Tachycardia R00.0
  atrial (paroxysmal) I47.1
  auricular I47.1
  AV nodal re-entry (re-entrant) I47.1
  junctional (paroxysmal) I47.1
  newborn P29.11
  nodal (paroxysmal) I47.1
  non-paroxysmal AV nodal I45.89
  paroxysmal (sustained) (nonsustained) I47.9
    with sinus bradycardia I49.5
    atrial (PAT) I47.1
    atrioventricular (AV) (re-entrant) I47.1
      psychogenic F54
    junctional I47.1
      ectopic I47.1
    nodal I47.1
    psychogenic (atrial) (supraventricular) (ventricular)
      F54
    supraventricular (sustained) I47.1
      psychogenic F54
    ventricular I47.2
      psychogenic F54
  psychogenic F45.8
  sick sinus I49.5
  sinoauricular NOS R00.0
    paroxysmal I47.1
  sinus [sinusal] NOS R00.0
    paroxysmal I47.1
  supraventricular I47.1
  ventricular (paroxysmal) (sustained) I47.2
    psychogenic F54
Tachygastria K31.89
Tachypnea R06.82
  hysterical F45.8
  newborn (idiopathic) (transitory) P22.1
  psychogenic F45.8
  transitory, of newborn P22.1
TACO (transfusion associated circulatory overload) E87.71
Taenia (infection) (infestation) B68.9
  diminuta B71.0
  echinococcal infestation B67.90
  mediocanellata B68.1

Taenia — *continued*
  nana B71.0
  saginata B68.1
  solium (intestinal form) B68.0
    larval form — *see* Cysticercosis
Taeniasis (intestine) — *see* Taenia
Tag (hypertrophied skin) (infected) L91.8
  adenoid J35.8
  anus K64.4
  hemorrhoidal K64.4
  hymen N89.8
  perineal N90.89
  preauricular Q17.0
  sentinel K64.4
  skin L91.8
    accessory (congenital) Q82.8
    anus K64.4
    congenital Q82.8
    preauricular Q17.0
  tonsil J35.8
  urethra, urethral N36.8
  vulva N90.89
Tahyna fever B33.8
Takahara's disease E80.3
Takayasu's disease or syndrome M31.4
Talcosis (pulmonary) J62.0
Talipes (congenital) Q66.89
  acquired, planus — *see* Deformity, limb, flat foot
  asymmetric Q66.89
  calcaneovalgus Q66.4-☑
  calcaneovarus Q66.1-☑
  calcaneus Q66.89
  cavus Q66.7-☑
  equinovalgus Q66.6
  equinovarus Q66.0-☑
  equinus Q66.89
  percavus Q66.7-☑
  planovalgus Q66.6
  planus (acquired) (any degree) — *see also* Deformity,
    limb, flat foot
    congenital Q66.5-☑
    due to rickets (sequelae) E64.3
  valgus Q66.6
  varus Q66.3-☑
Tall stature, constitutional E34.4
Talma's disease M62.89
Talon noir S90.3-☑
  hand S60.22-☑
  heel S90.3-☑
  toe S90.1-☑
Tamponade, heart I31.4
Tanapox (virus disease) B08.71
Tangier disease E78.6
Tantrum, child problem F91.8
Tapeworm (infection) (infestation) — *see* Infestation,
  tapeworm
Tapia's syndrome G52.7
TAR (thrombocytopenia with absent radius) **syndrome**
  Q87.2
Tarral-Besnier disease L44.0
Tarsal tunnel syndrome — *see* Syndrome, tarsal tunnel
Tarsalgia — *see* Pain, limb, lower
Tarsitis (eyelid) H01.8
  syphilitic A52.71
  tuberculous A18.4
Tartar (teeth) (dental calculus) K03.6
Tattoo (mark) L81.8
Tauri's disease E74.09
Taurodontism K00.2
Taussig-Bing syndrome Q20.1
Taybi's syndrome Q87.2
Tay-Sachs amaurotic familial idiocy or disease E75.02
TBI (traumatic brain injury) S06.9☑
Teacher's node or nodule J38.2
Tear, torn (traumatic) — *see also* Laceration
  with abortion — *see* Abortion
  annular fibrosis M51.35
  anus, anal (sphincter) S31.831☑
    complicating delivery
      with third degree perineal laceration — *see also*
        Delivery, complicated, by, laceration, per-
        ineum, third degree O70.20
        with mucosa O70.3
      without third degree perineal laceration O70.4
    nontraumatic (healed) (old) K62.81
  articular cartilage, old — *see* Derangement, joint, artic-
    ular cartilage, by site

Tear, torn — *continued*
  bladder
    with ectopic or molar pregnancy O08.6
    following ectopic or molar pregnancy O08.6
    obstetrical O71.5
    traumatic — *see* Injury, bladder
  bowel
    with ectopic or molar pregnancy O08.6
    following ectopic or molar pregnancy O08.6
    obstetrical trauma O71.5
  broad ligament
    with ectopic or molar pregnancy O08.6
    following ectopic or molar pregnancy O08.6
    obstetrical trauma O71.6
  bucket handle (knee) (meniscus) — *see* Tear, meniscus
  capsule, joint — *see* Sprain
  cartilage — *see also* Sprain
    articular, old — *see* Derangement, joint, articular
      cartilage, by site
  cervix
    with ectopic or molar pregnancy O08.6
    following ectopic or molar pregnancy O08.6
    obstetrical trauma (current) O71.3
    old N88.1
    traumatic — *see* Injury, uterus
  dural G97.41
    nontraumatic G96.11
  internal organ — *see* Injury, by site
  knee cartilage
    articular (current) S83.3-☑
    old — *see* Derangement, knee, meniscus, due to
      old tear
  ligament — *see* Sprain
  meniscus (knee) (current injury) S83.209☑
    bucket-handle S83.20-☑
    lateral
      bucket-handle S83.25-☑
      complex S83.27-☑
      peripheral S83.26-☑
      specified type NEC S83.28-☑
    medial
      bucket-handle S83.21-☑
      complex S83.23-☑
      peripheral S83.22-☑
      specified type NEC S83.24-☑
    old — *see* Derangement, knee, meniscus, due to
      old tear
    site other than knee — *code as* Sprain
    specified type NEC S83.20-☑
  muscle — *see* Strain
  pelvic
    floor, complicating delivery O70.1
    organ NEC, obstetrical trauma O71.5
      with ectopic or molar pregnancy O08.6
      following ectopic or molar pregnancy O08.6
  perineal, secondary O90.1
  periurethral tissue, obstetrical trauma O71.82
    with ectopic or molar pregnancy O08.6
    following ectopic or molar pregnancy O08.6
  rectovaginal septum — *see* Laceration, vagina
  retina, retinal (without detachment) (horseshoe) —
    see also Break, retina, horseshoe
    with detachment — *see* Detachment, retina, with
      retinal, break
  rotator cuff (nontraumatic) M75.10-☑
    complete M75.12-☑
    incomplete M75.11-☑
    traumatic S46.01-☑
      capsule S43.42-☑
  semilunar cartilage, knee — *see* Tear, meniscus
  supraspinatus (complete) (incomplete) (nontraumatic)
    — *see also* Tear, rotator cuff M75.10-☑
  tendon — *see* Strain
  tentorial, at birth P10.4
  umbilical cord
    complicating delivery O69.89☑
  urethra
    with ectopic or molar pregnancy O08.6
    following ectopic or molar pregnancy O08.6
    obstetrical trauma O71.5
  uterus — *see* Injury, uterus
  vagina — *see* Laceration, vagina
  vessel, from catheter — *see* Puncture, accidental
    complicating surgery
  vulva, complicating delivery O70.0
Tear-stone — *see* Dacryolith
Teeth — *see also* condition

Teeth — *continued*
grinding
psychogenic F45.8
sleep related G47.63
Teething (syndrome) K00.7
Telangiectasia, telangiectasis (verrucous) I78.1
ataxic (cerebellar) (Louis-Bar) G11.3
familial I78.0
hemorrhagic, hereditary (congenital) (senile) I78.0
hereditary, hemorrhagic (congenital) (senile) I78.0
juxtafoveal H35.07- ☑
macular H35.07- ☑
macularis eruptiva perstans D47.01
parafoveal H35.07- ☑
retinal (idiopathic) (juxtafoveal) (macular) (parafoveal)
H35.07- ☑
spider I78.1
Telephone scatologia F65.89
Telescoped bowel or intestine K56.1
congenital Q43.8
Temperature
body, high (of unknown origin) R50.9
cold, trauma from T69.9 ☑
newborn P80.0
specified effect NEC T69.8 ☑
Temple — *see* condition
Temporal — *see* condition
Temporomandibular joint pain-dysfunction syndrome M26.62- ☑
Temporosphenoidal — *see* condition
Tendency
bleeding — *see* Defect, coagulation
suicide
meaning personal history of attempted suicide Z91.5
meaning suicidal ideation — *see* Ideation, suicidal
to fall R29.6
Tenderness, abdominal R10.819
epigastric R10.816
generalized R10.817
left lower quadrant R10.814
left upper quadrant R10.812
periumbilic R10.815
rebound R10.829
epigastric R10.826
generalized R10.827
left lower quadrant R10.824
left upper quadrant R10.822
periumbilic R10.825
right lower quadrant R10.823
right upper quadrant R10.821
right lower quadrant R10.813
right upper quadrant R10.811
Tendinitis, tendonitis — *see also* Enthesopathy
Achilles M76.6- ☑
adhesive — *see* Tenosynovitis, specified type NEC
shoulder — *see* Capsulitis, adhesive
bicipital M75.2- ☑
calcific M65.2- ☑
ankle M65.27- ☑
foot M65.27- ☑
forearm M65.23- ☑
hand M65.24- ☑
lower leg M65.26- ☑
multiple sites M65.29
pelvic region M65.25- ☑
shoulder M75.3- ☑
specified site NEC M65.28
thigh M65.25- ☑
upper arm M65.22- ☑
due to use, overuse, pressure — *see also* Disorder, soft
tissue, due to use
specified NEC — *see* Disorder, soft tissue, due to
use, specified NEC
gluteal M76.0- ☑
patellar M76.5- ☑
peroneal M76.7- ☑
psoas M76.1- ☑
tibial (posterior) M76.82- ☑
anterior M76.81- ☑
trochanteric — *see* Bursitis, hip, trochanteric
Tendon — *see* condition
Tendosynovitis — *see* Tenosynovitis
Tenesmus (rectal) R19.8
vesical R30.1
Tennis elbow — *see* Epicondylitis, lateral
Tenonitis — *see also* Tenosynovitis
eye (capsule) H05.04- ☑

Tenontosynovitis — *see* Tenosynovitis
Tenontothecitis — *see* Tenosynovitis
Tenophyte — *see* Disorder, synovium, specified type NEC
Tenosynovitis — *see also* Synovitis M65.9
adhesive — *see* Tenosynovitis, specified type NEC
shoulder — *see* Capsulitis, adhesive
bicipital (calcifying) — *see* Tendinitis, bicipital
gonococcal A54.49
in (due to)
crystals M65.8- ☑
gonorrhea A54.49
syphilis (late) A52.78
use, overuse, pressure — *see also* Disorder, soft tissue, due to use
specified NEC — *see* Disorder, soft tissue, due to use, specified NEC
infective NEC M65.1- ☑
ankle M65.17- ☑
foot M65.17- ☑
forearm M65.13- ☑
hand M65.14- ☑
lower leg M65.16- ☑
multiple sites M65.19
pelvic region M65.15- ☑
shoulder region M65.11- ☑
specified site NEC M65.18
thigh M65.15- ☑
upper arm M65.12- ☑
radial styloid M65.4
shoulder region M65.81- ☑
adhesive — *see* Capsulitis, adhesive
specified type NEC M65.88
ankle M65.87- ☑
foot M65.87- ☑
forearm M65.83- ☑
hand M65.84- ☑
lower leg M65.86- ☑
multiple sites M65.89
pelvic region M65.85- ☑
shoulder region M65.81- ☑
specified site NEC M65.88
thigh M65.85- ☑
upper arm M65.82- ☑
tuberculous — *see* Tuberculosis, tenosynovitis
Tenovaginitis — *see* Tenosynovitis
Tension
arterial, high — *see also* Hypertension
without diagnosis of hypertension R03.0
headache G44.209
intractable G44.201
not intractable G44.209
nervous R45.0
pneumothorax J93.0
premenstrual N94.3
state (mental) F48.9
Tentorium — *see* condition
Teratencephalus Q89.8
Teratism Q89.7
Teratoblastoma (malignant) — *see* Neoplasm, malignant, by site
Teratocarcinoma — *see also* Neoplasm, malignant, by site
liver C22.7
Teratoma (solid) — *see also* Neoplasm, uncertain behavior, by site
with embryonal carcinoma, mixed — *see* Neoplasm, malignant, by site
with malignant transformation — *see* Neoplasm, malignant, by site
adult (cystic) — *see* Neoplasm, benign, by site
benign — *see* Neoplasm, benign, by site
combined with choriocarcinoma — *see* Neoplasm, malignant, by site
cystic (adult) — *see* Neoplasm, benign, by site
differentiated — *see* Neoplasm, benign, by site
embryonal — *see also* Neoplasm, malignant, by site
liver C22.7
immature — *see* Neoplasm, malignant, by site
liver C22.7
adult, benign, cystic, differentiated type or mature D13.4
malignant — *see also* Neoplasm, malignant, by site
anaplastic — *see* Neoplasm, malignant, by site
intermediate — *see* Neoplasm, malignant, by site
specified site — *see* Neoplasm, malignant, by site
unspecified site C62.90

Teratoma — *continued*
malignant — *see also* Neoplasm, malignant, by site — *continued*
undifferentiated — *see* Neoplasm, malignant, by site
mature — *see* Neoplasm, uncertain behavior, by site
malignant — *see* Neoplasm, by site, malignant, by site
ovary D27.- ☑
embryonal, immature or malignant C56- ☑
solid — *see* Neoplasm, uncertain behavior, by site
testis C62.9- ☑
adult, benign, cystic, differentiated type or mature D29.2- ☑
scrotal C62.1- ☑
undescended C62.0- ☑
Termination
anomalous — *see also* Malposition, congenital
right pulmonary vein Q26.3
pregnancy, elective Z33.2
Ternidens diminutus infestation B81.8
Ternidensiasis B81.8
Terror(s) night (child) F51.4
Terrorism, victim of Z65.4
Terry's syndrome — *see also* Myopia, degenerative
H44.2- ☑
Tertiary — *see* condition
Test, tests, testing (for)
adequacy (for dialysis)
hemodialysis Z49.31
peritoneal Z49.32
blood pressure Z01.30
abnormal reading — *see* Blood, pressure
blood typing Z01.83
Rh typing Z01.83
blood-alcohol Z04.89
positive — *see* Findings, abnormal, in blood
blood-drug Z04.89
positive — *see* Findings, abnormal, in blood
cardiac pulse generator (battery) Z45.010
fertility Z31.41
genetic
disease carrier status for procreative management
female Z31.430
male Z31.440
male partner of patient with recurrent pregnancy loss Z31.441
procreative management NEC
female Z31.438
male Z31.448
hearing Z01.10
with abnormal findings NEC Z01.118
infant or child (over 28 days old) Z00.129
with abnormal findings Z00.121
HIV (human immunodeficiency virus)
nonconclusive (in infants) R75
positive Z21
seropositive Z21
immunity status Z01.84
intelligence NEC Z01.89
laboratory (as part of a general medical examination) Z00.00
with abnormal finding Z00.01
for medicolegal reason NEC Z04.89
male partner of patient with recurrent pregnancy loss Z31.441
Mantoux (for tuberculosis) Z11.1
abnormal result R76.11
pregnancy, positive first pregnancy — *see* Pregnancy, normal, first
procreative Z31.49
fertility Z31.41
skin, diagnostic
allergy Z01.82
special screening examination — *see* Screening, by name of disease
Mantoux Z11.1
tuberculin Z11.1
specified NEC Z01.89
tuberculin Z11.1
abnormal result R76.11
vision Z01.00
with abnormal findings Z01.01
following failed vision screening Z01.020
with abnormal findings Z01.021
infant or child (over 28 days old) Z00.129
with abnormal findings Z00.121
Wassermann Z11.3

Test, tests, testing — *continued*
  Wassermann — *continued*
    positive — *see* Serology for syphilis, positive
Testicle, testicular, testis — *see also* condition
  feminization syndrome — *see also* Syndrome, androgen insensitivity E34.51
  migrans Q55.29
Tetanus, tetanic (cephalic) (convulsions) A35
  with
    abortion A34
    ectopic or molar pregnancy O08.0
  following ectopic or molar pregnancy O08.0
  inoculation reaction (due to serum) — *see* Complications, vaccination
  neonatorum A33
  obstetrical A34
  puerperal, postpartum, childbirth A34
Tetany (due to) R29.0
  alkalosis E87.3
  associated with rickets E55.0
  convulsions R29.0
    hysterical F44.5
  functional (hysterical) F44.5
  hyperkinetic R29.0
    hysterical F44.5
  hyperpnea R06.4
    hysterical F44.5
    psychogenic F45.8
  hyperventilation — *see also* Hyperventilation R06.4
    hysterical F44.5
  neonatal (without calcium or magnesium deficiency) P71.3
  parathyroid (gland) E20.9
  parathyroprival E89.2
  post- (para)thyroidectomy E89.2
  postoperative E89.2
  pseudotetany R29.0
  psychogenic (conversion reaction) F44.5
Tetralogy of Fallot Q21.3
Tetraplegia (chronic) — *see also* Quadriplegia G82.50
Thailand hemorrhagic fever A91
Thalassanemia — *see* Thalassemia
Thalassemia (anemia) (disease) D56.9
  with other hemoglobinopathy D56.8
  alpha (major) (severe) (triple gene defect) D56.0
    minor D56.3
    silent carrier D56.3
    trait D56.3
  beta (severe) D56.1
    homozygous D56.1
    major D56.1
    minor D56.3
    trait D56.3
  delta-beta (homozygous) D56.2
    minor D56.3
    trait D56.3
  dominant D56.8
  hemoglobin
    C D56.8
    E-beta D56.5
  intermedia D56.1
  major D56.1
  minor D56.3
  mixed D56.8
  sickle-cell — *see* Disease, sickle-cell, thalassemia
  specified type NEC D56.8
  trait D56.3
  variants D56.8
Thanatophoric dwarfism or short stature Q77.1
Thaysen-Gee disease (nontropical sprue) K90.0
Thaysen's disease K90.0
Thecoma D27- ☑
  luteinized D27- ☑
  malignant C56- ☑
Thelarche, premature E30.8
Thelaziasis B83.8
Thelitis N61.0
  puerperal, postpartum or gestational — *see* Infection, nipple
Therapeutic — *see* condition
Therapy
  drug, long-term (current) (prophylactic)
    agents affecting estrogen receptors and estrogen levels NEC Z79.818
    anastrozole (Arimidex) Z79.811
    antibiotics Z79.2
      short-term use — *omit code*
    anticoagulants Z79.01

Therapy — *continued*
  drug, long-term — *continued*
    anti-inflammatory Z79.1
    antiplatelet Z79.02
    antithrombotics Z79.02
    aromatase inhibitors Z79.811
    aspirin Z79.82
    birth control pill or patch Z79.3
    bisphosphonates Z79.83
    contraceptive, oral Z79.3
    drug, specified NEC Z79.899
    estrogen receptor downregulators Z79.818
    Evista Z79.810
    exemestane (Aromasin) Z79.811
    Fareston Z79.810
    fulvestrant (Faslodex) Z79.818
    gonadotropin-releasing hormone (GnRH) agonist Z79.818
    goserelin acetate (Zoladex) Z79.818
    hormone replacement Z79.890
    insulin Z79.4
    letrozole (Femara) Z79.811
    leuprolide acetate (leuprorelin) (Lupron) Z79.818
    megestrol acetate (Megace) Z79.818
    methadone
      for pain management Z79.891
      maintenance therapy F11.20
    Nolvadex Z79.810
    opiate analgesic Z79.891
    oral contraceptive Z79.3
    raloxifene (Evista) Z79.810
    selective estrogen receptor modulators (SERMs) Z79.810
    short term — *omit code*
    steroids
      inhaled Z79.51
      systemic Z79.52
    tamoxifen (Nolvadex) Z79.810
    toremifene (Fareston) Z79.810
Thermic — *see* condition
Thermography (abnormal) — *see also* Abnormal, diagnostic imaging R93.89
  breast R92.8
Thermoplegia T67.01 ☑
Thesaurismosis, glycogen — *see* Disease, glycogen storage
Thiamin deficiency E51.9
  specified NEC E51.8
Thiaminic deficiency with beriberi E51.11
Thibierge-Weissenbach syndrome — *see* Sclerosis, systemic
Thickening
  bone — *see* Hypertrophy, bone
  breast N64.59
  endometrium R93.89
  epidermal L85.9
    specified NEC L85.8
  hymen N89.6
  larynx J38.7
  nail L60.2
    congenital Q84.5
  periosteal — *see* Hypertrophy, bone
  pleura J92.9
    with asbestos J92.0
  skin R23.4
  subepiglottic J38.7
  tongue K14.8
  valve, heart — *see* Endocarditis
Thigh — *see* condition
Thinning vertebra — *see* Spondylopathy, specified NEC
Thirst, excessive R63.1
  due to deprivation of water T73.1 ☑
Thomsen disease G71.12
Thoracic — *see also* condition
  kidney Q63.2
  outlet syndrome G54.0
Thoracogastroschisis (congenital) Q79.8
Thoracopagus Q89.4
Thorax — *see* condition
Thorn's syndrome N28.89
Thorson-Björck syndrome E34.0
Threadworm (infection) (infestation) B80
Threatened
  abortion O20.0
    with subsequent abortion O03.9
  job loss, anxiety concerning Z56.2
  labor (without delivery) O47.9
    at or after 37 completed weeks of gestation O47.1

Threatened — *continued*
  labor — *continued*
    before 37 completed weeks of gestation O47.0- ☑
  loss of job, anxiety concerning Z56.2
  miscarriage O20.0
  unemployment, anxiety concerning Z56.2
Three-day fever A93.1
Threshers' lung J67.0
Thrix annulata (congenital) Q84.1
Throat — *see* condition
Thrombasthenia (Glanzmann) (hemorrhagic) (hereditary) D69.1
Thromboangiitis I73.1
  obliterans (general) I73.1
    cerebral I67.89
    vessels
      brain I67.89
      spinal cord I67.89
Thromboarteritis — *see* Arteritis
Thromboasthenia (Glanzmann) (hemorrhagic) (hereditary) D69.1
Thrombocytasthenia (Glanzmann) D69.1
Thrombocythemia (essential) (hemorrhagic) (idiopathic) (primary) D47.3
Thrombocytopathy (dystrophic) (granulopenic) D69.1
Thrombocytopenia, thrombocytopenic D69.6
  with absent radius (TAR) Q87.2
  congenital D69.42
  dilutional D69.59
  due to
    (massive) blood transfusion D69.59
    drugs D69.59
    extracorporeal circulation of blood D69.59
    platelet alloimmunization D69.59
  essential D69.3
  heparin induced (HIT) D75.82
  hereditary D69.42
  idiopathic D69.3
  neonatal, transitory P61.0
    due to
      exchange transfusion P61.0
      idiopathic maternal thrombocytopenia P61.0
      isoimmunization P61.0
  primary NEC D69.49
    idiopathic D69.3
  puerperal, postpartum O72.3
  secondary D69.59
  transient neonatal P61.0
Thrombocytosis, essential D47.3
  primary D47.3
Thromboembolism — *see* Embolism
Thrombopathy (Bernard-Soulier) D69.1
  constitutional D68.0
  Willebrand-Jurgens D68.0
Thrombopenia — *see* Thrombocytopenia
Thrombophilia D68.59
  primary NEC D68.59
  secondary NEC D68.69
  specified NEC D68.69
Thrombophlebitis I80.9
  antepartum O22.2- ☑
    deep O22.3- ☑
    superficial O22.2- ☑
  calf muscular vein (NOS) I80.25- ☑
  cavernous (venous) sinus G08
    complicating pregnancy O22.5- ☑
    nonpyogenic I67.6
  cerebral (sinus) (vein) G08
    nonpyogenic I67.6
    sequelae G09
  due to implanted device — *see* Complications, by site and type, specified NEC
  during or resulting from a procedure NEC T81.72 ☑
  femoral vein (superficial) I80.1- ☑
  femoropopliteal vein I80.0- ☑
  gastrocnemial vein I80.25- ☑
  hepatic (vein) I80.8
  idiopathic, recurrent I82.1
  iliac vein (common) (external) (internal) I80.21- ☑
  iliofemoral I80.1- ☑
  intracranial venous sinus (any) G08
    nonpyogenic I67.6
    sequelae G09
  intraspinal venous sinuses and veins G08
    nonpyogenic G95.19
  lateral (venous) sinus G08
    nonpyogenic I67.6
  leg I80.3

Thrombophlebitis — continued
  leg — continued
    superficial I80.0- ☑
  longitudinal (venous) sinus G08
    nonpyogenic I67.6
  lower extremity I80.299
  migrans, migrating I82.1
  pelvic
    with ectopic or molar pregnancy O08.0
    following ectopic or molar pregnancy O08.0
    puerperal O87.1
  peroneal vein I80.24- ☑
  popliteal vein — see Phlebitis, leg, deep, popliteal
  portal (vein) K75.1
  postoperative T81.72 ☑
  pregnancy — see Thrombophlebitis, antepartum
  puerperal, postpartum, childbirth O87.0
    deep O87.1
    pelvic O87.1
    septic O86.81
    superficial O87.0
  saphenous (greater) (lesser) I80.0- ☑
  sinus (intracranial) G08
    nonpyogenic I67.6
  soleal vein I80.25- ☑
  specified site NEC I80.8
  tibial vein (anterior) (posterior) I80.23- ☑

Thrombosis, thrombotic (bland) (multiple) (progressive)
    (silent) (vessel) I82.90
  anal K64.5
  antepartum — see Thrombophlebitis, antepartum
  aorta, aortic I74.10
    abdominal I74.09
      saddle I74.01
    bifurcation I74.09
    saddle I74.01
    specified site NEC I74.19
    terminal I74.09
    thoracic I74.11
    valve — see Endocarditis, aortic
  apoplexy I63.3- ☑
  artery, arteries (postinfectional) I74.9
    auditory, internal — see Occlusion, artery, precerebral, specified NEC
    basilar — see Occlusion, artery, basilar
    carotid (common) (internal) — see Occlusion, artery, carotid
    cerebellar (anterior inferior) (posterior inferior) (superior) — see Occlusion, artery, cerebellar
    cerebral — see Occlusion, artery, cerebral
    choroidal (anterior) — see Occlusion, artery, precerebral, specified NEC
    communicating, posterior — see Occlusion, artery, precerebral, specified NEC
    coronary — see also Infarct, myocardium
      not resulting in infarction I24.0
    hepatic I74.8
    hypophyseal — see Occlusion, artery, precerebral, specified NEC
    iliac I74.5
    limb I74.4
      lower I74.3
      upper I74.2
    meningeal, anterior or posterior — see Occlusion, artery, cerebral, specified NEC
    mesenteric (with gangrene) — see also Infarct, intestine K55.069
    ophthalmic — see Occlusion, artery, retina
    pontine — see Occlusion, artery, precerebral, specified NEC
    precerebral — see Occlusion, artery, precerebral
    pulmonary (iatrogenic) — see Embolism, pulmonary
    renal N28.0
    retinal — see Occlusion, artery, retina
    spinal, anterior or posterior G95.11
    traumatic NEC T14.8 ☑
    vertebral — see Occlusion, artery, vertebral
  atrium, auricular — see also Infarct, myocardium
    following acute myocardial infarction (current complication) I23.6
    not resulting in infarction I51.3
    old I51.3
  basilar (artery) — see Occlusion, artery, basilar
  brain (artery) (stem) — see also Occlusion, artery, cerebral
    due to syphilis A52.05
    puerperal O99.43
    sinus — see Thrombosis, intracranial venous sinus

Thrombosis, thrombotic — continued
  capillary I78.8
  cardiac — see also Infarct, myocardium
    not resulting in infarction I51.3
    old I51.3
    valve — see Endocarditis
  carotid (artery) (common) (internal) — see Occlusion, artery, carotid
  cavernous (venous) sinus — see Thrombosis, intracranial venous sinus
  cerebellar artery (anterior inferior) (posterior inferior) (superior) I66.3
  cerebral (artery) — see Occlusion, artery, cerebral
  cerebrovenous sinus — see also Thrombosis, intracranial venous sinus
    puerperium O87.3
  chronic I82.91
  coronary (artery) (vein) — see also Infarct, myocardium
    not resulting in infarction I24.0
  corpus cavernosum N48.89
  cortical I66.9
  deep — see Embolism, vein, lower extremity
  due to device, implant or graft — see also Complications, by site and type, specified NEC T85.868 ☑
    arterial graft NEC T82.868 ☑
    breast (implant) T85.868 ☑
    catheter NEC T85.868 ☑
      dialysis (renal) T82.868 ☑
        intraperitoneal T85.868 ☑
      infusion NEC T82.868 ☑
        spinal (epidural) (subdural) T85.860 ☑
      urinary (indwelling) T83.86 ☑
    electronic (electrode) (pulse generator) (stimulator)
      bone T84.86 ☑
      cardiac T82.867 ☑
      nervous system (brain) (peripheral nerve) (spinal) T85.860 ☑
      urinary T83.86 ☑
    fixation, internal (orthopedic) NEC T84.86 ☑
    gastrointestinal (bile duct) (esophagus) T85.868 ☑
    genital NEC T83.86 ☑
    heart T82.867 ☑
    joint prosthesis T84.86 ☑
    ocular (corneal graft) (orbital implant) NEC T85.868 ☑
    orthopedic NEC T84.86 ☑
    specified NEC T85.868 ☑
    urinary NEC T83.86 ☑
    vascular NEC T82.868 ☑
    ventricular intracranial shunt T85.860 ☑
  during the puerperium — see Thrombosis, puerperal
  endocardial — see also Infarct, myocardium
    not resulting in infarction I51.3
  eye — see Occlusion, retina
  genital organ
    female NEC N94.89
      pregnancy — see Thrombophlebitis, antepartum
    male N50.1
  gestational — see Phlebopathy, gestational
  heart (chamber) — see also Infarct, myocardium
    not resulting in infarction I51.3
    old I51.3
  hepatic (vein) I82.0
    artery I74.8
  history (of) Z86.718
  intestine (with gangrene) — see also Infarct, intestine K55.069
  intracardiac NEC (apical) (atrial) (auricular) (ventricular) (old) I51.3
  intracranial (arterial) I66.9
    venous sinus (any) G08
      nonpyogenic origin I67.6
      puerperium O87.3
  intramural — see also Infarct, myocardium
    not resulting in infarction I51.3
    old I51.3
  intraspinal venous sinuses and veins G08
    nonpyogenic G95.19
  kidney (artery) N28.0
  lateral (venous) sinus — see Thrombosis, intracranial venous sinus
  leg — see Thrombosis, vein, lower extremity
    arterial I74.3
  liver (venous) I82.0
    artery I74.8
    portal vein I81

Thrombosis, thrombotic — continued
  longitudinal (venous) sinus — see Thrombosis, intracranial venous sinus
  lower limb — see Thrombosis, vein, lower extremity
  lung (iatrogenic) (postoperative) — see Embolism, pulmonary
  meninges (brain) (arterial) I66.8
  mesenteric (artery) (with gangrene) — see also Infarct, intestine K55.069
    vein (inferior) (superior) K55.0 ☑
  mitral I34.8
  mural — see also Infarct, myocardium
    due to syphilis A52.06
    not resulting in infarction I51.3
    old I51.3
  omentum (with gangrene) — see also Infarct, intestine K55.069
  ophthalmic — see Occlusion, retina
  pampiniform plexus (male) N50.1
  parietal — see also Infarct, myocardium
    not resulting in infarction I24.0
  penis, superficial vein N48.81
  perianal venous K64.5
  peripheral arteries I74.4
    upper I74.2
  personal history (of) Z86.718
  portal I81
    due to syphilis A52.09
  precerebral artery — see Occlusion, artery, precerebral
  puerperal, postpartum O87.0
    brain (artery) O99.43
      venous (sinus) O87.3
    cardiac O99.43
    cerebral (artery) O99.43
      venous (sinus) O87.3
    superficial O87.0
  pulmonary (artery) (iatrogenic) (postoperative) (vein) — see Embolism, pulmonary
  renal (artery) N28.0
    vein I82.3
  resulting from presence of device, implant or graft — see Complications, by site and type, specified NEC
  retina, retinal — see Occlusion, retina
  scrotum N50.1
  seminal vesicle N50.1
  sigmoid (venous) sinus — see Thrombosis, intracranial venous sinus
  sinus, intracranial (any) — see Thrombosis, intracranial venous sinus
  specified site NEC I82.890
    chronic I82.891
  spermatic cord N50.1
  spinal cord (arterial) G95.11
    due to syphilis A52.09
    pyogenic origin G06.1
  spleen, splenic D73.5
    artery I74.8
  testis N50.1
  traumatic NEC T14.8 ☑
  tricuspid I07.8
  tumor — see Neoplasm, unspecified behavior, by site
  tunica vaginalis N50.1
  umbilical cord (vessels), complicating delivery O69.5 ☑
  vas deferens N50.1
  vein (acute) I82.90
    antecubital I82.61- ☑
      chronic I82.71- ☑
    axillary I82.A1- ☑ (following I82.7)
      chronic I82.A2- ☑ (following I82.7)
    basilic I82.61- ☑
      chronic I82.71- ☑
    brachial I82.62- ☑
      chronic I82.72- ☑
    brachiocephalic (innominate) I82.290
      chronic I82.291
    cephalic I82.61- ☑
      chronic I82.71- ☑
    cerebral, nonpyogenic I67.6
    chronic I82.91
    deep (DVT) I82.40- ☑
      calf I82.4Z- ☑
        chronic I82.5Z- ☑
      lower leg I82.4Z- ☑
        chronic I82.5Z- ☑
      thigh I82.4Y- ☑
        chronic I82.5Y- ☑

Thrombosis, thrombotic — *continued*
  vein — *continued*
    deep — *continued*
      upper leg I82.4Y ☑
        chronic I82.5Y- ☑
    femoral I82.41- ☑
      chronic I82.51- ☑
    iliac (iliofemoral) I82.42- ☑
      chronic I82.52- ☑
    innominate I82.290
      chronic I82.291
    internal jugular I82.C1- ☑ (*following* I82.7)
      chronic I82.C2- ☑ (*following* I82.7)
    lower extremity
      deep I82.40- ☑
        chronic I82.50- ☑
        specified NEC I82.49- ☑
          chronic NEC I82.59- ☑
      distal
        deep I82.4Z- ☑
      proximal
        deep I82.4Y- ☑
          chronic I82.5Y- ☑
      superficial I82.81- ☑
    perianal K64.5
    popliteal I82.43- ☑
      chronic I82.53- ☑
    radial I82.62- ☑
      chronic I82.72- ☑
    renal I82.3
    saphenous (greater) (lesser) I82.81- ☑
    specified NEC I82.890
      chronic NEC I82.891
    subclavian I82.B1- ☑ (*following* I82.7)
      chronic I82.B2- ☑ (*following* I82.7)
    thoracic NEC I82.290
      chronic I82.291
    tibial I82.44- ☑
      chronic I82.54- ☑
    ulnar I82.62- ☑
      chronic I82.72- ☑
    upper extremity I82.60- ☑
      chronic I82.70- ☑
      deep I82.62- ☑
        chronic I82.72- ☑
      superficial I82.61- ☑
        chronic I82.71- ☑
  vena cava
    inferior I82.220
      chronic I82.221
    superior I82.210
      chronic I82.211
  venous, perianal K64.5
  ventricle — *see also* Infarct, myocardium
    following acute myocardial infarction (current complication) I23.6
    not resulting in infarction I24.0
    old I51.3
Thrombus — *see* Thrombosis
Thrush — *see also* Candidiasis
  newborn P37.5
  oral B37.0
  vaginal B37.3
Thumb — *see also* condition
  sucking (child problem) F98.8
Thymitis E32.8
Thymoma (benign) D15.0
  malignant C37
Thymus, thymic (gland) — *see* condition
Thyrocele — *see* Goiter
Thyroglossal — *see also* condition
  cyst Q89.2
  duct, persistent Q89.2
Thyroid (gland) (body) — *see also* condition
  hormone resistance E07.89
  lingual Q89.2
  nodule (cystic) (nontoxic) (single) E04.1
Thyroiditis E06.9
  acute (nonsuppurative) (pyogenic) (suppurative) E06.0
  autoimmune E06.3
  chronic (nonspecific) (sclerosing) E06.5
    with thyrotoxicosis, transient E06.2
    fibrous E06.5
    lymphadenoid E06.3
    lymphocytic E06.3
    lymphoid E06.3
  de Quervain's E06.1

Thyroiditis — *continued*
  drug-induced E06.4
  fibrous (chronic) E06.5
  giant-cell (follicular) E06.1
  granulomatous (de Quervain) (subacute) E06.1
  Hashimoto's (struma lymphomatosa) E06.3
  iatrogenic E06.4
  ligneous E06.5
  lymphocytic (chronic) E06.3
  lymphoid E06.3
  lymphomatous E06.3
  nonsuppurative E06.1
  postpartum, puerperal O90.5
  pseudotuberculous E06.1
  pyogenic E06.0
  radiation E06.4
  Riedel's E06.5
  subacute (granulomatous) E06.1
  suppurative E06.0
  tuberculous A18.81
  viral E06.1
  woody E06.5
Thyrolingual duct, persistent Q89.2
Thyromegaly E01.0
Thyrotoxic
  crisis — *see* Thyrotoxicosis
  heart disease or failure — *see also* Thyrotoxicosis E05.90 *[I43]*
    with thyroid storm E05.91 *[I43]*
  storm — *see* Thyrotoxicosis
Thyrotoxicosis (recurrent) E05.90
  with
    goiter (diffuse) E05.00
      with thyroid storm E05.01
      adenomatous uninodular E05.10
        with thyroid storm E05.11
      multinodular E05.20
        with thyroid storm E05.21
      nodular E05.20
        with thyroid storm E05.21
      uninodular E05.10
        with thyroid storm E05.11
    infiltrative
      dermopathy E05.00
        with thyroid storm E05.01
      ophthalmopathy E05.00
        with thyroid storm E05.01
    single thyroid nodule E05.10
      with thyroid storm E05.11
    thyroid storm E05.91
  due to
    ectopic thyroid nodule or tissue E05.30
      with thyroid storm E05.31
    ingestion of (excessive) thyroid material E05.40
      with thyroid storm E05.41
    overproduction of thyroid-stimulating hormone E05.80
      with thyroid storm E05.81
    specified cause NEC E05.80
      with thyroid storm E05.81
  factitia E05.40
    with thyroid storm E05.41
  heart — *see also* Failure, heart, high-output E05.90 *[I43]*
    with thyroid storm — *see also* Failure, heart, high-output E05.91 *[I43]*
    failure — *see also* Failure, heart, high-output E05.90 *[I43]*
  neonatal (transient) P72.1
  transient with chronic thyroiditis E06.2
Tibia vara — *see* Osteochondrosis, juvenile, tibia
Tic (disorder) F95.9
  breathing F95.8
  child problem F95.0
  compulsive F95.1
  de la Tourette F95.2
  degenerative (generalized) (localized) G25.69
    facial G25.69
  disorder
    chronic
      motor F95.1
      vocal F95.1
    combined vocal and multiple motor F95.2
    transient F95.0
  douloureux G50.0
    atypical G50.1
    postherpetic, postzoster B02.22
  drug-induced G25.61
  eyelid F95.8

Tic — *continued*
  habit F95.9
    chronic F95.1
    transient of childhood F95.0
  lid, transient of childhood F95.0
  motor-verbal F95.2
  occupational F48.8
  orbicularis F95.8
    transient of childhood F95.0
  organic origin G25.69
  postchoreic G25.69
  provisional F95.0
  psychogenic, compulsive F95.1
  salaam R25.8
  spasm (motor or vocal) F95.9
    chronic F95.1
    transient of childhood F95.0
  specified NEC F95.8
Tick-borne — *see* condition
Tietze's disease or syndrome M94.0
Tight, tightness
  anus K62.89
  chest R07.89
  fascia (lata) M62.89
  foreskin (congenital) N47.1
  hymen, hymenal ring N89.6
  introitus (acquired) (congenital) N89.6
  rectal sphincter K62.89
  tendon — *see* Short, tendon
  urethral sphincter N35.919
Tilting vertebra — *see* Dorsopathy, deforming, specified NEC
Timidity, child F93.8
Tinea (intersecta) (tarsi) B35.9
  amiantacea L44.8
  asbestina B35.0
  barbae B35.0
  beard B35.0
  black dot B35.0
  blanca B36.2
  capitis B35.0
  corporis B35.4
  cruris B35.6
  flava B36.0
  foot B35.3
  furfuracea B36.0
  imbricata (Tokelau) B35.5
  kerion B35.0
  manuum B35.2
  microsporic — *see* Dermatophytosis
  nigra B36.1
  nodosa — *see* Piedra
  pedis B35.3
  scalp B35.0
  specified NEC B35.8
  sycosis B35.0
  tonsurans B35.0
  trichophytic — *see* Dermatophytosis
  unguium B35.1
  versicolor B36.0
Tingling sensation (skin) R20.2
Tin-miner's lung J63.5
Tinnitus NOS H93.1- ☑
  audible H93.1- ☑
  aurium H93.1- ☑
  pulsatile H93.A- ☑
  subjective H93.1- ☑
Tipped tooth (teeth) M26.33
Tipping
  pelvis M95.5
    with disproportion (fetopelvic) O33.0
      causing obstructed labor O65.0
  tooth (teeth), fully erupted M26.33
Tiredness R53.83
Tissue — *see* condition
Tobacco (nicotine)
  abuse — *see* Tobacco, use
  dependence — *see* Dependence, drug, nicotine
  harmful use Z72.0
  heart — *see* Tobacco, toxic effect
  maternal use, affecting newborn P04.2
  toxic effect — *see* Table of Drugs and Chemicals, by substance, poisoning
    chewing tobacco — *see* Table of Drugs and Chemicals, by substance, poisoning
    cigarettes — *see* Table of Drugs and Chemicals, by substance, poisoning
  use Z72.0

Tobacco — continued
   use — continued
      complicating
         childbirth O99.334
         pregnancy O99.33- ☑
         puerperium O99.335
      counseling and surveillance Z71.6
      history Z87.891
      withdrawal state — see also Dependence, drug, nicotine F17.203
Tocopherol deficiency E56.0
Todd's
   cirrhosis K74.3
   paralysis (postepileptic) (transitory) G83.84
Toe — see condition
Toilet, artificial opening — see Attention to, artificial, opening
Tokelau (ringworm) B35.5
Tollwut — see Rabies
Tommaselli's disease R31.9
   correct substance properly administered — see Table of Drugs and Chemicals, by drug, adverse effect
   overdose or wrong substance given or taken — see Table of Drugs and Chemicals, by drug, poisoning
Tongue — see also condition
   tie Q38.1
Tonic pupil — see Anomaly, pupil, function, tonic pupil
Toni-Fanconi syndrome (cystinosis) E72.09
   with cystinosis E72.04
Tonsil — see condition
Tonsillitis (acute) (catarrhal) (croupous) (follicular) (gangrenous) (infective) (lacunar) (lingual) (malignant) (membranous) (parenchymatous) (phlegmonous) (pseudomembranous) (purulent) (septic) (subacute) (suppurative) (toxic) (ulcerative) (vesicular) (viral) J03.90
   chronic J35.01
      with adenoiditis J35.03
   diphtheritic A36.0
   hypertrophic J35.01
      with adenoiditis J35.03
   recurrent J03.91
   specified organism NEC J03.80
      recurrent J03.81
   staphylococcal J03.80
      recurrent J03.81
   streptococcal J03.00
      recurrent J03.01
   tuberculous A15.8
   Vincent's A69.1
Tooth, teeth — see condition
Toothache K08.89
Topagnosis R20.8
Tophi — see Gout, chronic
TORCH infection — see Infection, congenital
   without active infection P00.2
Torn — see Tear
Tornwaldt's cyst or disease J39.2
Torsion
   accessory tube — see Torsion, fallopian tube
   adnexa (female) — see Torsion, fallopian tube
   aorta, acquired I77.1
   appendix epididymis N44.04
   appendix testis N44.03
   bile duct (common) (hepatic) K83.8
      congenital Q44.5
   bowel, colon or intestine K56.2
   cervix — see Malposition, uterus
   cystic duct K82.8
   dystonia — see Dystonia, torsion
   epididymis (appendix) N44.04
   fallopian tube N83.52- ☑
      with ovary N83.53
   gallbladder K82.8
      congenital Q44.1
   hydatid of Morgagni
      female N83.52- ☑
      male N44.03
   kidney (pedicle) (leading to infarction) N28.0
   Meckel's diverticulum (congenital) Q43.0
      malignant — see Table of Neoplasms, small intestine, malignant
   mesentery K56.2
   omentum K56.2
   organ or site, congenital NEC — see Anomaly, by site
   ovary (pedicle) N83.51- ☑
      with fallopian tube N83.53
      congenital Q50.2

Torsion — continued
   oviduct — see Torsion, fallopian tube
   penis (acquired) N48.82
      congenital Q55.63
   spasm — see Dystonia, torsion
   spermatic cord N44.02
      extravaginal N44.01
      intravaginal N44.02
   spleen D73.5
   testis, testicle N44.00
      appendix N44.03
   tibia — see Deformity, limb, specified type NEC, lower leg
   uterus — see Malposition, uterus
Torticollis (intermittent) (spastic) M43.6
   congenital (sternomastoid) Q68.0
   due to birth injury P15.8
   hysterical F44.4
   ocular R29.891
   psychogenic F45.8
      conversion reaction F44.4
   rheumatic M43.6
   rheumatoid M06.88
   spasmodic G24.3
   traumatic, current S13.4 ☑
Tortipelvis G24.1
Tortuous
   aortic arch Q25.46
   artery I77.1
   organ or site, congenital NEC — see Distortion
   retinal vessel, congenital Q14.1
   ureter N13.8
   urethra N36.8
   vein — see Varix
Torture, victim of Z65.4
Torula, torular (histolytica) (infection) — see Cryptococcosis
Torulosis — see Cryptococcosis
Torus (mandibularis) (palatinus) M27.0
   fracture — see Fracture, by site, torus
Touraine's syndrome Q79.8
Tourette's syndrome F95.2
Tourniquet syndrome — see Constriction, external, by site
Tower skull Q75.0
   with exophthalmos Q87.0
Toxemia R68.89
   bacterial — see Sepsis
   burn — see Burn
   eclamptic (with pre-existing hypertension) — see Eclampsia
   erysipelatous — see Erysipelas
   fatigue R68.89
   food — see Poisoning, food
   gastrointestinal K52.1
   intestinal K52.1
   kidney — see Uremia
   malarial — see Malaria
   myocardial — see Myocarditis, toxic
   of pregnancy — see Pre-eclampsia
   pre-eclamptic — see Pre-eclampsia
   small intestine K52.1
   staphylococcal, due to food A05.0
   stasis R68.89
   uremic — see Uremia
   urinary — see Uremia
Toxemica cerebropathia psychica (nonalcoholic) F04
   alcoholic — see Alcohol, amnestic disorder
Toxic (poisoning) — see also condition T65.91 ☑
   effect — see Table of Drugs and Chemicals, by substance, poisoning
   shock syndrome A48.3
   thyroid (gland) — see Thyrotoxicosis
Toxicemia — see Toxemia
Toxicity — see Table of Drugs and Chemicals, by substance, poisoning
   fava bean D55.0
   food, noxious — see Poisoning, food
   from drug or nonmedicinal substance — see Table of Drugs and Chemicals, by drug
Toxicosis — see also Toxemia
   capillary, hemorrhagic D69.0
Toxinfection, gastrointestinal K52.1
Toxocariasis B83.0
Toxoplasma, toxoplasmosis (acquired) B58.9
   with
      hepatitis B58.1

Toxoplasma, toxoplasmosis — continued
   with — continued
      meningoencephalitis B58.2
      ocular involvement B58.00
      other organ involvement B58.89
      pneumonia, pneumonitis B58.3
   congenital (acute) (subacute) (chronic) P37.1
   maternal, manifest toxoplasmosis in infant (acute) (subacute) (chronic) P37.1
tPA (rtPA) **administation in a different facility within the last 24 hours prior to admission to current facility** Z92.82
Trabeculation, bladder N32.89
Trachea — see condition
Tracheitis (catarrhal) (infantile) (membranous) (plastic) (septal) (suppurative) (viral) J04.10
   with
      bronchitis (15 years of age and above) J40
         acute or subacute — see Bronchitis, acute
         chronic J42
         tuberculous NEC A15.5
         under 15 years of age J20.9
      laryngitis (acute) J04.2
         chronic J37.1
         tuberculous NEC A15.5
   acute J04.10
      with obstruction J04.11
   chronic J42
      with
         bronchitis (chronic) J42
         laryngitis (chronic) J37.1
   diphtheritic (membranous) A36.89
   due to external agent — see Inflammation, respiratory, upper, due to
   syphilitic A52.73
   tuberculous A15.5
Trachelitis (nonvenereal) — see Cervicitis
Tracheobronchial — see condition
Tracheobronchitis (15 years of age and above) — see also Bronchitis
   due to
      Bordetella bronchiseptica A37.80
         with pneumonia A37.81
      Francisella tularensis A21.8
Tracheobronchomegaly Q32.4
   with bronchiectasis J47.9
      with
         exacerbation (acute) J47.1
         lower respiratory infection J47.0
   acquired J98.09
      with bronchiectasis J47.9
         with
            exacerbation (acute) J47.1
            lower respiratory infection J47.0
Tracheobronchopneumonitis — see Pneumonia, broncho-
Tracheocele (external) (internal) J39.8
   congenital Q32.1
Tracheomalacia J39.8
   congenital Q32.0
Tracheopharyngitis (acute) J06.9
   chronic J42
   due to external agent — see Inflammation, respiratory, upper, due to
Tracheostenosis J39.8
Tracheostomy
   complication — see Complication, tracheostomy
   status Z93.0
      attention to Z43.0
      malfunctioning J95.03
Trachoma, trachomatous A71.9
   active (stage) A71.1
   contraction of conjunctiva A71.1
   dubium A71.0
   healed or sequelae B94.0
   initial (stage) A71.0
   pannus A71.1
   Türck's J37.0
Traction, vitreomacular H43.82- ☑
Train sickness T75.3 ☑
Trait(s)
   Hb-S D57.3
   hemoglobin
      abnormal NEC D58.2
         with thalassemia D56.3
      C — see Disease, hemoglobin C
      S (Hb-S) D57.3
   Lepore D56.3

☑ **Additional Character Required** — **Refer to the Tabular List for Character Selection**   ▽ **Subterms under main terms may continue to next column or page**

Trait(s) — *continued*
 personality, accentuated Z73.1
 sickle-cell D57.3
  with elliptocytosis or spherocytosis D57.3
 type A personality Z73.1
Tramp Z59.0
Trance R41.89
 hysterical F44.89
Transaminasemia R74.0
Transection
 abdomen (partial) S38.3 ☑
 aorta (incomplete) — *see also* Injury, aorta
  complete — *see* Injury, aorta, laceration, major
 carotid artery (incomplete) — *see also* Injury, blood
  vessel, carotid, laceration
  complete — *see* Injury, blood vessel, carotid, laceration, major
 celiac artery (incomplete) S35.211 ☑
  branch (incomplete) S35.291 ☑
   complete S35.292 ☑
  complete S35.212 ☑
 innominate
  artery (incomplete) — *see also* Injury, blood vessel,
   thoracic, innominate, artery, laceration
   complete — *see* Injury, blood vessel, thoracic,
    innominate, artery, laceration, major
  vein (incomplete) — *see also* Injury, blood vessel,
   thoracic, innominate, vein, laceration
   complete — *see* Injury, blood vessel, thoracic,
    innominate, vein, laceration, major
 jugular vein (external) (incomplete) — *see also* Injury,
  blood vessel, jugular vein, laceration
  complete — *see* Injury, blood vessel, jugular vein,
   laceration, major
  internal (incomplete) — *see also* Injury, blood vessel,
   jugular vein, internal, laceration
   complete — *see* Injury, blood vessel, jugular vein,
    internal, laceration, major
 mesenteric artery (incomplete) — *see also* Injury,
  mesenteric, artery, laceration
  complete — *see* Injury, mesenteric artery, laceration,
   major
 pulmonary vessel (incomplete) — *see also* Injury, blood
  vessel, thoracic, pulmonary, laceration
  complete — *see* Injury, blood vessel, thoracic, pulmonary, laceration, major
 subclavian — *see* Transection, innominate
 vena cava (incomplete) — *see also* Injury, vena cava
  complete — *see* Injury, vena cava, laceration, major
 vertebral artery (incomplete) — *see also* Injury, blood
  vessel, vertebral, laceration
  complete — *see* Injury, blood vessel, vertebral, laceration, major
Transfusion
 associated (red blood cell) hemochromatosis E83.111
 blood
  ABO incompatible — *see* Complication(s), transfusion, incompatibility reaction, ABO
  minor blood group (Duffy) (E) (K) (Kell) (Kidd) (Lewis)
   (M) (N) (P) (S) T80.89 ☑
  reaction or complication — *see* Complications,
   transfusion
 fetomaternal (mother) — *see* Pregnancy, complicated
  by, placenta, transfusion syndrome
 maternofetal (mother) — *see* Pregnancy, complicated
  by, placenta, transfusion syndrome
 placental (syndrome) (mother) — *see* Pregnancy,
  complicated by, placenta, transfusion syndrome
 reaction (adverse) — *see* Complications, transfusion
 related acute lung injury (TRALI) J95.84
 twin-to-twin — *see* Pregnancy, complicated by, placenta, transfusion syndrome, fetus to fetus
Transient (meaning homeless) — *see also* condition Z59.0
Translocation
 balanced autosomal Q95.9
  in normal individual Q95.0
 chromosomes NEC Q99.8
  balanced and insertion in normal individual Q95.0
 Down syndrome Q90.2
 trisomy
  13 Q91.6
  18 Q91.2
  21 Q90.2
Translucency, iris — *see* Degeneration, iris
Transmission of chemical substances through the
 placenta — *see* Absorption, chemical, through
 placenta

Transparency, lung, unilateral J43.0
Transplant (ed) (status) Z94.9
 awaiting organ Z76.82
 bone Z94.6
  marrow Z94.81
 candidate Z76.82
 complication — *see* Complication, transplant
 cornea Z94.7
 heart Z94.1
  and lung(s) Z94.3
  valve Z95.2
   prosthetic Z95.2
   specified NEC Z95.4
   xenogenic Z95.3
 intestine Z94.82
 kidney Z94.0
 liver Z94.4
 lung(s) Z94.2
  and heart Z94.3
 organ (failure) (infection) (rejection) Z94.9
  removal status Z98.85
 pancreas Z94.83
 skin Z94.5
 social Z60.3
 specified organ or tissue NEC Z94.89
 stem cells Z94.84
 tissue Z94.9
Transplants, ovarian, endometrial N80.1
Transposed — *see* Transposition
Transposition (congenital) — *see also* Malposition,
 congenital
 abdominal viscera Q89.3
 aorta (dextra) Q20.3
 appendix Q43.8
 colon Q43.8
 corrected Q20.5
 great vessels (complete) (partial) Q20.3
 heart Q24.0
  with complete transposition of viscera Q89.3
 intestine (large) (small) Q43.8
 reversed jejunal (for bypass) (status) Z98.0
 scrotum Q55.23
 stomach Q40.2
  with general transposition of viscera Q89.3
 tooth, teeth, fully erupted M26.30
 vessels, great (complete) (partial) Q20.3
 viscera (abdominal) (thoracic) Q89.3
Transsexualism F64.0
Transverse — *see also* condition
 arrest (deep), in labor O64.0 ☑
 lie (mother) O32.2 ☑
  causing obstructed labor O64.8 ☑
Transvestism, transvestitism (dual-role) F64.1
 fetishistic F65.1
Trapped placenta (with hemorrhage) O72.0
 without hemorrhage O73.0
TRAPS (tumor necrosis factor receptor associated periodic
 syndrome) M04.1
Trauma, traumatism — *see also* Injury
 acoustic — *see* subcategory H83.3 ☑
 birth — *see* Birth, injury
 complicating ectopic or molar pregnancy O08.6
 during delivery O71.9
 following ectopic or molar pregnancy O08.6
 obstetric O71.9
  specified NEC O71.89
 occusal
  primary K08.81
  secondary K08.82
Traumatic — *see also* condition
 brain injury S06.9 ☑
Treacher Collins syndrome Q75.4
Treitz's hernia — *see* Hernia, abdomen, specified site
 NEC
Trematode infestation — *see* Infestation, fluke
Trematodiasis — *see* Infestation, fluke
Trembling paralysis — *see* Parkinsonism
Tremor(s) R25.1
 drug induced G25.1
 essential (benign) G25.0
 familial G25.0
 hereditary G25.0
 hysterical F44.4
 intention G25.2
 medication induced postural G25.1
 mercurial — *see* subcategory T56.1 ☑
 Parkinson's — *see* Parkinsonism
 psychogenic (conversion reaction) F44.4

Tremor(s) — *continued*
 senilis R54
 specified type NEC G25.2
Trench
 fever A79.0
 foot — *see* Immersion, foot
 mouth A69.1
Treponema pallidum infection — *see* Syphilis
Treponematosis
 due to
  T. pallidum — *see* Syphilis
  T. pertenue — *see* Yaws
Triad
 Hutchinson's (congenital syphilis) A50.53
 Kartagener's Q89.3
 Saint's — *see* Hernia, diaphragm
Trichiasis (eyelid) H02.059
 with entropion — *see* Entropion
 left H02.056
  lower H02.055
  upper H02.054
 right H02.053
  lower H02.052
  upper H02.051
Trichinella spiralis (infection) (infestation) B75
Trichinellosis, trichiniasis, trichinelliasis, trichinosis
 B75
 with muscle disorder B75 *[M63.80]*
  ankle B75 *[M63.87-]* ☑
  foot B75 *[M63.87-]* ☑
  forearm B75 *[M63.83-]* ☑
  hand B75 *[M63.84-]* ☑
  lower leg B75 *[M63.86-]* ☑
  multiple sites B75 *[M63.89]*
  pelvic region B75 *[M63.85-]* ☑
  shoulder region B75 *[M63.81-]* ☑
  specified site NEC B75 *[M63.88]*
  thigh B75 *[M63.85-]* ☑
  upper arm B75 *[M63.82-]* ☑
Trichobezoar T18.9 ☑
 intestine T18.3 ☑
 stomach T18.2 ☑
Trichocephaliasis, trichocephalosis B79
Trichocephalus infestation B79
Trichoclasis L67.8
Trichoepithelioma — *see also* Neoplasm, skin, benign
 malignant — *see* Neoplasm, skin, malignant
Trichofolliculoma — *see* Neoplasm, skin, benign
Tricholemmoma — *see* Neoplasm, skin, benign
Trichomoniasis A59.9
 bladder A59.03
 cervix A59.09
 intestinal A07.8
 prostate A59.02
 seminal vesicles A59.09
 specified site NEC A59.8
 urethra A59.03
 urogenitalis A59.00
 vagina A59.01
 vulva A59.01
Trichomycosis
 axillaris A48.8
 nodosa, nodularis B36.8
Trichonodosis L67.8
Trichophytid, trichophyton infection — *see* Dermato-
 phytosis
Trichophytobezoar T18.9 ☑
 intestine T18.3 ☑
 stomach T18.2 ☑
Trichophytosis — *see* Dermatophytosis
Trichoptilosis L67.8
Trichorrhexis (nodosa) (invaginata) L67.0
Trichosis axillaris A48.8
Trichosporosis nodosa B36.2
Trichostasis spinulosa (congenital) Q84.1
Trichostrongyliasis, trichostrongylosis (small intes-
 tine) B81.2
Trichostrongylus infection B81.2
Trichotillomania F63.3
Trichromat, trichromatopsia, anomalous (congenital)
 H53.55
Trichuriasis B79
Trichuris trichiura (infection) (infestation) (any site) B79
Tricuspid (valve) — *see* condition
Trifid — *see also* Accessory
 kidney (pelvis) Q63.8
 tongue Q38.3

▼ Subterms under main terms may continue to next column or page   ☑ Additional Character Required — Refer to the Tabular List for Character Selection   313

Trait — Trifid

Trigeminal neuralgia — see Neuralgia, trigeminal
Trigeminy R00.8
Trigger finger (acquired) M65.30
    congenital Q74.0
        index finger M65.32- ☑
        little finger M65.35- ☑
        middle finger M65.33- ☑
        ring finger M65.34- ☑
        thumb M65.31- ☑
Trigonitis (bladder) (chronic) (pseudomembranous)
    N30.30
    with hematuria N30.31
Trigonocephaly Q75.0
Trilocular heart — see Cor triloculare
Trimethylaminuria E72.52
Tripartite placenta O43.19- ☑
Triphalangeal thumb Q74.0
Triple — see also Accessory
    kidneys Q63.0
    uteri Q51.818
    X, female Q97.0
Triplegia G83.89
    congenital G80.8
Triplet (newborn) — see also Newborn, triplet
    complicating pregnancy — see Pregnancy, triplet
Triplication — see Accessory
Triploidy Q92.7
Trismus R25.2
    neonatorum A33
    newborn A33
Trisomy (syndrome) Q92.9
    13 (partial) Q91.7
        meiotic nondisjunction Q91.4
        mitotic nondisjunction Q91.5
        mosaicism Q91.5
        translocation Q91.6
    18 (partial) Q91.3
        meiotic nondisjunction Q91.0
        mitotic nondisjunction Q91.1
        mosaicism Q91.1
        translocation Q91.2
    20 Q92.8
    21 (partial) Q90.9
        meiotic nondisjunction Q90.0
        mitotic nondisjunction Q90.1
        mosaicism Q90.1
        translocation Q90.2
    22 Q92.8
    autosomes Q92.9
    chromosome specified NEC Q92.8
        partial Q92.2
            due to unbalanced translocation Q92.5
        specified NEC Q92.8
        whole (nonsex chromosome)
            meiotic nondisjunction Q92.0
            mitotic nondisjunction Q92.1
            mosaicism Q92.1
    due to
        dicentrics — see Extra, marker chromosomes
        extra rings — see Extra, marker chromosomes
        isochromosomes — see Extra, marker chromosomes
    specified NEC Q92.8
    whole chromosome Q92.9
        meiotic nondisjunction Q92.0
        mitotic nondisjunction Q92.1
        mosaicism Q92.1
        partial Q92.9
        specified NEC Q92.8
Tritanomaly, tritanopia H53.55
Trombiculosis, trombiculiasis, trombidiosis B88.0
Trophedema (congenital) (hereditary) Q82.0
Trophoblastic disease — see also Mole, hydatidiform
    O01.9
Tropholymphedema Q82.0
Trophoneurosis NEC G96.8
    disseminated M34.9
Tropical — see condition
Trouble — see also Disease
    heart — see Disease, heart
    kidney — see Disease, renal
    nervous R45.0
    sinus — see Sinusitis
Trousseau's syndrome (thrombophlebitis migrans) I82.1
Truancy, childhood
    from school Z72.810
Truncus
    arteriosus (persistent) Q20.0

Truncus — continued
    communis Q20.0
Trunk — see condition
Trypanosomiasis
    African B56.9
        by Trypanosoma brucei
            gambiense B56.0
            rhodesiense B56.1
    American — see Chagas' disease
    Brazilian — see Chagas' disease
    by Trypanosoma
        brucei gambiense B56.0
        brucei rhodesiense B56.1
        cruzi — see Chagas' disease
    gambiensis, Gambian B56.0
    rhodesiensis, Rhodesian B56.1
    South American — see Chagas' disease
    where
        African trypanosomiasis is prevalent B56.9
        Chagas' disease is prevalent B57.2
T-shaped incisors K00.2
Tsutsugamushi (disease) (fever) A75.3
Tube, tubal, tubular — see condition
Tubercle — see also Tuberculosis
    brain, solitary A17.81
    Darwin's Q17.8
    Ghon, primary infection A15.7
Tuberculid, tuberculide (indurating, subcutaneous)
    (lichenoid) (miliary) (papulonecrotic) (primary) (skin)
    A18.4
Tuberculoma — see also Tuberculosis
    brain A17.81
    meninges (cerebral) (spinal) A17.1
    spinal cord A17.81
Tuberculosis, tubercular, tuberculous (calcification)
    (calcified) (caseous) (chromogenic acid-fast bacilli)
    (degeneration) (fibrocaseous) (fistula) (interstitial)
    (isolated circumscribed lesions) (necrosis)
    (parenchymatous) (ulcerative) A15.9
    with pneumoconiosis (any condition in J60-J64) J65
    abdomen (lymph gland) A18.39
    abscess (respiratory) A15.9
        bone A18.03
            hip A18.02
            knee A18.02
            sacrum A18.01
            specified site NEC A18.03
            spinal A18.01
            vertebra A18.01
        brain A17.81
        breast A18.89
        Cowper's gland A18.15
        dura (mater) (cerebral) (spinal) A17.81
        epidural (cerebral) (spinal) A17.81
        female pelvis A18.17
        frontal sinus A15.8
        genital organs NEC A18.10
        genitourinary A18.10
        gland (lymphatic) — see Tuberculosis, lymph gland
        hip A18.02
        intestine A18.32
        ischiorectal A18.32
        joint NEC A18.02
            hip A18.02
            knee A18.02
            specified NEC A18.02
            vertebral A18.01
        kidney A18.11
        knee A18.02
        latent Z22.7
        lumbar (spine) A18.01
        lung — see Tuberculosis, pulmonary
        meninges (cerebral) (spinal) A17.0
        muscle A18.09
        perianal (fistula) A18.32
        perinephritic A18.11
        perirectal A18.32
        rectum A18.32
        retropharyngeal A15.8
        sacrum A18.01
        scrofulous A18.2
        scrotum A18.15
        skin (primary) A18.4
        spinal cord A17.81
        spine or vertebra (column) A18.01
        subdiaphragmatic A18.31
        testis A18.15
        urinary A18.13

Tuberculosis, tubercular, tuberculous — continued
    abscess — continued
        uterus A18.17
    accessory sinus — see Tuberculosis, sinus
    Addison's disease A18.7
    adenitis — see Tuberculosis, lymph gland
    adenoids A15.8
    adenopathy — see Tuberculosis, lymph gland
    adherent pericardium A18.84
    adnexa (uteri) A18.17
    adrenal (capsule) (gland) A18.7
    alimentary canal A18.32
    anemia A18.89
    ankle (joint) (bone) A18.02
    anus A18.32
    apex, apical — see Tuberculosis, pulmonary
    appendicitis, appendix A18.32
    arachnoid A17.0
    artery, arteritis A18.89
        cerebral A18.89
    arthritis (chronic) (synovial) A18.02
        spine or vertebra (column) A18.01
    articular — see Tuberculosis, joint
    ascites A18.31
    asthma — see Tuberculosis, pulmonary
    axilla, axillary (gland) A18.2
    bladder A18.12
    bone A18.03
        hip A18.02
        knee A18.02
        limb NEC A18.03
        sacrum A18.01
        spine or vertebral column A18.01
    bowel (miliary) A18.32
    brain A17.81
    breast A18.89
    broad ligament A18.17
    bronchi, bronchial, bronchus A15.5
        ectasia, ectasis (bronchiectasis) — see Tuberculosis,
            pulmonary
        fistula A15.5
            primary (progressive) A15.7
        gland or node A15.4
            primary (progressive) A15.7
        lymph gland or node A15.4
            primary (progressive) A15.7
    bronchiectasis — see Tuberculosis, pulmonary
    bronchitis A15.5
    bronchopleural A15.6
    bronchopneumonia, bronchopneumonic — see Tuber-
        culosis, pulmonary
    bronchorrhagia A15.5
    bronchotracheal A15.5
    bronze disease A18.7
    buccal cavity A18.83
    bulbourethral gland A18.15
    bursa A18.09
    cachexia A15.9
    cardiomyopathy A18.84
    caries — see Tuberculosis, bone
    cartilage A18.02
        intervertebral A18.01
    catarrhal — see Tuberculosis, respiratory
    cecum A18.32
    cellulitis (primary) A18.4
    cerebellum A17.81
    cerebral, cerebrum A17.81
    cerebrospinal A17.81
        meninges A17.0
    cervical (lymph gland or node) A18.2
    cervicitis, cervix (uteri) A18.16
    chest — see Tuberculosis, respiratory
    chorioretinitis A18.53
    choroid, choroiditis A18.53
    ciliary body A18.54
    colitis A18.32
    collier's J65
    colliquativa (primary) A18.4
    colon A18.32
    complex, primary A15.7
    congenital P37.0
    conjunctiva A18.59
    connective tissue (systemic) A18.89
    contact Z20.1
    cornea (ulcer) A18.52
    Cowper's gland A18.15
    coxae A18.02
    coxalgia A18.02

☑ **Additional Character Required** — **Refer to the Tabular List for Character Selection**   ▽ **Subterms under main terms may continue to next column or page**

Tuberculosis, tubercular, tuberculous — *continued*
cul-de-sac of Douglas A18.17
curvature, spine A18.01
cutis (colliquativa) (primary) A18.4
cyst, ovary A18.18
cystitis A18.12
dactylitis A18.03
diarrhea A18.32
diffuse — *see* Tuberculosis, miliary
digestive tract A18.32
disseminated — *see* Tuberculosis, miliary
duodenum A18.32
dura (mater) (cerebral) (spinal) A17.0
    abscess (cerebral) (spinal) A17.81
dysentery A18.32
ear (inner) (middle) A18.6
    bone A18.03
    external (primary) A18.4
    skin (primary) A18.4
elbow A18.02
emphysema — *see* Tuberculosis, pulmonary
empyema A15.6
encephalitis A17.82
endarteritis A18.89
endocarditis A18.84
    aortic A18.84
    mitral A18.84
    pulmonary A18.84
    tricuspid A18.84
endocrine glands NEC A18.82
endometrium A18.17
enteric, enterica, enteritis A18.32
enterocolitis A18.32
epididymis, epididymitis A18.15
epidural abscess (cerebral) (spinal) A17.81
epiglottis A15.5
episcleritis A18.51
erythema (induratum) (nodosum) (primary) A18.4
esophagus A18.83
eustachian tube A18.6
exposure (to) Z20.1
exudative — *see* Tuberculosis, pulmonary
eye A18.50
eyelid (primary) (lupus) A18.4
fallopian tube (acute) (chronic) A18.17
fascia A18.09
fauces A15.8
female pelvic inflammatory disease A18.17
finger A18.03
first infection A15.7
gallbladder A18.83
ganglion A18.09
gastritis A18.83
gastrocolic fistula A18.32
gastroenteritis A18.32
gastrointestinal tract A18.32
general, generalized — *see* Tuberculosis, miliary
genital organs A18.10
genitourinary A18.10
genu A18.02
glandula suprarenalis A18.7
glandular, general A18.2
glottis A15.5
grinder's J65
gum A18.83
hand A18.03
heart A18.84
hematogenous — *see* Tuberculosis, miliary
hemoptysis — *see* Tuberculosis, pulmonary
hemorrhage NEC — *see* Tuberculosis, pulmonary
hemothorax A15.6
hepatitis A18.83
hilar lymph nodes A15.4
    primary (progressive) A15.7
hip (joint) (disease) (bone) A18.02
hydropneumothorax A15.6
hydrothorax A15.6
hypoadrenalism A18.7
hypopharynx A15.8
ileocecal (hyperplastic) A18.32
ileocolitis A18.32
ileum A18.32
iliac spine (superior) A18.03
immunological findings only A15.7
indurativa (primary) A18.4
infantile A15.7
infection A15.9
    without clinical manifestations A15.7

Tuberculosis, tubercular, tuberculous — *continued*
infraclavicular gland A18.2
inguinal gland A18.2
inguinalis A18.2
intestine (any part) A18.32
iridocyclitis A18.54
iris, iritis A18.54
ischiorectal A18.32
jaw A18.03
jejunum A18.32
joint A18.02
    vertebral A18.01
keratitis (interstitial) A18.52
keratoconjunctivitis A18.52
kidney A18.11
knee (joint) A18.02
kyphosis, kyphoscoliosis A18.01
laryngitis A15.5
larynx A15.5
latent Z22.7
leptomeninges, leptomeningitis (cerebral) (spinal)
    A17.0
lichenoides (primary) A18.4
linguae A18.83
lip A18.83
liver A18.83
lordosis A18.01
lung — *see* Tuberculosis, pulmonary
lupus vulgaris A18.4
lymph gland or node (peripheral) A18.2
    abdomen A18.39
    bronchial A15.4
        primary (progressive) A15.7
    cervical A18.2
    hilar A15.4
        primary (progressive) A15.7
    intrathoracic A15.4
        primary (progressive) A15.7
    mediastinal A15.4
        primary (progressive) A15.7
    mesenteric A18.39
    retroperitoneal A18.39
    tracheobronchial A15.4
        primary (progressive) A15.7
lymphadenitis — *see* Tuberculosis, lymph gland
lymphangitis — *see* Tuberculosis, lymph gland
lymphatic (gland) (vessel) — *see* Tuberculosis, lymph
    gland
mammary gland A18.89
marasmus A15.9
mastoiditis A18.03
mediastinal lymph gland or node A15.4
    primary (progressive) A15.7
mediastinitis A15.8
    primary (progressive) A15.7
mediastinum A15.8
    primary (progressive) A15.7
medulla A17.81
melanosis, Addisonian A18.7
meninges, meningitis (basilar) (cerebral) (cerebrospinal)
    (spinal) A17.0
meningoencephalitis A17.82
mesentery, mesenteric (gland or node) A18.39
miliary A19.9
    acute A19.2
        multiple sites A19.1
        single specified site A19.0
    chronic A19.8
    specified NEC A19.8
millstone makers' J65
miner's J65
molder's J65
mouth A18.83
multiple A19.9
    acute A19.1
    chronic A19.8
muscle A18.09
myelitis A17.82
myocardium, myocarditis A18.84
nasal (passage) (sinus) A15.8
nasopharynx A15.8
neck gland A18.2
nephritis A18.11
nerve (mononeuropathy) A17.83
nervous system A17.9
nose (septum) A15.8
ocular A18.50
omentum A18.31
oophoritis (acute) (chronic) A18.17

Tuberculosis, tubercular, tuberculous — *continued*
optic (nerve trunk) (papilla) A18.59
orbit A18.59
orchitis A18.15
organ, specified NEC A18.89
osseous — *see* Tuberculosis, bone
osteitis — *see* Tuberculosis, bone
osteomyelitis — *see* Tuberculosis, bone
otitis media A18.6
ovary, ovaritis (acute) (chronic) A18.17
oviduct (acute) (chronic) A18.17
pachymeningitis A17.0
palate (soft) A18.83
pancreas A18.83
papulonecrotic (a) (primary) A18.4
parathyroid glands A18.82
paronychia (primary) A18.4
parotid gland or region A18.83
pelvis (bony) A18.03
penis A18.15
peribronchitis A15.5
pericardium, pericarditis A18.84
perichondritis, larynx A15.5
periostitis — *see* Tuberculosis, bone
perirectal fistula A18.32
peritoneum NEC A18.31
peritonitis A18.31
pharynx, pharyngitis A15.8
phlyctenulosis (keratoconjunctivitis) A18.52
phthisis NEC — *see* Tuberculosis, pulmonary
pituitary gland A18.82
pleura, pleural, pleurisy, pleuritis (fibrinous) (oblitera-
    tive) (purulent) (simple plastic) (with effusion)
    A15.6
    primary (progressive) A15.7
pneumonia, pneumonic — *see* Tuberculosis, pul-
    monary
pneumothorax (spontaneous) (tense valvular) — *see*
    Tuberculosis, pulmonary
polyneuropathy A17.89
polyserositis A19.9
    acute A19.1
    chronic A19.8
potter's J65
prepuce A18.15
primary (complex) A15.7
proctitis A18.32
prostate, prostatitis A18.14
pulmonalis — *see* Tuberculosis, pulmonary
pulmonary (cavitated) (fibrotic) (infiltrative) (nodular)
    A15.0
    childhood type or first infection A15.7
    primary (complex) A15.7
pyelitis A18.11
pyelonephritis A18.11
pyemia — *see* Tuberculosis, miliary
pyonephrosis A18.11
pyopneumothorax A15.6
pyothorax A15.6
rectum (fistula) (with abscess) A18.32
reinfection stage — *see* Tuberculosis, pulmonary
renal A18.11
renis A18.11
respiratory A15.9
    primary A15.7
    specified site NEC A15.8
retina, retinitis A18.53
retroperitoneal (lymph gland or node) A18.39
rheumatism NEC A18.09
rhinitis A15.8
sacroiliac (joint) A18.01
sacrum A18.01
salivary gland A18.83
salpingitis (acute) (chronic) A18.17
sandblaster's J65
sclera A18.51
scoliosis A18.01
scrofulous A18.2
scrotum A18.15
seminal tract or vesicle A18.15
senile A15.9
septic — *see* Tuberculosis, miliary
shoulder (joint) A18.02
    blade A18.03
sigmoid A18.32
sinus (any nasal) A15.8
    bone A18.03
    epididymis A18.15

Tuberculosis, tubercular, tuberculous — *continued*
- skeletal NEC A18.03
- skin (any site) (primary) A18.4
- small intestine A18.32
- soft palate A18.83
- spermatic cord A18.15
- spine, spinal (column) A18.01
  - cord A17.81
  - medulla A17.81
  - membrane A17.0
  - meninges A17.0
- spleen, splenitis A18.85
- spondylitis A18.01
- sternoclavicular joint A18.02
- stomach A18.83
- stonemason's J65
- subcutaneous tissue (cellular) (primary) A18.4
- subcutis (primary) A18.4
- subdeltoid bursa A18.83
- submaxillary (region) A18.83
- supraclavicular gland A18.2
- suprarenal (capsule) (gland) A18.7
- swelling, joint (see also category M01) — *see also* Tuberculosis, joint A18.02
- symphysis pubis A18.02
- synovitis A18.09
  - articular A18.02
  - spine or vertebra A18.01
- systemic — *see* Tuberculosis, miliary
- tarsitis A18.4
- tendon (sheath) — *see* Tuberculosis, tenosynovitis
- tenosynovitis A18.09
  - spine or vertebra A18.01
- testis A18.15
- throat A15.8
- thymus gland A18.82
- thyroid gland A18.81
- tongue A18.83
- tonsil, tonsillitis A15.8
- trachea, tracheal A15.5
  - lymph gland or node A15.4
    - primary (progressive) A15.7
- tracheobronchial A15.5
  - lymph gland or node A15.4
    - primary (progressive) A15.7
- tubal (acute) (chronic) A18.17
- tunica vaginalis A18.15
- ulcer (skin) (primary) A18.4
  - bowel or intestine A18.32
  - specified NEC — *see* Tuberculosis, by site
- unspecified site A15.9
- ureter A18.11
- urethra, urethral (gland) A18.13
- urinary organ or tract A18.13
- uterus A18.17
- uveal tract A18.54
- uvula A18.83
- vagina A18.18
- vas deferens A18.15
- verruca, verrucosa (cutis) (primary) A18.4
- vertebra (column) A18.01
- vesiculitis A18.15
- vulva A18.18
- wrist (joint) A18.02

Tuberculum
- Carabelli — *see* Excludes Note at K00.2
- occlusal — *see* Excludes Note at K00.2
- paramolare K00.2

Tuberosity, enitre maxillary M26.07
Tuberous sclerosis (brain) Q85.1
Tubo-ovarian — *see* condition
Tuboplasty, after previous sterilization Z31.0
- aftercare Z31.42
Tubotympanitis, catarrhal (chronic) — *see* Otitis, media, nonsuppurative, chronic, serous
Tularemia A21.9
- with
  - conjunctivitis A21.1
  - pneumonia A21.2
- abdominal A21.3
- bronchopneumonic A21.2
- conjunctivitis A21.1
- cryptogenic A21.3
- enteric A21.3
- gastrointestinal A21.3
- generalized A21.7
- ingestion A21.3
- intestinal A21.3

Tularemia — *continued*
- oculoglandular A21.1
- ophthalmic A21.1
- pneumonia (any), pneumonic A21.2
- pulmonary A21.2
- sepsis A21.7
- specified NEC A21.8
- typhoidal A21.7
- ulceroglandular A21.0
Tularensis conjunctivitis A21.1
Tumefaction — *see also* Swelling
- liver — *see* Hypertrophy, liver
Tumor — *see also* Neoplasm, unspecified behavior, by site
- acinar cell — *see* Neoplasm, uncertain behavior, by site
- acinic cell — *see* Neoplasm, uncertain behavior, by site
- adenocarcinoid — *see* Neoplasm, malignant, by site
- adenomatoid — *see also* Neoplasm, benign, by site
  - odontogenic — *see* Cyst, calcifying odontogenic
- adnexal (skin) — *see* Neoplasm, skin, benign, by site
- adrenal
  - cortical (benign) D35.0- ☑
    - malignant C74.0- ☑
  - rest — *see* Neoplasm, benign, by site
- alpha-cell
  - malignant
    - pancreas C25.4
    - specified site NEC — *see* Neoplasm, malignant, by site
    - unspecified site C25.4
  - pancreas D13.7
  - specified site NEC — *see* Neoplasm, benign, by site
  - unspecified site D13.7
- aneurysmal — *see* Aneurysm
- aortic body D44.7
  - malignant C75.5
- Askin's — *see* Neoplasm, connective tissue, malignant
- basal cell — *see also* Neoplasm, skin, uncertain behavior D48.5
- Bednar — *see* Neoplasm, skin, malignant
- benign (unclassified) — *see* Neoplasm, benign, by site
- beta-cell
  - malignant
    - pancreas C25.4
    - specified site NEC — *see* Neoplasm, malignant, by site
    - unspecified site C25.4
  - pancreas D13.7
  - specified site NEC — *see* Neoplasm, benign, by site
  - unspecified site D13.7
- Brenner D27.9
  - borderline malignancy D39.1- ☑
  - malignant C56- ☑
  - proliferating D39.1- ☑
- bronchial alveolar, intravascular D38.1
- Brooke's — *see* Neoplasm, skin, benign
- brown fat — *see* Lipoma
- Burkitt — *see* Lymphoma, Burkitt
- calcifying epithelial odontogenic — *see* Cyst, calcifying odontogenic
- carcinoid D3A.00 (following D36)
  - benign D3A.00 (following D36)
    - appendix D3A.020 (following D36)
    - ascending colon D3A.022 (following D36)
    - bronchus (lung) D3A.090 (following D36)
    - cecum D3A.021 (following D36)
    - colon D3A.029 (following D36)
    - descending colon D3A.024 (following D36)
    - duodenum D3A.010 (following D36)
    - foregut NOS D3A.094 (following D36)
    - hindgut NOS D3A.096 (following D36)
    - ileum D3A.012 (following D36)
    - jejunum D3A.011 (following D36)
    - kidney D3A.093 (following D36)
    - large intestine D3A.029 (following D36)
    - lung (bronchus) D3A.090 (following D36)
    - midgut NOS D3A.095 (following D36)
    - rectum D3A.026 (following D36)
    - sigmoid colon D3A.025 (following D36)
    - small intestine D3A.019 (following D36)
    - specified NEC D3A.098 (following D36)
    - stomach D3A.092 (following D36)
    - thymus D3A.091 (following D36)
    - transverse colon D3A.023 (following D36)
  - malignant C7A.00 (following C75)
    - appendix C7A.020 (following C75)
    - ascending colon C7A.022 (following C75)
    - bronchus (lung) C7A.090 (following C75)

Tumor — *continued*
- carcinoid — *continued*
  - malignant — *continued*
    - cecum C7A.021 (following C75)
    - colon C7A.029 (following C75)
    - descending colon C7A.024 (following C75)
    - duodenum C7A.010 (following C75)
    - foregut NOS C7A.094 (following C75)
    - hindgut NOS C7A.096 (following C75)
    - ileum C7A.012 (following C75)
    - jejunum C7A.011 (following C75)
    - kidney C7A.093 (following C75)
    - large intestine C7A.029 (following C75)
    - lung (bronchus) C7A.090 (following C75)
    - midgut NOS C7A.095 (following C75)
    - rectum C7A.026 (following C75)
    - sigmoid colon C7A.025 (following C75)
    - small intestine C7A.019 (following C75)
    - specified NEC C7A.098 (following C75)
    - stomach C7A.092 (following C75)
    - thymus C7A.091 (following C75)
    - transverse colon C7A.023 (following C75)
  - mesentery metastasis C7B.04 (following C75)
  - secondary C7B.00 (following C75)
    - bone C7B.03 (following C75)
    - distant lymph nodes C7B.01 (following C75)
    - liver C7B.02 (following C75)
    - peritoneum C7B.04 (following C75)
    - specified NEC C7B.09 (following C75)
- carotid body D44.6
  - malignant C75.4
- cells — *see also* Neoplasm, unspecified behavior, by site
  - benign — *see* Neoplasm, benign, by site
  - malignant — *see* Neoplasm, malignant, by site
  - uncertain whether benign or malignant — *see* Neoplasm, uncertain behavior, by site
- cervix, in pregnancy or childbirth — *see* Pregnancy, complicated by, tumor, cervix
- chondromatous giant cell — *see* Neoplasm, bone, benign
- chromaffin — *see also* Neoplasm, benign, by site
  - malignant — *see* Neoplasm, malignant, by site
- Cock's peculiar L72.3
- Codman's — *see* Neoplasm, bone, benign
- dentigerous, mixed — *see* Cyst, calcifying odontogenic
- dermoid — *see* Neoplasm, benign, by site
  - with malignant transformation C56- ☑
- desmoid (extra-abdominal) — *see also* Neoplasm, connective tissue, uncertain behavior
  - abdominal — *see* Neoplasm, connective tissue, uncertain behavior
- embolus — *see* Neoplasm, secondary, by site
- embryonal (mixed) — *see also* Neoplasm, uncertain behavior, by site
  - liver C22.7
- endodermal sinus
  - specified site — *see* Neoplasm, malignant, by site
  - unspecified site
    - female C56.- ☑
    - male C62.90
- epithelial
  - benign — *see* Neoplasm, benign, by site
  - malignant — *see* Neoplasm, malignant, by site
- Ewing's — *see* Neoplasm, bone, malignant, by site
- fatty — *see* Lipoma
- fibroid — *see* Leiomyoma
- G cell
  - malignant
    - pancreas C25.4
    - specified site NEC — *see* Neoplasm, malignant, by site
    - unspecified site C25.4
  - specified site — *see* Neoplasm, uncertain behavior, by site
  - unspecified site D37.8
- germ cell — *see also* Neoplasm, malignant, by site
  - mixed — *see* Neoplasm, malignant, by site
- ghost cell, odontogenic — *see* Cyst, calcifying odontogenic
- giant cell — *see also* Neoplasm, uncertain behavior, by site
  - bone D48.0
    - malignant — *see* Neoplasm, bone, malignant
    - chondromatous — *see* Neoplasm, bone, benign
    - malignant — *see* Neoplasm, malignant, by site
  - soft parts — *see* Neoplasm, connective tissue, uncertain behavior

Tumor — *continued*
  giant cell — *see also* Neoplasm, uncertain behavior,
    by site — *continued*
    soft parts — *see* Neoplasm, connective tissue, un-
      certain behavior — *continued*
      malignant — *see* Neoplasm, connective tissue,
        malignant
  glomus D18.00
    intra-abdominal D18.03
    intracranial D18.02
    jugulare D44.7
      malignant C75.5
    skin D18.01
    specified site NEC D18.09
  gonadal stromal — *see* Neoplasm, uncertain behavior,
    by site
  granular cell — *see also* Neoplasm, connective tissue,
    benign
    malignant — *see* Neoplasm, connective tissue, ma-
      lignant
  granulosa cell D39.1- ☑
    juvenile D39.1- ☑
    malignant C56- ☑
  granulosa cell-theca cell D39.1- ☑
    malignant C56- ☑
  Grawitz's C64- ☑
  hemorrhoidal — *see* Hemorrhoids
  hilar cell D27- ☑
  hilus cell D27- ☑
  Hurthle cell (benign) D34
    malignant C73
  hydatid — *see* Echinococcus
  hypernephroid — *see also* Neoplasm, uncertain behav-
    ior, by site
  interstitial cell — *see also* Neoplasm, uncertain behav-
    ior, by site
    benign — *see* Neoplasm, benign, by site
    malignant — *see* Neoplasm, malignant, by site
  intravascular bronchial alveolar D38.1
  islet cell — *see* Neoplasm, benign, by site
    malignant — *see* Neoplasm, malignant, by site
      pancreas C25.4
      specified site NEC — *see* Neoplasm, malignant,
        by site
      unspecified site C25.4
    pancreas D13.7
    specified site NEC — *see* Neoplasm, benign, by site
    unspecified site D13.7
  juxtaglomerular D41.0- ☑
  Klatskin's C22.1
  Krukenberg's C79.6- ☑
  Leydig cell — *see* Neoplasm, uncertain behavior, by
    site
    benign — *see* Neoplasm, benign, by site
      specified site — *see* Neoplasm, benign, by site
      unspecified site
        female D27.9
        male D29.20
    malignant — *see* Neoplasm, malignant, by site
      specified site — *see* Neoplasm, malignant, by
        site
      unspecified site
        female C56.9
        male C62.90
    specified site — *see* Neoplasm, uncertain behavior,
      by site
    unspecified site
      female D39.10
      male D40.10
  lipid cell, ovary D27- ☑
  lipoid cell, ovary D27- ☑
  malignant — *see also* Neoplasm, malignant, by site
    C80.1
    fusiform cell (type) C80.1
    giant cell (type) C80.1
    localized, plasma cell — *see* Plasmacytoma, solitary
    mixed NEC C80.1
    small cell (type) C80.1
    spindle cell (type) C80.1
    unclassified C80.1
  mast cell D47.09
  melanotic, neuroectodermal — *see* Neoplasm, benign,
    by site
  Merkel cell — *see* Carcinoma, Merkel cell
  mesenchymal
    malignant — *see* Neoplasm, connective tissue, ma-
      lignant

Tumor — *continued*
  mesenchymal — *continued*
    mixed — *see* Neoplasm, connective tissue, uncertain
      behavior
  mesodermal, mixed — *see also* Neoplasm, malignant,
    by site
    liver C22.4
  mesonephric — *see also* Neoplasm, uncertain behavior,
    by site
    malignant — *see* Neoplasm, malignant, by site
  metastatic
    from specified site — *see* Neoplasm, malignant, by
      site
    of specified site — *see* Neoplasm, malignant, by site
    to specified site — *see* Neoplasm, secondary, by site
  mixed NEC — *see also* Neoplasm, benign, by site
    malignant — *see* Neoplasm, malignant, by site
  mucinous of low malignant potential
    specified site — *see* Neoplasm, malignant, by site
    unspecified site C56.9
  mucocarcinoid
    specified site — *see* Neoplasm, malignant, by site
    unspecified site C18.1
  mucoepidermoid — *see* Neoplasm, uncertain behavior,
    by site
  Müllerian, mixed
    specified site — *see* Neoplasm, malignant, by site
    unspecified site C54.9
  myoepithelial — *see* Neoplasm, benign, by site
  neuroectodermal (peripheral) — *see* Neoplasm, malig-
    nant, by site
    primitive
      specified site — *see* Neoplasm, malignant, by
        site
      unspecified site C71.9
  neuroendocrine D3A.8 (*following* D36)
    malignant poorly differentiated C7A.1 (*following*
      C75)
    secondary NEC C7B.8 (*following* C75)
    specified NEC C7A.8 (*following* C75)
  neurogenic olfactory C30.0
  nonencapsulated sclerosing C73
  odontogenic (adenomatoid) (benign) (calcifying epithe-
    lial) (keratocystic) (squamous) — *see* Cyst, calci-
    fying odontogenic
    malignant C41.1
      upper jaw (bone) C41.0
  ovarian stromal D39.1- ☑
  ovary, in pregnancy — *see* Pregnancy, complicated by
  pacinian — *see* Neoplasm, skin, benign
  Pancoast's — *see* Pancoast's syndrome
  papillary — *see also* Papilloma
    cystic D37.9
    mucinous of low malignant potential C56- ☑
      specified site — *see* Neoplasm, malignant, by
        site
      unspecified site C56.9
    serous of low malignant potential
      specified site — *see* Neoplasm, malignant, by
        site
      unspecified site C56.9
  pelvic, in pregnancy or childbirth — *see* Pregnancy,
    complicated by
  phantom F45.8
  phyllodes D48.6- ☑
    benign D24- ☑
    malignant — *see* Neoplasm, breast, malignant
  Pindborg — *see* Cyst, calcifying odontogenic
  placental site trophoblastic D39.2
  plasma cell (malignant) (localized) — *see* Plasmacy-
    toma, solitary
  polyvesicular vitelline
    specified site — *see* Neoplasm, malignant, by site
    unspecified site
      female C56.9
      male C62.90
  Pott's puffy — *see* Osteomyelitis, specified NEC
  Rathke's pouch D44.3
  retinal anlage — *see* Neoplasm, benign, by site
  salivary gland type, mixed — *see* Neoplasm, salivary
    gland, benign
    malignant — *see* Neoplasm, salivary gland, malig-
      nant
  Sampson's N80.1
  Schmincke's — *see* Neoplasm, nasopharynx, malignant
  sclerosing stromal D27- ☑
  sebaceous — *see* Cyst, sebaceous

Tumor — *continued*
  secondary — *see* Neoplasm, secondary, by site
    carcinoid C7B.00 (*following* C75)
      bone C7B.03 (*following* C75)
      distant lymph nodes C7B.01 (*following* C75)
      liver C7B.02 (*following* C75)
      peritoneum C7B.04 (*following* C75)
      specified NEC C7B.09 (*following* C75)
    neuroendocrine NEC C7B.8 (*following* C75)
  serous of low malignant potential
    specified site — *see* Neoplasm, malignant, by site
    unspecified site C56.9
  Sertoli cell — *see* Neoplasm, benign, by site
    with lipid storage
      specified site — *see* Neoplasm, benign, by site
      unspecified site
        female D27.9
        male D29.20
    specified site — *see* Neoplasm, benign, by site
    unspecified site
      female D27.9
      male D29.20
  Sertoli-Leydig cell — *see* Neoplasm, benign, by site
    specified site — *see* Neoplasm, benign, by site
    unspecified site
      female D27.9
      male D29.20
  sex cord (-stromal) — *see* Neoplasm, uncertain behav-
    ior, by site
    with annular tubules D39.1- ☑
  skin appendage — *see* Neoplasm, skin, benign
  smooth muscle — *see* Neoplasm, connective tissue,
    uncertain behavior
  soft tissue
    benign — *see* Neoplasm, connective tissue, benign
    malignant — *see* Neoplasm, connective tissue, ma-
      lignant
  sternomastoid (congenital) Q68.0
  stromal
    endometrial D39.0
    gastric D48.1
      benign D21.4
      malignant C16.9
      uncertain behavior D48.1
    gastrointestinal C49.A- ☑
      benign D21.4
      esophagus C49.A1
      malignant C49.A0
        colon C49.A4
        duodenum C49.A3
        esophagus C49.A1
        ileum C49.A3
        jejunum C49.A3
        large intestine C49.A4
        Meckel diverticulum C49.A3
        omentum C49.A9
        peritoneum C49.A9
        rectum C49.A5
        small intestine C49.A3
        specified site NEC C49.A9
        stomach C49.A2
      rectum C49.A5
      small intestine C49.A3
      specified site NEC C49.A9
      stomach C49.A2
      uncertain behavior D48.1
    intestine
      benign D21.4
      malignant
        large C49.A4
        small C49.A3
      uncertain behavior D48.1
    ovarian D39.1- ☑
    stomach C49.A2
      benign D21.4
      malignant C49.A2
      uncertain behavior D48.1
  sweat gland — *see also* Neoplasm, skin, uncertain be-
    havior
    benign — *see* Neoplasm, skin, benign
    malignant — *see* Neoplasm, skin, malignant
  syphilitic, brain A52.17
  testicular D40.10
  testicular stromal D40.1- ☑
  theca cell D27.- ☑
  theca cell-granulosa cell D39.1- ☑
  Triton, malignant — *see* Neoplasm, nerve, malignant
  trophoblastic, placental site D39.2

Tumor — *continued*
  turban D23.4
  uterus (body), in pregnancy or childbirth — *see* Pregnancy, complicated by, tumor, uterus
  vagina, in pregnancy or childbirth — *see* Pregnancy, complicated by
  varicose — *see* Varix
  von Recklinghausen's — *see* Neurofibromatosis
  vulva or perineum, in pregnancy or childbirth — *see* Pregnancy, complicated by
    causing obstructed labor O65.5
  Warthin's — *see* Neoplasm, salivary gland, benign
  Wilms' C64- ☑
  yolk sac — *see* Neoplasm, malignant, by site
    specified site — *see* Neoplasm, malignant, by site
    unspecified site
      female C56.9
      male C62.90
Tumor lysis syndrome (following antineoplastic chemotherapy) (spontaneous) NEC E88.3
Tumorlet — *see* Neoplasm, uncertain behavior, by site
Tungiasis B88.1
Tunica vasculosa lentis Q12.2
Turban tumor D23.4
Türck's trachoma J37.0
Turner-Kieser syndrome Q87.2
Turner-like syndrome Q87.19
Turner's
  hypoplasia (tooth) K00.4
  syndrome Q96.9
    specified NEC Q96.8
  tooth K00.4
Turner-Ullrich syndrome Q96.9
Tussis convulsiva — *see* Whooping cough
Twiddler's syndrome (due to)
  automatic implantable defibrillator T82.198
  cardiac pacemaker T82.198 ☑
Twilight state
  epileptic F05
  psychogenic F44.89
Twin (newborn) — *see also* Newborn, twin
  conjoined Q89.4
  pregnancy — *see* Pregnancy, twin
Twinning, teeth K00.2
Twist, twisted
  bowel, colon or intestine K56.2
  hair (congenital) Q84.1
  mesentery K56.2
  omentum K56.2
  organ or site, congenital NEC — *see* Anomaly, by site
  ovarian pedicle — *see* Torsion, ovary
Twitching R25.3
Tylosis (acquired) L84
  buccalis K13.29
  linguae K13.29
  palmaris et plantaris (congenital) (inherited) Q82.8
    acquired L85.1
Tympanism R14.0
Tympanites (abdominal) (intestinal) R14.0
Tympanitis — *see* Myringitis
Tympanosclerosis H74.0 ☑
Tympanum — *see* condition
Tympany
  abdomen R14.0
  chest R09.89
Type A behavior pattern Z73.1
Typhlitis — *see* Appendicitis
Typhoenteritis — *see* Typhoid
Typhoid (abortive) (ambulant) (any site) (clinical) (fever) (hemorrhagic) (infection) (intermittent) (malignant) (rheumatic) (Widal negative) A01.00
  with pneumonia A01.03
  abdominal A01.09
  arthritis A01.04
  carrier (suspected) of Z22.0
  cholecystitis (current) A01.09
  endocarditis A01.02
  heart involvement A01.02
  inoculation reaction — *see* Complications, vaccination
  meningitis A01.01
  mesenteric lymph nodes A01.09
  myocarditis A01.02
  osteomyelitis A01.05
  perichondritis, larynx A01.09
  pneumonia A01.03
  specified NEC A01.09
  spine A01.05

Typhoid — *continued*
  ulcer (perforating) A01.09
Typhomalaria (fever) — *see* Malaria
Typhomania A01.00
Typhoperitonitis A01.09
Typhus (fever) A75.9
  abdominal, abdominalis — *see* Typhoid
  African tick A77.1
  amarillic A95.9
  brain A75.9 *[G94]*
  cerebral A75.9 *[G94]*
  classical A75.0
  due to Rickettsia
    prowazekii A75.0
      recrudescent A75.1
    tsutsugamushi A75.3
    typhi A75.2
  endemic (flea-borne) A75.2
  epidemic (louse-borne) A75.0
  exanthematicus SAI A75.0
    brillii SAI A75.1
    mexicanus SAI A75.2
    typhus murinus A75.2
  exanthematic NEC A75.0
  flea-borne A75.2
  India tick A77.1
  Kenya (tick) A77.1
  louse-borne A75.0
  Mexican A75.2
  mite-borne A75.3
  murine A75.2
  North Asian tick-borne A77.2
  petechial A75.9
  Queensland tick A77.3
  rat A75.2
  recrudescent A75.1
  recurrens — *see* Fever, relapsing
  Sao Paulo A77.0
  scrub (China) (India) (Malaysia) (New Guinea) A75.3
  shop (of Malaysia) A75.2
  Siberian tick A77.2
  tick-borne A77.9
  tropical (mite-borne) A75.3
Tyrosinemia E70.21
  newborn, transitory P74.5
Tyrosinosis E70.21
Tyrosinuria E70.29

U

Uhl's anomaly or disease Q24.8
Ulcer, ulcerated, ulcerating, ulceration, ulcerative
  alveolar process M27.3
  amebic (intestine) A06.1
    skin A06.7
  anastomotic — *see* Ulcer, gastrojejunal
  anorectal K62.6
  antral — *see* Ulcer, stomach
  anus (sphincter) (solitary) K62.6
  aorta — *see* Aneurysm
  aphthous (oral) (recurrent) K12.0
    genital organ(s)
      female N76.6
      male N50.89
  artery I77.2
  atrophic — *see* Ulcer, skin
    decubitus — *see* Ulcer, pressure, by site
  back L98.429
    with
      bone involvement without evidence of necrosis L98.426
      bone necrosis L98.424
      exposed fat layer L98.422
      muscle involvement without evidence of necrosis L98.425
      muscle necrosis L98.423
      skin breakdown only L98.421
      specified severity NEC L98.428
  Barrett's (esophagus) K22.10
    with bleeding K22.11
  bile duct (common) (hepatic) K83.8
  bladder (solitary) (sphincter) NEC N32.89
    bilharzial B65.9 *[N33]*
    in schistosomiasis (bilharzial) B65.9 *[N33]*
    submucosal — *see* Cystitis, interstitial
    tuberculous A18.12
  bleeding K27.4
  bone — *see* Osteomyelitis, specified type NEC

Ulcer, ulcerated, ulcerating, ulceration, ulcerative — *continued*
  bowel — *see* Ulcer, intestine
  breast N61.1
  bronchus J98.09
  buccal (cavity) (traumatic) K12.1
  Buruli A31.1
  buttock L98.419
    with
      bone involvement without evidence of necrosis L98.416
      bone necrosis L98.414
      exposed fat layer L98.412
      muscle involvement without evidence of necrosis L98.415
      muscle necrosis L98.413
      skin breakdown only L98.411
      specified severity NEC L98.418
  cancerous — *see* Neoplasm, malignant, by site
  cardia K22.10
    with bleeding K22.11
  cardioesophageal (peptic) K22.10
    with bleeding K22.11
  cecum — *see* Ulcer, intestine
  cervix (uteri) (decubitus) (trophic) N86
    with cervicitis N72
  chancroidal A57
  chiclero B55.1
  chronic (cause unknown) — *see* Ulcer, skin
  Cochin-China B55.1
  colon — *see* Ulcer, intestine
  conjunctiva H10.89
  cornea H16.00- ☑
    with hypopyon H16.03- ☑
    central H16.01- ☑
    dendritic (herpes simplex) B00.52
    marginal H16.04- ☑
    Mooren's H16.05- ☑
    mycotic H16.06- ☑
    perforated H16.07- ☑
    ring H16.02- ☑
    tuberculous (phlyctenular) A18.52
  corpus cavernosum (chronic) N48.5
  crural — *see* Ulcer, lower limb
  Curling's — *see* Ulcer, peptic, acute
  Cushing's — *see* Ulcer, peptic, acute
  cystic duct K82.8
  cystitis (interstitial) — *see* Cystitis, interstitial
  decubitus — *see* Ulcer, pressure, by site
  dendritic, cornea (herpes simplex) B00.52
  diabetes, diabetic — *see* Diabetes, ulcer
  Dieulafoy's K25.0
  due to
    infection NEC — *see* Ulcer, skin
    radiation NEC L59.8
    trophic disturbance (any region) — *see* Ulcer, skin
    X-ray L58.1
  duodenum, duodenal (eroded) (peptic) K26.9
    with
      hemorrhage K26.4
        and perforation K26.6
      perforation K26.5
    acute K26.3
      with
        hemorrhage K26.0
          and perforation K26.2
        perforation K26.1
    chronic K26.7
      with
        hemorrhage K26.4
          and perforation K26.6
        perforation K26.5
  dysenteric A09
  elusive — *see* Cystitis, interstitial
  endocarditis (acute) (chronic) (subacute) I28.8
  epiglottis J38.7
  esophagus (peptic) K22.10
    with bleeding K22.11
    due to
      aspirin K22.10
        with bleeding K22.11
      gastrointestinal reflux disease K21.0
      ingestion of chemical or medicament K22.10
        with bleeding K22.11
    fungal K22.10
      with bleeding K22.11
    infective K22.10
      with bleeding K22.11

Ulcer, ulcerated, ulcerating, ulceration, ulcerative
— *continued*
  esophagus — *continued*
    varicose — *see* Varix, esophagus
  eyelid (region) H01.8
  fauces J39.2
  Fenwick (-Hunner) (solitary) — *see* Cystitis, interstitial
  fistulous — *see* Ulcer, skin
  foot (indolent) (trophic) — *see* Ulcer, lower limb
  frambesial, initial A66.0
  frenum (tongue) K14.0
  gallbladder or duct K82.8
  gangrenous — *see* Gangrene
  gastric — *see* Ulcer, stomach
  gastrocolic — *see* Ulcer, gastrojejunal
  gastroduodenal — *see* Ulcer, peptic
  gastroesophageal — *see* Ulcer, stomach
  gastrointestinal — *see* Ulcer, gastrojejunal
  gastrojejunal (peptic) K28.9
    with
      hemorrhage K28.4
        and perforation K28.6
      perforation K28.5
    acute K28.3
      with
        hemorrhage K28.0
          and perforation K28.2
        perforation K28.1
    chronic K28.7
      with
        hemorrhage K28.4
          and perforation K28.6
        perforation K28.5
  gastrojejunocolic — *see* Ulcer, gastrojejunal
  gingiva K06.8
  gingivitis K05.10
    nonplaque induced K05.11
    plaque induced K05.10
  glottis J38.7
  granuloma of pudenda A58
  gum K06.8
  gumma, due to yaws A66.4
  heel — *see* Ulcer, lower limb
  hemorrhoid — *see also* Hemorrhoids, by degree K64.8
  Hunner's — *see* Cystitis, interstitial
  hypopharynx J39.2
  hypopyon (chronic) (subacute) — *see* Ulcer, cornea, with hypopyon
  hypostaticum — *see* Ulcer, varicose
  ileum — *see* Ulcer, intestine
  intestine, intestinal K63.3
    with perforation K63.1
    amebic A06.1
    duodenal — *see* Ulcer, duodenum
    granulocytopenic (with hemorrhage) — *see* Neutropenia
    marginal — *see* Ulcer, gastrojejunal
    perforating K63.1
      newborn P78.0
    primary, small intestine K63.3
    rectum K62.6
    stercoraceous, stercoral K63.3
    tuberculous A18.32
    typhoid (fever) — *see* Typhoid
    varicose I86.8
  jejunum, jejunal — *see* Ulcer, gastrojejunal
  keratitis — *see* Ulcer, cornea
  knee — *see* Ulcer, lower limb
  labium (majus) (minus) N76.6
  laryngitis — *see* Laryngitis
  larynx (aphthous) (contact) J38.7
    diphtheritic A36.2
  leg — *see* Ulcer, lower limb
  lip K13.0
  Lipschütz's N76.6
  lower limb (atrophic) (chronic) (neurogenic) (perforating) (pyogenic) (trophic) (tropical) L97.909
    with
      bone involvement without evidence of necrosis L97.906
      bone necrosis L97.904
      exposed fat layer L97.902
      muscle involvement without evidence of necrosis L97.905
      muscle necrosis L97.903
      skin breakdown only L97.901
      specified severity NEC L97.908
    ankle L97.309

Ulcer, ulcerated, ulcerating, ulceration, ulcerative
— *continued*
  lower limb — *continued*
    ankle — *continued*
      with
        bone involvement without evidence of necrosis L97.306
        bone necrosis L97.304
        exposed fat layer L97.302
        muscle involvement without evidence of necrosis L97.305
        muscle necrosis L97.303
        skin breakdown only L97.301
        specified severity NEC L97.308
      left L97.329
        with
          bone involvement without evidence of necrosis L97.326
          bone necrosis L97.324
          exposed fat layer L97.322
          muscle involvement without evidence of necrosis L97.325
          muscle necrosis L97.323
          skin breakdown only L97.321
          specified severity NEC L97.328
      right L97.319
        with
          bone involvement without evidence of necrosis L97.316
          bone necrosis L97.314
          exposed fat layer L97.312
          muscle involvement without evidence of necrosis L97.315
          muscle necrosis L97.313
          skin breakdown only L97.311
          specified severity NEC L97.318
    calf L97.209
      with
        bone involvement without evidence of necrosis L97.206
        bone necrosis L97.204
        exposed fat layer L97.202
        muscle involvement without evidence of necrosis L97.205
        muscle necrosis L97.203
        skin breakdown only L97.201
        specified severity NEC L97.208
      left L97.229
        with
          bone involvement without evidence of necrosis L97.226
          bone necrosis L97.224 •
          exposed fat layer L97.222
          muscle involvement without evidence of necrosis L97.225
          muscle necrosis L97.223
          skin breakdown only L97.221
          specified severity NEC L97.228
      right L97.219
        with
          bone involvement without evidence of necrosis L97.216
          bone necrosis L97.214
          exposed fat layer L97.212
          muscle involvement without evidence of necrosis L97.215
          muscle necrosis L97.213
          skin breakdown only L97.211
          specified severity NEC L97.218
    decubitus — *see* Ulcer, pressure, by site
    foot specified NEC L97.509
      with
        bone involvement without evidence of necrosis L97.506
        bone necrosis L97.504
        exposed fat layer L97.502
        muscle involvement without evidence of necrosis L97.505
        muscle necrosis L97.503
        skin breakdown only L97.501
        specified severity NEC L97.508
      left L97.529
        with
          bone involvement without evidence of necrosis L97.526
          bone necrosis L97.524
          exposed fat layer L97.522
          muscle involvement without evidence of necrosis L97.525

Ulcer, ulcerated, ulcerating, ulceration, ulcerative
— *continued*
  lower limb — *continued*
    foot specified — *continued*
      left — *continued*
        with — *continued*
          muscle necrosis L97.523
          skin breakdown only L97.521
          specified severity NEC L97.528
      right L97.519
        with
          bone involvement without evidence of necrosis L97.516
          bone necrosis L97.514
          exposed fat layer L97.512
          muscle involvement without evidence of necrosis L97.515
          muscle necrosis L97.513
          skin breakdown only L97.511
          specified severity NEC L97.518
    heel L97.409
      with
        bone involvement without evidence of necrosis L97.406
        bone necrosis L97.404
        exposed fat layer L97.402
        muscle involvement without evidence of necrosis L97.405
        muscle necrosis L97.403
        skin breakdown only L97.401
        specified severity NEC L97.408
      left L97.429
        with
          bone involvement without evidence of necrosis L97.426
          bone necrosis L97.424
          exposed fat layer L97.422
          muscle involvement without evidence of necrosis L97.425
          muscle necrosis L97.423
          skin breakdown only L97.421
          specified severity NEC L97.428
      right L97.419
        with
          bone involvement without evidence of necrosis L97.416
          bone necrosis L97.414
          exposed fat layer L97.412
          muscle involvement without evidence of necrosis L97.415
          muscle necrosis L97.413
          skin breakdown only L97.411
          specified severity NEC L97.418
    left L97.929
      with
        bone involvement without evidence of necrosis L97.926
        bone necrosis L97.924
        exposed fat layer L97.922
        muscle involvement without evidence of necrosis L97.925
        muscle necrosis L97.923
        skin breakdown only L97.921
        specified severity NEC L97.928
    leprous A30.1
    lower leg NOS L97.909
      with
        bone involvement without evidence of necrosis L97.906
        bone necrosis L97.904
        exposed fat layer L97.902
        muscle involvement without evidence of necrosis L97.905
        muscle necrosis L97.903
        skin breakdown only L97.901
        specified severity NEC L97.908
      left L97.929
        with
          bone involvement without evidence of necrosis L97.926
          bone necrosis L97.924
          exposed fat layer L97.922
          muscle involvement without evidence of necrosis L97.925
          muscle necrosis L97.923
          skin breakdown only L97.921
          specified severity NEC L97.928
      right L97.919

Index

Ulcer, ulcerated, ulcerating, ulceration, ulcerative

Ulcer, ulcerated, ulcerating, ulceration, ulcerative
— continued
lower limb — continued
lower leg — continued
right — continued
with
bone involvement without evidence of necrosis L97.916
bone necrosis L97.914
exposed fat layer L97.912
muscle involvement without evidence of necrosis L97.915
muscle necrosis L97.913
skin breakdown only L97.911
specified severity NEC L97.918
specified site NEC L97.809
with
bone involvement without evidence of necrosis L97.806
bone necrosis L97.804
exposed fat layer L97.802
muscle involvement without evidence of necrosis L97.805
muscle necrosis L97.803
skin breakdown only L97.801
specified severity NEC L97.808
left L97.829
with
bone involvement without evidence of necrosis L97.826
bone necrosis L97.824
exposed fat layer L97.822
muscle involvement without evidence of necrosis L97.825
muscle necrosis L97.823
skin breakdown only L97.821
specified severity NEC L97.828
right L97.819
with
bone involvement without evidence of necrosis L97.816
bone necrosis L97.814
exposed fat layer L97.812
muscle involvement without evidence of necrosis L97.815
muscle necrosis L97.813
skin breakdown only L97.811
specified severity NEC L97.818
midfoot L97.409
with
bone involvement without evidence of necrosis L97.406
bone necrosis L97.404
exposed fat layer L97.402
muscle involvement without evidence of necrosis L97.405
muscle necrosis L97.403
skin breakdown only L97.401
specified severity NEC L97.408
left L97.429
with
bone involvement without evidence of necrosis L97.426
bone necrosis L97.424
exposed fat layer L97.422
muscle involvement without evidence of necrosis L97.425
muscle necrosis L97.423
skin breakdown only L97.421
specified severity NEC L97.428
right L97.419
with
bone involvement without evidence of necrosis L97.416
bone necrosis L97.414
exposed fat layer L97.412
muscle involvement without evidence of necrosis L97.415
muscle necrosis L97.413
skin breakdown only L97.411
specified severity NEC L97.418
right L97.919
with
bone involvement without evidence of necrosis L97.916
bone necrosis L97.914
exposed fat layer L97.912
muscle involvement without evidence of necrosis L97.915

Ulcer, ulcerated, ulcerating, ulceration, ulcerative
— continued
lower limb — continued
right — continued
with — continued
muscle necrosis L97.913
skin breakdown only L97.911
specified severity NEC L97.918
syphilitic A52.19
thigh L97.109
with
bone involvement without evidence of necrosis L97.106
bone necrosis L97.104
exposed fat layer L97.102
muscle involvement without evidence of necrosis L97.105
muscle necrosis L97.103
skin breakdown only L97.101
specified severity NEC L97.108
left L97.129
with
bone involvement without evidence of necrosis L97.126
bone necrosis L97.124
exposed fat layer L97.122
muscle involvement without evidence of necrosis L97.125
muscle necrosis L97.123
skin breakdown only L97.121
specified severity NEC L97.128
right L97.119
with
bone involvement without evidence of necrosis L97.116
bone necrosis L97.114
exposed fat layer L97.112
muscle involvement without evidence of necrosis L97.115
muscle necrosis L97.113
skin breakdown only L97.111
specified severity NEC L97.118
toe L97.509
with
bone involvement without evidence of necrosis L97.506
bone necrosis L97.504
exposed fat layer L97.502
muscle involvement without evidence of necrosis L97.505
muscle necrosis L97.503
skin breakdown only L97.501
specified severity NEC L97.508
left L97.529
with
bone involvement without evidence of necrosis L97.526
bone necrosis L97.524
exposed fat layer L97.522
muscle involvement without evidence of necrosis L97.525
muscle necrosis L97.523
skin breakdown only L97.521
specified severity NEC L97.528
right L97.519
with
bone involvement without evidence of necrosis L97.516
bone necrosis L97.514
exposed fat layer L97.512
muscle involvement without evidence of necrosis L97.515
muscle necrosis L97.513
skin breakdown only L97.511
specified severity NEC L97.518
varicose — see Varix, leg, with, ulcer
luetic — see Ulcer, syphilitic
lung J98.4
tuberculous — see Tuberculosis, pulmonary
malignant — see Neoplasm, malignant, by site
marginal NEC — see Ulcer, gastrojejunal
meatus (urinarius) N34.2
Meckel's diverticulum Q43.0
malignant — see Table of Neoplasms, small intestine, malignant
Meleney's (chronic undermining) — see Ulcer, skin
Mooren's (cornea) — see Ulcer, cornea, Mooren's
mycobacterial (skin) A31.1

Ulcer, ulcerated, ulcerating, ulceration, ulcerative
— continued
nasopharynx J39.2
neck, uterus N86
neurogenic NEC — see Ulcer, skin
nose, nasal (passage) (infective) (septum) J34.0
skin — see Ulcer, skin
spirochetal A69.8
varicose (bleeding) I86.8
oral mucosa (traumatic) K12.1
palate (soft) K12.1
penis (chronic) N48.5
peptic (site unspecified) K27.9
with
hemorrhage K27.4
and perforation K27.6
perforation K27.5
acute K27.3
with
hemorrhage K27.0
and perforation K27.2
perforation K27.1
chronic K27.7
with
hemorrhage K27.4
and perforation K27.6
perforation K27.5
esophagus K22.10
with bleeding K22.11
newborn P78.82
perforating K27.5
skin — see Ulcer, skin
peritonsillar J35.8
phagedenic (tropical) — see Ulcer, skin
pharynx J39.2
phlebitis — see Phlebitis
plaster — see Ulcer, pressure, by site
popliteal space — see Ulcer, lower limb
postpyloric — see Ulcer, duodenum
prepuce N47.7
prepyloric — see Ulcer, stomach
pressure (pressure area) L89.9- ☑
ankle L89.5- ☑
back L89.1- ☑
buttock L89.3- ☑
coccyx L89.15- ☑
contiguous site of back, buttock, hip L89.4- ☑
elbow L89.0- ☑
face L89.81- ☑
head L89.81- ☑
heel L89.6- ☑
hip L89.2- ☑
sacral region (tailbone) L89.15- ☑
specified site NEC L89.89- ☑
stage 1 (healing) (pre-ulcer skin changes limited to persistent focal edema)
ankle L89.5- ☑
back L89.1- ☑
buttock L89.3- ☑
coccyx L89.15- ☑
contiguous site of back, buttock, hip L89.4- ☑
elbow L89.0- ☑
face L89.81- ☑
head L89.81- ☑
heel L89.6- ☑
hip L89.2- ☑
sacral region (tailbone) L89.15- ☑
specified site NEC L89.89- ☑
stage 2 (healing) (abrasion, blister, partial thickness skin loss involving epidermis and/or dermis)
ankle L89.5- ☑
back L89.1- ☑
buttock L89.3- ☑
coccyx L89.15- ☑
contiguous site of back, buttock, hip L89.4- ☑
elbow L89.0- ☑
face L89.81- ☑
head L89.81- ☑
heel L89.6- ☑
hip L89.2- ☑
sacral region (tailbone) L89.15- ☑
specified site NEC L89.89- ☑
stage 3 (healing) (full thickness skin loss involving damage or necrosis of subcutaneous tissue)
ankle L89.5- ☑
back L89.1- ☑
buttock L89.3- ☑

Ulcer, ulcerated, ulcerating, ulceration, ulcerative
— *continued*
pressure — *continued*
stage 3 — *continued*
coccyx L89.15- ☑
contiguous site of back, buttock, hip L89.4- ☑
elbow L89.0- ☑
face L89.81- ☑
head L89.81- ☑
heel L89.6- ☑
hip L89.2- ☑
sacral region (tailbone) L89.15- ☑
specified site NEC L89.89- ☑
stage 4 (healing) (necrosis of soft tissues through to underlying muscle, tendon, or bone)
ankle L89.5- ☑
back L89.1- ☑
buttock L89.3- ☑
coccyx L89.15- ☑
contiguous site of back, buttock, hip L89.4- ☑
elbow L89.0- ☑
face L89.81- ☑
head L89.81- ☑
heel L89.6- ☑
hip L89.2- ☑
sacral region (tailbone) L89.15- ☑
specified site NEC L89.89- ☑
unspecified stage
ankle L89.5- ☑
back L89.1- ☑
buttock L89.3- ☑
coccyx L89.15- ☑
contiguous site of back, buttock, hip L89.4- ☑
elbow L89.0- ☑
face L89.81- ☑
head L89.81- ☑
heel L89.6- ☑
hip L89.2- ☑
sacral region (tailbone) L89.15- ☑
specified site NEC L89.89- ☑
unstageable
ankle L89.5- ☑
back L89.1- ☑
buttock L89.3- ☑
coccyx L89.15- ☑
contiguous site of back, buttock, hip L89.4- ☑
elbow L89.0- ☑
face L89.81- ☑
head L89.81- ☑
heel L89.6- ☑
hip L89.2- ☑
sacral region (tailbone) L89.15- ☑
specified site NEC L89.89- ☑
primary of intestine K63.3
with perforation K63.1
prostate N41.9
pyloric — *see* Ulcer, stomach
rectosigmoid K63.3
with perforation K63.1
rectum (sphincter) (solitary) K62.6
stercoraceous, stercoral K62.6
retina — *see* Inflammation, chorioretinal
rodent — *see also* Neoplasm, skin, malignant
sclera — *see* Scleritis
scrofulous (tuberculous) A18.2
scrotum N50.89
tuberculous A18.15
varicose I86.1
seminal vesicle N50.89
sigmoid — *see* Ulcer, intestine
skin (atrophic) (chronic) (neurogenic) (non-healing) (perforating) (pyogenic) (trophic) (tropical) L98.499
with gangrene — *see* Gangrene
amebic A06.7
back — *see* Ulcer, back
buttock — *see* Ulcer, buttock
decubitus — *see* Ulcer, pressure
lower limb — *see* Ulcer, lower limb
mycobacterial A31.1
specified site NEC L98.499
with
bone involvement without evidence of necrosis L98.496
bone necrosis L98.494
exposed fat layer L98.492

Ulcer, ulcerated, ulcerating, ulceration, ulcerative
— *continued*
skin — *continued*
specified site — *continued*
with — *continued*
muscle involvement without evidence of necrosis L98.495
muscle necrosis L98.493
skin breakdown only L98.491
specified severity NEC L98.498
tuberculous (primary) A18.4
varicose — *see* Ulcer, varicose
sloughing — *see* Ulcer, skin
solitary, anus or rectum (sphincter) K62.6
sore throat J02.9
streptococcal J02.0
spermatic cord N50.89
spine (tuberculous) A18.01
stasis (venous) — *see* Varix, leg, with, ulcer
without varicose veins I87.2
stercoraceous, stercoral K63.3
with perforation K63.1
anus or rectum K62.6
stoma, stomal — *see* Ulcer, gastrojejunal
stomach (eroded) (peptic) (round) K25.9
with
hemorrhage K25.4
and perforation K25.6
perforation K25.5
acute K25.3
with
hemorrhage K25.0
and perforation K25.2
perforation K25.1
chronic K25.7
with
hemorrhage K25.4 *— blood loss*
and perforation K25.6
perforation K25.5
stomal — *see* Ulcer, gastrojejunal
stomatitis K12.1
stress — *see* Ulcer, peptic
strumous (tuberculous) A18.2
submucosal, bladder — *see* Cystitis, interstitial
syphilitic (any site) (early) (secondary) A51.39
late A52.79
perforating A52.79
foot A52.11
testis N50.89
thigh — *see* Ulcer, lower limb
throat J39.2
diphtheritic A36.0
toe — *see* Ulcer, lower limb
tongue (traumatic) K14.0
tonsil J35.8
diphtheritic A36.0
trachea J39.8
trophic — *see* Ulcer, skin
tropical — *see* Ulcer, skin
tuberculous — *see* Tuberculosis, ulcer
tunica vaginalis N50.89
turbinate J34.89
typhoid (perforating) — *see* Typhoid
unspecified site — *see* Ulcer, skin
urethra (meatus) — *see* Urethritis
uterus N85.8
cervix N86
with cervicitis N72
neck N86
with cervicitis N72
vagina N76.5
in Behçet's disease M35.2 [N77.0]
pessary N89.8
valve, heart I33.0
varicose (lower limb, any part) — *see also* Varix, leg, with, ulcer
broad ligament I86.2
esophagus — *see* Varix, esophagus
inflamed or infected — *see* Varix, leg, with ulcer, with inflammation
nasal septum I86.8
perineum I86.2
scrotum I86.1
specified site NEC I86.8
sublingual I86.0
vulva I86.3
vas deferens N50.89
vulva (acute) (infectional) N76.6

Ulcer, ulcerated, ulcerating, ulceration, ulcerative
— *continued*
vulva — *continued*
in (due to)
Behçet's disease M35.2 [N77.0]
herpesviral (herpes simplex) infection A60.04
tuberculosis A18.18
vulvobuccal, recurring N76.6
X-ray L58.1
yaws A66.4
Ulcerosa scarlatina A38.8
Ulcus — *see also* Ulcer
cutis tuberculosum A18.4
duodeni — *see* Ulcer, duodenum
durum (syphilitic) A51.0
extragenital A51.2
gastrojejunale — *see* Ulcer, gastrojejunal
hypostaticum — *see* Ulcer, varicose
molle (cutis) (skin) A57
serpens corneae — *see* Ulcer, cornea, central
ventriculi — *see* Ulcer, stomach
Ulegyria Q04.8
Ulerythema
ophryogenes, congenital Q84.2
sycosiforme L73.8
Ullrich (-Bonnevie)(-Turner) **syndrome** — *see also* Turner's syndrome Q87.19
Ullrich-Feichtiger syndrome Q87.0
Ulnar — *see* condition
Ulorrhagia, ulorrhea K06.8
Umbilicus, umbilical — *see* condition
Unacceptable
contours of tooth K08.54
morphology of tooth K08.54
Unavailability (of)
bed at medical facility Z75.1
health service-related agencies Z75.4
medical facilities (at) Z75.3
due to
investigation by social service agency Z75.2
lack of services at home Z75.0
remoteness from facility Z75.3
waiting list Z75.1
home Z75.0
outpatient clinic Z75.3
schooling Z55.1
social service agencies Z75.4
Uncinaria americana infestation B76.1
Uncinariasis B76.9
Uncongenial work Z56.5
Unconscious (ness) — *see* Coma
Under observation — *see* Observation
Underachievement in school Z55.3
Underdevelopment — *see also* Undeveloped
nose Q30.1
sexual E30.0
Underdosing — *see also* Table of Drugs and Chemicals, categories T36-T50, with final character 6 Z91.14
intentional NEC Z91.128
due to financial hardship of patient Z91.120
unintentional NEC Z91.138
due to patient's age related debility Z91.130
Underfeeding, newborn P92.3
Underfill, endodontic M27.53
Underimmunization status Z28.3
Undernourishment — *see* Malnutrition
Undernutrition — *see* Malnutrition
Underweight R63.6
for gestational age — *see* Light for dates
Underwood's disease P83.0
Undescended — *see also* Malposition, congenital
cecum Q43.3
colon Q43.3
testicle — *see* Cryptorchid
Undeveloped, undevelopment — *see also* Hypoplasia
brain (congenital) Q02
cerebral (congenital) Q02
heart Q24.8
lung Q33.6
testis E29.1
uterus E30.0
Undiagnosed (disease) R69
Undulant fever — *see* Brucellosis
Unemployment, anxiety concerning Z56.0
threatened Z56.2
Unequal length (acquired) (limb) — *see also* Deformity, limb, unequal length

▽ Subterms under main terms may continue to next column or page   ☑ Additional Character Required — Refer to the Tabular List for Character Selection   321

Ulcer, ulcerated, ulcerating, ulceration, ulcerative — Unequal length

Unequal length — *continued*
  leg — *see also* Deformity, limb, unequal length
    congenital Q72.9- ☑
Unextracted dental root K08.3
Unguis incarnatus L60.0
Unhappiness R45.2
Unicornate uterus Q51.4
  in pregnancy or childbirth O34.00
Unilateral — *see also* condition
  development, breast N64.89
  organ or site, congenital NEC — *see* Agenesis, by site
Unilocular heart Q20.8
Union, abnormal — *see also* Fusion
  larynx and trachea Q34.8
Universal mesentery Q43.3
Unrepairable overhanging of dental restorative materials K08.52
Unsatisfactory
  restoration of tooth K08.50
    specified NEC K08.59
  sample of cytologic smear
    anus R85.615
    cervix R87.615
    vagina R87.625
  surroundings Z59.1
  work Z56.5
Unsoundness of mind — *see* Psychosis
Unstable
  back NEC — *see* Instability, joint, spine
  hip (congenital) Q65.6
    acquired — *see* Derangement, joint, specified type NEC, hip
  joint — *see* Instability, joint
    secondary to removal of joint prosthesis M96.89
  lie (mother) O32.0 ☑
  lumbosacral joint (congenital) — *see* subcategory M53.2
  sacroiliac — *see* subcategory M53.2 ☑
  spine NEC — *see* Instability, joint, spine
Unsteadiness on feet R26.81
Untruthfulness, child problem F91.8
Unverricht (-Lundborg) disease or epilepsy — *see* Epilepsy, generalized, idiopathic
Unwanted pregnancy Z64.0
Upbringing, institutional Z62.22
  away from parents NEC Z62.29
  in care of non-parental family member Z62.21
  in foster care Z62.21
  in orphanage or group home Z62.22
  in welfare custody Z62.21
Upper respiratory — *see* condition
Upset
  gastric K30
  gastrointestinal K30
    psychogenic F45.8
  intestinal (large) (small) K59.9
    psychogenic F45.8
  menstruation N93.9
  mental F48.9
  stomach K30
    psychogenic F45.8
Urachus — *see also* condition
  patent or persistent Q64.4
Urbach-Oppenheim disease (necrobiosis lipoidica diabeticorum) — *see* E08-E13 with .620
Urbach's lipoid proteinosis E78.89
Urbach-Wiethe disease E78.89
Urban yellow fever A95.1
Urea
  blood, high — *see* Uremia
  cycle metabolism disorder — *see* Disorder, urea cycle metabolism
Uremia, uremic N19
  with
    ectopic or molar pregnancy O08.4
    polyneuropathy N18.9 *[G63]*
  chronic NOS — *see also* Disease, kidney, chronic N18.9
    due to hypertension — *see* Hypertensive, kidney
  complicating
    ectopic or molar pregnancy O08.4
  congenital P96.0
  extrarenal R39.2
  following ectopic or molar pregnancy O08.4
  newborn P96.0
  prerenal R39.2
Ureter, ureteral — *see* condition
Ureteralgia N23

Ureterectasis — *see* Hydroureter
Ureteritis N28.89
  cystica N28.86
  due to calculus N20.1
    with calculus, kidney N20.2
      with hydronephrosis N13.2
  gonococcal (acute) (chronic) A54.21
  nonspecific N28.89
Ureterocele N28.89
  congenital (orthotopic) Q62.31
    ectopic Q62.32
Ureterolith, ureterolithiasis — *see* Calculus, ureter
Ureterostomy
  attention to Z43.6
  status Z93.6
Urethra, urethral — *see* condition
Urethralgia R39.89
Urethritis (anterior) (posterior) N34.2
  calculous N21.1
  candidal B37.41
  chlamydial A56.01
  diplococcal (gonococcal) A54.01
    with abscess (accessory gland) (periurethral) A54.1
  gonococcal A54.01
    with abscess (accessory gland) (periurethral) A54.1
  nongonococcal N34.1
    Reiter's — *see* Reiter's disease
  nonspecific N34.1
  nonvenereal N34.1
  postmenopausal N34.2
  puerperal O86.22
  Reiter's — *see* Reiter's disease
  specified NEC N34.2
  trichomonal or due to Trichomonas (vaginalis) A59.03
Urethrocele N81.0
  with
    cystocele — *see* Cystocele
    prolapse of uterus — *see* Prolapse, uterus
Urethrolithiasis (with colic or infection) N21.1
Urethrorectal — *see* condition
Urethrorrhagia N36.8
Urethrorrhea R36.9
Urethrostomy
  attention to Z43.6
  status Z93.6
Urethrotrigonitis — *see* Trigonitis
Urethrovaginal — *see* condition
Urgency
  fecal R15.2
  hypertensive — *see* Hypertension
  urinary R39.15
Urhidrosis, uridrosis L74.8
Uric acid in blood (increased) E79.0
Uricacidemia (asymptomatic) E79.0
Uricemia (asymptomatic) E79.0
Uricosuria R82.998
Urinary — *see* condition
Urination
  frequent R35.0
  painful R30.9
Urine
  blood in — *see* Hematuria
  discharge, excessive R35.8
  enuresis, nonorganic origin F98.0
  extravasation R39.0
  frequency R35.0
  incontinence R32
    nonorganic origin F98.0
  intermittent stream R39.198
  pus in N39.0
  retention or stasis R33.9
    organic R33.8
      drug-induced R33.0
    psychogenic F45.8
  secretion
    deficient R34
    excessive R35.8
    frequency R35.0
  stream
    intermittent R39.198
    slowing R39.198
    splitting R39.13
    weak R39.12
Urinemia — *see* Uremia
Urinoma, urethra N36.8
Uroarthritis, infectious (Reiter's) — *see* Reiter's disease
Urodialysis R34
Urolithiasis — *see* Calculus, urinary

Uronephrosis — *see* Hydronephrosis
Uropathy N39.9
  obstructive N13.9
    specified NEC N13.8
  reflux N13.9
    specified NEC N13.8
  vesicoureteral reflux-associated — *see* Reflux, vesicoureteral
Urosepsis — *code to* condition
Urticaria L50.9
  with angioneurotic edema T78.3 ☑
    hereditary D84.1
  allergic L50.0
  cholinergic L50.5
  chronic L50.8
  cold, familial L50.2
  contact L50.6
  dermatographic L50.3
  due to
    cold or heat L50.2
    drugs L50.0
    food L50.0
    inhalants L50.0
    plants L50.6
    serum — *see also* Reaction, serum T80.69 ☑
  factitial L50.3
  familial cold M04.2
  giant T78.3 ☑
    hereditary D84.1
  gigantea T78.3 ☑
  idiopathic L50.1
  larynx T78.3 ☑
    hereditary D84.1
  neonatorum P83.88
  nonallergic L50.1
  papulosa (Hebra) L28.2
  pigmentosa D47.01
    congenital Q82.2
    of neonatal onset Q82.2
    of newborn onset Q82.2
  recurrent periodic L50.8
  serum — *see also* Reaction, serum T80.69 ☑
  solar L56.3
  specified type NEC L50.8
  thermal (cold) (heat) L50.2
  vibratory L50.4
  xanthelasmoidea — *see* Urticaria pigmentosa
Use (of)
  alcohol Z72.89
    with
      intoxication F10.929
      sleep disorder F10.982
    harmful — *see* Abuse, alcohol
  amphetamines — *see* Use, stimulant NEC
  caffeine — *see* Use, stimulant NEC
  cannabis F12.90
    with
      anxiety disorder F12.980
      intoxication F12.929
        with
          delirium F12.921
          perceptual disturbance F12.922
        uncomplicated F12.920
      other specified disorder F12.988
      psychosis F12.959
        delusions F12.950
        hallucinations F12.951
      unspecified disorder F12.99
      withdrawal F12.93
  cocaine F14.90
    with
      anxiety disorder F14.980
      intoxication F14.929
        with
          delirium F14.921
          perceptual disturbance F14.922
        uncomplicated F14.920
      other specified disorder F14.988
      psychosis F14.959
        delusions F14.950
        hallucinations F14.951
      sexual dysfunction F14.981
      sleep disorder F14.982
      unspecified disorder F14.99
    harmful — *see* Abuse, drug, cocaine
  drug(s) NEC F19.90
    with sleep disorder F19.982
    harmful — *see* Abuse, drug, by type

☑ **Additional Character Required — Refer to the Tabular List for Character Selection**   ▽ Subterms under main terms may continue to next column or page

Use — *continued*
  hallucinogen NEC F16.90
    with
      anxiety disorder F16.980
      intoxication F16.929
        with
          delirium F16.921
        uncomplicated F16.920
      mood disorder F16.94
      other specified disorder F16.988
      perception disorder (flashbacks) F16.983
      psychosis F16.959
        delusions F16.950
        hallucinations F16.951
      unspecified disorder F16.99
    harmful — *see* Abuse, drug, hallucinogen NEC
  inhalants F18.90
    with
      anxiety disorder F18.980
      intoxication F18.929
        with delirium F18.921
        uncomplicated F18.920
      mood disorder F18.94
      other specified disorder F18.988
      persisting dementia F18.97
      psychosis F18.959
        delusions F18.950
        hallucinations F18.951
      unspecified disorder F18.99
    harmful — *see* Abuse, drug, inhalant
  methadone — *see* Use, opioid
  nonprescribed drugs F19.90
    harmful — *see* Abuse, non-psychoactive substance
  opioid F11.90
    with
      disorder F11.99
        mood F11.94
        sleep F11.982
        specified type NEC F11.988
      intoxication F11.929
        with
          delirium F11.921
          perceptual disturbance F11.922
        uncomplicated F11.920
      withdrawal F11.93
    harmful — *see* Abuse, drug, opioid
  patent medicines F19.90
    harmful — *see* Abuse, non-psychoactive substance
  psychoactive drug NEC F19.90
    with
      anxiety disorder F19.980
      intoxication F19.929
        with
          delirium F19.921
          perceptual disturbance F19.922
        uncomplicated F19.920
      mood disorder F19.94
      other specified disorder F19.988
      persisting
        amnestic disorder F19.96
        dementia F19.97
      psychosis F19.959
        delusions F19.950
        hallucinations F19.951
      sexual dysfunction F19.981
      sleep disorder F19.982
      unspecified disorder F19.99
      withdrawal F19.939
        with
          delirium F19.931
          perceptual disturbance F19.932
        uncomplicated F19.930
    harmful — *see* Abuse, drug NEC, psychoactive NEC
  sedative, hypnotic, or anxiolytic F13.90
    with
      anxiety disorder F13.980
      intoxication F13.929
        with
          delirium F13.921
        uncomplicated F13.920
      other specified disorder F13.988
      persisting
        amnestic disorder F13.96
        dementia F13.97
      psychosis F13.959
        delusions F13.950
        hallucinations F13.951
      sexual dysfunction F13.981

Use — *continued*
  sedative, hypnotic, or anxiolytic — *continued*
    with — *continued*
      sleep disorder F13.982
      unspecified disorder F13.99
    harmful — *see* Abuse, drug, sedative, hypnotic, or
      anxiolytic
  stimulant NEC F15.90
    with
      anxiety disorder F15.980
      intoxication F15.929
        with
          delirium F15.921
          perceptual disturbance F15.922
        uncomplicated F15.920
      mood disorder F15.94
      other specified disorder F15.988
      psychosis F15.959
        delusions F15.950
        hallucinations F15.951
      sexual dysfunction F15.981
      sleep disorder F15.982
      unspecified disorder F15.99
      withdrawal F15.93
    harmful — *see* Abuse, drug, stimulant NEC
  tobacco Z72.0
    with dependence — *see* Dependence, drug, nicotine
  volatile solvents — *see also* Use, inhalant F18.90
    harmful — *see* Abuse, drug, inhalant
Usher-Senear disease or syndrome L10.4
Uta B55.1
Uteromegaly N85.2
Uterovaginal — *see condition*
Uterovesical — *see condition*
Uveal — *see condition*
Uveitis (anterior) — *see also* Iridocyclitis
  acute — *see* Iridocyclitis, acute
  chronic — *see* Iridocyclitis, chronic
  due to toxoplasmosis (acquired) B58.09
    congenital P37.1
  granulomatous — *see* Iridocyclitis, chronic
  heterochromic — *see* Cyclitis, Fuchs' heterochromic
  lens-induced — *see* Iridocyclitis, lens-induced
  posterior — *see* Chorioretinitis
  sympathetic H44.13- ☑
  syphilitic (secondary) A51.43
    congenital (early) A50.01
    late A52.71
  tuberculous A18.54
Uveoencephalitis — *see* Inflammation, chorioretinal
Uveokeratitis — *see* Iridocyclitis
Uveoparotitis D86.89
Uvula — *see condition*
Uvulitis (acute) (catarrhal) (chronic) (membranous)
  (suppurative) (ulcerative) K12.2

V

Vaccination (prophylactic)
  complication or reaction — *see* Complications, vacci-
    nation
  delayed Z28.9
  encounter for Z23
  not done — *see* Immunization, not done, because (of)
Vaccinia (generalized) (localized) T88.1 ☑
  congenital P35.8
  without vaccination B08.011
Vacuum, in sinus (accessory) (nasal) J34.89
Vagabond, vagabondage Z59.0
Vagabond's disease B85.1
Vagina, vaginal — *see condition*
Vaginalitis (tunica) (testis) N49.1
Vaginismus (reflex) N94.2
  functional F52.5
  nonorganic F52.5
  psychogenic F52.5
  secondary N94.2
Vaginitis (acute) (circumscribed) (diffuse) (emphysematous) (nonvenereal) (ulcerative) N76.0
  with ectopic or molar pregnancy O08.0
  amebic A06.82
  atrophic, postmenopausal N95.2
  bacterial N76.0
  blennorrhagic (gonococcal) A54.02
  candidal B37.3
  chlamydial A56.02
  chronic N76.1

Vaginitis — *continued*
  due to Trichomonas (vaginalis) A59.01
  following ectopic or molar pregnancy O08.0
  gonococcal A54.02
    with abscess (accessory gland) (periurethral) A54.1
  granuloma A58
  in (due to)
    candidiasis B37.3
    herpesviral (herpes simplex) infection A60.04
    pinworm infection B80 *[N77.1]*
  monilial B37.3
  mycotic (candidal) B37.3
  postmenopausal atrophic N95.2
  puerperal (postpartum) O86.13
  senile (atrophic) N95.2
  subacute or chronic N76.1
  syphilitic (early) A51.0
    late A52.76
  trichomonal A59.01
  tuberculous A18.18
Vaginosis — *see* Vaginitis
Vagotonia G52.2
Vagrancy Z59.0
VAIN — *see* Neoplasia, intraepithelial, vagina
Vallecula — *see condition*
Valley fever B38.0
Valsuani's disease — *see* Anemia, obstetric
Valve, valvular (formation) — *see also* condition
  cerebral ventricle (communicating) in situ Z98.2
  cervix, internal os Q51.828
  congenital NEC — *see* Atresia, by site
  ureter (pelvic junction) (vesical orifice) Q62.39
  urethra (congenital) (posterior) Q64.2
Valvulitis (chronic) — *see* Endocarditis
Valvulopathy — *see* Endocarditis
Van Bogaert's leukoencephalopathy (sclerosing)
  (subacute) A81.1
Van Bogaert-Scherer-Epstein disease or syndrome
  E75.5
Van Buchem's syndrome M85.2
Van Creveld-von Gierke disease E74.01
Van der Hoeve (-de Kleyn) **syndrome** Q78.0
Van der Woude's syndrome Q38.0
Van Neck's disease or osteochondrosis M91.0
Vanishing lung J44.9
Vapor asphyxia or suffocation T59.9 ☑
  specified agent — *see* Table of Drugs and Chemicals
Variance, lethal ball, prosthetic heart valve T82.09 ☑
Variants, thalassemic D56.8
Variations in hair color L67.1
Varicella B01.9
  with
    complications NEC B01.89
    encephalitis B01.11
    encephalomyelitis B01.11
    meningitis B01.0
    myelitis B01.12
    pneumonia B01.2
  congenital P35.8
Varices — *see* Varix
Varicocele (scrotum) (thrombosed) I86.1
  ovary I86.2
  perineum I86.3
  spermatic cord (ulcerated) I86.1
Varicose
  aneurysm (ruptured) I77.0
  dermatitis — *see* Varix, leg, with, inflammation
  eczema — *see* Varix, leg, with, inflammation
  phlebitis — *see* Varix, with, inflammation
  tumor — *see* Varix
  ulcer (lower limb, any part) — *see also* Varix, leg, with,
    ulcer
    anus — *see also* Hemorrhoids K64.8
    esophagus — *see* Varix, esophagus
    inflamed or infected — *see* Varix, leg, with ulcer,
      with inflammation
    nasal septum I86.8
    perineum I86.3
    scrotum I86.1
    specified site NEC I86.8
    vein — *see* Varix
    vessel — *see* Varix, leg
Varicosis, varicosities, varicosity — *see* Varix
Variola (major) (minor) B03
Varioloid B03
Varix (lower limb) I83.90

▽ Subterms under main terms may continue to next column or page   ☑ Additional Character Required — Refer to the Tabular List for Character Selection   323

Use — Varix

Varix — continued
- with
  - bleeding I83.899
  - edema I83.899
  - inflammation I83.10
    - with ulcer (venous) I83.209
  - pain I83.819
  - rupture I83.899
  - specified complication NEC I83.899
  - stasis dermatitis I83.10
    - with ulcer (venous) I83.209
  - swelling I83.899
  - ulcer I83.009
    - with inflammation I83.209
- aneurysmal I77.0
- asymptomatic I83.9- ☑
- bladder I86.2
- broad ligament I86.2
- complicating
  - childbirth (lower extremity) O87.4
    - anus or rectum O87.2
    - genital (vagina, vulva or perineum) O87.8
  - pregnancy (lower extremity) O22.0- ☑
    - anus or rectum O22.4- ☑
    - genital (vagina, vulva or perineum) O22.1- ☑
  - puerperium (lower extremity) O87.4
    - anus or rectum O87.2
    - genital (vagina, vulva, perineum) O87.8
- congenital (any site) Q27.8
- esophagus (idiopathic) (primary) (ulcerated) I85.00
  - bleeding I85.01
  - congenital Q27.8
  - in (due to)
    - alcoholic liver disease I85.10
      - bleeding I85.11
    - cirrhosis of liver I85.10
      - bleeding I85.11
    - portal hypertension I85.10
      - bleeding I85.11
    - schistosomiasis I85.10
      - bleeding I85.11
    - toxic liver disease I85.10
      - bleeding I85.11
  - secondary I85.10
    - bleeding I85.11
- gastric I86.4
- inflamed or infected I83.10
  - ulcerated I83.209
- labia (majora) I86.3
- leg (asymptomatic) I83.90
  - with
    - edema I83.899
    - inflammation I83.10
      - with ulcer — see Varix, leg, with, ulcer, with inflammation by site
    - pain I83.819
    - specified complication NEC I83.899
    - swelling I83.899
    - ulcer I83.009
      - with inflammation I83.209
      - ankle I83.003
        - with inflammation I83.203
      - calf I83.002
        - with inflammation I83.202
      - foot NEC I83.005
        - with inflammation I83.205
      - heel I83.004
        - with inflammation I83.204
      - lower leg NEC I83.008
        - with inflammation I83.208
      - midfoot I83.004
        - with inflammation I83.204
      - thigh I83.001
        - with inflammation I83.201
  - bilateral (asymptomatic) I83.93
    - with
      - edema I83.893
      - pain I83.813
      - specified complication NEC I83.893
      - swelling I83.893
      - ulcer I83.0- ☑
        - with inflammation I83.209
  - left (asymptomatic) I83.92
    - with
      - edema I83.892
      - inflammation I83.12
        - with ulcer — see Varix, leg, with, ulcer, with inflammation by site

Varix — continued
- leg — continued
  - left — continued
    - with — continued
      - pain I83.812
      - specified complication NEC I83.892
      - swelling I83.892
      - ulcer I83.029
        - with inflammation I83.229
        - ankle I83.023
          - with inflammation I83.223
        - calf I83.022
          - with inflammation I83.222
        - foot NEC I83.025
          - with inflammation I83.225
        - heel I83.024
          - with inflammation I83.224
        - lower leg NEC I83.028
          - with inflammation I83.228
        - midfoot I83.024
          - with inflammation I83.224
        - thigh I83.021
          - with inflammation I83.221
  - right (asymptomatic) I83.91
    - with
      - edema I83.891
      - inflammation I83.11
        - with ulcer — see Varix, leg, with, ulcer, with inflammation by site
      - pain I83.811
      - specified complication NEC I83.891
      - swelling I83.891
      - ulcer I83.019
        - with inflammation I83.219
        - ankle I83.013
          - with inflammation I83.213
        - calf I83.012
          - with inflammation I83.212
        - foot NEC I83.015
          - with inflammation I83.215
        - heel I83.014
          - with inflammation I83.214
        - lower leg NEC I83.018
          - with inflammation I83.218
        - midfoot I83.014
          - with inflammation I83.214
        - thigh I83.011
          - with inflammation I83.211
- nasal septum I86.8
- orbit I86.8
  - congenital Q27.8
- ovary I86.2
- papillary I78.1
- pelvis I86.2
- perineum I86.3
- pharynx I86.8
- placenta O43.89- ☑
- renal papilla I86.8
- retina H35.09
- scrotum (ulcerated) I86.1
- sigmoid colon I86.8
- specified site NEC I86.8
- spinal (cord) (vessels) I86.8
- spleen, splenic (vein) (with phlebolith) I86.8
- stomach I86.4
- sublingual I86.0
- ulcerated I83.009
  - inflamed or infected I83.209
- uterine ligament I86.2
- vagina I86.8
- vocal cord I86.8
- vulva I86.3

Vas deferens — see condition
Vas deferentitis N49.1
Vasa previa O69.4 ☑
- hemorrhage from, affecting newborn P50.0
Vascular — see also condition
- loop on optic papilla Q14.2
- spasm I73.9
- spider I78.1
Vascularization, cornea — see Neovascularization, cornea
Vasculitis I77.6
- allergic D69.0
- cryoglobulinemic D89.1
- disseminated I77.6
- hypocomplementemic M31.8
- kidney I77.89

Vasculitis — continued
- livedoid L95.0
- nodular L95.8
- retina H35.06- ☑
- rheumatic — see Fever, rheumatic
- rheumatoid — see Rheumatoid, vasculitis
- skin (limited to) L95.9
  - specified NEC L95.8
- systemic M31.8
Vasculopathy, necrotizing M31.9
- cardiac allograft T86.290
- specified NEC M31.8
Vasitis (nodosa) N49.1
- tuberculous A18.15
Vasodilation I73.9
Vasomotor — see condition
Vasoplasty, after previous sterilization Z31.0
- aftercare Z31.42
Vasospasm (vasoconstriction) I73.9
- cerebral (cerebrovascular) (artery) I67.848
  - reversible I67.841
- coronary I20.1
- nerve
  - arm — see Mononeuropathy, upper limb
  - brachial plexus G54.0
  - cervical plexus G54.2
  - leg — see Mononeuropathy, lower limb
- peripheral NOS I73.9
- retina (artery) — see Occlusion, artery, retina
Vasospastic — see condition
Vasovagal attack (paroxysmal) R55
- psychogenic F45.8
VATER syndrome Q87.2
Vater's ampulla — see condition
Vegetation, vegetative
- adenoid (nasal fossa) J35.8
- endocarditis (acute) (any valve) (subacute) I33.0
- heart (mycotic) (valve) I33.0
Veil
- Jackson's Q43.3
Vein, venous — see condition
Veldt sore — see Ulcer, skin
Velpeau's hernia — see Hernia, femoral
Venereal
- bubo A55
- disease A64
- granuloma inguinale A58
- lymphogranuloma (Durand-Nicolas-Favre) A55
Venofibrosis I87.8
Venom, venomous — see Table of Drugs and Chemicals, by animal or substance, poisoning
Venous — see condition
Ventilator lung, newborn P27.8
Ventral — see condition
Ventricle, ventricular — see also condition
- escape I49.3
- inversion Q20.5
Ventriculitis (cerebral) — see also Encephalitis G04.90
Ventriculostomy status Z98.2
Vernet's syndrome G52.7
Verneuil's disease (syphilitic bursitis) A52.78
Verruca (due to HPV) (filiformis) (simplex) (viral) (vulgaris) B07.9
- acuminata A63.0
- necrogenica (primary) (tuberculosa) A18.4
- plana B07.8
- plantaris B07.0
- seborrheica L82.1
  - inflamed L82.0
- senile (seborrheic) L82.1
  - inflamed L82.0
- tuberculosa (primary) A18.4
- venereal A63.0
Verrucosities — see Verruca
Verruga peruana, peruviana A44.1
Version
- with extraction
- cervix — see Malposition, uterus
- uterus (postinfectional) (postpartal, old) — see Malposition, uterus
Vertebra, vertebral — see condition
Vertical talus (congenital) Q66.80
- left foot Q66.82
- right foot Q66.81
Vertigo R42
- auditory — see Vertigo, aural
- aural H81.31- ☑

☑ **Additional Character Required** — Refer to the Tabular List for Character Selection   ▽ **Subterms under main terms may continue to next column or page**

Vertigo — continued
  benign paroxysmal (positional) H81.1- ☑
  central (origin) H81.4
  cerebral H81.4
  Dix and Hallpike (epidemic) — see Neuronitis, vestibular
  due to infrasound T75.23 ☑
  epidemic A88.1
    Dix and Hallpike — see Neuronitis, vestibular
    Pedersen's — see Neuronitis, vestibular
    vestibular neuronitis — see Neuronitis, vestibular
  hysterical F44.89
  infrasound T75.23 ☑
  labyrinthine — see subcategory H81.0 ☑
  laryngeal R05
  malignant positional H81.4
  Ménière's — see subcategory H81.0 ☑
  menopausal N95.1
  otogenic — see Vertigo, aural
  paroxysmal positional, benign — see Vertigo, benign paroxysmal
  Pedersen's (epidemic) — see Neuronitis, vestibular
  peripheral NEC H81.39- ☑
  positional
    benign paroxysmal — see Vertigo, benign paroxysmal
    malignant H81.4
Very-low-density-lipoprotein-type (VLDL) **hyperlipoproteinemia** E78.1
Vesania — see Psychosis
Vesical — see condition
Vesicle
  cutaneous R23.8
  seminal — see condition
  skin R23.8
Vesicocolic — see condition
Vesicoperineal — see condition
Vesicorectal — see condition
Vesicourethrorectal — see condition
Vesicovaginal — see condition
Vesicular — see condition
Vesiculitis (seminal) N49.0
  amebic A06.82
  gonorrheal (acute) (chronic) A54.23
  trichomonal A59.09
  tuberculous A18.15
Vestibulitis (ear) — see also subcategory H83.0 ☑
  nose (external) J34.89
  vulvar N94.810
Vestibulopathy , acute peripheral (recurrent) — see Neuronitis, vestibular
Vestige, vestigial — see also Persistence
  branchial Q18.0
  structures in vitreous Q14.0
Vibration
  adverse effects T75.20 ☑
    pneumatic hammer syndrome T75.21 ☑
    specified effect NEC T75.29 ☑
    vasospastic syndrome T75.22 ☑
    vertigo from infrasound T75.23 ☑
  exposure (occupational) Z57.7
  vertigo T75.23 ☑
Vibriosis A28.9
Victim (of)
  crime Z65.4
  disaster Z65.5
  terrorism Z65.4
  torture Z65.4
  war Z65.5
Vidal's disease L28.0
Villaret's syndrome G52.7
Villous — see condition
VIN — see Neoplasia, intraepithelial, vulva
Vincent's infection (angina) (gingivitis) A69.1
  stomatitis NEC A69.1
Vinson-Plummer syndrome D50.1
Violence, physical R45.6
Viosterol deficiency — see Deficiency, calciferol
Vipoma — see Neoplasm, malignant, by site
Viremia B34.9
Virilism (adrenal) E25.9
  congenital E25.0
Virilization (female) (suprarenal) E25.9
  congenital E25.0
  isosexual E28.2
Virulent bubo A57
Virus, viral — see also condition

Virus, viral — continued
  as cause of disease classified elsewhere B97.89
    respiratory syncytial virus (RSV) — see Virus, infection, respiratory syncytial (RSV)
  cytomegalovirus B25.9
  human immunodeficiency (HIV) — see Human, immunodeficiency virus (HIV) disease
  infection — see Infection, virus
  respiratory syncytial (RSV)
    as cause of disease classified elsewhere B97.4
    bronchiolitis J21.0
    bronchitis J20.5
    bronchopneumonia J12.1
    otitis media H65.- ☑ [B97.4]
    pneumonia J12.1
    upper respiratory infection J06.9 [B97.4]
  specified NEC B34.8
  swine influenza (viruses that normally cause infections in pigs) — see also Influenza, due to, identified novel influenza A virus J09.X2
  West Nile (fever) A92.30
    with
      complications NEC A92.39
      cranial nerve disorders A92.32
      encephalitis A92.31
      encephalomyelitis A92.31
      neurologic manifestation NEC A92.32
      optic neuritis A92.32
      polyradiculitis A92.32
Viscera, visceral — see condition
Visceroptosis K63.4
Visible peristalsis R19.2
Vision, visual
  binocular, suppression H53.34
  blurred, blurring H53.8
    hysterical F44.6
  defect, defective NEC H54.7
  disorientation (syndrome) H53.8
  disturbance H53.9
    hysterical F44.6
  double H53.2
  examination Z01.00
    with abnormal findings Z01.01
    following failed vision screening Z01.020
      with abnormal findings Z01.021
  field, limitation (defect) — see Defect, visual field
  hallucinations R44.1
  halos H53.19
  loss — see Loss, vision
    sudden — see Disturbance, vision, subjective, loss, sudden
  low (both eyes) — see Low, vision
  perception, simultaneous without fusion H53.33
Vitality, lack or want of R53.83
  newborn P96.89
Vitamin deficiency — see Deficiency, vitamin
Vitelline duct, persistent Q43.0
Vitiligo L80
  eyelid H02.739
    left H02.736
      lower H02.735
      upper H02.734
    right H02.733
      lower H02.732
      upper H02.731
  pinta A67.2
  vulva N90.89
Vitreal corneal syndrome H59.01- ☑
Vitreoretinopathy, proliferative — see also Retinopathy, proliferative
  with retinal detachment — see Detachment, retina, traction
Vitreous — see also condition
  touch syndrome — see Complication, postprocedural, following cataract surgery
Vocal cord — see condition
Vogt-Koyanagi syndrome H20.82- ☑
Vogt's disease or syndrome G80.3
Vogt-Spielmeyer amaurotic idiocy or disease E75.4
Voice
  change R49.9
    specified NEC R49.8
  loss — see Aphonia
Volhynian fever A79.0
Volkmann's ischemic contracture or paralysis (complicating trauma) T79.6 ☑
Volvulus (bowel) (colon) (intestine) K56.2
  with perforation K56.2

Volvulus — continued
  congenital Q43.8
  duodenum K31.5
  fallopian tube — see Torsion, fallopian tube
  oviduct — see Torsion, fallopian tube
  stomach (due to absence of gastrocolic ligament) K31.89
Vomiting R11.10
  with nausea R11.2
  asphyxia — see Foreign body, by site, causing asphyxia, gastric contents
  bilious (cause unknown) R11.14
    following gastro-intestinal surgery K91.0
    in newborn P92.01
  blood — see Hematemesis
  causing asphyxia, choking, or suffocation — see Foreign body, by site
  cyclical, in migraine G43.A0 (following G43.7)
    with refractory migraine G43.A1 (following G43.7)
    intractable G43.A1 (following G43.7)
    not intractable G43.A0 (following G43.7)
    psychogenic F50.89
    without refractory migraine G43.A0 (following G43.7)
  cyclical syndrome NOS (unrelated to migraine) R11.15
  fecal mater R11.13
  following gastrointestinal surgery K91.0
    psychogenic F50.89
  functional K31.89
  hysterical F50.89
  nervous F50.89
  neurotic F50.89
  newborn NEC P92.09
    bilious P92.01
  periodic R11.10
    psychogenic F50.89
  persistent R11.15
  projectile R11.12
  psychogenic F50.89
  uremic — see Uremia
  without nausea R11.11
Vomito negro — see Fever, yellow
Von Bezold's abscess — see Mastoiditis, acute
Von Economo-Cruchet disease A85.8
Von Eulenburg's disease G71.19
Von Gierke's disease E74.01
Von Hippel (-Lindau) **disease or syndrome** Q85.8
Von Jaksch's anemia or disease D64.89
Von Recklinghausen
  disease (neurofibromatosis) Q85.01
    bones E21.0
Von Schroetter's syndrome I82.890
Von Willebrand (-Jurgens)(-Minot) **disease or syndrome** D68.0
Von Zumbusch's disease L40.1
Voyeurism F65.3
Vrolik's disease Q78.0
Vulva — see condition
Vulvismus N94.2
Vulvitis (acute) (allergic) (atrophic) (hypertrophic) (intertriginous) (senile) N76.2
  with ectopic or molar pregnancy O08.0
  adhesive, congenital Q52.79
  blennorrhagic (gonococcal) A54.02
  candidal B37.3
  chlamydial A56.02
  due to Haemophilus ducreyi A57
  following ectopic or molar pregnancy O08.0
  gonococcal A54.02
    with abscess (accessory gland) (periurethral) A54.1
  herpesviral A60.04
  leukoplakic N90.4
  monilial B37.3
  puerperal (postpartum) O86.19
  subacute or chronic N76.3
  syphilitic (early) A51.0
    late A52.76
  trichomonal A59.01
  tuberculous A18.18
Vulvodynia N94.819
  specified NEC N94.818
Vulvorectal — see condition
Vulvovaginitis (acute) — see Vaginitis

W

Waiting list, person on Z75.1
  for organ transplant Z76.82
  undergoing social agency investigation Z75.2

▽ Subterms under main terms may continue to next column or page   ☑ Additional Character Required — Refer to the Tabular List for Character Selection   **325**

Vertigo — Waiting list, person on

Waldenström
- hypergammaglobulinemia D89.0
- syndrome or macroglobulinemia C88.0

Waldenström-Kjellberg syndrome D50.1

Walking
- difficulty R26.2
  - psychogenic F44.4
- sleep F51.3
  - hysterical F44.89

Wall, abdominal — see condition

Wallenberg's disease or syndrome G46.3

Wallgren's disease I87.8

Wandering
- gallbladder, congenital Q44.1
- in diseases classified elsewhere Z91.83
- kidney, congenital Q63.8
- organ or site, congenital NEC — see Malposition, congenital, by site
- pacemaker (heart) I49.8
- spleen D73.89

War neurosis F48.8

Wart (due to HPV) (filiform) (infectious) (viral) B07.9
- anogenital region (venereal) A63.0
- common B07.8
- external genital organs (venereal) A63.0
- flat B07.8
- Hassal-Henle's (of cornea) H18.49
- Peruvian A44.1
- plantar B07.0
- prosector (tuberculous) A18.4
- seborrheic L82.1
  - inflamed L82.0
- senile (seborrheic) L82.1
  - inflamed L82.0
- tuberculous A18.4
- venereal A63.0

Warthin's tumor — see Neoplasm, salivary gland, benign

Wassilieff's disease A27.0

Wasting
- disease R64
  - due to malnutrition E41
- extreme (due to malnutrition) E41
- muscle NEC — see Atrophy, muscle

Water
- clefts (senile cataract) — see Cataract, senile, incipient
- deprivation of T73.1 ☑
- intoxication E87.79
- itch B76.9
- lack of T73.1 ☑
- loading E87.70
- on
  - brain — see Hydrocephalus
  - chest J94.8
- poisoning E87.79

Waterbrash R12

Waterhouse (-Friderichsen) **syndrome or disease** (meningococcal) A39.1

Water-losing nephritis N25.89

Watermelon stomach K31.819
- with hemorrhage K31.811
- without hemorrhage K31.819

Watsoniasis B66.8

Wax in ear — see Impaction, cerumen

Weak, weakening, weakness (generalized) R53.1
- arches (acquired) — see also Deformity, limb, flat foot
- bladder (sphincter) R32
- facial R29.810
  - following
    - cerebrovascular disease I69.992
      - cerebral infarction I69.392
      - intracerebral hemorrhage I69.192
      - nontraumatic intracranial hemorrhage NEC I69.292
      - specified disease NEC I69.892
      - stroke I69.392
      - subarachnoid hemorrhage I69.092
- foot (double) — see also Weak, arches
- heart, cardiac — see Failure, heart
- mind F70
- muscle M62.81
- myocardium — see Failure, heart
- newborn P96.89
- pelvic fundus N81.89
- pubocervical tissue N81.82
- rectovaginal tissue N81.83
- senile R54
- urinary stream R39.12
- valvular — see Endocarditis

Wear, worn (with normal or routine use)
- articular bearing surface of internal joint prosthesis — see Complications, joint prosthesis, mechanical, wear of articular bearing surfaces, by site
- device, implant or graft — see Complications, by site, mechanical complication
- tooth, teeth (approximal) (hard tissues) (interproximal) (occlusal) K03.0

Weather, weathered
- effects of
  - cold T69.9 ☑
    - specified effect NEC T69.8 ☑
  - hot — see Heat
- skin L57.8

Weaver's syndrome Q87.3

Web, webbed (congenital)
- duodenal Q43.8
- esophagus Q39.4
- fingers Q70.1- ☑
- larynx (glottic) (subglottic) Q31.0
- neck (pterygium colli) Q18.3
- Paterson-Kelly D50.1
- popliteal syndrome Q87.89
- toes Q70.3- ☑

Weber-Christian disease M35.6

Weber-Cockayne syndrome (epidermolysis bullosa) Q81.8

Weber-Gubler syndrome G46.3

Weber-Leyden syndrome G46.3

Weber-Osler syndrome I78.0

Weber's paralysis or syndrome G46.3

Wedge-shaped or wedging vertebra — see Collapse, vertebra NEC

Wegener's granulomatosis or syndrome M31.30
- with
  - kidney involvement M31.31
  - lung involvement M31.30
    - with kidney involvement M31.31

Wegner's disease A50.02

Weight
- 1000-2499 grams at birth (low) — see Low, birthweight
- 999 grams or less at birth (extremely low) — see Low, birthweight, extreme
- and length below 10th percentile for gestational age P05.1- ☑
- below but length above 10th percentile for gestational age P05.0- ☑
- gain (abnormal) (excessive) R63.5
  - in pregnancy — see Pregnancy, complicated by, excessive weight gain
  - low — see Pregnancy, complicated by, insufficient, weight gain
- loss (abnormal) (cause unknown) R63.4

Weightlessness (effect of) T75.82 ☑

Weil (I)-**Marchesani syndrome** Q87.19

Weil's disease A27.0

Weingarten's syndrome J82

Weir Mitchell's disease I73.81

Weiss-Baker syndrome G90.09

Wells' disease L98.3

Wen — see Cyst, sebaceous

Wenckebach's block or phenomenon I44.1

Werdnig-Hoffmann syndrome (muscular atrophy) G12.0

Werlhof's disease D69.3

Wermer's disease or syndrome E31.21

Werner-His disease A79.0

Werner's disease or syndrome E34.8

Wernicke-Korsakoff's syndrome or psychosis (alcoholic) F10.96
- with dependence F10.26
- drug-induced
  - due to drug abuse — see Abuse, drug, by type, with amnestic disorder
  - due to drug dependence — see Dependence, drug, by type, with amnestic disorder
- nonalcoholic F04

Wernicke-Posadas disease B38.9

Wernicke's
- developmental aphasia F80.2
- disease or syndrome E51.2
- encephalopathy E51.2
- polioencephalitis, superior E51.2

West African fever B50.8

Westphal-Strümpell syndrome E83.01

West's syndrome — see Epilepsy, spasms

Wet
- feet, tropical (maceration) (syndrome) — see Immersion, foot
- lung (syndrome), newborn P22.1

Wharton's duct — see condition

Wheal — see Urticaria

Wheezing R06.2

Whiplash injury S13.4 ☑

Whipple's disease — see also subcategory M14.8- K90.81

Whipworm (disease) (infection) (infestation) B79

Whistling face Q87.0

White — see also condition
- kidney, small N03.9
- leg, puerperal, postpartum, childbirth O87.1
- mouth B37.0
- patches of mouth K13.29
- spot lesions, teeth
  - chewing surface K02.51
  - pit and fissure surface K02.51
  - smooth surface K02.61

Whitehead L70.0

Whitlow — see also Cellulitis, digit
- with lymphangitis — see Lymphangitis, acute, digit
- herpesviral B00.89

Whitmore's disease or fever — see Melioidosis

Whooping cough A37.90
- with pneumonia A37.91
  - due to Bordetella
    - bronchiseptica A37.81
    - parapertussis A37.11
    - pertussis A37.01
  - specified organism NEC A37.81
- due to
  - Bordetella
    - bronchiseptica A37.80
      - with pneumonia A37.81
    - parapertussis A37.10
      - with pneumonia A37.11
    - pertussis A37.00
      - with pneumonia A37.01
  - specified NEC A37.80
    - with pneumonia A37.81

Wichman's asthma J38.5

Wide cranial sutures, newborn P96.3

Widening aorta — see Ectasia, aorta
- with aneurysm — see Aneurysm, aorta

Wilkie's disease or syndrome K55.1

Wilkinson-Sneddon disease or syndrome L13.1

Willebrand (-Jürgens) **thrombopathy** D68.0

Williams syndrome Q93.82

Willige-Hunt disease or syndrome G23.1

Wilms' tumor C64- ☑

Wilson-Mikity syndrome P27.0

Wilson's
- disease or syndrome E83.01
- hepatolenticular degeneration E83.01
- lichen ruber L43.9

Window — see also Imperfect, closure
- aorticopulmonary Q21.4

Winter — see condition

Wiskott-Aldrich syndrome D82.0

Withdrawal state — see also Dependence, drug by type, with withdrawal
- alcohol
  - with perceptual disturbances F10.232
  - without perceptual disturbances F10.239
- caffeine F15.93
- cannabis F12.23
- newborn
  - correct therapeutic substance properly administered P96.2
  - infant of dependent mother P96.1
- therapeutic substance, neonatal P96.2

Witts' anemia D50.8

Witzelsucht F07.0

Woakes' ethmoiditis or syndrome J33.1

Wolff-Hirschorn syndrome Q93.3

Wolff-Parkinson-White syndrome I45.6

Wolhynian fever A79.0

Wolman's disease E75.5

Wood lung or pneumonitis J67.8

Woolly, wooly hair (congenital) (nevus) Q84.1

Woolsorter's disease A22.1

Word
- blindness (congenital) (developmental) F81.0
- deafness (congenital) (developmental) H93.25

326   ☑ **Additional Character Required** — Refer to the Tabular List for Character Selection   ▽ **Subterms under main terms may continue to next column or page**

Waldenström — Word

Worm(s) (infection) (infestation) — *see also* Infestation, helminth
  guinea B72
  in intestine NEC B82.0
Worm-eaten soles A66.3
Worn out — *see* Exhaustion
  cardiac
    defibrillator (with synchronous cardiac pacemaker) Z45.02
    pacemaker
      battery Z45.010
      lead Z45.018
  device, implant or graft — *see* Complications, by site, mechanical
Worried well Z71.1
Worries R45.82
Wound check Z48.0- ✓
  due to injury — *code to* Injury, by site, using appropriate seventh character for subsequent encounter
Wound, open T14.8- ✓
  abdomen, abdominal
    wall S31.109 ✓
      with penetration into peritoneal cavity S31.609 ✓
      bite — *see* Bite, abdomen, wall
      epigastric region S31.102 ✓
        with penetration into peritoneal cavity S31.602 ✓
        bite — *see* Bite, abdomen, wall, epigastric region
        laceration — *see* Laceration, abdomen, wall, epigastric region
        puncture — *see* Puncture, abdomen, wall, epigastric region
      laceration — *see* Laceration, abdomen, wall
      left
        lower quadrant S31.104 ✓
          with penetration into peritoneal cavity S31.604 ✓
          bite — *see* Bite, abdomen, wall, left, lower quadrant
          laceration — *see* Laceration, abdomen, wall, left, lower quadrant
          puncture — *see* Puncture, abdomen, wall, left, lower quadrant
        upper quadrant S31.101 ✓
          with penetration into peritoneal cavity S31.601 ✓
          bite — *see* Bite, abdomen, wall, left, upper quadrant
          laceration — *see* Laceration, abdomen, wall, left, upper quadrant
          puncture — *see* Puncture, abdomen, wall, left, upper quadrant
      periumbilic region S31.105 ✓
        with penetration into peritoneal cavity S31.605 ✓
        bite — *see* Bite, abdomen, wall, periumbilic region
        laceration — *see* Laceration, abdomen, wall, periumbilic region
        puncture — *see* Puncture, abdomen, wall, periumbilic region
      puncture — *see* Puncture, abdomen, wall
      right
        lower quadrant S31.103 ✓
          with penetration into peritoneal cavity S31.603 ✓
          bite — *see* Bite, abdomen, wall, right, lower quadrant
          laceration — *see* Laceration, abdomen, wall, right, lower quadrant
          puncture — *see* Puncture, abdomen, wall, right, lower quadrant
        upper quadrant S31.100 ✓
          with penetration into peritoneal cavity S31.600 ✓
          bite — *see* Bite, abdomen, wall, right, upper quadrant
          laceration — *see* Laceration, abdomen, wall, right, upper quadrant
          puncture — *see* Puncture, abdomen, wall, right, upper quadrant
    alveolar (process) — *see* Wound, open, oral cavity
    ankle S91.00- ✓
      bite — *see* Bite, ankle
      laceration — *see* Laceration, ankle

Wound, open — *continued*
  ankle — *continued*
    puncture — *see* Puncture, ankle
  antecubital space — *see* Wound, open, elbow
  anterior chamber, eye — *see* Wound, open, ocular
  anus S31.839 ✓
    bite S31.835 ✓
    laceration — *see* Laceration, anus
    puncture — *see* Puncture, anus
  arm (upper) S41.10- ✓
    with amputation — *see* Amputation, traumatic, arm
    bite — *see* Bite, arm
    forearm — *see* Wound, open, forearm
    laceration — *see* Laceration, arm
    puncture — *see* Puncture, arm
  auditory canal (external) (meatus) — *see* Wound, open, ear
  auricle, ear — *see* Wound, open, ear
  axilla — *see* Wound, open, arm
  back — *see also* Wound, open, thorax, back
    lower S31.000 ✓
      with penetration into retroperitoneal space S31.001 ✓
      bite — *see* Bite, back, lower
      laceration — *see* Laceration, back, lower
      puncture — *see* Puncture, back, lower
  bite — *see* Bite
  blood vessel — *see* Injury, blood vessel
  breast S21.00- ✓
    with amputation — *see* Amputation, traumatic, breast
    bite — *see* Bite, breast
    laceration — *see* Laceration, breast
    puncture — *see* Puncture, breast
  buttock S31.809 ✓
    bite — *see* Bite, buttock
    laceration — *see* Laceration, buttock
    left S31.829 ✓
    puncture — *see* Puncture, buttock
    right S31.819 ✓
  calf — *see* Wound, open, leg
  canaliculus lacrimalis — *see* Wound, open, eyelid
  canthus, eye — *see* Wound, open, eyelid
  cervical esophagus S11.20 ✓
    bite S11.25 ✓
    laceration — *see* Laceration, esophagus, traumatic, cervical
    puncture — *see* Puncture, cervical esophagus
  cheek (external) S01.40- ✓
    bite — *see* Bite, cheek
    internal — *see* Wound, open, oral cavity
    laceration — *see* Laceration, cheek
    puncture — *see* Puncture, cheek
  chest wall — *see* Wound, open, thorax
  chin — *see* Wound, open, head, specified site NEC
  choroid — *see* Wound, open, ocular
  ciliary body (eye) — *see* Wound, open, ocular
  clitoris S31.40 ✓
    with amputation — *see* Amputation, traumatic, clitoris
    bite S31.45 ✓
    laceration — *see* Laceration, vulva
    puncture — *see* Puncture, vulva
  conjunctiva — *see* Wound, open, ocular
  cornea — *see* Wound, open, ocular
  costal region — *see* Wound, open, thorax
  Descemet's membrane — *see* Wound, open, ocular
  digit(s)
    foot — *see* Wound, open, toe
    hand — *see* Wound, open, finger
  ear (canal) (external) S01.30- ✓
    with amputation — *see* Amputation, traumatic, ear
    bite — *see* Bite, ear
    drum S09.2- ✓
    laceration — *see* Laceration, ear
    puncture — *see* Puncture, ear
  elbow S51.00- ✓
    bite — *see* Bite, elbow
    laceration — *see* Laceration, elbow
    puncture — *see* Puncture, elbow
  epididymis — *see* Wound, open, testis
  epigastric region S31.102 ✓
    with penetration into peritoneal cavity S31.602 ✓
    bite — *see* Bite, abdomen, wall, epigastric region
    laceration — *see* Laceration, abdomen, wall, epigastric region

Wound, open — *continued*
  epigastric region — *continued*
    puncture — *see* Puncture, abdomen, wall, epigastric region
  epiglottis — *see* Wound, open, neck, specified site NEC
  esophagus (thoracic) S27.819 ✓
    cervical — *see* Wound, open, cervical esophagus
    laceration S27.813 ✓
    specified type NEC S27.818 ✓
  eye — *see* Wound, open, ocular
  eyeball — *see* Wound, open, ocular
  eyebrow — *see* Wound, open, eyelid
  eyelid S01.10- ✓
    bite — *see* Bite, eyelid
    laceration — *see* Laceration, eyelid
    puncture — *see* Puncture, eyelid
  face NEC — *see* Wound, open, head, specified site NEC
  finger(s) S61.209 ✓
    with
      amputation — *see* Amputation, traumatic, finger
      damage to nail S61.309 ✓
    bite — *see* Bite, finger
    index S61.208 ✓
      with
        damage to nail S61.308 ✓
      left S61.201 ✓
        with
          damage to nail S61.301 ✓
      right S61.200 ✓
        with
          damage to nail S61.300 ✓
    laceration — *see* Laceration, finger
    little S61.208 ✓
      with
        damage to nail S61.308 ✓
      left S61.207 ✓
        with damage to nail S61.307 ✓
      right S61.206 ✓
        with damage to nail S61.306 ✓
    middle S61.208 ✓
      with
        damage to nail S61.308 ✓
      left S61.203 ✓
        with damage to nail S61.303 ✓
      right S61.202 ✓
        with damage to nail S61.302 ✓
    puncture — *see* Puncture, finger
    ring S61.208 ✓
      with
        damage to nail S61.308 ✓
      left S61.205 ✓
        with damage to nail S61.305 ✓
      right S61.204 ✓
        with damage to nail S61.304 ✓
  flank — *see* Wound, open, abdomen, wall
  foot (except toe(s) alone) S91.30- ✓
    with amputation — *see* Amputation, traumatic, foot
    bite — *see* Bite, foot
    laceration — *see* Laceration, foot
    puncture — *see* Puncture, foot
    toe — *see* Wound, open, toe
  forearm S51.80- ✓
    with
      amputation — *see* Amputation, traumatic, forearm
    bite — *see* Bite, forearm
    elbow only — *see* Wound, open, elbow
    laceration — *see* Laceration, forearm
    puncture — *see* Puncture, forearm
  forehead — *see* Wound, open, head, specified site NEC
  genital organs, external
    with amputation — *see* Amputation, traumatic, genital organs
    bite — *see* Bite, genital organ
    female S31.502 ✓
      vagina S31.40 ✓
      vulva S31.40 ✓
    laceration — *see* Laceration, genital organ
    male S31.501 ✓
      penis S31.20 ✓
      scrotum S31.30 ✓
      testes S31.30 ✓
    puncture — *see* Puncture, genital organ
  globe (eye) — *see* Wound, open, ocular
  groin — *see* Wound, open, abdomen, wall
  gum — *see* Wound, open, oral cavity

▽ Subterms under main terms may continue to next column or page   ✓ **Additional Character Required — Refer to the Tabular List for Character Selection**   **327**

Worm(s) — Wound, open

Wound, open — *continued*
- hand S61.40- ☑
  - with
    - amputation — *see* Amputation, traumatic, hand
  - bite — *see* Bite, hand
  - finger(s) — *see* Wound, open, finger
  - laceration — *see* Laceration, hand
  - puncture — *see* Puncture, hand
  - thumb — *see* Wound, open, thumb
- head S01.90 ☑
  - bite — *see* Bite, head
  - cheek — *see* Wound, open, cheek
  - ear — *see* Wound, open, ear
  - eyelid — *see* Wound, open, eyelid
  - laceration — *see* Laceration, head
  - lip — *see* Wound, open, lip
  - nose S01.20 ☑
  - oral cavity — *see* Wound, open, oral cavity
  - puncture — *see* Puncture, head
  - scalp — *see* Wound, open, scalp
  - specified site NEC S01.80 ☑
  - temporomandibular area — *see* Wound, open, cheek
- heel — *see* Wound, open, foot
- hip S71.00- ☑
  - with amputation — *see* Amputation, traumatic, hip
  - bite — *see* Bite, hip
  - laceration — *see* Laceration, hip
  - puncture — *see* Puncture, hip
- hymen S31.40 ☑
  - bite — *see* Bite, vulva
  - laceration — *see* Laceration, vagina
  - puncture — *see* Puncture, vagina
- hypochondrium S31.109 ☑
  - bite — *see* Bite, hypochondrium
  - laceration — *see* Laceration, hypochondrium
  - puncture — *see* Puncture, hypochondrium
- hypogastric region S31.109 ☑
  - bite — *see* Bite, hypogastric region
  - laceration — *see* Laceration, hypogastric region
  - puncture — *see* Puncture, hypogastric region
- iliac (region) — *see* Wound, open, inguinal region
- inguinal region S31.109 ☑
  - bite — *see* Bite, abdomen, wall, lower quadrant
  - laceration — *see* Laceration, inguinal region
  - puncture — *see* Puncture, inguinal region
- instep — *see* Wound, open, foot
- interscapular region — *see* Wound, open, thorax, back
- intraocular — *see* Wound, open, ocular
- iris — *see* Wound, open, ocular
- jaw — *see* Wound, open, head, specified site NEC
- knee S81.00- ☑
  - bite — *see* Bite, knee
  - laceration — *see* Laceration, knee
  - puncture — *see* Puncture, knee
- labium (majus) (minus) — *see* Wound, open, vulva
- laceration — *see* Laceration, by site
- lacrimal duct — *see* Wound, open, eyelid
- larynx S11.019 ☑
  - bite — *see* Bite, larynx
  - laceration — *see* Laceration, larynx
  - puncture — *see* Puncture, larynx
- left
  - lower quadrant S31.104 ☑
    - with penetration into peritoneal cavity S31.604 ☑
    - bite — *see* Bite, abdomen, wall, left, lower quadrant
    - laceration — *see* Laceration, abdomen, wall, left, lower quadrant
    - puncture — *see* Puncture, abdomen, wall, left, lower quadrant
  - upper quadrant S31.101 ☑
    - with penetration into peritoneal cavity S31.601 ☑
    - bite — *see* Bite, abdomen, wall, left, upper quadrant
    - laceration — *see* Laceration, abdomen, wall, left, upper quadrant
    - puncture — *see* Puncture, abdomen, wall, left, upper quadrant
- leg (lower) S81.80- ☑
  - with amputation — *see* Amputation, traumatic, leg
  - ankle — *see* Wound, open, ankle
  - bite — *see* Bite, leg
  - foot — *see* Wound, open, foot

Wound, open — *continued*
- leg — *continued*
  - knee — *see* Wound, open, knee
  - laceration — *see* Laceration, leg
  - puncture — *see* Puncture, leg
  - toe — *see* Wound, open, toe
  - upper — *see* Wound, open, thigh
- lip S01.501 ☑
  - bite — *see* Bite, lip
  - laceration — *see* Laceration, lip
  - puncture — *see* Puncture, lip
- loin S31.109 ☑
  - bite — *see* Bite, abdomen, wall
  - laceration — *see* Laceration, loin
  - puncture — *see* Puncture, loin
- lower back — *see* Wound, open, back, lower
- lumbar region — *see* Wound, open, back, lower
- malar region — *see* Wound, open, head, specified site NEC
- mammary — *see* Wound, open, breast
- mastoid region — *see* Wound, open, head, specified site NEC
- mouth — *see* Wound, open, oral cavity
- nail
  - finger — *see* Wound, open, finger, with damage to nail
  - toe — *see* Wound, open, toe, with damage to nail
- nape (neck) — *see* Wound, open, neck
- nasal (septum) (sinus) — *see* Wound, open, nose
- nasopharynx — *see* Wound, open, head, specified site NEC
- neck S11.90 ☑
  - bite — *see* Bite, neck
  - involving
    - cervical esophagus S11.20 ☑
    - larynx — *see* Wound, open, larynx
    - pharynx S11.20 ☑
    - thyroid S11.10 ☑
    - trachea (cervical) S11.029 ☑
      - bite — *see* Bite, trachea
      - laceration S11.021 ☑
        - with foreign body S11.022 ☑
      - puncture S11.023 ☑
        - with foreign body S11.024 ☑
  - laceration — *see* Laceration, neck
  - puncture — *see* Puncture, neck
  - specified site NEC S11.80 ☑
    - specified type NEC S11.89 ☑
- nose (septum) (sinus) S01.20 ☑
  - with amputation — *see* Amputation, traumatic, nose
  - bite — *see* Bite, nose
  - laceration — *see* Laceration, nose
  - puncture — *see* Puncture, nose
- ocular S05.90 ☑
  - avulsion (traumatic enucleation) S05.7- ☑
  - eyeball S05.6- ☑
    - with foreign body S05.5- ☑
  - eyelid — *see* Wound, open, eyelid
  - laceration and rupture S05.3- ☑
    - with prolapse or loss of intraocular tissue S05.2- ☑
  - orbit (penetrating) (with or without foreign body) S05.4- ☑
  - periocular area — *see* Wound, open, eyelid
  - specified NEC S05.8X- ☑
- oral cavity S01.502 ☑
  - bite S01.552 ☑
  - laceration — *see* Laceration, oral cavity
  - puncture — *see* Puncture, oral cavity
- orbit — *see* Wound, open, ocular, orbit
- palate — *see* Wound, open, oral cavity
- palm — *see* Wound, open, hand
- pelvis, pelvic — *see also* Wound, open, back, lower
  - girdle — *see* Wound, open, hip
- penetrating — *see* Puncture, by site
- penis S31.20 ☑
  - with amputation — *see* Amputation, traumatic, penis
  - bite S31.25 ☑
  - laceration — *see* Laceration, penis
  - puncture — *see* Puncture, penis
- perineum
  - bite — *see* Bite, perineum
  - female S31.502 ☑
  - laceration — *see* Laceration, perineum

Wound, open — *continued*
- perineum — *continued*
  - male S31.501 ☑
  - puncture — *see* Puncture, perineum
- periocular area (with or without lacrimal passages) — *see* Wound, open, eyelid
- periumbilic region S31.105 ☑
  - with penetration into peritoneal cavity S31.605 ☑
  - bite — *see* Bite, abdomen, wall, periumbilic region
  - laceration — *see* Laceration, abdomen, wall, periumbilic region
  - puncture — *see* Puncture, abdomen, wall, periumbilic region
- phalanges
  - finger — *see* Wound, open, finger
  - toe — *see* Wound, open, toe
- pharynx S11.20 ☑
- pinna — *see* Wound, open, ear
- popliteal space — *see* Wound, open, knee
- prepuce — *see* Wound, open, penis
- pubic region — *see* Wound, open, back, lower
- pudendum — *see* Wound, open, genital organs, external
- puncture wound — *see* Puncture
- rectovaginal septum — *see* Wound, open, vagina
- right
  - lower quadrant S31.103 ☑
    - with penetration into peritoneal cavity S31.603 ☑
    - bite — *see* Bite, abdomen, wall, right, lower quadrant
    - laceration — *see* Laceration, abdomen, wall, right, lower quadrant
    - puncture — *see* Puncture, abdomen, wall, right, lower quadrant
  - upper quadrant S31.100 ☑
    - with penetration into peritoneal cavity S31.600 ☑
    - bite — *see* Bite, abdomen, wall, right, upper quadrant
    - laceration — *see* Laceration, abdomen, wall, right, upper quadrant
    - puncture — *see* Puncture, abdomen, wall, right, upper quadrant
- sacral region — *see* Wound, open, back, lower
- sacroiliac region — *see* Wound, open, back, lower
- salivary gland — *see* Wound, open, oral cavity
- scalp S01.00 ☑
  - bite S01.05 ☑
  - laceration — *see* Laceration, scalp
  - puncture — *see* Puncture, scalp
- scalpel, newborn (birth injury) P15.8
- scapular region — *see* Wound, open, shoulder
- sclera — *see* Wound, open, ocular
- scrotum S31.30 ☑
  - with amputation — *see* Amputation, traumatic, scrotum
  - bite S31.35 ☑
  - laceration — *see* Laceration, scrotum
  - puncture — *see* Puncture, scrotum
- shin — *see* Wound, open, leg
- shoulder S41.00- ☑
  - with amputation — *see* Amputation, traumatic, arm
  - bite — *see* Bite, shoulder
  - laceration — *see* Laceration, shoulder
  - puncture — *see* Puncture, shoulder
- skin NOS T14.8 ☑
- spermatic cord — *see* Wound, open, testis
- sternal region — *see* Wound, open, thorax, front wall
- submaxillary region — *see* Wound, open, head, specified site NEC
- submental region — *see* Wound, open, head, specified site NEC
- subungual
  - finger(s) — *see* Wound, open, finger
  - toe(s) — *see* Wound, open, toe
- supraclavicular region — *see* Wound, open, neck, specified site NEC
- temple, temporal region — *see* Wound, open, head, specified site NEC
- temporomandibular area — *see* Wound, open, cheek
- testis S31.30 ☑
  - with amputation — *see* Amputation, traumatic, testes
  - bite S31.35 ☑
  - laceration — *see* Laceration, testis
  - puncture — *see* Puncture, testis

☑ **Additional Character Required** — Refer to the Tabular List for Character Selection   ▽ **Subterms under main terms may continue to next column or page**

Wound, open — *continued*
  thigh S71.10- ☑
    with amputation — *see* Amputation, traumatic, hip
    bite — *see* Bite, thigh
    laceration — *see* Laceration, thigh
    puncture — *see* Puncture, thigh
  thorax, thoracic (wall) S21.90 ☑
    back S21.20- ☑
      with penetration S21.40 ☑
    bite — *see* Bite, thorax
    breast — *see* Wound, open, breast
    front S21.10- ☑
      with penetration S21.30 ☑
    laceration — *see* Laceration, thorax
    puncture — *see* Puncture, thorax
  throat — *see* Wound, open, neck
  thumb S61.009 ☑
    with
      amputation — *see* Amputation, traumatic, thumb
      damage to nail S61.109 ☑
    bite — *see* Bite, thumb
    laceration — *see* Laceration, thumb
    left S61.002 ☑
      with
        damage to nail S61.102 ☑
    puncture — *see* Puncture, thumb
    right S61.001 ☑
      with
        damage to nail S61.101 ☑
  thyroid (gland) — *see* Wound, open, neck, thyroid
  toe(s) S91.109 ☑
    with
      amputation — *see* Amputation, traumatic, toe
      damage to nail S91.209 ☑
    bite — *see* Bite, toe
    great S91.103 ☑
      with
        damage to nail S91.203 ☑
      left S91.102 ☑
        with
          damage to nail S91.202 ☑
      right S91.101 ☑
        with
          damage to nail S91.201 ☑
    laceration — *see* Laceration, toe
    lesser S91.106 ☑
      with
        damage to nail S91.206 ☑
      left S91.105 ☑
        with
          damage to nail S91.205 ☑
      right S91.104 ☑
        with
          damage to nail S91.204 ☑
    puncture — *see* Puncture, toe
  tongue — *see* Wound, open, oral cavity
  trachea (cervical region) — *see* Wound, open, neck, trachea
  tunica vaginalis — *see* Wound, open, testis
  tympanum, tympanic membrane S09.2- ☑
    laceration — *see* Laceration, ear, drum
    puncture — *see* Puncture, tympanum
  umbilical region — *see* Wound, open, abdomen, wall, periumbilic region
  uvula — *see* Wound, open, oral cavity
  vagina S31.40 ☑
    bite S31.45 ☑
    laceration — *see* Laceration, vagina
    puncture — *see* Puncture, vagina
  vitreous (humor) — *see* Wound, open, ocular
  vocal cord S11.039 ☑
    bite — *see* Bite, vocal cord
    laceration S11.031 ☑
      with foreign body S11.032 ☑
    puncture S11.033 ☑
      with foreign body S11.034 ☑
  vulva S31.40 ☑
    with amputation — *see* Amputation, traumatic, vulva
    bite S31.45 ☑
    laceration — *see* Laceration, vulva
    puncture — *see* Puncture, vulva
  wrist S61.50- ☑
    bite — *see* Bite, wrist

Wound, open — *continued*
  wrist — *continued*
    laceration — *see* Laceration, wrist
    puncture — *see* Puncture, wrist
Wound, superficial — *see* Injury — *see also* specified injury type
Wright's syndrome G54.0
Wrist — *see* condition
Wrong drug (by accident) (given in error) — *see* Table of Drugs and Chemicals, by drug, poisoning
Wry neck — *see* Torticollis
Wuchereria (bancrofti) **infestation** B74.0
Wuchereriasis B74.0
Wuchernde Struma Langhans C73

X

Xanthelasma (eyelid) (palpebrarum) H02.60
  left H02.66
    lower H02.65
    upper H02.64
  right H02.63
    lower H02.62
    upper H02.61
Xanthelasmatosis (essential) E78.2
Xanthinuria, hereditary E79.8
Xanthoastrocytoma
  specified site — *see* Neoplasm, malignant, by site
  unspecified site C71.9
Xanthofibroma — *see* Neoplasm, connective tissue, benign
Xanthogranuloma D76.3
Xanthoma(s), xanthomatosis (primary) (familial) (hereditary) E75.5
  with
    hyperlipoproteinemia
      Type I E78.3
      Type III E78.2
      Type IV E78.1
      Type V E78.3
  bone (generalisata) C96.5
  cerebrotendinous E75.5
  cutaneotendinous E75.5
  disseminatum (skin) E78.2
  eruptive E78.2
  hypercholesterinemic E78.00
  hypercholesterolemic E78.00
  hyperlipidemic E78.5
  joint E75.5
  multiple (skin) E78.2
  tendon (sheath) E75.5
  tuberosum E78.2
  tuberous E78.2
  tubo-eruptive E78.2
  verrucous, oral mucosa K13.4
Xanthosis R23.8
Xenophobia F40.10
Xeroderma — *see also* Ichthyosis
  acquired L85.0
    eyelid H01.149
      left H01.146
        lower H01.145
        upper H01.144
      right H01.143
        lower H01.142
        upper H01.141
  pigmentosum Q82.1
  vitamin A deficiency E50.8
Xerophthalmia (vitamin A deficiency) E50.7
  unrelated to vitamin A deficiency — *see* Keratoconjunctivitis
Xerosis
  conjunctiva H11.14- ☑
    with Bitot's spots — *see also* Pigmentation, conjunctiva
      vitamin A deficiency E50.1
    vitamin A deficiency E50.0
  cornea H18.89- ☑
    with ulceration — *see* Ulcer, cornea
      vitamin A deficiency E50.3
    vitamin A deficiency E50.2
  cutis L85.3
  skin L85.3
Xerostomia K11.7
Xiphopagus Q89.4
XO syndrome Q96.9

X-ray (of)
  abnormal findings — *see* Abnormal, diagnostic imaging
  breast (mammogram) (routine) Z12.31
  chest
    routine (as part of a general medical examination) Z00.00
      with abnormal findings Z00.01
  routine (as part of a general medical examination) Z00.00
    with abnormal findings Z00.01
XXXXY syndrome Q98.1
XXY syndrome Q98.0

Y

Yaba pox (virus disease) B08.72
Yatapoxvirus B08.70
  specified NEC B08.79
Yawning R06.89
  psychogenic F45.8
Yaws A66.9
  bone lesions A66.6
  butter A66.1
  chancre A66.0
  cutaneous, less than five years after infection A66.2
  early (cutaneous) (macular) (maculopapular) (micropapular) (papular) A66.2
    frambeside A66.2
    skin lesions NEC A66.2
  eyelid A66.2
  ganglion A66.6
  gangosis, gangosa A66.5
  gumma, gummata A66.4
    bone A66.6
  gummatous
    frambeside A66.4
    osteitis A66.6
    periostitis A66.6
  hydrarthrosis — *see also* subcategory M14.8- A66.6
  hyperkeratosis (early) (late) A66.3
  initial lesions A66.0
  joint lesions — *see also* subcategory M14.8- A66.6
  juxta-articular nodules A66.7
  late nodular (ulcerated) A66.4
  latent (without clinical manifestations) (with positive serology) A66.8
  mother A66.0
  mucosal A66.7
  multiple papillomata A66.1
  nodular, late (ulcerated) A66.4
  osteitis A66.6
  papilloma, plantar or palmar A66.1
  periostitis (hypertrophic) A66.6
  specified NEC A66.7
  ulcers A66.4
  wet crab A66.1
Yeast infection — *see also* Candidiasis B37.9
Yellow
  atrophy (liver) — *see* Failure, hepatic
  fever — *see* Fever, yellow
  jack — *see* Fever, yellow
  jaundice — *see* Jaundice
  nail syndrome L60.5
Yersiniosis — *see also* Infection, Yersinia
  extraintestinal A28.2
  intestinal A04.6

Z

Zahorsky's syndrome (herpangina) B08.5
Zellweger's syndrome E71.510
Zenker's diverticulum (esophagus) K22.5
Ziehen-Oppenheim disease G24.1
Zieve's syndrome K70.0
Zika NOS A92.5
  congenital P35.4
Zinc
  deficiency, dietary E60
  metabolism disorder E83.2
Zollinger-Ellison syndrome E16.4
Zona — *see* Herpes, zoster
Zoophobia F40.218
Zoster (herpes) — *see* Herpes, zoster
Zygomycosis B46.9
  specified NEC B46.8
Zymotic — *see* condition

▼ **Subterms under main terms may continue to next column or page**   ☑ **Additional Character Required — Refer to the Tabular List for Character Selection**   **329**

Wound, open — Zymotic

Note: The list below gives the code number for neoplasms by anatomical site. For each site there are six possible code numbers according to whether the neoplasm in question is malignant, benign, in situ, of uncertain behavior, or of unspecified nature. The description of the neoplasm will often indicate which of the six columns is appropriate; e.g., malignant melanoma of skin, benign fibroadenoma of breast, carcinoma in situ of cervix uteri. Where such descriptors are not present, the remainder of the Index should be consulted where guidance is given to the appropriate column for each morphological (histological) variety listed; e.g., Mesonephroma – see Neoplasm, malignant; Embryoma — see also Neoplasm, uncertain behavior; Disease, Bowen's – see Neoplasm, skin, in situ. However, the guidance in the Index can be overridden if one of the descriptors mentioned above is present; e.g., malignant adenoma of colon is coded to C18.9 and not to D12.6 as the adjective "malignant" overrides the Index entry "Adenoma — see also Neoplasm, benign, by site." Codes listed with a dash -, following the code have a required additional character for laterality. The tabular list must be reviewed for the complete code.

	Malignant Primary	Malignant Secondary	Ca in situ	Benign	Uncertain Behavior	Unspecified Behavior
Neoplasm, neoplastic	C80.1	C79.9	D09.9	D36.9	D48.9	D49.9
abdomen, abdominal	C76.2	C79.8-☑	D09.8	D36.7	D48.7	D49.89
cavity	C76.2	C79.8-☑	D09.8	D36.7	D48.7	D49.89
organ	C76.2	C79.8-☑	D09.8	D36.7	D48.7	D49.89
viscera	C76.2	C79.8-☑	D09.8	D36.7	D48.7	D49.89
wall — *see also* Neoplasm, abdomen, wall, skin	C44.509	C79.2	D04.5	D23.5	D48.5	D49.2
connective tissue	C49.4	C79.8-☑	—	D21.4	D48.1	D49.2
skin	C44.509	—	—	—	—	—
basal cell carcinoma	C44.519					
specified type NEC	C44.599	—	—	—	—	—
squamous cell carcinoma	C44.529					
abdominopelvic	C76.8	C79.8-☑	—	D36.7	D48.7	D49.89
accessory sinus — *see* Neoplasm, sinus						
acoustic nerve	C72.4-☑	C79.49	—	D33.3	D43.3	D49.7
adenoid (pharynx) (tissue)	C11.1	C79.89	D00.08	D10.6	D37.05	D49.0
adipose tissue — *see also* Neoplasm, connective tissue	C49.4	C79.89	—	D21.9	D48.1	D49.2
adnexa (uterine)	C57.4	C79.89	D07.39	D28.7	D39.8	D49.59
adrenal	C74.9-☑	C79.7-☑	D09.3	D35.0-☑	D44.1-☑	D49.7
capsule	C74.9-☑	C79.7-☑	D09.3	D35.0-☑	D44.1-☑	D49.7
cortex	C74.0-☑	C79.7-☑	D09.3	D35.0-☑	D44.1-☑	D49.7
gland	C74.9-☑	C79.7-☑	D09.3	D35.0-☑	D44.1-☑	D49.7
medulla	C74.1-☑	C79.7-☑	D09.3	D35.0-☑	D44.1-☑	D49.7
ala nasi (external) — *see also* Neoplasm, skin, nose	C44.301	C79.2	D04.39	D23.39	D48.5	D49.2
alimentary canal or tract NEC	C26.9	C78.80	D01.9	D13.9	D37.9	D49.0
alveolar	C03.9	C79.89	D00.03	D10.39	D37.09	D49.0
mucosa	C03.9	C79.89	D00.03	D10.39	D37.09	D49.0
lower	C03.1	C79.89	D00.03	D10.39	D37.09	D49.0
upper	C03.0	C79.89	D00.03	D10.39	D37.09	D49.0
ridge or process	C41.1	C79.51	—	D16.5	D48.0	D49.2
carcinoma	C03.9	C79.8-☑	—	—	—	—
lower	C03.1	C79.8-☑	—	—	—	—
upper	C03.0	C79.8-☑	—	—	—	—
lower	C41.1	C79.51	—	D16.5	D48.0	D49.2
mucosa	C03.9	C79.89	D00.03	D10.39	D37.09	D49.0
lower	C03.1	C79.89	D00.03	D10.39	D37.09	D49.0
upper	C03.0	C79.89	D00.03	D10.39	D37.09	D49.0
upper	C41.0	C79.51	—	D16.4	D48.0	D49.2
sulcus	C06.1	C79.89	D00.02	D10.39	D37.09	D49.0
alveolus	C03.9	C79.89	D00.03	D10.39	D37.09	D49.0
lower	C03.1	C79.89	D00.03	D10.39	D37.09	D49.0
upper	C03.0	C79.89	D00.03	D10.39	D37.09	D49.0
ampulla of Vater	C24.1	C78.89	D01.5	D13.5	D37.6	D49.0
ankle NEC	C76.5-☑	C79.89	D04.7-☑	D36.7	D48.7	D49.89
anorectum, anorectal (junction)	C21.8	C78.5	D01.3	D12.9	D37.8	D49.0
antecubital fossa or space	C76.4-☑	C79.89	D04.6-☑	D36.7	D48.7	D49.89

Neoplasm, neoplastic — continued	Malignant Primary	Malignant Secondary	Ca in situ	Benign	Uncertain Behavior	Unspecified Behavior
antrum (Highmore) (maxillary)	C31.0	C78.39	D02.3	D14.0	D38.5	D49.1
pyloric	C16.3	C78.89	D00.2	D13.1	D37.1	D49.0
tympanicum	C30.1	C78.39	D02.3	D14.0	D38.5	D49.1
anus, anal	C21.0	C78.5	D01.3	D12.9	D37.8	D49.0
canal	C21.1	C78.5	D01.3	D12.9	D37.8	D49.0
cloacogenic zone	C21.2	C78.5	D01.3	D12.9	D37.8	D49.0
margin — *see also* Neoplasm, anus, skin	C44.500	C79.2	D04.5	D23.5	D48.5	D49.2
overlapping lesion with rectosigmoid junction or rectum	C21.8	—	—	—	—	—
skin	C44.500	C79.2	D04.5	D23.5	D48.5	D49.2
basal cell carcinoma	C44.510					
specified type NEC	C44.590	—		—	—	—
squamous cell carcinoma	C44.520	—		—	—	—
sphincter	C21.1	C78.5	D01.3	D12.9	D37.8	D49.0
aorta (thoracic)	C49.3	C79.89	—	D21.3	D48.1	D49.2
abdominal	C49.4	C79.89	—	D21.4	D48.1	D49.2
aortic body	C75.5	C79.89	—	D35.6	D44.7	D49.7
aponeurosis	C49.9	C79.89	—	D21.9	D48.1	D49.2
palmar	C49.1-☑	C79.89	—	D21.1-☑	D48.1	D49.2
plantar	C49.2-☑	C79.89	—	D21.2-☑	D48.1	D49.2
appendix	C18.1	C78.5	D01.0	D12.1	D37.3	D49.0
arachnoid	C70.9	C79.49	—	D32.9	D42.9	D49.7
cerebral	C70.0	C79.32	—	D32.0	D42.0	D49.7
spinal	C70.1	C79.49	—	D32.1	D42.1	D49.7
areola	C50.0-☑	C79.81	D05-☑	D24-☑	D48.6-☑	D49.3
arm NEC	C76.4-☑	C79.89	D04.6-☑	D36.7	D48.7	D49.89
artery — *see* Neoplasm, connective tissue						
aryepiglottic fold	C13.1	C79.89	D00.08	D10.7	D37.05	D49.0
hypopharyngeal aspect	C13.1	C79.89	D00.08	D10.7	D37.05	D49.0
laryngeal aspect	C32.1	C78.39	D02.0	D14.1	D38.0	D49.1
marginal zone	C13.1	C79.89	D00.08	D10.7	D37.05	D49.0
arytenoid (cartilage)	C32.3	C78.39	D02.0	D14.1	D38.0	D49.1
fold — *see* Neoplasm, aryepiglottic						
associated with transplanted organ	C80.2	—	—	—	—	—
atlas	C41.2	C79.51	—	D16.6	D48.0	D49.2
atrium, cardiac	C38.0	C79.89	—	D15.1	D48.7	D49.89
auditory						
canal (external) (skin)	C44.20-☑	C79.2	D04.2-☑	D23.2-☑	D48.5	D49.2
internal	C30.1	C78.39	D02.3	D14.0	D38.5	D49.1
nerve	C72.4-☑	C79.49	—	D33.3	D43.3	D49.7
tube	C30.1	C78.39	D02.3	D14.0	D38.5	D49.1
opening	C11.2	C79.89	D00.08	D10.6	D37.05	D49.0
auricle, ear — *see also* Neoplasm, skin, ear	C44.20-☑	C79.2	D04.2-☑	D23.2-☑	D48.5	D49.2
auricular canal (external) — *see also* Neoplasm, skin, ear	C44.20-☑	C79.2	D04.2-☑	D23.2-☑	D48.5	D49.2
internal	C30.1	C78.39	D02.3	D14.0	D38.5	D49.2
autonomic nerve or nervous system NEC (see Neoplasm, nerve, peripheral)						
axilla, axillary	C76.1	C79.89	D09.8	D36.7	D48.7	D49.89
fold — *see also* Neoplasm, skin, trunk	C44.509	C79.2	D04.5	D23.5	D48.5	D49.2
back NEC	C76.8	C79.89	D04.5	D36.7	D48.7	D49.89
Bartholin's gland	C51.0	C79.82	D07.1	D28.0	D39.8	D49.59
basal ganglia	C71.0	C79.31	—	D33.0	D43.0	D49.6
basis pedunculi	C71.7	C79.31	—	D33.1	D43.1	D49.6
bile or biliary (tract)	C24.9	C78.89	D01.5	D13.5	D37.6	D49.0

Neoplasm, neoplastic
— continued
bile or biliary — continued

	Malignant Primary	Malignant Secondary	Ca in situ	Benign	Uncertain Behavior	Unspecified Behavior
canaliculi (biliferi) (intrahepatic)	C22.1	C78.7	D01.5	D13.4	D37.6	D49.0
canals, interlobular	C22.1	C78.89	D01.5	D13.4	D37.6	D49.0
duct or passage (common) (cystic) (extrahepatic)	C24.0	C78.89	D01.5	D13.5	D37.6	D49.0
interlobular	C22.1	C78.89	D01.5	D13.4	D37.6	D49.0
intrahepatic	C22.1	C78.7	D01.5	D13.4	D37.6	D49.0
and extrahepatic	C24.8	C78.89	D01.5	D13.5	D37.6	D49.0
bladder (urinary)	C67.9	C79.11	D09.0	D30.3	D41.4	D49.4
dome	C67.1	C79.11	D09.0	D30.3	D41.4	D49.4
neck	C67.5	C79.11	D09.0	D30.3	D41.4	D49.4
orifice	C67.9	C79.11	D09.0	D30.3	D41.4	D49.4
ureteric	C67.6	C79.11	D09.0	D30.3	D41.4	D49.4
urethral	C67.5	C79.11	D09.0	D30.3	D41.4	D49.4
overlapping lesion	C67.8	—	—	—	—	—
sphincter	C67.8	C79.11	D09.0	D30.3	D41.4	D49.4
trigone	C67.0	C79.11	D09.0	D30.3	D41.4	D49.4
urachus	C67.7	C79.11	D09.0	D30.3	D41.4	D49.4
wall	C67.9	C79.11	D09.0	D30.3	D41.4	D49.4
anterior	C67.3	C79.11	D09.0	D30.3	D41.4	D49.4
lateral	C67.2	C79.11	D09.0	D30.3	D41.4	D49.4
posterior	C67.4	C79.11	D09.0	D30.3	D41.4	D49.4
blood vessel — see Neoplasm, connective tissue						
bone (periosteum)	C41.9	C79.51	—	D16.9-	D48.0	D49.2
acetabulum						
ankle	C40.3-☑	C79.51	—	D16.3-☑	—	—
arm NEC	C40.0-☑	C79.51	—	D16.0-☑	—	—
astragalus	C40.3-☑	C79.51	—	D16.3-☑	—	—
atlas	C41.2	C79.51	—	D16.6	D48.0	D49.2
axis	C41.2	C79.51	—	D16.6	D48.0	D49.2
back NEC	C41.2	C79.51	—	D16.6	D48.0	D49.2
calcaneus	C40.3-☑	C79.51	—	D16.3-☑	—	—
calvarium	C41.0	C79.51	—	D16.4	D48.0	D49.2
carpus (any)	C40.1-☑	C79.51	—	D16.1-☑	—	—
cartilage NEC	C41.9	C79.51	—	D16.9	D48.0	D49.2
clavicle	C41.3	C79.51	—	D16.7	D48.0	D49.2
clivus	C41.0	C79.51	—	D16.4	D48.0	D49.2
coccygeal vertebra	C41.4	C79.51	—	D16.8	D48.0	D49.2
coccyx	C41.4	C79.51	—	D16.8	D48.0	D49.2
costal cartilage	C41.3	C79.51	—	D16.7	D48.0	D49.2
costovertebral joint	C41.3	C79.51	—	D16.7	D48.0	D49.2
cranial	C41.0	C79.51	—	D16.4	D48.0	D49.2
cuboid	C40.3-☑	C79.51	—	D16.3-☑	—	—
cuneiform	C41.9	C79.51	—	D16.9	D48.0	D49.2
elbow	C40.0-☑	C79.51	—	D16.0-☑	—	—
ethmoid (labyrinth)	C41.0	C79.51	—	D16.4	D48.0	D49.2
face	C41.0	C79.51	—	D16.4	D48.0	D49.2
femur (any part)	C40.2-☑	C79.51	—	D16.2-☑	—	—
fibula (any part)	C40.2-☑	C79.51	—	D16.2-☑	—	—
finger (any)	C40.1-☑	C79.51	—	D16.1-☑	—	—
foot	C40.3-☑	C79.51	—	D16.3-☑	—	—
forearm	C40.0-☑	C79.51	—	D16.0-☑	—	—
frontal	C41.0	C79.51	—	D16.4	D48.0	D49.2
hand	C40.1-☑	C79.51	—	D16.1-☑	—	—
heel	C40.3-☑	C79.51	—	D16.3-☑	—	—
hip	C41.4	C79.51	—	D16.8	D48.0	D49.2
humerus (any part)	C40.0-☑	C79.51	—	D16.0-☑	—	—
hyoid	C41.0	C79.51	—	D16.4	D48.0	D49.2
ilium	C41.4	C79.51	—	D16.8	D48.0	D49.2
innominate	C41.4	C79.51	—	D16.8	D48.0	D49.2
intervertebral cartilage or disc	C41.2	C79.51	—	D16.6	D48.0	D49.2
ischium	C41.4	C79.51	—	D16.8	D48.0	D49.2
jaw (lower)	C41.1	C79.51	—	D16.5	D48.0	D49.2
knee	C40.2-☑	C79.51	—	D16.2-☑	—	—
leg NEC	C40.2-☑	C79.51	—	D16.2-☑	—	—
limb NEC	C40.9-☑	C79.51	—	D16.9	—	—

Neoplasm, neoplastic
— continued
bone — continued
limb — continued

	Malignant Primary	Malignant Secondary	Ca in situ	Benign	Uncertain Behavior	Unspecified Behavior
lower (long bones)	C40.2-☑	C79.51	—	D16.2-☑	—	—
short bones	C40.3-☑	C79.51	—	D16.3-☑	—	—
upper (long bones)	C40.0-☑	C79.51	—	D16.0-☑	—	—
short bones	C40.1-☑	C79.51	—	D16.1-☑	—	—
malar	C41.0	C79.51	—	D16.4	D48.0	D49.2
mandible	C41.1	C79.51	—	D16.5	D48.0	D49.2
marrow NEC (any bone)	C96.9	C79.52	—	—	D47.9	D49.89
mastoid	C41.0	C79.51	—	D16.4	D48.0	D49.2
maxilla, maxillary (superior)	C41.0	C79.51	—	D16.4	D48.0	D49.2
inferior	C41.1	C79.51	—	D16.5	D48.0	D49.2
metacarpus (any)	C40.1-☑	C79.51	—	D16.1-☑	—	—
metatarsus (any)	C40.3-☑	C79.51	—	D16.3-☑	—	—
navicular						
ankle	C40.3-☑	C79.51	—	D16.3-☑	—	—
hand	C40.1-☑	C79.51	—	D16.1-☑	—	—
nose, nasal	C41.0	C79.51	—	D16.4	D48.0	D49.2
occipital	C41.0	C79.51	—	D16.4	D48.0	D49.2
orbit	C41.0	C79.51	—	D16.4	D48.0	D49.2
overlapping sites	C40.8-☑	—	—	—	—	—
parietal	C41.0	C79.51	—	D16.4	D48.0	D49.2
patella	C40.2-☑	C79.51	—	—	—	—
pelvic	C41.4	C79.51	—	D16.8	D48.0	D49.2
phalanges						
foot	C40.3-☑	C79.51	—	—	—	—
hand	C40.1-☑	C79.51	—	—	—	—
pubic	C41.4	C79.51	—	D16.8	D48.0	D49.2
radius (any part)	C40.0-☑	C79.51	—	D16.0-☑	—	—
rib	C41.3	C79.51	—	D16.7	D48.0	D49.2
sacral vertebra	C41.4	C79.51	—	D16.8	D48.0	D49.2
sacrum	C41.4	C79.51	—	D16.8	D48.0	D49.2
scaphoid						
of ankle	C40.3-☑	C79.51	—	—	—	—
of hand	C40.1-☑	C79.51	—	—	—	—
scapula (any part)	C40.0-☑	C79.51	—	D16.0-☑	—	—
sella turcica	C41.0	C79.51	—	D16.4	D48.0	D49.2
shoulder	C40.0-☑	C79.51	—	D16.0-☑	—	—
skull	C41.0	C79.51	—	D16.4	D48.0	D49.2
sphenoid	C41.0	C79.51	—	D16.4	D48.0	D49.2
spine, spinal (column)	C41.2	C79.51	—	D16.6	D48.0	D49.2
coccyx	C41.4	C79.51	—	D16.8	D48.0	D49.2
sacrum	C41.4	C79.51	—	D16.8	D48.0	D49.2
sternum	C41.3	C79.51	—	D16.7	D48.0	D49.2
tarsus (any)	C40.3-☑	C79.51	—	—	—	—
temporal	C41.0	C79.51	—	D16.4	D48.0	D49.2
thumb	C40.1-☑	C79.51	—	—	—	—
tibia (any part)	C40.2-☑	C79.51	—	—	—	—
toe (any)	C40.3-☑	C79.51	—	—	—	—
trapezium	C40.1-☑	C79.51	—	—	—	—
trapezoid	C40.1-☑	C79.51	—	—	—	—
turbinate	C41.0	C79.51	—	D16.4	D48.0	D49.2
ulna (any part)	C40.0-☑	C79.51	—	D16.0-☑	—	—
unciform	C40.1-☑	C79.51	—	—	—	—
vertebra (column)	C41.2	C79.51	—	D16.6	D48.0	D49.2
coccyx	C41.4	C79.51	—	D16.8	D48.0	D49.2
sacrum	C41.4	C79.51	—	D16.8	D48.0	D49.2
vomer	C41.0	C79.51	—	D16.4	D48.0	D49.2
wrist	C40.1-☑	C79.51	—	—	—	—
xiphoid process	C41.3	C79.51	—	D16.7	D48.0	D49.2
zygomatic	C41.0	C79.51	—	D16.4	D48.0	D49.2
book-leaf (mouth) — ventral surface of tongue and floor of mouth	C06.89	C79.89	D00.00	D10.39	D37.09	D49.0
bowel — see Neoplasm, intestine						
brachial plexus	C47.1-☑	C79.89	—	D36.12	D48.2	D49.2
brain NEC	C71.9	C79.31	—	D33.2	D43.2	D49.6

Neoplasm, neoplastic — continued
brain — continued

	Malignant Primary	Malignant Secondary	Ca in situ	Benign	Uncertain Behavior	Unspecified Behavior
basal ganglia	C71.0	C79.31	—	D33.0	D43.0	D49.6
cerebellopontine angle	C71.6	C79.31	—	D33.1	D43.1	D49.6
cerebellum NOS	C71.6	C79.31	—	D33.1	D43.1	D49.6
cerebrum	C71.0	C79.31	—	D33.0	D43.0	D49.6
choroid plexus	C71.7	C79.31	—	D33.1	D43.1	D49.6
corpus callosum	C71.8	C79.31	—	D33.2	D43.2	D49.6
corpus striatum	C71.0	C79.31	—	D33.0	D43.0	D49.6
cortex (cerebral)	C71.0	C79.31	—	D33.0	D43.0	D49.6
frontal lobe	C71.1	C79.31	—	D33.0	D43.0	D49.6
globus pallidus	C71.0	C79.31	—	D33.0	D43.0	D49.6
hippocampus	C71.2	C79.31	—	D33.0	D43.0	D49.6
hypothalamus	C71.0	C79.31	—	D33.0	D43.0	D49.6
internal capsule	C71.0	C79.31	—	D33.0	D43.0	D49.6
medulla oblongata	C71.7	C79.31	—	D33.1	D43.1	D49.6
meninges	C70.0	C79.32	—	D32.0	D42.0	D49.7
midbrain	C71.7	C79.31	—	D33.1	D43.1	D49.6
occipital lobe	C71.4	C79.31	—	D33.0	D43.0	D49.6
overlapping lesion	C71.8	C79.31	—	—	—	—
parietal lobe	C71.3	C79.31	—	D33.0	D43.0	D49.6
peduncle	C71.7	C79.31	—	D33.1	D43.1	D49.6
pons	C71.7	C79.31	—	D33.1	D43.1	D49.6
stem	C71.7	C79.31	—	D33.1	D43.1	D49.6
tapetum	C71.8	C79.31	—	D33.2	D43.2	D49.6
temporal lobe	C71.2	C79.31	—	D33.0	D43.0	D49.6
thalamus	C71.0	C79.31	—	D33.0	D43.0	D49.6
uncus	C71.2	C79.31	—	D33.0	D43.0	D49.6
ventricle (floor)	C71.5	C79.31	—	D33.0	D43.0	D49.6
fourth	C71.7	C79.31	—	D33.1	D43.1	D49.6
branchial (cleft) (cyst) (vestiges)	C10.4	C79.89	D00.08	D10.5	D37.05	D49.0
breast (connective tissue) (glandular tissue) (soft parts)	C50.9-☑	C79.81	D05.-☑	D24.-☑	D48.6-☑	D49.3
areola	C50.0-☑	C79.81	D05.-☑	D24.-☑	D48.6-☑	D49.3
axillary tail	C50.6-☑	C79.81	D05.-☑	D24.-☑	D48.6-☑	D49.3
central portion	C50.1-☑	C79.81	D05.-☑	D24.-☑	D48.6-☑	D49.3
inner	C50.8-☑	C79.81	D05.-☑	D24.-☑	D48.6-☑	D49.3
lower	C50.8-☑	C79.81	D05.-☑	D24.-☑	D48.6-☑	D49.3
lower-inner quadrant	C50.3-☑	C79.81	D05.-☑	D24.-☑	D48.6-☑	D49.3
lower-outer quadrant	C50.5-☑	C79.81	D05.-☑	D24.-☑	D48.6-☑	D49.3
mastectomy site (skin) — see also Neoplasm, breast, skin	C44.501	C79.2	—	—	—	—
specified as breast tissue	C50.8-☑	C79.81	—	—	—	—
midline	C50.8-☑	C79.81	D05.-☑	D24.-☑	D48.6-☑	D49.3
nipple	C50.0-☑	C79.81	D05.-☑	D24.-☑	D48.6-☑	D49.3
outer	C50.8-☑	C79.81	D05.-☑	D24.-☑	D48.6-☑	D49.3
overlapping lesion	C50.8-☑	—	—	—	—	—
skin	C44.501	C79.2	D04.5	D23.5	D48.5	D49.2
basal cell carcinoma	C44.511	—	—	—	—	—
specified type NEC	C44.591	—	—	—	—	—
squamous cell carcinoma	C44.521	—	—	—	—	—
tail (axillary)	C50.6-☑	C79.81	D05.-☑	D24.-☑	D48.6-☑	D49.3
upper	C50.8-☑	C79.81	D05.-☑	D24.-☑	D48.6-☑	D49.3
upper-inner quadrant	C50.2-☑	C79.81	D05.-☑	D24.-☑	D48.6-☑	D49.3
upper-outer quadrant	C50.4-☑	C79.81	D05.-☑	D24.-☑	D48.6-☑	D49.3
broad ligament	C57.1-☑	C79.82	D07.39	D28.2	D39.8	D49.59
bronchiogenic, bronchogenic (lung)	C34.9-☑	C78.0-☑	D02.2-☑	D14.3-☑	D38.1	D49.1
bronchiole	C34.9-☑	C78.0-☑	D02.2-☑	D14.3-☑	D38.1	D49.1
bronchus	C34.9-☑	C78.0-☑	D02.2-☑	D14.3-☑	D38.1	D49.1
carina	C34.0-☑	C78.0-☑	D02.2-☑	D14.3-☑	D38.1	D49.1
lower lobe of lung	C34.3-☑	C78.0-☑	D02.2-☑	D14.3-☑	D38.1	D49.1

Neoplasm, neoplastic — continued
bronchus — continued

	Malignant Primary	Malignant Secondary	Ca in situ	Benign	Uncertain Behavior	Unspecified Behavior
main	C34.0-☑	C78.0-☑	D02.2-☑	D14.3-☑	D38.1	D49.1
middle lobe of lung	C34.2	C78.0-☑	D02.21	D14.31	D38.1	D49.1
overlapping lesion	C34.8-☑	—	—	—	—	—
upper lobe of lung	C34.1-☑	C78.0-☑	D02.2-☑	D14.3-☑	D38.1	D49.1
brow	C44.309	C79.2	D04.39	D23.39	D48.5	D49.2
basal cell carcinoma	C44.319	—	—	—	—	—
specified type NEC	C44.399	—	—	—	—	—
squamous cell carcinoma	C44.329	—	—	—	—	—
buccal (cavity)	C06.9	C79.89	D00.00	D10.39	D37.09	D49.0
commissure	C06.0	C79.89	D00.02	D10.39	D37.09	D49.0
groove (lower) (upper)	C06.1	C79.89	D00.02	D10.39	D37.09	D49.0
mucosa	C06.0	C79.89	D00.02	D10.39	D37.09	D49.0
sulcus (lower) (upper)	C06.1	C79.89	D00.02	D10.39	D37.09	D49.0
bulbourethral gland	C68.0	C79.19	D09.19	D30.4	D41.3	D49.59
bursa — see Neoplasm, connective tissue						
buttock NEC	C76.3	C79.89	D04.5	D36.7	D48.7	D49.89
calf	C76.5-☑	C79.89	D04.7-☑	D36.7	D48.7	D49.89
calvarium	C41.0	C79.51	—	D16.4	D48.0	D49.2
calyx, renal	C65.-☑	C79.0-☑	D09.19	D30.1-☑	D41.1-☑	D49.51-☑
canal anal	C21.1	C78.5	D01.3	D12.9	D37.8	D49.0
auditory (external) — see also Neoplasm, skin, ear	C44.20-☑	C79.2	D04.2-☑	D23.2-☑	D48.5	D49.2
auricular (external) — see also Neoplasm, skin, ear	C44.20-☑	C79.2	D04.2-☑	D23.2-☑	D48.5	D49.2
canaliculi, biliary (biliferi) (intrahepatic)	C22.1	C78.7	D01.5	D13.4	D37.6	D49.0
canthus (eye) (inner) (outer)	C44.10-☑	C79.2	D04.1-☑	D23.1-☑	D48.5	D49.2
basal cell carcinoma	C44.11-☑	—	—	—	—	—
sebaceous cell	C44.13-☑	—	—	—	—	—
specified type NEC	C44.19-☑	—	—	—	—	—
squamous cell carcinoma	C44.12-☑	—	—	—	—	—
capillary — see Neoplasm, connective tissue						
caput coli	C18.0	C78.5	D01.0	D12.0	D37.4	D49.0
carcinoid — see Tumor, carcinoid						
cardia (gastric)	C16.0	C78.89	D00.2	D13.1	D37.1	D49.0
cardiac orifice (stomach)	C16.0	C78.89	D00.2	D13.1	D37.1	D49.0
cardio-esophageal junction	C16.0	C78.89	D00.2	D13.1	D37.1	D49.0
cardio-esophagus	C16.0	C78.89	D00.2	D13.1	D37.1	D49.0
carina (bronchus)	C34.0-☑	C78.0-☑	D02.2-☑	D14.3-☑	D38.1	D49.1
carotid (artery)	C49.0	C79.89	—	D21.0	D48.1	D49.2
body	C75.4	C79.89	—	D35.5	D44.6	D49.7
carpus (any bone)	C40.1-☑	C79.51	—	D16.1-☑	—	—
cartilage (articular) (joint) NEC — see also Neoplasm, bone						
arytenoid	C32.3	C78.39	D02.0	D14.1	D38.0	D49.1
auricular	C49.0	C79.89	—	D21.0	D48.1	D49.2
bronchi	C34.0-☑	C78.39	—	D14.3-☑	D38.1	D49.1
costal	C41.3	C79.51	—	D16.7	D48.0	D49.2
cricoid	C32.3	C78.39	D02.0	D14.1	D38.0	D49.1
cuneiform	C32.3	C78.39	D02.0	D14.1	D38.0	D49.1
ear (external)	C49.0	C79.89	—	D21.0	D48.1	D49.2
ensiform	C41.3	C79.51	—	D16.7	D48.0	D49.2
epiglottis	C32.1	C78.39	D02.0	D14.1	D38.0	D49.1

	Malignant Primary	Malignant Secondary	Ca in situ	Benign	Uncertain Behavior	Unspecified Behavior
Neoplasm, neoplastic						
— continued						
cartilage — see also						
Neoplasm, bone —						
continued						
epiglottis —						
continued						
anterior						
surface	C10.1	C79.89	D00.08	D10.5	D37.05	D49.0
eyelid	C49.0	C79.89	—	D21.0	D48.1	D49.2
intervertebral	C41.2	C79.51	—	D16.6	D48.0	D49.2
larynx, laryngeal	C32.3	C78.39	D02.0	D14.1	D38.0	D49.1
nose, nasal	C30.0	C78.39	D02.3	D14.0	D38.5	D49.1
pinna	C49.0	C79.89	—	D21.0	D48.1	D49.2
rib	C41.3	C79.51	—	D16.7	D48.0	D49.2
semilunar						
(knee)	C40.2-☑	C79.51	—	D16.2-☑	D48.0	D49.2
thyroid	C32.3	C78.39	D02.0	D14.1	D38.0	D49.1
trachea	C33	C78.39	D02.1	D14.2	D38.1	D49.1
cauda equina	C72.1	C79.49	—	D33.4	D43.4	D49.7
cavity						
buccal	C06.9	C79.89	D00.00	D10.30	D37.09	D49.0
nasal	C30.0	C78.39	D02.3	D14.0	D38.5	D49.1
oral	C06.9	C79.89	D00.00	D10.30	D37.09	D49.0
peritoneal	C48.2	C78.6	—	D20.1	D48.4	D49.0
tympanic	C30.1	C78.39	D02.3	D14.0	D38.5	D49.1
cecum	C18.0	C78.5	D01.0	D12.0	D37.4	D49.0
central nervous						
system	C72.9	C79.40	—	—	—	—
cerebellopontine						
(angle)	C71.6	C79.31		D33.1	D43.1	D49.6
cerebellum,						
cerebellar	C71.6	C79.31		D33.1	D43.1	D49.6
cerebrum, cerebra						
(cortex)						
(hemisphere)						
(white matter)	C71.0	C79.31	—	D33.0	D43.0	D49.6
meninges	C70.0	C79.32	—	D32.0	D42.0	D49.7
peduncle	C71.7	C79.31	—	D33.1	D43.1	D49.6
ventricle	C71.5	C79.31	—	D33.0	D43.0	D49.6
fourth	C71.7	C79.31	—	D33.1	D43.1	D49.6
cervical region	C76.0	C79.89	D09.8	D36.7	D48.7	D49.89
cervix (cervical) (uteri)						
(uterus)	C53.9	C79.82	D06.9	D26.0	D39.0	D49.59
canal	C53.0	C79.82	D06.0	D26.0	D39.0	D49.59
endocervix (canal)						
(gland)	C53.0	C79.82	D06.0	D26.0	D39.0	D49.59
exocervix	C53.1	C79.82	D06.1	D26.0	D39.0	D49.59
external os	C53.1	C79.82	D06.1	D26.0	D39.0	D49.59
internal os	C53.0	C79.82	D06.0	D26.0	D39.0	D49.59
nabothian gland	C53.0	C79.82	D06.0	D26.0	D39.0	D49.59
overlapping						
lesion	C53.8	—	—	—	—	—
squamocolumnar						
junction	C53.8	C79.82	D06.7	D26.0	D39.0	D49.59
stump	C53.8	C79.82	D06.7	D26.0	D39.0	D49.59
cheek	C76.0	C79.89	D09.8	D36.7	D48.7	D49.89
external	C44.309	C79.2	D04.39	D23.39	D48.5	D49.2
basal cell						
carcinoma	C44.319	—	—	—	—	—
specified type						
NEC	C44.399	—	—	—	—	—
squamous cell						
carcinoma	C44.329	—	—	—	—	—
inner aspect	C06.0	C79.89	D00.02	D10.39	D37.09	D49.0
internal	C06.0	C79.89	D00.02	D10.39	D37.09	D49.0
mucosa	C06.0	C79.89	D00.02	D10.39	D37.09	D49.0
chest (wall) NEC	C76.1	C79.89	D09.8	D36.7	D48.7	D49.89
chiasma opticum	C72.3-☑	C79.49	—	D33.3	D43.3	D49.7
chin	C44.309	C79.2	D04.39	D23.39	D48.5	D49.2
basal cell						
carcinoma	C44.319	—	—	—	—	—
specified type						
NEC	C44.399	—	—	—	—	—
squamous cell						
carcinoma	C44.329	—	—	—	—	—
choana	C11.3	C79.89	D00.08	D10.6	D37.05	D49.0
cholangiole	C22.1	C78.89	D01.5	D13.4	D37.6	D49.0
choledochal duct	C24.0	C78.89	D01.5	D13.5	D37.6	D49.0
choroid	C69.3-☑	C79.49	D09.2-☑	D31.3-☑	D48.7	D49.81
plexus	C71.5	C79.31	—	D33.0	D43.0	D49.6
ciliary body	C69.4-☑	C79.49	D09.2-☑	D31.4-☑	D48.7	D49.89
clavicle	C41.3	C79.51	—	D16.7	D48.0	D49.2

	Malignant Primary	Malignant Secondary	Ca in situ	Benign	Uncertain Behavior	Unspecified Behavior
Neoplasm, neoplastic						
— continued						
clitoris	C51.2	C79.82	D07.1	D28.0	D39.8	D49.59
clivus	C41.0	C79.51	—	D16.4	D48.0	D49.2
cloacogenic zone	C21.2	C78.5	D01.3	D12.9	D37.8	D49.0
coccygeal						
body or glomus	C49.5	C79.89	—	D21.5	D48.1	D49.2
vertebra	C41.4	C79.51	—	D16.8	D48.0	D49.2
coccyx	C41.4	C79.51	—	D16.8	D48.0	D49.2
colon — see also						
Neoplasm,						
intestine,						
large	C18.9	C78.5		—	—	—
with rectum	C19	C78.5	D01.1	D12.7	D37.5	D49.0
columnella — see also						
Neoplasm, skin,						
face	C44.390	C79.2	D04.39	D23.39	D48.5	D49.2
column, spinal — see						
Neoplasm, spine						
commissure						
labial, lip	C00.6	C79.89	D00.01	D10.39	D37.01	D49.0
laryngeal	C32.0	C78.39	D02.0	D14.1	D38.0	D49.1
common (bile)						
duct	C24.0	C78.89	D01.5	D13.5	D37.6	D49.0
concha — see also						
Neoplasm, skin,						
ear	C44.20-☑	C79.2	D04.2-☑	D23.2-☑	D48.5	D49.2
nose	C30.0	C78.39	D02.3	D14.0	D38.5	D49.1
conjunctiva	C69.0-☑	C79.49	D09.2-☑	D31.0-☑	D48.7	D49.89
connective tissue						
NEC	C49.9	C79.89		D21.9	D48.1	D49.2

Note: For neoplasms of connective tissue (blood vessel, bursa, fascia, ligament, muscle, peripheral nerves, sympathetic and parasympathetic nerves and ganglia, synovia, tendon, etc.) or of morphological types that indicate connective tissue, code according to the list under "Neoplasm, connective tissue". For sites that do not appear in this list, code to neoplasm of that site; e.g., fibrosarcoma, pancreas (C25.9)

Note: Morphological types that indicate connective tissue appear in their proper place in the alphabetic index with the instruction "see Neoplasm, connective tissue ...."

	Malignant Primary	Malignant Secondary	Ca in situ	Benign	Uncertain Behavior	Unspecified Behavior
abdomen	C49.4	C79.89	—	D21.4	D48.1	D49.2
abdominal wall	C49.4	C79.89	—	D21.4	D48.1	D49.2
ankle	C49.2-☑	C79.89	—	D21.2-☑	D48.1	D49.2
antecubital fossa or						
space	C49.1-☑	C79.89	—	D21.1-☑	D48.1	D49.2
arm	C49.1-☑	C79.89	—	D21.1-☑	D48.1	D49.2
auricle (ear)	C49.0	C79.89	—	D21.0	D48.1	D49.2
axilla	C49.3	C79.89	—	D21.3	D48.1	D49.2
back	C49.6	C79.89	—	D21.6	D48.1	D49.2
breast — see						
Neoplasm,						
breast						
buttock	C49.5	C79.89	—	D21.5	D48.1	D49.2
calf	C49.2-☑	C79.89	—	D21.2-☑	D48.1	D49.2
cervical region	C49.0	C79.89	—	D21.0	D48.1	D49.2
cheek	C49.0	C79.89	—	D21.0	D48.1	D49.2
chest (wall)	C49.3	C79.89	—	D21.3	D48.1	D49.2
chin	C49.0	C79.89	—	D21.0	D48.1	D49.2
diaphragm	C49.3	C79.89	—	D21.3	D48.1	D49.2
ear (external)	C49.0	C79.89	—	D21.0	D48.1	D49.2
elbow	C49.1-☑	C79.89	—	D21.1-☑	D48.1	D49.2
extrarectal	C49.5	C79.89	—	D21.5	D48.1	D49.2
extremity	C49.9	C79.89	—	D21.9	D48.1	D49.2
lower	C49.2-☑	C79.89	—	D21.2-☑	D48.1	D49.2
upper	C49.1-☑	C79.89	—	D21.1-☑	D48.1	D49.2
eyelid	C49.0	C79.89	—	D21.0	D48.1	D49.2
face	C49.0	C79.89	—	D21.0	D48.1	D49.2
finger	C49.1-☑	C79.89	—	D21.1-☑	D48.1	D49.2
flank	C49.6	C79.89	—	D21.6	D48.1	D49.2
foot	C49.2-☑	C79.89	—	D21.2-☑	D48.1	D49.2
forearm	C49.1-☑	C79.89	—	D21.1-☑	D48.1	D49.2
forehead	C49.0	C79.89	—	D21.0	D48.1	D49.2
gastric	C49.4	C79.89	—	D21.4	D48.1	D49.2
gastrointestinal	C49.4	C79.89	—	D21.4	D48.1	D49.2
gluteal region	C49.5	C79.89	—	D21.5	D48.1	D49.2
great vessels						
NEC	C49.3	C79.89	—	D21.3	D48.1	D49.2
groin	C49.5	C79.89	—	D21.5	D48.1	D49.2
hand	C49.1-☑	C79.89	—	D21.1-☑	D48.1	D49.2
head	C49.0	C79.89	—	D21.0	D48.1	D49.2

Neoplasm, neoplastic
— *continued*
connective tissue — *continued*

	Malignant Primary	Malignant Secondary	Ca in situ	Benign	Uncertain Behavior	Unspecified Behavior
heel	C49.2-☑	C79.89	—	D21.2-☑	D48.1	D49.2
hip	C49.2-☑	C79.89	—	D21.2-☑	D48.1	D49.2
hypochondrium	C49.4	C79.89	—	D21.4	D48.1	D49.2
iliopsoas muscle	C49.5	C79.89	—	D21.5	D48.1	D49.2
infraclavicular region	C49.3	C79.89	—	D21.3	D48.1	D49.2
inguinal (canal) (region)	C49.5	C79.89	—	D21.5	D48.1	D49.2
intestinal	C49.4	C79.89	—	D21.4	D48.1	D49.2
intrathoracic	C49.3	C79.89	—	D21.3	D48.1	D49.2
ischiorectal fossa	C49.5	C79.89	—	D21.5	D48.1	D49.2
jaw	C03.9	C79.89	D00.03	D10.39	D48.1	D49.0
knee	C49.2-☑	C79.89	—	D21.2-☑	D48.1	D49.2
leg	C49.2-☑	C79.89	—	D21.2-☑	D48.1	D49.2
limb NEC	C49.9	C79.89	—	D21.9	D48.1	D49.2
lower	C49.2-☑	C79.89	—	D21.2-☑	D48.1	D49.2
upper	C49.1-☑	C79.89	—	D21.1-☑	D48.1	D49.2
nates	C49.5	C79.89	—	D21.5	D48.1	D49.2
neck	C49.0	C79.89	—	D21.0	D48.1	D49.2
orbit	C69.6-☑	C79.49	D09.2-☑	D31.6-☑	D48.1	D49.89
overlapping lesion	C49.8	—	—	—	—	—
pararectal	C49.5	C79.89	—	D21.5	D48.1	D49.2
para-urethral	C49.5	C79.89	—	D21.5	D48.1	D49.2
paravaginal	C49.5	C79.89	—	D21.5	D48.1	D49.2
pelvis (floor)	C49.5	C79.89	—	D21.5	D48.1	D49.2
pelvo-abdominal	C49.8	C79.89	—	D21.6	D48.1	D49.2
perineum	C49.5	C79.89	—	D21.5	D48.1	D49.2
perirectal (tissue)	C49.5	C79.89	—	D21.5	D48.1	D49.2
periurethral (tissue)	C49.5	C79.89	—	D21.5	D48.1	D49.2
popliteal fossa or space	C49.2-☑	C79.89	—	D21.2-☑	D48.1	D49.2
presacral	C49.5	C79.89	—	D21.5	D48.1	D49.2
psoas muscle	C49.4	C79.89	—	D21.4	D48.1	D49.2
pterygoid fossa	C49.0	C79.89	—	D21.0	D48.1	D49.2
rectovaginal septum or wall	C49.5	C79.89	—	D21.5	D48.1	D49.2
rectovesical	C49.5	C79.89	—	D21.5	D48.1	D49.2
retroperitoneum	C48.0	C78.6	—	D20.0	D48.3	D49.0
sacrococcygeal region	C49.5	C79.89	—	D21.5	D48.1	D49.2
scalp	C49.0	C79.89	—	D21.0	D48.1	D49.2
scapular region	C49.3	C79.89	—	D21.3	D48.1	D49.2
shoulder	C49.1-☑	C79.89	—	D21.1-☑	D48.1	D49.2
skin (dermis) NEC — see also Neoplasm, skin, by site	C44.90	C79.2	D04.9	D23.9	D48.5	D49.2
stomach	C49.4	C79.89	—	D21.4	D48.1	D49.2
submental	C49.0	C79.89	—	D21.0	D48.1	D49.2
supraclavicular region	C49.0	C79.89	—	D21.0	D48.1	D49.2
temple	C49.0	C79.89	—	D21.0	D48.1	D49.2
temporal region	C49.0	C79.89	—	D21.0	D48.1	D49.2
thigh	C49.2-☑	C79.89	—	D21.2-☑	D48.1	D49.2
thoracic (duct) (wall)	C49.3	C79.89	—	D21.3	D48.1	D49.2
thorax	C49.3	C79.89	—	D21.3	D48.1	D49.2
thumb	C49.1-☑	C79.89	—	D21.1-☑	D48.1	D49.2
toe	C49.2-☑	C79.89	—	D21.2-☑	D48.1	D49.2
trunk	C49.6	C79.89	—	D21.6	D48.1	D49.2
umbilicus	C49.4	C79.89	—	D21.4	D48.1	D49.2
vesicorectal	C49.5	C79.89	—	D21.5	D48.1	D49.2
wrist	C49.1-☑	C79.89	—	D21.1-☑	D48.1	D49.2
conus medullaris	C72.0	C79.49	—	D33.4	D43.4	D49.7
cord (true) (vocal)	C32.0	C78.39	D02.0	D14.1	D38.0	D49.1
false	C32.1	C78.39	D02.0	D14.1	D38.0	D49.1
spermatic	C63.1-☑	C79.82	D07.69	D29.8	D40.8	D49.59
spinal (cervical) (lumbar) (thoracic)	C72.0	C79.49	—	D33.4	D43.4	D49.7
cornea (limbus)	C69.1-☑	C79.49	D09.2-☑	D31.1-☑	D48.7	D49.89
corpus						
albicans	C56.-☑	C79.6-☑	D07.39	D27.-☑	D39.1-☑	D49.59
callosum, brain	C71.0	C79.31	—	D33.2	D43.2	D49.6

Neoplasm, neoplastic
— *continued*
corpus — *continued*

	Malignant Primary	Malignant Secondary	Ca in situ	Benign	Uncertain Behavior	Unspecified Behavior
cavernosum	C60.2	C79.82	D07.4	D29.0	D40.8	D49.59
gastric	C16.2	C78.89	D00.2	D13.1	D37.1	D49.0
overlapping sites	C54.8	—	—	—	—	—
penis	C60.2	C79.82	D07.4	D29.0	D40.8	D49.59
striatum, cerebrum	C71.0	C79.31	—	D33.0	D43.0	D49.6
uteri	C54.9	C79.82	D07.0	D26.1	D39.0	D49.59
isthmus	C54.0	C79.82	D07.0	D26.1	D39.0	D49.59
cortex						
adrenal	C74.0-☑	C79.7-☑	D09.3	D35.0-☑	D44.1-☑	D49.7
cerebral	C71.0	C79.31	—	D33.0	D43.0	D49.6
costal cartilage	C41.3	C79.51	—	D16.7	D48.0	D49.2
costovertebral joint	C41.3	C79.51	—	D16.7	D48.0	D49.2
Cowper's gland	C68.0	C79.19	D09.19	D30.4	D41.3	D49.59
cranial (fossa, any)	C71.9	C79.31	—	D33.2	D43.2	D49.6
meninges	C70.0	C79.32	—	D32.0	D42.0	D49.7
nerve	C72.50	C79.49	—	D33.3	D43.3	D49.7
specified NEC	C72.59	C79.49	—	D33.3	D43.3	D49.7
craniobuccal pouch	C75.2	C79.89	D09.3	D35.2	D44.3	D49.7
craniopharyngeal (duct) (pouch)	C75.2	C79.89	D09.3	D35.3	D44.4	D49.7
cricoid	C13.0	C79.89	D00.08	D10.7	D37.05	D49.0
cartilage	C32.3	C78.39	D02.0	D14.1	D38.0	D49.1
cricopharynx	C13.0	C79.89	D00.08	D10.7	D37.05	D49.0
crypt of Morgagni	C21.8	C78.5	D01.3	D12.9	D37.8	D49.0
crystalline lens	C69.4-☑	C79.49	D09.2-☑	D31.4-☑	D48.7	D49.89
cul-de-sac (Douglas')	C48.1	C78.6	—	D20.1	D48.4	D49.0
cuneiform cartilage	C32.3	C78.39	D02.0	D14.1	D38.0	D49.1
cutaneous — see Neoplasm, skin						
cutis — see Neoplasm, skin						
cystic (bile) duct (common)	C24.0	C78.89	D01.5	D13.5	D37.6	D49.0
dermis — see Neoplasm, skin						
diaphragm	C49.3	C79.89	—	D21.3	D48.1	D49.2
digestive organs, system, tube, or tract NEC	C26.9	C78.89	D01.9	D13.9	D37.9	D49.0
disc, intervertebral	C41.2	C79.51	—	D16.6	D48.0	D49.2
disease, generalized	C80.0	—	—	—	—	—
disseminated	C80.0	—	—	—	—	—
Douglas' cul-de-sac or pouch	C48.1	C78.6	—	D20.1	D48.4	D49.0
duodenojejunal junction	C17.8	C78.4	D01.49	D13.39	D37.2	D49.0
duodenum	C17.0	C78.4	D01.49	D13.2	D37.2	D49.0
dura (cranial) (mater)	C70.9	C79.49	—	D32.9	D42.9	D49.7
cerebral	C70.0	C79.32	—	D32.0	D42.0	D49.7
spinal	C70.1	C79.49	—	D32.1	D42.1	D49.7
ear (external) — see also Neoplasm, skin, ear	C44.20-☑	C79.2	D04.2-☑	D23.2-☑	D48.5	D49.2
auricle or auris — see also Neoplasm, skin, ear	C44.20-☑	C79.2	D04.2-☑	D23.2-☑	D48.5	D49.2
canal, external — see also Neoplasm, skin, ear	C44.20-☑	C79.2	D04.2-☑	D23.2-☑	D48.5	D49.2
cartilage	C49.0	C79.89	—	D21.0	D48.1	D49.2
external meatus — see also Neoplasm, skin, ear	C44.20-☑	C79.2	D04.2-☑	D23.2-☑	D48.5	D49.2
inner	C30.1	C78.39	D02.3	D14.0	D38.5	D49.1
lobule — see also Neoplasm, skin, ear	C44.20-☑	C79.2	D04.2-☑	D23.2-☑	D48.5	D49.2
middle	C30.1	C78.39	D02.3	D14.0	D38.5	D49.1
overlapping lesion with accessory sinuses	C31.8	—	—	—	—	—

☑ Additional Character Required — Refer to the Tabular List for Character Selection   ⓥ Subterms under main terms may continue to next column or page

Neoplasm, neoplastic — continued

	Malignant Primary	Malignant Secondary	Ca in situ	Benign	Uncertain Behavior	Unspecified Behavior
Neoplasm, neoplastic						
— *continued*						
ear — *see also*						
Neoplasm, skin, ear						
— *continued*						
skin	C44.20-☑	C79.2	D04.2-☑	D23.2-☑	D48.5	D49.2
basal cell						
carcinoma	C44.21-☑	—	—	—	—	—
specified type						
NEC	C44.29-☑	—	—	—	—	—
squamous cell						
carcinoma	C44.22-☑	—	—	—	—	—
earlobe	C44.20-☑	C79.2	D04.2-☑	D23.2-☑	D48.5	D49.2
basal cell						
carcinoma	C44.21-☑	—	—	—	—	—
specified type						
NEC	C44.29-☑	—	—	—	—	—
squamous cell						
carcinoma	C44.22-☑	—	—	—	—	—
ejaculatory duct	C63.7	C79.82	D07.69	D29.8	D40.8	D49.59
elbow NEC	C76.4-☑	C79.89	D04.6-☑	D36.7	D48.7	D49.89
endocardium	C38.0	C79.89		D15.1	D48.7	D49.89
endocervix (canal)						
(gland)	C53.0	C79.82	D06.0	D26.0	D39.0	D49.59
endocrine gland						
NEC	C75.9	C79.89	D09.3	D35.9	D44.9	D49.7
pluriglandular	C75.8	C79.89	D09.3	D35.7	D44.9	D49.7
endometrium (gland)						
(stroma)	C54.1	C79.82	D07.0	D26.1	D39.0	D49.59
ensiform cartilage	C41.3	C79.51	—	D16.7	D48.0	D49.2
enteric — *see*						
Neoplasm,						
intestine						
ependyma (brain)	C71.5	C79.31	—	D33.0	D43.0	D49.6
fourth ventricle	C71.7	C79.31	—	D33.1	D43.1	D49.6
epicardium	C38.0	C79.89		D15.1	D48.7	D49.89
epididymis	C63.0-☑	C79.82	D07.69	D29.3-☑	D40.8	D49.59
epidural	C72.9	C79.49		D33.9	D43.9	D49.7
epiglottis	C32.1	C78.39	D02.0	D14.1	D38.0	D49.1
anterior aspect or						
surface	C10.1	C79.89	D00.08	D10.5	D37.05	D49.0
cartilage	C32.3	C78.39	D02.0	D14.1	D38.0	D49.1
free border						
(margin)	C10.1	C79.89	D00.08	D10.5	D37.05	D49.0
junctional						
region	C10.8	C79.89	D00.08	D10.5	D37.05	D49.0
posterior (laryngeal)						
surface	C32.1	C78.39	D02.0	D14.1	D38.0	D49.1
suprahyoid						
portion	C32.1	C78.39	D02.0	D14.1	D38.0	D49.1
esophagogastric						
junction	C16.0	C78.89	D00.2	D13.1	D37.1	D49.0
esophagus	C15.9	C78.89	D00.1	D13.0	D37.8	D49.0
abdominal	C15.5	C78.89	D00.1	D13.0	D37.8	D49.0
cervical	C15.3	C78.89	D00.1	D13.0	D37.8	D49.0
distal (third)	C15.5	C78.89	D00.1	D13.0	D37.8	D49.0
lower (third)	C15.5	C78.89	D00.1	D13.0	D37.8	D49.0
middle (third)	C15.4	C78.89	D00.1	D13.0	D37.8	D49.0
overlapping						
lesion	C15.8	—	—	—	—	—
proximal (third)	C15.3	C78.89	D00.1	D13.0	D37.8	D49.0
thoracic	C15.4	C78.89	D00.1	D13.0	D37.8	D49.0
upper (third)	C15.3	C78.89	D00.1	D13.0	D37.8	D49.0
ethmoid (sinus)	C31.1	C78.39	D02.3	D14.0	D38.5	D49.1
bone or						
labyrinth	C41.0	C79.51	—	D16.4	D48.0	D49.2
eustachian tube	C30.1	C78.39	D02.3	D14.0	D38.5	D49.1
exocervix	C53.1	C79.82	D06.1	D26.0	D39.0	D49.59
external						
meatus (ear) — *see*						
also Neoplasm,						
skin, ear	C44.20-☑	C79.2	D04.2-☑	D23.2-☑	D48.5	D49.2
os, cervix uteri	C53.1	C79.82	D06.1	D26.0	D39.0	D49.59
extradural	C72.9	C79.49	—	D33.9	D43.9	D49.7
extrahepatic (bile)						
duct	C24.0	C78.89	D01.5	D13.5	D37.6	D49.0
overlapping lesion						
with						
gallbladder	C24.8	—	—	—	—	—
extraocular						
muscle	C69.6-☑	C79.49	D09.2-☑	D31.6-☑	D48.7	D49.89
extrarectal	C76.3	C79.89	D09.8	D36.7	D48.7	D49.89
extremity	C76.8	C79.89	D04.8	D36.7	D48.7	D49.89

Neoplasm, neoplastic — continued

	Malignant Primary	Malignant Secondary	Ca in situ	Benign	Uncertain Behavior	Unspecified Behavior
Neoplasm, neoplastic						
— *continued*						
extremity — *continued*						
lower	C76.5-☑	C79.89	D04.7-☑	D36.7	D48.7	D49.89
upper	C76.4-☑	C79.89	D04.6-☑	D36.7	D48.7	D49.89
eyeball	C69.9-☑	C79.49	D09.2-☑	D31.9-☑	D48.7	D49.89
eyebrow	C44.309	C79.2	D04.39	D23.39	D48.5	D49.2
basal cell						
carcinoma	C44.319	—	—	—	—	—
specified type						
NEC	C44.399	—	—	—	—	—
squamous cell						
carcinoma	C44.329	—	—	—	—	—
eyelid (lower) (skin)						
(upper)	C44.10-☑	—	—	—	—	—
basal cell						
carcinoma	C44.11-☑	—	—	—	—	—
cartilage	C49.0	C79.89	—	D21.0	D48.1	D49.2
sebaceous cell	C44.13-☑	—	—	—	—	—
specified type						
NEC	C44.19-☑	—	—	—	—	—
squamous cell						
carcinoma	C44.12-☑	—	—	—	—	—
eye NEC	C69.9-☑	C79.49	D09.2-☑	D31.9-☑	D48.7	D49.89
overlapping						
sites	C69.8-☑	—	—	—	—	—
face NEC	C76.0	C79.89	D04.39	D36.7	D48.7	D49.89
fallopian tube						
(accessory)	C57.0-☑	C79.82	D07.39	D28.2	D39.8	D49.59
falx (cerebella)						
(cerebri)	C70.0	C79.32	—	D32.0	D42.0	D49.7
fascia — *see also*						
Neoplasm,						
connective tissue						
palmar	C49.1-☑	C79.89	—	D21.1-☑	D48.1	D49.2
plantar	C49.2-☑	C79.89	—	D21.2-☑	D48.1	D49.2
fatty tissue — *see*						
Neoplasm,						
connective tissue						
fauces, faucial NEC	C10.9	C79.89	D00.08	D10.5	D37.05	D49.0
pillars	C09.1	C79.89	D00.08	D10.5	D37.05	D49.0
tonsil	C09.9	C79.89	D00.08	D10.4	D37.05	D49.0
femur (any part)	C40.2-☑	—	—	D16.2-☑	—	—
fetal membrane	C58	C79.82	D07.0	D26.7	D39.2	D49.59
fibrous tissue — *see*						
Neoplasm,						
connective tissue						
fibula (any part)	C40.2-☑	C79.51	—	D16.2-☑	—	—
filum terminale	C72.0	C79.49	—	D33.4	D43.4	D49.7
finger NEC	C76.4-☑	C79.89	D04.6-☑	D36.7	D48.7	D49.89
flank NEC	C76.8	C79.89	D04.5	D36.7	D48.7	D49.89
follicle, nabothian	C53.0	C79.82	D06.0	D26.0	D39.0	D49.59
foot NEC	C76.5-☑	C79.89	D04.7-☑	D36.7	D48.7	D49.89
forearm NEC	C76.4-☑	C79.89	D04.6-☑	D36.7	D48.7	D49.89
forehead (skin)	C44.309	C79.2	D04.39	D23.39	D48.5	D49.2
basal cell						
carcinoma	C44.319	—	—	—	—	—
specified type						
NEC	C44.399	—	—	—	—	—
squamous cell						
carcinoma	C44.329	—	—	—	—	—
foreskin	C60.0	C79.82	D07.4	D29.0	D40.8	D49.59
fornix						
pharyngeal	C11.3	C79.89	D00.08	D10.6	D37.05	D49.0
vagina	C52	C79.82	D07.2	D28.1	D39.8	D49.59
fossa (of)						
anterior (cranial)	C71.9	C79.31	—	D33.2	D43.2	D49.6
cranial	C71.9	C79.31	—	D33.2	D43.2	D49.6
ischiorectal	C76.3	C79.89	D09.8	D36.7	D48.7	D49.89
middle (cranial)	C71.9	C79.31	—	D33.2	D43.2	D49.6
piriform	C12	C79.89	D00.08	D10.7	D37.05	D49.0
pituitary	C75.1	C79.89	D09.3	D35.2	D44.3	D49.7
posterior						
(cranial)	C71.9	C79.31	—	D33.2	D43.2	D49.6
pterygoid	C49.0	C79.89	—	D21.0	D48.1	D49.2
pyriform	C12	C79.89	D00.08	D10.7	D37.05	D49.0
Rosenmuller	C11.2	C79.89	D00.08	D10.6	D37.05	D49.0
tonsillar	C09.9	C79.89	D00.08	D10.5	D37.05	D49.0
fourchette	C51.9	C79.82	D07.1	D28.0	D39.8	D49.59
frenulum						
labii — *see*						
Neoplasm, lip,						
internal						

	Malignant Primary	Malignant Secondary	Ca in situ	Benign	Uncertain Behavior	Unspecified Behavior
Neoplasm, neoplastic						
— *continued*						
frenulum — *continued*						
linguae	C02.2	C79.89	D00.07	D10.1	D37.02	D49.0
frontal						
bone	C41.0	C79.51	—	D16.4	D48.0	D49.2
lobe, brain	C71.1	C79.31	—	D33.0	D43.0	D49.6
pole	C71.1	C79.31	—	D33.0	D43.0	D49.6
sinus	C31.2	C78.39	D02.3	D14.0	D38.5	D49.1
fundus						
stomach	C16.1	C78.89	D00.2	D13.1	D37.1	D49.0
uterus	C54.3	C79.82	D07.0	D26.1	D39.0	D49.59
gallbladder	C23	C78.89	D01.5	D13.5	D37.6	D49.0
overlapping lesion with extrahepatic bile ducts	C24.8	—	—	—	—	—
gall duct (extrahepatic)	C24.0	C78.89	D01.5	D13.5	D37.6	D49.0
intrahepatic	C22.1	C78.7	D01.5	D13.4	D37.6	D49.0
ganglia — *see also* Neoplasm, nerve, peripheral	C47.9	C79.89	—	D36.10	D48.2	D49.2
basal	C71.0	C79.31	—	D33.0	D43.0	D49.6
cranial nerve	C72.50	C79.49	—	D33.3	D43.3	D49.7
Gartner's duct	C52	C79.82	D07.2	D28.1	D39.8	D49.59
gastric — *see* Neoplasm, stomach						
gastrocolic	C26.9	C78.89	D01.9	D13.9	D37.9	D49.0
gastroesophageal junction	C16.0	C78.89	D00.2	D13.1	D37.1	D49.0
gastrointestinal (tract) NEC	C26.9	C78.89	D01.9	D13.9	D37.9	D49.0
generalized	C80.0	—	—	—	—	—
genital organ or tract						
female NEC	C57.9	C79.82	D07.30	D28.9	D39.9	D49.59
overlapping lesion	C57.8	—	—	—	—	—
specified site NEC	C57.7	C79.82	D07.39	D28.7	D39.8	D49.59
male NEC	C63.9	C79.82	D07.60	D29.9	D40.9	D49.59
overlapping lesion	C63.8	—	—	—	—	—
specified site NEC	C63.7	C79.82	D07.69	D29.8	D40.8	D49.59
genitourinary tract						
female	C57.9	C79.82	D07.30	D28.9	D39.9	D49.59
male	C63.9	C79.82	D07.60	D29.9	D40.9	D49.59
gingiva (alveolar) (marginal)	C03.9	C79.89	D00.03	D10.39	D37.09	D49.0
lower	C03.1	C79.89	D00.03	D10.39	D37.09	D49.0
mandibular	C03.1	C79.89	D00.03	D10.39	D37.09	D49.0
maxillary	C03.0	C79.89	D00.03	D10.39	D37.09	D49.0
upper	C03.0	C79.89	D00.03	D10.39	D37.09	D49.0
gland, glandular (lymphatic) (system) — *see also* Neoplasm, lymph gland						
endocrine NEC	C75.9	C79.89	D09.3	D35.9	D44.9	D49.7
salivary — *see* Neoplasm, salivary gland						
glans penis	C60.1	C79.82	D07.4	D29.0	D40.8	D49.59
globus pallidus	C71.0	C79.31	—	D33.0	D43.0	D49.6
glomus						
coccygeal	C49.5	C79.89	—	D21.5	D48.1	D49.2
jugularis	C75.5	C79.89	—	D35.6	D44.7	D49.7
glosso-epiglottic fold(s)	C10.1	C79.89	D00.08	D10.5	D37.05	D49.0
glossopalatine fold	C09.1	C79.89	D00.08	D10.5	D37.05	D49.0
glossopharyngeal sulcus	C09.0	C79.89	D00.08	D10.5	D37.05	D49.0
glottis	C32.0	C78.39	D02.0	D14.1	D38.0	D49.1
gluteal region	C76.3	C79.89	D04.5	D36.7	D48.7	D49.89
great vessels NEC	C49.3	C79.89	—	D21.3	D48.1	D49.2
groin NEC	C76.3	C79.89	D04.5	D36.7	D48.7	D49.89
gum	C03.9	C79.89	D00.03	D10.39	D37.09	D49.0
lower	C03.1	C79.89	D00.03	D10.39	D37.09	D49.0
upper	C03.0	C79.89	D00.03	D10.39	D37.09	D49.0
hand NEC	C76.4-☑	C79.89	D04.6-☑	D36.7	D48.7	D49.89
head NEC	C76.0	C79.89	D04.4	D36.7	D48.7	D49.89
heart	C38.0	C79.89	—	D15.1	D48.7	D49.89

	Malignant Primary	Malignant Secondary	Ca in situ	Benign	Uncertain Behavior	Unspecified Behavior
Neoplasm, neoplastic						
— *continued*						
heel NEC	C76.5-☑	C79.89	D04.7-☑	D36.7	D48.7	D49.89
helix — *see also* Neoplasm, skin, ear	C44.20-☑	C79.2	D04.2-☑	D23.2-☑	D48.5	D49.2
hematopoietic, hemopoietic tissue NEC	C96.9	—	—	—	—	—
specified NEC	C96.Z	—	—	—	—	—
hemisphere, cerebral	C71.0	C79.31	—	D33.0	D43.0	D49.6
hemorrhoidal zone	C21.1	C78.5	D01.3	D12.9	D37.8	D49.0
hepatic — *see also* Index to disease, by histology	C22.9	C78.7	D01.5	D13.4	D37.6	D49.0
duct (bile)	C24.0	C78.89	D01.5	D13.5	D37.6	D49.0
flexure (colon)	C18.3	C78.5	D01.0	D12.3	D37.4	D49.0
primary	C22.8	C78.7	D01.5	D13.4	D37.6	D49.0
hepatobiliary	C24.9	C78.89	D01.5	D13.5	D37.6	D49.0
hepatoblastoma	C22.2	C78.7	D01.5	D13.4	D37.6	D49.0
hepatoma	C22.0	C78.7	D01.5	D13.4	D37.6	D49.0
hilus of lung	C34.0-☑	C78.0-☑	D02.2-☑	D14.3-☑	D38.1	D49.1
hippocampus, brain	C71.2	C79.31	—	D33.0	D43.0	D49.6
hip NEC	C76.5-☑	C79.89	D04.7-☑	D36.7	D48.7	D49.89
humerus (any part)	C40.0-☑	C79.51	—	D16.0-☑	—	—
hymen	C52	C79.82	D07.2	D28.1	D39.8	D49.59
hypopharynx, hypopharyngeal NEC	C13.9	C79.89	D00.08	D10.7	D37.05	D49.0
overlapping lesion	C13.8	—	—	—	—	—
postcricoid region	C13.0	C79.89	D00.08	D10.7	D37.05	D49.0
posterior wall	C13.2	C79.89	D00.08	D10.7	D37.05	D49.0
pyriform fossa (sinus)	C12	C79.89	D00.08	D10.7	D37.05	D49.0
hypophysis	C75.1	C79.89	D09.3	D35.2	D44.3	D49.7
hypothalamus	C71.0	C79.31	—	D33.0	D43.0	D49.6
ileocecum, ileocecal (coil) (junction) (valve)	C18.0	C78.5	D01.0	D12.0	D37.4	D49.0
ileum	C17.2	C78.4	D01.49	D13.39	D37.2	D49.0
ilium	C41.4	C79.51	—	D16.8	D48.0	D49.2
immunoproliferative NEC	C88.9	—	—	—	—	—
infraclavicular (region)	C76.1	C79.89	D04.5	D36.7	D48.7	D49.89
inguinal (region)	C76.3	C79.89	D04.5	D36.7	D48.7	D49.89
insula	C71.0	C79.31	—	D33.0	D43.0	D49.6
insular tissue (pancreas)	C25.4	C78.89	D01.7	D13.7	D37.8	D49.0
brain	C71.0	C79.31	—	D33.0	D43.0	D49.6
interarytenoid fold	C13.1	C78.39	D00.08	D10.7	D37.05	D49.0
hypopharyngeal aspect	C13.1	C79.89	D00.08	D10.7	D37.05	D49.0
laryngeal aspect	C32.1	C78.39	D02.0	D14.1	D38.0	D49.1
marginal zone	C13.1	C79.89	D00.08	D10.7	D37.05	D49.0
interdental papillae	C03.9	C79.89	D00.03	D10.39	D37.09	D49.0
lower	C03.1	C79.89	D00.03	D10.39	D37.09	D49.0
upper	C03.0	C79.89	D00.03	D10.39	D37.09	D49.0
internal						
capsule	C71.0	C79.31	—	D33.0	D43.0	D49.6
os (cervix)	C53.0	C79.82	D06.0	D26.0	D39.0	D49.59
intervertebral cartilage or disc	C41.2	C79.51	—	D16.6	D48.0	D49.2
intestine, intestinal	C26.0	C78.80	D01.40	D13.9	D37.8	D49.0
large	C18.9	C78.5	D01.0	D12.6	D37.4	D49.0
appendix	C18.1	C78.5	D01.0	D12.1	D37.3	D49.0
caput coli	C18.0	C78.5	D01.0	D12.0	D37.4	D49.0
cecum	C18.0	C78.5	D01.0	D12.0	D37.4	D49.0
colon	C18.9	C78.5	D01.0	D12.6	D37.4	D49.0
and rectum	C19	C78.5	D01.1	D12.7	D37.5	D49.0
ascending	C18.2	C78.5	D01.0	D12.2	D37.4	D49.0
caput	C18.0	C78.5	D01.0	D12.0	D37.4	D49.0
descending	C18.6	C78.5	D01.0	D12.4	D37.4	D49.0
distal	C18.6	C78.5	D01.0	D12.4	D37.4	D49.0

☑ **Additional Character Required — Refer to the Tabular List for Character Selection** ▽ **Subterms under main terms may continue to next column or page**

Neoplasm, neoplastic — continued

intestine, intestinal — continued / large — continued / colon — continued

	Malignant Primary	Malignant Secondary	Ca in situ	Benign	Uncertain Behavior	Unspecified Behavior
left	C18.6	C78.5	D01.0	D12.4	D37.4	D49.0
overlapping lesion	C18.8	—	—	—	—	—
pelvic	C18.7	C78.5	D01.0	D12.5	D37.4	D49.0
right	C18.2	C78.5	D01.0	D12.2	D37.4	D49.0
sigmoid (flexure)	C18.7	C78.5	D01.0	D12.5	D37.4	D49.0
transverse	C18.4	C78.5	D01.0	D12.3	D37.4	D49.0
hepatic flexure	C18.3	C78.5	D01.0	D12.3	D37.4	D49.0
ileocecum, ileocecal (coil) (valve)	C18.0	C78.5	D01.0	D12.0	D37.4	D49.0
overlapping lesion	C18.8	—	—	—	—	—
sigmoid flexure (lower) (upper)	C18.7	C78.5	D01.0	D12.5	D37.4	D49.0
splenic flexure	C18.5	C78.5	D01.0	D12.3	D37.4	D49.0
small	C17.9	C78.4	D01.40	D13.30	D37.2	D49.0
duodenum	C17.0	C78.4	D01.49	D13.2	D37.2	D49.0
ileum	C17.2	C78.4	D01.49	D13.39	D37.2	D49.0
jejunum	C17.1	C78.4	D01.49	D13.39	D37.2	D49.0
overlapping lesion	C17.8	—	—	—	—	—
tract NEC	C26.0	C78.89	D01.40	D13.9	D37.8	D49.0
intra-abdominal	C76.2	C79.89	D09.8	D36.7	D48.7	D49.89
intracranial NEC	C71.9	C79.31	—	D33.2	D43.2	D49.6
intrahepatic (bile) duct	C22.1	C78.7	D01.5	D13.4	D37.6	D49.0
intraocular	C69.9-☑	C79.49	D09.2-☑	D31.9-☑	D48.7	D49.89
intraorbital	C69.6-☑	C79.49	D09.2-☑	D31.6-☑	D48.7	D49.89
intrasellar	C75.1	C79.89	D09.3	D35.2	D44.3	D49.7
intrathoracic (cavity) (organs)	C76.1	C79.89	D09.8	D15.9	D48.7	D49.89
specified NEC	C76.1	C79.89	D09.8	D15.7	—	—
iris	C69.4-☑	C79.49	D09.2-☑	D31.4-☑	D48.7	D49.89
ischiorectal (fossa)	C76.3	C79.89	D09.8	D36.7	D48.7	D49.89
ischium	C41.4	C79.51	—	D16.8	D48.0	D49.2
island of Reil	C71.0	C79.31	—	D33.0	D43.0	D49.6
islands or islets of Langerhans	C25.4	C78.89	D01.7	D13.7	D37.8	D49.0
isthmus uteri	C54.0	C79.82	D07.0	D26.1	D39.0	D49.59
jaw	C76.0	C79.89	D09.8	D36.7	D48.7	D49.89
bone	C41.1	C79.51	—	D16.5	D48.0	D49.2
lower	C41.1	C79.51	—	D16.5	—	—
upper	C41.0	C79.51	—	D16.4	—	—
carcinoma (any type) (lower)						
(upper)	C76.0	C79.89	—	—	—	—
skin — see also Neoplasm, skin, face	C44.309	C79.2	D04.39	D23.39	D48.5	D49.2
soft tissues	C03.9	C79.89	D00.03	D10.39	D37.09	D49.0
lower	C03.1	C79.89	D00.03	D10.39	D37.09	D49.0
upper	C03.0	C79.89	D00.03	D10.39	D37.09	D49.0
jejunum	C17.1	C78.4	D01.49	D13.39	D37.2	D49.0
joint NEC — see also Neoplasm, bone	C41.9	C79.51	—	D16.9	D48.0	D49.2
acromioclavicular	C40.0-☑	C79.51	—	D16.0-☑	—	—
bursa or synovial membrane — see Neoplasm, connective tissue						
costovertebral	C41.3	C79.51	—	D16.7	D48.0	D49.2
sternocostal	C41.3	C79.51	—	D16.7	D48.0	D49.2
temporomandibular	C41.1	C79.51	—	D16.5	D48.0	D49.2
junction						
anorectal	C21.8	C78.5	D01.3	D12.9	D37.8	D49.0
cardioesophageal	C16.0	C78.89	D00.2	D13.1	D37.1	D49.0
esophagogastric	C16.0	C78.89	D00.2	D13.1	D37.1	D49.0
gastroesophageal	C16.0	C78.89	D00.2	D13.1	D37.1	D49.0
hard and soft palate	C05.9	C79.89	D00.00	D10.39	D37.09	D49.0
ileocecal	C18.0	C78.5	D01.0	D12.0	D37.4	D49.0

Neoplasm, neoplastic — continued

junction — continued

	Malignant Primary	Malignant Secondary	Ca in situ	Benign	Uncertain Behavior	Unspecified Behavior
pelvirectal	C19	C78.5	D01.1	D12.7	D37.5	D49.0
pelviureteric	C65.-☑	C79.0-☑	D09.19	D30.1-☑	D41.1-☑	D49.59
rectosigmoid	C19	C78.5	D01.1	D12.7	D37.5	D49.0
squamocolumnar, of cervix	C53.8	C79.82	D06.7	D26.0	D39.0	D49.59
Kaposi's sarcoma — see Kaposi's, sarcoma						
kidney (parenchymal)	C64.-☑	C79.0-☑	D09.19	D30.0-☑	D41.0-☑	D49.51-☑
calyx	C65.-☑	C79.0-☑	D09.19	D30.1-☑	D41.1-☑	D49.51-☑
hilus	C65.-☑	C79.0-☑	D09.19	D30.1-☑	D41.1-☑	D49.51-☑
pelvis	C65.-☑	C79.0-☑	D09.19	D30.1-☑	D41.1-☑	D49.51-☑
knee NEC	C76.5-☑	C79.89	D04.7-☑	D36.7	D48.7	D49.89
labia (skin)	C51.9	C79.82	D07.1	D28.0	D39.8	D49.59
majora	C51.0	C79.82	D07.1	D28.0	D39.8	D49.59
minora	C51.1	C79.82	D07.1	D28.0	D39.8	D49.59
labial — see also Neoplasm, lip	C00.9	C79.89	D00.01	D10.0	D37.01	D49.0
sulcus (lower) (upper)	C06.1	C79.89	D00.02	D10.39	D37.09	D49.0
labium (skin)	C51.9	C79.82	D07.1	D28.0	D39.8	D49.59
majus	C51.0	C79.82	D07.1	D28.0	D39.8	D49.59
minus	C51.1	C79.82	D07.1	D28.0	D39.8	D49.59
lacrimal canaliculi	C69.5-☑	C79.49	D09.2-☑	D31.5-☑	D48.7	D49.89
duct (nasal)	C69.5-☑	C79.49	D09.2-☑	D31.5-☑	D48.7	D49.89
gland	C69.5-☑	C79.49	D09.2-☑	D31.5-☑	D48.7	D49.89
punctum	C69.5-☑	C79.49	D09.2-☑	D31.5-☑	D48.7	D49.89
sac	C69.5-☑	C79.49	D09.2-☑	D31.5-☑	D48.7	D49.89
Langerhans, islands or islets	C25.4	C78.89	D01.7	D13.7	D37.8	D49.0
laryngopharynx	C13.9	C79.89	D00.08	D10.7	D37.05	D49.0
larynx, laryngeal NEC	C32.9	C78.39	D02.0	D14.1	D38.0	D49.1
aryepiglottic fold	C32.1	C78.39	D02.0	D14.1	D38.0	D49.1
cartilage (arytenoid) (cricoid) (cuneiform) (thyroid)	C32.3	C78.39	D02.0	D14.1	D38.0	D49.1
commissure (anterior) (posterior)	C32.0	C78.39	D02.0	D14.1	D38.0	D49.1
extrinsic NEC	C32.1	C78.39	D02.0	D14.1	D38.0	D49.1
meaning hypopharynx	C13.9	C79.89	D00.08	D10.7	D37.05	D49.0
interarytenoid fold	C32.1	C78.39	D02.0	D14.1	D38.0	D49.1
intrinsic	C32.0	C78.39	D02.0	D14.1	D38.0	D49.1
overlapping lesion	C32.8	—	—	—	—	—
ventricular band	C32.1	C78.39	D02.0	D14.1	D38.0	D49.1
leg NEC	C76.5-☑	C79.89	D04.7-☑	D36.7	D48.7	D49.89
lens, crystalline	C69.4-☑	C79.49	D09.2-☑	D31.4-☑	D48.7	D49.89
lid (lower) (upper)	C44.10-☑	C79.2	D04.1-☑	D23.1-☑	D48.5	D49.2
basal cell carcinoma	C44.11-☑	—	—	—	—	—
sebaceous cell specified type	C44.13-☑	—	—	—	—	—
specified type NEC	C44.19-☑	—	—	—	—	—
squamous cell carcinoma	C44.12-☑	—	—	—	—	—
ligament — see also Neoplasm, connective tissue						
broad	C57.1-☑	C79.82	D07.39	D28.2	D39.8	D49.59
Mackenrodt's	C57.7	C79.82	D07.39	D28.7	D39.8	D49.59
non-uterine — see Neoplasm, connective tissue						
round	C57.2-☑	C79.82	—	D28.2	D39.8	D49.59
sacro-uterine	C57.3	C79.82	—	D28.2	D39.8	D49.59
uterine	C57.3	C79.82	—	D28.2	D39.8	D49.59
utero-ovarian	C57.7	C79.82	D07.39	D28.2	D39.8	D49.59
uterosacral	C57.3	C79.82	—	D28.2	D39.8	D49.59
limb	C76.8	C79.89	D04.8	D36.7	D48.7	D49.89
lower	C76.5-☑	C79.89	D04.7-☑	D36.7	D48.7	D49.89
upper	C76.4-☑	C79.89	D04.6-☑	D36.7	D48.7	D49.89
limbus of cornea	C69.1-☑	C79.49	D09.2-☑	D31.1-☑	D48.7	D49.89

Neoplasm, neoplastic	Malignant Primary	Malignant Secondary	Ca in situ	Benign	Uncertain Behavior	Unspecified Behavior
— continued						
lingual NEC — see also Neoplasm,						
tongue	C02.9	C79.89	D00.07	D10.1	D37.02	D49.0
lingula, lung	C34.1-☑	C78.0-☑	D02.2-☑	D14.3-☑	D38.1	D49.1
lip	C00.9	C79.89	D00.01	D10.0	D37.01	D49.0
buccal aspect — see Neoplasm, lip, internal						
commissure	C00.6	C79.89	D00.01	D10.0	D37.01	D49.0
external	C00.2	C79.89	D00.01	D10.0	D37.01	D49.0
lower	C00.1	C79.89	D00.01	D10.0	D37.01	D49.0
upper	C00.0	C79.89	D00.01	D10.0	D37.01	D49.0
frenulum — see Neoplasm, lip, internal						
inner aspect — see Neoplasm, lip, internal						
internal	C00.5	C79.89	D00.01	D10.0	D37.01	D49.0
lower	C00.4	C79.89	D00.01	D10.0	D37.01	D49.0
upper	C00.3	C79.89	D00.01	D10.0	D37.01	D49.0
lipstick area	C00.2	C79.89	D00.01	D10.0	D37.01	D49.0
lower	C00.1	C79.89	D00.01	D10.0	D37.01	D49.0
upper	C00.0	C79.89	D00.01	D10.0	D37.01	D49.0
lower	C00.1	C79.89	D00.01	D10.0	D37.01	D49.0
internal	C00.4	C79.89	D00.01	D10.0	D37.01	D49.0
mucosa — see Neoplasm, lip, internal						
oral aspect — see Neoplasm, lip, internal						
overlapping						
lesion	C00.8	—	—	—	—	—
with oral cavity or pharynx	C14.8	—	—	—	—	—
skin (commissure) (lower)						
(upper)	C44.00	C79.2	D04.0	D23.0	D48.5	D49.2
basal cell carcinoma	C44.01	—	—	—	—	—
specified type NEC	C44.09	—	—	—	—	—
squamous cell carcinoma	C44.02	—	—	—	—	—
upper	C00.0	C79.89	D00.01	D10.0	D37.01	D49.0
internal	C00.3	C79.89	D00.01	D10.0	D37.01	D49.0
vermilion						
border	C00.2	C79.89	D00.01	D10.0	D37.01	D49.0
lower	C00.1	C79.89	D00.01	D10.0	D37.01	D49.0
upper	C00.0	C79.89	D00.01	D10.0	D37.01	D49.0
lipomatous — see Lipoma, by site						
liver — see also Index to disease, by						
histology	C22.9	C78.7	D01.5	D13.4	D37.6	D49.0
primary	C22.8	C78.7	D01.5	D13.4	D37.6	D49.0
lumbosacral plexus	C47.5	C79.89	—	D36.16	D48.2	D49.2
lung	C34.9-☑	C78.0-☑	D02.2-☑	D14.3-☑	D38.1	D49.1
azygos lobe	C34.1-☑	C78.0-☑	D02.2-☑	D14.3-☑	D38.1	D49.1
carina	C34.0-☑	C78.0-☑	D02.2-☑	D14.3-☑	D38.1	D49.1
hilus	C34.0-☑	C78.0-☑	D02.2-☑	D14.3-☑	D38.1	D49.1
lingula	C34.1-☑	C78.0-☑	D02.2-☑	D14.3-☑	D38.1	D49.1
lobe NEC	C34.9-☑	C78.0-☑	D02.2-☑	D14.3-☑	D38.1	D49.1
lower lobe	C34.3-☑	C78.0-☑	D02.2-☑	D14.3-☑	D38.1	D49.1
main bronchus	C34.0-☑	C78.0-☑	D02.2-☑	D14.3-☑	D38.1	D49.1
mesothelioma — see Mesothelioma						
middle lobe	C34.2	C78.0-☑	D02.21	D14.31	D38.1	D49.1
overlapping lesion	C34.8-☑	—	—	—	—	—
upper lobe	C34.1-☑	C78.0-☑	D02.2-☑	D14.3-☑	D38.1	D49.1
lymph, lymphatic channel NEC	C49.9	C79.89		D21.9	D48.1	D49.2
gland						
(secondary)	—	C77.9		D36.0	D48.7	D49.89
abdominal	—	C77.2		D36.0	D48.7	D49.89
aortic	—	C77.2		D36.0	D48.7	D49.89
arm	—	C77.3		D36.0	D48.7	D49.89

Neoplasm, neoplastic	Malignant Primary	Malignant Secondary	Ca in situ	Benign	Uncertain Behavior	Unspecified Behavior
— continued						
lymph, lymphatic channel — continued						
gland — continued						
auricular (anterior) (posterior)	—	C77.0	—	D36.0	D48.7	D49.89
axilla, axillary	—	C77.3	—	D36.0	D48.7	D49.89
brachial	—	C77.3	—	D36.0	D48.7	D49.89
bronchial	—	C77.1	—	D36.0	D48.7	D49.89
bronchopulmonary	—	C77.1	—	D36.0	D48.7	D49.89
celiac	—	C77.2	—	D36.0	D48.7	D49.89
cervical	—	C77.0	—	D36.0	D48.7	D49.89
cervicofacial	—	C77.0	—	D36.0	D48.7	D49.89
Cloquet	—	C77.4	—	D36.0	D48.7	D49.89
colic	—	C77.2	—	D36.0	D48.7	D49.89
common duct	—	C77.2	—	D36.0	D48.7	D49.89
cubital	—	C77.3	—	D36.0	D48.7	D49.89
diaphragmatic	—	C77.1	—	D36.0	D48.7	D49.89
epigastric, inferior	—	C77.1	—	D36.0	D48.7	D49.89
epitrochlear	—	C77.3	—	D36.0	D48.7	D49.89
esophageal	—	C77.1	—	D36.0	D48.7	D49.89
face	—	C77.0	—	D36.0	D48.7	D49.89
femoral	—	C77.4	—	D36.0	D48.7	D49.89
gastric	—	C77.2	—	D36.0	D48.7	D49.89
groin	—	C77.4	—	D36.0	D48.7	D49.89
head	—	C77.0	—	D36.0	D48.7	D49.89
hepatic	—	C77.2	—	D36.0	D48.7	D49.89
hilar (pulmonary)	—	C77.1	—	D36.0	D48.7	D49.89
splenic	—	C77.2	—	D36.0	D48.7	D49.89
hypogastric	—	C77.5	—	D36.0	D48.7	D49.89
ileocolic	—	C77.2	—	D36.0	D48.7	D49.89
iliac	—	C77.5	—	D36.0	D48.7	D49.89
infraclavicular	—	C77.3	—	D36.0	D48.7	D49.89
inguina, inguinal	—	C77.4	—	D36.0	D48.7	D49.89
innominate	—	C77.1	—	D36.0	D48.7	D49.89
intercostal	—	C77.1	—	D36.0	D48.7	D49.89
intestinal	—	C77.2	—	D36.0	D48.7	D49.89
intrabdominal	—	C77.2	—	D36.0	D48.7	D49.89
intrapelvic	—	C77.5	—	D36.0	D48.7	D49.89
intrathoracic	—	C77.1	—	D36.0	D48.7	D49.89
jugular	—	C77.0	—	D36.0	D48.7	D49.89
leg	—	C77.4	—	D36.0	D48.7	D49.89
limb						
lower	—	C77.4	—	D36.0	D48.7	D49.89
upper	—	C77.3	—	D36.0	D48.7	D49.89
lower limb	—	C77.4	—	D36.0	D48.7	D49.89
lumbar	—	C77.2	—	D36.0	D48.7	D49.89
mandibular	—	C77.0	—	D36.0	D48.7	D49.89
mediastinal	—	C77.1	—	D36.0	D48.7	D49.89
mesenteric (inferior) (superior)	—	C77.2	—	D36.0	D48.7	D49.89
midcolic	—	C77.2	—	D36.0	D48.7	D49.89
multiple sites in categories C77.0 - C77.5	—	C77.8	—	D36.0	D48.7	D49.89
neck	—	C77.0	—	D36.0	D48.7	D49.89
obturator	—	C77.5	—	D36.0	D48.7	D49.89
occipital	—	C77.0	—	D36.0	D48.7	D49.89
pancreatic	—	C77.2	—	D36.0	D48.7	D49.89
para-aortic	—	C77.2	—	D36.0	D48.7	D49.89
paracervical	—	C77.5	—	D36.0	D48.7	D49.89
parametrial	—	C77.5	—	D36.0	D48.7	D49.89
parasternal	—	C77.1	—	D36.0	D48.7	D49.89
parotid	—	C77.0	—	D36.0	D48.7	D49.89
pectoral	—	C77.3	—	D36.0	D48.7	D49.89
pelvic	—	C77.5	—	D36.0	D48.7	D49.89
peri-aortic	—	C77.2	—	D36.0	D48.7	D49.89
peripancreatic	—	C77.2	—	D36.0	D48.7	D49.89
popliteal	—	C77.4	—	D36.0	D48.7	D49.89
porta hepatis	—	C77.2	—	D36.0	D48.7	D49.89
portal	—	C77.2	—	D36.0	D48.7	D49.89
preauricular	—	C77.0	—	D36.0	D48.7	D49.89
prelaryngeal	—	C77.0	—	D36.0	D48.7	D49.89
presymphysial	—	C77.5	—	D36.0	D48.7	D49.89
pretracheal	—	C77.0	—	D36.0	D48.7	D49.89
primary (any site) NEC	C96.9	—	—	—	—	—

☑ Additional Character Required — Refer to the Tabular List for Character Selection   Subterms under main terms may continue to next column or page

Neoplasm, neoplastic — continued

	Malignant Primary	Malignant Secondary	Ca in situ	Benign	Uncertain Behavior	Unspecified Behavior
lymph, lymphatic channel — continued						
gland — continued						
pulmonary (hiler)	—	C77.1	—	D36.0	D48.7	D49.89
pyloric	—	C77.2	—	D36.0	D48.7	D49.89
retroperitoneal	—	C77.2	—	D36.0	D48.7	D49.89
retropharyngeal	—	C77.0	—	D36.0	D48.7	D49.89
Rosenmuller's	—	C77.4	—	D36.0	D48.7	D49.89
sacral	—	C77.5	—	D36.0	D48.7	D49.89
scalene	—	C77.0	—	D36.0	D48.7	D49.89
site NEC	—	C77.9	—	D36.0	D48.7	D49.89
splenic (hilar)	—	C77.2	—	D36.0	D48.7	D49.89
subclavicular	—	C77.3	—	D36.0	D48.7	D49.89
subinguinal	—	C77.4	—	D36.0	D48.7	D49.89
sublingual	—	C77.0	—	D36.0	D48.7	D49.89
submandibular	—	C77.0	—	D36.0	D48.7	D49.89
submaxillary	—	C77.0	—	D36.0	D48.7	D49.89
submental	—	C77.0	—	D36.0	D48.7	D49.89
subscapular	—	C77.3	—	D36.0	D48.7	D49.89
supraclavicular	—	C77.0	—	D36.0	D48.7	D49.89
thoracic	—	C77.1	—	D36.0	D48.7	D49.89
tibial	—	C77.4	—	D36.0	D48.7	D49.89
tracheal	—	C77.1	—	D36.0	D48.7	D49.89
tracheobronchial	—	C77.1	—	D36.0	D48.7	D49.89
upper limb	—	C77.3	—	D36.0	D48.7	D49.89
Virchow's	—	C77.0	—	D36.0	D48.7	D49.89
node — see also Neoplasm, lymph gland						
primary NEC	C96.9	—	—	—	—	—
vessel — see also Neoplasm, connective tissue	C49.9	C79.89	—	D21.9	D48.1	D49.2
Mackenrodt's ligament	C57.7	C79.82	D07.39	D28.7	D39.8	D49.59
malar	C41.0	C79.51	—	D16.4	D48.0	D49.2
region — see Neoplasm, cheek						
mammary gland — see Neoplasm, breast						
mandible	C41.1	C79.51	—	D16.5	D48.0	D49.2
alveolar						
mucosa (carcinoma)	C03.1	C79.89	D00.03	D10.39	D37.09	D49.0
ridge or process	C41.1	C79.51	—	D16.5	D48.0	D49.2
marrow (bone) NEC	C96.9	C79.52	—	—	D47.9	D49.89
mastectomy site (skin) — see also Neoplasm, breast, skin	C44.501	C79.2	—	—	—	—
specified as breast tissue	C50.8-☑	C79.81	—	—	—	—
mastoid (air cells) (antrum) (cavity)	C30.1	C78.39	D02.3	D14.0	D38.5	D49.1
bone or process	C41.0	C79.51	—	D16.4	D48.0	D49.2
maxilla, maxillary (superior)	C41.0	C79.51	—	D16.4	D48.0	D49.2
alveolar						
mucosa	C03.0	C79.89	D00.03	D10.39	D37.09	D49.0
ridge or process (carcinoma)	C41.0	C79.51	—	D16.4	D48.0	D49.2
antrum	C31.0	C78.39	D02.3	D14.0	D38.5	D49.1
carcinoma	C03.0	C79.51	—	—	—	—
inferior — see Neoplasm, mandible						
sinus	C31.0	C78.39	D02.3	D14.0	D38.5	D49.1
meatus external (ear) — see also Neoplasm, skin, ear	C44.20-☑	C79.2	D04.2-☑	D23.2-☑	D48.5	D49.2
Meckel diverticulum, malignant	C17.3	C78.4	D01.49	D13.39	D37.2	D49.0
mediastinum, mediastinal	C38.3	C78.1	—	D15.2	D38.3	D49.89
anterior	C38.1	C78.1	—	D15.2	D38.3	D49.89

Neoplasm, neoplastic — continued

	Malignant Primary	Malignant Secondary	Ca in situ	Benign	Uncertain Behavior	Unspecified Behavior
mediastinum, mediastinal — continued						
posterior	C38.2	C78.1	—	D15.2	D38.3	D49.89
medulla						
adrenal	C74.1-☑	C79.7-☑	D09.3	D35.0-☑	D44.1-☑	D49.7
oblongata	C71.7	C79.31	—	D33.1	D43.1	D49.6
meibomian gland	C44.10-☑	C79.2	D04.1-☑	D23.1-☑	D48.5	D49.2
basal cell carcinoma	C44.11-☑	—	—	—	—	—
sebaceous cell	C44.13-☑	—	—	—	—	—
specified type NEC	C44.19-☑	—	—	—	—	—
squamous cell carcinoma	C44.12-☑	—	—	—	—	—
melanoma — see Melanoma						
meninges	C70.9	C79.49	—	D32.9	D42.9	D49.7
brain	C70.0	C79.32	—	D32.0	D42.0	D49.7
cerebral	C70.0	C79.32	—	D32.0	D42.0	D49.7
crainial	C70.0	C79.32	—	D32.0	D42.0	D49.7
intracranial	C70.0	C79.32	—	D32.0	D42.0	D49.7
spinal (cord)	C70.1	C79.49	—	D32.1	D42.1	D49.7
meniscus, knee joint (lateral) (medial)	C40.2-☑	C79.51	—	D16.2-☑	D48.0	D49.2
Merkel cell — see Carcinoma, Merkel cell						
mesentery, mesenteric	C48.1	C78.6	—	D20.1	D48.4	D49.0
mesoappendix	C48.1	C78.6	—	D20.1	D48.4	D49.0
mesocolon	C48.1	C78.6	—	D20.1	D48.4	D49.0
mesopharynx — see Neoplasm, oropharynx						
mesosalpinx	C57.1-☑	C79.82	D07.39	D28.2	D39.8	D49.59
mesothelial tissue — see Mesothelioma						
mesothelioma — see Mesothelioma						
mesovarium	C57.1-☑	C79.82	D07.39	D28.2	D39.8	D49.59
metacarpus (any bone)	C40.1-☑	C79.51	—	D16.1-☑	—	—
metastatic NEC — see also Neoplasm, by site, secondary	—	C79.9	—	—	—	—
metatarsus (any bone)	C40.3-☑	C79.51	—	D16.3-☑	—	—
midbrain	C71.7	C79.31	—	D33.1	D43.1	D49.6
milk duct — see Neoplasm, breast						
mons						
pubis	C51.9	C79.82	D07.1	D28.0	D39.8	D49.59
veneris	C51.9	C79.82	D07.1	D28.0	D39.8	D49.59
motor tract	C72.9	C79.49	—	D33.9	D43.9	D49.7
brain	C71.9	C79.31	—	D33.2	D43.2	D49.6
cauda equina	C72.1	C79.49	—	D33.4	D43.4	D49.7
spinal	C72.0	C79.49	—	D33.4	D43.4	D49.7
mouth	C06.9	C79.89	D00.00	D10.30	D37.09	D49.0
book-leaf	C06.89	C79.89	—	—	—	—
floor	C04.9	C79.89	D00.06	D10.2	D37.09	D49.0
anterior portion	C04.0	C79.89	D00.06	D10.2	D37.09	D49.0
lateral portion	C04.1	C79.89	D00.06	D10.2	D37.09	D49.0
overlapping lesion	C04.8	—	—	—	—	—
overlapping NEC	C06.80	—	—	—	—	—
roof	C05.9	C79.89	D00.00	D10.39	D37.09	D49.0
specified part NEC	C06.89	C79.89	D00.00	D10.39	D37.09	D49.0
vestibule	C06.1	C79.89	D00.00	D10.39	D37.09	D49.0
mucosa						
alveolar (ridge or process)	C03.9	C79.89	D00.03	D10.39	D37.09	D49.0
lower	C03.1	C79.89	D00.03	D10.39	D37.09	D49.0
upper	C03.0	C79.89	D00.03	D10.39	D37.09	D49.0
buccal	C06.0	C79.89	D00.02	D10.39	D37.09	D49.0
cheek	C06.0	C79.89	D00.02	D10.39	D37.09	D49.0

Neoplasm, neoplastic	Malignant Primary	Malignant Secondary	Ca in situ	Benign	Uncertain Behavior	Unspecified Behavior
— continued						
mucosa — continued						
lip — see Neoplasm, lip, internal						
nasal	C30.0	C78.39	D02.3	D14.0	D38.5	D49.1
oral	C06.0	C79.89	D00.02	D10.39	D37.09	D49.0
Mullerian duct						
female	C57.7	C79.82	D07.39	D28.7	D39.8	D49.59
male	C63.7	C79.82	D07.69	D29.8	D40.8	D49.59
muscle — see also Neoplasm, connective tissue						
extraocular	C69.6-☑	C79.49	D09.2-☑	D31.6-☑	D48.7	D49.89
myocardium	C38.0	C79.89	—	D15.1	D48.7	D49.89
myometrium	C54.2	C79.82	D07.0	D26.1	D39.0	D49.59
myopericardium	C38.0	C79.89	—	D15.1	D48.7	D49.89
nabothian gland (follicle)	C53.0	C79.82	D06.0	D26.0	D39.0	D49.59
nail — see also Neoplasm, skin, limb	C44.90	C79.2	D04.9	D23.9	D48.5	D49.2
finger — see also Neoplasm, skin, limb, upper	C44.60-☑	C79.2	D04.6-☑	D23.6-☑	D48.5	D49.2
toe — see also Neoplasm, skin, limb, lower	C44.70-☑	C79.2	D04.7-☑	D23.7-☑	D48.5	D49.2
nares, naris (anterior) (posterior)	C30.0	C78.39	D02.3	D14.0	D38.5	D49.1
nasal — see Neoplasm, nose						
nasolabial groove — see also Neoplasm, skin, face	C44.309	C79.2	D04.39	D23.39	D48.5	D49.2
nasolacrimal duct	C69.5-☑	C79.49	D09.2-☑	D31.5-☑	D48.7	D49.89
nasopharynx, nasopharyngeal	C11.9	C79.89	D00.08	D10.6	D37.05	D49.0
floor	C11.3	C79.89	D00.08	D10.6	D37.05	D49.0
overlapping lesion	C11.8	—	—	—	—	—
roof	C11.0	C79.89	D00.08	D10.6	D37.05	D49.0
wall	C11.9	C79.89	D00.08	D10.6	D37.05	D49.0
anterior	C11.3	C79.89	D00.08	D10.6	D37.05	D49.0
lateral	C11.2	C79.89	D00.08	D10.6	D37.05	D49.0
posterior	C11.1	C79.89	D00.08	D10.6	D37.05	D49.0
superior	C11.0	C79.89	D00.08	D10.6	D37.05	D49.0
nates — see also Neoplasm, skin, trunk	C44.509	C79.2	D04.5	D23.5	D48.5	D49.2
neck NEC	C76.0	C79.89	D09.8	D36.7	D48.7	D49.89
skin	C44.40	—	—	—	—	—
basal cell carcinoma	C44.41	—	—	—	—	—
specified type NEC	C44.49	—	—	—	—	—
squamous cell carcinoma	C44.42	—	—	—	—	—
nerve (ganglion)	C47.9	C79.89		D36.10	D48.2	D49.2
abducens	C72.59	C79.49		D33.3	D43.3	D49.7
accessory (spinal)	C72.59	C79.49		D33.3	D43.3	D49.7
acoustic	C72.4-☑	C79.49		D33.3	D43.3	D49.7
auditory	C72.4-☑	C79.49		D33.3	D43.3	D49.7
autonomic NEC — see also Neoplasm, nerve, peripheral	C47.9	C79.89		D36.10	D48.2	D49.2
brachial	C47.1-☑	C79.89		D36.12	D48.2	D49.2
cranial	C72.50	C79.49		D33.3	D43.3	D49.7
specified NEC	C72.59	C79.49		D33.3	D43.3	D49.7
facial	C72.59	C79.49		D33.3	D43.3	D49.7
femoral	C47.2-☑	C79.89		D36.13	D48.2	D49.2
ganglion NEC — see also Neoplasm, nerve, peripheral	C47.9	C79.89	—	D36.10	D48.2	D49.2
glossopharyngeal	C72.59	C79.49	—	D33.3	D43.3	D49.7
hypoglossal	C72.59	C79.49	—	D33.3	D43.3	D49.7
intercostal	C47.3	C79.89		D36.14	D48.2	D49.2
lumbar	C47.6	C79.89		D36.17	D48.2	D49.2
median	C47.1-☑	C79.89	—	D36.12	D48.2	D49.2
obturator	C47.2-☑	C79.89	—	D36.13	D48.2	D49.2

Neoplasm, neoplastic	Malignant Primary	Malignant Secondary	Ca in situ	Benign	Uncertain Behavior	Unspecified Behavior
— continued						
nerve — continued						
oculomotor	C72.59	C79.49	—	D33.3	D43.3	D49.7
olfactory	C47.2-☑	C79.49	—	D33.3	D43.3	D49.7
optic	C72.3-☑	C79.49	—	D33.3	D43.3	D49.7
parasympathetic NEC	C47.9	C79.89	—	D36.10	D48.2	D49.2
peripheral NEC	C47.9	C79.89	—	D36.10	D48.2	D49.2
abdomen	C47.4	C79.89	—	D36.15	D48.2	D49.2
abdominal wall	C47.4	C79.89	—	D36.15	D48.2	D49.2
ankle	C47.2-☑	C79.89	—	D36.13	D48.2	D49.2
antecubital fossa or space	C47.1-☑	C79.89	—	D36.12	D48.2	D49.2
arm	C47.1-☑	C79.89	—	D36.12	D48.2	D49.2
auricle (ear)	C47.0	C79.89	—	D36.11	D48.2	D49.2
axilla	C47.3	C79.89	—	D36.12	D48.2	D49.2
back	C47.6	C79.89	—	D36.17	D48.2	D49.2
buttock	C47.5	C79.89	—	D36.16	D48.2	D49.2
calf	C47.2-☑	C79.89	—	D36.13	D48.2	D49.2
cervical region	C47.0	C79.89	—	D36.11	D48.2	D49.2
cheek	C47.0	C79.89	—	D36.11	D48.2	D49.2
chest (wall)	C47.3	C79.89	—	D36.14	D48.2	D49.2
chin	C47.0	C79.89	—	D36.11	D48.2	D49.2
ear (external)	C47.0	C79.89	—	D36.11	D48.2	D49.2
elbow	C47.1-☑	C79.89	—	D36.12	D48.2	D49.2
extrarectal	C47.5	C79.89	—	D36.16	D48.2	D49.2
extremity	C47.9	C79.89	—	D36.10	D48.2	D49.2
lower	C47.2-☑	C79.89	—	D36.13	D48.2	D49.2
upper	C47.1-☑	C79.89	—	D36.12	D48.2	D49.2
eyelid	C47.0	C79.89	—	D36.11	D48.2	D49.2
face	C47.0	C79.89	—	D36.11	D48.2	D49.2
finger	C47.1-☑	C79.89	—	D36.12	D48.2	D49.2
flank	C47.6	C79.89	—	D36.17	D48.2	D49.2
foot	C47.2-☑	C79.89	—	D36.13	D48.2	D49.2
forearm	C47.1-☑	C79.89	—	D36.12	D48.2	D49.2
forehead	C47.0	C79.89	—	D36.11	D48.2	D49.2
gluteal region	C47.5	C79.89	—	D36.16	D48.2	D49.2
groin	C47.5	C79.89	—	D36.16	D48.2	D49.2
hand	C47.1-☑	C79.89	—	D36.12	D48.2	D49.2
head	C47.0	C79.89	—	D36.11	D48.2	D49.2
heel	C47.2-☑	C79.89	—	D36.13	D48.2	D49.2
hip	C47.2-☑	C79.89	—	D36.13	D48.2	D49.2
infraclavicular region	C47.3	C79.89	—	D36.14	D48.2	D49.2
inguinal (canal) (region)	C47.5	C79.89	—	D36.16	D48.2	D49.2
intrathoracic	C47.3	C79.89	—	D36.14	D48.2	D49.2
ischiorectal fossa	C47.5	C79.89	—	D36.16	D48.2	D49.2
knee	C47.2-☑	C79.89	—	D36.13	D48.2	D49.2
leg	C47.2-☑	C79.89	—	D36.13	D48.2	D49.2
limb NEC	C47.9	C79.89	—	D36.10	D48.2	D49.2
lower	C47.2-☑	C79.89	—	D36.13	D48.2	D49.2
upper	C47.1-☑	C79.89	—	D36.12	D48.2	D49.2
nates	C47.5	C79.89	—	D36.16	D48.2	D49.2
neck	C47.0	C79.89	—	D36.11	D48.2	D49.2
orbit	C69.6-☑	C79.49	—	D31.6-☑	D48.7	D49.2
pararectal	C47.5	C79.89	—	D36.16	D48.2	D49.2
paraurethral	C47.5	C79.89	—	D36.16	D48.2	D49.2
paravaginal	C47.5	C79.89	—	D36.16	D48.2	D49.2
pelvis (floor)	C47.5	C79.89	—	D36.16	D48.2	D49.2
pelvoabdominal	C47.8	C79.89	—	D36.17	D48.2	D49.2
perineum	C47.5	C79.89	—	D36.16	D48.2	D49.2
perirectal (tissue)	C47.5	C79.89	—	D36.16	D48.2	D49.2
periurethral (tissue)	C47.5	C79.89	—	D36.16	D48.2	D49.2
popliteal fossa or space	C47.2-☑	C79.89	—	D36.13	D48.2	D49.2
presacral	C47.5	C79.89	—	D36.16	D48.2	D49.2
pterygoid fossa	C47.0	C79.89	—	D36.11	D48.2	D49.2
rectovaginal septum or wall	C47.5	C79.89	—	D36.16	D48.2	D49.2
rectovesical	C47.5	C79.89	—	D36.16	D48.2	D49.2
sacrococcygeal region	C47.5	C79.89	—	D36.16	D48.2	D49.2
scalp	C47.0	C79.89	—	D36.11	D48.2	D49.2

Neoplasm, neoplastic — continued (left column)

Term	Malignant Primary	Malignant Secondary	Ca in situ	Benign	Uncertain Behavior	Unspecified Behavior
nerve — continued						
peripheral — continued						
scapular region	C47.3	C79.89	—	D36.14	D48.2	D49.2
shoulder	C47.1-☑	C79.89	—	D36.12	D48.2	D49.2
submental	C47.0	C79.89	—	D36.11	D48.2	D49.2
supraclavicular region	C47.0	C79.89	—	D36.11	D48.2	D49.2
temple	C47.0	C79.89	—	D36.11	D48.2	D49.2
temporal region	C47.0	C79.89	—	D36.11	D48.2	D49.2
thigh	C47.2-☑	C79.89	—	D36.13	D48.2	D49.2
thoracic (duct) (wall)	C47.3	C79.89	—	D36.14	D48.2	D49.2
thorax	C47.3	C79.89	—	D36.14	D48.2	D49.2
thumb	C47.1-☑	C79.89	—	D36.12	D48.2	D49.2
toe	C47.2-☑	C79.89	—	D36.13	D48.2	D49.2
trunk	C47.6	C79.89	—	D36.17	D48.2	D49.2
umbilicus	C47.4	C79.89	—	D36.15	D48.2	D49.2
vesicorectal	C47.5	C79.89	—	D36.16	D48.2	D49.2
wrist	C47.1-☑	C79.89	—	D36.12	D48.2	D49.2
radial	C47.1-☑	C79.89	—	D36.12	D48.2	D49.2
sacral	C47.5	C79.89	—	D36.16	D48.2	D49.2
sciatic	C47.2-☑	C79.89	—	D36.13	D48.2	D49.2
spinal NEC	C47.9	C79.89	—	D36.10	D48.2	D49.2
accessory	C72.59	C79.49	—	D33.3	D43.3	D49.7
sympathetic NEC — see also Neoplasm, nerve, peripheral	C47.9	C79.89	—	D36.10	D48.2	D49.2
trigeminal	C72.59	C79.49	—	D33.3	D43.3	D49.7
trochlear	C72.59	C79.49	—	D33.3	D43.3	D49.7
ulnar	C47.1-☑	C79.89	—	D36.12	D48.2	D49.2
vagus	C72.59	C79.49	—	D33.3	D43.3	D49.7
nervous system (central)	C72.9	C79.40	—	D33.9	D43.9	D49.7
autonomic — see Neoplasm, nerve, peripheral						
parasympathetic — see Neoplasm, nerve, peripheral						
specified site NEC	—	C79.49	—	D33.7	D43.8	
sympathetic — see Neoplasm, nerve, peripheral						
nevus — see Nevus						
nipple	C50.0-☑	C79.81	D05.-☑	D24.-☑	—	—
nose, nasal	C76.0	C79.89	D09.8	D36.7	D48.7	D49.89
ala (external) (nasi) — see also Neoplasm, nose, skin	C44.301	C79.2	D04.39	D23.39	D48.5	D49.2
bone	C41.0	C79.51	—	D16.4	D48.0	D49.2
cartilage	C30.0	C78.39	D02.3	D14.0	D38.5	D49.1
cavity	C30.0	C78.39	D02.3	D14.0	D38.5	D49.1
choana	C11.3	C79.89	D00.08	D10.6	D37.05	D49.0
external (skin) — see also Neoplasm, nose, skin	C44.301	C79.2	D04.39	D23.39	D48.5	D49.2
fossa	C30.0	C78.39	D02.3	D14.0	D38.5	D49.1
internal	C30.0	C78.39	D02.3	D14.0	D38.5	D49.1
mucosa	C30.0	C78.39	D02.3	D14.0	D38.5	D49.1
septum	C30.0	C78.39	D02.3	D14.0	D38.5	D49.1
posterior margin	C11.3	C79.89	D00.08	D10.6	D37.05	D49.0
sinus — see Neoplasm, sinus						
skin	C44.301	C79.2	D04.39	D23.39	D48.5	D49.2
basal cell carcinoma	C44.311	—	—	—	—	—
specified type NEC	C44.391	—	—	—	—	—
squamous cell carcinoma	C44.321	—	—	—	—	—
turbinate (mucosa)	C30.0	C78.39	D02.3	D14.0	D38.5	D49.1
bone	C41.0	C79.51	—	D16.4	D48.0	D49.2
vestibule	C30.0	C78.39	D02.3	D14.0	D38.5	D49.1

Neoplasm, neoplastic — continued (right column)

Term	Malignant Primary	Malignant Secondary	Ca in situ	Benign	Uncertain Behavior	Unspecified Behavior
nostril	C30.0	C78.39	D02.3	D14.0	D38.5	D49.1
nucleus pulposus	C41.2	C79.51	—	D16.6	D48.0	D49.2
occipital bone	C41.0	C79.51	—	D16.4	D48.0	D49.2
lobe or pole, brain	C71.4	C79.31	—	D33.0	D43.0	D49.6
odontogenic — see Neoplasm, jaw bone						
olfactory nerve or bulb	C72.2-☑	C79.49	—	D33.3	D43.3	D49.7
olive (brain)	C71.7	C79.31	—	D33.1	D43.1	D49.6
omentum	C48.1	C78.6	—	D20.1	D48.4	D49.0
operculum (brain)	C71.0	C79.31	—	D33.0	D43.0	D49.6
optic nerve, chiasm, or tract	C72.3-☑	C79.49	—	D33.3	D43.3	D49.7
oral (cavity)	C06.9	C79.89	D00.00	D10.30	D37.09	D49.0
ill-defined	C14.8	C79.89	D00.00	D10.30	D37.09	D49.0
mucosa	C06.0	C79.89	D00.02	D10.39	D37.09	D49.0
orbit	C69.6-☑	C79.49	D09.2-☑	D31.6-☑	D48.7	D49.89
autonomic nerve	C69.6-☑	C79.49	—	D31.6-☑	D48.7	D49.2
bone	C41.0	C79.51	—	D16.4	D48.0	D49.2
eye	C69.6-☑	C79.49	D09.2-☑	D31.6-☑	D48.7	D49.89
peripheral nerves	C69.6-☑	C79.49	—	D31.6-☑	D48.7	D49.2
soft parts	C69.6-☑	C79.49	D09.2-☑	D31.6-☑	D48.7	D49.89
organ of Zuckerkandl	C75.5	C79.89	—	D35.6	D44.7	D49.7
oropharynx	C10.9	C79.89	D00.08	D10.5	D37.05	D49.0
branchial cleft (vestige)	C10.4	C79.89	D00.08	D10.5	D37.05	D49.0
junctional region	C10.8	C79.89	D00.08	D10.5	D37.05	D49.0
lateral wall	C10.2	C79.89	D00.08	D10.5	D37.05	D49.0
overlapping lesion	C10.8	—	—	—	—	—
pillars or fauces	C09.1	C79.89	D00.08	D10.5	D37.05	D49.0
posterior wall	C10.3	C79.89	D00.08	D10.5	D37.05	D49.0
vallecula	C10.0	C79.89	D00.08	D10.5	D37.05	D49.0
os external	C53.1	C79.82	D06.1	D26.0	D39.0	D49.59
internal	C53.0	C79.82	D06.0	D26.0	D39.0	D49.59
ovary	C56.-☑	C79.6-☑	D07.39	D27.-☑	D39.1-☑	D49.59
oviduct	C57.0-☑	C79.82	D07.39	D28.2	D39.8	D49.59
palate	C05.9	C79.89	D00.00	D10.39	D37.09	D49.0
hard	C05.0	C79.89	D00.05	D10.39	D37.09	D49.0
junction of hard and soft palate	C05.9	C79.89	D00.00	D10.39	D37.09	D49.0
overlapping lesions	C05.8	—	—	—	—	—
soft	C05.1	C79.89	D00.04	D10.39	D37.09	D49.0
nasopharyngeal surface	C11.3	C79.89	D00.08	D10.6	D37.05	D49.0
posterior surface	C11.3	C79.89	D00.08	D10.6	D37.05	D49.0
superior surface	C11.3	C79.89	D00.08	D10.6	D37.05	D49.0
palatoglossal arch	C09.1	C79.89	D00.00	D10.5	D37.09	D49.0
palatopharyngeal arch	C09.1	C79.89	D00.00	D10.5	D37.09	D49.0
pallium	C71.0	C79.31	—	D33.0	D43.0	D49.6
palpebra	C44.10-☑	C79.2	D04.1-☑	D23.1-☑	D48.5	D49.2
basal cell carcinoma	C44.11-☑	—	—	—	—	—
sebaceous cell	C44.13-☑	—	—	—	—	—
specified type NEC	C44.19-☑	—	—	—	—	—
squamous cell carcinoma	C44.12-☑	—	—	—	—	—
pancreas	C25.9	C78.89	D01.7	D13.6	D37.8	D49.0
body	C25.1	C78.89	D01.7	D13.6	D37.8	D49.0
duct (of Santorini) (of Wirsung)	C25.3	C78.89	D01.7	D13.6	D37.8	D49.0
ectopic tissue	C25.7	C78.89	—	D13.6	D37.8	D49.0
head	C25.0	C78.89	D01.7	D13.6	D37.8	D49.0
islet cells	C25.4	C78.89	D01.7	D13.7	D37.8	D49.0
neck	C25.7	C78.89	D01.7	D13.6	D37.8	D49.0
overlapping lesion	C25.8	—	—	—	—	—
tail	C25.2	C78.89	D01.7	D13.6	D37.8	D49.0

Neoplasm, neoplastic	Malignant Primary	Malignant Secondary	Ca in situ	Benign	Uncertain Behavior	Unspecified Behavior
— continued						
para-aortic body	C75.5	C79.89	—	D35.6	D44.7	D49.7
paraganglion NEC	C75.5	C79.89	—	D35.6	D44.7	D49.7
parametrium	C57.3	C79.82	—	D28.2	D39.8	D49.59
paranephric	C48.0	C78.6	—	D20.0	D48.3	D49.0
pararectal	C76.3	C79.89	—	D36.7	D48.7	D49.89
parasagittal (region)	C76.0	C79.89	D09.8	D36.7	D48.7	D49.89
parasellar	C72.9	C79.49	—	D33.9	D43.8	D49.7
parathyroid (gland)	C75.0	C79.89	D09.3	D35.1	D44.2	D49.7
paraurethral	C76.3	C79.89	—	D36.7	D48.7	D49.89
gland	C68.1	C79.19	D09.19	D30.8	D41.8	D49.59
paravaginal	C76.3	C79.89	—	D36.7	D48.7	D49.89
parenchyma, kidney	C64.-☑	C79.0-☑	D09.19	D30.0-☑	D41.0-☑	D49.51-☑
parietal						
bone	C41.0	C79.51	—	D16.4	D48.0	D49.2
lobe, brain	C71.3	C79.31	—	D33.0	D43.0	D49.6
paroophoron	C57.1-☑	C79.82	D07.39	D28.2	D39.8	D49.59
parotid (duct) (gland)	C07	C79.89	D00.00	D11.0	D37.030	D49.0
parovarium	C57.1-☑	C79.82	D07.39	D28.2	D39.8	D49.59
patella	C40.20	C79.51	—	—	—	—
peduncle, cerebral	C71.7	C79.31	—	D33.1	D43.1	D49.6
pelvirectal junction	C19	C78.5	D01.1	D12.7	D37.5	D49.0
pelvis, pelvic	C76.3	C79.89	D09.8	D36.7	D48.7	D49.89
bone	C41.4	C79.51	—	D16.8	D48.0	D49.2
floor	C76.3	C79.89	D09.8	D36.7	D48.7	D49.89
renal	C65.-☑	C79.0-☑	D09.19	D30.1-☑	D41.1-☑	D49.51-☑
viscera	C76.3	C79.89	D09.8	D36.7	D48.7	D49.89
wall	C76.3	C79.89	D09.8	D36.7	D48.7	D49.89
pelvo-abdominal	C76.8	C79.89	D09.8	D36.7	D48.7	D49.89
penis	C60.9	C79.82	D07.4	D29.0	D40.8	D49.59
body	C60.2	C79.82	D07.4	D29.0	D40.8	D49.59
corpus (cavernosum)	C60.2	C79.82	D07.4	D29.0	D40.8	D49.59
glans	C60.1	C79.82	D07.4	D29.0	D40.8	D49.59
overlapping sites	C60.8	—	—	—	—	—
skin NEC	C60.9	C79.82	D07.4	D29.0	D40.8	D49.59
periadrenal (tissue)	C48.0	C78.6	—	D20.0	D48.3	D49.0
perianal (skin) — see also Neoplasm, anus, skin	C44.500	C79.2	D04.5	D23.5	D48.5	D49.2
pericardium	C38.0	C79.89	—	D15.1	D48.7	D49.89
perinephric	C48.0	C78.6	—	D20.0	D48.3	D49.0
perineum	C76.3	C79.89	D09.8	D36.7	D48.7	D49.89
periodontal tissue NEC	C03.9	C79.89	D00.03	D10.39	D37.09	D49.0
periosteum — see Neoplasm, bone						
peripancreatic	C48.0	C78.6	—	D20.0	D48.3	D49.0
peripheral nerve NEC	C47.9	C79.89	—	D36.10	D48.2	D49.2
perirectal (tissue)	C76.3	C79.89	—	D36.7	D48.7	D49.89
perirenal (tissue)	C48.0	C78.6	—	D20.0	D48.3	D49.0
peritoneum, peritoneal (cavity)	C48.2	C78.6	—	D20.1	D48.4	D49.0
benign mesothelial tissue — see Mesothelioma, benign						
overlapping lesion with digestive organs	C26.9	—	—	—	—	—
parietal	C48.1	C78.6	—	D20.1	D48.4	D49.0
pelvic	C48.1	C78.6	—	D20.1	D48.4	D49.0
specified part NEC	C48.1	C78.6	—	D20.1	D48.4	D49.0
peritonsillar (tissue)	C76.0	C79.89	D09.8	D36.7	D48.7	D49.89
periurethral tissue	C76.3	C79.89	—	D36.7	D48.7	D49.89
phalanges						
foot	C40.3-☑	C79.51	—	D16.3-☑	—	—
hand	C40.1-☑	C79.51	—	D16.1-☑	—	—
pharynx, pharyngeal	C14.0	C79.89	D00.08	D10.9	D37.05	D49.0
bursa	C11.1	C79.89	D00.08	D10.6	D37.05	D49.0

Neoplasm, neoplastic	Malignant Primary	Malignant Secondary	Ca in situ	Benign	Uncertain Behavior	Unspecified Behavior
— continued						
pharynx, pharyngeal — continued						
fornix	C11.3	C79.89	D00.08	D10.6	D37.05	D49.0
recess	C11.2	C79.89	D00.08	D10.6	D37.05	D49.0
region	C14.0	C79.89	D00.08	D10.9	D37.05	D49.0
tonsil	C11.1	C79.89	D00.08	D10.6	D37.05	D49.0
wall (lateral) (posterior)	C14.0	C79.89	D00.08	D10.9	D37.05	D49.0
pia mater	C70.9	C79.40	—	D32.9	D42.9	D49.7
cerebral	C70.0	C79.32	—	D32.0	D42.0	D49.7
cranial	C70.0	C79.32	—	D32.0	D42.0	D49.7
spinal	C70.1	C79.49	—	D32.1	D42.1	D49.7
pillars of fauces	C09.1	C79.89	D00.08	D10.5	D37.05	D49.0
pineal (body) (gland)	C75.3	C79.89	D09.3	D35.4	D44.5	D49.7
pinna (ear) NEC — see also Neoplasm, skin, ear	C44.20-☑	C79.2	D04.2-☑	D23.2-☑	D48.5	D49.2
piriform fossa or sinus	C12	C79.89	D00.08	D10.7	D37.05	D49.0
pituitary (body) (fossa) (gland) (lobe)	C75.1	C79.89	D09.3	D35.2	D44.3	D49.7
placenta	C58	C79.82	D07.0	D26.7	D39.2	D49.59
pleura, pleural (cavity)	C38.4	C78.2	—	D19.0	D38.2	D49.1
overlapping lesion with heart or mediastinum	C38.8	—	—	—	—	—
parietal	C38.4	C78.2	—	D19.0	D38.2	D49.1
visceral	C38.4	C78.2	—	D19.0	D38.2	D49.1
plexus						
brachial	C47.1-☑	C79.89	—	D36.12	D48.2	D49.2
cervical	C47.0	C79.89	—	D36.11	D48.2	D49.2
choroid	C71.5	C79.31	—	D33.0	D43.0	D49.6
lumbosacral	C47.5	C79.89	—	D36.16	D48.2	D49.2
sacral	C47.5	C79.89	—	D36.16	D48.2	D49.2
pluriendocrine	C75.8	C79.89	D09.3	D35.7	D44.9	D49.7
pole						
frontal	C71.1	C79.31	—	D33.0	D43.0	D49.6
occipital	C71.4	C79.31	—	D33.0	D43.0	D49.6
pons (varolii)	C71.7	C79.31	—	D33.1	D43.1	D49.6
popliteal fossa or space	C76.5-☑	C79.89	D04.7-☑	D36.7	D48.7	D49.89
postcricoid (region)	C13.0	C79.89	D00.08	D10.7	D37.05	D49.0
posterior fossa (cranial)	C71.9	C79.31	—	D33.2	D43.2	D49.6
postnasal space	C11.9	C79.89	D00.08	D10.6	D37.05	D49.0
prepuce	C60.0	C79.82	D07.4	D29.0	D40.8	D49.59
prepylorus	C16.4	C78.89	D00.2	D13.1	D37.1	D49.0
presacral (region)	C76.3	C79.89	—	D36.7	D48.7	D49.89
prostate (gland)	C61	C79.82	D07.5	D29.1	D40.0	D49.59
utricle	C68.0	C79.19	D09.19	D30.4	D41.3	D49.59
pterygoid fossa	C49.0	C79.89	—	D21.0	D48.1	D49.2
pubic bone	C41.4	C79.51	—	D16.8	D48.0	D49.2
pudenda, pudendum (female)	C51.9	C79.82	D07.1	D28.0	D39.8	D49.59
pulmonary — see also Neoplasm, lung	C34.9-☑	C78.0-☑	D02.2-☑	D14.3-☑	D38.1	D49.1
putamen	C71.0	C79.31	—	D33.0	D43.0	D49.6
pyloric						
antrum	C16.3	C78.89	D00.2	D13.1	D37.1	D49.0
canal	C16.4	C78.89	D00.2	D13.1	D37.1	D49.0
pylorus	C16.4	C78.89	D00.2	D13.1	D37.1	D49.0
pyramid (brain)	C71.7	C79.31	—	D33.1	D43.1	D49.6
pyriform fossa or sinus	C12	C79.89	D00.08	D10.7	D37.05	D49.0
radius (any part)	C40.0-☑	C79.51	—	D16.0-☑	—	—
Rathke's pouch	C75.1	C79.89	D09.3	D35.2	D44.3	D49.7
rectosigmoid (junction)	C19	C78.5	D01.1	D12.7	D37.5	D49.0
overlapping lesion with anus or rectum	C21.8	—	—	—	—	—
rectouterine pouch	C48.1	C78.6	—	D20.1	D48.4	D49.0
rectovaginal septum or wall	C76.3	C79.89	D09.8	D36.7	D48.7	D49.89
rectovesical septum	C76.3	C79.89	D09.8	D36.7	D48.7	D49.89
rectum (ampulla)	C20	C78.5	D01.2	D12.8	D37.5	D49.0

☑ Additional Character Required — Refer to the Tabular List for Character Selection ▽ Subterms under main terms may continue to next column or page

Neoplasm, neoplastic	Malignant Primary	Malignant Secondary	Ca in situ	Benign	Uncertain Behavior	Unspecified Behavior
— continued						
rectum — continued						
and colon	C19	C78.5	D01.1	D12.7	D37.5	D49.0
overlapping lesion with anus or rectosigmoid junction	C21.8	—	—	—	—	—
renal	C64.-☑	C79.0-☑	D09.19	D30.0-☑	D41.0-☑	D49.51-☑
calyx	C65.-☑	C79.0-☑	D09.19	D30.1-☑	D41.1-☑	D49.51-☑
hilus	C65.-☑	C79.0-☑	D09.19	D30.1-☑	D41.1-☑	D49.51-☑
parenchyma	C64.-☑	C79.0-☑	D09.19	D30.0-☑	D41.0-☑	D49.51-☑
pelvis	C65.-☑	C79.0-☑	D09.19	D30.1-☑	D41.1-☑	D49.51-☑
respiratory						
organs or system NEC	C39.9	C78.30	D02.4	D14.4	D38.6	D49.1
tract NEC	C39.9	C78.30	D02.4	D14.4	D38.5	D49.1
upper	C39.0	C78.30	D02.4	D14.4	D38.5	D49.1
retina	C69.2-☑	C79.49	D09.2-☑	D31.2-☑	D48.7	D49.81
retrobulbar	C69.6-☑	C79.49	—	D31.6-☑	D48.7	D49.89
retrocecal	C48.0	C78.6	—	D20.0	D48.3	D49.0
retromolar (area) (triangle)						
(trigone)	C06.2	C79.89	D00.00	D10.39	D37.09	D49.0
retro-orbital	C76.0	C79.89	D09.8	D36.7	D48.7	D49.89
retroperitoneal (space) (tissue)	C48.0	C78.6	—	D20.0	D48.3	D49.0
retroperitoneum	C48.0	C78.6	—	D20.0	D48.3	D49.0
retropharyngeal	C14.0	C79.89	D00.08	D10.9	D37.05	D49.0
retrovesical (septum)	C76.3	C79.89	D09.8	D36.7	D48.7	D49.89
rhinencephalon	C71.0	C79.31	—	D33.0	D43.0	D49.6
rib	C41.3	C79.51	—	D16.7	D48.0	D49.2
Rosenmuller's fossa	C11.2	C79.89	D00.08	D10.6	D37.05	D49.0
round ligament	C57.2-☑	C79.82	—	D28.2	D39.8	D49.59
sacrococcyx, sacrococcygeal region	C41.4	C79.51	—	D16.8	D48.0	D49.2
	C76.3	C79.89	D09.8	D36.7	D48.7	D49.89
sacrouterine ligament	C57.3	C79.82	—	D28.2	D39.8	D49.59
sacrum, sacral (vertebra)	C41.4	C79.51	—	D16.8	D48.0	D49.2
salivary gland or duct (major)	C08.9	C79.89	D00.00	D11.9	D37.039	D49.0
minor NEC	C06.9	C79.89	D00.00	D10.39	D37.04	D49.0
overlapping lesion	C08.9	—	—	—	—	—
parotid	C07	C79.89	D00.00	D11.0	D37.030	D49.0
pluriglandular	C08.9	C79.89	D00.00	D11.9	D37.039	D49.0
sublingual	C08.1	C79.89	D00.00	D11.7	D37.031	D49.0
submandibular	C08.0	C79.89	D00.00	D11.7	D37.032	D49.0
submaxillary	C08.0	C79.89	D00.00	D11.7	D37.032	D49.0
salpinx (uterine)	C57.0-☑	C79.82	D07.39	D28.2	D39.8	D49.59
Santorini's duct	C25.3	C78.89	D01.7	D13.6	D37.8	D49.0
scalp	C44.40	C79.2	D04.4	D23.4	D48.5	D49.2
basal cell carcinoma	C44.41	—	—	—	—	—
specified type NEC	C44.49	—	—	—	—	—
squamous cell carcinoma	C44.42	—	—	—	—	—
scapula (any part)	C40.0-☑	C79.51	—	D16.0-☑	D48.0	D49.2
scapular region	C76.1	C79.89	D09.8	D36.7	D48.7	D49.89
scar NEC — see also Neoplasm, skin, by site	C44.90	C79.2	D04.9	D23.9	D48.5	D49.2
sciatic nerve	C47.2-☑	C79.89	—	D36.13	D48.2	D49.2
sclera	C69.4-☑	C79.49	D09.2-☑	D31.4-☑	D48.7	D49.89
scrotum (skin)	C63.2	C79.82	D07.61	D29.4	D40.8	D49.59
sebaceous gland — see Neoplasm, skin						
sella turcica	C75.1	C79.89	D09.3	D35.2	D44.3	D49.7
bone	C41.0	C79.51	—	D16.4	D48.0	D49.2
semilunar cartilage (knee)	C40.2-☑	C79.51	—	D16.2-☑	D48.0	D49.2
seminal vesicle	C63.7	C79.82	D07.69	D29.8	D40.8	D49.59
septum						
nasal	C30.0	C78.39	D02.3	D14.0	D38.5	D49.1
posterior margin	C11.3	C79.89	D00.08	D10.6	D37.05	D49.0
rectovaginal	C76.3	C79.89	D09.8	D36.7	D48.7	D49.89
rectovesical	C76.3	C79.89	D09.8	D36.7	D48.7	D49.89

Neoplasm, neoplastic	Malignant Primary	Malignant Secondary	Ca in situ	Benign	Uncertain Behavior	Unspecified Behavior
— continued						
septum — continued						
urethrovaginal	C57.9	C79.82	D07.30	D28.9	D39.9	D49.59
vesicovaginal	C57.9	C79.82	D07.30	D28.9	D39.9	D49.59
shoulder NEC	C76.4-☑	C79.89	D04.6-☑	D36.7	D48.7	D49.89
sigmoid flexure (lower) (upper)	C18.7	C78.5	D01.0	D12.5	D37.4	D49.0
sinus (accessory)	C31.9	C78.39	D02.3	D14.0	D38.5	D49.1
bone (any)	C41.0	C79.51	—	D16.4	D48.0	D49.2
ethmoidal	C31.1	C78.39	D02.3	D14.0	D38.5	D49.1
frontal	C31.2	C78.39	D02.3	D14.0	D38.5	D49.1
maxillary	C31.0	C78.39	D02.3	D14.0	D38.5	D49.1
nasal, paranasal NEC	C31.9	C78.39	D02.3	D14.0	D38.5	D49.1
overlapping lesion	C31.8	—	—	—	—	—
pyriform	C12	C79.89	D00.08	D10.7	D37.05	D49.0
sphenoid	C31.3	C78.39	D02.3	D14.0	D38.5	D49.1
skeleton, skeletal NEC	C41.9	C79.51	—	D16.9	D48.0	D49.2
Skene's gland	C68.1	C79.19	D09.19	D30.8	D41.8	D49.59
skin NOS	C44.90	C79.2	D04.9	D23.9	D48.5	D49.2
abdominal wall	C44.509	C79.2	D04.5	D23.5	D48.5	D49.2
basal cell carcinoma	C44.519	—	—	—	—	—
specified type NEC	C44.599	—	—	—	—	—
squamous cell carcinoma	C44.529	—	—	—	—	—
ala nasi — see also Neoplasm, nose, skin	C44.301	C79.2	D04.39	D23.39	D48.5	D49.2
ankle — see also Neoplasm, skin, limb, lower	C44.70-☑	C79.2	D04.7-☑	D23.7-☑	D48.5	D49.2
antecubital space — see also Neoplasm, skin, limb, upper	C44.60-☑	C79.2	D04.6-☑	D23.6-☑	D48.5	D49.2
anus	C44.500	C79.2	D04.5	D23.5	D48.5	D49.2
basal cell carcinoma	C44.510	—	—	—	—	—
specified type NEC	C44.590	—	—	—	—	—
squamous cell carcinoma	C44.520	—	—	—	—	—
arm — see also Neoplasm, skin, limb, upper	C44.60-☑	C79.2	D04.6-☑	D23.6-☑	D48.5	D49.2
auditory canal (external) — see also Neoplasm, skin, ear	C44.20-☑	C79.2	D04.2-☑	D23.2-☑	D48.5	D49.2
auricle (ear) — see also Neoplasm, skin, ear	C44.20-☑	C79.2	D04.2-☑	D23.2-☑	D48.5	D49.2
auricular canal (external) — see also Neoplasm, skin, ear	C44.20-☑	C79.2	D04.2-☑	D23.2-☑	D48.5	D49.2
axilla, axillary fold — see also Neoplasm, skin, trunk	C44.509	C79.2	D04.5	D23.5	D48.5	D49.2
back — see also Neoplasm, skin, trunk	C44.509	C79.2	D04.5	D23.5	D48.5	D49.2
basal cell carcinoma	C44.91	—	—	—	—	—
breast	C44.501	C79.2	D04.5	D23.5	D48.5	D49.2
basal cell carcinoma	C44.511	—	—	—	—	—
specified type NEC	C44.591	—	—	—	—	—
squamous cell carcinoma	C44.521	—	—	—	—	—
brow — see also Neoplasm, skin, face	C44.309	C79.2	D04.39	D23.39	D48.5	D49.2
buttock — see also Neoplasm, skin, trunk	C44.509	C79.2	D04.5	D23.5	D48.5	D49.2

	Malignant Primary	Malignant Secondary	Ca in situ	Benign	Uncertain Behavior	Unspecified Behavior
Neoplasm, neoplastic						
— *continued*						
skin — *continued*						
calf — *see also*						
Neoplasm, skin,						
limb, lower	C44.70-☑	C79.2	D04.7-☑	D23.7-☑	D48.5	D49.2
canthus (eye) (inner)						
(outer)	C44.10-☑	C79.2	D04.1-☑	D23.1-☑	D48.5	D49.2
basal cell						
carcinoma	C44.11-☑	—	—	—	—	—
sebaceous cell	C44.13-☑	—	—	—	—	—
specified type						
NEC	C44.19-☑	—	—	—	—	—
squamous cell						
carcinoma	C44.12-☑	—	—	—	—	—
cervical region — *see*						
also Neoplasm,						
skin, neck	C44.40	C79.2	D04.4	D23.4	D48.5	D49.2
cheek (external) —						
see also						
Neoplasm, skin,						
face	C44.309	C79.2	D04.39	D23.39	D48.5	D49.2
chest (wall) — *see*						
also Neoplasm,						
skin, trunk	C44.509	C79.2	D04.5	D23.5	D48.5	D49.2
chin — *see also*						
Neoplasm, skin,						
face	C44.309	C79.2	D04.39	D23.39	D48.5	D49.2
clavicular area — *see*						
also Neoplasm,						
skin, trunk	C44.509	C79.2	D04.5	D23.5	D48.5	D49.2
clitoris	C51.2	C79.82	D07.1	D28.0	D39.8	D49.59
columnella — *see*						
also Neoplasm,						
skin, face	C44.309	C79.2	D04.39	D23.39	D48.5	D49.2
concha — *see also*						
Neoplasm, skin,						
ear	C44.20-☑	C79.2	D04.2-☑	D23.2-☑	D48.5	D49.2
ear (external)	C44.20-☑	C79.2	D04.2-☑	D23.2-☑	D48.5	D49.2
basal cell						
carcinoma	C44.21-☑	—	—	—	—	—
specified type						
NEC	C44.29-☑	—	—	—	—	—
squamous cell						
carcinoma	C44.22-☑	—	—	—	—	—
elbow — *see also*						
Neoplasm, skin,						
limb, upper	C44.60-☑	C79.2	D04.6-☑	D23.6-☑	D48.5	D49.2
eyebrow — *see also*						
Neoplasm, skin,						
face	C44.309	C79.2	D04.39	D23.39	D48.5	D49.2
eyelid	C44.10-☑	C79.2	D04.1-☑	D23.1-☑	D48.5	D49.2
basal cell						
carcinoma	C44.11-☑	—	—	—	—	—
sebaceous cell	C44.13-☑	—	—	—	—	—
specified type						
NEC	C44.19-☑	—	—	—	—	—
squamous cell						
carcinoma	C44.12-☑	—	—	—	—	—
face NOS	C44.300	C79.2	D04.30	D23.30	D48.5	D49.2
basal cell						
carcinoma	C44.310	—	—	—	—	—
specified type						
NEC	C44.390	—	—	—	—	—
squamous cell						
carcinoma	C44.320	—	—	—	—	—
female genital organs						
(external)	C51.9	C79.82	D07.1	D28.0	D39.8	D49.59
clitoris	C51.2	C79.82	D07.1	D28.0	D39.8	D49.59
labium NEC	C51.9	C79.82	D07.1	D28.0	D39.8	D49.59
majus	C51.0	C79.82	D07.1	D28.0	D39.8	D49.59
minus	C51.1	C79.82	D07.1	D28.0	D39.8	D49.59
pudendum	C51.9	C79.82	D07.1	D28.0	D39.8	D49.59
vulva	C51.9	C79.82	D07.1	D28.0	D39.8	D49.59
finger — *see also*						
Neoplasm, skin,						
limb, upper	C44.60-☑	C79.2	D04.6-☑	D23.6-☑	D48.5	D49.2
flank — *see also*						
Neoplasm, skin,						
trunk	C44.509	C79.2	D04.5	D23.5	D48.5	D49.2
foot — *see also*						
Neoplasm, skin,						
limb, lower	C44.70-☑	C79.2	D04.7-☑	D23.7-☑	D48.5	D49.2

	Malignant Primary	Malignant Secondary	Ca in situ	Benign	Uncertain Behavior	Unspecified Behavior
Neoplasm, neoplastic						
— *continued*						
skin — *continued*						
forearm — *see also*						
Neoplasm, skin,						
limb, upper	C44.60-☑	C79.2	D04.6-☑	D23.6-☑	D48.5	D49.2
forehead — *see also*						
Neoplasm, skin,						
face	C44.309	C79.2	D04.39	D23.39	D48.5	D49.2
glabella — *see also*						
Neoplasm, skin,						
face	C44.309	C79.2	D04.39	D23.39	D48.5	D49.2
gluteal region — *see*						
also Neoplasm,						
skin, trunk	C44.509	C79.2	D04.5	D23.5	D48.5	D49.2
groin — *see also*						
Neoplasm, skin,						
trunk	C44.509	C79.2	D04.5	D23.5	D48.5	D49.2
hand — *see also*						
Neoplasm, skin,						
limb, upper	C44.60-☑	C79.2	D04.6-☑	D23.6-☑	D48.5	D49.2
head NEC — *see also*						
Neoplasm, skin,						
scalp	C44.40	C79.2	D04.4	D23.4	D48.5	D49.2
heel — *see also*						
Neoplasm, skin,						
limb, lower	C44.70-☑	C79.2	D04.7-☑	D23.7-☑	D48.5	D49.2
helix — *see also*						
Neoplasm, skin,						
ear	C44.20-☑	C79.2	D04.2-☑	D23.2-☑	D48.5	D49.2
hip — *see also*						
Neoplasm, skin,						
limb, lower	C44.70-☑	C79.2	D04.7-☑	D23.7-☑	D48.5	D49.2
infraclavicular region						
— *see also*						
Neoplasm, skin,						
trunk	C44.509	C79.2	D04.5	D23.5	D48.5	D49.2
inguinal region — *see*						
also Neoplasm,						
skin, trunk	C44.509	C79.2	D04.5	D23.5	D48.5	D49.2
jaw — *see also*						
Neoplasm, skin,						
face	C44.309	C79.2	D04.39	D23.39	D48.5	D49.2
Kaposi's sarcoma —						
see Kaposi's,						
sarcoma, skin						
knee — *see also*						
Neoplasm, skin,						
limb, lower	C44.70-☑	C79.2	D04.7-☑	D23.7-☑	D48.5	D49.2
labia						
majora	C51.0	C79.82	D07.1	D28.0	D39.8	D49.59
minora	C51.1	C79.82	D07.1	D28.0	D39.8	D49.59
leg — *see also*						
Neoplasm, skin,						
limb, lower	C44.70-☑	C79.2	D04.7-☑	D23.7-☑	D48.5	D49.2
lid (lower)						
(upper)	C44.10-☑	C79.2	D04.1-☑	D23.1-☑	D48.5	D49.2
basal cell						
carcinoma	C44.11-☑	—	—	—	—	—
sebaceous cell	C44.13-☑	—	—	—	—	—
specified type						
NEC	C44.19-☑	—	—	—	—	—
squamous cell						
carcinoma	C44.12-☑	—	—	—	—	—
limb NEC	C44.90	C79.2	D04.9	D23.9	D48.5	D49.2
basal cell						
carcinoma	C44.91	—	—	—	—	—
lower	C44.70-☑	C79.2	D04.7-☑	D23.7-☑	D48.5	D49.2
basal cell						
carcinoma	C44.71-☑	—	—	—	—	—
specified type						
NEC	C44.79-☑	—	—	—	—	—
squamous cell						
carcinoma	C44.72-☑	—	—	—	—	—
upper	C44.60-☑	C79.2	D04.6-☑	D23.6-☑	D48.5	D49.2
basal cell						
carcinoma	C44.61-☑	—	—	—	—	—
specified type						
NEC	C44.69-☑	—	—	—	—	—
squamous cell						
carcinoma	C44.62-☑	—	—	—	—	—
lip (lower)						
(upper)	C44.00	C79.2	D04.0	D23.0	D48.5	D49.2

   ☑ **Additional Character Required — Refer to the Tabular List for Character Selection**   ▽ Subterms under main terms may continue to next column or page

Neoplasm, neoplastic — continued
skin — continued

	Malignant Primary	Malignant Secondary	Ca in situ	Benign	Uncertain Behavior	Unspecified Behavior
lip — continued						
basal cell carcinoma	C44.01	—	—	—	—	—
specified type NEC	C44.09	—	—	—	—	—
squamous cell carcinoma	C44.02	—	—	—	—	—
male genital organs	C63.9	C79.82	D07.60	D29.9	D40.8	D49.59
penis	C60.9	C79.82	D07.4	D29.0	D40.8	D49.59
prepuce	C60.0	C79.82	D07.4	D29.0	D40.8	D49.59
scrotum	C63.2	C79.82	D07.61	D29.4	D40.8	D49.59
mastectomy site (skin) — see also Neoplasm, skin, breast	C44.501	C79.2				
specified as breast tissue	C50.8-☑	C79.81	—	—	—	—
meatus, acoustic (external) — see also Neoplasm, skin, ear	C44.20-☑	C79.2	D04.2-☑	D23.2-☑	D48.5	D49.2
melanotic — see Melanoma						
Merkel cell — see Carcinoma, Merkel cell						
nates — see also Neoplasm, skin, trunk	C44.509	C79.2	D04.5	D23.5	D48.5	D49.2
neck	C44.40	C79.2	D04.4	D23.4	D48.5	D49.2
basal cell carcinoma	C44.41	—	—	—	—	—
specified type NEC	C44.49	—	—	—	—	—
squamous cell carcinoma	C44.42	—	—	—	—	—
nevus — see Nevus, skin						
nose (external) — see also Neoplasm, nose, skin	C44.301	C79.2	D04.39	D23.39	D48.5	D49.2
overlapping lesion	C44.80	—	—	—	—	—
basal cell carcinoma	C44.81	—	—	—	—	—
specified type NEC	C44.89	—	—	—	—	—
squamous cell carcinoma	C44.82	—	—	—	—	—
palm — see also Neoplasm, skin, limb, upper	C44.60-☑	C79.2	D04.6-☑	D23.6-☑	D48.5	D49.2
palpebra	C44.10-☑	C79.2	D04.1-☑	D23.1-☑	D48.5	D49.2
basal cell carcinoma	C44.11-☑	—	—	—	—	—
sebaceous cell	C44.13-☑	—	—	—	—	—
specified type NEC	C44.19-☑	—	—	—	—	—
squamous cell carcinoma	C44.12-☑	—	—	—	—	—
penis NEC	C60.9	C79.82	D07.4	D29.0	D40.8	D49.59
perianal — see also Neoplasm, skin, anus	C44.500	C79.2	D04.5	D23.5	D48.5	D49.2
perineum — see also Neoplasm, skin, anus	C44.500	C79.2	D04.5	D23.5	D48.5	D49.2
pinna — see also Neoplasm, skin, ear	C44.20-☑	C79.2	D04.2-☑	D23.2-☑	D48.5	D49.2
plantar — see also Neoplasm, skin, limb, lower	C44.70-☑	C79.2	D04.7-☑	D23.7-☑	D48.5	D49.2
popliteal fossa or space — see also Neoplasm, skin, limb, lower	C44.70-☑	C79.2	D04.7-☑	D23.7-☑	D48.5	D49.2
prepuce	C60.0	C79.82	D07.4	D29.0	D40.8	D49.59

Neoplasm, neoplastic — continued
skin — continued

	Malignant Primary	Malignant Secondary	Ca in situ	Benign	Uncertain Behavior	Unspecified Behavior
pubes — see also Neoplasm, skin, trunk	C44.509	C79.2	D04.5	D23.5	D48.5	D49.2
sacrococcygeal region — see also Neoplasm, skin, trunk	C44.509	C79.2	D04.5	D23.5	D48.5	D49.2
scalp	C44.40	C79.2	D04.4	D23.4	D48.5	D49.2
basal cell carcinoma	C44.41	—	—	—	—	—
specified type NEC	C44.49	—	—	—	—	—
squamous cell carcinoma	C44.42	—	—	—	—	—
scapular region — see also Neoplasm, skin, trunk	C44.509	C79.2	D04.5	D23.5	D48.5	D49.2
scrotum	C63.2	C79.82	D07.61	D29.4	D40.8	D49.59
shoulder — see also Neoplasm, skin, limb, upper	C44.60-☑	C79.2	D04.6-☑	D23.6-☑	D48.5	D49.2
sole (foot) — see also Neoplasm, skin, limb, lower	C44.70-☑	C79.2	D04.7-☑	D23.7-☑	D48.5	D49.2
specified sites NEC	C44.80	C79.2	D04.8	D23.9	D48.5	D49.2
basal cell carcinoma	C44.81	—	—	—	—	—
specified type NEC	C44.89	—	—	—	—	—
squamous cell carcinoma	C44.82	—	—	—	—	—
specified type NEC	C44.99	—	—	—	—	—
squamous cell carcinoma	C44.92	—	—	—	—	—
submammary fold — see also Neoplasm, skin, trunk	C44.509	C79.2	D04.5	D23.5	D48.5	D49.2
supraclavicular region — see also Neoplasm, skin, neck	C44.40	C79.2	D04.4	D23.4	D48.5	D49.2
temple — see also Neoplasm, skin, face	C44.309	C79.2	D04.39	D23.39	D48.5	D49.2
thigh — see also Neoplasm, skin, limb, lower	C44.70-☑	C79.2	D04.7-☑	D23.7-☑	D48.5	D49.2
thoracic wall — see also Neoplasm, skin, trunk	C44.509	C79.2	D04.5	D23.5	D48.5	D49.2
thumb — see also Neoplasm, skin, limb, upper	C44.60-☑	C79.2	D04.6-☑	D23.6-☑	D48.5	D49.2
toe — see also Neoplasm, skin, limb, lower	C44.70-☑	C79.2	D04.7-☑	D23.7-☑	D48.5	D49.2
tragus — see also Neoplasm, skin, ear	C44.20-☑	C79.2	D04.2-☑	D23.2-☑	D48.5	D49.2
trunk	C44.509	C79.2	D04.5	D23.5	D48.5	D49.2
basal cell carcinoma	C44.519	—	—	—	—	—
specified type NEC	C44.599	—	—	—	—	—
squamous cell carcinoma	C44.529	—	—	—	—	—
umbilicus — see also Neoplasm, skin, trunk	C44.509	C79.2	D04.5	D23.5	D48.5	D49.2
vulva	C51.9	C79.82	D07.1	D28.0	D39.8	D49.59
overlapping lesion	C51.8					
wrist — see also Neoplasm, skin, limb, upper	C44.60-☑	C79.2	D04.6-☑	D23.6-☑	D48.5	D49.2
skull	C41.0	C79.51	—	D16.4	D48.0	D49.2

Neoplasm, neoplastic	Malignant Primary	Malignant Secondary	Ca in situ	Benign	Uncertain Behavior	Unspecified Behavior
— continued						
soft parts or tissues —						
see Neoplasm,						
connective tissue						
specified site NEC	C76.8	C79.89	D09.8	D36.7	D48.7	D49.89
spermatic cord	C63.1-☑	C79.82	D07.69	D29.8	D40.8	D49.59
sphenoid	C31.3	C78.39	D02.3	D14.0	D38.5	D49.1
bone	C41.0	C79.51	—	D16.4	D48.0	D49.2
sinus	C31.3	C78.39	D02.3	D14.0	D38.5	D49.1
sphincter						
anal	C21.1	C78.5	D01.3	D12.9	D37.8	D49.0
of Oddi	C24.0	C78.89	D01.5	D13.5	D37.6	D49.0
spine, spinal						
(column)	C41.2	C79.51	—	D16.6	D48.0	D49.2
bulb	C71.7	C79.31	—	D33.1	D43.1	D49.6
coccyx	C41.4	C79.51	—	D16.8	D48.0	D49.2
cord (cervical)						
(lumbar) (sacral)						
(thoracic)	C72.0	C79.49	—	D33.4	D43.4	D49.7
dura mater	C70.1	C79.49	—	D32.1	D42.1	D49.7
lumbosacral	C41.2	C79.51	—	D16.6	D48.0	D49.2
marrow NEC	C96.9	C79.52	—	—	D47.9	D49.89
membrane	C70.1	C79.49	—	D32.1	D42.1	D49.7
meninges	C70.1	C79.49	—	D32.1	D42.1	D49.7
nerve (root)	C47.9	C79.89	—	D36.10	D48.2	D49.2
pia mater	C70.1	C79.49	—	D32.1	D42.1	D49.7
root	C47.9	C79.89	—	D36.10	D48.2	D49.2
sacrum	C41.4	C79.51	—	D16.8	D48.0	D49.2
spleen, splenic						
NEC	C26.1	C78.89	D01.7	D13.9	D37.8	D49.0
flexure (colon)	C18.5	C78.5	D01.0	D12.3	D37.4	D49.0
stem, brain	C71.7	C79.31	—	D33.1	D43.1	D49.6
Stensen's duct	C07	C79.89	D00.00	D11.0	D37.030	D49.0
sternum	C41.3	C79.51	—	D16.7	D48.0	D49.2
stomach	C16.9	C78.89	D00.2	D13.1	D37.1	D49.0
antrum (pyloric)	C16.3	C78.89	D00.2	D13.1	D37.1	D49.0
body	C16.2	C78.89	D00.2	D13.1	D37.1	D49.0
cardia	C16.0	C78.89	D00.2	D13.1	D37.1	D49.0
cardiac orifice	C16.0	C78.82	D00.2	D13.1	D37.1	D49.0
corpus	C16.2	C78.89	D00.2	D13.1	D37.1	D49.0
fundus	C16.1	C78.89	D00.2	D13.1	D37.1	D49.0
greater curvature						
NEC	C16.6	C78.89	D00.2	D13.1	D37.1	D49.0
lesser curvature						
NEC	C16.5	C78.89	D00.2	D13.1	D37.1	D49.0
overlapping						
lesion	C16.8	—	—	—	—	—
prepylorus	C16.4	C78.89	D00.2	D13.1	D37.1	D49.0
pylorus	C16.4	C78.89	D00.2	D13.1	D37.1	D49.0
wall NEC	C16.9	C78.89	D00.2	D13.1	D37.1	D49.0
anterior NEC	C16.8	C78.89	D00.2	D13.1	D37.1	D49.0
posterior NEC	C16.8	C78.89	D00.2	D13.1	D37.1	D49.0
stroma,						
endometrial	C54.1	C79.82	D07.0	D26.1	D39.0	D49.59
stump, cervical	C53.8	C79.82	D06.7	D26.1	D39.0	D49.59
subcutaneous (nodule)						
(tissue) NEC — *see*						
Neoplasm,						
connective tissue						
subdural	C70.9	C79.32	—	D32.9	D42.9	D49.7
subglottis,						
subglottic	C32.2	C78.39	D02.0	D14.1	D38.0	D49.1
sublingual	C04.9	C79.89	D00.06	D10.2	D37.09	D49.0
gland or duct	C08.1	C79.89	D00.00	D11.7	D37.031	D49.0
submandibular						
gland	C08.0	C79.89	D00.00	D11.7	D37.032	D49.0
submaxillary gland or						
duct	C08.0	C79.89	D00.00	D11.7	D37.032	D49.0
submental	C76.0	C79.89	D09.8	D36.7	D48.7	D49.89
subpleural	C34.9-☑	C78.0-☑	D02.2-☑	D14.3-☑	D38.1	D49.1
substernal	C38.1	C78.1	—	D15.2	D38.3	D49.89
sudoriferous,						
sudoriparous gland,						
site						
unspecified	C44.90	C79.2	D04.9	D23.9	D48.5	D49.2
specified site — *see*						
Neoplasm, skin						
supraclavicular						
region	C76.0	C79.89	D09.8	D36.7	D48.7	D49.89
supraglottis	C32.1	C78.39	D02.0	D14.1	D38.0	D49.1
suprarenal	C74.9-☑	C79.7-☑	D09.3	D35.0-☑	D44.1-☑	D49.7
capsule	C74.9-☑	C79.7-☑	D09.3	D35.0-☑	D44.1-☑	D49.7

Neoplasm, neoplastic	Malignant Primary	Malignant Secondary	Ca in situ	Benign	Uncertain Behavior	Unspecified Behavior
— continued						
suprarenal —						
continued						
cortex	C74.0-☑	C79.7-☑	D09.3	D35.0-☑	D44.1-☑	D49.7
gland	C74.9-☑	C79.7-☑	D09.3	D35.0-☑	D44.1-☑	D49.7
medulla	C74.1-☑	C79.7-☑	D09.3	D35.0-☑	D44.1-☑	D49.7
suprasellar						
(region)	C71.9	C79.31	—	D33.2	D43.2	D49.6
supratentorial (brain)						
NEC	C71.0	C79.31	—	D33.0	D43.0	D49.6
sweat gland (apocrine)						
(eccrine), site						
unspecified	C44.90	C79.2	D04.9	D23.9	D48.5	D49.2
specified site — *see*						
Neoplasm, skin						
sympathetic nerve or						
nervous system						
NEC	C47.9	C79.89	—	D36.10	D48.2	D49.2
symphysis pubis	C41.4	C79.51	—	D16.8	D48.0	D49.2
synovial membrane —						
see Neoplasm,						
connective tissue						
tapetum, brain	C71.8	C79.31	—	D33.2	D43.2	D49.6
tarsus (any bone)	C40.3-☑	C79.51	—	D16.3-☑	—	—
temple (skin) — *see*						
also Neoplasm, skin,						
face	C44.309	C79.2	D04.39	D23.39	D48.5	D49.2
temporal						
bone	C41.0	C79.51	—	D16.4	D48.0	D49.2
lobe or pole	C71.2	C79.31	—	D33.0	D43.0	D49.6
region	C76.0	C79.89	D09.8	D36.7	D48.7	D49.89
skin — *see also*						
Neoplasm, skin,						
face	C44.309	C79.2	D04.39	D23.39	D48.5	D49.2
tendon (sheath) — *see*						
Neoplasm,						
connective tissue						
tentorium						
(cerebelli)	C70.0	C79.32	—	D32.0	D42.0	D49.7
testis, testes	C62.9-☑	C79.82	D07.69	D29.2-☑	D40.1-☑	D49.59
descended	C62.1-☑	C79.82	D07.69	D29.2-☑	D40.1-☑	D49.59
ectopic	C62.0-☑	C79.82	D07.69	D29.2-☑	D40.1-☑	D49.59
retained	C62.0-☑	C79.82	D07.69	D29.2-☑	D40.1-☑	D49.59
scrotal	C62.1-☑	C79.82	D07.69	D29.2-☑	D40.1-☑	D49.59
undescended	C62.0-☑	C79.82	D07.69	D29.2-☑	D40.1-☑	D49.59
unspecified whether						
descended or						
undescended	C62.9-☑	C79.82	D07.69	D29.2-☑	D40.1-☑	D49.59
thalamus	C71.0	C79.31	—	D33.0	D43.0	D49.6
thigh NEC	C76.5-☑	C79.89	D04.7-☑	D36.7	D48.7	D49.89
thorax, thoracic (cavity)						
(organs NEC)	C76.1	C79.89	D09.8	D36.7	D48.7	D49.89
duct	C49.3	C79.89	—	D21.3	D48.1	D49.2
wall NEC	C76.1	C79.89	D09.8	D36.7	D48.7	D49.89
throat	C14.0	C79.89	D00.08	D10.9	D37.05	D49.0
thumb NEC	C76.4-☑	C79.89	D04.6-☑	D36.7	D48.7	D49.89
thymus (gland)	C37	C79.89	D09.3	D15.0	D38.4	D49.89
thyroglossal duct	C73	C79.89	D09.3	D34	D44.0	D49.7
thyroid (gland)	C73	C79.89	D09.3	D34	D44.0	D49.7
cartilage	C32.3	C78.39	D02.0	D14.1	D38.0	D49.1
tibia (any part)	C40.2-☑	C79.51	—	D16.2-☑	—	—
toe NEC	C76.5-☑	C79.89	D04.7-☑	D36.7	D48.7	D49.89
tongue	C02.9	C79.89	D00.07	D10.1	D37.02	D49.0
anterior (two-thirds)						
NEC	C02.3	C79.89	D00.07	D10.1	D37.02	D49.0
dorsal surface	C02.0	C79.89	D00.07	D10.1	D37.02	D49.0
ventral surface	C02.2	C79.89	D00.07	D10.1	D37.02	D49.0
base (dorsal						
surface)	C01	C79.89	D00.07	D10.1	D37.02	D49.0
border (lateral)	C02.1	C79.89	D00.07	D10.1	D37.02	D49.0
dorsal surface						
NEC	C02.0	C79.89	D00.07	D10.1	D37.02	D49.0
fixed part NEC	C01	C79.89	D00.07	D10.1	D37.02	D49.0
foreamen						
cecum	C02.0	C79.89	D00.07	D10.1	D37.02	D49.0
frenulum						
linguae	C02.2	C79.89	D00.07	D10.1	D37.02	D49.0
junctional zone	C02.8	C79.89	D00.07	D10.1	D37.02	D49.0
margin (lateral)	C02.1	C79.89	D00.07	D10.1	D37.02	D49.0
midline NEC	C02.0	C79.89	D00.07	D10.1	D37.02	D49.0
mobile part NEC	C02.3	C79.89	D00.07	D10.1	D37.02	D49.0

☑ Additional Character Required — Refer to the Tabular List for Character Selection · Subterms under main terms may continue to next column or page

Neoplasm, neoplastic — continued

	Malignant Primary	Malignant Secondary	Ca in situ	Benign	Uncertain Behavior	Unspecified Behavior
tongue — continued						
overlapping lesion	C02.8	—	—	—	—	—
posterior (third)	C01	C79.89	D00.07	D10.1	D37.02	D49.0
root	C01	C79.89	D00.07	D10.1	D37.02	D49.0
surface (dorsal)	C02.0	C79.89	D00.07	D10.1	D37.02	D49.0
base	C01	C79.89	D00.07	D10.1	D37.02	D49.0
ventral	C02.2	C79.89	D00.07	D10.1	D37.02	D49.0
tip	C02.1	C79.89	D00.07	D10.1	D37.02	D49.0
tonsil	C02.4	C79.89	D00.07	D10.1	D37.02	D49.0
tonsil	C09.9	C79.89	D00.08	D10.4	D37.05	D49.0
fauces, faucial	C09.9	C79.89	D00.08	D10.4	D37.05	D49.0
lingual	C02.4	C79.89	D00.07	D10.1	D37.02	D49.0
overlapping sites	C09.8	—	—	—	—	—
palatine	C09.9	C79.89	D00.08	D10.4	D37.05	D49.0
pharyngeal	C11.1	C79.89	D00.08	D10.6	D37.05	D49.0
pillar (anterior) (posterior)	C09.1	C79.89	D00.08	D10.5	D37.05	D49.0
tonsillar fossa	C09.0	C79.89	D00.08	D10.5	D37.05	D49.0
tooth socket NEC	C03.9	C79.89	D00.03	D10.39	D37.09	D49.0
trachea (cartilage) (mucosa)	C33	C78.39	D02.1	D14.2	D38.1	D49.1
overlapping lesion with bronchus or lung	C34.8-☑	—	—	—	—	—
tracheobronchial	C34.8-☑	C78.39	D02.1	D14.2	D38.1	D49.1
overlapping lesion with lung	C34.8-☑	—	—	—	—	—
tragus — see also Neoplasm, skin, ear	C44.20-☑	C79.2	D04.2-☑	D23.2-☑	D48.5	D49.2
trunk NEC	C76.8	C79.89	D04.5	D36.7	D48.7	D49.89
tubo-ovarian	C57.8	C79.82	D07.39	D28.7	D39.8	D49.59
tunica vaginalis	C63.7	C79.82	D07.69	D29.8	D40.8	D49.59
turbinate (bone)	C41.0	C79.51		D16.4	D48.0	D49.2
nasal	C30.0	C78.39	D02.3	D14.0	D38.5	D49.1
tympanic cavity	C30.1	C78.39	D02.3	D14.0	D38.5	D49.1
ulna (any part)	C40.0-☑	C79.51		D16.0-☑	—	—
umbilicus, umbilical — see also Neoplasm, skin, trunk	C44.509	C79.2	D04.5	D23.5	D48.5	D49.2
uncus, brain	C71.2	C79.31		D33.0	D43.0	D49.6
unknown site or unspecified	C80.1	C79.9	D09.9	D36.9	D48.9	D49.9
urachus	C67.7	C79.11	D09.0	D30.3	D41.4	D49.4
ureter-bladder (junction)	C67.6	C79.11	D09.0	D30.3	D41.4	D49.4
ureter, ureteral	C66.-☑	C79.19	D09.19	D30.2-☑	D41.2-☑	D49.59
orifice (bladder)	C67.6	C79.11	D09.0	D30.3	D41.4	D49.4
urethra, urethral (gland)	C68.0	C79.19	D09.19	D30.4	D41.3	D49.59
orifice, internal	C67.5	C79.11	D09.0	D30.3	D41.4	D49.4
urethrovaginal (septum)	C57.9	C79.82	D07.30	D28.9	D39.8	D49.59
urinary organ or system	C68.9	C79.10	D09.10	D30.9	D41.9	D49.59
bladder — see Neoplasm, bladder						
overlapping lesion	C68.8	—	—	—	—	—
specified sites NEC	C68.8	C79.19	D09.19	D30.8	D41.8	D49.59
utero-ovarian	C57.8	C79.82	D07.39	D28.7	D39.8	D49.59
ligament	C57.1-☑	C79.82	D07.39	D28.2	D39.8	D49.59
uterosacral ligament	C57.3	C79.82	—	D28.2	D39.8	D49.59
uterus, uteri, uterine	C55	C79.82	D07.0	D26.9	D39.0	D49.59
adnexa NEC	C57.4	C79.82	D07.39	D28.7	D39.8	D49.59
body	C54.9	C79.82	D07.0	D26.1	D39.0	D49.59
cervix	C53.9	C79.82	D06.9	D26.0	D39.0	D49.59
cornu	C54.9	C79.82	D07.0	D26.1	D39.0	D49.59
corpus	C54.9	C79.82	D07.0	D26.1	D39.0	D49.59
endocervix (canal) (gland)	C53.0	C79.82	D06.0	D26.0	D39.0	D49.59
endometrium	C54.1	C79.82	D07.0	D26.1	D39.0	D49.59
exocervix	C53.1	C79.82	D06.1	D26.0	D39.0	D49.59
external os	C53.1	C79.82	D06.1	D26.0	D39.0	D49.59
fundus	C54.3	C79.82	D07.0	D26.1	D39.0	D49.59

Neoplasm, neoplastic — continued

	Malignant Primary	Malignant Secondary	Ca in situ	Benign	Uncertain Behavior	Unspecified Behavior
uterus, uteri, uterine — continued						
internal os	C53.0	C79.82	D06.0	D26.0	D39.0	D49.59
isthmus	C54.0	C79.82	D07.0	D26.1	D39.0	D49.59
ligament	C57.3	C79.82	—	D28.2	D39.8	D49.59
broad	C57.1-☑	C79.82	D07.39	D28.2	D39.8	D49.59
round	C57.2-☑	C79.82		D28.2	D39.8	D49.59
lower segment	C54.0	C79.82	D07.0	D26.1	D39.0	D49.59
myometrium	C54.2	C79.82	D07.0	D26.1	D39.0	D49.59
overlapping sites	C54.8	—	—	—	—	—
squamocolumnar junction	C53.8	C79.82	D06.7	D26.0	D39.0	D49.59
tube	C57.0-☑	C79.82	D07.39	D28.2	D39.8	D49.59
utricle, prostatic	C68.0	C79.19	D09.19	D30.4	D41.3	D49.59
uveal tract	C69.4-☑	C79.49	D09.2-☑	D31.4-☑	D48.7	D49.89
uvula	C05.2	C79.89	D00.04	D10.39	D37.09	D49.0
vagina, vaginal (fornix) (vault) (wall)	C52	C79.82	D07.2	D28.1	D39.8	D49.59
vaginovesical	C57.9	C79.82	D07.30	D28.9	D39.9	D49.59
septum	C57.9	C79.82	D07.30	D28.9	D39.9	D49.59
vallecula (epiglottis)	C10.0	C79.89	D00.08	D10.5	D37.05	D49.0
vascular — see Neoplasm, connective tissue						
vas deferens	C63.1-☑	C79.82	D07.69	D29.8	D40.8	D49.59
Vater's ampulla	C24.1	C78.89	D01.5	D13.5	D37.6	D49.0
vein, venous — see Neoplasm, connective tissue						
vena cava (abdominal) (inferior)	C49.4	C79.89	—	D21.4	D48.1	D49.2
superior	C49.3	C79.89	—	D21.3	D48.1	D49.2
ventricle (cerebral) (floor) (lateral) (third)	C71.5	C79.31	—	D33.0	D43.0	D49.6
cardiac (left) (right)	C38.0	C79.89	—	D15.1	D48.7	D49.89
fourth	C71.7	C79.31	—	D33.1	D43.1	D49.6
ventricular band of larynx	C32.1	C78.39	D02.0	D14.1	D38.0	D49.1
ventriculus — see Neoplasm, stomach						
vermillion border — see Neoplasm, lip						
vermis, cerebellum	C71.6	C79.31	—	D33.1	D43.1	D49.6
vertebra (column)	C41.2	C79.51	—	D16.6	D48.0	D49.2
coccyx	C41.4	C79.51	—	D16.8	D48.0	D49.2
marrow NEC	C96.9	C79.52	—	—	D47.9	D49.89
sacrum	C41.4	C79.51	—	D16.8	D48.0	D49.2
vesical — see Neoplasm, bladder						
vesicle, seminal	C63.7	C79.82	D07.69	D29.8	D40.8	D49.59
vesicocervical tissue	C57.9	C79.82	D07.30	D28.9	D39.9	D49.59
vesicorectal	C76.3	C79.82	D09.8	D36.7	D48.7	D49.89
vesicovaginal	C57.9	C79.82	D07.30	D28.9	D39.9	D49.59
septum	C57.9	C79.82	D07.30	D28.9	D39.9	D49.59
vessel (blood) — see Neoplasm, connective tissue						
vestibular gland, greater	C51.0	C79.82	D07.1	D28.0	D39.8	D49.59
vestibule mouth	C06.1	C79.89	D00.00	D10.39	D37.09	D49.0
nose	C30.0	C78.39	D02.3	D14.0	D38.5	D49.1
Virchow's gland	C77.0	C77.0	—	D36.0	D48.7	D49.89
viscera NEC	C76.8	C79.89	D09.8	D36.7	D48.7	D49.89
vocal cords (true)	C32.0	C78.39	D02.0	D14.1	D38.0	D49.1
false	C32.1	C78.39	D02.0	D14.1	D38.0	D49.1
vomer	C41.0	C79.51	—	D16.4	D48.0	D49.2
vulva	C51.9	C79.82	D07.1	D28.0	D39.8	D49.59
vulvovaginal gland	C51.0	C79.82	D07.1	D28.0	D39.8	D49.59
Waldeyer's ring	C14.2	C79.89	D00.08	D10.9	D37.05	D49.0
Wharton's duct	C08.0	C79.89	D00.00	D11.7	D37.032	D49.0
white matter (central) (cerebral)	C71.0	C79.31	—	D33.0	D43.0	D49.6

	Malignant Primary	Malignant Secondary	Ca in situ	Benign	Uncertain Behavior	Unspecified Behavior
Neoplasm, neoplastic						
— *continued*						
windpipe	C33	C78.39	D02.1	D14.2	D38.1	D49.1
Wirsung's duct	C25.3	C78.89	D01.7	D13.6	D37.8	D49.0
wolffian (body) (duct)						
female	C57.7	C79.82	D07.39	D28.7	D39.8	D49.59
male	C63.7	C79.82	D07.69	D29.8	D40.8	D49.59
womb — *see*						
Neoplasm, uterus						
wrist NEC	C76.4-☑	C79.89	D04.6-☑	D36.7	D48.7	D49.89
xiphoid process	C41.3	C79.51	—	D16.7	D48.0	D49.2
Zuckerkandl						
organ	C75.5	C79.89	—	D35.6	D44.7	D49.7

Substance	Poisoning, Accidental (unintentional)	Poisoning, Intentional Self-harm	Poisoning, Assault	Poisoning, Undetermined	Adverse Effect	Under-dosing
14-Hydroxydihydromorphinone	T40.2X1	T40.2X2	T40.2X3	T40.2X4	T40.2X5	T40.2X6
1-Propanol	T51.3X1	T51.3X2	T51.3X3	T51.3X4	—	—
2,3,7,8-Tetrachlorodibenzo-p-dioxin	T53.7X1	T53.7X2	T53.7X3	T53.7X4	—	—
2,4,5-T (trichlorophenoxyacetic acid)	T60.1X1	T60.1X2	T60.1X3	T60.1X4	—	—
2,4,5-Trichlorophenoxyacetic acid	T60.3X1	T60.3X2	T60.3X3	T60.3X4	—	—
2,4-D (dichlorophenoxyacetic acid)	T60.3X1	T60.3X2	T60.3X3	T60.3X4	—	—
2,4-Toluene diisocyanate	T65.0X1	T65.0X2	T65.0X3	T65.0X4	—	—
2-Deoxy-5-fluorouridine	T45.1X1	T45.1X2	T45.1X3	T45.1X4	T45.1X5	T45.1X6
2-Ethoxyethanol	T52.3X1	T52.3X2	T52.3X3	T52.3X4	—	—
2-Methoxyethanol	T52.3X1	T52.3X2	T52.3X3	T52.3X4	—	—
2-Propanol	T51.2X1	T51.2X2	T51.2X3	T51.2X4	—	—
3,4-methylenedioxymeth-amphetamine	T43.641	T43.642	T43.643	T43.644	—	—
4-Aminobutyric acid	T43.8X1	T43.8X2	T43.8X3	T43.8X4	T43.8X5	T43.8X6
4-Aminophenol derivatives	T39.1X1	T39.1X2	T39.1X3	T39.1X4	T39.1X5	T39.1X6
5-Deoxy-5-fluorouridine	T45.1X1	T45.1X2	T45.1X3	T45.1X4	T45.1X5	T45.1X6
5-Methoxypsoralen (5-MOP)	T50.991	T50.992	T50.993	T50.994	T50.995	T50.996
8-Aminoquinoline drugs	T37.2X1	T37.2X2	T37.2X3	T37.2X4	T37.2X5	T37.2X6
8-Methoxypsoralen (8-MOP)	T50.991	T50.992	T50.993	T50.994	T50.995	T50.996
ABOB	T37.5X1	T37.5X2	T37.5X3	T37.5X4	T37.5X5	T37.5X6
Abrine	T62.2X1	T62.2X2	T62.2X3	T62.2X4	—	—
Abrus (seed)	T62.2X1	T62.2X2	T62.2X3	T62.2X4	—	—
Absinthe	T51.0X1	T51.0X2	T51.0X3	T51.0X4	—	—
beverage	T51.0X1	T51.0X2	T51.0X3	T51.0X4	—	—
Acaricide	T60.8X1	T60.8X2	T60.8X3	T60.8X4	—	—
Acebutolol	T44.7X1	T44.7X2	T44.7X3	T44.7X4	T44.7X5	T44.7X6
Acecarbromal	T42.6X1	T42.6X2	T42.6X3	T42.6X4	T42.6X5	T42.6X6
Aceclidine	T44.1X1	T44.1X2	T44.1X3	T44.1X4	T44.1X5	T44.1X6
Acedapsone	T37.0X1	T37.0X2	T37.0X3	T37.0X4	T37.0X5	T37.0X6
Acefylline piperazine	T48.6X1	T48.6X2	T48.6X3	T48.6X4	T48.6X5	T48.6X6
Acemorphan	T40.2X1	T40.2X2	T40.2X3	T40.2X4	T40.2X5	T40.2X6
Acenocoumarin	T45.511	T45.512	T45.513	T45.514	T45.515	T45.516
Acenocoumarol	T45.511	T45.512	T45.513	T45.514	T45.515	T45.516
Acepifylline	T48.6X1	T48.6X2	T48.6X3	T48.6X4	T48.6X5	T48.6X6
Acepromazine	T43.3X1	T43.3X2	T43.3X3	T43.3X4	T43.3X5	T43.3X6
Acesulfamethoxypyridazine	T37.0X1	T37.0X2	T37.0X3	T37.0X4	T37.0X5	T37.0X6
Acetal	T52.8X1	T52.8X2	T52.8X3	T52.8X4	—	—
Acetaldehyde (vapor)	T52.8X1	T52.8X2	T52.8X3	T52.8X4	—	—
liquid	T65.891	T65.892	T65.893	T65.894	—	—
Acetaminophen	T39.1X1	T39.1X2	T39.1X3	T39.1X4	T39.1X5	T39.1X6
Acetaminosalol	T39.1X1	T39.1X2	T39.1X3	T39.1X4	T39.1X5	T39.1X6
Acetanilide	T39.1X1	T39.1X2	T39.1X3	T39.1X4	T39.1X5	T39.1X6
Acetarsol	T37.3X1	T37.3X2	T37.3X3	T37.3X4	T37.3X5	T37.3X6
Acetazolamide	T50.2X1	T50.2X2	T50.2X3	T50.2X4	T50.2X5	T50.2X6
Acetiamine	T45.2X1	T45.2X2	T45.2X3	T45.2X4	T45.2X5	T45.2X6
Acetic						
acid	T54.2X1	T54.2X2	T54.2X3	T54.2X4	—	—
with sodium acetate (ointment)	T49.3X1	T49.3X2	T49.3X3	T49.3X4	T49.3X5	T49.3X6
ester (solvent)(vapor)	T52.8X1	T52.8X2	T52.8X3	T52.8X4	—	—
irrigating solution	T50.3X1	T50.3X2	T50.3X3	T50.3X4	T50.3X5	T50.3X6
medicinal (lotion)	T49.2X1	T49.2X2	T49.2X3	T49.2X4	T49.2X5	T49.2X6
anhydride	T65.891	T65.892	T65.893	T65.894	—	—
ether (vapor)	T52.8X1	T52.8X2	T52.8X3	T52.8X4	—	—
Acetohexamide	T38.3X1	T38.3X2	T38.3X3	T38.3X4	T38.3X5	T38.3X6
Acetohydroxamic acid	T50.991	T50.992	T50.993	T50.994	T50.995	T50.996
Acetomenaphthone	T45.7X1	T45.7X2	T45.7X3	T45.7X4	T45.7X5	T45.7X6
Acetomorphine	T40.1X1	T40.1X2	T40.1X3	T40.1X4	—	—
Acetone (oils)	T52.4X1	T52.4X2	T52.4X3	T52.4X4	—	—
chlorinated	T52.4X1	T52.4X2	T52.4X3	T52.4X4	—	—
vapor	T52.4X1	T52.4X2	T52.4X3	T52.4X4	—	—
Acetonitrile	T52.8X1	T52.8X2	T52.8X3	T52.8X4	—	—
Acetophenazine	T43.3X1	T43.3X2	T43.3X3	T43.3X4	T43.3X5	T43.3X6
Acetophenetedin	T39.1X1	T39.1X2	T39.1X3	T39.1X4	T39.1X5	T39.1X6
Acetophenone	T52.4X1	T52.4X2	T52.4X3	T52.4X4	—	—
Acetorphine	T40.2X1	T40.2X2	T40.2X3	T40.2X4	—	—
Acetosulfone (sodium)	T37.1X1	T37.1X2	T37.1X3	T37.1X4	T37.1X5	T37.1X6
Acetrizoate (sodium)	T50.8X1	T50.8X2	T50.8X3	T50.8X4	T50.8X5	T50.8X6
Acetrizoic acid	T50.8X1	T50.8X2	T50.8X3	T50.8X4	T50.8X5	T50.8X6
Acetyl						
bromide	T53.6X1	T53.6X2	T53.6X3	T53.6X4	—	—
chloride	T53.6X1	T53.6X2	T53.6X3	T53.6X4	—	—
Acetylcarbromal	T42.6X1	T42.6X2	T42.6X3	T42.6X4	T42.6X5	T42.6X6
Acetylcholine						
chloride	T44.1X1	T44.1X2	T44.1X3	T44.1X4	T44.1X5	T44.1X6
derivative	T44.1X1	T44.1X2	T44.1X3	T44.1X4	T44.1X5	T44.1X6
Acetylcysteine	T48.4X1	T48.4X2	T48.4X3	T48.4X4	T48.4X5	T48.4X6
Acetyldigitoxin	T46.0X1	T46.0X2	T46.0X3	T46.0X4	T46.0X5	T46.0X6
Acetyldigoxin	T46.0X1	T46.0X2	T46.0X3	T46.0X4	T46.0X5	T46.0X6
Acetyldihydrocodeine	T40.2X1	T40.2X2	T40.2X3	T40.2X4	—	—
Acetyldihydrocodeinone	T40.2X1	T40.2X2	T40.2X3	T40.2X4	—	—
Acetylene (gas)	T59.891	T59.892	T59.893	T59.894	—	—
dichloride	T53.6X1	T53.6X2	T53.6X3	T53.6X4	—	—
incomplete combustion of	T58.11	T58.12	T58.13	T58.14	—	—
industrial	T59.891	T59.892	T59.893	T59.894	—	—
tetrachloride	T53.6X1	T53.6X2	T53.6X3	T53.6X4	—	—
vapor	T53.6X1	T53.6X2	T53.6X3	T53.6X4	—	—
Acetylpheneturide	T42.6X1	T42.6X2	T42.6X3	T42.6X4	T42.6X5	T42.6X6
Acetylphenylhydrazine	T39.8X1	T39.8X2	T39.8X3	T39.8X4	T39.8X5	T39.8X6
Acetylsalicylic acid (salts)	T39.011	T39.012	T39.013	T39.014	T39.015	T39.016
enteric coated	T39.011	T39.012	T39.013	T39.014	T39.015	T39.016
Acetylsulfamethoxypyridazine	T37.0X1	T37.0X2	T37.0X3	T37.0X4	T37.0X5	T37.0X6
Achromycin	T36.4X1	T36.4X2	T36.4X3	T36.4X4	T36.4X5	T36.4X6
ophthalmic preparation	T49.5X1	T49.5X2	T49.5X3	T49.5X4	T49.5X5	T49.5X6
topical NEC	T49.0X1	T49.0X2	T49.0X3	T49.0X4	T49.0X5	T49.0X6
Aciclovir	T37.5X1	T37.5X2	T37.5X3	T37.5X4	T37.5X5	T37.5X6
Acidifying agent NEC	T50.901	T50.902	T50.903	T50.904	T50.905	T50.906
Acid (corrosive) NEC	T54.2X1	T54.2X2	T54.2X3	T54.2X4	—	—
Acipimox	T46.6X1	T46.6X2	T46.6X3	T46.6X4	T46.6X5	T46.6X6
Acitretin	T50.991	T50.992	T50.993	T50.994	T50.995	T50.996
Aclarubicin	T45.1X1	T45.1X2	T45.1X3	T45.1X4	T45.1X5	T45.1X6
Aclatonium napadisilate	T48.1X1	T48.1X2	T48.1X3	T48.1X4	T48.1X5	T48.1X6
Aconite (wild)	T46.991	T46.992	T46.993	T46.994	T46.995	T46.996
Aconitine	T46.991	T46.992	T46.993	T46.994	T46.995	T46.996
Aconitum ferox	T46.991	T46.992	T46.993	T46.994	T46.995	T46.996
Acridine	T65.6X1	T65.6X2	T65.6X3	T65.6X4	—	—
vapor	T59.891	T59.892	T59.893	T59.894	—	—
Acriflavine	T37.91	T37.92	T37.93	T37.94	T37.95	T37.96
Acriflavinium chloride	T49.0X1	T49.0X2	T49.0X3	T49.0X4	T49.0X5	T49.0X6
Acrinol	T49.0X1	T49.0X2	T49.0X3	T49.0X4	T49.0X5	T49.0X6
Acrisorcin	T49.0X1	T49.0X2	T49.0X3	T49.0X4	T49.0X5	T49.0X6
Acrivastine	T45.0X1	T45.0X2	T45.0X3	T45.0X4	T45.0X5	T45.0X6
Acrolein (gas)	T59.891	T59.892	T59.893	T59.894	—	—
liquid	T54.1X1	T54.1X2	T54.1X3	T54.1X4	—	—
Acrylamide	T65.891	T65.892	T65.893	T65.894	—	—
Acrylic resin	T49.3X1	T49.3X2	T49.3X3	T49.3X4	T49.3X5	T49.3X6
Acrylonitrile	T65.891	T65.892	T65.893	T65.894	—	—
Actaea spicata	T62.2X1	T62.2X2	T62.2X3	T62.2X4	—	—
berry	T62.1X1	T62.1X2	T62.1X3	T62.1X4	—	—
Acterol	T37.3X1	T37.3X2	T37.3X3	T37.3X4	T37.3X5	T37.3X6
ACTH	T38.811	T38.812	T38.813	T38.814	T38.815	T38.816
Actinomycin C	T45.1X1	T45.1X2	T45.1X3	T45.1X4	T45.1X5	T45.1X6
Actinomycin D	T45.1X1	T45.1X2	T45.1X3	T45.1X4	T45.1X5	T45.1X6
Activated charcoal — see also Charcoal, medicinal	T47.6X1	T47.6X2	T47.6X3	T47.6X4	T47.6X5	T47.6X6
Acyclovir	T37.5X1	T37.5X2	T37.5X3	T37.5X4	T37.5X5	T37.5X6
Adenine	T45.2X1	T45.2X2	T45.2X3	T45.2X4	T45.2X5	T45.2X6
arabinoside	T37.5X1	T37.5X2	T37.5X3	T37.5X4	T37.5X5	T37.5X6
Adenosine (phosphate)	T46.2X1	T46.2X2	T46.2X3	T46.2X4	T46.2X5	T46.2X6
ADH	T38.891	T38.892	T38.893	T38.894	T38.895	T38.896
Adhesive NEC	T65.891	T65.892	T65.893	T65.894	—	—
Adicillin	T36.0X1	T36.0X2	T36.0X3	T36.0X4	T36.0X5	T36.0X6
Adiphenine	T44.3X1	T44.3X2	T44.3X3	T44.3X4	T44.3X5	T44.3X6
Adipiodone	T50.8X1	T50.8X2	T50.8X3	T50.8X4	T50.8X5	T50.8X6
Adjunct, pharmaceutical	T50.901	T50.902	T50.903	T50.904	T50.905	T50.906
Adrenal (extract, cortex or medulla) (glucocorticoids) (hormones) (mineralocorticoids)	T38.0X1	T38.0X2	T38.0X3	T38.0X4	T38.0X5	T38.0X6
ENT agent	T49.6X1	T49.6X2	T49.6X3	T49.6X4	T49.6X5	T49.6X6
ophthalmic preparation	T49.5X1	T49.5X2	T49.5X3	T49.5X4	T49.5X5	T49.5X6
topical NEC	T49.0X1	T49.0X2	T49.0X3	T49.0X4	T49.0X5	T49.0X6
Adrenalin — see Adrenaline						
Adrenaline	T44.5X1	T44.5X2	T44.5X3	T44.5X4	T44.5X5	T44.5X6
Adrenergic NEC	T44.901	T44.902	T44.903	T44.904	T44.905	T44.906
blocking agent NEC	T44.8X1	T44.8X2	T44.8X3	T44.8X4	T44.8X5	T44.8X6
beta, heart	T44.7X1	T44.7X2	T44.7X3	T44.7X4	T44.7X5	T44.7X6
specified NEC	T44.991	T44.992	T44.993	T44.994	T44.995	T44.996
Adrenochrome						
derivative	T46.991	T46.992	T46.993	T46.994	T46.995	T46.996
(mono) semicarbazone	T46.991	T46.992	T46.993	T46.994	T46.995	T46.996
Adrenocorticotrophic hormone	T38.811	T38.812	T38.813	T38.814	T38.815	T38.816
Adrenocorticotrophin	T38.811	T38.812	T38.813	T38.814	T38.815	T38.816
Adriamycin	T45.1X1	T45.1X2	T45.1X3	T45.1X4	T45.1X5	T45.1X6
Aerosol spray NEC	T65.91	T65.92	T65.93	T65.94	—	—
Aerosporin	T36.8X1	T36.8X2	T36.8X3	T36.8X4	T36.8X5	T36.8X6
ENT agent	T49.6X1	T49.6X2	T49.6X3	T49.6X4	T49.6X5	T49.6X6
ophthalmic preparation	T49.5X1	T49.5X2	T49.5X3	T49.5X4	T49.5X5	T49.5X6

Table of Drugs and Chemicals

Aerosporin — Aluminium, aluminum

Substance	Poisoning, Accidental (unintentional)	Poisoning, Intentional Self-harm	Poisoning, Assault	Poisoning, Undetermined	Adverse Effect	Under-dosing
Aerosporin — *continued*						
topical NEC	T49.0X1	T49.0X2	T49.0X3	T49.0X4	T49.0X5	T49.0X6
Aethusa cynapium	T62.2X1	T62.2X2	T62.2X3	T62.2X4	—	—
Afghanistan black	T40.7X1	T40.7X2	T40.7X3	T40.7X4	T40.7X5	T40.7X6
Aflatoxin	T64.01	T64.02	T64.03	T64.04		
Afloqualone	T42.8X1	T42.8X2	T42.8X3	T42.8X4	T42.8X5	T42.8X6
African boxwood	T62.2X1	T62.2X2	T62.2X3	T62.2X4	—	—
Agar	T47.4X1	T47.4X2	T47.4X3	T47.4X4	T47.4X5	T47.4X6
Agonist						
predominantly						
alpha-adrenoreceptor	T44.4X1	T44.4X2	T44.4X3	T44.4X4	T44.4X5	T44.4X6
beta-adrenoreceptor	T44.5X1	T44.5X2	T44.5X3	T44.5X4	T44.5X5	T44.5X6
Agricultural agent NEC	T65.91	T65.92	T65.93	T65.94		
Agrypnal	T42.3X1	T42.3X2	T42.3X3	T42.3X4	T42.3X5	T42.3X6
AHLG	T50.Z11	T50.Z12	T50.Z13	T50.Z14	T50.Z15	T50.Z16
Air contaminant(s), source/type NOS	T65.91	T65.92	T65.93	T65.94		
Ajmaline	T46.2X1	T46.2X2	T46.2X3	T46.2X4	T46.2X5	T46.2X6
Akee	T62.1X1	T62.1X2	T62.1X3	T62.1X4	—	—
Akrinol	T49.0X1	T49.0X2	T49.0X3	T49.0X4	T49.0X5	T49.0X6
Akritoin	T37.8X1	T37.8X2	T37.8X3	T37.8X4	T37.8X5	T37.8X6
Alacepril	T46.4X1	T46.4X2	T46.4X3	T46.4X4	T46.4X5	T46.4X6
Alantolactone	T37.4X1	T37.4X2	T37.4X3	T37.4X4	T37.4X5	T37.4X6
Albamycin	T36.8X1	T36.8X2	T36.8X3	T36.8X4	T36.8X5	T36.8X6
Albendazole	T37.4X1	T37.4X2	T37.4X3	T37.4X4	T37.4X5	T37.4X6
Albumin						
bovine	T45.8X1	T45.8X2	T45.8X3	T45.8X4	T45.8X5	T45.8X6
human serum	T45.8X1	T45.8X2	T45.8X3	T45.8X4	T45.8X5	T45.8X6
salt-poor	T45.8X1	T45.8X2	T45.8X3	T45.8X4	T45.8X5	T45.8X6
normal human serum	T45.8X1	T45.8X2	T45.8X3	T45.8X4	T45.8X5	T45.8X6
Albuterol	T48.6X1	T48.6X2	T48.6X3	T48.6X4	T48.6X5	T48.6X6
Albutoin	T42.0X1	T42.0X2	T42.0X3	T42.0X4	T42.0X5	T42.0X6
Alclometasone	T49.0X1	T49.0X2	T49.0X3	T49.0X4	T49.0X5	T49.0X6
Alcohol	T51.91	T51.92	T51.93	T51.94	—	—
absolute	T51.0X1	T51.0X2	T51.0X3	T51.0X4	—	—
beverage	T51.0X1	T51.0X2	T51.0X3	T51.0X4	—	—
allyl	T51.8X1	T51.8X2	T51.8X3	T51.8X4	—	—
amyl	T51.3X1	T51.3X2	T51.3X3	T51.3X4	—	—
antifreeze	T51.1X1	T51.1X2	T51.1X3	T51.1X4	—	—
beverage	T51.0X1	T51.0X2	T51.0X3	T51.0X4	—	—
butyl	T51.3X1	T51.3X2	T51.3X3	T51.3X4	—	—
dehydrated	T51.0X1	T51.0X2	T51.0X3	T51.0X4	—	—
beverage	T51.0X1	T51.0X2	T51.0X3	T51.0X4	—	—
denatured	T51.0X1	T51.0X2	T51.0X3	T51.0X4	—	—
deterrent NEC	T50.6X1	T50.6X2	T50.6X3	T50.6X4	T50.6X5	T50.6X6
diagnostic (gastric function)	T50.8X1	T50.8X2	T50.8X3	T50.8X4	T50.8X5	T50.8X6
ethyl	T51.0X1	T51.0X2	T51.0X3	T51.0X4	—	—
beverage	T51.0X1	T51.0X2	T51.0X3	T51.0X4	—	—
grain	T51.0X1	T51.0X2	T51.0X3	T51.0X4	—	—
beverage	T51.0X1	T51.0X2	T51.0X3	T51.0X4	—	—
industrial	T51.0X1	T51.0X2	T51.0X3	T51.0X4	—	—
isopropyl	T51.2X1	T51.2X2	T51.2X3	T51.2X4	—	—
methyl	T51.1X1	T51.1X2	T51.1X3	T51.1X4	—	—
preparation for consumption	T51.0X1	T51.0X2	T51.0X3	T51.0X4	—	—
propyl	T51.3X1	T51.3X2	T51.3X3	T51.3X4	—	—
secondary	T51.2X1	T51.2X2	T51.2X3	T51.2X4	—	—
radiator	T51.1X1	T51.1X2	T51.1X3	T51.1X4	—	—
rubbing	T51.2X1	T51.2X2	T51.2X3	T51.2X4	—	—
specified type NEC	T51.8X1	T51.8X2	T51.8X3	T51.8X4	—	—
surgical	T51.0X1	T51.0X2	T51.0X3	T51.0X4	—	—
vapor (from any type of Alcohol)	T59.891	T59.892	T59.893	T59.894	—	—
wood	T51.1X1	T51.1X2	T51.1X3	T51.1X4	—	—
Alcuronium (chloride)	T48.1X1	T48.1X2	T48.1X3	T48.1X4	T48.1X5	T48.1X6
Aldactone	T50.0X1	T50.0X2	T50.0X3	T50.0X4	T50.0X5	T50.0X6
Aldesulfone sodium	T37.1X1	T37.1X2	T37.1X3	T37.1X4	T37.1X5	T37.1X6
Aldicarb	T60.0X1	T60.0X2	T60.0X3	T60.0X4	—	—
Aldomet	T46.5X1	T46.5X2	T46.5X3	T46.5X4	T46.5X5	T46.5X6
Aldosterone	T50.0X1	T50.0X2	T50.0X3	T50.0X4	T50.0X5	T50.0X6
Aldrin (dust)	T60.1X1	T60.1X2	T60.1X3	T60.1X4	—	—
Aleve — *see* Naproxen						
Alexitol sodium	T47.1X1	T47.1X2	T47.1X3	T47.1X4	T47.1X5	T47.1X6
Alfacalcidol	T45.2X1	T45.2X2	T45.2X3	T45.2X4	T45.2X5	T45.2X6
Alfadolone	T41.1X1	T41.1X2	T41.1X3	T41.1X4	T41.1X5	T41.1X6
Alfaxalone	T41.1X1	T41.1X2	T41.1X3	T41.1X4	T41.1X5	T41.1X6
Alfentanil	T40.4X1	T40.4X2	T40.4X3	T40.4X4	T40.4X5	T40.4X6
Alfuzosin (hydrochloride)	T44.8X1	T44.8X2	T44.8X3	T44.8X4	T44.8X5	T44.8X6
Algae (harmful) (toxin)	T65.821	T65.822	T65.823	T65.824	—	—
Algeldrate	T47.1X1	T47.1X2	T47.1X3	T47.1X4	T47.1X5	T47.1X6
Algin	T47.8X1	T47.8X2	T47.8X3	T47.8X4	T47.8X5	T47.8X6
Alglucerase	T45.3X1	T45.3X2	T45.3X3	T45.3X4	T45.3X5	T45.3X6

Substance	Poisoning, Accidental (unintentional)	Poisoning, Intentional Self-harm	Poisoning, Assault	Poisoning, Undetermined	Adverse Effect	Under-dosing
Alidase	T45.3X1	T45.3X2	T45.3X3	T45.3X4	T45.3X5	T45.3X6
Alimemazine	T43.3X1	T43.3X2	T43.3X3	T43.3X4	T43.3X5	T43.3X6
Aliphatic thiocyanates	T65.0X1	T65.0X2	T65.0X3	T65.0X4	—	—
Alizapride	T45.0X1	T45.0X2	T45.0X3	T45.0X4	T45.0X5	T45.0X6
Alkali (caustic)	T54.3X1	T54.3X2	T54.3X3	T54.3X4		
Alkaline antiseptic solution (aromatic)	T49.6X1	T49.6X2	T49.6X3	T49.6X4	T49.6X5	T49.6X6
Alkalinizing agents (medicinal)	T50.901	T50.902	T50.903	T50.904	T50.905	T50.906
Alkalizing agent NEC	T50.901	T50.902	T50.903	T50.904	T50.905	T50.906
Alka-seltzer	T39.011	T39.012	T39.013	T39.014	T39.015	T39.016
Alkavervir	T46.5X1	T46.5X2	T46.5X3	T46.5X4	T46.5X5	T46.5X6
Alkonium (bromide)	T49.0X1	T49.0X2	T49.0X3	T49.0X4	T49.0X5	T49.0X6
Alkylating drug NEC	T45.1X1	T45.1X2	T45.1X3	T45.1X4	T45.1X5	T45.1X6
antimyeloproliferative	T45.1X1	T45.1X2	T45.1X3	T45.1X4	T45.1X5	T45.1X6
lymphatic	T45.1X1	T45.1X2	T45.1X3	T45.1X4	T45.1X5	T45.1X6
Alkylisocyanate	T65.0X1	T65.0X2	T65.0X3	T65.0X4	—	—
Allantoin	T49.4X1	T49.4X2	T49.4X3	T49.4X4	T49.4X5	T49.4X6
Allegron	T43.011	T43.012	T43.013	T43.014	T43.015	T43.016
Allethrin	T49.0X1	T49.0X2	T49.0X3	T49.0X4	T49.0X5	T49.0X6
Allobarbital	T42.3X1	T42.3X2	T42.3X3	T42.3X4	T42.3X5	T42.3X6
Allopurinol	T50.4X1	T50.4X2	T50.4X3	T50.4X4	T50.4X5	T50.4X6
Allyl						
alcohol	T51.8X1	T51.8X2	T51.8X3	T51.8X4	—	—
disulfide	T46.6X1	T46.6X2	T46.6X3	T46.6X4	T46.6X5	T46.6X6
Allylestrenol	T38.5X1	T38.5X2	T38.5X3	T38.5X4	T38.5X5	T38.5X6
Allylisopropylacetylurea	T42.6X1	T42.6X2	T42.6X3	T42.6X4	T42.6X5	T42.6X6
Allylisopropylmalonylurea	T42.3X1	T42.3X2	T42.3X3	T42.3X4	T42.3X5	T42.3X6
Allylthiourea	T49.3X1	T49.3X2	T49.3X3	T49.3X4	T49.3X5	T49.3X6
Allyltribromide	T42.6X1	T42.6X2	T42.6X3	T42.6X4	T42.6X5	T42.6X6
Allypropymal	T42.3X1	T42.3X2	T42.3X3	T42.3X4	T42.3X5	T42.3X6
Almagate	T47.1X1	T47.1X2	T47.1X3	T47.1X4	T47.1X5	T47.1X6
Almasilate	T47.1X1	T47.1X2	T47.1X3	T47.1X4	T47.1X5	T47.1X6
Almitrine	T50.7X1	T50.7X2	T50.7X3	T50.7X4	T50.7X5	T50.7X6
Aloes	T47.2X1	T47.2X2	T47.2X3	T47.2X4	T47.2X5	T47.2X6
Aloglutamol	T47.1X1	T47.1X2	T47.1X3	T47.1X4	T47.1X5	T47.1X6
Aloin	T47.2X1	T47.2X2	T47.2X3	T47.2X4	T47.2X5	T47.2X6
Aloxidone	T42.2X1	T42.2X2	T42.2X3	T42.2X4	T42.2X5	T42.2X6
Alpha						
acetyldigoxin	T46.0X1	T46.0X2	T46.0X3	T46.0X4	T46.0X5	T46.0X6
adrenergic blocking drug	T44.6X1	T44.6X2	T44.6X3	T44.6X4	T44.6X5	T44.6X6
amylase	T45.3X1	T45.3X2	T45.3X3	T45.3X4	T45.3X5	T45.3X6
tocoferol (acetate)	T45.2X1	T45.2X2	T45.2X3	T45.2X4	T45.2X5	T45.2X6
tocopherol	T45.2X1	T45.2X2	T45.2X3	T45.2X4	T45.2X5	T45.2X6
Alphadolone	T41.1X1	T41.1X2	T41.1X3	T41.1X4	T41.1X5	T41.1X6
Alphaprodine	T40.4X1	T40.4X2	T40.4X3	T40.4X4	T40.4X5	T40.4X6
Alphaxalone	T41.1X1	T41.1X2	T41.1X3	T41.1X4	T41.1X5	T41.1X6
Alprazolam	T42.4X1	T42.4X2	T42.4X3	T42.4X4	T42.4X5	T42.4X6
Alprenolol	T44.7X1	T44.7X2	T44.7X3	T44.7X4	T44.7X5	T44.7X6
Alprostadil	T46.7X1	T46.7X2	T46.7X3	T46.7X4	T46.7X5	T46.7X6
Alsactide	T38.811	T38.812	T38.813	T38.814	T38.815	T38.816
Alseroxylon	T46.5X1	T46.5X2	T46.5X3	T46.5X4	T46.5X5	T46.5X6
Alteplase	T45.611	T45.612	T45.613	T45.614	T45.615	T45.616
Altizide	T50.2X1	T50.2X2	T50.2X3	T50.2X4	T50.2X5	T50.2X6
Altretamine	T45.1X1	T45.1X2	T45.1X3	T45.1X4	T45.1X5	T45.1X6
Alum (medicinal)	T49.4X1	T49.4X2	T49.4X3	T49.4X4	T49.4X5	T49.4X6
nonmedicinal (ammonium) (potassium)	T56.891	T56.892	T56.893	T56.894	—	—
Aluminium, aluminum						
acetate	T49.2X1	T49.2X2	T49.2X3	T49.2X4	T49.2X5	T49.2X6
solution	T49.0X1	T49.0X2	T49.0X3	T49.0X4	T49.0X5	T49.0X6
aspirin	T39.011	T39.012	T39.013	T39.014	T39.015	T39.016
bis (acetylsalicylate)	T39.011	T39.012	T39.013	T39.014	T39.015	T39.016
carbonate (gel, basic)	T47.1X1	T47.1X2	T47.1X3	T47.1X4	T47.1X5	T47.1X6
chlorhydroxide-complex	T47.1X1	T47.1X2	T47.1X3	T47.1X4	T47.1X5	T47.1X6
chloride	T49.2X1	T49.2X2	T49.2X3	T49.2X4	T49.2X5	T49.2X6
clofibrate	T46.6X1	T46.6X2	T46.6X3	T46.6X4	T46.6X5	T46.6X6
diacetate	T49.2X1	T49.2X2	T49.2X3	T49.2X4	T49.2X5	T49.2X6
glycinate	T47.1X1	T47.1X2	T47.1X3	T47.1X4	T47.1X5	T47.1X6
hydroxide (gel)	T47.1X1	T47.1X2	T47.1X3	T47.1X4	T47.1X5	T47.1X6
hydroxide-magnesium carb. gel	T47.1X1	T47.1X2	T47.1X3	T47.1X4	T47.1X5	T47.1X6
magnesium silicate	T47.1X1	T47.1X2	T47.1X3	T47.1X4	T47.1X5	T47.1X6
nicotinate	T46.7X1	T46.7X2	T46.7X3	T46.7X4	T46.7X5	T46.7X6
ointment (surgical) (topical)	T49.3X1	T49.3X2	T49.3X3	T49.3X4	T49.3X5	T49.3X6
phosphate	T47.1X1	T47.1X2	T47.1X3	T47.1X4	T47.1X5	T47.1X6
salicylate	T39.091	T39.092	T39.093	T39.094	T39.095	T39.096
silicate	T47.1X1	T47.1X2	T47.1X3	T47.1X4	T47.1X5	T47.1X6
sodium silicate	T47.1X1	T47.1X2	T47.1X3	T47.1X4	T47.1X5	T47.1X6
subacetate	T49.2X1	T49.2X2	T49.2X3	T49.2X4	T49.2X5	T49.2X6
sulfate	T49.0X1	T49.0X2	T49.0X3	T49.0X4	T49.0X5	T49.0X6
tannate	T47.6X1	T47.6X2	T47.6X3	T47.6X4	T47.6X5	T47.6X6

Substance	Poisoning, Accidental (unintentional)	Poisoning, Intentional Self-harm	Poisoning, Assault	Poisoning, Undetermined	Adverse Effect	Under-dosing
Aluminium, aluminum — *continued*						
topical NEC	T49.3X1	T49.3X2	T49.3X3	T49.3X4	T49.3X5	T49.3X6
Alurate	T42.3X1	T42.3X2	T42.3X3	T42.3X4	T42.3X5	T42.3X6
Alverine	T44.3X1	T44.3X2	T44.3X3	T44.3X4	T44.3X5	T44.3X6
Alvodine	T40.2X1	T40.2X2	T40.2X3	T40.2X4	T40.2X5	T40.2X6
Amanita phalloides	T62.0X1	T62.0X2	T62.0X3	T62.0X4	—	—
Amanitine	T62.0X1	T62.0X2	T62.0X3	T62.0X4	—	—
Amantadine	T42.8X1	T42.8X2	T42.8X3	T42.8X4	T42.8X5	T42.8X6
Ambazone	T49.6X1	T49.6X2	T49.6X3	T49.6X4	T49.6X5	T49.6X6
Ambenonium (chloride)	T44.0X1	T44.0X2	T44.0X3	T44.0X4	T44.0X5	T44.0X6
Ambroxol	T48.4X1	T48.4X2	T48.4X3	T48.4X4	T48.4X5	T48.4X6
Ambuphylline	T48.6X1	T48.6X2	T48.6X3	T48.6X4	T48.6X5	T48.6X6
Ambutonium bromide	T44.3X1	T44.3X2	T44.3X3	T44.3X4	T44.3X5	T44.3X6
Amcinonide	T49.0X1	T49.0X2	T49.0X3	T49.0X4	T49.0X5	T49.0X6
Amdinocilline	T36.0X1	T36.0X2	T36.0X3	T36.0X4	T36.0X5	T36.0X6
Ametazole	T50.8X1	T50.8X2	T50.8X3	T50.8X4	T50.8X5	T50.8X6
Amethocaine	T41.3X1	T41.3X2	T41.3X3	T41.3X4	T41.3X5	T41.3X6
regional	T41.3X1	T41.3X2	T41.3X3	T41.3X4	T41.3X5	T41.3X6
spinal	T41.3X1	T41.3X2	T41.3X3	T41.3X4	T41.3X5	T41.3X6
Amethopterin	T45.1X1	T45.1X2	T45.1X3	T45.1X4	T45.1X5	T45.1X6
Amezinium metilsulfate	T44.991	T44.992	T44.993	T44.994	T44.995	T44.996
Amfebutamone	T43.291	T43.292	T43.293	T43.294	T43.295	T43.296
Amfepramone	T50.5X1	T50.5X2	T50.5X3	T50.5X4	T50.5X5	T50.5X6
Amfetamine	T43.621	T43.622	T43.623	T43.624	T43.625	T43.626
Amfetaminil	T43.621	T43.622	T43.623	T43.624	T43.625	T43.626
Amfomycin	T36.8X1	T36.8X2	T36.8X3	T36.8X4	T36.8X5	T36.8X6
Amidefrine mesilate	T48.5X1	T48.5X2	T48.5X3	T48.5X4	T48.5X5	T48.5X6
Amidone	T40.3X1	T40.3X2	T40.3X3	T40.3X4	T40.3X5	T40.3X6
Amidopyrine	T39.2X1	T39.2X2	T39.2X3	T39.2X4	T39.2X5	T39.2X6
Amidotrizoate	T50.8X1	T50.8X2	T50.8X3	T50.8X4	T50.8X5	T50.8X6
Amiflamine	T43.1X1	T43.1X2	T43.1X3	T43.1X4	T43.1X5	T43.1X6
Amikacin	T36.5X1	T36.5X2	T36.5X3	T36.5X4	T36.5X5	T36.5X6
Amikhelline	T46.3X1	T46.3X2	T46.3X3	T46.3X4	T46.3X5	T46.3X6
Amiloride	T50.2X1	T50.2X2	T50.2X3	T50.2X4	T50.2X5	T50.2X6
Aminacrine	T49.0X1	T49.0X2	T49.0X3	T49.0X4	T49.0X5	T49.0X6
Amineptine	T43.011	T43.012	T43.013	T43.014	T43.015	T43.016
Aminitrozole	T37.3X1	T37.3X2	T37.3X3	T37.3X4	T37.3X5	T37.3X6
Aminoacetic acid (derivatives)	T50.3X1	T50.3X2	T50.3X3	T50.3X4	T50.3X5	T50.3X6
Amino acids	T50.3X1	T50.3X2	T50.3X3	T50.3X4	T50.3X5	T50.3X6
Aminoacridine	T49.0X1	T49.0X2	T49.0X3	T49.0X4	T49.0X5	T49.0X6
Aminobenzoic acid (-p)	T49.3X1	T49.3X2	T49.3X3	T49.3X4	T49.3X5	T49.3X6
Aminocaproic acid	T45.621	T45.622	T45.623	T45.624	T45.625	T45.626
Aminoethylisothiourium	T45.8X1	T45.8X2	T45.8X3	T45.8X4	T45.8X5	T45.8X6
Aminofenazone	T39.2X1	T39.2X2	T39.2X3	T39.2X4	T39.2X5	T39.2X6
Aminoglutethimide	T45.1X1	T45.1X2	T45.1X3	T45.1X4	T45.1X5	T45.1X6
Aminohippuric acid	T50.8X1	T50.8X2	T50.8X3	T50.8X4	T50.8X5	T50.8X6
Aminomethylbenzoic acid	T45.691	T45.692	T45.693	T45.694	T45.695	T45.696
Aminometradine	T50.2X1	T50.2X2	T50.2X3	T50.2X4	T50.2X5	T50.2X6
Aminopentamide	T44.3X1	T44.3X2	T44.3X3	T44.3X4	T44.3X5	T44.3X6
Aminophenazone	T39.2X1	T39.2X2	T39.2X3	T39.2X4	T39.2X5	T39.2X6
Aminophenol	T54.0X1	T54.0X2	T54.0X3	T54.0X4	—	—
Aminophenylpyridone	T43.591	T43.592	T43.593	T43.594	T43.595	T43.596
Aminophylline	T48.6X1	T48.6X2	T48.6X3	T48.6X4	T48.6X5	T48.6X6
Aminopterin sodium	T45.1X1	T45.1X2	T45.1X3	T45.1X4	T45.1X5	T45.1X6
Aminopyrine	T39.2X1	T39.2X2	T39.2X3	T39.2X4	T39.2X5	T39.2X6
Aminorex	T50.5X1	T50.5X2	T50.5X3	T50.5X4	T50.5X5	T50.5X6
Aminosalicylic acid	T37.1X1	T37.1X2	T37.1X3	T37.1X4	T37.1X5	T37.1X6
Aminosalylum	T37.1X1	T37.1X2	T37.1X3	T37.1X4	T37.1X5	T37.1X6
Amiodarone	T46.2X1	T46.2X2	T46.2X3	T46.2X4	T46.2X5	T46.2X6
Amiphenazole	T50.7X1	T50.7X2	T50.7X3	T50.7X4	T50.7X5	T50.7X6
Amiquinsin	T46.5X1	T46.5X2	T46.5X3	T46.5X4	T46.5X5	T46.5X6
Amisometradine	T50.2X1	T50.2X2	T50.2X3	T50.2X4	T50.2X5	T50.2X6
Amisulpride	T43.591	T43.592	T43.593	T43.594	T43.595	T43.596
Amitriptyline	T43.011	T43.012	T43.013	T43.014	T43.015	T43.016
Amitriptylinoxide	T43.011	T43.012	T43.013	T43.014	T43.015	T43.016
Amlexanox	T48.6X1	T48.6X2	T48.6X3	T48.6X4	T48.6X5	T48.6X6
Ammonia (fumes) (gas)	T59.891	T59.892	T59.893	T59.894	—	—
(vapor)						
aromatic spirit	T48.991	T48.992	T48.993	T48.994	T48.995	T48.996
liquid (household)	T54.3X1	T54.3X2	T54.3X3	T54.3X4	—	—
Ammoniated mercury	T49.0X1	T49.0X2	T49.0X3	T49.0X4	T49.0X5	T49.0X6
Ammonium						
acid tartrate	T49.5X1	T49.5X2	T49.5X3	T49.5X4	T49.5X5	T49.5X6
bromide	T42.6X1	T42.6X2	T42.6X3	T42.6X4	T42.6X5	T42.6X6
carbonate	T54.3X1	T54.3X2	T54.3X3	T54.3X4	—	—
chloride	T50.991	T50.992	T50.993	T50.994	T50.995	T50.996
expectorant	T48.4X1	T48.4X2	T48.4X3	T48.4X4	T48.4X5	T48.4X6
compounds (household) NEC	T54.3X1	T54.3X2	T54.3X3	T54.3X4	—	—
fumes (any usage)	T59.891	T59.892	T59.893	T59.894	—	—
industrial	T54.3X1	T54.3X2	T54.3X3	T54.3X4	—	—

Substance	Poisoning, Accidental (unintentional)	Poisoning, Intentional Self-harm	Poisoning, Assault	Poisoning, Undetermined	Adverse Effect	Under-dosing
Ammonium — *continued*						
ichthyosulronate	T49.4X1	T49.4X2	T49.4X3	T49.4X4	T49.4X5	T49.4X6
mandelate	T37.91	T37.92	T37.93	T37.94	T37.95	T37.96
sulfamate	T60.3X1	T60.3X2	T60.3X3	T60.3X4		
sulfonate resin	T47.8X1	T47.8X2	T47.8X3	T47.8X4	T47.8X5	T47.8X6
Amobarbital (sodium)	T42.3X1	T42.3X2	T42.3X3	T42.3X4	T42.3X5	T42.3X6
Amodiaquine	T37.2X1	T37.2X2	T37.2X3	T37.2X4	T37.2X5	T37.2X6
Amopyroquin (e)	T37.2X1	T37.2X2	T37.2X3	T37.2X4	T37.2X5	T37.2X6
Amoxapine	T43.011	T43.012	T43.013	T43.014	T43.015	T43.016
Amoxicillin	T36.0X1	T36.0X2	T36.0X3	T36.0X4	T36.0X5	T36.0X6
Amperozide	T43.591	T43.592	T43.593	T43.594	T43.595	T43.596
Amphenidone	T43.591	T43.592	T43.593	T43.594	T43.595	T43.596
Amphetamine NEC	T43.621	T43.622	T43.623	T43.624	T43.625	T43.626
Amphomycin	T36.8X1	T36.8X2	T36.8X3	T36.8X4	T36.8X5	T36.8X6
Amphotalide	T37.4X1	T37.4X2	T37.4X3	T37.4X4	T37.4X5	T37.4X6
Amphotericin B	T36.7X1	T36.7X2	T36.7X3	T36.7X4	T36.7X5	T36.7X6
topical	T49.0X1	T49.0X2	T49.0X3	T49.0X4	T49.0X5	T49.0X6
Ampicillin	T36.0X1	T36.0X2	T36.0X3	T36.0X4	T36.0X5	T36.0X6
Amprotropine	T44.3X1	T44.3X2	T44.3X3	T44.3X4	T44.3X5	T44.3X6
Amsacrine	T45.1X1	T45.1X2	T45.1X3	T45.1X4	T45.1X5	T45.1X6
Amygdaline	T62.2X1	T62.2X2	T62.2X3	T62.2X4	—	—
Amyl						
acetate	T52.8X1	T52.8X2	T52.8X3	T52.8X4		
vapor	T59.891	T59.892	T59.893	T59.894		
alcohol	T51.3X1	T51.3X2	T51.3X3	T51.3X4		
chloride	T53.6X1	T53.6X2	T53.6X3	T53.6X4		
formate	T52.8X1	T52.8X2	T52.8X3	T52.8X4		
nitrite	T46.3X1	T46.3X2	T46.3X3	T46.3X4	T46.3X5	T46.3X6
propionate	T65.891	T65.892	T65.893	T65.894		
Amylase	T47.5X1	T47.5X2	T47.5X3	T47.5X4	T47.5X5	T47.5X6
Amyleine, regional	T41.3X1	T41.3X2	T41.3X3	T41.3X4	T41.3X5	T41.3X6
Amylene						
dichloride	T53.6X1	T53.6X2	T53.6X3	T53.6X4	—	—
hydrate	T51.3X1	T51.3X2	T51.3X3	T51.3X4	—	—
Amylmetacresol	T49.6X1	T49.6X2	T49.6X3	T49.6X4	T49.6X5	T49.6X6
Amylobarbitone	T42.3X1	T42.3X2	T42.3X3	T42.3X4	T42.3X5	T42.3X6
Amylocaine, regional	T41.3X1	T41.3X2	T41.3X3	T41.3X4	T41.3X5	T41.3X6
infiltration (subcutaneous)	T41.3X1	T41.3X2	T41.3X3	T41.3X4	T41.3X5	T41.3X6
nerve block (peripheral) (plexus)	T41.3X1	T41.3X2	T41.3X3	T41.3X4	T41.3X5	T41.3X6
spinal	T41.3X1	T41.3X2	T41.3X3	T41.3X4	T41.3X5	T41.3X6
topical (surface)	T41.3X1	T41.3X2	T41.3X3	T41.3X4	T41.3X5	T41.3X6
Amylopectin	T47.6X1	T47.6X2	T47.6X3	T47.6X4	T47.6X5	T47.6X6
Amytal (sodium)	T42.3X1	T42.3X2	T42.3X3	T42.3X4	T42.3X5	T42.3X6
Anabolic steroid	T38.7X1	T38.7X2	T38.7X3	T38.7X4	T38.7X5	T38.7X6
Analeptic NEC	T50.7X1	T50.7X2	T50.7X3	T50.7X4	T50.7X5	T50.7X6
Analgesic	T39.91	T39.92	T39.93	T39.94	T39.95	T39.96
anti-inflammatory NEC	T39.91	T39.92	T39.93	T39.94	T39.95	T39.96
propionic acid derivative	T39.311	T39.312	T39.313	T39.314	T39.315	T39.316
antirheumatic NEC	T39.4X1	T39.4X2	T39.4X3	T39.4X4	T39.4X5	T39.4X6
aromatic NEC	T39.1X1	T39.1X2	T39.1X3	T39.1X4	T39.1X5	T39.1X6
narcotic NEC	T40.601	T40.602	T40.603	T40.604	T40.605	T40.606
combination	T40.601	T40.602	T40.603	T40.604	T40.605	T40.606
obstetric	T40.601	T40.602	T40.603	T40.604	T40.605	T40.606
non-narcotic NEC	T39.91	T39.92	T39.93	T39.94	T39.95	T39.96
combination	T39.91	T39.92	T39.93	T39.94	T39.95	T39.96
pyrazole	T39.2X1	T39.2X2	T39.2X3	T39.2X4	T39.2X5	T39.2X6
specified NEC	T39.8X1	T39.8X2	T39.8X3	T39.8X4	T39.8X5	T39.8X6
Analgin	T39.2X1	T39.2X2	T39.2X3	T39.2X4	T39.2X5	T39.2X6
Anamirta cocculus	T62.1X1	T62.1X2	T62.1X3	T62.1X4		
Ancillin	T36.0X1	T36.0X2	T36.0X3	T36.0X4	T36.0X5	T36.0X6
Ancrod	T45.691	T45.692	T45.693	T45.694	T45.695	T45.696
Androgen	T38.7X1	T38.7X2	T38.7X3	T38.7X4	T38.7X5	T38.7X6
Androgen-estrogen mixture	T38.7X1	T38.7X2	T38.7X3	T38.7X4	T38.7X5	T38.7X6
Androstalone	T38.7X1	T38.7X2	T38.7X3	T38.7X4	T38.7X5	T38.7X6
Androstanolone	T38.7X1	T38.7X2	T38.7X3	T38.7X4	T38.7X5	T38.7X6
Androsterone	T38.7X1	T38.7X2	T38.7X3	T38.7X4	T38.7X5	T38.7X6
Anemone pulsatilla	T62.2X1	T62.2X2	T62.2X3	T62.2X4		
Anesthesia						
caudal	T41.3X1	T41.3X2	T41.3X3	T41.3X4	T41.3X5	T41.3X6
endotracheal	T41.0X1	T41.0X2	T41.0X3	T41.0X4	T41.0X5	T41.0X6
epidural	T41.3X1	T41.3X2	T41.3X3	T41.3X4	T41.3X5	T41.3X6
inhalation	T41.0X1	T41.0X2	T41.0X3	T41.0X4	T41.0X5	T41.0X6
local	T41.3X1	T41.3X2	T41.3X3	T41.3X4	T41.3X5	T41.3X6
mucosal	T41.3X1	T41.3X2	T41.3X3	T41.3X4	T41.3X5	T41.3X6
muscle relaxation	T48.1X1	T48.1X2	T48.1X3	T48.1X4	T48.1X5	T48.1X6
nerve blocking	T41.3X1	T41.3X2	T41.3X3	T41.3X4	T41.3X5	T41.3X6
plexus blocking	T41.3X1	T41.3X2	T41.3X3	T41.3X4	T41.3X5	T41.3X6
potentiated	T41.201	T41.202	T41.203	T41.204	T41.205	T41.206
rectal	T41.201	T41.202	T41.203	T41.204	T41.205	T41.206
general	T41.201	T41.202	T41.203	T41.204	T41.205	T41.206
local	T41.3X1	T41.3X2	T41.3X3	T41.3X4	T41.3X5	T41.3X6

Substance	Poisoning, Accidental (unintentional)	Poisoning, Intentional Self-harm	Poisoning, Assault	Poisoning, Undetermined	Adverse Effect	Under-dosing
Anesthesia — *continued*						
regional	T41.3X1	T41.3X2	T41.3X3	T41.3X4	T41.3X5	T41.3X6
surface	T41.3X1	T41.3X2	T41.3X3	T41.3X4	T41.3X5	T41.3X6
Anesthetic NEC — *see also*	T41.41	T41.42	T41.43	T41.44	T41.45	T41.46
Anesthesia						
with muscle relaxant	T41.201	T41.202	T41.203	T41.204	T41.205	T41.206
general	T41.201	T41.202	T41.203	T41.204	T41.205	T41.206
local	T41.3X1	T41.3X2	T41.3X3	T41.3X4	T41.3X5	T41.3X6
gaseous NEC	T41.0X1	T41.0X2	T41.0X3	T41.0X4	T41.0X5	T41.0X6
general NEC	T41.201	T41.202	T41.203	T41.204	T41.205	T41.206
halogenated hydrocarbon derivatives NEC	T41.0X1	T41.0X2	T41.0X3	T41.0X4	T41.0X5	T41.0X6
infiltration NEC	T41.3X1	T41.3X2	T41.3X3	T41.3X4	T41.3X5	T41.3X6
intravenous NEC	T41.1X1	T41.1X2	T41.1X3	T41.1X4	T41.1X5	T41.1X6
local NEC	T41.3X1	T41.3X2	T41.3X3	T41.3X4	T41.3X5	T41.3X6
rectal	T41.201	T41.202	T41.203	T41.204	T41.205	T41.206
general	T41.201	T41.202	T41.203	T41.204	T41.205	T41.206
local	T41.3X1	T41.3X2	T41.3X3	T41.3X4	T41.3X5	T41.3X6
regional NEC	T41.3X1	T41.3X2	T41.3X3	T41.3X4	T41.3X5	T41.3X6
spinal NEC	T41.3X1	T41.3X2	T41.3X3	T41.3X4	T41.3X5	T41.3X6
thiobarbiturate	T41.1X1	T41.1X2	T41.1X3	T41.1X4	T41.1X5	T41.1X6
topical	T41.3X1	T41.3X2	T41.3X3	T41.3X4	T41.3X5	T41.3X6
Aneurine	T45.2X1	T45.2X2	T45.2X3	T45.2X4	T45.2X5	T45.2X6
Angio-Conray	T50.8X1	T50.8X2	T50.8X3	T50.8X4	T50.8X5	T50.8X6
Angiotensin	T44.5X1	T44.5X2	T44.5X3	T44.5X4	T44.5X5	T44.5X6
Angiotensinamide	T44.991	T44.992	T44.993	T44.994	T44.995	T44.996
Anhydrohydroxy-progesterone	T38.5X1	T38.5X2	T38.5X3	T38.5X4	T38.5X5	T38.5X6
Anhydron	T50.2X1	T50.2X2	T50.2X3	T50.2X4	T50.2X5	T50.2X6
Anileridine	T40.4X1	T40.4X2	T40.4X3	T40.4X4	T40.4X5	T40.4X6
Aniline (dye) (liquid)	T65.3X1	T65.3X2	T65.3X3	T65.3X4		
analgesic	T39.1X1	T39.1X2	T39.1X3	T39.1X4	T39.1X5	T39.1X6
derivatives, therapeutic NEC	T39.1X1	T39.1X2	T39.1X3	T39.1X4	T39.1X5	T39.1X6
vapor	T65.3X1	T65.3X2	T65.3X3	T65.3X4		
Aniscoropine	T44.3X1	T44.3X2	T44.3X3	T44.3X4	T44.3X5	T44.3X6
Anise oil	T47.5X1	T47.5X2	T47.5X3	T47.5X4	T47.5X5	T47.5X6
Anisidine	T65.3X1	T65.3X2	T65.3X3	T65.3X4		
Anisindione	T45.511	T45.512	T45.513	T45.514	T45.515	T45.516
Anisotropine methyl-bromide	T44.3X1	T44.3X2	T44.3X3	T44.3X4	T44.3X5	T44.3X6
Anistreplase	T45.611	T45.612	T45.613	T45.614	T45.615	T45.616
Anorexiant (central)	T50.5X1	T50.5X2	T50.5X3	T50.5X4	T50.5X5	T50.5X6
Anorexic agents	T50.5X1	T50.5X2	T50.5X3	T50.5X4	T50.5X5	T50.5X6
Ansamycin	T36.6X1	T36.6X2	T36.6X3	T36.6X4	T36.6X5	T36.6X6
Ant (bite) (sting)	T63.421	T63.422	T63.423	T63.424		
Antabuse	T50.6X1	T50.6X2	T50.6X3	T50.6X4	T50.6X5	T50.6X6
Antacid NEC	T47.1X1	T47.1X2	T47.1X3	T47.1X4	T47.1X5	T47.1X6
Antagonist						
Aldosterone	T50.0X1	T50.0X2	T50.0X3	T50.0X4	T50.0X5	T50.0X6
alpha-adrenoreceptor	T44.6X1	T44.6X2	T44.6X3	T44.6X4	T44.6X5	T44.6X6
anticoagulant	T45.7X1	T45.7X2	T45.7X3	T45.7X4	T45.7X5	T45.7X6
beta-adrenoreceptor	T44.7X1	T44.7X2	T44.7X3	T44.7X4	T44.7X5	T44.7X6
extrapyramidal NEC	T44.3X1	T44.3X2	T44.3X3	T44.3X4	T44.3X5	T44.3X6
folic acid	T45.1X1	T45.1X2	T45.1X3	T45.1X4	T45.1X5	T45.1X6
H2 receptor	T47.0X1	T47.0X2	T47.0X3	T47.0X4	T47.0X5	T47.0X6
heavy metal	T45.8X1	T45.8X2	T45.8X3	T45.8X4	T45.8X5	T45.8X6
narcotic analgesic	T50.7X1	T50.7X2	T50.7X3	T50.7X4	T50.7X5	T50.7X6
opiate	T50.7X1	T50.7X2	T50.7X3	T50.7X4	T50.7X5	T50.7X6
pyrimidine	T45.1X1	T45.1X2	T45.1X3	T45.1X4	T45.1X5	T45.1X6
serotonin	T46.5X1	T46.5X2	T46.5X3	T46.5X4	T46.5X5	T46.5X6
Antazolin (e)	T45.0X1	T45.0X2	T45.0X3	T45.0X4	T45.0X5	T45.0X6
Anterior pituitary hormone NEC	T38.811	T38.812	T38.813	T38.814	T38.815	T38.816
Anthelmintic NEC	T37.4X1	T37.4X2	T37.4X3	T37.4X4	T37.4X5	T37.4X6
Anthiolimine	T37.4X1	T37.4X2	T37.4X3	T37.4X4	T37.4X5	T37.4X6
Anthralin	T49.4X1	T49.4X2	T49.4X3	T49.4X4	T49.4X5	T49.4X6
Anthramycin	T45.1X1	T45.1X2	T45.1X3	T45.1X4	T45.1X5	T45.1X6
Antiadrenergic NEC	T44.8X1	T44.8X2	T44.8X3	T44.8X4	T44.8X5	T44.8X6
Antiallergic NEC	T45.0X1	T45.0X2	T45.0X3	T45.0X4	T45.0X5	T45.0X6
Antiandrogen NEC	T38.6X1	T38.6X2	T38.6X3	T38.6X4	T38.6X5	T38.6X6
Anti-anemic (drug) (preparation)	T45.8X1	T45.8X2	T45.8X3	T45.8X4	T45.8X5	T45.8X6
Antianxiety drug NEC	T43.501	T43.502	T43.503	T43.504	T43.505	T43.506
Antiaris toxicaria	T65.891	T65.892	T65.893	T65.894		
Antiarteriosclerotic drug	T46.6X1	T46.6X2	T46.6X3	T46.6X4	T46.6X5	T46.6X6
Antiasthmatic drug NEC	T48.6X1	T48.6X2	T48.6X3	T48.6X4	T48.6X5	T48.6X6
Antibiotic NEC	T36.91	T36.92	T36.93	T36.94	T36.95	T36.96
aminoglycoside	T36.5X1	T36.5X2	T36.5X3	T36.5X4	T36.5X5	T36.5X6
anticancer	T45.1X1	T45.1X2	T45.1X3	T45.1X4	T45.1X5	T45.1X6
antifungal	T36.7X1	T36.7X2	T36.7X3	T36.7X4	T36.7X5	T36.7X6
antimycobacterial	T36.5X1	T36.5X2	T36.5X3	T36.5X4	T36.5X5	T36.5X6
antineoplastic	T45.1X1	T45.1X2	T45.1X3	T45.1X4	T45.1X5	T45.1X6
b-lactam NEC	T36.1X1	T36.1X2	T36.1X3	T36.1X4	T36.1X5	T36.1X6
Antibiotic — *continued*						
cephalosporin (group)	T36.1X1	T36.1X2	T36.1X3	T36.1X4	T36.1X5	T36.1X6
chloramphenicol (group)	T36.2X1	T36.2X2	T36.2X3	T36.2X4	T36.2X5	T36.2X6
ENT	T49.6X1	T49.6X2	T49.6X3	T49.6X4	T49.6X5	T49.6X6
eye	T49.5X1	T49.5X2	T49.5X3	T49.5X4	T49.5X5	T49.5X6
fungicidal (local)	T49.0X1	T49.0X2	T49.0X3	T49.0X4	T49.0X5	T49.0X6
intestinal	T36.8X1	T36.8X2	T36.8X3	T36.8X4	T36.8X5	T36.8X6
local	T49.0X1	T49.0X2	T49.0X3	T49.0X4	T49.0X5	T49.0X6
macrolides	T36.3X1	T36.3X2	T36.3X3	T36.3X4	T36.3X5	T36.3X6
polypeptide	T36.8X1	T36.8X2	T36.8X3	T36.8X4	T36.8X5	T36.8X6
specified NEC	T36.8X1	T36.8X2	T36.8X3	T36.8X4	T36.8X5	T36.8X6
tetracycline (group)	T36.4X1	T36.4X2	T36.4X3	T36.4X4	T36.4X5	T36.4X6
throat	T49.6X1	T49.6X2	T49.6X3	T49.6X4	T49.6X5	T49.6X6
Anticancer agents NEC	T45.1X1	T45.1X2	T45.1X3	T45.1X4	T45.1X5	T45.1X6
Anticholesterolemic drug NEC	T46.6X1	T46.6X2	T46.6X3	T46.6X4	T46.6X5	T46.6X6
Anticholinergic NEC	T44.3X1	T44.3X2	T44.3X3	T44.3X4	T44.3X5	T44.3X6
Anticholinesterase	T44.0X1	T44.0X2	T44.0X3	T44.0X4	T44.0X5	T44.0X6
organophosphorus	T44.0X1	T44.0X2	T44.0X3	T44.0X4	T44.0X5	T44.0X6
insecticide	T60.0X1	T60.0X2	T60.0X3	T60.0X4	—	—
nerve gas	T59.891	T59.892	T59.893	T59.894	—	—
reversible	T44.0X1	T44.0X2	T44.0X3	T44.0X4	T44.0X5	T44.0X6
ophthalmological	T49.5X1	T49.5X2	T49.5X3	T49.5X4	T49.5X5	T49.5X6
Anticoagulant NEC	T45.511	T45.512	T45.513	T45.514	T45.515	T45.516
Antagonist	T45.7X1	T45.7X2	T45.7X3	T45.7X4	T45.7X5	T45.7X6
Anti-common-cold drug NEC	T48.5X1	T48.5X2	T48.5X3	T48.5X4	T48.5X5	T48.5X6
Anticonvulsant	T42.71	T42.72	T42.73	T42.74	T42.75	T42.76
barbiturate	T42.3X1	T42.3X2	T42.3X3	T42.3X4	T42.3X5	T42.3X6
combination (with barbiturate)	T42.3X1	T42.3X2	T42.3X3	T42.3X4	T42.3X5	T42.3X6
hydantoin	T42.0X1	T42.0X2	T42.0X3	T42.0X4	T42.0X5	T42.0X6
hypnotic NEC	T42.6X1	T42.6X2	T42.6X3	T42.6X4	T42.6X5	T42.6X6
oxazolidinedione	T42.2X1	T42.2X2	T42.2X3	T42.2X4	T42.2X5	T42.2X6
pyrimidinedione	T42.6X1	T42.6X2	T42.6X3	T42.6X4	T42.6X5	T42.6X6
specified NEC	T42.6X1	T42.6X2	T42.6X3	T42.6X4	T42.6X5	T42.6X6
succinimide	T42.2X1	T42.2X2	T42.2X3	T42.2X4	T42.2X5	T42.2X6
Antidepressant	T43.201	T43.202	T43.203	T43.204	T43.205	T43.206
monoamine oxidase inhibitor	T43.1X1	T43.1X2	T43.1X3	T43.1X4	T43.1X5	T43.1X6
selective serotonin norepinephrine reuptake inhibitor	T43.211	T43.212	T43.213	T43.214	T43.215	T43.216
selective serotonin reuptake inhibitor	T43.221	T43.222	T43.223	T43.224	T43.225	T43.226
specified NEC	T43.291	T43.292	T43.293	T43.294	T43.295	T43.296
tetracyclic	T43.021	T43.022	T43.023	T43.024	T43.025	T43.026
triazolopyridine	T43.211	T43.212	T43.213	T43.214	T43.215	T43.216
tricyclic	T43.011	T43.012	T43.013	T43.014	T43.015	T43.016
Antidiabetic NEC	T38.3X1	T38.3X2	T38.3X3	T38.3X4	T38.3X5	T38.3X6
biguanide	T38.3X1	T38.3X2	T38.3X3	T38.3X4	T38.3X5	T38.3X6
and sulfonyl combined	T38.3X1	T38.3X2	T38.3X3	T38.3X4	T38.3X5	T38.3X6
combined	T38.3X1	T38.3X2	T38.3X3	T38.3X4	T38.3X5	T38.3X6
sulfonylurea	T38.3X1	T38.3X2	T38.3X3	T38.3X4	T38.3X5	T38.3X6
Antidiarrheal drug NEC	T47.6X1	T47.6X2	T47.6X3	T47.6X4	T47.6X5	T47.6X6
absorbent	T47.6X1	T47.6X2	T47.6X3	T47.6X4	T47.6X5	T47.6X6
Anti-D immunoglobulin (human)	T50.Z11	T50.Z12	T50.Z13	T50.Z14	T50.Z15	T50.Z16
Antidiphtheria serum	T50.Z11	T50.Z12	T50.Z13	T50.Z14	T50.Z15	T50.Z16
Antidiuretic hormone	T38.891	T38.892	T38.893	T38.894	T38.895	T38.896
Antidote NEC	T50.6X1	T50.6X2	T50.6X3	T50.6X4	T50.6X5	T50.6X6
heavy metal	T45.8X1	T45.8X2	T45.8X3	T45.8X4	T45.8X5	T45.8X6
Antidysrhythmic NEC	T46.2X1	T46.2X2	T46.2X3	T46.2X4	T46.2X5	T46.2X6
Antiemetic drug	T45.0X1	T45.0X2	T45.0X3	T45.0X4	T45.0X5	T45.0X6
Antiepilepsy agent	T42.71	T42.72	T42.73	T42.74	T42.75	T42.76
combination	T42.5X1	T42.5X2	T42.5X3	T42.5X4	T42.5X5	T42.5X6
mixed	T42.5X1	T42.5X2	T42.5X3	T42.5X4	T42.5X5	T42.5X6
specified, NEC	T42.6X1	T42.6X2	T42.6X3	T42.6X4	T42.6X5	T42.6X6
Antiestrogen NEC	T38.6X1	T38.6X2	T38.6X3	T38.6X4	T38.6X5	T38.6X6
Antifertility pill	T38.4X1	T38.4X2	T38.4X3	T38.4X4	T38.4X5	T38.4X6
Antifibrinolytic drug	T45.621	T45.622	T45.623	T45.624	T45.625	T45.626
Antifilarial drug	T37.4X1	T37.4X2	T37.4X3	T37.4X4	T37.4X5	T37.4X6
Antiflatulent	T47.5X1	T47.5X2	T47.5X3	T47.5X4	T47.5X5	T47.5X6
Antifreeze	T65.91	T65.92	T65.93	T65.94	—	—
alcohol	T51.1X1	T51.1X2	T51.1X3	T51.1X4	—	—
ethylene glycol	T51.8X1	T51.8X2	T51.8X3	T51.8X4	—	—
Antifungal						
antibiotic (systemic)	T36.7X1	T36.7X2	T36.7X3	T36.7X4	T36.7X5	T36.7X6
anti-infective NEC	T37.91	T37.92	T37.93	T37.94	T37.95	T37.96
disinfectant, local	T49.0X1	T49.0X2	T49.0X3	T49.0X4	T49.0X5	T49.0X6
nonmedicinal (spray)	T60.3X1	T60.3X2	T60.3X3	T60.3X4	—	—
topical	T49.0X1	T49.0X2	T49.0X3	T49.0X4	T49.0X5	T49.0X6

Additional Character May Be Required — Refer to the Tabular List for Character Selection ▽ **Subterms under main terms may continue to next column or page**

Substance	Poisoning, Accidental (unintentional)	Poisoning, Intentional Self-harm	Poisoning, Assault	Poisoning, Undetermined	Adverse Effect	Underdosing
Anti-gastric-secretion drug NEC	T47.1X1	T47.1X2	T47.1X3	T47.1X4	T47.1X5	T47.1X6
Antigonadotrophin NEC	T38.6X1	T38.6X2	T38.6X3	T38.6X4	T38.6X5	T38.6X6
Antihallucinogen	T43.501	T43.502	T43.503	T43.504	T43.505	T43.506
Antihelmintics	T37.4X1	T37.4X2	T37.4X3	T37.4X4	T37.4X5	T37.4X6
Antihemophilic						
factor	T45.8X1	T45.8X2	T45.8X3	T45.8X4	T45.8X5	T45.8X6
fraction	T45.8X1	T45.8X2	T45.8X3	T45.8X4	T45.8X5	T45.8X6
globulin concentrate	T45.7X1	T45.7X2	T45.7X3	T45.7X4	T45.7X5	T45.7X6
human plasma	T45.8X1	T45.8X2	T45.8X3	T45.8X4	T45.8X5	T45.8X6
plasma, dried	T45.7X1	T45.7X2	T45.7X3	T45.7X4	T45.7X5	T45.7X6
Antihemorrhoidal preparation	T49.2X1	T49.2X2	T49.2X3	T49.2X4	T49.2X5	T49.2X6
Antiheparin drug	T45.7X1	T45.7X2	T45.7X3	T45.7X4	T45.7X5	T45.7X6
Antihistamine	T45.0X1	T45.0X2	T45.0X3	T45.0X4	T45.0X5	T45.0X6
Antihookworm drug	T37.4X1	T37.4X2	T37.4X3	T37.4X4	T37.4X5	T37.4X6
Anti-human lymphocyte globulin	T50.Z11	T50.Z12	T50.Z13	T50.Z14	T50.Z15	T50.Z16
Antihyperlipidemic drug	T46.6X1	T46.6X2	T46.6X3	T46.6X4	T46.6X5	T46.6X6
Antihypertensive drug NEC	T46.5X1	T46.5X2	T46.5X3	T46.5X4	T46.5X5	T46.5X6
Anti-infective NEC	T37.91	T37.92	T37.93	T37.94	T37.95	T37.96
anthelmintic	T37.4X1	T37.4X2	T37.4X3	T37.4X4	T37.4X5	T37.4X6
antibiotics	T36.91	T36.92	T36.93	T36.94	T36.95	T36.96
specified NEC	T36.8X1	T36.8X2	T36.8X3	T36.8X4	T36.8X5	T36.8X6
antimalarial	T37.2X1	T37.2X2	T37.2X3	T37.2X4	T37.2X5	T37.2X6
antimycobacterial NEC	T37.1X1	T37.1X2	T37.1X3	T37.1X4	T37.1X5	T37.1X6
antibiotics	T36.5X1	T36.5X2	T36.5X3	T36.5X4	T36.5X5	T36.5X6
antiprotozoal NEC	T37.3X1	T37.3X2	T37.3X3	T37.3X4	T37.3X5	T37.3X6
blood	T37.2X1	T37.2X2	T37.2X3	T37.2X4	T37.2X5	T37.2X6
antiviral	T37.5X1	T37.5X2	T37.5X3	T37.5X4	T37.5X5	T37.5X6
arsenical	T37.8X1	T37.8X2	T37.8X3	T37.8X4	T37.8X5	T37.8X6
bismuth, local	T49.0X1	T49.0X2	T49.0X3	T49.0X4	T49.0X5	T49.0X6
ENT	T49.6X1	T49.6X2	T49.6X3	T49.6X4	T49.6X5	T49.6X6
eye NEC	T49.5X1	T49.5X2	T49.5X3	T49.5X4	T49.5X5	T49.5X6
heavy metals NEC	T37.8X1	T37.8X2	T37.8X3	T37.8X4	T37.8X5	T37.8X6
local NEC	T49.0X1	T49.0X2	T49.0X3	T49.0X4	T49.0X5	T49.0X6
specified NEC	T49.0X1	T49.0X2	T49.0X3	T49.0X4	T49.0X5	T49.0X6
mixed	T37.91	T37.92	T37.93	T37.94	T37.95	T37.96
ophthalmic preparation	T49.5X1	T49.5X2	T49.5X3	T49.5X4	T49.5X5	T49.5X6
topical NEC	T49.0X1	T49.0X2	T49.0X3	T49.0X4	T49.0X5	T49.0X6
Anti-inflammatory drug NEC	T39.391	T39.392	T39.393	T39.394	T39.395	T39.396
local	T49.0X1	T49.0X2	T49.0X3	T49.0X4	T49.0X5	T49.0X6
nonsteroidal NEC	T39.391	T39.392	T39.393	T39.394	T39.395	T39.396
propionic acid derivative	T39.311	T39.312	T39.313	T39.314	T39.315	T39.316
specified NEC	T39.391	T39.392	T39.393	T39.394	T39.395	T39.396
Antikaluretic	T50.3X1	T50.3X2	T50.3X3	T50.3X4	T50.3X5	T50.3X6
Antiknock (tetraethyl lead)	T56.0X1	T56.0X2	T56.0X3	T56.0X4	—	—
Antilipemic drug NEC	T46.6X1	T46.6X2	T46.6X3	T46.6X4	T46.6X5	T46.6X6
Antimalarial	T37.2X1	T37.2X2	T37.2X3	T37.2X4	T37.2X5	T37.2X6
prophylactic NEC	T37.2X1	T37.2X2	T37.2X3	T37.2X4	T37.2X5	T37.2X6
pyrimidine derivative	T37.2X1	T37.2X2	T37.2X3	T37.2X4	T37.2X5	T37.2X6
Antimetabolite	T45.1X1	T45.1X2	T45.1X3	T45.1X4	T45.1X5	T45.1X6
Antimitotic agent	T45.1X1	T45.1X2	T45.1X3	T45.1X4	T45.1X5	T45.1X6
Antimony (compounds) (vapor) NEC	T56.891	T56.892	T56.893	T56.894	—	—
anti-infectives	T37.8X1	T37.8X2	T37.8X3	T37.8X4	T37.8X5	T37.8X6
dimercaptosuccinate	T37.3X1	T37.3X2	T37.3X3	T37.3X4	T37.3X5	T37.3X6
hydride	T56.891	T56.892	T56.893	T56.894	—	—
pesticide (vapor)	T60.8X1	T60.8X2	T60.8X3	T60.8X4	—	—
potassium (sodium) tartrate	T37.8X1	T37.8X2	T37.8X3	T37.8X4	T37.8X5	T37.8X6
sodium	T37.3X1	T37.3X2	T37.3X3	T37.3X4	T37.3X5	T37.3X6
dimercaptosuccinate						
tartrated	T37.8X1	T37.8X2	T37.8X3	T37.8X4	T37.8X5	T37.8X6
Antimuscarinic NEC	T44.3X1	T44.3X2	T44.3X3	T44.3X4	T44.3X5	T44.3X6
Antimycobacterial drug NEC	T37.1X1	T37.1X2	T37.1X3	T37.1X4	T37.1X5	T37.1X6
antibiotics	T36.5X1	T36.5X2	T36.5X3	T36.5X4	T36.5X5	T36.5X6
combination	T37.1X1	T37.1X2	T37.1X3	T37.1X4	T37.1X5	T37.1X6
Antinausea drug	T45.0X1	T45.0X2	T45.0X3	T45.0X4	T45.0X5	T45.0X6
Antinematode drug	T37.4X1	T37.4X2	T37.4X3	T37.4X4	T37.4X5	T37.4X6
Antineoplastic NEC	T45.1X1	T45.1X2	T45.1X3	T45.1X4	T45.1X5	T45.1X6
alkaloidal	T45.1X1	T45.1X2	T45.1X3	T45.1X4	T45.1X5	T45.1X6
antibiotics	T45.1X1	T45.1X2	T45.1X3	T45.1X4	T45.1X5	T45.1X6
combination	T45.1X1	T45.1X2	T45.1X3	T45.1X4	T45.1X5	T45.1X6
estrogen	T38.5X1	T38.5X2	T38.5X3	T38.5X4	T38.5X5	T38.5X6
steroid	T38.7X1	T38.7X2	T38.7X3	T38.7X4	T38.7X5	T38.7X6
Antiparasitic drug (systemic)	T37.91	T37.92	T37.93	T37.94	T37.95	T37.96
local	T49.0X1	T49.0X2	T49.0X3	T49.0X4	T49.0X5	T49.0X6
specified NEC	T37.8X1	T37.8X2	T37.8X3	T37.8X4	T37.8X5	T37.8X6

Substance	Poisoning, Accidental (unintentional)	Poisoning, Intentional Self-harm	Poisoning, Assault	Poisoning, Undetermined	Adverse Effect	Underdosing
Antiparkinsonism drug NEC	T42.8X1	T42.8X2	T42.8X3	T42.8X4	T42.8X5	T42.8X6
Antiperspirant NEC	T49.2X1	T49.2X2	T49.2X3	T49.2X4	T49.2X5	T49.2X6
Antiphlogistic NEC	T39.4X1	T39.4X2	T39.4X3	T39.4X4	T39.4X5	T39.4X6
Antiplatyhelmintic drug	T37.4X1	T37.4X2	T37.4X3	T37.4X4	T37.4X5	T37.4X6
Antiprotozoal drug NEC	T37.3X1	T37.3X2	T37.3X3	T37.3X4	T37.3X5	T37.3X6
blood	T37.2X1	T37.2X2	T37.2X3	T37.2X4	T37.2X5	T37.2X6
local	T49.0X1	T49.0X2	T49.0X3	T49.0X4	T49.0X5	T49.0X6
Antipruritic drug NEC	T49.1X1	T49.1X2	T49.1X3	T49.1X4	T49.1X5	T49.1X6
Antipsychotic drug	T43.501	T43.502	T43.503	T43.504	T43.505	T43.506
specified NEC	T43.591	T43.592	T43.593	T43.594	T43.595	T43.596
Antipyretic	T39.91	T39.92	T39.93	T39.94	T39.95	T39.96
specified NEC	T39.8X1	T39.8X2	T39.8X3	T39.8X4	T39.8X5	T39.8X6
Antipyrine	T39.2X1	T39.2X2	T39.2X3	T39.2X4	T39.2X5	T39.2X6
Antirabies hyperimmune serum	T50.Z11	T50.Z12	T50.Z13	T50.Z14	T50.Z15	T50.Z16
Antirheumatic NEC	T39.4X1	T39.4X2	T39.4X3	T39.4X4	T39.4X5	T39.4X6
Antirigidity drug NEC	T42.8X1	T42.8X2	T42.8X3	T42.8X4	T42.8X5	T42.8X6
Antischistosomal drug	T37.4X1	T37.4X2	T37.4X3	T37.4X4	T37.4X5	T37.4X6
Antiscorpion sera	T50.Z11	T50.Z12	T50.Z13	T50.Z14	T50.Z15	T50.Z16
Antiseborrheics	T49.4X1	T49.4X2	T49.4X3	T49.4X4	T49.4X5	T49.4X6
Antiseptics (external) (medicinal)	T49.0X1	T49.0X2	T49.0X3	T49.0X4	T49.0X5	T49.0X6
Antistine	T45.0X1	T45.0X2	T45.0X3	T45.0X4	T45.0X5	T45.0X6
Antitapeworm drug	T37.4X1	T37.4X2	T37.4X3	T37.4X4	T37.4X5	T37.4X6
Antitetanus immunoglobulin	T50.Z11	T50.Z12	T50.Z13	T50.Z14	T50.Z15	T50.Z16
Antithrombotic	T45.521	T45.522	T45.523	T45.524	T45.525	T45.526
Antithyroid drug NEC	T38.2X1	T38.2X2	T38.2X3	T38.2X4	T38.2X5	T38.2X6
Antitoxin	T50.Z11	T50.Z12	T50.Z13	T50.Z14	T50.Z15	T50.Z16
diphtheria	T50.Z11	T50.Z12	T50.Z13	T50.Z14	T50.Z15	T50.Z16
gas gangrene	T50.Z11	T50.Z12	T50.Z13	T50.Z14	T50.Z15	T50.Z16
tetanus	T50.Z11	T50.Z12	T50.Z13	T50.Z14	T50.Z15	T50.Z16
Antitrichomonal drug	T37.3X1	T37.3X2	T37.3X3	T37.3X4	T37.3X5	T37.3X6
Antituberculars	T37.1X1	T37.1X2	T37.1X3	T37.1X4	T37.1X5	T37.1X6
antibiotics	T36.5X1	T36.5X2	T36.5X3	T36.5X4	T36.5X5	T36.5X6
Antitussive NEC	T48.3X1	T48.3X2	T48.3X3	T48.3X4	T48.3X5	T48.3X6
codeine mixture	T40.2X1	T40.2X2	T40.2X3	T40.2X4	T40.2X5	T40.2X6
opiate	T40.2X1	T40.2X2	T40.2X3	T40.2X4	T40.2X5	T40.2X6
Antivaricose drug	T46.8X1	T46.8X2	T46.8X3	T46.8X4	T46.8X5	T46.8X6
Antivenin, antivenom (sera)						
crotaline	T50.Z11	T50.Z12	T50.Z13	T50.Z14	T50.Z15	T50.Z16
spider bite	T50.Z11	T50.Z12	T50.Z13	T50.Z14	T50.Z15	T50.Z16
Antivertigo drug	T45.0X1	T45.0X2	T45.0X3	T45.0X4	T45.0X5	T45.0X6
Antiviral drug NEC	T37.5X1	T37.5X2	T37.5X3	T37.5X4	T37.5X5	T37.5X6
eye	T49.5X1	T49.5X2	T49.5X3	T49.5X4	T49.5X5	T49.5X6
Antiwhipworm drug	T37.4X1	T37.4X2	T37.4X3	T37.4X4	T37.4X5	T37.4X6
Ant poison — see Insecticide						
Antrol — see also by specific chemical substance	T60.91	T60.92	T60.93	T60.94	—	—
fungicide	T60.91	T60.92	T60.93	T60.94	—	—
ANTU (alpha naphthylthiourea)	T60.4X1	T60.4X2	T60.4X3	T60.4X4	—	—
Apalcillin	T36.0X1	T36.0X2	T36.0X3	T36.0X4	T36.0X5	T36.0X6
APC	T48.5X1	T48.5X2	T48.5X3	T48.5X4	T48.5X5	T48.5X6
Aplonidine	T44.4X1	T44.4X2	T44.4X3	T44.4X4	T44.4X5	T44.4X6
Apomorphine	T47.7X1	T47.7X2	T47.7X3	T47.7X4	T47.7X5	T47.7X6
Appetite depressants, central	T50.5X1	T50.5X2	T50.5X3	T50.5X4	T50.5X5	T50.5X6
Apraclonidine (hydrochloride)	T44.4X1	T44.4X2	T44.4X3	T44.4X4	T44.4X5	T44.4X6
Apresoline	T46.5X1	T46.5X2	T46.5X3	T46.5X4	T46.5X5	T46.5X6
Aprindine	T46.2X1	T46.2X2	T46.2X3	T46.2X4	T46.2X5	T46.2X6
Aprobarbital	T42.3X1	T42.3X2	T42.3X3	T42.3X4	T42.3X5	T42.3X6
Apronalide	T42.6X1	T42.6X2	T42.6X3	T42.6X4	T42.6X5	T42.6X6
Aprotinin	T45.621	T45.622	T45.623	T45.624	T45.625	T45.626
Aptocaine	T41.3X1	T41.3X2	T41.3X3	T41.3X4	T41.3X5	T41.3X6
Aqua fortis	T54.2X1	T54.2X2	T54.2X3	T54.2X4	—	—
Ara-A	T37.5X1	T37.5X2	T37.5X3	T37.5X4	T37.5X5	T37.5X6
Ara-C	T45.1X1	T45.1X2	T45.1X3	T45.1X4	T45.1X5	T45.1X6
Arachis oil	T49.3X1	T49.3X2	T49.3X3	T49.3X4	T49.3X5	T49.3X6
cathartic	T47.4X1	T47.4X2	T47.4X3	T47.4X4	T47.4X5	T47.4X6
Aralen	T37.2X1	T37.2X2	T37.2X3	T37.2X4	T37.2X5	T37.2X6
Arecoline	T44.1X1	T44.1X2	T44.1X3	T44.1X4	T44.1X5	T44.1X6
Arginine	T50.991	T50.992	T50.993	T50.994	T50.995	T50.996
glutamate	T50.991	T50.992	T50.993	T50.994	T50.995	T50.996
Argyrol	T49.0X1	T49.0X2	T49.0X3	T49.0X4	T49.0X5	T49.0X6
ENT agent	T49.6X1	T49.6X2	T49.6X3	T49.6X4	T49.6X5	T49.6X6
ophthalmic preparation	T49.5X1	T49.5X2	T49.5X3	T49.5X4	T49.5X5	T49.5X6
Aristocort	T38.0X1	T38.0X2	T38.0X3	T38.0X4	T38.0X5	T38.0X6
ENT agent	T49.6X1	T49.6X2	T49.6X3	T49.6X4	T49.6X5	T49.6X6
ophthalmic preparation	T49.5X1	T49.5X2	T49.5X3	T49.5X4	T49.5X5	T49.5X6

Table of Drugs and Chemicals

Aristocort — Benzamine

Substance	Poisoning, Accidental (unintentional)	Poisoning, Intentional Self-harm	Poisoning, Assault	Poisoning, Undetermined	Adverse Effect	Under-dosing
Aristocort — *continued*						
topical NEC	T49.0X1	T49.0X2	T49.0X3	T49.0X4	T49.0X5	T49.0X6
Aromatics, corrosive	T54.1X1	T54.1X2	T54.1X3	T54.1X4	—	—
disinfectants	T54.1X1	T54.1X2	T54.1X3	T54.1X4	—	—
Arsenate of lead	T57.0X1	T57.0X2	T57.0X3	T57.0X4	—	—
herbicide	T57.0X1	T57.0X2	T57.0X3	T57.0X4	—	—
Arsenic, arsenicals (compounds) (dust) (vapor) **NEC**	T57.0X1	T57.0X2	T57.0X3	T57.0X4	—	—
anti-infectives	T37.8X1	T37.8X2	T37.8X3	T37.8X4	T37.8X5	T37.8X6
pesticide (dust) (fumes)	T57.0X1	T57.0X2	T57.0X3	T57.0X4	—	—
Arsine (gas)	T57.0X1	T57.0X2	T57.0X3	T57.0X4	—	—
Arsphenamine (silver)	T37.8X1	T37.8X2	T37.8X3	T37.8X4	T37.8X5	T37.8X6
Arsthinol	T37.3X1	T37.3X2	T37.3X3	T37.3X4	T37.3X5	T37.3X6
Artane	T44.3X1	T44.3X2	T44.3X3	T44.3X4	T44.3X5	T44.3X6
Arthropod (venomous) **NEC**	T63.481	T63.482	T63.483	T63.484		
Articaine	T41.3X1	T41.3X2	T41.3X3	T41.3X4	T41.3X5	T41.3X6
Asbestos	T57.8X1	T57.8X2	T57.8X3	T57.8X4	—	—
Ascaridole	T37.4X1	T37.4X2	T37.4X3	T37.4X4	T37.4X5	T37.4X6
Ascorbic acid	T45.2X1	T45.2X2	T45.2X3	T45.2X4	T45.2X5	T45.2X6
Asiaticoside	T49.0X1	T49.0X2	T49.0X3	T49.0X4	T49.0X5	T49.0X6
Asparaginase	T45.1X1	T45.1X2	T45.1X3	T45.1X4	T45.1X5	T45.1X6
Aspidium (oleoresin)	T37.4X1	T37.4X2	T37.4X3	T37.4X4	T37.4X5	T37.4X6
Aspirin (aluminum)	T39.011	T39.012	T39.013	T39.014	T39.015	T39.016
(soluble)	T39.011	T39.012	T39.013	T39.014	T39.015	T39.016
Aspoxicillin	T36.0X1	T36.0X2	T36.0X3	T36.0X4	T36.0X5	T36.0X6
Astemizole	T45.0X1	T45.0X2	T45.0X3	T45.0X4	T45.0X5	T45.0X6
Astringent (local)	T49.2X1	T49.2X2	T49.2X3	T49.2X4	T49.2X5	T49.2X6
specified NEC	T49.2X1	T49.2X2	T49.2X3	T49.2X4	T49.2X5	T49.2X6
Astromicin	T36.5X1	T36.5X2	T36.5X3	T36.5X4	T36.5X5	T36.5X6
Ataractic drug NEC	T43.501	T43.502	T43.503	T43.504	T43.505	T43.506
Atenolol	T44.7X1	T44.7X2	T44.7X3	T44.7X4	T44.7X5	T44.7X6
Atonia drug, intestinal	T47.4X1	T47.4X2	T47.4X3	T47.4X4	T47.4X5	T47.4X6
Atophan	T50.4X1	T50.4X2	T50.4X3	T50.4X4	T50.4X5	T50.4X6
Atracurium besilate	T48.1X1	T48.1X2	T48.1X3	T48.1X4	T48.1X5	T48.1X6
Atropine	T44.3X1	T44.3X2	T44.3X3	T44.3X4	T44.3X5	T44.3X6
derivative	T44.3X1	T44.3X2	T44.3X3	T44.3X4	T44.3X5	T44.3X6
methonitrate	T44.3X1	T44.3X2	T44.3X3	T44.3X4	T44.3X5	T44.3X6
Attapulgite	T47.6X1	T47.6X2	T47.6X3	T47.6X4	T47.6X5	T47.6X6
Auramine	T65.891	T65.892	T65.893	T65.894	—	—
dye	T65.6X1	T65.6X2	T65.6X3	T65.6X4	—	—
fungicide	T60.3X1	T60.3X2	T60.3X3	T60.3X4	—	—
Auranofin	T39.4X1	T39.4X2	T39.4X3	T39.4X4	T39.4X5	T39.4X6
Aurantiin	T46.991	T46.992	T46.993	T46.994	T46.995	T46.996
Aureomycin	T36.4X1	T36.4X2	T36.4X3	T36.4X4	T36.4X5	T36.4X6
ophthalmic preparation	T49.5X1	T49.5X2	T49.5X3	T49.5X4	T49.5X5	T49.5X6
topical NEC	T49.0X1	T49.0X2	T49.0X3	T49.0X4	T49.0X5	T49.0X6
Aurothioglucose	T39.4X1	T39.4X2	T39.4X3	T39.4X4	T39.4X5	T39.4X6
Aurothioglycanide	T39.4X1	T39.4X2	T39.4X3	T39.4X4	T39.4X5	T39.4X6
Aurothiomalate sodium	T39.4X1	T39.4X2	T39.4X3	T39.4X4	T39.4X5	T39.4X6
Aurotioprol	T39.4X1	T39.4X2	T39.4X3	T39.4X4	T39.4X5	T39.4X6
Automobile fuel	T52.0X1	T52.0X2	T52.0X3	T52.0X4	—	—
Autonomic nervous system agent NEC	T44.901	T44.902	T44.903	T44.904	T44.905	T44.906
Avlosulfon	T37.1X1	T37.1X2	T37.1X3	T37.1X4	T37.1X5	T37.1X6
Avomine	T42.6X1	T42.6X2	T42.6X3	T42.6X4	T42.6X5	T42.6X6
Axerophthol	T45.2X1	T45.2X2	T45.2X3	T45.2X4	T45.2X5	T45.2X6
Azacitidine	T45.1X1	T45.1X2	T45.1X3	T45.1X4	T45.1X5	T45.1X6
Azacyclonol	T43.591	T43.592	T43.593	T43.594	T43.595	T43.596
Azadirachta	T60.2X1	T60.2X2	T60.2X3	T60.2X4	—	—
Azanidazole	T37.3X1	T37.3X2	T37.3X3	T37.3X4	T37.3X5	T37.3X6
Azapetine	T46.7X1	T46.7X2	T46.7X3	T46.7X4	T46.7X5	T46.7X6
Azapropazone	T39.2X1	T39.2X2	T39.2X3	T39.2X4	T39.2X5	T39.2X6
Azaribine	T45.1X1	T45.1X2	T45.1X3	T45.1X4	T45.1X5	T45.1X6
Azaserine	T45.1X1	T45.1X2	T45.1X3	T45.1X4	T45.1X5	T45.1X6
Azatadine	T45.0X1	T45.0X2	T45.0X3	T45.0X4	T45.0X5	T45.0X6
Azatepa	T45.1X1	T45.1X2	T45.1X3	T45.1X4	T45.1X5	T45.1X6
Azathioprine	T45.1X1	T45.1X2	T45.1X3	T45.1X4	T45.1X5	T45.1X6
Azelaic acid	T49.0X1	T49.0X2	T49.0X3	T49.0X4	T49.0X5	T49.0X6
Azelastine	T45.0X1	T45.0X2	T45.0X3	T45.0X4	T45.0X5	T45.0X6
Azidocillin	T36.0X1	T36.0X2	T36.0X3	T36.0X4	T36.0X5	T36.0X6
Azidothymidine	T37.5X1	T37.5X2	T37.5X3	T37.5X4	T37.5X5	T37.5X6
Azinphos (ethyl) (methyl)	T60.0X1	T60.0X2	T60.0X3	T60.0X4	—	—
Aziridine (chelating)	T54.1X1	T54.1X2	T54.1X3	T54.1X4	—	—
Azithromycin	T36.3X1	T36.3X2	T36.3X3	T36.3X4	T36.3X5	T36.3X6
Azlocillin	T36.0X1	T36.0X2	T36.0X3	T36.0X4	T36.0X5	T36.0X6
Azobenzene smoke	T65.3X1	T65.3X2	T65.3X3	T65.3X4	—	—
acaricide	T60.8X1	T60.8X2	T60.8X3	T60.8X4	—	—
Azosulfamide	T37.0X1	T37.0X2	T37.0X3	T37.0X4	T37.0X5	T37.0X6
AZT	T37.5X1	T37.5X2	T37.5X3	T37.5X4	T37.5X5	T37.5X6
Aztreonam	T36.1X1	T36.1X2	T36.1X3	T36.1X4	T36.1X5	T36.1X6
Azulfidine	T37.0X1	T37.0X2	T37.0X3	T37.0X4	T37.0X5	T37.0X6
Azuresin	T50.8X1	T50.8X2	T50.8X3	T50.8X4	T50.8X5	T50.8X6
b-acetyldigoxin	T46.0X1	T46.0X2	T46.0X3	T46.0X4	T46.0X5	T46.0X6
P-Acetamidophenol	T39.1X1	T39.1X2	T39.1X3	T39.1X4	T39.1X5	T39.1X6
Bacampicillin	T36.0X1	T36.0X2	T36.0X3	T36.0X4	T36.0X5	T36.0X6
Bacillus						
lactobacillus	T47.8X1	T47.8X2	T47.8X3	T47.8X4	T47.8X5	T47.8X6
subtilis	T47.6X1	T47.6X2	T47.6X3	T47.6X4	T47.6X5	T47.6X6
Bacimycin	T49.0X1	T49.0X2	T49.0X3	T49.0X4	T49.0X5	T49.0X6
ophthalmic preparation	T49.5X1	T49.5X2	T49.5X3	T49.5X4	T49.5X5	T49.5X6
Bacitracin zinc	T49.0X1	T49.0X2	T49.0X3	T49.0X4	T49.0X5	T49.0X6
with neomycin	T49.0X1	T49.0X2	T49.0X3	T49.0X4	T49.0X5	T49.0X6
ENT agent	T49.6X1	T49.6X2	T49.6X3	T49.6X4	T49.6X5	T49.6X6
ophthalmic preparation	T49.5X1	T49.5X2	T49.5X3	T49.5X4	T49.5X5	T49.5X6
topical NEC	T49.0X1	T49.0X2	T49.0X3	T49.0X4	T49.0X5	T49.0X6
Baclofen	T42.8X1	T42.8X2	T42.8X3	T42.8X4	T42.8X5	T42.8X6
Baking soda	T50.991	T50.992	T50.993	T50.994	T50.995	T50.996
BAL	T45.8X1	T45.8X2	T45.8X3	T45.8X4	T45.8X5	T45.8X6
Bambuterol	T48.6X1	T48.6X2	T48.6X3	T48.6X4	T48.6X5	T48.6X6
Bamethan (sulfate)	T46.7X1	T46.7X2	T46.7X3	T46.7X4	T46.7X5	T46.7X6
Bamifylline	T48.6X1	T48.6X2	T48.6X3	T48.6X4	T48.6X5	T48.6X6
Bamipine	T45.0X1	T45.0X2	T45.0X3	T45.0X4	T45.0X5	T45.0X6
Baneberry — *see Actaea spicata*						
Banewort — *see Belladonna*						
Barbenyl	T42.3X1	T42.3X2	T42.3X3	T42.3X4	T42.3X5	T42.3X6
Barbexaclone	T42.6X1	T42.6X2	T42.6X3	T42.6X4	T42.6X5	T42.6X6
Barbital	T42.3X1	T42.3X2	T42.3X3	T42.3X4	T42.3X5	T42.3X6
sodium	T42.3X1	T42.3X2	T42.3X3	T42.3X4	T42.3X5	T42.3X6
Barbitone	T42.3X1	T42.3X2	T42.3X3	T42.3X4	T42.3X5	T42.3X6
Barbiturate NEC	T42.3X1	T42.3X2	T42.3X3	T42.3X4	T42.3X5	T42.3X6
with tranquilizer	T42.3X1	T42.3X2	T42.3X3	T42.3X4	T42.3X5	T42.3X6
anesthetic (intravenous)	T41.1X1	T41.1X2	T41.1X3	T41.1X4	T41.1X5	T41.1X6
Barium (carbonate) (chloride)	T57.8X1	T57.8X2	T57.8X3	T57.8X4	—	—
(sulfite)						
diagnostic agent	T50.8X1	T50.8X2	T50.8X3	T50.8X4	T50.8X5	T50.8X6
pesticide	T60.4X1	T60.4X2	T60.4X3	T60.4X4	—	—
rodenticide	T60.4X1	T60.4X2	T60.4X3	T60.4X4	—	—
sulfate (medicinal)	T50.8X1	T50.8X2	T50.8X3	T50.8X4	T50.8X5	T50.8X6
Barrier cream	T49.3X1	T49.3X2	T49.3X3	T49.3X4	T49.3X5	T49.3X6
Basic fuchsin	T49.0X1	T49.0X2	T49.0X3	T49.0X4	T49.0X5	T49.0X6
Battery acid or fluid	T54.2X1	T54.2X2	T54.2X3	T54.2X4	—	—
Bay rum	T51.8X1	T51.8X2	T51.8X3	T51.8X4	—	—
b-benzalbutyramide	T46.6X1	T46.6X2	T46.6X3	T46.6X4	T46.6X5	T46.6X6
BCG (vaccine)	T50.A91	T50.A92	T50.A93	T50.A94	T50.A95	T50.A96
BCNU	T45.1X1	T45.1X2	T45.1X3	T45.1X4	T45.1X5	T45.1X6
Bearsfoot	T62.2X1	T62.2X2	T62.2X3	T62.2X4	—	—
Beclamide	T42.6X1	T42.6X2	T42.6X3	T42.6X4	T42.6X5	T42.6X6
Beclomethasone	T44.5X1	T44.5X2	T44.5X3	T44.5X4	T44.5X5	T44.5X6
Bee (sting) (venom)	T63.441	T63.442	T63.443	T63.444		
Befunolol	T49.5X1	T49.5X2	T49.5X3	T49.5X4	T49.5X5	T49.5X6
Bekanamycin	T36.5X1	T36.5X2	T36.5X3	T36.5X4	T36.5X5	T36.5X6
Belladonna — *see also Nightshade*						
alkaloids	T44.3X1	T44.3X2	T44.3X3	T44.3X4	T44.3X5	T44.3X6
extract	T44.3X1	T44.3X2	T44.3X3	T44.3X4	T44.3X5	T44.3X6
herb	T44.3X1	T44.3X2	T44.3X3	T44.3X4	T44.3X5	T44.3X6
Bemegride	T50.7X1	T50.7X2	T50.7X3	T50.7X4	T50.7X5	T50.7X6
Benactyzine	T44.3X1	T44.3X2	T44.3X3	T44.3X4	T44.3X5	T44.3X6
Benadryl	T45.0X1	T45.0X2	T45.0X3	T45.0X4	T45.0X5	T45.0X6
Benaprizine	T44.3X1	T44.3X2	T44.3X3	T44.3X4	T44.3X5	T44.3X6
Benazepril	T46.4X1	T46.4X2	T46.4X3	T46.4X4	T46.4X5	T46.4X6
Bencyclane	T46.7X1	T46.7X2	T46.7X3	T46.7X4	T46.7X5	T46.7X6
Bendazol	T46.3X1	T46.3X2	T46.3X3	T46.3X4	T46.3X5	T46.3X6
Bendrofluazide	T50.2X1	T50.2X2	T50.2X3	T50.2X4	T50.2X5	T50.2X6
Bendroflumethiazide	T50.2X1	T50.2X2	T50.2X3	T50.2X4	T50.2X5	T50.2X6
Benemid	T50.4X1	T50.4X2	T50.4X3	T50.4X4	T50.4X5	T50.4X6
Benethamine penicillin	T36.0X1	T36.0X2	T36.0X3	T36.0X4	T36.0X5	T36.0X6
Benexate	T47.1X1	T47.1X2	T47.1X3	T47.1X4	T47.1X5	T47.1X6
Benfluorex	T46.6X1	T46.6X2	T46.6X3	T46.6X4	T46.6X5	T46.6X6
Benfotiamine	T45.2X1	T45.2X2	T45.2X3	T45.2X4	T45.2X5	T45.2X6
Benisone	T49.0X1	T49.0X2	T49.0X3	T49.0X4	T49.0X5	T49.0X6
Benomyl	T60.0X1	T60.0X2	T60.0X3	T60.0X4	—	—
Benoquin	T49.8X1	T49.8X2	T49.8X3	T49.8X4	T49.8X5	T49.8X6
Benoxinate	T41.3X1	T41.3X2	T41.3X3	T41.3X4	T41.3X5	T41.3X6
Benperidol	T43.4X1	T43.4X2	T43.4X3	T43.4X4	T43.4X5	T43.4X6
Benproperine	T48.3X1	T48.3X2	T48.3X3	T48.3X4	T48.3X5	T48.3X6
Benserazide	T42.8X1	T42.8X2	T42.8X3	T42.8X4	T42.8X5	T42.8X6
Bentazepam	T42.4X1	T42.4X2	T42.4X3	T42.4X4	T42.4X5	T42.4X6
Bentiromide	T50.8X1	T50.8X2	T50.8X3	T50.8X4	T50.8X5	T50.8X6
Bentonite	T49.3X1	T49.3X2	T49.3X3	T49.3X4	T49.3X5	T49.3X6
Benzalbutyramide	T46.6X1	T46.6X2	T46.6X3	T46.6X4	T46.6X5	T46.6X6
Benzalkonium (chloride)	T49.0X1	T49.0X2	T49.0X3	T49.0X4	T49.0X5	T49.0X6
ophthalmic preparation	T49.5X1	T49.5X2	T49.5X3	T49.5X4	T49.5X5	T49.5X6
Benzamidosalicylate (calcium)	T37.1X1	T37.1X2	T37.1X3	T37.1X4	T37.1X5	T37.1X6
Benzamine	T41.3X1	T41.3X2	T41.3X3	T41.3X4	T41.3X5	T41.3X6

354

Additional Character May Be Required — Refer to the Tabular List for Character Selection ▽ Subterms under main terms may continue to next column or page

Substance	Poisoning, Accidental (unintentional)	Poisoning, Intentional Self-harm	Poisoning, Assault	Poisoning, Undetermined	Adverse Effect	Under-dosing
Benzamine — *continued*						
lactate	T49.1X1	T49.1X2	T49.1X3	T49.1X4	T49.1X5	T49.1X6
Benzamphetamine	T50.5X1	T50.5X2	T50.5X3	T50.5X4	T50.5X5	T50.5X6
Benzapril hydrochloride	T46.5X1	T46.5X2	T46.5X3	T46.5X4	T46.5X5	T46.5X6
Benzathine	T36.0X1	T36.0X2	T36.0X3	T36.0X4	T36.0X5	T36.0X6
benzylpenicillin						
Benzathine penicillin	T36.0X1	T36.0X2	T36.0X3	T36.0X4	T36.0X5	T36.0X6
Benzatropine	T42.8X1	T42.8X2	T42.8X3	T42.8X4	T42.8X5	T42.8X6
Benzbromarone	T50.4X1	T50.4X2	T50.4X3	T50.4X4	T50.4X5	T50.4X6
Benzcarbimine	T45.1X1	T45.1X2	T45.1X3	T45.1X4	T45.1X5	T45.1X6
Benzedrex	T44.991	T44.992	T44.993	T44.994	T44.995	T44.996
Benzedrine (amphetamine)	T43.621	T43.622	T43.623	T43.624	T43.625	T43.626
Benzenamine	T65.3X1	T65.3X2	T65.3X3	T65.3X4	—	—
Benzene	T52.1X1	T52.1X2	T52.1X3	T52.1X4	—	—
homologues (acetyl) (dimethyl)	T52.2X1	T52.2X2	T52.2X3	T52.2X4	—	—
(methyl) (solvent)						
Benzethonium (chloride)	T49.0X1	T49.0X2	T49.0X3	T49.0X4	T49.0X5	T49.0X6
Benzfetamine	T50.5X1	T50.5X2	T50.5X3	T50.5X4	T50.5X5	T50.5X6
Benzhexol	T44.3X1	T44.3X2	T44.3X3	T44.3X4	T44.3X5	T44.3X6
Benzhydramine (chloride)	T45.0X1	T45.0X2	T45.0X4	T45.0X4	T45.0X5	T45.0X6
Benzidine	T65.891	T65.892	T65.893	T65.894	—	—
Benzilonium bromide	T44.3X1	T44.3X2	T44.3X3	T44.3X4	T44.3X5	T44.3X6
Benzimidazole	T60.3X1	T60.3X2	T60.3X3	T60.3X4	—	—
Benzin (e) — *see* Ligroin						
Benziodarone	T46.3X1	T46.3X2	T46.3X3	T46.3X4	T46.3X5	T46.3X6
Benznidazole	T37.3X1	T37.3X2	T37.3X3	T37.3X4	T37.3X5	T37.3X6
Benzocaine	T41.3X1	T41.3X2	T41.3X3	T41.3X4	T41.3X5	T41.3X6
Benzodiapin	T42.4X1	T42.4X2	T42.4X3	T42.4X4	T42.4X5	T42.4X6
Benzodiazepine NEC	T42.4X1	T42.4X2	T42.4X3	T42.4X4	T42.4X5	T42.4X6
Benzoic acid	T49.0X1	T49.0X2	T49.0X3	T49.0X4	T49.0X5	T49.0X6
with salicylic acid	T49.0X1	T49.0X2	T49.0X3	T49.0X4	T49.0X5	T49.0X6
Benzoin (tincture)	T48.5X1	T48.5X2	T48.5X3	T48.5X4	T48.5X5	T48.5X6
Benzol (benzene)	T52.1X1	T52.1X2	T52.1X3	T52.1X4	—	—
vapor	T52.0X1	T52.0X2	T52.0X3	T52.0X4	—	—
Benzomorphan	T40.2X1	T40.2X2	T40.2X3	T40.2X4	T40.2X5	T40.2X6
Benzonatate	T48.3X1	T48.3X2	T48.3X3	T48.3X4	T48.3X5	T48.3X6
Benzophenones	T49.3X1	T49.3X2	T49.3X3	T49.3X4	T49.3X5	T49.3X6
Benzopyrone	T46.991	T46.992	T46.993	T46.994	T46.995	T46.996
Benzothiadiazides	T50.2X1	T50.2X2	T50.2X3	T50.2X4	T50.2X5	T50.2X6
Benzoxonium chloride	T49.0X1	T49.0X2	T49.0X3	T49.0X4	T49.0X5	T49.0X6
Benzoylpas calcium	T37.1X1	T37.1X2	T37.1X3	T37.1X4	T37.1X5	T37.1X6
Benzoyl peroxide	T49.0X1	T49.0X2	T49.0X3	T49.0X4	T49.0X5	T49.0X6
Benzperidin	T43.591	T43.592	T43.593	T43.594	T43.595	T43.596
Benzperidol	T43.591	T43.592	T43.593	T43.594	T43.595	T43.596
Benzphetamine	T50.5X1	T50.5X2	T50.5X3	T50.5X4	T50.5X5	T50.5X6
Benzpyrinium bromide	T44.1X1	T44.1X2	T44.1X3	T44.1X4	T44.1X5	T44.1X6
Benzquinamide	T45.0X1	T45.0X2	T45.0X3	T45.0X4	T45.0X5	T45.0X6
Benzthiazide	T50.2X1	T50.2X2	T50.2X3	T50.2X4	T50.2X5	T50.2X6
Benztropine						
anticholinergic	T44.3X1	T44.3X2	T44.3X3	T44.3X4	T44.3X5	T44.3X6
antiparkinson	T42.8X1	T42.8X2	T42.8X3	T42.8X4	T42.8X5	T42.8X6
Benzydamine	T49.0X1	T49.0X2	T49.0X3	T49.0X4	T49.0X5	T49.0X6
Benzyl						
acetate	T52.8X1	T52.8X2	T52.8X3	T52.8X4	—	—
alcohol	T49.0X1	T49.0X2	T49.0X3	T49.0X4	T49.0X5	T49.0X6
benzoate	T49.0X1	T49.0X2	T49.0X3	T49.0X4	T49.0X5	T49.0X6
Benzoic acid	T49.0X1	T49.0X2	T49.0X3	T49.0X4	T49.0X5	T49.0X6
morphine	T40.2X1	T40.2X2	T40.2X3	T40.2X4	—	—
nicotinate	T46.6X1	T46.6X2	T46.6X3	T46.6X4	T46.6X5	T46.6X6
penicillin	T36.0X1	T36.0X2	T36.0X3	T36.0X4	T36.0X5	T36.0X6
Benzylhydrochlorthiazide	T50.2X1	T50.2X2	T50.2X3	T50.2X4	T50.2X5	T50.2X6
Benzylpenicillin	T36.0X1	T36.0X2	T36.0X3	T36.0X4	T36.0X5	T36.0X6
Benzylthiouracil	T38.2X1	T38.2X2	T38.2X3	T38.2X4	T38.2X5	T38.2X6
Bephenium	T37.4X1	T37.4X2	T37.4X3	T37.4X4	T37.4X5	T37.4X6
hydroxynaphthoate						
Bepridil	T46.1X1	T46.1X2	T46.1X3	T46.1X4	T46.1X5	T46.1X6
Bergamot oil	T65.891	T65.892	T65.893	T65.894	—	—
Bergapten	T50.991	T50.992	T50.993	T50.994	T50.995	T50.996
Berries, poisonous	T62.1X1	T62.1X2	T62.1X3	T62.1X4	—	—
Beryllium (compounds)	T56.7X1	T56.7X2	T56.7X3	T56.7X4	—	—
beta adrenergic blocking agent, heart	T44.7X1	T44.7X2	T44.7X3	T44.7X4	T44.7X5	T44.7X6
Betacarotene	T45.2X1	T45.2X2	T45.2X3	T45.2X4	T45.2X5	T45.2X6
Beta-Chlor	T42.6X1	T42.6X2	T42.6X3	T42.6X4	T42.6X5	T42.6X6
Betahistine	T46.7X1	T46.7X2	T46.7X3	T46.7X4	T46.7X5	T46.7X6
Betaine	T47.5X1	T47.5X2	T47.5X3	T47.5X4	T47.5X5	T47.5X6
Betamethasone	T49.0X1	T49.0X2	T49.0X3	T49.0X4	T49.0X5	T49.0X6
topical	T49.0X1	T49.0X2	T49.0X3	T49.0X4	T49.0X5	T49.0X6
Betamicin	T36.8X1	T36.8X2	T36.8X3	T36.8X4	T36.8X5	T36.8X6
Betanidine	T46.5X1	T46.5X2	T46.5X3	T46.5X4	T46.5X5	T46.5X6
Betaxolol	T44.7X1	T44.7X2	T44.7X3	T44.7X4	T44.7X5	T44.7X6
Betazole	T50.8X1	T50.8X2	T50.8X3	T50.8X4	T50.8X5	T50.8X6
Bethanechol	T44.1X1	T44.1X2	T44.1X3	T44.1X4	T44.1X5	T44.1X6
Bethanechol — *continued*						
chloride	T44.1X1	T44.1X2	T44.1X3	T44.1X4	T44.1X5	T44.1X6
Bethanidine	T46.5X1	T46.5X2	T46.5X3	T46.5X4	T46.5X5	T46.5X6
Betoxycaine	T41.3X1	T41.3X2	T41.3X3	T41.3X4	T41.3X5	T41.3X6
Betula oil	T49.3X1	T49.3X2	T49.3X3	T49.3X4	T49.3X5	T49.3X6
Bevantolol	T44.7X1	T44.7X2	T44.7X3	T44.7X4	T44.7X5	T44.7X6
Bevonium metilsulfate	T44.3X1	T44.3X2	T44.3X3	T44.3X4	T44.3X5	T44.3X6
Bezafibrate	T46.6X1	T46.6X2	T46.6X3	T46.6X4	T46.6X5	T46.6X6
Bezitramide	T40.4X1	T40.4X2	T40.4X3	T40.4X4	T40.4X5	T40.4X6
BHA	T50.991	T50.992	T50.993	T50.994	T50.995	T50.996
Bhang	T40.7X1	T40.7X2	T40.7X3	T40.7X4	T40.7X5	T40.7X6
BHC (medicinal)	T49.0X1	T49.0X2	T49.0X3	T49.0X4	T49.0X5	T49.0X6
nonmedicinal (vapor)	T53.6X1	T53.6X2	T53.6X3	T53.6X4	—	—
Bialamicol	T37.3X1	T37.3X2	T37.3X3	T37.3X4	T37.3X5	T37.3X6
Bibenzonium bromide	T48.3X1	T48.3X2	T48.3X3	T48.3X4	T48.3X5	T48.3X6
Bibrocathol	T49.5X1	T49.5X2	T49.5X3	T49.5X4	T49.5X5	T49.5X6
Bichloride of mercury — *see* Mercury, chloride						
Bichromates (calcium) (potassium)(sodium) (crystals)	T57.8X1	T57.8X2	T57.8X3	T57.8X4	—	—
fumes	T56.2X1	T56.2X2	T56.2X3	T56.2X4	—	—
Biclotymol	T49.6X1	T49.6X2	T49.6X3	T49.6X4	T49.6X5	T49.6X6
Bicucculine	T50.7X1	T50.7X2	T50.7X3	T50.7X4	T50.7X5	T50.7X6
Bifemelane	T43.291	T43.292	T43.293	T43.294	T43.295	T43.296
Biguanide derivatives, oral	T38.3X1	T38.3X2	T38.3X3	T38.3X4	T38.3X5	T38.3X6
Bile salts	T47.5X1	T47.5X2	T47.5X3	T47.5X4	T47.5X5	T47.5X6
Biligrafin	T50.8X1	T50.8X2	T50.8X3	T50.8X4	T50.8X5	T50.8X6
Bilopaque	T50.8X1	T50.8X2	T50.8X3	T50.8X4	T50.8X5	T50.8X6
Binifibrate	T46.6X1	T46.6X2	T46.6X3	T46.6X4	T46.6X5	T46.6X6
Binitrobenzol	T65.3X1	T65.3X2	T65.3X3	T65.3X4	—	—
Bioflavonoid(s)	T46.991	T46.992	T46.993	T46.994	T46.995	T46.996
Biological substance NEC	T50.901	T50.902	T50.903	T50.904	T50.905	T50.906
Biotin	T45.2X1	T45.2X2	T45.2X3	T45.2X4	T45.2X5	T45.2X6
Biperiden	T44.3X1	T44.3X2	T44.3X3	T44.3X4	T44.3X5	T44.3X6
Bisacodyl	T47.2X1	T47.2X2	T47.2X3	T47.2X4	T47.2X5	T47.2X6
Bisbentiamine	T45.2X1	T45.2X2	T45.2X3	T45.2X4	T45.2X5	T45.2X6
Bisbutiamine	T45.2X1	T45.2X2	T45.2X3	T45.2X4	T45.2X5	T45.2X6
Bisdequalinium (salts) (diacetate)	T49.6X1	T49.6X2	T49.6X3	T49.6X4	T49.6X5	T49.6X6
Bishydroxycoumarin	T45.511	T45.512	T45.513	T45.514	T45.515	T45.516
Bismarsen	T37.8X1	T37.8X2	T37.8X3	T37.8X4	T37.8X5	T37.8X6
Bismuth salts	T47.6X1	T47.6X2	T47.6X3	T47.6X4	T47.6X5	T47.6X6
aluminate	T47.1X1	T47.1X2	T47.1X3	T47.1X4	T47.1X5	T47.1X6
anti-infectives	T37.8X1	T37.8X2	T37.8X3	T37.8X4	T37.8X5	T37.8X6
formic iodide	T49.0X1	T49.0X2	T49.0X3	T49.0X4	T49.0X5	T49.0X6
glycolylarsenate	T49.0X1	T49.0X2	T49.0X3	T49.0X4	T49.0X5	T49.0X6
nonmedicinal (compounds) NEC	T65.91	T65.92	T65.93	T65.94	—	—
subcarbonate	T47.6X1	T47.6X2	T47.6X3	T47.6X4	T47.6X5	T47.6X6
subsalicylate	T37.8X1	T37.8X2	T37.8X3	T37.8X4	T37.8X5	T37.8X6
sulfarsphenamine	T37.8X1	T37.8X2	T37.8X3	T37.8X4	T37.8X5	T37.8X6
Bisoprolol	T44.7X1	T44.7X2	T44.7X3	T44.7X4	T44.7X5	T44.7X6
Bisoxatin	T47.2X1	T47.2X2	T47.2X3	T47.2X4	T47.2X5	T47.2X6
Bisulepin (hydrochloride)	T45.0X1	T45.0X2	T45.0X3	T45.0X4	T45.0X5	T45.0X6
Bithionol	T37.8X1	T37.8X2	T37.8X3	T37.8X4	T37.8X5	T37.8X6
anthelminthic	T37.4X1	T37.4X2	T37.4X3	T37.4X4	T37.4X5	T37.4X6
Bitolterol	T48.6X1	T48.6X2	T48.6X3	T48.6X4	T48.6X5	T48.6X6
Bitoscanate	T37.4X1	T37.4X2	T37.4X3	T37.4X4	T37.4X5	T37.4X6
Bitter almond oil	T62.8X1	T62.8X2	T62.8X3	T62.8X4	—	—
Bittersweet	T62.2X1	T62.2X2	T62.2X3	T62.2X4	—	—
Black						
flag	T60.91	T60.92	T60.93	T60.94	—	—
henbane	T62.2X1	T62.2X2	T62.2X3	T62.2X4	—	—
leaf (40)	T60.91	T60.92	T60.93	T60.94	—	—
widow spider (bite)	T63.311	T63.312	T63.313	T63.314	—	—
antivenin	T50.Z11	T50.Z12	T50.Z13	T50.Z14	T50.Z15	T50.Z16
Blast furnace gas (carbon monoxide from)	T58.8X1	T58.8X2	T58.8X3	T58.8X4	—	—
Bleach	T54.91	T54.92	T54.93	T54.94	—	—
Bleaching agent (medicinal)	T49.4X1	T49.4X2	T49.4X3	T49.4X4	T49.4X5	T49.4X6
Bleomycin	T45.1X1	T45.1X2	T45.1X3	T45.1X4	T45.1X5	T45.1X6
Blockain	T41.3X1	T41.3X2	T41.3X3	T41.3X4	T41.3X5	T41.3X6
infiltration (subcutaneous)	T41.3X1	T41.3X2	T41.3X3	T41.3X4	T41.3X5	T41.3X6
nerve block (peripheral) (plexus)	T41.3X1	T41.3X2	T41.3X3	T41.3X4	T41.3X5	T41.3X6
topical (surface)	T41.3X1	T41.3X2	T41.3X3	T41.3X4	T41.3X5	T41.3X6
Blockers, calcium channel	T46.1X1	T46.1X2	T46.1X3	T46.1X4	T46.1X5	T46.1X6
Blood (derivatives) (natural) (plasma) (whole)	T45.8X1	T45.8X2	T45.8X3	T45.8X4	T45.8X5	T45.8X6
dried	T45.8X1	T45.8X2	T45.8X3	T45.8X4	T45.8X5	T45.8X6

▽ Subterms under main terms may continue to next column or page   Additional Character May Be Required — Refer to the Tabular List for Character Selection   355

Benzamine — Blood

Substance	Poisoning, Accidental (unintentional)	Poisoning, Intentional Self-harm	Poisoning, Assault	Poisoning, Undetermined	Adverse Effect	Under-dosing
Blood — *continued*						
drug affecting NEC	T45.91	T45.92	T45.93	T45.94	T45.95	T45.96
expander NEC	T45.8X1	T45.8X2	T45.8X3	T45.8X4	T45.8X5	T45.8X6
fraction NEC	T45.8X1	T45.8X2	T45.8X3	T45.8X4	T45.8X5	T45.8X6
substitute	T45.8X1	T45.8X2	T45.8X3	T45.8X4	T45.8X5	T45.8X6
(macromolecular)						
Blue velvet	T40.2X1	T40.2X2	T40.2X3	T40.2X4	—	—
Bone meal	T62.8X1	T62.8X2	T62.8X3	T62.8X4	—	—
Bonine	T45.0X1	T45.0X2	T45.0X3	T45.0X4	T45.0X5	T45.0X6
Bopindolol	T44.7X1	T44.7X2	T44.7X3	T44.7X4	T44.7X5	T44.7X6
Boracic acid	T49.0X1	T49.0X2	T49.0X3	T49.0X4	T49.0X5	T49.0X6
ENT agent	T49.6X1	T49.6X2	T49.6X3	T49.6X4	T49.6X5	T49.6X6
ophthalmic preparation	T49.5X1	T49.5X2	T49.5X3	T49.5X4	T49.5X5	T49.5X6
Borane complex	T57.8X1	T57.8X2	T57.8X3	T57.8X4	—	—
Borate(s)	T57.8X1	T57.8X2	T57.8X3	T57.8X4	—	—
buffer	T50.991	T50.992	T50.993	T50.994	T50.995	T50.996
cleanser	T54.91	T54.92	T54.93	T54.94	—	—
sodium	T57.8X1	T57.8X2	T57.8X3	T57.8X4	—	—
Borax (cleanser)	T54.91	T54.92	T54.93	T54.94	—	—
Bordeaux mixture	T60.3X1	T60.3X2	T60.3X3	T60.3X4	—	—
Boric acid	T49.0X1	T49.0X2	T49.0X3	T49.0X4	T49.0X5	T49.0X6
ENT agent	T49.6X1	T49.6X2	T49.6X3	T49.6X4	T49.6X5	T49.6X6
ophthalmic preparation	T49.5X1	T49.5X2	T49.5X3	T49.5X4	T49.5X5	T49.5X6
Bornaprine	T44.3X1	T44.3X2	T44.3X3	T44.3X4	T44.3X5	T44.3X6
Boron	T57.8X1	T57.8X2	T57.8X3	T57.8X4	—	—
hydride NEC	T57.8X1	T57.8X2	T57.8X3	T57.8X4	—	—
fumes or gas	T57.8X1	T57.8X2	T57.8X3	T57.8X4	—	—
trifluoride	T59.891	T59.892	T59.893	T59.894	—	—
Botox	T48.291	T48.292	T48.293	T48.294	T48.295	T48.296
Botulinus anti-toxin (type A, B)	T50.Z11	T50.Z12	T50.Z13	T50.Z14	T50.Z15	T50.Z16
Brake fluid vapor	T59.891	T59.892	T59.893	T59.894	—	—
Brallobarbital	T42.3X1	T42.3X2	T42.3X3	T42.3X4	T42.3X5	T42.3X6
Bran (wheat)	T47.4X1	T47.4X2	T47.4X3	T47.4X4	T47.4X5	T47.4X6
Brass (fumes)	T56.891	T56.892	T56.893	T56.894	—	—
Brasso	T52.0X1	T52.0X2	T52.0X3	T52.0X4	—	—
Bretylium tosilate	T46.2X1	T46.2X2	T46.2X3	T46.2X4	T46.2X5	T46.2X6
Brevital (sodium)	T41.1X1	T41.1X2	T41.1X3	T41.1X4	T41.1X5	T41.1X6
Brinase	T45.3X1	T45.3X2	T45.3X3	T45.3X4	T45.3X5	T45.3X6
British antilewisite	T45.8X1	T45.8X2	T45.8X3	T45.8X4	—	T45.8X6
Brodifacoum	T60.4X1	T60.4X2	T60.4X3	T60.4X4	—	—
Bromal (hydrate)	T42.6X1	T42.6X2	T42.6X3	T42.6X4	T42.6X5	T42.6X6
Bromazepam	T42.4X1	T42.4X2	T42.4X3	T42.4X4	T42.4X5	T42.4X6
Bromazine	T45.0X1	T45.0X2	T45.0X3	T45.0X4	T45.0X5	T45.0X6
Brombenzylcyanide	T59.3X1	T59.3X2	T59.3X3	T59.3X4	—	—
Bromelains	T45.3X1	T45.3X2	T45.3X3	T45.3X4	T45.3X5	T45.3X6
Bromethalin	T60.4X1	T60.4X2	T60.4X3	T60.4X4	—	—
Bromhexine	T48.4X1	T48.4X2	T48.4X3	T48.4X4	T48.4X5	T48.4X6
Bromide salts	T42.6X1	T42.6X2	T42.6X3	T42.6X4	T42.6X5	T42.6X6
Bromindione	T45.511	T45.512	T45.513	T45.514	T45.515	T45.516
Bromine	T42.6X1	T42.6X2	T42.6X3	T42.6X4	T42.6X5	T42.6X6
compounds (medicinal)	T42.6X1	T42.6X2	T42.6X3	T42.6X4	T42.6X5	T42.6X6
sedative	T42.6X1	T42.6X2	T42.6X3	T42.6X4	T42.6X5	T42.6X6
vapor	T59.891	T59.892	T59.893	T59.894	—	—
Bromisoval	T42.6X1	T42.6X2	T42.6X3	T42.6X4	T42.6X5	T42.6X6
Bromisovalum	T42.6X1	T42.6X2	T42.6X3	T42.6X4	T42.6X5	T42.6X6
Bromobenzylcyanide	T59.3X1	T59.3X2	T59.3X3	T59.3X4	—	—
Bromochlorosalicylani-lide	T49.0X1	T49.0X2	T49.0X3	T49.0X4	T49.0X5	T49.0X6
Bromocriptine	T42.8X1	T42.8X2	T42.8X3	T42.8X4	T42.8X5	T42.8X6
Bromodiphenhydramine	T45.0X1	T45.0X2	T45.0X3	T45.0X4	T45.0X5	T45.0X6
Bromoform	T42.6X1	T42.6X2	T42.6X3	T42.6X4	T42.6X5	T42.6X6
Bromophenol blue reagent	T50.991	T50.992	T50.993	T50.994	T50.995	T50.996
Bromopride	T47.8X1	T47.8X2	T47.8X3	T47.8X4	T47.8X5	T47.8X6
Bromosalicylchloranitide	T49.0X1	T49.0X2	T49.0X3	T49.0X4	T49.0X5	T49.0X6
Bromosalicylhydroxamic acid	T37.1X1	T37.1X2	T37.1X3	T37.1X4	T37.1X5	T37.1X6
Bromo-seltzer	T39.1X1	T39.1X2	T39.1X3	T39.1X4	T39.1X5	T39.1X6
Bromoxynil	T60.3X1	T60.3X2	T60.3X3	T60.3X4	—	—
Bromperidol	T43.4X1	T43.4X2	T43.4X3	T43.4X4	T43.4X5	T43.4X6
Brompheniramine	T45.0X1	T45.0X2	T45.0X3	T45.0X4	T45.0X5	T45.0X6
Bromsulfophthalein	T50.8X1	T50.8X2	T50.8X3	T50.8X4	T50.8X5	T50.8X6
Bromural	T42.6X1	T42.6X2	T42.6X3	T42.6X4	T42.6X5	T42.6X6
Bromvaletone	T42.6X1	T42.6X2	T42.6X3	T42.6X4	T42.6X5	T42.6X6
Bronchodilator NEC	T48.6X1	T48.6X2	T48.6X3	T48.6X4	T48.6X5	T48.6X6
Brotizolam	T42.4X1	T42.4X2	T42.4X3	T42.4X4	T42.4X5	T42.4X6
Brovincamine	T46.7X1	T46.7X2	T46.7X3	T46.7X4	T46.7X5	T46.7X6
Brown recluse spider (bite) (venom)	T63.331	T63.332	T63.333	T63.334	—	—
Brown spider (bite) (venom)	T63.391	T63.392	T63.393	T63.394	—	—
Broxaterol	T48.6X1	T48.6X2	T48.6X3	T48.6X4	T48.6X5	T48.6X6
Broxuridine	T45.1X1	T45.1X2	T45.1X3	T45.1X4	T45.1X5	T45.1X6
Broxyquinoline	T37.8X1	T37.8X2	T37.8X3	T37.8X4	T37.8X5	T37.8X6
Bruceine	T48.291	T48.292	T48.293	T48.294	T48.295	T48.296
Brucia	T62.2X1	T62.2X2	T62.2X3	T62.2X4	—	—
Brucine	T65.1X1	T65.1X2	T65.1X3	T65.1X4	—	—
Brunswick green — *see* Copper						
Bruten — *see* Ibuprofen						
Bryonia	T47.2X1	T47.2X2	T47.2X3	T47.2X4	T47.2X5	T47.2X6
Buclizine	T45.0X1	T45.0X2	T45.0X3	T45.0X4	T45.0X5	T45.0X6
Buclosamide	T49.0X1	T49.0X2	T49.0X3	T49.0X4	T49.0X5	T49.0X6
Budesonide	T44.5X1	T44.5X2	T44.5X3	T44.5X4	T44.5X5	T44.5X6
Budralazine	T46.5X1	T46.5X2	T46.5X3	T46.5X4	T46.5X5	T46.5X6
Bufferin	T39.011	T39.012	T39.013	T39.014	T39.015	T39.016
Buflomedil	T46.7X1	T46.7X2	T46.7X3	T46.7X4	T46.7X5	T46.7X6
Buformin	T38.3X1	T38.3X2	T38.3X3	T38.3X4	T38.3X5	T38.3X6
Bufotenine	T40.991	T40.992	T40.993	T40.994	—	—
Bufrolin	T48.6X1	T48.6X2	T48.6X3	T48.6X4	T48.6X5	T48.6X6
Bufylline	T48.6X1	T48.6X2	T48.6X3	T48.6X4	T48.6X5	T48.6X6
Bulk filler	T50.5X1	T50.5X2	T50.5X3	T50.5X4	T50.5X5	T50.5X6
cathartic	T47.4X1	T47.4X2	T47.4X3	T47.4X4	T47.4X5	T47.4X6
Bumetanide	T50.1X1	T50.1X2	T50.1X3	T50.1X4	T50.1X5	T50.1X6
Bunaftine	T46.2X1	T46.2X2	T46.2X3	T46.2X4	T46.2X5	T46.2X6
Bunamiodyl	T50.8X1	T50.8X2	T50.8X3	T50.8X4	T50.8X5	T50.8X6
Bunazosin	T44.6X1	T44.6X2	T44.6X3	T44.6X4	T44.6X5	T44.6X6
Bunitrolol	T44.7X1	T44.7X2	T44.7X3	T44.7X4	T44.7X5	T44.7X6
Buphenine	T46.7X1	T46.7X2	T46.7X3	T46.7X4	T46.7X5	T46.7X6
Bupivacaine	T41.3X1	T41.3X2	T41.3X3	T41.3X4	T41.3X5	T41.3X6
infiltration (subcutaneous)	T41.3X1	T41.3X2	T41.3X3	T41.3X4	T41.3X5	T41.3X6
nerve block (peripheral) (plexus)	T41.3X1	T41.3X2	T41.3X3	T41.3X4	T41.3X5	T41.3X6
spinal	T41.3X1	T41.3X2	T41.3X3	T41.3X4	T41.3X5	T41.3X6
Bupranolol	T44.7X1	T44.7X2	T44.7X3	T44.7X4	T44.7X5	T44.7X6
Buprenorphine	T40.4X1	T40.4X2	T40.4X3	T40.4X4	T40.4X5	T40.4X6
Bupropion	T43.291	T43.292	T43.293	T43.294	T43.295	T43.296
Burimamide	T47.1X1	T47.1X2	T47.1X3	T47.1X4	T47.1X5	T47.1X6
Buserelin	T38.891	T38.892	T38.893	T38.894	T38.895	T38.896
Buspirone	T43.591	T43.592	T43.593	T43.594	T43.595	T43.596
Busulfan, busulphan	T45.1X1	T45.1X2	T45.1X3	T45.1X4	T45.1X5	T45.1X6
Butabarbital (sodium)	T42.3X1	T42.3X2	T42.3X3	T42.3X4	T42.3X5	T42.3X6
Butabarbitone	T42.3X1	T42.3X2	T42.3X3	T42.3X4	T42.3X5	T42.3X6
Butabarpal	T42.3X1	T42.3X2	T42.3X3	T42.3X4	T42.3X5	T42.3X6
Butacaine	T41.3X1	T41.3X2	T41.3X3	T41.3X4	T41.3X5	T41.3X6
Butalamine	T46.7X1	T46.7X2	T46.7X3	T46.7X4	T46.7X5	T46.7X6
Butalbital	T42.3X1	T42.3X2	T42.3X3	T42.3X4	T42.3X5	T42.3X6
Butallylonal	T42.3X1	T42.3X2	T42.3X3	T42.3X4	T42.3X5	T42.3X6
Butamben	T41.3X1	T41.3X2	T41.3X3	T41.3X4	T41.3X5	T41.3X6
Butamirate	T48.3X1	T48.3X2	T48.3X3	T48.3X4	T48.3X5	T48.3X6
Butane (distributed in mobile container)	T59.891	T59.892	T59.893	T59.894	—	—
distributed through pipes	T59.891	T59.892	T59.893	T59.894	—	—
incomplete combustion	T58.11	T58.12	T58.13	T58.14	—	—
Butanilicaine	T41.3X1	T41.3X2	T41.3X3	T41.3X4	T41.3X5	T41.3X6
Butanol	T51.3X1	T51.3X2	T51.3X3	T51.3X4	—	—
Butanone, 2-butanone	T52.4X1	T52.4X2	T52.4X3	T52.4X4	—	—
Butantrone	T49.4X1	T49.4X2	T49.4X3	T49.4X4	T49.4X5	T49.4X6
Butaperazine	T43.3X1	T43.3X2	T43.3X3	T43.3X4	T43.3X5	T43.3X6
Butazolidin	T39.2X1	T39.2X2	T39.2X3	T39.2X4	T39.2X5	T39.2X6
Butetamate	T48.6X1	T48.6X2	T48.6X3	T48.6X4	T48.6X5	T48.6X6
Butethal	T42.3X1	T42.3X2	T42.3X3	T42.3X4	T42.3X5	T42.3X6
Butethamate	T44.3X1	T44.3X2	T44.3X3	T44.3X4	T44.3X5	T44.3X6
Buthalitone (sodium)	T41.1X1	T41.1X2	T41.1X3	T41.1X4	T41.1X5	T41.1X6
Butisol (sodium)	T42.3X1	T42.3X2	T42.3X3	T42.3X4	T42.3X5	T42.3X6
Butizide	T50.2X1	T50.2X2	T50.2X3	T50.2X4	T50.2X5	T50.2X6
Butobarbital	T42.3X1	T42.3X2	T42.3X3	T42.3X4	T42.3X5	T42.3X6
sodium	T42.3X1	T42.3X2	T42.3X3	T42.3X4	T42.3X5	T42.3X6
Butobarbitone	T42.3X1	T42.3X2	T42.3X3	T42.3X4	T42.3X5	T42.3X6
Butoconazole (nitrate)	T49.0X1	T49.0X2	T49.0X3	T49.0X4	T49.0X5	T49.0X6
Butorphanol	T40.4X1	T40.4X2	T40.4X3	T40.4X4	T40.4X5	T40.4X6
Butriptyline	T43.011	T43.012	T43.013	T43.014	T43.015	T43.016
Butropium bromide	T44.3X1	T44.3X2	T44.3X3	T44.3X4	T44.3X5	T44.3X6
Buttercups	T62.2X1	T62.2X2	T62.2X3	T62.2X4	—	—
Butter of antimony — *see* Antimony						
Butyl						
acetate (secondary)	T52.8X1	T52.8X2	T52.8X3	T52.8X4	—	—
alcohol	T51.3X1	T51.3X2	T51.3X3	T51.3X4	—	—
aminobenzoate	T41.3X1	T41.3X2	T41.3X3	T41.3X4	T41.3X5	T41.3X6
butyrate	T52.8X1	T52.8X2	T52.8X3	T52.8X4	—	—
carbinol	T51.3X1	T51.3X2	T51.3X3	T51.3X4	—	—
carbitol	T52.3X1	T52.3X2	T52.3X3	T52.3X4	—	—
cellosolve	T52.3X1	T52.3X2	T52.3X3	T52.3X4	—	—
chloral (hydrate)	T42.6X1	T42.6X2	T42.6X3	T42.6X4	T42.6X5	T42.6X6
formate	T52.8X1	T52.8X2	T52.8X3	T52.8X4	—	—
lactate	T52.8X1	T52.8X2	T52.8X3	T52.8X4	—	—

Additional Character May Be Required — Refer to the Tabular List for Character Selection   ▽ Subterms under main terms may continue to next column or page

Substance	Poisoning, Accidental (unintentional)	Poisoning, Intentional Self-harm	Poisoning, Assault	Poisoning, Undetermined	Adverse Effect	Under-dosing
Butyl — *continued*						
propionate	T52.8X1	T52.8X2	T52.8X3	T52.8X4	—	—
scopolamine bromide	T44.3X1	T44.3X2	T44.3X3	T44.3X4	T44.3X5	T44.3X6
thiobarbital sodium	T41.1X1	T41.1X2	T41.1X3	T41.1X4	T41.1X5	T41.1X6
Butylated hydroxyanisole	T50.991	T50.992	T50.993	T50.994	T50.995	T50.996
Butylchloral hydrate	T42.6X1	T42.6X2	T42.6X3	T42.6X4	T42.6X5	T42.6X6
Butyltoluene	T52.2X1	T52.2X2	T52.2X3	T52.2X4	—	—
Butyn	T41.3X1	T41.3X2	T41.3X3	T41.3X4	T41.3X5	T41.3X6
Butyrophenone (-based tranquilizers)	T43.4X1	T43.4X2	T43.4X3	T43.4X4	T43.4X5	T43.4X6
Cabergoline	T42.8X1	T42.8X2	T42.8X3	T42.8X4	T42.8X5	T42.8X6
Cacodyl, cacodylic acid	T57.0X1	T57.0X2	T57.0X3	T57.0X4	—	—
Cactinomycin	T45.1X1	T45.1X2	T45.1X3	T45.1X4	T45.1X5	T45.1X6
Cade oil	T49.4X1	T49.4X2	T49.4X3	T49.4X4	T49.4X5	T49.4X6
Cadexomer iodine	T49.0X1	T49.0X2	T49.0X3	T49.0X4	T49.0X5	T49.0X6
Cadmium (chloride) (fumes) (oxide)	T56.3X1	T56.3X2	T56.3X3	T56.3X4		
sulfide (medicinal) NEC	T49.4X1	T49.4X2	T49.4X3	T49.4X4	T49.4X5	T49.4X6
Cadralazine	T46.5X1	T46.5X2	T46.5X3	T46.5X4	T46.5X5	T46.5X6
Caffeine	T43.611	T43.612	T43.613	T43.614	T43.615	T43.616
Calabar bean	T62.2X1	T62.2X2	T62.2X3	T62.2X4	—	—
Caladium seguinum	T62.2X1	T62.2X2	T62.2X3	T62.2X4	—	—
Calamine (lotion)	T49.3X1	T49.3X2	T49.3X3	T49.3X4	T49.3X5	T49.3X6
Calcifediol	T45.2X1	T45.2X2	T45.2X3	T45.2X4	T45.2X5	T45.2X6
Calciferol	T45.2X1	T45.2X2	T45.2X3	T45.2X4	T45.2X5	T45.2X6
Calcitonin	T50.991	T50.992	T50.993	T50.994	T50.995	T50.996
Calcitriol	T45.2X1	T45.2X2	T45.2X3	T45.2X4	T45.2X5	T45.2X6
Calcium	T50.3X1	T50.3X2	T50.3X3	T50.3X4	T50.3X5	T50.3X6
actylsalicylate	T39.011	T39.012	T39.013	T39.014	T39.015	T39.016
benzamidosalicylate	T37.1X1	T37.1X2	T37.1X3	T37.1X4	T37.1X5	T37.1X6
bromide	T42.6X1	T42.6X2	T42.6X3	T42.6X4	T42.6X5	T42.6X6
bromolactobionate	T42.6X1	T42.6X2	T42.6X3	T42.6X4	T42.6X5	T42.6X6
carbaspirin	T39.011	T39.012	T39.013	T39.014	T39.015	T39.016
carbimide	T50.6X1	T50.6X2	T50.6X3	T50.6X4	T50.6X5	T50.6X6
carbonate	T47.1X1	T47.1X2	T47.1X3	T47.1X4	T47.1X5	T47.1X6
chloride	T50.991	T50.992	T50.993	T50.994	T50.995	T50.996
anhydrous	T50.991	T50.992	T50.993	T50.994	T50.995	T50.996
cyanide	T57.8X1	T57.8X2	T57.8X3	T57.8X4	—	—
dioctyl sulfosuccinate	T47.4X1	T47.4X2	T47.4X3	T47.4X4	T47.4X5	T47.4X6
disodium edathamil	T45.8X1	T45.8X2	T45.8X3	T45.8X4	T45.8X5	T45.8X6
disodium edetate	T45.8X1	T45.8X2	T45.8X3	T45.8X4	T45.8X5	T45.8X6
dobesilate	T46.991	T46.992	T46.993	T46.994	T46.995	T46.996
EDTA	T45.8X1	T45.8X2	T45.8X3	T45.8X4	T45.8X5	T45.8X6
ferrous citrate	T45.4X1	T45.4X2	T45.4X3	T45.4X4	T45.4X5	T45.4X6
folinate	T45.8X1	T45.8X2	T45.8X3	T45.8X4	T45.8X5	T45.8X6
glubionate	T50.3X1	T50.3X2	T50.3X3	T50.3X4	T50.3X5	T50.3X6
gluconate	T50.3X1	T50.3X2	T50.3X3	T50.3X4	T50.3X5	T50.3X6
gluconogalactogluconate	T50.3X1	T50.3X2	T50.3X3	T50.3X4	T50.3X5	T50.3X6
hydrate, hydroxide	T54.3X1	T54.3X2	T54.3X3	T54.3X4	—	—
hypochlorite	T54.3X1	T54.3X2	T54.3X3	T54.3X4	—	—
iodide	T48.4X1	T48.4X2	T48.4X3	T48.4X4	T48.4X5	T48.4X6
ipodate	T50.8X1	T50.8X2	T50.8X3	T50.8X4	T50.8X5	T50.8X6
lactate	T50.3X1	T50.3X2	T50.3X3	T50.3X4	T50.3X5	T50.3X6
leucovorin	T45.8X1	T45.8X2	T45.8X3	T45.8X4	T45.8X5	T45.8X6
mandelate	T37.91	T37.92	T37.93	T37.94	T37.95	T37.96
oxide	T54.3X1	T54.3X2	T54.3X3	T54.3X4	—	—
pantothenate	T45.2X1	T45.2X2	T45.2X3	T45.2X4	T45.2X5	T45.2X6
phosphate	T50.3X1	T50.3X2	T50.3X3	T50.3X4	T50.3X5	T50.3X6
salicylate	T39.091	T39.092	T39.093	T39.094	T39.095	T39.096
salts	T50.3X1	T50.3X2	T50.3X3	T50.3X4.	T50.3X5	T50.3X6
Calculus-dissolving drug	T50.991	T50.992	T50.993	T50.994	T50.995	T50.996
Calomel	T49.0X1	T49.0X2	T49.0X3	T49.0X4	T49.0X5	T49.0X6
Caloric agent	T50.3X1	T50.3X2	T50.3X3	T50.3X4	T50.3X5	T50.3X6
Calusterone	T38.7X1	T38.7X2	T38.7X3	T38.7X4	T38.7X5	T38.7X6
Camazepam	T42.4X1	T42.4X2	T42.4X3	T42.4X4	T42.4X5	T42.4X6
Camomile	T49.0X1	T49.0X2	T49.0X3	T49.0X4	T49.0X5	T49.0X6
Camoquin	T37.2X1	T37.2X2	T37.2X3	T37.2X4	T37.2X5	T37.2X6
Camphor						
insecticide	T60.2X1	T60.2X2	T60.2X3	T60.2X4	—	—
medicinal	T49.8X1	T49.8X2	T49.8X3	T49.8X4	T49.8X5	T49.8X6
Camylofin	T44.3X1	T44.3X2	T44.3X3	T44.3X4	T44.3X5	T44.3X6
Cancer chemotherapy drug regimen	T45.1X1	T45.1X2	T45.1X3	T45.1X4	T45.1X5	T45.1X6
Candeptin	T49.0X1	T49.0X2	T49.0X3	T49.0X4	T49.0X5	T49.0X6
Candicidin	T49.0X1	T49.0X2	T49.0X3	T49.0X4	T49.0X5	T49.0X6
Cannabinol	T40.7X1	T40.7X2	T40.7X3	T40.7X4	T40.7X5	T40.7X6
Cannabis (derivatives)	T40.7X1	T40.7X2	T40.7X3	T40.7X4	T40.7X5	T40.7X6
Canned heat	T51.1X1	T51.1X2	T51.1X3	T51.1X4	—	—
Canrenoic acid	T50.0X1	T50.0X2	T50.0X3	T50.0X4	T50.0X5	T50.0X6
Canrenone	T50.0X1	T50.0X2	T50.0X3	T50.0X4	T50.0X5	T50.0X6
Cantharides, cantharidin, cantharis	T49.8X1	T49.8X2	T49.8X3	T49.8X4	T49.8X5	T49.8X6
Canthaxanthin	T50.991	T50.992	T50.993	T50.994	T50.995	T50.996

Substance	Poisoning, Accidental (unintentional)	Poisoning, Intentional Self-harm	Poisoning, Assault	Poisoning, Undetermined	Adverse Effect	Under-dosing
Capillary-active drug NEC	T46.901	T46.902	T46.903	T46.904	T46.905	T46.906
Capreomycin	T36.8X1	T36.8X2	T36.8X3	T36.8X4	T36.8X5	T36.8X6
Capsicum	T49.4X1	T49.4X2	T49.4X3	T49.4X4	T49.4X5	T49.4X6
Captafol	T60.3X1	T60.3X2	T60.3X3	T60.3X4	—	—
Captan	T60.3X1	T60.3X2	T60.3X3	T60.3X4	—	—
Captodiame, captodiamine	T43.591	T43.592	T43.593	T43.594	T43.595	T43.596
Captopril	T46.4X1	T46.4X2	T46.4X3	T46.4X4	T46.4X5	T46.4X6
Caramiphen	T44.3X1	T44.3X2	T44.3X3	T44.3X4	T44.3X5	T44.3X6
Carazolol	T44.7X1	T44.7X2	T44.7X3	T44.7X4	T44.7X5	T44.7X6
Carbachol	T44.1X1	T44.1X2	T44.1X3	T44.1X4	T44.1X5	T44.1X6
Carbacrylamine (resin)	T50.3X1	T50.3X2	T50.3X3	T50.3X4	T50.3X5	T50.3X6
Carbamate (insecticide)	T60.0X1	T60.0X2	T60.0X3	T60.0X4	—	—
Carbamate (sedative)	T42.6X1	T42.6X2	T42.6X3	T42.6X4	T42.6X5	T42.6X6
herbicide	T60.0X1	T60.0X2	T60.0X3	T60.0X4	—	—
insecticide	T60.0X1	T60.0X2	T60.0X3	T60.0X4	—	—
Carbamazepine	T42.1X1	T42.1X2	T42.1X3	T42.1X4	T42.1X5	T42.1X6
Carbamide	T47.3X1	T47.3X2	T47.3X3	T47.3X4	T47.3X5	T47.3X6
peroxide	T49.0X1	T49.0X2	T49.0X3	T49.0X4	T49.0X5	T49.0X6
topical	T49.8X1	T49.8X2	T49.8X3	T49.8X4	T49.8X5	T49.8X6
Carbamylcholine chloride	T44.1X1	T44.1X2	T44.1X3	T44.1X4	T44.1X5	T44.1X6
Carbaril	T60.0X1	T60.0X2	T60.0X3	T60.0X4	—	—
Carbarsone	T37.3X1	T37.3X2	T37.3X3	T37.3X4	T37.3X5	T37.3X6
Carbaryl	T60.0X1	T60.0X2	T60.0X3	T60.0X4	—	—
Carbaspirin	T39.011	T39.012	T39.013	T39.014	T39.015	T39.016
Carbazochrome (salicylate) (sodium sulfonate)	T49.4X1	T49.4X2	T49.4X3	T49.4X4	T49.4X5	T49.4X6
Carbenicillin	T36.0X1	T36.0X2	T36.0X3	T36.0X4	T36.0X5	T36.0X6
Carbenoxolone	T47.1X1	T47.1X2	T47.1X3	T47.1X4	T47.1X5	T47.1X6
Carbetapentane	T48.3X1	T48.3X2	T48.3X3	T48.3X4	T48.3X5	T48.3X6
Carbethyl salicylate	T39.091	T39.092	T39.093	T39.094	T39.095	T39.096
Carbidopa (with levodopa)	T42.8X1	T42.8X2	T42.8X3	T42.8X4	T42.8X5	T42.8X6
Carbimazole	T38.2X1	T38.2X2	T38.2X3	T38.2X4	T38.2X5	T38.2X6
Carbinol	T51.1X1	T51.1X2	T51.1X3	T51.1X4	—	—
Carbinoxamine	T45.0X1	T45.0X2	T45.0X3	T45.0X4	T45.0X5	T45.0X6
Carbiphene	T39.8X1	T39.8X2	T39.8X3	T39.8X4	T39.8X5	T39.8X6
Carbitol	T52.3X1	T52.3X2	T52.3X3	T52.3X4	—	—
Carbocaine	T41.3X1	T41.3X2	T41.3X3	T41.3X4	T41.3X5	T41.3X6
infiltration (subcutaneous)	T41.3X1	T41.3X2	T41.3X3	T41.3X4	T41.3X5	T41.3X6
nerve block (peripheral) (plexus)	T41.3X1	T41.3X2	T41.3X3	T41.3X4	T41.3X5	T41.3X6
topical (surface)	T41.3X1	T41.3X2	T41.3X3	T41.3X4	T41.3X5	T41.3X6
Carbocisteine	T48.4X1	T48.4X2	T48.4X3	T48.4X4	T48.4X5	T48.4X6
Carbocromen	T46.3X1	T46.3X2	T46.3X3	T46.3X4	T46.3X5	T46.3X6
Carbol fuchsin	T49.0X1	T49.0X2	T49.0X3	T49.0X4	T49.0X5	T49.0X6
Carbolic acid — *see also* Phenol	T54.0X1	T54.0X2	T54.0X3	T54.0X4	—	—
Carbolonium (bromide)	T48.1X1	T48.1X2	T48.1X3	T48.1X4	T48.1X5	T48.1X6
Carbo medicinalis	T47.6X1	T47.6X2	T47.6X3	T47.6X4	T47.6X5	T47.6X6
Carbomycin	T36.8X1	T36.8X2	T36.8X3	T36.8X4	T36.8X5	T36.8X6
Carbon						
bisulfide (liquid)	T65.4X1	T65.4X2	T65.4X3	T65.4X4	—	—
vapor	T65.4X1	T65.4X2	T65.4X3	T65.4X4	—	—
dioxide (gas)	T59.7X1	T59.7X2	T59.7X3	T59.7X4	—	—
medicinal	T41.5X1	T41.5X2	T41.5X3	T41.5X4	T41.5X5	T41.5X6
nonmedicinal	T59.7X1	T59.7X2	T59.7X3	T59.7X4	—	—
snow	T49.4X1	T49.4X2	T49.4X3	T49.4X4	T49.4X5	T49.4X6
disulfide (liquid)	T65.4X1	T65.4X2	T65.4X3	T65.4X4	—	—
vapor	T65.4X1	T65.4X2	T65.4X3	T65.4X4	—	—
monoxide (from incomplete combustion)	T58.91	T58.92	T58.93	T58.94	—	—
blast furnace gas	T58.8X1	T58.8X2	T58.8X3	T58.8X4	—	—
butane (distributed in mobile container)	T58.11	T58.12	T58.13	T58.14	—	—
distributed through pipes	T58.11	T58.12	T58.13	T58.14	—	—
charcoal fumes	T58.2X1	T58.2X2	T58.2X3	T58.2X4	—	—
coal	T58.2X1	T58.2X2	T58.2X3	T58.2X4	—	—
coke (in domestic stoves, fireplaces)	T58.2X1	T58.2X2	T58.2X3	T58.2X4	—	—
exhaust gas (motor) not in transit	T58.01	T58.02	T58.03	T58.04	—	—
combustion engine, any not in watercraft	T58.01	T58.02	T58.03	T58.04	—	—
farm tractor, not in transit	T58.01	T58.02	T58.03	T58.04	—	—
gas engine	T58.01	T58.02	T58.03	T58.04	—	—
motor pump	T58.01	T58.02	T58.03	T58.04	—	—
motor vehicle, not in transit	T58.01	T58.02	T58.03	T58.04	—	—
fuel (in domestic use)	T58.2X1	T58.2X2	T58.2X3	T58.2X4	—	—
gas (piped)	T58.11	T58.12	T58.13	T58.14	—	—
in mobile container	T58.11	T58.12	T58.13	T58.14	—	—

▽ Subterms under main terms may continue to next column or page　　　Additional Character May Be Required — Refer to the Tabular List for Character Selection　　　357

Butyl — Carbon

Left sidebar: Table of Drugs and Chemicals — Carbon — Central nervous system

Substance	Poisoning, Accidental (unintentional)	Poisoning, Intentional Self-harm	Poisoning, Assault	Poisoning, Undetermined	Adverse Effect	Under-dosing
Carbon — *continued*						
monoxide — *continued*						
fuel — *continued*						
piped (natural)	T58.11	T58.12	T58.13	T58.14	—	—
utility	T58.11	T58.12	T58.13	T58.14	—	—
in mobile container	T58.11	T58.12	T58.13	T58.14	—	—
gas (piped)	T58.11	T58.12	T58.13	T58.14	—	—
illuminating gas	T58.11	T58.12	T58.13	T58.14	—	—
industrial fuels or gases, any	T58.8X1	T58.8X2	T58.8X3	T58.8X4	—	—
kerosene (in domestic stoves, fireplaces)	T58.2X1	T58.2X2	T58.2X3	T58.2X4	—	—
kiln gas or vapor	T58.8X1	T58.8X2	T58.8X3	T58.8X4	—	—
motor exhaust gas, not in transit	T58.01	T58.02	T58.03	T58.04	—	—
piped gas (manufactured) (natural)	T58.11	T58.12	T58.13	T58.14	—	—
producer gas	T58.8X1	T58.8X2	T58.8X3	T58.8X4	—	—
propane (distributed in mobile container)	T58.11	T58.12	T58.13	T58.14	—	—
distributed through pipes	T58.11	T58.12	T58.13	T58.14	—	—
solid (in domestic stoves, fireplaces)	T58.2X1	T58.2X2	T58.2X3	T58.2X4	—	—
specified source NEC	T58.8X1	T58.8X2	T58.8X3	T58.8X4	—	—
stove gas	T58.11	T58.12	T58.13	T58.14	—	—
piped	T58.11	T58.12	T58.13	T58.14	—	—
utility gas	T58.11	T58.12	T58.13	T58.14	—	—
piped	T58.11	T58.12	T58.13	T58.14	—	—
water gas	T58.11	T58.12	T58.13	T58.14	—	—
wood (in domestic stoves, fireplaces)	T58.2X1	T58.2X2	T58.2X3	T58.2X4	—	—
tetrachloride (vapor) NEC	T53.0X1	T53.0X2	T53.0X3	T53.0X4	—	—
liquid (cleansing agent) NEC	T53.0X1	T53.0X2	T53.0X3	T53.0X4	—	—
solvent	T53.0X1	T53.0X2	T53.0X3	T53.0X4	—	—
Carbonic acid gas	T59.7X1	T59.7X2	T59.7X3	T59.7X4	—	—
anhydrase inhibitor NEC	T50.2X1	T50.2X2	T50.2X3	T50.2X4	T50.2X5	T50.2X6
Carbophenothion	T60.0X1	T60.0X2	T60.0X3	T60.0X4	—	—
Carboplatin	T45.1X1	T45.1X2	T45.1X3	T45.1X4	T45.1X5	T45.1X6
Carboprost	T48.0X1	T48.0X2	T48.0X3	T48.0X4	T48.0X5	T48.0X6
Carboquone	T45.1X1	T45.1X2	T45.1X3	T45.1X4	T45.1X5	T45.1X6
Carbowax	T49.3X1	T49.3X2	T49.3X3	T49.3X4	T49.3X5	T49.3X6
Carboxymethylcellulose	T47.4X1	T47.4X2	T47.4X3	T47.4X4	T47.4X5	T47.4X6
Carbrital	T42.3X1	T42.3X2	T42.3X3	T42.3X4	T42.3X5	T42.3X6
Carbromal	T42.6X1	T42.6X2	T42.6X3	T42.6X4	T42.6X5	T42.6X6
Carbutamide	T38.3X1	T38.3X2	T38.3X3	T38.3X4	T38.3X5	T38.3X6
Carbuterol	T48.6X1	T48.6X2	T48.6X3	T48.6X4	T48.6X5	T48.6X6
Cardiac						
depressants	T46.2X1	T46.2X2	T46.2X3	T46.2X4	T46.2X5	T46.2X6
rhythm regulator	T46.2X1	T46.2X2	T46.2X3	T46.2X4	T46.2X5	T46.2X6
specified NEC	T46.2X1	T46.2X2	T46.2X3	T46.2X4	T46.2X5	T46.2X6
Cardiografin	T50.8X1	T50.8X2	T50.8X3	T50.8X4	T50.8X5	T50.8X6
Cardiogreen	T50.8X1	T50.8X2	T50.8X3	T50.8X4	T50.8X5	T50.8X6
Cardiotonic (glycoside) **NEC**	T46.0X1	T46.0X2	T46.0X3	T46.0X4	T46.0X5	T46.0X6
Cardiovascular drug NEC	T46.901	T46.902	T46.903	T46.904	T46.905	T46.906
Cardrase	T50.2X1	T50.2X2	T50.2X3	T50.2X4	T50.2X5	T50.2X6
Carfecillin	T36.0X1	T36.0X2	T36.0X3	T36.0X4	T36.0X5	T36.0X6
Carfenazine	T43.3X1	T43.3X2	T43.3X3	T43.3X4	T43.3X5	T43.3X6
Carfusin	T49.0X1	T49.0X2	T49.0X3	T49.0X4	T49.0X5	T49.0X6
Carindacillin	T36.0X1	T36.0X2	T36.0X3	T36.0X4	T36.0X5	T36.0X6
Carisoprodol	T42.8X1	T42.8X2	T42.8X3	T42.8X4	T42.8X5	T42.8X6
Carmellose	T47.4X1	T47.4X2	T47.4X3	T47.4X4	T47.4X5	T47.4X6
Carminative	T47.5X1	T47.5X2	T47.5X3	T47.5X4	T47.5X5	T47.5X6
Carmofur	T45.1X1	T45.1X2	T45.1X3	T45.1X4	T45.1X5	T45.1X6
Carmustine	T45.1X1	T45.1X2	T45.1X3	T45.1X4	T45.1X5	T45.1X6
Carotene	T45.2X1	T45.2X2	T45.2X3	T45.2X4	T45.2X5	T45.2X6
Carphenazine	T43.3X1	T43.3X2	T43.3X3	T43.3X4	T43.3X5	T43.3X6
Carpipramine	T42.4X1	T42.4X2	T42.4X3	T42.4X4	T42.4X5	T42.4X6
Carprofen	T39.311	T39.312	T39.313	T39.314	T39.315	T39.316
Carpronium chloride	T44.3X1	T44.3X2	T44.3X3	T44.3X4	T44.3X5	T44.3X6
Carrageenan	T47.8X1	T47.8X2	T47.8X3	T47.8X4	T47.8X5	T47.8X6
Carteolol	T44.7X1	T44.7X2	T44.7X3	T44.7X4	T44.7X5	T44.7X6
Carter's Little Pills	T47.2X1	T47.2X2	T47.2X3	T47.2X4	T47.2X5	T47.2X6
Cascara (sagrada)	T47.2X1	T47.2X2	T47.2X3	T47.2X4	T47.2X5	T47.2X6
Cassava	T62.2X1	T62.2X2	T62.2X3	T62.2X4	—	—
Castellani's paint	T49.0X1	T49.0X2	T49.0X3	T49.0X4	T49.0X5	T49.0X6
Castor						
bean	T62.2X1	T62.2X2	T62.2X3	T62.2X4	—	—
oil	T47.2X1	T47.2X2	T47.2X3	T47.2X4	T47.2X5	T47.2X6
Catalase	T45.3X1	T45.3X2	T45.3X3	T45.3X4	T45.3X5	T45.3X6
Caterpillar (sting)	T63.431	T63.432	T63.433	T63.434	—	—
Catha (edulis) (tea)	T43.691	T43.692	T43.693	T43.694	—	—

Substance	Poisoning, Accidental (unintentional)	Poisoning, Intentional Self-harm	Poisoning, Assault	Poisoning, Undetermined	Adverse Effect	Under-dosing
Cathartic NEC	T47.4X1	T47.4X2	T47.4X3	T47.4X4	T47.4X5	T47.4X6
anthacene derivative	T47.2X1	T47.2X2	T47.2X3	T47.2X4	T47.2X5	T47.2X6
bulk	T47.4X1	T47.4X2	T47.4X3	T47.4X4	T47.4X5	T47.4X6
contact	T47.2X1	T47.2X2	T47.2X3	T47.2X4	T47.2X5	T47.2X6
emollient NEC	T47.4X1	T47.4X2	T47.4X3	T47.4X4	T47.4X5	T47.4X6
irritant NEC	T47.2X1	T47.2X2	T47.2X3	T47.2X4	T47.2X5	T47.2X6
mucilage	T47.4X1	T47.4X2	T47.4X3	T47.4X4	T47.4X5	T47.4X6
saline	T47.3X1	T47.3X2	T47.3X3	T47.3X4	T47.3X5	T47.3X6
vegetable	T47.2X1	T47.2X2	T47.2X3	T47.2X4	T47.2X5	T47.2X6
Cathine	T50.5X1	T50.5X2	T50.5X3	T50.5X4	T50.5X5	T50.5X6
Cathomycin	T36.8X1	T36.8X2	T36.8X3	T36.8X4	T36.8X5	T36.8X6
Cation exchange resin	T50.3X1	T50.3X2	T50.3X3	T50.3X4	T50.3X5	T50.3X6
Caustic(s) **NEC**	T54.91	T54.92	T54.93	T54.94	—	—
alkali	T54.3X1	T54.3X2	T54.3X3	T54.3X4	—	—
hydroxide	T54.3X1	T54.3X2	T54.3X3	T54.3X4	—	—
potash	T54.3X1	T54.3X2	T54.3X3	T54.3X4	—	—
soda	T54.3X1	T54.3X2	T54.3X3	T54.3X4	—	—
specified NEC	T54.91	T54.92	T54.93	T54.94	—	—
Ceepryn	T49.0X1	T49.0X2	T49.0X3	T49.0X4	T49.0X5	T49.0X6
ENT agent	T49.6X1	T49.6X2	T49.6X3	T49.6X4	T49.6X5	T49.6X6
lozenges	T49.6X1	T49.6X2	T49.6X3	T49.6X4	T49.6X5	T49.6X6
Cefacetrile	T36.1X1	T36.1X2	T36.1X3	T36.1X4	T36.1X5	T36.1X6
Cefaclor	T36.1X1	T36.1X2	T36.1X3	T36.1X4	T36.1X5	T36.1X6
Cefadroxil	T36.1X1	T36.1X2	T36.1X3	T36.1X4	T36.1X5	T36.1X6
Cefalexin	T36.1X1	T36.1X2	T36.1X3	T36.1X4	T36.1X5	T36.1X6
Cefaloglycin	T36.1X1	T36.1X2	T36.1X3	T36.1X4	T36.1X5	T36.1X6
Cefaloridine	T36.1X1	T36.1X2	T36.1X3	T36.1X4	T36.1X5	T36.1X6
Cefalosporins	T36.1X1	T36.1X2	T36.1X3	T36.1X4	T36.1X5	T36.1X6
Cefalotin	T36.1X1	T36.1X2	T36.1X3	T36.1X4	T36.1X5	T36.1X6
Cefamandole	T36.1X1	T36.1X2	T36.1X3	T36.1X4	T36.1X5	T36.1X6
Cefamycin antibiotic	T36.1X1	T36.1X2	T36.1X3	T36.1X4	T36.1X5	T36.1X6
Cefapirin	T36.1X1	T36.1X2	T36.1X3	T36.1X4	T36.1X5	T36.1X6
Cefatrizine	T36.1X1	T36.1X2	T36.1X3	T36.1X4	T36.1X5	T36.1X6
Cefazedone	T36.1X1	T36.1X2	T36.1X3	T36.1X4	T36.1X5	T36.1X6
Cefazolin	T36.1X1	T36.1X2	T36.1X3	T36.1X4	T36.1X5	T36.1X6
Cefbuperazone	T36.1X1	T36.1X2	T36.1X3	T36.1X4	T36.1X5	T36.1X6
Cefetamet	T36.1X1	T36.1X2	T36.1X3	T36.1X4	T36.1X5	T36.1X6
Cefixime	T36.1X1	T36.1X2	T36.1X3	T36.1X4	T36.1X5	T36.1X6
Cefmenoxime	T36.1X1	T36.1X2	T36.1X3	T36.1X4	T36.1X5	T36.1X6
Cefmetazole	T36.1X1	T36.1X2	T36.1X3	T36.1X4	T36.1X5	T36.1X6
Cefminox	T36.1X1	T36.1X2	T36.1X3	T36.1X4	T36.1X5	T36.1X6
Cefonicid	T36.1X1	T36.1X2	T36.1X3	T36.1X4	T36.1X5	T36.1X6
Cefoperazone	T36.1X1	T36.1X2	T36.1X3	T36.1X4	T36.1X5	T36.1X6
Ceforanide	T36.1X1	T36.1X2	T36.1X3	T36.1X4	T36.1X5	T36.1X6
Cefotaxime	T36.1X1	T36.1X2	T36.1X3	T36.1X4	T36.1X5	T36.1X6
Cefotetan	T36.1X1	T36.1X2	T36.1X3	T36.1X4	T36.1X5	T36.1X6
Cefotiam	T36.1X1	T36.1X2	T36.1X3	T36.1X4	T36.1X5	T36.1X6
Cefoxitin	T36.1X1	T36.1X2	T36.1X3	T36.1X4	T36.1X5	T36.1X6
Cefpimizole	T36.1X1	T36.1X2	T36.1X3	T36.1X4	T36.1X5	T36.1X6
Cefpiramide	T36.1X1	T36.1X2	T36.1X3	T36.1X4	T36.1X5	T36.1X6
Cefradine	T36.1X1	T36.1X2	T36.1X3	T36.1X4	T36.1X5	T36.1X6
Cefroxadine	T36.1X1	T36.1X2	T36.1X3	T36.1X4	T36.1X5	T36.1X6
Cefsulodin	T36.1X1	T36.1X2	T36.1X3	T36.1X4	T36.1X5	T36.1X6
Ceftazidime	T36.1X1	T36.1X2	T36.1X3	T36.1X4	T36.1X5	T36.1X6
Cefteram	T36.1X1	T36.1X2	T36.1X3	T36.1X4	T36.1X5	T36.1X6
Ceftezole	T36.1X1	T36.1X2	T36.1X3	T36.1X4	T36.1X5	T36.1X6
Ceftizoxime	T36.1X1	T36.1X2	T36.1X3	T36.1X4	T36.1X5	T36.1X6
Ceftriaxone	T36.1X1	T36.1X2	T36.1X3	T36.1X4	T36.1X5	T36.1X6
Cefuroxime	T36.1X1	T36.1X2	T36.1X3	T36.1X4	T36.1X5	T36.1X6
Cefuzonam	T36.1X1	T36.1X2	T36.1X3	T36.1X4	T36.1X5	T36.1X6
Celestone	T38.0X1	T38.0X2	T38.0X3	T38.0X4	T38.0X5	T38.0X6
topical	T49.0X1	T49.0X2	T49.0X3	T49.0X4	T49.0X5	T49.0X6
Celiprolol	T44.7X1	T44.7X2	T44.7X3	T44.7X4	T44.7X5	T44.7X6
Cellosolve	T52.91	T52.92	T52.93	T52.94	—	—
Cell stimulants and proliferants	T49.8X1	T49.8X2	T49.8X3	T49.8X4	T49.8X5	T49.8X6
Cellulose						
cathartic	T47.4X1	T47.4X2	T47.4X3	T47.4X4	T47.4X5	T47.4X6
hydroxyethyl	T47.4X1	T47.4X2	T47.4X3	T47.4X4	T47.4X5	T47.4X6
nitrates (topical)	T49.3X1	T49.3X2	T49.3X3	T49.3X4	T49.3X5	T49.3X6
oxidized	T49.4X1	T49.4X2	T49.4X3	T49.4X4	T49.4X5	T49.4X6
Centipede (bite)	T63.411	T63.412	T63.413	T63.414	—	—
Central nervous system						
depressants	T42.71	T42.72	T42.73	T42.74	T42.75	T42.76
anesthetic (general) NEC	T41.201	T41.202	T41.203	T41.204	T41.205	T41.206
gases NEC	T41.0X1	T41.0X2	T41.0X3	T41.0X4	T41.0X5	T41.0X6
intravenous	T41.1X1	T41.1X2	T41.1X3	T41.1X4	T41.1X5	T41.1X6
barbiturates	T42.3X1	T42.3X2	T42.3X3	T42.3X4	T42.3X5	T42.3X6
benzodiazepines	T42.4X1	T42.4X2	T42.4X3	T42.4X4	T42.4X5	T42.4X6
bromides	T42.6X1	T42.6X2	T42.6X3	T42.6X4	T42.6X5	T42.6X6
cannabis sativa	T40.7X1	T40.7X2	T40.7X3	T40.7X4	T40.7X5	T40.7X6
chloral hydrate	T42.6X1	T42.6X2	T42.6X3	T42.6X4	T42.6X5	T42.6X6
ethanol	T51.0X1	T51.0X2	T51.0X3	T51.0X4	—	—

358
Additional Character May Be Required — Refer to the Tabular List for Character Selection
▽ Subterms under main terms may continue to next column or page

Table of Drugs and Chemicals

Substance	Poisoning, Accidental (unintentional)	Poisoning, Intentional Self-harm	Poisoning, Assault	Poisoning, Undetermined	Adverse Effect	Under-dosing
Central nervous system —						
continued						
depressants — *continued*						
hallucinogenics	T40.901	T40.902	T40.903	T40.904	T40.905	T40.906
hypnotics	T42.71	T42.72	T42.73	T42.74	T42.75	T42.76
specified NEC	T42.6X1	T42.6X2	T42.6X3	T42.6X4	T42.6X5	T42.6X6
muscle relaxants	T42.8X1	T42.8X2	T42.8X3	T42.8X4	T42.8X5	T42.8X6
paraldehyde	T42.6X1	T42.6X2	T42.6X3	T42.6X4	T42.6X5	T42.6X6
sedatives;	T42.71	T42.72	T42.73	T42.74	T42.75	T42.76
sedative-hypnotics						
mixed NEC	T42.6X1	T42.6X2	T42.6X3	T42.6X4	T42.6X5	T42.6X6
specified NEC	T42.6X1	T42.6X2	T42.6X3	T42.6X4	T42.6X5	T42.6X6
muscle-tone depressants	T42.8X1	T42.8X2	T42.8X3	T42.8X4	T42.8X5	T42.8X6
stimulants	T43.601	T43.602	T43.603	T43.604	T43.605	T43.606
amphetamines	T43.621	T43.622	T43.623	T43.624	T43.625	T43.626
analeptics	T50.7X1	T50.7X2	T50.7X3	T50.7X4	T50.7X5	T50.7X6
antidepressants	T43.201	T43.202	T43.203	T43.204	T43.205	T43.206
opiate antagonists	T50.7X1	T50.7X2	T50.7X3	T50.7X4	T50.7X5	T50.7X6
specified NEC	T43.691	T43.692	T43.693	T43.694	T43.695	T43.696
Cephalexin	T36.1X1	T36.1X2	T36.1X3	T36.1X4	T36.1X5	T36.1X6
Cephaloglycin	T36.1X1	T36.1X2	T36.1X3	T36.1X4	T36.1X5	T36.1X6
Cephaloridine	T36.1X1	T36.1X2	T36.1X3	T36.1X4	T36.1X5	T36.1X6
Cephalosporins	T36.1X1	T36.1X2	T36.1X3	T36.1X4	T36.1X5	T36.1X6
N (adicillin)	T36.0X1	T36.0X2	T36.0X3	T36.0X4	T36.0X5	T36.0X6
Cephalothin	T36.1X1	T36.1X2	T36.1X3	T36.1X4	T36.1X5	T36.1X6
Cephalotin	T36.1X1	T36.1X2	T36.1X3	T36.1X4	T36.1X5	T36.1X6
Cephradine	T36.1X1	T36.1X2	T36.1X3	T36.1X4	T36.1X5	T36.1X6
Cerbera (odallam)	T62.2X1	T62.2X2	T62.2X3	T62.2X4	—	—
Cerberin	T46.0X1	T46.0X2	T46.0X3	T46.0X4	T46.0X5	T46.0X6
Cerebral stimulants	T43.601	T43.602	T43.603	T43.604	T43.605	T43.606
psychotherapeutic	T43.601	T43.602	T43.603	T43.604	T43.605	T43.606
specified NEC	T43.691	T43.692	T43.693	T43.694	T43.695	T43.696
Cerium oxalate	T45.0X1	T45.0X2	T45.0X3	T45.0X4	T45.0X5	T45.0X6
Cerous oxalate	T45.0X1	T45.0X2	T45.0X3	T45.0X4	T45.0X5	T45.0X6
Ceruletide	T50.8X1	T50.8X2	T50.8X3	T50.8X4	T50.8X5	T50.8X6
Cetalkonium (chloride)	T49.0X1	T49.0X2	T49.0X3	T49.0X4	T49.0X5	T49.0X6
Cethexonium chloride	T49.0X1	T49.0X2	T49.0X3	T49.0X4	T49.0X5	T49.0X6
Cetiedil	T46.7X1	T46.7X2	T46.7X3	T46.7X4	T46.7X5	T46.7X6
Cetirizine	T45.0X1	T45.0X2	T45.0X3	T45.0X4	T45.0X5	T45.0X6
Cetomacrogol	T50.991	T50.992	T50.993	T50.994	T50.995	T50.996
Cetotiamine	T45.2X1	T45.2X2	T45.2X3	T45.2X4	T45.2X5	T45.2X6
Cetoxime	T45.0X1	T45.0X2	T45.0X3	T45.0X4	T45.0X5	T45.0X6
Cetraxate	T47.1X1	T47.1X2	T47.1X3	T47.1X4	T47.1X5	T47.1X6
Cetrimide	T49.0X1	T49.0X2	T49.0X3	T49.0X4	T49.0X5	T49.0X6
Cetrimonium (bromide)	T49.0X1	T49.0X2	T49.0X3	T49.0X4	T49.0X5	T49.0X6
Cetylpyridinium chloride	T49.0X1	T49.0X2	T49.0X3	T49.0X4	T49.0X5	T49.0X6
ENT agent	T49.6X1	T49.6X2	T49.6X3	T49.6X4	T49.6X5	T49.6X6
lozenges	T49.6X1	T49.6X2	T49.6X3	T49.6X4	T49.6X5	T49.6X6
Cevadilla — *see* Sabadilla						
Cevitamic acid	T45.2X1	T45.2X2	T45.2X3	T45.2X4	T45.2X5	T45.2X6
Chalk, precipitated	T47.1X1	T47.1X2	T47.1X3	T47.1X4	T47.1X5	T47.1X6
Chamomile	T49.0X1	T49.0X2	T49.0X3	T49.0X4	T49.0X5	T49.0X6
Ch'an su	T46.0X1	T46.0X2	T46.0X3	T46.0X4	T46.0X5	T46.0X6
Charcoal	T47.6X1	T47.6X2	T47.6X3	T47.6X4	T47.6X5	T47.6X6
activated — *see also* Charcoal, medicinal	T47.6X1	T47.6X2	T47.6X3	T47.6X4	T47.6X5	T47.6X6
fumes (Carbon monoxide)	T58.2X1	T58.2X2	T58.2X3	T58.2X4	—	—
industrial	T58.8X1	T58.8X2	T58.8X3	T58.8X4	—	—
medicinal (activated)	T47.6X1	T47.6X2	T47.6X3	T47.6X4	T47.6X5	T47.6X6
antidiarrheal	T47.6X1	T47.6X2	T47.6X3	T47.6X4	T47.6X5	T47.6X6
poison control	T47.8X1	T47.8X2	T47.8X3	T47.8X4	T47.8X5	T47.8X6
specified use other than for diarrhea	T47.8X1	T47.8X2	T47.8X3	T47.8X4	T47.8X5	T47.8X6
topical	T49.8X1	T49.8X2	T49.8X3	T49.8X4	T49.8X5	T49.8X6
Chaulmosulfone	T37.1X1	T37.1X2	T37.1X3	T37.1X4	T37.1X5	T37.1X6
Chelating agent NEC	T50.6X1	T50.6X2	T50.6X3	T50.6X4	T50.6X5	T50.6X6
Chelidonium majus	T62.2X1	T62.2X2	T62.2X3	T62.2X4	—	—
Chemical substance NEC	T65.91	T65.92	T65.93	T65.94		
Chenodeoxycholic acid	T47.5X1	T47.5X2	T47.5X3	T47.5X4	T47.5X5	T47.5X6
Chenodiol	T47.5X1	T47.5X2	T47.5X3	T47.5X4	T47.5X5	T47.5X6
Chenopodium	T37.4X1	T37.4X2	T37.4X3	T37.4X4	T37.4X5	T37.4X6
Cherry laurel	T62.2X1	T62.2X2	T62.2X3	T62.2X4	—	—
Chinidin (e)	T46.2X1	T46.2X2	T46.2X3	T46.2X4	T46.2X5	T46.2X6
Chiniofon	T37.8X1	T37.8X2	T37.8X3	T37.8X4	T37.8X5	T37.8X6
Chlophedianol	T48.3X1	T48.3X2	T48.3X3	T48.3X4	T48.3X5	T48.3X6
Chloral	T42.6X1	T42.6X2	T42.6X3	T42.6X4	T42.6X5	T42.6X6
derivative	T42.6X1	T42.6X2	T42.6X3	T42.6X4	T42.6X5	T42.6X6
hydrate	T42.6X1	T42.6X2	T42.6X3	T42.6X4	T42.6X5	T42.6X6
Chloralamide	T42.6X1	T42.6X2	T42.6X3	T42.6X4	T42.6X5	T42.6X6
Chloralodol	T42.6X1	T42.6X2	T42.6X3	T42.6X4	T42.6X5	T42.6X6
Chloralose	T60.4X1	T60.4X2	T60.4X3	T60.4X4		
Chlorambucil	T45.1X1	T45.1X2	T45.1X3	T45.1X4	T45.1X5	T45.1X6
Chloramine	T57.8X1	T57.8X2	T57.8X3	T57.8X4	—	—

Substance	Poisoning, Accidental (unintentional)	Poisoning, Intentional Self-harm	Poisoning, Assault	Poisoning, Undetermined	Adverse Effect	Under-dosing
Chloramine — *continued*						
T	T49.0X1	T49.0X2	T49.0X3	T49.0X4	T49.0X5	T49.0X6
topical	T49.0X1	T49.0X2	T49.0X3	T49.0X4	T49.0X5	T49.0X6
Chloramphenicol	T36.2X1	T36.2X2	T36.2X3	T36.2X4	T36.2X5	T36.2X6
ENT agent	T49.6X1	T49.6X2	T49.6X3	T49.6X4	T49.6X5	T49.6X6
ophthalmic preparation	T49.5X1	T49.5X2	T49.5X3	T49.5X4	T49.5X5	T49.5X6
topical NEC	T49.0X1	T49.0X2	T49.0X3	T49.0X4	T49.0X5	T49.0X6
Chlorate (potassium) (sodium) **NEC**	T60.3X1	T60.3X2	T60.3X3	T60.3X4	—	—
herbicide	T60.3X1	T60.3X2	T60.3X3	T60.3X4	—	—
Chlorazanil	T50.2X1	T50.2X2	T50.2X3	T50.2X4	T50.2X5	T50.2X6
Chlorbenzene, chlorbenzol	T53.7X1	T53.7X2	T53.7X3	T53.7X4	—	—
Chlorbenzoxamine	T44.3X1	T44.3X2	T44.3X3	T44.3X4	T44.3X5	T44.3X6
Chlorbutol	T42.6X1	T42.6X2	T42.6X3	T42.6X4	T42.6X5	T42.6X6
Chlorcyclizine	T45.0X1	T45.0X2	T45.0X3	T45.0X4	T45.0X5	T45.0X6
Chlordan (e) (dust)	T60.1X1	T60.1X2	T60.1X3	T60.1X4		
Chlordantoin	T49.0X1	T49.0X2	T49.0X3	T49.0X4	T49.0X5	T49.0X6
Chlordiazepoxide	T42.4X1	T42.4X2	T42.4X3	T42.4X4	T42.4X5	T42.4X6
Chlordiethyl benzamide	T49.3X1	T49.3X2	T49.3X3	T49.3X4	T49.3X5	T49.3X6
Chloresium	T49.8X1	T49.8X2	T49.8X3	T49.8X4	T49.8X5	T49.8X6
Chlorethiazol	T42.6X1	T42.6X2	T42.6X3	T42.6X4	T42.6X5	T42.6X6
Chlorethyl — *see* Ethyl chloride						
Chloretone	T42.6X1	T42.6X2	T42.6X3	T42.6X4	T42.6X5	T42.6X6
Chlorex	T53.6X1	T53.6X2	T53.6X3	T53.6X4	—	—
insecticide	T60.1X1	T60.1X2	T60.1X3	T60.1X4	—	—
Chlorfenvinphos	T60.0X1	T60.0X2	T60.0X3	T60.0X4	—	—
Chlorhexadol	T42.6X1	T42.6X2	T42.6X3	T42.6X4	T42.6X5	T42.6X6
Chlorhexamide	T45.1X1	T45.1X2	T45.1X3	T45.1X4	T45.1X5	T45.1X6
Chlorhexidine	T49.0X1	T49.0X2	T49.0X3	T49.0X4	T49.0X5	T49.0X6
Chlorhydroxyquinolin	T49.0X1	T49.0X2	T49.0X3	T49.0X4	T49.0X5	T49.0X6
Chloride of lime (bleach)	T54.3X1	T54.3X2	T54.3X3	T54.3X4	—	—
Chlorimipramine	T43.011	T43.012	T43.013	T43.014	T43.015	T43.016
Chlorinated						
camphene	T53.6X1	T53.6X2	T53.6X3	T53.6X4	—	—
diphenyl	T53.7X1	T53.7X2	T53.7X3	T53.7X4	—	—
hydrocarbons NEC	T53.91	T53.92	T53.93	T53.94	—	—
solvents	T53.91	T53.92	T53.93	T53.94	—	—
lime (bleach)	T54.3X1	T54.3X2	T54.3X3	T54.3X4	—	—
and boric acid solution	T49.0X1	T49.0X2	T49.0X3	T49.0X4	T49.0X5	T49.0X6
naphthalene (insecticide)	T60.1X1	T60.1X2	T60.1X3	T60.1X4	—	—
industrial (non-pesticide)	T53.7X1	T53.7X2	T53.7X3	T53.7X4	—	—
pesticide NEC	T60.8X1	T60.8X2	T60.8X3	T60.8X4	—	—
soda — *see also* sodium hypochlorite						
solution	T49.0X1	T49.0X2	T49.0X3	T49.0X4	T49.0X5	T49.0X6
Chlorine (fumes) (gas)	T59.4X1	T59.4X2	T59.4X3	T59.4X4	—	—
bleach	T54.3X1	T54.3X2	T54.3X3	T54.3X4	—	—
compound gas NEC	T59.4X1	T59.4X2	T59.4X3	T59.4X4	—	—
disinfectant	T59.4X1	T59.4X2	T59.4X3	T59.4X4	—	—
releasing agents NEC	T59.4X1	T59.4X2	T59.4X3	T59.4X4	—	—
Chlorisondamine chloride	T46.991	T46.992	T46.993	T46.994	T46.995	T46.996
Chlormadinone	T38.5X1	T38.5X2	T38.5X3	T38.5X4	T38.5X5	T38.5X6
Chlormephos	T60.0X1	T60.0X2	T60.0X3	T60.0X4	—	—
Chlormerodrin	T50.2X1	T50.2X2	T50.2X3	T50.2X4	T50.2X5	T50.2X6
Chlormethiazole	T42.6X1	T42.6X2	T42.6X3	T42.6X4	T42.6X5	T42.6X6
Chlormethine	T45.1X1	T45.1X2	T45.1X3	T45.1X4	T45.1X5	T45.1X6
Chlormethylenecycline	T36.4X1	T36.4X2	T36.4X3	T36.4X4	T36.4X5	T36.4X6
Chlormezanone	T42.6X1	T42.6X2	T42.6X3	T42.6X4	T42.6X5	T42.6X6
Chloroacetic acid	T60.3X1	T60.3X2	T60.3X3	T60.3X4	—	—
Chloroacetone	T59.3X1	T59.3X2	T59.3X3	T59.3X4	—	—
Chloroacetophenone	T59.3X1	T59.3X2	T59.3X3	T59.3X4	—	—
Chloroaniline	T53.7X1	T53.7X2	T53.7X3	T53.7X4	—	—
Chlorobenzene, chlorobenzol	T53.7X1	T53.7X2	T53.7X3	T53.7X4	—	—
Chlorobromomethane (fire extinguisher)	T53.6X1	T53.6X2	T53.6X3	T53.6X4	—	—
Chlorobutanol	T49.0X1	T49.0X2	T49.0X3	T49.0X4	T49.0X5	T49.0X6
Chlorocresol	T49.0X1	T49.0X2	T49.0X3	T49.0X4	T49.0X5	T49.0X6
Chlorodehydromethyltestosterone	T38.7X1	T38.7X2	T38.7X3	T38.7X4	T38.7X5	T38.7X6
Chlorodinitrobenzene	T53.7X1	T53.7X2	T53.7X3	T53.7X4	—	—
dust or vapor	T53.7X1	T53.7X2	T53.7X3	T53.7X4	—	—
Chlorodiphenyl	T53.7X1	T53.7X2	T53.7X3	T53.7X4	—	—
Chloroethane — *see* Ethyl chloride						
Chloroethylene	T53.6X1	T53.6X2	T53.6X3	T53.6X4	—	—
Chlorofluorocarbons	T53.5X1	T53.5X2	T53.5X3	T53.5X4	—	—
Chloroform (fumes) (vapor)	T53.1X1	T53.1X2	T53.1X3	T53.1X4	—	—
anesthetic	T41.0X1	T41.0X2	T41.0X3	T41.0X4	T41.0X5	T41.0X6
solvent	T53.1X1	T53.1X2	T53.1X3	T53.1X4	—	—
water, concentrated	T41.0X1	T41.0X2	T41.0X3	T41.0X4	T41.0X5	T41.0X6
Chloroguanide	T37.2X1	T37.2X2	T37.2X3	T37.2X4	T37.2X5	T37.2X6

Central nervous system — Chloroguanide

Substance	Poisoning, Accidental (unintentional)	Poisoning, Intentional Self-harm	Poisoning, Assault	Poisoning, Undetermined	Adverse Effect	Under-dosing
Chloromycetin	T36.2X1	T36.2X2	T36.2X3	T36.2X4	T36.2X5	T36.2X6
ENT agent	T49.6X1	T49.6X2	T49.6X3	T49.6X4	T49.6X5	T49.6X6
ophthalmic preparation	T49.5X1	T49.5X2	T49.5X3	T49.5X4	T49.5X5	T49.5X6
otic solution	T49.6X1	T49.6X2	T49.6X3	T49.6X4	T49.6X5	T49.6X6
topical NEC	T49.0X1	T49.0X2	T49.0X3	T49.0X4	T49.0X5	T49.0X6
Chloronitrobenzene	T53.7X1	T53.7X2	T53.7X3	T53.7X4	—	—
dust or vapor	T53.7X1	T53.7X2	T53.7X3	T53.7X4	—	—
Chlorophacinone	T60.4X1	T60.4X2	T60.4X3	T60.4X4	—	—
Chlorophenol	T53.7X1	T53.7X2	T53.7X3	T53.7X4	—	—
Chlorophenothane	T60.1X1	T60.1X2	T60.1X3	T60.1X4	—	—
Chlorophyll	T50.991	T50.992	T50.993	T50.994	T50.995	T50.996
Chloropicrin (fumes)	T53.6X1	T53.6X2	T53.6X3	T53.6X4	—	—
fumigant	T60.8X1	T60.8X2	T60.8X3	T60.8X4	—	—
fungicide	T60.3X1	T60.3X2	T60.3X3	T60.3X4	—	—
pesticide	T60.8X1	T60.8X2	T60.8X3	T60.8X4	—	—
Chloroprocaine	T41.3X1	T41.3X2	T41.3X3	T41.3X4	T41.3X5	T41.3X6
infiltration (subcutaneous)	T41.3X1	T41.3X2	T41.3X3	T41.3X4	T41.3X5	T41.3X6
nerve block (peripheral) (plexus)	T41.3X1	T41.3X2	T41.3X3	T41.3X4	T41.3X5	T41.3X6
spinal	T41.3X1	T41.3X2	T41.3X3	T41.3X4	T41.3X5	T41.3X6
Chloroptic	T49.5X1	T49.5X2	T49.5X3	T49.5X4	T49.5X5	T49.5X6
Chloropurine	T45.1X1	T45.1X2	T45.1X3	T45.1X4	T45.1X5	T45.1X6
Chloropyramine	T45.0X1	T45.0X2	T45.0X3	T45.0X4	T45.0X5	T45.0X6
Chloropyrifos	T60.0X1	T60.0X2	T60.0X3	T60.0X4	—	—
Chloropyrilene	T45.0X1	T45.0X2	T45.0X3	T45.0X4	T45.0X5	T45.0X6
Chloroquine	T37.2X1	T37.2X2	T37.2X3	T37.2X4	T37.2X5	T37.2X6
Chlorothalonil	T60.3X1	T60.3X2	T60.3X3	T60.3X4	—	—
Chlorothen	T45.0X1	T45.0X2	T45.0X3	T45.0X4	T45.0X5	T45.0X6
Chlorothiazide	T50.2X1	T50.2X2	T50.2X3	T50.2X4	T50.2X5	T50.2X6
Chlorothymol	T49.4X1	T49.4X2	T49.4X3	T49.4X4	T49.4X5	T49.4X6
Chlorotrianisene	T38.5X1	T38.5X2	T38.5X3	T38.5X4	T38.5X5	T38.5X6
Chlorovinyldichloroarsine, not in war	T57.0X1	T57.0X2	T57.0X3	T57.0X4	—	—
Chloroxine	T49.4X1	T49.4X2	T49.4X3	T49.4X4	T49.4X5	T49.4X6
Chloroxylenol	T49.0X1	T49.0X2	T49.0X3	T49.0X4	T49.0X5	T49.0X6
Chlorphenamine	T45.0X1	T45.0X2	T45.0X3	T45.0X4	T45.0X5	T45.0X6
Chlorphenesin	T42.8X1	T42.8X2	T42.8X3	T42.8X4	T42.8X5	T42.8X6
topical (antifungal)	T49.0X1	T49.0X2	T49.0X3	T49.0X4	T49.0X5	T49.0X6
Chlorpheniramine	T45.0X1	T45.0X2	T45.0X3	T45.0X4	T45.0X5	T45.0X6
Chlorphenoxamine	T45.0X1	T45.0X2	T45.0X3	T45.0X4	T45.0X5	T45.0X6
Chlorphentermine	T50.5X1	T50.5X2	T50.5X3	T50.5X4	T50.5X5	T50.5X6
Chlorprocaine — see Chloroprocaine						
Chlorproguanil	T37.2X1	T37.2X2	T37.2X3	T37.2X4	T37.2X5	T37.2X6
Chlorpromazine	T43.3X1	T43.3X2	T43.3X3	T43.3X4	T43.3X5	T43.3X6
Chlorpropamide	T38.3X1	T38.3X2	T38.3X3	T38.3X4	T38.3X5	T38.3X6
Chlorprothixene	T43.4X1	T43.4X2	T43.4X3	T43.4X4	T43.4X5	T43.4X6
Chlorquinaldol	T49.0X1	T49.0X2	T49.0X3	T49.0X4	T49.0X5	T49.0X6
Chlorquinol	T49.0X1	T49.0X2	T49.0X3	T49.0X4	T49.0X5	T49.0X6
Chlortalidone	T50.2X1	T50.2X2	T50.2X3	T50.2X4	T50.2X5	T50.2X6
Chlortetracycline	T36.4X1	T36.4X2	T36.4X3	T36.4X4	T36.4X5	T36.4X6
Chlorthalidone	T50.2X1	T50.2X2	T50.2X3	T50.2X4	T50.2X5	T50.2X6
Chlorthion	T60.0X1	T60.0X2	T60.0X3	T60.0X4	—	—
Chlorthiophos	T60.0X1	T60.0X2	T60.0X3	T60.0X4	—	—
Chlortrianisene	T38.5X1	T38.5X2	T38.5X3	T38.5X4	T38.5X5	T38.5X6
Chlor-Trimeton	T45.0X1	T45.0X2	T45.0X3	T45.0X4	T45.0X5	T45.0X6
Chlorzoxazone	T42.8X1	T42.8X2	T42.8X3	T42.8X4	T42.8X5	T42.8X6
Choke damp	T59.7X1	T59.7X2	T59.7X3	T59.7X4	—	—
Cholagogues	T47.5X1	T47.5X2	T47.5X3	T47.5X4	T47.5X5	T47.5X6
Cholebrine	T50.8X1	T50.8X2	T50.8X3	T50.8X4	T50.8X5	T50.8X6
Cholecalciferol	T45.2X1	T45.2X2	T45.2X3	T45.2X4	T45.2X5	T45.2X6
Cholecystokinin	T50.8X1	T50.8X2	T50.8X3	T50.8X4	T50.8X5	T50.8X6
Cholera vaccine	T50.A91	T50.A92	T50.A93	T50.A94	T50.A95	T50.A96
Choleretic	T47.5X1	T47.5X2	T47.5X3	T47.5X4	T47.5X5	T47.5X6
Cholesterol-lowering agents	T46.6X1	T46.6X2	T46.6X3	T46.6X4	T46.6X5	T46.6X6
Cholestyramine (resin)	T46.6X1	T46.6X2	T46.6X3	T46.6X4	T46.6X5	T46.6X6
Cholic acid	T47.5X1	T47.5X2	T47.5X3	T47.5X4	T47.5X5	T47.5X6
Choline	T48.6X1	T48.6X2	T48.6X3	T48.6X4	T48.6X5	T48.6X6
chloride	T50.991	T50.992	T50.993	T50.994	T50.995	T50.996
dihydrogen citrate	T50.991	T50.992	T50.993	T50.994	T50.995	T50.996
salicylate	T39.091	T39.092	T39.093	T39.094	T39.095	T39.096
theophyllinate	T48.6X1	T48.6X2	T48.6X3	T48.6X4	T48.6X5	T48.6X6
Cholinergic (drug) **NEC**	T44.1X1	T44.1X2	T44.1X3	T44.1X4	T44.1X5	T44.1X6
muscle tone enhancer	T44.1X1	T44.1X2	T44.1X3	T44.1X4	T44.1X5	T44.1X6
organophosphorus	T44.0X1	T44.0X2	T44.0X3	T44.0X4	T44.0X5	T44.0X6
insecticide	T60.0X1	T60.0X2	T60.0X3	T60.0X4	—	—
nerve gas	T59.891	T59.892	T59.893	T59.894	—	—
trimethyl ammonium propanediol	T44.1X1	T44.1X2	T44.1X3	T44.1X4	T44.1X5	T44.1X6
Cholinesterase reactivator	T50.6X1	T50.6X2	T50.6X3	T50.6X4	T50.6X5	T50.6X6
Cholografin	T50.8X1	T50.8X2	T50.8X3	T50.8X4	T50.8X5	T50.8X6
Chorionic gonadotropin	T38.891	T38.892	T38.893	T38.894	T38.895	T38.896
Chromate	T56.2X1	T56.2X2	T56.2X3	T56.2X4	—	—
dust or mist	T56.2X1	T56.2X2	T56.2X3	T56.2X4	—	—
lead — see also lead	T56.0X1	T56.0X2	T56.0X3	T56.0X4	—	—
paint	T56.0X1	T56.0X2	T56.0X3	T56.0X4	—	—
Chromic						
acid	T56.2X1	T56.2X2	T56.2X3	T56.2X4	—	—
dust or mist	T56.2X1	T56.2X2	T56.2X3	T56.2X4	—	—
phosphate 32P	T45.1X1	T45.1X2	T45.1X3	T45.1X4	T45.1X5	T45.1X6
Chromium	T56.2X1	T56.2X2	T56.2X3	T56.2X4	—	—
compounds — see Chromate						
sesquioxide	T50.8X1	T50.8X2	T50.8X3	T50.8X4	T50.8X5	T50.8X6
Chromomycin A3	T45.1X1	T45.1X2	T45.1X3	T45.1X4	T45.1X5	T45.1X6
Chromonar	T46.3X1	T46.3X2	T46.3X3	T46.3X4	T46.3X5	T46.3X6
Chromyl chloride	T56.2X1	T56.2X2	T56.2X3	T56.2X4	—	—
Chrysarobin	T49.4X1	T49.4X2	T49.4X3	T49.4X4	T49.4X5	T49.4X6
Chrysazin	T47.2X1	T47.2X2	T47.2X3	T47.2X4	T47.2X5	T47.2X6
Chymar	T45.3X1	T45.3X2	T45.3X3	T45.3X4	T45.3X5	T45.3X6
ophthalmic preparation	T49.5X1	T49.5X2	T49.5X3	T49.5X4	T49.5X5	T49.5X6
Chymopapain	T45.3X1	T45.3X2	T45.3X3	T45.3X4	T45.3X5	T45.3X6
Chymotrypsin	T45.3X1	T45.3X2	T45.3X3	T45.3X4	T45.3X5	T45.3X6
ophthalmic preparation	T49.5X1	T49.5X2	T49.5X3	T49.5X4	T49.5X5	T49.5X6
Cianidanol	T50.991	T50.992	T50.993	T50.994	T50.995	T50.996
Cianopramine	T43.011	T43.012	T43.013	T43.014	T43.015	T43.016
Cibenzoline	T46.2X1	T46.2X2	T46.2X3	T46.2X4	T46.2X5	T46.2X6
Ciclacillin	T36.0X1	T36.0X2	T36.0X3	T36.0X4	T36.0X5	T36.0X6
Ciclobarbital — see Hexobarbital						
Ciclonicate	T46.7X1	T46.7X2	T46.7X3	T46.7X4	T46.7X5	T46.7X6
Ciclopirox (olamine)	T49.0X1	T49.0X2	T49.0X3	T49.0X4	T49.0X5	T49.0X6
Ciclosporin	T45.1X1	T45.1X2	T45.1X3	T45.1X4	T45.1X5	T45.1X6
Cicuta maculata or virosa	T62.2X1	T62.2X2	T62.2X3	T62.2X4	—	—
Cicutoxin	T62.2X1	T62.2X2	T62.2X3	T62.2X4	—	—
Cigarette lighter fluid	T52.0X1	T52.0X2	T52.0X3	T52.0X4	—	—
Cigarettes (tobacco)	T65.221	T65.222	T65.223	T65.224	—	—
Ciguatoxin	T61.01	T61.02	T61.03	T61.04	—	—
Cilazapril	T46.4X1	T46.4X2	T46.4X3	T46.4X4	T46.4X5	T46.4X6
Cimetidine	T47.0X1	T47.0X2	T47.0X3	T47.0X4	T47.0X5	T47.0X6
Cimetropium bromide	T44.3X1	T44.3X2	T44.3X3	T44.3X4	T44.3X5	T44.3X6
Cinchocaine	T41.3X1	T41.3X2	T41.3X3	T41.3X4	T41.3X5	T41.3X6
topical (surface)	T41.3X1	T41.3X2	T41.3X3	T41.3X4	T41.3X5	T41.3X6
Cinchona	T37.2X1	T37.2X2	T37.2X3	T37.2X4	T37.2X5	T37.2X6
Cinchonine alkaloids	T37.2X1	T37.2X2	T37.2X3	T37.2X4	T37.2X5	T37.2X6
Cinchophen	T50.4X1	T50.4X2	T50.4X3	T50.4X4	T50.4X5	T50.4X6
Cinepazide	T46.7X1	T46.7X2	T46.7X3	T46.7X4	T46.7X5	T46.7X6
Cinnamedrine	T48.5X1	T48.5X2	T48.5X3	T48.5X4	T48.5X5	T48.5X6
Cinnarizine	T45.0X1	T45.0X2	T45.0X3	T45.0X4	T45.0X5	T45.0X6
Cinoxacin	T37.8X1	T37.8X2	T37.8X3	T37.8X4	T37.8X5	T37.8X6
Ciprofibrate	T46.6X1	T46.6X2	T46.6X3	T46.6X4	T46.6X5	T46.6X6
Ciprofloxacin	T36.8X1	T36.8X2	T36.8X3	T36.8X4	T36.8X5	T36.8X6
Cisapride	T47.8X1	T47.8X2	T47.8X3	T47.8X4	T47.8X5	T47.8X6
Cisplatin	T45.1X1	T45.1X2	T45.1X3	T45.1X4	T45.1X5	T45.1X6
Citalopram	T43.221	T43.222	T43.223	T43.224	T43.225	T43.226
Citanest	T41.3X1	T41.3X2	T41.3X3	T41.3X4	T41.3X5	T41.3X6
infiltration (subcutaneous)	T41.3X1	T41.3X2	T41.3X3	T41.3X4	T41.3X5	T41.3X6
nerve block (peripheral) (plexus)	T41.3X1	T41.3X2	T41.3X3	T41.3X4	T41.3X5	T41.3X6
Citric acid	T47.5X1	T47.5X2	T47.5X3	T47.5X4	T47.5X5	T47.5X6
Citrovorum (factor)	T45.8X1	T45.8X2	T45.8X3	T45.8X4	T45.8X5	T45.8X6
Claviceps purpurea	T62.2X1	T62.2X2	T62.2X3	T62.2X4	—	—
Clavulanic acid	T36.1X1	T36.1X2	T36.1X3	T36.1X4	T36.1X5	T36.1X6
Cleaner, cleansing agent, type not specified	T65.891	T65.892	T65.893	T65.894	—	—
of paint or varnish	T52.91	T52.92	T52.93	T52.94	—	—
specified type NEC	T65.891	T65.892	T65.893	T65.894	—	—
Clebopride	T47.8X1	T47.8X2	T47.8X3	T47.8X4	T47.8X5	T47.8X6
Clefamide	T37.3X1	T37.3X2	T37.3X3	T37.3X4	T37.3X5	T37.3X6
Clemastine	T45.0X1	T45.0X2	T45.0X3	T45.0X4	T45.0X5	T45.0X6
Clematis vitalba	T62.2X1	T62.2X2	T62.2X3	T62.2X4	—	—
Clemizole	T45.0X1	T45.0X2	T45.0X3	T45.0X4	T45.0X5	T45.0X6
penicillin	T36.0X1	T36.0X2	T36.0X3	T36.0X4	T36.0X5	T36.0X6
Clenbuterol	T48.6X1	T48.6X2	T48.6X3	T48.6X4	T48.6X5	T48.6X6
Clidinium bromide	T44.3X1	T44.3X2	T44.3X3	T44.3X4	T44.3X5	T44.3X6
Clindamycin	T36.8X1	T36.8X2	T36.8X3	T36.8X4	T36.8X5	T36.8X6
Clinofibrate	T46.6X1	T46.6X2	T46.6X3	T46.6X4	T46.6X5	T46.6X6
Clioquinol	T37.8X1	T37.8X2	T37.8X3	T37.8X4	T37.8X5	T37.8X6
Cliradon	T40.2X1	T40.2X2	T40.2X3	T40.2X4	—	—
Clobazam	T42.4X1	T42.4X2	T42.4X3	T42.4X4	T42.4X5	T42.4X6
Clobenzorex	T50.5X1	T50.5X2	T50.5X3	T50.5X4	T50.5X5	T50.5X6
Clobetasol	T49.0X1	T49.0X2	T49.0X3	T49.0X4	T49.0X5	T49.0X6
Clobetasone	T49.0X1	T49.0X2	T49.0X3	T49.0X4	T49.0X5	T49.0X6
Clobutinol	T48.3X1	T48.3X2	T48.3X3	T48.3X4	T48.3X5	T48.3X6
Clocortolone	T38.0X1	T38.0X2	T38.0X3	T38.0X4	T38.0X5	T38.0X6
Clodantoin	T49.0X1	T49.0X2	T49.0X3	T49.0X4	T49.0X5	T49.0X6

Substance	Poisoning, Accidental (unintentional)	Poisoning, Intentional Self-harm	Poisoning, Assault	Poisoning, Undetermined	Adverse Effect	Under-dosing
Clodronic acid	T50.991	T50.992	T50.993	T50.994	T50.995	T50.996
Clofazimine	T37.1X1	T37.1X2	T37.1X3	T37.1X4	T37.1X5	T37.1X6
Clofedanol	T48.3X1	T48.3X2	T48.3X3	T48.3X4	T48.3X5	T48.3X6
Clofenamide	T50.2X1	T50.2X2	T50.2X3	T50.2X4	T50.2X5	T50.2X6
Clofenotane	T49.0X1	T49.0X2	T49.0X3	T49.0X4	T49.0X5	T49.0X6
Clofezone	T39.2X1	T39.2X2	T39.2X3	T39.2X4	T39.2X5	T39.2X6
Clofibrate	T46.6X1	T46.6X2	T46.6X3	T46.6X4	T46.6X5	T46.6X6
Clofibride	T46.6X1	T46.6X2	T46.6X3	T46.6X4	T46.6X5	T46.6X6
Cloforex	T50.5X1	T50.5X2	T50.5X3	T50.5X4	T50.5X5	T50.5X6
Clomethiazole	T42.6X1	T42.6X2	T42.6X3	T42.6X4	T42.6X5	T42.6X6
Clometocillin	T36.0X1	T36.0X2	T36.0X3	T36.0X4	T36.0X5	T36.0X6
Clomifene	T38.5X1	T38.5X2	T38.5X3	T38.5X4	T38.5X5	T38.5X6
Clomiphene	T38.5X1	T38.5X2	T38.5X3	T38.5X4	T38.5X5	T38.5X6
Clomipramine	T43.011	T43.012	T43.013	T43.014	T43.015	T43.016
Clomocycline	T36.4X1	T36.4X2	T36.4X3	T36.4X4	T36.4X5	T36.4X6
Clonazepam	T42.4X1	T42.4X2	T42.4X3	T42.4X4	T42.4X5	T42.4X6
Clonidine	T46.5X1	T46.5X2	T46.5X3	T46.5X4	T46.5X5	T46.5X6
Clonixin	T39.8X1	T39.8X2	T39.8X3	T39.8X4	T39.8X5	T39.8X6
Clopamide	T50.2X1	T50.2X2	T50.2X3	T50.2X4	T50.2X5	T50.2X6
Clopenthixol	T43.4X1	T43.4X2	T43.4X3	T43.4X4	T43.4X5	T43.4X6
Cloperastine	T48.3X1	T48.3X2	T48.3X3	T48.3X4	T48.3X5	T48.3X6
Clophedianol	T48.3X1	T48.3X2	T48.3X3	T48.3X4	T48.3X5	T48.3X6
Cloponone	T36.2X1	T36.2X2	T36.2X3	T36.2X4	T36.2X5	T36.2X6
Cloprednol	T38.0X1	T38.0X2	T38.0X3	T38.0X4	T38.0X5	T38.0X6
Cloral betaine	T42.6X1	T42.6X2	T42.6X3	T42.6X4	T42.6X5	T42.6X6
Cloramfenicol	T36.2X1	T36.2X2	T36.2X3	T36.2X4	T36.2X5	T36.2X6
Clorazepate (dipotassium)	T42.4X1	T42.4X2	T42.4X3	T42.4X4	T42.4X5	T42.4X6
Clorexolone	T50.2X1	T50.2X2	T50.2X3	T50.2X4	T50.2X5	T50.2X6
Clorfenamine	T45.0X1	T45.0X2	T45.0X3	T45.0X4	T45.0X5	T45.0X6
Clorgiline	T43.1X1	T43.1X2	T43.1X3	T43.1X4	T43.1X5	T43.1X6
Clorotepine	T44.3X1	T44.3X2	T44.3X3	T44.3X4	T44.3X5	T44.3X6
Clorox (bleach)	T54.91	T54.92	T54.93	T54.94	—	—
Clorprenaline	T48.6X1	T48.6X2	T48.6X3	T48.6X4	T48.6X5	T48.6X6
Clortermine	T50.5X1	T50.5X2	T50.5X3	T50.5X4	T50.5X5	T50.5X6
Clotiapine	T43.591	T43.592	T43.593	T43.594	T43.595	T43.596
Clotiazepam	T42.4X1	T42.4X2	T42.4X3	T42.4X4	T42.4X5	T42.4X6
Clotibric acid	T46.6X1	T46.6X2	T46.6X3	T46.6X4	T46.6X5	T46.6X6
Clotrimazole	T49.0X1	T49.0X2	T49.0X3	T49.0X4	T49.0X5	T49.0X6
Cloxacillin	T36.0X1	T36.0X2	T36.0X3	T36.0X4	T36.0X5	T36.0X6
Cloxazolam	T42.4X1	T42.4X2	T42.4X3	T42.4X4	T42.4X5	T42.4X6
Cloxiquine	T49.0X1	T49.0X2	T49.0X3	T49.0X4	T49.0X5	T49.0X6
Clozapine	T42.4X1	T42.4X2	T42.4X3	T42.4X4	T42.4X5	T42.4X6
Coagulant NEC	T45.7X1	T45.7X2	T45.7X3	T45.7X4	T45.7X5	T45.7X6
Coal (carbon monoxide from) — see also Carbon, monoxide, coal	T58.2X1	T58.2X2	T58.2X3	T58.2X4	—	—
oil — see Kerosene						
tar	T49.1X1	T49.1X2	T49.1X3	T49.1X4	T49.1X5	T49.1X6
fumes	T59.891	T59.892	T59.893	T59.894	—	—
medicinal (ointment)	T49.4X1	T49.4X2	T49.4X3	T49.4X4	T49.4X5	T49.4X6
analgesics NEC	T39.2X1	T39.2X2	T39.2X3	T39.2X4	T39.2X5	T39.2X6
naphtha (solvent)	T52.0X1	T52.0X2	T52.0X3	T52.0X4	—	—
Cobalamine	T45.2X1	T45.2X2	T45.2X3	T45.2X4	T45.2X5	T45.2X6
Cobalt (nonmedicinal) (fumes) (industrial)	T56.891	T56.892	T56.893	T56.894	—	—
medicinal (trace) (chloride)	T45.8X1	T45.8X2	T45.8X3	T45.8X4	T45.8X5	T45.8X6
Cobra (venom)	T63.041	T63.042	T63.043	T63.044	—	—
Coca (leaf)	T40.5X1	T40.5X2	T40.5X3	T40.5X4	T40.5X5	T40.5X6
Cocaine	T40.5X1	T40.5X2	T40.5X3	T40.5X4	T40.5X5	T40.5X6
topical anesthetic	T41.3X1	T41.3X2	T41.3X3	T41.3X4	T41.3X5	T41.3X6
Cocarboxylase	T45.3X1	T45.3X2	T45.3X3	T45.3X4	T45.3X5	T45.3X6
Coccidioidin	T50.8X1	T50.8X2	T50.8X3	T50.8X4	T50.8X5	T50.8X6
Cocculus indicus	T62.1X1	T62.1X2	T62.1X3	T62.1X4	—	—
Cochineal	T65.6X1	T65.6X2	T65.6X3	T65.6X4	—	—
medicinal products	T50.991	T50.992	T50.993	T50.994	T50.995	T50.996
Codeine	T40.2X1	T40.2X2	T40.2X3	T40.2X4	T40.2X5	T40.2X6
Cod-liver oil	T45.2X1	T45.2X2	T45.2X3	T45.2X4	T45.2X5	T45.2X6
Coenzyme A	T50.991	T50.992	T50.993	T50.994	T50.995	T50.996
Coffee	T62.8X1	T62.8X2	T62.8X3	T62.8X4	—	—
Cogalactoisomerase	T50.991	T50.992	T50.993	T50.994	T50.995	T50.996
Cogentin	T44.3X1	T44.3X2	T44.3X3	T44.3X4	T44.3X5	T44.3X6
Coke fumes or gas (carbon monoxide)	T58.2X1	T58.2X2	T58.2X3	T58.2X4	—	—
industrial use	T58.8X1	T58.8X2	T58.8X3	T58.8X4	—	—
Colace	T47.4X1	T47.4X2	T47.4X3	T47.4X4	T47.4X5	T47.4X6
Colaspase	T45.1X1	T45.1X2	T45.1X3	T45.1X4	T45.1X5	T45.1X6
Colchicine	T50.4X1	T50.4X2	T50.4X3	T50.4X4	T50.4X5	T50.4X6
Colchicum	T62.2X1	T62.2X2	T62.2X3	T62.2X4	—	—
Cold cream	T49.3X1	T49.3X2	T49.3X3	T49.3X4	T49.3X5	T49.3X6
Colecalciferol	T45.2X1	T45.2X2	T45.2X3	T45.2X4	T45.2X5	T45.2X6
Colestipol	T46.6X1	T46.6X2	T46.6X3	T46.6X4	T46.6X5	T46.6X6
Colestyramine	T46.6X1	T46.6X2	T46.6X3	T46.6X4	T46.6X5	T46.6X6
Colimycin	T36.8X1	T36.8X2	T36.8X3	T36.8X4	T36.8X5	T36.8X6

Substance	Poisoning, Accidental (unintentional)	Poisoning, Intentional Self-harm	Poisoning, Assault	Poisoning, Undetermined	Adverse Effect	Under-dosing
Colistimethate	T36.8X1	T36.8X2	T36.8X3	T36.8X4	T36.8X5	T36.8X6
Colistin	T36.8X1	T36.8X2	T36.8X3	T36.8X4	T36.8X5	T36.8X6
sulfate (eye preparation)	T49.5X1	T49.5X2	T49.5X3	T49.5X4	T49.5X5	T49.5X6
Collagen	T50.991	T50.992	T50.993	T50.994	T50.995	T50.996
Collagenase	T49.4X1	T49.4X2	T49.4X3	T49.4X4	T49.4X5	T49.4X6
Collodion	T49.3X1	T49.3X2	T49.3X3	T49.3X4	T49.3X5	T49.3X6
Colocynth	T47.2X1	T47.2X2	T47.2X3	T47.2X4	T47.2X5	T47.2X6
Colophony adhesive	T49.3X1	T49.3X2	T49.3X3	T49.3X4	T49.3X5	T49.3X6
Colorant — see Dye	T50.991	T50.992	T50.993	T50.994	T50.995	T50.996
Coloring matter — see Dye(s)						
Combustion gas (after combustion) — see Carbon, monoxide						
prior to combustion	T59.891	T59.892	T59.893	T59.894	—	—
Compazine	T43.3X1	T43.3X2	T43.3X3	T43.3X4	T43.3X5	T43.3X6
Compound						
1080 (sodium fluoroacetate)	T60.4X1	T60.4X2	T60.4X3	T60.4X4	—	—
269 (endrin)	T60.1X1	T60.1X2	T60.1X3	T60.1X4	—	—
3422 (parathion)	T60.0X1	T60.0X2	T60.0X3	T60.0X4	—	—
3911 (phorate)	T60.0X1	T60.0X2	T60.0X3	T60.0X4	—	—
3956 (toxaphene)	T60.1X1	T60.1X2	T60.1X3	T60.1X4	—	—
4049 (malathion)	T60.0X1	T60.0X2	T60.0X3	T60.0X4	—	—
4069 (malathion)	T60.0X1	T60.0X2	T60.0X3	T60.0X4	—	—
4124 (dicapthon)	T60.0X1	T60.0X2	T60.0X3	T60.0X4	—	—
42 (warfarin)	T60.4X1	T60.4X2	T60.4X3	T60.4X4	—	—
497 (dieldrin)	T60.1X1	T60.1X2	T60.1X3	T60.1X4	—	—
E (cortisone)	T38.0X1	T38.0X2	T38.0X3	T38.0X4	T38.0X5	T38.0X6
F (hydrocortisone)	T38.0X1	T38.0X2	T38.0X3	T38.0X4	T38.0X5	T38.0X6
Congener, anabolic	T38.7X1	T38.7X2	T38.7X3	T38.7X4	T38.7X5	T38.7X6
Congo red	T50.8X1	T50.8X2	T50.8X3	T50.8X4	T50.8X5	T50.8X6
Coniine, conine	T62.2X1	T62.2X2	T62.2X3	T62.2X4	—	—
Conium (maculatum)	T62.2X1	T62.2X2	T62.2X3	T62.2X4	—	—
Conjugated estrogenic substances	T38.5X1	T38.5X2	T38.5X3	T38.5X4	T38.5X5	T38.5X6
Contac	T48.5X1	T48.5X2	T48.5X3	T48.5X4	T48.5X5	T48.5X6
Contact lens solution	T49.5X1	T49.5X2	T49.5X3	T49.5X4	T49.5X5	T49.5X6
Contraceptive (oral)	T38.4X1	T38.4X2	T38.4X3	T38.4X4	T38.4X5	T38.4X6
vaginal	T49.8X1	T49.8X2	T49.8X3	T49.8X4	T49.8X5	T49.8X6
Contrast medium, radiography	T50.8X1	T50.8X2	T50.8X3	T50.8X4	T50.8X5	T50.8X6
Convallaria glycosides	T46.0X1	T46.0X2	T46.0X3	T46.0X4	T46.0X5	T46.0X6
Convallaria majalis	T62.2X1	T62.2X2	T62.2X3	T62.2X4	—	—
berry	T62.1X1	T62.1X2	T62.1X3	T62.1X4	—	—
Copperhead snake (bite) (venom)	T63.061	T63.062	T63.063	T63.064	—	—
Copper (dust) (fumes) (nonmedicinal) NEC	T56.4X1	T56.4X2	T56.4X3	T56.4X4	—	—
arsenate, arsenite	T57.0X1	T57.0X2	T57.0X3	T57.0X4	—	—
insecticide	T60.2X1	T60.2X2	T60.2X3	T60.2X4	—	—
emetic	T47.7X1	T47.7X2	T47.7X3	T47.7X4	T47.7X5	T47.7X6
fungicide	T60.3X1	T60.3X2	T60.3X3	T60.3X4	—	—
gluconate	T49.0X1	T49.0X2	T49.0X3	T49.0X4	T49.0X5	T49.0X6
insecticide	T60.2X1	T60.2X2	T60.2X3	T60.2X4	—	—
medicinal (trace)	T45.8X1	T45.8X2	T45.8X3	T45.8X4	T45.8X5	T45.8X6
oleate	T49.0X1	T49.0X2	T49.0X3	T49.0X4	T49.0X5	T49.0X6
sulfate	T56.4X1	T56.4X2	T56.4X3	T56.4X4	—	—
cupric	T56.4X1	T56.4X2	T56.4X3	T56.4X4	—	—
fungicide	T60.3X1	T60.3X2	T60.3X3	T60.3X4	—	—
medicinal						
ear	T49.6X1	T49.6X2	T49.6X3	T49.6X4	T49.6X5	T49.6X6
emetic	T47.7X1	T47.7X2	T47.7X3	T47.7X4	T47.7X5	T47.7X6
eye	T49.5X1	T49.5X2	T49.5X3	T49.5X4	T49.5X5	T49.5X6
cuprous	T56.4X1	T56.4X2	T56.4X3	T56.4X4	—	—
fungicide	T60.3X1	T60.3X2	T60.3X3	T60.3X4	—	—
medicinal						
ear	T49.6X1	T49.6X2	T49.6X3	T49.6X4	T49.6X5	T49.6X6
emetic	T47.7X1	T47.7X2	T47.7X3	T47.7X4	T47.7X5	T47.7X6
eye	T49.5X1	T49.5X2	T49.5X3	T49.5X4	T49.5X5	T49.5X6
Coral (sting)	T63.691	T63.692	T63.693	T63.694	—	—
snake (bite) (venom)	T63.021	T63.022	T63.023	T63.024	—	—
Corbadrine	T49.6X1	T49.6X2	T49.6X3	T49.6X4	T49.6X5	T49.6X6
Cordite	T65.891	T65.892	T65.893	T65.894	—	—
vapor	T59.891	T59.892	T59.893	T59.894	—	—
Cordran	T49.0X1	T49.0X2	T49.0X3	T49.0X4	T49.0X5	T49.0X6
Corn cures	T49.4X1	T49.4X2	T49.4X3	T49.4X4	T49.4X5	T49.4X6
Cornhusker's lotion	T49.3X1	T49.3X2	T49.3X3	T49.3X4	T49.3X5	T49.3X6
Corn starch	T49.3X1	T49.3X2	T49.3X3	T49.3X4	T49.3X5	T49.3X6
Coronary vasodilator NEC	T46.3X1	T46.3X2	T46.3X3	T46.3X4	T46.3X5	T46.3X6
Corrosive NEC	T54.91	T54.92	T54.93	T54.94	—	—
acid NEC	T54.2X1	T54.2X2	T54.2X3	T54.2X4	—	—
aromatics	T54.1X1	T54.1X2	T54.1X3	T54.1X4	—	—
disinfectant	T54.1X1	T54.1X2	T54.1X3	T54.1X4	—	—

Substance	Poisoning, Accidental (unintentional)	Poisoning, Intentional Self-harm	Poisoning, Assault	Poisoning, Undetermined	Adverse Effect	Under-dosing
Corrosive — *continued*						
fumes NEC	T54.91	T54.92	T54.93	T54.94	—	—
specified NEC	T54.91	T54.92	T54.93	T54.94	—	—
sublimate	T56.1X1	T56.1X2	T56.1X3	T56.1X4	—	—
Cortate	T38.0X1	T38.0X2	T38.0X3	T38.0X4	T38.0X5	T38.0X6
Cort-Dome	T38.0X1	T38.0X2	T38.0X3	T38.0X4	T38.0X5	T38.0X6
ENT agent	T49.6X1	T49.6X2	T49.6X3	T49.6X4	T49.6X5	T49.6X6
ophthalmic preparation	T49.5X1	T49.5X2	T49.5X3	T49.5X4	T49.5X5	T49.5X6
topical NEC	T49.0X1	T49.0X2	T49.0X3	T49.0X4	T49.0X5	T49.0X6
Cortef	T38.0X1	T38.0X2	T38.0X3	T38.0X4	T38.0X5	T38.0X6
ENT agent	T49.6X1	T49.6X2	T49.6X3	T49.6X4	T49.6X5	T49.6X6
ophthalmic preparation	T49.5X1	T49.5X2	T49.5X3	T49.5X4	T49.5X5	T49.5X6
topical NEC	T49.0X1	T49.0X2	T49.0X3	T49.0X4	T49.0X5	T49.0X6
Corticosteroid	T38.0X1	T38.0X2	T38.0X3	T38.0X4	T38.0X5	T38.0X6
ENT agent	T49.6X1	T49.6X2	T49.6X3	T49.6X4	T49.6X5	T49.6X6
mineral	T50.0X1	T50.0X2	T50.0X3	T50.0X4	T50.0X5	T50.0X6
ophthalmic	T49.5X1	T49.5X2	T49.5X3	T49.5X4	T49.5X5	T49.5X6
topical NEC	T49.0X1	T49.0X2	T49.0X3	T49.0X4	T49.0X5	T49.0X6
Corticotropin	T38.811	T38.812	T38.813	T38.814	T38.815	T38.816
Cortisol	T49.0X1	T49.0X2	T49.0X3	T49.0X4	T49.0X5	T49.0X6
ENT agent	T49.6X1	T49.6X2	T49.6X3	T49.6X4	T49.6X5	T49.6X6
ophthalmic preparation	T49.5X1	T49.5X2	T49.5X3	T49.5X4	T49.5X5	T49.5X6
topical NEC	T49.0X1	T49.0X2	T49.0X3	T49.0X4	T49.0X5	T49.0X6
Cortisone (acetate)	T38.0X1	T38.0X2	T38.0X3	T38.0X4	T38.0X5	T38.0X6
ENT agent	T49.6X1	T49.6X2	T49.6X3	T49.6X4	T49.6X5	T49.6X6
ophthalmic preparation	T49.5X1	T49.5X2	T49.5X3	T49.5X4	T49.5X5	T49.5X6
topical NEC	T49.0X1	T49.0X2	T49.0X3	T49.0X4	T49.0X5	T49.0X6
Cortivazol	T38.0X1	T38.0X2	T38.0X3	T38.0X4	T38.0X5	T38.0X6
Cortogen	T38.0X1	T38.0X2	T38.0X3	T38.0X4	T38.0X5	T38.0X6
ENT agent	T49.6X1	T49.6X2	T49.6X3	T49.6X4	T49.6X5	T49.6X6
ophthalmic preparation	T49.5X1	T49.5X2	T49.5X3	T49.5X4	T49.5X5	T49.5X6
Cortone	T38.0X1	T38.0X2	T38.0X3	T38.0X4	T38.0X5	T38.0X6
ENT agent	T49.6X1	T49.6X2	T49.6X3	T49.6X4	T49.6X5	T49.6X6
ophthalmic preparation	T49.5X1	T49.5X2	T49.5X3	T49.5X4	T49.5X5	T49.5X6
Cortril	T38.0X1	T38.0X2	T38.0X3	T38.0X4	T38.0X5	T38.0X6
ENT agent	T49.6X1	T49.6X2	T49.6X3	T49.6X4	T49.6X5	T49.6X6
ophthalmic preparation	T49.5X1	T49.5X2	T49.5X3	T49.5X4	T49.5X5	T49.5X6
topical NEC	T49.0X1	T49.0X2	T49.0X3	T49.0X4	T49.0X5	T49.0X6
Corynebacterium parvum	T45.1X1	T45.1X2	T45.1X3	T45.1X4	T45.1X5	T45.1X6
Cosmetic preparation	T49.8X1	T49.8X2	T49.8X3	T49.8X4	T49.8X5	T49.8X6
Cosmetics	T49.8X1	T49.8X2	T49.8X3	T49.8X4	T49.8X5	T49.8X6
Cosyntropin	T38.811	T38.812	T38.813	T38.814	T38.815	T38.816
Cotarnine	T45.7X1	T45.7X2	T45.7X3	T45.7X4	T45.7X5	T45.7X6
Co-trimoxazole	T36.8X1	T36.8X2	T36.8X3	T36.8X4	T36.8X5	T36.8X6
Cottonseed oil	T49.3X1	T49.3X2	T49.3X3	T49.3X4	T49.3X5	T49.3X6
Cough mixture (syrup)	T48.4X1	T48.4X2	T48.4X3	T48.4X4	T48.4X5	T48.4X6
containing opiates	T40.2X1	T40.2X2	T40.2X3	T40.2X4	T40.2X5	T40.2X6
expectorants	T48.4X1	T48.4X2	T48.4X3	T48.4X4	T48.4X5	T48.4X6
Coumadin	T45.511	T45.512	T45.513	T45.514	T45.515	T45.516
rodenticide	T60.4X1	T60.4X2	T60.4X3	T60.4X4	—	—
Coumaphos	T60.0X1	T60.0X2	T60.0X3	T60.0X4	—	—
Coumarin	T45.511	T45.512	T45.513	T45.514	T45.515	T45.516
Coumetarol	T45.511	T45.512	T45.513	T45.514	T45.515	T45.516
Cowbane	T62.2X1	T62.2X2	T62.2X3	T62.2X4	—	—
Cozyme	T45.2X1	T45.2X2	T45.2X3	T45.2X4	T45.2X5	T45.2X6
Crack	T40.5X1	T40.5X2	T40.5X3	T40.5X4	—	—
Crataegus extract	T46.0X1	T46.0X2	T46.0X3	T46.0X4	T46.0X5	T46.0X6
Creolin	T54.1X1	T54.1X2	T54.1X3	T54.1X4	—	—
disinfectant	T54.1X1	T54.1X2	T54.1X3	T54.1X4	—	—
Creosol (compound)	T49.0X1	T49.0X2	T49.0X3	T49.0X4	T49.0X5	T49.0X6
Creosote (coal tar)	T49.0X1	T49.0X2	T49.0X3	T49.0X4	T49.0X5	T49.0X6
(beechwood)						
medicinal (expectorant)	T48.4X1	T48.4X2	T48.4X3	T48.4X4	T48.4X5	T48.4X6
syrup	T48.4X1	T48.4X2	T48.4X3	T48.4X4	T48.4X5	T48.4X6
Cresol(s)	T49.0X1	T49.0X2	T49.0X3	T49.0X4	T49.0X5	T49.0X6
and soap solution	T49.0X1	T49.0X2	T49.0X3	T49.0X4	T49.0X5	T49.0X6
Cresyl acetate	T49.0X1	T49.0X2	T49.0X3	T49.0X4	T49.0X5	T49.0X6
Cresylic acid	T49.0X1	T49.0X2	T49.0X3	T49.0X4	T49.0X5	T49.0X6
Crimidine	T60.4X1	T60.4X2	T60.4X3	T60.4X4	—	—
Croconazole	T37.8X1	T37.8X2	T37.8X3	T37.8X4	T37.8X5	T37.8X6
Cromoglicic acid	T48.6X1	T48.6X2	T48.6X3	T48.6X4	T48.6X5	T48.6X6
Cromolyn	T48.6X1	T48.6X2	T48.6X3	T48.6X4	T48.6X5	T48.6X6
Cromonar	T46.3X1	T46.3X2	T46.3X3	T46.3X4	T46.3X5	T46.3X6
Cropropamide	T39.8X1	T39.8X2	T39.8X3	T39.8X4	T39.8X5	T39.8X6
with crotethamide	T50.7X1	T50.7X2	T50.7X3	T50.7X4	T50.7X5	T50.7X6
Crotamiton	T49.0X1	T49.0X2	T49.0X3	T49.0X4	T49.0X5	T49.0X6
Crotethamide	T39.8X1	T39.8X2	T39.8X3	T39.8X4	T39.8X5	T39.8X6
with cropropamide	T50.7X1	T50.7X2	T50.7X3	T50.7X4	T50.7X5	T50.7X6
Croton (oil)	T47.2X1	T47.2X2	T47.2X3	T47.2X4	T47.2X5	T47.2X6
chloral	T42.6X1	T42.6X2	T42.6X3	T42.6X4	T42.6X5	T42.6X6
Crude oil	T52.0X1	T52.0X2	T52.0X3	T52.0X4	—	—
Cryogenine	T39.8X1	T39.8X2	T39.8X3	T39.8X4	T39.8X5	T39.8X6
Cryolite (vapor)	T60.1X1	T60.1X2	T60.1X3	T60.1X4	—	—

Substance	Poisoning, Accidental (unintentional)	Poisoning, Intentional Self-harm	Poisoning, Assault	Poisoning, Undetermined	Adverse Effect	Under-dosing
Cryolite — *continued*						
insecticide	T60.1X1	T60.1X2	T60.1X3	T60.1X4	—	—
Cryptenamine (tannates)	T46.5X1	T46.5X2	T46.5X3	T46.5X4	T46.5X5	T46.5X6
Crystal violet	T49.0X1	T49.0X2	T49.0X3	T49.0X4	T49.0X5	T49.0X6
Cuckoopint	T62.2X1	T62.2X2	T62.2X3	T62.2X4	—	—
Cumetharol	T45.511	T45.512	T45.513	T45.514	T45.515	T45.516
Cupric						
acetate	T60.3X1	T60.3X2	T60.3X3	T60.3X4	—	—
acetoarsenite	T57.0X1	T57.0X2	T57.0X3	T57.0X4	—	—
arsenate	T57.0X1	T57.0X2	T57.0X3	T57.0X4	—	—
gluconate	T49.0X1	T49.0X2	T49.0X3	T49.0X4	T49.0X5	T49.0X6
oleate	T49.0X1	T49.0X2	T49.0X3	T49.0X4	T49.0X5	T49.0X6
sulfate	T56.4X1	T56.4X2	T56.4X3	T56.4X4	—	—
Cuprous sulfate — *see also*	T56.4X1	T56.4X2	T56.4X3	T56.4X4	—	—
Copper sulfate						
Curare, curarine	T48.1X1	T48.1X2	T48.1X3	T48.1X4	T48.1X5	T48.1X6
Cyamemazine	T43.3X1	T43.3X2	T43.3X3	T43.3X4	T43.3X5	T43.3X6
Cyamopsis tetragonoloba	T46.6X1	T46.6X2	T46.6X3	T46.6X4	T46.6X5	T46.6X6
Cyanacetyl hydrazide	T37.1X1	T37.1X2	T37.1X3	T37.1X4	T37.1X5	T37.1X6
Cyanic acid (gas)	T59.891	T59.892	T59.893	T59.894	—	—
Cyanide(s) (compounds)	T65.0X1	T65.0X2	T65.0X3	T65.0X4	—	—
(potassium) (sodium)						
NEC						
dust or gas (inhalation)	T57.3X1	T57.3X2	T57.3X3	T57.3X4	—	—
NEC						
fumigant	T65.0X1	T65.0X2	T65.0X3	T65.0X4	—	—
hydrogen	T57.3X1	T57.3X2	T57.3X3	T57.3X4	—	—
mercuric — *see* Mercury						
pesticide (dust) (fumes)	T65.0X1	T65.0X2	T65.0X3	T65.0X4	—	—
Cyanoacrylate adhesive	T49.3X1	T49.3X2	T49.3X3	T49.3X4	T49.3X5	T49.3X6
Cyanocobalamin	T45.8X1	T45.8X2	T45.8X3	T45.8X4	T45.8X5	T45.8X6
Cyanogen (chloride) (gas)	T59.891	T59.892	T59.893	T59.894	—	—
NEC						
Cyclacillin	T36.0X1	T36.0X2	T36.0X3	T36.0X4	T36.0X5	T36.0X6
Cyclaine	T41.3X1	T41.3X2	T41.3X3	T41.3X4	T41.3X5	T41.3X6
Cyclamate	T50.991	T50.992	T50.993	T50.994	T50.995	T50.996
Cyclamen europaeum	T62.2X1	T62.2X2	T62.2X3	T62.2X4	—	—
Cyclandelate	T46.7X1	T46.7X2	T46.7X3	T46.7X4	T46.7X5	T46.7X6
Cyclazocine	T50.7X1	T50.7X2	T50.7X3	T50.7X4	T50.7X5	T50.7X6
Cyclizine	T45.0X1	T45.0X2	T45.0X3	T45.0X4	T45.0X5	T45.0X6
Cyclobarbital	T42.3X1	T42.3X2	T42.3X3	T42.3X4	T42.3X5	T42.3X6
Cyclobarbitone	T42.3X1	T42.3X2	T42.3X3	T42.3X4	T42.3X5	T42.3X6
Cyclobenzaprine	T48.1X1	T48.1X2	T48.1X3	T48.1X4	T48.1X5	T48.1X6
Cyclodrine	T44.3X1	T44.3X2	T44.3X3	T44.3X4	T44.3X5	T44.3X6
Cycloguanil embonate	T37.2X1	T37.2X2	T37.2X3	T37.2X4	T37.2X5	T37.2X6
Cyclohexane	T52.8X1	T52.8X2	T52.8X3	T52.8X4	—	—
Cyclohexanol	T51.8X1	T51.8X2	T51.8X3	T51.8X4	—	—
Cyclohexanone	T52.4X1	T52.4X2	T52.4X3	T52.4X4	—	—
Cycloheximide	T60.3X1	T60.3X2	T60.3X3	T60.3X4	—	—
Cyclohexyl acetate	T52.8X1	T52.8X2	T52.8X3	T52.8X4	—	—
Cycloleucine	T45.1X1	T45.1X2	T45.1X3	T45.1X4	T45.1X5	T45.1X6
Cyclomethycaine	T41.3X1	T41.3X2	T41.3X3	T41.3X4	T41.3X5	T41.3X6
Cyclopentamine	T44.4X1	T44.4X2	T44.4X3	T44.4X4	T44.4X5	T44.4X6
Cyclopenthiazide	T50.2X1	T50.2X2	T50.2X3	T50.2X4	T50.2X5	T50.2X6
Cyclopentolate	T44.3X1	T44.3X2	T44.3X3	T44.3X4	T44.3X5	T44.3X6
Cyclophosphamide	T45.1X1	T45.1X2	T45.1X3	T45.1X4	T45.1X5	T45.1X6
Cycloplegic drug	T49.5X1	T49.5X2	T49.5X3	T49.5X4	T49.5X5	T49.5X6
Cyclopropane	T41.291	T41.292	T41.293	T41.294	T41.295	T41.296
Cyclopyrabital	T39.8X1	T39.8X2	T39.8X3	T39.8X4	T39.8X5	T39.8X6
Cycloserine	T37.1X1	T37.1X2	T37.1X3	T37.1X4	T37.1X5	T37.1X6
Cyclosporin	T45.1X1	T45.1X2	T45.1X3	T45.1X4	T45.1X5	T45.1X6
Cyclothiazide	T50.2X1	T50.2X2	T50.2X3	T50.2X4	T50.2X5	T50.2X6
Cycrimine	T44.3X1	T44.3X2	T44.3X3	T44.3X4	T44.3X5	T44.3X6
Cyhalothrin	T60.1X1	T60.1X2	T60.1X3	T60.1X4	—	—
Cymarin	T46.0X1	T46.0X2	T46.0X3	T46.0X4	T46.0X5	T46.0X6
Cypermethrin	T60.1X1	T60.1X2	T60.1X3	T60.1X4	—	—
Cyphenothrin	T60.2X1	T60.2X2	T60.2X3	T60.2X4	—	—
Cyproheptadine	T45.0X1	T45.0X2	T45.0X3	T45.0X4	T45.0X5	T45.0X6
Cyproterone	T38.6X1	T38.6X2	T38.6X3	T38.6X4	T38.6X5	T38.6X6
Cysteamine	T50.6X1	T50.6X2	T50.6X3	T50.6X4	T50.6X5	T50.6X6
Cytarabine	T45.1X1	T45.1X2	T45.1X3	T45.1X4	T45.1X5	T45.1X6
Cytisus						
laburnum	T62.2X1	T62.2X2	T62.2X3	T62.2X4	—	—
scoparius	T62.2X1	T62.2X2	T62.2X3	T62.2X4	—	—
Cytochrome C	T47.5X1	T47.5X2	T47.5X3	T47.5X4	T47.5X5	T47.5X6
Cytomel	T38.1X1	T38.1X2	T38.1X3	T38.1X4	T38.1X5	T38.1X6
Cytosine arabinoside	T45.1X1	T45.1X2	T45.1X3	T45.1X4	T45.1X5	T45.1X6
Cytoxan	T45.1X1	T45.1X2	T45.1X3	T45.1X4	T45.1X5	T45.1X6
Cytozyme	T45.7X1	T45.7X2	T45.7X3	T45.7X4	T45.7X5	T45.7X6
S-Carboxymethylcysteine	T48.4X1	T48.4X2	T48.4X3	T48.4X4	T48.4X5	T48.4X6
Dacarbazine	T45.1X1	T45.1X2	T45.1X3	T45.1X4	T45.1X5	T45.1X6
Dactinomycin	T45.1X1	T45.1X2	T45.1X3	T45.1X4	T45.1X5	T45.1X6
DADPS	T37.1X1	T37.1X2	T37.1X3	T37.1X4	T37.1X5	T37.1X6

Substance	Poisoning, Accidental (unintentional)	Poisoning, Intentional Self-harm	Poisoning, Assault	Poisoning, Undetermined	Adverse Effect	Under-dosing
Dakin's solution	T49.0X1	T49.0X2	T49.0X3	T49.0X4	T49.0X5	T49.0X6
Dalapon (sodium)	T60.3X1	T60.3X2	T60.3X3	T60.3X4	—	—
Dalmane	T42.4X1	T42.4X2	T42.4X3	T42.4X4	T42.4X5	T42.4X6
Danazol	T38.6X1	T38.6X2	T38.6X3	T38.6X4	T38.6X5	T38.6X6
Danilone	T45.511	T45.512	T45.513	T45.514	T45.515	T45.516
Danthron	T47.2X1	T47.2X2	T47.2X3	T47.2X4	T47.2X5	T47.2X6
Dantrolene	T42.8X1	T42.8X2	T42.8X3	T42.8X4	T42.8X5	T42.8X6
Dantron	T47.2X1	T47.2X2	T47.2X3	T47.2X4	T47.2X5	T47.2X6
Daphne (gnidium) (mezereum)	T62.2X1	T62.2X2	T62.2X3	T62.2X4	—	—
berry	T62.1X1	T62.1X2	T62.1X3	T62.1X4	—	—
Dapsone	T37.1X1	T37.1X2	T37.1X3	T37.1X4	T37.1X5	T37.1X6
Daraprim	T37.2X1	T37.2X2	T37.2X3	T37.2X4	T37.2X5	T37.2X6
Darnel	T62.2X1	T62.2X2	T62.2X3	T62.2X4	—	—
Darvon	T39.8X1	T39.8X2	T39.8X3	T39.8X4	T39.8X5	T39.8X6
Daunomycin	T45.1X1	T45.1X2	T45.1X3	T45.1X4	T45.1X5	T45.1X6
Daunorubicin	T45.1X1	T45.1X2	T45.1X3	T45.1X4	T45.1X5	T45.1X6
DBI	T38.3X1	T38.3X2	T38.3X3	T38.3X4	T38.3X5	T38.3X6
D-Con	T60.91	T60.92	T60.93	T60.94	—	—
insecticide	T60.2X1	T60.2X2	T60.2X3	T60.2X4	—	—
rodenticide	T60.4X1	T60.4X2	T60.4X3	T60.4X4	—	—
DDAVP	T38.891	T38.892	T38.893	T38.894	T38.895	T38.896
DDE (bis(chlorophenyl)- dichloroethylene)	T60.2X1	T60.2X2	T60.2X3	T60.2X4	—	—
DDS	T37.1X1	T37.1X2	T37.1X3	T37.1X4	T37.1X5	T37.1X6
DDT (dust)	T60.1X1	T60.1X2	T60.1X3	T60.1X4	—	—
Deadly nightshade — see also Belladonna	T62.2X1	T62.2X2	T62.2X3	T62.2X4	—	—
berry	T62.1X1	T62.1X2	T62.1X3	T62.1X4	—	—
Deamino-D-arginine vasopressin	T38.891	T38.892	T38.893	T38.894	T38.895	T38.896
Deanol (aceglumate)	T50.991	T50.992	T50.993	T50.994	T50.995	T50.996
Debrisoquine	T46.5X1	T46.5X2	T46.5X3	T46.5X4	T46.5X5	T46.5X6
Decaborane	T57.8X1	T57.8X2	T57.8X3	T57.8X4	—	—
fumes	T59.891	T59.892	T59.893	T59.894	—	—
Decadron	T38.0X1	T38.0X2	T38.0X3	T38.0X4	T38.0X5	T38.0X6
ENT agent	T49.6X1	T49.6X2	T49.6X3	T49.6X4	T49.6X5	T49.6X6
ophthalmic preparation	T49.5X1	T49.5X2	T49.5X3	T49.5X4	T49.5X5	T49.5X6
topical NEC	T49.0X1	T49.0X2	T49.0X3	T49.0X4	T49.0X5	T49.0X6
Decahydronaphthalene	T52.8X1	T52.8X2	T52.8X3	T52.8X4	—	—
Decalin	T52.8X1	T52.8X2	T52.8X3	T52.8X4	—	—
Decamethonium (bromide)	T48.1X1	T48.1X2	T48.1X3	T48.1X4	T48.1X5	T48.1X6
Decholin	T47.5X1	T47.5X2	T47.5X3	T47.5X4	T47.5X5	T47.5X6
Declomycin	T36.4X1	T36.4X2	T36.4X3	T36.4X4	T36.4X5	T36.4X6
Decongestant, nasal (mucosa)	T48.5X1	T48.5X2	T48.5X3	T48.5X4	T48.5X5	T48.5X6
combination	T48.5X1	T48.5X2	T48.5X3	T48.5X4	T48.5X5	T48.5X6
Deet	T60.8X1	T60.8X2	T60.8X3	T60.8X4	—	—
Deferoxamine	T45.8X1	T45.8X2	T45.8X3	T45.8X4	T45.8X5	T45.8X6
Deflazacort	T38.0X1	T38.0X2	T38.0X3	T38.0X4	T38.0X5	T38.0X6
Deglycyrrhizinized extract of licorice	T48.4X1	T48.4X2	T48.4X3	T48.4X4	T48.4X5	T48.4X6
Dehydrocholic acid	T47.5X1	T47.5X2	T47.5X3	T47.5X4	T47.5X5	T47.5X6
Dehydroemetine	T37.3X1	T37.3X2	T37.3X3	T37.3X4	T37.3X5	T37.3X6
Dekalin	T52.8X1	T52.8X2	T52.8X3	T52.8X4	—	—
Delalutin	T38.5X1	T38.5X2	T38.5X3	T38.5X4	T38.5X5	T38.5X6
Delorazepam	T42.4X1	T42.4X2	T42.4X3	T42.4X4	T42.4X5	T42.4X6
Delphinium	T62.2X1	T62.2X2	T62.2X3	T62.2X4	—	—
Deltamethrin	T60.1X1	T60.1X2	T60.1X3	T60.1X4	—	—
Deltasone	T38.0X1	T38.0X2	T38.0X3	T38.0X4	T38.0X5	T38.0X6
Delta	T38.0X1	T38.0X2	T38.0X3	T38.0X4	T38.0X5	T38.0X6
Delvinal	T42.3X1	T42.3X2	T42.3X3	T42.3X4	T42.3X5	T42.3X6
Demecarium (bromide)	T49.5X1	T49.5X2	T49.5X3	T49.5X4	T49.5X5	T49.5X6
Demeclocycline	T36.4X1	T36.4X2	T36.4X3	T36.4X4	T36.4X5	T36.4X6
Demecolcine	T45.1X1	T45.1X2	T45.1X3	T45.1X4	T45.1X5	T45.1X6
Demegestone	T38.5X1	T38.5X2	T38.5X3	T38.5X4	T38.5X5	T38.5X6
Demelanizing agents	T49.8X1	T49.8X2	T49.8X3	T49.8X4	T49.8X5	T49.8X6
Demephion -O and -S	T60.0X1	T60.0X2	T60.0X3	T60.0X4	—	—
Demerol	T40.2X1	T40.2X2	T40.2X3	T40.2X4	T40.2X5	T40.2X6
Demethylchlortetracycline	T36.4X1	T36.4X2	T36.4X3	T36.4X4	T36.4X5	T36.4X6
Demethyltetracycline	T36.4X1	T36.4X2	T36.4X3	T36.4X4	T36.4X5	T36.4X6
Demeton -O and -S	T60.0X1	T60.0X2	T60.0X3	T60.0X4	—	—
Demulcent (external)	T49.3X1	T49.3X2	T49.3X3	T49.3X4	T49.3X5	T49.3X6
specified NEC	T49.3X1	T49.3X2	T49.3X3	T49.3X4	T49.3X5	T49.3X6
Demulen	T38.4X1	T38.4X2	T38.4X3	T38.4X4	T38.4X5	T38.4X6
Denatured alcohol	T51.0X1	T51.0X2	T51.0X3	T51.0X4	—	—
Dendrid	T49.5X1	T49.5X2	T49.5X3	T49.5X4	T49.5X5	T49.5X6
Dental drug, topical application NEC	T49.7X1	T49.7X2	T49.7X3	T49.7X4	T49.7X5	T49.7X6
Dentifrice	T49.7X1	T49.7X2	T49.7X3	T49.7X4	T49.7X5	T49.7X6
Deodorant spray (feminine hygiene)	T49.8X1	T49.8X2	T49.8X3	T49.8X4	T49.8X5	T49.8X6
Deoxycortone	T50.0X1	T50.0X2	T50.0X3	T50.0X4	T50.0X5	T50.0X6

Substance	Poisoning, Accidental (unintentional)	Poisoning, Intentional Self-harm	Poisoning, Assault	Poisoning, Undetermined	Adverse Effect	Under-dosing
Deoxyribonuclease (pancreatic)	T45.3X1	T45.3X2	T45.3X3	T45.3X4	T45.3X5	T45.3X6
Depilatory	T49.4X1	T49.4X2	T49.4X3	T49.4X4	T49.4X5	T49.4X6
Deprenalin	T42.8X1	T42.8X2	T42.8X3	T42.8X4	T42.8X5	T42.8X6
Deprenyl	T42.8X1	T42.8X2	T42.8X3	T42.8X4	T42.8X5	T42.8X6
Depressant						
appetite (central)	T50.5X1	T50.5X2	T50.5X3	T50.5X4	T50.5X5	T50.5X6
cardiac	T46.2X1	T46.2X2	T46.2X3	T46.2X4	T46.2X5	T46.2X6
central nervous system (anesthetic) — see also Central nervous system, depressants	T42.71	T42.72	T42.73	T42.74	T42.75	T42.76
general anesthetic	T41.201	T41.202	T41.203	T41.204	T41.205	T41.206
muscle tone	T42.8X1	T42.8X2	T42.8X3	T42.8X4	T42.8X5	T42.8X6
muscle tone, central	T42.8X1	T42.8X2	T42.8X3	T42.8X4	T42.8X5	T42.8X6
psychotherapeutic	T43.501	T43.502	T43.503	T43.504	T43.505	T43.506
Depressant, appetite	T50.5X1	T50.5X2	T50.5X3	T50.5X4	T50.5X5	T50.5X6
Deptropine	T45.0X1	T45.0X2	T45.0X3	T45.0X4	T45.0X5	T45.0X6
Dequalinium (chloride)	T49.0X1	T49.0X2	T49.0X3	T49.0X4	T49.0X5	T49.0X6
Derris root	T60.2X1	T60.2X2	T60.2X3	T60.2X4	—	—
Deserpidine	T46.5X1	T46.5X2	T46.5X3	T46.5X4	T46.5X5	T46.5X6
Desferrioxamine	T45.8X1	T45.8X2	T45.8X3	T45.8X4	T45.8X5	T45.8X6
Desipramine	T43.011	T43.012	T43.013	T43.014	T43.015	T43.016
Deslanoside	T46.0X1	T46.0X2	T46.0X3	T46.0X4	T46.0X5	T46.0X6
Desloughing agent	T49.4X1	T49.4X2	T49.4X3	T49.4X4	T49.4X5	T49.4X6
Desmethylimipramine	T43.011	T43.012	T43.013	T43.014	T43.015	T43.016
Desmopressin	T38.891	T38.892	T38.893	T38.894	T38.895	T38.896
Desocodeine	T40.2X1	T40.2X2	T40.2X3	T40.2X4	T40.2X5	T40.2X6
Desogestrel	T38.5X1	T38.5X2	T38.5X3	T38.5X4	T38.5X5	T38.5X6
Desomorphine	T40.2X1	T40.2X2	T40.2X3	T40.2X4	—	—
Desonide	T49.0X1	T49.0X2	T49.0X3	T49.0X4	T49.0X5	T49.0X6
Desoximetasone	T49.0X1	T49.0X2	T49.0X3	T49.0X4	T49.0X5	T49.0X6
Desoxycorticosteroid	T50.0X1	T50.0X2	T50.0X3	T50.0X4	T50.0X5	T50.0X6
Desoxycortone	T50.0X1	T50.0X2	T50.0X3	T50.0X4	T50.0X5	T50.0X6
Desoxyephedrine	T43.621	T43.622	T43.623	T43.624	T43.625	T43.626
Detaxtran	T46.6X1	T46.6X2	T46.6X3	T46.6X4	T46.6X5	T46.6X6
Detergent	T49.2X1	T49.2X2	T49.2X3	T49.2X4	T49.2X5	T49.2X6
external medication	T49.2X1	T49.2X2	T49.2X3	T49.2X4	T49.2X5	T49.2X6
local	T49.2X1	T49.2X2	T49.2X3	T49.2X4	T49.2X5	T49.2X6
medicinal	T49.2X1	T49.2X2	T49.2X3	T49.2X4	T49.2X5	T49.2X6
nonmedicinal	T55.1X1	T55.1X2	T55.1X3	T55.1X4	—	—
specified NEC	T55.1X1	T55.1X2	T55.1X3	T55.1X4	—	—
Deterrent, alcohol	T50.6X1	T50.6X2	T50.6X3	T50.6X4	T50.6X5	T50.6X6
Detoxifying agent	T50.6X1	T50.6X2	T50.6X3	T50.6X4	T50.6X5	T50.6X6
Detrothyronine	T38.1X1	T38.1X2	T38.1X3	T38.1X4	T38.1X5	T38.1X6
Dettol (external medication)	T49.0X1	T49.0X2	T49.0X3	T49.0X4	T49.0X5	T49.0X6
Dexamethasone	T38.0X1	T38.0X2	T38.0X3	T38.0X4	T38.0X5	T38.0X6
ENT agent	T49.6X1	T49.6X2	T49.6X3	T49.6X4	T49.6X5	T49.6X6
ophthalmic preparation	T49.5X1	T49.5X2	T49.5X3	T49.5X4	T49.5X5	T49.5X6
topical NEC	T49.0X1	T49.0X2	T49.0X3	T49.0X4	T49.0X5	T49.0X6
Dexamfetamine	T43.621	T43.622	T43.623	T43.624	T43.625	T43.626
Dexamphetamine	T43.621	T43.622	T43.623	T43.624	T43.625	T43.626
Dexbrompheniramine	T45.0X1	T45.0X2	T45.0X3	T45.0X4	T45.0X5	T45.0X6
Dexchlorpheniramine	T45.0X1	T45.0X2	T45.0X3	T45.0X4	T45.0X5	T45.0X6
Dexedrine	T43.621	T43.622	T43.623	T43.624	T43.625	T43.626
Dexetimide	T44.3X1	T44.3X2	T44.3X3	T44.3X4	T44.3X5	T44.3X6
Dexfenfluramine	T50.5X1	T50.5X2	T50.5X3	T50.5X4	T50.5X5	T50.5X6
Dexpanthenol	T45.2X1	T45.2X2	T45.2X3	T45.2X4	T45.2X5	T45.2X6
Dextran (40) (70) (150)	T45.8X1	T45.8X2	T45.8X3	T45.8X4	T45.8X5	T45.8X6
Dextriferron	T45.4X1	T45.4X2	T45.4X3	T45.4X4	T45.4X5	T45.4X6
Dextroamphetamine	T43.621	T43.622	T43.623	T43.624	T43.625	T43.626
Dextro calcium pantothenate	T45.2X1	T45.2X2	T45.2X3	T45.2X4	T45.2X5	T45.2X6
Dextromethorphan	T48.3X1	T48.3X2	T48.3X3	T48.3X4	T48.3X5	T48.3X6
Dextromoramide	T40.4X1	T40.4X2	T40.4X3	T40.4X4	—	—
topical	T49.8X1	T49.8X2	T49.8X3	T49.8X4	T49.8X5	T49.8X6
Dextro pantothenyl alcohol	T45.2X1	T45.2X2	T45.2X3	T45.2X4	T45.2X5	T45.2X6
Dextropropoxyphene	T40.4X1	T40.4X2	T40.4X3	T40.4X4	T40.4X5	T40.4X6
Dextrorphan	T40.2X1	T40.2X2	T40.2X3	T40.2X4	T40.2X5	T40.2X6
Dextrose	T50.3X1	T50.3X2	T50.3X3	T50.3X4	T50.3X5	T50.3X6
concentrated solution, intravenous	T46.8X1	T46.8X2	T46.8X3	T46.8X4	T46.8X5	T46.8X6
Dextrothyroxin	T38.1X1	T38.1X2	T38.1X3	T38.1X4	T38.1X5	T38.1X6
Dextrothyroxine sodium	T38.1X1	T38.1X2	T38.1X3	T38.1X4	T38.1X5	T38.1X6
DFP	T44.0X1	T44.0X2	T44.0X3	T44.0X4	T44.0X5	T44.0X6
DHE	T37.3X1	T37.3X2	T37.3X3	T37.3X4	T37.3X5	T37.3X6
45	T46.5X1	T46.5X2	T46.5X3	T46.5X4	T46.5X5	T46.5X6
Diabinese	T38.3X1	T38.3X2	T38.3X3	T38.3X4	T38.3X5	T38.3X6
Diacetone alcohol	T52.4X1	T52.4X2	T52.4X3	T52.4X4	—	—
Diacetyl monoxime	T50.991	T50.992	T50.993	T50.994	—	—
Diacetylmorphine	T40.1X1	T40.1X2	T40.1X3	T40.1X4	—	—
Diachylon plaster	T49.4X1	T49.4X2	T49.4X3	T49.4X4	T49.4X5	T49.4X6

Table of Drugs and Chemicals

Substance	Poisoning, Accidental (unintentional)	Poisoning, Intentional Self-harm	Poisoning, Assault	Poisoning, Undetermined	Adverse Effect	Under-dosing
Diaethylstilboestrolum	T38.5X1	T38.5X2	T38.5X3	T38.5X4	T38.5X5	T38.5X6
Diagnostic agent NEC	T50.8X1	T50.8X2	T50.8X3	T50.8X4	T50.8X5	T50.8X6
Dial (soap)	T49.2X1	T49.2X2	T49.2X3	T49.2X4	T49.2X5	T49.2X6
sedative	T42.3X1	T42.3X2	T42.3X3	T42.3X4	T42.3X5	T42.3X6
Dialkyl carbonate	T52.91	T52.92	T52.93	T52.94	—	—
Diallylbarbituric acid	T42.3X1	T42.3X2	T42.3X3	T42.3X4	T42.3X5	T42.3X6
Diallymal	T42.3X1	T42.3X2	T42.3X3	T42.3X4	T42.3X5	T42.3X6
Dialysis solution (intraperitoneal)	T50.3X1	T50.3X2	T50.3X3	T50.3X4	T50.3X5	T50.3X6
Diaminodiphenylsulfone	T37.1X1	T37.1X2	T37.1X3	T37.1X4	T37.1X5	T37.1X6
Diamorphine	T40.1X1	T40.1X2	T40.1X3	T40.1X4	—	—
Diamox	T50.2X1	T50.2X2	T50.2X3	T50.2X4	T50.2X5	T50.2X6
Diamthazole	T49.0X1	T49.0X2	T49.0X3	T49.0X4	T49.0X5	T49.0X6
Dianthone	T47.2X1	T47.2X2	T47.2X3	T47.2X4	T47.2X5	T47.2X6
Diaphenylsulfone	T37.0X1	T37.0X2	T37.0X3	T37.0X4	T37.0X5	T37.0X6
Diasone (sodium)	T37.1X1	T37.1X2	T37.1X3	T37.1X4	T37.1X5	T37.1X6
Diastase	T47.5X1	T47.5X2	T47.5X3	T47.5X4	T47.5X5	T47.5X6
Diatrizoate	T50.8X1	T50.8X2	T50.8X3	T50.8X4	T50.8X5	T50.8X6
Diazepam	T42.4X1	T42.4X2	T42.4X3	T42.4X4	T42.4X5	T42.4X6
Diazinon	T60.0X1	T60.0X2	T60.0X3	T60.0X4	—	—
Diazomethane (gas)	T59.891	T59.892	T59.893	T59.894		
Diazoxide	T46.5X1	T46.5X2	T46.5X3	T46.5X4	T46.5X5	T46.5X6
Dibekacin	T36.5X1	T36.5X2	T36.5X3	T36.5X4	T36.5X5	T36.5X6
Dibenamine	T44.6X1	T44.6X2	T44.6X3	T44.6X4	T44.6X5	T44.6X6
Dibenzepin	T43.011	T43.012	T43.013	T43.014	T43.015	T43.016
Dibenzheptropine	T45.0X1	T45.0X2	T45.0X3	T45.0X4	T45.0X5	T45.0X6
Dibenzyline	T44.6X1	T44.6X2	T44.6X3	T44.6X4	T44.6X5	T44.6X6
Diborane (gas)	T59.891	T59.892	T59.893	T59.894	—	—
Dibromochloropropane	T60.8X1	T60.8X2	T60.8X3	T60.8X4	—	—
Dibromodulcitol	T45.1X1	T45.1X2	T45.1X3	T45.1X4	T45.1X5	T45.1X6
Dibromoethane	T53.6X1	T53.6X2	T53.6X3	T53.6X4	—	—
Dibromomannitol	T45.1X1	T45.1X2	T45.1X3	T45.1X4	T45.1X5	T45.1X6
Dibromopropamidine isethionate	T49.0X1	T49.0X2	T49.0X3	T49.0X4	T49.0X5	T49.0X6
Dibrompropamidine	T49.0X1	T49.0X2	T49.0X3	T49.0X4	T49.0X5	T49.0X6
Dibucaine	T41.3X1	T41.3X2	T41.3X3	T41.3X4	T41.3X5	T41.3X6
topical (surface)	T41.3X1	T41.3X2	T41.3X3	T41.3X4	T41.3X5	T41.3X6
Dibunate sodium	T48.3X1	T48.3X2	T48.3X3	T48.3X4	T48.3X5	T48.3X6
Dibutoline sulfate	T44.3X1	T44.3X2	T44.3X3	T44.3X4	T44.3X5	T44.3X6
Dicamba	T60.3X1	T60.3X2	T60.3X3	T60.3X4	—	—
Dicapthon	T60.0X1	T60.0X2	T60.0X3	T60.0X4	—	—
Dichlobenil	T60.3X1	T60.3X2	T60.3X3	T60.3X4	—	—
Dichlone	T60.3X1	T60.3X2	T60.3X3	T60.3X4	—	—
Dichloralphenozone	T42.6X1	T42.6X2	T42.6X3	T42.6X4	T42.6X5	T42.6X6
Dichlorbenzidine	T65.3X1	T65.3X2	T65.3X3	T65.3X4	—	—
Dichlorhydrin	T52.8X1	T52.8X2	T52.8X3	T52.8X4	—	—
Dichlorhydroxyquinoline	T37.8X1	T37.8X2	T37.8X3	T37.8X4	T37.8X5	T37.8X6
Dichlorobenzene	T53.7X1	T53.7X2	T53.7X3	T53.7X4	—	—
Dichlorobenzyl alcohol	T49.6X1	T49.6X2	T49.6X3	T49.6X4	T49.6X5	T49.6X6
Dichlorodifluoromethane	T53.5X1	T53.5X2	T53.5X3	T53.5X4	—	—
Dichloroethane	T52.8X1	T52.8X2	T52.8X3	T52.8X4	—	—
Dichloroethylene	T53.6X1	T53.6X2	T53.6X3	T53.6X4	—	—
Dichloroethyl sulfide, not in war	T59.891	T59.892	T59.893	T59.894	—	—
Dichloroformoxime, not in war	T59.891	T59.892	T59.893	T59.894	—	—
Dichlorohydrin, alpha-dichlorohydrin	T52.8X1	T52.8X2	T52.8X3	T52.8X4	—	—
Dichloromethane (solvent)	T53.4X1	T53.4X2	T53.4X3	T53.4X4	—	—
vapor	T53.4X1	T53.4X2	T53.4X3	T53.4X4	—	—
Dichloronaphthoquinone	T60.3X1	T60.3X2	T60.3X3	T60.3X4	—	—
Dichlorophen	T37.4X1	T37.4X2	T37.4X3	T37.4X4	T37.4X5	T37.4X6
Dichloropropene	T60.3X1	T60.3X2	T60.3X3	T60.3X4	—	—
Dichloropropionic acid	T60.3X1	T60.3X2	T60.3X3	T60.3X4	—	—
Dichlorphenamide	T50.2X1	T50.2X2	T50.2X3	T50.2X4	T50.2X5	T50.2X6
Dichlorvos	T60.0X1	T60.0X2	T60.0X3	T60.0X4	—	—
Diclofenac	T39.391	T39.392	T39.393	T39.394	T39.395	T39.396
Diclofenamide	T50.2X1	T50.2X2	T50.2X3	T50.2X4	T50.2X5	T50.2X6
Diclofensine	T43.291	T43.292	T43.293	T43.294	T43.295	T43.296
Diclonixine	T39.8X1	T39.8X2	T39.8X3	T39.8X4	T39.8X5	T39.8X6
Dicloxacillin	T36.0X1	T36.0X2	T36.0X3	T36.0X4	T36.0X5	T36.0X6
Dicophane	T49.0X1	T49.0X2	T49.0X3	T49.0X4	T49.0X5	T49.0X6
Dicoumarol, dicoumarin, dicumarol	T45.511	T45.512	T45.513	T45.514	T45.515	T45.516
Dicrotophos	T60.0X1	T60.0X2	T60.0X3	T60.0X4	—	—
Dicyanogen (gas)	T65.0X1	T65.0X2	T65.0X3	T65.0X4	—	—
Dicyclomine	T44.3X1	T44.3X2	T44.3X3	T44.3X4	T44.3X5	T44.3X6
Dicycloverine	T44.3X1	T44.3X2	T44.3X3	T44.3X4	T44.3X5	T44.3X6
Dideoxycytidine	T37.5X1	T37.5X2	T37.5X3	T37.5X4	T37.5X5	T37.5X6
Dideoxyinosine	T37.5X1	T37.5X2	T37.5X3	T37.5X4	T37.5X5	T37.5X6
Dieldrin (vapor)	T60.1X1	T60.1X2	T60.1X3	T60.1X4	—	—
Diemal	T42.3X1	T42.3X2	T42.3X3	T42.3X4	T42.3X5	T42.3X6
Dienestrol	T38.5X1	T38.5X2	T38.5X3	T38.5X4	T38.5X5	T38.5X6
Dienoestrol	T38.5X1	T38.5X2	T38.5X3	T38.5X4	T38.5X5	T38.5X6
Dietetic drug NEC	T50.901	T50.902	T50.903	T50.904	T50.905	T50.906
Diethazine	T42.8X1	T42.8X2	T42.8X3	T42.8X4	T42.8X5	T42.8X6
Diethyl						
barbituric acid	T42.3X1	T42.3X2	T42.3X3	T42.3X4	T42.3X5	T42.3X6
carbamazine	T37.4X1	T37.4X2	T37.4X3	T37.4X4	T37.4X5	T37.4X6
carbinol	T51.3X1	T51.3X2	T51.3X3	T51.3X4	—	—
carbonate	T52.8X1	T52.8X2	T52.8X3	T52.8X4	—	—
ether (vapor) — see also ether	T41.0X1	T41.0X2	T41.0X3	T41.0X4	T41.0X5	T41.0X6
oxide	T52.8X1	T52.8X2	T52.8X3	T52.8X4	—	—
propion	T50.5X1	T50.5X2	T50.5X3	T50.5X4	T50.5X5	T50.5X6
stilbestrol	T38.5X1	T38.5X2	T38.5X3	T38.5X4	T38.5X5	T38.5X6
toluamide (nonmedicinal)	T60.8X1	T60.8X2	T60.8X3	T60.8X4	—	—
medicinal	T49.3X1	T49.3X2	T49.3X3	T49.3X4	T49.3X5	T49.3X6
Diethylcarbamazine	T37.4X1	T37.4X2	T37.4X3	T37.4X4	T37.4X5	T37.4X6
Diethylene						
dioxide	T52.8X1	T52.8X2	T52.8X3	T52.8X4	—	—
glycol (monoacetate) (monobutyl ether) (monoethyl ether)	T52.3X1	T52.3X2	T52.3X3	T52.3X4	—	—
Diethylhexylphthalate	T65.891	T65.892	T65.893	T65.894	—	—
Diethylpropion	T50.5X1	T50.5X2	T50.5X3	T50.5X4	T50.5X5	T50.5X6
Diethylstilbestrol	T38.5X1	T38.5X2	T38.5X3	T38.5X4	T38.5X5	T38.5X6
Diethylstilboestrol	T38.5X1	T38.5X2	T38.5X3	T38.5X4	T38.5X5	T38.5X6
Diethylsulfone-diethylmethane	T42.6X1	T42.6X2	T42.6X3	T42.6X4	T42.6X5	T42.6X6
Diethyltoluamide	T49.0X1	T49.0X2	T49.0X3	T49.0X4	T49.0X5	T49.0X6
Diethyltryptamine (DET)	T40.991	T40.992	T40.993	T40.994	—	—
Difebarbamate	T42.3X1	T42.3X2	T42.3X3	T42.3X4	T42.3X5	T42.3X6
Difencloxazine	T40.2X1	T40.2X2	T40.2X3	T40.2X4	T40.2X5	T40.2X6
Difenidol	T45.0X1	T45.0X2	T45.0X3	T45.0X4	T45.0X5	T45.0X6
Difenoxin	T47.6X1	T47.6X2	T47.6X3	T47.6X4	T47.6X5	T47.6X6
Difetarsone	T37.3X1	T37.3X2	T37.3X3	T37.3X4	T37.3X5	T37.3X6
Diffusin	T45.3X1	T45.3X2	T45.3X3	T45.3X4	T45.3X5	T45.3X6
Diflorasone	T49.0X1	T49.0X2	T49.0X3	T49.0X4	T49.0X5	T49.0X6
Diflos	T44.0X1	T44.0X2	T44.0X3	T44.0X4	T44.0X5	T44.0X6
Diflubenzuron	T60.1X1	T60.1X2	T60.1X3	T60.1X4	—	—
Diflucortolone	T49.0X1	T49.0X2	T49.0X3	T49.0X4	T49.0X5	T49.0X6
Diflunisal	T39.091	T39.092	T39.093	T39.094	T39.095	T39.096
Difluoromethyldopa	T42.8X1	T42.8X2	T42.8X3	T42.8X4	T42.8X5	T42.8X6
Difluorophate	T44.0X1	T44.0X2	T44.0X3	T44.0X4	T44.0X5	T44.0X6
Digestant NEC	T47.5X1	T47.5X2	T47.5X3	T47.5X4	T47.5X5	T47.5X6
Digitalin (e)(yl)	T46.0X1	T46.0X2	T46.0X3	T46.0X4	T46.0X5	T46.0X6
Digitalis (leaf)(glycoside)	T46.0X1	T46.0X2	T46.0X3	T46.0X4	T46.0X5	T46.0X6
lanata	T46.0X1	T46.0X2	T46.0X3	T46.0X4	T46.0X5	T46.0X6
purpurea	T46.0X1	T46.0X2	T46.0X3	T46.0X4	T46.0X5	T46.0X6
Digitoxin	T46.0X1	T46.0X2	T46.0X3	T46.0X4	T46.0X5	T46.0X6
Digitoxose	T46.0X1	T46.0X2	T46.0X3	T46.0X4	T46.0X5	T46.0X6
Digoxin	T46.0X1	T46.0X2	T46.0X3	T46.0X4	T46.0X5	T46.0X6
Digoxine	T46.0X1	T46.0X2	T46.0X3	T46.0X4	T46.0X5	T46.0X6
Dihydralazine	T46.5X1	T46.5X2	T46.5X3	T46.5X4	T46.5X5	T46.5X6
Dihydrazine	T46.5X1	T46.5X2	T46.5X3	T46.5X4	T46.5X5	T46.5X6
Dihydrocodeine	T40.2X1	T40.2X2	T40.2X3	T40.2X4	T40.2X5	T40.2X6
Dihydrocodeinone	T40.2X1	T40.2X2	T40.2X3	T40.2X4	T40.2X5	T40.2X6
Dihydroergocornine	T46.7X1	T46.7X2	T46.7X3	T46.7X4	T46.7X5	T46.7X6
Dihydroergocristine (mesilate)	T46.7X1	T46.7X2	T46.7X3	T46.7X4	T46.7X5	T46.7X6
Dihydroergokryptine	T46.7X1	T46.7X2	T46.7X3	T46.7X4	T46.7X5	T46.7X6
Dihydroergotamine	T46.5X1	T46.5X2	T46.5X3	T46.5X4	T46.5X5	T46.5X6
Dihydroergotoxine	T46.7X1	T46.7X2	T46.7X3	T46.7X4	T46.7X5	T46.7X6
mesilate	T46.7X1	T46.7X2	T46.7X3	T46.7X4	T46.7X5	T46.7X6
Dihydrohydroxycodeinone	T40.2X1	T40.2X2	T40.2X3	T40.2X4	T40.2X5	T40.2X6
Dihydrohydroxymorphinone	T40.2X1	T40.2X2	T40.2X3	T40.2X4	T40.2X5	T40.2X6
Dihydroisocodeine	T40.2X1	T40.2X2	T40.2X3	T40.2X4	T40.2X5	T40.2X6
Dihydromorphine	T40.2X1	T40.2X2	T40.2X3	T40.2X4	—	—
Dihydromorphinone	T40.2X1	T40.2X2	T40.2X3	T40.2X4	T40.2X5	T40.2X6
Dihydrostreptomycin	T36.5X1	T36.5X2	T36.5X3	T36.5X4	T36.5X5	T36.5X6
Dihydrotachysterol	T45.2X1	T45.2X2	T45.2X3	T45.2X4	T45.2X5	T45.2X6
Dihydroxyaluminum aminoacetate	T47.1X1	T47.1X2	T47.1X3	T47.1X4	T47.1X5	T47.1X6
Dihydroxyaluminum sodium carbonate	T47.1X1	T47.1X2	T47.1X3	T47.1X4	T47.1X5	T47.1X6
Dihydroxyanthraquinone	T47.2X1	T47.2X2	T47.2X3	T47.2X4	T47.2X5	T47.2X6
Dihydroxycodeinone	T40.2X1	T40.2X2	T40.2X3	T40.2X4	T40.2X5	T40.2X6
Dihydroxypropyl theophylline	T50.2X1	T50.2X2	T50.2X3	T50.2X4	T50.2X5	T50.2X6
Diiodohydroxyquin	T37.8X1	T37.8X2	T37.8X3	T37.8X4	T37.8X5	T37.8X6
topical	T49.0X1	T49.0X2	T49.0X3	T49.0X4	T49.0X5	T49.0X6
Diiodohydroxyquinoline	T37.8X1	T37.8X2	T37.8X3	T37.8X4	T37.8X5	T37.8X6
Diiodotyrosine	T38.2X1	T38.2X2	T38.2X3	T38.2X4	T38.2X5	T38.2X6
Diisopromine	T44.3X1	T44.3X2	T44.3X3	T44.3X4	T44.3X5	T44.3X6
Diisopropylamine	T46.3X1	T46.3X2	T46.3X3	T46.3X4	T46.3X5	T46.3X6
Diisopropylfluorophosphonate	T44.0X1	T44.0X2	T44.0X3	T44.0X4	T44.0X5	T44.0X6

Additional Character May Be Required — Refer to the Tabular List for Character Selection Subterms under main terms may continue to next column or page

Substance	Poisoning, Accidental (unintentional)	Poisoning, Intentional Self-harm	Poisoning, Assault	Poisoning, Undetermined	Adverse Effect	Under-dosing
Dilantin	T42.0X1	T42.0X2	T42.0X3	T42.0X4	T42.0X5	T42.0X6
Dilaudid	T40.2X1	T40.2X2	T40.2X3	T40.2X4	T40.2X5	T40.2X6
Dilazep	T46.3X1	T46.3X2	T46.3X3	T46.3X4	T46.3X5	T46.3X6
Dill	T47.5X1	T47.5X2	T47.5X3	T47.5X4	T47.5X5	T47.5X6
Diloxanide	T37.3X1	T37.3X2	T37.3X3	T37.3X4	T37.3X5	T37.3X6
Diltiazem	T46.1X1	T46.1X2	T46.1X3	T46.1X4	T46.1X5	T46.1X6
Dimazole	T49.0X1	T49.0X2	T49.0X3	T49.0X4	T49.0X5	T49.0X6
Dimefline	T50.7X1	T50.7X2	T50.7X3	T50.7X4	T50.7X5	T50.7X6
Dimefox	T60.0X1	T60.0X2	T60.0X3	T60.0X4	—	—
Dimemorfan	T48.3X1	T48.3X2	T48.3X3	T48.3X4	T48.3X5	T48.3X6
Dimenhydrinate	T45.0X1	T45.0X2	T45.0X3	T45.0X4	T45.0X5	T45.0X6
Dimercaprol (British anti-lewisite)	T45.8X1	T45.8X2	T45.8X3	T45.8X4	T45.8X5	T45.8X6
Dimercaptopropanol	T45.8X1	T45.8X2	T45.8X3	T45.8X4	T45.8X5	T45.8X6
Dimestrol	T38.5X1	T38.5X2	T38.5X3	T38.5X4	T38.5X5	T38.5X6
Dimetane	T45.0X1	T45.0X2	T45.0X3	T45.0X4	T45.0X5	T45.0X6
Dimethicone	T47.1X1	T47.1X2	T47.1X3	T47.1X4	T47.1X5	T47.1X6
Dimethindene	T45.0X1	T45.0X2	T45.0X3	T45.0X4	T45.0X5	T45.0X6
Dimethisoquin	T49.1X1	T49.1X2	T49.1X3	T49.1X4	T49.1X5	T49.1X6
Dimethisterone	T38.5X1	T38.5X2	T38.5X3	T38.5X4	T38.5X5	T38.5X6
Dimethoate	T60.0X1	T60.0X2	T60.0X3	T60.0X4	—	—
Dimethocaine	T41.3X1	T41.3X2	T41.3X3	T41.3X4	T41.3X5	T41.3X6
Dimethoxanate	T48.3X1	T48.3X2	T48.3X3	T48.3X4	T48.3X5	T48.3X6
Dimethyl						
arsine, arsinic acid	T57.0X1	T57.0X2	T57.0X3	T57.0X4	—	—
carbinol	T51.2X1	T51.2X2	T51.2X3	T51.2X4	—	—
carbonate	T52.8X1	T52.8X2	T52.8X3	T52.8X4	—	—
diguanide	T38.3X1	T38.3X2	T38.3X3	T38.3X4	T38.3X5	T38.3X6
ketone	T52.4X1	T52.4X2	T52.4X3	T52.4X4	—	—
vapor	T52.4X1	T52.4X2	T52.4X3	T52.4X4	—	—
meperidine	T40.2X1	T40.2X2	T40.2X3	T40.2X4	T40.2X5	T40.2X6
parathion	T60.0X1	T60.0X2	T60.0X3	T60.0X4	—	—
phthlate	T49.3X1	T49.3X2	T49.3X3	T49.3X4	T49.3X5	T49.3X6
polysiloxane	T47.8X1	T47.8X2	T47.8X3	T47.8X4	T47.8X5	T47.8X6
sulfate (fumes)	T59.891	T59.892	T59.893	T59.894	—	—
liquid	T65.891	T65.892	T65.893	T65.894	—	—
sulfoxide (nonmedicinal)	T52.8X1	T52.8X2	T52.8X3	T52.8X4	—	—
medicinal	T49.4X1	T49.4X2	T49.4X3	T49.4X4	T49.4X5	T49.4X6
tryptamine	T40.991	T40.992	T40.993	T40.994	—	—
tubocurarine	T48.1X1	T48.1X2	T48.1X3	T48.1X4	T48.1X5	T48.1X6
Dimethylamine sulfate	T49.4X1	T49.4X2	T49.4X3	T49.4X4	T49.4X5	T49.4X6
Dimethylformamide	T52.8X1	T52.8X2	T52.8X3	T52.8X4	—	—
Dimethyltubocurarinium chloride	T48.1X1	T48.1X2	T48.1X3	T48.1X4	T48.1X5	T48.1X6
Dimeticone	T47.1X1	T47.1X2	T47.1X3	T47.1X4	T47.1X5	T47.1X6
Dimetilan	T60.0X1	T60.0X2	T60.0X3	T60.0X4	—	—
Dimetindene	T45.0X1	T45.0X2	T45.0X3	T45.0X4	T45.0X5	T45.0X6
Dimetotiazine	T43.3X1	T43.3X2	T43.3X3	T43.3X4	T43.3X5	T43.3X6
Dimorpholamine	T50.7X1	T50.7X2	T50.7X3	T50.7X4	T50.7X5	T50.7X6
Dimoxyline	T46.3X1	T46.3X2	T46.3X3	T46.3X4	T46.3X5	T46.3X6
Dinitrobenzene	T65.3X1	T65.3X2	T65.3X3	T65.3X4	—	—
vapor	T59.891	T59.892	T59.893	T59.894	—	—
Dinitrobenzol	T65.3X1	T65.3X2	T65.3X3	T65.3X4	—	—
vapor	T59.891	T59.892	T59.893	T59.894	—	—
Dinitrobutylphenol	T65.3X1	T65.3X2	T65.3X3	T65.3X4	—	—
Dinitro (-ortho-)cresol (pesticide) (spray)	T65.3X1	T65.3X2	T65.3X3	T65.3X4	—	—
Dinitrocyclohexylphenol	T65.3X1	T65.3X2	T65.3X3	T65.3X4	—	—
Dinitrophenol	T65.3X1	T65.3X2	T65.3X3	T65.3X4	—	—
Dinoprost	T48.0X1	T48.0X2	T48.0X3	T48.0X4	T48.0X5	T48.0X6
Dinoprostone	T48.0X1	T48.0X2	T48.0X3	T48.0X4	T48.0X5	T48.0X6
Dinoseb	T60.3X1	T60.3X2	T60.3X3	T60.3X4	—	—
Dioctyl sulfosuccinate (calcium) (sodium)	T47.4X1	T47.4X2	T47.4X3	T47.4X4	T47.4X5	T47.4X6
Diodone	T50.8X1	T50.8X2	T50.8X3	T50.8X4	T50.8X5	T50.8X6
Diodoquin	T37.8X1	T37.8X2	T37.8X3	T37.8X4	T37.8X5	T37.8X6
Dionin	T40.2X1	T40.2X2	T40.2X3	T40.2X4	T40.2X5	T40.2X6
Diosmin	T46.991	T46.992	T46.993	T46.994	T46.995	T46.996
Dioxane	T52.8X1	T52.8X2	T52.8X3	T52.8X4	—	—
Dioxathion	T60.0X1	T60.0X2	T60.0X3	T60.0X4	—	—
Dioxin	T53.7X1	T53.7X2	T53.7X3	T53.7X4	—	—
Dioxopromethazine	T43.3X1	T43.3X2	T43.3X3	T43.3X4	T43.3X5	T43.3X6
Dioxyline	T46.3X1	T46.3X2	T46.3X3	T46.3X4	T46.3X5	T46.3X6
Dipentene	T52.8X1	T52.8X2	T52.8X3	T52.8X4	—	—
Diperodon	T41.3X1	T41.3X2	T41.3X3	T41.3X4	T41.3X5	T41.3X6
Diphacinone	T60.4X1	T60.4X2	T60.4X3	T60.4X4	—	—
Diphemanil	T44.3X1	T44.3X2	T44.3X3	T44.3X4	T44.3X5	T44.3X6
metilsulfate	T44.3X1	T44.3X2	T44.3X3	T44.3X4	T44.3X5	T44.3X6
Diphenadione	T45.511	T45.512	T45.513	T45.514	T45.515	T45.516
rodenticide	T60.4X1	T60.4X2	T60.4X3	T60.4X4	—	—
Diphenhydramine	T45.0X1	T45.0X2	T45.0X3	T45.0X4	T45.0X5	T45.0X6
Diphenidol	T45.0X1	T45.0X2	T45.0X3	T45.0X4	T45.0X5	T45.0X6
Diphenoxylate	T47.6X1	T47.6X2	T47.6X3	T47.6X4	T47.6X5	T47.6X6
Diphenylamine	T65.3X1	T65.3X2	T65.3X3	T65.3X4	—	—
Diphenylbutazone	T39.2X1	T39.2X2	T39.2X3	T39.2X4	T39.2X5	T39.2X6
Diphenylchloroarsine, not in war	T57.0X1	T57.0X2	T57.0X3	T57.0X4	—	—
Diphenylhydantoin	T42.0X1	T42.0X2	T42.0X3	T42.0X4	T42.0X5	T42.0X6
Diphenylmethane dye	T52.1X1	T52.1X2	T52.1X3	T52.1X4	—	—
Diphenylpyraline	T45.0X1	T45.0X2	T45.0X3	T45.0X4	T45.0X5	T45.0X6
Diphtheria						
antitoxin	T50.Z11	T50.Z12	T50.Z13	T50.Z14	T50.Z15	T50.Z16
toxoid	T50.A91	T50.A92	T50.A93	T50.A94	T50.A95	T50.A96
with tetanus toxoid	T50.A21	T50.A22	T50.A23	T50.A24	T50.A25	T50.A26
with pertussis component	T50.A11	T50.A12	T50.A13	T50.A14	T50.A15	T50.A16
vaccine	T50.A91	T50.A92	T50.A93	T50.A94	T50.A95	T50.A96
combination						
without pertussis	T50.A21	T50.A22	T50.A23	T50.A24	T50.A25	T50.A26
including pertussis	T50.A11	T50.A12	T50.A13	T50.A14	T50.A15	T50.A16
Diphylline	T50.2X1	T50.2X2	T50.2X3	T50.2X4	T50.2X5	T50.2X6
Dipipanone	T40.4X1	T40.4X2	T40.4X3	T40.4X4	—	—
Dipivefrine	T49.5X1	T49.5X2	T49.5X3	T49.5X4	T49.5X5	T49.5X6
Diplovax	T50.B91	T50.B92	T50.B93	T50.B94	T50.B95	T50.B96
Diprophylline	T48.291	T48.292	T48.293	T48.294	T48.295	T48.296
Dipropyline	T48.291	T48.292	T48.293	T48.294	T48.295	T48.296
Dipyridamole	T46.3X1	T46.3X2	T46.3X3	T46.3X4	T46.3X5	T46.3X6
Dipyrone	T39.2X1	T39.2X2	T39.2X3	T39.2X4	T39.2X5	T39.2X6
Diquat (dibromide)	T60.3X1	T60.3X2	T60.3X3	T60.3X4	—	—
Disinfectant	T65.891	T65.892	T65.893	T65.894	—	—
alkaline	T54.3X1	T54.3X2	T54.3X3	T54.3X4	—	—
aromatic	T54.1X1	T54.1X2	T54.1X3	T54.1X4	—	—
intestinal	T37.8X1	T37.8X2	T37.8X3	T37.8X4	T37.8X5	T37.8X6
Disipal	T42.8X1	T42.8X2	T42.8X3	T42.8X4	T42.8X5	T42.8X6
Disodium edetate	T50.6X1	T50.6X2	T50.6X3	T50.6X4	T50.6X5	T50.6X6
Disoprofol	T41.291	T41.292	T41.293	T41.294	T41.295	T41.296
Disopyramide	T46.2X1	T46.2X2	T46.2X3	T46.2X4	T46.2X5	T46.2X6
Distigmine (bromide)	T44.0X1	T44.0X2	T44.0X3	T44.0X4	T44.0X5	T44.0X6
Disulfamide	T50.2X1	T50.2X2	T50.2X3	T50.2X4	T50.2X5	T50.2X6
Disulfanilamide	T37.0X1	T37.0X2	T37.0X3	T37.0X4	T37.0X5	T37.0X6
Disulfiram	T50.6X1	T50.6X2	T50.6X3	T50.6X4	T50.6X5	T50.6X6
Disulfoton	T60.0X1	T60.0X2	T60.0X3	T60.0X4	—	—
Dithiazanine iodide	T37.4X1	T37.4X2	T37.4X3	T37.4X4	T37.4X5	T37.4X6
Dithiocarbamate	T60.0X1	T60.0X2	T60.0X3	T60.0X4	—	—
Dithranol	T49.4X1	T49.4X2	T49.4X3	T49.4X4	T49.4X5	T49.4X6
Diucardin	T50.2X1	T50.2X2	T50.2X3	T50.2X4	T50.2X5	T50.2X6
Diupres	T50.2X1	T50.2X2	T50.2X3	T50.2X4	T50.2X5	T50.2X6
Diuretic NEC	T50.2X1	T50.2X2	T50.2X3	T50.2X4	T50.2X5	T50.2X6
benzothiadiazine	T50.2X1	T50.2X2	T50.2X3	T50.2X4	T50.2X5	T50.2X6
carbonic acid anhydrase inhibitors	T50.2X1	T50.2X2	T50.2X3	T50.2X4	T50.2X5	T50.2X6
furfuryl NEC	T50.2X1	T50.2X2	T50.2X3	T50.2X4	T50.2X5	T50.2X6
loop (high-ceiling)	T50.1X1	T50.1X2	T50.1X3	T50.1X4	T50.1X5	T50.1X6
mercurial NEC	T50.2X1	T50.2X2	T50.2X3	T50.2X4	T50.2X5	T50.2X6
osmotic	T50.2X1	T50.2X2	T50.2X3	T50.2X4	T50.2X5	T50.2X6
purine NEC	T50.2X1	T50.2X2	T50.2X3	T50.2X4	T50.2X5	T50.2X6
saluretic NEC	T50.2X1	T50.2X2	T50.2X3	T50.2X4	T50.2X5	T50.2X6
sulfonamide	T50.2X1	T50.2X2	T50.2X3	T50.2X4	T50.2X5	T50.2X6
thiazide NEC	T50.2X1	T50.2X2	T50.2X3	T50.2X4	T50.2X5	T50.2X6
xanthine	T50.2X1	T50.2X2	T50.2X3	T50.2X4	T50.2X5	T50.2X6
Diurgin	T50.2X1	T50.2X2	T50.2X3	T50.2X4	T50.2X5	T50.2X6
Diuril	T50.2X1	T50.2X2	T50.2X3	T50.2X4	T50.2X5	T50.2X6
Diuron	T60.3X1	T60.3X2	T60.3X3	T60.3X4	—	—
Divalproex	T42.6X1	T42.6X2	T42.6X3	T42.6X4	T42.6X5	T42.6X6
Divinyl ether	T41.0X1	T41.0X2	T41.0X3	T41.0X4	T41.0X5	T41.0X6
Dixanthogen	T49.0X1	T49.0X2	T49.0X3	T49.0X4	T49.0X5	T49.0X6
Dixyrazine	T43.3X1	T43.3X2	T43.3X3	T43.3X4	T43.3X5	T43.3X6
D-lysergic acid diethylamide	T40.8X1	T40.8X2	T40.8X3	T40.8X4	—	—
DMCT	T36.4X1	T36.4X2	T36.4X3	T36.4X4	T36.4X5	T36.4X6
DMSO — see Dimethyl sulfoxide						
DNBP	T60.3X1	T60.3X2	T60.3X3	T60.3X4	—	—
DNOC	T65.3X1	T65.3X2	T65.3X3	T65.3X4	—	—
Dobutamine	T44.5X1	T44.5X2	T44.5X3	T44.5X4	T44.5X5	T44.5X6
DOCA	T38.0X1	T38.0X2	T38.0X3	T38.0X4	T38.0X5	T38.0X6
Docusate sodium	T47.4X1	T47.4X2	T47.4X3	T47.4X4	T47.4X5	T47.4X6
Dodicin	T49.0X1	T49.0X2	T49.0X3	T49.0X4	T49.0X5	T49.0X6
Dofamium chloride	T49.0X1	T49.0X2	T49.0X3	T49.0X4	T49.0X5	T49.0X6
Dolophine	T40.3X1	T40.3X2	T40.3X3	T40.3X4	T40.3X5	T40.3X6
Doloxene	T39.8X1	T39.8X2	T39.8X3	T39.8X4	T39.8X5	T39.8X6
Domestic gas (after combustion) — see Gas, utility						
prior to combustion	T59.891	T59.892	T59.893	T59.894	—	—
Domiodol	T48.4X1	T48.4X2	T48.4X3	T48.4X4	T48.4X5	T48.4X6
Domiphen (bromide)	T49.0X1	T49.0X2	T49.0X3	T49.0X4	T49.0X5	T49.0X6
Domperidone	T45.0X1	T45.0X2	T45.0X3	T45.0X4	T45.0X5	T45.0X6

▼ Subterms under main terms may continue to next column or page   Additional Character May Be Required — Refer to the Tabular List for Character Selection

Substance	Poisoning, Accidental (unintentional)	Poisoning, Intentional Self-harm	Poisoning, Assault	Poisoning, Undetermined	Adverse Effect	Under-dosing
Dopa	T42.8X1	T42.8X2	T42.8X3	T42.8X4	T42.8X5	T42.8X6
Dopamine	T44.991	T44.992	T44.993	T44.994	T44.995	T44.996
Doriden	T42.6X1	T42.6X2	T42.6X3	T42.6X4	T42.6X5	T42.6X6
Dormiral	T42.3X1	T42.3X2	T42.3X3	T42.3X4	T42.3X5	T42.3X6
Dormison	T42.6X1	T42.6X2	T42.6X3	T42.6X4	T42.6X5	T42.6X6
Dornase	T48.4X1	T48.4X2	T48.4X3	T48.4X4	T48.4X5	T48.4X6
Dorsacaine	T41.3X1	T41.3X2	T41.3X3	T41.3X4	T41.3X5	T41.3X6
Dosulepin	T43.011	T43.012	T43.013	T43.014	T43.015	T43.016
Dothiepin	T43.011	T43.012	T43.013	T43.014	T43.015	T43.016
Doxantrazole	T48.6X1	T48.6X2	T48.6X3	T48.6X4	T48.6X5	T48.6X6
Doxapram	T50.7X1	T50.7X2	T50.7X3	T50.7X4	T50.7X5	T50.7X6
Doxazosin	T44.6X1	T44.6X2	T44.6X3	T44.6X4	T44.6X5	T44.6X6
Doxepin	T43.011	T43.012	T43.013	T43.014	T43.015	T43.016
Doxifluridine	T45.1X1	T45.1X2	T45.1X3	T45.1X4	T45.1X5	T45.1X6
Doxorubicin	T45.1X1	T45.1X2	T45.1X3	T45.1X4	T45.1X5	T45.1X6
Doxycycline	T36.4X1	T36.4X2	T36.4X3	T36.4X4	T36.4X5	T36.4X6
Doxylamine	T45.0X1	T45.0X2	T45.0X3	T45.0X4	T45.0X5	T45.0X6
Dramamine	T45.0X1	T45.0X2	T45.0X3	T45.0X4	T45.0X5	T45.0X6
Drano (drain cleaner)	T54.3X1	T54.3X2	T54.3X3	T54.3X4	—	—
Dressing, live pulp	T49.7X1	T49.7X2	T49.7X3	T49.7X4	T49.7X5	T49.7X6
Drocode	T40.2X1	T40.2X2	T40.2X3	T40.2X4	T40.2X5	T40.2X6
Dromoran	T40.2X1	T40.2X2	T40.2X3	T40.2X4	T40.2X5	T40.2X6
Dromostanolone	T38.7X1	T38.7X2	T38.7X3	T38.7X4	T38.7X5	T38.7X6
Dronabinol	T40.7X1	T40.7X2	T40.7X3	T40.7X4	T40.7X5	T40.7X6
Droperidol	T43.591	T43.592	T43.593	T43.594	T43.595	T43.596
Dropropizine	T48.3X1	T48.3X2	T48.3X3	T48.3X4	T48.3X5	T48.3X6
Drostanolone	T38.7X1	T38.7X2	T38.7X3	T38.7X4	T38.7X5	T38.7X6
Drotaverine	T44.3X1	T44.3X2	T44.3X3	T44.3X4	T44.3X5	T44.3X6
Drotrecogin alfa	T45.511	T45.512	T45.513	T45.514	T45.515	T45.516
Drug NEC	T50.901	T50.902	T50.903	T50.904	T50.905	T50.906
specified NEC	T50.991	T50.992	T50.993	T50.994	T50.995	T50.996
DTIC	T45.1X1	T45.1X2	T45.1X3	T45.1X4	T45.1X5	T45.1X6
Duboisine	T44.3X1	T44.3X2	T44.3X3	T44.3X4	T44.3X5	T44.3X6
Dulcolax	T47.2X1	T47.2X2	T47.2X3	T47.2X4	T47.2X5	T47.2X6
Duponol (C) (EP)	T49.2X1	T49.2X2	T49.2X3	T49.2X4	T49.2X5	T49.2X6
Durabolin	T38.7X1	T38.7X2	T38.7X3	T38.7X4	T38.7X5	T38.7X6
Dyclone	T41.3X1	T41.3X2	T41.3X3	T41.3X4	T41.3X5	T41.3X6
Dyclonine	T41.3X1	T41.3X2	T41.3X3	T41.3X4	T41.3X5	T41.3X6
Dydrogesterone	T38.5X1	T38.5X2	T38.5X3	T38.5X4	T38.5X5	T38.5X6
Dye NEC	T65.6X1	T65.6X2	T65.6X3	T65.6X4	—	—
antiseptic	T49.0X1	T49.0X2	T49.0X3	T49.0X4	T49.0X5	T49.0X6
diagnostic agents	T50.8X1	T50.8X2	T50.8X3	T50.8X4	T50.8X5	T50.8X6
pharmaceutical NEC	T50.901	T50.902	T50.903	T50.904	T50.905	T50.906
Dyflos	T44.0X1	T44.0X2	T44.0X3	T44.0X4	T44.0X5	T44.0X6
Dymelor	T38.3X1	T38.3X2	T38.3X3	T38.3X4	T38.3X5	T38.3X6
Dynamite	T65.3X1	T65.3X2	T65.3X3	T65.3X4	—	—
fumes	T59.891	T59.892	T59.893	T59.894	—	—
Dyphylline	T44.3X1	T44.3X2	T44.3X3	T44.3X4	T44.3X5	T44.3X6
b-eucaine	T49.1X1	T49.1X2	T49.1X3	T49.1X4	T49.1X5	T49.1X6
Ear drug NEC	T49.6X1	T49.6X2	T49.6X3	T49.6X4	T49.6X5	T49.6X6
Ear preparations	T49.6X1	T49.6X2	T49.6X3	T49.6X4	T49.6X5	T49.6X6
Echothiophate, echothiopate, ecothiophate	T49.5X1	T49.5X2	T49.5X3	T49.5X4	T49.5X5	T49.5X6
Econazole	T49.0X1	T49.0X2	T49.0X3	T49.0X4	T49.0X5	T49.0X6
Ecothiopate iodide	T49.5X1	T49.5X2	T49.5X3	T49.5X4	T49.5X5	T49.5X6
Ecstasy	T43.641	T43.642	T43.643	T43.644		
Ectylurea	T42.6X1	T42.6X2	T42.6X3	T42.6X4	T42.6X5	T42.6X6
Edathamil disodium	T45.8X1	T45.8X2	T45.8X3	T45.8X4	T45.8X5	T45.8X6
Edecrin	T50.1X1	T50.1X2	T50.1X3	T50.1X4	T50.1X5	T50.1X6
Edetate, disodium	T45.8X1	T45.8X2	T45.8X3	T45.8X4	T45.8X5	T45.8X6
(calcium)						
Edoxudine	T49.5X1	T49.5X2	T49.5X3	T49.5X4	T49.5X5	T49.5X6
Edrophonium	T44.0X1	T44.0X2	T44.0X3	T44.0X4	T44.0X5	T44.0X6
chloride	T44.0X1	T44.0X2	T44.0X3	T44.0X4	T44.0X5	T44.0X6
EDTA	T50.6X1	T50.6X2	T50.6X3	T50.6X4	T50.6X5	T50.6X6
Eflornithine	T37.2X1	T37.2X2	T37.2X3	T37.2X4	T37.2X5	T37.2X6
Efloxate	T46.3X1	T46.3X2	T46.3X3	T46.3X4	T46.3X5	T46.3X6
Elase	T49.8X1	T49.8X2	T49.8X3	T49.8X4	T49.8X5	T49.8X6
Elastase	T47.5X1	T47.5X2	T47.5X3	T47.5X4	T47.5X5	T47.5X6
Elaterium	T47.2X1	T47.2X2	T47.2X3	T47.2X4	T47.2X5	T47.2X6
Elcatonin	T50.991	T50.992	T50.993	T50.994	T50.995	T50.996
Elder	T62.2X1	T62.2X2	T62.2X3	T62.2X4	—	—
berry, (unripe)	T62.1X1	T62.1X2	T62.1X3	T62.1X4	—	—
Electrolyte balance drug	T50.3X1	T50.3X2	T50.3X3	T50.3X4	T50.3X5	T50.3X6
Electrolytes NEC	T50.3X1	T50.3X2	T50.3X3	T50.3X4	T50.3X5	T50.3X6
Electrolytic agent NEC	T50.3X1	T50.3X2	T50.3X3	T50.3X4	T50.3X5	T50.3X6
Elemental diet	T50.901	T50.902	T50.903	T50.904	T50.905	T50.906
Elliptinium acetate	T45.1X1	T45.1X2	T45.1X3	T45.1X4	T45.1X5	T45.1X6
Embramine	T45.0X1	T45.0X2	T45.0X3	T45.0X4	T45.0X5	T45.0X6
Emepronium (salts)	T44.3X1	T44.3X2	T44.3X3	T44.3X4	T44.3X5	T44.3X6
bromide	T44.3X1	T44.3X2	T44.3X3	T44.3X4	T44.3X5	T44.3X6
Emetic NEC	T47.7X1	T47.7X2	T47.7X3	T47.7X4	T47.7X5	T47.7X6
Emetine	T37.3X1	T37.3X2	T37.3X3	T37.3X4	T37.3X5	T37.3X6
Emollient NEC	T49.3X1	T49.3X2	T49.3X3	T49.3X4	T49.3X5	T49.3X6
Emorfazone	T39.8X1	T39.8X2	T39.8X3	T39.8X4	T39.8X5	T39.8X6
Emylcamate	T43.591	T43.592	T43.593	T43.594	T43.595	T43.596
Enalapril	T46.4X1	T46.4X2	T46.4X3	T46.4X4	T46.4X5	T46.4X6
Enalaprilat	T46.4X1	T46.4X2	T46.4X3	T46.4X4	T46.4X5	T46.4X6
Encainide	T46.2X1	T46.2X2	T46.2X3	T46.2X4	T46.2X5	T46.2X6
Endocaine	T41.3X1	T41.3X2	T41.3X3	T41.3X4	T41.3X5	T41.3X6
Endosulfan	T60.2X1	T60.2X2	T60.2X3	T60.2X4	—	—
Endothall	T60.3X1	T60.3X2	T60.3X3	T60.3X4	—	—
Endralazine	T46.5X1	T46.5X2	T46.5X3	T46.5X4	T46.5X5	T46.5X6
Endrin	T60.1X1	T60.1X2	T60.1X3	T60.1X4	—	—
Enflurane	T41.0X1	T41.0X2	T41.0X3	T41.0X4	T41.0X5	T41.0X6
Enhexymal	T42.3X1	T42.3X2	T42.3X3	T42.3X4	T42.3X5	T42.3X6
Enocitabine	T45.1X1	T45.1X2	T45.1X3	T45.1X4	T45.1X5	T45.1X6
Enovid	T38.4X1	T38.4X2	T38.4X3	T38.4X4	T38.4X5	T38.4X6
Enoxacin	T36.8X1	T36.8X2	T36.8X3	T36.8X4	T36.8X5	T36.8X6
Enoxaparin (sodium)	T45.511	T45.512	T45.513	T45.514	T45.515	T45.516
Enpiprazole	T43.591	T43.592	T43.593	T43.594	T43.595	T43.596
Enprofylline	T48.6X1	T48.6X2	T48.6X3	T48.6X4	T48.6X5	T48.6X6
Enprostil	T47.1X1	T47.1X2	T47.1X3	T47.1X4	T47.1X5	T47.1X6
Enterogastrone	T38.891	T38.892	T38.893	T38.894	T38.895	T38.896
ENT preparations (anti-infectives)	T49.6X1	T49.6X2	T49.6X3	T49.6X4	T49.6X5	T49.6X6
Enviomycin	T36.8X1	T36.8X2	T36.8X3	T36.8X4	T36.8X5	T36.8X6
Enzodase	T45.3X1	T45.3X2	T45.3X3	T45.3X4	T45.3X5	T45.3X6
Enzyme NEC	T45.3X1	T45.3X2	T45.3X3	T45.3X4	T45.3X5	T45.3X6
depolymerizing	T49.8X1	T49.8X2	T49.8X3	T49.8X4	T49.8X5	T49.8X6
fibrolytic	T45.3X1	T45.3X2	T45.3X3	T45.3X4	T45.3X5	T45.3X6
gastric	T47.5X1	T47.5X2	T47.5X3	T47.5X4	T47.5X5	T47.5X6
intestinal	T47.5X1	T47.5X2	T47.5X3	T47.5X4	T47.5X5	T47.5X6
local action	T49.4X1	T49.4X2	T49.4X3	T49.4X4	T49.4X5	T49.4X6
proteolytic	T49.4X1	T49.4X2	T49.4X3	T49.4X4	T49.4X5	T49.4X6
thrombolytic	T45.3X1	T45.3X2	T45.3X3	T45.3X4	T45.3X5	T45.3X6
EPAB	T41.3X1	T41.3X2	T41.3X3	T41.3X4	T41.3X5	T41.3X6
Epanutin	T42.0X1	T42.0X2	T42.0X3	T42.0X4	T42.0X5	T42.0X6
Ephedra	T44.991	T44.992	T44.993	T44.994	T44.995	T44.996
Ephedrine	T44.991	T44.992	T44.993	T44.994	T44.995	T44.996
Epichlorhydrin, epichlorohydrin	T52.8X1	T52.8X2	T52.8X3	T52.8X4	—	—
Epicillin	T36.0X1	T36.0X2	T36.0X3	T36.0X4	T36.0X5	T36.0X6
Epiestriol	T38.5X1	T38.5X2	T38.5X3	T38.5X4	T38.5X5	T38.5X6
Epilim — see Sodium valproate						
Epimestrol	T38.5X1	T38.5X2	T38.5X3	T38.5X4	T38.5X5	T38.5X6
Epinephrine	T44.5X1	T44.5X2	T44.5X3	T44.5X4	T44.5X5	T44.5X6
Epirubicin	T45.1X1	T45.1X2	T45.1X3	T45.1X4	T45.1X5	T45.1X6
Epitiostanol	T38.7X1	T38.7X2	T38.7X3	T38.7X4	T38.7X5	T38.7X6
Epitizide	T50.2X1	T50.2X2	T50.2X3	T50.2X4	T50.2X5	T50.2X6
EPN	T60.0X1	T60.0X2	T60.0X3	T60.0X4	—	—
EPO	T45.8X1	T45.8X2	T45.8X3	T45.8X4	T45.8X5	T45.8X6
Epoetin alpha	T45.8X1	T45.8X2	T45.8X3	T45.8X4	T45.8X5	T45.8X6
Epomediol	T50.991	T50.992	T50.993	T50.994	T50.995	T50.996
Epoprostenol	T45.521	T45.522	T45.523	T45.524	T45.525	T45.526
Epoxy resin	T65.891	T65.892	T65.893	T65.894	—	—
Eprazinone	T48.4X1	T48.4X2	T48.4X3	T48.4X4	T48.4X5	T48.4X6
Epsilon aminocaproic acid	T45.621	T45.622	T45.623	T45.624	T45.625	T45.626
Epsom salt	T47.3X1	T47.3X2	T47.3X3	T47.3X4	T47.3X5	T47.3X6
Eptazocine	T40.4X1	T40.4X2	T40.4X3	T40.4X4	T40.4X5	T40.4X6
Equanil	T43.591	T43.592	T43.593	T43.594	T43.595	T43.596
Equisetum	T62.2X1	T62.2X2	T62.2X3	T62.2X4	—	—
diuretic	T50.2X1	T50.2X2	T50.2X3	T50.2X4	T50.2X5	T50.2X6
Ergobasine	T48.0X1	T48.0X2	T48.0X3	T48.0X4	T48.0X5	T48.0X6
Ergocalciferol	T45.2X1	T45.2X2	T45.2X3	T45.2X4	T45.2X5	T45.2X6
Ergoloid mesylates	T46.7X1	T46.7X2	T46.7X3	T46.7X4	T46.7X5	T46.7X6
Ergometrine	T48.0X1	T48.0X2	T48.0X3	T48.0X4	T48.0X5	T48.0X6
Ergonovine	T48.0X1	T48.0X2	T48.0X3	T48.0X4	T48.0X5	T48.0X6
Ergotamine	T46.5X1	T46.5X2	T46.5X3	T46.5X4	T46.5X5	T46.5X6
Ergotocine	T48.0X1	T48.0X2	T48.0X3	T48.0X4	T48.0X5	T48.0X6
Ergotrate	T48.0X1	T48.0X2	T48.0X3	T48.0X4	T48.0X5	T48.0X6
Ergot NEC	T64.81	T64.82	T64.83	T64.84	—	—
derivative	T48.0X1	T48.0X2	T48.0X3	T48.0X4	T48.0X5	T48.0X6
medicinal (alkaloids)	T48.0X1	T48.0X2	T48.0X3	T48.0X4	T48.0X5	T48.0X6
prepared	T48.0X1	T48.0X2	T48.0X3	T48.0X4	T48.0X5	T48.0X6
Eritrityl tetranitrate	T46.3X1	T46.3X2	T46.3X3	T46.3X4	T46.3X5	T46.3X6
Erythrityl tetranitrate	T46.3X1	T46.3X2	T46.3X3	T46.3X4	T46.3X5	T46.3X6
Erythrol tetranitrate	T46.3X1	T46.3X2	T46.3X3	T46.3X4	T46.3X5	T46.3X6
Erythromycin (salts)	T36.3X1	T36.3X2	T36.3X3	T36.3X4	T36.3X5	T36.3X6
ophthalmic preparation	T49.5X1	T49.5X2	T49.5X3	T49.5X4	T49.5X5	T49.5X6
topical NEC	T49.0X1	T49.0X2	T49.0X3	T49.0X4	T49.0X5	T49.0X6
Erythropoietin	T45.8X1	T45.8X2	T45.8X3	T45.8X4	T45.8X5	T45.8X6
human	T45.8X1	T45.8X2	T45.8X3	T45.8X4	T45.8X5	T45.8X6
Escin	T46.991	T46.992	T46.993	T46.994	T46.995	T46.996
Esculin	T45.2X1	T45.2X2	T45.2X3	T45.2X4	T45.2X5	T45.2X6
Esculoside	T45.2X1	T45.2X2	T45.2X3	T45.2X4	T45.2X5	T45.2X6

Additional Character May Be Required — Refer to the Tabular List for Character Selection

Subterms under main terms may continue to next column or page

Substance	Poisoning, Accidental (unintentional)	Poisoning, Intentional Self-harm	Poisoning, Assault	Poisoning, Undetermined	Adverse Effect	Under-dosing
ESDT (ether-soluble tar distillate)	T49.1X1	T49.1X2	T49.1X3	T49.1X4	T49.1X5	T49.1X6
Eserine	T49.5X1	T49.5X2	T49.5X3	T49.5X4	T49.5X5	T49.5X6
Esflurbiprofen	T39.311	T39.312	T39.313	T39.314	T39.315	T39.316
Eskabarb	T42.3X1	T42.3X2	T42.3X3	T42.3X4	T42.3X5	T42.3X6
Eskalith	T43.8X1	T43.8X2	T43.8X3	T43.8X4	T43.8X5	T43.8X6
Esmolol	T44.7X1	T44.7X2	T44.7X3	T44.7X4	T44.7X5	T44.7X6
Estanozolol	T38.7X1	T38.7X2	T38.7X3	T38.7X4	T38.7X5	T38.7X6
Estazolam	T42.4X1	T42.4X2	T42.4X3	T42.4X4	T42.4X5	T42.4X6
Estradiol	T38.5X1	T38.5X2	T38.5X3	T38.5X4	T38.5X5	T38.5X6
with testosterone	T38.7X1	T38.7X2	T38.7X3	T38.7X4	T38.7X5	T38.7X6
benzoate	T38.5X1	T38.5X2	T38.5X3	T38.5X4	T38.5X5	T38.5X6
Estramustine	T45.1X1	T45.1X2	T45.1X3	T45.1X4	T45.1X5	T45.1X6
Estriol	T38.5X1	T38.5X2	T38.5X3	T38.5X4	T38.5X5	T38.5X6
Estrogen	T38.5X1	T38.5X2	T38.5X3	T38.5X4	T38.5X5	T38.5X6
with progesterone	T38.5X1	T38.5X2	T38.5X3	T38.5X4	T38.5X5	T38.5X6
conjugated	T38.5X1	T38.5X2	T38.5X3	T38.5X4	T38.5X5	T38.5X6
Estrone	T38.5X1	T38.5X2	T38.5X3	T38.5X4	T38.5X5	T38.5X6
Estropipate	T38.5X1	T38.5X2	T38.5X3	T38.5X4	T38.5X5	T38.5X6
Etacrynate sodium	T50.1X1	T50.1X2	T50.1X3	T50.1X4	T50.1X5	T50.1X6
Etacrynic acid	T50.1X1	T50.1X2	T50.1X3	T50.1X4	T50.1X5	T50.1X6
Etafedrine	T48.6X1	T48.6X2	T48.6X3	T48.6X4	T48.6X5	T48.6X6
Etafenone	T46.3X1	T46.3X2	T46.3X3	T46.3X4	T46.3X5	T46.3X6
Etambutol	T37.1X1	T37.1X2	T37.1X3	T37.1X4	T37.1X5	T37.1X6
Etamiphyllin	T48.6X1	T48.6X2	T48.6X3	T48.6X4	T48.6X5	T48.6X6
Etamivan	T50.7X1	T50.7X2	T50.7X3	T50.7X4	T50.7X5	T50.7X6
Etamsylate	T45.7X1	T45.7X2	T45.7X3	T45.7X4	T45.7X5	T45.7X6
Etebenecid	T50.4X1	T50.4X2	T50.4X3	T50.4X4	T50.4X5	T50.4X6
Ethacridine	T49.0X1	T49.0X2	T49.0X3	T49.0X4	T49.0X5	T49.0X6
Ethacrynic acid	T50.1X1	T50.1X2	T50.1X3	T50.1X4	T50.1X5	T50.1X6
Ethadione	T42.2X1	T42.2X2	T42.2X3	T42.2X4	T42.2X5	T42.2X6
Ethambutol	T37.1X1	T37.1X2	T37.1X3	T37.1X4	T37.1X5	T37.1X6
Ethamide	T50.2X1	T50.2X2	T50.2X3	T50.2X4	T50.2X5	T50.2X6
Ethamivan	T50.7X1	T50.7X2	T50.7X3	T50.7X4	T50.7X5	T50.7X6
Ethamsylate	T45.7X1	T45.7X2	T45.7X3	T45.7X4	T45.7X5	T45.7X6
Ethanol	T51.0X1	T51.0X2	T51.0X3	T51.0X4	—	—
beverage	T51.0X1	T51.0X2	T51.0X3	T51.0X4	—	—
Ethanolamine oleate	T46.8X1	T46.8X2	T46.8X3	T46.8X4	T46.8X5	T46.8X6
Ethaverine	T44.3X1	T44.3X2	T44.3X3	T44.3X4	T44.3X5	T44.3X6
Ethchlorvynol	T42.6X1	T42.6X2	T42.6X3	T42.6X4	T42.6X5	T42.6X6
Ethebenecid	T50.4X1	T50.4X2	T50.4X3	T50.4X4	T50.4X5	T50.4X6
Ether (vapor)	T41.0X1	T41.0X2	T41.0X3	T41.0X4	T41.0X5	T41.0X6
anesthetic	T41.0X1	T41.0X2	T41.0X3	T41.0X4	T41.0X5	T41.0X6
divinyl	T41.0X1	T41.0X2	T41.0X3	T41.0X4	T41.0X5	T41.0X6
ethyl (medicinal)	T41.0X1	T41.0X2	T41.0X3	T41.0X4	T41.0X5	T41.0X6
nonmedicinal	T52.8X1	T52.8X2	T52.8X3	T52.8X4	—	—
petroleum — see Ligroin						
solvent	T52.8X1	T52.8X2	T52.8X3	T52.8X4	—	—
Ethiazide	T50.2X1	T50.2X2	T50.2X3	T50.2X4	T50.2X5	T50.2X6
Ethidium chloride (vapor)	T59.891	T59.892	T59.893	T59.894		
Ethinamate	T42.6X1	T42.6X2	T42.6X3	T42.6X4	T42.6X5	T42.6X6
Ethinylestradiol, ethinyloestradiol	T38.5X1	T38.5X2	T38.5X3	T38.5X4	T38.5X5	T38.5X6
with						
levonorgestrel	T38.4X1	T38.4X2	T38.4X3	T38.4X4	T38.4X5	T38.4X6
norethisterone	T38.4X1	T38.4X2	T38.4X3	T38.4X4	T38.4X5	T38.4X6
Ethiodized oil (131 I)	T50.8X1	T50.8X2	T50.8X3	T50.8X4	T50.8X5	T50.8X6
Ethion	T60.0X1	T60.0X2	T60.0X3	T60.0X4	—	—
Ethionamide	T37.1X1	T37.1X2	T37.1X3	T37.1X4	T37.1X5	T37.1X6
Ethioniamide	T37.1X1	T37.1X2	T37.1X3	T37.1X4	T37.1X5	T37.1X6
Ethisterone	T38.5X1	T38.5X2	T38.5X3	T38.5X4	T38.5X5	T38.5X6
Ethobral	T42.3X1	T42.3X2	T42.3X3	T42.3X4	T42.3X5	T42.3X6
Ethocaine (infiltration) (topical)	T41.3X1	T41.3X2	T41.3X3	T41.3X4	T41.3X5	T41.3X6
nerve block (peripheral) (plexus)	T41.3X1	T41.3X2	T41.3X3	T41.3X4	T41.3X5	T41.3X6
spinal	T41.3X1	T41.3X2	T41.3X3	T41.3X4	T41.3X5	T41.3X6
Ethoheptazine	T40.4X1	T40.4X2	T40.4X3	T40.4X4	T40.4X5	T40.4X6
Ethopropazine	T44.3X1	T44.3X2	T44.3X3	T44.3X4	T44.3X5	T44.3X6
Ethosuximide	T42.2X1	T42.2X2	T42.2X3	T42.2X4	T42.2X5	T42.2X6
Ethotoin	T42.0X1	T42.0X2	T42.0X3	T42.0X4	T42.0X5	T42.0X6
Ethoxazene	T37.91	T37.92	T37.93	T37.94	T37.95	T37.96
Ethoxazorutoside	T46.991	T46.992	T46.993	T46.994	T46.995	T46.996
Ethoxzolamide	T50.2X1	T50.2X2	T50.2X3	T50.2X4	T50.2X5	T50.2X6
Ethyl						
acetate	T52.8X1	T52.8X2	T52.8X3	T52.8X4	—	—
alcohol	T51.0X1	T51.0X2	T51.0X3	T51.0X4	—	—
beverage	T51.0X1	T51.0X2	T51.0X3	T51.0X4	—	—
aldehyde (vapor)	T59.891	T59.892	T59.893	T59.894	—	—
liquid	T52.8X1	T52.8X2	T52.8X3	T52.8X4	—	—
aminobenzoate	T41.3X1	T41.3X2	T41.3X3	T41.3X4	T41.3X5	T41.3X6
aminophenothiazine	T43.3X1	T43.3X2	T43.3X3	T43.3X4	T43.3X5	T43.3X6
benzoate	T52.8X1	T52.8X2	T52.8X3	T52.8X4	—	—
Ethyl — continued						
biscoumacetate	T45.511	T45.512	T45.513	T45.514	T45.515	T45.516
bromide (anesthetic)	T41.0X1	T41.0X2	T41.0X3	T41.0X4	T41.0X5	T41.0X6
carbamate	T45.1X1	T45.1X2	T45.1X3	T45.1X4	T45.1X5	T45.1X6
carbinol	T51.3X1	T51.3X2	T51.3X3	T51.3X4	—	—
carbonate	T52.8X1	T52.8X2	T52.8X3	T52.8X4	—	—
chaulmoograte	T37.1X1	T37.1X2	T37.1X3	T37.1X4	T37.1X5	T37.1X6
chloride (anesthetic)	T41.0X1	T41.0X2	T41.0X3	T41.0X4	T41.0X5	T41.0X6
anesthetic (local)	T41.3X1	T41.3X2	T41.3X3	T41.3X4	T41.3X5	T41.3X6
inhaled	T41.0X1	T41.0X2	T41.0X3	T41.0X4	T41.0X5	T41.0X6
local	T49.4X1	T49.4X2	T49.4X3	T49.4X4	T49.4X5	T49.4X6
solvent	T53.6X1	T53.6X2	T53.6X3	T53.6X4	—	—
dibunate	T48.3X1	T48.3X2	T48.3X3	T48.3X4	T48.3X5	T48.3X6
dichloroarsine (vapor)	T57.0X1	T57.0X2	T57.0X3	T57.0X4	—	—
estranol	T38.7X1	T38.7X2	T38.7X3	T38.7X4	T38.7X5	T38.7X6
ether — see also ether						
formate NEC (solvent)	T52.0X1	T52.0X2	T52.0X3	T52.0X4	—	—
fumarate	T49.4X1	T49.4X2	T49.4X3	T49.4X4	T49.4X5	T49.4X6
hydroxyisobutyrate NEC (solvent)	T52.8X1	T52.8X2	T52.8X3	T52.8X4		
iodoacetate	T59.3X1	T59.3X2	T59.3X3	T59.3X4	—	—
lactate NEC (solvent)	T52.8X1	T52.8X2	T52.8X3	T52.8X4	—	—
loflazepate	T42.4X1	T42.4X2	T42.4X3	T42.4X4	T42.4X5	T42.4X6
mercuric chloride	T56.1X1	T56.1X2	T56.1X3	T56.1X4	—	—
methylcarbinol	T51.8X1	T51.8X2	T51.8X3	T51.8X4	—	—
morphine	T40.2X1	T40.2X2	T40.2X3	T40.2X4	T40.2X5	T40.2X6
noradrenaline	T48.6X1	T48.6X2	T48.6X3	T48.6X4	T48.6X5	T48.6X6
oxybutyrate NEC (solvent)	T52.8X1	T52.8X2	T52.8X3	T52.8X4	—	—
Ethylene (gas)	T59.891	T59.892	T59.893	T59.894	—	—
anesthetic (general)	T41.0X1	T41.0X2	T41.0X3	T41.0X4	T41.0X5	T41.0X6
chlorohydrin	T52.8X1	T52.8X2	T52.8X3	T52.8X4	—	—
vapor	T53.6X1	T53.6X2	T53.6X3	T53.6X4	—	—
dichloride	T52.8X1	T52.8X2	T52.8X3	T52.8X4	—	—
vapor	T53.6X1	T53.6X2	T53.6X3	T53.6X4	—	—
dinitrate	T52.3X1	T52.3X2	T52.3X3	T52.3X4	—	—
glycol(s)	T52.8X1	T52.8X2	T52.8X3	T52.8X4	—	—
dinitrate	T52.3X1	T52.3X2	T52.3X3	T52.3X4	—	—
monobutyl ether	T52.3X1	T52.3X2	T52.3X3	T52.3X4	—	—
imine	T54.1X1	T54.1X2	T54.1X3	T54.1X4	—	—
oxide (fumigant) (nonmedicinal)	T59.891	T59.892	T59.893	T59.894	—	—
medicinal	T49.0X1	T49.0X2	T49.0X3	T49.0X4	T49.0X5	T49.0X6
Ethylenediaminetetra-acetic acid	T50.6X1	T50.6X2	T50.6X3	T50.6X4	T50.6X5	T50.6X6
Ethylenediamine theophylline	T48.6X1	T48.6X2	T48.6X3	T48.6X4	T48.6X5	T48.6X6
Ethylenedinitrilotetra-acetate	T50.6X1	T50.6X2	T50.6X3	T50.6X4	T50.6X5	T50.6X6
Ethylestrenol	T38.7X1	T38.7X2	T38.7X3	T38.7X4	T38.7X5	T38.7X6
Ethylhydroxycellulose	T47.4X1	T47.4X2	T47.4X3	T47.4X4	T47.4X5	T47.4X6
Ethylidene						
chloride NEC	T53.6X1	T53.6X2	T53.6X3	T53.6X4	—	—
diacetate	T60.3X1	T60.3X2	T60.3X3	T60.3X4	—	—
dicoumarin	T45.511	T45.512	T45.513	T45.514	T45.515	T45.516
dicoumarol	T45.511	T45.512	T45.513	T45.514	T45.515	T45.516
diethyl ether	T52.0X1	T52.0X2	T52.0X3	T52.0X4	—	—
Ethylmorphine	T40.2X1	T40.2X2	T40.2X3	T40.2X4	T40.2X5	T40.2X6
Ethylnorepinephrine	T48.6X1	T48.6X2	T48.6X3	T48.6X4	T48.6X5	T48.6X6
Ethylparachlorophen-oxyisobutyrate	T46.6X1	T46.6X2	T46.6X3	T46.6X4	T46.6X5	T46.6X6
Ethynodiol	T38.4X1	T38.4X2	T38.4X3	T38.4X4	T38.4X5	T38.4X6
with mestranol diacetate	T38.4X1	T38.4X2	T38.4X3	T38.4X4	T38.4X5	T38.4X6
Etidocaine	T41.3X1	T41.3X2	T41.3X3	T41.3X4	T41.3X5	T41.3X6
infiltration (subcutaneous)	T41.3X1	T41.3X2	T41.3X3	T41.3X4	T41.3X5	T41.3X6
nerve (peripheral) (plexus)	T41.3X1	T41.3X2	T41.3X3	T41.3X4	T41.3X5	T41.3X6
Etidronate	T50.991	T50.992	T50.993	T50.994	T50.995	T50.996
Etidronic acid (disodium salt)	T50.991	T50.992	T50.993	T50.994	T50.995	T50.996
Etifoxine	T42.6X1	T42.6X2	T42.6X3	T42.6X4	T42.6X5	T42.6X6
Etilefrine	T44.4X1	T44.4X2	T44.4X3	T44.4X4	T44.4X5	T44.4X6
Etilfen	T42.3X1	T42.3X2	T42.3X3	T42.3X4	T42.3X5	T42.3X6
Etinodiol	T38.4X1	T38.4X2	T38.4X3	T38.4X4	T38.4X5	T38.4X6
Etiroxate	T46.6X1	T46.6X2	T46.6X3	T46.6X4	T46.6X5	T46.6X6
Etizolam	T42.4X1	T42.4X2	T42.4X3	T42.4X4	T42.4X5	T42.4X6
Etodolac	T39.391	T39.392	T39.393	T39.394	T39.395	T39.396
Etofamide	T37.3X1	T37.3X2	T37.3X3	T37.3X4	T37.3X5	T37.3X6
Etofibrate	T46.6X1	T46.6X2	T46.6X3	T46.6X4	T46.6X5	T46.6X6
Etofylline	T46.7X1	T46.7X2	T46.7X3	T46.7X4	T46.7X5	T46.7X6
clofibrate	T46.6X1	T46.6X2	T46.6X3	T46.6X4	T46.6X5	T46.6X6
Etoglucid	T45.1X1	T45.1X2	T45.1X3	T45.1X4	T45.1X5	T45.1X6
Etomidate	T41.1X1	T41.1X2	T41.1X3	T41.1X4	T41.1X5	T41.1X6
Etomide	T39.8X1	T39.8X2	T39.8X3	T39.8X4	T39.8X5	T39.8X6
Etomidoline	T44.3X1	T44.3X2	T44.3X3	T44.3X4	T44.3X5	T44.3X6
Etoposide	T45.1X1	T45.1X2	T45.1X3	T45.1X4	T45.1X5	T45.1X6

Table of Drugs and Chemicals

Etorphine — Flumidin

Substance	Poisoning, Accidental (unintentional)	Poisoning, Intentional Self-harm	Poisoning, Assault	Poisoning, Undetermined	Adverse Effect	Under-dosing
Etorphine	T40.2X1	T40.2X2	T40.2X3	T40.2X4	T40.2X5	T40.2X6
Etoval	T42.3X1	T42.3X2	T42.3X3	T42.3X4	T42.3X5	T42.3X6
Etozolin	T50.1X1	T50.1X2	T50.1X3	T50.1X4	T50.1X5	T50.1X6
Etretinate	T50.991	T50.992	T50.993	T50.994	T50.995	T50.996
Etryptamine	T43.691	T43.692	T43.693	T43.694	T43.695	T43.696
Etybenzatropine	T44.3X1	T44.3X2	T44.3X3	T44.3X4	T44.3X5	T44.3X6
Etynodiol	T38.4X1	T38.4X2	T38.4X3	T38.4X4	T38.4X5	T38.4X6
Eucaine	T41.3X1	T41.3X2	T41.3X3	T41.3X4	T41.3X5	T41.3X6
Eucalyptus oil	T49.7X1	T49.7X2	T49.7X3	T49.7X4	T49.7X5	T49.7X6
Eucatropine	T49.5X1	T49.5X2	T49.5X3	T49.5X4	T49.5X5	T49.5X6
Eucodal	T40.2X1	T40.2X2	T40.2X3	T40.2X4	T40.2X5	T40.2X6
Euneryl	T42.3X1	T42.3X2	T42.3X3	T42.3X4	T42.3X5	T42.3X6
Euphthalmine	T44.3X1	T44.3X2	T44.3X3	T44.3X4	T44.3X5	T44.3X6
Eurax	T49.0X1	T49.0X2	T49.0X3	T49.0X4	T49.0X5	T49.0X6
Euresol	T49.4X1	T49.4X2	T49.4X3	T49.4X4	T49.4X5	T49.4X6
Euthroid	T38.1X1	T38.1X2	T38.1X3	T38.1X4	T38.1X5	T38.1X6
Evans blue	T50.8X1	T50.8X2	T50.8X3	T50.8X4	T50.8X5	T50.8X6
Evipal	T42.3X1	T42.3X2	T42.3X3	T42.3X4	T42.3X5	T42.3X6
sodium	T41.1X1	T41.1X2	T41.1X3	T41.1X4	T41.1X5	T41.1X6
Evipan	T42.3X1	T42.3X2	T42.3X3	T42.3X4	T42.3X5	T42.3X6
sodium	T41.1X1	T41.1X2	T41.1X3	T41.1X4	T41.1X5	T41.1X6
Exalamide	T49.0X1	T49.0X2	T49.0X3	T49.0X4	T49.0X5	T49.0X6
Exalgin	T39.1X1	T39.1X2	T39.1X3	T39.1X4	T39.1X5	T39.1X6
Excipients, pharmaceutical	T50.901	T50.902	T50.903	T50.904	T50.905	T50.906
Exhaust gas (engine) (motor vehicle)	T58.01	T58.02	T58.03	T58.04	—	—
Ex-Lax (phenolphthalein)	T47.2X1	T47.2X2	T47.2X3	T47.2X4	T47.2X5	T47.2X6
Expectorant NEC	T48.4X1	T48.4X2	T48.4X3	T48.4X4	T48.4X5	T48.4X6
Extended insulin zinc suspension	T38.3X1	T38.3X2	T38.3X3	T38.3X4	T38.3X5	T38.3X6
External medications (skin) (mucous membrane)	T49.91	T49.92	T49.93	T49.94	T49.95	T49.96
dental agent	T49.7X1	T49.7X2	T49.7X3	T49.7X4	T49.7X5	T49.7X6
ENT agent	T49.6X1	T49.6X2	T49.6X3	T49.6X4	T49.6X5	T49.6X6
ophthalmic preparation	T49.5X1	T49.5X2	T49.5X3	T49.5X4	T49.5X5	T49.5X6
specified NEC	T49.8X1	T49.8X2	T49.8X3	T49.8X4	T49.8X5	T49.8X6
Extrapyramidal antagonist NEC	T44.3X1	T44.3X2	T44.3X3	T44.3X4	T44.3X5	T44.3X6
Eye agents (anti-infective)	T49.5X1	T49.5X2	T49.5X3	T49.5X4	T49.5X5	T49.5X6
Eye drug NEC	T49.5X1	T49.5X2	T49.5X3	T49.5X4	T49.5X5	T49.5X6
FAC (fluorouracil + doxorubicin + cyclophosphamide)	T45.1X1	T45.1X2	T45.1X3	T45.1X4	T45.1X5	T45.1X6
Factor						
I (fibrinogen)	T45.8X1	T45.8X2	T45.8X3	T45.8X4	T45.8X5	T45.8X6
III (thromboplastin)	T45.8X1	T45.8X2	T45.8X3	T45.8X4	T45.8X5	T45.8X6
IX complex	T45.7X1	T45.7X2	T45.7X3	T45.7X4	T45.7X5	T45.7X6
human	T45.8X1	T45.8X2	T45.8X3	T45.8X4	T45.8X5	T45.8X6
VIII (antihemophilic Factor) (concentrate)	T45.8X1	T45.8X2	T45.8X3	T45.8X4	T45.8X5	T45.8X6
Famotidine	T47.0X1	T47.0X2	T47.0X3	T47.0X4	T47.0X5	T47.0X6
Fat suspension, intravenous	T50.991	T50.992	T50.993	T50.994	T50.995	T50.996
Fazadinium bromide	T48.1X1	T48.1X2	T48.1X3	T48.1X4	T48.1X5	T48.1X6
Febarbamate	T42.3X1	T42.3X2	T42.3X3	T42.3X4	T42.3X5	T42.3X6
Fecal softener	T47.4X1	T47.4X2	T47.4X3	T47.4X4	T47.4X5	T47.4X6
Fedrilate	T48.3X1	T48.3X2	T48.3X3	T48.3X4	T48.3X5	T48.3X6
Felodipine	T46.1X1	T46.1X2	T46.1X3	T46.1X4	T46.1X5	T46.1X6
Felypressin	T38.891	T38.892	T38.893	T38.894	T38.895	T38.896
Femoxetine	T43.221	T43.222	T43.223	T43.224	T43.225	T43.226
Fenalcomine	T46.3X1	T46.3X2	T46.3X3	T46.3X4	T46.3X5	T46.3X6
Fenamisal	T37.1X1	T37.1X2	T37.1X3	T37.1X4	T37.1X5	T37.1X6
Fenazone	T39.2X1	T39.2X2	T39.2X3	T39.2X4	T39.2X5	T39.2X6
Fenbendazole	T37.4X1	T37.4X2	T37.4X3	T37.4X4	T37.4X5	T37.4X6
Fenbutrazate	T50.5X1	T50.5X2	T50.5X3	T50.5X4	T50.5X5	T50.5X6
Fencamfamine	T43.691	T43.692	T43.693	T43.694	T43.695	T43.696
Fendiline	T46.1X1	T46.1X2	T46.1X3	T46.1X4	T46.1X5	T46.1X6
Fenetylline	T43.691	T43.692	T43.693	T43.694	T43.695	T43.696
Fenflumizole	T39.391	T39.392	T39.393	T39.394	T39.395	T39.396
Fenfluramine	T50.5X1	T50.5X2	T50.5X3	T50.5X4	T50.5X5	T50.5X6
Fenobarbital	T42.3X1	T42.3X2	T42.3X3	T42.3X4	T42.3X5	T42.3X6
Fenofibrate	T46.6X1	T46.6X2	T46.6X3	T46.6X4	T46.6X5	T46.6X6
Fenoprofen	T39.311	T39.312	T39.313	T39.314	T39.315	T39.316
Fenoterol	T48.6X1	T48.6X2	T48.6X3	T48.6X4	T48.6X5	T48.6X6
Fenoverine	T44.3X1	T44.3X2	T44.3X3	T44.3X4	T44.3X5	T44.3X6
Fenoxazoline	T48.5X1	T48.5X2	T48.5X3	T48.5X4	T48.5X5	T48.5X6
Fenproporex	T50.5X1	T50.5X2	T50.5X3	T50.5X4	T50.5X5	T50.5X6
Fenquizone	T50.2X1	T50.2X2	T50.2X3	T50.2X4	T50.2X5	T50.2X6
Fentanyl	T40.4X1	T40.4X2	T40.4X3	T40.4X4	T40.4X5	T40.4X6
Fentazin	T43.3X1	T43.3X2	T43.3X3	T43.3X4	T43.3X5	T43.3X6
Fenthion	T60.0X1	T60.0X2	T60.0X3	T60.0X4		
Fenticlor	T49.0X1	T49.0X2	T49.0X3	T49.0X4	T49.0X5	T49.0X6
Fenylbutazone	T39.2X1	T39.2X2	T39.2X3	T39.2X4	T39.2X5	T39.2X6

Substance	Poisoning, Accidental (unintentional)	Poisoning, Intentional Self-harm	Poisoning, Assault	Poisoning, Undetermined	Adverse Effect	Under-dosing
Feprazone	T39.2X1	T39.2X2	T39.2X3	T39.2X4	T39.2X5	T39.2X6
Fer de lance (bite) (venom)	T63.061	T63.062	T63.063	T63.064		
Ferric — see also Iron						
chloride	T45.4X1	T45.4X2	T45.4X3	T45.4X4	T45.4X5	T45.4X6
citrate	T45.4X1	T45.4X2	T45.4X3	T45.4X4	T45.4X5	T45.4X6
hydroxide						
colloidal	T45.4X1	T45.4X2	T45.4X3	T45.4X4	T45.4X5	T45.4X6
polymaltose	T45.4X1	T45.4X2	T45.4X3	T45.4X4	T45.4X5	T45.4X6
pyrophosphate	T45.4X1	T45.4X2	T45.4X3	T45.4X4	T45.4X5	T45.4X6
Ferritin	T45.4X1	T45.4X2	T45.4X3	T45.4X4	T45.4X5	T45.4X6
Ferrocholinate	T45.4X1	T45.4X2	T45.4X3	T45.4X4	T45.4X5	T45.4X6
Ferrodextrane	T45.4X1	T45.4X2	T45.4X3	T45.4X4	T45.4X5	T45.4X6
Ferropolimaler	T45.4X1	T45.4X2	T45.4X3	T45.4X4	T45.4X5	T45.4X6
Ferrous — see also Iron						
phosphate	T45.4X1	T45.4X2	T45.4X3	T45.4X4	T45.4X5	T45.4X6
salt	T45.4X1	T45.4X2	T45.4X3	T45.4X4	T45.4X5	T45.4X6
with folic acid	T45.4X1	T45.4X2	T45.4X3	T45.4X4	T45.4X5	T45.4X6
Ferrous fumerate, gluconate, lactate, salt NEC, sulfate (medicinal)	T45.4X1	T45.4X2	T45.4X3	T45.4X4	T45.4X5	T45.4X6
Ferrovanadium (fumes)	T59.891	T59.892	T59.893	T59.894	—	—
Ferrum — see Iron						
Fertilizers NEC	T65.891	T65.892	T65.893	T65.894	—	—
with herbicide mixture	T60.3X1	T60.3X2	T60.3X3	T60.3X4	—	—
Fetoxilate	T47.6X1	T47.6X2	T47.6X3	T47.6X4	T47.6X5	T47.6X6
Fiber, dietary	T47.4X1	T47.4X2	T47.4X3	T47.4X4	T47.4X5	T47.4X6
Fiberglass	T65.831	T65.832	T65.833	T65.834		
Fibrinogen (human)	T45.8X1	T45.8X2	T45.8X3	T45.8X4	T45.8X5	T45.8X6
Fibrinolysin (human)	T45.691	T45.692	T45.693	T45.694	T45.695	T45.696
Fibrinolysis						
affecting drug	T45.601	T45.602	T45.603	T45.604	T45.605	T45.606
inhibitor NEC	T45.621	T45.622	T45.623	T45.624	T45.625	T45.626
Fibrinolytic drug	T45.611	T45.612	T45.613	T45.614	T45.615	T45.616
Filix mas	T37.4X1	T37.4X2	T37.4X3	T37.4X4	T37.4X5	T37.4X6
Filtering cream	T49.3X1	T49.3X2	T49.3X3	T49.3X4	T49.3X5	T49.3X6
Fiorinal	T39.011	T39.012	T39.013	T39.014	T39.015	T39.016
Firedamp	T59.891	T59.892	T59.893	T59.894	—	—
Fish, noxious, nonbacterial	T61.91	T61.92	T61.93	T61.94	—	—
ciguatera	T61.01	T61.02	T61.03	T61.04	—	—
scombroid	T61.11	T61.12	T61.13	T61.14	—	—
shell	T61.781	T61.782	T61.783	T61.784	—	—
specified NEC	T61.771	T61.772	T61.773	T61.774	—	—
Flagyl	T37.3X1	T37.3X2	T37.3X3	T37.3X4	T37.3X5	T37.3X6
Flavine adenine dinucleotide	T45.2X1	T45.2X2	T45.2X3	T45.2X4	T45.2X5	T45.2X6
Flavodic acid	T46.991	T46.992	T46.993	T46.994	T46.995	T46.996
Flavoxate	T44.3X1	T44.3X2	T44.3X3	T44.3X4	T44.3X5	T44.3X6
Flaxedil	T48.1X1	T48.1X2	T48.1X3	T48.1X4	T48.1X5	T48.1X6
Flaxseed (medicinal)	T49.3X1	T49.3X2	T49.3X3	T49.3X4	T49.3X5	T49.3X6
Flecainide	T46.2X1	T46.2X2	T46.2X3	T46.2X4	T46.2X5	T46.2X6
Fleroxacin	T36.8X1	T36.8X2	T36.8X3	T36.8X4	T36.8X5	T36.8X6
Floctafenine	T39.8X1	T39.8X2	T39.8X3	T39.8X4	T39.8X5	T39.8X6
Flomax	T44.6X1	T44.6X2	T44.6X3	T44.6X4	T44.6X5	T44.6X6
Flomoxef	T36.1X1	T36.1X2	T36.1X3	T36.1X4	T36.1X5	T36.1X6
Flopropione	T44.3X1	T44.3X2	T44.3X3	T44.3X4	T44.3X5	T44.3X6
Florantyrone	T47.5X1	T47.5X2	T47.5X3	T47.5X4	T47.5X5	T47.5X6
Floraquin	T37.8X1	T37.8X2	T37.8X3	T37.8X4	T37.8X5	T37.8X6
Florinef	T38.0X1	T38.0X2	T38.0X3	T38.0X4	T38.0X5	T38.0X6
ENT agent	T49.6X1	T49.6X2	T49.6X3	T49.6X4	T49.6X5	T49.6X6
ophthalmic preparation	T49.5X1	T49.5X2	T49.5X3	T49.5X4	T49.5X5	T49.5X6
topical NEC	T49.0X1	T49.0X2	T49.0X3	T49.0X4	T49.0X5	T49.0X6
Flowers of sulfur	T49.4X1	T49.4X2	T49.4X3	T49.4X4	T49.4X5	T49.4X6
Floxuridine	T45.1X1	T45.1X2	T45.1X3	T45.1X4	T45.1X5	T45.1X6
Fluanisone	T43.4X1	T43.4X2	T43.4X3	T43.4X4	T43.4X5	T43.4X6
Flubendazole	T37.4X1	T37.4X2	T37.4X3	T37.4X4	T37.4X5	T37.4X6
Fluclorolone acetonide	T49.0X1	T49.0X2	T49.0X3	T49.0X4	T49.0X5	T49.0X6
Flucloxacillin	T36.0X1	T36.0X2	T36.0X3	T36.0X4	T36.0X5	T36.0X6
Fluconazole	T37.8X1	T37.8X2	T37.8X3	T37.8X4	T37.8X5	T37.8X6
Flucytosine	T37.8X1	T37.8X2	T37.8X3	T37.8X4	T37.8X5	T37.8X6
Fludeoxyglucose (18F)	T50.8X1	T50.8X2	T50.8X3	T50.8X4	T50.8X5	T50.8X6
Fludiazepam	T42.4X1	T42.4X2	T42.4X3	T42.4X4	T42.4X5	T42.4X6
Fludrocortisone	T50.0X1	T50.0X2	T50.0X3	T50.0X4	T50.0X5	T50.0X6
ENT agent	T49.6X1	T49.6X2	T49.6X3	T49.6X4	T49.6X5	T49.6X6
ophthalmic preparation	T49.5X1	T49.5X2	T49.5X3	T49.5X4	T49.5X5	T49.5X6
topical NEC	T49.0X1	T49.0X2	T49.0X3	T49.0X4	T49.0X5	T49.0X6
Fludroxycortide	T49.0X1	T49.0X2	T49.0X3	T49.0X4	T49.0X5	T49.0X6
Flufenamic acid	T39.391	T39.392	T39.393	T39.394	T39.395	T39.396
Fluindione	T45.511	T45.512	T45.513	T45.514	T45.515	T45.516
Flumequine	T37.8X1	T37.8X2	T37.8X3	T37.8X4	T37.8X5	T37.8X6
Flumethasone	T49.0X1	T49.0X2	T49.0X3	T49.0X4	T49.0X5	T49.0X6
Flumethiazide	T50.2X1	T50.2X2	T50.2X3	T50.2X4	T50.2X5	T50.2X6
Flumidin	T37.5X1	T37.5X2	T37.5X3	T37.5X4	T37.5X5	T37.5X6

Substance	Poisoning, Accidental (unintentional)	Poisoning, Intentional Self-harm	Poisoning, Assault	Poisoning, Undetermined	Adverse Effect	Under-dosing
Flunarizine	T46.7X1	T46.7X2	T46.7X3	T46.7X4	T46.7X5	T46.7X6
Flunidazole	T37.8X1	T37.8X2	T37.8X3	T37.8X4	T37.8X5	T37.8X6
Flunisolide	T48.6X1	T48.6X2	T48.6X3	T48.6X4	T48.6X5	T48.6X6
Flunitrazepam	T42.4X1	T42.4X2	T42.4X3	T42.4X4	T42.4X5	T42.4X6
Fluocinolone (acetonide)	T49.0X1	T49.0X2	T49.0X3	T49.0X4	T49.0X5	T49.0X6
Fluocinonide	T49.0X1	T49.0X2	T49.0X3	T49.0X4	T49.0X5	T49.0X6
Fluocortin (butyl)	T49.0X1	T49.0X2	T49.0X3	T49.0X4	T49.0X5	T49.0X6
Fluocortolone	T49.0X1	T49.0X2	T49.0X3	T49.0X4	T49.0X5	T49.0X6
Fluohydrocortisone	T38.0X1	T38.0X2	T38.0X3	T38.0X4	T38.0X5	T38.0X6
ENT agent	T49.6X1	T49.6X2	T49.6X3	T49.6X4	T49.6X5	T49.6X6
ophthalmic preparation	T49.5X1	T49.5X2	T49.5X3	T49.5X4	T49.5X5	T49.5X6
topical NEC	T49.0X1	T49.0X2	T49.0X3	T49.0X4	T49.0X5	T49.0X6
Fluonid	T49.0X1	T49.0X2	T49.0X3	T49.0X4	T49.0X5	T49.0X6
Fluopromazine	T43.3X1	T43.3X2	T43.3X3	T43.3X4	T43.3X5	T43.3X6
Fluoracetate	T60.8X1	T60.8X2	T60.8X3	T60.8X4	—	—
Fluorescein	T50.8X1	T50.8X2	T50.8X3	T50.8X4	T50.8X5	T50.8X6
Fluorhydrocortisone	T50.0X1	T50.0X2	T50.0X3	T50.0X4	T50.0X5	T50.0X6
Fluoride (nonmedicinal) (pesticide) (sodium) NEC	T60.8X1	T60.8X2	T60.8X3	T60.8X4	—	—
hydrogen — see Hydrofluoric acid						
medicinal NEC	T50.991	T50.992	T50.993	T50.994	T50.995	T50.996
dental use	T49.7X1	T49.7X2	T49.7X3	T49.7X4	T49.7X5	T49.7X6
not pesticide NEC	T54.91	T54.92	T54.93	T54.94	—	—
stannous	T49.7X1	T49.7X2	T49.7X3	T49.7X4	T49.7X5	T49.7X6
Fluorinated corticosteroids	T38.0X1	T38.0X2	T38.0X3	T38.0X4	T38.0X5	T38.0X6
Fluorine (gas)	T59.5X1	T59.5X2	T59.5X3	T59.5X4	—	—
salt — see Fluoride(s)						
Fluoristan	T49.7X1	T49.7X2	T49.7X3	T49.7X4	T49.7X5	T49.7X6
Fluormetholone	T49.0X1	T49.0X2	T49.0X3	T49.0X4	T49.0X5	T49.0X6
Fluoroacetate	T60.8X1	T60.8X2	T60.8X3	T60.8X4	—	—
Fluorocarbon monomer	T53.6X1	T53.6X2	T53.6X3	T53.6X4	—	—
Fluorocytosine	T37.8X1	T37.8X2	T37.8X3	T37.8X4	T37.8X5	T37.8X6
Fluorodeoxyuridine	T45.1X1	T45.1X2	T45.1X3	T45.1X4	T45.1X5	T45.1X6
Fluorometholone	T49.0X1	T49.0X2	T49.0X3	T49.0X4	T49.0X5	T49.0X6
ophthalmic preparation	T49.5X1	T49.5X2	T49.5X3	T49.5X4	T49.5X5	T49.5X6
Fluorophosphate insecticide	T60.0X1	T60.0X2	T60.0X3	T60.0X4	—	—
Fluorosol	T46.3X1	T46.3X2	T46.3X3	T46.3X4	T46.3X5	T46.3X6
Fluorouracil	T45.1X1	T45.1X2	T45.1X3	T45.1X4	T45.1X5	T45.1X6
Fluorphenylalanine	T49.5X1	T49.5X2	T49.5X3	T49.5X4	T49.5X5	T49.5X6
Fluothane	T41.0X1	T41.0X2	T41.0X3	T41.0X4	T41.0X5	T41.0X6
Fluoxetine	T43.221	T43.222	T43.223	T43.224	T43.225	T43.226
Fluoxymesterone	T38.7X1	T38.7X2	T38.7X3	T38.7X4	T38.7X5	T38.7X6
Flupenthixol	T43.4X1	T43.4X2	T43.4X3	T43.4X4	T43.4X5	T43.4X6
Flupentixol	T43.4X1	T43.4X2	T43.4X3	T43.4X4	T43.4X5	T43.4X6
Fluphenazine	T43.3X1	T43.3X2	T43.3X3	T43.3X4	T43.3X5	T43.3X6
Fluprednidene	T49.0X1	T49.0X2	T49.0X3	T49.0X4	T49.0X5	T49.0X6
Fluprednisolone	T38.0X1	T38.0X2	T38.0X3	T38.0X4	T38.0X5	T38.0X6
Fluradoline	T39.8X1	T39.8X2	T39.8X3	T39.8X4	T39.8X5	T39.8X6
Flurandrenolide	T49.0X1	T49.0X2	T49.0X3	T49.0X4	T49.0X5	T49.0X6
Flurandrenolone	T49.0X1	T49.0X2	T49.0X3	T49.0X4	T49.0X5	T49.0X6
Flurazepam	T42.4X1	T42.4X2	T42.4X3	T42.4X4	T42.4X5	T42.4X6
Flurbiprofen	T39.311	T39.312	T39.313	T39.314	T39.315	T39.316
Flurobate	T49.0X1	T49.0X2	T49.0X3	T49.0X4	T49.0X5	T49.0X6
Fluroxene	T41.0X1	T41.0X2	T41.0X3	T41.0X4	T41.0X5	T41.0X6
Fluspirilene	T43.591	T43.592	T43.593	T43.594	T43.595	T43.596
Flutamide	T38.6X1	T38.6X2	T38.6X3	T38.6X4	T38.6X5	T38.6X6
Flutazolam	T38.0X1	T38.0X2	T38.0X3	T38.0X4	T38.0X5	T38.0X6
Fluticasone propionate	T38.0X1	T38.0X2	T38.0X3	T38.0X4	T38.0X5	T38.0X6
Flutoprazepam	T42.4X1	T42.4X2	T42.4X3	T42.4X4	T42.4X5	T42.4X6
Flutropium bromide	T48.6X1	T48.6X2	T48.6X3	T48.6X4	T48.6X5	T48.6X6
Fluvoxamine	T43.221	T43.222	T43.223	T43.224	T43.225	T43.226
Folacin	T45.8X1	T45.8X2	T45.8X3	T45.8X4	T45.8X5	T45.8X6
Folic acid	T45.8X1	T45.8X2	T45.8X3	T45.8X4	T45.8X5	T45.8X6
with ferrous salt	T45.2X1	T45.2X2	T45.2X3	T45.2X4	T45.2X5	T45.2X6
antagonist	T45.1X1	T45.1X2	T45.1X3	T45.1X4	T45.1X5	T45.1X6
Folinic acid	T45.8X1	T45.8X2	T45.8X3	T45.8X4	T45.8X5	T45.8X6
Folium stramoniae	T48.6X1	T48.6X2	T48.6X3	T48.6X4	T48.6X5	T48.6X6
Follicle-stimulating hormone, human	T38.811	T38.812	T38.813	T38.814	T38.815	T38.816
Folpet	T60.3X1	T60.3X2	T60.3X3	T60.3X4	—	—
Fominoben	T48.3X1	T48.3X2	T48.3X3	T48.3X4	T48.3X5	T48.3X6
Food, foodstuffs, noxious, nonbacterial, NEC	T62.91	T62.92	T62.93	T62.94	—	—
berries	T62.1X1	T62.1X2	T62.1X3	T62.1X4	—	—
fish — see also Fish	T61.91	T61.92	T61.93	T61.94	—	—
mushrooms	T62.0X1	T62.0X2	T62.0X3	T62.0X4	—	—
plants	T62.2X1	T62.2X2	T62.2X3	T62.2X4	—	—
seafood	T61.91	T61.92	T61.93	T61.94	—	—
specified NEC	T61.8X1	T61.8X2	T61.8X3	T61.8X4	—	—
seeds	T62.2X1	T62.2X2	T62.2X3	T62.2X4	—	—
Food, foodstuffs, noxious, nonbacterial, — continued						
shellfish	T61.781	T61.782	T61.783	T61.784	—	—
specified NEC	T62.8X1	T62.8X2	T62.8X3	T62.8X4	—	—
Fool's parsley	T62.2X1	T62.2X2	T62.2X3	T62.2X4	—	—
Formaldehyde (solution), gas or vapor	T59.2X1	T59.2X2	T59.2X3	T59.2X4	—	—
fungicide	T60.3X1	T60.3X2	T60.3X3	T60.3X4	—	—
Formalin	T59.2X1	T59.2X2	T59.2X3	T59.2X4	—	—
fungicide	T60.3X1	T60.3X2	T60.3X3	T60.3X4	—	—
vapor	T59.2X1	T59.2X2	T59.2X3	T59.2X4	—	—
Formic acid	T54.2X1	T54.2X2	T54.2X3	T54.2X4	—	—
vapor	T59.891	T59.892	T59.893	T59.894	—	—
Foscarnet sodium	T37.5X1	T37.5X2	T37.5X3	T37.5X4	T37.5X5	T37.5X6
Fosfestrol	T38.5X1	T38.5X2	T38.5X3	T38.5X4	T38.5X5	T38.5X6
Fosfomycin	T36.8X1	T36.8X2	T36.8X3	T36.8X4	T36.8X5	T36.8X6
Fosfonet sodium	T37.5X1	T37.5X2	T37.5X3	T37.5X4	T37.5X5	T37.5X6
Fosinopril	T46.4X1	T46.4X2	T46.4X3	T46.4X4	T46.4X5	T46.4X6
sodium	T46.4X1	T46.4X2	T46.4X3	T46.4X4	T46.4X5	T46.4X6
Fowler's solution	T57.0X1	T57.0X2	T57.0X3	T57.0X4	—	—
Foxglove	T62.2X1	T62.2X2	T62.2X3	T62.2X4	—	—
Framycetin	T36.5X1	T36.5X2	T36.5X3	T36.5X4	T36.5X5	T36.5X6
Frangula	T47.2X1	T47.2X2	T47.2X3	T47.2X4	T47.2X5	T47.2X6
extract	T47.2X1	T47.2X2	T47.2X3	T47.2X4	T47.2X5	T47.2X6
Frei antigen	T50.8X1	T50.8X2	T50.8X3	T50.8X4	T50.8X5	T50.8X6
Freon	T53.5X1	T53.5X2	T53.5X3	T53.5X4	—	—
Fructose	T50.3X1	T50.3X2	T50.3X3	T50.3X4	T50.3X5	T50.3X6
Frusemide	T50.1X1	T50.1X2	T50.1X3	T50.1X4	T50.1X5	T50.1X6
FSH	T38.811	T38.812	T38.813	T38.814	T38.815	T38.816
Ftorafur	T45.1X1	T45.1X2	T45.1X3	T45.1X4	T45.1X5	T45.1X6
Fuel						
automobile	T52.0X1	T52.0X2	T52.0X3	T52.0X4	—	—
exhaust gas, not in transit	T58.01	T58.02	T58.03	T58.04	—	—
vapor NEC	T52.0X1	T52.0X2	T52.0X3	T52.0X4	—	—
gas (domestic use) — see also Carbon, monoxide, fuel, utility	T59.891	T59.892	T59.893	T59.894	—	—
utility	T59.891	T59.892	T59.893	T59.894	—	—
incomplete combustion of — see Carbon, monoxide, fuel, utility						
in mobile container	T59.891	T59.892	T59.893	T59.894	—	—
piped (natural)	T59.891	T59.892	T59.893	T59.894	—	—
industrial, incomplete combustion	T58.8X1	T58.8X2	T58.8X3	T58.8X4	—	—
Fugillin	T36.8X1	T36.8X2	T36.8X3	T36.8X4	T36.8X5	T36.8X6
Fulminate of mercury	T56.1X1	T56.1X2	T56.1X3	T56.1X4	—	—
Fulvicin	T36.7X1	T36.7X2	T36.7X3	T36.7X4	T36.7X5	T36.7X6
Fumadil	T36.8X1	T36.8X2	T36.8X3	T36.8X4	T36.8X5	T36.8X6
Fumagillin	T36.8X1	T36.8X2	T36.8X3	T36.8X4	T36.8X5	T36.8X6
Fumaric acid	T49.4X1	T49.4X2	T49.4X3	T49.4X4	T49.4X5	T49.4X6
Fumes (from)	T59.91	T59.92	T59.93	T59.94	—	—
carbon monoxide — see Carbon, monoxide						
charcoal (domestic use) — see Charcoal, fumes						
chloroform — see Chloroform						
coke (in domestic stoves, fireplaces) — see Coke fumes						
corrosive NEC	T54.91	T54.92	T54.93	T54.94	—	—
ether — see ether						
freons	T53.5X1	T53.5X2	T53.5X3	T53.5X4	—	—
hydrocarbons	T59.891	T59.892	T59.893	T59.894	—	—
petroleum (liquefied)	T59.891	T59.892	T59.893	T59.894	—	—
distributed through pipes (pure or mixed with air)	T59.891	T59.892	T59.893	T59.894	—	—
lead — see lead						
metal — see Metals, or the specified metal						
nitrogen dioxide	T59.0X1	T59.0X2	T59.0X3	T59.0X4	—	—
pesticides — see Pesticides						
petroleum (liquefied)	T59.891	T59.892	T59.893	T59.894	—	—
distributed through pipes (pure or mixed with air)	T59.891	T59.892	T59.893	T59.894	—	—
polyester	T59.891	T59.892	T59.893	T59.894	—	—
specified source NEC — see also substance specified	T59.891	T59.892	T59.893	T59.894	—	—
sulfur dioxide	T59.1X1	T59.1X2	T59.1X3	T59.1X4	—	—
Fumigant NEC	T60.91	T60.92	T60.93	T60.94	—	—

Subterms under main terms may continue to next column or page   Additional Character May Be Required — Refer to the Tabular List for Character Selection   369

Flunarizine — Fumigant NEC

Substance	Poisoning, Accidental (unintentional)	Poisoning, Intentional Self-harm	Poisoning, Assault	Poisoning, Undetermined	Adverse Effect	Under-dosing
Fungicide NEC (nonmedicinal)	T60.3X1	T60.3X2	T60.3X3	T60.3X4	—	—
Fungi, noxious, used as food	T62.0X1	T62.0X2	T62.0X3	T62.0X4	—	—
Fungizone	T36.7X1	T36.7X2	T36.7X3	T36.7X4	T36.7X5	T36.7X6
topical	T49.0X1	T49.0X2	T49.0X3	T49.0X4	T49.0X5	T49.0X6
Furacin	T49.0X1	T49.0X2	T49.0X3	T49.0X4	T49.0X5	T49.0X6
Furadantin	T37.91	T37.92	T37.93	T37.94	T37.95	T37.96
Furazolidone	T37.8X1	T37.8X2	T37.8X3	T37.8X4	T37.8X5	T37.8X6
Furazolium chloride	T49.0X1	T49.0X2	T49.0X3	T49.0X4	T49.0X5	T49.0X6
Furfural	T52.8X1	T52.8X2	T52.8X3	T52.8X4	—	—
Furnace (coal burning) (domestic), gas from	T58.2X1	T58.2X2	T58.2X3	T58.2X4	—	—
industrial	T58.8X1	T58.8X2	T58.8X3	T58.8X4	—	—
Furniture polish	T65.891	T65.892	T65.893	T65.894	—	—
Furosemide	T50.1X1	T50.1X2	T50.1X3	T50.1X4	T50.1X5	T50.1X6
Furoxone	T37.91	T37.92	T37.93	T37.94	T37.95	T37.96
Fursultiamine	T45.2X1	T45.2X2	T45.2X3	T45.2X4	T45.2X5	T45.2X6
Fusafungine	T36.8X1	T36.8X2	T36.8X3	T36.8X4	T36.8X5	T36.8X6
Fusel oil (any) (amyl) (butyl) (propyl), vapor	T51.3X1	T51.3X2	T51.3X3	T51.3X4	—	—
Fusidate (ethanolamine) (sodium)	T36.8X1	T36.8X2	T36.8X3	T36.8X4	T36.8X5	T36.8X6
Fusidic acid	T36.8X1	T36.8X2	T36.8X3	T36.8X4	T36.8X5	T36.8X6
Fytic acid, nonasodium	T50.6X1	T50.6X2	T50.6X3	T50.6X4	T50.6X5	T50.6X6
b-Galactosidase	T47.5X1	T47.5X2	T47.5X3	T47.5X4	T47.5X5	T47.5X6
GABA	T43.8X1	T43.8X2	T43.8X3	T43.8X4	T43.8X5	T43.8X6
Gadopentetic acid	T50.8X1	T50.8X2	T50.8X3	T50.8X4	T50.8X5	T50.8X6
Galactose	T50.3X1	T50.3X2	T50.3X3	T50.3X4	T50.3X5	T50.3X6
Galantamine	T44.0X1	T44.0X2	T44.0X3	T44.0X4	T44.0X5	T44.0X6
Gallamine (triethiodide)	T48.1X1	T48.1X2	T48.1X3	T48.1X4	T48.1X5	T48.1X6
Gallium citrate	T50.991	T50.992	T50.993	T50.994	T50.995	T50.996
Gallopamil	T46.1X1	T46.1X2	T46.1X3	T46.1X4	T46.1X5	T46.1X6
Gamboge	T47.2X1	T47.2X2	T47.2X3	T47.2X4	T47.2X5	T47.2X6
Gamimune	T50.Z11	T50.Z12	T50.Z13	T50.Z14	T50.Z15	T50.Z16
Gamma-aminobutyric acid	T43.8X1	T43.8X2	T43.8X3	T43.8X4	T43.8X5	T43.8X6
Gamma-benzene hexachloride (medicinal)	T49.0X1	T49.0X2	T49.0X3	T49.0X4	T49.0X5	T49.0X6
nonmedicinal, vapor	T53.6X1	T53.6X2	T53.6X3	T53.6X4	—	—
Gamma-BHC (medicinal) — see also Gamma-benzene hexachloride	T49.0X1	T49.0X2	T49.0X3	T49.0X4	T49.0X5	T49.0X6
Gamma globulin	T50.Z11	T50.Z12	T50.Z13	T50.Z14	T50.Z15	T50.Z16
Gamulin	T50.Z11	T50.Z12	T50.Z13	T50.Z14	T50.Z15	T50.Z16
Ganciclovir (sodium)	T37.5X1	T37.5X2	T37.5X3	T37.5X4	T37.5X5	T37.5X6
Ganglionic blocking drug NEC	T44.2X1	T44.2X2	T44.2X3	T44.2X4	T44.2X5	T44.2X6
specified NEC	T44.2X1	T44.2X2	T44.2X3	T44.2X4	T44.2X5	T44.2X6
Ganja	T40.7X1	T40.7X2	T40.7X3	T40.7X4	T40.7X5	T40.7X6
Garamycin	T36.5X1	T36.5X2	T36.5X3	T36.5X4	T36.5X5	T36.5X6
ophthalmic preparation	T49.5X1	T49.5X2	T49.5X3	T49.5X4	T49.5X5	T49.5X6
topical NEC	T49.0X1	T49.0X2	T49.0X3	T49.0X4	T49.0X5	T49.0X6
Gardenal	T42.3X1	T42.3X2	T42.3X3	T42.3X4	T42.3X5	T42.3X6
Gardepanyl	T42.3X1	T42.3X2	T42.3X3	T42.3X4	T42.3X5	T42.3X6
Gaseous substance — see Gas						
Gasoline	T52.0X1	T52.0X2	T52.0X3	T52.0X4	—	—
vapor	T52.0X1	T52.0X2	T52.0X3	T52.0X4	—	—
Gastric enzymes	T47.5X1	T47.5X2	T47.5X3	T47.5X4	T47.5X5	T47.5X6
Gastrografin	T50.8X1	T50.8X2	T50.8X3	T50.8X4	T50.8X5	T50.8X6
Gastrointestinal drug	T47.91	T47.92	T47.93	T47.94	T47.95	T47.96
biological	T47.8X1	T47.8X2	T47.8X3	T47.8X4	T47.8X5	T47.8X6
specified NEC	T47.8X1	T47.8X2	T47.8X3	T47.8X4	T47.8X5	T47.8X6
Gas NEC	T59.91	T59.92	T59.93	T59.94	—	—
acetylene	T59.891	T59.892	T59.893	T59.894	—	—
incomplete combustion of	T58.11	T58.12	T58.13	T58.14	—	—
air contaminants, source or type not specified	T59.91	T59.92	T59.93	T59.94	—	—
anesthetic	T41.0X1	T41.0X2	T41.0X3	T41.0X4	T41.0X5	T41.0X6
blast furnace	T58.8X1	T58.8X2	T58.8X3	T58.8X4	—	—
butane — see butane						
carbon monoxide — see Carbon, monoxide						
chlorine	T59.4X1	T59.4X2	T59.4X3	T59.4X4	—	—
coal	T58.2X1	T58.2X2	T58.2X3	T58.2X4	—	—
cyanide	T57.3X1	T57.3X2	T57.3X3	T57.3X4	—	—
dicyanogen	T65.0X1	T65.0X2	T65.0X3	T65.0X4	—	—
domestic — see Domestic gas						
exhaust	T58.01	T58.02	T58.03	T58.04	—	—
from utility (for cooking, heating, or lighting) (after combustion) — see Carbon, monoxide, fuel, utility						
Gas — continued						
from utility — see Carbon, monoxide, fuel, utility — continued						
prior to combustion	T59.891	T59.892	T59.893	T59.894	—	—
from wood- or coal-burning stove or fireplace	T58.2X1	T58.2X2	T58.2X3	T58.2X4	—	—
fuel (domestic use) (after combustion) — see also Carbon, monoxide, fuel						
industrial use	T58.8X1	T58.8X2	T58.8X3	T58.8X4	—	—
prior to combustion	T59.891	T59.892	T59.893	T59.894	—	—
utility	T59.891	T59.892	T59.893	T59.894	—	—
incomplete combustion of — see Carbon, monoxide, fuel, utility						
in mobile container	T59.891	T59.892	T59.893	T59.894	—	—
piped (natural)	T59.891	T59.892	T59.893	T59.894	—	—
garage	T58.01	T58.02	T58.03	T58.04	—	—
hydrocarbon NEC	T59.891	T59.892	T59.893	T59.894	—	—
incomplete combustion of — see Carbon, monoxide, fuel, utility						
liquefied — see butane						
piped	T59.891	T59.892	T59.893	T59.894	—	—
hydrocyanic acid	T65.0X1	T65.0X2	T65.0X3	T65.0X4	—	—
illuminating (after combustion)	T58.11	T58.12	T58.13	T58.14	—	—
prior to combustion	T59.891	T59.892	T59.893	T59.894	—	—
incomplete combustion, any — see Carbon, monoxide						
kiln	T58.8X1	T58.8X2	T58.8X3	T58.8X4	—	—
lacrimogenic	T59.3X1	T59.3X2	T59.3X3	T59.3X4	—	—
liquefied petroleum — see butane						
marsh	T59.891	T59.892	T59.893	T59.894	—	—
motor exhaust, not in transit	T58.01	T58.02	T58.03	T58.04	—	—
mustard, not in war	T59.891	T59.892	T59.893	T59.894	—	—
natural	T59.891	T59.892	T59.893	T59.894	—	—
nerve, not in war	T59.91	T59.92	T59.93	T59.94	—	—
oil	T52.0X1	T52.0X2	T52.0X3	T52.0X4	—	—
petroleum (liquefied) (distributed in mobile containers)	T59.891	T59.892	T59.893	T59.894	—	—
piped (pure or mixed with air)	T59.891	T59.892	T59.893	T59.894	—	—
piped (manufactured) (natural) NEC	T59.891	T59.892	T59.893	T59.894	—	—
producer	T58.8X1	T58.8X2	T58.8X3	T58.8X4	—	—
propane — see propane						
refrigerant (chlorofluoro-carbon)	T53.5X1	T53.5X2	T53.5X3	T53.5X4	—	—
not chlorofluoro-carbon	T59.891	T59.892	T59.893	T59.894	—	—
sewer	T59.91	T59.92	T59.93	T59.94	—	—
specified source NEC	T59.91	T59.92	T59.93	T59.94	—	—
stove (after combustion)	T58.11	T58.12	T58.13	T58.14	—	—
prior to combustion	T59.891	T59.892	T59.893	T59.894	—	—
tear	T59.3X1	T59.3X2	T59.3X3	T59.3X4	—	—
therapeutic	T41.5X1	T41.5X2	T41.5X3	T41.5X4	T41.5X5	T41.5X6
utility (for cooking, heating, or lighting) (piped) NEC	T59.891	T59.892	T59.893	T59.894	—	—
incomplete combustion of — see Carbon, monoxide, fuel, utilty						
in mobile container	T59.891	T59.892	T59.893	T59.894	—	—
piped (natural)	T59.891	T59.892	T59.893	T59.894	—	—
water	T58.11	T58.12	T58.13	T58.14	—	—
incomplete combustion of — see Carbon, monoxide, fuel, utility						
Gaultheria procumbens	T62.2X1	T62.2X2	T62.2X3	T62.2X4	—	—
Gefarnate	T44.3X1	T44.3X2	T44.3X3	T44.3X4	T44.3X5	T44.3X6
Gelatin (intravenous)	T45.8X1	T45.8X2	T45.8X3	T45.8X4	T45.8X5	T45.8X6
absorbable (sponge)	T45.7X1	T45.7X2	T45.7X3	T45.7X4	T45.7X5	T45.7X6
Gelfilm	T49.8X1	T49.8X2	T49.8X3	T49.8X4	T49.8X5	T49.8X6
Gelfoam	T45.7X1	T45.7X2	T45.7X3	T45.7X4	T45.7X5	T45.7X6
Gelsemine	T50.991	T50.992	T50.993	T50.994	T50.995	T50.996
Gelsemium (sempervirens)	T62.2X1	T62.2X2	T62.2X3	T62.2X4	—	—
Gemeprost	T48.0X1	T48.0X2	T48.0X3	T48.0X4	T48.0X5	T48.0X6
Gemfibrozil	T46.6X1	T46.6X2	T46.6X3	T46.6X4	T46.6X5	T46.6X6
Gemonil	T42.3X1	T42.3X2	T42.3X3	T42.3X4	T42.3X5	T42.3X6
Gentamicin	T36.5X1	T36.5X2	T36.5X3	T36.5X4	T36.5X5	T36.5X6

Substance	Poisoning, Accidental (unintentional)	Poisoning, Intentional Self-harm	Poisoning, Assault	Poisoning, Undetermined	Adverse Effect	Under-dosing
Gentamicin — *continued*						
ophthalmic preparation	T49.5X1	T49.5X2	T49.5X3	T49.5X4	T49.5X5	T49.5X6
topical NEC	T49.0X1	T49.0X2	T49.0X3	T49.0X4	T49.0X5	T49.0X6
Gentian	T47.5X1	T47.5X2	T47.5X3	T47.5X4	T47.5X5	T47.5X6
violet	T49.0X1	T49.0X2	T49.0X3	T49.0X4	T49.0X5	T49.0X6
Gepefrine	T44.4X1	T44.4X2	T44.4X3	T44.4X4	T44.4X5	T44.4X6
Gestonorone caproate	T38.5X1	T38.5X2	T38.5X3	T38.5X4	T38.5X5	T38.5X6
Gexane	T49.0X1	T49.0X2	T49.0X3	T49.0X4	T49.0X5	T49.0X6
Gila monster (venom)	T63.111	T63.112	T63.113	T63.114	—	—
Ginger	T47.5X1	T47.5X2	T47.5X3	T47.5X4	T47.5X5	T47.5X6
Jamaica — *see* Jamaica, ginger						
Gitalin	T46.0X1	T46.0X2	T46.0X3	T46.0X4	T46.0X5	T46.0X6
amorphous	T46.0X1	T46.0X2	T46.0X3	T46.0X4	T46.0X5	T46.0X6
Gitaloxin	T46.0X1	T46.0X2	T46.0X3	T46.0X4	T46.0X5	T46.0X6
Gitoxin	T46.0X1	T46.0X2	T46.0X3	T46.0X4	T46.0X5	T46.0X6
Glafenine	T39.8X1	T39.8X2	T39.8X3	T39.8X4	T39.8X5	T39.8X6
Glandular extract (medicinal) **NEC**	T50.Z91	T50.Z92	T50.Z93	T50.Z94	T50.Z95	T50.Z96
Glaucarubin	T37.3X1	T37.3X2	T37.3X3	T37.3X4	T37.3X5	T37.3X6
Glibenclamide	T38.3X1	T38.3X2	T38.3X3	T38.3X4	T38.3X5	T38.3X6
Glibornuride	T38.3X1	T38.3X2	T38.3X3	T38.3X4	T38.3X5	T38.3X6
Gliclazide	T38.3X1	T38.3X2	T38.3X3	T38.3X4	T38.3X5	T38.3X6
Glimidine	T38.3X1	T38.3X2	T38.3X3	T38.3X4	T38.3X5	T38.3X6
Glipizide	T38.3X1	T38.3X2	T38.3X3	T38.3X4	T38.3X5	T38.3X6
Gliquidone	T38.3X1	T38.3X2	T38.3X3	T38.3X4	T38.3X5	T38.3X6
Glisolamide	T38.3X1	T38.3X2	T38.3X3	T38.3X4	T38.3X5	T38.3X6
Glisoxepide	T38.3X1	T38.3X2	T38.3X3	T38.3X4	T38.3X5	T38.3X6
Globin zinc insulin	T38.3X1	T38.3X2	T38.3X3	T38.3X4	T38.3X5	T38.3X6
Globulin						
antilymphocytic	T50.Z11	T50.Z12	T50.Z13	T50.Z14	T50.Z15	T50.Z16
antirhesus	T50.Z11	T50.Z12	T50.Z13	T50.Z14	T50.Z15	T50.Z16
antivenin	T50.Z11	T50.Z12	T50.Z13	T50.Z14	T50.Z15	T50.Z16
antiviral	T50.Z11	T50.Z12	T50.Z13	T50.Z14	T50.Z15	T50.Z16
Glucagon	T38.3X1	T38.3X2	T38.3X3	T38.3X4	T38.3X5	T38.3X6
Glucocorticoids	T38.0X1	T38.0X2	T38.0X3	T38.0X4	T38.0X5	T38.0X6
Glucocorticosteroid	T38.0X1	T38.0X2	T38.0X3	T38.0X4	T38.0X5	T38.0X6
Gluconic acid	T50.991	T50.992	T50.993	T50.994	T50.995	T50.996
Glucosamine sulfate	T39.4X1	T39.4X2	T39.4X3	T39.4X4	T39.4X5	T39.4X6
Glucose	T50.3X1	T50.3X2	T50.3X3	T50.3X4	T50.3X5	T50.3X6
with sodium chloride	T50.3X1	T50.3X2	T50.3X3	T50.3X4	T50.3X5	T50.3X6
Glucosulfone sodium	T37.1X1	T37.1X2	T37.1X3	T37.1X4	T37.1X5	T37.1X6
Glucurolactone	T47.8X1	T47.8X2	T47.8X3	T47.8X4	T47.8X5	T47.8X6
Glue NEC	T52.8X1	T52.8X2	T52.8X3	T52.8X4	—	—
Glutamic acid	T47.5X1	T47.5X2	T47.5X3	T47.5X4	T47.5X5	T47.5X6
Glutaral (medicinal)	T49.0X1	T49.0X2	T49.0X3	T49.0X4	T49.0X5	T49.0X6
nonmedicinal	T65.891	T65.892	T65.893	T65.894	—	—
Glutaraldehyde (nonmedicinal)	T65.891	T65.892	T65.893	T65.894	—	—
medicinal	T49.0X1	T49.0X2	T49.0X3	T49.0X4	T49.0X5	T49.0X6
Glutathione	T50.6X1	T50.6X2	T50.6X3	T50.6X4	T50.6X5	T50.6X6
Glutethimide	T42.6X1	T42.6X2	T42.6X3	T42.6X4	T42.6X5	T42.6X6
Glyburide	T38.3X1	T38.3X2	T38.3X3	T38.3X4	T38.3X5	T38.3X6
Glycerin	T47.4X1	T47.4X2	T47.4X3	T47.4X4	T47.4X5	T47.4X6
Glycerol	T47.4X1	T47.4X2	T47.4X3	T47.4X4	T47.4X5	T47.4X6
borax	T49.6X1	T49.6X2	T49.6X3	T49.6X4	T49.6X5	T49.6X6
intravenous	T50.3X1	T50.3X2	T50.3X3	T50.3X4	T50.3X5	T50.3X6
iodinated	T48.4X1	T48.4X2	T48.4X3	T48.4X4	T48.4X5	T48.4X6
Glycerophosphate	T50.991	T50.992	T50.993	T50.994	T50.995	T50.996
Glyceryl						
gualacolate	T48.4X1	T48.4X2	T48.4X3	T48.4X4	T48.4X5	T48.4X6
nitrate	T46.3X1	T46.3X2	T46.3X3	T46.3X4	T46.3X5	T46.3X6
triacetate (topical)	T49.0X1	T49.0X2	T49.0X3	T49.0X4	T49.0X5	T49.0X6
trinitrate	T46.3X1	T46.3X2	T46.3X3	T46.3X4	T46.3X5	T46.3X6
Glycine	T50.3X1	T50.3X2	T50.3X3	T50.3X4	T50.3X5	T50.3X6
Glyclopyramide	T38.3X1	T38.3X2	T38.3X3	T38.3X4	T38.3X5	T38.3X6
Glycobiarsol	T37.3X1	T37.3X2	T37.3X3	T37.3X4	T37.3X5	T37.3X6
Glycols (ether)	T52.3X1	T52.3X2	T52.3X3	T52.3X4	—	—
Glyconiazide	T37.1X1	T37.1X2	T37.1X3	T37.1X4	T37.1X5	T37.1X6
Glycopyrrolate	T44.3X1	T44.3X2	T44.3X3	T44.3X4	T44.3X5	T44.3X6
Glycopyrronium	T44.3X1	T44.3X2	T44.3X3	T44.3X4	T44.3X5	T44.3X6
bromide	T44.3X1	T44.3X2	T44.3X3	T44.3X4	T44.3X5	T44.3X6
Glycoside, cardiac (stimulant)	T46.0X1	T46.0X2	T46.0X3	T46.0X4	T46.0X5	T46.0X6
Glycyclamide	T38.3X1	T38.3X2	T38.3X3	T38.3X4	T38.3X5	T38.3X6
Glycyrrhiza extract	T48.4X1	T48.4X2	T48.4X3	T48.4X4	T48.4X5	T48.4X6
Glycyrrhizic acid	T48.4X1	T48.4X2	T48.4X3	T48.4X4	T48.4X5	T48.4X6
Glycyrrhizinate potassium	T48.4X1	T48.4X2	T48.4X3	T48.4X4	T48.4X5	T48.4X6
Glymidine sodium	T38.3X1	T38.3X2	T38.3X3	T38.3X4	T38.3X5	T38.3X6
Glyphosate	T60.3X1	T60.3X2	T60.3X3	T60.3X4	—	—
Glyphylline	T48.6X1	T48.6X2	T48.6X3	T48.6X4	T48.6X5	T48.6X6
Gold						
colloidal (l98Au)	T45.1X1	T45.1X2	T45.1X3	T45.1X4	T45.1X5	T45.1X6
salts	T39.4X1	T39.4X2	T39.4X3	T39.4X4	T39.4X5	T39.4X6

Substance	Poisoning, Accidental (unintentional)	Poisoning, Intentional Self-harm	Poisoning, Assault	Poisoning, Undetermined	Adverse Effect	Under-dosing
Golden sulfide of antimony	T56.891	T56.892	T56.893	T56.894	—	—
Goldylocks	T62.2X1	T62.2X2	T62.2X3	T62.2X4	—	—
Gonadal tissue extract	T38.901	T38.902	T38.903	T38.904	T38.905	T38.906
female	T38.5X1	T38.5X2	T38.5X3	T38.5X4	T38.5X5	T38.5X6
male	T38.7X1	T38.7X2	T38.7X3	T38.7X4	T38.7X5	T38.7X6
Gonadorelin	T38.891	T38.892	T38.893	T38.894	T38.895	T38.896
Gonadotropin	T38.891	T38.892	T38.893	T38.894	T38.895	T38.896
chorionic	T38.891	T38.892	T38.893	T38.894	T38.895	T38.896
pituitary	T38.811	T38.812	T38.813	T38.814	T38.815	T38.816
Goserelin	T45.1X1	T45.1X2	T45.1X3	T45.1X4	T45.1X5	T45.1X6
Grain alcohol	T51.0X1	T51.0X2	T51.0X3	T51.0X4	—	—
Gramicidin	T49.0X1	T49.0X2	T49.0X3	T49.0X4	T49.0X5	T49.0X6
Granisetron	T45.0X1	T45.0X2	T45.0X3	T45.0X4	T45.0X5	T45.0X6
Gratiola officinalis	T62.2X1	T62.2X2	T62.2X3	T62.2X4	—	—
Grease	T65.891	T65.892	T65.893	T65.894	—	—
Green hellebore	T62.2X1	T62.2X2	T62.2X3	T62.2X4	—	—
Green soap	T49.2X1	T49.2X2	T49.2X3	T49.2X4	T49.2X5	T49.2X6
Grifulvin	T36.7X1	T36.7X2	T36.7X3	T36.7X4	T36.7X5	T36.7X6
Griseofulvin	T36.7X1	T36.7X2	T36.7X3	T36.7X4	T36.7X5	T36.7X6
Growth hormone	T38.811	T38.812	T38.813	T38.814	T38.815	T38.816
Guaiacol derivatives	T48.4X1	T48.4X2	T48.4X3	T48.4X4	T48.4X5	T48.4X6
Guaiac reagent	T50.991	T50.992	T50.993	T50.994	T50.995	T50.996
Guaifenesin	T48.4X1	T48.4X2	T48.4X3	T48.4X4	T48.4X5	T48.4X6
Guaimesal	T48.4X1	T48.4X2	T48.4X3	T48.4X4	T48.4X5	T48.4X6
Guaiphenesin	T48.4X1	T48.4X2	T48.4X3	T48.4X4	T48.4X5	T48.4X6
Guamecycline	T36.4X1	T36.4X2	T36.4X3	T36.4X4	T36.4X5	T36.4X6
Guanabenz	T46.5X1	T46.5X2	T46.5X3	T46.5X4	T46.5X5	T46.5X6
Guanacline	T46.5X1	T46.5X2	T46.5X3	T46.5X4	T46.5X5	T46.5X6
Guanadrel	T46.5X1	T46.5X2	T46.5X3	T46.5X4	T46.5X5	T46.5X6
Guanatol	T37.2X1	T37.2X2	T37.2X3	T37.2X4	T37.2X5	T37.2X6
Guanethidine	T46.5X1	T46.5X2	T46.5X3	T46.5X4	T46.5X5	T46.5X6
Guanfacine	T46.5X1	T46.5X2	T46.5X3	T46.5X4	T46.5X5	T46.5X6
Guano	T65.891	T65.892	T65.893	T65.894	—	—
Guanochlor	T46.5X1	T46.5X2	T46.5X3	T46.5X4	T46.5X5	T46.5X6
Guanoclor	T46.5X1	T46.5X2	T46.5X3	T46.5X4	T46.5X5	T46.5X6
Guanoctine	T46.5X1	T46.5X2	T46.5X3	T46.5X4	T46.5X5	T46.5X6
Guanoxabenz	T46.5X1	T46.5X2	T46.5X3	T46.5X4	T46.5X5	T46.5X6
Guanoxan	T46.5X1	T46.5X2	T46.5X3	T46.5X4	T46.5X5	T46.5X6
Guar gum (medicinal)	T46.6X1	T46.6X2	T46.6X3	T46.6X4	T46.6X5	T46.6X6
Hachimycin	T36.7X1	T36.7X2	T36.7X3	T36.7X4	T36.7X5	T36.7X6
Hair						
dye	T49.4X1	T49.4X2	T49.4X3	T49.4X4	T49.4X5	T49.4X6
preparation NEC	T49.4X1	T49.4X2	T49.4X3	T49.4X4	T49.4X5	T49.4X6
Halazepam	T42.4X1	T42.4X2	T42.4X3	T42.4X4	T42.4X5	T42.4X6
Halcinolone	T49.0X1	T49.0X2	T49.0X3	T49.0X4	T49.0X5	T49.0X6
Halcinonide	T49.0X1	T49.0X2	T49.0X3	T49.0X4	T49.0X5	T49.0X6
Halethazole	T49.0X1	T49.0X2	T49.0X3	T49.0X4	T49.0X5	T49.0X6
Hallucinogen NOS	T40.901	T40.902	T40.903	T40.904	T40.905	T40.906
specified NEC	T40.991	T40.992	T40.993	T40.994	T40.995	T40.996
Halofantrine	T37.2X1	T37.2X2	T37.2X3	T37.2X4	T37.2X5	T37.2X6
Halofenate	T46.6X1	T46.6X2	T46.6X3	T46.6X4	T46.6X5	T46.6X6
Halometasone	T49.0X1	T49.0X2	T49.0X3	T49.0X4	T49.0X5	T49.0X6
Haloperidol	T43.4X1	T43.4X2	T43.4X3	T43.4X4	T43.4X5	T43.4X6
Haloprogin	T49.0X1	T49.0X2	T49.0X3	T49.0X4	T49.0X5	T49.0X6
Halotex	T49.0X1	T49.0X2	T49.0X3	T49.0X4	T49.0X5	T49.0X6
Halothane	T41.0X1	T41.0X2	T41.0X3	T41.0X4	T41.0X5	T41.0X6
Haloxazolam	T42.4X1	T42.4X2	T42.4X3	T42.4X4	T42.4X5	T42.4X6
Halquinols	T49.0X1	T49.0X2	T49.0X3	T49.0X4	T49.0X5	T49.0X6
Hamamelis	T49.2X1	T49.2X2	T49.2X3	T49.2X4	T49.2X5	T49.2X6
Haptendextran	T45.8X1	T45.8X2	T45.8X3	T45.8X4	T45.8X5	T45.8X6
Harmonyl	T46.5X1	T46.5X2	T46.5X3	T46.5X4	T46.5X5	T46.5X6
Hartmann's solution	T50.3X1	T50.3X2	T50.3X3	T50.3X4	T50.3X5	T50.3X6
Hashish	T40.7X1	T40.7X2	T40.7X3	T40.7X4	T40.7X5	T40.7X6
Hawaiian Woodrose seeds	T40.991	T40.992	T40.993	T40.994	—	—
HCB	T60.3X1	T60.3X2	T60.3X3	T60.3X4	—	—
HCH	T53.6X1	T53.6X2	T53.6X3	T53.6X4	—	—
medicinal	T49.0X1	T49.0X2	T49.0X3	T49.0X4	T49.0X5	T49.0X6
HCN	T57.3X1	T57.3X2	T57.3X3	T57.3X4	—	—
Headache cures, drugs, powders NEC	T50.901	T50.902	T50.903	T50.904	T50.905	T50.906
Heavenly Blue (morning glory)	T40.991	T40.992	T40.993	T40.994	—	—
Heavy metal antidote	T45.8X1	T45.8X2	T45.8X3	T45.8X4	T45.8X5	T45.8X6
Hedaquinium	T49.0X1	T49.0X2	T49.0X3	T49.0X4	T49.0X5	T49.0X6
Hedge hyssop	T62.2X1	T62.2X2	T62.2X3	T62.2X4	—	—
Heet	T49.8X1	T49.8X2	T49.8X3	T49.8X4	T49.8X5	T49.8X6
Helenin	T37.4X1	T37.4X2	T37.4X3	T37.4X4	T37.4X5	T37.4X6
Helium (nonmedicinal) **NEC**	T59.891	T59.892	T59.893	T59.894	—	—
medicinal	T48.991	T48.992	T48.993	T48.994	T48.995	T48.996
Hellebore (black) (green) (white)	T62.2X1	T62.2X2	T62.2X3	T62.2X4	—	—
Hematin	T45.8X1	T45.8X2	T45.8X3	T45.8X4	T45.8X5	T45.8X6

▽ Subterms under main terms may continue to next column or page   Additional Character May Be Required — Refer to the Tabular List for Character Selection   371

Gentamicin — Hematin

Table of Drugs and Chemicals

Substance	Poisoning, Accidental (unintentional)	Poisoning, Intentional Self-harm	Poisoning, Assault	Poisoning, Undetermined	Adverse Effect	Under-dosing
Hematinic preparation	T45.8X1	T45.8X2	T45.8X3	T45.8X4	T45.8X5	T45.8X6
Hematological agent	T45.91	T45.92	T45.93	T45.94	T45.95	T45.96
specified NEC	T45.8X1	T45.8X2	T45.8X3	T45.8X4	T45.8X5	T45.8X6
Hemlock	T62.2X1	T62.2X2	T62.2X3	T62.2X4	—	—
Hemostatic	T45.621	T45.622	T45.623	T45.624	T45.625	T45.626
drug, systemic	T45.621	T45.622	T45.623	T45.624	T45.625	T45.626
Hemostyptic	T49.4X1	T49.4X2	T49.4X3	T49.4X4	T49.4X5	T49.4X6
Henbane	T62.2X1	T62.2X2	T62.2X3	T62.2X4	—	—
Heparin (sodium)	T45.511	T45.512	T45.513	T45.514	T45.515	T45.516
action reverser	T45.7X1	T45.7X2	T45.7X3	T45.7X4	T45.7X5	T45.7X6
Heparin-fraction	T45.511	T45.512	T45.513	T45.514	T45.515	T45.516
Heparinoid (systemic)	T45.511	T45.512	T45.513	T45.514	T45.515	T45.516
Hepatic secretion stimulant	T47.8X1	T47.8X2	T47.8X3	T47.8X4	T47.8X5	T47.8X6
Hepatitis B						
immune globulin	T50.Z11	T50.Z12	T50.Z13	T50.Z14	T50.Z15	T50.Z16
vaccine	T50.B91	T50.B92	T50.B93	T50.B94	T50.B95	T50.B96
Hepronicate	T46.7X1	T46.7X2	T46.7X3	T46.7X4	T46.7X5	T46.7X6
Heptabarb	T42.3X1	T42.3X2	T42.3X3	T42.3X4	T42.3X5	T42.3X6
Heptabarbital	T42.3X1	T42.3X2	T42.3X3	T42.3X4	T42.3X5	T42.3X6
Heptabarbitone	T42.3X1	T42.3X2	T42.3X3	T42.3X4	T42.3X5	T42.3X6
Heptachlor	T60.1X1	T60.1X2	T60.1X3	T60.1X4	—	—
Heptalgin	T40.2X1	T40.2X2	T40.2X3	T40.2X4	T40.2X5	T40.2X6
Heptaminol	T46.3X1	T46.3X2	T46.3X3	T46.3X4	T46.3X5	T46.3X6
Herbicide NEC	T60.3X1	T60.3X2	T60.3X3	T60.3X4	—	—
Heroin	T40.1X1	T40.1X2	T40.1X3	T40.1X4	—	—
Herplex	T49.5X1	T49.5X2	T49.5X3	T49.5X4	T49.5X5	T49.5X6
HES	T45.8X1	T45.8X2	T45.8X3	T45.8X4	T45.8X5	T45.8X6
Hesperidin	T46.991	T46.992	T46.993	T46.994	T46.995	T46.996
Hetacillin	T36.0X1	T36.0X2	T36.0X3	T36.0X4	T36.0X5	T36.0X6
Hetastarch	T45.8X1	T45.8X2	T45.8X3	T45.8X4	T45.8X5	T45.8X6
HETP	T60.0X1	T60.0X2	T60.0X3	T60.0X4	—	—
Hexachlorobenzene (vapor)	T60.3X1	T60.3X2	T60.3X3	T60.3X4	—	—
Hexachlorocyclohexane	T53.6X1	T53.6X2	T53.6X3	T53.6X4	—	—
Hexachlorophene	T49.0X1	T49.0X2	T49.0X3	T49.0X4	T49.0X5	T49.0X6
Hexadiline	T46.3X1	T46.3X2	T46.3X3	T46.3X4	T46.3X5	T46.3X6
Hexadimethrine (bromide)	T45.7X1	T45.7X2	T45.7X3	T45.7X4	T45.7X5	T45.7X6
Hexadylamine	T46.3X1	T46.3X2	T46.3X3	T46.3X4	T46.3X5	T46.3X6
Hexaethyl tetraphosphate	T60.0X1	T60.0X2	T60.0X3	T60.0X4	—	—
Hexafluorenium bromide	T48.1X1	T48.1X2	T48.1X3	T48.1X4	T48.1X5	T48.1X6
Hexafluronium (bromide)	T48.1X1	T48.1X2	T48.1X3	T48.1X4	T48.1X5	T48.1X6
Hexa-germ	T49.2X1	T49.2X2	T49.2X3	T49.2X4	T49.2X5	T49.2X6
Hexahydrobenzol	T52.8X1	T52.8X2	T52.8X3	T52.8X4	—	—
Hexahydrocresol(s)	T51.8X1	T51.8X2	T51.8X3	T51.8X4	—	—
arsenide	T57.0X1	T57.0X2	T57.0X3	T57.0X4	—	—
arseniurated	T57.0X1	T57.0X2	T57.0X3	T57.0X4	—	—
cyanide	T57.3X1	T57.3X2	T57.3X3	T57.3X4	—	—
gas	T59.891	T59.892	T59.893	T59.894	—	—
Fluoride (liquid)	T57.8X1	T57.8X2	T57.8X3	T57.8X4	—	—
vapor	T59.891	T59.892	T59.893	T59.894	—	—
phophorated	T60.0X1	T60.0X2	T60.0X3	T60.0X4	—	—
sulfate	T57.8X1	T57.8X2	T57.8X3	T57.8X4	—	—
sulfide (gas)	T59.6X1	T59.6X2	T59.6X3	T59.6X4	—	—
arseniurated	T57.0X1	T57.0X2	T57.0X3	T57.0X4	—	—
sulfurated	T57.8X1	T57.8X2	T57.8X3	T57.8X4	—	—
Hexahydrophenol	T51.8X1	T51.8X2	T51.8X3	T51.8X4	—	—
Hexalen	T51.8X1	T51.8X2	T51.8X3	T51.8X4	—	—
Hexamethonium bromide	T44.2X1	T44.2X2	T44.2X3	T44.2X4	T44.2X5	T44.2X6
Hexamethylene	T52.8X1	T52.8X2	T52.8X3	T52.8X4	—	—
Hexamethylmelamine	T45.1X1	T45.1X2	T45.1X3	T45.1X4	T45.1X5	T45.1X6
Hexamidine	T49.0X1	T49.0X2	T49.0X3	T49.0X4	T49.0X5	T49.0X6
Hexamine (mandelate)	T37.8X1	T37.8X2	T37.8X3	T37.8X4	T37.8X5	T37.8X6
Hexanone, 2-hexanone	T52.4X1	T52.4X2	T52.4X3	T52.4X4	—	—
Hexanuorenium	T48.1X1	T48.1X2	T48.1X3	T48.1X4	T48.1X5	T48.1X6
Hexapropymate	T42.6X1	T42.6X2	T42.6X3	T42.6X4	T42.6X5	T42.6X6
Hexasonium iodide	T44.3X1	T44.3X2	T44.3X3	T44.3X4	T44.3X5	T44.3X6
Hexcarbacholine bromide	T48.1X1	T48.1X2	T48.1X3	T48.1X4	T48.1X5	T48.1X6
Hexemal	T42.3X1	T42.3X2	T42.3X3	T42.3X4	T42.3X5	T42.3X6
Hexestrol	T38.5X1	T38.5X2	T38.5X3	T38.5X4	T38.5X5	T38.5X6
Hexethal (sodium)	T42.3X1	T42.3X2	T42.3X3	T42.3X4	T42.3X5	T42.3X6
Hexetidine	T37.8X1	T37.8X2	T37.8X3	T37.8X4	T37.8X5	T37.8X6
Hexobarbital	T42.3X1	T42.3X2	T42.3X3	T42.3X4	T42.3X5	T42.3X6
rectal	T41.291	T41.292	T41.293	T41.294	T41.295	T41.296
sodium	T41.1X1	T41.1X2	T41.1X3	T41.1X4	T41.1X5	T41.1X6
Hexobendine	T46.3X1	T46.3X2	T46.3X3	T46.3X4	T46.3X5	T46.3X6
Hexocyclium	T44.3X1	T44.3X2	T44.3X3	T44.3X4	T44.3X5	T44.3X6
metilsulfate	T44.3X1	T44.3X2	T44.3X3	T44.3X4	T44.3X5	T44.3X6
Hexoestrol	T38.5X1	T38.5X2	T38.5X3	T38.5X4	T38.5X5	T38.5X6
Hexone	T52.4X1	T52.4X2	T52.4X3	T52.4X4	—	—
Hexoprenaline	T48.6X1	T48.6X2	T48.6X3	T48.6X4	T48.6X5	T48.6X6
Hexylcaine	T41.3X1	T41.3X2	T41.3X3	T41.3X4	T41.3X5	T41.3X6
Hexylresorcinol	T52.2X1	T52.2X2	T52.2X3	T52.2X4	—	—

Substance	Poisoning, Accidental (unintentional)	Poisoning, Intentional Self-harm	Poisoning, Assault	Poisoning, Undetermined	Adverse Effect	Under-dosing
HGH (human growth hormone)	T38.811	T38.812	T38.813	T38.814	T38.815	T38.816
Hinkle's pills	T47.2X1	T47.2X2	T47.2X3	T47.2X4	T47.2X5	T47.2X6
Histalog	T50.8X1	T50.8X2	T50.8X3	T50.8X4	T50.8X5	T50.8X6
Histamine (phosphate)	T50.8X1	T50.8X2	T50.8X3	T50.8X4	T50.8X5	T50.8X6
Histoplasmin	T50.8X1	T50.8X2	T50.8X3	T50.8X4	T50.8X5	T50.8X6
Holly berries	T62.2X1	T62.2X2	T62.2X3	T62.2X4	—	—
Homatropine	T44.3X1	T44.3X2	T44.3X3	T44.3X4	T44.3X5	T44.3X6
methylbromide	T44.3X1	T44.3X2	T44.3X3	T44.3X4	T44.3X5	T44.3X6
Homochlorcyclizine	T45.0X1	T45.0X2	T45.0X3	T45.0X4	T45.0X5	T45.0X6
Homosalate	T49.3X1	T49.3X2	T49.3X3	T49.3X4	T49.3X5	T49.3X6
Homo-tet	T50.Z11	T50.Z12	T50.Z13	T50.Z14	T50.Z15	T50.Z16
Hormone	T38.801	T38.802	T38.803	T38.804	T38.805	T38.806
adrenal cortical steroids	T38.0X1	T38.0X2	T38.0X3	T38.0X4	T38.0X5	T38.0X6
androgenic	T38.7X1	T38.7X2	T38.7X3	T38.7X4	T38.7X5	T38.7X6
anterior pituitary NEC	T38.811	T38.812	T38.813	T38.814	T38.815	T38.816
antidiabetic agents	T38.3X1	T38.3X2	T38.3X3	T38.3X4	T38.3X5	T38.3X6
antidiuretic	T38.891	T38.892	T38.893	T38.894	T38.895	T38.896
cancer therapy	T45.1X1	T45.1X2	T45.1X3	T45.1X4	T45.1X5	T45.1X6
follicle stimulating	T38.811	T38.812	T38.813	T38.814	T38.815	T38.816
gonadotropic	T38.891	T38.892	T38.893	T38.894	T38.895	T38.896
pituitary	T38.811	T38.812	T38.813	T38.814	T38.815	T38.816
growth	T38.811	T38.812	T38.813	T38.814	T38.815	T38.816
luteinizing	T38.811	T38.812	T38.813	T38.814	T38.815	T38.816
ovarian	T38.5X1	T38.5X2	T38.5X3	T38.5X4	T38.5X5	T38.5X6
oxytocic	T48.0X1	T48.0X2	T48.0X3	T48.0X4	T48.0X5	T48.0X6
parathyroid (derivatives)	T50.991	T50.992	T50.993	T50.994	T50.995	T50.996
pituitary (posterior) NEC	T38.891	T38.892	T38.893	T38.894	T38.895	T38.896
anterior	T38.811	T38.812	T38.813	T38.814	T38.815	T38.816
specified, NEC	T38.891	T38.892	T38.893	T38.894	T38.895	T38.896
thyroid	T38.1X1	T38.1X2	T38.1X3	T38.1X4	T38.1X5	T38.1X6
Hornet (sting)	T63.451	T63.452	T63.453	T63.454	—	—
Horse anti-human lymphocytic serum	T50.Z11	T50.Z12	T50.Z13	T50.Z14	T50.Z15	T50.Z16
Horticulture agent NEC	T65.91	T65.92	T65.93	T65.94	—	—
with pesticide	T60.91	T60.92	T60.93	T60.94	—	—
Human						
albumin	T45.8X1	T45.8X2	T45.8X3	T45.8X4	T45.8X5	T45.8X6
growth hormone (HGH)	T38.811	T38.812	T38.813	T38.814	T38.815	T38.816
immune serum	T50.Z11	T50.Z12	T50.Z13	T50.Z14	T50.Z15	T50.Z16
Hyaluronidase	T45.3X1	T45.3X2	T45.3X3	T45.3X4	T45.3X5	T45.3X6
Hyazyme	T45.3X1	T45.3X2	T45.3X3	T45.3X4	T45.3X5	T45.3X6
Hycodan	T40.2X1	T40.2X2	T40.2X3	T40.2X4	T40.2X5	T40.2X6
Hydantoin derivative NEC	T42.0X1	T42.0X2	T42.0X3	T42.0X4	T42.0X5	T42.0X6
Hydeltra	T38.0X1	T38.0X2	T38.0X3	T38.0X4	T38.0X5	T38.0X6
Hydergine	T44.6X1	T44.6X2	T44.6X3	T44.6X4	T44.6X5	T44.6X6
Hydrabamine penicillin	T36.0X1	T36.0X2	T36.0X3	T36.0X4	T36.0X5	T36.0X6
Hydralazine	T46.5X1	T46.5X2	T46.5X3	T46.5X4	T46.5X5	T46.5X6
Hydrargaphen	T49.0X1	T49.0X2	T49.0X3	T49.0X4	T49.0X5	T49.0X6
Hydrargyri aminochloridum	T49.0X1	T49.0X2	T49.0X3	T49.0X4	T49.0X5	T49.0X6
Hydrastine	T48.291	T48.292	T48.293	T48.294	T48.295	T48.296
Hydrazine	T54.1X1	T54.1X2	T54.1X3	T54.1X4	—	—
monoamine oxidase inhibitors	T43.1X1	T43.1X2	T43.1X3	T43.1X4	T43.1X5	T43.1X6
Hydrazoic acid, azides	T54.2X1	T54.2X2	T54.2X3	T54.2X4	—	—
Hydriodic acid	T48.4X1	T48.4X2	T48.4X3	T48.4X4	T48.4X5	T48.4X6
Hydrocarbon gas	T59.891	T59.892	T59.893	T59.894	—	—
incomplete combustion of — see Carbon, monoxide, fuel, utility						
liquefied (mobile container)	T59.891	T59.892	T59.893	T59.894	—	—
piped (natural)	T59.891	T59.892	T59.893	T59.894	—	—
Hydrochloric acid (liquid)	T54.2X1	T54.2X2	T54.2X3	T54.2X4	—	—
medicinal (digestant)	T47.5X1	T47.5X2	T47.5X3	T47.5X4	T47.5X5	T47.5X6
vapor	T59.891	T59.892	T59.893	T59.894	—	—
Hydrochlorothiazide	T50.2X1	T50.2X2	T50.2X3	T50.2X4	T50.2X5	T50.2X6
Hydrocodone	T40.2X1	T40.2X2	T40.2X3	T40.2X4	T40.2X5	T40.2X6
Hydrocortisone (derivatives)	T38.0X1	T38.0X2	T38.0X3	T38.0X4	T38.0X5	T38.0X6
aceponate	T49.0X1	T49.0X2	T49.0X3	T49.0X4	T49.0X5	T49.0X6
ENT agent	T49.6X1	T49.6X2	T49.6X3	T49.6X4	T49.6X5	T49.6X6
ophthalmic preparation	T49.5X1	T49.5X2	T49.5X3	T49.5X4	T49.5X5	T49.5X6
topical NEC	T49.0X1	T49.0X2	T49.0X3	T49.0X4	T49.0X5	T49.0X6
Hydrocortone	T38.0X1	T38.0X2	T38.0X3	T38.0X4	T38.0X5	T38.0X6
ENT agent	T49.6X1	T49.6X2	T49.6X3	T49.6X4	T49.6X5	T49.6X6
ophthalmic preparation	T49.5X1	T49.5X2	T49.5X3	T49.5X4	T49.5X5	T49.5X6
topical NEC	T49.0X1	T49.0X2	T49.0X3	T49.0X4	T49.0X5	T49.0X6
Hydrocyanic acid (liquid)	T57.3X1	T57.3X2	T57.3X3	T57.3X4	—	—
gas	T65.0X1	T65.0X2	T65.0X3	T65.0X4	—	—
Hydroflumethiazide	T50.2X1	T50.2X2	T50.2X3	T50.2X4	T50.2X5	T50.2X6
Hydrofluoric acid (liquid)	T54.2X1	T54.2X2	T54.2X3	T54.2X4	—	—

Table of Drugs and Chemicals

Substance	Poisoning, Accidental (unintentional)	Poisoning, Intentional Self-harm	Poisoning, Assault	Poisoning, Undetermined	Adverse Effect	Under-dosing
Hydrofluoric acid — *continued*						
vapor	T59.891	T59.892	T59.893	T59.894	—	—
Hydrogen	T59.891	T59.892	T59.893	T59.894	—	—
arsenide	T57.0X1	T57.0X2	T57.0X3	T57.0X4	—	—
arseniureted	T57.0X1	T57.0X2	T57.0X3	T57.0X4	—	—
chloride	T57.8X1	T57.8X2	T57.8X3	T57.8X4	—	—
cyanide (salts)	T57.3X1	T57.3X2	T57.3X3	T57.3X4	—	—
gas	T57.3X1	T57.3X2	T57.3X3	T57.3X4	—	—
Fluoride	T59.5X1	T59.5X2	T59.5X3	T59.5X4	—	—
vapor	T59.5X1	T59.5X2	T59.5X3	T59.5X4	—	—
peroxide	T49.0X1	T49.0X2	T49.0X3	T49.0X4	T49.0X5	T49.0X6
phosphureted	T57.1X1	T57.1X2	T57.1X3	T57.1X4	—	—
sulfide	T59.6X1	T59.6X2	T59.6X3	T59.6X4	—	—
arseniureted	T57.0X1	T57.0X2	T57.0X3	T57.0X4	—	—
sulfureted	T59.6X1	T59.6X2	T59.6X3	T59.6X4	—	—
Hydromethylpyridine	T46.7X1	T46.7X2	T46.7X3	T46.7X4	T46.7X5	T46.7X6
Hydromorphinol	T40.2X1	T40.2X2	T40.2X3	T40.2X4		
Hydromorphinone	T40.2X1	T40.2X2	T40.2X3	T40.2X4	T40.2X5	T40.2X6
Hydromorphone	T40.2X1	T40.2X2	T40.2X3	T40.2X4	T40.2X5	T40.2X6
Hydromox	T50.2X1	T50.2X2	T50.2X3	T50.2X4	T50.2X5	T50.2X6
Hydrophilic lotion	T49.3X1	T49.3X2	T49.3X3	T49.3X4	T49.3X5	T49.3X6
Hydroquinidine	T46.2X1	T46.2X2	T46.2X3	T46.2X4	T46.2X5	T46.2X6
Hydroquinone	T52.2X1	T52.2X2	T52.2X3	T52.2X4	—	—
vapor	T59.891	T59.892	T59.893	T59.894	—	—
Hydrosulfuric acid (gas)	T59.6X1	T59.6X2	T59.6X3	T59.6X4	—	—
Hydrotalcite	T47.1X1	T47.1X2	T47.1X3	T47.1X4	T47.1X5	T47.1X6
Hydrous wool fat	T49.3X1	T49.3X2	T49.3X3	T49.3X4	T49.3X5	T49.3X6
Hydroxide, caustic	T54.3X1	T54.3X2	T54.3X3	T54.3X4	—	—
Hydroxocobalamin	T45.8X1	T45.8X2	T45.8X3	T45.8X4	T45.8X5	T45.8X6
Hydroxyamphetamine	T49.5X1	T49.5X2	T49.5X3	T49.5X4	T49.5X5	T49.5X6
Hydroxycarbamide	T45.1X1	T45.1X2	T45.1X3	T45.1X4	T45.1X5	T45.1X6
Hydroxychloroquine	T37.8X1	T37.8X2	T37.8X3	T37.8X4	T37.8X5	T37.8X6
Hydroxydihydrocodeinone	T40.2X1	T40.2X2	T40.2X3	T40.2X4	T40.2X5	T40.2X6
Hydroxyestrone	T38.5X1	T38.5X2	T38.5X3	T38.5X4	T38.5X5	T38.5X6
Hydroxyethyl starch	T45.8X1	T45.8X2	T45.8X3	T45.8X4	T45.8X5	T45.8X6
Hydroxymethylpentanone	T52.4X1	T52.4X2	T52.4X3	T52.4X4	—	—
Hydroxyphenamate	T43.591	T43.592	T43.593	T43.594	T43.595	T43.596
Hydroxyphenylbutazone	T39.2X1	T39.2X2	T39.2X3	T39.2X4	T39.2X5	T39.2X6
Hydroxyprogesterone	T38.5X1	T38.5X2	T38.5X3	T38.5X4	T38.5X5	T38.5X6
caproate	T38.5X1	T38.5X2	T38.5X3	T38.5X4	T38.5X5	T38.5X6
Hydroxyquinoline (derivatives) NEC	T37.8X1	T37.8X2	T37.8X3	T37.8X4	T37.8X5	T37.8X6
Hydroxystilbamidine	T37.3X1	T37.3X2	T37.3X3	T37.3X4	T37.3X5	T37.3X6
Hydroxytoluene (nonmedicinal)	T54.0X1	T54.0X2	T54.0X3	T54.0X4	—	—
medicinal	T49.0X1	T49.0X2	T49.0X3	T49.0X4	T49.0X5	T49.0X6
Hydroxyurea	T45.1X1	T45.1X2	T45.1X3	T45.1X4	T45.1X5	T45.1X6
Hydroxyzine	T43.591	T43.592	T43.593	T43.594	T43.595	T43.596
Hyoscine	T44.3X1	T44.3X2	T44.3X3	T44.3X4	T44.3X5	T44.3X6
Hyoscyamine	T44.3X1	T44.3X2	T44.3X3	T44.3X4	T44.3X5	T44.3X6
Hyoscyamus	T44.3X1	T44.3X2	T44.3X3	T44.3X4	T44.3X5	T44.3X6
dry extract	T44.3X1	T44.3X2	T44.3X3	T44.3X4	T44.3X5	T44.3X6
Hypaque	T50.8X1	T50.8X2	T50.8X3	T50.8X4	T50.8X5	T50.8X6
Hypertussis	T50.Z11	T50.Z12	T50.Z13	T50.Z14	T50.Z15	T50.Z16
Hypnotic	T42.71	T42.72	T42.73	T42.74	T42.75	T42.76
anticonvulsant	T42.71	T42.72	T42.73	T42.74	T42.75	T42.76
specified NEC	T42.6X1	T42.6X2	T42.6X3	T42.6X4	T42.6X5	T42.6X6
Hypochlorite	T49.0X1	T49.0X2	T49.0X3	T49.0X4	T49.0X5	T49.0X6
Hypophysis, posterior	T38.891	T38.892	T38.893	T38.894	T38.895	T38.896
Hypotensive NEC	T46.5X1	T46.5X2	T46.5X3	T46.5X4	T46.5X5	T46.5X6
Hypromellose	T49.5X1	T49.5X2	T49.5X3	T49.5X4	T49.5X5	T49.5X6
Ibacitabine	T37.5X1	T37.5X2	T37.5X3	T37.5X4	T37.5X5	T37.5X6
Ibopamine	T44.991	T44.992	T44.993	T44.994	T44.995	T44.996
Ibufenac	T39.311	T39.312	T39.313	T39.314	T39.315	T39.316
Ibuprofen	T39.311	T39.312	T39.313	T39.314	T39.315	T39.316
Ibuproxam	T39.311	T39.312	T39.313	T39.314	T39.315	T39.316
Ibuterol	T48.6X1	T48.6X2	T48.6X3	T48.6X4	T48.6X5	T48.6X6
Ichthammol	T49.0X1	T49.0X2	T49.0X3	T49.0X4	T49.0X5	T49.0X6
Ichthyol	T49.4X1	T49.4X2	T49.4X3	T49.4X4	T49.4X5	T49.4X6
Idarubicin	T45.1X1	T45.1X2	T45.1X3	T45.1X4	T45.1X5	T45.1X6
Idrocilamide	T42.8X1	T42.8X2	T42.8X3	T42.8X4	T42.8X5	T42.8X6
Ifenprodil	T46.7X1	T46.7X2	T46.7X3	T46.7X4	T46.7X5	T46.7X6
Ifosfamide	T45.1X1	T45.1X2	T45.1X3	T45.1X4	T45.1X5	T45.1X6
Iletin	T38.3X1	T38.3X2	T38.3X3	T38.3X4	T38.3X5	T38.3X6
Ilex	T62.2X1	T62.2X2	T62.2X3	T62.2X4	—	—
Illuminating gas (after combustion)	T58.11	T58.12	T58.13	T58.14	—	—
prior to combustion	T59.891	T59.892	T59.893	T59.894	—	—
Ilopan	T45.2X1	T45.2X2	T45.2X3	T45.2X4	T45.2X5	T45.2X6
Iloprost	T46.7X1	T46.7X2	T46.7X3	T46.7X4	T46.7X5	T46.7X6
Ilotycin	T36.3X1	T36.3X2	T36.3X3	T36.3X4	T36.3X5	T36.3X6
ophthalmic preparation	T49.5X1	T49.5X2	T49.5X3	T49.5X4	T49.5X5	T49.5X6
topical NEC	T49.0X1	T49.0X2	T49.0X3	T49.0X4	T49.0X5	T49.0X6

Substance	Poisoning, Accidental (unintentional)	Poisoning, Intentional Self-harm	Poisoning, Assault	Poisoning, Undetermined	Adverse Effect	Under-dosing
Imidazole-4-carboxamide	T45.1X1	T45.1X2	T45.1X3	T45.1X4	T45.1X5	T45.1X6
Iminostilbene	T42.1X1	T42.1X2	T42.1X3	T42.1X4	T42.1X5	T42.1X6
Imipenem	T36.0X1	T36.0X2	T36.0X3	T36.0X4	T36.0X5	T36.0X6
Imipramine	T43.011	T43.012	T43.013	T43.014	T43.015	T43.016
Immu-G	T50.Z11	T50.Z12	T50.Z13	T50.Z14	T50.Z15	T50.Z16
Immuglobin	T50.Z11	T50.Z12	T50.Z13	T50.Z14	T50.Z15	T50.Z16
Immune						
globulin	T50.Z11	T50.Z12	T50.Z13	T50.Z14	T50.Z15	T50.Z16
serum globulin	T50.Z11	T50.Z12	T50.Z13	T50.Z14	T50.Z15	T50.Z16
Immunoglobin human (intravenous) (normal)	T50.Z11	T50.Z12	T50.Z13	T50.Z14	T50.Z15	T50.Z16
unmodified	T50.Z11	T50.Z12	T50.Z13	T50.Z14	T50.Z15	T50.Z16
Immunosuppressive drug	T45.1X1	T45.1X2	T45.1X3	T45.1X4	T45.1X5	T45.1X6
Immu-tetanus	T50.Z11	T50.Z12	T50.Z13	T50.Z14	T50.Z15	T50.Z16
Indalpine	T43.221	T43.222	T43.223	T43.224	T43.225	T43.226
Indanazoline	T48.5X1	T48.5X2	T48.5X3	T48.5X4	T48.5X5	T48.5X6
Indandione (derivatives)	T45.511	T45.512	T45.513	T45.514	T45.515	T45.516
Indapamide	T46.5X1	T46.5X2	T46.5X3	T46.5X4	T46.5X5	T46.5X6
Indendione (derivatives)	T45.511	T45.512	T45.513	T45.514	T45.515	T45.516
Indenolol	T44.7X1	T44.7X2	T44.7X3	T44.7X4	T44.7X5	T44.7X6
Inderal	T44.7X1	T44.7X2	T44.7X3	T44.7X4	T44.7X5	T44.7X6
Indian						
hemp	T40.7X1	T40.7X2	T40.7X3	T40.7X4	T40.7X5	T40.7X6
tobacco	T62.2X1	T62.2X2	T62.2X3	T62.2X4	—	—
Indigo carmine	T50.8X1	T50.8X2	T50.8X3	T50.8X4	T50.8X5	T50.8X6
Indobufen	T45.521	T45.522	T45.523	T45.524	T45.525	T45.526
Indocin	T39.2X1	T39.2X2	T39.2X3	T39.2X4	T39.2X5	T39.2X6
Indocyanine green	T50.8X1	T50.8X2	T50.8X3	T50.8X4	T50.8X5	T50.8X6
Indometacin	T39.391	T39.392	T39.393	T39.394	T39.395	T39.396
Indomethacin	T39.391	T39.392	T39.393	T39.394	T39.395	T39.396
farnesil	T39.4X1	T39.4X2	T39.4X3	T39.4X4	T39.4X5	T39.4X6
Indoramin	T44.6X1	T44.6X2	T44.6X3	T44.6X4	T44.6X5	T44.6X6
Industrial						
alcohol	T51.0X1	T51.0X2	T51.0X3	T51.0X4	—	—
fumes	T59.891	T59.892	T59.893	T59.894	—	—
solvents (fumes) (vapors)	T52.91	T52.92	T52.93	T52.94	—	—
Influenza vaccine	T50.B91	T50.B92	T50.B93	T50.B94	T50.B95	T50.B96
Ingested substance NEC	T65.91	T65.92	T65.93	T65.94	—	—
INH	T37.1X1	T37.1X2	T37.1X3	T37.1X4	T37.1X5	T37.1X6
Inhalation, gas (noxious) — *see* Gas						
Inhibitor						
angiotensin-converting enzyme	T46.4X1	T46.4X2	T46.4X3	T46.4X4	T46.4X5	T46.4X6
carbonic anhydrase	T50.2X1	T50.2X2	T50.2X3	T50.2X4	T50.2X5	T50.2X6
fibrinolysis	T45.621	T45.622	T45.623	T45.624	T45.625	T45.626
monoamine oxidase NEC	T43.1X1	T43.1X2	T43.1X3	T43.1X4	T43.1X5	T43.1X6
hydrazine	T43.1X1	T43.1X2	T43.1X3	T43.1X4	T43.1X5	T43.1X6
postsynaptic	T43.8X1	T43.8X2	T43.8X3	T43.8X4	T43.8X5	T43.8X6
prothrombin synthesis	T45.511	T45.512	T45.513	T45.514	T45.515	T45.516
Ink	T65.891	T65.892	T65.893	T65.894	—	—
Inorganic substance NEC	T57.91	T57.92	T57.93	T57.94	—	—
Inosine pranobex	T37.5X1	T37.5X2	T37.5X3	T37.5X4	T37.5X5	T37.5X6
Inositol	T50.991	T50.992	T50.993	T50.994	T50.995	T50.996
nicotinate	T46.7X1	T46.7X2	T46.7X3	T46.7X4	T46.7X5	T46.7X6
Inproquone	T45.1X1	T45.1X2	T45.1X3	T45.1X4	T45.1X5	T45.1X6
Insecticide NEC	T60.91	T60.92	T60.93	T60.94	—	—
carbamate	T60.0X1	T60.0X2	T60.0X3	T60.0X4	—	—
chlorinated	T60.1X1	T60.1X2	T60.1X3	T60.1X4	—	—
mixed	T60.91	T60.92	T60.93	T60.94	—	—
organochlorine	T60.1X1	T60.1X2	T60.1X3	T60.1X4	—	—
organophosphorus	T60.0X1	T60.0X2	T60.0X3	T60.0X4	—	—
Insect (sting), venomous	T63.481	T63.482	T63.483	T63.484	—	—
ant	T63.421	T63.422	T63.423	T63.424	—	—
bee	T63.441	T63.442	T63.443	T63.444	—	—
caterpillar	T63.431	T63.432	T63.433	T63.434	—	—
hornet	T63.451	T63.452	T63.453	T63.454	—	—
wasp	T63.461	T63.462	T63.463	T63.464	—	—
Insular tissue extract	T38.3X1	T38.3X2	T38.3X3	T38.3X4	T38.3X5	T38.3X6
Insulin (amorphous) (globin) (isophane) (Lente) (NPH) (Semilente) (Ultralente)	T38.3X1	T38.3X2	T38.3X3	T38.3X4	T38.3X5	T38.3X6
defalan	T38.3X1	T38.3X2	T38.3X3	T38.3X4	T38.3X5	T38.3X6
human	T38.3X1	T38.3X2	T38.3X3	T38.3X4	T38.3X5	T38.3X6
injection, soluble	T38.3X1	T38.3X2	T38.3X3	T38.3X4	T38.3X5	T38.3X6
biphasic	T38.3X1	T38.3X2	T38.3X3	T38.3X4	T38.3X5	T38.3X6
intermediate acting	T38.3X1	T38.3X2	T38.3X3	T38.3X4	T38.3X5	T38.3X6
protamine zinc	T38.3X1	T38.3X2	T38.3X3	T38.3X4	T38.3X5	T38.3X6
slow acting	T38.3X1	T38.3X2	T38.3X3	T38.3X4	T38.3X5	T38.3X6
zinc						
protamine injection	T38.3X1	T38.3X2	T38.3X3	T38.3X4	T38.3X5	T38.3X6
suspension (amorphous) (crystalline)	T38.3X1	T38.3X2	T38.3X3	T38.3X4	T38.3X5	T38.3X6

Hydrofluoric acid — Insulin

Substance	Poisoning, Accidental (unintentional)	Poisoning, Intentional Self-harm	Poisoning, Assault	Poisoning, Undetermined	Adverse Effect	Under-dosing
Interferon (alpha) (beta) (gamma)	T37.5X1	T37.5X2	T37.5X3	T37.5X4	T37.5X5	T37.5X6
Intestinal motility control drug	T47.6X1	T47.6X2	T47.6X3	T47.6X4	T47.6X5	T47.6X6
biological	T47.8X1	T47.8X2	T47.8X3	T47.8X4	T47.8X5	T47.8X6
Intranarcon	T41.1X1	T41.1X2	T41.1X3	T41.1X4	T41.1X5	T41.1X6
Intravenous						
amino acids	T50.991	T50.992	T50.993	T50.994	T50.995	T50.996
fat suspension	T50.991	T50.992	T50.993	T50.994	T50.995	T50.996
Inulin	T50.8X1	T50.8X2	T50.8X3	T50.8X4	T50.8X5	T50.8X6
Invert sugar	T50.3X1	T50.3X2	T50.3X3	T50.3X4	T50.3X5	T50.3X6
Inza — see Naproxen						
Iobenzamic acid	T50.8X1	T50.8X2	T50.8X3	T50.8X4	T50.8X5	T50.8X6
Iocarmic acid	T50.8X1	T50.8X2	T50.8X3	T50.8X4	T50.8X5	T50.8X6
Iocetamic acid	T50.8X1	T50.8X2	T50.8X3	T50.8X4	T50.8X5	T50.8X6
Iodamide	T50.8X1	T50.8X2	T50.8X3	T50.8X4	T50.8X5	T50.8X6
Iodide NEC — see also	T49.0X1	T49.0X2	T49.0X3	T49.0X4	T49.0X5	T49.0X6
Iodine						
mercury (ointment)	T49.0X1	T49.0X2	T49.0X3	T49.0X4	T49.0X5	T49.0X6
methylate	T49.0X1	T49.0X2	T49.0X3	T49.0X4	T49.0X5	T49.0X6
potassium (expectorant) NEC	T48.4X1	T48.4X2	T48.4X3	T48.4X4	T48.4X5	T48.4X6
Iodinated						
contrast medium	T50.8X1	T50.8X2	T50.8X3	T50.8X4	T50.8X5	T50.8X6
glycerol	T48.4X1	T48.4X2	T48.4X3	T48.4X4	T48.4X5	T48.4X6
human serum albumin (131I)	T50.8X1	T50.8X2	T50.8X3	T50.8X4	T50.8X5	T50.8X6
Iodine (antiseptic, external) (tincture) **NEC**	T49.0X1	T49.0X2	T49.0X3	T49.0X4	T49.0X5	T49.0X6
125 — see also Radiation sickness, and Exposure to radioactive isotopes						
therapeutic	T50.8X1	T50.8X2	T50.8X3	T50.8X4	T50.8X5	T50.8X6
131 — see also Radiation sickness, and Exposure to radioactive isotopes						
therapeutic	T38.2X1	T38.2X2	T38.2X3	T38.2X4	T38.2X5	T38.2X6
diagnostic	T50.8X1	T50.8X2	T50.8X3	T50.8X4	T50.8X5	T50.8X6
for thyroid conditions (antithyroid)	T38.2X1	T38.2X2	T38.2X3	T38.2X4	T38.2X5	T38.2X6
solution	T49.0X1	T49.0X2	T49.0X3	T49.0X4	T49.0X5	T49.0X6
vapor	T59.891	T59.892	T59.893	T59.894	—	—
Iodipamide	T50.8X1	T50.8X2	T50.8X3	T50.8X4	T50.8X5	T50.8X6
Iodized (poppy seed) oil	T50.8X1	T50.8X2	T50.8X3	T50.8X4	T50.8X5	T50.8X6
Iodobismitol	T37.8X1	T37.8X2	T37.8X3	T37.8X4	T37.8X5	T37.8X6
Iodochlorhydroxyquin	T37.8X1	T37.8X2	T37.8X3	T37.8X4	T37.8X5	T37.8X6
topical	T49.0X1	T49.0X2	T49.0X3	T49.0X4	T49.0X5	T49.0X6
Iodochlorhydroxyquinoline	T37.8X1	T37.8X2	T37.8X3	T37.8X4	T37.8X5	T37.8X6
Iodocholesterol (131I)	T50.8X1	T50.8X2	T50.8X3	T50.8X4	T50.8X5	T50.8X6
Iodoform	T49.0X1	T49.0X2	T49.0X3	T49.0X4	T49.0X5	T49.0X6
Iodohippuric acid	T50.8X1	T50.8X2	T50.8X3	T50.8X4	T50.8X5	T50.8X6
Iodopanoic acid	T50.8X1	T50.8X2	T50.8X3	T50.8X4	T50.8X5	T50.8X6
Iodophthalein (sodium)	T50.8X1	T50.8X2	T50.8X3	T50.8X4	T50.8X5	T50.8X6
Iodopyracet	T50.8X1	T50.8X2	T50.8X3	T50.8X4	T50.8X5	T50.8X6
Iodoquinol	T37.8X1	T37.8X2	T37.8X3	T37.8X4	T37.8X5	T37.8X6
Iodoxamic acid	T50.8X1	T50.8X2	T50.8X3	T50.8X4	T50.8X5	T50.8X6
Iofendylate	T50.8X1	T50.8X2	T50.8X3	T50.8X4	T50.8X5	T50.8X6
Ioglycamic acid	T50.8X1	T50.8X2	T50.8X3	T50.8X4	T50.8X5	T50.8X6
Iohexol	T50.8X1	T50.8X2	T50.8X3	T50.8X4	T50.8X5	T50.8X6
Ion exchange resin						
anion	T47.8X1	T47.8X2	T47.8X3	T47.8X4	T47.8X5	T47.8X6
cation	T50.3X1	T50.3X2	T50.3X3	T50.3X4	T50.3X5	T50.3X6
cholestyramine	T46.6X1	T46.6X2	T46.6X3	T46.6X4	T46.6X5	T46.6X6
intestinal	T47.8X1	T47.8X2	T47.8X3	T47.8X4	T47.8X5	T47.8X6
Iopamidol	T50.8X1	T50.8X2	T50.8X3	T50.8X4	T50.8X5	T50.8X6
Iopanoic acid	T50.8X1	T50.8X2	T50.8X3	T50.8X4	T50.8X5	T50.8X6
Iophenoic acid	T50.8X1	T50.8X2	T50.8X3	T50.8X4	T50.8X5	T50.8X6
Iopodate, sodium	T50.8X1	T50.8X2	T50.8X3	T50.8X4	T50.8X5	T50.8X6
Iopodic acid	T50.8X1	T50.8X2	T50.8X3	T50.8X4	T50.8X5	T50.8X6
Iopromide	T50.8X1	T50.8X2	T50.8X3	T50.8X4	T50.8X5	T50.8X6
Iopydol	T50.8X1	T50.8X2	T50.8X3	T50.8X4	T50.8X5	T50.8X6
Iotalamic acid	T50.8X1	T50.8X2	T50.8X3	T50.8X4	T50.8X5	T50.8X6
Iothalamate	T50.8X1	T50.8X2	T50.8X3	T50.8X4	T50.8X5	T50.8X6
Iothiouracil	T38.2X1	T38.2X2	T38.2X3	T38.2X4	T38.2X5	T38.2X6
Iotrol	T50.8X1	T50.8X2	T50.8X3	T50.8X4	T50.8X5	T50.8X6
Iotrolan	T50.8X1	T50.8X2	T50.8X3	T50.8X4	T50.8X5	T50.8X6
Iotroxate	T50.8X1	T50.8X2	T50.8X3	T50.8X4	T50.8X5	T50.8X6
Iotroxic acid	T50.8X1	T50.8X2	T50.8X3	T50.8X4	T50.8X5	T50.8X6
Ioversol	T50.8X1	T50.8X2	T50.8X3	T50.8X4	T50.8X5	T50.8X6
Ioxaglate	T50.8X1	T50.8X2	T50.8X3	T50.8X4	T50.8X5	T50.8X6
Ioxaglic acid	T50.8X1	T50.8X2	T50.8X3	T50.8X4	T50.8X5	T50.8X6
Ioxitalamic acid	T50.8X1	T50.8X2	T50.8X3	T50.8X4	T50.8X5	T50.8X6
Ipecac	T47.7X1	T47.7X2	T47.7X3	T47.7X4	T47.7X5	T47.7X6
Ipecacuanha	T48.4X1	T48.4X2	T48.4X3	T48.4X4	T48.4X5	T48.4X6
Ipodate, calcium	T50.8X1	T50.8X2	T50.8X3	T50.8X4	T50.8X5	T50.8X6
Ipral	T42.3X1	T42.3X2	T42.3X3	T42.3X4	T42.3X5	T42.3X6
Ipratropium (bromide)	T48.6X1	T48.6X2	T48.6X3	T48.6X4	T48.6X5	T48.6X6
Ipriflavone	T46.3X1	T46.3X2	T46.3X3	T46.3X4	T46.3X5	T46.3X6
Iprindole	T43.011	T43.012	T43.013	T43.014	T43.015	T43.016
Iproclozide	T43.1X1	T43.1X2	T43.1X3	T43.1X4	T43.1X5	T43.1X6
Iprofenin	T50.8X1	T50.8X2	T50.8X3	T50.8X4	T50.8X5	T50.8X6
Iproheptine	T49.2X1	T49.2X2	T49.2X3	T49.2X4	T49.2X5	T49.2X6
Iproniazid	T43.1X1	T43.1X2	T43.1X3	T43.1X4	T43.1X5	T43.1X6
Iproplatin	T45.1X1	T45.1X2	T45.1X3	T45.1X4	T45.1X5	T45.1X6
Iproveratril	T46.1X1	T46.1X2	T46.1X3	T46.1X4	T46.1X5	T46.1X6
Iron (compounds) (medicinal) **NEC**	T45.4X1	T45.4X2	T45.4X3	T45.4X4	T45.4X5	T45.4X6
ammonium	T45.4X1	T45.4X2	T45.4X3	T45.4X4	T45.4X5	T45.4X6
dextran injection	T45.4X1	T45.4X2	T45.4X3	T45.4X4	T45.4X5	T45.4X6
nonmedicinal	T56.891	T56.892	T56.893	T56.894	—	—
salts	T45.4X1	T45.4X2	T45.4X3	T45.4X4	T45.4X5	T45.4X6
sorbitex	T45.4X1	T45.4X2	T45.4X3	T45.4X4	T45.4X5	T45.4X6
sorbitol citric acid complex	T45.4X1	T45.4X2	T45.4X3	T45.4X4	T45.4X5	T45.4X6
Irrigating fluid (vaginal)	T49.8X1	T49.8X2	T49.8X3	T49.8X4	T49.8X5	T49.8X6
eye	T49.5X1	T49.5X2	T49.5X3	T49.5X4	T49.5X5	T49.5X6
Isepamicin	T36.5X1	T36.5X2	T36.5X3	T36.5X4	T36.5X5	T36.5X6
Isoaminile (citrate)	T48.3X1	T48.3X2	T48.3X3	T48.3X4	T48.3X5	T48.3X6
Isoamyl nitrite	T46.3X1	T46.3X2	T46.3X3	T46.3X4	T46.3X5	T46.3X6
Isobenzan	T60.1X1	T60.1X2	T60.1X3	T60.1X4	—	—
Isobutyl acetate	T52.8X1	T52.8X2	T52.8X3	T52.8X4	—	—
Isocarboxazid	T43.1X1	T43.1X2	T43.1X3	T43.1X4	T43.1X5	T43.1X6
Isoconazole	T49.0X1	T49.0X2	T49.0X3	T49.0X4	T49.0X5	T49.0X6
Isocyanate	T65.0X1	T65.0X2	T65.0X3	T65.0X4	—	—
Isoephedrine	T44.991	T44.992	T44.993	T44.994	T44.995	T44.996
Isoetarine	T48.6X1	T48.6X2	T48.6X3	T48.6X4	T48.6X5	T48.6X6
Isoethadione	T42.2X1	T42.2X2	T42.2X3	T42.2X4	T42.2X5	T42.2X6
Isoetharine	T44.5X1	T44.5X2	T44.5X3	T44.5X4	T44.5X5	T44.5X6
Isoflurane	T41.0X1	T41.0X2	T41.0X3	T41.0X4	T41.0X5	T41.0X6
Isoflurophate	T44.0X1	T44.0X2	T44.0X3	T44.0X4	T44.0X5	T44.0X6
Isomaltose, ferric complex	T45.4X1	T45.4X2	T45.4X3	T45.4X4	T45.4X5	T45.4X6
Isometheptene	T44.3X1	T44.3X2	T44.3X3	T44.3X4	T44.3X5	T44.3X6
Isoniazid	T37.1X1	T37.1X2	T37.1X3	T37.1X4	T37.1X5	T37.1X6
with						
rifampicin	T36.6X1	T36.6X2	T36.6X3	T36.6X4	T36.6X5	T36.6X6
thioacetazone	T37.1X1	T37.1X2	T37.1X3	T37.1X4	T37.1X5	T37.1X6
Isonicotinic acid hydrazide	T37.1X1	T37.1X2	T37.1X3	T37.1X4	T37.1X5	T37.1X6
Isonipecaine	T40.4X1	T40.4X2	T40.4X3	T40.4X4	T40.4X5	T40.4X6
Isopentaquine	T37.2X1	T37.2X2	T37.2X3	T37.2X4	T37.2X5	T37.2X6
Isophane insulin	T38.3X1	T38.3X2	T38.3X3	T38.3X4	T38.3X5	T38.3X6
Isophorone	T65.891	T65.892	T65.893	T65.894	—	—
Isophosphamide	T45.1X1	T45.1X2	T45.1X3	T45.1X4	T45.1X5	T45.1X6
Isopregnenone	T38.5X1	T38.5X2	T38.5X3	T38.5X4	T38.5X5	T38.5X6
Isoprenaline	T48.6X1	T48.6X2	T48.6X3	T48.6X4	T48.6X5	T48.6X6
Isopromethazine	T43.3X1	T43.3X2	T43.3X3	T43.3X4	T43.3X5	T43.3X6
Isopropamide	T44.3X1	T44.3X2	T44.3X3	T44.3X4	T44.3X5	T44.3X6
iodide	T44.3X1	T44.3X2	T44.3X3	T44.3X4	T44.3X5	T44.3X6
Isopropanol	T51.2X1	T51.2X2	T51.2X3	T51.2X4	—	—
Isopropyl						
acetate	T52.8X1	T52.8X2	T52.8X3	T52.8X4	—	—
alcohol	T51.2X1	T51.2X2	T51.2X3	T51.2X4	—	—
medicinal	T49.4X1	T49.4X2	T49.4X3	T49.4X4	T49.4X5	T49.4X6
ether	T52.8X1	T52.8X2	T52.8X3	T52.8X4	—	—
Isopropylaminophenazone	T39.2X1	T39.2X2	T39.2X3	T39.2X4	T39.2X5	T39.2X6
Isoproterenol	T48.6X1	T48.6X2	T48.6X3	T48.6X4	T48.6X5	T48.6X6
Isosorbide dinitrate	T46.3X1	T46.3X2	T46.3X3	T46.3X4	T46.3X5	T46.3X6
Isothipendyl	T45.0X1	T45.0X2	T45.0X3	T45.0X4	T45.0X5	T45.0X6
Isotretinoin	T50.991	T50.992	T50.993	T50.994	T50.995	T50.996
Isoxazolyl penicillin	T36.0X1	T36.0X2	T36.0X3	T36.0X4	T36.0X5	T36.0X6
Isoxicam	T39.391	T39.392	T39.393	T39.394	T39.395	T39.396
Isoxsuprine	T46.7X1	T46.7X2	T46.7X3	T46.7X4	T46.7X5	T46.7X6
Ispagula	T47.4X1	T47.4X2	T47.4X3	T47.4X4	T47.4X5	T47.4X6
husk	T47.4X1	T47.4X2	T47.4X3	T47.4X4	T47.4X5	T47.4X6
Isradipine	T46.1X1	T46.1X2	T46.1X3	T46.1X4	T46.1X5	T46.1X6
I-thyroxine sodium	T38.1X1	T38.1X2	T38.1X3	T38.1X4	T38.1X5	T38.1X6
Itraconazole	T37.8X1	T37.8X2	T37.8X3	T37.8X4	T37.8X5	T37.8X6
Itramin tosilate	T46.3X1	T46.3X2	T46.3X3	T46.3X4	T46.3X5	T46.3X6
Ivermectin	T37.4X1	T37.4X2	T37.4X3	T37.4X4	T37.4X5	T37.4X6
Izoniazid	T37.1X1	T37.1X2	T37.1X3	T37.1X4	T37.1X5	T37.1X6
with thioacetazone	T37.1X1	T37.1X2	T37.1X3	T37.1X4	T37.1X5	T37.1X6
Jalap	T47.2X1	T47.2X2	T47.2X3	T47.2X4	T47.2X5	T47.2X6
Jamaica						
dogwood (bark)	T39.8X1	T39.8X2	T39.8X3	T39.8X4	T39.8X5	T39.8X6
ginger	T65.891	T65.892	T65.893	T65.894	—	—
root	T62.2X1	T62.2X2	T62.2X3	T62.2X4	—	—
Jatropha	T62.2X1	T62.2X2	T62.2X3	T62.2X4	—	—
curcas	T62.2X1	T62.2X2	T62.2X3	T62.2X4	—	—

Additional Character May Be Required — Refer to the Tabular List for Character Selection   ▽ **Subterms under main terms may continue to next column or page**

Substance	Poisoning, Accidental (unintentional)	Poisoning, Intentional Self-harm	Poisoning, Assault	Poisoning, Undetermined	Adverse Effect	Under-dosing
Jectofer	T45.4X1	T45.4X2	T45.4X3	T45.4X4	T45.4X5	T45.4X6
Jellyfish (sting)	T63.621	T63.622	T63.623	T63.624	—	—
Jequirity (bean)	T62.2X1	T62.2X2	T62.2X3	T62.2X4	—	—
Jimson weed (stramonium)	T62.2X1	T62.2X2	T62.2X3	T62.2X4	—	—
seeds	T62.2X1	T62.2X2	T62.2X3	T62.2X4	—	—
Josamycin	T36.3X1	T36.3X2	T36.3X3	T36.3X4	T36.3X5	T36.3X6
Juniper tar	T49.1X1	T49.1X2	T49.1X3	T49.1X4	T49.1X5	T49.1X6
Kallidinogenase	T46.7X1	T46.7X2	T46.7X3	T46.7X4	T46.7X5	T46.7X6
Kallikrein	T46.7X1	T46.7X2	T46.7X3	T46.7X4	T46.7X5	T46.7X6
Kanamycin	T36.5X1	T36.5X2	T36.5X3	T36.5X4	T36.5X5	T36.5X6
Kantrex	T36.5X1	T36.5X2	T36.5X3	T36.5X4	T36.5X5	T36.5X6
Kaolin	T47.6X1	T47.6X2	T47.6X3	T47.6X4	T47.6X5	T47.6X6
light	T47.6X1	T47.6X2	T47.6X3	T47.6X4	T47.6X5	T47.6X6
Karaya (gum)	T47.4X1	T47.4X2	T47.4X3	T47.4X4	T47.4X5	T47.4X6
Kebuzone	T39.2X1	T39.2X2	T39.2X3	T39.2X4	T39.2X5	T39.2X6
Kelevan	T60.1X1	T60.1X2	T60.1X3	T60.1X4	—	—
Kemithal	T41.1X1	T41.1X2	T41.1X3	T41.1X4	T41.1X5	T41.1X6
Kenacort	T38.0X1	T38.0X2	T38.0X3	T38.0X4	T38.0X5	T38.0X6
Keratolytic drug NEC	T49.4X1	T49.4X2	T49.4X3	T49.4X4	T49.4X5	T49.4X6
anthracene	T49.4X1	T49.4X2	T49.4X3	T49.4X4	T49.4X5	T49.4X6
Keratoplastic NEC	T49.4X1	T49.4X2	T49.4X3	T49.4X4	T49.4X5	T49.4X6
Kerosene, kerosine (fuel) (solvent) NEC	T52.0X1	T52.0X2	T52.0X3	T52.0X4	—	—
insecticide	T52.0X1	T52.0X2	T52.0X3	T52.0X4	—	—
vapor	T52.0X1	T52.0X2	T52.0X3	T52.0X4	—	—
Ketamine	T41.291	T41.292	T41.293	T41.294	T41.295	T41.296
Ketazolam	T42.4X1	T42.4X2	T42.4X3	T42.4X4	T42.4X5	T42.4X6
Ketazon	T39.2X1	T39.2X2	T39.2X3	T39.2X4	T39.2X5	T39.2X6
Ketobemidone	T40.4X1	T40.4X2	T40.4X3	T40.4X4	—	—
Ketoconazole	T49.0X1	T49.0X2	T49.0X3	T49.0X4	T49.0X5	T49.0X6
Ketols	T52.4X1	T52.4X2	T52.4X3	T52.4X4	—	—
Ketone oils	T52.4X1	T52.4X2	T52.4X3	T52.4X4	—	—
Ketoprofen	T39.311	T39.312	T39.313	T39.314	T39.315	T39.316
Ketorolac	T39.8X1	T39.8X2	T39.8X3	T39.8X4	T39.8X5	T39.8X6
Ketotifen	T45.0X1	T45.0X2	T45.0X3	T45.0X4	T45.0X5	T45.0X6
Khat	T43.691	T43.692	T43.693	T43.694	—	—
Khellin	T46.3X1	T46.3X2	T46.3X3	T46.3X4	T46.3X5	T46.3X6
Khelloside	T46.3X1	T46.3X2	T46.3X3	T46.3X4	T46.3X5	T46.3X6
Kiln gas or vapor (carbon monoxide)	T58.8X1	T58.8X2	T58.8X3	T58.8X4	—	—
Kitasamycin	T36.3X1	T36.3X2	T36.3X3	T36.3X4	T36.3X5	T36.3X6
Konsyl	T47.4X1	T47.4X2	T47.4X3	T47.4X4	T47.4X5	T47.4X6
Kosam seed	T62.2X1	T62.2X2	T62.2X3	T62.2X4	—	—
Krait (venom)	T63.091	T63.092	T63.093	T63.094	—	—
Kwell (insecticide)	T60.1X1	T60.1X2	T60.1X3	T60.1X4	—	—
anti-infective (topical)	T49.0X1	T49.0X2	T49.0X3	T49.0X4	T49.0X5	T49.0X6
Labetalol	T44.8X1	T44.8X2	T44.8X3	T44.8X4	T44.8X5	T44.8X6
Laburnum (seeds)	T62.2X1	T62.2X2	T62.2X3	T62.2X4	—	—
leaves	T62.2X1	T62.2X2	T62.2X3	T62.2X4	—	—
Lachesine	T49.5X1	T49.5X2	T49.5X3	T49.5X4	T49.5X5	T49.5X6
Lacidipine	T46.5X1	T46.5X2	T46.5X3	T46.5X4	T46.5X5	T46.5X6
Lacquer	T65.6X1	T65.6X2	T65.6X3	T65.6X4	—	—
Lacrimogenic gas	T59.3X1	T59.3X2	T59.3X3	T59.3X4	—	—
Lactated potassic saline	T50.3X1	T50.3X2	T50.3X3	T50.3X4	T50.3X5	T50.3X6
Lactic acid	T49.8X1	T49.8X2	T49.8X3	T49.8X4	T49.8X5	T49.8X6
Lactobacillus						
acidophilus	T47.6X1	T47.6X2	T47.6X3	T47.6X4	T47.6X5	T47.6X6
compound	T47.6X1	T47.6X2	T47.6X3	T47.6X4	T47.6X5	T47.6X6
bifidus, lyophilized	T47.6X1	T47.6X2	T47.6X3	T47.6X4	T47.6X5	T47.6X6
bulgaricus	T47.6X1	T47.6X2	T47.6X3	T47.6X4	T47.6X5	T47.6X6
sporogenes	T47.6X1	T47.6X2	T47.6X3	T47.6X4	T47.6X5	T47.6X6
Lactoflavin	T45.2X1	T45.2X2	T45.2X3	T45.2X4	T45.2X5	T45.2X6
Lactose (as excipient)	T50.901	T50.902	T50.903	T50.904	T50.905	T50.906
Lactuca (virosa) (extract)	T42.6X1	T42.6X2	T42.6X3	T42.6X4	T42.6X5	T42.6X6
Lactucarium	T42.6X1	T42.6X2	T42.6X3	T42.6X4	T42.6X5	T42.6X6
Lactulose	T47.3X1	T47.3X2	T47.3X3	T47.3X4	T47.3X5	T47.3X6
Laevo — *see* Levo-						
Lanatosides	T46.0X1	T46.0X2	T46.0X3	T46.0X4	T46.0X5	T46.0X6
Lanolin	T49.3X1	T49.3X2	T49.3X3	T49.3X4	T49.3X5	T49.3X6
Largactil	T43.3X1	T43.3X2	T43.3X3	T43.3X4	T43.3X5	T43.3X6
Larkspur	T62.2X1	T62.2X2	T62.2X3	T62.2X4	—	—
Laroxyl	T43.011	T43.012	T43.013	T43.014	T43.015	T43.016
Lasix	T50.1X1	T50.1X2	T50.1X3	T50.1X4	T50.1X5	T50.1X6
Lassar's paste	T49.4X1	T49.4X2	T49.4X3	T49.4X4	T49.4X5	T49.4X6
Latamoxef	T36.1X1	T36.1X2	T36.1X3	T36.1X4	T36.1X5	T36.1X6
Latex	T65.811	T65.812	T65.813	T65.814	—	—
Lathyrus (seed)	T62.2X1	T62.2X2	T62.2X3	T62.2X4	—	—
Laudanum	T40.0X1	T40.0X2	T40.0X3	T40.0X4	T40.0X5	T40.0X6
Laudexium	T48.1X1	T48.1X2	T48.1X3	T48.1X4	T48.1X5	T48.1X6
Laughing gas	T41.0X1	T41.0X2	T41.0X3	T41.0X4	T41.0X5	T41.0X6
Laurel, black or cherry	T62.2X1	T62.2X2	T62.2X3	T62.2X4	—	—
Laurolinium	T49.0X1	T49.0X2	T49.0X3	T49.0X4	T49.0X5	T49.0X6
Lauryl sulfoacetate	T49.2X1	T49.2X2	T49.2X3	T49.2X4	T49.2X5	T49.2X6

Substance	Poisoning, Accidental (unintentional)	Poisoning, Intentional Self-harm	Poisoning, Assault	Poisoning, Undetermined	Adverse Effect	Under-dosing
Laxative NEC	T47.4X1	T47.4X2	T47.4X3	T47.4X4	T47.4X5	T47.4X6
osmotic	T47.3X1	T47.3X2	T47.3X3	T47.3X4	T47.3X5	T47.3X6
saline	T47.3X1	T47.3X2	T47.3X3	T47.3X4	T47.3X5	T47.3X6
stimulant	T47.2X1	T47.2X2	T47.2X3	T47.2X4	T47.2X5	T47.2X6
L-dopa	T42.8X1	T42.8X2	T42.8X3	T42.8X4	T42.8X5	T42.8X6
Lead (dust) (fumes) (vapor)	T56.0X1	T56.0X2	T56.0X3	T56.0X4	—	—
NEC						
acetate	T49.2X1	T49.2X2	T49.2X3	T49.2X4	T49.2X5	T49.2X6
alkyl (fuel additive)	T56.0X1	T56.0X2	T56.0X3	T56.0X4	—	—
anti-infectives	T37.8X1	T37.8X2	T37.8X3	T37.8X4	T37.8X5	T37.8X6
antiknock compound (tetraethyl)	T56.0X1	T56.0X2	T56.0X3	T56.0X4	—	—
arsenate, arsenite (dust)(herbicide) (insecticide) (vapor)	T57.0X1	T57.0X2	T57.0X3	T57.0X4	—	—
carbonate	T56.0X1	T56.0X2	T56.0X3	T56.0X4	—	—
paint	T56.0X1	T56.0X2	T56.0X3	T56.0X4	—	—
chromate	T56.0X1	T56.0X2	T56.0X3	T56.0X4	—	—
paint	T56.0X1	T56.0X2	T56.0X3	T56.0X4	—	—
dioxide	T56.0X1	T56.0X2	T56.0X3	T56.0X4	—	—
inorganic	T56.0X1	T56.0X2	T56.0X3	T56.0X4	—	—
iodide	T56.0X1	T56.0X2	T56.0X3	T56.0X4	—	—
pigment (paint)	T56.0X1	T56.0X2	T56.0X3	T56.0X4	—	—
monoxide (dust)	T56.0X1	T56.0X2	T56.0X3	T56.0X4	—	—
paint	T56.0X1	T56.0X2	T56.0X3	T56.0X4	—	—
organic	T56.0X1	T56.0X2	T56.0X3	T56.0X4	—	—
oxide	T56.0X1	T56.0X2	T56.0X3	T56.0X4	—	—
paint	T56.0X1	T56.0X2	T56.0X3	T56.0X4	—	—
paint	T56.0X1	T56.0X2	T56.0X3	T56.0X4	—	—
salts	T56.0X1	T56.0X2	T56.0X3	T56.0X4	—	—
specified compound NEC	T56.0X1	T56.0X2	T56.0X3	T56.0X4	—	—
tetra-ethyl	T56.0X1	T56.0X2	T56.0X3	T56.0X4	—	—
Lebanese red	T40.7X1	T40.7X2	T40.7X3	T40.7X4	T40.7X5	T40.7X6
Lefetamine	T39.8X1	T39.8X2	T39.8X3	T39.8X4	T39.8X5	T39.8X6
Lenperone	T43.4X1	T43.4X2	T43.4X3	T43.4X4	T43.4X5	T43.4X6
Lente lietin (insulin)	T38.3X1	T38.3X2	T38.3X3	T38.3X4	T38.3X5	T38.3X6
Leptazol	T50.7X1	T50.7X2	T50.7X3	T50.7X4	T50.7X5	T50.7X6
Leptophos	T60.0X1	T60.0X2	T60.0X3	T60.0X4	—	—
Leritine	T40.2X1	T40.2X2	T40.2X3	T40.2X4	T40.2X5	T40.2X6
Letosteine	T48.4X1	T48.4X2	T48.4X3	T48.4X4	T48.4X5	T48.4X6
Letter	T38.1X1	T38.1X2	T38.1X3	T38.1X4	T38.1X5	T38.1X6
Lettuce opium	T42.6X1	T42.6X2	T42.6X3	T42.6X4	T42.6X5	T42.6X6
Leucinocaine	T41.3X1	T41.3X2	T41.3X3	T41.3X4	T41.3X5	T41.3X6
Leucocianidol	T46.991	T46.992	T46.993	T46.994	T46.995	T46.996
Leucovorin (factor)	T45.8X1	T45.8X2	T45.8X3	T45.8X4	T45.8X5	T45.8X6
Leukeran	T45.1X1	T45.1X2	T45.1X3	T45.1X4	T45.1X5	T45.1X6
Leuprolide	T38.891	T38.892	T38.893	T38.894	T38.895	T38.896
Levalbuterol	T48.6X1	T48.6X2	T48.6X3	T48.6X4	T48.6X5	T48.6X6
Levallorphan	T50.7X1	T50.7X2	T50.7X3	T50.7X4	T50.7X5	T50.7X6
Levamisole	T37.4X1	T37.4X2	T37.4X3	T37.4X4	T37.4X5	T37.4X6
Levanil	T42.6X1	T42.6X2	T42.6X3	T42.6X4	T42.6X5	T42.6X6
Levarterenol	T44.4X1	T44.4X2	T44.4X3	T44.4X4	T44.4X5	T44.4X6
Levdropropizine	T48.3X1	T48.3X2	T48.3X3	T48.3X4	T48.3X5	T48.3X6
Levobunolol	T49.5X1	T49.5X2	T49.5X3	T49.5X4	T49.5X5	T49.5X6
Levocabastine (hydrochloride)	T45.0X1	T45.0X2	T45.0X3	T45.0X4	T45.0X5	T45.0X6
Levocarnitine	T50.991	T50.992	T50.993	T50.994	T50.995	T50.996
Levodopa	T42.8X1	T42.8X2	T42.8X3	T42.8X4	T42.8X5	T42.8X6
with carbidopa	T42.8X1	T42.8X2	T42.8X3	T42.8X4	T42.8X5	T42.8X6
Levo-dromoran	T40.2X1	T40.2X2	T40.2X3	T40.2X4	T40.2X5	T40.2X6
Levoglutamide	T50.991	T50.992	T50.993	T50.994	T50.995	T50.996
Levoid	T38.1X1	T38.1X2	T38.1X3	T38.1X4	T38.1X5	T38.1X6
Levo-isomethadone	T40.3X1	T40.3X2	T40.3X3	T40.3X4	T40.3X5	T40.3X6
Levomepromazine	T43.3X1	T43.3X2	T43.3X3	T43.3X4	T43.3X5	T43.3X6
Levonordefrin	T49.6X1	T49.6X2	T49.6X3	T49.6X4	T49.6X5	T49.6X6
Levonorgestrel	T38.4X1	T38.4X2	T38.4X3	T38.4X4	T38.4X5	T38.4X6
with ethinylestradiol	T38.5X1	T38.5X2	T38.5X3	T38.5X4	T38.5X5	T38.5X6
Levopromazine	T43.3X1	T43.3X2	T43.3X3	T43.3X4	T43.3X5	T43.3X6
Levoprome	T42.6X1	T42.6X2	T42.6X3	T42.6X4	T42.6X5	T42.6X6
Levopropoxyphene	T40.4X1	T40.4X2	T40.4X3	T40.4X4	T40.4X5	T40.4X6
Levopropylhexedrine	T50.5X1	T50.5X2	T50.5X3	T50.5X4	T50.5X5	T50.5X6
Levoproxyphylline	T48.6X1	T48.6X2	T48.6X3	T48.6X4	T48.6X5	T48.6X6
Levorphanol	T40.4X1	T40.4X2	T40.4X3	T40.4X4	T40.4X5	T40.4X6
Levothyroxine	T38.1X1	T38.1X2	T38.1X3	T38.1X4	T38.1X5	T38.1X6
sodium	T38.1X1	T38.1X2	T38.1X3	T38.1X4	T38.1X5	T38.1X6
Levsin	T44.3X1	T44.3X2	T44.3X3	T44.3X4	T44.3X5	T44.3X6
Levulose	T50.3X1	T50.3X2	T50.3X3	T50.3X4	T50.3X5	T50.3X6
Lewisite (gas), not in war	T57.0X1	T57.0X2	T57.0X3	T57.0X4	—	—
Librium	T42.4X1	T42.4X2	T42.4X3	T42.4X4	T42.4X5	T42.4X6
Lidex	T49.0X1	T49.0X2	T49.0X3	T49.0X4	T49.0X5	T49.0X6
Lidocaine	T41.3X1	T41.3X2	T41.3X3	T41.3X4	T41.3X5	T41.3X6
regional	T41.3X1	T41.3X2	T41.3X3	T41.3X4	T41.3X5	T41.3X6
spinal	T41.3X1	T41.3X2	T41.3X3	T41.3X4	T41.3X5	T41.3X6

Table of Drugs and Chemicals

Lidofenin — Mecamylamine

Substance	Poisoning, Accidental (unintentional)	Poisoning, Intentional Self-harm	Poisoning, Assault	Poisoning, Undetermined	Adverse Effect	Under-dosing
Lidofenin	T50.8X1	T50.8X2	T50.8X3	T50.8X4	T50.8X5	T50.8X6
Lidoflazine	T46.1X1	T46.1X2	T46.1X3	T46.1X4	T46.1X5	T46.1X6
Lighter fluid	T52.0X1	T52.0X2	T52.0X3	T52.0X4	—	—
Lignin hemicellulose	T47.6X1	T47.6X2	T47.6X3	T47.6X4	T47.6X5	T47.6X6
Lignocaine	T41.3X1	T41.3X2	T41.3X3	T41.3X4	T41.3X5	T41.3X6
regional	T41.3X1	T41.3X2	T41.3X3	T41.3X4	T41.3X5	T41.3X6
spinal	T41.3X1	T41.3X2	T41.3X3	T41.3X4	T41.3X5	T41.3X6
Ligroin (e) (solvent)	T52.0X1	T52.0X2	T52.0X3	T52.0X4	—	—
vapor	T59.891	T59.892	T59.893	T59.894	—	—
Ligustrum vulgare	T62.2X1	T62.2X2	T62.2X3	T62.2X4	—	—
Lily of the valley	T62.2X1	T62.2X2	T62.2X3	T62.2X4	—	—
Lime (chloride)	T54.3X1	T54.3X2	T54.3X3	T54.3X4	—	—
Limonene	T52.8X1	T52.8X2	T52.8X3	T52.8X4	—	—
Lincomycin	T36.8X1	T36.8X2	T36.8X3	T36.8X4	T36.8X5	T36.8X6
Lindane (insecticide) (nonmedicinal) (vapor)	T53.6X1	T53.6X2	T53.6X3	T53.6X4	—	—
medicinal	T49.0X1	T49.0X2	T49.0X3	T49.0X4	T49.0X5	T49.0X6
Liniments NEC	T49.91	T49.92	T49.93	T49.94	T49.95	T49.96
Linoleic acid	T46.6X1	T46.6X2	T46.6X3	T46.6X4	T46.6X5	T46.6X6
Linolenic acid	T46.6X1	T46.6X2	T46.6X3	T46.6X4	T46.6X5	T46.6X6
Linseed	T47.4X1	T47.4X2	T47.4X3	T47.4X4	T47.4X5	T47.4X6
Liothyronine	T38.1X1	T38.1X2	T38.1X3	T38.1X4	T38.1X5	T38.1X6
Liotrix	T38.1X1	T38.1X2	T38.1X3	T38.1X4	T38.1X5	T38.1X6
Lipancreatin	T47.5X1	T47.5X2	T47.5X3	T47.5X4	T47.5X5	T47.5X6
Lipo-alprostadil	T46.7X1	T46.7X2	T46.7X3	T46.7X4	T46.7X5	T46.7X6
Lipo-Lutin	T38.5X1	T38.5X2	T38.5X3	T38.5X4	T38.5X5	T38.5X6
Lipotropic drug NEC	T50.901	T50.902	T50.903	T50.904	T50.905	T50.906
Liquefied petroleum gases	T59.891	T59.892	T59.893	T59.894	—	—
piped (pure or mixed with air)	T59.891	T59.892	T59.893	T59.894	—	—
Liquid						
paraffin	T47.4X1	T47.4X2	T47.4X3	T47.4X4	T47.4X5	T47.4X6
petrolatum	T47.4X1	T47.4X2	T47.4X3	T47.4X4	T47.4X5	T47.4X6
topical	T49.3X1	T49.3X2	T49.3X3	T49.3X4	T49.3X5	T49.3X6
specified NEC	T65.891	T65.892	T65.893	T65.894	—	—
substance	T65.91	T65.92	T65.93	T65.94	—	—
Liquor creosolis compositus	T65.891	T65.892	T65.893	T65.894	—	—
Liquorice	T48.4X1	T48.4X2	T48.4X3	T48.4X4	T48.4X5	T48.4X6
extract	T47.8X1	T47.8X2	T47.8X3	T47.8X4	T47.8X5	T47.8X6
Lisinopril	T46.4X1	T46.4X2	T46.4X3	T46.4X4	T46.4X5	T46.4X6
Lisuride	T42.8X1	T42.8X2	T42.8X3	T42.8X4	T42.8X5	T42.8X6
Lithane	T43.8X1	T43.8X2	T43.8X3	T43.8X4	T43.8X5	T43.8X6
Lithium	T56.891	T56.892	T56.893	T56.894	—	—
gluconate	T43.591	T43.592	T43.593	T43.594	T43.595	T43.596
salts (carbonate)	T43.591	T43.592	T43.593	T43.594	T43.595	T43.596
Lithonate	T43.8X1	T43.8X2	T43.8X3	T43.8X4	T43.8X5	T43.8X6
Liver						
extract	T45.8X1	T45.8X2	T45.8X3	T45.8X4	T45.8X5	T45.8X6
for parenteral use	T45.8X1	T45.8X2	T45.8X3	T45.8X4	T45.8X5	T45.8X6
fraction 1	T45.8X1	T45.8X2	T45.8X3	T45.8X4	T45.8X5	T45.8X6
hydrolysate	T45.8X1	T45.8X2	T45.8X3	T45.8X4	T45.8X5	T45.8X6
Lizard (bite) (venom)	T63.121	T63.122	T63.123	T63.124	—	—
LMD	T45.8X1	T45.8X2	T45.8X3	T45.8X4	T45.8X5	T45.8X6
Lobelia	T62.2X1	T62.2X2	T62.2X3	T62.2X4	—	—
Lobeline	T50.7X1	T50.7X2	T50.7X3	T50.7X4	T50.7X5	T50.7X6
Local action drug NEC	T49.8X1	T49.8X2	T49.8X3	T49.8X4	T49.8X5	T49.8X6
Locorten	T49.0X1	T49.0X2	T49.0X3	T49.0X4	T49.0X5	T49.0X6
Lofepramine	T43.011	T43.012	T43.013	T43.014	T43.015	T43.016
Lolium temulentum	T62.2X1	T62.2X2	T62.2X3	T62.2X4	—	—
Lomotil	T47.6X1	T47.6X2	T47.6X3	T47.6X4	T47.6X5	T47.6X6
Lomustine	T45.1X1	T45.1X2	T45.1X3	T45.1X4	T45.1X5	T45.1X6
Lonidamine	T45.1X1	T45.1X2	T45.1X3	T45.1X4	T45.1X5	T45.1X6
Loperamide	T47.6X1	T47.6X2	T47.6X3	T47.6X4	T47.6X5	T47.6X6
Loprazolam	T42.4X1	T42.4X2	T42.4X3	T42.4X4	T42.4X5	T42.4X6
Lorajmine	T46.2X1	T46.2X2	T46.2X3	T46.2X4	T46.2X5	T46.2X6
Loratidine	T45.0X1	T45.0X2	T45.0X3	T45.0X4	T45.0X5	T45.0X6
Lorazepam	T42.4X1	T42.4X2	T42.4X3	T42.4X4	T42.4X5	T42.4X6
Lorcainide	T46.2X1	T46.2X2	T46.2X3	T46.2X4	T46.2X5	T46.2X6
Lormetazepam	T42.4X1	T42.4X2	T42.4X3	T42.4X4	T42.4X5	T42.4X6
Lotions NEC	T49.91	T49.92	T49.93	T49.94	T49.95	T49.96
Lotusate	T42.3X1	T42.3X2	T42.3X3	T42.3X4	T42.3X5	T42.3X6
Lovastatin	T46.6X1	T46.6X2	T46.6X3	T46.6X4	T46.6X5	T46.6X6
Lowila	T49.2X1	T49.2X2	T49.2X3	T49.2X4	T49.2X5	T49.2X6
Loxapine	T43.591	T43.592	T43.593	T43.594	T43.595	T43.596
Lozenges (throat)	T49.6X1	T49.6X2	T49.6X3	T49.6X4	T49.6X5	T49.6X6
LSD	T40.8X1	T40.8X2	T40.8X3	T40.8X4	—	—
L-Tryptophan — *see* amino acid						
Lubricant, eye	T49.5X1	T49.5X2	T49.5X3	T49.5X4	T49.5X5	T49.5X6
Lubricating oil NEC	T52.0X1	T52.0X2	T52.0X3	T52.0X4	—	—
Lucanthone	T37.4X1	T37.4X2	T37.4X3	T37.4X4	T37.4X5	T37.4X6
Luminal	T42.3X1	T42.3X2	T42.3X3	T42.3X4	T42.3X5	T42.3X6
Lung irritant (gas) **NEC**	T59.91	T59.92	T59.93	T59.94		

Substance	Poisoning, Accidental (unintentional)	Poisoning, Intentional Self-harm	Poisoning, Assault	Poisoning, Undetermined	Adverse Effect	Under-dosing
Luteinizing hormone	T38.811	T38.812	T38.813	T38.814	T38.815	T38.816
Lutocylol	T38.5X1	T38.5X2	T38.5X3	T38.5X4	T38.5X5	T38.5X6
Lutromone	T38.5X1	T38.5X2	T38.5X3	T38.5X4	T38.5X5	T38.5X6
Lututrin	T48.291	T48.292	T48.293	T48.294	T48.295	T48.296
Lye (concentrated)	T54.3X1	T54.3X2	T54.3X3	T54.3X4	—	—
Lygranum (skin test)	T50.8X1	T50.8X2	T50.8X3	T50.8X4	T50.8X5	T50.8X6
Lymecycline	T36.4X1	T36.4X2	T36.4X3	T36.4X4	T36.4X5	T36.4X6
Lymphogranuloma venereum antigen	T50.8X1	T50.8X2	T50.8X3	T50.8X4	T50.8X5	T50.8X6
Lynestrenol	T38.4X1	T38.4X2	T38.4X3	T38.4X4	T38.4X5	T38.4X6
Lyovac Sodium Edecrin	T50.1X1	T50.1X2	T50.1X3	T50.1X4	T50.1X5	T50.1X6
Lypressin	T38.891	T38.892	T38.893	T38.894	T38.895	T38.896
Lysergic acid diethylamide	T40.8X1	T40.8X2	T40.8X3	T40.8X4	—	—
Lysergide	T40.8X1	T40.8X2	T40.8X3	T40.8X4	—	—
Lysine vasopressin	T38.891	T38.892	T38.893	T38.894	T38.895	T38.896
Lysol	T54.1X1	T54.1X2	T54.1X3	T54.1X4	—	—
Lysozyme	T49.0X1	T49.0X2	T49.0X3	T49.0X4	T49.0X5	T49.0X6
Lytta (vitatta)	T49.8X1	T49.8X2	T49.8X3	T49.8X4	T49.8X5	T49.8X6
Mace	T59.3X1	T59.3X2	T59.3X3	T59.3X4	—	—
Macrogol	T50.991	T50.992	T50.993	T50.994	T50.995	T50.996
Macrolide						
anabolic drug	T38.7X1	T38.7X2	T38.7X3	T38.7X4	T38.7X5	T38.7X6
antibiotic	T36.3X1	T36.3X2	T36.3X3	T36.3X4	T36.3X5	T36.3X6
Mafenide	T49.0X1	T49.0X2	T49.0X3	T49.0X4	T49.0X5	T49.0X6
Magaldrate	T47.1X1	T47.1X2	T47.1X3	T47.1X4	T47.1X5	T47.1X6
Magic mushroom	T40.991	T40.992	T40.993	T40.994	—	—
Magnamycin	T36.8X1	T36.8X2	T36.8X3	T36.8X4	T36.8X5	T36.8X6
Magnesia magma	T47.1X1	T47.1X2	T47.1X3	T47.1X4	T47.1X5	T47.1X6
Magnesium NEC	T56.891	T56.892	T56.893	T56.894	—	—
carbonate	T47.1X1	T47.1X2	T47.1X3	T47.1X4	T47.1X5	T47.1X6
citrate	T47.4X1	T47.4X2	T47.4X3	T47.4X4	T47.4X5	T47.4X6
hydroxide	T47.1X1	T47.1X2	T47.1X3	T47.1X4	T47.1X5	T47.1X6
oxide	T47.1X1	T47.1X2	T47.1X3	T47.1X4	T47.1X5	T47.1X6
peroxide	T49.0X1	T49.0X2	T49.0X3	T49.0X4	T49.0X5	T49.0X6
salicylate	T39.091	T39.092	T39.093	T39.094	T39.095	T39.096
silicofluoride	T50.3X1	T50.3X2	T50.3X3	T50.3X4	T50.3X5	T50.3X6
sulfate	T47.4X1	T47.4X2	T47.4X3	T47.4X4	T47.4X5	T47.4X6
thiosulfate	T45.0X1	T45.0X2	T45.0X3	T45.0X4	T45.0X5	T45.0X6
trisilicate	T47.1X1	T47.1X2	T47.1X3	T47.1X4	T47.1X5	T47.1X6
Malathion (medicinal)	T49.0X1	T49.0X2	T49.0X3	T49.0X4	T49.0X5	T49.0X6
insecticide	T60.0X1	T60.0X2	T60.0X3	T60.0X4	—	—
Male fern extract	T37.4X1	T37.4X2	T37.4X3	T37.4X4	T37.4X5	T37.4X6
M-AMSA	T45.1X1	T45.1X2	T45.1X3	T45.1X4	T45.1X5	T45.1X6
Mandelic acid	T37.8X1	T37.8X2	T37.8X3	T37.8X4	T37.8X5	T37.8X6
Manganese (dioxide) (salts)	T57.2X1	T57.2X2	T57.2X3	T57.2X4	—	—
medicinal	T50.991	T50.992	T50.993	T50.994	T50.995	T50.996
Mannitol	T47.3X1	T47.3X2	T47.3X3	T47.3X4	T47.3X5	T47.3X6
hexanitrate	T46.3X1	T46.3X2	T46.3X3	T46.3X4	T46.3X5	T46.3X6
Mannomustine	T45.1X1	T45.1X2	T45.1X3	T45.1X4	T45.1X5	T45.1X6
MAO inhibitors	T43.1X1	T43.1X2	T43.1X3	T43.1X4	T43.1X5	T43.1X6
Mapharsen	T37.8X1	T37.8X2	T37.8X3	T37.8X4	T37.8X5	T37.8X6
Maphenide	T49.0X1	T49.0X2	T49.0X3	T49.0X4	T49.0X5	T49.0X6
Maprotiline	T43.021	T43.022	T43.023	T43.024	T43.025	T43.026
Marcaine	T41.3X1	T41.3X2	T41.3X3	T41.3X4	T41.3X5	T41.3X6
infiltration (subcutaneous)	T41.3X1	T41.3X2	T41.3X3	T41.3X4	T41.3X5	T41.3X6
nerve block (peripheral) (plexus)	T41.3X1	T41.3X2	T41.3X3	T41.3X4	T41.3X5	T41.3X6
Marezine	T45.0X1	T45.0X2	T45.0X3	T45.0X4	T45.0X5	T45.0X6
Marihuana	T40.7X1	T40.7X2	T40.7X3	T40.7X4	T40.7X5	T40.7X6
Marijuana	T40.7X1	T40.7X2	T40.7X3	T40.7X4	T40.7X5	T40.7X6
Marine (sting)	T63.691	T63.692	T63.693	T63.694	—	—
animals (sting)	T63.691	T63.692	T63.693	T63.694	—	—
plants (sting)	T63.711	T63.712	T63.713	T63.714	—	—
Marplan	T43.1X1	T43.1X2	T43.1X3	T43.1X4	T43.1X5	T43.1X6
Marsh gas	T59.891	T59.892	T59.893	T59.894	—	—
Marsilid	T43.1X1	T43.1X2	T43.1X3	T43.1X4	T43.1X5	T43.1X6
Matulane	T45.1X1	T45.1X2	T45.1X3	T45.1X4	T45.1X5	T45.1X6
Mazindol	T50.5X1	T50.5X2	T50.5X3	T50.5X4	T50.5X5	T50.5X6
MCPA	T60.3X1	T60.3X2	T60.3X3	T60.3X4	—	—
MDMA	T43.641	T43.642	T43.643	T43.644	—	—
Meadow saffron	T62.2X1	T62.2X2	T62.2X3	T62.2X4	—	—
Measles virus vaccine (attenuated)	T50.B91	T50.B92	T50.B93	T50.B94	T50.B95	T50.B96
Meat, noxious	T62.8X1	T62.8X2	T62.8X3	T62.8X4	—	—
Meballymal	T42.3X1	T42.3X2	T42.3X3	T42.3X4	T42.3X5	T42.3X6
Mebanazine	T43.1X1	T43.1X2	T43.1X3	T43.1X4	T43.1X5	T43.1X6
Mebaral	T42.3X1	T42.3X2	T42.3X3	T42.3X4	T42.3X5	T42.3X6
Mebendazole	T37.4X1	T37.4X2	T37.4X3	T37.4X4	T37.4X5	T37.4X6
Mebeverine	T44.3X1	T44.3X2	T44.3X3	T44.3X4	T44.3X5	T44.3X6
Mebhydrolin	T45.0X1	T45.0X2	T45.0X3	T45.0X4	T45.0X5	T45.0X6
Mebumal	T42.3X1	T42.3X2	T42.3X3	T42.3X4	T42.3X5	T42.3X6
Mebutamate	T43.591	T43.592	T43.593	T43.594	T43.595	T43.596
Mecamylamine	T44.2X1	T44.2X2	T44.2X3	T44.2X4	T44.2X5	T44.2X6

Additional Character May Be Required — Refer to the Tabular List for Character Selection ▽ Subterms under main terms may continue to next column or page

Substance	Poisoning, Accidental (unintentional)	Poisoning, Intentional Self-harm	Poisoning, Assault	Poisoning, Undetermined	Adverse Effect	Under-dosing
Mechlorethamine	T45.1X1	T45.1X2	T45.1X3	T45.1X4	T45.1X5	T45.1X6
Mecillinam	T36.0X1	T36.0X2	T36.0X3	T36.0X4	T36.0X5	T36.0X6
Meclizine (hydrochloride)	T45.0X1	T45.0X2	T45.0X3	T45.0X4	T45.0X5	T45.0X6
Meclocycline	T36.4X1	T36.4X2	T36.4X3	T36.4X4	T36.4X5	T36.4X6
Meclofenamate	T39.391	T39.392	T39.393	T39.394	T39.395	T39.396
Meclofenamic acid	T39.391	T39.392	T39.393	T39.394	T39.395	T39.396
Meclofenoxate	T43.691	T43.692	T43.693	T43.694	T43.695	T43.696
Meclozine	T45.0X1	T45.0X2	T45.0X3	T45.0X4	T45.0X5	T45.0X6
Mecobalamin	T45.8X1	T45.8X2	T45.8X3	T45.8X4	T45.8X5	T45.8X6
Mecoprop	T60.3X1	T60.3X2	T60.3X3	T60.3X4	—	—
Mecrilate	T49.3X1	T49.3X2	T49.3X3	T49.3X4	T49.3X5	T49.3X6
Mecysteine	T48.4X1	T48.4X2	T48.4X3	T48.4X4	T48.4X5	T48.4X6
Medazepam	T42.4X1	T42.4X2	T42.4X3	T42.4X4	T42.4X5	T42.4X6
Medicament NEC	T50.901	T50.902	T50.903	T50.904	T50.905	T50.906
Medinal	T42.3X1	T42.3X2	T42.3X3	T42.3X4	T42.3X5	T42.3X6
Medomin	T42.3X1	T42.3X2	T42.3X3	T42.3X4	T42.3X5	T42.3X6
Medrogestone	T38.5X1	T38.5X2	T38.5X3	T38.5X4	T38.5X5	T38.5X6
Medroxalol	T44.8X1	T44.8X2	T44.8X3	T44.8X4	T44.8X5	T44.8X6
Medroxyprogesterone acetate (depot)	T38.5X1	T38.5X2	T38.5X3	T38.5X4	T38.5X5	T38.5X6
Medrysone	T49.0X1	T49.0X2	T49.0X3	T49.0X4	T49.0X5	T49.0X6
Mefenamic acid	T39.391	T39.392	T39.393	T39.394	T39.395	T39.396
Mefenorex	T50.5X1	T50.5X2	T50.5X3	T50.5X4	T50.5X5	T50.5X6
Mefloquine	T37.2X1	T37.2X2	T37.2X3	T37.2X4	T37.2X5	T37.2X6
Mefruside	T50.2X1	T50.2X2	T50.2X3	T50.2X4	T50.2X5	T50.2X6
Megahallucinogen	T40.901	T40.902	T40.903	T40.904	T40.905	T40.906
Megestrol	T38.5X1	T38.5X2	T38.5X3	T38.5X4	T38.5X5	T38.5X6
Meglumine						
antimoniate	T37.8X1	T37.8X2	T37.8X3	T37.8X4	T37.8X5	T37.8X6
diatrizoate	T50.8X1	T50.8X2	T50.8X3	T50.8X4	T50.8X5	T50.8X6
iodipamide	T50.8X1	T50.8X2	T50.8X3	T50.8X4	T50.8X5	T50.8X6
iotroxate	T50.8X1	T50.8X2	T50.8X3	T50.8X4	T50.8X5	T50.8X6
MEK (methyl ethyl ketone)	T52.4X1	T52.4X2	T52.4X3	T52.4X4	—	—
Meladinin	T49.3X1	T49.3X2	T49.3X3	T49.3X4	T49.3X5	T49.3X6
Meladrazine	T44.3X1	T44.3X2	T44.3X3	T44.3X4	T44.3X5	T44.3X6
Melaleuca alternifolia oil	T49.0X1	T49.0X2	T49.0X3	T49.0X4	T49.0X5	T49.0X6
Melanizing agents	T49.3X1	T49.3X2	T49.3X3	T49.3X4	T49.3X5	T49.3X6
Melanocyte-stimulating hormone	T38.891	T38.892	T38.893	T38.894	T38.895	T38.896
Melarsonyl potassium	T37.3X1	T37.3X2	T37.3X3	T37.3X4	T37.3X5	T37.3X6
Melarsoprol	T37.3X1	T37.3X2	T37.3X3	T37.3X4	T37.3X5	T37.3X6
Melia azedarach	T62.2X1	T62.2X2	T62.2X3	T62.2X4	—	—
Melitracen	T43.011	T43.012	T43.013	T43.014	T43.015	T43.016
Mellaril	T43.3X1	T43.3X2	T43.3X3	T43.3X4	T43.3X5	T43.3X6
Meloxine	T49.3X1	T49.3X2	T49.3X3	T49.3X4	T49.3X5	T49.3X6
Melperone	T43.4X1	T43.4X2	T43.4X3	T43.4X4	T43.4X5	T43.4X6
Melphalan	T45.1X1	T45.1X2	T45.1X3	T45.1X4	T45.1X5	T45.1X6
Memantine	T43.8X1	T43.8X2	T43.8X3	T43.8X4	T43.8X5	T43.8X6
Menadiol	T45.7X1	T45.7X2	T45.7X3	T45.7X4	T45.7X5	T45.7X6
sodium sulfate	T45.7X1	T45.7X2	T45.7X3	T45.7X4	T45.7X5	T45.7X6
Menadione	T45.7X1	T45.7X2	T45.7X3	T45.7X4	T45.7X5	T45.7X6
sodium bisulfite	T45.7X1	T45.7X2	T45.7X3	T45.7X4	T45.7X5	T45.7X6
Menaphthone	T45.7X1	T45.7X2	T45.7X3	T45.7X4	T45.7X5	T45.7X6
Menaquinone	T45.7X1	T45.7X2	T45.7X3	T45.7X4	T45.7X5	T45.7X6
Menatetrenone	T45.7X1	T45.7X2	T45.7X3	T45.7X4	T45.7X5	T45.7X6
Meningococcal vaccine	T50.A91	T50.A92	T50.A93	T50.A94	T50.A95	T50.A96
Menningovax (-AC) (-C)	T50.A91	T50.A92	T50.A93	T50.A94	T50.A95	T50.A96
Menotropins	T38.811	T38.812	T38.813	T38.814	T38.815	T38.816
Menthol	T48.5X1	T48.5X2	T48.5X3	T48.5X4	T48.5X5	T48.5X6
Mepacrine	T37.2X1	T37.2X2	T37.2X3	T37.2X4	T37.2X5	T37.2X6
Meparfynol	T42.6X1	T42.6X2	T42.6X3	T42.6X4	T42.6X5	T42.6X6
Mepartricin	T36.7X1	T36.7X2	T36.7X3	T36.7X4	T36.7X5	T36.7X6
Mepazine	T43.3X1	T43.3X2	T43.3X3	T43.3X4	T43.3X5	T43.3X6
Mepenzolate	T44.3X1	T44.3X2	T44.3X3	T44.3X4	T44.3X5	T44.3X6
bromide	T44.3X1	T44.3X2	T44.3X3	T44.3X4	T44.3X5	T44.3X6
Meperidine	T40.4X1	T40.4X2	T40.4X3	T40.4X4	T40.4X5	T40.4X6
Mephebarbital	T42.3X1	T42.3X2	T42.3X3	T42.3X4	T42.3X5	T42.3X6
Mephenamin (e)	T42.8X1	T42.8X2	T42.8X3	T42.8X4	T42.8X5	T42.8X6
Mephenesin	T42.8X1	T42.8X2	T42.8X3	T42.8X4	T42.8X5	T42.8X6
Mephenhydramine	T45.0X1	T45.0X2	T45.0X3	T45.0X4	T45.0X5	T45.0X6
Mephenoxalone	T42.8X1	T42.8X2	T42.8X3	T42.8X4	T42.8X5	T42.8X6
Mephentermine	T44.991	T44.992	T44.993	T44.994	T44.995	T44.996
Mephenytoin	T42.0X1	T42.0X2	T42.0X3	T42.0X4	T42.0X5	T42.0X6
with phenobarbital	T42.3X1	T42.3X2	T42.3X3	T42.3X4	T42.3X5	T42.3X6
Mephobarbital	T42.3X1	T42.3X2	T42.3X3	T42.3X4	T42.3X5	T42.3X6
Mephosfolan	T60.0X1	T60.0X2	T60.0X3	T60.0X4	—	—
Mepindolol	T44.7X1	T44.7X2	T44.7X3	T44.7X4	T44.7X5	T44.7X6
Mepiperphenidol	T44.3X1	T44.3X2	T44.3X3	T44.3X4	T44.3X5	T44.3X6
Mepitiostane	T38.7X1	T38.7X2	T38.7X3	T38.7X4	T38.7X5	T38.7X6
Mepivacaine	T41.3X1	T41.3X2	T41.3X3	T41.3X4	T41.3X5	T41.3X6
epidural	T41.3X1	T41.3X2	T41.3X3	T41.3X4	T41.3X5	T41.3X6
Meprednisone	T38.0X1	T38.0X2	T38.0X3	T38.0X4	T38.0X5	T38.0X6
Meprobam	T43.591	T43.592	T43.593	T43.594	T43.595	T43.596

Substance	Poisoning, Accidental (unintentional)	Poisoning, Intentional Self-harm	Poisoning, Assault	Poisoning, Undetermined	Adverse Effect	Under-dosing
Meprobamate	T43.591	T43.592	T43.593	T43.594	T43.595	T43.596
Meproscillarin	T46.0X1	T46.0X2	T46.0X3	T46.0X4	T46.0X5	T46.0X6
Meprylcaine	T41.3X1	T41.3X2	T41.3X3	T41.3X4	T41.3X5	T41.3X6
Meptazinol	T39.8X1	T39.8X2	T39.8X3	T39.8X4	T39.8X5	T39.8X6
Mepyramine	T45.0X1	T45.0X2	T45.0X3	T45.0X4	T45.0X5	T45.0X6
Mequitazine	T43.3X1	T43.3X2	T43.3X3	T43.3X4	T43.3X5	T43.3X6
Meralluride	T50.2X1	T50.2X2	T50.2X3	T50.2X4	T50.2X5	T50.2X6
Merbaphen	T50.2X1	T50.2X2	T50.2X3	T50.2X4	T50.2X5	T50.2X6
Merbromin	T49.0X1	T49.0X2	T49.0X3	T49.0X4	T49.0X5	T49.0X6
Mercaptobenzothiazole salts	T49.0X1	T49.0X2	T49.0X3	T49.0X4	T49.0X5	T49.0X6
Mercaptomerin	T50.2X1	T50.2X2	T50.2X3	T50.2X4	T50.2X5	T50.2X6
Mercaptopurine	T45.1X1	T45.1X2	T45.1X3	T45.1X4	T45.1X5	T45.1X6
Mercumatilin	T50.2X1	T50.2X2	T50.2X3	T50.2X4	T50.2X5	T50.2X6
Mercuramide	T50.2X1	T50.2X2	T50.2X3	T50.2X4	T50.2X5	T50.2X6
Mercurochrome	T49.0X1	T49.0X2	T49.0X3	T49.0X4	T49.0X5	T49.0X6
Mercurophylline	T50.2X1	T50.2X2	T50.2X3	T50.2X4	T50.2X5	T50.2X6
Mercury, mercurial, mercuric, mercurous (compounds) (cyanide) (fumes) (nonmedicinal) (vapor) NEC	T56.1X1	T56.1X2	T56.1X3	T56.1X4	—	—
ammoniated	T49.0X1	T49.0X2	T49.0X3	T49.0X4	T49.0X5	T49.0X6
anti-infective						
local	T49.0X1	T49.0X2	T49.0X3	T49.0X4	T49.0X5	T49.0X6
systemic	T37.8X1	T37.8X2	T37.8X3	T37.8X4	T37.8X5	T37.8X6
topical	T49.0X1	T49.0X2	T49.0X3	T49.0X4	T49.0X5	T49.0X6
chloride (ammoniated)	T49.0X1	T49.0X2	T49.0X3	T49.0X4	T49.0X5	T49.0X6
fungicide	T56.1X1	T56.1X2	T56.1X3	T56.1X4	—	—
diuretic NEC	T50.2X1	T50.2X2	T50.2X3	T50.2X4	T50.2X5	T50.2X6
fungicide	T56.1X1	T56.1X2	T56.1X3	T56.1X4	—	—
organic (fungicide)	T56.1X1	T56.1X2	T56.1X3	T56.1X4	—	—
oxide, yellow	T49.0X1	T49.0X2	T49.0X3	T49.0X4	T49.0X5	T49.0X6
Mersalyl	T50.2X1	T50.2X2	T50.2X3	T50.2X4	T50.2X5	T50.2X6
Merthiolate	T49.0X1	T49.0X2	T49.0X3	T49.0X4	T49.0X5	T49.0X6
ophthalmic preparation	T49.5X1	T49.5X2	T49.5X3	T49.5X4	T49.5X5	T49.5X6
Meruvax	T50.B91	T50.B92	T50.B93	T50.B94	T50.B95	T50.B96
Mesalazine	T47.8X1	T47.8X2	T47.8X3	T47.8X4	T47.8X5	T47.8X6
Mescal buttons	T40.991	T40.992	T40.993	T40.994	—	—
Mescaline	T40.991	T40.992	T40.993	T40.994	—	—
Mesna	T48.4X1	T48.4X2	T48.4X3	T48.4X4	T48.4X5	T48.4X6
Mesoglycan	T46.6X1	T46.6X2	T46.6X3	T46.6X4	T46.6X5	T46.6X6
Mesoridazine	T43.3X1	T43.3X2	T43.3X3	T43.3X4	T43.3X5	T43.3X6
Mestanolone	T38.7X1	T38.7X2	T38.7X3	T38.7X4	T38.7X5	T38.7X6
Mesterolone	T38.7X1	T38.7X2	T38.7X3	T38.7X4	T38.7X5	T38.7X6
Mestranol	T38.5X1	T38.5X2	T38.5X3	T38.5X4	T38.5X5	T38.5X6
Mesulergine	T42.8X1	T42.8X2	T42.8X3	T42.8X4	T42.8X5	T42.8X6
Mesulfen	T49.0X1	T49.0X2	T49.0X3	T49.0X4	T49.0X5	T49.0X6
Mesuximide	T42.2X1	T42.2X2	T42.2X3	T42.2X4	T42.2X5	T42.2X6
Metabutethamine	T41.3X1	T41.3X2	T41.3X3	T41.3X4	T41.3X5	T41.3X6
Metacesylacetate	T49.0X1	T49.0X2	T49.0X3	T49.0X4	T49.0X5	T49.0X6
Metacycline	T36.4X1	T36.4X2	T36.4X3	T36.4X4	T36.4X5	T36.4X6
Metaldehyde (snail killer) NEC	T60.8X1	T60.8X2	T60.8X3	T60.8X4	—	—
Metals (heavy) (nonmedicinal)	T56.91	T56.92	T56.93	T56.94	—	—
dust, fumes, or vapor NEC	T56.91	T56.92	T56.93	T56.94	—	—
light NEC	T56.91	T56.92	T56.93	T56.94	—	—
dust, fumes, or vapor NEC	T56.91	T56.92	T56.93	T56.94	—	—
specified NEC	T56.891	T56.892	T56.893	T56.894	—	—
thallium	T56.811	T56.812	T56.813	T56.814	—	—
Metamfetamine	T43.621	T43.622	T43.623	T43.624	T43.625	T43.626
Metamizole sodium	T39.2X1	T39.2X2	T39.2X3	T39.2X4	T39.2X5	T39.2X6
Metampicillin	T36.0X1	T36.0X2	T36.0X3	T36.0X4	T36.0X5	T36.0X6
Metamucil	T47.4X1	T47.4X2	T47.4X3	T47.4X4	T47.4X5	T47.4X6
Metandienone	T38.7X1	T38.7X2	T38.7X3	T38.7X4	T38.7X5	T38.7X6
Metandrostenolone	T38.7X1	T38.7X2	T38.7X3	T38.7X4	T38.7X5	T38.7X6
Metaphen	T49.0X1	T49.0X2	T49.0X3	T49.0X4	T49.0X5	T49.0X6
Metaphos	T60.0X1	T60.0X2	T60.0X3	T60.0X4	—	—
Metapramine	T43.011	T43.012	T43.013	T43.014	T43.015	T43.016
Metaproterenol	T48.291	T48.292	T48.293	T48.294	T48.295	T48.296
Metaraminol	T44.4X1	T44.4X2	T44.4X3	T44.4X4	T44.4X5	T44.4X6
Metaxalone	T42.8X1	T42.8X2	T42.8X3	T42.8X4	T42.8X5	T42.8X6
Metenolone	T38.7X1	T38.7X2	T38.7X3	T38.7X4	T38.7X5	T38.7X6
Metergoline	T42.8X1	T42.8X2	T42.8X3	T42.8X4	T42.8X5	T42.8X6
Metescufylline	T46.991	T46.992	T46.993	T46.994	T46.995	T46.996
Metetoin	T42.0X1	T42.0X2	T42.0X3	T42.0X4	T42.0X5	T42.0X6
Metformin	T38.3X1	T38.3X2	T38.3X3	T38.3X4	T38.3X5	T38.3X6
Methacholine	T44.1X1	T44.1X2	T44.1X3	T44.1X4	T44.1X5	T44.1X6
Methacycline	T36.4X1	T36.4X2	T36.4X3	T36.4X4	T36.4X5	T36.4X6
Methadone	T40.3X1	T40.3X2	T40.3X3	T40.3X4	T40.3X5	T40.3X6
Methallenestril	T38.5X1	T38.5X2	T38.5X3	T38.5X4	T38.5X5	T38.5X6

Substance	Poisoning, Accidental (unintentional)	Poisoning, Intentional Self-harm	Poisoning, Assault	Poisoning, Undetermined	Adverse Effect	Under-dosing
Methallenoestril	T38.5X1	T38.5X2	T38.5X3	T38.5X4	T38.5X5	T38.5X6
Methamphetamine	T43.621	T43.622	T43.623	T43.624	T43.625	T43.626
Methampyrone	T39.2X1	T39.2X2	T39.2X3	T39.2X4	T39.2X5	T39.2X6
Methandienone	T38.7X1	T38.7X2	T38.7X3	T38.7X4	T38.7X5	T38.7X6
Methandriol	T38.7X1	T38.7X2	T38.7X3	T38.7X4	T38.7X5	T38.7X6
Methandrostenolone	T38.7X1	T38.7X2	T38.7X3	T38.7X4	T38.7X5	T38.7X6
Methane	T59.891	T59.892	T59.893	T59.894	—	—
Methanethiol	T59.891	T59.892	T59.893	T59.894	—	—
Methaniazide	T37.1X1	T37.1X2	T37.1X3	T37.1X4	T37.1X5	T37.1X6
Methanol (vapor)	T51.1X1	T51.1X2	T51.1X3	T51.1X4	—	—
Methantheline	T44.3X1	T44.3X2	T44.3X3	T44.3X4	T44.3X5	T44.3X6
Methanthelinium bromide	T44.3X1	T44.3X2	T44.3X3	T44.3X4	T44.3X5	T44.3X6
Methaphenilene	T45.0X1	T45.0X2	T45.0X3	T45.0X4	T45.0X5	T45.0X6
Methapyrilene	T45.0X1	T45.0X2	T45.0X3	T45.0X4	T45.0X5	T45.0X6
Methaqualone (compound)	T42.6X1	T42.6X2	T42.6X3	T42.6X4	T42.6X5	T42.6X6
Metharbital	T42.3X1	T42.3X2	T42.3X3	T42.3X4	T42.3X5	T42.3X6
Methazolamide	T50.2X1	T50.2X2	T50.2X3	T50.2X4	T50.2X5	T50.2X6
Methdilazine	T43.3X1	T43.3X2	T43.3X3	T43.3X4	T43.3X5	T43.3X6
Methedrine	T43.621	T43.622	T43.623	T43.624	T43.625	T43.626
Methenamine (mandelate)	T37.8X1	T37.8X2	T37.8X3	T37.8X4	T37.8X5	T37.8X6
Methenolone	T38.7X1	T38.7X2	T38.7X3	T38.7X4	T38.7X5	T38.7X6
Methergine	T48.0X1	T48.0X2	T48.0X3	T48.0X4	T48.0X5	T48.0X6
Methetoin	T42.0X1	T42.0X2	T42.0X3	T42.0X4	T42.0X5	T42.0X6
Methiacil	T38.2X1	T38.2X2	T38.2X3	T38.2X4	T38.2X5	T38.2X6
Methicillin	T36.0X1	T36.0X2	T36.0X3	T36.0X4	T36.0X5	T36.0X6
Methimazole	T38.2X1	T38.2X2	T38.2X3	T38.2X4	T38.2X5	T38.2X6
Methiodal sodium	T50.8X1	T50.8X2	T50.8X3	T50.8X4	T50.8X5	T50.8X6
Methionine	T50.991	T50.992	T50.993	T50.994	T50.995	T50.996
Methisazone	T37.5X1	T37.5X2	T37.5X3	T37.5X4	T37.5X5	T37.5X6
Methisoprinol	T37.5X1	T37.5X2	T37.5X3	T37.5X4	T37.5X5	T37.5X6
Methitural	T42.3X1	T42.3X2	T42.3X3	T42.3X4	T42.3X5	T42.3X6
Methixene	T44.3X1	T44.3X2	T44.3X3	T44.3X4	T44.3X5	T44.3X6
Methobarbital, methobarbitone	T42.3X1	T42.3X2	T42.3X3	T42.3X4	T42.3X5	T42.3X6
Methocarbamol	T42.8X1	T42.8X2	T42.8X3	T42.8X4	T42.8X5	T42.8X6
skeletal muscle relaxant	T48.1X1	T48.1X2	T48.1X3	T48.1X4	T48.1X5	T48.1X6
Methohexital	T41.1X1	T41.1X2	T41.1X3	T41.1X4	T41.1X5	T41.1X6
Methohexitone	T41.1X1	T41.1X2	T41.1X3	T41.1X4	T41.1X5	T41.1X6
Methoin	T42.0X1	T42.0X2	T42.0X3	T42.0X4	T42.0X5	T42.0X6
Methopholine	T39.8X1	T39.8X2	T39.8X3	T39.8X4	T39.8X5	T39.8X6
Methopromazine	T43.3X1	T43.3X2	T43.3X3	T43.3X4	T43.3X5	T43.3X6
Methorate	T48.3X1	T48.3X2	T48.3X3	T48.3X4	T48.3X5	T48.3X6
Methoserpidine	T46.5X1	T46.5X2	T46.5X3	T46.5X4	T46.5X5	T46.5X6
Methotrexate	T45.1X1	T45.1X2	T45.1X3	T45.1X4	T45.1X5	T45.1X6
Methotrimeprazine	T43.3X1	T43.3X2	T43.3X3	T43.3X4	T43.3X5	T43.3X6
Methoxa-Dome	T49.3X1	T49.3X2	T49.3X3	T49.3X4	T49.3X5	T49.3X6
Methoxamine	T44.4X1	T44.4X2	T44.4X3	T44.4X4	T44.4X5	T44.4X6
Methoxsalen	T50.991	T50.992	T50.993	T50.994	T50.995	T50.996
Methoxyaniline	T65.3X1	T65.3X2	T65.3X3	T65.3X4	—	—
Methoxybenzyl penicillin	T36.0X1	T36.0X2	T36.0X3	T36.0X4	T36.0X5	T36.0X6
Methoxychlor	T53.7X1	T53.7X2	T53.7X3	T53.7X4	—	—
Methoxy-DDT	T53.7X1	T53.7X2	T53.7X3	T53.7X4	—	—
Methoxyflurane	T41.0X1	T41.0X2	T41.0X3	T41.0X4	T41.0X5	T41.0X6
Methoxyphenamine	T48.6X1	T48.6X2	T48.6X3	T48.6X4	T48.6X5	T48.6X6
Methoxypromazine	T43.3X1	T43.3X2	T43.3X3	T43.3X4	T43.3X5	T43.3X6
Methscopolamine bromide	T44.3X1	T44.3X2	T44.3X3	T44.3X4	T44.3X5	T44.3X6
Methsuximide	T42.2X1	T42.2X2	T42.2X3	T42.2X4	T42.2X5	T42.2X6
Methyclothiazide	T50.2X1	T50.2X2	T50.2X3	T50.2X4	T50.2X5	T50.2X6
Methyl						
acetate	T52.4X1	T52.4X2	T52.4X3	T52.4X4	—	—
acetone	T52.4X1	T52.4X2	T52.4X3	T52.4X4	—	—
acrylate	T65.891	T65.892	T65.893	T65.894	—	—
alcohol	T51.1X1	T51.1X2	T51.1X3	T51.1X4	—	—
aminophenol	T65.3X1	T65.3X2	T65.3X3	T65.3X4	—	—
amphetamine	T43.621	T43.622	T43.623	T43.624	T43.625	T43.626
androstanolone	T38.7X1	T38.7X2	T38.7X3	T38.7X4	T38.7X5	T38.7X6
atropine	T44.3X1	T44.3X2	T44.3X3	T44.3X4	T44.3X5	T44.3X6
benzene	T52.2X1	T52.2X2	T52.2X3	T52.2X4	—	—
benzoate	T52.8X1	T52.8X2	T52.8X3	T52.8X4	—	—
benzol	T52.2X1	T52.2X2	T52.2X3	T52.2X4	—	—
bromide (gas)	T59.891	T59.892	T59.893	T59.894	—	—
fumigant	T60.8X1	T60.8X2	T60.8X3	T60.8X4	—	—
butanol	T51.3X1	T51.3X2	T51.3X3	T51.3X4	—	—
carbinol	T51.1X1	T51.1X2	T51.1X3	T51.1X4	—	—
carbonate	T52.8X1	T52.8X2	T52.8X3	T52.8X4	—	—
CCNU	T45.1X1	T45.1X2	T45.1X3	T45.1X4	T45.1X5	T45.1X6
cellosolve	T52.91	T52.92	T52.93	T52.94	—	—
cellulose	T47.4X1	T47.4X2	T47.4X3	T47.4X4	T47.4X5	T47.4X6
chloride (gas)	T59.891	T59.892	T59.893	T59.894	—	—
chloroformate	T59.3X1	T59.3X2	T59.3X3	T59.3X4	—	—
cyclohexane	T52.8X1	T52.8X2	T52.8X3	T52.8X4	—	—
cyclohexanol	T51.8X1	T51.8X2	T51.8X3	T51.8X4	—	—

Substance	Poisoning, Accidental (unintentional)	Poisoning, Intentional Self-harm	Poisoning, Assault	Poisoning, Undetermined	Adverse Effect	Under-dosing
Methyl — continued						
cyclohexanone	T52.8X1	T52.8X2	T52.8X3	T52.8X4	—	—
cyclohexyl acetate	T52.8X1	T52.8X2	T52.8X3	T52.8X4	—	—
demeton	T60.0X1	T60.0X2	T60.0X3	T60.0X4	—	—
dihydromorphinone	T40.2X1	T40.2X2	T40.2X3	T40.2X4	T40.2X5	T40.2X6
ergometrine	T48.0X1	T48.0X2	T48.0X3	T48.0X4	T48.0X5	T48.0X6
ergonovine	T48.0X1	T48.0X2	T48.0X3	T48.0X4	T48.0X5	T48.0X6
ethyl ketone	T52.4X1	T52.4X2	T52.4X3	T52.4X4	—	—
glucamine antimonate	T37.8X1	T37.8X2	T37.8X3	T37.8X4	T37.8X5	T37.8X6
hydrazine	T65.891	T65.892	T65.893	T65.894	—	—
iodide	T65.891	T65.892	T65.893	T65.894	—	—
isobutyl ketone	T52.4X1	T52.4X2	T52.4X3	T52.4X4	—	—
isothiocyanate	T60.3X1	T60.3X2	T60.3X3	T60.3X4	—	—
mercaptan	T59.891	T59.892	T59.893	T59.894	—	—
morphine NEC	T40.2X1	T40.2X2	T40.2X3	T40.2X4	T40.2X5	T40.2X6
nicotinate	T49.4X1	T49.4X2	T49.4X3	T49.4X4	T49.4X5	T49.4X6
paraben	T49.0X1	T49.0X2	T49.0X3	T49.0X4	T49.0X5	T49.0X6
parafynol	T42.6X1	T42.6X2	T42.6X3	T42.6X4	T42.6X5	T42.6X6
parathion	T60.0X1	T60.0X2	T60.0X3	T60.0X4	—	—
peridol	T43.4X1	T43.4X2	T43.4X3	T43.4X4	T43.4X5	T43.4X6
phenidate	T43.631	T43.632	T43.633	T43.634	T43.635	T43.636
prednisolone	T38.0X1	T38.0X2	T38.0X3	T38.0X4	T38.0X5	T38.0X6
ENT agent	T49.6X1	T49.6X2	T49.6X3	T49.6X4	T49.6X5	T49.6X6
ophthalmic preparation	T49.5X1	T49.5X2	T49.5X3	T49.5X4	T49.5X5	T49.5X6
topical NEC	T49.0X1	T49.0X2	T49.0X3	T49.0X4	T49.0X5	T49.0X6
propylcarbinol	T51.3X1	T51.3X2	T51.3X3	T51.3X4	—	—
rosaniline NEC	T49.0X1	T49.0X2	T49.0X3	T49.0X4	T49.0X5	T49.0X6
salicylate	T49.2X1	T49.2X2	T49.2X3	T49.2X4	T49.2X5	T49.2X6
sulfate (fumes)	T59.891	T59.892	T59.893	T59.894	—	—
liquid	T52.8X1	T52.8X2	T52.8X3	T52.8X4	—	—
sulfonal	T42.6X1	T42.6X2	T42.6X3	T42.6X4	T42.6X5	T42.6X6
testosterone	T38.7X1	T38.7X2	T38.7X3	T38.7X4	T38.7X5	T38.7X6
thiouracil	T38.2X1	T38.2X2	T38.2X3	T38.2X4	T38.2X5	T38.2X6
Methylamphetamine	T43.621	T43.622	T43.623	T43.624	T43.625	T43.626
Methylated spirit	T51.1X1	T51.1X2	T51.1X3	T51.1X4	—	—
Methylatropine nitrate	T44.3X1	T44.3X2	T44.3X3	T44.3X4	T44.3X5	T44.3X6
Methylbenactyzium bromide	T44.3X1	T44.3X2	T44.3X3	T44.3X4	T44.3X5	T44.3X6
Methylbenzethonium chloride	T49.0X1	T49.0X2	T49.0X3	T49.0X4	T49.0X5	T49.0X6
Methylcellulose	T47.4X1	T47.4X2	T47.4X3	T47.4X4	T47.4X5	T47.4X6
laxative	T47.4X1	T47.4X2	T47.4X3	T47.4X4	T47.4X5	T47.4X6
Methylchlorophenoxyacetic acid	T60.3X1	T60.3X2	T60.3X3	T60.3X4	—	—
Methyldopa	T46.5X1	T46.5X2	T46.5X3	T46.5X4	T46.5X5	T46.5X6
Methyldopate	T46.5X1	T46.5X2	T46.5X3	T46.5X4	T46.5X5	T46.5X6
Methylene						
blue	T50.6X1	T50.6X2	T50.6X3	T50.6X4	T50.6X5	T50.6X6
chloride or dichloride (solvent) NEC	T53.4X1	T53.4X2	T53.4X3	T53.4X4	—	—
Methylenedioxyamphetamine	T43.621	T43.622	T43.623	T43.624	T43.625	T43.626
Methylenedioxymeth-amphetamine	T43.641	T43.642	T43.643	T43.644	—	—
Methylergometrine	T48.0X1	T48.0X2	T48.0X3	T48.0X4	T48.0X5	T48.0X6
Methylergonovine	T48.0X1	T48.0X2	T48.0X3	T48.0X4	T48.0X5	T48.0X6
Methylestrenolone	T38.5X1	T38.5X2	T38.5X3	T38.5X4	T38.5X5	T38.5X6
Methylethyl cellulose	T50.991	T50.992	T50.993	T50.994	T50.995	T50.996
Methylhexabital	T42.3X1	T42.3X2	T42.3X3	T42.3X4	T42.3X5	T42.3X6
Methylmorphine	T40.2X1	T40.2X2	T40.2X3	T40.2X4	T40.2X5	T40.2X6
Methylparaben (ophthalmic)	T49.5X1	T49.5X2	T49.5X3	T49.5X4	T49.5X5	T49.5X6
Methylparafynol	T42.6X1	T42.6X2	T42.6X3	T42.6X4	T42.6X5	T42.6X6
Methylpentynol, methylpenthynol	T42.6X1	T42.6X2	T42.6X3	T42.6X4	T42.6X5	T42.6X6
Methylphenidate	T43.631	T43.632	T43.633	T43.634	T43.635	T43.636
Methylphenobarbital	T42.3X1	T42.3X2	T42.3X3	T42.3X4	T42.3X5	T42.3X6
Methylpolysiloxane	T47.1X1	T47.1X2	T47.1X3	T47.1X4	T47.1X5	T47.1X6
Methylprednisolone — see Methyl, prednisolone						
Methylrosaniline	T49.0X1	T49.0X2	T49.0X3	T49.0X4	T49.0X5	T49.0X6
Methylrosanilinium chloride	T49.0X1	T49.0X2	T49.0X3	T49.0X4	T49.0X5	T49.0X6
Methyltestosterone	T38.7X1	T38.7X2	T38.7X3	T38.7X4	T38.7X5	T38.7X6
Methylthionine chloride	T50.6X1	T50.6X2	T50.6X3	T50.6X4	T50.6X5	T50.6X6
Methylthioninium chloride	T50.6X1	T50.6X2	T50.6X3	T50.6X4	T50.6X5	T50.6X6
Methylthiouracil	T38.2X1	T38.2X2	T38.2X3	T38.2X4	T38.2X5	T38.2X6
Methyprylon	T42.6X1	T42.6X2	T42.6X3	T42.6X4	T42.6X5	T42.6X6
Methysergide	T46.5X1	T46.5X2	T46.5X3	T46.5X4	T46.5X5	T46.5X6
Metiamide	T47.1X1	T47.1X2	T47.1X3	T47.1X4	T47.1X5	T47.1X6
Meticillin	T36.0X1	T36.0X2	T36.0X3	T36.0X4	T36.0X5	T36.0X6
Meticrane	T50.2X1	T50.2X2	T50.2X3	T50.2X4	T50.2X5	T50.2X6
Metildigoxin	T46.0X1	T46.0X2	T46.0X3	T46.0X4	T46.0X5	T46.0X6

378
Additional Character May Be Required — Refer to the Tabular List for Character Selection
Subterms under main terms may continue to next column or page

Table of Drugs and Chemicals

Substance	Poisoning, Accidental (unintentional)	Poisoning, Intentional Self-harm	Poisoning, Assault	Poisoning, Undetermined	Adverse Effect	Under-dosing
Metipranolol	T49.5X1	T49.5X2	T49.5X3	T49.5X4	T49.5X5	T49.5X6
Metirosine	T46.5X1	T46.5X2	T46.5X3	T46.5X4	T46.5X5	T46.5X6
Metisazone	T37.5X1	T37.5X2	T37.5X3	T37.5X4	T37.5X5	T37.5X6
Metixene	T44.3X1	T44.3X2	T44.3X3	T44.3X4	T44.3X5	T44.3X6
Metizoline	T48.5X1	T48.5X2	T48.5X3	T48.5X4	T48.5X5	T48.5X6
Metoclopramide	T45.0X1	T45.0X2	T45.0X3	T45.0X4	T45.0X5	T45.0X6
Metofenazate	T43.3X1	T43.3X2	T43.3X3	T43.3X4	T43.3X5	T43.3X6
Metofoline	T39.8X1	T39.8X2	T39.8X3	T39.8X4	T39.8X5	T39.8X6
Metolazone	T50.2X1	T50.2X2	T50.2X3	T50.2X4	T50.2X5	T50.2X6
Metopon	T40.2X1	T40.2X2	T40.2X3	T40.2X4	T40.2X5	T40.2X6
Metoprine	T45.1X1	T45.1X2	T45.1X3	T45.1X4	T45.1X5	T45.1X6
Metoprolol	T44.7X1	T44.7X2	T44.7X3	T44.7X4	T44.7X5	T44.7X6
Metrifonate	T60.0X1	T60.0X2	T60.0X3	T60.0X4	—	—
Metrizamide	T50.8X1	T50.8X2	T50.8X3	T50.8X4	T50.8X5	T50.8X6
Metrizoic acid	T50.8X1	T50.8X2	T50.8X3	T50.8X4	T50.8X5	T50.8X6
Metronidazole	T37.8X1	T37.8X2	T37.8X3	T37.8X4	T37.8X5	T37.8X6
Metycaine						
infiltration (subcutaneous)	T41.3X1	T41.3X2	T41.3X3	T41.3X4	T41.3X5	T41.3X6
nerve block (peripheral) (plexus)	T41.3X1	T41.3X2	T41.3X3	T41.3X4	T41.3X5	T41.3X6
topical (surface)	T41.3X1	T41.3X2	T41.3X3	T41.3X4	T41.3X5	T41.3X6
Metyrapone	T50.8X1	T50.8X2	T50.8X3	T50.8X4	T50.8X5	T50.8X6
Mevinphos	T60.0X1	T60.0X2	T60.0X3	T60.0X4	—	—
Mexazolam	T42.4X1	T42.4X2	T42.4X3	T42.4X4	T42.4X5	T42.4X6
Mexenone	T49.3X1	T49.3X2	T49.3X3	T49.3X4	T49.3X5	T49.3X6
Mexiletine	T46.2X1	T46.2X2	T46.2X3	T46.2X4	T46.2X5	T46.2X6
Mezereon	T62.2X1	T62.2X2	T62.2X3	T62.2X4	—	—
berries	T62.1X1	T62.1X2	T62.1X3	T62.1X4	—	—
Mezlocillin	T36.0X1	T36.0X2	T36.0X3	T36.0X4	T36.0X5	T36.0X6
Mianserin	T43.021	T43.022	T43.023	T43.024	T43.025	T43.026
Micatin	T49.0X1	T49.0X2	T49.0X3	T49.0X4	T49.0X5	T49.0X6
Miconazole	T49.0X1	T49.0X2	T49.0X3	T49.0X4	T49.0X5	T49.0X6
Micronomicin	T36.5X1	T36.5X2	T36.5X3	T36.5X4	T36.5X5	T36.5X6
Midazolam	T42.4X1	T42.4X2	T42.4X3	T42.4X4	T42.4X5	T42.4X6
Midecamycin	T36.3X1	T36.3X2	T36.3X3	T36.3X4	T36.3X5	T36.3X6
Mifepristone	T38.6X1	T38.6X2	T38.6X3	T38.6X4	T38.6X5	T38.6X6
Milk of magnesia	T47.1X1	T47.1X2	T47.1X3	T47.1X4	T47.1X5	T47.1X6
Millipede (tropical) (venomous)	T63.411	T63.412	T63.413	T63.414	—	—
Miltown	T43.591	T43.592	T43.593	T43.594	T43.595	T43.596
Milverine	T44.3X1	T44.3X2	T44.3X3	T44.3X4	T44.3X5	T44.3X6
Minaprine	T43.291	T43.292	T43.293	T43.294	T43.295	T43.296
Minaxolone	T41.291	T41.292	T41.293	T41.294	T41.295	T41.296
Mineral						
acids	T54.2X1	T54.2X2	T54.2X3	T54.2X4	—	—
oil (laxative)(medicinal)	T47.4X1	T47.4X2	T47.4X3	T47.4X4	T47.4X5	T47.4X6
emulsion	T47.2X1	T47.2X2	T47.2X3	T47.2X4	T47.2X5	T47.2X6
nonmedicinal	T52.0X1	T52.0X2	T52.0X3	T52.0X4	—	—
topical	T49.3X1	T49.3X2	T49.3X3	T49.3X4	T49.3X5	T49.3X6
salt NEC	T50.3X1	T50.3X2	T50.3X3	T50.3X4	T50.3X5	T50.3X6
spirits	T52.0X1	T52.0X2	T52.0X3	T52.0X4	—	—
Mineralocorticosteroid	T50.0X1	T50.0X2	T50.0X3	T50.0X4	T50.0X5	T50.0X6
Minocycline	T36.4X1	T36.4X2	T36.4X3	T36.4X4	T36.4X5	T36.4X6
Minoxidil	T46.7X1	T46.7X2	T46.7X3	T46.7X4	T46.7X5	T46.7X6
Miokamycin	T36.3X1	T36.3X2	T36.3X3	T36.3X4	T36.3X5	T36.3X6
Miotic drug	T49.5X1	T49.5X2	T49.5X3	T49.5X4	T49.5X5	T49.5X6
Mipafox	T60.0X1	T60.0X2	T60.0X3	T60.0X4	—	—
Mirex	T60.1X1	T60.1X2	T60.1X3	T60.1X4	—	—
Mirtazapine	T43.021	T43.022	T43.023	T43.024	T43.025	T43.026
Misonidazole	T37.3X1	T37.3X2	T37.3X3	T37.3X4	T37.3X5	T37.3X6
Misoprostol	T47.1X1	T47.1X2	T47.1X3	T47.1X4	T47.1X5	T47.1X6
Mithramycin	T45.1X1	T45.1X2	T45.1X3	T45.1X4	T45.1X5	T45.1X6
Mitobronitol	T45.1X1	T45.1X2	T45.1X3	T45.1X4	T45.1X5	T45.1X6
Mitoguazone	T45.1X1	T45.1X2	T45.1X3	T45.1X4	T45.1X5	T45.1X6
Mitolactol	T45.1X1	T45.1X2	T45.1X3	T45.1X4	T45.1X5	T45.1X6
Mitomycin	T45.1X1	T45.1X2	T45.1X3	T45.1X4	T45.1X5	T45.1X6
Mitopodozide	T45.1X1	T45.1X2	T45.1X3	T45.1X4	T45.1X5	T45.1X6
Mitotane	T45.1X1	T45.1X2	T45.1X3	T45.1X4	T45.1X5	T45.1X6
Mitoxantrone	T45.1X1	T45.1X2	T45.1X3	T45.1X4	T45.1X5	T45.1X6
Mivacurium chloride	T48.1X1	T48.1X2	T48.1X3	T48.1X4	T48.1X5	T48.1X6
Miyari bacteria	T47.6X1	T47.6X2	T47.6X3	T47.6X4	T47.6X5	T47.6X6
Moclobemide	T43.1X1	T43.1X2	T43.1X3	T43.1X4	T43.1X5	T43.1X6
Moderil	T46.5X1	T46.5X2	T46.5X3	T46.5X4	T46.5X5	T46.5X6
Mofebutazone	T39.2X1	T39.2X2	T39.2X3	T39.2X4	T39.2X5	T39.2X6
Mogadon — see Nitrazepam						
Molindone	T43.591	T43.592	T43.593	T43.594	T43.595	T43.596
Molsidomine	T46.3X1	T46.3X2	T46.3X3	T46.3X4	T46.3X5	T46.3X6
Mometasone	T49.0X1	T49.0X2	T49.0X3	T49.0X4	T49.0X5	T49.0X6
Monistat	T49.0X1	T49.0X2	T49.0X3	T49.0X4	T49.0X5	T49.0X6
Monkshood	T62.2X1	T62.2X2	T62.2X3	T62.2X4	—	—
Monoamine oxidase inhibitor NEC	T43.1X1	T43.1X2	T43.1X3	T43.1X4	T43.1X5	T43.1X6
hydrazine	T43.1X1	T43.1X2	T43.1X3	T43.1X4	T43.1X5	T43.1X6

Substance	Poisoning, Accidental (unintentional)	Poisoning, Intentional Self-harm	Poisoning, Assault	Poisoning, Undetermined	Adverse Effect	Under-dosing
Monobenzone	T49.4X1	T49.4X2	T49.4X3	T49.4X4	T49.4X5	T49.4X6
Monochloroacetic acid	T60.3X1	T60.3X2	T60.3X3	T60.3X4	—	—
Monochlorobenzene	T53.7X1	T53.7X2	T53.7X3	T53.7X4	—	—
Monoethanolamine	T46.8X1	T46.8X2	T46.8X3	T46.8X4	T46.8X5	T46.8X6
oleate	T46.8X1	T46.8X2	T46.8X3	T46.8X4	T46.8X5	T46.8X6
Monooctanoin	T50.991	T50.992	T50.993	T50.994	T50.995	T50.996
Monophenylbutazone	T39.2X1	T39.2X2	T39.2X3	T39.2X4	T39.2X5	T39.2X6
Monosodium glutamate	T65.891	T65.892	T65.893	T65.894	—	—
Monosulfiram	T49.0X1	T49.0X2	T49.0X3	T49.0X4	T49.0X5	T49.0X6
Monoxide, carbon — see Carbon, monoxide						
Monoxidine hydrochloride	T46.1X1	T46.1X2	T46.1X3	T46.1X4	T46.1X5	T46.1X6
Monuron	T60.3X1	T60.3X2	T60.3X3	T60.3X4	—	—
Moperone	T43.4X1	T43.4X2	T43.4X3	T43.4X4	T43.4X5	T43.4X6
Mopidamol	T45.1X1	T45.1X2	T45.1X3	T45.1X4	T45.1X5	T45.1X6
MOPP (mechloreth-amine + vincristine + prednisone + procarba-zine)	T45.1X1	T45.1X2	T45.1X3	T45.1X4	T45.1X5	T45.1X6
Morfin	T40.2X1	T40.2X2	T40.2X3	T40.2X4	T40.2X5	T40.2X6
Morinamide	T37.1X1	T37.1X2	T37.1X3	T37.1X4	T37.1X5	T37.1X6
Morning glory seeds	T40.991	T40.992	T40.993	T40.994	—	—
Moroxydine	T37.5X1	T37.5X2	T37.5X3	T37.5X4	T37.5X5	T37.5X6
Morphazinamide	T37.1X1	T37.1X2	T37.1X3	T37.1X4	T37.1X5	T37.1X6
Morphine	T40.2X1	T40.2X2	T40.2X3	T40.2X4	T40.2X5	T40.2X6
antagonist	T50.7X1	T50.7X2	T50.7X3	T50.7X4	T50.7X5	T50.7X6
Morpholinylethylmorphine	T40.2X1	T40.2X2	T40.2X3	T40.2X4	—	—
Morsuximide	T42.2X1	T42.2X2	T42.2X3	T42.2X4	T42.2X5	T42.2X6
Mosapramine	T43.591	T43.592	T43.593	T43.594	T43.595	T43.596
Moth balls — see also Pesticides	T60.2X1	T60.2X2	T60.2X3	T60.2X4	—	—
naphthalene	T60.2X1	T60.2X2	T60.2X3	T60.2X4	—	—
paradichlorobenzene	T60.1X1	T60.1X2	T60.1X3	T60.1X4	—	—
Motor exhaust gas	T58.01	T58.02	T58.03	T58.04	—	—
Mouthwash (antiseptic) (zinc chloride)	T49.6X1	T49.6X2	T49.6X3	T49.6X4	T49.6X5	T49.6X6
Moxastine	T45.0X1	T45.0X2	T45.0X3	T45.0X4	T45.0X5	T45.0X6
Moxaverine	T44.3X1	T44.3X2	T44.3X3	T44.3X4	T44.3X5	T44.3X6
Moxisylyte	T46.7X1	T46.7X2	T46.7X3	T46.7X4	T46.7X5	T46.7X6
Mucilage, plant	T47.4X1	T47.4X2	T47.4X3	T47.4X4	T47.4X5	T47.4X6
Mucolytic drug	T48.4X1	T48.4X2	T48.4X3	T48.4X4	T48.4X5	T48.4X6
Mucomyst	T48.4X1	T48.4X2	T48.4X3	T48.4X4	T48.4X5	T48.4X6
Mucous membrane agents (external)	T49.91	T49.92	T49.93	T49.94	T49.95	T49.96
specified NEC	T49.8X1	T49.8X2	T49.8X3	T49.8X4	T49.8X5	T49.8X6
Multiple unspecified drugs, medicaments and biological substances	T50.911	T50.912	T50.913	T50.914	T50.915	T50.916
Mumps						
immune globulin (human)	T50.Z11	T50.Z12	T50.Z13	T50.Z14	T50.Z15	T50.Z16
skin test antigen	T50.8X1	T50.8X2	T50.8X3	T50.8X4	T50.8X5	T50.8X6
vaccine	T50.B91	T50.B92	T50.B93	T50.B94	T50.B95	T50.B96
Mumpsvax	T50.B91	T50.B92	T50.B93	T50.B94	T50.B95	T50.B96
Mupirocin	T49.0X1	T49.0X2	T49.0X3	T49.0X4	T49.0X5	T49.0X6
Muriatic acid — see Hydrochloric acid						
Muromonab-CD3	T45.1X1	T45.1X2	T45.1X3	T45.1X4	T45.1X5	T45.1X6
Muscle-action drug NEC	T48.201	T48.202	T48.203	T48.204	T48.205	T48.206
Muscle affecting agents NEC	T48.201	T48.202	T48.203	T48.204	T48.205	T48.206
oxytocic	T48.0X1	T48.0X2	T48.0X3	T48.0X4	T48.0X5	T48.0X6
relaxants	T48.201	T48.202	T48.203	T48.204	T48.205	T48.206
central nervous system	T42.8X1	T42.8X2	T42.8X3	T42.8X4	T42.8X5	T42.8X6
skeletal	T48.1X1	T48.1X2	T48.1X3	T48.1X4	T48.1X5	T48.1X6
smooth	T44.3X1	T44.3X2	T44.3X3	T44.3X4	T44.3X5	T44.3X6
Muscle relaxant — see Relaxant, muscle						
Muscle-tone depressant, central NEC	T42.8X1	T42.8X2	T42.8X3	T42.8X4	T42.8X5	T42.8X6
specified NEC	T42.8X1	T42.8X2	T42.8X3	T42.8X4	T42.8X5	T42.8X6
Mushroom, noxious	T62.0X1	T62.0X2	T62.0X3	T62.0X4	—	—
Mussel, noxious	T61.781	T61.782	T61.783	T61.784	—	—
Mustard (emetic)	T47.7X1	T47.7X2	T47.7X3	T47.7X4	T47.7X5	T47.7X6
black	T47.7X1	T47.7X2	T47.7X3	T47.7X4	T47.7X5	T47.7X6
gas, not in war	T59.91	T59.92	T59.93	T59.94	—	—
nitrogen	T45.1X1	T45.1X2	T45.1X3	T45.1X4	T45.1X5	T45.1X6
Mustine	T45.1X1	T45.1X2	T45.1X3	T45.1X4	T45.1X5	T45.1X6
M-vac	T45.1X1	T45.1X2	T45.1X3	T45.1X4	T45.1X5	T45.1X6
Mycifradin	T36.5X1	T36.5X2	T36.5X3	T36.5X4	T36.5X5	T36.5X6
topical	T49.0X1	T49.0X2	T49.0X3	T49.0X4	T49.0X5	T49.0X6
Mycitracin	T36.8X1	T36.8X2	T36.8X3	T36.8X4	T36.8X5	T36.8X6
ophthalmic preparation	T49.5X1	T49.5X2	T49.5X3	T49.5X4	T49.5X5	T49.5X6
Mycostatin	T36.7X1	T36.7X2	T36.7X3	T36.7X4	T36.7X5	T36.7X6
topical	T49.0X1	T49.0X2	T49.0X3	T49.0X4	T49.0X5	T49.0X6

Metipranolol — Mycostatin

Table of Drugs and Chemicals

Mycotoxins — Nitrobenzene, nitrobenzol

Substance	Poisoning, Accidental (unintentional)	Poisoning, Intentional Self-harm	Poisoning, Assault	Poisoning, Undetermined	Adverse Effect	Under-dosing
Mycotoxins	T64.81	T64.82	T64.83	T64.84	—	—
aflatoxin	T64.01	T64.02	T64.03	T64.04	—	—
specified NEC	T64.81	T64.82	T64.83	T64.84	—	—
Mydriacyl	T44.3X1	T44.3X2	T44.3X3	T44.3X4	T44.3X5	T44.3X6
Mydriatic drug	T49.5X1	T49.5X2	T49.5X3	T49.5X4	T49.5X5	T49.5X6
Myelobromal	T45.1X1	T45.1X2	T45.1X3	T45.1X4	T45.1X5	T45.1X6
Myleran	T45.1X1	T45.1X2	T45.1X3	T45.1X4	T45.1X5	T45.1X6
Myochrysin (e)	T39.2X1	T39.2X2	T39.2X3	T39.2X4	T39.2X5	T39.2X6
Myoneural blocking agents	T48.1X1	T48.1X2	T48.1X3	T48.1X4	T48.1X5	T48.1X6
Myralact	T49.0X1	T49.0X2	T49.0X3	T49.0X4	T49.0X5	T49.0X6
Myristica fragrans	T62.2X1	T62.2X2	T62.2X3	T62.2X4	—	—
Myristicin	T65.891	T65.892	T65.893	T65.894	—	—
Mysoline	T42.3X1	T42.3X2	T42.3X3	T42.3X4	T42.3X5	T42.3X6
Nabilone	T40.7X1	T40.7X2	T40.7X3	T40.7X4	T40.7X5	T40.7X6
Nabumetone	T39.391	T39.392	T39.393	T39.394	T39.395	T39.396
Nadolol	T44.7X1	T44.7X2	T44.7X3	T44.7X4	T44.7X5	T44.7X6
Nafcillin	T36.0X1	T36.0X2	T36.0X3	T36.0X4	T36.0X5	T36.0X6
Nafoxidine	T38.6X1	T38.6X2	T38.6X3	T38.6X4	T38.6X5	T38.6X6
Naftazone	T46.991	T46.992	T46.993	T46.994	T46.995	T46.996
Naftidrofuryl (oxalate)	T46.7X1	T46.7X2	T46.7X3	T46.7X4	T46.7X5	T46.7X6
Naftifine	T49.0X1	T49.0X2	T49.0X3	T49.0X4	T49.0X5	T49.0X6
Nail polish remover	T52.91	T52.92	T52.93	T52.94	—	—
Nalbuphine	T40.4X1	T40.4X2	T40.4X3	T40.4X4	T40.4X5	T40.4X6
Naled	T60.0X1	T60.0X2	T60.0X3	T60.0X4	—	—
Nalidixic acid	T37.8X1	T37.8X2	T37.8X3	T37.8X4	T37.8X5	T37.8X6
Nalorphine	T50.7X1	T50.7X2	T50.7X3	T50.7X4	T50.7X5	T50.7X6
Naloxone	T50.7X1	T50.7X2	T50.7X3	T50.7X4	T50.7X5	T50.7X6
Naltrexone	T50.7X1	T50.7X2	T50.7X3	T50.7X4	T50.7X5	T50.7X6
Namenda	T43.8X1	T43.8X2	T43.8X3	T43.8X4	T43.8X5	T43.8X6
Nandrolone	T38.7X1	T38.7X2	T38.7X3	T38.7X4	T38.7X5	T38.7X6
Naphazoline	T48.5X1	T48.5X2	T48.5X3	T48.5X4	T48.5X5	T48.5X6
Naphtha (painters') (petroleum)	T52.0X1	T52.0X2	T52.0X3	T52.0X4	—	—
solvent	T52.0X1	T52.0X2	T52.0X3	T52.0X4	—	—
vapor	T52.0X1	T52.0X2	T52.0X3	T52.0X4	—	—
Naphthalene (non-chlorinated)	T60.2X1	T60.2X2	T60.2X3	T60.2X4	—	—
chlorinated	T60.1X1	T60.1X2	T60.1X3	T60.1X4	—	—
vapor	T60.1X1	T60.1X2	T60.1X3	T60.1X4	—	—
insecticide or moth repellent	T60.2X1	T60.2X2	T60.2X3	T60.2X4	—	—
chlorinated	T60.1X1	T60.1X2	T60.1X3	T60.1X4	—	—
vapor	T60.2X1	T60.2X2	T60.2X3	T60.2X4	—	—
chlorinated	T60.1X1	T60.1X2	T60.1X3	T60.1X4	—	—
Naphthol	T65.891	T65.892	T65.893	T65.894	—	—
Naphthylamine	T65.891	T65.892	T65.893	T65.894	—	—
Naphthylthiourea (ANTU)	T60.4X1	T60.4X2	T60.4X3	T60.4X4	—	—
Naprosyn — *see* Naproxen						
Naproxen	T39.311	T39.312	T39.313	T39.314	T39.315	T39.316
Narcotic (drug)	T40.601	T40.602	T40.603	T40.604	T40.605	T40.606
analgesic NEC	T40.601	T40.602	T40.603	T40.604	T40.605	T40.606
antagonist	T50.7X1	T50.7X2	T50.7X3	T50.7X4	T50.7X5	T50.7X6
specified NEC	T40.691	T40.692	T40.693	T40.694	T40.695	T40.696
synthetic	T40.4X1	T40.4X2	T40.4X3	T40.4X4	T40.4X5	T40.4X6
Narcotine	T48.3X1	T48.3X2	T48.3X3	T48.3X4	T48.3X5	T48.3X6
Nardil	T43.1X1	T43.1X2	T43.1X3	T43.1X4	T43.1X5	T43.1X6
Nasal drug NEC	T49.6X1	T49.6X2	T49.6X3	T49.6X4	T49.6X5	T49.6X6
Natamycin	T49.0X1	T49.0X2	T49.0X3	T49.0X4	T49.0X5	T49.0X6
Natrium cyanide — *see* Cyanide(s)						
Natural						
blood (product)	T45.8X1	T45.8X2	T45.8X3	T45.8X4	T45.8X5	T45.8X6
gas (piped)	T59.891	T59.892	T59.893	T59.894	—	—
incomplete combustion	T58.11	T58.12	T58.13	T58.14	—	—
Nealbarbital	T42.3X1	T42.3X2	T42.3X3	T42.3X4	T42.3X5	T42.3X6
Nectadon	T48.3X1	T48.3X2	T48.3X3	T48.3X4	T48.3X5	T48.3X6
Nedocromil	T48.6X1	T48.6X2	T48.6X3	T48.6X4	T48.6X5	T48.6X6
Nefopam	T39.8X1	T39.8X2	T39.8X3	T39.8X4	T39.8X5	T39.8X6
Nematocyst (sting)	T63.691	T63.692	T63.693	T63.694	—	—
Nembutal	T42.3X1	T42.3X2	T42.3X3	T42.3X4	T42.3X5	T42.3X6
Nemonapride	T43.591	T43.592	T43.593	T43.594	T43.595	T43.596
Neoarsphenamine	T37.8X1	T37.8X2	T37.8X3	T37.8X4	T37.8X5	T37.8X6
Neocinchophen	T50.4X1	T50.4X2	T50.4X3	T50.4X4	T50.4X5	T50.4X6
Neomycin (derivatives)	T36.5X1	T36.5X2	T36.5X3	T36.5X4	T36.5X5	T36.5X6
with						
bacitracin	T49.0X1	T49.0X2	T49.0X3	T49.0X4	T49.0X5	T49.0X6
neostigmine	T44.0X1	T44.0X2	T44.0X3	T44.0X4	T44.0X5	T44.0X6
ENT agent	T49.6X1	T49.6X2	T49.6X3	T49.6X4	T49.6X5	T49.6X6
ophthalmic preparation	T49.5X1	T49.5X2	T49.5X3	T49.5X4	T49.5X5	T49.5X6
topical NEC	T49.0X1	T49.0X2	T49.0X3	T49.0X4	T49.0X5	T49.0X6
Neonal	T42.3X1	T42.3X2	T42.3X3	T42.3X4	T42.3X5	T42.3X6
Neoprontosil	T37.0X1	T37.0X2	T37.0X3	T37.0X4	T37.0X5	T37.0X6
Neosalvarsan	T37.8X1	T37.8X2	T37.8X3	T37.8X4	T37.8X5	T37.8X6
Neosilversalvarsan	T37.8X1	T37.8X2	T37.8X3	T37.8X4	T37.8X5	T37.8X6
Neosporin	T36.8X1	T36.8X2	T36.8X3	T36.8X4	T36.8X5	T36.8X6
ENT agent	T49.6X1	T49.6X2	T49.6X3	T49.6X4	T49.6X5	T49.6X6
opthalmic preparation	T49.5X1	T49.5X2	T49.5X3	T49.5X4	T49.5X5	T49.5X6
topical NEC	T49.0X1	T49.0X2	T49.0X3	T49.0X4	T49.0X5	T49.0X6
Neostigmine bromide	T44.0X1	T44.0X2	T44.0X3	T44.0X4	T44.0X5	T44.0X6
Neraval	T42.3X1	T42.3X2	T42.3X3	T42.3X4	T42.3X5	T42.3X6
Neravan	T42.3X1	T42.3X2	T42.3X3	T42.3X4	T42.3X5	T42.3X6
Nerium oleander	T62.2X1	T62.2X2	T62.2X3	T62.2X4	—	—
Nerve gas, not in war	T59.91	T59.92	T59.93	T59.94	—	—
Nesacaine	T41.3X1	T41.3X2	T41.3X3	T41.3X4	T41.3X5	T41.3X6
infiltration (subcutaneous)	T41.3X1	T41.3X2	T41.3X3	T41.3X4	T41.3X5	T41.3X6
nerve block (peripheral) (plexus)	T41.3X1	T41.3X2	T41.3X3	T41.3X4	T41.3X5	T41.3X6
Netilmicin	T36.5X1	T36.5X2	T36.5X3	T36.5X4	T36.5X5	T36.5X6
Neurobarb	T42.3X1	T42.3X2	T42.3X3	T42.3X4	T42.3X5	T42.3X6
Neuroleptic drug NEC	T43.501	T43.502	T43.503	T43.504	T43.505	T43.506
Neuromuscular blocking drug	T48.1X1	T48.1X2	T48.1X3	T48.1X4	T48.1X5	T48.1X6
Neutral insulin injection	T38.3X1	T38.3X2	T38.3X3	T38.3X4	T38.3X5	T38.3X6
Neutral spirits	T51.0X1	T51.0X2	T51.0X3	T51.0X4	—	—
beverage	T51.0X1	T51.0X2	T51.0X3	T51.0X4	—	—
Niacin	T46.7X1	T46.7X2	T46.7X3	T46.7X4	T46.7X5	T46.7X6
Niacinamide	T45.2X1	T45.2X2	T45.2X3	T45.2X4	T45.2X5	T45.2X6
Nialamide	T43.1X1	T43.1X2	T43.1X3	T43.1X4	T43.1X5	T43.1X6
Niaprazine	T42.6X1	T42.6X2	T42.6X3	T42.6X4	T42.6X5	T42.6X6
Nicametate	T46.7X1	T46.7X2	T46.7X3	T46.7X4	T46.7X5	T46.7X6
Nicardipine	T46.1X1	T46.1X2	T46.1X3	T46.1X4	T46.1X5	T46.1X6
Nicergoline	T46.7X1	T46.7X2	T46.7X3	T46.7X4	T46.7X5	T46.7X6
Nickel (carbonyl) (tetra-carbonyl) (fumes) (vapor)	T56.891	T56.892	T56.893	T56.894	—	—
Nickelocene	T56.891	T56.892	T56.893	T56.894	—	—
Niclosamide	T37.4X1	T37.4X2	T37.4X3	T37.4X4	T37.4X5	T37.4X6
Nicofuranose	T46.7X1	T46.7X2	T46.7X3	T46.7X4	T46.7X5	T46.7X6
Nicomorphine	T40.2X1	T40.2X2	T40.2X3	T40.2X4	—	—
Nicorandil	T46.3X1	T46.3X2	T46.3X3	T46.3X4	T46.3X5	T46.3X6
Nicotiana (plant)	T62.2X1	T62.2X2	T62.2X3	T62.2X4	—	—
Nicotinamide	T45.2X1	T45.2X2	T45.2X3	T45.2X4	T45.2X5	T45.2X6
Nicotine (insecticide) (spray) (sulfate) **NEC**	T60.2X1	T60.2X2	T60.2X3	T60.2X4	—	—
from tobacco	T65.291	T65.292	T65.293	T65.294	—	—
cigarettes	T65.221	T65.222	T65.223	T65.224	—	—
not insecticide	T65.291	T65.292	T65.293	T65.294	—	—
Nicotinic acid	T46.7X1	T46.7X2	T46.7X3	T46.7X4	T46.7X5	T46.7X6
Nicotinyl alcohol	T46.7X1	T46.7X2	T46.7X3	T46.7X4	T46.7X5	T46.7X6
Nicoumalone	T45.511	T45.512	T45.513	T45.514	T45.515	T45.516
Nifedipine	T46.1X1	T46.1X2	T46.1X3	T46.1X4	T46.1X5	T46.1X6
Nifenazone	T39.2X1	T39.2X2	T39.2X3	T39.2X4	T39.2X5	T39.2X6
Nifuraldezone	T37.91	T37.92	T37.93	T37.94	T37.95	T37.96
Nifuratel	T37.8X1	T37.8X2	T37.8X3	T37.8X4	T37.8X5	T37.8X6
Nifurtimox	T37.3X1	T37.3X2	T37.3X3	T37.3X4	T37.3X5	T37.3X6
Nifurtoinol	T37.8X1	T37.8X2	T37.8X3	T37.8X4	T37.8X5	T37.8X6
Nightshade, deadly (solanum) — *see also* Belladonna	T62.2X1	T62.2X2	T62.2X3	T62.2X4	—	—
berry	T62.1X1	T62.1X2	T62.1X3	T62.1X4	—	—
Nikethamide	T50.7X1	T50.7X2	T50.7X3	T50.7X4	T50.7X5	T50.7X6
Nilstat	T36.7X1	T36.7X2	T36.7X3	T36.7X4	T36.7X5	T36.7X6
topical	T49.0X1	T49.0X2	T49.0X3	T49.0X4	T49.0X5	T49.0X6
Nilutamide	T38.6X1	T38.6X2	T38.6X3	T38.6X4	T38.6X5	T38.6X6
Nimesulide	T39.391	T39.392	T39.393	T39.394	T39.395	T39.396
Nimetazepam	T42.4X1	T42.4X2	T42.4X3	T42.4X4	T42.4X5	T42.4X6
Nimodipine	T46.1X1	T46.1X2	T46.1X3	T46.1X4	T46.1X5	T46.1X6
Nimorazole	T37.3X1	T37.3X2	T37.3X3	T37.3X4	T37.3X5	T37.3X6
Nimustine	T45.1X1	T45.1X2	T45.1X3	T45.1X4	T45.1X5	T45.1X6
Niridazole	T37.4X1	T37.4X2	T37.4X3	T37.4X4	T37.4X5	T37.4X6
Nisentil	T40.2X1	T40.2X2	T40.2X3	T40.2X4	T40.2X5	T40.2X6
Nisoldipine	T46.1X1	T46.1X2	T46.1X3	T46.1X4	T46.1X5	T46.1X6
Nitramine	T65.3X1	T65.3X2	T65.3X3	T65.3X4	—	—
Nitrate, organic	T46.3X1	T46.3X2	T46.3X3	T46.3X4	T46.3X5	T46.3X6
Nitrazepam	T42.4X1	T42.4X2	T42.4X3	T42.4X4	T42.4X5	T42.4X6
Nitrefazole	T50.6X1	T50.6X2	T50.6X3	T50.6X4	T50.6X5	T50.6X6
Nitrendipine	T46.1X1	T46.1X2	T46.1X3	T46.1X4	T46.1X5	T46.1X6
Nitric						
acid (liquid)	T54.2X1	T54.2X2	T54.2X3	T54.2X4	—	—
vapor	T59.891	T59.892	T59.893	T59.894	—	—
oxide (gas)	T59.0X1	T59.0X2	T59.0X3	T59.0X4	—	—
Nitrimidazine	T37.3X1	T37.3X2	T37.3X3	T37.3X4	T37.3X5	T37.3X6
Nitrite, amyl (medicinal) (vapor)	T46.3X1	T46.3X2	T46.3X3	T46.3X4	T46.3X5	T46.3X6
Nitroaniline	T65.3X1	T65.3X2	T65.3X3	T65.3X4	—	—
vapor	T59.891	T59.892	T59.893	T59.894	—	—
Nitrobenzene, nitrobenzol	T65.3X1	T65.3X2	T65.3X3	T65.3X4	—	—

380

Additional Character May Be Required — Refer to the Tabular List for Character Selection · Subterms under main terms may continue to next column or page

Substance	Poisoning, Accidental (unintentional)	Poisoning, Intentional Self-harm	Poisoning, Assault	Poisoning, Undetermined	Adverse Effect	Under-dosing
Nitrobenzene, nitrobenzol — continued						
vapor	T65.3X1	T65.3X2	T65.3X3	T65.3X4	—	—
Nitrocellulose	T65.891	T65.892	T65.893	T65.894	—	—
lacquer	T65.891	T65.892	T65.893	T65.894	—	—
Nitrodiphenyl	T65.3X1	T65.3X2	T65.3X3	T65.3X4	—	—
Nitrofural	T49.0X1	T49.0X2	T49.0X3	T49.0X4	T49.0X5	T49.0X6
Nitrofurantoin	T37.8X1	T37.8X2	T37.8X3	T37.8X4	T37.8X5	T37.8X6
Nitrofurazone	T49.0X1	T49.0X2	T49.0X3	T49.0X4	T49.0X5	T49.0X6
Nitrogen	T59.0X1	T59.0X2	T59.0X3	T59.0X4	—	—
mustard	T45.1X1	T45.1X2	T45.1X3	T45.1X4	T45.1X5	T45.1X6
Nitroglycerin, nitroglycerol (medicinal)	T46.3X1	T46.3X2	T46.3X3	T46.3X4	T46.3X5	T46.3X6
nonmedicinal	T65.5X1	T65.5X2	T65.5X3	T65.5X4	—	—
fumes	T65.5X1	T65.5X2	T65.5X3	T65.5X4	—	—
Nitroglycol	T52.3X1	T52.3X2	T52.3X3	T52.3X4	—	—
Nitrohydrochloric acid	T54.2X1	T54.2X2	T54.2X3	T54.2X4	—	—
Nitromersol	T49.0X1	T49.0X2	T49.0X3	T49.0X4	T49.0X5	T49.0X6
Nitronaphthalene	T65.891	T65.892	T65.893	T65.894	—	—
Nitrophenol	T54.0X1	T54.0X2	T54.0X3	T54.0X4	—	—
Nitropropane	T52.8X1	T52.8X2	T52.8X3	T52.8X4	—	—
Nitroprusside	T46.5X1	T46.5X2	T46.5X3	T46.5X4	T46.5X5	T46.5X6
Nitrosodimethylamine	T65.3X1	T65.3X2	T65.3X3	T65.3X4	—	—
Nitrothiazol	T37.4X1	T37.4X2	T37.4X3	T37.4X4	T37.4X5	T37.4X6
Nitrotoluene, nitrotoluol	T65.3X1	T65.3X2	T65.3X3	T65.3X4	—	—
vapor	T65.3X1	T65.3X2	T65.3X3	T65.3X4	—	—
Nitrous						
acid (liquid)	T54.2X1	T54.2X2	T54.2X3	T54.2X4	—	—
fumes	T59.891	T59.892	T59.893	T59.894	—	—
ether spirit	T46.3X1	T46.3X2	T46.3X3	T46.3X4	T46.3X5	T46.3X6
oxide	T41.0X1	T41.0X2	T41.0X3	T41.0X4	T41.0X5	T41.0X6
Nitroxoline	T37.8X1	T37.8X2	T37.8X3	T37.8X4	T37.8X5	T37.8X6
Nitrozone	T49.0X1	T49.0X2	T49.0X3	T49.0X4	T49.0X5	T49.0X6
Nizatidine	T47.0X1	T47.0X2	T47.0X3	T47.0X4	T47.0X5	T47.0X6
Nizofenone	T43.8X1	T43.8X2	T43.8X3	T43.8X4	T43.8X5	T43.8X6
Noctec	T42.6X1	T42.6X2	T42.6X3	T42.6X4	T42.6X5	T42.6X6
Noludar	T42.6X1	T42.6X2	T42.6X3	T42.6X4	T42.6X5	T42.6X6
Nomegestrol	T38.5X1	T38.5X2	T38.5X3	T38.5X4	T38.5X5	T38.5X6
Nomifensine	T43.291	T43.292	T43.293	T43.294	T43.295	T43.296
Nonoxinol	T49.8X1	T49.8X2	T49.8X3	T49.8X4	T49.8X5	T49.8X6
Nonylphenoxy (polyethoxyethanol)	T49.8X1	T49.8X2	T49.8X3	T49.8X4	T49.8X5	T49.8X6
Noptil	T42.3X1	T42.3X2	T42.3X3	T42.3X4	T42.3X5	T42.3X6
Noradrenaline	T44.4X1	T44.4X2	T44.4X3	T44.4X4	T44.4X5	T44.4X6
Noramidopyrine	T39.2X1	T39.2X2	T39.2X3	T39.2X4	T39.2X5	T39.2X6
methanesulfonate sodium	T39.2X1	T39.2X2	T39.2X3	T39.2X4	T39.2X5	T39.2X6
Norbormide	T60.4X1	T60.4X2	T60.4X3	T60.4X4	—	—
Nordazepam	T42.4X1	T42.4X2	T42.4X3	T42.4X4	T42.4X5	T42.4X6
Norepinephrine	T44.4X1	T44.4X2	T44.4X3	T44.4X4	T44.4X5	T44.4X6
Norethandrolone	T38.7X1	T38.7X2	T38.7X3	T38.7X4	T38.7X5	T38.7X6
Norethindrone	T38.4X1	T38.4X2	T38.4X3	T38.4X4	T38.4X5	T38.4X6
Norethisterone (acetate) (enantate)	T38.4X1	T38.4X2	T38.4X3	T38.4X4	T38.4X5	T38.4X6
with ethinylestradiol	T38.5X1	T38.5X2	T38.5X3	T38.5X4	T38.5X5	T38.5X6
Noretynodrel	T38.5X1	T38.5X2	T38.5X3	T38.5X4	T38.5X5	T38.5X6
Norfenefrine	T44.4X1	T44.4X2	T44.4X3	T44.4X4	T44.4X5	T44.4X6
Norfloxacin	T36.8X1	T36.8X2	T36.8X3	T36.8X4	T36.8X5	T36.8X6
Norgestrel	T38.4X1	T38.4X2	T38.4X3	T38.4X4	T38.4X5	T38.4X6
Norgestrienone	T38.4X1	T38.4X2	T38.4X3	T38.4X4	T38.4X5	T38.4X6
Norlestrin	T38.4X1	T38.4X2	T38.4X3	T38.4X4	T38.4X5	T38.4X6
Norlutin	T38.4X1	T38.4X2	T38.4X3	T38.4X4	T38.4X5	T38.4X6
Normal serum albumin (human), salt-poor	T45.8X1	T45.8X2	T45.8X3	T45.8X4	T45.8X5	T45.8X6
Normethandrone	T38.5X1	T38.5X2	T38.5X3	T38.5X4	T38.5X5	T38.5X6
Normison — see Benzodiazepines						
Normorphine	T40.2X1	T40.2X2	T40.2X3	T40.2X4	—	—
Norpseudoephedrine	T50.5X1	T50.5X2	T50.5X3	T50.5X4	T50.5X5	T50.5X6
Nortestosterone (furanpropionate)	T38.7X1	T38.7X2	T38.7X3	T38.7X4	T38.7X5	T38.7X6
Nortriptyline	T43.011	T43.012	T43.013	T43.014	T43.015	T43.016
Noscapine	T48.3X1	T48.3X2	T48.3X3	T48.3X4	T48.3X5	T48.3X6
Nose preparations	T49.6X1	T49.6X2	T49.6X3	T49.6X4	T49.6X5	T49.6X6
Novobiocin	T36.5X1	T36.5X2	T36.5X3	T36.5X4	T36.5X5	T36.5X6
Novocain (infiltration) (topical)	T41.3X1	T41.3X2	T41.3X3	T41.3X4	T41.3X5	T41.3X6
nerve block (peripheral) (plexus)	T41.3X1	T41.3X2	T41.3X3	T41.3X4	T41.3X5	T41.3X6
spinal	T41.3X1	T41.3X2	T41.3X3	T41.3X4	T41.3X5	T41.3X6
Noxious foodstuff	T62.91	T62.92	T62.93	T62.94	—	—
specified NEC	T62.8X1	T62.8X2	T62.8X3	T62.8X4	—	—
Noxiptiline	T43.011	T43.012	T43.013	T43.014	T43.015	T43.016
Noxytiolin	T49.0X1	T49.0X2	T49.0X3	T49.0X4	T49.0X5	T49.0X6

Substance	Poisoning, Accidental (unintentional)	Poisoning, Intentional Self-harm	Poisoning, Assault	Poisoning, Undetermined	Adverse Effect	Under-dosing
NPH Iletin (insulin)	T38.3X1	T38.3X2	T38.3X3	T38.3X4	T38.3X5	T38.3X6
Numorphan	T40.2X1	T40.2X2	T40.2X3	T40.2X4	T40.2X5	T40.2X6
Nunol	T42.3X1	T42.3X2	T42.3X3	T42.3X4	T42.3X5	T42.3X6
Nupercaine (spinal anesthetic)	T41.3X1	T41.3X2	T41.3X3	T41.3X4	T41.3X5	T41.3X6
topical (surface)	T41.3X1	T41.3X2	T41.3X3	T41.3X4	T41.3X5	T41.3X6
Nutmeg oil (liniment)	T49.3X1	T49.3X2	T49.3X3	T49.3X4	T49.3X5	T49.3X6
Nutritional supplement	T50.901	T50.902	T50.903	T50.904	T50.905	T50.906
Nux vomica	T65.1X1	T65.1X2	T65.1X3	T65.1X4	—	—
Nydrazid	T37.1X1	T37.1X2	T37.1X3	T37.1X4	T37.1X5	T37.1X6
Nylidrin	T46.7X1	T46.7X2	T46.7X3	T46.7X4	T46.7X5	T46.7X6
Nystatin	T36.7X1	T36.7X2	T36.7X3	T36.7X4	T36.7X5	T36.7X6
topical	T49.0X1	T49.0X2	T49.0X3	T49.0X4	T49.0X5	T49.0X6
Nytol	T45.0X1	T45.0X2	T45.0X3	T45.0X4	T45.0X5	T45.0X6
Obidoxime chloride	T50.6X1	T50.6X2	T50.6X3	T50.6X4	T50.6X5	T50.6X6
Octafonium (chloride)	T49.3X1	T49.3X2	T49.3X3	T49.3X4	T49.3X5	T49.3X6
Octamethyl pyrophosphoramide	T60.0X1	T60.0X2	T60.0X3	T60.0X4	—	—
Octanoin	T50.991	T50.992	T50.993	T50.994	T50.995	T50.996
Octatropine methylbromide	T44.3X1	T44.3X2	T44.3X3	T44.3X4	T44.3X5	T44.3X6
Octotiamine	T45.2X1	T45.2X2	T45.2X3	T45.2X4	T45.2X5	T45.2X6
Octoxinol (9)	T49.8X1	T49.8X2	T49.8X3	T49.8X4	T49.8X5	T49.8X6
Octreotide	T38.991	T38.992	T38.993	T38.994	T38.995	T38.996
Octyl nitrite	T46.3X1	T46.3X2	T46.3X3	T46.3X4	T46.3X5	T46.3X6
Oestradiol	T38.5X1	T38.5X2	T38.5X3	T38.5X4	T38.5X5	T38.5X6
Oestriol	T38.5X1	T38.5X2	T38.5X3	T38.5X4	T38.5X5	T38.5X6
Oestrogen	T38.5X1	T38.5X2	T38.5X3	T38.5X4	T38.5X5	T38.5X6
Oestrone	T38.5X1	T38.5X2	T38.5X3	T38.5X4	T38.5X5	T38.5X6
Ofloxacin	T36.8X1	T36.8X2	T36.8X3	T36.8X4	T36.8X5	T36.8X6
Oil (of)	T65.891	T65.892	T65.893	T65.894	—	—
bitter almond	T62.8X1	T62.8X2	T62.8X3	T62.8X4	—	—
cloves	T49.7X1	T49.7X2	T49.7X3	T49.7X4	T49.7X5	T49.7X6
colors	T65.6X1	T65.6X2	T65.6X3	T65.6X4	—	—
fumes	T59.891	T59.892	T59.893	T59.894	—	—
lubricating	T52.0X1	T52.0X2	T52.0X3	T52.0X4	—	—
Niobe	T52.8X1	T52.8X2	T52.8X3	T52.8X4	—	—
vitriol (liquid)	T54.2X1	T54.2X2	T54.2X3	T54.2X4	—	—
fumes	T54.2X1	T54.2X2	T54.2X3	T54.2X4	—	—
wintergreen (bitter) NEC	T49.3X1	T49.3X2	T49.3X3	T49.3X4	T49.3X5	T49.3X6
Oily preparation (for skin)	T49.3X1	T49.3X2	T49.3X3	T49.3X4	T49.3X5	T49.3X6
Ointment NEC	T49.3X1	T49.3X2	T49.3X3	T49.3X4	T49.3X5	T49.3X6
Olanzapine	T43.591	T43.592	T43.593	T43.594	T43.595	T43.596
Oleander	T62.2X1	T62.2X2	T62.2X3	T62.2X4	—	—
Oleandomycin	T36.3X1	T36.3X2	T36.3X3	T36.3X4	T36.3X5	T36.3X6
Oleandrin	T46.0X1	T46.0X2	T46.0X3	T46.0X4	T46.0X5	T46.0X6
Oleic acid	T46.6X1	T46.6X2	T46.6X3	T46.6X4	T46.6X5	T46.6X6
Oleovitamin A	T45.2X1	T45.2X2	T45.2X3	T45.2X4	T45.2X5	T45.2X6
Oleum ricini	T47.2X1	T47.2X2	T47.2X3	T47.2X4	T47.2X5	T47.2X6
Olive oil (medicinal) NEC	T47.4X1	T47.4X2	T47.4X3	T47.4X4	T47.4X5	T47.4X6
Olivomycin	T45.1X1	T45.1X2	T45.1X3	T45.1X4	T45.1X5	T45.1X6
Olsalazine	T47.8X1	T47.8X2	T47.8X3	T47.8X4	T47.8X5	T47.8X6
Omeprazole	T47.1X1	T47.1X2	T47.1X3	T47.1X4	T47.1X5	T47.1X6
OMPA	T60.0X1	T60.0X2	T60.0X3	T60.0X4	—	—
Oncovin	T45.1X1	T45.1X2	T45.1X3	T45.1X4	T45.1X5	T45.1X6
Ondansetron	T45.0X1	T45.0X2	T45.0X3	T45.0X4	T45.0X5	T45.0X6
Ophthaine	T41.3X1	T41.3X2	T41.3X3	T41.3X4	T41.3X5	T41.3X6
Ophthetic	T41.3X1	T41.3X2	T41.3X3	T41.3X4	T41.3X5	T41.3X6
Opiate NEC	T40.601	T40.602	T40.603	T40.604	T40.605	T40.606
antagonists	T50.7X1	T50.7X2	T50.7X3	T50.7X4	T50.7X5	T50.7X6
Opioid NEC	T40.2X1	T40.2X2	T40.2X3	T40.2X4	T40.2X5	T40.2X6
Opipramol	T43.011	T43.012	T43.013	T43.014	T43.015	T43.016
Opium alkaloids (total)	T40.0X1	T40.0X2	T40.0X3	T40.0X4	T40.0X5	T40.0X6
standardized powdered	T40.0X1	T40.0X2	T40.0X3	T40.0X4	T40.0X5	T40.0X6
tincture (camphorated)	T40.0X1	T40.0X2	T40.0X3	T40.0X4	T40.0X5	T40.0X6
Oracon	T38.4X1	T38.4X2	T38.4X3	T38.4X4	T38.4X5	T38.4X6
Oragrafin	T50.8X1	T50.8X2	T50.8X3	T50.8X4	T50.8X5	T50.8X6
Oral contraceptives	T38.4X1	T38.4X2	T38.4X3	T38.4X4	T38.4X5	T38.4X6
Oral rehydration salts	T50.3X1	T50.3X2	T50.3X3	T50.3X4	T50.3X5	T50.3X6
Orazamide	T50.991	T50.992	T50.993	T50.994	T50.995	T50.996
Orciprenaline	T48.291	T48.292	T48.293	T48.294	T48.295	T48.296
Organidin	T48.4X1	T48.4X2	T48.4X3	T48.4X4	T48.4X5	T48.4X6
Organonitrate NEC	T46.3X1	T46.3X2	T46.3X3	T46.3X4	T46.3X5	T46.3X6
Organophosphates	T60.0X1	T60.0X2	T60.0X3	T60.0X4	—	—
Orimune	T50.B91	T50.B92	T50.B93	T50.B94	T50.B95	T50.B96
Orinase	T38.3X1	T38.3X2	T38.3X3	T38.3X4	T38.3X5	T38.3X6
Ormeloxifene	T38.6X1	T38.6X2	T38.6X3	T38.6X4	T38.6X5	T38.6X6
Ornidazole	T37.3X1	T37.3X2	T37.3X3	T37.3X4	T37.3X5	T37.3X6
Ornithine aspartate	T50.991	T50.992	T50.993	T50.994	T50.995	T50.996
Ornoprostil	T47.1X1	T47.1X2	T47.1X3	T47.1X4	T47.1X5	T47.1X6
Orphenadrine (hydrochloride)	T42.8X1	T42.8X2	T42.8X3	T42.8X4	T42.8X5	T42.8X6
Ortal (sodium)	T42.3X1	T42.3X2	T42.3X3	T42.3X4	T42.3X5	T42.3X6

Table of Drugs and Chemicals

Orthoboric acid — Peanut oil

Substance	Poisoning, Accidental (unintentional)	Poisoning, Intentional Self-harm	Poisoning, Assault	Poisoning, Undetermined	Adverse Effect	Under-dosing
Orthoboric acid	T49.0X1	T49.0X2	T49.0X3	T49.0X4	T49.0X5	T49.0X6
ENT agent	T49.6X1	T49.6X2	T49.6X3	T49.6X4	T49.6X5	T49.6X6
ophthalmic preparation	T49.5X1	T49.5X2	T49.5X3	T49.5X4	T49.5X5	T49.5X6
Orthocaine	T41.3X1	T41.3X2	T41.3X3	T41.3X4	T41.3X5	T41.3X6
Orthodichlorobenzene	T53.7X1	T53.7X2	T53.7X3	T53.7X4	—	—
Ortho-Novum	T38.4X1	T38.4X2	T38.4X3	T38.4X4	T38.4X5	T38.4X6
Orthotolidine (reagent)	T54.2X1	T54.2X2	T54.2X3	T54.2X4	—	—
Osmic acid (liquid)	T54.2X1	T54.2X2	T54.2X3	T54.2X4	—	—
fumes	T54.2X1	T54.2X2	T54.2X3	T54.2X4	—	—
Osmotic diuretics	T50.2X1	T50.2X2	T50.2X3	T50.2X4	T50.2X5	T50.2X6
Otilonium bromide	T44.3X1	T44.3X2	T44.3X3	T44.3X4	T44.3X5	T44.3X6
Otorhinolaryngological drug NEC	T49.6X1	T49.6X2	T49.6X3	T49.6X4	T49.6X5	T49.6X6
Ouabain (e)	T46.0X1	T46.0X2	T46.0X3	T46.0X4	T46.0X5	T46.0X6
Ovarian						
hormone	T38.5X1	T38.5X2	T38.5X3	T38.5X4	T38.5X5	T38.5X6
stimulant	T38.5X1	T38.5X2	T38.5X3	T38.5X4	T38.5X5	T38.5X6
Ovral	T38.4X1	T38.4X2	T38.4X3	T38.4X4	T38.4X5	T38.4X6
Ovulen	T38.4X1	T38.4X2	T38.4X3	T38.4X4	T38.4X5	T38.4X6
Oxacillin	T36.0X1	T36.0X2	T36.0X3	T36.0X4	T36.0X5	T36.0X6
Oxalic acid	T54.2X1	T54.2X2	T54.2X3	T54.2X4	—	—
ammonium salt	T50.991	T50.992	T50.993	T50.994	T50.995	T50.996
Oxamniquine	T37.4X1	T37.4X2	T37.4X3	T37.4X4	T37.4X5	T37.4X6
Oxanamide	T43.591	T43.592	T43.593	T43.594	T43.595	T43.596
Oxandrolone	T38.7X1	T38.7X2	T38.7X3	T38.7X4	T38.7X5	T38.7X6
Oxantel	T37.4X1	T37.4X2	T37.4X3	T37.4X4	T37.4X5	T37.4X6
Oxapium iodide	T44.3X1	T44.3X2	T44.3X3	T44.3X4	T44.3X5	T44.3X6
Oxaprotiline	T43.021	T43.022	T43.023	T43.024	T43.025	T43.026
Oxaprozin	T39.311	T39.312	T39.313	T39.314	T39.315	T39.316
Oxatomide	T45.0X1	T45.0X2	T45.0X3	T45.0X4	T45.0X5	T45.0X6
Oxazepam	T42.4X1	T42.4X2	T42.4X3	T42.4X4	T42.4X5	T42.4X6
Oxazimedrine	T50.5X1	T50.5X2	T50.5X3	T50.5X4	T50.5X5	T50.5X6
Oxazolam	T42.4X1	T42.4X2	T42.4X3	T42.4X4	T42.4X5	T42.4X6
Oxazolidine derivatives	T42.2X1	T42.2X2	T42.2X3	T42.2X4	T42.2X5	T42.2X6
Oxazolidinedione (derivative)	T42.2X1	T42.2X2	T42.2X3	T42.2X4	T42.2X5	T42.2X6
Ox bile extract	T47.5X1	T47.5X2	T47.5X3	T47.5X4	T47.5X5	T47.5X6
Oxcarbazepine	T42.1X1	T42.1X2	T42.1X3	T42.1X4	T42.1X5	T42.1X6
Oxedrine	T44.4X1	T44.4X2	T44.4X3	T44.4X4	T44.4X5	T44.4X6
Oxeladin (citrate)	T48.3X1	T48.3X2	T48.3X3	T48.3X4	T48.3X5	T48.3X6
Oxendolone	T38.5X1	T38.5X2	T38.5X3	T38.5X4	T38.5X5	T38.5X6
Oxetacaine	T41.3X1	T41.3X2	T41.3X3	T41.3X4	T41.3X5	T41.3X6
Oxethazine	T41.3X1	T41.3X2	T41.3X3	T41.3X4	T41.3X5	T41.3X6
Oxetorone	T39.8X1	T39.8X2	T39.8X3	T39.8X4	T39.8X5	T39.8X6
Oxiconazole	T49.0X1	T49.0X2	T49.0X3	T49.0X4	T49.0X5	T49.0X6
Oxidizing agent NEC	T54.91	T54.92	T54.93	T54.94	—	—
Oxipurinol	T50.4X1	T50.4X2	T50.4X3	T50.4X4	T50.4X5	T50.4X6
Oxitriptan	T43.291	T43.292	T43.293	T43.294	T43.295	T43.296
Oxitropium bromide	T48.6X1	T48.6X2	T48.6X3	T48.6X4	T48.6X5	T48.6X6
Oxodipine	T46.1X1	T46.1X2	T46.1X3	T46.1X4	T46.1X5	T46.1X6
Oxolamine	T48.3X1	T48.3X2	T48.3X3	T48.3X4	T48.3X5	T48.3X6
Oxolinic acid	T37.8X1	T37.8X2	T37.8X3	T37.8X4	T37.8X5	T37.8X6
Oxomemazine	T43.3X1	T43.3X2	T43.3X3	T43.3X4	T43.3X5	T43.3X6
Oxophenarsine	T37.3X1	T37.3X2	T37.3X3	T37.3X4	T37.3X5	T37.3X6
Oxprenolol	T44.7X1	T44.7X2	T44.7X3	T44.7X4	T44.7X5	T44.7X6
Oxsoralen	T49.3X1	T49.3X2	T49.3X3	T49.3X4	T49.3X5	T49.3X6
Oxtriphylline	T48.6X1	T48.6X2	T48.6X3	T48.6X4	T48.6X5	T48.6X6
Oxybate sodium	T41.291	T41.292	T41.293	T41.294	T41.295	T41.296
Oxybuprocaine	T41.3X1	T41.3X2	T41.3X3	T41.3X4	T41.3X5	T41.3X6
Oxybutynin	T44.3X1	T44.3X2	T44.3X3	T44.3X4	T44.3X5	T44.3X6
Oxychlorosene	T49.0X1	T49.0X2	T49.0X3	T49.0X4	T49.0X5	T49.0X6
Oxycodone	T40.2X1	T40.2X2	T40.2X3	T40.2X4	T40.2X5	T40.2X6
Oxyfedrine	T46.3X1	T46.3X2	T46.3X3	T46.3X4	T46.3X5	T46.3X6
Oxygen	T41.5X1	T41.5X2	T41.5X3	T41.5X4	T41.5X5	T41.5X6
Oxylone	T49.0X1	T49.0X2	T49.0X3	T49.0X4	T49.0X5	T49.0X6
ophthalmic preparation	T49.5X1	T49.5X2	T49.5X3	T49.5X4	T49.5X5	T49.5X6
Oxymesterone	T38.7X1	T38.7X2	T38.7X3	T38.7X4	T38.7X5	T38.7X6
Oxymetazoline	T48.5X1	T48.5X2	T48.5X3	T48.5X4	T48.5X5	T48.5X6
Oxymetholone	T38.7X1	T38.7X2	T38.7X3	T38.7X4	T38.7X5	T38.7X6
Oxymorphone	T40.2X1	T40.2X2	T40.2X3	T40.2X4	T40.2X5	T40.2X6
Oxypertine	T43.591	T43.592	T43.593	T43.594	T43.595	T43.596
Oxyphenbutazone	T39.2X1	T39.2X2	T39.2X3	T39.2X4	T39.2X5	T39.2X6
Oxyphencyclimine	T44.3X1	T44.3X2	T44.3X3	T44.3X4	T44.3X5	T44.3X6
Oxyphenisatine	T47.2X1	T47.2X2	T47.2X3	T47.2X4	T47.2X5	T47.2X6
Oxyphenonium bromide	T44.3X1	T44.3X2	T44.3X3	T44.3X4	T44.3X5	T44.3X6
Oxypolygelatin	T45.8X1	T45.8X2	T45.8X3	T45.8X4	T45.8X5	T45.8X6
Oxyquinoline (derivatives)	T37.8X1	T37.8X2	T37.8X3	T37.8X4	T37.8X5	T37.8X6
Oxytetracycline	T36.4X1	T36.4X2	T36.4X3	T36.4X4	T36.4X5	T36.4X6
Oxytocic drug NEC	T48.0X1	T48.0X2	T48.0X3	T48.0X4	T48.0X5	T48.0X6
Oxytocin (synthetic)	T48.0X1	T48.0X2	T48.0X3	T48.0X4	T48.0X5	T48.0X6
Ozone	T59.891	T59.892	T59.893	T59.894	—	—
PABA	T49.3X1	T49.3X2	T49.3X3	T49.3X4	T49.3X5	T49.3X6
Packed red cells	T45.8X1	T45.8X2	T45.8X3	T45.8X4	T45.8X5	T45.8X6
Padimate	T49.3X1	T49.3X2	T49.3X3	T49.3X4	T49.3X5	T49.3X6
Paint NEC	T65.6X1	T65.6X2	T65.6X3	T65.6X4	—	—
cleaner	T52.91	T52.92	T52.93	T52.94	—	—
fumes NEC	T59.891	T59.892	T59.893	T59.894	—	—
lead (fumes)	T56.0X1	T56.0X2	T56.0X3	T56.0X4	—	—
solvent NEC	T52.8X1	T52.8X2	T52.8X3	T52.8X4	—	—
stripper	T52.8X1	T52.8X2	T52.8X3	T52.8X4	—	—
Palfium	T40.2X1	T40.2X2	T40.2X3	T40.2X4	—	—
Palm kernel oil	T50.991	T50.992	T50.993	T50.994	T50.995	T50.996
Paludrine	T37.2X1	T37.2X2	T37.2X3	T37.2X4	T37.2X5	T37.2X6
PAM (pralidoxime)	T50.6X1	T50.6X2	T50.6X3	T50.6X4	T50.6X5	T50.6X6
Pamaquine (naphthoute)	T37.2X1	T37.2X2	T37.2X3	T37.2X4	T37.2X5	T37.2X6
Panadol	T39.1X1	T39.1X2	T39.1X3	T39.1X4	T39.1X5	T39.1X6
Pancreatic						
digestive secretion stimulant	T47.8X1	T47.8X2	T47.8X3	T47.8X4	T47.8X5	T47.8X6
dornase	T45.3X1	T45.3X2	T45.3X3	T45.3X4	T45.3X5	T45.3X6
Pancreatin	T47.5X1	T47.5X2	T47.5X3	T47.5X4	T47.5X5	T47.5X6
Pancrelipase	T47.5X1	T47.5X2	T47.5X3	T47.5X4	T47.5X5	T47.5X6
Pancuronium (bromide)	T48.1X1	T48.1X2	T48.1X3	T48.1X4	T48.1X5	T48.1X6
Pangamic acid	T45.2X1	T45.2X2	T45.2X3	T45.2X4	T45.2X5	T45.2X6
Panthenol	T45.2X1	T45.2X2	T45.2X3	T45.2X4	T45.2X5	T45.2X6
topical	T49.8X1	T49.8X2	T49.8X3	T49.8X4	T49.8X5	T49.8X6
Pantopon	T40.0X1	T40.0X2	T40.0X3	T40.0X4	T40.0X5	T40.0X6
Pantothenic acid	T45.2X1	T45.2X2	T45.2X3	T45.2X4	T45.2X5	T45.2X6
Panwarfin	T45.511	T45.512	T45.513	T45.514	T45.515	T45.516
Papain	T47.5X1	T47.5X2	T47.5X3	T47.5X4	T47.5X5	T47.5X6
digestant	T47.5X1	T47.5X2	T47.5X3	T47.5X4	T47.5X5	T47.5X6
Papaveretum	T40.0X1	T40.0X2	T40.0X3	T40.0X4	T40.0X5	T40.0X6
Papaverine	T44.3X1	T44.3X2	T44.3X3	T44.3X4	T44.3X5	T44.3X6
Para-acetamidophenol	T39.1X1	T39.1X2	T39.1X3	T39.1X4	T39.1X5	T39.1X6
Para-aminobenzoic acid	T49.3X1	T49.3X2	T49.3X3	T49.3X4	T49.3X5	T49.3X6
Para-aminophenol derivatives	T39.1X1	T39.1X2	T39.1X3	T39.1X4	T39.1X5	T39.1X6
Para-aminosalicylic acid	T37.1X1	T37.1X2	T37.1X3	T37.1X4	T37.1X5	T37.1X6
Paracetaldehyde	T42.6X1	T42.6X2	T42.6X3	T42.6X4	T42.6X5	T42.6X6
Paracetamol	T39.1X1	T39.1X2	T39.1X3	T39.1X4	T39.1X5	T39.1X6
Parachlorophenol (camphorated)	T49.0X1	T49.0X2	T49.0X3	T49.0X4	T49.0X5	T49.0X6
Paracodin	T40.2X1	T40.2X2	T40.2X3	T40.2X4	T40.2X5	T40.2X6
Paradione	T42.2X1	T42.2X2	T42.2X3	T42.2X4	T42.2X5	T42.2X6
Paraffin(s) (wax)	T52.0X1	T52.0X2	T52.0X3	T52.0X4	—	—
liquid (medicinal)	T47.4X1	T47.4X2	T47.4X3	T47.4X4	T47.4X5	T47.4X6
nonmedicinal	T52.0X1	T52.0X2	T52.0X3	T52.0X4	—	—
Paraformaldehyde	T60.3X1	T60.3X2	T60.3X3	T60.3X4	—	—
Paraldehyde	T42.6X1	T42.6X2	T42.6X3	T42.6X4	T42.6X5	T42.6X6
Paramethadione	T42.2X1	T42.2X2	T42.2X3	T42.2X4	T42.2X5	T42.2X6
Paramethasone	T38.0X1	T38.0X2	T38.0X3	T38.0X4	T38.0X5	T38.0X6
acetate	T49.0X1	T49.0X2	T49.0X3	T49.0X4	T49.0X5	T49.0X6
Paraoxon	T60.0X1	T60.0X2	T60.0X3	T60.0X4	—	—
Paraquat	T60.3X1	T60.3X2	T60.3X3	T60.3X4	—	—
Parasympatholytic NEC	T44.3X1	T44.3X2	T44.3X3	T44.3X4	T44.3X5	T44.3X6
Parasympathomimetic drug NEC	T44.1X1	T44.1X2	T44.1X3	T44.1X4	T44.1X5	T44.1X6
Parathion	T60.0X1	T60.0X2	T60.0X3	T60.0X4	—	—
Parathormone	T50.991	T50.992	T50.993	T50.994	T50.995	T50.996
Parathyroid extract	T50.991	T50.992	T50.993	T50.994	T50.995	T50.996
Paratyphoid vaccine	T50.A91	T50.A92	T50.A93	T50.A94	T50.A95	T50.A96
Paredrine	T44.4X1	T44.4X2	T44.4X3	T44.4X4	T44.4X5	T44.4X6
Paregoric	T40.0X1	T40.0X2	T40.0X3	T40.0X4	T40.0X5	T40.0X6
Pargyline	T46.5X1	T46.5X2	T46.5X3	T46.5X4	T46.5X5	T46.5X6
Paris green	T57.0X1	T57.0X2	T57.0X3	T57.0X4	—	—
insecticide	T57.0X1	T57.0X2	T57.0X3	T57.0X4	—	—
Parnate	T43.1X1	T43.1X2	T43.1X3	T43.1X4	T43.1X5	T43.1X6
Paromomycin	T36.5X1	T36.5X2	T36.5X3	T36.5X4	T36.5X5	T36.5X6
Paroxypropione	T45.1X1	T45.1X2	T45.1X3	T45.1X4	T45.1X5	T45.1X6
Parzone	T40.2X1	T40.2X2	T40.2X3	T40.2X4	T40.2X5	T40.2X6
PAS	T37.1X1	T37.1X2	T37.1X3	T37.1X4	T37.1X5	T37.1X6
Pasiniazid	T37.1X1	T37.1X2	T37.1X3	T37.1X4	T37.1X5	T37.1X6
PBB (polybrominated biphenyls)	T65.891	T65.892	T65.893	T65.894	—	—
PCB	T65.891	T65.892	T65.893	T65.894	—	—
PCP						
meaning pentachlorophenol	T60.1X1	T60.1X2	T60.1X3	T60.1X4	—	—
fungicide	T60.3X1	T60.3X2	T60.3X3	T60.3X4	—	—
herbicide	T60.3X1	T60.3X2	T60.3X3	T60.3X4	—	—
insecticide	T60.1X1	T60.1X2	T60.1X3	T60.1X4	—	—
meaning phencyclidine	T40.991	T40.992	T40.993	T40.994	—	—
Peach kernel oil (emulsion)	T47.4X1	T47.4X2	T47.4X3	T47.4X4	T47.4X5	T47.4X6
Peanut oil (emulsion) NEC	T47.4X1	T47.4X2	T47.4X3	T47.4X4	T47.4X5	T47.4X6
topical	T49.3X1	T49.3X2	T49.3X3	T49.3X4	T49.3X5	T49.3X6

Substance	Poisoning, Accidental (unintentional)	Poisoning, Intentional Self-harm	Poisoning, Assault	Poisoning, Undetermined	Adverse Effect	Under-dosing
Pearly Gates (morning glory seeds)	T40.991	T40.992	T40.993	T40.994	—	—
Pecazine	T43.3X1	T43.3X2	T43.3X3	T43.3X4	T43.3X5	T43.3X6
Pectin	T47.6X1	T47.6X2	T47.6X3	T47.6X4	T47.6X5	T47.6X6
Pefloxacin	T37.8X1	T37.8X2	T37.8X3	T37.8X4	T37.8X5	T37.8X6
Pegademase, bovine	T50.Z91	T50.Z92	T50.Z93	T50.Z94	T50.Z95	T50.Z96
Pelletierine tannate	T37.4X1	T37.4X2	T37.4X3	T37.4X4	T37.4X5	T37.4X6
Pemirolast (potassium)	T48.6X1	T48.6X2	T48.6X3	T48.6X4	T48.6X5	T48.6X6
Pemoline	T50.7X1	T50.7X2	T50.7X3	T50.7X4	T50.7X5	T50.7X6
Pempidine	T44.2X1	T44.2X2	T44.2X3	T44.2X4	T44.2X5	T44.2X6
Penamecillin	T36.0X1	T36.0X2	T36.0X3	T36.0X4	T36.0X5	T36.0X6
Penbutolol	T44.7X1	T44.7X2	T44.7X3	T44.7X4	T44.7X5	T44.7X6
Penethamate	T36.0X1	T36.0X2	T36.0X3	T36.0X4	T36.0X5	T36.0X6
Penfluridol	T43.591	T43.592	T43.593	T43.594	T43.595	T43.596
Penflutizide	T50.2X1	T50.2X2	T50.2X3	T50.2X4	T50.2X5	T50.2X6
Pengitoxin	T46.0X1	T46.0X2	T46.0X3	T46.0X4	T46.0X5	T46.0X6
Penicillamine	T50.6X1	T50.6X2	T50.6X3	T50.6X4	T50.6X5	T50.6X6
Penicillin (any)	T36.0X1	T36.0X2	T36.0X3	T36.0X4	T36.0X5	T36.0X6
Penicillinase	T45.3X1	T45.3X2	T45.3X3	T45.3X4	T45.3X5	T45.3X6
Penicilloyl polylysine	T50.8X1	T50.8X2	T50.8X3	T50.8X4	T50.8X5	T50.8X6
Penimepicycline	T36.4X1	T36.4X2	T36.4X3	T36.4X4	T36.4X5	T36.4X6
Pentachloroethane	T53.6X1	T53.6X2	T53.6X3	T53.6X4	—	—
Pentachloronaphthalene	T53.7X1	T53.7X2	T53.7X3	T53.7X4	—	—
Pentachlorophenol (pesticide)	T60.1X1	T60.1X2	T60.1X3	T60.1X4	—	—
fungicide	T60.3X1	T60.3X2	T60.3X3	T60.3X4	—	—
herbicide	T60.3X1	T60.3X2	T60.3X3	T60.3X4	—	—
insecticide	T60.1X1	T60.1X2	T60.1X3	T60.1X4	—	—
Pentaerythritol	T46.3X1	T46.3X2	T46.3X3	T46.3X4	T46.3X5	T46.3X6
chloral	T42.6X1	T42.6X2	T42.6X3	T42.6X4	T42.6X5	T42.6X6
tetranitrate NEC	T46.3X1	T46.3X2	T46.3X3	T46.3X4	T46.3X5	T46.3X6
Pentaerythrityl tetranitrate	T46.3X1	T46.3X2	T46.3X3	T46.3X4	T46.3X5	T46.3X6
Pentagastrin	T50.8X1	T50.8X2	T50.8X3	T50.8X4	T50.8X5	T50.8X6
Pentalin	T53.6X1	T53.6X2	T53.6X3	T53.6X4	—	—
Pentamethonium bromide	T44.2X1	T44.2X2	T44.2X3	T44.2X4	T44.2X5	T44.2X6
Pentamidine	T37.3X1	T37.3X2	T37.3X3	T37.3X4	T37.3X5	T37.3X6
Pentanol	T51.3X1	T51.3X2	T51.3X3	T51.3X4	—	—
Pentapyrrolinium (bitartrate)	T44.2X1	T44.2X2	T44.2X3	T44.2X4	T44.2X5	T44.2X6
Pentaquine	T37.2X1	T37.2X2	T37.2X3	T37.2X4	T37.2X5	T37.2X6
Pentazocine	T40.4X1	T40.4X2	T40.4X3	T40.4X4	T40.4X5	T40.4X6
Pentetrazole	T50.7X1	T50.7X2	T50.7X3	T50.7X4	T50.7X5	T50.7X6
Penthienate bromide	T44.3X1	T44.3X2	T44.3X3	T44.3X4	T44.3X5	T44.3X6
Pentifylline	T46.7X1	T46.7X2	T46.7X3	T46.7X4	T46.7X5	T46.7X6
Pentobarbital	T42.3X1	T42.3X2	T42.3X3	T42.3X4	T42.3X5	T42.3X6
sodium	T42.3X1	T42.3X2	T42.3X3	T42.3X4	T42.3X5	T42.3X6
Pentobarbitone	T42.3X1	T42.3X2	T42.3X3	T42.3X4	T42.3X5	T42.3X6
Pentolonium tartrate	T44.2X1	T44.2X2	T44.2X3	T44.2X4	T44.2X5	T44.2X6
Pentosan polysulfate (sodium)	T39.8X1	T39.8X2	T39.8X3	T39.8X4	T39.8X5	T39.8X6
Pentostatin	T45.1X1	T45.1X2	T45.1X3	T45.1X4	T45.1X5	T45.1X6
Pentothal	T41.1X1	T41.1X2	T41.1X3	T41.1X4	T41.1X5	T41.1X6
Pentoxifylline	T46.7X1	T46.7X2	T46.7X3	T46.7X4	T46.7X5	T46.7X6
Pentoxyverine	T48.3X1	T48.3X2	T48.3X3	T48.3X4	T48.3X5	T48.3X6
Pentrinat	T46.3X1	T46.3X2	T46.3X3	T46.3X4	T46.3X5	T46.3X6
Pentylenetetrazole	T50.7X1	T50.7X2	T50.7X3	T50.7X4	T50.7X5	T50.7X6
Pentylsalicylamide	T37.1X1	T37.1X2	T37.1X3	T37.1X4	T37.1X5	T37.1X6
Pentymal	T42.3X1	T42.3X2	T42.3X3	T42.3X4	T42.3X5	T42.3X6
Peplomycin	T45.1X1	T45.1X2	T45.1X3	T45.1X4	T45.1X5	T45.1X6
Peppermint (oil)	T47.5X1	T47.5X2	T47.5X3	T47.5X4	T47.5X5	T47.5X6
Pepsin	T47.5X1	T47.5X2	T47.5X3	T47.5X4	T47.5X5	T47.5X6
digestant	T47.5X1	T47.5X2	T47.5X3	T47.5X4	T47.5X5	T47.5X6
Pepstatin	T47.1X1	T47.1X2	T47.1X3	T47.1X4	T47.1X5	T47.1X6
Peptavlon	T50.8X1	T50.8X2	T50.8X3	T50.8X4	T50.8X5	T50.8X6
Perazine	T43.3X1	T43.3X2	T43.3X3	T43.3X4	T43.3X5	T43.3X6
Percaine (spinal)	T41.3X1	T41.3X2	T41.3X3	T41.3X4	T41.3X5	T41.3X6
topical (surface)	T41.3X1	T41.3X2	T41.3X3	T41.3X4	T41.3X5	T41.3X6
Perchloroethylene	T53.3X1	T53.3X2	T53.3X3	T53.3X4	—	—
medicinal	T37.4X1	T37.4X2	T37.4X3	T37.4X4	T37.4X5	T37.4X6
vapor	T53.3X1	T53.3X2	T53.3X3	T53.3X4	—	—
Percodan	T40.2X1	T40.2X2	T40.2X3	T40.2X4	T40.2X5	T40.2X6
Percogesic — *see also* acetaminophen	T45.0X1	T45.0X2	T45.0X3	T45.0X4	T45.0X5	T45.0X6
Percorten	T38.0X1	T38.0X2	T38.0X3	T38.0X4	T38.0X5	T38.0X6
Pergolide	T42.8X1	T42.8X2	T42.8X3	T42.8X4	T42.8X5	T42.8X6
Pergonal	T38.811	T38.812	T38.813	T38.814	T38.815	T38.816
Perhexilene	T46.3X1	T46.3X2	T46.3X3	T46.3X4	T46.3X5	T46.3X6
Perhexiline (maleate)	T46.3X1	T46.3X2	T46.3X3	T46.3X4	T46.3X5	T46.3X6
Periactin	T45.0X1	T45.0X2	T45.0X3	T45.0X4	T45.0X5	T45.0X6
Periciazine	T43.3X1	T43.3X2	T43.3X3	T43.3X4	T43.3X5	T43.3X6
Periclor	T42.6X1	T42.6X2	T42.6X3	T42.6X4	T42.6X5	T42.6X6
Perindopril	T46.4X1	T46.4X2	T46.4X3	T46.4X4	T46.4X5	T46.4X6

Substance	Poisoning, Accidental (unintentional)	Poisoning, Intentional Self-harm	Poisoning, Assault	Poisoning, Undetermined	Adverse Effect	Under-dosing
Perisoxal	T39.8X1	T39.8X2	T39.8X3	T39.8X4	T39.8X5	T39.8X6
Peritoneal dialysis solution	T50.3X1	T50.3X2	T50.3X3	T50.3X4	T50.3X5	T50.3X6
Peritrate	T46.3X1	T46.3X2	T46.3X3	T46.3X4	T46.3X5	T46.3X6
Perlapine	T42.4X1	T42.4X2	T42.4X3	T42.4X4	T42.4X5	T42.4X6
Permanganate	T65.891	T65.892	T65.893	T65.894	—	—
Permethrin	T60.1X1	T60.1X2	T60.1X3	T60.1X4	—	—
Pernocton	T42.3X1	T42.3X2	T42.3X3	T42.3X4	T42.3X5	T42.3X6
Pernoston	T42.3X1	T42.3X2	T42.3X3	T42.3X4	T42.3X5	T42.3X6
Peronine	T40.2X1	T40.2X2	T40.2X3	T40.2X4	—	—
Perphenazine	T43.3X1	T43.3X2	T43.3X3	T43.3X4	T43.3X5	T43.3X6
Pertofrane	T43.011	T43.012	T43.013	T43.014	T43.015	T43.016
Pertussis						
immune serum (human)	T50.Z11	T50.Z12	T50.Z13	T50.Z14	T50.Z15	T50.Z16
vaccine (with diphtheria toxoid) (with tetanus toxoid)	T50.A11	T50.A12	T50.A13	T50.A14	T50.A15	T50.A16
Peruvian balsam	T49.0X1	T49.0X2	T49.0X3	T49.0X4	T49.0X5	T49.0X6
Peruvoside	T46.0X1	T46.0X2	T46.0X3	T46.0X4	T46.0X5	T46.0X6
Pesticide (dust) (fumes) (vapor) **NEC**	T60.91	T60.92	T60.93	T60.94	—	—
arsenic	T57.0X1	T57.0X2	T57.0X3	T57.0X4	—	—
chlorinated	T60.1X1	T60.1X2	T60.1X3	T60.1X4	—	—
cyanide	T65.0X1	T65.0X2	T65.0X3	T65.0X4	—	—
kerosene	T52.0X1	T52.0X2	T52.0X3	T52.0X4	—	—
mixture (of compounds)	T60.91	T60.92	T60.93	T60.94	—	—
naphthalene	T60.2X1	T60.2X2	T60.2X3	T60.2X4	—	—
organochlorine (compounds)	T60.1X1	T60.1X2	T60.1X3	T60.1X4	—	—
petroleum (distillate) (products) NEC	T60.8X1	T60.8X2	T60.8X3	T60.8X4	—	—
specified ingredient NEC	T60.8X1	T60.8X2	T60.8X3	T60.8X4	—	—
strychnine	T65.1X1	T65.1X2	T65.1X3	T65.1X4	—	—
thallium	T60.4X1	T60.4X2	T60.4X3	T60.4X4	—	—
Pethidine	T40.4X1	T40.4X2	T40.4X3	T40.4X4	T40.4X5	T40.4X6
Petrichloral	T42.6X1	T42.6X2	T42.6X3	T42.6X4	T42.6X5	T42.6X6
Petrol	T52.0X1	T52.0X2	T52.0X3	T52.0X4	—	—
vapor	T52.0X1	T52.0X2	T52.0X3	T52.0X4	—	—
Petrolatum	T49.3X1	T49.3X2	T49.3X3	T49.3X4	T49.3X5	T49.3X6
hydrophilic	T49.3X1	T49.3X2	T49.3X3	T49.3X4	T49.3X5	T49.3X6
liquid	T47.4X1	T47.4X2	T47.4X3	T47.4X4	T47.4X5	T47.4X6
topical	T49.3X1	T49.3X2	T49.3X3	T49.3X4	T49.3X5	T49.3X6
nonmedicinal	T52.0X1	T52.0X2	T52.0X3	T52.0X4	—	—
red veterinary	T49.3X1	T49.3X2	T49.3X3	T49.3X4	T49.3X5	T49.3X6
white	T49.3X1	T49.3X2	T49.3X3	T49.3X4	T49.3X5	T49.3X6
Petroleum (products) **NEC**	T52.0X1	T52.0X2	T52.0X3	T52.0X4	—	—
benzine(s) — *see* Ligroin						
ether — *see* Ligroin						
jelly — *see* Petrolatum						
naphtha — *see* Ligroin						
pesticide	T60.8X1	T60.8X2	T60.8X3	T60.8X4	—	—
solids	T52.0X1	T52.0X2	T52.0X3	T52.0X4	—	—
solvents	T52.0X1	T52.0X2	T52.0X3	T52.0X4	—	—
vapor	T52.0X1	T52.0X2	T52.0X3	T52.0X4	—	—
Peyote	T40.991	T40.992	T40.993	T40.994	—	—
Phanodorm, phanodorn	T42.3X1	T42.3X2	T42.3X3	T42.3X4	T42.3X5	T42.3X6
Phanquinone	T37.3X1	T37.3X2	T37.3X3	T37.3X4	T37.3X5	T37.3X6
Phanquone	T37.3X1	T37.3X2	T37.3X3	T37.3X4	T37.3X5	T37.3X6
Pharmaceutical						
adjunct NEC	T50.901	T50.902	T50.903	T50.904	T50.905	T50.906
excipient NEC	T50.901	T50.902	T50.903	T50.904	T50.905	T50.906
sweetener	T50.901	T50.902	T50.903	T50.904	T50.905	T50.906
viscous agent	T50.901	T50.902	T50.903	T50.904	T50.905	T50.906
Phemitone	T42.3X1	T42.3X2	T42.3X3	T42.3X4	T42.3X5	T42.3X6
Phenacaine	T41.3X1	T41.3X2	T41.3X3	T41.3X4	T41.3X5	T41.3X6
Phenacemide	T42.6X1	T42.6X2	T42.6X3	T42.6X4	T42.6X5	T42.6X6
Phenacetin	T39.1X1	T39.1X2	T39.1X3	T39.1X4	T39.1X5	T39.1X6
Phenadoxone	T40.2X1	T40.2X2	T40.2X3	T40.2X4	—	—
Phenaglycodol	T43.591	T43.592	T43.593	T43.594	T43.595	T43.596
Phenantoin	T42.0X1	T42.0X2	T42.0X3	T42.0X4	T42.0X5	T42.0X6
Phenaphthazine reagent	T50.991	T50.992	T50.993	T50.994	T50.995	T50.996
Phenazocine	T40.4X1	T40.4X2	T40.4X3	T40.4X4	T40.4X5	T40.4X6
Phenazone	T39.2X1	T39.2X2	T39.2X3	T39.2X4	T39.2X5	T39.2X6
Phenazopyridine	T39.8X1	T39.8X2	T39.8X3	T39.8X4	T39.8X5	T39.8X6
Phenbenicillin	T36.0X1	T36.0X2	T36.0X3	T36.0X4	T36.0X5	T36.0X6
Phenbutrazate	T50.5X1	T50.5X2	T50.5X3	T50.5X4	T50.5X5	T50.5X6
Phencyclidine	T40.991	T40.992	T40.993	T40.994	T40.995	T40.996
Phendimetrazine	T50.5X1	T50.5X2	T50.5X3	T50.5X4	T50.5X5	T50.5X6
Phenelzine	T43.1X1	T43.1X2	T43.1X3	T43.1X4	T43.1X5	T43.1X6
Phenemal	T42.3X1	T42.3X2	T42.3X3	T42.3X4	T42.3X5	T42.3X6
Phenergan	T42.6X1	T42.6X2	T42.6X3	T42.6X4	T42.6X5	T42.6X6
Pheneticillin	T36.0X1	T36.0X2	T36.0X3	T36.0X4	T36.0X5	T36.0X6
Pheneturide	T42.6X1	T42.6X2	T42.6X3	T42.6X4	T42.6X5	T42.6X6
Phenformin	T38.3X1	T38.3X2	T38.3X3	T38.3X4	T38.3X5	T38.3X6

Substance	Poisoning, Accidental (unintentional)	Poisoning, Intentional Self-harm	Poisoning, Assault	Poisoning, Undetermined	Adverse Effect	Under-dosing
Phenglutarimide	T44.3X1	T44.3X2	T44.3X3	T44.3X4	T44.3X5	T44.3X6
Phenicarbazide	T39.8X1	T39.8X2	T39.8X3	T39.8X4	T39.8X5	T39.8X6
Phenindamine	T45.0X1	T45.0X2	T45.0X3	T45.0X4	T45.0X5	T45.0X6
Phenindione	T45.511	T45.512	T45.513	T45.514	T45.515	T45.516
Pheniprazine	T43.1X1	T43.1X2	T43.1X3	T43.1X4	T43.1X5	T43.1X6
Pheniramine	T45.0X1	T45.0X2	T45.0X3	T45.0X4	T45.0X5	T45.0X6
Phenisatin	T47.2X1	T47.2X2	T47.2X3	T47.2X4	T47.2X5	T47.2X6
Phenmetrazine	T50.5X1	T50.5X2	T50.5X3	T50.5X4	T50.5X5	T50.5X6
Phenobal	T42.3X1	T42.3X2	T42.3X3	T42.3X4	T42.3X5	T42.3X6
Phenobarbital	T42.3X1	T42.3X2	T42.3X3	T42.3X4	T42.3X5	T42.3X6
with						
mephenytoin	T42.3X1	T42.3X2	T42.3X3	T42.3X4	T42.3X5	T42.3X6
phenytoin	T42.3X1	T42.3X2	T42.3X3	T42.3X4	T42.3X5	T42.3X6
sodium	T42.3X1	T42.3X2	T42.3X3	T42.3X4	T42.3X5	T42.3X6
Phenobarbitone	T42.3X1	T42.3X2	T42.3X3	T42.3X4	T42.3X5	T42.3X6
Phenobutiodil	T50.8X1	T50.8X2	T50.8X3	T50.8X4	T50.8X5	T50.8X6
Phenoctide	T49.0X1	T49.0X2	T49.0X3	T49.0X4	T49.0X5	T49.0X6
Phenol	T49.0X1	T49.0X2	T49.0X3	T49.0X4	T49.0X5	T49.0X6
disinfectant	T54.0X1	T54.0X2	T54.0X3	T54.0X4	—	—
in oil injection	T46.8X1	T46.8X2	T46.8X3	T46.8X4	T46.8X5	T46.8X6
medicinal	T49.1X1	T49.1X2	T49.1X3	T49.1X4	T49.1X5	T49.1X6
nonmedicinal NEC	T54.0X1	T54.0X2	T54.0X3	T54.0X4	—	—
pesticide	T60.8X1	T60.8X2	T60.8X3	T60.8X4	—	—
red	T50.8X1	T50.8X2	T50.8X3	T50.8X4	T50.8X5	T50.8X6
Phenolic preparation	T49.1X1	T49.1X2	T49.1X3	T49.1X4	T49.1X5	T49.1X6
Phenolphthalein	T47.2X1	T47.2X2	T47.2X3	T47.2X4	T47.2X5	T47.2X6
Phenolsulfonphthalein	T50.8X1	T50.8X2	T50.8X3	T50.8X4	T50.8X5	T50.8X6
Phenomorphan	T40.2X1	T40.2X2	T40.2X3	T40.2X4	T40.2X5	T40.2X6
Phenonyl	T42.3X1	T42.3X2	T42.3X3	T42.3X4	T42.3X5	T42.3X6
Phenoperidine	T40.4X1	T40.4X2	T40.4X3	T40.4X4	T40.4X5	T40.4X6
Phenopyrazone	T46.991	T46.992	T46.993	T46.994	T46.995	T46.996
Phenoquin	T50.4X1	T50.4X2	T50.4X3	T50.4X4	T50.4X5	T50.4X6
Phenothiazine (psychotropic)	T43.3X1	T43.3X2	T43.3X3	T43.3X4	T43.3X5	T43.3X6
NEC						
insecticide	T60.2X1	T60.2X2	T60.2X3	T60.2X4	—	—
Phenothrin	T49.0X1	T49.0X2	T49.0X3	T49.0X4	T49.0X5	T49.0X6
Phenoxybenzamine	T46.7X1	T46.7X2	T46.7X3	T46.7X4	T46.7X5	T46.7X6
Phenoxyethanol	T49.0X1	T49.0X2	T49.0X3	T49.0X4	T49.0X5	T49.0X6
Phenoxymethyl penicillin	T36.0X1	T36.0X2	T36.0X3	T36.0X4	T36.0X5	T36.0X6
Phenprobamate	T42.8X1	T42.8X2	T42.8X3	T42.8X4	T42.8X5	T42.8X6
Phenprocoumon	T45.511	T45.512	T45.513	T45.514	T45.515	T45.516
Phensuximide	T42.2X1	T42.2X2	T42.2X3	T42.2X4	T42.2X5	T42.2X6
Phentermine	T50.5X1	T50.5X2	T50.5X3	T50.5X4	T50.5X5	T50.5X6
Phenthicillin	T36.0X1	T36.0X2	T36.0X3	T36.0X4	T36.0X5	T36.0X6
Phentolamine	T46.7X1	T46.7X2	T46.7X3	T46.7X4	T46.7X5	T46.7X6
Phenyl						
butazone	T39.2X1	T39.2X2	T39.2X3	T39.2X4	T39.2X5	T39.2X6
enediamine	T65.3X1	T65.3X2	T65.3X3	T65.3X4	—	—
hydrazine	T65.3X1	T65.3X2	T65.3X3	T65.3X4	—	—
antineoplastic	T45.1X1	T45.1X2	T45.1X3	T45.1X4	T45.1X5	T45.1X6
mercuric compounds — *see* Mercury						
salicylate	T49.3X1	T49.3X2	T49.3X3	T49.3X4	T49.3X5	T49.3X6
Phenylalanine mustard	T45.1X1	T45.1X2	T45.1X3	T45.1X4	T45.1X5	T45.1X6
Phenylbutazone	T39.2X1	T39.2X2	T39.2X3	T39.2X4	T39.2X5	T39.2X6
Phenylenediamine	T65.3X1	T65.3X2	T65.3X3	T65.3X4	—	—
Phenylephrine	T44.4X1	T44.4X2	T44.4X3	T44.4X4	T44.4X5	T44.4X6
Phenylethylbiguanide	T38.3X1	T38.3X2	T38.3X3	T38.3X4	T38.3X5	T38.3X6
Phenylmercuric						
acetate	T49.0X1	T49.0X2	T49.0X3	T49.0X4	T49.0X5	T49.0X6
borate	T49.0X1	T49.0X2	T49.0X3	T49.0X4	T49.0X5	T49.0X6
nitrate	T49.0X1	T49.0X2	T49.0X3	T49.0X4	T49.0X5	T49.0X6
Phenylmethylbarbitone	T42.3X1	T42.3X2	T42.3X3	T42.3X4	T42.3X5	T42.3X6
Phenylpropanol	T47.5X1	T47.5X2	T47.5X3	T47.5X4	T47.5X5	T47.5X6
Phenylpropanolamine	T44.991	T44.992	T44.993	T44.994	T44.995	T44.996
Phenylsulfthion	T60.0X1	T60.0X2	T60.0X3	T60.0X4	—	—
Phenyltoloxamine	T45.0X1	T45.0X2	T45.0X3	T45.0X4	T45.0X5	T45.0X6
Phenyramidol, phenyramidon	T39.8X1	T39.8X2	T39.8X3	T39.8X4	T39.8X5	T39.8X6
Phenytoin	T42.0X1	T42.0X2	T42.0X3	T42.0X4	T42.0X5	T42.0X6
with Phenobarbital	T42.3X1	T42.3X2	T42.3X3	T42.3X4	T42.3X5	T42.3X6
pHisoHex	T49.2X1	T49.2X2	T49.2X3	T49.2X4	T49.2X5	T49.2X6
Pholcodine	T48.3X1	T48.3X2	T48.3X3	T48.3X4	T48.3X5	T48.3X6
Pholedrine	T46.991	T46.992	T46.993	T46.994	T46.995	T46.996
Phorate	T60.0X1	T60.0X2	T60.0X3	T60.0X4	—	—
Phosdrin	T60.0X1	T60.0X2	T60.0X3	T60.0X4	—	—
Phosfolan	T60.0X1	T60.0X2	T60.0X3	T60.0X4	—	—
Phosgene (gas)	T59.891	T59.892	T59.893	T59.894	—	—
Phosphamidon	T60.0X1	T60.0X2	T60.0X3	T60.0X4	—	—
Phosphate	T65.891	T65.892	T65.893	T65.894	—	—
laxative	T47.4X1	T47.4X2	T47.4X3	T47.4X4	T47.4X5	T47.4X6
organic	T60.0X1	T60.0X2	T60.0X3	T60.0X4	—	—
solvent	T52.91	T52.92	T52.93	T52.94	—	—
Phosphate — *continued*						
tricresyl	T65.891	T65.892	T65.893	T65.894	—	—
Phosphine	T57.1X1	T57.1X2	T57.1X3	T57.1X4	—	—
fumigant	T57.1X1	T57.1X2	T57.1X3	T57.1X4	—	—
Phospholine	T49.5X1	T49.5X2	T49.5X3	T49.5X4	T49.5X5	T49.5X6
Phosphoric acid	T54.2X1	T54.2X2	T54.2X3	T54.2X4	—	—
Phosphorus (compound) **NEC**	T57.1X1	T57.1X2	T57.1X3	T57.1X4	—	—
pesticide	T60.0X1	T60.0X2	T60.0X3	T60.0X4	—	—
Phthalates	T65.891	T65.892	T65.893	T65.894	—	—
Phthalic anhydride	T65.891	T65.892	T65.893	T65.894	—	—
Phthalimidoglutarimide	T42.6X1	T42.6X2	T42.6X3	T42.6X4	T42.6X5	T42.6X6
Phthalylsulfathiazole	T37.0X1	T37.0X2	T37.0X3	T37.0X4	T37.0X5	T37.0X6
Phylloquinone	T45.7X1	T45.7X2	T45.7X3	T45.7X4	T45.7X5	T45.7X6
Physeptone	T40.3X1	T40.3X2	T40.3X3	T40.3X4	T40.3X5	T40.3X6
Physostigma venenosum	T62.2X1	T62.2X2	T62.2X3	T62.2X4	—	—
Physostigmine	T49.5X1	T49.5X2	T49.5X3	T49.5X4	T49.5X5	T49.5X6
Phytolacca decandra	T62.2X1	T62.2X2	T62.2X3	T62.2X4	—	—
berries	T62.1X1	T62.1X2	T62.1X3	T62.1X4	—	—
Phytomenadione	T45.7X1	T45.7X2	T45.7X3	T45.7X4	T45.7X5	T45.7X6
Phytonadione	T45.7X1	T45.7X2	T45.7X3	T45.7X4	T45.7X5	T45.7X6
Picoperine	T48.3X1	T48.3X2	T48.3X3	T48.3X4	T48.3X5	T48.3X6
Picosulfate (sodium)	T47.2X1	T47.2X2	T47.2X3	T47.2X4	T47.2X5	T47.2X6
Picric (acid)	T54.2X1	T54.2X2	T54.2X3	T54.2X4	—	—
Picrotoxin	T50.7X1	T50.7X2	T50.7X3	T50.7X4	T50.7X5	T50.7X6
Piketoprofen	T49.0X1	T49.0X2	T49.0X3	T49.0X4	T49.0X5	T49.0X6
Pilocarpine	T44.1X1	T44.1X2	T44.1X3	T44.1X4	T44.1X5	T44.1X6
Pilocarpus (jaborandi) extract	T44.1X1	T44.1X2	T44.1X3	T44.1X4	T44.1X5	T44.1X6
Pilsicainide (hydrochloride)	T46.2X1	T46.2X2	T46.2X3	T46.2X4	T46.2X5	T46.2X6
Pimaricin	T36.7X1	T36.7X2	T36.7X3	T36.7X4	T36.7X5	T36.7X6
Pimeclone	T50.7X1	T50.7X2	T50.7X3	T50.7X4	T50.7X5	T50.7X6
Pimelic ketone	T52.8X1	T52.8X2	T52.8X3	T52.8X4	—	—
Pimethixene	T45.0X1	T45.0X2	T45.0X3	T45.0X4	T45.0X5	T45.0X6
Piminodine	T40.2X1	T40.2X2	T40.2X3	T40.2X4	T40.2X5	T40.2X6
Pimozide	T43.591	T43.592	T43.593	T43.594	T43.595	T43.596
Pinacidil	T46.5X1	T46.5X2	T46.5X3	T46.5X4	T46.5X5	T46.5X6
Pinaverium bromide	T44.3X1	T44.3X2	T44.3X3	T44.3X4	T44.3X5	T44.3X6
Pinazepam	T42.4X1	T42.4X2	T42.4X3	T42.4X4	T42.4X5	T42.4X6
Pindolol	T44.7X1	T44.7X2	T44.7X3	T44.7X4	T44.7X5	T44.7X6
Pindone	T60.4X1	T60.4X2	T60.4X3	T60.4X4	—	—
Pine oil (disinfectant)	T65.891	T65.892	T65.893	T65.894	—	—
Pinkroot	T37.4X1	T37.4X2	T37.4X3	T37.4X4	T37.4X5	T37.4X6
Pipadone	T40.2X1	T40.2X2	T40.2X3	T40.2X4	—	—
Pipamazine	T45.0X1	T45.0X2	T45.0X3	T45.0X4	T45.0X5	T45.0X6
Pipamperone	T43.4X1	T43.4X2	T43.4X3	T43.4X4	T43.4X5	T43.4X6
Pipazetate	T48.3X1	T48.3X2	T48.3X3	T48.3X4	T48.3X5	T48.3X6
Pipemidic acid	T37.8X1	T37.8X2	T37.8X3	T37.8X4	T37.8X5	T37.8X6
Pipenzolate bromide	T44.3X1	T44.3X2	T44.3X3	T44.3X4	T44.3X5	T44.3X6
Piperacetazine	T43.3X1	T43.3X2	T43.3X3	T43.3X4	T43.3X5	T43.3X6
Piperacillin	T36.0X1	T36.0X2	T36.0X3	T36.0X4	T36.0X5	T36.0X6
Piperazine	T37.4X1	T37.4X2	T37.4X3	T37.4X4	T37.4X5	T37.4X6
estrone sulfate	T38.5X1	T38.5X2	T38.5X3	T38.5X4	T38.5X5	T38.5X6
Piper cubeba	T62.2X1	T62.2X2	T62.2X3	T62.2X4	—	—
Piperidione	T48.3X1	T48.3X2	T48.3X3	T48.3X4	T48.3X5	T48.3X6
Piperidolate	T44.3X1	T44.3X2	T44.3X3	T44.3X4	T44.3X5	T44.3X6
Piperocaine	T41.3X1	T41.3X2	T41.3X3	T41.3X4	T41.3X5	T41.3X6
infiltration (subcutaneous)	T41.3X1	T41.3X2	T41.3X3	T41.3X4	T41.3X5	T41.3X6
nerve block (peripheral) (plexus)	T41.3X1	T41.3X2	T41.3X3	T41.3X4	T41.3X5	T41.3X6
topical (surface)	T41.3X1	T41.3X2	T41.3X3	T41.3X4	T41.3X5	T41.3X6
Piperonyl butoxide	T60.8X1	T60.8X2	T60.8X3	T60.8X4	—	—
Pipethanate	T44.3X1	T44.3X2	T44.3X3	T44.3X4	T44.3X5	T44.3X6
Pipobroman	T45.1X1	T45.1X2	T45.1X3	T45.1X4	T45.1X5	T45.1X6
Pipotiazine	T43.3X1	T43.3X2	T43.3X3	T43.3X4	T43.3X5	T43.3X6
Pipoxizine	T45.0X1	T45.0X2	T45.0X3	T45.0X4	T45.0X5	T45.0X6
Pipradrol	T43.691	T43.692	T43.693	T43.694	T43.695	T43.696
Piprinhydrinate	T45.0X1	T45.0X2	T45.0X3	T45.0X4	T45.0X5	T45.0X6
Pirarubicin	T45.1X1	T45.1X2	T45.1X3	T45.1X4	T45.1X5	T45.1X6
Pirazinamide	T37.1X1	T37.1X2	T37.1X3	T37.1X4	T37.1X5	T37.1X6
Pirbuterol	T48.6X1	T48.6X2	T48.6X3	T48.6X4	T48.6X5	T48.6X6
Pirenzepine	T47.1X1	T47.1X2	T47.1X3	T47.1X4	T47.1X5	T47.1X6
Piretanide	T50.1X1	T50.1X2	T50.1X3	T50.1X4	T50.1X5	T50.1X6
Piribedil	T42.8X1	T42.8X2	T42.8X3	T42.8X4	T42.8X5	T42.8X6
Piridoxilate	T46.3X1	T46.3X2	T46.3X3	T46.3X4	T46.3X5	T46.3X6
Piritramide	T40.4X1	T40.4X2	T40.4X3	T40.4X4	—	—
Piromidic acid	T37.8X1	T37.8X2	T37.8X3	T37.8X4	T37.8X5	T37.8X6
Piroxicam	T39.391	T39.392	T39.393	T39.394	T39.395	T39.396
beta-cyclodextrin complex	T39.8X1	T39.8X2	T39.8X3	T39.8X4	T39.8X5	T39.8X6
Pirozadil	T46.6X1	T46.6X2	T46.6X3	T46.6X4	T46.6X5	T46.6X6
Piscidia (bark) (erythrina)	T39.8X1	T39.8X2	T39.8X3	T39.8X4	T39.8X5	T39.8X6
Pitch	T65.891	T65.892	T65.893	T65.894	—	—
Pitkin's solution	T41.3X1	T41.3X2	T41.3X3	T41.3X4	T41.3X5	T41.3X6

Substance	Poisoning, Accidental (unintentional)	Poisoning, Intentional Self-harm	Poisoning, Assault	Poisoning, Undetermined	Adverse Effect	Under-dosing
Pitocin	T48.0X1	T48.0X2	T48.0X3	T48.0X4	T48.0X5	T48.0X6
Pitressin (tannate)	T38.891	T38.892	T38.893	T38.894	T38.895	T38.896
Pituitary extracts	T38.891	T38.892	T38.893	T38.894	T38.895	T38.896
(posterior)						
anterior	T38.811	T38.812	T38.813	T38.814	T38.815	T38.816
Pituitrin	T38.891	T38.892	T38.893	T38.894	T38.895	T38.896
Pivampicillin	T36.0X1	T36.0X2	T36.0X3	T36.0X4	T36.0X5	T36.0X6
Pivmecillinam	T36.0X1	T36.0X2	T36.0X3	T36.0X4	T36.0X5	T36.0X6
Placental hormone	T38.891	T38.892	T38.893	T38.894	T38.895	T38.896
Placidyl	T42.6X1	T42.6X2	T42.6X3	T42.6X4	T42.6X5	T42.6X6
Plague vaccine	T50.A91	T50.A92	T50.A93	T50.A94	T50.A95	T50.A96
Plant						
food or fertilizer NEC	T65.891	T65.892	T65.893	T65.894	—	—
containing herbicide	T60.3X1	T60.3X2	T60.3X3	T60.3X4	—	—
noxious, used as food	T62.2X1	T62.2X2	T62.2X3	T62.2X4	—	—
berries	T62.1X1	T62.1X2	T62.1X3	T62.1X4	—	—
seeds	T62.2X1	T62.2X2	T62.2X3	T62.2X4	—	—
specified type NEC	T62.2X1	T62.2X2	T62.2X3	T62.2X4	—	—
Plasma	T45.8X1	T45.8X2	T45.8X3	T45.8X4	T45.8X5	T45.8X6
expander NEC	T45.8X1	T45.8X2	T45.8X3	T45.8X4	T45.8X5	T45.8X6
protein fraction (human)	T45.8X1	T45.8X2	T45.8X3	T45.8X4	T45.8X5	T45.8X6
Plasmanate	T45.8X1	T45.8X2	T45.8X3	T45.8X4	T45.8X5	T45.8X6
Plasminogen (tissue)	T45.611	T45.612	T45.613	T45.614	T45.615	T45.616
activator						
Plaster dressing	T49.3X1	T49.3X2	T49.3X3	T49.3X4	T49.3X5	T49.3X6
Plastic dressing	T49.3X1	T49.3X2	T49.3X3	T49.3X4	T49.3X5	T49.3X6
Plegicil	T43.3X1	T43.3X2	T43.3X3	T43.3X4	T43.3X5	T43.3X6
Plicamycin	T45.1X1	T45.1X2	T45.1X3	T45.1X4	T45.1X5	T45.1X6
Podophyllotoxin	T49.8X1	T49.8X2	T49.8X3	T49.8X4	T49.8X5	T49.8X6
Podophyllum (resin)	T49.4X1	T49.4X2	T49.4X3	T49.4X4	T49.4X5	T49.4X6
Poisonous berries	T62.1X1	T62.1X2	T62.1X3	T62.1X4	—	—
Poison NEC	T65.91	T65.92	T65.93	T65.94	—	—
Pokeweed (any part)	T62.2X1	T62.2X2	T62.2X3	T62.2X4	—	—
Poldine metilsulfate	T44.3X1	T44.3X2	T44.3X3	T44.3X4	T44.3X5	T44.3X6
Polidexide (sulfate)	T46.6X1	T46.6X2	T46.6X3	T46.6X4	T46.6X5	T46.6X6
Polidocanol	T46.8X1	T46.8X2	T46.8X3	T46.8X4	T46.8X5	T46.8X6
Poliomyelitis vaccine	T50.B91	T50.B92	T50.B93	T50.B94	T50.B95	T50.B96
Polish (car) (floor) (furniture)	T65.891	T65.892	T65.893	T65.894	—	—
(metal) (porcelain)						
(silver)						
abrasive	T65.891	T65.892	T65.893	T65.894	—	—
porcelain	T65.891	T65.892	T65.893	T65.894	—	—
Poloxalkol	T47.4X1	T47.4X2	T47.4X3	T47.4X4	T47.4X5	T47.4X6
Poloxamer	T47.4X1	T47.4X2	T47.4X3	T47.4X4	T47.4X5	T47.4X6
Polyaminostyrene resins	T50.3X1	T50.3X2	T50.3X3	T50.3X4	T50.3X5	T50.3X6
Polycarbophil	T47.4X1	T47.4X2	T47.4X3	T47.4X4	T47.4X5	T47.4X6
Polychlorinated biphenyl	T65.891	T65.892	T65.893	T65.894	—	—
Polycycline	T36.4X1	T36.4X2	T36.4X3	T36.4X4	T36.4X5	T36.4X6
Polyester fumes	T59.891	T59.892	T59.893	T59.894	—	—
Polyester resin hardener	T52.91	T52.92	T52.93	T52.94	—	—
fumes	T59.891	T59.892	T59.893	T59.894	—	—
Polyestradiol phosphate	T38.5X1	T38.5X2	T38.5X3	T38.5X4	T38.5X5	T38.5X6
Polyethanolamine alkyl	T49.2X1	T49.2X2	T49.2X3	T49.2X4	T49.2X5	T49.2X6
sulfate						
Polyethylene adhesive	T49.3X1	T49.3X2	T49.3X3	T49.3X4	T49.3X5	T49.3X6
Polyferose	T45.4X1	T45.4X2	T45.4X3	T45.4X4	T45.4X5	T45.4X6
Polygeline	T45.8X1	T45.8X2	T45.8X3	T45.8X4	T45.8X5	T45.8X6
Polymyxin	T36.8X1	T36.8X2	T36.8X3	T36.8X4	T36.8X5	T36.8X6
B	T36.8X1	T36.8X2	T36.8X3	T36.8X4	T36.8X5	T36.8X6
ENT agent	T49.6X1	T49.6X2	T49.6X3	T49.6X4	T49.6X5	T49.6X6
ophthalmic preparation	T49.5X1	T49.5X2	T49.5X3	T49.5X4	T49.5X5	T49.5X6
topical NEC	T49.0X1	T49.0X2	T49.0X3	T49.0X4	T49.0X5	T49.0X6
E sulfate (eye preparation)	T49.5X1	T49.5X2	T49.5X3	T49.5X4	T49.5X5	T49.5X6
Polynoxylin	T49.0X1	T49.0X2	T49.0X3	T49.0X4	T49.0X5	T49.0X6
Polyoestradiol phosphate	T38.5X1	T38.5X2	T38.5X3	T38.5X4	T38.5X5	T38.5X6
Polyoxymethyleneurea	T49.0X1	T49.0X2	T49.0X3	T49.0X4	T49.0X5	T49.0X6
Polysilane	T47.8X1	T47.8X2	T47.8X3	T47.8X4	T47.8X5	T47.8X6
Polytetrafluoroethylene	T59.891	T59.892	T59.893	T59.894	—	—
(inhaled)						
Polythiazide	T50.2X1	T50.2X2	T50.2X3	T50.2X4	T50.2X5	T50.2X6
Polyvidone	T45.8X1	T45.8X2	T45.8X3	T45.8X4	T45.8X5	T45.8X6
Polyvinylpyrrolidone	T45.8X1	T45.8X2	T45.8X3	T45.8X4	T45.8X5	T45.8X6
Pontocaine (hydrochloride)	T41.3X1	T41.3X2	T41.3X3	T41.3X4	T41.3X5	T41.3X6
(infiltration) (topical)						
nerve block (peripheral)	T41.3X1	T41.3X2	T41.3X3	T41.3X4	T41.3X5	T41.3X6
(plexus)						
spinal	T41.3X1	T41.3X2	T41.3X3	T41.3X4	T41.3X5	T41.3X6
Porfiromycin	T45.1X1	T45.1X2	T45.1X3	T45.1X4	T45.1X5	T45.1X6
Posterior pituitary hormone NEC	T38.891	T38.892	T38.893	T38.894	T38.895	T38.896
Pot	T40.7X1	T40.7X2	T40.7X3	T40.7X4	T40.7X5	T40.7X6
Potash (caustic)	T54.3X1	T54.3X2	T54.3X3	T54.3X4	—	—

Substance	Poisoning, Accidental (unintentional)	Poisoning, Intentional Self-harm	Poisoning, Assault	Poisoning, Undetermined	Adverse Effect	Under-dosing
Potassic saline injection	T50.3X1	T50.3X2	T50.3X3	T50.3X4	T50.3X5	T50.3X6
(lactated)						
Potassium (salts) **NEC**	T50.3X1	T50.3X2	T50.3X3	T50.3X4	T50.3X5	T50.3X6
aminobenzoate	T45.8X1	T45.8X2	T45.8X3	T45.8X4	T45.8X5	T45.8X6
aminosalicylate	T37.1X1	T37.1X2	T37.1X3	T37.1X4	T37.1X5	T37.1X6
antimony ' tartrate'	T37.8X1	T37.8X2	T37.8X3	T37.8X4	T37.8X5	T37.8X6
arsenite (solution)	T57.0X1	T57.0X2	T57.0X3	T57.0X4	—	—
bichromate	T56.2X1	T56.2X2	T56.2X3	T56.2X4	—	—
bisulfate	T47.3X1	T47.3X2	T47.3X3	T47.3X4	T47.3X5	T47.3X6
bromide	T42.6X1	T42.6X2	T42.6X3	T42.6X4	T42.6X5	T42.6X6
canrenoate	T50.0X1	T50.0X2	T50.0X3	T50.0X4	T50.0X5	T50.0X6
carbonate	T54.3X1	T54.3X2	T54.3X3	T54.3X4	—	—
chlorate NEC	T65.891	T65.892	T65.893	T65.894	—	—
chloride	T50.3X1	T50.3X2	T50.3X3	T50.3X4	T50.3X5	T50.3X6
citrate	T50.991	T50.992	T50.993	T50.994	T50.995	T50.996
cyanide	T65.0X1	T65.0X2	T65.0X3	T65.0X4	—	—
ferric hexacyanoferrate	T50.6X1	T50.6X2	T50.6X3	T50.6X4	T50.6X5	T50.6X6
(medicinal)						
nonmedicinal	T65.891	T65.892	T65.893	T65.894	—	—
Fluoride	T57.8X1	T57.8X2	T57.8X3	T57.8X4	—	—
glucaldrate	T47.1X1	T47.1X2	T47.1X3	T47.1X4	T47.1X5	T47.1X6
hydroxide	T54.3X1	T54.3X2	T54.3X3	T54.3X4	—	—
iodate	T49.0X1	T49.0X2	T49.0X3	T49.0X4	T49.0X5	T49.0X6
iodide	T48.4X1	T48.4X2	T48.4X3	T48.4X4	T48.4X5	T48.4X6
nitrate	T57.8X1	T57.8X2	T57.8X3	T57.8X4	—	—
oxalate	T65.891	T65.892	T65.893	T65.894	—	—
perchlorate (nonmedicinal) NEC	T65.891	T65.892	T65.893	T65.894	—	—
antithyroid	T38.2X1	T38.2X2	T38.2X3	T38.2X4	T38.2X5	T38.2X6
medicinal	T38.2X1	T38.2X2	T38.2X3	T38.2X4	T38.2X5	T38.2X6
Permanganate (nonmedicinal)	T65.891	T65.892	T65.893	T65.894	—	—
medicinal	T49.0X1	T49.0X2	T49.0X3	T49.0X4	T49.0X5	T49.0X6
sulfate	T47.2X1	T47.2X2	T47.2X3	T47.2X4	T47.2X5	T47.2X6
Potassium-removing resin	T50.3X1	T50.3X2	T50.3X3	T50.3X4	T50.3X5	T50.3X6
Potassium-retaining drug	T50.3X1	T50.3X2	T50.3X3	T50.3X4	T50.3X5	T50.3X6
Povidone	T45.8X1	T45.8X2	T45.8X3	T45.8X4	T45.8X5	T45.8X6
iodine	T49.0X1	T49.0X2	T49.0X3	T49.0X4	T49.0X5	T49.0X6
Practolol	T44.7X1	T44.7X2	T44.7X3	T44.7X4	T44.7X5	T44.7X6
Prajmalium bitartrate	T46.2X1	T46.2X2	T46.2X3	T46.2X4	T46.2X5	T46.2X6
Pralidoxime (iodide)	T50.6X1	T50.6X2	T50.6X3	T50.6X4	T50.6X5	T50.6X6
chloride	T50.6X1	T50.6X2	T50.6X3	T50.6X4	T50.6X5	T50.6X6
Pramiverine	T44.3X1	T44.3X2	T44.3X3	T44.3X4	T44.3X5	T44.3X6
Pramocaine	T49.1X1	T49.1X2	T49.1X3	T49.1X4	T49.1X5	T49.1X6
Pramoxine	T49.1X1	T49.1X2	T49.1X3	T49.1X4	T49.1X5	T49.1X6
Prasterone	T38.7X1	T38.7X2	T38.7X3	T38.7X4	T38.7X5	T38.7X6
Pravastatin	T46.6X1	T46.6X2	T46.6X3	T46.6X4	T46.6X5	T46.6X6
Prazepam	T42.4X1	T42.4X2	T42.4X3	T42.4X4	T42.4X5	T42.4X6
Praziquantel	T37.4X1	T37.4X2	T37.4X3	T37.4X4	T37.4X5	T37.4X6
Prazitone	T43.291	T43.292	T43.293	T43.294	T43.295	T43.296
Prazosin	T44.6X1	T44.6X2	T44.6X3	T44.6X4	T44.6X5	T44.6X6
Prednicarbate	T49.0X1	T49.0X2	T49.0X3	T49.0X4	T49.0X5	T49.0X6
Prednimustine	T45.1X1	T45.1X2	T45.1X3	T45.1X4	T45.1X5	T45.1X6
Prednisolone	T38.0X1	T38.0X2	T38.0X3	T38.0X4	T38.0X5	T38.0X6
ENT agent	T49.6X1	T49.6X2	T49.6X3	T49.6X4	T49.6X5	T49.6X6
ophthalmic preparation	T49.5X1	T49.5X2	T49.5X3	T49.5X4	T49.5X5	T49.5X6
steaglate	T49.0X1	T49.0X2	T49.0X3	T49.0X4	T49.0X5	T49.0X6
topical NEC	T49.0X1	T49.0X2	T49.0X3	T49.0X4	T49.0X5	T49.0X6
Prednisone	T38.0X1	T38.0X2	T38.0X3	T38.0X4	T38.0X5	T38.0X6
Prednylidene	T38.0X1	T38.0X2	T38.0X3	T38.0X4	T38.0X5	T38.0X6
Pregnandiol	T38.5X1	T38.5X2	T38.5X3	T38.5X4	T38.5X5	T38.5X6
Pregneninolone	T38.5X1	T38.5X2	T38.5X3	T38.5X4	T38.5X5	T38.5X6
Preludin	T43.691	T43.692	T43.693	T43.694	T43.695	T43.696
Premarin	T38.5X1	T38.5X2	T38.5X3	T38.5X4	T38.5X5	T38.5X6
Premedication anesthetic	T41.201	T41.202	T41.203	T41.204	T41.205	T41.206
Prenalterol	T44.5X1	T44.5X2	T44.5X3	T44.5X4	T44.5X5	T44.5X6
Prenoxdiazine	T48.3X1	T48.3X2	T48.3X3	T48.3X4	T48.3X5	T48.3X6
Prenylamine	T46.3X1	T46.3X2	T46.3X3	T46.3X4	T46.3X5	T46.3X6
Preparation H	T49.8X1	T49.8X2	T49.8X3	T49.8X4	T49.8X5	T49.8X6
Preparation, local	T49.4X1	T49.4X2	T49.4X3	T49.4X4	T49.4X5	T49.4X6
Preservative (nonmedicinal)	T65.891	T65.892	T65.893	T65.894	—	—
medicinal	T50.901	T50.902	T50.903	T50.904	T50.905	T50.906
wood	T60.91	T60.92	T60.93	T60.94	—	—
Prethcamide	T50.7X1	T50.7X2	T50.7X3	T50.7X4	T50.7X5	T50.7X6
Pride of China	T62.2X1	T62.2X2	T62.2X3	T62.2X4	—	—
Pridinol	T44.3X1	T44.3X2	T44.3X3	T44.3X4	T44.3X5	T44.3X6
Prifinium bromide	T44.3X1	T44.3X2	T44.3X3	T44.3X4	T44.3X5	T44.3X6
Prilocaine	T41.3X1	T41.3X2	T41.3X3	T41.3X4	T41.3X5	T41.3X6
infiltration (subcutaneous)	T41.3X1	T41.3X2	T41.3X3	T41.3X4	T41.3X5	T41.3X6
nerve block (peripheral) (plexus)	T41.3X1	T41.3X2	T41.3X3	T41.3X4	T41.3X5	T41.3X6
regional	T41.3X1	T41.3X2	T41.3X3	T41.3X4	T41.3X5	T41.3X6

▽ Subterms under main terms may continue to next column or page   Additional Character May Be Required — Refer to the Tabular List for Character Selection   385

Pitocin — Prilocaine

Substance	Poisoning, Accidental (unintentional)	Poisoning, Intentional Self-harm	Poisoning, Assault	Poisoning, Undetermined	Adverse Effect	Under-dosing
Primaquine	T37.2X1	T37.2X2	T37.2X3	T37.2X4	T37.2X5	T37.2X6
Primidone	T42.6X1	T42.6X2	T42.6X3	T42.6X4	T42.6X5	T42.6X6
Primula (veris)	T62.2X1	T62.2X2	T62.2X3	T62.2X4	—	—
Prinadol	T40.2X1	T40.2X2	T40.2X3	T40.2X4	T40.2X5	T40.2X6
Priscol, Priscoline	T44.6X1	T44.6X2	T44.6X3	T44.6X4	T44.6X5	T44.6X6
Pristinamycin	T36.3X1	T36.3X2	T36.3X3	T36.3X4	T36.3X5	T36.3X6
Privet	T62.2X1	T62.2X2	T62.2X3	T62.2X4	—	—
berries	T62.1X1	T62.1X2	T62.1X3	T62.1X4	—	—
Privine	T44.4X1	T44.4X2	T44.4X3	T44.4X4	T44.4X5	T44.4X6
Pro-Banthine	T44.3X1	T44.3X2	T44.3X3	T44.3X4	T44.3X5	T44.3X6
Probarbital	T42.3X1	T42.3X2	T42.3X3	T42.3X4	T42.3X5	T42.3X6
Probenecid	T50.4X1	T50.4X2	T50.4X3	T50.4X4	T50.4X5	T50.4X6
Probucol	T46.6X1	T46.6X2	T46.6X3	T46.6X4	T46.6X5	T46.6X6
Procainamide	T46.2X1	T46.2X2	T46.2X3	T46.2X4	T46.2X5	T46.2X6
Procaine	T41.3X1	T41.3X2	T41.3X3	T41.3X4	T41.3X5	T41.3X6
benzylpenicillin	T36.0X1	T36.0X2	T36.0X3	T36.0X4	T36.0X5	T36.0X6
nerve block (periphreal) (plexus)	T41.3X1	T41.3X2	T41.3X3	T41.3X4	T41.3X5	T41.3X6
penicillin G	T36.0X1	T36.0X2	T36.0X3	T36.0X4	T36.0X5	T36.0X6
regional	T41.3X1	T41.3X2	T41.3X3	T41.3X4	T41.3X5	T41.3X6
spinal	T41.3X1	T41.3X2	T41.3X3	T41.3X4	T41.3X5	T41.3X6
Procalmidol	T43.591	T43.592	T43.593	T43.594	T43.595	T43.596
Procarbazine	T45.1X1	T45.1X2	T45.1X3	T45.1X4	T45.1X5	T45.1X6
Procaterol	T44.5X1	T44.5X2	T44.5X3	T44.5X4	T44.5X5	T44.5X6
Prochlorperazine	T43.3X1	T43.3X2	T43.3X3	T43.3X4	T43.3X5	T43.3X6
Procyclidine	T44.3X1	T44.3X2	T44.3X3	T44.3X4	T44.3X5	T44.3X6
Producer gas	T58.8X1	T58.8X2	T58.8X3	T58.8X4	—	—
Profadol	T40.4X1	T40.4X2	T40.4X3	T40.4X4	T40.4X5	T40.4X6
Profenamine	T44.3X1	T44.3X2	T44.3X3	T44.3X4	T44.3X5	T44.3X6
Profenil	T44.3X1	T44.3X2	T44.3X3	T44.3X4	T44.3X5	T44.3X6
Proflavine	T49.0X1	T49.0X2	T49.0X3	T49.0X4	T49.0X5	T49.0X6
Progabide	T42.6X1	T42.6X2	T42.6X3	T42.6X4	T42.6X5	T42.6X6
Progesterone	T38.5X1	T38.5X2	T38.5X3	T38.5X4	T38.5X5	T38.5X6
Progestin	T38.5X1	T38.5X2	T38.5X3	T38.5X4	T38.5X5	T38.5X6
oral contraceptive	T38.4X1	T38.4X2	T38.4X3	T38.4X4	T38.4X5	T38.4X6
Progestogen NEC	T38.5X1	T38.5X2	T38.5X3	T38.5X4	T38.5X5	T38.5X6
Progestone	T38.5X1	T38.5X2	T38.5X3	T38.5X4	T38.5X5	T38.5X6
Proglumide	T47.1X1	T47.1X2	T47.1X3	T47.1X4	T47.1X5	T47.1X6
Proguanil	T37.2X1	T37.2X2	T37.2X3	T37.2X4	T37.2X5	T37.2X6
Prolactin	T38.811	T38.812	T38.813	T38.814	T38.815	T38.816
Prolintane	T43.691	T43.692	T43.693	T43.694	T43.695	T43.696
Proloid	T38.1X1	T38.1X2	T38.1X3	T38.1X4	T38.1X5	T38.1X6
Proluton	T38.5X1	T38.5X2	T38.5X3	T38.5X4	T38.5X5	T38.5X6
Promacetin	T37.1X1	T37.1X2	T37.1X3	T37.1X4	T37.1X5	T37.1X6
Promazine	T43.3X1	T43.3X2	T43.3X3	T43.3X4	T43.3X5	T43.3X6
Promedol	T40.2X1	T40.2X2	T40.2X3	T40.2X4	—	—
Promegestone	T38.5X1	T38.5X2	T38.5X3	T38.5X4	T38.5X5	T38.5X6
Promethazine (teoclate)	T43.3X1	T43.3X2	T43.3X3	T43.3X4	T43.3X5	T43.3X6
Promin	T37.1X1	T37.1X2	T37.1X3	T37.1X4	T37.1X5	T37.1X6
Pronase	T45.3X1	T45.3X2	T45.3X3	T45.3X4	T45.3X5	T45.3X6
Pronestyl (hydrochloride)	T46.2X1	T46.2X2	T46.2X3	T46.2X4	T46.2X5	T46.2X6
Pronetalol	T44.7X1	T44.7X2	T44.7X3	T44.7X4	T44.7X5	T44.7X6
Prontosil	T37.0X1	T37.0X2	T37.0X3	T37.0X4	T37.0X5	T37.0X6
Propachlor	T60.3X1	T60.3X2	T60.3X3	T60.3X4	—	—
Propafenone	T46.2X1	T46.2X2	T46.2X3	T46.2X4	T46.2X5	T46.2X6
Propallylonal	T42.3X1	T42.3X2	T42.3X3	T42.3X4	T42.3X5	T42.3X6
Propamidine	T49.0X1	T49.0X2	T49.0X3	T49.0X4	T49.0X5	T49.0X6
Propane (distributed in mobile container)	T59.891	T59.892	T59.893	T59.894	—	—
distributed through pipes	T59.891	T59.892	T59.893	T59.894	—	—
incomplete combustion	T58.11	T58.12	T58.13	T58.14	—	—
Propanidid	T41.291	T41.292	T41.293	T41.294	T41.295	T41.296
Propanil	T60.3X1	T60.3X2	T60.3X3	T60.3X4	—	—
Propantheline	T44.3X1	T44.3X2	T44.3X3	T44.3X4	T44.3X5	T44.3X6
bromide	T44.3X1	T44.3X2	T44.3X3	T44.3X4	T44.3X5	T44.3X6
Proparacaine	T41.3X1	T41.3X2	T41.3X3	T41.3X4	T41.3X5	T41.3X6
Propatylnitrate	T46.3X1	T46.3X2	T46.3X3	T46.3X4	T46.3X5	T46.3X6
Propicillin	T36.0X1	T36.0X2	T36.0X3	T36.0X4	T36.0X5	T36.0X6
Propiolactone	T49.0X1	T49.0X2	T49.0X3	T49.0X4	T49.0X5	T49.0X6
Propiomazine	T45.0X1	T45.0X2	T45.0X3	T45.0X4	T45.0X5	T45.0X6
Propionaldehyde (medicinal)	T42.6X1	T42.6X2	T42.6X3	T42.6X4	T42.6X5	T42.6X6
Propionate (calcium) (sodium)	T49.0X1	T49.0X2	T49.0X3	T49.0X4	T49.0X5	T49.0X6
Propion gel	T49.0X1	T49.0X2	T49.0X3	T49.0X4	T49.0X5	T49.0X6
Propitocaine	T41.3X1	T41.3X2	T41.3X3	T41.3X4	T41.3X5	T41.3X6
infiltration (subcutaneous)	T41.3X1	T41.3X2	T41.3X3	T41.3X4	T41.3X5	T41.3X6
nerve block (peripheral) (plexus)	T41.3X1	T41.3X2	T41.3X3	T41.3X4	T41.3X5	T41.3X6
Propofol	T41.291	T41.292	T41.293	T41.294	T41.295	T41.296
Propoxur	T60.0X1	T60.0X2	T60.0X3	T60.0X4	—	—
Propoxycaine	T41.3X1	T41.3X2	T41.3X3	T41.3X4	T41.3X5	T41.3X6
infiltration (subcutaneous)	T41.3X1	T41.3X2	T41.3X3	T41.3X4	T41.3X5	T41.3X6

Substance	Poisoning, Accidental (unintentional)	Poisoning, Intentional Self-harm	Poisoning, Assault	Poisoning, Undetermined	Adverse Effect	Under-dosing
Propoxycaine — continued						
nerve block (peripheral) (plexus)	T41.3X1	T41.3X2	T41.3X3	T41.3X4	T41.3X5	T41.3X6
topical (surface)	T41.3X1	T41.3X2	T41.3X3	T41.3X4	T41.3X5	T41.3X6
Propoxyphene	T40.4X1	T40.4X2	T40.4X3	T40.4X4	T40.4X5	T40.4X6
Propranolol	T44.7X1	T44.7X2	T44.7X3	T44.7X4	T44.7X5	T44.7X6
Propyl						
alcohol	T51.3X1	T51.3X2	T51.3X3	T51.3X4	—	—
carbinol	T51.3X1	T51.3X2	T51.3X3	T51.3X4	—	—
hexadrine	T44.4X1	T44.4X2	T44.4X3	T44.4X4	T44.4X5	T44.4X6
iodone	T50.8X1	T50.8X2	T50.8X3	T50.8X4	T50.8X5	T50.8X6
thiouracil	T38.2X1	T38.2X2	T38.2X3	T38.2X4	T38.2X5	T38.2X6
Propylaminophenothiazine	T43.3X1	T43.3X2	T43.3X3	T43.3X4	T43.3X5	T43.3X6
Propylene	T59.891	T59.892	T59.893	T59.894	—	—
Propylhexedrine	T48.5X1	T48.5X2	T48.5X3	T48.5X4	T48.5X5	T48.5X6
Propyliodone	T50.8X1	T50.8X2	T50.8X3	T50.8X4	T50.8X5	T50.8X6
Propylparaben (ophthalmic)	T49.5X1	T49.5X2	T49.5X3	T49.5X4	T49.5X5	T49.5X6
Propylthiouracil	T38.2X1	T38.2X2	T38.2X3	T38.2X4	T38.2X5	T38.2X6
Propyphenazone	T39.2X1	T39.2X2	T39.2X3	T39.2X4	T39.2X5	T39.2X6
Proquazone	T39.391	T39.392	T39.393	T39.394	T39.395	T39.396
Proscillaridin	T46.0X1	T46.0X2	T46.0X3	T46.0X4	T46.0X5	T46.0X6
Prostacyclin	T45.521	T45.522	T45.523	T45.524	T45.525	T45.526
Prostaglandin (I2)	T45.521	T45.522	T45.523	T45.524	T45.525	T45.526
E1	T46.7X1	T46.7X2	T46.7X3	T46.7X4	T46.7X5	T46.7X6
E2	T48.0X1	T48.0X2	T48.0X3	T48.0X4	T48.0X5	T48.0X6
F2 alpha	T48.0X1	T48.0X2	T48.0X3	T48.0X4	T48.0X5	T48.0X6
Prostigmin	T44.0X1	T44.0X2	T44.0X3	T44.0X4	T44.0X5	T44.0X6
Prosultiamine	T45.2X1	T45.2X2	T45.2X3	T45.2X4	T45.2X5	T45.2X6
Protamine sulfate	T45.7X1	T45.7X2	T45.7X3	T45.7X4	T45.7X5	T45.7X6
zinc insulin	T38.3X1	T38.3X2	T38.3X3	T38.3X4	T38.3X5	T38.3X6
Protease	T47.5X1	T47.5X2	T47.5X3	T47.5X4	T47.5X5	T47.5X6
Protectant, skin NEC	T49.3X1	T49.3X2	T49.3X3	T49.3X4	T49.3X5	T49.3X6
Protein hydrolysate	T50.991	T50.992	T50.993	T50.994	T50.995	T50.996
Prothiaden — see Dothiepin hydrochloride						
Prothionamide	T37.1X1	T37.1X2	T37.1X3	T37.1X4	T37.1X5	T37.1X6
Prothipendyl	T43.591	T43.592	T43.593	T43.594	T43.595	T43.596
Prothoate	T60.0X1	T60.0X2	T60.0X3	T60.0X4	—	—
Prothrombin						
activator	T45.7X1	T45.7X2	T45.7X3	T45.7X4	T45.7X5	T45.7X6
synthesis inhibitor	T45.511	T45.512	T45.513	T45.514	T45.515	T45.516
Protionamide	T37.1X1	T37.1X2	T37.1X3	T37.1X4	T37.1X5	T37.1X6
Protirelin	T38.891	T38.892	T38.893	T38.894	T38.895	T38.896
Protokylol	T48.6X1	T48.6X2	T48.6X3	T48.6X4	T48.6X5	T48.6X6
Protopam	T50.6X1	T50.6X2	T50.6X3	T50.6X4	T50.6X5	T50.6X6
Protoveratrine(s) (A) (B)	T46.5X1	T46.5X2	T46.5X3	T46.5X4	T46.5X5	T46.5X6
Protriptyline	T43.011	T43.012	T43.013	T43.014	T43.015	T43.016
Provera	T38.5X1	T38.5X2	T38.5X3	T38.5X4	T38.5X5	T38.5X6
Provitamin A	T45.2X1	T45.2X2	T45.2X3	T45.2X4	T45.2X5	T45.2X6
Proxibarbal	T42.3X1	T42.3X2	T42.3X3	T42.3X4	T42.3X5	T42.3X6
Proxymetacaine	T41.3X1	T41.3X2	T41.3X3	T41.3X4	T41.3X5	T41.3X6
Proxyphylline	T48.6X1	T48.6X2	T48.6X3	T48.6X4	T48.6X5	T48.6X6
Prozac — see Fluoxetine hydrochloride						
Prunus						
laurocerasus	T62.2X1	T62.2X2	T62.2X3	T62.2X4	—	—
virginiana	T62.2X1	T62.2X2	T62.2X3	T62.2X4	—	—
Prussian blue						
commercial	T65.891	T65.892	T65.893	T65.894	—	—
therapeutic	T50.6X1	T50.6X2	T50.6X3	T50.6X4	T50.6X5	T50.6X6
Prussic acid	T65.0X1	T65.0X2	T65.0X3	T65.0X4	—	—
vapor	T57.3X1	T57.3X2	T57.3X3	T57.3X4	—	—
Pseudoephedrine	T44.991	T44.992	T44.993	T44.994	T44.995	T44.996
Psilocin	T40.991	T40.992	T40.993	T40.994	—	—
Psilocybin	T40.991	T40.992	T40.993	T40.994	—	—
Psilocybine	T40.991	T40.992	T40.993	T40.994	—	—
Psoralene (nonmedicinal)	T65.891	T65.892	T65.893	T65.894	—	—
Psoralens (medicinal)	T50.991	T50.992	T50.993	T50.994	T50.995	T50.996
PSP (phenolsulfonphthalein)	T50.8X1	T50.8X2	T50.8X3	T50.8X4	T50.8X5	T50.8X6
Psychodysleptic drug NOS	T40.901	T40.902	T40.903	T40.904	T40.905	T40.906
specified NEC	T40.991	T40.992	T40.993	T40.994	T40.995	T40.996
Psychostimulant	T43.601	T43.602	T43.603	T43.604	T43.605	T43.606
amphetamine	T43.621	T43.622	T43.623	T43.624	T43.625	T43.626
caffeine	T43.611	T43.612	T43.613	T43.614	T43.615	T43.616
methylphenidate	T43.631	T43.632	T43.633	T43.634	T43.635	T43.636
specified NEC	T43.691	T43.692	T43.693	T43.694	T43.695	T43.696
Psychotherapeutic drug NEC	T43.91	T43.92	T43.93	T43.94	T43.95	T43.96
antidepressants — see also Antidepressant	T43.201	T43.202	T43.203	T43.204	T43.205	T43.206
specified NEC	T43.8X1	T43.8X2	T43.8X3	T43.8X4	T43.8X5	T43.8X6

Additional Character May Be Required — Refer to the Tabular List for Character Selection   ▽ Subterms under main terms may continue to next column or page

Substance	Poisoning, Accidental (unintentional)	Poisoning, Intentional Self-harm	Poisoning, Assault	Poisoning, Undetermined	Adverse Effect	Under-dosing
Psychotherapeutic drug —						
continued						
tranquilizers NEC	T43.501	T43.502	T43.503	T43.504	T43.505	T43.506
Psychotomimetic agents	T40.901	T40.902	T40.903	T40.904	T40.905	T40.906
Psychotropic drug NEC	T43.91	T43.92	T43.93	T43.94	T43.95	T43.96
specified NEC	T43.8X1	T43.8X2	T43.8X3	T43.8X4	T43.8X5	T43.8X6
Psyllium hydrophilic	T47.4X1	T47.4X2	T47.4X3	T47.4X4	T47.4X5	T47.4X6
mucilloid						
Pteroylglutamic acid	T45.8X1	T45.8X2	T45.8X3	T45.8X4	T45.8X5	T45.8X6
Pteroyltriglutamate	T45.1X1	T45.1X2	T45.1X3	T45.1X4	T45.1X5	T45.1X6
PTFE — *see*						
Polytetrafluoroethylene						
Pulp						
devitalizing paste	T49.7X1	T49.7X2	T49.7X3	T49.7X4	T49.7X5	T49.7X6
dressing	T49.7X1	T49.7X2	T49.7X3	T49.7X4	T49.7X5	T49.7X6
Pulsatilla	T62.2X1	T62.2X2	T62.2X3	T62.2X4	—	—
Pumpkin seed extract	T37.4X1	T37.4X2	T37.4X3	T37.4X4	T37.4X5	T37.4X6
Purex (bleach)	T54.91	T54.92	T54.93	T54.94	—	—
Purgative NEC — *see also*	T47.4X1	T47.4X2	T47.4X3	T47.4X4	T47.4X5	T47.4X6
Cathartic						
Purine analogue	T45.1X1	T45.1X2	T45.1X3	T45.1X4	T45.1X5	T45.1X6
(antineoplastic)						
Purine diuretics	T50.2X1	T50.2X2	T50.2X3	T50.2X4	T50.2X5	T50.2X6
Purinethol	T45.1X1	T45.1X2	T45.1X3	T45.1X4	T45.1X5	T45.1X6
PVP	T45.8X1	T45.8X2	T45.8X3	T45.8X4	T45.8X5	T45.8X6
Pyrabital	T39.8X1	T39.8X2	T39.8X3	T39.8X4	T39.8X5	T39.8X6
Pyramidon	T39.2X1	T39.2X2	T39.2X3	T39.2X4	T39.2X5	T39.2X6
Pyrantel	T37.4X1	T37.4X2	T37.4X3	T37.4X4	T37.4X5	T37.4X6
Pyrathiazine	T45.0X1	T45.0X2	T45.0X3	T45.0X4	T45.0X5	T45.0X6
Pyrazinamide	T37.1X1	T37.1X2	T37.1X3	T37.1X4	T37.1X5	T37.1X6
Pyrazinoic acid (amide)	T37.1X1	T37.1X2	T37.1X3	T37.1X4	T37.1X5	T37.1X6
Pyrazole (derivatives)	T39.2X1	T39.2X2	T39.2X3	T39.2X4	T39.2X5	T39.2X6
Pyrazolone analgesic NEC	T39.2X1	T39.2X2	T39.2X3	T39.2X4	T39.2X5	T39.2X6
Pyrethrin, pyrethrum	T60.2X1	T60.2X2	T60.2X3	T60.2X4	—	—
(nonmedicinal)						
Pyrethrum extract	T49.0X1	T49.0X2	T49.0X3	T49.0X4	T49.0X5	T49.0X6
Pyribenzamine	T45.0X1	T45.0X2	T45.0X3	T45.0X4	T45.0X5	T45.0X6
Pyridine	T52.8X1	T52.8X2	T52.8X3	T52.8X4		
aldoxime methiodide	T50.6X1	T50.6X2	T50.6X3	T50.6X4	T50.6X5	T50.6X6
aldoxime methyl chloride	T50.6X1	T50.6X2	T50.6X3	T50.6X4	T50.6X5	T50.6X6
vapor	T59.891	T59.892	T59.893	T59.894	—	—
Pyridium	T39.8X1	T39.8X2	T39.8X3	T39.8X4	T39.8X5	T39.8X6
Pyridostigmine bromide	T44.0X1	T44.0X2	T44.0X3	T44.0X4	T44.0X5	T44.0X6
Pyridoxal phosphate	T45.2X1	T45.2X2	T45.2X3	T45.2X4	T45.2X5	T45.2X6
Pyridoxine	T45.2X1	T45.2X2	T45.2X3	T45.2X4	T45.2X5	T45.2X6
Pyrilamine	T45.0X1	T45.0X2	T45.0X3	T45.0X4	T45.0X5	T45.0X6
Pyrimethamine	T37.2X1	T37.2X2	T37.2X3	T37.2X4	T37.2X5	T37.2X6
with sulfadoxine	T37.2X1	T37.2X2	T37.2X3	T37.2X4	T37.2X5	T37.2X6
Pyrimidine antagonist	T45.1X1	T45.1X2	T45.1X3	T45.1X4	T45.1X5	T45.1X6
Pyriminil	T60.4X1	T60.4X2	T60.4X3	T60.4X4		
Pyrithione zinc	T49.4X1	T49.4X2	T49.4X3	T49.4X4	T49.4X5	T49.4X6
Pyrithyldione	T42.6X1	T42.6X2	T42.6X3	T42.6X4	T42.6X5	T42.6X6
Pyrogallic acid	T49.0X1	T49.0X2	T49.0X3	T49.0X4	T49.0X5	T49.0X6
Pyrogallol	T49.0X1	T49.0X2	T49.0X3	T49.0X4	T49.0X5	T49.0X6
Pyroxylin	T49.3X1	T49.3X2	T49.3X3	T49.3X4	T49.3X5	T49.3X6
Pyrrobutamine	T45.0X1	T45.0X2	T45.0X3	T45.0X4	T45.0X5	T45.0X6
Pyrrolizidine alkaloids	T62.8X1	T62.8X2	T62.8X3	T62.8X4	—	—
Pyrvinium chloride	T37.4X1	T37.4X2	T37.4X3	T37.4X4	T37.4X5	T37.4X6
PZI	T38.3X1	T38.3X2	T38.3X3	T38.3X4	T38.3X5	T38.3X6
Quaalude	T42.6X1	T42.6X2	T42.6X3	T42.6X4	T42.6X5	T42.6X6
Quarternary ammonium						
anti-infective	T49.0X1	T49.0X2	T49.0X3	T49.0X4	T49.0X5	T49.0X6
ganglion blocking	T44.2X1	T44.2X2	T44.2X3	T44.2X4	T44.2X5	T44.2X6
parasympatholytic	T44.3X1	T44.3X2	T44.3X3	T44.3X4	T44.3X5	T44.3X6
Quazepam	T42.4X1	T42.4X2	T42.4X3	T42.4X4	T42.4X5	T42.4X6
Quicklime	T54.3X1	T54.3X2	T54.3X3	T54.3X4	—	—
Quillaja extract	T48.4X1	T48.4X2	T48.4X3	T48.4X4	T48.4X5	T48.4X6
Quinacrine	T37.2X1	T37.2X2	T37.2X3	T37.2X4	T37.2X5	T37.2X6
Quinaglute	T46.2X1	T46.2X2	T46.2X3	T46.2X4	T46.2X5	T46.2X6
Quinalbarbital	T42.3X1	T42.3X2	T42.3X3	T42.3X4	T42.3X5	T42.3X6
Quinalbarbitone sodium	T42.3X1	T42.3X2	T42.3X3	T42.3X4	T42.3X5	T42.3X6
Quinalphos	T60.0X1	T60.0X2	T60.0X3	T60.0X4	—	—
Quinapril	T46.4X1	T46.4X2	T46.4X3	T46.4X4	T46.4X5	T46.4X6
Quinestradiol	T38.5X1	T38.5X2	T38.5X3	T38.5X4	T38.5X5	T38.5X6
Quinestradol	T38.5X1	T38.5X2	T38.5X3	T38.5X4	T38.5X5	T38.5X6
Quinestrol	T38.5X1	T38.5X2	T38.5X3	T38.5X4	T38.5X5	T38.5X6
Quinethazone	T50.2X1	T50.2X2	T50.2X3	T50.2X4	T50.2X5	T50.2X6
Quingestanol	T38.4X1	T38.4X2	T38.4X3	T38.4X4	T38.4X5	T38.4X6
Quinidine	T46.2X1	T46.2X2	T46.2X3	T46.2X4	T46.2X5	T46.2X6
Quinine	T37.2X1	T37.2X2	T37.2X3	T37.2X4	T37.2X5	T37.2X6
Quiniobine	T37.8X1	T37.8X2	T37.8X3	T37.8X4	T37.8X5	T37.8X6
Quinisocaine	T49.1X1	T49.1X2	T49.1X3	T49.1X4	T49.1X5	T49.1X6
Quinocide	T37.2X1	T37.2X2	T37.2X3	T37.2X4	T37.2X5	T37.2X6

Substance	Poisoning, Accidental (unintentional)	Poisoning, Intentional Self-harm	Poisoning, Assault	Poisoning, Undetermined	Adverse Effect	Under-dosing
Quinoline (derivatives) **NEC**	T37.8X1	T37.8X2	T37.8X3	T37.8X4	T37.8X5	T37.8X6
Quinupramine	T43.011	T43.012	T43.013	T43.014	T43.015	T43.016
Quotane	T41.3X1	T41.3X2	T41.3X3	T41.3X4	T41.3X5	T41.3X6
Rabies						
immune globulin (human)	T50.Z11	T50.Z12	T50.Z13	T50.Z14	T50.Z15	T50.Z16
vaccine	T50.B91	T50.B92	T50.B93	T50.B94	T50.B95	T50.B96
Racemoramide	T40.2X1	T40.2X2	T40.2X3	T40.2X4	—	—
Racemorphan	T40.2X1	T40.2X2	T40.2X3	T40.2X4	T40.2X5	T40.2X6
Racepinefrin	T44.5X1	T44.5X2	T44.5X3	T44.5X4	T44.5X5	T44.5X6
Raclopride	T43.591	T43.592	T43.593	T43.594	T43.595	T43.596
Radiator alcohol	T51.1X1	T51.1X2	T51.1X3	T51.1X4	—	—
Radioactive drug NEC	T50.8X1	T50.8X2	T50.8X3	T50.8X4	T50.8X5	T50.8X6
Radio-opaque (drugs)	T50.8X1	T50.8X2	T50.8X3	T50.8X4	T50.8X5	T50.8X6
(materials)						
Ramifenazone	T39.2X1	T39.2X2	T39.2X3	T39.2X4	T39.2X5	T39.2X6
Ramipril	T46.4X1	T46.4X2	T46.4X3	T46.4X4	T46.4X5	T46.4X6
Ranitidine	T47.0X1	T47.0X2	T47.0X3	T47.0X4	T47.0X5	T47.0X6
Ranunculus	T62.2X1	T62.2X2	T62.2X3	T62.2X4	—	—
Rat poison NEC	T60.4X1	T60.4X2	T60.4X3	T60.4X4	—	—
Rattlesnake (venom)	T63.011	T63.012	T63.013	T63.014	—	—
Raubasine	T46.7X1	T46.7X2	T46.7X3	T46.7X4	T46.7X5	T46.7X6
Raudixin	T46.5X1	T46.5X2	T46.5X3	T46.5X4	T46.5X5	T46.5X6
Rautensin	T46.5X1	T46.5X2	T46.5X3	T46.5X4	T46.5X5	T46.5X6
Rautina	T46.5X1	T46.5X2	T46.5X3	T46.5X4	T46.5X5	T46.5X6
Rautotal	T46.5X1	T46.5X2	T46.5X3	T46.5X4	T46.5X5	T46.5X6
Rauwiloid	T46.5X1	T46.5X2	T46.5X3	T46.5X4	T46.5X5	T46.5X6
Rauwoldin	T46.5X1	T46.5X2	T46.5X3	T46.5X4	T46.5X5	T46.5X6
Rauwolfia (alkaloids)	T46.5X1	T46.5X2	T46.5X3	T46.5X4	T46.5X5	T46.5X6
Razoxane	T45.1X1	T45.1X2	T45.1X3	T45.1X4	T45.1X5	T45.1X6
Realgar	T57.0X1	T57.0X2	T57.0X3	T57.0X4		
Recombinant (R) — *see* specific						
protein						
Red blood cells, packed	T45.8X1	T45.8X2	T45.8X3	T45.8X4	T45.8X5	T45.8X6
Red squill (scilliroside)	T60.4X1	T60.4X2	T60.4X3	T60.4X4	—	—
Reducing agent, industrial	T65.891	T65.892	T65.893	T65.894	—	—
NEC						
Refrigerant gas	T53.5X1	T53.5X2	T53.5X3	T53.5X4	—	—
(chlorofluorocarbon)						
not chlorofluorocarbon	T59.891	T59.892	T59.893	T59.894	—	—
Regroton	T50.2X1	T50.2X2	T50.2X3	T50.2X4	T50.2X5	T50.2X6
Rehydration salts (oral)	T50.3X1	T50.3X2	T50.3X3	T50.3X4	T50.3X5	T50.3X6
Rela	T42.8X1	T42.8X2	T42.8X3	T42.8X4	T42.8X5	T42.8X6
Relaxant, muscle						
anesthetic	T48.1X1	T48.1X2	T48.1X3	T48.1X4	T48.1X5	T48.1X6
central nervous system	T42.8X1	T42.8X2	T42.8X3	T42.8X4	T42.8X5	T42.8X6
skeletal NEC	T48.1X1	T48.1X2	T48.1X3	T48.1X4	T48.1X5	T48.1X6
smooth NEC	T44.3X1	T44.3X2	T44.3X3	T44.3X4	T44.3X5	T44.3X6
Remoxipride	T43.591	T43.592	T43.593	T43.594	T43.595	T43.596
Renese	T50.2X1	T50.2X2	T50.2X3	T50.2X4	T50.2X5	T50.2X6
Renografin	T50.8X1	T50.8X2	T50.8X3	T50.8X4	T50.8X5	T50.8X6
Replacement solution	T50.3X1	T50.3X2	T50.3X3	T50.3X4	T50.3X5	T50.3X6
Reproterol	T48.6X1	T48.6X2	T48.6X3	T48.6X4	T48.6X5	T48.6X6
Rescinnamine	T46.5X1	T46.5X2	T46.5X3	T46.5X4	T46.5X5	T46.5X6
Reserpin (e)	T46.5X1	T46.5X2	T46.5X3	T46.5X4	T46.5X5	T46.5X6
Resorcin, resorcinol	T65.891	T65.892	T65.893	T65.894	—	—
(nonmedicinal)						
medicinal	T49.4X1	T49.4X2	T49.4X3	T49.4X4	T49.4X5	T49.4X6
Respaire	T48.4X1	T48.4X2	T48.4X3	T48.4X4	T48.4X5	T48.4X6
Respiratory drug NEC	T48.901	T48.902	T48.903	T48.904	T48.905	T48.906
antiasthmatic NEC	T48.6X1	T48.6X2	T48.6X3	T48.6X4	T48.6X5	T48.6X6
anti-common-cold NEC	T48.5X1	T48.5X2	T48.5X3	T48.5X4	T48.5X5	T48.5X6
expectorant NEC	T48.4X1	T48.4X2	T48.4X3	T48.4X4	T48.4X5	T48.4X6
stimulant	T48.901	T48.902	T48.903	T48.904	T48.905	T48.906
Retinoic acid	T49.0X1	T49.0X2	T49.0X3	T49.0X4	T49.0X5	T49.0X6
Retinol	T45.2X1	T45.2X2	T45.2X3	T45.2X4	T45.2X5	T45.2X6
Rh (D) immune globulin	T50.Z11	T50.Z12	T50.Z13	T50.Z14	T50.Z15	T50.Z16
(human)						
Rhodine	T39.011	T39.012	T39.013	T39.014	T39.015	T39.016
RhoGAM	T50.Z11	T50.Z12	T50.Z13	T50.Z14	T50.Z15	T50.Z16
Rhubarb						
dry extract	T47.2X1	T47.2X2	T47.2X3	T47.2X4	T47.2X5	T47.2X6
tincture, compound	T47.2X1	T47.2X2	T47.2X3	T47.2X4	T47.2X5	T47.2X6
Ribavirin	T37.5X1	T37.5X2	T37.5X3	T37.5X4	T37.5X5	T37.5X6
Riboflavin	T45.2X1	T45.2X2	T45.2X3	T45.2X4	T45.2X5	T45.2X6
Ribostamycin	T36.5X1	T36.5X2	T36.5X3	T36.5X4	T36.5X5	T36.5X6
Ricin	T62.2X1	T62.2X2	T62.2X3	T62.2X4	—	—
Ricinus communis	T62.2X1	T62.2X2	T62.2X3	T62.2X4	—	—
Rickettsial vaccine NEC	T50.A91	T50.A92	T50.A93	T50.A94	T50.A95	T50.A96
Rifabutin	T36.6X1	T36.6X2	T36.6X3	T36.6X4	T36.6X5	T36.6X6
Rifamide	T36.6X1	T36.6X2	T36.6X3	T36.6X4	T36.6X5	T36.6X6
Rifampicin	T36.6X1	T36.6X2	T36.6X3	T36.6X4	T36.6X5	T36.6X6
with isoniazid	T37.1X1	T37.1X2	T37.1X3	T37.1X4	T37.1X5	T37.1X6
Rifampin	T36.6X1	T36.6X2	T36.6X3	T36.6X4	T36.6X5	T36.6X6

Table of Drugs and Chemicals

Rifamycin — Shellfish, noxious, nonbacterial

Substance	Poisoning, Accidental (unintentional)	Poisoning, Intentional Self-harm	Poisoning, Assault	Poisoning, Undetermined	Adverse Effect	Under-dosing
Rifamycin	T36.6X1	T36.6X2	T36.6X3	T36.6X4	T36.6X5	T36.6X6
Rifaximin	T36.6X1	T36.6X2	T36.6X3	T36.6X4	T36.6X5	T36.6X6
Rimantadine	T37.5X1	T37.5X2	T37.5X3	T37.5X4	T37.5X5	T37.5X6
Rimazolium metilsulfate	T39.8X1	T39.8X2	T39.8X3	T39.8X4	T39.8X5	T39.8X6
Rimifon	T37.1X1	T37.1X2	T37.1X3	T37.1X4	T37.1X5	T37.1X6
Rimiterol	T48.6X1	T48.6X2	T48.6X3	T48.6X4	T48.6X5	T48.6X6
Ringer (lactate) solution	T50.3X1	T50.3X2	T50.3X3	T50.3X4	T50.3X5	T50.3X6
Ristocetin	T36.8X1	T36.8X2	T36.8X3	T36.8X4	T36.8X5	T36.8X6
Ritalin	T43.631	T43.632	T43.633	T43.634	T43.635	T43.636
Ritodrine	T44.5X1	T44.5X2	T44.5X3	T44.5X4	T44.5X5	T44.5X6
Roach killer — see Insecticide						
Rociverine	T44.3X1	T44.3X2	T44.3X3	T44.3X4	T44.3X5	T44.3X6
Rocky Mountain spotted fever vaccine	T50.A91	T50.A92	T50.A93	T50.A94	T50.A95	T50.A96
Rodenticide NEC	T60.4X1	T60.4X2	T60.4X3	T60.4X4	—	—
Rohypnol	T42.4X1	T42.4X2	T42.4X3	T42.4X4	T42.4X5	T42.4X6
Rokitamycin	T36.3X1	T36.3X2	T36.3X3	T36.3X4	T36.3X5	T36.3X6
Rolaids	T47.1X1	T47.1X2	T47.1X3	T47.1X4	T47.1X5	T47.1X6
Rolitetracycline	T36.4X1	T36.4X2	T36.4X3	T36.4X4	T36.4X5	T36.4X6
Romilar	T48.3X1	T48.3X2	T48.3X3	T48.3X4	T48.3X5	T48.3X6
Ronifibrate	T46.6X1	T46.6X2	T46.6X3	T46.6X4	T46.6X5	T46.6X6
Rosaprostol	T47.1X1	T47.1X2	T47.1X3	T47.1X4	T47.1X5	T47.1X6
Rose bengal sodium (131I)	T50.8X1	T50.8X2	T50.8X3	T50.8X4	T50.8X5	T50.8X6
Rose water ointment	T49.3X1	T49.3X2	T49.3X3	T49.3X4	T49.3X5	T49.3X6
Rosoxacin	T37.8X1	T37.8X2	T37.8X3	T37.8X4	T37.8X5	T37.8X6
Rotenone	T60.2X1	T60.2X2	T60.2X3	T60.2X4	—	—
Rotoxamine	T45.0X1	T45.0X2	T45.0X3	T45.0X4	T45.0X5	T45.0X6
Rough-on-rats	T60.4X1	T60.4X2	T60.4X3	T60.4X4	—	—
Roxatidine	T47.0X1	T47.0X2	T47.0X3	T47.0X4	T47.0X5	T47.0X6
Roxithromycin	T36.3X1	T36.3X2	T36.3X3	T36.3X4	T36.3X5	T36.3X6
Rt-PA	T45.611	T45.612	T45.613	T45.614	T45.615	T45.616
Rubbing alcohol	T51.2X1	T51.2X2	T51.2X3	T51.2X4	—	—
Rubefacient	T49.4X1	T49.4X2	T49.4X3	T49.4X4	T49.4X5	T49.4X6
Rubella vaccine	T50.B91	T50.B92	T50.B93	T50.B94	T50.B95	T50.B96
Rubeola vaccine	T50.B91	T50.B92	T50.B93	T50.B94	T50.B95	T50.B96
Rubidium chloride Rb82	T50.8X1	T50.8X2	T50.8X3	T50.8X4	T50.8X5	T50.8X6
Rubidomycin	T45.1X1	T45.1X2	T45.1X3	T45.1X4	T45.1X5	T45.1X6
Rue	T62.2X1	T62.2X2	T62.2X3	T62.2X4	—	—
Rufocromomycin	T45.1X1	T45.1X2	T45.1X3	T45.1X4	T45.1X5	T45.1X6
Russel's viper venin	T45.7X1	T45.7X2	T45.7X3	T45.7X4	T45.7X5	T45.7X6
Ruta (graveolens)	T62.2X1	T62.2X2	T62.2X3	T62.2X4	—	—
Rutinum	T46.991	T46.992	T46.993	T46.994	T46.995	T46.996
Rutoside	T46.991	T46.992	T46.993	T46.994	T46.995	T46.996
b-sitosterol(s)	T46.6X1	T46.6X2	T46.6X3	T46.6X4	T46.6X5	T46.6X6
Sabadilla (plant)	T62.2X1	T62.2X2	T62.2X3	T62.2X4	—	—
pesticide	T60.2X1	T60.2X2	T60.2X3	T60.2X4	—	—
Saccharated iron oxide	T45.8X1	T45.8X2	T45.8X3	T45.8X4	T45.8X5	T45.8X6
Saccharin	T50.901	T50.902	T50.903	T50.904	T50.905	T50.906
Saccharomyces boulardii	T47.6X1	T47.6X2	T47.6X3	T47.6X4	T47.6X5	T47.6X6
Safflower oil	T46.6X1	T46.6X2	T46.6X3	T46.6X4	T46.6X5	T46.6X6
Safrazine	T43.1X1	T43.1X2	T43.1X3	T43.1X4	T43.1X5	T43.1X6
Salazosulfapyridine	T37.0X1	T37.0X2	T37.0X3	T37.0X4	T37.0X5	T37.0X6
Salbutamol	T48.6X1	T48.6X2	T48.6X3	T48.6X4	T48.6X5	T48.6X6
Salicylamide	T39.091	T39.092	T39.093	T39.094	T39.095	T39.096
Salicylate NEC	T39.091	T39.092	T39.093	T39.094	T39.095	T39.096
methyl	T49.3X1	T49.3X2	T49.3X3	T49.3X4	T49.3X5	T49.3X6
theobromine calcium	T50.2X1	T50.2X2	T50.2X3	T50.2X4	T50.2X5	T50.2X6
Salicylazosulfapyridine	T37.0X1	T37.0X2	T37.0X3	T37.0X4	T37.0X5	T37.0X6
Salicylhydroxamic acid	T49.0X1	T49.0X2	T49.0X3	T49.0X4	—	T49.0X6
Salicylic acid	T49.4X1	T49.4X2	T49.4X3	T49.4X4	T49.4X5	T49.4X6
with benzoic acid	T49.4X1	T49.4X2	T49.4X3	T49.4X4	T49.4X5	T49.4X6
congeners	T39.091	T39.092	T39.093	T39.094	T39.095	T39.096
derivative	T39.091	T39.092	T39.093	T39.094	T39.095	T39.096
salts	T39.091	T39.092	T39.093	T39.094	T39.095	T39.096
Salinazid	T37.1X1	T37.1X2	T37.1X3	T37.1X4	T37.1X5	T37.1X6
Salmeterol	T48.6X1	T48.6X2	T48.6X3	T48.6X4	T48.6X5	T48.6X6
Salol	T49.3X1	T49.3X2	T49.3X3	T49.3X4	T49.3X5	T49.3X6
Salsalate	T39.091	T39.092	T39.093	T39.094	T39.095	T39.096
Salt-replacing drug	T50.901	T50.902	T50.903	T50.904	T50.905	T50.906
Salt-retaining mineralocorticoid	T50.0X1	T50.0X2	T50.0X3	T50.0X4	T50.0X5	T50.0X6
Salt substitute	T50.901	T50.902	T50.903	T50.904	T50.905	T50.906
Saluretic NEC	T50.2X1	T50.2X2	T50.2X3	T50.2X4	T50.2X5	T50.2X6
Saluron	T50.2X1	T50.2X2	T50.2X3	T50.2X4	T50.2X5	T50.2X6
Salvarsan 606 (neosilver) (silver)	T37.8X1	T37.8X2	T37.8X3	T37.8X4	T37.8X5	T37.8X6
Sambucus canadensis	T62.2X1	T62.2X2	T62.2X3	T62.2X4	—	—
berry	T62.1X1	T62.1X2	T62.1X3	T62.1X4	—	—
Sandril	T46.5X1	T46.5X2	T46.5X3	T46.5X4	T46.5X5	T46.5X6
Sanguinaria canadensis	T62.2X1	T62.2X2	T62.2X3	T62.2X4	—	—
Saniflush (cleaner)	T54.2X1	T54.2X2	T54.2X3	T54.2X4	—	—
Santonin	T37.4X1	T37.4X2	T37.4X3	T37.4X4	T37.4X5	T37.4X6
Santyl	T49.8X1	T49.8X2	T49.8X3	T49.8X4	T49.8X5	T49.8X6
Saralasin	T46.5X1	T46.5X2	T46.5X3	T46.5X4	T46.5X5	T46.5X6
Sarcolysin	T45.1X1	T45.1X2	T45.1X3	T45.1X4	T45.1X5	T45.1X6
Sarkomycin	T45.1X1	T45.1X2	T45.1X3	T45.1X4	T45.1X5	T45.1X6
Saroten	T43.011	T43.012	T43.013	T43.014	T43.015	T43.016
Saturnine — see Lead						
Savin (oil)	T49.4X1	T49.4X2	T49.4X3	T49.4X4	T49.4X5	T49.4X6
Scammony	T47.2X1	T47.2X2	T47.2X3	T47.2X4	T47.2X5	T47.2X6
Scarlet red	T49.8X1	T49.8X2	T49.8X3	T49.8X4	T49.8X5	T49.8X6
Scheele's green	T57.0X1	T57.0X2	T57.0X3	T57.0X4	—	—
insecticide	T57.0X1	T57.0X2	T57.0X3	T57.0X4	—	—
Schizontozide (blood) (tissue)	T37.2X1	T37.2X2	T37.2X3	T37.2X4	T37.2X5	T37.2X6
Schradan	T60.0X1	T60.0X2	T60.0X3	T60.0X4	—	—
Schweinfurth green	T57.0X1	T57.0X2	T57.0X3	T57.0X4	—	—
insecticide	T57.0X1	T57.0X2	T57.0X3	T57.0X4	—	—
Scilla, rat poison	T60.4X1	T60.4X2	T60.4X3	T60.4X4	—	—
Scillaren	T60.4X1	T60.4X2	T60.4X3	T60.4X4	—	—
Sclerosing agent	T46.8X1	T46.8X2	T46.8X3	T46.8X4	T46.8X5	T46.8X6
Scombrotoxin	T61.11	T61.12	T61.13	T61.14	—	—
Scopolamine	T44.3X1	T44.3X2	T44.3X3	T44.3X4	T44.3X5	T44.3X6
Scopolia extract	T44.3X1	T44.3X2	T44.3X3	T44.3X4	T44.3X5	T44.3X6
Scouring powder	T65.891	T65.892	T65.893	T65.894	—	—
Sea						
anemone (sting)	T63.631	T63.632	T63.633	T63.634	—	—
cucumber (sting)	T63.691	T63.692	T63.693	T63.694	—	—
snake (bite) (venom)	T63.091	T63.092	T63.093	T63.094	—	—
urchin spine (puncture)	T63.691	T63.692	T63.693	T63.694	—	—
Seafood	T61.91	T61.92	T61.93	T61.94	—	—
specified NEC	T61.8X1	T61.8X2	T61.8X3	T61.8X4	—	—
Secbutabarbital	T42.3X1	T42.3X2	T42.3X3	T42.3X4	T42.3X5	T42.3X6
Secbutabarbitone	T42.3X1	T42.3X2	T42.3X3	T42.3X4	T42.3X5	T42.3X6
Secnidazole	T37.3X1	T37.3X2	T37.3X3	T37.3X4	T37.3X5	T37.3X6
Secobarbital	T42.3X1	T42.3X2	T42.3X3	T42.3X4	T42.3X5	T42.3X6
Seconal	T42.3X1	T42.3X2	T42.3X3	T42.3X4	T42.3X5	T42.3X6
Secretin	T50.8X1	T50.8X2	T50.8X3	T50.8X4	T50.8X5	T50.8X6
Sedative NEC	T42.71	T42.72	T42.73	T42.74	T42.75	T42.76
mixed NEC	T42.6X1	T42.6X2	T42.6X3	T42.6X4	T42.6X5	T42.6X6
Sedormid	T42.6X1	T42.6X2	T42.6X3	T42.6X4	T42.6X5	T42.6X6
Seed disinfectant or dressing	T60.8X1	T60.8X2	T60.8X3	T60.8X4	—	—
Seeds (poisonous)	T62.2X1	T62.2X2	T62.2X3	T62.2X4	—	—
Selegiline	T42.8X1	T42.8X2	T42.8X3	T42.8X4	T42.8X5	T42.8X6
Selenium NEC	T56.891	T56.892	T56.893	T56.894	—	—
disulfide or sulfide	T49.4X1	T49.4X2	T49.4X3	T49.4X4	T49.4X5	T49.4X6
fumes	T59.891	T59.892	T59.893	T59.894	—	—
sulfide	T49.4X1	T49.4X2	T49.4X3	T49.4X4	T49.4X5	T49.4X6
Selenomethionine (75Se)	T50.8X1	T50.8X2	T50.8X3	T50.8X4	T50.8X5	T50.8X6
Selsun	T49.4X1	T49.4X2	T49.4X3	T49.4X4	T49.4X5	T49.4X6
Semustine	T45.1X1	T45.1X2	T45.1X3	T45.1X4	T45.1X5	T45.1X6
Senega syrup	T48.4X1	T48.4X2	T48.4X3	T48.4X4	T48.4X5	T48.4X6
Senna	T47.2X1	T47.2X2	T47.2X3	T47.2X4	T47.2X5	T47.2X6
Sennoside A+B	T47.2X1	T47.2X2	T47.2X3	T47.2X4	T47.2X5	T47.2X6
Septisol	T49.2X1	T49.2X2	T49.2X3	T49.2X4	T49.2X5	T49.2X6
Seractide	T38.811	T38.812	T38.813	T38.814	T38.815	T38.816
Serax	T42.4X1	T42.4X2	T42.4X3	T42.4X4	T42.4X5	T42.4X6
Serenesil	T42.6X1	T42.6X2	T42.6X3	T42.6X4	T42.6X5	T42.6X6
Serenium (hydrochloride)	T37.91	T37.92	T37.93	T37.94	T37.95	T37.96
Serepax — see Oxazepam						
Sermorelin	T38.891	T38.892	T38.893	T38.894	T38.895	T38.896
Sernyl	T41.1X1	T41.1X2	T41.1X3	T41.1X4	T41.1X5	T41.1X6
Serotonin	T50.991	T50.992	T50.993	T50.994	T50.995	T50.996
Serpasil	T46.5X1	T46.5X2	T46.5X3	T46.5X4	T46.5X5	T46.5X6
Serrapeptase	T45.3X1	T45.3X2	T45.3X3	T45.3X4	T45.3X5	T45.3X6
Serum						
antibotulinus	T50.Z11	T50.Z12	T50.Z13	T50.Z14	T50.Z15	T50.Z16
anticytotoxic	T50.Z11	T50.Z12	T50.Z13	T50.Z14	T50.Z15	T50.Z16
antidiphtheria	T50.Z11	T50.Z12	T50.Z13	T50.Z14	T50.Z15	T50.Z16
antimeningococcus	T50.Z11	T50.Z12	T50.Z13	T50.Z14	T50.Z15	T50.Z16
anti-Rh	T50.Z11	T50.Z12	T50.Z13	T50.Z14	T50.Z15	T50.Z16
anti-snake-bite	T50.Z11	T50.Z12	T50.Z13	T50.Z14	T50.Z15	T50.Z16
antitetanic	T50.Z11	T50.Z12	T50.Z13	T50.Z14	T50.Z15	T50.Z16
antitoxic	T50.Z11	T50.Z12	T50.Z13	T50.Z14	T50.Z15	T50.Z16
complement (inhibitor)	T45.8X1	T45.8X2	T45.8X3	T45.8X4	T45.8X5	T45.8X6
convalescent	T50.Z11	T50.Z12	T50.Z13	T50.Z14	T50.Z15	T50.Z16
hemolytic complement	T45.8X1	T45.8X2	T45.8X3	T45.8X4	T45.8X5	T45.8X6
immune (human)	T50.Z11	T50.Z12	T50.Z13	T50.Z14	T50.Z15	T50.Z16
protective NEC	T50.Z11	T50.Z12	T50.Z13	T50.Z14	T50.Z15	T50.Z16
Setastine	T45.0X1	T45.0X2	T45.0X3	T45.0X4	T45.0X5	T45.0X6
Setoperone	T43.591	T43.592	T43.593	T43.594	T43.595	T43.596
Sewer gas	T59.91	T59.92	T59.93	T59.94	—	—
Shampoo	T55.0X1	T55.0X2	T55.0X3	T55.0X4	—	—
Shellfish, noxious, nonbacterial	T61.781	T61.782	T61.783	T61.784	—	—

Substance	Poisoning, Accidental (unintentional)	Poisoning, Intentional Self-harm	Poisoning, Assault	Poisoning, Undetermined	Adverse Effect	Under-dosing
Sildenafil	T46.7X1	T46.7X2	T46.7X3	T46.7X4	T46.7X5	T46.7X6
Silibinin	T50.991	T50.992	T50.993	T50.994	T50.995	T50.996
Silicone NEC	T65.891	T65.892	T65.893	T65.894	—	—
medicinal	T49.3X1	T49.3X2	T49.3X3	T49.3X4	T49.3X5	T49.3X6
Silvadene	T49.0X1	T49.0X2	T49.0X3	T49.0X4	T49.0X5	T49.0X6
Silver	T49.0X1	T49.0X2	T49.0X3	T49.0X4	T49.0X5	T49.0X6
anti-infectives	T49.0X1	T49.0X2	T49.0X3	T49.0X4	T49.0X5	T49.0X6
arsphenamine	T37.8X1	T37.8X2	T37.8X3	T37.8X4	T37.8X5	T37.8X6
colloidal	T49.0X1	T49.0X2	T49.0X3	T49.0X4	T49.0X5	T49.0X6
nitrate	T49.0X1	T49.0X2	T49.0X3	T49.0X4	T49.0X5	T49.0X6
ophthalmic preparation	T49.5X1	T49.5X2	T49.5X3	T49.5X4	T49.5X5	T49.5X6
toughened (keratolytic)	T49.4X1	T49.4X2	T49.4X3	T49.4X4	T49.4X5	T49.4X6
nonmedicinal (dust)	T56.891	T56.892	T56.893	T56.894	—	—
protein	T49.5X1	T49.5X2	T49.5X3	T49.5X4	T49.5X5	T49.5X6
salvarsan	T37.8X1	T37.8X2	T37.8X3	T37.8X4	T37.8X5	T37.8X6
sulfadiazine	T49.4X1	T49.4X2	T49.4X3	T49.4X4	T49.4X5	T49.4X6
Silymarin	T50.991	T50.992	T50.993	T50.994	T50.995	T50.996
Simaldrate	T47.1X1	T47.1X2	T47.1X3	T47.1X4	T47.1X5	T47.1X6
Simazine	T60.3X1	T60.3X2	T60.3X3	T60.3X4	—	—
Simethicone	T47.1X1	T47.1X2	T47.1X3	T47.1X4	T47.1X5	T47.1X6
Simfibrate	T46.6X1	T46.6X2	T46.6X3	T46.6X4	T46.6X5	T46.6X6
Simvastatin	T46.6X1	T46.6X2	T46.6X3	T46.6X4	T46.6X5	T46.6X6
Sincalide	T50.8X1	T50.8X2	T50.8X3	T50.8X4	T50.8X5	T50.8X6
Sinequan	T43.011	T43.012	T43.013	T43.014	T43.015	T43.016
Singoserp	T46.5X1	T46.5X2	T46.5X3	T46.5X4	T46.5X5	T46.5X6
Sintrom	T45.511	T45.512	T45.513	T45.514	T45.515	T45.516
Sisomicin	T36.5X1	T36.5X2	T36.5X3	T36.5X4	T36.5X5	T36.5X6
Sitosterols	T46.6X1	T46.6X2	T46.6X3	T46.6X4	T46.6X5	T46.6X6
Skeletal muscle relaxants	T48.1X1	T48.1X2	T48.1X3	T48.1X4	T48.1X5	T48.1X6
Skin						
agents (external)	T49.91	T49.92	T49.93	T49.94	T49.95	T49.96
specified NEC	T49.8X1	T49.8X2	T49.8X3	T49.8X4	T49.8X5	T49.8X6
test antigen	T50.8X1	T50.8X2	T50.8X3	T50.8X4	T50.8X5	T50.8X6
Sleep-eze	T45.0X1	T45.0X2	T45.0X3	T45.0X4	T45.0X5	T45.0X6
Sleeping draught, pill	T42.71	T42.72	T42.73	T42.74	T42.75	T42.76
Smallpox vaccine	T50.B11	T50.B12	T50.B13	T50.B14	T50.B15	T50.B16
Smelter fumes NEC	T56.91	T56.92	T56.93	T56.94	—	—
Smog	T59.1X1	T59.1X2	T59.1X3	T59.1X4	—	—
Smoke NEC	T59.811	T59.812	T59.813	T59.814	—	—
Smooth muscle relaxant	T44.3X1	T44.3X2	T44.3X3	T44.3X4	T44.3X5	T44.3X6
Snail killer NEC	T60.8X1	T60.8X2	T60.8X3	T60.8X4	—	—
Snake venom or bite	T63.001	T63.002	T63.003	T63.004	—	—
hemocoagulase	T45.7X1	T45.7X2	T45.7X3	T45.7X4	T45.7X5	T45.7X6
Snuff	T65.211	T65.212	T65.213	T65.214	—	—
Soap (powder) (product)	T55.0X1	T55.0X2	T55.0X3	T55.0X4	—	—
enema	T47.4X1	T47.4X2	T47.4X3	T47.4X4	T47.4X5	T47.4X6
medicinal, soft	T49.2X1	T49.2X2	T49.2X3	T49.2X4	T49.2X5	T49.2X6
superfatted	T49.2X1	T49.2X2	T49.2X3	T49.2X4	T49.2X5	T49.2X6
Sobrerol	T48.4X1	T48.4X2	T48.4X3	T48.4X4	T48.4X5	T48.4X6
Soda (caustic)	T54.3X1	T54.3X2	T54.3X3	T54.3X4	—	—
bicarb	T47.1X1	T47.1X2	T47.1X3	T47.1X4	T47.1X5	T47.1X6
chlorinated — see Sodium, hypochlorite						
Sodium						
acetosulfone	T37.1X1	T37.1X2	T37.1X3	T37.1X4	T37.1X5	T37.1X6
acetrizoate	T50.8X1	T50.8X2	T50.8X3	T50.8X4	T50.8X5	T50.8X6
acid phosphate	T50.3X1	T50.3X2	T50.3X3	T50.3X4	T50.3X5	T50.3X6
alginate	T47.8X1	T47.8X2	T47.8X3	T47.8X4	T47.8X5	T47.8X6
amidotrizoate	T50.8X1	T50.8X2	T50.8X3	T50.8X4	T50.8X5	T50.8X6
aminopterin	T45.1X1	T45.1X2	T45.1X3	T45.1X4	T45.1X5	T45.1X6
amylosulfate	T47.8X1	T47.8X2	T47.8X3	T47.8X4	T47.8X5	T47.8X6
amytal	T42.3X1	T42.3X2	T42.3X3	T42.3X4	T42.3X5	T42.3X6
antimony gluconate	T37.3X1	T37.3X2	T37.3X3	T37.3X4	T37.3X5	T37.3X6
arsenate	T57.0X1	T57.0X2	T57.0X3	T57.0X4	—	—
aurothiomalate	T39.4X1	T39.4X2	T39.4X3	T39.4X4	T39.4X5	T39.4X6
aurothiosulfate	T39.4X1	T39.4X2	T39.4X3	T39.4X4	T39.4X5	T39.4X6
barbiturate	T42.3X1	T42.3X2	T42.3X3	T42.3X4	T42.3X5	T42.3X6
basic phosphate	T47.4X1	T47.4X2	T47.4X3	T47.4X4	T47.4X5	T47.4X6
bicarbonate	T47.1X1	T47.1X2	T47.1X3	T47.1X4	T47.1X5	T47.1X6
bichromate	T57.8X1	T57.8X2	T57.8X3	T57.8X4	—	—
biphosphate	T50.3X1	T50.3X2	T50.3X3	T50.3X4	T50.3X5	T50.3X6
bisulfate	T65.891	T65.892	T65.893	T65.894	—	—
borate						
cleanser	T57.8X1	T57.8X2	T57.8X3	T57.8X4	—	—
eye	T49.5X1	T49.5X2	T49.5X3	T49.5X4	T49.5X5	T49.5X6
therapeutic	T49.8X1	T49.8X2	T49.8X3	T49.8X4	T49.8X5	T49.8X6
bromide	T42.6X1	T42.6X2	T42.6X3	T42.6X4	T42.6X5	T42.6X6
cacodylate (nonmedicinal) NEC	T50.8X1	T50.8X2	T50.8X3	T50.8X4	T50.8X5	T50.8X6
anti-infective	T37.8X1	T37.8X2	T37.8X3	T37.8X4	T37.8X5	T37.8X6
herbicide	T60.3X1	T60.3X2	T60.3X3	T60.3X4	—	—
calcium edetate	T45.8X1	T45.8X2	T45.8X3	T45.8X4	T45.8X5	T45.8X6
carbonate NEC	T54.3X1	T54.3X2	T54.3X3	T54.3X4	—	—

Substance	Poisoning, Accidental (unintentional)	Poisoning, Intentional Self-harm	Poisoning, Assault	Poisoning, Undetermined	Adverse Effect	Under-dosing
Sodium — *continued*						
chlorate NEC	T65.891	T65.892	T65.893	T65.894	—	—
herbicide	T54.91	T54.92	T54.93	T54.94	—	—
chloride	T50.3X1	T50.3X2	T50.3X3	T50.3X4	T50.3X5	T50.3X6
with glucose	T50.3X1	T50.3X2	T50.3X3	T50.3X4	T50.3X5	T50.3X6
chromate	T65.891	T65.892	T65.893	T65.894	—	—
citrate	T50.991	T50.992	T50.993	T50.994	T50.995	T50.996
cromoglicate	T48.6X1	T48.6X2	T48.6X3	T48.6X4	T48.6X5	T48.6X6
cyanide	T65.0X1	T65.0X2	T65.0X3	T65.0X4	—	—
cyclamate	T50.3X1	T50.3X2	T50.3X3	T50.3X4	T50.3X5	T50.3X6
dehydrocholate	T45.8X1	T45.8X2	T45.8X3	T45.8X4	T45.8X5	T45.8X6
diatrizoate	T50.8X1	T50.8X2	T50.8X3	T50.8X4	T50.8X5	T50.8X6
dibunate	T48.4X1	T48.4X2	T48.4X3	T48.4X4	T48.4X5	T48.4X6
dioctyl sulfosuccinate	T47.4X1	T47.4X2	T47.4X3	T47.4X4	T47.4X5	T47.4X6
dipantoyl ferrate	T45.8X1	T45.8X2	T45.8X3	T45.8X4	T45.8X5	T45.8X6
edetate	T45.8X1	T45.8X2	T45.8X3	T45.8X4	T45.8X5	T45.8X6
ethacrynate	T50.1X1	T50.1X2	T50.1X3	T50.1X4	T50.1X5	T50.1X6
feredetate	T45.8X1	T45.8X2	T45.8X3	T45.8X4	T45.8X5	T45.8X6
Fluoride — *see* Fluoride						
fluoroacetate (dust) (pesticide)	T60.4X1	T60.4X2	T60.4X3	T60.4X4	—	—
free salt	T50.3X1	T50.3X2	T50.3X3	T50.3X4	T50.3X5	T50.3X6
fusidate	T36.8X1	T36.8X2	T36.8X3	T36.8X4	T36.8X5	T36.8X6
glucaldrate	T47.1X1	T47.1X2	T47.1X3	T47.1X4	T47.1X5	T47.1X6
glucosulfone	T37.1X1	T37.1X2	T37.1X3	T37.1X4	T37.1X5	T37.1X6
glutamate	T45.8X1	T45.8X2	T45.8X3	T45.8X4	T45.8X5	T45.8X6
hydrogen carbonate	T50.3X1	T50.3X2	T50.3X3	T50.3X4	T50.3X5	T50.3X6
hydroxide	T54.3X1	T54.3X2	T54.3X3	T54.3X4	—	—
hypochlorite (bleach) NEC	T54.3X1	T54.3X2	T54.3X3	T54.3X4	—	—
disinfectant	T54.3X1	T54.3X2	T54.3X3	T54.3X4	—	—
medicinal (anti-infective) (external)	T49.0X1	T49.0X2	T49.0X3	T49.0X4	T49.0X5	T49.0X6
vapor	T54.3X1	T54.3X2	T54.3X3	T54.3X4	—	—
hyposulfite	T49.0X1	T49.0X2	T49.0X3	T49.0X4	T49.0X5	T49.0X6
indigotin disulfonate	T50.8X1	T50.8X2	T50.8X3	T50.8X4	T50.8X5	T50.8X6
iodide	T50.991	T50.992	T50.993	T50.994	T50.995	T50.996
I-131	T50.8X1	T50.8X2	T50.8X3	T50.8X4	T50.8X5	T50.8X6
therapeutic	T38.2X1	T38.2X2	T38.2X3	T38.2X4	T38.2X5	T38.2X6
iodohippurate (131I)	T50.8X1	T50.8X2	T50.8X3	T50.8X4	T50.8X5	T50.8X6
iopodate	T50.8X1	T50.8X2	T50.8X3	T50.8X4	T50.8X5	T50.8X6
iothalamate	T50.8X1	T50.8X2	T50.8X3	T50.8X4	T50.8X5	T50.8X6
iron edetate	T45.4X1	T45.4X2	T45.4X3	T45.4X4	T45.4X5	T45.4X6
lactate (compound solution)	T45.8X1	T45.8X2	T45.8X3	T45.8X4	T45.8X5	T45.8X6
lauryl (sulfate)	T49.2X1	T49.2X2	T49.2X3	T49.2X4	T49.2X5	T49.2X6
L-triiodothyronine	T38.1X1	T38.1X2	T38.1X3	T38.1X4	T38.1X5	T38.1X6
magnesium citrate	T50.991	T50.992	T50.993	T50.994	T50.995	T50.996
mersalate	T50.2X1	T50.2X2	T50.2X3	T50.2X4	T50.2X5	T50.2X6
metasilicate	T65.891	T65.892	T65.893	T65.894	—	—
metrizoate	T50.8X1	T50.8X2	T50.8X3	T50.8X4	T50.8X5	T50.8X6
monofluoroacetate (pesticide)	T60.1X1	T60.1X2	T60.1X3	T60.1X4	—	—
morrhuate	T46.8X1	T46.8X2	T46.8X3	T46.8X4	T46.8X5	T46.8X6
nafcillin	T36.0X1	T36.0X2	T36.0X3	T36.0X4	T36.0X5	T36.0X6
nitrate (oxidizing agent)	T65.891	T65.892	T65.893	T65.894	—	—
nitrite	T50.6X1	T50.6X2	T50.6X3	T50.6X4	T50.6X5	T50.6X6
nitroferricyanide	T46.5X1	T46.5X2	T46.5X3	T46.5X4	T46.5X5	T46.5X6
nitroprusside	T46.5X1	T46.5X2	T46.5X3	T46.5X4	T46.5X5	T46.5X6
oxalate	T65.891	T65.892	T65.893	T65.894	—	—
oxide/peroxide	T65.891	T65.892	T65.893	T65.894	—	—
oxybate	T41.291	T41.292	T41.293	T41.294	T41.295	T41.296
para-aminohippurate	T50.8X1	T50.8X2	T50.8X3	T50.8X4	T50.8X5	T50.8X6
perborate (nonmedicinal) NEC	T65.891	T65.892	T65.893	T65.894	—	—
medicinal	T49.0X1	T49.0X2	T49.0X3	T49.0X4	T49.0X5	T49.0X6
soap	T55.0X1	T55.0X2	T55.0X3	T55.0X4	—	—
percarbonate — *see* Sodium, perborate						
pertechnetate Tc99m	T50.8X1	T50.8X2	T50.8X3	T50.8X4	T50.8X5	T50.8X6
phosphate						
cellulose	T45.8X1	T45.8X2	T45.8X3	T45.8X4	T45.8X5	T45.8X6
dibasic	T47.2X1	T47.2X2	T47.2X3	T47.2X4	T47.2X5	T47.2X6
monobasic	T47.2X1	T47.2X2	T47.2X3	T47.2X4	T47.2X5	T47.2X6
phytate	T50.6X1	T50.6X2	T50.6X3	T50.6X4	T50.6X5	T50.6X6
picosulfate	T47.2X1	T47.2X2	T47.2X3	T47.2X4	T47.2X5	T47.2X6
polyhydroxyaluminium monocarbonate	T47.1X1	T47.1X2	T47.1X3	T47.1X4	T47.1X5	T47.1X6
polystyrene sulfonate	T50.3X1	T50.3X2	T50.3X3	T50.3X4	T50.3X5	T50.3X6
propionate	T49.0X1	T49.0X2	T49.0X3	T49.0X4	T49.0X5	T49.0X6
propyl hydroxybenzoate	T50.991	T50.992	T50.993	T50.994	T50.995	T50.996
psylliate	T46.8X1	T46.8X2	T46.8X3	T46.8X4	T46.8X5	T46.8X6
removing resins	T50.3X1	T50.3X2	T50.3X3	T50.3X4	T50.3X5	T50.3X6
salicylate	T39.091	T39.092	T39.093	T39.094	T39.095	T39.096

Table of Drugs and Chemicals

Sodium — Strychnine

Substance	Poisoning, Accidental (unintentional)	Poisoning, Intentional Self-harm	Poisoning, Assault	Poisoning, Undetermined	Adverse Effect	Under-dosing
Sodium — *continued*						
salt NEC	T50.3X1	T50.3X2	T50.3X3	T50.3X4	T50.3X5	T50.3X6
selenate	T60.2X1	T60.2X2	T60.2X3	T60.2X4	—	—
stibogluconate	T37.3X1	T37.3X2	T37.3X3	T37.3X4	T37.3X5	T37.3X6
sulfate	T47.4X1	T47.4X2	T47.4X3	T47.4X4	T47.4X5	T47.4X6
sulfoxone	T37.1X1	T37.1X2	T37.1X3	T37.1X4	T37.1X5	T37.1X6
tetradecyl sulfate	T46.8X1	T46.8X2	T46.8X3	T46.8X4	T46.8X5	T46.8X6
thiopental	T41.1X1	T41.1X2	T41.1X3	T41.1X4	T41.1X5	T41.1X6
thiosalicylate	T39.091	T39.092	T39.093	T39.094	T39.095	T39.096
thiosulfate	T50.6X1	T50.6X2	T50.6X3	T50.6X4	T50.6X5	T50.6X6
tolbutamide	T38.3X1	T38.3X2	T38.3X3	T38.3X4	T38.3X5	T38.3X6
(L)-triiodothyronine	T38.1X1	T38.1X2	T38.1X3	T38.1X4	T38.1X5	T38.1X6
tyropanoate	T50.8X1	T50.8X2	T50.8X3	T50.8X4	T50.8X5	T50.8X6
valproate	T42.6X1	T42.6X2	T42.6X3	T42.6X4	T42.6X5	T42.6X6
versenate	T50.6X1	T50.6X2	T50.6X3	T50.6X4	T50.6X5	T50.6X6
Sodium-free salt	T50.901	T50.902	T50.903	T50.904	T50.905	T50.906
Sodium-removing resin	T50.3X1	T50.3X2	T50.3X3	T50.3X4	T50.3X5	T50.3X6
Soft soap	T55.0X1	T55.0X2	T55.0X3	T55.0X4	—	—
Solanine	T62.2X1	T62.2X2	T62.2X3	T62.2X4	—	—
berries	T62.1X1	T62.1X2	T62.1X3	T62.1X4	—	—
Solanum dulcamara	T62.2X1	T62.2X2	T62.2X3	T62.2X4	—	—
berries	T62.1X1	T62.1X2	T62.1X3	T62.1X4	—	—
Solapsone	T37.1X1	T37.1X2	T37.1X3	T37.1X4	T37.1X5	T37.1X6
Solar lotion	T49.3X1	T49.3X2	T49.3X3	T49.3X4	T49.3X5	T49.3X6
Solasulfone	T37.1X1	T37.1X2	T37.1X3	T37.1X4	T37.1X5	T37.1X6
Soldering fluid	T65.891	T65.892	T65.893	T65.894	—	—
Solid substance	T65.91	T65.92	T65.93	T65.94	—	—
specified NEC	T65.891	T65.892	T65.893	T65.894	—	—
Solvent, industrial NEC	T52.91	T52.92	T52.93	T52.94	—	—
naphtha	T52.0X1	T52.0X2	T52.0X3	T52.0X4	—	—
petroleum	T52.0X1	T52.0X2	T52.0X3	T52.0X4	—	—
specified NEC	T52.8X1	T52.8X2	T52.8X3	T52.8X4	—	—
Soma	T42.8X1	T42.8X2	T42.8X3	T42.8X4	T42.8X5	T42.8X6
Somatorelin	T38.891	T38.892	T38.893	T38.894	T38.895	T38.896
Somatostatin	T38.991	T38.992	T38.993	T38.994	T38.995	T38.996
Somatotropin	T38.811	T38.812	T38.813	T38.814	T38.815	T38.816
Somatrem	T38.811	T38.812	T38.813	T38.814	T38.815	T38.816
Somatropin	T38.811	T38.812	T38.813	T38.814	T38.815	T38.816
Sominex	T45.0X1	T45.0X2	T45.0X3	T45.0X4	T45.0X5	T45.0X6
Somnos	T42.6X1	T42.6X2	T42.6X3	T42.6X4	T42.6X5	T42.6X6
Somonal	T42.3X1	T42.3X2	T42.3X3	T42.3X4	T42.3X5	T42.3X6
Soneryl	T42.3X1	T42.3X2	T42.3X3	T42.3X4	T42.3X5	T42.3X6
Soothing syrup	T50.901	T50.902	T50.903	T50.904	T50.905	T50.906
Sopor	T42.6X1	T42.6X2	T42.6X3	T42.6X4	T42.6X5	T42.6X6
Soporific	T42.71	T42.72	T42.73	T42.74	T42.75	T42.76
Soporific drug	T42.71	T42.72	T42.73	T42.74	T42.75	T42.76
specified type NEC	T42.6X1	T42.6X2	T42.6X3	T42.6X4	T42.6X5	T42.6X6
Sorbide nitrate	T46.3X1	T46.3X2	T46.3X3	T46.3X4	T46.3X5	T46.3X6
Sorbitol	T47.4X1	T47.4X2	T47.4X3	T47.4X4	T47.4X5	T47.4X6
Sotalol	T44.7X1	T44.7X2	T44.7X3	T44.7X4	T44.7X5	T44.7X6
Sotradecol	T46.8X1	T46.8X2	T46.8X3	T46.8X4	T46.8X5	T46.8X6
Soysterol	T46.6X1	T46.6X2	T46.6X3	T46.6X4	T46.6X5	T46.6X6
Spacoline	T44.3X1	T44.3X2	T44.3X3	T44.3X4	T44.3X5	T44.3X6
Spanish fly	T49.8X1	T49.8X2	T49.8X3	T49.8X4	T49.8X5	T49.8X6
Sparine	T43.3X1	T43.3X2	T43.3X3	T43.3X4	T43.3X5	T43.3X6
Sparteine	T48.0X1	T48.0X2	T48.0X3	T48.0X4	T48.0X5	T48.0X6
Spasmolytic						
anticholinergics	T44.3X1	T44.3X2	T44.3X3	T44.3X4	T44.3X5	T44.3X6
autonomic	T44.3X1	T44.3X2	T44.3X3	T44.3X4	T44.3X5	T44.3X6
bronchial NEC	T48.6X1	T48.6X2	T48.6X3	T48.6X4	T48.6X5	T48.6X6
quaternary ammonium	T44.3X1	T44.3X2	T44.3X3	T44.3X4	T44.3X5	T44.3X6
skeletal muscle NEC	T48.1X1	T48.1X2	T48.1X3	T48.1X4	T48.1X5	T48.1X6
Spectinomycin	T36.5X1	T36.5X2	T36.5X3	T36.5X4	T36.5X5	T36.5X6
Speed	T43.621	T43.622	T43.623	T43.624	T43.625	T43.626
Spermicide	T49.8X1	T49.8X2	T49.8X3	T49.8X4	T49.8X5	T49.8X6
Spider (bite) (venom)	T63.391	T63.392	T63.393	T63.394	—	—
antivenin	T50.Z11	T50.Z12	T50.Z13	T50.Z14	T50.Z15	T50.Z16
Spigelia (root)	T37.4X1	T37.4X2	T37.4X3	T37.4X4	T37.4X5	T37.4X6
Spindle inactivator	T50.4X1	T50.4X2	T50.4X3	T50.4X4	T50.4X5	T50.4X6
Spiperone	T43.4X1	T43.4X2	T43.4X3	T43.4X4	T43.4X5	T43.4X6
Spiramycin	T36.3X1	T36.3X2	T36.3X3	T36.3X4	T36.3X5	T36.3X6
Spirapril	T46.4X1	T46.4X2	T46.4X3	T46.4X4	T46.4X5	T46.4X6
Spirilene	T43.591	T43.592	T43.593	T43.594	T43.595	T43.596
Spirit(s) (neutral) **NEC**	T51.0X1	T51.0X2	T51.0X3	T51.0X4	—	—
beverage	T51.0X1	T51.0X2	T51.0X3	T51.0X4	—	—
industrial	T51.0X1	T51.0X2	T51.0X3	T51.0X4	—	—
mineral	T52.0X1	T52.0X2	T52.0X3	T52.0X4	—	—
of salt — *see* Hydrochloric acid						
surgical	T51.0X1	T51.0X2	T51.0X3	T51.0X4	—	—
Spironolactone	T50.0X1	T50.0X2	T50.0X3	T50.0X4	T50.0X5	T50.0X6
Spiroperidol	T43.4X1	T43.4X2	T43.4X3	T43.4X4	T43.4X5	T43.4X6
Sponge, absorbable	T45.7X1	T45.7X2	T45.7X3	T45.7X4	T45.7X5	T45.7X6
(gelatin)						
Sporostacin	T49.0X1	T49.0X2	T49.0X3	T49.0X4	T49.0X5	T49.0X6
Spray (aerosol)	T65.91	T65.92	T65.93	T65.94	—	—
cosmetic	T65.891	T65.892	T65.893	T65.894	—	—
medicinal NEC	T50.901	T50.902	T50.903	T50.904	T50.905	T50.906
pesticides — *see* Pesticides						
specified content — *see* specific substance						
Spurge flax	T62.2X1	T62.2X2	T62.2X3	T62.2X4	—	—
Spurges	T62.2X1	T62.2X2	T62.2X3	T62.2X4	—	—
Sputum viscosity-lowering drug	T48.4X1	T48.4X2	T48.4X3	T48.4X4	T48.4X5	T48.4X6
Squill	T46.0X1	T46.0X2	T46.0X3	T46.0X4	T46.0X5	T46.0X6
rat poison	T60.4X1	T60.4X2	T60.4X3	T60.4X4	—	—
Squirting cucumber (cathartic)	T47.2X1	T47.2X2	T47.2X3	T47.2X4	T47.2X5	T47.2X6
Stains	T65.6X1	T65.6X2	T65.6X3	T65.6X4	—	—
Stannous fluoride	T49.7X1	T49.7X2	T49.7X3	T49.7X4	T49.7X5	T49.7X6
Stanolone	T38.7X1	T38.7X2	T38.7X3	T38.7X4	T38.7X5	T38.7X6
Stanozolol	T38.7X1	T38.7X2	T38.7X3	T38.7X4	T38.7X5	T38.7X6
Staphisagria or stavesacre (pediculicide)	T49.0X1	T49.0X2	T49.0X3	T49.0X4	T49.0X5	T49.0X6
Starch	T50.901	T50.902	T50.903	T50.904	T50.905	T50.906
Stelazine	T43.3X1	T43.3X2	T43.3X3	T43.3X4	T43.3X5	T43.3X6
Stemetil	T43.3X1	T43.3X2	T43.3X3	T43.3X4	T43.3X5	T43.3X6
Stepronin	T48.4X1	T48.4X2	T48.4X3	T48.4X4	T48.4X5	T48.4X6
Sterculia	T47.4X1	T47.4X2	T47.4X3	T47.4X4	T47.4X5	T47.4X6
Sternutator gas	T59.891	T59.892	T59.893	T59.894	—	—
Steroid	T38.0X1	T38.0X2	T38.0X3	T38.0X4	T38.0X5	T38.0X6
anabolic	T38.7X1	T38.7X2	T38.7X3	T38.7X4	T38.7X5	T38.7X6
androgenic	T38.7X1	T38.7X2	T38.7X3	T38.7X4	T38.7X5	T38.7X6
antineoplastic, hormone	T38.7X1	T38.7X2	T38.7X3	T38.7X4	T38.7X5	T38.7X6
estrogen	T38.5X1	T38.5X2	T38.5X3	T38.5X4	T38.5X5	T38.5X6
ENT agent	T49.6X1	T49.6X2	T49.6X3	T49.6X4	T49.6X5	T49.6X6
ophthalmic preparation	T49.5X1	T49.5X2	T49.5X3	T49.5X4	T49.5X5	T49.5X6
topical NEC	T49.0X1	T49.0X2	T49.0X3	T49.0X4	T49.0X5	T49.0X6
Stibine	T56.891	T56.892	T56.893	T56.894	—	—
Stibogluconate	T37.3X1	T37.3X2	T37.3X3	T37.3X4	T37.3X5	T37.3X6
Stibophen	T37.4X1	T37.4X2	T37.4X3	T37.4X4	T37.4X5	T37.4X6
Stilbamidine (isetionate)	T37.3X1	T37.3X2	T37.3X3	T37.3X4	T37.3X5	T37.3X6
Stilbestrol	T38.5X1	T38.5X2	T38.5X3	T38.5X4	T38.5X5	T38.5X6
Stilboestrol	T38.5X1	T38.5X2	T38.5X3	T38.5X4	T38.5X5	T38.5X6
Stimulant						
central nervous system — *see also* Psychostimulant	T43.601	T43.602	T43.603	T43.604	T43.605	T43.606
analeptics	T50.7X1	T50.7X2	T50.7X3	T50.7X4	T50.7X5	T50.7X6
opiate antagonist	T50.7X1	T50.7X2	T50.7X3	T50.7X4	T50.7X5	T50.7X6
psychotherapeutic NEC — *see also* Psychotherapeutic drug	T43.601	T43.602	T43.603	T43.604	T43.605	T43.606
specified NEC	T43.691	T43.692	T43.693	T43.694	T43.695	T43.696
respiratory	T48.901	T48.902	T48.903	T48.904	T48.905	T48.906
Stone-dissolving drug	T50.901	T50.902	T50.903	T50.904	T50.905	T50.906
Storage battery (cells) (acid)	T54.2X1	T54.2X2	T54.2X3	T54.2X4	—	—
Stovaine	T41.3X1	T41.3X2	T41.3X3	T41.3X4	T41.3X5	T41.3X6
infiltration (subcutaneous)	T41.3X1	T41.3X2	T41.3X3	T41.3X4	T41.3X5	T41.3X6
nerve block (peripheral) (plexus)	T41.3X1	T41.3X2	T41.3X3	T41.3X4	T41.3X5	T41.3X6
spinal	T41.3X1	T41.3X2	T41.3X3	T41.3X4	T41.3X5	T41.3X6
topical (surface)	T41.3X1	T41.3X2	T41.3X3	T41.3X4	T41.3X5	T41.3X6
Stovarsal	T37.8X1	T37.8X2	T37.8X3	T37.8X4	T37.8X5	T37.8X6
Stove gas — *see* Gas, stove						
Stoxil	T49.5X1	T49.5X2	T49.5X3	T49.5X4	T49.5X5	T49.5X6
Stramonium	T48.6X1	T48.6X2	T48.6X3	T48.6X4	T48.6X5	T48.6X6
natural state	T62.2X1	T62.2X2	T62.2X3	T62.2X4	—	—
Streptodornase	T45.3X1	T45.3X2	T45.3X3	T45.3X4	T45.3X5	T45.3X6
Streptoduocin	T36.5X1	T36.5X2	T36.5X3	T36.5X4	T36.5X5	T36.5X6
Streptokinase	T45.611	T45.612	T45.613	T45.614	T45.615	T45.616
Streptomycin (derivative)	T36.5X1	T36.5X2	T36.5X3	T36.5X4	T36.5X5	T36.5X6
Streptonivicin	T36.5X1	T36.5X2	T36.5X3	T36.5X4	T36.5X5	T36.5X6
Streptovarycin	T36.5X1	T36.5X2	T36.5X3	T36.5X4	T36.5X5	T36.5X6
Streptozocin	T45.1X1	T45.1X2	T45.1X3	T45.1X4	T45.1X5	T45.1X6
Streptozotocin	T45.1X1	T45.1X2	T45.1X3	T45.1X4	T45.1X5	T45.1X6
Stripper (paint) (solvent)	T52.8X1	T52.8X2	T52.8X3	T52.8X4	—	—
Strobane	T60.1X1	T60.1X2	T60.1X3	T60.1X4	—	—
Strofantina	T46.0X1	T46.0X2	T46.0X3	T46.0X4	T46.0X5	T46.0X6
Strophanthin (g) (k)	T46.0X1	T46.0X2	T46.0X3	T46.0X4	T46.0X5	T46.0X6
Strophanthus	T46.0X1	T46.0X2	T46.0X3	T46.0X4	T46.0X5	T46.0X6
Strophantin	T46.0X1	T46.0X2	T46.0X3	T46.0X4	T46.0X5	T46.0X6
Strophantin-g	T46.0X1	T46.0X2	T46.0X3	T46.0X4	T46.0X5	T46.0X6
Strychnine (nonmedicinal) (pesticide) (salts)	T65.1X1	T65.1X2	T65.1X3	T65.1X4	—	—
medicinal	T48.291	T48.292	T48.293	T48.294	T48.295	T48.296

Substance	Poisoning, Accidental (unintentional)	Poisoning, Intentional Self-harm	Poisoning, Assault	Poisoning, Undetermined	Adverse Effect	Underdosing
Strychnos (ignatii) — *see* Strychnine						
Styramate	T42.8X1	T42.8X2	T42.8X3	T42.8X4	T42.8X5	T42.8X6
Styrene	T65.891	T65.892	T65.893	T65.894	—	—
Succinimide, antiepileptic or anticonvulsant	T42.2X1	T42.2X2	T42.2X3	T42.2X4	T42.2X5	T42.2X6
mercuric — *see* Mercury						
Succinylcholine	T48.1X1	T48.1X2	T48.1X3	T48.1X4	T48.1X5	T48.1X6
Succinylsulfathiazole	T37.0X1	T37.0X2	T37.0X3	T37.0X5	T37.0X6	
Sucralfate	T47.1X1	T47.1X2	T47.1X3	T47.1X4	T47.1X5	T47.1X6
Sucrose	T50.3X1	T50.3X2	T50.3X3	T50.3X4	T50.3X5	T50.3X6
Sufentanil	T40.4X1	T40.4X2	T40.4X3	T40.4X4	T40.4X5	T40.4X6
Sulbactam	T36.0X1	T36.0X2	T36.0X3	T36.0X4	T36.0X5	T36.0X6
Sulbenicillin	T36.0X1	T36.0X2	T36.0X3	T36.0X4	T36.0X5	T36.0X6
Sulbentine	T49.0X1	T49.0X2	T49.0X3	T49.0X4	T49.0X5	T49.0X6
Sulfacetamide	T49.0X1	T49.0X2	T49.0X3	T49.0X4	T49.0X5	T49.0X6
ophthalmic preparation	T49.5X1	T49.5X2	T49.5X3	T49.5X4	T49.5X5	T49.5X6
Sulfachlorpyridazine	T37.0X1	T37.0X2	T37.0X3	T37.0X4	T37.0X5	T37.0X6
Sulfacitine	T37.0X1	T37.0X2	T37.0X3	T37.0X4	T37.0X5	T37.0X6
Sulfadiasulfone sodium	T37.0X1	T37.0X2	T37.0X3	T37.0X4	T37.0X5	T37.0X6
Sulfadiazine	T37.0X1	T37.0X2	T37.0X3	T37.0X4	T37.0X5	T37.0X6
silver (topical)	T49.0X1	T49.0X2	T49.0X3	T49.0X4	T49.0X5	T49.0X6
Sulfadimethoxine	T37.0X1	T37.0X2	T37.0X3	T37.0X4	T37.0X5	T37.0X6
Sulfadimidine	T37.0X1	T37.0X2	T37.0X3	T37.0X4	T37.0X5	T37.0X6
Sulfadoxine	T37.0X1	T37.0X2	T37.0X3	T37.0X4	T37.0X5	T37.0X6
with pyrimethamine	T37.2X1	T37.2X2	T37.2X3	T37.2X4	T37.2X5	T37.2X6
Sulfaethidole	T37.0X1	T37.0X2	T37.0X3	T37.0X4	T37.0X5	T37.0X6
Sulfafurazole	T37.0X1	T37.0X2	T37.0X3	T37.0X4	T37.0X5	T37.0X6
Sulfaguanidine	T37.0X1	T37.0X2	T37.0X3	T37.0X4	T37.0X5	T37.0X6
Sulfalene	T37.0X1	T37.0X2	T37.0X3	T37.0X4	T37.0X5	T37.0X6
Sulfaloxate	T37.0X1	T37.0X2	T37.0X3	T37.0X4	T37.0X5	T37.0X6
Sulfaloxic acid	T37.0X1	T37.0X2	T37.0X3	T37.0X4	T37.0X5	T37.0X6
Sulfamazone	T39.2X1	T39.2X2	T39.2X3	T39.2X4	T39.2X5	T39.2X6
Sulfamerazine	T37.0X1	T37.0X2	T37.0X3	T37.0X4	T37.0X5	T37.0X6
Sulfameter	T37.0X1	T37.0X2	T37.0X3	T37.0X4	T37.0X5	T37.0X6
Sulfamethazine	T37.0X1	T37.0X2	T37.0X3	T37.0X4	T37.0X5	T37.0X6
Sulfamethizole	T37.0X1	T37.0X2	T37.0X3	T37.0X4	T37.0X5	T37.0X6
Sulfamethoxazole	T37.0X1	T37.0X2	T37.0X3	T37.0X4	T37.0X5	T37.0X6
with trimethoprim	T36.8X1	T36.8X2	T36.8X3	T36.8X4	T36.8X5	T36.8X6
Sulfamethoxydiazine	T37.0X1	T37.0X2	T37.0X3	T37.0X4	T37.0X5	T37.0X6
Sulfamethoxypyridazine	T37.0X1	T37.0X2	T37.0X3	T37.0X4	T37.0X5	T37.0X6
Sulfamethylthiazole	T37.0X1	T37.0X2	T37.0X3	T37.0X4	T37.0X5	T37.0X6
Sulfametoxydiazine	T37.0X1	T37.0X2	T37.0X3	T37.0X4	T37.0X5	T37.0X6
Sulfamidopyrine	T39.2X1	T39.2X2	T39.2X3	T39.2X4	T39.2X5	T39.2X6
Sulfamonomethoxine	T37.0X1	T37.0X2	T37.0X3	T37.0X4	T37.0X5	T37.0X6
Sulfamoxole	T37.0X1	T37.0X2	T37.0X3	T37.0X4	T37.0X5	T37.0X6
Sulfamylon	T49.0X1	T49.0X2	T49.0X3	T49.0X4	T49.0X5	T49.0X6
Sulfan blue (diagnostic dye)	T50.8X1	T50.8X2	T50.8X3	T50.8X4	T50.8X5	T50.8X6
Sulfanilamide	T37.0X1	T37.0X2	T37.0X3	T37.0X4	T37.0X5	T37.0X6
Sulfanilylguanidine	T37.0X1	T37.0X2	T37.0X3	T37.0X4	T37.0X5	T37.0X6
Sulfaperin	T37.0X1	T37.0X2	T37.0X3	T37.0X4	T37.0X5	T37.0X6
Sulfaphenazole	T37.0X1	T37.0X2	T37.0X3	T37.0X4	T37.0X5	T37.0X6
Sulfaphenylthiazole	T37.0X1	T37.0X2	T37.0X3	T37.0X4	T37.0X5	T37.0X6
Sulfaproxyline	T37.0X1	T37.0X2	T37.0X3	T37.0X4	T37.0X5	T37.0X6
Sulfapyridine	T37.0X1	T37.0X2	T37.0X3	T37.0X4	T37.0X5	T37.0X6
Sulfapyrimidine	T37.0X1	T37.0X2	T37.0X3	T37.0X4	T37.0X5	T37.0X6
Sulfarsphenamine	T37.8X1	T37.8X2	T37.8X3	T37.8X4	T37.8X5	T37.8X6
Sulfasalazine	T37.0X1	T37.0X2	T37.0X3	T37.0X4	T37.0X5	T37.0X6
Sulfasuxidine	T37.0X1	T37.0X2	T37.0X3	T37.0X4	T37.0X5	T37.0X6
Sulfasymazine	T37.0X1	T37.0X2	T37.0X3	T37.0X4	T37.0X5	T37.0X6
Sulfated amylopectin	T47.8X1	T47.8X2	T47.8X3	T47.8X4	T47.8X5	T47.8X6
Sulfathiazole	T37.0X1	T37.0X2	T37.0X3	T37.0X4	T37.0X5	T37.0X6
Sulfatostearate	T49.2X1	T49.2X2	T49.2X3	T49.2X4	T49.2X5	T49.2X6
Sulfinpyrazone	T50.4X1	T50.4X2	T50.4X3	T50.4X4	T50.4X5	T50.4X6
Sulfiram	T49.0X1	T49.0X2	T49.0X3	T49.0X4	T49.0X5	T49.0X6
Sulfisomidine	T37.0X1	T37.0X2	T37.0X3	T37.0X4	T37.0X5	T37.0X6
Sulfisoxazole	T37.0X1	T37.0X2	T37.0X3	T37.0X4	T37.0X5	T37.0X6
ophthalmic preparation	T49.5X1	T49.5X2	T49.5X3	T49.5X4	T49.5X5	T49.5X6
Sulfobromophthalein (sodium)	T50.8X1	T50.8X2	T50.8X3	T50.8X4	T50.8X5	T50.8X6
Sulfobromphthalein	T50.8X1	T50.8X2	T50.8X3	T50.8X4	T50.8X5	T50.8X6
Sulfogaiacol	T48.4X1	T48.4X2	T48.4X3	T48.4X4	T48.4X5	T48.4X6
Sulfomyxin	T36.8X1	T36.8X2	T36.8X3	T36.8X4	T36.8X5	T36.8X6
Sulfonal	T42.6X1	T42.6X2	T42.6X3	T42.6X4	T42.6X5	T42.6X6
Sulfonamide NEC	T37.0X1	T37.0X2	T37.0X3	T37.0X4	T37.0X5	T37.0X6
eye	T49.5X1	T49.5X2	T49.5X3	T49.5X4	T49.5X5	T49.5X6
Sulfonazide	T37.1X1	T37.1X2	T37.1X3	T37.1X4	T37.1X5	T37.1X6
Sulfones	T37.1X1	T37.1X2	T37.1X3	T37.1X4	T37.1X5	T37.1X6
Sulfonethylmethane	T42.6X1	T42.6X2	T42.6X3	T42.6X4	T42.6X5	T42.6X6
Sulfonmethane	T42.6X1	T42.6X2	T42.6X3	T42.6X4	T42.6X5	T42.6X6
Sulfonphthal, sulfonphthol	T50.8X1	T50.8X2	T50.8X3	T50.8X4	T50.8X5	T50.8X6
Sulfonylurea derivatives, oral	T38.3X1	T38.3X2	T38.3X3	T38.3X4	T38.3X5	T38.3X6
Sulforidazine	T43.3X1	T43.3X2	T43.3X3	T43.3X4	T43.3X5	T43.3X6
Sulfoxone	T37.1X1	T37.1X2	T37.1X3	T37.1X4	T37.1X5	T37.1X6
Sulfuric acid	T54.2X1	T54.2X2	T54.2X3	T54.2X4	—	—
Sulfur, sulfurated, sulfuric, sulfurous, sulfuryl (compounds NEC) (medicinal)						
acid	T54.2X1	T54.2X2	T54.2X3	T54.2X4	—	—
dioxide (gas)	T59.1X1	T59.1X2	T59.1X3	T59.1X4	—	—
ether — *see* Ether(s)						
hydrogen	T59.6X1	T59.6X2	T59.6X3	T59.6X4	—	—
medicinal (keratolytic) (ointment) NEC	T49.4X1	T49.4X2	T49.4X3	T49.4X4	T49.4X5	T49.4X6
ointment	T49.0X1	T49.0X2	T49.0X3	T49.0X4	T49.0X5	T49.0X6
pesticide (vapor)	T60.91	T60.92	T60.93	T60.94	—	—
vapor NEC	T59.891	T59.892	T59.893	T59.894	—	—
Sulglicotide	T47.1X1	T47.1X2	T47.1X3	T47.1X4	T47.1X5	T47.1X6
Sulindac	T39.391	T39.392	T39.393	T39.394	T39.395	T39.396
Sulisatin	T47.2X1	T47.2X2	T47.2X3	T47.2X4	T47.2X5	T47.2X6
Sulisobenzone	T49.3X1	T49.3X2	T49.3X3	T49.3X4	T49.3X5	T49.3X6
Sulkowitch's reagent	T50.8X1	T50.8X2	T50.8X3	T50.8X4	T50.8X5	T50.8X6
Sulmetozine	T44.3X1	T44.3X2	T44.3X3	T44.3X4	T44.3X5	T44.3X6
Suloctidil	T46.7X1	T46.7X2	T46.7X3	T46.7X4	T46.7X5	T46.7X6
Sulph- — *see also* Sulf-						
Sulphadiazine	T37.0X1	T37.0X2	T37.0X3	T37.0X4	T37.0X5	T37.0X6
Sulphadimethoxine	T37.0X1	T37.0X2	T37.0X3	T37.0X4	T37.0X5	T37.0X6
Sulphadimidine	T37.0X1	T37.0X2	T37.0X3	T37.0X4	T37.0X5	T37.0X6
Sulphadione	T37.1X1	T37.1X2	T37.1X3	T37.1X4	T37.1X5	T37.1X6
Sulphafurazole	T37.0X1	T37.0X2	T37.0X3	T37.0X4	T37.0X5	T37.0X6
Sulphamethizole	T37.0X1	T37.0X2	T37.0X3	T37.0X4	T37.0X5	T37.0X6
Sulphamethoxazole	T37.0X1	T37.0X2	T37.0X3	T37.0X4	T37.0X5	T37.0X6
Sulphan blue	T50.8X1	T50.8X2	T50.8X3	T50.8X4	T50.8X5	T50.8X6
Sulphaphenazole	T37.0X1	T37.0X2	T37.0X3	T37.0X4	T37.0X5	T37.0X6
Sulphapyridine	T37.0X1	T37.0X2	T37.0X3	T37.0X4	T37.0X5	T37.0X6
Sulphasalazine	T37.0X1	T37.0X2	T37.0X3	T37.0X4	T37.0X5	T37.0X6
Sulphinpyrazone	T50.4X1	T50.4X2	T50.4X3	T50.4X4	T50.4X5	T50.4X6
Sulpiride	T43.591	T43.592	T43.593	T43.594	T43.595	T43.596
Sulprostone	T48.0X1	T48.0X2	T48.0X3	T48.0X4	T48.0X5	T48.0X6
Sulpyrine	T39.2X1	T39.2X2	T39.2X3	T39.2X4	T39.2X5	T39.2X6
Sultamicillin	T36.0X1	T36.0X2	T36.0X3	T36.0X4	T36.0X5	T36.0X6
Sulthiame	T42.6X1	T42.6X2	T42.6X3	T42.6X4	T42.6X5	T42.6X6
Sultiame	T42.6X1	T42.6X2	T42.6X3	T42.6X4	T42.6X5	T42.6X6
Sultopride	T43.591	T43.592	T43.593	T43.594	T43.595	T43.596
Sumatriptan	T39.8X1	T39.8X2	T39.8X3	T39.8X4	T39.8X5	T39.8X6
Sunflower seed oil	T46.6X1	T46.6X2	T46.6X3	T46.6X4	T46.6X5	T46.6X6
Superinone	T48.4X1	T48.4X2	T48.4X3	T48.4X4	T48.4X5	T48.4X6
Suprofen	T39.311	T39.312	T39.313	T39.314	T39.315	T39.316
Suramin (sodium)	T37.4X1	T37.4X2	T37.4X3	T37.4X4	T37.4X5	T37.4X6
Surfacaine	T41.3X1	T41.3X2	T41.3X3	T41.3X4	T41.3X5	T41.3X6
Surital	T41.1X1	T41.1X2	T41.1X3	T41.1X4	T41.1X5	T41.1X6
Sutilains	T45.3X1	T45.3X2	T45.3X3	T45.3X4	T45.3X5	T45.3X6
Suxamethonium (chloride)	T48.1X1	T48.1X2	T48.1X3	T48.1X4	T48.1X5	T48.1X6
Suxethonium (chloride)	T48.1X1	T48.1X2	T48.1X3	T48.1X4	T48.1X5	T48.1X6
Suxibuzone	T39.2X1	T39.2X2	T39.2X3	T39.2X4	T39.2X5	T39.2X6
Sweetener	T50.901	T50.902	T50.903	T50.904	T50.905	T50.906
Sweet niter spirit	T46.3X1	T46.3X2	T46.3X3	T46.3X4	T46.3X5	T46.3X6
Sweet oil (birch)	T49.3X1	T49.3X2	T49.3X3	T49.3X4	T49.3X5	T49.3X6
Sym-dichloroethyl ether	T53.6X1	T53.6X2	T53.6X3	T53.6X4	—	—
Sympatholytic NEC	T44.8X1	T44.8X2	T44.8X3	T44.8X4	T44.8X5	T44.8X6
haloalkylamine	T44.8X1	T44.8X2	T44.8X3	T44.8X4	T44.8X5	T44.8X6
Sympathomimetic NEC	T44.901	T44.902	T44.903	T44.904	T44.905	T44.906
anti-common-cold	T48.5X1	T48.5X2	T48.5X3	T48.5X4	T48.5X5	T48.5X6
bronchodilator	T48.6X1	T48.6X2	T48.6X3	T48.6X4	T48.6X5	T48.6X6
specified NEC	T44.991	T44.992	T44.993	T44.994	T44.995	T44.996
Synagis	T50.B91	T50.B92	T50.B93	T50.B94	T50.B95	T50.B96
Synalar	T49.0X1	T49.0X2	T49.0X3	T49.0X4	T49.0X5	T49.0X6
Synthroid	T38.1X1	T38.1X2	T38.1X3	T38.1X4	T38.1X5	T38.1X6
Syntocinon	T48.0X1	T48.0X2	T48.0X3	T48.0X4	T48.0X5	T48.0X6
Syrosingopine	T46.5X1	T46.5X2	T46.5X3	T46.5X4	T46.5X5	T46.5X6
Systemic drug	T45.91	T45.92	T45.93	T45.94	T45.95	T45.96
specified NEC	T45.8X1	T45.8X2	T45.8X3	T45.8X4	T45.8X5	T45.8X6
Tablets — *see also* specified substance	T50.901	T50.902	T50.903	T50.904	T50.905	T50.906
Tace	T38.5X1	T38.5X2	T38.5X3	T38.5X4	T38.5X5	T38.5X6
Tacrine	T44.0X1	T44.0X2	T44.0X3	T44.0X4	T44.0X5	T44.0X6
Tadalafil	T46.7X1	T46.7X2	T46.7X3	T46.7X4	T46.7X5	T46.7X6
Talampicillin	T36.0X1	T36.0X2	T36.0X3	T36.0X4	T36.0X5	T36.0X6
Talbutal	T42.3X1	T42.3X2	T42.3X3	T42.3X4	T42.3X5	T42.3X6
Talc powder	T49.3X1	T49.3X2	T49.3X3	T49.3X4	T49.3X5	T49.3X6
Talcum	T49.3X1	T49.3X2	T49.3X3	T49.3X4	T49.3X5	T49.3X6
Taleranol	T38.6X1	T38.6X2	T38.6X3	T38.6X4	T38.6X5	T38.6X6

Substance	Poisoning, Accidental (unintentional)	Poisoning, Intentional Self-harm	Poisoning, Assault	Poisoning, Undetermined	Adverse Effect	Under-dosing
Tamoxifen	T38.6X1	T38.6X2	T38.6X3	T38.6X4	T38.6X5	T38.6X6
Tamsulosin	T44.6X1	T44.6X2	T44.6X3	T44.6X4	T44.6X5	T44.6X6
Tandearil, tanderil	T39.2X1	T39.2X2	T39.2X3	T39.2X4	T39.2X5	T39.2X6
Tannic acid	T49.2X1	T49.2X2	T49.2X3	T49.2X4	T49.2X5	T49.2X6
medicinal (astringent)	T49.2X1	T49.2X2	T49.2X3	T49.2X4	T49.2X5	T49.2X6
Tannin — see Tannic acid						
Tansy	T62.2X1	T62.2X2	T62.2X3	T62.2X4	—	—
TAO	T36.3X1	T36.3X2	T36.3X3	T36.3X4	T36.3X5	T36.3X6
Tapazole	T38.2X1	T38.2X2	T38.2X3	T38.2X4	T38.2X5	T38.2X6
Taractan	T43.591	T43.592	T43.593	T43.594	T43.595	T43.596
Tarantula (venomous)	T63.321	T63.322	T63.323	T63.324	—	—
Tartar emetic	T37.8X1	T37.8X2	T37.8X3	T37.8X4	T37.8X5	T37.8X6
Tartaric acid	T65.891	T65.892	T65.893	T65.894	—	—
Tartrated antimony (anti-infective)	T37.8X1	T37.8X2	T37.8X3	T37.8X4	T37.8X5	T37.8X6
Tartrate, laxative	T47.4X1	T47.4X2	T47.4X3	T47.4X4	T47.4X5	T47.4X6
Tar NEC	T52.0X1	T52.0X2	T52.0X3	T52.0X4	—	—
camphor	T60.1X1	T60.1X2	T60.1X3	T60.1X4	—	—
distillate	T49.1X1	T49.1X2	T49.1X3	T49.1X4	T49.1X5	T49.1X6
fumes	T59.891	T59.892	T59.893	T59.894	—	—
medicinal	T49.1X1	T49.1X2	T49.1X3	T49.1X4	T49.1X5	T49.1X6
ointment	T49.1X1	T49.1X2	T49.1X3	T49.1X4	T49.1X5	T49.1X6
Tauromustine	T45.1X1	T45.1X2	T45.1X3	T45.1X4	T45.1X5	T45.1X6
TCA — see Trichloroacetic acid						
TCDD	T53.7X1	T53.7X2	T53.7X3	T53.7X4	—	—
TDI (vapor)	T65.0X1	T65.0X2	T65.0X3	T65.0X4	—	—
Tear						
gas	T59.3X1	T59.3X2	T59.3X3	T59.3X4	—	—
solution	T49.5X1	T49.5X2	T49.5X3	T49.5X4	T49.5X5	T49.5X6
Teclothiazide	T50.2X1	T50.2X2	T50.2X3	T50.2X4	T50.2X5	T50.2X6
Teclozan	T37.3X1	T37.3X2	T37.3X3	T37.3X4	T37.3X5	T37.3X6
Tegafur	T45.1X1	T45.1X2	T45.1X3	T45.1X4	T45.1X5	T45.1X6
Tegretol	T42.1X1	T42.1X2	T42.1X3	T42.1X4	T42.1X5	T42.1X6
Teicoplanin	T36.8X1	T36.8X2	T36.8X3	T36.8X4	T36.8X5	T36.8X6
Telepaque	T50.8X1	T50.8X2	T50.8X3	T50.8X4	T50.8X5	T50.8X6
Tellurium	T56.891	T56.892	T56.893	T56.894	—	—
fumes	T56.891	T56.892	T56.893	T56.894	—	—
TEM	T45.1X1	T45.1X2	T45.1X3	T45.1X4	T45.1X5	T45.1X6
Temazepam	T42.4X1	T42.4X2	T42.4X3	T42.4X4	T42.4X5	T42.4X6
Temocillin	T36.0X1	T36.0X2	T36.0X3	T36.0X4	T36.0X5	T36.0X6
Tenamfetamine	T43.621	T43.622	T43.623	T43.624	T43.625	T43.626
Teniposide	T45.1X1	T45.1X2	T45.1X3	T45.1X4	T45.1X5	T45.1X6
Tenitramine	T46.3X1	T46.3X2	T46.3X3	T46.3X4	T46.3X5	T46.3X6
Tenoglicin	T48.4X1	T48.4X2	T48.4X3	T48.4X4	T48.4X5	T48.4X6
Tenonitrozole	T37.3X1	T37.3X2	T37.3X3	T37.3X4	T37.3X5	T37.3X6
Tenoxicam	T39.391	T39.392	T39.393	T39.394	T39.395	T39.396
TEPA	T45.1X1	T45.1X2	T45.1X3	T45.1X4	T45.1X5	T45.1X6
TEPP	T60.0X1	T60.0X2	T60.0X3	T60.0X4	—	—
Teprotide	T46.5X1	T46.5X2	T46.5X3	T46.5X4	T46.5X5	T46.5X6
Terazosin	T44.6X1	T44.6X2	T44.6X3	T44.6X4	T44.6X5	T44.6X6
Terbufos	T60.0X1	T60.0X2	T60.0X3	T60.0X4	—	—
Terbutaline	T48.6X1	T48.6X2	T48.6X3	T48.6X4	T48.6X5	T48.6X6
Terconazole	T49.0X1	T49.0X2	T49.0X3	T49.0X4	T49.0X5	T49.0X6
Terfenadine	T45.0X1	T45.0X2	T45.0X3	T45.0X4	T45.0X5	T45.0X6
Teriparatide (acetate)	T50.991	T50.992	T50.993	T50.994	T50.995	T50.996
Terizidone	T37.1X1	T37.1X2	T37.1X3	T37.1X4	T37.1X5	T37.1X6
Terlipressin	T38.891	T38.892	T38.893	T38.894	T38.895	T38.896
Terodiline	T46.3X1	T46.3X2	T46.3X3	T46.3X4	T46.3X5	T46.3X6
Teroxalene	T37.4X1	T37.4X2	T37.4X3	T37.4X4	T37.4X5	T37.4X6
Terpin (cis) hydrate	T48.4X1	T48.4X2	T48.4X3	T48.4X4	T48.4X5	T48.4X6
Terramycin	T36.4X1	T36.4X2	T36.4X3	T36.4X4	T36.4X5	T36.4X6
Tertatolol	T44.7X1	T44.7X2	T44.7X3	T44.7X4	T44.7X5	T44.7X6
Tessalon	T48.3X1	T48.3X2	T48.3X3	T48.3X4	T48.3X5	T48.3X6
Testolactone	T38.7X1	T38.7X2	T38.7X3	T38.7X4	T38.7X5	T38.7X6
Testosterone	T38.7X1	T38.7X2	T38.7X3	T38.7X4	T38.7X5	T38.7X6
Tetanus toxoid or vaccine	T50.A91	T50.A92	T50.A93	T50.A94	T50.A95	T50.A96
antitoxin	T50.Z11	T50.Z12	T50.Z13	T50.Z14	T50.Z15	T50.Z16
immune globulin (human)	T50.Z11	T50.Z12	T50.Z13	T50.Z14	T50.Z15	T50.Z16
toxoid	T50.A91	T50.A92	T50.A93	T50.A94	T50.A95	T50.A96
with diphtheria toxoid	T50.A21	T50.A22	T50.A23	T50.A24	T50.A25	T50.A26
with pertussis	T50.A11	T50.A12	T50.A13	T50.A14	T50.A15	T50.A16
Tetrabenazine	T43.591	T43.592	T43.593	T43.594	T43.595	T43.596
Tetracaine	T41.3X1	T41.3X2	T41.3X3	T41.3X4	T41.3X5	T41.3X6
nerve block (peripheral) (plexus)	T41.3X1	T41.3X2	T41.3X3	T41.3X4	T41.3X5	T41.3X6
regional	T41.3X1	T41.3X2	T41.3X3	T41.3X4	T41.3X5	T41.3X6
spinal	T41.3X1	T41.3X2	T41.3X3	T41.3X4	T41.3X5	T41.3X6
Tetrachlorethylene — see Tetrachloroethylene						
Tetrachlormethiazide	T50.2X1	T50.2X2	T50.2X3	T50.2X4	T50.2X5	T50.2X6
Tetrachloroethane	T53.6X1	T53.6X2	T53.6X3	T53.6X4	—	—
vapor	T53.6X1	T53.6X2	T53.6X3	T53.6X4	—	—
paint or varnish	T53.6X1	T53.6X2	T53.6X3	T53.6X4	—	—

Substance	Poisoning, Accidental (unintentional)	Poisoning, Intentional Self-harm	Poisoning, Assault	Poisoning, Undetermined	Adverse Effect	Under-dosing
Tetrachloroethylene (liquid)	T53.3X1	T53.3X2	T53.3X3	T53.3X4	—	—
medicinal	T37.4X1	T37.4X2	T37.4X3	T37.4X4	T37.4X5	T37.4X6
vapor	T53.3X1	T53.3X2	T53.3X3	T53.3X4	—	—
Tetrachloromethane — see Carbon tetrachloride						
Tetracosactide	T38.811	T38.812	T38.813	T38.814	T38.815	T38.816
Tetracosactrin	T38.811	T38.812	T38.813	T38.814	T38.815	T38.816
Tetracycline	T36.4X1	T36.4X2	T36.4X3	T36.4X4	T36.4X5	T36.4X6
ophthalmic preparation	T49.5X1	T49.5X2	T49.5X3	T49.5X4	T49.5X5	T49.5X6
topical NEC	T49.0X1	T49.0X2	T49.0X3	T49.0X4	T49.0X5	T49.0X6
Tetradifon	T60.8X1	T60.8X2	T60.8X3	T60.8X4	—	—
Tetradotoxin	T61.771	T61.772	T61.773	T61.774	—	—
Tetraethyl						
lead	T56.0X1	T56.0X2	T56.0X3	T56.0X4	—	—
pyrophosphate	T60.0X1	T60.0X2	T60.0X3	T60.0X4	—	—
Tetraethylammonium chloride	T44.2X1	T44.2X2	T44.2X3	T44.2X4	T44.2X5	T44.2X6
Tetraethylthiuram disulfide	T50.6X1	T50.6X2	T50.6X3	T50.6X4	T50.6X5	T50.6X6
Tetrahydroaminoacridine	T44.0X1	T44.0X2	T44.0X3	T44.0X4	T44.0X5	T44.0X6
Tetrahydrocannabinol	T40.7X1	T40.7X2	T40.7X3	T40.7X4	T40.7X5	T40.7X6
Tetrahydrofuran	T52.8X1	T52.8X2	T52.8X3	T52.8X4	—	—
Tetrahydronaphthalene	T52.8X1	T52.8X2	T52.8X3	T52.8X4	—	—
Tetrahydrozoline	T49.5X1	T49.5X2	T49.5X3	T49.5X4	T49.5X5	T49.5X6
Tetralin	T52.8X1	T52.8X2	T52.8X3	T52.8X4	—	—
Tetramethrin	T60.2X1	T60.2X2	T60.2X3	T60.2X4	—	—
Tetramethylthiuram (disulfide) NEC	T60.3X1	T60.3X2	T60.3X3	T60.3X4	—	—
medicinal	T49.0X1	T49.0X2	T49.0X3	T49.0X4	T49.0X5	T49.0X6
Tetramisole	T37.4X1	T37.4X2	T37.4X3	T37.4X4	T37.4X5	T37.4X6
Tetranicotinoyl fructose	T46.7X1	T46.7X2	T46.7X3	T46.7X4	T46.7X5	T46.7X6
Tetrazepam	T42.4X1	T42.4X2	T42.4X3	T42.4X4	T42.4X5	T42.4X6
Tetronal	T42.6X1	T42.6X2	T42.6X3	T42.6X4	T42.6X5	T42.6X6
Tetryl	T65.3X1	T65.3X2	T65.3X3	T65.3X4	—	—
Tetrylammonium chloride	T44.2X1	T44.2X2	T44.2X3	T44.2X4	T44.2X5	T44.2X6
Tetryzoline	T49.5X1	T49.5X2	T49.5X3	T49.5X4	T49.5X5	T49.5X6
Thalidomide	T45.1X1	T45.1X2	T45.1X3	T45.1X4	T45.1X5	T45.1X6
Thallium (compounds) (dust)	T56.811	T56.812	T56.813	T56.814	—	—
NEC						
pesticide	T60.4X1	T60.4X2	T60.4X3	T60.4X4	—	—
THC	T40.7X1	T40.7X2	T40.7X3	T40.7X4	T40.7X5	T40.7X6
Thebacon	T48.3X1	T48.3X2	T48.3X3	T48.3X4	T48.3X5	T48.3X6
Thebaine	T40.2X1	T40.2X2	T40.2X3	T40.2X4	T40.2X5	T40.2X6
Thenoic acid	T49.6X1	T49.6X2	T49.6X3	T49.6X4	T49.6X5	T49.6X6
Thenyldiamine	T45.0X1	T45.0X2	T45.0X3	T45.0X4	T45.0X5	T45.0X6
Theobromine (calcium salicylate)	T48.6X1	T48.6X2	T48.6X3	T48.6X4	T48.6X5	T48.6X6
sodium salicylate	T48.6X1	T48.6X2	T48.6X3	T48.6X4	T48.6X5	T48.6X6
Theophyllamine	T48.6X1	T48.6X2	T48.6X3	T48.6X4	T48.6X5	T48.6X6
Theophylline	T48.6X1	T48.6X2	T48.6X3	T48.6X4	T48.6X5	T48.6X6
aminobenzoic acid	T48.6X1	T48.6X2	T48.6X3	T48.6X4	T48.6X5	T48.6X6
ethylenediamine	T48.6X1	T48.6X2	T48.6X3	T48.6X4	T48.6X5	T48.6X6
piperazine	T48.6X1	T48.6X2	T48.6X3	T48.6X4	T48.6X5	T48.6X6
p-amino-benzoate						
Thiabendazole	T37.4X1	T37.4X2	T37.4X3	T37.4X4	T37.4X5	T37.4X6
Thialbarbital	T41.1X1	T41.1X2	T41.1X3	T41.1X4	T41.1X5	T41.1X6
Thiamazole	T38.2X1	T38.2X2	T38.2X3	T38.2X4	T38.2X5	T38.2X6
Thiambutosine	T37.1X1	T37.1X2	T37.1X3	T37.1X4	T37.1X5	T37.1X6
Thiamine	T45.2X1	T45.2X2	T45.2X3	T45.2X4	T45.2X5	T45.2X6
Thiamphenicol	T36.2X1	T36.2X2	T36.2X3	T36.2X4	T36.2X5	T36.2X6
Thiamylal	T41.1X1	T41.1X2	T41.1X3	T41.1X4	T41.1X5	T41.1X6
sodium	T41.1X1	T41.1X2	T41.1X3	T41.1X4	T41.1X5	T41.1X6
Thiazesim	T43.291	T43.292	T43.293	T43.294	T43.295	T43.296
Thiazides (diuretics)	T50.2X1	T50.2X2	T50.2X3	T50.2X4	T50.2X5	T50.2X6
Thiazinamium metilsulfate	T43.3X1	T43.3X2	T43.3X3	T43.3X4	T43.3X5	T43.3X6
Thiethylperazine	T43.3X1	T43.3X2	T43.3X3	T43.3X4	T43.3X5	T43.3X6
Thimerosal	T49.0X1	T49.0X2	T49.0X3	T49.0X4	T49.0X5	T49.0X6
ophthalmic preparation	T49.5X1	T49.5X2	T49.5X3	T49.5X4	T49.5X5	T49.5X6
Thioacetazone	T37.1X1	T37.1X2	T37.1X3	T37.1X4	T37.1X5	T37.1X6
with isoniazid	T37.1X1	T37.1X2	T37.1X3	T37.1X4	T37.1X5	T37.1X6
Thiobarbital sodium	T41.1X1	T41.1X2	T41.1X3	T41.1X4	T41.1X5	T41.1X6
Thiobarbiturate anesthetic	T41.1X1	T41.1X2	T41.1X3	T41.1X4	T41.1X5	T41.1X6
Thiobismol	T37.8X1	T37.8X2	T37.8X3	T37.8X4	T37.8X5	T37.8X6
Thiobutabarbital sodium	T41.1X1	T41.1X2	T41.1X3	T41.1X4	T41.1X5	T41.1X6
Thiocarbamate (insecticide)	T60.0X1	T60.0X2	T60.0X3	T60.0X4	—	—
Thiocarbamide	T38.2X1	T38.2X2	T38.2X3	T38.2X4	T38.2X5	T38.2X6
Thiocarbarsone	T37.8X1	T37.8X2	T37.8X3	T37.8X4	T37.8X5	T37.8X6
Thiocarlide	T37.1X1	T37.1X2	T37.1X3	T37.1X4	T37.1X5	T37.1X6
Thioctamide	T50.991	T50.992	T50.993	T50.994	T50.995	T50.996

Substance	Poisoning, Accidental (unintentional)	Poisoning, Intentional Self-harm	Poisoning, Assault	Poisoning, Undetermined	Adverse Effect	Under-dosing
Thioctic acid	T50.991	T50.992	T50.993	T50.994	T50.995	T50.996
Thiofos	T60.0X1	T60.0X2	T60.0X3	T60.0X4	—	—
Thioglycolate	T49.4X1	T49.4X2	T49.4X3	T49.4X4	T49.4X5	T49.4X6
Thioglycolic acid	T65.891	T65.892	T65.893	T65.894	—	—
Thioguanine	T45.1X1	T45.1X2	T45.1X3	T45.1X4	T45.1X5	T45.1X6
Thiomercaptomerin	T50.2X1	T50.2X2	T50.2X3	T50.2X4	T50.2X5	T50.2X6
Thiomerin	T50.2X1	T50.2X2	T50.2X3	T50.2X4	T50.2X5	T50.2X6
Thiomersal	T49.0X1	T49.0X2	T49.0X3	T49.0X4	T49.0X5	T49.0X6
Thionazin	T60.0X1	T60.0X2	T60.0X3	T60.0X4	—	—
Thiopental (sodium)	T41.1X1	T41.1X2	T41.1X3	T41.1X4	T41.1X5	T41.1X6
Thiopentone (sodium)	T41.1X1	T41.1X2	T41.1X3	T41.1X4	T41.1X5	T41.1X6
Thiopropazate	T43.3X1	T43.3X2	T43.3X3	T43.3X4	T43.3X5	T43.3X6
Thioproperazine	T43.3X1	T43.3X2	T43.3X3	T43.3X4	T43.3X5	T43.3X6
Thioridazine	T43.3X1	T43.3X2	T43.3X3	T43.3X4	T43.3X5	T43.3X6
Thiosinamine	T49.3X1	T49.3X2	T49.3X3	T49.3X4	T49.3X5	T49.3X6
Thiotepa	T45.1X1	T45.1X2	T45.1X3	T45.1X4	T45.1X5	T45.1X6
Thiothixene	T43.4X1	T43.4X2	T43.4X3	T43.4X4	T43.4X5	T43.4X6
Thiouracil (benzyl) (methyl) (propyl)	T38.2X1	T38.2X2	T38.2X3	T38.2X4	T38.2X5	T38.2X6
Thiourea	T38.2X1	T38.2X2	T38.2X3	T38.2X4	T38.2X5	T38.2X6
Thiphenamil	T44.3X1	T44.3X2	T44.3X3	T44.3X4	T44.3X5	T44.3X6
Thiram	T60.3X1	T60.3X2	T60.3X3	T60.3X4	—	—
medicinal	T49.2X1	T49.2X2	T49.2X3	T49.2X4	T49.2X5	T49.2X6
Thonzylamine (systemic)	T45.0X1	T45.0X2	T45.0X3	T45.0X4	T45.0X5	T45.0X6
mucosal decongestant	T48.5X1	T48.5X2	T48.5X3	T48.5X4	T48.5X5	T48.5X6
Thorazine	T43.3X1	T43.3X2	T43.3X3	T43.3X4	T43.3X5	T43.3X6
Thorium dioxide suspension	T50.8X1	T50.8X2	T50.8X3	T50.8X4	T50.8X5	T50.8X6
Thornapple	T62.2X1	T62.2X2	T62.2X3	T62.2X4	—	—
Throat drug NEC	T49.6X1	T49.6X2	T49.6X3	T49.6X4	T49.6X5	T49.6X6
Thrombin	T45.7X1	T45.7X2	T45.7X3	T45.7X4	T45.7X5	T45.7X6
Thrombolysin	T45.611	T45.612	T45.613	T45.614	T45.615	T45.616
Thromboplastin	T45.7X1	T45.7X2	T45.7X3	T45.7X4	T45.7X5	T45.7X6
Thurfyl nicotinate	T46.7X1	T46.7X2	T46.7X3	T46.7X4	T46.7X5	T46.7X6
Thymol	T49.0X1	T49.0X2	T49.0X3	T49.0X4	T49.0X5	T49.0X6
Thymopentin	T37.5X1	T37.5X2	T37.5X3	T37.5X4	T37.5X5	T37.5X6
Thymoxamine	T46.7X1	T46.7X2	T46.7X3	T46.7X4	T46.7X5	T46.7X6
Thymus extract	T38.891	T38.892	T38.893	T38.894	T38.895	T38.896
Thyreotrophic hormone	T38.811	T38.812	T38.813	T38.814	T38.815	T38.816
Thyroglobulin	T38.1X1	T38.1X2	T38.1X3	T38.1X4	T38.1X5	T38.1X6
Thyroid (hormone)	T38.1X1	T38.1X2	T38.1X3	T38.1X4	T38.1X5	T38.1X6
Thyrolar	T38.1X1	T38.1X2	T38.1X3	T38.1X4	T38.1X5	T38.1X6
Thyrotrophin	T38.811	T38.812	T38.813	T38.814	T38.815	T38.816
Thyrotropic hormone	T38.811	T38.812	T38.813	T38.814	T38.815	T38.816
Thyroxine	T38.1X1	T38.1X2	T38.1X3	T38.1X4	T38.1X5	T38.1X6
Tiabendazole	T37.4X1	T37.4X2	T37.4X3	T37.4X4	T37.4X5	T37.4X6
Tiamizide	T50.2X1	T50.2X2	T50.2X3	T50.2X4	T50.2X5	T50.2X6
Tianeptine	T43.291	T43.292	T43.293	T43.294	T43.295	T43.296
Tiapamil	T46.1X1	T46.1X2	T46.1X3	T46.1X4	T46.1X5	T46.1X6
Tiapride	T43.591	T43.592	T43.593	T43.594	T43.595	T43.596
Tiaprofenic acid	T39.311	T39.312	T39.313	T39.314	T39.315	T39.316
Tiaramide	T39.8X1	T39.8X2	T39.8X3	T39.8X4	T39.8X5	T39.8X6
Ticarcillin	T36.0X1	T36.0X2	T36.0X3	T36.0X4	T36.0X5	T36.0X6
Ticlatone	T49.0X1	T49.0X2	T49.0X3	T49.0X4	T49.0X5	T49.0X6
Ticlopidine	T45.521	T45.522	T45.523	T45.524	T45.525	T45.526
Ticrynafen	T50.1X1	T50.1X2	T50.1X3	T50.1X4	T50.1X5	T50.1X6
Tidiacic	T50.991	T50.992	T50.993	T50.994	T50.995	T50.996
Tiemonium	T44.3X1	T44.3X2	T44.3X3	T44.3X4	T44.3X5	T44.3X6
iodide	T44.3X1	T44.3X2	T44.3X3	T44.3X4	T44.3X5	T44.3X6
Tienilic acid	T50.1X1	T50.1X2	T50.1X3	T50.1X4	T50.1X5	T50.1X6
Tifenamil	T44.3X1	T44.3X2	T44.3X3	T44.3X4	T44.3X5	T44.3X6
Tigan	T45.0X1	T45.0X2	T45.0X3	T45.0X4	T45.0X5	T45.0X6
Tigloidine	T44.3X1	T44.3X2	T44.3X3	T44.3X4	T44.3X5	T44.3X6
Tilactase	T47.5X1	T47.5X2	T47.5X3	T47.5X4	T47.5X5	T47.5X6
Tiletamine	T41.291	T41.292	T41.293	T41.294	T41.295	T41.296
Tilidine	T40.4X1	T40.4X2	T40.4X3	T40.4X4	—	—
Timepidium bromide	T44.3X1	T44.3X2	T44.3X3	T44.3X4	T44.3X5	T44.3X6
Timiperone	T43.4X1	T43.4X2	T43.4X3	T43.4X4	T43.4X5	T43.4X6
Timolol	T44.7X1	T44.7X2	T44.7X3	T44.7X4	T44.7X5	T44.7X6
Tincture, iodine — *see* Iodine						
Tindal	T43.3X1	T43.3X2	T43.3X3	T43.3X4	T43.3X5	T43.3X6
Tinidazole	T37.3X1	T37.3X2	T37.3X3	T37.3X4	T37.3X5	T37.3X6
Tin (chloride) (dust) (oxide)	T56.6X1	T56.6X2	T56.6X3	T56.6X4	—	—
NEC						
anti-infectives	T37.8X1	T37.8X2	T37.8X3	T37.8X4	T37.8X5	T37.8X6
Tinoridine	T39.8X1	T39.8X2	T39.8X3	T39.8X4	T39.8X5	T39.8X6
Tiocarlide	T37.1X1	T37.1X2	T37.1X3	T37.1X4	T37.1X5	T37.1X6
Tioclomarol	T45.511	T45.512	T45.513	T45.514	T45.515	T45.516
Tioconazole	T49.0X1	T49.0X2	T49.0X3	T49.0X4	T49.0X5	T49.0X6
Tioguanine	T45.1X1	T45.1X2	T45.1X3	T45.1X4	T45.1X5	T45.1X6
Tiopronin	T50.991	T50.992	T50.993	T50.994	T50.995	T50.996
Tiotixene	T43.4X1	T43.4X2	T43.4X3	T43.4X4	T43.4X5	T43.4X6
Tioxolone	T49.4X1	T49.4X2	T49.4X3	T49.4X4	T49.4X5	T49.4X6
Tipepidine	T48.3X1	T48.3X2	T48.3X3	T48.3X4	T48.3X5	T48.3X6
Tiquizium bromide	T44.3X1	T44.3X2	T44.3X3	T44.3X4	T44.3X5	T44.3X6
Tiratricol	T38.1X1	T38.1X2	T38.1X3	T38.1X4	T38.1X5	T38.1X6
Tisopurine	T50.4X1	T50.4X2	T50.4X3	T50.4X4	T50.4X5	T50.4X6
Titanium (compounds) (vapor)	T56.891	T56.892	T56.893	T56.894	—	—
dioxide	T49.3X1	T49.3X2	T49.3X3	T49.3X4	T49.3X5	T49.3X6
ointment	T49.3X1	T49.3X2	T49.3X3	T49.3X4	T49.3X5	T49.3X6
oxide	T49.3X1	T49.3X2	T49.3X3	T49.3X4	T49.3X5	T49.3X6
tetrachloride	T56.891	T56.892	T56.893	T56.894	—	—
Titanocene	T56.891	T56.892	T56.893	T56.894	—	—
Titroid	T38.1X1	T38.1X2	T38.1X3	T38.1X4	T38.1X5	T38.1X6
Tizanidine	T42.8X1	T42.8X2	T42.8X3	T42.8X4	T42.8X5	T42.8X6
TMTD	T60.3X1	T60.3X2	T60.3X3	T60.3X4	—	—
TNT (fumes)	T65.3X1	T65.3X2	T65.3X3	T65.3X4	—	—
Toadstool	T62.0X1	T62.0X2	T62.0X3	T62.0X4	—	—
Tobacco NEC	T65.291	T65.292	T65.293	T65.294	—	—
cigarettes	T65.221	T65.222	T65.223	T65.224	—	—
Indian	T62.2X1	T62.2X2	T62.2X3	T62.2X4	—	—
smoke, second-hand	T65.221	T65.222	T65.223	T65.224	—	—
Tobramycin	T36.5X1	T36.5X2	T36.5X3	T36.5X4	T36.5X5	T36.5X6
Tocainide	T46.2X1	T46.2X2	T46.2X3	T46.2X4	T46.2X5	T46.2X6
Tocoferol	T45.2X1	T45.2X2	T45.2X3	T45.2X4	T45.2X5	T45.2X6
Tocopherol	T45.2X1	T45.2X2	T45.2X3	T45.2X4	T45.2X5	T45.2X6
acetate	T45.2X1	T45.2X2	T45.2X3	T45.2X4	T45.2X5	T45.2X6
Tocosamine	T48.0X1	T48.0X2	T48.0X3	T48.0X4	T48.0X5	T48.0X6
Todralazine	T46.5X1	T46.5X2	T46.5X3	T46.5X4	T46.5X5	T46.5X6
Tofisopam	T42.4X1	T42.4X2	T42.4X3	T42.4X4	T42.4X5	T42.4X6
Tofranil	T43.011	T43.012	T43.013	T43.014	T43.015	T43.016
Toilet deodorizer	T65.891	T65.892	T65.893	T65.894	—	—
Tolamolol	T44.7X1	T44.7X2	T44.7X3	T44.7X4	T44.7X5	T44.7X6
Tolazamide	T38.3X1	T38.3X2	T38.3X3	T38.3X4	T38.3X5	T38.3X6
Tolazoline	T46.7X1	T46.7X2	T46.7X3	T46.7X4	T46.7X5	T46.7X6
Tolbutamide (sodium)	T38.3X1	T38.3X2	T38.3X3	T38.3X4	T38.3X5	T38.3X6
Tolciclate	T49.0X1	T49.0X2	T49.0X3	T49.0X4	T49.0X5	T49.0X6
Tolmetin	T39.391	T39.392	T39.393	T39.394	T39.395	T39.396
Tolnaftate	T49.0X1	T49.0X2	T49.0X3	T49.0X4	T49.0X5	T49.0X6
Tolonidine	T46.5X1	T46.5X2	T46.5X3	T46.5X4	T46.5X5	T46.5X6
Toloxatone	T42.6X1	T42.6X2	T42.6X3	T42.6X4	T42.6X5	T42.6X6
Tolperisone	T44.3X1	T44.3X2	T44.3X3	T44.3X4	T44.3X5	T44.3X6
Tolserol	T42.8X1	T42.8X2	T42.8X3	T42.8X4	T42.8X5	T42.8X6
Toluene (liquid)	T52.2X1	T52.2X2	T52.2X3	T52.2X4	—	—
diisocyanate	T65.0X1	T65.0X2	T65.0X3	T65.0X4	—	—
Toluidine	T65.891	T65.892	T65.893	T65.894	—	—
vapor	T59.891	T59.892	T59.893	T59.894	—	—
Toluol (liquid)	T52.2X1	T52.2X2	T52.2X3	T52.2X4	—	—
vapor	T52.2X1	T52.2X2	T52.2X3	T52.2X4	—	—
Toluylenediamine	T65.3X1	T65.3X2	T65.3X3	T65.3X4	—	—
Tolylene-2,4-diisocyanate	T65.0X1	T65.0X2	T65.0X3	T65.0X4	—	—
Tonic NEC	T50.901	T50.902	T50.903	T50.904	T50.905	T50.906
Topical action drug NEC	T49.91	T49.92	T49.93	T49.94	T49.95	T49.96
ear, nose or throat	T49.6X1	T49.6X2	T49.6X3	T49.6X4	T49.6X5	T49.6X6
eye	T49.5X1	T49.5X2	T49.5X3	T49.5X4	T49.5X5	T49.5X6
skin	T49.91	T49.92	T49.93	T49.94	T49.95	T49.96
specified NEC	T49.8X1	T49.8X2	T49.8X3	T49.8X4	T49.8X5	T49.8X6
Toquizine	T44.3X1	T44.3X2	T44.3X3	T44.3X4	T44.3X5	T44.3X6
Toremifene	T38.6X1	T38.6X2	T38.6X3	T38.6X4	T38.6X5	T38.6X6
Tosylchloramide sodium	T49.8X1	T49.8X2	T49.8X3	T49.8X4	T49.8X5	T49.8X6
Toxaphene (dust) (spray)	T60.1X1	T60.1X2	T60.1X3	T60.1X4	—	—
Toxin, diphtheria (Schick Test)	T50.8X1	T50.8X2	T50.8X3	T50.8X4	T50.8X5	T50.8X6
Toxoid						
combined	T50.A21	T50.A22	T50.A23	T50.A24	T50.A25	T50.A26
diphtheria	T50.A91	T50.A92	T50.A93	T50.A94	T50.A95	T50.A96
tetanus	T50.A91	T50.A92	T50.A93	T50.A94	T50.A95	T50.A96
Trace element NEC	T45.8X1	T45.8X2	T45.8X3	T45.8X4	T45.8X5	T45.8X6
Tractor fuel NEC	T52.0X1	T52.0X2	T52.0X3	T52.0X4	—	—
Tragacanth	T50.991	T50.992	T50.993	T50.994	T50.995	T50.996
Tramadol	T40.4X1	T40.4X2	T40.4X3	T40.4X4	T40.4X5	T40.4X6
Tramazoline	T48.5X1	T48.5X2	T48.5X3	T48.5X4	T48.5X5	T48.5X6
Tranexamic acid	T45.621	T45.622	T45.623	T45.624	T45.625	T45.626
Tranilast	T45.0X1	T45.0X2	T45.0X3	T45.0X4	T45.0X5	T45.0X6
Tranquilizer NEC	T43.501	T43.502	T43.503	T43.504	T43.505	T43.506
with hypnotic or sedative	T42.6X1	T42.6X2	T42.6X3	T42.6X4	T42.6X5	T42.6X6
benzodiazepine NEC	T42.4X1	T42.4X2	T42.4X3	T42.4X4	T42.4X5	T42.4X6
butyrophenone NEC	T43.4X1	T43.4X2	T43.4X3	T43.4X4	T43.4X5	T43.4X6
carbamate	T43.591	T43.592	T43.593	T43.594	T43.595	T43.596
dimethylamine	T43.3X1	T43.3X2	T43.3X3	T43.3X4	T43.3X5	T43.3X6
ethylamine	T43.3X1	T43.3X2	T43.3X3	T43.3X4	T43.3X5	T43.3X6
hydroxyzine	T43.591	T43.592	T43.593	T43.594	T43.595	T43.596
major NEC	T43.501	T43.502	T43.503	T43.504	T43.505	T43.506
penothiazine NEC	T43.3X1	T43.3X2	T43.3X3	T43.3X4	T43.3X5	T43.3X6
phenothiazine-based	T43.3X1	T43.3X2	T43.3X3	T43.3X4	T43.3X5	T43.3X6

▽ Subterms under main terms may continue to next column or page   Additional Character May Be Required — Refer to the Tabular List for Character Selection   **393**

Thioctic acid — Tranquilizer NEC

Table of Drugs and Chemicals

Substance	Poisoning, Accidental (unintentional)	Poisoning, Intentional Self-harm	Poisoning, Assault	Poisoning, Undetermined	Adverse Effect	Under-dosing
Tranquilizer — *continued*						
piperazine NEC	T43.3X1	T43.3X2	T43.3X3	T43.3X4	T43.3X5	T43.3X6
piperidine	T43.3X1	T43.3X2	T43.3X3	T43.3X4	T43.3X5	T43.3X6
propylamine	T43.3X1	T43.3X2	T43.3X3	T43.3X4	T43.3X5	T43.3X6
specified NEC	T43.591	T43.592	T43.593	T43.594	T43.595	T43.596
thioxanthene NEC	T43.591	T43.592	T43.593	T43.594	T43.595	T43.596
Tcanxene	T42.4X1	T42.4X2	T42.4X3	T42.4X4	T42.4X5	T42.4X6
Tranylcypromine	T43.1X1	T43.1X2	T43.1X3	T43.1X4	T43.1X5	T43.1X6
Trapidil	T46.3X1	T46.3X2	T46.3X3	T46.3X4	T46.3X5	T46.3X6
Trasentine	T44.3X1	T44.3X2	T44.3X3	T44.3X4	T44.3X5	T44.3X6
Travert	T50.3X1	T50.3X2	T50.3X3	T50.3X4	T50.3X5	T50.3X6
Trazodone	T43.211	T43.212	T43.213	T43.214	T43.215	T43.216
Trecator	T37.1X1	T37.1X2	T37.1X3	T37.1X4	T37.1X5	T37.1X6
Treosulfan	T45.1X1	T45.1X2	T45.1X3	T45.1X4	T45.1X5	T45.1X6
Tretamine	T45.1X1	T45.1X2	T45.1X3	T45.1X4	T45.1X5	T45.1X6
Tretinoin	T49.0X1	T49.0X2	T49.0X3	T49.0X4	T49.0X5	T49.0X6
Tretoquinol	T48.6X1	T48.6X2	T48.6X3	T48.6X4	T48.6X5	T48.6X6
Triacetin	T49.0X1	T49.0X2	T49.0X3	T49.0X4	T49.0X5	T49.0X6
Triacetoxyanthracene	T49.4X1	T49.4X2	T49.4X3	T49.4X4	T49.4X5	T49.4X6
Triacetyloleandomycin	T36.3X1	T36.3X2	T36.3X3	T36.3X4	T36.3X5	T36.3X6
Triamcinolone	T38.0X1	T38.0X2	T38.0X3	T38.0X4	T38.0X5	T38.0X6
ENT agent	T49.6X1	T49.6X2	T49.6X3	T49.6X4	T49.6X5	T49.6X6
hexacetonide	T49.0X1	T49.0X2	T49.0X3	T49.0X4	T49.0X5	T49.0X6
ophthalmic preparation	T49.5X1	T49.5X2	T49.5X3	T49.5X4	T49.5X5	T49.5X6
topical NEC	T49.0X1	T49.0X2	T49.0X3	T49.0X4	T49.0X5	T49.0X6
Triampyzine	T44.3X1	T44.3X2	T44.3X3	T44.3X4	T44.3X5	T44.3X6
Triamterene	T50.2X1	T50.2X2	T50.2X3	T50.2X4	T50.2X5	T50.2X6
Triazine (herbicide)	T60.3X1	T60.3X2	T60.3X3	T60.3X4	—	—
Triaziquone	T45.1X1	T45.1X2	T45.1X3	T45.1X4	T45.1X5	T45.1X6
Triazolam	T42.4X1	T42.4X2	T42.4X3	T42.4X4	T42.4X5	T42.4X6
Triazole (herbicide)	T60.3X1	T60.3X2	T60.3X3	T60.3X4	—	—
Tribenoside	T46.991	T46.992	T46.993	T46.994	T46.995	T46.996
Tribromacetaldehyde	T42.6X1	T42.6X2	T42.6X3	T42.6X4	T42.6X5	T42.6X6
Tribromoethanol, rectal	T41.291	T41.292	T41.293	T41.294	T41.295	T41.296
Tribromomethane	T42.6X1	T42.6X2	T42.6X3	T42.6X4	T42.6X5	T42.6X6
Trichlorethane	T53.2X1	T53.2X2	T53.2X3	T53.2X4	—	—
Trichlorethylene	T53.2X1	T53.2X2	T53.2X3	T53.2X4	—	—
Trichlorfon	T60.0X1	T60.0X2	T60.0X3	T60.0X4	—	—
Trichlormethiazide	T50.2X1	T50.2X2	T50.2X3	T50.2X4	T50.2X5	T50.2X6
Trichlormethine	T45.1X1	T45.1X2	T45.1X3	T45.1X4	T45.1X5	T45.1X6
Trichloroacetic acid, Trichloracetic acid	T54.2X1	T54.2X2	T54.2X3	T54.2X4	—	—
medicinal	T49.4X1	T49.4X2	T49.4X3	T49.4X4	T49.4X5	T49.4X6
Trichloroethane	T53.2X1	T53.2X2	T53.2X3	T53.2X4	—	—
Trichloroethanol	T42.6X1	T42.6X2	T42.6X3	T42.6X4	T42.6X5	T42.6X6
Trichloroethylene (liquid)	T53.2X1	T53.2X2	T53.2X3	T53.2X4	—	—
(vapor)						
anesthetic (gas)	T41.0X1	T41.0X2	T41.0X3	T41.0X4	T41.0X5	T41.0X6
vapor NEC	T53.2X1	T53.2X2	T53.2X3	T53.2X4	—	—
Trichloroethyl phosphate	T42.6X1	T42.6X2	T42.6X3	T42.6X4	T42.6X5	T42.6X6
Trichlorofluoromethane NEC	T53.5X1	T53.5X2	T53.5X3	T53.5X4	—	—
Trichloronate	T60.0X1	T60.0X2	T60.0X3	T60.0X4	—	—
Trichloropropane	T53.6X1	T53.6X2	T53.6X3	T53.6X4	—	—
Trichlorotriethylamine	T45.1X1	T45.1X2	T45.1X3	T45.1X4	T45.1X5	T45.1X6
Trichomonacides NEC	T37.3X1	T37.3X2	T37.3X3	T37.3X4	T37.3X5	T37.3X6
Trichomycin	T36.7X1	T36.7X2	T36.7X3	T36.7X4	T36.7X5	T36.7X6
Triclobisonium chloride	T49.0X1	T49.0X2	T49.0X3	T49.0X4	T49.0X5	T49.0X6
Triclocarban	T49.0X1	T49.0X2	T49.0X3	T49.0X4	T49.0X5	T49.0X6
Triclofos	T42.6X1	T42.6X2	T42.6X3	T42.6X4	T42.6X5	T42.6X6
Triclosan	T49.0X1	T49.0X2	T49.0X3	T49.0X4	T49.0X5	T49.0X6
Tricresyl phosphate	T65.891	T65.892	T65.893	T65.894	—	—
solvent	T52.91	T52.92	T52.93	T52.94	—	—
Tricyclamol chloride	T44.3X1	T44.3X2	T44.3X3	T44.3X4	T44.3X5	T44.3X6
Tridesilon	T49.0X1	T49.0X2	T49.0X3	T49.0X4	T49.0X5	T49.0X6
Tridihexethyl iodide	T44.3X1	T44.3X2	T44.3X3	T44.3X4	T44.3X5	T44.3X6
Tridione	T42.2X1	T42.2X2	T42.2X3	T42.2X4	T42.2X5	T42.2X6
Trientine	T45.8X1	T45.8X2	T45.8X3	T45.8X4	T45.8X5	T45.8X6
Triethanolamine NEC	T54.3X1	T54.3X2	T54.3X3	T54.3X4	—	—
detergent	T54.3X1	T54.3X2	T54.3X3	T54.3X4	—	—
trinitrate (biphosphate)	T46.3X1	T46.3X2	T46.3X3	T46.3X4	T46.3X5	T46.3X6
Triethanomelamine	T45.1X1	T45.1X2	T45.1X3	T45.1X4	T45.1X5	T45.1X6
Triethylenemelamine	T45.1X1	T45.1X2	T45.1X3	T45.1X4	T45.1X5	T45.1X6
Triethylenephosphoramide	T45.1X1	T45.1X2	T45.1X3	T45.1X4	T45.1X5	T45.1X6
Triethylenethiophosphoramide	T45.1X1	T45.1X2	T45.1X3	T45.1X4	T45.1X5	T45.1X6
Trifluoperazine	T43.3X1	T43.3X2	T43.3X3	T43.3X4	T43.3X5	T43.3X6
Trifluoroethyl vinyl ether	T41.0X1	T41.0X2	T41.0X3	T41.0X4	T41.0X5	T41.0X6
Trifluperidol	T43.4X1	T43.4X2	T43.4X3	T43.4X4	T43.4X5	T43.4X6
Triflupromazine	T43.3X1	T43.3X2	T43.3X3	T43.3X4	T43.3X5	T43.3X6
Trifluridine	T37.5X1	T37.5X2	T37.5X3	T37.5X4	T37.5X5	T37.5X6
Triflusal	T45.521	T45.522	T45.523	T45.524	T45.525	T45.526
Trihexyphenidyl	T44.3X1	T44.3X2	T44.3X3	T44.3X4	T44.3X5	T44.3X6
Triiodothyronine	T38.1X1	T38.1X2	T38.1X3	T38.1X4	T38.1X5	T38.1X6

Substance	Poisoning, Accidental (unintentional)	Poisoning, Intentional Self-harm	Poisoning, Assault	Poisoning, Undetermined	Adverse Effect	Under-dosing
Trilene	T41.0X1	T41.0X2	T41.0X3	T41.0X4	T41.0X5	T41.0X6
Trilostane	T38.991	T38.992	T38.993	T38.994	T38.995	T38.996
Trimebutine	T44.3X1	T44.3X2	T44.3X3	T44.3X4	T44.3X5	T44.3X6
Trimecaine	T41.3X1	T41.3X2	T41.3X3	T41.3X4	T41.3X5	T41.3X6
Trimeprazine (tartrate)	T44.3X1	T44.3X2	T44.3X3	T44.3X4	T44.3X5	T44.3X6
Trimetaphan camsilate	T44.2X1	T44.2X2	T44.2X3	T44.2X4	T44.2X5	T44.2X6
Trimetazidine	T46.7X1	T46.7X2	T46.7X3	T46.7X4	T46.7X5	T46.7X6
Trimethadione	T42.2X1	T42.2X2	T42.2X3	T42.2X4	T42.2X5	T42.2X6
Trimethaphan	T44.2X1	T44.2X2	T44.2X3	T44.2X4	T44.2X5	T44.2X6
Trimethidinium	T44.2X1	T44.2X2	T44.2X3	T44.2X4	T44.2X5	T44.2X6
Trimethobenzamide	T45.0X1	T45.0X2	T45.0X3	T45.0X4	T45.0X5	T45.0X6
Trimethoprim	T37.8X1	T37.8X2	T37.8X3	T37.8X4	T37.8X5	T37.8X6
with sulfamethoxazole	T36.8X1	T36.8X2	T36.8X3	T36.8X4	T36.8X5	T36.8X6
Trimethylcarbinol	T51.3X1	T51.3X2	T51.3X3	T51.3X4	—	—
Trimethylpsoralen	T49.3X1	T49.3X2	T49.3X3	T49.3X4	T49.3X5	T49.3X6
Trimeton	T45.0X1	T45.0X2	T45.0X3	T45.0X4	T45.0X5	T45.0X6
Trimetrexate	T45.1X1	T45.1X2	T45.1X3	T45.1X4	T45.1X5	T45.1X6
Trimipramine	T43.011	T43.012	T43.013	T43.014	T43.015	T43.016
Trimustine	T45.1X1	T45.1X2	T45.1X3	T45.1X4	T45.1X5	T45.1X6
Trinitrine	T46.3X1	T46.3X2	T46.3X3	T46.3X4	T46.3X5	T46.3X6
Trinitrobenzol	T65.3X1	T65.3X2	T65.3X3	T65.3X4	—	—
Trinitrophenol	T65.3X1	T65.3X2	T65.3X3	T65.3X4	—	—
Trinitrotoluene (fumes)	T65.3X1	T65.3X2	T65.3X3	T65.3X4	—	—
Trional	T42.6X1	T42.6X2	T42.6X3	T42.6X4	T42.6X5	T42.6X6
Triorthocresyl phosphate	T65.891	T65.892	T65.893	T65.894	—	—
Trioxide of arsenic	T57.0X1	T57.0X2	T57.0X3	T57.0X4	—	—
Trioxysalen	T49.4X1	T49.4X2	T49.4X3	T49.4X4	T49.4X5	T49.4X6
Tripamide	T50.2X1	T50.2X2	T50.2X3	T50.2X4	T50.2X5	T50.2X6
Triparanol	T46.6X1	T46.6X2	T46.6X3	T46.6X4	T46.6X5	T46.6X6
Tripelennamine	T45.0X1	T45.0X2	T45.0X3	T45.0X4	T45.0X5	T45.0X6
Triperiden	T44.3X1	T44.3X2	T44.3X3	T44.3X4	T44.3X5	T44.3X6
Triperidol	T43.4X1	T43.4X2	T43.4X3	T43.4X4	T43.4X5	T43.4X6
Triphenylphosphate	T65.891	T65.892	T65.893	T65.894	—	—
Triple						
bromides	T42.6X1	T42.6X2	T42.6X3	T42.6X4	T42.6X5	T42.6X6
carbonate	T47.1X1	T47.1X2	T47.1X3	T47.1X4	T47.1X5	T47.1X6
vaccine						
DPT	T50.A11	T50.A12	T50.A13	T50.A14	T50.A15	T50.A16
including pertussis	T50.A11	T50.A12	T50.A13	T50.A14	T50.A15	T50.A16
MMR	T50.B91	T50.B92	T50.B93	T50.B94	T50.B95	T50.B96
Triprolidine	T45.0X1	T45.0X2	T45.0X3	T45.0X4	T45.0X5	T45.0X6
Trisodium hydrogen edetate	T50.6X1	T50.6X2	T50.6X3	T50.6X4	T50.6X5	T50.6X6
Trisoralen	T49.3X1	T49.3X2	T49.3X3	T49.3X4	T49.3X5	T49.3X6
Trisulfapyrimidines	T37.0X1	T37.0X2	T37.0X3	T37.0X4	T37.0X5	T37.0X6
Trithiozine	T44.3X1	T44.3X2	T44.3X3	T44.3X4	T44.3X5	T44.3X6
Tritiozine	T44.3X1	T44.3X2	T44.3X3	T44.3X4	T44.3X5	T44.3X6
Tritoqualine	T45.0X1	T45.0X2	T45.0X3	T45.0X4	T45.0X5	T45.0X6
Trofosfamide	T45.1X1	T45.1X2	T45.1X3	T45.1X4	T45.1X5	T45.1X6
Troleandomycin	T36.3X1	T36.3X2	T36.3X3	T36.3X4	T36.3X5	T36.3X6
Trolnitrate (phosphate)	T46.3X1	T46.3X2	T46.3X3	T46.3X4	T46.3X5	T46.3X6
Tromantadine	T37.5X1	T37.5X2	T37.5X3	T37.5X4	T37.5X5	T37.5X6
Trometamol	T50.2X1	T50.2X2	T50.2X3	T50.2X4	T50.2X5	T50.2X6
Tromethamine	T50.2X1	T50.2X2	T50.2X3	T50.2X4	T50.2X5	T50.2X6
Tronothane	T41.3X1	T41.3X2	T41.3X3	T41.3X4	T41.3X5	T41.3X6
Tropacine	T44.3X1	T44.3X2	T44.3X3	T44.3X4	T44.3X5	T44.3X6
Tropatepine	T44.3X1	T44.3X2	T44.3X3	T44.3X4	T44.3X5	T44.3X6
Tropicamide	T44.3X1	T44.3X2	T44.3X3	T44.3X4	T44.3X5	T44.3X6
Trospium chloride	T44.3X1	T44.3X2	T44.3X3	T44.3X4	T44.3X5	T44.3X6
Troxerutin	T46.991	T46.992	T46.993	T46.994	T46.995	T46.996
Troxidone	T42.2X1	T42.2X2	T42.2X3	T42.2X4	T42.2X5	T42.2X6
Tryparsamide	T37.3X1	T37.3X2	T37.3X3	T37.3X4	T37.3X5	T37.3X6
Trypsin	T45.3X1	T45.3X2	T45.3X3	T45.3X4	T45.3X5	T45.3X6
Tryptizol	T43.011	T43.012	T43.013	T43.014	T43.015	T43.016
TSH	T38.811	T38.812	T38.813	T38.814	T38.815	T38.816
Tuaminoheptane	T48.5X1	T48.5X2	T48.5X3	T48.5X4	T48.5X5	T48.5X6
Tuberculin, purified protein derivative (PPD)	T50.8X1	T50.8X2	T50.8X3	T50.8X4	T50.8X5	T50.8X6
Tubocurare	T48.1X1	T48.1X2	T48.1X3	T48.1X4	T48.1X5	T48.1X6
Tubocurarine (chloride)	T48.1X1	T48.1X2	T48.1X3	T48.1X4	T48.1X5	T48.1X6
Tulobuterol	T48.6X1	T48.6X2	T48.6X3	T48.6X4	T48.6X5	T48.6X6
Turpentine (spirits of)	T52.8X1	T52.8X2	T52.8X3	T52.8X4	—	—
vapor	T52.8X1	T52.8X2	T52.8X3	T52.8X4	—	—
Tybamate	T43.591	T43.592	T43.593	T43.594	T43.595	T43.596
Tyloxapol	T48.4X1	T48.4X2	T48.4X3	T48.4X4	T48.4X5	T48.4X6
Tymazoline	T48.5X1	T48.5X2	T48.5X3	T48.5X4	T48.5X5	T48.5X6
Typhoid-paratyphoid vaccine	T50.A91	T50.A92	T50.A93	T50.A94	T50.A95	T50.A96
Typhus vaccine	T50.A91	T50.A92	T50.A93	T50.A94	T50.A95	T50.A96
Tyropanoate	T50.8X1	T50.8X2	T50.8X3	T50.8X4	T50.8X5	T50.8X6
Tyrothricin	T49.6X1	T49.6X2	T49.6X3	T49.6X4	T49.6X5	T49.6X6
ENT agent	T49.6X1	T49.6X2	T49.6X3	T49.6X4	T49.6X5	T49.6X6
ophthalmic preparation	T49.5X1	T49.5X2	T49.5X3	T49.5X4	T49.5X5	T49.5X6

Additional Character May Be Required — Refer to the Tabular List for Character Selection   ▽ Subterms under main terms may continue to next column or page

Table of Drugs and Chemicals

Tranquilizer NEC — Tyrothricin

Substance	Poisoning, Accidental (unintentional)	Poisoning, Intentional Self-harm	Poisoning, Assault	Poisoning, Undetermined	Adverse Effect	Under-dosing
Ufenamate	T39.391	T39.392	T39.393	T39.394	T39.395	T39.396
Ultraviolet light	T49.3X1	T49.3X2	T49.3X3	T49.3X4	T49.3X5	T49.3X6
protectant						
Undecenoic acid	T49.0X1	T49.0X2	T49.0X3	T49.0X4	T49.0X5	T49.0X6
Undecoylium	T49.0X1	T49.0X2	T49.0X3	T49.0X4	T49.0X5	T49.0X6
Undecylenic acid	T49.0X1	T49.0X2	T49.0X3	T49.0X4	T49.0X5	T49.0X6
(derivatives)						
Unna's boot	T49.3X1	T49.3X2	T49.3X3	T49.3X4	T49.3X5	T49.3X6
Unsaturated fatty acid	T46.6X1	T46.6X2	T46.6X3	T46.6X4	T46.6X5	T46.6X6
Uracil mustard	T45.1X1	T45.1X2	T45.1X3	T45.1X4	T45.1X5	T45.1X6
Uramustine	T45.1X1	T45.1X2	T45.1X3	T45.1X4	T45.1X5	T45.1X6
Urapidil	T46.5X1	T46.5X2	T46.5X3	T46.5X4	T46.5X5	T46.5X6
Urari	T48.1X1	T48.1X2	T48.1X3	T48.1X4	T48.1X5	T48.1X6
Urate oxidase	T50.4X1	T50.4X2	T50.4X3	T50.4X4	T50.4X5	T50.4X6
Urea	T47.3X1	T47.3X2	T47.3X3	T47.3X4	T47.3X5	T47.3X6
peroxide	T49.0X1	T49.0X2	T49.0X3	T49.0X4	T49.0X5	T49.0X6
stibamine	T37.4X1	T37.4X2	T37.4X3	T37.4X4	T37.4X5	T37.4X6
topical	T49.8X1	T49.8X2	T49.8X3	T49.8X4	T49.8X5	T49.8X6
Urethane	T45.1X1	T45.1X2	T45.1X3	T45.1X4	T45.1X5	T45.1X6
Urginea (maritima) (scilla) — *see* Squill						
Uric acid metabolism drug NEC	T50.4X1	T50.4X2	T50.4X3	T50.4X4	T50.4X5	T50.4X6
Uricosuric agent	T50.4X1	T50.4X2	T50.4X3	T50.4X4	T50.4X5	T50.4X6
Urinary anti-infective	T37.8X1	T37.8X2	T37.8X3	T37.8X4	T37.8X5	T37.8X6
Urofollitropin	T38.811	T38.812	T38.813	T38.814	T38.815	T38.816
Urokinase	T45.611	T45.612	T45.613	T45.614	T45.615	T45.616
Urokon	T50.8X1	T50.8X2	T50.8X3	T50.8X4	T50.8X5	T50.8X6
Ursodeoxycholic acid	T50.991	T50.992	T50.993	T50.994	T50.995	T50.996
Ursodiol	T50.991	T50.992	T50.993	T50.994	T50.995	T50.996
Urtica	T62.2X1	T62.2X2	T62.2X3	T62.2X4	—	—
Utility gas — *see* Gas, utility						
Vaccine NEC	T50.Z91	T50.Z92	T50.Z93	T50.Z94	T50.Z95	T50.Z96
antineoplastic	T50.Z91	T50.Z92	T50.Z93	T50.Z94	T50.Z95	T50.Z96
bacterial NEC	T50.A91	T50.A92	T50.A93	T50.A94	T50.A95	T50.A96
with						
other bacterial component	T50.A21	T50.A22	T50.A23	T50.A24	T50.A25	T50.A26
pertussis component	T50.A11	T50.A12	T50.A13	T50.A14	T50.A15	T50.A16
viral-rickettsial component	T50.A21	T50.A22	T50.A23	T50.A24	T50.A25	T50.A26
mixed NEC	T50.A21	T50.A22	T50.A23	T50.A24	T50.A25	T50.A26
BCG	T50.A91	T50.A92	T50.A93	T50.A94	T50.A95	T50.A96
cholera	T50.A91	T50.A92	T50.A93	T50.A94	T50.A95	T50.A96
diphtheria	T50.A91	T50.A92	T50.A93	T50.A94	T50.A95	T50.A96
with tetanus	T50.A21	T50.A22	T50.A23	T50.A24		T50.A26
and pertussis	T50.A11	T50.A12	T50.A13	T50.A14	T50.A15	T50.A16
influenza	T50.B91	T50.B92	T50.B93	T50.B94	T50.B95	T50.B96
measles	T50.B91	T50.B92	T50.B93	T50.B94	T50.B95	T50.B96
with mumps and rubella	T50.B91	T50.B92	T50.B93	T50.B94	T50.B95	T50.B96
meningococcal	T50.A91	T50.A92	T50.A93	T50.A94	T50.A95	T50.A96
mumps	T50.B91	T50.B92	T50.B93	T50.B94	T50.B95	T50.B96
paratyphoid	T50.A91	T50.A92	T50.A93	T50.A94	T50.A95	T50.A96
pertussis	T50.A11	T50.A12	T50.A13	T50.A14	T50.A15	T50.A16
with diphtheria	T50.A11	T50.A12	T50.A13	T50.A14	T50.A15	T50.A16
and tetanus	T50.A11	T50.A12	T50.A13	T50.A14	T50.A15	T50.A16
with other component	T50.A11	T50.A12	T50.A13	T50.A14	T50.A15	T50.A16
plague	T50.A91	T50.A92	T50.A93	T50.A94	T50.A95	T50.A96
poliomyelitis	T50.B91	T50.B92	T50.B93	T50.B94	T50.B95	T50.B96
poliovirus	T50.B91	T50.B92	T50.B93	T50.B94	T50.B95	T50.B96
rabies	T50.B91	T50.B92	T50.B93	T50.B94	T50.B95	T50.B96
respiratory syncytial virus	T50.B91	T50.B92	T50.B93	T50.B94	T50.B95	T50.B96
rickettsial NEC	T50.A91	T50.A92	T50.A93	T50.A94	T50.A95	T50.A96
with bacterial component	T50.A21	T50.A22	T50.A23	T50.A24	T50.A25	T50.A26
Rocky Mountain spotted fever	T50.A91	T50.A92	T50.A93	T50.A94	T50.A95	T50.A96
rubella	T50.B91	T50.B92	T50.B93	T50.B94	T50.B95	T50.B96
sabin oral	T50.B91	T50.B92	T50.B93	T50.B94	T50.B95	T50.B96
smallpox	T50.B11	T50.B12	T50.B13	T50.B14	T50.B15	T50.B16
TAB	T50.A91	T50.A92	T50.A93	T50.A94	T50.A95	T50.A96
tetanus	T50.A91	T50.A92	T50.A93	T50.A94	T50.A95	T50.A96
typhoid	T50.A91	T50.A92	T50.A93	T50.A94	T50.A95	T50.A96
typhus	T50.A91	T50.A92	T50.A93	T50.A94	T50.A95	T50.A96
viral NEC	T50.B91	T50.B92	T50.B93	T50.B94	T50.B95	T50.B96
yellow fever	T50.B91	T50.B92	T50.B93	T50.B94	T50.B95	T50.B96
Vaccinia immune globulin	T50.Z11	T50.Z12	T50.Z13	T50.Z14	T50.Z15	T50.Z16
Vaginal contraceptives	T49.8X1	T49.8X2	T49.8X3	T49.8X4	T49.8X5	T49.8X6
Valerian						
root	T42.6X1	T42.6X2	T42.6X3	T42.6X4	T42.6X5	T42.6X6
tincture	T42.6X1	T42.6X2	T42.6X3	T42.6X4	T42.6X5	T42.6X6
Valethamate bromide	T44.3X1	T44.3X2	T44.3X3	T44.3X4	T44.3X5	T44.3X6
Valisone	T49.0X1	T49.0X2	T49.0X3	T49.0X4	T49.0X5	T49.0X6
Valium	T42.4X1	T42.4X2	T42.4X3	T42.4X4	T42.4X5	T42.4X6
Valmid	T42.6X1	T42.6X2	T42.6X3	T42.6X4	T42.6X5	T42.6X6
Valnoctamide	T42.6X1	T42.6X2	T42.6X3	T42.6X4	T42.6X5	T42.6X6
Valproate (sodium)	T42.6X1	T42.6X2	T42.6X3	T42.6X4	T42.6X5	T42.6X6
Valproic acid	T42.6X1	T42.6X2	T42.6X3	T42.6X4	T42.6X5	T42.6X6
Valpromide	T42.6X1	T42.6X2	T42.6X3	T42.6X4	T42.6X5	T42.6X6
Vanadium	T56.891	T56.892	T56.893	T56.894	—	—
Vancomycin	T36.8X1	T36.8X2	T36.8X3	T36.8X4	T36.8X5	T36.8X6
Vapor — *see also* Gas	T59.91	T59.92	T59.93	T59.94	—	—
kiln (carbon monoxide)	T58.8X1	T58.8X2	T58.8X3	T58.8X4	—	—
lead — *see* lead						
specified source NEC	T59.891	T59.892	T59.893	T59.894	—	—
Vardenafil	T46.7X1	T46.7X2	T46.7X3	T46.7X4	T46.7X5	T46.7X6
Varicose reduction drug	T46.8X1	T46.8X2	T46.8X3	T46.8X4	T46.8X5	T46.8X6
Varnish	T65.4X1	T65.4X2	T65.4X3	T65.4X4	—	—
cleaner	T52.91	T52.92	T52.93	T52.94	—	—
Vaseline	T49.3X1	T49.3X2	T49.3X3	T49.3X4	T49.3X5	T49.3X6
Vasodilan	T46.7X1	T46.7X2	T46.7X3	T46.7X4	T46.7X5	T46.7X6
Vasodilator						
coronary NEC	T46.3X1	T46.3X2	T46.3X3	T46.3X4	T46.3X5	T46.3X6
peripheral NEC	T46.7X1	T46.7X2	T46.7X3	T46.7X4	T46.7X5	T46.7X6
Vasopressin	T38.891	T38.892	T38.893	T38.894	T38.895	T38.896
Vasopressor drugs	T38.891	T38.892	T38.893	T38.894	T38.895	T38.896
Vecuronium bromide	T48.1X1	T48.1X2	T48.1X3	T48.1X4	T48.1X5	T48.1X6
Vegetable extract, astringent	T49.2X1	T49.2X2	T49.2X3	T49.2X4	T49.2X5	T49.2X6
Venlafaxine	T43.211	T43.212	T43.213	T43.214	T43.215	T43.216
Venom, venomous (bite) (sting)	T63.91	T63.92	T63.93	T63.94	—	—
amphibian NEC	T63.831	T63.832	T63.833	T63.834	—	—
animal NEC	T63.891	T63.892	T63.893	T63.894	—	—
ant	T63.421	T63.422	T63.423	T63.424	—	—
arthropod NEC	T63.481	T63.482	T63.483	T63.484	—	—
bee	T63.441	T63.442	T63.443	T63.444	—	—
centipede	T63.411	T63.412	T63.413	T63.414	—	—
fish	T63.591	T63.592	T63.593	T63.594	—	—
frog	T63.811	T63.812	T63.813	T63.814	—	—
hornet	T63.451	T63.452	T63.453	T63.454	—	—
insect NEC	T63.481	T63.482	T63.483	T63.484	—	—
lizard	T63.121	T63.122	T63.123	T63.124	—	—
marine						
animals	T63.691	T63.692	T63.693	T63.694	—	—
bluebottle	T63.611	T63.612	T63.613	T63.614	—	—
jellyfish NEC	T63.621	T63.622	T63.623	T63.624	—	—
Portugese Man-o-war	T63.611	T63.612	T63.613	T63.614	—	—
sea anemone	T63.631	T63.632	T63.633	T63.634	—	—
specified NEC	T63.691	T63.692	T63.693	T63.694	—	—
fish	T63.591	T63.592	T63.593	T63.594	—	—
plants	T63.711	T63.712	T63.713	T63.714	—	—
sting ray	T63.511	T63.512	T63.513	T63.514	—	—
millipede (tropical)	T63.411	T63.412	T63.413	T63.414	—	—
plant NEC	T63.791	T63.792	T63.793	T63.794	—	—
marine	T63.711	T63.712	T63.713	T63.714	—	—
reptile	T63.191	T63.192	T63.193	T63.194	—	—
gila monster	T63.111	T63.112	T63.113	T63.114	—	—
lizard NEC	T63.121	T63.122	T63.123	T63.124	—	—
scorpion	T63.2X1	T63.2X2	T63.2X3	T63.2X4	—	—
snake	T63.001	T63.002	T63.003	T63.004	—	—
African NEC	T63.081	T63.082	T63.083	T63.084	—	—
American (North) (South) NEC	T63.061	T63.062	T63.063	T63.064	—	—
Asian	T63.081	T63.082	T63.083	T63.084	—	—
Australian	T63.071	T63.072	T63.073	T63.074	—	—
cobra	T63.041	T63.042	T63.043	T63.044	—	—
coral snake	T63.021	T63.022	T63.023	T63.024	—	—
rattlesnake	T63.011	T63.012	T63.013	T63.014	—	—
specified NEC	T63.091	T63.092	T63.093	T63.094	—	—
taipan	T63.031	T63.032	T63.033	T63.034	—	—
specified NEC	T63.891	T63.892	T63.893	T63.894	—	—
spider	T63.301	T63.302	T63.303	T63.304	—	—
black widow	T63.311	T63.312	T63.313	T63.314	—	—
brown recluse	T63.331	T63.332	T63.333	T63.334	—	—
specified NEC	T63.391	T63.392	T63.393	T63.394	—	—
tarantula	T63.321	T63.322	T63.323	T63.324	—	—
sting ray	T63.511	T63.512	T63.513	T63.514	—	—
toad	T63.821	T63.822	T63.823	T63.824	—	—
wasp	T63.461	T63.462	T63.463	T63.464	—	—
Venous sclerosing drug NEC	T46.8X1	T46.8X2	T46.8X3	T46.8X4	T46.8X5	T46.8X6
Ventolin — *see* Albuterol						
Veramon	T42.3X1	T42.3X2	T42.3X3	T42.3X4	T42.3X5	T42.3X6
Verapamil	T46.1X1	T46.1X2	T46.1X3	T46.1X4	T46.1X5	T46.1X6
Veratrine	T46.5X1	T46.5X2	T46.5X3	T46.5X4	T46.5X5	T46.5X6

Table of Drugs and Chemicals

Veratrum — Zinc

Substance	Poisoning, Accidental (unintentional)	Poisoning, Intentional Self-harm	Poisoning, Assault	Poisoning, Undetermined	Adverse Effect	Under-dosing
Veratrum						
album	T62.2X1	T62.2X2	T62.2X3	T62.2X4	—	—
alkaloids	T46.5X1	T46.5X2	T46.5X3	T46.5X4	T46.5X5	T46.5X6
viride	T62.2X1	T62.2X2	T62.2X3	T62.2X4	—	—
Verdigris	T60.3X1	T60.3X2	T60.3X3	T60.3X4	—	—
Veronal	T42.3X1	T42.3X2	T42.3X3	T42.3X4	T42.3X5	T42.3X6
Veroxil	T37.4X1	T37.4X2	T37.4X3	T37.4X4	T37.4X5	T37.4X6
Versenate	T50.6X1	T50.6X2	T50.6X3	T50.6X4	T50.6X5	T50.6X6
Versidyne	T39.8X1	T39.8X2	T39.8X3	T39.8X4	T39.8X5	T39.8X6
Vetrabutine	T48.0X1	T48.0X2	T48.0X3	T48.0X4	T48.0X5	T48.0X6
Vidarabine	T37.5X1	T37.5X2	T37.5X3	T37.5X4	T37.5X5	T37.5X6
Vienna						
green	T57.0X1	T57.0X2	T57.0X3	T57.0X4	—	—
insecticide	T60.2X1	T60.2X2	T60.2X3	T60.2X4	—	—
red	T57.0X1	T57.0X2	T57.0X3	T57.0X4	—	—
pharmaceutical dye	T50.991	T50.992	T50.993	T50.994	T50.995	T50.996
Vigabatrin	T42.6X1	T42.6X2	T42.6X3	T42.6X4	T42.6X5	T42.6X6
Viloxazine	T43.291	T43.292	T43.293	T43.294	T43.295	T43.296
Viminol	T39.8X1	T39.8X2	T39.8X3	T39.8X4	T39.8X5	T39.8X6
Vinbarbital, vinbarbitone	T42.3X1	T42.3X2	T42.3X3	T42.3X4	T42.3X5	T42.3X6
Vinblastine	T45.1X1	T45.1X2	T45.1X3	T45.1X4	T45.1X5	T45.1X6
Vinburnine	T46.7X1	T46.7X2	T46.7X3	T46.7X4	T46.7X5	T46.7X6
Vincamine	T45.1X1	T45.1X2	T45.1X3	T45.1X4	T45.1X5	T45.1X6
Vincristine	T45.1X1	T45.1X2	T45.1X3	T45.1X4	T45.1X5	T45.1X6
Vindesine	T45.1X1	T45.1X2	T45.1X3	T45.1X4	T45.1X5	T45.1X6
Vinesthene, vinethene	T41.0X1	T41.0X2	T41.0X3	T41.0X4	T41.0X5	T41.0X6
Vinorelbine tartrate	T45.1X1	T45.1X2	T45.1X3	T45.1X4	T45.1X5	T45.1X6
Vinpocetine	T46.7X1	T46.7X2	T46.7X3	T46.7X4	T46.7X5	T46.7X6
Vinyl						
acetate	T65.891	T65.892	T65.893	T65.894	—	—
bital	T42.3X1	T42.3X2	T42.3X3	T42.3X4	T42.3X5	T42.3X6
bromide	T65.891	T65.892	T65.893	T65.894	—	—
chloride	T59.891	T59.892	T59.893	T59.894	—	—
ether	T41.0X1	T41.0X2	T41.0X3	T41.0X4	T41.0X5	T41.0X6
Vinylbital	T42.3X1	T42.3X2	T42.3X3	T42.3X4	T42.3X5	T42.3X6
Vinylidene chloride	T65.891	T65.892	T65.893	T65.894	—	—
Vioform	T37.8X1	T37.8X2	T37.8X3	T37.8X4	T37.8X5	T37.8X6
topical	T49.0X1	T49.0X2	T49.0X3	T49.0X4	T49.0X5	T49.0X6
Viomycin	T36.8X1	T36.8X2	T36.8X3	T36.8X4	T36.8X5	T36.8X6
Viosterol	T45.2X1	T45.2X2	T45.2X3	T45.2X4	T45.2X5	T45.2X6
Viper (venom)	T63.091	T63.092	T63.093	T63.094	—	—
Viprynium	T37.4X1	T37.4X2	T37.4X3	T37.4X4	T37.4X5	T37.4X6
Viquidil	T46.7X1	T46.7X2	T46.7X3	T46.7X4	T46.7X5	T46.7X6
Viral vaccine NEC	T50.B91	T50.B92	T50.B93	T50.B94	T50.B95	T50.B96
Virginiamycin	T36.8X1	T36.8X2	T36.8X3	T36.8X4	T36.8X5	T36.8X6
Virugon	T37.5X1	T37.5X2	T37.5X3	T37.5X4	T37.5X5	T37.5X6
Viscous agent	T50.901	T50.902	T50.903	T50.904	T50.905	T50.906
Visine	T49.5X1	T49.5X2	T49.5X3	T49.5X4	T49.5X5	T49.5X6
Visnadine	T46.3X1	T46.3X2	T46.3X3	T46.3X4	T46.3X5	T46.3X6
Vitamin NEC	T45.2X1	T45.2X2	T45.2X3	T45.2X4	T45.2X5	T45.2X6
A	T45.2X1	T45.2X2	T45.2X3	T45.2X4	T45.2X5	T45.2X6
B1	T45.2X1	T45.2X2	T45.2X3	T45.2X4	T45.2X5	T45.2X6
B2	T45.2X1	T45.2X2	T45.2X3	T45.2X4	T45.2X5	T45.2X6
B6	T45.2X1	T45.2X2	T45.2X3	T45.2X4	T45.2X5	T45.2X6
B12	T45.2X1	T45.2X2	T45.2X3	T45.2X4	T45.2X5	T45.2X6
B15	T45.2X1	T45.2X2	T45.2X3	T45.2X4	T45.2X5	T45.2X6
B NEC	T45.2X1	T45.2X2	T45.2X3	T45.2X4	T45.2X5	T45.2X6
nicotinic acid	T46.7X1	T46.7X2	T46.7X3	T46.7X4	T46.7X5	T46.7X6
C	T45.2X1	T45.2X2	T45.2X3	T45.2X4	T45.2X5	T45.2X6
D	T45.2X1	T45.2X2	T45.2X3	T45.2X4	T45.2X5	T45.2X6
D2	T45.2X1	T45.2X2	T45.2X3	T45.2X4	T45.2X5	T45.2X6
D3	T45.2X1	T45.2X2	T45.2X3	T45.2X4	T45.2X5	T45.2X6
E	T45.2X1	T45.2X2	T45.2X3	T45.2X4	T45.2X5	T45.2X6
E acetate	T45.2X1	T45.2X2	T45.2X3	T45.2X4	T45.2X5	T45.2X6
hematopoietic	T45.8X1	T45.8X2	T45.8X3	T45.8X4	T45.8X5	T45.8X6
K1	T45.7X1	T45.7X2	T45.7X3	T45.7X4	T45.7X5	T45.7X6
K2	T45.7X1	T45.7X2	T45.7X3	T45.7X4	T45.7X5	T45.7X6
K NEC	T45.7X1	T45.7X2	T45.7X3	T45.7X4	T45.7X5	T45.7X6
PP	T45.2X1	T45.2X2	T45.2X3	T45.2X4	T45.2X5	T45.2X6
ulceroprotectant	T47.1X1	T47.1X2	T47.1X3	T47.1X4	T47.1X5	T47.1X6
Vleminckx's solution	T49.4X1	T49.4X2	T49.4X3	T49.4X4	T49.4X5	T49.4X6
Voltaren — *see* Diclofenac						
sodium						
Warfarin	T45.511	T45.512	T45.513	T45.514	T45.515	T45.516
rodenticide	T60.4X1	T60.4X2	T60.4X3	T60.4X4	—	—
sodium	T45.511	T45.512	T45.513	T45.514	T45.515	T45.516
Wasp (sting)	T63.461	T63.462	T63.463	T63.464	—	—
Water						
balance drug	T50.3X1	T50.3X2	T50.3X3	T50.3X4	T50.3X5	T50.3X6
distilled	T50.3X1	T50.3X2	T50.3X3	T50.3X4	T50.3X5	T50.3X6
gas — *see* Gas, water						

Substance	Poisoning, Accidental (unintentional)	Poisoning, Intentional Self-harm	Poisoning, Assault	Poisoning, Undetermined	Adverse Effect	Under-dosing
Water — *continued*						
gas — *see* Gas, water — *continued*						
incomplete combustion of — *see* Carbon, monoxide, fuel, utility						
hemlock	T62.2X1	T62.2X2	T62.2X3	T62.2X4	—	—
moccasin (venom)	T63.061	T63.062	T63.063	T63.064	—	—
purified	T50.3X1	T50.3X2	T50.3X3	T50.3X4	T50.3X5	T50.3X6
Wax (paraffin) (petroleum)	T52.0X1	T52.0X2	T52.0X3	T52.0X4	—	—
automobile	T65.891	T65.892	T65.893	T65.894	—	—
floor	T52.0X1	T52.0X2	T52.0X3	T52.0X4	—	—
Weed killers NEC	T60.3X1	T60.3X2	T60.3X3	T60.3X4	—	—
Welldorm	T42.6X1	T42.6X2	T42.6X3	T42.6X4	T42.6X5	T42.6X6
White						
arsenic	T57.0X1	T57.0X2	T57.0X3	T57.0X4	—	—
hellebore	T62.2X1	T62.2X2	T62.2X3	T62.2X4	—	—
lotion (keratolytic)	T49.4X1	T49.4X2	T49.4X3	T49.4X4	T49.4X5	T49.4X6
spirit	T52.0X1	T52.0X2	T52.0X3	T52.0X4	—	—
Whitewash	T65.891	T65.892	T65.893	T65.894	—	—
Whole blood (human)	T45.8X1	T45.8X2	T45.8X3	T45.8X4	T45.8X5	T45.8X6
Wild						
black cherry	T62.2X1	T62.2X2	T62.2X3	T62.2X4	—	—
poisonous plants NEC	T62.2X1	T62.2X2	T62.2X3	T62.2X4	—	—
Window cleaning fluid	T65.891	T65.892	T65.893	T65.894	—	—
Wintergreen (oil)	T49.3X1	T49.3X2	T49.3X3	T49.3X4	T49.3X5	T49.3X6
Wisterine	T62.2X1	T62.2X2	T62.2X3	T62.2X4	—	—
Witch hazel	T49.2X1	T49.2X2	T49.2X3	T49.2X4	T49.2X5	T49.2X6
Wood alcohol or spirit	T51.1X1	T51.1X2	T51.1X3	T51.1X4	—	—
Wool fat (hydrous)	T49.3X1	T49.3X2	T49.3X3	T49.3X4	T49.3X5	T49.3X6
Woorali	T48.1X1	T48.1X2	T48.1X3	T48.1X4	T48.1X5	T48.1X6
Wormseed, American	T37.4X1	T37.4X2	T37.4X3	T37.4X4	T37.4X5	T37.4X6
Xamoterol	T44.5X1	T44.5X2	T44.5X3	T44.5X4	T44.5X5	T44.5X6
Xanthine diuretics	T50.2X1	T50.2X2	T50.2X3	T50.2X4	T50.2X5	T50.2X6
Xanthinol nicotinate	T46.7X1	T46.7X2	T46.7X3	T46.7X4	T46.7X5	T46.7X6
Xanthotoxin	T49.3X1	T49.3X2	T49.3X3	T49.3X4	T49.3X5	T49.3X6
Xantinol nicotinate	T46.7X1	T46.7X2	T46.7X3	T46.7X4	T46.7X5	T46.7X6
Xantocillin	T36.0X1	T36.0X2	T36.0X3	T36.0X4	T36.0X5	T36.0X6
Xenon (127Xe) (133Xe)	T50.8X1	T50.8X2	T50.8X3	T50.8X4	T50.8X5	T50.8X6
Xenysalate	T49.4X1	T49.4X2	T49.4X3	T49.4X4	T49.4X5	T49.4X6
Xibornol	T37.8X1	T37.8X2	T37.8X3	T37.8X4	T37.8X5	T37.8X6
Xigris	T45.511	T45.512	T45.513	T45.514	T45.515	T45.516
Xipamide	T50.2X1	T50.2X2	T50.2X3	T50.2X4	T50.2X5	T50.2X6
Xylene (vapor)	T52.2X1	T52.2X2	T52.2X3	T52.2X4	—	—
Xylocaine (infiltration)	T41.3X1	T41.3X2	T41.3X3	T41.3X4	T41.3X5	T41.3X6
(topical)						
nerve block (peripheral) (plexus)	T41.3X1	T41.3X2	T41.3X3	T41.3X4	T41.3X5	T41.3X6
spinal	T41.3X1	T41.3X2	T41.3X3	T41.3X4	T41.3X5	T41.3X6
Xylol (vapor)	T52.2X1	T52.2X2	T52.2X3	T52.2X4	—	—
Xylometazoline	T48.5X1	T48.5X2	T48.5X3	T48.5X4	T48.5X5	T48.5X6
Yeast	T45.2X1	T45.2X2	T45.2X3	T45.2X4	T45.2X5	T45.2X6
dried	T45.2X1	T45.2X2	T45.2X3	T45.2X4	T45.2X5	T45.2X6
Yellow						
fever vaccine	T50.B91	T50.B92	T50.B93	T50.B94	T50.B95	T50.B96
jasmine	T62.2X1	T62.2X2	T62.2X3	T62.2X4	—	—
phenolphthalein	T47.2X1	T47.2X2	T47.2X3	T47.2X4	T47.2X5	T47.2X6
Yew	T62.2X1	T62.2X2	T62.2X3	T62.2X4	—	—
Yohimbic acid	T40.991	T40.992	T40.993	T40.994	T40.995	T40.996
Zactane	T39.8X1	T39.8X2	T39.8X3	T39.8X4	T39.8X5	T39.8X6
Zalcitabine	T37.5X1	T37.5X2	T37.5X3	T37.5X4	T37.5X5	T37.5X6
Zaroxolyn	T50.2X1	T50.2X2	T50.2X3	T50.2X4	T50.2X5	T50.2X6
Zephiran (topical)	T49.0X1	T49.0X2	T49.0X3	T49.0X4	T49.0X5	T49.0X6
ophthalmic preparation	T49.5X1	T49.5X2	T49.5X3	T49.5X4	T49.5X5	T49.5X6
Zeranol	T38.7X1	T38.7X2	T38.7X3	T38.7X4	T38.7X5	T38.7X6
Zerone	T51.1X1	T51.1X2	T51.1X3	T51.1X4	—	—
Zidovudine	T37.5X1	T37.5X2	T37.5X3	T37.5X4	T37.5X5	T37.5X6
Zimeldine	T43.221	T43.222	T43.223	T43.224	T43.225	T43.226
Zinc (compounds) (fumes) (vapor)	T56.5X1	T56.5X2	T56.5X3	T56.5X4	—	—
NEC	T49.0X1	T49.0X2	T49.0X3	T49.0X4	T49.0X5	T49.0X6
anti-infectives	T49.0X1	T49.0X2	T49.0X3	T49.0X4	T49.0X5	T49.0X6
antivaricose	T46.8X1	T46.8X2	T46.8X3	T46.8X4	T46.8X5	T46.8X6
bacitracin	T49.0X1	T49.0X2	T49.0X3	T49.0X4	T49.0X5	T49.0X6
chloride (mouthwash)	T49.6X1	T49.6X2	T49.6X3	T49.6X4	T49.6X5	T49.6X6
chromate	T56.5X1	T56.5X2	T56.5X3	T56.5X4	—	—
gelatin	T49.3X1	T49.3X2	T49.3X3	T49.3X4	T49.3X5	T49.3X6
oxide	T49.3X1	T49.3X2	T49.3X3	T49.3X4	T49.3X5	T49.3X6
plaster	T49.3X1	T49.3X2	T49.3X3	T49.3X4	T49.3X5	T49.3X6
peroxide	T49.0X1	T49.0X2	T49.0X3	T49.0X4	T49.0X5	T49.0X6
pesticides	T56.5X1	T56.5X2	T56.5X3	T56.5X4	—	—
phosphide	T60.4X1	T60.4X2	T60.4X3	T60.4X4	—	—
pyrithionate	T49.4X1	T49.4X2	T49.4X3	T49.4X4	T49.4X5	T49.4X6
stearate	T49.3X1	T49.3X2	T49.3X3	T49.3X4	T49.3X5	T49.3X6

Additional Character May Be Required — Refer to the Tabular List for Character Selection   ▽ Subterms under main terms may continue to next column or page

Substance	Poisoning, Accidental (unintentional)	Poisoning, Intentional Self-harm	Poisoning, Assault	Poisoning, Undetermined	Adverse Effect	Under-dosing
Zinc (compounds) (fumes) (vapor)						
NEC — *continued*						
sulfate	T49.5X1	T49.5X2	T49.5X3	T49.5X4	T49.5X5	T49.5X6
ENT agent	T49.6X1	T49.6X2	T49.6X3	T49.6X4	T49.6X5	T49.6X6
ophthalmic solution	T49.5X1	T49.5X2	T49.5X3	T49.5X4	T49.5X5	T49.5X6
topical NEC	T49.0X1	T49.0X2	T49.0X3	T49.0X4	T49.0X5	T49.0X6
undecylenate	T49.0X1	T49.0X2	T49.0X3	T49.0X4	T49.0X5	T49.0X6
Zineb	T60.0X1	T60.0X2	T60.0X3	T60.0X4	—	—
Zinostatin	T45.1X1	T45.1X2	T45.1X3	T45.1X4	T45.1X5	T45.1X6
Zipeprol	T48.3X1	T48.3X2	T48.3X3	T48.3X4	T48.3X5	T48.3X6
Zofenopril	T46.4X1	T46.4X2	T46.4X3	T46.4X4	T46.4X5	T46.4X6
Zolpidem	T42.6X1	T42.6X2	T42.6X3	T42.6X4	T42.6X5	T42.6X6
Zomepirac	T39.391	T39.392	T39.393	T39.394	T39.395	T39.396
Zopiclone	T42.6X1	T42.6X2	T42.6X3	T42.6X4	T42.6X5	T42.6X6
Zorubicin	T45.1X1	T45.1X2	T45.1X3	T45.1X4	T45.1X5	T45.1X6
Zotepine	T43.591	T43.592	T43.593	T43.594	T43.595	T43.596
Zovant	T45.511	T45.512	T45.513	T45.514	T45.515	T45.516
Zoxazolamine	T42.8X1	T42.8X2	T42.8X3	T42.8X4	T42.8X5	T42.8X6
Zuclopenthixol	T43.4X1	T43.4X2	T43.4X3	T43.4X4	T43.4X5	T43.4X6
Zygadenus (venenosus)	T62.2X1	T62.2X2	T62.2X3	T62.2X4	—	—
Zyprexa	T43.591	T43.592	T43.593	T43.594	T43.595	T43.596

▽ **Subterms under main terms may continue to next column or page**   **Additional Character May Be Required — Refer to the Tabular List for Character Selection**

A

Abandonment (causing exposure to weather conditions) (with intent to injure or kill) NEC X58 ☑
Abuse (adult) (child) (mental) (physical) (sexual) X58 ☑
Accident (to) X58 ☑
  aircraft (in transit) (powered) — *see also* Accident, transport, aircraft
    due to, caused by cataclysm — *see* Forces of nature, by type
  animal-drawn vehicle — *see* Accident, transport, animal-drawn vehicle occupant
  animal-rider — *see* Accident, transport, animal-rider
  automobile — *see* Accident, transport, car occupant
  bare foot water skier V94.4 ☑
  boat, boating — *see also* Accident, watercraft
    striking swimmer
      powered V94.11 ☑
      unpowered V94.12 ☑
  bus — *see* Accident, transport, bus occupant
  cable car, not on rails V98.0 ☑
    on rails — *see* Accident, transport, streetcar occupant
  car — *see* Accident, transport, car occupant
  caused by, due to
    animal NEC W64 ☑
    chain hoist W24.0 ☑
    cold (excessive) — *see* Exposure, cold
    corrosive liquid, substance — *see* Table of Drugs and Chemicals
    cutting or piercing instrument — *see* Contact, with, by type of instrument
    drive belt W24.0 ☑
    electric
      current — *see* Exposure, electric current
      motor — *see also* Contact, with, by type of machine W31.3 ☑
      current (of) W86.8 ☑
    environmental factor NEC X58 ☑
    explosive material — *see* Explosion
    fire, flames — *see* Exposure, fire
    firearm missile — *see* Discharge, firearm by type
    heat (excessive) — *see* Heat
    hot — *see* Contact, with, hot
    ignition — *see* Ignition
    lifting device W24.0 ☑
    lightning — *see* subcategory T75.0 ☑
      causing fire — *see* Exposure, fire
    machine, machinery — *see* Contact, with, by type of machine
    natural factor NEC X58 ☑
    pulley (block) W24.0 ☑
    radiation — *see* Radiation
    steam X13.1 ☑
      inhalation X13.0 ☑
      pipe X16 ☑
    thunderbolt — *see* subcategory T75.0 ☑
      causing fire — *see* Exposure, fire
    transmission device W24.1 ☑
  coach — *see* Accident, transport, bus occupant
  coal car — *see* Accident, transport, industrial vehicle occupant
  diving — *see also* Fall, into, water
    with
      drowning or submersion — *see* Drowning
  forklift — *see* Accident, transport, industrial vehicle occupant
  heavy transport vehicle NOS — *see* Accident, transport, truck occupant
  ice yacht V98.2 ☑
  in
    medical, surgical procedure
      as, or due to misadventure — *see* Misadventure
      causing an abnormal reaction or later complication without mention of misadventure — *see also* Complication of or following, by type of procedure Y84.9
  land yacht V98.1 ☑
  late effect of — *see* W00-X58 with 7th character S
  logging car — *see* Accident, transport, industrial vehicle occupant
  machine, machinery — *see also* Contact, with, by type of machine
    on board watercraft V93.69 ☑
      explosion — *see* Explosion, in, watercraft

Accident — *continued*
  machine, machinery — *see also* Contact, with, by type of machine — *continued*
    on board watercraft — *continued*
      fire — *see* Burn, on board watercraft
      powered craft V93.63 ☑
        ferry boat V93.61 ☑
        fishing boat V93.62 ☑
        jetskis V93.63 ☑
        liner V93.61 ☑
        merchant ship V93.60 ☑
        passenger ship V93.61 ☑
        sailboat V93.64 ☑
  mine tram — *see* Accident, transport, industrial vehicle occupant
  mobility scooter (motorized) — *see* Accident, transport, pedestrian, conveyance, specified type NEC
  motor scooter — *see* Accident, transport, motorcyclist
  motor vehicle NOS (traffic) — *see also* Accident, transport V89.2 ☑
    nontraffic V89.0 ☑
    three-wheeled NOS — *see* Accident, transport, three-wheeled motor vehicle occupant
  motorcycle NOS — *see* Accident, transport, motorcyclist
  nonmotor vehicle NOS (nontraffic) — *see also* Accident, transport V89.1 ☑
    traffic NOS V89.3 ☑
  nontraffic (victim's mode of transport NOS) V88.9 ☑
    collision (between) V88.7 ☑
      bus and truck V88.5 ☑
      car and:
        bus V88.3 ☑
        pickup V88.2 ☑
        three-wheeled motor vehicle V88.0 ☑
        train V88.6 ☑
        truck V88.4 ☑
        two-wheeled motor vehicle V88.0 ☑
        van V88.2 ☑
      specified vehicle NEC and:
        three-wheeled motor vehicle V88.1 ☑
        two-wheeled motor vehicle V88.1 ☑
    known mode of transport — *see* Accident, transport, by type of vehicle
    noncollision V88.8 ☑
  on board watercraft V93.89 ☑
    powered craft V93.83 ☑
      ferry boat V93.81 ☑
      fishing boat V93.82 ☑
      jetskis V93.83 ☑
      liner V93.81 ☑
      merchant ship V93.80 ☑
      passenger ship V93.81 ☑
    unpowered craft V93.88 ☑
      canoe V93.85 ☑
      inflatable V93.86 ☑
        in tow
          recreational V94.31 ☑
          specified NEC V94.32 ☑
      kayak V93.85 ☑
      sailboat V93.84 ☑
      surf-board V93.88 ☑
      water skis V93.87 ☑
      windsurfer V93.88 ☑
  parachutist V97.29 ☑
    entangled in object V97.21 ☑
    injured on landing V97.22 ☑
  pedal cycle — *see* Accident, transport, pedal cyclist
  pedestrian (on foot)
    with
      another pedestrian W51 ☑
        on pedestrian conveyance NEC V00.09 ☑
        with fall W03 ☑
          due to ice or snow W00.0 ☑
      roller skater (in-line) V00.01 ☑
      skate boarder V00.02 ☑
      transport vehicle — *see* Accident, transport
    on pedestrian conveyance — *see* Accident, transport, pedestrian, conveyance
  pick-up truck or van — *see* Accident, transport, pickup truck occupant
  quarry truck — *see* Accident, transport, industrial vehicle occupant
  railway vehicle (any) (in motion) — *see* Accident, transport, railway vehicle occupant
    due to cataclysm — *see* Forces of nature, by type

Accident — *continued*
  scooter (non-motorized) — *see* Accident, transport, pedestrian, conveyance, scooter
  sequelae of — *see* categories W00-X58 with 7th character S
  skateboard — *see* Accident, transport, pedestrian, conveyance, skateboard
  ski(ing) — *see* Accident, transport, pedestrian, conveyance
    lift V98.3 ☑
  specified cause NEC X58 ☑
  streetcar — *see* Accident, transport, streetcar occupant
  traffic (victim's mode of transport NOS) V87.9 ☑
    collision (between) V87.7 ☑
      bus and truck V87.5 ☑
      car and:
        bus V87.3 ☑
        pickup V87.2 ☑
        three-wheeled motor vehicle V87.0 ☑
        train V87.6 ☑
        truck V87.4 ☑
        two-wheeled motor vehicle V87.0 ☑
        van V87.2 ☑
      specified vehicle NEC V86.39 ☑
        and
          three-wheeled motor vehicle V87.1 ☑
          two-wheeled motor vehicle V87.1 ☑
        driver V86.09 ☑
        passenger V86.19 ☑
        person on outside V86.29 ☑
        while boarding or alighting V86.49 ☑
    known mode of transport — *see* Accident, transport, by type of vehicle
    noncollision V87.8 ☑
  transport (involving injury to) V99 ☑
    18 wheeler — *see* Accident, transport, truck occupant
    agricultural vehicle occupant (nontraffic) V84.9 ☑
      driver V84.5 ☑
      hanger-on V84.7 ☑
      passenger V84.6 ☑
      traffic V84.3 ☑
        driver V84.0 ☑
        hanger-on V84.2 ☑
        passenger V84.1 ☑
      while boarding or alighting V84.4 ☑
    aircraft NEC V97.89 ☑
      military NEC V97.818 ☑
        civilian injured by V97.811 ☑
        with civilian aircraft V97.810 ☑
      occupant injured (in)
        nonpowered craft accident V96.9 ☑
          balloon V96.00 ☑
            collision V96.03 ☑
            crash V96.01 ☑
            explosion V96.05 ☑
            fire V96.04 ☑
            forced landing V96.02 ☑
            specified type NEC V96.09 ☑
          glider V96.20 ☑
            collision V96.23 ☑
            crash V96.21 ☑
            explosion V96.25 ☑
            fire V96.24 ☑
            forced landing V96.22 ☑
            specified type NEC V96.29 ☑
          hang glider V96.10 ☑
            collision V96.13 ☑
            crash V96.11 ☑
            explosion V96.15 ☑
            fire V96.14 ☑
            forced landing V96.12 ☑
            specified type NEC V96.19 ☑
          specified craft NEC V96.8 ☑
        powered craft accident V95.9 ☑
          fixed wing NEC
            commercial V95.30 ☑
              collision V95.33 ☑
              crash V95.31 ☑
              explosion V95.35 ☑
              fire V95.34 ☑
              forced landing V95.32 ☑
              specified type NEC V95.39 ☑
            private V95.20 ☑
              collision V95.23 ☑
              crash V95.21 ☑

Accident — *continued*
  transport — *continued*
    aircraft — *continued*
      occupant injured — *continued*
        powered craft accident — *continued*
          fixed wing — *continued*
            private — *continued*
              explosion V95.25 ☑
              fire V95.24 ☑
              forced landing V95.22 ☑
              specified type NEC V95.29 ☑
          glider V95.10 ☑
            collision V95.13 ☑
            crash V95.11 ☑
            explosion V95.15 ☑
            fire V95.14 ☑
            forced landing V95.12 ☑
            specified type NEC V95.19 ☑
          helicopter V95.00 ☑
            collision V95.03 ☑
            crash V95.01 ☑
            explosion V95.05 ☑
            fire V95.04 ☑
            forced landing V95.02 ☑
            specified type NEC V95.09 ☑
          spacecraft V95.40 ☑
            collision V95.43 ☑
            crash V95.41 ☑
            explosion V95.45 ☑
            fire V95.44 ☑
            forced landing V95.42 ☑
            specified type NEC V95.49 ☑
          specified craft NEC V95.8 ☑
          ultralight V95.10 ☑
            collision V95.13 ☑
            crash V95.11 ☑
            explosion V95.15 ☑
            fire V95.14 ☑
            forced landing V95.12 ☑
            specified type NEC V95.19 ☑
        specified accident NEC V97.0 ☑
        while boarding or alighting V97.1 ☑
      person (injured by)
        falling from, in or on aircraft V97.0 ☑
        machinery on aircraft V97.89 ☑
        on ground with aircraft involvement
          V97.39 ☑
        rotating propeller V97.32 ☑
        struck by object falling from aircraft V97.31 ☑
        sucked into aircraft jet V97.33 ☑
        while boarding or alighting aircraft V97.1 ☑
    airport (battery-powered) passenger vehicle — *see*
      Accident, transport, industrial vehicle occu-
      pant
    all-terrain vehicle occupant (nontraffic) V86.95 ☑
      driver V86.55 ☑
      dune buggy — *see* Accident, transport, dune
        buggy occupant
      hanger-on V86.75 ☑
      passenger V86.65 ☑
      snowmobile — *see* Accident, transport, snowmo-
        bile occupant
      specified type NEC V86.99 ☑
        driver V86.59 ☑
        passenger V86.69 ☑
        person on outside V86.79 ☑
      traffic V86.35 ☑
        driver V86.05 ☑
        hanger-on V86.25 ☑
        passenger V86.15 ☑
      while boarding or alighting V86.45 ☑
    ambulance occupant (traffic) V86.31 ☑
      driver V86.01 ☑
      hanger-on V86.21 ☑
      nontraffic V86.91 ☑
        driver V86.51 ☑
        hanger-on V86.71 ☑
        passenger V86.61 ☑
      passenger V86.11 ☑
      while boarding or alighting V86.41 ☑
    animal-drawn vehicle occupant (in) V80.929 ☑
      collision (with)
        animal V80.12 ☑
          being ridden V80.711 ☑
        animal-drawn vehicle V80.721 ☑
        bus V80.42 ☑

Accident — *continued*
  transport — *continued*
    animal-drawn vehicle occupant — *continued*
      collision — *continued*
        car V80.42 ☑
        fixed or stationary object V80.82 ☑
        military vehicle V80.920 ☑
        nonmotor vehicle V80.791 ☑
        pedal cycle V80.22 ☑
        pedestrian V80.12 ☑
        pickup V80.42 ☑
        railway train or vehicle V80.62 ☑
        specified motor vehicle NEC V80.52 ☑
        streetcar V80.731 ☑
        truck V80.42 ☑
        two- or three-wheeled motor vehicle
          V80.32 ☑
        van V80.42 ☑
      noncollision V80.02 ☑
      specified circumstance NEC V80.928 ☑
    animal-rider V80.919 ☑
      collision (with)
        animal V80.11 ☑
          being ridden V80.710 ☑
        animal-drawn vehicle V80.720 ☑
        bus V80.41 ☑
        car V80.41 ☑
        fixed or stationary object V80.81 ☑
        military vehicle V80.910 ☑
        nonmotor vehicle V80.790 ☑
        pedal cycle V80.21 ☑
        pedestrian V80.11 ☑
        pickup V80.41 ☑
        railway train or vehicle V80.61 ☑
        specified motor vehicle NEC V80.51 ☑
        streetcar V80.730 ☑
        truck V80.41 ☑
        two- or three-wheeled motor vehicle
          V80.31 ☑
        van V80.41 ☑
      noncollision V80.018 ☑
        specified as horse rider V80.010 ☑
      specified circumstance NEC V80.918 ☑
    armored car — *see* Accident, transport, truck occu-
      pant
    battery-powered truck (baggage) (mail) — *see* Ac-
      cident, transport, industrial vehicle occupant
    bus occupant V79.9 ☑
      collision (with)
        animal (traffic) V70.9 ☑
          being ridden (traffic) V76.9 ☑
            nontraffic V76.3 ☑
            while boarding or alighting V76.4 ☑
          nontraffic V70.3 ☑
          while boarding or alighting V70.4 ☑
        animal-drawn vehicle (traffic) V76.9 ☑
          nontraffic V76.3 ☑
          while boarding or alighting V76.4 ☑
        bus (traffic) V74.9 ☑
          nontraffic V74.3 ☑
          while boarding or alighting V74.4 ☑
        car (traffic) V73.9 ☑
          nontraffic V73.3 ☑
          while boarding or alighting V73.4 ☑
        motor vehicle NOS (traffic) V79.60 ☑
          nontraffic V79.20 ☑
          specified type NEC (traffic) V79.69 ☑
            nontraffic V79.29 ☑
        pedal cycle (traffic) V71.9 ☑
          nontraffic V71.3 ☑
          while boarding or alighting V71.4 ☑
        pickup truck (traffic) V73.9 ☑
          nontraffic V73.3 ☑
          while boarding or alighting V73.4 ☑
        railway vehicle (traffic) V75.9 ☑
          nontraffic V75.3 ☑
          while boarding or alighting V75.4 ☑
        specified vehicle NEC (traffic) V76.9 ☑
          nontraffic V76.3 ☑
          while boarding or alighting V76.4 ☑
        stationary object (traffic) V77.9 ☑
          nontraffic V77.3 ☑
          while boarding or alighting V77.4 ☑
        streetcar (traffic) V76.9 ☑
          nontraffic V76.3 ☑
          while boarding or alighting V76.4 ☑

Accident — *continued*
  transport — *continued*
    bus occupant — *continued*
      collision — *continued*
        three wheeled motor vehicle (traffic) V72.9 ☑
          nontraffic V72.3 ☑
          while boarding or alighting V72.4 ☑
        truck (traffic) V74.9 ☑
          nontraffic V74.3 ☑
          while boarding or alighting V74.4 ☑
        two wheeled motor vehicle (traffic) V72.9 ☑
          nontraffic V72.3 ☑
          while boarding or alighting V72.4 ☑
        van (traffic) V73.9 ☑
          nontraffic V73.3 ☑
          while boarding or alighting V73.4 ☑
      driver
        collision (with)
          animal (traffic) V70.5 ☑
            being ridden (traffic) V76.5 ☑
              nontraffic V76.0 ☑
            nontraffic V70.0 ☑
          animal-drawn vehicle (traffic) V76.5 ☑
            nontraffic V76.0 ☑
          bus (traffic) V74.5 ☑
            nontraffic V74.0 ☑
          car (traffic) V73.5 ☑
            nontraffic V73.0 ☑
          motor vehicle NOS (traffic) V79.40 ☑
            nontraffic V79.00 ☑
            specified type NEC (traffic) V79.49 ☑
              nontraffic V79.09 ☑
          pedal cycle (traffic) V71.5 ☑
            nontraffic V71.0 ☑
          pickup truck (traffic) V73.5 ☑
            nontraffic V73.0 ☑
          railway vehicle (traffic) V75.5 ☑
            nontraffic V75.0 ☑
          specified vehicle NEC (traffic) V76.5 ☑
            nontraffic V76.0 ☑
          stationary object (traffic) V77.5 ☑
            nontraffic V77.0 ☑
          streetcar (traffic) V76.5 ☑
            nontraffic V76.0 ☑
          three wheeled motor vehicle (traffic)
            V72.5 ☑
            nontraffic V72.0 ☑
          truck (traffic) V74.5 ☑
            nontraffic V74.0 ☑
          two wheeled motor vehicle (traffic)
            V72.5 ☑
            nontraffic V72.0 ☑
          van (traffic) V73.5 ☑
            nontraffic V73.0 ☑
        noncollision accident (traffic) V78.5 ☑
          nontraffic V78.0 ☑
      hanger-on
        collision (with)
          animal (traffic) V70.7 ☑
            being ridden (traffic) V76.7 ☑
              nontraffic V76.2 ☑
            nontraffic V70.2 ☑
          animal-drawn vehicle (traffic) V76.7 ☑
            nontraffic V76.2 ☑
          bus (traffic) V74.7 ☑
            nontraffic V74.2 ☑
          car (traffic) V73.7 ☑
            nontraffic V73.2 ☑
          pedal cycle (traffic) V71.7 ☑
            nontraffic V71.2 ☑
          pickup truck (traffic) V73.7 ☑
            nontraffic V73.2 ☑
          railway vehicle (traffic) V75.7 ☑
            nontraffic V75.2 ☑
          specified vehicle NEC (traffic) V76.7 ☑
            nontraffic V76.2 ☑
          stationary object (traffic) V77.7 ☑
            nontraffic V77.2 ☑
          streetcar (traffic) V76.7 ☑
            nontraffic V76.2 ☑
          three wheeled motor vehicle (traffic)
            V72.7 ☑
            nontraffic V72.2 ☑
          truck (traffic) V74.7 ☑
            nontraffic V74.2 ☑

Accident — *continued*
  transport — *continued*
    bus occupant — *continued*
      hanger-on — *continued*
        collision — *continued*
          two wheeled motor vehicle (traffic) V72.7 ☑
            nontraffic V72.2 ☑
          van (traffic) V73.7 ☑
            nontraffic V73.2 ☑
          noncollision accident (traffic) V78.7 ☑
            nontraffic V78.2 ☑
        noncollision accident (traffic) V78.9 ☑
          nontraffic V78.3 ☑
          while boarding or alighting V78.4 ☑
        nontraffic V79.3 ☑
      passenger
        collision (with)
          animal (traffic) V70.6 ☑
            being ridden (traffic) V76.6 ☑
              nontraffic V76.1 ☑
            nontraffic V70.1 ☑
          animal-drawn vehicle (traffic) V76.6 ☑
            nontraffic V76.1 ☑
          bus (traffic) V74.6 ☑
            nontraffic V74.1 ☑
          car (traffic) V73.6 ☑
            nontraffic V73.1 ☑
          motor vehicle NOS (traffic) V79.50 ☑
            nontraffic V79.10 ☑
            specified type NEC (traffic) V79.59 ☑
              nontraffic V79.19 ☑
          pedal cycle (traffic) V71.6 ☑
            nontraffic V71.1 ☑
          pickup truck (traffic) V73.6 ☑
            nontraffic V73.1 ☑
          railway vehicle (traffic) V75.6 ☑
            nontraffic V75.1 ☑
          specified vehicle NEC (traffic) V76.6 ☑
            nontraffic V76.1 ☑
          stationary object (traffic) V77.6 ☑
            nontraffic V77.1 ☑
          streetcar (traffic) V76.6 ☑
            nontraffic V76.1 ☑
          three wheeled motor vehicle (traffic) V72.6 ☑
            nontraffic V72.1 ☑
          truck (traffic) V74.6 ☑
            nontraffic V74.1 ☑
          two wheeled motor vehicle (traffic) V72.6 ☑
            nontraffic V72.1 ☑
          van (traffic) V73.6 ☑
            nontraffic V73.1 ☑
        noncollision accident (traffic) V78.6 ☑
          nontraffic V78.1 ☑
      specified type NEC V79.88 ☑
      military vehicle V79.81 ☑
    cable car, not on rails V98.0 ☑
      on rails — *see* Accident, transport, streetcar occupant
    car occupant V49.9 ☑
      ambulance occupant — *see* Accident, transport, ambulance occupant
      collision (with)
        animal (traffic) V40.9 ☑
          being ridden (traffic) V46.9 ☑
            nontraffic V46.3 ☑
            while boarding or alighting V46.4 ☑
          nontraffic V40.3 ☑
          while boarding or alighting V40.4 ☑
        animal-drawn vehicle (traffic) V46.9 ☑
          nontraffic V46.3 ☑
          while boarding or alighting V46.4 ☑
        bus (traffic) V44.9 ☑
          nontraffic V44.3 ☑
          while boarding or alighting V44.4 ☑
        car (traffic) V43.92 ☑
          nontraffic V43.32 ☑
          while boarding or alighting V43.42 ☑
        motor vehicle NOS (traffic) V49.60 ☑
          nontraffic V49.20 ☑
          specified type NEC (traffic) V49.69 ☑
            nontraffic V49.29 ☑
        pedal cycle (traffic) V41.9 ☑
          nontraffic V41.3 ☑

Accident — *continued*
  transport — *continued*
    car occupant — *continued*
      collision — *continued*
        pedal cycle — *continued*
          while boarding or alighting V41.4 ☑
        pickup truck (traffic) V43.93 ☑
          nontraffic V43.33 ☑
          while boarding or alighting V43.43 ☑
        railway vehicle (traffic) V45.9 ☑
          nontraffic V45.3 ☑
          while boarding or alighting V45.4 ☑
        specified vehicle NEC (traffic) V46.9 ☑
          nontraffic V46.3 ☑
          while boarding or alighting V46.4 ☑
        sport utility vehicle (traffic) V43.91 ☑
          nontraffic V43.31 ☑
          while boarding or alighting V43.41 ☑
        stationary object (traffic) V47.9 ☑
          nontraffic V47.3 ☑
          while boarding or alighting V47.4 ☑
        streetcar (traffic) V46.9 ☑
          nontraffic V46.3 ☑
          while boarding or alighting V46.4 ☑
        three wheeled motor vehicle (traffic) V42.9 ☑
          nontraffic V42.3 ☑
          while boarding or alighting V42.4 ☑
        truck (traffic) V44.9 ☑
          nontraffic V44.3 ☑
          while boarding or alighting V44.4 ☑
        two wheeled motor vehicle (traffic) V42.9 ☑
          nontraffic V42.3 ☑
          while boarding or alighting V42.4 ☑
        van (traffic) V43.94 ☑
          nontraffic V43.34 ☑
          while boarding or alighting V43.44 ☑
      driver
        collision (with)
          animal (traffic) V40.5 ☑
            being ridden (traffic) V46.5 ☑
              nontraffic V46.0 ☑
            nontraffic V40.0 ☑
          animal-drawn vehicle (traffic) V46.5 ☑
            nontraffic V46.0 ☑
          bus (traffic) V44.5 ☑
            nontraffic V44.0 ☑
          car (traffic) V43.52 ☑
            nontraffic V43.02 ☑
          motor vehicle NOS (traffic) V49.40 ☑
            nontraffic V49.00 ☑
            specified type NEC (traffic) V49.49 ☑
              nontraffic V49.09 ☑
          pedal cycle (traffic) V41.5 ☑
            nontraffic V41.0 ☑
          pickup truck (traffic) V43.53 ☑
            nontraffic V43.03 ☑
          railway vehicle (traffic) V45.5 ☑
            nontraffic V45.0 ☑
          specified vehicle NEC (traffic) V46.5 ☑
            nontraffic V46.0 ☑
          sport utility vehicle (traffic) V43.51 ☑
            nontraffic V43.01 ☑
          stationary object (traffic) V47.5 ☑
            nontraffic V47.0 ☑
          streetcar (traffic) V46.5 ☑
            nontraffic V46.0 ☑
          three wheeled motor vehicle (traffic) V42.5 ☑
            nontraffic V42.0 ☑
          truck (traffic) V44.5 ☑
            nontraffic V44.0 ☑
          two wheeled motor vehicle (traffic) V42.5 ☑
            nontraffic V42.0 ☑
          van (traffic) V43.54 ☑
            nontraffic V43.04 ☑
        noncollision accident (traffic) V48.5 ☑
          nontraffic V48.0 ☑
      hanger-on
        collision (with)
          animal (traffic) V40.7 ☑
            being ridden (traffic) V46.7 ☑
              nontraffic V46.2 ☑
            nontraffic V40.2 ☑
          animal-drawn vehicle (traffic) V46.7 ☑
            nontraffic V46.2 ☑

Accident — *continued*
  transport — *continued*
    car occupant — *continued*
      hanger-on — *continued*
        collision — *continued*
          bus (traffic) V44.7 ☑
            nontraffic V44.2 ☑
          car (traffic) V43.72 ☑
            nontraffic V43.22 ☑
          pedal cycle (traffic) V41.7 ☑
            nontraffic V41.2 ☑
          pickup truck (traffic) V43.73 ☑
            nontraffic V43.23 ☑
          railway vehicle (traffic) V45.7 ☑
            nontraffic V45.2 ☑
          specified vehicle NEC (traffic) V46.7 ☑
            nontraffic V46.2 ☑
          sport utility vehicle (traffic) V43.71 ☑
            nontraffic V43.21 ☑
          stationary object (traffic) V47.7 ☑
            nontraffic V47.2 ☑
          streetcar (traffic) V46.7 ☑
            nontraffic V46.2 ☑
          three wheeled motor vehicle (traffic) V42.7 ☑
            nontraffic V42.2 ☑
          truck (traffic) V44.7 ☑
            nontraffic V44.2 ☑
          two wheeled motor vehicle (traffic) V42.7 ☑
            nontraffic V42.2 ☑
          van (traffic) V43.74 ☑
            nontraffic V43.24 ☑
        noncollision accident (traffic) V48.7 ☑
          nontraffic V48.2 ☑
      noncollision accident (traffic) V48.9 ☑
        nontraffic V48.3 ☑
        while boarding or alighting V48.4 ☑
      nontraffic V49.3 ☑
      passenger
        collision (with)
          animal (traffic) V40.6 ☑
            being ridden (traffic) V46.6 ☑
              nontraffic V46.1 ☑
            nontraffic V40.1 ☑
          animal-drawn vehicle (traffic) V46.6 ☑
            nontraffic V46.1 ☑
          bus (traffic) V44.6 ☑
            nontraffic V44.1 ☑
          car (traffic) V43.62 ☑
            nontraffic V43.12 ☑
          motor vehicle NOS (traffic) V49.50 ☑
            nontraffic V49.10 ☑
            specified type NEC (traffic) V49.59 ☑
              nontraffic V49.19 ☑
          pedal cycle (traffic) V41.6 ☑
            nontraffic V41.1 ☑
          pickup truck (traffic) V43.63 ☑
            nontraffic V43.13 ☑
          railway vehicle (traffic) V45.6 ☑
            nontraffic V45.1 ☑
          specified vehicle NEC (traffic) V46.6 ☑
            nontraffic V46.1 ☑
          sport utility vehicle (traffic) V43.61 ☑
            nontraffic V43.11 ☑
          stationary object (traffic) V47.6 ☑
            nontraffic V47.1 ☑
          streetcar (traffic) V46.6 ☑
            nontraffic V46.1 ☑
          three wheeled motor vehicle (traffic) V42.6 ☑
            nontraffic V42.1 ☑
          truck (traffic) V44.6 ☑
            nontraffic V44.1 ☑
          two wheeled motor vehicle (traffic) V42.6 ☑
            nontraffic V42.1 ☑
          van (traffic) V43.64 ☑
            nontraffic V43.14 ☑
        noncollision accident (traffic) V48.6 ☑
          nontraffic V48.1 ☑
      specified type NEC V49.88 ☑
      military vehicle V49.81 ☑
    coal car — *see* Accident, transport, industrial vehicle occupant
    construction vehicle occupant (nontraffic) V85.9 ☑

Accident — *continued*
  transport — *continued*
    construction vehicle occupant — *continued*
      driver V85.5
      hanger-on V85.7 ☑
      passenger V85.6 ☑
      traffic V85.3 ☑
        driver V85.0 ☑
        hanger-on V85.2 ☑
        passenger V85.1 ☑
      while boarding or alighting V85.4 ☑
    dirt bike rider (nontraffic) V86.96 ☑
      driver V86.56 ☑
      hanger-on V86.76 ☑
      passenger V86.66 ☑
      traffic V86.36 ☑
        driver V86.06 ☑
        hanger-on V86.26 ☑
        passenger V86.16 ☑
      while boarding or alighting V86.46 ☑
    due to cataclysm — *see* Forces of nature, by type
    dune buggy occupant (nontraffic) V86.93 ☑
      driver V86.53 ☑
      hanger-on V86.73 ☑
      passenger V86.63 ☑
      traffic V86.33 ☑
        driver V86.03 ☑
        hanger-on V86.23 ☑
        passenger V86.13 ☑
      while boarding or alighting V86.43 ☑
    forklift — *see* Accident, transport, industrial vehicle occupant
    go cart — *see* Accident, transport, all-terrain vehicle occupant
    golf cart — *see* Accident, transport, all-terrain vehicle occupant
    heavy transport vehicle occupant — *see* Accident, transport, truck occupant
    ice yacht V98.2 ☑
    industrial vehicle occupant (nontraffic) V83.9 ☑
      driver V83.5 ☑
      hanger-on V83.7 ☑
      passenger V83.6 ☑
      traffic V83.3 ☑
        driver V83.0 ☑
        hanger-on V83.2 ☑
        passenger V83.1 ☑
      while boarding or alighting V83.4 ☑
    interurban electric car — *see* Accident, transport, streetcar
    land yacht V98.1 ☑
    logging car — *see* Accident, transport, industrial vehicle occupant
    military vehicle occupant (traffic) V86.34 ☑
      driver V86.04 ☑
      hanger-on V86.24 ☑
      nontraffic V86.94 ☑
        driver V86.54 ☑
        hanger-on V86.74 ☑
        passenger V86.64 ☑
      passenger V86.14 ☑
      while boarding or alighting V86.44 ☑
    mine tram — *see* Accident, transport, industrial vehicle occupant
    motor vehicle NEC occupant (traffic) V89.2 ☑
    motorcoach — *see* Accident, transport, bus occupant
    motor/cross bike rider — *see also* Accident, transport, dirt bike rider V86.96 ☑
    motorcyclist V29.9 ☑
      collision (with)
        animal (traffic) V20.9 ☑
          being ridden (traffic) V26.9 ☑
            nontraffic V26.2 ☑
            while boarding or alighting V26.3 ☑
          nontraffic V20.2 ☑
          while boarding or alighting V20.3 ☑
        animal-drawn vehicle (traffic) V26.9 ☑
          nontraffic V26.2 ☑
          while boarding or alighting V26.3 ☑
        bus (traffic) V24.9 ☑
          nontraffic V24.2 ☑
          while boarding or alighting V24.3 ☑
        car (traffic) V23.9 ☑
          nontraffic V23.2 ☑
          while boarding or alighting V23.3 ☑

Accident — *continued*
  transport — *continued*
    motorcyclist — *continued*
      collision — *continued*
        motor vehicle NOS (traffic) V29.60 ☑
          nontraffic V29.20 ☑
          specified type NEC (traffic) V29.69 ☑
            nontraffic V29.29 ☑
        pedal cycle (traffic) V21.9 ☑
          nontraffic V21.2 ☑
          while boarding or alighting V21.3 ☑
        pickup truck (traffic) V23.9 ☑
          nontraffic V23.2 ☑
          while boarding or alighting V23.3 ☑
        railway vehicle (traffic) V25.9 ☑
          nontraffic V25.2 ☑
          while boarding or alighting V25.3 ☑
        specified vehicle NEC (traffic) V26.9 ☑
          nontraffic V26.2 ☑
          while boarding or alighting V26.3 ☑
        stationary object (traffic) V27.9 ☑
          nontraffic V27.2 ☑
          while boarding or alighting V27.3 ☑
        streetcar (traffic) V26.9 ☑
          nontraffic V26.2 ☑
          while boarding or alighting V26.3 ☑
        three wheeled motor vehicle (traffic) V22.9 ☑
          nontraffic V22.2 ☑
          while boarding or alighting V22.3 ☑
        truck (traffic) V24.9 ☑
          nontraffic V24.2 ☑
          while boarding or alighting V24.3 ☑
        two wheeled motor vehicle (traffic) V22.9 ☑
          nontraffic V22.2 ☑
          while boarding or alighting V22.3 ☑
        van (traffic) V23.9 ☑
          nontraffic V23.2 ☑
          while boarding or alighting V23.3 ☑
      driver
        collision (with)
          animal (traffic) V20.4 ☑
            being ridden (traffic) V26.4 ☑
              nontraffic V26.0 ☑
            nontraffic V20.0 ☑
          animal-drawn vehicle (traffic) V26.4 ☑
            nontraffic V26.0 ☑
          bus (traffic) V24.4 ☑
            nontraffic V24.0 ☑
          car (traffic) V23.4 ☑
            nontraffic V23.0 ☑
          motor vehicle NOS (traffic) V29.40 ☑
            nontraffic V29.00 ☑
            specified type NEC (traffic) V29.49 ☑
              nontraffic V29.09 ☑
          pedal cycle (traffic) V21.4 ☑
            nontraffic V21.0 ☑
          pickup truck (traffic) V23.4 ☑
            nontraffic V23.0 ☑
          railway vehicle (traffic) V25.4 ☑
            nontraffic V25.0 ☑
          specified vehicle NEC (traffic) V26.4 ☑
            nontraffic V26.0 ☑
          stationary object (traffic) V27.4 ☑
            nontraffic V27.0 ☑
          streetcar (traffic) V26.4 ☑
            nontraffic V26.0 ☑
          three wheeled motor vehicle (traffic) V22.4 ☑
            nontraffic V22.0 ☑
          truck (traffic) V24.4 ☑
            nontraffic V24.0 ☑
          two wheeled motor vehicle (traffic) V22.4 ☑
            nontraffic V22.0 ☑
          van (traffic) V23.4 ☑
            nontraffic V23.0 ☑
        noncollision accident (traffic) V28.4 ☑
          nontraffic V28.0 ☑
      noncollision accident (traffic) V28.9 ☑
        nontraffic V28.2 ☑
        while boarding or alighting V28.3 ☑
      nontraffic V29.3 ☑
      passenger
        collision (with)
          animal (traffic) V20.5 ☑
            being ridden (traffic) V26.5 ☑

Accident — *continued*
  transport — *continued*
    motorcyclist — *continued*
      passenger — *continued*
        collision — *continued*
          animal — *continued*
            being ridden — *continued*
              nontraffic V26.1 ☑
            nontraffic V20.1 ☑
          animal-drawn vehicle (traffic) V26.5 ☑
            nontraffic V26.1 ☑
          bus (traffic) V24.5 ☑
            nontraffic V24.1 ☑
          car (traffic) V23.5 ☑
            nontraffic V23.1 ☑
          motor vehicle NOS (traffic) V29.50 ☑
            nontraffic V29.10 ☑
            specified type NEC (traffic) V29.59 ☑
              nontraffic V29.19 ☑
          pedal cycle (traffic) V21.5 ☑
            nontraffic V21.1 ☑
          pickup truck (traffic) V23.5 ☑
            nontraffic V23.1 ☑
          railway vehicle (traffic) V25.5 ☑
            nontraffic V25.1 ☑
          specified vehicle NEC (traffic) V26.5 ☑
            nontraffic V26.1 ☑
          stationary object (traffic) V27.5 ☑
            nontraffic V27.1 ☑
          streetcar (traffic) V26.5 ☑
            nontraffic V26.1 ☑
          three wheeled motor vehicle (traffic) V22.5 ☑
            nontraffic V22.1 ☑
          truck (traffic) V24.5 ☑
            nontraffic V24.1 ☑
          two wheeled motor vehicle (traffic) V22.5 ☑
            nontraffic V22.1 ☑
          van (traffic) V23.5 ☑
            nontraffic V23.1 ☑
        noncollision accident (traffic) V28.5 ☑
          nontraffic V28.1 ☑
    specified type NEC V29.88 ☑
    military vehicle V29.81 ☑
  occupant (of)
    aircraft (powered) V95.9 ☑
      fixed wing
        commercial — *see* Accident, transport, aircraft, occupant, powered, fixed wing, commercial
        private — *see* Accident, transport, aircraft, occupant, powered, fixed wing, private
      nonpowered V96.9 ☑
      specified NEC V95.8 ☑
    airport battery-powered vehicle — *see* Accident, transport, industrial vehicle occupant
    all-terrain vehicle (ATV) — *see* Accident, transport, all-terrain vehicle occupant
    animal-drawn vehicle — *see* Accident, transport, animal-drawn vehicle occupant
    automobile — *see* Accident, transport, car occupant
    balloon V96.00 ☑
    battery-powered vehicle — *see* Accident, transport, industrial vehicle occupant
    bicycle — *see* Accident, transport, pedal cyclist
      motorized — *see* Accident, transport, motorcycle rider
    boat NEC — *see* Accident, watercraft
    bulldozer — *see* Accident, transport, construction vehicle occupant
    bus — *see* Accident, transport, bus occupant
    cable car (on rails) — *see also* Accident, transport, streetcar occupant
      not on rails V98.0 ☑
    car — *see also* Accident, transport, car occupant
      cable (on rails) — *see also* Accident, transport, streetcar occupant
      not on rails V98.0 ☑
    coach — *see* Accident, transport, bus occupant
    coal-car — *see* Accident, transport, industrial vehicle occupant
    digger — *see* Accident, transport, construction vehicle occupant

External Causes I

Accident — Accident

Accident — continued
  transport — continued
    occupant — continued
      dump truck — see Accident, transport, construction vehicle occupant
      earth-leveler — see Accident, transport, construction vehicle occupant
      farm machinery (self-propelled) — see Accident, transport, agricultural vehicle occupant
      forklift — see Accident, transport, industrial vehicle occupant
      glider (unpowered) V96.20 ☑
        hang V96.10 ☑
        powered (microlight) (ultralight) — see Accident, transport, aircraft, occupant, powered, glider
      glider (unpowered) NEC V96.20 ☑
      hang-glider V96.10 ☑
      harvester — see Accident, transport, agricultural vehicle occupant
      heavy (transport) vehicle — see Accident, transport, truck occupant
      helicopter — see Accident, transport, aircraft, occupant, helicopter
      ice-yacht V98.2 ☑
      kite (carrying person) V96.8 ☑
      land-yacht V98.1 ☑
      logging car — see Accident, transport, industrial vehicle occupant
      mechanical shovel — see Accident, transport, construction vehicle occupant
      microlight — see Accident, transport, aircraft, occupant, powered, glider
      minibus — see Accident, transport, pickup truck occupant
      minivan — see Accident, transport, pickup truck occupant
      moped — see Accident, transport, motorcycle
      motor scooter — see Accident, transport, motorcycle
      motorcycle (with sidecar) — see Accident, transport, motorcycle
      off-road motor-vehicle — see also Accident, transport, all-terrain vehicle occupant V86.99 ☑
      pedal cycle — see also Accident, transport, pedal cyclist
      pick-up (truck) — see Accident, transport, pickup truck occupant
      railway (train) (vehicle) (subterranean) (elevated) — see Accident, transport, railway vehicle occupant
      rickshaw — see Accident, transport, pedal cycle
        motorized — see Accident, transport, three-wheeled motor vehicle
        pedal driven — see Accident, transport, pedal cyclist
      road-roller — see Accident, transport, construction vehicle occupant
      ship NOS V94.9 ☑
      ski-lift (chair) (gondola) V98.3 ☑
      snowmobile — see Accident, transport, snowmobile occupant
      spacecraft, spaceship — see Accident, transport, aircraft, occupant, spacecraft
      sport utility vehicle — see Accident, transport, pickup truck occupant
      streetcar (interurban) (operating on public street or highway) — see Accident, transport, streetcar occupant
      SUV — see Accident, transport, pickup truck occupant
      téléférique V98.0 ☑
      three-wheeled vehicle (motorized) — see also Accident, transport, three-wheeled motor vehicle occupant
        nonmotorized — see Accident, transport, pedal cycle
      tractor (farm) (and trailer) — see Accident, transport, agricultural vehicle occupant
      train — see Accident, transport, railway vehicle occupant
      tram — see Accident, transport, streetcar occupant
        in mine or quarry — see Accident, transport, industrial vehicle occupant
      tricycle — see Accident, transport, pedal cycle

Accident — continued
  transport — continued
    occupant — continued
      tricycle — see Accident, transport, pedal cycle — continued
        motorized — see Accident, transport, three-wheeled motor vehicle
      trolley — see Accident, transport, streetcar occupant
        in mine or quarry — see Accident, transport, industrial vehicle occupant
      tub, in mine or quarry — see Accident, transport, industrial vehicle occupant
      ultralight — see Accident, transport, aircraft, occupant, powered, glider
      van — see Accident, transport, van occupant
      vehicle NEC V89.9 ☑
        heavy transport — see Accident, transport, truck occupant
        motor (traffic) NEC V89.2 ☑
        nontraffic NEC V89.0 ☑
      watercraft NOS V94.9 ☑
        causing drowning — see Drowning, resulting from accident to boat
    off-road motor-vehicle — see also Accident, transport, all-terrain vehicle occupant V86.99 ☑
    parachutist V97.29 ☑
      after accident to aircraft — see Accident, transport, aircraft
      entangled in object V97.21 ☑
      injured on landing V97.22 ☑
    pedal cyclist V19.9 ☑
      collision (with)
        animal (traffic) V10.9 ☑
          being ridden (traffic) V16.9 ☑
            nontraffic V16.2 ☑
            while boarding or alighting V16.3 ☑
          nontraffic V10.2 ☑
          while boarding or alighting V10.3 ☑
        animal-drawn vehicle (traffic) V16.9 ☑
          nontraffic V16.2 ☑
          while boarding or alighting V16.3 ☑
        bus (traffic) V14.9 ☑
          nontraffic V14.2 ☑
          while boarding or alighting V14.3 ☑
        car (traffic) V13.9 ☑
          nontraffic V13.2 ☑
          while boarding or alighting V13.3 ☑
        motor vehicle NOS (traffic) V19.60 ☑
          nontraffic V19.20 ☑
          specified type NEC (traffic) V19.69 ☑
            nontraffic V19.29 ☑
        pedal cycle (traffic) V11.9 ☑
          nontraffic V11.2 ☑
          while boarding or alighting V11.3 ☑
        pickup truck (traffic) V13.9 ☑
          nontraffic V13.2 ☑
          while boarding or alighting V13.3 ☑
        railway vehicle (traffic) V15.9 ☑
          nontraffic V15.2 ☑
          while boarding or alighting V15.3 ☑
        specified vehicle NEC (traffic) V16.9 ☑
          nontraffic V16.2 ☑
          while boarding or alighting V16.3 ☑
        stationary object (traffic) V17.9 ☑
          nontraffic V17.2 ☑
          while boarding or alighting V17.3 ☑
        streetcar (traffic) V16.9 ☑
          nontraffic V16.2 ☑
          while boarding or alighting V16.3 ☑
        three wheeled motor vehicle (traffic) V12.9 ☑
          nontraffic V12.2 ☑
          while boarding or alighting V12.3 ☑
        truck (traffic) V14.9 ☑
          nontraffic V14.2 ☑
          while boarding or alighting V14.3 ☑
        two wheeled motor vehicle (traffic) V12.9 ☑
          nontraffic V12.2 ☑
          while boarding or alighting V12.3 ☑
        van (traffic) V13.9 ☑
          nontraffic V13.2 ☑
          while boarding or alighting V13.3 ☑
      driver
        collision (with)
          animal (traffic) V10.4 ☑
            being ridden (traffic) V16.4 ☑

Accident — continued
  transport — continued
    pedal cyclist — continued
      driver — continued
        collision — continued
          animal — continued
            being ridden — continued
              nontraffic V16.0 ☑
            nontraffic V10.0 ☑
          animal-drawn vehicle (traffic) V16.4 ☑
            nontraffic V16.0 ☑
          bus (traffic) V14.4 ☑
            nontraffic V14.0 ☑
          car (traffic) V13.4 ☑
            nontraffic V13.0 ☑
          motor vehicle NOS (traffic) V19.40 ☑
            nontraffic V19.00 ☑
            specified type NEC (traffic) V19.49 ☑
              nontraffic V19.09 ☑
          pedal cycle (traffic) V11.4 ☑
            nontraffic V11.0 ☑
          pickup truck (traffic) V13.4 ☑
            nontraffic V13.0 ☑
          railway vehicle (traffic) V15.4 ☑
            nontraffic V15.0 ☑
          specified vehicle NEC (traffic) V16.4 ☑
            nontraffic V16.0 ☑
          stationary object (traffic) V17.4 ☑
            nontraffic V17.0 ☑
          streetcar (traffic) V16.4 ☑
            nontraffic V16.0 ☑
          three wheeled motor vehicle (traffic) V12.4 ☑
            nontraffic V12.0 ☑
          truck (traffic) V14.4 ☑
            nontraffic V14.0 ☑
          two wheeled motor vehicle (traffic) V12.4 ☑
            nontraffic V12.0 ☑
          van (traffic) V13.4 ☑
            nontraffic V13.0 ☑
        noncollision accident (traffic) V18.4 ☑
          nontraffic V18.0 ☑
      noncollision accident (traffic) V18.9 ☑
        nontraffic V18.2 ☑
        while boarding or alighting V18.3 ☑
      nontraffic V19.3 ☑
      passenger
        collision (with)
          animal (traffic) V10.5 ☑
            being ridden (traffic) V16.5 ☑
              nontraffic V16.1 ☑
            nontraffic V10.1 ☑
          animal-drawn vehicle (traffic) V16.5 ☑
            nontraffic V16.1 ☑
          bus (traffic) V14.5 ☑
            nontraffic V14.1 ☑
          car (traffic) V13.5 ☑
            nontraffic V13.1 ☑
          motor vehicle NOS (traffic) V19.50 ☑
            nontraffic V19.10 ☑
            specified type NEC (traffic) V19.59 ☑
              nontraffic V19.19 ☑
          pedal cycle (traffic) V11.5 ☑
            nontraffic V11.1 ☑
          pickup truck (traffic) V13.5 ☑
            nontraffic V13.1 ☑
          railway vehicle (traffic) V15.5 ☑
            nontraffic V15.1 ☑
          specified vehicle NEC (traffic) V16.5 ☑
            nontraffic V16.1 ☑
          stationary object (traffic) V17.5 ☑
            nontraffic V17.1 ☑
          streetcar (traffic) V16.5 ☑
            nontraffic V16.1 ☑
          three wheeled motor vehicle (traffic) V12.5 ☑
            nontraffic V12.1 ☑
          truck (traffic) V14.5 ☑
            nontraffic V14.1 ☑
          two wheeled motor vehicle (traffic) V12.5 ☑
            nontraffic V12.1 ☑
          van (traffic) V13.5 ☑
            nontraffic V13.1 ☑
        noncollision accident (traffic) V18.5 ☑

☑ Additional Character Required — Refer to the Tabular List for Character Selection   ▽ Subterms under main terms may continue to next column or page

Accident — *continued*
  transport — *continued*
    pedal cyclist — *continued*
      passenger — *continued*
        noncollision accident — *continued*
          nontraffic V18.1 ☑
      specified type NEC V19.88 ☑
      military vehicle V19.81 ☑
    pedestrian
      conveyance (occupant) V09.9 ☑
        baby stroller V00.828 ☑
          collision (with) V09.9 ☑
            animal being ridden or animal drawn
              vehicle V06.99 ☑
              nontraffic V06.09 ☑
              traffic V06.19 ☑
            bus or heavy transport V04.99 ☑
              nontraffic V04.09 ☑
              traffic V04.19 ☑
            car V03.99 ☑
              nontraffic V03.09 ☑
              traffic V03.19 ☑
            pedal cycle V01.99 ☑
              nontraffic V01.09 ☑
              traffic V01.19 ☑
            pick-up truck or van V03.99 ☑
              nontraffic V03.09 ☑
              traffic V03.19 ☑
            railway (train) (vehicle) V05.99 ☑
              nontraffic V05.09 ☑
              traffic V05.19 ☑
            stationary object V00.822 ☑
            streetcar V06.99 ☑
              nontraffic V06.09 ☑
              traffic V06.19 ☑
            two- or three-wheeled motor vehicle
              V02.99 ☑
              nontraffic V02.09 ☑
              traffic V02.19 ☑
            vehicle V09.9 ☑
              animal-drawn V06.99 ☑
                nontraffic V06.09 ☑
                traffic V06.19 ☑
              motor
                nontraffic V09.00 ☑
                traffic V09.20 ☑
        fall V00.821 ☑
        nontraffic V09.1 ☑
          involving motor vehicle NEC V09.00 ☑
        traffic V09.3 ☑
          involving motor vehicle NEC V09.20 ☑
        flat-bottomed NEC V00.388 ☑
          collision (with) V09.9 ☑
            animal being ridden or animal drawn
              vehicle V06.99 ☑
              nontraffic V06.09 ☑
              traffic V06.19 ☑
            bus or heavy transport V04.99 ☑
              nontraffic V04.09 ☑
              traffic V04.19 ☑
            car V03.99 ☑
              nontraffic V03.09 ☑
              traffic V03.19 ☑
            pedal cycle V01.99 ☑
              nontraffic V01.09 ☑
              traffic V01.19 ☑
            pick-up truck or van V03.99 ☑
              nontraffic V03.09 ☑
              traffic V03.19 ☑
            railway (train) (vehicle) V05.99 ☑
              nontraffic V05.09 ☑
              traffic V05.19 ☑
            stationary object V00.382 ☑
            streetcar V06.99 ☑
              nontraffic V06.09 ☑
              traffic V06.19 ☑
            two- or three-wheeled motor vehicle
              V02.99 ☑
              nontraffic V02.09 ☑
              traffic V02.19 ☑
            vehicle V09.9 ☑
              animal-drawn V06.99 ☑
                nontraffic V06.09 ☑
                traffic V06.19 ☑
              motor
                nontraffic V09.00 ☑

Accident — *continued*
  transport — *continued*
    pedestrian — *continued*
      conveyance — *continued*
        flat-bottomed — *continued*
          collision — *continued*
            vehicle — *continued*
              motor — *continued*
                traffic V09.20 ☑
        fall V00.381 ☑
        nontraffic V09.1 ☑
          involving motor vehicle NEC V09.00 ☑
        snow
          board — *see* Accident, transport,
            pedestrian, conveyance, snow
            board
          ski — *see* Accident, transport, pedes-
            trian, conveyance, skis (snow)
        traffic V09.3 ☑
          involving motor vehicle NEC V09.20 ☑
        gliding type NEC V00.288 ☑
          collision (with) V09.9 ☑
            animal being ridden or animal drawn
              vehicle V06.99 ☑
              nontraffic V06.09 ☑
              traffic V06.19 ☑
            bus or heavy transport V04.99 ☑
              nontraffic V04.09 ☑
              traffic V04.19 ☑
            car V03.99 ☑
              nontraffic V03.09 ☑
              traffic V03.19 ☑
            pedal cycle V01.99 ☑
              nontraffic V01.09 ☑
              traffic V01.19 ☑
            pick-up truck or van V03.99 ☑
              nontraffic V03.09 ☑
              traffic V03.19 ☑
            railway (train) (vehicle) V05.99 ☑
              nontraffic V05.09 ☑
              traffic V05.19 ☑
            stationary object V00.282 ☑
            streetcar V06.99 ☑
              nontraffic V06.09 ☑
              traffic V02.19 ☑
            two- or three-wheeled motor vehicle
              V02.99 ☑
              nontraffic V02.09 ☑
              traffic V02.19 ☑
            vehicle V09.9 ☑
              animal-drawn V06.99 ☑
                nontraffic V06.09 ☑
                traffic V06.19 ☑
              motor
                nontraffic V09.00 ☑
                traffic V09.20 ☑
        fall V00.281 ☑
        heelies — *see* Accident, transport,
          pedestrian, conveyance, heelies
        ice skate — *see* Accident, transport,
          pedestrian, conveyance, ice skate
        nontraffic V09.1 ☑
          involving motor vehicle NEC V09.00 ☑
        sled — *see* Accident, transport, pedestri-
          an, conveyance, sled
        traffic V09.3 ☑
          involving motor vehicle NEC V09.20 ☑
          wheelies — *see* Accident, transport,
            pedestrian, conveyance, heelies
        heelies V00.158 ☑
          colliding with stationary object
            V00.152 ☑
          fall V00.151 ☑
        ice skates V00.218 ☑
          collision (with) V09.9 ☑
            animal being ridden or animal drawn
              vehicle V06.99 ☑
              nontraffic V06.09 ☑
              traffic V06.19 ☑
            bus or heavy transport V04.99 ☑
              nontraffic V04.09 ☑
              traffic V04.19 ☑
            car V03.99 ☑
              nontraffic V03.09 ☑
              traffic V03.19 ☑
            pedal cycle V01.99 ☑

Accident — *continued*
  transport — *continued*
    pedestrian — *continued*
      conveyance — *continued*
        ice skates — *continued*
          collision — *continued*
            pedal cycle — *continued*
              nontraffic V01.09 ☑
              traffic V01.19 ☑
            pick-up truck or van V03.99 ☑
              nontraffic V03.09 ☑
              traffic V03.19 ☑
            railway (train) (vehicle) V05.99 ☑
              nontraffic V05.09 ☑
              traffic V05.19 ☑
            stationary object V00.212 ☑
            streetcar V06.99 ☑
              nontraffic V06.09 ☑
              traffic V06.19 ☑
            two- or three-wheeled motor vehicle
              V02.99 ☑
              nontraffic V02.09 ☑
              traffic V02.19 ☑
            vehicle V09.9 ☑
              animal-drawn V06.99 ☑
                nontraffic V06.09 ☑
                traffic V06.19 ☑
              motor
                nontraffic V09.00 ☑
                traffic V09.20 ☑
        fall V00.211 ☑
        nontraffic V09.1 ☑
          involving motor vehicle NEC V09.00 ☑
        traffic V09.3 ☑
          involving motor vehicle NEC V09.20 ☑
        motorized mobility scooter V00.838 ☑
          collision with stationary object
            V00.832 ☑
          fall from V00.831 ☑
        nontraffic V09.1 ☑
          involving motor vehicle V09.00 ☑
            military V09.01 ☑
            specified type NEC V09.09 ☑
        roller skates (non in-line) V00.128 ☑
          collision (with) V09.9 ☑
            animal being ridden or animal drawn
              vehicle V06.91 ☑
              nontraffic V06.01 ☑
              traffic V06.11 ☑
            bus or heavy transport V04.91 ☑
              nontraffic V04.01 ☑
              traffic V04.11 ☑
            car V03.91 ☑
              nontraffic V03.01 ☑
              traffic V03.11 ☑
            pedal cycle V01.91 ☑
              nontraffic V01.01 ☑
              traffic V01.11 ☑
            pick-up truck or van V03.91 ☑
              nontraffic V03.01 ☑
              traffic V03.11 ☑
            railway (train) (vehicle) V05.91 ☑
              nontraffic V05.01 ☑
              traffic V05.11 ☑
            stationary object V00.122 ☑
            streetcar V06.91 ☑
              nontraffic V06.01 ☑
              traffic V06.11 ☑
            two- or three-wheeled motor vehicle
              V02.91 ☑
              nontraffic V02.01 ☑
              traffic V02.11 ☑
            vehicle V09.9 ☑
              animal-drawn V06.91 ☑
                nontraffic V06.01 ☑
                traffic V06.11 ☑
              motor
                nontraffic V09.00 ☑
                traffic V09.20 ☑
        fall V00.121 ☑
        in-line V00.118 ☑
          collision — *see also* Accident, trans-
            port, pedestrian, conveyance
            occupant, roller skates, collision
            with stationary object V00.112 ☑
          fall V00.111 ☑

Accident — *continued*
  transport — *continued*
    pedestrian — *continued*
      conveyance — *continued*
        roller skates — *continued*
          nontraffic V09.1
            involving motor vehicle NEC V09.00 ☑
          traffic V09.3 ☑
            involving motor vehicle NEC V09.20 ☑
        rolling shoes V00.158 ☑
          colliding with stationary object
            V00.152 ☑
          fall V00.151 ☑
        rolling type NEC V00.188 ☑
          collision (with) V09.9 ☑
            animal being ridden or animal drawn
              vehicle V06.99 ☑
              nontraffic V06.09 ☑
              traffic V06.19 ☑
            bus or heavy transport V04.99 ☑
              nontraffic V04.09 ☑
              traffic V04.19 ☑
            car V03.99 ☑
              nontraffic V03.09 ☑
              traffic V03.19 ☑
            pedal cycle V01.99 ☑
              nontraffic V01.09 ☑
              traffic V01.19 ☑
            pick-up truck or van V03.99 ☑
              nontraffic V03.09 ☑
              traffic V03.19 ☑
            railway (train) (vehicle) V05.99 ☑
              nontraffic V05.09 ☑
              traffic V05.19 ☑
            stationary object V00.182 ☑
            streetcar V06.99 ☑
              nontraffic V06.09 ☑
              traffic V06.19 ☑
            two- or three-wheeled motor vehicle
              V02.99 ☑
              nontraffic V02.09 ☑
              traffic V02.19 ☑
            vehicle V09.9 ☑
              animal-drawn V06.99 ☑
                nontraffic V06.09 ☑
                traffic V06.19 ☑
              motor
                nontraffic V09.00 ☑
                traffic V09.20 ☑
        fall V00.181 ☑
        in-line roller skate — *see* Accident,
          transport, pedestrian, conveyance,
          roller skate, in-line
        nontraffic V09.1 ☑
          involving motor vehicle NEC V09.00 ☑
        roller skate — *see* Accident, transport,
          pedestrian, conveyance, roller
          skate
        scooter (non-motorized) — *see* Accident,
          transport, pedestrian, conveyance,
          scooter
        skateboard — *see* Accident, transport,
          pedestrian, conveyance, skate-
          board
        traffic V09.3 ☑
          involving motor vehicle NEC V09.20 ☑
      scooter (non-motorized) V00.148 ☑
        collision (with) V09.9 ☑
          animal being ridden or animal drawn
            vehicle V06.99 ☑
              nontraffic V06.09 ☑
              traffic V06.19 ☑
          bus or heavy transport V04.99 ☑
            nontraffic V04.09 ☑
            traffic V04.19 ☑
          car V03.99 ☑
            nontraffic V03.09 ☑
            traffic V03.19 ☑
          pedal cycle V01.99 ☑
            nontraffic V01.09 ☑
            traffic V01.19 ☑
          pick-up truck or van V03.99 ☑
            nontraffic V03.09 ☑
            traffic V03.19 ☑
          railway (train) (vehicle) V05.99 ☑
            nontraffic V05.09 ☑

Accident — *continued*
  transport — *continued*
    pedestrian — *continued*
      conveyance — *continued*
        scooter — *continued*
          collision — *continued*
            railway — *continued*
              traffic V05.19 ☑
            stationary object V00.142 ☑
            streetcar V06.99 ☑
              nontraffic V06.09 ☑
              traffic V06.19 ☑
            two- or three-wheeled motor vehicle
              V02.99 ☑
              nontraffic V02.09 ☑
              traffic V02.19 ☑
            vehicle V09.9 ☑
              animal-drawn V06.99 ☑
                nontraffic V06.09 ☑
                traffic V06.19 ☑
              motor
                nontraffic V09.00 ☑
                traffic V09.20 ☑
          fall V00.141 ☑
          nontraffic V09.1 ☑
            involving motor vehicle NEC V09.00 ☑
          traffic V09.3 ☑
            involving motor vehicle NEC V09.20 ☑
       skate board V00.138 ☑
        collision (with) V09.9 ☑
          animal being ridden or animal drawn
            vehicle V06.92 ☑
              nontraffic V06.02 ☑
              traffic V06.12 ☑
          bus or heavy transport V04.92 ☑
            nontraffic V04.02 ☑
            traffic V04.12 ☑
          car V03.92 ☑
            nontraffic V03.02 ☑
            traffic V03.12 ☑
          pedal cycle V01.92 ☑
            nontraffic V01.02 ☑
            traffic V01.12 ☑
          pick-up truck or van V03.92 ☑
            nontraffic V03.02 ☑
            traffic V03.12 ☑
          railway (train) (vehicle) V05.92 ☑
            nontraffic V05.02 ☑
            traffic V05.12 ☑
          stationary object V00.132 ☑
          streetcar V06.92 ☑
            nontraffic V06.02 ☑
            traffic V06.12 ☑
          two- or three-wheeled motor vehicle
            V02.92 ☑
            nontraffic V02.02 ☑
            traffic V02.12 ☑
          vehicle V09.9 ☑
            animal-drawn V06.92 ☑
              nontraffic V06.02 ☑
              traffic V06.12 ☑
            motor
              nontraffic V09.00 ☑
              traffic V09.20 ☑
        fall V00.131 ☑
        nontraffic V09.1 ☑
          involving motor vehicle NEC V09.00 ☑
        traffic V09.3 ☑
          involving motor vehicle NEC V09.20 ☑
      skis (snow) V00.328 ☑
        collision (with) V09.9 ☑
          animal being ridden or animal drawn
            vehicle V06.99 ☑
              nontraffic V06.09 ☑
              traffic V06.19 ☑
          bus or heavy transport V04.99 ☑
            nontraffic V04.09 ☑
            traffic V04.19 ☑
          car V03.99 ☑
            nontraffic V03.09 ☑
            traffic V03.19 ☑
          pedal cycle V01.99 ☑
            nontraffic V01.09 ☑
            traffic V01.19 ☑
          pick-up truck or van V03.99 ☑
            nontraffic V03.09 ☑

Accident — *continued*
  transport — *continued*
    pedestrian — *continued*
      conveyance — *continued*
        skis — *continued*
          collision — *continued*
            pick-up truck or van — *continued*
              traffic V03.19 ☑
            railway (train) (vehicle) V05.99 ☑
              nontraffic V05.09 ☑
              traffic V05.19 ☑
            stationary object V00.322 ☑
            streetcar V06.99 ☑
              nontraffic V06.09 ☑
              traffic V06.19 ☑
            two- or three-wheeled motor vehicle
              V02.99 ☑
              nontraffic V02.09 ☑
              traffic V02.19 ☑
            vehicle V09.9 ☑
              animal-drawn V06.99 ☑
                nontraffic V06.09 ☑
                traffic V06.19 ☑
              motor
                nontraffic V09.00 ☑
                traffic V09.20 ☑
        fall V00.321 ☑
        nontraffic V09.1 ☑
          involving motor vehicle NEC V09.00 ☑
        traffic V09.3 ☑
          involving motor vehicle NEC V09.20 ☑
      sled V00.228 ☑
        collision (with) V09.9 ☑
          animal being ridden or animal drawn
            vehicle V06.99 ☑
              nontraffic V06.09 ☑
              traffic V06.19 ☑
          bus or heavy transport V04.99 ☑
            nontraffic V04.09 ☑
            traffic V04.19 ☑
          car V03.99 ☑
            nontraffic V03.09 ☑
            traffic V03.19 ☑
          pedal cycle V01.99 ☑
            nontraffic V01.09 ☑
            traffic V01.19 ☑
          pick-up truck or van V03.99 ☑
            nontraffic V03.09 ☑
            traffic V03.19 ☑
          railway (train) (vehicle) V05.99 ☑
            nontraffic V05.09 ☑
            traffic V05.19 ☑
          stationary object V00.222 ☑
          streetcar V06.99 ☑
            nontraffic V06.09 ☑
            traffic V06.19 ☑
          two- or three-wheeled motor vehicle
            V02.99 ☑
            nontraffic V02.09 ☑
            traffic V02.19 ☑
          vehicle V09.9 ☑
            animal-drawn V06.99 ☑
              nontraffic V06.09 ☑
              traffic V06.19 ☑
            motor
              nontraffic V09.00 ☑
              traffic V09.20 ☑
        fall V00.221 ☑
        nontraffic V09.1 ☑
          involving motor vehicle NEC V09.00 ☑
        traffic V09.3 ☑
          involving motor vehicle NEC V09.20 ☑
      snow board V00.318 ☑
        collision (with) V09.9 ☑
          animal being ridden or animal drawn
            vehicle V06.99 ☑
              nontraffic V06.09 ☑
              traffic V06.19 ☑
          bus or heavy transport V04.99 ☑
            nontraffic V04.09 ☑
            traffic V04.19 ☑
          car V03.99 ☑
            nontraffic V03.09 ☑
            traffic V03.19 ☑
          pedal cycle V01.99 ☑
            nontraffic V01.09 ☑

    ☑ **Additional Character Required — Refer to the Tabular List for Character Selection**   ▽ Subterms under main terms may continue to next column or page

Accident — *continued*
  transport — *continued*
    pedestrian — *continued*
      conveyance — *continued*
        snow board — *continued*
          collision — *continued*
            pedal cycle — *continued*
              traffic V01.19
            pick-up truck or van V03.99 ☑
              nontraffic V03.09 ☑
              traffic V03.19 ☑
            railway (train) (vehicle) V05.99 ☑
              nontraffic V05.09 ☑
              traffic V05.19 ☑
            stationary object V00.312 ☑
            streetcar V06.99 ☑
              nontraffic V06.09 ☑
              traffic V06.19 ☑
            two- or three-wheeled motor vehicle
              V02.99 ☑
              nontraffic V02.09 ☑
              traffic V02.19 ☑
            vehicle V09.9 ☑
              animal-drawn V06.99 ☑
                nontraffic V06.09 ☑
                traffic V06.19 ☑
              motor
                nontraffic V09.00 ☑
                traffic V09.20 ☑
           fall V00.311 ☑
          nontraffic V09.1 ☑
            involving motor vehicle NEC V09.00 ☑
          traffic V09.3 ☑
            involving motor vehicle NEC V09.20 ☑
         specified type NEC V00.898 ☑
          collision (with) V09.9 ☑
            animal being ridden or animal drawn
              vehicle V06.99 ☑
              nontraffic V06.09 ☑
              traffic V06.19 ☑
            bus or heavy transport V04.99 ☑
              nontraffic V04.09 ☑
              traffic V04.19 ☑
            car V03.99 ☑
              nontraffic V03.09 ☑
              traffic V03.19 ☑
            pedal cycle V01.99 ☑
              nontraffic V01.09 ☑
              traffic V01.19 ☑
            pick-up truck or van V03.99 ☑
              nontraffic V03.09 ☑
              traffic V03.19 ☑
            railway (train) (vehicle) V05.99 ☑
              nontraffic V05.09 ☑
              traffic V05.19 ☑
            stationary object V00.892 ☑
            streetcar V06.99 ☑
              nontraffic V06.09 ☑
              traffic V06.19 ☑
            two- or three-wheeled motor vehicle
              V02.99 ☑
              nontraffic V02.09 ☑
              traffic V02.19 ☑
            vehicle V09.9 ☑
              animal-drawn V06.99 ☑
                nontraffic V06.09 ☑
                traffic V06.19 ☑
              motor
                nontraffic V09.00 ☑
                traffic V09.20 ☑
           fall V00.891 ☑
          nontraffic V09.1 ☑
            involving motor vehicle NEC V09.00 ☑
          traffic V09.3 ☑
            involving motor vehicle NEC V09.20 ☑
        traffic V09.3 ☑
          involving motor vehicle V09.20 ☑
            military V09.21 ☑
            specified type NEC V09.29 ☑
        wheelchair (powered) V00.818 ☑
          collision (with) V09.9 ☑
            animal being ridden or animal drawn
              vehicle V06.99 ☑
              nontraffic V06.09 ☑
              traffic V06.19 ☑
            bus or heavy transport V04.99 ☑

Accident — *continued*
  transport — *continued*
    pedestrian — *continued*
      conveyance — *continued*
        wheelchair — *continued*
          collision — *continued*
            bus or heavy transport — *contin-ued*
              nontraffic V04.09 ☑
              traffic V04.19 ☑
            car V03.99 ☑
              nontraffic V03.09 ☑
              traffic V03.19 ☑
            pedal cycle V01.99 ☑
              nontraffic V01.09 ☑
              traffic V01.19 ☑
            pick-up truck or van V03.99 ☑
              nontraffic V03.09 ☑
              traffic V03.19 ☑
            railway (train) (vehicle) V05.99 ☑
              nontraffic V05.09 ☑
              traffic V05.19 ☑
            stationary object V00.812 ☑
            streetcar V06.99 ☑
              nontraffic V06.09 ☑
              traffic V06.19 ☑
            two- or three-wheeled motor vehicle
              V02.99 ☑
              nontraffic V02.09 ☑
              traffic V02.19 ☑
            vehicle V09.9 ☑
              animal-drawn V06.99 ☑
                nontraffic V06.09 ☑
                traffic V06.19 ☑
              motor
                nontraffic V09.00 ☑
                traffic V09.20 ☑
           fall V00.811 ☑
          nontraffic V09.1 ☑
            involving motor vehicle NEC V09.00 ☑
          traffic V09.3 ☑
            involving motor vehicle NEC V09.20 ☑
        wheeled shoe V00.158 ☑
          colliding with stationary object
            V00.152 ☑
          fall V00.151 ☑
      on foot — *see also* Accident, pedestrian
        collision (with)
          animal being ridden or animal drawn ve-
            hicle V06.90 ☑
            nontraffic V06.00 ☑
            traffic V06.10 ☑
          bus or heavy transport V04.90 ☑
            nontraffic V04.00 ☑
            traffic V04.10 ☑
          car V03.90 ☑
            nontraffic V03.00 ☑
            traffic V03.10 ☑
          pedal cycle V01.90 ☑
            nontraffic V01.00 ☑
            traffic V01.10 ☑
          pick-up truck or van V03.90 ☑
            nontraffic V03.00 ☑
            traffic V03.10 ☑
          railway (train) (vehicle) V05.90 ☑
            nontraffic V05.00 ☑
            traffic V05.10 ☑
          streetcar V06.90 ☑
            nontraffic V06.00 ☑
            traffic V06.10 ☑
          two- or three-wheeled motor vehicle
            V02.90 ☑
            nontraffic V02.00 ☑
            traffic V02.10 ☑
          vehicle V09.9 ☑
            animal-drawn V06.90 ☑
              nontraffic V06.00 ☑
              traffic V06.10 ☑
            motor
        nontraffic V09.1 ☑
          involving motor vehicle V09.00 ☑
            military V09.01 ☑
            specified type NEC V09.09 ☑
        traffic V09.3 ☑
          involving motor vehicle V09.20 ☑
            military V09.21 ☑

Accident — *continued*
  transport — *continued*
    pedestrian — *continued*
      on foot — *see also* Accident, pedestrian — *con-tinued*
        traffic — *continued*
          involving motor vehicle — *continued*
            specified type NEC V09.29 ☑
      person NEC (unknown way or transportation) V99
        collision (between)
          bus (with)
            heavy transport vehicle (traffic) V87.5 ☑
            nontraffic V88.5 ☑
          car (with)
            bus (traffic) V87.3 ☑
            nontraffic V88.3 ☑
            heavy transport vehicle (traffic) V87.4 ☑
            nontraffic V88.4 ☑
            nontraffic V88.5 ☑
            pick-up truck or van (traffic) V87.2 ☑
            nontraffic V88.2 ☑
            train or railway vehicle (traffic) V87.6 ☑
            nontraffic V88.6 ☑
            two-or three-wheeled motor vehicle
              (traffic) V87.0 ☑
            nontraffic V88.0 ☑
            motor vehicle (traffic) NEC V87.7 ☑
            nontraffic V88.7 ☑
          two-or three-wheeled vehicle (with) (traffic)
            motor vehicle NEC V87.1 ☑
            nontraffic V88.1 ☑
          nonmotor vehicle (collision) (noncollision) (traf-
            fic) V87.9 ☑
          nontraffic V88.9 ☑
      pickup truck occupant V59.9 ☑
        collision (with)
          animal (traffic) V50.9 ☑
            being ridden (traffic) V56.9 ☑
              nontraffic V56.3 ☑
              while boarding or alighting V56.4 ☑
            nontraffic V50.3 ☑
            while boarding or alighting V50.4 ☑
          animal-drawn vehicle (traffic) V56.9 ☑
            nontraffic V56.3 ☑
            while boarding or alighting V56.4 ☑
          bus (traffic) V54.9 ☑
            nontraffic V54.3 ☑
            while boarding or alighting V54.4 ☑
          car (traffic) V53.9 ☑
            nontraffic V53.3 ☑
            while boarding or alighting V53.4 ☑
          motor vehicle NOS (traffic) V59.60 ☑
            nontraffic V59.20 ☑
            specified type NEC (traffic) V59.69 ☑
              nontraffic V59.29 ☑
          pedal cycle (traffic) V51.9 ☑
            nontraffic V51.3 ☑
            while boarding or alighting V51.4 ☑
          pickup truck (traffic) V53.9 ☑
            nontraffic V53.3 ☑
            while boarding or alighting V53.4 ☑
          railway vehicle (traffic) V55.9 ☑
            nontraffic V55.3 ☑
            while boarding or alighting V55.4 ☑
          specified vehicle NEC (traffic) V56.9 ☑
            nontraffic V56.3 ☑
            while boarding or alighting V56.4 ☑
          stationary object (traffic) V57.9 ☑
            nontraffic V57.3 ☑
            while boarding or alighting V57.4 ☑
          streetcar (traffic) V56.9 ☑
            nontraffic V56.3 ☑
            while boarding or alighting V56.4 ☑
          three wheeled motor vehicle (traffic) V52.9 ☑
            nontraffic V52.3 ☑
            while boarding or alighting V52.4 ☑
          truck (traffic) V54.9 ☑
            nontraffic V54.3 ☑
            while boarding or alighting V54.4 ☑
          two wheeled motor vehicle (traffic) V52.9 ☑
            nontraffic V52.3 ☑
            while boarding or alighting V52.4 ☑
          van (traffic) V53.9 ☑
            nontraffic V53.3 ☑
            while boarding or alighting V53.4 ☑

Accident — *continued*
  transport — *continued*
    pickup truck occupant — *continued*
      driver
        collision (with)
          animal (traffic) V50.5 ☑
            being ridden (traffic) V56.5 ☑
              nontraffic V56.0 ☑
            nontraffic V50.0 ☑
          animal-drawn vehicle (traffic) V56.5 ☑
            nontraffic V56.0 ☑
          bus (traffic) V54.5 ☑
            nontraffic V54.0 ☑
          car (traffic) V53.5 ☑
            nontraffic V53.0 ☑
          motor vehicle NOS (traffic) V59.40 ☑
            nontraffic V59.00 ☑
            specified type NEC (traffic) V59.49 ☑
              nontraffic V59.09 ☑
          pedal cycle (traffic) V51.5 ☑
            nontraffic V51.0 ☑
          pickup truck (traffic) V53.5 ☑
            nontraffic V53.0 ☑
          railway vehicle (traffic) V55.5 ☑
            nontraffic V55.0 ☑
          specified vehicle NEC (traffic) V56.5 ☑
            nontraffic V56.0 ☑
          stationary object (traffic) V57.5 ☑
            nontraffic V57.0 ☑
          streetcar (traffic) V56.5 ☑
            nontraffic V56.0 ☑
          three wheeled motor vehicle (traffic)
            V52.5 ☑
            nontraffic V52.0 ☑
          truck (traffic) V54.5 ☑
            nontraffic V54.0 ☑
          two wheeled motor vehicle (traffic)
            V52.5 ☑
            nontraffic V52.0 ☑
          van (traffic) V53.5 ☑
            nontraffic V53.0 ☑
        noncollision accident (traffic) V58.5 ☑
          nontraffic V58.0 ☑
      hanger-on
        collision (with)
          animal (traffic) V50.7 ☑
            being ridden (traffic) V56.7 ☑
              nontraffic V56.2 ☑
            nontraffic V50.2 ☑
          animal-drawn vehicle (traffic) V56.7 ☑
            nontraffic V56.2 ☑
          bus (traffic) V54.7 ☑
            nontraffic V54.2 ☑
          car (traffic) V53.7 ☑
            nontraffic V53.2 ☑
          pedal cycle (traffic) V51.7 ☑
            nontraffic V51.2 ☑
          pickup truck (traffic) V53.7 ☑
            nontraffic V53.2 ☑
          railway vehicle (traffic) V55.7 ☑
            nontraffic V55.2 ☑
          specified vehicle NEC (traffic) V56.7 ☑
            nontraffic V56.2 ☑
          stationary object (traffic) V57.7 ☑
            nontraffic V57.2 ☑
          streetcar (traffic) V56.7 ☑
            nontraffic V56.2 ☑
          three wheeled motor vehicle (traffic)
            V52.7 ☑
            nontraffic V52.2 ☑
          truck (traffic) V54.7 ☑
            nontraffic V54.2 ☑
          two wheeled motor vehicle (traffic)
            V52.7 ☑
            nontraffic V52.2 ☑
          van (traffic) V53.7 ☑
            nontraffic V53.2 ☑
        noncollision accident (traffic) V58.7 ☑
          nontraffic V58.2 ☑
      noncollision accident (traffic) V58.9 ☑
        nontraffic V58.3 ☑
        while boarding or alighting V58.4 ☑
      nontraffic V59.3 ☑
      passenger
        collision (with)
          animal (traffic) V50.6 ☑

Accident — *continued*
  transport — *continued*
    pickup truck occupant — *continued*
      passenger — *continued*
        collision — *continued*
          animal — *continued*
            being ridden (traffic) V56.6 ☑
              nontraffic V56.1 ☑
            nontraffic V50.1 ☑
          animal-drawn vehicle (traffic) V56.6 ☑
            nontraffic V56.1 ☑
          bus (traffic) V54.6 ☑
            nontraffic V54.1 ☑
          car (traffic) V53.6 ☑
            nontraffic V53.1 ☑
          motor vehicle NOS (traffic) V59.50 ☑
            nontraffic V59.10 ☑
            specified type NEC (traffic) V59.59 ☑
              nontraffic V59.19 ☑
          pedal cycle (traffic) V51.6 ☑
            nontraffic V51.1 ☑
          pickup truck (traffic) V53.6 ☑
            nontraffic V53.1 ☑
          railway vehicle (traffic) V55.6 ☑
            nontraffic V55.1 ☑
          specified vehicle NEC (traffic) V56.6 ☑
            nontraffic V56.1 ☑
          stationary object (traffic) V57.6 ☑
            nontraffic V57.1 ☑
          streetcar (traffic) V56.6 ☑
            nontraffic V56.1 ☑
          three wheeled motor vehicle (traffic)
            V52.6 ☑
            nontraffic V52.1 ☑
          truck (traffic) V54.6 ☑
            nontraffic V54.1 ☑
          two wheeled motor vehicle (traffic)
            V52.6 ☑
            nontraffic V52.1 ☑
          van (traffic) V53.6 ☑
            nontraffic V53.1 ☑
        noncollision accident (traffic) V58.6 ☑
          nontraffic V58.1 ☑
      specified type NEC V59.88 ☑
      military vehicle V59.81 ☑
    quarry truck — *see* Accident, transport, industrial
      vehicle occupant
    race car — *see* Accident, transport, motor vehicle
      NEC occupant
    railway vehicle occupant V81.9 ☑
      collision (with) V81.3 ☑
        motor vehicle (non-military) (traffic) V81.1 ☑
          military V81.83 ☑
          nontraffic V81.0 ☑
        rolling stock V81.2 ☑
        specified object NEC V81.3 ☑
      during derailment V81.7 ☑
        with antecedent collision — *see* Accident,
          transport, railway vehicle occupant,
          collision
      explosion V81.81 ☑
      fall (in railway vehicle) V81.5 ☑
        during derailment V81.7 ☑
          with antecedent collision — *see* Accident,
            transport, railway vehicle occupant,
            collision
        from railway vehicle V81.6 ☑
          during derailment V81.7 ☑
            with antecedent collision — *see* Acci-
              dent, transport, railway vehicle
              occupant, collision
        while boarding or alighting V81.4 ☑
      fire V81.81 ☑
      object falling onto train V81.82 ☑
      specified type NEC V81.89 ☑
      while boarding or alighting V81.4 ☑
    ski lift V98.3 ☑
    snowmobile occupant (nontraffic) V86.92 ☑
      driver V86.52 ☑
      hanger-on V86.72 ☑
      passenger V86.62 ☑
      traffic V86.32 ☑
        driver V86.02 ☑
        hanger-on V86.22 ☑
        passenger V86.12 ☑
      while boarding or alighting V86.42 ☑

Accident — *continued*
  transport — *continued*
    specified NEC V98.8 ☑
    sport utility vehicle occupant — *see also* Accident,
      transport, pickup truck occupant
    streetcar occupant V82.9 ☑
      collision (with) V82.3 ☑
        motor vehicle (traffic) V82.1 ☑
          nontraffic V82.0 ☑
        rolling stock V82.2 ☑
      during derailment V82.7 ☑
        with antecedent collision — *see* Accident,
          transport, streetcar occupant, collision
      fall (in streetcar) V82.5 ☑
        during derailment V82.7 ☑
          with antecedent collision — *see* Accident,
            transport, streetcar occupant, colli-
            sion
        from streetcar V82.6 ☑
          during derailment V82.7 ☑
            with antecedent collision — *see* Acci-
              dent, transport, streetcar occu-
              pant, collision
          while boarding or alighting V82.4 ☑
        while boarding or alighting V82.4 ☑
      specified type NEC V82.8 ☑
      while boarding or alighting V82.4 ☑
    three-wheeled motor vehicle occupant V39.9 ☑
      collision (with)
        animal (traffic) V30.9 ☑
          being ridden (traffic) V36.9 ☑
            nontraffic V36.3 ☑
              while boarding or alighting V36.4 ☑
          nontraffic V30.3 ☑
            while boarding or alighting V30.4 ☑
        animal-drawn vehicle (traffic) V36.9 ☑
          nontraffic V36.3 ☑
            while boarding or alighting V36.4 ☑
        bus (traffic) V34.9 ☑
          nontraffic V34.3 ☑
            while boarding or alighting V34.4 ☑
        car (traffic) V33.9 ☑
          nontraffic V33.3 ☑
            while boarding or alighting V33.4 ☑
        motor vehicle NOS (traffic) V39.60 ☑
          nontraffic V39.20 ☑
          specified type NEC (traffic) V39.69 ☑
            nontraffic V39.29 ☑
        pedal cycle (traffic) V31.9 ☑
          nontraffic V31.3 ☑
            while boarding or alighting V31.4 ☑
        pickup truck (traffic) V33.9 ☑
          nontraffic V33.3 ☑
            while boarding or alighting V33.4 ☑
        railway vehicle (traffic) V35.9 ☑
          nontraffic V35.3 ☑
            while boarding or alighting V35.4 ☑
        specified vehicle NEC (traffic) V36.9 ☑
          nontraffic V36.3 ☑
            while boarding or alighting V36.4 ☑
        stationary object (traffic) V37.9 ☑
          nontraffic V37.3 ☑
            while boarding or alighting V37.4 ☑
        streetcar (traffic) V36.9 ☑
          nontraffic V36.3 ☑
            while boarding or alighting V36.4 ☑
        three wheeled motor vehicle (traffic) V32.9 ☑
          nontraffic V32.3 ☑
            while boarding or alighting V32.4 ☑
        truck (traffic) V34.9 ☑
          nontraffic V34.3 ☑
            while boarding or alighting V34.4 ☑
        two wheeled motor vehicle (traffic) V32.9 ☑
          nontraffic V32.3 ☑
            while boarding or alighting V32.4 ☑
        van (traffic) V33.9 ☑
          nontraffic V33.3 ☑
            while boarding or alighting V33.4 ☑
      driver
        collision (with)
          animal (traffic) V30.5 ☑
            being ridden (traffic) V36.5 ☑
              nontraffic V36.0 ☑
            nontraffic V30.0 ☑
          animal-drawn vehicle (traffic) V36.5 ☑
            nontraffic V36.0 ☑

Accident — *continued*
  transport — *continued*
    three-wheeled motor vehicle occupant — *continued*
      driver — *continued*
        collision — *continued*
          bus (traffic) V34.5 ☑
            nontraffic V34.0 ☑
          car (traffic) V33.5 ☑
            nontraffic V33.0 ☑
          motor vehicle NOS (traffic) V39.40 ☑
            nontraffic V39.00 ☑
            specified type NEC (traffic) V39.49 ☑
              nontraffic V39.09 ☑
          pedal cycle (traffic) V31.5 ☑
            nontraffic V31.0 ☑
          pickup truck (traffic) V33.5 ☑
            nontraffic V33.0 ☑
          railway vehicle (traffic) V35.5 ☑
            nontraffic V35.0 ☑
          specified vehicle NEC (traffic) V36.5 ☑
            nontraffic V36.0 ☑
          stationary object (traffic) V37.5 ☑
            nontraffic V37.0 ☑
          streetcar (traffic) V36.5 ☑
            nontraffic V36.0 ☑
          three wheeled motor vehicle (traffic)
            V32.5 ☑
            nontraffic V32.0 ☑
          truck (traffic) V34.5 ☑
            nontraffic V34.0 ☑
          two wheeled motor vehicle (traffic)
            V32.5 ☑
            nontraffic V32.0 ☑
          van (traffic) V33.5 ☑
            nontraffic V33.0 ☑
        noncollision accident (traffic) V38.5 ☑
          nontraffic V38.0 ☑
      hanger-on
        collision (with)
          animal (traffic) V30.7 ☑
            being ridden (traffic) V36.7 ☑
              nontraffic V36.2 ☑
            nontraffic V30.2 ☑
          animal-drawn vehicle (traffic) V36.7 ☑
            nontraffic V36.2 ☑
          bus (traffic) V34.7 ☑
            nontraffic V34.2 ☑
          car (traffic) V33.7 ☑
            nontraffic V33.2 ☑
          pedal cycle (traffic) V31.7 ☑
            nontraffic V31.2 ☑
          pickup truck (traffic) V33.7 ☑
            nontraffic V33.2 ☑
          railway vehicle (traffic) V35.7 ☑
            nontraffic V35.2 ☑
          specified vehicle NEC (traffic) V36.7 ☑
            nontraffic V36.2 ☑
          stationary object (traffic) V37.7 ☑
            nontraffic V37.2 ☑
          streetcar (traffic) V36.7 ☑
            nontraffic V36.2 ☑
          three wheeled motor vehicle (traffic)
            V32.7 ☑
            nontraffic V32.2 ☑
          truck (traffic) V34.7 ☑
            nontraffic V34.2 ☑
          two wheeled motor vehicle (traffic)
            V32.7 ☑
            nontraffic V32.2 ☑
          van (traffic) V33.7 ☑
            nontraffic V33.2 ☑
        noncollision accident (traffic) V38.7 ☑
          nontraffic V38.2 ☑
      noncollision accident (traffic) V38.9 ☑
        nontraffic V38.3 ☑
        while boarding or alighting V38.4 ☑
      nontraffic V39.3 ☑
      passenger
        collision (with)
          animal (traffic) V30.6 ☑
            being ridden (traffic) V36.6 ☑
              nontraffic V36.1 ☑
            nontraffic V30.1 ☑
          animal-drawn vehicle (traffic) V36.6 ☑
            nontraffic V36.1 ☑

Accident — *continued*
  transport — *continued*
    three-wheeled motor vehicle occupant — *continued*
      passenger — *continued*
        collision — *continued*
          bus (traffic) V34.6 ☑
            nontraffic V34.1 ☑
          car (traffic) V33.6 ☑
            nontraffic V33.1 ☑
          motor vehicle NOS (traffic) V39.50 ☑
            nontraffic V39.10 ☑
            specified type NEC (traffic) V39.59 ☑
              nontraffic V39.19 ☑
          pedal cycle (traffic) V31.6 ☑
            nontraffic V31.1 ☑
          pickup truck (traffic) V33.6 ☑
            nontraffic V33.1 ☑
          railway vehicle (traffic) V35.6 ☑
            nontraffic V35.1 ☑
          specified vehicle NEC (traffic) V36.6 ☑
            nontraffic V36.1 ☑
          stationary object (traffic) V37.6 ☑
            nontraffic V37.1 ☑
          streetcar (traffic) V36.6 ☑
            nontraffic V36.1 ☑
          three wheeled motor vehicle (traffic)
            V32.6 ☑
            nontraffic V32.1 ☑
          truck (traffic) V34.6 ☑
            nontraffic V34.1 ☑
          two wheeled motor vehicle (traffic)
            V32.6 ☑
            nontraffic V32.1 ☑
          van (traffic) V33.6 ☑
            nontraffic V33.1 ☑
        noncollision accident (traffic) V38.6 ☑
          nontraffic V38.1 ☑
      specified type NEC V39.89 ☑
      military vehicle V39.81
    tractor (farm) (and trailer) — *see* Accident, transport,
      agricultural vehicle occupant
    tram — *see* Accident, transport, streetcar
      in mine or quarry — *see* Accident, transport, in-
      dustrial vehicle occupant
    trolley — *see* Accident, transport, streetcar
      in mine or quarry — *see* Accident, transport, in-
      dustrial vehicle occupant
    truck (heavy) occupant V69.9 ☑
      collision (with)
        animal (traffic) V60.9 ☑
          being ridden (traffic) V66.9 ☑
            nontraffic V66.3 ☑
            while boarding or alighting V66.4 ☑
          nontraffic V60.3 ☑
          while boarding or alighting V60.4 ☑
        animal-drawn vehicle (traffic) V66.9 ☑
          nontraffic V66.3 ☑
          while boarding or alighting V66.4 ☑
        bus (traffic) V64.9 ☑
          nontraffic V64.3 ☑
          while boarding or alighting V64.4 ☑
        car (traffic) V63.9 ☑
          nontraffic V63.3 ☑
          while boarding or alighting V63.4 ☑
        motor vehicle NOS (traffic) V69.60 ☑
          nontraffic V69.20 ☑
          specified type NEC (traffic) V69.69 ☑
            nontraffic V69.29 ☑
        pedal cycle (traffic) V61.9 ☑
          nontraffic V61.3 ☑
          while boarding or alighting V61.4 ☑
        pickup truck (traffic) V63.9 ☑
          nontraffic V63.3 ☑
          while boarding or alighting V63.4 ☑
        railway vehicle (traffic) V65.9 ☑
          nontraffic V65.3 ☑
          while boarding or alighting V65.4 ☑
        specified vehicle NEC (traffic) V66.9 ☑
          nontraffic V66.3 ☑
          while boarding or alighting V66.4 ☑
        stationary object (traffic) V67.9 ☑
          nontraffic V67.3 ☑
          while boarding or alighting V67.4 ☑
        streetcar (traffic) V66.9 ☑
          nontraffic V66.3 ☑

Accident — *continued*
  transport — *continued*
    truck occupant — *continued*
      collision — *continued*
        streetcar — *continued*
          while boarding or alighting V66.4 ☑
        three wheeled motor vehicle (traffic) V62.9 ☑
          nontraffic V62.3 ☑
          while boarding or alighting V62.4 ☑
        truck (traffic) V64.9 ☑
          nontraffic V64.3 ☑
          while boarding or alighting V64.4 ☑
        two wheeled motor vehicle (traffic) V62.9 ☑
          nontraffic V62.3 ☑
          while boarding or alighting V62.4 ☑
        van (traffic) V63.9 ☑
          nontraffic V63.3 ☑
          while boarding or alighting V63.4 ☑
      driver
        collision (with)
          animal (traffic) V60.5 ☑
            being ridden (traffic) V66.5 ☑
              nontraffic V66.0 ☑
            nontraffic V60.0 ☑
          animal-drawn vehicle (traffic) V66.5 ☑
            nontraffic V66.0 ☑
          bus (traffic) V64.5 ☑
            nontraffic V64.0 ☑
          car (traffic) V63.5 ☑
            nontraffic V63.0 ☑
          motor vehicle NOS (traffic) V69.40 ☑
            nontraffic V69.00 ☑
            specified type NEC (traffic) V69.49 ☑
              nontraffic V69.09 ☑
          pedal cycle (traffic) V61.5 ☑
            nontraffic V61.0 ☑
          pickup truck (traffic) V63.5 ☑
            nontraffic V63.0 ☑
          railway vehicle (traffic) V65.5 ☑
            nontraffic V65.0 ☑
          specified vehicle NEC (traffic) V66.5 ☑
            nontraffic V66.0 ☑
          stationary object (traffic) V67.5 ☑
            nontraffic V67.0 ☑
          streetcar (traffic) V66.5 ☑
            nontraffic V66.0 ☑
          three wheeled motor vehicle (traffic)
            V62.5 ☑
            nontraffic V62.0 ☑
          truck (traffic) V64.5 ☑
            nontraffic V64.0 ☑
          two wheeled motor vehicle (traffic)
            V62.5 ☑
            nontraffic V62.0 ☑
          van (traffic) V63.5 ☑
            nontraffic V63.0 ☑
        noncollision accident (traffic) V68.5 ☑
          nontraffic V68.0 ☑
      dump — *see* Accident, transport, construction
        vehicle occupant
      hanger-on
        collision (with)
          animal (traffic) V60.7 ☑
            being ridden (traffic) V66.7 ☑
              nontraffic V66.2 ☑
            nontraffic V60.2 ☑
          animal-drawn vehicle (traffic) V66.7 ☑
            nontraffic V66.2 ☑
          bus (traffic) V64.7 ☑
            nontraffic V64.2 ☑
          car (traffic) V63.7 ☑
            nontraffic V63.2 ☑
          pedal cycle (traffic) V61.7 ☑
            nontraffic V61.2 ☑
          pickup truck (traffic) V63.7 ☑
            nontraffic V63.2 ☑
          railway vehicle (traffic) V65.7 ☑
            nontraffic V65.2 ☑
          specified vehicle NEC (traffic) V66.7 ☑
            nontraffic V66.2 ☑
          stationary object (traffic) V67.7 ☑
            nontraffic V67.2 ☑
          streetcar (traffic) V66.7 ☑
            nontraffic V66.2 ☑
          three wheeled motor vehicle (traffic)
            V62.7 ☑

Accident — *continued*
　transport — *continued*
　　truck occupant — *continued*
　　　hanger-on — *continued*
　　　　collision — *continued*
　　　　　three wheeled motor vehicle — *continued*
　　　　　　nontraffic V62.2 ☑
　　　　　truck (traffic) V64.7 ☑
　　　　　　nontraffic V64.2 ☑
　　　　　two wheeled motor vehicle (traffic)
　　　　　　V62.7 ☑
　　　　　　nontraffic V62.2 ☑
　　　　　van (traffic) V63.7 ☑
　　　　　　nontraffic V63.2 ☑
　　　　noncollision accident (traffic) V68.7 ☑
　　　　　nontraffic V68.2 ☑
　　　noncollision accident (traffic) V68.9 ☑
　　　　nontraffic V68.3 ☑
　　　　while boarding or alighting V68.4 ☑
　　　nontraffic V69.3 ☑
　　passenger
　　　collision (with)
　　　　animal (traffic) V60.6 ☑
　　　　　being ridden (traffic) V66.6 ☑
　　　　　　nontraffic V66.1-
　　　　　nontraffic V60.1 ☑
　　　　animal-drawn vehicle (traffic) V66.6 ☑
　　　　　nontraffic V66.1 ☑
　　　　bus (traffic) V64.6 ☑
　　　　　nontraffic V64.1 ☑
　　　　car (traffic) V63.6 ☑
　　　　　nontraffic V63.1 ☑
　　　　motor vehicle NOS (traffic) V69.50 ☑
　　　　　nontraffic V69.10 ☑
　　　　　specified type NEC (traffic) V69.59 ☑
　　　　　　nontraffic V69.19 ☑
　　　　pedal cycle (traffic) V61.6 ☑
　　　　　nontraffic V61.1 ☑
　　　　pickup truck (traffic) V63.6 ☑
　　　　　nontraffic V63.1 ☑
　　　　railway vehicle (traffic) V65.6 ☑
　　　　　nontraffic V65.1 ☑
　　　　specified vehicle NEC (traffic) V66.6 ☑
　　　　　nontraffic V66.1 ☑
　　　　stationary object (traffic) V67.6 ☑
　　　　　nontraffic V67.1 ☑
　　　　streetcar (traffic) V66.6 ☑
　　　　　nontraffic V66.1 ☑
　　　　three wheeled motor vehicle (traffic)
　　　　　V62.6 ☑
　　　　　nontraffic V62.1 ☑
　　　　truck (traffic) V64.6 ☑
　　　　　nontraffic V64.1 ☑
　　　　two wheeled motor vehicle (traffic)
　　　　　V62.6 ☑
　　　　　nontraffic V62.1 ☑
　　　　van (traffic) V63.6 ☑
　　　　　nontraffic V63.1 ☑
　　　　noncollision accident (traffic) V68.6 ☑
　　　　　nontraffic V68.1 ☑
　　　pickup — *see* Accident, transport, pickup truck
　　　　occupant
　　　specified type NEC V69.88 ☑
　　　　military vehicle V69.81 ☑
　van occupant V59.9 ☑
　　collision (with)
　　　animal (traffic) V50.9 ☑
　　　　being ridden (traffic) V56.9 ☑
　　　　　nontraffic V56.3 ☑
　　　　　while boarding or alighting V56.4 ☑
　　　　nontraffic V50.3 ☑
　　　　while boarding or alighting V50.4 ☑
　　　animal-drawn vehicle (traffic) V56.9 ☑
　　　　nontraffic V56.3 ☑
　　　　while boarding or alighting V56.4 ☑
　　　bus (traffic) V54.9 ☑
　　　　nontraffic V54.3 ☑
　　　　while boarding or alighting V54.4 ☑
　　　car (traffic) V53.9 ☑
　　　　nontraffic V53.3 ☑
　　　　while boarding or alighting V53.4 ☑
　　　motor vehicle NOS (traffic) V59.60 ☑
　　　　nontraffic V59.20 ☑
　　　　specified type NEC (traffic) V59.69 ☑
　　　　　nontraffic V59.29 ☑

Accident — *continued*
　transport — *continued*
　　van occupant — *continued*
　　　collision — *continued*
　　　　pedal cycle (traffic) V51.9 ☑
　　　　　nontraffic V51.3 ☑
　　　　　while boarding or alighting V51.4 ☑
　　　　pickup truck (traffic) V53.9 ☑
　　　　　nontraffic V53.3 ☑
　　　　　while boarding or alighting V53.4 ☑
　　　　railway vehicle (traffic) V55.9 ☑
　　　　　nontraffic V55.3 ☑
　　　　　while boarding or alighting V55.4 ☑
　　　　specified vehicle NEC (traffic) V56.9 ☑
　　　　　nontraffic V56.3 ☑
　　　　　while boarding or alighting V56.4 ☑
　　　　stationary object (traffic) V57.9 ☑
　　　　　nontraffic V57.3 ☑
　　　　　while boarding or alighting V57.4 ☑
　　　　streetcar (traffic) V56.9 ☑
　　　　　nontraffic V56.3 ☑
　　　　　while boarding or alighting V56.4 ☑
　　　　three wheeled motor vehicle (traffic) V52.9 ☑
　　　　　nontraffic V52.3 ☑
　　　　　while boarding or alighting V52.4 ☑
　　　　truck (traffic) V54.9 ☑
　　　　　nontraffic V54.3 ☑
　　　　　while boarding or alighting V54.4 ☑
　　　　two wheeled motor vehicle (traffic) V52.9 ☑
　　　　　nontraffic V52.3 ☑
　　　　　while boarding or alighting V52.4 ☑
　　　　van (traffic) V53.9 ☑
　　　　　nontraffic V53.3 ☑
　　　　　while boarding or alighting V53.4 ☑
　　　driver
　　　　collision (with)
　　　　　animal (traffic) V50.5 ☑
　　　　　　being ridden (traffic) V56.5 ☑
　　　　　　　nontraffic V56.0 ☑
　　　　　　nontraffic V50.0 ☑
　　　　　animal-drawn vehicle (traffic) V56.5 ☑
　　　　　　nontraffic V56.0 ☑
　　　　　bus (traffic) V54.5 ☑
　　　　　　nontraffic V54.0 ☑
　　　　　car (traffic) V53.5 ☑
　　　　　　nontraffic V53.0 ☑
　　　　　motor vehicle NOS (traffic) V59.40 ☑
　　　　　　nontraffic V59.00 ☑
　　　　　　specified type NEC (traffic) V59.49 ☑
　　　　　　　nontraffic V59.09 ☑
　　　　　pedal cycle (traffic) V51.5 ☑
　　　　　　nontraffic V51.0 ☑
　　　　　pickup truck (traffic) V53.5 ☑
　　　　　　nontraffic V53.0 ☑
　　　　　railway vehicle (traffic) V55.5 ☑
　　　　　　nontraffic V55.0 ☑
　　　　　specified vehicle NEC (traffic) V56.5 ☑
　　　　　　nontraffic V56.0 ☑
　　　　　stationary object (traffic) V57.5 ☑
　　　　　　nontraffic V57.0 ☑
　　　　　streetcar (traffic) V56.5 ☑
　　　　　　nontraffic V56.0 ☑
　　　　　three wheeled motor vehicle (traffic)
　　　　　　V52.5 ☑
　　　　　　nontraffic V52.0 ☑
　　　　　truck (traffic) V54.5 ☑
　　　　　　nontraffic V54.0 ☑
　　　　　two wheeled motor vehicle (traffic)
　　　　　　V52.5 ☑
　　　　　　nontraffic V52.0 ☑
　　　　　van (traffic) V53.5 ☑
　　　　　　nontraffic V53.0 ☑
　　　　noncollision accident (traffic) V58.5 ☑
　　　　　nontraffic V58.0 ☑
　　　hanger-on
　　　　collision (with)
　　　　　animal (traffic) V50.7 ☑
　　　　　　being ridden (traffic) V56.7 ☑
　　　　　　　nontraffic V56.2 ☑
　　　　　　nontraffic V50.2 ☑
　　　　　animal-drawn vehicle (traffic) V56.7 ☑
　　　　　　nontraffic V56.2 ☑
　　　　　bus (traffic) V54.7 ☑
　　　　　　nontraffic V54.2 ☑
　　　　　car (traffic) V53.7 ☑
　　　　　　nontraffic V53.2 ☑

Accident — *continued*
　transport — *continued*
　　van occupant — *continued*
　　　hanger-on — *continued*
　　　　collision — *continued*
　　　　　pedal cycle (traffic) V51.7 ☑
　　　　　　nontraffic V51.2 ☑
　　　　　pickup truck (traffic) V53.7 ☑
　　　　　　nontraffic V53.2 ☑
　　　　　railway vehicle (traffic) V55.7 ☑
　　　　　　nontraffic V55.2 ☑
　　　　　specified vehicle NEC (traffic) V56.7 ☑
　　　　　　nontraffic V56.2 ☑
　　　　　stationary object (traffic) V57.7 ☑
　　　　　　nontraffic V57.2 ☑
　　　　　streetcar (traffic) V56.7 ☑
　　　　　　nontraffic V56.2 ☑
　　　　　three wheeled motor vehicle (traffic)
　　　　　　V52.7 ☑
　　　　　　nontraffic V52.2 ☑
　　　　　truck (traffic) V54.7 ☑
　　　　　　nontraffic V54.2 ☑
　　　　　two wheeled motor vehicle (traffic)
　　　　　　V52.7 ☑
　　　　　　nontraffic V52.2 ☑
　　　　　van (traffic) V53.7 ☑
　　　　　　nontraffic V53.2 ☑
　　　　noncollision accident (traffic) V58.7 ☑
　　　　　nontraffic V58.2 ☑
　　　noncollision accident (traffic) V58.9 ☑
　　　　nontraffic V58.3 ☑
　　　　while boarding or alighting V58.4 ☑
　　　nontraffic V59.3 ☑
　　　passenger
　　　　collision (with)
　　　　　animal (traffic) V50.6 ☑
　　　　　　being ridden (traffic) V56.6 ☑
　　　　　　　nontraffic V56.1 ☑
　　　　　　nontraffic V50.1 ☑
　　　　　animal-drawn vehicle (traffic) V56.6 ☑
　　　　　　nontraffic V56.1 ☑
　　　　　bus (traffic) V54.6 ☑
　　　　　　nontraffic V54.1 ☑
　　　　　car (traffic) V53.6 ☑
　　　　　　nontraffic V53.1 ☑
　　　　　motor vehicle NOS (traffic) V59.50 ☑
　　　　　　nontraffic V59.10 ☑
　　　　　　specified type NEC (traffic) V59.59 ☑
　　　　　　　nontraffic V59.19 ☑
　　　　　pedal cycle (traffic) V51.6 ☑
　　　　　　nontraffic V51.1 ☑
　　　　　pickup truck (traffic) V53.6 ☑
　　　　　　nontraffic V53.1 ☑
　　　　　railway vehicle (traffic) V55.6 ☑
　　　　　　nontraffic V55.1 ☑
　　　　　specified vehicle NEC (traffic) V56.6 ☑
　　　　　　nontraffic V56.1 ☑
　　　　　stationary object (traffic) V57.6 ☑
　　　　　　nontraffic V57.1 ☑
　　　　　streetcar (traffic) V56.6 ☑
　　　　　　nontraffic V56.1 ☑
　　　　　three wheeled motor vehicle (traffic)
　　　　　　V52.6 ☑
　　　　　　nontraffic V52.1 ☑
　　　　　truck (traffic) V54.6 ☑
　　　　　　nontraffic V54.1 ☑
　　　　　two wheeled motor vehicle (traffic)
　　　　　　V52.6 ☑
　　　　　　nontraffic V52.1 ☑
　　　　　van (traffic) V53.6 ☑
　　　　　　nontraffic V53.1 ☑
　　　　noncollision accident (traffic) V58.6 ☑
　　　　　nontraffic V58.1 ☑
　　　specified type NEC V59.88 ☑
　　　　military vehicle V59.81 ☑
　　watercraft occupant — *see* Accident, watercraft
　vehicle NEC V89.9 ☑
　　animal-drawn NEC — *see* Accident, transport, animal-drawn vehicle occupant
　　special
　　　agricultural — *see* Accident, transport, agricultural vehicle occupant
　　　construction — *see* Accident, transport, construction vehicle occupant
　　　industrial — *see* Accident, transport, industrial vehicle occupant

Accident — *continued*
  vehicle — *continued*
    three-wheeled NEC (motorized) — *see* Accident, transport, three-wheeled motor vehicle occupant
    watercraft V94.9 ☑
      causing
        drowning — *see* Drowning, due to, accident to, watercraft
        injury NEC V91.89 ☑
          crushed between craft and object V91.19 ☑
            powered craft V91.13 ☑
              ferry boat V91.11 ☑
              fishing boat V91.12 ☑
              jetskis V91.13 ☑
              liner V91.11 ☑
              merchant ship V91.10 ☑
              passenger ship V91.11 ☑
            unpowered craft V91.18 ☑
              canoe V91.15 ☑
              inflatable V91.16 ☑
              kayak V91.15 ☑
              sailboat V91.14 ☑
              surf-board V91.18 ☑
              windsurfer V91.18 ☑
          fall on board V91.29 ☑
            powered craft V91.23 ☑
              ferry boat V91.21 ☑
              fishing boat V91.22 ☑
              jetskis V91.23 ☑
              liner V91.21 ☑
              merchant ship V91.20 ☑
              passenger ship V91.21 ☑
            unpowered craft
              canoe V91.25 ☑
              inflatable V91.26 ☑
              kayak V91.25 ☑
              sailboat V91.24 ☑
          fire on board causing burn V91.09 ☑
            powered craft V91.03 ☑
              ferry boat V91.01 ☑
              fishing boat V91.02 ☑
              jetskis V91.03 ☑
              liner V91.01 ☑
              merchant ship V91.00 ☑
              passenger ship V91.01 ☑
            unpowered craft V91.08 ☑
              canoe V91.05 ☑
              inflatable V91.06 ☑
              kayak V91.05 ☑
              sailboat V91.04 ☑
              surf-board V91.08 ☑
              water skis V91.07 ☑
              windsurfer V91.08 ☑
          hit by falling object V91.39 ☑
            powered craft V91.33 ☑
              ferry boat V91.31 ☑
              fishing boat V91.32 ☑
              jetskis V91.33 ☑
              liner V91.31 ☑
              merchant ship V91.30 ☑
              passenger ship V91.31 ☑
            unpowered craft V91.38 ☑
              canoe V91.35 ☑
              inflatable V91.36 ☑
              kayak V91.35 ☑
              sailboat V91.34 ☑
              surf-board V91.38 ☑
              water skis V91.37 ☑
              windsurfer V91.38 ☑
          specified type NEC V91.89 ☑
            powered craft V91.83 ☑
              ferry boat V91.81 ☑
              fishing boat V91.82 ☑
              jetskis V91.83 ☑
              liner V91.81 ☑
              merchant ship V91.80 ☑
              passenger ship V91.81 ☑
            unpowered craft V91.88 ☑
              canoe V91.85 ☑
              inflatable V91.86 ☑
              kayak V91.85 ☑
              sailboat V91.84 ☑
              surf-board V91.88 ☑
              water skis V91.87 ☑
              windsurfer V91.88 ☑

Accident — *continued*
  watercraft — *continued*
    due to, caused by cataclysm — *see* Forces of nature, by type
    military NEC V94.818 ☑
      civilian in water injured by V94.811 ☑
      with civilian watercraft V94.810 ☑
    nonpowered, struck by
      nonpowered vessel V94.22 ☑
      powered vessel V94.21 ☑
    specified type NEC V94.89 ☑
    striking swimmer
      powered V94.11 ☑
      unpowered V94.12 ☑
Acid throwing (assault) Y08.89 ☑
Activity (involving) (of victim at time of event) Y93.9
  aerobic and step exercise (class) Y93.A3 (*following* Y93.7)
  alpine skiing Y93.23
  animal care NEC Y93.K9 (*following* Y93.7)
  arts and handcrafts NEC Y93.D9 (*following* Y93.7)
  athletics played as a team or group NEC Y93.69
  athletics played individually NEC Y93.59
  athletics NEC Y93.79
  baking Y93.G3 (*following* Y93.7)
  ballet Y93.41
  barbells Y93.B3 (*following* Y93.7)
  BASE (Building, Antenna, Span, Earth) jumping Y93.33
  baseball Y93.64
  basketball Y93.67
  bathing (personal) Y93.E1 (*following* Y93.7)
  beach volleyball Y93.68
  bike riding Y93.55
  blackout game Y93.85
  boogie boarding Y93.18
  bowling Y93.54
  boxing Y93.71
  brass instrument playing Y93.J4 (*following* Y93.7)
  building construction Y93.H3 (*following* Y93.7)
  bungee jumping Y93.34
  calisthenics Y93.A2 (*following* Y93.7)
  canoeing (in calm and turbulent water) Y93.16
  capture the flag Y93.6A
  cardiorespiratory exercise NEC Y93.A9 (*following* Y93.7)
  caregiving (providing) NEC Y93.F9 (*following* Y93.7)
    bathing Y93.F1 (*following* Y93.7)
    lifting Y93.F2 (*following* Y93.7)
  cellular
    communication device Y93.C2 (*following* Y93.7)
    telephone Y93.C2 (*following* Y93.7)
  challenge course Y93.A5 (*following* Y93.7)
  cheerleading Y93.45
  choking game Y93.85
  circuit training Y93.A4 (*following* Y93.7)
  cleaning
    floor Y93.E5 (*following* Y93.7)
  climbing NEC Y93.39
    mountain Y93.31
    rock Y93.31
    wall Y93.31
  clothing care and maintenance NEC Y93.E9 (*following* Y93.7)
  combatives Y93.75
  computer
    keyboarding Y93.C1 (*following* Y93.7)
    technology NEC Y93.C9 (*following* Y93.7)
  confidence course Y93.A5 (*following* Y93.7)
  construction (building) Y93.H3 (*following* Y93.7)
  cooking and baking Y93.G3 (*following* Y93.7)
  cool down exercises Y93.A2 (*following* Y93.7)
  cricket Y93.69
  crocheting Y93.D1 (*following* Y93.7)
  cross country skiing Y93.24
  dancing (all types) Y93.41
  digging
    dirt Y93.H1 (*following* Y93.7)
  dirt digging Y93.H1 (*following* Y93.7)
  dishwashing Y93.G1 (*following* Y93.7)
  diving (platform) (springboard) Y93.12
    underwater Y93.15
  dodge ball Y93.6A
  downhill skiing Y93.23
  drum playing Y93.J2 (*following* Y93.7)
  dumbbells Y93.B3 (*following* Y93.7)
  electronic
    devices NEC Y93.C9 (*following* Y93.7)
      hand held interactive Y93.C2 (*following* Y93.7)

Activity — *continued*
  electronic — *continued*
    game playing (using) (with)
      interactive device Y93.C2 (*following* Y93.7)
      keyboard or other stationary device Y93.C1 (*following* Y93.7)
  elliptical machine Y93.A1 (*following* Y93.7)
  exercise(s)
    machines ((primarily) for)
      cardiorespiratory conditioning Y93.A1 (*following* Y93.7)
      muscle strengthening Y93.B1 (*following* Y93.7)
    muscle strengthening (non-machine) NEC Y93.B9 (*following* Y93.7)
  external motion NEC Y93.I9 (*following* Y93.7)
    rollercoaster Y93.I1 (*following* Y93.7)
  fainting game Y93.85
  field hockey Y93.65
  figure skating (pairs) (singles) Y93.21
  flag football Y93.62
  floor mopping and cleaning Y93.E5 (*following* Y93.7)
  food preparation and clean up Y93.G1 (*following* Y93.7)
  football (American) NOS Y93.61
    flag Y93.62
    tackle Y93.61
    touch Y93.62
  four square Y93.6A
  free weights Y93.B3 (*following* Y93.7)
  frisbee (ultimate) Y93.74
  furniture
    building Y93.D3 (*following* Y93.7)
    finishing Y93.D3 (*following* Y93.7)
    repair Y93.D3 (*following* Y93.7)
  game playing (electronic)
    using interactive device Y93.C2 (*following* Y93.7)
    using keyboard or other stationary device Y93.C1 (*following* Y93.7)
  gardening Y93.H2 (*following* Y93.7)
  golf Y93.53
  grass drills Y93.A6 (*following* Y93.7)
  grilling and smoking food Y93.G2 (*following* Y93.7)
  grooming and shearing an animal Y93.K3 (*following* Y93.7)
  guerilla drills Y93.A6 (*following* Y93.7)
  gymnastics (rhythmic) Y93.43
  hand held interactive electronic device Y93.C2 (*following* Y93.7)
  handball Y93.73
  handcrafts NEC Y93.D9 (*following* Y93.7)
  hang gliding Y93.35
  hiking (on level or elevated terrain) Y93.01
  hockey (ice) Y93.22
    field Y93.65
  horseback riding Y93.52
  household (interior) maintenance NEC Y93.E9 (*following* Y93.7)
  ice NEC Y93.29
    dancing Y93.21
    hockey Y93.22
    skating Y93.21
  inline roller skating Y93.51
  ironing Y93.E4 (*following* Y93.7)
  judo Y93.75
  jumping jacks Y93.A2 (*following* Y93.7)
  jumping rope Y93.56
  jumping (off) NEC Y93.39
    BASE (Building, Antenna, Span, Earth) Y93.33
    bungee Y93.34
    jacks Y93.A2 (*following* Y93.7)
    rope Y93.56
  karate Y93.75
  kayaking (in calm and turbulent water) Y93.16
  keyboarding (computer) Y93.C1 (*following* Y93.7)
  kickball Y93.6A
  knitting Y93.D1 (*following* Y93.7)
  lacrosse Y93.65
  land maintenance NEC Y93.H9 (*following* Y93.7)
  landscaping Y93.H2 (*following* Y93.7)
  laundry Y93.E2 (*following* Y93.7)
  machines (exercise)
    primarily for cardiorespiratory conditioning Y93.A1 (*following* Y93.7)
    primarily for muscle strengthening Y93.B1 (*following* Y93.7)
  maintenance
    exterior building NEC Y93.H9 (*following* Y93.7)
    household (interior) NEC Y93.E9 (*following* Y93.7)
    land Y93.H9 (*following* Y93.7)
    property Y93.H9 (*following* Y93.7)

Activity — *continued*
   marching (on level or elevated terrain) Y93.01
   martial arts Y93.75
   microwave oven Y93.G3 *(following* Y93.7*)*
   milking an animal Y93.K2 *(following* Y93.7*)*
   mopping (floor) Y93.E5 *(following* Y93.7*)*
   mountain climbing Y93.31
   muscle strengthening
      exercises (non-machine) NEC Y93.B9 *(following* Y93.7*)*
      machines Y93.B1 *(following* Y93.7*)*
   musical keyboard (electronic) playing Y93.J1 *(following* Y93.7*)*
   nordic skiing Y93.24
   obstacle course Y93.A5 *(following* Y93.7*)*
   oven (microwave) Y93.G3 *(following* Y93.7*)*
   packing up and unpacking in moving to a new residence Y93.E6 *(following* Y93.7*)*
   parasailing Y93.19
   pass out game Y93.85
   percussion instrument playing NEC Y93.J2 *(following* Y93.7*)*
   personal
      bathing and showering Y93.E1 *(following* Y93.7*)*
      hygiene NEC Y93.E8 *(following* Y93.7*)*
      showering Y93.E1 *(following* Y93.7*)*
   physical games generally associated with school recess, summer camp and children Y93.6A
   physical training NEC Y93.A9 *(following* Y93.7*)*
   piano playing Y93.J1 *(following* Y93.7*)*
   pilates Y93.B4 *(following* Y93.7*)*
   platform diving Y93.12
   playing musical instrument
      brass instrument Y93.J4 *(following* Y93.7*)*
      drum Y93.J2 *(following* Y93.7*)*
      musical keyboard (electronic) Y93.J1 *(following* Y93.7*)*
      percussion instrument NEC Y93.J2 *(following* Y93.7*)*
      piano Y93.J1 *(following* Y93.7*)*
      string instrument Y93.J3 *(following* Y93.7*)*
      winds instrument Y93.J4 *(following* Y93.7*)*
   property maintenance
      exterior NEC Y93.H9 *(following* Y93.7*)*
      interior NEC Y93.E9 *(following* Y93.7*)*
   pruning (garden and lawn) Y93.H2 *(following* Y93.7*)*
   pull-ups Y93.B2 *(following* Y93.7*)*
   push-ups Y93.B2 *(following* Y93.7*)*
   racquetball Y93.73
   rafting (in calm and turbulent water) Y93.16
   raking (leaves) Y93.H1 *(following* Y93.7*)*
   rappelling Y93.32
   refereeing a sports activity Y93.81
   residential relocation Y93.E6 *(following* Y93.7*)*
   rhythmic gymnastics Y93.43
   rhythmic movement NEC Y93.49
   riding
      horseback Y93.52
      rollercoaster Y93.I1 *(following* Y93.7*)*
   rock climbing Y93.31
   roller skating (inline) Y93.51
   rollercoaster riding Y93.I1 *(following* Y93.7*)*
   rough housing and horseplay Y93.83
   rowing (in calm and turbulent water) Y93.16
   rugby Y93.63
   running Y93.02
   SCUBA diving Y93.15
   sewing Y93.D2 *(following* Y93.7*)*
   shoveling Y93.H1 *(following* Y93.7*)*
      dirt Y93.H1 *(following* Y93.7*)*
      snow Y93.H1 *(following* Y93.7*)*
   showering (personal) Y93.E1 *(following* Y93.7*)*
   sit-ups Y93.B2 *(following* Y93.7*)*
   skateboarding Y93.51
   skating (ice) Y93.21
      roller Y93.51
   skiing (alpine) (downhill) Y93.23
      cross country Y93.24
      nordic Y93.24
      water Y93.17
   sledding (snow) Y93.23
   sleeping (sleep) Y93.84
   smoking and grilling food Y93.G2 *(following* Y93.7*)*
   snorkeling Y93.15
   snow NEC Y93.29
      boarding Y93.23
      shoveling Y93.H1 *(following* Y93.7*)*
      sledding Y93.23
      tubing Y93.23
   soccer Y93.66

Activity — *continued*
   softball Y93.64
   specified NEC Y93.89
   spectator at an event Y93.82
   sports NEC Y93.79
      sports played as a team or group NEC Y93.69
      sports played individually NEC Y93.59
   springboard diving Y93.12
   squash Y93.73
   stationary bike Y93.A1 *(following* Y93.7*)*
   step (stepping) exercise (class) Y93.A3 *(following* Y93.7*)*
   stepper machine Y93.A1 *(following* Y93.7*)*
   stove Y93.G3 *(following* Y93.7*)*
   string instrument playing Y93.J3 *(following* Y93.7*)*
   surfing Y93.18
      wind Y93.18
   swimming Y93.11
   tackle football Y93.61
   tap dancing Y93.41
   tennis Y93.73
   tobogganing Y93.23
   touch football Y93.62
   track and field events (non-running) Y93.57
      running Y93.02
   trampoline Y93.44
   treadmill Y93.A1 *(following* Y93.7*)*
   trimming shrubs Y93.H2 *(following* Y93.7*)*
   tubing (in calm and turbulent water) Y93.16
      snow Y93.23
   ultimate frisbee Y93.74
   underwater diving Y93.15
   unpacking in moving to a new residence Y93.E6 *(following* Y93.7*)*
   use of stove, oven and microwave oven Y93.G3 *(following* Y93.7*)*
   vacuuming Y93.E3 *(following* Y93.7*)*
   volleyball (beach) (court) Y93.68
   wake boarding Y93.17
   walking (on level or elevated terrain) Y93.01
      an animal Y93.K1 *(following* Y93.7*)*
   walking an animal Y93.K1 *(following* Y93.7*)*
   wall climbing Y93.31
   warm up and cool down exercises Y93.A2 *(following* Y93.7*)*
   water NEC Y93.19
      aerobics Y93.14
      craft NEC Y93.19
      exercise Y93.14
      polo Y93.13
      skiing Y93.17
      sliding Y93.18
      survival training and testing Y93.19
   weeding (garden and lawn) Y93.H2 *(following* Y93.7*)*
   wind instrument playing Y93.J4 *(following* Y93.7*)*
   windsurfing Y93.18
   wrestling Y93.72
   yoga Y93.42
Adverse effect of drugs — *see* Table of Drugs and Chemicals
Aerosinusitis — *see* Air, pressure
After-effect, late — *see* Sequelae
Air
   blast in war operations — *see* War operations, air blast
   pressure
      change, rapid
         during
            ascent W94.29 ☑
            while (in) (surfacing from)
               aircraft W94.23 ☑
               deep water diving W94.21 ☑
               underground W94.22 ☑
            descent W94.39 ☑
            in
               aircraft W94.31 ☑
               water W94.32 ☑
      high, prolonged W94.0 ☑
      low, prolonged W94.12 ☑
         due to residence or long visit at high altitude W94.11 ☑
Alpine sickness W94.11 ☑
Altitude sickness W94.11 ☑
Anaphylactic shock, anaphylaxis — *see* Table of Drugs and Chemicals
Andes disease W94.11 ☑
Arachnidism, arachnoidism X58 ☑
Arson (with intent to injure or kill) X97 ☑

Asphyxia, asphyxiation
   by
      food (bone) (seed) — *see* categories T17 and T18 ☑
      gas — *see also* Table of Drugs and Chemicals
         legal
            execution — *see* Legal, intervention, gas
            intervention — *see* Legal, intervention, gas
   from
      fire — *see also* Exposure, fire
         in war operations — *see* War operations, fire
      ignition — *see* Ignition
      vomitus T17.81 ☑
   in war operations — *see* War operations, restriction of airway
Aspiration
   food (any type) (into respiratory tract) (with asphyxia, obstruction respiratory tract, suffocation) — *see* categories T17 and T18 ☑
   foreign body — *see* Foreign body, aspiration
   vomitus (with asphyxia, obstruction respiratory tract, suffocation) T17.81 ☑
Assassination (attempt) — *see* Assault
Assault (homicidal) (by) (in) Y09
   arson X97 ☑
   bite (of human being) Y04.1 ☑
   bodily force Y04.8 ☑
      bite Y04.1 ☑
      bumping into Y04.2 ☑
      sexual — *see* subcategories T74.0, T76.0 ☑
      unarmed fight Y04.0 ☑
   bomb X96.9 ☑
      antipersonnel X96.0 ☑
      fertilizer X96.3 ☑
      gasoline X96.1 ☑
      letter X96.2 ☑
      petrol X96.1 ☑
      pipe X96.3 ☑
      specified NEC X96.8 ☑
   brawl (hand) (fists) (foot) (unarmed) Y04.0 ☑
   burning, burns (by fire) NEC X97 ☑
      acid Y08.89 ☑
      caustic, corrosive substance Y08.89 ☑
      chemical from swallowing caustic, corrosive substance — *see* Table of Drugs and Chemicals
      cigarette(s) X97 ☑
      hot object X98.9 ☑
         fluid NEC X98.2 ☑
         household appliance X98.3 ☑
         specified NEC X98.8 ☑
         steam X98.0 ☑
         tap water X98.1 ☑
         vapors X98.0 ☑
      scalding — *see* Assault, burning
      steam X98.0 ☑
      vitriol Y08.89 ☑
   caustic, corrosive substance (gas) Y08.89 ☑
   crashing of
      aircraft Y08.81 ☑
      motor vehicle Y03.8 ☑
         pushed in front of Y02.0 ☑
         run over Y03.0 ☑
         specified NEC Y03.8 ☑
   cutting or piercing instrument X99.9 ☑
      dagger X99.2 ☑
      glass X99.0 ☑
      knife X99.1 ☑
      specified NEC X99.8 ☑
      sword X99.2 ☑
   dagger X99.2 ☑
   drowning (in) X92.9 ☑
      bathtub X92.0 ☑
      natural water X92.3 ☑
      specified NEC X92.8 ☑
      swimming pool X92.1 ☑
         following fall X92.2 ☑
   dynamite X96.8 ☑
   explosive(s) (material) X96.9 ☑
   fight (hand) (fists) (foot) (unarmed) Y04.0 ☑
      with weapon — *see* Assault, by type of weapon
   fire X97 ☑
   firearm X95.9 ☑
      airgun X95.01 ☑
      handgun X93 ☑
      hunting rifle X94.1 ☑
      larger X94.9 ☑
         specified NEC X94.8 ☑

Assault — *continued*
 firearm — *continued*
  machine gun X94.2 ☑
  shotgun X94.0 ☑
  specified NEC X95.8 ☑
 from high place Y01 ☑
 gunshot (wound) NEC — *see* Assault, firearm, by type
 incendiary device X97 ☑
 injury Y09
  to child due to criminal abortion attempt NEC Y08.89 ☑
 knife X99.1 ☑
 late effect of — *see* categories X92-Y08 with 7th character S
 placing before moving object NEC Y02.8 ☑
  motor vehicle Y02.0 ☑
 poisoning — *see* categories T36-T65 with 7th character S
 puncture, any part of body — *see* Assault, cutting or piercing instrument
 pushing
  before moving object NEC Y02.8 ☑
   motor vehicle Y02.0 ☑
   subway train Y02.1 ☑
   train Y02.1 ☑
  from high place Y01 ☑
 rape T74.2- ☑
 scalding — *see* Assault, burning
 sequelae of — *see* categories X92-Y08 with 7th character S
 sexual (by bodily force) T74.2- ☑
 shooting — *see* Assault, firearm
 specified means NEC Y08.89 ☑
 stab, any part of body — *see* Assault, cutting or piercing instrument
 steam X98.0 ☑
 striking against
  other person Y04.2 ☑
  sports equipment Y08.09 ☑
   baseball bat Y08.02 ☑
   hockey stick Y08.01 ☑
 struck by
  sports equipment Y08.09 ☑
   baseball bat Y08.02 ☑
   hockey stick Y08.01 ☑
 submersion — *see* Assault, drowning
 violence Y09
 weapon Y09
  blunt Y00 ☑
  cutting or piercing — *see* Assault, cutting or piercing instrument
  firearm — *see* Assault, firearm
 wound Y09
  cutting — *see* Assault, cutting or piercing instrument
  gunshot — *see* Assault, firearm
  knife X99.1 ☑
  piercing — *see* Assault, cutting or piercing instrument
  puncture — *see* Assault, cutting or piercing instrument
  stab — *see* Assault, cutting or piercing instrument
Attack by mammals NEC W55.89 ☑
Avalanche — *see* Landslide
Aviator's disease — *see* Air, pressure

B

Barotitis, barodontalgia, barosinusitis, barotrauma (otitic) (sinus) — *see* Air, pressure
Battered (baby) (child) (person) (syndrome) X58 ☑
Bayonet wound W26.1 ☑
 in
  legal intervention — *see* Legal, intervention, sharp object, bayonet
  war operations — *see* War operations, combat
 stated as undetermined whether accidental or intentional Y28.8 ☑
 suicide (attempt) X78.2 ☑
Bean in nose — *see* categories T17 and T18 ☑
Bed set on fire NEC — *see* Exposure, fire, uncontrolled, building, bed
Beheading (by guillotine)
 homicide X99.9 ☑
 legal execution — *see* Legal, intervention
Bending, injury in (prolonged) (static) X50.1 ☑

Bends — *see* Air, pressure, change
Bite, bitten by
 alligator W58.01 ☑
 arthropod (nonvenomous) NEC W57 ☑
 bull W55.21 ☑
 cat W55.01 ☑
 cow W55.21 ☑
 crocodile W58.11 ☑
 dog W54.0 ☑
 goat W55.31 ☑
 hoof stock NEC W55.31 ☑
 horse W55.11 ☑
 human being (accidentally) W50.3 ☑
  with intent to injure or kill Y04.1 ☑
  as, or caused by, a crowd or human stampede (with fall) W52 ☑
  assault Y04.1 ☑
  homicide (attempt) Y04.1 ☑
  in
   fight Y04.1 ☑
 insect (nonvenomous) W57 ☑
 lizard (nonvenomous) W59.01 ☑
 mammal NEC W55.81 ☑
  marine W56.31 ☑
 marine animal (nonvenomous) W56.81 ☑
 millipede W57 ☑
 moray eel W56.51 ☑
 mouse W53.01 ☑
 person(s) (accidentally) W50.3 ☑
  with intent to injure or kill Y04.1 ☑
  as, or caused by, a crowd or human stampede (with fall) W52 ☑
  assault Y04.1 ☑
  homicide (attempt) Y04.1 ☑
  in
   fight Y04.1 ☑
 pig W55.41 ☑
 raccoon W55.51 ☑
 rat W53.11 ☑
 reptile W59.81 ☑
  lizard W59.01 ☑
  snake W59.11 ☑
  turtle W59.21 ☑
   terrestrial W59.81 ☑
 rodent W53.81 ☑
  mouse W53.01 ☑
  rat W53.11 ☑
  specified NEC W53.81 ☑
  squirrel W53.21 ☑
 shark W56.41 ☑
 sheep W55.31 ☑
 snake (nonvenomous) W59.11 ☑
 spider (nonvenomous) W57 ☑
 squirrel W53.21 ☑
Blast (air) in war operations — *see* War operations, blast
Blizzard X37.2 ☑
Blood alcohol level Y90.9
 less than 20mg/100ml Y90.0
 presence in blood, level not specified Y90.9
 20-39mg/100ml Y90.1
 40-59mg/100ml Y90.2
 60-79mg/100ml Y90.3
 80-99mg/100ml Y90.4
 100-119mg/100ml Y90.5
 120-199mg/100ml Y90.6
 200-239mg/100ml Y90.7
Blow X58 ☑
 by law-enforcing agent, police (on duty) — *see* Legal, intervention, manhandling
 blunt object — *see* Legal, intervention, blunt object
Blowing up — *see* Explosion
Brawl (hand) (fists) (foot) Y04.0 ☑
Breakage (accidental) (part of)
 ladder (causing fall) W11 ☑
 scaffolding (causing fall) W12 ☑
Broken
 glass, contact with — *see* Contact, with, glass
 power line (causing electric shock) W85 ☑
Bumping against, into (accidentally)
 object NEC W22.8 ☑
  caused by crowd or human stampede (with fall) W52 ☑
  sports equipment W21.9 ☑
  with fall — *see* Fall, due to, bumping against, object
 person(s) W51 ☑
  with fall W03 ☑

Bumping against, into — *continued*
 person(s) — *continued*
  with fall — *continued*
   due to ice or snow W00.0 ☑
  assault Y04.2 ☑
  caused by, a crowd or human stampede (with fall) W52 ☑
  homicide (attempt) Y04.2 ☑
 sports equipment W21.9 ☑
Burn, burned, burning (accidental) (by) (from) (on)
 acid NEC — *see* Table of Drugs and Chemicals
 bed linen — *see* Exposure, fire, uncontrolled, in building, bed
 blowtorch X08.8 ☑
  with ignition of clothing NEC X06.2 ☑
  nightwear X05 ☑
 bonfire, campfire (controlled) — *see also* Exposure, fire, controlled, not in building)
  uncontrolled — *see* Exposure, fire, uncontrolled, not in building
 candle X08.8 ☑
  with ignition of clothing NEC X06.2 ☑
  nightwear X05 ☑
 caustic liquid, substance (external) (internal) NEC — *see* Table of Drugs and Chemicals
 chemical (external) (internal) — *see also* Table of Drugs and Chemicals
  in war operations — *see* War operations. fire
 cigar(s) or cigarette(s) X08.8 ☑
  with ignition of clothing NEC X06.2 ☑
  nightwear X05 ☑
 clothes, clothing NEC (from controlled fire) X06.2 ☑
  with conflagration — *see* Exposure, fire, uncontrolled, building
  not in building or structure — *see* Exposure, fire, uncontrolled, not in building
 cooker (hot) X15.8 ☑
  stated as undetermined whether accidental or intentional Y27.3 ☑
  suicide (attempt) X77.3 ☑
 electric blanket X16 ☑
 engine (hot) X17 ☑
 fire, flames — *see* Exposure, fire
 flare, Very pistol — *see* Discharge, firearm NEC
 heat
  from appliance (electrical) (household) X15.8 ☑
   cooker X15.8 ☑
   hotplate X15.2 ☑
   kettle X15.8 ☑
   light bulb X15.8 ☑
   saucepan X15.3 ☑
   skillet X15.3 ☑
   stated as undetermined whether accidental or intentional Y27.3 ☑
   stove X15.0 ☑
   suicide (attempt) X77.3 ☑
   toaster X15.1 ☑
  in local application or packing during medical or surgical procedure Y63.5
 heating
  appliance, radiator or pipe X16 ☑
 homicide (attempt) — *see* Assault, burning
 hot
  air X14.1 ☑
  cooker X15.8 ☑
  drink X10.0 ☑
  engine X17 ☑
  fat X10.2 ☑
  fluid NEC X12 ☑
  food X10.1 ☑
  gases X14.1 ☑
  heating appliance X16 ☑
  household appliance NEC X15.8 ☑
  kettle X15.8 ☑
  liquid NEC X12 ☑
  machinery X17 ☑
  metal (molten) (liquid) NEC X18 ☑
  object (not producing fire or flames) NEC X19 ☑
  oil (cooking) X10.2 ☑
  pipe(s) X16 ☑
  radiator X16 ☑
  saucepan (glass) (metal) X15.3 ☑
  stove (kitchen) X15.0 ☑
  substance NEC X19 ☑
   caustic or corrosive NEC — *see* Table of Drugs and Chemicals

Burn, burned, burning — continued
- hot — continued
  - toaster X15.1 ☑
  - tool X17 ☑
  - vapor X13.1 ☑
  - water (tap) — see Contact, with, hot, tap water
- hotplate X15.2 ☑
  - suicide (attempt) X77.3 ☑
- ignition — see Ignition
- in war operations — see War operations, fire
- inflicted by other person X97 ☑
  - by hot objects, hot vapor, and steam — see Assault, burning, hot object
- internal, from swallowed caustic, corrosive liquid, substance — see Table of Drugs and Chemicals
- iron (hot) X15.8 ☑
  - stated as undetermined whether accidental or intentional Y27.3 ☑
  - suicide (attempt) X77.3 ☑
- kettle (hot) X15.8 ☑
  - stated as undetermined whether accidental or intentional Y27.3 ☑
  - suicide (attempt) X77.3 ☑
- lamp (flame) X08.8 ☑
  - with ignition of clothing NEC X06.2 ☑
    - nightwear X05 ☑
- lighter (cigar) (cigarette) X08.8 ☑
  - with ignition of clothing NEC X06.2 ☑
    - nightwear X05 ☑
- lightning — see subcategory T75.0 ☑
  - causing fire — see Exposure, fire
- liquid (boiling) (hot) NEC X12 ☑
  - stated as undetermined whether accidental or intentional Y27.2 ☑
  - suicide (attempt) X77.2 ☑
- local application of externally applied substance in medical or surgical care Y63.5
- machinery (hot) X17 ☑
- matches X08.8 ☑
  - with ignition of clothing NEC X06.2 ☑
    - nightwear X05 ☑
- mattress — see Exposure, fire, uncontrolled, building, bed
- medicament, externally applied Y63.5
- metal (hot) (liquid) (molten) NEC X18 ☑
- nightwear (nightclothes, nightdress, gown, pajamas, robe) X05 ☑
- object (hot) NEC X19 ☑
- on board watercraft
  - due to
    - accident to watercraft V91.09 ☑
      - powered craft V91.03 ☑
        - ferry boat V91.01 ☑
        - fishing boat V91.02 ☑
        - jetskis V91.03 ☑
        - liner V91.01 ☑
        - merchant ship V91.00 ☑
        - passenger ship V91.01 ☑
      - unpowered craft V91.08 ☑
        - canoe V91.05 ☑
        - inflatable V91.06 ☑
        - kayak V91.05 ☑
        - sailboat V91.04 ☑
        - surf-board V91.08 ☑
        - water skis V91.07 ☑
        - windsurfer V91.08 ☑
    - fire on board V93.09 ☑
      - ferry boat V93.01 ☑
      - fishing boat V93.02 ☑
      - jetskis V93.03 ☑
      - liner V93.01 ☑
      - merchant ship V93.00 ☑
      - passenger ship V93.01 ☑
      - powered craft NEC V93.03 ☑
      - sailboat V93.04 ☑
    - specified heat source NEC on board V93.19 ☑
      - ferry boat V93.11 ☑
      - fishing boat V93.12 ☑
      - jetskis V93.13 ☑
      - liner V93.11 ☑
      - merchant ship V93.10 ☑
      - passenger ship V93.11 ☑
      - powered craft NEC V93.13 ☑
      - sailboat V93.14 ☑
- pipe (hot) X16 ☑
  - smoking X08.8 ☑

Burn, burned, burning — continued
- pipe — continued
  - smoking — continued
    - with ignition of clothing NEC X06.2 ☑
      - nightwear X05 ☑
- powder — see Powder burn
- radiator (hot) X16 ☑
- saucepan (hot) (glass) (metal) X15.3 ☑
  - stated as undetermined whether accidental or intentional Y27.3 ☑
  - suicide (attempt) X77.3 ☑
- self-inflicted X76 ☑
  - stated as undetermined whether accidental or intentional Y26 ☑
- stated as undetermined whether accidental or intentional Y27.0 ☑
- steam X13.1 ☑
  - pipe X16 ☑
    - stated as undetermined whether accidental or intentional Y27.8 ☑
  - stated as undetermined whether accidental or intentional Y27.0 ☑
  - suicide (attempt) X77.0 ☑
- stove (hot) (kitchen) X15.0 ☑
  - stated as undetermined whether accidental or intentional Y27.3 ☑
  - suicide (attempt) X77.3 ☑
- substance (hot) NEC X19 ☑
  - boiling X12 ☑
    - stated as undetermined whether accidental or intentional Y27.2 ☑
    - suicide (attempt) X77.2 ☑
  - molten (metal) X18 ☑
- suicide (attempt) NEC X76 ☑
  - hot
    - household appliance X77.3 ☑
    - object X77.9 ☑
- therapeutic misadventure
  - heat in local application or packing during medical or surgical procedure Y63.5
  - overdose of radiation Y63.2
- toaster (hot) X15.1 ☑
  - stated as undetermined whether accidental or intentional Y27.3 ☑
  - suicide (attempt) X77.3 ☑
- tool (hot) X17 ☑
- torch, welding X08.8 ☑
  - with ignition of clothing NEC X06.2 ☑
    - nightwear X05 ☑
- trash fire (controlled) — see Exposure, fire, controlled, not in building
  - uncontrolled — see Exposure, fire, uncontrolled, not in building
- vapor (hot) X13.1 ☑
  - stated as undetermined whether accidental or intentional Y27.0 ☑
  - suicide (attempt) X77.0 ☑
- Very pistol — see Discharge, firearm NEC
Butted by animal W55.82 ☑
- bull W55.22 ☑
- cow W55.22 ☑
- goat W55.32 ☑
- horse W55.12 ☑
- pig W55.42 ☑
- sheep W55.32 ☑

C

Caisson disease — see Air, pressure, change
Campfire (exposure to) (controlled) — see also Exposure, fire, controlled, not in building
- uncontrolled — see Exposure, fire, uncontrolled, not in building
Capital punishment (any means) — see Legal, intervention
Car sickness T75.3 ☑
Casualty (not due to war) NEC X58 ☑
- war — see War operations
Cat
- bite W55.01 ☑
- scratch W55.03 ☑
Cataclysm, cataclysmic (any injury) NEC — see Forces of nature
Catching fire — see Exposure, fire

Caught
- between
  - folding object W23.0 ☑
  - objects (moving) (stationary and moving) W23.0 ☑
    - and machinery — see Contact, with, by type of machine
      - stationary W23.1 ☑
  - sliding door and door frame W23.0 ☑
- by, in
  - machinery (moving parts of) — see Contact, with, by type of machine
  - washing-machine wringer W23.0 ☑
- under packing crate (due to losing grip) W23.1 ☑
Cave-in caused by cataclysmic earth surface movement or eruption — see Landslide
Change(s) in air pressure — see Air, pressure, change
Choked, choking (on) (any object except food or vomitus)
- food (bone) (seed) — see categories T17 and T18 ☑
- vomitus T17.81- ☑
Civil insurrection — see War operations
Cloudburst (any injury) X37.8 ☑
Cold, exposure to (accidental) (excessive) (extreme) (natural) (place) NEC — see Exposure, cold
Collapse
- building W20.1 ☑
  - burning (uncontrolled fire) X00.2 ☑
- dam or man-made structure (causing earth movement) X36.0 ☑
- machinery — see Contact, with, by type of machine
- structure W20.1 ☑
  - burning (uncontrolled fire) X00.2 ☑
Collision (accidental) NEC — see also Accident, transport V89.9 ☑
- pedestrian W51 ☑
  - with fall W03 ☑
    - due to ice or snow W00.0 ☑
      - involving pedestrian conveyance — see Accident, transport, pedestrian, conveyance
    - and
      - crowd or human stampede (with fall) W52 ☑
        - object W22.8 ☑
          - with fall — see Fall, due to, bumping against, object
- person(s) — see Collision, pedestrian
- transport vehicle NEC V89.9 ☑
  - and
    - avalanche, fallen or not moving — see Accident, transport
      - falling or moving — see Landslide
    - landslide, fallen or not moving — see Accident, transport
      - falling or moving — see Landslide
  - due to cataclysm — see Forces of nature, by type
  - intentional, purposeful suicide (attempt) — see Suicide, collision
Combustion, spontaneous — see Ignition
Complication (delayed) **of or following** (medical or surgical procedure) Y84.9
- with misadventure — see Misadventure
- amputation of limb(s) Y83.5
- anastomosis (arteriovenous) (blood vessel) (gastrojejunal) (tendon) (natural or artificial material) Y83.2
- aspiration (of fluid) Y84.4
  - tissue Y84.8
- biopsy Y84.8
- blood
  - sampling Y84.7
  - transfusion
    - procedure Y84.8
- bypass Y83.2
- catheterization (urinary) Y84.6
  - cardiac Y84.0
- colostomy Y83.3
- cystostomy Y83.3
- dialysis (kidney) Y84.1
- drug — see Table of Drugs and Chemicals
- due to misadventure — see Misadventure
- duodenostomy Y83.3
- electroshock therapy Y84.3
- external stoma, creation of Y83.3
- formation of external stoma Y83.3
- gastrostomy Y83.3
- graft Y83.2
- hypothermia (medically-induced) Y84.8

Complication (delayed) of or following —
    continued
  implant, implantation (of)
    artificial
      internal device (cardiac pacemaker) (electrodes
        in brain) (heart valve prosthesis) (orthope-
        dic) Y83.1
      material or tissue (for anastomosis or bypass)
        Y83.2
        with creation of external stoma Y83.3
    natural tissues (for anastomosis or bypass) Y83.2
      with creation of external stoma Y83.3
  infusion
    procedure Y84.8
  injection — *see* Table of Drugs and Chemicals
    procedure Y84.8
  insertion of gastric or duodenal sound Y84.5
  insulin-shock therapy Y84.3
  paracentesis (abdominal) (thoracic) (aspirative) Y84.4
  procedures other than surgical operation — *see* Com-
    plication of or following, by type of procedure
  radiological procedure or therapy Y84.2
  removal of organ (partial) (total) NEC Y83.6
  sampling
    blood Y84.7
    fluid NEC Y84.4
    tissue Y84.8
  shock therapy Y84.3
  surgical operation NEC — *see also* Complication of or
    following, by type of operation Y83.9
    reconstructive NEC Y83.4
      with
        anastomosis, bypass or graft Y83.2
        formation of external stoma Y83.3
    specified NEC Y83.8
  transfusion — *see also* Table of Drugs and Chemicals
    procedure Y84.8
  transplant, transplantation (heart) (kidney) (liver)
    (whole organ, any) Y83.0
    partial organ Y83.4
  ureterostomy Y83.3
  vaccination — *see also* Table of Drugs and Chemicals
    procedure Y84.8

Compression
  divers' squeeze — *see* Air, pressure, change
  trachea by
    food (lodged in esophagus) — *see* categories T17
      and T18 ☑
    vomitus (lodged in esophagus) T17.81-

Conflagration — *see* Exposure, fire, uncontrolled

Constriction (external)
  hair W49.01 ☑
  jewelry W49.04 ☑
  ring W49.04 ☑
  rubber band W49.03 ☑
  specified item NEC W49.09 ☑
  string W49.02 ☑
  thread W49.02 ☑

Contact (accidental)
  with
    abrasive wheel (metalworking) W31.1 ☑
    alligator W58.09 ☑
      bite W58.01 ☑
      crushing W58.03 ☑
      strike W58.02 ☑
    amphibian W62.9 ☑
      frog W62.0 ☑
      toad W62.1 ☑
    animal (nonvenomous) NEC W64 ☑
      marine W56.89 ☑
        bite W56.81 ☑
        dolphin — *see* Contact, with, dolphin
        fish NEC — *see* Contact, with, fish
        mammal — *see* Contact, with, mammal, ma-
          rine
        orca — *see* Contact, with, orca
        sea lion — *see* Contact, with, sea lion
        shark — *see* Contact, with, shark
        strike W56.82 ☑
    animate mechanical force NEC W64 ☑
    arrow W21.89 ☑
      not thrown, projected or falling W45.8 ☑
    arthropods (nonvenomous) W57 ☑
    axe W27.0 ☑
    band-saw (industrial) W31.2 ☑
    bayonet — *see* Bayonet wound
    bee(s) X58 ☑

Contact — *continued*
  with — *continued*
    bench-saw (industrial) W31.2 ☑
    bird W61.99 ☑
      bite W61.91 ☑
      chicken — *see* Contact, with, chicken
      duck — *see* Contact, with, duck
      goose — *see* Contact, with, goose
      macaw — *see* Contact, with, macaw
      parrot — *see* Contact, with, parrot
      psittacine — *see* Contact, with, psittacine
      strike W61.92 ☑
      turkey — *see* Contact, with, turkey
    blender W29.0 ☑
    boiling water X12 ☑
      stated as undetermined whether accidental or
        intentional Y27.2 ☑
      suicide (attempt) X77.2 ☑
    bore, earth-drilling or mining (land) (seabed)
      W31.0 ☑
    buffalo — *see* Contact, with, hoof stock NEC
    bull W55.29 ☑
      bite W55.21 ☑
      gored W55.22 ☑
      strike W55.22 ☑
    bumper cars W31.81 ☑
    camel — *see* Contact, with, hoof stock NEC
    can
      lid W26.8 ☑
      opener W27.4 ☑
        powered W29.0 ☑
    cat W55.09 ☑
      bite W55.01 ☑
      scratch W55.03 ☑
    caterpillar (venomous) X58 ☑
    centipede (venomous) X58 ☑
    chain
      hoist W24.0 ☑
        agricultural operations W30.89 ☑
      saw W29.3 ☑
    chicken W61.39 ☑
      peck W61.33 ☑
      strike W61.32 ☑
    chisel W27.0 ☑
    circular saw W31.2 ☑
    cobra X58 ☑
    combine (harvester) W30.0 ☑
    conveyer belt W24.1 ☑
    cooker (hot) X15.8 ☑
      stated as undetermined whether accidental or
        intentional Y27.3 ☑
      suicide (attempt) X77.3 ☑
    coral X58 ☑
    cotton gin W31.82 ☑
    cow W55.29 ☑
      bite W55.21 ☑
      strike W55.22 ☑
    crane W24.0 ☑
      agricultural operations W30.89 ☑
    crocodile W58.19 ☑
      bite W58.11 ☑
      crushing W58.13 ☑
      strike W58.12 ☑
    dagger W26.1 ☑
      stated as undetermined whether accidental or
        intentional Y28.2 ☑
      suicide (attempt) X78.2 ☑
    dairy equipment W31.82 ☑
    dart W21.89 ☑
      not thrown, projected or falling W45.8 ☑
    deer — *see* Contact, with, hoof stock NEC
    derrick W24.0 ☑
      agricultural operations W30.89 ☑
      hay W30.2 ☑
    dog W54.8 ☑
      bite W54.0 ☑
      strike W54.1 ☑
    dolphin W56.09 ☑
      bite W56.01 ☑
      strike W56.02 ☑
    donkey — *see* Contact, with, hoof stock NEC
    drill (powered) W29.8 ☑
      earth (land) (seabed) W31.0 ☑
      nonpowered W27.8 ☑
    drive belt W24.0 ☑
      agricultural operations W30.89 ☑

Contact — *continued*
  with — *continued*
    dry ice — *see* Exposure, cold, man-made
    dryer (clothes) (powered) (spin) W29.2 ☑
    duck W61.69 ☑
      bite W61.61 ☑
      strike W61.62 ☑
    earth (-)
      drilling machine (industrial) W31.0 ☑
      scraping machine in stationary use W31.83 ☑
    edge of stiff paper W26.2 ☑
    electric
      beater W29.0 ☑
      blanket X16 ☑
      fan W29.2 ☑
        commercial W31.82 ☑
      knife W29.1 ☑
      mixer W29.0 ☑
    elevator (building) W24.0 ☑
      agricultural operations W30.89 ☑
        grain W30.3 ☑
    engine(s), hot NEC X17 ☑
    excavating machine W31.0 ☑
    farm machine W30.9 ☑
    feces — *see* Contact, with, by type of animal
    fer de lance X58 ☑
    fish W56.59 ☑
      bite W56.51 ☑
      shark — *see* Contact, with, shark
      strike W56.52 ☑
    flying horses W31.81 ☑
    forging (metalworking) machine W31.1 ☑
    fork W27.4 ☑
    forklift (truck) W24.0 ☑
      agricultural operations W30.89 ☑
    frog W62.0 ☑
    garden
      cultivator (powered) W29.3 ☑
        riding W30.89 ☑
      fork W27.1 ☑
    gas turbine W31.3 ☑
    Gila monster X58 ☑
    giraffe — *see* Contact, with, hoof stock NEC
    glass (sharp) (broken) W25 ☑
      assault X99.0 ☑
      due to fall — *see* Fall, by type
      stated as undetermined whether accidental or
        intentional Y28.0 ☑
      suicide (attempt) X78.0 ☑
      with subsequent fall W18.02 ☑
    goat W55.39 ☑
      bite W55.31 ☑
      strike W55.32 ☑
    goose W61.59 ☑
      bite W61.51 ☑
      strike W61.52 ☑
    hand
      saw W27.0 ☑
      tool (not powered) NEC W27.8 ☑
        powered W29.8 ☑
    harvester W30.0 ☑
    hay-derrick W30.2 ☑
    heating
      appliance (hot) X16 ☑
      pad (electric) X16 ☑
    heat NEC X19 ☑
      from appliance (electrical) (household) —
        see Contact, with, hot, household appliance
      heating appliance X16 ☑
    hedge-trimmer (powered) W29.3 ☑
    hoe W27.1 ☑
    hoist (chain) (shaft) NEC W24.0 ☑
      agricultural W30.89 ☑
    hoof stock NEC W55.39 ☑
      bite W55.31 ☑
      strike W55.32 ☑
    hornet(s) X58 ☑
    horse W55.19 ☑
      bite W55.11 ☑
      strike W55.12 ☑
    hot
      air X14.1 ☑
        inhalation X14.0 ☑
      cooker X15.8 ☑
      drinks X10.0 ☑
      engine X17 ☑

Contact — *continued*
 with — *continued*
  hot — *continued*
   fats X10.2 ☑
   fluids NEC X12 ☑
    assault X98.2 ☑
    suicide (attempt) X77.2 ☑
    undetermined whether accidental or intentional Y27.2 ☑
   food X10.1 ☑
   gases X14.1 ☑
    inhalation X14.0 ☑
   heating appliance X16 ☑
   household appliance X15.8 ☑
    assault X98.3 ☑
    cooker X15.8 ☑
    hotplate X15.2 ☑
    kettle X15.8 ☑
    light bulb X15.8 ☑
    object NEC X19 ☑
     assault X98.8 ☑
     stated as undetermined whether accidental or intentional Y27.9 ☑
     suicide (attempt) X77.8 ☑
    saucepan X15.3 ☑
    skillet X15.3 ☑
    stated as undetermined whether accidental or intentional Y27.3 ☑
    stove X15.0 ☑
    suicide (attempt) X77.3 ☑
    toaster X15.1 ☑
   kettle X15.8 ☑
   light bulb X15.8 ☑
   liquid NEC — *see also* Burn X12 ☑
    drinks X10.0 ☑
    stated as undetermined whether accidental or intentional Y27.2 ☑
    suicide (attempt) X77.2 ☑
    tap water X11.8 ☑
     stated as undetermined whether accidental or intentional Y27.1 ☑
     suicide (attempt) X77.1 ☑
   machinery X17 ☑
   metal (molten) (liquid) NEC X18 ☑
   object (not producing fire or flames) NEC X19 ☑
   oil (cooking) X10.2 ☑
   pipe X16 ☑
   plate X15.2 ☑
   radiator X16 ☑
   saucepan (glass) (metal) X15.3 ☑
   skillet X15.3 ☑
   stove (kitchen) X15.0 ☑
   substance NEC X19 ☑
   tap-water X11.8 ☑
    assault X98.1 ☑
    heated on stove X12 ☑
     stated as undetermined whether accidental or intentional Y27.2 ☑
     suicide (attempt) X77.2 ☑
    in bathtub X11.0 ☑
    running X11.1 ☑
     stated as undetermined whether accidental or intentional Y27.1 ☑
     suicide (attempt) X77.1 ☑
   toaster X15.1 ☑
   tool X17 ☑
   vapors X13.1 ☑
    inhalation X13.0 ☑
   water (tap) X11.8 ☑
    boiling X12 ☑
     stated as undetermined whether accidental or intentional Y27.2 ☑
     suicide (attempt) X77.2 ☑
    heated on stove X12 ☑
     stated as undetermined whether accidental or intentional Y27.2 ☑
     suicide (attempt) X77.2 ☑
    in bathtub X11.0 ☑
    running X11.1 ☑
     stated as undetermined whether accidental or intentional Y27.1 ☑
     suicide (attempt) X77.1 ☑
  hotplate X15.2 ☑
  ice-pick W27.4 ☑
  insect (nonvenomous) NEC W57 ☑
  kettle (hot) X15.8 ☑

Contact — *continued*
 with — *continued*
  knife W26.0 ☑
   assault X99.1 ☑
   electric W29.1 ☑
   stated as undetermined whether accidental or intentional Y28.1 ☑
   suicide (attempt) X78.1 ☑
  lathe (metalworking) W31.1 ☑
   turnings W45.8 ☑
   woodworking W31.2 ☑
  lawnmower (powered) (ridden) W28 ☑
   causing electrocution W86.8 ☑
    suicide (attempt) X83.1 ☑
   unpowered W27.1 ☑
  lift, lifting (devices) W24.0 ☑
   agricultural operations W30.89 ☑
   shaft W24.0 ☑
  liquefied gas — *see* Exposure, cold, man-made
  liquid air, hydrogen, nitrogen — *see* Exposure, cold, man-made
  lizard (nonvenomous) W59.09 ☑
   bite W59.01 ☑
   strike W59.02 ☑
  llama — *see* Contact, with, hoof stock NEC
  macaw W61.19 ☑
   bite W61.11 ☑
   strike W61.12 ☑
  machine, machinery W31.9 ☑
   abrasive wheel W31.1 ☑
   agricultural including animal-powered W30.9 ☑
    combine harvester W30.0 ☑
    grain storage elevator W30.3 ☑
    hay derrick W30.2 ☑
    power take-off device W30.1 ☑
    reaper W30.0 ☑
    specified NEC W30.89 ☑
    thresher W30.0 ☑
    transport vehicle, stationary W30.81 ☑
   band saw W31.2 ☑
   bench saw W31.2 ☑
   circular saw W31.2 ☑
   commercial NEC W31.82 ☑
   drilling, metal (industrial) W31.1 ☑
   earth-drilling W31.0 ☑
   earthmoving or scraping W31.89 ☑
   excavating W31.89 ☑
   forging machine W31.1 ☑
   gas turbine W31.3 ☑
   hot X17 ☑
   internal combustion engine W31.3 ☑
   land drill W31.0 ☑
   lathe W31.1 ☑
   lifting (devices) W24.0 ☑
   metal drill W31.1 ☑
   metalworking (industrial) W31.1 ☑
   milling, metal W31.1 ☑
   mining W31.0 ☑
   molding W31.2 ☑
   overhead plane W31.2 ☑
   power press, metal W31.1 ☑
   prime mover W31.3 ☑
   printing W31.89 ☑
   radial saw W31.2 ☑
   recreational W31.81 ☑
   roller-coaster W31.81 ☑
   rolling mill, metal W31.1 ☑
   sander W31.2 ☑
   seabed drill W31.0 ☑
   shaft
    hoist W31.0 ☑
    lift W31.0 ☑
   specified NEC W31.89 ☑
   spinning W31.89 ☑
   steam engine W31.3 ☑
   transmission W24.1 ☑
   undercutter W31.0 ☑
   water driven turbine W31.3 ☑
   weaving W31.89 ☑
   woodworking or forming (industrial) W31.2 ☑
  mammal (feces) (urine) W55.89 ☑
   bull — *see* Contact, with, bull
   cat — *see* Contact, with, cat
   cow — *see* Contact, with, cow
   goat — *see* Contact, with, goat
   hoof stock — *see* Contact, with, hoof stock

Contact — *continued*
 with — *continued*
  mammal — *continued*
   horse — *see* Contact, with, horse
   marine W56.39 ☑
    dolphin — *see* Contact, with, dolphin
    orca — *see* Contact, with, orca
    sea lion — *see* Contact, with, sea lion
    specified NEC W56.39 ☑
     bite W56.31 ☑
     strike W56.32 ☑
   pig — *see* Contact, with, pig
   raccoon — *see* Contact, with, raccoon
   rodent — *see* Contact, with, rodent
   sheep — *see* Contact, with, sheep
   specified NEC W55.89 ☑
    bite W55.81 ☑
    strike W55.82 ☑
  marine
   animal W56.89 ☑
    bite W56.81 ☑
    dolphin — *see* Contact, with, dolphin
    fish NEC — *see* Contact, with, fish
    mammal — *see* Contact, with, mammal, marine
    orca — *see* Contact, with, orca
    sea lion — *see* Contact, with, sea lion
    shark — *see* Contact, with, shark
    strike W56.82 ☑
  meat
   grinder (domestic) W29.0 ☑
    industrial W31.82 ☑
    nonpowered W27.4 ☑
   slicer (domestic) W29.0 ☑
    industrial W31.82 ☑
  merry go round W31.81 ☑
  metal, hot (liquid) (molten) NEC X18 ☑
  millipede W57 ☑
  nail W45.0 ☑
   gun W29.4 ☑
  needle (sewing) W27.3 ☑
   hypodermic W46.0 ☑
    contaminated W46.1 ☑
  object (blunt) NEC
   hot NEC X19 ☑
   legal intervention — *see* Legal, intervention, blunt object
   sharp NEC W45.8 ☑
    inflicted by other person NEC W45.8 ☑
     stated as
      intentional homicide (attempt) — *see* Assault, cutting or piercing instrument
     legal intervention — *see* Legal, intervention, sharp object
    self-inflicted X78.9 ☑
  orca W56.29 ☑
   bite W56.21 ☑
   strike W56.22 ☑
  overhead plane W31.2 ☑
  paper (as sharp object) W26.2 ☑
  paper-cutter W27.5 ☑
  parrot W61.09 ☑
   bite W61.01 ☑
   strike W61.02 ☑
  pig W55.49 ☑
   bite W55.41 ☑
   strike W55.42 ☑
  pipe, hot X16 ☑
  pitchfork W27.1 ☑
  plane (metal) (wood) W27.0 ☑
   overhead W31.2 ☑
  plant thorns, spines, sharp leaves or other mechanisms W60 ☑
  powered
   garden cultivator W29.3 ☑
   household appliance, implement, or machine W29.8 ☑
   saw (industrial) W31.2 ☑
    hand W29.8 ☑
  printing machine W31.89 ☑
  psittacine bird W61.29 ☑
   bite W61.21 ☑
   macaw — *see* Contact, with, macaw
   parrot — *see* Contact, with, parrot
   strike W61.22 ☑

Contact — *continued*
  with — *continued*
    pulley (block) (transmission) W24.0 ☑
      agricultural operations W30.89 ☑
    raccoon W55.59 ☑
      bite W55.51 ☑
      strike W55.52 ☑
    radial-saw (industrial) W31.2 ☑
    radiator (hot) X16 ☑
    rake W27.1 ☑
    rattlesnake X58 ☑
    reaper W30.0 ☑
    reptile W59.89 ☑
      lizard — *see* Contact, with, lizard
      snake — *see* Contact, with, snake
      specified NEC W59.89 ☑
        bite W59.81 ☑
        crushing W59.83 ☑
        strike W59.82 ☑
      turtle — *see* Contact, with, turtle
    rivet gun (powered) W29.4 ☑
    road scraper — *see* Accident, transport, construction vehicle
    rodent (feces) (urine) W53.89 ☑
      bite W53.81 ☑
      mouse W53.09 ☑
        bite W53.01 ☑
      rat W53.19 ☑
        bite W53.11 ☑
      specified NEC W53.89 ☑
        bite W53.81 ☑
      squirrel W53.29 ☑
        bite W53.21 ☑
    roller coaster W31.81 ☑
    rope NEC W24.0 ☑
      agricultural operations W30.89 ☑
    saliva — *see* Contact, with, by type of animal
    sander W29.8 ☑
      industrial W31.2 ☑
    saucepan (hot) (glass) (metal) X15.3 ☑
    saw W27.0 ☑
      band (industrial) W31.2 ☑
      bench (industrial) W31.2 ☑
      chain W29.3 ☑
      hand W27.0 ☑
    sawing machine, metal W31.1 ☑
    scissors W27.2 ☑
    scorpion X58 ☑
    screwdriver W27.0 ☑
      powered W29.8 ☑
    sea
      anemone, cucumber or urchin (spine) X58 ☑
      lion W56.19 ☑
        bite W56.11 ☑
        strike W56.12 ☑
    serpent — *see* Contact, with, snake, by type
    sewing-machine (electric) (powered) W29.2 ☑
      not powered W27.8 ☑
    shaft (hoist) (lift) (transmission) NEC W24.0 ☑
      agricultural W30.89 ☑
    shark W56.49 ☑
      bite W56.41 ☑
      strike W56.42 ☑
    sharp object(s) W26.9 ☑
      specified NEC W26.8 ☑
    shears (hand) W27.2 ☑
      powered (industrial) W31.1 ☑
        domestic W29.2 ☑
    sheep W55.39 ☑
      bite W55.31 ☑
      strike W55.32 ☑
    shovel W27.8 ☑
      steam — *see* Accident, transport, construction vehicle
    snake (nonvenomous) W59.19 ☑
      bite W59.11 ☑
      crushing W59.13 ☑
      strike W59.12 ☑
    spade W27.1 ☑
    spider (venomous) X58 ☑
    spin-drier W29.2 ☑
    spinning machine W31.89 ☑
    splinter W45.8 ☑
    sports equipment W21.9 ☑
    staple gun (powered) W29.8 ☑
    steam X13.1 ☑

Contact — *continued*
  with — *continued*
    steam — *continued*
      engine W31.3 ☑
      inhalation X13.0 ☑
      pipe X16 ☑
      shovel W31.89 ☑
    stove (hot) (kitchen) X15.0 ☑
    substance, hot NEC X19 ☑
      molten (metal) X18 ☑
    sword W26.1 ☑
      assault X99.2 ☑
      stated as undetermined whether accidental or intentional Y28.2 ☑
      suicide (attempt) X78.2 ☑
    tarantula X58 ☑
    thresher W30.0 ☑
    tin can lid W26.8 ☑
    toad W62.1 ☑
    toaster (hot) X15.1 ☑
    tool W27.8 ☑
      hand (not powered) W27.8 ☑
        auger W27.0 ☑
        axe W27.0 ☑
        can opener W27.4 ☑
        chisel W27.0 ☑
        fork W27.4 ☑
        garden W27.1 ☑
        handsaw W27.0 ☑
        hoe W27.1 ☑
        ice-pick W27.4 ☑
        kitchen utensil W27.4 ☑
        manual
          lawn mower W27.1 ☑
          sewing machine W27.8 ☑
        meat grinder W27.4 ☑
        needle (sewing) W27.3 ☑
          hypodermic W46.0 ☑
            contaminated W46.1 ☑
        paper cutter W27.5 ☑
        pitchfork W27.1 ☑
        rake W27.1 ☑
        scissors W27.2 ☑
        screwdriver W27.0 ☑
        specified NEC W27.8 ☑
        workbench W27.0 ☑
      hot X17 ☑
      powered W29.8 ☑
        blender W29.0 ☑
          commercial W31.82 ☑
        can opener W29.0 ☑
          commercial W31.82 ☑
        chainsaw W29.3 ☑
        clothes dryer W29.2 ☑
          commercial W31.82 ☑
        dishwasher W29.2 ☑
          commercial W31.82 ☑
        edger W29.3 ☑
        electric fan W29.2 ☑
          commercial W31.82 ☑
        electric knife W29.1 ☑
        food processor W29.0 ☑
          commercial W31.82 ☑
        garbage disposal W29.0 ☑
          commercial W31.82 ☑
        garden tool W29.3 ☑
        hedge trimmer W29.3 ☑
        ice maker W29.0 ☑
          commercial W31.82 ☑
        kitchen appliance W29.0 ☑
          commercial W31.82 ☑
        lawn mower W28 ☑
        meat grinder W29.0 ☑
          commercial W31.82 ☑
        mixer W29.0 ☑
          commercial W31.82 ☑
        rototiller W29.3 ☑
        sewing machine W29.2 ☑
          commercial W31.82 ☑
        washing machine W29.2 ☑
          commercial W31.82 ☑
    transmission device (belt, cable, chain, gear, pinion, shaft) W24.1 ☑
      agricultural operations W30.89 ☑
    turbine (gas) (water-driven) W31.3 ☑
    turkey W61.49 ☑

Contact — *continued*
  with — *continued*
    turkey — *continued*
      peck W61.43 ☑
      strike W61.42 ☑
    turtle (nonvenomous) W59.29 ☑
      bite W59.21 ☑
      strike W59.22 ☑
      terrestrial W59.89 ☑
        bite W59.81 ☑
        crushing W59.83 ☑
        strike W59.82 ☑
    under-cutter W31.0 ☑
    urine — *see* Contact, with, by type of animal
    vehicle
      agricultural use (transport) — *see* Accident, transport, agricultural vehicle
      not on public highway W30.81 ☑
      industrial use (transport) — *see* Accident, transport, industrial vehicle
      not on public highway W31.83 ☑
      off-road use (transport) — *see* Accident, transport, all-terrain or off-road vehicle
      not on public highway W31.83 ☑
      special construction use (transport) — *see* Accident, transport, construction vehicle
      not on public highway W31.83 ☑
    venomous
      animal X58 ☑
      arthropods X58 ☑
      lizard X58 ☑
      marine animal NEC X58 ☑
      marine plant NEC X58 ☑
      millipedes (tropical) X58 ☑
      plant(s) X58 ☑
      snake X58 ☑
      spider X58 ☑
      viper X58 ☑
    washing-machine (powered) W29.2 ☑
    wasp X58 ☑
    weaving-machine W31.89 ☑
    winch W24.0 ☑
      agricultural operations W30.89 ☑
    wire NEC W24.0 ☑
      agricultural operations W30.89 ☑
    wood slivers W45.8 ☑
    yellow jacket X58 ☑
    zebra — *see* Contact, with, hoof stock NEC
  pressure X50.9 ☑
  stress X50.9 ☑
Coup de soleil X32 ☑
Crash
  aircraft (in transit) (powered) V95.9 ☑
    balloon V96.01 ☑
    fixed wing NEC (private) V95.21 ☑
      commercial V95.31 ☑
    glider V96.21 ☑
      hang V96.11 ☑
      powered V95.11 ☑
    helicopter V95.01 ☑
    in war operations — *see* War operations, destruction of aircraft
    microlight V95.11 ☑
    nonpowered V96.9 ☑
      specified NEC V96.8 ☑
    powered NEC V95.8 ☑
    stated as
      homicide (attempt) Y08.81 ☑
      suicide (attempt) X83.0 ☑
    ultralight V95.11 ☑
  spacecraft V95.41 ☑
  transport vehicle NEC — *see also* Accident, transport V89.9 ☑
    homicide (attempt) Y03.8 ☑
    motor NEC (traffic) V89.2 ☑
      homicide (attempt) Y03.8 ☑
      suicide (attempt) — *see* Suicide, collision
Cruelty (mental) (physical) (sexual) X58 ☑
Crushed (accidentally) X58 ☑
  between objects (moving) (stationary and moving) W23.0 ☑
    stationary W23.1 ☑
  by
    alligator W58.03 ☑
    avalanche NEC — *see* Landslide
    cave-in W20.0 ☑

Crushed — *continued*
  by — *continued*
    cave-in — *continued*
      caused by cataclysmic earth surface movement — *see* Landslide
    crocodile W58.13
    crowd or human stampede W52 ☑
    falling
      aircraft V97.39 ☑
        in war operations — *see* War operations, destruction of aircraft
      earth, material W20.0 ☑
        caused by cataclysmic earth surface movement — *see* Landslide
      object NEC W20.8 ☑
    landslide NEC — *see* Landslide
    lizard (nonvenomous) W59.09 ☑
    machinery — *see* Contact, with, by type of machine
    reptile NEC W59.89 ☑
    snake (nonvenomous) W59.13 ☑
  in
    machinery — *see* Contact, with, by type of machine

Cut, cutting (any part of body) (accidental) — *see also* Contact, with, by object or machine
  during medical or surgical treatment as misadventure — *see* Index to Diseases and Injuries, Complications
  homicide (attempt) — *see* Assault, cutting or piercing instrument
  inflicted by other person — *see* Assault, cutting or piercing instrument
  legal
    execution — *see* Legal, intervention
    intervention — *see* Legal, intervention, sharp object
  machine NEC — *see also* Contact, with, by type of machine W31.9
  self-inflicted — *see* Suicide, cutting or piercing instrument
  suicide (attempt) — *see* Suicide, cutting or piercing instrument
Cyclone (any injury) X37.1 ☑

D

Decapitation (accidental circumstances) NEC X58 ☑
  homicide X99.9 ☑
  legal execution — *see* Legal, intervention
Dehydration from lack of water X58 ☑
Deprivation X58 ☑
Derailment (accidental)
  railway (rolling stock) (train) (vehicle) (without antecedent collision) V81.7 ☑
    with antecedent collision — *see* Accident, transport, railway vehicle occupant
  streetcar (without antecedent collision) V82.7 ☑
    with antecedent collision — *see* Accident, transport, streetcar occupant
Descent
  parachute (voluntary) (without accident to aircraft) V97.29 ☑
    due to accident to aircraft — *see* Accident, transport, aircraft
Desertion X58 ☑
Destitution X58 ☑
Disability, late effect or sequela of injury — *see* Sequelae
Discharge (accidental)
  airgun W34.010 ☑
    assault X95.01 ☑
    homicide (attempt) X95.01 ☑
    stated as undetermined whether accidental or intentional Y24.0 ☑
    suicide (attempt) X74.01 ☑
  BB gun — *see* Discharge, airgun
  firearm (accidental) W34.00 ☑
    assault X95.9 ☑
    handgun (pistol) (revolver) W32.0 ☑
      assault X93
      homicide (attempt) X93 ☑
      legal intervention — *see* Legal, intervention, firearm, handgun
      stated as undetermined whether accidental or intentional Y22 ☑
      suicide (attempt) X72 ☑
    homicide (attempt) X95.9 ☑
    hunting rifle W33.02 ☑

Discharge — *continued*
  firearm — *continued*
    hunting rifle — *continued*
      assault X94.1 ☑
      homicide (attempt) X94.1 ☑
      legal intervention
        injuring
          bystander Y35.032 ☑
          law enforcement personnel Y35.031 ☑
          suspect Y35.033 ☑
          unspecified person Y35.039 ☑
      stated as undetermined whether accidental or intentional Y23.1 ☑
      suicide (attempt) X73.1 ☑
    larger W33.00 ☑
      assault X94.9 ☑
      homicide (attempt) X94.9 ☑
      hunting rifle — *see* Discharge, firearm, hunting rifle
      legal intervention — *see* Legal, intervention, firearm by type of firearm
      machine gun — *see* Discharge, firearm, machine gun
      shotgun — *see* Discharge, firearm, shotgun
      specified NEC W33.09 ☑
        assault X94.8 ☑
        homicide (attempt) X94.8 ☑
        legal intervention
          injuring
            bystander Y35.092 ☑
            law enforcement personnel Y35.091 ☑
            suspect Y35.093 ☑
            unspecified person Y35.099 ☑
        stated as undetermined whether accidental or intentional Y23.8 ☑
        suicide (attempt) X73.8 ☑
      stated as undetermined whether accidental or intentional Y23.9 ☑
      suicide (attempt) X73.9 ☑
    legal intervention
      injuring
        bystander Y35.002 ☑
        law enforcement personnel Y35.001 ☑
        suspect Y35.03 ☑
        unspecified person Y35.009 ☑
      using rubber bullet
        injuring
          bystander Y35.042 ☑
          law enforcement personnel Y35.041 ☑
          suspect Y35.043 ☑
          unspecified person Y35.049 ☑
    machine gun W33.03 ☑
      assault X94.2 ☑
      homicide (attempt) X94.2 ☑
      legal intervention — *see* Legal, intervention, firearm, machine gun
      stated as undetermined whether accidental or intentional Y23.3 ☑
      suicide (attempt) X73.2 ☑
    pellet gun — *see* Discharge, airgun
    shotgun W33.01 ☑
      assault X94.0 ☑
      homicide (attempt) X94.0 ☑
      legal intervention — *see* Legal, intervention, firearm, specified NEC
      stated as undetermined whether accidental or intentional Y23.0 ☑
      suicide (attempt) X73.0 ☑
    specified NEC W34.09 ☑
      assault X95.8 ☑
      homicide (attempt) X95.8 ☑
      legal intervention — *see* Legal, intervention, firearm, specified NEC
      stated as undetermined whether accidental or intentional Y24.8 ☑
      suicide (attempt) X74.8 ☑
    stated as undetermined whether accidental or intentional Y24.9 ☑
    suicide (attempt) X74.9 ☑
    Very pistol W34.09 ☑
      assault X95.8 ☑
      homicide (attempt) X95.8 ☑
      stated as undetermined whether accidental or intentional Y24.8 ☑
      suicide (attempt) X74.8 ☑

Discharge — *continued*
  firework(s) W39 ☑
    stated as undetermined whether accidental or intentional Y25 ☑
  gas-operated gun NEC W34.018 ☑
    airgun — *see* Discharge, airgun
    assault X95.09 ☑
    homicide (attempt) X95.09 ☑
    paintball gun — *see* Discharge, paintball gun
    stated as undetermined whether accidental or intentional Y24.8 ☑
    suicide (attempt) X74.09 ☑
  gun NEC — *see also* Discharge, firearm NEC
    air — *see* Discharge, airgun
    BB — *see* Discharge, airgun
    for single hand use — *see* Discharge, firearm, handgun
    hand — *see* Discharge, firearm, handgun
    machine — *see* Discharge, firearm, machine gun
    other specified — *see* Discharge, firearm NEC
    paintball — *see* Discharge, paintball gun
    pellet — *see* Discharge, airgun
  handgun — *see* Discharge, firearm, handgun
  machine gun — *see* Discharge, firearm, machine gun
  paintball gun W34.011 ☑
    assault X95.02 ☑
    homicide (attempt) X95.02 ☑
    stated as undetermined whether accidental or intentional Y24.8 ☑
    suicide (attempt) X74.02 ☑
  pistol — *see* Discharge, firearm, handgun
    flare — *see* Discharge, firearm, Very pistol
    pellet — *see* Discharge, airgun
    Very — *see* Discharge, firearm, Very pistol
  revolver — *see* Discharge, firearm, handgun
  rifle (hunting) — *see* Discharge, firearm, hunting rifle
  shotgun — *see* Discharge, firearm, shotgun
  spring-operated gun NEC W34.018 ☑
    assault X95.09 ☑
    homicide (attempt) X95.09 ☑
    stated as undetermined whether accidental or intentional Y24.8 ☑
    suicide (attempt) X74.09 ☑
Disease
  Andes W94.11 ☑
  aviator's — *see* Air, pressure
  range W94.11 ☑
Diver's disease, palsy, paralysis, squeeze — *see* Air, pressure
Diving (into water) — *see* Accident, diving
Dog bite W54.0 ☑
Dragged by transport vehicle NEC — *see also* Accident, transport V09.9 ☑
Drinking poison (accidental) — *see* Table of Drugs and Chemicals
Dropped (accidentally) **while being carried or supported by other person** W04 ☑
Drowning (accidental) W74 ☑
  assault X92.9 ☑
  due to
    accident (to)
      machinery — *see* Contact, with, by type of machine
      watercraft V90.89 ☑
        burning V90.29 ☑
          powered V90.23 ☑
            fishing boat V90.22 ☑
            jetskis V90.23 ☑
            merchant ship V90.20 ☑
            passenger ship V90.21 ☑
          unpowered V90.28 ☑
            canoe V90.25 ☑
            inflatable V90.26 ☑
            kayak V90.25 ☑
            sailboat V90.24 ☑
            water skis V90.27 ☑
        crushed V90.39 ☑
          powered V90.33 ☑
            fishing boat V90.32 ☑
            jetskis V90.33 ☑
            merchant ship V90.30 ☑
            passenger ship V90.31 ☑
          unpowered V90.38 ☑
            canoe V90.35 ☑
            inflatable V90.36 ☑
            kayak V90.35 ☑

Drowning — *continued*
  due to — *continued*
    accident — *continued*
      watercraft — *continued*
        crushed — *continued*
          unpowered — *continued*
            sailboat V90.34 ☑
            water skis V90.37 ☑
        overturning V90.09 ☑
          powered V90.03 ☑
            fishing boat V90.02 ☑
            jetskis V90.03 ☑
            merchant ship V90.00 ☑
            passenger ship V90.01 ☑
          unpowered V90.08 ☑
            canoe V90.05 ☑
            inflatable V90.06 ☑
            kayak V90.05 ☑
            sailboat V90.04 ☑
        sinking V90.19 ☑
          powered V90.13 ☑
            fishing boat V90.12 ☑
            jetskis V90.13 ☑
            merchant ship V90.10 ☑
            passenger ship V90.11 ☑
          unpowered V90.18 ☑
            canoe V90.15 ☑
            inflatable V90.16 ☑
            kayak V90.15 ☑
            sailboat V90.14 ☑
        specified type NEC V90.89 ☑
          powered V90.83 ☑
            fishing boat V90.82 ☑
            jetskis V90.83 ☑
            merchant ship V90.80 ☑
            passenger ship V90.81 ☑
          unpowered V90.88 ☑
            canoe V90.85 ☑
            inflatable V90.86 ☑
            kayak V90.85 ☑
            sailboat V90.84 ☑
            water skis V90.87 ☑
    avalanche — *see* Landslide
    cataclysmic
      earth surface movement NEC — *see* Forces of nature, earth movement
      storm — *see* Forces of nature, cataclysmic storm
    cloudburst X37.8 ☑
    cyclone X37.1 ☑
    fall overboard (from) V92.09 ☑
      powered craft V92.03 ☑
        ferry boat V92.01 ☑
        fishing boat V92.02 ☑
        jetskis V92.03 ☑
        liner V92.01 ☑
        merchant ship V92.00 ☑
        passenger ship V92.01 ☑
      resulting from
        accident to watercraft — *see* Drowning, due to, accident to, watercraft
        being washed overboard (from) V92.29 ☑
          powered craft V92.23 ☑
            ferry boat V92.21 ☑
            fishing boat V92.22 ☑
            jetskis V92.23 ☑
            liner V92.21 ☑
            merchant ship V92.20 ☑
            passenger ship V92.21 ☑
          unpowered craft V92.28 ☑
            canoe V92.25 ☑
            inflatable V92.26 ☑
            kayak V92.25 ☑
            sailboat V92.24 ☑
            surf-board V92.28 ☑
            water skis V92.27 ☑
            windsurfer V92.28 ☑
        motion of watercraft V92.19 ☑
          powered craft V92.13 ☑
            ferry boat V92.11 ☑
            fishing boat V92.12 ☑
            jetskis V92.13 ☑
            liner V92.11 ☑
            merchant ship V92.10 ☑
            passenger ship V92.11 ☑
          unpowered craft
            canoe V92.15 ☑

Drowning — *continued*
  due to — *continued*
    fall overboard — *continued*
      resulting from — *continued*
        motion of watercraft — *continued*
          unpowered craft — *continued*
            inflatable V92.16 ☑
            kayak V92.15 ☑
            sailboat V92.14 ☑
        unpowered craft V92.08 ☑
          canoe V92.05 ☑
          inflatable V92.06 ☑
          kayak V92.05 ☑
          sailboat V92.04 ☑
          surf-board V92.08 ☑
          water skis V92.07 ☑
          windsurfer V92.08 ☑
    hurricane X37.0 ☑
    jumping into water from watercraft (involved in accident) — *see also* Drowning, due to, accident to, watercraft
      without accident to or on watercraft W16.711 ☑
    tidal wave NEC — *see* Forces of nature, tidal wave
    torrential rain X37.8 ☑
  following
    fall
      into
        bathtub W16.211 ☑
        bucket W16.221 ☑
        fountain — *see* Drowning, following, fall, into, water, specified NEC
        quarry — *see* Drowning, following, fall, into, water, specified NEC
        reservoir — *see* Drowning, following, fall, into, water, specified NEC
        swimming-pool W16.011 ☑
          stated as undetermined whether accidental or intentional Y21.3 ☑
          striking
            bottom W16.021 ☑
            wall W16.031 ☑
          suicide (attempt) X71.2 ☑
        water NOS W16.41 ☑
          natural (lake) (open sea) (river) (stream) (pond) W16.111 ☑
            striking
              bottom W16.121 ☑
              side W16.131 ☑
          specified NEC W16.311 ☑
            striking
              bottom W16.321 ☑
              wall W16.331 ☑
      overboard NEC — *see* Drowning, due to, fall overboard
    jump or dive
      from boat W16.711 ☑
        striking bottom W16.721 ☑
      into
        fountain — *see* Drowning, following, jump or dive, into, water, specified NEC
        quarry — *see* Drowning, following, jump or dive, into, water, specified NEC
        reservoir — *see* Drowning, following, jump or dive, into, water, specified NEC
        swimming-pool W16.511 ☑
          striking
            bottom W16.521 ☑
            wall W16.531 ☑
          suicide (attempt) X71.2 ☑
        water NOS W16.91 ☑
          natural (lake) (open sea) (river) (stream) (pond) W16.611 ☑
          specified NEC W16.811 ☑
            bottom W16.821 ☑
            striking
              bottom W16.821 ☑
              wall W16.831 ☑
            striking
              bottom W16.821 ☑
              wall W16.831 ☑
            striking bottom W16.621 ☑
  homicide (attempt) X92.9 ☑
  in
    bathtub (accidental) W65 ☑
      assault X92.0 ☑
      following fall W16.211 ☑

Drowning — *continued*
  in — *continued*
    bathtub — *continued*
      following fall — *continued*
        stated as undetermined whether accidental or intentional Y21.1 ☑
      stated as undetermined whether accidental or intentional Y21.0 ☑
      suicide (attempt) X71.0 ☑
    lake — *see* Drowning, in, natural water
    natural water (lake) (open sea) (river) (stream) (pond) W69 ☑
      assault X92.3 ☑
      following
        dive or jump W16.611 ☑
          striking bottom W16.621 ☑
        fall W16.111 ☑
          striking
            bottom W16.121 ☑
            side W16.131 ☑
      stated as undetermined whether accidental or intentional Y21.4 ☑
      suicide (attempt) X71.3 ☑
    quarry — *see* Drowning, in, specified place NEC
    quenching tank — *see* Drowning, in, specified place NEC
    reservoir — *see* Drowning, in, specified place NEC
    river — *see* Drowning, in, natural water
    sea — *see* Drowning, in, natural water
    specified place NEC W73 ☑
      assault X92.8 ☑
      following
        dive or jump W16.811 ☑
          striking
            bottom W16.821 ☑
            wall W16.831 ☑
        fall W16.311 ☑
          striking
            bottom W16.321 ☑
            wall W16.331 ☑
      stated as undetermined whether accidental or intentional Y21.8 ☑
      suicide (attempt) X71.8 ☑
    stream — *see* Drowning, in, natural water
    swimming-pool W67 ☑
      assault X92.1 ☑
        following fall X92.2 ☑
      following
        dive or jump W16.511 ☑
          striking
            bottom W16.521 ☑
            wall W16.531 ☑
        fall W16.011 ☑
          striking
            bottom W16.021 ☑
            wall W16.031 ☑
      stated as undetermined whether accidental or intentional Y21.2 ☑
        following fall Y21.3 ☑
      suicide (attempt) X71.1 ☑
        following fall X71.2 ☑
    war operations — *see* War operations, restriction of airway
  resulting from accident to watercraft — *see* Drowning, due to, accident, watercraft
  self-inflicted X71.9 ☑
  stated as undetermined whether accidental or intentional Y21.9 ☑
  suicide (attempt) X71.9 ☑

E

Earth falling (on) W20.0 ☑
  caused by cataclysmic earth surface movement or eruption — *see* Landslide
Earth (surface) **movement NEC** — *see* Forces of nature, earth movement
Earthquake (any injury) X34 ☑
Effect(s) (adverse) **of**
  air pressure (any) — *see* Air, pressure
  cold, excessive (exposure to) — *see* Exposure, cold
  heat (excessive) — *see* Heat
  hot place (weather) — *see* Heat
  insolation X30 ☑
  late — *see* Sequelae
  motion — *see* Motion

External Causes Index

Effect(s) (adverse) **of** — *continued*
  nuclear explosion or weapon in war operations — *see*
    War operations, nuclear weapon
  radiation — *see* Radiation
  travel — *see* Travel
Electric shock (accidental) (by) (in) — *see* Exposure,
    electric current
Electrocution (accidental) — *see* Exposure, electric cur-
    rent
Endotracheal tube wrongly placed during anesthetic
    procedure
Entanglement
  in
    bed linen, causing suffocation T71 ☑
    wheel of pedal cycle V19.88 ☑
Entry of foreign body or material — *see* Foreign body
Environmental pollution related condition — *see*
    category Z57 ☑
Execution, legal (any method) — *see* Legal, intervention
Exhaustion
  cold — *see* Exposure, cold
  due to excessive exertion — *see also* Overexertion
    X50.9 ☑
  heat — *see* Heat
Explosion (accidental) (of) (with secondary fire) W40.9 ☑
  acetylene W40.1 ☑
  aerosol can W36.1 ☑
  air tank (compressed) (in machinery) W36.2 ☑
  aircraft (in transit) (powered) NEC V95.9 ☑
    balloon V96.05 ☑
    fixed wing NEC (private) V95.25 ☑
      commercial V95.35 ☑
    glider V96.25 ☑
      hang V96.15 ☑
      powered V95.15 ☑
    helicopter V95.05 ☑
    in war operations — *see* War operations, destruction
      of aircraft
    microlight V95.15 ☑
    nonpowered V96.9 ☑
      specified NEC V96.8 ☑
    powered NEC V95.8 ☑
    stated as
      homicide (attempt) Y03.8 ☑
      suicide (attempt) X83.0 ☑
    ultralight V95.15 ☑
  anesthetic gas in operating room W40.1 ☑
  antipersonnel bomb W40.8 ☑
    assault X96.0 ☑
    homicide (attempt) X96.0 ☑
    suicide (attempt) X75 ☑
  assault X96.9 ☑
  bicycle tire W37.0 ☑
  blasting (cap) (materials) W40.0 ☑
  boiler (machinery), not on transport vehicle W35 ☑
    on watercraft — *see* Explosion, in, watercraft
  butane W40.1 ☑
  caused by other person X96.9 ☑
  coal gas W40.1 ☑
  detonator W40.0 ☑
  dump (munitions) W40.8 ☑
  dynamite W40.0 ☑
    in
      assault X96.8 ☑
      homicide (attempt) X96.8 ☑
      legal intervention
        injuring
          bystander Y35.112 ☑
          law enforcement personnel Y35.111 ☑
          suspect Y35.113 ☑
          unspecified person Y35.119 ☑
      suicide (attempt) X75 ☑
  explosive (material) W40.9 ☑
    gas W40.1 ☑
    in blasting operation W40.0 ☑
    specified NEC W40.8 ☑
      in
        assault X96.8 ☑
        homicide (attempt) X96.8 ☑
        legal intervention
          injuring
            bystander Y35.192 ☑
            law enforcement personnel
              Y35.191 ☑
            suspect Y35.193 ☑
            unspecified person Y35.199 ☑

Explosion — *continued*
  explosive — *continued*
    specified — *continued*
      in — *continued*
        suicide (attempt) X75 ☑
  factory (munitions) W40.8 ☑
  fertilizer bomb W40.8 ☑
    assault X96.3 ☑
    homicide (attempt) X96.3 ☑
    suicide (attempt) X75 ☑
  firearm (parts) NEC W34.19 ☑
    airgun W34.110 ☑
    BB gun W34.110 ☑
    gas, air or spring-operated gun NEC W34.118 ☑
    hangun W32.1 ☑
    hunting rifle W33.12 ☑
    larger firearm W33.10 ☑
      specified NEC W33.19 ☑
    machine gun W33.13 ☑
    paintball gun W34.111 ☑
    pellet gun W34.110 ☑
    shotgun W33.11 ☑
    Very pistol [flare] W34.19 ☑
  fire-damp W40.1 ☑
  fireworks W39 ☑
  gas (coal) (explosive) W40.1 ☑
    cylinder W36.9 ☑
      aerosol can W36.1 ☑
      air tank W36.2 ☑
      pressurized W36.3 ☑
      specified NEC W36.8 ☑
  gasoline (fumes) (tank) not in moving motor vehicle
    W40.1 ☑
    bomb W40.8 ☑
      assault X96.1 ☑
      homicide (attempt) X96.1 ☑
      suicide (attempt) X75 ☑
    in motor vehicle — *see* Accident, transport, by type
      of vehicle
  grain store W40.8 ☑
  grenade W40.8 ☑
    in
      assault X96.8 ☑
      homicide (attempt) X96.8 ☑
      legal intervention
        injuring
          bystander Y35.192 ☑
          law enforcement personnel Y35.191 ☑
          suspect Y35.193 ☑
          unspecified person Y35.199 ☑
      suicide (attempt) X75 ☑
  handgun (parts) — *see* Explosion, firearm, hangun
    (parts)
  homicide (attempt) X96.9 ☑
    antipersonnel bomb — *see* Explosion, antipersonnel
      bomb
    fertilizer bomb — *see* Explosion, fertilizer bomb
    gasoline bomb — *see* Explosion, gasoline bomb
    letter bomb — *see* Explosion, letter bomb
    pipe bomb — *see* Explosion, pipe bomb
    specified NEC X96.8 ☑
  hose, pressurized W37.8 ☑
  hot water heater, tank (in machinery) W35 ☑
    on watercraft — *see* Explosion, in, watercraft
  in, on
    dump W40.8 ☑
    factory W40.8 ☑
    mine (of explosive gases) NEC W40.1 ☑
    watercraft V93.59 ☑
      powered craft V93.53 ☑
        ferry boat V93.51 ☑
        fishing boat V93.52 ☑
        jetskis V93.53 ☑
        liner V93.51 ☑
        merchant ship V93.50 ☑
        passenger ship V93.51 ☑
        sailboat V93.54 ☑
  letter bomb W40.8 ☑
    assault X96.2 ☑
    homicide (attempt) X96.2 ☑
    suicide (attempt) X75 ☑
  machinery — *see also* Contact, with, by type of ma-
    chine
    on board watercraft — *see* Explosion, in, watercraft
    pressure vessel — *see* Explosion, by type of vessel
  methane W40.1 ☑

Explosion — *continued*
  mine W40.1 ☑
  missile NEC W40.8 ☑
  mortar bomb W40.8 ☑
    in
      assault X96.8 ☑
      homicide (attempt) X96.8 ☑
      legal intervention
        injuring
          bystander Y35.192 ☑
          law enforcement personnel Y35.191 ☑
          suspect Y35.193 ☑
          unspecified person Y35.199 ☑
      suicide (attempt) X75 ☑
  munitions (dump) (factory) W40.8 ☑
  pipe, pressurized W37.8 ☑
    bomb W40.8 ☑
      assault X96.4 ☑
      homicide (attempt) X96.4 ☑
      suicide (attempt) X75 ☑
  pressure, pressurized
    cooker W38 ☑
    gas tank (in machinery) W36.3 ☑
    hose W37.8 ☑
    pipe W37.8 ☑
    specified device NEC W38 ☑
    tire W37.8 ☑
      bicycle W37.0 ☑
    vessel (in machinery) W38 ☑
  propane W40.1 ☑
  self-inflicted X75 ☑
  shell (artillery) NEC W40.8 ☑
    during war operations — *see* War operations, explo-
      sion
    in
      legal intervention
        injuring
          bystander Y35.122 ☑
          law enforcement personnel Y35.121 ☑
          suspect Y35.123 ☑
          unspecified person Y35.129 ☑
    war — *see* War operations, explosion
  spacecraft V95.45 ☑
  stated as undetermined whether accidental or inten-
    tional Y25 ☑
  steam or water lines (in machinery) W37.8 ☑
  stove W40.9 ☑
  suicide (attempt) X75 ☑
  tire, pressurized W37.8 ☑
    bicycle W37.0 ☑
  undetermined whether accidental or intentional Y25 ☑
  vehicle tire NEC W37.8 ☑
    bicycle W37.0 ☑
  war operations — *see* War operations, explosion
Exposure (to) X58 ☑
  air pressure change — *see* Air, pressure
  cold (accidental) (excessive) (extreme) (natural) (place)
    X31 ☑
    assault Y08.89 ☑
    due to
      man-made conditions W93.8 ☑
        dry ice (contact) W93.01 ☑
          inhalation W93.02 ☑
        liquid air (contact) (hydrogen) (nitrogen)
          W93.11 ☑
          inhalation W93.12 ☑
        refrigeration unit (deep freeze) W93.2 ☑
        suicide (attempt) X83.2 ☑
      weather (conditions) X31 ☑
    homicide (attempt) Y08.89 ☑
    self-inflicted X83.2 ☑
  due to abandonment or neglect X58 ☑
  electric current W86.8 ☑
    appliance (faulty) W86.8 ☑
      domestic W86.0 ☑
    caused by other person Y08.89 ☑
    conductor (faulty) W86.1 ☑
    control apparatus (faulty) W86.1 ☑
    electric power generating plant, distribution station
      W86.1 ☑
    electroshock gun — *see* Exposure, electric current,
      taser
    high-voltage cable W85 ☑
    homicide (attempt) Y08.89 ☑
    legal execution — *see* Legal, intervention, specified
      means NEC

Effect — Exposure

Exposure — *continued*
  electric current — *continued*
    lightning — *see* subcategory T75.0 ☑
    live rail W86.8 ☑
    misadventure in medical or surgical procedure in electroshock therapy Y63.4
    motor (electric) (faulty) W86.8 ☑
      domestic W86.0 ☑
    self-inflicted X83.1 ☑
    specified NEC W86.8 ☑
      domestic W86.0 ☑
    stun gun — *see* Exposure, electric current, taser
    suicide (attempt) X83.1 ☑
    taser W86.8 ☑
      assault Y08.89 ☑
      legal intervention — *see* category Y35 ☑
      self-harm (intentional) X83.8 ☑
      undetermined intent Y33 ☑
    third rail W86.8 ☑
    transformer (faulty) W86.1 ☑
    transmission lines W85 ☑
  environmental tobacco smoke X58 ☑
  excessive
    cold — *see* Exposure, cold
    heat (natural) NEC X30 ☑
      man-made W92 ☑
  factor(s) NOS X58 ☑
    environmental NEC X58 ☑
      man-made NEC W99 ☑
      natural NEC — *see* Forces of nature
    specified NEC X58 ☑
  fire, flames (accidental) X08.8 ☑
    assault X97 ☑
    campfire — *see* Exposure, fire, controlled, not in building
    controlled (in)
      with ignition (of) clothing — *see also* Ignition, clothes X06.2 ☑
        nightwear X05 ☑
      bonfire — *see* Exposure, fire, controlled, not in building
      brazier (in building or structure) — *see also* Exposure, fire, controlled, building
        not in building or structure — *see* Exposure, fire, controlled, not in building
      building or structure X02.0 ☑
        with
          fall from building X02.3 ☑
          from building X02.5 ☑
          injury due to building collapse X02.2 ☑
          smoke inhalation X02.1 ☑
          hit by object from building X02.4 ☑
          specified mode of injury NEC X02.8 ☑
      fireplace, furnace or stove — *see* Exposure, fire, controlled, building
      not in building or structure X03.0 ☑
        with
          fall X03.3 ☑
          smoke inhalation X03.1 ☑
          hit by object X03.4 ☑
          specified mode of injury NEC X03.8 ☑
      trash — *see* Exposure, fire, controlled, not in building
    fireplace — *see* Exposure, fire, controlled, building
    fittings or furniture (in building or structure) (uncontrolled) — *see* Exposure, fire, uncontrolled, building
    forest (uncontrolled) — *see* Exposure, fire, uncontrolled, not in building
    grass (uncontrolled) — *see* Exposure, fire, uncontrolled, not in building
    hay (uncontrolled) — *see* Exposure, fire, uncontrolled, not in building
    homicide (attempt) X97 ☑
    ignition of highly flammable material X04 ☑
    in, of, on, starting in
      machinery — *see* Contact, with, by type of machine
      motor vehicle (in motion) — *see also* Accident, transport, occupant by type of vehicle V87.8 ☑
        with collision — *see* Collision
      railway rolling stock, train, vehicle V81.81 ☑
        with collision — *see* Accident, transport, railway vehicle occupant
      street car (in motion) V82.8 ☑

Exposure — *continued*
  fire, flames — *continued*
    in, of, on, starting in — *continued*
      street car — *continued*
        with collision — *see* Accident, transport, streetcar occupant
      transport vehicle NEC — *see also* Accident, transport
        with collision — *see* Collision
      war operations — *see also* War operations, fire
        from nuclear explosion — *see* War operations, nuclear weapons
      watercraft (in transit) (not in transit) V91.09 ☑
        localized — *see* Burn, on board watercraft, due to, fire on board
        powered craft V91.03 ☑
          ferry boat V91.01 ☑
          fishing boat V91.02 ☑
          jet skis V91.03 ☑
          liner V91.01 ☑
          merchant ship V91.00 ☑
          passenger ship V91.01 ☑
        unpowered craft V91.08 ☑
          canoe V91.05 ☑
          inflatable V91.06 ☑
          kayak V91.05 ☑
          sailboat V91.04 ☑
          surf-board V91.08 ☑
          waterskis V91.07 ☑
          windsurfer V91.08 ☑
    lumber (uncontrolled) — *see* Exposure, fire, uncontrolled, not in building
    mine (uncontrolled) — *see* Exposure, fire, uncontrolled, not in building
    prairie (uncontrolled) — *see* Exposure, fire, uncontrolled, not in building
    resulting from
      explosion — *see* Explosion
      lightning X08.8 ☑
    self-inflicted X76 ☑
    specified NEC X08.8 ☑
    started by other person X97 ☑
    stated as undetermined whether accidental or intentional Y26 ☑
    stove — *see* Exposure, fire, controlled, building
    suicide (attempt) X76 ☑
    tunnel (uncontrolled) — *see* Exposure, fire, uncontrolled, not in building
    uncontrolled
      in building or structure X00.0 ☑
        with
          fall from building X00.3 ☑
          injury due to building collapse X00.2 ☑
          jump from building X00.5 ☑
          smoke inhalation X00.1 ☑
        bed X08.00 ☑
          due to
            cigarette X08.01 ☑
            specified material NEC X08.09 ☑
        furniture NEC X08.20 ☑
          due to
            cigarette X08.21 ☑
            specified material NEC X08.29 ☑
        hit by object from building X00.4 ☑
        sofa X08.10 ☑
          due to
            cigarette X08.11 ☑
            specified material NEC X08.19 ☑
        specified mode of injury NEC X00.8 ☑
      not in building or structure (any) X01.0 ☑
        with
          fall X01.3 ☑
          smoke inhalation X01.1 ☑
          hit by object X01.4 ☑
          specified mode of injury NEC X01.8 ☑
    undetermined whether accidental or intentional Y26 ☑
  forces of nature NEC — *see* Forces of nature
  G-forces (abnormal) W49.9 ☑
  gravitational forces (abnormal) W49.9 ☑
  heat (natural) NEC — *see* Heat
  high-pressure jet (hydraulic) (pneumatic) W49.9 ☑
  hydraulic jet W49.9 ☑
  inanimate mechanical force W49.9 ☑
  jet, high-pressure (hydraulic) (pneumatic) W49.9 ☑
  lightning — *see* subcategory T75.0 ☑

Exposure — *continued*
  lightning — *see* subcategory — *continued*
    causing fire — *see* Exposure, fire
  mechanical forces NEC W49.9 ☑
    animate NEC W64 ☑
    inanimate NEC W49.9 ☑
  noise W42.9 ☑
    supersonic W42.0 ☑
  noxious substance — *see* Table of Drugs and Chemicals
  pneumatic jet W49.9 ☑
  prolonged in deep-freeze unit or refrigerator W93.2 ☑
  radiation — *see* Radiation
  smoke — *see also* Exposure, fire
    tobacco, second hand Z77.22
  specified factors NEC X58 ☑
  sunlight X32 ☑
    man-made (sun lamp) W89.8 ☑
    tanning bed W89.1 ☑
  supersonic waves W42.0 ☑
  transmission line(s), electric W85 ☑
  vibration W49.9 ☑
  waves
    infrasound W49.9 ☑
    sound W42.9 ☑
    supersonic W42.0 ☑
  weather NEC — *see* Forces of nature
External cause status Y99.9
  child assisting in compensated work for family Y99.8
  civilian activity done for financial or other compensation Y99.0
  civilian activity done for income or pay Y99.0
  family member assisting in compensated work for other family member Y99.8
  hobby not done for income Y99.8
  leisure activity Y99.8
  military activity Y99.1
  off-duty activity of military personnel Y99.8
  recreation or sport not for income or while a student Y99.8
  specified NEC Y99.8
  student activity Y99.8
  volunteer activity Y99.2

F

Factors, supplemental
  alcohol
    blood level
      less than 20mg/100ml Y90.0
      presence in blood, level not specified Y90.9
      20-39mg/100ml Y90.1
      40-59mg/100ml Y90.2
      60-79mg/100ml Y90.3
      80-99mg/100ml Y90.4
      100-119mg/100ml Y90.5
      120-199mg/100ml Y90.6
      200-239mg/100ml Y90.7
      240mg/100ml or more Y90.8
    presence in blood, but level not specified Y90.9
  environmental-pollution-related condition- *see* Z57 ☑
  nosocomial condition Y95
  work-related condition Y99.0
Failure
  in suture or ligature during surgical procedure Y65.2
  mechanical, of instrument or apparatus (any) (during any medical or surgical procedure) Y65.8
  sterile precautions (during medical and surgical care) — *see* Misadventure, failure, sterile precautions, by type of procedure
  to
    introduce tube or instrument Y65.4
      endotracheal tube during anesthesia Y65.3
    make curve (transport vehicle) NEC — *see* Accident, transport
    remove tube or instrument Y65.4
Fall, falling (accidental) W19 ☑
  building W20.1 ☑
    burning (uncontrolled fire) X00.3 ☑
  down
    embankment W17.81 ☑
    escalator W10.0 ☑
    hill W17.81 ☑
    ladder W11 ☑
    ramp W10.2 ☑
    stairs, steps W10.9 ☑

Fall, falling — *continued*
- due to
  - bumping against
    - object W18.00 ☑
      - sharp glass W18.02 ☑
      - specified NEC W18.09 ☑
      - sports equipment W18.01 ☑
    - person W03 ☑
      - due to ice or snow W00.0 ☑
      - on pedestrian conveyance — *see* Accident, transport, pedestrian, conveyance
  - collision with another person W03 ☑
    - due to ice or snow W00.0 ☑
    - involving pedestrian conveyance — *see* Accident, transport, pedestrian, conveyance
  - grocery cart tipping over W17.82 ☑
  - ice or snow W00.9 ☑
    - from one level to another W00.2 ☑
      - on stairs or steps W00.1 ☑
    - involving pedestrian conveyance — *see* Accident, transport, pedestrian, conveyance
    - on same level W00.0 ☑
  - slipping (on moving sidewalk) W01.0 ☑
    - with subsequent striking against object W01.10 ☑
      - furniture W01.190 ☑
      - sharp object W01.119 ☑
        - glass W01.110 ☑
        - power tool or machine W01.111 ☑
        - specified NEC W01.118 ☑
      - specified NEC W01.198 ☑
  - striking against
    - object W18.00 ☑
      - sharp glass W18.02 ☑
      - specified NEC W18.09 ☑
      - sports equipment W18.01 ☑
    - person W03 ☑
      - due to ice or snow W00.0 ☑
      - on pedestrian conveyance — *see* Accident, transport, pedestrian, conveyance
- earth (with asphyxia or suffocation (by pressure)) — *see* Earth, falling
- from, off, out of
  - aircraft NEC (with accident to aircraft NEC) V97.0 ☑
    - while boarding or alighting V97.1 ☑
  - balcony W13.0 ☑
  - bed W06 ☑
  - boat, ship, watercraft NEC (with drowning or submersion) — *see* Drowning, due to, fall overboard
    - with hitting bottom or object V94.0 ☑
  - bridge W13.1 ☑
  - building W13.9 ☑
    - burning (uncontrolled fire) X00.3 ☑
  - cavity W17.2 ☑
  - chair W07 ☑
  - cherry picker W17.89 ☑
  - cliff W15 ☑
  - dock W17.4 ☑
  - embankment W17.81 ☑
  - escalator W10.0 ☑
  - flagpole W13.8 ☑
  - furniture NEC W08 ☑
  - grocery cart W17.82 ☑
  - haystack W17.89 ☑
  - high place NEC W17.89 ☑
    - stated as undetermined whether accidental or intentional Y30 ☑
  - hole W17.2 ☑
  - incline W10.2 ☑
  - ladder W11 ☑
  - lifting device W17.89 ☑
  - machine, machinery — *see also* Contact, with, by type of machine
    - not in operation W17.89 ☑
  - manhole W17.1 ☑
  - mobile elevated work platform [MEWP] W17.89 ☑
  - motorized mobility scooter W05.2 ☑
  - one level to another NEC W17.89 ☑
    - intentional, purposeful, suicide (attempt) X80 ☑
    - stated as undetermined whether accidental or intentional Y30 ☑
  - pit W17.2 ☑
  - playground equipment W09.8 ☑
    - jungle gym W09.2 ☑
    - slide W09.0 ☑

Fall, falling — *continued*
- from, off, out of — *continued*
  - playground equipment — *continued*
    - swing W09.1 ☑
  - quarry W17.89 ☑
  - railing W13.9 ☑
  - ramp W10.2 ☑
  - roof W13.2 ☑
  - scaffolding W12 ☑
  - scooter (nonmotorized) W05.1 ☑
    - motorized mobility W05.2 ☑
  - sky lift W17.89 ☑
  - stairs, steps W10.9 ☑
    - curb W10.1 ☑
    - due to ice or snow W00.1 ☑
    - escalator W10.0 ☑
    - incline W10.2 ☑
    - ramp W10.2 ☑
    - sidewalk curb W10.1 ☑
    - specified NEC W10.8 ☑
  - stepladder W11 ☑
  - storm drain W17.1 ☑
  - streetcar NEC V82.6 ☑
    - while boarding or alighting V82.4 ☑
    - with antecedent collision — *see* Accident, transport, streetcar occupant
  - structure NEC W13.8 ☑
    - burning (uncontrolled fire) X00.3 ☑
  - table W08 ☑
  - toilet W18.11 ☑
    - with subsequent striking against object W18.12 ☑
  - train NEC V81.6 ☑
    - during derailment (without antecedent collision) V81.7 ☑
      - with antecedent collision — *see* Accident, transport, railway vehicle occupant
    - while boarding or alighting V81.4 ☑
  - transport vehicle after collision — *see* Accident, transport, by type of vehicle, collision
  - tree W14 ☑
  - vehicle (in motion) NEC — *see also* Accident, transport V89.9 ☑
    - motor NEC — *see also* Accident, transport, occupant, by type of vehicle V87.8 ☑
    - stationary W17.89 ☑
      - while boarding or alighting — *see* Accident, transport, by type of vehicle, while boarding or alighting
  - viaduct W13.8 ☑
  - wall W13.8 ☑
  - watercraft — *see also* Drowning, due to, fall overboard
    - with hitting bottom or object V94.0 ☑
  - well W17.0 ☑
  - wheelchair, non-moving W05.0 ☑
    - powered — *see* Accident, transport, pedestrian, conveyance occupant, specified type NEC
  - window W13.4 ☑
- in, on
  - aircraft NEC V97.0 ☑
    - while boarding or alighting V97.1 ☑
    - with accident to aircraft V97.0 ☑
  - bathtub (empty) W18.2 ☑
    - filled W16.212 ☑
      - causing drowning W16.211 ☑
  - escalator W10.0 ☑
  - incline W10.2 ☑
  - ladder W11 ☑
  - machine, machinery — *see* Contact, with, by type of machine
  - object, edged, pointed or sharp (with cut) — *see* Fall, by type
  - playground equipment W09.8 ☑
    - jungle gym W09.2 ☑
    - slide W09.0 ☑
    - swing W09.1 ☑
  - ramp W10.2 ☑
  - scaffolding W12 ☑
  - shower W18.2 ☑
    - causing drowning W16.211 ☑
  - staircase, stairs, steps W10.9 ☑
    - curb W10.1 ☑
    - due to ice or snow W00.1 ☑
    - escalator W10.0 ☑
    - incline W10.2 ☑

Fall, falling — *continued*
- in, on — *continued*
  - staircase, stairs, steps — *continued*
    - specified NEC W10.8 ☑
  - streetcar (without antecedent collision) V82.5 ☑
    - with antecedent collision — *see* Accident, transport, streetcar occupant
    - while boarding or alighting V82.4 ☑
  - train (without antecedent collision) V81.5 ☑
    - with antecedent collision — *see* Accident, transport, railway vehicle occupant
    - during derailment (without antecedent collision) V81.7 ☑
      - with antecedent collision — *see* Accident, transport, railway vehicle occupant
    - while boarding or alighting V81.4 ☑
  - transport vehicle after collision — *see* Accident, transport, by type of vehicle, collision
  - watercraft V93.39 ☑
    - due to
      - accident to craft V91.29 ☑
        - powered craft V91.23 ☑
          - ferry boat V91.21 ☑
          - fishing boat V91.22 ☑
          - jetskis V91.23 ☑
          - liner V91.21 ☑
          - merchant ship V91.20 ☑
          - passenger ship V91.21 ☑
        - unpowered craft
          - canoe V91.25 ☑
          - inflatable V91.26 ☑
          - kayak V91.25 ☑
          - sailboat V91.24 ☑
      - powered craft V93.33 ☑
        - ferry boat V93.31 ☑
        - fishing boat V93.32 ☑
        - jetskis V93.33 ☑
        - liner V93.31 ☑
        - merchant ship V93.30 ☑
        - passenger ship V93.31 ☑
      - unpowered craft V93.38 ☑
        - canoe V93.35 ☑
        - inflatable V93.36 ☑
        - kayak V93.35 ☑
        - sailboat V93.34 ☑
        - surf-board V93.38 ☑
        - windsurfer V93.38 ☑
- into
  - cavity W17.2 ☑
  - dock W17.4 ☑
  - fire — *see* Exposure, fire, by type
  - haystack W17.89 ☑
  - hole W17.2 ☑
  - lake — *see* Fall, into, water
  - manhole W17.1 ☑
  - moving part of machinery — *see* Contact, with, by type of machine
  - ocean — *see* Fall, into, water
  - opening in surface NEC W17.89 ☑
  - pit W17.2 ☑
  - pond — *see* Fall, into, water
  - quarry W17.89 ☑
  - river — *see* Fall, into, water
  - shaft W17.89 ☑
  - storm drain W17.1 ☑
  - stream — *see* Fall, into, water
  - swimming pool — *see also* Fall, into, water, in, swimming pool
    - empty W17.3 ☑
  - tank W17.89 ☑
  - water W16.42 ☑
    - causing drowning W16.41 ☑
    - from watercraft — *see* Drowning, due to, fall overboard
    - hitting diving board W21.4 ☑
    - in
      - bathtub W16.212 ☑
        - causing drowning W16.211 ☑
      - bucket W16.222 ☑
        - causing drowning W16.221 ☑
      - natural body of water W16.112 ☑
        - causing drowning W16.111 ☑
        - striking
          - bottom W16.122 ☑
            - causing drowning W16.121 ☑
          - side W16.132 ☑

Fall, falling — *continued*
　into — *continued*
　　water — *continued*
　　　in — *continued*
　　　　natural body of water — *continued*
　　　　　striking — *continued*
　　　　　　side — *continued*
　　　　　　　causing drowning W16.131 ☑
　　　　　specified water NEC W16.312 ☑
　　　　　　causing drowning W16.311 ☑
　　　　　　striking
　　　　　　　bottom W16.322 ☑
　　　　　　　　causing drowning W16.321 ☑
　　　　　　　wall W16.332 ☑
　　　　　　　　causing drowning W16.331 ☑
　　　　　swimming pool W16.012 ☑
　　　　　　causing drowning W16.011 ☑
　　　　　　striking
　　　　　　　bottom W16.022 ☑
　　　　　　　　causing drowning W16.031 ☑
　　　　　　　wall W16.032 ☑
　　　　　　　　causing drowning W16.021 ☑
　　　　　utility bucket W16.222 ☑
　　　　　　causing drowning W16.221 ☑
　　　　well W17.0 ☑
　involving
　　bed W06 ☑
　　chair W07 ☑
　　furniture NEC W08 ☑
　　glass — *see* Fall, by type
　　playground equipment W09.8 ☑
　　　jungle gym W09.2 ☑
　　　slide W09.0 ☑
　　　swing W09.1 ☑
　　roller blades — *see* Accident, transport, pedestrian, conveyance
　　skateboard(s) — *see* Accident, transport, pedestrian, conveyance
　　skates (ice) (in line) (roller) — *see* Accident, transport, pedestrian, conveyance
　　skis — *see* Accident, transport, pedestrian, conveyance
　　table W08 ☑
　　wheelchair, non-moving W05.0 ☑
　　　powered — *see* Accident, transport, pedestrian, conveyance, specified type NEC
　object — *see* Struck by, object, falling
　off
　　toilet W18.11 ☑
　　　with subsequent striking against object W18.12 ☑
　on same level W18.30 ☑
　　due to
　　　specified NEC W18.39 ☑
　　　stepping on an object W18.31 ☑
　out of
　　bed W06 ☑
　　building NEC W13.8 ☑
　　chair W07 ☑
　　furniture NEC W08 ☑
　　wheelchair, non-moving W05.0 ☑
　　　powered — *see* Accident, transport, pedestrian, conveyance, specified type NEC
　　window W13.4 ☑
　over
　　animal W01.0 ☑
　　cliff W15 ☑
　　embankment W17.81 ☑
　　small object W01.0 ☑
　rock W20.8 ☑
　same level W18.30 ☑
　　from
　　　being crushed, pushed, or stepped on by a crowd or human stampede W52 ☑
　　　collision, pushing, shoving, by or with other person W03 ☑
　　　slipping, stumbling, tripping W01.0 ☑
　　involving ice or snow W00.0 ☑
　　　involving skates (ice) (roller), skateboard, skis — *see* Accident, transport, pedestrian, conveyance
　snowslide (avalanche) — *see* Landslide
　stone W20.8 ☑
　structure W20.1 ☑
　　burning (uncontrolled fire) X00.3 ☑

Fall, falling — *continued*
　through
　　bridge W13.1 ☑
　　floor W13.3 ☑
　　roof W13.2 ☑
　　wall W13.8 ☑
　　window W13.4 ☑
　　timber W20.8 ☑
　　tree (caused by lightning) W20.8 ☑
　while being carried or supported by other person(s) W04 ☑
Fallen on by
　animal (not being ridden) NEC W55.89 ☑
Felo-de-se — *see* Suicide
Fight (hand) (fists) (foot) — *see* Assault, fight
Fire (accidental) — *see* Exposure, fire
Firearm discharge — *see* Discharge, firearm
Fireball effects from nuclear explosion in war operations — *see* War operations, nuclear weapons
Fireworks (explosion) W39 ☑
Flash burns from explosion — *see* Explosion
Flood (any injury) (caused by) X38 ☑
　collapse of man-made structure causing earth movement X36.0 ☑
　tidal wave — *see* Forces of nature, tidal wave
Food (any type) in
　air passages (with asphyxia, obstruction, or suffocation) — *see* categories T17 and T18 ☑
　alimentary tract causing asphyxia (due to compression of trachea) — *see* categories T17 and T18 ☑
Forces of nature X39.8 ☑
　avalanche X36.1 ☑
　　causing transport accident — *see* Accident, transport, by type of vehicle
　blizzard X37.2 ☑
　cataclysmic storm X37.9 ☑
　　with flood X38 ☑
　　blizzard X37.2 ☑
　　cloudburst X37.8 ☑
　　cyclone X37.1 ☑
　　dust storm X37.3 ☑
　　hurricane X37.0 ☑
　　specified storm NEC X37.8 ☑
　　storm surge X37.0 ☑
　　tornado X37.1 ☑
　　twister X37.1 ☑
　　typhoon X37.0 ☑
　cloudburst X37.8 ☑
　cold (natural) X31 ☑
　cyclone X37.1 ☑
　dam collapse causing earth movement X36.0 ☑
　dust storm X37.3 ☑
　earth movement X36.1 ☑
　　caused by dam or structure collapse X36.0 ☑
　　earthquake X34 ☑
　earthquake X34 ☑
　flood (caused by) X38 ☑
　　dam collapse X36.0 ☑
　　tidal wave — *see* Forces of nature, tidal wave
　heat (natural) X30 ☑
　hurricane X37.0 ☑
　landslide X36.1 ☑
　　causing transport accident — *see* Accident, transport, by type of vehicle
　lightning — *see* subcategory T75.0 ☑
　　causing fire — *see* Exposure, fire
　mudslide X36.1 ☑
　　causing transport accident — *see* Accident, transport, by type of vehicle
　radiation (natural) X39.08 ☑
　　radon X39.01 ☑
　radon X39.01 ☑
　specified force NEC X39.8 ☑
　storm surge X37.0 ☑
　structure collapse causing earth movement X36.0 ☑
　sunlight X32 ☑
　tidal wave X37.41 ☑
　　due to
　　　earthquake X37.41 ☑
　　　landslide X37.43 ☑
　　　storm X37.42 ☑
　　　volcanic eruption X37.41 ☑
　tornado X37.1 ☑
　tsunami X37.41 ☑
　twister X37.1 ☑
　typhoon X37.0 ☑

Forces of nature — *continued*
　volcanic eruption X35 ☑
Foreign body
　aspiration — *see* Index to Diseases and Injuries, Foreign body, respiratory tract
　embedded in skin W45 ☑
　entering through skin W45.8 ☑
　　can lid W26.8 ☑
　　nail W45.0 ☑
　　paper W26.2 ☑
　　specified NEC W45.8 ☑
　　splinter W45.8 ☑
Forest fire (exposure to) — *see* Exposure, fire, uncontrolled, not in building
Found injured X58 ☑
　from exposure (to) — *see* Exposure
　on
　　highway, road(way), street V89.9 ☑
　　railway right of way V81.9 ☑
Fracture (circumstances unknown or unspecified) X58 ☑
　due to specified cause NEC X58 ☑
Freezing — *see* Exposure, cold
Frostbite X31 ☑
　due to man-made conditions — *see* Exposure, cold, man-made
Frozen — *see* Exposure, cold

G

Gored by bull W55.22 ☑
Gunshot wound W34.00 ☑

H

Hailstones, injured by X39.8 ☑
Hanged herself or himself — *see* Hanging, self-inflicted
Hanging (accidental) — *see also* category T71 ☑
　legal execution — *see* Legal, intervention, specified means NEC
Heat (effects of) (excessive) X30 ☑
　due to
　　man-made conditions W92 ☑
　　　on board watercraft V93.29 ☑
　　　　fishing boat V93.22 ☑
　　　　merchant ship V93.20 ☑
　　　　passenger ship V93.21 ☑
　　　　sailboat V93.24 ☑
　　　　specified powered craft NEC V93.23 ☑
　　weather (conditions) X30 ☑
　from
　　electric heating apparatus causing burning X16 ☑
　　nuclear explosion in war operations — *see* War operations, nuclear weapons
　inappropriate in local application or packing in medical or surgical procedure Y63.5
Hemorrhage
　delayed following medical or surgical treatment without mention of misadventure — *see* Index to Diseases and Injuries, Complication(s)
　during medical or surgical treatment as misadventure — *see* Index to Diseases and Injuries, Complication(s)
High
　altitude (effects) — *see* Air, pressure, low
　level of radioactivity, effects — *see* Radiation
　pressure (effects) — *see* Air, pressure, high
　temperature, effects — *see* Heat
Hit, hitting (accidental) by — *see* Struck by
Hitting against — *see* Striking against
Homicide (attempt) (justifiable) — *see* Assault
Hot
　place, effects — *see also* Heat
　weather, effects X30 ☑
House fire (uncontrolled) — *see* Exposure, fire, uncontrolled, building
Humidity, causing problem X39.8 ☑
Hunger X58 ☑
Hurricane (any injury) X37.0 ☑
Hypobarism, hypobaropathy — *see* Air, pressure, low

I

Ictus
　caloris — *see also* Heat
　solaris X30 ☑
Ignition (accidental) — *see also* Exposure, fire X08.8 ☑

Ignition — continued
  anesthetic gas in operating room W40.1 ☑
  apparel X06.2 ☑
    from highly flammable material X04 ☑
    nightwear X05 ☑
  bed linen (sheets) (spreads) (pillows) (mattress) — see
      Exposure, fire, uncontrolled, building, bed
  benzine X04 ☑
  clothes, clothing NEC (from controlled fire) X06.2 ☑
    from
      highly flammable material X04 ☑
  ether X04 ☑
    in operating room W40.1 ☑
  explosive material — see Explosion
  gasoline X04 ☑
  jewelry (plastic) (any) X06.0 ☑
  kerosene X04 ☑
  material
    explosive — see Explosion
    highly flammable with secondary explosion X04 ☑
  nightwear X05 ☑
  paraffin X04 ☑
  petrol X04 ☑
Immersion (accidental) — see also Drowning
  hand or foot due to cold (excessive) X31 ☑
Implantation of quills of porcupine W55.89 ☑
Inanition (from) (hunger) X58 ☑
  thirst X58 ☑
Inappropriate operation performed
  correct operation on wrong side or body part (wrong
      side) (wrong site) Y65.53
  operation intended for another patient done on wrong
      patient Y65.52
  wrong operation performed on correct patient Y65.51
Inattention after, at birth (homicidal intent) (infanticidal
    intent) X58 ☑
Incident, adverse
  device
    anesthesiology Y70.8
      accessory Y70.2
      diagnostic Y70.0
      miscellaneous Y70.8
      monitoring Y70.0
      prosthetic Y70.2
      rehabilitative Y70.1
      surgical Y70.3
      therapeutic Y70.1
    cardiovascular Y71.8
      accessory Y71.2
      diagnostic Y71.2
      miscellaneous Y71.8
      monitoring Y71.0
      prosthetic Y71.2
      rehabilitative Y71.1
      surgical Y71.3
      therapeutic Y71.1
    gastroenterology Y73.8
      accessory Y73.2
      diagnostic Y73.0
      miscellaneous Y73.8
      monitoring Y73.0
      prosthetic Y73.2
      rehabilitative Y73.1
      surgical Y73.3
      therapeutic Y73.1
    general
      hospital Y74.8
        accessory Y74.2
        diagnostic Y74.0
        miscellaneous Y74.8
        monitoring Y74.0
        prosthetic Y74.2
        rehabilitative Y74.1
        surgical Y74.3
        therapeutic Y74.1
      surgical Y81.8
        accessory Y81.2
        diagnostic Y81.0
        miscellaneous Y81.8
        monitoring Y81.0
        prosthetic Y81.2
        rehabilitative Y81.1
        surgical Y81.3
        therapeutic Y81.1
    gynecological Y76.8
      accessory Y76.2
      diagnostic Y76.0
      miscellaneous Y76.8

Incident, adverse — continued
  device — continued
    gynecological — continued
      monitoring Y76.0
      prosthetic Y76.2
      rehabilitative Y76.1
      surgical Y76.3
      therapeutic Y76.1
    medical Y82.9
      specified type NEC Y82.8
    neurological Y75.8
      accessory Y75.2
      diagnostic Y75.0
      miscellaneous Y75.8
      monitoring Y75.0
      prosthetic Y75.2
      rehabilitative Y75.1
      surgical Y75.3
      therapeutic Y75.1
    obstetrical Y76.8
      accessory Y76.2
      diagnostic Y76.0
      miscellaneous Y76.8
      monitoring Y76.0
      prosthetic Y76.2
      rehabilitative Y76.1
      surgical Y76.3
      therapeutic Y76.1
    ophthalmic Y77.8
      accessory Y77.2
      diagnostic Y77.0
      miscellaneous Y77.8
      monitoring Y77.0
      prosthetic Y77.2
      rehabilitative Y77.1
      surgical Y77.3
      therapeutic Y77.1
    orthopedic Y79.8
      accessory Y79.2
      diagnostic Y79.0
      miscellaneous Y79.8
      monitoring Y79.0
      prosthetic Y79.2
      rehabilitative Y79.1
      surgical Y79.3
      therapeutic Y79.1
    otorhinolaryngological Y72.8
      accessory Y72.2
      diagnostic Y72.0
      miscellaneous Y72.8
      monitoring Y72.0
      prosthetic Y72.2
      rehabilitative Y72.1
      surgical Y72.3
      therapeutic Y72.1
    personal use Y74.8
      accessory Y74.2
      diagnostic Y74.0
      miscellaneous Y74.8
      monitoring Y74.0
      prosthetic Y74.2
      rehabilitative Y74.1
      surgical Y74.3
      therapeutic Y74.1
    physical medicine Y80.8
      accessory Y80.2
      diagnostic Y80.0
      miscellaneous Y80.8
      monitoring Y80.0
      prosthetic Y80.2
      rehabilitative Y80.1
      surgical Y80.3
      therapeutic Y80.1
    plastic surgical Y81.8
      accessory Y81.2
      diagnostic Y81.0
      miscellaneous Y81.8
      monitoring Y81.0
      prosthetic Y81.2
      rehabilitative Y81.1
      surgical Y81.3
      therapeutic Y81.1
    radiological Y78.8
      accessory Y78.2
      diagnostic Y78.0
      miscellaneous Y78.8
      monitoring Y78.0
      prosthetic Y78.2
      rehabilitative Y78.1

Incident, adverse — continued
  device — continued
    radiological — continued
      surgical Y78.3
      therapeutic Y78.1
    urology Y73.8
      accessory Y73.2
      diagnostic Y73.0
      miscellaneous Y73.8
      monitoring Y73.0
      prosthetic Y73.2
      rehabilitative Y73.1
      surgical Y73.3
      therapeutic Y73.1
Incineration (accidental) — see Exposure, fire
Infanticide — see Assault
Infrasound waves (causing injury) W49.9 ☑
Ingestion
  foreign body (causing injury) (with obstruction) — see
      Foreign body, alimentary canal
  poisonous
    plant(s) X58 ☑
    substance NEC — see Table of Drugs and Chemicals
Inhalation
  excessively cold substance, man-made — see Exposure,
      cold, man-made
  food (any type) (into respiratory tract) (with asphyxia,
      obstruction respiratory tract, suffocation) — see
      categories T17 and T18 ☑
  foreign body — see Foreign body, aspiration
  gastric contents (with asphyxia, obstruction respiratory
      passage, suffocation) T17.81- ☑
  hot air or gases X14.0 ☑
  liquid air, hydrogen, nitrogen W93.12 ☑
    suicide (attempt) X83.2 ☑
  steam X13.0 ☑
    assault X98.0 ☑
    stated as undetermined whether accidental or inten-
        tional Y27.0 ☑
    suicide (attempt) X77.0 ☑
  toxic gas — see Table of Drugs and Chemicals
  vomitus (with asphyxia, obstruction respiratory pas-
      sage, suffocation) T17.81- ☑
Injury, injured (accidental(ly)) NOS X58 ☑
  by, caused by, from
    assault — see Assault
    law-enforcing agent, police, in course of legal inter-
        vention — see Legal intervention
    suicide (attempt) X83.8 ☑
  due to, in
    civil insurrection — see War operations
    fight — see also Assault, fight Y04.0 ☑
    war operations — see War operations
  homicide — see also Assault Y09
  inflicted (by)
    in course of arrest (attempted), suppression of dis-
        turbance, maintenance of order, by law-en-
        forcing agents — see Legal intervention
    other person
      stated as
        accidental X58 ☑
        intentional, homicide (attempt) — see Assault
        undetermined whether accidental or inten-
            tional Y33 ☑
  purposely (inflicted) by other person(s) — see Assault
  self-inflicted X83.8 ☑
    stated as accidental X58 ☑
  specified cause NEC X58 ☑
  undetermined whether accidental or intentional Y33 ☑
Insolation, effects X30 ☑
Insufficient nourishment X58 ☑
Interruption of respiration (by)
  food (lodged in esophagus) — see categories T17 and
      T18 ☑
  vomitus (lodged in esophagus) T17.81- ☑
Intervention, legal — see Legal intervention
Intoxication
  drug — see Table of Drugs and Chemicals
  poison — see Table of Drugs and Chemicals

J

Jammed (accidentally)
  between objects (moving) (stationary and moving)
      W23.0 ☑
    stationary W23.1 ☑

Jumped, jumping
  before moving object NEC X81.8 ☑
    motor vehicle X81.0 ☑
    subway train X81.1 ☑
    train X81.1 ☑
    undetermined whether accidental or intentional
      Y31 ☑
  from
    boat (into water) voluntarily, without accident (to
      or on boat) W16.712 ☑
      striking bottom W16.722 ☑
        causing drowning W16.721 ☑
      with
        accident to or on boat — *see* Accident, water-
          craft
        drowning or submersion W16.711 ☑
          suicide (attempt) X71.3 ☑
    building — *see also* Jumped, from, high place
      W13.9 ☑
      burning (uncontrolled fire) X00.5 ☑
    high place NEC W17.89 ☑
      suicide (attempt) X80 ☑
      undetermined whether accidental or intentional
        Y30 ☑
    structure — *see also* Jumped, from, high place
      W13.9 ☑
      burning (uncontrolled fire) X00.5 ☑
  into water W16.92 ☑
    causing drowning W16.91 ☑
    from, off watercraft — *see* Jumped, from, boat
    in
      natural body W16.612 ☑
        causing drowning W16.611 ☑
        striking bottom W16.622 ☑
          causing drowning W16.621 ☑
      specified place NEC W16.812 ☑
        causing drowning W16.811 ☑
        striking
          bottom W16.822 ☑
            causing drowning W16.821 ☑
          wall W16.832 ☑
            causing drowning W16.831 ☑
      swimming pool W16.512 ☑
        causing drowning W16.511 ☑
        striking
          bottom W16.522 ☑
            causing drowning W16.521 ☑
          wall W16.532 ☑
            causing drowning W16.531 ☑
  suicide (attempt) X71.3 ☑

K

Kicked by
  animal NEC W55.82 ☑
  person(s) (accidentally) W50.1 ☑
    with intent to injure or kill Y04.0 ☑
    as, or caused by, a crowd or human stampede (with
      fall) W52 ☑
    assault Y04.0 ☑
    homicide (attempt) Y04.0 ☑
    in
      fight Y04.0 ☑
      legal intervention
        injuring
          bystander Y35.812 ☑
          law enforcement personnel Y35.811 ☑
          suspect Y35.813 ☑
          unspecified person Y35.819 ☑
Kicking
  against
    object W22.8 ☑
      sports equipment W21.9 ☑
      stationary W22.09 ☑
        sports equipment W21.89 ☑
    person — *see* Striking against, person
    sports equipment W21.9 ☑
  carpet stretcher with knee X50.3 ☑
Killed, killing (accidentally) NOS — *see also* Injury X58 ☑
  in
    action — *see* War operations
    brawl, fight (hand) (fists) (foot) Y04.0 ☑
      by weapon — *see also* Assault
        cutting, piercing — *see* Assault, cutting or
          piercing instrument

Killed, killing — *continued*
  in — *continued*
    brawl, fight — *continued*
      by weapon — *see also* Assault — *continued*
        firearm — *see* Discharge, firearm, by type,
          homicide
  self
    stated as
      accident NOS X58 ☑
      suicide — *see* Suicide
      undetermined whether accidental or intentional
        Y33 ☑
Kneeling (prolonged (static)) X50.1 ☑
Knocked down (accidentally) (by) NOS X58 ☑
  animal (not being ridden) NEC — *see also* Struck by,
    by type of animal
  crowd or human stampede W52 ☑
  person W51 ☑
    in brawl, fight Y04.0 ☑
  transport vehicle NEC — *see also* Accident, transport
    V09.9 ☑

L

Laceration NEC — *see* Injury
Lack of
  care (helpless person) (infant) (newborn) X58 ☑
  food except as result of abandonment or neglect
    X58 ☑
    due to abandonment or neglect X58 ☑
  water except as result of transport accident X58 ☑
    due to transport accident — *see* Accident, transport,
      by type
    helpless person, infant, newborn X58 ☑
Landslide (falling on transport vehicle) X36.1 ☑
  caused by collapse of man-made structure X36.0 ☑
Late effect — *see* Sequelae
Legal
  execution (any method) — *see* Legal, intervention
  intervention (by)
    baton — *see* Legal, intervention, blunt object, baton
    bayonet — *see* Legal, intervention, sharp object,
      bayonet
    blow — *see* Legal, intervention, manhandling
    blunt object
      baton
        injuring
          bystander Y35.312 ☑
          law enforcement personnel Y35.311 ☑
          suspect Y35.313 ☑
          unspecified person Y35.319 ☑
      injuring
        bystander Y35.302 ☑
        law enforcement personnel Y35.301 ☑
        suspect Y35.303 ☑
        unspecified person Y35.309 ☑
      specified NEC
        injuring
          bystander Y35.392 ☑
          law enforcement personnel Y35.391 ☑
          suspect Y35.393 ☑
          unspecified person Y35.399 ☑
      stave
        injuring
          bystander Y35.392 ☑
          law enforcement personnel Y35.391 ☑
          suspect Y35.393 ☑
          unspecified person Y35.399 ☑
    bomb — *see* Legal, intervention, explosive
    conducted energy device
      injuring
        bystander Y35.832 ☑
        law enforcement personnel Y35.831 ☑
        suspect Y35.833 ☑
        unspecified person Y35.839 ☑
    cutting or piercing instrument — *see* Legal, inter-
      vention, sharp object
    dynamite — *see* Legal, intervention, explosive, dy-
      namite
    electroshock device (taser)
      injuring
        bystander Y35.832 ☑
        law enforcement personnel Y35.831 ☑
        suspect Y35.833 ☑
        unspecified person Y35.839 ☑

Legal — *continued*
  intervention — *continued*
    explosive(s)
      dynamite
        injuring
          bystander Y35.112 ☑
          law enforcement personnel Y35.111 ☑
          suspect Y35.113 ☑
          unspecified person Y35.119 ☑
      grenade
        injuring
          bystander Y35.192 ☑
          law enforcement personnel Y35.191 ☑
          suspect Y35.193 ☑
          unspecified person Y35.199 ☑
      injuring
        bystander Y35.102 ☑
        law enforcement personnel Y35.101 ☑
        suspect Y35.103 ☑
        unspecified person Y35.109 ☑
      mortar bomb
        injuring
          bystander Y35.192 ☑
          law enforcement personnel Y35.191 ☑
          suspect Y35.193 ☑
          unspecified person Y35.199 ☑
      shell
        injuring
          bystander Y35.122 ☑
          law enforcement personnel Y35.121 ☑
          suspect Y35.123 ☑
          unspecified person Y35.129 ☑
      specified NEC
        injuring
          bystander Y35.192 ☑
          law enforcement personnel Y35.191 ☑
          suspect Y35.193 ☑
          unspecified person Y35.199 ☑
    firearm(s) (discharge)
      handgun
        injuring
          bystander Y35.022 ☑
          law enforcement personnel Y35.021 ☑
          suspect Y35.023 ☑
          unspecified person Y35.029 ☑
      injuring
        bystander Y35.002 ☑
        law enforcement personnel Y35.001 ☑
        suspect Y35.003 ☑
        unspecified person Y35.009 ☑
      machine gun
        injuring
          bystander Y35.012 ☑
          law enforcement personnel Y35.011 ☑
          suspect Y35.013 ☑
          unspecified person Y35.019 ☑
      rifle pellet
        injuring
          bystander Y35.032 ☑
          law enforcement personnel Y35.031 ☑
          suspect Y35.033 ☑
          unspecified person Y35.039 ☑
      rubber bullet
        injuring
          bystander Y35.042 ☑
          law enforcement personnel Y35.041 ☑
          suspect Y35.043 ☑
          unspecified person Y35.049 ☑
      shotgun — *see* Legal, intervention, firearm,
        specified NEC
      specified NEC
        injuring
          bystander Y35.092 ☑
          law enforcement personnel Y35.091 ☑
          suspect Y35.093 ☑
          unspecified person Y35.099 ☑
    gas (asphyxiation) (poisoning)
      injuring
        bystander Y35.202 ☑
        law enforcement personnel Y35.201 ☑
        suspect Y35.203 ☑
        unspecified person Y35.209 ☑
      specified NEC
        injuring
          bystander Y35.292 ☑
          law enforcement personnel Y35.291 ☑
          suspect Y35.293 ☑

External Causes Index (side tab)

Legal — *continued*
  intervention — *continued*
    gas — *continued*
      specified — *continued*
        injuring — *continued*
          unspecified person Y35.299 ☑
        tear gas
          injuring
            bystander Y35.212 ☑
            law enforcement personnel Y35.211 ☑
            suspect Y35.213 ☑
            unspecified person Y35.219 ☑
    grenade — *see* Legal, intervention, explosive, grenade
    injuring
      bystander Y35.92 ☑
      law enforcement personnel Y35.91 ☑
      suspect Y35.93 ☑
      unspecified person Y35.99 ☑
    late effect (of) — *see* with 7th character S Y35 ☑
    manhandling
      injuring
        bystander Y35.812 ☑
        law enforcement personnel Y35.811 ☑
        suspect Y35.813 ☑
        unspecified person Y35.819 ☑
    sequelae (of) — *see* with 7th character S Y35 ☑
    sharp objects
      bayonet
        injuring
          bystander Y35.412 ☑
          law enforcement personnel Y35.411 ☑
          suspect Y35.413 ☑
          unspecified person Y35.419 ☑
      injuring
        bystander Y35.402 ☑
        law enforcement personnel Y35.401 ☑
        suspect Y35.403 ☑
        unspecified person Y35.409 ☑
      specified NEC
        injuring
          bystander Y35.492 ☑
          law enforcement personnel Y35.491 ☑
          suspect Y35.493 ☑
          unspecified person Y35.499 ☑
    specified means NEC
      injuring
        bystander Y35.892 ☑
        law enforcement personnel Y35.891 ☑
        suspect Y35.893 ☑
    stabbing — *see* Legal, intervention, sharp object
    stave — *see* Legal, intervention, blunt object, stave
    stun gun
      injuring
        bystander Y35.832 ☑
        law enforcement personnel Y35.831 ☑
        suspect Y35.833 ☑
        unspecified person Y35.839 ☑
    taser
      injuring
        bystander Y35.832 ☑
        law enforcement personnel Y35.831 ☑
        suspect Y35.833 ☑
        unspecified person Y35.839 ☑
    tear gas — *see* Legal, intervention, gas, tear gas
    truncheon — *see* Legal, intervention, blunt object, stave

Lifting — *see also* Overexertion
  heavy objects X50.0 ☑
  weights X50.0 ☑
Lightning (shock) (stroke) (struck by) — *see* subcategory T75.0 ☑
  causing fire — *see* Exposure, fire
Loss of control (transport vehicle) NEC — *see* Accident, transport
Lost at sea NOS — *see* Drowning, due to, fall overboard
Low
  pressure (effects) — *see* Air, pressure, low
  temperature (effects) — *see* Exposure, cold
Lying before train, vehicle or other moving object X81.8 ☑
  subway train X81.1 ☑
  train X81.1 ☑
  undetermined whether accidental or intentional Y31 ☑
Lynching — *see* Assault

M

Malfunction (mechanism or component) (of)
  firearm W34.10 ☑
    airgun W34.110 ☑
    BB gun W34.110 ☑
    gas, air or spring-operated gun NEC W34.118 ☑
    handgun W32.1 ☑
    hunting rifle W33.12 ☑
    larger firearm W33.10 ☑
      specified NEC W33.19 ☑
    machine gun W33.13 ☑
    paintball gun W34.111 ☑
    pellet gun W34.110 ☑
    shotgun W33.11 ☑
    specified NEC W34.19 ☑
    Very pistol [flare] W34.19 ☑
  handgun — *see* Malfunction, firearm, handgun
Maltreatment — *see* Perpetrator
Mangled (accidentally) NOS X58 ☑
Manhandling (in brawl, fight) Y04.0 ☑
  legal intervention — *see* Legal, intervention, manhandling
Manslaughter (nonaccidental) — *see* Assault
Mauled by animal NEC W55.89 ☑
Medical procedure, complication of (delayed or as an abnormal reaction without mention of misadventure) — *see* Complication of or following, by specified type of procedure
  due to or as a result of misadventure — *see* Misadventure
Melting (due to fire) — *see also* Exposure, fire
  apparel NEC X06.3 ☑
  clothes, clothing NEC X06.3 ☑
    nightwear X05 ☑
  fittings or furniture (burning building) (uncontrolled fire) X00.8 ☑
  nightwear X05 ☑
  plastic jewelry X06.1 ☑
Mental cruelty X58 ☑
Military operations (injuries to military and civilians occuring during peacetime on military property and during routine military exercises and operations) (by) (from) (involving) Y37.90- ☑
  air blast Y37.20- ☑
  aircraft
    destruction — *see* Military operations, destruction of aircraft
    airway restriction — *see* Military operations, restriction of airways
    asphyxiation — *see* Military operations, restriction of airways
  biological weapons Y37.6X- ☑
  blast Y37.20- ☑
  blast fragments Y37.20- ☑
  blast wave Y37.20- ☑
  blast wind Y37.20- ☑
  bomb Y37.20- ☑
    dirty Y37.50- ☑
    gasoline Y37.31- ☑
    incendiary Y37.31- ☑
    petrol Y37.31- ☑
  bullet Y37.43- ☑
    incendiary Y37.32- ☑
    rubber Y37.41- ☑
  chemical weapons Y37.7X- ☑
  combat
    hand to hand (unarmed) combat Y37.44- ☑
    using blunt or piercing object Y37.45- ☑
  conflagration — *see* Military operations, fire
  conventional warfare NEC Y37.49- ☑
  depth-charge Y37.01- ☑
  destruction of aircraft Y37.10- ☑
    due to
      air to air missile Y37.11- ☑
      collision with other aircraft Y37.12- ☑
      detonation (accidental) of onboard munitions and explosives Y37.14- ☑
      enemy fire or explosives Y37.11- ☑
      explosive placed on aircraft Y37.11- ☑
      onboard fire Y37.13- ☑
      rocket propelled grenade [RPG] Y37.11- ☑
      small arms fire Y37.11- ☑
      surface to air missile Y37.11- ☑
    specified NEC Y37.19- ☑

Military operations — *continued*
  detonation (accidental) of
    onboard marine weapons Y37.05- ☑
    own munitions or munitions launch device Y37.24- ☑
  dirty bomb Y37.50- ☑
  explosion (of) Y37.20- ☑
    aerial bomb Y37.21- ☑
    bomb NOS — *see also* Military operations, bomb(s) Y37.20- ☑
    fragments Y37.20- ☑
    grenade Y37.29- ☑
    guided missile Y37.22- ☑
    improvised explosive device [IED] (person-borne) (roadside) (vehicle-borne) Y37.23- ☑
    land mine Y37.29- ☑
    marine mine (at sea) (in harbor) Y37.02- ☑
    marine weapon Y37.00- ☑
      specified NEC Y37.09- ☑
    own munitions or munitions launch device (accidental) Y37.24- ☑
    sea-based artillery shell Y37.03- ☑
    specified NEC Y37.29- ☑
    torpedo Y37.04- ☑
  fire Y37.30- ☑
    specified NEC Y37.39- ☑
  firearms
    discharge Y37.43- ☑
    pellets Y37.42- ☑
  flamethrower Y37.33- ☑
  fragments (from) (of)
    improvised explosive device [IED] (person-borne) (roadside) (vehicle-borne) Y37.26- ☑
    munitions Y37.25- ☑
    specified NEC Y37.29- ☑
    weapons Y37.27- ☑
  friendly fire Y37.92- ☑
  hand to hand (unarmed) combat Y37.44- ☑
  hot substances — *see* Military operations, fire
  incendiary bullet Y37.32- ☑
  nuclear weapon (effects of) Y37.50- ☑
    acute radiation exposure Y37.54- ☑
    blast pressure Y37.51- ☑
    direct blast Y37.51- ☑
    direct heat Y37.53- ☑
    fallout exposure Y37.54- ☑
    fireball Y37.53- ☑
    indirect blast (struck or crushed by blast debris) (being thrown by blast) Y37.52- ☑
    ionizing radiation (immediate exposure) Y37.54- ☑
    nuclear radiation Y37.54- ☑
    radiation
      ionizing (immediate exposure) Y37.54- ☑
      nuclear Y37.54- ☑
      thermal Y37.53- ☑
    secondary effects Y37.54- ☑
    specified NEC Y37.59- ☑
    thermal radiation Y37.53- ☑
  restriction of air (airway)
    intentional Y37.46- ☑
    unintentional Y37.47- ☑
  rubber bullets Y37.41- ☑
  shrapnel NOS Y37.29- ☑
  suffocation — *see* Military operations, restriction of airways
  unconventional warfare NEC Y37.7X- ☑
  underwater blast NOS Y37.00- ☑
  warfare
    conventional NEC Y37.49- ☑
    unconventional NEC Y37.7X- ☑
  weapon of mass destruction [WMD] Y37.91- ☑
  weapons
    biological weapons Y37.6X- ☑
    chemical Y37.7X- ☑
    nuclear (effects of) Y37.50- ☑
      acute radiation exposure Y37.54- ☑
      blast pressure Y37.51- ☑
      direct blast Y37.51- ☑
      direct heat Y37.53- ☑
      fallout exposure Y37.54- ☑
      fireball Y37.53- ☑
      radiation
        ionizing (immediate exposure) Y37.54- ☑
        nuclear Y37.54- ☑
        thermal Y37.53- ☑
      secondary effects Y37.54- ☑

(side tab) Legal — Military operations

Military operations — *continued*
  weapons — *continued*
    nuclear — *continued*
      specified NEC Y37.59- ☑
    of mass destruction [WMD] Y37.91- ☑
Misadventure(s) **to patient**(s) **during surgical or medical care** Y69
  contaminated medical or biological substance (blood, drug, fluid) Y64.9
    administered (by) NEC Y64.9
      immunization Y64.1
      infusion Y64.0
      injection Y64.1
      specified means NEC Y64.8
      transfusion Y64.0
      vaccination Y64.1
  excessive amount of blood or other fluid during transfusion or infusion Y63.0
  failure
    in dosage Y63.9
      electroshock therapy Y63.4
      inappropriate temperature (too hot or too cold) in local application and packing Y63.5
      infusion
        excessive amount of fluid Y63.0
        incorrect dilution of fluid Y63.1
      insulin-shock therapy Y63.4
      nonadministration of necessary drug or biological substance Y63.6
      overdose — *see* Table of Drugs and Chemicals
        radiation, in therapy Y63.2
      radiation
        overdose Y63.2
      specified procedure NEC Y63.8
      transfusion
        excessive amount of blood Y63.0
  mechanical, of instrument or apparatus (any) (during any procedure) Y65.8
  sterile precautions (during procedure) Y62.9
    aspiration of fluid or tissue (by puncture or catheterization, except heart) Y62.6
    biopsy (except needle aspiration) Y62.8
      needle (aspirating) Y62.6
    blood sampling Y62.6
    catheterization Y62.6
      heart Y62.5
    dialysis (kidney) Y62.2
    endoscopic examination Y62.4
    enema Y62.8
    immunization Y62.3
    infusion Y62.1
    injection Y62.3
    needle biopsy Y62.6
    paracentesis (abdominal) (thoracic) Y62.6
    perfusion Y62.2
    puncture (lumbar) Y62.6
    removal of catheter or packing Y62.8
    specified procedure NEC Y62.8
    surgical operation Y62.0
    transfusion Y62.1
    vaccination Y62.3
  suture or ligature during surgical procedure Y65.2
  to introduce or to remove tube or instrument — *see* Failure, to
  hemorrhage — *see* Index to Diseases and Injuries, Complication(s)
  inadvertent exposure of patient to radiation Y63.3
  inappropriate
    operation performed — *see* Inappropriate operation performed
    temperature (too hot or too cold) in local application or packing Y63.5
  infusion — *see also* Misadventure, by type, infusion Y69
    excessive amount of fluid Y63.0
    incorrect dilution of fluid Y63.1
    wrong fluid Y65.1
  mismatched blood in transfusion Y65.0
  nonadministration of necessary drug or biological substance Y63.6
  overdose — *see* Table of Drugs and Chemicals
    radiation (in therapy) Y63.2
  perforation — *see* Index to Diseases and Injuries, Complication(s)
  performance of inappropriate operation — *see* Inappropriate operation performed
  puncture — *see* Index to Diseases and Injuries, Complication(s)

Misadventure(s) **to patient**(s) **during surgical or medical care** — *continued*
  specified type NEC Y65.8
    failure
      suture or ligature during surgical operation Y65.2
      to introduce or to remove tube or instrument — *see* Failure, to
    infusion of wrong fluid Y65.1
    performance of inappropriate operation — *see* Inappropriate operation performed
    transfusion of mismatched blood Y65.0
    wrong
      fluid in infusion Y65.1
      placement of endotracheal tube during anesthetic procedure Y65.3
  transfusion — *see* Misadventure, by type, transfusion
    excessive amount of blood Y63.0
    mismatched blood Y65.0
  wrong
    drug given in error — *see* Table of Drugs and Chemicals
    fluid in infusion Y65.1
    placement of endotracheal tube during anesthetic procedure Y65.3
Mismatched blood in transfusion Y65.0
Motion sickness T75.3 ☑
Mountain sickness W94.11 ☑
Mudslide (of cataclysmic nature) — *see* Landslide
Murder (attempt) — *see* Assault

N

Nail
  contact with W45.0 ☑
    gun W29.4 ☑
  embedded in skin W45.0 ☑
Neglect (criminal) (homicidal intent) X58 ☑
Noise (causing injury) (pollution) W42.9 ☑
  supersonic W42.0 ☑
Nonadministration (of)
  drug or biological substance (necessary) Y63.6
  surgical and medical care Y66
Nosocomial condition Y95

O

Object
  falling
    from, in, on, hitting
      machinery — *see* Contact, with, by type of machine
    set in motion by
      accidental explosion or rupture of pressure vessel W38 ☑
      firearm — *see* Discharge, firearm, by type
      machine(ry) — *see* Contact, with, by type of machine
Overdose (drug) — *see* Table of Drugs and Chemicals
  radiation Y63.2
Overexertion X50.9 ☑
  from
    prolonged static or awkward postures X50.1 ☑
    repetitive movements X50.3 ☑
    specified strenuous movements or postures NEC X50.9 ☑
    strenuous movement or load X50.0 ☑
Overexposure (accidental) (to)
  cold — *see also* Exposure, cold X31 ☑
    due to man-made conditions — *see* Exposure, cold, man-made
  heat — *see also* Heat X30 ☑
  radiation — *see* Radiation
  radioactivity W88.0 ☑
  sun (sunburn) X32 ☑
  weather NEC — *see* Forces of nature
  wind NEC — *see* Forces of nature
Overheated — *see* Heat
Overturning (accidental)
  machinery — *see* Contact, with, by type of machine
  transport vehicle NEC — *see also* Accident, transport V89.9 ☑
  watercraft (causing drowning, submersion) — *see also* Drowning, due to, accident to, watercraft, overturning
    causing injury except drowning or submersion — *see* Accident, watercraft, causing, injury NEC

P

Parachute descent (voluntary) (without accident to aircraft) V97.29 ☑
  due to accident to aircraft — *see* Accident, transport, aircraft
Pecked by bird W61.99 ☑
Perforation during medical or surgical treatment as misadventure — *see* Index to Diseases and Injuries, Complication(s)
Perpetrator, perpetration, of assault, maltreatment and neglect (by) Y07.9
  boyfriend Y07.03
  brother Y07.410
    stepbrother Y07.435
  coach Y07.53
  cousin
    female Y07.491
    male Y07.490
  daycare provider Y07.519
    at-home
      adult care Y07.512
      childcare Y07.510
    care center
      adult care Y07.513
      childcare Y07.511
  family member NEC Y07.499
  father Y07.11
    adoptive Y07.13
    foster Y07.420
    stepfather Y07.430
  foster father Y07.420
  foster mother Y07.421
  girl friend Y07.04
  healthcare provider Y07.529
    mental health Y07.521
    specified NEC Y07.528
  husband Y07.01
  instructor Y07.53
  mother Y07.12
    adoptive Y07.14
    foster Y07.421
    stepmother Y07.433
  multiple perpetrators Y07.6
  nonfamily member Y07.50
    specified NEC Y07.59
  nurse Y07.528
  occupational therapist Y07.528
  partner of parent
    female Y07.434
    male Y07.432
  physical therapist Y07.528
  sister Y07.411
  speech therapist Y07.528
  stepbrother Y07.435
  stepfather Y07.430
  stepmother Y07.433
  stepsister Y07.436
  teacher Y07.53
  wife Y07.02
Piercing — *see* Contact, with, by type of object or machine
Pinched
  between objects (moving) (stationary and moving) W23.0 ☑
  stationary W23.1 ☑
Pinned under machine(ry) — *see* Contact, with, by type of machine
Place of occurrence Y92.9
  abandoned house Y92.89
  airplane Y92.813
  airport Y92.520
  ambulatory health services establishment NEC Y92.538
  ambulatory surgery center Y92.530
  amusement park Y92.831
  apartment (co-op) — *see* Place of occurrence, residence, apartment
  assembly hall Y92.29
  bank Y92.510
  barn Y92.71
  baseball field Y92.320
  basketball court Y92.310
  beach Y92.832
  boarding house — *see* Place of occurrence, residence, boarding house
  boat Y92.814
  bowling alley Y92.39

Place of occurrence — *continued*
- bridge Y92.89
- building under construction Y92.61
- bus Y92.811
  - station Y92.521
- cafe Y92.511
- campsite Y92.833
- campus — *see* Place of occurrence, school
- canal Y92.89
- car Y92.810
- casino Y92.59
- children's home — *see* Place of occurrence, residence, institutional, orphanage
- church Y92.22
- cinema Y92.26
- clubhouse Y92.29
- coal pit Y92.64
- college (community) Y92.214
- condominium — *see* Place of occurrence, residence, apartment
- construction area — *see* Place of occurrence, industrial and construction area
- convalescent home — *see* Place of occurrence, residence, institutional, nursing home
- court-house Y92.240
- cricket ground Y92.328
- cultural building Y92.258
  - art gallery Y92.250
  - museum Y92.251
  - music hall Y92.252
  - opera house Y92.253
  - specified NEC Y92.258
  - theater Y92.254
- dancehall Y92.252
- day nursery Y92.210
- dentist office Y92.531
- derelict house Y92.89
- desert Y92.820
- dockyard Y92.62
- dock NOS Y92.89
- doctor's office Y92.531
- dormitory — *see* Place of occurrence, residence, institutional, school dormitory
- dry dock Y92.62
- factory (building) (premises) Y92.63
- farm (land under cultivation) (outbuildings) Y92.79
  - barn Y92.71
  - chicken coop Y92.72
  - field Y92.73
  - hen house Y92.72
  - house — *see* Place of occurrence, residence, house
  - orchard Y92.74
  - specified NEC Y92.79
- football field Y92.321
- forest Y92.821
- freeway Y92.411
- gallery Y92.250
- garage (commercial) Y92.59
  - boarding house Y92.044
  - military base Y92.135
  - mobile home Y92.025
  - nursing home Y92.124
  - orphanage Y92.114
  - private house Y92.015
  - reform school Y92.155
- gas station Y92.524
- gasworks Y92.69
- golf course Y92.39
- gravel pit Y92.64
- grocery Y92.512
- gymnasium Y92.39
- handball court Y92.318
- harbor Y92.89
- harness racing course Y92.39
- healthcare provider office Y92.531
- highway (interstate) Y92.411
- hill Y92.828
- hockey rink Y92.330
- home — *see* Place of occurrence, residence
- hospice — *see* Place of occurrence, residence, institutional, nursing home
- hospital Y92.239
  - cafeteria Y92.233
  - corridor Y92.232
  - operating room Y92.234
  - patient
    - bathroom Y92.231
    - room Y92.230

Place of occurrence — *continued*
- hospital — *continued*
  - specified NEC Y92.238
- hotel Y92.59
- house — *see also* Place of occurrence, residence
  - abandoned Y92.89
  - under construction Y92.61
- industrial and construction area (yard) Y92.69
  - building under construction Y92.61
  - dock Y92.62
  - dry dock Y92.62
  - factory Y92.63
  - gasworks Y92.69
  - mine Y92.64
  - oil rig Y92.65
  - pit Y92.64
  - power station Y92.69
  - shipyard Y92.62
  - specified NEC Y92.69
  - tunnel under construction Y92.69
  - workshop Y92.69
- kindergarten Y92.211
- lacrosse field Y92.328
- lake Y92.828
- library Y92.241
- mall Y92.59
- market Y92.512
- marsh Y92.828
- military
  - base — *see* Place of occurrence, residence, institutional, military base
  - training ground Y92.84
- mine Y92.64
- mosque Y92.22
- motel Y92.59
- motorway (interstate) Y92.411
- mountain Y92.828
- movie-house Y92.26
- museum Y92.251
- music-hall Y92.252
- not applicable Y92.9
- nuclear power station Y92.69
- nursing home — *see* Place of occurrence, residence, institutional, nursing home
- office building Y92.59
- offshore installation Y92.65
- oil rig Y92.65
- old people's home — *see* Place of occurrence, residence, institutional, specified NEC
- opera-house Y92.253
- orphanage — *see* Place of occurrence, residence, institutional, orphanage
- outpatient surgery center Y92.530
- park (public) Y92.830
  - amusement Y92.831
- parking garage Y92.89
  - lot Y92.481
- pavement Y92.480
- physician office Y92.531
- polo field Y92.328
- pond Y92.828
- post office Y92.242
- power station Y92.69
- prairie Y92.828
- prison — *see* Place of occurrence, residence, institutional, prison
- public
  - administration building Y92.248
    - city hall Y92.243
    - courthouse Y92.240
    - library Y92.241
    - post office Y92.242
    - specified NEC Y92.248
  - building NEC Y92.29
  - hall Y92.29
  - place NOS Y92.89
- race course Y92.39
- radio station Y92.59
- railway line (bridge) Y92.85
- ranch (outbuildings) — *see* Place of occurrence, farm
- recreation area Y92.838
  - amusement park Y92.831
  - beach Y92.832
  - campsite Y92.833
  - park (public) Y92.830
  - seashore Y92.832
  - specified NEC Y92.838

Place of occurrence — *continued*
- reform school - — *see* Place of occurrence, residence, institutional, reform school
- religious institution Y92.22
- residence (non-institutional) (private) Y92.009
  - apartment Y92.039
    - bathroom Y92.031
    - bedroom Y92.032
    - kitchen Y92.030
    - specified NEC Y92.038
  - bathroom Y92.002
  - bedroom Y92.003
  - boarding house Y92.049
    - bathroom Y92.041
    - bedroom Y92.042
    - driveway Y92.043
    - garage Y92.044
    - garden Y92.046
    - kitchen Y92.040
    - specified NEC Y92.048
    - swimming pool Y92.045
    - yard Y92.046
  - dining room Y92.001
  - garden Y92.007
  - home Y92.009
  - house, single family Y92.019
    - bathroom Y92.012
    - bedroom Y92.013
    - dining room Y92.011
    - driveway Y92.014
    - garage Y92.015
    - garden Y92.017
    - kitchen Y92.010
    - specified NEC Y92.018
    - swimming pool Y92.016
    - yard Y92.017
  - institutional Y92.10
    - children's home — *see* Place of occurrence, residence, institutional, orphanage
    - hospice — *see* Place of occurrence, residence, institutional, nursing home
    - military base Y92.139
      - barracks Y92.133
      - garage Y92.135
      - garden Y92.137
      - kitchen Y92.130
      - mess hall Y92.131
      - specified NEC Y92.138
      - swimming pool Y92.136
      - yard Y92.137
    - nursing home Y92.129
      - bathroom Y92.121
      - bedroom Y92.122
      - driveway Y92.123
      - garage Y92.124
      - garden Y92.126
      - kitchen Y92.120
      - specified NEC Y92.128
      - swimming pool Y92.125
      - yard Y92.126
    - orphanage Y92.119
      - bathroom Y92.111
      - bedroom Y92.112
      - driveway Y92.113
      - garage Y92.114
      - garden Y92.116
      - kitchen Y92.110
      - specified NEC Y92.118
      - swimming pool Y92.115
      - yard Y92.116
    - prison Y92.149
      - bathroom Y92.142
      - cell Y92.143
      - courtyard Y92.147
      - dining room Y92.141
      - kitchen Y92.140
      - specified NEC Y92.148
      - swimming pool Y92.146
    - reform school Y92.159
      - bathroom Y92.152
      - bedroom Y92.153
      - dining room Y92.151
      - driveway Y92.154
      - garage Y92.155
      - garden Y92.157
      - kitchen Y92.150
      - specified NEC Y92.158
      - swimming pool Y92.156
      - yard Y92.157

Place of occurrence — continued
  residence — continued
    institutional — continued
      school dormitory Y92.169
        bathroom Y92.162
        bedroom Y92.163
        dining room Y92.161
        kitchen Y92.160
        specified NEC Y92.168
      specified NEC Y92.199
        bathroom Y92.192
        bedroom Y92.193
        dining room Y92.191
        driveway Y92.194
        garage Y92.195
        garden Y92.197
        kitchen Y92.190
        specified NEC Y92.198
        swimming pool Y92.196
        yard Y92.197
    kitchen Y92.000
    mobile home Y92.029
      bathroom Y92.022
      bedroom Y92.023
      dining room Y92.021
      driveway Y92.024
      garage Y92.025
      garden Y92.027
      kitchen Y92.020
      specified NEC Y92.028
      swimming pool Y92.026
      yard Y92.027
    specified place in residence NEC Y92.008
    specified residence type NEC Y92.099
      bathroom Y92.091
      bedroom Y92.092
      driveway Y92.093
      garage Y92.094
      garden Y92.096
      kitchen Y92.090
      specified NEC Y92.098
      swimming pool Y92.095
      yard Y92.096
  restaurant Y92.511
  riding school Y92.39
  river Y92.828
  road Y92.410
  rodeo ring Y92.39
  rugby field Y92.328
  same day surgery center Y92.530
  sand pit Y92.64
  school (private) (public) (state) Y92.219
    college Y92.214
    daycare center Y92.210
    elementary school Y92.211
    high school Y92.213
    kindergarten Y92.211
    middle school Y92.212
    specified NEC Y92.218
    trace school Y92.215
    university Y92.214
    vocational school Y92.215
  sea (shore) Y92.832
  senior citizen center Y92.29
  service area
    airport Y92.520
    bus station Y92.521
    gas station Y92.524
    highway rest stop Y92.523
    railway station Y92.522
  shipyard Y92.62
  shop (commercial) Y92.513
  sidewalk Y92.480
  silo Y92.79
  skating rink (roller) Y92.331
    ice Y92.330
  slaughter house Y92.86
  soccer field Y92.322
  specified place NEC Y92.89
  sports area Y92.39
    athletic
      court Y92.318
        basketball Y92.310
        specified NEC Y92.318
        squash Y92.311
        tennis Y92.312
      field Y92.328
        baseball Y92.320
        cricket ground Y92.328

Place of occurrence — continued
  sports area — continued
    athletic — continued
      field — continued
        football Y92.321
        hockey Y92.328
        soccer Y92.322
        specified NEC Y92.328
    golf course Y92.39
    gymnasium Y92.39
    riding school Y92.39
    skating rink (roller) Y92.331
      ice Y92.330
    stadium Y92.39
    swimming pool Y92.34
  squash court Y92.311
  stadium Y92.39
  steeplechasing course Y92.39
  store Y92.512
  stream Y92.828
  street and highway Y92.410
    bike path Y92.482
    freeway Y92.411
    highway ramp Y92.415
    interstate highway Y92.411
    local residential or business street Y92.414
    motorway Y92.411
    parking lot Y92.481
    parkway Y92.412
    sidewalk Y92.480
    specified NEC Y92.488
    state road Y92.413
  subway car Y92.816
  supermarket Y92.512
  swamp Y92.828
  swimming pool (public) Y92.34
    private (at) Y92.095
      boarding house Y92.045
      military base Y92.136
      mobile home Y92.026
      nursing home Y92.125
      orphanage Y92.115
      prison Y92.146
      reform school Y92.156
      single family residence Y92.016
  synagogue Y92.22
  television station Y92.59
  tennis court Y92.312
  theater Y92.254
  trade area Y92.59
    bank Y92.510
    cafe Y92.511
    casino Y92.59
    garage Y92.59
    hotel Y92.59
    market Y92.512
    office building Y92.59
    radio station Y92.59
    restaurant Y92.511
    shop Y92.513
    shopping mall Y92.59
    store Y92.512
    supermarket Y92.512
    television station Y92.59
    warehouse Y92.59
  trailer park, residential — see Place of occurrence, residence, mobile home
  trailer site NOS Y92.89
  train Y92.815
    station Y92.522
  truck Y92.812
  tunnel under construction Y92.69
  university Y92.214
  urgent (health) care center Y92.532
  vehicle (transport) Y92.818
    airplane Y92.813
    boat Y92.814
    bus Y92.811
    car Y92.810
    specified NEC Y92.818
    subway car Y92.816
    train Y92.815
    truck Y92.812
  warehouse Y92.59
  water reservoir Y92.89
  wilderness area Y92.828
    desert Y92.820
    forest Y92.821
    marsh Y92.828

Place of occurrence — continued
  wilderness area — continued
    mountain Y92.828
    prairie Y92.828
    specified NEC Y92.828
    swamp Y92.828
  workshop Y92.69
  yard, private Y92.096
    boarding house Y92.046
    mobile home Y92.027
    single family house Y92.017
  youth center Y92.29
  zoo (zoological garden) Y92.834
Plumbism — see Table of Drugs and Chemicals, lead
Poisoning (accidental) (by) — see also Table of Drugs and Chemicals
  by plant, thorns, spines, sharp leaves or other mechanisms NEC X58 ☑
  carbon monoxide
    generated by
      motor vehicle — see Accident, transport
      watercraft (in transit) (not in transit) V93.89 ☑
        ferry boat V93.81 ☑
        fishing boat V93.82 ☑
        jet skis V93.83 ☑
        liner V93.81 ☑
        merchant ship V93.80 ☑
        passenger ship V93.81 ☑
        powered craft NEC V93.83 ☑
  caused by injection of poisons into skin by plant thorns, spines, sharp leaves X58 ☑
  marine or sea plants (venomous) X58 ☑
  execution — see Legal, intervention, gas
  intervention
    by gas — see Legal, intervention, gas
    other specified means — see Legal, intervention, specified means NEC
  exhaust gas
    generated by
      motor vehicle — see Accident, transport
      watercraft (in transit) (not in transit) V93.89 ☑
        ferry boat V93.81 ☑
        fishing boat V93.82 ☑
        jet skis V93.83 ☑
        liner V93.81 ☑
        merchant ship V93.80 ☑
        passenger ship V93.81 ☑
        powered craft NEC V93.83 ☑
  fumes or smoke due to
    explosion — see also Explosion W40.9 ☑
    fire — see Exposure, fire
    ignition — see Ignition
  gas
    in legal intervention — see Legal, intervention, gas
    legal execution — see Legal, intervention, gas
  in war operations — see War operations
  legal
Powder burn (by) (from)
  airgun W34.110 ☑
  BB gun W34.110 ☑
  firearm NEC W34.19 ☑
  gas, air or spring-operated gun NEC W34.118 ☑
  handgun W32.1 ☑
  hunting rifle W33.12 ☑
  larger firearm W33.10 ☑
    specified NEC W33.19 ☑
  machine gun W33.13 ☑
  paintball gun W34.111 ☑
  pellet gun W34.110 ☑
  shotgun W33.11 ☑
  Very pistol [flare] W34.19 ☑
Premature cessation (of) **surgical and medical care** Y66
Privation (food) (water) X58 ☑
Procedure (operation)
  correct, on wrong side or body part (wrong side) (wrong site) Y65.53
  intended for another patient done on wrong patient Y65.52
  performed on patient not scheduled for surgery Y65.52
  performed on wrong patient Y65.52
  wrong, performed on correct patient Y65.51
Prolonged
  sitting in transport vehicle — see Travel, by type of vehicle

Prolonged — *continued*
  stay in
    high altitude as cause of anoxia, barodontalgia, barotitis or hypoxia W94.11 ☑
    weightless environment X52 ☑
Pulling, excessive — *see also* Overexertion X50.9- ☑
Puncture, puncturing — *see also* Contact, with, by type of object or machine
  by
    plant thorns, spines, sharp leaves or other mechanisms NEC W60 ☑
  during medical or surgical treatment as misadventure — *see* Index to Diseases and Injuries, Complication(s)
Pushed, pushing (accidental) (injury in)
  by other person(s) (accidental) W51 ☑
    as, or caused by, a crowd or human stampede (with fall) W52 ☑
    before moving object NEC Y02.8 ☑
      motor vehicle Y02.0 ☑
      subway train Y02.1 ☑
      train Y02.1 ☑
    from
      high place NEC
        in accidental circumstances W17.89 ☑
        stated as
          intentional, homicide (attempt) Y01 ☑
          undetermined whether accidental or intentional Y30 ☑
      transport vehicle NEC — *see also* Accident, transport V89.9 ☑
        stated as
          intentional, homicide (attempt) Y08.89 ☑
    with fall W03 ☑
      due to ice or snow W00.0 ☑
  overexertion X50.9 ☑

R

Radiation (exposure to)
  arc lamps W89.0 ☑
  atomic power plant (malfunction) NEC W88.1 ☑
  complication of or abnormal reaction to medical radiotherapy Y84.2
  electromagnetic, ionizing W88.0 ☑
  gamma rays W88.1 ☑
  in
    war operations (from or following nuclear explosion) — *see* War operations
  inadvertent exposure of patient (receiving test or therapy) Y63.3
  infrared (heaters and lamps) W90.1 ☑
    excessive heat from W92 ☑
  ionized, ionizing (particles, artificially accelerated)
    radioisotopes W88.1 ☑
    specified NEC W88.8 ☑
    x-rays W88.0 ☑
  isotopes, radioactive — *see* Radiation, radioactive isotopes
  laser(s) W90.2 ☑
    in war operations — *see* War operations
    misadventure in medical care Y63.2
  light sources (man-made visible and ultraviolet) W89.9 ☑
    natural X32 ☑
    specified NEC W89.8 ☑
    tanning bed W89.1 ☑
    welding light W89.0 ☑
  man-made visible light W89.9 ☑
    specified NEC W89.8 ☑
    tanning bed W89.1 ☑
    welding light W89.0 ☑
  microwave W90.8 ☑
  misadventure in medical or surgical procedure Y63.2
  natural NEC X39.08 ☑
    radon X39.01 ☑
  overdose (in medical or surgical procedure) Y63.2
  radar W90.0 ☑
  radioactive isotopes (any) W88.1 ☑
    atomic power plant malfunction W88.1 ☑
    misadventure in medical or surgical treatment Y63.2
  radiofrequency W90.0 ☑
  radium NEC W88.1 ☑
  sun X32 ☑
  ultraviolet (light) (man-made) W89.9 ☑
    natural X32 ☑

Radiation — *continued*
  ultraviolet — *continued*
    specified NEC W89.8 ☑
    tanning bed W89.1 ☑
    welding light W89.0 ☑
  welding arc, torch, or light W89.0 ☑
    excessive heat from W92 ☑
  x-rays (hard) (soft) W88.0 ☑
Range disease W94.11
Rape (attempted) T74.2- ☑
Rat bite W53.11 ☑
Reaching (prolonged) (static) X50.1 ☑
Reaction, abnormal to medical procedure — *see also* Complication of or following, by type of procedure Y84.9
  biologicals — *see* Table of Drugs and Chemicals
  drugs — *see* Table of Drugs and Chemicals
  vaccine — *see* Table of Drugs and Chemicals
  with misadventure — *see* Misadventure
Recoil
  airgun W34.110 ☑
  BB gun W34.110 ☑
  firearm NEC W34.19 ☑
  gas, air or spring-operated gun NEC W34.118 ☑
  handgun W32.1 ☑
  hunting rifle W33.12 ☑
  larger firearm W33.10 ☑
    specified NEC W33.19 ☑
  machine gun W33.13 ☑
  paintball gun W34.111 ☑
  pellet W34.110 ☑
  shotgun W33.11 ☑
  Very pistol [flare] W34.19 ☑
Reduction in
  atmospheric pressure — *see* Air, pressure, change
Rock falling on or hitting (accidentally) (person) W20.8 ☑
  in cave-in W20.0 ☑
Run over (accidentally) (by)
  animal (not being ridden) NEC W55.89 ☑
  machinery — *see* Contact, with, by specified type of machine
  transport vehicle NEC — *see also* Accident, transport V09.9 ☑
    intentional homicide (attempt) Y03.0 ☑
    motor NEC V09.20 ☑
      intentional homicide (attempt) Y03.0 ☑
Running
  before moving object X81.8 ☑
    motor vehicle X81.0 ☑
Running off, away
  animal (being ridden) — *see also* Accident, transport V80.918 ☑
    not being ridden W55.89 ☑
  animal-drawn vehicle NEC — *see also* Accident, transport V80.928 ☑
  highway, road(way), street
    transport vehicle NEC — *see also* Accident, transport V89.9 ☑
Rupture pressurized devices — *see* Explosion, by type of device

S

Saturnism — *see* Table of Drugs and Chemicals, lead
Scald, scalding (accidental) (by) (from) (in) X19 ☑
  air (hot) X14.1 ☑
  gases (hot) X14.1 ☑
  homicide (attempt) — *see* Assault, burning, hot object inflicted by other person
    stated as intentional, homicide (attempt) — *see* Assault, burning, hot object
  liquid (boiling) (hot) NEC X12 ☑
    stated as undetermined whether accidental or intentional Y27.2 ☑
    suicide (attempt) X77.2 ☑
  local application of externally applied substance in medical or surgical care Y63.5
  metal (molten) (liquid) (hot) NEC X18 ☑
  self-inflicted X77.9 ☑
  stated as undetermined whether accidental or intentional Y27.8 ☑
  steam X13.1 ☑
    assault X98.0 ☑
    stated as undetermined whether accidental or intentional Y27.0 ☑

Scald, scalding — *continued*
  steam — *continued*
    suicide (attempt) X77.0 ☑
  suicide (attempt) X77.9 ☑
  vapor (hot) X13.1 ☑
    assault X98.0 ☑
    stated as undetermined whether accidental or intentional Y27.0 ☑
    suicide (attempt) X77.0 ☑
Scratched by
  cat W55.03 ☑
  person(s) (accidentally) W50.4 ☑
    with intent to injure or kill Y04.0 ☑
    as, or caused by, a crowd or human stampede (with fall) W52 ☑
    assault Y04.0 ☑
    homicide (attempt) Y04.0 ☑
    in
      fight Y04.0 ☑
      legal intervention
        injuring
          bystander Y35.892 ☑
          law enforcement personnel Y35.891 ☑
          suspect Y35.893 ☑
Seasickness T75.3
Self-harm NEC — *see also* External cause by type, undetermined whether accidental or intentional
  intentional — *see* Suicide
  poisoning NEC — *see* Table of Drugs and Chemicals, poisoning, accidental
Self-inflicted (injury) **NEC** — *see also* External cause by type, undetermined whether accidental or intentional
  intentional — *see* Suicide
  poisoning NEC — *see* Table of Drugs and Chemicals, poisoning, accidental
Sequelae (of)
  accident NEC — *see* W00-X58 with 7th character S
  assault (homicidal) (any means) — *see* X92-Y08 with 7th character S
  homicide, attempt (any means) — *see* X92-Y08 with 7th character S
  injury undetermined whether accidentally or purposely inflicted — *see* Y21-Y33 with 7th character S
  intentional self-harm (classifiable to X71-X83) — *see* X71-X83 with 7th character S
  legal intervention — *see* with 7th character S Y35 ☑
  motor vehicle accident — *see* V00-V99 with 7th character S
  suicide, attempt (any means) — *see* X71-X83 with 7th character S
  transport accident — *see* V00-V99 with 7th character S
  war operations — *see* War operations
Shock
  electric — *see* Exposure, electric current
  from electric appliance (any) (faulty) W86.8 ☑
    domestic W86.0 ☑
    suicide (attempt) X83.1 ☑
Shooting, shot (accidental(ly)) — *see also* Discharge, firearm, by type
  herself or himself — *see* Discharge, firearm by type, self-inflicted
  homicide (attempt) — *see* Discharge, firearm by type, homicide
  in war operations — *see* War operations
  inflicted by other person — *see* Discharge, firearm by type, homicide
    accidental — *see* Discharge, firearm, by type of firearm
  legal
    execution — *see* Legal, intervention, firearm
    intervention — *see* Legal, intervention, firearm
  self-inflicted — *see* Discharge, firearm by type, suicide
    accidental — *see* Discharge, firearm, by type of firearm
  suicide (attempt) — *see* Discharge, firearm by type, suicide
Shoving (accidentally) **by other person** — *see* Pushed, by other person
Sickness
  alpine W94.11 ☑
  motion — *see* Motion
  mountain W94.11 ☑
Sinking (accidental)
  watercraft (causing drowning, submersion) — *see also* Drowning, due to, accident to, watercraft, sinking

Sinking — continued

watercraft — see also Drowning, due to, accident to, watercraft, sinking — continued

causing injury except drowning or submersion — see Accident, watercraft, causing, injury NEC

Siriasis X32 ☑

Sitting (prolonged) (static) X50.1 ☑

Slashed wrists — see Cut, self-inflicted

Slipping (accidental) (on same level) (with fall) W01.0 ☑

on

ice W00.0 ☑

with skates — see Accident, transport, pedestrian, conveyance

mud W01.0 ☑

oil W01.0 ☑

snow W00.0 ☑

with skis — see Accident, transport, pedestrian, conveyance

surface (slippery) (wet) NEC W01.0 ☑

without fall W18.40 ☑

due to

specified NEC W18.49 ☑

stepping from one level to another W18.43 ☑

stepping into hole or opening W18.42 ☑

stepping on object W18.41 ☑

Sliver, wood, contact with W45.8 ☑

Smoldering (due to fire) — see Exposure, fire

Sodomy (attempted) **by force** T74.2 ☑

Sound waves (causing injury) W42.9 ☑

supersonic W42.0 ☑

Splinter, contact with W45.8 ☑

Stab, stabbing — see Cut

Standing (prolonged) (static) X50.1 ☑

Starvation X58 ☑

Status of external cause Y99.9

child assisting in compensated work for family Y99.8

civilian activity done for financial or other compensation Y99.0

civilian activity done for income or pay Y99.0

family member assisting in compensated work for other family member Y99.8

hobby not done for income Y99.8

leisure activity Y99.8

military activity Y99.1

off-duty activity of military personnel Y99.8

recreation or sport not for income or while a student Y99.8

specified NEC Y99.8

student activity Y99.8

volunteer activity Y99.2

Stepped on

by

animal (not being ridden) NEC W55.89 ☑

crowd or human stampede W52 ☑

person W50.0 ☑

Stepping on

object W22.8 ☑

sports equipment W21.9 ☑

stationary W22.09 ☑

sports equipment W21.89 ☑

with fall W18.31 ☑

person W51 ☑

by crowd or human stampede W52 ☑

sports equipment W21.9 ☑

Sting

arthropod, nonvenomous W57 ☑

insect, nonvenomous W57 ☑

Storm (cataclysmic) — see Forces of nature, cataclysmic storm

Straining, excessive — see also Overexertion X50.9 ☑

Strangling — see Strangulation

Strangulation (accidental) T71 ☑

Strenuous movements — see also Overexertion X50.9 ☑

Striking against

airbag (automobile) W22.10 ☑

driver side W22.11 ☑

front passenger side W22.12 ☑

specified NEC W22.19 ☑

bottom when

diving or jumping into water (in) W16.822 ☑

causing drowning W16.821 ☑

from boat W16.722 ☑

causing drowning W16.721 ☑

natural body W16.622 ☑

causing drowning W16.821 ☑

Striking against — continued

bottom when — continued

diving or jumping into water — continued

swimming pool W16.522 ☑

causing drowning W16.521 ☑

falling into water (in) W16.322 ☑

causing drowning W16.321 ☑

fountain — see Striking against, bottom when, falling into water, specified NEC

natural body W16.122 ☑

causing drowning W16.121 ☑

reservoir — see Striking against, bottom when, falling into water, specified NEC

specified NEC W16.322 ☑

causing drowning W16.321 ☑

swimming pool W16.022 ☑

causing drowning W16.021 ☑

diving board (swimming-pool) W21.4 ☑

object W22.8 ☑

caused by crowd or human stampede (with fall) W52 ☑

furniture W22.03 ☑

lamppost W22.02 ☑

sports equipment W21.9 ☑

stationary W22.09 ☑

sports equipment W21.89 ☑

wall W22.01 ☑

with

drowning or submersion — see Drowning

fall — see Fall, due to, bumping against, object

person(s) W51 ☑

as, or caused by, a crowd or human stampede (with fall) W52 ☑

assault Y04.2 ☑

homicide (attempt) Y04.2 ☑

with fall W03 ☑

due to ice or snow W00.0 ☑

sports equipment W21.9 ☑

wall (when) W22.01 ☑

diving or jumping into water (in) W16.832 ☑

causing drowning W16.831 ☑

swimming pool W16.532 ☑

causing drowning W16.531 ☑

falling into water (in) W16.332 ☑

causing drowning W16.331 ☑

fountain — see Striking against, wall when, falling into water, specified NEC

natural body W16.132 ☑

causing drowning W16.131 ☑

reservoir — see Striking against, wall when, falling into water, specified NEC

specified NEC W16.332 ☑

causing drowning W16.331 ☑

swimming pool W16.032 ☑

causing drowning W16.031 ☑

swimming pool (when) W22.042 ☑

causing drowning W22.041 ☑

diving or jumping into water W16.532 ☑

causing drowning W16.531 ☑

falling into water W16.032 ☑

causing drowning W16.031 ☑

Struck (accidentally) **by**

airbag (automobile) W22.10 ☑

driver side W22.11 ☑

front passenger side W22.12 ☑

specified NEC W22.19 ☑

alligator W58.02 ☑

animal (not being ridden) NEC W55.89 ☑

avalanche — see Landslide

ball (hit) (thrown) W21.00 ☑

assault Y08.09 ☑

baseball W21.03 ☑

basketball W21.05 ☑

football W21.01 ☑

golf ball W21.04 ☑

soccer W21.02 ☑

softball W21.07 ☑

specified NEC W21.09 ☑

volleyball W21.06 ☑

bat or racquet

baseball bat W21.11 ☑

assault Y08.02 ☑

golf club W21.13 ☑

assault Y08.09 ☑

specified NEC W21.19 ☑

assault Y08.09 ☑

Struck (accidentally) **by** — continued

bat or racquet — continued

tennis racquet W21.12 ☑

assault Y08.09 ☑

bullet — see also Discharge, firearm by type

in war operations — see War operations

crocodile W58.12 ☑

dog W54.1 ☑

flare, Very pistol — see Discharge, firearm NEC

hailstones X39.8 ☑

hockey (ice)

field

puck W21.221 ☑

stick W21.211 ☑

puck W21.220 ☑

stick W21.210 ☑

assault Y08.01 ☑

landslide — see Landslide

law-enforcement agent (on duty) — see Legal, intervention, manhandling

with blunt object — see Legal, intervention, blunt object

lightning T75.0 ☑

causing fire — see Exposure, fire

machine — see Contact, with, by type of machine

mammal NEC W55.89 ☑

marine W56.32 ☑

marine animal W56.82 ☑

missile

firearm — see Discharge, firearm by type

in war operations — see War operations, missile

object W22.8 ☑

blunt W22.8 ☑

assault Y00 ☑

suicide (attempt) X79 ☑

undetermined whether accidental or intentional Y29 ☑

falling W20.8 ☑

from, in, on

building W20.1 ☑

burning (uncontrolled fire) X00.4 ☑

cataclysmic

earth surface movement NEC — see Landslide

storm — see Forces of nature, cataclysmic storm

cave-in W20.0 ☑

earthquake X34 ☑

machine (in operation) — see Contact, with, by type of machine

structure W20.1 ☑

burning X00.4 ☑

transport vehicle (in motion) — see Accident, transport, by type of vehicle

watercraft V93.49 ☑

due to

accident to craft V91.39 ☑

powered craft V91.33 ☑

ferry boat V91.31 ☑

fishing boat V91.32 ☑

jetskis V91.33 ☑

liner V91.31 ☑

merchant ship V91.30 ☑

passenger ship V91.31 ☑

unpowered craft V91.38 ☑

canoe V91.35 ☑

inflatable V91.36 ☑

kayak V91.35 ☑

sailboat V91.34 ☑

surf-board V91.38 ☑

windsurfer V91.38 ☑

powered craft V93.43 ☑

ferry boat V93.41 ☑

fishing boat V93.42 ☑

jetskis V93.43 ☑

liner V93.41 ☑

merchant ship V93.40 ☑

passenger ship V93.41 ☑

unpowered craft V93.48 ☑

sailboat V93.44 ☑

surf-board V93.48 ☑

windsurfer V93.48 ☑

moving NEC W20.8 ☑

projected W20.8 ☑

assault Y00 ☑

in sports W21.9 ☑

Struck (accidentally) **by** — *continued*
object — *continued*
  projected — *continued*
   in sports — *continued*
    assault Y08.09 ☑
    ball W21.00 ☑
     baseball W21.03 ☑
     basketball W21.05 ☑
     football W21.01 ☑
     golf ball W21.04 ☑
     soccer W21.02 ☑
     softball W21.07 ☑
     specified NEC W21.09 ☑
     volleyball W21.06 ☑
    bat or racquet
     baseball bat W21.11 ☑
      assault Y08.02 ☑
     golf club W21.13 ☑
      assault Y08.09 ☑
     specified NEC W21.19 ☑
      assault Y08.09 ☑
     tennis racquet W21.12 ☑
      assault Y08.09 ☑
    hockey (ice)
     field
      puck W21.221 ☑
      stick W21.211 ☑
     puck W21.220 ☑
     stick W21.210 ☑
      assault Y08.01 ☑
    specified NEC W21.89 ☑
  set in motion by explosion — *see* Explosion
  thrown W20.8 ☑
   assault Y00 ☑
   in sports W21.9 ☑
    assault Y08.09 ☑
    ball W21.00 ☑
     baseball W21.03 ☑
     basketball W21.05 ☑
     football W21.01 ☑
     golf ball W21.04 ☑
     soccer W21.02 ☑
     soft ball W21.07 ☑
     specified NEC W21.09 ☑
     volleyball W21.06 ☑
    bat or racquet
     baseball bat W21.11 ☑
      assault Y08.02 ☑
     golf club W21.13 ☑
      assault Y08.09 ☑
     specified NEC W21.19 ☑
      assault Y08.09 ☑
     tennis racquet W21.12 ☑
      assault Y08.09 ☑
    hockey (ice)
     field
      puck W21.221 ☑
      stick W21.211 ☑
     puck W21.220 ☑
     stick W21.210 ☑
      assault Y08.01 ☑
    specified NEC W21.89 ☑
  other person(s) W50.0 ☑
   with
    blunt object W22.8 ☑
     intentional, homicide (attempt) Y00 ☑
     sports equipment W21.9 ☑
     undetermined whether accidental or intentional Y29 ☑
    fall W03 ☑
     due to ice or snow W00.0 ☑
   as, or caused by, a crowd or human stampede (with fall) W52 ☑
   assault Y04.2 ☑
   homicide (attempt) Y04.2 ☑
   in legal intervention
    injuring
     bystander Y35.812 ☑
     law enforcement personnel Y35.811 ☑
     suspect Y35.813 ☑
     unspecified person Y35.819 ☑
    sports equipment W21.9 ☑
  police (on duty) — *see* Legal, intervention, manhandling
   with blunt object — *see* Legal, intervention, blunt object

Struck (accidentally) **by** — *continued*
sports equipment W21.9 ☑
  assault Y08.09 ☑
  ball W21.00 ☑
   baseball W21.03 ☑
   basketball W21.05 ☑
   football W21.01 ☑
   golf ball W21.04 ☑
   soccer W21.02 ☑
   soft ball W21.07 ☑
   specified NEC W21.09 ☑
   volleyball W21.06 ☑
  bat or racquet
   baseball bat W21.11 ☑
    assault Y08.02 ☑
   golf club W21.13 ☑
    assault Y08.09 ☑
   specified NEC W21.19 ☑
   tennis racquet W21.12 ☑
    assault Y08.09 ☑
  cleats (shoe) W21.31 ☑
  foot wear NEC W21.39 ☑
  football helmet W21.81 ☑
  hockey (ice)
   field
    puck W21.221 ☑
    stick W21.211 ☑
   puck W21.220 ☑
   stick W21.210 ☑
    assault Y08.01 ☑
  skate blades W21.32 ☑
  specified NEC W21.89 ☑
   assault Y08.09 ☑
thunderbolt — *see* subcategory T75.0 ☑
  causing fire — *see* Exposure, fire
transport vehicle NEC — *see also* Accident, transport V09.9 ☑
  intentional, homicide (attempt) Y03.0 ☑
  motor NEC — *see also* Accident, transport V09.20 ☑
   homicide Y03.0 ☑
vehicle (transport) NEC — *see* Accident, transport, by type of vehicle
  stationary (falling from jack, hydraulic lift, ramp) W20.8 ☑

Stumbling
over
  animal NEC W01.0 ☑
   with fall W18.09 ☑
  carpet, rug or (small) object W22.8 ☑
   with fall W18.09 ☑
  person W51 ☑
   with fall W03 ☑
    due to ice or snow W00.0 ☑
without fall W18.40 ☑
  due to
   specified NEC W18.49 ☑
   stepping from one level to another W18.43 ☑
   stepping into hole or opening W18.42 ☑
   stepping on object W18.41 ☑
Submersion (accidental) — *see* Drowning
Suffocation (accidental) (by external means) (by pressure) (mechanical) — *see also* category T71 ☑
due to, by
  avalanche — *see* Landslide
  explosion — *see* Explosion
  fire — *see* Exposure, fire
  food, any type (aspiration) (ingestion) (inhalation) — *see* categories T17 and T18 ☑
  ignition — *see* Ignition
  landslide — *see* Landslide
  machine(ry) — *see* Contact, with, by type of machine
  vomitus (aspiration) (inhalation) T17.81- ☑
in
  burning building X00.8 ☑
Suicide, suicidal (attempted) (by) X83.8 ☑
blunt object X79 ☑
burning, burns X76 ☑
  hot object X77.9 ☑
   fluid NEC X77.2 ☑
   household appliance X77.3 ☑
   specified NEC X77.8 ☑
   steam X77.0 ☑
   tap water X77.1 ☑
   vapors X77.0 ☑
caustic substance — *see* Table of Drugs and Chemicals

Suicide, suicidal — *continued*
cold, extreme X83.2 ☑
collision of motor vehicle with
  motor vehicle X82.0 ☑
  specified NEC X82.8 ☑
  train X82.1 ☑
  tree X82.2 ☑
crashing of aircraft X83.0 ☑
cut (any part of body) X78.9 ☑
cutting or piercing instrument X78.9 ☑
  dagger X78.2 ☑
  glass X78.0 ☑
  knife X78.1 ☑
  specified NEC X78.8 ☑
  sword X78.2 ☑
drowning (in) X71.9 ☑
  bathtub X71.0 ☑
  natural water X71.3 ☑
  specified NEC X71.8 ☑
  swimming pool X71.1 ☑
   following fall X71.2 ☑
electrocution X83.1 ☑
explosive(s) (material) X75 ☑
fire, flames X76 ☑
firearm X74.9 ☑
  airgun X74.01 ☑
  handgun X72 ☑
  hunting rifle X73.1 ☑
  larger X73.9 ☑
   specified NEC X73.8 ☑
  machine gun X73.2 ☑
  shotgun X73.0 ☑
  specified NEC X74.8 ☑
hanging X83.8 ☑
hot object — *see* Suicide, burning, hot object
jumping
  before moving object X81.8 ☑
   motor vehicle X81.0 ☑
   subway train X81.1 ☑
   train X81.1 ☑
  from high place X80 ☑
late effect of attempt — *see* X71-X83 with 7th character S
lying before moving object, train, vehicle X81.8 ☑
poisoning — *see* Table of Drugs and Chemicals
puncture (any part of body) — *see* Suicide, cutting or piercing instrument
scald — *see* Suicide, burning, hot object
sequelae of attempt — *see* X71-X83 with 7th character S
sharp object (any) — *see* Suicide, cutting or piercing instrument
shooting — *see* Suicide, firearm
specified means NEC X83.8 ☑
stab (any part of body) — *see* Suicide, cutting or piercing instrument
steam, hot vapors X77.0 ☑
strangulation X83.8 ☑
submersion — *see* Suicide, drowning
suffocation X83.8 ☑
wound NEC X83.8 ☑
Sunstroke X32 ☑
Supersonic waves (causing injury) W42.0 ☑
Surgical procedure, complication of (delayed or as an abnormal reaction without mention of misadventure) — *see also* Complication of or following, by type of procedure
due to or as a result of misadventure — *see* Misadventure
Swallowed, swallowing
foreign body — *see* Foreign body, alimentary canal
poison — *see* Table of Drugs and Chemicals
substance
  caustic or corrosive — *see* Table of Drugs and Chemicals
  poisonous — *see* Table of Drugs and Chemicals

T

Tackle in sport W03 ☑
Terrorism (involving) Y38.80 ☑
biological weapons Y38.6X- ☑
chemical weapons Y38.7X- ☑
conflagration Y38.3X- ☑
drowning and submersion Y38.89- ☑
explosion Y38.2X- ☑

Terrorism — *continued*
  explosion — *continued*
    destruction of aircraft Y38.1X- ☑
    marine weapons Y38.0X- ☑
  fire Y38.3X- ☑
  firearms Y38.4X- ☑
  hot substances Y38.3X- ☑
  lasers Y38.89- ☑
  nuclear weapons Y38.5X- ☑
  piercing or stabbing instruments Y38.89- ☑
  secondary effects Y38.9X- ☑
  specified method NEC Y38.89- ☑
  suicide bomber Y38.81- ☑
Thirst X58 ☑
Threat to breathing
  aspiration — *see* Aspiration
  due to cave-in, falling earth or substance NEC T71 ☑
Thrown (accidentally)
  against part (any) of or object in transport vehicle (in motion) NEC — *see also* Accident, transport
  from
    high place, homicide (attempt) Y01 ☑
    machinery — *see* Contact, with, by type of machine
    transport vehicle NEC — *see also* Accident, transport V89.9 ☑
  off — *see* Thrown, from
Thunderbolt — *see* subcategory T75.0 ☑
  causing fire — *see* Exposure, fire
Tidal wave (any injury) **NEC** — *see* Forces of nature, tidal wave
Took
  overdose (drug) — *see* Table of Drugs and Chemicals
  poison — *see* Table of Drugs and Chemicals
Tornado (any injury) X37.1 ☑
Torrential rain (any injury) X37.8 ☑
Torture X58 ☑
Trampled by animal NEC W55.89 ☑
Trapped (accidentally)
  between objects (moving) (stationary and moving) — *see* Caught
  by part (any) of
    motorcycle V29.88 ☑
    pedal cycle V19.88 ☑
    transport vehicle NEC — *see also* Accident, transport V89.9 ☑
Travel (effects) (sickness) T75.3 ☑
Tree falling on or hitting (accidentally) (person) W20.8 ☑
Tripping
  over
    animal W01.0 ☑
      with fall W01.0 ☑
    carpet, rug or (small) object W22.8 ☑
      with fall W18.09 ☑
    person W51 ☑
      with fall W03 ☑
        due to ice or snow W00.0 ☑
  without fall W18.40 ☑
    due to
      specified NEC W18.49 ☑
      stepping from one level to another W18.43 ☑
      stepping into hole or opening W18.42 ☑
      stepping on object W18.41 ☑
Twisted by person(s) (accidentally) W50.2 ☑
  with intent to injure or kill Y04.0 ☑
  as, or caused by, a crowd or human stampede (with fall) W52 ☑
  assault Y04.0 ☑
  homicide (attempt) Y04.0 ☑
  in
    fight Y04.0 ☑
    legal intervention — *see* Legal, intervention, manhandling
Twisting (prolonged) (static) X50.1- ☑

U

Underdosing of necessary drugs, medicaments or biological substances Y63.6
Undetermined intent (contact) (exposure)
  automobile collision Y32 ☑
  blunt object Y29 ☑
  drowning (submersion) (in) Y21.9 ☑
    bathtub Y21.0 ☑
      after fall Y21.1 ☑

Undetermined intent — *continued*
  drowning — *continued*
    natural water (lake) (ocean) (pond) (river) (stream) Y21.4 ☑
    specified place NEC Y21.8 ☑
    swimming pool Y21.2 ☑
      after fall Y21.3 ☑
  explosive material Y25 ☑
  fall, jump or push from high place Y30 ☑
  falling, lying or running before moving object Y31 ☑
  fire Y26 ☑
  firearm discharge Y24.9 ☑
    airgun (BB) (pellet) Y24.0 ☑
    handgun (pistol) (revolver) Y22 ☑
    hunting rifle Y23.1 ☑
    larger Y23.9 ☑
      hunting rifle Y23.1 ☑
      machine gun Y23.3 ☑
      military Y23.2 ☑
      shotgun Y23.0 ☑
      specified type NEC Y23.8 ☑
    machine gun Y23.3 ☑
    military Y23.2 ☑
    shotgun Y23.0 ☑
    specified type NEC Y24.8 ☑
    Very pistol Y24.8 ☑
  hot object Y27.9 ☑
    fluid NEC Y27.2 ☑
    household appliance Y27.3 ☑
    specified object NEC Y27.8 ☑
    steam Y27.0 ☑
    tap water Y27.1 ☑
    vapor Y27.0 ☑
  jump, fall or push from high place Y30 ☑
  lying, falling or running before moving object Y31 ☑
  motor vehicle crash Y32 ☑
  push, fall or jump from high place Y30 ☑
  running, falling or lying before moving object Y31 ☑
  sharp object Y28.9 ☑
    dagger Y28.2 ☑
    glass Y28.0 ☑
    knife Y28.1 ☑
    specified object NEC Y28.8 ☑
    sword Y28.2 ☑
  smoke Y26 ☑
  specified event NEC Y33 ☑
Use of hand as hammer X50.3 ☑

V

Vibration (causing injury) W49.9 ☑
Victim (of)
  avalanche — *see* Landslide
  earth movements NEC — *see* Forces of nature, earth movement
  earthquake X34 ☑
  flood — *see* Flood
  landslide — *see* Landslide
  lightning — *see* subcategory T75.0 ☑
    causing fire — *see* Exposure, fire
  storm (cataclysmic) NEC — *see* Forces of nature, cataclysmic storm
  volcanic eruption X35 ☑
Volcanic eruption (any injury) X35 ☑
Vomitus, gastric contents in air passages (with asphyxia, obstruction or suffocation) T17.81- ☑

W

Walked into stationary object (any) W22.09 ☑
  furniture W22.03 ☑
  lamppost W22.02 ☑
  wall W22.01 ☑
War operations (injuries to military personnel and civilians during war, civil insurrection and peacekeeping missions) (by) (from) (involving) Y36.90 ☑
  after cessation of hostilities Y36.89- ☑
    explosion (of)
      bomb placed during war operations Y36.82- ☑
      mine placed during war operations Y36.81- ☑
    specified NEC Y36.88- ☑
  air blast Y36.20- ☑
  aircraft
    destruction — *see* War operations, destruction of aircraft

War operations — *continued*
  airway restriction — *see* War operations, restriction of airways
  asphyxiation — *see* War operations, restriction of airways
  biological weapons Y36.6X- ☑
  blast Y36.20- ☑
  blast fragments Y36.20- ☑
  blast wave Y36.20- ☑
  blast wind Y36.20- ☑
  bomb Y36.20- ☑
    dirty Y36.50- ☑
    gasoline Y36.31- ☑
    incendiary Y36.31- ☑
    petrol Y36.31- ☑
  bullet Y36.43- ☑
    incendiary Y36.32- ☑
    rubber Y36.41- ☑
  chemical weapons Y36.7X- ☑
  combat
    hand to hand (unarmed) combat Y36.44- ☑
    using blunt or piercing object Y36.45- ☑
  conflagration — *see* War operations, fire
  conventional warfare NEC Y36.49- ☑
  depth-charge Y36.01- ☑
  destruction of aircraft Y36.10- ☑
    due to
      air to air missile Y36.11- ☑
      collision with other aircraft Y36.12- ☑
      detonation (accidental) of onboard munitions and explosives Y36.14- ☑
      enemy fire or explosives Y36.11- ☑
      explosive placed on aircraft Y36.11- ☑
      onboard fire Y36.13- ☑
      rocket propelled grenade [RPG] Y36.11- ☑
      small arms fire Y36.11- ☑
      surface to air missile Y36.11- ☑
    specified NEC Y36.19- ☑
  detonation (accidental) of
    onboard marine weapons Y36.05- ☑
    own munitions or munitions launch device Y36.24- ☑
  dirty bomb Y36.50- ☑
  explosion (of) Y36.20- ☑
    aerial bomb Y36.21- ☑
    after cessation of hostilities
      bomb placed during war operations Y36.82- ☑
      mine placed during war operations Y36.81- ☑
    bomb NOS — *see also* War operations, bomb(s) Y36.20- ☑
    fragments Y36.20- ☑
    grenade Y36.29- ☑
    guided missile Y36.22- ☑
    improvised explosive device [IED] (person-borne) (roadside) (vehicle-borne) Y36.23- ☑
    land mine Y36.29- ☑
    marine mine (at sea) (in harbor) Y36.02- ☑
    marine weapon Y36.00- ☑
      specified NEC Y36.09- ☑
    own munitions or munitions launch device (accidental) Y36.24- ☑
    sea-based artillery shell Y36.03- ☑
    specified NEC Y36.29- ☑
    torpedo Y36.04- ☑
  fire Y36.30- ☑
    specified NEC Y36.39- ☑
  firearms
    discharge Y36.43- ☑
    pellets Y36.42- ☑
  flamethrower Y36.33- ☑
  fragments (from) (of)
    improvised explosive device [IED] (person-borne) (roadside) (vehicle-borne) Y36.26- ☑
    munitions Y36.25- ☑
    specified NEC Y36.29- ☑
    weapons Y36.27- ☑
  friendly fire Y36.92 ☑
  hand to hand (unarmed) combat Y36.44- ☑
  hot substances — *see* War operations, fire
  incendiary bullet Y36.32- ☑
  nuclear weapon (effects of) Y36.50- ☑
    acute radiation exposure Y36.54- ☑
    blast pressure Y36.51- ☑
    direct blast Y36.51- ☑
    direct heat Y36.53- ☑
    fallout exposure Y36.54- ☑

War operations — *continued*
  nuclear weapon — *continued*
    fireball Y36.53- ☑
    indirect blast (struck or crushed by blast debris)
      (being thrown by blast) Y36.52- ☑
    ionizing radiation (immediate exposure) Y36.54- ☑
    nuclear radiation Y36.54- ☑
    radiation
      ionizing (immediate exposure) Y36.54- ☑
      nuclear Y36.54- ☑
      thermal Y36.53- ☑
    secondary effects Y36.54- ☑
    specified NEC Y36.59- ☑
    thermal radiation Y36.53- ☑
  restriction of air (airway)
    intentional Y36.46- ☑
    unintentional Y36.47- ☑
  rubber bullets Y36.41- ☑
  shrapnel NOS Y36.29- ☑
  suffocation — *see* War operations, restriction of airways
  unconventional warfare NEC Y36.7X- ☑
  underwater blast NOS Y36.00- ☑

War operations — *continued*
  warfare
    conventional NEC Y36.49- ☑
    unconventional NEC Y36.7X- ☑
  weapon of mass destruction [WMD] Y36.91 ☑
  weapons
    biological weapons Y36.6X- ☑
    chemical Y36.7X- ☑
    nuclear (effects of) Y36.50- ☑
      acute radiation exposure Y36.54- ☑
      blast pressure Y36.51- ☑
      direct blast Y36.51- ☑
      direct heat Y36.53- ☑
      fallout exposure Y36.54- ☑
      fireball Y36.53- ☑
      radiation
        ionizing (immediate exposure) Y36.54- ☑
        nuclear Y36.54- ☑
        thermal Y36.53- ☑
      secondary effects Y36.54- ☑
      specified NEC Y36.59- ☑

War operations — *continued*
  weapons — *continued*
    of mass destruction [WMD] Y36.91 ☑
Washed
  away by flood — *see* Flood
  off road by storm (transport vehicle) — *see* Forces of
    nature, cataclysmic storm
Weather exposure NEC — *see* Forces of nature
Weightlessness (causing injury) (effects of) (in spacecraft,
  real or simulated) X52 ☑
Work related condition Y99.0
Wound (accidental) NEC — *see also* Injury X58 ☑
  battle — *see also* War operations Y36.90 ☑
  gunshot — *see* Discharge, firearm by type
Wreck transport vehicle NEC — *see also* Accident,
  transport V89.9 ☑
Wrong
  device implanted into correct surgical site Y65.51
  fluid in infusion Y65.1
  patient, procedure performed on Y65.52
  procedure (operation) on correct patient Y65.51

ICD-10-CM Tabular List of Diseases and Injuries

Chapter 1. Certain Infectious and Parasitic Diseases (A00–B99)

Chapter-specific Guidelines with Coding Examples

The chapter-specific guidelines from the ICD-10-CM Official Guidelines for Coding and Reporting have been provided below. Along with these guidelines are coding examples, contained in the shaded boxes, that have been developed to help illustrate the coding and/or sequencing guidance found in these guidelines.

a. Human immunodeficiency virus (HIV) infections

1) Code only confirmed cases

Code only confirmed cases of HIV infection/illness. This is an exception to the hospital inpatient guideline Section II, H.

In this context, "confirmation" does not require documentation of positive serology or culture for HIV; the provider's diagnostic statement that the patient is HIV positive, or has an HIV-related illness is sufficient.

> Patient admitted with anemia with possible HIV infection
>
> **D64.9   Anemia, unspecified**
>
> *Explanation:* Only the anemia is coded in this scenario because it has not been confirmed that an HIV infection is present. This is an exception to the guideline Section II, H for hospital inpatient coding.

2) Selection and sequencing of HIV codes

(a) Patient admitted for HIV-related condition

If a patient is admitted for an HIV-related condition, the principal diagnosis should be B20, Human immunodeficiency virus [HIV] disease followed by additional diagnosis codes for all reported HIV-related conditions.

> HIV with PCP
>
> **B20   Human immunodeficiency virus [HIV] disease**
>
> **B59   Pneumocystosis**
>
> *Explanation:* Pneumonia due to *Pneumocystis carinii* is an HIV related condition, so the HIV diagnosis code is reported first, followed by the code for the pneumonia.

(b) Patient with HIV disease admitted for unrelated condition

If a patient with HIV disease is admitted for an unrelated condition (such as a traumatic injury), the code for the unrelated condition (e.g., the nature of injury code) should be the principal diagnosis. Other diagnoses would be B20 followed by additional diagnosis codes for all reported HIV-related conditions.

> Unstable angina, native coronary artery atherosclerosis, HIV
>
> **I25.110   Atherosclerotic heart disease of native coronary artery with unstable angina pectoris**
>
> **B20   Human immunodeficiency virus [HIV] disease**
>
> *Explanation:* The arteriosclerotic coronary artery disease and the unstable angina are not related to HIV, so those conditions are reported first using a combination code, and HIV is reported secondarily.

(c) Whether the patient is newly diagnosed

Whether the patient is newly diagnosed or has had previous admissions/encounters for HIV conditions is irrelevant to the sequencing decision.

> Newly diagnosed multiple cutaneous Kaposi's sarcoma lesions in previously diagnosed HIV disease
>
> **B20   Human immunodeficiency virus [HIV] disease**
>
> **C46.0   Kaposi's sarcoma of skin**
>
> *Explanation:* Even though the HIV was diagnosed on a previous encounter, it is still sequenced first when coded with an HIV related condition. Kaposi's sarcoma is an HIV-related condition.

(d) Asymptomatic human immunodeficiency virus

Z21, Asymptomatic human immunodeficiency virus [HIV] infection status, is to be applied when the patient without any documentation of symptoms is listed as being "HIV positive," "known HIV," "HIV test positive," or similar terminology. Do not use this code if the term "AIDS" is used or if the patient is treated for any HIV-related illness or is described as having any condition(s) resulting from his/her HIV positive status; use B20 in these cases.

> Patient admitted with acute appendicitis. Status positive HIV test on Atripla, with no prior symptoms
>
> **K35.80   Unspecified acute appendicitis**
>
> **Z21   Asymptomatic human immunodeficiency virus [HIV] infection status**
>
> *Explanation:* Code Z21 is sequenced second since documentation indicates that the patient has had a positive HIV test but has been asymptomatic. Being on medication for HIV is not an indication that code B20 is used instead of Z21. Unless there has been documentation that the patient has had current or prior symptoms or HIV-related complications, code B20 is not used. The appendicitis is not an AIDS-related complication and is sequenced first.

(e) Patients with inconclusive HIV serology

Patients with inconclusive HIV serology, but no definitive diagnosis or manifestations of the illness, may be assigned code R75, Inconclusive laboratory evidence of human immunodeficiency virus [HIV].

(f) Previously diagnosed HIV-related illness

Patients with any known prior diagnosis of an HIV-related illness should be coded to B20. Once a patient has developed an HIV-related illness, the patient should always be assigned code B20 on every subsequent admission/encounter. Patients previously diagnosed with any HIV illness (B20) should never be assigned to R75 or Z21, Asymptomatic human immunodeficiency virus [HIV] infection status.

(g) HIV infection in pregnancy, childbirth and the puerperium

During pregnancy, childbirth or the puerperium, a patient admitted (or presenting for a health care encounter) because of an HIV-related illness should receive a principal diagnosis code of O98.7-, Human immunodeficiency [HIV] disease complicating pregnancy, childbirth and the puerperium, followed by B20 and the code(s) for the HIV-related illness(es). Codes from Chapter 15 always take sequencing priority.

Patients with asymptomatic HIV infection status admitted (or presenting for a health care encounter) during pregnancy, childbirth, or the puerperium should receive codes of O98.7- and Z21.

(h) Encounters for testing for HIV

If a patient is being seen to determine his/her HIV status, use code Z11.4, Encounter for screening for human immunodeficiency virus [HIV]. Use additional codes for any associated high risk behavior.

If a patient with signs or symptoms is being seen for HIV testing, code the signs and symptoms. An additional counseling code Z71.7, Human immunodeficiency virus [HIV] counseling, may be used if counseling is provided during the encounter for the test.

When a patient returns to be informed of his/her HIV test results and the test result is negative, use code Z71.7, Human immunodeficiency virus [HIV] counseling.

If the results are positive, see previous guidelines and assign codes as appropriate.

b. Infectious agents as the cause of diseases classified to other chapters

Certain infections are classified in chapters other than Chapter 1 and no organism is identified as part of the infection code. In these instances, it is necessary to use an additional code from Chapter 1 to identify the organism. A code from category B95, Streptococcus, Staphylococcus, and Enterococcus as the cause of diseases classified to other chapters, B96, Other bacterial agents as the cause of diseases classified to other chapters, or B97, Viral agents as the cause of diseases classified to other chapters, is to be used as an additional code to identify the organism. An instructional note will be found at the infection code advising that an additional organism code is required.

E. coli UTI

N39.0	**Urinary tract infection, site not specified**
B96.20	**Unspecified Escherichia coli [E.coli] as the cause of diseases classified elsewhere**

Explanation: An instructional note under the code for the urinary tract infection indicates to code also the specific organism.

c. Infections resistant to antibiotics

Many bacterial infections are resistant to current antibiotics. It is necessary to identify all infections documented as antibiotic resistant. Assign a code from category Z16, Resistance to antimicrobial drugs, following the infection code only if the infection code does not identify drug resistance.

d. Sepsis, severe sepsis, and septic shock

1) Coding of sepsis and severe sepsis

(a) Sepsis

For a diagnosis of sepsis, assign the appropriate code for the underlying systemic infection. If the type of infection or causal organism is not further specified, assign code A41.9, Sepsis, unspecified organism.

A code from subcategory R65.2, Severe sepsis, should not be assigned unless severe sepsis or an associated acute organ dysfunction is documented.

(i) Negative or inconclusive blood cultures and sepsis

Negative or inconclusive blood cultures do not preclude a diagnosis of sepsis in patients with clinical evidence of the condition; however, the provider should be queried.

(ii) Urosepsis

The term urosepsis is a nonspecific term. It is not to be considered synonymous with sepsis. It has no default code in the Alphabetic Index. Should a provider use this term, he/she must be queried for clarification.

(iii) Sepsis with organ dysfunction

If a patient has sepsis and associated acute organ dysfunction or multiple organ dysfunction (MOD), follow the instructions for coding severe sepsis.

(iv) Acute organ dysfunction that is not clearly associated with the sepsis

If a patient has sepsis and an acute organ dysfunction, but the medical record documentation indicates that the acute organ dysfunction is related to a medical condition other than the sepsis, do not assign a code from subcategory R65.2, Severe sepsis. An acute organ dysfunction must be associated with the sepsis in order to assign the severe sepsis code. If the documentation is not clear as to whether an acute organ dysfunction is related to the sepsis or another medical condition, query the provider.

Sepsis and acute respiratory failure due to COPD exacerbation

A41.9	**Sepsis, unspecified organism**
J44.1	**Chronic obstructive pulmonary disease with (acute) exacerbation**
J96.00	**Acute respiratory failure, unspecified whether with hypoxia or hypercapnia**

Explanation: Although acute organ dysfunction is present in the form of acute respiratory failure, severe sepsis (R65.2) is not coded in this example, as the acute respiratory failure is attributed to the COPD exacerbation rather than the sepsis. Sequencing of these codes would be determined by the circumstances of the admission.

(b) Severe sepsis

The coding of severe sepsis requires a minimum of 2 codes: first a code for the underlying systemic infection, followed by a code from subcategory R65.2, Severe sepsis. If the causal organism is not documented, assign code A41.9, Sepsis, unspecified organism, for the infection. Additional code(s) for the associated acute organ dysfunction are also required.

Due to the complex nature of severe sepsis, some cases may require querying the provider prior to assignment of the codes.

2) Septic shock

(a) Septic shock generally refers to circulatory failure associated with severe sepsis, and therefore, it represents a type of acute organ dysfunction.

For cases of septic shock, the code for the systemic infection should be sequenced first, followed by code R65.21, Severe sepsis with septic shock or code T81.12, Postprocedural septic shock. Any additional codes for the other acute organ dysfunctions should also be assigned. As noted in the sequencing instructions in the Tabular List, the code for septic shock cannot be assigned as a principal diagnosis.

Sepsis with septic shock

A41.9	**Sepsis, unspecified organism**
R65.21	**Severe sepsis with septic shock**

Explanation: Documentation of septic shock automatically implies severe sepsis as it is a form of acute organ dysfunction. Septic shock is not coded as the principal diagnosis; it is always preceded by the code for the systemic infection.

3) Sequencing of severe sepsis

If severe sepsis is present on admission, and meets the definition of principal diagnosis, the underlying systemic infection should be assigned as principal diagnosis followed by the appropriate code from subcategory R65.2 as required by the sequencing rules in the Tabular List. A code from subcategory R65.2 can never be assigned as a principal diagnosis. When severe sepsis develops during an encounter (it was not present on admission), the underlying systemic infection and the appropriate code from subcategory R65.2 should be assigned as secondary diagnoses. Severe sepsis may be present on admission, but the diagnosis may not be confirmed until sometime after admission. If the documentation is not clear whether severe sepsis was present on admission, the provider should be queried.

4) Sepsis *or* severe sepsis with a localized infection

If the reason for admission is sepsis or severe sepsis and a localized infection, such as pneumonia or cellulitis, a code(s) for the underlying systemic infection should be assigned first and the code for the localized infection should be assigned as a secondary diagnosis. If the patient has severe sepsis, a code from subcategory R65.2 should also be assigned as a secondary diagnosis. If the patient is admitted with a localized infection, such as pneumonia, and sepsis/severe sepsis doesn't develop until after admission, the localized infection should be assigned first, followed by the appropriate sepsis/severe sepsis codes.

Patient presents with acute renal failure due to severe sepsis from *Pseudomonas* pneumonia

A41.52	**Sepsis due to Pseudomonas**
J15.1	**Pneumonia due to Pseudomonas**
R65.20	**Severe sepsis without septic shock**
N17.9	**Acute kidney failure, unspecified**

Explanation: If all conditions are present on admission, the systemic infection (sepsis) is sequenced first followed by the codes for the localized infection (pneumonia), severe sepsis and any organ dysfunction. If only the pneumonia was present on admission with the sepsis and resulting renal failure developing later in the admission, then the pneumonia would be sequenced first.

5) Sepsis due to a postprocedural infection

(a) Documentation of causal relationship

As with all postprocedural complications, code assignment is based on the provider's documentation of the relationship between the infection and the procedure.

(b) Sepsis due to a postprocedural infection

For infections following a procedure, a code from T81.40, to T81.43 Infection following a procedure, or a code from O86.00 to O86.03, Infection of obstetric surgical wound, that identifies the site of the infection should be coded first, if known. Assign an additional code for sepsis following a procedure (T81.44) or sepsis following an obstetrical procedure (O86.04). Use an additional code to identify the infectious agent. If the patient has severe sepsis, the appropriate code from subcategory R65.2 should also be assigned with the additional code(s) for any acute organ dysfunction.

For infections following infusion, transfusion, therapeutic injection, or immunization, a code from subcategory T80.2, Infections following infusion, transfusion, and therapeutic injection, or code T88.0-, Infection following immunization, should be coded first, followed by the code for the specific infection. If the patient has severe sepsis, the appropriate code from subcategory R65.2 should also be assigned, with the additional codes(s) for any acute organ dysfunction.

(c) Postprocedural infection and postprocedural septic shock

If a postprocedural infection has resulted in postprocedural septic shock, assign the codes indicated above for sepsis due to a postprocedural infection, followed by code T81.12-, Postprocedural septic shock. Do not assign code R65.21, Severe sepsis with septic shock. Additional code(s) should be assigned for any acute organ dysfunction.

Septic shock following abdominal procedure with intramuscular abscess

T81.42XA	**Infection following a procedure, deep incisional surgical site, initial encounter**
T81.44XA	**Sepsis following a procedure, initial encounter**
A41.9	**Sepsis, unspecified organism**
T81.12XA	**Postprocedural septic shock, initial encounter**

Explanation: The first code reported identifies the site of the postprocedural infection with intramuscular abscess coded to "deep incisional surgical site." If sepsis occurred as a result of the postprocedural infection, code T81.44- should be coded as a secondary diagnosis, followed by a code for the specific type of sepsis. Postprocedural septic shock is captured by code T81.12- and not with code R65.21. If any other acute organ dysfunction was documented as associated with the postprocedural sepsis, additional codes could be assigned to represent those conditions.

6) Sepsis and severe sepsis associated with a noninfectious process (condition)

In some cases a noninfectious process (condition), such as trauma, may lead to an infection which can result in sepsis or severe sepsis. If sepsis or severe sepsis is documented as associated with a noninfectious condition, such as a burn or serious injury, and this condition meets the definition for principal diagnosis, the code for the noninfectious condition should be sequenced first, followed by the code for the resulting infection. If severe sepsis is present, a code from subcategory R65.2 should also be assigned with any associated organ dysfunction(s) codes. It is not necessary to assign a code from subcategory R65.1, Systemic inflammatory response syndrome (SIRS) of non-infectious origin, for these cases.

If the infection meets the definition of principal diagnosis, it should be sequenced before the non-infectious condition. When both the associated non-infectious condition and the infection meet the definition of principal diagnosis, either may be assigned as principal diagnosis.

Only one code from category R65, Symptoms and signs specifically associated with systemic inflammation and infection, should be assigned. Therefore, when a non-infectious condition leads to an infection resulting in severe sepsis, assign the appropriate code from subcategory R65.2, Severe sepsis. Do not additionally assign a code from subcategory R65.1, Systemic inflammatory response syndrome (SIRS) of non-infectious origin.

See Section I.C.18. SIRS due to non-infectious process

Patient admitted with multiple third-degree burns of right upper arm develops severe MSSA sepsis with septic shock, three days into admission

T22.391A	**Burn of third degree of multiple sites of right shoulder and upper arm limb, except wrist and hand, initial encounter**
A41.01	**Sepsis due to Methicillin susceptible Staphylococcus aureus**
R65.21	**Severe sepsis with septic shock**

Explanation: Severe sepsis is coded rather than SIRS from R65 because it is documented as a severe systemic infectious response with septic shock to a noninfectious condition. The code for the systemic infection is not used as the principal diagnosis because it was not present on admission. The patient was admitted for the burn injury.

7) Sepsis and septic shock complicating abortion, pregnancy, childbirth, and the puerperium

See Section I.C.15. Sepsis and septic shock complicating abortion, pregnancy, childbirth and the puerperium

8) Newborn sepsis

See Section I.C.16. f. Bacterial sepsis of Newborn

e. Methicillin resistant Staphylococcus aureus (MRSA) conditions

1) Selection and sequencing of MRSA codes

(a) Combination codes for MRSA infection

When a patient is diagnosed with an infection that is due to methicillin resistant *Staphylococcus aureus* (MRSA), and that infection has a combination code that includes the causal organism (e.g., sepsis, pneumonia) assign the appropriate combination code for the condition (e.g., code A41.02, Sepsis due to Methicillin resistant Staphylococcus aureus or code J15.212, Pneumonia due to Methicillin resistant Staphylococcus aureus). Do not assign code B95.62, Methicillin resistant Staphylococcus aureus infection as the cause of diseases classified elsewhere, as an additional code, because the combination code includes the type of infection and the MRSA organism. Do not assign a code from subcategory Z16.11, Resistance to penicillins, as an additional diagnosis.

See Section C.1. for instructions on coding and sequencing of sepsis and severe sepsis.

(b) Other codes for MRSA infection

When there is documentation of a current infection (e.g., wound infection, stitch abscess, urinary tract infection) due to MRSA, and that infection does not have a combination code that includes the causal organism, assign the appropriate code to identify the condition along with code B95.62, Methicillin resistant Staphylococcus aureus infection as the cause of diseases classified elsewhere for the MRSA infection. Do not assign a code from subcategory Z16.11, Resistance to penicillins.

(c) Methicillin susceptible Staphylococcus aureus (MSSA) and MRSA colonization

The condition or state of being colonized or carrying MSSA or MRSA is called colonization or carriage, while an individual person is described as being colonized or being a carrier. Colonization means that MSSA or MSRA is present on or in the body without necessarily causing illness. A positive MRSA colonization test might be documented by the provider as "MRSA screen positive" or "MRSA nasal swab positive".

Assign code Z22.322, Carrier or suspected carrier of Methicillin resistant Staphylococcus aureus, for patients documented as having MRSA colonization. Assign code Z22.321, Carrier or suspected carrier of Methicillin susceptible Staphylococcus aureus, for patients documented as having MSSA colonization. Colonization is not necessarily indicative of a disease process or as the cause of a specific condition the patient may have unless documented as such by the provider.

(d) MRSA colonization and infection

If a patient is documented as having both MRSA colonization and infection during a hospital admission, code Z22.322, Carrier or suspected carrier of Methicillin resistant Staphylococcus aureus, and a code for the MRSA infection may both be assigned.

f. Zika virus infections

1) Code only confirmed cases

Code only a confirmed diagnosis of Zika virus (A92.5, Zika virus disease) as documented by the provider. This is an exception to the hospital inpatient guideline Section II, H. In this context, "confirmation" does not require documentation of the type of test performed; the **provider's** diagnostic statement that the condition is confirmed is sufficient. This code should be assigned regardless of the stated mode of transmission.

If the provider documents "suspected", "possible" or "probable" Zika, do not assign code A92.5. Assign a code(s) explaining the reason for encounter (such as fever, rash, or joint pain) or Z20.821, Contact with and (suspected) exposure to Zika virus.

A 45-year-old female recently returned from a Caribbean vacation complaining of fever, headache, joint and muscle aches and is admitted for suspected influenza. Infectious Disease consult diagnoses Zika virus. Patient discharged with Zika virus disease and instructions for hydration, rest, acetaminophen, and follow-up with Infectious Disease.

A92.5	**Zika virus disease**

Explanation: Although only a confirmed diagnosis should be coded, when a provider documents a diagnosis of Zika virus, code A92.5 Zika virus disease, is reported whether or not there is any indication of the type of tests performed. If the patient is pregnant, code first a code from category O98.5- Other viral diseases complicating pregnancy, childbirth and the puerperium, followed by code (A92.5) for the confirmed Zika virus. See also guideline 1.C.15.a.1.

Chapter 1. Certain Infectious and Parasitic Diseases (A00-B99)

INCLUDES diseases generally recognized as communicable or transmissible
Use additional code to identify resistance to antimicrobial drugs (Z16.-)
EXCLUDES 1 certain localized infections — see body system-related chapters
EXCLUDES 2 carrier or suspected carrier of infectious disease (Z22.-)
infectious and parasitic diseases complicating pregnancy, childbirth and the puerperium (O98.-)
infectious and parasitic diseases specific to the perinatal period (P35-P39)
influenza and other acute respiratory infections (J00-J22)

This chapter contains the following blocks:

A00-A09 Intestinal infectious diseases
A15-A19 Tuberculosis
A20-A28 Certain zoonotic bacterial diseases
A30-A49 Other bacterial diseases
A50-A64 Infections with a predominantly sexual mode of transmission
A65-A69 Other spirochetal diseases
A70-A74 Other diseases caused by chlamydiae
A75-A79 Rickettsioses
A80-A89 Viral and prion infections of the central nervous system
A90-A99 Arthropod-borne viral fevers and viral hemorrhagic fevers
B00-B09 Viral infections characterized by skin and mucous membrane lesions
B10 Other human herpesviruses
B15-B19 Viral hepatitis
B20 Human immunodeficiency virus [HIV] disease
B25-B34 Other viral diseases
B35-B49 Mycoses
B50-B64 Protozoal diseases
B65-B83 Helminthiases
B85-B89 Pediculosis, acariasis and other infestations
B90-B94 Sequelae of infectious and parasitic diseases
B95-B97 Bacterial and viral infectious agents
B99 Other infectious diseases

Intestinal infectious diseases (A00-A09)

✓4ᵗʰ A00 Cholera

DEF: Acute infection of the bowel due to vibrio cholerae that presents with profuse diarrhea, cramps, and vomiting, resulting in severe dehydration, electrolyte imbalance, and death. It is spread through ingestion of food or water contaminated with feces of infected persons.
CC Excl: For CC codes in category A00: PDX collection 2

A00.0 Cholera due to Vibrio cholerae 01, biovar cholerae CC
Classical cholera

A00.1 Cholera due to Vibrio cholerae 01, biovar eltor CC
Cholera eltor

A00.9 Cholera, unspecified CC

✓4ᵗʰ A01 Typhoid and paratyphoid fevers

DEF: Typhoid fever: Acute generalized illness caused by *Salmonella typhi*. Clinical features include fever, headache, abdominal pain, cough, toxemia, leukopenia, abnormal pulse, rose spots on the skin, bacteremia, hyperplasia of intestinal lymph nodes, mesentery lymphadenopathy, and Peyer's patches in the intestines.
DEF: Paratyphoid fever: Prolonged febrile illness, caused by *Salmonella* serotypes other than *S. typhi*, especially *S. enterica* serotypes paratyphi A, B, and C.
CC Excl: For CC codes in category A01: PDX collection 3

✓5ᵗʰ A01.0 Typhoid fever
Infection due to Salmonella typhi

A01.00 Typhoid fever, unspecified CC

A01.01 Typhoid meningitis CC

A01.02 Typhoid fever with heart involvement CC
Typhoid endocarditis
Typhoid myocarditis

A01.03 Typhoid pneumonia CC HCC

A01.04 Typhoid arthritis CC HCC

A01.05 Typhoid osteomyelitis CC HCC

A01.09 Typhoid fever with other complications CC

A01.1 Paratyphoid fever A CC

A01.2 Paratyphoid fever B CC

A01.3 Paratyphoid fever C CC

A01.4 Paratyphoid fever, unspecified CC
Infection due to Salmonella paratyphi NOS

✓4ᵗʰ A02 Other salmonella infections

INCLUDES infection or foodborne intoxication due to any Salmonella species other than S. typhi and S. paratyphi

A02.0 Salmonella enteritis CC
Salmonellosis
TIP: Dehydration (E86.0) is a complication of salmonella enteritis and may be reported separately.
CC Excl: PDX collection 4

A02.1 Salmonella sepsis HIV MCC HCC
CC Excl: PDX collection 5

✓5ᵗʰ A02.2 Localized salmonella infections

A02.20 Localized salmonella infection, unspecified HIV

A02.21 Salmonella meningitis HIV MCC
CC Excl: PDX collection 6

A02.22 Salmonella pneumonia HIV MCC HCC
CC Excl: PDX collection 7

A02.23 Salmonella arthritis HIV CC HCC
CC Excl: PDX collection 8

A02.24 Salmonella osteomyelitis HIV CC HCC
CC Excl: PDX collection 9

A02.25 Salmonella pyelonephritis HIV CC
Salmonella tubulo-interstitial nephropathy
CC Excl: PDX collection 10

A02.29 Salmonella with other localized infection HIV CC
CC Excl: PDX collection 10

A02.8 Other specified salmonella infections HIV CC
CC Excl: PDX collection 11

A02.9 Salmonella infection, unspecified HIV CC
CC Excl: PDX collection 12

✓4ᵗʰ A03 Shigellosis

DEF: Infection caused by the genus the *Shigella*, of the family *Enterobacteriaceae* that is known to cause an acute dysenteric infection of the bowel with fever, drowsiness, anorexia, nausea, vomiting, bloody diarrhea, abdominal cramps, and distention.

A03.0 Shigellosis due to Shigella dysenteriae CC
Group A shigellosis [Shiga-Kruse dysentery]
CC Excl: PDX collection 13

A03.1 Shigellosis due to Shigella flexneri
Group B shigellosis

A03.2 Shigellosis due to Shigella boydii
Group C shigellosis

A03.3 Shigellosis due to Shigella sonnei
Group D shigellosis

A03.8 Other shigellosis

A03.9 Shigellosis, unspecified
Bacillary dysentery NOS

✓4ᵗʰ A04 Other bacterial intestinal infections

EXCLUDES 1 bacterial foodborne intoxications, NEC (A05.-)
tuberculous enteritis (A18.32)
DEF: Escherichia coli: Gram negative, anaerobic of the family *Enterobacteriaceae* found in the large intestine of warm-blooded animals, generally as a nonpathologic entity aiding in digestion. They become pathogenic when an opportunity to grow somewhere outside this relationship presents itself, such as ingestion of fecal contaminated food or water.
CC Excl: For CC codes in category A04, unless otherwise noted:
For codes A04.0-A04.4: PDX collection 14
For codes A04.5-A04.8: PDX collection 15

A04.0 Enteropathogenic Escherichia coli infection CC

A04.1 Enterotoxigenic Escherichia coli infection CC

A04.2 Enteroinvasive Escherichia coli infection CC

A04.3 Enterohemorrhagic Escherichia coli infection CC
DEF: *E. coli* infection penetrating the intestinal mucosa, producing microscopic ulceration and bleeding.

A04.4 Other intestinal Escherichia coli infections CC
Escherichia coli enteritis NOS

A04.5 Campylobacter enteritis CC
TIP: For Guillain-Barre syndrome occurring as a sequela of *Campylobacter enteritis*, assign code G61.0 as the first-listed diagnosis followed by B94.8 for the sequelae.

A04.6 Enteritis due to Yersinia enterocolitica CC
EXCLUDES 1 extraintestinal yersiniosis (A28.2)

✓5ᵗʰ **A04.7 Enterocolitis due to Clostridium difficile**

Foodborne intoxication by Clostridium difficile
Pseudomembraneous colitis
AHA: 2017,4Q,4

A04.71   Enterocolitis due to Clostridium   `CC`
difficile, recurrent

A04.72   Enterocolitis due to Clostridium   `CC`
difficile, not specified as recurrent

A04.8 Other specified bacterial intestinal infections   `CC`

A04.9 Bacterial intestinal infection, unspecified   `CC`

Bacterial enteritis NOS
CC Excl: PDX collection 16

✓4ᵗʰ **A05 Other bacterial foodborne intoxications, not elsewhere classified**

EXCLUDES 1   *Clostridium difficile foodborne intoxication and infection*
(A04.7-)
Escherichia coli infection (A04.0-A04.4)
listeriosis (A32.-)
salmonella foodborne intoxication and infection (A02.-)
toxic effect of noxious foodstuffs (T61-T62)

CC Excl: For CC codes in category A05, unless ortherwise noted: PDX
collection 17

A05.0 Foodborne staphylococcal intoxication   `CC`

TIP: Assign code A04.8 to report a staphylococcal infection when
it is caused by the ingestion of contaminated food but not caused
by *S. aureus* toxins.

A05.1 Botulism food poisoning   `CC`

Botulism NOS
Classical foodborne intoxication due to Clostridium botulinum
EXCLUDES 1   *infant botulism (A48.51)*
wound botulism (A48.52)
DEF: Muscle-paralyzing neurotoxic disease caused by ingesting
pre-formed toxin from the bacterium *Clostridium botulinum*. It
causes vomiting and diarrhea, vision problems, slurred speech,
difficulty swallowing, paralysis, and death.
CC Excl: PDX collection 18

A05.2 Foodborne Clostridium perfringens   `CC`
[Clostridium welchii] intoxication

Enteritis necroticans
Pig-bel
CC Excl: PDX collection 19

A05.3 Foodborne Vibrio parahaemolyticus   `CC`
intoxication

A05.4 Foodborne Bacillus cereus intoxication   `CC`

A05.5 Foodborne Vibrio vulnificus intoxication   `CC`

A05.8 Other specified bacterial foodborne   `CC`
intoxications

A05.9 Bacterial foodborne intoxication, unspecified

✓4ᵗʰ **A06 Amebiasis**

INCLUDES   infection due to Entamoeba histolytica
EXCLUDES 1   *other protozoal intestinal diseases (A07.-)*
EXCLUDES 2   *acanthamebiasis (B60.1-)*
Naegleriasis (B60.2)

DEF: Infection with a single cell protozoan known as the amoeba.
Transmission occurs through ingestion of feces, contaminated food or
water, use of human feces as fertilizer, or person-to-person contact.

A06.0 Acute amebic dysentery   `CC`

Acute amebiasis
Intestinal amebiasis NOS
CC Excl: PDX collection 20

A06.1 Chronic intestinal amebiasis   `CC`

CC Excl: PDX collection 20

A06.2 Amebic nondysenteric colitis   `CC`

CC Excl: PDX collection 21

A06.3 Ameboma of intestine   `CC`

Ameboma NOS
CC Excl: PDX collection 22

A06.4 Amebic liver abscess   `MCC`

Hepatic amebiasis
CC Excl: PDX collection 23

A06.5 Amebic lung abscess   `MCC` `HCC`

Amebic abscess of lung (and liver)
CC Excl: PDX collection 24

A06.6 Amebic brain abscess   `MCC`

Amebic abscess of brain (and liver) (and lung)
CC Excl: PDX collection 25

A06.7 Cutaneous amebiasis

✓5ᵗʰ **A06.8 Amebic infection of other sites**

CC Excl: For CC codes in subcategory A06.8: PDX collection 22

A06.81   Amebic cystitis   `CC`

A06.82   Other amebic genitourinary   `CC`
infections

Amebic balanitis
Amebic vesiculitis
Amebic vulvovaginitis

A06.89   Other amebic infections   `CC`

Amebic appendicitis
Amebic splenic abscess

A06.9 Amebiasis, unspecified

✓4ᵗʰ **A07 Other protozoal intestinal diseases**

DEF: Protozoa: Group comprised of the simplest, single celled organisms,
ranging in size from micro to macroscopic. They can live alone or in
colonies, and do not show any differentiation in tissues. Most are motile
and can live free in nature, but some are parasitic, causing disease in the
variety of hosts they inhabit.

CC Excl: For CC codes in category A07, unless otherwise noted: PDX
collection 26

A07.0 Balantidiasis

Balantidial dysentery

A07.1 Giardiasis [lambliasis]   `CC`

DEF: Infection caused by the flagellate protozoan *Giardia lamblia*
causing gastrointestinal problems such as vomiting, chronic
diarrhea, and weight loss. The most common parasite in the US,
this is usually transmitted by ingesting contaminated water while
in the cyst state and latches onto the wall of the small intestine.

A07.2 Cryptosporidiosis   `CC` `HCC`

DEF: Microscopic parasite found in water and one of the most
common causes of waterborne gastrointestinal infectious disease
in the United States. It is usually transmitted by ingesting
contaminated drinking water or recreational water and causes
profuse watery diarrhea, flatulence, abdominal pain, and
cramping.

A07.3 Isosporiasis   `HIV` `CC`

Infection due to Isospora belli and Isospora hominis
Intestinal coccidiosis
Isosporosis

A07.4 Cyclosporiasis   `CC`

CC Excl: PDX collection 27

A07.8 Other specified protozoal intestinal diseases   `CC`

Intestinal microsporidiosis
Intestinal trichomoniasis
Sarcocystosis
Sarcosporidiosis

A07.9 Protozoal intestinal disease, unspecified   `CC`

Flagellate diarrhea
Protozoal colitis
Protozoal diarrhea
Protozoal dysentery

✓4ᵗʰ **A08 Viral and other specified intestinal infections**

EXCLUDES 1   *influenza with involvement of gastrointestinal tract (J09.X3,*
J10.2, J11.2)

CC Excl: For CC codes in category A08: PDX collection 28

A08.0 Rotaviral enteritis   `CC`

✓5ᵗʰ **A08.1 Acute gastroenteropathy due to Norwalk agent and other**
small round viruses

A08.11   Acute gastroenteropathy due to   `CC`
Norwalk agent

Acute gastroenteropathy due to Norovirus
Acute gastroenteropathy due to Norwalk-like agent

A08.19   Acute gastroenteropathy due to   `CC`
other small round viruses

Acute gastroenteropathy due to small round virus
[SRV] NOS

A08.2 Adenoviral enteritis   `CC`

✓5ᵗʰ **A08.3 Other viral enteritis**

A08.31   Calicivirus enteritis   `CC`

A08.32   Astrovirus enteritis   `CC`

A08.39　Other viral enteritis `CC`
Coxsackie virus enteritis
Echovirus enteritis
Enterovirus enteritis NEC
Torovirus enteritis

A08.4　Viral intestinal infection, unspecified
Viral enteritis NOS
Viral gastroenteritis NOS
Viral gastroenteropathy NOS
AHA: 2016,3Q,12

A08.8　Other specified intestinal infections

A09　Infectious gastroenteritis and colitis, unspecified
Infectious colitis NOS
Infectious enteritis NOS
Infectious gastroenteritis NOS
EXCLUDES 1　colitis NOS (K52.9)
　　　　　　diarrhea NOS (R19.7)
　　　　　　enteritis NOS (K52.9)
　　　　　　gastroenteritis NOS (K52.9)
　　　　　　noninfective gastroenteritis and colitis, unspecified (K52.9)
DEF: Colitis: Inflammation of mucous membranes of the colon.
DEF: Enteritis: Inflammation of mucous membranes of the small intestine.
DEF: Gastroenteritis: Inflammation of mucous membranes of the stomach and intestines.

Tuberculosis (A15-A19)

INCLUDES　infections due to Mycobacterium tuberculosis and Mycobacterium bovis
EXCLUDES 1　congenital tuberculosis (P37.0)
　　　　　　nonspecific reaction to test for tuberculosis without active tuberculosis (R76.1-)
　　　　　　pneumoconiosis associated with tuberculosis, any type in A15 (J65)
　　　　　　positive PPD (R76.11)
　　　　　　positive tuberculin skin test without active tuberculosis (R76.11)
　　　　　　sequelae of tuberculosis (B90.-)
　　　　　　silicotuberculosis (J65)
DEF: Bacterial infection that typically spreads by inhalation of an airborne agent that usually attacks the lungs, but may also affect other organs.

✓4ᵗʰ A15　Respiratory tuberculosis
CC Excl: For CC codes in category A15, unless otherwise noted: PDX collection 29

A15.0　Tuberculosis of lung `HIV` `CC`
Tuberculous bronchiectasis
Tuberculous fibrosis of lung
Tuberculous pneumonia
Tuberculous pneumothorax

Tuberculosis of Lung

Granulomas from Mycobacterium tuberculosis

A15.4　Tuberculosis of intrathoracic lymph nodes `HIV` `CC`
Tuberculosis of hilar lymph nodes
Tuberculosis of mediastinal lymph nodes
Tuberculosis of tracheobronchial lymph nodes
EXCLUDES 1　tuberculosis specified as primary (A15.7)

A15.5　Tuberculosis of larynx, trachea and bronchus `HIV` `CC`
Tuberculosis of bronchus
Tuberculosis of glottis
Tuberculosis of larynx
Tuberculosis of trachea

A15.6　Tuberculous pleurisy `HIV` `CC`
Tuberculosis of pleura Tuberculous empyema
EXCLUDES 1　primary respiratory tuberculosis (A15.7)

A15.7　Primary respiratory tuberculosis `HIV` `CC`
CC Excl: PDX collection 30

A15.8　Other respiratory tuberculosis `HIV` `CC`
Mediastinal tuberculosis
Nasopharyngeal tuberculosis
Tuberculosis of nose
Tuberculosis of sinus [any nasal]
CC Excl: PDX collection 31

A15.9　Respiratory tuberculosis unspecified `HIV` `CC`
CC Excl: PDX collection 31

✓4ᵗʰ A17　Tuberculosis of nervous system

A17.0　Tuberculous meningitis `HIV` `MCC`
Tuberculosis of meninges (cerebral)(spinal)
Tuberculous leptomeningitis
EXCLUDES 1　tuberculous meningoencephalitis (A17.82)
CC Excl: PDX collection 32

A17.1　Meningeal tuberculoma `HIV` `MCC`
Tuberculoma of meninges (cerebral) (spinal)
EXCLUDES 2　tuberculoma of brain and spinal cord (A17.81)
CC Excl: PDX collection 32

✓5ᵗʰ A17.8　Other tuberculosis of nervous system

A17.81　Tuberculoma of brain and spinal cord `HIV` `MCC`
Tuberculous abscess of brain and spinal cord
CC Excl: PDX collection 33

A17.82　Tuberculous meningoencephalitis `HIV` `MCC`
Tuberculous myelitis
CC Excl: PDX collection 33

A17.83　Tuberculous neuritis `HIV` `MCC`
Tuberculous mononeuropathy
CC Excl: No Excl

A17.89　Other tuberculosis of nervous system `HIV` `MCC`
Tuberculous polyneuropathy
CC Excl: PDX collection 34

A17.9　Tuberculosis of nervous system, unspecified `HIV` `CC`
CC Excl: PDX collection 35

✓4ᵗʰ A18　Tuberculosis of other organs

✓5ᵗʰ A18.0　Tuberculosis of bones and joints

A18.01　Tuberculosis of spine `HIV` `CC`
Pott's disease or curvature of spine
Tuberculous arthritis
Tuberculous osteomyelitis of spine
Tuberculous spondylitis
CC Excl: PDX collection 36

A18.02　Tuberculous arthritis of other joints `HIV` `CC`
Tuberculosis of hip (joint)
Tuberculosis of knee (joint)
CC Excl: PDX collection 37

A18.03　Tuberculosis of other bones `HIV` `CC`
Tuberculous mastoiditis
Tuberculous osteomyelitis
CC Excl: PDX collection 38

A18.09　Other musculoskeletal tuberculosis `HIV` `CC`
Tuberculous myositis
Tuberculous synovitis
Tuberculous tenosynovitis
CC Excl: PDX collection 39

✓5ᵗʰ A18.1　Tuberculosis of genitourinary system

A18.10　Tuberculosis of genitourinary system, unspecified `HIV` `CC`
CC Excl: PDX collection 40

A18.11　Tuberculosis of kidney and ureter `HIV` `CC`
CC Excl: PDX collection 41

A18.12 Tuberculosis of bladder   HIV CC
CC Excl: PDX collection 41

A18.13 Tuberculosis of other urinary organs   HIV CC
Tuberculous urethritis
CC Excl: PDX collection 41

A18.14 Tuberculosis of prostate   HIV CC A ♂
CC Excl: PDX collection 42

A18.15 Tuberculosis of other male genital organs   HIV CC ♂
CC Excl: PDX collection 42

A18.16 Tuberculosis of cervix   HIV CC ♀
CC Excl: PDX collection 43

A18.17 Tuberculous female pelvic inflammatory disease   HIV CC ♀
Tuberculous endometritis
Tuberculous oophoritis and salpingitis
CC Excl: PDX collection 43

A18.18 Tuberculosis of other female genital organs   HIV CC ♀
Tuberculous ulceration of vulva
CC Excl: PDX collection 43

A18.2 Tuberculous peripheral lymphadenopathy   HIV CC
Tuberculous adenitis
EXCLUDES 2   tuberculosis of bronchial and mediastinal lymph nodes (A15.4)
tuberculosis of mesenteric and retroperitoneal lymph nodes (A18.39)
tuberculous tracheobronchial adenopathy (A15.4)
CC Excl: PDX collection 44

√5ᵗʰ A18.3 Tuberculosis of intestines, peritoneum and mesenteric glands
CC Excl: For CC/MCC codes in subcategory A18.3: PDX collection 45

A18.31 Tuberculous peritonitis   HIV MCC
Tuberculous ascites
DEF: Tuberculous inflammation of the membrane lining the abdomen.

A18.32 Tuberculous enteritis   HIV CC
Tuberculosis of anus and rectum
Tuberculosis of intestine (large) (small)

A18.39 Retroperitoneal tuberculosis   HIV CC
Tuberculosis of mesenteric glands
Tuberculosis of retroperitoneal (lymph glands)

A18.4 Tuberculosis of skin and subcutaneous tissue   HIV CC
Erythema induratum, tuberculous
Lupus excedens
Lupus vulgaris NOS
Lupus vulgaris of eyelid
Scrofuloderma
Tuberculosis of external ear
EXCLUDES 2   lupus erythematosus (L93.-)
~~lupus NOS (M32.9)~~
▶systemic lupus erythematosus◀ (M32.-)
CC Excl: PDX collection 30

√5ᵗʰ A18.5 Tuberculosis of eye
EXCLUDES 2   lupus vulgaris of eyelid (A18.4)
CC Excl: For CC codes in subcategory A18.5: PDX collection 46

A18.50 Tuberculosis of eye, unspecified   HIV CC

A18.51 Tuberculous episcleritis   HIV CC

A18.52 Tuberculous keratitis   HIV CC
Tuberculous interstitial keratitis
Tuberculous keratoconjunctivitis (interstitial) (phlyctenular)

A18.53 Tuberculous chorioretinitis   HIV CC

A18.54 Tuberculous iridocyclitis   HIV CC

A18.59 Other tuberculosis of eye   HIV CC
Tuberculous conjunctivitis

A18.6 Tuberculosis of (inner) (middle) ear   HIV CC
Tuberculous otitis media
EXCLUDES 2   tuberculosis of external ear (A18.4)
tuberculous mastoiditis (A18.03)
CC Excl: PDX collection 47

A18.7 Tuberculosis of adrenal glands   HIV CC
Tuberculous Addison's disease
CC Excl: PDX collection 48

√5ᵗʰ A18.8 Tuberculosis of other specified organs

A18.81 Tuberculosis of thyroid gland   HIV CC
CC Excl: PDX collection 49

A18.82 Tuberculosis of other endocrine glands   HIV CC
Tuberculosis of pituitary gland
Tuberculosis of thymus gland
CC Excl: PDX collection 35

A18.83 Tuberculosis of digestive tract organs, not elsewhere classified   HIV CC
EXCLUDES 1   tuberculosis of intestine (A18.32)
CC Excl: PDX collection 45

A18.84 Tuberculosis of heart   HIV CC
Tuberculous cardiomyopathy
Tuberculous endocarditis
Tuberculous myocarditis
Tuberculous pericarditis
CC Excl: PDX collection 35

A18.85 Tuberculosis of spleen   HIV CC
CC Excl: PDX collection 50

A18.89 Tuberculosis of other sites   HIV CC
Tuberculosis of muscle
Tuberculous cerebral arteritis
CC Excl: PDX collection 35

√4ᵗʰ A19 Miliary tuberculosis
INCLUDES   disseminated tuberculosis
generalized tuberculosis
tuberculous polyserositis
CC Excl: For MCC codes in category A19: PDX collection 51

A19.0 Acute miliary tuberculosis of a single specified site   HIV MCC

A19.1 Acute miliary tuberculosis of multiple sites   HIV MCC

A19.2 Acute miliary tuberculosis, unspecified   HIV MCC

A19.8 Other miliary tuberculosis   HIV MCC

A19.9 Miliary tuberculosis, unspecified   HIV MCC

Certain zoonotic bacterial diseases (A20-A28)

√4ᵗʰ A20 Plague
INCLUDES   infection due to Yersinia pestis

A20.0 Bubonic plague   MCC
CC Excl: PDX collection 52

A20.1 Cellulocutaneous plague   MCC
CC Excl: PDX collection 52

A20.2 Pneumonic plague   MCC HCC
CC Excl: PDX collection 53

A20.3 Plague meningitis   MCC
CC Excl: PDX collection 54

A20.7 Septicemic plague   MCC HCC
CC Excl: PDX collection 55

A20.8 Other forms of plague   MCC
Abortive plague
Asymptomatic plague
Pestis minor
CC Excl: PDX collection 54

A20.9 Plague, unspecified   MCC
CC Excl: PDX collection 56

√4ᵗʰ A21 Tularemia
INCLUDES   deer-fly fever
infection due to Francisella tularensis
rabbit fever
DEF: Febrile disease transmitted to humans by the bites of deer flies, fleas, and ticks, by inhaling aerosolized *F. tularensis*, or by ingesting contaminated food or water. Patients quickly develop fever, chills, weakness, headache, backache, and malaise.

A21.0 Ulceroglandular tularemia   CC
CC Excl: PDX collection 57

A21.1 Oculoglandular tularemia   CC
Ophthalmic tularemia
CC Excl: PDX collection 58

A21.2 Pulmonary tularemia `CC` `HCC`
     CC Excl: PDX collection 59

A21.3 Gastrointestinal tularemia `CC`
     Abdominal tularemia
     CC Excl: PDX collection 60

A21.7 Generalized tularemia `CC`
     CC Excl: PDX collection 61

A21.8 Other forms of tularemia `CC`
     CC Excl: PDX collection 61

A21.9 Tularemia, unspecified `CC`
     CC Excl: PDX collection 61

✓4ᵗʰ **A22 Anthrax**
     INCLUDES   infection due to Bacillus anthracis

A22.0 Cutaneous anthrax `CC`
     Malignant carbuncle
     Malignant pustule
     CC Excl: PDX collection 62

A22.1 Pulmonary anthrax `MCC` `HCC`
     Inhalation anthrax
     Ragpicker's disease
     Woolsorter's disease
     CC Excl: PDX collection 63

A22.2 Gastrointestinal anthrax `CC`
     CC Excl: PDX collection 64

A22.7 Anthrax sepsis `MCC` `HCC`
     CC Excl: PDX collection 5

A22.8 Other forms of anthrax `CC`
     Anthrax meningitis
     CC Excl: PDX collection 65

A22.9 Anthrax, unspecified `CC`
     CC Excl: PDX collection 66

✓4ᵗʰ **A23 Brucellosis**
     INCLUDES   Malta fever
             Mediterranean fever
             undulant fever

A23.0 Brucellosis due to Brucella melitensis

A23.1 Brucellosis due to Brucella abortus

A23.2 Brucellosis due to Brucella suis

A23.3 Brucellosis due to Brucella canis

A23.8 Other brucellosis `CC`
     CC Excl: PDX collection 67

A23.9 Brucellosis, unspecified `CC`
     CC Excl: PDX collection 67

✓4ᵗʰ **A24 Glanders and melioidosis**
     CC Excl: For CC codes in category A24, unless otherwise noted: PDX collection 69

A24.0 Glanders `CC`
     Infection due to Pseudomonas mallei
     Malleus
     CC Excl: PDX collection 68

A24.1 Acute and fulminating melioidosis `CC`
     Melioidosis pneumonia
     Melioidosis sepsis

A24.2 Subacute and chronic melioidosis `CC`

A24.3 Other melioidosis `CC`

A24.9 Melioidosis, unspecified `CC`
     Infection due to Pseudomonas pseudomallei NOS
     Whitmore's disease

✓4ᵗʰ **A25 Rat-bite fevers**
     CC Excl: For CC codes in category A25: PDX collection 70

A25.0 Spirillosis `CC`
     Sodoku

A25.1 Streptobacillosis `CC`
     Epidemic arthritic erythema
     Haverhill fever
     Streptobacillary rat-bite fever

A25.9 Rat-bite fever, unspecified `CC`

✓4ᵗʰ **A26 Erysipeloid**
     DEF: Acute cutaneous infection typically caused by trauma to the skin. Presenting as cellulitis, it may become systemic affecting other organs. It is gram positive bacillus and mainly acquired by those who routinely handle meat.

A26.0 Cutaneous erysipeloid
     Erythema migrans

A26.7 Erysipelothrix sepsis `MCC` `HCC`
     CC Excl: PDX collection 71

A26.8 Other forms of erysipeloid

A26.9 Erysipeloid, unspecified

✓4ᵗʰ **A27 Leptospirosis**
     CC Excl: For CC codes in category A27: PDX collection 72

A27.0 Leptospirosis icterohemorrhagica `CC`
     Leptospiral or spirochetal jaundice (hemorrhagic)
     Weil's disease

✓5ᵗʰ **A27.8 Other forms of leptospirosis**

     A27.81 Aseptic meningitis in leptospirosis `MCC`
         CC Excl: PDX collection 73

     A27.89 Other forms of leptospirosis `CC`

A27.9 Leptospirosis, unspecified `CC`

✓4ᵗʰ **A28 Other zoonotic bacterial diseases, not elsewhere classified**
     CC Excl: For CC codes in category A28, unless otherwise noted: PDX collection 74

A28.0 Pasteurellosis `CC`

A28.1 Cat-scratch disease `CC`
     Cat-scratch fever
     CC Excl: PDX collection 75

A28.2 Extraintestinal yersiniosis `CC`
     EXCLUDES 1   enteritis due to Yersinia enterocolitica (A04.6)
                 plague (A20.-)

A28.8 Other specified zoonotic bacterial diseases, not elsewhere classified `CC`

A28.9 Zoonotic bacterial disease, unspecified `CC`

Other bacterial diseases (A30-A49)

AHA: 2016,3Q,8-14

✓4ᵗʰ **A30 Leprosy [Hansen's disease]**
     INCLUDES   infection due to Mycobacterium leprae
     EXCLUDES 1   sequelae of leprosy (B92)

A30.0 Indeterminate leprosy `CC`
     I leprosy
     CC Excl: PDX collection 76

A30.1 Tuberculoid leprosy `CC`
     TT leprosy
     CC Excl: PDX collection 77

A30.2 Borderline tuberculoid leprosy `CC`
     BT leprosy
     CC Excl: PDX collection 78

A30.3 Borderline leprosy `CC`
     BB leprosy
     CC Excl: PDX collection 78

A30.4 Borderline lepromatous leprosy `CC`
     BL leprosy
     CC Excl: PDX collection 78

A30.5 Lepromatous leprosy `CC`
     LL leprosy
     CC Excl: PDX collection 79

A30.8 Other forms of leprosy `CC`
     CC Excl: PDX collection 80

A30.9 Leprosy, unspecified `CC`
     CC Excl: PDX collection 81

N Newborn: 0   P Pediatric: 0-17   M Maternity: 9-64   A Adult: 15-124   **MCC** Major Complication/Comorbidity   **CC** Complication/Comorbidity   **SW** Severe Wound Dx

440   ICD-10-CM 2020

✓4th **A31 Infection due to other mycobacteria**

     EXCLUDES 2   leprosy (A30.-)
                  tuberculosis (A15-A19)

     CC Excl: For CC codes in category A31, unless otherwise noted: PDX collection 83

   A31.0 Pulmonary mycobacterial infection   CC HCC

     Infection due to Mycobacterium avium
     Infection due to Mycobacterium intracellulare [Battey bacillus]
     Infection due to Mycobacterium kansasii
     CC Excl: PDX collection 82

   A31.1 Cutaneous mycobacterial infection   CC

     Buruli ulcer
     Infection due to Mycobacterium marinum
     Infection due to Mycobacterium ulcerans

   A31.2 Disseminated mycobacterium avium-intracellulare complex (DMAC)   HIV CC HCC
     MAC sepsis

   A31.8 Other mycobacterial infections   HIV CC

   A31.9 Mycobacterial infection, unspecified   HIV CC

     Atypical mycobacterial infection NOS
     Mycobacteriosis NOS

✓4th **A32 Listeriosis**

     INCLUDES   listerial foodborne infection
     EXCLUDES 1   neonatal (disseminated) listeriosis (P37.2)
     CC Excl: For CC codes in category A32: PDX collection 74

   A32.0 Cutaneous listeriosis   CC

✓5th **A32.1 Listerial meningitis and meningoencephalitis**

     A32.11 Listerial meningitis   CC

     A32.12 Listerial meningoencephalitis   CC

   A32.7 Listerial sepsis   MCC HCC
     CC Excl: PDX collection 71

✓5th **A32.8 Other forms of listeriosis**

     A32.81 Oculoglandular listeriosis   CC

     A32.82 Listerial endocarditis   CC

     A32.89 Other forms of listeriosis   CC
         Listerial cerebral arteritis

   A32.9 Listeriosis, unspecified   CC

   A33 Tetanus neonatorum   MCC N
     CC Excl: PDX collection 84

   A34 Obstetrical tetanus   CC M ♀
     CC Excl: PDX collection 85

   A35 Other tetanus   MCC
     Tetanus NOS
     EXCLUDES 1   obstetrical tetanus (A34)
              tetanus neonatorum (A33)

     DEF: Tetanus: Acute, often fatal, infectious disease caused by the anaerobic, spore-forming bacillus *Clostridium tetani*. The bacillus enters the body through a contaminated wound, burns, surgical wounds, or cutaneous ulcers. Symptoms include lockjaw, spasms, seizures, and paralysis.
     CC Excl: PDX collection 86

✓4th **A36 Diphtheria**

     CC Excl: For CC codes in category A36, unless otherwise noted: PDX collection 87

   A36.0 Pharyngeal diphtheria   CC
     Diphtheritic membranous angina
     Tonsillar diphtheria

   A36.1 Nasopharyngeal diphtheria   CC

   A36.2 Laryngeal diphtheria   CC
     Diphtheritic laryngotracheitis

   A36.3 Cutaneous diphtheria   CC
     EXCLUDES 2   erythrasma (L08.1)

✓5th **A36.8 Other diphtheria**

     A36.81 Diphtheritic cardiomyopathy   CC HCC
         Diphtheritic myocarditis
         CC Excl: PDX collection 88

     A36.82 Diphtheritic radiculomyelitis   CC

     A36.83 Diphtheritic polyneuritis   CC

     A36.84 Diphtheritic tubulo-interstitial nephropathy   CC

     A36.85 Diphtheritic cystitis   CC

     A36.86 Diphtheritic conjunctivitis   CC

     A36.89 Other diphtheritic complications   CC
         Diphtheritic peritonitis

   A36.9 Diphtheria, unspecified   CC

✓4th **A37 Whooping cough**

     DEF: Acute, highly contagious respiratory tract infection caused by *Bordetella pertussis* and *B. bronchiseptica*. Whooping cough is known by its characteristic paroxysmal cough.
     CC Excl: For codes in category A37:
     For MCC codes: PDX collection 90
     For CC codes: PDX collection 89

✓5th **A37.0 Whooping cough due to Bordetella pertussis**

     A37.00 Whooping cough due to Bordetella pertussis without pneumonia   CC

     A37.01 Whooping cough due to Bordetella pertussis with pneumonia   MCC

✓5th **A37.1 Whooping cough due to Bordetella parapertussis**

     A37.10 Whooping cough due to Bordetella parapertussis without pneumonia   CC

     A37.11 Whooping cough due to Bordetella parapertussis with pneumonia   MCC

✓5th **A37.8 Whooping cough due to other Bordetella species**

     A37.80 Whooping cough due to other Bordetella species without pneumonia   CC

     A37.81 Whooping cough due to other Bordetella species with pneumonia   MCC

✓5th **A37.9 Whooping cough, unspecified species**

     A37.90 Whooping cough, unspecified species without pneumonia   CC

     A37.91 Whooping cough, unspecified species with pneumonia   MCC

✓4th **A38 Scarlet fever**

     INCLUDES   scarlatina
     EXCLUDES 2   streptococcal sore throat (J02.0)
     DEF: Acute contagious disease caused by Group A bacteria, the same bacterium that causes strep throat. Individuals with strep throat can develop scarlet fever particularly if the infection is not treated with antibiotics. It is characterized by a red blush to the skin of the chest and abdomen and swelling of the nose, throat, and mouth.
     CC Excl: For CC codes in category A38: PDX collection 91

   A38.0 Scarlet fever with otitis media   CC

   A38.1 Scarlet fever with myocarditis   CC

   A38.8 Scarlet fever with other complications   CC

   A38.9 Scarlet fever, uncomplicated   CC
     Scarlet fever, NOS

✓4th **A39 Meningococcal infection**

     DEF: Condition caused by *Neisseria meningitidis*, a bacteria that may invade the spinal cord, brain, heart, joints, optic nerve, or bloodstream.

   A39.0 Meningococcal meningitis   MCC
     CC Excl: PDX collection 92

   A39.1 Waterhouse-Friderichsen syndrome   MCC HCC
     Meningococcal hemorrhagic adrenalitis
     Meningococcic adrenal syndrome
     CC Excl: PDX collection 93

   A39.2 Acute meningococcemia   MCC HCC
     CC Excl: PDX collection 94

   A39.3 Chronic meningococcemia   MCC HCC
     CC Excl: PDX collection 94

   A39.4 Meningococcemia, unspecified   MCC HCC
     CC Excl: PDX collection 94

✓5th **A39.5 Meningococcal heart disease**

     A39.50 Meningococcal carditis, unspecified   MCC
         CC Excl: PDX collection 95

     A39.51 Meningococcal endocarditis   MCC
         CC Excl: PDX collection 96

     A39.52 Meningococcal myocarditis   MCC
         CC Excl: PDX collection 97

     A39.53 Meningococcal pericarditis   MCC
         CC Excl: PDX collection 98

✓ Additional Character Required   ✓x7th Placeholder   Unacceptable PDx   Questionable PDx   Manifestation   Unspecified Dx   H1-H14 HAC   HCC CMS-HCC Dx   HIV HIV Dx

☑5ᵗʰ A39.8 Other meningococcal infections

    A39.81 Meningococcal encephalitis `MCC`
        CC Excl: PDX collection 99

    A39.82 Meningococcal retrobulbar neuritis `CC`
        CC Excl: PDX collection 100

    A39.83 Meningococcal arthritis `CC` `HCC`
        CC Excl: PDX collection 101

    A39.84 Postmeningococcal arthritis `CC` `HCC`
        CC Excl: PDX collection 101

    A39.89 Other meningococcal infections `CC`
        Meningococcal conjunctivitis
        CC Excl: PDX collection 102

A39.9 Meningococcal infection, unspecified `CC`
    Meningococcal disease NOS
    CC Excl: PDX collection 102

☑4ᵗʰ A40 Streptococcal sepsis
    Code first:
        postprocedural streptococcal sepsis (T81.4-)
        streptococcal sepsis during labor (O75.3)
        streptococcal sepsis following abortion or ectopic or molar pregnancy (O03-O07, O08.0)
        streptococcal sepsis following immunization (T88.0)
        streptococcal sepsis following infusion, transfusion or therapeutic injection (T80.2-)
    EXCLUDES 1   neonatal (P36.0-P36.1)
            puerperal sepsis (O85)
            sepsis due to Streptococcus, group D (A41.81)
    AHA: 2018,4Q,89; 2018,1Q,16; 2016,1Q,32
    CC Excl: For MCC codes in category A40, unless otherwise noted: PDX collection 71

    A40.0 Sepsis due to streptococcus, group A `MCC` `HCC`

    A40.1 Sepsis due to streptococcus, group B `MCC` `HCC`
        AHA: 2019,1Q,14

    A40.3 Sepsis due to Streptococcus pneumoniae `MCC` `HCC`
        Pneumococcal sepsis
        CC Excl: No Excl

    A40.8 Other streptococcal sepsis `MCC` `HCC`

    A40.9 Streptococcal sepsis, unspecified `HIV` `MCC` `HCC`

☑4ᵗʰ A41 Other sepsis
    Code first:
        postprocedural sepsis (T81.4-)
        sepsis during labor (O75.3)
        sepsis following abortion, ectopic or molar pregnancy (O03-O07, O08.0)
        sepsis following immunization (T88.0)
        sepsis following infusion, transfusion or therapeutic injection (T80.2-)
    EXCLUDES 1   bacteremia NOS (R78.81)
            neonatal (P36.-)
            puerperal sepsis (O85)
            streptococcal sepsis (A40.-)
    EXCLUDES 2   sepsis (due to) (in) actinomycotic (A42.7)
            sepsis (due to) (in) anthrax (A22.7)
            sepsis (due to) (in) candidal (B37.7)
            sepsis (due to) (in) Erysipelothrix (A26.7)
            sepsis (due to) (in) extraintestinal yersiniosis (A28.2)
            sepsis (due to) (in) gonococcal (A54.86)
            sepsis (due to) (in) herpesviral (B00.7)
            sepsis (due to) (in) listerial (A32.7)
            sepsis (due to) (in) melioidosis (A24.1)
            sepsis (due to) (in) meningococcal (A39.2-A39.4)
            sepsis (due to) (in) plague (A20.7)
            sepsis (due to) (in) tularemia (A21.7)
            toxic shock syndrome (A48.3)
    AHA: 2018,4Q,18; 2018,1Q,16; 2016,1Q,32; 2014,2Q,13
    CC Excl: For MCC codes in category A41: PDX collection 71

    ☑5ᵗʰ A41.0 Sepsis due to Staphylococcus aureus

        A41.01 Sepsis due to Methicillin susceptible Staphylococcus aureus `HIV` `MCC` `HCC`
            MSSA sepsis
            Staphylococcus aureus sepsis NOS

        A41.02 Sepsis due to Methicillin resistant Staphylococcus aureus `HIV` `MCC` `HCC`

A41.1 Sepsis due to other specified staphylococcus `HIV` `MCC` `HCC`
    Coagulase negative staphylococcus sepsis

A41.2 Sepsis due to unspecified staphylococcus `HIV` `MCC` `HCC`

A41.3 Sepsis due to Hemophilus influenzae `HIV` `MCC` `HCC`

A41.4 Sepsis due to anaerobes `HIV` `MCC` `HCC`
    EXCLUDES 1   gas gangrene (A48.0)

☑5ᵗʰ A41.5 Sepsis due to other Gram-negative organisms

    A41.50 Gram-negative sepsis, unspecified `HIV` `MCC` `HCC`
        Gram-negative sepsis NOS

    A41.51 Sepsis due to Escherichia coli [E. coli] `HIV` `MCC` `HCC`

    A41.52 Sepsis due to Pseudomonas `HIV` `MCC` `HCC`
        Pseudomonas aeroginosa

    A41.53 Sepsis due to Serratia `HIV` `MCC` `HCC`

    A41.59 Other Gram-negative sepsis `HIV` `MCC` `HCC`

☑5ᵗʰ A41.8 Other specified sepsis

    A41.81 Sepsis due to Enterococcus `HIV` `MCC` `HCC`
        TIP: *E. faecium,* is a species of *Enterococcus* that is highly resistant to multiple antibiotics. Assign a code from category Z16 when resistance to antimicrobial drugs is documented.

    A41.89 Other specified sepsis `HIV` `MCC` `HCC`
        AHA: 2017,1Q,51; 2016,3Q,8-14
        TIP: Viral sepsis is coded here; assign an additional code to identify the specific viral agent or illness.

A41.9 Sepsis, unspecified organism `HIV` `MCC` `HCC`
    Septicemia NOS

☑4ᵗʰ A42 Actinomycosis
    EXCLUDES 1   actinomycetoma (B47.1)

    A42.0 Pulmonary actinomycosis `HIV` `CC` `HCC`
        CC Excl: PDX collection 103

    A42.1 Abdominal actinomycosis `HIV` `CC`
        CC Excl: PDX collection 104

    A42.2 Cervicofacial actinomycosis `HIV` `CC`
        CC Excl: PDX collection 105

    A42.7 Actinomycotic sepsis `HIV` `MCC` `HCC`
        CC Excl: PDX collection 71

    ☑5ᵗʰ A42.8 Other forms of actinomycosis
        CC Excl: For CC codes in subcategory A42.8: PDX collection 106

        A42.81 Actinomycotic meningitis `HIV` `CC`

        A42.82 Actinomycotic encephalitis `HIV` `CC`

        A42.89 Other forms of actinomycosis `HIV` `CC`

    A42.9 Actinomycosis, unspecified `HIV` `CC`
        CC Excl: PDX collection 106

☑4ᵗʰ A43 Nocardiosis
    DEF: Rare bacterial infection occurring most often in those with weakened immune systems. Can be acquired in soil, decaying plants, or standing water. It typically begins in the lungs and has a tendency to spread to other body systems.

    A43.0 Pulmonary nocardiosis `HIV` `CC` `HCC`
        CC Excl: PDX collection 103

    A43.1 Cutaneous nocardiosis `HIV` `CC`
        CC Excl: PDX collection 107

    A43.8 Other forms of nocardiosis `HIV` `CC`
        CC Excl: PDX collection 106

    A43.9 Nocardiosis, unspecified `HIV` `CC`
        CC Excl: PDX collection 106

☑4ᵗʰ A44 Bartonellosis
    CC Excl: For CC codes in category A44: PDX collection 108

    A44.0 Systemic bartonellosis `CC`
        Oroya fever

    A44.1 Cutaneous and mucocutaneous bartonellosis `CC`
        Verruga peruana

    A44.8 Other forms of bartonellosis `CC`

    A44.9 Bartonellosis, unspecified `CC`

A46 Erysipelas
    EXCLUDES 1   postpartum or puerperal erysipelas (O86.89)
    DEF: Skin infection affecting the upper dermis and superficial dermal lymphatics. Lesion edges are well-demarcated with distinct raised borders. It is often caused by group A *Streptococci.*

N Newborn: 0   **P** Pediatric: 0-17   **M** Maternity: 9-64   **A** Adult: 15-124   **MCC** Major Complication/Comorbidity   **CC** Complication/Comorbidity   **SW** Severe Wound Dx

442   ICD-10-CM 2020

✓4ᵗʰ **A48 Other bacterial diseases, not elsewhere classified**

     EXCLUDES 1   *actinomycetoma (B47.1)*

A48.0 Gas gangrene   MCC HCC

     Clostridial cellulitis

     Clostridial myonecrosis

     AHA: 2017,4Q,102

     CC Excl: PDX collection 109

A48.1 Legionnaires' disease   HIV MCC HCC

     DEF: Severe and often fatal infection by *Legionella pneumophila.* Symptoms include high fever, gastrointestinal pain, headache, myalgia, dry cough, and pneumonia and it is usually transmitted through airborne water droplets via air conditioning systems or hot tubs.

     CC Excl: PDX collection 110

A48.2 Nonpneumonic Legionnaires' disease [Pontiac fever]

A48.3 Toxic shock syndrome   MCC HCC

     Use additional code to identify the organism (B95, B96)

     EXCLUDES 1   *endotoxic shock NOS (R57.8)*

                 sepsis NOS (A41.9)

     DEF: Bacteria producing an endotoxin, such as *Staphylococci,* flood the body with the toxins producing a high fever, vomiting and diarrhea, decreasing blood pressure, a skin rash, and shock.

     Synonym(s): TSS.

     CC Excl: PDX collection 111

A48.4 Brazilian purpuric fever

     Systemic Hemophilus aegyptius infection

✓5ᵗʰ **A48.5 Other specified botulism**

     Non-foodborne intoxication due to toxins of Clostridium botulinum [C. botulinum]

     EXCLUDES 1   *food poisoning due to toxins of Clostridium botulinum (A05.1)*

     A48.51 Infant botulism   CC P

         CC Excl: PDX collection 18

     A48.52 Wound botulism   CC

         Non-foodborne botulism NOS

         Use additional code for associated wound

         CC Excl: PDX collection 18

A48.8 Other specified bacterial diseases

✓4ᵗʰ **A49 Bacterial infection of unspecified site**

     EXCLUDES 1   *bacterial agents as the cause of diseases classified elsewhere (B95-B96)*

                 chlamydial infection NOS (A74.9)

                 meningococcal infection NOS (A39.9)

                 rickettsial infection NOS (A79.9)

                 spirochetal infection NOS (A69.9)

✓5ᵗʰ **A49.0 Staphylococcal infection, unspecified site**

     A49.01 Methicillin susceptible Staphylococcus aureus infection, unspecified site

         Methicillin susceptible Staphylococcus aureus (MSSA) infection

         Staphylococcus aureus infection NOS

     A49.02 Methicillin resistant Staphylococcus aureus infection, unspecified site

         Methicillin resistant Staphylococcus aureus (MRSA) infection

A49.1 Streptococcal infection, unspecified site

A49.2 Hemophilus influenzae infection, unspecified site

A49.3 Mycoplasma infection, unspecified site

A49.8 Other bacterial infections of unspecified site

A49.9 Bacterial infection, unspecified

     EXCLUDES 1   *bacteremia NOS (R78.81)*

Infections with a predominantly sexual mode of transmission (A50-A64)

     EXCLUDES 1   *human immunodeficiency virus [HIV] disease (B20)*

                 nonspecific and nongonococcal urethritis (N34.1)

                 Reiter's disease (M02.3-)

✓4ᵗʰ **A50 Congenital syphilis**

     CC Excl: For CC/MCC codes in category A50, unless otherwise noted: PDX collection 112

✓5ᵗʰ **A50.0 Early congenital syphilis, symptomatic**

     Any congenital syphilitic condition specified as early or manifest less than two years after birth.

     A50.01 Early congenital syphilitic oculopathy   CC

     A50.02 Early congenital syphilitic osteochondropathy   CC

     A50.03 Early congenital syphilitic pharyngitis   CC

         Early congenital syphilitic laryngitis

     A50.04 Early congenital syphilitic pneumonia   CC

     A50.05 Early congenital syphilitic rhinitis   CC

     A50.06 Early cutaneous congenital syphilis   CC

     A50.07 Early mucocutaneous congenital syphilis   CC

     A50.08 Early visceral congenital syphilis   CC

     A50.09 Other early congenital syphilis, symptomatic   CC

A50.1 Early congenital syphilis, latent

     Congenital syphilis without clinical manifestations, with positive serological reaction and negative spinal fluid test, less than two years after birth.

A50.2 Early congenital syphilis, unspecified   CC

     Congenital syphilis NOS less than two years after birth.

     CC Excl: PDX collection 113

✓5ᵗʰ **A50.3 Late congenital syphilitic oculopathy**

     EXCLUDES 1   *Hutchinson's triad (A50.53)*

     A50.30 Late congenital syphilitic oculopathy, unspecified   CC

     A50.31 Late congenital syphilitic interstitial keratitis   CC

     A50.32 Late congenital syphilitic chorioretinitis   CC

     A50.39 Other late congenital syphilitic oculopathy   CC

✓5ᵗʰ **A50.4 Late congenital neurosyphilis [juvenile neurosyphilis]**

     Use additional code to identify any associated mental disorder

     EXCLUDES 1   *Hutchinson's triad (A50.53)*

     A50.40 Late congenital neurosyphilis, unspecified   CC

         Juvenile neurosyphilis NOS

         CC Excl: PDX collection 114

     A50.41 Late congenital syphilitic meningitis   MCC

         CC Excl: PDX collection 115

     A50.42 Late congenital syphilitic encephalitis   MCC

         CC Excl: PDX collection 114

     A50.43 Late congenital syphilitic polyneuropathy   CC

         CC Excl: PDX collection 114

     A50.44 Late congenital syphilitic optic nerve atrophy   CC

     A50.45 Juvenile general paresis   CC

         Dementia paralytica juvenilis

         Juvenile tabetoparetic neurosyphilis

         CC Excl: PDX collection 114

     A50.49 Other late congenital neurosyphilis   CC

         Juvenile tabes dorsalis

         CC Excl: PDX collection 114

✓5ᵗʰ **A50.5 Other late congenital syphilis, symptomatic**

     Any congenital syphilitic condition specified as late or manifest two years or more after birth.

     A50.51 Clutton's joints   CC

     A50.52 Hutchinson's teeth   CC

     A50.53 Hutchinson's triad   CC

     A50.54 Late congenital cardiovascular syphilis   CC

     A50.55 Late congenital syphilitic arthropathy   CC HCC

     A50.56 Late congenital syphilitic osteochondropathy   CC

     A50.57 Syphilitic saddle nose   CC

     A50.59 Other late congenital syphilis, symptomatic   CC

A50.6 Late congenital syphilis, latent

     Congenital syphilis without clinical manifestations, with positive serological reaction and negative spinal fluid test, two years or more after birth.

A50.7 Late congenital syphilis, unspecified

     Congenital syphilis NOS two years or more after birth.

A50.9 Congenital syphilis, unspecified

✓ Additional Character Required   ✓ˣ7ᵗʰ Placeholder   **Unacceptable PDx**   Questionable PDx   Manifestation   Unspecified Dx   H1-H14 HAC   HCC CMS-HCC Dx   HIV HIV Dx

✓4ᵗʰ A51 Early syphilis

DEF: Syphilis: Sexually transmitted disease caused by the treponema pallidum spirochete. Syphilis usually exhibits cutaneous manifestations and may exist for years without symptoms.

A51.Ø Primary genital syphilis
Syphilitic chancre NOS

A51.1 Primary anal syphilis

A51.2 Primary syphilis of other sites

✓5ᵗʰ A51.3 Secondary syphilis of skin and mucous membranes

DEF: Transitory or chronic cutaneous eruptions that present within two to 10 weeks following an initial syphilis infection that may include nontender lymphadenopathy along with alopecia and condylomata lata.

A51.31 Condyloma latum CC
CC Excl: PDX collection 112

A51.32 Syphilitic alopecia CC
CC Excl: PDX collection 116

A51.39 Other secondary syphilis of skin CC
Syphilitic leukoderma
Syphilitic mucous patch
EXCLUDES 1   late syphilitic leukoderma (A52.79)
CC Excl: PDX collection 112

✓5ᵗʰ A51.4 Other secondary syphilis

A51.41 Secondary syphilitic meningitis MCC
CC Excl: PDX collection 117

A51.42 Secondary syphilitic female pelvic disease CC ♀
CC Excl: PDX collection 113

A51.43 Secondary syphilitic oculopathy CC
Secondary syphilitic chorioretinitis
Secondary syphilitic iridocyclitis, iritis
Secondary syphilitic uveitis
CC Excl: PDX collection 112

A51.44 Secondary syphilitic nephritis CC
CC Excl: PDX collection 113

A51.45 Secondary syphilitic hepatitis CC
CC Excl: PDX collection 118

A51.46 Secondary syphilitic osteopathy CC
CC Excl: PDX collection 119

A51.49 Other secondary syphilitic conditions CC
Secondary syphilitic lymphadenopathy
Secondary syphilitic myositis
CC Excl: No Excl

A51.5 Early syphilis, latent
Syphilis (acquired) without clinical manifestations, with positive serological reaction and negative spinal fluid test, less than two years after infection.

A51.9 Early syphilis, unspecified

✓4ᵗʰ A52 Late syphilis

✓5ᵗʰ A52.Ø Cardiovascular and cerebrovascular syphilis
CC Excl: For CC codes in subcategory A52.Ø: PDX collection 114

A52.ØØ Cardiovascular syphilis, unspecified CC

A52.Ø1 Syphilitic aneurysm of aorta CC

A52.Ø2 Syphilitic aortitis CC

A52.Ø3 Syphilitic endocarditis CC
Syphilitic aortic valve incompetence or stenosis
Syphilitic mitral valve stenosis
Syphilitic pulmonary valve regurgitation

A52.Ø4 Syphilitic cerebral arteritis CC

A52.Ø5 Other cerebrovascular syphilis CC
Syphilitic cerebral aneurysm (ruptured) (non-ruptured)
Syphilitic cerebral thrombosis

A52.Ø6 Other syphilitic heart involvement CC
Syphilitic coronary artery disease
Syphilitic myocarditis
Syphilitic pericarditis

A52.Ø9 Other cardiovascular syphilis CC

✓5ᵗʰ A52.1 Symptomatic neurosyphilis
CC Excl: For CC/MCC codes in subcategory A52.1, unless otherwise noted: PDX collection 114

A52.1Ø Symptomatic neurosyphilis, unspecified CC

A52.11 Tabes dorsalis CC
Locomotor ataxia (progressive)
Tabetic neurosyphilis

A52.12 Other cerebrospinal syphilis CC

A52.13 Late syphilitic meningitis MCC
CC Excl: PDX collection 115

A52.14 Late syphilitic encephalitis MCC

A52.15 Late syphilitic neuropathy CC
Late syphilitic acoustic neuritis
Late syphilitic optic (nerve) atrophy
Late syphilitic polyneuropathy
Late syphilitic retrobulbar neuritis

A52.16 Charcôt's arthropathy (tabetic) CC
DEF: Progressive neurologic arthropathy in which chronic degeneration of joints in the weight-bearing areas with peripheral hypertrophy occurs as a complication of a neuropathy disorder. Supporting structures relax from a loss of sensation resulting in chronic joint instability.

A52.17 General paresis CC
Dementia paralytica

A52.19 Other symptomatic neurosyphilis CC
Syphilitic parkinsonism

A52.2 Asymptomatic neurosyphilis CC
CC Excl: PDX collection 114

A52.3 Neurosyphilis, unspecified CC
Gumma (syphilitic)
Syphilis (late)
Syphiloma
CC Excl: PDX collection 114

✓5ᵗʰ A52.7 Other symptomatic late syphilis
CC Excl: For CC codes in subcategory A52.7, unless otherwise noted: PDX collection 116

A52.71 Late syphilitic oculopathy CC
Late syphilitic chorioretinitis
Late syphilitic episcleritis
CC Excl: PDX collection 120

A52.72 Syphilis of lung and bronchus CC

A52.73 Symptomatic late syphilis of other respiratory organs CC

A52.74 Syphilis of liver and other viscera CC
Late syphilitic peritonitis

A52.75 Syphilis of kidney and ureter CC
Syphilitic glomerular disease

A52.76 Other genitourinary symptomatic late syphilis CC
Late syphilitic female pelvic inflammatory disease

A52.77 Syphilis of bone and joint CC

A52.78 Syphilis of other musculoskeletal tissue CC
Late syphilitic bursitis
Syphilis [stage unspecified] of bursa
Syphilis [stage unspecified] of muscle
Syphilis [stage unspecified] of synovium
Syphilis [stage unspecified] of tendon

A52.79 Other symptomatic late syphilis CC
Late syphilitic leukoderma
Syphilis of adrenal gland
Syphilis of pituitary gland
Syphilis of thyroid gland
Syphilitic splenomegaly
EXCLUDES 1   syphilitic leukoderma (secondary) (A51.39)

A52.8 Late syphilis, latent
Syphilis (acquired) without clinical manifestations, with positive serological reaction and negative spinal fluid test, two years or more after infection

A52.9 Late syphilis, unspecified

✓4ᵗʰ A53 Other and unspecified syphilis

A53.Ø Latent syphilis, unspecified as early or late
Latent syphilis NOS
Positive serological reaction for syphilis

A53.9   **Syphilis, unspecified**
Infection due to Treponema pallidum NOS
Syphilis (acquired) NOS
> **EXCLUDES 1**   *syphilis NOS under two years of age (A50.2)*

✓4ᵗʰ **A54**   **Gonococcal infection**
DEF: Sexually transmitted bacterial infection caused by *Neisseria gonorrhoeae.* Women are often asymptomatic, while men tend to develop urinary symptoms quickly.

✓5ᵗʰ **A54.0**   **Gonococcal infection of lower genitourinary tract without periurethral or accessory gland abscess**
> **EXCLUDES 1**   *gonococcal infection with genitourinary gland abscess (A54.1)*
> *gonococcal infection with periurethral abscess (A54.1)*
>
> **CC Excl:** For CC codes in subcategory A54.0: PDX collection 121

A54.00   **Gonococcal infection of lower genitourinary tract, unspecified**   `CC`

A54.01   **Gonococcal cystitis and urethritis, unspecified**   `CC`

A54.02   **Gonococcal vulvovaginitis, unspecified**   `CC` ♀

A54.03   **Gonococcal cervicitis, unspecified**   `CC` ♀

A54.09   **Other gonococcal infection of lower genitourinary tract**   `CC`

A54.1   **Gonococcal infection of lower genitourinary tract with periurethral and accessory gland abscess**   `CC`
Gonococcal Bartholin's gland abscess
CC Excl: PDX collection 121

✓5ᵗʰ **A54.2**   **Gonococcal pelviperitonitis and other gonococcal genitourinary infection**
CC Excl: For CC codes in subcategory A54.2: PDX collection 121

A54.21   **Gonococcal infection of kidney and ureter**   `CC`

A54.22   **Gonococcal prostatitis**   `CC` ♂

A54.23   **Gonococcal infection of other male genital organs**   `CC` ♂
Gonococcal epididymitis
Gonococcal orchitis

A54.24   **Gonococcal female pelvic inflammatory disease**   `CC` ♀
Gonococcal pelviperitonitis
> **EXCLUDES 1**   *gonococcal peritonitis (A54.85)*

A54.29   **Other gonococcal genitourinary infections**   `CC`

✓5ᵗʰ **A54.3**   **Gonococcal infection of eye**
CC Excl: For CC codes in subcategory A54.3: PDX collection 116

A54.30   **Gonococcal infection of eye, unspecified**   `CC`

A54.31   **Gonococcal conjunctivitis**   `CC`
Ophthalmia neonatorum due to gonococcus

A54.32   **Gonococcal iridocyclitis**   `CC`

A54.33   **Gonococcal keratitis**   `CC`

A54.39   **Other gonococcal eye infection**   `CC`
Gonococcal endophthalmia

✓5ᵗʰ **A54.4**   **Gonococcal infection of musculoskeletal system**
CC Excl: For CC codes in subcategory A54.4: PDX collection 122

A54.40   **Gonococcal infection of musculoskeletal system, unspecified**   `CC` `HCC`

A54.41   **Gonococcal spondylopathy**   `CC` `HCC`

A54.42   **Gonococcal arthritis**   `CC` `HCC`
> **EXCLUDES 2**   *gonococcal infection of spine (A54.41)*

A54.43   **Gonococcal osteomyelitis**   `CC` `HCC`
> **EXCLUDES 2**   *gonococcal infection of spine (A54.41)*

A54.49   **Gonococcal infection of other musculoskeletal tissue**   `CC` `HCC`
Gonococcal bursitis
Gonococcal myositis
Gonococcal synovitis
Gonococcal tenosynovitis

A54.5   **Gonococcal pharyngitis**

A54.6   **Gonococcal infection of anus and rectum**

✓5ᵗʰ **A54.8**   **Other gonococcal infections**

A54.81   **Gonococcal meningitis**   `MCC`
CC Excl: PDX collection 117

A54.82   **Gonococcal brain abscess**   `CC`
CC Excl: PDX collection 123

A54.83   **Gonococcal heart infection**   `CC`
Gonococcal endocarditis
Gonococcal myocarditis
Gonococcal pericarditis
CC Excl: PDX collection 124

A54.84   **Gonococcal pneumonia**   `CC` `HCC`
CC Excl: PDX collection 123

A54.85   **Gonococcal peritonitis**   `CC` `HCC`
> **EXCLUDES 1**   *gonococcal pelviperitonitis (A54.24)*
>
> **CC Excl:** PDX collection 125

A54.86   **Gonococcal sepsis**   `MCC` `HCC`
CC Excl: PDX collection 71

A54.89   **Other gonococcal infections**   `CC`
Gonococcal keratoderma
Gonococcal lymphadenitis
CC Excl: PDX collection 123

A54.9   **Gonococcal infection, unspecified**   `CC`
CC Excl: PDX collection 123

A55   **Chlamydial lymphogranuloma (venereum)**
Climatic or tropical bubo
Durand-Nicolas-Favre disease
Esthiomene
Lymphogranuloma inguinale

✓4ᵗʰ **A56**   **Other sexually transmitted chlamydial diseases**
> **INCLUDES**   sexually transmitted diseases due to Chlamydia trachomatis
> **EXCLUDES 1**   *neonatal chlamydial conjunctivitis (P39.1)*
> *neonatal chlamydial pneumonia (P23.1)*
> **EXCLUDES 2**   *chlamydial lymphogranuloma (A55)*
> *conditions classified to A74.-*

DEF: Chlamydia trachomatis: Bacterium that causes a common venereal disease. Symptoms of chlamydia are usually mild or absent, however, serious complications may cause irreversible damage, including cystitis, pelvic inflammatory disease, and infertility in women and discharge from the penis, prostatitis, and infertility in men. Genital chlamydial infection can cause arthritis, skin lesions, and inflammation of the eye and urethra. **Synonym(s):** *Reiter's syndrome.*

✓5ᵗʰ **A56.0**   **Chlamydial infection of lower genitourinary tract**

A56.00   **Chlamydial infection of lower genitourinary tract, unspecified**

A56.01   **Chlamydial cystitis and urethritis**

A56.02   **Chlamydial vulvovaginitis**   ♀

A56.09   **Other chlamydial infection of lower genitourinary tract**
Chlamydial cervicitis

✓5ᵗʰ **A56.1**   **Chlamydial infection of pelviperitoneum and other genitourinary organs**

A56.11   **Chlamydial female pelvic inflammatory disease**   ♀

A56.19   **Other chlamydial genitourinary infection**
Chlamydial epididymitis
Chlamydial orchitis

A56.2   **Chlamydial infection of genitourinary tract, unspecified**

A56.3   **Chlamydial infection of anus and rectum**

A56.4   **Chlamydial infection of pharynx**

A56.8   **Sexually transmitted chlamydial infection of other sites**

A57   **Chancroid**
Ulcus molle
DEF: Localized infection by *Haemophilus ducreyi,* causing genital ulcers and infecting the inguinal lymph nodes.

A58   **Granuloma inguinale**
Donovanosis

✓ Additional Character Required   ✓x7ᵗʰ Placeholder   Unacceptable PDx   Questionable PDx   Manifestation   Unspecified Dx   `H1`-`H14` HAC   `HCC` CMS-HCC Dx   `HIV` HIV Dx

ICD-10-CM 2020   **445**

✓4th **A59 Trichomoniasis**

> EXCLUDES 2   intestinal trichomoniasis (A07.8)
>
> **DEF:** Infection with the parasitic, flagellated protozoa of the genus *Trichomonas*. This protozoon is found in the intestinal and genitourinary tracts of humans and in the mouth around tartar, cavities, and areas of periodontal disease.

  ✓5th **A59.0 Urogenital trichomoniasis**

    A59.00 Urogenital trichomoniasis, unspecified
      Fluor (vaginalis) due to Trichomonas
      Leukorrhea (vaginalis) due to Trichomonas

    A59.01 Trichomonal vulvovaginitis ♀

    A59.02 Trichomonal prostatitis ♂

    A59.03 Trichomonal cystitis and urethritis

    A59.09 Other urogenital trichomoniasis
      Trichomonas cervicitis

  A59.8 Trichomoniasis of other sites

  A59.9 Trichomoniasis, unspecified

✓4th **A60 Anogenital herpesviral [herpes simplex] infections**

  ✓5th **A60.0 Herpesviral infection of genitalia and urogenital tract**

    A60.00 Herpesviral infection of urogenital system, unspecified HIV

    A60.01 Herpesviral infection of penis HIV ♂

    A60.02 Herpesviral infection of other male genital organs ♂

    A60.03 Herpesviral cervicitis ♀

    A60.04 Herpesviral vulvovaginitis HIV ♀
      Herpesviral [herpes simplex] ulceration
      Herpesviral [herpes simplex] vaginitis
      Herpesviral [herpes simplex] vulvitis

    A60.09 Herpesviral infection of other urogenital tract HIV

  A60.1 Herpesviral infection of perianal skin and rectum HIV

  A60.9 Anogenital herpesviral infection, unspecified HIV

✓4th **A63 Other predominantly sexually transmitted diseases, not elsewhere classified**

> EXCLUDES 2   molluscum contagiosum (B08.1)
>   papilloma of cervix (D26.0)

  A63.0 Anogenital (venereal) warts
    Anogenital warts due to (human) papillomavirus [HPV]
    Condyloma acuminatum

  A63.8 Other specified predominantly sexually transmitted diseases

A64 Unspecified sexually transmitted disease

Other spirochetal diseases (A65-A69)

> EXCLUDES 2   leptospirosis (A27.-)
>   syphilis (A50-A53)

> **CC Excl:** For CC codes in categories A65-A69, unless otherwise noted: PDX collection 108

A65 Nonvenereal syphilis
  Bejel
  Endemic syphilis
  Njovera

✓4th **A66 Yaws**

> INCLUDES   bouba
>   frambesia (tropica)
>   pian

  A66.0 Initial lesions of yaws
    Chancre of yaws
    Frambesia, initial or primary
    Initial frambesial ulcer
    Mother yaw

  A66.1 Multiple papillomata and wet crab yaws
    Frambesioma
    Pianoma
    Plantar or palmar papilloma of yaws

  A66.2 Other early skin lesions of yaws
    Cutaneous yaws, less than five years after infection
    Early yaws (cutaneous) (macular) (maculopapular) (micropapular) (papular)
    Frambeside of early yaws

  A66.3 Hyperkeratosis of yaws
    Ghoul hand
    Hyperkeratosis, palmar or plantar (early) (late) due to yaws
    Worm-eaten soles

  A66.4 Gummata and ulcers of yaws
    Gummatous frambeside
    Nodular late yaws (ulcerated)

  A66.5 Gangosa
    Rhinopharyngitis mutilans

  A66.6 Bone and joint lesions of yaws HCC
    Yaws ganglion
    Yaws goundou
    Yaws gumma, bone
    Yaws gummatous osteitis or periostitis
    Yaws hydrarthrosis
    Yaws osteitis
    Yaws periostitis (hypertrophic)

  A66.7 Other manifestations of yaws
    Juxta-articular nodules of yaws
    Mucosal yaws

  A66.8 Latent yaws
    Yaws without clinical manifestations, with positive serology

  A66.9 Yaws, unspecified

✓4th **A67 Pinta [carate]**

  A67.0 Primary lesions of pinta
    Chancre (primary) of pinta
    Papule (primary) of pinta

  A67.1 Intermediate lesions of pinta
    Erythematous plaques of pinta
    Hyperchromic lesions of pinta
    Hyperkeratosis of pinta
    Pintids

  A67.2 Late lesions of pinta
    Achromic skin lesions of pinta
    Cicatricial skin lesions of pinta
    Dyschromic skin lesions of pinta

  A67.3 Mixed lesions of pinta
    Achromic with hyperchromic skin lesions of pinta [carate]

  A67.9 Pinta, unspecified

✓4th **A68 Relapsing fevers**

> INCLUDES   recurrent fever
> EXCLUDES 2   Lyme disease (A69.2-)

  A68.0 Louse-borne relapsing fever CC
    Relapsing fever due to Borrelia recurrentis

  A68.1 Tick-borne relapsing fever CC
    Relapsing fever due to any Borrelia species other than Borrelia recurrentis

  A68.9 Relapsing fever, unspecified CC

✓4th **A69 Other spirochetal infections**

  A69.0 Necrotizing ulcerative stomatitis
    Cancrum oris
    Fusospirochetal gangrene
    Noma
    Stomatitis gangrenosa

  A69.1 Other Vincent's infections CC
    Fusospirochetal pharyngitis
    Necrotizing ulcerative (acute) gingivitis
    Necrotizing ulcerative (acute) gingivostomatitis
    Spirochetal stomatitis
    Trench mouth
    Vincent's angina
    Vincent's gingivitis
    CC Excl: PDX collection 126

  ✓5th **A69.2 Lyme disease**
    Erythema chronicum migrans due to Borrelia burgdorferi
    DEF: Recurrent multisystem disorder through tick bites that begins with lesions of erythema chronicum migrans and is followed by arthritis of the large joints, myalgia, malaise, and neurological and cardiac manifestations.

    A69.20 Lyme disease, unspecified

    A69.21 Meningitis due to Lyme disease CC

N Newborn: 0   P Pediatric: 0-17   M Maternity: 9-64   A Adult: 15-124   MCC Major Complication/Comorbidity   CC Complication/Comorbidity   SW Severe Wound Dx

446   ICD-10-CM 2020

A69.22 Other neurologic disorders in Lyme disease `CC`
Cranial neuritis
Meningoencephalitis
Polyneuropathy

A69.23 Arthritis due to Lyme disease `CC` `HCC`

A69.29 Other conditions associated with Lyme disease `CC`
Myopericarditis due to Lyme disease
AHA: 2016,3Q,12

A69.8 Other specified spirochetal infections

A69.9 Spirochetal infection, unspecified

Other diseases caused by chlamydiae (A70-A74)

EXCLUDES 1　sexually transmitted chlamydial diseases (A55-A56)

A70 Chlamydia psittaci infections `CC`
Ornithosis
Parrot fever
Psittacosis
CC Excl: PDX collection 127

✓4ᵗʰ **A71 Trachoma**
EXCLUDES 1　sequelae of trachoma (B94.0)

A71.0 Initial stage of trachoma
Trachoma dubium

A71.1 Active stage of trachoma
Granular conjunctivitis (trachomatous)
Trachomatous follicular conjunctivitis
Trachomatous pannus

A71.9 Trachoma, unspecified

✓4ᵗʰ **A74 Other diseases caused by chlamydiae**
EXCLUDES 1　neonatal chlamydial conjunctivitis (P39.1)
neonatal chlamydial pneumonia (P23.1)
Reiter's disease (M02.3-)
sexually transmitted chlamydial diseases (A55-A56)
EXCLUDES 2　chlamydial pneumonia (J16.0)

A74.0 Chlamydial conjunctivitis
Paratrachoma

✓5ᵗʰ **A74.8 Other chlamydial diseases**

A74.81 Chlamydial peritonitis
A74.89 Other chlamydial diseases

A74.9 Chlamydial infection, unspecified
Chlamydiosis NOS

Rickettsioses (A75-A79)

DEF: Rickettsia: Condition caused by bacteria that live in lice/ticks transmitted to humans through bites.
CC Excl: For CC codes in categories A75-A79, unless otherwise noted: PDX collection 108

✓4ᵗʰ **A75 Typhus fever**
EXCLUDES 1　rickettsiosis due to Ehrlichia sennetsu (A79.81)

A75.0 Epidemic louse-borne typhus fever due to Rickettsia prowazekii `CC`
Classical typhus (fever)
Epidemic (louse-borne) typhus

A75.1 Recrudescent typhus [Brill's disease] `CC`
Brill-Zinsser disease

A75.2 Typhus fever due to Rickettsia typhi `CC`
Murine (flea-borne) typhus

A75.3 Typhus fever due to Rickettsia tsutsugamushi `CC`
Scrub (mite-borne) typhus
Tsutsugamushi fever

A75.9 Typhus fever, unspecified `CC`
Typhus (fever) NOS
CC Excl: PDX collection 128

✓4ᵗʰ **A77 Spotted fever [tick-borne rickettsioses]**

A77.0 Spotted fever due to Rickettsia rickettsii `CC`
Rocky Mountain spotted fever
Sao Paulo fever

A77.1 Spotted fever due to Rickettsia conorii `CC`
African tick typhus
Boutonneuse fever
India tick typhus
Kenya tick typhus
Marseilles fever
Mediterranean tick fever

A77.2 Spotted fever due to Rickettsia siberica `CC`
North Asian tick fever
Siberian tick typhus

A77.3 Spotted fever due to Rickettsia australis `CC`
Queensland tick typhus

✓5ᵗʰ **A77.4 Ehrlichiosis**
EXCLUDES 1　Rickettsiosis due to Ehrlichia sennetsu (A79.81)

A77.40 Ehrlichiosis, unspecified `CC`
A77.41 Ehrlichiosis chafeensis [E. chafeensis] `CC`
A77.49 Other ehrlichiosis `CC`

A77.8 Other spotted fevers `CC`

A77.9 Spotted fever, unspecified `CC`
Tick-borne typhus NOS

A78 Q fever `CC`
Infection due to Coxiella burnetii
Nine Mile fever
Quadrilateral fever

✓4ᵗʰ **A79 Other rickettsioses**

A79.0 Trench fever `CC`
Quintan fever
Wolhynian fever

A79.1 Rickettsialpox due to Rickettsia akari `CC`
Kew Garden fever
Vesicular rickettsiosis
CC Excl: PDX collection 114

✓5ᵗʰ **A79.8 Other specified rickettsioses**

A79.81 Rickettsiosis due to Ehrlichia sennetsu `CC`
CC Excl: PDX collection 114

A79.89 Other specified rickettsioses `CC`
CC Excl: PDX collection 114

A79.9 Rickettsiosis, unspecified `CC`
Rickettsial infection NOS
CC Excl: PDX collection 114

Viral and prion infections of the central nervous system (A80-A89)

EXCLUDES 1　postpolio syndrome (G14)
sequelae of poliomyelitis (B91)
sequelae of viral encephalitis (B94.1)

✓4ᵗʰ **A80 Acute poliomyelitis**
CC Excl: For MCC codes in category A80: PDX collection 130

A80.0 Acute paralytic poliomyelitis, vaccine-associated `MCC`

A80.1 Acute paralytic poliomyelitis, wild virus, imported `MCC`

A80.2 Acute paralytic poliomyelitis, wild virus, indigenous `MCC`

✓5ᵗʰ **A80.3 Acute paralytic poliomyelitis, other and unspecified**

A80.30 Acute paralytic poliomyelitis, unspecified `MCC`

A80.39 Other acute paralytic poliomyelitis `MCC`

A80.4 Acute nonparalytic poliomyelitis

A80.9 Acute poliomyelitis, unspecified

Chapter 1. Certain Infectious and Parasitic Diseases

A81–A89

✔4ᵗʰ **A81 Atypical virus infections of central nervous system**

> **INCLUDES**   diseases of the central nervous system caused by prions
>
> Use additional code to identify:
> dementia with behavioral disturbance (F02.81)
> dementia without behavioral disturbance (F02.80)

✔5ᵗʰ **A81.0 Creutzfeldt-Jakob disease**

> **DEF:** Communicable, rare spongiform encephalopathy occurring later in life with progressive destruction of the pyramidal and extrapyramidal systems eventually leading to death. Progressive dementia, wasting of muscles, tremor, and other symptoms are present.
>
> **CC Excl: For CC codes in subcategory A81.0:** PDX collection 131

     A81.00 Creutzfeldt-Jakob disease, unspecified `CC` `HCC`

> Jakob-Creutzfeldt disease, unspecified

     A81.01 Variant Creutzfeldt-Jakob disease `CC` `HCC`

> vCJD

     A81.09 Other Creutzfeldt-Jakob disease `CC` `HCC`

> CJD
> Familial Creutzfeldt-Jakob disease
> Iatrogenic Creutzfeldt-Jakob disease
> Sporadic Creutzfeldt-Jakob disease
> Subacute spongiform encephalopathy (with dementia)

   A81.1 Subacute sclerosing panencephalitis `CC` `HCC`

> Dawson's inclusion body encephalitis
> Van Bogaert's sclerosing leukoencephalopathy
> **CC Excl:** PDX collection 132

   A81.2 Progressive multifocal leukoencephalopathy `HIV` `CC` `HCC`

> Multifocal leukoencephalopathy NOS
> **CC Excl:** PDX collection 133

✔5ᵗʰ **A81.8 Other atypical virus infections of central nervous system**

> **CC Excl: For CC codes in subcategory A81.8, unless otherwise noted:** PDX collection 135

     A81.81 Kuru `CC` `HCC`

> **CC Excl:** PDX collection 134

     A81.82 Gerstmann-Sträussler-Scheinker syndrome `HIV` `CC` `HCC`

> GSS syndrome

     A81.83 Fatal familial insomnia `HIV` `CC` `HCC`

> FFI

     A81.89 Other atypical virus infections of central nervous system `HIV` `CC` `HCC`

   A81.9 Atypical virus infection of central nervous system, unspecified `HIV` `CC` `HCC`

> Prion diseases of the central nervous system NOS
> **CC Excl:** PDX collection 134

✔4ᵗʰ **A82 Rabies**

> **CC Excl: For CC codes in category A82:** PDX collection 136

   A82.0 Sylvatic rabies `CC`

   A82.1 Urban rabies `CC`

   A82.9 Rabies, unspecified `CC`

✔4ᵗʰ **A83 Mosquito-borne viral encephalitis**

> **INCLUDES**   mosquito-borne viral meningoencephalitis
> **EXCLUDES 2**   Venezuelan equine encephalitis (A92.2)
> West Nile fever (A92.3-)
> West Nile virus (A92.3-)
>
> **CC Excl: For MCC codes in category A83:** PDX collection 137

   A83.0 Japanese encephalitis `MCC`

   A83.1 Western equine encephalitis `MCC`

   A83.2 Eastern equine encephalitis `MCC`

   A83.3 St Louis encephalitis `MCC`

   A83.4 Australian encephalitis `MCC`

> Kunjin virus disease

   A83.5 California encephalitis `MCC`

> California meningoencephalitis
> La Crosse encephalitis

   A83.6 Rocio virus disease `MCC`

   A83.8 Other mosquito-borne viral encephalitis `MCC`

   A83.9 Mosquito-borne viral encephalitis, unspecified `MCC`

✔4ᵗʰ **A84 Tick-borne viral encephalitis**

> **INCLUDES**   tick-borne viral meningoencephalitis
> **CC Excl: For MCC codes in category A84:** PDX collection 137

   A84.0 Far Eastern tick-borne encephalitis [Russian spring-summer encephalitis] `MCC`

   A84.1 Central European tick-borne encephalitis `MCC`

   A84.8 Other tick-borne viral encephalitis `MCC`

> Louping ill
> Powassan virus disease

   A84.9 Tick-borne viral encephalitis, unspecified `MCC`

✔4ᵗʰ **A85 Other viral encephalitis, not elsewhere classified**

> **INCLUDES**   specified viral encephalomyelitis NEC
> specified viral meningoencephalitis NEC
> **EXCLUDES 1**   benign myalgic encephalomyelitis (G93.3)
> encephalitis due to cytomegalovirus (B25.8)
> encephalitis due to herpesvirus NEC (B10.0-)
> encephalitis due to herpesvirus [herpes simplex] (B00.4)
> encephalitis due to measles virus (B05.0)
> encephalitis due to mumps virus (B26.2)
> encephalitis due to poliomyelitis virus (A80.-)
> encephalitis due to zoster (B02.0)
> lymphocytic choriomeningitis (A87.2)
>
> **CC Excl: For CC codes in category A85:** PDX collection 138

   A85.0 Enteroviral encephalitis `HIV` `CC`

> Enteroviral encephalomyelitis

   A85.1 Adenoviral encephalitis `HIV` `CC`

> Adenoviral meningoencephalitis

   A85.2 Arthropod-borne viral encephalitis, unspecified `MCC`

> **EXCLUDES 1**   West nile virus with encephalitis (A92.31)
> **CC Excl:** PDX collection 137

   A85.8 Other specified viral encephalitis `HIV` `CC`

> Encephalitis lethargica
> Von Economo-Cruchet disease

A86 Unspecified viral encephalitis `HIV` `CC`

> Viral encephalomyelitis NOS
> Viral meningoencephalitis NOS
> **CC Excl:** PDX collection 139

✔4ᵗʰ **A87 Viral meningitis**

> **EXCLUDES 1**   meningitis due to herpesvirus [herpes simplex] (B00.3)
> meningitis due to measles virus (B05.1)
> meningitis due to mumps virus (B26.1)
> meningitis due to poliomyelitis virus (A80.-)
> meningitis due to zoster (B02.1)
>
> **DEF:** Meningitis: Inflammation of the meningeal layers of the brain and spine.
>
> **CC Excl: For CC codes in category A87, unless otherwise noted:** PDX collection 140

   A87.0 Enteroviral meningitis `CC`

> Coxsackievirus meningitis
> Echovirus meningitis

   A87.1 Adenoviral meningitis `CC`

   A87.2 Lymphocytic choriomeningitis `CC`

> Lymphocytic meningoencephalitis
> **CC Excl:** PDX collection 141

   A87.8 Other viral meningitis `CC`

   A87.9 Viral meningitis, unspecified `CC`

✔4ᵗʰ **A88 Other viral infections of central nervous system, not elsewhere classified**

> **EXCLUDES 1**   viral encephalitis NOS (A86)
> viral meningitis NOS (A87.9)

   A88.0 Enteroviral exanthematous fever [Boston exanthem] `CC`

> **CC Excl:** PDX collection 137

   A88.1 Epidemic vertigo

   A88.8 Other specified viral infections of central nervous system `HIV` `CC`

> **CC Excl:** PDX collection 138

A89 Unspecified viral infection of central nervous system `HIV` `CC`

> **CC Excl:** PDX collection 139

N Newborn: 0   **P** Pediatric: 0-17   **M** Maternity: 9-64   **A** Adult: 15-124   **MCC** Major Complication/Comorbidity   **CC** Complication/Comorbidity   **SW** Severe Wound Dx

448   ICD-10-CM 2020

Arthropod-borne viral fevers and viral hemorrhagic fevers (A90-A99)

A90 Dengue fever [classical dengue] `CC`
> EXCLUDES 1   *dengue hemorrhagic fever (A91)*
AHA: 2016,3Q,13
CC Excl: PDX collection 142

A91 Dengue hemorrhagic fever `CC`
CC Excl: PDX collection 143

✓4th A92 Other mosquito-borne viral fevers
> EXCLUDES 1   *Ross River disease (B33.1)*
CC Excl: For codes in category A92:
For MCC codes: PDX collection 145
For CC codes, unless otherwise noted: PDX collection 144

A92.0 Chikungunya virus disease `CC`
Chikungunya (hemorrhagic) fever
CC Excl: PDX collection 143

A92.1 O'nyong-nyong fever `CC`

A92.2 Venezuelan equine fever `CC`
Venezuelan equine encephalitis
Venezuelan equine encephalomyelitis virus disease

✓5th A92.3 West Nile virus infection
West Nile fever
AHA: 2016,3Q,12

A92.30 West Nile virus infection, unspecified `MCC`
West Nile fever NOS
West Nile fever without complications
West Nile virus NOS

A92.31 West Nile virus infection with encephalitis `MCC`
West Nile encephalitis
West Nile encephalomyelitis

A92.32 West Nile virus infection with other neurologic manifestation `MCC`
Use additional code to specify the neurologic manifestation

A92.39 West Nile virus infection with other complications `MCC`
Use additional code to specify the other conditions

A92.4 Rift Valley fever `CC`

A92.5 Zika virus disease `CC`
Zika virus fever
Zika virus infection
Zika NOS
> EXCLUDES 1   *congenital Zika virus disease (P35.4)*
AHA: 2016,4Q,4-7
DEF: Virus transmitted via a bite from an infected Aedes species mosquito. Common symptoms of the virus include fever, rash, joint pain, and conjunctivitis; they are usually mild in nature and may last from several days to a week. Most people who have the Zika virus do not require medical attention; however, in pregnant women, the Zika virus can cause a serious birth defect called microcephaly, as well as other severe fetal brain defects.

A92.8 Other specified mosquito-borne viral fevers `CC`

A92.9 Mosquito-borne viral fever, unspecified `CC`
CC Excl: PDX collection 143

✓4th A93 Other arthropod-borne viral fevers, not elsewhere classified
CC Excl: For CC codes in category A93, unless otherwise noted: PDX collection 143

A93.0 Oropouche virus disease `CC`
Oropouche fever
CC Excl: PDX collection 144

A93.1 Sandfly fever `CC`
Pappataci fever
Phlebotomus fever

A93.2 Colorado tick fever `CC`

A93.8 Other specified arthropod-borne viral fevers `CC`
Piry virus disease
Vesicular stomatitis virus disease [Indiana fever]

A94 Unspecified arthropod-borne viral fever `CC`
Arboviral fever NOS
Arbovirus infection NOS
CC Excl: PDX collection 143

✓4th A95 Yellow fever
CC Excl: For CC codes in category A95: PDX collection 146

A95.0 Sylvatic yellow fever `CC`
Jungle yellow fever

A95.1 Urban yellow fever `CC`

A95.9 Yellow fever, unspecified `CC`

✓4th A96 Arenaviral hemorrhagic fever
CC Excl: For CC codes in category A96: PDX collection 147

A96.0 Junin hemorrhagic fever `CC`
Argentinian hemorrhagic fever

A96.1 Machupo hemorrhagic fever `CC`
Bolivian hemorrhagic fever

A96.2 Lassa fever

A96.8 Other arenaviral hemorrhagic fevers `CC`

A96.9 Arenaviral hemorrhagic fever, unspecified `CC`

✓4th A98 Other viral hemorrhagic fevers, not elsewhere classified
> EXCLUDES 1   *chikungunya hemorrhagic fever (A92.0)*
>   *dengue hemorrhagic fever (A91)*
CC Excl: For CC codes in category A98, unless otherwise noted: PDX collection 143

A98.0 Crimean-Congo hemorrhagic fever `CC`
Central Asian hemorrhagic fever

A98.1 Omsk hemorrhagic fever `CC`

A98.2 Kyasanur Forest disease `CC`

A98.3 Marburg virus disease

A98.4 Ebola virus disease

A98.5 Hemorrhagic fever with renal syndrome `CC`
Epidemic hemorrhagic fever
Korean hemorrhagic fever
Russian hemorrhagic fever
Hantaan virus disease
Hantavirus disease with renal manifestations
Nephropathia epidemica
Songo fever
> EXCLUDES 1   *hantavirus (cardio)-pulmonary syndrome (B33.4)*
CC Excl: PDX collection 148

A98.8 Other specified viral hemorrhagic fevers `CC`

A99 Unspecified viral hemorrhagic fever `CC`
CC Excl: PDX collection 143

Viral infections characterized by skin and mucous membrane lesions (B00-B09)

✓4th B00 Herpesviral [herpes simplex] infections
> EXCLUDES 1   *congenital herpesviral infections (P35.2)*
> EXCLUDES 2   *anogenital herpesviral infection (A60.-)*
>   *gammaherpesviral mononucleosis (B27.0-)*
>   *herpangina (B08.5)*

B00.0 Eczema herpeticum `HIV`
Kaposi's varicelliform eruption

B00.1 Herpesviral vesicular dermatitis `HIV`
Herpes simplex facialis
Herpes simplex labialis
Herpes simplex otitis externa
Vesicular dermatitis of ear
Vesicular dermatitis of lip

B00.2 Herpesviral gingivostomatitis and pharyngotonsillitis `HIV` `CC`
Herpesviral pharyngitis
CC Excl: PDX collection 149

B00.3 Herpesviral meningitis `HIV` `MCC`
CC Excl: PDX collection 150

B00.4 Herpesviral encephalitis `HIV` `MCC`

Herpesviral meningoencephalitis

Simian B disease

EXCLUDES 1   herpesviral encephalitis due to herpesvirus 6 and 7 (B10.01, B10.09)

non-simplex herpesviral encephalitis (B10.0-)

CC Excl: PDX collection 151

✓5ᵗʰ **B00.5 Herpesviral ocular disease**

CC Excl: For CC codes in subcategory B00.5: PDX collection 152

B00.50 Herpesviral ocular disease, unspecified `HIV` `CC`

B00.51 Herpesviral iridocyclitis `HIV` `CC`

Herpesviral iritis

Herpesviral uveitis, anterior

B00.52 Herpesviral keratitis `HIV` `CC`

Herpesviral keratoconjunctivitis

B00.53 Herpesviral conjunctivitis `HIV` `CC`

B00.59 Other herpesviral disease of eye `HIV` `CC`

Herpesviral dermatitis of eyelid

B00.7 Disseminated herpesviral disease `HIV` `MCC` `HCC`

Herpesviral sepsis

CC Excl: PDX collection 153

✓5ᵗʰ **B00.8 Other forms of herpesviral infections**

B00.81 Herpesviral hepatitis `HIV` `CC`

CC Excl: PDX collection 154

B00.82 Herpes simplex myelitis `MCC` `HCC`

CC Excl: PDX collection 155

B00.89 Other herpesviral infection `HIV` `CC`

Herpesviral whitlow

CC Excl: PDX collection 156

B00.9 Herpesviral infection, unspecified `HIV`

Herpes simplex infection NOS

✓4ᵗʰ **B01 Varicella [chickenpox]**

CC Excl: For CC codes in category B01: PDX collection 157

B01.0 Varicella meningitis `CC`

✓5ᵗʰ **B01.1 Varicella encephalitis, myelitis and encephalomyelitis**

Postchickenpox encephalitis, myelitis and encephalomyelitis

B01.11 Varicella encephalitis and encephalomyelitis `MCC`

Postchickenpox encephalitis and encephalomyelitis

CC Excl: PDX collection 158

B01.12 Varicella myelitis `MCC` `HCC`

Postchickenpox myelitis

CC Excl: PDX collection 159

B01.2 Varicella pneumonia `MCC`

CC Excl: PDX collection 160

✓5ᵗʰ **B01.8 Varicella with other complications**

B01.81 Varicella keratitis `CC`

B01.89 Other varicella complications `CC`

B01.9 Varicella without complication `CC`

Varicella NOS

✓4ᵗʰ **B02 Zoster [herpes zoster]**

INCLUDES   shingles

zona

B02.0 Zoster encephalitis `HIV` `CC`

Zoster meningoencephalitis

CC Excl: PDX collection 161

B02.1 Zoster meningitis `HIV` `MCC`

AHA: 2019,1Q,18

CC Excl: PDX collection 162

✓5ᵗʰ **B02.2 Zoster with other nervous system involvement**

CC Excl: For CC codes in subcategory B02.2: PDX collection 161

B02.21 Postherpetic geniculate ganglionitis `HIV` `CC`

B02.22 Postherpetic trigeminal neuralgia `HIV` `CC`

B02.23 Postherpetic polyneuropathy `HIV` `CC`

B02.24 Postherpetic myelitis `MCC` `HCC`

Herpes zoster myelitis

CC Excl: PDX collection 163

B02.29 Other postherpetic nervous system involvement `HIV` `CC`

Postherpetic radiculopathy

✓5ᵗʰ **B02.3 Zoster ocular disease**

CC Excl: For CC codes in subcategory B02.3: PDX collection 164

B02.30 Zoster ocular disease, unspecified `HIV` `CC`

B02.31 Zoster conjunctivitis `HIV` `CC`

B02.32 Zoster iridocyclitis `HIV` `CC`

B02.33 Zoster keratitis `HIV` `CC`

Herpes zoster keratoconjunctivitis

B02.34 Zoster scleritis `HIV` `CC`

B02.39 Other herpes zoster eye disease `HIV` `CC`

Zoster blepharitis

B02.7 Disseminated zoster `HIV` `CC`

CC Excl: PDX collection 165

B02.8 Zoster with other complications `HIV` `CC`

Herpes zoster otitis externa

CC Excl: PDX collection 165

B02.9 Zoster without complications `HIV`

Zoster NOS

B03 Smallpox `CC`

NOTE   In 1980 the 33rd World Health Assembly declared that smallpox had been eradicated.

The classification is maintained for surveillance purposes.

CC Excl: PDX collection 166

B04 Monkeypox `CC`

CC Excl: PDX collection 167

✓4ᵗʰ **B05 Measles**

INCLUDES   morbilli

EXCLUDES 1   subacute sclerosing panencephalitis (A81.1)

B05.0 Measles complicated by encephalitis `MCC`

Postmeasles encephalitis

CC Excl: PDX collection 168

B05.1 Measles complicated by meningitis `CC`

Postmeasles meningitis

CC Excl: PDX collection 169

B05.2 Measles complicated by pneumonia `MCC`

Postmeasles pneumonia

CC Excl: PDX collection 170

B05.3 Measles complicated by otitis media

Postmeasles otitis media

B05.4 Measles with intestinal complications `CC`

CC Excl: PDX collection 169

✓5ᵗʰ **B05.8 Measles with other complications**

B05.81 Measles keratitis and keratoconjunctivitis `CC`

CC Excl: PDX collection 171

B05.89 Other measles complications `CC`

CC Excl: PDX collection 169

B05.9 Measles without complication

Measles NOS

✓4ᵗʰ **B06 Rubella [German measles]**

EXCLUDES 1   congenital rubella (P35.0)

DEF: Highly contagious virus in which the symptoms are mild and short-lived in most people. Rubella during pregnancy, however, can result in abortion, stillbirth, or congenital defects.

CC Excl: For CC/MCC codes in category B06, unless otherwise noted: PDX collection 172

✓5ᵗʰ **B06.0 Rubella with neurological complications**

B06.00 Rubella with neurological complication, unspecified `CC`

B06.01 Rubella encephalitis `MCC`

Rubella meningoencephalitis

B06.02 Rubella meningitis `CC`

B06.09 Other neurological complications of rubella `CC`

✓5ᵗʰ **B06.8 Rubella with other complications**

B06.81 Rubella pneumonia `CC`

B06.82 Rubella arthritis `CC` `HCC`

CC Excl: PDX collection 173

B06.89 Other rubella complications `CC`

N Newborn: 0   P Pediatric: 0-17   M Maternity: 9-64   A Adult: 15-124   MCC Major Complication/Comorbidity   CC Complication/Comorbidity   SW Severe Wound Dx

450   ICD-10-CM 2020

B06.9 **Rubella without complication**
Rubella NOS

✓4ᵗʰ **B07** **Viral warts**

INCLUDES   verruca simplex
verruca vulgaris
viral warts due to human papillomavirus

EXCLUDES 2   *anogenital (venereal) warts (A63.0)*
papilloma of bladder (D41.4)
papilloma of cervix (D26.0)
papilloma larynx (D14.1)

B07.0 **Plantar wart**
Verruca plantaris

B07.8 **Other viral warts**
Common wart
Flat wart
Verruca plana

B07.9 **Viral wart, unspecified**

✓4ᵗʰ **B08** **Other viral infections characterized by skin and mucous membrane lesions, not elsewhere classified**
EXCLUDES 1   *vesicular stomatitis virus disease (A93.8)*

✓5ᵗʰ **B08.0** **Other orthopoxvirus infections**
EXCLUDES 2   *monkeypox (B04)*

✓6ᵗʰ **B08.01** **Cowpox and vaccinia not from vaccine**

B08.010 **Cowpox**
DEF: Disease contracted by milking infected cows. The vesicles usually appear on the fingers, hands, and adjacent areas and usually disappear without scarring. Other symptoms include local edema, lymphangitis, and regional lymphadenitis with or without fever.

B08.011 **Vaccinia not from vaccine**
EXCLUDES 1   *vaccinia (from vaccination) (generalized) (T88.1)*

B08.02 **Orf virus disease**
Contagious pustular dermatitis
Ecthyma contagiosum

B08.03 **Pseudocowpox [milker's node]**

B08.04 **Paravaccinia, unspecified**

B08.09 **Other orthopoxvirus infections**
Orthopoxvirus infection NOS

B08.1 **Molluscum contagiosum**
DEF: Benign poxvirus infection causing small bumps on the skin or conjunctiva and is transmitted by close contact.

✓5ᵗʰ **B08.2** **Exanthema subitum [sixth disease]**
Roseola infantum

B08.20 **Exanthema subitum [sixth disease], unspecified**   P
Roseola infantum, unspecified

B08.21 **Exanthema subitum [sixth disease] due to human herpesvirus 6**   P
Roseola infantum due to human herpesvirus 6

B08.22 **Exanthema subitum [sixth disease] due to human herpesvirus 7**   P
Roseola infantum due to human herpesvirus 7

B08.3 **Erythema infectiosum [fifth disease]**   CC
DEF: Infection with human parvovirus B19, mainly occurring in children. Symptoms include a low-grade fever, malaise, or a "cold" a few days before the appearance of a mild rash illness that presents as a "slapped-cheek" rash on the face and a lacy red rash on the trunk and limbs.
CC Excl: PDX collection 174

B08.4 **Enteroviral vesicular stomatitis with exanthem**
Hand, foot and mouth disease

B08.5 **Enteroviral vesicular pharyngitis**
Herpangina
DEF: Acute infectious Coxsackie virus infection causing throat lesions, fever, and vomiting that generally affects children in the summer.

✓5ᵗʰ **B08.6** **Parapoxvirus infections**

B08.60 **Parapoxvirus infection, unspecified**

B08.61 **Bovine stomatitis**

B08.62 **Sealpox**

B08.69 **Other parapoxvirus infections**

✓5ᵗʰ **B08.7** **Yatapoxvirus infections**

B08.70 **Yatapoxvirus infection, unspecified**

B08.71 **Tanapox virus disease**   CC
CC Excl: PDX collection 167

B08.72 **Yaba pox virus disease**
Yaba monkey tumor disease

B08.79 **Other yatapoxvirus infections**

B08.8 **Other specified viral infections characterized by skin and mucous membrane lesions**
Enteroviral lymphonodular pharyngitis
Foot-and-mouth disease
Poxvirus NEC

B09 **Unspecified viral infection characterized by skin and mucous membrane lesions**
Viral enanthema NOS
Viral exanthema NOS

Other human herpesviruses (B10)

✓4ᵗʰ **B10** **Other human herpesviruses**
EXCLUDES 2   *cytomegalovirus (B25.9)*
Epstein-Barr virus (B27.0-)
herpes NOS (B00.9)
herpes simplex (B00.-)
herpes zoster (B02.-)
human herpesvirus NOS (B00.-)
human herpesvirus 1 and 2 (B00.-)
human herpesvirus 3 (B01.-, B02.-)
human herpesvirus 4 (B27.0-)
human herpesvirus 5 (B25.-)
varicella (B01.-)
zoster (B02.-)

✓5ᵗʰ **B10.0** **Other human herpesvirus encephalitis**
EXCLUDES 2   *herpes encephalitis NOS (B00.4)*
herpes simplex encephalitis (B00.4)
human herpesvirus encephalitis (B00.4)
simian B herpes virus encephalitis (B00.4)

B10.01 **Human herpesvirus 6 encephalitis**   HIV MCC
CC Excl: PDX collection 151

B10.09 **Other human herpesvirus encephalitis**   HIV MCC
Human herpesvirus 7 encephalitis
CC Excl: PDX collection 151

✓5ᵗʰ **B10.8** **Other human herpesvirus infection**

B10.81 **Human herpesvirus 6 infection**

B10.82 **Human herpesvirus 7 infection**

B10.89 **Other human herpesvirus infection**
Human herpesvirus 8 infection
Kaposi's sarcoma-associated herpesvirus infection

Viral hepatitis (B15-B19)

EXCLUDES 1   *sequelae of viral hepatitis (B94.2)*
EXCLUDES 2   *cytomegaloviral hepatitis (B25.1)*
herpesviral [herpes simplex] hepatitis (B00.81)
DEF: Hepatitis A: HAV infection that is self-limiting with flulike symptoms. Transmission is fecal-oral.
DEF: Hepatitis B: HBV infection that can be chronic and systemic. Transmission is bodily fluids.
DEF: Hepatitis C: HCV infection that can be chronic and systemic. Transmission is blood transfusion and unidentified agents.
DEF: Hepatitis D (delta): HDV that occurs only in the presence of hepatitis B virus. Transmission is contaminated blood in contact with mucous membranes.
DEF: Hepatitis E: HEV is an epidemic form. Transmission is fecal-oral, most often from contaminated water.
CC Excl: For CC/MCC codes in categories B15-B19: PDX collection 175

✓4ᵗʰ **B15** **Acute hepatitis A**

B15.0 **Hepatitis A with hepatic coma**   MCC

B15.9 **Hepatitis A without hepatic coma**   CC
Hepatitis A (acute)(viral) NOS

✓4ᵗʰ **B16** **Acute hepatitis B**
AHA: 2016,3Q,13

B16.0 **Acute hepatitis B with delta-agent with hepatic coma**   MCC

B16.1 **Acute hepatitis B with delta-agent without hepatic coma**   CC

B16.2 **Acute hepatitis B without delta-agent with hepatic coma**   MCC

Chapter 1. Certain Infectious and Parasitic Diseases

B16.9 Acute hepatitis B without delta-agent and without hepatic coma   `CC`
Hepatitis B (acute) (viral) NOS

✓4ᵗʰ **B17 Other acute viral hepatitis**

B17.0 Acute delta-(super) infection of hepatitis B carrier   `CC`

✓5ᵗʰ **B17.1 Acute hepatitis C**

    B17.10 Acute hepatitis C without hepatic coma   `CC`
       Acute hepatitis C NOS

    B17.11 Acute hepatitis C with hepatic coma   `MCC`

B17.2 Acute hepatitis E   `CC`

B17.8 Other specified acute viral hepatitis   `CC`
Hepatitis non-A non-B (acute) (viral) NEC

B17.9 Acute viral hepatitis, unspecified   `CC`
Acute hepatitis NOS
Acute infectious hepatitis NOS

✓4ᵗʰ **B18 Chronic viral hepatitis**
INCLUDES carrier of viral hepatitis
AHA: 2017,1Q,41

B18.0 Chronic viral hepatitis B with delta-agent   `CC` `HCC`

B18.1 Chronic viral hepatitis B without delta-agent   `CC` `HCC`
Carrier of viral hepatitis B
Chronic (viral) hepatitis B

B18.2 Chronic viral hepatitis C   `HCC`
Carrier of viral hepatitis C
AHA: 2018,1Q,4

B18.8 Other chronic viral hepatitis   `CC` `HCC`
Carrier of other viral hepatitis

B18.9 Chronic viral hepatitis, unspecified   `CC` `HCC`
Carrier of unspecified viral hepatitis

✓4ᵗʰ **B19 Unspecified viral hepatitis**

B19.0 Unspecified viral hepatitis with hepatic coma   `MCC`

✓5ᵗʰ **B19.1 Unspecified viral hepatitis B**

    B19.10 Unspecified viral hepatitis B without hepatic coma   `CC`
       Unspecified viral hepatitis B NOS

    B19.11 Unspecified viral hepatitis B with hepatic coma   `MCC`

✓5ᵗʰ **B19.2 Unspecified viral hepatitis C**

    B19.20 Unspecified viral hepatitis C without hepatic coma
       Viral hepatitis C NOS

    B19.21 Unspecified viral hepatitis C with hepatic coma   `MCC`

B19.9 Unspecified viral hepatitis without hepatic coma   `CC`
Viral hepatitis NOS

Human immunodeficiency virus [HIV] disease (B20)

B20 Human immunodeficiency virus [HIV] disease   `CC` `HCC`
INCLUDES acquired immune deficiency syndrome [AIDS]
AIDS-related complex [ARC]
HIV infection, symptomatic
Code first Human immunodeficiency virus [HIV] disease complicating pregnancy, childbirth and the puerperium, if applicable (O98.7-)
Use additional code(s) to identify all manifestations of HIV infection
EXCLUDES 1 *asymptomatic human immunodeficiency virus [HIV] infection status (Z21)*
exposure to HIV virus (Z20.6)
inconclusive serologic evidence of HIV (R75)
AHA: 2019,1Q,8-11
CC Excl: PDX collection 176

Other viral diseases (B25-B34)

✓4ᵗʰ **B25 Cytomegaloviral disease**
EXCLUDES 1 *congenital cytomegalovirus infection (P35.1)*
cytomegaloviral mononucleosis (B27.1-)

B25.0 Cytomegaloviral pneumonitis   `MCC` `HCC`
CC Excl: PDX collection 110

B25.1 Cytomegaloviral hepatitis   `CC` `HCC`
CC Excl: No Excl

B25.2 Cytomegaloviral pancreatitis   `MCC` `HCC`
CC Excl: PDX collection 177

B25.8 Other cytomegaloviral diseases   `HIV` `CC` `HCC`
Cytomegaloviral encephalitis
CC Excl: PDX collection 178

B25.9 Cytomegaloviral disease, unspecified   `HIV` `CC` `HCC`
CC Excl: PDX collection 178

✓4ᵗʰ **B26 Mumps**
INCLUDES epidemic parotitis
infectious parotitis

B26.0 Mumps orchitis   `CC` ♂
CC Excl: PDX collection 179

B26.1 Mumps meningitis   `MCC`
CC Excl: PDX collection 180

B26.2 Mumps encephalitis   `MCC`
CC Excl: PDX collection 181

B26.3 Mumps pancreatitis   `CC`
CC Excl: PDX collection 182

✓5ᵗʰ **B26.8 Mumps with other complications**
CC Excl: For CC codes in subcategory B26.8, unless otherwise noted: PDX collection 184

    B26.81 Mumps hepatitis   `CC`
       CC Excl: PDX collection 183

    B26.82 Mumps myocarditis   `CC`

    B26.83 Mumps nephritis   `CC`

    B26.84 Mumps polyneuropathy   `CC`
       CC Excl: PDX collection 185

    B26.85 Mumps arthritis   `CC` `HCC`

    B26.89 Other mumps complications   `CC`

B26.9 Mumps without complication
Mumps NOS
Mumps parotitis NOS

✓4ᵗʰ **B27 Infectious mononucleosis**
INCLUDES glandular fever
monocytic angina
Pfeiffer's disease

✓5ᵗʰ **B27.0 Gammaherpesviral mononucleosis**
Mononucleosis due to Epstein-Barr virus

    B27.00 Gammaherpesviral mononucleosis without complication

    B27.01 Gammaherpesviral mononucleosis with polyneuropathy

    B27.02 Gammaherpesviral mononucleosis with meningitis

    B27.09 Gammaherpesviral mononucleosis with other complications
       Hepatomegaly in gammaherpesviral mononucleosis

✓5ᵗʰ **B27.1 Cytomegaloviral mononucleosis**

    B27.10 Cytomegaloviral mononucleosis without complications

    B27.11 Cytomegaloviral mononucleosis with polyneuropathy

    B27.12 Cytomegaloviral mononucleosis with meningitis

    B27.19 Cytomegaloviral mononucleosis with other complication
       Hepatomegaly in cytomegaloviral mononucleosis

✓5ᵗʰ **B27.8 Other infectious mononucleosis**

    B27.80 Other infectious mononucleosis without complication

    B27.81 Other infectious mononucleosis with polyneuropathy

    B27.82 Other infectious mononucleosis with meningitis

    B27.89 Other infectious mononucleosis with other complication
       Hepatomegaly in other infectious mononucleosis

✓5ᵗʰ **B27.9 Infectious mononucleosis, unspecified**

    B27.90 Infectious mononucleosis, unspecified without complication

    B27.91 Infectious mononucleosis, unspecified with polyneuropathy

    B27.92 Infectious mononucleosis, unspecified with meningitis

`N` Newborn: 0   `P` Pediatric: 0-17   `M` Maternity: 9-64   `A` Adult: 15-124   `MCC` Major Complication/Comorbidity   `CC` Complication/Comorbidity   `SW` Severe Wound Dx

452   ICD-10-CM 2020

B27.99 **Infectious mononucleosis, unspecified with other complication**
Hepatomegaly in unspecified infectious mononucleosis

☑4ᵗʰ **B30** **Viral conjunctivitis**
EXCLUDES 1   herpesviral [herpes simplex] ocular disease (B00.5)
ocular zoster (B02.3)

Viral Conjunctivitis

Normal conjunctiva

Inflamed conjunctiva

B30.0 **Keratoconjunctivitis due to adenovirus**
Epidemic keratoconjunctivitis
Shipyard eye

B30.1 **Conjunctivitis due to adenovirus**
Acute adenoviral follicular conjunctivitis
Swimming-pool conjunctivitis

B30.2 **Viral pharyngoconjunctivitis**

B30.3 **Acute epidemic hemorrhagic conjunctivitis (enteroviral)**
Conjunctivitis due to coxsackievirus 24
Conjunctivitis due to enterovirus 70
Hemorrhagic conjunctivitis (acute)(epidemic)

B30.8 **Other viral conjunctivitis**
Newcastle conjunctivitis

B30.9 **Viral conjunctivitis, unspecified**

☑4ᵗʰ **B33** **Other viral diseases, not elsewhere classified**

B33.0 **Epidemic myalgia**
Bornholm disease

B33.1 **Ross River disease**   CC
Epidemic polyarthritis and exanthema
Ross River fever
CC Excl: PDX collection 144

☑5ᵗʰ **B33.2** **Viral carditis**
Coxsackie (virus) carditis

   B33.20 **Viral carditis, unspecified**   CC
     CC Excl: PDX collection 186

   B33.21 **Viral endocarditis**   CC
     CC Excl: PDX collection 187

   B33.22 **Viral myocarditis**   CC
     CC Excl: PDX collection 186

   B33.23 **Viral pericarditis**   CC
     CC Excl: PDX collection 188

   B33.24 **Viral cardiomyopathy**   HCC

B33.3 **Retrovirus infections, not elsewhere classified**
Retrovirus infection NOS

B33.4 **Hantavirus (cardio)-pulmonary syndrome [HPS] [HCPS]**   CC
Hantavirus disease with pulmonary manifestations
Sin nombre virus disease
Use additional code to identify any associated acute kidney failure (N17.9)
EXCLUDES 1   hantavirus disease with renal manifestations (A98.5)
hemorrhagic fever with renal manifestations (A98.5)
CC Excl: PDX collection 189

B33.8 **Other specified viral diseases**
EXCLUDES 1   anogenital human papillomavirus infection (A63.0)
viral warts due to human papillomavirus infection (B07)

☑4ᵗʰ **B34** **Viral infection of unspecified site**
EXCLUDES 1   anogenital human papillomavirus infection (A63.0)
cytomegaloviral disease NOS (B25.9)
herpesvirus [herpes simplex] infection NOS (B00.9)
retrovirus infection NOS (B33.3)
viral agents as the cause of diseases classified elsewhere (B97.-)
viral warts due to human papillomavirus infection (B07)

B34.0 **Adenovirus infection, unspecified**

B34.1 **Enterovirus infection, unspecified**
Coxsackievirus infection NOS
Echovirus infection NOS

B34.2 **Coronavirus infection, unspecified**
EXCLUDES 1   pneumonia due to SARS-associated coronavirus (J12.81)

B34.3 **Parvovirus infection, unspecified**   CC
CC Excl: PDX collection 174

B34.4 **Papovavirus infection, unspecified**

B34.8 **Other viral infections of unspecified site**

B34.9 **Viral infection, unspecified**
Viremia NOS
AHA: 2016,3Q,10

Mycoses (B35-B49)

EXCLUDES 2   hypersensitivity pneumonitis due to organic dust (J67.-)
mycosis fungoides (C84.0-)

☑4ᵗʰ **B35** **Dermatophytosis**
INCLUDES   favus
infections due to species of Epidermophyton, Micro-sporum and Trichophyton
tinea, any type except those in B36.-
DEF: Contagious superficial fungal infection of the skin that invades and grows in dead keratin.

B35.0 **Tinea barbae and tinea capitis**
Beard ringworm
Kerion
Scalp ringworm
Sycosis, mycotic

B35.1 **Tinea unguium**
Dermatophytic onychia
Dermatophytosis of nail
Onychomycosis
Ringworm of nails

B35.2 **Tinea manuum**
Dermatophytosis of hand
Hand ringworm

B35.3 **Tinea pedis**
Athlete's foot
Dermatophytosis of foot
Foot ringworm

B35.4 **Tinea corporis**
Ringworm of the body

B35.5 **Tinea imbricata**
Tokelau

B35.6 **Tinea cruris**
Dhobi itch
Groin ringworm
Jock itch

B35.8 **Other dermatophytoses**
Disseminated dermatophytosis
Granulomatous dermatophytosis

B35.9 **Dermatophytosis, unspecified**
Ringworm NOS

☑4ᵗʰ **B36** **Other superficial mycoses**

B36.0 **Pityriasis versicolor**
Tinea flava
Tinea versicolor

Chapter 1. Certain Infectious and Parasitic Diseases

B36.1   Tinea nigra
Keratomycosis nigricans palmaris
Microsporosis nigra
Pityriasis nigra

B36.2   White piedra
Tinea blanca

B36.3   Black piedra

B36.8   Other specified superficial mycoses

B36.9   Superficial mycosis, unspecified

√4ᵗʰ **B37   Candidiasis**

INCLUDES   candidosis
      moniliasis
EXCLUDES 1   neonatal candidiasis (P37.5)
DEF: Candida: Genus of yeast-like fungi that are commonly found in the mouth, skin, intestinal tract, and vagina. It may cause a white, cheesy discharge.

B37.0   Candidal stomatitis   HIV CC
Oral thrush
CC Excl: PDX collection 190

B37.1   Pulmonary candidiasis   HIV MCC HCC
Candidal bronchitis
Candidal pneumonia
CC Excl: PDX collection 190

B37.2   Candidiasis of skin and nail   HIV
Candidal onychia
Candidal paronychia
EXCLUDES 2   diaper dermatitis (L22)

B37.3   Candidiasis of vulva and vagina   ♀
Candidal vulvovaginitis
Monilial vulvovaginitis
Vaginal thrush

√5ᵗʰ **B37.4   Candidiasis of other urogenital sites**

B37.41   Candidal cystitis and urethritis   CC H6
CC Excl: PDX collection 191

B37.42   Candidal balanitis   ♂

B37.49   Other urogenital candidiasis   CC H6
Candidal pyelonephritis
CC Excl: PDX collection 191

B37.5   Candidal meningitis   HIV MCC
CC Excl: PDX collection 192

B37.6   Candidal endocarditis   HIV MCC
CC Excl: PDX collection 190

B37.7   Candidal sepsis   MCC HCC
Disseminated candidiasis
Systemic candidiasis
AHA: 2014,4Q,46
TIP: This code is assigned when sepsis is documented as due to any *Candida* type. If non-*Candida albicans* is documented, code B48.8 Other specified mycoses, is assigned.
CC Excl: PDX collection 193

√5ᵗʰ **B37.8   Candidiasis of other sites**
CC Excl: For CC codes in subcategory B37.8, unless otherwise noted: PDX collection 190

B37.81   Candidal esophagitis   HIV MCC HCC

B37.82   Candidal enteritis   HIV MCC
Candidal proctitis

B37.83   Candidal cheilitis   HIV CC

B37.84   Candidal otitis externa   HIV CC

B37.89   Other sites of candidiasis   HIV CC
Candidal osteomyelitis
CC Excl: PDX collection 194

B37.9   Candidiasis, unspecified   HIV
Thrush NOS

√4ᵗʰ **B38   Coccidioidomycosis**

B38.0   Acute pulmonary coccidioidomycosis   HIV CC HCC
CC Excl: PDX collection 195

B38.1   Chronic pulmonary coccidioidomycosis   HIV CC HCC
CC Excl: PDX collection 196

B38.2   Pulmonary coccidioidomycosis, unspecified   HIV CC HCC
CC Excl: PDX collection 196

B38.3   Cutaneous coccidioidomycosis   HIV CC
CC Excl: PDX collection 197

B38.4   Coccidioidomycosis meningitis   HIV MCC
DEF: *Coccidioides immitis* infection of the lining of the brain and/or spinal cord.
CC Excl: PDX collection 198

B38.7   Disseminated coccidioidomycosis   HIV CC
Generalized coccidioidomycosis
CC Excl: PDX collection 199

√5ᵗʰ **B38.8   Other forms of coccidioidomycosis**

B38.81   Prostatic coccidioidomycosis   HIV CC ♂
CC Excl: PDX collection 197

B38.89   Other forms of coccidioidomycosis   HIV CC
CC Excl: PDX collection 199

B38.9   Coccidioidomycosis, unspecified   HIV CC
CC Excl: PDX collection 199

√4ᵗʰ **B39   Histoplasmosis**
Code first associated AIDS (B20)
Use additional code for any associated manifestations, such as:
   endocarditis (I39)
   meningitis (G02)
   pericarditis (I32)
   retinitis (H32)
DEF: Type of lung infection caused by breathing in fungal spores often found in the droppings of bats and birds or soil contaminated by their droppings.
CC Excl: For MCC codes in category B39: PDX collection 200

Histoplasmosis

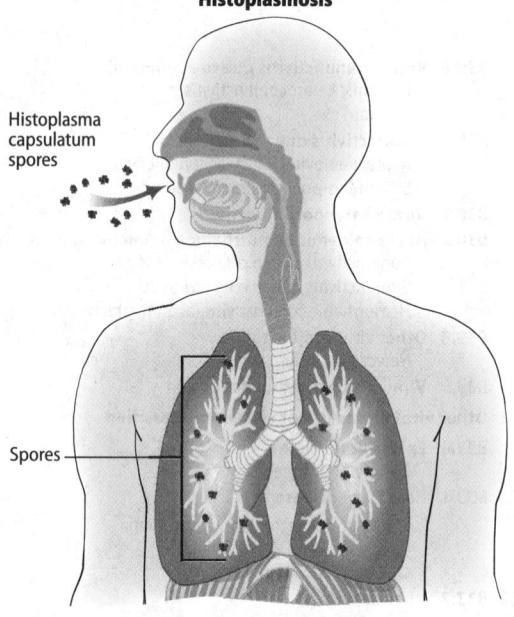

Histoplasma capsulatum spores

Spores

B39.0   Acute pulmonary histoplasmosis capsulati   HIV MCC HCC

B39.1   Chronic pulmonary histoplasmosis capsulati   HIV MCC HCC

B39.2   Pulmonary histoplasmosis capsulati, unspecified   HIV MCC HCC

B39.3   Disseminated histoplasmosis capsulati   HIV CC
Generalized histoplasmosis capsulati
CC Excl: PDX collection 201

B39.4   Histoplasmosis capsulati, unspecified   HIV
American histoplasmosis

B39.5   Histoplasmosis duboisii   HIV
African histoplasmosis

B39.9   Histoplasmosis, unspecified   HIV

√4ᵗʰ **B40   Blastomycosis**
EXCLUDES 1   Brazilian blastomycosis (B41.-)
        keloidal blastomycosis (B48.0)
CC Excl: For CC codes in category B40: PDX collection 202

B40.0   Acute pulmonary blastomycosis   CC HCC

B40.1   Chronic pulmonary blastomycosis   CC HCC

B40.2   Pulmonary blastomycosis, unspecified   CC HCC

B40.3   Cutaneous blastomycosis   CC

B40.7 Disseminated blastomycosis `CC`
    Generalized blastomycosis

√5ᵗʰ **B40.8 Other forms of blastomycosis**
     B40.81 Blastomycotic meningoencephalitis `CC`
       Meningomyelitis due to blastomycosis
     B40.89 Other forms of blastomycosis `CC`

B40.9 Blastomycosis, unspecified `CC`

√4ᵗʰ **B41 Paracoccidioidomycosis**
    `INCLUDES` Brazilian blastomycosis
          Lutz' disease
    CC Excl: For CC codes in category B41: PDX collection 203

B41.0 Pulmonary paracoccidioidomycosis `CC` `HCC`

B41.7 Disseminated paracoccidioidomycosis `CC`
    Generalized paracoccidioidomycosis

B41.8 Other forms of paracoccidioidomycosis `CC`

B41.9 Paracoccidioidomycosis, unspecified `CC`

√4ᵗʰ **B42 Sporotrichosis**

B42.0 Pulmonary sporotrichosis

B42.1 Lymphocutaneous sporotrichosis

B42.7 Disseminated sporotrichosis
    Generalized sporotrichosis

√5ᵗʰ **B42.8 Other forms of sporotrichosis**
     B42.81 Cerebral sporotrichosis
       Meningitis due to sporotrichosis
     B42.82 Sporotrichosis arthritis `HCC`
     B42.89 Other forms of sporotrichosis

B42.9 Sporotrichosis, unspecified

√4ᵗʰ **B43 Chromomycosis and pheomycotic abscess**

B43.0 Cutaneous chromomycosis
    Dermatitis verrucosa

B43.1 Pheomycotic brain abscess
    Cerebral chromomycosis

B43.2 Subcutaneous pheomycotic abscess and cyst

B43.8 Other forms of chromomycosis

B43.9 Chromomycosis, unspecified

√4ᵗʰ **B44 Aspergillosis**
    `INCLUDES` aspergilloma
    CC Excl: For CC codes in category B44, unless otherwise noted: PDX collection 204

B44.0 Invasive pulmonary aspergillosis `MCC` `HCC`
    CC Excl: PDX collection 110

B44.1 Other pulmonary aspergillosis `CC` `HCC`

B44.2 Tonsillar aspergillosis `CC` `HCC`

B44.7 Disseminated aspergillosis `CC` `HCC`
    Generalized aspergillosis

√5ᵗʰ **B44.8 Other forms of aspergillosis**
     B44.81 Allergic bronchopulmonary `CC` `HCC`
        aspergillosis
        CC Excl: PDX collection 205
     B44.89 Other forms of aspergillosis `CC` `HCC`

B44.9 Aspergillosis, unspecified `CC` `HCC`

√4ᵗʰ **B45 Cryptococcosis**
    CC Excl: For CC codes in category B45: PDX collection 206

B45.0 Pulmonary cryptococcosis `HIV` `CC` `HCC`

B45.1 Cerebral cryptococcosis `MCC` `HCC`
    Cryptococcal meningitis
    Cryptococcosis meningocerebralis
    CC Excl: PDX collection 207

B45.2 Cutaneous cryptococcosis `HIV` `CC` `HCC`

B45.3 Osseous cryptococcosis `HIV` `CC` `HCC`

B45.7 Disseminated cryptococcosis `HIV` `CC` `HCC`
    Generalized cryptococcosis

B45.8 Other forms of cryptococcosis `HIV` `CC` `HCC`

B45.9 Cryptococcosis, unspecified `HIV` `CC` `HCC`

√4ᵗʰ **B46 Zygomycosis**
    CC Excl: For MCC codes in category B46: PDX collection 208

B46.0 Pulmonary mucormycosis `MCC` `HCC`

B46.1 Rhinocerebral mucormycosis `MCC` `HCC`

B46.2 Gastrointestinal mucormycosis `MCC` `HCC`

B46.3 Cutaneous mucormycosis `MCC` `HCC`
    Subcutaneous mucormycosis

B46.4 Disseminated mucormycosis `MCC` `HCC`
    Generalized mucormycosis

B46.5 Mucormycosis, unspecified `MCC` `HCC`

B46.8 Other zygomycoses `MCC` `HCC`
    Entomophthoromycosis

B46.9 Zygomycosis, unspecified `MCC` `HCC`
    Phycomycosis NOS

√4ᵗʰ **B47 Mycetoma**

B47.0 Eumycetoma `CC`
    Madura foot, mycotic
    Maduromycosis
    CC Excl: PDX collection 209

B47.1 Actinomycetoma `HIV` `CC`
    CC Excl: PDX collection 106

B47.9 Mycetoma, unspecified `HIV` `CC`
    Madura foot NOS
    CC Excl: PDX collection 210

√4ᵗʰ **B48 Other mycoses, not elsewhere classified**

B48.0 Lobomycosis
    Keloidal blastomycosis
    Lobo's disease

B48.1 Rhinosporidiosis

B48.2 Allescheriasis `CC`
    Infection due to Pseudallescheria boydii
    `EXCLUDES 1` eumycetoma (B47.0)
    CC Excl: PDX collection 211

B48.3 Geotrichosis `CC`
    Geotrichum stomatitis
    CC Excl: PDX collection 212

B48.4 Penicillosis `CC` `HCC`
    CC Excl: PDX collection 204

B48.8 Other specified mycoses `HIV` `CC` `HCC`
    Adiaspiromycosis
    Infection of tissue and organs by Alternaria
    Infection of tissue and organs by Drechslera
    Infection of tissue and organs by Fusarium
    Infection of tissue and organs by saprophytic fungi NEC
    AHA: 2014,4Q,46; 2014,2Q,13
    TIP: This code is assigned when sepsis is documented as due to non-*Candida albicans*. If sepsis is due to any *Candida* type, code B37.7 Candidal sepsis, is assigned.
    CC Excl: PDX collection 213

B49 Unspecified mycosis `CC`
    Fungemia NOS
    CC Excl: PDX collection 212

Protozoal diseases (B50-B64)

`EXCLUDES 1` amebiasis (A06.-)
          other protozoal intestinal diseases (A07.-)

√4ᵗʰ **B50 Plasmodium falciparum malaria**
    `INCLUDES` mixed infections of Plasmodium falciparum with any other Plasmodium species
    CC Excl: For CC/MCC codes in category B50: PDX collection 214

B50.0 Plasmodium falciparum malaria with cerebral `CC`
    complications
    Cerebral malaria NOS

B50.8 Other severe and complicated Plasmodium `CC`
    falciparum malaria
    Severe or complicated Plasmodium falciparum malaria NOS

B50.9 Plasmodium falciparum malaria, unspecified `MCC`

√4ᵗʰ **B51 Plasmodium vivax malaria**
    `INCLUDES` mixed infections of Plasmodium vivax with other Plasmodium species, except Plasmodium falciparum
    `EXCLUDES 1` Plasmodium vivax with Plasmodium falciparum (B50.-)

B51.0 Plasmodium vivax malaria with rupture of `CC`
    spleen
    CC Excl: PDX collection 214

B51.8 **Plasmodium vivax malaria with other complications**   `CC`
     CC Excl: PDX collection 214

B51.9 **Plasmodium vivax malaria without complication**   `CC`
     Plasmodium vivax malaria NOS
     CC Excl: PDX collection 215

✓4ᵗʰ **B52** **Plasmodium malariae malaria**
     INCLUDES   mixed infections of Plasmodium malariae with other Plasmodium species, except Plasmodium falciparum and Plasmodium vivax
     EXCLUDES 1   *Plasmodium falciparum (B50.-)*
          Plasmodium vivax (B51.-)

     B52.0 **Plasmodium malariae malaria with nephropathy**   `CC`
         CC Excl: PDX collection 216

     B52.8 **Plasmodium malariae malaria with other complications**   `CC`
         CC Excl: PDX collection 214

     B52.9 **Plasmodium malariae malaria without complication**   `CC`
         Plasmodium malariae malaria NOS
         CC Excl: PDX collection 214

✓4ᵗʰ **B53** **Other specified malaria**
     CC Excl: For CC codes in subcategory B53: PDX collection 214

     B53.0 **Plasmodium ovale malaria**   `CC`
         EXCLUDES 1   *Plasmodium ovale with Plasmodium falciparum (B50.-)*
            Plasmodium ovale with Plasmodium malariae (B52.-)
            Plasmodium ovale with Plasmodium vivax (B51.-)

     B53.1 **Malaria due to simian plasmodia**   `CC`
         EXCLUDES 1   *malaria due to simian plasmodia with Plasmodium falciparum (B50.-)*
            malaria due to simian plasmodia with Plasmodium malariae (B52.-)
            malaria due to simian plasmodia with Plasmodium ovale (B53.0)
            malaria due to simian plasmodia with Plasmodium vivax (B51.-)

     B53.8 **Other malaria, not elsewhere classified**   `CC`

B54 **Unspecified malaria**   `CC`
     CC Excl: PDX collection 217

✓4ᵗʰ **B55** **Leishmaniasis**
     CC Excl: For CC codes in category B55: PDX collection 218

     B55.0 **Visceral leishmaniasis**   `CC`
         Kala-azar
         Post-kala-azar dermal leishmaniasis

     B55.1 **Cutaneous leishmaniasis**   `CC`

     B55.2 **Mucocutaneous leishmaniasis**   `CC`

     B55.9 **Leishmaniasis, unspecified**   `CC`

✓4ᵗʰ **B56** **African trypanosomiasis**
     CC Excl: For CC codes in category B56: PDX collection 218

     B56.0 **Gambiense trypanosomiasis**   `CC`
         Infection due to Trypanosoma brucei gambiense
         West African sleeping sickness

     B56.1 **Rhodesiense trypanosomiasis**   `CC`
         East African sleeping sickness
         Infection due to Trypanosoma brucei rhodesiense

     B56.9 **African trypanosomiasis, unspecified**   `CC`
         Sleeping sickness NOS

✓4ᵗʰ **B57** **Chagas' disease**
     INCLUDES   American trypanosomiasis
          infection due to Trypanosoma cruzi
     CC Excl: For CC codes in category B57, unless otherwise noted: PDX collection 218

     B57.0 **Acute Chagas' disease with heart involvement**   `CC`
         Acute Chagas' disease with myocarditis
         CC Excl: PDX collection 219

     B57.1 **Acute Chagas' disease without heart involvement**   `CC`
         Acute Chagas' disease NOS

B57.2 **Chagas' disease (chronic) with heart involvement**   `CC`
     American trypanosomiasis NOS
     Chagas' disease (chronic) NOS
     Chagas' disease (chronic) with myocarditis
     Trypanosomiasis NOS
     CC Excl: PDX collection 219

✓5ᵗʰ **B57.3** **Chagas' disease (chronic) with digestive system involvement**
     B57.30 **Chagas' disease with digestive system involvement, unspecified**   `CC`
     B57.31 **Megaesophagus in Chagas' disease**   `CC`
     B57.32 **Megacolon in Chagas' disease**   `CC`
     B57.39 **Other digestive system involvement in Chagas' disease**   `CC`

✓5ᵗʰ **B57.4** **Chagas' disease (chronic) with nervous system involvement**
     B57.40 **Chagas' disease with nervous system involvement, unspecified**   `CC`
     B57.41 **Meningitis in Chagas' disease**   `CC`
     B57.42 **Meningoencephalitis in Chagas' disease**   `CC`
     B57.49 **Other nervous system involvement in Chagas' disease**   `CC`

B57.5 **Chagas' disease (chronic) with other organ involvement**   `CC`

✓4ᵗʰ **B58** **Toxoplasmosis**
     INCLUDES   infection due to Toxoplasma gondii
     EXCLUDES 1   *congenital toxoplasmosis (P37.1)*

✓5ᵗʰ **B58.0** **Toxoplasma oculopathy**
     B58.00 **Toxoplasma oculopathy, unspecified**   `HIV` `CC`
         CC Excl: PDX collection 220
     B58.01 **Toxoplasma chorioretinitis**   `HIV` `CC`
         CC Excl: PDX collection 221
     B58.09 **Other toxoplasma oculopathy**   `HIV` `CC`
         Toxoplasma uveitis
         CC Excl: PDX collection 222

B58.1 **Toxoplasma hepatitis**   `HIV` `CC`
     CC Excl: PDX collection 223

B58.2 **Toxoplasma meningoencephalitis**   `HIV` `MCC` `HCC`
     CC Excl: PDX collection 224

B58.3 **Pulmonary toxoplasmosis**   `HIV` `MCC` `HCC`
     CC Excl: PDX collection 225

✓5ᵗʰ **B58.8** **Toxoplasmosis with other organ involvement**
     CC Excl: For CC codes in subcategory B58.8: PDX collection 220
     B58.81 **Toxoplasma myocarditis**   `HIV` `MCC`
         CC Excl: PDX collection 226
     B58.82 **Toxoplasma myositis**   `HIV` `CC`
     B58.83 **Toxoplasma tubulo-interstitial nephropathy**   `HIV` `CC`
         Toxoplasma pyelonephritis
     B58.89 **Toxoplasmosis with other organ involvement**   `HIV` `CC`

     B58.9 **Toxoplasmosis, unspecified**   `HIV` `CC`
         CC Excl: PDX collection 227

B59 **Pneumocystosis**   `HIV` `MCC` `HCC`
     Pneumonia due to Pneumocystis carinii
     Pneumonia due to Pneumocystis jiroveci
     CC Excl: PDX collection 228

✓4ᵗʰ **B60** **Other protozoal diseases, not elsewhere classified**
     EXCLUDES 1   *cryptosporidiosis (A07.2)*
          intestinal microsporidiosis (A07.8)
          isosporiasis (A07.3)
     CC Excl: For CC codes in category B60, unless otherwise noted: PDX collection 229

     B60.0 **Babesiosis**   `CC`
         Piroplasmosis
         CC Excl: PDX collection 218

✓5ᵗʰ **B60.1** **Acanthamebiasis**
     B60.10 **Acanthamebiasis, unspecified**   `CC`
     B60.11 **Meningoencephalitis due to Acanthamoeba (culbertsoni)**
     B60.12 **Conjunctivitis due to Acanthamoeba**
     B60.13 **Keratoconjunctivitis due to Acanthamoeba**
     B60.19 **Other acanthamebic disease**   `CC`

B60.2 Naegleriasis `CC`
     Primary amebic meningoencephalitis

B60.8 Other specified protozoal diseases `HIV`
     Microsporidiosis

B64 Unspecified protozoal disease

Helminthiases (B65-B83)

✓4ᵗʰ **B65 Schistosomiasis [bilharziasis]**
     `INCLUDES` snail fever
     CC Excl: For CC codes in category B65: PDX collection 230

B65.0 Schistosomiasis due to Schistosoma haematobium [urinary schistosomiasis] `CC`

B65.1 Schistosomiasis due to Schistosoma mansoni [intestinal schistosomiasis] `CC`

B65.2 Schistosomiasis due to Schistosoma japonicum `CC`
     Asiatic schistosomiasis

B65.3 Cercarial dermatitis `CC`
     Swimmer's itch

B65.8 Other schistosomiasis `CC`
     Infection due to Schistosoma intercalatum
     Infection due to Schistosoma mattheei
     Infection due to Schistosoma mekongi

B65.9 Schistosomiasis, unspecified `CC`

✓4ᵗʰ **B66 Other fluke infections**
     CC Excl: For CC codes in category B66: PDX collection 231

B66.0 Opisthorchiasis `CC`
     Infection due to cat liver fluke
     Infection due to Opisthorchis (felineus)(viverrini)

B66.1 Clonorchiasis `CC`
     Chinese liver fluke disease
     Infection due to Clonorchis sinensis
     Oriental liver fluke disease

B66.2 Dicroceliasis `CC`
     Infection due to Dicrocoelium dendriticum
     Lancet fluke infection

B66.3 Fascioliasis `CC`
     Infection due to Fasciola gigantica
     Infection due to Fasciola hepatica
     Infection due to Fasciola indica
     Sheep liver fluke disease

B66.4 Paragonimiasis `CC` `HCC`
     Infection due to Paragonimus species
     Lung fluke disease
     Pulmonary distomiasis

B66.5 Fasciolopsiasis `CC`
     Infection due to Fasciolopsis buski
     Intestinal distomiasis

B66.8 Other specified fluke infections `CC`
     Echinostomiasis
     Heterophyiasis
     Metagonimiasis
     Nanophyetiasis
     Watsoniasis

B66.9 Fluke infection, unspecified

✓4ᵗʰ **B67 Echinococcosis**
     `INCLUDES` hydatidosis

B67.0 Echinococcus granulosus infection of liver `CC`
     CC Excl: PDX collection 232

B67.1 Echinococcus granulosus infection of lung `CC` `HCC`
     CC Excl: PDX collection 233

B67.2 Echinococcus granulosus infection of bone `CC`
     CC Excl: PDX collection 234

✓5ᵗʰ **B67.3 Echinococcus granulosus infection, other and multiple sites**

B67.31 Echinococcus granulosus infection, thyroid gland `CC`
     CC Excl: PDX collection 235

B67.32 Echinococcus granulosus infection, multiple sites `CC`
     CC Excl: PDX collection 234

B67.39 Echinococcus granulosus infection, other sites `CC`
     CC Excl: PDX collection 234

B67.4 Echinococcus granulosus infection, unspecified `CC`
     Dog tapeworm (infection)
     CC Excl: PDX collection 236

B67.5 Echinococcus multilocularis infection of liver `CC`
     CC Excl: PDX collection 237

✓5ᵗʰ **B67.6 Echinococcus multilocularis infection, other and multiple sites**

B67.61 Echinococcus multilocularis infection, multiple sites `CC`
     CC Excl: PDX collection 238

B67.69 Echinococcus multilocularis infection, other sites `CC`
     CC Excl: PDX collection 238

B67.7 Echinococcus multilocularis infection, unspecified `CC`
     CC Excl: PDX collection 239

B67.8 Echinococcosis, unspecified, of liver `CC`
     CC Excl: PDX collection 240

✓5ᵗʰ **B67.9 Echinococcosis, other and unspecified**

B67.90 Echinococcosis, unspecified `CC`
     Echinococcosis NOS
     CC Excl: PDX collection 240

B67.99 Other echinococcosis `CC`
     CC Excl: PDX collection 240

✓4ᵗʰ **B68 Taeniasis**
     `EXCLUDES 1` cysticercosis (B69.-)

B68.0 Taenia solium taeniasis `CC`
     Pork tapeworm (infection)
     CC Excl: PDX collection 241

B68.1 Taenia saginata taeniasis `CC`
     Beef tapeworm (infection)
     Infection due to adult tapeworm Taenia saginata
     CC Excl: PDX collection 242

B68.9 Taeniasis, unspecified `CC`
     CC Excl: PDX collection 242

✓4ᵗʰ **B69 Cysticercosis**
     `INCLUDES` cysticerciasis infection due to larval form of Taenia solium
     DEF: Condition that is developed when larvae or eggs of the tapeworm *Taenia solium* are ingested, most commonly in fecally contaminated water or undercooked pork.
     CC Excl: For CC codes in category B69: PDX collection 242

B69.0 Cysticercosis of central nervous system `CC`

B69.1 Cysticercosis of eye `CC`

✓5ᵗʰ **B69.8 Cysticercosis of other sites**

B69.81 Myositis in cysticercosis `CC`

B69.89 Cysticercosis of other sites `CC`

B69.9 Cysticercosis, unspecified `CC`

✓4ᵗʰ **B70 Diphyllobothriasis and sparganosis**

B70.0 Diphyllobothriasis `CC`
     Diphyllobothrium (adult) (latum) (pacificum) infection
     Fish tapeworm (infection)
     `EXCLUDES 2` larval diphyllobothriasis (B70.1)
     CC Excl: PDX collcetion 242

B70.1 Sparganosis `CC`
     Infection due to Sparganum (mansoni) (proliferum)
     Infection due to Spirometra larva
     Larval diphyllobothriasis
     Spirometrosis
     CC Excl: PDX collection 242

✓4ᵗʰ **B71 Other cestode infections**
     CC Excl: For CC codes in category B71: PDX collection 242

B71.0 Hymenolepiasis `CC`
     Dwarf tapeworm infection
     Rat tapeworm (infection)

B71.1 Dipylidiasis `CC`

B71.8 Other specified cestode infections `CC`
     Coenurosis

☑ Additional Character Required   ✓x7ᵗʰ Placeholder   Unacceptable PDx   Questionable PDx   Manifestation   Unspecified Dx   H1-H14 HAC   HCC CMS-HCC Dx   HIV HIV Dx

ICD-10-CM 2020   457

B71.9 **Cestode infection, unspecified**
　　　Tapeworm (infection) NOS

B72 **Dracunculiasis** `CC`
　　INCLUDES　guinea worm infection
　　　　infection due to Dracunculus medinensis
　　CC Excl: PDX collection 243

✓4ᵗʰ B73 **Onchocerciasis**
　　INCLUDES　onchocerca volvulus infection
　　　　onchocercosis
　　　　river blindness
　　CC Excl: For CC codes in category B73: PDX collection 243

　　✓5ᵗʰ B73.0 **Onchocerciasis with eye disease**
　　　B73.00 **Onchocerciasis with eye** `CC`
　　　　　involvement, unspecified
　　　B73.01 **Onchocerciasis with** `CC`
　　　　　endophthalmitis
　　　B73.02 **Onchocerciasis with glaucoma** `CC`
　　　B73.09 **Onchocerciasis with other eye** `CC`
　　　　　involvement
　　　　　　Infestation of eyelid due to onchocerciasis
　　B73.1 **Onchocerciasis without eye disease** `CC`

✓4ᵗʰ B74 **Filariasis**
　　EXCLUDES 2　onchocerciasis (B73)
　　　　tropical (pulmonary) eosinophilia NOS (J82)
　　CC Excl: For CC codes in category B74: PDX collection 243

　　B74.0 **Filariasis due to Wuchereria bancrofti** `CC`
　　　　Bancroftian elephantiasis
　　　　Bancroftian filariasis
　　B74.1 **Filariasis due to Brugia malayi** `CC`
　　B74.2 **Filariasis due to Brugia timori** `CC`
　　B74.3 **Loiasis** `CC`
　　　　Calabar swelling
　　　　Eyeworm disease of Africa
　　　　Loa loa infection
　　B74.4 **Mansonelliasis** `CC`
　　　　Infection due to Mansonella ozzardi
　　　　Infection due to Mansonella perstans
　　　　Infection due to Mansonella streptocerca
　　B74.8 **Other filariases** `CC`
　　　　Dirofilariasis
　　B74.9 **Filariasis, unspecified** `CC`

B75 **Trichinellosis** `CC`
　　INCLUDES　infection due to Trichinella species
　　　　trichiniasis
　　DEF: Infection by *Trichinella spiralis*, the smallest of the parasitic
　　nematodes, that is transmitted by eating undercooked pork or bear meat.
　　Synonym(s): Trichinosis.
　　CC Excl: PDX collection 244

✓4ᵗʰ B76 **Hookworm diseases**
　　INCLUDES　uncinariasis
　　CC Excl: For CC codes in category B76: PDX collection 245

　　B76.0 **Ancylostomiasis** `CC`
　　　　Infection due to Ancylostoma species
　　B76.1 **Necatoriasis** `CC`
　　　　Infection due to Necator americanus
　　B76.8 **Other hookworm diseases** `CC`
　　B76.9 **Hookworm disease, unspecified** `CC`
　　　　Cutaneous larva migrans NOS

✓4ᵗʰ B77 **Ascariasis**
　　INCLUDES　ascaridiasis
　　　　roundworm infection
　　CC Excl: For CC codes in category B77: PDX collection 246

　　B77.0 **Ascariasis with intestinal complications** `CC`
　　✓5ᵗʰ B77.8 **Ascariasis with other complications**
　　　B77.81 **Ascariasis pneumonia** `MCC`
　　　　　CC Excl: PDX collection 247
　　　B77.89 **Ascariasis with other complications** `CC`
　　B77.9 **Ascariasis, unspecified** `CC`

✓4ᵗʰ B78 **Strongyloidiasis**
　　EXCLUDES 1　trichostrongyliasis (B81.2)
　　CC Excl: For CC codes in category B78: PDX collection 246

　　B78.0 **Intestinal strongyloidiasis** `HIV` `CC`
　　B78.1 **Cutaneous strongyloidiasis**
　　B78.7 **Disseminated strongyloidiasis** `HIV` `CC`
　　B78.9 **Strongyloidiasis, unspecified** `HIV` `CC`

B79 **Trichuriasis** `CC`
　　INCLUDES　trichocephaliasis
　　　　whipworm (disease)(infection)
　　CC Excl: PDX collection 246

B80 **Enterobiasis** `CC`
　　INCLUDES　oxyuriasis
　　　　pinworm infection
　　　　threadworm infection
　　CC Excl: PDX collection 246

✓4ᵗʰ B81 **Other intestinal helminthiases, not elsewhere classified**
　　EXCLUDES 1　angiostrongyliasis due to:
　　　　angiostrongylus cantonensis (B83.2)
　　　　parastrongylus cantonensis (B83.2)

　　B81.0 **Anisakiasis** `CC`
　　　　Infection due to Anisakis larva
　　　　CC Excl: PDX collection 246
　　B81.1 **Intestinal capillariasis** `CC`
　　　　Capillariasis NOS
　　　　Infection due to Capillaria philippinensis
　　　　EXCLUDES 2　hepatic capillariasis (B83.8)
　　　　CC Excl: PDX collection 246
　　B81.2 **Trichostrongyliasis** `CC`
　　　　CC Excl: PDX collection 246
　　B81.3 **Intestinal angiostrongyliasis** `CC`
　　　　Angiostrongyliasis due to:
　　　　angiostrongylus costaricensis
　　　　parastrongylus costaricensis
　　　　CC Excl: PDX collection 248
　　B81.4 **Mixed intestinal helminthiases** `CC`
　　　　Infection due to intestinal helminths classified to more than
　　　　　one of the categories B65.0-B81.3 and B81.8
　　　　Mixed helminthiasis NOS
　　　　CC Excl: PDX collection 248
　　B81.8 **Other specified intestinal helminthiases** `CC`
　　　　Infection due to Oesophagostomum species
　　　　　[esophagostomiasis]
　　　　Infection due to Ternidens diminutus [ternidensiasis]
　　　　CC Excl: PDX collection 248

✓4ᵗʰ B82 **Unspecified intestinal parasitism**
　　B82.0 **Intestinal helminthiasis, unspecified** `CC`
　　　　CC Excl: PDX collection 248
　　B82.9 **Intestinal parasitism, unspecified**

✓4ᵗʰ B83 **Other helminthiases**
　　EXCLUDES 1　capillariasis NOS (B81.1)
　　EXCLUDES 2　intestinal capillariasis (B81.1)

　　B83.0 **Visceral larva migrans**
　　　　Toxocariasis
　　B83.1 **Gnathostomiasis**
　　　　Wandering swelling
　　B83.2 **Angiostrongyliasis due to Parastrongylus cantonensis**
　　　　Eosinophilic meningoencephalitis due to Parastrongylus
　　　　　cantonensis
　　　　EXCLUDES 2　intestinal angiostrongyliasis (B81.3)
　　B83.3 **Syngamiasis**
　　　　Syngamosis
　　B83.4 **Internal hirudiniasis**
　　　　EXCLUDES 2　external hirudiniasis (B88.3)
　　B83.8 **Other specified helminthiases**
　　　　Acanthocephaliasis
　　　　Gongylonemiasis
　　　　Hepatic capillariasis
　　　　Metastrongyliasis
　　　　Thelaziasis

`N` Newborn: 0　`P` Pediatric: 0-17　`M` Maternity: 9-64　`A` Adult: 15-124　`MCC` Major Complication/Comorbidity　`CC` Complication/Comorbidity　`SW` Severe Wound Dx

458　　　　　　ICD-10-CM 2020

B83.9 **Helminthiasis, unspecified**
Worms NOS
EXCLUDES 1   *intestinal helminthiasis NOS (B82.0)*

Pediculosis, acariasis and other infestations (B85-B89)

√4ᵗʰ **B85** **Pediculosis and phthiriasis**

B85.0 **Pediculosis due to Pediculus humanus capitis**
Head-louse infestation

B85.1 **Pediculosis due to Pediculus humanus corporis**
Body-louse infestation

B85.2 **Pediculosis, unspecified**

B85.3 **Phthiriasis**
Infestation by crab-louse
Infestation by Phthirus pubis

B85.4 **Mixed pediculosis and phthiriasis**
Infestation classifiable to more than one of the categories
B85.0-B85.3

B86 **Scabies**
Sarcoptic itch
DEF: Mite infestation that is caused by *Sarcoptes scabiei*. Scabies causes intense itching and sometimes secondary infection.

√4ᵗʰ **B87** **Myiasis**
INCLUDES   infestation by larva of flies

B87.0 **Cutaneous myiasis**
Creeping myiasis

B87.1 **Wound myiasis**
Traumatic myiasis

B87.2 **Ocular myiasis**

B87.3 **Nasopharyngeal myiasis**
Laryngeal myiasis

B87.4 **Aural myiasis**

√5ᵗʰ **B87.8** **Myiasis of other sites**

B87.81 **Genitourinary myiasis**

B87.82 **Intestinal myiasis**

B87.89 **Myiasis of other sites**

B87.9 **Myiasis, unspecified**

√4ᵗʰ **B88** **Other infestations**

B88.0 **Other acariasis**
Acarine dermatitis
Dermatitis due to Demodex species
Dermatitis due to Dermanyssus gallinae
Dermatitis due to Liponyssoides sanguineus
Trombiculosis
EXCLUDES 2   *scabies (B86)*

B88.1 **Tungiasis [sandflea infestation]**

B88.2 **Other arthropod infestations**
Scarabiasis

B88.3 **External hirudiniasis**
Leech infestation NOS
EXCLUDES 2   *internal hirudiniasis (B83.4)*

B88.8 **Other specified infestations**
Ichthyoparasitism due to Vandellia cirrhosa
Linguatulosis
Porocephaliasis

B88.9 **Infestation, unspecified**
Infestation (skin) NOS
Infestation by mites NOS
Skin parasites NOS

B89 **Unspecified parasitic disease**

Sequelae of infectious and parasitic diseases (B90-B94)

NOTE   Categories B90-B94 are to be used to indicate conditions in categories A00-B89 as the cause of sequelae, which are themselves classified elsewhere. The "sequelae" include conditions specified as such; they also include residuals of diseases classifiable to the above categories if there is evidence that the disease itself is no longer present. Codes from these categories are not to be used for chronic infections. Code chronic current infections to active infectious disease as appropriate.

Code first condition resulting from (sequela) the infectious or parasitic disease

√4ᵗʰ **B90** **Sequelae of tuberculosis**

B90.0 **Sequelae of central nervous system tuberculosis**

B90.1 **Sequelae of genitourinary tuberculosis**

B90.2 **Sequelae of tuberculosis of bones and joints**

B90.8 **Sequelae of tuberculosis of other organs**
EXCLUDES 2   *sequelae of respiratory tuberculosis (B90.9)*

B90.9 **Sequelae of respiratory and unspecified tuberculosis**
Sequelae of tuberculosis NOS

B91 **Sequelae of poliomyelitis**
EXCLUDES 1   *postpolio syndrome (G14)*

B92 **Sequelae of leprosy**

√4ᵗʰ **B94** **Sequelae of other and unspecified infectious and parasitic diseases**

B94.0 **Sequelae of trachoma**

B94.1 **Sequelae of viral encephalitis**

B94.2 **Sequelae of viral hepatitis**

B94.8 **Sequelae of other specified infectious and parasitic diseases**
AHA: 2017,4Q,109

B94.9 **Sequelae of unspecified infectious and parasitic disease**

Bacterial and viral infectious agents (B95-B97)

NOTE   These categories are provided for use as supplementary or additional codes to identify the infectious agent(s) in diseases classified elsewhere.

AHA: 2018,4Q,34; 2018,1Q,16

√4ᵗʰ **B95** **Streptococcus, Staphylococcus, and Enterococcus as the cause of diseases classified elsewhere**

B95.0 **Streptococcus, group A, as the cause of diseases classified elsewhere**

B95.1 **Streptococcus, group B, as the cause of diseases classified elsewhere**
AHA: 2019,2Q,8-10

B95.2 **Enterococcus as the cause of diseases classified elsewhere**

B95.3 **Streptococcus pneumoniae as the cause of diseases classified elsewhere**

B95.4 **Other streptococcus as the cause of diseases classified elsewhere**

B95.5 **Unspecified streptococcus as the cause of diseases classified elsewhere**

√5ᵗʰ **B95.6** **Staphylococcus aureus as the cause of diseases classified elsewhere**

B95.61 **Methicillin susceptible Staphylococcus aureus infection as the cause of diseases classified elsewhere**
Methicillin susceptible Staphylococcus aureus (MSSA) infection as the cause of diseases classified elsewhere
Staphylococcus aureus infection NOS as the cause of diseases classified elsewhere

B95.62 **Methicillin resistant Staphylococcus aureus infection as the cause of diseases classified elsewhere**
Methicillin resistant staphylococcus aureus (MRSA) infection as the cause of diseases classified elsewhere
AHA: 2016,1Q,12

B95.7 **Other staphylococcus as the cause of diseases classified elsewhere**

B95.8 **Unspecified staphylococcus as the cause of diseases classified elsewhere**

√4ᵗʰ **B96** **Other bacterial agents as the cause of diseases classified elsewhere**

B96.0 **Mycoplasma pneumoniae [M. pneumoniae] as the cause of diseases classified elsewhere**
Pleuro-pneumonia-like-organism [PPLO]

B96.1 **Klebsiella pneumoniae [K. pneumoniae] as the cause of diseases classified elsewhere**

√5ᵗʰ **B96.2** **Escherichia coli [E. coli] as the cause of diseases classified elsewhere**

B96.20 **Unspecified Escherichia coli [E. coli] as the cause of diseases classified elsewhere**
Escherichia coli [E. coli] NOS

▲ **B96.21** **Shiga toxin-producing Escherichia coli [E. coli] [STEC] O157 as the cause of diseases classified elsewhere**

E. coli O157:H- (nonmotile) with confirmation of Shiga toxin

E. coli O157 with confirmation of Shiga toxin when H antigen is unknown, or is not H7

O157:H7 Escherichia coli [E.coli] with or without confirmation of Shiga toxin-production

Shiga toxin-producing Escherichia coli [E.coli] O157:H7 with or without confirmation of Shiga toxin-production

STEC O157:H7 with or without confirmation of Shiga toxin-production

▲ **B96.22** **Other specified Shiga toxin-producing Escherichia coli [E. coli] [STEC] as the cause of diseases classified elsewhere**

Non-O157 Shiga toxin-producing Escherichia coli [E.coli]

Non-O157 Shiga toxin-producing Escherichia coli [E.coli] with known O group

▲ **B96.23** **Unspecified Shiga toxin-producing Escherichia coli [E. coli] [STEC] as the cause of diseases classified elsewhere**

Shiga toxin-producing Escherichia coli [E. coli] with unspecified O group

STEC NOS

B96.29 **Other Escherichia coli [E. coli] as the cause of diseases classified elsewhere**

Non-Shiga toxin-producing E. coli

B96.3 **Hemophilus influenzae [H. influenzae] as the cause of diseases classified elsewhere**

B96.4 **Proteus (mirabilis) (morganii) as the cause of diseases classified elsewhere**

B96.5 **Pseudomonas (aeruginosa) (mallei) (pseudomallei) as the cause of diseases classified elsewhere**

AHA: 2015,1Q,18

B96.6 **Bacteroides fragilis [B. fragilis] as the cause of diseases classified elsewhere**

B96.7 **Clostridium perfringens [C. perfringens] as the cause of diseases classified elsewhere**

√5ᵗʰ **B96.8** **Other specified bacterial agents as the cause of diseases classified elsewhere**

B96.81 **Helicobacter pylori [H. pylori] as the cause of diseases classified elsewhere**

B96.82 **Vibrio vulnificus as the cause of diseases classified elsewhere**

B96.89 **Other specified bacterial agents as the cause of diseases classified elsewhere**

√4ᵗʰ **B97** **Viral agents as the cause of diseases classified elsewhere**

AHA: 2016,3Q,8-10,14

B97.0 **Adenovirus as the cause of diseases classified elsewhere**

√5ᵗʰ **B97.1** **Enterovirus as the cause of diseases classified elsewhere**

B97.10 **Unspecified enterovirus as the cause of diseases classified elsewhere**

B97.11 **Coxsackievirus as the cause of diseases classified elsewhere**

B97.12 **Echovirus as the cause of diseases classified elsewhere**

B97.19 **Other enterovirus as the cause of diseases classified elsewhere**

√5ᵗʰ **B97.2** **Coronavirus as the cause of diseases classified elsewhere**

B97.21 **SARS-associated coronavirus as the cause of diseases classified elsewhere** `CC`

EXCLUDES 1 pneumonia due to SARS-associated coronavirus (J12.81)

CC Excl: PDX collection 249

B97.29 **Other coronavirus as the cause of diseases classified elsewhere**

√5ᵗʰ **B97.3** **Retrovirus as the cause of diseases classified elsewhere**

EXCLUDES 1 human immunodeficiency virus [HIV] disease (B20)

B97.30 **Unspecified retrovirus as the cause of diseases classified elsewhere**

B97.31 **Lentivirus as the cause of diseases classified elsewhere**

B97.32 **Oncovirus as the cause of diseases classified elsewhere**

B97.33 **Human T-cell lymphotrophic virus, type I [HTLV-I] as the cause of diseases classified elsewhere** `CC`

CC Excl: PDX collection 250

B97.34 **Human T-cell lymphotrophic virus, type II [HTLV-II] as the cause of diseases classified elsewhere** `CC`

CC Excl: PDX collection 251

B97.35 **Human immunodeficiency virus, type 2 [HIV 2] as the cause of diseases classified elsewhere** `CC` `HCC`

CC Excl: PDX collection 252

B97.39 **Other retrovirus as the cause of diseases classified elsewhere**

B97.4 **Respiratory syncytial virus as the cause of diseases classified elsewhere**

▶RSV as the cause of diseases classified elsewhere◀

▶Code first related disorders, such as:◀

▶otitis media (H65.-)◀

▶upper respiratory infection (J06.9)◀

EXCLUDES 2 ▶acute bronchiolitis due to respiratory syncytial virus (RSV) (J21.0)◀

▶acute bronchitis due to respiratory syncytial virus (RSV) (J20.5)◀

▶respiratory syncytial virus (RSV) pneumonia (J12.1)◀

B97.5 **Reovirus as the cause of diseases classified elsewhere**

B97.6 **Parvovirus as the cause of diseases classified elsewhere**

B97.7 **Papillomavirus as the cause of diseases classified elsewhere**

√5ᵗʰ **B97.8** **Other viral agents as the cause of diseases classified elsewhere**

B97.81 **Human metapneumovirus as the cause of diseases classified elsewhere**

B97.89 **Other viral agents as the cause of diseases classified elsewhere**

Other infectious diseases (B99)

√4ᵗʰ **B99** **Other and unspecified infectious diseases**

B99.8 **Other infectious disease** `HIV`

B99.9 **Unspecified infectious disease**

Chapter 2. Neoplasms (C00–D49)

Chapter-specific Guidelines with Coding Examples

The chapter-specific guidelines from the ICD-10-CM Official Guidelines for Coding and Reporting have been provided below. Along with these guidelines are coding examples, contained in the shaded boxes, that have been developed to help illustrate the coding and/or sequencing guidance found in these guidelines.

General guidelines

Chapter 2 of the ICD-10-CM contains the codes for most benign and all malignant neoplasms. Certain benign neoplasms, such as prostatic adenomas, may be found in the specific body system chapters. To properly code a neoplasm it is necessary to determine from the record if the neoplasm is benign, in-situ, malignant, or of uncertain histologic behavior. If malignant, any secondary (metastatic) sites should also be determined.

Primary malignant neoplasms overlapping site boundaries

A primary malignant neoplasm that overlaps two or more contiguous (next to each other) sites should be classified to the subcategory/code .8 ('overlapping lesion'), unless the combination is specifically indexed elsewhere. For multiple neoplasms of the same site that are not contiguous such as tumors in different quadrants of the same breast, codes for each site should be assigned.

A 73-year-old white female with a large rapidly growing malignant tumor in the left breast extending from the upper outer quadrant into the axillary tail

C50.812   **Malignant neoplasm of overlapping sites of left female breast**

Explanation: Because this is a single large tumor that overlaps two contiguous sites, a single code for overlapping sites is assigned.

A 52-year old white female with two distinct lesions of the right breast, one (0.5 cm) in the upper outer quadrant and a second (1.5 cm) in the lower outer quadrant; path report indicates both lesions are malignant

C50.411   **Malignant neoplasm of upper-outer quadrant of right female breast**

C50.511   **Malignant neoplasm of lower-outer quadrant of right female breast**

Explanation: This patient has two distinct malignant lesions of right breast in adjacent quadrants. Because the lesions are not contiguous, two codes are reported.

Malignant neoplasm of ectopic tissue

Malignant neoplasms of ectopic tissue are to be coded to the site of origin mentioned, e.g., ectopic pancreatic malignant neoplasms involving the stomach are coded to malignant neoplasm of pancreas, unspecified (C25.9).

The neoplasm table in the Alphabetic Index should be referenced first. However, if the histological term is documented, that term should be referenced first, rather than going immediately to the Neoplasm Table, in order to determine which column in the Neoplasm Table is appropriate. For example, if the documentation indicates "adenoma," refer to the term in the Alphabetic Index to review the entries under this term and the instructional note to "see also neoplasm, by site, benign." The table provides the proper code based on the type of neoplasm and the site. It is important to select the proper column in the table that corresponds to the type of neoplasm. The Tabular List should then be referenced to verify that the correct code has been selected from the table and that a more specific site code does not exist.

See Section I.C.21. Factors influencing health status and contact with health services, Status, for information regarding Z15.0, codes for genetic susceptibility to cancer.

a. Treatment directed at the malignancy

If the treatment is directed at the malignancy, designate the malignancy as the principal diagnosis.

The only exception to this guideline is if a patient admission/encounter is solely for the administration of chemotherapy, immunotherapy or external beam radiation therapy, assign the appropriate Z51.-- code as the first-listed or principal diagnosis, and the diagnosis or problem for which the service is being performed as a secondary diagnosis.

b. Treatment of secondary site

When a patient is admitted because of a primary neoplasm with metastasis and treatment is directed toward the secondary site only, the secondary neoplasm is designated as the principal diagnosis even though the primary malignancy is still present.

Patient with primary prostate cancer with metastasis to lungs admitted for wedge resection of mass in right lung

C78.01   **Secondary malignant neoplasm of right lung**

C61   **Malignant neoplasm of prostate**

Explanation: Since the admission is for treatment of the lung metastasis, the secondary lung metastasis is sequenced before the primary prostate cancer.

c. Coding and sequencing of complications

Coding and sequencing of complications associated with the malignancies or with the therapy thereof are subject to the following guidelines:

1) Anemia associated with malignancy

When admission/encounter is for management of an anemia associated with the malignancy, and the treatment is only for anemia, the appropriate code for the malignancy is sequenced as the principal or first-listed diagnosis followed by the appropriate code for the anemia (such as code D63.0, Anemia in neoplastic disease).

Patient is admitted for treatment of anemia in advanced colon cancer

C18.9   **Malignant neoplasm of colon, unspecified**

D63.0   **Anemia in neoplastic disease**

Explanation: Even though the admission was solely to treat the anemia, this guideline indicates that the code for the malignancy is sequenced first.

2) Anemia associated with chemotherapy, immunotherapy and radiation therapy

When the admission/encounter is for management of an anemia associated with an adverse effect of the administration of chemotherapy or immunotherapy and the only treatment is for the anemia, the anemia code is sequenced first followed by the appropriate codes for the neoplasm and the adverse effect (T45.1X5, Adverse effect of antineoplastic and immunosuppressive drugs).

A 56-year-old Hispanic male with grade II follicular lymphoma involving multiple lymph node sites referred for blood transfusion to treat anemia due to chemotherapy

D64.81   **Anemia due to antineoplastic chemotherapy**

C82.18   **Follicular lymphoma grade II, lymph nodes of multiple sites**

T45.1X5A   **Adverse effect of antineoplastic and immunosuppressive drugs, initial encounter**

Explanation: The code for the anemia is sequenced first followed by the code for the malignant neoplasm and lastly the code for the adverse effect.

When the admission/encounter is for management of an anemia associated with an adverse effect of radiotherapy, the anemia code should be sequenced first, followed by the appropriate neoplasm code and code Y84.2, Radiological procedure and radiotherapy as the cause of abnormal reaction of the patient, or of later complication, without mention of misadventure at the time of the procedure.

A 55-year-old male with a large malignant rectal tumor has been receiving external radiation therapy to shrink the tumor prior to planned surgery. He is admitted today for a blood transfusion to treat anemia related to radiation therapy.

D64.89	Other specified anemias
C20	Malignant neoplasm of rectum
Y84.2	Radiological procedure and radiotherapy as the cause of abnormal reaction of the patient, or of later complication, without mention of misadventure at the time of the procedure

Explanation: The code for the anemia is sequenced first, followed by the code for the malignancy, and lastly the code for the abnormal reaction due to radiotherapy.

3) Management of dehydration due to the malignancy

When the admission/encounter is for management of dehydration due to the malignancy and only the dehydration is being treated (intravenous rehydration), the dehydration is sequenced first, followed by the code(s) for the malignancy.

4) Treatment of a complication resulting from a surgical procedure

When the admission/encounter is for treatment of a complication resulting from a surgical procedure, designate the complication as the principal or first-listed diagnosis if treatment is directed at resolving the complication.

d. Primary malignancy previously excised

When a primary malignancy has been previously excised or eradicated from its site and there is no further treatment directed to that site and there is no evidence of any existing primary malignancy at that site, a code from category Z85, Personal history of malignant neoplasm, should be used to indicate the former site of the malignancy. Any mention of extension, invasion, or metastasis to another site is coded as a secondary malignant neoplasm to that site. The secondary site may be the principal or first-listed **diagnosis** with the Z85 code used as a secondary code.

History of breast cancer, left radical mastectomy 18 months ago with no current treatment; bronchoscopy with lung biopsy shows metastatic disease in the right lung

C78.01	Secondary malignant neoplasm of right lung
Z85.3	Personal history of malignant neoplasm of breast

Explanation: The patient has undergone a diagnostic procedure that revealed metastatic breast cancer in the right lung. The code for the secondary (metastatic) site is sequenced first followed by a personal history code to identify the former site of the primary malignancy.

e. Admissions/encounters involving chemotherapy, immunotherapy and radiation therapy

1) Episode of care involves surgical removal of neoplasm

When an episode of care involves the surgical removal of a neoplasm, primary or secondary site, followed by adjunct chemotherapy or radiation treatment during the same episode of care, the code for the neoplasm should be assigned as principal or first-listed diagnosis.

2) Patient admission/encounter solely for administration of chemotherapy, immunotherapy and radiation therapy

If a patient admission/encounter is solely for the administration of chemotherapy, immunotherapy or external beam radiation therapy assign code Z51.0, Encounter for antineoplastic radiation therapy, or Z51.11, Encounter for antineoplastic chemotherapy, or Z51.12, Encounter for antineoplastic immunotherapy as the first-listed or principal diagnosis. If a patient receives more than one of these therapies during the same admission more than one of these codes may be assigned, in any sequence.

The malignancy for which the therapy is being administered should be assigned as a secondary diagnosis.

If a patient admission/encounter is for the insertion or implantation of radioactive elements (e.g., brachytherapy) the appropriate code for the malignancy is sequenced as the principal or first-listed diagnosis. Code Z51.0 should not be assigned.

3) Patient admitted for radiation therapy, chemotherapy or immunotherapy and develops complications

When a patient is admitted for the purpose of external beam radiotherapy, immunotherapy or chemotherapy and develops complications such as uncontrolled nausea and vomiting or dehydration, the principal or first-listed diagnosis is Z51.0, Encounter for antineoplastic radiation therapy, or Z51.11, Encounter for antineoplastic chemotherapy, or Z51.12, Encounter for antineoplastic immunotherapy followed by any codes for the complications.

When a patient is admitted for the purpose of insertion or implantation of radioactive elements (e.g., brachytherapy) and develops complications such as uncontrolled nausea and vomiting or dehydration, the principal or first-listed diagnosis is the appropriate code for the malignancy followed by any codes for the complications.

A patient with prostate cancer was admitted for brachytherapy seed implantation and consequently developed urinary retention.

C61	Malignant neoplasm of prostate
R33.9	Retention of urine, unspecified

Explanation: A code for the malignancy should be listed as the principal diagnosis when insertion of a radioactive element is the reason for admission, even when a complication related to that radioactive element occurs. Codes describing the complications should be listed as secondary codes.

f. Admission/encounter to determine extent of malignancy

When the reason for admission/encounter is to determine the extent of the malignancy, or for a procedure such as paracentesis or thoracentesis, the primary malignancy or appropriate metastatic site is designated as the principal or first-listed diagnosis, even though chemotherapy or radiotherapy is administered.

Patient with left lung cancer with malignant pleural effusion admitted for paracentesis and initiation/administration of chemotherapy

C34.92	Malignant neoplasm of unspecified part of left bronchus or lung
J91.0	Malignant pleural effusion
Z51.11	Encounter for antineoplastic chemotherapy

Explanation: The lung cancer is sequenced before the chemotherapy in this instance because the paracentesis for the malignant effusion is also being performed. An instructional note under the malignant effusion instructs that the lung cancer be sequenced first.

g. Symptoms, signs, and abnormal findings listed in Chapter 18 associated with neoplasms

Symptoms, signs, and ill-defined conditions listed in Chapter 18 characteristic of, or associated with, an existing primary or secondary site malignancy cannot be used to replace the malignancy as principal or first-listed diagnosis, regardless of the number of admissions or encounters for treatment and care of the neoplasm.

See Section I.C.21. Factors influencing health status and contact with health services, Encounter for prophylactic organ removal.

h. Admission/encounter for pain control/management

See Section I.C.6. for information on coding admission/encounter for pain control/management.

i. Malignancy in two or more noncontiguous sites

A patient may have more than one malignant tumor in the same organ. These tumors may represent different primaries or metastatic disease, depending on the site. Should the documentation be unclear, the provider should be queried as to the status of each tumor so that the correct codes can be assigned.

j. Disseminated malignant neoplasm, unspecified

Code C80.0, Disseminated malignant neoplasm, unspecified, is for use only in those cases where the patient has advanced metastatic disease and no known primary or secondary sites are specified. It should not be used in place of assigning codes for the primary site and all known secondary sites.

Patient who has had no medical care for many years is seen today and diagnosed with carcinomatosis

C80.0	Disseminated malignant neoplasm, unspecified

Explanation: Carcinomatosis NOS is an "includes" note under this code. Should seldom be used but is available for use in cases such as this.

k. Malignant neoplasm without specification of site

Code C80.1, Malignant (primary) neoplasm, unspecified, equates to Cancer, unspecified. This code should only be used when no determination can be made as to the primary site of a malignancy. This code should rarely be used in the inpatient setting.

l. Sequencing of neoplasm codes

1) Encounter for treatment of primary malignancy

If the reason for the encounter is for treatment of a primary malignancy, assign the malignancy as the principal/first-listed diagnosis. The primary site is to be sequenced first, followed by any metastatic sites.

2) Encounter for treatment of secondary malignancy

When an encounter is for a primary malignancy with metastasis and treatment is directed toward the metastatic (secondary) site(s) only, the metastatic site(s) is designated as the principal/first-listed diagnosis. The primary malignancy is coded as an additional code.

> Patient has primary colon cancer with metastasis to rib and is evaluated for possible excision of portion of rib bone
>
> **C79.51**　　**Secondary malignant neoplasm of bone**
>
> **C18.9**　　**Malignant neoplasm of colon, unspecified**
>
> *Explanation*: The treatment for this encounter is focused on the metastasis to the rib bone rather than the primary colon cancer, thus indicating that the bone metastasis is sequenced as the first-listed code.

3) Malignant neoplasm in a pregnant patient

When a pregnant woman has a malignant neoplasm, a code from subcategory O9A.1-, Malignant neoplasm complicating pregnancy, childbirth, and the puerperium, should be sequenced first, followed by the appropriate code from Chapter 2 to indicate the type of neoplasm.

> A 30-year-old pregnant female in second trimester evaluated for thyroid malignancy
>
> **O9A.112**　　**Malignant neoplasm complicating pregnancy, second trimester**
>
> **C73**　　**Malignant neoplasm of thyroid gland**
>
> *Explanation*: Codes from chapter 15 describing complications of pregnancy are sequenced as first-listed codes, further specified by codes from other chapters such as neoplastic, unless the pregnancy is documented as incidental to the condition. See also guideline 1.C.15.a.1.

4) Encounter for complication associated with a neoplasm

When an encounter is for management of a complication associated with a neoplasm, such as dehydration, and the treatment is only for the complication, the complication is coded first, followed by the appropriate code(s) for the neoplasm.

The exception to this guideline is anemia. When the admission/encounter is for management of an anemia associated with the malignancy, and the treatment is only for anemia, the appropriate code for the malignancy is sequenced as the principal or first-listed diagnosis followed by code D63.0, Anemia in neoplastic disease.

> Patient with pancreatic cancer is seen for initiation of TPN for cancer-related moderate protein-calorie malnutrition
>
> **E44.0**　　**Moderate protein-calorie malnutrition**
>
> **C25.9**　　**Malignant neoplasm of pancreas, unspecified**
>
> *Explanation*: The encounter is to initiate treatment for malnutrition, a common complication of many types of neoplasms, and is sequenced first.

5) Complication from surgical procedure for treatment of a neoplasm

When an encounter is for treatment of a complication resulting from a surgical procedure performed for the treatment of the neoplasm, designate the complication as the principal/first-listed diagnosis. See **the** guideline regarding the coding of a current malignancy versus personal history to determine if the code for the neoplasm should also be assigned.

6) Pathologic fracture due to a neoplasm

When an encounter is for a pathological fracture due to a neoplasm, and the focus of treatment is the fracture, a code from subcategory M84.5, Pathological fracture in neoplastic disease, should be sequenced first, followed by the code for the neoplasm.

If the focus of treatment is the neoplasm with an associated pathological fracture, the neoplasm code should be sequenced first, followed by a code from M84.5 for the pathological fracture.

m. Current malignancy versus personal history of malignancy

When a primary malignancy has been excised but further treatment, such as an additional surgery for the malignancy, radiation therapy or chemotherapy is directed to that site, the primary malignancy code should be used until treatment is completed.

> Female patient with ongoing chemotherapy after right mastectomy for breast cancer
>
> **C50.911**　　**Malignant neoplasm of unspecified site of right female breast**
>
> **Z90.11**　　**Acquired absence of right breast and nipple**
>
> *Explanation*: Even though the breast has been removed, the breast cancer is still being treated with chemotherapy and therefore is still coded as a current condition rather than personal history.

When a primary malignancy has been previously excised or eradicated from its site, there is no further treatment (of the malignancy) directed to that site, and there is no evidence of any existing primary malignancy at that site, a code from category Z85, Personal history of malignant neoplasm, should be used to indicate the former site of the malignancy.

Subcategories Z85.0 – Z85.7 should only be assigned for the former site of a primary malignancy, not the site of a secondary malignancy. Codes from subcategory Z85.8-, may be assigned for the former site(s) of either a primary or secondary malignancy included in this subcategory.

See Section I.C.21. Factors influencing health status and contact with health services, History (of)

n. Leukemia, multiple myeloma, and malignant plasma cell neoplasms in remission versus personal history

The categories for leukemia, and category C90, Multiple myeloma and malignant plasma cell neoplasms, have codes indicating whether or not the leukemia has achieved remission. There are also codes Z85.6, Personal history of leukemia, and Z85.79, Personal history of other malignant neoplasms of lymphoid, hematopoietic and related tissues. If the documentation is unclear as to whether the leukemia has achieved remission, the provider should be queried.

See Section I.C.21. Factors influencing health status and contact with health services, History (of)

o. Aftercare following surgery for neoplasm

See Section I.C.21. Factors influencing health status and contact with health services, Aftercare

p. Follow-up care for completed treatment of a malignancy

See Section I.C.21. Factors influencing health status and contact with health services, Follow-up

q. Prophylactic organ removal for prevention of malignancy

See Section I.C. 21, Factors influencing health status and contact with health services, Prophylactic organ removal

r. Malignant neoplasm associated with transplanted organ

A malignant neoplasm of a transplanted organ should be coded as a transplant complication. Assign first the appropriate code from category T86.-, Complications of transplanted organs and tissue, followed by code C80.2, Malignant neoplasm associated with transplanted organ. Use an additional code for the specific malignancy.

Chapter 2. Neoplasms (C00-D49)

> **NOTE**

Functional activity
All neoplasms are classified in this chapter, whether they are functionally active or not. An additional code from Chapter 4 may be used, to identify functional activity associated with any neoplasm.

Morphology [Histology]
Chapter 2 classifies neoplasms primarily by site (topography), with broad groupings for behavior, malignant, in situ, benign, etc. The Table of Neoplasms should be used to identify the correct topography code. In a few cases, such as for malignant melanoma and certain neuroendocrine tumors, the morphology (histologic type) is included in the category and codes.

Primary malignant neoplasms overlapping site boundaries
A primary malignant neoplasm that overlaps two or more contiguous (next to each other) sites should be classified to the subcategory/code .8 ("overlapping lesion"), unless the combination is specifically indexed elsewhere. For multiple neoplasms of the same site that are not contiguous, such as tumors in different quadrants of the same breast, codes for each site should be assigned.

Malignant neoplasm of ectopic tissue
Malignant neoplasms of ectopic tissue are to be coded to the site mentioned, e.g., ectopic pancreatic malignant neoplasms are coded to pancreas, unspecified (C25.9).

AHA: 2017,4Q,103; 2017,1Q,4,5-6,8

This chapter contains the following blocks:

C00-C14	Malignant neoplasms of lip, oral cavity and pharynx
C15-C26	Malignant neoplasms of digestive organs
C30-C39	Malignant neoplasms of respiratory and intrathoracic organs
C40-C41	Malignant neoplasms of bone and articular cartilage
C43-C44	Melanoma and other malignant neoplasms of skin
C45-C49	Malignant neoplasms of mesothelial and soft tissue
C50	Malignant neoplasms of breast
C51-C58	Malignant neoplasms of female genital organs
C60-C63	Malignant neoplasms of male genital organs
C64-C68	Malignant neoplasms of urinary tract
C69-C72	Malignant neoplasms of eye, brain and other parts of central nervous system
C73-C75	Malignant neoplasms of thyroid and other endocrine glands
C7A	Malignant neuroendocrine tumors
C7B	Secondary neuroendocrine tumors
C76-C80	Malignant neoplasms of ill-defined, other secondary and unspecified sites
C81-C96	Malignant neoplasms of lymphoid, hematopoietic and related tissue
D00-D09	In situ neoplasms
D10-D36	Benign neoplasms, except benign neuroendocrine tumors
D3A	Benign neuroendocrine tumors
D37-D48	Neoplasms of uncertain behavior, polycythemia vera and myelodysplastic syndromes
D49	Neoplasms of unspecified behavior

MALIGNANT NEOPLASMS(C00-C96)

Malignant neoplasms, stated or presumed to be primary (of specified sites), and certain specified histologies, except neuroendocrine, and of lymphoid, hematopoietic and related tissue (C00-C75)

Malignant neoplasms of lip, oral cavity and pharynx (C00-C14)

✓4ᵗʰ **C00**   **Malignant neoplasm of lip**
Use additional code to identify:
   alcohol abuse and dependence (F10.-)
   history of tobacco dependence (Z87.891)
   tobacco dependence (F17.-)
   tobacco use (Z72.0)
> **EXCLUDES 1**   malignant melanoma of lip (C43.0)
>   Merkel cell carcinoma of lip (C4A.0)
>   other and unspecified malignant neoplasm of skin of lip (C44.0-)

   C00.0   **Malignant neoplasm of external upper lip**
      Malignant neoplasm of lipstick area of upper lip
      Malignant neoplasm of upper lip NOS
      Malignant neoplasm of vermilion border of upper lip

   C00.1   **Malignant neoplasm of external lower lip**
      Malignant neoplasm of lower lip NOS
      Malignant neoplasm of lipstick area of lower lip
      Malignant neoplasm of vermilion border of lower lip

   C00.2   **Malignant neoplasm of external lip, unspecified**
      Malignant neoplasm of vermilion border of lip NOS

   C00.3   **Malignant neoplasm of upper lip, inner aspect**
      Malignant neoplasm of buccal aspect of upper lip
      Malignant neoplasm of frenulum of upper lip
      Malignant neoplasm of mucosa of upper lip
      Malignant neoplasm of oral aspect of upper lip

   C00.4   **Malignant neoplasm of lower lip, inner aspect**
      Malignant neoplasm of buccal aspect of lower lip
      Malignant neoplasm of frenulum of lower lip
      Malignant neoplasm of mucosa of lower lip
      Malignant neoplasm of oral aspect of lower lip

   C00.5   **Malignant neoplasm of lip, unspecified, inner aspect**
      Malignant neoplasm of buccal aspect of lip, unspecified
      Malignant neoplasm of frenulum of lip, unspecified
      Malignant neoplasm of mucosa of lip, unspecified
      Malignant neoplasm of oral aspect of lip, unspecified

   C00.6   **Malignant neoplasm of commissure of lip, unspecified**

   C00.8   **Malignant neoplasm of overlapping sites of lip**

   C00.9   **Malignant neoplasm of lip, unspecified**

C01   **Malignant neoplasm of base of tongue**   HCC
      Malignant neoplasm of dorsal surface of base of tongue
      Malignant neoplasm of fixed part of tongue NOS
      Malignant neoplasm of posterior third of tongue
      Use additional code to identify:
        alcohol abuse and dependence (F10.-)
        history of tobacco dependence (Z87.891)
        tobacco dependence (F17.-)
        tobacco use (Z72.0)

Malignant Neoplasm of Tongue

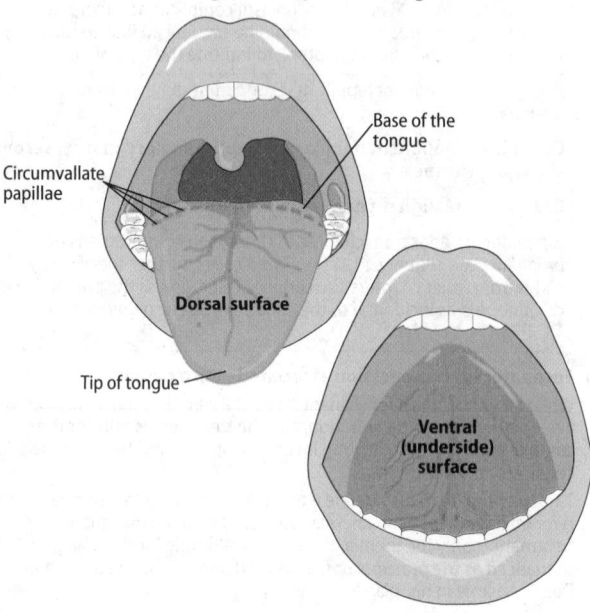

Labels: Base of the tongue; Circumvallate papillae; Dorsal surface; Tip of tongue; Ventral (underside) surface

✓4ᵗʰ **C02**   **Malignant neoplasm of other and unspecified parts of tongue**
      Use additional code to identify:
        alcohol abuse and dependence (F10.-)
        history of tobacco dependence (Z87.891)
        tobacco dependence (F17.-)
        tobacco use (Z72.0)

   C02.0   **Malignant neoplasm of dorsal surface of tongue**   HCC
      Malignant neoplasm of anterior two-thirds of tongue, dorsal surface
> **EXCLUDES 2**   malignant neoplasm of dorsal surface of base of tongue (C01)

   C02.1   **Malignant neoplasm of border of tongue**   HCC
      Malignant neoplasm of tip of tongue

   C02.2   **Malignant neoplasm of ventral surface of tongue**   HCC
      Malignant neoplasm of anterior two-thirds of tongue, ventral surface
      Malignant neoplasm of frenulum linguae

C02.3 **Malignant neoplasm of anterior two-thirds of tongue, part unspecified** `HCC`
> Malignant neoplasm of middle third of tongue NOS
> Malignant neoplasm of mobile part of tongue NOS

C02.4 **Malignant neoplasm of lingual tonsil** `HCC`
> **EXCLUDES 2** *malignant neoplasm of tonsil NOS (C09.9)*

C02.8 **Malignant neoplasm of overlapping sites of tongue** `HCC`
> Malignant neoplasm of two or more contiguous sites of tongue

C02.9 **Malignant neoplasm of tongue, unspecified** `HCC`

✓4ᵗʰ **C03** **Malignant neoplasm of gum**
> **INCLUDES** malignant neoplasm of alveolar (ridge) mucosa
> malignant neoplasm of gingiva
> Use additional code to identify:
> alcohol abuse and dependence (F10.-)
> history of tobacco dependence (Z87.891)
> tobacco dependence (F17.-)
> tobacco use (Z72.0)
> **EXCLUDES 2** *malignant odontogenic neoplasms (C41.0-C41.1)*

C03.0 **Malignant neoplasm of upper gum** `HCC`

C03.1 **Malignant neoplasm of lower gum** `HCC`

C03.9 **Malignant neoplasm of gum, unspecified** `HCC`

✓4ᵗʰ **C04** **Malignant neoplasm of floor of mouth**
> Use additional code to identify:
> alcohol abuse and dependence (F10.-)
> history of tobacco dependence (Z87.891)
> tobacco dependence (F17.-)
> tobacco use (Z72.0)

C04.0 **Malignant neoplasm of anterior floor of mouth** `HCC`
> Malignant neoplasm of anterior to the premolar-canine junction

C04.1 **Malignant neoplasm of lateral floor of mouth** `HCC`

C04.8 **Malignant neoplasm of overlapping sites of floor of mouth** `HCC`

C04.9 **Malignant neoplasm of floor of mouth, unspecified** `HCC`

✓4ᵗʰ **C05** **Malignant neoplasm of palate**
> Use additional code to identify:
> alcohol abuse and dependence (F10.-)
> history of tobacco dependence (Z87.891)
> tobacco dependence (F17.-)
> tobacco use (Z72.0)
> **EXCLUDES 1** *Kaposi's sarcoma of palate (C46.2)*

C05.0 **Malignant neoplasm of hard palate** `HCC`

C05.1 **Malignant neoplasm of soft palate** `HCC`
> **EXCLUDES 2** *malignant neoplasm of nasopharyngeal surface of soft palate (C11.3)*

C05.2 **Malignant neoplasm of uvula** `HCC`

C05.8 **Malignant neoplasm of overlapping sites of palate** `HCC`

C05.9 **Malignant neoplasm of palate, unspecified** `HCC`
> Malignant neoplasm of roof of mouth

✓4ᵗʰ **C06** **Malignant neoplasm of other and unspecified parts of mouth**
> Use additional code to identify:
> alcohol abuse and dependence (F10.-)
> history of tobacco dependence (Z87.891)
> tobacco dependence (F17.-)
> tobacco use (Z72.0)

C06.0 **Malignant neoplasm of cheek mucosa** `HCC`
> Malignant neoplasm of buccal mucosa NOS
> Malignant neoplasm of internal cheek

C06.1 **Malignant neoplasm of vestibule of mouth** `HCC`
> Malignant neoplasm of buccal sulcus (upper) (lower)
> Malignant neoplasm of labial sulcus (upper) (lower)

C06.2 **Malignant neoplasm of retromolar area** `HCC`

✓5ᵗʰ **C06.8** **Malignant neoplasm of overlapping sites of other and unspecified parts of mouth**

C06.80 **Malignant neoplasm of overlapping sites of unspecified parts of mouth** `HCC`

C06.89 **Malignant neoplasm of overlapping sites of other parts of mouth** `HCC`
> "book leaf" neoplasm [ventral surface of tongue and floor of mouth]

C06.9 **Malignant neoplasm of mouth, unspecified** `HCC`
> Malignant neoplasm of minor salivary gland, unspecified site
> Malignant neoplasm of oral cavity NOS

C07 **Malignant neoplasm of parotid gland** `HCC`
> Use additional code to identify:
> alcohol abuse and dependence (F10.-)
> exposure to environmental tobacco smoke (Z77.22)
> exposure to tobacco smoke in the perinatal period (P96.81)
> history of tobacco dependence (Z87.891)
> occupational exposure to environmental tobacco smoke (Z57.31)
> tobacco dependence (F17.-)
> tobacco use (Z72.0)

✓4ᵗʰ **C08** **Malignant neoplasm of other and unspecified major salivary glands**
> **INCLUDES** malignant neoplasm of salivary ducts
> Use additional code to identify:
> alcohol abuse and dependence (F10.-)
> exposure to environmental tobacco smoke (Z77.22)
> exposure to tobacco smoke in the perinatal period (P96.81)
> history of tobacco dependence (Z87.891)
> occupational exposure to environmental tobacco smoke (Z57.31)
> tobacco dependence (F17.-)
> tobacco use (Z72.0)
> **EXCLUDES 1** *malignant neoplasms of specified minor salivary glands which are classified according to their anatomical location*
> **EXCLUDES 2** *malignant neoplasms of minor salivary glands NOS (C06.9)*
> *malignant neoplasm of parotid gland (C07)*

C08.0 **Malignant neoplasm of submandibular gland** `HCC`
> Malignant neoplasm of submaxillary gland

C08.1 **Malignant neoplasm of sublingual gland** `HCC`

C08.9 **Malignant neoplasm of major salivary gland, unspecified** `HCC`
> Malignant neoplasm of salivary gland (major) NOS

✓4ᵗʰ **C09** **Malignant neoplasm of tonsil**
> Use additional code to identify:
> alcohol abuse and dependence (F10.-)
> exposure to environmental tobacco smoke (Z77.22)
> exposure to tobacco smoke in the perinatal period (P96.81)
> history of tobacco dependence (Z87.891)
> occupational exposure to environmental tobacco smoke (Z57.31)
> tobacco dependence (F17.-)
> tobacco use (Z72.0)
> **EXCLUDES 2** *malignant neoplasm of lingual tonsil (C02.4)*
> *malignant neoplasm of pharyngeal tonsil (C11.1)*

C09.0 **Malignant neoplasm of tonsillar fossa** `HCC`

C09.1 **Malignant neoplasm of tonsillar pillar (anterior) (posterior)** `HCC`

C09.8 **Malignant neoplasm of overlapping sites of tonsil** `HCC`

C09.9 **Malignant neoplasm of tonsil, unspecified** `HCC`
> Malignant neoplasm of tonsil NOS
> Malignant neoplasm of faucial tonsils
> Malignant neoplasm of palatine tonsils

✓4ᵗʰ **C10** **Malignant neoplasm of oropharynx**
> Use additional code to identify:
> alcohol abuse and dependence (F10.-)
> exposure to environmental tobacco smoke (Z77.22)
> exposure to tobacco smoke in the perinatal period (P96.81)
> history of tobacco dependence (Z87.891)
> occupational exposure to environmental tobacco smoke (Z57.31)
> tobacco dependence (F17.-)
> tobacco use (Z72.0)
> **EXCLUDES 2** *malignant neoplasm of tonsil (C09.-)*
> **DEF:** Oropharynx: Middle portion of pharynx (throat); communicates with the oral cavity, nasopharynx and laryngopharynx.

C10.0 **Malignant neoplasm of vallecula** `HCC`

C10.1 **Malignant neoplasm of anterior surface of epiglottis** `HCC`
> Malignant neoplasm of epiglottis, free border [margin]
> Malignant neoplasm of glossoepiglottic fold(s)
> **EXCLUDES 2** *malignant neoplasm of epiglottis (suprahyoid portion) NOS (C32.1)*

C10.2 **Malignant neoplasm of lateral wall of oropharynx** `HCC`

C10.3 **Malignant neoplasm of posterior wall of oropharynx** `HCC`

✓ Additional Character Required   ✓x7ᵗʰ Placeholder   Unacceptable PDx   Questionable PDx   Manifestation   Unspecified Dx   H1-H14 HAC   `HCC` CMS-HCC Dx   HIV HIV Dx

ICD-10-CM 2020   465

Chapter 2. Neoplasms

C02.3–C10.3

Chapter 2. Neoplasms

C10.4   **Malignant neoplasm of branchial cleft**   `HCC`

Malignant neoplasm of branchial cyst [site of neoplasm]

C10.8   **Malignant neoplasm of overlapping sites of oropharynx**   `HCC`

Malignant neoplasm of junctional region of oropharynx

C10.9   **Malignant neoplasm of oropharynx, unspecified**   `HCC`

√4ᵗʰ **C11**   **Malignant neoplasm of nasopharynx**

Use additional code to identify:

exposure to environmental tobacco smoke (Z77.22)

exposure to tobacco smoke in the perinatal period (P96.81)

history of tobacco dependence (Z87.891)

occupational exposure to environmental tobacco smoke (Z57.31)

tobacco dependence (F17.-)

tobacco use (Z72.0)

DEF: Nasopharynx: Upper portion of pharynx (throat); communicates with the nasal cavities, oropharynx and tympanic cavities.

C11.0   **Malignant neoplasm of superior wall of nasopharynx**   `HCC`

Malignant neoplasm of roof of nasopharynx

C11.1   **Malignant neoplasm of posterior wall of nasopharynx**   `HCC`

Malignant neoplasm of adenoid

Malignant neoplasm of pharyngeal tonsil

C11.2   **Malignant neoplasm of lateral wall of nasopharynx**   `HCC`

Malignant neoplasm of fossa of Rosenmüller

Malignant neoplasm of opening of auditory tube

Malignant neoplasm of pharyngeal recess

C11.3   **Malignant neoplasm of anterior wall of nasopharynx**   `HCC`

Malignant neoplasm of floor of nasopharynx

Malignant neoplasm of nasopharyngeal (anterior) (posterior) surface of soft palate

Malignant neoplasm of posterior margin of nasal choana

Malignant neoplasm of posterior margin of nasal septum

C11.8   **Malignant neoplasm of overlapping sites of nasopharynx**   `HCC`

C11.9   **Malignant neoplasm of nasopharynx, unspecified**   `HCC`

Malignant neoplasm of nasopharyngeal wall NOS

C12   **Malignant neoplasm of pyriform sinus**   `HCC`

Malignant neoplasm of pyriform fossa

Use additional code to identify:

exposure to environmental tobacco smoke (Z77.22)

exposure to tobacco smoke in the perinatal period (P96.81)

history of tobacco dependence (Z87.891)

occupational exposure to environmental tobacco smoke (Z57.31)

tobacco dependence (F17.-)

tobacco use (Z72.0)

√4ᵗʰ **C13**   **Malignant neoplasm of hypopharynx**

Use additional code to identify:

exposure to environmental tobacco smoke (Z77.22)

exposure to tobacco smoke in the perinatal period (P96.81)

history of tobacco dependence (Z87.891)

occupational exposure to environmental tobacco smoke (Z57.31)

tobacco dependence (F17.-)

tobacco use (Z72.0)

EXCLUDES 2   *malignant neoplasm of pyriform sinus (C12)*

DEF: Hypopharynx: Lower portion of pharynx (throat); communicates with the oropharynx and the esophagus. ***Synonyms:*** *laryngopharynx.*

C13.0   **Malignant neoplasm of postcricoid region**   `HCC`

C13.1   **Malignant neoplasm of aryepiglottic fold, hypopharyngeal aspect**   `HCC`

Malignant neoplasm of aryepiglottic fold, marginal zone

Malignant neoplasm of aryepiglottic fold NOS

Malignant neoplasm of interarytenoid fold, marginal zone

Malignant neoplasm of interarytenoid fold NOS

EXCLUDES 2   *malignant neoplasm of aryepiglottic fold or interarytenoid fold, laryngeal aspect (C32.1)*

C13.2   **Malignant neoplasm of posterior wall of hypopharynx**   `HCC`

C13.8   **Malignant neoplasm of overlapping sites of hypopharynx**   `HCC`

C13.9   **Malignant neoplasm of hypopharynx, unspecified**   `HCC`

Malignant neoplasm of hypopharyngeal wall NOS

√4ᵗʰ **C14**   **Malignant neoplasm of other and ill-defined sites in the lip, oral cavity and pharynx**

Use additional code to identify:

alcohol abuse and dependence (F10.-)

exposure to environmental tobacco smoke (Z77.22)

exposure to tobacco smoke in the perinatal period (P96.81)

history of tobacco dependence (Z87.891)

occupational exposure to environmental tobacco smoke (Z57.31)

tobacco dependence (F17.-)

tobacco use (Z72.0)

EXCLUDES 1   *malignant neoplasm of oral cavity NOS (C06.9)*

C14.0   **Malignant neoplasm of pharynx, unspecified**   `HCC`

C14.2   **Malignant neoplasm of Waldeyer's ring**   `HCC`

DEF: Waldeyer's ring: Ring of lymphoid tissue that is made up of the two palatine tonsils, the pharyngeal tonsil (adenoid), and the lingual tonsil. It functions as the defense against infection and assists with the development of the immune system.

C14.8   **Malignant neoplasm of overlapping sites of lip, oral cavity and pharynx**   `HCC`

Primary malignant neoplasm of two or more contiguous sites of lip, oral cavity and pharynx

EXCLUDES 1   *"book leaf" neoplasm [ventral surface of tongue and floor of mouth] (C06.89)*

Malignant neoplasms of digestive organs (C15-C26)

EXCLUDES 1   *Kaposi's sarcoma of gastrointestinal sites (C46.4)*

EXCLUDES 2   *gastrointestinal stromal tumors (C49.A-)*

√4ᵗʰ **C15**   **Malignant neoplasm of esophagus**

Use additional code to identify:

alcohol abuse and dependence (F10.-)

C15.3   **Malignant neoplasm of upper third of esophagus**   `HCC`

C15.4   **Malignant neoplasm of middle third of esophagus**   `HCC`

C15.5   **Malignant neoplasm of lower third of esophagus**   `HCC`

EXCLUDES 1   *malignant neoplasm of cardio-esophageal junction (C16.0)*

C15.8   **Malignant neoplasm of overlapping sites of esophagus**   `HCC`

C15.9   **Malignant neoplasm of esophagus, unspecified**   `HCC`

√4ᵗʰ **C16**   **Malignant neoplasm of stomach**

Use additional code to identify:

alcohol abuse and dependence (F10.-)

EXCLUDES 2   *malignant carcinoid tumor of the stomach (C7A.092)*

C16.0   **Malignant neoplasm of cardia**   `HCC`

Malignant neoplasm of cardiac orifice

Malignant neoplasm of cardio-esophageal junction

Malignant neoplasm of esophagus and stomach

Malignant neoplasm of gastro-esophageal junction

C16.1   **Malignant neoplasm of fundus of stomach**   `HCC`

C16.2   **Malignant neoplasm of body of stomach**   `HCC`

C16.3   **Malignant neoplasm of pyloric antrum**   `HCC`

Malignant neoplasm of gastric antrum

C16.4   **Malignant neoplasm of pylorus**   `HCC`

Malignant neoplasm of prepylorus

Malignant neoplasm of pyloric canal

C16.5   **Malignant neoplasm of lesser curvature of stomach, unspecified**   `HCC`

Malignant neoplasm of lesser curvature of stomach, not classifiable to C16.1-C16.4

C16.6   **Malignant neoplasm of greater curvature of stomach, unspecified**   `HCC`

Malignant neoplasm of greater curvature of stomach, not classifiable to C16.0-C16.4

C16.8   **Malignant neoplasm of overlapping sites of stomach**   `HCC`

C16.9   **Malignant neoplasm of stomach, unspecified**   `HCC`

Gastric cancer NOS

√4ᵗʰ **C17**   **Malignant neoplasm of small intestine**

EXCLUDES 1   *malignant carcinoid tumors of the small intestine (C7A.01)*

AHA: 2016,1Q,19

C17.0   **Malignant neoplasm of duodenum**   `HCC`

C17.1   **Malignant neoplasm of jejunum**   `HCC`

Ⓝ Newborn: 0   Ⓟ Pediatric: 0-17   Ⓜ Maternity: 9-64   Ⓐ Adult: 15-124   `MCC` Major Complication/Comorbidity   `CC` Complication/Comorbidity   `SW` Severe Wound Dx

466   ICD-10-CM 2020

C17.2 Malignant neoplasm of ileum   `HCC`
> *EXCLUDES 1*   *malignant neoplasm of ileocecal valve (C18.0)*

C17.3 Meckel's diverticulum, malignant   `HCC`
> *EXCLUDES 1*   *Meckel's diverticulum, congenital (Q43.0)*
> **DEF:** Congenital, abnormal remnant of embryonic digestive system development that leaves a sacculation or outpouching from the wall of the small intestine near the terminal part of the ileum made of acid-secreting tissue as in the stomach.

C17.8 Malignant neoplasm of overlapping sites of small intestine   `HCC`

C17.9 Malignant neoplasm of small intestine, unspecified   `HCC`

✓4ᵗʰ **C18 Malignant neoplasm of colon**
> *EXCLUDES 1*   *malignant carcinoid tumors of the colon (C7A.02-)*

Colon

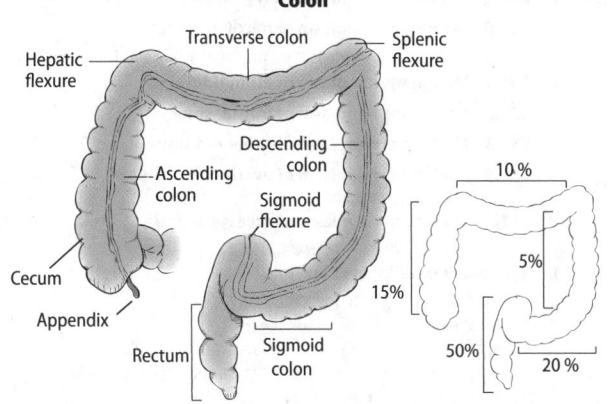

Transverse colon
Splenic flexure
Hepatic flexure
Descending colon
Ascending colon
Sigmoid flexure
Cecum
Appendix
Rectum
Sigmoid colon

10 %
5%
15%
50%
20 %

Anatomical distribution of large bowel cancers

C18.0 Malignant neoplasm of cecum   `HCC`
> Malignant neoplasm of ileocecal valve

C18.1 Malignant neoplasm of appendix   `HCC`

C18.2 Malignant neoplasm of ascending colon   `HCC`

C18.3 Malignant neoplasm of hepatic flexure   `HCC`

C18.4 Malignant neoplasm of transverse colon   `HCC`

C18.5 Malignant neoplasm of splenic flexure   `HCC`

C18.6 Malignant neoplasm of descending colon   `HCC`

C18.7 Malignant neoplasm of sigmoid colon   `HCC`
> Malignant neoplasm of sigmoid (flexure)
> *EXCLUDES 1*   *malignant neoplasm of rectosigmoid junction (C19)*

C18.8 Malignant neoplasm of overlapping sites of colon   `HCC`

C18.9 Malignant neoplasm of colon, unspecified   `HCC`
> Malignant neoplasm of large intestine NOS

C19 Malignant neoplasm of rectosigmoid junction   `HCC`
> Malignant neoplasm of colon with rectum
> Malignant neoplasm of rectosigmoid (colon)
> *EXCLUDES 1*   *malignant carcinoid tumors of the colon (C7A.02-)*

C20 Malignant neoplasm of rectum   `HCC`
> Malignant neoplasm of rectal ampulla
> *EXCLUDES 1*   *malignant carcinoid tumor of the rectum (C7A.026)*

✓4ᵗʰ **C21 Malignant neoplasm of anus and anal canal**
> *EXCLUDES 2*   *malignant carcinoid tumors of the colon (C7A.02-)*
> *malignant melanoma of anal margin (C43.51)*
> *malignant melanoma of anal skin (C43.51)*
> *malignant melanoma of perianal skin (C43.51)*
> *other and unspecified malignant neoplasm of anal margin (C44.500, C44.510, C44.520, C44.590)*
> *other and unspecified malignant neoplasm of anal skin (C44.500, C44.510, C44.520, C44.590)*
> *other and unspecified malignant neoplasm of perianal skin (C44.500, C44.510, C44.520, C44.590)*

C21.0 Malignant neoplasm of anus, unspecified   `HCC`

C21.1 Malignant neoplasm of anal canal   `HCC`
> Malignant neoplasm of anal sphincter

C21.2 Malignant neoplasm of cloacogenic zone   `HCC`

C21.8 Malignant neoplasm of overlapping sites of rectum, anus and anal canal   `HCC`
> Malignant neoplasm of anorectal junction
> Malignant neoplasm of anorectum
> Primary malignant neoplasm of two or more contiguous sites of rectum, anus and anal canal

✓4ᵗʰ **C22 Malignant neoplasm of liver and intrahepatic bile ducts**
> Use additional code to identify:
> alcohol abuse and dependence (F10.-)
> hepatitis B (B16.-, B18.0-B18.1)
> hepatitis C (B17.1-, B18.2)
> *EXCLUDES 1*   *malignant neoplasm of biliary tract NOS (C24.9)*
> *secondary malignant neoplasm of liver and intrahepatic bile duct (C78.7)*

C22.0 Liver cell carcinoma   `HCC`
> Hepatocellular carcinoma
> Hepatoma
> **AHA:** 2016,1Q,18

C22.1 Intrahepatic bile duct carcinoma   `HCC`
> Cholangiocarcinoma
> *EXCLUDES 1*   *malignant neoplasm of hepatic duct (C24.0)*

C22.2 Hepatoblastoma   `HCC`

C22.3 Angiosarcoma of liver   `HCC`
> Kupffer cell sarcoma

C22.4 Other sarcomas of liver   `HCC`

C22.7 Other specified carcinomas of liver   `HCC`

C22.8 Malignant neoplasm of liver, primary, unspecified as to type   `HCC`

C22.9 Malignant neoplasm of liver, not specified as primary or secondary   `HCC`

C23 Malignant neoplasm of gallbladder   `HCC`

✓4ᵗʰ **C24 Malignant neoplasm of other and unspecified parts of biliary tract**
> *EXCLUDES 1*   *malignant neoplasm of intrahepatic bile duct (C22.1)*

C24.0 Malignant neoplasm of extrahepatic bile duct   `HCC`
> Malignant neoplasm of biliary duct or passage NOS
> Malignant neoplasm of common bile duct
> Malignant neoplasm of cystic duct
> Malignant neoplasm of hepatic duct

C24.1 Malignant neoplasm of ampulla of Vater   `HCC`
> **DEF:** Malignant neoplasm in the area of dilation at the juncture of the common bile and pancreatic ducts near the opening into the lumen of the duodenum.

C24.8 Malignant neoplasm of overlapping sites of biliary tract   `HCC`
> Malignant neoplasm involving both intrahepatic and extrahepatic bile ducts
> Primary malignant neoplasm of two or more contiguous sites of biliary tract

C24.9 Malignant neoplasm of biliary tract, unspecified   `HCC`

Chapter 2. Neoplasms

C17.2–C24.9

Chapter 2. Neoplasms

C25-C33

✓4ᵗʰ C25 Malignant neoplasm of pancreas

Code also exocrine pancreatic insufficiency (K86.81)
Use additional code to identify:
alcohol abuse and dependence (F10.-)

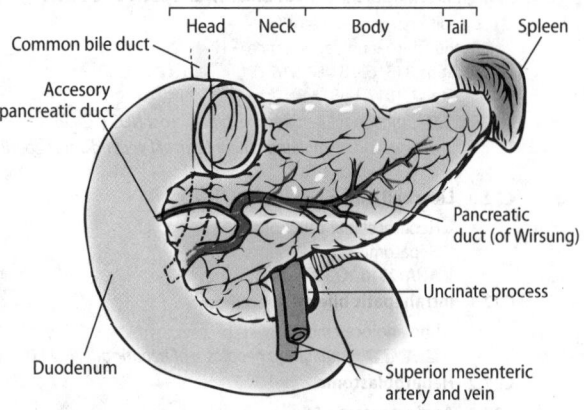

Pancreas

Head — Neck — Body — Tail — Spleen
Common bile duct
Accesory pancreatic duct
Pancreatic duct (of Wirsung)
Uncinate process
Duodenum
Superior mesenteric artery and vein

C25.0 Malignant neoplasm of head of pancreas HCC
C25.1 Malignant neoplasm of body of pancreas HCC
C25.2 Malignant neoplasm of tail of pancreas HCC
C25.3 Malignant neoplasm of pancreatic duct HCC
C25.4 Malignant neoplasm of endocrine pancreas HCC
  Malignant neoplasm of islets of Langerhans
  Use additional code to identify any functional activity
C25.7 Malignant neoplasm of other parts of pancreas HCC
  Malignant neoplasm of neck of pancreas
C25.8 Malignant neoplasm of overlapping sites of pancreas HCC
C25.9 Malignant neoplasm of pancreas, unspecified HCC

✓4ᵗʰ C26 Malignant neoplasm of other and ill-defined digestive organs

EXCLUDES 1 malignant neoplasm of peritoneum and retroperitoneum (C48.-)

C26.0 Malignant neoplasm of intestinal tract, part unspecified HCC
  Malignant neoplasm of intestine NOS
C26.1 Malignant neoplasm of spleen HCC
  EXCLUDES 1 Hodgkin lymphoma (C81.-)
    non-Hodgkin lymphoma (C82-C85)
C26.9 Malignant neoplasm of ill-defined sites within the digestive system HCC
  Malignant neoplasm of alimentary canal or tract NOS
  Malignant neoplasm of gastrointestinal tract NOS
  EXCLUDES 1 malignant neoplasm of abdominal NOS (C76.2)
    malignant neoplasm of intra-abdominal NOS (C76.2)

Malignant neoplasms of respiratory and intrathoracic organs (C30-C39)

INCLUDES malignant neoplasm of middle ear
EXCLUDES 1 mesothelioma (C45.-)

✓4ᵗʰ C30 Malignant neoplasm of nasal cavity and middle ear

C30.0 Malignant neoplasm of nasal cavity HCC
  Malignant neoplasm of cartilage of nose
  Malignant neoplasm of nasal concha
  Malignant neoplasm of internal nose
  Malignant neoplasm of septum of nose
  Malignant neoplasm of vestibule of nose
  EXCLUDES 1 malignant neoplasm of nasal bone (C41.0)
    malignant neoplasm of nose NOS (C76.0)
    malignant neoplasm of olfactory bulb (C72.2-)
    malignant neoplasm of posterior margin of nasal septum and choana (C11.3)
    malignant melanoma of skin of nose (C43.31)
    malignant neoplasm of turbinates (C41.0)
    other and unspecified malignant neoplasm of skin of nose (C44.301, C44.311, C44.321, C44.391)

C30.1 Malignant neoplasm of middle ear HCC
  Malignant neoplasm of antrum tympanicum
  Malignant neoplasm of auditory tube
  Malignant neoplasm of eustachian tube
  Malignant neoplasm of inner ear
  Malignant neoplasm of mastoid air cells
  Malignant neoplasm of tympanic cavity
  EXCLUDES 1 malignant neoplasm of auricular canal (external) (C43.2-,C44.2-)
    malignant neoplasm of bone of ear (meatus) (C41.0)
    malignant neoplasm of cartilage of ear (C49.0)
    malignant melanoma of skin of (external) ear (C43.2-)
    other and unspecified malignant neoplasm of skin of (external) ear (C44.2-)

✓4ᵗʰ C31 Malignant neoplasm of accessory sinuses

C31.0 Malignant neoplasm of maxillary sinus HCC
  Malignant neoplasm of antrum (Highmore) (maxillary)
C31.1 Malignant neoplasm of ethmoidal sinus HCC
C31.2 Malignant neoplasm of frontal sinus HCC
C31.3 Malignant neoplasm of sphenoid sinus HCC
C31.8 Malignant neoplasm of overlapping sites of accessory sinuses HCC
C31.9 Malignant neoplasm of accessory sinus, unspecified HCC

✓4ᵗʰ C32 Malignant neoplasm of larynx

Use additional code to identify:
alcohol abuse and dependence (F10.-)
exposure to environmental tobacco smoke (Z77.22)
exposure to tobacco smoke in the perinatal period (P96.81)
history of tobacco dependence (Z87.891)
occupational exposure to environmental tobacco smoke (Z57.31)
tobacco dependence (F17.-)
tobacco use (Z72.0)

C32.0 Malignant neoplasm of glottis HCC
  Malignant neoplasm of intrinsic larynx
  Malignant neoplasm of laryngeal commissure (anterior)(posterior)
  Malignant neoplasm of vocal cord (true) NOS
C32.1 Malignant neoplasm of supraglottis HCC
  Malignant neoplasm of aryepiglottic fold or interarytenoid fold, laryngeal aspect
  Malignant neoplasm of epiglottis (suprahyoid portion) NOS
  Malignant neoplasm of extrinsic larynx
  Malignant neoplasm of false vocal cord
  Malignant neoplasm of posterior (laryngeal) surface of epiglottis
  Malignant neoplasm of ventricular bands
  EXCLUDES 2 malignant neoplasm of anterior surface of epiglottis (C10.1)
    malignant neoplasm of aryepiglottic fold or interarytenoid fold, hypopharyngeal aspect (C13.1)
    malignant neoplasm of aryepiglottic fold or interarytenoid fold, marginal zone (C13.1)
    malignant neoplasm of aryepiglottic fold or interarytenoid fold NOS (C13.1)
C32.2 Malignant neoplasm of subglottis HCC
C32.3 Malignant neoplasm of laryngeal cartilage HCC
C32.8 Malignant neoplasm of overlapping sites of larynx HCC
C32.9 Malignant neoplasm of larynx, unspecified HCC

C33 Malignant neoplasm of trachea HCC

Use additional code to identify:
exposure to environmental tobacco smoke (Z77.22)
exposure to tobacco smoke in the perinatal period (P96.81)
history of tobacco dependence (Z87.891)
occupational exposure to environmental tobacco smoke (Z57.31)
tobacco dependence (F17.-)
tobacco use (Z72.0)

Chapter 2. Neoplasms

✓4ᵗʰ **C34 Malignant neoplasm of bronchus and lung**

Use additional code to identify:
exposure to environmental tobacco smoke (Z77.22)
exposure to tobacco smoke in the perinatal period (P96.81)
history of tobacco dependence (Z87.891)
occupational exposure to environmental tobacco smoke (Z57.31)
tobacco dependence (F17.-)
tobacco use (Z72.0)

EXCLUDES 1   Kaposi's sarcoma of lung (C46.5-)
malignant carcinoid tumor of the bronchus and lung (C7A.090)

AHA: 2019,1Q,16
TIP: When documented, assign code I31.3 for associated malignant pericardial effusion. If the sole reason for admission is to treat the effusion with no treatment of the lung malignancy rendered, code I31.3 may be sequenced first.

✓5ᵗʰ **C34.0 Malignant neoplasm of main bronchus**

Malignant neoplasm of carina
Malignant neoplasm of hilus (of lung)

     C34.00 Malignant neoplasm of unspecified main bronchus HCC
     C34.01 Malignant neoplasm of right main bronchus HCC
     C34.02 Malignant neoplasm of left main bronchus HCC

✓5ᵗʰ **C34.1 Malignant neoplasm of upper lobe, bronchus or lung**

     C34.10 Malignant neoplasm of upper lobe, unspecified bronchus or lung HCC
     C34.11 Malignant neoplasm of upper lobe, right bronchus or lung HCC
     C34.12 Malignant neoplasm of upper lobe, left bronchus or lung HCC

C34.2 Malignant neoplasm of middle lobe, bronchus or lung HCC

✓5ᵗʰ **C34.3 Malignant neoplasm of lower lobe, bronchus or lung**

     C34.30 Malignant neoplasm of lower lobe, unspecified bronchus or lung HCC
     C34.31 Malignant neoplasm of lower lobe, right bronchus or lung HCC
     C34.32 Malignant neoplasm of lower lobe, left bronchus or lung HCC

✓5ᵗʰ **C34.8 Malignant neoplasm of overlapping sites of bronchus and lung**

     C34.80 Malignant neoplasm of overlapping sites of unspecified bronchus and lung HCC
     C34.81 Malignant neoplasm of overlapping sites of right bronchus and lung HCC
     C34.82 Malignant neoplasm of overlapping sites of left bronchus and lung HCC

✓5ᵗʰ **C34.9 Malignant neoplasm of unspecified part of bronchus or lung**

     C34.90 Malignant neoplasm of unspecified part of unspecified bronchus or lung HCC
     Lung cancer NOS
     C34.91 Malignant neoplasm of unspecified part of right bronchus or lung HCC
     C34.92 Malignant neoplasm of unspecified part of left bronchus or lung HCC

C37 Malignant neoplasm of thymus HCC

EXCLUDES 1   malignant carcinoid tumor of the thymus (C7A.091)

✓4ᵗʰ **C38 Malignant neoplasm of heart, mediastinum and pleura**

EXCLUDES 1   mesothelioma (C45.-)

C38.0 Malignant neoplasm of heart HCC

Malignant neoplasm of pericardium
EXCLUDES 1   malignant neoplasm of great vessels (C49.3)

C38.1 Malignant neoplasm of anterior mediastinum HCC

C38.2 Malignant neoplasm of posterior mediastinum HCC

C38.3 Malignant neoplasm of mediastinum, part unspecified HCC

C38.4 Malignant neoplasm of pleura HCC

C38.8 Malignant neoplasm of overlapping sites of heart, mediastinum and pleura HCC

✓4ᵗʰ **C39 Malignant neoplasm of other and ill-defined sites in the respiratory system and intrathoracic organs**

Use additional code to identify:
exposure to environmental tobacco smoke (Z77.22)
exposure to tobacco smoke in the perinatal period (P96.81)
history of tobacco dependence (Z87.891)
occupational exposure to environmental tobacco smoke (Z57.31)
tobacco dependence (F17.-)
tobacco use (Z72.0)

EXCLUDES 1   intrathoracic malignant neoplasm NOS (C76.1)
thoracic malignant neoplasm NOS (C76.1)

C39.0 Malignant neoplasm of upper respiratory tract, part unspecified HCC

C39.9 Malignant neoplasm of lower respiratory tract, part unspecified HCC

Malignant neoplasm of respiratory tract NOS

Malignant neoplasms of bone and articular cartilage (C40-C41)

INCLUDES   malignant neoplasm of cartilage (articular) (joint)
     malignant neoplasm of periosteum
EXCLUDES 1   malignant neoplasm of bone marrow NOS (C96.9)
     malignant neoplasm of synovia (C49.-)

✓4ᵗʰ **C40 Malignant neoplasm of bone and articular cartilage of limbs**

Use additional code to identify major osseous defect, if applicable (M89.7-)

✓5ᵗʰ **C40.0 Malignant neoplasm of scapula and long bones of upper limb**

     C40.00 Malignant neoplasm of scapula and long bones of unspecified upper limb HCC
     C40.01 Malignant neoplasm of scapula and long bones of right upper limb HCC
     C40.02 Malignant neoplasm of scapula and long bones of left upper limb HCC

✓5ᵗʰ **C40.1 Malignant neoplasm of short bones of upper limb**

     C40.10 Malignant neoplasm of short bones of unspecified upper limb HCC
     C40.11 Malignant neoplasm of short bones of right upper limb HCC
     C40.12 Malignant neoplasm of short bones of left upper limb HCC

✓5ᵗʰ **C40.2 Malignant neoplasm of long bones of lower limb**

     C40.20 Malignant neoplasm of long bones of unspecified lower limb HCC
     C40.21 Malignant neoplasm of long bones of right lower limb HCC
     C40.22 Malignant neoplasm of long bones of left lower limb HCC

✓5ᵗʰ **C40.3 Malignant neoplasm of short bones of lower limb**

     C40.30 Malignant neoplasm of short bones of unspecified lower limb HCC
     C40.31 Malignant neoplasm of short bones of right lower limb HCC
     C40.32 Malignant neoplasm of short bones of left lower limb HCC

✓5ᵗʰ **C40.8 Malignant neoplasm of overlapping sites of bone and articular cartilage of limb**

     C40.80 Malignant neoplasm of overlapping sites of bone and articular cartilage of unspecified limb HCC
     C40.81 Malignant neoplasm of overlapping sites of bone and articular cartilage of right limb CC HCC
     CC Excl: PDX collection 293
     C40.82 Malignant neoplasm of overlapping sites of bone and articular cartilage of left limb HCC

✓5ᵗʰ **C40.9 Malignant neoplasm of unspecified bones and articular cartilage of limb**

     C40.90 Malignant neoplasm of unspecified bones and articular cartilage of unspecified limb HCC
     C40.91 Malignant neoplasm of unspecified bones and articular cartilage of right limb HCC
     C40.92 Malignant neoplasm of unspecified bones and articular cartilage of left limb HCC

Chapter 2. Neoplasms

C41–C4A.59

✓4ᵗʰ **C41 Malignant neoplasm of bone and articular cartilage of other and unspecified sites**

> EXCLUDES 1   malignant neoplasm of bones of limbs (C40.-)
> malignant neoplasm of cartilage of ear (C49.0)
> malignant neoplasm of cartilage of eyelid (C49.0)
> malignant neoplasm of cartilage of larynx (C32.3)
> malignant neoplasm of cartilage of limbs (C40.-)
> malignant neoplasm of cartilage of nose (C30.0)

C41.0 Malignant neoplasm of bones of skull and face   HCC

> Malignant neoplasm of maxilla (superior)
> Malignant neoplasm of orbital bone
> EXCLUDES 2   carcinoma, any type except intraosseous or odontogenic of:
> maxillary sinus (C31.0)
> upper jaw (C03.0)
> malignant neoplasm of jaw bone (lower) (C41.1)

C41.1 Malignant neoplasm of mandible   HCC

> Malignant neoplasm of inferior maxilla
> Malignant neoplasm of lower jaw bone
> EXCLUDES 2   carcinoma, any type except intraosseous or odontogenic of:
> jaw NOS (C03.9)
> lower (C03.1)
> malignant neoplasm of upper jaw bone (C41.0)

C41.2 Malignant neoplasm of vertebral column   HCC

> EXCLUDES 1   malignant neoplasm of sacrum and coccyx (C41.4)

C41.3 Malignant neoplasm of ribs, sternum and clavicle   HCC

C41.4 Malignant neoplasm of pelvic bones, sacrum and coccyx   HCC

C41.9 Malignant neoplasm of bone and articular cartilage, unspecified   HCC

Melanoma and other malignant neoplasms of skin (C43-C44)

✓4ᵗʰ **C43 Malignant melanoma of skin**

> EXCLUDES 1   melanoma in situ (D03.-)
> EXCLUDES 2   malignant melanoma of skin of genital organs (C51-C52, C60.-, C63.-)
> Merkel cell carcinoma (C4A.-)
> sites other than skin - code to malignant neoplasm of the site

C43.0 Malignant melanoma of lip   HCC

> EXCLUDES 1   malignant neoplasm of vermilion border of lip (C00.0-C00.2)

✓5ᵗʰ **C43.1 Malignant melanoma of eyelid, including canthus**

> AHA: 2018,4Q,4

C43.10 Malignant melanoma of unspecified eyelid, including canthus   HCC

✓6ᵗʰ **C43.11 Malignant melanoma of right eyelid, including canthus**

> **C43.111 Malignant melanoma of right upper eyelid, including canthus**   HCC
> **C43.112 Malignant melanoma of right lower eyelid, including canthus**   HCC

✓6ᵗʰ **C43.12 Malignant melanoma of left eyelid, including canthus**

> **C43.121 Malignant melanoma of left upper eyelid, including canthus**   HCC
> **C43.122 Malignant melanoma of left lower eyelid, including canthus**   HCC

✓5ᵗʰ **C43.2 Malignant melanoma of ear and external auricular canal**

C43.20 Malignant melanoma of unspecified ear and external auricular canal   HCC

C43.21 Malignant melanoma of right ear and external auricular canal   HCC

C43.22 Malignant melanoma of left ear and external auricular canal   HCC

✓5ᵗʰ **C43.3 Malignant melanoma of other and unspecified parts of face**

C43.30 Malignant melanoma of unspecified part of face   HCC

C43.31 Malignant melanoma of nose   HCC

C43.39 Malignant melanoma of other parts of face   HCC

C43.4 Malignant melanoma of scalp and neck   HCC

✓5ᵗʰ **C43.5 Malignant melanoma of trunk**

> EXCLUDES 2   malignant neoplasm of anus NOS (C21.0)
> malignant neoplasm of scrotum (C63.2)

C43.51 Malignant melanoma of anal skin   HCC

> Malignant melanoma of anal margin
> Malignant melanoma of perianal skin

C43.52 Malignant melanoma of skin of breast   HCC

C43.59 Malignant melanoma of other part of trunk   HCC

✓5ᵗʰ **C43.6 Malignant melanoma of upper limb, including shoulder**

C43.60 Malignant melanoma of unspecified upper limb, including shoulder   HCC

C43.61 Malignant melanoma of right upper limb, including shoulder   HCC

C43.62 Malignant melanoma of left upper limb, including shoulder   HCC

✓5ᵗʰ **C43.7 Malignant melanoma of lower limb, including hip**

C43.70 Malignant melanoma of unspecified lower limb, including hip   HCC

C43.71 Malignant melanoma of right lower limb, including hip   HCC

C43.72 Malignant melanoma of left lower limb, including hip   HCC

C43.8 Malignant melanoma of overlapping sites of skin   HCC

C43.9 Malignant melanoma of skin, unspecified   HCC

> Malignant melanoma of unspecified site of skin
> Melanoma (malignant) NOS

✓4ᵗʰ **C4A Merkel cell carcinoma**

> **DEF:** Malignant cutaneous cancer predominantly found in elderly patients with sun exposure that usually presents as a flesh-colored or bluish-red lump typically seen on the neck, head, and face.

C4A.0 Merkel cell carcinoma of lip   HCC

> EXCLUDES 1   malignant neoplasm of vermilion border of lip (C00.0-C00.2)

✓5ᵗʰ **C4A.1 Merkel cell carcinoma of eyelid, including canthus**

> AHA: 2018,4Q,4

C4A.10 Merkel cell carcinoma of unspecified eyelid, including canthus   HCC

✓6ᵗʰ **C4A.11 Merkel cell carcinoma of right eyelid, including canthus**

> **C4A.111 Merkel cell carcinoma of right upper eyelid, including canthus**   HCC
> **C4A.112 Merkel cell carcinoma of right lower eyelid, including canthus**   HCC

✓6ᵗʰ **C4A.12 Merkel cell carcinoma of left eyelid, including canthus**

> **C4A.121 Merkel cell carcinoma of left upper eyelid, including canthus**   HCC
> **C4A.122 Merkel cell carcinoma of left lower eyelid, including canthus**   HCC

✓5ᵗʰ **C4A.2 Merkel cell carcinoma of ear and external auricular canal**

C4A.20 Merkel cell carcinoma of unspecified ear and external auricular canal   HCC

C4A.21 Merkel cell carcinoma of right ear and external auricular canal   HCC

C4A.22 Merkel cell carcinoma of left ear and external auricular canal   HCC

✓5ᵗʰ **C4A.3 Merkel cell carcinoma of other and unspecified parts of face**

C4A.30 Merkel cell carcinoma of unspecified part of face   HCC

C4A.31 Merkel cell carcinoma of nose   HCC

C4A.39 Merkel cell carcinoma of other parts of face   HCC

C4A.4 Merkel cell carcinoma of scalp and neck   HCC

✓5ᵗʰ **C4A.5 Merkel cell carcinoma of trunk**

> EXCLUDES 2   malignant neoplasm of anus NOS (C21.0)
> malignant neoplasm of scrotum (C63.2)

C4A.51 Merkel cell carcinoma of anal skin   HCC

> Merkel cell carcinoma of anal margin
> Merkel cell carcinoma of perianal skin

C4A.52 Merkel cell carcinoma of skin of breast   HCC

C4A.59 Merkel cell carcinoma of other part of trunk   HCC

N Newborn: 0   P Pediatric: 0-17   M Maternity: 9-64   A Adult: 15-124   MCC Major Complication/Comorbidity   CC Complication/Comorbidity   SW Severe Wound Dx

470   ICD-10-CM 2020

√5ᵗʰ **C4A.6 Merkel cell carcinoma of upper limb, including shoulder**

    C4A.60 Merkel cell carcinoma of unspecified upper limb, including shoulder HCC

    C4A.61 Merkel cell carcinoma of right upper limb, including shoulder HCC

    C4A.62 Merkel cell carcinoma of left upper limb, including shoulder HCC

√5ᵗʰ **C4A.7 Merkel cell carcinoma of lower limb, including hip**

    C4A.70 Merkel cell carcinoma of unspecified lower limb, including hip HCC

    C4A.71 Merkel cell carcinoma of right lower limb, including hip HCC

    C4A.72 Merkel cell carcinoma of left lower limb, including hip HCC

C4A.8 Merkel cell carcinoma of overlapping sites HCC

C4A.9 Merkel cell carcinoma, unspecified HCC

    Merkel cell carcinoma of unspecified site

    Merkel cell carcinoma NOS

√4ᵗʰ **C44 Other and unspecified malignant neoplasm of skin**

    INCLUDES malignant neoplasm of sebaceous glands

             malignant neoplasm of sweat glands

    EXCLUDES 1 *Kaposi's sarcoma of skin (C46.0)*

             malignant melanoma of skin (C43.-)

             malignant neoplasm of skin of genital organs (C51-C52, C60.-, C63.2)

             Merkel cell carcinoma (C4A.-)

    DEF: Basal cell carcinoma: Abnormal growth of skin cells that arises from the deepest layer of the epidermis and may present as an open sore, red patches, pink growth, or scar. Typically caused by sun exposure, it is one of the most common forms of skin cancer.

    DEF: Squamous cell carcinoma: Uncontrolled growth of abnormal skin cells that arises from the outer layers of the skin (epidermis) and may present as an open sore. It is characterized by a firm, red nodule, elevated growth with a central depression, or a flat sore with a scaly crust.

√5ᵗʰ **C44.0 Other and unspecified malignant neoplasm of skin of lip**

    EXCLUDES 1 *malignant neoplasm of lip (C00.-)*

    C44.00 Unspecified malignant neoplasm of skin of lip

    C44.01 Basal cell carcinoma of skin of lip

    C44.02 Squamous cell carcinoma of skin of lip

    C44.09 Other specified malignant neoplasm of skin of lip

√5ᵗʰ **C44.1 Other and unspecified malignant neoplasm of skin of eyelid, including canthus**

    EXCLUDES 1 *connective tissue of eyelid (C49.0)*

    AHA: 2018,4Q,4

    √6ᵗʰ **C44.10 Unspecified malignant neoplasm of skin of eyelid, including canthus**

        C44.101 Unspecified malignant neoplasm of skin of unspecified eyelid, including canthus

        √7ᵗʰ **C44.102 Unspecified malignant neoplasm of skin of right eyelid, including canthus**

            C44.1021 Unspecified malignant neoplasm of skin of right upper eyelid, including canthus

            C44.1022 Unspecified malignant neoplasm of skin of right lower eyelid, including canthus

        √7ᵗʰ **C44.109 Unspecified malignant neoplasm of skin of left eyelid, including canthus**

            C44.1091 Unspecified malignant neoplasm of skin of left upper eyelid, including canthus

            C44.1092 Unspecified malignant neoplasm of skin of left lower eyelid, including canthus

    √6ᵗʰ **C44.11 Basal cell carcinoma of skin of eyelid, including canthus**

        C44.111 Basal cell carcinoma of skin of unspecified eyelid, including canthus

        √7ᵗʰ **C44.112 Basal cell carcinoma of skin of right eyelid, including canthus**

            C44.1121 Basal cell carcinoma of skin of right upper eyelid, including canthus

            C44.1122 Basal cell carcinoma of skin of right lower eyelid, including canthus

        √7ᵗʰ **C44.119 Basal cell carcinoma of skin of left eyelid, including canthus**

            C44.1191 Basal cell carcinoma of skin of left upper eyelid, including canthus

            C44.1192 Basal cell carcinoma of skin of left lower eyelid, including canthus

    √6ᵗʰ **C44.12 Squamous cell carcinoma of skin of eyelid, including canthus**

        C44.121 Squamous cell carcinoma of skin of unspecified eyelid, including canthus

        √7ᵗʰ **C44.122 Squamous cell carcinoma of skin of right eyelid, including canthus**

            C44.1221 Squamous cell carcinoma of skin of right upper eyelid, including canthus

            C44.1222 Squamous cell carcinoma of skin of right lower eyelid, including canthus

        √7ᵗʰ **C44.129 Squamous cell carcinoma of skin of left eyelid, including canthus**

            C44.1291 Squamous cell carcinoma of skin of left upper eyelid, including canthus

            C44.1292 Squamous cell carcinoma of skin of left lower eyelid, including canthus

    √6ᵗʰ **C44.13 Sebaceous cell carcinoma of skin of eyelid, including canthus**

        C44.131 Sebaceous cell carcinoma of skin of unspecified eyelid, including canthus

        √7ᵗʰ **C44.132 Sebaceous cell carcinoma of skin of right eyelid, including canthus**

            C44.1321 Sebaceous cell carcinoma of skin of right upper eyelid, including canthus

            C44.1322 Sebaceous cell carcinoma of skin of right lower eyelid, including canthus

        √7ᵗʰ **C44.139 Sebaceous cell carcinoma of skin of left eyelid, including canthus**

            C44.1391 Sebaceous cell carcinoma of skin of left upper eyelid, including canthus

            C44.1392 Sebaceous cell carcinoma of skin of left lower eyelid, including canthus

    √6ᵗʰ **C44.19 Other specified malignant neoplasm of skin of eyelid, including canthus**

        C44.191 Other specified malignant neoplasm of skin of unspecified eyelid, including canthus

        √7ᵗʰ **C44.192 Other specified malignant neoplasm of skin of right eyelid, including canthus**

            C44.1921 Other specified malignant neoplasm of skin of right upper eyelid, including canthus

            C44.1922 Other specified malignant neoplasm of skin of right lower eyelid, including canthus

        √7ᵗʰ **C44.199 Other specified malignant neoplasm of skin of left eyelid, including canthus**

            C44.1991 Other specified malignant neoplasm of skin of left upper eyelid, including canthus

            C44.1992 Other specified malignant neoplasm of skin of left lower eyelid, including canthus

√5ᵗʰ **C44.2 Other and unspecified malignant neoplasm of skin of ear and external auricular canal**

    EXCLUDES 1 *connective tissue of ear (C49.0)*

    √6ᵗʰ **C44.20 Unspecified malignant neoplasm of skin of ear and external auricular canal**

        C44.201 Unspecified malignant neoplasm of skin of unspecified ear and external auricular canal

        C44.202 Unspecified malignant neoplasm of skin of right ear and external auricular canal

        C44.209 Unspecified malignant neoplasm of skin of left ear and external auricular canal

    √6ᵗʰ **C44.21 Basal cell carcinoma of skin of ear and external auricular canal**

        C44.211 Basal cell carcinoma of skin of unspecified ear and external auricular canal

☑ Additional Character Required   √x7ᵗʰ Placeholder   Unacceptable PDx   Questionable PDx   Manifestation   Unspecified Dx   H1-H14 HAC   HCC CMS-HCC Dx   HIV HIV Dx

ICD-10-CM 2020   471

Chapter 2. Neoplasms

        C44.212   Basal cell carcinoma of skin of right ear and external auricular canal

        C44.219   Basal cell carcinoma of skin of left ear and external auricular canal

   ✓6ᵗʰ   **C44.22**   Squamous cell carcinoma of skin of ear and external auricular canal

        C44.221   Squamous cell carcinoma of skin of unspecified ear and external auricular canal

        C44.222   Squamous cell carcinoma of skin of right ear and external auricular canal

        C44.229   Squamous cell carcinoma of skin of left ear and external auricular canal

   ✓6ᵗʰ   **C44.29**   Other specified malignant neoplasm of skin of ear and external auricular canal

        C44.291   Other specified malignant neoplasm of skin of unspecified ear and external auricular canal

        C44.292   Other specified malignant neoplasm of skin of right ear and external auricular canal

        C44.299   Other specified malignant neoplasm of skin of left ear and external auricular canal

  ✓5ᵗʰ   **C44.3**   Other and unspecified malignant neoplasm of skin of other and unspecified parts of face

   ✓6ᵗʰ   **C44.30**   Unspecified malignant neoplasm of skin of other and unspecified parts of face

        C44.300   Unspecified malignant neoplasm of skin of unspecified part of face

        C44.301   Unspecified malignant neoplasm of skin of nose

        C44.309   Unspecified malignant neoplasm of skin of other parts of face

   ✓6ᵗʰ   **C44.31**   Basal cell carcinoma of skin of other and unspecified parts of face

        C44.310   Basal cell carcinoma of skin of unspecified parts of face

        C44.311   Basal cell carcinoma of skin of nose

        C44.319   Basal cell carcinoma of skin of other parts of face

   ✓6ᵗʰ   **C44.32**   Squamous cell carcinoma of skin of other and unspecified parts of face

        C44.320   Squamous cell carcinoma of skin of unspecified parts of face

        C44.321   Squamous cell carcinoma of skin of nose

        C44.329   Squamous cell carcinoma of skin of other parts of face

   ✓6ᵗʰ   **C44.39**   Other specified malignant neoplasm of skin of other and unspecified parts of face

        C44.390   Other specified malignant neoplasm of skin of unspecified parts of face

        C44.391   Other specified malignant neoplasm of skin of nose

        C44.399   Other specified malignant neoplasm of skin of other parts of face

  ✓5ᵗʰ   **C44.4**   Other and unspecified malignant neoplasm of skin of scalp and neck

     C44.40   Unspecified malignant neoplasm of skin of scalp and neck

     C44.41   Basal cell carcinoma of skin of scalp and neck

     C44.42   Squamous cell carcinoma of skin of scalp and neck

     C44.49   Other specified malignant neoplasm of skin of scalp and neck

  ✓5ᵗʰ   **C44.5**   Other and unspecified malignant neoplasm of skin of trunk

     EXCLUDES 1   *anus NOS (C21.0)*

                scrotum (C63.2)

   ✓6ᵗʰ   **C44.50**   Unspecified malignant neoplasm of skin of trunk

        C44.500   Unspecified malignant neoplasm of anal skin

            Unspecified malignant neoplasm of anal margin

            Unspecified malignant neoplasm of perianal skin

        C44.501   Unspecified malignant neoplasm of skin of breast

        C44.509   Unspecified malignant neoplasm of skin of other part of trunk

   ✓6ᵗʰ   **C44.51**   Basal cell carcinoma of skin of trunk

        C44.510   Basal cell carcinoma of anal skin

            Basal cell carcinoma of anal margin

            Basal cell carcinoma of perianal skin

        C44.511   Basal cell carcinoma of skin of breast

        C44.519   Basal cell carcinoma of skin of other part of trunk

   ✓6ᵗʰ   **C44.52**   Squamous cell carcinoma of skin of trunk

        C44.520   Squamous cell carcinoma of anal skin

            Squamous cell carcinoma of anal margin

            Squamous cell carcinoma of perianal skin

        C44.521   Squamous cell carcinoma of skin of breast

        C44.529   Squamous cell carcinoma of skin of other part of trunk

   ✓6ᵗʰ   **C44.59**   Other specified malignant neoplasm of skin of trunk

        C44.590   Other specified malignant neoplasm of anal skin

            Other specified malignant neoplasm of anal margin

            Other specified malignant neoplasm of perianal skin

        C44.591   Other specified malignant neoplasm of skin of breast

        C44.599   Other specified malignant neoplasm of skin of other part of trunk

  ✓5ᵗʰ   **C44.6**   Other and unspecified malignant neoplasm of skin of upper limb, including shoulder

   ✓6ᵗʰ   **C44.60**   Unspecified malignant neoplasm of skin of upper limb, including shoulder

        C44.601   Unspecified malignant neoplasm of skin of unspecified upper limb, including shoulder

        C44.602   Unspecified malignant neoplasm of skin of right upper limb, including shoulder

        C44.609   Unspecified malignant neoplasm of skin of left upper limb, including shoulder

   ✓6ᵗʰ   **C44.61**   Basal cell carcinoma of skin of upper limb, including shoulder

        C44.611   Basal cell carcinoma of skin of unspecified upper limb, including shoulder

        C44.612   Basal cell carcinoma of skin of right upper limb, including shoulder

        C44.619   Basal cell carcinoma of skin of left upper limb, including shoulder

   ✓6ᵗʰ   **C44.62**   Squamous cell carcinoma of skin of upper limb, including shoulder

        C44.621   Squamous cell carcinoma of skin of unspecified upper limb, including shoulder

        C44.622   Squamous cell carcinoma of skin of right upper limb, including shoulder

        C44.629   Squamous cell carcinoma of skin of left upper limb, including shoulder

   ✓6ᵗʰ   **C44.69**   Other specified malignant neoplasm of skin of upper limb, including shoulder

        C44.691   Other specified malignant neoplasm of skin of unspecified upper limb, including shoulder

        C44.692   Other specified malignant neoplasm of skin of right upper limb, including shoulder

        C44.699   Other specified malignant neoplasm of skin of left upper limb, including shoulder

  ✓5ᵗʰ   **C44.7**   Other and unspecified malignant neoplasm of skin of lower limb, including hip

   ✓6ᵗʰ   **C44.70**   Unspecified malignant neoplasm of skin of lower limb, including hip

        C44.701   Unspecified malignant neoplasm of skin of unspecified lower limb, including hip

        C44.702   Unspecified malignant neoplasm of skin of right lower limb, including hip

        C44.709   Unspecified malignant neoplasm of skin of left lower limb, including hip

   ✓6ᵗʰ   **C44.71**   Basal cell carcinoma of skin of lower limb, including hip

        C44.711   Basal cell carcinoma of skin of unspecified lower limb, including hip

        C44.712   Basal cell carcinoma of skin of right lower limb, including hip

        C44.719   Basal cell carcinoma of skin of left lower limb, including hip

N Newborn: 0   P Pediatric: 0-17   M Maternity: 9-64   A Adult: 15-124   MCC Major Complication/Comorbidity   CC Complication/Comorbidity   SW Severe Wound Dx

472   ICD-10-CM 2020

✓6ᵗʰ **C44.72** Squamous cell carcinoma of skin of lower limb, including hip

  C44.721 Squamous cell carcinoma of skin of unspecified lower limb, including hip

  C44.722 Squamous cell carcinoma of skin of right lower limb, including hip

  C44.729 Squamous cell carcinoma of skin of left lower limb, including hip

✓6ᵗʰ **C44.79** Other specified malignant neoplasm of skin of lower limb, including hip

  C44.791 Other specified malignant neoplasm of skin of unspecified lower limb, including hip

  C44.792 Other specified malignant neoplasm of skin of right lower limb, including hip

  C44.799 Other specified malignant neoplasm of skin of left lower limb, including hip

✓5ᵗʰ **C44.8** Other and unspecified malignant neoplasm of overlapping sites of skin

  C44.80 Unspecified malignant neoplasm of overlapping sites of skin

  C44.81 Basal cell carcinoma of overlapping sites of skin

  C44.82 Squamous cell carcinoma of overlapping sites of skin

  C44.89 Other specified malignant neoplasm of overlapping sites of skin

✓5ᵗʰ **C44.9** Other and unspecified malignant neoplasm of skin, unspecified

  C44.90 Unspecified malignant neoplasm of skin, unspecified

    Malignant neoplasm of unspecified site of skin

  C44.91 Basal cell carcinoma of skin, unspecified

  C44.92 Squamous cell carcinoma of skin, unspecified

  C44.99 Other specified malignant neoplasm of skin, unspecified

Malignant neoplasms of mesothelial and soft tissue (C45-C49)

✓4ᵗʰ **C45** **Mesothelioma**

  DEF: Rare type of cancer that forms in the thin layer of protective tissue that covers the majority of internal organs (mesothelium).

  C45.0 Mesothelioma of pleura   HCC

    EXCLUDES 1   *other malignant neoplasm of pleura (C38.4)*

    AHA: 2017,2Q,11

    TIP: For pleural mesothelioma that has metastasized to the chest wall, assign this code for the primary site along with C79.89 for metastatic cancer in the chest wall.

  C45.1 Mesothelioma of peritoneum   HCC

    Mesothelioma of cul-de-sac

    Mesothelioma of mesentery

    Mesothelioma of mesocolon

    Mesothelioma of omentum

    Mesothelioma of peritoneum (parietal) (pelvic)

    EXCLUDES 1   *other malignant neoplasm of soft tissue of peritoneum (C48.-)*

  C45.2 Mesothelioma of pericardium   HCC

    EXCLUDES 1   *other malignant neoplasm of pericardium (C38.0)*

  C45.7 Mesothelioma of other sites   HCC

  C45.9 Mesothelioma, unspecified   HCC

✓4ᵗʰ **C46** **Kaposi's sarcoma**

  Code first any human immunodeficiency virus [HIV] disease (B20)

  DEF: Malignant neoplasm that causes patches of abnormal tissue to grow under the skin, in the lining of the mouth, nose, and throat, in lymph nodes, or in other visceral organs. Kaposi's sarcoma is caused by human herpesvirus8 (HHV8).

  C46.0 Kaposi's sarcoma of skin   HIV HCC

  C46.1 Kaposi's sarcoma of soft tissue   HIV HCC

    Kaposi's sarcoma of blood vessel

    Kaposi's sarcoma of connective tissue

    Kaposi's sarcoma of fascia

    Kaposi's sarcoma of ligament

    Kaposi's sarcoma of lymphatic(s) NEC

    Kaposi's sarcoma of muscle

    EXCLUDES 2   *Kaposi's sarcoma of lymph glands and nodes (C46.3)*

  C46.2 Kaposi's sarcoma of palate   HIV HCC

  C46.3 Kaposi's sarcoma of lymph nodes   HIV HCC

  C46.4 Kaposi's sarcoma of gastrointestinal sites   HIV HCC

✓5ᵗʰ **C46.5** Kaposi's sarcoma of lung

  AHA: 2019,1Q,16

  TIP: When associated malignant pericardial effusion is documented, assign code I31.3. If the sole reason for admission is to treat the effusion with no treatment of the lung malignancy rendered, code I31.3 may be sequenced first.

  C46.50 Kaposi's sarcoma of unspecified lung   HIV HCC

  C46.51 Kaposi's sarcoma of right lung   HIV HCC

  C46.52 Kaposi's sarcoma of left lung   HIV HCC

  C46.7 Kaposi's sarcoma of other sites   HIV HCC

  C46.9 Kaposi's sarcoma, unspecified   HIV HCC

    Kaposi's sarcoma of unspecified site

✓4ᵗʰ **C47** **Malignant neoplasm of peripheral nerves and autonomic nervous system**

  INCLUDES   malignant neoplasm of sympathetic and parasympathetic nerves and ganglia

  EXCLUDES 1   *Kaposi's sarcoma of soft tissue (C46.1)*

  C47.0 Malignant neoplasm of peripheral nerves of head, face and neck   HCC

    EXCLUDES 1   *malignant neoplasm of peripheral nerves of orbit (C69.6-)*

✓5ᵗʰ **C47.1** Malignant neoplasm of peripheral nerves of upper limb, including shoulder

  C47.10 Malignant neoplasm of peripheral nerves of unspecified upper limb, including shoulder   HCC

  C47.11 Malignant neoplasm of peripheral nerves of right upper limb, including shoulder   HCC

  C47.12 Malignant neoplasm of peripheral nerves of left upper limb, including shoulder   HCC

✓5ᵗʰ **C47.2** Malignant neoplasm of peripheral nerves of lower limb, including hip

  C47.20 Malignant neoplasm of peripheral nerves of unspecified lower limb, including hip   HCC

  C47.21 Malignant neoplasm of peripheral nerves of right lower limb, including hip   HCC

  C47.22 Malignant neoplasm of peripheral nerves of left lower limb, including hip   HCC

  C47.3 Malignant neoplasm of peripheral nerves of thorax   HCC

  C47.4 Malignant neoplasm of peripheral nerves of abdomen   HCC

  C47.5 Malignant neoplasm of peripheral nerves of pelvis   HCC

  C47.6 Malignant neoplasm of peripheral nerves of trunk, unspecified   HCC

    Malignant neoplasm of peripheral nerves of unspecified part of trunk

  C47.8 Malignant neoplasm of overlapping sites of peripheral nerves and autonomic nervous system   HCC

  C47.9 Malignant neoplasm of peripheral nerves and autonomic nervous system, unspecified   HCC

    Malignant neoplasm of unspecified site of peripheral nerves and autonomic nervous system

✓4ᵗʰ **C48** **Malignant neoplasm of retroperitoneum and peritoneum**

  EXCLUDES 1   *Kaposi's sarcoma of connective tissue (C46.1)*
        mesothelioma (C45.-)

  C48.0 Malignant neoplasm of retroperitoneum   HCC

  C48.1 Malignant neoplasm of specified parts of peritoneum   HCC

    Malignant neoplasm of cul-de-sac

    Malignant neoplasm of mesentery

    Malignant neoplasm of mesocolon

    Malignant neoplasm of omentum

    Malignant neoplasm of parietal peritoneum

    Malignant neoplasm of pelvic peritoneum

  C48.2 Malignant neoplasm of peritoneum, unspecified   HCC

  C48.8 Malignant neoplasm of overlapping sites of retroperitoneum and peritoneum   HCC

✅ Additional Character Required   ✓x7ᵗʰ Placeholder   Unacceptable PDx   Questionable PDx   Manifestation   Unspecified Dx   H1-H14 HAC   HCC CMS-HCC Dx   HIV HIV Dx

Chapter 2. Neoplasms

✓4ᵗʰ **C49 Malignant neoplasm of other connective and soft tissue**

INCLUDES   malignant neoplasm of blood vessel
malignant neoplasm of bursa
malignant neoplasm of cartilage
malignant neoplasm of fascia
malignant neoplasm of fat
malignant neoplasm of ligament, except uterine
malignant neoplasm of lymphatic vessel
malignant neoplasm of muscle
malignant neoplasm of synovia
malignant neoplasm of tendon (sheath)

EXCLUDES 1   *malignant neoplasm of cartilage (of):*
articular (C40-C41)
larynx (C32.3)
nose (C30.0)
malignant neoplasm of connective tissue of breast (C50.-)

EXCLUDES 2   *Kaposi's sarcoma of soft tissue (C46.1)*
malignant neoplasm of heart (C38.0)
malignant neoplasm of peripheral nerves and autonomic nervous system (C47.-)
malignant neoplasm of peritoneum (C48.2)
malignant neoplasm of retroperitoneum (C48.0)
malignant neoplasm of uterine ligament (C57.3)
mesothelioma (C45.-)

C49.0 Malignant neoplasm of connective and soft tissue of head, face and neck   HCC
Malignant neoplasm of connective tissue of ear
Malignant neoplasm of connective tissue of eyelid
EXCLUDES 1   *connective tissue of orbit (C69.6-)*

✓5ᵗʰ **C49.1 Malignant neoplasm of connective and soft tissue of upper limb, including shoulder**
C49.10 Malignant neoplasm of connective and soft tissue of unspecified upper limb, including shoulder   HCC
C49.11 Malignant neoplasm of connective and soft tissue of right upper limb, including shoulder   HCC
C49.12 Malignant neoplasm of connective and soft tissue of left upper limb, including shoulder   HCC

✓5ᵗʰ **C49.2 Malignant neoplasm of connective and soft tissue of lower limb, including hip**
C49.20 Malignant neoplasm of connective and soft tissue of unspecified lower limb, including hip   HCC
C49.21 Malignant neoplasm of connective and soft tissue of right lower limb, including hip   HCC
C49.22 Malignant neoplasm of connective and soft tissue of left lower limb, including hip   HCC

C49.3 Malignant neoplasm of connective and soft tissue of thorax   HCC
Malignant neoplasm of axilla
Malignant neoplasm of diaphragm
Malignant neoplasm of great vessels
EXCLUDES 1   *malignant neoplasm of breast (C50.-)*
malignant neoplasm of heart (C38.0)
malignant neoplasm of mediastinum (C38.1-C38.3)
malignant neoplasm of thymus (C37)
AHA: 2015,3Q,19

C49.4 Malignant neoplasm of connective and soft tissue of abdomen   HCC
Malignant neoplasm of abdominal wall
Malignant neoplasm of hypochondrium

C49.5 Malignant neoplasm of connective and soft tissue of pelvis   HCC
Malignant neoplasm of buttock
Malignant neoplasm of groin
Malignant neoplasm of perineum

C49.6 Malignant neoplasm of connective and soft tissue of trunk, unspecified   HCC
Malignant neoplasm of back NOS

C49.8 Malignant neoplasm of overlapping sites of connective and soft tissue   HCC
Primary malignant neoplasm of two or more contiguous sites of connective and soft tissue

C49.9 Malignant neoplasm of connective and soft tissue, unspecified   HCC

✓5ᵗʰ **C49.A Gastrointestinal stromal tumor**
AHA: 2016,4Q,8
DEF: Uncommon malignant tumor found in the GI tract that originates from interstitial cells of the autonomic nervous system. Most occur in the stomach or small intestine but can originate anywhere in the GI tract.

C49.A0 Gastrointestinal stromal tumor, unspecified site   HCC
C49.A1 Gastrointestinal stromal tumor of esophagus   HCC
C49.A2 Gastrointestinal stromal tumor of stomach   HCC
C49.A3 Gastrointestinal stromal tumor of small intestine   HCC
C49.A4 Gastrointestinal stromal tumor of large intestine   HCC
C49.A5 Gastrointestinal stromal tumor of rectum   HCC
C49.A9 Gastrointestinal stromal tumor of other sites   HCC

Malignant neoplasms of breast (C50)

✓4ᵗʰ **C50 Malignant neoplasm of breast**
INCLUDES   connective tissue of breast
Paget's disease of breast
Paget's disease of nipple
Use additional code to identify estrogen receptor status (Z17.0, Z17.1)
EXCLUDES 1   *skin of breast (C44.501, C44.511, C44.521, C44.591)*
AHA: 2017,4Q,19

Female Breast

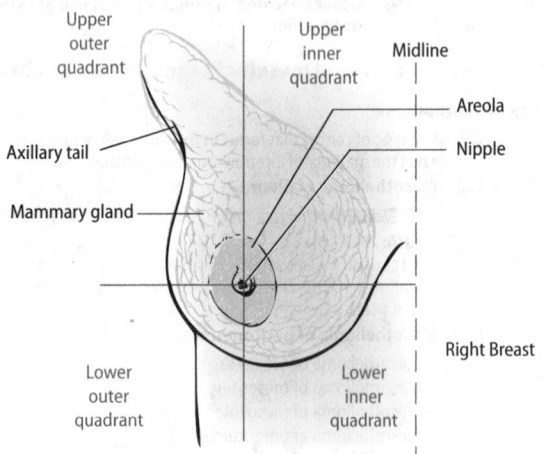

✓5ᵗʰ **C50.0 Malignant neoplasm of nipple and areola**
✓6ᵗʰ **C50.01 Malignant neoplasm of nipple and areola, female**
C50.011 Malignant neoplasm of nipple and areola, right female breast   HCC ♀
C50.012 Malignant neoplasm of nipple and areola, left female breast   HCC ♀
C50.019 Malignant neoplasm of nipple and areola, unspecified female breast   HCC ♀
✓6ᵗʰ **C50.02 Malignant neoplasm of nipple and areola, male**
C50.021 Malignant neoplasm of nipple and areola, right male breast   HCC ♂
C50.022 Malignant neoplasm of nipple and areola, left male breast   HCC ♂
C50.029 Malignant neoplasm of nipple and areola, unspecified male breast   HCC ♂

✓5ᵗʰ **C50.1 Malignant neoplasm of central portion of breast**
✓6ᵗʰ **C50.11 Malignant neoplasm of central portion of breast, female**
C50.111 Malignant neoplasm of central portion of right female breast   HCC ♀
C50.112 Malignant neoplasm of central portion of left female breast   HCC ♀

N Newborn: 0   P Pediatric: 0-17   M Maternity: 9-64   A Adult: 15-124   MCC Major Complication/Comorbidity   CC Complication/Comorbidity   SW Severe Wound Dx

	C50.119	Malignant neoplasm of central portion of unspecified female breast	HCC ♀

√6ᵗʰ **C50.12**   Malignant neoplasm of central portion of breast, male

	C50.121	Malignant neoplasm of central portion of right male breast	HCC ♂
	C50.122	Malignant neoplasm of central portion of left male breast	HCC ♂
	C50.129	Malignant neoplasm of central portion of unspecified male breast	HCC ♂

√5ᵗʰ **C50.2**   Malignant neoplasm of upper-inner quadrant of breast

√6ᵗʰ **C50.21**   Malignant neoplasm of upper-inner quadrant of breast, female

	C50.211	Malignant neoplasm of upper-inner quadrant of right female breast	HCC ♀
	C50.212	Malignant neoplasm of upper-inner quadrant of left female breast	HCC ♀
	C50.219	Malignant neoplasm of upper-inner quadrant of unspecified female breast	HCC ♀

√6ᵗʰ **C50.22**   Malignant neoplasm of upper-inner quadrant of breast, male

	C50.221	Malignant neoplasm of upper-inner quadrant of right male breast	HCC ♂
	C50.222	Malignant neoplasm of upper-inner quadrant of left male breast	HCC ♂
	C50.229	Malignant neoplasm of upper-inner quadrant of unspecified male breast	HCC ♂

√5ᵗʰ **C50.3**   Malignant neoplasm of lower-inner quadrant of breast

√6ᵗʰ **C50.31**   Malignant neoplasm of lower-inner quadrant of breast, female

	C50.311	Malignant neoplasm of lower-inner quadrant of right female breast	HCC ♀
	C50.312	Malignant neoplasm of lower-inner quadrant of left female breast	HCC ♀
	C50.319	Malignant neoplasm of lower-inner quadrant of unspecified female breast	HCC ♀

√6ᵗʰ **C50.32**   Malignant neoplasm of lower-inner quadrant of breast, male

	C50.321	Malignant neoplasm of lower-inner quadrant of right male breast	HCC ♂
	C50.322	Malignant neoplasm of lower-inner quadrant of left male breast	HCC ♂
	C50.329	Malignant neoplasm of lower-inner quadrant of unspecified male breast	HCC ♂

√5ᵗʰ **C50.4**   Malignant neoplasm of upper-outer quadrant of breast

√6ᵗʰ **C50.41**   Malignant neoplasm of upper-outer quadrant of breast, female

	C50.411	Malignant neoplasm of upper-outer quadrant of right female breast	HCC ♀
	C50.412	Malignant neoplasm of upper-outer quadrant of left female breast	HCC ♀
	C50.419	Malignant neoplasm of upper-outer quadrant of unspecified female breast	HCC ♀

√6ᵗʰ **C50.42**   Malignant neoplasm of upper-outer quadrant of breast, male

	C50.421	Malignant neoplasm of upper-outer quadrant of right male breast	HCC ♂
	C50.422	Malignant neoplasm of upper-outer quadrant of left male breast	HCC ♂
	C50.429	Malignant neoplasm of upper-outer quadrant of unspecified male breast	HCC ♂

√5ᵗʰ **C50.5**   Malignant neoplasm of lower-outer quadrant of breast

√6ᵗʰ **C50.51**   Malignant neoplasm of lower-outer quadrant of breast, female

	C50.511	Malignant neoplasm of lower-outer quadrant of right female breast	HCC ♀
	C50.512	Malignant neoplasm of lower-outer quadrant of left female breast	HCC ♀
	C50.519	Malignant neoplasm of lower-outer quadrant of unspecified female breast	HCC ♀

√6ᵗʰ **C50.52**   Malignant neoplasm of lower-outer quadrant of breast, male

	C50.521	Malignant neoplasm of lower-outer quadrant of right male breast	HCC ♂
	C50.522	Malignant neoplasm of lower-outer quadrant of left male breast	HCC ♂
	C50.529	Malignant neoplasm of lower-outer quadrant of unspecified male breast	HCC ♂

√5ᵗʰ **C50.6**   Malignant neoplasm of axillary tail of breast

√6ᵗʰ **C50.61**   Malignant neoplasm of axillary tail of breast, female

	C50.611	Malignant neoplasm of axillary tail of right female breast	HCC ♀
	C50.612	Malignant neoplasm of axillary tail of left female breast	HCC ♀
	C50.619	Malignant neoplasm of axillary tail of unspecified female breast	HCC ♀

√6ᵗʰ **C50.62**   Malignant neoplasm of axillary tail of breast, male

	C50.621	Malignant neoplasm of axillary tail of right male breast	HCC ♂
	C50.622	Malignant neoplasm of axillary tail of left male breast	HCC ♂
	C50.629	Malignant neoplasm of axillary tail of unspecified male breast	HCC ♂

√5ᵗʰ **C50.8**   Malignant neoplasm of overlapping sites of breast

√6ᵗʰ **C50.81**   Malignant neoplasm of overlapping sites of breast, female

	C50.811	Malignant neoplasm of overlapping sites of right female breast	HCC ♀
	C50.812	Malignant neoplasm of overlapping sites of left female breast	HCC ♀
	C50.819	Malignant neoplasm of overlapping sites of unspecified female breast	HCC ♀

√6ᵗʰ **C50.82**   Malignant neoplasm of overlapping sites of breast, male

	C50.821	Malignant neoplasm of overlapping sites of right male breast	HCC ♂
	C50.822	Malignant neoplasm of overlapping sites of left male breast	HCC ♂
	C50.829	Malignant neoplasm of overlapping sites of unspecified male breast	HCC ♂

√5ᵗʰ **C50.9**   Malignant neoplasm of breast of unspecified site

√6ᵗʰ **C50.91**   Malignant neoplasm of breast of unspecified site, female

	C50.911	Malignant neoplasm of unspecified site of right female breast	HCC ♀
	C50.912	Malignant neoplasm of unspecified site of left female breast	HCC ♀
	C50.919	Malignant neoplasm of unspecified site of unspecified female breast	HCC ♀

√6ᵗʰ **C50.92**   Malignant neoplasm of breast of unspecified site, male

	C50.921	Malignant neoplasm of unspecified site of right male breast	HCC ♂
	C50.922	Malignant neoplasm of unspecified site of left male breast	HCC ♂

✔ Additional Character Required   √x7ᵗʰ Placeholder   Unacceptable PDx   Questionable PDx   Manifestation   Unspecified Dx   H1-H14 HAC   HCC CMS-HCC Dx   HIV HIV Dx

ICD-10-CM 2020   475

Chapter 2. Neoplasms

C50.929   **Malignant neoplasm of**   HCC ♂
           unspecified site of unspecified
           male breast

Malignant neoplasms of female genital organs (C51-C58)

INCLUDES   malignant neoplasm of skin of female genital organs

√4ᵗʰ **C51 Malignant neoplasm of vulva**
        EXCLUDES 1   carcinoma in situ of vulva (D07.1)

      C51.0 Malignant neoplasm of labium majus   HCC ♀
             Malignant neoplasm of Bartholin's [greater vestibular] gland

      C51.1 Malignant neoplasm of labium minus   HCC ♀

      C51.2 Malignant neoplasm of clitoris   HCC ♀

      C51.8 Malignant neoplasm of overlapping sites of vulva   HCC ♀

      C51.9 Malignant neoplasm of vulva, unspecified   HCC ♀
             Malignant neoplasm of external female genitalia NOS
             Malignant neoplasm of pudendum

   C52 Malignant neoplasm of vagina   HCC ♀
        EXCLUDES 1   carcinoma in situ of vagina (D07.2)

√4ᵗʰ **C53 Malignant neoplasm of cervix uteri**
        EXCLUDES 1   carcinoma in situ of cervix uteri (D06.-)
        AHA: 2017,4Q,103

      C53.0 Malignant neoplasm of endocervix   HCC ♀

      C53.1 Malignant neoplasm of exocervix   HCC ♀

      C53.8 Malignant neoplasm of overlapping sites of cervix uteri   HCC ♀

      C53.9 Malignant neoplasm of cervix uteri, unspecified   HCC ♀

√4ᵗʰ **C54 Malignant neoplasm of corpus uteri**

      C54.0 Malignant neoplasm of isthmus uteri   HCC ♀
             Malignant neoplasm of lower uterine segment

      C54.1 Malignant neoplasm of endometrium   HCC ♀

      C54.2 Malignant neoplasm of myometrium   HCC ♀

      C54.3 Malignant neoplasm of fundus uteri   HCC ♀

      C54.8 Malignant neoplasm of overlapping sites of corpus uteri   HCC ♀

      C54.9 Malignant neoplasm of corpus uteri, unspecified   HCC ♀

   C55 Malignant neoplasm of uterus, part unspecified   HCC ♀

√4ᵗʰ **C56 Malignant neoplasm of ovary**
        Use additional code to identify any functional activity

      C56.1 Malignant neoplasm of right ovary   HCC ♀

      C56.2 Malignant neoplasm of left ovary   HCC ♀

      C56.9 Malignant neoplasm of unspecified ovary   HCC ♀

√4ᵗʰ **C57 Malignant neoplasm of other and unspecified female genital organs**

    √5ᵗʰ **C57.0 Malignant neoplasm of fallopian tube**
             Malignant neoplasm of oviduct
             Malignant neoplasm of uterine tube

          C57.00 Malignant neoplasm of unspecified fallopian tube   HCC ♀

          C57.01 Malignant neoplasm of right fallopian tube   HCC ♀

          C57.02 Malignant neoplasm of left fallopian tube   HCC ♀

    √5ᵗʰ **C57.1 Malignant neoplasm of broad ligament**

          C57.10 Malignant neoplasm of unspecified broad ligament   HCC ♀

          C57.11 Malignant neoplasm of right broad ligament   HCC ♀

          C57.12 Malignant neoplasm of left broad ligament   HCC ♀

    √5ᵗʰ **C57.2 Malignant neoplasm of round ligament**

          C57.20 Malignant neoplasm of unspecified round ligament   HCC ♀

          C57.21 Malignant neoplasm of right round ligament   HCC ♀

          C57.22 Malignant neoplasm of left round ligament   HCC ♀

      C57.3 Malignant neoplasm of parametrium   HCC ♀
             Malignant neoplasm of uterine ligament NOS

      C57.4 Malignant neoplasm of uterine adnexa, unspecified   HCC ♀

      C57.7 Malignant neoplasm of other specified female genital organs   HCC ♀
             Malignant neoplasm of wolffian body or duct

      C57.8 Malignant neoplasm of overlapping sites of female genital organs   HCC ♀
             Primary malignant neoplasm of two or more contiguous sites of the female genital organs whose point of origin cannot be determined
             Primary tubo-ovarian malignant neoplasm whose point of origin cannot be determined
             Primary utero-ovarian malignant neoplasm whose point of origin cannot be determined

      C57.9 Malignant neoplasm of female genital organ, unspecified   HCC ♀
             Malignant neoplasm of female genitourinary tract NOS

   C58 Malignant neoplasm of placenta   HCC M ♀
        INCLUDES   choriocarcinoma NOS
                    chorionepithelioma NOS
        EXCLUDES 1   chorioadenoma (destruens) (D39.2)
                     hydatidiform mole NOS (O01.9)
                     invasive hydatidiform mole (D39.2)
                     male choriocarcinoma NOS (C62.9-)
                     malignant hydatidiform mole (D39.2)

Malignant neoplasms of male genital organs (C60-C63)

INCLUDES   malignant neoplasm of skin of male genital organs

√4ᵗʰ **C60 Malignant neoplasm of penis**

      C60.0 Malignant neoplasm of prepuce   HCC ♂
             Malignant neoplasm of foreskin

      C60.1 Malignant neoplasm of glans penis   HCC ♂

      C60.2 Malignant neoplasm of body of penis   HCC ♂
             Malignant neoplasm of corpus cavernosum

      C60.8 Malignant neoplasm of overlapping sites of penis   HCC ♂

      C60.9 Malignant neoplasm of penis, unspecified   HCC ♂
             Malignant neoplasm of skin of penis NOS

   C61 Malignant neoplasm of prostate   HCC ♂
        Use additional code to identify:
          hormone sensitivity status (Z19.1-Z19.2)
          rising PSA following treatment for malignant neoplasm of prostate (R97.21)
        EXCLUDES 1   malignant neoplasm of seminal vesicle (C63.7)
        AHA: 2017,1Q,17

√4ᵗʰ **C62 Malignant neoplasm of testis**
        Use additional code to identify any functional activity

    √5ᵗʰ **C62.0 Malignant neoplasm of undescended testis**
             Malignant neoplasm of ectopic testis
             Malignant neoplasm of retained testis

          C62.00 Malignant neoplasm of unspecified undescended testis   HCC ♂

          C62.01 Malignant neoplasm of undescended right testis   HCC ♂

          C62.02 Malignant neoplasm of undescended left testis   HCC ♂

    √5ᵗʰ **C62.1 Malignant neoplasm of descended testis**
             Malignant neoplasm of scrotal testis

          C62.10 Malignant neoplasm of unspecified descended testis   HCC ♂

          C62.11 Malignant neoplasm of descended right testis   HCC ♂

          C62.12 Malignant neoplasm of descended left testis   HCC ♂

    √5ᵗʰ **C62.9 Malignant neoplasm of testis, unspecified whether descended or undescended**

          C62.90 Malignant neoplasm of unspecified testis, unspecified whether descended or undescended   HCC ♂
                 Malignant neoplasm of testis NOS

          C62.91 Malignant neoplasm of right testis, unspecified whether descended or undescended   HCC ♂

          C62.92 Malignant neoplasm of left testis, unspecified whether descended or undescended   HCC ♂

Chapter 2. Neoplasms (side tab)

✓4ᵗʰ **C63** **Malignant neoplasm of** other and unspecified male genital organs

  ✓5ᵗʰ **C63.0** **Malignant neoplasm of** epididymis

    C63.00 **Malignant neoplasm of unspecified epididymis**   HCC ♂

    C63.01 **Malignant neoplasm of** right **epididymis**   HCC ♂

    C63.02 **Malignant neoplasm of** left **epididymis**   HCC ♂

  ✓5ᵗʰ **C63.1** **Malignant neoplasm of** spermatic cord

    C63.10 **Malignant neoplasm of unspecified spermatic cord**   HCC ♂

    C63.11 **Malignant neoplasm of** right **spermatic cord**   HCC ♂

    C63.12 **Malignant neoplasm of** left **spermatic cord**   HCC ♂

  C63.2 **Malignant neoplasm of** scrotum   HCC ♂

    Malignant neoplasm of skin of scrotum

  C63.7 **Malignant neoplasm of other specified male genital organs**   HCC ♂

    Malignant neoplasm of seminal vesicle

    Malignant neoplasm of tunica vaginalis

  C63.8 **Malignant neoplasm of** overlapping sites **of male genital organs**   HCC ♂

    Primary malignant neoplasm of two or more contiguous sites of male genital organs whose point of origin cannot be determined

  C63.9 **Malignant neoplasm of male genital organ, unspecified**   HCC ♂

    Malignant neoplasm of male genitourinary tract NOS

Malignant neoplasms of urinary tract (C64-C68)

✓4ᵗʰ **C64** **Malignant neoplasm of** kidney, except renal pelvis

  EXCLUDES 1   malignant carcinoid tumor of the kidney (C7A.093)

    malignant neoplasm of renal calyces (C65.-)

    malignant neoplasm of renal pelvis (C65.-)

  C64.1 **Malignant neoplasm of** right **kidney, except renal pelvis**   HCC

  C64.2 **Malignant neoplasm of** left **kidney, except renal pelvis**   HCC

  C64.9 **Malignant neoplasm of unspecified kidney, except renal pelvis**   HCC

✓4ᵗʰ **C65** **Malignant neoplasm of** renal pelvis

  INCLUDES   malignant neoplasm of pelviureteric junction

    malignant neoplasm of renal calyces

  C65.1 **Malignant neoplasm of** right **renal pelvis**   HCC

  C65.2 **Malignant neoplasm of** left **renal pelvis**   HCC

  C65.9 **Malignant neoplasm of unspecified renal pelvis**   HCC

✓4ᵗʰ **C66** **Malignant neoplasm of** ureter

  EXCLUDES 1   malignant neoplasm of ureteric orifice of bladder (C67.6)

  C66.1 **Malignant neoplasm of** right **ureter**   HCC

  C66.2 **Malignant neoplasm of** left **ureter**   HCC

  C66.9 **Malignant neoplasm of unspecified ureter**   HCC

✓4ᵗʰ **C67** **Malignant neoplasm of** bladder

  C67.0 **Malignant neoplasm of** trigone **of bladder**   HCC

  C67.1 **Malignant neoplasm of** dome **of bladder**   HCC

  C67.2 **Malignant neoplasm of** lateral wall **of bladder**   HCC

  C67.3 **Malignant neoplasm of** anterior wall **of bladder**   HCC

  C67.4 **Malignant neoplasm of** posterior wall **of bladder**   HCC

  C67.5 **Malignant neoplasm of** bladder neck   HCC

    Malignant neoplasm of internal urethral orifice

  C67.6 **Malignant neoplasm of** ureteric orifice   HCC

  C67.7 **Malignant neoplasm of** urachus   HCC

  C67.8 **Malignant neoplasm of** overlapping sites **of bladder**   HCC

  C67.9 **Malignant neoplasm of bladder, unspecified**   HCC

    AHA: 2016,1Q,19

✓4ᵗʰ **C68** **Malignant neoplasm of other and unspecified** urinary organs

  EXCLUDES 1   malignant neoplasm of female genitourinary tract NOS (C57.9)

    malignant neoplasm of male genitourinary tract NOS (C63.9)

  AHA: 2016,1Q,14

  C68.0 **Malignant neoplasm of** urethra   HCC

    EXCLUDES 1   malignant neoplasm of urethral orifice of bladder (C67.5)

  C68.1 **Malignant neoplasm of** paraurethral glands   CC HCC

    CC Excl: PDX collection 312

  C68.8 **Malignant neoplasm of** overlapping sites of **urinary organs**   HCC

    Primary malignant neoplasm of two or more contiguous sites of urinary organs whose point of origin cannot be determined

  C68.9 **Malignant neoplasm of urinary organ, unspecified**   HCC

    Malignant neoplasm of urinary system NOS

Malignant neoplasms of eye, brain and other parts of central nervous system (C69-C72)

✓4ᵗʰ **C69** **Malignant neoplasm of** eye and adnexa

  EXCLUDES 1   malignant neoplasm of connective tissue of eyelid (C49.0)

    malignant neoplasm of eyelid (skin) (C43.1-, C44.1-)

    malignant neoplasm of optic nerve (C72.3-)

  ✓5ᵗʰ **C69.0** **Malignant neoplasm of** conjunctiva

    C69.00 **Malignant neoplasm of unspecified conjunctiva**   HCC

    C69.01 **Malignant neoplasm of** right **conjunctiva**   HCC

    C69.02 **Malignant neoplasm of** left **conjunctiva**   HCC

  ✓5ᵗʰ **C69.1** **Malignant neoplasm of** cornea

    C69.10 **Malignant neoplasm of unspecified cornea**   HCC

    C69.11 **Malignant neoplasm of** right **cornea**   HCC

    C69.12 **Malignant neoplasm of** left **cornea**   HCC

  ✓5ᵗʰ **C69.2** **Malignant neoplasm of** retina

    EXCLUDES 1   dark area on retina (D49.81)

     neoplasm of unspecified behavior of retina and choroid (D49.81)

     retinal freckle (D49.81)

    C69.20 **Malignant neoplasm of unspecified retina**   HCC

    C69.21 **Malignant neoplasm of** right **retina**   HCC

    C69.22 **Malignant neoplasm of** left **retina**   HCC

  ✓5ᵗʰ **C69.3** **Malignant neoplasm of** choroid

    C69.30 **Malignant neoplasm of unspecified choroid**   HCC

    C69.31 **Malignant neoplasm of** right **choroid**   HCC

    C69.32 **Malignant neoplasm of** left **choroid**   HCC

  ✓5ᵗʰ **C69.4** **Malignant neoplasm of** ciliary body

    C69.40 **Malignant neoplasm of unspecified ciliary body**   HCC

    C69.41 **Malignant neoplasm of** right **ciliary body**   HCC

    C69.42 **Malignant neoplasm of** left **ciliary body**   HCC

  ✓5ᵗʰ **C69.5** **Malignant neoplasm of** lacrimal gland and duct

    Malignant neoplasm of lacrimal sac

    Malignant neoplasm of nasolacrimal duct

    C69.50 **Malignant neoplasm of unspecified lacrimal gland and duct**   HCC

    C69.51 **Malignant neoplasm of** right **lacrimal gland and duct**   HCC

    C69.52 **Malignant neoplasm of** left **lacrimal gland and duct**   HCC

  ✓5ᵗʰ **C69.6** **Malignant neoplasm of** orbit

    Malignant neoplasm of connective tissue of orbit

    Malignant neoplasm of extraocular muscle

    Malignant neoplasm of peripheral nerves of orbit

    Malignant neoplasm of retrobulbar tissue

    Malignant neoplasm of retro-ocular tissue

    EXCLUDES 1   malignant neoplasm of orbital bone (C41.0)

    C69.60 **Malignant neoplasm of unspecified orbit**   HCC

    C69.61 **Malignant neoplasm of** right **orbit**   HCC

    C69.62 **Malignant neoplasm of** left **orbit**   HCC

☑ Additional Character Required   ✓x7ᵗʰ Placeholder   Unacceptable PDx   Questionable PDx   Manifestation   Unspecified Dx   H1-H14 HAC   HCC CMS-HCC Dx   HIV HIV Dx

ICD-10-CM 2020   477

C63–C69.62 (side tab)

Chapter 2. Neoplasms

✓5ᵗʰ **C69.8** **Malignant neoplasm of** overlapping sites **of eye and adnexa**

    C69.80 **Malignant neoplasm of overlapping sites of unspecified eye and adnexa** HCC

    C69.81 **Malignant neoplasm of overlapping sites of** right **eye and adnexa** HCC

    C69.82 **Malignant neoplasm of overlapping sites of** left **eye and adnexa** HCC

✓5ᵗʰ **C69.9** **Malignant neoplasm of unspecified site of eye**

    Malignant neoplasm of eyeball

    C69.90 **Malignant neoplasm of unspecified site of unspecified eye** HCC

    C69.91 **Malignant neoplasm of unspecified site of** right **eye** HCC

    C69.92 **Malignant neoplasm of unspecified site of** left **eye** HCC

✓4ᵗʰ **C70** **Malignant neoplasm of** meninges

    C70.0 **Malignant neoplasm of** cerebral **meninges** HCC

    C70.1 **Malignant neoplasm of** spinal **meninges** HCC

    C70.9 **Malignant neoplasm of meninges, unspecified** HCC

✓4ᵗʰ **C71** **Malignant neoplasm of** brain

    EXCLUDES 1 *malignant neoplasm of cranial nerves (C72.2-C72.5)*

               retrobulbar malignant neoplasm (C69.6-)

Lobes of the Brain

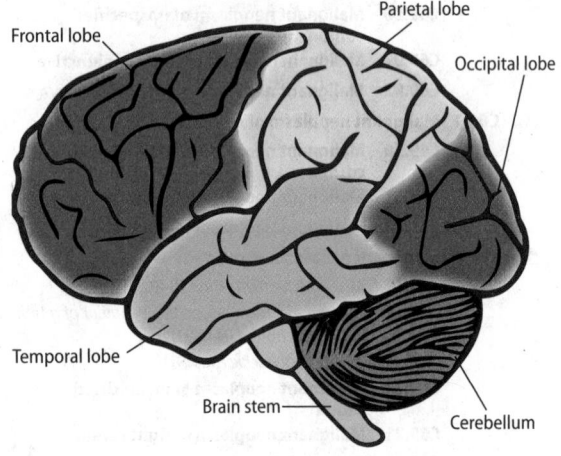

Frontal lobe — Parietal lobe — Occipital lobe — Temporal lobe — Brain stem — Cerebellum

    C71.0 **Malignant neoplasm of** cerebrum, except lobes **and ventricles** HCC

    Malignant neoplasm of supratentorial NOS

    C71.1 **Malignant neoplasm of** frontal **lobe** HCC

    C71.2 **Malignant neoplasm of** temporal **lobe** HCC

    C71.3 **Malignant neoplasm of** parietal **lobe** HCC

    C71.4 **Malignant neoplasm of** occipital **lobe** HCC

    C71.5 **Malignant neoplasm of** cerebral ventricle HCC

        EXCLUDES 1 *malignant neoplasm of fourth cerebral ventricle (C71.7)*

    C71.6 **Malignant neoplasm of** cerebellum HCC

    C71.7 **Malignant neoplasm of** brain stem HCC

    Malignant neoplasm of fourth cerebral ventricle

    Infratentorial malignant neoplasm NOS

    C71.8 **Malignant neoplasm of** overlapping sites **of brain** HCC

    C71.9 **Malignant neoplasm of brain, unspecified** HCC

        AHA: 2014,3Q,3

✓4ᵗʰ **C72** **Malignant neoplasm of** spinal cord, cranial nerves **and other parts of** central nervous system

    EXCLUDES 1 *malignant neoplasm of meninges (C70.-)*

               malignant neoplasm of peripheral nerves and autonomic nervous system (C47.-)

    C72.0 **Malignant neoplasm of** spinal cord HCC

    C72.1 **Malignant neoplasm of** cauda equina HCC

  ✓5ᵗʰ **C72.2** **Malignant neoplasm of** olfactory nerve

    Malignant neoplasm of olfactory bulb

    C72.20 **Malignant neoplasm of unspecified olfactory nerve** HCC

    C72.21 **Malignant neoplasm of** right **olfactory nerve** HCC

    C72.22 **Malignant neoplasm of** left **olfactory nerve** HCC

  ✓5ᵗʰ **C72.3** **Malignant neoplasm of** optic nerve

    C72.30 **Malignant neoplasm of unspecified optic nerve** HCC

    C72.31 **Malignant neoplasm of** right **optic nerve** HCC

    C72.32 **Malignant neoplasm of** left **optic nerve** HCC

  ✓5ᵗʰ **C72.4** **Malignant neoplasm of** acoustic nerve

    C72.40 **Malignant neoplasm of unspecified acoustic nerve** HCC

    C72.41 **Malignant neoplasm of** right **acoustic nerve** HCC

    C72.42 **Malignant neoplasm of** left **acoustic nerve** HCC

  ✓5ᵗʰ **C72.5** **Malignant neoplasm of other and unspecified** cranial nerves

    C72.50 **Malignant neoplasm of unspecified cranial nerve** HCC

    Malignant neoplasm of cranial nerve NOS

    C72.59 **Malignant neoplasm of other cranial nerves** HCC

    C72.9 **Malignant neoplasm of central nervous system, unspecified** HCC

    Malignant neoplasm of unspecified site of central nervous system

    Malignant neoplasm of nervous system NOS

Malignant neoplasms of thyroid and other endocrine glands (C73-C75)

C73 **Malignant neoplasm of** thyroid gland HCC

    Use additional code to identify any functional activity

✓4ᵗʰ **C74** **Malignant neoplasm of** adrenal gland

    TIP: If an adrenal gland tumor is described as functional (producing too much of a hormone), additional codes should be assigned to report the functional activity.

  ✓5ᵗʰ **C74.0** **Malignant neoplasm of** cortex of adrenal gland

    C74.00 **Malignant neoplasm of cortex of unspecified adrenal gland** HCC

    C74.01 **Malignant neoplasm of cortex of** right **adrenal gland** HCC

    C74.02 **Malignant neoplasm of cortex of** left **adrenal gland** HCC

  ✓5ᵗʰ **C74.1** **Malignant neoplasm of** medulla of adrenal gland

    C74.10 **Malignant neoplasm of medulla of unspecified adrenal gland** HCC

    C74.11 **Malignant neoplasm of medulla of** right **adrenal gland** HCC

    C74.12 **Malignant neoplasm of medulla of** left **adrenal gland** HCC

  ✓5ᵗʰ **C74.9** **Malignant neoplasm of unspecified part of adrenal gland**

    C74.90 **Malignant neoplasm of unspecified part of unspecified adrenal gland** HCC

    C74.91 **Malignant neoplasm of unspecified part of** right **adrenal gland** HCC

    C74.92 **Malignant neoplasm of unspecified part of** left **adrenal gland** HCC

✓4ᵗʰ **C75** **Malignant neoplasm of other endocrine glands and related structures**

    EXCLUDES 1 *malignant carcinoid tumors (C7A.0-)*

               malignant neoplasm of adrenal gland (C74.-)

               malignant neoplasm of endocrine pancreas (C25.4)

               malignant neoplasm of islets of Langerhans (C25.4)

               malignant neoplasm of ovary (C56.-)

               malignant neoplasm of testis (C62.-)

               malignant neoplasm of thymus (C37)

               malignant neoplasm of thyroid gland (C73)

               malignant neuroendocrine tumors (C7A.-)

    C75.0 **Malignant neoplasm of** parathyroid **gland** HCC

    C75.1 **Malignant neoplasm of** pituitary **gland** HCC

    C75.2 **Malignant neoplasm of** craniopharyngeal duct HCC

    C75.3 **Malignant neoplasm of** pineal **gland** HCC

    C75.4 **Malignant neoplasm of** carotid body HCC

    C75.5 **Malignant neoplasm of** aortic body **and other** paraganglia HCC

Ⓝ Newborn: 0   Ⓟ Pediatric: 0-17   Ⓜ Maternity: 9-64   Ⓐ Adult: 15-124   MCC Major Complication/Comorbidity   CC Complication/Comorbidity   SW Severe Wound Dx

478   ICD-10-CM 2020

C75.8 Malignant neoplasm with pluriglandular involvement, unspecified   HCC

C75.9 Malignant neoplasm of endocrine gland, unspecified   HCC

Malignant neuroendocrine tumors (C7A)

√4ᵗʰ **C7A Malignant neuroendocrine tumors**

Code also any associated multiple endocrine neoplasia [MEN] syndromes (E31.2-)

Use additional code to identify any associated endocrine syndrome, such as:

carcinoid syndrome (E34.0)

EXCLUDES 2   *malignant pancreatic islet cell tumors (C25.4)*
Merkel cell carcinoma (C4A.-)

DEF: Tumors comprised of cells that are capable of producing hormonal syndromes in which the normal hormonal balance required to support body system functions is adversely affected.

√5ᵗʰ **C7A.0 Malignant carcinoid tumors**

DEF: Specific type of slow-growing benign or malignant neuroendocrine tumors. Carcinoid tumors occur most commonly in the hormone producing cells of the gastrointestinal tracts and can also occur in the pancreas, testes, ovaries, or lungs.

C7A.00 Malignant carcinoid tumor of unspecified site   HCC

√6ᵗʰ **C7A.01** Malignant carcinoid tumors of the small intestine

     C7A.010 Malignant carcinoid tumor of the duodenum   HCC

     C7A.011 Malignant carcinoid tumor of the jejunum   HCC

     C7A.012 Malignant carcinoid tumor of the ileum   HCC

     C7A.019 Malignant carcinoid tumor of the small intestine, unspecified portion   HCC

√6ᵗʰ **C7A.02** Malignant carcinoid tumors of the appendix, large intestine, and rectum

     C7A.020 Malignant carcinoid tumor of the appendix   HCC

     C7A.021 Malignant carcinoid tumor of the cecum   HCC

     C7A.022 Malignant carcinoid tumor of the ascending colon   HCC

     C7A.023 Malignant carcinoid tumor of the transverse colon   HCC

     C7A.024 Malignant carcinoid tumor of the descending colon   HCC

     C7A.025 Malignant carcinoid tumor of the sigmoid colon   HCC

     C7A.026 Malignant carcinoid tumor of the rectum   HCC

     C7A.029 Malignant carcinoid tumor of the large intestine, unspecified portion   HCC

       Malignant carcinoid tumor of the colon NOS

√6ᵗʰ **C7A.09** Malignant carcinoid tumors of other sites

     C7A.090 Malignant carcinoid tumor of the bronchus and lung   HCC

       AHA: 2019,1Q,16

       TIP: When associated malignant pericardial effusion is documented, assign code I31.3. If the sole reason for admission is to treat the effusion with no treatment of the lung malignancy rendered, code I31.3 may be sequenced first.

     C7A.091 Malignant carcinoid tumor of the thymus   HCC

     C7A.092 Malignant carcinoid tumor of the stomach   HCC

     C7A.093 Malignant carcinoid tumor of the kidney   HCC

     C7A.094 Malignant carcinoid tumor of the foregut, unspecified   HCC

     C7A.095 Malignant carcinoid tumor of the midgut, unspecified   HCC

     C7A.096 Malignant carcinoid tumor of the hindgut, unspecified   HCC

     C7A.098 Malignant carcinoid tumors of other sites   HCC

C7A.1 Malignant poorly differentiated neuroendocrine tumors   HCC

     Malignant poorly differentiated neuroendocrine tumor NOS
     High grade neuroendocrine carcinoma, any site
     Malignant poorly differentiated neuroendocrine carcinoma, any site

C7A.8 Other malignant neuroendocrine tumors   HCC

Secondary neuroendocrine tumors (C7B)

√4ᵗʰ **C7B Secondary neuroendocrine tumors**

Use additional code to identify any functional activity

√5ᵗʰ **C7B.0 Secondary carcinoid tumors**

     C7B.00 Secondary carcinoid tumors, unspecified site   HCC

     C7B.01 Secondary carcinoid tumors of distant lymph nodes   HCC

     C7B.02 Secondary carcinoid tumors of liver   HCC

     C7B.03 Secondary carcinoid tumors of bone   HCC

     C7B.04 Secondary carcinoid tumors of peritoneum   HCC

       Mesentary metastasis of carcinoid tumor

     C7B.09 Secondary carcinoid tumors of other sites   HCC

C7B.1 Secondary Merkel cell carcinoma   HCC

     Merkel cell carcinoma nodal presentation
     Merkel cell carcinoma visceral metastatic presentation

C7B.8 Other secondary neuroendocrine tumors   HCC

Malignant neoplasms of ill-defined, other secondary and unspecified sites (C76-C80)

√4ᵗʰ **C76 Malignant neoplasm of other and ill-defined sites**

EXCLUDES 1   *malignant neoplasm of female genitourinary tract NOS (C57.9)*
malignant neoplasm of male genitourinary tract NOS (C63.9)
malignant neoplasm of lymphoid, hematopoietic and related tissue (C81-C96)
malignant neoplasm of skin (C44.-)
malignant neoplasm of unspecified site NOS (C80.1)

C76.0 Malignant neoplasm of head, face and neck   HCC

     Malignant neoplasm of cheek NOS
     Malignant neoplasm of nose NOS

C76.1 Malignant neoplasm of thorax   HCC

     Intrathoracic malignant neoplasm NOS
     Malignant neoplasm of axilla NOS
     Thoracic malignant neoplasm NOS

C76.2 Malignant neoplasm of abdomen   HCC

C76.3 Malignant neoplasm of pelvis   HCC

     Malignant neoplasm of groin NOS
     Malignant neoplasm of sites overlapping systems within the pelvis
     Rectovaginal (septum) malignant neoplasm
     Rectovesical (septum) malignant neoplasm

√5ᵗʰ **C76.4** Malignant neoplasm of upper limb

     C76.40 Malignant neoplasm of unspecified upper limb   HCC

     C76.41 Malignant neoplasm of right upper limb   HCC

     C76.42 Malignant neoplasm of left upper limb   HCC

√5ᵗʰ **C76.5** Malignant neoplasm of lower limb

     C76.50 Malignant neoplasm of unspecified lower limb   HCC

     C76.51 Malignant neoplasm of right lower limb   HCC

     C76.52 Malignant neoplasm of left lower limb   HCC

C76.8 Malignant neoplasm of other specified ill-defined sites   HCC

     Malignant neoplasm of overlapping ill-defined sites

☑ Additional Character Required   √x 7ᵗʰ Placeholder   Unacceptable PDx   Questionable PDx   Manifestation   Unspecified Dx   H1-H14 HAC   HCC CMS-HCC Dx   HIV HIV Dx

ICD-10-CM 2020   479

Chapter 2. Neoplasms

C77–C80.2

✓4ᵗʰ **C77 Secondary and unspecified malignant neoplasm of lymph nodes**

> *EXCLUDES 1*   malignant neoplasm of lymph nodes, specified as primary (C81-C86, C88, C96.-)
>
> mesentary metastasis of carcinoid tumor (C7B.04)
>
> secondary carcinoid tumors of distant lymph nodes (C7B.01)

C77.0 Secondary and unspecified malignant neoplasm of lymph nodes of head, face and neck   HCC

> Secondary and unspecified malignant neoplasm of supraclavicular lymph nodes

C77.1 Secondary and unspecified malignant neoplasm of intrathoracic lymph nodes   HCC

C77.2 Secondary and unspecified malignant neoplasm of intra-abdominal lymph nodes   HCC

C77.3 Secondary and unspecified malignant neoplasm of axilla and upper limb lymph nodes   HCC

> Secondary and unspecified malignant neoplasm of pectoral lymph nodes

C77.4 Secondary and unspecified malignant neoplasm of inguinal and lower limb lymph nodes   HCC

C77.5 Secondary and unspecified malignant neoplasm of intrapelvic lymph nodes

C77.8 Secondary and unspecified malignant neoplasm of lymph nodes of multiple regions   HCC

C77.9 Secondary and unspecified malignant neoplasm of lymph node, unspecified   HCC

✓4ᵗʰ **C78 Secondary malignant neoplasm of respiratory and digestive organs**

> *EXCLUDES 1*   secondary carcinoid tumors of liver (C7B.02)
>
> secondary carcinoid tumors of peritoneum (C7B.04)
>
> *EXCLUDES 2*   lymph node metastases (C77.0)

✓5ᵗʰ **C78.0 Secondary malignant neoplasm of lung**

> **AHA:** 2019,1Q,16

C78.00 Secondary malignant neoplasm of unspecified lung   HCC

C78.01 Secondary malignant neoplasm of right lung   HCC

C78.02 Secondary malignant neoplasm of left lung   HCC

C78.1 Secondary malignant neoplasm of mediastinum   HCC

C78.2 Secondary malignant neoplasm of pleura   HCC

✓5ᵗʰ **C78.3 Secondary malignant neoplasm of other and unspecified respiratory organs**

C78.30 Secondary malignant neoplasm of unspecified respiratory organ   HCC

C78.39 Secondary malignant neoplasm of other respiratory organs   HCC

C78.4 Secondary malignant neoplasm of small intestine   HCC

C78.5 Secondary malignant neoplasm of large intestine and rectum   HCC

C78.6 Secondary malignant neoplasm of retroperitoneum and peritoneum   HCC

> **AHA:** 2017,2Q,12

C78.7 Secondary malignant neoplasm of liver and intrahepatic bile duct   HCC

✓5ᵗʰ **C78.8 Secondary malignant neoplasm of other and unspecified digestive organs**

C78.80 Secondary malignant neoplasm of unspecified digestive organ   HCC

C78.89 Secondary malignant neoplasm of other digestive organs   HCC

> Code also exocrine pancreatic insufficiency (K86.81)

✓4ᵗʰ **C79 Secondary malignant neoplasm of other and unspecified sites**

> *EXCLUDES 1*   secondary carcinoid tumors (C7B.-)
>
> secondary neuroendocrine tumors (C7B.-)

✓5ᵗʰ **C79.0 Secondary malignant neoplasm of kidney and renal pelvis**

C79.00 Secondary malignant neoplasm of unspecified kidney and renal pelvis   HCC

C79.01 Secondary malignant neoplasm of right kidney and renal pelvis   HCC

C79.02 Secondary malignant neoplasm of left kidney and renal pelvis   HCC

✓5ᵗʰ **C79.1 Secondary malignant neoplasm of bladder and other and unspecified urinary organs**

C79.10 Secondary malignant neoplasm of unspecified urinary organs   HCC

C79.11 Secondary malignant neoplasm of bladder   HCC

> *EXCLUDES 2*   lymph node metastases (C77.0)

C79.19 Secondary malignant neoplasm of other urinary organs   HCC

C79.2 Secondary malignant neoplasm of skin   HCC

> *EXCLUDES 1*   secondary Merkel cell carcinoma (C7B.1)

✓5ᵗʰ **C79.3 Secondary malignant neoplasm of brain and cerebral meninges**

C79.31 Secondary malignant neoplasm of brain   HCC

C79.32 Secondary malignant neoplasm of cerebral meninges   HCC

✓5ᵗʰ **C79.4 Secondary malignant neoplasm of other and unspecified parts of nervous system**

C79.40 Secondary malignant neoplasm of unspecified part of nervous system   HCC

C79.49 Secondary malignant neoplasm of other parts of nervous system   HCC

✓5ᵗʰ **C79.5 Secondary malignant neoplasm of bone and bone marrow**

> *EXCLUDES 1*   secondary carcinoid tumors of bone (C7B.03)

C79.51 Secondary malignant neoplasm of bone   HCC

> **TIP:** Do not assign in addition to a code from subcategory C90.0 when multiple myeloma is described as metastatic to the bone; bone involvement is integral to multiple myeloma.

C79.52 Secondary malignant neoplasm of bone marrow   HCC

✓5ᵗʰ **C79.6 Secondary malignant neoplasm of ovary**

C79.60 Secondary malignant neoplasm of unspecified ovary   HCC ♀

C79.61 Secondary malignant neoplasm of right ovary   HCC ♀

C79.62 Secondary malignant neoplasm of left ovary   HCC ♀

✓5ᵗʰ **C79.7 Secondary malignant neoplasm of adrenal gland**

C79.70 Secondary malignant neoplasm of unspecified adrenal gland   HCC

C79.71 Secondary malignant neoplasm of right adrenal gland   HCC

C79.72 Secondary malignant neoplasm of left adrenal gland   HCC

✓5ᵗʰ **C79.8 Secondary malignant neoplasm of other specified sites**

C79.81 Secondary malignant neoplasm of breast   HCC

C79.82 Secondary malignant neoplasm of genital organs   HCC

C79.89 Secondary malignant neoplasm of other specified sites   HCC

> **AHA:** 2017,2Q,11

C79.9 Secondary malignant neoplasm of unspecified site   HCC

> Metastatic cancer NOS
>
> Metastatic disease NOS
>
> *EXCLUDES 1*   carcinomatosis NOS (C80.0)
>
> generalized cancer NOS (C80.0)
>
> malignant (primary) neoplasm of unspecified site (C80.1)

✓4ᵗʰ **C80 Malignant neoplasm without specification of site**

> *EXCLUDES 1*   malignant carcinoid tumor of unspecified site (C7A.00)
>
> malignant neoplasm of specified multiple sites — code to each site

C80.0 Disseminated malignant neoplasm, unspecified   HCC

> Carcinomatosis NOS
>
> Generalized cancer, unspecified site (primary) (secondary)
>
> Generalized malignancy, unspecified site (primary) (secondary)

C80.1 Malignant (primary) neoplasm, unspecified   HCC

> Cancer NOS
>
> Cancer unspecified site (primary)
>
> Carcinoma unspecified site (primary)
>
> Malignancy unspecified site (primary)
>
> *EXCLUDES 1*   secondary malignant neoplasm of unspecified site (C79.9)

C80.2 Malignant neoplasm associated with transplanted organ   HCC

> Code first complication of transplanted organ (T86.-)
>
> Use additional code to identify the specific malignancy

N Newborn: 0   **P** Pediatric: 0-17   **M** Maternity: 9-64   **A** Adult: 15-124   **MCC** Major Complication/Comorbidity   **CC** Complication/Comorbidity   **SW** Severe Wound Dx

480   ICD-10-CM 2020

Malignant neoplasms of lymphoid, hematopoietic and related tissue (C81-C96)

EXCLUDES 2   *Kaposi's sarcoma of lymph nodes (C46.3)*
secondary and unspecified neoplasm of lymph nodes (C77.-)
secondary neoplasm of bone marrow (C79.52)
secondary neoplasm of spleen (C78.89)

✓4th C81 Hodgkin lymphoma

EXCLUDES 1   *personal history of Hodgkin lymphoma (Z85.71)*

DEF: Malignant disorder of lymphoid cells characterized by the presence of progressively swollen lymph nodes and spleen that may also involve the liver. A diagnosis of Hodgkin's lymphoma can be confirmed by the presence of Reed-Sternberg cells. **Synonym(s):** *Hodgkin disease.*

✓5th C81.0 Nodular lymphocyte predominant Hodgkin lymphoma

C81.00	Nodular lymphocyte predominant Hodgkin lymphoma, unspecified site	HCC
C81.01	Nodular lymphocyte predominant Hodgkin lymphoma, lymph nodes of head, face, and neck	HCC
C81.02	Nodular lymphocyte predominant Hodgkin lymphoma, intrathoracic lymph nodes	HCC
C81.03	Nodular lymphocyte predominant Hodgkin lymphoma, intra-abdominal lymph nodes	HCC
C81.04	Nodular lymphocyte predominant Hodgkin lymphoma, lymph nodes of axilla and upper limb	HCC
C81.05	Nodular lymphocyte predominant Hodgkin lymphoma, lymph nodes of inguinal region and lower limb	HCC
C81.06	Nodular lymphocyte predominant Hodgkin lymphoma, intrapelvic lymph nodes	HCC
C81.07	Nodular lymphocyte predominant Hodgkin lymphoma, spleen	HCC
C81.08	Nodular lymphocyte predominant Hodgkin lymphoma, lymph nodes of multiple sites	HCC
C81.09	Nodular lymphocyte predominant Hodgkin lymphoma, extranodal and solid organ sites	HCC

✓5th C81.1 Nodular sclerosis Hodgkin lymphoma

Nodular sclerosis classical Hodgkin lymphoma

C81.10	Nodular sclerosis Hodgkin lymphoma, unspecified site	HCC
C81.11	Nodular sclerosis Hodgkin lymphoma, lymph nodes of head, face, and neck	HCC
C81.12	Nodular sclerosis Hodgkin lymphoma, intrathoracic lymph nodes	HCC
C81.13	Nodular sclerosis Hodgkin lymphoma, intra-abdominal lymph nodes	HCC
C81.14	Nodular sclerosis Hodgkin lymphoma, lymph nodes of axilla and upper limb	HCC
C81.15	Nodular sclerosis Hodgkin lymphoma, lymph nodes of inguinal region and lower limb	HCC
C81.16	Nodular sclerosis Hodgkin lymphoma, intrapelvic lymph nodes	HCC
C81.17	Nodular sclerosis Hodgkin lymphoma, spleen	HCC
C81.18	Nodular sclerosis Hodgkin lymphoma, lymph nodes of multiple sites	HCC
C81.19	Nodular sclerosis Hodgkin lymphoma, extranodal and solid organ sites	HCC

✓5th C81.2 Mixed cellularity Hodgkin lymphoma

Mixed cellularity classical Hodgkin lymphoma

C81.20	Mixed cellularity Hodgkin lymphoma, unspecified site	HCC
C81.21	Mixed cellularity Hodgkin lymphoma, lymph nodes of head, face, and neck	HCC
C81.22	Mixed cellularity Hodgkin lymphoma, intrathoracic lymph nodes	HCC
C81.23	Mixed cellularity Hodgkin lymphoma, intra-abdominal lymph nodes	HCC
C81.24	Mixed cellularity Hodgkin lymphoma, lymph nodes of axilla and upper limb	HCC
C81.25	Mixed cellularity Hodgkin lymphoma, lymph nodes of inguinal region and lower limb	HCC
C81.26	Mixed cellularity Hodgkin lymphoma, intrapelvic lymph nodes	HCC
C81.27	Mixed cellularity Hodgkin lymphoma, spleen	HCC
C81.28	Mixed cellularity Hodgkin lymphoma, lymph nodes of multiple sites	HCC
C81.29	Mixed cellularity Hodgkin lymphoma, extranodal and solid organ sites	HCC

✓5th C81.3 Lymphocyte depleted Hodgkin lymphoma

Lymphocyte depleted classical Hodgkin lymphoma

C81.30	Lymphocyte depleted Hodgkin lymphoma, unspecified site	HCC
C81.31	Lymphocyte depleted Hodgkin lymphoma, lymph nodes of head, face, and neck	HCC
C81.32	Lymphocyte depleted Hodgkin lymphoma, intrathoracic lymph nodes	HCC
C81.33	Lymphocyte depleted Hodgkin lymphoma, intra-abdominal lymph nodes	HCC
C81.34	Lymphocyte depleted Hodgkin lymphoma, lymph nodes of axilla and upper limb	HCC
C81.35	Lymphocyte depleted Hodgkin lymphoma, lymph nodes of inguinal region and lower limb	HCC
C81.36	Lymphocyte depleted Hodgkin lymphoma, intrapelvic lymph nodes	HCC
C81.37	Lymphocyte depleted Hodgkin lymphoma, spleen	HCC
C81.38	Lymphocyte depleted Hodgkin lymphoma, lymph nodes of multiple sites	HCC
C81.39	Lymphocyte depleted Hodgkin lymphoma, extranodal and solid organ sites	HCC

✓5th C81.4 Lymphocyte-rich Hodgkin lymphoma

Lymphocyte-rich classical Hodgkin lymphoma

EXCLUDES 1   *nodular lymphocyte predominant Hodgkin lymphoma (C81.0-)*

C81.40	Lymphocyte-rich Hodgkin lymphoma, unspecified site	HCC
C81.41	Lymphocyte-rich Hodgkin lymphoma, lymph nodes of head, face, and neck	HCC
C81.42	Lymphocyte-rich Hodgkin lymphoma, intrathoracic lymph nodes	HCC
C81.43	Lymphocyte-rich Hodgkin lymphoma, intra-abdominal lymph nodes	HCC
C81.44	Lymphocyte-rich Hodgkin lymphoma, lymph nodes of axilla and upper limb	HCC
C81.45	Lymphocyte-rich Hodgkin lymphoma, lymph nodes of inguinal region and lower limb	HCC
C81.46	Lymphocyte-rich Hodgkin lymphoma, intrapelvic lymph nodes	HCC
C81.47	Lymphocyte-rich Hodgkin lymphoma, spleen	HCC
C81.48	Lymphocyte-rich Hodgkin lymphoma, lymph nodes of multiple sites	HCC
C81.49	Lymphocyte-rich Hodgkin lymphoma, extranodal and solid organ sites	HCC

✓5th C81.7 Other Hodgkin lymphoma

Classical Hodgkin lymphoma NOS
Other classical Hodgkin lymphoma

C81.70	Other Hodgkin lymphoma, unspecified site	HCC
C81.71	Other Hodgkin lymphoma, lymph nodes of head, face, and neck	HCC
C81.72	Other Hodgkin lymphoma, intrathoracic lymph nodes	HCC
C81.73	Other Hodgkin lymphoma, intra-abdominal lymph nodes	HCC
C81.74	Other Hodgkin lymphoma, lymph nodes of axilla and upper limb	HCC
C81.75	Other Hodgkin lymphoma, lymph nodes of inguinal region and lower limb	HCC
C81.76	Other Hodgkin lymphoma, intrapelvic lymph nodes	HCC
C81.77	Other Hodgkin lymphoma, spleen	HCC
C81.78	Other Hodgkin lymphoma, lymph nodes of multiple sites	HCC

✓ Additional Character Required   ✓x7th Placeholder   Unacceptable PDx   Questionable PDx   Manifestation   Unspecified Dx   H1-H14 HAC   HCC CMS-HCC Dx   HIV HIV Dx

ICD-10-CM 2020   481

C81.79　Other Hodgkin lymphoma, extranodal and solid organ sites HCC

✓5th **C81.9　Hodgkin lymphoma, unspecified**

C81.90　Hodgkin lymphoma, unspecified, unspecified site HCC

C81.91　Hodgkin lymphoma, unspecified, lymph nodes of head, face, and neck HCC

C81.92　Hodgkin lymphoma, unspecified, intrathoracic lymph nodes HCC

C81.93　Hodgkin lymphoma, unspecified, intra-abdominal lymph nodes HCC

C81.94　Hodgkin lymphoma, unspecified, lymph nodes of axilla and upper limb HCC

C81.95　Hodgkin lymphoma, unspecified, lymph nodes of inguinal region and lower limb HCC

C81.96　Hodgkin lymphoma, unspecified, intrapelvic lymph nodes HCC

C81.97　Hodgkin lymphoma, unspecified, spleen HCC

C81.98　Hodgkin lymphoma, unspecified, lymph nodes of multiple sites HCC

C81.99　Hodgkin lymphoma, unspecified, extranodal and solid organ sites HCC

✓4th **C82　Follicular lymphoma**

INCLUDES　follicular lymphoma with or without diffuse areas

EXCLUDES 1　mature T/NK-cell lymphomas (C84.-)
　　　　　personal history of non-Hodgkin lymphoma (Z85.72)

DEF: Most common subgroup of non-Hodgkin lymphomas (NHL), accounting for 20 to 30 percent of all NHLs. NHL is a B-cell lymphoma that is slow growing and characterized by the circular pattern of malignant cell growth with the cells clustered into identifiable nodules or follicles.

✓5th **C82.0　Follicular lymphoma grade I**

C82.00　Follicular lymphoma grade I, unspecified site HCC

C82.01　Follicular lymphoma grade I, lymph nodes of head, face, and neck HCC

C82.02　Follicular lymphoma grade I, intrathoracic lymph nodes HCC

C82.03　Follicular lymphoma grade I, intra-abdominal lymph nodes HCC

C82.04　Follicular lymphoma grade I, lymph nodes of axilla and upper limb HCC

C82.05　Follicular lymphoma grade I, lymph nodes of inguinal region and lower limb HCC

C82.06　Follicular lymphoma grade I, intrapelvic lymph nodes HCC

C82.07　Follicular lymphoma grade I, spleen HCC

C82.08　Follicular lymphoma grade I, lymph nodes of multiple sites HCC

C82.09　Follicular lymphoma grade I, extranodal and solid organ sites HCC

✓5th **C82.1　Follicular lymphoma grade II**

C82.10　Follicular lymphoma grade II, unspecified site HCC

C82.11　Follicular lymphoma grade II, lymph nodes of head, face, and neck HCC

C82.12　Follicular lymphoma grade II, intrathoracic lymph nodes HCC

C82.13　Follicular lymphoma grade II, intra-abdominal lymph nodes HCC

C82.14　Follicular lymphoma grade II, lymph nodes of axilla and upper limb HCC

C82.15　Follicular lymphoma grade II, lymph nodes of inguinal region and lower limb HCC

C82.16　Follicular lymphoma grade II, intrapelvic lymph nodes HCC

C82.17　Follicular lymphoma grade II, spleen CC HCC
CC Excl: PDX collection 424

C82.18　Follicular lymphoma grade II, lymph nodes of multiple sites HCC

C82.19　Follicular lymphoma grade II, extranodal and solid organ sites HCC

✓5th **C82.2　Follicular lymphoma grade III, unspecified**

C82.20　Follicular lymphoma grade III, unspecified, unspecified site HCC

C82.21　Follicular lymphoma grade III, unspecified, lymph nodes of head, face, and neck HCC

C82.22　Follicular lymphoma grade III, unspecified, intrathoracic lymph nodes HCC

C82.23　Follicular lymphoma grade III, unspecified, intra-abdominal lymph nodes HCC

C82.24　Follicular lymphoma grade III, unspecified, lymph nodes of axilla and upper limb HCC

C82.25　Follicular lymphoma grade III, unspecified, lymph nodes of inguinal region and lower limb HCC

C82.26　Follicular lymphoma grade III, unspecified, intrapelvic lymph nodes HCC

C82.27　Follicular lymphoma grade III, unspecified, spleen HCC

C82.28　Follicular lymphoma grade III, unspecified, lymph nodes of multiple sites HCC

C82.29　Follicular lymphoma grade III, unspecified, extranodal and solid organ sites HCC

✓5th **C82.3　Follicular lymphoma grade IIIa**

C82.30　Follicular lymphoma grade IIIa, unspecified site HCC

C82.31　Follicular lymphoma grade IIIa, lymph nodes of head, face, and neck HCC

C82.32　Follicular lymphoma grade IIIa, intrathoracic lymph nodes HCC

C82.33　Follicular lymphoma grade IIIa, intra-abdominal lymph nodes HCC

C82.34　Follicular lymphoma grade IIIa, lymph nodes of axilla and upper limb HCC

C82.35　Follicular lymphoma grade IIIa, lymph nodes of inguinal region and lower limb HCC

C82.36　Follicular lymphoma grade IIIa, intrapelvic lymph nodes HCC

C82.37　Follicular lymphoma grade IIIa, spleen HCC

C82.38　Follicular lymphoma grade IIIa, lymph nodes of multiple sites HCC

C82.39　Follicular lymphoma grade IIIa, extranodal and solid organ sites HCC

✓5th **C82.4　Follicular lymphoma grade IIIb**

C82.40　Follicular lymphoma grade IIIb, unspecified site HCC

C82.41　Follicular lymphoma grade IIIb, lymph nodes of head, face, and neck HCC

C82.42　Follicular lymphoma grade IIIb, intrathoracic lymph nodes HCC

C82.43　Follicular lymphoma grade IIIb, intra-abdominal lymph nodes HCC

C82.44　Follicular lymphoma grade IIIb, lymph nodes of axilla and upper limb HCC

C82.45　Follicular lymphoma grade IIIb, lymph nodes of inguinal region and lower limb HCC

C82.46　Follicular lymphoma grade IIIb, intrapelvic lymph nodes HCC

C82.47　Follicular lymphoma grade IIIb, spleen HCC

C82.48　Follicular lymphoma grade IIIb, lymph nodes of multiple sites HCC

C82.49　Follicular lymphoma grade IIIb, extranodal and solid organ sites HCC

✓5th **C82.5　Diffuse follicle center lymphoma**

C82.50　Diffuse follicle center lymphoma, unspecified site HIV HCC

C82.51　Diffuse follicle center lymphoma, lymph nodes of head, face, and neck HIV HCC

C82.52　Diffuse follicle center lymphoma, intrathoracic lymph nodes HIV HCC

C82.53　Diffuse follicle center lymphoma, intra-abdominal lymph nodes HIV HCC

C82.54　Diffuse follicle center lymphoma, lymph nodes of axilla and upper limb HIV HCC

C82.55　Diffuse follicle center lymphoma, lymph nodes of inguinal region and lower limb HIV HCC

C82.56　Diffuse follicle center lymphoma, intrapelvic lymph nodes HIV HCC

C82.57　Diffuse follicle center lymphoma, spleen HIV HCC

C82.58　Diffuse follicle center lymphoma, lymph nodes of multiple sites HIV HCC

C82.59　Diffuse follicle center lymphoma, extranodal and solid organ sites HIV HCC

√5ᵗʰ **C82.6** **Cutaneous follicle center lymphoma**

C82.60 **Cutaneous follicle center lymphoma, unspecified site** `HCC`

C82.61 **Cutaneous follicle center lymphoma, lymph nodes of head, face, and neck** `HCC`

C82.62 **Cutaneous follicle center lymphoma, intrathoracic lymph nodes** `HCC`

C82.63 **Cutaneous follicle center lymphoma, intra-abdominal lymph nodes** `HCC`

C82.64 **Cutaneous follicle center lymphoma, lymph nodes of axilla and upper limb** `HCC`

C82.65 **Cutaneous follicle center lymphoma, lymph nodes of inguinal region and lower limb** `HCC`

C82.66 **Cutaneous follicle center lymphoma, intrapelvic lymph nodes** `HCC`

C82.67 **Cutaneous follicle center lymphoma, spleen** `HCC`

C82.68 **Cutaneous follicle center lymphoma, lymph nodes of multiple sites** `HCC`

C82.69 **Cutaneous follicle center lymphoma, extranodal and solid organ sites** `HCC`

√5ᵗʰ **C82.8** **Other types of follicular lymphoma**

C82.80 **Other types of follicular lymphoma, unspecified site** `HCC`

C82.81 **Other types of follicular lymphoma, lymph nodes of head, face, and neck** `HCC`

C82.82 **Other types of follicular lymphoma, intrathoracic lymph nodes** `HCC`

C82.83 **Other types of follicular lymphoma, intra-abdominal lymph nodes** `HCC`

C82.84 **Other types of follicular lymphoma, lymph nodes of axilla and upper limb** `HCC`

C82.85 **Other types of follicular lymphoma, lymph nodes of inguinal region and lower limb** `HCC`

C82.86 **Other types of follicular lymphoma, intrapelvic lymph nodes** `HCC`

C82.87 **Other types of follicular lymphoma, spleen** `HCC`

C82.88 **Other types of follicular lymphoma, lymph nodes of multiple sites** `HCC`

C82.89 **Other types of follicular lymphoma, extranodal and solid organ sites** `HCC`

√5ᵗʰ **C82.9** **Follicular lymphoma, unspecified**

C82.90 **Follicular lymphoma, unspecified, unspecified site** `HCC`

C82.91 **Follicular lymphoma, unspecified, lymph nodes of head, face, and neck** `HCC`

C82.92 **Follicular lymphoma, unspecified, intrathoracic lymph nodes** `HCC`

C82.93 **Follicular lymphoma, unspecified, intra-abdominal lymph nodes** `HCC`

C82.94 **Follicular lymphoma, unspecified, lymph nodes of axilla and upper limb** `HCC`

C82.95 **Follicular lymphoma, unspecified, lymph nodes of inguinal region and lower limb** `HCC`

C82.96 **Follicular lymphoma, unspecified, intrapelvic lymph nodes** `HCC`

C82.97 **Follicular lymphoma, unspecified, spleen** `HCC`

C82.98 **Follicular lymphoma, unspecified, lymph nodes of multiple sites** `HCC`

C82.99 **Follicular lymphoma, unspecified, extranodal and solid organ sites** `HCC`

√4ᵗʰ **C83** **Non-follicular lymphoma**

EXCLUDES 1   personal history of non-Hodgkin lymphoma (Z85.72)

√5ᵗʰ **C83.0** **Small cell B-cell lymphoma**

Lymphoplasmacytic lymphoma
Nodal marginal zone lymphoma
Non-leukemic variant of B-CLL
Splenic marginal zone lymphoma
EXCLUDES 1   chronic lymphocytic leukemia (C91.1)
           mature T/NK-cell lymphomas (C84.-)
           Waldenström macroglobulinemia (C88.0)
DEF: Nonfollicular lymphoma that is rare, slow growing, and usually found in the older population.

C83.00 **Small cell B-cell lymphoma, unspecified** `HIV` `CC` `HCC`
site
CC Excl: PDX collection 435

C83.01 **Small cell B-cell lymphoma, lymph nodes** `HIV` `CC` `HCC`
of head, face, and neck
CC Excl: PDX collection 436

C83.02 **Small cell B-cell lymphoma, intrathoracic lymph nodes** `HIV` `HCC`

C83.03 **Small cell B-cell lymphoma, intra-abdominal lymph nodes** `HIV` `HCC`

C83.04 **Small cell B-cell lymphoma, lymph nodes of axilla and upper limb** `HIV` `HCC`

C83.05 **Small cell B-cell lymphoma, lymph nodes of inguinal region and lower limb** `HIV` `HCC`

C83.06 **Small cell B-cell lymphoma, intrapelvic lymph nodes** `HIV` `HCC`

C83.07 **Small cell B-cell lymphoma, spleen** `HIV` `HCC`

C83.08 **Small cell B-cell lymphoma, lymph nodes of multiple sites** `HIV` `HCC`

C83.09 **Small cell B-cell lymphoma, extranodal and solid organ sites** `HIV` `HCC`

√5ᵗʰ **C83.1** **Mantle cell lymphoma**

Centrocytic lymphoma
Malignant lymphomatous polyposis
DEF: Rare form of B-cell non-Hodgkin lymphoma named for the location of the tumor cell production, the mantle zone of the lymph nodes.

C83.10 **Mantle cell lymphoma, unspecified site** `HIV` `HCC`

C83.11 **Mantle cell lymphoma, lymph nodes of head, face, and neck** `HIV` `HCC`

C83.12 **Mantle cell lymphoma, intrathoracic lymph nodes** `HIV` `HCC`

C83.13 **Mantle cell lymphoma, intra-abdominal lymph nodes** `HIV` `HCC`

C83.14 **Mantle cell lymphoma, lymph nodes of axilla and upper limb** `HIV` `HCC`

C83.15 **Mantle cell lymphoma, lymph nodes of inguinal region and lower limb** `HIV` `HCC`

C83.16 **Mantle cell lymphoma, intrapelvic lymph nodes** `HIV` `HCC`

C83.17 **Mantle cell lymphoma, spleen** `HIV` `HCC`

C83.18 **Mantle cell lymphoma, lymph nodes of multiple sites** `HIV` `HCC`

C83.19 **Mantle cell lymphoma, extranodal and solid organ sites** `HIV` `HCC`

√5ᵗʰ **C83.3** **Diffuse large B-cell lymphoma**

Anaplastic diffuse large B-cell lymphoma
CD30-positive diffuse large B-cell lymphoma
Centroblastic diffuse large B-cell lymphoma
Diffuse large B-cell lymphoma, subtype not specified
Immunoblastic diffuse large B-cell lymphoma
Plasmablastic diffuse large B-cell lymphoma
T-cell rich diffuse large B-cell lymphoma
EXCLUDES 1   mediastinal (thymic) large B-cell lymphoma (C85.2-)
           mature T/NK-cell lymphomas (C84.-)
DEF: Nonfollicular lymphoma that is one of the more common types of lymphoma. This cancer is fast growing and affects any age but is found mostly in the older population.

C83.30 **Diffuse large B-cell lymphoma, unspecified site** `HIV` `HCC`

C83.31 **Diffuse large B-cell lymphoma, lymph nodes of head, face, and neck** `HIV` `HCC`

C83.32 **Diffuse large B-cell lymphoma, intrathoracic lymph nodes** `HIV` `HCC`

C83.33 **Diffuse large B-cell lymphoma, intra-abdominal lymph nodes** `HIV` `HCC`

C83.34 **Diffuse large B-cell lymphoma, lymph nodes of axilla and upper limb** `HIV` `HCC`

C83.35 **Diffuse large B-cell lymphoma, lymph nodes of inguinal region and lower limb** `HIV` `HCC`

C83.36 **Diffuse large B-cell lymphoma, intrapelvic lymph nodes** `HIV` `HCC`

C83.37 **Diffuse large B-cell lymphoma, spleen** `HIV` `HCC`

C83.38 **Diffuse large B-cell lymphoma, lymph nodes of multiple sites** `HIV` `HCC`

C83.39 **Diffuse large B-cell lymphoma, extranodal and solid organ sites** `HIV` `HCC`

Chapter 2. Neoplasms

C83.5–C84.19

✓5ᵗʰ **C83.5** **Lymphoblastic (diffuse) lymphoma**
B-precursor lymphoma
Lymphoblastic B-cell lymphoma
Lymphoblastic lymphoma NOS
Lymphoblastic T-cell lymphoma
T-precursor lymphoma
DEF: Type of non-Hodgkin lymphoma considered lymphoma or leukemia—the determination is made based on the amount of bone marrow involvement. The cells are small to medium immature T-cells that often originate in the thymus where many of the T-cells are made.

C83.50 **Lymphoblastic (diffuse) lymphoma, unspecified site** HCC

C83.51 **Lymphoblastic (diffuse) lymphoma, lymph nodes of head, face, and neck** HCC

C83.52 **Lymphoblastic (diffuse) lymphoma, intrathoracic lymph nodes** HCC

C83.53 **Lymphoblastic (diffuse) lymphoma, intra-abdominal lymph nodes** HCC

C83.54 **Lymphoblastic (diffuse) lymphoma, lymph nodes of axilla and upper limb** HCC

C83.55 **Lymphoblastic (diffuse) lymphoma, lymph nodes of inguinal region and lower limb** HCC

C83.56 **Lymphoblastic (diffuse) lymphoma, intrapelvic lymph nodes** HCC

C83.57 **Lymphoblastic (diffuse) lymphoma, spleen** HCC

C83.58 **Lymphoblastic (diffuse) lymphoma, lymph nodes of multiple sites** HCC

C83.59 **Lymphoblastic (diffuse) lymphoma, extranodal and solid organ sites** HCC

✓5ᵗʰ **C83.7** **Burkitt lymphoma**
Atypical Burkitt lymphoma
Burkitt-like lymphoma
EXCLUDES 1   mature B-cell leukemia Burkitt type (C91.A-)
DEF: Malignancy of the lymphatic system, most often seen as a large bone-deteriorating lesion within the jaw or as an abdominal mass. It is a form of non-Hodgkin's lymphoma and is recognized as the fastest growing human tumor.

C83.70 **Burkitt lymphoma, unspecified site** HIV HCC

C83.71 **Burkitt lymphoma, lymph nodes of head, face, and neck** HIV HCC

C83.72 **Burkitt lymphoma, intrathoracic lymph nodes** HIV HCC

C83.73 **Burkitt lymphoma, intra-abdominal lymph nodes** HIV HCC

C83.74 **Burkitt lymphoma, lymph nodes of axilla and upper limb** HIV HCC

C83.75 **Burkitt lymphoma, lymph nodes of inguinal region and lower limb** HIV HCC

C83.76 **Burkitt lymphoma, intrapelvic lymph nodes** HIV HCC

C83.77 **Burkitt lymphoma, spleen** HIV HCC

C83.78 **Burkitt lymphoma, lymph nodes of multiple sites** HIV HCC

C83.79 **Burkitt lymphoma, extranodal and solid organ sites** HIV HCC

✓5ᵗʰ **C83.8** **Other non-follicular lymphoma**
Intravascular large B-cell lymphoma
Lymphoid granulomatosis
Primary effusion B-cell lymphoma
EXCLUDES 1   mediastinal (thymic) large B-cell lymphoma (C85.2-)
T-cell rich B-cell lymphoma (C83.3-)

C83.80 **Other non-follicular lymphoma, unspecified site** HIV HCC

C83.81 **Other non-follicular lymphoma, lymph nodes of head, face, and neck** HIV HCC

C83.82 **Other non-follicular lymphoma, intrathoracic lymph nodes** HIV HCC

C83.83 **Other non-follicular lymphoma, intra-abdominal lymph nodes** HIV HCC

C83.84 **Other non-follicular lymphoma, lymph nodes of axilla and upper limb** HIV HCC

C83.85 **Other non-follicular lymphoma, lymph nodes of inguinal region and lower limb** HIV HCC

C83.86 **Other non-follicular lymphoma, intrapelvic lymph nodes** HIV HCC

C83.87 **Other non-follicular lymphoma, spleen** HIV HCC

C83.88 **Other non-follicular lymphoma, lymph nodes of multiple sites** HIV HCC

C83.89 **Other non-follicular lymphoma, extranodal and solid organ sites** HIV HCC

✓5ᵗʰ **C83.9** **Non-follicular (diffuse) lymphoma, unspecified**

C83.90 **Non-follicular (diffuse) lymphoma, unspecified, unspecified site** HIV HCC

C83.91 **Non-follicular (diffuse) lymphoma, unspecified, lymph nodes of head, face, and neck** HIV HCC

C83.92 **Non-follicular (diffuse) lymphoma, unspecified, intrathoracic lymph nodes** HIV HCC

C83.93 **Non-follicular (diffuse) lymphoma, unspecified, intra-abdominal lymph nodes** HIV HCC

C83.94 **Non-follicular (diffuse) lymphoma, unspecified, lymph nodes of axilla and upper limb** HIV HCC

C83.95 **Non-follicular (diffuse) lymphoma, unspecified, lymph nodes of inguinal region and lower limb** HIV HCC

C83.96 **Non-follicular (diffuse) lymphoma, unspecified, intrapelvic lymph nodes** HIV HCC

C83.97 **Non-follicular (diffuse) lymphoma, unspecified, spleen** HIV HCC

C83.98 **Non-follicular (diffuse) lymphoma, unspecified, lymph nodes of multiple sites** HIV HCC

C83.99 **Non-follicular (diffuse) lymphoma, unspecified, extranodal and solid organ sites** HIV HCC

✓4ᵗʰ **C84** **Mature T/NK-cell lymphomas**
EXCLUDES 1   personal history of non-Hodgkin lymphoma (Z85.72)

✓5ᵗʰ **C84.0** **Mycosis fungoides**
EXCLUDES 1   peripheral T-cell lymphoma, not classified (C84.4-)
DEF: Most common form of cutaneous T-cell lymphoma. A type of non-Hodgkin lymphoma in which white blood cells become cancerous and affect the skin and sometimes internal organs.
Synonym(s): Alibert-Bazin syndrome.

C84.00 **Mycosis fungoides, unspecified site** HCC

C84.01 **Mycosis fungoides, lymph nodes of head, face, and neck** HCC

C84.02 **Mycosis fungoides, intrathoracic lymph nodes** HCC

C84.03 **Mycosis fungoides, intra-abdominal lymph nodes** HCC

C84.04 **Mycosis fungoides, lymph nodes of axilla and upper limb** HCC

C84.05 **Mycosis fungoides, lymph nodes of inguinal region and lower limb** HCC

C84.06 **Mycosis fungoides, intrapelvic lymph nodes** HCC

C84.07 **Mycosis fungoides, spleen** HCC

C84.08 **Mycosis fungoides, lymph nodes of multiple sites** HCC

C84.09 **Mycosis fungoides, extranodal and solid organ sites** HCC

✓5ᵗʰ **C84.1** **Sézary disease**
DEF: Extension of mycosis fungoides that affects the blood and all of the skin, appearing as sunburn, rather than patches. It spreads to the lymph nodes and is often linked to a weakened immune system.

C84.10 **Sézary disease, unspecified site** HCC

C84.11 **Sézary disease, lymph nodes of head, face, and neck** HCC

C84.12 **Sézary disease, intrathoracic lymph nodes** HCC

C84.13 **Sézary disease, intra-abdominal lymph nodes** HCC

C84.14 **Sézary disease, lymph nodes of axilla and upper limb** HCC

C84.15 **Sézary disease, lymph nodes of inguinal region and lower limb** HCC

C84.16 **Sézary disease, intrapelvic lymph nodes** HCC

C84.17 **Sézary disease, spleen** HCC

C84.18 **Sézary disease, lymph nodes of multiple sites** HCC

C84.19 **Sézary disease, extranodal and solid organ sites** HCC

Ⓝ Newborn: 0   Ⓟ Pediatric: 0-17   Ⓜ Maternity: 9-64   Ⓐ Adult: 15-124   MCC Major Complication/Comorbidity   CC Complication/Comorbidity   SW Severe Wound Dx

484   ICD-10-CM 2020

√5ᵗʰ **C84.4 Peripheral T-cell lymphoma, not classified**
Lennert's lymphoma
Lymphoepithelioid lymphoma
Mature T-cell lymphoma, not elsewhere classified

C84.40 Peripheral T-cell lymphoma, not classified, unspecified site `HIV` `HCC`

C84.41 Peripheral T-cell lymphoma, not classified, lymph nodes of head, face, and neck `HIV` `HCC`

C84.42 Peripheral T-cell lymphoma, not classified, intrathoracic lymph nodes `HIV` `HCC`

C84.43 Peripheral T-cell lymphoma, not classified, intra-abdominal lymph nodes `HIV` `HCC`

C84.44 Peripheral T-cell lymphoma, not classified, lymph nodes of axilla and upper limb `HIV` `HCC`

C84.45 Peripheral T-cell lymphoma, not classified, lymph nodes of inguinal region and lower limb `HIV` `HCC`

C84.46 Peripheral T-cell lymphoma, not classified, intrapelvic lymph nodes `HIV` `HCC`

C84.47 Peripheral T-cell lymphoma, not classified, spleen `HIV` `HCC`

C84.48 Peripheral T-cell lymphoma, not classified, lymph nodes of multiple sites `HIV` `HCC`

C84.49 Peripheral T-cell lymphoma, not classified, extranodal and solid organ sites `HIV` `HCC`

√5ᵗʰ **C84.6 Anaplastic large cell lymphoma, ALK-positive**
Anaplastic large cell lymphoma, CD30-positive

C84.60 Anaplastic large cell lymphoma, ALK-positive, unspecified site `HIV` `HCC`

C84.61 Anaplastic large cell lymphoma, ALK-positive, lymph nodes of head, face, and neck `HIV` `HCC`

C84.62 Anaplastic large cell lymphoma, ALK-positive, intrathoracic lymph nodes `HIV` `HCC`

C84.63 Anaplastic large cell lymphoma, ALK-positive, intra-abdominal lymph nodes `HIV` `HCC`

C84.64 Anaplastic large cell lymphoma, ALK-positive, lymph nodes of axilla and upper limb `HIV` `HCC`

C84.65 Anaplastic large cell lymphoma, ALK-positive, lymph nodes of inguinal region and lower limb `HIV` `HCC`

C84.66 Anaplastic large cell lymphoma, ALK-positive, intrapelvic lymph nodes `HIV` `HCC`

C84.67 Anaplastic large cell lymphoma, ALK-positive, spleen `HIV` `HCC`

C84.68 Anaplastic large cell lymphoma, ALK-positive, lymph nodes of multiple sites `HIV` `HCC`

C84.69 Anaplastic large cell lymphoma, ALK-positive, extranodal and solid organ sites `HIV` `HCC`

√5ᵗʰ **C84.7 Anaplastic large cell lymphoma, ALK-negative**
EXCLUDES 1   primary cutaneous CD30-positive T-cell proliferations (C86.6-)

C84.70 Anaplastic large cell lymphoma, ALK-negative, unspecified site `HIV` `HCC`

C84.71 Anaplastic large cell lymphoma, ALK-negative, lymph nodes of head, face, and neck `HIV` `HCC`

C84.72 Anaplastic large cell lymphoma, ALK-negative, intrathoracic lymph nodes `HIV` `HCC`

C84.73 Anaplastic large cell lymphoma, ALK-negative, intra-abdominal lymph nodes `HIV` `HCC`

C84.74 Anaplastic large cell lymphoma, ALK-negative, lymph nodes of axilla and upper limb `HIV` `HCC`

C84.75 Anaplastic large cell lymphoma, ALK-negative, lymph nodes of inguinal region and lower limb `HIV` `HCC`

C84.76 Anaplastic large cell lymphoma, ALK-negative, intrapelvic lymph nodes `HIV` `HCC`

C84.77 Anaplastic large cell lymphoma, ALK-negative, spleen `HIV` `HCC`

C84.78 Anaplastic large cell lymphoma, ALK-negative, lymph nodes of multiple sites `HIV` `HCC`

C84.79 Anaplastic large cell lymphoma, ALK-negative, extranodal and solid organ sites `HIV` `HCC`

√5ᵗʰ **C84.A Cutaneous T-cell lymphoma, unspecified**

C84.A0 Cutaneous T-cell lymphoma, unspecified, unspecified site `HIV` `HCC`

C84.A1 Cutaneous T-cell lymphoma, unspecified lymph nodes of head, face, and neck `HIV` `HCC`

C84.A2 Cutaneous T-cell lymphoma, unspecified, intrathoracic lymph nodes `HIV` `HCC`

C84.A3 Cutaneous T-cell lymphoma, unspecified, intra-abdominal lymph nodes `HIV` `HCC`

C84.A4 Cutaneous T-cell lymphoma, unspecified, lymph nodes of axilla and upper limb `HIV` `HCC`

C84.A5 Cutaneous T-cell lymphoma, unspecified, lymph nodes of inguinal region and lower limb `HIV` `HCC`

C84.A6 Cutaneous T-cell lymphoma, unspecified, intrapelvic lymph nodes `HIV` `HCC`

C84.A7 Cutaneous T-cell lymphoma, unspecified, spleen `HIV` `HCC`

C84.A8 Cutaneous T-cell lymphoma, unspecified, lymph nodes of multiple sites `HIV` `HCC`

C84.A9 Cutaneous T-cell lymphoma, unspecified, extranodal and solid organ sites `HIV` `HCC`

√5ᵗʰ **C84.Z Other mature T/NK-cell lymphomas**

NOTE   If T-cell lineage or involvement is mentioned in conjunction with a specific lymphoma, code to the more specific description.

EXCLUDES 1   angioimmunoblastic T-cell lymphoma (C86.5)
blastic NK-cell lymphoma (C86.4)
enteropathy-type T-cell lymphoma (C86.2)
extranodal NK-cell lymphoma, nasal type (C86.0)
hepatosplenic T-cell lymphoma (C86.1)
primary cutaneous CD30-positive T-cell proliferations (C86.6)
subcutaneous panniculitis-like T-cell lymphoma (C86.3)
T-cell leukemia (C91.1-)

C84.Z0 Other mature T/NK-cell lymphomas, unspecified site `HIV` `HCC`

C84.Z1 Other mature T/NK-cell lymphomas, lymph nodes of head, face, and neck `HIV` `HCC`

C84.Z2 Other mature T/NK-cell lymphomas, intrathoracic lymph nodes `HIV` `HCC`

C84.Z3 Other mature T/NK-cell lymphomas, intra-abdominal lymph nodes `HIV` `HCC`

C84.Z4 Other mature T/NK-cell lymphomas, lymph nodes of axilla and upper limb `HIV` `HCC`

C84.Z5 Other mature T/NK-cell lymphomas, lymph nodes of inguinal region and lower limb `HIV` `HCC`

C84.Z6 Other mature T/NK-cell lymphomas, intrapelvic lymph nodes `HIV` `HCC`

C84.Z7 Other mature T/NK-cell lymphomas, spleen `HIV` `HCC`

C84.Z8 Other mature T/NK-cell lymphomas, lymph nodes of multiple sites `HIV` `HCC`

C84.Z9 Other mature T/NK-cell lymphomas, extranodal and solid organ sites `HIV` `HCC`

√5ᵗʰ **C84.9 Mature T/NK-cell lymphomas, unspecified**
NK/T cell lymphoma NOS
EXCLUDES 1   mature T-cell lymphoma, not elsewhere classified (C84.4-)

C84.90 Mature T/NK-cell lymphomas, unspecified, unspecified site `HIV` `HCC`

C84.91 Mature T/NK-cell lymphomas, unspecified, lymph nodes of head, face, and neck `HIV` `HCC`

C84.92 Mature T/NK-cell lymphomas, unspecified, intrathoracic lymph nodes `HIV` `HCC`

C84.93 Mature T/NK-cell lymphomas, unspecified, intra-abdominal lymph nodes `HIV` `HCC`

C84.94 Mature T/NK-cell lymphomas, unspecified, lymph nodes of axilla and upper limb `HIV` `HCC`

C84.95 Mature T/NK-cell lymphomas, unspecified, lymph nodes of inguinal region and lower limb `HIV` `HCC`

✔ Additional Character Required   √7ᵗʰ Placeholder   Unacceptable PDx   Questionable PDx   Manifestation   Unspecified Dx   H1-H4 HAC   HCC CMS-HCC Dx   HIV HIV Dx
ICD-10-CM 2020   485

C84.4–C84.95

C84.96 Mature T/NK-cell lymphomas, unspecified, intrapelvic lymph nodes `HIV` `HCC`

C84.97 Mature T/NK-cell lymphomas, unspecified, spleen `HIV` `HCC`

C84.98 Mature T/NK-cell lymphomas, unspecified, lymph nodes of multiple sites `HIV` `HCC`

C84.99 Mature T/NK-cell lymphomas, unspecified, extranodal and solid organ sites `HIV` `HCC`

✓4ᵗʰ **C85 Other specified and unspecified types of non-Hodgkin lymphoma**

> **EXCLUDES 1** *other specified types of T/NK-cell lymphoma (C86.-)*
> *personal history of non-Hodgkin lymphoma (Z85.72)*

✓5ᵗʰ **C85.1 Unspecified B-cell lymphoma**

> **NOTE** If B-cell lineage or involvement is mentioned in conjunction with a specific lymphoma, code to the more specific description.

C85.10 Unspecified B-cell lymphoma, unspecified site `HIV` `HCC`

C85.11 Unspecified B-cell lymphoma, lymph nodes of head, face, and neck `HIV` `HCC`

C85.12 Unspecified B-cell lymphoma, intrathoracic lymph nodes `HIV` `HCC`

C85.13 Unspecified B-cell lymphoma, intra-abdominal lymph nodes `HIV` `HCC`

C85.14 Unspecified B-cell lymphoma, lymph nodes of axilla and upper limb `HIV` `HCC`

C85.15 Unspecified B-cell lymphoma, lymph nodes of inguinal region and lower limb `HIV` `HCC`

C85.16 Unspecified B-cell lymphoma, intrapelvic lymph nodes `HIV` `HCC`

C85.17 Unspecified B-cell lymphoma, spleen `HIV` `HCC`

C85.18 Unspecified B-cell lymphoma, lymph nodes of multiple sites `HIV` `HCC`

C85.19 Unspecified B-cell lymphoma, extranodal and solid organ sites `HIV` `HCC`

✓6ᵗʰ **C85.2 Mediastinal (thymic) large B-cell lymphoma**

C85.20 Mediastinal (thymic) large B-cell lymphoma, unspecified site `HIV` `HCC`

C85.21 Mediastinal (thymic) large B-cell lymphoma, lymph nodes of head, face, and neck `HIV` `HCC`

C85.22 Mediastinal (thymic) large B-cell lymphoma, intrathoracic lymph nodes `HIV` `HCC`

C85.23 Mediastinal (thymic) large B-cell lymphoma, intra-abdominal lymph nodes `HIV` `HCC`

C85.24 Mediastinal (thymic) large B-cell lymphoma, lymph nodes of axilla and upper limb `HIV` `HCC`

C85.25 Mediastinal (thymic) large B-cell lymphoma, lymph nodes of inguinal region and lower limb `HIV` `HCC`

C85.26 Mediastinal (thymic) large B-cell lymphoma, intrapelvic lymph nodes `HIV` `HCC`

C85.27 Mediastinal (thymic) large B-cell lymphoma, spleen `HIV` `HCC`

C85.28 Mediastinal (thymic) large B-cell lymphoma, lymph nodes of multiple sites `HIV` `HCC`

C85.29 Mediastinal (thymic) large B-cell lymphoma, extranodal and solid organ sites `HIV` `HCC`

✓5ᵗʰ **C85.8 Other specified types of non-Hodgkin lymphoma**

C85.80 Other specified types of non-Hodgkin lymphoma, unspecified site `HIV` `HCC`

C85.81 Other specified types of non-Hodgkin lymphoma, lymph nodes of head, face, and neck `HIV` `HCC`

C85.82 Other specified types of non-Hodgkin lymphoma, intrathoracic lymph nodes `HIV` `HCC`

C85.83 Other specified types of non-Hodgkin lymphoma, intra-abdominal lymph nodes `HIV` `HCC`

C85.84 Other specified types of non-Hodgkin lymphoma, lymph nodes of axilla and upper limb `HIV` `HCC`

C85.85 Other specified types of non-Hodgkin lymphoma, lymph nodes of inguinal region and lower limb `HIV` `HCC`

C85.86 Other specified types of non-Hodgkin lymphoma, intrapelvic lymph nodes `HIV` `HCC`

C85.87 Other specified types of non-Hodgkin lymphoma, spleen `HIV` `HCC`

C85.88 Other specified types of non-Hodgkin lymphoma, lymph nodes of multiple sites `HIV` `HCC`

C85.89 Other specified types of non-Hodgkin lymphoma, extranodal and solid organ sites `HIV` `HCC`

✓5ᵗʰ **C85.9 Non-Hodgkin lymphoma, unspecified**

Lymphoma NOS
Malignant lymphoma NOS
Non-Hodgkin lymphoma NOS

C85.90 Non-Hodgkin lymphoma, unspecified, unspecified site `HIV` `HCC`

C85.91 Non-Hodgkin lymphoma, unspecified, lymph nodes of head, face, and neck `HIV` `HCC`

C85.92 Non-Hodgkin lymphoma, unspecified, intrathoracic lymph nodes `HIV` `HCC`

C85.93 Non-Hodgkin lymphoma, unspecified, intra-abdominal lymph nodes `HIV` `HCC`

C85.94 Non-Hodgkin lymphoma, unspecified, lymph nodes of axilla and upper limb `HIV` `HCC`

C85.95 Non-Hodgkin lymphoma, unspecified, lymph nodes of inguinal region and lower limb `HIV` `HCC`

C85.96 Non-Hodgkin lymphoma, unspecified, intrapelvic lymph nodes `HIV` `HCC`

C85.97 Non-Hodgkin lymphoma, unspecified, spleen `HIV` `HCC`

C85.98 Non-Hodgkin lymphoma, unspecified, lymph nodes of multiple sites `HIV` `HCC`

C85.99 Non-Hodgkin lymphoma, unspecified, extranodal and solid organ sites `HIV` `HCC`

✓4ᵗʰ **C86 Other specified types of T/NK-cell lymphoma**

> **EXCLUDES 1** *anaplastic large cell lymphoma, ALK negative (C84.7-)*
> *anaplastic large cell lymphoma, ALK positive (C84.6-)*
> *mature T/NK-cell lymphomas (C84.-)*
> *other specified types of non-Hodgkin lymphoma (C85.8-)*

C86.0 Extranodal NK/T-cell lymphoma, nasal type `HIV` `HCC`

C86.1 Hepatosplenic T-cell lymphoma `HIV` `HCC`

Alpha-beta and gamma delta types

C86.2 Enteropathy-type (intestinal) T-cell lymphoma `HIV` `HCC`

Enteropathy associated T-cell lymphoma

C86.3 Subcutaneous panniculitis-like T-cell lymphoma `HIV` `HCC`

C86.4 Blastic NK-cell lymphoma `HIV` `HCC`

Blastic plasmacytoid dendritic cell neoplasm (BPDCN)

C86.5 Angioimmunoblastic T-cell lymphoma `HIV` `HCC`

Angioimmunoblastic lymphadenopathy with dysproteinemia (AILD)

C86.6 Primary cutaneous CD30-positive T-cell proliferations `HIV` `HCC`

Lymphomatoid papulosis
Primary cutaneous anaplastic large cell lymphoma
Primary cutaneous CD30-positive large T-cell lymphoma

✓4ᵗʰ **C88 Malignant immunoproliferative diseases and certain other B-cell lymphomas**

> **EXCLUDES 1** *B-cell lymphoma, unspecified (C85.1-)*
> *personal history of other malignant neoplasms of lymphoid, hematopoietic and related tissues (Z85.79)*

C88.0 Waldenström macroglobulinemia `HCC`

Lymphoplasmacytic lymphoma with IgM-production
Macroglobulinemia (idiopathic) (primary)
> **EXCLUDES 1** *small cell B-cell lymphoma (C83.0)*

C88.2 Heavy chain disease `HCC`

Franklin disease
Gamma heavy chain disease
Mu heavy chain disease

C88.3 Immunoproliferative small intestinal disease `HCC`

Alpha heavy chain disease
Mediterranean lymphoma

C88.4 **Extranodal marginal zone B-cell lymphoma of mucosa-associated lymphoid tissue [MALT-lymphoma]** `HIV` `HCC`

Lymphoma of skin-associated lymphoid tissue [SALT-lymphoma]

Lymphoma of bronchial-associated lymphoid tissue [BALT-lymphoma]

EXCLUDES 1   *high malignant (diffuse large B-cell) lymphoma (C83.3-)*

C88.8 **Other malignant immunoproliferative diseases** `HCC`

C88.9 **Malignant immunoproliferative disease, unspecified** `HCC`

Immunoproliferative disease NOS

✓4ᵗʰ **C90** **Multiple myeloma and malignant plasma cell neoplasms**

EXCLUDES 1   *personal history of other malignant neoplasms of lymphoid, hematopoietic and related tissues (Z85.79)*

AHA: 2019,2Q,30

✓5ᵗʰ **C90.0** **Multiple myeloma**

Kahler's disease

Medullary plasmacytoma

Myelomatosis

Plasma cell myeloma

EXCLUDES 1   *solitary myeloma (C90.3-)*

solitary plasmacytoma (C90.3-)

TIP: Do not assign an additional code for bone metastasis (C79.51) when multiple myeloma is described as metastatic to the bone; bone involvement is integral to this disease process.

C90.00 **Multiple myeloma not having achieved remission** `HCC`

Multiple myeloma with failed remission

Multiple myeloma NOS

C90.01 **Multiple myeloma in remission** `HCC`

C90.02 **Multiple myeloma in relapse** `HCC`

✓5ᵗʰ **C90.1** **Plasma cell leukemia**

Plasmacytic leukemia

AHA: 2019,2Q,30

C90.10 **Plasma cell leukemia not having achieved remission** `HCC`

Plasma cell leukemia with failed remission

Plasma cell leukemia NOS

C90.11 **Plasma cell leukemia in remission** `HCC`

C90.12 **Plasma cell leukemia in relapse** `HCC`

✓5ᵗʰ **C90.2** **Extramedullary plasmacytoma**

C90.20 **Extramedullary plasmacytoma not having achieved remission** `HCC`

Extramedullary plasmacytoma with failed remission

Extramedullary plasmacytoma NOS

C90.21 **Extramedullary plasmacytoma in remission** `HCC`

C90.22 **Extramedullary plasmacytoma in relapse** `HCC`

✓5ᵗʰ **C90.3** **Solitary plasmacytoma**

Localized malignant plasma cell tumor NOS

Plasmacytoma NOS

Solitary myeloma

C90.30 **Solitary plasmacytoma not having achieved remission** `HCC`

Solitary plasmacytoma with failed remission

Solitary plasmacytoma NOS

C90.31 **Solitary plasmacytoma in remission** `HCC`

C90.32 **Solitary plasmacytoma in relapse** `HCC`

✓4ᵗʰ **C91** **Lymphoid leukemia**

EXCLUDES 1   *personal history of leukemia (Z85.6)*

DEF: Malignant proliferation of immature lymphocytes (white blood cells that make up lymphoid tissue), called lymphoblasts, that originate in the bone marrow. Can be acute (ALL) or chronic (CLL).

✓5ᵗʰ **C91.0** **Acute lymphoblastic leukemia [ALL]**

NOTE   ▶Codes in subcategory C91.0- should only be used for T-cell and B-cell precursor leukemia◀

C91.00 **Acute lymphoblastic leukemia not having achieved remission** `HCC`

Acute lymphoblastic leukemia with failed remission

Acute lymphoblastic leukemia NOS

C91.01 **Acute lymphoblastic leukemia, in remission** `HCC`

C91.02 **Acute lymphoblastic leukemia, in relapse** `HCC`

✓5ᵗʰ **C91.1** **Chronic lymphocytic leukemia of B-cell type**

Lymphoplasmacytic leukemia

Richter syndrome

EXCLUDES 1   *lymphoplasmacytic lymphoma (C83.0-)*

C91.10 **Chronic lymphocytic leukemia of B-cell type not having achieved remission** `HCC`

Chronic lymphocytic leukemia of B-cell type with failed remission

Chronic lymphocytic leukemia of B-cell type NOS

C91.11 **Chronic lymphocytic leukemia of B-cell type in remission** `HCC`

C91.12 **Chronic lymphocytic leukemia of B-cell type in relapse** `HCC`

✓5ᵗʰ **C91.3** **Prolymphocytic leukemia of B-cell type**

C91.30 **Prolymphocytic leukemia of B-cell type not having achieved remission** `HCC`

Prolymphocytic leukemia of B-cell type with failed remission

Prolymphocytic leukemia of B-cell type NOS

C91.31 **Prolymphocytic leukemia of B-cell type, in remission** `HCC`

C91.32 **Prolymphocytic leukemia of B-cell type, in relapse** `HCC`

✓5ᵗʰ **C91.4** **Hairy cell leukemia**

Leukemic reticuloendotheliosis

DEF: Rare type of leukemia that is slow growing and often also considered a type of lymphoma. The small B-cell lymphocytes appear with "hairy" projections under a microscope and are found mostly in the bone marrow, spleen, and blood.

C91.40 **Hairy cell leukemia not having achieved remission** `HCC`

Hairy cell leukemia with failed remission

Hairy cell leukemia NOS

C91.41 **Hairy cell leukemia, in remission** `HCC`

C91.42 **Hairy cell leukemia, in relapse** `HCC`

✓5ᵗʰ **C91.5** **Adult T-cell lymphoma/leukemia (HTLV-1-associated)**

Acute variant of adult T-cell lymphoma/leukemia (HTLV-1-associated)

Chronic variant of adult T-cell lymphoma/leukemia (HTLV-1-associated)

Lymphomatoid variant of adult T-cell lymphoma/leukemia (HTLV-1-associated)

Smouldering variant of adult T-cell lymphoma/leukemia (HTLV-1-associated)

C91.50 **Adult T-cell lymphoma/leukemia (HTLV-1-associated) not having achieved remission** `HCC` `A`

Adult T-cell lymphoma/leukemia (HTLV-1-associated) with failed remission

Adult T-cell lymphoma/leukemia (HTLV-1-associated) NOS

C91.51 **Adult T-cell lymphoma/leukemia (HTLV-1-associated), in remission** `HCC` `A`

C91.52 **Adult T-cell lymphoma/leukemia (HTLV-1-associated), in relapse** `HCC` `A`

✓5ᵗʰ **C91.6** **Prolymphocytic leukemia of T-cell type**

C91.60 **Prolymphocytic leukemia of T-cell type not having achieved remission** `HCC`

Prolymphocytic leukemia of T-cell type with failed remission

Prolymphocytic leukemia of T-cell type NOS

C91.61 **Prolymphocytic leukemia of T-cell type, in remission** `HCC`

C91.62 **Prolymphocytic leukemia of T-cell type, in relapse** `HCC`

✓5ᵗʰ **C91.A** **Mature B-cell leukemia Burkitt-type**

EXCLUDES 1   *Burkitt lymphoma (C83.7-)*

C91.A0 **Mature B-cell leukemia Burkitt-type not having achieved remission** `HCC`

Mature B-cell leukemia Burkitt-type with failed remission

Mature B-cell leukemia Burkitt-type NOS

C91.A1 **Mature B-cell leukemia Burkitt-type, in remission** `HCC`

C91.A2 **Mature B-cell leukemia Burkitt-type, in relapse** `HCC`

☑ Additional Character Required   ✓x7ᵗʰ Placeholder   Unacceptable PDx   Questionable PDx   Manifestation   Unspecified Dx   H1-H14 HAC   HCC CMS-HCC Dx   HIV HIV Dx

ICD-10-CM 2020   487

Chapter 2. Neoplasms

√5ᵗʰ **C91.Z** **Other lymphoid leukemia**

T-cell large granular lymphocytic leukemia (associated with rheumatoid arthritis)

C91.ZØ **Other lymphoid leukemia** not having achieved remission   HCC

Other lymphoid leukemia with failed remission
Other lymphoid leukemia NOS

C91.Z1 **Other lymphoid leukemia, in remission**   HCC

C91.Z2 **Other lymphoid leukemia, in relapse**   HCC

√5ᵗʰ **C91.9** **Lymphoid leukemia, unspecified**

C91.9Ø **Lymphoid leukemia, unspecified** not having achieved remission   HCC

Lymphoid leukemia with failed remission
Lymphoid leukemia NOS

C91.91 **Lymphoid leukemia, unspecified, in remission**   HCC

C91.92 **Lymphoid leukemia, unspecified, in relapse**   HCC

√4ᵗʰ **C92** **Myeloid leukemia**

INCLUDES   granulocytic leukemia
                myelogenous leukemia

EXCLUDES 1   *personal history of leukemia (Z85.6)*

AHA: 2019,1Q,16

DEF: Cancer that develops in immature myelocytes called myeloblasts. These are the cells that become white blood cells (except lymphocytes), red blood cells, or platelet making cells. Can be acute (AML) or chronic (CML).

TIP: Pancytopenia, although common in some types of myeloid leukemia's, is not always inherent. When it is documented, code D61.818 can be assigned in addition to a code from this category.

√5ᵗʰ **C92.Ø** **Acute myeloblastic leukemia**

Acute myeloblastic leukemia, minimal differentiation
Acute myeloblastic leukemia (with maturation)
Acute myeloblastic leukemia 1/ETO
Acute myeloblastic leukemia MØ
Acute myeloblastic leukemia M1
Acute myeloblastic leukemia M2
Acute myeloblastic leukemia with t(8;21)
Acute myeloblastic leukemia (without a FAB classification) NOS
Refractory anemia with excess blasts in transformation [RAEBT]

EXCLUDES 1   *acute exacerbation of chronic myeloid leukemia (C92.1Ø)*
              refractory anemia with excess of blasts not in transformation (D46.2-)

AHA: 2018,4Q,87

C92.ØØ **Acute myeloblastic leukemia,** not having achieved remission   HCC

Acute myeloblastic leukemia with failed remission
Acute myeloblastic leukemia NOS

C92.Ø1 **Acute myeloblastic leukemia, in remission**   HCC

C92.Ø2 **Acute myeloblastic leukemia, in relapse**   HCC

√5ᵗʰ **C92.1** **Chronic myeloid leukemia, BCR/ABL-positive**

Chronic myelogenous leukemia, Philadelphia chromosome (Ph1) positive
Chronic myelogenous leukemia, t(9;22) (q34;q11)
Chronic myelogenous leukemia with crisis of blast cells

EXCLUDES 1   *atypical chronic myeloid leukemia BCR/ABL-negative (C92.2-)*
              chronic myelomonocytic leukemia (C93.1-)
              chronic myeloproliferative disease (D47.1)

C92.1Ø **Chronic myeloid leukemia, BCR/ABL-positive,** not having achieved remission   HCC

Chronic myeloid leukemia, BCR/ABL-positive with failed remission
Chronic myeloid leukemia, BCR/ABL-positive NOS

C92.11 **Chronic myeloid leukemia, BCR/ABL-positive, in remission**   HCC

C92.12 **Chronic myeloid leukemia, BCR/ABL-positive, in relapse**   HCC

√5ᵗʰ **C92.2** **Atypical chronic myeloid leukemia, BCR/ABL-negative**

C92.2Ø **Atypical chronic myeloid leukemia, BCR/ABL-negative,** not having achieved remission   HCC

Atypical chronic myeloid leukemia, BCR/ABL-negative with failed remission
Atypical chronic myeloid leukemia, BCR/ABL-negative NOS

C92.21 **Atypical chronic myeloid leukemia, BCR/ABL-negative, in remission**   HCC

C92.22 **Atypical chronic myeloid leukemia, BCR/ABL-negative, in relapse**   HCC

√5ᵗʰ **C92.3** **Myeloid sarcoma**

A malignant tumor of immature myeloid cells
Chloroma
Granulocytic sarcoma

C92.3Ø **Myeloid sarcoma,** not having achieved remission   HCC

Myeloid sarcoma with failed remission
Myeloid sarcoma NOS

C92.31 **Myeloid sarcoma, in remission**   HCC

C92.32 **Myeloid sarcoma, in relapse**   HCC

√5ᵗʰ **C92.4** **Acute promyelocytic leukemia**

AML M3
AML Me with t(15;17) and variants

C92.4Ø **Acute promyelocytic leukemia,** not having achieved remission   HCC

Acute promyelocytic leukemia with failed remission
Acute promyelocytic leukemia NOS

C92.41 **Acute promyelocytic leukemia, in remission**   HCC

C92.42 **Acute promyelocytic leukemia, in relapse**   HCC

√5ᵗʰ **C92.5** **Acute myelomonocytic leukemia**

AML M4
AML M4 Eo with inv(16) or t(16;16)

C92.5Ø **Acute myelomonocytic leukemia,** not having achieved remission   HCC

Acute myelomonocytic leukemia with failed remission
Acute myelomonocytic leukemia NOS

C92.51 **Acute myelomonocytic leukemia, in remission**   HCC

C92.52 **Acute myelomonocytic leukemia, in relapse**   HCC

√5ᵗʰ **C92.6** **Acute myeloid leukemia with 11q23-abnormality**

Acute myeloid leukemia with variation of MLL-gene

C92.6Ø **Acute myeloid leukemia with 11q23-abnormality** not having achieved remission   HCC

Acute myeloid leukemia with 11q23-abnormality with failed remission
Acute myeloid leukemia with 11q23-abnormality NOS

C92.61 **Acute myeloid leukemia with 11q23-abnormality** in remission   HCC

C92.62 **Acute myeloid leukemia with 11q23-abnormality** in relapse   HCC

√5ᵗʰ **C92.A** **Acute myeloid leukemia with multilineage dysplasia**

Acute myeloid leukemia with dysplasia of remaining hematopoesis and/or myelodysplastic disease in its history

C92.AØ **Acute myeloid leukemia with multilineage dysplasia,** not having achieved remission   HCC

Acute myeloid leukemia with multilineage dysplasia with failed remission
Acute myeloid leukemia with multilineage dysplasia NOS

C92.A1 **Acute myeloid leukemia with multilineage dysplasia, in remission**   HCC

C92.A2 **Acute myeloid leukemia with multilineage dysplasia, in relapse**   HCC

√5ᵗʰ **C92.Z** **Other myeloid leukemia**

C92.ZØ **Other myeloid leukemia** not having achieved remission   HCC

Myeloid leukemia NEC with failed remission
Myeloid leukemia NEC

C92.Z1 **Other myeloid leukemia, in remission**   HCC

C92.Z2 **Other myeloid leukemia, in relapse**   HCC

N Newborn: 0   P Pediatric: 0-17   M Maternity: 9-64   A Adult: 15-124   MCC Major Complication/Comorbidity   CC Complication/Comorbidity   SW Severe Wound Dx

488   ICD-10-CM 2020

✓5ᵗʰ **C92.9 Myeloid leukemia, unspecified**

C92.90 Myeloid leukemia, unspecified, not HCC
having achieved remission
Myeloid leukemia, unspecified with failed remission
Myeloid leukemia, unspecified NOS

C92.91 Myeloid leukemia, unspecified in HCC
remission

C92.92 Myeloid leukemia, unspecified in relapse HCC

✓4ᵗʰ **C93 Monocytic leukemia**

INCLUDES   monocytoid leukemia
EXCLUDES 1   personal history of leukemia (Z85.6)

✓5ᵗʰ **C93.0 Acute monoblastic/monocytic leukemia**

AML M5
AML M5a
AML M5b

C93.00 Acute monoblastic/monocytic leukemia, HCC
not having achieved remission
Acute monoblastic/monocytic leukemia with failed
remission
Acute monoblastic/monocytic leukemia NOS

C93.01 Acute monoblastic/monocytic leukemia, HCC
in remission

C93.02 Acute monoblastic/monocytic leukemia, HCC
in relapse

✓5ᵗʰ **C93.1 Chronic myelomonocytic leukemia**

Chronic monocytic leukemia
CMML-1
CMML-2
CMML with eosinophilia

C93.10 Chronic myelomonocytic leukemia not HCC
having achieved remission
Chronic myelomonocytic leukemia with failed
remission
Chronic myelomonocytic leukemia NOS

C93.11 Chronic myelomonocytic leukemia, in HCC
remission

C93.12 Chronic myelomonocytic leukemia, in HCC
relapse

✓5ᵗʰ **C93.3 Juvenile myelomonocytic leukemia**

C93.30 Juvenile myelomonocytic leukemia, not HCC P
having achieved remission
Juvenile myelomonocytic leukemia with failed
remission
Juvenile myelomonocytic leukemia NOS

C93.31 Juvenile myelomonocytic leukemia, in HCC P
remission

C93.32 Juvenile myelomonocytic leukemia, in HCC P
relapse

✓5ᵗʰ **C93.Z Other monocytic leukemia**

C93.Z0 Other monocytic leukemia, not having HCC
achieved remission
Other monocytic leukemia NOS

C93.Z1 Other monocytic leukemia, in remission HCC

C93.Z2 Other monocytic leukemia, in relapse HCC

✓5ᵗʰ **C93.9 Monocytic leukemia, unspecified**

C93.90 Monocytic leukemia, unspecified, not HCC
having achieved remission
Monocytic leukemia, unspecified with failed remission
Monocytic leukemia, unspecified NOS

C93.91 Monocytic leukemia, unspecified in HCC
remission

C93.92 Monocytic leukemia, unspecified in HCC
relapse

✓4ᵗʰ **C94 Other leukemias of specified cell type**

EXCLUDES 1   leukemic reticuloendotheliosis (C91.4-)
myelodysplastic syndromes (D46.-)
personal history of leukemia (Z85.6)
plasma cell leukemia (C90.1-)

✓5ᵗʰ **C94.0 Acute erythroid leukemia**

Acute myeloid leukemia M6(a)(b)
Erythroleukemia
DEF: Erythroleukemia: Malignant blood dyscrasia (a
myeloproliferative disorder).

C94.00 Acute erythroid leukemia, not having HCC
achieved remission
Acute erythroid leukemia with failed remission
Acute erythroid leukemia NOS

C94.01 Acute erythroid leukemia, in remission HCC

C94.02 Acute erythroid leukemia, in relapse HCC

✓5ᵗʰ **C94.2 Acute megakaryoblastic leukemia**

Acute myeloid leukemia M7
Acute megakaryocytic leukemia

C94.20 Acute megakaryoblastic leukemia not HCC
having achieved remission
Acute megakaryoblastic leukemia with failed
remission
Acute megakaryoblastic leukemia NOS

C94.21 Acute megakaryoblastic leukemia, in HCC
remission

C94.22 Acute megakaryoblastic leukemia, in HCC
relapse

✓5ᵗʰ **C94.3 Mast cell leukemia**

AHA: 2017,4Q,5

C94.30 Mast cell leukemia not having achieved HCC
remission
Mast cell leukemia with failed remission
Mast cell leukemia NOS

C94.31 Mast cell leukemia, in remission HCC

C94.32 Mast cell leukemia, in relapse HCC

✓5ᵗʰ **C94.4 Acute panmyelosis with myelofibrosis**

Acute myelofibrosis
EXCLUDES 1   myelofibrosis NOS (D75.81)
secondary myelofibrosis NOS (D75.81)

C94.40 Acute panmyelosis with myelofibrosis HCC
not having achieved remission
Acute myelofibrosis NOS
Acute panmyelosis with myelofibrosis with failed
remission
Acute panmyelosis NOS

C94.41 Acute panmyelosis with myelofibrosis, HCC
in remission

C94.42 Acute panmyelosis with myelofibrosis, HCC
in relapse

C94.6 Myelodysplastic disease, not classified HCC
Myeloproliferative disease, not classified

✓5ᵗʰ **C94.8 Other specified leukemias**

Aggressive NK-cell leukemia
Acute basophilic leukemia

C94.80 Other specified leukemias not having HCC
achieved remission
Other specified leukemia with failed remission
Other specified leukemias NOS

C94.81 Other specified leukemias, in remission HCC

C94.82 Other specified leukemias, in relapse HCC

Chapter 2. Neoplasms

✓4ᵗʰ **C95 Leukemia of unspecified** cell type

    EXCLUDES 1   *personal history of leukemia (Z85.6)*

  ✓5ᵗʰ **C95.0 Acute leukemia of unspecified cell type**

      Acute bilineal leukemia

      Acute mixed lineage leukemia

      Biphenotypic acute leukemia

      Stem cell leukemia of unclear lineage

      EXCLUDES 1   *acute exacerbation of unspecified chronic leukemia (C95.10)*

    C95.00 Acute leukemia of unspecified cell type not having achieved remission HCC

      Acute leukemia of unspecified cell type with failed remission

      Acute leukemia NOS

    C95.01 Acute leukemia of unspecified cell type, in remission HCC

    C95.02 Acute leukemia of unspecified cell type, in relapse HCC

  ✓5ᵗʰ **C95.1 Chronic leukemia of unspecified cell type**

    C95.10 Chronic leukemia of unspecified cell type not having achieved remission HCC

      Chronic leukemia of unspecified cell type with failed remission

      Chronic leukemia NOS

    C95.11 Chronic leukemia of unspecified cell type, in remission HCC

    C95.12 Chronic leukemia of unspecified cell type, in relapse HCC

  ✓5ᵗʰ **C95.9 Leukemia, unspecified**

    C95.90 Leukemia, unspecified not having achieved remission HCC

      Leukemia, unspecified with failed remission

      Leukemia NOS

    C95.91 Leukemia, unspecified, in remission HCC

    C95.92 Leukemia, unspecified, in relapse HCC

✓4ᵗʰ **C96 Other and unspecified malignant neoplasms of lymphoid, hematopoietic and related tissue**

    EXCLUDES 1   *personal history of other malignant neoplasms of lymphoid, hematopoietic and related tissues (Z85.79)*

  C96.0 Multifocal and multisystemic (disseminated) Langerhans-cell histiocytosis HCC

    Histiocytosis X, multisystemic

    Letterer-Siwe disease

    EXCLUDES 1   *adult pulmonary Langerhans cell histiocytosis (J84.82)*

        multifocal and unisystemic Langerhans-cell histiocytosis (C96.5)

        unifocal Langerhans-cell histiocytosis (C96.6)

  ✓5ᵗʰ **C96.2 Malignant mast cell neoplasm**

    EXCLUDES 1   *indolent mastocytosis (D47.02)*

        mast cell leukemia (C94.30)

        mastocytosis (congenital) (cutaneous) (Q82.2)

    AHA: 2017,4Q,5

    DEF: Mast cell: Type of white blood cell found in the loose connective tissue of blood vessels and bronchioles responsible for acute hypersensitivity reactions, including anaphylactic shock. The IgE receptors on these cells bind with allergens causing cell degranulation and diffuse, widespread histamine release that results in airway constriction and vasodilation with decreased systemic blood pressure.

    C96.20 Malignant mast cell neoplasm, unspecified HCC

    C96.21 Aggressive systemic mastocytosis HCC

    C96.22 Mast cell sarcoma HCC

    C96.29 Other malignant mast cell neoplasm HCC

  C96.4 Sarcoma of dendritic cells (accessory cells) HCC

    Follicular dendritic cell sarcoma

    Interdigitating dendritic cell sarcoma

    Langerhans cell sarcoma

  C96.5 Multifocal and unisystemic Langerhans-cell histiocytosis HCC

    Hand-Schüller-Christian disease

    Histiocytosis X, multifocal

    EXCLUDES 1   *multifocal and multisystemic (disseminated) Langerhans-cell histiocytosis (C96.0)*

        unifocal Langerhans-cell histiocytosis (C96.6)

  C96.6 Unifocal Langerhans-cell histiocytosis HCC

    Eosinophilic granuloma

    Histiocytosis X, unifocal

    Histiocytosis X NOS

    Langerhans-cell histiocytosis NOS

    EXCLUDES 1   *multifocal and multisysemic (disseminated) Langerhans-cell histiocytosis (C96.0)*

        multifocal and unisystemic Langerhans-cell histiocytosis (C96.5)

  C96.A Histiocytic sarcoma HCC

    Malignant histiocytosis

  C96.Z Other specified malignant neoplasms of lymphoid, hematopoietic and related tissue HCC

  C96.9 Malignant neoplasm of lymphoid, hematopoietic and related tissue, unspecified HCC

In situ neoplasms (D00-D09)

INCLUDES   Bowen's disease

           erythroplasia

           grade III intraepithelial neoplasia

           Queyrat's erythroplasia

✓4ᵗʰ **D00 Carcinoma in situ of** oral cavity, esophagus and stomach

    EXCLUDES 1   *melanoma in situ (D03.-)*

  ✓5ᵗʰ **D00.0 Carcinoma in situ of lip, oral cavity and pharynx**

    Use additional code to identify:

      exposure to environmental tobacco smoke (Z77.22)

      exposure to tobacco smoke in the perinatal period (P96.81)

      history of tobacco dependence (Z87.891)

      occupational exposure to environmental tobacco smoke (Z57.31)

      tobacco dependence (F17.-)

      tobacco use (Z72.0)

    EXCLUDES 1   *carcinoma in situ of aryepiglottic fold or interarytenoid fold, laryngeal aspect (D02.0)*

        carcinoma in situ of epiglottis NOS (D02.0)

        carcinoma in situ of epiglottis suprahyoid portion (D02.0)

        carcinoma in situ of skin of lip (D03.0, D04.0)

    D00.00 Carcinoma in situ of oral cavity, unspecified site

    D00.01 Carcinoma in situ of labial mucosa and vermilion border

    D00.02 Carcinoma in situ of buccal mucosa

    D00.03 Carcinoma in situ of gingiva and edentulous alveolar ridge

    D00.04 Carcinoma in situ of soft palate

    D00.05 Carcinoma in situ of hard palate

    D00.06 Carcinoma in situ of floor of mouth

    D00.07 Carcinoma in situ of tongue

    D00.08 Carcinoma in situ of pharynx

      Carcinoma in situ of aryepiglottic fold NOS

      Carcinoma in situ of hypopharyngeal aspect of aryepiglottic fold

      Carcinoma in situ of marginal zone of aryepiglottic fold

  D00.1 Carcinoma in situ of esophagus

  D00.2 Carcinoma in situ of stomach

✓4ᵗʰ **D01 Carcinoma in situ of other and unspecified digestive organs**

    EXCLUDES 1   *melanoma in situ (D03.-)*

  D01.0 Carcinoma in situ of colon

    EXCLUDES 1   *carcinoma in situ of rectosigmoid junction (D01.1)*

  D01.1 Carcinoma in situ of rectosigmoid junction

  D01.2 Carcinoma in situ of rectum

  D01.3 Carcinoma in situ of anus and anal canal

    Anal intraepithelial neoplasia III [AIN III]

    Severe dysplasia of anus

    EXCLUDES 1   *anal intraepithelial neoplasia I and II [AIN I and AIN II] (K62.82)*

        carcinoma in situ of anal margin (D04.5)

        carcinoma in situ of anal skin (D04.5)

        carcinoma in situ of perianal skin (D04.5)

  ✓5ᵗʰ **D01.4 Carcinoma in situ of other and unspecified parts of intestine**

    EXCLUDES 1   *carcinoma in situ of ampulla of Vater (D01.5)*

    D01.40 Carcinoma in situ of unspecified part of intestine

    D01.49 Carcinoma in situ of other parts of intestine

D01.5 **Carcinoma in situ of** liver, gallbladder and bile ducts
     Carcinoma in situ of ampulla of Vater

D01.7 **Carcinoma in situ of other specified digestive organs**
     Carcinoma in situ of pancreas

D01.9 **Carcinoma in situ of digestive organ, unspecified**

✓4ᵗʰ **D02** **Carcinoma in situ of** middle ear and respiratory system
     Use additional code to identify:
       exposure to environmental tobacco smoke (Z77.22)
       exposure to tobacco smoke in the perinatal period (P96.81)
       history of tobacco dependence (Z87.891)
       occupational exposure to environmental tobacco smoke (Z57.31)
       tobacco dependence (F17.-)
       tobacco use (Z72.0)
     EXCLUDES 1   *melanoma in situ (D03.-)*

D02.0 **Carcinoma in situ of** larynx
     Carcinoma in situ of aryepiglottic fold or interarytenoid fold,
       laryngeal aspect
     Carcinoma in situ of epiglottis (suprahyoid portion)
     EXCLUDES 1   *carcinoma in situ of aryepiglottic fold or*
               interarytenoid fold NOS (D00.08)
               carcinoma in situ of hypopharyngeal aspect (D00.08)
               carcinoma in situ of marginal zone (D00.08)

D02.1 **Carcinoma in situ of** trachea

✓5ᵗʰ **D02.2** **Carcinoma in situ of** bronchus and lung

     D02.20 **Carcinoma in situ of unspecified bronchus and lung**
     D02.21 **Carcinoma in situ of** right **bronchus and lung**
     D02.22 **Carcinoma in situ of** left **bronchus and lung**

D02.3 **Carcinoma in situ of other parts of respiratory system**
     Carcinoma in situ of accessory sinuses
     Carcinoma in situ of middle ear
     Carcinoma in situ of nasal cavities
     EXCLUDES 1   *carcinoma in situ of ear (external) (skin) (D04.2-)*
               carcinoma in situ of nose NOS (D09.8)
               carcinoma in situ of skin of nose (D04.3)

D02.4 **Carcinoma in situ of respiratory system, unspecified**

✓4ᵗʰ **D03** **Melanoma in situ**

D03.0 **Melanoma in situ of** lip   HCC

✓5ᵗʰ **D03.1** **Melanoma in situ of** eyelid, including canthus
     AHA: 2018,4Q,4

     D03.10 **Melanoma in situ of unspecified eyelid,**   HCC
             including canthus

   ✓6ᵗʰ **D03.11** **Melanoma in situ of** right **eyelid, including canthus**
         D03.111 **Melanoma in situ of right**   HCC
                upper eyelid, including
                canthus
         D03.112 **Melanoma in situ of right** lower   HCC
                eyelid, including canthus

   ✓6ᵗʰ **D03.12** **Melanoma in situ of** left **eyelid, including canthus**
         D03.121 **Melanoma in situ of left** upper   HCC
                eyelid, including canthus
         D03.122 **Melanoma in situ of left** lower   HCC
                eyelid, including canthus

✓5ᵗʰ **D03.2** **Melanoma in situ of** ear and external auricular canal

     D03.20 **Melanoma in situ of unspecified ear and**   HCC
             external auricular canal
     D03.21 **Melanoma in situ of** right **ear and**   HCC
             external auricular canal
     D03.22 **Melanoma in situ of** left **ear and external**   HCC
             auricular canal

✓5ᵗʰ **D03.3** **Melanoma in situ of other and unspecified parts of** face

     D03.30 **Melanoma in situ of unspecified part of**   HCC
             face
     D03.39 **Melanoma in situ of other parts of face**

D03.4 **Melanoma in situ of** scalp and neck   HCC

✓5ᵗʰ **D03.5** **Melanoma in situ of** trunk

     D03.51 **Melanoma in situ of** anal skin   HCC
         Melanoma in situ of anal margin
         Melanoma in situ of perianal skin
     D03.52 **Melanoma in situ of** breast (skin) (soft   HCC
             tissue)
     D03.59 **Melanoma in situ of other part of trunk**   HCC

✓5ᵗʰ **D03.6** **Melanoma in situ of** upper limb, including shoulder

     D03.60 **Melanoma in situ of unspecified upper**   HCC
             limb, including shoulder

     D03.61 **Melanoma in situ of** right **upper limb,**   HCC
             including shoulder
     D03.62 **Melanoma in situ of** left **upper limb,**   HCC
             including shoulder

✓5ᵗʰ **D03.7** **Melanoma in situ of** lower limb, including hip

     D03.70 **Melanoma in situ of unspecified lower**   HCC
             limb, including hip
     D03.71 **Melanoma in situ of** right **lower limb,**   HCC
             including hip
     D03.72 **Melanoma in situ of** left **lower limb,**   HCC
             including hip

D03.8 **Melanoma in situ of other sites**   HCC
     Melanoma in situ of scrotum
     EXCLUDES 1   *carcinoma in situ of scrotum (D07.61)*

D03.9 **Melanoma in situ, unspecified**   HCC

✓4ᵗʰ **D04** **Carcinoma in situ of** skin
     EXCLUDES 1   *erythroplasia of Queyrat (penis) NOS (D07.4)*
               melanoma in situ (D03.-)

D04.0 **Carcinoma in situ of skin of** lip
     EXCLUDES 1   *carcinoma in situ of vermilion border of lip (D00.01)*
     EXCLUDES 2   ▶*carcinoma in situ of vermilion border of lip (D00.01)*◀

✓5ᵗʰ **D04.1** **Carcinoma in situ of skin of** eyelid, including canthus
     AHA: 2018,4Q,4

     D04.10 **Carcinoma in situ of skin of unspecified eyelid,**
             including canthus

   ✓6ᵗʰ **D04.11** **Carcinoma in situ of skin of** right **eyelid, including**
             canthus
         D04.111 **Carcinoma in situ of skin of right** upper
                eyelid, including canthus
         D04.112 **Carcinoma in situ of skin of right** lower
                eyelid, including canthus

   ✓6ᵗʰ **D04.12** **Carcinoma in situ of skin of** left **eyelid, including**
             canthus
         D04.121 **Carcinoma in situ of skin of left** upper
                eyelid, including canthus
         D04.122 **Carcinoma in situ of skin of left** lower
                eyelid, including canthus

✓5ᵗʰ **D04.2** **Carcinoma in situ of skin of** ear and external auricular canal

     D04.20 **Carcinoma in situ of skin of unspecified ear and**
             external auricular canal
     D04.21 **Carcinoma in situ of skin of** right **ear and external**
             auricular canal
     D04.22 **Carcinoma in situ of skin of** left **ear and external**
             auricular canal

✓5ᵗʰ **D04.3** **Carcinoma in situ of skin of other and unspecified** parts of
     face
     D04.30 **Carcinoma in situ of skin of unspecified part of face**
     D04.39 **Carcinoma in situ of skin of other parts of face**

D04.4 **Carcinoma in situ of skin of** scalp and neck

D04.5 **Carcinoma in situ of skin of** trunk
     Carcinoma in situ of anal margin
     Carcinoma in situ of anal skin
     Carcinoma in situ of perianal skin
     Carcinoma in situ of skin of breast
     EXCLUDES 1   *carcinoma in situ of anus NOS (D01.3)*
               carcinoma in situ of scrotum (D07.61)
               carcinoma in situ of skin of genital organs (D07.-)

✓5ᵗʰ **D04.6** **Carcinoma in situ of skin of** upper limb, including shoulder

     D04.60 **Carcinoma in situ of skin of unspecified upper limb,**
             including shoulder
     D04.61 **Carcinoma in situ of skin of** right **upper limb,**
             including shoulder
     D04.62 **Carcinoma in situ of skin of** left **upper limb,**
             including shoulder

✓5ᵗʰ **D04.7** **Carcinoma in situ of skin of** lower limb, including hip

     D04.70 **Carcinoma in situ of skin of unspecified lower limb,**
             including hip
     D04.71 **Carcinoma in situ of skin of** right **lower limb,**
             including hip
     D04.72 **Carcinoma in situ of skin of** left **lower limb,**
             including hip

D04.8 **Carcinoma in situ of skin of other sites**

D04.9 **Carcinoma in situ of skin, unspecified**

☑ Additional Character Required   ✓ₓ7ᵗʰ Placeholder   <u>Unacceptable PDx</u>   Questionable PDx   Manifestation   Unspecified Dx   H1 - H1d HAC   HCC CMS-HCC Dx   HIV HIV Dx

Chapter 2. Neoplasms

✓4th **D05 Carcinoma in situ of breast**

    EXCLUDES 1   *carcinoma in situ of skin of breast (D04.5)*
            melanoma in situ of breast (skin) (D03.5)
            Paget's disease of breast or nipple (C50.-)

  ✓5th **D05.0 Lobular carcinoma in situ of breast**
    D05.00 Lobular carcinoma in situ of unspecified breast
    D05.01 Lobular carcinoma in situ of right breast
    D05.02 Lobular carcinoma in situ of left breast

  ✓5th **D05.1 Intraductal carcinoma in situ of breast**
    D05.10 Intraductal carcinoma in situ of unspecified breast
    D05.11 Intraductal carcinoma in situ of right breast
    D05.12 Intraductal carcinoma in situ of left breast

  ✓5th **D05.8 Other specified type of carcinoma in situ of breast**
    D05.80 Other specified type of carcinoma in situ of unspecified breast
    D05.81 Other specified type of carcinoma in situ of right breast
    D05.82 Other specified type of carcinoma in situ of left breast

  ✓5th **D05.9 Unspecified type of carcinoma in situ of breast**
    D05.90 Unspecified type of carcinoma in situ of unspecified breast
    D05.91 Unspecified type of carcinoma in situ of right breast
    D05.92 Unspecified type of carcinoma in situ of left breast

✓4th **D06 Carcinoma in situ of cervix uteri**

    INCLUDES   cervical adenocarcinoma in situ
            cervical intraepithelial glandular neoplasia
            cervical intraepithelial neoplasia III [CIN III]
            severe dysplasia of cervix uteri

    EXCLUDES 1   *cervical intraepithelial neoplasia II [CIN II] (N87.1)*
            cytologic evidence of malignancy of cervix without histologic confirmation (R87.614)
            high grade squamous intraepithelial lesion (HGSIL) of cervix (R87.613)
            melanoma in situ of cervix (D03.5)
            moderate cervical dysplasia (N87.1)

  D06.0 Carcinoma in situ of endocervix ♀
  D06.1 Carcinoma in situ of exocervix ♀
  D06.7 Carcinoma in situ of other parts of cervix ♀
  D06.9 Carcinoma in situ of cervix, unspecified ♀

✓4th **D07 Carcinoma in situ of other and unspecified genital organs**

    EXCLUDES 1   *melanoma in situ of trunk (D03.5)*

  D07.0 Carcinoma in situ of endometrium ♀
  D07.1 Carcinoma in situ of vulva ♀
    Severe dysplasia of vulva
    Vulvar intraepithelial neoplasia III [VIN III]
    EXCLUDES 1   *moderate dysplasia of vulva (N90.1)*
            vulvar intraepithelial neoplasia II [VIN II] (N90.1)

  D07.2 Carcinoma in situ of vagina ♀
    Severe dysplasia of vagina
    Vaginal intraepithelial neoplasia III [VAIN III]
    EXCLUDES 1   *moderate dysplasia of vagina (N89.1)*
            vaginal intraepithelial neoplasia II [VIN II] (N89.1)

  ✓5th **D07.3 Carcinoma in situ of other and unspecified female genital organs**
    D07.30 Carcinoma in situ of unspecified female genital organs ♀
    D07.39 Carcinoma in situ of other female genital organs ♀

  D07.4 Carcinoma in situ of penis ♂
    Erythroplasia of Queyrat NOS

  D07.5 Carcinoma in situ of prostate ♂
    Prostatic intraepithelial neoplasia III (PIN III)
    Severe dysplasia of prostate
    EXCLUDES 1   *dysplasia (mild) (moderate) of prostate (N42.3-)*
            prostatic intraepithelial neoplasia II [PIN II] (N42.3-)

  ✓5th **D07.6 Carcinoma in situ of other and unspecified male genital organs**
    D07.60 Carcinoma in situ of unspecified male genital organs ♂
    D07.61 Carcinoma in situ of scrotum ♂
    D07.69 Carcinoma in situ of other male genital organs ♂

✓4th **D09 Carcinoma in situ of other and unspecified sites**

    EXCLUDES 1   *melanoma in situ (D03.-)*

  D09.0 Carcinoma in situ of bladder

  ✓5th **D09.1 Carcinoma in situ of other and unspecified urinary organs**
    D09.10 Carcinoma in situ of unspecified urinary organ
    D09.19 Carcinoma in situ of other urinary organs

  ✓5th **D09.2 Carcinoma in situ of eye**
    EXCLUDES 1   *carcinoma in situ of skin of eyelid (D04.1-)*
    D09.20 Carcinoma in situ of unspecified eye
    D09.21 Carcinoma in situ of right eye
    D09.22 Carcinoma in situ of left eye

  D09.3 Carcinoma in situ of thyroid and other endocrine glands
    EXCLUDES 1   *carcinoma in situ of endocrine pancreas (D01.7)*
            carcinoma in situ of ovary (D07.39)
            carcinoma in situ of testis (D07.69)

  D09.8 Carcinoma in situ of other specified sites
  D09.9 Carcinoma in situ, unspecified

Benign neoplasms, except benign neuroendocrine tumors (D10-D36)

✓4th **D10 Benign neoplasm of mouth and pharynx**

  D10.0 Benign neoplasm of lip
    Benign neoplasm of lip (frenulum) (inner aspect) (mucosa) (vermilion border)
    EXCLUDES 1   *benign neoplasm of skin of lip (D22.0, D23.0)*

  D10.1 Benign neoplasm of tongue
    Benign neoplasm of lingual tonsil

  D10.2 Benign neoplasm of floor of mouth

  ✓5th **D10.3 Benign neoplasm of other and unspecified parts of mouth**
    D10.30 Benign neoplasm of unspecified part of mouth
    D10.39 Benign neoplasm of other parts of mouth
      Benign neoplasm of minor salivary gland NOS
      EXCLUDES 1   *benign odontogenic neoplasms (D16.4-D16.5)*
            benign neoplasm of mucosa of lip (D10.0)
            benign neoplasm of nasopharyngeal surface of soft palate (D10.6)

  D10.4 Benign neoplasm of tonsil
    Benign neoplasm of tonsil (faucial) (palatine)
    EXCLUDES 1   *benign neoplasm of lingual tonsil (D10.1)*
            benign neoplasm of pharyngeal tonsil (D10.6)
            benign neoplasm of tonsillar fossa (D10.5)
            benign neoplasm of tonsillar pillars (D10.5)

  D10.5 Benign neoplasm of other parts of oropharynx
    Benign neoplasm of epiglottis, anterior aspect
    Benign neoplasm of tonsillar fossa
    Benign neoplasm of tonsillar pillars
    Benign neoplasm of vallecula
    EXCLUDES 1   *benign neoplasm of epiglottis NOS (D14.1)*
            benign neoplasm of epiglottis, suprahyoid portion (D14.1)
    DEF: Oropharynx: Middle portion of pharynx (throat); communicates with the oral cavity, nasopharynx and laryngopharynx.

  D10.6 Benign neoplasm of nasopharynx
    Benign neoplasm of pharyngeal tonsil
    Benign neoplasm of posterior margin of septum and choanae
    DEF: Nasopharynx: Upper portion of pharynx (throat); communicates with the nasal cavities, oropharynx and tympanic cavities.

  D10.7 Benign neoplasm of hypopharynx
    DEF: Hypopharynx: Lower portion of pharynx (throat); communicates with the oropharynx and the esophagus.
    Synonyms: *laryngopharynx.*

  D10.9 Benign neoplasm of pharynx, unspecified

✓4th **D11 Benign neoplasm of major salivary glands**

    EXCLUDES 1   *benign neoplasms of specified minor salivary glands which are classified according to their anatomical location*
            benign neoplasms of minor salivary glands NOS (D10.39)

  D11.0 Benign neoplasm of parotid gland

  D11.7 Benign neoplasm of other major salivary glands
    Benign neoplasm of sublingual salivary gland
    Benign neoplasm of submandibular salivary gland

  D11.9 Benign neoplasm of major salivary gland, unspecified

N Newborn: 0   P Pediatric: 0-17   M Maternity: 9-64   A Adult: 15-124   MCC Major Complication/Comorbidity   CC Complication/Comorbidity   SW Severe Wound Dx

492   ICD-10-CM 2020

✓4ᵗʰ **D12 Benign neoplasm of colon, rectum, anus and anal canal**

     EXCLUDES 1   *benign carcinoid tumors of the large intestine, and rectum (D3A.Ø2-)*

         ▶*polyp of colon NOS (K63.5)*◀

     AHA: 2018,2Q,14; 2017,1Q,15; 2015,2Q,14

     TIP: Code K63.5 Polyp of colon, is assigned when documentation states hyperplastic colon polyps, regardless of the site in the colon. Slow-growing, hyperplastic polyps are not precancerous and are classified differently from benign or adenomatous polyps.

   D12.Ø Benign neoplasm of cecum
     Benign neoplasm of ileocecal valve

   D12.1 Benign neoplasm of appendix
     EXCLUDES 1   *benign carcinoid tumor of the appendix (D3A.Ø20)*

   D12.2 Benign neoplasm of ascending colon

   D12.3 Benign neoplasm of transverse colon
     Benign neoplasm of hepatic flexure
     Benign neoplasm of splenic flexure
     AHA: 2017,1Q,16

   D12.4 Benign neoplasm of descending colon

   D12.5 Benign neoplasm of sigmoid colon

   D12.6 Benign neoplasm of colon, unspecified
     Adenomatosis of colon
     Benign neoplasm of large intestine NOS
     Polyposis (hereditary) of colon
     EXCLUDES 1   *inflammatory polyp of colon (K51.4-)*
         polyp of colon NOS (K63.5)

   D12.7 Benign neoplasm of rectosigmoid junction

   D12.8 Benign neoplasm of rectum
     EXCLUDES 1   *benign carcinoid tumor of the rectum (D3A.Ø26)*
     AHA: 2018,1Q,6

   D12.9 Benign neoplasm of anus and anal canal
     Benign neoplasm of anus NOS
     EXCLUDES 1   *benign neoplasm of anal margin (D22.5, D23.5)*
         benign neoplasm of anal skin (D22.5, D23.5)
         benign neoplasm of perianal skin (D22.5, D23.5)

✓4ᵗʰ **D13 Benign neoplasm of other and ill-defined parts of digestive system**

     EXCLUDES 1   *benign stromal tumors of digestive system (D21.4)*

   D13.Ø Benign neoplasm of esophagus

   D13.1 Benign neoplasm of stomach
     EXCLUDES 1   *benign carcinoid tumor of the stomach (D3A.Ø92)*

   D13.2 Benign neoplasm of duodenum
     EXCLUDES 1   *benign carcinoid tumor of the duodenum (D3A.Ø1Ø)*

✓5ᵗʰ **D13.3 Benign neoplasm of other and unspecified parts of small intestine**
     EXCLUDES 1   *benign carcinoid tumors of the small intestine (D3A.Ø1-)*
         benign neoplasm of ileocecal valve (D12.Ø)

     D13.3Ø Benign neoplasm of unspecified part of small intestine

     D13.39 Benign neoplasm of other parts of small intestine

   D13.4 Benign neoplasm of liver
     Benign neoplasm of intrahepatic bile ducts

   D13.5 Benign neoplasm of extrahepatic bile ducts

   D13.6 Benign neoplasm of pancreas
     EXCLUDES 1   *benign neoplasm of endocrine pancreas (D13.7)*

   D13.7 Benign neoplasm of endocrine pancreas
     Benign neoplasm of islets of Langerhans
     Islet cell tumor
     Use additional code to identify any functional activity

   D13.9 Benign neoplasm of ill-defined sites within the digestive system
     Benign neoplasm of digestive system NOS
     Benign neoplasm of intestine NOS
     Benign neoplasm of spleen

✓4ᵗʰ **D14 Benign neoplasm of middle ear and respiratory system**

   D14.Ø Benign neoplasm of middle ear, nasal cavity and accessory sinuses
     Benign neoplasm of cartilage of nose
     EXCLUDES 1   *benign neoplasm of auricular canal (external) (D22.2-, D23.2-)*
         benign neoplasm of bone of ear (D16.4)
         benign neoplasm of bone of nose (D16.4)
         benign neoplasm of cartilage of ear (D21.Ø)
         benign neoplasm of ear (external)(skin) (D22.2-, D23.2-)
         benign neoplasm of nose NOS (D36.7)
         benign neoplasm of skin of nose (D22.39, D23.39)
         benign neoplasm of olfactory bulb (D33.3)
         benign neoplasm of posterior margin of septum and choanae (D1Ø.6)
         polyp of accessory sinus (J33.8)
         polyp of ear (middle) (H74.4)
         polyp of nasal (cavity) (J33.-)

   D14.1 Benign neoplasm of larynx
     Adenomatous polyp of larynx
     Benign neoplasm of epiglottis (suprahyoid portion)
     EXCLUDES 1   *benign neoplasm of epiglottis, anterior aspect (D1Ø.5)*
         polyp (nonadenomatous) of vocal cord or larynx (J38.1)

   D14.2 Benign neoplasm of trachea

✓5ᵗʰ **D14.3 Benign neoplasm of bronchus and lung**
     EXCLUDES 1   *benign carcinoid tumor of the bronchus and lung (D3A.Ø90)*

     D14.3Ø Benign neoplasm of unspecified bronchus and lung

     D14.31 Benign neoplasm of right bronchus and lung

     D14.32 Benign neoplasm of left bronchus and lung

   D14.4 Benign neoplasm of respiratory system, unspecified

✓4ᵗʰ **D15 Benign neoplasm of other and unspecified intrathoracic organs**

     EXCLUDES 1   *benign neoplasm of mesothelial tissue (D19.-)*

   D15.Ø Benign neoplasm of thymus
     EXCLUDES 1   *benign carcinoid tumor of the thymus (D3A.Ø91)*

   D15.1 Benign neoplasm of heart
     EXCLUDES 1   *benign neoplasm of great vessels (D21.3)*

   D15.2 Benign neoplasm of mediastinum

   D15.7 Benign neoplasm of other specified intrathoracic organs

   D15.9 Benign neoplasm of intrathoracic organ, unspecified

✓4ᵗʰ **D16 Benign neoplasm of bone and articular cartilage**

     EXCLUDES 1   *benign neoplasm of connective tissue of ear (D21.Ø)*
         benign neoplasm of connective tissue of eyelid (D21.Ø)
         benign neoplasm of connective tissue of larynx (D14.1)
         benign neoplasm of connective tissue of nose (D14.Ø)
         benign neoplasm of synovia (D21.-)

✓5ᵗʰ **D16.Ø Benign neoplasm of scapula and long bones of upper limb**

     D16.ØØ Benign neoplasm of scapula and long bones of unspecified upper limb

     D16.Ø1 Benign neoplasm of scapula and long bones of right upper limb

     D16.Ø2 Benign neoplasm of scapula and long bones of left upper limb

✓5ᵗʰ **D16.1 Benign neoplasm of short bones of upper limb**

     D16.1Ø Benign neoplasm of short bones of unspecified upper limb

     D16.11 Benign neoplasm of short bones of right upper limb

     D16.12 Benign neoplasm of short bones of left upper limb

✓5ᵗʰ **D16.2 Benign neoplasm of long bones of lower limb**

     D16.2Ø Benign neoplasm of long bones of unspecified lower limb

     D16.21 Benign neoplasm of long bones of right lower limb

     D16.22 Benign neoplasm of long bones of left lower limb

✓5ᵗʰ **D16.3 Benign neoplasm of short bones of lower limb**

     D16.3Ø Benign neoplasm of short bones of unspecified lower limb

     D16.31 Benign neoplasm of short bones of right lower limb

     D16.32 Benign neoplasm of short bones of left lower limb

☑ Additional Character Required   ✓x7ᵗʰ Placeholder   Unacceptable PDx   Questionable PDx   Manifestation   Unspecified Dx   **H1**-**H14** HAC   **HCC** CMS-HCC Dx   **HIV** HIV Dx

ICD-10-CM 2020   **493**

Chapter 2. Neoplasms

D16.4   **Benign neoplasm of bones of skull and face**
Benign neoplasm of maxilla (superior)
Benign neoplasm of orbital bone
Keratocyst of maxilla
Keratocystic odontogenic tumor of maxilla
EXCLUDES 2   *benign neoplasm of lower jaw bone (D16.5)*

D16.5   **Benign neoplasm of lower jaw bone**
Keratocyst of mandible
Keratocystic odontogenic tumor of mandible

D16.6   **Benign neoplasm of vertebral column**
EXCLUDES 1   *benign neoplasm of sacrum and coccyx (D16.8)*

D16.7   **Benign neoplasm of ribs, sternum and clavicle**

D16.8   **Benign neoplasm of pelvic bones, sacrum and coccyx**

D16.9   **Benign neoplasm of bone and articular cartilage, unspecified**

D17   **Benign lipomatous neoplasm**

D17.0   **Benign lipomatous neoplasm of skin and subcutaneous tissue of head, face and neck**

D17.1   **Benign lipomatous neoplasm of skin and subcutaneous tissue of trunk**

D17.2   **Benign lipomatous neoplasm of skin and subcutaneous tissue of limb**
   D17.20   Benign lipomatous neoplasm of skin and subcutaneous tissue of unspecified limb
   D17.21   Benign lipomatous neoplasm of skin and subcutaneous tissue of right arm
   D17.22   Benign lipomatous neoplasm of skin and subcutaneous tissue of left arm
   D17.23   Benign lipomatous neoplasm of skin and subcutaneous tissue of right leg
   D17.24   Benign lipomatous neoplasm of skin and subcutaneous tissue of left leg

D17.3   **Benign lipomatous neoplasm of skin and subcutaneous tissue of other and unspecified sites**
   D17.30   Benign lipomatous neoplasm of skin and subcutaneous tissue of unspecified sites
   D17.39   Benign lipomatous neoplasm of skin and subcutaneous tissue of other sites

D17.4   **Benign lipomatous neoplasm of intrathoracic organs**

D17.5   **Benign lipomatous neoplasm of intra-abdominal organs**
EXCLUDES 1   *benign lipomatous neoplasm of peritoneum and retroperitoneum (D17.79)*

D17.6   **Benign lipomatous neoplasm of spermatic cord**   ♂

D17.7   **Benign lipomatous neoplasm of other sites**
   D17.71   Benign lipomatous neoplasm of kidney
   D17.72   Benign lipomatous neoplasm of other genitourinary organ
   D17.79   Benign lipomatous neoplasm of other sites
     Benign lipomatous neoplasm of peritoneum
     Benign lipomatous neoplasm of retroperitoneum

D17.9   **Benign lipomatous neoplasm, unspecified**
Lipoma NOS

D18   **Hemangioma and lymphangioma, any site**
EXCLUDES 1   *benign neoplasm of glomus jugulare (D35.6)*
blue or pigmented nevus (D22.-)
nevus NOS (D22.-)
vascular nevus (Q82.5)

D18.0   **Hemangioma**
Angioma NOS
Cavernous nevus
DEF: Common benign tumor usually occurring in infancy that is composed of newly formed blood vessels due to malformation of the angioblastic tissue.
   D18.00   Hemangioma unspecified site
   D18.01   Hemangioma of skin and subcutaneous tissue
   D18.02   Hemangioma of intracranial structures   HCC
   D18.03   Hemangioma of intra-abdominal structures
   D18.09   Hemangioma of other sites

D18.1   **Lymphangioma, any site**
AHA: 2018,3Q,31; 2018,2Q,13

D19   **Benign neoplasm of mesothelial tissue**

D19.0   **Benign neoplasm of mesothelial tissue of pleura**

D19.1   **Benign neoplasm of mesothelial tissue of peritoneum**

D19.7   **Benign neoplasm of mesothelial tissue of other sites**

D19.9   **Benign neoplasm of mesothelial tissue, unspecified**
Benign mesothelioma NOS

D20   **Benign neoplasm of soft tissue of retroperitoneum and peritoneum**
EXCLUDES 1   *benign lipomatous neoplasm of peritoneum and retroperitoneum (D17.79)*
benign neoplasm of mesothelial tissue (D19.-)

D20.0   **Benign neoplasm of soft tissue of retroperitoneum**

D20.1   **Benign neoplasm of soft tissue of peritoneum**

D21   **Other benign neoplasms of connective and other soft tissue**
INCLUDES   benign neoplasm of blood vessel
benign neoplasm of bursa
benign neoplasm of cartilage
benign neoplasm of fascia
benign neoplasm of fat
benign neoplasm of ligament, except uterine
benign neoplasm of lymphatic channel
benign neoplasm of muscle
benign neoplasm of synovia
benign neoplasm of tendon (sheath)
benign stromal tumors
EXCLUDES 1   *benign neoplasm of articular cartilage (D16.-)*
benign neoplasm of cartilage of larynx (D14.1)
benign neoplasm of cartilage of nose (D14.0)
benign neoplasm of connective tissue of breast (D24.-)
benign neoplasm of peripheral nerves and autonomic nervous system (D36.1-)
benign neoplasm of peritoneum (D20.1)
benign neoplasm of retroperitoneum (D20.0)
benign neoplasm of uterine ligament, any (D28.2)
benign neoplasm of vascular tissue (D18.-)
hemangioma (D18.0-)
lipomatous neoplasm (D17.-)
lymphangioma (D18.1)
uterine leiomyoma (D25.-)

D21.0   **Benign neoplasm of connective and other soft tissue of head, face and neck**
Benign neoplasm of connective tissue of ear
Benign neoplasm of connective tissue of eyelid
EXCLUDES 1   *benign neoplasm of connective tissue of orbit (D31.6-)*

D21.1   **Benign neoplasm of connective and other soft tissue of upper limb, including shoulder**
   D21.10   Benign neoplasm of connective and other soft tissue of unspecified upper limb, including shoulder
   D21.11   Benign neoplasm of connective and other soft tissue of right upper limb, including shoulder
   D21.12   Benign neoplasm of connective and other soft tissue of left upper limb, including shoulder

D21.2   **Benign neoplasm of connective and other soft tissue of lower limb, including hip**
   D21.20   Benign neoplasm of connective and other soft tissue of unspecified lower limb, including hip
   D21.21   Benign neoplasm of connective and other soft tissue of right lower limb, including hip
   D21.22   Benign neoplasm of connective and other soft tissue of left lower limb, including hip

D21.3   **Benign neoplasm of connective and other soft tissue of thorax**
Benign neoplasm of axilla
Benign neoplasm of diaphragm
Benign neoplasm of great vessels
EXCLUDES 1   *benign neoplasm of heart (D15.1)*
benign neoplasm of mediastinum (D15.2)
benign neoplasm of thymus (D15.0)

D21.4   **Benign neoplasm of connective and other soft tissue of abdomen**
Benign stromal tumors of abdomen

D21.5   **Benign neoplasm of connective and other soft tissue of pelvis**
EXCLUDES 1   *benign neoplasm of any uterine ligament (D28.2)*
uterine leiomyoma (D25.-)

D21.6   **Benign neoplasm of connective and other soft tissue of trunk, unspecified**
▶Benign neoplasm of connective and other soft tissue back NOS◀

D21.9   **Benign neoplasm of connective and other soft tissue, unspecified**

✓4ᵗʰ D22 Melanocytic nevi

INCLUDES atypical nevus

      blue hairy pigmented nevus

      nevus NOS

D22.0 Melanocytic nevi of lip

✓5ᵗʰ D22.1 Melanocytic nevi of eyelid, including canthus

    AHA: 2018,4Q,4

    D22.10 Melanocytic nevi of unspecified eyelid, including canthus

    ✓6ᵗʰ D22.11 Melanocytic nevi of right eyelid, including canthus

        D22.111 Melanocytic nevi of right upper eyelid, including canthus

        D22.112 Melanocytic nevi of right lower eyelid, including canthus

    ✓6ᵗʰ D22.12 Melanocytic nevi of left eyelid, including canthus

        D22.121 Melanocytic nevi of left upper eyelid, including canthus

        D22.122 Melanocytic nevi of left lower eyelid, including canthus

✓5ᵗʰ D22.2 Melanocytic nevi of ear and external auricular canal

    D22.20 Melanocytic nevi of unspecified ear and external auricular canal

    D22.21 Melanocytic nevi of right ear and external auricular canal

    D22.22 Melanocytic nevi of left ear and external auricular canal

✓5ᵗʰ D22.3 Melanocytic nevi of other and unspecified parts of face

    D22.30 Melanocytic nevi of unspecified part of face

    D22.39 Melanocytic nevi of other parts of face

D22.4 Melanocytic nevi of scalp and neck

D22.5 Melanocytic nevi of trunk

    Melanocytic nevi of anal margin

    Melanocytic nevi of anal skin

    Melanocytic nevi of perianal skin

    Melanocytic nevi of skin of breast

✓5ᵗʰ D22.6 Melanocytic nevi of upper limb, including shoulder

    D22.60 Melanocytic nevi of unspecified upper limb, including shoulder

    D22.61 Melanocytic nevi of right upper limb, including shoulder

    D22.62 Melanocytic nevi of left upper limb, including shoulder

✓5ᵗʰ D22.7 Melanocytic nevi of lower limb, including hip

    D22.70 Melanocytic nevi of unspecified lower limb, including hip

    D22.71 Melanocytic nevi of right lower limb, including hip

    D22.72 Melanocytic nevi of left lower limb, including hip

D22.9 Melanocytic nevi, unspecified

✓4ᵗʰ D23 Other benign neoplasms of skin

INCLUDES benign neoplasm of hair follicles

      benign neoplasm of sebaceous glands

      benign neoplasm of sweat glands

EXCLUDES 1 *benign lipomatous neoplasms of skin (D17.0-D17.3)*

      melanocytic nevi (D22.-)

EXCLUDES 2 ▶*melanocytic nevi (D22.-)*◀

D23.0 Other benign neoplasm of skin of lip

    EXCLUDES 1 *benign neoplasm of vermilion border of lip (D10.0)*

✓5ᵗʰ D23.1 Other benign neoplasm of skin of eyelid, including canthus

    AHA: 2018,4Q,4

    D23.10 Other benign neoplasm of skin of unspecified eyelid, including canthus

    ✓6ᵗʰ D23.11 Other benign neoplasm of skin of right eyelid, including canthus

        D23.111 Other benign neoplasm of skin of right upper eyelid, including canthus

        D23.112 Other benign neoplasm of skin of right lower eyelid, including canthus

    ✓6ᵗʰ D23.12 Other benign neoplasm of skin of left eyelid, including canthus

        D23.121 Other benign neoplasm of skin of left upper eyelid, including canthus

        D23.122 Other benign neoplasm of skin of left lower eyelid, including canthus

✓5ᵗʰ D23.2 Other benign neoplasm of skin of ear and external auricular canal

    D23.20 Other benign neoplasm of skin of unspecified ear and external auricular canal

D23.21 Other benign neoplasm of skin of right ear and external auricular canal

D23.22 Other benign neoplasm of skin of left ear and external auricular canal

✓5ᵗʰ D23.3 Other benign neoplasm of skin of other and unspecified parts of face

    D23.30 Other benign neoplasm of skin of unspecified part of face

    D23.39 Other benign neoplasm of skin of other parts of face

D23.4 Other benign neoplasm of skin of scalp and neck

D23.5 Other benign neoplasm of skin of trunk

    Other benign neoplasm of anal margin

    Other benign neoplasm of anal skin

    Other benign neoplasm of perianal skin

    Other benign neoplasm of skin of breast

    EXCLUDES 1 *benign neoplasm of anus NOS (D12.9)*

✓5ᵗʰ D23.6 Other benign neoplasm of skin of upper limb, including shoulder

    D23.60 Other benign neoplasm of skin of unspecified upper limb, including shoulder

    D23.61 Other benign neoplasm of skin of right upper limb, including shoulder

    D23.62 Other benign neoplasm of skin of left upper limb, including shoulder

✓5ᵗʰ D23.7 Other benign neoplasm of skin of lower limb, including hip

    D23.70 Other benign neoplasm of skin of unspecified lower limb, including hip

    D23.71 Other benign neoplasm of skin of right lower limb, including hip

    D23.72 Other benign neoplasm of skin of left lower limb, including hip

D23.9 Other benign neoplasm of skin, unspecified

✓4ᵗʰ D24 Benign neoplasm of breast

INCLUDES benign neoplasm of connective tissue of breast

      benign neoplasm of soft parts of breast

      fibroadenoma of breast

EXCLUDES 2 *adenofibrosis of breast (N60.2)*

      benign cyst of breast (N60.-)

      benign mammary dysplasia (N60.-)

      benign neoplasm of skin of breast (D22.5, D23.5)

      fibrocystic disease of breast (N60.-)

D24.1 Benign neoplasm of right breast

D24.2 Benign neoplasm of left breast

D24.9 Benign neoplasm of unspecified breast

✓4ᵗʰ D25 Leiomyoma of uterus

INCLUDES uterine fibroid

      uterine fibromyoma

      uterine myoma

Uterine Leiomyomas (Fibroids)

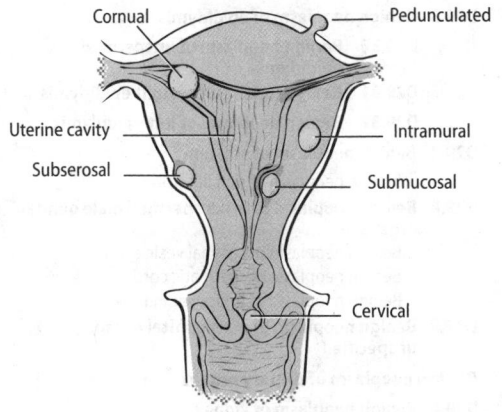

D25.0 Submucous leiomyoma of uterus   ♀

D25.1 Intramural leiomyoma of uterus   ♀

    Interstitial leiomyoma of uterus

☑ Additional Character Required   ✓x7ᵗʰ Placeholder   Unacceptable PDx   Questionable PDx   Manifestation   Unspecified Dx   H1-H4 HAC   HCC CMS-HCC Dx   HIV HIV Dx

ICD-10-CM 2020   495

Chapter 2. Neoplasms

D25.2–D32.0

D25.2   **Subserosal** leiomyoma of uterus   ♀
       Subperitoneal leiomyoma of uterus

D25.9   **Leiomyoma of uterus, unspecified**   ♀

✓4ᵗʰ **D26**   **Other benign neoplasms of uterus**

   D26.0   **Other benign neoplasm of cervix uteri**   ♀

   D26.1   **Other benign neoplasm of corpus uteri**   ♀

   D26.7   **Other benign neoplasm of other parts of uterus**   ♀

   D26.9   **Other benign neoplasm of uterus, unspecified**   ♀

✓4ᵗʰ **D27**   **Benign neoplasm of ovary**

      Use additional code to identify any functional activity

      EXCLUDES 2   *corpus albicans cyst (N83.2-)* ·
               corpus luteum cyst (N83.1-)
               endometrial cyst (N80.1)
               follicular (atretic) cyst (N83.0-)
               graafian follicle cyst (N83.0-)
               ovarian cyst NEC (N83.2-)
               ovarian retention cyst (N83.2-)

   D27.0   **Benign neoplasm of right ovary**   ♀

   D27.1   **Benign neoplasm of left ovary**   ♀

   D27.9   **Benign neoplasm of unspecified ovary**   ♀

✓4ᵗʰ **D28**   **Benign neoplasm of other and unspecified female genital organs**

      INCLUDES   adenomatous polyp
               benign neoplasm of skin of female genital organs
               benign teratoma

      EXCLUDES 1   *epoophoron cyst (Q50.5)*
               fimbrial cyst (Q50.4)
               Gartner's duct cyst (Q52.4)
               parovarian cyst (Q50.5)

   D28.0   **Benign neoplasm of vulva**   ♀

   D28.1   **Benign neoplasm of vagina**   ♀

   D28.2   **Benign neoplasm of uterine tubes and ligaments**   ♀
         Benign neoplasm of fallopian tube
         Benign neoplasm of uterine ligament (broad) (round)

   D28.7   **Benign neoplasm of other specified female genital organs**   ♀

   D28.9   **Benign neoplasm of female genital organ, unspecified**   ♀

✓4ᵗʰ **D29**   **Benign neoplasm of male genital organs**

      INCLUDES   benign neoplasm of skin of male genital organs

   D29.0   **Benign neoplasm of penis**   ♂

   D29.1   **Benign neoplasm of prostate**   ♂
         EXCLUDES 1   *enlarged prostate (N40.-)*

   ✓5ᵗʰ D29.2   **Benign neoplasm of testis**
         Use additional code to identify any functional activity

     D29.20   **Benign neoplasm of unspecified testis**   ♂

     D29.21   **Benign neoplasm of right testis**   ♂

     D29.22   **Benign neoplasm of left testis**   ♂

   ✓5ᵗʰ D29.3   **Benign neoplasm of epididymis**

     D29.30   **Benign neoplasm of unspecified epididymis**

     D29.31   **Benign neoplasm of right epididymis**   ♂

     D29.32   **Benign neoplasm of left epididymis**   ♂

   D29.4   **Benign neoplasm of scrotum**   ♂
         Benign neoplasm of skin of scrotum

   D29.8   **Benign neoplasm of other specified male genital organs**   ♂
         Benign neoplasm of seminal vesicle
         Benign neoplasm of spermatic cord
         Benign neoplasm of tunica vaginalis

   D29.9   **Benign neoplasm of male genital organ, unspecified**   ♂

✓4ᵗʰ **D30**   **Benign neoplasm of urinary organs**

   ✓5ᵗʰ D30.0   **Benign neoplasm of kidney**
         EXCLUDES 1   *benign carcinoid tumor of the kidney (D3A.093)*
               benign neoplasm of renal calyces (D30.1-)
               benign neoplasm of renal pelvis (D30.1-)

     D30.00   **Benign neoplasm of unspecified kidney**

     D30.01   **Benign neoplasm of right kidney**

     D30.02   **Benign neoplasm of left kidney**

   ✓5ᵗʰ D30.1   **Benign neoplasm of renal pelvis**

     D30.10   **Benign neoplasm of unspecified renal pelvis**

     D30.11   **Benign neoplasm of right renal pelvis**

     D30.12   **Benign neoplasm of left renal pelvis**

   ✓5ᵗʰ D30.2   **Benign neoplasm of ureter**
         EXCLUDES 1   *benign neoplasm of ureteric orifice of bladder (D30.3)*

     D30.20   **Benign neoplasm of unspecified ureter**

     D30.21   **Benign neoplasm of right ureter**

     D30.22   **Benign neoplasm of left ureter**

   D30.3   **Benign neoplasm of bladder**
         Benign neoplasm of ureteric orifice of bladder
         Benign neoplasm of urethral orifice of bladder

   D30.4   **Benign neoplasm of urethra**
         EXCLUDES 1   *benign neoplasm of urethral orifice of bladder (D30.3)*

   D30.8   **Benign neoplasm of other specified urinary organs**
         Benign neoplasm of paraurethral glands

   D30.9   **Benign neoplasm of urinary organ, unspecified**
         Benign neoplasm of urinary system NOS

✓4ᵗʰ **D31**   **Benign neoplasm of eye and adnexa**

      EXCLUDES 1   *benign neoplasm of connective tissue of eyelid (D21.0)*
               benign neoplasm of optic nerve (D33.3)
               benign neoplasm of skin of eyelid (D22.1-, D23.1-)

   ✓5ᵗʰ D31.0   **Benign neoplasm of conjunctiva**

     D31.00   **Benign neoplasm of unspecified conjunctiva**

     D31.01   **Benign neoplasm of right conjunctiva**

     D31.02   **Benign neoplasm of left conjunctiva**

   ✓5ᵗʰ D31.1   **Benign neoplasm of cornea**

     D31.10   **Benign neoplasm of unspecified cornea**

     D31.11   **Benign neoplasm of right cornea**

     D31.12   **Benign neoplasm of left cornea**

   ✓5ᵗʰ D31.2   **Benign neoplasm of retina**
         EXCLUDES 1   *dark area on retina (D49.81)*
               hemangioma of retina (D49.81)
               neoplasm of unspecified behavior of retina and choroid (D49.81)
               retinal freckle (D49.81)

     D31.20   **Benign neoplasm of unspecified retina**

     D31.21   **Benign neoplasm of right retina**

     D31.22   **Benign neoplasm of left retina**

   ✓5ᵗʰ D31.3   **Benign neoplasm of choroid**

     D31.30   **Benign neoplasm of unspecified choroid**

     D31.31   **Benign neoplasm of right choroid**

     D31.32   **Benign neoplasm of left choroid**

   ✓5ᵗʰ D31.4   **Benign neoplasm of ciliary body**

     D31.40   **Benign neoplasm of unspecified ciliary body**

     D31.41   **Benign neoplasm of right ciliary body**

     D31.42   **Benign neoplasm of left ciliary body**

   ✓5ᵗʰ D31.5   **Benign neoplasm of lacrimal gland and duct**
         Benign neoplasm of lacrimal sac
         Benign neoplasm of nasolacrimal duct

     D31.50   **Benign neoplasm of unspecified lacrimal gland and duct**

     D31.51   **Benign neoplasm of right lacrimal gland and duct**

     D31.52   **Benign neoplasm of left lacrimal gland and duct**

   ✓5ᵗʰ D31.6   **Benign neoplasm of unspecified site of orbit**
         Benign neoplasm of connective tissue of orbit
         Benign neoplasm of extraocular muscle
         Benign neoplasm of peripheral nerves of orbit
         Benign neoplasm of retrobulbar tissue
         Benign neoplasm of retro-ocular tissue
         EXCLUDES 1   *benign neoplasm of orbital bone (D16.4)*

     D31.60   **Benign neoplasm of unspecified site of unspecified orbit**

     D31.61   **Benign neoplasm of unspecified site of right orbit**

     D31.62   **Benign neoplasm of unspecified site of left orbit**

   ✓5ᵗʰ D31.9   **Benign neoplasm of unspecified part of eye**
         Benign neoplasm of eyeball

     D31.90   **Benign neoplasm of unspecified part of unspecified eye**

     D31.91   **Benign neoplasm of unspecified part of right eye**

     D31.92   **Benign neoplasm of unspecified part of left eye**

✓4ᵗʰ **D32**   **Benign neoplasm of meninges**

   D32.0   **Benign neoplasm of cerebral meninges**   HCC

N Newborn: 0   **P** Pediatric: 0-17   **M** Maternity: 9-64   **A** Adult: 15-124   **MCC** Major Complication/Comorbidity   **CC** Complication/Comorbidity   **SW** Severe Wound Dx

496   ICD-10-CM 2020

D32.1 Benign neoplasm of **spinal** meninges   `HCC`

D32.9 Benign neoplasm of meninges, unspecified   `HCC`
> Meningioma NOS

✓4ᵗʰ **D33** Benign neoplasm of **brain and other parts of central nervous system**
> `EXCLUDES 1`   angioma (D18.0-)
> benign neoplasm of meninges (D32.-)
> benign neoplasm of peripheral nerves and autonomic nervous system (D36.1-)
> hemangioma (D18.0-)
> neurofibromatosis (Q85.0-)
> retro-ocular benign neoplasm (D31.6-)

D33.0 Benign neoplasm of **brain, supratentorial**   `HCC`
> Benign neoplasm of cerebral ventricle
> Benign neoplasm of cerebrum
> Benign neoplasm of frontal lobe
> Benign neoplasm of occipital lobe
> Benign neoplasm of parietal lobe
> Benign neoplasm of temporal lobe
> `EXCLUDES 1`   benign neoplasm of fourth ventricle (D33.1)

D33.1 Benign neoplasm of **brain, infratentorial**   `HCC`
> Benign neoplasm of brain stem
> Benign neoplasm of cerebellum
> Benign neoplasm of fourth ventricle

D33.2 Benign neoplasm of **brain, unspecified**   `HCC`

D33.3 Benign neoplasm of **cranial nerves**   `HCC`
> Benign neoplasm of olfactory bulb

D33.4 Benign neoplasm of **spinal cord**   `HCC`

D33.7 Benign neoplasm of **other specified parts of central nervous system**   `HCC`

D33.9 Benign neoplasm of **central nervous system, unspecified**   `HCC`
> Benign neoplasm of nervous system (central) NOS

D34 Benign neoplasm of **thyroid gland**
> Use additional code to identify any functional activity

✓4ᵗʰ **D35** Benign neoplasm of **other and unspecified endocrine glands**
> Use additional code to identify any functional activity
> `EXCLUDES 1`   benign neoplasm of endocrine pancreas (D13.7)
> benign neoplasm of ovary (D27.-)
> benign neoplasm of testis (D29.2.-)
> benign neoplasm of thymus (D15.0)

✓5ᵗʰ **D35.0** Benign neoplasm of **adrenal gland**

> **D35.00** Benign neoplasm of **unspecified adrenal gland**
> **D35.01** Benign neoplasm of **right adrenal gland**
> **D35.02** Benign neoplasm of **left adrenal gland**

D35.1 Benign neoplasm of **parathyroid gland**

D35.2 Benign neoplasm of **pituitary gland**   `HCC`
> **AHA:** 2014,3Q,22

D35.3 Benign neoplasm of **craniopharyngeal duct**   `HCC`

D35.4 Benign neoplasm of **pineal gland**   `HCC`

D35.5 Benign neoplasm of **carotid body**

D35.6 Benign neoplasm of **aortic body and other paraganglia**
> Benign tumor of glomus jugulare

D35.7 Benign neoplasm of **other specified endocrine glands**

D35.9 Benign neoplasm of **endocrine gland, unspecified**
> Benign neoplasm of unspecified endocrine gland

✓4ᵗʰ **D36** Benign neoplasm of **other and unspecified sites**

D36.0 Benign neoplasm of **lymph nodes**
> `EXCLUDES 1`   lymphangioma (D18.1)

✓5ᵗʰ **D36.1** Benign neoplasm of **peripheral nerves and autonomic nervous system**
> `EXCLUDES 1`   benign neoplasm of peripheral nerves of orbit (D31.6-)
> neurofibromatosis (Q85.0-)

> **D36.10** Benign neoplasm of peripheral nerves and autonomic nervous system, **unspecified**
> **D36.11** Benign neoplasm of peripheral nerves and autonomic nervous system of **face, head, and neck**
> **D36.12** Benign neoplasm of peripheral nerves and autonomic nervous system, **upper limb, including shoulder**
> **D36.13** Benign neoplasm of peripheral nerves and autonomic nervous system of **lower limb, including hip**

D36.14 Benign neoplasm of peripheral nerves and autonomic nervous system of **thorax**

D36.15 Benign neoplasm of peripheral nerves and autonomic nervous system of **abdomen**

D36.16 Benign neoplasm of peripheral nerves and autonomic nervous system of **pelvis**

D36.17 Benign neoplasm of peripheral nerves and autonomic nervous system of **trunk, unspecified**

D36.7 Benign neoplasm of **other specified sites**
> ▶Benign neoplasm of back NOS◀
> Benign neoplasm of nose NOS

D36.9 Benign neoplasm, **unspecified site**

Benign neuroendocrine tumors (D3A)

✓4ᵗʰ **D3A** Benign neuroendocrine tumors
> Code also any associated multiple endocrine neoplasia [MEN] syndromes (E31.2-)
> Use additional code to identify any associated endocrine syndrome, such as:
> carcinoid syndrome (E34.0)
> `EXCLUDES 2`   benign pancreatic islet cell tumors (D13.7)

✓5ᵗʰ **D3A.0** Benign carcinoid tumors

> **D3A.00** Benign carcinoid tumor of **unspecified site**
> > Carcinoid tumor NOS

> ✓6ᵗʰ **D3A.01** Benign carcinoid tumors of the **small intestine**
> > **D3A.010** Benign carcinoid tumor of the **duodenum**
> > **D3A.011** Benign carcinoid tumor of the **jejunum**
> > **D3A.012** Benign carcinoid tumor of the **ileum**
> > **D3A.019** Benign carcinoid tumor of the **small intestine, unspecified portion**

> ✓6ᵗʰ **D3A.02** Benign carcinoid tumors of the **appendix, large intestine, and rectum**
> > **D3A.020** Benign carcinoid tumor of the **appendix**
> > **D3A.021** Benign carcinoid tumor of the **cecum**
> > **D3A.022** Benign carcinoid tumor of the **ascending colon**
> > **D3A.023** Benign carcinoid tumor of the **transverse colon**
> > **D3A.024** Benign carcinoid tumor of the **descending colon**
> > **D3A.025** Benign carcinoid tumor of the **sigmoid colon**
> > **D3A.026** Benign carcinoid tumor of the **rectum**
> > **D3A.029** Benign carcinoid tumor of the **large intestine, unspecified portion**
> > > Benign carcinoid tumor of the colon NOS

> ✓6ᵗʰ **D3A.09** Benign carcinoid tumors of **other sites**
> > **D3A.090** Benign carcinoid tumor of the **bronchus and lung**
> > **D3A.091** Benign carcinoid tumor of the **thymus**
> > **D3A.092** Benign carcinoid tumor of the **stomach**
> > **D3A.093** Benign carcinoid tumor of the **kidney**
> > **D3A.094** Benign carcinoid tumor of the **foregut, unspecified**
> > **D3A.095** Benign carcinoid tumor of the **midgut, unspecified**
> > **D3A.096** Benign carcinoid tumor of the **hindgut, unspecified**
> > **D3A.098** Benign carcinoid tumors of **other sites**

D3A.8 Other benign neuroendocrine tumors
> Neuroendocrine tumor NOS

✓ Additional Character Required   ✓x7ᵗʰ Placeholder   Unacceptable PDx   Questionable PDx   Manifestation   Unspecified Dx   H1-H14 HAC   HCC CMS-HCC Dx   HIV HIV Dx

ICD-10-CM 2020   497

Neoplasms of uncertain behavior, polycythemia vera and myelodysplastic syndromes (D37-D48)

NOTE Categories D37-D44, and D48 classify by site neoplasms of uncertain behavior, i.e., histologic confirmation whether the neoplasm is malignant or benign cannot be made.

EXCLUDES 1 *neoplasms of unspecified behavior (D49.-)*

✓4ᵗʰ **D37 Neoplasm of uncertain behavior of oral cavity and digestive organs**

EXCLUDES 1 *stromal tumors of uncertain behavior of digestive system (D48.1)*

✓5ᵗʰ **D37.0 Neoplasm of uncertain behavior of lip, oral cavity and pharynx**

EXCLUDES 1 *neoplasm of uncertain behavior of aryepiglottic fold or interarytenoid fold, laryngeal aspect (D38.0)*
neoplasm of uncertain behavior of epiglottis NOS (D38.0)
neoplasm of uncertain behavior of skin of lip (D48.5)
neoplasm of uncertain behavior of suprahyoid portion of epiglottis (D38.0)

D37.01 Neoplasm of uncertain behavior of lip
Neoplasm of uncertain behavior of vermilion border of lip

D37.02 Neoplasm of uncertain behavior of tongue

✓6ᵗʰ **D37.03 Neoplasm of uncertain behavior of the major salivary glands**

D37.030 Neoplasm of uncertain behavior of the parotid salivary glands

D37.031 Neoplasm of uncertain behavior of the sublingual salivary glands

D37.032 Neoplasm of uncertain behavior of the submandibular salivary glands

D37.039 Neoplasm of uncertain behavior of the major salivary glands, unspecified

D37.04 Neoplasm of uncertain behavior of the minor salivary glands
Neoplasm of uncertain behavior of submucosal salivary glands of lip
Neoplasm of uncertain behavior of submucosal salivary glands of cheek
Neoplasm of uncertain behavior of submucosal salivary glands of hard palate
Neoplasm of uncertain behavior of submucosal salivary glands of soft palate

D37.05 Neoplasm of uncertain behavior of pharynx
Neoplasm of uncertain behavior of aryepiglottic fold of pharynx NOS
Neoplasm of uncertain behavior of hypopharyngeal aspect of aryepiglottic fold of pharynx
Neoplasm of uncertain behavior of marginal zone of aryepiglottic fold of pharynx

D37.09 Neoplasm of uncertain behavior of other specified sites of the oral cavity

D37.1 Neoplasm of uncertain behavior of stomach

D37.2 Neoplasm of uncertain behavior of small intestine

D37.3 Neoplasm of uncertain behavior of appendix

D37.4 Neoplasm of uncertain behavior of colon

D37.5 Neoplasm of uncertain behavior of rectum
Neoplasm of uncertain behavior of rectosigmoid junction

D37.6 Neoplasm of uncertain behavior of liver, gallbladder and bile ducts
Neoplasm of uncertain behavior of ampulla of Vater

D37.8 Neoplasm of uncertain behavior of other specified digestive organs
Neoplasm of uncertain behavior of anal canal
Neoplasm of uncertain behavior of anal sphincter
Neoplasm of uncertain behavior of anus NOS
Neoplasm of uncertain behavior of esophagus
Neoplasm of uncertain behavior of intestine NOS
Neoplasm of uncertain behavior of pancreas

EXCLUDES 1 *neoplasm of uncertain behavior of anal margin (D48.5)*
neoplasm of uncertain behavior of anal skin (D48.5)
neoplasm of uncertain behavior of perianal skin (D48.5)

D37.9 Neoplasm of uncertain behavior of digestive organ, unspecified

✓4ᵗʰ **D38 Neoplasm of uncertain behavior of middle ear and respiratory and intrathoracic organs**

EXCLUDES 1 *neoplasm of uncertain behavior of heart (D48.7)*

D38.0 Neoplasm of uncertain behavior of larynx
Neoplasm of uncertain behavior of aryepiglottic fold or interarytenoid fold, laryngeal aspect
Neoplasm of uncertain behavior of epiglottis (suprahyoid portion)

EXCLUDES 1 *neoplasm of uncertain behavior of aryepiglottic fold or interarytenoid fold NOS (D37.05)*
neoplasm of uncertain behavior of hypopharyngeal aspect of aryepiglottic fold (D37.05)
neoplasm of uncertain behavior of marginal zone of aryepiglottic fold (D37.05)

D38.1 Neoplasm of uncertain behavior of trachea, bronchus and lung

D38.2 Neoplasm of uncertain behavior of pleura

D38.3 Neoplasm of uncertain behavior of mediastinum

D38.4 Neoplasm of uncertain behavior of thymus

D38.5 Neoplasm of uncertain behavior of other respiratory organs
Neoplasm of uncertain behavior of accessory sinuses
Neoplasm of uncertain behavior of cartilage of nose
Neoplasm of uncertain behavior of middle ear
Neoplasm of uncertain behavior of nasal cavities

EXCLUDES 1 *neoplasm of uncertain behavior of ear (external) (skin) (D48.5)*
neoplasm of uncertain behavior of nose NOS (D48.7)
neoplasm of uncertain behavior of skin of nose (D48.5)

D38.6 Neoplasm of uncertain behavior of respiratory organ, unspecified

✓4ᵗʰ **D39 Neoplasm of uncertain behavior of female genital organs**

D39.0 Neoplasm of uncertain behavior of uterus ♀

✓5ᵗʰ **D39.1 Neoplasm of uncertain behavior of ovary**
Use additional code to identify any functional activity

D39.10 Neoplasm of uncertain behavior of unspecified ovary ♀

D39.11 Neoplasm of uncertain behavior of right ovary ♀

D39.12 Neoplasm of uncertain behavior of left ovary ♀

D39.2 Neoplasm of uncertain behavior of placenta Ⓜ ♀
Chorioadenoma destruens
Invasive hydatidiform mole
Malignant hydatidiform mole

EXCLUDES 1 *hydatidiform mole NOS (O01.9)*

D39.8 Neoplasm of uncertain behavior of other specified female genital organs ♀
Neoplasm of uncertain behavior of skin of female genital organs

D39.9 Neoplasm of uncertain behavior of female genital organ, unspecified ♀

✓4ᵗʰ **D40 Neoplasm of uncertain behavior of male genital organs**

D40.0 Neoplasm of uncertain behavior of prostate ♂

✓5ᵗʰ **D40.1 Neoplasm of uncertain behavior of testis**

D40.10 Neoplasm of uncertain behavior of unspecified testis ♂

D40.11 Neoplasm of uncertain behavior of right testis ♂

D40.12 Neoplasm of uncertain behavior of left testis ♂

D40.8 Neoplasm of uncertain behavior of other specified male genital organs ♂
Neoplasm of uncertain behavior of skin of male genital organs

D40.9 Neoplasm of uncertain behavior of male genital organ, unspecified ♂

✓4ᵗʰ **D41 Neoplasm of uncertain behavior of urinary organs**

✓5ᵗʰ **D41.0 Neoplasm of uncertain behavior of kidney**

EXCLUDES 1 *neoplasm of uncertain behavior of renal pelvis (D41.1-)*

D41.00 Neoplasm of uncertain behavior of unspecified kidney

D41.01 Neoplasm of uncertain behavior of right kidney

D41.02 Neoplasm of uncertain behavior of left kidney

✓5ᵗʰ **D41.1 Neoplasm of uncertain behavior of renal pelvis**

D41.10 Neoplasm of uncertain behavior of unspecified renal pelvis

D41.11   Neoplasm of uncertain behavior of right renal pelvis

D41.12   Neoplasm of uncertain behavior of left renal pelvis

✓5ᵗʰ **D41.2**   **Neoplasm of uncertain behavior of ureter**

     D41.20   **Neoplasm of uncertain behavior of unspecified ureter**

     D41.21   Neoplasm of uncertain behavior of right ureter

     D41.22   Neoplasm of uncertain behavior of left ureter

D41.3   Neoplasm of uncertain behavior of urethra

D41.4   Neoplasm of uncertain behavior of bladder

D41.8   Neoplasm of uncertain behavior of other specified urinary organs

D41.9   Neoplasm of uncertain behavior of unspecified urinary organ

✓4ᵗʰ **D42**   **Neoplasm of uncertain behavior of meninges**

D42.0   Neoplasm of uncertain behavior of cerebral meninges   HCC

D42.1   Neoplasm of uncertain behavior of spinal meninges   HCC

D42.9   Neoplasm of uncertain behavior of meninges, unspecified   HCC

✓4ᵗʰ **D43**   **Neoplasm of uncertain behavior of brain and central nervous system**

     EXCLUDES 1   *neoplasm of uncertain behavior of peripheral nerves and autonomic nervous system (D48.2)*

D43.0   Neoplasm of uncertain behavior of brain, supratentorial   HCC

     Neoplasm of uncertain behavior of cerebral ventricle

     Neoplasm of uncertain behavior of cerebrum

     Neoplasm of uncertain behavior of frontal lobe

     Neoplasm of uncertain behavior of occipital lobe

     Neoplasm of uncertain behavior of parietal lobe

     Neoplasm of uncertain behavior of temporal lobe

     EXCLUDES 1   *neoplasm of uncertain behavior of fourth ventricle (D43.1)*

D43.1   Neoplasm of uncertain behavior of brain, infratentorial   HCC

     Neoplasm of uncertain behavior of brain stem

     Neoplasm of uncertain behavior of cerebellum

     Neoplasm of uncertain behavior of fourth ventricle

D43.2   Neoplasm of uncertain behavior of brain, unspecified   HCC

D43.3   Neoplasm of uncertain behavior of cranial nerves   HCC

D43.4   Neoplasm of uncertain behavior of spinal cord   HCC

D43.8   Neoplasm of uncertain behavior of other specified parts of central nervous system   HCC

D43.9   Neoplasm of uncertain behavior of central nervous system, unspecified   HCC

     Neoplasm of uncertain behavior of nervous system (central) NOS

✓4ᵗʰ **D44**   **Neoplasm of uncertain behavior of endocrine glands**

     EXCLUDES 1   *multiple endocrine adenomatosis (E31.2-)*

             multiple endocrine neoplasia (E31.2-)

             neoplasm of uncertain behavior of endocrine pancreas (D37.8)

             neoplasm of uncertain behavior of ovary (D39.1-)

             neoplasm of uncertain behavior of testis (D40.1-)

             neoplasm of uncertain behavior of thymus (D38.4)

D44.0   Neoplasm of uncertain behavior of thyroid gland

✓5ᵗʰ **D44.1**   **Neoplasm of uncertain behavior of adrenal gland**

     Use additional code to identify any functional activity

     D44.10   **Neoplasm of uncertain behavior of unspecified adrenal gland**

     D44.11   Neoplasm of uncertain behavior of right adrenal gland

     D44.12   Neoplasm of uncertain behavior of left adrenal gland

D44.2   Neoplasm of uncertain behavior of parathyroid gland

D44.3   Neoplasm of uncertain behavior of pituitary gland   HCC

     Use additional code to identify any functional activity

D44.4   Neoplasm of uncertain behavior of craniopharyngeal duct   HCC

D44.5   Neoplasm of uncertain behavior of pineal gland   HCC

D44.6   Neoplasm of uncertain behavior of carotid body   HCC

D44.7   Neoplasm of uncertain behavior of aortic body and other paraganglia   HCC

     AHA: 2016,4Q,26

D44.9   Neoplasm of uncertain behavior of unspecified endocrine gland

D45   **Polycythemia vera**   HCC

     EXCLUDES 1   *familial polycythemia (D75.0)*

             secondary polycythemia (D75.1)

     DEF: Abnormal proliferation of all bone marrow elements, increased red cell mass, and total blood volume. The etiology is unknown, but it is frequently associated with splenomegaly, leukocytosis, and thrombocythemia.

✓4ᵗʰ **D46**   **Myelodysplastic syndromes**

     Use additional code for adverse effect, if applicable, to identify drug (T36-T50 with fifth or sixth character 5)

     EXCLUDES 2   *drug-induced aplastic anemia (D61.1)*

D46.0   Refractory anemia without ring sideroblasts, so stated   HCC

     Refractory anemia without sideroblasts, without excess of blasts

D46.1   Refractory anemia with ring sideroblasts   HCC

     RARS

✓5ᵗʰ **D46.2**   **Refractory anemia with excess of blasts [RAEB]**

     D46.20   **Refractory anemia with excess of blasts, unspecified**   HCC

          RAEB NOS

     D46.21   **Refractory anemia with excess of blasts 1**   HCC

          RAEB 1

     D46.22   **Refractory anemia with excess of blasts 2**   HCC

          RAEB 2

D46.A   Refractory cytopenia with multilineage dysplasia   HCC

D46.B   Refractory cytopenia with multilineage dysplasia and ring sideroblasts   HCC

     RCMD RS

D46.C   Myelodysplastic syndrome with isolated del(5q) chromosomal abnormality   HCC

     Myelodysplastic syndrome with 5q deletion

     5q minus syndrome NOS

D46.4   Refractory anemia, unspecified   HCC

D46.Z   Other myelodysplastic syndromes   HCC

     EXCLUDES 1   *chronic myelomonocytic leukemia (C93.1-)*

D46.9   Myelodysplastic syndrome, unspecified   HCC

     Myelodysplasia NOS

✓4ᵗʰ **D47**   **Other neoplasms of uncertain behavior of lymphoid, hematopoietic and related tissue**

✓5ᵗʰ **D47.0**   **Mast cell neoplasms of uncertain behavior**

     EXCLUDES 1   *congenital cutaneous mastocytosis (Q82.2)*

             histiocytic neoplasms of uncertain behavior (D47.Z9)

             malignant mast cell neoplasm (C96.2-)

     AHA: 2017,4Q,5

     D47.01   **Cutaneous mastocytosis**

          Diffuse cutaneous mastocytosis

          Maculopapular cutaneous mastocytosis

          Solitary mastocytoma

          Telangiectasia macularis eruptiva perstans

          Urticaria pigmentosa

          EXCLUDES 1   *congenital (diffuse) (maculopapular) cutaneous mastocytosis (Q82.2)*

                congenital urticaria pigmentosa (Q82.2)

                extracutaneous mastocytoma (D47.09)

Chapter 2. Neoplasms

D47.02   Systemic mastocytosis
Indolent systemic mastocytosis
Isolated bone marrow mastocytosis
Smoldering systemic mastocytosis
Systemic mastocytosis, with an associated
    hematological non-mast cell lineage disease
    (SM-AHNMD)
Code also, if applicable, any associated hematological
    non-mast cell lineage disease, such as:
    acute myeloid leukemia (C92.6-, C92.A-)
    chronic myelomonocytic leukemia (C93.1-)
    essential thrombocytosis (D47.3)
    hypereosinophilic syndrome (D72.1)
    myelodysplastic syndrome (D46.9)
    myeloproliferative syndrome (D47.1)
    non-Hodgkin lymphoma (C82-C85)
    plasma cell myeloma (C90.0-)
    polycythemia vera (D45)
    EXCLUDES 1   *aggressive systemic mastocytosis (C96.21)*
                mast cell leukemia (C94.3-)

D47.09   Other mast cell neoplasms of uncertain behavior
Extracutaneous mastocytoma
Mast cell tumor NOS
Mastocytoma NOS
Mastocytosis NOS

D47.1   Chronic myeloproliferative disease   `HCC`
Chronic neutrophilic leukemia
Myeloproliferative disease, unspecified
   EXCLUDES 1   *atypical chronic myeloid leukemia BCR/ABL-negative*
            (C92.2-)
           chronic myeloid leukemia BCR/ABL-positive (C92.1-)
           myelofibrosis NOS (D75.81)
           myelophthisic anemia (D61.82)
           myelophthisis (D61.82)
           secondary myelofibrosis NOS (D75.81)

D47.2   Monoclonal gammopathy
Monoclonal gammopathy of undetermined significance [MGUS]

D47.3   Essential (hemorrhagic) thrombocythemia   `HCC`
Essential thrombocytosis
Idiopathic hemorrhagic thrombocythemia
DEF: Chronic myeloproliferative neoplasm involving production
of excess blood platelets that may result in abnormal clotting or
hemorrhaging.

D47.4   Osteomyelofibrosis   `HCC`
Chronic idiopathic myelofibrosis
Myelofibrosis (idiopathic) (with myeloid metaplasia)
Myelosclerosis (megakaryocytic) with myeloid metaplasia
Secondary myelofibrosis in myeloproliferative disease
   EXCLUDES 1   *acute myelofibrosis (C94.4-)*

✓5ᵗʰ **D47.Z   Other specified neoplasms of uncertain behavior of
lymphoid, hematopoietic and related tissue**
AHA: 2016,4Q,8

**D47.Z1   Post-transplant lymphoproliferative
disorder (PTLD)**   `HCC`
Code first complications of transplanted organs and
    tissue (T86.-)
DEF: Excessive proliferation of B-cell lymphocytes
following Epstein-Barr virus infection in organ
transplant patients. It may progress to non-Hodgkin
lymphoma.

D47.Z2   Castleman disease   `HCC`
Code also if applicable human herpesvirus 8 infection
    (B10.89)
   EXCLUDES 2   *Kaposi's sarcoma (C46-)*
DEF: Rare disease of the lymph nodes and lymphoid
tissues that closely mimics lymphoma.

**D47.Z9   Other specified neoplasms of uncertain
behavior of lymphoid, hematopoietic
and related tissue**   `HCC`
Histiocytic tumors of uncertain behavior

D47.9   Neoplasm of uncertain behavior of lymphoid,   `HCC`
hematopoietic and related tissue, unspecified
Lymphoproliferative disease NOS

✓4ᵗʰ **D48   Neoplasm of uncertain behavior of other and unspecified sites**
   EXCLUDES 1   *neurofibromatosis (nonmalignant) (Q85.0-)*

**D48.0   Neoplasm of uncertain behavior of bone and articular
cartilage**
   EXCLUDES 1   *neoplasm of uncertain behavior of cartilage of ear*
            (D48.1)
           neoplasm of uncertain behavior of cartilage of larynx
            (D38.0)
           neoplasm of uncertain behavior of cartilage of nose
            (D38.5)
           neoplasm of uncertain behavior of connective tissue
            of eyelid (D48.1)
           neoplasm of uncertain behavior of synovia (D48.1)

**D48.1   Neoplasm of uncertain behavior of connective and other
soft tissue**
Neoplasm of uncertain behavior of connective tissue of ear
Neoplasm of uncertain behavior of connective tissue of eyelid
Stromal tumors of uncertain behavior of digestive system
   EXCLUDES 1   *neoplasm of uncertain behavior of articular cartilage*
            (D48.0)
           neoplasm of uncertain behavior of cartilage of larynx
            (D38.0)
           neoplasm of uncertain behavior of cartilage of nose
            (D38.5)
           neoplasm of uncertain behavior of connective tissue
            of breast (D48.6-)

**D48.2   Neoplasm of uncertain behavior of peripheral nerves and
autonomic nervous system**
   EXCLUDES 1   *neoplasm of uncertain behavior of peripheral nerves*
            of orbit (D48.7)

D48.3   Neoplasm of uncertain behavior of retroperitoneum

D48.4   Neoplasm of uncertain behavior of peritoneum

D48.5   Neoplasm of uncertain behavior of skin
Neoplasm of uncertain behavior of anal margin
Neoplasm of uncertain behavior of anal skin
Neoplasm of uncertain behavior of perianal skin
Neoplasm of uncertain behavior of skin of breast
   EXCLUDES 1   *neoplasm of uncertain behavior of anus NOS (D37.8)*
           neoplasm of uncertain behavior of skin of genital
            organs (D39.8, D40.8)
           neoplasm of uncertain behavior of vermilion border
            of lip (D37.0)

✓5ᵗʰ **D48.6   Neoplasm of uncertain behavior of breast**
Neoplasm of uncertain behavior of connective tissue of breast
Cystosarcoma phyllodes
   EXCLUDES 1   *neoplasm of uncertain behavior of skin of breast*
            (D48.5)

**D48.60   Neoplasm of uncertain behavior of unspecified
breast**
D48.61   Neoplasm of uncertain behavior of right breast
D48.62   Neoplasm of uncertain behavior of left breast

D48.7   Neoplasm of uncertain behavior of other specified sites
Neoplasm of uncertain behavior of eye
Neoplasm of uncertain behavior of heart
Neoplasm of uncertain behavior of peripheral nerves of orbit
   EXCLUDES 1   *neoplasm of uncertain behavior of connective tissue*
            (D48.1)
           neoplasm of uncertain behavior of skin of eyelid
            (D48.5)

D48.9   Neoplasm of uncertain behavior, unspecified

ℕ Newborn: 0   ℙ Pediatric: 0-17   Ⅿ Maternity: 9-64   Ⓐ Adult: 15-124   `MCC` Major Complication/Comorbidity   `CC` Complication/Comorbidity   `SW` Severe Wound Dx

500   ICD-10-CM 2020

Neoplasms of unspecified behavior (D49)

✓4ᵗʰ D49 Neoplasms of unspecified behavior

> **NOTE** Category D49 classifies by site neoplasms of unspecified morphology and behavior. The term "mass", unless otherwise stated, is not to be regarded as a neoplastic growth.

> **INCLUDES** "growth" NOS
> neoplasm NOS
> new growth NOS
> tumor NOS

> **EXCLUDES 1** *neoplasms of uncertain behavior (D37-D44, D48)*

D49.0 Neoplasm of unspecified behavior of digestive system

> **EXCLUDES 1** *neoplasm of unspecified behavior of margin of anus (D49.2)*
> *neoplasm of unspecified behavior of perianal skin (D49.2)*
> *neoplasm of unspecified behavior of skin of anus (D49.2)*

D49.1 Neoplasm of unspecified behavior of respiratory system

D49.2 Neoplasm of unspecified behavior of bone, soft tissue, and skin

> **EXCLUDES 1** *neoplasm of unspecified behavior of anal canal (D49.0)*
> *neoplasm of unspecified behavior of anus NOS (D49.0)*
> *neoplasm of unspecified behavior of bone marrow (D49.89)*
> *neoplasm of unspecified behavior of cartilage of larynx (D49.1)*
> *neoplasm of unspecified behavior of cartilage of nose (D49.1)*
> *neoplasm of unspecified behavior of connective tissue of breast (D49.3)*
> *neoplasm of unspecified behavior of skin of genital organs (D49.59)*
> *neoplasm of unspecified behavior of vermilion border of lip (D49.0)*

D49.3 Neoplasm of unspecified behavior of breast

> **EXCLUDES 1** *neoplasm of unspecified behavior of skin of breast (D49.2)*

D49.4 Neoplasm of unspecified behavior of bladder

✓5ᵗʰ D49.5 Neoplasm of unspecified behavior of other genitourinary organs

> **AHA:** 2016,4Q,9

> **✓6ᵗʰ D49.51 Neoplasm of unspecified behavior of kidney**
>> **D49.511 Neoplasm of unspecified behavior of right kidney**
>> **D49.512 Neoplasm of unspecified behavior of left kidney**
>> **D49.519 Neoplasm of unspecified behavior of unspecified kidney**
>
> **D49.59 Neoplasm of unspecified behavior of other genitourinary organ**

D49.6 Neoplasm of unspecified behavior of brain   HCC

> **EXCLUDES 1** *neoplasm of unspecified behavior of cerebral meninges (D49.7)*
> *neoplasm of unspecified behavior of cranial nerves (D49.7)*

D49.7 Neoplasm of unspecified behavior of endocrine glands and other parts of nervous system

> **EXCLUDES 1** *neoplasm of unspecified behavior of peripheral, sympathetic, and parasympathetic nerves and ganglia (D49.2)*

✓5ᵗʰ D49.8 Neoplasm of unspecified behavior of other specified sites

> **EXCLUDES 1** *neoplasm of unspecified behavior of eyelid (skin) (D49.2)*
> *neoplasm of unspecified behavior of eyelid cartilage (D49.2)*
> *neoplasm of unspecified behavior of great vessels (D49.2)*
> *neoplasm of unspecified behavior of optic nerve (D49.7)*

> **D49.81 Neoplasm of unspecified behavior of retina and choroid**
>> Dark area on retina
>> Retinal freckle

> **D49.89 Neoplasm of unspecified behavior of other specified sites**

D49.9 Neoplasm of unspecified behavior of unspecified site

Chapter 3. Diseases of the Blood and Blood-forming Organs and Certain Disorders Involving the Immune Mechanism (D5Ø–D89)

Chapter-specific Guidelines with Coding Examples
Reserved for future guideline expansion

Chapter 3. Diseases of the Blood and Blood-forming Organs and Certain Disorders Involving the Immune Mechanism (D50-D89)

EXCLUDES 2   *autoimmune disease (systemic) NOS (M35.9)*
certain conditions originating in the perinatal period (P00-P96)
complications of pregnancy, childbirth and the puerperium (O00-O9A)
congenital malformations, deformations and chromosomal abnormalities (Q00-Q99)
endocrine, nutritional and metabolic diseases (E00-E88)
human immunodeficiency virus [HIV] disease (B20)
injury, poisoning and certain other consequences of external causes (S00-T88)
neoplasms (C00-D49)
symptoms, signs and abnormal clinical and laboratory findings, not elsewhere classified (R00-R94)

This chapter contains the following blocks:

D50-D53	Nutritional anemias
D55-D59	Hemolytic anemias
D60-D64	Aplastic and other anemias and other bone marrow failure syndromes
D65-D69	Coagulation defects, purpura and other hemorrhagic conditions
D70-D77	Other disorders of blood and blood-forming organs
D78	Intraoperative and postprocedural complications of the spleen
D80-D89	Certain disorders involving the immune mechanism

Nutritional anemias (D50-D53)

DEF: Nutritional anemia: The result of inadequate intake or absorption of a vitamin or mineral that impacts the production of red blood cells or causes them to develop abnormally affecting the size and shape.

TIP: Documentation must identify a link between anemia and the nutritional deficiency; low levels of a particular nutrient may occur concurrently with anemia but not cause the anemia.

✓4ᵗʰ D50   Iron deficiency anemia

    INCLUDES   asiderotic anemia
               hypochromic anemia

D50.0   **Iron deficiency anemia secondary to blood loss (chronic)**
Posthemorrhagic anemia (chronic)
    EXCLUDES 1   *acute posthemorrhagic anemia (D62)*
                   congenital anemia from fetal blood loss (P61.3)

D50.1   **Sideropenic dysphagia**
Kelly-Paterson syndrome
Plummer-Vinson syndrome

D50.8   **Other iron deficiency anemias**
Iron deficiency anemia due to inadequate dietary iron intake

D50.9   **Iron deficiency anemia, unspecified**

✓4ᵗʰ D51   Vitamin B12 deficiency anemia

    EXCLUDES 1   *vitamin B12 deficiency (E53.8)*

D51.0   **Vitamin B12 deficiency anemia due to intrinsic factor deficiency**
Addison anemia
Biermer anemia
Pernicious (congenital) anemia
Congenital intrinsic factor deficiency
DEF: Chronic progressive anemia due to vitamin B12 malabsorption, caused by lack of secretion of intrinsic factor, which is produced by the gastric mucosa of the stomach.

D51.1   **Vitamin B12 deficiency anemia due to selective vitamin B12 malabsorption with proteinuria**
Imerslund (Gräsbeck) syndrome
Megaloblastic hereditary anemia

D51.2   **Transcobalamin II deficiency**

D51.3   **Other dietary vitamin B12 deficiency anemia**
Vegan anemia

D51.8   **Other vitamin B12 deficiency anemias**

D51.9   **Vitamin B12 deficiency anemia, unspecified**

✓4ᵗʰ D52   Folate deficiency anemia

    EXCLUDES 1   *folate deficiency without anemia (E53.8)*
DEF: Deficiency in a B complex vitamin needed for the production of healthy red blood cells. Lack of folate, or folic acid, and other absorption conditions can cause anemia resulting in large, misshapen red blood cells called megaloblasts.

D52.0   **Dietary folate deficiency anemia**
Nutritional megaloblastic anemia
DEF: Result of a poor diet with inadequate intake of folate, which is needed to produce healthy red blood cells.

D52.1   **Drug-induced folate deficiency anemia**
Use additional code for adverse effect, if applicable, to identify drug (T36-T50 with fifth or sixth character 5)

D52.8   **Other folate deficiency anemias**

D52.9   **Folate deficiency anemia, unspecified**
Folic acid deficiency anemia NOS

✓4ᵗʰ D53   Other nutritional anemias

    INCLUDES   megaloblastic anemia unresponsive to vitamin B12 or folate therapy

D53.0   **Protein deficiency anemia**
Amino-acid deficiency anemia
Orotaciduric anemia
    EXCLUDES 1   *Lesch-Nyhan syndrome (E79.1)*

D53.1   **Other megaloblastic anemias, not elsewhere classified**
Megaloblastic anemia NOS
    EXCLUDES 1   *Di Guglielmo's disease (C94.0)*

D53.2   **Scorbutic anemia**
    EXCLUDES 1   *scurvy (E54)*

D53.8   **Other specified nutritional anemias**
Anemia associated with deficiency of copper
Anemia associated with deficiency of molybdenum
Anemia associated with deficiency of zinc
    EXCLUDES 1   *nutritional deficiencies without anemia, such as:*
                 copper deficiency NOS (E61.0)
                 molybdenum deficiency NOS (E61.5)
                 zinc deficiency NOS (E60)

D53.9   **Nutritional anemia, unspecified**
Simple chronic anemia
    EXCLUDES 1   *anemia NOS (D64.9)*
AHA: 2018,4Q,88

Hemolytic anemias (D55-D59)

✓4ᵗʰ D55   Anemia due to enzyme disorders

    EXCLUDES 1   *drug-induced enzyme deficiency anemia (D59.2)*

D55.0   **Anemia due to glucose-6-phosphate dehydrogenase [G6PD] deficiency**   **HCC**
Favism
G6PD deficiency anemia
    EXCLUDES 1   ▶*glucose-6-phosphate dehydrogenase (G6PD) deficiency without anemia (D75.A)*◀

D55.1   **Anemia due to other disorders of glutathione metabolism**   **HCC**
Anemia (due to) enzyme deficiencies, except G6PD, related to the hexose monophosphate [HMP] shunt pathway
Anemia (due to) hemolytic nonspherocytic (hereditary), type I

D55.2   **Anemia due to disorders of glycolytic enzymes**   **HCC**
Hemolytic nonspherocytic (hereditary) anemia, type II
Hexokinase deficiency anemia
Pyruvate kinase [PK] deficiency anemia
Triose-phosphate isomerase deficiency anemia
    EXCLUDES 1   *disorders of glycolysis not associated with anemia (E74.8)*

D55.3   **Anemia due to disorders of nucleotide metabolism**   **HCC**

D55.8   **Other anemias due to enzyme disorders**   **HCC**

D55.9   **Anemia due to enzyme disorder, unspecified**   **HCC**

✓4ᵗʰ **D56 Thalassemia**

EXCLUDES 1   sickle-cell thalassemia (D57.4-)

DEF: Group of inherited disorders of hemoglobin metabolism causing mild to severe anemia. It is usually found in people of Mediterranean, African, Chinese, or Asian descent.

Thalassemia

Misshapen RBC

Misshapen RBC

Healthy RBC

D56.0 Alpha thalassemia   HCC

Alpha thalassemia major
Hemoglobin H Constant Spring
Hemoglobin H disease
Hydrops fetalis due to alpha thalassemia
Severe alpha thalassemia
Triple gene defect alpha thalassemia
Use additional code, if applicable, for hydrops fetalis due to alpha thalassemia (P56.99)

EXCLUDES 1   alpha thalassemia trait or minor (D56.3)
       asymptomatic alpha thalassemia (D56.3)
       hydrops fetalis due to isoimmunization (P56.0)
       hydrops fetalis not due to immune hemolysis (P83.2)

DEF: HBA1 and HBA2 genetic variant of chromosome 16 prevalent among those of African and Southeast Asian descent. Alpha thalassemia is associated with a wide spectrum of anemic presentation and includes hemoglobin H disease subtypes.

D56.1 Beta thalassemia   HCC

Beta thalassemia major
Cooley's anemia
Homozygous beta thalassemia
Severe beta thalassemia
Thalassemia intermedia
Thalassemia major

EXCLUDES 1   beta thalassemia minor (D56.3)
       beta thalassemia trait (D56.3)
       delta-beta thalassemia (D56.2)
       hemoglobin E-beta thalassemia (D56.5)
       sickle-cell beta thalassemia (D57.4-)

D56.2 Delta-beta thalassemia   HCC

Homozygous delta-beta thalassemia

EXCLUDES 1   delta-beta thalassemia minor (D56.3)
       delta-beta thalassemia trait (D56.3)

D56.3 Thalassemia minor

Alpha thalassemia minor
Alpha thalassemia silent carrier
Alpha thalassemia trait
Beta thalassemia minor
Beta thalassemia trait
Delta-beta thalassemia minor
Delta-beta thalassemia trait
Thalassemia trait NOS

EXCLUDES 1   alpha thalassemia (D56.0)
       beta thalassemia (D56.1)
       delta-beta thalassemia (D56.2)
       hemoglobin E-beta thalassemia (D56.5)
       sickle-cell trait (D57.3)

DEF: Solitary abnormal gene that identifies a carrier of the disease, yet with an absence of symptoms or a clinically mild anemic presentation.

D56.4 Hereditary persistence of fetal hemoglobin [HPFH]   HCC

D56.5 Hemoglobin E-beta thalassemia   HCC

EXCLUDES 1   beta thalassemia (D56.1)
       beta thalassemia minor (D56.3)
       beta thalassemia trait (D56.3)
       delta-beta thalassemia (D56.2)
       delta-beta thalassemia trait (D56.3)
       hemoglobin E disease (D58.2)
       other hemoglobinopathies (D58.2)
       sickle-cell beta thalassemia (D57.4-)

D56.8 Other thalassemias   HCC

Dominant thalassemia
Hemoglobin C thalassemia
Mixed thalassemia
Thalassemia with other hemoglobinopathy

EXCLUDES 1   hemoglobin C disease (D58.2)
       hemoglobin E disease (D58.2)
       other hemoglobinopathies (D58.2)
       sickle-cell anemia (D57.-)
       sickle-cell thalassemia (D57.4)

D56.9 Thalassemia, unspecified

Mediterranean anemia (with other hemoglobinopathy)

✓4ᵗʰ **D57 Sickle-cell disorders** — Hb~SS

Use additional code for any associated fever (R50.81)

EXCLUDES 1   other hemoglobinopathies (D58.-)

DEF: Severe, chronic inherited diseases caused by a genetic variation in hemoglobin protein of the red blood cell. The gene mutation causes the red blood cell to become hard, sticky, and crescent or sickle shaped making it harder for red blood cells to travel through the bloodstream disrupting blood flow and decreasing oxygen transport to tissues.

Sickle cell

Sickle cells

Normal RBCs

Hb-SS = sickle cell

✓5ᵗʰ **D57.0 Hb-SS disease with crisis**

Sickle-cell disease NOS with crisis
Hb-SS disease with vasoocclusive pain

D57.00 Hb-SS disease with crisis, unspecified   HCC

D57.01 Hb-SS disease with acute chest syndrome   HCC

D57.02 Hb-SS disease with splenic sequestration   HCC

✓ Additional Character Required   ✓x7ᵗʰ Placeholder   Unacceptable PDx   Questionable PDx   Manifestation   Unspecified Dx   H1 - H14 HAC   HCC CMS-HCC Dx   HIV HIV Dx

ICD-10-CM 2020   505

D57.1 Sickle-cell disease without crisis HCC
  Hb-SS disease without crisis
  Sickle-cell anemia NOS
  Sickle-cell disease NOS
  Sickle-cell disorder NOS

✓5ᵗʰ **D57.2 Sickle-cell/Hb-C disease**
  Hb-SC disease
  Hb-S/Hb-C disease

  D57.20 Sickle-cell/Hb-C disease without crisis HCC

✓6ᵗʰ **D57.21 Sickle-cell/Hb-C disease with crisis**

  D57.211 Sickle-cell/Hb-C disease with acute chest syndrome HCC

  D57.212 Sickle-cell/Hb-C disease with splenic sequestration MCC HCC
    CC Excl: PDX collection 496

  D57.219 Sickle-cell/Hb-C disease with crisis, unspecified HCC
    Sickle-cell/Hb-C disease with crisis NOS

D57.3 Sickle-cell trait HCC
  Hb-S trait
  Heterozygous hemoglobin S
  DEF: Heterozygous genetic makeup characterized by one gene for normal hemoglobin and one for sickle-cell hemoglobin. The clinical disease is rarely present.

✓5ᵗʰ **D57.4 Sickle-cell thalassemia**
  Sickle-cell beta thalassemia
  Thalassemia Hb-S disease

  D57.40 Sickle-cell thalassemia without crisis HCC
    Microdrepanocytosis
    Sickle-cell thalassemia NOS

✓6ᵗʰ **D57.41 Sickle-cell thalassemia with crisis**
    Sickle-cell thalassemia with vasoocclusive pain

  D57.411 Sickle-cell thalassemia with acute chest syndrome HCC

  D57.412 Sickle-cell thalassemia with splenic sequestration MCC HCC
    CC Excl: PDX collection 496

  D57.419 Sickle-cell thalassemia with crisis, unspecified HCC
    Sickle-cell thalassemia with crisis NOS

✓5ᵗʰ **D57.8 Other sickle-cell disorders**
  Hb-SD disease
  Hb-SE disease

  D57.80 Other sickle-cell disorders without crisis HCC

✓6ᵗʰ **D57.81 Other sickle-cell disorders with crisis**

  D57.811 Other sickle-cell disorders with acute chest syndrome HCC

  D57.812 Other sickle-cell disorders with splenic sequestration HCC

  D57.819 Other sickle-cell disorders with crisis, unspecified HCC
    Other sickle-cell disorders with crisis NOS

✓4ᵗʰ **D58 Other hereditary hemolytic anemias**
  EXCLUDES 1   hemolytic anemia of the newborn (P55.-)

D58.0 Hereditary spherocytosis HCC
  Acholuric (familial) jaundice
  Congenital (spherocytic) hemolytic icterus
  Minkowski-Chauffard syndrome
  DEF: Inherited condition caused by mutations to genes responsible for the production of proteins that form the membranes of red blood cells. The shape and flexibility of the red blood cell membrane is altered diminishing the cells ability to traverse the spleen, therefore becoming trapped and destroyed before the red blood cell has reached maturity.

D58.1 Hereditary elliptocytosis HCC
  Elliptocytosis (congenital)
  Ovalocytosis (congenital) (hereditary)

D58.2 Other hemoglobinopathies HCC
  Abnormal hemoglobin NOS
  Congenital Heinz body anemia
  Hb-C disease
  Hb-D disease
  Hb-E disease
  Hemoglobinopathy NOS
  Unstable hemoglobin hemolytic disease
  EXCLUDES 1   familial polycythemia (D75.0)
        Hb-M disease (D74.0)
        hemoglobin E-beta thalassemia (D56.5)
        hereditary persistence of fetal hemoglobin [HPFH] (D56.4)
        high-altitude polycythemia (D75.1)
        methemoglobinemia (D74.-)
        other hemoglobinopathies with thalassemia (D56.8)

D58.8 Other specified hereditary hemolytic anemias HCC
  Stomatocytosis

D58.9 Hereditary hemolytic anemia, unspecified HCC

✓4ᵗʰ **D59 Acquired hemolytic anemia**
  DEF: Non-hereditary anemia characterized by premature destruction of red blood cells caused by infectious organisms, poisons, and physical agents.
  CC Excl: For CC/MCC codes in category D59: PDX collection 496

D59.0 Drug-induced autoimmune hemolytic anemia HCC
  Use additional code for adverse effect, if applicable, to identify drug (T36-T50 with fifth or sixth character 5)

D59.1 Other autoimmune hemolytic anemias HCC
  Autoimmune hemolytic disease (cold type) (warm type)
  Chronic cold hemagglutinin disease
  Cold agglutinin disease
  Cold agglutinin hemoglobinuria
  Cold type (secondary) (symptomatic) hemolytic anemia
  Warm type (secondary) (symptomatic) hemolytic anemia
  EXCLUDES 1   Evans syndrome (D69.41)
        hemolytic disease of newborn (P55.-)
        paroxysmal cold hemoglobinuria (D59.6)

D59.2 Drug-induced nonautoimmune hemolytic anemia HCC
  Drug-induced enzyme deficiency anemia
  Use additional code for adverse effect, if applicable, to identify drug (T36-T50 with fifth or sixth character 5)

D59.3 Hemolytic-uremic syndrome MCC HCC
  Use additional code to identify associated:
    E. coli infection (B96.2-)
    Pneumococcal pneumonia (J13)
    Shigella dysenteriae (A03.9)
  DEF: Condition typically precipitated by infection causing low platelets and destruction of red blood cells resulting in hemolytic anemia. This cell damage and blockage of renal capillaries lead to kidney failure. Mainly affects children.

D59.4 Other nonautoimmune hemolytic anemias CC HCC
  Mechanical hemolytic anemia
  Microangiopathic hemolytic anemia
  Toxic hemolytic anemia

D59.5 Paroxysmal nocturnal hemoglobinuria [Marchiafava-Micheli] HCC
  EXCLUDES 1   hemoglobinuria NOS (R82.3)

D59.6 Hemoglobinuria due to hemolysis from other external causes HCC
  Hemoglobinuria from exertion
  March hemoglobinuria
  Paroxysmal cold hemoglobinuria
  Use additional code (Chapter 20) to identify external cause
  EXCLUDES 1   hemoglobinuria NOS (R82.3)

D59.8 Other acquired hemolytic anemias HCC

D59.9 Acquired hemolytic anemia, unspecified CC HCC
  Idiopathic hemolytic anemia, chronic

N Newborn: 0   P Pediatric: 0-17   M Maternity: 9-64   A Adult: 15-124   MCC Major Complication/Comorbidity   CC Complication/Comorbidity   SW Severe Wound Dx

506   ICD-10-CM 2020

Aplastic and other anemias and other bone marrow failure syndromes (D60-D64)

✓4ᵗʰ D60 Acquired pure red cell aplasia [erythroblastopenia]

INCLUDES   red cell aplasia (acquired) (adult) (with thymoma)

EXCLUDES 1   congenital red cell aplasia (D61.01)

DEF: Bone marrow failure characterized by underproduction of red blood cells while white blood cell and platelet production remains normal.

CC Excl: For MCC codes in category D60: PDX collection 496

D60.0   Chronic acquired pure red cell aplasia   MCC HCC

D60.1   Transient acquired pure red cell aplasia   MCC HCC

D60.8   Other acquired pure red cell aplasias   MCC HCC

D60.9   Acquired pure red cell aplasia, unspecified   MCC HCC

✓4ᵗʰ D61 Other aplastic anemias and other bone marrow failure syndromes

EXCLUDES 1   neutropenia (D70.-)

AHA: 2014,4Q,22

DEF: Aplastic anemia: Bone marrow failure characterized by underproduction of red bloods cells, white blood cells and platelets.

CC Excl: For CC/MCC codes in category D61, unless otherwise noted: PDX collection 496

✓5ᵗʰ D61.0 Constitutional aplastic anemia

D61.01   Constitutional (pure) red blood cell aplasia   CC HCC

Blackfan-Diamond syndrome
Congenital (pure) red cell aplasia
Familial hypoplastic anemia
Primary (pure) red cell aplasia
Red cell (pure) aplasia of infants

EXCLUDES 1   acquired red cell aplasia (D60.9)

CC Excl: PDX collection 498

D61.09   Other constitutional aplastic anemia   CC HCC

Fanconi's anemia
Pancytopenia with malformations

CC Excl: PDX collection 499

D61.1 Drug-induced aplastic anemia   MCC HCC

(handwritten: drug ✗)

Use additional code for adverse effect, if applicable, to identify drug (T36-T50 with fifth or sixth character 5)

D61.2 Aplastic anemia due to other external agents   MCC HCC

(handwritten: external ✗)

Code first, if applicable, toxic effects of substances chiefly nonmedicinal as to source (T51-T65)

D61.3 Idiopathic aplastic anemia   MCC HCC

✓5ᵗʰ D61.8 Other specified aplastic anemias and other bone marrow failure syndromes

CC Excl: For CC codes in subcategory D61.8: PDX collection 500

✓6ᵗʰ D61.81 Pancytopenia

EXCLUDES 1   pancytopenia (due to) (with) aplastic anemia (D61.9)
pancytopenia (due to) (with) bone marrow infiltration (D61.82)
pancytopenia (due to) (with) congenital (pure) red cell aplasia (D61.01)
pancytopenia (due to) (with) hairy cell leukemia (C91.4-)
pancytopenia (due to) (with) human immunodeficiency virus disease (B20)
pancytopenia (due to) (with) leukoerythroblastic anemia (D61.82)
pancytopenia (due to) (with) myeloproliferative disease (D47.1)

EXCLUDES 2   pancytopenia (due to) (with) myelodysplastic syndromes (D46.-)

DEF: Shortage of all three blood cells: white, red, and platelets.

D61.810 Antineoplastic chemotherapy induced pancytopenia   CC HCC

EXCLUDES 2   aplastic anemia due to antineoplastic chemotherapy (D61.1)

D61.811 Other drug-induced pancytopenia   CC HCC

EXCLUDES 2   aplastic anemia due to drugs (D61.1)

D61.818 Other pancytopenia   CC HCC

AHA: 2019,1Q,16

TIP: Assign this code in addition to myeloid leukemia codes (C92.-) when pancytopenia is documented. Although common in some types of myeloid leukemia, pancytopenia is not always inherent.

D61.82 Myelophthisis   CC HCC

Leukoerythroblastic anemia
Myelophthisic anemia
Panmyelophthisis

Code also the underlying disorder, such as:
   malignant neoplasm of breast (C50.-)
   tuberculosis (A15.-)

EXCLUDES 1   idiopathic myelofibrosis (D47.1)
myelofibrosis NOS (D75.81)
myelofibrosis with myeloid metaplasia (D47.4)
primary myelofibrosis (D47.1)
secondary myelofibrosis (D75.81)

DEF: Condition that occurs when normal hematopoietic tissue in the bone marrow is replaced with abnormal tissue, such as fibrous tissue or tumors. Most commonly seen during the advanced stages of cancer.

D61.89 Other specified aplastic anemias and other bone marrow failure syndromes   MCC HCC

CC Excl: PDX collection 496

D61.9 Aplastic anemia, unspecified   HCC

Hypoplastic anemia NOS
Medullary hypoplasia

D62 Acute posthemorrhagic anemia

EXCLUDES 1   anemia due to chronic blood loss (D50.0)
blood loss anemia NOS (D50.0)
congenital anemia from fetal blood loss (P61.3)

✓4ᵗʰ D63 Anemia in chronic diseases classified elsewhere

D63.0 Anemia in neoplastic disease

Code first neoplasm (C00-D49)

EXCLUDES 1   aplastic anemia due to antineoplastic chemotherapy (D61.1)

EXCLUDES 2   anemia due to antineoplastic chemotherapy (D64.81)

D63.1 Anemia in chronic kidney disease

Erythropoietin resistant anemia (EPO resistant anemia)
Code first underlying chronic kidney disease (CKD) (N18.-)

D63.8 Anemia in other chronic diseases classified elsewhere

Code first underlying disease, such as:
   diphyllobothriasis (B70.0)
   hookworm disease (B76.0-B76.9)
   hypothyroidism (E00.0-E03.9)
   malaria (B50.0-B54)
   symptomatic late syphilis (A52.79)
   tuberculosis (A18.89)

✓4ᵗʰ D64 Other anemias

EXCLUDES 1   refractory anemia (D46.-)
refractory anemia with excess blasts in transformation [RAEB T] (C92.0-)

DEF: Sideroblastic anemia: Hereditary or secondary disorder in which the red blood cells cannot effectively use iron, a nutrient needed to make hemoglobin. Although the iron can enter the red blood cell it is not assimilated into the hemoglobin molecule and builds up ringed sideroblasts around the cell nucleus.

D64.0 Hereditary sideroblastic anemia   HCC

Sex-linked hypochromic sideroblastic anemia

D64.1 Secondary sideroblastic anemia due to disease   HCC

Code first underlying disease

D64.2 Secondary sideroblastic anemia due to drugs and toxins   HCC

Code first poisoning due to drug or toxin, if applicable (T36-T65 with fifth or sixth character 1-4 or 6)
Use additional code for adverse effect, if applicable, to identify drug (T36-T50 with fifth or sixth character 5)

D64.3 Other sideroblastic anemias   HCC

Sideroblastic anemia NOS
Pyridoxine-responsive sideroblastic anemia NEC

✔ Additional Character Required   ✓ˣ7ᵗʰ Placeholder   Unacceptable PDx   Questionable PDx   Manifestation   Unspecified Dx   H1-H14 HAC   HCC CMS-HCC Dx   HIV HIV Dx

ICD-10-CM 2020   507

Chapter 3. Diseases of the Blood and Blood-forming Organs

D64.4   **Congenital dyserythropoietic anemia**
Dyshematopoietic anemia (congenital)
> EXCLUDES 1   *Blackfan-Diamond syndrome (D61.Ø1)*
> *Di Guglielmo's disease (C94.Ø)*

√5ᵗʰ **D64.8**   **Other specified anemias**

D64.81   **Anemia due to antineoplastic chemotherapy**
Antineoplastic chemotherapy induced anemia
> EXCLUDES 1   *aplastic anemia due to antineoplastic chemotherapy (D61.1)*
> EXCLUDES 2   *anemia in neoplastic disease (D63.Ø)*

AHA: 2014,4Q,22
DEF: Reversible adverse effect of chemotherapy, causing inhibition of bone marrow production. A decrease in red blood cell production prevents adequate oxygenation of the tissues and organs causing fatigue, shortness of breath (SOB), and exacerbation of other medical conditions.

D64.89   **Other specified anemias**
Infantile pseudoleukemia

D64.9   **Anemia, unspecified**
AHA: 2018,4Q,88; 2017,1Q,7

Coagulation defects, purpura and other hemorrhagic conditions (D65-D69)

D65   **Disseminated intravascular coagulation [defibrination syndrome]**   MCC HCC
Afibrinogenemia, acquired
Consumption coagulopathy
Diffuse or disseminated intravascular coagulation [DIC]
Fibrinolytic hemorrhage, acquired
Fibrinolytic purpura
Purpura fulminans
> EXCLUDES 1   *disseminated intravascular coagulation (complicating):*
> *abortion or ectopic or molar pregnancy (OØØ-OØ7, OØ8.1)*
> *in newborn (P6Ø)*
> *pregnancy, childbirth and the puerperium (O45.Ø, O46.Ø, O67.Ø, O72.3)*

CC Excl: PDX collection 502

Coagulation

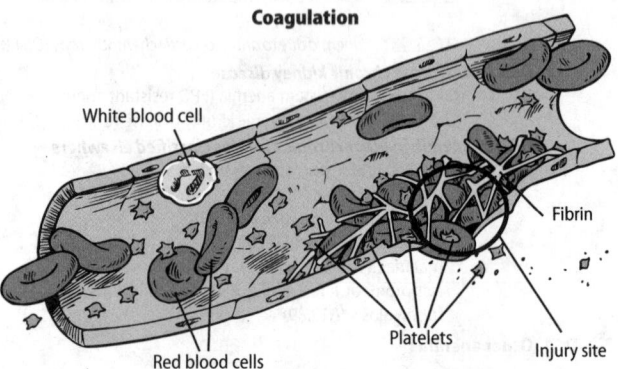

White blood cell
Fibrin
Platelets
Injury site
Red blood cells

D66   **Hereditary factor VIII deficiency**   MCC HCC
Classical hemophilia
Deficiency factor VIII (with functional defect)
Hemophilia A
Hemophilia NOS
> EXCLUDES 1   *factor VIII deficiency with vascular defect (D68.Ø)*

DEF: Hereditary, sex-linked lack of antihemophilic globulin (AHG) (factor VIII) that causes abnormal coagulation characterized by increased bleeding; large bruises of skin; bleeding in the mouth, nose, and gastrointestinal tract; and hemorrhages into joints, resulting in swelling and impaired function.
CC Excl: PDX collection 502

D67   **Hereditary factor IX deficiency**   MCC HCC
Christmas disease
Factor IX deficiency (with functional defect)
Hemophilia B
Plasma thromboplastin component [PTC] deficiency
CC Excl: PDX collection 502

√4ᵗʰ **D68**   **Other coagulation defects**
> EXCLUDES 1   *abnormal coagulation profile (R79.1)*
> *coagulation defects complicating abortion or ectopic or molar pregnancy (OØØ-OØ7, OØ8.1)*
> *coagulation defects complicating pregnancy, childbirth and the puerperium (O45.Ø, O46.Ø, O67.Ø, O72.3)*

AHA: 2016,1Q,14
CC Excl: For CC codes in category D68, unless otherwise noted: PDX collection 502

D68.Ø   **Von Willebrand's disease**   CC HCC
Angiohemophilia
Factor VIII deficiency with vascular defect
Vascular hemophilia
> EXCLUDES 1   *capillary fragility (hereditary) (D69.8)*
> *factor VIII deficiency NOS (D66)*
> *factor VIII deficiency with functional defect (D66)*

DEF: Congenital, abnormal blood coagulation caused by deficient blood factor VII. Symptoms include excess or prolonged bleeding.

D68.1   **Hereditary factor XI deficiency**   CC HCC
Hemophilia C
Plasma thromboplastin antecedent [PTA] deficiency
Rosenthal's disease

D68.2   **Hereditary deficiency of other clotting factors**   CC HCC
AC globulin deficiency
Congenital afibrinogenemia
Deficiency of factor I [fibrinogen]
Deficiency of factor II [prothrombin]
Deficiency of factor V [labile]
Deficiency of factor VII [stable]
Deficiency of factor X [Stuart-Prower]
Deficiency of factor XII [Hageman]
Deficiency of factor XIII [fibrin stabilizing]
Dysfibrinogenemia (congenital)
Hypoproconvertinemia
Owren's disease
Proaccelerin deficiency

√5ᵗʰ **D68.3**   **Hemorrhagic disorder due to circulating anticoagulants**

√6ᵗʰ **D68.31**   **Hemorrhagic disorder due to intrinsic circulating anticoagulants, antibodies, or inhibitors**

D68.311   **Acquired hemophilia**   CC HCC
Autoimmune hemophilia
Autoimmune inhibitors to clotting factors
Secondary hemophilia
CC Excl: PDX collection 503

D68.312   **Antiphospholipid antibody with hemorrhagic disorder**
Lupus anticoagulant (LAC) with hemorrhagic disorder
Systemic lupus erythematosus [SLE] inhibitor with hemorrhagic disorder
> EXCLUDES 1   *antiphospholipid antibody, finding without diagnosis (R76.Ø)*
> *antiphospholipid antibody syndrome (D68.61)*
> *antiphospholipid antibody with hypercoagulable state (D68.61)*
> *lupus anticoagulant (LAC) finding without diagnosis (R76.Ø)*
> *lupus anticoagulant (LAC) with hypercoagulable state (D68.62)*
> *systemic lupus erythematosus [SLE] inhibitor finding without diagnosis (R76.Ø)*
> *systemic lupus erythematosus [SLE] inhibitor with hypercoagulable state (D68.62)*

CC Excl: PDX collection 504

D68.318 Other hemorrhagic disorder due to intrinsic circulating anticoagulants, antibodies, or inhibitors `CC` `HCC`

Antithromboplastinemia

Antithromboplastinogenemia

Hemorrhagic disorder due to intrinsic increase in antithrombin

Hemorrhagic disorder due to intrinsic increase in anti-VIIIa

Hemorrhagic disorder due to intrinsic increase in anti-IXa

Hemorrhagic disorder due to intrinsic increase in anti-XIa

CC Excl: PDX collection 503

D68.32 Hemorrhagic disorder due to extrinsic circulating anticoagulants `CC` `HCC`

Drug-induced hemorrhagic disorder

Hemorrhagic disorder due to increase in anti-IIa

Hemorrhagic disorder due to increase in anti-Xa

Hyperheparinemia

Use additional code for adverse effect, if applicable, to identify drug (T45.515, T45.525)

AHA: 2016,1Q,14-15

TIP: Do not assign to identify routine therapeutic anticoagulation effects; assign only for documented adverse effects.

D68.4 Acquired coagulation factor deficiency `CC` `HCC`

Deficiency of coagulation factor due to liver disease

Deficiency of coagulation factor due to vitamin K deficiency

EXCLUDES 1   *vitamin K deficiency of newborn (P53)*

√5ᵗʰ **D68.5 Primary thrombophilia**

Primary hypercoagulable states

EXCLUDES 1   *antiphospholipid syndrome (D68.61)*

lupus anticoagulant (D68.62)

secondary activated protein C resistance (D68.69)

secondary antiphospholipid antibody syndrome (D68.69)

secondary lupus anticoagulant with hypercoagulable state (D68.69)

secondary systemic lupus erythematosus [SLE] inhibitor with hypercoagulable state (D68.69)

systemic lupus erythematosus [SLE] inhibitor finding without diagnosis (R76.0)

systemic lupus erythematosus [SLE] inhibitor with hemorrhagic disorder (D68.312)

thrombotic thrombocytopenic purpura (M31.1)

DEF: Thrombophilia: Increased tendency of the blood to clot, which can lead to thrombus or embolus formation.

D68.51 Activated protein C resistance `HCC`

Factor V Leiden mutation

D68.52 Prothrombin gene mutation `HCC`

D68.59 Other primary thrombophilia `HCC`

Antithrombin III deficiency

Hypercoagulable state NOS

Primary hypercoagulable state NEC

Primary thrombophilia NEC

Protein C deficiency

Protein S deficiency

Thrombophilia NOS

√5ᵗʰ **D68.6 Other thrombophilia**

Other hypercoagulable states

EXCLUDES 1   *diffuse or disseminated intravascular coagulation [DIC] (D65)*

heparin induced thrombocytopenia (HIT) (D75.82)

hyperhomocysteinemia (E72.11)

D68.61 Antiphospholipid syndrome `HCC`

Anticardiolipin syndrome

Antiphospholipid antibody syndrome

EXCLUDES 1   *anti-phospholipid antibody, finding without diagnosis (R76.0)*

anti-phospholipid antibody with hemorrhagic disorder (D68.312)

lupus anticoagulant syndrome (D68.62)

D68.62 Lupus anticoagulant syndrome `HCC`

Lupus anticoagulant

Presence of systemic lupus erythematosus [SLE] inhibitor

EXCLUDES 1   *anticardiolipin syndrome (D68.61)*

antiphospholipid syndrome (D68.61)

lupus anticoagulant (LAC) finding without diagnosis (R76.0)

lupus anticoagulant (LAC) with hemorrhagic disorder (D68.312)

D68.69 Other thrombophilia `HCC`

Hypercoagulable states NEC

Secondary hypercoagulable state NOS

D68.8 Other specified coagulation defects `CC` `HCC`

EXCLUDES 1   *hemorrhagic disease of newborn (P53)*

D68.9 Coagulation defect, unspecified `CC` `HCC`

√4ᵗʰ **D69 Purpura and other hemorrhagic conditions**

EXCLUDES 1   *benign hypergammaglobulinemic purpura (D89.0)*

cryoglobulinemic purpura (D89.1)

essential (hemorrhagic) thrombocythemia (D47.3)

hemorrhagic thrombocythemia (D47.3)

purpura fulminans (D65)

thrombotic thrombocytopenic purpura (M31.1)

Waldenström hypergammaglobulinemic purpura (D89.0)

CC Excl: For CC codes in category D69: PDX collection 502

D69.0 Allergic purpura `CC` `HCC`

Allergic vasculitis

Nonthrombocytopenic hemorrhagic purpura

Nonthrombocytopenic idiopathic purpura

Purpura anaphylactoid

Purpura Henoch(-Schönlein)

Purpura rheumatica

Vascular purpura

EXCLUDES 1   *thrombocytopenic hemorrhagic purpura (D69.3)*

DEF: Any hemorrhagic condition, thrombocytic or nonthrombocytopenic in origin, caused by a presumed allergic reaction.

D69.1 Qualitative platelet defects `CC` `HCC`

Bernard-Soulier [giant platelet] syndrome

Glanzmann's disease

Grey platelet syndrome

Thromboasthenia (hemorrhagic) (hereditary)

Thrombocytopathy

EXCLUDES 1   *von Willebrand's disease (D68.0)*

D69.2 Other nonthrombocytopenic purpura `HCC`

Purpura NOS

Purpura simplex

Senile purpura

D69.3 Immune thrombocytopenic purpura `CC` `HCC`

Hemorrhagic (thrombocytopenic) purpura

Idiopathic thrombocytopenic purpura

Tidal platelet dysgenesis

DEF: Tidal platelet dysgenesis: Fluctuation of platelet counts from normal to very low within periods of 20 to 40 days and may involve autoimmune platelet destruction.

√5ᵗʰ **D69.4 Other primary thrombocytopenia**

EXCLUDES 1   *transient neonatal thrombocytopenia (P61.0)*

Wiskott-Aldrich syndrome (D82.0)

D69.41 Evans syndrome `CC` `HCC`

D69.42 Congenital and hereditary thrombocytopenia purpura `CC` `HCC`

Congenital thrombocytopenia

Hereditary thrombocytopenia

Code first congenital or hereditary disorder, such as: thrombocytopenia with absent radius (TAR syndrome) (Q87.2)

D69.49 Other primary thrombocytopenia `HCC`

Megakaryocytic hypoplasia

Primary thrombocytopenia NOS

☑ Additional Character Required   √x7ᵗʰ Placeholder   Unacceptable PDx   Questionable PDx   Manifestation   Unspecified Dx   H1-H14 HAC   HCC CMS-HCC Dx   HIV HIV Dx

ICD-10-CM 2020   509

Chapter 3. Diseases of the Blood and Blood-forming Organs

D69.5–D73.4

✓5ᵗʰ **D69.5 Secondary thrombocytopenia**

> **EXCLUDES 1** *heparin induced thrombocytopenia (HIT) (D75.82)*
> *transient thrombocytopenia of newborn (P61.0)*

     D69.51 Posttransfusion purpura
Posttransfusion purpura from whole blood (fresh) or blood products
PTP

     D69.59 Other secondary thrombocytopenia
AHA: 2014,4Q,22

D69.6 Thrombocytopenia, unspecified   HCC

D69.8 Other specified hemorrhagic conditions   HCC
Capillary fragility (hereditary)
Vascular pseudohemophilia

D69.9 Hemorrhagic condition, unspecified   HCC

Other disorders of blood and blood-forming organs (D70-D77)

✓4ᵗʰ **D70 Neutropenia**

> **INCLUDES** agranulocytosis
> decreased absolute neurophile count (ANC)

Use additional code for any associated:
fever (R50.81)
mucositis (J34.81, K12.3-, K92.81, N76.81)

> **EXCLUDES 1** *neutropenic splenomegaly (D73.81)*
> *transient neonatal neutropenia (P61.5)*

DEF: Abnormally low number of neutrophils. Neutrophils are phagocytic, meaning they surround and consume harmful pathogens, primarily bacteria. When neutrophil counts decrease the risk of infection increases.

D70.0 Congenital agranulocytosis   CC   HCC
Congenital neutropenia
Infantile genetic agranulocytosis
Kostmann's disease

D70.1 Agranulocytosis secondary to cancer chemotherapy   CC   HCC
Code also underlying neoplasm
Use additional code for adverse effect, if applicable, to identify drug (T45.1X5)
AHA: 2014,4Q,22

D70.2 Other drug-induced agranulocytosis   CC   HCC
Use additional code for adverse effect, if applicable, to identify drug (T36-T50 with fifth or sixth character 5)

D70.3 Neutropenia due to infection   CC   HCC

D70.4 Cyclic neutropenia   CC   HCC
Cyclic hematopoiesis
Periodic neutropenia

D70.8 Other neutropenia   CC   HCC

D70.9 Neutropenia, unspecified   CC   HCC

D71 Functional disorders of polymorphonuclear neutrophils   CC   HCC
Cell membrane receptor complex [CR3] defect
Chronic (childhood) granulomatous disease
Congenital dysphagocytosis
Progressive septic granulomatosis

✓4ᵗʰ **D72 Other disorders of white blood cells**

> **EXCLUDES 1** *basophilia (D72.824)*
> *immunity disorders (D80–D89)*
> *neutropenia (D70)*
> *preleukemia (syndrome) (D46.9)*

D72.0 Genetic anomalies of leukocytes   HCC
Alder (granulation) (granulocyte) anomaly
Alder syndrome
Hereditary leukocytic hypersegmentation
Hereditary leukocytic hyposegmentation
Hereditary leukomelanopathy
May-Hegglin (granulation) (granulocyte) anomaly
May-Hegglin syndrome
Pelger-Huët (granulation) (granulocyte) anomaly
Pelger-Huët syndrome

> **EXCLUDES 1** *Chédiak (-Steinbrinck)-Higashi syndrome (E70.330)*

D72.1 Eosinophilia
Allergic eosinophilia
Hereditary eosinophilia

> **EXCLUDES 1** *Löffler's syndrome (J82)*
> *pulmonary eosinophilia (J82)*

✓5ᵗʰ **D72.8 Other specified disorders of white blood cells**

> **EXCLUDES 1** *leukemia (C91-C95)*

✓6ᵗʰ **D72.81 Decreased white blood cell count**

> **EXCLUDES 1** *neutropenia (D70.-)*

D72.810 Lymphocytopenia
Decreased lymphocytes

D72.818 Other decreased white blood cell count
Basophilic leukopenia
Eosinophilic leukopenia
Monocytopenia
Other decreased leukocytes
Plasmacytopenia

D72.819 Decreased white blood cell count, unspecified
Decreased leukocytes, unspecified
Leukocytopenia, unspecified
Leukopenia

> **EXCLUDES 1** *malignant leukopenia (D70.9)*

✓6ᵗʰ **D72.82 Elevated white blood cell count**

> **EXCLUDES 1** *eosinophilia (D72.1)*

D72.820 Lymphocytosis (symptomatic)
Elevated lymphocytes

D72.821 Monocytosis (symptomatic)

> **EXCLUDES 1** *infectious mononucleosis (B27.-)*

D72.822 Plasmacytosis

D72.823 Leukemoid reaction
Basophilic leukemoid reaction
Leukemoid reaction NOS
Lymphocytic leukemoid reaction
Monocytic leukemoid reaction
Myelocytic leukemoid reaction
Neutrophilic leukemoid reaction

D72.824 Basophilia
DEF: Increase in the basophils of the blood, a type of white blood cell, often seen in conjunction with neoplastic disorders.

D72.825 Bandemia
Bandemia without diagnosis of specific infection

> **EXCLUDES 1** *confirmed infection — code to infection*
> *leukemia (C91.-, C92.-, C93.-, C94.-, C95.-)*

DEF: Increase in early neutrophil cells, called band cells that may indicate infection.

D72.828 Other elevated white blood cell count

D72.829 Elevated white blood cell count, unspecified
Elevated leukocytes, unspecified
Leukocytosis, unspecified

D72.89 Other specified disorders of white blood cells
Abnormality of white blood cells NEC

D72.9 Disorder of white blood cells, unspecified
Abnormal leukocyte differential NOS

✓4ᵗʰ **D73 Diseases of spleen**

D73.0 Hyposplenism
Atrophy of spleen

> **EXCLUDES 1** *asplenia (congenital) (Q89.01)*
> *postsurgical absence of spleen (Z90.81)*

D73.1 Hypersplenism

> **EXCLUDES 1** *neutropenic splenomegaly (D73.81)*
> *primary splenic neutropenia (D73.81)*
> *splenitis, splenomegaly in late syphilis (A52.79)*
> *splenitis, splenomegaly in tuberculosis (A18.85)*
> *splenomegaly NOS (R16.1)*
> *splenomegaly congenital (Q89.0)*

D73.2 Chronic congestive splenomegaly

D73.3 Abscess of spleen

D73.4 Cyst of spleen

D73.5 Infarction of spleen
Splenic rupture, nontraumatic
Torsion of spleen
> EXCLUDES 1   rupture of spleen due to Plasmodium vivax malaria (B51.0)
> traumatic rupture of spleen (S36.03-)

√5ᵗʰ **D73.8 Other diseases of spleen**

D73.81 Neutropenic splenomegaly
Werner-Schultz disease

D73.89 Other diseases of spleen
Fibrosis of spleen NOS
Perisplenitis
Splenitis NOS

D73.9 Disease of spleen, unspecified

√4ᵗʰ **D74 Methemoglobinemia**

> CC Excl: For CC codes in category D74: PDX collection 506

D74.0 Congenital methemoglobinemia   CC
Congenital NADH-methemoglobin reductase deficiency
Hemoglobin-M [Hb-M] disease
Methemoglobinemia, hereditary

D74.8 Other methemoglobinemias   CC
Acquired methemoglobinemia (with sulfhemoglobinemia)
Toxic methemoglobinemia

D74.9 Methemoglobinemia, unspecified   CC

√4ᵗʰ **D75 Other and unspecified diseases of blood and blood-forming organs**

> EXCLUDES 2   acute lymphadenitis (L04.-)
> chronic lymphadenitis (I88.1)
> enlarged lymph nodes (R59.-)
> hypergammaglobulinemia NOS (D89.2)
> lymphadenitis NOS (I88.9)
> mesenteric lymphadenitis (acute) (chronic) (I88.0)

D75.0 Familial erythrocytosis
Benign polycythemia
Familial polycythemia
> EXCLUDES 1   hereditary ovalocytosis (D58.1)

D75.1 Secondary polycythemia
Acquired polycythemia
Emotional polycythemia
Erythrocytosis NOS
Hypoxemic polycythemia
Nephrogenous polycythemia
Polycythemia due to erythropoietin
Polycythemia due to fall in plasma volume
Polycythemia due to high altitude
Polycythemia due to stress
Polycythemia NOS
Relative polycythemia
> EXCLUDES 1   polycythemia neonatorum (P61.1)
> polycythemia vera (D45)

DEF: Elevated number of red blood cells in circulating blood as a result of reduced oxygen supply to the tissues.

√5ᵗʰ **D75.8 Other specified diseases of blood and blood-forming organs**

D75.81 Myelofibrosis   CC HCC
Myelofibrosis NOS
Secondary myelofibrosis NOS
Code first the underlying disorder, such as:
   malignant neoplasm of breast (C50.-)
Use additional code, if applicable, for associated therapy-related myelodysplastic syndrome (D46.-)
Use additional code for adverse effect, if applicable, to identify drug (T45.1X5)
> EXCLUDES 1   acute myelofibrosis (C94.4-)
> idiopathic myelofibrosis (D47.1)
> leukoerythroblastic anemia (D61.82)
> myelofibrosis with myeloid metaplasia (D47.4)
> myelophthisic anemia (D61.82)
> myelophthisis (D61.82)
> primary myelofibrosis (D47.1)
CC Excl: PDX collection 488

D75.82 Heparin induced thrombocytopenia (HIT)   CC HCC
DEF: Immune-mediated reaction to heparin therapy causing an abrupt fall in platelet count and serious complications such as pulmonary embolism, stroke, AMI, or DVT.

D75.89 Other specified diseases of blood and blood-forming organs

D75.9 Disease of blood and blood-forming organs, unspecified

D75.A Glucose-6-phosphate dehydrogenase (G6PD) deficiency without anemia
> EXCLUDES 1   glucose-6-phosphate dehydrogenase (G6PD) deficiency with anemia (D55.0)

√4ᵗʰ **D76 Other specified diseases with participation of lymphoreticular and reticulohistiocytic tissue**
> EXCLUDES 1   (Abt-) Letterer-Siwe disease (C96.0)
> eosinophilic granuloma (C96.6)
> Hand-Schüller-Christian disease (C96.5)
> histiocytic medullary reticulosis (C96.9)
> histiocytic sarcoma (C96.A)
> histiocytosis X, multifocal (C96.5)
> histiocytosis X, unifocal (C96.6)
> Langerhans-cell histiocytosis, multifocal (C96.5)
> Langerhans-cell histiocytosis NOS (C96.6)
> Langerhans-cell histiocytosis, unifocal (C96.6)
> leukemic reticuloendotheliosis (C91.4-)
> lipomelanotic reticulosis (I89.8)
> malignant histiocytosis (C96.A)
> malignant reticulosis (C86.0)
> nonlipid reticuloendotheliosis (C96.0)

> CC Excl: For CC codes in category D76: PDX collection 507

D76.1 Hemophagocytic lymphohistiocytosis   CC HCC
Familial hemophagocytic reticulosis
Histiocytoses of mononuclear phagocytes

D76.2 Hemophagocytic syndrome, infection-associated   CC HCC
Use additional code to identify infectious agent or disease

D76.3 Other histiocytosis syndromes   CC HCC
Reticulohistiocytoma (giant-cell)
Sinus histiocytosis with massive lymphadenopathy
Xanthogranuloma

D77 Other disorders of blood and blood-forming organs in diseases classified elsewhere
Code first underlying disease, such as:
   amyloidosis (E85.-)
   congenital early syphilis (A50.0)
   echinococcosis (B67.0-B67.9)
   malaria (B50.0-B54)
   schistosomiasis [bilharziasis] (B65.0-B65.9)
   vitamin C deficiency (E54)
> EXCLUDES 1   rupture of spleen due to Plasmodium vivax malaria (B51.0)
> splenitis, splenomegaly in late syphilis (A52.79)
> splenitis, splenomegaly in tuberculosis (A18.85)

Intraoperative and postprocedural complications of the spleen (D78)

> CC Excl: For CC codes in category D78, unless otherwise noted: PDX collection 508

√4ᵗʰ **D78 Intraoperative and postprocedural complications of the spleen**
AHA: 2016,4Q,9-10

√5ᵗʰ **D78.0 Intraoperative hemorrhage and hematoma of the spleen complicating a procedure**
> EXCLUDES 1   intraoperative hemorrhage and hematoma of the spleen due to accidental puncture or laceration during a procedure (D78.1-)

D78.01 Intraoperative hemorrhage and hematoma of the spleen complicating a procedure on the spleen   CC

D78.02 Intraoperative hemorrhage and hematoma of the spleen complicating other procedure   CC

√5ᵗʰ **D78.1** **Accidental puncture and laceration of the spleen during a procedure**

     D78.11 **Accidental puncture and laceration of the spleen during a** procedure on the spleen   CC
       CC Excl: PDX collection 509

     D78.12 **Accidental puncture and laceration of the spleen during other procedure**   CC
       CC Excl: PDX collection 509

√5ᵗʰ **D78.2** **Postprocedural hemorrhage of the spleen following a procedure**

     D78.21 **Postprocedural hemorrhage of the spleen following a** procedure on the spleen   CC

     D78.22 **Postprocedural hemorrhage of the spleen following other procedure**   CC

√5ᵗʰ **D78.3** **Postprocedural hematoma and seroma of the spleen following a procedure**

     D78.31 **Postprocedural hematoma of the spleen following a** procedure on the spleen   CC

     D78.32 **Postprocedural hematoma of the spleen following other procedure**   CC

     D78.33 **Postprocedural seroma of the spleen following a** procedure on the spleen   CC

     D78.34 **Postprocedural seroma of the spleen following other procedure**   CC

√5ᵗʰ **D78.8** **Other intraoperative and postprocedural complications of the spleen**
     Use additional code, if applicable, to further specify disorder

     D78.81 **Other intraoperative complications of the spleen**   CC
       CC Excl: PDX collection 510

     D78.89 **Other postprocedural complications of the spleen**   CC
       CC Excl: PDX collection 510

Certain disorders involving the immune mechanism (D80-D89)

INCLUDES   defects in the complement system
      immunodeficiency disorders, except human immunodeficiency virus [HIV] disease
      sarcoidosis

EXCLUDES 1   *autoimmune disease (systemic) NOS (M35.9)*
      functional disorders of polymorphonuclear neutrophils (D71)
      human immunodeficiency virus [HIV] disease (B20)

CC Excl: For CC codes in categories D80-D89 unless otherwise noted: PDX collection 511

√4ᵗʰ **D80** **Immunodeficiency with predominantly antibody defects**

     D80.0 **Hereditary hypogammaglobulinemia**   CC HCC
       Autosomal recessive agammaglobulinemia (Swiss type)
       X-linked agammaglobulinemia [Bruton] (with growth hormone deficiency)

     D80.1 **Nonfamilial hypogammaglobulinemia**   CC HCC
       Agammaglobulinemia with immunoglobulin-bearing B-lymphocytes
       Common variable agammaglobulinemia [CVAgamma]
       Hypogammaglobulinemia NOS
       CC Excl: PDX collection 512

     D80.2 **Selective deficiency of immunoglobulin A [IgA]**   CC HCC
       CC Excl: PDX collection 512

     D80.3 **Selective deficiency of immunoglobulin G [IgG] subclasses**   CC HCC

     D80.4 **Selective deficiency of immunoglobulin M [IgM]**   CC HCC

     D80.5 **Immunodeficiency with increased immunoglobulin M [IgM]**   CC HCC

     D80.6 **Antibody deficiency with near-normal immunoglobulins or with hyperimmunoglobulinemia**   CC HCC

     D80.7 **Transient hypogammaglobulinemia of infancy**   CC HCC

     D80.8 **Other immunodeficiencies with predominantly antibody defects**   CC HCC
       Kappa light chain deficiency

     D80.9 **Immunodeficiency with predominantly antibody defects, unspecified**   CC HCC

√4ᵗʰ **D81** **Combined immunodeficiencies**

     EXCLUDES 1   *autosomal recessive agammaglobulinemia (Swiss type) (D80.0)*

     D81.0 **Severe combined immunodeficiency [SCID] with reticular dysgenesis**   CC HCC

     D81.1 **Severe combined immunodeficiency [SCID] with low T- and B-cell numbers**   CC HCC

     D81.2 **Severe combined immunodeficiency [SCID] with low or normal B-cell numbers**   CC HCC

▲ √5ᵗʰ **D81.3** **Adenosine deaminase [ADA] deficiency**

       ● **D81.30** **Adenosine deaminase deficiency, unspecified**   CC
         ADA deficiency NOS

       ● **D81.31** **Severe combined immunodeficiency due to adenosine deaminase deficiency**   CC
         ADA deficiency with SCID
         Adenosine deaminase [ADA] deficiency with severe combined immunodeficiency

       ● **D81.32** **Adenosine deaminase 2 deficiency**   CC
         ADA2 deficiency
         Adenosine deaminase deficiency type 2
         Code also, if applicable, any associated manifestations, such as:
           polyarteritis nodosa (M30.0)
           stroke (I63.-)

       ● **D81.39** **Other adenosine deaminase deficiency**   CC
         Adenosine deaminase [ADA] deficiency type 1, NOS
         Adenosine deaminase [ADA] deficiency type 1, without SCID
         Adenosine deaminase [ADA] deficiency type 1, without severe combined immunodeficiency
         Partial ADA deficiency (type 1)
         Partial adenosine deaminase deficiency (type 1)

     D81.4 **Nezelof's syndrome**   CC HCC

     D81.5 **Purine nucleoside phosphorylase [PNP] deficiency**   CC HCC
       CC Excl: PDX collection 513

     D81.6 **Major histocompatibility complex class I deficiency**   CC HCC
       Bare lymphocyte syndrome

     D81.7 **Major histocompatibility complex class II deficiency**   CC HCC

√5ᵗʰ **D81.8** **Other combined immunodeficiencies**

     √6ᵗʰ **D81.81** **Biotin-dependent carboxylase deficiency**
       Multiple carboxylase deficiency
       EXCLUDES 1   *biotin-dependent carboxylase deficiency due to dietary deficiency of biotin (E53.8)*

       D81.810 **Biotinidase deficiency**

       D81.818 **Other biotin-dependent carboxylase deficiency**
         Holocarboxylase synthetase deficiency
         Other multiple carboxylase deficiency

       D81.819 **Biotin-dependent carboxylase deficiency, unspecified**
         Multiple carboxylase deficiency, unspecified

     D81.89 **Other combined immunodeficiencies**   CC HCC

     D81.9 **Combined immunodeficiency, unspecified**   CC HCC
       Severe combined immunodeficiency disorder [SCID] NOS

√4ᵗʰ **D82** **Immunodeficiency associated with other major defects**

     EXCLUDES 1   *ataxia telangiectasia [Louis-Bar] (G11.3)*

     D82.0 **Wiskott-Aldrich syndrome**   CC HCC
       Immunodeficiency with thrombocytopenia and eczema

     D82.1 **Di George's syndrome**   CC HCC
       Pharyngeal pouch syndrome
       Thymic alymphoplasia
       Thymic aplasia or hypoplasia with immunodeficiency

     D82.2 **Immunodeficiency with short-limbed stature**   HCC

     D82.3 **Immunodeficiency following hereditary defective response to Epstein-Barr virus**   HCC
       X-linked lymphoproliferative disease

     D82.4 **Hyperimmunoglobulin E [IgE] syndrome**   HCC

N Newborn: 0   P Pediatric: 0-17   M Maternity: 9-64   A Adult: 15-124   MCC Major Complication/Comorbidity   CC Complication/Comorbidity   SW Severe Wound Dx

512   ICD-10-CM 2020

D82.8   **Immunodeficiency associated with other specified major defects**   `HCC`

D82.9   **Immunodeficiency associated with major defect, unspecified**   `HCC`

☑4ᵗʰ **D83**   **Common variable immunodeficiency**

D83.0   **Common variable immunodeficiency with predominant abnormalities of B-cell numbers and function**   `CC` `HCC`

D83.1   **Common variable immunodeficiency with predominant immunoregulatory T-cell disorders**   `CC` `HCC`

D83.2   **Common variable immunodeficiency with autoantibodies to B- or T-cells**   `CC` `HCC`

D83.8   **Other common variable immunodeficiencies**   `CC` `HCC`

D83.9   **Common variable immunodeficiency, unspecified**   `CC` `HCC`

☑4ᵗʰ **D84**   **Other immunodeficiencies**

D84.0   **Lymphocyte function antigen-1 [LFA-1] defect**   `HCC`

D84.1   **Defects in the complement system**   `HCC`
     C1 esterase inhibitor [C1-INH] deficiency

D84.8   **Other specified immunodeficiencies**   `CC` `HCC`

D84.9   **Immunodeficiency, unspecified**   `CC` `HCC`

☑4ᵗʰ **D86**   **Sarcoidosis**
     DEF: Clustering of immune cells resulting in granuloma formation. Often affects the lungs and lymphatic system but can occur in other body sites.

D86.0   **Sarcoidosis of lung**   `HCC`

D86.1   **Sarcoidosis of lymph nodes**

D86.2   **Sarcoidosis of lung with sarcoidosis of lymph nodes**   `HCC`

D86.3   **Sarcoidosis of skin**

☑5ᵗʰ **D86.8**   **Sarcoidosis of other sites**

     D86.81   **Sarcoid meningitis**

     D86.82   **Multiple cranial nerve palsies in sarcoidosis**   `HCC`

     D86.83   **Sarcoid iridocyclitis**

     D86.84   **Sarcoid pyelonephritis**
         Tubulo-interstitial nephropathy in sarcoidosis

     D86.85   **Sarcoid myocarditis**

     D86.86   **Sarcoid arthropathy**
         Polyarthritis in sarcoidosis

     D86.87   **Sarcoid myositis**

     D86.89   **Sarcoidosis of other sites**
         Hepatic granuloma
         Uveoparotid fever [Heerfordt]

D86.9   **Sarcoidosis, unspecified**

☑4ᵗʰ **D89**   **Other disorders involving the immune mechanism, not elsewhere classified**
     EXCLUDES 1   hyperglobulinemia NOS (R77.1)
         monoclonal gammopathy (of undetermined significance) (D47.2)
     EXCLUDES 2   transplant failure and rejection (T86.-)

D89.0   **Polyclonal hypergammaglobulinemia**
     Benign hypergammaglobulinemic purpura
     Polyclonal gammopathy NOS

D89.1   **Cryoglobulinemia**   `HCC`
     Cryoglobulinemic purpura
     Cryoglobulinemic vasculitis
     Essential cryoglobulinemia
     Idiopathic cryoglobulinemia
     Mixed cryoglobulinemia
     Primary cryoglobulinemia
     Secondary cryoglobulinemia

D89.2   **Hypergammaglobulinemia, unspecified**

D89.3   **Immune reconstitution syndrome**   `HCC`
     Immune reconstitution inflammatory syndrome [IRIS]
     Use additional code for adverse effect, if applicable, to identify drug (T36-T50 with fifth or sixth character 5)

☑5ᵗʰ **D89.4**   **Mast cell activation syndrome and related disorders**
     EXCLUDES 1   aggressive systemic mastocytosis (C96.21)
         congenital cutaneous mastocytosis (Q82.2)
         (non-congenital) cutaneous mastocytosis (D47.01)
         (indolent) systemic mastocytosis (D47.02)
         malignant mast cell neoplasm (C96.2-)
         malignant mastocytoma (C96.29)
         mast cell leukemia (C94.3-)
         mast cell sarcoma (C96.22)
         mastocytoma NOS (D47.09)
         other mast cell neoplasms of uncertain behavior (D47.09)
         systemic mastocytosis associated with a clonal hematologic non-mast cell lineage disease (SM-AHNMD) (D47.02)
     AHA: 2016,4Q,11

D89.40   **Mast cell activation, unspecified**   `HCC`
     Mast cell activation disorder, unspecified
     Mast cell activation syndrome, NOS

D89.41   **Monoclonal mast cell activation syndrome**   `HCC`

D89.42   **Idiopathic mast cell activation syndrome**   `HCC`

D89.43   **Secondary mast cell activation**   `HCC`
     Secondary mast cell activation syndrome
     Code also underlying etiology, if known

D89.49   **Other mast cell activation disorder**   `HCC`
     Other mast cell activation syndrome

☑5ᵗʰ **D89.8**   **Other specified disorders involving the immune mechanism, not elsewhere classified**

☑6ᵗʰ **D89.81**   **Graft-versus-host disease**
     Code first underlying cause, such as:
         complications of transplanted organs and tissue (T86.-)
         complications of blood transfusion (T80.89)
     Use additional code to identify associated manifestations, such as:
         desquamative dermatitis (L30.8)
         diarrhea (R19.7)
         elevated bilirubin (R17)
         hair loss (L65.9)
     CC Excl: For CC codes in subcategory D89.81: PDX collection 514

     D89.810   **Acute graft-versus-host disease**   `CC` `HCC`

     D89.811   **Chronic graft-versus-host disease**   `CC` `HCC`

     D89.812   **Acute on chronic graft-versus-host disease**   `CC` `HCC`

     D89.813   **Graft-versus-host disease, unspecified**   `CC` `HCC`

D89.82   **Autoimmune lymphoproliferative syndrome [ALPS]**   `HCC`
     DEF: Rare genetic alteration of the Fas protein that impairs normal cellular apoptosis (normal cell death), causing abnormal accumulation of lymphocytes in the lymph glands, liver, and spleen. Symptoms include neutropenia, anemia, and thrombocytopenia.

D89.89   **Other specified disorders involving the immune mechanism, not elsewhere classified**   `HCC`
     EXCLUDES 1   human immunodeficiency virus disease (B20)
     AHA: 2017,4Q,109

D89.9   **Disorder involving the immune mechanism, unspecified**   `HCC`
     Immune disease NOS
     AHA: 2015,3Q,22

☑ Additional Character Required   ☑x7ᵗʰ Placeholder   Unacceptable PDx   Questionable PDx   Manifestation   Unspecified Dx   `H1`-`H14` HAC   `HCC` CMS-HCC Dx   `HIV` HIV Dx

ICD-10-CM 2020   **513**

Chapter 4. Endocrine, Nutritional and Metabolic Diseases (E00–E89)

Chapter-specific Guidelines with Coding Examples

The chapter-specific guidelines from the ICD-10-CM Official Guidelines for Coding and Reporting have been provided below. Along with these guidelines are coding examples, contained in the shaded boxes, that have been developed to help illustrate the coding and/or sequencing guidance found in these guidelines.

a. Diabetes mellitus

The diabetes mellitus codes are combination codes that include the type of diabetes mellitus, the body system affected, and the complications affecting that body system. As many codes within a particular category as are necessary to describe all of the complications of the disease may be used. They should be sequenced based on the reason for a particular encounter. Assign as many codes from categories E08–E13 as needed to identify all of the associated conditions that the patient has.

> Patient is seen for poorly controlled diabetes, type 2, with diabetic polyneuropathy and diabetic retinopathy with macular edema
>
> **E11.65**   **Type 2 diabetes mellitus with hyperglycemia**
>
> **E11.311**   **Type 2 diabetes mellitus with unspecified diabetic retinopathy with macular edema**
>
> **E11.42**   **Type 2 diabetes mellitus with diabetic polyneuropathy**
>
> *Explanation*: Use as many codes to describe the diabetic complications as needed. Many are combination codes that describe more than one condition. Code first the reason for the encounter. "Poorly controlled" is described as "with hyperglycemia." Diabetes documented as "uncontrolled" is not assumed to be hyperglycemic but can be classified to either hyperglycemia or hypoglycemia. If documentation is not clear, the provider must be queried so that the appropriate code can be reported.

1) Type of diabetes

The age of a patient is not the sole determining factor, though most type 1 diabetics develop the condition before reaching puberty. For this reason type 1 diabetes mellitus is also referred to as juvenile diabetes.

> A 45-year-old patient is diagnosed with type 1 diabetes
>
> **E10.9**   **Type 1 diabetes mellitus without complications**
>
> *Explanation*: Although most type 1 diabetics are diagnosed in childhood or adolescence, it can also begin in adults.

2) Type of diabetes mellitus not documented

If the type of diabetes mellitus is not documented in the medical record the default is E11.-, Type 2 diabetes mellitus.

> H & P lists diabetes and hypertension on patient problem list
>
> **E11.9**   **Type 2 diabetes mellitus without complications**
>
> **I10**   **Essential (primary) hypertension**
>
> *Explanation*: Since the type of diabetes was not documented and no complications were noted, the default code is E11.9.

3) Diabetes mellitus and the use of insulin and oral hypoglycemics

If the documentation in a medical record does not indicate the type of diabetes but does indicate that the patient uses insulin, code E11-, Type 2 diabetes mellitus, should be assigned. An additional code should be assigned from category Z79 to identify the long-term (current) use of insulin or oral hypoglycemic drugs. If the patient is treated with both oral medications and insulin, only the code for long-term (current) use of insulin should be assigned. Code Z79.4 should not be assigned if insulin is given temporarily to bring a type 2 patient's blood sugar under control during an encounter.

> Diabetic patient on daily metformin is admitted in ketoacidosis; insulin given to stabilize blood sugars and discontinued at discharge
>
> **E11.10**   **Type 2 diabetes mellitus with ketoacidosis without coma**
>
> **Z79.84**   **Long term (current) use of oral hypoglycemic drugs**
>
> *Explanation*: Type 2 is the default for diabetes when not further specified in the documentation. Although insulin was given to the patient during the encounter, it was discontinued at discharge, indicating that the patient does not regularly use insulin. Applying code Z79.4 to represent long-term use of insulin would be inappropriate.

4) Diabetes mellitus in pregnancy and gestational diabetes

See Section I.C.15. Diabetes mellitus in pregnancy.

See Section I.C.15. Gestational (pregnancy induced) diabetes

5) Complications due to insulin pump malfunction

(a) Underdose of insulin due to insulin pump failure

An underdose of insulin due to an insulin pump failure should be assigned to a code from subcategory T85.6, Mechanical complication of other specified internal and external prosthetic devices, implants and grafts, that specifies the type of pump malfunction, as the principal or first-listed code, followed by code T38.3X6-, Underdosing of insulin and oral hypoglycemic [antidiabetic] drugs. Additional codes for the type of diabetes mellitus and any associated complications due to the underdosing should also be assigned.

> A 24-year-old type 1 diabetic male treated in ED for hyperglycemia; insulin pump found to be malfunctioning and underdosing
>
> **T85.614A**   **Breakdown (mechanical) of insulin pump, initial encounter**
>
> **T38.3X6A**   **Underdosing of insulin and oral hypoglycemic [antidiabetic] drugs, initial encounter**
>
> **E10.65**   **Type 1 diabetes mellitus with hyperglycemia**
>
> *Explanation*: The complication code for the mechanical breakdown of the pump is sequenced first, followed by the underdosing code and type of diabetes with complication. Code all other diabetic complication codes necessary to describe the patient's condition.

(b) Overdose of insulin due to insulin pump failure

The principal or first-listed code for an encounter due to an insulin pump malfunction resulting in an overdose of insulin, should also be T85.6-, Mechanical complication of other specified internal and external prosthetic devices, implants and grafts, followed by code T38.3X1-, Poisoning by insulin and oral hypoglycemic [antidiabetic] drugs, accidental (unintentional).

> A 24-year-old type 1 diabetic male found down with diabetic coma, brought into ED and treated for hypoglycemia; insulin pump found to be malfunctioning and overdosing
>
> **T85.614A**   **Breakdown (mechanical) of insulin pump, initial encounter**
>
> **T38.3X1A**   **Poisoning by insulin and oral hypoglycemic [antidiabetic] drugs, accidental (unintentional), initial encounter**
>
> **E10.641**   **Type 1 diabetes mellitus with hypoglycemia with coma**
>
> *Explanation*: The complication code for the mechanical breakdown of the pump is sequenced first, followed by the poisoning code and type of diabetes with complication. All the characters in the combination code must be used to form a valid code and to fully describe the type of diabetes, the hypoglycemia, and the coma.

Chapter 4. Endocrine, Nutritional and Metabolic Diseases

6) Secondary diabetes mellitus

Codes under categories E08, Diabetes mellitus due to underlying condition, E09, Drug or chemical induced diabetes mellitus, and E13, Other specified diabetes mellitus, identify complications/manifestations associated with secondary diabetes mellitus. Secondary diabetes is always caused by another condition or event (e.g., cystic fibrosis, malignant neoplasm of pancreas, pancreatectomy, adverse effect of drug, or poisoning).

(a) Secondary diabetes mellitus and the use of insulin or oral hypoglycemic drugs

For patients with secondary diabetes mellitus who routinely use insulin or oral hypoglycemic drugs, an additional code from category Z79 should be assigned to identify the long-term (current) use of insulin or oral hypoglycemic drugs. If the patient is treated with both oral medications and insulin, only the code for long-term (current) use of insulin should be assigned. Code Z79.4 should not be assigned if insulin is given temporarily to bring a secondary diabetic patient's blood sugar under control during an encounter.

The patient, maintained on metformin and insulin, was admitted for treatment of diabetic gangrene. The patient developed diabetes secondary to Nelson's syndrome.

E24.1   **Nelson's syndrome**

E08.52   **Diabetes mellitus due to underlying condition with diabetic peripheral angiopathy with gangrene**

Z79.4   **Long term (current) use of insulin**

Explanation: When diabetes is caused by an underlying condition, the underlying condition should always be sequenced before any codes representing the diabetes. Patients with secondary diabetes may be maintained on both insulin and an oral hypoglycemic. Report only the code for the long-term use of insulin when both oral hypoglycemic and insulin are prescribed.

(b) Assigning and sequencing secondary diabetes codes and its causes

The sequencing of the secondary diabetes codes in relationship to codes for the cause of the diabetes is based on the Tabular List instructions for categories E08, E09 and E13.

(i) Secondary diabetes mellitus due to pancreatectomy

For postpancreatectomy diabetes mellitus (lack of insulin due to the surgical removal of all or part of the pancreas), assign code E89.1, Postprocedural hypoinsulinemia. Assign a code from category E13 and a code from subcategory Z90.41, Acquired absence of pancreas, as additional codes.

Patient with newly diagnosed diabetes after surgical removal of part of pancreas is discharged with referral for consult to initiate insulin.

E89.1   **Postprocedural hypoinsulinemia**

E13.9   **Other specified diabetes mellitus without complications**

Z90.411   **Acquired partial absence of pancreas**

Explanation: Sequence the postprocedural complication of the hypoinsulinemia due to the partial removal of the pancreas as the first-listed code, followed by the other specified diabetes (NEC) with or without complications and the partial or total acquired absence of the pancreas. Code Z79.4 Long term (current) use of insulin, is not added because the insulin has not yet been started.

(ii) Secondary diabetes due to drugs

Secondary diabetes may be caused by an adverse effect of correctly administered medications, poisoning or sequela of poisoning.

See section I.C.19.e for coding of adverse effects and poisoning, and section I.C.20 for external cause code reporting.

Initial encounter for corticosteroid-induced diabetes mellitus

E09.9   **Drug or chemical induced diabetes mellitus without complications**

T38.0X5A   **Adverse effect of glucocorticoids and synthetic analogues, initial encounter**

Explanation: If the diabetes is caused by an adverse effect of a drug, the diabetic condition is coded first. If it occurs from a poisoning or overdose, the poisoning code causing the diabetes is sequenced first.

Chapter 4. Endocrine, Nutritional and Metabolic Diseases (E00-E89)

> **NOTE** All neoplasms, whether functionally active or not, are classified in Chapter 2. Appropriate codes in this chapter (i.e. E05.8, E07.0, E16-E31, E34.-) may be used as additional codes to indicate either functional activity by neoplasms and ectopic endocrine tissue or hyperfunction and hypofunction of endocrine glands associated with neoplasms and other conditions classified elsewhere.

> *EXCLUDES 1*   transitory endocrine and metabolic disorders specific to newborn (P70-P74)

AHA: 2018,2Q,6

This chapter contains the following blocks:

E00-E07   Disorders of thyroid gland
E08-E13   Diabetes mellitus
E15-E16   Other disorders of glucose regulation and pancreatic internal secretion
E20-E35   Disorders of other endocrine glands
E36   Intraoperative complications of endocrine system
E40-E46   Malnutrition
E50-E64   Other nutritional deficiencies
E65-E68   Overweight, obesity and other hyperalimentation
E70-E88   Metabolic disorders
E89   Postprocedural endocrine and metabolic complications and disorders, not elsewhere classified

Disorders of thyroid gland (E00-E07)

✓4th E00 Congenital iodine-deficiency syndrome

Use additional code (F70-F79) to identify associated intellectual disabilities

> *EXCLUDES 1*   subclinical iodine-deficiency hypothyroidism (E02)

E00.0 Congenital iodine-deficiency syndrome, neurological type
Endemic cretinism, neurological type

E00.1 Congenital iodine-deficiency syndrome, myxedematous type
Endemic hypothyroid cretinism
Endemic cretinism, myxedematous type

E00.2 Congenital iodine-deficiency syndrome, mixed type
Endemic cretinism, mixed type

E00.9 Congenital iodine-deficiency syndrome, unspecified
Congenital iodine-deficiency hypothyroidism NOS
Endemic cretinism NOS

✓4th E01 Iodine-deficiency related thyroid disorders and allied conditions

> *EXCLUDES 1*   congenital iodine-deficiency syndrome (E00.-)
> subclinical iodine-deficiency hypothyroidism (E02)

E01.0 Iodine-deficiency related diffuse (endemic) goiter

E01.1 Iodine-deficiency related multinodular (endemic) goiter
Iodine-deficiency related nodular goiter

E01.2 Iodine-deficiency related (endemic) goiter, unspecified
Endemic goiter NOS

E01.8 Other iodine-deficiency related thyroid disorders and allied conditions
Acquired iodine-deficiency hypothyroidism NOS

E02 Subclinical iodine-deficiency hypothyroidism

✓4th E03 Other hypothyroidism

> *EXCLUDES 1*   iodine-deficiency related hypothyroidism (E00-E02)
> postprocedural hypothyroidism (E89.0)

DEF: Hypothyroidism: Underproduction of thyroid hormone.

E03.0 Congenital hypothyroidism with diffuse goiter
Congenital parenchymatous goiter (nontoxic)
Congenital goiter (nontoxic) NOS

> *EXCLUDES 1*   transitory congenital goiter with normal function (P72.0)

E03.1 Congenital hypothyroidism without goiter
Aplasia of thyroid (with myxedema)
Congenital atrophy of thyroid
Congenital hypothyroidism NOS

E03.2 Hypothyroidism due to medicaments and other exogenous substances
Code first poisoning due to drug or toxin, if applicable (T36-T65 with fifth or sixth character 1-4 or 6)
Use additional code for adverse effect, if applicable, to identify drug (T36-T50 with fifth or sixth character 5)

E03.3 Postinfectious hypothyroidism

E03.4 Atrophy of thyroid (acquired)
> *EXCLUDES 1*   congenital atrophy of thyroid (E03.1)

E03.5 Myxedema coma   `MCC` `HCC`
CC Excl: PDX collection 515

E03.8 Other specified hypothyroidism

E03.9 Hypothyroidism, unspecified
Myxedema NOS

✓4th E04 Other nontoxic goiter

> *EXCLUDES 1*   congenital goiter (NOS) (diffuse) (parenchymatous) (E03.0)
> iodine-deficiency related goiter (E00-E02)

E04.0 Nontoxic diffuse goiter
Diffuse (colloid) nontoxic goiter
Simple nontoxic goiter

E04.1 Nontoxic single thyroid nodule
Colloid nodule (cystic) (thyroid)
Nontoxic uninodular goiter
Thyroid (cystic) nodule NOS
DEF: Enlarged thyroid, commonly due to decreased thyroid production, with a single nodule. No clinical hypothyroidism.

E04.2 Nontoxic multinodular goiter
Cystic goiter NOS
Multinodular (cystic) goiter NOS
DEF: Enlarged thyroid, commonly due to decreased thyroid production with multiple nodules. No clinical hypothyroidism.

E04.8 Other specified nontoxic goiter

E04.9 Nontoxic goiter, unspecified
Goiter NOS
Nodular goiter (nontoxic) NOS

✓4th E05 Thyrotoxicosis [hyperthyroidism]

> *EXCLUDES 1*   chronic thyroiditis with transient thyrotoxicosis (E06.2)
> neonatal thyrotoxicosis (P72.1)

DEF: Excessive quantities of hormones from the thyroid gland caused by overproduction or loss of storage ability.
CC Excl: For MCC codes in category E05: PDX collection 516

✓5th E05.0 Thyrotoxicosis with diffuse goiter
Exophthalmic or toxic goiter NOS
Graves' disease
Toxic diffuse goiter
DEF: Diffuse thyroid enlargement accompanied by hyperthyroidism, bulging eyes, and dermopathy.

E05.00 Thyrotoxicosis with diffuse goiter without thyrotoxic crisis or storm

E05.01 Thyrotoxicosis with diffuse goiter with thyrotoxic crisis or storm   `MCC`

Goiter

Pyramidal lobe
Thyroid cartilage
(- - - -) Healthy thyroid
Goiter (hyperfunctioning thyroid)

✓5th E05.1 Thyrotoxicosis with toxic single thyroid nodule
Thyrotoxicosis with toxic uninodular goiter
DEF: Symptomatic hyperthyroidism with a single nodule on the enlarged thyroid gland. Onset of symptoms can be abrupt and include extreme nervousness, insomnia, weight loss, tremors, and psychosis or coma.

uninodular

E05.10 Thyrotoxicosis with toxic single thyroid nodule without thyrotoxic crisis or storm

E05.11 Thyrotoxicosis with toxic single thyroid nodule with thyrotoxic crisis or storm   `MCC`

✓5th E05.2 Thyrotoxicosis with toxic multinodular goiter
Toxic nodular goiter NOS

E05.20 Thyrotoxicosis with toxic multinodular goiter without thyrotoxic crisis or storm

multinodular

E05.21 Thyrotoxicosis with toxic multinodular goiter with thyrotoxic crisis or storm   `MCC`

✔ Additional Character Required   ✓x7th Placeholder   Unacceptable PDx   Questionable PDx   Manifestation   Unspecified Dx   H1-H14 HAC   HCC CMS-HCC Dx   HIV HIV Dx

ICD-10-CM 2020   517

√5th **E05.3 Thyrotoxicosis from ectopic thyroid tissue**

    E05.30 Thyrotoxicosis from ectopic thyroid tissue without thyrotoxic crisis or storm

    E05.31 Thyrotoxicosis from ectopic thyroid tissue with thyrotoxic crisis or storm   MCC

√5th **E05.4 Thyrotoxicosis factitia**

    E05.40 Thyrotoxicosis factitia without thyrotoxic crisis or storm

    E05.41 Thyrotoxicosis factitia with thyrotoxic crisis or storm   MCC

√5th **E05.8 Other thyrotoxicosis**

    Overproduction of thyroid-stimulating hormone

    E05.80 Other thyrotoxicosis without thyrotoxic crisis or storm

    E05.81 Other thyrotoxicosis with thyrotoxic crisis or storm   MCC

√5th **E05.9 Thyrotoxicosis, unspecified**

    Hyperthyroidism NOS

    E05.90 Thyrotoxicosis, unspecified without thyrotoxic crisis or storm

    E05.91 Thyrotoxicosis, unspecified with thyrotoxic crisis or storm   MCC

√4th **E06 Thyroiditis**

    EXCLUDES 1   postpartum thyroiditis (O90.5)

    DEF: Inflammation of the thyroid gland.

    E06.0 Acute thyroiditis   CC

      Abscess of thyroid

      Pyogenic thyroiditis

      Suppurative thyroiditis

      Use additional code (B95-B97) to identify infectious agent

      CC Excl: PDX collection 517

    E06.1 Subacute thyroiditis

      de Quervain thyroiditis

      Giant-cell thyroiditis

      Granulomatous thyroiditis

      Nonsuppurative thyroiditis

      Viral thyroiditis

      EXCLUDES 1   autoimmune thyroiditis (E06.3)

    E06.2 Chronic thyroiditis with transient thyrotoxicosis

      EXCLUDES 1   autoimmune thyroiditis (E06.3)

    E06.3 Autoimmune thyroiditis

      Hashimoto's thyroiditis

      Hashitoxicosis (transient)

      Lymphadenoid goiter

      Lymphocytic thyroiditis

      Struma lymphomatosa

    E06.4 Drug-induced thyroiditis

      Use additional code for adverse effect, if applicable, to identify drug (T36-T50 with fifth or sixth character 5)

    E06.5 Other chronic thyroiditis

      Chronic fibrous thyroiditis

      Chronic thyroiditis NOS

      Ligneous thyroiditis

      Riedel thyroiditis

    E06.9 Thyroiditis, unspecified

√4th **E07 Other disorders of thyroid**

    E07.0 Hypersecretion of calcitonin

      C-cell hyperplasia of thyroid

      Hypersecretion of thyrocalcitonin

    E07.1 Dyshormogenetic goiter

      Familial dyshormogenetic goiter

      Pendred's syndrome

      EXCLUDES 1   transitory congenital goiter with normal function (P72.0)

√5th **E07.8 Other specified disorders of thyroid**

    E07.81 Sick-euthyroid syndrome   CC

      Euthyroid sick-syndrome

      DEF: Thyroid dysfunction caused by abnormal levels of thyroid hormones T3 and/or T4. This syndrome is often associated with starvation or critical illness.

    E07.89 Other specified disorders of thyroid

      Abnormality of thyroid-binding globulin

      Hemorrhage of thyroid

      Infarction of thyroid

    E07.9 Disorder of thyroid, unspecified

Diabetes mellitus (E08-E13)

AHA: 2018,4Q,88; 2018,3Q,3-4; 2018,2Q,6; 2017,4Q,6; 2017,1Q,42; 2016,4Q,11-13; 2016,2Q,36; 2016,1Q,11-13

√4th **E08 Diabetes mellitus due to underlying condition**

    Code first the underlying condition, such as:

      congenital rubella (P35.0)

      Cushing's syndrome (E24.-)

      cystic fibrosis (E84.-)

      malignant neoplasm (C00-C96)

      malnutrition (E40-E46)

      pancreatitis and other diseases of the pancreas (K85-K86.-)

    Use additional code to identify control using:

      insulin (Z79.4)

      oral antidiabetic drugs (Z79.84)

      oral hypoglycemic drugs (Z79.84)

    EXCLUDES 1   drug or chemical induced diabetes mellitus (E09.-)

      gestational diabetes (O24.4-)

      neonatal diabetes mellitus (P70.2)

      postpancreatectomy diabetes mellitus (E13.-)

      postprocedural diabetes mellitus (E13.-)

      secondary diabetes mellitus NEC (E13.-)

      type 1 diabetes mellitus (E10.-)

      type 2 diabetes mellitus (E11.-)

    AHA: 2013,4Q,114; 2013,3Q,20

    CC Excl: For MCC codes in category E08: PDX collection 518

√5th **E08.0 Diabetes mellitus due to underlying condition with hyperosmolarity**

    DEF: Diabetic hyperosmolarity: Extremely high levels of glucose in the blood without ketones.

    E08.00 Diabetes mellitus due to underlying condition with hyperosmolarity without nonketotic hyperglycemic-hyperosmolar coma (NKHHC)   MCC H9 HCC

    E08.01 Diabetes mellitus due to underlying condition with hyperosmolarity with coma   MCC H9 HCC

√5th **E08.1 Diabetes mellitus due to underlying condition with ketoacidosis**

    DEF: Diabetic ketoacidosis: Potentially life-threatening complication due to a shortage of insulin in which the body switches to burning fatty acids and producing acidic ketone bodies.

    E08.10 Diabetes mellitus due to underlying condition with ketoacidosis without coma   MCC H9 HCC

    E08.11 Diabetes mellitus due to underlying condition with ketoacidosis with coma   MCC HCC

√5th **E08.2 Diabetes mellitus due to underlying condition with kidney complications**

    E08.21 Diabetes mellitus due to underlying condition with diabetic nephropathy   HCC

      Diabetes mellitus due to underlying condition with intercapillary glomerulosclerosis

      Diabetes mellitus due to underlying condition with intracapillary glomerulonephrosis

      Diabetes mellitus due to underlying condition with Kimmelstiel-Wilson disease

    E08.22 Diabetes mellitus due to underlying condition with diabetic chronic kidney disease   HCC

      Use additional code to identify stage of chronic kidney disease (N18.1-N18.6)

    E08.29 Diabetes mellitus due to underlying condition with other diabetic kidney complication   HCC

      Renal tubular degeneration in diabetes mellitus due to underlying condition

N Newborn: 0   P Pediatric: 0-17   M Maternity: 9-64   A Adult: 15-124   MCC Major Complication/Comorbidity   CC Complication/Comorbidity   SW Severe Wound Dx

518   ICD-10-CM 2020

☑5ᵗʰ **E08.3 Diabetes mellitus due to underlying condition with ophthalmic complications**

> One of the following 7th characters is to be assigned to codes in subcategories E08.32, E08.33, E08.34, E08.35, and E08.37 to designate laterality of the disease:
> 1   right eye
> 2   left eye
> 3   bilateral
> 9   unspecified eye

☑6ᵗʰ **E08.31 Diabetes mellitus due to underlying condition with unspecified diabetic retinopathy**

> **DEF:** Diabetic retinopathy: Diabetic complication from damage to the retinal vessels resulting in vision problems that can progress to blindness.

E08.311 Diabetes mellitus due to underlying condition with unspecified diabetic retinopathy with macular edema   HCC

E08.319 Diabetes mellitus due to underlying condition with unspecified diabetic retinopathy without macular edema   HCC

☑6ᵗʰ **E08.32 Diabetes mellitus due to underlying condition with mild nonproliferative diabetic retinopathy**

> Diabetes mellitus due to underlying condition with nonproliferative diabetic retinopathy NOS

☑7ᵗʰ **E08.321 Diabetes mellitus due to underlying condition with mild nonproliferative diabetic retinopathy with macular edema**   HCC

☑7ᵗʰ **E08.329 Diabetes mellitus due to underlying condition with mild nonproliferative diabetic retinopathy without macular edema**   HCC

☑6ᵗʰ **E08.33 Diabetes mellitus due to underlying condition with moderate nonproliferative diabetic retinopathy**

☑7ᵗʰ **E08.331 Diabetes mellitus due to underlying condition with moderate nonproliferative diabetic retinopathy with macular edema**   HCC

☑7ᵗʰ **E08.339 Diabetes mellitus due to underlying condition with moderate nonproliferative diabetic retinopathy without macular edema**   HCC

☑6ᵗʰ **E08.34 Diabetes mellitus due to underlying condition with severe nonproliferative diabetic retinopathy**

☑7ᵗʰ **E08.341 Diabetes mellitus due to underlying condition with severe nonproliferative diabetic retinopathy with macular edema**   HCC

☑7ᵗʰ **E08.349 Diabetes mellitus due to underlying condition with severe nonproliferative diabetic retinopathy without macular edema**   HCC

☑6ᵗʰ **E08.35 Diabetes mellitus due to underlying condition with proliferative diabetic retinopathy**

☑7ᵗʰ **E08.351 Diabetes mellitus due to underlying condition with proliferative diabetic retinopathy with macular edema**   HCC

☑7ᵗʰ **E08.352 Diabetes mellitus due to underlying condition with proliferative diabetic retinopathy with traction retinal detachment involving the macula**   HCC

☑7ᵗʰ **E08.353 Diabetes mellitus due to underlying condition with proliferative diabetic retinopathy with traction retinal detachment not involving the macula**   HCC

☑7ᵗʰ **E08.354 Diabetes mellitus due to underlying condition with proliferative diabetic retinopathy with combined traction retinal detachment and rhegmatogenous retinal detachment**   HCC

☑7ᵗʰ **E08.355 Diabetes mellitus due to underlying condition with stable proliferative diabetic retinopathy**   HCC

☑7ᵗʰ **E08.359 Diabetes mellitus due to underlying condition with proliferative diabetic retinopathy without macular edema**   HCC

E08.36 Diabetes mellitus due to underlying condition with diabetic cataract   HCC

> **AHA:** 2019,2Q,30-31; 2016,4Q,142

☑x7ᵗʰ **E08.37 Diabetes mellitus due to underlying condition with diabetic macular edema, resolved following treatment**   HCC

E08.39 Diabetes mellitus due to underlying condition with other diabetic ophthalmic complication   HCC

> Use additional code to identify manifestation, such as:
> diabetic glaucoma (H40-H42)

☑5ᵗʰ **E08.4 Diabetes mellitus due to underlying condition with neurological complications**

E08.40 Diabetes mellitus due to underlying condition with diabetic neuropathy, unspecified   HCC

E08.41 Diabetes mellitus due to underlying condition with diabetic mononeuropathy   HCC

E08.42 Diabetes mellitus due to underlying condition with diabetic polyneuropathy   HCC

> Diabetes mellitus due to underlying condition with diabetic neuralgia

E08.43 Diabetes mellitus due to underlying condition with diabetic autonomic (poly)neuropathy   HCC

> Diabetes mellitus due to underlying condition with diabetic gastroparesis
> **AHA:** 2013,4Q,114

E08.44 Diabetes mellitus due to underlying condition with diabetic amyotrophy   HCC

E08.49 Diabetes mellitus due to underlying condition with other diabetic neurological complication   HCC

☑5ᵗʰ **E08.5 Diabetes mellitus due to underlying condition with circulatory complications**

E08.51 Diabetes mellitus due to underlying condition with diabetic peripheral angiopathy without gangrene   HCC

> **AHA:** 2018,2Q,7

E08.52 Diabetes mellitus due to underlying condition with diabetic peripheral angiopathy with gangrene   CC HCC

> Diabetes mellitus due to underlying condition with diabetic gangrene
> **AHA:** 2018,2Q,7; 2017,4Q,102
> **CC Excl:** PDX collection 519

E08.59 Diabetes mellitus due to underlying condition with other circulatory complications   HCC

☑ Additional Character Required   ☑x7ᵗʰ Placeholder   Unacceptable PDx   Questionable PDx   Manifestation   Unspecified Dx   H1-H4 HAC   HCC CMS-HCC Dx   HIV HIV Dx

√5ᵗʰ **E08.6 Diabetes mellitus due to underlying condition with other specified complications**

√6ᵗʰ **E08.61 Diabetes mellitus due to underlying condition with diabetic arthropathy**

E08.610 Diabetes mellitus due to underlying condition with diabetic neuropathic arthropathy   HCC

Diabetes mellitus due to underlying condition with Charcôt's joints

DEF: Charcot's joint: Progressive neurologic arthropathy in which chronic degeneration of joints in the weight-bearing areas with peripheral hypertrophy occurs as a complication of a neuropathy disorder. Supporting structures relax from a loss of sensation resulting in chronic joint instability.

E08.618 Diabetes mellitus due to underlying condition with other diabetic arthropathy   HCC

AHA: 2018,2Q,6

√6ᵗʰ **E08.62 Diabetes mellitus due to underlying condition with skin complications**

E08.620 Diabetes mellitus due to underlying condition with diabetic dermatitis   HCC

Diabetes mellitus due to underlying condition with diabetic necrobiosis lipoidica

E08.621 Diabetes mellitus due to underlying condition with foot ulcer   HCC

Use additional code to identify site of ulcer (L97.4-, L97.5-)

E08.622 Diabetes mellitus due to underlying condition with other skin ulcer   HCC

Use additional code to identify site of ulcer (L97.1-L97.9, L98.41-L98.49)

AHA: 2017,4Q,17

E08.628 Diabetes mellitus due to underlying condition with other skin complications   HCC

AHA: 2017,4Q,100-101

√6ᵗʰ **E08.63 Diabetes mellitus due to underlying condition with oral complications**

E08.630 Diabetes mellitus due to underlying condition with periodontal disease   HCC

E08.638 Diabetes mellitus due to underlying condition with other oral complications   HCC

√6ᵗʰ **E08.64 Diabetes mellitus due to underlying condition with hypoglycemia**

E08.641 Diabetes mellitus due to underlying condition with hypoglycemia with coma   MCC HCC

E08.649 Diabetes mellitus due to underlying condition with hypoglycemia without coma   HCC

AHA: 2016,3Q,42; 2015,3Q,21

E08.65 Diabetes mellitus due to underlying condition with hyperglycemia   HCC

E08.69 Diabetes mellitus due to underlying condition with other specified complication   HCC

Use additional code to identify complication

AHA: 2016,4Q,141; 2016,1Q,13

E08.8 Diabetes mellitus due to underlying condition with unspecified complications   HCC

E08.9 Diabetes mellitus due to underlying condition without complications   HCC

√4ᵗʰ **E09 Drug or chemical induced diabetes mellitus**

Code first poisoning due to drug or toxin, if applicable (T36-T65 with fifth or sixth character 1-4 or 6)

Use additional code for adverse effect, if applicable, to identify drug (T36-T50 with fifth or sixth character 5)

Use additional code to identify control using:
insulin (Z79.4)
oral antidiabetic drugs (Z79.84)
oral hypoglycemic drugs (Z79.84)

EXCLUDES 1   diabetes mellitus due to underlying condition (E08.-)
gestational diabetes (O24.4-)
neonatal diabetes mellitus (P70.2)
postpancreatectomy diabetes mellitus (E13.-)
postprocedural diabetes mellitus (E13.-)
secondary diabetes mellitus NEC (E13.-)
type 1 diabetes mellitus (E10.-)
type 2 diabetes mellitus (E11.-)

AHA: 2013,4Q,114; 2013,3Q,20

CC Excl: For MCC codes in category E09: PDX collection 518

√5ᵗʰ **E09.0 Drug or chemical induced diabetes mellitus with hyperosmolarity**

DEF: Diabetic hyperosmolarity: Extremely high levels of glucose in the blood without ketones.

E09.00 Drug or chemical induced diabetes mellitus with hyperosmolarity without nonketotic hyperglycemic-hyperosmolar coma (NKHHC)   MCC H9 HCC

E09.01 Drug or chemical induced diabetes mellitus with hyperosmolarity with coma   MCC H9 HCC

√5ᵗʰ **E09.1 Drug or chemical induced diabetes mellitus with ketoacidosis**

DEF: Diabetic ketoacidosis: Potentially life-threatening complication due to a shortage of insulin in which the body switches to burning fatty acids and producing acidic ketone bodies.

E09.10 Drug or chemical induced diabetes mellitus with ketoacidosis without coma   MCC H9 HCC

E09.11 Drug or chemical induced diabetes mellitus with ketoacidosis with coma   MCC HCC

√5ᵗʰ **E09.2 Drug or chemical induced diabetes mellitus with kidney complications**

E09.21 Drug or chemical induced diabetes mellitus with diabetic nephropathy   HCC

Drug or chemical induced diabetes mellitus with intercapillary glomerulosclerosis

Drug or chemical induced diabetes mellitus with intracapillary glomerulonephrosis

Drug or chemical induced diabetes mellitus with Kimmelstiel-Wilson disease

E09.22 Drug or chemical induced diabetes mellitus with diabetic chronic kidney disease   HCC

Use additional code to identify stage of chronic kidney disease (N18.1-N18.6)

E09.29 Drug or chemical induced diabetes mellitus with other diabetic kidney complication   HCC

Drug or chemical induced diabetes mellitus with renal tubular degeneration

√5ᵗʰ **E09.3 Drug or chemical induced diabetes mellitus with ophthalmic complications**

One of the following 7th characters is to be assigned to codes in subcategories E09.32, E09.33, E09.34, E09.35, and E09.37 to designate laterality of the disease:
1   right eye
2   left eye
3   bilateral
9   unspecified eye

√6ᵗʰ **E09.31 Drug or chemical induced diabetes mellitus with unspecified diabetic retinopathy**

DEF: Diabetic retinopathy: Diabetic complication from damage to the retinal vessels resulting in vision problems that can progress to blindness.

E09.311 Drug or chemical induced diabetes mellitus with unspecified diabetic retinopathy with macular edema   HCC

N Newborn: 0   P Pediatric: 0-17   M Maternity: 9-64   A Adult: 15-124   MCC Major Complication/Comorbidity   CC Complication/Comorbidity   SW Severe Wound Dx

520   ICD-10-CM 2020

E09.319   Drug or chemical induced diabetes mellitus with unspecified diabetic retinopathy without macular edema   HCC

√6ᵗʰ E09.32   Drug or chemical induced diabetes mellitus with mild nonproliferative diabetic retinopathy

Drug or chemical induced diabetes mellitus with nonproliferative diabetic retinopathy NOS

√7ᵗʰ E09.321   Drug or chemical induced diabetes mellitus with mild nonproliferative diabetic retinopathy with macular edema   HCC

√7ᵗʰ E09.329   Drug or chemical induced diabetes mellitus with mild nonproliferative diabetic retinopathy without macular edema   HCC

√6ᵗʰ E09.33   Drug or chemical induced diabetes mellitus with moderate nonproliferative diabetic retinopathy

√7ᵗʰ E09.331   Drug or chemical induced diabetes mellitus with moderate nonproliferative diabetic retinopathy with macular edema   HCC

√7ᵗʰ E09.339   Drug or chemical induced diabetes mellitus with moderate nonproliferative diabetic retinopathy without macular edema   HCC

√6ᵗʰ E09.34   Drug or chemical induced diabetes mellitus with severe nonproliferative diabetic retinopathy

√7ᵗʰ E09.341   Drug or chemical induced diabetes mellitus with severe nonproliferative diabetic retinopathy with macular edema   HCC

√7ᵗʰ E09.349   Drug or chemical induced diabetes mellitus with severe nonproliferative diabetic retinopathy without macular edema   HCC

√6ᵗʰ E09.35   Drug or chemical induced diabetes mellitus with proliferative diabetic retinopathy

√7ᵗʰ E09.351   Drug or chemical induced diabetes mellitus with proliferative diabetic retinopathy with macular edema   HCC

√7ᵗʰ E09.352   Drug or chemical induced diabetes mellitus with proliferative diabetic retinopathy with traction retinal detachment involving the macula   HCC

√7ᵗʰ E09.353   Drug or chemical induced diabetes mellitus with proliferative diabetic retinopathy with traction retinal detachment not involving the macula   HCC

√7ᵗʰ E09.354   Drug or chemical induced diabetes mellitus with proliferative diabetic retinopathy with combined traction retinal detachment and rhegmatogenous retinal detachment   HCC

√7ᵗʰ E09.355   Drug or chemical induced diabetes mellitus with stable proliferative diabetic retinopathy   HCC

√7ᵗʰ E09.359   Drug or chemical induced diabetes mellitus with proliferative diabetic retinopathy without macular edema   HCC

E09.36   Drug or chemical induced diabetes mellitus with diabetic cataract   HCC

AHA: 2019,2Q,30-31; 2016,4Q,142

√x 7ᵗʰ E09.37   Drug or chemical induced diabetes mellitus with diabetic macular edema, resolved following treatment   HCC

E09.39   Drug or chemical induced diabetes mellitus with other diabetic ophthalmic complication   HCC

Use additional code to identify manifestation, such as:

diabetic glaucoma (H40-H42)

√5ᵗʰ E09.4   Drug or chemical induced diabetes mellitus with neurological complications

E09.40   Drug or chemical induced diabetes mellitus with neurological complications with diabetic neuropathy, unspecified   HCC

E09.41   Drug or chemical induced diabetes mellitus with neurological complications with diabetic mononeuropathy   HCC

E09.42   Drug or chemical induced diabetes mellitus with neurological complications with diabetic polyneuropathy   HCC

Drug or chemical induced diabetes mellitus with diabetic neuralgia

E09.43   Drug or chemical induced diabetes mellitus with neurological complications with diabetic autonomic (poly)neuropathy   HCC

Drug or chemical induced diabetes mellitus with diabetic gastroparesis

AHA: 2013,4Q,114

E09.44   Drug or chemical induced diabetes mellitus with neurological complications with diabetic amyotrophy   HCC

E09.49   Drug or chemical induced diabetes mellitus with neurological complications with other diabetic neurological complication   HCC

√5ᵗʰ E09.5   Drug or chemical induced diabetes mellitus with circulatory complications

E09.51   Drug or chemical induced diabetes mellitus with diabetic peripheral angiopathy without gangrene   HCC

AHA: 2018,2Q,7

E09.52   Drug or chemical induced diabetes mellitus with diabetic peripheral angiopathy with gangrene   CC   HCC

Drug or chemical induced diabetes mellitus with diabetic gangrene

AHA: 2018,2Q,7; 2017,4Q,102

CC Excl: PDX collection 519

E09.59   Drug or chemical induced diabetes mellitus with other circulatory complications   HCC

√5ᵗʰ E09.6   Drug or chemical induced diabetes mellitus with other specified complications

√6ᵗʰ E09.61   Drug or chemical induced diabetes mellitus with diabetic arthropathy

E09.610   Drug or chemical induced diabetes mellitus with diabetic neuropathic arthropathy   HCC

Drug or chemical induced diabetes mellitus with Charcôt's joints

DEF: Charcot's joint: Progressive neurologic arthropathy in which chronic degeneration of joints in the weight-bearing areas with peripheral hypertrophy occurs as a complication of a neuropathy disorder. Supporting structures relax from a loss of sensation resulting in chronic joint instability.

E09.618   Drug or chemical induced diabetes mellitus with other diabetic arthropathy   HCC

AHA: 2018,2Q,6

✔ Additional Character Required   √x 7ᵗʰ Placeholder   Unacceptable PDx   Questionable PDx   Manifestation   Unspecified Dx   H1 - H14 HAC   HCC CMS-HCC Dx   HIV HIV Dx

ICD-10-CM 2020   521

Chapter 4. Endocrine, Nutritional and Metabolic Diseases

E09.62–E10.349

√6th **E09.62 Drug or chemical induced diabetes mellitus with skin complications**

    E09.620 Drug or chemical induced diabetes mellitus with diabetic dermatitis `HCC`

        Drug or chemical induced diabetes mellitus with diabetic necrobiosis lipoidica

    E09.621 Drug or chemical induced diabetes mellitus with foot ulcer `HCC`

        Use additional code to identify site of ulcer (L97.4-, L97.5-)

    E09.622 Drug or chemical induced diabetes mellitus with other skin ulcer `HCC`

        Use additional code to identify site of ulcer (L97.1-L97.9, L98.41-L98.49)

        AHA: 2017,4Q,17

    E09.628 Drug or chemical induced diabetes mellitus with other skin complications `HCC`

        AHA: 2017,4Q,100-101

√6th **E09.63 Drug or chemical induced diabetes mellitus with oral complications**

    E09.630 Drug or chemical induced diabetes mellitus with periodontal disease `HCC`

    E09.638 Drug or chemical induced diabetes mellitus with other oral complications `HCC`

√6th **E09.64 Drug or chemical induced diabetes mellitus with hypoglycemia**

    E09.641 Drug or chemical induced diabetes mellitus with hypoglycemia with coma `MCC` `HCC`

    E09.649 Drug or chemical induced diabetes mellitus with hypoglycemia without coma `HCC`

        AHA: 2016,3Q,42; 2015,3Q,21

    E09.65 Drug or chemical induced diabetes mellitus with hyperglycemia `CC` `HCC`

    E09.69 Drug or chemical induced diabetes mellitus with other specified complication `CC` `HCC`

        Use additional code to identify complication

        AHA: 2016,4Q,141; 2016,1Q,13

E09.8 Drug or chemical induced diabetes mellitus with unspecified complications `CC` `HCC`

E09.9 Drug or chemical induced diabetes mellitus without complications `CC` `HCC`

√4th **E10 Type 1 diabetes mellitus**

    `INCLUDES` brittle diabetes (mellitus)

        diabetes (mellitus) due to autoimmune process

        diabetes (mellitus) due to immune mediated pancreatic islet beta-cell destruction

        idiopathic diabetes (mellitus)

        juvenile onset diabetes (mellitus)

        ketosis-prone diabetes (mellitus)

    `EXCLUDES 1` *diabetes mellitus due to underlying condition (E08.-)*

        drug or chemical induced diabetes mellitus (E09.-)

        gestational diabetes (O24.4-)

        hyperglycemia NOS (R73.9)

        neonatal diabetes mellitus (P70.2)

        postpancreatectomy diabetes mellitus (E13.-)

        postprocedural diabetes mellitus (E13.-)

        secondary diabetes mellitus NEC (E13.-)

        type 2 diabetes mellitus (E11.-)

    AHA: 2013,4Q,114; 2013,3Q,20

    CC Excl: For MCC codes in category E10: PDX collection 520

√5th **E10.1 Type 1 diabetes mellitus with ketoacidosis**

    AHA: 2013,3Q,20

    DEF: Diabetic ketoacidosis: Potentially life-threatening complication due to a shortage of insulin in which the body switches to burning fatty acids and producing acidic ketone bodies.

    E10.10 Type 1 diabetes mellitus with ketoacidosis without coma `MCC` `H9` `HCC`

    E10.11 Type 1 diabetes mellitus with ketoacidosis with coma `MCC` `HCC`

√5th **E10.2 Type 1 diabetes mellitus with kidney complications**

    E10.21 Type 1 diabetes mellitus with diabetic nephropathy `HCC`

        Type 1 diabetes mellitus with intercapillary glomerulosclerosis

        Type 1 diabetes mellitus with intracapillary glomerulonephrosis

        Type 1 diabetes mellitus with Kimmelstiel-Wilson disease

    E10.22 Type 1 diabetes mellitus with diabetic chronic kidney disease `HCC`

        Use additional code to identify stage of chronic kidney disease (N18.1-N18.6)

    E10.29 Type 1 diabetes mellitus with other diabetic kidney complication `HCC`

        Type 1 diabetes mellitus with renal tubular degeneration

        AHA: 2016,1Q,13

√5th **E10.3 Type 1 diabetes mellitus with ophthalmic complications**

    One of the following 7th characters is to be assigned to codes in subcategories E10.32, E10.33, E10.34, E10.35, and E10.37 to designate laterality of the disease:

    1   right eye

    2   left eye

    3   bilateral

    9   unspecified eye

√6th **E10.31 Type 1 diabetes mellitus with unspecified diabetic retinopathy**

    DEF: Diabetic retinopathy: Diabetic complication from damage to the retinal vessels resulting in vision problems that can progress to blindness.

    E10.311 Type 1 diabetes mellitus with unspecified diabetic retinopathy with macular edema `HCC`

    E10.319 Type 1 diabetes mellitus with unspecified diabetic retinopathy without macular edema `HCC`

√6th **E10.32 Type 1 diabetes mellitus with mild nonproliferative diabetic retinopathy**

    Type 1 diabetes mellitus with nonproliferative diabetic retinopathy NOS

    √7th **E10.321 Type 1 diabetes mellitus with mild nonproliferative diabetic retinopathy with macular edema** `HCC`

    √7th **E10.329 Type 1 diabetes mellitus with mild nonproliferative diabetic retinopathy without macular edema** `HCC`

√6th **E10.33 Type 1 diabetes mellitus with moderate nonproliferative diabetic retinopathy**

    √7th **E10.331 Type 1 diabetes mellitus with moderate nonproliferative diabetic retinopathy with macular edema** `HCC`

    √7th **E10.339 Type 1 diabetes mellitus with moderate nonproliferative diabetic retinopathy without macular edema** `HCC`

√6th **E10.34 Type 1 diabetes mellitus with severe nonproliferative diabetic retinopathy**

    √7th **E10.341 Type 1 diabetes mellitus with severe nonproliferative diabetic retinopathy with macular edema** `HCC`

    √7th **E10.349 Type 1 diabetes mellitus with severe nonproliferative diabetic retinopathy without macular edema** `HCC`

`N` Newborn: 0   `P` Pediatric: 0-17   `M` Maternity: 9-64   `A` Adult: 15-124   `MCC` Major Complication/Comorbidity   `CC` Complication/Comorbidity   `SW` Severe Wound Dx

522   ICD-10-CM 2020

√6ᵗʰ **E10.35** **Type 1 diabetes mellitus with proliferative diabetic retinopathy**

    √7ᵗʰ **E10.351** **Type 1 diabetes mellitus with proliferative diabetic retinopathy with macular edema** `HCC`

    √7ᵗʰ **E10.352** **Type 1 diabetes mellitus with proliferative diabetic retinopathy with traction retinal detachment involving the macula** `HCC`

    √7ᵗʰ **E10.353** **Type 1 diabetes mellitus with proliferative diabetic retinopathy with traction retinal detachment not involving the macula** `HCC`

    √7ᵗʰ **E10.354** **Type 1 diabetes mellitus with proliferative diabetic retinopathy with combined traction retinal detachment and rhegmatogenous retinal detachment** `HCC`

    √7ᵗʰ **E10.355** **Type 1 diabetes mellitus with stable proliferative diabetic retinopathy** `HCC`

    √7ᵗʰ **E10.359** **Type 1 diabetes mellitus with proliferative diabetic retinopathy without macular edema** `HCC`

E10.36 **Type 1 diabetes mellitus with diabetic cataract** `HCC`
    AHA: 2019,2Q,30-31; 2016,4Q,142

√x7ᵗʰ **E10.37** **Type 1 diabetes mellitus with diabetic macular edema, resolved following treatment** `HCC`

E10.39 **Type 1 diabetes mellitus with other diabetic ophthalmic complication** `HCC`
    Use additional code to identify manifestation, such as:
      diabetic glaucoma (H40-H42)

√5ᵗʰ **E10.4** **Type 1 diabetes mellitus with neurological complications**

E10.40 **Type 1 diabetes mellitus with diabetic neuropathy, unspecified** `HCC`

E10.41 **Type 1 diabetes mellitus with diabetic mononeuropathy** `HCC`

E10.42 **Type 1 diabetes mellitus with diabetic polyneuropathy** `HCC`
    Type 1 diabetes mellitus with diabetic neuralgia

E10.43 **Type 1 diabetes mellitus with diabetic autonomic (poly)neuropathy** `HCC`
    Type 1 diabetes mellitus with diabetic gastroparesis
    AHA: 2013,4Q,114

E10.44 **Type 1 diabetes mellitus with diabetic amyotrophy** `HCC`

E10.49 **Type 1 diabetes mellitus with other diabetic neurological complication** `HCC`

√5ᵗʰ **E10.5** **Type 1 diabetes mellitus with circulatory complications**

E10.51 **Type 1 diabetes mellitus with diabetic peripheral angiopathy without gangrene** `HCC`
    AHA: 2018,2Q,7

E10.52 **Type 1 diabetes mellitus with diabetic peripheral angiopathy with gangrene** `CC` `HCC`
    Type 1 diabetes mellitus with diabetic gangrene
    AHA: 2018,2Q,7; 2017,4Q,102
    CC Excl: PDX collection 519

E10.59 **Type 1 diabetes mellitus with other circulatory complications** `HCC`

√5ᵗʰ **E10.6** **Type 1 diabetes mellitus with other specified complications**

    √6ᵗʰ **E10.61** **Type 1 diabetes mellitus with diabetic arthropathy**

      E10.610 **Type 1 diabetes mellitus with diabetic neuropathic arthropathy** `HCC`
       Type 1 diabetes mellitus with Charcôt's joints
       DEF: Charcot's joint: Progressive neurologic arthropathy in which chronic degeneration of joints in the weight-bearing areas with peripheral hypertrophy occurs as a complication of a neuropathy disorder. Supporting structures relax from a loss of sensation resulting in chronic joint instability.

      E10.618 **Type 1 diabetes mellitus with other diabetic arthropathy** `HCC`
       AHA: 2018,2Q,6

    √6ᵗʰ **E10.62** **Type 1 diabetes mellitus with skin complications**

      E10.620 **Type 1 diabetes mellitus with diabetic dermatitis** `HCC`
       Type 1 diabetes mellitus with diabetic necrobiosis lipoidica

      E10.621 **Type 1 diabetes mellitus with foot ulcer** `HCC`
       Use additional code to identify site of ulcer (L97.4-, L97.5-)

      E10.622 **Type 1 diabetes mellitus with other skin ulcer** `HCC`
       Use additional code to identify site of ulcer (L97.1-L97.9, L98.41-L98.49)
       AHA: 2017,4Q,17

      E10.628 **Type 1 diabetes mellitus with other skin complications** `HCC`
       AHA: 2017,4Q,100-101

    √6ᵗʰ **E10.63** **Type 1 diabetes mellitus with oral complications**

      E10.630 **Type 1 diabetes mellitus with periodontal disease** `HCC`

      E10.638 **Type 1 diabetes mellitus with other oral complications** `HCC`

    √6ᵗʰ **E10.64** **Type 1 diabetes mellitus with hypoglycemia**

      E10.641 **Type 1 diabetes mellitus with hypoglycemia with coma** `MCC` `HCC`

      E10.649 **Type 1 diabetes mellitus with hypoglycemia without coma** `HCC`
       AHA: 2016,3Q,42; 2016,1Q,13; 2015,3Q,21

    E10.65 **Type 1 diabetes mellitus with hyperglycemia** `HCC`
      AHA: 2013,3Q,20

    E10.69 **Type 1 diabetes mellitus with other specified complication** `HCC`
      Use additional code to identify complication
      AHA: 2016,4Q,141; 2016,1Q,13

E10.8 **Type 1 diabetes mellitus with unspecified complications** `HCC`

E10.9 **Type 1 diabetes mellitus without complications** `HCC`

√4ᵗʰ **E11 Type 2 diabetes mellitus**

INCLUDES diabetes (mellitus) due to insulin secretory defect
diabetes NOS
insulin resistant diabetes (mellitus)

Use additional code to identify control using:
insulin (Z79.4)
oral antidiabetic drugs (Z79.84)
oral hypoglycemic drugs (Z79.84)

EXCLUDES 1 *diabetes mellitus due to underlying condition (E08.-)*
drug or chemical induced diabetes mellitus (E09.-)
gestational diabetes (O24.4-)
neonatal diabetes mellitus (P70.2)
postpancreatectomy diabetes mellitus (E13.-)
postprocedural diabetes mellitus (E13.-)
secondary diabetes mellitus NEC (E13.-)
type 1 diabetes mellitus (E10.-)

AHA: 2016,2Q,10; 2013,4Q,114; 2013,3Q,20; 2013,1Q,26
CC Excl: For MCC codes in category E11: PDX collection 518

√5ᵗʰ **E11.0 Type 2 diabetes mellitus with hyperosmolarity**
DEF: Diabetic hyperosmolarity: Extremely high levels of glucose in the blood without ketones.

E11.00 Type 2 diabetes mellitus with hyperosmolarity without nonketotic hyperglycemic-hyperosmolar coma (NKHHC) H9 HCC

E11.01 Type 2 diabetes mellitus with hyperosmolarity with coma MCC H9 HCC

√5ᵗʰ **E11.1 Type 2 diabetes mellitus with ketoacidosis**
DEF: Diabetic ketoacidosis: Potentially life-threatening complication due to a shortage of insulin in which the body switches to burning fatty acids and producing acidic ketone bodies.

E11.10 Type 2 diabetes mellitus with ketoacidosis without coma MCC HCC

E11.11 Type 2 diabetes mellitus with ketoacidosis with coma MCC HCC

√5ᵗʰ **E11.2 Type 2 diabetes mellitus with kidney complications**

E11.21 Type 2 diabetes mellitus with diabetic nephropathy HCC
Type 2 diabetes mellitus with intercapillary glomerulosclerosis
Type 2 diabetes mellitus with intracapillary glomerulonephrosis
Type 2 diabetes mellitus with Kimmelstiel-Wilson disease

E11.22 Type 2 diabetes mellitus with diabetic chronic kidney disease HCC
Use additional code to identify stage of chronic kidney disease (N18.1-N18.6)
AHA: 2016,1Q,12

E11.29 Type 2 diabetes mellitus with other diabetic kidney complication HCC
Type 2 diabetes mellitus with renal tubular degeneration

√5ᵗʰ **E11.3 Type 2 diabetes mellitus with ophthalmic complications**

One of the following 7th characters is to be assigned to codes in subcategories E11.32, E11.33, E11.34, E11.35, and E11.37 to designate laterality of the disease:
1 right eye
2 left eye
3 bilateral
9 unspecified eye

√6ᵗʰ **E11.31 Type 2 diabetes mellitus with unspecified diabetic retinopathy**
DEF: Diabetic retinopathy: Diabetic complication from damage to the retinal vessels resulting in vision problems that can progress to blindness.

E11.311 Type 2 diabetes mellitus with unspecified diabetic retinopathy with macular edema HCC

E11.319 Type 2 diabetes mellitus with unspecified diabetic retinopathy without macular edema HCC

√6ᵗʰ **E11.32 Type 2 diabetes mellitus with mild nonproliferative diabetic retinopathy**
Type 2 diabetes mellitus with nonproliferative diabetic retinopathy NOS

E11.321 Type 2 diabetes mellitus with mild nonproliferative diabetic retinopathy with macular edema HCC

E11.329 Type 2 diabetes mellitus with mild nonproliferative diabetic retinopathy without macular edema HCC

√6ᵗʰ **E11.33 Type 2 diabetes mellitus with moderate nonproliferative diabetic retinopathy**

E11.331 Type 2 diabetes mellitus with moderate nonproliferative diabetic retinopathy with macular edema HCC

E11.339 Type 2 diabetes mellitus with moderate nonproliferative diabetic retinopathy without macular edema HCC

√6ᵗʰ **E11.34 Type 2 diabetes mellitus with severe nonproliferative diabetic retinopathy**

E11.341 Type 2 diabetes mellitus with severe nonproliferative diabetic retinopathy with macular edema HCC

E11.349 Type 2 diabetes mellitus with severe nonproliferative diabetic retinopathy without macular edema HCC

√6ᵗʰ **E11.35 Type 2 diabetes mellitus with proliferative diabetic retinopathy**

E11.351 Type 2 diabetes mellitus with proliferative diabetic retinopathy with macular edema HCC

E11.352 Type 2 diabetes mellitus with proliferative diabetic retinopathy with traction retinal detachment involving the macula HCC

E11.353 Type 2 diabetes mellitus with proliferative diabetic retinopathy with traction retinal detachment not involving the macula HCC

E11.354 Type 2 diabetes mellitus with proliferative diabetic retinopathy with combined traction retinal detachment and rhegmatogenous retinal detachment HCC

E11.355 Type 2 diabetes mellitus with stable proliferative diabetic retinopathy HCC

E11.359 Type 2 diabetes mellitus with proliferative diabetic retinopathy without macular edema HCC

E11.36 Type 2 diabetes mellitus with diabetic cataract HCC
AHA: 2019,2Q,30-31; 2016,4Q,142

√x7ᵗʰ **E11.37 Type 2 diabetes mellitus with diabetic macular edema, resolved following treatment** HCC

E11.39 Type 2 diabetes mellitus with other diabetic ophthalmic complication HCC
Use additional code to identify manifestation, such as:
diabetic glaucoma (H40-H42)

√5ᵗʰ **E11.4 Type 2 diabetes mellitus with neurological complications**

E11.40 Type 2 diabetes mellitus with diabetic neuropathy, unspecified HCC
AHA: 2013,4Q,129

E11.41 Type 2 diabetes mellitus with diabetic mononeuropathy HCC

E11.42   **Type 2 diabetes mellitus with diabetic polyneuropathy**   `HCC`
Type 2 diabetes mellitus with diabetic neuralgia
AHA: 2016,1Q,12

E11.43   **Type 2 diabetes mellitus with diabetic autonomic (poly)neuropathy**   `HCC`
Type 2 diabetes mellitus with diabetic gastroparesis
AHA: 2013,4Q,114

E11.44   **Type 2 diabetes mellitus with diabetic amyotrophy**   `HCC`

E11.49   **Type 2 diabetes mellitus with other diabetic neurological complication**   `HCC`

✓5ᵗʰ **E11.5**   **Type 2 diabetes mellitus with circulatory complications**

E11.51   **Type 2 diabetes mellitus with diabetic peripheral angiopathy without gangrene**   `HCC`
AHA: 2018,2Q,7

E11.52   **Type 2 diabetes mellitus with diabetic peripheral angiopathy with gangrene**   `CC` `HCC`
Type 2 diabetes mellitus with diabetic gangrene
AHA: 2018,2Q,7; 2017,4Q,102
CC Excl: PDX collection 519

E11.59   **Type 2 diabetes mellitus with other circulatory complications**   `HCC`

✓5ᵗʰ **E11.6**   **Type 2 diabetes mellitus with other specified complications**

✓6ᵗʰ **E11.61**   **Type 2 diabetes mellitus with diabetic arthropathy**

E11.610   **Type 2 diabetes mellitus with diabetic neuropathic arthropathy**   `HCC`
Type 2 diabetes mellitus with Charcôt's joints
DEF: Charcot's joint: Progressive neurologic arthropathy in which chronic degeneration of joints in the weight-bearing areas with peripheral hypertrophy occurs as a complication of a neuropathy disorder. Supporting structures relax from a loss of sensation resulting in chronic joint instability.

E11.618   **Type 2 diabetes mellitus with other diabetic arthropathy**   `HCC`
AHA: 2018,2Q,6

✓6ᵗʰ **E11.62**   **Type 2 diabetes mellitus with skin complications**

E11.620   **Type 2 diabetes mellitus with diabetic dermatitis**   `HCC`
Type 2 diabetes mellitus with diabetic necrobiosis lipoidica

E11.621   **Type 2 diabetes mellitus with foot ulcer**   `HCC`
Use additional code to identify site of ulcer (L97.4-, L97.5-)
AHA: 2016,1Q,12

E11.622   **Type 2 diabetes mellitus with other skin ulcer**   `HCC`
Use additional code to identify site of ulcer (L97.1-L97.9, L98.41-L98.49)
AHA: 2017,4Q,17

E11.628   **Type 2 diabetes mellitus with other skin complications**   `HCC`
AHA: 2017,4Q,100-101

✓6ᵗʰ **E11.63**   **Type 2 diabetes mellitus with oral complications**

E11.630   **Type 2 diabetes mellitus with periodontal disease**   `HCC`

E11.638   **Type 2 diabetes mellitus with other oral complications**   `HCC`

✓6ᵗʰ **E11.64**   **Type 2 diabetes mellitus with hypoglycemia**

E11.641   **Type 2 diabetes mellitus with hypoglycemia with coma**   `MCC` `HCC`

E11.649   **Type 2 diabetes mellitus with hypoglycemia without coma**   `HCC`
AHA: 2016,3Q,42; 2015,3Q,21

E11.65   **Type 2 diabetes mellitus with hyperglycemia**   `HCC`
AHA: 2013,3Q,20

E11.69   **Type 2 diabetes mellitus with other specified complication**   `HCC`
Use additional code to identify complication
AHA: 2016,4Q,141; 2016,1Q,13

E11.8   **Type 2 diabetes mellitus with unspecified complications**   `HCC`

E11.9   **Type 2 diabetes mellitus without complications**   `HCC`

✓4ᵗʰ **E13**   **Other specified diabetes mellitus**

> `INCLUDES` diabetes mellitus due to genetic defects of beta-cell function
> diabetes mellitus due to genetic defects in insulin action
> postpancreatectomy diabetes mellitus
> postprocedural diabetes mellitus
> secondary diabetes mellitus NEC

Use additional code to identify control using:
   insulin (Z79.4)
   oral antidiabetic drugs (Z79.84)
   oral hypoglycemic drugs (Z79.84)

> `EXCLUDES 1` diabetes (mellitus) due to autoimmune process (E10.-)
> diabetes (mellitus) due to immune mediated pancreatic islet beta-cell destruction (E10.-)
> diabetes mellitus due to underlying condition (E08.-)
> drug or chemical induced diabetes mellitus (E09.-)
> gestational diabetes (O24.4-)
> neonatal diabetes mellitus (P70.2)
> type 1 diabetes mellitus (E10.-)

AHA: 2018,3Q,4; 2016,1Q,11-13; 2013,4Q,114; 2013,3Q,20
TIP: Use this category when the diabetes is documented as diabetes type 1.5. Synonymous terms used in the documentation may also include combined diabetes type 1 and type 2, latent autoimmune diabetes of adults (LADA), slow-progressing type 1 diabetes, or double diabetes.
TIP: When postprocedural or postpancreatectomy hypoinsulinemia (E89.1) is documented with postprocedural or postpancreatectomy diabetes mellitus (E13.-), code E89.1 should be sequenced first.
CC Excl: For MCC codes in category E13: PDX collection 518

✓5ᵗʰ **E13.0**   **Other specified diabetes mellitus with hyperosmolarity**
DEF: Diabetic hyperosmolarity: Extremely high levels of glucose in the blood without ketones.

E13.00   **Other specified diabetes mellitus with hyperosmolarity without nonketotic hyperglycemic-hyperosmolar coma (NKHHC)**   `MCC` `H9` `HCC`
> `EXCLUDES 2` type 2 diabetes mellitus (E11.-)

E13.01   **Other specified diabetes mellitus with hyperosmolarity with coma**   `MCC` `H9` `HCC`

✓5ᵗʰ **E13.1**   **Other specified diabetes mellitus with ketoacidosis**
AHA: 2016,2Q,10; 2013,1Q,26
DEF: Diabetic ketoacidosis: Potentially life-threatening complication due to a shortage of insulin in which the body switches to burning fatty acids and producing acidic ketone bodies.

E13.10   **Other specified diabetes mellitus with ketoacidosis without coma**   `MCC` `H9` `HCC`

E13.11   **Other specified diabetes mellitus with ketoacidosis with coma**   `MCC` `HCC`

✓5ᵗʰ **E13.2**   **Other specified diabetes mellitus with kidney complications**

E13.21   **Other specified diabetes mellitus with diabetic nephropathy**   `HCC`
Other specified diabetes mellitus with intercapillary glomerulosclerosis
Other specified diabetes mellitus with intracapillary glomerulonephrosis
Other specified diabetes mellitus with Kimmelstiel-Wilson disease

E13.22   **Other specified diabetes mellitus with diabetic chronic kidney disease**   `HCC`
Use additional code to identify stage of chronic kidney disease (N18.1-N18.6)

E13.29   **Other specified diabetes mellitus with other diabetic kidney complication**   `HCC`
Other specified diabetes mellitus with renal tubular degeneration

---

Chapter 4. Endocrine, Nutritional and Metabolic Diseases

√5ᵗʰ **E13.3** **Other specified diabetes mellitus with ophthalmic complications**

One of the following 7th characters is to be assigned to codes in subcategories E13.32, E13.33, E13.34, E13.35, and E13.37 to designate laterality of the disease:
1 right eye
2 left eye
3 bilateral
9 unspecified eye

√6ᵗʰ **E13.31** **Other specified diabetes mellitus with unspecified diabetic retinopathy**
DEF: Diabetic retinopathy: Diabetic complication from damage to the retinal vessels resulting in vision problems that can progress to blindness.

E13.311 Other specified diabetes mellitus with unspecified diabetic retinopathy with macular edema HCC

E13.319 Other specified diabetes mellitus with unspecified diabetic retinopathy without macular edema HCC

√6ᵗʰ **E13.32** **Other specified diabetes mellitus with mild nonproliferative diabetic retinopathy**
Other specified diabetes mellitus with nonproliferative diabetic retinopathy NOS

√7ᵗʰ **E13.321** Other specified diabetes mellitus with mild nonproliferative diabetic retinopathy with macular edema HCC

√7ᵗʰ **E13.329** Other specified diabetes mellitus with mild nonproliferative diabetic retinopathy without macular edema HCC

√6ᵗʰ **E13.33** **Other specified diabetes mellitus with moderate nonproliferative diabetic retinopathy**

√7ᵗʰ **E13.331** Other specified diabetes mellitus with moderate nonproliferative diabetic retinopathy with macular edema HCC

√7ᵗʰ **E13.339** Other specified diabetes mellitus with moderate nonproliferative diabetic retinopathy without macular edema HCC

√6ᵗʰ **E13.34** **Other specified diabetes mellitus with severe nonproliferative diabetic retinopathy**

√7ᵗʰ **E13.341** Other specified diabetes mellitus with severe nonproliferative diabetic retinopathy with macular edema HCC

√7ᵗʰ **E13.349** Other specified diabetes mellitus with severe nonproliferative diabetic retinopathy without macular edema HCC

√6ᵗʰ **E13.35** **Other specified diabetes mellitus with proliferative diabetic retinopathy**

√7ᵗʰ **E13.351** Other specified diabetes mellitus with proliferative diabetic retinopathy with macular edema HCC

√7ᵗʰ **E13.352** Other specified diabetes mellitus with proliferative diabetic retinopathy with traction retinal detachment involving the macula HCC

√7ᵗʰ **E13.353** Other specified diabetes mellitus with proliferative diabetic retinopathy with traction retinal detachment not involving the macula HCC

√7ᵗʰ **E13.354** Other specified diabetes mellitus with proliferative diabetic retinopathy with combined traction retinal detachment and rhegmatogenous retinal detachment HCC

√7ᵗʰ **E13.355** Other specified diabetes mellitus with stable proliferative diabetic retinopathy HCC

√7ᵗʰ **E13.359** Other specified diabetes mellitus with proliferative diabetic retinopathy without macular edema HCC

E13.36 Other specified diabetes mellitus with diabetic cataract HCC
AHA: 2019,2Q,30-31; 2016,4Q,142

√x7ᵗʰ **E13.37** Other specified diabetes mellitus with diabetic macular edema, resolved following treatment HCC

E13.39 Other specified diabetes mellitus with other diabetic ophthalmic complication HCC
Use additional code to identify manifestation, such as:
diabetic glaucoma (H40-H42)

√5ᵗʰ **E13.4** **Other specified diabetes mellitus with neurological complications**

E13.40 Other specified diabetes mellitus with diabetic neuropathy, unspecified HCC

E13.41 Other specified diabetes mellitus with diabetic mononeuropathy HCC

E13.42 Other specified diabetes mellitus with diabetic polyneuropathy HCC
Other specified diabetes mellitus with diabetic neuralgia

E13.43 Other specified diabetes mellitus with diabetic autonomic (poly)neuropathy HCC
Other specified diabetes mellitus with diabetic gastroparesis
AHA: 2013,4Q,114

E13.44 Other specified diabetes mellitus with diabetic amyotrophy HCC

E13.49 Other specified diabetes mellitus with other diabetic neurological complication HCC

√5ᵗʰ **E13.5** **Other specified diabetes mellitus with circulatory complications**

E13.51 Other specified diabetes mellitus with diabetic peripheral angiopathy without gangrene HCC
AHA: 2018,2Q,7

E13.52 Other specified diabetes mellitus with diabetic peripheral angiopathy with gangrene CC HCC
Other specified diabetes mellitus with diabetic gangrene
AHA: 2018,2Q,7; 2017,4Q,102
CC Excl: PDX collection 519

E13.59 Other specified diabetes mellitus with other circulatory complications HCC

√5ᵗʰ **E13.6** **Other specified diabetes mellitus with other specified complications**

√6ᵗʰ **E13.61** **Other specified diabetes mellitus with diabetic arthropathy**

E13.610 Other specified diabetes mellitus with diabetic neuropathic arthropathy HCC
Other specified diabetes mellitus with Charcôt's joints
DEF: Charcot's joint: Progressive neurologic arthropathy in which chronic degeneration of joints in the weight-bearing areas with peripheral hypertrophy occurs as a complication of a neuropathy disorder. Supporting structures relax from a loss of sensation resulting in chronic joint instability.

E13.618 Other specified diabetes mellitus with other diabetic arthropathy HCC
AHA: 2018,2Q,6

✓6ᵗʰ **E13.62** **Other specified diabetes mellitus with skin complications**

  E13.620 **Other specified diabetes mellitus with diabetic dermatitis** `HCC`
    Other specified diabetes mellitus with diabetic necrobiosis lipoidica

  E13.621 **Other specified diabetes mellitus with foot ulcer** `HCC`
    Use additional code to identify site of ulcer (L97.4-, L97.5-)

  E13.622 **Other specified diabetes mellitus with other skin ulcer** `HCC`
    Use additional code to identify site of ulcer (L97.1-L97.9, L98.41-L98.49)
    AHA: 2017,4Q,17

  E13.628 **Other specified diabetes mellitus with other skin complications** `HCC`
    AHA: 2017,4Q,100-101

✓6ᵗʰ **E13.63** **Other specified diabetes mellitus with oral complications**

  E13.630 **Other specified diabetes mellitus with periodontal disease** `HCC`

  E13.638 **Other specified diabetes mellitus with other oral complications** `HCC`

✓6ᵗʰ **E13.64** **Other specified diabetes mellitus with hypoglycemia**

  E13.641 **Other specified diabetes mellitus with hypoglycemia with coma** `MCC` `HCC`

  E13.649 **Other specified diabetes mellitus with hypoglycemia without coma** `HCC`
    AHA: 2016,3Q,42; 2015,3Q,21

E13.65 **Other specified diabetes mellitus with hyperglycemia** `HCC`

E13.69 **Other specified diabetes mellitus with other specified complication** `HCC`
  Use additional code to identify complication
  AHA: 2016,4Q,141; 2016,1Q,13

E13.8 **Other specified diabetes mellitus with unspecified complications** `HCC`

E13.9 **Other specified diabetes mellitus without complications** `HCC`

Other disorders of glucose regulation and pancreatic internal secretion (E15-E16)

E15 **Nondiabetic hypoglycemic coma** `CC` `H9` `HCC`
  INCLUDES drug-induced insulin coma in nondiabetic
    hyperinsulinism with hypoglycemic coma
    hypoglycemic coma NOS
  CC Excl: PDX collection 520

✓4ᵗʰ **E16** **Other disorders of pancreatic internal secretion**

E16.0 **Drug-induced hypoglycemia without coma**
  Use additional code for adverse effect, if applicable, to identify drug (T36-T50 with fifth or sixth character 5)
  EXCLUDES 1 diabetes with hypoglycemia without coma (E09.649)

E16.1 **Other hypoglycemia**
  Functional hyperinsulinism
  Functional nonhyperinsulinemic hypoglycemia
  Hyperinsulinism NOS
  Hyperplasia of pancreatic islet beta cells NOS
  EXCLUDES 1 diabetes with hypoglycemia (E08.649, E10.649, E11.649, E13.649)
    hypoglycemia in infant of diabetic mother (P70.1)
    neonatal hypoglycemia (P70.4)

E16.2 **Hypoglycemia, unspecified**
  EXCLUDES 1 diabetes with hypoglycemia (E08.649, E10.649, E11.649, E13.649)
  AHA: 2016,3Q,42
  TIP: Assign for nondiabetic hypoglycemic encephalopathy not further clarified in the documentation.

E16.3 **Increased secretion of glucagon**
  Hyperplasia of pancreatic endocrine cells with glucagon excess

E16.4 **Increased secretion of gastrin**
  Hypergastrinemia
  Hyperplasia of pancreatic endocrine cells with gastrin excess
  Zollinger-Ellison syndrome

E16.8 **Other specified disorders of pancreatic internal secretion**
  Increased secretion from endocrine pancreas of growth hormone-releasing hormone
  Increased secretion from endocrine pancreas of pancreatic polypeptide
  Increased secretion from endocrine pancreas of somatostatin
  Increased secretion from endocrine pancreas of vasoactive-intestinal polypeptide

E16.9 **Disorder of pancreatic internal secretion, unspecified**
  Islet-cell hyperplasia NOS
  Pancreatic endocrine cell hyperplasia NOS

Disorders of other endocrine glands (E20-E35)

EXCLUDES 1 galactorrhea (N64.3)
  gynecomastia (N62)

✓4ᵗʰ **E20** **Hypoparathyroidism**
  EXCLUDES 1 Di George's syndrome (D82.1)
    postprocedural hypoparathyroidism (E89.2)
    tetany NOS (R29.0)
    transitory neonatal hypoparathyroidism (P71.4)

E20.0 **Idiopathic hypoparathyroidism** `HCC`
  DEF: Abnormally low secretion of parathyroid hormones, with unknown cause, which causes decreased calcium and increased phosphorus in the blood, resulting in muscle cramps, tetany, tingling, or burning in the lips, fingers, and toes, and cataracts.

E20.1 **Pseudohypoparathyroidism**

E20.8 **Other hypoparathyroidism** `HCC`

E20.9 **Hypoparathyroidism, unspecified** `HCC`
  Parathyroid tetany

✓4ᵗʰ **E21** **Hyperparathyroidism and other disorders of parathyroid gland**
  EXCLUDES 1 adult osteomalacia (M83.-)
    ectopic hyperparathyroidism (E34.2)
    familial hypocalciuric hypercalcemia (E83.52)
    hungry bone syndrome (E83.81)
    infantile and juvenile osteomalacia (E55.0)

E21.0 **Primary hyperparathyroidism** `HCC`
  Hyperplasia of parathyroid
  Osteitis fibrosa cystica generalisata [von Recklinghausen's disease of bone]
  DEF: Parathyroid dysfunction commonly caused by hyperplasia of two or more glands. Symptoms include hypercalcemia and increased parathyroid hormone levels.

E21.1 **Secondary hyperparathyroidism, not elsewhere classified** `HCC`
  EXCLUDES 1 secondary hyperparathyroidism of renal origin (N25.81)

E21.2 **Other hyperparathyroidism** `HCC`
  Tertiary hyperparathyroidism
  EXCLUDES 1 familial hypocalciuric hypercalcemia (E83.52)

E21.3 **Hyperparathyroidism, unspecified** `HCC`

E21.4 **Other specified disorders of parathyroid gland** `HCC`

E21.5 **Disorder of parathyroid gland, unspecified** `HCC`

Chapter 4. Endocrine, Nutritional and Metabolic Diseases

E22–E27.1

✓4ᵗʰ **E22 Hyperfunction of pituitary gland**

> *EXCLUDES 1*   *Cushing's syndrome (E24.-)*
> *Nelson's syndrome (E24.1)*
> *overproduction of ACTH not associated with Cushing's disease (E27.0)*
> *overproduction of pituitary ACTH (E24.0)*
> *overproduction of thyroid-stimulating hormone (E05.8-)*

CC Excl: For CC codes in category E22, unless otherwise noted: PDX collection 521

E22.0 Acromegaly and pituitary gigantism   HCC

Overproduction of growth hormone

> *EXCLUDES 1*   *constitutional gigantism (E34.4)*
> *constitutional tall stature (E34.4)*
> *increased secretion from endocrine pancreas of growth hormone-releasing hormone (E16.8)*

DEF: Acromegaly: Chronic condition caused by overproduction of the pituitary growth hormone resulting in enlarged skeletal parts and facial features.

E22.1 Hyperprolactinemia   CC HCC

Use additional code for adverse effect, if applicable, to identify drug (T36-T50 with fifth or sixth character 5)

E22.2 Syndrome of inappropriate secretion of antidiuretic hormone   CC HCC

CC Excl: PDX collection 522

E22.8 Other hyperfunction of pituitary gland   CC HCC

Central precocious puberty

E22.9 Hyperfunction of pituitary gland, unspecified   CC HCC

✓4ᵗʰ **E23 Hypofunction and other disorders of the pituitary gland**

> *INCLUDES*   the listed conditions whether the disorder is in the pituitary or the hypothalamus
> *EXCLUDES 1*   *postprocedural hypopituitarism (E89.3)*

E23.0 Hypopituitarism   HCC

Fertile eunuch syndrome
Hypogonadotropic hypogonadism
Idiopathic growth hormone deficiency
Isolated deficiency of gonadotropin
Isolated deficiency of growth hormone
Isolated deficiency of pituitary hormone
Kallmann's syndrome
Lorain-Levi short stature
Necrosis of pituitary gland (postpartum)
Panhypopituitarism
Pituitary cachexia
Pituitary insufficiency NOS
Pituitary short stature
Sheehan's syndrome
Simmonds' disease

E23.1 Drug-induced hypopituitarism   HCC

Use additional code for adverse effect, if applicable, to identify drug (T36-T50 with fifth or sixth character 5)

E23.2 Diabetes insipidus   CC HCC

> *EXCLUDES 1*   *nephrogenic diabetes insipidus (N25.1)*

CC Excl: PDX collection 524

E23.3 Hypothalamic dysfunction, not elsewhere classified   HCC

> *EXCLUDES 1*   *Prader-Willi syndrome ▶(Q87.11)◀*
> *Russell-Silver syndrome ▶(Q87.19)◀*

E23.6 Other disorders of pituitary gland   HCC

Abscess of pituitary
Adiposogenital dystrophy

E23.7 Disorder of pituitary gland, unspecified   HCC

✓4ᵗʰ **E24 Cushing's syndrome**

> *EXCLUDES 1*   *congenital adrenal hyperplasia (E25.0)*

DEF: Abdominal striae, acne, hypertension, decreased carbohydrate tolerance, moon face, obesity, protein catabolism, and psychiatric disturbances resulting from increased adrenocortical secretion of cortisol caused by ACTH-dependent adrenocortical hyperplasia or tumor, or by steroid effects.

CC Excl: For CC codes in category E24: PDX collection 525

E24.0 Pituitary-dependent Cushing's disease   CC HCC

Overproduction of pituitary ACTH
Pituitary-dependent hypercorticalism

E24.1 Nelson's syndrome   HCC

E24.2 Drug-induced Cushing's syndrome   CC HCC

Use additional code for adverse effect, if applicable, to identify drug (T36-T50 with fifth or sixth character 5)

E24.3 Ectopic ACTH syndrome   CC HCC

E24.4 Alcohol-induced pseudo-Cushing's syndrome   CC HCC

E24.8 Other Cushing's syndrome   CC HCC

E24.9 Cushing's syndrome, unspecified   CC HCC

✓4ᵗʰ **E25 Adrenogenital disorders**

> *INCLUDES*   adrenogenital syndromes, virilizing or feminizing, whether acquired or due to adrenal hyperplasia consequent on inborn enzyme defects in hormone synthesis
> female adrenal pseudohermaphroditism
> female heterosexual precocious pseudopuberty
> male isosexual precocious pseudopuberty
> male macrogenitosomia praecox
> male sexual precocity with adrenal hyperplasia
> male virilization (female)
> *EXCLUDES 1*   *indeterminate sex and pseudohermaphroditism (Q56)*
> *chromosomal abnormalities (Q90-Q99)*

E25.0 Congenital adrenogenital disorders associated with enzyme deficiency   HCC

Congenital adrenal hyperplasia
21-Hydroxylase deficiency
Salt-losing congenital adrenal hyperplasia

E25.8 Other adrenogenital disorders   HCC

Idiopathic adrenogenital disorder
Use additional code for adverse effect, if applicable, to identify drug (T36-T50 with fifth or sixth character 5)

E25.9 Adrenogenital disorder, unspecified   HCC

Adrenogenital syndrome NOS

✓4ᵗʰ **E26 Hyperaldosteronism**

✓5ᵗʰ **E26.0 Primary hyperaldosteronism**

E26.01 Conn's syndrome   HCC

Code also adrenal adenoma (D35.0-)

E26.02 Glucocorticoid-remediable aldosteronism   HCC

Familial aldosteronism type I

DEF: Rare autosomal dominant familial form of primary aldosteronism in which the secretion of aldosterone is under the influence of adrenocorticotrophic hormone (ACTH) rather than the renin-angiotensin mechanism. Moderate hypersecretion of aldosterone and suppressed plasma renin activity that are rapidly reversed by administration of glucosteroids. Symptoms include hypertension and mild hypokalemia.

E26.09 Other primary hyperaldosteronism   HCC

Primary aldosteronism due to adrenal hyperplasia (bilateral)

E26.1 Secondary hyperaldosteronism   HCC

✓5ᵗʰ **E26.8 Other hyperaldosteronism**

E26.81 Bartter's syndrome   HCC

E26.89 Other hyperaldosteronism   HCC

E26.9 Hyperaldosteronism, unspecified   HCC

Aldosteronism NOS
Hyperaldosteronism NOS

✓4ᵗʰ **E27 Other disorders of adrenal gland**

CC Excl: For CC codes in category E27: PDX collection 526

E27.0 Other adrenocortical overactivity   CC HCC

Overproduction of ACTH, not associated with Cushing's disease
Premature adrenarche

> *EXCLUDES 1*   *Cushing's syndrome (E24.-)*

E27.1 Primary adrenocortical insufficiency   CC HCC

Addison's disease
Autoimmune adrenalitis

> *EXCLUDES 1*   *Addison only phenotype adrenoleukodystrophy (E71.528)*
> *amyloidosis (E85.-)*
> *tuberculous Addison's disease (A18.7)*
> *Waterhouse-Friderichsen syndrome (A39.1)*

N Newborn: 0   P Pediatric: 0-17   M Maternity: 9-64   A Adult: 15-124   MCC Major Complication/Comorbidity   CC Complication/Comorbidity   SW Severe Wound Dx

528   ICD-10-CM 2020

E27.2 Addisonian crisis `CC` `HCC`
Adrenal crisis
Adrenocortical crisis
DEF: Life-threatening condition that occurs when there is not enough cortisol excreted from the adrenal glands. This condition may be due to injury to the adrenal glands or to the pituitary gland, which controls adrenal hormone secretion, or when a patient stops hydrocortisone treatment too quickly or too early.

E27.3 Drug-induced adrenocortical insufficiency `CC` `HCC`
Use additional code for adverse effect, if applicable, to identify drug (T36-T50 with fifth or sixth character 5)

√5ᵗʰ **E27.4 Other and unspecified adrenocortical insufficiency**
EXCLUDES 1   adrenoleukodystrophy [Addison-Schilder] (E71.528)
Waterhouse-Friderichsen syndrome (A39.1)

E27.40 Unspecified adrenocortical insufficiency `CC` `HCC`
Adrenocortical insufficiency NOS
Hypoaldosteronism

E27.49 Other adrenocortical insufficiency `CC` `HCC`
Adrenal hemorrhage
Adrenal infarction

E27.5 Adrenomedullary hyperfunction `CC` `HCC`
Adrenomedullary hyperplasia
Catecholamine hypersecretion

E27.8 Other specified disorders of adrenal gland `HCC`
Abnormality of cortisol-binding globulin

E27.9 Disorder of adrenal gland, unspecified `HCC`

√4ᵗʰ **E28 Ovarian dysfunction**
EXCLUDES 1   isolated gonadotropin deficiency (E23.0)
postprocedural ovarian failure (E89.4-)

E28.0 Estrogen excess ♀
Use additional code for adverse effect, if applicable, to identify drug (T36-T50 with fifth or sixth character 5)

E28.1 Androgen excess ♀
Hypersecretion of ovarian androgens
Use additional code for adverse effect, if applicable, to identify drug (T36-T50 with fifth or sixth character 5)

E28.2 Polycystic ovarian syndrome ♀
Sclerocystic ovary syndrome
Stein-Leventhal syndrome
DEF: Common hormonal disorder among women of reproductive age that involves enlarged ovaries with numerous small cysts located along the outer ovarian edge.

√5ᵗʰ **E28.3 Primary ovarian failure**
EXCLUDES 1   pure gonadal dysgenesis (Q99.1)
Turner's syndrome (Q96.-)

√6ᵗʰ **E28.31 Premature menopause**
E28.310 Symptomatic premature menopause `A` ♀
Symptoms such as flushing, sleeplessness, headache, lack of concentration, associated with premature menopause

E28.319 Asymptomatic premature menopause `A` ♀
Premature menopause NOS

E28.39 Other primary ovarian failure ♀
Decreased estrogen
Resistant ovary syndrome

E28.8 Other ovarian dysfunction ♀
Ovarian hyperfunction NOS
EXCLUDES 1   postprocedural ovarian failure (E89.4-)

E28.9 Ovarian dysfunction, unspecified ♀

√4ᵗʰ **E29 Testicular dysfunction**
EXCLUDES 1   androgen insensitivity syndrome (E34.5-)
azoospermia or oligospermia NOS (N46.0-N46.1)
isolated gonadotropin deficiency (E23.0)
Klinefelter's syndrome (Q98.0-Q98.1, Q98.4)

E29.0 Testicular hyperfunction ♂
Hypersecretion of testicular hormones

E29.1 Testicular hypofunction ♂
Defective biosynthesis of testicular androgen NOS
5-delta-Reductase deficiency (with male pseudohermaphroditism)
Testicular hypogonadism NOS
Use additional code for adverse effect, if applicable, to identify drug (T36-T50 with fifth or sixth character 5)
EXCLUDES 1   postprocedural testicular hypofunction (E89.5)

E29.8 Other testicular dysfunction ♂
E29.9 Testicular dysfunction, unspecified ♂

√4ᵗʰ **E30 Disorders of puberty, not elsewhere classified**
E30.0 Delayed puberty
Constitutional delay of puberty
Delayed sexual development

E30.1 Precocious puberty `P`
Precocious menstruation
EXCLUDES 1   Albright (-McCune) (-Sternberg) syndrome (Q78.1)
central precocious puberty (E22.8)
congenital adrenal hyperplasia (E25.0)
female heterosexual precocious pseudopuberty (E25.-)
male isosexual precocious pseudopuberty (E25.-)

E30.8 Other disorders of puberty `P`
Premature thelarche

E30.9 Disorder of puberty, unspecified

√4ᵗʰ **E31 Polyglandular dysfunction**
EXCLUDES 1   ataxia telangiectasia [Louis-Bar] (G11.3)
dystrophia myotonica [Steinert] (G71.11)
pseudohypoparathyroidism (E20.1)

E31.0 Autoimmune polyglandular failure `HCC`
Schmidt's syndrome

E31.1 Polyglandular hyperfunction `HCC`
EXCLUDES 1   multiple endocrine adenomatosis (E31.2-)
multiple endocrine neoplasia (E31.2-)

√5ᵗʰ **E31.2 Multiple endocrine neoplasia [MEN] syndromes**
Multiple endocrine adenomatosis
Code also any associated malignancies and other conditions associated with the syndromes
DEF: Group of conditions in which several endocrine glands grow excessively (such as in adenomatous hyperplasia) and/or develop benign or malignant tumors. Tumors and hyperplasia associated with MEN often produce excess hormones, which impede normal physiology. There is no comprehensive cure known for MEN syndrome. Treatment is directed at the hyperplasia or tumors in each individual gland. Tumors are usually surgically removed and oral medications or hormonal injections are used to correct hormone imbalances.

E31.20 Multiple endocrine neoplasia [MEN] syndrome, unspecified `HCC`
Multiple endocrine adenomatosis NOS
Multiple endocrine neoplasia [MEN] syndrome NOS

E31.21 Multiple endocrine neoplasia [MEN] type I `HCC`
Wermer's syndrome

E31.22 Multiple endocrine neoplasia [MEN] type IIA `HCC`
Sipple's syndrome

E31.23 Multiple endocrine neoplasia [MEN] type IIB `HCC`

E31.8 Other polyglandular dysfunction `HCC`
E31.9 Polyglandular dysfunction, unspecified `HCC`

√4ᵗʰ **E32 Diseases of thymus**
EXCLUDES 1   aplasia or hypoplasia of thymus with immunodeficiency (D82.1)
myasthenia gravis (G70.0)

E32.0 Persistent hyperplasia of thymus `HCC`
Hypertrophy of thymus

E32.1 Abscess of thymus `CC` `HCC`
CC Excl: PDX collection 527

E32.8 Other diseases of thymus `HCC`
EXCLUDES 1   aplasia or hypoplasia with immunodeficiency (D82.1)
thymoma (D15.0)

E32.9 Disease of thymus, unspecified `HCC`

Chapter 4. Endocrine, Nutritional and Metabolic Diseases

E34–E45

✓4th **E34 Other endocrine disorders**
> EXCLUDES 1   *pseudohypoparathyroidism (E20.1)*

E34.0 Carcinoid syndrome   CC   HCC
> NOTE   May be used as an additional code to identify functional activity associated with a carcinoid tumor.
> **CC Excl:** PDX collection 528

E34.1 Other hypersecretion of intestinal hormones

E34.2 Ectopic hormone secretion, not elsewhere classified
> EXCLUDES 1   *ectopic ACTH syndrome (E24.3)*

E34.3 Short stature due to endocrine disorder
> Constitutional short stature
> Laron-type short stature
> EXCLUDES 1   *achondroplastic short stature (Q77.4)*
>   *hypochondroplastic short stature (Q77.4)*
>   *nutritional short stature (E45)*
>   *pituitary short stature (E23.0)*
>   *progeria (E34.8)*
>   *renal short stature (N25.0)*
>   *Russell-Silver syndrome ▶(Q87.19)◀*
>   *short-limbed stature with immunodeficiency (D82.2)*
>   *short stature in specific dysmorphic syndromes —*
>   *code to syndrome — see Alphabetical Index*
>   *short stature NOS (R62.52)*

E34.4 Constitutional tall stature   HCC
> Constitutional gigantism

✓5th **E34.5 Androgen insensitivity syndrome**
> **DEF:** X-linked recessive condition in which individuals that are chromosomally male fail to develop normal male external genitalia due to an abnormality on the X chromosome that prohibits the body, completely or in part, from recognizing the androgens produced. *Synonym(s): AIS*

E34.50 Androgen insensitivity syndrome, unspecified
> Androgen insensitivity NOS

E34.51 Complete androgen insensitivity syndrome
> Complete androgen insensitivity
> de Quervain syndrome
> Goldberg-Maxwell syndrome

E34.52 Partial androgen insensitivity syndrome
> Partial androgen insensitivity
> Reifenstein syndrome

E34.8 Other specified endocrine disorders
> Pineal gland dysfunction
> Progeria
> EXCLUDES 2   *pseudohypoparathyroidism (E20.1)*

E34.9 Endocrine disorder, unspecified
> Endocrine disturbance NOS
> Hormone disturbance NOS

E35 *Disorders of endocrine glands in diseases classified elsewhere*
> Code first underlying disease, such as:
>   late congenital syphilis of thymus gland [Dubois disease] (A50.5)
> Use additional code, if applicable, to identify:
>   sequelae of tuberculosis of other organs (B90.8)
> EXCLUDES 1   *Echinococcus granulosus infection of thyroid gland (B67.3)*
>   *meningococcal hemorrhagic adrenalitis (A39.1)*
>   *syphilis of endocrine gland (A52.79)*
>   *tuberculosis of adrenal gland, except calcification (A18.7)*
>   *tuberculosis of endocrine gland NEC (A18.82)*
>   *tuberculosis of thyroid gland (A18.81)*
>   *Waterhouse-Friderichsen syndrome (A39.1)*

Intraoperative complications of endocrine system (E36)

✓4th **E36 Intraoperative complications of endocrine system**
> EXCLUDES 2   *postprocedural endocrine and metabolic complications and disorders, not elsewhere classified (E89.-)*

✓5th **E36.0 Intraoperative hemorrhage and hematoma of an endocrine system organ or structure complicating a procedure**
> EXCLUDES 1   *intraoperative hemorrhage and hematoma of an endocrine system organ or structure due to accidental puncture or laceration during a procedure (E36.1-)*

E36.01 Intraoperative hemorrhage and hematoma of an endocrine system organ or structure complicating an endocrine system procedure   CC
> **CC Excl:** PDX collection 529

E36.02 Intraoperative hemorrhage and hematoma of an endocrine system organ or structure complicating other procedure   CC
> **CC Excl:** PDX collection 529

✓5th **E36.1 Accidental puncture and laceration of an endocrine system organ or structure during a procedure**

E36.11 Accidental puncture and laceration of an endocrine system organ or structure during an endocrine system procedure   CC
> **CC Excl:** PDX collection 509

E36.12 Accidental puncture and laceration of an endocrine system organ or structure during other procedure   CC
> **CC Excl:** PDX collection 509

E36.8 Other intraoperative complications of endocrine system
> Use additional code, if applicable, to further specify disorder

Malnutrition (E40-E46)

> EXCLUDES 1   *intestinal malabsorption (K90.-)*
>   *sequelae of protein-calorie malnutrition (E64.0)*
> EXCLUDES 2   *nutritional anemias (D50-D53)*
>   *starvation (T73.0)*
> **AHA:** 2017,4Q,108; 2017,3Q,25
> **TIP:** Assign additional code for BMI from category Z68, when documented. BMI can be based on documentation from clinicians who are not the patient's provider.
> **CC Excl: For CC/MCC codes in categories E40-E46:** PDX collection 530

E40 Kwashiorkor   MCC   HCC
> Severe malnutrition with nutritional edema with dyspigmentation of skin and hair
> EXCLUDES 1   *marasmic kwashiorkor (E42)*

E41 Nutritional marasmus   MCC   HCC
> Severe malnutrition with marasmus
> EXCLUDES 1   *marasmic kwashiorkor (E42)*
> **AHA:** 2017,3Q,24
> **DEF:** Protein-calorie malabsorption or malnutrition in children characterized by tissue wasting, dehydration, and subcutaneous fat depletion. It may occur with infectious disease.

E42 Marasmic kwashiorkor   CC   HCC
> Intermediate form severe protein-calorie malnutrition
> Severe protein-calorie malnutrition with signs of both kwashiorkor and marasmus

E43 Unspecified severe protein-calorie malnutrition   CC   HCC
> Starvation edema
> **AHA:** 2017,4Q,108

✓4th **E44 Protein-calorie malnutrition of moderate and mild degree**

E44.0 Moderate protein-calorie malnutrition   MCC   HCC

E44.1 Mild protein-calorie malnutrition   CC   HCC

E45 Retarded development following protein-calorie malnutrition   CC   HCC
> Nutritional short stature
> Nutritional stunting
> Physical retardation due to malnutrition

N Newborn: 0   P Pediatric: 0-17   M Maternity: 9-64   A Adult: 15-124   MCC Major Complication/Comorbidity   CC Complication/Comorbidity   SW Severe Wound Dx

530   ICD-10-CM 2020

E46   **Unspecified protein-calorie malnutrition**   `CC` `HCC`
Malnutrition NOS
Protein-calorie imbalance NOS
EXCLUDES 1   *nutritional deficiency NOS (E63.9)*
AHA: 2018,4Q,82

Other nutritional deficiencies (E50-E64)

EXCLUDES 2   *nutritional anemias (D50-D53)*
CC Excl: For CC codes in categories E50-E64, unless otherwise noted: PDX collection 531

✓4ᵗʰ **E50**   **Vitamin A deficiency**
EXCLUDES 1   *sequelae of vitamin A deficiency (E64.1)*

E50.0   **Vitamin A deficiency with conjunctival xerosis**
E50.1   **Vitamin A deficiency with Bitot's spot and conjunctival xerosis**
Bitot's spot in the young child
DEF: Vitamin A deficiency with conjunctival dryness and superficial spots of keratinized epithelium.
E50.2   **Vitamin A deficiency with corneal xerosis**
E50.3   **Vitamin A deficiency with corneal ulceration and xerosis**
E50.4   **Vitamin A deficiency with keratomalacia**
DEF: Vitamin A deficiency creating corneal dryness that progresses to corneal insensitivity, softness, and necrosis. It is usually bilateral.
E50.5   **Vitamin A deficiency with night blindness**
E50.6   **Vitamin A deficiency with xerophthalmic scars of cornea**
E50.7   **Other ocular manifestations of vitamin A deficiency**
Xerophthalmia NOS
E50.8   **Other manifestations of vitamin A deficiency**
Follicular keratosis
Xeroderma
E50.9   **Vitamin A deficiency, unspecified**
Hypovitaminosis A NOS

✓4ᵗʰ **E51**   **Thiamine deficiency**
EXCLUDES 1   *sequelae of thiamine deficiency (E64.8)*

✓5ᵗʰ **E51.1**   **Beriberi**

E51.11   **Dry beriberi**   `CC`
Beriberi NOS
Beriberi with polyneuropathy
E51.12   **Wet beriberi**   `CC`
Beriberi with cardiovascular manifestations
Cardiovascular beriberi
Shoshin disease

E51.2   **Wernicke's encephalopathy**   `MCC`
DEF: Deficiency of vitamin B1 resulting in a triad of acute mental confusion, ataxia, and ophthalmoplegia. The vast majority of affected patients are alcoholics.
E51.8   **Other manifestations of thiamine deficiency**   `CC`
E51.9   **Thiamine deficiency, unspecified**   `CC`

E52   **Niacin deficiency [pellagra]**
Niacin (-tryptophan) deficiency
Nicotinamide deficiency
Pellagra (alcoholic)
EXCLUDES 1   *sequelae of niacin deficiency (E64.8)*

✓4ᵗʰ **E53**   **Deficiency of other B group vitamins**
EXCLUDES 1   *sequelae of vitamin B deficiency (E64.8)*

E53.0   **Riboflavin deficiency**   `CC`
Ariboflavinosis
Vitamin B2 deficiency
E53.1   **Pyridoxine deficiency**
Vitamin B6 deficiency
EXCLUDES 1   *pyridoxine-responsive sideroblastic anemia (D64.3)*
E53.8   **Deficiency of other specified B group vitamins**
Biotin deficiency
Cyanocobalamin deficiency
Folate deficiency
Folic acid deficiency
Pantothenic acid deficiency
Vitamin B12 deficiency
EXCLUDES 1   *folate deficiency anemia (D52.-)*
     vitamin B12 deficiency anemia (D51.-)
E53.9   **Vitamin B deficiency, unspecified**

E54   **Ascorbic acid deficiency**
Deficiency of vitamin C
Scurvy
EXCLUDES 1   *scorbutic anemia (D53.2)*
     sequelae of vitamin C deficiency (E64.2)
DEF: Vitamin C deficiency causing swollen gums, myalgia, weight loss, and weakness.

✓4ᵗʰ **E55**   **Vitamin D deficiency**
EXCLUDES 1   *adult osteomalacia (M83.-)*
     osteoporosis (M80.-)
     sequelae of rickets (E64.3)

E55.0   **Rickets, active**   `CC`
Infantile osteomalacia
Juvenile osteomalacia
EXCLUDES 1   *celiac rickets (K90.0)*
     Crohn's rickets (K50.-)
     hereditary vitamin D-dependent rickets (E83.32)
     inactive rickets (E64.3)
     renal rickets (N25.0)
     sequelae of rickets (E64.3)
     vitamin D-resistant rickets (E83.31)
DEF: Rickets: Softening or weakening of the bones due to a lack of vitamin D, calcium, and phosphate.
CC Excl: PDX collection 532
E55.9   **Vitamin D deficiency, unspecified**
Avitaminosis D

✓4ᵗʰ **E56**   **Other vitamin deficiencies**
EXCLUDES 1   *sequelae of other vitamin deficiencies (E64.8)*

E56.0   **Deficiency of vitamin E**
E56.1   **Deficiency of vitamin K**
EXCLUDES 1   *deficiency of coagulation factor due to vitamin K deficiency (D68.4)*
     vitamin K deficiency of newborn (P53)
E56.8   **Deficiency of other vitamins**
E56.9   **Vitamin deficiency, unspecified**

E58   **Dietary calcium deficiency**
EXCLUDES 1   *disorders of calcium metabolism (E83.5-)*
     sequelae of calcium deficiency (E64.8)

E59   **Dietary selenium deficiency**
Keshan disease
EXCLUDES 1   *sequelae of selenium deficiency (E64.8)*

E60   **Dietary zinc deficiency**

✓4ᵗʰ **E61**   **Deficiency of other nutrient elements**
Use additional code for adverse effect, if applicable, to identify drug (T36-T50 with fifth or sixth character 5)
EXCLUDES 1   *disorders of mineral metabolism (E83.-)*
     iodine deficiency related thyroid disorders (E00-E02)
     sequelae of malnutrition and other nutritional deficiencies (E64.-)

E61.0   **Copper deficiency**
E61.1   **Iron deficiency**
EXCLUDES 1   *iron deficiency anemia (D50.-)*
E61.2   **Magnesium deficiency**
E61.3   **Manganese deficiency**
E61.4   **Chromium deficiency**
E61.5   **Molybdenum deficiency**
E61.6   **Vanadium deficiency**
E61.7   **Deficiency of multiple nutrient elements**
E61.8   **Deficiency of other specified nutrient elements**
E61.9   **Deficiency of nutrient element, unspecified**

✓4ᵗʰ **E63**   **Other nutritional deficiencies**
EXCLUDES 1   *dehydration (E86.0)*
     failure to thrive, adult (R62.7)
     failure to thrive, child (R62.51)
     feeding problems in newborn (P92.-)
     sequelae of malnutrition and other nutritional deficiencies (E64.-)

E63.0   **Essential fatty acid [EFA] deficiency**
E63.1   **Imbalance of constituents of food intake**
E63.8   **Other specified nutritional deficiencies**
E63.9   **Nutritional deficiency, unspecified**

☑4ᵗʰ **E64 Sequelae of malnutrition and other nutritional deficiencies**

> **NOTE** This category is to be used to indicate conditions in categories E43, E44, E46, E50-E63 as the cause of sequelae, which are themselves classified elsewhere. The 'sequelae' include conditions specified as such; they also include the late effects of diseases classifiable to the above categories if the disease itself is no longer present
>
> Code first condition resulting from (sequela) of malnutrition and other nutritional deficiencies

E64.0 Sequelae of protein-calorie malnutrition CC HCC
> EXCLUDES 2   retarded development following protein-calorie malnutrition (E45)
>
> CC Excl: PDX collection 530

E64.1 Sequelae of vitamin A deficiency

E64.2 Sequelae of vitamin C deficiency

E64.3 Sequelae of rickets

E64.8 Sequelae of other nutritional deficiencies

E64.9 Sequelae of unspecified nutritional deficiency

Overweight, obesity and other hyperalimentation (E65-E68)

E65 Localized adiposity
> Fat pad

☑4ᵗʰ **E66 Overweight and obesity**
> Code first obesity complicating pregnancy, childbirth and the puerperium, if applicable (O99.21-)
> Use additional code to identify body mass index (BMI), if known (Z68.-)
> EXCLUDES 1   adiposogenital dystrophy (E23.6)
>   lipomatosis NOS (E88.2)
>   lipomatosis dolorosa [Dercum] (E88.2)
>   Prader-Willi syndrome ▶(Q87.11)◀
>
> AHA: 2018,4Q,77,79-80
> TIP: Do not assign a BMI code (Z68.-) when a pregnant patient is documented as being overweight or obese. Only a code from subcategory O99.21- and a code from this category should be assigned.

☑5ᵗʰ **E66.0 Obesity due to excess calories**

E66.01 Morbid (severe) obesity due to excess calories H11 HCC
> EXCLUDES 1   morbid (severe) obesity with alveolar hypoventilation (E66.2)

[handwritten: morbidly obese]

E66.09 Other obesity due to excess calories

E66.1 Drug-induced obesity
> Use additional code for adverse effect, if applicable, to identify drug (T36-T50 with fifth or sixth character 5)

E66.2 Morbid (severe) obesity with alveolar hypoventilation CC HCC
> Obesity hypoventilation syndrome (OHS)
> Pickwickian syndrome
> CC Excl: PDX collection 533

E66.3 Overweight
> AHA: 2018,4Q,78

E66.8 Other obesity

E66.9 Obesity, unspecified
> Obesity NOS

☑4ᵗʰ **E67 Other hyperalimentation**
> EXCLUDES 1   hyperalimentation NOS (R63.2)
>   sequelae of hyperalimentation (E68)

E67.0 Hypervitaminosis A

E67.1 Hypercarotenemia
> DEF: Elevated blood carotene level as a result of excessive carotenoid ingestion or an inability to convert carotenoids to vitamin A. Characteristics often include yellow discoloration of the skin, which may follow overeating of carotenoid-rich foods such as carrots, sweet potatoes, or squash.

E67.2 Megavitamin-B6 syndrome

E67.3 Hypervitaminosis D

E67.8 Other specified hyperalimentation

E68 Sequelae of hyperalimentation
> Code first condition resulting from (sequela) of hyperalimentation

Metabolic disorders (E70-E88)

> EXCLUDES 1   androgen insensitivity syndrome (E34.5-)
>   congenital adrenal hyperplasia (E25.0)
>   Ehlers-Danlos syndrome ▶(Q79.6-)◀
>   hemolytic anemias attributable to enzyme disorders (D55.-)
>   Marfan's syndrome (Q87.4)
>   5-alpha-reductase deficiency (E29.1)
>
> AHA: 2018,2Q,6

☑4ᵗʰ **E70 Disorders of aromatic amino-acid metabolism**

> CC Excl: For CC codes in category E70: PDX collection 534

E70.0 Classical phenylketonuria CC HCC

E70.1 Other hyperphenylalaninemias CC HCC

☑5ᵗʰ **E70.2 Disorders of tyrosine metabolism**
> EXCLUDES 1   transitory tyrosinemia of newborn (P74.5)

E70.20 Disorder of tyrosine metabolism, unspecified CC HCC

E70.21 Tyrosinemia CC HCC
> Hypertyrosinemia

E70.29 Other disorders of tyrosine metabolism CC HCC
> Alkaptonuria
> Ochronosis

☑5ᵗʰ **E70.3 Albinism**
> DEF: Absence of pigment in skin, hair, and eyes. This genetic condition is often accompanied by astigmatism, photophobia, and nystagmus.

E70.30 Albinism, unspecified CC HCC

☑6ᵗʰ **E70.31 Ocular albinism**

E70.310 X-linked ocular albinism CC HCC

E70.311 Autosomal recessive ocular albinism CC HCC

E70.318 Other ocular albinism

E70.319 Ocular albinism, unspecified CC HCC

☑6ᵗʰ **E70.32 Oculocutaneous albinism**
> EXCLUDES 1   Chediak-Higashi syndrome (E70.330)
>   Hermansky-Pudlak syndrome (E70.331)

E70.320 Tyrosinase negative oculocutaneous albinism CC HCC
> Albinism I
> Oculocutaneous albinism ty-neg

E70.321 Tyrosinase positive oculocutaneous albinism CC HCC
> Albinism II
> Oculocutaneous albinism ty-pos

E70.328 Other oculocutaneous albinism CC HCC
> Cross syndrome

E70.329 Oculocutaneous albinism, unspecified CC HCC

☑6ᵗʰ **E70.33 Albinism with hematologic abnormality**

E70.330 Chediak-Higashi syndrome CC HCC

E70.331 Hermansky-Pudlak syndrome CC HCC

E70.338 Other albinism with hematologic abnormality CC HCC

E70.339 Albinism with hematologic abnormality, unspecified CC HCC

E70.39 Other specified albinism CC HCC
> Piebaldism

☑5ᵗʰ **E70.4 Disorders of histidine metabolism**

E70.40 Disorders of histidine metabolism, unspecified CC HCC

E70.41 Histidinemia CC HCC

E70.49 Other disorders of histidine metabolism CC HCC

E70.5 Disorders of tryptophan metabolism CC HCC

E70.8 Other disorders of aromatic amino-acid metabolism CC HCC

E70.9 Disorder of aromatic amino-acid metabolism, unspecified CC HCC

Ⓝ Newborn: 0   Ⓟ Pediatric: 0-17   Ⓜ Maternity: 9-64   Ⓐ Adult: 15-124   MCC Major Complication/Comorbidity   CC Complication/Comorbidity   SW Severe Wound Dx

532   ICD-10-CM 2020

✓4th **E71 Disorders of branched-chain amino-acid metabolism and fatty-acid metabolism**

    E71.0 Maple-syrup-urine disease `CC` `HCC`
        CC Excl: PDX collection 534

✓5th **E71.1 Other disorders of branched-chain amino-acid metabolism**
        CC Excl: For CC codes in subcategory E71.1: PDX collection 534

    ✓6th **E71.11 Branched-chain organic acidurias**
        E71.110 Isovaleric acidemia `CC` `HCC`
        E71.111 3-methylglutaconic aciduria `CC` `HCC`
        E71.118 Other branched-chain organic acidurias `CC` `HCC`

    ✓6th **E71.12 Disorders of propionate metabolism**
        E71.120 Methylmalonic acidemia `CC` `HCC`
        E71.121 Propionic acidemia `CC` `HCC`
        E71.128 Other disorders of propionate metabolism `CC` `HCC`

    E71.19 Other disorders of branched-chain amino-acid metabolism `CC` `HCC`
        Hyperleucine-isoleucinemia
        Hypervalinemia

  E71.2 Disorder of branched-chain amino-acid metabolism, unspecified `CC` `HCC`
        CC Excl: PDX collection 534

✓5th **E71.3 Disorders of fatty-acid metabolism**
    EXCLUDES 1   peroxisomal disorders (E71.5)
        Refsum's disease (G60.1)
        Schilder's disease (G37.0)
    EXCLUDES 2   carnitine deficiency due to inborn error of metabolism (E71.42)

    CC Excl: For CC codes in subcategory E71.3, unless otherwise noted: PDX collection 535

    E71.30 Disorder of fatty-acid metabolism, unspecified

    ✓6th **E71.31 Disorders of fatty-acid oxidation**
        E71.310 Long chain/very long chain acyl CoA dehydrogenase deficiency `CC` `HCC`
            LCAD
            VLCAD
        E71.311 Medium chain acyl CoA dehydrogenase deficiency `CC` `HCC`
            MCAD
        E71.312 Short chain acyl CoA dehydrogenase deficiency `CC` `HCC`
            SCAD
        E71.313 Glutaric aciduria type II `CC` `HCC`
            Glutaric aciduria type II A
            Glutaric aciduria type II B
            Glutaric aciduria type II C
            EXCLUDES 1 glutaric aciduria (type 1) NOS (E72.3)
        E71.314 Muscle carnitine palmitoyltransferase deficiency `CC` `HCC`
        E71.318 Other disorders of fatty-acid oxidation `CC` `HCC`

    E71.32 Disorders of ketone metabolism `CC` `HCC`

    E71.39 Other disorders of fatty-acid metabolism `CC` `HCC`
        CC Excl: PDX collection 492

✓5th **E71.4 Disorders of carnitine metabolism**
    EXCLUDES 1   muscle carnitine palmitoyltransferase deficiency (E71.314)

    E71.40 Disorder of carnitine metabolism, unspecified `HCC`

    E71.41 Primary carnitine deficiency `HCC`

    E71.42 Carnitine deficiency due to inborn errors of metabolism `HCC`
        Code also associated inborn error or metabolism

    E71.43 Iatrogenic carnitine deficiency `HCC`
        Carnitine deficiency due to hemodialysis
        Carnitine deficiency due to Valproic acid therapy

    ✓6th **E71.44 Other secondary carnitine deficiency**
        E71.440 Ruvalcaba-Myhre-Smith syndrome `HCC`
        E71.448 Other secondary carnitine deficiency `HCC`

✓5th **E71.5 Peroxisomal disorders**
    EXCLUDES 1   Schilder's disease (G37.0)
    CC Excl: For CC codes in subcategory E71.5: PDX collection 536

    E71.50 Peroxisomal disorder, unspecified `CC` `HCC`

    ✓6th **E71.51 Disorders of peroxisome biogenesis**
        Group 1 peroxisomal disorders
        EXCLUDES 1 Refsum's disease (G60.1)
        E71.510 Zellweger syndrome `CC` `HCC`
        E71.511 Neonatal adrenoleukodystrophy `CC` `HCC`
          EXCLUDES 1 X-linked adrenoleukodystrophy (E71.42-)
        E71.518 Other disorders of peroxisome biogenesis `CC` `HCC`

    ✓6th **E71.52 X-linked adrenoleukodystrophy**
        E71.520 Childhood cerebral X-linked adrenoleukodystrophy `CC` `HCC`
        E71.521 Adolescent X-linked adrenoleukodystrophy `CC` `HCC`
        E71.522 Adrenomyeloneuropathy `CC` `HCC`
        E71.528 Other X-linked adrenoleukodystrophy `CC` `HCC`
          Addison only phenotype adrenoleukodystrophy
          Addison-Schilder adrenoleukodystrophy
        E71.529 X-linked adrenoleukodystrophy, unspecified type `CC` `HCC`

    E71.53 Other group 2 peroxisomal disorders `CC` `HCC`

    ✓6th **E71.54 Other peroxisomal disorders**
        E71.540 Rhizomelic chondrodysplasia punctata `CC` `HCC`
          EXCLUDES 1 chondrodysplasia punctata NOS (Q77.3)
        E71.541 Zellweger-like syndrome `CC` `HCC`
        E71.542 Other group 3 peroxisomal disorders `CC` `HCC`
        E71.548 Other peroxisomal disorders `CC` `HCC`

✓4th **E72 Other disorders of amino-acid metabolism**
    EXCLUDES 1   disorders of:
        aromatic amino-acid metabolism (E70.-)
        branched-chain amino-acid metabolism (E71.0-E71.2)
        fatty-acid metabolism (E71.3)
        purine and pyrimidine metabolism (E79.-)
        gout (M1A.-, M10.-)
    CC Excl: For CC codes in category E72, unless otherwise noted: PDX collection 534

✓5th **E72.0 Disorders of amino-acid transport**
    EXCLUDES 1   disorders of tryptophan metabolism (E70.5)

    E72.00 Disorders of amino-acid transport, unspecified `CC` `HCC`

    E72.01 Cystinuria `CC` `HCC`

    E72.02 Hartnup's disease `CC` `HCC`

    E72.03 Lowe's syndrome `CC` `HCC`
        Use additional code for associated glaucoma (H42)
        CC Excl: No Excl

    E72.04 Cystinosis `CC` `HCC`
        Fanconi (-de Toni) (-Debré) syndrome with cystinosis
        EXCLUDES 1 Fanconi (-de Toni) (-Debré) syndrome without cystinosis (E72.09)

    E72.09 Other disorders of amino-acid transport `CC` `HCC`
        Fanconi (-de Toni) (-Debré) syndrome, unspecified

✓5th **E72.1 Disorders of sulfur-bearing amino-acid metabolism**
    EXCLUDES 1   cystinosis (E72.04)
        cystinuria (E72.01)
        transcobalamin II deficiency (D51.2)

    E72.10 Disorders of sulfur-bearing amino-acid metabolism, unspecified `CC` `HCC`

    E72.11 Homocystinuria `CC` `HCC`
        Cystathionine synthase deficiency

✓ Additional Character Required   ✓x7th Placeholder   Unacceptable PDx   Questionable PDx   Manifestation   Unspecified Dx   H1-H14 HAC   `HCC` CMS-HCC Dx   HIV HIV Dx

Chapter 4. Endocrine, Nutritional and Metabolic Diseases

E72.12–E74.9

E72.12	**Methylenetetrahydrofolate reductase deficiency**	CC HCC
E72.19	**Other disorders of sulfur-bearing amino-acid metabolism**	CC HCC
	Cystathioninuria	
	Methioninemia	
	Sulfite oxidase deficiency	

√5ᵗʰ **E72.2** **Disorders of urea cycle metabolism**

EXCLUDES 1   *disorders of ornithine metabolism (E72.4)*

E72.20 **Disorder of urea cycle metabolism, unspecified**   CC HCC
     Hyperammonemia

     EXCLUDES 1   *hyperammonemia- hyperornithinemia-homocitrullinemia syndrome E72.4*
         transient hyperammonemia of newborn (P74.6)

E72.21 **Argininemia**   CC HCC

E72.22 **Arginosuccinic aciduria**   CC HCC

E72.23 **Citrullinemia**   CC HCC

E72.29 **Other disorders of urea cycle metabolism**   CC HCC

E72.3 **Disorders of lysine and hydroxylysine metabolism**   CC HCC
     Glutaric aciduria NOS
     Glutaric aciduria (type I)
     Hydroxylysinemia
     Hyperlysinemia

     EXCLUDES 1   *glutaric aciduria type II (E71.313)*
         Refsum's disease (G60.1)
         Zellweger syndrome (E71.510)

E72.4 **Disorders of ornithine metabolism**   CC HCC
     Hyperammonemia-Hyperornithinemia-Homocitrullinemia syndrome
     Ornithinemia (types I, II)
     Ornithine transcarbamylase deficiency

     EXCLUDES 1   *hereditary choroidal dystrophy (H31.2-)*

√5ᵗʰ **E72.5** **Disorders of glycine metabolism**

E72.50 **Disorder of glycine metabolism, unspecified**   CC HCC

E72.51 **Non-ketotic hyperglycinemia**   CC HCC

E72.52 **Trimethylaminuria**   CC HCC

E72.53 **Primary hyperoxaluria**   CC HCC
     Oxalosis
     Oxaluria
     AHA: 2018,4Q,29

E72.59 **Other disorders of glycine metabolism**   CC HCC
     D-glycericacidemia
     Hyperhydroxyprolinemia
     Hyperprolinemia (types I, II)
     Sarcosinemia

√5ᵗʰ **E72.8** **Other specified disorders of amino-acid metabolism**
     AHA: 2018,4Q,5

E72.81 **Disorders of gamma aminobutyric acid metabolism**   CC HCC
     4-hydroxybutyric aciduria
     Disorders of GABA metabolism
     GABA metabolic defect
     GABA transaminase deficiency
     GABA-T deficiency
     Gamma-hydroxybutyric aciduria
     SSADHD
     Succinic semialdehyde dehydrogenase deficiency

E72.89 **Other specified disorders of amino-acid metabolism**   CC HCC
     Disorders of beta-amino-acid metabolism
     Disorders of gamma-glutamyl cycle

E72.9 **Disorder of amino-acid metabolism, unspecified**   CC HCC

√4ᵗʰ **E73** **Lactose intolerance**

     DEF: Inability to break down sugar in dairy products due to a deficiency in the enzyme lactase.

E73.0 **Congenital lactase deficiency**

E73.1 **Secondary lactase deficiency**

E73.8 **Other lactose intolerance**

E73.9 **Lactose intolerance, unspecified**

√4ᵗʰ **E74** **Other disorders of carbohydrate metabolism**

     EXCLUDES 1   *diabetes mellitus (E08-E13)*
         hypoglycemia NOS (E16.2)
         increased secretion of glucagon (E16.3)
         mucopolysaccharidosis (E76.0-E76.3)

     CC Excl: For CC codes in category E74: PDX collection 534

√5ᵗʰ **E74.0** **Glycogen storage disease**

E74.00 **Glycogen storage disease, unspecified**   CC HCC

E74.01 **von Gierke disease**   CC HCC
     Type I glycogen storage disease

E74.02 **Pompe disease**   CC HCC
     Cardiac glycogenosis
     Type II glycogen storage disease

E74.03 **Cori disease**   CC HCC
     Forbes disease
     Type III glycogen storage disease

E74.04 **McArdle disease**   CC HCC
     Type V glycogen storage disease

E74.09 **Other glycogen storage disease**   CC HCC
     Andersen disease
     Hers disease
     Tauri disease
     Glycogen storage disease, types Ø, IV, VI-XI
     Liver phosphorylase deficiency
     Muscle phosphofructokinase deficiency

√5ᵗʰ **E74.1** **Disorders of fructose metabolism**

     EXCLUDES 1   *muscle phosphofructokinase deficiency (E74.09)*

E74.10 **Disorder of fructose metabolism, unspecified**

E74.11 **Essential fructosuria**
     Fructokinase deficiency

E74.12 **Hereditary fructose intolerance**
     Fructosemia

E74.19 **Other disorders of fructose metabolism**
     Fructose-1, 6-diphosphatase deficiency

√5ᵗʰ **E74.2** **Disorders of galactose metabolism**

E74.20 **Disorders of galactose metabolism, unspecified**   CC HCC

E74.21 **Galactosemia**   CC HCC
     DEF: Any of three genetic disorders caused by a defective galactose metabolism. Symptoms include failure to thrive in infancy, jaundice, liver and spleen damage, cataracts, and mental retardation.

E74.29 **Other disorders of galactose metabolism**   CC HCC
     Galactokinase deficiency

√5ᵗʰ **E74.3** **Other disorders of intestinal carbohydrate absorption**

     EXCLUDES 2   *lactose intolerance (E73.-)*

E74.31 **Sucrase-isomaltase deficiency**

E74.39 **Other disorders of intestinal carbohydrate absorption**
     Disorder of intestinal carbohydrate absorption NOS
     Glucose-galactose malabsorption
     Sucrase deficiency

E74.4 **Disorders of pyruvate metabolism and gluconeogenesis**   CC HCC
     Deficiency of phosphoenolpyruvate carboxykinase
     Deficiency of pyruvate carboxylase
     Deficiency of pyruvate dehydrogenase

     EXCLUDES 1   *disorders of pyruvate metabolism and gluconeogenesis with anemia (D55.-)*
         Leigh's syndrome (G31.82)

E74.8 **Other specified disorders of carbohydrate metabolism**   CC HCC
     Essential pentosuria
     Renal glycosuria

E74.9 **Disorder of carbohydrate metabolism, unspecified**   HCC

N Newborn: 0   P Pediatric: 0-17   M Maternity: 9-64   A Adult: 15-124   MCC Major Complication/Comorbidity   CC Complication/Comorbidity   SW Severe Wound Dx

534   ICD-10-CM 2020

✓4ᵗʰ **E75 Disorders of sphingolipid metabolism and other lipid storage disorders**

> EXCLUDES 1   *mucolipidosis, types I-III (E77.0-E77.1)*
>   *Refsum's disease (G60.1)*

> **CC Excl:** For CC codes in category E75, unless otherwise noted: PDX collection 537

✓5ᵗʰ **E75.0 GM2 gangliosidosis**

    E75.00   GM2 gangliosidosis, unspecified   `CC` `HCC`

    E75.01   Sandhoff disease   `CC` `HCC`

    E75.02   Tay-Sachs disease   `CC` `HCC`

> **DEF:** Genetic mutation of the HEXA gene that inhibits the breakdown of a toxic substance called ganglioside. The accumulation of ganglioside results in destruction of the neurons in the brain and spinal cord.

Tay-Sachs Disease

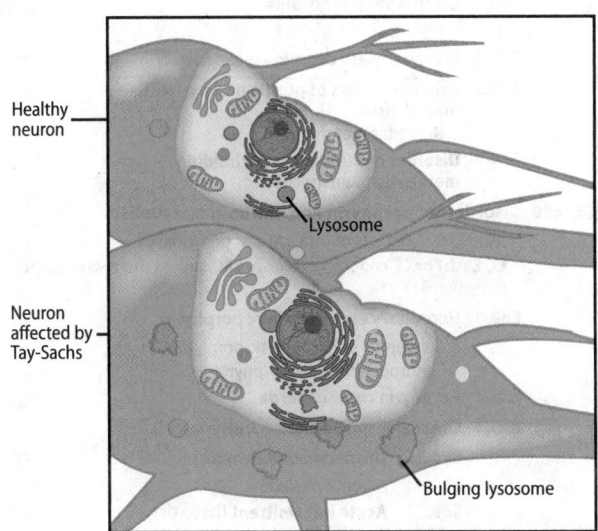

Healthy neuron

Lysosome

Neuron affected by Tay-Sachs

Bulging lysosome

    E75.09   Other GM2 gangliosidosis   `CC` `HCC`

       Adult GM2 gangliosidosis
       Juvenile GM2 gangliosidosis

✓5ᵗʰ **E75.1 Other and unspecified gangliosidosis**

    E75.10   Unspecified gangliosidosis   `CC` `HCC`

       Gangliosidosis NOS

    E75.11   Mucolipidosis IV   `CC` `HCC`

    E75.19   Other gangliosidosis   `CC` `HCC`

       GM1 gangliosidosis
       GM3 gangliosidosis

✓5ᵗʰ **E75.2 Other sphingolipidosis**

> EXCLUDES 1   *adrenoleukodystrophy [Addison-Schilder] (E71.528)*

> **CC Excl:** For CC codes in subcategory E75.2: PDX collection 538

    E75.21   Fabry (-Anderson) disease   `HCC`

    E75.22   Gaucher disease   `HCC`

    E75.23   Krabbe disease   `CC` `HCC`

✓6ᵗʰ   **E75.24   Niemann-Pick disease**

       E75.240   Niemann-Pick disease type A   `HCC`

       E75.241   Niemann-Pick disease type B   `HCC`

       E75.242   Niemann-Pick disease type C   `HCC`

       E75.243   Niemann-Pick disease type D   `HCC`

       E75.248   Other Niemann-Pick disease   `HCC`

       E75.249   Niemann-Pick disease, unspecified   `HCC`

    E75.25   Metachromatic leukodystrophy   `CC` `HCC`

    E75.26   Sulfatase deficiency   `CC` `HCC`

       Multiple sulfatase deficiency (MSD)

       AHA: 2018,4Q,5-6

    E75.29   Other sphingolipidosis   `CC` `HCC`

       Farber's syndrome
       Sulfatide lipidosis

E75.3   Sphingolipidosis, unspecified   `HCC`

E75.4   Neuronal ceroid lipofuscinosis   `CC` `HCC`

       Batten disease
       Bielschowsky-Jansky disease
       Kufs disease
       Spielmeyer-Vogt disease

E75.5   Other lipid storage disorders

       Cerebrotendinous cholesterosis [van Bogaert-Scherer-Epstein]
       Wolman's disease

E75.6   Lipid storage disorder, unspecified

✓4ᵗʰ **E76 Disorders of glycosaminoglycan metabolism**

> **CC Excl:** For CC codes in category E76: PDX collection 539

✓5ᵗʰ **E76.0 Mucopolysaccharidosis, type I**

    E76.01   Hurler's syndrome   `CC` `HCC`

    E76.02   Hurler-Scheie syndrome   `CC` `HCC`

    E76.03   Scheie's syndrome   `CC` `HCC`

E76.1   Mucopolysaccharidosis, type II   `CC` `HCC`

       Hunter's syndrome

✓5ᵗʰ **E76.2 Other mucopolysaccharidoses**

✓6ᵗʰ   **E76.21   Morquio mucopolysaccharidoses**

       E76.210   Morquio A mucopolysaccharidoses   `CC` `HCC`

          Classic Morquio syndrome
          Morquio syndrome A
          Mucopolysaccharidosis, type IVA

       E76.211   Morquio B mucopolysaccharidoses   `CC` `HCC`

          Morquio-like mucopolysaccharidoses
          Morquio-like syndrome
          Morquio syndrome B
          Mucopolysaccharidosis, type IVB

       E76.219   Morquio mucopolysaccharidoses, unspecified   `CC` `HCC`

          Morquio syndrome
          Mucopolysaccharidosis, type IV

    E76.22   Sanfilippo mucopolysaccharidoses   `CC` `HCC`

       Mucopolysaccharidosis, type III (A) (B) (C) (D)
       Sanfilippo A syndrome
       Sanfilippo B syndrome
       Sanfilippo C syndrome
       Sanfilippo D syndrome

    E76.29   Other mucopolysaccharidoses   `CC` `HCC`

       beta-Glucuronidase deficiency
       Maroteaux-Lamy (mild) (severe) syndrome
       Mucopolysaccharidosis, types VI, VII

E76.3   Mucopolysaccharidosis, unspecified   `CC` `HCC`

E76.8   Other disorders of glucosaminoglycan metabolism   `CC` `HCC`

E76.9   Glucosaminoglycan metabolism disorder, unspecified   `CC` `HCC`

✓4ᵗʰ **E77 Disorders of glycoprotein metabolism**

E77.0   Defects in post-translational modification of lysosomal enzymes   `HCC`

       Mucolipidosis II [I-cell disease]
       Mucolipidosis III [pseudo-Hurler polydystrophy]

E77.1   Defects in glycoprotein degradation   `HCC`

       Aspartylglucosaminuria
       Fucosidosis
       Mannosidosis
       Sialidosis [mucolipidosis I]

E77.8   Other disorders of glycoprotein metabolism   `HCC`

E77.9   Disorder of glycoprotein metabolism, unspecified   `HCC`

✓ Additional Character Required   ✓x7ᵗʰ Placeholder   Unacceptable PDx   Questionable PDx   Manifestation   Unspecified Dx   `H1`-`H14` HAC   `HCC` CMS-HCC Dx   `HIV` HIV Dx

ICD-10-CM 2020   535

E78 Disorders of lipoprotein metabolism and other lipidemias
EXCLUDES 1   sphingolipidosis (E75.0-E75.3)

E78.0 Pure hypercholesterolemia
AHA: 2016,4Q,13-14

E78.00 Pure hypercholesterolemia, unspecified
Fredrickson's hyperlipoproteinemia, type IIa
Hyperbetalipoproteinemia
Low-density-lipoprotein-type [LDL] hyperlipoproteinemia
(Pure) hypercholesterolemia NOS

E78.01 Familial hypercholesterolemia

E78.1 Pure hyperglyceridemia
Elevated fasting triglycerides
Endogenous hyperglyceridemia
Fredrickson's hyperlipoproteinemia, type IV
Hyperlipidemia, group B
Hyperprebetalipoproteinemia
Very-low-density-lipoprotein-type [VLDL] hyperlipoproteinemia

E78.2 Mixed hyperlipidemia
Broad- or floating-betalipoproteinemia
Combined hyperlipidemia NOS
Elevated cholesterol with elevated triglycerides NEC
Fredrickson's hyperlipoproteinemia, type IIb or III
Hyperbetalipoproteinemia with prebetalipoproteinemia
Hypercholesteremia with endogenous hyperglyceridemia
Hyperlipidemia, group C
Tubo-eruptive xanthoma
Xanthoma tuberosum
EXCLUDES 1   cerebrotendinous cholesterosis [van Bogaert-Scherer-Epstein] (E75.5)
familial combined hyperlipidemia (E78.49)

E78.3 Hyperchylomicronemia
Chylomicron retention disease
Fredrickson's hyperlipoproteinemia, type I or V
Hyperlipidemia, group D
Mixed hyperglyceridemia

E78.4 Other hyperlipidemia
AHA: 2018,4Q,6

E78.41 Elevated Lipoprotein(a)
Elevated Lp(a)

E78.49 Other hyperlipidemia
Familial combined hyperlipidemia

E78.5 Hyperlipidemia, unspecified

E78.6 Lipoprotein deficiency
Abetalipoproteinemia
Depressed HDL cholesterol
High-density lipoprotein deficiency
Hypoalphalipoproteinemia
Hypobetalipoproteinemia (familial)
Lecithin cholesterol acyltransferase deficiency
Tangier disease

E78.7 Disorders of bile acid and cholesterol metabolism
EXCLUDES 1   Niemann-Pick disease type C (E75.242)

E78.70 Disorder of bile acid and cholesterol metabolism, unspecified

E78.71 Barth syndrome CC
CC Excl: PDX collection 540

E78.72 Smith-Lemli-Opitz syndrome CC
CC Excl: PDX collection 540

E78.79 Other disorders of bile acid and cholesterol metabolism

E78.8 Other disorders of lipoprotein metabolism
E78.81 Lipoid dermatoarthritis
E78.89 Other lipoprotein metabolism disorders

E78.9 Disorder of lipoprotein metabolism, unspecified

E79 Disorders of purine and pyrimidine metabolism
EXCLUDES 1   Ataxia-telangiectasia ►(Q87.19)◄
Bloom's syndrome (Q82.8)
Cockayne's syndrome ►(Q87.19)◄
calculus of kidney (N20.0)
combined immunodeficiency disorders (D81.-)
Fanconi's anemia (D61.09)
gout (M1A.-, M10.-)
orotaciduric anemia (D53.0)
progeria (E34.8)
Werner's syndrome (E34.8)
xeroderma pigmentosum (Q82.1)

CC Excl: For CC codes in category E79: PDX collection 513

E79.0 Hyperuricemia without signs of inflammatory arthritis and tophaceous disease
Asymptomatic hyperuricemia

E79.1 Lesch-Nyhan syndrome CC HCC
HGPRT deficiency

E79.2 Myoadenylate deaminase deficiency CC HCC

E79.8 Other disorders of purine and pyrimidine metabolism CC HCC
Hereditary xanthinuria

E79.9 Disorder of purine and pyrimidine metabolism, unspecified CC HCC

E80 Disorders of porphyrin and bilirubin metabolism
INCLUDES   defects of catalase and peroxidase
CC Excl: For CC codes in category E80, unless otherwise noted: PDX collection 513

E80.0 Hereditary erythropoietic porphyria CC HCC
Congenital erythropoietic porphyria
Erythropoietic protoporphyria

E80.1 Porphyria cutanea tarda CC HCC

E80.2 Other and unspecified porphyria
E80.20 Unspecified porphyria CC HCC
Porphyria NOS

E80.21 Acute intermittent (hepatic) porphyria CC HCC

E80.29 Other porphyria CC HCC
Hereditary coproporphyria

E80.3 Defects of catalase and peroxidase CC HCC
Acatalasia [Takahara]
CC Excl: PDX collection 492

E80.4 Gilbert syndrome

E80.5 Crigler-Najjar syndrome

E80.6 Other disorders of bilirubin metabolism
Dubin-Johnson syndrome
Rotor's syndrome

E80.7 Disorder of bilirubin metabolism, unspecified

E83 Disorders of mineral metabolism
EXCLUDES 1   dietary mineral deficiency (E58-E61)
parathyroid disorders (E20-E21)
vitamin D deficiency (E55.-)

E83.0 Disorders of copper metabolism
E83.00 Disorder of copper metabolism, unspecified
E83.01 Wilson's disease
Code also associated Kayser Fleischer ring (H18.04-)
E83.09 Other disorders of copper metabolism
Menkes' (kinky hair) (steely hair) disease

E83.1 Disorders of iron metabolism
EXCLUDES 1   iron deficiency anemia (D50.-)
sideroblastic anemia (D64.0-D64.3)

E83.10 Disorder of iron metabolism, unspecified

E83.11 Hemochromatosis
EXCLUDES 1   GALD (P78.84)
gestational alloimmune liver disease (P78.84)
neonatal hemochromatosis (P78.84)

E83.110 Hereditary hemochromatosis HCC
Bronzed diabetes
Pigmentary cirrhosis (of liver)
Primary (hereditary) hemochromatosis

E83.111 Hemochromatosis due to repeated red blood cell transfusions `CC`

Iron overload due to repeated red blood cell transfusions

Transfusion (red blood cell) associated hemochromatosis

E83.118 Other hemochromatosis

E83.119 Hemochromatosis, unspecified

E83.19 Other disorders of iron metabolism

Use additional code, if applicable, for idiopathic pulmonary hemosiderosis (J84.03)

E83.2 Disorders of zinc metabolism

Acrodermatitis enteropathica

✓5ᵗʰ **E83.3 Disorders of phosphorus metabolism and phosphatases**

EXCLUDES 1   *adult osteomalacia (M83.-)*

osteoporosis (M80.-)

E83.30 Disorder of phosphorus metabolism, unspecified

E83.31 Familial hypophosphatemia

Vitamin D-resistant osteomalacia

Vitamin D-resistant rickets

EXCLUDES 1   *vitamin D-deficiency rickets (E55.0)*

E83.32 Hereditary vitamin D-dependent rickets (type 1) (type 2)

25-hydroxyvitamin D 1-alpha-hydroxylase deficiency

Pseudovitamin D deficiency

Vitamin D receptor defect

E83.39 Other disorders of phosphorus metabolism `CC`

Acid phosphatase deficiency

Hypophosphatasia

✓5ᵗʰ **E83.4 Disorders of magnesium metabolism**

E83.40 Disorders of magnesium metabolism, unspecified

E83.41 Hypermagnesemia

AHA: 2016,4Q,54

E83.42 Hypomagnesemia

E83.49 Other disorders of magnesium metabolism

✓5ᵗʰ **E83.5 Disorders of calcium metabolism**

EXCLUDES 1   *chondrocalcinosis (M11.1-M11.2)*

hungry bone syndrome (E83.81)

hyperparathyroidism (E21.0-E21.3)

E83.50 Unspecified disorder of calcium metabolism

E83.51 Hypocalcemia `CC`

E83.52 Hypercalcemia

Familial hypocalciuric hypercalcemia

E83.59 Other disorders of calcium metabolism

✓5ᵗʰ **E83.8 Other disorders of mineral metabolism**

E83.81 Hungry bone syndrome

E83.89 Other disorders of mineral metabolism

E83.9 Disorder of mineral metabolism, unspecified

✓4ᵗʰ **E84 Cystic fibrosis**

INCLUDES   mucoviscidosis

Code also exocrine pancreatic insufficiency (K86.81)

DEF: Genetic disorder affecting the respiratory, digestive, and reproductive systems in infants to young adults by disturbing exocrine gland function and causing chronic pulmonary disease with excess mucus production and pancreatic deficiency.

CC Excl: For CC/MC codes in category E84: PDX collection 541

E84.0 Cystic fibrosis with pulmonary manifestations `MCC` `HCC`

Use additional code to identify any infectious organism present, such as:

Pseudomonas (B96.5)

✓5ᵗʰ **E84.1 Cystic fibrosis with intestinal manifestations**

E84.11 Meconium ileus in cystic fibrosis `MCC` `HCC` `N`

EXCLUDES 1   *meconium ileus not due to cystic fibrosis (P76.0)*

E84.19 Cystic fibrosis with other intestinal manifestations `CC` `HCC`

Distal intestinal obstruction syndrome

E84.8 Cystic fibrosis with other manifestations `CC` `HCC`

E84.9 Cystic fibrosis, unspecified `CC` `HCC`

✓4ᵗʰ **E85 Amyloidosis**

EXCLUDES 2   *Alzheimer's disease (G30.0-)*

DEF: Conditions of diverse etiologies characterized by the accumulation of insoluble fibrillar proteins (amyloid) in various organs and tissues of the body, compromising vital functions.

CC Excl: For CC codes in category E85: PDX collection 542

E85.0 Non-neuropathic heredofamilial amyloidosis `CC` `HCC`

Hereditary amyloid nephropathy

Code also associated disorders, such as:

autoinflammatory syndromes (M04.-)

EXCLUDES 2   *transthyretin-related (ATTR) familial amyloid cardiomyopathy (E85.4)*

E85.1 Neuropathic heredofamilial amyloidosis `CC` `HCC`

Amyloid polyneuropathy (Portuguese)

Transthyretin-related (ATTR) familial amyloid polyneuropathy

AHA: 2012,4Q,99

E85.2 Heredofamilial amyloidosis, unspecified `CC` `HCC`

E85.3 Secondary systemic amyloidosis `CC` `HCC`

Hemodialysis-associated amyloidosis

E85.4 Organ-limited amyloidosis `CC` `HCC`

Localized amyloidosis

Transthyretin-related (ATTR) familial amyloid cardiomyopathy

✓5ᵗʰ **E85.8 Other amyloidosis**

AHA: 2017,4Q,7

E85.81 Light chain (AL) amyloidosis `CC` `HCC`

E85.82 Wild-type transthyretin-related (ATTR) amyloidosis `CC` `HCC`

Senile systemic amyloidosis (SSA)

E85.89 Other amyloidosis `CC` `HCC`

E85.9 Amyloidosis, unspecified `CC` `HCC`

✓4ᵗʰ **E86 Volume depletion**

Use additional code(s) for any associated disorders of electrolyte and acid-base balance (E87.-)

EXCLUDES 1   *dehydration of newborn (P74.1)*

hypovolemic shock NOS (R57.1)

postprocedural hypovolemic shock (T81.19)

traumatic hypovolemic shock (T79.4)

AHA: 2019,2Q,7; 2018,2Q,6

E86.0 Dehydration

AHA: 2019,2Q,7; 2019,1Q,12; 2014,1Q,7

TIP: Can be assigned in addition to hypernatremia (E87.0) or hyponatremia (E87.1), when documented.

E86.1 Hypovolemia

Depletion of volume of plasma

E86.9 Volume depletion, unspecified

DEF: Depletion of total body water (dehydration) and/or contraction of total intravascular plasma (hypovolemia).

✓4ᵗʰ **E87 Other disorders of fluid, electrolyte and acid-base balance**

EXCLUDES 1   *diabetes insipidus (E23.2)*

electrolyte imbalance associated with hyperemesis gravidarum (O21.1)

electrolyte imbalance following ectopic or molar pregnancy (O08.5)

familial periodic paralysis (G72.3)

AHA: 2018,2Q,6

CC Excl: For CC codes in category E87: PDX collection 543

E87.0 Hyperosmolality and hypernatremia `CC`

Sodium [Na] excess

Sodium [Na] overload

AHA: 2014,1Q,7

TIP: Assign an additional code for dehydration (E86.0), when documented.

E87.1 Hypo-osmolality and hyponatremia `CC`

Sodium [Na] deficiency

EXCLUDES 1   *syndrome of inappropriate secretion of antidiuretic hormone (E22.2)*

AHA: 2014,1Q,7

TIP: Assign an additional code for dehydration (E86.0), when documented.

Chapter 4. Endocrine, Nutritional and Metabolic Diseases

E83.111–E87.1

✓ Additional Character Required   ✓x7ᵗʰ Placeholder   Unacceptable PDx   Questionable PDx   Manifestation   Unspecified Dx   H1-H14 HAC   HCC CMS-HCC Dx   HIV HIV Dx

ICD-10-CM 2020   537

Chapter 4. Endocrine, Nutritional and Metabolic Diseases

E87.2 Acidosis `CC`
Acidosis NOS
Lactic acidosis
Metabolic acidosis
Respiratory acidosis
EXCLUDES 1 *diabetic acidosis — see categories E08-E10, E13 with ketoacidosis*
DEF: Reduction of alkaline in the blood and tissues caused by an increase in acid and decrease in bicarbonate.

E87.3 Alkalosis `CC`
Alkalosis NOS
Metabolic alkalosis
Respiratory alkalosis

E87.4 Mixed disorder of acid-base balance `CC`

E87.5 Hyperkalemia
Potassium [K] excess
Potassium [K] overload

E87.6 Hypokalemia
Potassium [K] deficiency

E87.7 Fluid overload √5ᵗʰ
EXCLUDES 1 *edema NOS (R60.9)*
fluid retention (R60.9)
E87.70 Fluid overload, unspecified
E87.71 Transfusion associated circulatory overload
Fluid overload due to transfusion (blood) (blood components)
TACO
E87.79 Other fluid overload

E87.8 Other disorders of electrolyte and fluid balance, not elsewhere classified
Electrolyte imbalance NOS
Hyperchloremia
Hypochloremia

E88 Other and unspecified metabolic disorders √4ᵗʰ
Use additional codes for associated conditions
EXCLUDES 1 *histiocytosis X (chronic) (C96.6)*

E88.0 Disorders of plasma-protein metabolism, not elsewhere classified √5ᵗʰ
EXCLUDES 1 *disorder of lipoprotein metabolism (E78.-)*
monoclonal gammopathy (of undetermined significance) (D47.2)
polyclonal hypergammaglobulinemia (D89.0)
Waldenström macroglobulinemia (C88.0)
E88.01 Alpha-1-antitrypsin deficiency `HCC`
AAT deficiency
E88.02 Plasminogen deficiency `CC`
Dysplasminogenemia
Hypoplasminogenemia
Type 1 plasminogen deficiency
Type 2 plasminogen deficiency
Code also, if applicable, ligneous conjunctivitis (H10.51)
Use additional code for associated findings, such as:
hydrocephalus (G91.4)
ligneous conjunctivitis (H10.51)
otitis media (H67.-)
respiratory disorder related to plasminogen deficiency (J99)
AHA: 2018,4Q,6-7
CC Excl: PDX collection 2034
E88.09 Other disorders of plasma-protein metabolism, not elsewhere classified
Bisalbuminemia

E88.1 Lipodystrophy, not elsewhere classified
Lipodystrophy NOS
EXCLUDES 1 *Whipple's disease (K90.81)*

E88.2 Lipomatosis, not elsewhere classified
Lipomatosis NOS
Lipomatosis (Check) dolorosa [Dercum]

E88.3 Tumor lysis syndrome `MCC`
Tumor lysis syndrome (spontaneous)
Tumor lysis syndrome following antineoplastic drug chemotherapy
Use additional code for adverse effect, if applicable, to identify drug (T45.1X5)
AHA: 2019,2Q,24
DEF: Potentially fatal metabolic complication of tumor necrosis caused by spontaneous or treatment-related accumulation of byproducts from dying cancer cells. Symptoms include hyperkalemia, hyperphosphatemia, hypocalcemia, hyperuricemia, and hyperuricosuria.
CC Excl: PDX collection 544

E88.4 Mitochondrial metabolism disorders √5ᵗʰ
EXCLUDES 1 *disorders of pyruvate metabolism (E74.4)*
Kearns-Sayre syndrome (H49.81)
Leber's disease (H47.22)
Leigh's encephalopathy (G31.82)
mitochondrial myopathy, NEC (G71.3)
Reye's syndrome (G93.7)
CC Excl: For CC codes in subcategory E88.4: PDX collection 545
E88.40 Mitochondrial metabolism disorder, unspecified `CC` `HCC`
E88.41 MELAS syndrome `CC` `HCC`
Mitochondrial myopathy, encephalopathy, lactic acidosis and stroke-like episodes
E88.42 MERRF syndrome `CC` `HCC`
Myoclonic epilepsy associated with ragged-red fibers
Code also progressive myoclonic epilepsy (G40.3-)
E88.49 Other mitochondrial metabolism disorders `CC` `HCC`

E88.8 Other specified metabolic disorders √5ᵗʰ
E88.81 Metabolic syndrome
Dysmetabolic syndrome X
Use additional codes for associated manifestations, such as:
obesity (E66.-)
DEF: Group of health risks that increase the likelihood of developing heart disease, stroke, and diabetes. These risks include certain parameters for blood pressure, cholesterol, and glucose levels.
E88.89 Other specified metabolic disorders `HCC`
Launois-Bensaude adenolipomatosis
EXCLUDES 1 *adult pulmonary Langerhans cell histiocytosis (J84.82)*

E88.9 Metabolic disorder, unspecified

Postprocedural endocrine and metabolic complications and disorders, not elsewhere classified (E89)

CC Excl: For CC codes in category E89, unless otherwise noted: PDX collection 546

E89 Postprocedural endocrine and metabolic complications and disorders, not elsewhere classified √4ᵗʰ
EXCLUDES 2 *intraoperative complications of endocrine system organ or structure (E36.0-, E36.1-, E36.8)*

E89.0 Postprocedural hypothyroidism
Postirradiation hypothyroidism
Postsurgical hypothyroidism

E89.1 Postprocedural hypoinsulinemia `CC`
Postpancreatectomy hyperglycemia
Postsurgical hypoinsulinemia
Use additional code, if applicable, to identify:
acquired absence of pancreas (Z90.41-)
diabetes mellitus (postpancreatectomy) (postprocedural) (E13.-)
insulin use (Z79.4)
EXCLUDES 1 *transient postprocedural hyperglycemia (R73.9)*
transient postprocedural hypoglycemia (E16.2)
CC Excl: PDX collection 520

E89.2 Postprocedural hypoparathyroidism `HCC`
Parathyroprival tetany

E89.3 Postprocedural hypopituitarism `HCC`
Postirradiation hypopituitarism

✓5ᵗʰ **E89.4 Postprocedural ovarian failure**

    E89.40 Asymptomatic postprocedural ♀
        ovarian failure
        Postprocedural ovarian failure NOS

    E89.41 Symptomatic postprocedural ♀
        ovarian failure
        Symptoms such as flushing, sleeplessness, headache,
        lack of concentration, associated with
        postprocedural menopause

E89.5 Postprocedural testicular hypofunction ♂

E89.6 Postprocedural adrenocortical (-medullary) `CC` `HCC`
    hypofunction
      CC Excl: PDX collection 526

✓5ᵗʰ **E89.8 Other postprocedural endocrine and metabolic complications**
    and disorders
      AHA: 2016,4Q,9-10

    ✓6ᵗʰ **E89.81 Postprocedural hemorrhage of an endocrine system**
        organ or structure following a procedure

        E89.810 Postprocedural `CC`
            hemorrhage of an
            endocrine system organ
            or structure following an
            endocrine system
            procedure

        E89.811 Postprocedural `CC`
            hemorrhage of an
            endocrine system organ
            or structure following
            other procedure

    ✓6ᵗʰ **E89.82 Postprocedural hematoma and seroma of an**
        endocrine system organ or structure

        E89.820 Postprocedural hematoma `CC`
            of an endocrine system
            organ or structure
            following an endocrine
            system procedure

        E89.821 Postprocedural hematoma `CC`
            of an endocrine system
            organ or structure
            following other procedure

        E89.822 Postprocedural seroma of `CC`
            an endocrine system
            organ or structure
            following an endocrine
            system procedure

        E89.823 Postprocedural seroma of `CC`
            an endocrine system
            organ or structure
            following other procedure

    E89.89 Other postprocedural endocrine and `CC`
        metabolic complications and
        disorders
           Use additional code, if applicable, to further specify
           disorder

Chapter 5. Mental, Behavioral and Neurodevelopmental Disorders (F01–F99)

Chapter-specific Guidelines with Coding Examples

The chapter-specific guidelines from the ICD-10-CM Official Guidelines for Coding and Reporting have been provided below. Along with these guidelines are coding examples, contained in the shaded boxes, that have been developed to help illustrate the coding and/or sequencing guidance found in these guidelines.

a. Pain disorders related to psychological factors

Assign code F45.41, for pain that is exclusively related to psychological disorders. As indicated by the Excludes 1 note under category G89, a code from category G89 should not be assigned with code F45.41.

> Perceived abdominal pain determined to be persistent somatoform pain disorder
>
> **F45.41   Pain disorder exclusively related to psychological factors**
>
> *Explanation*: This pain was diagnosed as being exclusively psychological; therefore, no code from category G89 is added.

Code F45.42, Pain disorders with related psychological factors, should be used with a code from category G89, Pain, not elsewhere classified, if there is documentation of a psychological component for a patient with acute or chronic pain.

See Section I.C.6. Pain

b. Mental and behavioral disorders due to psychoactive substance use

1) In remission

Selection of codes for "in remission" for categories F10-F19, Mental and behavioral disorders due to psychoactive substance use (categories F10-F19 with -11, -.21) requires the provider's clinical judgment. The appropriate codes for "in remission" are assigned only on the basis of provider documentation (as defined in the Official Guidelines for Coding and Reporting), unless otherwise instructed by the classification.

Mild substance use disorders in early or sustained remission are classified to the appropriate codes for substance abuse in remission, and moderate or severe substance use disorders in early or sustained remission are classified to the appropriate codes for substance dependence in remission.

> Insomnia in patient with history of methamphetamine abuse; lab results indicate no current drug use
>
> **G47.00   Insomnia, unspecified**
>
> **F15.10   Other stimulant abuse, uncomplicated**
>
> *Explanation*: Insomnia is a common side-effect of stimulant use, such as methamphetamines. Although lab tests do not indicate that the patient is currently using methamphetamines, there is no specific documentation stating that the stimulant abuse is in remission. "History of" abuse does not equate to "in remission" in this instance.

2) Psychoactive substance use, abuse and dependence

When the provider documentation refers to use, abuse and dependence of the same substance (e.g. alcohol, opioid, cannabis, etc.), only one code should be assigned to identify the pattern of use based on the following hierarchy:

- If both use and abuse are documented, assign only the code for abuse
- If both abuse and dependence are documented, assign only the code for dependence
- If use, abuse and dependence are all documented, assign only the code for dependence
- If both use and dependence are documented, assign only the code for dependence.

> History and physical notes cannabis dependence; progress note says cannabis abuse
>
> **F12.20   Cannabis dependence, uncomplicated**
>
> *Explanation*: In the hierarchy, the dependence code is used if both abuse and dependence are documented.

> Discharge summary says cocaine abuse; progress notes list cocaine use
>
> **F14.10   Cocaine abuse, uncomplicated**
>
> *Explanation*: In the hierarchy, the abuse code is used if both abuse and use are documented.

3) Psychoactive substance use, unspecified

As with all other unspecified diagnoses, the codes for unspecified psychoactive substance use disorders (F10.9-, F11.9-, F12.9-, F13.9-, F14.9-, F15.9-, F16.9-, F18.9-, F19.9-) should only be assigned based on provider documentation and when they meet the definition of a reportable diagnosis (see Section III, Reporting Additional Diagnoses). These codes are to be used only when the psychoactive substance use is associated with a physical, mental or behavioral disorder, and such a relationship is documented by the provider.

c. Factitious disorder

Factitious disorder imposed on self or Munchausen's syndrome is a disorder in which a person falsely reports or causes his or her own physical or psychological signs or symptoms. For patients with documented factitious disorder on self or Munchausen's syndrome, assign the appropriate code from subcategory F68.1-, Factitious disorder imposed on self.

Munchausen's syndrome by proxy (MSBP) is a disorder in which a caregiver (perpetrator) falsely reports or causes an illness or injury in another person (victim) under his or her care, such as a child, an elderly adult, or a person who has a disability. The condition is also referred to as "factitious disorder imposed on another" or "factitious disorder by proxy." The perpetrator, not the victim, receives this diagnosis. Assign code F68.A, Factitious disorder imposed on another, to the perpetrator's record. For the victim of a patient suffering from MSBP, assign the appropriate code from categories T74, Adult and child abuse, neglect and other maltreatment, confirmed, or T76, Adult and child abuse, neglect and other maltreatment, suspected.

See Section I.C.19.f. Adult and child abuse, neglect and other maltreatment

Chapter 5. Mental, Behavioral and Neurodevelopmental Disorders (F01-F99)

INCLUDES   disorders of psychological development

EXCLUDES 2   *symptoms, signs and abnormal clinical laboratory findings, not elsewhere classified (R00-R99)*

This chapter contains the following blocks:

F01-F09   Mental disorders due to known physiological conditions
F10-F19   Mental and behavioral disorders due to psychoactive substance use
F20-F29   Schizophrenia, schizotypal, delusional, and other non-mood psychotic disorders
F30-F39   Mood [affective] disorders
F40-F48   Anxiety, dissociative, stress-related, somatoform and other nonpsychotic mental disorders
F50-F59   Behavioral syndromes associated with physiological disturbances and physical factors
F60-F69   Disorders of adult personality and behavior
F70-F79   Intellectual disabilities
F80-F89   Pervasive and specific developmental disorders
F90-F98   Behavioral and emotional disorders with onset usually occurring in childhood and adolescence
F99   Unspecified mental disorder

Mental disorders due to known physiological conditions (F01-F09)

NOTE   This block comprises a range of mental disorders grouped together on the basis of their having in common a demonstrable etiology in cerebral disease, brain injury, or other insult leading to cerebral dysfunction. The dysfunction may be primary, as in diseases, injuries, and insults that affect the brain directly and selectively; or secondary, as in systemic diseases and disorders that attack the brain only as one of the multiple organs or systems of the body that are involved.

✓4ᵗʰ F01   Vascular dementia

Vascular dementia as a result of infarction of the brain due to vascular disease, including hypertensive cerebrovascular disease.

INCLUDES   arteriosclerotic dementia

Code first the underlying physiological condition or sequelae of cerebrovascular disease.

✓5ᵗʰ F01.5   Vascular dementia

F01.50   Vascular dementia without behavioral disturbance   HCC A

Major neurocognitive disorder without behavioral disturbance

F01.51   Vascular dementia with behavioral disturbance   CC HCC A

Major neurocognitive disorder due to vascular disease, with behavioral disturbance
Major neurocognitive disorder with aggressive behavior
Major neurocognitive disorder with combative behavior
Major neurocognitive disorder with violent behavior
Vascular dementia with aggressive behavior
Vascular dementia with combative behavior
Vascular dementia with violent behavior
Use additional code, if applicable, to identify wandering in vascular dementia (Z91.83)

CC Excl: PDX collection 547

✓4ᵗʰ F02   Dementia in other diseases classified elsewhere

INCLUDES   major neurocognitive disorder in other diseases classified elsewhere

Code first the underlying physiological condition, such as:
Alzheimer's (G30.-)
cerebral lipidosis (E75.4)
Creutzfeldt-Jakob disease (A81.0-)
dementia with Lewy bodies (G31.83)
dementia with Parkinsonism (G31.83)
epilepsy and recurrent seizures (G40.-)
frontotemporal dementia (G31.09)
hepatolenticular degeneration (E83.0)
human immunodeficiency virus [HIV] disease (B20)
Huntington's disease (G10)
hypercalcemia (E83.52)
hypothyroidism, acquired (E00-E03.-)
intoxications (T36-T65)
Jakob-Creutzfeldt disease (A81.0-)
multiple sclerosis (G35)
neurosyphilis (A52.17)
niacin deficiency [pellagra] (E52)
Parkinson's disease (G20)
Pick's disease (G31.01)
polyarteritis nodosa (M30.0)
prion disease (A81.9)
systemic lupus erythematosus (M32.-)
traumatic brain injury (S06.-)
trypanosomiasis (B56.-, B57.-)
vitamin B deficiency (E53.8)

EXCLUDES 2   *dementia in alcohol and psychoactive substance disorders (F10-F19, with .17, .27, .97)*
vascular dementia (F01.5-)

✓5ᵗʰ F02.8   Dementia in other diseases classified elsewhere

AHA: 2017,2Q,7; 2016,4Q,141; 2016,2Q,6

TIP: A code from this subcategory should always be assigned with a code from category G30 when Alzheimer's disease is documented, even in the absence of documented dementia.

F02.80   *Dementia in other diseases classified elsewhere without behavioral disturbance*   HCC

Dementia in other diseases classified elsewhere NOS
Major neurocognitive disorder in other diseases classified elsewhere

F02.81   *Dementia in other diseases classified elsewhere with behavioral disturbance*   CC HCC

Dementia in other diseases classified elsewhere with aggressive behavior
Dementia in other diseases classified elsewhere with combative behavior
Dementia in other diseases classified elsewhere with violent behavior
Major neurocognitive disorder in other diseases classified elsewhere with aggressive behavior
Major neurocognitive disorder in other diseases classified elsewhere with combative behavior
Major neurocognitive disorder in other diseases classified elsewhere with violent behavior
Use additional code, if applicable, to identify wandering in dementia in conditions classified elsewhere (Z91.83)

CC Excl: PDX collection 548

[handwritten: Code G30.8 or G30.]

[handwritten: Always code with G30]

N Newborn: 0   **P** Pediatric: 0-17   **M** Maternity: 9-64   **A** Adult: 15-124   **MCC** Major Complication/Comorbidity   **CC** Complication/Comorbidity   **SW** Severe Wound Dx

542   ICD-10-CM 2020

☑4ᵗʰ **F03　Unspecified dementia**

Presenile dementia NOS
Presenile psychosis NOS
Primary degenerative dementia NOS
Senile dementia NOS
Senile dementia depressed or paranoid type
Senile psychosis NOS

EXCLUDES 1　*senility NOS (R41.81)*

EXCLUDES 2　*mild memory disturbance due to known physiological condition (F06.8)*
　　　　　senile dementia with delirium or acute confusional state (F05)

☑5ᵗʰ **F03.9　Unspecified dementia**

F03.90　Unspecified dementia without behavioral disturbance　HIV HCC A
Dementia NOS
AHA: 2012,4Q,92

F03.91　Unspecified dementia with behavioral disturbance　CC HCC A
Unspecified dementia with aggressive behavior
Unspecified dementia with combative behavior
Unspecified dementia with violent behavior
Use additional code, if applicable, to identify wandering in unspecified dementia (Z91.83)
CC Excl: PDX collection 548

F04　Amnestic disorder due to known physiological condition　HCC

Korsakov's psychosis or syndrome, nonalcoholic
Code first the underlying physiological condition

EXCLUDES 1　*amnesia NOS (R41.3)*
　　　　　anterograde amnesia (R41.1)
　　　　　dissociative amnesia (F44.0)
　　　　　retrograde amnesia (R41.2)

EXCLUDES 2　*alcohol-induced or unspecified Korsakov's syndrome (F10.26, F10.96)*
　　　　　Korsakov's syndrome induced by other psychoactive substances (F13.26, F13.96, F19.16, F19.26, F19.96)

F05　Delirium due to known physiological condition　CC

Acute or subacute brain syndrome
Acute or subacute confusional state (nonalcoholic)
Acute or subacute infective psychosis
Acute or subacute organic reaction
Acute or subacute psycho-organic syndrome
Delirium of mixed etiology
Delirium superimposed on dementia
Sundowning
Code first the underlying physiological condition

EXCLUDES 1　*delirium NOS (R41.0)*

EXCLUDES 2　*delirium tremens alcohol-induced or unspecified (F10.231, F10.921)*

AHA: 2019,2Q,34
CC Excl: PDX collection 549

☑4ᵗʰ **F06　Other mental disorders due to known physiological condition**

INCLUDES　mental disorders due to endocrine disorder
mental disorders due to exogenous hormone
mental disorders due to exogenous toxic substance
mental disorders due to primary cerebral disease
mental disorders due to somatic illness
mental disorders due to systemic disease affecting the brain
Code first the underlying physiological condition

EXCLUDES 1　*unspecified dementia (F03)*

EXCLUDES 2　*delirium due to known physiological condition (F05)*
　　　　　dementia as classified in F01-F02
　　　　　other mental disorders associated with alcohol and other psychoactive substances (F10-F19)

F06.0　Psychotic disorder with hallucinations due to known physiological condition　CC

Organic hallucinatory state (nonalcoholic)

EXCLUDES 2　*hallucinations and perceptual disturbance induced by alcohol and other psychoactive substances (F10-F19 with .151, .251, .951)*
　　　　　schizophrenia (F20.-)

CC Excl: PDX collection 550

F06.1　Catatonic disorder due to known physiological condition

Catatonia associated with another mental disorder
Catatonia NOS

EXCLUDES 1　*catatonic stupor (R40.1)*
　　　　　stupor NOS (R40.1)

EXCLUDES 2　*catatonic schizophrenia (F20.2)*
　　　　　dissociative stupor (F44.2)

DEF: Catatonic: Abnormal neuropsychiatric state characterized by stupor, immobility or purposeless movements, or unresponsiveness in a person who otherwise appears awake.

F06.2　Psychotic disorder with delusions due to known physiological condition　CC

Paranoid and paranoid-hallucinatory organic states
Schizophrenia-like psychosis in epilepsy

EXCLUDES 2　*alcohol and drug-induced psychotic disorder (F10-F19 with .150, .250, .950)*
　　　　　brief psychotic disorder (F23)
　　　　　delusional disorder (F22)
　　　　　schizophrenia (F20.-)

CC Excl: PDX collection 550

☑5ᵗʰ **F06.3　Mood disorder due to known physiological condition**

EXCLUDES 2　*mood disorders due to alcohol and other psychoactive substances (F10-F19 with .14, .24, .94)*
　　　　　mood disorders, not due to known physiological condition or unspecified (F30-F39)

F06.30　Mood disorder due to known physiological condition, unspecified　CC

F06.31　Mood disorder due to known physiological condition with depressive features　CC
Depressive disorder due to known physiological condition, with depressive features

F06.32　Mood disorder due to known physiological condition with major depressive-like episode
Depressive disorder due to known physiological condition, with major depressive-like episode

F06.33　Mood disorder due to known physiological condition with manic features
Bipolar and related disorder due to a known physiological condition, with manic features
Bipolar and related disorder due to known physiological condition, with manic- or hypomanic-like episodes

F06.34　Mood disorder due to known physiological condition with mixed features
Bipolar and related disorder due to known physiological condition, with mixed features
Depressive disorder due to known physiological condition, with mixed features

F06.4　Anxiety disorder due to known physiological condition　CC

EXCLUDES 2　*anxiety disorders due to alcohol and other psychoactive substances (F10-F19 with .180, .280, .980)*
　　　　　anxiety disorders, not due to known physiological condition or unspecified (F40.-, F41.-)

F06.8　Other specified mental disorders due to known physiological condition　HIV

Epileptic psychosis NOS
Obsessive-compulsive and related disorder due to a known physiological condition
Organic dissociative disorder
Organic emotionally labile [asthenic] disorder

Chapter 5. Mental, Behavioral and Neurodevelopmental Disorders

F07–F10.239

√4ᵗʰ **F07** **Personality and behavioral disorders due to known physiological condition**
Code first the underlying physiological condition

F07.0 **Personality change due to known physiological condition**
Frontal lobe syndrome
Limbic epilepsy personality syndrome
Lobotomy syndrome
Organic personality disorder
Organic pseudopsychopathic personality
Organic pseudoretarded personality
Postleucotomy syndrome
Code first underlying physiological condition
EXCLUDES 1   *mild cognitive impairment (G31.84)*
postconcussional syndrome (F07.81)
postencephalitic syndrome (F07.89)
signs and symptoms involving emotional state (R45.-)
EXCLUDES 2   *specific personality disorder (F60.-)*

√5ᵗʰ **F07.8** **Other personality and behavioral disorders due to known physiological condition**

F07.81 **Postconcussional syndrome**   CC
Postcontusional syndrome (encephalopathy)
Post-traumatic brain syndrome, nonpsychotic
Use additional code to identify associated
post-traumatic headache, if applicable (G44.3-)
EXCLUDES 1   *current concussion (brain) (S06.0-)*
postencephalitic syndrome (F07.89)
DEF: Concussion symptoms that persist for weeks or months after a head injury. These symptoms may include headache, giddiness, fatigue, insomnia, mood fluctuation, and a subjective feeling of impaired intellectual function with extreme reaction to normal stressors.

F07.89 **Other personality and behavioral disorders due to known physiological condition**
Postencephalitic syndrome
Right hemispheric organic affective disorder

F07.9 **Unspecified personality and behavioral disorder due to known physiological condition**   HIV
Organic psychosyndrome

F09 **Unspecified mental disorder due to known physiological condition**   HIV CC
Mental disorder NOS due to known physiological condition
Organic brain syndrome NOS
Organic mental disorder NOS
Organic psychosis NOS
Symptomatic psychosis NOS
Code first the underlying physiological condition
EXCLUDES 1   *psychosis NOS (F29)*

Mental and behavioral disorders due to psychoactive substance use (F10-F19)

AHA: 2018,4Q,69-70; 2017,4Q,8; 2017,2Q,27
CC Excl: For CC codes in categories F10-F19, unless otherwise noted: PDX collection 550

√4ᵗʰ **F10** **Alcohol related disorders**
Use additional code for blood alcohol level, if applicable (Y90.-)

√5ᵗʰ **F10.1** **Alcohol abuse**
EXCLUDES 1   *alcohol dependence (F10.2-)*
alcohol use, unspecified (F10.9-)
AHA: 2018,1Q,16; 2015,2Q,15
TIP: Alcohol withdrawal is classified to dependence only (F10.23-); there is no combination code for alcohol abuse with withdrawal. When alcohol abuse and alcohol withdrawal are documented for the same encounter, query the provider for clarification.
TIP: Assign when documentation indicates alcohol withdrawal without dependence; do not assign an additional code for withdrawal.

F10.10 **Alcohol abuse, uncomplicated**
Alcohol use disorder, mild

F10.11 **Alcohol abuse, in remission**
Alcohol use disorder, mild, in early remission
Alcohol use disorder, mild, in sustained remission

√6ᵗʰ **F10.12** **Alcohol abuse with intoxication**

F10.120 **Alcohol abuse with intoxication, uncomplicated**   HCC

F10.121 **Alcohol abuse with intoxication delirium**   CC HCC

F10.129 **Alcohol abuse with intoxication, unspecified**   HCC

F10.14 **Alcohol abuse with alcohol-induced mood disorder**   CC HCC
Alcohol use disorder, mild, with alcohol-induced bipolar or related disorder
Alcohol use disorder, mild, with alcohol-induced depressive disorder

√6ᵗʰ **F10.15** **Alcohol abuse with alcohol-induced psychotic disorder**

F10.150 **Alcohol abuse with alcohol-induced psychotic disorder with delusions**   HCC

F10.151 **Alcohol abuse with alcohol-induced psychotic disorder with hallucinations**   CC HCC
DEF: Psychosis lasting less than six months with slight or no clouding of consciousness in which auditory hallucinations predominate.

F10.159 **Alcohol abuse with alcohol-induced psychotic disorder, unspecified**   CC HCC

√6ᵗʰ **F10.18** **Alcohol abuse with other alcohol-induced disorders**

F10.180 **Alcohol abuse with alcohol-induced anxiety disorder**   CC HCC

F10.181 **Alcohol abuse with alcohol-induced sexual dysfunction**   CC HCC

F10.182 **Alcohol abuse with alcohol-induced sleep disorder**   HCC

F10.188 **Alcohol abuse with other alcohol-induced disorder**   CC HCC

F10.19 **Alcohol abuse with unspecified alcohol-induced disorder**   HCC

√5ᵗʰ **F10.2** **Alcohol dependence**
EXCLUDES 1   *alcohol abuse (F10.1-)*
alcohol use, unspecified (F10.9-)
EXCLUDES 2   *toxic effect of alcohol (T51.0-)*

F10.20 **Alcohol dependence, uncomplicated**   HCC
Alcohol use disorder, moderate
Alcohol use disorder, severe

F10.21 **Alcohol dependence, in remission**   HCC
Alcohol use disorder, moderate, in early remission
Alcohol use disorder, moderate, in sustained remission
Alcohol use disorder, severe, in early remission
Alcohol use disorder, severe, in sustained remission

√6ᵗʰ **F10.22** **Alcohol dependence with intoxication**
Acute drunkenness (in alcoholism)
EXCLUDES 2   *alcohol dependence with withdrawal (F10.23-)*

F10.220 **Alcohol dependence with intoxication, uncomplicated**   HCC

F10.221 **Alcohol dependence with intoxication delirium**   CC HCC

F10.229 **Alcohol dependence with intoxication, unspecified**   HCC

√6ᵗʰ **F10.23** **Alcohol dependence with withdrawal**
EXCLUDES 2   *alcohol dependence with intoxication (F10.22-)*
AHA: 2018,1Q,16; 2015,2Q,15
TIP: Do not assign a code from this subcategory when documentation indicates alcohol withdrawal without dependence.

F10.230 **Alcohol dependence with withdrawal, uncomplicated**   CC HCC

F10.231 **Alcohol dependence with withdrawal delirium**   CC HCC

F10.232 **Alcohol dependence with withdrawal with perceptual disturbance**   CC HCC

F10.239 **Alcohol dependence with withdrawal, unspecified**   CC HCC

F10.24 Alcohol dependence with alcohol-induced mood disorder `CC` `HCC`
Alcohol use disorder, moderate, with alcohol-induced bipolar or related disorder
Alcohol use disorder, moderate, with alcohol-induced depressive disorder
Alcohol use disorder, severe, with alcohol-induced bipolar or related disorder
Alcohol use disorder, severe, with alcohol-induced depressive disorder

√6th **F10.25 Alcohol dependence with alcohol-induced psychotic disorder**
  F10.250 Alcohol dependence with alcohol-induced psychotic disorder with delusions `HCC`
  F10.251 Alcohol dependence with alcohol-induced psychotic disorder with hallucinations `CC` `HCC`
  F10.259 Alcohol dependence with alcohol-induced psychotic disorder, unspecified `CC` `HCC`

F10.26 Alcohol dependence with alcohol-induced persisting amnestic disorder `HCC`
Alcohol use disorder, moderate, with alcohol-induced major neurocognitive disorder, amnestic-confabulatory type
Alcohol use disorder, severe, with alcohol-induced major neurocognitive disorder, amnestic-confabulatory type
DEF: Prominent and lasting reduced memory span and disordered time appreciation and confabulation that occurs in alcoholics as sequel to acute alcoholic psychosis.

F10.27 Alcohol dependence with alcohol-induced persisting dementia `CC` `HCC`
Alcohol use disorder, moderate, with alcohol-induced major neurocognitive disorder, nonamnestic-confabulatory type
Alcohol use disorder, severe, with alcohol-induced major neurocognitive disorder, nonamnestic-confabulatory type

√6th **F10.28 Alcohol dependence with other alcohol-induced disorders**
  F10.280 Alcohol dependence with alcohol-induced anxiety disorder `CC` `HCC`
  F10.281 Alcohol dependence with alcohol-induced sexual dysfunction `CC` `HCC`
  F10.282 Alcohol dependence with alcohol-induced sleep disorder `HCC`
  F10.288 Alcohol dependence with other alcohol-induced disorder `CC` `HCC`
    Alcohol use disorder, moderate, with alcohol-induced mild neurocognitive disorder
    Alcohol use disorder, severe, with alcohol-induced mild neurocognitive disorder

F10.29 Alcohol dependence with unspecified alcohol-induced disorder `CC` `HCC`

√5th **F10.9 Alcohol use, unspecified**
  EXCLUDES 1   alcohol abuse (F10.1-)
         alcohol dependence (F10.2-)
  AHA: 2018,2Q,10-11
  TIP: Assign a substance use code only when the provider documents a relationship between the use and an associated physical, mental, or behavioral disorder. As with all diagnoses, substance use codes must meet the definition of a reportable diagnosis.
√6th **F10.92 Alcohol use, unspecified with intoxication**
  F10.920 Alcohol use, unspecified with intoxication, uncomplicated `HCC`
    AHA: 2018,2Q,10-11
  F10.921 Alcohol use, unspecified with intoxication delirium `CC` `HCC`

F10.929 Alcohol use, unspecified with intoxication, unspecified `HCC`

F10.94 Alcohol use, unspecified with alcohol-induced mood disorder `CC` `HCC`
Alcohol induced bipolar or related disorder, without use disorder
Alcohol induced depressive disorder, without use disorder

√6th **F10.95 Alcohol use, unspecified with alcohol-induced psychotic disorder**
  F10.950 Alcohol use, unspecified with alcohol-induced psychotic disorder with delusions `HCC`
  F10.951 Alcohol use, unspecified with alcohol-induced psychotic disorder with hallucinations `CC` `HCC`
  F10.959 Alcohol use, unspecified with alcohol-induced psychotic disorder, unspecified `CC` `HCC`
    Alcohol-induced psychotic disorder without use disorder

F10.96 Alcohol use, unspecified with alcohol-induced persisting amnestic disorder `HCC`
Alcohol-induced major neurocognitive disorder, amnestic-confabulatory type, without use disorder

F10.97 Alcohol use, unspecified with alcohol-induced persisting dementia `HCC`
Alcohol-induced major neurocognitive disorder, nonamnestic-confabulatory type, without use disorder

√6th **F10.98 Alcohol use, unspecified with other alcohol-induced disorders**
  F10.980 Alcohol use, unspecified with alcohol-induced anxiety disorder `CC` `HCC`
    Alcohol induced anxiety disorder, without use disorder
  F10.981 Alcohol use, unspecified with alcohol-induced sexual dysfunction `CC` `HCC`
    Alcohol induced sexual dysfunction, without use disorder
  F10.982 Alcohol use, unspecified with alcohol-induced sleep disorder `HCC`
    Alcohol induced sleep disorder, without use disorder
  F10.988 Alcohol use, unspecified with other alcohol-induced disorder `CC` `HCC`
    Alcohol induced mild neurocognitive disorder, without use disorder

F10.99 Alcohol use, unspecified with unspecified alcohol-induced disorder `HCC`

√4th **F11 Opioid related disorders**
√5th **F11.1 Opioid abuse**
  EXCLUDES 1   opioid dependence (F11.2-)
         opioid use, unspecified (F11.9-)
  F11.10 Opioid abuse, uncomplicated `HCC`
    Opioid use disorder, mild
  F11.11 Opioid abuse, in remission `HCC`
    Opioid use disorder, mild, in early remission
    Opioid use disorder, mild, in sustained remission
√6th **F11.12 Opioid abuse with intoxication**
  F11.120 Opioid abuse with intoxication, uncomplicated `HCC`
  F11.121 Opioid abuse with intoxication delirium `CC` `HCC`
  F11.122 Opioid abuse with intoxication with perceptual disturbance `HCC`
  F11.129 Opioid abuse with intoxication, unspecified `HCC`

Chapter 5. Mental, Behavioral and Neurodevelopmental Disorders

F11.14 **Opioid abuse with opioid-induced mood disorder** HCC
     Opioid use disorder, mild, with opioid-induced depressive disorder

√6th **F11.15** **Opioid abuse with opioid-induced psychotic disorder**
     F11.150 **Opioid abuse with opioid-induced psychotic disorder with delusions** CC HCC
     F11.151 **Opioid abuse with opioid-induced psychotic disorder with hallucinations** CC HCC
     F11.159 **Opioid abuse with opioid-induced psychotic disorder, unspecified** HCC

√6th **F11.18** **Opioid abuse with other opioid-induced disorder**
     F11.181 **Opioid abuse with opioid-induced sexual dysfunction** HCC
     F11.182 **Opioid abuse with opioid-induced sleep disorder** HCC
     F11.188 **Opioid abuse with other opioid-induced disorder** HCC

F11.19 **Opioid abuse with unspecified opioid-induced disorder** HCC

√5th **F11.2** **Opioid dependence**
     EXCLUDES 1   opioid abuse (F11.1-)
             opioid use, unspecified (F11.9-)
     EXCLUDES 2   opioid poisoning (T40.0-T40.2-)

F11.20 **Opioid dependence, uncomplicated** CC HCC
     Opioid use disorder, moderate
     Opioid use disorder, severe
     CC Excl: No Excl

F11.21 **Opioid dependence, in remission** HCC
     Opioid use disorder, moderate, in early remission
     Opioid use disorder, moderate, in sustained remission
     Opioid use disorder, severe, in early remission
     Opioid use disorder, severe, in sustained remission

√6th **F11.22** **Opioid dependence with intoxication**
     EXCLUDES 1   opioid dependence with withdrawal (F11.23)
     F11.220 **Opioid dependence with intoxication, uncomplicated** HCC
     F11.221 **Opioid dependence with intoxication delirium** CC HCC
     F11.222 **Opioid dependence with intoxication with perceptual disturbance** CC HCC
          CC Excl: No Excl
     F11.229 **Opioid dependence with intoxication, unspecified** HCC

F11.23 **Opioid dependence with withdrawal** CC HCC
     EXCLUDES 1   opioid dependence with intoxication (F11.22-)

F11.24 **Opioid dependence with opioid-induced mood disorder** HCC
     Opioid use disorder, moderate, with opioid induced depressive disorder

√6th **F11.25** **Opioid dependence with opioid-induced psychotic disorder**
     F11.250 **Opioid dependence with opioid-induced psychotic disorder with delusions** CC HCC
     F11.251 **Opioid dependence with opioid-induced psychotic disorder with hallucinations** CC HCC
     F11.259 **Opioid dependence with opioid-induced psychotic disorder, unspecified** CC HCC
          CC Excl: No Excl

√6th **F11.28** **Opioid dependence with other opioid-induced disorder**
     F11.281 **Opioid dependence with opioid-induced sexual dysfunction** CC HCC
          CC Excl: No Excl

F11.282 **Opioid dependence with opioid-induced sleep disorder** CC HCC
     CC Excl: No Excl

F11.288 **Opioid dependence with other opioid-induced disorder** CC HCC
     CC Excl: No Excl

F11.29 **Opioid dependence with unspecified opioid-induced disorder** HCC

√5th **F11.9** **Opioid use, unspecified**
     EXCLUDES 1   opioid abuse (F11.1-)
             opioid dependence (F11.2-)
     TIP: Assign a substance use code only when the provider documents a relationship between the use and an associated physical, mental, or behavioral disorder. As with all diagnoses, substance use codes must meet the definition of a reportable diagnosis.

F11.90 **Opioid use, unspecified, uncomplicated**
     AHA: 2018,2Q,10-11

√6th **F11.92** **Opioid use, unspecified with intoxication**
     EXCLUDES 1   opioid use, unspecified with withdrawal (F11.93)
     F11.920 **Opioid use, unspecified with intoxication, uncomplicated** HCC
     F11.921 **Opioid use, unspecified with intoxication delirium** CC HCC
          Opioid-induced delirium
     F11.922 **Opioid use, unspecified with intoxication with perceptual disturbance** HCC
     F11.929 **Opioid use, unspecified with intoxication, unspecified** HCC

F11.93 **Opioid use, unspecified with withdrawal** CC HCC
     EXCLUDES 1   opioid use, unspecified with intoxication (F11.92-)

F11.94 **Opioid use, unspecified with opioid-induced mood disorder** HCC
     Opioid induced depressive disorder, without use disorder

√6th **F11.95** **Opioid use, unspecified with opioid-induced psychotic disorder**
     F11.950 **Opioid use, unspecified with opioid-induced psychotic disorder with delusions** CC HCC
     F11.951 **Opioid use, unspecified with opioid-induced psychotic disorder with hallucinations** CC HCC
     F11.959 **Opioid use, unspecified with opioid-induced psychotic disorder, unspecified** HCC

√6th **F11.98** **Opioid use, unspecified with other specified opioid-induced disorder**
     F11.981 **Opioid use, unspecified with opioid-induced sexual dysfunction** HCC
          Opioid induced sexual dysfunction, without use disorder
     F11.982 **Opioid use, unspecified with opioid-induced sleep disorder** HCC
          Opioid induced sleep disorder, without use disorder
     F11.988 **Opioid use, unspecified with other opioid-induced disorder** HCC
          Opioid induced anxiety disorder, without use disorder

F11.99 **Opioid use, unspecified with unspecified opioid-induced disorder** HCC

√4ᵗʰ **F12**   **Cannabis related disorders**

> **INCLUDES**   marijuana

√5ᵗʰ **F12.1**   **Cannabis abuse**

> **EXCLUDES 1**   *cannabis dependence (F12.2-)*
> *cannabis use, unspecified (F12.9-)*

     F12.10   **Cannabis abuse, uncomplicated**
         Cannabis use disorder, mild

     F12.11   **Cannabis abuse, in remission**
         Cannabis use disorder, mild, in early remission
         Cannabis use disorder, mild, in sustained remission

√6ᵗʰ **F12.12**   **Cannabis abuse with intoxication**

         F12.120   **Cannabis abuse with intoxication, uncomplicated**   `HCC`

         F12.121   **Cannabis abuse with intoxication delirium**   `CC` `HCC`

         F12.122   **Cannabis abuse with intoxication with perceptual disturbance**   `HCC`

         F12.129   **Cannabis abuse with intoxication, unspecified**   `HCC`

√6ᵗʰ **F12.15**   **Cannabis abuse with psychotic disorder**

         F12.150   **Cannabis abuse with psychotic disorder with delusions**   `CC` `HCC`

         F12.151   **Cannabis abuse with psychotic disorder with hallucinations**   `CC` `HCC`

         F12.159   **Cannabis abuse with psychotic disorder, unspecified**   `HCC`

√6ᵗʰ **F12.18**   **Cannabis abuse with other cannabis-induced disorder**

         F12.180   **Cannabis abuse with cannabis-induced anxiety disorder**   `HCC`

         F12.188   **Cannabis abuse with other cannabis-induced disorder**   `HCC`
            Cannabis use disorder, mild, with cannabis-induced sleep disorder

     F12.19   **Cannabis abuse with unspecified cannabis-induced disorder**   `HCC`

√5ᵗʰ **F12.2**   **Cannabis dependence**

> **EXCLUDES 1**   *cannabis abuse (F12.1-)*
> *cannabis use, unspecified (F12.9-)*
> **EXCLUDES 2**   *cannabis poisoning (T40.7-)*

     F12.20   **Cannabis dependence, uncomplicated**   `HCC`
         Cannabis use disorder, moderate
         Cannabis use disorder, severe

     F12.21   **Cannabis dependence, in remission**   `HCC`
         Cannabis use disorder, moderate, in early remission
         Cannabis use disorder, moderate, in sustained remission
         Cannabis use disorder, severe, in early remission
         Cannabis use disorder, severe, in sustained remission

√6ᵗʰ **F12.22**   **Cannabis dependence with intoxication**

         F12.220   **Cannabis dependence with intoxication, uncomplicated**   `HCC`

         F12.221   **Cannabis dependence with intoxication delirium**   `CC` `HCC`

         F12.222   **Cannabis dependence with intoxication with perceptual disturbance**   `HCC`

         F12.229   **Cannabis dependence with intoxication, unspecified**   `HCC`

     F12.23   **Cannabis dependence with withdrawal**   `HCC`
         AHA: 2018,4Q,7

√6ᵗʰ **F12.25**   **Cannabis dependence with psychotic disorder**

         F12.250   **Cannabis dependence with psychotic disorder with delusions**   `CC` `HCC`

         F12.251   **Cannabis dependence with psychotic disorder with hallucinations**   `CC` `HCC`

         F12.259   **Cannabis dependence with psychotic disorder, unspecified**   `HCC`

√6ᵗʰ **F12.28**   **Cannabis dependence with other cannabis-induced disorder**

         F12.280   **Cannabis dependence with cannabis-induced anxiety disorder**   `HCC`

         F12.288   **Cannabis dependence with other cannabis-induced disorder**   `HCC`
            Cannabis use disorder, moderate, with cannabis-induced sleep disorder
            Cannabis use disorder, severe, with cannabis-induced sleep disorder

     F12.29   **Cannabis dependence with unspecified cannabis-induced disorder**   `HCC`

√5ᵗʰ **F12.9**   **Cannabis use, unspecified**

> **EXCLUDES 1**   *cannabis abuse (F12.1-)*
> *cannabis dependence (F12.2-)*

> **TIP:** Assign a substance use code only when the provider documents a relationship between the use and an associated physical, mental, or behavioral disorder. As with all diagnoses, substance use codes must meet the definition of a reportable diagnosis.

     F12.90   **Cannabis use, unspecified, uncomplicated**
         AHA: 2018,2Q,10-11

√6ᵗʰ **F12.92**   **Cannabis use, unspecified with intoxication**

         F12.920   **Cannabis use, unspecified, with intoxication, uncomplicated**   `HCC`

         F12.921   **Cannabis use, unspecified with intoxication delirium**   `CC` `HCC`

         F12.922   **Cannabis use, unspecified with intoxication with perceptual disturbance**   `HCC`

         F12.929   **Cannabis use, unspecified with intoxication, unspecified**   `HCC`

     F12.93   **Cannabis use, unspecified with withdrawal**   `HCC`
         AHA: 2018,4Q,7

√6ᵗʰ **F12.95**   **Cannabis use, unspecified with psychotic disorder**

         F12.950   **Cannabis use, unspecified with psychotic disorder with delusions**   `CC` `HCC`

         F12.951   **Cannabis use, unspecified with psychotic disorder with hallucinations**   `CC` `HCC`

         F12.959   **Cannabis use, unspecified with psychotic disorder, unspecified**   `HCC`
            Cannabis induced psychotic disorder, without use disorder

√6ᵗʰ **F12.98**   **Cannabis use, unspecified with other cannabis-induced disorder**

         F12.980   **Cannabis use, unspecified with anxiety disorder**   `HCC`
            Cannabis induced anxiety disorder, without use disorder

         F12.988   **Cannabis use, unspecified with other cannabis-induced disorder**   `HCC`
            Cannabis induced sleep disorder, without use disorder

     F12.99   **Cannabis use, unspecified with unspecified cannabis-induced disorder**   `HCC`

√4ᵗʰ **F13**   **Sedative, hypnotic, or anxiolytic related disorders**

√5ᵗʰ **F13.1**   **Sedative, hypnotic or anxiolytic-related abuse**

> **EXCLUDES 1**   *sedative, hypnotic or anxiolytic-related dependence (F13.2-)*
> *sedative, hypnotic, or anxiolytic use, unspecified (F13.9-)*

     F13.10   **Sedative, hypnotic or anxiolytic abuse, uncomplicated**   `HCC`
         Sedative, hypnotic, or anxiolytic use disorder, mild

F13.11 Sedative, hypnotic or anxiolytic **abuse, in remission** `HCC`
- Sedative, hypnotic or anxiolytic use disorder, mild, in early remission
- Sedative, hypnotic or anxiolytic use disorder, mild, in sustained remission

√6ᵗʰ **F13.12** Sedative, hypnotic or anxiolytic abuse with intoxication
- **F13.120** Sedative, hypnotic or anxiolytic abuse with intoxication, uncomplicated `HCC`
- **F13.121** Sedative, hypnotic or anxiolytic abuse with intoxication delirium `CC` `HCC`
- **F13.129** Sedative, hypnotic or anxiolytic abuse with intoxication, unspecified `HCC`

F13.14 Sedative, hypnotic or anxiolytic abuse with sedative, hypnotic or anxiolytic-induced mood disorder `HCC`
- Sedative, hypnotic, or anxiolytic use disorder, mild, with sedative, hypnotic, or anxiolytic-induced bipolar or related disorder
- Sedative, hypnotic, or anxiolytic use disorder, mild, with sedative, hypnotic, or anxiolytic-induced depressive disorder

√6ᵗʰ **F13.15** Sedative, hypnotic or anxiolytic abuse with sedative, hypnotic or anxiolytic-induced psychotic disorder
- **F13.150** Sedative, hypnotic or anxiolytic abuse with sedative, hypnotic or anxiolytic-induced psychotic disorder with delusions `CC` `HCC`
- **F13.151** Sedative, hypnotic or anxiolytic abuse with sedative, hypnotic or anxiolytic-induced psychotic disorder with hallucinations `CC` `HCC`
- **F13.159** Sedative, hypnotic or anxiolytic abuse with sedative, hypnotic or anxiolytic-induced psychotic disorder, unspecified `HCC`

√6ᵗʰ **F13.18** Sedative, hypnotic or anxiolytic abuse with other sedative, hypnotic or anxiolytic-induced disorders
- **F13.180** Sedative, hypnotic or anxiolytic abuse with sedative, hypnotic or anxiolytic-induced anxiety disorder `HCC`
- **F13.181** Sedative, hypnotic or anxiolytic abuse with sedative, hypnotic or anxiolytic-induced sexual dysfunction `HCC`
- **F13.182** Sedative, hypnotic or anxiolytic abuse with sedative, hypnotic or anxiolytic-induced sleep disorder `HCC`
- **F13.188** Sedative, hypnotic or anxiolytic abuse with other sedative, hypnotic or anxiolytic-induced disorder `HCC`

F13.19 Sedative, hypnotic or anxiolytic abuse with unspecified sedative, hypnotic or anxiolytic-induced disorder `HCC`

√5ᵗʰ **F13.2** Sedative, hypnotic or anxiolytic-related dependence
- **EXCLUDES 1**   sedative, hypnotic or anxiolytic-related abuse (F13.1-)
  - sedative, hypnotic, or anxiolytic use, unspecified (F13.9-)
- **EXCLUDES 2**   sedative, hypnotic, or anxiolytic poisoning (T42.-)

F13.20 Sedative, hypnotic or anxiolytic dependence, uncomplicated `CC` `HCC`
- **CC Excl:** No Excl

F13.21 Sedative, hypnotic or anxiolytic dependence, in remission `HCC`
- Sedative, hypnotic or anxiolytic use disorder, moderate, in early remission
- Sedative, hypnotic or anxiolytic use disorder, moderate, in sustained remission
- Sedative, hypnotic or anxiolytic use disorder, severe, in early remission
- Sedative, hypnotic or anxiolytic use disorder, severe, in sustained remission

√6ᵗʰ **F13.22** Sedative, hypnotic or anxiolytic dependence with intoxication
- **EXCLUDES 1**   sedative, hypnotic or anxiolytic dependence with withdrawal (F13.23-)
- **F13.220** Sedative, hypnotic or anxiolytic dependence with intoxication, uncomplicated `HCC`
- **F13.221** Sedative, hypnotic or anxiolytic dependence with intoxication delirium `CC` `HCC`
- **F13.229** Sedative, hypnotic or anxiolytic dependence with intoxication, unspecified `HCC`

√6ᵗʰ **F13.23** Sedative, hypnotic or anxiolytic dependence with withdrawal
- Sedative, hypnotic, or anxiolytic use disorder, moderate
- Sedative, hypnotic, or anxiolytic use disorder, severe
- **EXCLUDES 1**   sedative, hypnotic or anxiolytic dependence with intoxication (F13.22-)
- **F13.230** Sedative, hypnotic or anxiolytic dependence with withdrawal, uncomplicated `CC` `HCC`
- **F13.231** Sedative, hypnotic or anxiolytic dependence with withdrawal delirium `CC` `HCC`
- **F13.232** Sedative, hypnotic or anxiolytic dependence with withdrawal with perceptual disturbance `CC` `HCC`
  - Sedative, hypnotic, or anxiolytic withdrawal with perceptual disturbances
- **F13.239** Sedative, hypnotic or anxiolytic dependence with withdrawal, unspecified `CC` `HCC`
  - Sedative, hypnotic, or anxiolytic withdrawal without perceptual disturbances

F13.24 Sedative, hypnotic or anxiolytic dependence with sedative, hypnotic or anxiolytic-induced mood disorder `HCC`
- Sedative, hypnotic, or anxiolytic use disorder, moderate, with sedative, hypnotic, or anxiolytic-induced bipolar or related disorder
- Sedative, hypnotic, or anxiolytic use disorder, moderate, with sedative, hypnotic, or anxiolytic-induced depressive disorder
- Sedative, hypnotic, or anxiolytic use disorder, severe, with sedative, hypnotic, or anxiolytic-induced bipolar or related disorder
- Sedative, hypnotic, or anxiolytic use disorder, severe, with sedative, hypnotic, or anxiolytic-induced depressive disorder

√6ᵗʰ **F13.25** Sedative, hypnotic or anxiolytic dependence with sedative, hypnotic or anxiolytic-induced psychotic disorder
- **F13.250** Sedative, hypnotic or anxiolytic dependence with sedative, hypnotic or anxiolytic-induced psychotic disorder with delusions `CC` `HCC`

N Newborn: 0   P Pediatric: 0-17   M Maternity: 9-64   A Adult: 15-124   MCC Major Complication/Comorbidity   CC Complication/Comorbidity   SW Severe Wound Dx

548   ICD-10-CM 2020

F13.251 Sedative, hypnotic or anxiolytic dependence with sedative, hypnotic or anxiolytic-induced psychotic disorder with hallucinations　CC HCC

F13.259 Sedative, hypnotic or anxiolytic dependence with sedative, hypnotic or anxiolytic-induced psychotic disorder, unspecified　CC HCC
CC Excl: No Excl

F13.26 Sedative, hypnotic or anxiolytic dependence with sedative, hypnotic or anxiolytic-induced persisting amnestic disorder　CC HCC
CC Excl: No Excl

F13.27 Sedative, hypnotic or anxiolytic dependence with sedative, hypnotic or anxiolytic-induced persisting dementia　CC HCC
Sedative, hypnotic, or anxiolytic use disorder, moderate, with sedative, hypnotic, or anxiolytic induced major neurocognitive disorder
Sedative, hypnotic, or anxiolytic use disorder, severe, with sedative, hypnotic, or anxiolytic-induced major neurocognitive disorder

√6ᵗʰ **F13.28** Sedative, hypnotic or anxiolytic dependence with other sedative, hypnotic or anxiolytic-induced disorders

F13.280 Sedative, hypnotic or anxiolytic dependence with sedative, hypnotic or anxiolytic-induced anxiety disorder　CC HCC
CC Excl: No Excl

F13.281 Sedative, hypnotic or anxiolytic dependence with sedative, hypnotic or anxiolytic-induced sexual dysfunction　CC HCC
CC Excl: No Excl

F13.282 Sedative, hypnotic or anxiolytic dependence with sedative, hypnotic or anxiolytic-induced sleep disorder　CC HCC
CC Excl: No Excl

F13.288 Sedative, hypnotic or anxiolytic dependence with other sedative, hypnotic or anxiolytic-induced disorder　CC HCC
Sedative, hypnotic, or anxiolytic use disorder, moderate, with sedative, hypnotic, or anxiolytic-induced mild neurocognitive disorder
Sedative, hypnotic, or anxiolytic use disorder, severe, with sedative, hypnotic, or anxiolytic-induced mild neurocognitive disorder
CC Excl: No Excl

F13.29 Sedative, hypnotic or anxiolytic dependence with unspecified sedative, hypnotic or anxiolytic-induced disorder　HCC

√5ᵗʰ **F13.9** Sedative, hypnotic or anxiolytic-related use, unspecified
EXCLUDES 1　sedative, hypnotic or anxiolytic-related abuse (F13.1-)
sedative, hypnotic or anxiolytic-related dependence (F13.2-)
TIP: Assign a substance use code only when the provider documents a relationship between the use and an associated physical, mental, or behavioral disorder. As with all diagnoses, substance use codes must meet the definition of a reportable diagnosis.

F13.90 Sedative, hypnotic, or anxiolytic use, unspecified, uncomplicated
AHA: 2018,2Q,10-11

√6ᵗʰ **F13.92** Sedative, hypnotic or anxiolytic use, unspecified with intoxication
EXCLUDES 1　sedative, hypnotic or anxiolytic use, unspecified with withdrawal (F13.93-)

F13.920 Sedative, hypnotic or anxiolytic use, unspecified with intoxication, uncomplicated　HCC

F13.921 Sedative, hypnotic or anxiolytic use, unspecified with intoxication delirium　CC HCC
Sedative, hypnotic, or anxiolytic-induced delirium

F13.929 Sedative, hypnotic or anxiolytic use, unspecified with intoxication, unspecified　HCC

√6ᵗʰ **F13.93** Sedative, hypnotic or anxiolytic use, unspecified with withdrawal
EXCLUDES 1　sedative, hypnotic or anxiolytic use, unspecified with intoxication (F13.92-)

F13.930 Sedative, hypnotic or anxiolytic use, unspecified with withdrawal, uncomplicated　CC HCC

F13.931 Sedative, hypnotic or anxiolytic use, unspecified with withdrawal delirium　CC HCC

F13.932 Sedative, hypnotic or anxiolytic use, unspecified with withdrawal with perceptual disturbances　CC HCC

F13.939 Sedative, hypnotic or anxiolytic use, unspecified with withdrawal, unspecified　CC HCC

F13.94 Sedative, hypnotic or anxiolytic use, unspecified with sedative, hypnotic or anxiolytic-induced mood disorder　HCC
Sedative, hypnotic, or anxiolytic-induced bipolar or related disorder, without use disorder
Sedative, hypnotic, or anxiolytic-induced depressive disorder, without use disorder

√6ᵗʰ **F13.95** Sedative, hypnotic or anxiolytic use, unspecified with sedative, hypnotic or anxiolytic-induced psychotic disorder

F13.950 Sedative, hypnotic or anxiolytic use, unspecified with sedative, hypnotic or anxiolytic-induced psychotic disorder with delusions　CC HCC

F13.951 Sedative, hypnotic or anxiolytic use, unspecified with sedative, hypnotic or anxiolytic-induced psychotic disorder with hallucinations　CC HCC

F13.959 Sedative, hypnotic or anxiolytic use, unspecified with sedative, hypnotic or anxiolytic-induced psychotic disorder, unspecified　HCC
Sedative, hypnotic, or anxiolytic-induced psychotic disorder, without use disorder

F13.96 Sedative, hypnotic or anxiolytic use, unspecified with sedative, hypnotic or anxiolytic-induced persisting amnestic disorder　HCC

F13.97 Sedative, hypnotic or anxiolytic use, unspecified with sedative, hypnotic or anxiolytic-induced persisting dementia　CC HCC
Sedative, hypnotic, or anxiolytic-induced major neurocognitive disorder, without use disorder

Chapter 5. Mental, Behavioral and Neurodevelopmental Disorders

✓6ᵗʰ **F13.98** Sedative, hypnotic or anxiolytic use, unspecified with other sedative, hypnotic or anxiolytic-induced disorders

F13.980 Sedative, hypnotic or anxiolytic use, unspecified with sedative, hypnotic or anxiolytic-induced anxiety disorder   HCC

Sedative, hypnotic, or anxiolytic-induced anxiety disorder, without use disorder

F13.981 Sedative, hypnotic or anxiolytic use, unspecified with sedative, hypnotic or anxiolytic-induced sexual dysfunction   HCC

Sedative, hypnotic, or anxiolytic-induced sexual dysfunction disorder, without use disorder

F13.982 Sedative, hypnotic or anxiolytic use, unspecified with sedative, hypnotic or anxiolytic-induced sleep disorder   HCC

Sedative, hypnotic, or anxiolytic-induced sleep disorder, without use disorder

F13.988 Sedative, hypnotic or anxiolytic use, unspecified with other sedative, hypnotic or anxiolytic-induced disorder   HCC

Sedative, hypnotic, or anxiolytic-induced mild neurocognitive disorder

F13.99 Sedative, hypnotic or anxiolytic use, unspecified with unspecified sedative, hypnotic or anxiolytic-induced disorder   HCC

✓4ᵗʰ **F14** Cocaine related disorders

EXCLUDES 2   other stimulant-related disorders (F15.-)

✓5ᵗʰ **F14.1** Cocaine abuse

EXCLUDES 1   cocaine dependence (F14.2-)
         cocaine use, unspecified (F14.9-)

F14.10 Cocaine abuse, uncomplicated   HCC

Cocaine use disorder, mild

F14.11 Cocaine abuse, in remission   HCC

Cocaine use disorder, mild, in early remission
Cocaine use disorder, mild, in sustained remission

✓6ᵗʰ **F14.12** Cocaine abuse with intoxication

F14.120 Cocaine abuse with intoxication, uncomplicated   HCC

F14.121 Cocaine abuse with intoxication with delirium   CC HCC

F14.122 Cocaine abuse with intoxication with perceptual disturbance   HCC

F14.129 Cocaine abuse with intoxication, unspecified   HCC

F14.14 Cocaine abuse with cocaine-induced mood disorder   HCC

Cocaine use disorder, mild, with cocaine-induced bipolar or related disorder
Cocaine use disorder, mild, with cocaine-induced depressive disorder

✓6ᵗʰ **F14.15** Cocaine abuse with cocaine-induced psychotic disorder

F14.150 Cocaine abuse with cocaine-induced psychotic disorder with delusions   CC HCC

F14.151 Cocaine abuse with cocaine-induced psychotic disorder with hallucinations   CC HCC

F14.159 Cocaine abuse with cocaine-induced psychotic disorder, unspecified   HCC

✓6ᵗʰ **F14.18** Cocaine abuse with other cocaine-induced disorder

F14.180 Cocaine abuse with cocaine-induced anxiety disorder   HCC

F14.181 Cocaine abuse with cocaine-induced sexual dysfunction   HCC

F14.182 Cocaine abuse with cocaine-induced sleep disorder   HCC

F14.188 Cocaine abuse with other cocaine-induced disorder   HCC

Cocaine use disorder, mild, with cocaine-induced obsessive compulsive or related disorder

F14.19 Cocaine abuse with unspecified cocaine-induced disorder   HCC

✓5ᵗʰ **F14.2** Cocaine dependence

EXCLUDES 1   cocaine abuse (F14.1-)
         cocaine use, unspecified (F14.9-)
EXCLUDES 2   cocaine poisoning (T40.5-)

F14.20 Cocaine dependence, uncomplicated   HCC

Cocaine use disorder, moderate
Cocaine use disorder, severe

F14.21 Cocaine dependence, in remission   HCC

Cocaine use disorder, moderate, in early remission
Cocaine use disorder, moderate, in sustained remission
Cocaine use disorder, severe, in early remission
Cocaine use disorder, severe, in sustained remission

✓6ᵗʰ **F14.22** Cocaine dependence with intoxication

EXCLUDES 1   cocaine dependence with withdrawal (F14.23)

F14.220 Cocaine dependence with intoxication, uncomplicated   HCC

F14.221 Cocaine dependence with intoxication delirium   CC HCC

F14.222 Cocaine dependence with intoxication with perceptual disturbance   CC HCC
     CC Excl: No Excl

F14.229 Cocaine dependence with intoxication, unspecified   CC HCC
     CC Excl: No Excl

F14.23 Cocaine dependence with withdrawal   CC HCC

EXCLUDES 1   cocaine dependence with intoxication (F14.22-)

F14.24 Cocaine dependence with cocaine-induced mood disorder   HCC

Cocaine use disorder, moderate, with cocaine-induced bipolar or related disorder
Cocaine use disorder, moderate, with cocaine-induced depressive disorder
Cocaine use disorder, severe, with cocaine-induced bipolar or related disorder
Cocaine use disorder, severe, with cocaine-induced depressive disorder

✓6ᵗʰ **F14.25** Cocaine dependence with cocaine-induced psychotic disorder

F14.250 Cocaine dependence with cocaine-induced psychotic disorder with delusions   CC HCC

F14.251 Cocaine dependence with cocaine-induced psychotic disorder with hallucinations   CC HCC

F14.259 Cocaine dependence with cocaine-induced psychotic disorder, unspecified   CC HCC
     CC Excl: No Excl

✓6ᵗʰ **F14.28** Cocaine dependence with other cocaine-induced disorder

F14.280 Cocaine dependence with cocaine-induced anxiety disorder   CC HCC
     CC Excl: No Excl

F14.281 Cocaine dependence with cocaine-induced sexual dysfunction   CC HCC
     CC Excl: No Excl

N Newborn: 0   P Pediatric: 0-17   M Maternity: 9-64   A Adult: 15-124   HCC Major Complication/Comorbidity   CC Complication/Comorbidity   SW Severe Wound Dx

550   ICD-10-CM 2020

F14.282 Cocaine dependence with cocaine-induced sleep disorder `CC` `HCC`
CC Excl: No Excl

F14.288 Cocaine dependence with other cocaine-induced disorder `CC` `HCC`
Cocaine use disorder, moderate, with cocaine-induced obsessive compulsive or related disorder
Cocaine use disorder, severe, with cocaine-induced obsessive compulsive or related disorder
CC Excl: No Excl

F14.29 Cocaine dependence with unspecified cocaine-induced disorder `HCC`

F14.9 Cocaine use, unspecified
EXCLUDES 1   cocaine abuse (F14.1-)
   cocaine dependence (F14.2-)
TIP: Assign a substance use code only when the provider documents a relationship between the use and an associated physical, mental, or behavioral disorder. As with all diagnoses, substance use codes must meet the definition of a reportable diagnosis.

F14.90 Cocaine use, unspecified, uncomplicated
AHA: 2018,2Q,10-11

F14.92 Cocaine use, unspecified with intoxication
F14.920 Cocaine use, unspecified with intoxication, uncomplicated `HCC`
F14.921 Cocaine use, unspecified with intoxication delirium `CC` `HCC`
F14.922 Cocaine use, unspecified with intoxication with perceptual disturbance `HCC`
F14.929 Cocaine use, unspecified with intoxication, unspecified `HCC`

F14.94 Cocaine use, unspecified with cocaine-induced mood disorder `HCC`
Cocaine induced bipolar or related disorder, without use disorder
Cocaine induced depressive disorder, without use disorder

F14.95 Cocaine use, unspecified with cocaine-induced psychotic disorder
F14.950 Cocaine use, unspecified with cocaine-induced psychotic disorder with delusions `CC` `HCC`
F14.951 Cocaine use, unspecified with cocaine-induced psychotic disorder with hallucinations `CC` `HCC`
F14.959 Cocaine use, unspecified with cocaine-induced psychotic disorder, unspecified `HCC`
Cocaine induced psychotic disorder, without use disorder

F14.98 Cocaine use, unspecified with other specified cocaine-induced disorder
F14.980 Cocaine use, unspecified with cocaine-induced anxiety disorder `HCC`
Cocaine induced anxiety disorder, without use disorder
F14.981 Cocaine use, unspecified with cocaine-induced sexual dysfunction `HCC`
Cocaine induced sexual dysfunction, without use disorder
F14.982 Cocaine use, unspecified with cocaine-induced sleep disorder `HCC`
Cocaine induced sleep disorder, without use disorder

F14.988 Cocaine use, unspecified with other cocaine-induced disorder `HCC`
Cocaine induced obsessive compulsive or related disorder

F14.99 Cocaine use, unspecified with unspecified cocaine-induced disorder `HCC`

F15 Other stimulant related disorders
INCLUDES   amphetamine-related disorders
   caffeine
EXCLUDES 2   cocaine-related disorders (F14.-)

F15.1 Other stimulant abuse
EXCLUDES 1   other stimulant dependence (F15.2-)
   other stimulant use, unspecified (F15.9-)

F15.10 Other stimulant abuse, uncomplicated `HCC`
Amphetamine type substance use disorder, mild
Other or unspecified stimulant use disorder, mild

F15.11 Other stimulant abuse, in remission `HCC`
Amphetamine type substance use disorder, mild, in early remission
Amphetamine type substance use disorder, mild, in sustained remission
Other or unspecified stimulant use disorder, mild, in early remission
Other or unspecified stimulant use disorder, mild, in sustained remission

F15.12 Other stimulant abuse with intoxication
F15.120 Other stimulant abuse with intoxication, uncomplicated `HCC`
F15.121 Other stimulant abuse with intoxication delirium `CC` `HCC`
F15.122 Other stimulant abuse with intoxication with perceptual disturbance `HCC`
Amphetamine or other stimulant use disorder, mild, with amphetamine or other stimulant intoxication, with perceptual disturbances
F15.129 Other stimulant abuse with intoxication, unspecified `HCC`
Amphetamine or other stimulant use disorder, mild, with amphetamine or other stimulant intoxication, without perceptual disturbances

F15.14 Other stimulant abuse with stimulant-induced mood disorder `HCC`
Amphetamine or other stimulant use disorder, mild, with amphetamine or other stimulant induced bipolar or related disorder
Amphetamine or other stimulant use disorder, mild, with amphetamine or other stimulant induced depressive disorder

F15.15 Other stimulant abuse with stimulant-induced psychotic disorder
F15.150 Other stimulant abuse with stimulant-induced psychotic disorder with delusions `CC` `HCC`
F15.151 Other stimulant abuse with stimulant-induced psychotic disorder with hallucinations `CC` `HCC`
F15.159 Other stimulant abuse with stimulant-induced psychotic disorder, unspecified `HCC`

F15.18 Other stimulant abuse with other stimulant-induced disorder
F15.180 Other stimulant abuse with stimulant-induced anxiety disorder `HCC`
F15.181 Other stimulant abuse with stimulant-induced sexual dysfunction `HCC`

Chapter 5. Mental, Behavioral and Neurodevelopmental Disorders

F15.182-F15.90

F15.182   **Other stimulant abuse with stimulant-induced sleep disorder**   HCC

F15.188   **Other stimulant abuse with other stimulant-induced disorder**   HCC

Amphetamine or other stimulant use disorder, mild, with amphetamine or other stimulant induced obsessive-compulsive or related disorder

F15.19   **Other stimulant abuse with unspecified stimulant-induced disorder**   HCC

✓5ᵗʰ **F15.2**   **Other stimulant dependence**

EXCLUDES 1   *other stimulant abuse (F15.1-)*

               other stimulant use, unspecified (F15.9-)

F15.20   **Other stimulant dependence, uncomplicated**   CC   HCC

Amphetamine type substance use disorder, moderate

Amphetamine type substance use disorder, severe

Other or unspecified stimulant use disorder, moderate

Other or unspecified stimulant use disorder, severe

CC Excl: No Excl

F15.21   **Other stimulant dependence, in remission**   HCC

Amphetamine type substance use disorder, moderate, in early remission

Amphetamine type substance use disorder, moderate, in sustained remission

Amphetamine type substance use disorder, severe, in early remission

Amphetamine type substance use disorder, severe, in sustained remission

Other or unspecified stimulant use disorder, moderate, in early remission

Other or unspecified stimulant use disorder, moderate, in sustained remission

Other or unspecified stimulant use disorder, severe, in early remission

Other or unspecified stimulant use disorder, severe, in sustained remission

✓6ᵗʰ **F15.22**   **Other stimulant dependence with intoxication**

EXCLUDES 1   *other stimulant dependence with withdrawal (F15.23)*

F15.220   **Other stimulant dependence with intoxication, uncomplicated**   HCC

F15.221   **Other stimulant dependence with intoxication delirium**   CC   HCC

F15.222   **Other stimulant dependence with intoxication with perceptual disturbance**   CC   HCC

Amphetamine or other stimulant use disorder, moderate, with amphetamine or other stimulant intoxication, with perceptual disturbances

Amphetamine or other stimulant use disorder, severe, with amphetamine or other stimulant intoxication, with perceptual disturbances

CC Excl: No Excl

F15.229   **Other stimulant dependence with intoxication, unspecified**   HCC

Amphetamine or other stimulant use disorder, moderate, with amphetamine or other stimulant intoxication, without perceptual disturbances

Amphetamine or other stimulant use disorder, severe, with amphetamine or other stimulant intoxication, without perceptual disturbances

F15.23   **Other stimulant dependence with withdrawal**   CC   HCC

Amphetamine or other stimulant withdrawal

EXCLUDES 1   *other stimulant dependence with intoxication (F15.22-)*

F15.24   **Other stimulant dependence with stimulant-induced mood disorder**   HCC

Amphetamine or other stimulant use disorder, moderate, with amphetamine or other stimulant-induced bipolar or related disorder

Amphetamine or other stimulant use disorder, moderate, with amphetamine or other stimulant induced depressive disorder

Amphetamine or other stimulant use disorder, severe, with amphetamine or other stimulant-induced bipolar or related disorder

Amphetamine or other stimulant use disorder, severe, with amphetamine or other stimulant-induced depressive disorder

✓6ᵗʰ **F15.25**   **Other stimulant dependence with stimulant-induced psychotic disorder**

F15.250   **Other stimulant dependence with stimulant-induced psychotic disorder with delusions**   CC   HCC

F15.251   **Other stimulant dependence with stimulant-induced psychotic disorder with hallucinations**   CC   HCC

F15.259   **Other stimulant dependence with stimulant-induced psychotic disorder, unspecified**   CC   HCC

CC Excl: No Excl

✓6ᵗʰ **F15.28**   **Other stimulant dependence with other stimulant-induced disorder**

F15.280   **Other stimulant dependence with stimulant-induced anxiety disorder**   CC   HCC

CC Excl: No Excl

F15.281   **Other stimulant dependence with stimulant-induced sexual dysfunction**   CC   HCC

CC Excl: No Excl

F15.282   **Other stimulant dependence with stimulant-induced sleep disorder**   CC   HCC

CC Excl: No Excl

F15.288   **Other stimulant dependence with other stimulant-induced disorder**   CC   HCC

Amphetamine or other stimulant use disorder, moderate, with amphetamine orother stimulant induced obsessive compulsive or related disorder

Amphetamine or other stimulant use disorder, severe, with amphetamine or otherstimulant induced obsessive compulsive or related disorder

CC Excl: No Excl

F15.29   **Other stimulant dependence with unspecified stimulant-induced disorder**   HCC

✓5ᵗʰ **F15.9**   **Other stimulant use, unspecified**

EXCLUDES 1   *other stimulant abuse (F15.1-)*

               other stimulant dependence (F15.2-)

TIP: Assign a substance use code only when the provider documents a relationship between the use and an associated physical, mental, or behavioral disorder. As with all diagnoses, substance use codes must meet the definition of a reportable diagnosis.

F15.90   **Other stimulant use, unspecified, uncomplicated**

AHA: 2018,2Q,10-11

N Newborn: 0   P Pediatric: 0-17   M Maternity: 9-64   A Adult: 15-124   MCC Major Complication/Comorbidity   CC Complication/Comorbidity   SW Severe Wound Dx

552

ICD-10-CM 2020

☑6ᵗʰ **F15.92** **Other stimulant use, unspecified with intoxication**
> *EXCLUDES 1* — *other stimulant use, unspecified with withdrawal (F15.93)*

　　F15.920 **Other stimulant use, unspecified with intoxication, uncomplicated** ᴴᶜᶜ

　　F15.921 **Other stimulant use, unspecified with intoxication delirium** ᶜᶜ ᴴᶜᶜ
> Amphetamine or other stimulant-induced delirium

　　F15.922 **Other stimulant use, unspecified with intoxication with perceptual disturbance** ᴴᶜᶜ

　　F15.929 **Other stimulant use, unspecified with intoxication, unspecified** ᴴᶜᶜ
> Caffeine intoxication

F15.93 **Other stimulant use, unspecified with withdrawal** ᶜᶜ ᴴᶜᶜ
> Caffeine withdrawal
> *EXCLUDES 1* — *other stimulant use, unspecified with intoxication (F15.92-)*

F15.94 **Other stimulant use, unspecified with stimulant-induced mood disorder** ᴴᶜᶜ
> Amphetamine or other stimulant-induced bipolar or related disorder, without use disorder
> Amphetamine or other stimulant-induced depressive disorder, without use disorder

☑6ᵗʰ **F15.95** **Other stimulant use, unspecified with stimulant-induced psychotic disorder**

　　F15.950 **Other stimulant use, unspecified with stimulant-induced psychotic disorder with delusions** ᶜᶜ ᴴᶜᶜ

　　F15.951 **Other stimulant use, unspecified with stimulant-induced psychotic disorder with hallucinations** ᶜᶜ ᴴᶜᶜ

　　F15.959 **Other stimulant use, unspecified with stimulant-induced psychotic disorder, unspecified** ᴴᶜᶜ
> Amphetamine or other stimulant-induced psychotic disorder, without use disorder

☑6ᵗʰ **F15.98** **Other stimulant use, unspecified with other stimulant-induced disorder**

　　F15.980 **Other stimulant use, unspecified with stimulant-induced anxiety disorder** ᴴᶜᶜ
> Amphetamine or other stimulant-induced anxiety disorder, without use disorder
> Caffeine induced anxiety disorder, without use disorder

　　F15.981 **Other stimulant use, unspecified with stimulant-induced sexual dysfunction** ᴴᶜᶜ
> Amphetamine or other stimulant-induced sexual dysfunction, without use disorder

　　F15.982 **Other stimulant use, unspecified with stimulant-induced sleep disorder** ᴴᶜᶜ
> Amphetamine or other stimulant-induced sleep disorder, without use disorder
> Caffeine induced sleep disorder, without use disorder

　　F15.988 **Other stimulant use, unspecified with other stimulant-induced disorder** ᴴᶜᶜ
> Amphetamine or other stimulant-induced obsessive compulsive or related disorder, without use disorder

F15.99 **Other stimulant use, unspecified with unspecified stimulant-induced disorder** ᴴᶜᶜ

☑4ᵗʰ **F16** **Hallucinogen related disorders**
> *INCLUDES* — ecstasy
> PCP
> phencyclidine
> **AHA:** 2018,4Q,31

☑5ᵗʰ **F16.1** **Hallucinogen abuse**
> *EXCLUDES 1* — *hallucinogen dependence (F16.2-)*
> *hallucinogen use, unspecified (F16.9-)*

　　F16.10 **Hallucinogen abuse, uncomplicated** ᴴᶜᶜ
> Other hallucinogen use disorder, mild
> Phencyclidine use disorder, mild

　　F16.11 **Hallucinogen abuse, in remission** ᴴᶜᶜ
> Other hallucinogen use disorder, mild, in early remission
> Other hallucinogen use disorder, mild, in sustained remission
> Phencyclidine use disorder, mild, in early remission
> Phencyclidine use disorder, mild, in sustained remission

☑6ᵗʰ **F16.12** **Hallucinogen abuse with intoxication**

　　F16.120 **Hallucinogen abuse with intoxication, uncomplicated** ᴴᶜᶜ

　　F16.121 **Hallucinogen abuse with intoxication with delirium** ᶜᶜ ᴴᶜᶜ

　　F16.122 **Hallucinogen abuse with intoxication with perceptual disturbance** ᴴᶜᶜ

　　F16.129 **Hallucinogen abuse with intoxication, unspecified** ᴴᶜᶜ

　　F16.14 **Hallucinogen abuse with hallucinogen-induced mood disorder** ᴴᶜᶜ
> Other hallucinogen use disorder, mild, with other hallucinogen induced bipolar or related disorder
> Other hallucinogen use disorder, mild, with other hallucinogen induced depressive disorder
> Phencyclidine use disorder, mild, with phencyclidine induced bipolar or related disorder
> Phencyclidine use disorder, mild, with phencyclidine induced depressive disorder

☑6ᵗʰ **F16.15** **Hallucinogen abuse with hallucinogen-induced psychotic disorder**

　　F16.150 **Hallucinogen abuse with hallucinogen-induced psychotic disorder with delusions** ᶜᶜ ᴴᶜᶜ

　　F16.151 **Hallucinogen abuse with hallucinogen-induced psychotic disorder with hallucinations** ᶜᶜ ᴴᶜᶜ

　　F16.159 **Hallucinogen abuse with hallucinogen-induced psychotic disorder, unspecified** ᴴᶜᶜ

☑6ᵗʰ **F16.18** **Hallucinogen abuse with other hallucinogen-induced disorder**

　　F16.180 **Hallucinogen abuse with hallucinogen-induced anxiety disorder** ᴴᶜᶜ

　　F16.183 **Hallucinogen abuse with hallucinogen persisting perception disorder (flashbacks)** ᴴᶜᶜ

　　F16.188 **Hallucinogen abuse with other hallucinogen-induced disorder** ᴴᶜᶜ

F16.19 **Hallucinogen abuse with unspecified hallucinogen-induced disorder** ᴴᶜᶜ

✓5ᵗʰ **F16.2 Hallucinogen** dependence

    EXCLUDES 1   hallucinogen abuse (F16.1-)

                  hallucinogen use, unspecified (F16.9-)

    F16.20 Hallucinogen dependence,   CC HCC
uncomplicated

        Other hallucinogen use disorder, moderate

        Other hallucinogen use disorder, severe

        Phencyclidine use disorder, moderate

        Phencyclidine use disorder, severe

        CC Excl: No Excl

    F16.21 Hallucinogen dependence, in   HCC
remission

        Other hallucinogen use disorder, moderate, in early
remission

        Other hallucinogen use disorder, moderate, in
sustained remission

        Other hallucinogen use disorder, severe, in early
remission

        Other hallucinogen use disorder, severe, in sustained
remission

        Phencyclidine use disorder, moderate, in early
remission

        Phencyclidine use disorder, moderate, in sustained
remission

        Phencyclidine use disorder, severe, in early remission

        Phencyclidine use disorder, severe, in sustained
remission

✓6ᵗʰ   **F16.22 Hallucinogen dependence with** intoxication

        F16.220 Hallucinogen dependence   HCC
**with intoxication,
uncomplicated**

        F16.221 Hallucinogen dependence   CC HCC
**with intoxication with
delirium**

        F16.229 Hallucinogen dependence   HCC
**with intoxication,
unspecified**

    F16.24 Hallucinogen dependence with   HCC
hallucinogen-induced mood
disorder

        Other hallucinogen use disorder, moderate, with
other hallucinogen induced bipolar or related
disorder

        Other hallucinogen use disorder, moderate, with
other hallucinogen induced depressive disorder

        Other hallucinogen use disorder, severe, with other
hallucinogen-induced bipolar or related disorder

        Other hallucinogen use disorder, severe, with other
hallucinogen-induced depressive disorder

        Phencyclidine use disorder, moderate, with
phencyclidine induced bipolar or related disorder

        Phencyclidine use disorder, moderate, with
phencyclidine induced depressive disorder

        Phencyclidine use disorder, severe, with
phencyclidine induced bipolar or related disorder

        Phencyclidine use disorder, severe, with
phencyclidine-induced depressive disorder

✓6ᵗʰ   **F16.25 Hallucinogen dependence with**
hallucinogen-induced psychotic disorder

        F16.250 Hallucinogen dependence   CC HCC
**with
hallucinogen-induced
psychotic disorder with
delusions**

        F16.251 Hallucinogen dependence   CC HCC
**with
hallucinogen-induced
psychotic disorder with
hallucinations**

        F16.259 Hallucinogen dependence   CC HCC
**with
hallucinogen-induced
psychotic disorder,
unspecified**

            CC Excl: No Excl

✓6ᵗʰ   **F16.28 Hallucinogen dependence with** other
hallucinogen-induced disorder

    F16.280 Hallucinogen dependence   CC HCC
**with
hallucinogen-induced
anxiety disorder**

        CC Excl: No Excl

    F16.283 Hallucinogen dependence   CC HCC
**with hallucinogen
persisting perception
disorder (flashbacks)**

        CC Excl: No Excl

    F16.288 Hallucinogen dependence   CC HCC
**with other
hallucinogen-induced
disorder**

        CC Excl: No Excl

  F16.29 Hallucinogen dependence with   HCC
**unspecified hallucinogen-induced
disorder**

✓5ᵗʰ **F16.9 Hallucinogen use, unspecified**

    EXCLUDES 1   hallucinogen abuse (F16.1-)

                  hallucinogen dependence (F16.2-)

    TIP: Assign a substance use code only when the provider
documents a relationship between the use and an associated
physical, mental, or behavioral disorder. As with all diagnoses,
substance use codes must meet the definition of a reportable
diagnosis.

  F16.90 Hallucinogen use, unspecified, uncomplicated

        AHA: 2018,2Q,10-11

✓6ᵗʰ   **F16.92 Hallucinogen use, unspecified with** intoxication

    F16.920 Hallucinogen use,   HCC
**unspecified with
intoxication,
uncomplicated**

    F16.921 Hallucinogen use,   CC HCC
**unspecified with
intoxication with** delirium

        Other hallucinogen intoxication delirium

    F16.929 Hallucinogen use,   HCC
**unspecified with
intoxication, unspecified**

  F16.94 Hallucinogen use, unspecified with   HCC
hallucinogen-induced mood
disorder

        Other hallucinogen induced bipolar or related
disorder, without use disorder

        Other hallucinogen induced depressive disorder,
without use disorder

        Phencyclidine induced bipolar or related disorder,
without use disorder

        Phencyclidine induced depressive disorder, without
use disorder

✓6ᵗʰ   **F16.95 Hallucinogen use, unspecified with**
hallucinogen-induced psychotic disorder

    F16.950 Hallucinogen use,   CC HCC
**unspecified with
hallucinogen-induced
psychotic disorder with
delusions**

    F16.951 Hallucinogen use,   CC HCC
**unspecified with
hallucinogen-induced
psychotic disorder with
hallucinations**

    F16.959 Hallucinogen use,   HCC
**unspecified with
hallucinogen-induced
psychotic disorder,
unspecified**

        Other hallucinogen induced psychotic
disorder, without use disorder

        Phencyclidine induced psychotic disorder,
without use disorder

N Newborn: 0   P Pediatric: 0-17   M Maternity: 9-64   A Adult: 15-124   MCC Major Complication/Comorbidity   CC Complication/Comorbidity   SW Severe Wound Dx

554   ICD-10-CM 2020

√6ᵗʰ **F16.98 Hallucinogen use, unspecified with other specified hallucinogen-induced disorder**

    F16.980 Hallucinogen use, unspecified with hallucinogen-induced anxiety disorder   `HCC`

      Other hallucinogen-induced anxiety disorder, without use disorder

      Phencyclidine induced anxiety disorder, without use disorder

    F16.983 Hallucinogen use, unspecified with hallucinogen persisting perception disorder (flashbacks)   `HCC`

    F16.988 Hallucinogen use, unspecified with other hallucinogen-induced disorder   `HCC`

F16.99 Hallucinogen use, unspecified with unspecified hallucinogen-induced disorder   `HCC`

√4ᵗʰ **F17 Nicotine dependence**

   `EXCLUDES 1`   history of tobacco dependence (Z87.891)

           tobacco use NOS (Z72.0)

   `EXCLUDES 2`   tobacco use (smoking) during pregnancy, childbirth and the puerperium (O99.33-)

           toxic effect of nicotine (T65.2-)

   AHA: 2013,4Q,108-109

   √5ᵗʰ **F17.2 Nicotine dependence**

     √6ᵗʰ **F17.20 Nicotine dependence, unspecified**

       F17.200 Nicotine dependence, unspecified, uncomplicated

         Tobacco use disorder, mild

         Tobacco use disorder, moderate

         Tobacco use disorder, severe

         AHA: 2016,1Q,36

         TIP: Assign when provider documentation indicates "smoker" without further specification.

       F17.201 Nicotine dependence, unspecified, in remission

         Tobacco use disorder, mild, in early remission

         Tobacco use disorder, mild, in sustained remission

         Tobacco use disorder, moderate, in early remission

         Tobacco use disorder, moderate, in sustained remission

         Tobacco use disorder, severe, in early remission

         Tobacco use disorder, severe, in sustained remission

       F17.203 Nicotine dependence unspecified, with withdrawal   `CC`

         Tobacco withdrawal

       F17.208 Nicotine dependence, unspecified, with other nicotine-induced disorders

       F17.209 Nicotine dependence, unspecified, with unspecified nicotine-induced disorders

     √6ᵗʰ **F17.21 Nicotine dependence, cigarettes**

       F17.210 Nicotine dependence, cigarettes, uncomplicated

         AHA: 2017,2Q,28-29

       F17.211 Nicotine dependence, cigarettes, in remission

         Tobacco use disorder, cigarettes, mild, in early remission

         Tobacco use disorder, cigarettes, mild, in sustained remission

         Tobacco use disorder, cigarettes, moderate, in early remission

         Tobacco use disorder, cigarettes, moderate, in sustained remission

         Tobacco use disorder, cigarettes, severe, in early remission

         Tobacco use disorder, cigarettes, severe, in sustained remission

       F17.213 Nicotine dependence, cigarettes, with withdrawal   `CC`

       F17.218 Nicotine dependence, cigarettes, with other nicotine-induced disorders

       F17.219 Nicotine dependence, cigarettes, with unspecified nicotine-induced disorders

     √6ᵗʰ **F17.22 Nicotine dependence, chewing tobacco**

       F17.220 Nicotine dependence, chewing tobacco, uncomplicated

       F17.221 Nicotine dependence, chewing tobacco, in remission

         Tobacco use disorder, chewing tobacco, mild, in early remission

         Tobacco use disorder, chewing tobacco, mild, in sustained remission

         Tobacco use disorder, chewing tobacco, moderate, in early remission

         Tobacco use disorder, chewing tobacco, moderate, in sustained remission

         Tobacco use disorder, chewing tobacco, severe, in early remission

         Tobacco use disorder, chewing tobacco, severe, in sustained remission

       F17.223 Nicotine dependence, chewing tobacco, with withdrawal   `CC`

       F17.228 Nicotine dependence, chewing tobacco, with other nicotine-induced disorders

       F17.229 Nicotine dependence, chewing tobacco, with unspecified nicotine-induced disorders

     √6ᵗʰ **F17.29 Nicotine dependence, other tobacco product**

       F17.290 Nicotine dependence, other tobacco product, uncomplicated

         AHA: 2017,2Q,28-29

       F17.291 Nicotine dependence, other tobacco product, in remission

         Tobacco use disorder, other tobacco product, mild, in early remission

         Tobacco use disorder, other tobacco product, mild, in sustained remission

         Tobacco use disorder, other tobacco product, moderate, in early remission

         Tobacco use disorder, other tobacco product, moderate, in sustained remission

         Tobacco use disorder, other tobacco product, severe, in early remission

         Tobacco use disorder, other tobacco product, severe, in sustained remission

       F17.293 Nicotine dependence, other tobacco product, with withdrawal   `CC`

       F17.298 Nicotine dependence, other tobacco product, with other nicotine-induced disorders

       F17.299 Nicotine dependence, other tobacco product, with unspecified nicotine-induced disorders

✔ Additional Character Required   √x7ᵗʰ Placeholder   Unacceptable PDx   Questionable PDx   Manifestation   Unspecified Dx   H1–H14 HAC   HCC CMS-HCC Dx   HIV HIV Dx

ICD-10-CM 2020   555

Chapter 5. Mental, Behavioral and Neurodevelopmental Disorders

F18–F18.959

✓4ᵗʰ **F18 Inhalant related disorders**
  INCLUDES volatile solvents

✓5ᵗʰ **F18.1 Inhalant abuse**
  EXCLUDES 1 *inhalant dependence (F18.2-)*
              inhalant use, unspecified (F18.9-)

  F18.10 Inhalant abuse, uncomplicated   HCC
    Inhalant use disorder, mild

  F18.11 Inhalant abuse, in remission   HCC
    Inhalant use disorder, mild, in early remission
    Inhalant use disorder, mild, in sustained remission

  ✓6ᵗʰ **F18.12 Inhalant abuse with intoxication**
    F18.120 Inhalant abuse with   HCC
              intoxication,
              uncomplicated
    F18.121 Inhalant abuse with   CC HCC
              intoxication delirium
    F18.129 Inhalant abuse with   HCC
              intoxication, unspecified

  F18.14 Inhalant abuse with   HCC
          inhalant-induced mood disorder
    Inhalant use disorder, mild, with inhalant induced
      depressive disorder

  ✓6ᵗʰ **F18.15 Inhalant abuse with inhalant-induced psychotic**
          disorder
    F18.150 Inhalant abuse with   CC HCC
              inhalant-induced
              psychotic disorder with
              delusions
    F18.151 Inhalant abuse with   CC HCC
              inhalant-induced
              psychotic disorder with
              hallucinations
    F18.159 Inhalant abuse with   HCC
              inhalant-induced
              psychotic disorder,
              unspecified

  F18.17 Inhalant abuse with   CC HCC
          inhalant-induced dementia
    Inhalant use disorder, mild, with inhalant induced
      major neurocognitive disorder

  ✓6ᵗʰ **F18.18 Inhalant abuse with other inhalant-induced**
          disorders
    F18.180 Inhalant abuse with   HCC
              inhalant-induced anxiety
              disorder
    F18.188 Inhalant abuse with other   HCC
              inhalant-induced disorder
      Inhalant use disorder, mild, with inhalant
        induced mild neurocognitive disorder

  F18.19 Inhalant abuse with unspecified   HCC
          inhalant-induced disorder

✓5ᵗʰ **F18.2 Inhalant dependence**
  EXCLUDES 1 *inhalant abuse (F18.1-)*
              inhalant use, unspecified (F18.9-)

  F18.20 Inhalant dependence,   CC HCC
          uncomplicated
    Inhalant use disorder, moderate
    Inhalant use disorder, severe
    CC Excl: No Excl

  F18.21 Inhalant dependence, in remission   HCC
    Inhalant use disorder, moderate, in early remission
    Inhalant use disorder, moderate, in sustained
      remission
    Inhalant use disorder, severe, in early remission
    Inhalant use disorder, severe, in sustained remission

  ✓6ᵗʰ **F18.22 Inhalant dependence with intoxication**
    F18.220 Inhalant dependence with   HCC
              intoxication,
              uncomplicated
    F18.221 Inhalant dependence with   CC HCC
              intoxication delirium
    F18.229 Inhalant dependence with   HCC
              intoxication, unspecified

  F18.24 Inhalant dependence with   HCC
          inhalant-induced mood disorder
    Inhalant use disorder, moderate, with inhalant
      induced depressive disorder
    Inhalant use disorder, severe, with inhalant induced
      depressive disorder

  ✓6ᵗʰ **F18.25 Inhalant dependence with inhalant-induced**
          psychotic disorder
    F18.250 Inhalant dependence with   CC HCC
              inhalant-induced
              psychotic disorder with
              delusions
    F18.251 Inhalant dependence with   CC HCC
              inhalant-induced
              psychotic disorder with
              hallucinations
    F18.259 Inhalant dependence with   CC HCC
              inhalant-induced
              psychotic disorder,
              unspecified
      CC Excl: No Excl

  F18.27 Inhalant dependence with   CC HCC
          inhalant-induced dementia
    Inhalant use disorder, moderate, with inhalant
      induced major neurocognitive disorder
    Inhalant use disorder, severe, with inhalant induced
      major neurocognitive disorder

  ✓6ᵗʰ **F18.28 Inhalant dependence with other inhalant-induced**
          disorders
    F18.280 Inhalant dependence with   CC HCC
              inhalant-induced anxiety
              disorder
      CC Excl: No Excl
    F18.288 Inhalant dependence with   CC HCC
              other inhalant-induced
              disorder
      Inhalant use disorder, moderate, with
        inhalant-induced mild neurocognitive
        disorder
      Inhalant use disorder, severe, with
        inhalant-induced mild neurocognitive
        disorder
      CC Excl: No Excl

  F18.29 Inhalant dependence with   HCC
          unspecified inhalant-induced
          disorder

✓5ᵗʰ **F18.9 Inhalant use, unspecified**
  EXCLUDES 1 *inhalant abuse (F18.1-)*
              inhalant dependence (F18.2-)

  F18.90 Inhalant use, unspecified, uncomplicated
    AHA: 2018,2Q,10-11

  ✓6ᵗʰ **F18.92 Inhalant use, unspecified with intoxication**
    F18.920 Inhalant use, unspecified   HCC
              with intoxication,
              uncomplicated
    F18.921 Inhalant use, unspecified   CC HCC
              with intoxication with
              delirium
    F18.929 Inhalant use, unspecified   HCC
              with intoxication,
              unspecified

  F18.94 Inhalant use, unspecified with   HCC
          inhalant-induced mood disorder
    Inhalant induced depressive disorder

  ✓6ᵗʰ **F18.95 Inhalant use, unspecified with inhalant-induced**
          psychotic disorder
    F18.950 Inhalant use, unspecified   CC HCC
              with inhalant-induced
              psychotic disorder with
              delusions
    F18.951 Inhalant use, unspecified   CC HCC
              with inhalant-induced
              psychotic disorder with
              hallucinations
    F18.959 Inhalant use, unspecified   HCC
              with inhalant-induced
              psychotic disorder,
              unspecified

F18.97 Inhalant use, unspecified with inhalant-induced persisting dementia `CC` `HCC`

    Inhalant-induced major neurocognitive disorder

✓6ᵗʰ **F18.98 Inhalant use, unspecified with other inhalant-induced disorders**

    F18.980 Inhalant use, unspecified with inhalant-induced anxiety disorder `HCC`

    F18.988 Inhalant use, unspecified with other inhalant-induced disorder `HCC`

        Inhalant-induced mild neurocognitive disorder

    F18.99 Inhalant use, unspecified with unspecified inhalant-induced disorder `HCC`

✓4ᵗʰ **F19 Other psychoactive substance related disorders**

    `INCLUDES` polysubstance drug use (indiscriminate drug use)

✓5ᵗʰ **F19.1 Other psychoactive substance abuse**

    `EXCLUDES 1` *other psychoactive substance dependence (F19.2-)*

        other psychoactive substance use, unspecified (F19.9-)

    F19.10 Other psychoactive substance abuse, uncomplicated `HCC`

        Other (or unknown) substance use disorder, mild

    F19.11 Other psychoactive substance abuse, in remission `HCC`

        Other (or unknown) substance use disorder, mild, in early remission

        Other (or unknown) substance use disorder, mild, in sustained remission

✓6ᵗʰ **F19.12 Other psychoactive substance abuse with intoxication**

    F19.120 Other psychoactive substance abuse with intoxication, uncomplicated `HCC`

    F19.121 Other psychoactive substance abuse with intoxication delirium `CC` `HCC`

    F19.122 Other psychoactive substance abuse with intoxication with perceptual disturbances `HCC`

    F19.129 Other psychoactive substance abuse with intoxication, unspecified `HCC`

    F19.14 Other psychoactive substance abuse with psychoactive substance-induced mood disorder `HCC`

        Other (or unknown) substance use disorder, mild, with other (or unknown) substance-induced bipolar or related disorder

        Other (or unknown) substance use disorder, mild, with other (or unknown) substance-induced depressive disorder

✓6ᵗʰ **F19.15 Other psychoactive substance abuse with psychoactive substance-induced psychotic disorder**

    F19.150 Other psychoactive substance abuse with psychoactive substance-induced psychotic disorder with delusions `CC` `HCC`

    F19.151 Other psychoactive substance abuse with psychoactive substance-induced psychotic disorder with hallucinations `CC` `HCC`

    F19.159 Other psychoactive substance abuse with psychoactive substance-induced psychotic disorder, unspecified `HCC`

    F19.16 Other psychoactive substance abuse with psychoactive substance-induced persisting amnestic disorder `HCC`

F19.17 Other psychoactive substance abuse with psychoactive substance-induced persisting dementia `CC` `HCC`

    Other (or unknown) substance use disorder, mild, with other (or unknown) substance-induced major neurocognitive disorder

✓6ᵗʰ **F19.18 Other psychoactive substance abuse with other psychoactive substance-induced disorders**

    F19.180 Other psychoactive substance abuse with psychoactive substance-induced anxiety disorder `HCC`

    F19.181 Other psychoactive substance abuse with psychoactive substance-induced sexual dysfunction `HCC`

    F19.182 Other psychoactive substance abuse with psychoactive substance-induced sleep disorder `HCC`

    F19.188 Other psychoactive substance abuse with other psychoactive substance-induced disorder `HCC`

        Other (or unknown) substance use disorder, mild, with other (or unknown) substance induced mild neurocognitive disorder

        Other (or unknown) substance use disorder, mild, with other (or unknown) substance induced obsessive-compulsive or related disorder

F19.19 Other psychoactive substance abuse with unspecified psychoactive substance-induced disorder `HCC`

✓5ᵗʰ **F19.2 Other psychoactive substance dependence**

    `EXCLUDES 1` *other psychoactive substance abuse (F19.1-)*

        other psychoactive substance use, unspecified (F19.9-)

    F19.20 Other psychoactive substance dependence, uncomplicated `CC` `HCC`

        Other (or unknown) substance use disorder, moderate

        Other (or unknown) substance use disorder, severe

        CC Excl: No Excl

    F19.21 Other psychoactive substance dependence, in remission `HCC`

        Other (or unknown) substance use disorder, moderate, in early remission

        Other (or unknown) substance use disorder, moderate, in sustained remission

        Other (or unknown) substance use disorder, severe, in early remission

        Other (or unknown) substance use disorder, severe, in sustained remission

✓6ᵗʰ **F19.22 Other psychoactive substance dependence with intoxication**

    `EXCLUDES 1` *other psychoactive substance dependence with withdrawal (F19.23-)*

    F19.220 Other psychoactive substance dependence with intoxication, uncomplicated `HCC`

    F19.221 Other psychoactive substance dependence with intoxication delirium `CC` `HCC`

    F19.222 Other psychoactive substance dependence with intoxication with perceptual disturbance `CC` `HCC`

        CC Excl: No Excl

    F19.229 Other psychoactive substance dependence with intoxication, unspecified `HCC`

✔ Additional Character Required   ✓x7ᵗʰ Placeholder   Unacceptable PDx   Questionable PDx   Manifestation   Unspecified Dx   H1-H14 HAC   HCC CMS-HCC Dx   HIV HIV Dx

ICD-10-CM 2020

557

√6ᵗʰ **F19.23 Other psychoactive substance dependence with withdrawal**

> EXCLUDES 1   *other psychoactive substance dependence with intoxication (F19.22-)*

     F19.230 Other psychoactive substance dependence with withdrawal, uncomplicated

     F19.231 Other psychoactive substance dependence with withdrawal delirium CC HCC

     F19.232 Other psychoactive substance dependence with withdrawal with perceptual disturbance CC HCC

     F19.239 Other psychoactive substance dependence with withdrawal, unspecified CC HCC

F19.24 Other psychoactive substance dependence with psychoactive substance-induced mood disorder HCC

> Other (or unknown) substance use disorder, moderate, with other (or unknown) substance induced bipolar or related disorder
> Other (or unknown) substance use disorder, moderate, with other (or unknown) substance induced depressive disorder
> Other (or unknown) substance use disorder, severe, with other (or unknown) substance induced bipolar or related disorder
> Other (or unknown) substance use disorder, severe, with other (or unknown) substance induced depressive disorder

√6ᵗʰ **F19.25 Other psychoactive substance dependence with psychoactive substance-induced psychotic disorder**

     F19.250 Other psychoactive substance dependence with psychoactive substance-induced psychotic disorder with delusions CC HCC

     F19.251 Other psychoactive substance dependence with psychoactive substance-induced psychotic disorder with hallucinations CC HCC

     F19.259 Other psychoactive substance dependence with psychoactive substance-induced psychotic disorder, unspecified CC HCC
>   **CC Excl:** No Excl

F19.26 Other psychoactive substance dependence with psychoactive substance-induced persisting amnestic disorder CC HCC
>   **CC Excl:** No Excl

F19.27 Other psychoactive substance dependence with psychoactive substance-induced persisting dementia CC HCC
> Other (or unknown) substance use disorder, moderate, with other (or unknown) substance induced major neurocognitive disorder
> Other (or unknown) substance use disorder, severe, with other (or unknown) substance induced major neurocognitive disorder

√6ᵗʰ **F19.28 Other psychoactive substance dependence with other psychoactive substance-induced disorders**

     F19.280 Other psychoactive substance dependence with psychoactive substance-induced anxiety disorder CC HCC
>   **CC Excl:** No Excl

     F19.281 Other psychoactive substance dependence with psychoactive substance-induced sexual dysfunction CC HCC
>   **CC Excl:** No Excl

     F19.282 Other psychoactive substance dependence with psychoactive substance-induced sleep disorder CC HCC
>   **CC Excl:** No Excl

     F19.288 Other psychoactive substance dependence with other psychoactive substance-induced disorder CC HCC
> Other (or unknown) substance use disorder, moderate, with other (or unknown) substance induced mild neurocognitive disorder
> Other (or unknown) substance use disorder, severe, with other (or unknown) substance induced mild neurocognitive disorder
> Other (or unknown) substance use disorder, moderate, with other (or unknown) substance induced obsessive compulsive or related disorder
> Other (or unknown) substance use disorder, severe, with other (or unknown) substance induced obsessive-compulsive or related disorder
>   **CC Excl:** No Excl

F19.29 Other psychoactive substance dependence with unspecified psychoactive substance-induced disorder HCC

√5ᵗʰ **F19.9 Other psychoactive substance use, unspecified**

> EXCLUDES 1   *other psychoactive substance abuse (F19.1-)*
>   *other psychoactive substance dependence (F19.2-)*

   F19.90 Other psychoactive substance use, unspecified, uncomplicated
>   **AHA:** 2018,2Q,10-11

√6ᵗʰ **F19.92 Other psychoactive substance use, unspecified with intoxication**

> EXCLUDES 1   *other psychoactive substance use, unspecified with withdrawal (F19.93)*

     F19.920 Other psychoactive substance use, unspecified with intoxication, uncomplicated HCC

     F19.921 Other psychoactive substance use, unspecified with intoxication with delirium CC HCC
> Other (or unknown) substance-induced delirium

     F19.922 Other psychoactive substance use, unspecified with intoxication with perceptual disturbance HCC

     F19.929 Other psychoactive substance use, unspecified with intoxication, unspecified HCC

√6ᵗʰ **F19.93 Other psychoactive substance use, unspecified with withdrawal**

> EXCLUDES 1   *other psychoactive substance use, unspecified with intoxication (F19.92-)*

     F19.930 Other psychoactive substance use, unspecified with withdrawal, uncomplicated CC HCC

     F19.931 Other psychoactive substance use, unspecified with withdrawal delirium CC HCC

F19.932 Other psychoactive substance use, unspecified with withdrawal with perceptual disturbance   `CC` `HCC`

F19.939 Other psychoactive substance use, unspecified with withdrawal, unspecified   `CC` `HCC`

F19.94 Other psychoactive substance use, unspecified with psychoactive substance-induced mood disorder   `HCC`

Other (or unknown) substance-induced bipolar or related disorder, without use disorder

Other (or unknown) substance-induced depressive disorder, without use disorder

√6ᵗʰ **F19.95** Other psychoactive substance use, unspecified with psychoactive substance-induced psychotic disorder

F19.950 Other psychoactive substance use, unspecified with psychoactive substance-induced psychotic disorder with delusions   `CC` `HCC`

F19.951 Other psychoactive substance use, unspecified with psychoactive substance-induced psychotic disorder with hallucinations   `CC` `HCC`

F19.959 Other psychoactive substance use, unspecified with psychoactive substance-induced psychotic disorder, unspecified   `HCC`

Other or unknown substance-induced psychotic disorder, without use disorder

F19.96 Other psychoactive substance use, unspecified with psychoactive substance-induced persisting amnestic disorder   `HCC`

F19.97 Other psychoactive substance use, unspecified with psychoactive substance-induced persisting dementia   `CC` `HCC`

Other (or unknown) substance-induced major neurocognitive disorder, without use disorder

√6ᵗʰ **F19.98** Other psychoactive substance use, unspecified with other psychoactive substance-induced disorders

F19.980 Other psychoactive substance use, unspecified with psychoactive substance-induced anxiety disorder   `HCC`

Other (or unknown) substance-induced anxiety disorder, without use disorder

F19.981 Other psychoactive substance use, unspecified with psychoactive substance-induced sexual dysfunction   `HCC`

Other (or unknown) substance-induced sexual dysfunction, without use disorder

F19.982 Other psychoactive substance use, unspecified with psychoactive substance-induced sleep disorder   `HCC`

Other (or unknown) substance-induced sleep disorder, without use disorder

F19.988 Other psychoactive substance use, unspecified with other psychoactive substance-induced disorder   `HCC`

Other (or unknown) substance-induced mild neurocognitive disorder, without use disorder

Other (or unknown) substance-induced obsessive-compulsive or related disorder, without use disorder

F19.99 Other psychoactive substance use, unspecified with unspecified psychoactive substance-induced disorder   `HCC`

Schizophrenia, schizotypal, delusional, and other non-mood psychotic disorders (F20-F29)

√4ᵗʰ **F20 Schizophrenia**

EXCLUDES 1   brief psychotic disorder (F23)

cyclic schizophrenia (F25.0)

mood [affective] disorders with psychotic symptoms (F30.2, F31.2, F31.5, F31.64, F32.3, F33.3)

schizoaffective disorder (F25.-)

schizophrenic reaction NOS (F23)

EXCLUDES 2   schizophrenic reaction in:

alcoholism (F10.15-, F10.25-, F10.95-)

brain disease (F06.2)

epilepsy (F06.2)

psychoactive drug use (F11-F19 with .15. .25, .95)

schizotypal disorder (F21)

DEF: Group of disorders with disturbances in thought (delusions, hallucinations), mood (blunted, flattened, inappropriate affect), and sense of self. Schizophrenia also includes bizarre, purposeless behavior, repetitious activity, or inactivity.

CC Excl: For CC codes in category F20: PDX collection 551

F20.0 Paranoid schizophrenia   `CC` `HCC`

Paraphrenic schizophrenia

EXCLUDES 1   involutional paranoid state (F22)

paranoia (F22)

DEF: Preoccupied with delusional suspicions and auditory hallucinations related to a single theme. This type of schizophrenia is usually hostile, grandiose, threatening, persecutory, and occasionally hypochondriacal.

F20.1 Disorganized schizophrenia   `CC` `HCC`

Hebephrenic schizophrenia

Hebephrenia

F20.2 Catatonic schizophrenia   `CC` `HCC`

Schizophrenic catalepsy

Schizophrenic catatonia

Schizophrenic flexibilitas cerea

EXCLUDES 1   catatonic stupor (R40.1)

DEF: Extreme changes in motor activity. One extreme is a decreased response or reaction to the environment and the other is spontaneous activity.

F20.3 Undifferentiated schizophrenia   `HCC`

Atypical schizophrenia

EXCLUDES 1   acute schizophrenia-like psychotic disorder (F23)

EXCLUDES 2   post-schizophrenic depression (F32.89)

F20.5 Residual schizophrenia   `CC` `HCC`

Restzustand (schizophrenic)

Schizophrenic residual state

√5ᵗʰ **F20.8 Other schizophrenia**

F20.81 Schizophreniform disorder   `CC` `HCC`

Schizophreniform psychosis NOS

F20.89 Other schizophrenia   `CC` `HCC`

Cenesthopathic schizophrenia

Simple schizophrenia

F20.9 Schizophrenia, unspecified   `HCC`

AHA: 2019,2Q,32

F21 Schizotypal disorder   `HCC`

Borderline schizophrenia

Latent schizophrenia

Latent schizophrenic reaction

Prepsychotic schizophrenia

Prodromal schizophrenia

Pseudoneurotic schizophrenia

Pseudopsychopathic schizophrenia

Schizotypal personality disorder

EXCLUDES 2   Asperger's syndrome (F84.5)

schizoid personality disorder (F60.1)

DEF: Disorder characterized by various oddities of thinking, perception, communication, and behavior that may be manifested as magical thinking, ideas of reference, paranoid ideation, recurrent illusions and derealization (depersonalization), or social isolation.

☑ Additional Character Required   √×7ᵗʰ Placeholder   Unacceptable PDx   Questionable PDx   Manifestation   Unspecified Dx   `H1`-`H14` HAC   `HCC` CMS-HCC Dx   `HIV` HIV Dx

ICD-10-CM 2020   559

F22 Delusional disorders `CC` `HCC`
Delusional dysmorphophobia
Involutional paranoid state
Paranoia
Paranoia querulans
Paranoid psychosis
Paranoid state
Paraphrenia (late)
Sensitiver Beziehungswahn
EXCLUDES 1   *mood [affective] disorders with psychotic symptoms (F30.2,*
F31.2, F31.5, F31.64, F32.3, F33.3)
paranoid schizophrenia (F20.0)
EXCLUDES 2   *paranoid personality disorder (F60.0)*
paranoid psychosis, psychogenic (F23)
paranoid reaction (F23)

F23 Brief psychotic disorder `CC` `HCC`
Paranoid reaction
Psychogenic paranoid psychosis
EXCLUDES 2   *mood [affective] disorders with psychotic symptoms (F30.2,*
F31.2, F31.5, F31.64, F32.3, F33.3)
AHA: 2019,2Q,32
CC Excl: No Excl

F24 Shared psychotic disorder `HCC`
Folie à deux
Induced paranoid disorder
Induced psychotic disorder

✓4ᵗʰ **F25 Schizoaffective disorders**
EXCLUDES 1   *mood [affective] disorders with psychotic symptoms (F30.2,*
F31.2, F31.5, F31.64, F32.3, F33.3)
schizophrenia (F20.-)

   F25.0 Schizoaffective disorder, bipolar type `HCC`
Cyclic schizophrenia
Schizoaffective disorder, manic type
Schizoaffective disorder, mixed type
Schizoaffective psychosis, bipolar type

   F25.1 Schizoaffective disorder, depressive type `HCC`
Schizoaffective psychosis, depressive type

   F25.8 Other schizoaffective disorders `HCC`

   F25.9 Schizoaffective disorder, unspecified `HCC`
Schizoaffective psychosis NOS

F28 Other psychotic disorder not due to a substance or `HIV` `CC` `HCC`
known physiological condition
Chronic hallucinatory psychosis
Other specified schizophrenia spectrum and other psychotic disorder

F29 Unspecified psychosis not due to a substance or `HIV` `CC` `HCC`
known physiological condition
Psychosis NOS
Unspecified schizophrenia spectrum and other psychotic disorder
EXCLUDES 1   *mental disorder NOS (F99)*
unspecified mental disorder due to known physiological
condition (F09)

Mood [affective] disorders (F30-F39)

✓4ᵗʰ **F30 Manic episode**
INCLUDES   bipolar disorder, single manic episode
        mixed affective episode
EXCLUDES 1   *bipolar disorder (F31.-)*
major depressive disorder, recurrent (F33.-)
major depressive disorder, single episode (F32.-)
DEF: Mania: Characterized by abnormal states of elation or excitement
out of keeping with the individual's circumstances and varying from
enhanced liveliness (hypomania) to violent, almost uncontrollable,
excitement. Aggression and anger, flight of ideas, distractibility, impaired
judgment, and grandiose ideas are common.
CC Excl: For CC codes in category F30, unless otherwise noted: PDX
collection 551

  ✓5ᵗʰ **F30.1 Manic episode without psychotic symptoms**
     F30.10 Manic episode without psychotic `CC` `HCC`
symptoms, unspecified
     F30.11 Manic episode without psychotic `CC` `HCC`
symptoms, mild
     F30.12 Manic episode without psychotic `CC` `HCC`
symptoms, moderate

     F30.13 Manic episode, severe, without `CC` `HCC`
psychotic symptoms
CC Excl: PDX collection 552

  F30.2 Manic episode, severe with psychotic `CC` `HCC`
symptoms
Manic stupor
Mania with mood-congruent psychotic symptoms
Mania with mood-incongruent psychotic symptoms

  F30.3 Manic episode in partial remission `HCC`

  F30.4 Manic episode in full remission `HCC`

  F30.8 Other manic episodes `HCC`
Hypomania

  F30.9 Manic episode, unspecified `CC` `HCC`
Mania NOS

✓4ᵗʰ **F31 Bipolar disorder**
INCLUDES   bipolar I disorder
        bipolar type I disorder
        manic-depressive illness
        manic-depressive psychosis
        manic-depressive reaction
EXCLUDES 1   *bipolar disorder, single manic episode (F30.-)*
major depressive disorder, recurrent (F33.-)
major depressive disorder, single episode (F32.-)
EXCLUDES 2   *cyclothymia (F34.0)*
CC Excl: For CC codes in category F31, unless otherwise noted: PDX
collection 551

  F31.0 Bipolar disorder, current episode hypomanic `CC` `HCC`

  ✓5ᵗʰ **F31.1 Bipolar disorder, current episode manic without psychotic**
features
     F31.10 Bipolar disorder, current episode `CC` `HCC`
manic without psychotic features,
unspecified
     F31.11 Bipolar disorder, current episode `CC` `HCC`
manic without psychotic features,
mild
     F31.12 Bipolar disorder, current episode `CC` `HCC`
manic without psychotic features,
moderate
     F31.13 Bipolar disorder, current episode `CC` `HCC`
manic without psychotic features,
severe
CC Excl: PDX collection 553

  F31.2 Bipolar disorder, current episode manic `CC` `HCC`
severe with psychotic features
Bipolar disorder, current episode manic with mood-congruent
psychotic symptoms
Bipolar disorder, current episode manic with mood-incongruent
psychotic symptoms
Bipolar I disorder, current or most recent episode manic with
psychotic features

  ✓5ᵗʰ **F31.3 Bipolar disorder, current episode depressed, mild or**
moderate severity
     F31.30 Bipolar disorder, current episode `CC` `HCC`
depressed, mild or moderate
severity, unspecified
     F31.31 Bipolar disorder, current episode `CC` `HCC`
depressed, mild
     F31.32 Bipolar disorder, current episode `CC` `HCC`
depressed, moderate

  F31.4 Bipolar disorder, current episode depressed, `CC` `HCC`
severe, without psychotic features
CC Excl: PDX collection 554

  F31.5 Bipolar disorder, current episode depressed, `CC` `HCC`
severe, with psychotic features
Bipolar disorder, current episode depressed with
mood-congruent psychotic symptoms
Bipolar disorder, current episode depressed with
mood-incongruent psychotic symptoms
Bipolar I disorder, current or most recent episode depressed,
with psychotic features

  ✓5ᵗʰ **F31.6 Bipolar disorder, current episode mixed**
     F31.60 Bipolar disorder, current episode `CC` `HCC`
mixed, unspecified
     F31.61 Bipolar disorder, current episode `CC` `HCC`
mixed, mild
     F31.62 Bipolar disorder, current episode `CC` `HCC`
mixed, moderate

F31.63 **Bipolar disorder, current episode mixed, severe, without psychotic features** `CC` `HCC`
     CC Excl: PDX collection 554

F31.64 **Bipolar disorder, current episode mixed, severe, with psychotic features** `CC` `HCC`
     Bipolar disorder, current episode mixed with mood-congruent psychotic symptoms
     Bipolar disorder, current episode mixed with mood-incongruent psychotic symptoms

✓5ᵗʰ **F31.7 Bipolar disorder, currently in remission**

F31.70 **Bipolar disorder, currently in remission, most recent episode unspecified** `HCC`

F31.71 **Bipolar disorder, in partial remission, most recent episode hypomanic** `HCC`

F31.72 **Bipolar disorder, in full remission, most recent episode hypomanic** `HCC`

F31.73 **Bipolar disorder, in partial remission, most recent episode manic** `HCC`

F31.74 **Bipolar disorder, in full remission, most recent episode manic** `HCC`

F31.75 **Bipolar disorder, in partial remission, most recent episode depressed** `HCC`

F31.76 **Bipolar disorder, in full remission, most recent episode depressed** `HCC`

F31.77 **Bipolar disorder, in partial remission, most recent episode mixed** `HCC`

F31.78 **Bipolar disorder, in full remission, most recent episode mixed** `HCC`

✓5ᵗʰ **F31.8 Other bipolar disorders**

F31.81 **Bipolar II disorder** `HCC`
     Bipolar disorder, type 2

F31.89 **Other bipolar disorder** `HCC`
     Recurrent manic episodes NOS

F31.9 Bipolar disorder, unspecified `HCC`
     Manic depression

✓4ᵗʰ **F32 Major depressive disorder, single episode**

     INCLUDES   single episode of agitated depression
     single episode of depressive reaction
     single episode of major depression
     single episode of psychogenic depression
     single episode of reactive depression
     single episode of vital depression
     EXCLUDES 1   *bipolar disorder (F31.-)*
     manic episode (F30.-)
     recurrent depressive disorder (F33.-)
     EXCLUDES 2   *adjustment disorder (F43.2)*
     DEF: Mood disorder that produces depression that may exhibit as sadness, low self-esteem, or guilt feelings. Other manifestations may be withdrawal from friends and family and interrupted sleep.
     CC Excl: For CC codes in category F32: PDX collection 555

F32.0 Major depressive disorder, single episode, mild `HCC`

F32.1 Major depressive disorder, single episode, moderate `CC` `HCC`

F32.2 Major depressive disorder, single episode, severe without psychotic features `CC` `HCC`

F32.3 Major depressive disorder, single episode, severe with psychotic features `CC` `HCC`
     Single episode of major depression with mood-congruent psychotic symptoms
     Single episode of major depression with mood-incongruent psychotic symptoms
     Single episode of major depression with psychotic symptoms
     Single episode of psychogenic depressive psychosis
     Single episode of psychotic depression
     Single episode of reactive depressive psychosis

F32.4 Major depressive disorder, single episode, in partial remission `HCC`

F32.5 Major depressive disorder, single episode, in full remission `HCC`

✓5ᵗʰ **F32.8 Other depressive episodes**
     AHA: 2016,4Q,14

F32.81 **Premenstrual dysphoric disorder** ♀
     EXCLUDES 1   *premenstrual tension syndrome (N94.3)*
     DEF: Severe manifestation of premenstrual syndrome (PMS) that can be disabling and destructive to day-to-day activities. It can exacerbate pre-existing emotional disorders, like depression and anxiety, and cause feelings of loss of control, fatigue, and irritability.

F32.89 **Other specified depressive episodes**
     Atypical depression
     Post-schizophrenic depression
     Single episode of 'masked' depression NOS

F32.9 Major depressive disorder, single episode, unspecified
     Depression NOS
     Depressive disorder NOS
     Major depression NOS
     AHA: 2013,4Q,107

✓4ᵗʰ **F33 Major depressive disorder, recurrent**

     INCLUDES   recurrent episodes of depressive reaction
     recurrent episodes of endogenous depression
     recurrent episodes of major depression
     recurrent episodes of psychogenic depression
     recurrent episodes of reactive depression
     recurrent episodes of seasonal depressive disorder
     recurrent episodes of vital depression
     EXCLUDES 1   *bipolar disorder (F31.-)*
     manic episode (F30.-)
     DEF: Mood disorder that produces depression that may exhibit as sadness, low self-esteem, or guilt feelings. Other manifestations may be withdrawal from friends and family and interrupted sleep.
     CC Excl: For CC codes in category F33, unless otherwise noted: PDX collection 555

F33.0 Major depressive disorder, recurrent, mild `HCC`

F33.1 Major depressive disorder, recurrent, moderate `CC` `HCC`

F33.2 Major depressive disorder, recurrent, severe without psychotic features `CC` `HCC`

F33.3 Major depressive disorder, recurrent, severe with psychotic symptoms `CC` `HCC`
     Endogenous depression with psychotic symptoms
     Major depressive disorder, recurrent, with psychotic features
     Recurrent severe episodes of major depression with mood-congruent psychotic symptoms
     Recurrent severe episodes of major depression with mood-incongruent psychotic symptoms
     Recurrent severe episodes of major depression with psychotic symptoms
     Recurrent severe episodes of psychogenic depressive psychosis
     Recurrent severe episodes of psychotic depression
     Recurrent severe episodes of reactive depressive psychosis
     CC Excl: PDX collection 551

✓5ᵗʰ **F33.4 Major depressive disorder, recurrent, in remission**

F33.40 **Major depressive disorder, recurrent, in remission, unspecified** `CC` `HCC`

F33.41 **Major depressive disorder, recurrent, in partial remission** `HCC`

F33.42 **Major depressive disorder, recurrent, in full remission** `HCC`

F33.8 Other recurrent depressive disorders `CC` `HCC`
     Recurrent brief depressive episodes
     CC Excl: PDX collection 551

F33.9 Major depressive disorder, recurrent, unspecified `CC` `HCC`
     Monopolar depression NOS

✓4ᵗʰ **F34 Persistent mood [affective] disorders**

F34.0 Cyclothymic disorder
     Affective personality disorder
     Cycloid personality
     Cyclothymia
     Cyclothymic personality
     DEF: Mood disorder characterized by fast and repeated alterations between hypomanic and depressed moods.

Chapter 5. Mental, Behavioral and Neurodevelopmental Disorders *(left margin)*

F34.1 Dysthymic disorder
Depressive neurosis
Depressive personality disorder
Dysthymia
Neurotic depression
Persistent anxiety depression
Persistent depressive disorder
EXCLUDES 2   *anxiety depression (mild or not persistent) (F41.8)*
DEF: Depression without psychosis. It is a less severe but persistent depression and is considered a mild to moderate chronic form of depression.

√5th **F34.8 Other persistent mood [affective] disorders**
AHA: 2016,4Q,14

    F34.81 Disruptive mood dysregulation disorder `CC` `HCC`
      CC Excl: PDX collection 551

    F34.89 Other specified persistent mood disorders `CC` `HCC`
      CC Excl: PDX collection 551

F34.9 Persistent mood [affective] disorder, unspecified `CC` `HCC`
    CC Excl: PDX collection 551

F39 Unspecified mood [affective] disorder `HCC`
Affective psychosis NOS

Anxiety, dissociative, stress-related, somatoform and other nonpsychotic mental disorders (F40-F48)

√4th **F40 Phobic anxiety disorders**
DEF: Phobia: Broad-range anxiety with abnormally intense dread of certain objects or specific situations that would not normally have that effect.

√5th **F40.0 Agoraphobia**
DEF: Profound anxiety or fear of leaving familiar settings like home, or being in unfamiliar locations or with strangers or crowds. Agoraphobia may or may not be preceded by recurrent panic attacks.

    F40.00 Agoraphobia, unspecified
    F40.01 Agoraphobia with panic disorder
Panic disorder with agoraphobia
EXCLUDES 1   *panic disorder without agoraphobia (F41.0)*

    F40.02 Agoraphobia without panic disorder

√5th **F40.1 Social phobias**
Anthropophobia
Social anxiety disorder
Social anxiety disorder of childhood
Social neurosis
    F40.10 Social phobia, unspecified
    F40.11 Social phobia, generalized

√5th **F40.2 Specific (isolated) phobias**
EXCLUDES 2   *dysmorphophobia (nondelusional) (F45.22)*
      nosophobia (F45.22)

   √6th **F40.21 Animal type phobia**
      F40.210 Arachnophobia
        Fear of spiders
      F40.218 Other animal type phobia

   √6th **F40.22 Natural environment type phobia**
      F40.220 Fear of thunderstorms
      F40.228 Other natural environment type phobia

   √6th **F40.23 Blood, injection, injury type phobia**
      F40.230 Fear of blood
      F40.231 Fear of injections and transfusions
      F40.232 Fear of other medical care
      F40.233 Fear of injury

   √6th **F40.24 Situational type phobia**
      F40.240 Claustrophobia
      F40.241 Acrophobia
      F40.242 Fear of bridges
      F40.243 Fear of flying
      F40.248 Other situational type phobia

   √6th **F40.29 Other specified phobia**
      F40.290 Androphobia
        Fear of men
      F40.291 Gynephobia
        Fear of women
      F40.298 Other specified phobia

F40.8 Other phobic anxiety disorders
Phobic anxiety disorder of childhood

F40.9 Phobic anxiety disorder, unspecified
Phobia NOS
Phobic state NOS

√4th **F41 Other anxiety disorders**
EXCLUDES 2   *anxiety in:*
    acute stress reaction (F43.0)
    neurasthenia (F48.8)
    psychophysiologic disorders (F45.-)
    transient adjustment reaction (F43.2)
    separation anxiety (F93.0)

F41.0 Panic disorder [episodic paroxysmal anxiety]
Panic attack
Panic state
EXCLUDES 1   *panic disorder with agoraphobia (F40.01)*
DEF: Neurotic disorder characterized by recurrent panic or anxiety, apprehension, fear, or terror. Symptoms include shortness of breath, palpitations, dizziness, and shakiness; fear of dying may persist.

F41.1 Generalized anxiety disorder
Anxiety neurosis
Anxiety reaction
Anxiety state
Overanxious disorder
EXCLUDES 2   *neurasthenia (F48.8)*

F41.3 Other mixed anxiety disorders

F41.8 Other specified anxiety disorders
Anxiety depression (mild or not persistent)
Anxiety hysteria
Mixed anxiety and depressive disorder

F41.9 Anxiety disorder, unspecified
Anxiety NOS

√4th **F42 Obsessive-compulsive disorder**
EXCLUDES 2   *obsessive-compulsive personality (disorder) (F60.5)*
    obsessive-compulsive symptoms occurring in depression (F32-F33)
    obsessive-compulsive symptoms occurring in schizophrenia (F20.-)
AHA: 2016,4Q,14-15

F42.2 Mixed obsessional thoughts and acts

F42.3 Hoarding disorder

F42.4 Excoriation (skin-picking) disorder
EXCLUDES 1   *factitial dermatitis (L98.1)*
    other specified behavioral and emotional disorders with onset usually occurring in early childhood and adolescence (F98.8)

F42.8 Other obsessive-compulsive disorder
Anancastic neurosis
Obsessive-compulsive neurosis

F42.9 Obsessive-compulsive disorder, unspecified

√4th **F43 Reaction to severe stress, and adjustment disorders**

F43.0 Acute stress reaction
Acute crisis reaction
Acute reaction to stress
Combat and operational stress reaction
Combat fatigue
Crisis state
Psychic shock

√5th **F43.1 Post-traumatic stress disorder (PTSD)**
Traumatic neurosis
DEF: Preoccupation with traumatic events beyond normal experience (i.e., rape, personal assault, etc.) that may also include recurring flashbacks of the trauma. Symptoms include difficulty remembering, sleeping, or concentrating, and guilt feelings for surviving.

    F43.10 Post-traumatic stress disorder, unspecified
    F43.11 Post-traumatic stress disorder, acute
    F43.12 Post-traumatic stress disorder, chronic

√5th **F43.2 Adjustment disorders**
Culture shock
Grief reaction
Hospitalism in children
EXCLUDES 2   *separation anxiety disorder of childhood (F93.0)*

    F43.20 Adjustment disorder, unspecified

F43.21 Adjustment disorder with depressed mood
AHA: 2014,1Q,25
F43.22 Adjustment disorder with anxiety
F43.23 Adjustment disorder with mixed anxiety and depressed mood
F43.24 Adjustment disorder with disturbance of conduct
F43.25 Adjustment disorder with mixed disturbance of emotions and conduct
F43.29 Adjustment disorder with other symptoms
F43.8 Other reactions to severe stress
Other specified trauma and stressor-related disorder
F43.9 Reaction to severe stress, unspecified
Trauma and stressor-related disorder, NOS

F44 Dissociative and conversion disorders
INCLUDES   conversion hysteria
conversion reaction
hysteria
hysterical psychosis
EXCLUDES 2   malingering [conscious simulation] (Z76.5)
F44.0 Dissociative amnesia   HCC
EXCLUDES 1   amnesia NOS (R41.3)
anterograde amnesia (R41.1)
dissociative amnesia with dissociative fugue (F44.1)
retrograde amnesia (R41.2)
EXCLUDES 2   alcohol-or other psychoactive substance-induced amnestic disorder (F10, F13, F19 with .26, .96)
amnestic disorder due to known physiological condition (F04)
postictal amnesia in epilepsy (G40.-)
F44.1 Dissociative fugue   HCC
Dissociative amnesia with dissociative fugue
EXCLUDES 2   postictal fugue in epilepsy (G40.-)
DEF: Dissociative hysteria identified by memory loss and flight from familiar surroundings to a completely separate environment. Episodes may last hours or days. Conscious activity is not associated with perception of surroundings and there is no later memory of the episode.
F44.2 Dissociative stupor
EXCLUDES 1   catatonic stupor (R40.1)
stupor NOS (R40.1)
EXCLUDES 2   catatonic disorder due to known physiological condition (F06.1)
depressive stupor (F32, F33)
manic stupor (F30, F31)
F44.4 Conversion disorder with motor symptom or deficit
Conversion disorder with abnormal movement
Conversion disorder with speech symptoms
Conversion disorder with swallowing symptoms
Conversion disorder with weakness/paralysis
Dissociative motor disorders
Psychogenic aphonia
Psychogenic dysphonia
F44.5 Conversion disorder with seizures or convulsions
Conversion disorder with attacks or seizures
Dissociative convulsions
AHA: 2019,1Q,19
F44.6 Conversion disorder with sensory symptom or deficit
Conversion disorder with anesthesia or sensory loss
Conversion disorder with special sensory symptoms
Dissociative anesthesia and sensory loss
Psychogenic deafness
F44.7 Conversion disorder with mixed symptom presentation
F44.8 Other dissociative and conversion disorders
F44.81 Dissociative identity disorder   HCC
Multiple personality disorder
F44.89 Other dissociative and conversion disorders
Ganser's syndrome
Psychogenic confusion
Psychogenic twilight state
Trance and possession disorders
F44.9 Dissociative and conversion disorder, unspecified
Dissociative disorder NOS

F45 Somatoform disorders
EXCLUDES 2   dissociative and conversion disorders (F44.-)
factitious disorders (F68.1-, F68.A)
hair-plucking (F63.3)
lalling (F80.0)
lisping (F80.0)
malingering [conscious simulation] (Z76.5)
nail-biting (F98.8)
psychological or behavioral factors associated with disorders or diseases classified elsewhere (F54)
sexual dysfunction, not due to a substance or known physiological condition (F52.-)
thumb-sucking (F98.8)
tic disorders (in childhood and adolescence) (F95.-)
Tourette's syndrome (F95.2)
trichotillomania (F63.3)
DEF: Types of disorders causing inconsistent physical symptoms that cannot be explained.
F45.0 Somatization disorder
Briquet's disorder
Multiple psychosomatic disorder
F45.1 Undifferentiated somatoform disorder
Somatic symptom disorder
Undifferentiated psychosomatic disorder
F45.2 Hypochondriacal disorders
EXCLUDES 2   delusional dysmorphophobia (F22)
fixed delusions about bodily functions or shape (F22)
F45.20 Hypochondriacal disorder, unspecified
F45.21 Hypochondriasis
Hypochondriacal neurosis
Illness anxiety disorder
F45.22 Body dysmorphic disorder
Dysmorphophobia (nondelusional)
Nosophobia
F45.29 Other hypochondriacal disorders
F45.4 Pain disorders related to psychological factors
EXCLUDES 1   pain NOS (R52)
F45.41 Pain disorder exclusively related to psychological factors
Somatoform pain disorder (persistent)
F45.42 Pain disorder with related psychological factors
Code also associated acute or chronic pain (G89.-)
F45.8 Other somatoform disorders
Psychogenic dysmenorrhea
Psychogenic dysphagia, including 'globus hystericus'
Psychogenic pruritus
Psychogenic torticollis
Somatoform autonomic dysfunction
Teeth grinding
EXCLUDES 1   sleep related teeth grinding (G47.63)
F45.9 Somatoform disorder, unspecified
Psychosomatic disorder NOS

F48 Other nonpsychotic mental disorders
F48.1 Depersonalization-derealization syndrome   HCC
F48.2 Pseudobulbar affect
Involuntary emotional expression disorder
Code first underlying cause, if known, such as:
amyotrophic lateral sclerosis (G12.21)
multiple sclerosis (G35)
sequelae of cerebrovascular disease (I69.-)
sequelae of traumatic intracranial injury (S06.-)
F48.8 Other specified nonpsychotic mental disorders
Dhat syndrome
Neurasthenia
Occupational neurosis, including writer's cramp
Psychasthenia
Psychasthenic neurosis
Psychogenic syncope
F48.9 Nonpsychotic mental disorder, unspecified
Neurosis NOS

Chapter 5. Mental, Behavioral and Neurodevelopmental Disorders

Behavioral syndromes associated with physiological disturbances and physical factors (F50-F59)

✓4ᵗʰ **F50 Eating disorders**

EXCLUDES 1   anorexia NOS (R63.0)

         feeding difficulties (R63.3)

         feeding problems of newborn (P92.-)

         polyphagia (R63.2)

EXCLUDES 2   feeding disorder in infancy or childhood (F98.2-)

AHA: 2018,4Q,82

TIP: Assign additional code for BMI from category Z68, when documented. BMI can be based on documentation from clinicians who are not the patient's provider.

CC Excl: For CC codes in category F50, unless otherwise noted: PDX collection 556

✓5ᵗʰ **F50.0 Anorexia nervosa**

EXCLUDES 1   loss of appetite (R63.0)

         psychogenic loss of appetite (F50.89)

DEF: Psychological eating disorder characterized by an intense fear of gaining weight and an unrealistic perception of body image that perpetuates the feeling of being fat or having too much fat. Avoidance of food and restrictive or unhealthy eating are common.

   F50.00 Anorexia nervosa, unspecified `CC`

   F50.01 Anorexia nervosa, restricting type `CC`

   F50.02 Anorexia nervosa, binge eating/purging type `CC`

     EXCLUDES 1   bulimia nervosa (F50.2)

   F50.2 Bulimia nervosa `CC`

Bulimia NOS

Hyperorexia nervosa

EXCLUDES 1   anorexia nervosa, binge eating/purging type (F50.02)

DEF: Episodic pattern of overeating (binge eating) followed by purging or extreme exercise accompanied by an awareness of the abnormal eating pattern with a fear of not being able to stop eating.

CC Excl: PDX collection 557

✓5ᵗʰ **F50.8 Other eating disorders**

EXCLUDES 2   pica of infancy and childhood (F98.3)

AHA: 2017,4Q,9; 2016,4Q,15-16

   F50.81 Binge eating disorder

   F50.82 Avoidant/restrictive food intake disorder

   F50.89 Other specified eating disorder

     Pica in adults

     Psychogenic loss of appetite

   F50.9 Eating disorder, unspecified

Atypical anorexia nervosa

Atypical bulimia nervosa

Feeding or eating disorder, unspecified

Other specified feeding disorder

✓4ᵗʰ **F51 Sleep disorders not due to a substance or known physiological condition**

EXCLUDES 2   organic sleep disorders (G47.-)

✓5ᵗʰ **F51.0 Insomnia not due to a substance or known physiological condition**

EXCLUDES 2   alcohol related insomnia (F10.182, F10.282, F10.982)

         drug-related insomnia (F11.182, F11.282, F11.982, F13.182, F13.282, F13.982, F14.182, F14.282, F14.982, F15.182, F15.282, F15.982, F19.182, F19.282, F19.982)

         insomnia NOS (G47.0-)

         insomnia due to known physiological condition (G47.0-)

         organic insomnia (G47.0-)

         sleep deprivation (Z72.820)

   F51.01 Primary insomnia

     Idiopathic insomnia

   F51.02 Adjustment insomnia

   F51.03 Paradoxical insomnia

   F51.04 Psychophysiologic insomnia

   F51.05 Insomnia due to other mental disorder

     Code also associated mental disorder

   F51.09 Other insomnia not due to a substance or known physiological condition

✓5ᵗʰ **F51.1 Hypersomnia not due to a substance or known physiological condition**

EXCLUDES 2   alcohol related hypersomnia (F10.182, F10.282, F10.982)

         drug-related hypersomnia (F11.182, F11.282, F11.982, F13.182, F13.282, F13.982, F14.182, F14.282, F14.982, F15.182, F15.282, F15.982, F19.182, F19.282, F19.982)

         hypersomnia NOS (G47.10)

         hypersomnia due to known physiological condition (G47.10)

         idiopathic hypersomnia (G47.11, G47.12)

         narcolepsy (G47.4-)

   F51.11 Primary hypersomnia

   F51.12 Insufficient sleep syndrome

     EXCLUDES 1   sleep deprivation (Z72.820)

   F51.13 Hypersomnia due to other mental disorder

     Code also associated mental disorder

   F51.19 Other hypersomnia not due to a substance or known physiological condition

   F51.3 Sleepwalking [somnambulism]

Non-rapid eye movement sleep arousal disorders, sleepwalking type

   F51.4 Sleep terrors [night terrors]

Non-rapid eye movement sleep arousal disorders, sleep terror type

   F51.5 Nightmare disorder

Dream anxiety disorder

   F51.8 Other sleep disorders not due to a substance or known physiological condition

   F51.9 Sleep disorder not due to a substance or known physiological condition, unspecified

Emotional sleep disorder NOS

✓4ᵗʰ **F52 Sexual dysfunction not due to a substance or known physiological condition**

EXCLUDES 2   Dhat syndrome (F48.8)

   F52.0 Hypoactive sexual desire disorder

Lack or loss of sexual desire

Male hypoactive sexual desire disorder

Sexual anhedonia

EXCLUDES 1   decreased libido (R68.82)

   F52.1 Sexual aversion disorder

Sexual aversion and lack of sexual enjoyment

✓5ᵗʰ **F52.2 Sexual arousal disorders**

Failure of genital response

   F52.21 Male erectile disorder ♂

     Erectile disorder

     Psychogenic impotence

     EXCLUDES 1   impotence of organic origin (N52.-)

             impotence NOS (N52.-)

   F52.22 Female sexual arousal disorder ♀

     Female sexual interest/arousal disorder

✓5ᵗʰ **F52.3 Orgasmic disorder**

Inhibited orgasm

Psychogenic anorgasmy

   F52.31 Female orgasmic disorder ♀

   F52.32 Male orgasmic disorder ♂

     Delayed ejaculation

   F52.4 Premature ejaculation ♂

   F52.5 Vaginismus not due to a substance or known physiological condition ♀

Psychogenic vaginismus

EXCLUDES 2   vaginismus (due to a known physiological condition) (N94.2)

DEF: Psychogenic response resulting in painful contractions of the vaginal canal muscles. This condition can be severe enough to prevent sexual intercourse.

   F52.6 Dyspareunia not due to a substance or known physiological condition

Genito-pelvic pain penetration disorder

Psychogenic dyspareunia

EXCLUDES 2   dyspareunia (due to a known physiological condition) (N94.1-)

N Newborn: 0   P Pediatric: 0-17   M Maternity: 9-64   A Adult: 15-124   MCC Major Complication/Comorbidity   CC Complication/Comorbidity   SW Severe Wound Dx

564   ICD-10-CM 2020

F52.8   **Other sexual dysfunction not due to a substance or known physiological condition**
> Excessive sexual drive
> Nymphomania
> Satyriasis

F52.9   **Unspecified sexual dysfunction not due to a substance or known physiological condition**
> Sexual dysfunction NOS

√4th **F53**   **Mental and behavioral disorders associated with the puerperium, not elsewhere classified**
> EXCLUDES 1   mood disorders with psychotic features (F30.2, F31.2, F31.5, F31.64, F32.3, F33.3)
> postpartum dysphoria (O90.6)
> psychosis in schizophrenia, schizotypal, delusional, and other psychotic disorders (F20-F29)

> AHA: 2018,4Q,8

F53.0   **Postpartum depression**   M ♀
> Postnatal depression, NOS
> Postpartum depression, NOS

F53.1   **Puerperal psychosis**   HCC M ♀
> Postpartum psychosis
> Puerperal psychosis, NOS

F54   *Psychological and behavioral factors associated with disorders or diseases classified elsewhere*
> Psychological factors affecting physical conditions
> Code first the associated physical disorder, such as:
>   asthma (J45.-)
>   dermatitis (L23-L25)
>   gastric ulcer (K25.-)
>   mucous colitis (K58.-)
>   ulcerative colitis (K51.-)
>   urticaria (L50.-)
> EXCLUDES 2   tension-type headache (G44.2)

√4th **F55**   **Abuse of non-psychoactive substances**
> EXCLUDES 2   abuse of psychoactive substances (F10-F19)

F55.0   **Abuse of antacids**

F55.1   **Abuse of herbal or folk remedies**

F55.2   **Abuse of laxatives**

F55.3   **Abuse of steroids or hormones**

F55.4   **Abuse of vitamins**

F55.8   **Abuse of other non-psychoactive substances**

F59   **Unspecified behavioral syndromes associated with physiological disturbances and physical factors**
> Psychogenic physiological dysfunction NOS

Disorders of adult personality and behavior (F60-F69)

√4th **F60**   **Specific personality disorders**

F60.0   **Paranoid personality disorder**   HCC
> Expansive paranoid personality (disorder)
> Fanatic personality (disorder)
> Paranoid personality (disorder)
> Querulant personality (disorder)
> Sensitive paranoid personality (disorder)
> EXCLUDES 2   paranoia (F22)
>   paranoia querulans (F22)
>   paranoid psychosis (F22)
>   paranoid schizophrenia (F20.0)
>   paranoid state (F22)

F60.1   **Schizoid personality disorder**   HCC
> EXCLUDES 2   Asperger's syndrome (F84.5)
>   delusional disorder (F22)
>   schizoid disorder of childhood (F84.5)
>   schizophrenia (F20.-)
>   schizotypal disorder (F21)

F60.2   **Antisocial personality disorder**   HCC
> Amoral personality (disorder)
> Asocial personality (disorder)
> Dissocial personality disorder
> Psychopathic personality (disorder)
> Sociopathic personality (disorder)
> EXCLUDES 1   conduct disorders (F91.-)
> EXCLUDES 2   borderline personality disorder (F60.3)

F60.3   **Borderline personality disorder**   HCC
> Aggressive personality (disorder)
> Emotionally unstable personality disorder
> Explosive personality (disorder)
> EXCLUDES 2   antisocial personality disorder (F60.2)

F60.4   **Histrionic personality disorder**   HCC
> Hysterical personality (disorder)
> Psychoinfantile personality (disorder)

F60.5   **Obsessive-compulsive personality disorder**   HCC
> Anankastic personality (disorder)
> Compulsive personality (disorder)
> Obsessional personality (disorder)
> EXCLUDES 2   obsessive-compulsive disorder (F42-)

F60.6   **Avoidant personality disorder**   HCC
> Anxious personality disorder

F60.7   **Dependent personality disorder**   HCC
> Asthenic personality (disorder)
> Inadequate personality (disorder)
> Passive personality (disorder)
> **DEF:** Lack of self-confidence, fear of abandonment, and an obsessive need to be taken care of.

√5th **F60.8**   **Other specific personality disorders**

     F60.81   **Narcissistic personality disorder**   HCC

     F60.89   **Other specific personality disorders**   HCC
>   Eccentric personality disorder
>   "Haltlose" type personality disorder
>   Immature personality disorder
>   Passive-aggressive personality disorder
>   Psychoneurotic personality disorder
>   Self-defeating personality disorder

F60.9   **Personality disorder, unspecified**   HCC
> Character disorder NOS
> Character neurosis NOS
> Pathological personality NOS

√4th **F63**   **Impulse disorders**
> EXCLUDES 2   habitual excessive use of alcohol or psychoactive substances (F10-F19)
>   impulse disorders involving sexual behavior (F65.-)

F63.0   **Pathological gambling**
> Compulsive gambling
> Gambling disorder
> EXCLUDES 1   gambling and betting NOS (Z72.6)
> EXCLUDES 2   excessive gambling by manic patients (F30, F31)
>   gambling in antisocial personality disorder (F60.2)

F63.1   **Pyromania**
> Pathological fire-setting
> EXCLUDES 2   fire-setting (by) (in):
>   adult with antisocial personality disorder (F60.2)
>   alcohol or psychoactive substance intoxication (F10-F19)
>   conduct disorders (F91.-)
>   mental disorders due to known physiological condition (F01-F09)
>   schizophrenia (F20.-)

F63.2   **Kleptomania**
> Pathological stealing
> EXCLUDES 1   shoplifting as the reason for observation for suspected mental disorder (Z03.8)
> EXCLUDES 2   depressive disorder with stealing (F31-F33)
>   stealing due to underlying mental condition - code to mental condition
>   stealing in mental disorders due to known physiological condition (F01-F09)

F63.3   **Trichotillomania**
> Hair plucking
> EXCLUDES 2   other stereotyped movement disorder (F98.4)

√5th **F63.8**   **Other impulse disorders**

     F63.81   **Intermittent explosive disorder**

     F63.89   **Other impulse disorders**   CC

F63.9   **Impulse disorder, unspecified**   CC
> Impulse control disorder NOS

✔ Additional Character Required   √x7th Placeholder   Unacceptable PDx   Questionable PDx   Manifestation   Unspecified Dx   H1-H14 HAC   HCC CMS-HCC Dx   HIV HIV Dx

ICD-10-CM 2020   565

Chapter 5. Mental, Behavioral and Neurodevelopmental Disorders

F64–F80.4

✓4ᵗʰ F64 Gender identity disorders
AHA: 2016,4Q,16

F64.0 Transsexualism
Gender identity disorder in adolescence and adulthood
Gender dysphoria in adolescents and adults

F64.1 Dual role transvestism
Use additional code to identify sex reassignment status (Z87.890)
> EXCLUDES 1   *gender identity disorder in childhood (F64.2)*
> EXCLUDES 2   *fetishistic transvestism (F65.1)*

F64.2 Gender identity disorder of childhood   P
Gender dysphoria in children
> EXCLUDES 1   *gender identity disorder in adolescence and adulthood (F64.0)*
> EXCLUDES 2   *sexual maturation disorder (F66)*

F64.8 Other gender identity disorders
Other specified gender dysphoria

F64.9 Gender identity disorder, unspecified
Gender dysphoria, unspecified
Gender-role disorder NOS

✓4ᵗʰ F65 Paraphilias

F65.0 Fetishism
Fetishistic disorder

F65.1 Transvestic fetishism
Fetishistic transvestism
Transvestic disorder

F65.2 Exhibitionism
Exhibitionistic disorder

F65.3 Voyeurism
Voyeuristic disorder

F65.4 Pedophilia
Pedophilic disorder

✓5ᵗʰ **F65.5 Sadomasochism**

     F65.50 Sadomasochism, unspecified

     F65.51 Sexual masochism
         Sexual masochism disorder

     F65.52 Sexual sadism
         Sexual sadism disorder

✓5ᵗʰ **F65.8 Other paraphilias**

     F65.81 Frotteurism
         Frotteuristic disorder

     F65.89 Other paraphilias
         Necrophilia
         Other specified paraphilic disorder

F65.9 Paraphilia, unspecified
Paraphilic disorder, unspecified
Sexual deviation NOS

F66 Other sexual disorders
Sexual maturation disorder
Sexual relationship disorder

✓4ᵗʰ F68 Other disorders of adult personality and behavior
AHA: 2018,4Q,9,65
CC Excl: For CC codes in category F68: PDX collection 551

✓5ᵗʰ **F68.1 Factitious disorder imposed on self**
Compensation neurosis
Elaboration of physical symptoms for psychological reasons
Hospital hopper syndrome
Münchausen's syndrome
Peregrinating patient
> EXCLUDES 2   *factitial dermatitis (L98.1)*
>   *person feigning illness (with obvious motivation) (Z76.5)*

     F68.10 Factitious disorder imposed on self, unspecified   CC

     F68.11 Factitious disorder imposed on self, with predominantly psychological signs and symptoms

     F68.12 Factitious disorder imposed on self, with predominantly physical signs and symptoms   CC

     F68.13 Factitious disorder imposed on self, with combined psychological and physical signs and symptoms

F68.A Factitious disorder imposed on another   CC
Factitious disorder by proxy
Münchausen's by proxy

F68.8 Other specified disorders of adult personality and behavior

F69 Unspecified disorder of adult personality and behavior   A

Intellectual disabilities (F70-F79)
Code first any associated physical or developmental disorders
> EXCLUDES 1   *borderline intellectual functioning, IQ above 70 to 84 (R41.83)*

F70 Mild intellectual disabilities
IQ level 50-55 to approximately 70
Mild mental subnormality

F71 Moderate intellectual disabilities
IQ level 35-40 to 50-55
Moderate mental subnormality

F72 Severe intellectual disabilities
IQ 20-25 to 35-40
Severe mental subnormality

F73 Profound intellectual disabilities
IQ level below 20-25
Profound mental subnormality

F78 Other intellectual disabilities

F79 Unspecified intellectual disabilities
Mental deficiency NOS
Mental subnormality NOS

Pervasive and specific developmental disorders (F80-F89)

✓4ᵗʰ F80 Specific developmental disorders of speech and language

F80.0 Phonological disorder
Dyslalia
Functional speech articulation disorder
Lalling
Lisping
Phonological developmental disorder
Speech articulation developmental disorder
Speech-sound disorder
> EXCLUDES 1   *speech articulation impairment due to aphasia NOS (R47.01)*
>   *speech articulation impairment due to apraxia (R48.2)*
> EXCLUDES 2   *speech articulation impairment due to hearing loss (F80.4)*
>   *speech articulation impairment due to intellectual disabilities (F70-F79)*
>   *speech articulation impairment with expressive language developmental disorder (F80.1)*
>   *speech articulation impairment with mixed receptive expressive language developmental disorder (F80.2)*

F80.1 Expressive language disorder
Developmental dysphasia or aphasia, expressive type
> EXCLUDES 1   *mixed receptive-expressive language disorder (F80.2)*
>   *dysphasia and aphasia NOS (R47.-)*
> EXCLUDES 2   *acquired aphasia with epilepsy [Landau-Kleffner] (G40.80-)*
>   *selective mutism (F94.0)*
>   *intellectual disabilities (F70-F79)*
>   *pervasive developmental disorders (F84.-)*

F80.2 Mixed receptive-expressive language disorder
Developmental dysphasia or aphasia, receptive type
Developmental Wernicke's aphasia
> EXCLUDES 1   *central auditory processing disorder (H93.25)*
>   *dysphasia or aphasia NOS (R47.-)*
>   *expressive language disorder (F80.1)*
>   *expressive type dysphasia or aphasia (F80.1)*
>   *word deafness (H93.25)*
> EXCLUDES 2   *acquired aphasia with epilepsy [Landau-Kleffner] (G40.80-)*
>   *pervasive developmental disorders (F84.-)*
>   *selective mutism (F94.0)*
>   *intellectual disabilities (F70-F79)*

F80.4 Speech and language development delay due to hearing loss
Code also type of hearing loss (H90.-, H91.-)

N Newborn: 0   P Pediatric: 0-17   M Maternity: 9-64   A Adult: 15-124   MCC Major Complication/Comorbidity   CC Complication/Comorbidity   SW Severe Wound Dx

566   ICD-10-CM 2020

✓5ᵗʰ F80.8 Other developmental disorders of speech and language
> AHA: 2017,1Q,27

> **F80.81 Childhood onset fluency disorder**
> > Cluttering NOS
> > Stuttering NOS
> > EXCLUDES 1   *adult onset fluency disorder (F98.5)*
> > > *fluency disorder in conditions classified elsewhere (R47.82)*
> > > *fluency disorder (stuttering) following cerebrovascular disease (I69. with final characters -23)*

> **F80.82 Social pragmatic communication disorder**
> > EXCLUDES 1   *Asperger's syndrome (F84.5)*
> > > *autistic disorder (F84.0)*
> > AHA: 2016,4Q,16

> **F80.89 Other developmental disorders of speech and language**

F80.9 Developmental disorder of speech and language, unspecified
> Communication disorder NOS
> Language disorder NOS

✓4ᵗʰ F81 Specific developmental disorders of scholastic skills

> **F81.0 Specific reading disorder**
> > "Backward reading"
> > Developmental dyslexia
> > Specific learning disorder, with impairment in reading
> > Specific reading retardation
> > EXCLUDES 1   *alexia NOS (R48.0)*
> > > *dyslexia NOS (R48.0)*
> > DEF: Serious impairment of reading skills unexplained in relation to general intelligence and teaching processes.

> **F81.2 Mathematics disorder**
> > Developmental acalculia
> > Developmental arithmetical disorder
> > Developmental Gerstmann's syndrome
> > Specific learning disorder, with impairment in mathematics
> > EXCLUDES 1   *acalculia NOS (R48.8)*
> > EXCLUDES 2   *arithmetical difficulties associated with a reading disorder (F81.0)*
> > > *arithmetical difficulties associated with a spelling disorder (F81.81)*
> > > *arithmetical difficulties due to inadequate teaching (Z55.8)*

> **✓5ᵗʰ F81.8 Other developmental disorders of scholastic skills**
> > **F81.81 Disorder of written expression**
> > > Specific learning disorder, with impairment in written expression
> > > Specific spelling disorder
> > **F81.89 Other developmental disorders of scholastic skills**

F81.9 Developmental disorder of scholastic skills, unspecified
> Knowledge acquisition disability NOS
> Learning disability NOS
> Learning disorder NOS

F82 Specific developmental disorder of motor function
> Clumsy child syndrome
> Developmental coordination disorder
> Developmental dyspraxia
> EXCLUDES 1   *abnormalities of gait and mobility (R26.-)*
> > *lack of coordination (R27.-)*
> EXCLUDES 2   *lack of coordination secondary to intellectual disabilities (F70-F79)*

✓4ᵗʰ F84 Pervasive developmental disorders
> Use additional code to identify any associated medical condition and intellectual disabilities.

> **F84.0 Autistic disorder**
> > Autism spectrum disorder
> > Infantile autism
> > Infantile psychosis
> > Kanner's syndrome
> > EXCLUDES 1   *Asperger's syndrome (F84.5)*
> > AHA: 2017,1Q,27

> **F84.2 Rett's syndrome**
> > EXCLUDES 1   *Asperger's syndrome (F84.5)*
> > > *autistic disorder (F84.0)*
> > > *other childhood disintegrative disorder (F84.3)*

F84.3 Other childhood disintegrative disorder   CC P
> Dementia infantilis
> Disintegrative psychosis
> Heller's syndrome
> Symbiotic psychosis
> Use additional code to identify any associated neurological condition
> EXCLUDES 1   *Asperger's syndrome (F84.5)*
> > *autistic disorder (F84.0)*
> > *Rett's syndrome (F84.2)*
> CC Excl: PDX collection 551

F84.5 Asperger's syndrome
> Asperger's disorder
> Autistic psychopathy
> Schizoid disorder of childhood
> DEF: High-functioning form of autism. Children with this syndrome usually develop speech on schedule, are generally very intelligent, and communicate well, but have considerable social shortcomings. *Synonym(s): AS.*

F84.8 Other pervasive developmental disorders
> Overactive disorder associated with intellectual disabilities and stereotyped movements

F84.9 Pervasive developmental disorder, unspecified
> Atypical autism

F88 Other disorders of psychological development
> Developmental agnosia
> Global developmental delay
> Other specified neurodevelopmental disorder

F89 Unspecified disorder of psychological development
> Developmental disorder NOS
> Neurodevelopmental disorder NOS

Behavioral and emotional disorders with onset usually occurring in childhood and adolescence (F90-F98)

> NOTE   Codes within categories F90-F98 may be used regardless of the age of a patient. These disorders generally have onset within the childhood or adolescent years, but may continue throughout life or not be diagnosed until adulthood

✓4ᵗʰ F90 Attention-deficit hyperactivity disorders
> INCLUDES   attention deficit disorder with hyperactivity
> > attention deficit syndrome with hyperactivity
> EXCLUDES 2   *anxiety disorders (F40.-, F41.-)*
> > *mood [affective] disorders (F30-F39)*
> > *pervasive developmental disorders (F84.-)*
> > *schizophrenia (F20.-)*

> **F90.0 Attention-deficit hyperactivity disorder, predominantly inattentive type**
> > Attention-deficit/hyperactivity disorder, predominantly inattentive presentation

> **F90.1 Attention-deficit hyperactivity disorder, predominantly hyperactive type**
> > Attention-deficit/hyperactivity disorder, predominantly hyperactive impulsive presentation

> **F90.2 Attention-deficit hyperactivity disorder, combined type**
> > Attention-deficit/hyperactivity disorder, combined presentation

> **F90.8 Attention-deficit hyperactivity disorder, other type**

F90.9 Attention-deficit hyperactivity disorder, unspecified type
> Attention-deficit hyperactivity disorder of childhood or adolescence NOS
> Attention-deficit hyperactivity disorder NOS

✓4ᵗʰ F91 Conduct disorders
> EXCLUDES 1   *antisocial behavior (Z72.81-)*
> > *antisocial personality disorder (F60.2)*
> EXCLUDES 2   *conduct problems associated with attention-deficit hyperactivity disorder (F90.-)*
> > *mood [affective] disorders (F30-F39)*
> > *pervasive developmental disorders (F84.-)*
> > *schizophrenia (F20.-)*

> **F91.0 Conduct disorder confined to family context**
> **F91.1 Conduct disorder, childhood-onset type**
> > Unsocialized conduct disorder
> > Conduct disorder, solitary aggressive type
> > Unsocialized aggressive disorder

✓ Additional Character Required   ✓x7ᵗʰ Placeholder   Unacceptable PDx   Questionable PDx   Manifestation   Unspecified Dx   H1-H14 HAC   HCC CMS-HCC Dx   HIV HIV Dx

ICD-10-CM 2020   567

Chapter 5. Mental, Behavioral and Neurodevelopmental Disorders

F91.2   Conduct disorder, adolescent-onset type
Socialized conduct disorder
Conduct disorder, group type

F91.3   Oppositional defiant disorder

F91.8   Other conduct disorders
Other specified conduct disorder
Other specified disruptive disorder

F91.9   Conduct disorder, unspecified
Behavioral disorder NOS
Conduct disorder NOS
Disruptive behavior disorder NOS
Disruptive disorder NOS

✓4ᵗʰ **F93   Emotional disorders with onset specific to childhood**

F93.0   Separation anxiety disorder of childhood
     EXCLUDES 2   mood [affective] disorders (F30-F39)
                nonpsychotic mental disorders (F40-F48)
                phobic anxiety disorder of childhood (F40.8)
                social phobia (F40.1)

F93.8   Other childhood emotional disorders
Identity disorder
     EXCLUDES 2   gender identity disorder of childhood (F64.2)

F93.9   Childhood emotional disorder, unspecified

✓4ᵗʰ **F94   Disorders of social functioning with onset specific to childhood and adolescence**

F94.0   Selective mutism
Elective mutism
     EXCLUDES 2   pervasive developmental disorders (F84.-)
                schizophrenia (F20.-)
                specific developmental disorders of speech and language (F80.-)
                transient mutism as part of separation anxiety in young children (F93.0)

F94.1   Reactive attachment disorder of childhood
Use additional code to identify any associated failure to thrive or growth retardation
     EXCLUDES 1   disinhibited attachment disorder of childhood (F94.2)
                normal variation in pattern of selective attachment
     EXCLUDES 2   Asperger's syndrome (F84.5)
                maltreatment syndromes (T74.-)
                sexual or physical abuse in childhood, resulting in psychosocial problems (Z62.81-)

F94.2   Disinhibited attachment disorder of childhood
Affectionless psychopathy
Institutional syndrome
     EXCLUDES 1   reactive attachment disorder of childhood (F94.1)
     EXCLUDES 2   Asperger's syndrome (F84.5)
                attention-deficit hyperactivity disorders (F90.-)
                hospitalism in children (F43.2-)

F94.8   Other childhood disorders of social functioning

F94.9   Childhood disorder of social functioning, unspecified

✓4ᵗʰ **F95   Tic disorder**

F95.0   Transient tic disorder
Provisional tic disorder

F95.1   Chronic motor or vocal tic disorder

F95.2   Tourette's disorder
Combined vocal and multiple motor tic disorder [de la Tourette]
Tourette's syndrome

F95.8   Other tic disorders

F95.9   Tic disorder, unspecified
Tic NOS

✓4ᵗʰ **F98   Other behavioral and emotional disorders with onset usually occurring in childhood and adolescence**
     EXCLUDES 2   breath-holding spells (R06.89)
                gender identity disorder of childhood (F64.2)
                Kleine-Levin syndrome (G47.13)
                obsessive-compulsive disorder (F42-)
                sleep disorders not due to a substance or known physiological condition (F51.-)

F98.0   Enuresis not due to a substance or known physiological condition
Enuresis (primary) (secondary) of nonorganic origin
Functional enuresis
Psychogenic enuresis
Urinary incontinence of nonorganic origin
     EXCLUDES 1   enuresis NOS (R32)

F98.1   Encopresis not due to a substance or known physiological condition
Functional encopresis
Incontinence of feces of nonorganic origin
Psychogenic encopresis
Use additional code to identify the cause of any coexisting constipation
     EXCLUDES 1   encopresis NOS (R15.-)

✓5ᵗʰ **F98.2   Other feeding disorders of infancy and childhood**
     EXCLUDES 1   feeding difficulties (R63.3)
     EXCLUDES 2   anorexia nervosa and other eating disorders (F50.-)
                feeding problems of newborn (P92.-)
                pica of infancy or childhood (F98.3)

F98.21   Rumination disorder of infancy

F98.29   Other feeding disorders of infancy and early childhood

F98.3   Pica of infancy and childhood

F98.4   Stereotyped movement disorders
Stereotype/habit disorder
     EXCLUDES 1   abnormal involuntary movements (R25.-)
     EXCLUDES 2   compulsions in obsessive-compulsive disorder (F42-)
                hair plucking (F63.3)
                movement disorders of organic origin (G20-G25)
                nail-biting (F98.8)
                nose-picking (F98.8)
                stereotypies that are part of a broader psychiatric condition (F01-F95)
                thumb-sucking (F98.8)
                tic disorders (F95.-)
                trichotillomania (F63.3)

F98.5   Adult onset fluency disorder
     EXCLUDES 1   childhood onset fluency disorder (F80.81)
                dysphasia (R47.02)
                fluency disorder in conditions classified elsewhere (R47.82)
                fluency disorder (stuttering) following cerebrovascular disease (I69. with final characters -23)
                tic disorders (F95.-)

F98.8   Other specified behavioral and emotional disorders with onset usually occurring in childhood and adolescence
Excessive masturbation
Nail-biting
Nose-picking
Thumb-sucking

F98.9   Unspecified behavioral and emotional disorders with onset usually occurring in childhood and adolescence

Unspecified mental disorder (F99)

F99   Mental disorder, not otherwise specified
Mental illness NOS
     EXCLUDES 1   unspecified mental disorder due to known physiological condition (F09)

Ⓝ Newborn: 0   Ⓟ Pediatric: 0-17   Ⓜ Maternity: 9-64   Ⓐ Adult: 15-124   **MCC** Major Complication/Comorbidity   **CC** Complication/Comorbidity   **SW** Severe Wound Dx

568   ICD-10-CM 2020

Chapter 6. Diseases of the Nervous System (G00-G99)

Chapter-specific Guidelines with Coding Examples

The chapter-specific guidelines from the ICD-10-CM Official Guidelines for Coding and Reporting have been provided below. Along with these guidelines are coding examples, contained in the shaded boxes, that have been developed to help illustrate the coding and/or sequencing guidance found in these guidelines.

a. Dominant/nondominant side

Codes from category G81, Hemiplegia and hemiparesis, and subcategories G83.1, Monoplegia of lower limb, G83.2, Monoplegia of upper limb, and G83.3, Monoplegia, unspecified, identify whether the dominant or nondominant side is affected. Should the affected side be documented, but not specified as dominant or nondominant, and the classification system does not indicate a default, code selection is as follows:

- For ambidextrous patients, the default should be dominant.
- If the left side is affected, the default is non-dominant.
- If the right side is affected, the default is dominant.

> Hemiplegia affecting left side of ambidextrous patient
>
> **G81.92   Hemiplegia, unspecified affecting left dominant side**
>
> *Explanation*: Documentation states that the left side is affected and dominant is used for ambidextrous persons.

> Right spastic hemiplegia, unknown whether patient is right- or left-handed
>
> **G81.11   Spastic hemiplegia affecting right dominant side**
>
> *Explanation*: Since it is unknown whether the patient is right- or left-handed, if the right side is affected, the default is dominant.

b. Pain—category G89

1) General coding information

Codes in category G89, Pain, not elsewhere classified, may be used in conjunction with codes from other categories and chapters to provide more detail about acute or chronic pain and neoplasm-related pain, unless otherwise indicated below.

If the pain is not specified as acute or chronic, post-thoracotomy, postprocedural, or neoplasm-related, do not assign codes from category G89.

A code from category G89 should not be assigned if the underlying (definitive) diagnosis is known, unless the reason for the encounter is pain control/management and not management of the underlying condition.

When an admission or encounter is for a procedure aimed at treating the underlying condition (e.g., spinal fusion, kyphoplasty), a code for the underlying condition (e.g., vertebral fracture, spinal stenosis) should be assigned as the principal diagnosis. No code from category G89 should be assigned.

> Elderly patient with back pain is admitted for kyphoplasty for age-related osteopathic compression fracture at vertebra T3
>
> **M80.08XA   Age-related osteoporosis with current pathological fracture, vertebra(e), initial encounter for fracture**
>
> *Explanation*: No code is assigned for the pain as it is inherent in the underlying condition being treated.

(a) Category G89 codes as principal or first-listed diagnosis

Category G89 codes are acceptable as principal diagnosis or the first-listed code:

- When pain control or pain management is the reason for the admission/encounter (e.g., a patient with displaced intervertebral disc, nerve impingement and severe back pain presents for injection of steroid into the spinal canal). The underlying cause of the pain should be reported as an additional diagnosis, if known.

- When a patient is admitted for the insertion of a neurostimulator for pain control, assign the appropriate pain code as the principal or first-listed diagnosis. When an admission or encounter is for a procedure aimed at treating the underlying condition and a neurostimulator is inserted for pain control during the same admission/encounter, a code for the underlying condition should be assigned as the principal diagnosis and the appropriate pain code should be assigned as a secondary diagnosis.

> Patient with chronic pain from lumbar spondylosis with radiculopathy not relieved by surgery is admitted for insertion of neurostimulator.
>
> **G89.29   Other chronic pain**
>
> **M47.26   Other spondylosis with radiculopathy, lumbar region**
>
> *Explanation*: Since the patient is admitted specifically for a neurostimulator implantation for pain management and not to treat the underlying spondylosis, the chronic pain code is sequenced first, followed by the underlying condition. Neither code M54.16 nor M54.5 is necessary because M47.26 describes the radiculopathy and the site.

(b) Use of category G89 codes in conjunction with site specific pain codes

(i) Assigning category G89 and site-specific pain codes

Codes from category G89 may be used in conjunction with codes that identify the site of pain (including codes from chapter 18) if the category G89 code provides additional information. For example, if the code describes the site of the pain, but does not fully describe whether the pain is acute or chronic, then both codes should be assigned.

> During hospital stay, patient is seen by orthopaedics to evaluate chronic left shoulder pain.
>
> **M25.512   Pain in left shoulder**
>
> **G89.29   Other chronic pain**
>
> *Explanation*: No underlying condition has been determined yet so the pain would be the reason for the visit. The M25 code in this instance does not fully describe the condition as it does not represent that the pain is chronic. The G89 chronic pain code is assigned to provide specificity.

(ii) Sequencing of category G89 codes with site-specific pain codes

The sequencing of category G89 codes with site-specific pain codes (including chapter 18 codes), is dependent on the circumstances of the encounter/admission as follows:

- If the encounter is for pain control or pain management, assign the code from category G89 followed by the code identifying the specific site of pain (e.g., encounter for pain management for acute neck pain from trauma is assigned code G89.11, Acute pain due to trauma, followed by code M54.2, Cervicalgia, to identify the site of pain).

> Management of acute, traumatic right knee pain
>
> **G89.11   Acute pain due to trauma**
>
> **M25.561   Pain in right knee**
>
> *Explanation*: The reason for the encounter is to manage or control the pain, not to treat or evaluate an underlying condition. The G89 pain code is assigned as the principal diagnosis but in this instance does not fully describe the condition as it does not include the site and laterality. The M25 pain code is added to provide this information.

Chapter 6. Diseases of the Nervous System

- If the encounter is for any other reason except pain control or pain management, and a related definitive diagnosis has not been established (confirmed) by the provider, assign the code for the specific site of pain first, followed by the appropriate code from category G89.

> Tests are performed to investigate the source of the patient's chronic epigastric abdominal pain
>
> **R10.13   Epigastric pain**
>
> **G89.29   Other chronic pain**
>
> *Explanation*: In this instance the patient's epigastric pain is not being treated; rather the source of the pain is being investigated. A code from chapter 18 for epigastric pain is sequenced before the additional specificity of the G89 code for the chronic pain.

2) Pain due to devices, implants and grafts
See Section I.C.19. Pain due to medical devices

3) Postoperative pain
The provider's documentation should be used to guide the coding of postoperative pain, as well as *Section III. Reporting Additional Diagnoses* and *Section IV. Diagnostic Coding and Reporting in the Outpatient Setting.*

The default for post-thoracotomy and other postoperative pain not specified as acute or chronic is the code for the acute form.

Routine or expected postoperative pain immediately after surgery should not be coded.

> Pain pump dose is increased for the patient's unexpected, extreme pain post-thoracotomy
>
> **G89.12   Acute post-thoracotomy pain**
>
> *Explanation*: When acute or chronic is not documented, default to acute. The use of "unexpected, extreme" and the increase of medication dosage indicate that the pain was more than routine or expected.

(a) Postoperative pain not associated with specific postoperative complication

Postoperative pain not associated with a specific postoperative complication is assigned to the appropriate postoperative pain code in category G89.

(b) Postoperative pain associated with specific postoperative complication

Postoperative pain associated with a specific postoperative complication (such as painful wire sutures) is assigned to the appropriate code(s) found in Chapter 19, Injury, poisoning, and certain other consequences of external causes. If appropriate, use additional code(s) from category G89 to identify acute or chronic pain (G89.18 or G89.28).

4) Chronic pain
Chronic pain is classified to subcategory G89.2. There is no time frame defining when pain becomes chronic pain. The provider's documentation should be used to guide use of these codes.

5) Neoplasm related pain
Code G89.3 is assigned to pain documented as being related, associated or due to cancer, primary or secondary malignancy, or tumor. This code is assigned regardless of whether the pain is acute or chronic.

This code may be assigned as the principal or first-listed code when the stated reason for the admission/encounter is documented as pain control/pain management. The underlying neoplasm should be reported as an additional diagnosis.

> Pain medication adjustment for chronic pain from bone metastasis
>
> **G89.3   Neoplasm related pain (acute)(chronic)**
>
> **C79.51   Secondary malignant neoplasm of bone**
>
> *Explanation*: Since the encounter was for pain medication management, the pain, rather than the neoplasm, was the reason for the encounter and is sequenced first. This "neoplasm-related pain" code includes both acute and chronic pain.

When the reason for the admission/encounter is management of the neoplasm and the pain associated with the neoplasm is also documented, code G89.3 may be assigned as an additional diagnosis. It is not necessary to assign an additional code for the site of the pain.

See Section I.C.2 for instructions on the sequencing of neoplasms for all other stated reasons for the admission/encounter (except for pain control/pain management).

> Patient with lung cancer presents with acute hip pain and is evaluated and found to have iliac bone metastasis
>
> **C79.51   Secondary malignant neoplasm of bone**
>
> **C34.90   Malignant neoplasm of unspecified part of unspecified bronchus or lung**
>
> **G89.3   Neoplasm related pain (acute)(chronic)**
>
> *Explanation*: The reason for the encounter was the evaluation and diagnosis of the bone metastasis, whose code would be assigned as first-listed, followed by codes for the primary neoplasm and the pain due to the iliac bone metastasis.

6) Chronic pain syndrome
Central pain syndrome (G89.0) and chronic pain syndrome (G89.4) are different than the term "chronic pain," and therefore codes should only be used when the provider has specifically documented this condition.

See Section I.C.5. Pain disorders related to psychological factors

Chapter 6. Diseases of the Nervous System (G00–G99)

EXCLUDES 2   *certain conditions originating in the perinatal period (P04-P96)*
certain infectious and parasitic diseases (A00-B99)
complications of pregnancy, childbirth and the puerperium (O00-O9A)
congenital malformations, deformations, and chromosomal abnormalities (Q00-Q99)
endocrine, nutritional and metabolic diseases (E00-E88)
injury, poisoning and certain other consequences of external causes (S00-T88)
neoplasms (C00-D49)
symptoms, signs and abnormal clinical and laboratory findings, not elsewhere classified (R00-R94)

This chapter contains the following blocks:

G00-G09   Inflammatory diseases of the central nervous system
G10-G14   Systemic atrophies primarily affecting the central nervous system
G20-G26   Extrapyramidal and movement disorders
G30-G32   Other degenerative diseases of the nervous system
G35-G37   Demyelinating diseases of the central nervous system
G40-G47   Episodic and paroxysmal disorders
G50-G59   Nerve, nerve root and plexus disorders
G60-G65   Polyneuropathies and other disorders of the peripheral nervous system
G70-G73   Diseases of myoneural junction and muscle
G80-G83   Cerebral palsy and other paralytic syndromes
G89-G99   Other disorders of the nervous system

Inflammatory diseases of the central nervous system (G00–G09)

✓4ᵗʰ G00   Bacterial meningitis, not elsewhere classified

INCLUDES   bacterial arachnoiditis
bacterial leptomeningitis
bacterial meningitis
bacterial pachymeningitis
EXCLUDES 1   *bacterial meningoencephalitis (G04.2)*
bacterial meningomyelitis (G04.2)
DEF: Inflammation of meningeal layers of the brain and spinal cord due to a bacterial infection.
CC Excl: For MCC codes in category G00: PDX collection 207

G00.0   Hemophilus meningitis   MCC
Meningitis due to Hemophilus influenzae

G00.1   Pneumococcal meningitis   MCC
Meningtitis due to Streptococcal pneumoniae

G00.2   Streptococcal meningitis   MCC
Use additional code to further identify organism (B95.0-B95.5)

G00.3   Staphylococcal meningitis   MCC
Use additional code to further identify organism (B95.61-B95.8)

G00.8   Other bacterial meningitis   MCC
Meningitis due to Escherichia coli
Meningitis due to Friedländer's bacillus
Meningitis due to Klebsiella
Use additional code to further identify organism (B96.-)

G00.9   Bacterial meningitis, unspecified   MCC
Meningitis due to gram-negative bacteria, unspecified
Purulent meningitis NOS
Pyogenic meningitis NOS
Suppurative meningitis NOS

G01   Meningitis in bacterial diseases classified elsewhere   MCC

Code first underlying disease
EXCLUDES 1   *meningitis (in):*
gonococcal (A54.81)
leptospirosis (A27.81)
listeriosis (A32.11)
Lyme disease (A69.21)
meningococcal (A39.0)
neurosyphilis (A52.13)
tuberculosis (A17.0)
meningoencephalitis and meningomyelitis in bacterial diseases classified elsewhere (G05)
CC Excl: PDX collection 207

G02   Meningitis in other infectious and parasitic diseases classified elsewhere   MCC

Code first underlying disease, such as:
African trypanosomiasis (B56.-)
poliovirus infection (A80.-)
EXCLUDES 1   *candidal meningitis (B37.5)*
coccidioidomycosis meningitis (B38.4)
cryptococcal meningitis (B45.1)
herpesviral [herpes simplex] meningitis (B00.3)
infectious mononucleosis complicated by meningitis (B27.- with fourth character 2)
measles complicated by meningitis (B05.1)
meningoencephalitis and meningomyelitis in other infectious and parasitic diseases classified elsewhere (G05)
mumps meningitis (B26.1)
rubella meningitis (B06.02)
varicella [chickenpox] meningitis (B01.0)
zoster meningitis (B02.1)
CC Excl: PDX collection 559

✓4ᵗʰ G03   Meningitis due to other and unspecified causes

INCLUDES   arachnoiditis NOS
leptomeningitis NOS
meningitis NOS
pachymeningitis NOS
EXCLUDES 1   *meningoencephalitis (G04.-)*
meningomyelitis (G04.-)
CC Excl: For CC/MCC codes in category G03, unless otherwise noted: PDX collection 207

G03.0   Nonpyogenic meningitis   MCC
Aseptic meningitis
Nonbacterial meningitis
DEF: Type of meningitis where no bacterial, viral, or other infectious source exists that explains the meningitis symptomology.

G03.1   Chronic meningitis   CC

G03.2   Benign recurrent meningitis [Mollaret]   CC
DEF: Aseptic or noninfectious inflammation of the meninges with the presence of Mollaret cells in the spinal fluid. The patient experiences recurrent bouts of inflammation, lasting anywhere from two to five days.
CC Excl: PDX collection 140

G03.8   Meningitis due to other specified causes   MCC

G03.9   Meningitis, unspecified   MCC
Arachnoiditis (spinal) NOS

✓4ᵗʰ G04   Encephalitis, myelitis and encephalomyelitis

INCLUDES   acute ascending myelitis
meningoencephalitis
meningomyelitis
EXCLUDES 1   *encephalopathy NOS (G93.40)*
EXCLUDES 2   *acute transverse myelitis (G37.3-)*
alcoholic encephalopathy (G31.2)
benign myalgic encephalomyelitis (G93.3)
multiple sclerosis (G35)
subacute necrotizing myelitis (G37.4)
toxic encephalitis (G92)
toxic encephalopathy (G92)
DEF: Encephalitis: Inflammation of the brain, often caused by viral or bacterial infection.
DEF: Encephalomyelitis: Inflammatory disease, often viral in nature, that affects the brain and spinal cord.
DEF: Myelitis: Inflammation of the spinal cord.
CC Excl: For CC/MCC codes in category G04, unless otherwise noted: PDX collection 560

✓5ᵗʰ G04.0   Acute disseminated encephalitis and encephalomyelitis (ADEM)
EXCLUDES 1   *acute necrotizing hemorrhagic encephalopathy (G04.3-)*
other noninfectious acute disseminated encephalomyelitis (noninfectious ADEM) (G04.81)

G04.00   Acute disseminated encephalitis and encephalomyelitis, unspecified   MCC

G04.01   **Postinfectious** acute disseminated encephalitis and encephalomyelitis (postinfectious ADEM)   `MCC`
> **EXCLUDES 1**   post chickenpox encephalitis (B01.1)
> post measles encephalitis (B05.0)
> post measles myelitis (B05.1)

G04.02   **Postimmunization** acute disseminated encephalitis, myelitis and encephalomyelitis   `MCC`
> Encephalitis, post immunization
> Encephalomyelitis, post immunization
> Use additional code to identify the vaccine (T50.A-, T50.B-, T50.Z-)
> **CC Excl:** No Excl

G04.1   **Tropical spastic paraplegia**   `CC` `HCC`
> **CC Excl:** PDX collection 561

G04.2   **Bacterial meningoencephalitis and meningomyelitis, not elsewhere classified**   `MCC`
> **CC Excl:** PDX collection 207

`✓5ᵗʰ` **G04.3**   **Acute necrotizing hemorrhagic encephalopathy**
> **EXCLUDES 1**   acute disseminated encephalitis and encephalomyelitis (G04.0-)

G04.30   **Acute necrotizing hemorrhagic encephalopathy, unspecified**   `MCC`
> **CC Excl:** No Excl

G04.31   **Postinfectious** acute necrotizing hemorrhagic encephalopathy   `MCC`

G04.32   **Postimmunization** acute necrotizing hemorrhagic encephalopathy   `MCC`
> Use additional code to identify the vaccine (T50.A-, T50.B-, T50.Z-)
> **CC Excl:** No Excl

G04.39   **Other acute necrotizing hemorrhagic encephalopathy**   `MCC`
> Code also underlying etiology, if applicable
> **CC Excl:** No Excl

`✓5ᵗʰ` **G04.8**   **Other encephalitis, myelitis and encephalomyelitis**
> Code also any associated seizure (G40.-, R56.9)

G04.81   **Other encephalitis and encephalomyelitis**   `HIV` `MCC`
> Noninfectious acute disseminated encephalomyelitis (noninfectious ADEM)

G04.89   **Other myelitis**   `HIV` `MCC` `HCC`

`✓5ᵗʰ` **G04.9**   **Encephalitis, myelitis and encephalomyelitis, unspecified**

G04.90   **Encephalitis and encephalomyelitis, unspecified**   `HIV` `MCC`
> Ventriculitis (cerebral) NOS
> **CC Excl:** PDX collection 562

G04.91   **Myelitis, unspecified**   `HIV` `MCC` `HCC`
> **CC Excl:** PDX collection 562

`✓4ᵗʰ` **G05**   **Encephalitis, myelitis and encephalomyelitis in diseases classified elsewhere**
> Code first underlying disease, such as:
> human immunodeficiency virus [HIV] disease (B20)
> poliovirus (A80.-)
> suppurative otitis media (H66.01-H66.4)
> trichinellosis (B75)
> **EXCLUDES 1**   adenoviral encephalitis, myelitis and encephalomyelitis (A85.1)
> congenital toxoplasmosis encephalitis, myelitis and encephalomyelitis (P37.1)
> cytomegaloviral encephalitis, myelitis and encephalomyelitis (B25.8)
> encephalitis, myelitis and encephalomyelitis (in) measles (B05.0)
> encephalitis, myelitis and encephalomyelitis (in) systemic lupus erythematosus (M32.19)
> enteroviral encephalitis, myelitis and encephalomyelitis (A85.0)
> eosinophilic meningoencephalitis (B83.2)
> herpesviral [herpes simplex] encephalitis, myelitis and encephalomyelitis (B00.4)
> listerial encephalitis, myelitis and encephalomyelitis (A32.12)
> meningococcal encephalitis, myelitis and encephalomyelitis (A39.81)
> mumps encephalitis, myelitis and encephalomyelitis (B26.2)
> postchickenpox encephalitis, myelitis and encephalomyelitis (B01.1-)
> rubella encephalitis, myelitis and encephalomyelitis (B06.01)
> toxoplasmosis encephalitis, myelitis and encephalomyelitis (B58.2)
> zoster encephalitis, myelitis and encephalomyelitis (B02.0)

G05.3   *Encephalitis and encephalomyelitis in diseases classified elsewhere*   `MCC`
> Meningoencephalitis in diseases classified elsewhere
> **CC Excl:** PDX collection 560

G05.4   *Myelitis in diseases classified elsewhere*   `MCC` `HCC`
> Meningomyelitis in diseases classified elsewhere
> **CC Excl:** PDX collection 560

`✓4ᵗʰ` **G06**   **Intracranial and intraspinal abscess and granuloma**
> Use additional code (B95-B97) to identify infectious agent
> **DEF:** Abscess: Circumscribed collection of pus resulting from bacteria, frequently associated with swelling and other signs of inflammation.
> **DEF:** Granuloma: Abnormal, dense collections or cells forming a mass or nodule of chronically inflamed tissue with granulations that is usually associated with an infective process.

G06.0   **Intracranial abscess and granuloma**   `MCC`
> Brain [any part] abscess (embolic)
> Cerebellar abscess (embolic)
> Cerebral abscess (embolic)
> Intracranial epidural abscess or granuloma
> Intracranial extradural abscess or granuloma
> Intracranial subdural abscess or granuloma
> Otogenic abscess (embolic)
> **EXCLUDES 1**   tuberculous intracranial abscess and granuloma (A17.81)
> **CC Excl:** PDX collection 563

G06.1   **Intraspinal abscess and granuloma**   `MCC`
> Abscess (embolic) of spinal cord [any part]
> Intraspinal epidural abscess or granuloma
> Intraspinal extradural abscess or granuloma
> Intraspinal subdural abscess or granuloma
> **EXCLUDES 1**   tuberculous intraspinal abscess and granuloma (A17.81)
> **CC Excl:** PDX collection 564

G06.2   **Extradural and subdural abscess, unspecified**   `MCC`
> **CC Excl:** PDX collection 565

`N` Newborn: 0   `P` Pediatric: 0-17   `M` Maternity: 9-64   `A` Adult: 15-124   `MCC` Major Complication/Comorbidity   `CC` Complication/Comorbidity   `SW` Severe Wound Dx

572   ICD-10-CM 2020

G07 *Intracranial and intraspinal abscess and granuloma in diseases classified elsewhere* `MCC`

Code first underlying disease, such as:
schistosomiasis granuloma of brain (B65.-)

> EXCLUDES 1   abscess of brain:
> amebic (A06.6)
> chromomycotic (B43.1)
> gonococcal (A54.82)
> tuberculous (A17.81)
> tuberculoma of meninges (A17.1)

CC Excl: PDX collection 565

G08 **Intracranial and intraspinal phlebitis and thrombophlebitis** `MCC`

Septic embolism of intracranial or intraspinal venous sinuses and veins
Septic endophlebitis of intracranial or intraspinal venous sinuses and veins
Septic phlebitis of intracranial or intraspinal venous sinuses and veins
Septic thrombophlebitis of intracranial or intraspinal venous sinuses and veins
Septic thrombosis of intracranial or intraspinal venous sinuses and veins

> EXCLUDES 1   intracranial phlebitis and thrombophlebitis complicating:
> abortion, ectopic or molar pregnancy (O00-O07, O08.7)
> pregnancy, childbirth and the puerperium (O22.5, O87.3)
> nonpyogenic intracranial phlebitis and thrombophlebitis (I67.6)

> EXCLUDES 2   intracranial phlebitis and thrombophlebitis complicating nonpyogenic intraspinal phlebitis and thrombophlebitis (G95.1)

DEF: Inflammation and formation of a blood clot in a vein within the brain or spine, or their linings.
CC Excl: PDX collection 565

G09 **Sequelae of inflammatory diseases of central nervous system**

> NOTE   Category G09 is to be used to indicate conditions whose primary classification is to G00-G08 as the cause of sequelae, themselves classifiable elsewhere. The "sequelae" include conditions specified as residuals.

Code first condition resulting from (sequela) of inflammatory diseases of central nervous system

Systemic atrophies primarily affecting the central nervous system (G10-G14)

G10 **Huntington's disease** `HCC`

Huntington's chorea
Huntington's dementia
Code also dementia in other diseases classified elsewhere without behavioral disturbance (F02.80)
DEF: Genetic disease caused by degeneration of nerve cells in the brain, characterized by chronic progressive mental deterioration. Dementia and death occur within 15 to 20 years of onset.

√4ᵗʰ **G11** **Hereditary ataxia**

> EXCLUDES 2   cerebral palsy (G80.-)
> hereditary and idiopathic neuropathy (G60.-)
> metabolic disorders (E70-E88)

DEF: Ataxia: Defect in muscular control or coordination due to a central nervous system disorder, particularly when voluntary muscular movements are attempted.

G11.0 **Congenital nonprogressive ataxia** `HCC`

G11.1 **Early-onset cerebellar ataxia** `HCC`

Early-onset cerebellar ataxia with essential tremor
Early-onset cerebellar ataxia with myoclonus [Hunt's ataxia]
Early-onset cerebellar ataxia with retained tendon reflexes
Friedreich's ataxia (autosomal recessive)
X-linked recessive spinocerebellar ataxia

G11.2 **Late-onset cerebellar ataxia** `HCC` `A`

G11.3 **Cerebellar ataxia with defective DNA repair** `HCC`

Ataxia telangiectasia [Louis-Bar]

> EXCLUDES 2   Cockayne's syndrome ▶(Q87.19)◀
> other disorders of purine and pyrimidine metabolism (E79.-)
> xeroderma pigmentosum (Q82.1)

G11.4 **Hereditary spastic paraplegia** `HCC`

G11.8 **Other hereditary ataxias** `HCC`

G11.9 **Hereditary ataxia, unspecified** `HCC`

Hereditary cerebellar ataxia NOS
Hereditary cerebellar degeneration
Hereditary cerebellar disease
Hereditary cerebellar syndrome

√4ᵗʰ **G12** **Spinal muscular atrophy and related syndromes**

G12.0 **Infantile spinal muscular atrophy, type I [Werdnig-Hoffman]** `HCC`

G12.1 **Other inherited spinal muscular atrophy** `HCC`

Adult form spinal muscular atrophy
Childhood form, type II spinal muscular atrophy
Distal spinal muscular atrophy
Juvenile form, type III spinal muscular atrophy [Kugelberg-Welander]
Progressive bulbar palsy of childhood [Fazio-Londe]
Scapuloperoneal form spinal muscular atrophy

√5ᵗʰ **G12.2** **Motor neuron disease**

AHA: 2017,4Q,9-10
For CC codes in subcategory G12.2: PDX collection 570

   G12.20 **Motor neuron disease, unspecified** `HCC`

   G12.21 **Amyotrophic lateral sclerosis** `HCC` `A`

   G12.22 **Progressive bulbar palsy** `HCC`

   G12.23 **Primary lateral sclerosis** `CC` `HCC`

   G12.24 **Familial motor neuron disease** `CC` `HCC`

   G12.25 **Progressive spinal muscle atrophy** `CC` `HCC`

   G12.29 **Other motor neuron disease** `HCC`

G12.8 **Other spinal muscular atrophies and related syndromes** `HCC`

G12.9 **Spinal muscular atrophy, unspecified** `HCC`

√4ᵗʰ **G13** **Systemic atrophies primarily affecting central nervous system in diseases classified elsewhere**

G13.0 *Paraneoplastic neuromyopathy and neuropathy* `HCC`

Carcinomatous neuromyopathy
Sensorial paraneoplastic neuropathy [Denny Brown]
Code first underlying neoplasm (C00-D49)

G13.1 *Other systemic atrophy primarily affecting central nervous system in neoplastic disease* `HCC`

Paraneoplastic limbic encephalopathy
Code first underlying neoplasm (C00-D49)

G13.2 *Systemic atrophy primarily affecting the central nervous system in myxedema* `HCC`

Code first underlying disease, such as:
hypothyroidism (E03.-)
myxedematous congenital iodine deficiency (E00.1)

G13.8 *Systemic atrophy primarily affecting central nervous system in other diseases classified elsewhere* `HCC`

Code first underlying disease

G14 **Postpolio syndrome**

> INCLUDES   postpolio myelitic syndrome
> EXCLUDES 1   sequelae of poliomyelitis (B91)

Extrapyramidal and movement disorders (G20-G26)

G20 **Parkinson's disease** `HCC`

Hemiparkinsonism
Idiopathic Parkinsonism or Parkinson's disease
Paralysis agitans
Parkinsonism or Parkinson's disease NOS
Primary Parkinsonism or Parkinson's disease

> EXCLUDES 1   dementia with Parkinsonism (G31.83)

AHA: 2017,2Q,7; 2016,2Q,6
TIP: Repeated falls (R29.6) are not integral to Parkinson's disease and can be separately coded.

√4ᵗʰ **G21 Secondary parkinsonism**

     EXCLUDES 1   dementia with Parkinsonism (G31.83)
           Huntington's disease (G10)
           Shy-Drager syndrome (G90.3)
           syphilitic Parkinsonism (A52.19)

     CC Excl: For CC/MCC codes in category G21, unless otherwise noted: PDX collection 572

G21.0 Malignant neuroleptic syndrome   MCC
     Use additional code for adverse effect, if applicable, to identify drug (T43.3X5, T43.4X5, T43.505, T43.595)
     EXCLUDES 1   neuroleptic induced parkinsonism (G21.11)
     CC Excl: PDX collection 571

√5ᵗʰ **G21.1 Other drug-induced secondary parkinsonism**

     G21.11 Neuroleptic induced parkinsonism   CC HCC
         Use additional code for adverse effect, if applicable, to identify drug (T43.3X5, T43.4X5, T43.505, T43.595)
         EXCLUDES 1   malignant neuroleptic syndrome (G21.0)

     G21.19 Other drug induced secondary parkinsonism   CC HCC
         Other medication-induced parkinsonism
         Use additional code for adverse effect, if applicable, to identify drug (T36-T50 with fifth or sixth character 5)

G21.2 Secondary parkinsonism due to other external agents   CC HCC
     Code first (T51-T65) to identify external agent

G21.3 Postencephalitic parkinsonism   CC HCC

G21.4 Vascular parkinsonism   HCC

G21.8 Other secondary parkinsonism   CC HCC

G21.9 Secondary parkinsonism, unspecified   CC HCC

√4ᵗʰ **G23 Other degenerative diseases of basal ganglia**

     EXCLUDES 2   multi-system degeneration of the autonomic nervous system (G90.3)

     CC Excl: For CC codes in category G23: PDX collection 573

G23.0 Hallervorden-Spatz disease   CC HCC
     Pigmentary pallidal degeneration

G23.1 Progressive supranuclear ophthalmoplegia [Steele-Richardson-Olszewski]   HCC
     Progressive supranuclear palsy

G23.2 Striatonigral degeneration   HCC

G23.8 Other specified degenerative diseases of basal ganglia   CC HCC
     Calcification of basal ganglia

G23.9 Degenerative disease of basal ganglia, unspecified   CC HCC

√4ᵗʰ **G24 Dystonia**

     INCLUDES   dyskinesia
     EXCLUDES 2   athetoid cerebral palsy (G80.3)

     DEF: Disorder of abnormal muscle tone, excessive or inadequate. Involuntary movements and prolonged muscle contractions result in tremors, abnormalities in posture, and twisting body motions that affect an isolated area or the whole body.

     CC Excl: For CC codes in category G24: PDX collection 574

√5ᵗʰ **G24.0 Drug induced dystonia**
     Use additional code for adverse effect, if applicable, to identify drug (T36-T50 with fifth or sixth character 5)

     G24.01 Drug induced subacute dyskinesia   CC
         Drug induced blepharospasm
         Drug induced orofacial dyskinesia
         Neuroleptic induced tardive dyskinesia
         Tardive dyskinesia

     G24.02 Drug induced acute dystonia   CC
         Acute dystonic reaction to drugs
         Neuroleptic induced acute dystonia

     G24.09 Other drug induced dystonia   CC

G24.1 Genetic torsion dystonia
     Dystonia deformans progressiva
     Dystonia musculorum deformans
     Familial torsion dystonia
     Idiopathic familial dystonia
     Idiopathic (torsion) dystonia NOS
     (Schwalbe-) Ziehen-Oppenheim disease

G24.2 Idiopathic nonfamilial dystonia   CC

G24.3 Spasmodic torticollis

     EXCLUDES 1   congenital torticollis (Q68.0)
           hysterical torticollis (F44.4)
           ocular torticollis (R29.891)
           psychogenic torticollis (F45.8)
           torticollis NOS (M43.6)
           traumatic recurrent torticollis (S13.4)

     DEF: Twisted, unnatural position of the neck due to contracted cervical muscles that pull the head to one side or cause involuntary shaking of the head.

G24.4 Idiopathic orofacial dystonia
     Orofacial dyskinesia
     EXCLUDES 1   drug induced orofacial dyskinesia (G24.01)

G24.5 Blepharospasm
     EXCLUDES 1   drug induced blepharospasm (G24.01)
     DEF: Involuntary contraction of the orbicularis oculi muscle, resulting in the eyelids being completely closed.

G24.8 Other dystonia
     Acquired torsion dystonia NOS

G24.9 Dystonia, unspecified
     Dyskinesia NOS

√4ᵗʰ **G25 Other extrapyramidal and movement disorders**

     EXCLUDES 2   sleep related movement disorders (G47.6-)

G25.0 Essential tremor
     Familial tremor
     EXCLUDES 1   tremor NOS (R25.1)

G25.1 Drug-induced tremor
     Use additional code for adverse effect, if applicable, to identify drug (T36-T50 with fifth or sixth character 5)

G25.2 Other specified forms of tremor
     Intention tremor

G25.3 Myoclonus
     Drug-induced myoclonus
     Palatal myoclonus
     Use additional code for adverse effect, if applicable, to identify drug (T36-T50 with fifth or sixth character 5)
     EXCLUDES 1   facial myokymia (G51.4)
           myoclonic epilepsy (G40.-)
     DEF: Spasmodic, brief, involuntary muscle contractions that can be due to an undetermined etiology, drug-induced, or caused by a disease process.

G25.4 Drug-induced chorea
     Use additional code for adverse effect, if applicable, to identify drug (T36-T50 with fifth or sixth character 5)

G25.5 Other chorea
     Chorea NOS
     EXCLUDES 1   chorea NOS with heart involvement (I02.0)
           Huntington's chorea (G10)
           rheumatic chorea (I02.-)
           Sydenham's chorea (I02.-)

√5ᵗʰ **G25.6 Drug induced tics and other tics of organic origin**

     G25.61 Drug induced tics
         Use additional code for adverse effect, if applicable, to identify drug (T36-T50 with fifth or sixth character 5)

     G25.69 Other tics of organic origin
         EXCLUDES 1   habit spasm (F95.9)
               tic NOS (F95.9)
               Tourette's syndrome (F95.2)

√5ᵗʰ **G25.7 Other and unspecified drug induced movement disorders**
     Use additional code for adverse effect, if applicable, to identify drug (T36-T50 with fifth or sixth character 5)

     G25.70 Drug induced movement disorder, unspecified
     G25.71 Drug induced akathisia
         Drug induced acathisia
         Neuroleptic induced acute akathisia
         Tardive akathisia

     G25.79 Other drug induced movement disorders

√5ᵗʰ **G25.8 Other specified extrapyramidal and movement disorders**

     G25.81 Restless legs syndrome
         DEF: Neurological disorder of unknown etiology creating an irresistible urge to move the legs, which may temporarily relieve the symptoms. This syndrome is accompanied by motor restlessness and sensations of pain, burning, prickling, or tingling.

N Newborn: 0   P Pediatric: 0-17   M Maternity: 9-64   A Adult: 15-124   MCC Major Complication/Comorbidity   CC Complication/Comorbidity   SW Severe Wound Dx

G25.82 Stiff-man syndrome `CC`
    CC Excl: PDX collection 575

G25.83 Benign shuddering attacks

G25.89 Other specified extrapyramidal and movement disorders

G25.9 Extrapyramidal and movement disorder, unspecified `CC`
    CC Excl: PDX collection 575

G26 *Extrapyramidal and movement disorders in diseases classified elsewhere*
    Code first underlying disease

Other degenerative diseases of the nervous system (G30-G32)

✓4ᵗʰ G30 Alzheimer's disease
    INCLUDES Alzheimer's dementia senile and presenile forms
    Use additional code to identify:
      delirium, if applicable (F05)
      dementia with behavioral disturbance (F02.81)
      dementia without behavioral disturbance (F02.80)
    EXCLUDES 1 *senile degeneration of brain NEC (G31.1)*
        senile dementia NOS (F03)
        senility NOS (R41.81)

[handwritten: Always code with F02]

    AHA: 2017,1Q,43
    TIP: A code from subcategory F02.8 should always be assigned with a code from this category, even in the absence of documented dementia.
    TIP: Functional quadriplegia (R53.2) is not integral to Alzheimer's disease and can be coded in addition to codes from category G30.

G30.0 Alzheimer's disease with early onset `HCC`

G30.1 Alzheimer's disease with late onset `HCC` `A`

G30.8 Other Alzheimer's disease `HCC`

G30.9 Alzheimer's disease, unspecified `HCC`
    AHA: 2016,2Q,6; 2012,4Q,95

✓4ᵗʰ G31 Other degenerative diseases of nervous system, not elsewhere classified
    ▶For codes G31.0–G31.83, G31.85–G31.9, use additional code to identify:◀
      dementia with behavioral disturbance (F02.81)
      dementia without behavioral disturbance (F02.80)
    EXCLUDES 2 *Reye's syndrome (G93.7)*

✓5ᵗʰ G31.0 Frontotemporal dementia

    G31.01 Pick's disease `HCC`
        Primary progressive aphasia
        Progressive isolated aphasia
        DEF: Progressive frontotemporal dementia with asymmetrical atrophy of the frontal and temporal regions of the cerebral cortex and abnormal rounded brain cells called Pick cells with the presence of abnormal staining of protein (called tau). Symptoms include prominent apathy, behavioral changes such as disinhibition and restlessness, echolalia, impairment of language, memory, and intellect, increased carelessness, poor personal hygiene, and decreased attention span.

    G31.09 Other frontotemporal dementia `HCC`
        Frontal dementia

G31.1 Senile degeneration of brain, not elsewhere classified `HCC`
    EXCLUDES 1 *Alzheimer's disease (G30.-)*
        senility NOS (R41.81)

G31.2 Degeneration of nervous system due to alcohol `CC` `HCC`
    Alcoholic cerebellar ataxia
    Alcoholic cerebellar degeneration
    Alcoholic cerebral degeneration
    Alcoholic encephalopathy
    Dysfunction of the autonomic nervous system due to alcohol
    Code also associated alcoholism (F10.-)

✓5ᵗʰ G31.8 Other specified degenerative diseases of nervous system

    G31.81 Alpers disease `CC` `HCC`
        Grey-matter degeneration
        CC Excl: PDX collection 537

    G31.82 Leigh's disease `CC` `HCC`
        Subacute necrotizing encephalopathy
        CC Excl: PDX collection 537

G31.83 Dementia with Lewy bodies `HCC`
    Dementia with Parkinsonism
    Lewy body dementia
    Lewy body disease
    AHA: 2017,2Q,7; 2016,4Q,141
    DEF: Cerebral dementia with neurophysiologic changes, increased hippocampal volume, hypoperfusion in the occipital lobes, beta amyloid deposits with neurofibrillary tangles, and atrophy of the cortex and brainstem. Hallmark neuropsychological characteristics include fluctuating cognition with pronounced variation in attention and alertness, recurrent hallucinations, and Parkinsonism.

G31.84 Mild cognitive impairment, so stated
    Mild neurocognitive disorder
    EXCLUDES 1 *age related cognitive decline (R41.81)*
        altered mental status (R41.82)
        cerebral degeneration (G31.9)
        change in mental status (R41.82)
        cognitive deficits following (sequelae of) cerebral hemorrhage or infarction (I69.01-, I69.11-, I69.21-, I69.31-, I69.81-, I69.91-)
        cognitive impairment due to intracranial or head injury (S06.-)
        dementia (F01.-, F02.-, F03)
        mild memory disturbance (F06.8)
        neurologic neglect syndrome (R41.4)
        personality change, nonpsychotic (F68.8)

G31.85 Corticobasal degeneration `HCC`

G31.89 Other specified degenerative diseases of nervous system `HCC`

G31.9 Degenerative disease of nervous system, unspecified `HCC`

✓4ᵗʰ G32 Other degenerative disorders of nervous system in diseases classified elsewhere

    G32.0 *Subacute combined degeneration of spinal cord in diseases classified elsewhere* `CC` `HCC`
      Dana-Putnam syndrome
      Sclerosis of spinal cord (combined) (dorsolateral) (posterolateral)
      Code first underlying disease, such as:
        anemia (D51.9)
        dietary (D51.3)
        pernicious (D51.0)
        vitamin B12 deficiency (E53.8)
      EXCLUDES 1 *syphilitic combined degeneration of spinal cord (A52.11)*
      CC Excl: PDX collection 576

✓5ᵗʰ G32.8 Other specified degenerative disorders of nervous system in diseases classified elsewhere
    Code first underlying disease, such as:
      amyloidosis cerebral degeneration (E85.-)
      cerebral degeneration (due to) hypothyroidism (E00.0-E03.9)
      cerebral degeneration (due to) neoplasm (C00-D49)
      cerebral degeneration (due to) vitamin B deficiency, except thiamine (E52-E53.-)
    EXCLUDES 1 *superior hemorrhagic polioencephalitis [Wernicke's encephalopathy] (E51.2)*

    G32.81 *Cerebellar ataxia in diseases classified elsewhere* `CC` `HCC`
        Code first underlying disease, such as:
          celiac disease (with gluten ataxia) (K90.0)
          cerebellar ataxia (in) neoplastic disease (paraneoplastic cerebellar degeneration) (C00-D49)
          non-celiac gluten ataxia (M35.9)
        EXCLUDES 1 *systemic atrophy primarily affecting the central nervous system in alcoholic cerebellar ataxia (G31.2)*
          systemic atrophy primarily affecting the central nervous system in myxedema (G13.2)
        CC Excl: PDX collection 567

    G32.89 *Other specified degenerative disorders of nervous system in diseases classified elsewhere*
        Degenerative encephalopathy in diseases classified elsewhere

---

✅ Additional Character Required   ✓x7ᵗʰ Placeholder   **Unacceptable PDx**   Questionable PDx   Manifestation   Unspecified Dx   M1-H14 HAC   HCC CMS-HCC Dx   HIV HIV Dx

Chapter 6. Diseases of the Nervous System

Demyelinating diseases of the central nervous system (G35-G37)

CC Excl: For CC codes in categories G35-G37, unless otherwise noted: PDX collection 578

G35 Multiple sclerosis `HCC`
Disseminated multiple sclerosis
Generalized multiple sclerosis
Multiple sclerosis NOS
Multiple sclerosis of brain stem
Multiple sclerosis of cord

✓4ᵗʰ G36 Other acute disseminated demyelination
EXCLUDES 1 postinfectious encephalitis and encephalomyelitis NOS (GØ4.Ø1)

DEF: Demyelination: Abnormal loss of myelin, the protective white matter that insulates nerve endings and facilitates neuroreception and neurotransmission. When this substance is damaged, the nerve is short-circuited, resulting in impaired or loss of function.

G36.Ø Neuromyelitis optica [Devic] `CC` `HCC`
Demyelination in optic neuritis
EXCLUDES 1 optic neuritis NOS (H46)
CC Excl: PDX collection 577

G36.1 Acute and subacute hemorrhagic leukoencephalitis [Hurst] `CC` `HCC`

G36.8 Other specified acute disseminated demyelination `CC` `HCC`

G36.9 Acute disseminated demyelination, unspecified `HIV` `CC` `HCC`

✓4ᵗʰ G37 Other demyelinating diseases of central nervous system

G37.Ø Diffuse sclerosis of central nervous system `CC` `HCC`
Periaxial encephalitis
Schilder's disease
EXCLUDES 1 X linked adrenoleukodystrophy (E71.52-)
CC Excl: PDX collection 579

G37.1 Central demyelination of corpus callosum `CC` `HCC`

G37.2 Central pontine myelinolysis `CC` `HCC`

G37.3 Acute transverse myelitis in demyelinating disease of central nervous system `CC` `HCC`
Acute transverse myelitis NOS
Acute transverse myelopathy
EXCLUDES 1 multiple sclerosis (G35)
neuromyelitis optica [Devic] (G36.Ø)
CC Excl: PDX collection 580

G37.4 Subacute necrotizing myelitis of central nervous system `HIV` `MCC` `HCC`
CC Excl: PDX collection 562

G37.5 Concentric sclerosis [Balo] of central nervous system `CC` `HCC`
CC Excl: PDX collection 579

G37.8 Other specified demyelinating diseases of central nervous system `CC` `HCC`

G37.9 Demyelinating disease of central nervous system, unspecified `HIV` `CC` `HCC`

Episodic and paroxysmal disorders (G40-G47)

✓4ᵗʰ G40 Epilepsy and recurrent seizures
NOTE The following terms are to be considered equivalent to intractable: pharmacoresistant (pharmacologically resistant), treatment resistant, refractory (medically) and poorly controlled

EXCLUDES 1 conversion disorder with seizures (F44.5)
convulsions NOS (R56.9)
post traumatic seizures (R56.1)
seizure (convulsive) NOS (R56.9)
seizure of newborn (P90)

EXCLUDES 2 hippocampal sclerosis (G93.81)
mesial temporal sclerosis (G93.81)
temporal sclerosis (G93.81)
Todd's paralysis (G83.84)

CC Excl: For codes in category G40:
For MCC codes: PDX collection 583
For CC codes, unless otherwise noted: PDX collection 582

✓5ᵗʰ G40.Ø Localization-related (focal) (partial) idiopathic epilepsy and epileptic syndromes with seizures of localized onset
Benign childhood epilepsy with centrotemporal EEG spikes
Childhood epilepsy with occipital EEG paroxysms
EXCLUDES 1 adult onset localization-related epilepsy (G40.1-, G40.2-)

✓6ᵗʰ G40.ØØ Localization-related (focal) (partial) idiopathic epilepsy and epileptic syndromes with seizures of localized onset, not intractable
Localization-related (focal) (partial) idiopathic epilepsy and epileptic syndromes with seizures of localized onset without intractability

G40.ØØ1 Localization-related (focal) (partial) idiopathic epilepsy and epileptic syndromes with seizures of localized onset, not intractable, with status epilepticus `CC` `HCC`
CC Excl: PDX collection 581

G40.ØØ9 Localization-related (focal) (partial) idiopathic epilepsy and epileptic syndromes with seizures of localized onset, not intractable, without status epilepticus `CC` `HCC`
Localization-related (focal) (partial) idiopathic epilepsy and epileptic syndromes with seizures of localized onset NOS
CC Excl: PDX collection 581

✓6ᵗʰ G40.Ø1 Localization-related (focal) (partial) idiopathic epilepsy and epileptic syndromes with seizures of localized onset, intractable

G40.Ø11 Localization-related (focal) (partial) idiopathic epilepsy and epileptic syndromes with seizures of localized onset, intractable, with status epilepticus `CC` `HCC`

G40.Ø19 Localization-related (focal) (partial) idiopathic epilepsy and epileptic syndromes with seizures of localized onset, intractable, without status epilepticus `CC` `HCC`

N Newborn: 0   **P** Pediatric: 0-17   **M** Maternity: 9-64   **A** Adult: 15-124   **MCC** Major Complication/Comorbidity   **CC** Complication/Comorbidity   **SW** Severe Wound Dx

576   ICD-10-CM 2020

✓5th **G40.1** **Localization-related (focal) (partial) symptomatic epilepsy and epileptic syndromes with simple partial seizures**
    Attacks without alteration of consciousness
    Epilepsia partialis continua [Kozhevnikof]
    Simple partial seizures developing into secondarily generalized seizures

✓6th **G40.10** **Localization-related (focal) (partial) symptomatic epilepsy and epileptic syndromes with simple partial seizures, not intractable**
    Localization-related (focal) (partial) symptomatic epilepsy and epileptic syndromes with simple partial seizures without intractability

    G40.101 **Localization-related (focal) (partial) symptomatic epilepsy and epileptic syndromes with simple partial seizures, not intractable, with status epilepticus** `CC` `HCC`
        CC Excl: PDX collection 581

    G40.109 **Localization-related (focal) (partial) symptomatic epilepsy and epileptic syndromes with simple partial seizures, not intractable, without status epilepticus** `CC` `HCC`
        Localization-related (focal) (partial) symptomatic epilepsy and epileptic syndromes with simple partial seizures NOS
        CC Excl: PDX collection 581

✓6th **G40.11** **Localization-related (focal) (partial) symptomatic epilepsy and epileptic syndromes with simple partial seizures, intractable**

    G40.111 **Localization-related (focal) (partial) symptomatic epilepsy and epileptic syndromes with simple partial seizures, intractable, with status epilepticus** `CC` `HCC`

    G40.119 **Localization-related (focal) (partial) symptomatic epilepsy and epileptic syndromes with simple partial seizures, intractable, without status epilepticus** `CC` `HCC`

✓5th **G40.2** **Localization-related (focal) (partial) symptomatic epilepsy and epileptic syndromes with complex partial seizures**
    Attacks with alteration of consciousness, often with automatisms
    Complex partial seizures developing into secondarily generalized seizures

✓6th **G40.20** **Localization-related (focal) (partial) symptomatic epilepsy and epileptic syndromes with complex partial seizures, not intractable**
    Localization-related (focal) (partial) symptomatic epilepsy and epileptic syndromes with complex partial seizures without intractability

    G40.201 **Localization-related (focal) (partial) symptomatic epilepsy and epileptic syndromes with complex partial seizures, not intractable, with status epilepticus** `CC` `HCC`
        CC Excl: PDX collection 581

    G40.209 **Localization-related (focal) (partial) symptomatic epilepsy and epileptic syndromes with complex partial seizures, not intractable, without status epilepticus** `CC` `HCC`
        Localization-related (focal) (partial) symptomatic epilepsy and epileptic syndromes with complex partial seizures NOS
        CC Excl: PDX collection 581

✓6th **G40.21** **Localization-related (focal) (partial) symptomatic epilepsy and epileptic syndromes with complex partial seizures, intractable**

    G40.211 **Localization-related (focal) (partial) symptomatic epilepsy and epileptic syndromes with complex partial seizures, intractable, with status epilepticus** `CC` `HCC`

    G40.219 **Localization-related (focal) (partial) symptomatic epilepsy and epileptic syndromes with complex partial seizures, intractable, without status epilepticus** `CC` `HCC`

✓5th **G40.3** **Generalized idiopathic epilepsy and epileptic syndromes**
    Code also MERRF syndrome, if applicable (E88.42)

✓6th **G40.30** **Generalized idiopathic epilepsy and epileptic syndromes, not intractable**
    Generalized idiopathic epilepsy and epileptic syndromes without intractability

    G40.301 **Generalized idiopathic epilepsy and epileptic syndromes, not intractable, with status epilepticus** `MCC` `HCC`

    G40.309 **Generalized idiopathic epilepsy and epileptic syndromes, not intractable, without status epilepticus** `HCC`
        Generalized idiopathic epilepsy and epileptic syndromes NOS

✓6th **G40.31** **Generalized idiopathic epilepsy and epileptic syndromes, intractable**

    G40.311 **Generalized idiopathic epilepsy and epileptic syndromes, intractable, with status epilepticus** `MCC` `HCC`

    G40.319 **Generalized idiopathic epilepsy and epileptic syndromes, intractable, without status epilepticus** `MCC` `HCC`

✓5th **G40.A** **Absence epileptic syndrome**
    Childhood absence epilepsy [pyknolepsy]
    Juvenile absence epilepsy
    Absence epileptic syndrome, NOS

✓6th **G40.A0** **Absence epileptic syndrome, not intractable**

    G40.A01 **Absence epileptic syndrome, not intractable, with status epilepticus** `HCC`

    G40.A09 **Absence epileptic syndrome, not intractable, without status epilepticus** `HCC`

✓6th **G40.A1** **Absence epileptic syndrome, intractable**

    G40.A11 **Absence epileptic syndrome, intractable, with status epilepticus** `CC` `HCC`

    G40.A19 **Absence epileptic syndrome, intractable, without status epilepticus** `CC` `HCC`

✓5th **G40.B** **Juvenile myoclonic epilepsy [impulsive petit mal]**

✓6th **G40.B0** **Juvenile myoclonic epilepsy, not intractable**

    G40.B01 **Juvenile myoclonic epilepsy, not intractable, with status epilepticus** `CC` `HCC`

    G40.B09 **Juvenile myoclonic epilepsy, not intractable, without status epilepticus** `CC` `HCC`

✓6th **G40.B1** **Juvenile myoclonic epilepsy, intractable**

    G40.B11 **Juvenile myoclonic epilepsy, intractable, with status epilepticus** `CC` `HCC`

    G40.B19 **Juvenile myoclonic epilepsy, intractable, without status epilepticus** `CC` `HCC`

☑ Additional Character Required   ✓x7th Placeholder   Unacceptable PDx   Questionable PDx   Manifestation   Unspecified Dx   `H1`-`H14` HAC   `HCC` CMS-HCC Dx   `HIV` HIV Dx

√5ᵗʰ G40.4 Other generalized epilepsy and epileptic syndromes
Epilepsy with grand mal seizures on awakening
Epilepsy with myoclonic absences
Epilepsy with myoclonic-astatic seizures
Grand mal seizure NOS
Nonspecific atonic epileptic seizures
Nonspecific clonic epileptic seizures
Nonspecific myoclonic epileptic seizures
Nonspecific tonic epileptic seizures
Nonspecific tonic-clonic epileptic seizures
Symptomatic early myoclonic encephalopathy

√6ᵗʰ G40.40 Other generalized epilepsy and epileptic syndromes, not intractable
Other generalized epilepsy and epileptic syndromes without intractability
Other generalized epilepsy and epileptic syndromes NOS

G40.401 Other generalized epilepsy and epileptic syndromes, not intractable, with status epilepticus HCC

G40.409 Other generalized epilepsy and epileptic syndromes, not intractable, without status epilepticus HCC

√6ᵗʰ G40.41 Other generalized epilepsy and epileptic syndromes, intractable

G40.411 Other generalized epilepsy and epileptic syndromes, intractable, with status epilepticus CC HCC

G40.419 Other generalized epilepsy and epileptic syndromes, intractable, without status epilepticus CC HCC

√5ᵗʰ G40.5 Epileptic seizures related to external causes
Epileptic seizures related to alcohol
Epileptic seizures related to drugs
Epileptic seizures related to hormonal changes
Epileptic seizures related to sleep deprivation
Epileptic seizures related to stress
Code also, if applicable, associated epilepsy and recurrent seizures (G40.-)
Use additional code for adverse effect, if applicable, to identify drug (T36-T50 with fifth or sixth character 5)

√6ᵗʰ G40.50 Epileptic seizures related to external causes, not intractable

G40.501 Epileptic seizures related to external causes, not intractable, with status epilepticus CC HCC

G40.509 Epileptic seizures related to external causes, not intractable, without status epilepticus CC HCC
Epileptic seizures related to external causes, NOS

√5ᵗʰ G40.8 Other epilepsy and recurrent seizures
Epilepsies and epileptic syndromes undetermined as to whether they are focal or generalized
Landau-Kleffner syndrome

√6ᵗʰ G40.80 Other epilepsy

G40.801 Other epilepsy, not intractable, with status epilepticus CC HCC
Other epilepsy without intractability with status epilepticus

G40.802 Other epilepsy, not intractable, without status epilepticus CC HCC
Other epilepsy NOS
Other epilepsy without intractability without status epilepticus

G40.803 Other epilepsy, intractable, with status epilepticus CC HCC

G40.804 Other epilepsy, intractable, without status epilepticus CC HCC

√6ᵗʰ G40.81 Lennox-Gastaut syndrome
DEF: Severe form of epilepsy with usual onset in early childhood. Seizures are frequent and difficult to treat, causing falls and intellectual impairment.

G40.811 Lennox-Gastaut syndrome, not intractable, with status epilepticus CC HCC

G40.812 Lennox-Gastaut syndrome, not intractable, without status epilepticus CC HCC

G40.813 Lennox-Gastaut syndrome, intractable, with status epilepticus CC HCC

G40.814 Lennox-Gastaut syndrome, intractable, without status epilepticus CC HCC

√6ᵗʰ G40.82 Epileptic spasms
Infantile spasms
Salaam attacks
West's syndrome

G40.821 Epileptic spasms, not intractable, with status epilepticus CC HCC
CC Excl: PDX collection 581

G40.822 Epileptic spasms, not intractable, without status epilepticus CC HCC
CC Excl: PDX collection 581

G40.823 Epileptic spasms, intractable, with status epilepticus CC HCC

G40.824 Epileptic spasms, intractable, without status epilepticus CC HCC

G40.89 Other seizures CC HCC
EXCLUDES 1   post traumatic seizures (R56.1)
recurrent seizures NOS (G40.909)
seizure NOS (R56.9)

√5ᵗʰ G40.9 Epilepsy, unspecified
AHA: 2019,1Q,19

√6ᵗʰ G40.90 Epilepsy, unspecified, not intractable
Epilepsy, unspecified, without intractability

G40.901 Epilepsy, unspecified, not intractable, with status epilepticus HCC

G40.909 Epilepsy, unspecified, not intractable, without status epilepticus HCC
Epilepsy NOS
Epileptic convulsions NOS
Epileptic fits NOS
Epileptic seizures NOS
Recurrent seizures NOS
Seizure disorder NOS

√6ᵗʰ G40.91 Epilepsy, unspecified, intractable
Intractable seizure disorder NOS

G40.911 Epilepsy, unspecified, intractable, with status epilepticus CC HCC

G40.919 Epilepsy, unspecified, intractable, without status epilepticus CC HCC

√4ᵗʰ **G43 Migraine**

NOTE   The following terms are to be considered equivalent to intractable: pharmacoresistant (pharmacologically resistant), treatment resistant, refractory (medically) and poorly controlled

Use additional code for adverse effect, if applicable, to identify drug (T36-T50 with fifth or sixth character 5)

EXCLUDES 1   headache NOS (R51)
           lower half migraine (G44.00)
EXCLUDES 2   headache syndromes (G44.-)

DEF: Headaches that occur periodically on one or both sides of the head that may be associated with nausea and vomiting, sensitivity to light and sound, dizziness, distorted vision, and cognitive disturbances.

√5ᵗʰ **G43.0 Migraine without aura**

Common migraine

EXCLUDES 1   chronic migraine without aura (G43.7-)

√6ᵗʰ **G43.00 Migraine without aura, not intractable**

Migraine without aura without mention of refractory migraine

G43.001 Migraine without aura, not intractable, with status migrainosus

G43.009 Migraine without aura, not intractable, without status migrainosus

Migraine without aura NOS

√6ᵗʰ **G43.01 Migraine without aura, intractable**

Migraine without aura with refractory migraine

G43.011 Migraine without aura, intractable, with status migrainosus

G43.019 Migraine without aura, intractable, without status migrainosus

√5ᵗʰ **G43.1 Migraine with aura**

Basilar migraine
Classical migraine
Migraine equivalents
Migraine preceded or accompanied by transient focal neurological phenomena
Migraine triggered seizures
Migraine with acute-onset aura
Migraine with aura without headache (migraine equivalents)
Migraine with prolonged aura
Migraine with typical aura
Retinal migraine

Code also any associated seizure (G40.-, R56.9)

EXCLUDES 1   persistent migraine aura (G43.5-, G43.6-)

√6ᵗʰ **G43.10 Migraine with aura, not intractable**

Migraine with aura without mention of refractory migraine

G43.101 Migraine with aura, not intractable, with status migrainosus

G43.109 Migraine with aura, not intractable, without status migrainosus

Migraine with aura NOS

√6ᵗʰ **G43.11 Migraine with aura, intractable**

Migraine with aura with refractory migraine

G43.111 Migraine with aura, intractable, with status migrainosus

G43.119 Migraine with aura, intractable, without status migrainosus

√5ᵗʰ **G43.4 Hemiplegic migraine**

Familial migraine
Sporadic migraine

√6ᵗʰ **G43.40 Hemiplegic migraine, not intractable**

Hemiplegic migraine without refractory migraine

G43.401 Hemiplegic migraine, not intractable, with status migrainosus

G43.409 Hemiplegic migraine, not intractable, without status migrainosus

Hemiplegic migraine NOS

√6ᵗʰ **G43.41 Hemiplegic migraine, intractable**

Hemiplegic migraine with refractory migraine

G43.411 Hemiplegic migraine, intractable, with status migrainosus

G43.419 Hemiplegic migraine, intractable, without status migrainosus

√5ᵗʰ **G43.5 Persistent migraine aura without cerebral infarction**

√6ᵗʰ **G43.50 Persistent migraine aura without cerebral infarction, not intractable**

Persistent migraine aura without cerebral infarction, without refractory migraine

G43.501 Persistent migraine aura without cerebral infarction, not intractable, with status migrainosus

G43.509 Persistent migraine aura without cerebral infarction, not intractable, without status migrainosus

Persistent migraine aura NOS

√6ᵗʰ **G43.51 Persistent migraine aura without cerebral infarction, intractable**

Persistent migraine aura without cerebral infarction, with refractory migraine

G43.511 Persistent migraine aura without cerebral infarction, intractable, with status migrainosus

G43.519 Persistent migraine aura without cerebral infarction, intractable, without status migrainosus

√5ᵗʰ **G43.6 Persistent migraine aura with cerebral infarction**

Code also the type of cerebral infarction (I63.-)

CC Excl: For CC codes in subcategory G43.6, unless otherwise noted: PDX collection 584

√6ᵗʰ **G43.60 Persistent migraine aura with cerebral infarction, not intractable**

Persistent migraine aura with cerebral infarction, without refractory migraine

G43.601 Persistent migraine aura with cerebral infarction, not intractable, with status migrainosus   CC

G43.609 Persistent migraine aura with cerebral infarction, not intractable, without status migrainosus   CC

CC Excl: PDX collection 585

√6ᵗʰ **G43.61 Persistent migraine aura with cerebral infarction, intractable**

Persistent migraine aura with cerebral infarction, with refractory migraine

G43.611 Persistent migraine aura with cerebral infarction, intractable, with status migrainosus   CC

G43.619 Persistent migraine aura with cerebral infarction, intractable, without status migrainosus   CC

√5ᵗʰ **G43.7 Chronic migraine without aura**

Transformed migraine

EXCLUDES 1   migraine without aura (G43.0-)

√6ᵗʰ **G43.70 Chronic migraine without aura, not intractable**

Chronic migraine without aura, without refractory migraine

G43.701 Chronic migraine without aura, not intractable, with status migrainosus

G43.709 Chronic migraine without aura, not intractable, without status migrainosus

Chronic migraine without aura NOS

√6ᵗʰ **G43.71 Chronic migraine without aura, intractable**

Chronic migraine without aura, with refractory migraine

G43.711 Chronic migraine without aura, intractable, with status migrainosus

G43.719 Chronic migraine without aura, intractable, without status migrainosus

√5ᵗʰ **G43.A Cyclical vomiting**

EXCLUDES 1   ►cyclical vomiting syndrome unrelated to migraine (R11.15)◄

▲ **G43.A0 Cyclical vomiting, in migraine, not intractable**

Cyclical vomiting, without refractory migraine

▲ **G43.A1 Cyclical vomiting, in migraine, intractable**

Cyclical vomiting, with refractory migraine

✓5ᵗʰ **G43.B** **Ophthalmoplegic** migraine

G43.B0 **Ophthalmoplegic migraine,** not intractable
Ophthalmoplegic migraine, without refractory migraine

G43.B1 **Ophthalmoplegic migraine,** intractable
Ophthalmoplegic migraine, with refractory migraine

✓5ᵗʰ **G43.C** **Periodic headache** syndromes in child or adult

G43.C0 **Periodic headache syndromes in child or adult,** not intractable
Periodic headache syndromes in child or adult, without refractory migraine

G43.C1 **Periodic headache syndromes in child or adult,** intractable
Periodic headache syndromes in child or adult, with refractory migraine

✓5ᵗʰ **G43.D** **Abdominal** migraine

G43.D0 **Abdominal migraine,** not intractable
Abdominal migraine, without refractory migraine

G43.D1 **Abdominal migraine,** intractable
Abdominal migraine, with refractory migraine

✓5ᵗʰ **G43.8** **Other migraine**

✓6ᵗʰ **G43.80** **Other migraine,** not intractable
Other migraine, without refractory migraine

G43.801 **Other migraine, not intractable,** with status migrainosus

G43.809 **Other migraine, not intractable,** without status migrainosus

✓6ᵗʰ **G43.81** **Other migraine,** intractable
Other migraine, with refractory migraine

G43.811 **Other migraine, intractable,** with status migrainosus

G43.819 **Other migraine, intractable,** without status migrainosus

✓6ᵗʰ **G43.82** **Menstrual** migraine, not intractable
Menstrual headache, not intractable
Menstrual migraine, without refractory migraine
Menstrually related migraine, not intractable
Pre-menstrual headache, not intractable
Pre-menstrual migraine, not intractable
Pure menstrual migraine, not intractable
Code also associated premenstrual tension syndrome (N94.3)

G43.821 **Menstrual migraine, not intractable,** with status migrainosus ♀

G43.829 **Menstrual migraine, not intractable,** without status migrainosus ♀
Menstrual migraine NOS

✓6ᵗʰ **G43.83** **Menstrual** migraine, intractable
Menstrual headache, intractable
Menstrual migraine, with refractory migraine
Menstrually related migraine, intractable
Pre-menstrual headache, intractable
Pre-menstrual migraine, intractable
Pure menstrual migraine, intractable
Code also associated premenstrual tension syndrome (N94.3)

G43.831 **Menstrual migraine, intractable,** with status migrainosus ♀

G43.839 **Menstrual migraine, intractable,** without status migrainosus ♀

✓5ᵗʰ **G43.9** **Migraine, unspecified**

✓6ᵗʰ **G43.90** **Migraine, unspecified,** not intractable
Migraine, unspecified, without refractory migraine

G43.901 **Migraine, unspecified, not intractable, with status migrainosus**
Status migrainosus NOS

G43.909 **Migraine, unspecified, not intractable, without status migrainosus**
Migraine NOS

✓6ᵗʰ **G43.91** **Migraine, unspecified,** intractable
Migraine, unspecified, with refractory migraine

G43.911 **Migraine, unspecified, intractable, with status migrainosus**

G43.919 **Migraine, unspecified, intractable, without status migrainosus**

✓4ᵗʰ **G44** **Other** headache **syndromes**

EXCLUDES 1   headache NOS (R51)
EXCLUDES 2   atypical facial pain (G50.1)
headache due to lumbar puncture (G97.1)
migraines (G43.-)
trigeminal neuralgia (G50.0)

✓5ᵗʰ **G44.0** **Cluster headaches** and other trigeminal autonomic cephalgias (TAC)
DEF: Cluster headache: Characteristic grouping or clustering of headaches that can last for a number of weeks or months and then completely disappear for months or years. They are typically not associated with gastrointestinal upset or light sensitivity as experienced in migraines.

✓6ᵗʰ **G44.00** **Cluster headache syndrome, unspecified**
Ciliary neuralgia
Cluster headache NOS
Histamine cephalgia
Lower half migraine
Migrainous neuralgia

G44.001 **Cluster headache syndrome, unspecified, intractable**

G44.009 **Cluster headache syndrome, unspecified, not intractable**
Cluster headache syndrome NOS

✓6ᵗʰ **G44.01** **Episodic** cluster headache
G44.011 **Episodic cluster headache,** intractable
G44.019 **Episodic cluster headache,** not intractable
Episodic cluster headache NOS

✓6ᵗʰ **G44.02** **Chronic** cluster headache
G44.021 **Chronic cluster headache,** intractable
G44.029 **Chronic cluster headache,** not intractable
Chronic cluster headache NOS

✓6ᵗʰ **G44.03** **Episodic paroxysmal hemicrania**
Paroxysmal hemicrania NOS
G44.031 **Episodic paroxysmal hemicrania, intractable**
G44.039 **Episodic paroxysmal hemicrania, not intractable**
Episodic paroxysmal hemicrania NOS

✓6ᵗʰ **G44.04** **Chronic** paroxysmal hemicrania
G44.041 **Chronic paroxysmal hemicrania, intractable**
G44.049 **Chronic paroxysmal hemicrania, not intractable**
Chronic paroxysmal hemicrania NOS

✓6ᵗʰ **G44.05** **Short lasting unilateral** neuralgiform headache with conjunctival injection and tearing (SUNCT)
G44.051 **Short lasting unilateral neuralgiform headache with conjunctival injection and tearing (SUNCT),** intractable
G44.059 **Short lasting unilateral neuralgiform headache with conjunctival injection and tearing (SUNCT),** not intractable
Short lasting unilateral neuralgiform headache with conjunctival injection and tearing (SUNCT) NOS

✓6ᵗʰ **G44.09** **Other** trigeminal autonomic cephalgias **(TAC)**
G44.091 **Other trigeminal autonomic cephalgias (TAC),** intractable
G44.099 **Other trigeminal autonomic cephalgias (TAC),** not intractable

G44.1 **Vascular** headache, not elsewhere classified
EXCLUDES 2   cluster headache (G44.0)
complicated headache syndromes (G44.5-)
drug-induced headache (G44.4-)
migraine (G43.-)
other specified headache syndromes (G44.8-)
post-traumatic headache (G44.3-)
tension-type headache (G44.2-)

✓5ᵗʰ **G44.2** **Tension-type** headache
✓6ᵗʰ **G44.20** **Tension-type headache, unspecified**
G44.201 **Tension-type headache, unspecified, intractable**

      G44.209 **Tension-type headache, unspecified, not intractable**
          Tension headache NOS

√6th G44.21 **Episodic tension-type headache**
      G44.211 **Episodic tension-type headache, intractable**
      G44.219 **Episodic tension-type headache, not intractable**
          Episodic tension-type headache NOS

√6th G44.22 **Chronic tension-type headache**
      G44.221 **Chronic tension-type headache, intractable**
      G44.229 **Chronic tension-type headache, not intractable**
          Chronic tension-type headache NOS

√5th **G44.3** **Post-traumatic headache**

  √6th **G44.30** **Post-traumatic headache, unspecified**
      G44.301 **Post-traumatic headache, unspecified, intractable**
      G44.309 **Post-traumatic headache, unspecified, not intractable**
          Post-traumatic headache NOS

  √6th **G44.31** **Acute post-traumatic headache**
      G44.311 **Acute post-traumatic headache, intractable**
      G44.319 **Acute post-traumatic headache, not intractable**
          Acute post-traumatic headache NOS

  √6th **G44.32** **Chronic post-traumatic headache**
      G44.321 **Chronic post-traumatic headache, intractable**
      G44.329 **Chronic post-traumatic headache, not intractable**
          Chronic post-traumatic headache NOS

√5th **G44.4** **Drug-induced headache, not elsewhere classified**
    Medication overuse headache
    Use additional code for adverse effect, if applicable, to identify drug (T36-T50 with fifth or sixth character 5)

      G44.40 **Drug-induced headache, not elsewhere classified, not intractable**
      G44.41 **Drug-induced headache, not elsewhere classified, intractable**

√5th **G44.5** **Complicated headache syndromes**

      G44.51 **Hemicrania continua**
          DEF: Persistent primary headache of unknown causation occurring on one side of the face and head. May last for more than three months, with daily and continuous pain of moderate intensity with severe exacerbations.
      G44.52 **New daily persistent headache (NDPH)**
      G44.53 **Primary thunderclap headache**
      G44.59 **Other complicated headache syndrome**

√5th **G44.8** **Other specified headache syndromes**
      G44.81 **Hypnic headache**
      G44.82 **Headache associated with sexual activity**
          Orgasmic headache
          Preorgasmic headache
      G44.83 **Primary cough headache**
      G44.84 **Primary exertional headache**
      G44.85 **Primary stabbing headache**
      G44.89 **Other headache syndrome**

√4th **G45** **Transient cerebral ischemic attacks and related syndromes**
    EXCLUDES 1 neonatal cerebral ischemia (P91.0)
          transient retinal artery occlusion (H34.0-)
    AHA: 2018,2Q,9
    DEF: Transient cerebral ischemic attack: Intermittent or brief cerebral dysfunction from lack of oxygenation with no persistent neurological deficits associated with occlusive vascular disease. TIA may denote an impending cerebrovascular accident.

    G45.0 **Vertebro-basilar artery syndrome**
    G45.1 **Carotid artery syndrome (hemispheric)**
    G45.2 **Multiple and bilateral precerebral artery syndromes**
    G45.3 **Amaurosis fugax**
    G45.4 **Transient global amnesia**
        EXCLUDES 1 amnesia NOS (R41.3)

    G45.8 **Other transient cerebral ischemic attacks and related syndromes** CC
        CC Excl: PDX collection 586

    G45.9 **Transient cerebral ischemic attack, unspecified** CC
        Spasm of cerebral artery
        TIA
        Transient cerebral ischemia NOS
        CC Excl: PDX collection 586

√4th **G46** **Vascular syndromes of brain in cerebrovascular diseases**
    Code first underlying cerebrovascular disease (I60-I69)
    CC Excl: For CC codes in category G46: PDX collection 586

    G46.0 **Middle cerebral artery syndrome** CC
    G46.1 **Anterior cerebral artery syndrome** CC
    G46.2 **Posterior cerebral artery syndrome** CC
    G46.3 **Brain stem stroke syndrome**
        Benedikt syndrome
        Claude syndrome
        Foville syndrome
        Millard-Gubler syndrome
        Wallenberg syndrome
        Weber syndrome
    G46.4 **Cerebellar stroke syndrome**
    G46.5 **Pure motor lacunar syndrome**
    G46.6 **Pure sensory lacunar syndrome**
    G46.7 **Other lacunar syndromes**
    G46.8 **Other vascular syndromes of brain in cerebrovascular diseases**

√4th **G47** **Sleep disorders**
    EXCLUDES 2 nightmares (F51.5)
          nonorganic sleep disorders (F51.-)
          sleep terrors (F51.4)
          sleepwalking (F51.3)

  √5th **G47.0** **Insomnia**
      EXCLUDES 2 alcohol related insomnia (F10.182, F10.282, F10.982)
          drug-related insomnia (F11.182, F11.282, F11.982, F13.182, F13.282, F13.982, F14.182, F14.282, F14.982, F15.182, F15.282, F15.982, F19.182, F19.282, F19.982)
          idiopathic insomnia (F51.01)
          insomnia due to a mental disorder (F51.05)
          insomnia not due to a substance or known physiological condition (F51.0-)
          nonorganic insomnia (F51.0-)
          primary insomnia (F51.01)
          sleep apnea (G47.3-)
      G47.00 **Insomnia, unspecified**
          Insomnia NOS
      G47.01 **Insomnia due to medical condition**
          Code also associated medical condition
      G47.09 **Other insomnia**

  √5th **G47.1** **Hypersomnia**
      EXCLUDES 2 alcohol-related hypersomnia (F10.182, F10.282, F10.982)
          drug-related hypersomnia (F11.182, F11.282, F11.982, F13.182, F13.282, F13.982, F14.182, F14.282, F14.982, F15.182, F15.282, F15.982, F19.182, F19.282, F19.982)
          hypersomnia due to a mental disorder (F51.13)
          hypersomnia not due to a substance or known physiological condition (F51.1-)
          primary hypersomnia (F51.11)
          sleep apnea (G47.3-)
      G47.10 **Hypersomnia, unspecified**
          Hypersomnia NOS
      G47.11 **Idiopathic hypersomnia with long sleep time**
          Idiopathic hypersomnia NOS
      G47.12 **Idiopathic hypersomnia without long sleep time**
      G47.13 **Recurrent hypersomnia**
          Kleine-Levin syndrome
          Menstrual related hypersomnia
      G47.14 **Hypersomnia due to medical condition**
          Code also associated medical condition
      G47.19 **Other hypersomnia**

☑ Additional Character Required   √x7th Placeholder   Unacceptable PDx   Questionable PDx   Manifestation   Unspecified Dx   H1-H14 HAC   HCC CMS-HCC Dx   HIV HIV Dx

ICD-10-CM 2020   **581**

Chapter 6. Diseases of the Nervous System

G47.2–G51.9

✓5ᵗʰ **G47.2 Circadian rhythm sleep disorders**

Disorders of the sleep wake schedule

Inversion of nyctohemeral rhythm

Inversion of sleep rhythm

DEF: Circadian rhythm: Daily cycle (24-hour period) of physical, mental and behavioral changes. It is largely influenced by environmental ques, such as changes in light or temperature. *Synonyms: sleep/wake cycle.*

G47.20 Circadian rhythm sleep disorder, unspecified type

Sleep wake schedule disorder NOS

G47.21 Circadian rhythm sleep disorder, delayed sleep phase type

Delayed sleep phase syndrome

G47.22 Circadian rhythm sleep disorder, advanced sleep phase type

G47.23 Circadian rhythm sleep disorder, irregular sleep wake type

Irregular sleep-wake pattern

G47.24 Circadian rhythm sleep disorder, free running type

Circadian rhythm sleep disorder, non-24-hour sleep-wake type

G47.25 Circadian rhythm sleep disorder, jet lag type

G47.26 Circadian rhythm sleep disorder, shift work type

G47.27 Circadian rhythm sleep disorder in conditions classified elsewhere

Code first underlying condition

G47.29 Other circadian rhythm sleep disorder

✓5ᵗʰ **G47.3 Sleep apnea**

Code also any associated underlying condition

EXCLUDES 1   apnea NOS (R06.81)

Cheyne-Stokes breathing (R06.3)

pickwickian syndrome (E66.2)

sleep apnea of newborn (P28.3)

G47.30 Sleep apnea, unspecified

Sleep apnea NOS

G47.31 Primary central sleep apnea

Idiopathic central sleep apnea

G47.32 High altitude periodic breathing

G47.33 Obstructive sleep apnea (adult) (pediatric)

Obstructive sleep apnea hypopnea

EXCLUDES 1   obstructive sleep apnea of newborn (P28.3)

G47.34 Idiopathic sleep related nonobstructive alveolar hypoventilation

Sleep related hypoxia

G47.35 Congenital central alveolar hypoventilation syndrome

G47.36 Sleep related hypoventilation in conditions classified elsewhere

Sleep related hypoxemia in conditions classified elsewhere

Code first underlying condition

G47.37 Central sleep apnea in conditions classified elsewhere

Code first underlying condition

G47.39 Other sleep apnea

✓5ᵗʰ **G47.4 Narcolepsy and cataplexy**

✓6ᵗʰ **G47.41 Narcolepsy**

G47.411 Narcolepsy with cataplexy

G47.419 Narcolepsy without cataplexy

Narcolepsy NOS

✓6ᵗʰ **G47.42 Narcolepsy in conditions classified elsewhere**

Code first underlying condition

G47.421 Narcolepsy in conditions classified elsewhere with cataplexy

G47.429 Narcolepsy in conditions classified elsewhere without cataplexy

✓5ᵗʰ **G47.5 Parasomnia**

EXCLUDES 1   alcohol induced parasomnia (F10.182, F10.282, F10.982)

drug induced parasomnia (F11.182, F11.282, F11.982, F13.182, F13.282, F13.982, F14.182, F14.282, F14.982, F15.182, F15.282, F15.982, F19.182, F19.282, F19.982)

parasomnia not due to a substance or known physiological condition (F51.8)

G47.50 Parasomnia, unspecified

Parasomnia NOS

G47.51 Confusional arousals

G47.52 REM sleep behavior disorder

G47.53 Recurrent isolated sleep paralysis

G47.54 Parasomnia in conditions classified elsewhere

Code first underlying condition

G47.59 Other parasomnia

✓5ᵗʰ **G47.6 Sleep related movement disorders**

EXCLUDES 2   restless legs syndrome (G25.81)

G47.61 Periodic limb movement disorder

G47.62 Sleep related leg cramps

G47.63 Sleep related bruxism

EXCLUDES 1   psychogenic bruxism (F45.8)

G47.69 Other sleep related movement disorders

G47.8 Other sleep disorders

Other specified sleep-wake disorder

G47.9 Sleep disorder, unspecified

Sleep disorder NOS

Unspecified sleep-wake disorder

Nerve, nerve root and plexus disorders (G50-G59)

EXCLUDES 1   current traumatic nerve, nerve root and plexus disorders — see Injury, nerve by body region

neuralgia NOS (M79.2)

neuritis NOS (M79.2)

peripheral neuritis in pregnancy (O26.82-)

radiculitis NOS (M54.1-)

✓4ᵗʰ **G50 Disorders of trigeminal nerve**

INCLUDES   disorders of 5th cranial nerve

Trigeminal and Facial Nerve Branches

Supratrochlear nerve

Supraorbital nerve

V2 branch

Infraorbital nerve

V1 branch

Trigeminal nerve (CN V) branches in infratemporal fossa

V3 branch

Mental nerve

Mental foramen

G50.0 Trigeminal neuralgia

Syndrome of paroxysmal facial pain

Tic douloureux

G50.1 Atypical facial pain

G50.8 Other disorders of trigeminal nerve

G50.9 Disorder of trigeminal nerve, unspecified

✓4ᵗʰ **G51 Facial nerve disorders**

INCLUDES   disorders of 7th cranial nerve

G51.0 Bell's palsy

Facial palsy

G51.1 Geniculate ganglionitis

EXCLUDES 1   postherpetic geniculate ganglionitis (B02.21)

G51.2 Melkersson's syndrome

Melkersson-Rosenthal syndrome

✓5ᵗʰ **G51.3 Clonic hemifacial spasm**

AHA: 2018,4Q,10

G51.31 Clonic hemifacial spasm, right

G51.32 Clonic hemifacial spasm, left

G51.33 Clonic hemifacial spasm, bilateral

G51.39 Clonic hemifacial spasm, unspecified

G51.4 Facial myokymia

G51.8 Other disorders of facial nerve

G51.9 Disorder of facial nerve, unspecified

N Newborn: 0   P Pediatric: 0-17   M Maternity: 9-64   A Adult: 15-124   MCC Major Complication/Comorbidity   CC Complication/Comorbidity   SW Severe Wound Dx

582   ICD-10-CM 2020

☑️4ᵗʰ **G52** **Disorders of other cranial nerves**
> **EXCLUDES 2**   *disorders of acoustic [8th] nerve (H93.3)*
> *disorders of optic [2nd] nerve (H46, H47.0)*
> *paralytic strabismus due to nerve palsy (H49.0-H49.2)*

G52.0 **Disorders of olfactory nerve**
> Disorders of 1st cranial nerve

G52.1 **Disorders of glossopharyngeal nerve**
> Disorder of 9th cranial nerve
> Glossopharyngeal neuralgia

G52.2 **Disorders of vagus nerve**
> Disorders of pneumogastric [10th] nerve

G52.3 **Disorders of hypoglossal nerve**
> Disorders of 12th cranial nerve

G52.7 **Disorders of multiple cranial nerves**
> Polyneuritis cranialis

G52.8 **Disorders of other specified cranial nerves**

G52.9 **Cranial nerve disorder, unspecified**

G53 *Cranial nerve disorders in diseases classified elsewhere*
> Code first underlying disease, such as:
> neoplasm (C00-D49)
> **EXCLUDES 1**   *multiple cranial nerve palsy in sarcoidosis (D86.82)*
> *multiple cranial nerve palsy in syphilis (A52.15)*
> *postherpetic geniculate ganglionitis (B02.21)*
> *postherpetic trigeminal neuralgia (B02.22)*

☑️4ᵗʰ **G54** **Nerve root and plexus disorders**
> **EXCLUDES 1**   *current traumatic nerve root and plexus disorders — see nerve injury by body region*
> *intervertebral disc disorders (M50-M51)*
> *neuralgia or neuritis NOS (M79.2)*
> *neuritis or radiculitis brachial NOS (M54.13)*
> *neuritis or radiculitis lumbar NOS (M54.16)*
> *neuritis or radiculitis lumbosacral NOS (M54.17)*
> *neuritis or radiculitis thoracic NOS (M54.14)*
> *radiculitis NOS (M54.10)*
> *radiculopathy NOS (M54.10)*
> *spondylosis (M47.-)*

G54.0 **Brachial plexus disorders**
> Thoracic outlet syndrome
> **DEF:** Acquired disorder affecting the spinal nerves that send signals to the shoulder, arm, and hand, causing corresponding motor and sensory dysfunction. This disorder is characterized by regional paresthesia, pain, muscle weakness, and in severe cases paralysis.

G54.1 **Lumbosacral plexus disorders**

G54.2 **Cervical root disorders, not elsewhere classified**

G54.3 **Thoracic root disorders, not elsewhere classified**

G54.4 **Lumbosacral root disorders, not elsewhere classified**

G54.5 **Neuralgic amyotrophy**
> Parsonage-Aldren-Turner syndrome
> Shoulder-girdle neuritis
> **EXCLUDES 1**   *neuralgic amyotrophy in diabetes mellitus (E08-E13 with .44)*

G54.6 **Phantom limb syndrome with pain**   HCC

G54.7 **Phantom limb syndrome without pain**   HCC
> Phantom limb syndrome NOS

G54.8 **Other nerve root and plexus disorders**

G54.9 **Nerve root and plexus disorder, unspecified**

G55 *Nerve root and plexus compressions in diseases classified elsewhere*
> Code first underlying disease, such as:
> neoplasm (C00-D49)
> **EXCLUDES 1**   *nerve root compression (due to) (in) ankylosing spondylitis (M45.-)*
> *nerve root compression (due to) (in) dorsopathies (M53.-, M54.-)*
> *nerve root compression (due to) (in) intervertebral disc disorders (M50.1.-, M51.1.-)*
> *nerve root compression (due to) (in) spondylopathies (M46.-, M48.-)*
> *nerve root compression (due to) (in) spondylosis (M47.0-M47.2-)*

☑️4ᵗʰ **G56** **Mononeuropathies of upper limb**
> **EXCLUDES 1**   *current traumatic nerve disorder — see nerve injury by body region*
> **AHA:** 2016,4Q,17-18

Nerves of Upper Limb

Radial
Deep branch of radial
Ulnar
Superficial branch of radial
Median

☑️5ᵗʰ **G56.0** **Carpal tunnel syndrome**
> **DEF:** Swelling and inflammation in the tendons or bursa surrounding the median nerve caused by repetitive activity. The resulting compression on the nerve causes pain, numbness, and tingling especially to the palm, index, middle finger, and thumb.

G56.00 **Carpal tunnel syndrome, unspecified upper limb**

G56.01 **Carpal tunnel syndrome, right upper limb**

G56.02 **Carpal tunnel syndrome, left upper limb**

G56.03 **Carpal tunnel syndrome, bilateral upper limbs**

☑️5ᵗʰ **G56.1** **Other lesions of median nerve**

G56.10 **Other lesions of median nerve, unspecified upper limb**

G56.11 **Other lesions of median nerve, right upper limb**

G56.12 **Other lesions of median nerve, left upper limb**

G56.13 **Other lesions of median nerve, bilateral upper limbs**

☑️5ᵗʰ **G56.2** **Lesion of ulnar nerve**
> Tardy ulnar nerve palsy

G56.20 **Lesion of ulnar nerve, unspecified upper limb**

G56.21 **Lesion of ulnar nerve, right upper limb**

G56.22 **Lesion of ulnar nerve, left upper limb**

G56.23 **Lesion of ulnar nerve, bilateral upper limbs**

☑️5ᵗʰ **G56.3** **Lesion of radial nerve**

G56.30 **Lesion of radial nerve, unspecified upper limb**

G56.31 **Lesion of radial nerve, right upper limb**

G56.32 **Lesion of radial nerve, left upper limb**

G56.33 **Lesion of radial nerve, bilateral upper limbs**

☑️5ᵗʰ **G56.4** **Causalgia of upper limb**
> Complex regional pain syndrome II of upper limb
> **EXCLUDES 1**   *complex regional pain syndrome I of lower limb (G90.52-)*
> *complex regional pain syndrome I of upper limb (G90.51-)*
> *complex regional pain syndrome II of lower limb (G57.7-)*
> *reflex sympathetic dystrophy of lower limb (G90.52-)*
> *reflex sympathetic dystrophy of upper limb (G90.51-)*

G56.40 **Causalgia of unspecified upper limb**

G56.41 **Causalgia of right upper limb**

G56.42 **Causalgia of left upper limb**

G56.43 **Causalgia of bilateral upper limbs**

☑️5ᵗʰ **G56.8** **Other specified mononeuropathies of upper limb**
> Interdigital neuroma of upper limb

G56.80 **Other specified mononeuropathies of unspecified upper limb**

☑️ Additional Character Required   ☑️x7ᵗʰ Placeholder   Unacceptable PDx   Questionable PDx   Manifestation   Unspecified Dx   H1-H14 HAC   HCC CMS-HCC Dx   HIV HIV Dx

ICD-10-CM 2020   583

G56.81   Other specified mononeuropathies of right upper limb
G56.82   Other specified mononeuropathies of left upper limb
G56.83   Other specified mononeuropathies of bilateral upper limbs

√5ᵗʰ G56.9   Unspecified mononeuropathy of upper limb
G56.90   Unspecified mononeuropathy of unspecified upper limb
G56.91   Unspecified mononeuropathy of right upper limb
G56.92   Unspecified mononeuropathy of left upper limb
G56.93   Unspecified mononeuropathy of bilateral upper limbs

√4ᵗʰ G57   Mononeuropathies of lower limb
EXCLUDES 1   current traumatic nerve disorder — see nerve injury by body region
AHA: 2016,4Q,17-18

Nerves of Lower Limb

Obturator nerve
Sciatic nerve
Femoral nerve
Saphenous nerve
Common fibular (peroneal) nerve
Deep fibular (peroneal) nerve
Tibial nerve
Superficial fibular (peroneal) nerve

√5ᵗʰ G57.0   Lesion of sciatic nerve
EXCLUDES 1   sciatica NOS (M54.3-)
EXCLUDES 2   sciatica attributed to intervertebral disc disorder (M51.1.-)
G57.00   Lesion of sciatic nerve, unspecified lower limb
G57.01   Lesion of sciatic nerve, right lower limb
G57.02   Lesion of sciatic nerve, left lower limb
G57.03   Lesion of sciatic nerve, bilateral lower limbs

√5ᵗʰ G57.1   Meralgia paresthetica
Lateral cutaneous nerve of thigh syndrome
G57.10   Meralgia paresthetica, unspecified lower limb
G57.11   Meralgia paresthetica, right lower limb
G57.12   Meralgia paresthetica, left lower limb
G57.13   Meralgia paresthetica, bilateral lower limbs

√5ᵗʰ G57.2   Lesion of femoral nerve
G57.20   Lesion of femoral nerve, unspecified lower limb
G57.21   Lesion of femoral nerve, right lower limb
G57.22   Lesion of femoral nerve, left lower limb
G57.23   Lesion of femoral nerve, bilateral lower limbs

√5ᵗʰ G57.3   Lesion of lateral popliteal nerve
Peroneal nerve palsy
G57.30   Lesion of lateral popliteal nerve, unspecified lower limb
G57.31   Lesion of lateral popliteal nerve, right lower limb
G57.32   Lesion of lateral popliteal nerve, left lower limb
G57.33   Lesion of lateral popliteal nerve, bilateral lower limbs

√5ᵗʰ G57.4   Lesion of medial popliteal nerve
G57.40   Lesion of medial popliteal nerve, unspecified lower limb
G57.41   Lesion of medial popliteal nerve, right lower limb
G57.42   Lesion of medial popliteal nerve, left lower limb
G57.43   Lesion of medial popliteal nerve, bilateral lower limbs

√5ᵗʰ G57.5   Tarsal tunnel syndrome
G57.50   Tarsal tunnel syndrome, unspecified lower limb
G57.51   Tarsal tunnel syndrome, right lower limb
G57.52   Tarsal tunnel syndrome, left lower limb
G57.53   Tarsal tunnel syndrome, bilateral lower limbs

√5ᵗʰ G57.6   Lesion of plantar nerve
Morton's metatarsalgia
G57.60   Lesion of plantar nerve, unspecified lower limb
G57.61   Lesion of plantar nerve, right lower limb
G57.62   Lesion of plantar nerve, left lower limb
G57.63   Lesion of plantar nerve, bilateral lower limbs

√5ᵗʰ G57.7   Causalgia of lower limb
Complex regional pain syndrome II of lower limb
EXCLUDES 1   complex regional pain syndrome I of lower limb (G90.52-)
complex regional pain syndrome I of upper limb (G90.51-)
complex regional pain syndrome II of upper limb (G56.4-)
reflex sympathetic dystrophy of lower limb (G90.52-)
reflex sympathetic dystrophy of upper limb (G90.51-)
G57.70   Causalgia of unspecified lower limb
G57.71   Causalgia of right lower limb
G57.72   Causalgia of left lower limb
G57.73   Causalgia of bilateral lower limbs

√5ᵗʰ G57.8   Other specified mononeuropathies of lower limb
Interdigital neuroma of lower limb
G57.80   Other specified mononeuropathies of unspecified lower limb
G57.81   Other specified mononeuropathies of right lower limb
G57.82   Other specified mononeuropathies of left lower limb
G57.83   Other specified mononeuropathies of bilateral lower limbs

√5ᵗʰ G57.9   Unspecified mononeuropathy of lower limb
G57.90   Unspecified mononeuropathy of unspecified lower limb
G57.91   Unspecified mononeuropathy of right lower limb
G57.92   Unspecified mononeuropathy of left lower limb
G57.93   Unspecified mononeuropathy of bilateral lower limbs

√4ᵗʰ G58   Other mononeuropathies
G58.0   Intercostal neuropathy
G58.7   Mononeuritis multiplex
G58.8   Other specified mononeuropathies
G58.9   Mononeuropathy, unspecified

G59   **Mononeuropathy in diseases classified elsewhere**
Code first underlying disease
EXCLUDES 1   diabetic mononeuropathy (E08-E13 with .41)
syphilitic nerve paralysis (A52.19)
syphilitic neuritis (A52.15)
tuberculous mononeuropathy (A17.83)

Polyneuropathies and other disorders of the peripheral nervous system (G60-G65)

> **EXCLUDES 1**   neuralgia NOS (M79.2)
> neuritis NOS (M79.2)
> peripheral neuritis in pregnancy (O26.82-)
> radiculitis NOS (M54.10)

✓4ᵗʰ G60   Hereditary and idiopathic neuropathy

G60.0   **Hereditary motor and sensory neuropathy**
Charcôt-Marie-Tooth disease
Déjérine-Sottas disease
Hereditary motor and sensory neuropathy, types I-IV
Hypertrophic neuropathy of infancy
Peroneal muscular atrophy (axonal type) (hypertrophic type)
Roussy-Levy syndrome

G60.1   **Refsum's disease**   `CC`
Infantile Refsum disease
DEF: Genetic disorder of the lipid metabolism characterized by retinitis pigmentosa, degenerative nerve disease, ataxia, and dry, rough, scaly skin.
CC Excl: PDX collection 588

G60.2   **Neuropathy in association with hereditary ataxia**

G60.3   **Idiopathic progressive neuropathy**

G60.8   **Other hereditary and idiopathic neuropathies**
Dominantly inherited sensory neuropathy
Morvan's disease
Nelaton's syndrome
Recessively inherited sensory neuropathy

G60.9   **Hereditary and idiopathic neuropathy, unspecified**

✓4ᵗʰ G61   Inflammatory polyneuropathy

G61.0   **Guillain-Barre syndrome**   `CC` `HCC`
Acute (post-)infective polyneuritis
Miller Fisher syndrome
AHA: 2014,2Q,4
DEF: Autoimmune disorder due to an immune response to foreign antigens with paraplegia of limbs, flaccid paralysis, ophthalmoplegia, ataxia, and areflexia. In most cases, this disorder is triggered by a mild viral infection, surgery, or following an immunization.
TIP: Guillain-Barre syndrome can occur as a sequela of *Campylobacter enteritis.* Assign code B94.8 for the sequelae as an additional diagnosis.
CC Excl: PDX collection 92

G61.1   **Serum neuropathy**   `HCC`
Use additional code for adverse effect, if applicable, to identify serum (T50.-)

✓5ᵗʰ G61.8   **Other inflammatory polyneuropathies**

    G61.81   **Chronic inflammatory demyelinating polyneuritis**   `CC` `HCC`
       CC Excl: PDX collection 589

    G61.82   **Multifocal motor neuropathy**   `HCC`
       MMN
       AHA: 2016,4Q,18

    G61.89   **Other inflammatory polyneuropathies**   `HCC`

G61.9   **Inflammatory polyneuropathy, unspecified**   `HCC`

✓4ᵗʰ G62   Other and unspecified polyneuropathies

G62.0   **Drug-induced polyneuropathy**   `HCC`
Use additional code for adverse effect, if applicable, to identify drug (T36-T50 with fifth or sixth character 5)

G62.1   **Alcoholic polyneuropathy**   `HCC`

G62.2   **Polyneuropathy due to other toxic agents**   `HCC`
Code first (T51-T65) to identify toxic agent

✓5ᵗʰ G62.8   **Other specified polyneuropathies**

    G62.81   **Critical illness polyneuropathy**   `CC` `HCC`
       Acute motor neuropathy
       CC Excl: PDX collection 590

    G62.82   **Radiation-induced polyneuropathy**   `HCC`
       Use additional external cause code (W88-W90, X39.0-) to identify cause

    G62.89   **Other specified polyneuropathies**
       AHA: 2016,2Q,11

G62.9   **Polyneuropathy, unspecified**
Neuropathy NOS

G63   *Polyneuropathy in diseases classified elsewhere*   `HCC`
Code first underlying disease, such as:
    amyloidosis (E85.-)
    endocrine disease, except diabetes (E00-E07, E15-E16, E20-E34)
    metabolic diseases (E70-E88)
    neoplasm (C00-D49)
    nutritional deficiency (E40-E64)

> **EXCLUDES 1**   polyneuropathy (in):
>   diabetes mellitus (E08-E13 with .42)
>   diphtheria (A36.83)
>   infectious mononucleosis (B27.0-B27.9 with 1)
>   Lyme disease (A69.22)
>   mumps (B26.84)
>   postherpetic (B02.23)
>   rheumatoid arthritis ▶(M05.5-)◀
>   scleroderma (M34.83)
>   systemic lupus erythematosus (M32.19)

    AHA: 2012,4Q,99

G64   Other disorders of peripheral nervous system
Disorder of peripheral nervous system NOS

✓4ᵗʰ G65   Sequelae of inflammatory and toxic polyneuropathies
Code first condition resulting from (sequela) of inflammatory and toxic polyneuropathies

G65.0   **Sequelae of Guillain-Barré syndrome**   `HCC`

G65.1   **Sequelae of other inflammatory polyneuropathy**   `HCC`

G65.2   **Sequelae of toxic polyneuropathy**   `HCC`

Diseases of myoneural junction and muscle (G70-G73)

✓4ᵗʰ G70   Myasthenia gravis and other myoneural disorders

> **EXCLUDES 1**   botulism (A05.1, A48.51-A48.52)
> transient neonatal myasthenia gravis (P94.0)

CC Excl: For CC/MCC codes in category G70: PDX collection 591

✓5ᵗʰ G70.0   **Myasthenia gravis**
DEF: Autoimmune neuromuscular disorder caused by antibodies to the acetylcholine receptors at the neuromuscular junction, interfering with proper binding of the neurotransmitter from the neuron to the target muscle, causing muscle weakness, fatigue, and exhaustion, without pain or atrophy.

    G70.00   **Myasthenia gravis without (acute) exacerbation**   `HCC`
       Myasthenia gravis NOS

    G70.01   **Myasthenia gravis with (acute) exacerbation**   `MCC` `HCC`
       Myasthenia gravis in crisis

G70.1   **Toxic myoneural disorders**   `HCC`
Code first (T51-T65) to identify toxic agent

G70.2   **Congenital and developmental myasthenia**   `HCC`

✓5ᵗʰ G70.8   **Other specified myoneural disorders**

    G70.80   **Lambert-Eaton syndrome, unspecified**   `CC` `HCC`
       Lambert-Eaton syndrome NOS

    G70.81   ***Lambert-Eaton syndrome in disease classified elsewhere***   `CC` `HCC`
       Code first underlying disease
>   **EXCLUDES 1**   Lambert-Eaton syndrome in neoplastic disease (G73.1)

    G70.89   **Other specified myoneural disorders**   `HCC`

G70.9   **Myoneural disorder, unspecified**   `HCC`

✓4ᵗʰ G71   Primary disorders of muscles

> **EXCLUDES 2**   arthrogryposis multiplex congenita (Q74.3)
> metabolic disorders (E70-E88)
> myositis (M60.-)

✓5ᵗʰ G71.0   **Muscular dystrophy**
AHA: 2018,4Q,11-12

    G71.00   **Muscular dystrophy, unspecified**   `HCC`

    G71.01   **Duchenne or Becker muscular dystrophy**   `HCC`
       Autosomal recessive, childhood type, muscular dystrophy resembling Duchenne or Becker muscular dystrophy
       Benign [Becker] muscular dystrophy
       Severe [Duchenne] muscular dystrophy

G71.02 **Facioscapulohumeral muscular dystrophy** `HCC`
Scapulohumeral muscular dystrophy

G71.09 **Other specified muscular dystrophies** `HCC`
Benign scapuloperoneal muscular dystrophy with early contractures [Emery-Dreifuss]
Congenital muscular dystrophy NOS
Congenital muscular dystrophy with specific morphological abnormalities of the muscle fiber
Distal muscular dystrophy
Limb-girdle muscular dystrophy
Ocular muscular dystrophy
Oculopharyngeal muscular dystrophy
Scapuloperoneal muscular dystrophy

✓5ᵗʰ **G71.1** **Myotonic disorders**

G71.11 **Myotonic muscular dystrophy** `HCC`
Dystrophia myotonica [Steinert]
Myotonia atrophica
Myotonic dystrophy
Proximal myotonic myopathy (PROMM)
Steinert disease

G71.12 **Myotonia congenita**
Acetazolamide responsive myotonia congenita
Dominant myotonia congenita [Thomsen disease]
Myotonia levior
Recessive myotonia congenita [Becker disease]

G71.13 **Myotonic chondrodystrophy**
Chondrodystrophic myotonia
Congenital myotonic chondrodystrophy
Schwartz-Jampel disease

G71.14 **Drug induced myotonia**
Use additional code for adverse effect, if applicable, to identify drug (T36-T50 with fifth or sixth character 5)

G71.19 **Other specified myotonic disorders**
Myotonia fluctuans
Myotonia permanens
Neuromyotonia [Isaacs]
Paramyotonia congenita (of von Eulenburg)
Pseudomyotonia
Symptomatic myotonia

G71.2 **Congenital myopathies** `CC` `HCC`
Central core disease
Fiber-type disproportion
Minicore disease
Multicore disease
Myotubular (centronuclear) myopathy
Nemaline myopathy
EXCLUDES 1 arthrogryposis multiplex congenita (Q74.3)
CC Excl: PDX collection 592

G71.3 **Mitochondrial myopathy, not elsewhere classified**
EXCLUDES 1 Kearns-Sayre syndrome (H49.81)
Leber's disease (H47.21)
Leigh's encephalopathy (G31.82)
mitochondrial metabolism disorders (E88.4.-)
Reye's syndrome (G93.7)

G71.8 **Other primary disorders of muscles**

G71.9 **Primary disorder of muscle, unspecified**
Hereditary myopathy NOS

✓4ᵗʰ **G72** **Other and unspecified myopathies**
EXCLUDES 1 arthrogryposis multiplex congenita (Q74.3)
dermatopolymyositis (M33.-)
ischemic infarction of muscle (M62.2-)
myositis (M60.-)
polymyositis (M33.2.-)

CC Excl: For CC codes in category G72, unless otherwise noted: PDX collection 593

G72.0 **Drug-induced myopathy** `CC`
Use additional code for adverse effect, if applicable, to identify drug (T36-T50 with fifth or sixth character 5)

G72.1 **Alcoholic myopathy** `CC`
Use additional code to identify alcoholism (F10.-)

G72.2 **Myopathy due to other toxic agents** `CC`
Code first (T51-T65) to identify toxic agent

G72.3 **Periodic paralysis**
Familial periodic paralysis
Hyperkalemic periodic paralysis (familial)
Hypokalemic periodic paralysis (familial)
Myotonic periodic paralysis (familial)
Normokalemic paralysis (familial)
Potassium sensitive periodic paralysis
EXCLUDES 1 paramyotonia congenita (of von Eulenburg) (G71.19)

✓5ᵗʰ **G72.4** **Inflammatory and immune myopathies, not elsewhere classified**

G72.41 **Inclusion body myositis [IBM]**

G72.49 **Other inflammatory and immune myopathies, not elsewhere classified**
Inflammatory myopathy NOS

✓5ᵗʰ **G72.8** **Other specified myopathies**

G72.81 **Critical illness myopathy** `CC`
Acute necrotizing myopathy
Acute quadriplegic myopathy
Intensive care (ICU) myopathy
Myopathy of critical illness
CC Excl: PDX collection 594

G72.89 **Other specified myopathies**

G72.9 **Myopathy, unspecified**

✓4ᵗʰ **G73** **Disorders of myoneural junction and muscle in diseases classified elsewhere**

G73.1 *Lambert-Eaton syndrome in neoplastic disease* `CC` `HCC`
Code first underlying neoplasm (C00-D49)
EXCLUDES 1 Lambert-Eaton syndrome not associated with neoplasm (G70.80-G70.81)
CC Excl: PDX collection 591

G73.3 *Myasthenic syndromes in other diseases classified elsewhere* `CC` `HCC`
Code first underlying disease, such as:
neoplasm (C00-D49)
thyrotoxicosis (E05.-)
CC Excl: PDX collection 591

G73.7 *Myopathy in diseases classified elsewhere*
Code first underlying disease, such as:
hyperparathyroidism (E21.0, E21.3)
hypoparathyroidism (E20.-)
glycogen storage disease (E74.0)
lipid storage disorders (E75.-)
EXCLUDES 1 myopathy in:
rheumatoid arthritis (M05.32)
sarcoidosis (D86.87)
scleroderma (M34.82)
sicca syndrome [Sjögren] (M35.03)
systemic lupus erythematosus (M32.19)

Cerebral palsy and other paralytic syndromes (G80-G83)

✓4ᵗʰ **G80** **Cerebral palsy**
EXCLUDES 1 hereditary spastic paraplegia (G11.4)

G80.0 **Spastic quadriplegic cerebral palsy** `CC` `HCC`
Congenital spastic paralysis (cerebral)

G80.1 **Spastic diplegic cerebral palsy** `HCC`
Spastic cerebral palsy NOS

G80.2 **Spastic hemiplegic cerebral palsy** `HCC`

G80.3 **Athetoid cerebral palsy** `HCC`
Double athetosis (syndrome)
Dyskinetic cerebral palsy
Dystonic cerebral palsy
Vogt disease

G80.4 **Ataxic cerebral palsy** `HCC`

G80.8 **Other cerebral palsy** `HCC`
Mixed cerebral palsy syndromes

G80.9 **Cerebral palsy, unspecified** `HCC`
Cerebral palsy NOS

✓4th **G81 Hemiplegia and hemiparesis**

> NOTE   This category is to be used only when hemiplegia (complete)(incomplete) is reported without further specification, or is stated to be old or longstanding but of unspecified cause. The category is also for use in multiple coding to identify these types of hemiplegia resulting from any cause.
>
> EXCLUDES 1   congenital cerebral palsy (G80.-)
> hemiplegia and hemiparesis due to sequela of cerebrovascular disease (I69.05-, I69.15-, I69.25-, I69.35-, I69.85-, I69.95-)

AHA: 2015, 1Q, 25

TIP: If the documentation specifies the affected side but not whether it is the dominant or nondominant side, the default is as follows: for ambidextrous patients, the default is dominant; when the left side is affected, the default is nondominant; and when the right side is affected, the default is dominant.

CC Excl: For CC codes in category G81: PDX collection 561

✓5th **G81.0 Flaccid hemiplegia**

G81.00	Flaccid hemiplegia affecting unspecified side	CC HCC
G81.01	Flaccid hemiplegia affecting right dominant side	CC HCC
G81.02	Flaccid hemiplegia affecting left dominant side	CC HCC
G81.03	Flaccid hemiplegia affecting right nondominant side	CC HCC
G81.04	Flaccid hemiplegia affecting left nondominant side	CC HCC

✓5th **G81.1 Spastic hemiplegia**

G81.10	Spastic hemiplegia affecting unspecified side	CC HCC
G81.11	Spastic hemiplegia affecting right dominant side	CC HCC
G81.12	Spastic hemiplegia affecting left dominant side	CC HCC
G81.13	Spastic hemiplegia affecting right nondominant side	CC HCC
G81.14	Spastic hemiplegia affecting left nondominant side	CC HCC

✓5th **G81.9 Hemiplegia, unspecified**

AHA: 2014, 1Q, 23

G81.90	Hemiplegia, unspecified affecting unspecified side	CC HCC
G81.91	Hemiplegia, unspecified affecting right dominant side	CC HCC
G81.92	Hemiplegia, unspecified affecting left dominant side	CC HCC
G81.93	Hemiplegia, unspecified affecting right nondominant side	CC HCC
G81.94	Hemiplegia, unspecified affecting left nondominant side	CC HCC

✓4th **G82 Paraplegia (paraparesis) and quadriplegia (quadriparesis)**

> NOTE   This category is to be used only when the listed conditions are reported without further specification, or are stated to be old or longstanding but of unspecified cause. The category is also for use in multiple coding to identify these conditions resulting from any cause
>
> EXCLUDES 1   congenital cerebral palsy (G80.-)
> functional quadriplegia (R53.2)
> hysterical paralysis (F44.4)

✓5th **G82.2 Paraplegia**

Paralysis of both lower limbs NOS
Paraparesis (lower) NOS
Paraplegia (lower) NOS

AHA: 2017, 3Q, 3

CC Excl: For CC codes in subcategory G82.2: PDX collection 561

G82.20	Paraplegia, unspecified	CC HCC
G82.21	Paraplegia, complete	CC HCC
G82.22	Paraplegia, incomplete	CC HCC

✓5th **G82.5 Quadriplegia**

CC Excl: For MCC codes in subcategory G82.5: PDX collection 595

G82.50	Quadriplegia, unspecified	MCC HCC
G82.51	Quadriplegia, C1-C4 complete	MCC HCC
G82.52	Quadriplegia, C1-C4 incomplete	MCC HCC

| G82.53 | Quadriplegia, C5-C7 complete | MCC HCC |
| G82.54 | Quadriplegia, C5-C7 incomplete | MCC HCC |

✓4th **G83 Other paralytic syndromes**

> NOTE   This category is to be used only when the listed conditions are reported without further specification, or are stated to be old or longstanding but of unspecified cause. The category is also for use in multiple coding to identify these conditions resulting from any cause.
>
> INCLUDES   paralysis (complete) (incomplete), except as in G80-G82

G83.0 Diplegia of upper limbs   CC HCC

Diplegia (upper)
Paralysis of both upper limbs
CC Excl: PDX collection 599

✓5th **G83.1 Monoplegia of lower limb**

Paralysis of lower limb

> EXCLUDES 1   monoplegia of lower limbs due to sequela of cerebrovascular disease (I69.04-, I69.14-, I69.24-, I69.34-, I69.84-, I69.94-)

TIP: If the documentation specifies the affected side but not whether it is the dominant or nondominant side, the default is as follows: for ambidextrous patients, the default is dominant; when the left side is affected, the default is nondominant; and when the right side is affected, the default is dominant.

G83.10	Monoplegia of lower limb affecting unspecified side	HCC
G83.11	Monoplegia of lower limb affecting right dominant side	HCC
G83.12	Monoplegia of lower limb affecting left dominant side	HCC
G83.13	Monoplegia of lower limb affecting right nondominant side	HCC
G83.14	Monoplegia of lower limb affecting left nondominant side	HCC

✓5th **G83.2 Monoplegia of upper limb**

Paralysis of upper limb

> EXCLUDES 1   monoplegia of upper limbs due to sequela of cerebrovascular disease (I69.03-, I69.13-, I69.23-, I69.33-, I69.83-, I69.93-)

TIP: If the documentation specifies the affected side but not whether it is the dominant or nondominant side, the default is as follows: for ambidextrous patients, the default is dominant; when the left side is affected, the default is nondominant; and when the right side is affected, the default is dominant.

G83.20	Monoplegia of upper limb affecting unspecified side	HCC
G83.21	Monoplegia of upper limb affecting right dominant side	HCC
G83.22	Monoplegia of upper limb affecting left dominant side	HCC
G83.23	Monoplegia of upper limb affecting right nondominant side	HCC
G83.24	Monoplegia of upper limb affecting left nondominant side	HCC

✓5th **G83.3 Monoplegia, unspecified**

TIP: If the documentation specifies the affected side but not whether it is the dominant or nondominant side, the default is as follows: for ambidextrous patients, the default is dominant; when the left side is affected, the default is nondominant; and when the right side is affected, the default is dominant.

G83.30	Monoplegia, unspecified affecting unspecified side	HCC
G83.31	Monoplegia, unspecified affecting right dominant side	HCC
G83.32	Monoplegia, unspecified affecting left dominant side	HCC
G83.33	Monoplegia, unspecified affecting right nondominant side	HCC
G83.34	Monoplegia, unspecified affecting left nondominant side	HCC

☑ Additional Character Required   ✓x7th Placeholder   Unacceptable PDx   Questionable PDx   Manifestation   Unspecified Dx   H1-H14 HAC   HCC CMS-HCC Dx   HIV HIV Dx

ICD-10-CM 2020   587

Chapter 6. Diseases of the Nervous System

G83.4 Cauda equina syndrome `CC` `HCC`

Neurogenic bladder due to cauda equina syndrome

EXCLUDES 1   cord bladder NOS (G95.89)

neurogenic bladder NOS (N31.9)

DEF: Compression of the spinal nerve roots presenting with pain and tingling radiating down the buttocks, back of the thigh and calf, and into the foot in a sciatic manner with aching in the bladder, perineum, and sacrum. Loss of bowel and bladder control may also occur.

CC Excl: PDX collection 600

G83.5 Locked-in state `MCC` `HCC`

CC Excl: PDX collection 601

√5th **G83.8 Other specified paralytic syndromes**

EXCLUDES 1   paralytic syndromes due to current spinal cord injury — code to spinal cord injury (S14, S24, S34)

G83.81 Brown-Séquard syndrome `HCC`

G83.82 Anterior cord syndrome `HCC`

G83.83 Posterior cord syndrome `HCC`

G83.84 Todd's paralysis (postepileptic) `HCC`

G83.89 Other specified paralytic syndromes `HCC`

G83.9 Paralytic syndrome, unspecified `HCC`

Other disorders of the nervous system (G89-G99)

√4th **G89 Pain, not elsewhere classified**

Code also related psychological factors associated with pain (F45.42)

EXCLUDES 1   generalized pain NOS (R52)

pain disorders exclusively related to psychological factors (F45.41)

pain NOS (R52)

EXCLUDES 2   atypical face pain (G50.1)

headache syndromes (G44.-)

localized pain, unspecified type — code to pain by site, such as:

abdomen pain (R10.-)

back pain (M54.9)

breast pain (N64.4)

chest pain (R07.1-R07.9)

ear pain (H92.0-)

eye pain (H57.1)

headache (R51)

joint pain (M25.5-)

limb pain (M79.6-)

lumbar region pain (M54.5)

painful urination (R30.9)

pelvic and perineal pain (R10.2)

renal colic (N23)

shoulder pain (M25.51-)

spine pain (M54.-)

throat pain (R07.0)

tongue pain (K14.6)

tooth pain (K08.8)

migraines (G43.-)

myalgia (M79.1-)

pain from prosthetic devices, implants, and grafts (T82.84, T83.84, T84.84, T85.84-)

phantom limb syndrome with pain (G54.6)

vulvar vestibulitis (N94.810)

vulvodynia (N94.81-)

G89.0 Central pain syndrome

Déjérine-Roussy syndrome

Myelopathic pain syndrome

Thalamic pain syndrome (hyperesthetic)

√5th **G89.1 Acute pain, not elsewhere classified**

G89.11 Acute pain due to trauma

G89.12 Acute post-thoracotomy pain

Post-thoracotomy pain NOS

G89.18 Other acute postprocedural pain

Postoperative pain NOS

Postprocedural pain NOS

√5th **G89.2 Chronic pain, not elsewhere classified**

EXCLUDES 1   causalgia, lower limb (G57.7-)

causalgia, upper limb (G56.4-)

central pain syndrome (G89.0)

chronic pain syndrome (G89.4)

complex regional pain syndrome II, lower limb (G57.7-)

complex regional pain syndrome II, upper limb (G56.4-)

neoplasm related chronic pain (G89.3)

reflex sympathetic dystrophy (G90.5-)

G89.21 Chronic pain due to trauma

G89.22 Chronic post-thoracotomy pain

G89.28 Other chronic postprocedural pain

Other chronic postoperative pain

G89.29 Other chronic pain

G89.3 Neoplasm related pain (acute) (chronic)

Cancer associated pain

Pain due to malignancy (primary) (secondary)

Tumor associated pain

G89.4 Chronic pain syndrome

Chronic pain associated with significant psychosocial dysfunction

√4th **G90 Disorders of autonomic nervous system**

EXCLUDES 1   dysfunction of the autonomic nervous system due to alcohol (G31.2)

√5th **G90.0 Idiopathic peripheral autonomic neuropathy**

G90.01 Carotid sinus syncope

Carotid sinus syndrome

DEF: Vagal activation caused by pressure on the carotid sinus baroreceptors. Sympathetic nerve impulses may cause sinus arrest or AV block.

G90.09 Other idiopathic peripheral autonomic neuropathy

Idiopathic peripheral autonomic neuropathy NOS

G90.1 Familial dysautonomia [Riley-Day] `CC` `HCC`

G90.2 Horner's syndrome

Bernard(-Horner) syndrome

Cervical sympathetic dystrophy or paralysis

G90.3 Multi-system degeneration of the autonomic `CC` `HCC`
nervous system

Neurogenic orthostatic hypotension [Shy-Drager]

EXCLUDES 1   orthostatic hypotension NOS (I95.1)

CC Excl: PDX collection 573

G90.4 Autonomic dysreflexia

Use additional code to identify the cause, such as:

fecal impaction (K56.41)

pressure ulcer (pressure area) (L89.-)

urinary tract infection (N39.0)

√5th **G90.5 Complex regional pain syndrome I (CRPS I)**

Reflex sympathetic dystrophy

EXCLUDES 1   causalgia of lower limb (G57.7-)

causalgia of upper limb (G56.4-)

complex regional pain syndrome II of lower limb (G57.7-)

complex regional pain syndrome II of upper limb (G56.4-)

CC Excl: For CC codes in subcategory G90.5, unless otherwise noted: PDX collection 603

G90.50 Complex regional pain syndrome I, `CC`
unspecified

CC Excl: PDX collection 602

√6th **G90.51 Complex regional pain syndrome I of upper limb**

G90.511 Complex regional pain `CC`
syndrome I of right upper limb

G90.512 Complex regional pain `CC`
syndrome I of left upper limb

G90.513 Complex regional pain `CC`
syndrome I of upper limb, bilateral

G90.519 Complex regional pain `CC`
syndrome I of unspecified upper limb

N Newborn: 0   P Pediatric: 0-17   M Maternity: 9-64   A Adult: 15-124   `MCC` Major Complication/Comorbidity   `CC` Complication/Comorbidity   `SW` Severe Wound Dx

588

ICD-10-CM 2020

√6ᵗʰ **G90.52   Complex regional pain syndrome I of** lower limb

      G90.521   Complex regional pain syndrome I of right **lower limb** `CC`

      G90.522   Complex regional pain syndrome I of left **lower limb** `CC`

      G90.523   Complex regional pain syndrome I of lower limb, bilateral

      G90.529   Complex regional pain syndrome I of unspecified lower limb `CC`

   G90.59   Complex regional pain syndrome I of other specified site `CC`

  G90.8   Other disorders of autonomic nervous system

  G90.9   Disorder of the autonomic nervous system, unspecified

√4ᵗʰ **G91   Hydrocephalus**

    `INCLUDES`   acquired hydrocephalus

    `EXCLUDES 1` *Arnold-Chiari syndrome with hydrocephalus (Q07.-)*
          congenital hydrocephalus (Q03.-)
          spina bifida with hydrocephalus (Q05.-)

    DEF: Abnormal buildup of cerebrospinal fluid in the brain causing dilation of the ventricles.

    CC Excl: For CC codes in category G91, unless otherwise noted: PDX collection 605

Hydrocephalus (Acquired)

Normal ventricles   Hydrocephalic ventricles

G91.0   Communicating hydrocephalus `CC` `HCC`

    Secondary normal pressure hydrocephalus
    CC Excl: PDX collection 604

G91.1   Obstructive hydrocephalus `CC` `HCC`

    DEF: Obstruction of the cerebrospinal fluid passage from the brain into the spinal canal characterized by headaches, drowsiness, poor coordination, urinary incontinence, nausea, vomiting, and papilledema.

G91.2   (Idiopathic) normal pressure hydrocephalus `CC` `HCC`

    Normal pressure hydrocephalus NOS
    CC Excl: PDX collection 604

G91.3   Post-traumatic hydrocephalus, unspecified `CC` `HCC`

G91.4   *Hydrocephalus in diseases classified elsewhere* `HCC`

    Code first underlying condition, such as:
      congenital syphilis (A50.4-)
      neoplasm (C00-D49)
      plasminogen deficiency (E88.02)
    `EXCLUDES 1` *hydrocephalus due to congenital toxoplasmosis (P37.1)*
    AHA: 2014,3Q,3

G91.8   Other hydrocephalus `CC` `HCC`

G91.9   Hydrocephalus, unspecified `CC` `HCC`

G92   Toxic encephalopathy `MCC`

  Toxic encephalitis
  Toxic metabolic encephalopathy
  Code first, if applicable, drug induced (T36-T50)
  Code first (T51-T65) to identify toxic agent
  AHA: 2017,1Q,39-40
  DEF: Brain tissue degeneration due to a toxic substance.
  CC Excl: PDX collection 606

√4ᵗʰ **G93   Other disorders of brain**

  G93.0   Cerebral cysts

    Arachnoid cyst
    Porencephalic cyst, acquired
    `EXCLUDES 1` *acquired periventricular cysts of newborn (P91.1)*
          congenital cerebral cysts (Q04.6)

  G93.1   Anoxic brain damage, not elsewhere classified `CC` `HCC`

    `EXCLUDES 1` *cerebral anoxia due to anesthesia during labor and delivery (O74.3)*
          cerebral anoxia due to anesthesia during the puerperium (O89.2)
          neonatal anoxia (P84)

    DEF: Brain injury not resulting from birth trauma that is due to lack of oxygen. Brain cells, when deprived of oxygen; begin to expire after 4 minutes.
    CC Excl: PDX collection 607

  G93.2   Benign intracranial hypertension

    `EXCLUDES 1` *hypertensive encephalopathy (I67.4)*

  G93.3   Postviral fatigue syndrome

    Benign myalgic encephalomyelitis
    `EXCLUDES 1` *chronic fatigue syndrome NOS (R53.82)*

√5ᵗʰ **G93.4   Other and unspecified encephalopathy**

    `EXCLUDES 1` *alcoholic encephalopathy (G31.2)*
          encephalopathy in diseases classified elsewhere (G94)
          hypertensive encephalopathy (I67.4)
          toxic (metabolic) encephalopathy (G92)

    G93.40   Encephalopathy, unspecified `HIV` `CC`

      AHA: 2017,2Q,8
      CC Excl: PDX collection 608

    G93.41   Metabolic encephalopathy `HIV` `MCC`

      Septic encephalopathy
      AHA: 2017,2Q,8; 2016,3Q,42; 2015,3Q,21
      TIP: Assign separately when documented with diabetic hypoglycemia (E08.649, E09.649, E10.649, E11.649, E13.649).
      CC Excl: PDX collection 609

    G93.49   Other encephalopathy `HIV` `CC`

      Encephalopathy NEC
      AHA: 2018,4Q,16; 2018,2Q,22,24; 2017,2Q,9
      CC Excl: PDX collection 610

  G93.5   Compression of brain `CC` `HCC`

    Arnold-Chiari type 1 compression of brain
    Compression of brain (stem)
    Herniation of brain (stem)
    `EXCLUDES 1` *diffuse traumatic compression of brain (S06.2-)*
          focal traumatic compression of brain (S06.3-)

  G93.6   Cerebral edema `MCC` `HCC`

    `EXCLUDES 1` *cerebral edema due to birth injury (P11.0)*
          traumatic cerebral edema (S06.1-)
    CC Excl: PDX collection 612

  G93.7   Reye's syndrome `MCC` `HCC` `P`

    Code first poisoning due to salicylates, if applicable (T39.0-, with sixth character 1-4)
    Use additional code for adverse effect due to salicylates, if applicable (T39.0-, with sixth character 5)
    DEF: Rare childhood illness often developed after a viral upper respiratory infection. Symptoms include vomiting, elevated serum transaminase, brain swelling, disturbances of consciousness, seizures, and changes in liver and other viscera and it can be fatal.
    CC Excl: PDX collection 613

√5ᵗʰ **G93.8   Other specified disorders of brain**

    G93.81   Temporal sclerosis

      Hippocampal sclerosis
      Mesial temporal sclerosis

    G93.82   Brain death `CC`

✔ Additional Character Required   √x7ᵗʰ Placeholder   Unacceptable PDx   Questionable PDx   Manifestation   Unspecified Dx   `H1`-`H14` HAC   `HCC` CMS-HCC Dx   `HIV` HIV Dx

ICD-10-CM 2020   **589**

G93.89 **Other specified disorders of brain**
Postradiation encephalopathy

G93.9 **Disorder of brain, unspecified** `HIV`

G94 *Other disorders of brain in diseases classified elsewhere*
Code first underlying disease
EXCLUDES 1 encephalopathy in congenital syphilis (A50.49)
encephalopathy in influenza (J09.X9, J10.81, J11.81)
encephalopathy in syphilis (A52.19)
hydrocephalus in diseases classified elsewhere (G91.4)
AHA: 2018,2Q,22; 2017,2Q,8-9

✓4ᵗʰ **G95** **Other and unspecified diseases of spinal cord**
EXCLUDES 2 myelitis (G04.-)

G95.0 **Syringomyelia and syringobulbia** `CC` `HCC`
CC Excl: PDX collection 614

✓5ᵗʰ **G95.1** **Vascular myelopathies**
EXCLUDES 2 intraspinal phlebitis and thrombophlebitis, except non-pyogenic (G08)

G95.11 **Acute infarction of spinal cord (embolic) (nonembolic)** `MCC` `HCC`
Anoxia of spinal cord
Arterial thrombosis of spinal cord
CC Excl: PDX collection 603

G95.19 **Other vascular myelopathies** `CC` `HCC`
Edema of spinal cord
Hematomyelia
Nonpyogenic intraspinal phlebitis and thrombophlebitis
Subacute necrotic myelopathy

✓5ᵗʰ **G95.2** **Other and unspecified cord compression**

G95.20 **Unspecified cord compression** `HIV` `CC` `HCC`
CC Excl: PDX collection 615

G95.29 **Other cord compression** `HIV` `CC` `HCC`
CC Excl: PDX collection 615

✓5ᵗʰ **G95.8** **Other specified diseases of spinal cord**
EXCLUDES 1 neurogenic bladder NOS (N31.9)
neurogenic bladder due to cauda equina syndrome (G83.4)
neuromuscular dysfunction of bladder without spinal cord lesion (N31.-)

G95.81 **Conus medullaris syndrome** `CC` `HCC`
CC Excl: PDX collection 603

G95.89 **Other specified diseases of spinal cord** `CC` `HCC`
Cord bladder NOS
Drug-induced myelopathy
Radiation-induced myelopathy
EXCLUDES 1 myelopathy NOS (G95.9)
CC Excl: PDX collection 603

G95.9 **Disease of spinal cord, unspecified** `HIV` `CC` `HCC`
Myelopathy NOS
CC Excl: PDX collection 615

✓4ᵗʰ **G96** **Other disorders of central nervous system**

G96.0 **Cerebrospinal fluid leak** `CC`
EXCLUDES 1 cerebrospinal fluid leak from spinal puncture (G97.0)
AHA: 2018,2Q,13
DEF: Cerebrospinal fluid discharging from the nose or the ear caused by a fracture of the frontal bone with tearing of dura mater and arachnoid. It is characterized by watery drainage usually from only one side of the nose or one ear, headache, vision changes, and hearing loss.
CC Excl: PDX collection 616

✓5ᵗʰ **G96.1** **Disorders of meninges, not elsewhere classified**

G96.11 **Dural tear** `CC`
EXCLUDES 1 accidental puncture or laceration of dura during a procedure (G97.41)
AHA: 2014,4Q,24
CC Excl: PDX collection 509

G96.12 **Meningeal adhesions (cerebral) (spinal)**

G96.19 **Other disorders of meninges, not elsewhere classified**

G96.8 **Other specified disorders of central nervous system**

G96.9 **Disorder of central nervous system, unspecified** `HIV`

✓4ᵗʰ **G97** **Intraoperative and postprocedural complications and disorders of nervous system, not elsewhere classified**
EXCLUDES 2 intraoperative and postprocedural cerebrovascular infarction (I97.81-, I97.82-)
AHA: 2016,4Q,9-10

G97.0 **Cerebrospinal fluid leak from spinal puncture** `CC`
CC Excl: PDX collection 617

Spinal Puncture

- Spinal cord
- Epidural space
- Subarachnoid space
- Vertebra
- Spinal needle

Lumbar area

G97.1 **Other reaction to spinal and lumbar puncture**
Headache due to lumbar puncture

G97.2 **Intracranial hypotension following ventricular shunting** `CC`
CC Excl: PDX collection 617

✓5ᵗʰ **G97.3** **Intraoperative hemorrhage and hematoma of a nervous system organ or structure complicating a procedure**
EXCLUDES 1 intraoperative hemorrhage and hematoma of a nervous system organ or structure due to accidental puncture and laceration during a procedure (G97.4-)

G97.31 **Intraoperative hemorrhage and hematoma of a nervous system organ or structure complicating a nervous system procedure** `CC`
CC Excl: PDX collection 618

G97.32 **Intraoperative hemorrhage and hematoma of a nervous system organ or structure complicating other procedure** `CC`
CC Excl: PDX collection 618

✓5ᵗʰ **G97.4** **Accidental puncture and laceration of a nervous system organ or structure during a procedure**
CC Excl: For CC codes in subcategory G97.4: PDX collection 509

G97.41 **Accidental puncture or laceration of dura during a procedure** `CC`
Incidental (inadvertent) durotomy
AHA: 2014,4Q,24

G97.48 **Accidental puncture and laceration of other nervous system organ or structure during a nervous system procedure** `CC`

G97.49 **Accidental puncture and laceration of other nervous system organ or structure during other procedure** `CC`

✓5ᵗʰ **G97.5** **Postprocedural hemorrhage of a nervous system organ or structure following a procedure**

G97.51 **Postprocedural hemorrhage of a nervous system organ or structure following a nervous system procedure** `CC`
CC Excl: PDX collection 619

G97.52 **Postprocedural hemorrhage of a nervous system organ or structure following other procedure** `CC`
CC Excl: PDX collection 619

√5ᵗʰ **G97.6** Postprocedural hematoma and seroma **of a nervous system organ or structure following a procedure**
     CC Excl: For CC codes in subcategory G97.6: PDX collection 619

     G97.61 **Postprocedural** hematoma **of a nervous system organ or structure following a nervous system procedure** `CC`

     G97.62 **Postprocedural** hematoma **of a nervous system organ or structure following** other procedure `CC`

     G97.63 **Postprocedural** seroma **of a nervous system organ or structure following a nervous system procedure** `CC`

     G97.64 **Postprocedural** seroma **of a nervous system organ or structure following** other procedure `CC`

√5ᵗʰ **G97.8** **Other intraoperative and postprocedural complications and disorders of nervous system**
     Use additional code to further specify disorder

     G97.81 **Other intraoperative complications of nervous system** `CC`
         CC Excl: PDX collection 617

     G97.82 **Other postprocedural complications and disorders of nervous system** `CC`
         CC Excl: PDX collection 617

√4ᵗʰ **G98** **Other disorders of nervous system not elsewhere classified**
     `INCLUDES` nervous system disorder NOS

     G98.0 **Neurogenic arthritis, not elsewhere classified**
         Nonsyphilitic neurogenic arthropathy NEC
         Nonsyphilitic neurogenic spondylopathy NEC
         `EXCLUDES 1` *spondylopathy (in):*
            syringomyelia and syringobulbia (G95.0)
            tabes dorsalis (A52.11)

     G98.8 **Other disorders of nervous system** `HIV`
         Nervous system disorder NOS

√4ᵗʰ **G99** **Other disorders of nervous system in diseases classified elsewhere**

     G99.0 *Autonomic neuropathy in diseases classified elsewhere* `CC`
         Code first underlying disease, such as:
            amyloidosis (E85.-)
            gout (M1A.-, M10.-)
            hyperthyroidism (E05.-)
         `EXCLUDES 1` *diabetic autonomic neuropathy (E08-E13 with .43)*
         CC Excl: PDX collection 620

     G99.2 *Myelopathy in diseases classified elsewhere* `CC` `HCC`
         Code first underlying disease, such as:
            neoplasm (C00-D49)
         `EXCLUDES 1` *myelopathy in:*
            intervertebral disease (M50.0-, M51.0-)
            spondylosis (M47.0-, M47.1-)
         AHA: 2018,3Q,18-19
         TIP: Use this code in addition to a spondylolisthesis code (M43.1-) or a spinal stenosis code (M48.0-) when either of these disorders is documented as the cause of the myelopathy.
         CC Excl: PDX collection 603

     G99.8 *Other specified disorders of nervous system in diseases classified elsewhere*
         Code first underlying disorder, such as:
            amyloidosis (E85.-) .
            avitaminosis (E56.9)
         `EXCLUDES 1` *nervous system involvement in:*
            cysticercosis (B69.0)
            rubella (B06.0-)
            syphilis (A52.1-)

Chapter 6. Diseases of the Nervous System

G97.6–G99.8

Chapter 7. Diseases of the Eye and Adnexa (H00–H59)

Chapter-specific Guidelines with Coding Examples

The chapter-specific guidelines from the ICD-10-CM Official Guidelines for Coding and Reporting have been provided below. Along with these guidelines are coding examples, contained in the shaded boxes, that have been developed to help illustrate the coding and/or sequencing guidance found in these guidelines.

a. Glaucoma

1) Assigning glaucoma codes
Assign as many codes from category H40, Glaucoma, as needed to identify the type of glaucoma, the affected eye, and the glaucoma stage.

2) Bilateral glaucoma with same type and stage
When a patient has bilateral glaucoma and both eyes are documented as being the same type and stage, and there is a code for bilateral glaucoma, report only the code for the type of glaucoma, bilateral, with the seventh character for the stage.

> Bilateral severe stage pigmentary glaucoma
>
> **H40.1333   Pigmentary glaucoma, bilateral, severe stage**
>
> *Explanation*: In this scenario, the patient has the same type and stage of glaucoma in both eyes. As this type of glaucoma has a code for bilateral, assign only the code for the bilateral glaucoma with the seventh character for the stage.

When a patient has bilateral glaucoma and both eyes are documented as being the same type and stage, and the classification does not provide a code for bilateral glaucoma (i.e. subcategories H40.10 and H40.20) report only one code for the type of glaucoma with the appropriate seventh character for the stage.

> Bilateral open-angle glaucoma; not specified as to type and stage indeterminate in both eyes
>
> **H40.10X4   Unspecified open-angle glaucoma, indeterminate stage**
>
> *Explanation*: In this scenario, the patient has glaucoma of the same type and stage of both eyes, but there is no code specifically for bilateral glaucoma. Only one code is assigned with the appropriate seventh character for the stage.

3) Bilateral glaucoma stage with different types or stages
When a patient has bilateral glaucoma and each eye is documented as having a different type or stage, and the classification distinguishes laterality, assign the appropriate code for each eye rather than the code for bilateral glaucoma.

When a patient has bilateral glaucoma and each eye is documented as having a different type, and the classification does not distinguish laterality (i.e. subcategories H40.10 and H40.20), assign one code for each type of glaucoma with the appropriate seventh character for the stage.

> Documentation relates mild, unspecified primary angle-closure glaucoma of the left eye with mild unspecified open-angle glaucoma of the right eye
>
> **H40.20X1   Unspecified primary angle-closure glaucoma, mild stage**
>
> **H40.10X1   Unspecified open-angle glaucoma, mild stage**
>
> *Explanation*: In this scenario the patient has a different type of glaucoma in each eye and the classification does not distinguish laterality. A code for each type of glaucoma is assigned, each with the appropriate seventh character for the stage.

When a patient has bilateral glaucoma and each eye is documented as having the same type, but different stage, and the classification does not distinguish laterality (i.e. subcategories H40.10 and H40.20), assign a code for the type of glaucoma for each eye with the seventh character for the specific glaucoma stage documented for each eye.

> Bilateral open-angle glaucoma, not specified as to type; the right eye is documented to be in mild stage and the left eye as being in moderate stage
>
> **H40.10X1   Unspecified open-angle glaucoma, mild stage**
>
> **H40.10X2   Unspecified open-angle glaucoma, moderate stage**
>
> *Explanation*: In this scenario the patient has the same type of glaucoma in each eye but each eye is at a different stage, and the classification does not distinguish laterality at this subcategory level. Two codes are assigned; both codes represent the same type of glaucoma but each has a different seventh character identifying the appropriate stage for each eye.

4) Patient admitted with glaucoma and stage evolves during the admission
If a patient is admitted with glaucoma and the stage progresses during the admission, assign the code for highest stage documented.

> Patient admitted with mild low-tension glaucoma of the right eye, which progresses to moderate stage during the patient's stay
>
> **H40.1212   Low-tension glaucoma, right eye, moderate stage**
>
> *Explanation*: When the glaucoma stage progresses during an admission, assign only the code for the highest stage documented.

5) Indeterminate stage glaucoma
Assignment of the seventh character "4" for "indeterminate stage" should be based on the clinical documentation. The seventh character "4" is used for glaucomas whose stage cannot be clinically determined. This seventh character should not be confused with the seventh character "0", unspecified, which should be assigned when there is no documentation regarding the stage of the glaucoma.

b. Blindness
If "blindness" or "low vision" of both eyes is documented but the visual impairment category is not documented, assign code H54.3, Unqualified visual loss, both eyes. If "blindness" or "low vision" in one eye is documented but the visual impairment category is not documented, assign a code from H54.6-, Unqualified visual loss, one eye. If "blindness" or "visual loss" is documented without any information about whether one or both eyes are affected, assign code H54.7, Unspecified visual loss.

> Blindness in 89-year-old male
>
> **H54.7   Unspecified visual loss**
>
> *Explanation*: Blindness is stated, but there is no mention of whether one or both eyes are affected or the severity of this visual impairment.

Chapter 7. Diseases of the Eye and Adnexa (H00-H59)

NOTE   Use an external cause code following the code for the eye condition, if applicable, to identify the cause of the eye condition

EXCLUDES 2   certain conditions originating in the perinatal period (P04-P96)
certain infectious and parasitic diseases (A00-B99)
complications of pregnancy, childbirth and the puerperium (O00-O9A)
congenital malformations, deformations, and chromosomal abnormalities (Q00-Q99)
diabetes mellitus related eye conditions (E09.3-, E10.3-, E11.3-, E13.3-)
endocrine, nutritional and metabolic diseases (E00-E88)
injury (trauma) of eye and orbit (S05.-)
injury, poisoning and certain other consequences of external causes (S00-T88)
neoplasms (C00-D49)
symptoms, signs and abnormal clinical and laboratory findings, not elsewhere classified (R00-R94)
syphilis related eye disorders (A50.01, A50.3-, A51.43, A52.71)

This chapter contains the following blocks:

H00-H05   Disorders of eyelid, lacrimal system and orbit
H10-H11   Disorders of conjunctiva
H15-H22   Disorders of sclera, cornea, iris and ciliary body
H25-H28   Disorders of lens
H30-H36   Disorders of choroid and retina
H40-H42   Glaucoma
H43-H44   Disorders of vitreous body and globe
H46-H47   Disorders of optic nerve and visual pathways
H49-H52   Disorders of ocular muscles, binocular movement, accommodation and refraction
H53-H54   Visual disturbances and blindness
H55-H57   Other disorders of eye and adnexa
H59   Intraoperative and postprocedural complications and disorders of eye and adnexa, not elsewhere classified

Disorders of eyelid, lacrimal system and orbit (H00-H05)

EXCLUDES 2   open wound of eyelid (S01.1-)
superficial injury of eyelid (S00.1-, S00.2-)

✓4ᵗʰ **H00**   **Hordeolum and chalazion**

   ✓5ᵗʰ **H00.0**   **Hordeolum (externum) (internum) of eyelid**

     DEF: Acute localized infection of the gland of Zeis (external hordeolum) or Molt or of the meibomian glands (internal hordeolum) of the orbit.

     ✓6ᵗʰ **H00.01**   **Hordeolum externum**
       Hordeolum NOS
       Stye
       H00.011   **Hordeolum externum right upper eyelid**
       H00.012   **Hordeolum externum right lower eyelid**
       H00.013   **Hordeolum externum right eye, unspecified eyelid**
       H00.014   **Hordeolum externum left upper eyelid**
       H00.015   **Hordeolum externum left lower eyelid**
       H00.016   **Hordeolum externum left eye, unspecified eyelid**
       H00.019   **Hordeolum externum unspecified eye, unspecified eyelid**

     ✓6ᵗʰ **H00.02**   **Hordeolum internum**
       Infection of meibomian gland
       H00.021   **Hordeolum internum right upper eyelid**
       H00.022   **Hordeolum internum right lower eyelid**
       H00.023   **Hordeolum internum right eye, unspecified eyelid**
       H00.024   **Hordeolum internum left upper eyelid**
       H00.025   **Hordeolum internum left lower eyelid**
       H00.026   **Hordeolum internum left eye, unspecified eyelid**
       H00.029   **Hordeolum internum unspecified eye, unspecified eyelid**

     ✓6ᵗʰ **H00.03**   **Abscess of eyelid**
       Furuncle of eyelid
       H00.031   **Abscess of right upper eyelid**
       H00.032   **Abscess of right lower eyelid**
       H00.033   **Abscess of eyelid right eye, unspecified eyelid**
       H00.034   **Abscess of left upper eyelid**
       H00.035   **Abscess of left lower eyelid**
       H00.036   **Abscess of eyelid left eye, unspecified eyelid**
       H00.039   **Abscess of eyelid unspecified eye, unspecified eyelid**

   ✓5ᵗʰ **H00.1**   **Chalazion**
     Meibomian (gland) cyst
     EXCLUDES 2   infected meibomian gland (H00.02-)
     DEF: Noninfectious, obstructive mass in the oil gland of the eyelid that results in a small chronic lump or inflammation.
     H00.11   **Chalazion right upper eyelid**
     H00.12   **Chalazion right lower eyelid**
     H00.13   **Chalazion right eye, unspecified eyelid**
     H00.14   **Chalazion left upper eyelid**
     H00.15   **Chalazion left lower eyelid**
     H00.16   **Chalazion left eye, unspecified eyelid**
     H00.19   **Chalazion unspecified eye, unspecified eyelid**

✓4ᵗʰ **H01**   **Other inflammation of eyelid**

   ✓5ᵗʰ **H01.0**   **Blepharitis**
     EXCLUDES 1   blepharoconjunctivitis (H10.5-)

     ✓6ᵗʰ **H01.00**   **Unspecified blepharitis**
       AHA: 2018,4Q,13
       H01.001   **Unspecified blepharitis right upper eyelid**
       H01.002   **Unspecified blepharitis right lower eyelid**
       H01.003   **Unspecified blepharitis right eye, unspecified eyelid**
       H01.004   **Unspecified blepharitis left upper eyelid**
       H01.005   **Unspecified blepharitis left lower eyelid**
       H01.006   **Unspecified blepharitis left eye, unspecified eyelid**
       H01.009   **Unspecified blepharitis unspecified eye, unspecified eyelid**
       H01.00A   **Unspecified blepharitis right eye, upper and lower eyelids**
       H01.00B   **Unspecified blepharitis left eye, upper and lower eyelids**

     ✓6ᵗʰ **H01.01**   **Ulcerative blepharitis**
       AHA: 2018,4Q,13
       H01.011   **Ulcerative blepharitis right upper eyelid**
       H01.012   **Ulcerative blepharitis right lower eyelid**
       H01.013   **Ulcerative blepharitis right eye, unspecified eyelid**
       H01.014   **Ulcerative blepharitis left upper eyelid**
       H01.015   **Ulcerative blepharitis left lower eyelid**
       H01.016   **Ulcerative blepharitis left eye, unspecified eyelid**
       H01.019   **Ulcerative blepharitis unspecified eye, unspecified eyelid**
       H01.01A   **Ulcerative blepharitis right eye, upper and lower eyelids**
       H01.01B   **Ulcerative blepharitis left eye, upper and lower eyelids**

     ✓6ᵗʰ **H01.02**   **Squamous blepharitis**
       AHA: 2018,4Q,13
       H01.021   **Squamous blepharitis right upper eyelid**
       H01.022   **Squamous blepharitis right lower eyelid**
       H01.023   **Squamous blepharitis right eye, unspecified eyelid**
       H01.024   **Squamous blepharitis left upper eyelid**
       H01.025   **Squamous blepharitis left lower eyelid**
       H01.026   **Squamous blepharitis left eye, unspecified eyelid**
       H01.029   **Squamous blepharitis unspecified eye, unspecified eyelid**
       H01.02A   **Squamous blepharitis right eye, upper and lower eyelids**
       H01.02B   **Squamous blepharitis left eye, upper and lower eyelids**

   ✓5ᵗʰ **H01.1**   **Noninfectious dermatoses of eyelid**

     ✓6ᵗʰ **H01.11**   **Allergic dermatitis of eyelid**
       Contact dermatitis of eyelid
       H01.111   **Allergic dermatitis of right upper eyelid**
       H01.112   **Allergic dermatitis of right lower eyelid**
       H01.113   **Allergic dermatitis of right eye, unspecified eyelid**
       H01.114   **Allergic dermatitis of left upper eyelid**
       H01.115   **Allergic dermatitis of left lower eyelid**
       H01.116   **Allergic dermatitis of left eye, unspecified eyelid**
       H01.119   **Allergic dermatitis of unspecified eye, unspecified eyelid**

√6ᵗʰ **H01.12　Discoid lupus erythematosus of eyelid**

　　H01.121　**Discoid lupus erythematosus of right upper eyelid**

　　H01.122　**Discoid lupus erythematosus of right lower eyelid**

　　H01.123　**Discoid lupus erythematosus of right eye, unspecified eyelid**

　　H01.124　**Discoid lupus erythematosus of left upper eyelid**

　　H01.125　**Discoid lupus erythematosus of left lower eyelid**

　　H01.126　**Discoid lupus erythematosus of left eye, unspecified eyelid**

　　H01.129　**Discoid lupus erythematosus of unspecified eye, unspecified eyelid**

√6ᵗʰ **H01.13　Eczematous dermatitis of eyelid**

　　H01.131　**Eczematous dermatitis of right upper eyelid**

　　H01.132　**Eczematous dermatitis of right lower eyelid**

　　H01.133　**Eczematous dermatitis of right eye, unspecified eyelid**

　　H01.134　**Eczematous dermatitis of left upper eyelid**

　　H01.135　**Eczematous dermatitis of left lower eyelid**

　　H01.136　**Eczematous dermatitis of left eye, unspecified eyelid**

　　H01.139　**Eczematous dermatitis of unspecified eye, unspecified eyelid**

√6ᵗʰ **H01.14　Xeroderma of eyelid**

　　H01.141　**Xeroderma of right upper eyelid**

　　H01.142　**Xeroderma of right lower eyelid**

　　H01.143　**Xeroderma of right eye, unspecified eyelid**

　　H01.144　**Xeroderma of left upper eyelid**

　　H01.145　**Xeroderma of left lower eyelid**

　　H01.146　**Xeroderma of left eye, unspecified eyelid**

　　H01.149　**Xeroderma of unspecified eye, unspecified eyelid**

H01.8　Other specified inflammations of eyelid

H01.9　Unspecified inflammation of eyelid
　　Inflammation of eyelid NOS

√4ᵗʰ **H02　Other disorders of eyelid**

　　EXCLUDES 1　*congenital malformations of eyelid (Q10.0-Q10.3)*

Entropion and Ectropion

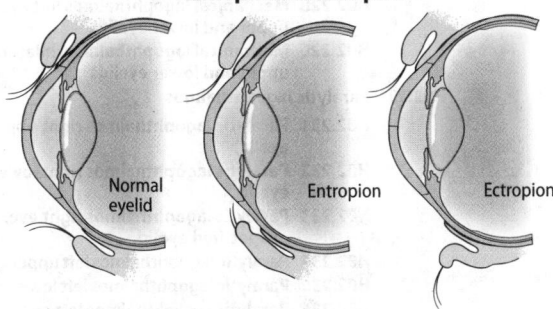

Normal eyelid　　Entropion　　Ectropion

√5ᵗʰ **H02.0　Entropion and trichiasis of eyelid**

　　DEF: Entropion: Inversion of the eyelid, turning the edge in toward the eyeball and causing irritation from contact of the lashes with the surface of the eye.
　　DEF: Trichiasis: Condition wherein the eyelid is in a normal position but lashes are ingrown or misdirected in their growth so that they irritate the tissues of the eye.

√6ᵗʰ **H02.00　Unspecified entropion of eyelid**

　　H02.001　**Unspecified entropion of right upper eyelid**

　　H02.002　**Unspecified entropion of right lower eyelid**

　　H02.003　**Unspecified entropion of right eye, unspecified eyelid**

　　H02.004　**Unspecified entropion of left upper eyelid**

　　H02.005　**Unspecified entropion of left lower eyelid**

　　H02.006　**Unspecified entropion of left eye, unspecified eyelid**

　　H02.009　**Unspecified entropion of unspecified eye, unspecified eyelid**

√6ᵗʰ **H02.01　Cicatricial entropion of eyelid**

　　H02.011　**Cicatricial entropion of right upper eyelid**

　　H02.012　**Cicatricial entropion of right lower eyelid**

　　H02.013　**Cicatricial entropion of right eye, unspecified eyelid**

　　H02.014　**Cicatricial entropion of left upper eyelid**

　　H02.015　**Cicatricial entropion of left lower eyelid**

　　H02.016　**Cicatricial entropion of left eye, unspecified eyelid**

　　H02.019　**Cicatricial entropion of unspecified eye, unspecified eyelid**

√6ᵗʰ **H02.02　Mechanical entropion of eyelid**

　　H02.021　**Mechanical entropion of right upper eyelid**

　　H02.022　**Mechanical entropion of right lower eyelid**

　　H02.023　**Mechanical entropion of right eye, unspecified eyelid**

　　H02.024　**Mechanical entropion of left upper eyelid**

　　H02.025　**Mechanical entropion of left lower eyelid**

　　H02.026　**Mechanical entropion of left eye, unspecified eyelid**

　　H02.029　**Mechanical entropion of unspecified eye, unspecified eyelid**

√6ᵗʰ **H02.03　Senile entropion of eyelid**

　　H02.031　**Senile entropion of right upper eyelid**　Ⓐ

　　H02.032　**Senile entropion of right lower eyelid**　Ⓐ

　　H02.033　**Senile entropion of right eye, unspecified eyelid**　Ⓐ

　　H02.034　**Senile entropion of left upper eyelid**　Ⓐ

　　H02.035　**Senile entropion of left lower eyelid**　Ⓐ

　　H02.036　**Senile entropion of left eye, unspecified eyelid**　Ⓐ

　　H02.039　**Senile entropion of unspecified eye, unspecified eyelid**　Ⓐ

√6ᵗʰ **H02.04　Spastic entropion of eyelid**

　　H02.041　**Spastic entropion of right upper eyelid**

　　H02.042　**Spastic entropion of right lower eyelid**

　　H02.043　**Spastic entropion of right eye, unspecified eyelid**

　　H02.044　**Spastic entropion of left upper eyelid**

　　H02.045　**Spastic entropion of left lower eyelid**

　　H02.046　**Spastic entropion of left eye, unspecified eyelid**

　　H02.049　**Spastic entropion of unspecified eye, unspecified eyelid**

√6ᵗʰ **H02.05　Trichiasis without entropion**

　　H02.051　**Trichiasis without entropion right upper eyelid**

　　H02.052　**Trichiasis without entropion right lower eyelid**

　　H02.053　**Trichiasis without entropion right eye, unspecified eyelid**

　　H02.054　**Trichiasis without entropion left upper eyelid**

　　H02.055　**Trichiasis without entropion left lower eyelid**

　　H02.056　**Trichiasis without entropion left eye, unspecified eyelid**

　　H02.059　**Trichiasis without entropion unspecified eye, unspecified eyelid**

√5ᵗʰ **H02.1　Ectropion of eyelid**

　　DEF: Drooping of the lower eyelid away from the eye or outward turning or eversion of the edge of the eyelid, exposing the palpebral conjunctiva and causing irritation.

√6ᵗʰ **H02.10　Unspecified ectropion of eyelid**

　　H02.101　**Unspecified ectropion of right upper eyelid**

　　H02.102　**Unspecified ectropion of right lower eyelid**

　　H02.103　**Unspecified ectropion of right eye, unspecified eyelid**

　　H02.104　**Unspecified ectropion of left upper eyelid**

　　H02.105　**Unspecified ectropion of left lower eyelid**

Chapter 7. Diseases of the Eye and Adnexa

H02.106–H02.34

H02.106 Unspecified ectropion of left eye, unspecified eyelid
H02.109 Unspecified ectropion of unspecified eye, unspecified eyelid

√6ᵗʰ **H02.11** Cicatricial ectropion of eyelid
    H02.111 Cicatricial ectropion of right upper eyelid
    H02.112 Cicatricial ectropion of right lower eyelid
    H02.113 Cicatricial ectropion of right eye, unspecified eyelid
    H02.114 Cicatricial ectropion of left upper eyelid
    H02.115 Cicatricial ectropion of left lower eyelid
    H02.116 Cicatricial ectropion of left eye, unspecified eyelid
    H02.119 Cicatricial ectropion of unspecified eye, unspecified eyelid

√6ᵗʰ **H02.12** Mechanical ectropion of eyelid
    H02.121 Mechanical ectropion of right upper eyelid
    H02.122 Mechanical ectropion of right lower eyelid
    H02.123 Mechanical ectropion of right eye, unspecified eyelid
    H02.124 Mechanical ectropion of left upper eyelid
    H02.125 Mechanical ectropion of left lower eyelid
    H02.126 Mechanical ectropion of left eye, unspecified eyelid
    H02.129 Mechanical ectropion of unspecified eye, unspecified eyelid

√6ᵗʰ **H02.13** Senile ectropion of eyelid
    H02.131 Senile ectropion of right upper eyelid   🅰
    H02.132 Senile ectropion of right lower eyelid   🅰
    H02.133 Senile ectropion of right eye, unspecified eyelid   🅰
    H02.134 Senile ectropion of left upper eyelid   🅰
    H02.135 Senile ectropion of left lower eyelid   🅰
    H02.136 Senile ectropion of left eye, unspecified eyelid   🅰
    H02.139 Senile ectropion of unspecified eye, unspecified eyelid   🅰

√6ᵗʰ **H02.14** Spastic ectropion of eyelid
    H02.141 Spastic ectropion of right upper eyelid
    H02.142 Spastic ectropion of right lower eyelid
    H02.143 Spastic ectropion of right eye, unspecified eyelid
    H02.144 Spastic ectropion of left upper eyelid
    H02.145 Spastic ectropion of left lower eyelid
    H02.146 Spastic ectropion of left eye, unspecified eyelid
    H02.149 Spastic ectropion of unspecified eye, unspecified eyelid

√6ᵗʰ **H02.15** Paralytic ectropion of eyelid
    AHA: 2018,4Q,13
    H02.151 Paralytic ectropion of right upper eyelid
    H02.152 Paralytic ectropion of right lower eyelid
    H02.153 Paralytic ectropion of right eye, unspecified eyelid
    H02.154 Paralytic ectropion of left upper eyelid
    H02.155 Paralytic ectropion of left lower eyelid
    H02.156 Paralytic ectropion of left eye, unspecified eyelid
    H02.159 Paralytic ectropion of unspecified eye, unspecified eyelid

√5ᵗʰ **H02.2** Lagophthalmos
    AHA: 2018,4Q,14
    DEF: Condition of the eye that prevents it from closing completely.

√6ᵗʰ **H02.20** Unspecified lagophthalmos
    H02.201 Unspecified lagophthalmos right upper eyelid
    H02.202 Unspecified lagophthalmos right lower eyelid
    H02.203 Unspecified lagophthalmos right eye, unspecified eyelid
    H02.204 Unspecified lagophthalmos left upper eyelid
    H02.205 Unspecified lagophthalmos left lower eyelid

H02.206 Unspecified lagophthalmos left eye, unspecified eyelid
H02.209 Unspecified lagophthalmos unspecified eye, unspecified eyelid
H02.20A Unspecified lagophthalmos right eye, upper and lower eyelids
H02.20B Unspecified lagophthalmos left eye, upper and lower eyelids
H02.20C Unspecified lagophthalmos, bilateral, upper and lower eyelids

√6ᵗʰ **H02.21** Cicatricial lagophthalmos
    H02.211 Cicatricial lagophthalmos right upper eyelid
    H02.212 Cicatricial lagophthalmos right lower eyelid
    H02.213 Cicatricial lagophthalmos right eye, unspecified eyelid
    H02.214 Cicatricial lagophthalmos left upper eyelid
    H02.215 Cicatricial lagophthalmos left lower eyelid
    H02.216 Cicatricial lagophthalmos left eye, unspecified eyelid
    H02.219 Cicatricial lagophthalmos unspecified eye, unspecified eyelid
    H02.21A Cicatricial lagophthalmos right eye, upper and lower eyelids
    H02.21B Cicatricial lagophthalmos left eye, upper and lower eyelids
    H02.21C Cicatricial lagophthalmos, bilateral, upper and lower eyelids

√6ᵗʰ **H02.22** Mechanical lagophthalmos
    H02.221 Mechanical lagophthalmos right upper eyelid
    H02.222 Mechanical lagophthalmos right lower eyelid
    H02.223 Mechanical lagophthalmos right eye, unspecified eyelid
    H02.224 Mechanical lagophthalmos left upper eyelid
    H02.225 Mechanical lagophthalmos left lower eyelid
    H02.226 Mechanical lagophthalmos left eye, unspecified eyelid
    H02.229 Mechanical lagophthalmos unspecified eye, unspecified eyelid
    H02.22A Mechanical lagophthalmos right eye, upper and lower eyelids
    H02.22B Mechanical lagophthalmos left eye, upper and lower eyelids
    H02.22C Mechanical lagophthalmos, bilateral, upper and lower eyelids

√6ᵗʰ **H02.23** Paralytic lagophthalmos
    H02.231 Paralytic lagophthalmos right upper eyelid
    H02.232 Paralytic lagophthalmos right lower eyelid
    H02.233 Paralytic lagophthalmos right eye, unspecified eyelid
    H02.234 Paralytic lagophthalmos left upper eyelid
    H02.235 Paralytic lagophthalmos left lower eyelid
    H02.236 Paralytic lagophthalmos left eye, unspecified eyelid
    H02.239 Paralytic lagophthalmos unspecified eye, unspecified eyelid
    H02.23A Paralytic lagophthalmos right eye, upper and lower eyelids
    H02.23B Paralytic lagophthalmos left eye, upper and lower eyelids
    H02.23C Paralytic lagophthalmos, bilateral, upper and lower eyelids

√5ᵗʰ **H02.3** Blepharochalasis
    Pseudoptosis
    DEF: Loss of elasticity and relaxation of skin of the eyelid, thickened or indurated skin on the eyelid associated with recurrent episodes of edema, and intracellular atrophy.
    H02.30 Blepharochalasis unspecified eye, unspecified eyelid
    H02.31 Blepharochalasis right upper eyelid
    H02.32 Blepharochalasis right lower eyelid
    H02.33 Blepharochalasis right eye, unspecified eyelid
    H02.34 Blepharochalasis left upper eyelid

🅝 Newborn: 0   🅟 Pediatric: 0-17   🅜 Maternity: 9-64   🅰 Adult: 15-124   **MCC** Major Complication/Comorbidity   **CC** Complication/Comorbidity   **SW** Severe Wound Dx

596   ICD-10-CM 2020

H02.35   **Blepharochalasis** left lower eyelid

H02.36   **Blepharochalasis** left eye, unspecified eyelid

√5ᵗʰ **H02.4**   **Ptosis of eyelid**

√6ᵗʰ   **H02.40**   **Unspecified ptosis of eyelid**

H02.401   **Unspecified ptosis of** right **eyelid**

H02.402   **Unspecified ptosis of** left **eyelid**

H02.403   **Unspecified ptosis of** bilateral **eyelids**

H02.409   **Unspecified ptosis of unspecified eyelid**

√6ᵗʰ   **H02.41**   **Mechanical ptosis of eyelid**

H02.411   **Mechanical ptosis of** right **eyelid**

H02.412   **Mechanical ptosis of** left **eyelid**

H02.413   **Mechanical ptosis of** bilateral **eyelids**

H02.419   **Mechanical ptosis of unspecified eyelid**

√6ᵗʰ   **H02.42**   **Myogenic ptosis of eyelid**

H02.421   **Myogenic ptosis of** right **eyelid**

H02.422   **Myogenic ptosis of** left **eyelid**

H02.423   **Myogenic ptosis of** bilateral **eyelids**

H02.429   **Myogenic ptosis of unspecified eyelid**

√6ᵗʰ   **H02.43**   **Paralytic ptosis of eyelid**

Neurogenic ptosis of eyelid

H02.431   **Paralytic ptosis of** right **eyelid**

H02.432   **Paralytic ptosis of** left **eyelid**

H02.433   **Paralytic ptosis of** bilateral **eyelids**

H02.439   **Paralytic ptosis unspecified eyelid**

√5ᵗʰ **H02.5**   **Other disorders affecting eyelid function**

EXCLUDES 2   *blepharospasm (G24.5)*

organic tic (G25.69)

psychogenic tic (F95.-)

√6ᵗʰ   **H02.51**   **Abnormal innervation syndrome**

H02.511   **Abnormal innervation syndrome** right upper **eyelid**

H02.512   **Abnormal innervation syndrome** right lower **eyelid**

H02.513   **Abnormal innervation syndrome** right eye, unspecified **eyelid**

H02.514   **Abnormal innervation syndrome** left upper **eyelid**

H02.515   **Abnormal innervation syndrome** left lower **eyelid**

H02.516   **Abnormal innervation syndrome** left eye, unspecified **eyelid**

H02.519   **Abnormal innervation syndrome** unspecified eye, unspecified **eyelid**

√6ᵗʰ   **H02.52**   **Blepharophimosis**

Ankyloblepharon

H02.521   **Blepharophimosis** right upper **eyelid**

H02.522   **Blepharophimosis** right lower **eyelid**

H02.523   **Blepharophimosis** right eye, unspecified **eyelid**

H02.524   **Blepharophimosis** left upper **eyelid**

H02.525   **Blepharophimosis** left lower **eyelid**

H02.526   **Blepharophimosis** left eye, unspecified **eyelid**

H02.529   **Blepharophimosis** unspecified eye, unspecified **lid**

√6ᵗʰ   **H02.53**   **Eyelid retraction**

Eyelid lag

H02.531   **Eyelid retraction** right upper **eyelid**

H02.532   **Eyelid retraction** right lower **eyelid**

H02.533   **Eyelid retraction** right eye, unspecified **eyelid**

H02.534   **Eyelid retraction** left upper **eyelid**

H02.535   **Eyelid retraction** left lower **eyelid**

H02.536   **Eyelid retraction** left eye, unspecified **eyelid**

H02.539   **Eyelid retraction** unspecified eye, unspecified **lid**

H02.59   **Other disorders affecting eyelid function**

Deficient blink reflex

Sensory disorders

√5ᵗʰ **H02.6**   **Xanthelasma of eyelid**

DEF: Condition in which there are small yellow tumors that occur on the eyelid, usually appearing near the nose.

H02.60   **Xanthelasma of unspecified eye, unspecified eyelid**

H02.61   **Xanthelasma of** right upper **eyelid**

H02.62   **Xanthelasma of** right lower **eyelid**

H02.63   **Xanthelasma of** right eye, unspecified **eyelid**

H02.64   **Xanthelasma of** left upper **eyelid**

H02.65   **Xanthelasma of** left lower **eyelid**

H02.66   **Xanthelasma of** left eye, unspecified **eyelid**

√5ᵗʰ **H02.7**   **Other and unspecified degenerative disorders of eyelid and periocular area**

H02.70   **Unspecified degenerative disorders of eyelid and periocular area**

√6ᵗʰ   **H02.71**   **Chloasma of eyelid and periocular area**

Dyspigmentation of eyelid

Hyperpigmentation of eyelid

H02.711   **Chloasma of** right upper **eyelid and periocular area**

H02.712   **Chloasma of** right lower **eyelid and periocular area**

H02.713   **Chloasma of** right eye, unspecified **eyelid and periocular area**

H02.714   **Chloasma of** left upper **eyelid and periocular area**

H02.715   **Chloasma of** left lower **eyelid and periocular area**

H02.716   **Chloasma of** left eye, unspecified **eyelid and periocular area**

H02.719   **Chloasma of unspecified eye, unspecified eyelid and periocular area**

√6ᵗʰ   **H02.72**   **Madarosis of eyelid and periocular area**

Hypotrichosis of eyelid

H02.721   **Madarosis of** right upper **eyelid and periocular area**

H02.722   **Madarosis of** right lower **eyelid and periocular area**

H02.723   **Madarosis of** right eye, unspecified **eyelid and periocular area**

H02.724   **Madarosis of** left upper **eyelid and periocular area**

H02.725   **Madarosis of** left lower **eyelid and periocular area**

H02.726   **Madarosis of** left eye, unspecified **eyelid and periocular area**

H02.729   **Madarosis of unspecified eye, unspecified eyelid and periocular area**

√6ᵗʰ   **H02.73**   **Vitiligo of eyelid and periocular area**

Hypopigmentation of eyelid

H02.731   **Vitiligo of** right upper **eyelid and periocular area**

H02.732   **Vitiligo of** right lower **eyelid and periocular area**

H02.733   **Vitiligo of** right eye, unspecified **eyelid and periocular area**

H02.734   **Vitiligo of** left upper **eyelid and periocular area**

H02.735   **Vitiligo of** left lower **eyelid and periocular area**

H02.736   **Vitiligo of** left eye, unspecified **eyelid and periocular area**

H02.739   **Vitiligo of unspecified eye, unspecified eyelid and periocular area**

H02.79   **Other degenerative disorders of eyelid and periocular area**

√5ᵗʰ **H02.8**   **Other specified disorders of eyelid**

√6ᵗʰ   **H02.81**   **Retained foreign body in eyelid**

Use additional code to identify the type of retained foreign body (Z18.-)

EXCLUDES 1   *laceration of eyelid with foreign body (S01.12-)*

retained intraocular foreign body (H44.6-, H44.7-)

superficial foreign body of eyelid and periocular area (S00.25-)

H02.811   **Retained foreign body in** right upper **eyelid**

H02.812   **Retained foreign body in** right lower **eyelid**

H02.813   **Retained foreign body in** right eye, unspecified **eyelid**

H02.814   **Retained foreign body in** left upper **eyelid**

H02.815   **Retained foreign body in** left lower **eyelid**

H02.816   **Retained foreign body in** left eye, unspecified **eyelid**

H02.819   **Retained foreign body in unspecified eye, unspecified eyelid**

☑ Additional Character Required   √x7ᵗʰ Placeholder   Unacceptable PDx   Questionable PDx   Manifestation   Unspecified Dx   H1-H14 HAC   HCC CMS-HCC Dx   HIV HIV Dx

ICD-10-CM 2020   597

Chapter 7. Diseases of the Eye and Adnexa

H02.35–H02.819

Chapter 7. Diseases of the Eye and Adnexa

√6ᵗʰ **H02.82 Cysts** of eyelid

Sebaceous cyst of eyelid

H02.821 Cysts of **right upper eyelid**

H02.822 Cysts of **right lower eyelid**

H02.823 Cysts of **right eye, unspecified eyelid**

H02.824 Cysts of **left upper eyelid**

H02.825 Cysts of **left lower eyelid**

H02.826 Cysts of **left eye, unspecified eyelid**

H02.829 Cysts of **unspecified eye, unspecified eyelid**

√6ᵗʰ **H02.83 Dermatochalasis** of eyelid

DEF: Acquired form of connective tissue disorder associated with decreased elastic tissue and abnormal elastin formation, resulting in loss of elasticity of the skin of the eyelid. It is generally associated with aging.

H02.831 Dermatochalasis of **right upper eyelid**

H02.832 Dermatochalasis of **right lower eyelid**

H02.833 Dermatochalasis of **right eye, unspecified eyelid**

H02.834 Dermatochalasis of **left upper eyelid**

H02.835 Dermatochalasis of **left lower eyelid**

H02.836 Dermatochalasis of **left eye, unspecified eyelid**

H02.839 Dermatochalasis of **unspecified eye, unspecified eyelid**

√6ᵗʰ **H02.84 Edema** of eyelid

Hyperemia of eyelid

H02.841 Edema of **right upper eyelid**

H02.842 Edema of **right lower eyelid**

H02.843 Edema of **right eye, unspecified eyelid**

H02.844 Edema of **left upper eyelid**

H02.845 Edema of **left lower eyelid**

H02.846 Edema of **left eye, unspecified eyelid**

H02.849 Edema of **unspecified eye, unspecified eyelid**

√6ᵗʰ **H02.85 Elephantiasis** of eyelid

H02.851 Elephantiasis of **right upper eyelid**

H02.852 Elephantiasis of **right lower eyelid**

H02.853 Elephantiasis of **right eye, unspecified eyelid**

H02.854 Elephantiasis of **left upper eyelid**

H02.855 Elephantiasis of **left lower eyelid**

H02.856 Elephantiasis of **left eye, unspecified eyelid**

H02.859 Elephantiasis of **unspecified eye, unspecified eyelid**

√6ᵗʰ **H02.86 Hypertrichosis** of eyelid

H02.861 Hypertrichosis of **right upper eyelid**

H02.862 Hypertrichosis of **right lower eyelid**

H02.863 Hypertrichosis of **right eye, unspecified eyelid**

H02.864 Hypertrichosis of **left upper eyelid**

H02.865 Hypertrichosis of **left lower eyelid**

H02.866 Hypertrichosis of **left eye, unspecified eyelid**

H02.869 Hypertrichosis of **unspecified eye, unspecified eyelid**

√6ᵗʰ **H02.87 Vascular anomalies** of eyelid

H02.871 Vascular anomalies of **right upper eyelid**

H02.872 Vascular anomalies of **right lower eyelid**

H02.873 Vascular anomalies of **right eye, unspecified eyelid**

H02.874 Vascular anomalies of **left upper eyelid**

H02.875 Vascular anomalies of **left lower eyelid**

H02.876 Vascular anomalies of **left eye, unspecified eyelid**

H02.879 Vascular anomalies of **unspecified eye, unspecified eyelid**

√6ᵗʰ **H02.88 Meibomian gland dysfunction** of eyelid

AHA: 2018,4Q,14-15

H02.881 Meibomian gland dysfunction right upper eyelid

H02.882 Meibomian gland dysfunction right lower eyelid

H02.883 Meibomian gland dysfunction of **right eye, unspecified eyelid**

H02.884 Meibomian gland dysfunction left upper eyelid

H02.885 Meibomian gland dysfunction left lower eyelid

H02.886 Meibomian gland dysfunction of left eye, unspecified eyelid

H02.889 Meibomian gland dysfunction of unspecified eye, unspecified eyelid

H02.88A Meibomian gland dysfunction right eye, upper and lower eyelids

H02.88B Meibomian gland dysfunction left eye, upper and lower eyelids

H02.89 Other specified disorders of eyelid

Hemorrhage of eyelid

H02.9 Unspecified disorder of eyelid

Disorder of eyelid NOS

√4ᵗʰ **H04 Disorders of lacrimal system**

EXCLUDES 1 *congenital malformations of lacrimal system (Q10.4-Q10.6)*

√5ᵗʰ **H04.0 Dacryoadenitis**

DEF: Inflammation of the lacrimal gland.

√6ᵗʰ **H04.00 Unspecified dacryoadenitis**

H04.001 Unspecified dacryoadenitis, right lacrimal gland

H04.002 Unspecified dacryoadenitis, left lacrimal gland

H04.003 Unspecified dacryoadenitis, bilateral lacrimal glands

H04.009 Unspecified dacryoadenitis, unspecified lacrimal gland

√6ᵗʰ **H04.01 Acute dacryoadenitis**

H04.011 Acute dacryoadenitis, right lacrimal gland

H04.012 Acute dacryoadenitis, left lacrimal gland

H04.013 Acute dacryoadenitis, bilateral lacrimal glands

H04.019 Acute dacryoadenitis, unspecified lacrimal gland

√6ᵗʰ **H04.02 Chronic dacryoadenitis**

H04.021 Chronic dacryoadenitis, right lacrimal gland

H04.022 Chronic dacryoadenitis, left lacrimal gland

H04.023 Chronic dacryoadenitis, bilateral lacrimal gland

H04.029 Chronic dacryoadenitis, unspecified lacrimal gland

√6ᵗʰ **H04.03 Chronic enlargement of lacrimal gland**

H04.031 Chronic enlargement of right lacrimal gland

H04.032 Chronic enlargement of left lacrimal gland

H04.033 Chronic enlargement of bilateral lacrimal glands

H04.039 Chronic enlargement of unspecified lacrimal gland

√5ᵗʰ **H04.1 Other disorders of lacrimal gland**

√6ᵗʰ **H04.11 Dacryops**

H04.111 Dacryops of right lacrimal gland

H04.112 Dacryops of left lacrimal gland

H04.113 Dacryops of bilateral lacrimal glands

H04.119 Dacryops of unspecified lacrimal gland

√6ᵗʰ **H04.12 Dry eye syndrome**

Tear film insufficiency, NOS

H04.121 Dry eye syndrome of right lacrimal gland

H04.122 Dry eye syndrome of left lacrimal gland

H04.123 Dry eye syndrome of bilateral lacrimal glands

H04.129 Dry eye syndrome of unspecified lacrimal gland

√6ᵗʰ **H04.13 Lacrimal cyst**

Lacrimal cystic degeneration

H04.131 Lacrimal cyst, right lacrimal gland

H04.132 Lacrimal cyst, left lacrimal gland

H04.133 Lacrimal cyst, bilateral lacrimal glands

H04.139 Lacrimal cyst, unspecified lacrimal gland

√6ᵗʰ **H04.14 Primary lacrimal gland atrophy**

H04.141 Primary lacrimal gland atrophy, right lacrimal gland

H04.142 Primary lacrimal gland atrophy, left lacrimal gland

H04.143 Primary lacrimal gland atrophy, bilateral lacrimal glands

H04.149 Primary lacrimal gland atrophy, unspecified lacrimal gland

N Newborn: 0   P Pediatric: 0-17   M Maternity: 9-64   A Adult: 15-124   MCC Major Complication/Comorbidity   CC Complication/Comorbidity   SW Severe Wound Dx

598

ICD-10-CM 2020

✓6ᵗʰ **H04.15** **Secondary** lacrimal gland atrophy

     H04.151 **Secondary lacrimal gland atrophy, right lacrimal gland**

     H04.152 **Secondary lacrimal gland atrophy, left lacrimal gland**

     H04.153 **Secondary lacrimal gland atrophy, bilateral lacrimal glands**

     H04.159 **Secondary lacrimal gland atrophy, unspecified lacrimal gland**

✓6ᵗʰ **H04.16** **Lacrimal gland dislocation**

     H04.161 **Lacrimal gland dislocation, right lacrimal gland**

     H04.162 **Lacrimal gland dislocation, left lacrimal gland**

     H04.163 **Lacrimal gland dislocation, bilateral lacrimal glands**

     H04.169 **Lacrimal gland dislocation, unspecified lacrimal gland**

     H04.19 **Other specified disorders of lacrimal gland**

✓5ᵗʰ **H04.2** **Epiphora**

     DEF: Excessive tearing or overflow of tears down the cheeks often due to a stricture in the lacrimal passages but can be caused by other conditions.

     ✓6ᵗʰ **H04.20** **Unspecified epiphora**

         H04.201 **Unspecified epiphora, right side**

         H04.202 **Unspecified epiphora, left side**

         H04.203 **Unspecified epiphora, bilateral**

         H04.209 **Unspecified epiphora, unspecified side**

     ✓6ᵗʰ **H04.21** **Epiphora due to excess lacrimation**

         H04.211 **Epiphora due to excess lacrimation, right lacrimal gland**

         H04.212 **Epiphora due to excess lacrimation, left lacrimal gland**

         H04.213 **Epiphora due to excess lacrimation, bilateral lacrimal glands**

         H04.219 **Epiphora due to excess lacrimation, unspecified lacrimal gland**

     ✓6ᵗʰ **H04.22** **Epiphora due to insufficient drainage**

         H04.221 **Epiphora due to insufficient drainage, right side**

         H04.222 **Epiphora due to insufficient drainage, left side**

         H04.223 **Epiphora due to insufficient drainage, bilateral**

         H04.229 **Epiphora due to insufficient drainage, unspecified side**

✓5ᵗʰ **H04.3** **Acute and unspecified inflammation of lacrimal passages**

     EXCLUDES 1   neonatal dacryocystitis (P39.1)

     ✓6ᵗʰ **H04.30** **Unspecified dacryocystitis**

         H04.301 **Unspecified dacryocystitis of right lacrimal passage**

         H04.302 **Unspecified dacryocystitis of left lacrimal passage**

         H04.303 **Unspecified dacryocystitis of bilateral lacrimal passages**

         H04.309 **Unspecified dacryocystitis of unspecified lacrimal passage**

     ✓6ᵗʰ **H04.31** **Phlegmonous dacryocystitis**

         H04.311 **Phlegmonous dacryocystitis of right lacrimal passage**

         H04.312 **Phlegmonous dacryocystitis of left lacrimal passage**

         H04.313 **Phlegmonous dacryocystitis of bilateral lacrimal passages**

         H04.319 **Phlegmonous dacryocystitis of unspecified lacrimal passage**

     ✓6ᵗʰ **H04.32** **Acute dacryocystitis**

         Acute dacryopericystitis

         H04.321 **Acute dacryocystitis of right lacrimal passage**

         H04.322 **Acute dacryocystitis of left lacrimal passage**

         H04.323 **Acute dacryocystitis of bilateral lacrimal passages**

         H04.329 **Acute dacryocystitis of unspecified lacrimal passage**

     ✓6ᵗʰ **H04.33** **Acute lacrimal canaliculitis**

         H04.331 **Acute lacrimal canaliculitis of right lacrimal passage**

         H04.332 **Acute lacrimal canaliculitis of left lacrimal passage**

         H04.333 **Acute lacrimal canaliculitis of bilateral lacrimal passages**

         H04.339 **Acute lacrimal canaliculitis of unspecified lacrimal passage**

✓5ᵗʰ **H04.4** **Chronic inflammation of lacrimal passages**

     ✓6ᵗʰ **H04.41** **Chronic dacryocystitis**

         H04.411 **Chronic dacryocystitis of right lacrimal passage**

         H04.412 **Chronic dacryocystitis of left lacrimal passage**

         H04.413 **Chronic dacryocystitis of bilateral lacrimal passages**

         H04.419 **Chronic dacryocystitis of unspecified lacrimal passage**

     ✓6ᵗʰ **H04.42** **Chronic lacrimal canaliculitis**

         H04.421 **Chronic lacrimal canaliculitis of right lacrimal passage**

         H04.422 **Chronic lacrimal canaliculitis of left lacrimal passage**

         H04.423 **Chronic lacrimal canaliculitis of bilateral lacrimal passages**

         H04.429 **Chronic lacrimal canaliculitis of unspecified lacrimal passage**

     ✓6ᵗʰ **H04.43** **Chronic lacrimal mucocele**

         H04.431 **Chronic lacrimal mucocele of right lacrimal passage**

         H04.432 **Chronic lacrimal mucocele of left lacrimal passage**

         H04.433 **Chronic lacrimal mucocele of bilateral lacrimal passages**

         H04.439 **Chronic lacrimal mucocele of unspecified lacrimal passage**

✓5ᵗʰ **H04.5** **Stenosis and insufficiency of lacrimal passages**

     ✓6ᵗʰ **H04.51** **Dacryolith**

         H04.511 **Dacryolith of right lacrimal passage**

         H04.512 **Dacryolith of left lacrimal passage**

         H04.513 **Dacryolith of bilateral lacrimal passages**

         H04.519 **Dacryolith of unspecified lacrimal passage**

     ✓6ᵗʰ **H04.52** **Eversion of lacrimal punctum**

         H04.521 **Eversion of right lacrimal punctum**

         H04.522 **Eversion of left lacrimal punctum**

         H04.523 **Eversion of bilateral lacrimal punctum**

         H04.529 **Eversion of unspecified lacrimal punctum**

     ✓6ᵗʰ **H04.53** **Neonatal obstruction of nasolacrimal duct**

         EXCLUDES 1   congenital stenosis and stricture of lacrimal duct (Q10.5)

         H04.531 **Neonatal obstruction of right nasolacrimal duct** N

         H04.532 **Neonatal obstruction of left nasolacrimal duct** N

         H04.533 **Neonatal obstruction of bilateral nasolacrimal duct** N

         H04.539 **Neonatal obstruction of unspecified nasolacrimal duct** N

     ✓6ᵗʰ **H04.54** **Stenosis of lacrimal canaliculi**

         H04.541 **Stenosis of right lacrimal canaliculi**

         H04.542 **Stenosis of left lacrimal canaliculi**

         H04.543 **Stenosis of bilateral lacrimal canaliculi**

         H04.549 **Stenosis of unspecified lacrimal canaliculi**

     ✓6ᵗʰ **H04.55** **Acquired stenosis of nasolacrimal duct**

         H04.551 **Acquired stenosis of right nasolacrimal duct**

         H04.552 **Acquired stenosis of left nasolacrimal duct**

         H04.553 **Acquired stenosis of bilateral nasolacrimal duct**

         H04.559 **Acquired stenosis of unspecified nasolacrimal duct**

     ✓6ᵗʰ **H04.56** **Stenosis of lacrimal punctum**

         H04.561 **Stenosis of right lacrimal punctum**

         H04.562 **Stenosis of left lacrimal punctum**

         H04.563 **Stenosis of bilateral lacrimal punctum**

         H04.569 **Stenosis of unspecified lacrimal punctum**

     ✓6ᵗʰ **H04.57** **Stenosis of lacrimal sac**

         H04.571 **Stenosis of right lacrimal sac**

Chapter 7. Diseases of the Eye and Adnexa

H04.572 Stenosis of left lacrimal sac
H04.573 Stenosis of bilateral lacrimal sac
H04.579 Stenosis of unspecified lacrimal sac

✓5th H04.6 Other changes of lacrimal passages

✓6th H04.61 Lacrimal fistula

H04.611 Lacrimal fistula right lacrimal passage   SW
H04.612 Lacrimal fistula left lacrimal passage   SW
H04.613 Lacrimal fistula bilateral lacrimal passages   SW
H04.619 Lacrimal fistula unspecified lacrimal passage   SW

H04.69 Other changes of lacrimal passages

✓5th H04.8 Other disorders of lacrimal system

✓6th H04.81 Granuloma of lacrimal passages

H04.811 Granuloma of right lacrimal passage
H04.812 Granuloma of left lacrimal passage
H04.813 Granuloma of bilateral lacrimal passages
H04.819 Granuloma of unspecified lacrimal passage

H04.89 Other disorders of lacrimal system

H04.9 Disorder of lacrimal system, unspecified

✓4th H05 Disorders of orbit

EXCLUDES 1   congenital malformation of orbit (Q10.7)

✓5th H05.0 Acute inflammation of orbit

H05.00 Unspecified acute inflammation of orbit

✓6th H05.01 Cellulitis of orbit

Abscess of orbit
CC Excl: For CC codes in subcategory H05.01: PDX collection 621

H05.011 Cellulitis of right orbit   CC
H05.012 Cellulitis of left orbit   CC
H05.013 Cellulitis of bilateral orbits   CC
H05.019 Cellulitis of unspecified orbit   CC

✓6th H05.02 Osteomyelitis of orbit

CC Excl: For CC codes in subcategory H05.02: PDX collection 622

H05.021 Osteomyelitis of right orbit   CC
H05.022 Osteomyelitis of left orbit   CC
H05.023 Osteomyelitis of bilateral orbits   CC
H05.029 Osteomyelitis of unspecified orbit   CC

✓6th H05.03 Periostitis of orbit

CC Excl: For CC codes in subcategory H05.03: PDX collection 623

H05.031 Periostitis of right orbit   CC
H05.032 Periostitis of left orbit   CC
H05.033 Periostitis of bilateral orbits   CC
H05.039 Periostitis of unspecified orbit   CC

✓6th H05.04 Tenonitis of orbit

H05.041 Tenonitis of right orbit
H05.042 Tenonitis of left orbit
H05.043 Tenonitis of bilateral orbits
H05.049 Tenonitis of unspecified orbit

✓5th H05.1 Chronic inflammatory disorders of orbit

H05.10 Unspecified chronic inflammatory disorders of orbit

✓6th H05.11 Granuloma of orbit

Pseudotumor (inflammatory) of orbit
H05.111 Granuloma of right orbit
H05.112 Granuloma of left orbit
H05.113 Granuloma of bilateral orbits
H05.119 Granuloma of unspecified orbit

✓6th H05.12 Orbital myositis

H05.121 Orbital myositis, right orbit
H05.122 Orbital myositis, left orbit
H05.123 Orbital myositis, bilateral
H05.129 Orbital myositis, unspecified orbit

✓5th H05.2 Exophthalmic conditions

H05.20 Unspecified exophthalmos

✓6th H05.21 Displacement (lateral) of globe

H05.211 Displacement (lateral) of globe, right eye
H05.212 Displacement (lateral) of globe, left eye
H05.213 Displacement (lateral) of globe, bilateral
H05.219 Displacement (lateral) of globe, unspecified eye

✓6th H05.22 Edema of orbit

Orbital congestion
H05.221 Edema of right orbit
H05.222 Edema of left orbit
H05.223 Edema of bilateral orbit
H05.229 Edema of unspecified orbit

✓6th H05.23 Hemorrhage of orbit

H05.231 Hemorrhage of right orbit
H05.232 Hemorrhage of left orbit
H05.233 Hemorrhage of bilateral orbit
H05.239 Hemorrhage of unspecified orbit

✓6th H05.24 Constant exophthalmos

H05.241 Constant exophthalmos, right eye
H05.242 Constant exophthalmos, left eye
H05.243 Constant exophthalmos, bilateral
H05.249 Constant exophthalmos, unspecified eye

✓6th H05.25 Intermittent exophthalmos

H05.251 Intermittent exophthalmos, right eye
H05.252 Intermittent exophthalmos, left eye
H05.253 Intermittent exophthalmos, bilateral
H05.259 Intermittent exophthalmos, unspecified eye

✓6th H05.26 Pulsating exophthalmos

H05.261 Pulsating exophthalmos, right eye
H05.262 Pulsating exophthalmos, left eye
H05.263 Pulsating exophthalmos, bilateral
H05.269 Pulsating exophthalmos, unspecified eye

✓5th H05.3 Deformity of orbit

EXCLUDES 1   congenital deformity of orbit (Q10.7)
hypertelorism (Q75.2)

H05.30 Unspecified deformity of orbit

✓6th H05.31 Atrophy of orbit

H05.311 Atrophy of right orbit
H05.312 Atrophy of left orbit
H05.313 Atrophy of bilateral orbit
H05.319 Atrophy of unspecified orbit

✓6th H05.32 Deformity of orbit due to bone disease

Code also associated bone disease
H05.321 Deformity of right orbit due to bone disease
H05.322 Deformity of left orbit due to bone disease
H05.323 Deformity of bilateral orbits due to bone disease
H05.329 Deformity of unspecified orbit due to bone disease

✓6th H05.33 Deformity of orbit due to trauma or surgery

H05.331 Deformity of right orbit due to trauma or surgery
H05.332 Deformity of left orbit due to trauma or surgery
H05.333 Deformity of bilateral orbits due to trauma or surgery
H05.339 Deformity of unspecified orbit due to trauma or surgery

✓6th H05.34 Enlargement of orbit

H05.341 Enlargement of right orbit
H05.342 Enlargement of left orbit
H05.343 Enlargement of bilateral orbits
H05.349 Enlargement of unspecified orbit

✓6th H05.35 Exostosis of orbit

H05.351 Exostosis of right orbit
H05.352 Exostosis of left orbit
H05.353 Exostosis of bilateral orbits
H05.359 Exostosis of unspecified orbit

✓5th H05.4 Enophthalmos

✓6th H05.40 Unspecified enophthalmos

H05.401 Unspecified enophthalmos, right eye

H05.402   Unspecified enophthalmos, left eye
H05.403   Unspecified enophthalmos, bilateral
H05.409   Unspecified enophthalmos, unspecified eye

✓6ᵗʰ H05.41   Enophthalmos due to atrophy of orbital tissue
H05.411   Enophthalmos due to atrophy of orbital tissue, right eye
H05.412   Enophthalmos due to atrophy of orbital tissue, left eye
H05.413   Enophthalmos due to atrophy of orbital tissue, bilateral
H05.419   Enophthalmos due to atrophy of orbital tissue, unspecified eye

✓6ᵗʰ H05.42   Enophthalmos due to trauma or surgery
H05.421   Enophthalmos due to trauma or surgery, right eye
H05.422   Enophthalmos due to trauma or surgery, left eye
H05.423   Enophthalmos due to trauma or surgery, bilateral
H05.429   Enophthalmos due to trauma or surgery, unspecified eye

✓5ᵗʰ H05.5   Retained (old) foreign body following penetrating wound of orbit
Retrobulbar foreign body
Use additional code to identify the type of retained foreign body (Z18.-)
EXCLUDES 1   current penetrating wound of orbit (S05.4-)
EXCLUDES 2   retained foreign body of eyelid (H02.81-)
retained intraocular foreign body (H44.6-, H44.7-)
H05.50   Retained (old) foreign body following penetrating wound of unspecified orbit
H05.51   Retained (old) foreign body following penetrating wound of right orbit
H05.52   Retained (old) foreign body following penetrating wound of left orbit
H05.53   Retained (old) foreign body following penetrating wound of bilateral orbits

✓5ᵗʰ H05.8   Other disorders of orbit
✓6ᵗʰ H05.81   Cyst of orbit
Encephalocele of orbit
H05.811   Cyst of right orbit
H05.812   Cyst of left orbit
H05.813   Cyst of bilateral orbits
H05.819   Cyst of unspecified orbit
✓6ᵗʰ H05.82   Myopathy of extraocular muscles
H05.821   Myopathy of extraocular muscles, right orbit
H05.822   Myopathy of extraocular muscles, left orbit
H05.823   Myopathy of extraocular muscles, bilateral
H05.829   Myopathy of extraocular muscles, unspecified orbit
H05.89   Other disorders of orbit
H05.9   Unspecified disorder of orbit

Disorders of conjunctiva (H10-H11)

✓4ᵗʰ H10   Conjunctivitis
EXCLUDES 1   keratoconjunctivitis (H16.2-)

✓5ᵗʰ H10.0   Mucopurulent conjunctivitis
✓6ᵗʰ H10.01   Acute follicular conjunctivitis
H10.011   Acute follicular conjunctivitis, right eye
H10.012   Acute follicular conjunctivitis, left eye
H10.013   Acute follicular conjunctivitis, bilateral
H10.019   Acute follicular conjunctivitis, unspecified eye
✓6ᵗʰ H10.02   Other mucopurulent conjunctivitis
H10.021   Other mucopurulent conjunctivitis, right eye
H10.022   Other mucopurulent conjunctivitis, left eye
H10.023   Other mucopurulent conjunctivitis, bilateral
H10.029   Other mucopurulent conjunctivitis, unspecified eye

✓5ᵗʰ H10.1   Acute atopic conjunctivitis
Acute papillary conjunctivitis
H10.10   Acute atopic conjunctivitis, unspecified eye
H10.11   Acute atopic conjunctivitis, right eye
H10.12   Acute atopic conjunctivitis, left eye
H10.13   Acute atopic conjunctivitis, bilateral

✓5ᵗʰ H10.2   Other acute conjunctivitis
✓6ᵗʰ H10.21   Acute toxic conjunctivitis
Acute chemical conjunctivitis
Code first (T51-T65) to identify chemical and intent
EXCLUDES 1   burn and corrosion of eye and adnexa (T26.-)
H10.211   Acute toxic conjunctivitis, right eye
H10.212   Acute toxic conjunctivitis, left eye
H10.213   Acute toxic conjunctivitis, bilateral
H10.219   Acute toxic conjunctivitis, unspecified eye
✓6ᵗʰ H10.22   Pseudomembranous conjunctivitis
H10.221   Pseudomembranous conjunctivitis, right eye
H10.222   Pseudomembranous conjunctivitis, left eye
H10.223   Pseudomembranous conjunctivitis, bilateral
H10.229   Pseudomembranous conjunctivitis, unspecified eye
✓6ᵗʰ H10.23   Serous conjunctivitis, except viral
EXCLUDES 1   viral conjunctivitis (B30.-)
H10.231   Serous conjunctivitis, except viral, right eye
H10.232   Serous conjunctivitis, except viral, left eye
H10.233   Serous conjunctivitis, except viral, bilateral
H10.239   Serous conjunctivitis, except viral, unspecified eye

✓5ᵗʰ H10.3   Unspecified acute conjunctivitis
EXCLUDES 1   ophthalmia neonatorum NOS (P39.1)
H10.30   Unspecified acute conjunctivitis, unspecified eye
H10.31   Unspecified acute conjunctivitis, right eye
H10.32   Unspecified acute conjunctivitis, left eye
H10.33   Unspecified acute conjunctivitis, bilateral

✓5ᵗʰ H10.4   Chronic conjunctivitis
✓6ᵗʰ H10.40   Unspecified chronic conjunctivitis
H10.401   Unspecified chronic conjunctivitis, right eye
H10.402   Unspecified chronic conjunctivitis, left eye
H10.403   Unspecified chronic conjunctivitis, bilateral
H10.409   Unspecified chronic conjunctivitis, unspecified eye
✓6ᵗʰ H10.41   Chronic giant papillary conjunctivitis
H10.411   Chronic giant papillary conjunctivitis, right eye
H10.412   Chronic giant papillary conjunctivitis, left eye
H10.413   Chronic giant papillary conjunctivitis, bilateral
H10.419   Chronic giant papillary conjunctivitis, unspecified eye
✓6ᵗʰ H10.42   Simple chronic conjunctivitis
H10.421   Simple chronic conjunctivitis, right eye
H10.422   Simple chronic conjunctivitis, left eye
H10.423   Simple chronic conjunctivitis, bilateral
H10.429   Simple chronic conjunctivitis, unspecified eye
✓6ᵗʰ H10.43   Chronic follicular conjunctivitis
H10.431   Chronic follicular conjunctivitis, right eye
H10.432   Chronic follicular conjunctivitis, left eye
H10.433   Chronic follicular conjunctivitis, bilateral
H10.439   Chronic follicular conjunctivitis, unspecified eye
H10.44   Vernal conjunctivitis
EXCLUDES 1   vernal keratoconjunctivitis with limbar and corneal involvement (H16.26-)
H10.45   Other chronic allergic conjunctivitis

✓5ᵗʰ **H10.5** **Blepharoconjunctivitis**

  ✓6ᵗʰ **H10.50** **Unspecified blepharoconjunctivitis**

    H10.501 Unspecified blepharoconjunctivitis, right eye

    H10.502 Unspecified blepharoconjunctivitis, left eye

    H10.503 Unspecified blepharoconjunctivitis, bilateral

    H10.509 Unspecified blepharoconjunctivitis, unspecified eye

  ✓6ᵗʰ **H10.51** **Ligneous conjunctivitis**

    Code also underlying condition if known, such as: plasminogen deficiency (E88.02)

    H10.511 Ligneous conjunctivitis, right eye

    H10.512 Ligneous conjunctivitis, left eye

    H10.513 Ligneous conjunctivitis, bilateral

    H10.519 Ligneous conjunctivitis, unspecified eye

  ✓6ᵗʰ **H10.52** **Angular blepharoconjunctivitis**

    H10.521 Angular blepharoconjunctivitis, right eye

    H10.522 Angular blepharoconjunctivitis, left eye

    H10.523 Angular blepharoconjunctivitis, bilateral

    H10.529 Angular blepharoconjunctivitis, unspecified eye

  ✓6ᵗʰ **H10.53** **Contact blepharoconjunctivitis**

    H10.531 Contact blepharoconjunctivitis, right eye

    H10.532 Contact blepharoconjunctivitis, left eye

    H10.533 Contact blepharoconjunctivitis, bilateral

    H10.539 Contact blepharoconjunctivitis, unspecified eye

✓5ᵗʰ **H10.8** **Other conjunctivitis**

  ✓6ᵗʰ **H10.81** **Pingueculitis**

    EXCLUDES 1   *pinguecula (H11.15-)*

    H10.811 Pingueculitis, right eye

    H10.812 Pingueculitis, left eye

    H10.813 Pingueculitis, bilateral

    H10.819 Pingueculitis, unspecified eye

  ✓6ᵗʰ **H10.82** **Rosacea conjunctivitis**

    Code first underlying rosacea dermatitis (L71.-)

    AHA: 2018,4Q,15

    H10.821 Rosacea conjunctivitis, right eye

    H10.822 Rosacea conjunctivitis, left eye

    H10.823 Rosacea conjunctivitis, bilateral

    H10.829 Rosacea conjunctivitis, unspecified eye

  H10.89 **Other conjunctivitis**

  H10.9 **Unspecified conjunctivitis**

✓4ᵗʰ **H11** **Other disorders of conjunctiva**

  EXCLUDES 1   *keratoconjunctivitis (H16.2-)*

  ✓5ᵗʰ **H11.0** **Pterygium of eye**

    EXCLUDES 1   *pseudopterygium (H11.81-)*

    DEF: Benign, wedge-shaped, conjunctival thickening that advances from the inner corner of the eye toward the cornea.

Pterygium

Pterygium

  ✓6ᵗʰ **H11.00** **Unspecified pterygium of eye**

    H11.001 Unspecified pterygium of right eye

    H11.002 Unspecified pterygium of left eye

    H11.003 Unspecified pterygium of eye, bilateral

    H11.009 Unspecified pterygium of unspecified eye

  ✓6ᵗʰ **H11.01** **Amyloid pterygium**

    H11.011 Amyloid pterygium of right eye

    H11.012 Amyloid pterygium of left eye

    H11.013 Amyloid pterygium of eye, bilateral

    H11.019 Amyloid pterygium of unspecified eye

  ✓6ᵗʰ **H11.02** **Central pterygium of eye**

    H11.021 Central pterygium of right eye

    H11.022 Central pterygium of left eye

    H11.023 Central pterygium of eye, bilateral

    H11.029 Central pterygium of unspecified eye

  ✓6ᵗʰ **H11.03** **Double pterygium of eye**

    H11.031 Double pterygium of right eye

    H11.032 Double pterygium of left eye

    H11.033 Double pterygium of eye, bilateral

    H11.039 Double pterygium of unspecified eye

  ✓6ᵗʰ **H11.04** **Peripheral pterygium of eye, stationary**

    H11.041 Peripheral pterygium, stationary, right eye

    H11.042 Peripheral pterygium, stationary, left eye

    H11.043 Peripheral pterygium, stationary, bilateral

    H11.049 Peripheral pterygium, stationary, unspecified eye

  ✓6ᵗʰ **H11.05** **Peripheral pterygium of eye, progressive**

    H11.051 Peripheral pterygium, progressive, right eye

    H11.052 Peripheral pterygium, progressive, left eye

    H11.053 Peripheral pterygium, progressive, bilateral

    H11.059 Peripheral pterygium, progressive, unspecified eye

  ✓6ᵗʰ **H11.06** **Recurrent pterygium of eye**

    H11.061 Recurrent pterygium of right eye

    H11.062 Recurrent pterygium of left eye

    H11.063 Recurrent pterygium of eye, bilateral

    H11.069 Recurrent pterygium of unspecified eye

✓5ᵗʰ **H11.1** **Conjunctival degenerations and deposits**

    EXCLUDES 2   *pseudopterygium (H11.81)*

  H11.10 **Unspecified conjunctival degenerations**

  ✓6ᵗʰ **H11.11** **Conjunctival deposits**

    H11.111 Conjunctival deposits, right eye

    H11.112 Conjunctival deposits, left eye

    H11.113 Conjunctival deposits, bilateral

    H11.119 Conjunctival deposits, unspecified eye

  ✓6ᵗʰ **H11.12** **Conjunctival concretions**

    H11.121 Conjunctival concretions, right eye

    H11.122 Conjunctival concretions, left eye

    H11.123 Conjunctival concretions, bilateral

    H11.129 Conjunctival concretions, unspecified eye

  ✓6ᵗʰ **H11.13** **Conjunctival pigmentations**

    Conjunctival argyrosis [argyria]

    H11.131 Conjunctival pigmentations, right eye

    H11.132 Conjunctival pigmentations, left eye

    H11.133 Conjunctival pigmentations, bilateral

    H11.139 Conjunctival pigmentations, unspecified eye

  ✓6ᵗʰ **H11.14** **Conjunctival xerosis, unspecified**

    EXCLUDES 1   *xerosis of conjunctiva due to vitamin A deficiency (E50.0, E50.1)*

    DEF: Abnormal dryness of the conjunctiva due to lack of insufficient tears or conjunctival secretions.

    H11.141 Conjunctival xerosis, unspecified, right eye

    H11.142 Conjunctival xerosis, unspecified, left eye

    H11.143 Conjunctival xerosis, unspecified, bilateral

    H11.149 Conjunctival xerosis, unspecified, unspecified eye

Ⓝ Newborn: 0   Ⓟ Pediatric: 0-17   Ⓜ Maternity: 9-64   Ⓐ Adult: 15-124   **MCC** Major Complication/Comorbidity   **CC** Complication/Comorbidity   **SW** Severe Wound Dx

602   ICD-10-CM 2020

√6ᵗʰ **H11.15 Pinguecula**

> **EXCLUDES 1**   pingueculitis (H10.81-)
>
> **DEF:** Proliferation on the conjunctiva near the sclerocorneal junction, usually of the side of the nose and usually in older patients.

Pinguecula

Pinguecula

     H11.151   Pinguecula, right eye
     H11.152   Pinguecula, left eye
     H11.153   Pinguecula, bilateral
     H11.159   Pinguecula, unspecified eye

√5ᵗʰ **H11.2 Conjunctival scars**

√6ᵗʰ   **H11.21   Conjunctival adhesions and strands (localized)**

     H11.211   Conjunctival adhesions and strands (localized), right eye
     H11.212   Conjunctival adhesions and strands (localized), left eye
     H11.213   Conjunctival adhesions and strands (localized), bilateral
     H11.219   Conjunctival adhesions and strands (localized), unspecified eye

√6ᵗʰ   **H11.22   Conjunctival granuloma**

     H11.221   Conjunctival granuloma, right eye
     H11.222   Conjunctival granuloma, left eye
     H11.223   Conjunctival granuloma, bilateral
     H11.229   Conjunctival granuloma, unspecified

√6ᵗʰ   **H11.23   Symblepharon**

     H11.231   Symblepharon, right eye
     H11.232   Symblepharon, left eye
     H11.233   Symblepharon, bilateral
     H11.239   Symblepharon, unspecified eye

√6ᵗʰ   **H11.24   Scarring of conjunctiva**

     H11.241   Scarring of conjunctiva, right eye
     H11.242   Scarring of conjunctiva, left eye
     H11.243   Scarring of conjunctiva, bilateral
     H11.249   Scarring of conjunctiva, unspecified eye

√5ᵗʰ **H11.3 Conjunctival hemorrhage**

     Subconjunctival hemorrhage

     H11.30   Conjunctival hemorrhage, unspecified eye
     H11.31   Conjunctival hemorrhage, right eye
     H11.32   Conjunctival hemorrhage, left eye
     H11.33   Conjunctival hemorrhage, bilateral

√5ᵗʰ **H11.4 Other conjunctival vascular disorders and cysts**

√6ᵗʰ   **H11.41   Vascular abnormalities of conjunctiva**

     Conjunctival aneurysm

     H11.411   Vascular abnormalities of conjunctiva, right eye
     H11.412   Vascular abnormalities of conjunctiva, left eye
     H11.413   Vascular abnormalities of conjunctiva, bilateral
     H11.419   Vascular abnormalities of conjunctiva, unspecified eye

√6ᵗʰ   **H11.42   Conjunctival edema**

     H11.421   Conjunctival edema, right eye
     H11.422   Conjunctival edema, left eye
     H11.423   Conjunctival edema, bilateral
     H11.429   Conjunctival edema, unspecified eye

√6ᵗʰ   **H11.43   Conjunctival hyperemia**

     H11.431   Conjunctival hyperemia, right eye
     H11.432   Conjunctival hyperemia, left eye
     H11.433   Conjunctival hyperemia, bilateral
     H11.439   Conjunctival hyperemia, unspecified eye

√6ᵗʰ   **H11.44   Conjunctival cysts**

     H11.441   Conjunctival cysts, right eye
     H11.442   Conjunctival cysts, left eye
     H11.443   Conjunctival cysts, bilateral
     H11.449   Conjunctival cysts, unspecified eye

√5ᵗʰ **H11.8 Other specified disorders of conjunctiva**

√6ᵗʰ   **H11.81   Pseudopterygium of conjunctiva**

     H11.811   Pseudopterygium of conjunctiva, right eye
     H11.812   Pseudopterygium of conjunctiva, left eye
     H11.813   Pseudopterygium of conjunctiva, bilateral
     H11.819   Pseudopterygium of conjunctiva, unspecified eye

√6ᵗʰ   **H11.82   Conjunctivochalasis**

     H11.821   Conjunctivochalasis, right eye
     H11.822   Conjunctivochalasis, left eye
     H11.823   Conjunctivochalasis, bilateral
     H11.829   Conjunctivochalasis, unspecified eye

   H11.89   Other specified disorders of conjunctiva

H11.9 Unspecified disorder of conjunctiva

Disorders of sclera, cornea, iris and ciliary body (H15-H22)

√4ᵗʰ **H15 Disorders of sclera**

√5ᵗʰ **H15.0 Scleritis**

√6ᵗʰ   **H15.00   Unspecified scleritis**

     H15.001   Unspecified scleritis, right eye
     H15.002   Unspecified scleritis, left eye
     H15.003   Unspecified scleritis, bilateral
     H15.009   Unspecified scleritis, unspecified eye

√6ᵗʰ   **H15.01   Anterior scleritis**

     H15.011   Anterior scleritis, right eye
     H15.012   Anterior scleritis, left eye
     H15.013   Anterior scleritis, bilateral
     H15.019   Anterior scleritis, unspecified eye

√6ᵗʰ   **H15.02   Brawny scleritis**

     H15.021   Brawny scleritis, right eye
     H15.022   Brawny scleritis, left eye
     H15.023   Brawny scleritis, bilateral
     H15.029   Brawny scleritis, unspecified eye

√6ᵗʰ   **H15.03   Posterior scleritis**

     Sclerotenonitis

     H15.031   Posterior scleritis, right eye
     H15.032   Posterior scleritis, left eye
     H15.033   Posterior scleritis, bilateral
     H15.039   Posterior scleritis, unspecified eye

√6ᵗʰ   **H15.04   Scleritis with corneal involvement**

     H15.041   Scleritis with corneal involvement, right eye
     H15.042   Scleritis with corneal involvement, left eye
     H15.043   Scleritis with corneal involvement, bilateral
     H15.049   Scleritis with corneal involvement, unspecified eye

√6ᵗʰ   **H15.05   Scleromalacia perforans**

     H15.051   Scleromalacia perforans, right eye
     H15.052   Scleromalacia perforans, left eye
     H15.053   Scleromalacia perforans, bilateral
     H15.059   Scleromalacia perforans, unspecified eye

√6ᵗʰ   **H15.09   Other scleritis**

     Scleral abscess

     H15.091   Other scleritis, right eye
     H15.092   Other scleritis, left eye
     H15.093   Other scleritis, bilateral
     H15.099   Other scleritis, unspecified eye

√5ᵗʰ **H15.1 Episcleritis**

√6ᵗʰ   **H15.10   Unspecified episcleritis**

     H15.101   Unspecified episcleritis, right eye
     H15.102   Unspecified episcleritis, left eye
     H15.103   Unspecified episcleritis, bilateral
     H15.109   Unspecified episcleritis, unspecified eye

☑ Additional Character Required   √x7ᵗʰ Placeholder   Unacceptable PDx   Questionable PDx   Manifestation   Unspecified Dx   H1-H14 HAC   HCC CMS-HCC Dx   HIV HIV Dx

ICD-10-CM 2020   603

✓6ᵗʰ **H15.11** **Episcleritis** periodica fugax

    H15.111 **Episcleritis periodica fugax,** right **eye**

    H15.112 **Episcleritis periodica fugax,** left **eye**

    H15.113 **Episcleritis periodica fugax,** bilateral

    H15.119 **Episcleritis periodica fugax, unspecified eye**

✓6ᵗʰ **H15.12** **Nodular episcleritis**

    H15.121 **Nodular episcleritis,** right **eye**

    H15.122 **Nodular episcleritis,** left **eye**

    H15.123 **Nodular episcleritis,** bilateral

    H15.129 **Nodular episcleritis, unspecified eye**

✓5ᵗʰ **H15.8** **Other disorders of sclera**

    EXCLUDES 2   blue sclera (Q13.5)

                 degenerative myopia (H44.2-)

  ✓6ᵗʰ **H15.81** **Equatorial staphyloma**

    H15.811 **Equatorial staphyloma,** right **eye**

    H15.812 **Equatorial staphyloma,** left **eye**

    H15.813 **Equatorial staphyloma,** bilateral

    H15.819 **Equatorial staphyloma, unspecified eye**

  ✓6ᵗʰ **H15.82** **Localized anterior staphyloma**

    H15.821 **Localized anterior staphyloma,** right **eye**

    H15.822 **Localized anterior staphyloma,** left **eye**

    H15.823 **Localized anterior staphyloma,** bilateral

    H15.829 **Localized anterior staphyloma, unspecified eye**

  ✓6ᵗʰ **H15.83** **Staphyloma posticum**

    H15.831 **Staphyloma posticum,** right **eye**

    H15.832 **Staphyloma posticum,** left **eye**

    H15.833 **Staphyloma posticum,** bilateral

    H15.839 **Staphyloma posticum, unspecified eye**

  ✓6ᵗʰ **H15.84** **Scleral ectasia**

    H15.841 **Scleral ectasia,** right **eye**

    H15.842 **Scleral ectasia,** left **eye**

    H15.843 **Scleral ectasia,** bilateral

    H15.849 **Scleral ectasia, unspecified eye**

  ✓6ᵗʰ **H15.85** **Ring staphyloma**

    H15.851 **Ring staphyloma,** right **eye**

    H15.852 **Ring staphyloma,** left **eye**

    H15.853 **Ring staphyloma,** bilateral

    H15.859 **Ring staphyloma, unspecified eye**

  H15.89 **Other disorders of sclera**

 H15.9 **Unspecified disorder of sclera**

✓4ᵗʰ **H16** **Keratitis**

  DEF: Condition in which the cornea becomes inflamed and irritated.

 ✓5ᵗʰ **H16.0** **Corneal ulcer**

  ✓6ᵗʰ **H16.00** **Unspecified corneal ulcer**

    H16.001 **Unspecified corneal ulcer,** right **eye**

    H16.002 **Unspecified corneal ulcer,** left **eye**

    H16.003 **Unspecified corneal ulcer,** bilateral

    H16.009 **Unspecified corneal ulcer, unspecified eye**

  ✓6ᵗʰ **H16.01** **Central corneal ulcer**

    H16.011 **Central corneal ulcer,** right **eye**

    H16.012 **Central corneal ulcer,** left **eye**

    H16.013 **Central corneal ulcer,** bilateral

    H16.019 **Central corneal ulcer, unspecified eye**

  ✓6ᵗʰ **H16.02** **Ring corneal ulcer**

    H16.021 **Ring corneal ulcer,** right **eye**

    H16.022 **Ring corneal ulcer,** left **eye**

    H16.023 **Ring corneal ulcer,** bilateral

    H16.029 **Ring corneal ulcer, unspecified eye**

  ✓6ᵗʰ **H16.03** **Corneal ulcer** with hypopyon

    H16.031 **Corneal ulcer with hypopyon,** right **eye**

    H16.032 **Corneal ulcer with hypopyon,** left **eye**

    H16.033 **Corneal ulcer with hypopyon,** bilateral

    H16.039 **Corneal ulcer with hypopyon, unspecified eye**

  ✓6ᵗʰ **H16.04** **Marginal corneal ulcer**

    H16.041 **Marginal corneal ulcer,** right **eye**

    H16.042 **Marginal corneal ulcer,** left **eye**

    H16.043 **Marginal corneal ulcer,** bilateral

    H16.049 **Marginal corneal ulcer, unspecified eye**

  ✓6ᵗʰ **H16.05** **Mooren's corneal ulcer**

    H16.051 **Mooren's corneal ulcer,** right **eye**

    H16.052 **Mooren's corneal ulcer,** left **eye**

    H16.053 **Mooren's corneal ulcer,** bilateral

    H16.059 **Mooren's corneal ulcer, unspecified eye**

  ✓6ᵗʰ **H16.06** **Mycotic corneal ulcer**

    H16.061 **Mycotic corneal ulcer,** right **eye**

    H16.062 **Mycotic corneal ulcer,** left **eye**

    H16.063 **Mycotic corneal ulcer,** bilateral

    H16.069 **Mycotic corneal ulcer, unspecified eye**

  ✓6ᵗʰ **H16.07** **Perforated corneal ulcer**

    H16.071 **Perforated corneal ulcer,** right **eye**

    H16.072 **Perforated corneal ulcer,** left **eye**

    H16.073 **Perforated corneal ulcer,** bilateral

    H16.079 **Perforated corneal ulcer, unspecified eye**

 ✓5ᵗʰ **H16.1** **Other and unspecified superficial keratitis without conjunctivitis**

  ✓6ᵗʰ **H16.10** **Unspecified superficial keratitis**

    H16.101 **Unspecified superficial keratitis,** right **eye**

    H16.102 **Unspecified superficial keratitis,** left **eye**

    H16.103 **Unspecified superficial keratitis,** bilateral

    H16.109 **Unspecified superficial keratitis, unspecified eye**

  ✓6ᵗʰ **H16.11** **Macular keratitis**

    Areolar keratitis

    Nummular keratitis

    Stellate keratitis

    Striate keratitis

    H16.111 **Macular keratitis,** right **eye**

    H16.112 **Macular keratitis,** left **eye**

    H16.113 **Macular keratitis,** bilateral

    H16.119 **Macular keratitis, unspecified eye**

  ✓6ᵗʰ **H16.12** **Filamentary keratitis**

    H16.121 **Filamentary keratitis,** right **eye**

    H16.122 **Filamentary keratitis,** left **eye**

    H16.123 **Filamentary keratitis,** bilateral

    H16.129 **Filamentary keratitis, unspecified eye**

  ✓6ᵗʰ **H16.13** **Photokeratitis**

    Snow blindness

    Welders keratitis

    H16.131 **Photokeratitis,** right **eye**

    H16.132 **Photokeratitis,** left **eye**

    H16.133 **Photokeratitis,** bilateral

    H16.139 **Photokeratitis, unspecified eye**

  ✓6ᵗʰ **H16.14** **Punctate keratitis**

    H16.141 **Punctate keratitis,** right **eye**

    H16.142 **Punctate keratitis,** left **eye**

    H16.143 **Punctate keratitis,** bilateral

    H16.149 **Punctate keratitis, unspecified eye**

 ✓5ᵗʰ **H16.2** **Keratoconjunctivitis**

  ✓6ᵗʰ **H16.20** **Unspecified keratoconjunctivitis**

    Superficial keratitis with conjunctivitis NOS

    H16.201 **Unspecified keratoconjunctivitis,** right **eye**

    H16.202 **Unspecified keratoconjunctivitis,** left **eye**

    H16.203 **Unspecified keratoconjunctivitis,** bilateral

    H16.209 **Unspecified keratoconjunctivitis, unspecified eye**

  ✓6ᵗʰ **H16.21** **Exposure keratoconjunctivitis**

    H16.211 **Exposure keratoconjunctivitis,** right **eye**

    H16.212 **Exposure keratoconjunctivitis,** left **eye**

    H16.213 **Exposure keratoconjunctivitis,** bilateral

    H16.219 **Exposure keratoconjunctivitis, unspecified eye**

  ✓6ᵗʰ **H16.22** **Keratoconjunctivitis** sicca, **not specified as Sjögren's**

    EXCLUDES 1   Sjögren's syndrome (M35.01)

    H16.221 **Keratoconjunctivitis sicca, not specified as Sjögren's,** right **eye**

    H16.222 **Keratoconjunctivitis sicca, not specified as Sjögren's,** left **eye**

    H16.223 **Keratoconjunctivitis sicca, not specified as Sjögren's,** bilateral

    H16.229 **Keratoconjunctivitis sicca, not specified as Sjögren's, unspecified eye**

  ✓6ᵗʰ **H16.23** **Neurotrophic keratoconjunctivitis**

    H16.231 **Neurotrophic keratoconjunctivitis,** right **eye**

    H16.232 **Neurotrophic keratoconjunctivitis,** left **eye**

N Newborn: 0 P Pediatric: 0-17 M Maternity: 9-64 A Adult: 15-124 MCC Major Complication/Comorbidity CC Complication/Comorbidity SW Severe Wound Dx

604   ICD-10-CM 2020

H16.233 Neurotrophic keratoconjunctivitis, bilateral

H16.239 Neurotrophic keratoconjunctivitis, unspecified eye

√6ᵗʰ **H16.24 Ophthalmia nodosa**

H16.241 Ophthalmia nodosa, right eye

H16.242 Ophthalmia nodosa, left eye

H16.243 Ophthalmia nodosa, bilateral

H16.249 Ophthalmia nodosa, unspecified eye

√6ᵗʰ **H16.25 Phlyctenular keratoconjunctivitis**

H16.251 Phlyctenular keratoconjunctivitis, right eye

H16.252 Phlyctenular keratoconjunctivitis, left eye

H16.253 Phlyctenular keratoconjunctivitis, bilateral

H16.259 Phlyctenular keratoconjunctivitis, unspecified eye

√6ᵗʰ **H16.26 Vernal keratoconjunctivitis, with limbar and corneal involvement**

> EXCLUDES 1   *vernal conjunctivitis without limbar and corneal involvement (H10.44)*

H16.261 Vernal keratoconjunctivitis, with limbar and corneal involvement, right eye

H16.262 Vernal keratoconjunctivitis, with limbar and corneal involvement, left eye

H16.263 Vernal keratoconjunctivitis, with limbar and corneal involvement, bilateral

H16.269 Vernal keratoconjunctivitis, with limbar and corneal involvement, unspecified eye

√6ᵗʰ **H16.29 Other keratoconjunctivitis**

H16.291 Other keratoconjunctivitis, right eye

H16.292 Other keratoconjunctivitis, left eye

H16.293 Other keratoconjunctivitis, bilateral

H16.299 Other keratoconjunctivitis, unspecified eye

√5ᵗʰ **H16.3 Interstitial and deep keratitis**

√6ᵗʰ **H16.30 Unspecified interstitial keratitis**

H16.301 Unspecified interstitial keratitis, right eye

H16.302 Unspecified interstitial keratitis, left eye

H16.303 Unspecified interstitial keratitis, bilateral

H16.309 Unspecified interstitial keratitis, unspecified eye

√6ᵗʰ **H16.31 Corneal abscess**

H16.311 Corneal abscess, right eye

H16.312 Corneal abscess, left eye

H16.313 Corneal abscess, bilateral

H16.319 Corneal abscess, unspecified eye

√6ᵗʰ **H16.32 Diffuse interstitial keratitis**

Cogan's syndrome

H16.321 Diffuse interstitial keratitis, right eye

H16.322 Diffuse interstitial keratitis, left eye

H16.323 Diffuse interstitial keratitis, bilateral

H16.329 Diffuse interstitial keratitis, unspecified eye

√6ᵗʰ **H16.33 Sclerosing keratitis**

H16.331 Sclerosing keratitis, right eye

H16.332 Sclerosing keratitis, left eye

H16.333 Sclerosing keratitis, bilateral

H16.339 Sclerosing keratitis, unspecified eye

√6ᵗʰ **H16.39 Other interstitial and deep keratitis**

H16.391 Other interstitial and deep keratitis, right eye

H16.392 Other interstitial and deep keratitis, left eye

H16.393 Other interstitial and deep keratitis, bilateral

H16.399 Other interstitial and deep keratitis, unspecified eye

√5ᵗʰ **H16.4 Corneal neovascularization**

√6ᵗʰ **H16.40 Unspecified corneal neovascularization**

H16.401 Unspecified corneal neovascularization, right eye

H16.402 Unspecified corneal neovascularization, left eye

H16.403 Unspecified corneal neovascularization, bilateral

H16.409 Unspecified corneal neovascularization, unspecified eye

√6ᵗʰ **H16.41 Ghost vessels (corneal)**

H16.411 Ghost vessels (corneal), right eye

H16.412 Ghost vessels (corneal), left eye

H16.413 Ghost vessels (corneal), bilateral

H16.419 Ghost vessels (corneal), unspecified eye

√6ᵗʰ **H16.42 Pannus (corneal)**

H16.421 Pannus (corneal), right eye

H16.422 Pannus (corneal), left eye

H16.423 Pannus (corneal), bilateral

H16.429 Pannus (corneal), unspecified eye

√6ᵗʰ **H16.43 Localized vascularization of cornea**

H16.431 Localized vascularization of cornea, right eye

H16.432 Localized vascularization of cornea, left eye

H16.433 Localized vascularization of cornea, bilateral

H16.439 Localized vascularization of cornea, unspecified eye

√6ᵗʰ **H16.44 Deep vascularization of cornea**

H16.441 Deep vascularization of cornea, right eye

H16.442 Deep vascularization of cornea, left eye

H16.443 Deep vascularization of cornea, bilateral

H16.449 Deep vascularization of cornea, unspecified eye

H16.8 Other keratitis

H16.9 Unspecified keratitis

√4ᵗʰ **H17 Corneal scars and opacities**

√5ᵗʰ **H17.0 Adherent leukoma**

H17.00 Adherent leukoma, unspecified eye

H17.01 Adherent leukoma, right eye

H17.02 Adherent leukoma, left eye

H17.03 Adherent leukoma, bilateral

√5ᵗʰ **H17.1 Central corneal opacity**

H17.10 Central corneal opacity, unspecified eye

H17.11 Central corneal opacity, right eye

H17.12 Central corneal opacity, left eye

H17.13 Central corneal opacity, bilateral

√5ᵗʰ **H17.8 Other corneal scars and opacities**

√6ᵗʰ **H17.81 Minor opacity of cornea**

Corneal nebula

H17.811 Minor opacity of cornea, right eye

H17.812 Minor opacity of cornea, left eye

H17.813 Minor opacity of cornea, bilateral

H17.819 Minor opacity of cornea, unspecified eye

√6ᵗʰ **H17.82 Peripheral opacity of cornea**

H17.821 Peripheral opacity of cornea, right eye

H17.822 Peripheral opacity of cornea, left eye

H17.823 Peripheral opacity of cornea, bilateral

H17.829 Peripheral opacity of cornea, unspecified eye

H17.89 Other corneal scars and opacities

H17.9 Unspecified corneal scar and opacity

√4ᵗʰ **H18 Other disorders of cornea**

√5ᵗʰ **H18.0 Corneal pigmentations and deposits**

√6ᵗʰ **H18.00 Unspecified corneal deposit**

H18.001 Unspecified corneal deposit, right eye

H18.002 Unspecified corneal deposit, left eye

H18.003 Unspecified corneal deposit, bilateral

H18.009 Unspecified corneal deposit, unspecified eye

√6ᵗʰ **H18.01 Anterior corneal pigmentations**

Staehli's line

H18.011 Anterior corneal pigmentations, right eye

H18.012 Anterior corneal pigmentations, left eye

H18.013 Anterior corneal pigmentations, bilateral

H18.019 Anterior corneal pigmentations, unspecified eye

√6ᵗʰ **H18.02 Argentous corneal deposits**

H18.021 Argentous corneal deposits, right eye

H18.022 Argentous corneal deposits, left eye

H18.023 Argentous corneal deposits, bilateral

H18.029 Argentous corneal deposits, unspecified eye

☑ Additional Character Required   √x7ᵗʰ Placeholder   Unacceptable PDx   Questionable PDx   Manifestation   Unspecified Dx   H1-H14 HAC   HCC CMS-HCC Dx   HIV HIV Dx

ICD-10-CM 2020   605

Chapter 7. Diseases of the Eye and Adnexa

H16.233–H18.029

✓6ᵗʰ **H18.03** **Corneal deposits in** metabolic disorders
  Code also associated metabolic disorder
  H18.031 **Corneal deposits in metabolic disorders, right eye**
  H18.032 **Corneal deposits in metabolic disorders, left eye**
  H18.033 **Corneal deposits in metabolic disorders, bilateral**
  H18.039 **Corneal deposits in metabolic disorders, unspecified eye**

✓6ᵗʰ **H18.04** Kayser-Fleischer ring
  Code also associated Wilson's disease (E83.01)
  H18.041 **Kayser-Fleischer ring, right eye**
  H18.042 **Kayser-Fleischer ring, left eye**
  H18.043 **Kayser-Fleischer ring, bilateral**
  H18.049 **Kayser-Fleischer ring, unspecified eye**

✓6ᵗʰ **H18.05** **Posterior** corneal pigmentations
  Krukenberg's spindle
  H18.051 **Posterior corneal pigmentations, right eye**
  H18.052 **Posterior corneal pigmentations, left eye**
  H18.053 **Posterior corneal pigmentations, bilateral**
  H18.059 **Posterior corneal pigmentations, unspecified eye**

✓6ᵗʰ **H18.06** **Stromal** corneal pigmentations
  Hematocornea
  H18.061 **Stromal corneal pigmentations, right eye**
  H18.062 **Stromal corneal pigmentations, left eye**
  H18.063 **Stromal corneal pigmentations, bilateral**
  H18.069 **Stromal corneal pigmentations, unspecified eye**

✓5ᵗʰ **H18.1** **Bullous keratopathy**
  DEF: Corneal swelling due to a damaged corneal endothelium. Bullous keratopathy is characterized by recurring, rupturing epithelial blisters causing glaucoma, iridocyclitis, and Fuchs dystrophy.
  H18.10 **Bullous keratopathy, unspecified eye**
  H18.11 **Bullous keratopathy, right eye**
  H18.12 **Bullous keratopathy, left eye**
  H18.13 **Bullous keratopathy, bilateral**

✓5ᵗʰ **H18.2** **Other and unspecified corneal edema**
  H18.20 **Unspecified corneal edema**

✓6ᵗʰ **H18.21** **Corneal edema** secondary to contact lens
  EXCLUDES 2   other corneal disorders due to contact lens (H18.82-)
  H18.211 **Corneal edema secondary to contact lens, right eye**
  H18.212 **Corneal edema secondary to contact lens, left eye**
  H18.213 **Corneal edema secondary to contact lens, bilateral**
  H18.219 **Corneal edema secondary to contact lens, unspecified eye**

✓6ᵗʰ **H18.22** **Idiopathic** corneal edema
  H18.221 **Idiopathic corneal edema, right eye**
  H18.222 **Idiopathic corneal edema, left eye**
  H18.223 **Idiopathic corneal edema, bilateral**
  H18.229 **Idiopathic corneal edema, unspecified eye**

✓6ᵗʰ **H18.23** **Secondary** corneal edema
  H18.231 **Secondary corneal edema, right eye**
  H18.232 **Secondary corneal edema, left eye**
  H18.233 **Secondary corneal edema, bilateral**
  H18.239 **Secondary corneal edema, unspecified eye**

✓5ᵗʰ **H18.3** **Changes of corneal membranes**
  H18.30 **Unspecified corneal membrane change**

✓6ᵗʰ **H18.31** **Folds and rupture in** Bowman's membrane
  H18.311 **Folds and rupture in Bowman's membrane, right eye**
  H18.312 **Folds and rupture in Bowman's membrane, left eye**
  H18.313 **Folds and rupture in Bowman's membrane, bilateral**
  H18.319 **Folds and rupture in Bowman's membrane, unspecified eye**

✓6ᵗʰ **H18.32** **Folds in** Descemet's membrane
  H18.321 **Folds in Descemet's membrane, right eye**

H18.322 **Folds in Descemet's membrane, left eye**
H18.323 **Folds in Descemet's membrane, bilateral**
H18.329 **Folds in Descemet's membrane, unspecified eye**

✓6ᵗʰ **H18.33** **Rupture in** Descemet's membrane
  H18.331 **Rupture in Descemet's membrane, right eye**
  H18.332 **Rupture in Descemet's membrane, left eye**
  H18.333 **Rupture in Descemet's membrane, bilateral**
  H18.339 **Rupture in Descemet's membrane, unspecified eye**

✓5ᵗʰ **H18.4** **Corneal degeneration**
  EXCLUDES 1   Mooren's ulcer (H16.0-)
        recurrent erosion of cornea (H18.83-)
  H18.40 **Unspecified corneal degeneration**

✓6ᵗʰ **H18.41** **Arcus senilis**
  Senile corneal changes
  H18.411 **Arcus senilis, right eye**
  H18.412 **Arcus senilis, left eye**
  H18.413 **Arcus senilis, bilateral**
  H18.419 **Arcus senilis, unspecified eye**

✓6ᵗʰ **H18.42** **Band** keratopathy
  H18.421 **Band keratopathy, right eye**
  H18.422 **Band keratopathy, left eye**
  H18.423 **Band keratopathy, bilateral**
  H18.429 **Band keratopathy, unspecified eye**

H18.43 **Other calcerous corneal degeneration**

✓6ᵗʰ **H18.44** **Keratomalacia**
  EXCLUDES 1   keratomalacia due to vitamin A deficiency (E50.4)
  H18.441 **Keratomalacia, right eye**
  H18.442 **Keratomalacia, left eye**
  H18.443 **Keratomalacia, bilateral**
  H18.449 **Keratomalacia, unspecified eye**

✓6ᵗʰ **H18.45** **Nodular** corneal degeneration
  H18.451 **Nodular corneal degeneration, right eye**
  H18.452 **Nodular corneal degeneration, left eye**
  H18.453 **Nodular corneal degeneration, bilateral**
  H18.459 **Nodular corneal degeneration, unspecified eye**

✓6ᵗʰ **H18.46** **Peripheral** corneal degeneration
  H18.461 **Peripheral corneal degeneration, right eye**
  H18.462 **Peripheral corneal degeneration, left eye**
  H18.463 **Peripheral corneal degeneration, bilateral**
  H18.469 **Peripheral corneal degeneration, unspecified eye**

H18.49 **Other corneal degeneration**

✓5ᵗʰ **H18.5** **Hereditary corneal dystrophies**
  H18.50 **Unspecified hereditary corneal dystrophies**
  H18.51 **Endothelial** corneal dystrophy
    Fuchs' dystrophy
  H18.52 **Epithelial (juvenile) corneal dystrophy**
  H18.53 **Granular** corneal dystrophy
  H18.54 **Lattice** corneal dystrophy
  H18.55 **Macular** corneal dystrophy
  H18.59 **Other** hereditary corneal dystrophies

✓5ᵗʰ **H18.6** **Keratoconus**
  ✓6ᵗʰ **H18.60** **Keratoconus, unspecified**
    H18.601 **Keratoconus, unspecified, right eye**
    H18.602 **Keratoconus, unspecified, left eye**
    H18.603 **Keratoconus, unspecified, bilateral**
    H18.609 **Keratoconus, unspecified, unspecified eye**
  ✓6ᵗʰ **H18.61** **Keratoconus, stable**
    H18.611 **Keratoconus, stable, right eye**
    H18.612 **Keratoconus, stable, left eye**
    H18.613 **Keratoconus, stable, bilateral**
    H18.619 **Keratoconus, stable, unspecified eye**
  ✓6ᵗʰ **H18.62** **Keratoconus, unstable**
    Acute hydrops
    H18.621 **Keratoconus, unstable, right eye**
    H18.622 **Keratoconus, unstable, left eye**
    H18.623 **Keratoconus, unstable, bilateral**

H18.629   Keratoconus, unstable, unspecified eye

√5ᵗʰ **H18.7**   **Other and unspecified corneal deformities**

     EXCLUDES 1   *congenital malformations of cornea (Q13.3-Q13.4)*

     H18.70   **Unspecified corneal deformity**

     √6ᵗʰ **H18.71**   **Corneal** ectasia

       H18.711   **Corneal ectasia, right eye**

       H18.712   **Corneal ectasia, left eye**

       H18.713   **Corneal ectasia, bilateral**

       H18.719   **Corneal ectasia, unspecified eye**

     √6ᵗʰ **H18.72**   **Corneal** staphyloma

       H18.721   **Corneal staphyloma, right eye**

       H18.722   **Corneal staphyloma, left eye**

       H18.723   **Corneal staphyloma, bilateral**

       H18.729   **Corneal staphyloma, unspecified eye**

     √6ᵗʰ **H18.73**   **Descemetocele**

       H18.731   **Descemetocele, right eye**

       H18.732   **Descemetocele, left eye**

       H18.733   **Descemetocele, bilateral**

       H18.739   **Descemetocele, unspecified eye**

     √6ᵗʰ **H18.79**   **Other corneal deformities**

       H18.791   **Other corneal deformities, right eye**

       H18.792   **Other corneal deformities, left eye**

       H18.793   **Other corneal deformities, bilateral**

       H18.799   **Other corneal deformities, unspecified eye**

√5ᵗʰ **H18.8**   **Other specified disorders of cornea**

     √6ᵗʰ **H18.81**   **Anesthesia and hypoesthesia of cornea**

       H18.811   **Anesthesia and hypoesthesia of cornea, right eye**

       H18.812   **Anesthesia and hypoesthesia of cornea, left eye**

       H18.813   **Anesthesia and hypoesthesia of cornea, bilateral**

       H18.819   **Anesthesia and hypoesthesia of cornea, unspecified eye**

     √6ᵗʰ **H18.82**   **Corneal disorder due to contact lens**

       EXCLUDES 2   *corneal edema due to contact lens (H18.21-)*

       H18.821   **Corneal disorder due to contact lens, right eye**

       H18.822   **Corneal disorder due to contact lens, left eye**

       H18.823   **Corneal disorder due to contact lens, bilateral**

       H18.829   **Corneal disorder due to contact lens, unspecified eye**

     √6ᵗʰ **H18.83**   **Recurrent erosion of cornea**

       H18.831   **Recurrent erosion of cornea, right eye**

       H18.832   **Recurrent erosion of cornea, left eye**

       H18.833   **Recurrent erosion of cornea, bilateral**

       H18.839   **Recurrent erosion of cornea, unspecified eye**

     √6ᵗʰ **H18.89**   **Other specified disorders of cornea**

       H18.891   **Other specified disorders of cornea, right eye**

       H18.892   **Other specified disorders of cornea, left eye**

       H18.893   **Other specified disorders of cornea, bilateral**

       H18.899   **Other specified disorders of cornea, unspecified eye**

H18.9   **Unspecified disorder of cornea**

√4ᵗʰ **H20**   **Iridocyclitis**

     CC Excl: For CC codes in category H20: PDX collection 624

     √5ᵗʰ **H20.0**   **Acute and subacute iridocyclitis**

       Acute anterior uveitis

       Acute cyclitis

       Acute iritis

       Subacute anterior uveitis

       Subacute cyclitis

       Subacute iritis

       EXCLUDES 1   *iridocyclitis, iritis, uveitis (due to) (in) diabetes mellitus (E08-E13 with .39)*

         iridocyclitis, iritis, uveitis (due to) (in) diphtheria (A36.89)

         iridocyclitis, iritis, uveitis (due to) (in) gonococcal (A54.32)

         iridocyclitis, iritis, uveitis (due to) (in) herpes (simplex) (B00.51)

         iridocyclitis, iritis, uveitis (due to) (in) herpes zoster (B02.32)

         iridocyclitis, iritis, uveitis (due to) (in) late congenital syphilis (A50.39)

         iridocyclitis, iritis, uveitis (due to) (in) late syphilis (A52.71)

         iridocyclitis, iritis, uveitis (due to) (in) sarcoidosis (D86.83)

         iridocyclitis, iritis, uveitis (due to) (in) syphilis (A51.43)

         iridocyclitis, iritis, uveitis (due to) (in) toxoplasmosis (B58.09)

         iridocyclitis, iritis, uveitis (due to) (in) tuberculosis (A18.54)

       H20.00   **Unspecified acute and subacute iridocyclitis**   `CC`

       √6ᵗʰ **H20.01**   **Primary iridocyclitis**

         H20.011   **Primary iridocyclitis, right eye**   `CC`

         H20.012   **Primary iridocyclitis, left eye**   `CC`

         H20.013   **Primary iridocyclitis, bilateral**   `CC`

         H20.019   **Primary iridocyclitis, unspecified eye**   `CC`

       √6ᵗʰ **H20.02**   **Recurrent acute iridocyclitis**

         H20.021   **Recurrent acute iridocyclitis, right eye**   `CC`

         H20.022   **Recurrent acute iridocyclitis, left eye**   `CC`

         H20.023   **Recurrent acute iridocyclitis, bilateral**   `CC`

         H20.029   **Recurrent acute iridocyclitis, unspecified eye**   `CC`

       √6ᵗʰ **H20.03**   **Secondary infectious iridocyclitis**

         H20.031   **Secondary infectious iridocyclitis, right eye**   `CC`

         H20.032   **Secondary infectious iridocyclitis, left eye**   `CC`

         H20.033   **Secondary infectious iridocyclitis, bilateral**   `CC`

         H20.039   **Secondary infectious iridocyclitis, unspecified eye**   `CC`

       √6ᵗʰ **H20.04**   **Secondary noninfectious iridocyclitis**

         H20.041   **Secondary noninfectious iridocyclitis, right eye**

         H20.042   **Secondary noninfectious iridocyclitis, left eye**

         H20.043   **Secondary noninfectious iridocyclitis, bilateral**

         H20.049   **Secondary noninfectious iridocyclitis, unspecified eye**

       √6ᵗʰ **H20.05**   **Hypopyon**

         H20.051   **Hypopyon, right eye**

         H20.052   **Hypopyon, left eye**

         H20.053   **Hypopyon, bilateral**

         H20.059   **Hypopyon, unspecified eye**

☑ Additional Character Required   √x7ᵗʰ Placeholder   Unacceptable PDx   Questionable PDx   Manifestation   Unspecified Dx   H1-H14 HAC   HCC CMS-HCC Dx   HIV HIV Dx

ICD-10-CM 2020   607

Chapter 7. Diseases of the Eye and Adnexa

✓5ᵗʰ **H20.1 Chronic iridocyclitis**
Use additional code for any associated cataract (H26.21-)
EXCLUDES 2   *posterior cyclitis (H30.2-)*
H20.10 Chronic iridocyclitis, unspecified eye
H20.11 Chronic iridocyclitis, right eye
H20.12 Chronic iridocyclitis, left eye
H20.13 Chronic iridocyclitis, bilateral

✓5ᵗʰ **H20.2 Lens-induced iridocyclitis**
H20.20 Lens-induced iridocyclitis, unspecified eye
H20.21 Lens-induced iridocyclitis, right eye
H20.22 Lens-induced iridocyclitis, left eye
H20.23 Lens-induced iridocyclitis, bilateral

✓5ᵗʰ **H20.8 Other iridocyclitis**
EXCLUDES 2   *glaucomatocyclitis crises (H40.4-)*
posterior cyclitis (H30.2-)
sympathetic uveitis (H44.13-)
✓6ᵗʰ **H20.81 Fuchs' heterochromic cyclitis**
H20.811 Fuchs' heterochromic cyclitis, right eye
H20.812 Fuchs' heterochromic cyclitis, left eye
H20.813 Fuchs' heterochromic cyclitis, bilateral
H20.819 Fuchs' heterochromic cyclitis, unspecified eye
✓6ᵗʰ **H20.82 Vogt-Koyanagi syndrome**
H20.821 Vogt-Koyanagi syndrome, right eye
H20.822 Vogt-Koyanagi syndrome, left eye
H20.823 Vogt-Koyanagi syndrome, bilateral
H20.829 Vogt-Koyanagi syndrome, unspecified eye

H20.9 Unspecified iridocyclitis   CC
Uveitis NOS

✓4ᵗʰ **H21 Other disorders of iris and ciliary body**
EXCLUDES 2   *sympathetic uveitis (H44.1-)*

✓5ᵗʰ **H21.0 Hyphema**
EXCLUDES 1   *traumatic hyphema (S05.1-)*

Hyphema

H21.00 Hyphema, unspecified eye
H21.01 Hyphema, right eye
H21.02 Hyphema, left eye
H21.03 Hyphema, bilateral

✓5ᵗʰ **H21.1 Other vascular disorders of iris and ciliary body**
Neovascularization of iris or ciliary body
Rubeosis iridis
Rubeosis of iris
✓6ᵗʰ **H21.1X Other vascular disorders of iris and ciliary body**
H21.1X1 Other vascular disorders of iris and ciliary body, right eye
H21.1X2 Other vascular disorders of iris and ciliary body, left eye
H21.1X3 Other vascular disorders of iris and ciliary body, bilateral
H21.1X9 Other vascular disorders of iris and ciliary body, unspecified eye

✓5ᵗʰ **H21.2 Degeneration of iris and ciliary body**
✓6ᵗʰ **H21.21 Degeneration of chamber angle**
H21.211 Degeneration of chamber angle, right eye
H21.212 Degeneration of chamber angle, left eye
H21.213 Degeneration of chamber angle, bilateral
H21.219 Degeneration of chamber angle, unspecified eye

✓6ᵗʰ **H21.22 Degeneration of ciliary body**
H21.221 Degeneration of ciliary body, right eye
H21.222 Degeneration of ciliary body, left eye
H21.223 Degeneration of ciliary body, bilateral
H21.229 Degeneration of ciliary body, unspecified eye
✓6ᵗʰ **H21.23 Degeneration of iris (pigmentary)**
Translucency of iris
H21.231 Degeneration of iris (pigmentary), right eye
H21.232 Degeneration of iris (pigmentary), left eye
H21.233 Degeneration of iris (pigmentary), bilateral
H21.239 Degeneration of iris (pigmentary), unspecified eye
✓6ᵗʰ **H21.24 Degeneration of pupillary margin**
H21.241 Degeneration of pupillary margin, right eye
H21.242 Degeneration of pupillary margin, left eye
H21.243 Degeneration of pupillary margin, bilateral
H21.249 Degeneration of pupillary margin, unspecified eye
✓6ᵗʰ **H21.25 Iridoschisis**
H21.251 Iridoschisis, right eye
H21.252 Iridoschisis, left eye
H21.253 Iridoschisis, bilateral
H21.259 Iridoschisis, unspecified eye
✓6ᵗʰ **H21.26 Iris atrophy (essential) (progressive)**
H21.261 Iris atrophy (essential) (progressive), right eye
H21.262 Iris atrophy (essential) (progressive), left eye
H21.263 Iris atrophy (essential) (progressive), bilateral
H21.269 Iris atrophy (essential) (progressive), unspecified eye
✓6ᵗʰ **H21.27 Miotic pupillary cyst**
H21.271 Miotic pupillary cyst, right eye
H21.272 Miotic pupillary cyst, left eye
H21.273 Miotic pupillary cyst, bilateral
H21.279 Miotic pupillary cyst, unspecified eye
H21.29 Other iris atrophy

✓5ᵗʰ **H21.3 Cyst of iris, ciliary body and anterior chamber**
EXCLUDES 2   *miotic pupillary cyst (H21.27-)*
✓6ᵗʰ **H21.30 Idiopathic cysts of iris, ciliary body or anterior chamber**
Cyst of iris, ciliary body or anterior chamber NOS
H21.301 Idiopathic cysts of iris, ciliary body or anterior chamber, right eye
H21.302 Idiopathic cysts of iris, ciliary body or anterior chamber, left eye
H21.303 Idiopathic cysts of iris, ciliary body or anterior chamber, bilateral
H21.309 Idiopathic cysts of iris, ciliary body or anterior chamber, unspecified eye
✓6ᵗʰ **H21.31 Exudative cysts of iris or anterior chamber**
H21.311 Exudative cysts of iris or anterior chamber, right eye
H21.312 Exudative cysts of iris or anterior chamber, left eye
H21.313 Exudative cysts of iris or anterior chamber, bilateral
H21.319 Exudative cysts of iris or anterior chamber, unspecified eye
✓6ᵗʰ **H21.32 Implantation cysts of iris, ciliary body or anterior chamber**
H21.321 Implantation cysts of iris, ciliary body or anterior chamber, right eye
H21.322 Implantation cysts of iris, ciliary body or anterior chamber, left eye
H21.323 Implantation cysts of iris, ciliary body or anterior chamber, bilateral
H21.329 Implantation cysts of iris, ciliary body or anterior chamber, unspecified eye

√6th H21.33 Parasitic cyst of iris, ciliary body or anterior chamber

> **CC Excl:** For CC codes in subcategory H21.33: PDX collection 625

    H21.331 Parasitic cyst of iris, ciliary body or anterior chamber, right eye   `CC`

    H21.332 Parasitic cyst of iris, ciliary body or anterior chamber, left eye   `CC`

    H21.333 Parasitic cyst of iris, ciliary body or anterior chamber, bilateral   `CC`

    H21.339 Parasitic cyst of iris, ciliary body or anterior chamber, unspecified eye   `CC`

√6th H21.34 Primary cyst of pars plana

    H21.341 Primary cyst of pars plana, right eye

    H21.342 Primary cyst of pars plana, left eye

    H21.343 Primary cyst of pars plana, bilateral

    H21.349 Primary cyst of pars plana, unspecified eye

√6th H21.35 Exudative cyst of pars plana

> **DEF:** Protein, fatty-filled bullous elevation of the nonpigmented outermost ciliary epithelium of pars plana, due to fluid leak from blood vessels.

    H21.351 Exudative cyst of pars plana, right eye

    H21.352 Exudative cyst of pars plana, left eye

    H21.353 Exudative cyst of pars plana, bilateral

    H21.359 Exudative cyst of pars plana, unspecified eye

√5th H21.4 Pupillary membranes

Iris bombé
Pupillary occlusion
Pupillary seclusion

> *EXCLUDES 1*   congenital pupillary membranes (Q13.8)

    H21.40 Pupillary membranes, unspecified eye

    H21.41 Pupillary membranes, right eye

    H21.42 Pupillary membranes, left eye

    H21.43 Pupillary membranes, bilateral

√5th H21.5 Other and unspecified adhesions and disruptions of iris and ciliary body

> *EXCLUDES 1*   corectopia (Q13.2)

√6th H21.50 Unspecified adhesions of iris

Synechia (iris) NOS

    H21.501 Unspecified adhesions of iris, right eye

    H21.502 Unspecified adhesions of iris, left eye

    H21.503 Unspecified adhesions of iris, bilateral

    H21.509 Unspecified adhesions of iris and ciliary body, unspecified eye

√6th H21.51 Anterior synechiae (iris)

    H21.511 Anterior synechiae (iris), right eye

    H21.512 Anterior synechiae (iris), left eye

    H21.513 Anterior synechiae (iris), bilateral

    H21.519 Anterior synechiae (iris), unspecified eye

√6th H21.52 Goniosynechiae

    H21.521 Goniosynechiae, right eye

    H21.522 Goniosynechiae, left eye

    H21.523 Goniosynechiae, bilateral

    H21.529 Goniosynechiae, unspecified eye

√6th H21.53 Iridodialysis

    H21.531 Iridodialysis, right eye

    H21.532 Iridodialysis, left eye

    H21.533 Iridodialysis, bilateral

    H21.539 Iridodialysis, unspecified eye

√6th H21.54 Posterior synechiae (iris)

    H21.541 Posterior synechiae (iris), right eye

    H21.542 Posterior synechiae (iris), left eye

    H21.543 Posterior synechiae (iris), bilateral

    H21.549 Posterior synechiae (iris), unspecified eye

√6th H21.55 Recession of chamber angle

    H21.551 Recession of chamber angle, right eye

    H21.552 Recession of chamber angle, left eye

    H21.553 Recession of chamber angle, bilateral

    H21.559 Recession of chamber angle, unspecified eye

√6th H21.56 Pupillary abnormalities

Deformed pupil
Ectopic pupil
Rupture of sphincter, pupil

> *EXCLUDES 1*   congenital deformity of pupil (Q13.2-)

    H21.561 Pupillary abnormality, right eye

    H21.562 Pupillary abnormality, left eye

    H21.563 Pupillary abnormality, bilateral

    H21.569 Pupillary abnormality, unspecified eye

√5th H21.8 Other specified disorders of iris and ciliary body

    H21.81 Floppy iris syndrome

Intraoperative floppy iris syndrome (IFIS)

Use additional code for adverse effect, if applicable, to identify drug (T36-T50 with fifth or sixth character 5)

    H21.82 Plateau iris syndrome (post-iridectomy) (postprocedural)

    H21.89 Other specified disorders of iris and ciliary body

H21.9 Unspecified disorder of iris and ciliary body

H22 Disorders of iris and ciliary body in diseases classified elsewhere

Code first underlying disease, such as:
    gout (M1A.-, M10.-)
    leprosy (A30.-)
    parasitic disease (B89)

Disorders of lens (H25-H28)

√4th H25 Age-related cataract

Senile cataract

> *EXCLUDES 2*   capsular glaucoma with pseudoexfoliation of lens (H40.1-)

Cataracts

Vitreous
Iris
Cornea
Retina
Pupil
Lens
Normal lens
Clouded lens

Lens affected by cataracts

√5th H25.0 Age-related incipient cataract

√6th H25.01 Cortical age-related cataract

    H25.011 Cortical age-related cataract, right eye   `A`

    H25.012 Cortical age-related cataract, left eye   `A`

    H25.013 Cortical age-related cataract, bilateral   `A`

    H25.019 Cortical age-related cataract, unspecified eye   `A`

√6th H25.03 Anterior subcapsular polar age-related cataract

    H25.031 Anterior subcapsular polar age-related cataract, right eye   `A`

    H25.032 Anterior subcapsular polar age-related cataract, left eye   `A`

    H25.033 Anterior subcapsular polar age-related cataract, bilateral   `A`

    H25.039 Anterior subcapsular polar age-related cataract, unspecified eye   `A`

☑ Additional Character Required   √x7th Placeholder   Unacceptable PDx   Questionable PDx   Manifestation   Unspecified Dx   **H1**-**H14** HAC   **HCC** CMS-HCC Dx   **HIV** HIV Dx

ICD-10-CM 2020   609

√6ᵗʰ **H25.04** Posterior subcapsular polar **age-related cataract**

   H25.041 Posterior subcapsular polar age-related cataract, **right eye** Ⓐ

   H25.042 Posterior subcapsular polar age-related cataract, **left eye** Ⓐ

   H25.043 Posterior subcapsular polar age-related cataract, **bilateral** Ⓐ

   H25.049 Posterior subcapsular polar age-related cataract, **unspecified eye** Ⓐ

√6ᵗʰ **H25.09** Other age-related incipient cataract

   Coronary age-related cataract
   Punctate age-related cataract
   Water clefts

   H25.091 Other age-related incipient cataract, **right eye** Ⓐ

   H25.092 Other age-related incipient cataract, **left eye** Ⓐ

   H25.093 Other age-related incipient cataract, **bilateral** Ⓐ

   H25.099 Other age-related incipient cataract, **unspecified eye** Ⓐ

√5ᵗʰ **H25.1** **Age-related nuclear cataract**

   Cataracta brunescens
   Nuclear sclerosis cataract
   AHA: 2019,2Q,31; 2016,1Q,32

   H25.10 Age-related nuclear cataract, **unspecified eye** Ⓐ

   H25.11 Age-related nuclear cataract, **right eye** Ⓐ

   H25.12 Age-related nuclear cataract, **left eye** Ⓐ

   H25.13 Age-related nuclear cataract, **bilateral** Ⓐ

√5ᵗʰ **H25.2** **Age-related cataract, morgagnian type**

   Age-related hypermature cataract

   H25.20 Age-related cataract, morgagnian type, **unspecified eye** Ⓐ

   H25.21 Age-related cataract, morgagnian type, **right eye** Ⓐ

   H25.22 Age-related cataract, morgagnian type, **left eye** Ⓐ

   H25.23 Age-related cataract, morgagnian type, **bilateral** Ⓐ

√5ᵗʰ **H25.8** **Other age-related cataract**

√6ᵗʰ **H25.81** Combined forms of age-related cataract

   AHA: 2019,2Q,30

   H25.811 Combined forms of age-related cataract, **right eye** Ⓐ

   H25.812 Combined forms of age-related cataract, **left eye** Ⓐ

   H25.813 Combined forms of age-related cataract, **bilateral** Ⓐ

   H25.819 Combined forms of age-related cataract, **unspecified eye** Ⓐ

   H25.89 Other age-related cataract Ⓐ

H25.9 Unspecified age-related cataract Ⓐ

√4ᵗʰ **H26** **Other cataract**

   EXCLUDES 1   congenital cataract (Q12.0)

√5ᵗʰ **H26.0** Infantile and juvenile cataract

√6ᵗʰ **H26.00** Unspecified infantile and juvenile cataract

   H26.001 Unspecified infantile and juvenile cataract, **right eye** Ⓟ

   H26.002 Unspecified infantile and juvenile cataract, **left eye** Ⓟ

   H26.003 Unspecified infantile and juvenile cataract, **bilateral** Ⓟ

   H26.009 Unspecified infantile and juvenile cataract, **unspecified eye** Ⓟ

√6ᵗʰ **H26.01** Infantile and juvenile **cortical, lamellar, or zonular cataract**

   H26.011 Infantile and juvenile cortical, lamellar, or zonular cataract, **right eye** Ⓟ

   H26.012 Infantile and juvenile cortical, lamellar, or zonular cataract, **left eye** Ⓟ

   H26.013 Infantile and juvenile cortical, lamellar, or zonular cataract, **bilateral** Ⓟ

   H26.019 Infantile and juvenile cortical, lamellar, or zonular cataract, **unspecified eye** Ⓟ

√6ᵗʰ **H26.03** Infantile and juvenile **nuclear cataract**

   H26.031 Infantile and juvenile nuclear cataract, **right eye** Ⓟ

   H26.032 Infantile and juvenile nuclear cataract, **left eye** Ⓟ

   H26.033 Infantile and juvenile nuclear cataract, **bilateral** Ⓟ

   H26.039 Infantile and juvenile nuclear cataract, **unspecified eye** Ⓟ

√6ᵗʰ **H26.04** Anterior subcapsular polar **infantile and juvenile cataract**

   H26.041 Anterior subcapsular polar infantile and juvenile cataract, **right eye** Ⓟ

   H26.042 Anterior subcapsular polar infantile and juvenile cataract, **left eye** Ⓟ

   H26.043 Anterior subcapsular polar infantile and juvenile cataract, **bilateral** Ⓟ

   H26.049 Anterior subcapsular polar infantile and juvenile cataract, **unspecified eye** Ⓟ

√6ᵗʰ **H26.05** Posterior subcapsular polar **infantile and juvenile cataract**

   H26.051 Posterior subcapsular polar infantile and juvenile cataract, **right eye** Ⓟ

   H26.052 Posterior subcapsular polar infantile and juvenile cataract, **left eye** Ⓟ

   H26.053 Posterior subcapsular polar infantile and juvenile cataract, **bilateral** Ⓟ

   H26.059 Posterior subcapsular polar infantile and juvenile cataract, **unspecified eye** Ⓟ

√6ᵗʰ **H26.06** Combined forms **of infantile and juvenile cataract**

   H26.061 Combined forms of infantile and juvenile cataract, **right eye** Ⓟ

   H26.062 Combined forms of infantile and juvenile cataract, **left eye** Ⓟ

   H26.063 Combined forms of infantile and juvenile cataract, **bilateral** Ⓟ

   H26.069 Combined forms of infantile and juvenile cataract, **unspecified eye** Ⓟ

   H26.09 Other infantile and juvenile cataract Ⓟ

√5ᵗʰ **H26.1** Traumatic cataract

   Use additional code (Chapter 20) to identify external cause

√6ᵗʰ **H26.10** Unspecified traumatic cataract

   H26.101 Unspecified traumatic cataract, **right eye**

   H26.102 Unspecified traumatic cataract, **left eye**

   H26.103 Unspecified traumatic cataract, **bilateral**

   H26.109 Unspecified traumatic cataract, **unspecified eye**

√6ᵗʰ **H26.11** Localized traumatic opacities

   H26.111 Localized traumatic opacities, **right eye**

   H26.112 Localized traumatic opacities, **left eye**

   H26.113 Localized traumatic opacities, **bilateral**

   H26.119 Localized traumatic opacities, **unspecified eye**

Chapter 7. Diseases of the Eye and Adnexa

✓6ᵗʰ **H26.12** Partially resolved **traumatic cataract**

     H26.121 **Partially resolved traumatic cataract, right eye**

     H26.122 **Partially resolved traumatic cataract, left eye**

     H26.123 **Partially resolved traumatic cataract, bilateral**

     H26.129 **Partially resolved traumatic cataract, unspecified eye**

✓6ᵗʰ **H26.13** Total **traumatic cataract**

     H26.131 **Total traumatic cataract, right eye**

     H26.132 **Total traumatic cataract, left eye**

     H26.133 **Total traumatic cataract, bilateral**

     H26.139 **Total traumatic cataract, unspecified eye**

✓5ᵗʰ **H26.2** Complicated **cataract**

     H26.20 **Unspecified complicated cataract**

         Cataracta complicata NOS

✓6ᵗʰ   **H26.21** **Cataract with neovascularization**

         Code also associated condition, such as:

            chronic iridocyclitis (H20.1-)

     H26.211 **Cataract with neovascularization, right eye**

     H26.212 **Cataract with neovascularization, left eye**

     H26.213 **Cataract with neovascularization, bilateral**

     H26.219 **Cataract with neovascularization, unspecified eye**

✓6ᵗʰ   **H26.22** **Cataract secondary to ocular disorders (degenerative) (inflammatory)**

         Code also associated ocular disorder

     H26.221 **Cataract secondary to ocular disorders (degenerative) (inflammatory), right eye**

     H26.222 **Cataract secondary to ocular disorders (degenerative) (inflammatory), left eye**

     H26.223 **Cataract secondary to ocular disorders (degenerative) (inflammatory), bilateral**

     H26.229 **Cataract secondary to ocular disorders (degenerative) (inflammatory), unspecified eye**

✓6ᵗʰ   **H26.23** **Glaucomatous flecks (subcapsular)**

         Code first underlying glaucoma (H40-H42)

     H26.231 **Glaucomatous flecks (subcapsular), right eye**

     H26.232 **Glaucomatous flecks (subcapsular), left eye**

     H26.233 **Glaucomatous flecks (subcapsular), bilateral**

     H26.239 **Glaucomatous flecks (subcapsular), unspecified eye**

✓5ᵗʰ **H26.3** Drug-induced **cataract**

     Toxic cataract

     Use additional code for adverse effect, if applicable, to identify drug (T36-T50 with fifth or sixth character 5)

     H26.30 **Drug-induced cataract, unspecified eye**

     H26.31 **Drug-induced cataract, right eye**

     H26.32 **Drug-induced cataract, left eye**

     H26.33 **Drug-induced cataract, bilateral**

✓5ᵗʰ **H26.4** Secondary **cataract**

     H26.40 **Unspecified secondary cataract**

✓6ᵗʰ   **H26.41** **Soemmering's ring**

     H26.411 **Soemmering's ring, right eye**

     H26.412 **Soemmering's ring, left eye**

     H26.413 **Soemmering's ring, bilateral**

     H26.419 **Soemmering's ring, unspecified eye**

✓6ᵗʰ   **H26.49** **Other secondary cataract**

         AHA: 2018,2Q,14

     H26.491 **Other secondary cataract, right eye**

     H26.492 **Other secondary cataract, left eye**

     H26.493 **Other secondary cataract, bilateral**

     H26.499 **Other secondary cataract, unspecified eye**

H26.8 Other specified **cataract**

H26.9 Unspecified **cataract**

✓4ᵗʰ **H27** **Other disorders of lens**

     EXCLUDES 1   congenital lens malformations (Q12.-)

            mechanical complications of intraocular lens implant (T85.2)

            pseudophakia (Z96.1)

✓5ᵗʰ **H27.0** Aphakia

     Acquired absence of lens

     Acquired aphakia

     Aphakia due to trauma

     EXCLUDES 1   cataract extraction status (Z98.4-)

            congenital absence of lens (Q12.3)

            congenital aphakia (Q12.3)

     H27.00 **Aphakia, unspecified eye**

     H27.01 **Aphakia, right eye**

     H27.02 **Aphakia, left eye**

     H27.03 **Aphakia, bilateral**

✓5ᵗʰ **H27.1** Dislocation of lens

     H27.10 **Unspecified dislocation of lens**

✓6ᵗʰ   **H27.11** **Subluxation of lens**

     H27.111 **Subluxation of lens, right eye**

     H27.112 **Subluxation of lens, left eye**

     H27.113 **Subluxation of lens, bilateral**

     H27.119 **Subluxation of lens, unspecified eye**

✓6ᵗʰ   **H27.12** **Anterior dislocation of lens**

     H27.121 **Anterior dislocation of lens, right eye**

     H27.122 **Anterior dislocation of lens, left eye**

     H27.123 **Anterior dislocation of lens, bilateral**

     H27.129 **Anterior dislocation of lens, unspecified eye**

✓6ᵗʰ   **H27.13** **Posterior dislocation of lens**

     H27.131 **Posterior dislocation of lens, right eye**

     H27.132 **Posterior dislocation of lens, left eye**

     H27.133 **Posterior dislocation of lens, bilateral**

     H27.139 **Posterior dislocation of lens, unspecified eye**

H27.8 Other specified **disorders of lens**

H27.9 Unspecified **disorder of lens**

H28 *Cataract in diseases classified elsewhere*

     Code first underlying disease, such as:

         hypoparathyroidism (E20.-)

         myotonia (G71.1-)

         myxedema (E03.-)

         protein-calorie malnutrition (E40-E46)

     EXCLUDES 1   cataract in diabetes mellitus (E08.36, E09.36, E10.36, E11.36, E13.36)

Disorders of choroid and retina (H30-H36)

✓4ᵗʰ **H30** **Chorioretinal inflammation**

     CC Excl: For CC codes in category H30: PDX collection 626

✓5ᵗʰ **H30.0** Focal **chorioretinal inflammation**

     Focal chorioretinitis

     Focal choroiditis

     Focal retinitis

     Focal retinochoroiditis

✓6ᵗʰ   **H30.00** **Unspecified focal chorioretinal inflammation**

     Focal chorioretinitis NOS

     Focal choroiditis NOS

     Focal retinitis NOS

     Focal retinochoroiditis NOS

     H30.001 **Unspecified focal chorioretinal inflammation, right eye**

     H30.002 **Unspecified focal chorioretinal inflammation, left eye**

     H30.003 **Unspecified focal chorioretinal inflammation, bilateral**

     H30.009 **Unspecified focal chorioretinal inflammation, unspecified eye**

✓6ᵗʰ   **H30.01** **Focal chorioretinal inflammation, juxtapapillary**

     H30.011 **Focal chorioretinal inflammation, juxtapapillary, right eye**

     H30.012 **Focal chorioretinal inflammation, juxtapapillary, left eye**

     H30.013 **Focal chorioretinal inflammation, juxtapapillary, bilateral**

     H30.019 **Focal chorioretinal inflammation, juxtapapillary, unspecified eye**

☑ Additional Character Required   ✓x7ᵗʰ Placeholder   Unacceptable PDx   Questionable PDx   Manifestation   Unspecified Dx   H1-H14 HAC   HCC CMS-HCC Dx   HIV HIV Dx

ICD-10-CM 2020   611

H26.12–H30.019

√6ᵗʰ **H30.02 Focal chorioretinal inflammation of** posterior pole

    H30.021 Focal chorioretinal inflammation of posterior pole, right eye

    H30.022 Focal chorioretinal inflammation of posterior pole, left eye

    H30.023 Focal chorioretinal inflammation of posterior pole, bilateral

    H30.029 Focal chorioretinal inflammation of posterior pole, unspecified eye

√6ᵗʰ **H30.03 Focal chorioretinal inflammation,** peripheral

    H30.031 Focal chorioretinal inflammation, peripheral, right eye

    H30.032 Focal chorioretinal inflammation, peripheral, left eye

    H30.033 Focal chorioretinal inflammation, peripheral, bilateral

    H30.039 Focal chorioretinal inflammation, peripheral, unspecified eye

√6ᵗʰ **H30.04 Focal chorioretinal inflammation,** macular or paramacular

    H30.041 Focal chorioretinal inflammation, macular or paramacular, right eye

    H30.042 Focal chorioretinal inflammation, macular or paramacular, left eye

    H30.043 Focal chorioretinal inflammation, macular or paramacular, bilateral

    H30.049 Focal chorioretinal inflammation, macular or paramacular, unspecified eye

√5ᵗʰ **H30.1 Disseminated chorioretinal inflammation**

    Disseminated chorioretinitis
    Disseminated choroiditis
    Disseminated retinitis
    Disseminated retinochoroiditis
    EXCLUDES 2   exudative retinopathy (H35.02-)

√6ᵗʰ **H30.10 Unspecified disseminated chorioretinal inflammation**

    Disseminated chorioretinitis NOS
    Disseminated choroiditis NOS
    Disseminated retinitis NOS
    Disseminated retinochoroiditis NOS

    H30.101 Unspecified disseminated chorioretinal inflammation, right eye CC

    H30.102 Unspecified disseminated chorioretinal inflammation, left eye CC

    H30.103 Unspecified disseminated chorioretinal inflammation, bilateral CC

    H30.109 Unspecified disseminated chorioretinal inflammation, unspecified eye CC

√6ᵗʰ **H30.11 Disseminated chorioretinal inflammation of** posterior pole

    H30.111 Disseminated chorioretinal inflammation of posterior pole, right eye CC

    H30.112 Disseminated chorioretinal inflammation of posterior pole, left eye CC

    H30.113 Disseminated chorioretinal inflammation of posterior pole, bilateral CC

    H30.119 Disseminated chorioretinal inflammation of posterior pole, unspecified eye CC

√6ᵗʰ **H30.12 Disseminated chorioretinal inflammation,** peripheral

    H30.121 Disseminated chorioretinal inflammation, peripheral right eye CC

    H30.122 Disseminated chorioretinal inflammation, peripheral, left eye CC

    H30.123 Disseminated chorioretinal inflammation, peripheral, bilateral CC

    H30.129 Disseminated chorioretinal inflammation, peripheral, unspecified eye CC

√6ᵗʰ **H30.13 Disseminated chorioretinal inflammation, generalized**

    H30.131 Disseminated chorioretinal inflammation, generalized, right eye CC

    H30.132 Disseminated chorioretinal inflammation, generalized, left eye CC

    H30.133 Disseminated chorioretinal inflammation, generalized, bilateral CC

    H30.139 Disseminated chorioretinal inflammation, generalized, unspecified eye CC

√6ᵗʰ **H30.14 Acute posterior multifocal placoid pigment epitheliopathy**

    H30.141 Acute posterior multifocal placoid pigment epitheliopathy, right eye CC

    H30.142 Acute posterior multifocal placoid pigment epitheliopathy, left eye CC

    H30.143 Acute posterior multifocal placoid pigment epitheliopathy, bilateral CC

    H30.149 Acute posterior multifocal placoid pigment epitheliopathy, unspecified eye CC

√5ᵗʰ **H30.2 Posterior cyclitis**

    Pars planitis

    H30.20 Posterior cyclitis, unspecified eye

    H30.21 Posterior cyclitis, right eye

    H30.22 Posterior cyclitis, left eye

    H30.23 Posterior cyclitis, bilateral

√5ᵗʰ **H30.8 Other chorioretinal inflammations**

√6ᵗʰ **H30.81 Harada's disease**

    H30.811 Harada's disease, right eye

    H30.812 Harada's disease, left eye

    H30.813 Harada's disease, bilateral

    H30.819 Harada's disease, unspecified eye

√6ᵗʰ **H30.89 Other chorioretinal inflammations**

    H30.891 Other chorioretinal inflammations, right eye CC

    H30.892 Other chorioretinal inflammations, left eye CC

    H30.893 Other chorioretinal inflammations, bilateral CC

    H30.899 Other chorioretinal inflammations, unspecified eye CC

√5ᵗʰ **H30.9 Unspecified chorioretinal inflammation**

    Chorioretinitis NOS
    Choroiditis NOS
    Neuroretinitis NOS
    Retinitis NOS
    Retinochoroiditis NOS

    H30.90 Unspecified chorioretinal inflammation, unspecified eye CC

    H30.91 Unspecified chorioretinal inflammation, right eye CC

    H30.92 Unspecified chorioretinal inflammation, left eye CC

    H30.93 Unspecified chorioretinal inflammation, bilateral CC

N Newborn: 0   P Pediatric: 0-17   M Maternity: 9-64   A Adult: 15-124   MCC Major Complication/Comorbidity   CC Complication/Comorbidity   SW Severe Wound Dx

612   ICD-10-CM 2020

Chapter 7. Diseases of the Eye and Adnexa

✓4ᵗʰ **H31 Other disorders of choroid**

> **CC Excl: For CC codes in category H31:** PDX collection 627

✓5ᵗʰ **H31.0 Chorioretinal scars**

> EXCLUDES 2   *postsurgical chorioretinal scars (H59.81-)*

✓6ᵗʰ **H31.00 Unspecified chorioretinal scars**

- **H31.001 Unspecified chorioretinal scars, right eye**
- **H31.002 Unspecified chorioretinal scars, left eye**
- **H31.003 Unspecified chorioretinal scars, bilateral**
- **H31.009 Unspecified chorioretinal scars, unspecified eye**

✓6ᵗʰ **H31.01 Macula scars of posterior pole (postinflammatory) (post-traumatic)**

> EXCLUDES 1   *postprocedural chorioretinal scar (H59.81-)*

- **H31.011 Macula scars of posterior pole (postinflammatory) (post-traumatic), right eye**
- **H31.012 Macula scars of posterior pole (postinflammatory) (post-traumatic), left eye**
- **H31.013 Macula scars of posterior pole (postinflammatory) (post-traumatic), bilateral**
- **H31.019 Macula scars of posterior pole (postinflammatory) (post-traumatic), unspecified eye**

✓6ᵗʰ **H31.02 Solar retinopathy**

- **H31.021 Solar retinopathy, right eye**
- **H31.022 Solar retinopathy, left eye**
- **H31.023 Solar retinopathy, bilateral**
- **H31.029 Solar retinopathy, unspecified eye**

✓6ᵗʰ **H31.09 Other chorioretinal scars**

- **H31.091 Other chorioretinal scars, right eye**
- **H31.092 Other chorioretinal scars, left eye**
- **H31.093 Other chorioretinal scars, bilateral**
- **H31.099 Other chorioretinal scars, unspecified eye**

✓5ᵗʰ **H31.1 Choroidal degeneration**

> EXCLUDES 2   *angioid streaks of macula (H35.33)*

✓6ᵗʰ **H31.10 Unspecified choroidal degeneration**

Choroidal sclerosis NOS

- **H31.101 Choroidal degeneration, unspecified, right eye**
- **H31.102 Choroidal degeneration, unspecified, left eye**
- **H31.103 Choroidal degeneration, unspecified, bilateral**
- **H31.109 Choroidal degeneration, unspecified, unspecified eye**

✓6ᵗʰ **H31.11 Age-related choroidal atrophy**

- **H31.111 Age-related choroidal atrophy, right eye** Ⓐ
- **H31.112 Age-related choroidal atrophy, left eye** Ⓐ
- **H31.113 Age-related choroidal atrophy, bilateral** Ⓐ
- **H31.119 Age-related choroidal atrophy, unspecified eye** Ⓐ

✓6ᵗʰ **H31.12 Diffuse secondary atrophy of choroid**

- **H31.121 Diffuse secondary atrophy of choroid, right eye**
- **H31.122 Diffuse secondary atrophy of choroid, left eye**
- **H31.123 Diffuse secondary atrophy of choroid, bilateral**
- **H31.129 Diffuse secondary atrophy of choroid, unspecified eye**

✓5ᵗʰ **H31.2 Hereditary choroidal dystrophy**

> EXCLUDES 2   *hyperornithinemia (E72.4)*
> *ornithinemia (E72.4)*

- **H31.20 Hereditary choroidal dystrophy, unspecified**
- **H31.21 Choroideremia**
- **H31.22 Choroidal dystrophy (central areolar) (generalized) (peripapillary)**
- **H31.23 Gyrate atrophy, choroid**
- **H31.29 Other hereditary choroidal dystrophy**

✓5ᵗʰ **H31.3 Choroidal hemorrhage and rupture**

✓6ᵗʰ **H31.30 Unspecified choroidal hemorrhage**

- **H31.301 Unspecified choroidal hemorrhage, right eye**
- **H31.302 Unspecified choroidal hemorrhage, left eye**
- **H31.303 Unspecified choroidal hemorrhage, bilateral**
- **H31.309 Unspecified choroidal hemorrhage, unspecified eye**

✓6ᵗʰ **H31.31 Expulsive choroidal hemorrhage**

- **H31.311 Expulsive choroidal hemorrhage, right eye**
- **H31.312 Expulsive choroidal hemorrhage, left eye**
- **H31.313 Expulsive choroidal hemorrhage, bilateral**
- **H31.319 Expulsive choroidal hemorrhage, unspecified eye**

✓6ᵗʰ **H31.32 Choroidal rupture**

- **H31.321 Choroidal rupture, right eye** CC
- **H31.322 Choroidal rupture, left eye** CC
- **H31.323 Choroidal rupture, bilateral** CC
- **H31.329 Choroidal rupture, unspecified eye** CC

✓5ᵗʰ **H31.4 Choroidal detachment**

✓6ᵗʰ **H31.40 Unspecified choroidal detachment**

- **H31.401 Unspecified choroidal detachment, right eye** CC
- **H31.402 Unspecified choroidal detachment, left eye** CC
- **H31.403 Unspecified choroidal detachment, bilateral** CC
- **H31.409 Unspecified choroidal detachment, unspecified eye** CC

✓6ᵗʰ **H31.41 Hemorrhagic choroidal detachment**

- **H31.411 Hemorrhagic choroidal detachment, right eye** CC
- **H31.412 Hemorrhagic choroidal detachment, left eye** CC
- **H31.413 Hemorrhagic choroidal detachment, bilateral** CC
- **H31.419 Hemorrhagic choroidal detachment, unspecified eye** CC

✓6ᵗʰ **H31.42 Serous choroidal detachment**

- **H31.421 Serous choroidal detachment, right eye** CC
- **H31.422 Serous choroidal detachment, left eye** CC
- **H31.423 Serous choroidal detachment, bilateral** CC
- **H31.429 Serous choroidal detachment, unspecified eye** CC

H31.8 Other specified disorders of choroid

H31.9 Unspecified disorder of choroid

H32 Chorioretinal disorders in diseases classified elsewhere

Code first underlying disease, such as:
- congenital toxoplasmosis (P37.1)
- histoplasmosis (B39.-)
- leprosy (A30.-)

> EXCLUDES 1   *chorioretinitis (in):*
> *toxoplasmosis (acquired) (B58.01)*
> *tuberculosis (A18.53)*

✓ Additional Character Required ✓x7ᵗʰ Placeholder Unacceptable PDx Questionable PDx Manifestation Unspecified Dx H1-H14 HAC HCC CMS-HCC Dx HIV HIV Dx

Chapter 7. Diseases of the Eye and Adnexa

✓4ᵗʰ H33 Retinal detachments and breaks

EXCLUDES 1   detachment of retinal pigment epithelium (H35.72-, H35.73-)

CC Excl: For CC codes in category H33, unless otherwise noted: PDX collection 628

Retinal Detachment

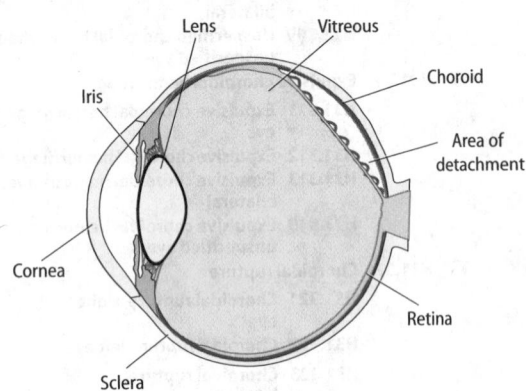

✓5ᵗʰ H33.0 Retinal detachment with retinal break

Rhegmatogenous retinal detachment

EXCLUDES 1   serous retinal detachment (without retinal break) (H33.2-)

✓6ᵗʰ H33.00 Unspecified retinal detachment with retinal break

- **H33.001** Unspecified retinal detachment with retinal break, **right eye**
- **H33.002** Unspecified retinal detachment with retinal break, **left eye**
- **H33.003** Unspecified retinal detachment with retinal break, **bilateral**
- **H33.009** Unspecified retinal detachment with retinal break, **unspecified eye**

✓6ᵗʰ H33.01 Retinal detachment with single break

- **H33.011** Retinal detachment with single break, **right eye**
- **H33.012** Retinal detachment with single break, **left eye**
- **H33.013** Retinal detachment with single break, **bilateral**
- **H33.019** Retinal detachment with single break, **unspecified eye**

✓6ᵗʰ H33.02 Retinal detachment with multiple breaks

- **H33.021** Retinal detachment with multiple breaks, **right eye**
- **H33.022** Retinal detachment with multiple breaks, **left eye**
- **H33.023** Retinal detachment with multiple breaks, **bilateral**
- **H33.029** Retinal detachment with multiple breaks, **unspecified eye**

✓6ᵗʰ H33.03 Retinal detachment with giant retinal tear

- **H33.031** Retinal detachment with giant retinal tear, **right eye**
- **H33.032** Retinal detachment with giant retinal tear, **left eye**
- **H33.033** Retinal detachment with giant retinal tear, **bilateral**
- **H33.039** Retinal detachment with giant retinal tear, **unspecified eye**

✓6ᵗʰ H33.04 Retinal detachment with retinal dialysis

- **H33.041** Retinal detachment with retinal dialysis, **right eye**
- **H33.042** Retinal detachment with retinal dialysis, **left eye**
- **H33.043** Retinal detachment with retinal dialysis, **bilateral**
- **H33.049** Retinal detachment with retinal dialysis, **unspecified eye**

✓6ᵗʰ H33.05 Total retinal detachment

- **H33.051** Total retinal detachment, **right eye**
- **H33.052** Total retinal detachment, **left eye**
- **H33.053** Total retinal detachment, **bilateral**
- **H33.059** Total retinal detachment, **unspecified eye**

✓5ᵗʰ H33.1 Retinoschisis and retinal cysts

EXCLUDES 1   congenital retinoschisis (Q14.1)

       microcystoid degeneration of retina (H35.42-)

✓6ᵗʰ H33.10 Unspecified retinoschisis

- **H33.101** Unspecified retinoschisis, **right eye**
- **H33.102** Unspecified retinoschisis, **left eye**
- **H33.103** Unspecified retinoschisis, **bilateral**
- **H33.109** Unspecified retinoschisis, **unspecified eye**

✓6ᵗʰ H33.11 Cyst of ora serrata

- **H33.111** Cyst of ora serrata, **right eye**
- **H33.112** Cyst of ora serrata, **left eye**
- **H33.113** Cyst of ora serrata, **bilateral**
- **H33.119** Cyst of ora serrata, **unspecified eye**

✓6ᵗʰ H33.12 Parasitic cyst of retina

CC Excl: For CC codes in subcategory H33.12: PDX collection 625

- **H33.121** Parasitic cyst of retina, **right eye** `CC`
- **H33.122** Parasitic cyst of retina, **left eye** `CC`
- **H33.123** Parasitic cyst of retina, **bilateral** `CC`
- **H33.129** Parasitic cyst of retina, **unspecified eye** `CC`

✓6ᵗʰ H33.19 Other retinoschisis and retinal cysts

Pseudocyst of retina

- **H33.191** Other retinoschisis and retinal cysts, **right eye**
- **H33.192** Other retinoschisis and retinal cysts, **left eye**
- **H33.193** Other retinoschisis and retinal cysts, **bilateral**
- **H33.199** Other retinoschisis and retinal cysts, **unspecified eye**

✓5ᵗʰ H33.2 Serous retinal detachment

Retinal detachment NOS

Retinal detachment without retinal break

EXCLUDES 1   central serous chorioretinopathy (H35.71-)

- **H33.20** Serous retinal detachment, **unspecified eye** `CC`
- **H33.21** Serous retinal detachment, **right eye** `CC`
- **H33.22** Serous retinal detachment, **left eye** `CC`
- **H33.23** Serous retinal detachment, **bilateral** `CC`

✓5ᵗʰ H33.3 Retinal breaks without detachment

EXCLUDES 1   chorioretinal scars after surgery for detachment (H59.81-)

       peripheral retinal degeneration without break (H35.4-)

✓6ᵗʰ H33.30 Unspecified retinal break

- **H33.301** Unspecified retinal break, **right eye**
- **H33.302** Unspecified retinal break, **left eye**
- **H33.303** Unspecified retinal break, **bilateral**
- **H33.309** Unspecified retinal break, **unspecified eye**

✓6ᵗʰ H33.31 Horseshoe tear of retina without detachment

Operculum of retina without detachment

- **H33.311** Horseshoe tear of retina without detachment, **right eye**
- **H33.312** Horseshoe tear of retina without detachment, **left eye**
- **H33.313** Horseshoe tear of retina without detachment, **bilateral**
- **H33.319** Horseshoe tear of retina without detachment, **unspecified eye**

✓6ᵗʰ H33.32 Round hole of retina without detachment

- **H33.321** Round hole, **right eye**
- **H33.322** Round hole, **left eye**
- **H33.323** Round hole, **bilateral**
- **H33.329** Round hole, **unspecified eye**

✓6ᵗʰ H33.33 Multiple defects of retina without detachment

- **H33.331** Multiple defects of retina without detachment, **right eye**
- **H33.332** Multiple defects of retina without detachment, **left eye**
- **H33.333** Multiple defects of retina without detachment, **bilateral**

N Newborn: 0   **P** Pediatric: 0-17   **M** Maternity: 9-64   **A** Adult: 15-124   **MCC** Major Complication/Comorbidity   **CC** Complication/Comorbidity   **SW** Severe Wound Dx

614   ICD-10-CM 2020

H33–H33.333

H33.339   Multiple defects of retina without detachment, unspecified eye

√5th **H33.4**   Traction detachment of retina

    Proliferative vitreo-retinopathy with retinal detachment

    H33.40   Traction detachment of retina, unspecified eye   `CC`

    H33.41   Traction detachment of retina, right eye   `CC`

    H33.42   Traction detachment of retina, left eye   `CC`

    H33.43   Traction detachment of retina, bilateral   `CC`

H33.8   Other retinal detachments   `CC`

√4th **H34**   Retinal vascular occlusions

    EXCLUDES 1   *amaurosis fugax (G45.3)*

    CC Excl: For CC codes in category H34: PDX collection 587

√5th **H34.0**   Transient retinal artery occlusion

    H34.00   Transient retinal artery occlusion, unspecified eye   `CC`

    H34.01   Transient retinal artery occlusion, right eye   `CC`

    H34.02   Transient retinal artery occlusion, left eye   `CC`

    H34.03   Transient retinal artery occlusion, bilateral   `CC`

√5th **H34.1**   Central retinal artery occlusion

    H34.10   Central retinal artery occlusion, unspecified eye   `CC`

    H34.11   Central retinal artery occlusion, right eye   `CC`

    H34.12   Central retinal artery occlusion, left eye   `CC`

    H34.13   Central retinal artery occlusion, bilateral   `CC`

√5th **H34.2**   Other retinal artery occlusions

    √6th **H34.21**   Partial retinal artery occlusion

      Hollenhorst's plaque

      Retinal microembolism

      H34.211   Partial retinal artery occlusion, right eye   `CC`

      H34.212   Partial retinal artery occlusion, left eye   `CC`

      H34.213   Partial retinal artery occlusion, bilateral   `CC`

      H34.219   Partial retinal artery occlusion, unspecified eye   `CC`

    √6th **H34.23**   Retinal artery branch occlusion

      H34.231   Retinal artery branch occlusion, right eye   `CC`

      H34.232   Retinal artery branch occlusion, left eye   `CC`

      H34.233   Retinal artery branch occlusion, bilateral   `CC`

      H34.239   Retinal artery branch occlusion, unspecified eye   `CC`

√5th **H34.8**   Other retinal vascular occlusions

    AHA: 2016,4Q,19

    √6th **H34.81**   Central retinal vein occlusion

      One of the following 7th characters is to be assigned to codes in subcategory H34.81 to designate the severity of the occlusion:
      0   with macular edema
      1   with retinal neovascularization
      2   stable
        old central retinal vein occlusion

      √7th H34.811   Central retinal vein occlusion, right eye   `CC`

      √7th H34.812   Central retinal vein occlusion, left eye   `CC`

      √7th H34.813   Central retinal vein occlusion, bilateral   `CC`

      √7th **H34.819**   Central retinal vein occlusion, unspecified eye   `CC`

    √6th **H34.82**   Venous engorgement

      Incipient retinal vein occlusion

      Partial retinal vein occlusion

      H34.821   Venous engorgement, right eye

      H34.822   Venous engorgement, left eye

      H34.823   Venous engorgement, bilateral

      H34.829   Venous engorgement, unspecified eye

    √6th **H34.83**   Tributary (branch) retinal vein occlusion

      One of the following 7th characters is to be assigned to codes in subcategory H34.83 to designate the severity of the occlusion:
      0   with macular edema
      1   with retinal neovascularization
      2   stable
        old tributary (branch) retinal vein occlusion

      √7th H34.831   Tributary (branch) retinal vein occlusion, right eye

      √7th H34.832   Tributary (branch) retinal vein occlusion, left eye

      √7th H34.833   Tributary (branch) retinal vein occlusion, bilateral

      √7th **H34.839**   Tributary (branch) retinal vein occlusion, unspecified eye

H34.9   Unspecified retinal vascular occlusion

√4th **H35**   Other retinal disorders

    EXCLUDES 2   *diabetic retinal disorders (E08.311-E08.359, E09.311-E09.359, E10.311-E10.359, E11.311-E11.359, E13.311-E13.359)*

    √5th **H35.0**   Background retinopathy and retinal vascular changes

      Code also any associated hypertension (I10.-)

      H35.00   Unspecified background retinopathy

      √6th **H35.01**   Changes in retinal vascular appearance

        Retinal vascular sheathing

        H35.011   Changes in retinal vascular appearance, right eye

        H35.012   Changes in retinal vascular appearance, left eye

        H35.013   Changes in retinal vascular appearance, bilateral

        H35.019   Changes in retinal vascular appearance, unspecified eye

      √6th **H35.02**   Exudative retinopathy

        Coats retinopathy

        H35.021   Exudative retinopathy, right eye

        H35.022   Exudative retinopathy, left eye

        H35.023   Exudative retinopathy, bilateral

        H35.029   Exudative retinopathy, unspecified eye

      √6th **H35.03**   Hypertensive retinopathy

        H35.031   Hypertensive retinopathy, right eye

        H35.032   Hypertensive retinopathy, left eye

        H35.033   Hypertensive retinopathy, bilateral

        H35.039   Hypertensive retinopathy, unspecified eye

      √6th **H35.04**   Retinal micro-aneurysms, unspecified

        H35.041   Retinal micro-aneurysms, unspecified, right eye

        H35.042   Retinal micro-aneurysms, unspecified, left eye

        H35.043   Retinal micro-aneurysms, unspecified, bilateral

        H35.049   Retinal micro-aneurysms, unspecified, unspecified eye

      √6th **H35.05**   Retinal neovascularization, unspecified

        H35.051   Retinal neovascularization, unspecified, right eye

        H35.052   Retinal neovascularization, unspecified, left eye

        H35.053   Retinal neovascularization, unspecified, bilateral

        H35.059   Retinal neovascularization, unspecified, unspecified eye

      √6th **H35.06**   Retinal vasculitis

        Eales disease

        Retinal perivasculitis

        DEF: Sight-threatening intraocular inflammation of the retinal blood vessels that causes minimal, partial, or even complete blindness.

        H35.061   Retinal vasculitis, right eye

        H35.062   Retinal vasculitis, left eye

        H35.063   Retinal vasculitis, bilateral

        H35.069   Retinal vasculitis, unspecified eye

      √6th **H35.07**   Retinal telangiectasis

        H35.071   Retinal telangiectasis, right eye

        H35.072   Retinal telangiectasis, left eye

☑ Additional Character Required   √x7th Placeholder   Unacceptable PDx   Questionable PDx   Manifestation   Unspecified Dx   `H1`-`H14` HAC   `HCC` CMS-HCC Dx   `HIV` HIV Dx

ICD-10-CM 2020   615

      H35.073 **Retinal telangiectasis,** bilateral
      H35.079 Retinal telangiectasis, unspecified eye
   H35.09 **Other intraretinal microvascular abnormalities**
      Retinal varices

✓5ᵗʰ **H35.1 Retinopathy of prematurity**

✓6ᵗʰ H35.10 **Retinopathy of prematurity, unspecified**
      Retinopathy of prematurity NOS
      H35.101 Retinopathy of prematurity, unspecified, right eye
      H35.102 Retinopathy of prematurity, unspecified, left eye
      H35.103 Retinopathy of prematurity, unspecified, bilateral
      H35.109 Retinopathy of prematurity, unspecified, unspecified eye

✓6ᵗʰ H35.11 **Retinopathy of prematurity,** stage 0
      H35.111 Retinopathy of prematurity, stage 0, right eye
      H35.112 Retinopathy of prematurity, stage 0, left eye
      H35.113 Retinopathy of prematurity, stage 0, bilateral
      H35.119 Retinopathy of prematurity, stage 0, unspecified eye

✓6ᵗʰ H35.12 **Retinopathy of prematurity,** stage 1
      H35.121 Retinopathy of prematurity, stage 1, right eye
      H35.122 Retinopathy of prematurity, stage 1, left eye
      H35.123 Retinopathy of prematurity, stage 1, bilateral
      H35.129 Retinopathy of prematurity, stage 1, unspecified eye

✓6ᵗʰ H35.13 **Retinopathy of prematurity,** stage 2
      H35.131 Retinopathy of prematurity, stage 2, right eye
      H35.132 Retinopathy of prematurity, stage 2, left eye
      H35.133 Retinopathy of prematurity, stage 2, bilateral
      H35.139 Retinopathy of prematurity, stage 2, unspecified eye

✓6ᵗʰ H35.14 **Retinopathy of prematurity,** stage 3
      H35.141 Retinopathy of prematurity, stage 3, right eye
      H35.142 Retinopathy of prematurity, stage 3, left eye
      H35.143 Retinopathy of prematurity, stage 3, bilateral
      H35.149 Retinopathy of prematurity, stage 3, unspecified eye

✓6ᵗʰ H35.15 **Retinopathy of prematurity,** stage 4
      H35.151 Retinopathy of prematurity, stage 4, right eye
      H35.152 Retinopathy of prematurity, stage 4, left eye
      H35.153 Retinopathy of prematurity, stage 4, bilateral
      H35.159 Retinopathy of prematurity, stage 4, unspecified eye

✓6ᵗʰ H35.16 **Retinopathy of prematurity,** stage 5
      H35.161 Retinopathy of prematurity, stage 5, right eye
      H35.162 Retinopathy of prematurity, stage 5, left eye
      H35.163 Retinopathy of prematurity, stage 5, bilateral
      H35.169 Retinopathy of prematurity, stage 5, unspecified eye

✓6ᵗʰ H35.17 **Retrolental fibroplasia**
      H35.171 Retrolental fibroplasia, right eye
      H35.172 Retrolental fibroplasia, left eye
      H35.173 Retrolental fibroplasia, bilateral
      H35.179 Retrolental fibroplasia, unspecified eye

✓5ᵗʰ **H35.2 Other non-diabetic proliferative retinopathy**
      Proliferative vitreo-retinopathy
      EXCLUDES 1   *proliferative vitreo-retinopathy with retinal detachment (H33.4-)*
   H35.20 **Other non-diabetic proliferative retinopathy, unspecified**

H35.21 **Other non-diabetic proliferative retinopathy,** right eye
H35.22 **Other non-diabetic proliferative retinopathy,** left eye
H35.23 **Other non-diabetic proliferative retinopathy,** bilateral

✓5ᵗʰ **H35.3 Degeneration of macula and posterior pole**

   H35.30 **Unspecified macular degeneration**   A
      Age-related macular degeneration

✓6ᵗʰ H35.31 **Nonexudative age-related macular degeneration**
      Atrophic age-related macular degeneration
      Dry age-related macular degeneration
      AHA: 2016,4Q,20-21

> One of the following 7th characters is to be assigned to each code in subcategory H35.31 to designate the stage of the disease:
> 0   stage unspecified
> 1   early dry stage
> 2   intermediate dry stage
> 3   advanced atrophic without subfoveal involvement
>   advanced dry stage
> 4   advanced atrophic with subfoveal involvement

      ✓7ᵗʰ **H35.311 Nonexudative age-related macular degeneration, right** eye   A
      ✓7ᵗʰ **H35.312 Nonexudative age-related macular degeneration, left** eye   A
      ✓7ᵗʰ **H35.313 Nonexudative age-related macular degeneration, bilateral**   A
      ✓7ᵗʰ **H35.319 Nonexudative age-related macular degeneration, unspecified eye**   A

✓6ᵗʰ H35.32 **Exudative age-related macular degeneration**
      Wet age-related macular degeneration
      AHA: 2016,4Q,20-21

> One of the following 7th characters is to be assigned to each code in subcategory H35.32 to designate the stage of the disease:
> 0   stage unspecified
> 1   with active choroidal neovascularization
> 2   with inactive choroidal neovascularization
>   with involuted or regressed neovascularization
> 3   with inactive scar

      ✓7ᵗʰ **H35.321 Exudative age-related macular degeneration, right** eye   HCC A
      ✓7ᵗʰ **H35.322 Exudative age-related macular degeneration, left** eye   HCC A
      ✓7ᵗʰ **H35.323 Exudative age-related macular degeneration, bilateral**   HCC A
      ✓7ᵗʰ **H35.329 Exudative age-related macular degeneration, unspecified eye**   HCC A

   H35.33 **Angioid streaks of macula**
      DEF: Degeneration of the choroid; characterized by broad, irregular, dark brown streaks radiating from optic disc; occurs with pseudoxanthoma elasticum or Paget's disease.

✓6ᵗʰ H35.34 **Macular cyst, hole, or pseudohole**
      H35.341 Macular cyst, hole, or pseudohole, right eye
      H35.342 Macular cyst, hole, or pseudohole, left eye
      H35.343 Macular cyst, hole, or pseudohole, bilateral
      H35.349 Macular cyst, hole, or pseudohole, unspecified eye

✓6ᵗʰ H35.35 **Cystoid macular degeneration**
      EXCLUDES 1   *cystoid macular edema following cataract surgery (H59.03-)*
      H35.351 Cystoid macular degeneration, right eye
      H35.352 Cystoid macular degeneration, left eye
      H35.353 Cystoid macular degeneration, bilateral

H35.359 Cystoid macular degeneration, unspecified eye

✓6ᵗʰ **H35.36 Drusen (degenerative) of macula**

AHA: 2017,1Q,51; 2016,4Q,21

H35.361 Drusen (degenerative) of macula, right eye
H35.362 Drusen (degenerative) of macula, left eye
H35.363 Drusen (degenerative) of macula, bilateral
H35.369 Drusen (degenerative) of macula, unspecified eye

✓6ᵗʰ **H35.37 Puckering of macula**

H35.371 Puckering of macula, right eye
H35.372 Puckering of macula, left eye
H35.373 Puckering of macula, bilateral
H35.379 Puckering of macula, unspecified eye

✓6ᵗʰ **H35.38 Toxic maculopathy**

Code first poisoning due to drug or toxin, if applicable (T36-T65 with fifth or sixth character 1-4 or 6)
Use additional code for adverse effect, if applicable, to identify drug (T36-T50 with fifth or sixth character 5)

H35.381 Toxic maculopathy, right eye
H35.382 Toxic maculopathy, left eye
H35.383 Toxic maculopathy, bilateral
H35.389 Toxic maculopathy, unspecified eye

✓5ᵗʰ **H35.4 Peripheral retinal degeneration**

EXCLUDES 1   hereditary retinal degeneration (dystrophy) (H35.5-)
peripheral retinal degeneration with retinal break (H33.3-)

H35.40 Unspecified peripheral retinal degeneration

✓6ᵗʰ **H35.41 Lattice degeneration of retina**

Palisade degeneration of retina
DEF: Degeneration of the retina, often bilateral, that is usually benign. It is characterized by lines intersecting at irregular intervals in the peripheral retina. Retinal thinning and retinal holes may occur.

H35.411 Lattice degeneration of retina, right eye
H35.412 Lattice degeneration of retina, left eye
H35.413 Lattice degeneration of retina, bilateral
H35.419 Lattice degeneration of retina, unspecified eye

✓6ᵗʰ **H35.42 Microcystoid degeneration of retina**

H35.421 Microcystoid degeneration of retina, right eye
H35.422 Microcystoid degeneration of retina, left eye
H35.423 Microcystoid degeneration of retina, bilateral
H35.429 Microcystoid degeneration of retina, unspecified eye

✓6ᵗʰ **H35.43 Paving stone degeneration of retina**

H35.431 Paving stone degeneration of retina, right eye
H35.432 Paving stone degeneration of retina, left eye
H35.433 Paving stone degeneration of retina, bilateral
H35.439 Paving stone degeneration of retina, unspecified eye

✓6ᵗʰ **H35.44 Age-related reticular degeneration of retina**

H35.441 Age-related reticular degeneration of retina, right eye Ⓐ
H35.442 Age-related reticular degeneration of retina, left eye Ⓐ
H35.443 Age-related reticular degeneration of retina, bilateral Ⓐ
H35.449 Age-related reticular degeneration of retina, unspecified eye Ⓐ

✓6ᵗʰ **H35.45 Secondary pigmentary degeneration**

H35.451 Secondary pigmentary degeneration, right eye
H35.452 Secondary pigmentary degeneration, left eye
H35.453 Secondary pigmentary degeneration, bilateral

H35.459 Secondary pigmentary degeneration, unspecified eye

✓6ᵗʰ **H35.46 Secondary vitreoretinal degeneration**

H35.461 Secondary vitreoretinal degeneration, right eye
H35.462 Secondary vitreoretinal degeneration, left eye
H35.463 Secondary vitreoretinal degeneration, bilateral
H35.469 Secondary vitreoretinal degeneration, unspecified eye

✓5ᵗʰ **H35.5 Hereditary retinal dystrophy**

EXCLUDES 1   dystrophies primarily involving Bruch's membrane (H31.1-)

H35.50 Unspecified hereditary retinal dystrophy
H35.51 Vitreoretinal dystrophy
H35.52 Pigmentary retinal dystrophy
Albipunctate retinal dystrophy
Retinitis pigmentosa
Tapetoretinal dystrophy
H35.53 Other dystrophies primarily involving the sensory retina
Stargardt's disease
H35.54 Dystrophies primarily involving the retinal pigment epithelium
Vitelliform retinal dystrophy

✓5ᵗʰ **H35.6 Retinal hemorrhage**

H35.60 Retinal hemorrhage, unspecified eye
H35.61 Retinal hemorrhage, right eye
H35.62 Retinal hemorrhage, left eye
H35.63 Retinal hemorrhage, bilateral

✓5ᵗʰ **H35.7 Separation of retinal layers**

EXCLUDES 1   retinal detachment (serous) (H33.2-)
rhegmatogenous retinal detachment (H33.0-)

CC Excl: For CC codes in subcategory H35.7: PDX collection 628

H35.70 Unspecified separation of retinal layers CC

✓6ᵗʰ **H35.71 Central serous chorioretinopathy**

H35.711 Central serous chorioretinopathy, right eye
H35.712 Central serous chorioretinopathy, left eye
H35.713 Central serous chorioretinopathy, bilateral
H35.719 Central serous chorioretinopathy, unspecified eye

✓6ᵗʰ **H35.72 Serous detachment of retinal pigment epithelium**

H35.721 Serous detachment of retinal pigment epithelium, right eye CC
H35.722 Serous detachment of retinal pigment epithelium, left eye CC
H35.723 Serous detachment of retinal pigment epithelium, bilateral CC
H35.729 Serous detachment of retinal pigment epithelium, unspecified eye CC

✓6ᵗʰ **H35.73 Hemorrhagic detachment of retinal pigment epithelium**

H35.731 Hemorrhagic detachment of retinal pigment epithelium, right eye CC
H35.732 Hemorrhagic detachment of retinal pigment epithelium, left eye CC
H35.733 Hemorrhagic detachment of retinal pigment epithelium, bilateral CC
H35.739 Hemorrhagic detachment of retinal pigment epithelium, unspecified eye CC

✓5ᵗʰ **H35.8 Other specified retinal disorders**

EXCLUDES 2   retinal hemorrhage (H35.6-)

H35.81 Retinal edema
Retinal cotton wool spots

H35.82   **Retinal ischemia**   CC
     CC Excl: PDX collection 629

H35.89   **Other specified retinal disorders**

H35.9   **Unspecified retinal disorder**

H36   *Retinal disorders in diseases classified elsewhere*
     Code first underlying disease, such as:
       lipid storage disorders (E75.-)
       sickle-cell disorders (D57.-)
     EXCLUDES 1   arteriosclerotic retinopathy (H35.0-)
           diabetic retinopathy (E08.3-, E09.3-, E10.3-, E11.3-, E13.3-)

Glaucoma (H40-H42)

H40   **Glaucoma**   √4th
     EXCLUDES 1   absolute glaucoma (H44.51-)
           congenital glaucoma (Q15.0)
           traumatic glaucoma due to birth injury (P15.3)

Open Angle/Angle Closure Glaucoma

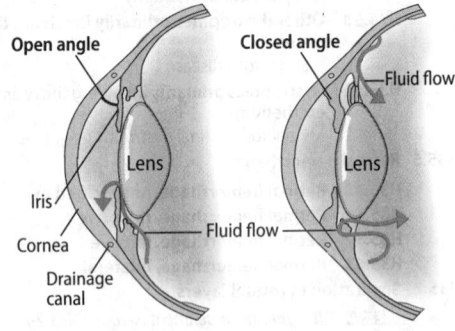

H40.0   **Glaucoma suspect**   √5th

   H40.00   **Preglaucoma, unspecified**   √6th
     H40.001   Preglaucoma, unspecified, **right eye**
     H40.002   Preglaucoma, unspecified, **left eye**
     H40.003   Preglaucoma, unspecified, **bilateral**
     H40.009   Preglaucoma, unspecified, **unspecified eye**

   H40.01   **Open angle with borderline findings, low risk**   √6th
     Open angle, low risk
     H40.011   Open angle with borderline findings, low risk, **right eye**
     H40.012   Open angle with borderline findings, low risk, **left eye**
     H40.013   Open angle with borderline findings, low risk, **bilateral**
     H40.019   Open angle with borderline findings, low risk, **unspecified eye**

   H40.02   **Open angle with borderline findings, high risk**   √6th
     Open angle, high risk
     H40.021   Open angle with borderline findings, high risk, **right eye**
     H40.022   Open angle with borderline findings, high risk, **left eye**
     H40.023   Open angle with borderline findings, high risk, **bilateral**
     H40.029   Open angle with borderline findings, high risk, **unspecified eye**

   H40.03   **Anatomical narrow angle**   √6th
     Primary angle closure suspect
     H40.031   Anatomical narrow angle, **right eye**
     H40.032   Anatomical narrow angle, **left eye**
     H40.033   Anatomical narrow angle, **bilateral**
     H40.039   Anatomical narrow angle, **unspecified eye**

   H40.04   **Steroid responder**   √6th
     H40.041   Steroid responder, **right eye**
     H40.042   Steroid responder, **left eye**
     H40.043   Steroid responder, **bilateral**
     H40.049   Steroid responder, **unspecified eye**

   H40.05   **Ocular hypertension**   √6th
     H40.051   Ocular hypertension, **right eye**
     H40.052   Ocular hypertension, **left eye**
     H40.053   Ocular hypertension, **bilateral**
     H40.059   Ocular hypertension, **unspecified eye**

   H40.06   **Primary angle closure without glaucoma damage**   √6th
     H40.061   Primary angle closure without glaucoma damage, **right eye**
     H40.062   Primary angle closure without glaucoma damage, **left eye**
     H40.063   Primary angle closure without glaucoma damage, **bilateral**
     H40.069   Primary angle closure without glaucoma damage, **unspecified eye**

H40.1   **Open-angle glaucoma**   √5th

   One of the following 7th characters is to be assigned to each code in subcategories H40.10, H40.11, H40.12, H40.13, and H40.14 to designate the stage of glaucoma.
   0   stage unspecified
   1   mild stage
   2   moderate stage
   3   severe stage
   4   indeterminate stage

   H40.10   **Unspecified open-angle glaucoma**   √x7th
     TIP: Only one code from this subcategory should be assigned when both left and right eyes are the same stage.

   H40.11   **Primary open-angle glaucoma**   √6th
     Chronic simple glaucoma
     AHA: 2016,4Q,22
     H40.111   Primary open-angle glaucoma, **right eye**   √7th
     H40.112   Primary open-angle glaucoma, **left eye**   √7th
     H40.113   Primary open-angle glaucoma, **bilateral**   √7th
     H40.119   Primary open-angle glaucoma, **unspecified eye**   √7th

   H40.12   **Low-tension glaucoma**   √6th
     H40.121   Low-tension glaucoma, **right eye**   √7th
     H40.122   Low-tension glaucoma, **left eye**   √7th
     H40.123   Low-tension glaucoma, **bilateral**   √7th
     H40.129   Low-tension glaucoma, **unspecified eye**   √7th

   H40.13   **Pigmentary glaucoma**   √6th
     H40.131   Pigmentary glaucoma, **right eye**   √7th
     H40.132   Pigmentary glaucoma, **left eye**   √7th
     H40.133   Pigmentary glaucoma, **bilateral**   √7th
     H40.139   Pigmentary glaucoma, **unspecified eye**   √7th

   H40.14   **Capsular glaucoma with pseudoexfoliation of lens**   √6th
     H40.141   Capsular glaucoma with pseudoexfoliation of lens, **right eye**   √7th
     H40.142   Capsular glaucoma with pseudoexfoliation of lens, **left eye**   √7th
     H40.143   Capsular glaucoma with pseudoexfoliation of lens, **bilateral**   √7th
     H40.149   Capsular glaucoma with pseudoexfoliation of lens, **unspecified eye**   √7th

   H40.15   **Residual stage of open-angle glaucoma**   √6th
     H40.151   Residual stage of open-angle glaucoma, **right eye**
     H40.152   Residual stage of open-angle glaucoma, **left eye**
     H40.153   Residual stage of open-angle glaucoma, **bilateral**
     H40.159   Residual stage of open-angle glaucoma, **unspecified eye**

H40.2   **Primary angle-closure glaucoma**   √5th
     EXCLUDES 1   aqueous misdirection (H40.83-)
           malignant glaucoma (H40.83-)

   One of the following 7th characters is to be assigned to code H40.20 and H40.22- to designate the stage of glaucoma.
   0   stage unspecified
   1   mild stage
   2   moderate stage
   3   severe stage
   4   indeterminate stage

   H40.20   **Unspecified primary angle-closure glaucoma**   √x7th
     TIP: Only one code from this subcategory should be assigned when both left and right eyes are the same stage.

N Newborn: 0   P Pediatric: 0-17   M Maternity: 9-64   A Adult: 15-124   MCC Major Complication/Comorbidity   CC Complication/Comorbidity   SW Severe Wound Dx

618   ICD-10-CM 2020

√6ᵗʰ **H40.21** **Acute angle-closure glaucoma**

Acute angle-closure glaucoma attack
Acute angle-closure glaucoma crisis
CC Excl: For CC codes in subcategory H40.21: PDX collection 630

H40.211 **Acute angle-closure glaucoma, right eye** `CC`

H40.212 **Acute angle-closure glaucoma, left eye** `CC`

H40.213 **Acute angle-closure glaucoma, bilateral** `CC`

H40.219 **Acute angle-closure glaucoma, unspecified eye** `CC`

√6ᵗʰ **H40.22** **Chronic angle-closure glaucoma**

Chronic primary angle closure glaucoma

√7ᵗʰ **H40.221** **Chronic angle-closure glaucoma, right eye**

√7ᵗʰ **H40.222** **Chronic angle-closure glaucoma, left eye**

√7ᵗʰ **H40.223** **Chronic angle-closure glaucoma, bilateral**

√7ᵗʰ **H40.229** **Chronic angle-closure glaucoma, unspecified eye**

√6ᵗʰ **H40.23** **Intermittent angle-closure glaucoma**

H40.231 **Intermittent angle-closure glaucoma, right eye**

H40.232 **Intermittent angle-closure glaucoma, left eye**

H40.233 **Intermittent angle-closure glaucoma, bilateral**

H40.239 **Intermittent angle-closure glaucoma, unspecified eye**

√6ᵗʰ **H40.24** **Residual stage of angle-closure glaucoma**

H40.241 **Residual stage of angle-closure glaucoma, right eye**

H40.242 **Residual stage of angle-closure glaucoma, left eye**

H40.243 **Residual stage of angle-closure glaucoma, bilateral**

H40.249 **Residual stage of angle-closure glaucoma, unspecified eye**

√5ᵗʰ **H40.3** **Glaucoma secondary to eye trauma**

Code also underlying condition

One of the following 7th characters is to be assigned to each code in subcategory H40.3- to designate the stage of glaucoma.
Ø   stage unspecified
1   mild stage
2   moderate stage
3   severe stage
4   indeterminate stage

√x7ᵗʰ **H40.30** **Glaucoma secondary to eye trauma, unspecified eye**

√x7ᵗʰ **H40.31** **Glaucoma secondary to eye trauma, right eye**

√x7ᵗʰ **H40.32** **Glaucoma secondary to eye trauma, left eye**

√x7ᵗʰ **H40.33** **Glaucoma secondary to eye trauma, bilateral**

√5ᵗʰ **H40.4** **Glaucoma secondary to eye inflammation**

Code also underlying condition

One of the following 7th characters is to be assigned to each code in subcategory H40.4- to designate the stage of glaucoma.
Ø   stage unspecified
1   mild stage
2   moderate stage
3   severe stage
4   indeterminate stage

√x7ᵗʰ **H40.40** **Glaucoma secondary to eye inflammation, unspecified eye**

√x7ᵗʰ **H40.41** **Glaucoma secondary to eye inflammation, right eye**

√x7ᵗʰ **H40.42** **Glaucoma secondary to eye inflammation, left eye**

√x7ᵗʰ **H40.43** **Glaucoma secondary to eye inflammation, bilateral**

√5ᵗʰ **H40.5** **Glaucoma secondary to other eye disorders**

Code also underlying eye disorder

One of the following 7th characters is to be assigned to each code in subcategory H40.5- to designate the stage of glaucoma.
Ø   stage unspecified
1   mild stage
2   moderate stage
3   severe stage
4   indeterminate stage

√x7ᵗʰ **H40.50** **Glaucoma secondary to other eye disorders, unspecified eye**

√x7ᵗʰ **H40.51** **Glaucoma secondary to other eye disorders, right eye**

√x7ᵗʰ **H40.52** **Glaucoma secondary to other eye disorders, left eye**

√x7ᵗʰ **H40.53** **Glaucoma secondary to other eye disorders, bilateral**

√5ᵗʰ **H40.6** **Glaucoma secondary to drugs**

Use additional code for adverse effect, if applicable, to identify drug (T36-T50 with fifth or sixth character 5)

One of the following 7th characters is to be assigned to each code in subcategory H40.6- to designate the stage of glaucoma
Ø   stage unspecified
1   mild stage
2   moderate stage
3   severe stage
4   indeterminate stage

√x7ᵗʰ **H40.60** **Glaucoma secondary to drugs, unspecified eye**

√x7ᵗʰ **H40.61** **Glaucoma secondary to drugs, right eye**

√x7ᵗʰ **H40.62** **Glaucoma secondary to drugs, left eye**

√x7ᵗʰ **H40.63** **Glaucoma secondary to drugs, bilateral**

√5ᵗʰ **H40.8** **Other glaucoma**

√6ᵗʰ **H40.81** **Glaucoma with increased episcleral venous pressure**

H40.811 **Glaucoma with increased episcleral venous pressure, right eye**

H40.812 **Glaucoma with increased episcleral venous pressure, left eye**

H40.813 **Glaucoma with increased episcleral venous pressure, bilateral**

H40.819 **Glaucoma with increased episcleral venous pressure, unspecified eye**

√6ᵗʰ **H40.82** **Hypersecretion glaucoma**

H40.821 **Hypersecretion glaucoma, right eye**

H40.822 **Hypersecretion glaucoma, left eye**

H40.823 **Hypersecretion glaucoma, bilateral**

H40.829 **Hypersecretion glaucoma, unspecified eye**

√6ᵗʰ **H40.83** **Aqueous misdirection**

Malignant glaucoma

H40.831 **Aqueous misdirection, right eye**

H40.832 **Aqueous misdirection, left eye**

H40.833 **Aqueous misdirection, bilateral**

H40.839 **Aqueous misdirection, unspecified eye**

H40.89 **Other specified glaucoma**

H40.9 **Unspecified glaucoma**

H42 *Glaucoma in diseases classified elsewhere*

Code first underlying condition, such as:
amyloidosis (E85.-)
aniridia (Q13.1)
glaucoma (in) diabetes mellitus (E08.39, E09.39, E10.39, E11.39, E13.39)
Lowe's syndrome (E72.03)
Reiger's anomaly (Q13.81)
specified metabolic disorder (E70-E88)
EXCLUDES 1   glaucoma (in) onchocerciasis (B73.02)
     glaucoma (in) syphilis (A52.71)
     glaucoma (in) tuberculous (A18.59)

✔ Additional Character Required   √x7ᵗʰ Placeholder   Unacceptable PDx   Questionable PDx   Manifestation   Unspecified Dx   H1-H14 HAC   HCC CMS-HCC Dx   HIV HIV Dx

ICD-10-CM 2020

619

Disorders of vitreous body and globe (H43-H44)

✓4ᵗʰ H43 Disorders of vitreous body

✓5ᵗʰ H43.Ø Vitreous prolapse

EXCLUDES 1   *traumatic vitreous prolapse (SØ5.2-)*
            vitreous syndrome following cataract surgery (H59.Ø-)

H43.ØØ Vitreous prolapse, unspecified eye
H43.Ø1 Vitreous prolapse, right eye
H43.Ø2 Vitreous prolapse, left eye
H43.Ø3 Vitreous prolapse, bilateral

✓5ᵗʰ H43.1 Vitreous hemorrhage

H43.1Ø Vitreous hemorrhage, unspecified eye   HCC
H43.11 Vitreous hemorrhage, right eye   HCC
H43.12 Vitreous hemorrhage, left eye   HCC
H43.13 Vitreous hemorrhage, bilateral   HCC

✓5ᵗʰ H43.2 Crystalline deposits in vitreous body

H43.2Ø Crystalline deposits in vitreous body, unspecified eye
H43.21 Crystalline deposits in vitreous body, right eye
H43.22 Crystalline deposits in vitreous body, left eye
H43.23 Crystalline deposits in vitreous body, bilateral

✓5ᵗʰ H43.3 Other vitreous opacities

✓6ᵗʰ H43.31 Vitreous membranes and strands

H43.311 Vitreous membranes and strands, right eye
H43.312 Vitreous membranes and strands, left eye
H43.313 Vitreous membranes and strands, bilateral
H43.319 Vitreous membranes and strands, unspecified eye

✓6ᵗʰ H43.39 Other vitreous opacities

Vitreous floaters

H43.391 Other vitreous opacities, right eye
H43.392 Other vitreous opacities, left eye
H43.393 Other vitreous opacities, bilateral
H43.399 Other vitreous opacities, unspecified eye

✓5ᵗʰ H43.8 Other disorders of vitreous body

EXCLUDES 1   *proliferative vitreo-retinopathy with retinal detachment (H33.4-)*
EXCLUDES 2   *vitreous abscess (H44.Ø2-)*

✓6ᵗʰ H43.81 Vitreous degeneration

Vitreous detachment

H43.811 Vitreous degeneration, right eye
H43.812 Vitreous degeneration, left eye
H43.813 Vitreous degeneration, bilateral
H43.819 Vitreous degeneration, unspecified eye

✓6ᵗʰ H43.82 Vitreomacular adhesion

Vitreomacular traction

H43.821 Vitreomacular adhesion, right eye   A
H43.822 Vitreomacular adhesion, left eye   A
H43.823 Vitreomacular adhesion, bilateral   A
H43.829 Vitreomacular adhesion, unspecified eye   A

H43.89 Other disorders of vitreous body
H43.9 Unspecified disorder of vitreous body

✓4ᵗʰ H44 Disorders of globe

INCLUDES   disorders affecting multiple structures of eye

CC Excl: For CC codes in category H44, unless otherwise noted: PDX collection 625

✓5ᵗʰ H44.Ø Purulent endophthalmitis

Use additional code to identify organism
EXCLUDES 1   *bleb associated endophthalmitis (H59.4-)*

✓6ᵗʰ H44.ØØ Unspecified purulent endophthalmitis

H44.ØØ1 Unspecified purulent endophthalmitis, right eye   CC
H44.ØØ2 Unspecified purulent endophthalmitis, left eye   CC
H44.ØØ3 Unspecified purulent endophthalmitis, bilateral   CC

H44.ØØ9 Unspecified purulent endophthalmitis, unspecified eye   CC

✓6ᵗʰ H44.Ø1 Panophthalmitis (acute)

H44.Ø11 Panophthalmitis (acute), right eye   CC
H44.Ø12 Panophthalmitis (acute), left eye   CC
H44.Ø13 Panophthalmitis (acute), bilateral   CC
H44.Ø19 Panophthalmitis (acute), unspecified eye   CC

✓6ᵗʰ H44.Ø2 Vitreous abscess (chronic)

CC Excl: For CC codes in subcategory H44.Ø2: PDX collection 631

H44.Ø21 Vitreous abscess (chronic), right eye   CC
H44.Ø22 Vitreous abscess (chronic), left eye   CC
H44.Ø23 Vitreous abscess (chronic), bilateral   CC
H44.Ø29 Vitreous abscess (chronic), unspecified eye   CC

✓5ᵗʰ H44.1 Other endophthalmitis

EXCLUDES 1   *bleb associated endophthalmitis (H59.4-)*
EXCLUDES 2   *ophthalmia nodosa (H16.2-)*

✓6ᵗʰ H44.11 Panuveitis

DEF: Inflammation of all layers of the uvea of the eye, including the choroid, iris, and ciliary body. It also typically involves the lens, retina, optic nerve, and vitreous and causes reduced vision or blindness.
CC Excl: For CC codes in subcategory H44.11: PDX collection 632

H44.111 Panuveitis, right eye   CC
H44.112 Panuveitis, left eye   CC
H44.113 Panuveitis, bilateral   CC
H44.119 Panuveitis, unspecified eye   CC

✓6ᵗʰ H44.12 Parasitic endophthalmitis, unspecified

H44.121 Parasitic endophthalmitis, unspecified, right eye   CC
H44.122 Parasitic endophthalmitis, unspecified, left eye   CC
H44.123 Parasitic endophthalmitis, unspecified, bilateral   CC
H44.129 Parasitic endophthalmitis, unspecified, unspecified eye   CC

✓6ᵗʰ H44.13 Sympathetic uveitis

CC Excl: For CC codes in subcategory H44.13: PDX collection 632

H44.131 Sympathetic uveitis, right eye   CC
H44.132 Sympathetic uveitis, left eye   CC
H44.133 Sympathetic uveitis, bilateral   CC
H44.139 Sympathetic uveitis, unspecified eye   CC

H44.19 Other endophthalmitis   CC

✓5ᵗʰ H44.2 Degenerative myopia

Malignant myopia
AHA: 2017,4Q,10-11

H44.2Ø Degenerative myopia, unspecified eye
H44.21 Degenerative myopia, right eye
H44.22 Degenerative myopia, left eye
H44.23 Degenerative myopia, bilateral

✓6ᵗʰ H44.2A Degenerative myopia with choroidal neovascularization

Use additional code for any associated choroid disorders (H31.-)

H44.2A1 Degenerative myopia with choroidal neovascularization, right eye
H44.2A2 Degenerative myopia with choroidal neovascularization, left eye
H44.2A3 Degenerative myopia with choroidal neovascularization, bilateral eye
H44.2A9 Degenerative myopia with choroidal neovascularization, unspecified eye

---

N Newborn: 0   P Pediatric: 0-17   M Maternity: 9-64   A Adult: 15-124   MCC Major Complication/Comorbidity   CC Complication/Comorbidity   SW Severe Wound Dx

620   ICD-10-CM 2020

√6ᵗʰ **H44.2B** Degenerative myopia with macular hole

    H44.2B1 Degenerative myopia with macular hole, **right eye**

    H44.2B2 Degenerative myopia with macular hole, **left eye**

    H44.2B3 Degenerative myopia with macular hole, **bilateral eye**

    H44.2B9 Degenerative myopia with macular hole, **unspecified eye**

√6ᵗʰ **H44.2C** Degenerative myopia with retinal detachment

    Use additional code to identify the retinal detachment (H33.-)

    H44.2C1 Degenerative myopia with retinal detachment, **right eye**

    H44.2C2 Degenerative myopia with retinal detachment, **left eye**

    H44.2C3 Degenerative myopia with retinal detachment, **bilateral eye**

    H44.2C9 Degenerative myopia with retinal detachment, **unspecified eye**

√6ᵗʰ **H44.2D** Degenerative myopia with foveoschisis

    H44.2D1 Degenerative myopia with foveoschisis, **right eye**

    H44.2D2 Degenerative myopia with foveoschisis, **left eye**

    H44.2D3 Degenerative myopia with foveoschisis, **bilateral eye**

    H44.2D9 Degenerative myopia with foveoschisis, **unspecified eye**

√6ᵗʰ **H44.2E** Degenerative myopia with other maculopathy

    H44.2E1 Degenerative myopia with other maculopathy, **right eye**

    H44.2E2 Degenerative myopia with other maculopathy, **left eye**

    H44.2E3 Degenerative myopia with other maculopathy, **bilateral eye**

    H44.2E9 Degenerative myopia with other maculopathy, **unspecified eye**

√5ᵗʰ **H44.3** Other and unspecified degenerative disorders of globe

    H44.30 Unspecified degenerative disorder of globe

√6ᵗʰ **H44.31** Chalcosis

    H44.311 Chalcosis, **right eye**

    H44.312 Chalcosis, **left eye**

    H44.313 Chalcosis, **bilateral**

    H44.319 Chalcosis, **unspecified eye**

√6ᵗʰ **H44.32** Siderosis of eye

    DEF: Iron pigment deposits within tissue of the eyeball caused by high iron content of the blood. Symptoms include cataracts, rust-colored anterior subcapsular deposits, iris heterochromia, pupillary mydriasis, and depressed electroretinogram amplitudes.

    H44.321 Siderosis of eye, **right eye**

    H44.322 Siderosis of eye, **left eye**

    H44.323 Siderosis of eye, **bilateral**

    H44.329 Siderosis of eye, **unspecified eye**

√6ᵗʰ **H44.39** Other degenerative disorders of globe

    H44.391 Other degenerative disorders of globe, **right eye**

    H44.392 Other degenerative disorders of globe, **left eye**

    H44.393 Other degenerative disorders of globe, **bilateral**

    H44.399 Other degenerative disorders of globe, **unspecified eye**

√5ᵗʰ **H44.4** Hypotony of eye

    H44.40 Unspecified hypotony of eye

√6ᵗʰ **H44.41** Flat anterior chamber hypotony of eye

    H44.411 Flat anterior chamber hypotony of **right eye**

    H44.412 Flat anterior chamber hypotony of **left eye**

    H44.413 Flat anterior chamber hypotony of eye, **bilateral**

    H44.419 Flat anterior chamber hypotony of **unspecified eye**

√6ᵗʰ **H44.42** Hypotony of eye due to ocular fistula

    H44.421 Hypotony of **right eye** due to ocular fistula

    H44.422 Hypotony of **left eye** due to ocular fistula

    H44.423 Hypotony of eye due to ocular fistula, **bilateral**

    H44.429 Hypotony of unspecified eye due to ocular fistula

√6ᵗʰ **H44.43** Hypotony of eye due to other ocular disorders

    H44.431 Hypotony of eye due to other ocular disorders, **right eye**

    H44.432 Hypotony of eye due to other ocular disorders, **left eye**

    H44.433 Hypotony of eye due to other ocular disorders, **bilateral**

    H44.439 Hypotony of eye due to other ocular disorders, **unspecified eye**

√6ᵗʰ **H44.44** Primary hypotony of eye

    H44.441 Primary hypotony of **right eye**

    H44.442 Primary hypotony of **left eye**

    H44.443 Primary hypotony of eye, **bilateral**

    H44.449 Primary hypotony of unspecified eye

√5ᵗʰ **H44.5** Degenerated conditions of globe

    H44.50 Unspecified degenerated conditions of globe

√6ᵗʰ **H44.51** Absolute glaucoma

    H44.511 Absolute glaucoma, **right eye**

    H44.512 Absolute glaucoma, **left eye**

    H44.513 Absolute glaucoma, **bilateral**

    H44.519 Absolute glaucoma, **unspecified eye**

√6ᵗʰ **H44.52** Atrophy of globe

    Phthisis bulbi

    H44.521 Atrophy of globe, **right eye**

    H44.522 Atrophy of globe, **left eye**

    H44.523 Atrophy of globe, **bilateral**

    H44.529 Atrophy of globe, **unspecified eye**

√6ᵗʰ **H44.53** Leucocoria

    H44.531 Leucocoria, **right eye**

    H44.532 Leucocoria, **left eye**

    H44.533 Leucocoria, **bilateral**

    H44.539 Leucocoria, **unspecified eye**

√5ᵗʰ **H44.6** Retained (old) intraocular foreign body, **magnetic**

    Use additional code to identify magnetic foreign body (Z18.11)

    EXCLUDES 1 current intraocular foreign body (S05.-)

    EXCLUDES 2 retained foreign body in eyelid (H02.81-)

        retained (old) foreign body following penetrating wound of orbit (H05.5-)

        retained (old) intraocular foreign body, nonmagnetic (H44.7-)

√6ᵗʰ **H44.60** Unspecified retained (old) intraocular foreign body, magnetic

    H44.601 Unspecified retained (old) intraocular foreign body, magnetic, **right eye**

    H44.602 Unspecified retained (old) intraocular foreign body, magnetic, **left eye**

    H44.603 Unspecified retained (old) intraocular foreign body, magnetic, **bilateral**

    H44.609 Unspecified retained (old) intraocular foreign body, magnetic, **unspecified eye**

√6ᵗʰ **H44.61** Retained (old) magnetic foreign body in **anterior chamber**

    H44.611 Retained (old) magnetic foreign body in anterior chamber, **right eye**

    H44.612 Retained (old) magnetic foreign body in anterior chamber, **left eye**

    H44.613 Retained (old) magnetic foreign body in anterior chamber, **bilateral**

    H44.619 Retained (old) magnetic foreign body in anterior chamber, **unspecified eye**

√6ᵗʰ **H44.62** Retained (old) magnetic foreign body in **iris or ciliary body**

    H44.621 Retained (old) magnetic foreign body in iris or ciliary body, **right eye**

    H44.622 Retained (old) magnetic foreign body in iris or ciliary body, **left eye**

    H44.623 Retained (old) magnetic foreign body in iris or ciliary body, **bilateral**

    H44.629 Retained (old) magnetic foreign body in iris or ciliary body, **unspecified eye**

√6ᵗʰ **H44.63** Retained (old) magnetic foreign body in **lens**

    H44.631 Retained (old) magnetic foreign body in lens, **right eye**

    H44.632 Retained (old) magnetic foreign body in lens, **left eye**

☑ Additional Character Required   √x7ᵗʰ Placeholder   Unacceptable PDx   Questionable PDx   Manifestation   Unspecified Dx   H1 - H4 HAC   HCC CMS-HCC Dx   HIV HIV Dx

ICD-10-CM 2020   621

Chapter 7. Diseases of the Eye and Adnexa

H44.633–H46.12

H44.633 Retained (old) magnetic foreign body in lens, **bilateral**

H44.639 Retained (old) magnetic foreign body in lens, **unspecified eye**

✓6ᵗʰ **H44.64** Retained (old) magnetic foreign body in **posterior wall of globe**

H44.641 Retained (old) magnetic foreign body in posterior wall of globe, **right eye**

H44.642 Retained (old) magnetic foreign body in posterior wall of globe, **left eye**

H44.643 Retained (old) magnetic foreign body in posterior wall of globe, **bilateral**

H44.649 Retained (old) magnetic foreign body in posterior wall of globe, **unspecified eye**

✓6ᵗʰ **H44.65** Retained (old) magnetic foreign body in **vitreous body**

H44.651 Retained (old) magnetic foreign body in vitreous body, **right eye**

H44.652 Retained (old) magnetic foreign body in vitreous body, **left eye**

H44.653 Retained (old) magnetic foreign body in vitreous body, **bilateral**

H44.659 Retained (old) magnetic foreign body in vitreous body, **unspecified eye**

✓6ᵗʰ **H44.69** Retained (old) intraocular foreign body, magnetic, **in other or multiple sites**

H44.691 Retained (old) intraocular foreign body, magnetic, in other or multiple sites, **right eye**

H44.692 Retained (old) intraocular foreign body, magnetic, in other or multiple sites, **left eye**

H44.693 Retained (old) intraocular foreign body, magnetic, in other or multiple sites, **bilateral**

H44.699 Retained (old) intraocular foreign body, magnetic, in other or multiple sites, **unspecified eye**

✓5ᵗʰ **H44.7** Retained (old) intraocular foreign body, **nonmagnetic**

Use additional code to identify nonmagnetic foreign body (Z18.01-Z18.10, Z18.12, Z18.2-Z18.9)

EXCLUDES 1 current intraocular foreign body (S05.-)

EXCLUDES 2 retained foreign body in eyelid (H02.81-)

retained (old) foreign body following penetrating wound of orbit (H05.5-)

retained (old) intraocular foreign body, magnetic (H44.6-)

✓6ᵗʰ **H44.70** Unspecified retained (old) intraocular foreign body, **nonmagnetic**

H44.701 Unspecified retained (old) intraocular foreign body, nonmagnetic, **right eye**

H44.702 Unspecified retained (old) intraocular foreign body, nonmagnetic, **left eye**

H44.703 Unspecified retained (old) intraocular foreign body, nonmagnetic, **bilateral**

H44.709 Unspecified retained (old) intraocular foreign body, nonmagnetic, **unspecified eye**

Retained (old) intraocular foreign body NOS

✓6ᵗʰ **H44.71** Retained (nonmagnetic) (old) foreign body in **anterior chamber**

H44.711 Retained (nonmagnetic) (old) foreign body in anterior chamber, **right eye**

H44.712 Retained (nonmagnetic) (old) foreign body in anterior chamber, **left eye**

H44.713 Retained (nonmagnetic) (old) foreign body in anterior chamber, **bilateral**

H44.719 Retained (nonmagnetic) (old) foreign body in anterior chamber, **unspecified eye**

✓6ᵗʰ **H44.72** Retained (nonmagnetic) (old) foreign body in **iris or ciliary body**

H44.721 Retained (nonmagnetic) (old) foreign body in iris or ciliary body, **right eye**

H44.722 Retained (nonmagnetic) (old) foreign body in iris or ciliary body, **left eye**

H44.723 Retained (nonmagnetic) (old) foreign body in iris or ciliary body, **bilateral**

H44.729 Retained (nonmagnetic) (old) foreign body in iris or ciliary body, **unspecified eye**

✓6ᵗʰ **H44.73** Retained (nonmagnetic) (old) foreign body in **lens**

H44.731 Retained (nonmagnetic) (old) foreign body in lens, **right eye**

H44.732 Retained (nonmagnetic) (old) foreign body in lens, **left eye**

H44.733 Retained (nonmagnetic) (old) foreign body in lens, **bilateral**

H44.739 Retained (nonmagnetic) (old) foreign body in lens, **unspecified eye**

✓6ᵗʰ **H44.74** Retained (nonmagnetic) (old) foreign body in **posterior wall of globe**

H44.741 Retained (nonmagnetic) (old) foreign body in posterior wall of globe, **right eye**

H44.742 Retained (nonmagnetic) (old) foreign body in posterior wall of globe, **left eye**

H44.743 Retained (nonmagnetic) (old) foreign body in posterior wall of globe, **bilateral**

H44.749 Retained (nonmagnetic) (old) foreign body in posterior wall of globe, **unspecified eye**

✓6ᵗʰ **H44.75** Retained (nonmagnetic) (old) foreign body in **vitreous body**

H44.751 Retained (nonmagnetic) (old) foreign body in vitreous body, **right eye**

H44.752 Retained (nonmagnetic) (old) foreign body in vitreous body, **left eye**

H44.753 Retained (nonmagnetic) (old) foreign body in vitreous body, **bilateral**

H44.759 Retained (nonmagnetic) (old) foreign body in vitreous body, **unspecified eye**

✓6ᵗʰ **H44.79** Retained (old) intraocular foreign body, **nonmagnetic, in other or multiple sites**

H44.791 Retained (old) intraocular foreign body, nonmagnetic, in other or multiple sites, **right eye**

H44.792 Retained (old) intraocular foreign body, nonmagnetic, in other or multiple sites, **left eye**

H44.793 Retained (old) intraocular foreign body, nonmagnetic, in other or multiple sites, **bilateral**

H44.799 Retained (old) intraocular foreign body, nonmagnetic, in other or multiple sites, **unspecified eye**

✓5ᵗʰ **H44.8** Other disorders of globe

✓6ᵗʰ **H44.81** Hemophthalmos

DEF: Pool of blood within the eyeball, not from a current injury.

H44.811 Hemophthalmos, **right eye**

H44.812 Hemophthalmos, **left eye**

H44.813 Hemophthalmos, **bilateral**

H44.819 Hemophthalmos, **unspecified eye**

✓6ᵗʰ **H44.82** Luxation of globe

H44.821 Luxation of globe, **right eye**

H44.822 Luxation of globe, **left eye**

H44.823 Luxation of globe, **bilateral**

H44.829 Luxation of globe, **unspecified eye**

H44.89 Other disorders of globe

H44.9 Unspecified disorder of globe

Disorders of optic nerve and visual pathways (H46-H47)

✓4ᵗʰ **H46** Optic neuritis

EXCLUDES 2 ischemic optic neuropathy (H47.01-)

neuromyelitis optica [Devic] (G36.0)

CC Excl: For CC codes in category H46: PDX collection 633

✓5ᵗʰ **H46.0** Optic papillitis

H46.00 Optic papillitis, **unspecified eye** — CC

H46.01 Optic papillitis, **right eye** — CC

H46.02 Optic papillitis, **left eye** — CC

H46.03 Optic papillitis, **bilateral** — CC

✓5ᵗʰ **H46.1** Retrobulbar neuritis

Retrobulbar neuritis NOS

EXCLUDES 1 syphilitic retrobulbar neuritis (A52.15)

H46.10 Retrobulbar neuritis, **unspecified eye** — CC

H46.11 Retrobulbar neuritis, **right eye** — CC

H46.12 Retrobulbar neuritis, **left eye** — CC

N Newborn: 0   P Pediatric: 0-17   M Maternity: 9-64   A Adult: 15-124   **MCC** Major Complication/Comorbidity   **CC** Complication/Comorbidity   **SW** Severe Wound Dx

622   ICD-10-CM 2020

H46.13   **Retrobulbar neuritis,** bilateral   `CC`

H46.2   **Nutritional** optic neuropathy

H46.3   **Toxic** optic neuropathy
    Code first (T51-T65) to identify cause

H46.8   **Other optic neuritis**   `CC`

H46.9   **Unspecified optic neuritis**   `CC`

√4ᵗʰ **H47**   **Other disorders of optic [2nd] nerve and visual pathways**

   √5ᵗʰ **H47.0**   **Disorders of optic nerve, not elsewhere classified**

     √6ᵗʰ **H47.01**   **Ischemic** optic neuropathy

       H47.011   **Ischemic optic neuropathy,** right eye
       H47.012   **Ischemic optic neuropathy,** left eye
       H47.013   **Ischemic optic neuropathy,** bilateral
       H47.019   **Ischemic optic neuropathy, unspecified eye**

     √6ᵗʰ **H47.02**   **Hemorrhage** in optic nerve sheath

       H47.021   **Hemorrhage in optic nerve sheath,** right eye
       H47.022   **Hemorrhage in optic nerve sheath,** left eye
       H47.023   **Hemorrhage in optic nerve sheath,** bilateral
       H47.029   **Hemorrhage in optic nerve sheath, unspecified eye**

     √6ᵗʰ **H47.03**   **Optic nerve** hypoplasia

       H47.031   **Optic nerve hypoplasia,** right eye
       H47.032   **Optic nerve hypoplasia,** left eye
       H47.033   **Optic nerve hypoplasia,** bilateral
       H47.039   **Optic nerve hypoplasia, unspecified eye**

     √6ᵗʰ **H47.09**   **Other disorders of optic nerve, not elsewhere classified**
       Compression of optic nerve
       H47.091   **Other disorders of optic nerve, not elsewhere classified,** right eye
       H47.092   **Other disorders of optic nerve, not elsewhere classified,** left eye
       H47.093   **Other disorders of optic nerve, not elsewhere classified,** bilateral
       H47.099   **Other disorders of optic nerve, not elsewhere classified, unspecified eye**

   √5ᵗʰ **H47.1**   **Papilledema**

     DEF: Swelling of the optic papilla, the raised area connected to the optic disk made up of nerves that enter the eyeball. It may be caused by increased intracranial pressure, decreased ocular pressure, or a retinal disorder.

     H47.10   **Unspecified papilledema**   `CC`
       CC Excl: PDX collection 634

     H47.11   **Papilledema associated with increased intracranial pressure**   `CC`
       CC Excl: PDX collection 634

     H47.12   **Papilledema associated with** decreased ocular pressure

     H47.13   **Papilledema associated with** retinal disorder

     √6ᵗʰ **H47.14**   **Foster-Kennedy syndrome**

       H47.141   **Foster-Kennedy syndrome,** right eye
       H47.142   **Foster-Kennedy syndrome,** left eye
       H47.143   **Foster-Kennedy syndrome,** bilateral
       H47.149   **Foster-Kennedy syndrome, unspecified eye**

   √5ᵗʰ **H47.2**   **Optic atrophy**

     H47.20   **Unspecified optic atrophy**

     √6ᵗʰ **H47.21**   **Primary optic atrophy**

       H47.211   **Primary optic atrophy,** right eye
       H47.212   **Primary optic atrophy,** left eye
       H47.213   **Primary optic atrophy,** bilateral
       H47.219   **Primary optic atrophy, unspecified eye**

     H47.22   **Hereditary** optic atrophy
       Leber's optic atrophy

     √6ᵗʰ **H47.23**   **Glaucomatous** optic atrophy

       H47.231   **Glaucomatous optic atrophy,** right eye
       H47.232   **Glaucomatous optic atrophy,** left eye
       H47.233   **Glaucomatous optic atrophy,** bilateral
       H47.239   **Glaucomatous optic atrophy, unspecified eye**

     √6ᵗʰ **H47.29**   **Other optic atrophy**
       Temporal pallor of optic disc
       H47.291   **Other optic atrophy,** right eye
       H47.292   **Other optic atrophy,** left eye

       H47.293   **Other optic atrophy,** bilateral
       H47.299   **Other optic atrophy, unspecified eye**

   √5ᵗʰ **H47.3**   **Other disorders of optic disc**

     √6ᵗʰ **H47.31**   **Coloboma** of optic disc

       H47.311   **Coloboma of optic disc,** right eye
       H47.312   **Coloboma of optic disc,** left eye
       H47.313   **Coloboma of optic disc,** bilateral
       H47.319   **Coloboma of optic disc, unspecified eye**

     √6ᵗʰ **H47.32**   **Drusen** of optic disc

       H47.321   **Drusen of optic disc,** right eye
       H47.322   **Drusen of optic disc,** left eye
       H47.323   **Drusen of optic disc,** bilateral
       H47.329   **Drusen of optic disc, unspecified eye**

     √6ᵗʰ **H47.33**   **Pseudopapilledema** of optic disc

       H47.331   **Pseudopapilledema of optic disc,** right eye
       H47.332   **Pseudopapilledema of optic disc,** left eye
       H47.333   **Pseudopapilledema of optic disc,** bilateral
       H47.339   **Pseudopapilledema of optic disc, unspecified eye**

     √6ᵗʰ **H47.39**   **Other disorders of optic disc**

       H47.391   **Other disorders of optic disc,** right eye
       H47.392   **Other disorders of optic disc,** left eye
       H47.393   **Other disorders of optic disc,** bilateral
       H47.399   **Other disorders of optic disc, unspecified eye**

   √5ᵗʰ **H47.4**   **Disorders of optic chiasm**
     Code also underlying condition
     CC Excl: For CC codes in subcategory H47.4: PDX collection 635

     H47.41   **Disorders of optic chiasm in (due to) inflammatory disorders**   `CC`

     H47.42   **Disorders of optic chiasm in (due to) neoplasm**   `CC`

     H47.43   **Disorders of optic chiasm in (due to) vascular disorders**   `CC`

     H47.49   **Disorders of optic chiasm in (due to) other disorders**   `CC`

   √5ᵗʰ **H47.5**   **Disorders of other visual pathways**
     Disorders of optic tracts, geniculate nuclei and optic radiations
     Code also underlying condition
     CC Excl: For CC codes in subcategory H47.5: PDX collection 635

     √6ᵗʰ **H47.51**   **Disorders of visual pathways in (due to) inflammatory disorders**

       H47.511   **Disorders of visual pathways in (due to) inflammatory disorders, right side**   `CC`
       H47.512   **Disorders of visual pathways in (due to) inflammatory disorders, left side**   `CC`
       H47.519   **Disorders of visual pathways in (due to) inflammatory disorders, unspecified side**   `CC`

     √6ᵗʰ **H47.52**   **Disorders of visual pathways in (due to) neoplasm**

       H47.521   **Disorders of visual pathways in (due to) neoplasm, right side**   `CC`
       H47.522   **Disorders of visual pathways in (due to) neoplasm, left side**   `CC`
       H47.529   **Disorders of visual pathways in (due to) neoplasm, unspecified side**   `CC`

     √6ᵗʰ **H47.53**   **Disorders of visual pathways in (due to)** vascular disorders

       H47.531   **Disorders of visual pathways in (due to) vascular disorders, right side**   `CC`
       H47.532   **Disorders of visual pathways in (due to) vascular disorders, left side**   `CC`

☑ Additional Character Required   √x7ᵗʰ Placeholder   Unacceptable PDx   Questionable PDx   Manifestation   Unspecified Dx   H1-H4 HAC   HCC CMS-HCC Dx   HIV HIV Dx

ICD-10-CM 2020

623

Chapter 7. Diseases of the Eye and Adnexa

H47.539 Disorders of visual pathways in (due to) vascular disorders, unspecified side `CC`

✓5ᵗʰ **H47.6 Disorders of visual cortex**

Code also underlying condition

`EXCLUDES 1` injury to visual cortex ▶S04.04-◀

CC Excl: For CC codes in subcategory H47.6: PDX collection 636

✓6ᵗʰ **H47.61 Cortical blindness**

H47.611 Cortical blindness, right side of brain
H47.612 Cortical blindness, left side of brain
H47.619 Cortical blindness, unspecified side of brain

✓6ᵗʰ **H47.62 Disorders of visual cortex in (due to) inflammatory disorders**

H47.621 Disorders of visual cortex in (due to) inflammatory disorders, right side of brain `CC`
H47.622 Disorders of visual cortex in (due to) inflammatory disorders, left side of brain `CC`
H47.629 Disorders of visual cortex in (due to) inflammatory disorders, unspecified side of brain `CC`

✓6ᵗʰ **H47.63 Disorders of visual cortex in (due to) neoplasm**

H47.631 Disorders of visual cortex in (due to) neoplasm, right side of brain `CC`
H47.632 Disorders of visual cortex in (due to) neoplasm, left side of brain `CC`
H47.639 Disorders of visual cortex in (due to) neoplasm, unspecified side of brain `CC`

✓6ᵗʰ **H47.64 Disorders of visual cortex in (due to) vascular disorders**

H47.641 Disorders of visual cortex in (due to) vascular disorders, right side of brain `CC`
H47.642 Disorders of visual cortex in (due to) vascular disorders, left side of brain `CC`
H47.649 Disorders of visual cortex in (due to) vascular disorders, unspecified side of brain `CC`

H47.9 Unspecified disorder of visual pathways

Disorders of ocular muscles, binocular movement, accommodation and refraction (H49-H52)

`EXCLUDES 2` nystagmus and other irregular eye movements (H55)

✓4ᵗʰ **H49 Paralytic strabismus**

`EXCLUDES 2` internal ophthalmoplegia (H52.51-)
internuclear ophthalmoplegia (H51.2-)
progressive supranuclear ophthalmoplegia (G23.1)

DEF: Strabismus: Misalignment of the eyes with the inability to move and focus in the same direction due to conditions affecting the muscles controlling them.

✓5ᵗʰ **H49.0 Third [oculomotor] nerve palsy**

H49.00 Third [oculomotor] nerve palsy, unspecified eye
H49.01 Third [oculomotor] nerve palsy, right eye
H49.02 Third [oculomotor] nerve palsy, left eye
H49.03 Third [oculomotor] nerve palsy, bilateral

✓5ᵗʰ **H49.1 Fourth [trochlear] nerve palsy**

H49.10 Fourth [trochlear] nerve palsy, unspecified eye
H49.11 Fourth [trochlear] nerve palsy, right eye
H49.12 Fourth [trochlear] nerve palsy, left eye
H49.13 Fourth [trochlear] nerve palsy, bilateral

✓5ᵗʰ **H49.2 Sixth [abducent] nerve palsy**

H49.20 Sixth [abducent] nerve palsy, unspecified eye
H49.21 Sixth [abducent] nerve palsy, right eye
H49.22 Sixth [abducent] nerve palsy, left eye
H49.23 Sixth [abducent] nerve palsy, bilateral

✓5ᵗʰ **H49.3 Total (external) ophthalmoplegia**

H49.30 Total (external) ophthalmoplegia, unspecified eye

H49.31 Total (external) ophthalmoplegia, right eye
H49.32 Total (external) ophthalmoplegia, left eye
H49.33 Total (external) ophthalmoplegia, bilateral

✓5ᵗʰ **H49.4 Progressive external ophthalmoplegia**

`EXCLUDES 1` Kearns-Sayre syndrome (H49.81-)

H49.40 Progressive external ophthalmoplegia, unspecified eye
H49.41 Progressive external ophthalmoplegia, right eye
H49.42 Progressive external ophthalmoplegia, left eye
H49.43 Progressive external ophthalmoplegia, bilateral

✓5ᵗʰ **H49.8 Other paralytic strabismus**

✓6ᵗʰ **H49.81 Kearns-Sayre syndrome**

Progressive external ophthalmoplegia with pigmentary retinopathy

Use additional code for other manifestation, such as: heart block (I45.9)

CC Excl: For CC codes in subcategory H49.81: PDX collection 545

H49.811 Kearns-Sayre syndrome, right eye `CC` `HCC`
H49.812 Kearns-Sayre syndrome, left eye `CC` `HCC`
H49.813 Kearns-Sayre syndrome, bilateral `CC` `HCC`
H49.819 Kearns-Sayre syndrome, unspecified eye `CC` `HCC`

✓6ᵗʰ **H49.88 Other paralytic strabismus**

External ophthalmoplegia NOS

H49.881 Other paralytic strabismus, right eye
H49.882 Other paralytic strabismus, left eye
H49.883 Other paralytic strabismus, bilateral
H49.889 Other paralytic strabismus, unspecified eye

H49.9 Unspecified paralytic strabismus

✓4ᵗʰ **H50 Other strabismus**

DEF: Strabismus: Misalignment of the eyes with the inability to move and focus in the same direction due to conditions affecting the muscles controlling them.

✓5ᵗʰ **H50.0 Esotropia**

Convergent concomitant strabismus

`EXCLUDES 1` intermittent esotropia (H50.31-, H50.32)

H50.00 Unspecified esotropia

✓6ᵗʰ **H50.01 Monocular esotropia**

H50.011 Monocular esotropia, right eye
H50.012 Monocular esotropia, left eye

✓6ᵗʰ **H50.02 Monocular esotropia with A pattern**

H50.021 Monocular esotropia with A pattern, right eye
H50.022 Monocular esotropia with A pattern, left eye

✓6ᵗʰ **H50.03 Monocular esotropia with V pattern**

H50.031 Monocular esotropia with V pattern, right eye
H50.032 Monocular esotropia with V pattern, left eye

✓6ᵗʰ **H50.04 Monocular esotropia with other noncomitancies**

H50.041 Monocular esotropia with other noncomitancies, right eye
H50.042 Monocular esotropia with other noncomitancies, left eye

H50.05 Alternating esotropia
H50.06 Alternating esotropia with A pattern
H50.07 Alternating esotropia with V pattern

Ⓝ Newborn: 0   Ⓟ Pediatric: 0-17   Ⓜ Maternity: 9-64   Ⓐ Adult: 15-124   `MCC` Major Complication/Comorbidity   `CC` Complication/Comorbidity   `SW` Severe Wound Dx

624   ICD-10-CM 2020

H50.08   Alternating esotropia with other noncomitancies

Eye Muscle Diseases

R.   L.
Monocular (one eye only) esotropia (inward)

Monocular exotropia (outward)

Monocular hypertropia (upward)

✓5ᵗʰ **H50.1   Exotropia**

Divergent concomitant strabismus

EXCLUDES 1   *intermittent exotropia (H50.33-, H50.34)*

H50.10   Unspecified exotropia

✓6ᵗʰ **H50.11   Monocular exotropia**

H50.111   Monocular exotropia, right eye
H50.112   Monocular exotropia, left eye

✓6ᵗʰ **H50.12   Monocular exotropia with A pattern**

H50.121   Monocular exotropia with A pattern, right eye
H50.122   Monocular exotropia with A pattern, left eye

✓6ᵗʰ **H50.13   Monocular exotropia with V pattern**

H50.131   Monocular exotropia with V pattern, right eye
H50.132   Monocular exotropia with V pattern, left eye

✓6ᵗʰ **H50.14   Monocular exotropia with other noncomitancies**

H50.141   Monocular exotropia with other noncomitancies, right eye
H50.142   Monocular exotropia with other noncomitancies, left eye

H50.15   Alternating exotropia
H50.16   Alternating exotropia with A pattern
H50.17   Alternating exotropia with V pattern
H50.18   Alternating exotropia with other noncomitancies

✓5ᵗʰ **H50.2   Vertical strabismus**

Hypertropia

H50.21   Vertical strabismus, right eye
H50.22   Vertical strabismus, left eye

✓5ᵗʰ **H50.3   Intermittent heterotropia**

H50.30   Unspecified intermittent heterotropia

✓6ᵗʰ **H50.31   Intermittent monocular esotropia**

H50.311   Intermittent monocular esotropia, right eye
H50.312   Intermittent monocular esotropia, left eye

H50.32   Intermittent alternating esotropia

✓6ᵗʰ **H50.33   Intermittent monocular exotropia**

H50.331   Intermittent monocular exotropia, right eye
H50.332   Intermittent monocular exotropia, left eye

H50.34   Intermittent alternating exotropia

✓5ᵗʰ **H50.4   Other and unspecified heterotropia**

H50.40   Unspecified heterotropia

✓6ᵗʰ **H50.41   Cyclotropia**

H50.411   Cyclotropia, right eye
H50.412   Cyclotropia, left eye

H50.42   Monofixation syndrome

H50.43   Accommodative component in esotropia

✓5ᵗʰ **H50.5   Heterophoria**

H50.50   Unspecified heterophoria
H50.51   Esophoria
H50.52   Exophoria
H50.53   Vertical heterophoria
H50.54   Cyclophoria
H50.55   Alternating heterophoria

✓5ᵗʰ **H50.6   Mechanical strabismus**

H50.60   Mechanical strabismus, unspecified

✓6ᵗʰ **H50.61   Brown's sheath syndrome**

H50.611   Brown's sheath syndrome, right eye
H50.612   Brown's sheath syndrome, left eye

H50.69   Other mechanical strabismus

Strabismus due to adhesions
Traumatic limitation of duction of eye muscle

✓5ᵗʰ **H50.8   Other specified strabismus**

✓6ᵗʰ **H50.81   Duane's syndrome**

H50.811   Duane's syndrome, right eye
H50.812   Duane's syndrome, left eye

H50.89   Other specified strabismus

H50.9   Unspecified strabismus

✓4ᵗʰ **H51   Other disorders of binocular movement**

H51.0   Palsy (spasm) of conjugate gaze

✓5ᵗʰ **H51.1   Convergence insufficiency and excess**

H51.11   Convergence insufficiency
H51.12   Convergence excess

✓5ᵗʰ **H51.2   Internuclear ophthalmoplegia**

H51.20   Internuclear ophthalmoplegia, unspecified eye
H51.21   Internuclear ophthalmoplegia, right eye
H51.22   Internuclear ophthalmoplegia, left eye
H51.23   Internuclear ophthalmoplegia, bilateral

H51.8   Other specified disorders of binocular movement
H51.9   Unspecified disorder of binocular movement

✓4ᵗʰ **H52   Disorders of refraction and accommodation**

✓5ᵗʰ **H52.0   Hypermetropia**

H52.00   Hypermetropia, unspecified eye
H52.01   Hypermetropia, right eye
H52.02   Hypermetropia, left eye
H52.03   Hypermetropia, bilateral

✓5ᵗʰ **H52.1   Myopia**

EXCLUDES 1   *degenerative myopia (H44.2-)*

H52.10   Myopia, unspecified eye
H52.11   Myopia, right eye
H52.12   Myopia, left eye
H52.13   Myopia, bilateral

✓5ᵗʰ **H52.2   Astigmatism**

✓6ᵗʰ **H52.20   Unspecified astigmatism**

H52.201   Unspecified astigmatism, right eye
H52.202   Unspecified astigmatism, left eye
H52.203   Unspecified astigmatism, bilateral
H52.209   Unspecified astigmatism, unspecified eye

✓6ᵗʰ **H52.21   Irregular astigmatism**

H52.211   Irregular astigmatism, right eye
H52.212   Irregular astigmatism, left eye
H52.213   Irregular astigmatism, bilateral
H52.219   Irregular astigmatism, unspecified eye

✓6ᵗʰ **H52.22   Regular astigmatism**

H52.221   Regular astigmatism, right eye
H52.222   Regular astigmatism, left eye
H52.223   Regular astigmatism, bilateral
H52.229   Regular astigmatism, unspecified eye

✓5ᵗʰ **H52.3   Anisometropia and aniseikonia**

H52.31   Anisometropia
H52.32   Aniseikonia

H52.4   Presbyopia

✓5ᵗʰ **H52.5   Disorders of accommodation**

✓6ᵗʰ **H52.51   Internal ophthalmoplegia (complete) (total)**

H52.511   Internal ophthalmoplegia (complete) (total), right eye
H52.512   Internal ophthalmoplegia (complete) (total), left eye

Chapter 7. Diseases of the Eye and Adnexa

H52.513   Internal ophthalmoplegia (complete) (total), **bilateral**

H52.519   Internal ophthalmoplegia (complete) (total), **unspecified eye**

✓6ᵗʰ **H52.52   Paresis of accommodation**

H52.521   Paresis of accommodation, **right eye**
H52.522   Paresis of accommodation, **left eye**
H52.523   Paresis of accommodation, **bilateral**
H52.529   Paresis of accommodation, **unspecified eye**

✓6ᵗʰ **H52.53   Spasm of accommodation**

H52.531   Spasm of accommodation, **right eye**
H52.532   Spasm of accommodation, **left eye**
H52.533   Spasm of accommodation, **bilateral**
H52.539   Spasm of accommodation, **unspecified eye**

H52.6   **Other disorders of refraction**

H52.7   **Unspecified disorder of refraction**

Visual disturbances and blindness (H53-H54)

✓4ᵗʰ **H53   Visual disturbances**

✓5ᵗʰ **H53.0   Amblyopia ex anopsia**

    EXCLUDES 1   *amblyopia due to vitamin A deficiency (E50.5)*

✓6ᵗʰ **H53.00   Unspecified amblyopia**

H53.001   Unspecified amblyopia, **right eye**
H53.002   Unspecified amblyopia, **left eye**
H53.003   Unspecified amblyopia, **bilateral**
H53.009   Unspecified amblyopia, **unspecified eye**

✓6ᵗʰ **H53.01   Deprivation amblyopia**

H53.011   Deprivation amblyopia, **right eye**
H53.012   Deprivation amblyopia, **left eye**
H53.013   Deprivation amblyopia, **bilateral**
H53.019   Deprivation amblyopia, **unspecified eye**

✓6ᵗʰ **H53.02   Refractive amblyopia**

H53.021   Refractive amblyopia, **right eye**
H53.022   Refractive amblyopia, **left eye**
H53.023   Refractive amblyopia, **bilateral**
H53.029   Refractive amblyopia, **unspecified eye**

✓6ᵗʰ **H53.03   Strabismic amblyopia**

    EXCLUDES 1   *strabismus (H50.-)*

H53.031   Strabismic amblyopia, **right eye**
H53.032   Strabismic amblyopia, **left eye**
H53.033   Strabismic amblyopia, **bilateral**
H53.039   Strabismic amblyopia, **unspecified eye**

✓6ᵗʰ **H53.04   Amblyopia suspect**

    AHA: 2016,4Q,22-23

H53.041   Amblyopia suspect, **right eye**
H53.042   Amblyopia suspect, **left eye**
H53.043   Amblyopia suspect, **bilateral**
H53.049   Amblyopia suspect, **unspecified eye**

✓5ᵗʰ **H53.1   Subjective visual disturbances**

    EXCLUDES 1   *subjective visual disturbances due to vitamin A deficiency (E50.5)*
                  visual hallucinations (R44.1)

    CC Excl: CC codes in subcategory H53.1: PDX collection 637

H53.10   **Unspecified subjective visual disturbances**

H53.11   **Day blindness**
          Hemeralopia

✓6ᵗʰ **H53.12   Transient visual loss**

          Scintillating scotoma
    EXCLUDES 1   *amaurosis fugax (G45.3-)*
                  transient retinal artery occlusion (H34.0-)

H53.121   Transient visual loss, **right eye**   cc
H53.122   Transient visual loss, **left eye**   cc
H53.123   Transient visual loss, **bilateral**   cc
H53.129   Transient visual loss, **unspecified eye**   cc

✓6ᵗʰ **H53.13   Sudden visual loss**

H53.131   Sudden visual loss, **right eye**   cc
H53.132   Sudden visual loss, **left eye**   cc

H53.133   Sudden visual loss, **bilateral**   cc

H53.139   Sudden visual loss, **unspecified eye**   cc

✓6ᵗʰ **H53.14   Visual discomfort**

          Asthenopia
          Photophobia

H53.141   Visual discomfort, **right eye**
H53.142   Visual discomfort, **left eye**
H53.143   Visual discomfort, **bilateral**
H53.149   Visual discomfort, **unspecified**

H53.15   **Visual distortions of shape and size**
          Metamorphopsia

H53.16   **Psychophysical visual disturbances**

H53.19   **Other subjective visual disturbances**
          Visual halos

H53.2   **Diplopia**
         Double vision

✓5ᵗʰ **H53.3   Other and unspecified disorders of binocular vision**

H53.30   **Unspecified disorder of binocular vision**
H53.31   **Abnormal retinal correspondence**
H53.32   **Fusion with defective stereopsis**
H53.33   **Simultaneous visual perception without fusion**
H53.34   **Suppression of binocular vision**

✓5ᵗʰ **H53.4   Visual field defects**

H53.40   **Unspecified visual field defects**

✓6ᵗʰ **H53.41   Scotoma involving central area**

          Central scotoma

H53.411   Scotoma involving central area, **right eye**
H53.412   Scotoma involving central area, **left eye**
H53.413   Scotoma involving central area, **bilateral**
H53.419   Scotoma involving central area, **unspecified eye**

✓6ᵗʰ **H53.42   Scotoma of blind spot area**

          Enlarged blind spot

H53.421   Scotoma of blind spot area, **right eye**
H53.422   Scotoma of blind spot area, **left eye**
H53.423   Scotoma of blind spot area, **bilateral**
H53.429   Scotoma of blind spot area, **unspecified eye**

✓6ᵗʰ **H53.43   Sector or arcuate defects**

          Arcuate scotoma
          Bjerrum scotoma

H53.431   Sector or arcuate defects, **right eye**
H53.432   Sector or arcuate defects, **left eye**
H53.433   Sector or arcuate defects, **bilateral**
H53.439   Sector or arcuate defects, **unspecified eye**

✓6ᵗʰ **H53.45   Other localized visual field defect**

          Peripheral visual field defect
          Ring scotoma NOS
          Scotoma NOS

H53.451   Other localized visual field defect, **right eye**
H53.452   Other localized visual field defect, **left eye**
H53.453   Other localized visual field defect, **bilateral**
H53.459   Other localized visual field defect, **unspecified eye**

✓6ᵗʰ **H53.46   Homonymous bilateral field defects**

          Homonymous hemianopia
          Homonymous hemianopsia
          Quadrant anopia
          Quadrant anopsia

H53.461   Homonymous bilateral field defects, **right side**
H53.462   Homonymous bilateral field defects, **left side**
H53.469   Homonymous bilateral field defects, **unspecified side**
          Homonymous bilateral field defects NOS

H53.47   **Heteronymous bilateral field defects**
          Heteronymous hemianop(s)ia

✓6ᵗʰ **H53.48   Generalized contraction of visual field**

H53.481   Generalized contraction of visual field, **right eye**
H53.482   Generalized contraction of visual field, **left eye**

N Newborn: 0   P Pediatric: 0-17   M Maternity: 9-64   A Adult: 15-124   MCC Major Complication/Comorbidity   CC Complication/Comorbidity   SW Severe Wound Dx

626   ICD-10-CM 2020

H53.483 **Generalized contraction of visual field, bilateral**

H53.489 **Generalized contraction of visual field, unspecified eye**

√5th **H53.5** **Color vision deficiencies**
Color blindness
EXCLUDES 2   *day blindness (H53.11)*

H53.50 **Unspecified color vision deficiencies**
Color blindness NOS

H53.51 **Achromatopsia**
DEF: Nonprogressive genetic visual disorder characterized by complete color blindness, decreased vision, and light sensitivity.

H53.52 **Acquired color vision deficiency**

H53.53 **Deuteranomaly**
Deuteranopia
DEF: Male-only genetic disorder causing difficulty in distinguishing green and red; no shortened spectrum.

H53.54 **Protanomaly**
Protanopia

H53.55 **Tritanomaly**
Tritanopia

H53.59 **Other color vision deficiencies**

√5th **H53.6** **Night blindness**
EXCLUDES 1   *night blindness due to vitamin A deficiency (E50.5)*

H53.60 **Unspecified night blindness**

H53.61 **Abnormal dark adaptation curve**

H53.62 **Acquired night blindness**

H53.63 **Congenital night blindness**

H53.69 **Other night blindness**

√5th **H53.7** **Vision sensitivity deficiencies**

H53.71 **Glare sensitivity**

H53.72 **Impaired contrast sensitivity**

H53.8 **Other visual disturbances**

H53.9 **Unspecified visual disturbance**

√4th **H54** **Blindness and low vision**

NOTE   For definition of visual impairment categories see table below

Code first any associated underlying cause of the blindness
EXCLUDES 1   *amaurosis fugax (G45.3)*
AHA: 2017,4Q,11-12

√5th **H54.0** **Blindness, both eyes**
Visual impairment categories 3, 4, 5 in both eyes.

√6th **H54.0X** **Blindness, both eyes, different category levels**

√7th **H54.0X3** **Blindness right eye, category 3**

H54.0X33 **Blindness right eye category 3, blindness left eye category 3**

H54.0X34 **Blindness right eye category 3, blindness left eye category 4**

H54.0X35 **Blindness right eye category 3, blindness left eye category 5**

√7th **H54.0X4** **Blindness right eye, category 4**

H54.0X43 **Blindness right eye category 4, blindness left eye category 3**

H54.0X44 **Blindness right eye category 4, blindness left eye category 4**

H54.0X45 **Blindness right eye category 4, blindness left eye category 5**

√7th **H54.0X5** **Blindness right eye, category 5**

H54.0X53 **Blindness right eye category 5, blindness left eye category 3**

H54.0X54 **Blindness right eye category 5, blindness left eye category 4**

H54.0X55 **Blindness right eye category 5, blindness left eye category 5**

√5th **H54.1** **Blindness, one eye, low vision other eye**
Visual impairment categories 3, 4, 5 in one eye, with categories 1 or 2 in the other eye.

H54.10 **Blindness, one eye, low vision other eye, unspecified eyes**

√6th **H54.11** **Blindness, right eye, low vision left eye**

√7th **H54.113** **Blindness right eye category 3, low vision left eye**

H54.1131 **Blindness right eye category 3, low vision left eye category 1**

H54.1132 **Blindness right eye category 3, low vision left eye category 2**

√7th **H54.114** **Blindness right eye category 4, low vision left eye**

H54.1141 **Blindness right eye category 4, low vision left eye category 1**

H54.1142 **Blindness right eye category 4, low vision left eye category 2**

√7th **H54.115** **Blindness right eye category 5, low vision left eye**

H54.1151 **Blindness right eye category 5, low vision left eye category 1**

H54.1152 **Blindness right eye category 5, low vision left eye category 2**

√6th **H54.12** **Blindness, left eye, low vision right eye**

√7th **H54.121** **Low vision right eye category 1, blindness left eye**

H54.1213 **Low vision right eye category 1, blindness left eye category 3**

H54.1214 **Low vision right eye category 1, blindness left eye category 4**

H54.1215 **Low vision right eye category 1, blindness left eye category 5**

√7th **H54.122** **Low vision right eye category 2, blindness left eye**

H54.1223 **Low vision right eye category 2, blindness left eye category 3**

H54.1224 **Low vision right eye category 2, blindness left eye category 4**

H54.1225 **Low vision right eye category 2, blindness left eye category 5**

√5th **H54.2** **Low vision, both eyes**
Visual impairment categories 1 or 2 in both eyes.

√6th **H54.2X** **Low vision, both eyes, different category levels**

√7th **H54.2X1** **Low vision, right eye, category 1**

H54.2X11 **Low vision right eye category 1, low vision left eye category 1**

H54.2X12 **Low vision right eye category 1, low vision left eye category 2**

√7th **H54.2X2** **Low vision, right eye, category 2**

H54.2X21 **Low vision right eye category 2, low vision left eye category 1**

H54.2X22 **Low vision right eye category 2, low vision left eye category 2**

H54.3 **Unqualified visual loss, both eyes**
Visual impairment category 9 in both eyes.
TIP: Assign only when both eyes are documented as affected by blindness or low vision but the visual impairment category is not documented.

√5th **H54.4** **Blindness, one eye**
Visual impairment categories 3, 4, 5 in one eye [normal vision in other eye]

H54.40 **Blindness, one eye, unspecified eye**

√6th **H54.41** **Blindness, right eye, normal vision left eye**

√7th **H54.413** **Blindness, right eye, category 3**

H54.413A **Blindness right eye category 3, normal vision left eye**

√7th **H54.414** **Blindness, right eye, category 4**

H54.414A **Blindness right eye category 4, normal vision left eye**

√7th **H54.415** **Blindness, right eye, category 5**

H54.415A **Blindness right eye category 5, normal vision left eye**

√6th **H54.42** **Blindness, left eye, normal vision right eye**

√7th **H54.42A** **Blindness, left eye, category 3-5**

H54.42A3 **Blindness left eye category 3, normal vision right eye**

H54.42A4 **Blindness left eye category 4, normal vision right eye**

H54.42A5 **Blindness left eye category 5, normal vision right eye**

☑ Additional Character Required   √x7th Placeholder   Unacceptable PDx   Questionable PDx   Manifestation   Unspecified Dx   H1-H14 HAC   HCC CMS-HCC Dx   HIV HIV Dx

Chapter 7. Diseases of the Eye and Adnexa

✓5ʰ **H54.5** **Low vision, one eye**

Visual impairment categories 1 or 2 in one eye [normal vision in other eye].

H54.50 **Low vision, one eye, unspecified**

✓6ʰ **H54.51** **Low vision, right eye, normal vision left eye**

✓7ʰ **H54.511** **Low vision, right eye, category 1-2**

     H54.511A **Low vision right eye category 1, normal vision left eye**

     H54.512A **Low vision right eye category 2, normal vision left eye**

✓7ʰ **H54.52** **Low vision, left eye, normal vision right eye**

✓7ʰ **H54.52A** **Low vision, left eye, category 1-2**

     H54.52A1 **Low vision left eye category 1, normal vision right eye**

     H54.52A2 **Low vision left eye category 2, normal vision right eye**

✓5ʰ **H54.6** **Unqualified visual loss, one eye**

Visual impairment category 9 in one eye [normal vision in other eye].

TIP: Assign a code from this category only when one eye is documented as affected by blindness or low vision but the visual impairment category is not documented.

H54.60 **Unqualified visual loss, one eye, unspecified**

H54.61 **Unqualified visual loss, right eye, normal vision left eye**

H54.62 **Unqualified visual loss, left eye, normal vision right eye**

H54.7 **Unspecified visual loss**

Visual impairment category 9 NOS

TIP: Assign only when documentation specifies blindness, visual loss, or low vision but not whether one or both eyes are affected or the visual impairment category.

H54.8 **Legal blindness, as defined in USA**

Blindness NOS according to USA definition

EXCLUDES 1   *legal blindness with specification of impairment level (H54.0-H54.7)*

NOTE   The table below gives a classification of severity of visual impairment recommended by a WHO Study Group on the Prevention of Blindness, Geneva, 6-10 November 1972.

The term "low vision" in category H54 comprises categories 1 and 2 of the table, the term "blindness" categories 3, 4 and 5, and the term "unqualified visual loss" category 9.

If the extent of the visual field is taken into account, patients with a field no greater than 10 but greater than 5 around central fixation should be placed in category 3 and patients with a field no greater than 5 around central fixation should be placed in category 4, even if the central acuity is not impaired.

Category of visual impairment	Visual acuity with best possible correction	
	Maximum less than:	**Minimum equal to or better than:**
1	6/18 3/10 (0.3) 20/70	6/60 1/10 (0.1) 20/200
2	6/60 1/10 (0.1) 20/200	3/60 1/20 (0.05) 20/400
3	3/60 1/200 (0.05) 20/400	1/60 (finger counting at one meter) 1/50 (0.02) 5/300 (20/1200)
4	1/60 (finger counting at one meter) 1/50 (0.02) 5/300	Light perception
5	No light perception	
9	Undetermined or unspecified	

Other disorders of eye and adnexa (H55-H57)

✓4ʰ **H55** **Nystagmus and other irregular eye movements**

✓5ʰ **H55.0** **Nystagmus**

DEF: Rapid, rhythmic, involuntary movements of the eyeball in vertical, horizontal, rotational, or mixed directions.

H55.00 **Unspecified nystagmus**

H55.01 **Congenital nystagmus**

H55.02 **Latent nystagmus**

H55.03 **Visual deprivation nystagmus**

H55.04 **Dissociated nystagmus**

H55.09 **Other forms of nystagmus**

✓5ʰ **H55.8** **Other irregular eye movements**

H55.81 **Saccadic eye movements**

H55.89 **Other irregular eye movements**

✓4ʰ **H57** **Other disorders of eye and adnexa**

✓5ʰ **H57.0** **Anomalies of pupillary function**

H57.00 **Unspecified anomaly of pupillary function**

H57.01 **Argyll Robertson pupil, atypical**

EXCLUDES 1   *syphilitic Argyll Robertson pupil (A52.19)*

H57.02 **Anisocoria**

H57.03 **Miosis**

H57.04 **Mydriasis**

✓6ʰ **H57.05** **Tonic pupil**

H57.051 **Tonic pupil, right eye**

H57.052 **Tonic pupil, left eye**

H57.053 **Tonic pupil, bilateral**

H57.059 **Tonic pupil, unspecified eye**

H57.09 **Other anomalies of pupillary function**

✓5ʰ **H57.1** **Ocular pain**

H57.10 **Ocular pain, unspecified eye**

H57.11 **Ocular pain, right eye**

H57.12 **Ocular pain, left eye**

H57.13 **Ocular pain, bilateral**

✓5ʰ **H57.8** **Other specified disorders of eye and adnexa**

AHA: 2018,4Q,15-16

✓6ʰ **H57.81** **Brow ptosis**

H57.811 **Brow ptosis, right**

H57.812 **Brow ptosis, left**

H57.813 **Brow ptosis, bilateral**

H57.819 **Brow ptosis, unspecified**

H57.89 **Other specified disorders of eye and adnexa**

H57.9 **Unspecified disorder of eye and adnexa**

Intraoperative and postprocedural complications and disorders of eye and adnexa, not elsewhere classified (H59)

✓4ʰ **H59** **Intraoperative and postprocedural complications and disorders of eye and adnexa, not elsewhere classified**

EXCLUDES 1   *mechanical complication of intraocular lens (T85.2)*

mechanical complication of other ocular prosthetic devices, implants and grafts (T85.3)

pseudophakia (Z96.1)

secondary cataracts (H26.4-)

✓5ʰ **H59.0** **Disorders of the eye following cataract surgery**

CC Excl: For CC codes in subcategory H59.0: PDX collection 638

✓6ʰ **H59.01** **Keratopathy (bullous aphakic) following cataract surgery**

Vitreal corneal syndrome

Vitreous (touch) syndrome

H59.011 **Keratopathy (bullous aphakic) following cataract surgery, right eye**   `CC`

H59.012 **Keratopathy (bullous aphakic) following cataract surgery, left eye**   `CC`

H59.013 **Keratopathy (bullous aphakic) following cataract surgery, bilateral**   `CC`

H59.019 **Keratopathy (bullous aphakic) following cataract surgery, unspecified eye**   `CC`

N Newborn: 0   P Pediatric: 0-17   M Maternity: 9-64   A Adult: 15-124   **MCC** Major Complication/Comorbidity   **CC** Complication/Comorbidity   **SW** Severe Wound Dx

628

ICD-10-CM 2020

  ✓6ᵗʰ **H59.02** Cataract (lens) fragments in eye following cataract surgery

      H59.021 Cataract (lens) fragments in eye following cataract surgery, right eye

      H59.022 Cataract (lens) fragments in eye following cataract surgery, left eye

      H59.023 Cataract (lens) fragments in eye following cataract surgery, bilateral

      H59.029 Cataract (lens) fragments in eye following cataract surgery, unspecified eye

  ✓6ᵗʰ **H59.03** Cystoid macular edema following cataract surgery

      H59.031 Cystoid macular edema following cataract surgery, right eye   `CC`

      H59.032 Cystoid macular edema following cataract surgery, left eye   `CC`

      H59.033 Cystoid macular edema following cataract surgery, bilateral   `CC`

      H59.039 Cystoid macular edema following cataract surgery, unspecified eye   `CC`

  ✓6ᵗʰ **H59.09** Other disorders of the eye following cataract surgery

      H59.091 Other disorders of the right eye following cataract surgery   `CC`

      H59.092 Other disorders of the left eye following cataract surgery   `CC`

      H59.093 Other disorders of the eye following cataract surgery, bilateral   `CC`

      H59.099 Other disorders of unspecified eye following cataract surgery   `CC`

✓5ᵗʰ **H59.1** Intraoperative hemorrhage and hematoma of eye and adnexa complicating a procedure

     EXCLUDES 1   intraoperative hemorrhage and hematoma of eye and adnexa due to accidental puncture or laceration during a procedure (H59.2-)

     CC Excl: For CC codes in subcategory H59.1: PDX collection 639

  ✓6ᵗʰ **H59.11** Intraoperative hemorrhage and hematoma of eye and adnexa complicating an ophthalmic procedure

      H59.111 Intraoperative hemorrhage and hematoma of right eye and adnexa complicating an ophthalmic procedure   `CC`

      H59.112 Intraoperative hemorrhage and hematoma of left eye and adnexa complicating an ophthalmic procedure   `CC`

      H59.113 Intraoperative hemorrhage and hematoma of eye and adnexa complicating an ophthalmic procedure, bilateral   `CC`

      H59.119 Intraoperative hemorrhage and hematoma of unspecified eye and adnexa complicating an ophthalmic procedure   `CC`

  ✓6ᵗʰ **H59.12** Intraoperative hemorrhage and hematoma of eye and adnexa complicating other procedure

      H59.121 Intraoperative hemorrhage and hematoma of right eye and adnexa complicating other procedure   `CC`

      H59.122 Intraoperative hemorrhage and hematoma of left eye and adnexa complicating other procedure   `CC`

      H59.123 Intraoperative hemorrhage and hematoma of eye and adnexa complicating other procedure, bilateral   `CC`

      H59.129 Intraoperative hemorrhage and hematoma of unspecified eye and adnexa complicating other procedure   `CC`

✓5ᵗʰ **H59.2** Accidental puncture and laceration of eye and adnexa during a procedure

     CC Excl: For CC codes in subcategory H59.2: PDX collection 509

  ✓6ᵗʰ **H59.21** Accidental puncture and laceration of eye and adnexa during an ophthalmic procedure

      H59.211 Accidental puncture and laceration of right eye and adnexa during an ophthalmic procedure   `CC`

      H59.212 Accidental puncture and laceration of left eye and adnexa during an ophthalmic procedure   `CC`

      H59.213 Accidental puncture and laceration of eye and adnexa during an ophthalmic procedure, bilateral   `CC`

      H59.219 Accidental puncture and laceration of unspecified eye and adnexa during an ophthalmic procedure   `CC`

  ✓6ᵗʰ **H59.22** Accidental puncture and laceration of eye and adnexa during other procedure

      H59.221 Accidental puncture and laceration of right eye and adnexa during other procedure   `CC`

      H59.222 Accidental puncture and laceration of left eye and adnexa during other procedure   `CC`

      H59.223 Accidental puncture and laceration of eye and adnexa during other procedure, bilateral   `CC`

      H59.229 Accidental puncture and laceration of unspecified eye and adnexa during other procedure   `CC`

✓5ᵗʰ **H59.3** Postprocedural hemorrhage, hematoma, and seroma of eye and adnexa following a procedure

     AHA: 2016,4Q,9-10

     CC Excl: For CC codes in subcategory H59.3: PDX collection 639

  ✓6ᵗʰ **H59.31** Postprocedural hemorrhage of eye and adnexa following an ophthalmic procedure

      H59.311 Postprocedural hemorrhage of right eye and adnexa following an ophthalmic procedure   `CC`

      H59.312 Postprocedural hemorrhage of left eye and adnexa following an ophthalmic procedure   `CC`

      H59.313 Postprocedural hemorrhage of eye and adnexa following an ophthalmic procedure, bilateral   `CC`

      H59.319 Postprocedural hemorrhage of unspecified eye and adnexa following an ophthalmic procedure   `CC`

  ✓6ᵗʰ **H59.32** Postprocedural hemorrhage of eye and adnexa following other procedure

      H59.321 Postprocedural hemorrhage of right eye and adnexa following other procedure   `CC`

      H59.322 Postprocedural hemorrhage of left eye and adnexa following other procedure   `CC`

✔ Additional Character Required   ✔x7ᵗʰ Placeholder   Unacceptable PDx   Questionable PDx   Manifestation   Unspecified Dx   H1-H14 HAC   HCC CMS-HCC Dx   HIV HIV Dx

ICD-10-CM 2020   629

Chapter 7. Diseases of the Eye and Adnexa

H59.323–H59.89

        H59.323   Postprocedural hemorrhage of eye and adnexa following other procedure, **bilateral**   `CC`

        H59.329   Postprocedural hemorrhage of unspecified eye and adnexa following other procedure   `CC`

   ✓6th **H59.33**   Postprocedural **hematoma** of eye and adnexa following an **ophthalmic procedure**

        H59.331   Postprocedural hematoma of **right** eye and adnexa following an ophthalmic procedure   `CC`

        H59.332   Postprocedural hematoma of **left** eye and adnexa following an ophthalmic procedure   `CC`

        H59.333   Postprocedural hematoma of eye and adnexa following an ophthalmic procedure, **bilateral**   `CC`

        H59.339   Postprocedural hematoma of unspecified eye and adnexa following an ophthalmic procedure   `CC`

   ✓6th **H59.34**   Postprocedural **hematoma** of eye and adnexa following **other procedure**

        H59.341   Postprocedural hematoma of **right** eye and adnexa following other procedure   `CC`

        H59.342   Postprocedural hematoma of **left** eye and adnexa following other procedure   `CC`

        H59.343   Postprocedural hematoma of eye and adnexa following other procedure, **bilateral**   `CC`

        H59.349   Postprocedural hematoma of unspecified eye and adnexa following other procedure   `CC`

   ✓6th **H59.35**   Postprocedural **seroma** of eye and adnexa following an **ophthalmic procedure**

        H59.351   Postprocedural seroma of **right** eye and adnexa following an ophthalmic procedure   `CC`

        H59.352   Postprocedural seroma of **left** eye and adnexa following an ophthalmic procedure   `CC`

        H59.353   Postprocedural seroma of eye and adnexa following an ophthalmic procedure, **bilateral**   `CC`

        H59.359   Postprocedural seroma of unspecified eye and adnexa following an ophthalmic procedure   `CC`

   ✓6th **H59.36**   Postprocedural **seroma** of eye and adnexa following **other procedure**

        H59.361   Postprocedural seroma of **right** eye and adnexa following other procedure   `CC`

        H59.362   Postprocedural seroma of **left** eye and adnexa following other procedure   `CC`

        H59.363   Postprocedural seroma of eye and adnexa following other procedure, **bilateral**   `CC`

        H59.369   Postprocedural seroma of unspecified eye and adnexa following other procedure   `CC`

 ✓5th **H59.4**   Inflammation (infection) of **postprocedural bleb**

     Postprocedural blebitis

     EXCLUDES 1   *filtering (vitreous) bleb after glaucoma surgery status (Z98.83)*

     H59.40   Inflammation (infection) of postprocedural bleb, unspecified

     H59.41   Inflammation (infection) of postprocedural bleb, stage 1

     H59.42   Inflammation (infection) of postprocedural bleb, stage 2

     H59.43   Inflammation (infection) of postprocedural bleb, stage 3

         Bleb endophthalmitis

 ✓5th **H59.8**   Other intraoperative and postprocedural complications and disorders of eye and adnexa, not elsewhere classified

     CC Excl: For CC codes in subcategory H59.8: PDX collection 638

   ✓6th **H59.81**   Chorioretinal scars after surgery for detachment

     H59.811   Chorioretinal scars after surgery for detachment, **right** eye   `CC`

     H59.812   Chorioretinal scars after surgery for detachment, **left** eye   `CC`

     H59.813   Chorioretinal scars after surgery for detachment, **bilateral**   `CC`

     H59.819   Chorioretinal scars after surgery for detachment, unspecified eye   `CC`

     H59.88   Other intraoperative complications of eye and adnexa, not elsewhere classified   `CC`

     H59.89   Other postprocedural complications and disorders of eye and adnexa, not elsewhere classified   `CC`

N Newborn: 0   P Pediatric: 0-17   M Maternity: 9-64   A Adult: 15-124   MCC Major Complication/Comorbidity   CC Complication/Comorbidity   SW Severe Wound Dx

630   ICD-10-CM 2020

Chapter 8. Diseases of the Ear and Mastoid Process (H60–H95)

Chapter-specific Guidelines with Coding Examples
Reserved for future guideline expansion.

Chapter 8. Diseases of the Ear and Mastoid Process

Chapter 8. Diseases of the Ear and Mastoid Process

H60–H60.91

Chapter 8. Diseases of the Ear and Mastoid Process (H60-H95)

NOTE Use an external cause code following the code for the ear condition, if applicable, to identify the cause of the ear condition

EXCLUDES 2 *certain conditions originating in the perinatal period (P04-P96)*
certain infectious and parasitic diseases (A00-B99)
complications of pregnancy, childbirth and the puerperium (O00-O9A)
congenital malformations, deformations and chromosomal abnormalities (Q00-Q99)
endocrine, nutritional and metabolic diseases (E00-E88)
injury, poisoning and certain other consequences of external causes (S00-T88)
neoplasms (C00-D49)
symptoms, signs and abnormal clinical and laboratory findings, not elsewhere classified (R00-R94)

This chapter contains the following blocks:
H60-H62   Diseases of external ear
H65-H75   Diseases of middle ear and mastoid
H80-H83   Diseases of inner ear
H90-H94   Other disorders of ear
H95   Intraoperative and postprocedural complications and disorders of ear and mastoid process, not elsewhere classified

Diseases of external ear (H60-H62)

✓4ᵗʰ H60 Otitis externa

TIP: When the specific infectious agent is identified, a code from Chapter 1 is assigned instead of a code from this category.

✓5ᵗʰ H60.0 Abscess of external ear
Boil of external ear
Carbuncle of auricle or external auditory canal
Furuncle of external ear
   H60.00 Abscess of external ear, unspecified ear
   H60.01 Abscess of right external ear
   H60.02 Abscess of left external ear
   H60.03 Abscess of external ear, bilateral

✓5ᵗʰ H60.1 Cellulitis of external ear
Cellulitis of auricle
Cellulitis of external auditory canal
   H60.10 Cellulitis of external ear, unspecified ear
   H60.11 Cellulitis of right external ear
   H60.12 Cellulitis of left external ear
   H60.13 Cellulitis of external ear, bilateral

✓5ᵗʰ H60.2 Malignant otitis externa

CC Excl: For CC codes in subcategory H60.2: PDX collection 640

   H60.20 Malignant otitis externa, unspecified ear   **CC**
   H60.21 Malignant otitis externa, right ear   **CC**
   H60.22 Malignant otitis externa, left ear   **CC**
   H60.23 Malignant otitis externa, bilateral   **CC**

✓5ᵗʰ H60.3 Other infective otitis externa

✓6ᵗʰ H60.31 Diffuse otitis externa
   H60.311 Diffuse otitis externa, right ear
   H60.312 Diffuse otitis externa, left ear
   H60.313 Diffuse otitis externa, bilateral
   H60.319 Diffuse otitis externa, unspecified ear

✓6ᵗʰ H60.32 Hemorrhagic otitis externa
   H60.321 Hemorrhagic otitis externa, right ear
   H60.322 Hemorrhagic otitis externa, left ear
   H60.323 Hemorrhagic otitis externa, bilateral
   H60.329 Hemorrhagic otitis externa, unspecified ear

✓6ᵗʰ H60.33 Swimmer's ear
DEF: Commonly occurs when water gets trapped in the ear after swimming.
   H60.331 Swimmer's ear, right ear
   H60.332 Swimmer's ear, left ear
   H60.333 Swimmer's ear, bilateral
   H60.339 Swimmer's ear, unspecified ear

✓6ᵗʰ H60.39 Other infective otitis externa
   H60.391 Other infective otitis externa, right ear
   H60.392 Other infective otitis externa, left ear
   H60.393 Other infective otitis externa, bilateral
   H60.399 Other infective otitis externa, unspecified ear

✓5ᵗʰ H60.4 Cholesteatoma of external ear
Keratosis obturans of external ear (canal)
EXCLUDES 2 *cholesteatoma of middle ear (H71.-)*
recurrent cholesteatoma of postmastoidectomy cavity (H95.0-)
DEF: Cholesteatoma: Noncancerous cyst-like mass of cell debris, including cholesterol and epithelial cells resulting from trauma, repeated or improperly healed infections, and congenital enclosure of epidermal cells.
   H60.40 Cholesteatoma of external ear, unspecified ear
   H60.41 Cholesteatoma of right external ear
   H60.42 Cholesteatoma of left external ear
   H60.43 Cholesteatoma of external ear, bilateral

✓5ᵗʰ H60.5 Acute noninfective otitis externa

✓6ᵗʰ H60.50 Unspecified acute noninfective otitis externa
Acute otitis externa NOS
   H60.501 Unspecified acute noninfective otitis externa, right ear
   H60.502 Unspecified acute noninfective otitis externa, left ear
   H60.503 Unspecified acute noninfective otitis externa, bilateral
   H60.509 Unspecified acute noninfective otitis externa, unspecified ear

✓6ᵗʰ H60.51 Acute actinic otitis externa
   H60.511 Acute actinic otitis externa, right ear
   H60.512 Acute actinic otitis externa, left ear
   H60.513 Acute actinic otitis externa, bilateral
   H60.519 Acute actinic otitis externa, unspecified ear

✓6ᵗʰ H60.52 Acute chemical otitis externa
   H60.521 Acute chemical otitis externa, right ear
   H60.522 Acute chemical otitis externa, left ear
   H60.523 Acute chemical otitis externa, bilateral
   H60.529 Acute chemical otitis externa, unspecified ear

✓6ᵗʰ H60.53 Acute contact otitis externa
   H60.531 Acute contact otitis externa, right ear
   H60.532 Acute contact otitis externa, left ear
   H60.533 Acute contact otitis externa, bilateral
   H60.539 Acute contact otitis externa, unspecified ear

✓6ᵗʰ H60.54 Acute eczematoid otitis externa
   H60.541 Acute eczematoid otitis externa, right ear
   H60.542 Acute eczematoid otitis externa, left ear
   H60.543 Acute eczematoid otitis externa, bilateral
   H60.549 Acute eczematoid otitis externa, unspecified ear

✓6ᵗʰ H60.55 Acute reactive otitis externa
   H60.551 Acute reactive otitis externa, right ear
   H60.552 Acute reactive otitis externa, left ear
   H60.553 Acute reactive otitis externa, bilateral
   H60.559 Acute reactive otitis externa, unspecified ear

✓6ᵗʰ H60.59 Other noninfective acute otitis externa
   H60.591 Other noninfective acute otitis externa, right ear
   H60.592 Other noninfective acute otitis externa, left ear
   H60.593 Other noninfective acute otitis externa, bilateral
   H60.599 Other noninfective acute otitis externa, unspecified ear

✓5ᵗʰ H60.6 Unspecified chronic otitis externa
   H60.60 Unspecified chronic otitis externa, unspecified ear
   H60.61 Unspecified chronic otitis externa, right ear
   H60.62 Unspecified chronic otitis externa, left ear
   H60.63 Unspecified chronic otitis externa, bilateral

✓5ᵗʰ H60.8 Other otitis externa

✓6ᵗʰ H60.8X Other otitis externa
   H60.8X1 Other otitis externa, right ear
   H60.8X2 Other otitis externa, left ear
   H60.8X3 Other otitis externa, bilateral
   H60.8X9 Other otitis externa, unspecified ear

✓5ᵗʰ H60.9 Unspecified otitis externa
   H60.90 Unspecified otitis externa, unspecified ear
   H60.91 Unspecified otitis externa, right ear

N Newborn: 0   **P** Pediatric: 0-17   **M** Maternity: 9-64   **A** Adult: 15-124   **MCC** Major Complication/Comorbidity   **CC** Complication/Comorbidity   **SW** Severe Wound Dx

632   ICD-10-CM 2020

H60.92   **Unspecified otitis externa, left** ear

H60.93   **Unspecified otitis externa, bilateral**

✓4ᵗʰ **H61**   **Other disorders of external ear**

   ✓5ᵗʰ **H61.0**   **Chondritis and perichondritis of external ear**

     Chondrodermatitis nodularis chronica helicis

     Perichondritis of auricle

     Perichondritis of pinna

     ✓6ᵗʰ **H61.00**   **Unspecified perichondritis of external ear**

       H61.001   **Unspecified perichondritis of right external ear**

       H61.002   **Unspecified perichondritis of left external ear**

       H61.003   **Unspecified perichondritis of external ear, bilateral**

       H61.009   **Unspecified perichondritis of external ear, unspecified ear**

     ✓6ᵗʰ **H61.01**   **Acute perichondritis of external ear**

       H61.011   **Acute perichondritis of right external ear**

       H61.012   **Acute perichondritis of left external ear**

       H61.013   **Acute perichondritis of external ear, bilateral**

       H61.019   **Acute perichondritis of external ear, unspecified ear**

     ✓6ᵗʰ **H61.02**   **Chronic perichondritis of external ear**

       H61.021   **Chronic perichondritis of right external ear**

       H61.022   **Chronic perichondritis of left external ear**

       H61.023   **Chronic perichondritis of external ear, bilateral**

       H61.029   **Chronic perichondritis of external ear, unspecified ear**

     ✓6ᵗʰ **H61.03**   **Chondritis of external ear**

       Chondritis of auricle

       Chondritis of pinna

       AHA: 2015, 1Q, 18

       DEF: Infection that has progressed into the cartilage and presents as indurated and edematous skin over the pinna. Vascular compromise occurs with tissue necrosis and deformity.

       H61.031   **Chondritis of right external ear**

       H61.032   **Chondritis of left external ear**

       H61.033   **Chondritis of external ear, bilateral**

       H61.039   **Chondritis of external ear, unspecified ear**

   ✓5ᵗʰ **H61.1**   **Noninfective disorders of pinna**

     EXCLUDES 2   cauliflower ear (M95.1-)

         gouty tophi of ear (M1A.-)

     ✓6ᵗʰ **H61.10**   **Unspecified noninfective disorders of pinna**

       Disorder of pinna NOS

       H61.101   **Unspecified noninfective disorders of pinna, right ear**

       H61.102   **Unspecified noninfective disorders of pinna, left ear**

       H61.103   **Unspecified noninfective disorders of pinna, bilateral**

       H61.109   **Unspecified noninfective disorders of pinna, unspecified ear**

     ✓6ᵗʰ **H61.11**   **Acquired deformity of pinna**

       Acquired deformity of auricle

       EXCLUDES 2   cauliflower ear (M95.1-)

       H61.111   **Acquired deformity of pinna, right ear**

       H61.112   **Acquired deformity of pinna, left ear**

       H61.113   **Acquired deformity of pinna, bilateral**

       H61.119   **Acquired deformity of pinna, unspecified ear**

     ✓6ᵗʰ **H61.12**   **Hematoma of pinna**

       Hematoma of auricle

       H61.121   **Hematoma of pinna, right ear**

       H61.122   **Hematoma of pinna, left ear**

       H61.123   **Hematoma of pinna, bilateral**

       H61.129   **Hematoma of pinna, unspecified ear**

     ✓6ᵗʰ **H61.19**   **Other noninfective disorders of pinna**

       H61.191   **Noninfective disorders of pinna, right ear**

       H61.192   **Noninfective disorders of pinna, left ear**

       H61.193   **Noninfective disorders of pinna, bilateral**

       H61.199   **Noninfective disorders of pinna, unspecified ear**

   ✓5ᵗʰ **H61.2**   **Impacted cerumen**

     Wax in ear

     H61.20   **Impacted cerumen, unspecified ear**

     H61.21   **Impacted cerumen, right ear**

     H61.22   **Impacted cerumen, left ear**

     H61.23   **Impacted cerumen, bilateral**

   ✓5ᵗʰ **H61.3**   **Acquired stenosis of external ear canal**

     Collapse of external ear canal

     EXCLUDES 1   postprocedural stenosis of external ear canal (H95.81-)

     ✓6ᵗʰ **H61.30**   **Acquired stenosis of external ear canal, unspecified**

       H61.301   **Acquired stenosis of right external ear canal, unspecified**

       H61.302   **Acquired stenosis of left external ear canal, unspecified**

       H61.303   **Acquired stenosis of external ear canal, unspecified, bilateral**

       H61.309   **Acquired stenosis of external ear canal, unspecified, unspecified ear**

     ✓6ᵗʰ **H61.31**   **Acquired stenosis of external ear canal secondary to trauma**

       H61.311   **Acquired stenosis of right external ear canal secondary to trauma**

       H61.312   **Acquired stenosis of left external ear canal secondary to trauma**

       H61.313   **Acquired stenosis of external ear canal secondary to trauma, bilateral**

       H61.319   **Acquired stenosis of external ear canal secondary to trauma, unspecified ear**

     ✓6ᵗʰ **H61.32**   **Acquired stenosis of external ear canal secondary to inflammation and infection**

       DEF: Narrowing of the external ear canal due to chronic inflammation or infection.

       H61.321   **Acquired stenosis of right external ear canal secondary to inflammation and infection**

       H61.322   **Acquired stenosis of left external ear canal secondary to inflammation and infection**

       H61.323   **Acquired stenosis of external ear canal secondary to inflammation and infection, bilateral**

       H61.329   **Acquired stenosis of external ear canal secondary to inflammation and infection, unspecified ear**

     ✓6ᵗʰ **H61.39**   **Other acquired stenosis of external ear canal**

       H61.391   **Other acquired stenosis of right external ear canal**

       H61.392   **Other acquired stenosis of left external ear canal**

       H61.393   **Other acquired stenosis of external ear canal, bilateral**

       H61.399   **Other acquired stenosis of external ear canal, unspecified ear**

   ✓5ᵗʰ **H61.8**   **Other specified disorders of external ear**

     ✓6ᵗʰ **H61.81**   **Exostosis of external canal**

       H61.811   **Exostosis of right external canal**

       H61.812   **Exostosis of left external canal**

       H61.813   **Exostosis of external canal, bilateral**

       H61.819   **Exostosis of external canal, unspecified ear**

     ✓6ᵗʰ **H61.89**   **Other specified disorders of external ear**

       H61.891   **Other specified disorders of right external ear**

       H61.892   **Other specified disorders of left external ear**

       H61.893   **Other specified disorders of external ear, bilateral**

       H61.899   **Other specified disorders of external ear, unspecified ear**

   ✓5ᵗʰ **H61.9**   **Disorder of external ear, unspecified**

     H61.90   **Disorder of external ear, unspecified, unspecified ear**

     H61.91   **Disorder of right external ear, unspecified**

     H61.92   **Disorder of left external ear, unspecified**

     H61.93   **Disorder of external ear, unspecified, bilateral**

✔ Additional Character Required   ✓x7ᵗʰ Placeholder   Unacceptable PDx   Questionable PDx   Manifestation   Unspecified Dx   H1-H15 HAC   HCC CMS-HCC Dx   HIV HIV Dx

ICD-10-CM 2020   633

Chapter 8. Diseases of the Ear and Mastoid Process

H62–H65.93

✓4ᵗʰ **H62 Disorders of external ear in diseases classified elsewhere**

  ✓5ᵗʰ **H62.4 Otitis externa in other diseases classified elsewhere**

    Code first underlying disease, such as:
      erysipelas (A46)
      impetigo (L01.0)

    EXCLUDES 1   otitis externa (in):
        candidiasis (B37.84)
        herpes viral [herpes simplex] (B00.1)
        herpes zoster (B02.8)

    H62.40 *Otitis externa in other diseases classified elsewhere, unspecified ear*

    H62.41 *Otitis externa in other diseases classified elsewhere, right ear*

    H62.42 *Otitis externa in other diseases classified elsewhere, left ear*

    H62.43 *Otitis externa in other diseases classified elsewhere, bilateral*

  ✓5ᵗʰ **H62.8 Other disorders of external ear in diseases classified elsewhere**

    Code first underlying disease, such as:
      gout (M1A.-, M10.-)

    ✓6ᵗʰ **H62.8X Other disorders of external ear in diseases classified elsewhere**

      H62.8X1 *Other disorders of right external ear in diseases classified elsewhere*

      H62.8X2 *Other disorders of left external ear in diseases classified elsewhere*

      H62.8X3 *Other disorders of external ear in diseases classified elsewhere, bilateral*

      H62.8X9 *Other disorders of external ear in diseases classified elsewhere, unspecified ear*

Diseases of middle ear and mastoid (H65-H75)

✓4ᵗʰ **H65 Nonsuppurative otitis media**

  INCLUDES   nonsuppurative otitis media with myringitis

  Use additional code for any associated perforated tympanic membrane (H72.-)

  ▶Use additional code, if applicable, to identify:◀
    exposure to environmental tobacco smoke (Z77.22)
    exposure to tobacco smoke in the perinatal period (P96.81)
    history of tobacco dependence (Z87.891)
    ▶infectious agent (B95-B97)◀
    occupational exposure to environmental tobacco smoke (Z57.31)
    tobacco dependence (F17.-)
    tobacco use (Z72.0)

  ✓5ᵗʰ **H65.0 Acute serous otitis media**

    Acute and subacute secretory otitis

    H65.00 Acute serous otitis media, unspecified ear
    H65.01 Acute serous otitis media, right ear
    H65.02 Acute serous otitis media, left ear
    H65.03 Acute serous otitis media, bilateral
    H65.04 Acute serous otitis media, recurrent, right ear
    H65.05 Acute serous otitis media, recurrent, left ear
    H65.06 Acute serous otitis media, recurrent, bilateral
    H65.07 Acute serous otitis media, recurrent, unspecified ear

  ✓5ᵗʰ **H65.1 Other acute nonsuppurative otitis media**

    EXCLUDES 1   otitic barotrauma (T70.0)
        otitis media (acute) NOS (H66.9)

    ✓6ᵗʰ **H65.11 Acute and subacute allergic otitis media (mucoid) (sanguinous) (serous)**

      H65.111 Acute and subacute allergic otitis media (mucoid) (sanguinous) (serous), right ear
      H65.112 Acute and subacute allergic otitis media (mucoid) (sanguinous) (serous), left ear
      H65.113 Acute and subacute allergic otitis media (mucoid) (sanguinous) (serous), bilateral
      H65.114 Acute and subacute allergic otitis media (mucoid) (sanguinous) (serous), recurrent, right ear
      H65.115 Acute and subacute allergic otitis media (mucoid) (sanguinous) (serous), recurrent, left ear
      H65.116 Acute and subacute allergic otitis media (mucoid) (sanguinous) (serous), recurrent, bilateral
      H65.117 Acute and subacute allergic otitis media (mucoid) (sanguinous) (serous), recurrent, unspecified ear

      H65.119 Acute and subacute allergic otitis media (mucoid) (sanguinous) (serous), unspecified ear

    ✓6ᵗʰ **H65.19 Other acute nonsuppurative otitis media**

      Acute and subacute mucoid otitis media
      Acute and subacute nonsuppurative otitis media NOS
      Acute and subacute sanguinous otitis media
      Acute and subacute seromucinous otitis media

      H65.191 Other acute nonsuppurative otitis media, right ear
      H65.192 Other acute nonsuppurative otitis media, left ear
      H65.193 Other acute nonsuppurative otitis media, bilateral
      H65.194 Other acute nonsuppurative otitis media, recurrent, right ear
      H65.195 Other acute nonsuppurative otitis media, recurrent, left ear
      H65.196 Other acute nonsuppurative otitis media, recurrent, bilateral
      H65.197 Other acute nonsuppurative otitis media, recurrent, unspecified ear
      H65.199 Other acute nonsuppurative otitis media, unspecified ear

  ✓5ᵗʰ **H65.2 Chronic serous otitis media**

    Chronic tubotympanal catarrh

    H65.20 Chronic serous otitis media, unspecified ear
    H65.21 Chronic serous otitis media, right ear
    H65.22 Chronic serous otitis media, left ear
    H65.23 Chronic serous otitis media, bilateral

  ✓5ᵗʰ **H65.3 Chronic mucoid otitis media**

    Chronic mucinous otitis media
    Chronic secretory otitis media
    Chronic transudative otitis media
    Glue ear

    EXCLUDES 1   adhesive middle ear disease (H74.1)

    H65.30 Chronic mucoid otitis media, unspecified ear
    H65.31 Chronic mucoid otitis media, right ear
    H65.32 Chronic mucoid otitis media, left ear
    H65.33 Chronic mucoid otitis media, bilateral

  ✓5ᵗʰ **H65.4 Other chronic nonsuppurative otitis media**

    ✓6ᵗʰ **H65.41 Chronic allergic otitis media**

      H65.411 Chronic allergic otitis media, right ear
      H65.412 Chronic allergic otitis media, left ear
      H65.413 Chronic allergic otitis media, bilateral
      H65.419 Chronic allergic otitis media, unspecified ear

    ✓6ᵗʰ **H65.49 Other chronic nonsuppurative otitis media**

      Chronic exudative otitis media
      Chronic nonsuppurative otitis media NOS
      Chronic otitis media with effusion (nonpurulent)
      Chronic seromucinous otitis media

      H65.491 Other chronic nonsuppurative otitis media, right ear
      H65.492 Other chronic nonsuppurative otitis media, left ear
      H65.493 Other chronic nonsuppurative otitis media, bilateral
      H65.499 Other chronic nonsuppurative otitis media, unspecified ear

  ✓5ᵗʰ **H65.9 Unspecified nonsuppurative otitis media**

    Allergic otitis media NOS
    Catarrhal otitis media NOS
    Exudative otitis media NOS
    Mucoid otitis media NOS
    Otitis media with effusion (nonpurulent) NOS
    Secretory otitis media NOS
    Seromucinous otitis media NOS
    Serous otitis media NOS
    Transudative otitis media NOS

    H65.90 Unspecified nonsuppurative otitis media, unspecified ear
    H65.91 Unspecified nonsuppurative otitis media, right ear
    H65.92 Unspecified nonsuppurative otitis media, left ear
    H65.93 Unspecified nonsuppurative otitis media, bilateral

N Newborn: 0   P Pediatric: 0-17   M Maternity: 9-64   A Adult: 15-124   MCC Major Complication/Comorbidity   CC Complication/Comorbidity   SW Severe Wound Dx

634   ICD-10-CM 2020

✓4ᵗʰ H66 Suppurative and unspecified otitis media

INCLUDES   suppurative and unspecified otitis media with myringitis

Use additional code to identify:

exposure to environmental tobacco smoke (Z77.22)

exposure to tobacco smoke in the perinatal period (P96.81)

history of tobacco dependence (Z87.891)

occupational exposure to environmental tobacco smoke (Z57.31)

tobacco dependence (F17.-)

tobacco use (Z72.0)

AHA: 2016,1Q,34

✓5ᵗʰ H66.0 Acute suppurative otitis media

✓6ᵗʰ H66.00 Acute suppurative otitis media without spontaneous rupture of ear drum

H66.001   Acute suppurative otitis media without spontaneous rupture of ear drum, right ear

H66.002   Acute suppurative otitis media without spontaneous rupture of ear drum, left ear

H66.003   Acute suppurative otitis media without spontaneous rupture of ear drum, bilateral

H66.004   Acute suppurative otitis media without spontaneous rupture of ear drum, recurrent, right ear

H66.005   Acute suppurative otitis media without spontaneous rupture of ear drum, recurrent, left ear

H66.006   Acute suppurative otitis media without spontaneous rupture of ear drum, recurrent, bilateral

H66.007   Acute suppurative otitis media without spontaneous rupture of ear drum, recurrent, unspecified ear

H66.009   Acute suppurative otitis media without spontaneous rupture of ear drum, unspecified ear

✓6ᵗʰ H66.01 Acute suppurative otitis media with spontaneous rupture of ear drum

DEF: Sudden, severe inflammation of the middle ear, causing pressure that perforates the ear drum tissue.

H66.011   Acute suppurative otitis media with spontaneous rupture of ear drum, right ear

H66.012   Acute suppurative otitis media with spontaneous rupture of ear drum, left ear

H66.013   Acute suppurative otitis media with spontaneous rupture of ear drum, bilateral

H66.014   Acute suppurative otitis media with spontaneous rupture of ear drum, recurrent, right ear

H66.015   Acute suppurative otitis media with spontaneous rupture of ear drum, recurrent, left ear

H66.016   Acute suppurative otitis media with spontaneous rupture of ear drum, recurrent, bilateral

H66.017   Acute suppurative otitis media with spontaneous rupture of ear drum, recurrent, unspecified ear

H66.019   Acute suppurative otitis media with spontaneous rupture of ear drum, unspecified ear

✓5ᵗʰ H66.1 Chronic tubotympanic suppurative otitis media

Benign chronic suppurative otitis media

Chronic tubotympanic disease

Use additional code for any associated perforated tympanic membrane (H72.-)

H66.10   Chronic tubotympanic suppurative otitis media, unspecified

H66.11   Chronic tubotympanic suppurative otitis media, right ear

H66.12   Chronic tubotympanic suppurative otitis media, left ear

H66.13   Chronic tubotympanic suppurative otitis media, bilateral

✓5ᵗʰ H66.2 Chronic atticoantral suppurative otitis media

Chronic atticoantral disease

Use additional code for any associated perforated tympanic membrane (H72.-)

H66.20   Chronic atticoantral suppurative otitis media, unspecified ear

H66.21   Chronic atticoantral suppurative otitis media, right ear

H66.22   Chronic atticoantral suppurative otitis media, left ear

H66.23   Chronic atticoantral suppurative otitis media, bilateral

✓5ᵗʰ H66.3 Other chronic suppurative otitis media

Chronic suppurative otitis media NOS

Use additional code for any associated perforated tympanic membrane (H72.-)

EXCLUDES 1   tuberculous otitis media (A18.6)

✓6ᵗʰ H66.3X Other chronic suppurative otitis media

H66.3X1   Other chronic suppurative otitis media, right ear

H66.3X2   Other chronic suppurative otitis media, left ear

H66.3X3   Other chronic suppurative otitis media, bilateral

H66.3X9   Other chronic suppurative otitis media, unspecified ear

✓5ᵗʰ H66.4 Suppurative otitis media, unspecified

Purulent otitis media NOS

Use additional code for any associated perforated tympanic membrane (H72.-)

H66.40   Suppurative otitis media, unspecified, unspecified ear

H66.41   Suppurative otitis media, unspecified, right ear

H66.42   Suppurative otitis media, unspecified, left ear

H66.43   Suppurative otitis media, unspecified, bilateral

✓5ᵗʰ H66.9 Otitis media, unspecified

Otitis media NOS

Acute otitis media NOS

Chronic otitis media NOS

Use additional code for any associated perforated tympanic membrane (H72.-)

H66.90   Otitis media, unspecified, unspecified ear

H66.91   Otitis media, unspecified, right ear

H66.92   Otitis media, unspecified, left ear

H66.93   Otitis media, unspecified, bilateral

✓4ᵗʰ H67 Otitis media in diseases classified elsewhere

Code first underlying disease, such as:

plasminogen deficiency (E88.02)

viral disease NEC (B00-B34)

Use additional code for any associated perforated tympanic membrane (H72.-)

EXCLUDES 1   otitis media in:

influenza (J09.X9, J10.83, J11.83)

measles (B05.3)

scarlet fever (A38.0)

tuberculosis (A18.6)

H67.1   Otitis media in diseases classified elsewhere, right ear

H67.2   Otitis media in diseases classified elsewhere, left ear

H67.3   Otitis media in diseases classified elsewhere, bilateral

H67.9   Otitis media in diseases classified elsewhere, unspecified ear

✓4ᵗʰ H68 Eustachian salpingitis and obstruction

DEF: Eustachian tube: Internal channel between the tympanic cavity and the nasopharynx that equalizes internal pressure to the outside pressure and drains mucous production from the middle ear.

✓5ᵗʰ H68.0 Eustachian salpingitis

✓6ᵗʰ H68.00 Unspecified Eustachian salpingitis

H68.001   Unspecified Eustachian salpingitis, right ear

H68.002   Unspecified Eustachian salpingitis, left ear

H68.003   Unspecified Eustachian salpingitis, bilateral

H68.009   Unspecified Eustachian salpingitis, unspecified ear

✓6ᵗʰ H68.01 Acute Eustachian salpingitis

H68.011   Acute Eustachian salpingitis, right ear

H68.012   Acute Eustachian salpingitis, left ear

H68.013   Acute Eustachian salpingitis, bilateral

H68.019   Acute Eustachian salpingitis, unspecified ear

✓6ᵗʰ H68.02 Chronic Eustachian salpingitis

H68.021   Chronic Eustachian salpingitis, right ear

H68.022   Chronic Eustachian salpingitis, left ear

✔ Additional Character Required   ✔×7ᵗʰ Placeholder   Unacceptable PDx   Questionable PDx   Manifestation   Unspecified Dx   H1-H14 HAC   HCC CMS-HCC Dx   HIV HIV Dx

ICD-10-CM 2020   635

Chapter 8. Diseases of the Ear and Mastoid Process

         H68.023 **Chronic Eustachian salpingitis,** bilateral

         H68.029 **Chronic Eustachian salpingitis,** unspecified ear

✓5ᵗʰ **H68.1** **Obstruction of Eustachian tube**

     Stenosis of Eustachian tube

     Stricture of Eustachian tube

   ✓6ᵗʰ **H68.10** **Unspecified obstruction of Eustachian tube**

         H68.101 **Unspecified obstruction of Eustachian tube,** right **ear**

         H68.102 **Unspecified obstruction of Eustachian tube,** left **ear**

         H68.103 **Unspecified obstruction of Eustachian tube,** bilateral

         H68.109 **Unspecified obstruction of Eustachian tube,** unspecified **ear**

   ✓6ᵗʰ **H68.11** **Osseous obstruction of Eustachian tube**

         H68.111 **Osseous obstruction of Eustachian tube,** right **ear**

         H68.112 **Osseous obstruction of Eustachian tube,** left **ear**

         H68.113 **Osseous obstruction of Eustachian tube,** bilateral

         H68.119 **Osseous obstruction of Eustachian tube,** unspecified **ear**

   ✓6ᵗʰ **H68.12** **Intrinsic cartilagenous obstruction of Eustachian tube**

         H68.121 **Intrinsic cartilagenous obstruction of Eustachian tube,** right **ear**

         H68.122 **Intrinsic cartilagenous obstruction of Eustachian tube,** left **ear**

         H68.123 **Intrinsic cartilagenous obstruction of Eustachian tube,** bilateral

         H68.129 **Intrinsic cartilagenous obstruction of Eustachian tube,** unspecified **ear**

   ✓6ᵗʰ **H68.13** **Extrinsic cartilagenous obstruction of Eustachian tube**

     Compression of Eustachian tube

         H68.131 **Extrinsic cartilagenous obstruction of Eustachian tube,** right **ear**

         H68.132 **Extrinsic cartilagenous obstruction of Eustachian tube,** left **ear**

         H68.133 **Extrinsic cartilagenous obstruction of Eustachian tube,** bilateral

         H68.139 **Extrinsic cartilagenous obstruction of Eustachian tube,** unspecified **ear**

✓4ᵗʰ **H69** **Other and unspecified disorders of Eustachian tube**

     DEF: Eustachian tube: Internal channel between the tympanic cavity and the nasopharynx that equalizes internal pressure to the outside pressure and drains mucous production from the middle ear.

   ✓5ᵗʰ **H69.0** **Patulous Eustachian tube**

       H69.00 **Patulous Eustachian tube,** unspecified **ear**

       H69.01 **Patulous Eustachian tube,** right **ear**

       H69.02 **Patulous Eustachian tube,** left **ear**

       H69.03 **Patulous Eustachian tube,** bilateral

   ✓5ᵗʰ **H69.8** **Other specified disorders of Eustachian tube**

       H69.80 **Other specified disorders of Eustachian tube,** unspecified **ear**

       H69.81 **Other specified disorders of Eustachian tube,** right **ear**

       H69.82 **Other specified disorders of Eustachian tube,** left **ear**

       H69.83 **Other specified disorders of Eustachian tube,** bilateral

   ✓5ᵗʰ **H69.9** **Unspecified Eustachian tube disorder**

       H69.90 **Unspecified Eustachian tube disorder,** unspecified **ear**

       H69.91 **Unspecified Eustachian tube disorder,** right **ear**

       H69.92 **Unspecified Eustachian tube disorder,** left **ear**

       H69.93 **Unspecified Eustachian tube disorder,** bilateral

✓4ᵗʰ **H70** **Mastoiditis and related conditions**

   ✓5ᵗʰ **H70.0** **Acute mastoiditis**

     Abscess of mastoid

     Empyema of mastoid

     CC Excl: For CC codes in subcategory H70.0: PDX collection 641

   ✓6ᵗʰ **H70.00** **Acute mastoiditis** without complications

         H70.001 **Acute mastoiditis without complications,** right **ear**   `CC`

         H70.002 **Acute mastoiditis without complications,** left **ear**   `CC`

         H70.003 **Acute mastoiditis without complications,** bilateral   `CC`

         H70.009 **Acute mastoiditis without complications,** unspecified **ear**   `CC`

   ✓6ᵗʰ **H70.01** **Subperiosteal abscess** of mastoid

         H70.011 **Subperiosteal abscess of mastoid,** right **ear**   `CC`

         H70.012 **Subperiosteal abscess of mastoid,** left **ear**   `CC`

         H70.013 **Subperiosteal abscess of mastoid,** bilateral   `CC`

         H70.019 **Subperiosteal abscess of mastoid,** unspecified **ear**   `CC`

   ✓6ᵗʰ **H70.09** **Acute mastoiditis with other complications**

         H70.091 **Acute mastoiditis with other complications,** right **ear**   `CC`

         H70.092 **Acute mastoiditis with other complications,** left **ear**   `CC`

         H70.093 **Acute mastoiditis with other complications,** bilateral   `CC`

         H70.099 **Acute mastoiditis with other complications,** unspecified **ear**   `CC`

   ✓5ᵗʰ **H70.1** **Chronic mastoiditis**

     Caries of mastoid

     Fistula of mastoid

     EXCLUDES 1   *tuberculous mastoiditis (A18.03)*

       H70.10 **Chronic mastoiditis,** unspecified **ear**

       H70.11 **Chronic mastoiditis,** right **ear**

       H70.12 **Chronic mastoiditis,** left **ear**

       H70.13 **Chronic mastoiditis,** bilateral

   ✓5ᵗʰ **H70.2** **Petrositis**

     Inflammation of petrous bone

   ✓6ᵗʰ **H70.20** **Unspecified petrositis**

         H70.201 **Unspecified petrositis,** right **ear**

         H70.202 **Unspecified petrositis,** left **ear**

         H70.203 **Unspecified petrositis,** bilateral

         H70.209 **Unspecified petrositis,** unspecified **ear**

   ✓6ᵗʰ **H70.21** **Acute petrositis**

     DEF: Sudden, severe inflammation of the petrous temporal bone behind the ear, associated with a middle ear infection.

         H70.211 **Acute petrositis,** right **ear**

         H70.212 **Acute petrositis,** left **ear**

         H70.213 **Acute petrositis,** bilateral

         H70.219 **Acute petrositis,** unspecified **ear**

   ✓6ᵗʰ **H70.22** **Chronic petrositis**

         H70.221 **Chronic petrositis,** right **ear**

         H70.222 **Chronic petrositis,** left **ear**

         H70.223 **Chronic petrositis,** bilateral

         H70.229 **Chronic petrositis,** unspecified **ear**

   ✓5ᵗʰ **H70.8** **Other mastoiditis and related conditions**

     EXCLUDES 1   *preauricular sinus and cyst (Q18.1)*

           sinus, fistula, and cyst of branchial cleft (Q18.0)

   ✓6ᵗʰ **H70.81** **Postauricular fistula**

         H70.811 **Postauricular fistula,** right **ear**   `SW`

         H70.812 **Postauricular fistula,** left **ear**   `SW`

         H70.813 **Postauricular fistula,** bilateral   `SW`

         H70.819 **Postauricular fistula,** unspecified **ear**   `SW`

   ✓6ᵗʰ **H70.89** **Other mastoiditis and related conditions**

         H70.891 **Other mastoiditis and related conditions,** right **ear**

         H70.892 **Other mastoiditis and related conditions,** left **ear**

         H70.893 **Other mastoiditis and related conditions,** bilateral

         H70.899 **Other mastoiditis and related conditions,** unspecified **ear**

N Newborn: 0   P Pediatric: 0-17   M Maternity: 9-64   A Adult: 15-124   MCC Major Complication/Comorbidity   CC Complication/Comorbidity   SW Severe Wound Dx

636   **ICD-10-CM 2020**

√5ᵗʰ **H70.9 Unspecified mastoiditis**

    H70.90 Unspecified mastoiditis, unspecified ear

    H70.91 Unspecified mastoiditis, right ear

    H70.92 Unspecified mastoiditis, left ear

    H70.93 Unspecified mastoiditis, bilateral

√4ᵗʰ **H71 Cholesteatoma of middle ear**

    EXCLUDES 2   *cholesteatoma of external ear (H60.4-)*

          recurrent cholesteatoma of postmastoidectomy cavity (H95.0-)

    DEF: Cholesteatoma: Noncancerous cyst-like mass of cell debris, including cholesterol and epithelial cells resulting from trauma, repeated or improperly healed infections, and congenital enclosure of epidermal cells.

Cholesteatoma of Middle Ear

Middle ear chamber

Ear drum

Cholesteatoma sac

√5ᵗʰ **H71.0 Cholesteatoma of attic**

    H71.00 Cholesteatoma of attic, unspecified ear

    H71.01 Cholesteatoma of attic, right ear

    H71.02 Cholesteatoma of attic, left ear

    H71.03 Cholesteatoma of attic, bilateral

√5ᵗʰ **H71.1 Cholesteatoma of tympanum**

    H71.10 Cholesteatoma of tympanum, unspecified ear

    H71.11 Cholesteatoma of tympanum, right ear

    H71.12 Cholesteatoma of tympanum, left ear

    H71.13 Cholesteatoma of tympanum, bilateral

√5ᵗʰ **H71.2 Cholesteatoma of mastoid**

    H71.20 Cholesteatoma of mastoid, unspecified ear

    H71.21 Cholesteatoma of mastoid, right ear

    H71.22 Cholesteatoma of mastoid, left ear

    H71.23 Cholesteatoma of mastoid, bilateral

√5ᵗʰ **H71.3 Diffuse cholesteatosis**

    H71.30 Diffuse cholesteatosis, unspecified ear

    H71.31 Diffuse cholesteatosis, right ear

    H71.32 Diffuse cholesteatosis, left ear

    H71.33 Diffuse cholesteatosis, bilateral

√5ᵗʰ **H71.9 Unspecified cholesteatoma**

    H71.90 Unspecified cholesteatoma, unspecified ear

    H71.91 Unspecified cholesteatoma, right ear

    H71.92 Unspecified cholesteatoma, left ear

    H71.93 Unspecified cholesteatoma, bilateral

√4ᵗʰ **H72 Perforation of tympanic membrane**

    INCLUDES   persistent post-traumatic perforation of ear drum

          postinflammatory perforation of ear drum

    Code first any associated otitis media (H65.-, H66.1-, H66.2-, H66.3-, H66.4-, H66.9-, H67.-)

    EXCLUDES 1   *acute suppurative otitis media with rupture of the tympanic membrane (H66.01-)*

          traumatic rupture of ear drum (S09.2-)

√5ᵗʰ **H72.0 Central perforation of tympanic membrane**

    H72.00 Central perforation of tympanic membrane, unspecified ear

    H72.01 Central perforation of tympanic membrane, right ear

    H72.02 Central perforation of tympanic membrane, left ear

    H72.03 Central perforation of tympanic membrane, bilateral

√5ᵗʰ **H72.1 Attic perforation of tympanic membrane**

    Perforation of pars flaccida

    H72.10 Attic perforation of tympanic membrane, unspecified ear

    H72.11 Attic perforation of tympanic membrane, right ear

    H72.12 Attic perforation of tympanic membrane, left ear

    H72.13 Attic perforation of tympanic membrane, bilateral

√5ᵗʰ **H72.2 Other marginal perforations of tympanic membrane**

    √6ᵗʰ **H72.2X Other marginal perforations of tympanic membrane**

        H72.2X1 Other marginal perforations of tympanic membrane, right ear

        H72.2X2 Other marginal perforations of tympanic membrane, left ear

        H72.2X3 Other marginal perforations of tympanic membrane, bilateral

        H72.2X9 Other marginal perforations of tympanic membrane, unspecified ear

√5ᵗʰ **H72.8 Other perforations of tympanic membrane**

    √6ᵗʰ **H72.81 Multiple perforations of tympanic membrane**

        H72.811 Multiple perforations of tympanic membrane, right ear

        H72.812 Multiple perforations of tympanic membrane, left ear

        H72.813 Multiple perforations of tympanic membrane, bilateral

        H72.819 Multiple perforations of tympanic membrane, unspecified ear

    √6ᵗʰ **H72.82 Total perforations of tympanic membrane**

        H72.821 Total perforations of tympanic membrane, right ear

        H72.822 Total perforations of tympanic membrane, left ear

        H72.823 Total perforations of tympanic membrane, bilateral

        H72.829 Total perforations of tympanic membrane, unspecified ear

√5ᵗʰ **H72.9 Unspecified perforation of tympanic membrane**

    H72.90 Unspecified perforation of tympanic membrane, unspecified ear

    H72.91 Unspecified perforation of tympanic membrane, right ear

    H72.92 Unspecified perforation of tympanic membrane, left ear

    H72.93 Unspecified perforation of tympanic membrane, bilateral

√4ᵗʰ **H73 Other disorders of tympanic membrane**

    √5ᵗʰ **H73.0 Acute myringitis**

        EXCLUDES 1   *acute myringitis with otitis media (H65, H66)*

        √6ᵗʰ **H73.00 Unspecified acute myringitis**

            Acute tympanitis NOS

            H73.001 Acute myringitis, right ear

            H73.002 Acute myringitis, left ear

            H73.003 Acute myringitis, bilateral

            H73.009 Acute myringitis, unspecified ear

        √6ᵗʰ **H73.01 Bullous myringitis**

            DEF: Bacterial or viral otitis media that is characterized by the appearance of serous or hemorrhagic blebs on the ear drum and sudden onset of severe pain in ear.

            H73.011 Bullous myringitis, right ear

            H73.012 Bullous myringitis, left ear

            H73.013 Bullous myringitis, bilateral

            H73.019 Bullous myringitis, unspecified ear

        √6ᵗʰ **H73.09 Other acute myringitis**

            H73.091 Other acute myringitis, right ear

            H73.092 Other acute myringitis, left ear

            H73.093 Other acute myringitis, bilateral

            H73.099 Other acute myringitis, unspecified ear

    √5ᵗʰ **H73.1 Chronic myringitis**

        Chronic tympanitis

        EXCLUDES 1   *chronic myringitis with otitis media (H65, H66)*

        H73.10 Chronic myringitis, unspecified ear

        H73.11 Chronic myringitis, right ear

        H73.12 Chronic myringitis, left ear

        H73.13 Chronic myringitis, bilateral

    √5ᵗʰ **H73.2 Unspecified myringitis**

        H73.20 Unspecified myringitis, unspecified ear

        H73.21 Unspecified myringitis, right ear

☑ Additional Character Required   √x7ᵗʰ Placeholder   Unacceptable PDx   Questionable PDx   Manifestation   Unspecified Dx   H1 -H14 HAC   HCC CMS-HCC Dx   HIV HIV Dx

ICD-10-CM 2020   637

H73.22 Unspecified myringitis, left ear
H73.23 Unspecified myringitis, bilateral

✓5ᵗʰ **H73.8** Other specified disorders of tympanic membrane

✓6ᵗʰ **H73.81** Atrophic flaccid tympanic membrane
H73.811 Atrophic flaccid tympanic membrane, right ear
H73.812 Atrophic flaccid tympanic membrane, left ear
H73.813 Atrophic flaccid tympanic membrane, bilateral
H73.819 Atrophic flaccid tympanic membrane, unspecified ear

✓6ᵗʰ **H73.82** Atrophic nonflaccid tympanic membrane
H73.821 Atrophic nonflaccid tympanic membrane, right ear
H73.822 Atrophic nonflaccid tympanic membrane, left ear
H73.823 Atrophic nonflaccid tympanic membrane, bilateral
H73.829 Atrophic nonflaccid tympanic membrane, unspecified ear

✓6ᵗʰ **H73.89** Other specified disorders of tympanic membrane
H73.891 Other specified disorders of tympanic membrane, right ear
H73.892 Other specified disorders of tympanic membrane, left ear
H73.893 Other specified disorders of tympanic membrane, bilateral
H73.899 Other specified disorders of tympanic membrane, unspecified ear

✓5ᵗʰ **H73.9** Unspecified disorder of tympanic membrane
H73.90 Unspecified disorder of tympanic membrane, unspecified ear
H73.91 Unspecified disorder of tympanic membrane, right ear
H73.92 Unspecified disorder of tympanic membrane, left ear
H73.93 Unspecified disorder of tympanic membrane, bilateral

✓4ᵗʰ **H74** Other disorders of middle ear mastoid
EXCLUDES 2   mastoiditis (H70.-)

✓5ᵗʰ **H74.0** Tympanosclerosis
DEF: Calcification of tissue in the ear drum, middle ear bones, and middle ear canal.
H74.01 Tympanosclerosis, right ear
H74.02 Tympanosclerosis, left ear
H74.03 Tympanosclerosis, bilateral
H74.09 Tympanosclerosis, unspecified ear

✓5ᵗʰ **H74.1** Adhesive middle ear disease
Adhesive otitis
EXCLUDES 1   glue ear (H65.3-)
H74.11 Adhesive right middle ear disease
H74.12 Adhesive left middle ear disease
H74.13 Adhesive middle ear disease, bilateral
H74.19 Adhesive middle ear disease, unspecified ear

✓5ᵗʰ **H74.2** Discontinuity and dislocation of ear ossicles
H74.20 Discontinuity and dislocation of ear ossicles, unspecified ear
H74.21 Discontinuity and dislocation of right ear ossicles
H74.22 Discontinuity and dislocation of left ear ossicles
H74.23 Discontinuity and dislocation of ear ossicles, bilateral

✓5ᵗʰ **H74.3** Other acquired abnormalities of ear ossicles

✓6ᵗʰ **H74.31** Ankylosis of ear ossicles
H74.311 Ankylosis of ear ossicles, right ear
H74.312 Ankylosis of ear ossicles, left ear
H74.313 Ankylosis of ear ossicles, bilateral
H74.319 Ankylosis of ear ossicles, unspecified ear

✓6ᵗʰ **H74.32** Partial loss of ear ossicles
H74.321 Partial loss of ear ossicles, right ear
H74.322 Partial loss of ear ossicles, left ear
H74.323 Partial loss of ear ossicles, bilateral
H74.329 Partial loss of ear ossicles, unspecified ear

✓6ᵗʰ **H74.39** Other acquired abnormalities of ear ossicles
H74.391 Other acquired abnormalities of right ear ossicles

H74.392 Other acquired abnormalities of left ear ossicles
H74.393 Other acquired abnormalities of ear ossicles, bilateral
H74.399 Other acquired abnormalities of ear ossicles, unspecified ear

✓5ᵗʰ **H74.4** Polyp of middle ear
H74.40 Polyp of middle ear, unspecified ear
H74.41 Polyp of right middle ear
H74.42 Polyp of left middle ear
H74.43 Polyp of middle ear, bilateral

✓5ᵗʰ **H74.8** Other specified disorders of middle ear and mastoid

✓6ᵗʰ **H74.8X** Other specified disorders of middle ear and mastoid
H74.8X1 Other specified disorders of right middle ear and mastoid
H74.8X2 Other specified disorders of left middle ear and mastoid
H74.8X3 Other specified disorders of middle ear and mastoid, bilateral
H74.8X9 Other specified disorders of middle ear and mastoid, unspecified ear

✓5ᵗʰ **H74.9** Unspecified disorder of middle ear and mastoid
H74.90 Unspecified disorder of middle ear and mastoid, unspecified ear
H74.91 Unspecified disorder of right middle ear and mastoid
H74.92 Unspecified disorder of left middle ear and mastoid
H74.93 Unspecified disorder of middle ear and mastoid, bilateral

✓4ᵗʰ **H75** Other disorders of middle ear and mastoid in diseases classified elsewhere
Code first underlying disease

✓5ᵗʰ **H75.0** Mastoiditis in infectious and parasitic diseases classified elsewhere
EXCLUDES 1   mastoiditis (in):
syphilis (A52.77)
tuberculosis (A18.03)
H75.00 Mastoiditis in infectious and parasitic diseases classified elsewhere, unspecified ear
H75.01 Mastoiditis in infectious and parasitic diseases classified elsewhere, right ear
H75.02 Mastoiditis in infectious and parasitic diseases classified elsewhere, left ear
H75.03 Mastoiditis in infectious and parasitic diseases classified elsewhere, bilateral

✓5ᵗʰ **H75.8** Other specified disorders of middle ear and mastoid in diseases classified elsewhere
H75.80 Other specified disorders of middle ear and mastoid in diseases classified elsewhere, unspecified ear
H75.81 Other specified disorders of right middle ear and mastoid in diseases classified elsewhere
H75.82 Other specified disorders of left middle ear and mastoid in diseases classified elsewhere
H75.83 Other specified disorders of middle ear and mastoid in diseases classified elsewhere, bilateral

Diseases of inner ear (H80-H83)

✓4ᵗʰ **H80** Otosclerosis
INCLUDES   otospongiosis

✓5ᵗʰ **H80.0** Otosclerosis involving oval window, nonobliterative
H80.00 Otosclerosis involving oval window, nonobliterative, unspecified ear
H80.01 Otosclerosis involving oval window, nonobliterative, right ear
H80.02 Otosclerosis involving oval window, nonobliterative, left ear
H80.03 Otosclerosis involving oval window, nonobliterative, bilateral

✓5ᵗʰ **H80.1** Otosclerosis involving oval window, obliterative
H80.10 Otosclerosis involving oval window, obliterative, unspecified ear
H80.11 Otosclerosis involving oval window, obliterative, right ear
H80.12 Otosclerosis involving oval window, obliterative, left ear
H80.13 Otosclerosis involving oval window, obliterative, bilateral

Chapter 8. Diseases of the Ear and Mastoid Process

✓5ᵗʰ **H80.2 Cochlear otosclerosis**
  Otosclerosis involving otic capsule
  Otosclerosis involving round window
  H80.20 Cochlear otosclerosis, unspecified ear
  H80.21 Cochlear otosclerosis, right ear
  H80.22 Cochlear otosclerosis, left ear
  H80.23 Cochlear otosclerosis, bilateral
✓5ᵗʰ **H80.8 Other otosclerosis**
  H80.80 Other otosclerosis, unspecified ear
  H80.81 Other otosclerosis, right ear
  H80.82 Other otosclerosis, left ear
  H80.83 Other otosclerosis, bilateral
✓5ᵗʰ **H80.9 Unspecified otosclerosis**
  H80.90 Unspecified otosclerosis, unspecified ear
  H80.91 Unspecified otosclerosis, right ear
  H80.92 Unspecified otosclerosis, left ear
  H80.93 Unspecified otosclerosis, bilateral

✓4ᵗʰ **H81 Disorders of vestibular function**
  EXCLUDES 1 epidemic vertigo (A88.1)
    vertigo NOS (R42)
✓5ᵗʰ **H81.0 Ménière's disease**
  Labyrinthine hydrops
  Ménière's syndrome or vertigo
  DEF: Distended membranous labyrinth of the middle ear from fluctuating pressure of fluid (hydrops) that causes vertigo, tinnitus, pressure, and hearing loss that may last on and off for several hours. Episodes may occur in clusters or may subside for weeks, months, or even years.
  H81.01 Ménière's disease, right ear
  H81.02 Ménière's disease, left ear
  H81.03 Ménière's disease, bilateral
  H81.09 Ménière's disease, unspecified ear
✓5ᵗʰ **H81.1 Benign paroxysmal vertigo**
  H81.10 Benign paroxysmal vertigo, unspecified ear
  H81.11 Benign paroxysmal vertigo, right ear
  H81.12 Benign paroxysmal vertigo, left ear
  H81.13 Benign paroxysmal vertigo, bilateral
✓5ᵗʰ **H81.2 Vestibular neuronitis**
  DEF: Transient benign vertigo caused by inflammation of the vestibular nerve. It is characterized by response to caloric stimulation on one side and nystagmus with rhythmic movement of the eyes. Normal auditory function is present.
  H81.20 Vestibular neuronitis, unspecified ear
  H81.21 Vestibular neuronitis, right ear
  H81.22 Vestibular neuronitis, left ear
  H81.23 Vestibular neuronitis, bilateral
✓5ᵗʰ **H81.3 Other peripheral vertigo**
  ✓6ᵗʰ **H81.31 Aural vertigo**
    H81.311 Aural vertigo, right ear
    H81.312 Aural vertigo, left ear
    H81.313 Aural vertigo, bilateral
    H81.319 Aural vertigo, unspecified ear
  ✓6ᵗʰ **H81.39 Other peripheral vertigo**
    Lermoyez' syndrome
    Otogenic vertigo
    Peripheral vertigo NOS
    H81.391 Other peripheral vertigo, right ear
    H81.392 Other peripheral vertigo, left ear
    H81.393 Other peripheral vertigo, bilateral
    H81.399 Other peripheral vertigo, unspecified ear
▲ **H81.4 Vertigo of central origin**
  Central positional nystagmus
  ~~H81.41 Vertigo of central origin, right ear~~
  ~~H81.42 Vertigo of central origin, left ear~~
  ~~H81.43 Vertigo of central origin, bilateral~~
  ~~H81.49 Vertigo of central origin, unspecified ear~~
✓5ᵗʰ **H81.8 Other disorders of vestibular function**
  ✓6ᵗʰ **H81.8X Other disorders of vestibular function**
    H81.8X1 Other disorders of vestibular function, right ear
    H81.8X2 Other disorders of vestibular function, left ear
    H81.8X3 Other disorders of vestibular function, bilateral
    H81.8X9 Other disorders of vestibular function, unspecified ear

✓5ᵗʰ **H81.9 Unspecified disorder of vestibular function**
  Vertiginous syndrome NOS
  H81.90 Unspecified disorder of vestibular function, unspecified ear
  H81.91 Unspecified disorder of vestibular function, right ear
  H81.92 Unspecified disorder of vestibular function, left ear
  H81.93 Unspecified disorder of vestibular function, bilateral
✓4ᵗʰ **H82 Vertiginous syndromes in diseases classified elsewhere**
  Code first underlying disease
  EXCLUDES 1 epidemic vertigo (A88.1)
  H82.1 Vertiginous syndromes in diseases classified elsewhere, right ear
  H82.2 Vertiginous syndromes in diseases classified elsewhere, left ear
  H82.3 Vertiginous syndromes in diseases classified elsewhere, bilateral
  H82.9 Vertiginous syndromes in diseases classified elsewhere, unspecified ear
✓4ᵗʰ **H83 Other diseases of inner ear**
✓5ᵗʰ **H83.0 Labyrinthitis**
  DEF: Inflammation of the inner ear, or labyrinth, characterized by pus, vertigo, dizziness, nausea, and hearing loss.
  H83.01 Labyrinthitis, right ear
  H83.02 Labyrinthitis, left ear
  H83.03 Labyrinthitis, bilateral
  H83.09 Labyrinthitis, unspecified ear
✓5ᵗʰ **H83.1 Labyrinthine fistula**
  H83.11 Labyrinthine fistula, right ear
  H83.12 Labyrinthine fistula, left ear SW
  H83.13 Labyrinthine fistula, bilateral SW
  H83.19 Labyrinthine fistula, unspecified ear SW
✓5ᵗʰ **H83.2 Labyrinthine dysfunction**
  Labyrinthine hypersensitivity
  Labyrinthine hypofunction
  Labyrinthine loss of function
  DEF: Decreased function of the labyrinth sensors.
  ✓6ᵗʰ **H83.2X Labyrinthine dysfunction**
    H83.2X1 Labyrinthine dysfunction, right ear
    H83.2X2 Labyrinthine dysfunction, left ear
    H83.2X3 Labyrinthine dysfunction, bilateral
    H83.2X9 Labyrinthine dysfunction, unspecified ear
✓5ᵗʰ **H83.3 Noise effects on inner ear**
  Acoustic trauma of inner ear
  Noise-induced hearing loss of inner ear
  ✓6ᵗʰ **H83.3X Noise effects on inner ear**
    H83.3X1 Noise effects on right inner ear
    H83.3X2 Noise effects on left inner ear
    H83.3X3 Noise effects on inner ear, bilateral
    H83.3X9 Noise effects on inner ear, unspecified ear
✓5ᵗʰ **H83.8 Other specified diseases of inner ear**
  ✓6ᵗʰ **H83.8X Other specified diseases of inner ear**
    H83.8X1 Other specified diseases of right inner ear
    H83.8X2 Other specified diseases of left inner ear
    H83.8X3 Other specified diseases of inner ear, bilateral
    H83.8X9 Other specified diseases of inner ear, unspecified ear
✓5ᵗʰ **H83.9 Unspecified disease of inner ear**
  H83.90 Unspecified disease of inner ear, unspecified ear
  H83.91 Unspecified disease of right inner ear
  H83.92 Unspecified disease of left inner ear
  H83.93 Unspecified disease of inner ear, bilateral

Chapter 8. Diseases of the Ear and Mastoid Process

Other disorders of ear (H90–H94)

✓4ᵗʰ H90 Conductive and sensorineural hearing loss

EXCLUDES 1   *deaf nonspeaking NEC (H91.3)*
deafness NOS (H91.9-)
hearing loss NOS (H91.9-)
noise-induced hearing loss (H83.3-)
ototoxic hearing loss (H91.Ø-)
sudden (idiopathic) hearing loss (H91.2-)

AHA: 2015,2Q,7

DEF: Conductive hearing loss: Hearing Loss due to the inability of sound waves to move from the outer (external ear) to the inner ear.

DEF: Sensorineural hearing loss: Hearing loss that occurs from damage to the hair cells of the inner ear or problems with the nerve pathways from the inner ear to the brain.

H90.Ø   Conductive hearing loss, bilateral

✓5ᵗʰ **H90.1**   Conductive hearing loss, unilateral with unrestricted hearing on the contralateral side

     H90.11   Conductive hearing loss, unilateral, right ear, with unrestricted hearing on the contralateral side

     H90.12   Conductive hearing loss, unilateral, left ear, with unrestricted hearing on the contralateral side

H90.2   Conductive hearing loss, unspecified

     Conductive deafness NOS

H90.3   Sensorineural hearing loss, bilateral

✓5ᵗʰ **H90.4**   Sensorineural hearing loss, unilateral with unrestricted hearing on the contralateral side

     H90.41   Sensorineural hearing loss, unilateral, right ear, with unrestricted hearing on the contralateral side

     H90.42   Sensorineural hearing loss, unilateral, left ear, with unrestricted hearing on the contralateral side

H90.5   Unspecified sensorineural hearing loss

     Central hearing loss NOS
     Congenital deafness NOS
     Neural hearing loss NOS
     Perceptive hearing loss NOS
     Sensorineural deafness NOS
     Sensory hearing loss NOS

     EXCLUDES 1   *abnormal auditory perception (H93.2-)*
         psychogenic deafness (F44.6)

H90.6   Mixed conductive and sensorineural hearing loss, bilateral

     AHA: 2015,2Q,7

✓5ᵗʰ **H90.7**   Mixed conductive and sensorineural hearing loss, unilateral with unrestricted hearing on the contralateral side

     H90.71   Mixed conductive and sensorineural hearing loss, unilateral, right ear, with unrestricted hearing on the contralateral side

     H90.72   Mixed conductive and sensorineural hearing loss, unilateral, left ear, with unrestricted hearing on the contralateral side

H90.8   Mixed conductive and sensorineural hearing loss, unspecified

✓5ᵗʰ **H90.A**   Conductive and sensorineural hearing loss with restricted hearing on the contralateral side

     AHA: 2016,4Q,23-25

     ✓6ᵗʰ **H90.A1**   Conductive hearing loss, unilateral, with restricted hearing on the contralateral side

         H90.A11   Conductive hearing loss, unilateral, right ear with restricted hearing on the contralateral side

         H90.A12   Conductive hearing loss, unilateral, left ear with restricted hearing on the contralateral side

     ✓6ᵗʰ **H90.A2**   Sensorineural hearing loss, unilateral, with restricted hearing on the contralateral side

         H90.A21   Sensorineural hearing loss, unilateral, right ear, with restricted hearing on the contralateral side

         H90.A22   Sensorineural hearing loss, unilateral, left ear, with restricted hearing on the contralateral side

     ✓6ᵗʰ **H90.A3**   Mixed conductive and sensorineural hearing loss, unilateral with restricted hearing on the contralateral side

         H90.A31   Mixed conductive and sensorineural hearing loss, unilateral, right ear with restricted hearing on the contralateral side

         H90.A32   Mixed conductive and sensorineural hearing, unilateral, left ear with restricted hearing on the contralateral side

✓4ᵗʰ H91 Other and unspecified hearing loss

EXCLUDES 1   *abnormal auditory perception (H93.2-)*
hearing loss as classified in H90.-
impacted cerumen (H61.2-)
noise-induced hearing loss (H83.3-)
psychogenic deafness (F44.6)
transient ischemic deafness (H93.Ø1-)

✓5ᵗʰ **H91.Ø**   Ototoxic hearing loss

     Code first poisoning due to drug or toxin, if applicable (T36-T65 with fifth or sixth character 1-4 or 6)

     Use additional code for adverse effect, if applicable, to identify drug (T36-T5Ø with fifth or sixth character 5)

     H91.Ø1   Ototoxic hearing loss, right ear

     H91.Ø2   Ototoxic hearing loss, left ear

     H91.Ø3   Ototoxic hearing loss, bilateral

     H91.Ø9   Ototoxic hearing loss, unspecified ear

✓5ᵗʰ **H91.1**   Presbycusis

     Presbyacusia

     H91.10   Presbycusis, unspecified ear

     H91.11   Presbycusis, right ear

     H91.12   Presbycusis, left ear

     H91.13   Presbycusis, bilateral

✓5ᵗʰ **H91.2**   Sudden idiopathic hearing loss

     Sudden hearing loss NOS

     H91.20   Sudden idiopathic hearing loss, unspecified ear

     H91.21   Sudden idiopathic hearing loss, right ear

     H91.22   Sudden idiopathic hearing loss, left ear

     H91.23   Sudden idiopathic hearing loss, bilateral

H91.3   Deaf nonspeaking, not elsewhere classified

✓5ᵗʰ **H91.8**   Other specified hearing loss

     ✓6ᵗʰ **H91.8X**   Other specified hearing loss

         H91.8X1   Other specified hearing loss, right ear

         H91.8X2   Other specified hearing loss, left ear

         H91.8X3   Other specified hearing loss, bilateral

         H91.8X9   Other specified hearing loss, unspecified ear

✓5ᵗʰ **H91.9**   Unspecified hearing loss

     Deafness NOS
     High frequency deafness
     Low frequency deafness

     H91.90   Unspecified hearing loss, unspecified ear

     H91.91   Unspecified hearing loss, right ear

     H91.92   Unspecified hearing loss, left ear

     H91.93   Unspecified hearing loss, bilateral

✓4ᵗʰ H92 Otalgia and effusion of ear

✓5ᵗʰ **H92.Ø**   Otalgia

     H92.Ø1   Otalgia, right ear

     H92.Ø2   Otalgia, left ear

     H92.Ø3   Otalgia, bilateral

     H92.Ø9   Otalgia, unspecified ear

✓5ᵗʰ **H92.1**   Otorrhea

     EXCLUDES 1   *leakage of cerebrospinal fluid through ear (G96.Ø)*

     H92.10   Otorrhea, unspecified ear

     H92.11   Otorrhea, right ear

     H92.12   Otorrhea, left ear

     H92.13   Otorrhea, bilateral

✓5ᵗʰ **H92.2**   Otorrhagia

     EXCLUDES 1   *traumatic otorrhagia — code to injury*

     H92.20   Otorrhagia, unspecified ear

     H92.21   Otorrhagia, right ear

     H92.22   Otorrhagia, left ear

     H92.23   Otorrhagia, bilateral

✓4ᵗʰ H93 Other disorders of ear, not elsewhere classified

✓5ᵗʰ **H93.Ø**   Degenerative and vascular disorders of ear

     EXCLUDES 1   *presbycusis (H91.1)*

     ✓6ᵗʰ **H93.Ø1**   Transient ischemic deafness

         H93.Ø11   Transient ischemic deafness, right ear

         H93.Ø12   Transient ischemic deafness, left ear

         H93.Ø13   Transient ischemic deafness, bilateral

         H93.Ø19   Transient ischemic deafness, unspecified ear

N Newborn: 0   **P** Pediatric: 0-17   **M** Maternity: 9-64   **A** Adult: 15-124   **MCC** Major Complication/Comorbidity   **CC** Complication/Comorbidity   **SW** Severe Wound Dx

640   ICD-10-CM 2020

√6ᵗʰ **H93.09** **Unspecified degenerative and vascular disorders of ear**

     H93.091 Unspecified degenerative and vascular disorders of **right** ear

     H93.092 Unspecified degenerative and vascular disorders of **left** ear

     H93.093 Unspecified degenerative and vascular disorders of ear, **bilateral**

     H93.099 Unspecified degenerative and vascular disorders of **unspecified** ear

√5ᵗʰ **H93.1** **Tinnitus**

     H93.11 Tinnitus, **right** ear

     H93.12 Tinnitus, **left** ear

     H93.13 Tinnitus, **bilateral**

     H93.19 Tinnitus, **unspecified** ear

√5ᵗʰ **H93.A** **Pulsatile tinnitus**

     AHA: 2016,4Q,25-26

     H93.A1 Pulsatile tinnitus, **right** ear

     H93.A2 Pulsatile tinnitus, **left** ear

     H93.A3 Pulsatile tinnitus, **bilateral**

     H93.A9 Pulsatile tinnitus, **unspecified** ear

√5ᵗʰ **H93.2** **Other abnormal auditory perceptions**

     EXCLUDES 2   auditory hallucinations (R44.0)

√6ᵗʰ **H93.21** **Auditory recruitment**

     H93.211 Auditory recruitment, **right** ear

     H93.212 Auditory recruitment, **left** ear

     H93.213 Auditory recruitment, **bilateral**

     H93.219 Auditory recruitment, **unspecified** ear

√6ᵗʰ **H93.22** **Diplacusis**

     H93.221 Diplacusis, **right** ear

     H93.222 Diplacusis, **left** ear

     H93.223 Diplacusis, **bilateral**

     H93.229 Diplacusis, **unspecified** ear

√6ᵗʰ **H93.23** **Hyperacusis**

     DEF: Exceptionally acute sense of hearing caused by such conditions as Bell's palsy. This term may also refer to painful sensitivity to sounds.

     H93.231 Hyperacusis, **right** ear

     H93.232 Hyperacusis, **left** ear

     H93.233 Hyperacusis, **bilateral**

     H93.239 Hyperacusis, **unspecified** ear

√6ᵗʰ **H93.24** **Temporary auditory threshold shift**

     H93.241 Temporary auditory threshold shift, **right** ear

     H93.242 Temporary auditory threshold shift, **left** ear

     H93.243 Temporary auditory threshold shift, **bilateral**

     H93.249 Temporary auditory threshold shift, **unspecified** ear

H93.25 **Central auditory processing disorder**

     Congenital auditory imperception

     Word deafness

     EXCLUDES 1   mixed receptive-expressive language disorder (F80.2)

√6ᵗʰ **H93.29** **Other abnormal auditory perceptions**

     H93.291 Other abnormal auditory perceptions, **right** ear

     H93.292 Other abnormal auditory perceptions, **left** ear

     H93.293 Other abnormal auditory perceptions, **bilateral**

     H93.299 Other abnormal auditory perceptions, **unspecified** ear

√5ᵗʰ **H93.3** **Disorders of acoustic nerve**

     Disorder of 8th cranial nerve

     EXCLUDES 1   acoustic neuroma (D33.3)

                 syphilitic acoustic neuritis (A52.15)

√6ᵗʰ **H93.3X** **Disorders of acoustic nerve**

     H93.3X1 Disorders of **right** acoustic nerve

     H93.3X2 Disorders of **left** acoustic nerve

     H93.3X3 Disorders of **bilateral** acoustic nerves

     H93.3X9 Disorders of **unspecified** acoustic nerve

√5ᵗʰ **H93.8** **Other specified disorders of ear**

√6ᵗʰ **H93.8X** **Other specified disorders of ear**

     H93.8X1 Other specified disorders of **right** ear

     H93.8X2 Other specified disorders of **left** ear

     H93.8X3 Other specified disorders of ear, **bilateral**

     H93.8X9 Other specified disorders of ear, **unspecified** ear

√5ᵗʰ **H93.9** **Unspecified disorder of ear**

     H93.90 Unspecified disorder of ear, **unspecified** ear

     H93.91 Unspecified disorder of **right** ear

     H93.92 Unspecified disorder of **left** ear

     H93.93 Unspecified disorder of ear, **bilateral**

√4ᵗʰ **H94** **Other disorders of ear in diseases classified elsewhere**

√5ᵗʰ **H94.0** **Acoustic neuritis in infectious and parasitic diseases classified elsewhere**

     Code first underlying disease, such as:

     parasitic disease (B65-B89)

     EXCLUDES 1   acoustic neuritis (in):

                 herpes zoster (B02.29)

                 syphilis (A52.15)

     H94.00 *Acoustic neuritis in infectious and parasitic diseases classified elsewhere, unspecified ear*

     H94.01 *Acoustic neuritis in infectious and parasitic diseases classified elsewhere, right ear*

     H94.02 *Acoustic neuritis in infectious and parasitic diseases classified elsewhere, left ear*

     H94.03 *Acoustic neuritis in infectious and parasitic diseases classified elsewhere, bilateral*

√5ᵗʰ **H94.8** **Other specified disorders of ear in diseases classified elsewhere**

     Code first underlying disease, such as:

     congenital syphilis (A50.0)

     EXCLUDES 1   aural myiasis (B87.4)

                 syphilitic labyrinthitis (A52.79)

     H94.80 *Other specified disorders of ear in diseases classified elsewhere, unspecified ear*

     H94.81 *Other specified disorders of right ear in diseases classified elsewhere*

     H94.82 *Other specified disorders of left ear in diseases classified elsewhere*

     H94.83 *Other specified disorders of ear in diseases classified elsewhere, bilateral*

Intraoperative and postprocedural complications and disorders of ear and mastoid process, not elsewhere classified (H95)

CC Excl: For CC codes in category H95, unless otherwise noted: PDX collection 642

√4ᵗʰ **H95** **Intraoperative and postprocedural complications and disorders of ear and mastoid process, not elsewhere classified**

     AHA: 2016,4Q,9-10

√5ᵗʰ **H95.0** **Recurrent cholesteatoma of postmastoidectomy cavity**

     H95.00 Recurrent cholesteatoma of postmastoidectomy cavity, **unspecified** ear

     H95.01 Recurrent cholesteatoma of postmastoidectomy cavity, **right** ear

     H95.02 Recurrent cholesteatoma of postmastoidectomy cavity, **left** ear

     H95.03 Recurrent cholesteatoma of postmastoidectomy cavity, **bilateral** ears

√5ᵗʰ **H95.1** **Other disorders of ear and mastoid process following mastoidectomy**

√6ᵗʰ **H95.11** **Chronic inflammation of postmastoidectomy cavity**

     H95.111 Chronic inflammation of postmastoidectomy cavity, **right** ear

     H95.112 Chronic inflammation of postmastoidectomy cavity, **left** ear

     H95.113 Chronic inflammation of postmastoidectomy cavity, **bilateral** ears

     H95.119 Chronic inflammation of postmastoidectomy cavity, **unspecified** ear

√6ᵗʰ **H95.12** **Granulation of postmastoidectomy cavity**

     H95.121 Granulation of postmastoidectomy cavity, **right** ear

     H95.122 Granulation of postmastoidectomy cavity, **left** ear

     H95.123 Granulation of postmastoidectomy cavity, **bilateral** ears

     H95.129 Granulation of postmastoidectomy cavity, **unspecified** ear

☑ Additional Character Required   √x7ᵗʰ Placeholder   Unacceptable PDx   Questionable PDx   Manifestation   Unspecified Dx   H1-H14 HAC   HCC CMS-HCC Dx   HIV HIV Dx

ICD-10-CM 2020   641

Chapter 8. Diseases of the Ear and Mastoid Process

H95.13–H95.89

√6ᵗʰ **H95.13** Mucosal cyst of postmastoidectomy cavity

  H95.131 Mucosal cyst of postmastoidectomy cavity, **right** ear

  H95.132 Mucosal cyst of postmastoidectomy cavity, **left** ear

  H95.133 Mucosal cyst of postmastoidectomy cavity, **bilateral ears**

  H95.139 Mucosal cyst of postmastoidectomy cavity, **unspecified** ear

√6ᵗʰ **H95.19** Other disorders following mastoidectomy

  H95.191 Other disorders following mastoidectomy, **right** ear

  H95.192 Other disorders following mastoidectomy, **left** ear

  H95.193 Other disorders following mastoidectomy, **bilateral** ears

  H95.199 Other disorders following mastoidectomy, **unspecified** ear

√5ᵗʰ **H95.2** Intraoperative hemorrhage and hematoma of ear and mastoid process complicating a procedure

  EXCLUDES 1   intraoperative hemorrhage and hematoma of ear and mastoid process due to accidental puncture or laceration during a procedure (H95.3-)

  H95.21 Intraoperative hemorrhage and hematoma of ear and mastoid process complicating a **procedure** on the ear and mastoid process   CC

  H95.22 Intraoperative hemorrhage and hematoma of ear and mastoid process complicating **other** procedure   CC

√5ᵗʰ **H95.3** Accidental puncture and laceration of ear and mastoid process during a procedure

  H95.31 Accidental puncture and laceration of the ear and mastoid process during a **procedure** on the ear and mastoid process   CC
    CC Excl: PDX collection 509

  H95.32 Accidental puncture and laceration of the ear and mastoid process during **other** procedure   CC
    CC Excl: PDX collection 509

√5ᵗʰ **H95.4** Postprocedural hemorrhage of ear and mastoid process following a procedure

  H95.41 Postprocedural hemorrhage of ear and mastoid process following a procedure on the ear and mastoid process   CC

  H95.42 Postprocedural hemorrhage of ear and mastoid process following **other** procedure   CC

√5ᵗʰ **H95.5** Postprocedural hematoma and seroma of ear and mastoid process following a procedure

  H95.51 Postprocedural **hematoma** of ear and mastoid process following a procedure on the ear and mastoid process   CC

  H95.52 Postprocedural **hematoma** of ear and mastoid process following **other** procedure   CC

  H95.53 Postprocedural **seroma** of ear and mastoid process following a procedure on the ear and mastoid process   CC

  H95.54 Postprocedural **seroma** of ear and mastoid process following **other** procedure   CC

√5ᵗʰ **H95.8** Other intraoperative and postprocedural complications and disorders of the ear and mastoid process, not elsewhere classified

  EXCLUDES 2   postprocedural complications and disorders following mastoidectomy (H95.0-, H95.1-)

  For CC codes in subcategory H95.8: PDX collection 643

√6ᵗʰ **H95.81** Postprocedural stenosis of external ear canal

  H95.811 Postprocedural stenosis of **right** external ear canal   CC

  H95.812 Postprocedural stenosis of **left** external ear canal   CC

  H95.813 Postprocedural stenosis of external ear canal, **bilateral**   CC

  H95.819 Postprocedural stenosis of unspecified external ear canal   CC

H95.88 Other intraoperative complications and disorders of the ear and mastoid process, not elsewhere classified   CC
  Use additional code, if applicable, to further specify disorder

H95.89 Other postprocedural complications and disorders of the ear and mastoid process, not elsewhere classified   CC
  Use additional code, if applicable, to further specify disorder

N Newborn: 0   P Pediatric: 0-17   M Maternity: 9-64   A Adult: 15-124   MCC Major Complication/Comorbidity   CC Complication/Comorbidity   SW Severe Wound Dx

642   ICD-10-CM 2020

Chapter 9. Diseases of the Circulatory System (I00–I99)

Chapter-specific Guidelines with Coding Examples

The chapter-specific guidelines from the ICD-10-CM Official Guidelines for Coding and Reporting have been provided below. Along with these guidelines are coding examples, contained in the shaded boxes, that have been developed to help illustrate the coding and/or sequencing guidance found in these guidelines.

a. Hypertension

The classification presumes a causal relationship between hypertension and heart involvement and between hypertension and kidney involvement, as the two conditions are linked by the term "with" in the Alphabetic Index. These conditions should be coded as related even in the absence of provider documentation explicitly linking them, unless the documentation clearly states the conditions are unrelated.

For hypertension and conditions not specifically linked by relational terms such as "with," "associated with" or "due to" in the classification, provider documentation must link the conditions in order to code them as related.

1) Hypertension with heart disease

Hypertension with heart conditions classified to I50.- or I51.4-I51.7, I51.89, I51.9, are assigned to a code from category I11, Hypertensive heart disease. Use additional code(s) from category I50, Heart failure, to identify the type(s) of heart failure in those patients with heart failure.

The same heart conditions (I50.-, I51.4-I51.7, I51.89, I51.9) with hypertension are coded separately if the provider has documented they are unrelated to the hypertension. Sequence according to the circumstances of the admission/encounter.

> Patient is admitted in left heart failure. Patient also has a history of hypertension managed by medication.
>
> **I11.0**   **Hypertensive heart disease with heart failure**
>
> **I50.1**   **Left ventricular failure, unspecified**
>
> *Explanation*: Without a diagnostic statement to the contrary, hypertension and heart failure have an assumed causal relationship, and a combination code should be used. An additional code to identify the type of heart failure (I50.-) should also be provided.

2) Hypertensive chronic kidney disease

Assign codes from category I12, Hypertensive chronic kidney disease, when both hypertension and a condition classifiable to category N18, Chronic kidney disease (CKD), are present. CKD should not be coded as hypertensive if the provider indicates the CKD is not related to the hypertension.

The appropriate code from category N18 should be used as a secondary code with a code from category I12 to identify the stage of chronic kidney disease.

See Section I.C.14. Chronic kidney disease.

If a patient has hypertensive chronic kidney disease and acute renal failure, an additional code for the acute renal failure is required.

> Patient is admitted with stage IV chronic kidney disease (CKD) due to polycystic kidney disease. Patient also is on lisinopril for hypertension.
>
> **N18.4**   **Chronic kidney disease, stage 4 (severe)**
>
> **Q61.3**   **Polycystic kidney, unspecified**
>
> **I10**   **Essential (primary) hypertension**
>
> *Explanation*: A combination code describing a relationship between hypertension and CKD is not used because the physician documentation identifies the polycystic kidney disease as the cause for the CKD.

3) Hypertensive heart and chronic kidney disease

Assign codes from combination category I13, Hypertensive heart and chronic kidney disease, when there is hypertension with both heart and kidney involvement. If heart failure is present, assign an additional code from category I50 to identify the type of heart failure.

The appropriate code from category N18, Chronic kidney disease, should be used as a secondary code with a code from category I13 to identify the stage of chronic kidney disease.

See Section I.C.14. Chronic kidney disease.

The codes in category I13, Hypertensive heart and chronic kidney disease, are combination codes that include hypertension, heart disease and chronic kidney disease. The Includes note at I13 specifies that the conditions included at I11 and I12 are included together in I13. If a patient has hypertension, heart disease and chronic kidney disease, then a code from I13 should be used, not individual codes for hypertension, heart disease and chronic kidney disease, or codes from I11 or I12.

For patients with both acute renal failure and chronic kidney disease, an additional code for acute renal failure is required.

> Hypertensive heart and kidney disease with congestive heart failure and stage 2 chronic kidney disease
>
> **I13.0**   **Hypertensive heart and chronic kidney disease with heart failure and stage 1 through stage 4 chronic kidney disease, or unspecified chronic kidney disease**
>
> **I50.9**   **Heart failure, unspecified**
>
> **N18.2**   **Chronic kidney disease, stage 2 (mild)**
>
> *Explanation*: Combination codes in category I13 are used to report conditions classifiable to *both* categories I11 and I12. Do not report conditions classifiable to I11 and I12 separately. Use additional codes to report type of heart failure and stage of CKD.

4) Hypertensive cerebrovascular disease

For hypertensive cerebrovascular disease, first assign the appropriate code from categories I60-I69, followed by the appropriate hypertension code.

> Rupture of cerebral aneurysm caused by malignant hypertension
>
> **I60.7**   **Nontraumatic subarachnoid hemorrhage from unspecified intracranial artery**
>
> **I10**   **Essential (primary) hypertension**
>
> *Explanation*: Hypertensive cerebrovascular disease requires two codes: the appropriate I60–I69 code followed by the appropriate hypertension code.

5) Hypertensive retinopathy

Subcategory H35.0, Background retinopathy and retinal vascular changes, should be used with a code from category I10 – I15, Hypertensive disease to include the systemic hypertension. The sequencing is based on the reason for the encounter.

6) Hypertension, secondary

Secondary hypertension is due to an underlying condition. Two codes are required: one to identify the underlying etiology and one from category I15 to identify the hypertension. Sequencing of codes is determined by the reason for admission/encounter.

> Renovascular hypertension due to renal artery atherosclerosis
>
> **I15.0**   **Renovascular hypertension**
>
> **I70.1**   **Atherosclerosis of renal artery**
>
> *Explanation*: Secondary hypertension requires two codes: a code to identify the etiology and the appropriate I15 code.

7) Hypertension, transient

Assign code R03.0, Elevated blood pressure reading without diagnosis of hypertension, unless patient has an established diagnosis of hypertension. Assign code O13.-, Gestational [pregnancy-induced] hypertension without significant proteinuria, or O14.-, Pre-eclampsia, for transient hypertension of pregnancy.

8) Hypertension, controlled

This diagnostic statement usually refers to an existing state of hypertension under control by therapy. Assign the appropriate code from categories I10-I15, Hypertensive diseases.

9) Hypertension, uncontrolled

Uncontrolled hypertension may refer to untreated hypertension or hypertension not responding to current therapeutic regimen. In either case, assign the appropriate code from categories I10-I15, Hypertensive diseases.

10) Hypertensive crisis

Assign a code from category I16, Hypertensive crisis, for documented hypertensive urgency, hypertensive emergency or unspecified hypertensive crisis. Code also any identified hypertensive disease (I10-I15). The sequencing is based on the reason for the encounter.

11) Pulmonary hypertension

Pulmonary hypertension is classified to category I27, Other pulmonary heart diseases. For secondary pulmonary hypertension (I27.1, I27.2-), code also any associated conditions or adverse effects of drugs or toxins.

The sequencing is based on the reason for the encounter, except for adverse effects of drugs (See Section I.C.19.e.).

b. Atherosclerotic coronary artery disease and angina

ICD-10-CM has combination codes for atherosclerotic heart disease with angina pectoris. The subcategories for these codes are I25.11, Atherosclerotic heart disease of native coronary artery with angina pectoris and I25.7, Atherosclerosis of coronary artery bypass graft(s) and coronary artery of transplanted heart with angina pectoris.

When using one of these combination codes it is not necessary to use an additional code for angina pectoris. A causal relationship can be assumed in a patient with both atherosclerosis and angina pectoris, unless the documentation indicates the angina is due to something other than the atherosclerosis.

If a patient with coronary artery disease is admitted due to an acute myocardial infarction (AMI), the AMI should be sequenced before the coronary artery disease.

See Section I.C.9. Acute myocardial infarction (AMI)

c. Intraoperative and postprocedural cerebrovascular accident

Medical record documentation should clearly specify the cause- and- effect relationship between the medical intervention and the cerebrovascular accident in order to assign a code for intraoperative or postprocedural cerebrovascular accident.

Proper code assignment depends on whether it was an infarction or hemorrhage and whether it occurred intraoperatively or postoperatively. If it was a cerebral hemorrhage, code assignment depends on the type of procedure performed.

> Embolic cerebral infarction of the right middle cerebral artery that occurred during hip replacement surgery. The surgeon documented as due to the surgery.
>
> | I97.811 | Intraoperative cerebrovascular infarction during other surgery |
> |---|---|
> | I63.411 | Cerebral infarction due to embolism of right middle cerebral artery |
>
> *Explanation*: Code assignment for intraoperative or postprocedural cerebrovascular accident is based on the provider's documentation of a cause-and-effect relationship between the condition and the procedure. Proper code assignment also depends on whether the cerebrovascular accident was an infarction or hemorrhage, occurred intraoperatively or postoperatively, and the type of procedure performed.

d. Sequelae of cerebrovascular disease

1) Category I69, Sequelae of cerebrovascular disease

Category I69 is used to indicate conditions classifiable to categories I60-I67 as the causes of sequela (neurologic deficits), themselves classified elsewhere. These "late effects" include neurologic deficits that persist after initial onset of conditions classifiable to categories I60-I67. The neurologic deficits caused by cerebrovascular disease may be present from the onset or may arise at any time after the onset of the condition classifiable to categories I60-I67.

Codes from category I69, Sequelae of cerebrovascular disease, that specify hemiplegia, hemiparesis and monoplegia identify whether the dominant or nondominant side is affected. Should the affected side be documented, but not specified as dominant or nondominant, and the classification system does not indicate a default, code selection is as follows:

- For ambidextrous patients, the default should be dominant.
- If the left side is affected, the default is non-dominant.
- If the right side is affected, the default is dominant.

2) Codes from category I69 with codes from I60–I67

Codes from category I69 may be assigned on a health care record with codes from I60-I67, if the patient has a current cerebrovascular disease and deficits from an old cerebrovascular disease.

3) Codes from category I69 and personal history of transient ischemic attack (TIA) and cerebral infarction (Z86.73)

Codes from category I69 should not be assigned if the patient does not have neurologic deficits.

See Section I.C.21. 4. History (of) for use of personal history codes

e. Acute myocardial infarction (AMI)

1) Type 1 ST elevation myocardial infarction (STEMI) and non ST elevation myocardial infarction (NSTEMI)

The ICD-10-CM codes for type 1 acute myocardial infarction (AMI) identify the site, such as anterolateral wall or true posterior wall. Subcategories I21.0-I21.2 and code I21.3 are used for type 1 ST elevation myocardial infarction (STEMI). Code I21.4, Non-ST elevation (NSTEMI) myocardial

infarction, is used for type 1 non ST elevation myocardial infarction (NSTEMI) and nontransmural MIs.

If a type 1 NSTEMI evolves to STEMI, assign the STEMI code. If a type 1 STEMI converts to NSTEMI due to thrombolytic therapy, it is still coded as STEMI.

For encounters occurring while the myocardial infarction is equal to, or less than, four weeks old, including transfers to another acute setting or a postacute setting, and the myocardial infarction meets the definition for "other diagnoses" (see Section III, Reporting Additional Diagnoses), codes from category I21 may continue to be reported. For encounters after the 4 week time frame and the patient is still receiving care related to the myocardial infarction, the appropriate aftercare code should be assigned, rather than a code from category I21. For old or healed myocardial infarctions not requiring further care, code I25.2, Old myocardial infarction, may be assigned.

2) Acute myocardial infarction, unspecified

Code I21.9, Acute myocardial infarction, unspecified, is the default for unspecified acute myocardial infarction or unspecified type. If only type 1 STEMI or transmural MI without the site is documented, assign code I21.3, ST elevation (STEMI) myocardial infarction of unspecified site.

3) AMI documented as nontransmural or subendocardial but site provided

If an AMI is documented as nontransmural or subendocardial, but the site is provided, it is still coded as a subendocardial AMI.

See Section I.C.21.3 for information on coding status post administration of tPA in a different facility within the last 24 hours.

4) Subsequent acute myocardial infarction

A code from category I22, Subsequent ST elevation (STEMI) and non-ST elevation (NSTEMI) myocardial infarction, is to be used when a patient who has suffered a type 1 or unspecified AMI has a new AMI within the 4 week time frame of the initial AMI. A code from category I22 must be used in conjunction with a code from category I21. The sequencing of the I22 and I21 codes depends on the circumstances of the encounter.

Do not assign code I22 for subsequent myocardial infarctions other than type 1 or unspecified. For subsequent type 2 AMI assign only code I21.A1. For subsequent type 4 or type 5 AMI, assign only code I21.A9.

If a subsequent myocardial infarction of one type occurs within 4 weeks of a myocardial infarction of a different type, assign the appropriate codes from category I21 to identify each type. Do not assign a code from I22. Codes from category I22 should only be assigned if both the initial and subsequent myocardial infarctions are type 1 or unspecified.

5) Other types of myocardial infarction

The ICD-10-CM provides codes for different types of myocardial infarction. Type 1 myocardial infarctions are assigned to codes I21.0-I21.4.

Type 2 myocardial infarction (myocardial infarction due to demand ischemia or secondary to ischemic **im**balance) is assigned to code I21.A1, Myocardial infarction type 2 with the underlying cause **coded first**. Do not assign code I24.8, Other forms of acute ischemic heart disease, for the demand ischemia. **If** a type 2 AMI is described as NSTEMI or STEMI, only assign code I21.A1. Codes I21.01-I21.4 should only be assigned for type 1 AMIs.

Acute myocardial infarctions type 3, 4a, 4b, 4c and 5 are assigned to code I21.A9, Other myocardial infarction type.

The "Code also" and "Code first" notes should be followed related to complications, and for coding of postprocedural myocardial infarctions during or following cardiac surgery.

> Myocardial infarction involving the left circumflex artery occurring during PTCA with stent insertion to treat coronary artery disease
>
> | I25.10 | Atherosclerotic heart disease of native coronary artery without angina pectoris |
> |---|---|
> | I97.790 | Other intraoperative cardiac functional disturbances during cardiac surgery |
> | I21.A9 | Other myocardial infarction type |
>
> *Explanation*: A myocardial infarction occurring during a revascularization procedure is not considered a type 1 myocardial infarction (MI) and should not be coded to a type 1 MI code (I21.0-, I21.1-, I21.2-, I21.3) even when the specific site of the MI is documented. According to the code first instruction at I21.A9, the complication code (I97.790) should be sequenced before code I21.A9.

Chapter 9. Diseases of the Circulatory System (I00-I99)

EXCLUDES 2   *certain conditions originating in the perinatal period (P04-P96)*
certain infectious and parasitic diseases (A00-B99)
complications of pregnancy, childbirth and the puerperium (O00-O9A)
congenital malformations, deformations, and chromosomal abnormalities (Q00-Q99)
endocrine, nutritional and metabolic diseases (E00-E88)
injury, poisoning and certain other consequences of external causes (S00-T88)
neoplasms (C00-D49)
symptoms, signs and abnormal clinical and laboratory findings, not elsewhere classified (R00-R94)
systemic connective tissue disorders (M30-M36)
transient cerebral ischemic attacks and related syndromes (G45.-)

This chapter contains the following blocks:

I00-I02	Acute rheumatic fever
I05-I09	Chronic rheumatic heart diseases
I10-I16	Hypertensive diseases
I20-I25	Ischemic heart diseases
I26-I28	Pulmonary heart disease and diseases of pulmonary circulation
I30-I52	Other forms of heart disease
I60-I69	Cerebrovascular diseases
I70-I79	Diseases of arteries, arterioles and capillaries
I80-I89	Diseases of veins, lymphatic vessels and lymph nodes, not elsewhere classified
I95-I99	Other and unspecified disorders of the circulatory system

Acute rheumatic fever (I00-I02)

DEF: Inflammatory disease that can follow a throat infection by group A streptococci. Complications can involve the joints (arthritis), subcutaneous tissue (nodules), skin (erythema marginatum), heart (carditis), or brain (chorea).

I00   Rheumatic fever without heart involvement
     INCLUDES   arthritis, rheumatic, acute or subacute
     EXCLUDES 1   *rheumatic fever with heart involvement (I01.0-I01.9)*

✓4ᵗʰ **I01   Rheumatic fever with heart involvement**
     EXCLUDES 1   *chronic diseases of rheumatic origin (I05-I09) unless rheumatic fever is also present or there is evidence of reactivation or activity of the rheumatic process*

     I01.0   Acute rheumatic pericarditis   `CC`
         Any condition in I00 with pericarditis
         Rheumatic pericarditis (acute)
         EXCLUDES 1   *acute pericarditis not specified as rheumatic (I30.-)*
         CC Excl: PDX collection 188

     I01.1   Acute rheumatic endocarditis   `CC`
         Any condition in I00 with endocarditis or valvulitis
         Acute rheumatic valvulitis
         CC Excl: PDX collection 644

     I01.2   Acute rheumatic myocarditis   `CC`
         Any condition in I00 with myocarditis
         CC Excl: PDX collection 186

     I01.8   Other acute rheumatic heart disease   `CC`
         Any condition in I00 with other or multiple types of heart involvement
         Acute rheumatic pancarditis
         CC Excl: PDX collection 645

     I01.9   Acute rheumatic heart disease, unspecified   `CC`
         Any condition in I00 with unspecified type of heart involvement
         Rheumatic carditis, acute
         Rheumatic heart disease, active or acute
         CC Excl: PDX collection 646

✓4ᵗʰ **I02   Rheumatic chorea**
     INCLUDES   Sydenham's chorea
     EXCLUDES 1   *chorea NOS (G25.5)*
                   Huntington's chorea (G10)

     I02.0   Rheumatic chorea with heart involvement   `CC`
         Chorea NOS with heart involvement
         Rheumatic chorea with heart involvement of any type classifiable under I01.-
         CC Excl: PDX collection 645

     I02.9   Rheumatic chorea without heart involvement   `CC`
         Rheumatic chorea NOS
         CC Excl: PDX collection 646

Chronic rheumatic heart diseases (I05-I09)

✓4ᵗʰ **I05   Rheumatic mitral valve diseases**
     INCLUDES   conditions classifiable to both I05.0 and I05.2-I05.9, whether specified as rheumatic or not
     EXCLUDES 1   *mitral valve disease specified as nonrheumatic (I34.-)*
                   mitral valve disease with aortic and/or tricuspid valve involvement (I08.-)

     I05.0   Rheumatic mitral stenosis
         Mitral (valve) obstruction (rheumatic)
         DEF: Narrowing of the mitral valve between the left atrium and left ventricle due to rheumatic fever. Symptoms include shortness of breath during or after exercise, fatigue, palpitations, chest discomfort, and swelling of feet or legs.

     I05.1   Rheumatic mitral insufficiency
         Rheumatic mitral incompetence
         Rheumatic mitral regurgitation
         EXCLUDES 1   *mitral insufficiency not specified as rheumatic (I34.0)*

     I05.2   Rheumatic mitral stenosis with insufficiency
         Rheumatic mitral stenosis with incompetence or regurgitation

     I05.8   Other rheumatic mitral valve diseases
         Rheumatic mitral (valve) failure

     I05.9   Rheumatic mitral valve disease, unspecified
         Rheumatic mitral (valve) disorder (chronic) NOS

✓4ᵗʰ **I06   Rheumatic aortic valve diseases**
     EXCLUDES 1   *aortic valve disease not specified as rheumatic (I35.-)*
                   aortic valve disease with mitral and/or tricuspid valve involvement (I08.-)

     I06.0   Rheumatic aortic stenosis
         Rheumatic aortic (valve) obstruction

     I06.1   Rheumatic aortic insufficiency
         Rheumatic aortic incompetence
         Rheumatic aortic regurgitation

     I06.2   Rheumatic aortic stenosis with insufficiency
         Rheumatic aortic stenosis with incompetence or regurgitation

     I06.8   Other rheumatic aortic valve diseases

     I06.9   Rheumatic aortic valve disease, unspecified
         Rheumatic aortic (valve) disease NOS

✓4ᵗʰ **I07   Rheumatic tricuspid valve diseases**
     INCLUDES   rheumatic tricuspid valve diseases specified as rheumatic or unspecified
     EXCLUDES 1   *tricuspid valve disease specified as nonrheumatic (I36.-)*
                   tricuspid valve disease with aortic and/or mitral valve involvement (I08.-)

     I07.0   Rheumatic tricuspid stenosis
         Tricuspid (valve) stenosis (rheumatic)

     I07.1   Rheumatic tricuspid insufficiency
         Tricuspid (valve) insufficiency (rheumatic)

     I07.2   Rheumatic tricuspid stenosis and insufficiency

     I07.8   Other rheumatic tricuspid valve diseases

     I07.9   Rheumatic tricuspid valve disease, unspecified
         Rheumatic tricuspid valve disorder NOS

✓4ᵗʰ **I08   Multiple valve diseases**
     INCLUDES   multiple valve diseases specified as rheumatic or unspecified
     EXCLUDES 1   *endocarditis, valve unspecified (I38)*
                   multiple valve disease specified a nonrheumatic (I34.-, I35.-, I36.-, I37.-, I38.-, Q22.-, Q23.-, Q24.8-)
                   rheumatic valve disease NOS (I09.1)

     I08.0   Rheumatic disorders of both mitral and aortic valves
         Involvement of both mitral and aortic valves specified as rheumatic or unspecified
         AHA: 2019,2Q,5

     I08.1   Rheumatic disorders of both mitral and tricuspid valves

     I08.2   Rheumatic disorders of both aortic and tricuspid valves

     I08.3   Combined rheumatic disorders of mitral, aortic and tricuspid valves

     I08.8   Other rheumatic multiple valve diseases

     I08.9   Rheumatic multiple valve disease, unspecified

✓4ᵗʰ **I09   Other rheumatic heart diseases**

     I09.0   Rheumatic myocarditis   `CC`
         EXCLUDES 1   *myocarditis not specified as rheumatic (I51.4)*
         CC Excl: PDX collection 647

☑ Additional Character Required   ✓x7ᵗʰ Placeholder   Unacceptable PDx   Questionable PDx   Manifestation   Unspecified Dx   **H1**-**H14** HAC   **HCC** CMS-HCC Dx   **HIV** HIV Dx

ICD-10-CM 2020   645

Chapter 9. Diseases of the Circulatory System

I09.1   Rheumatic diseases of endocardium, valve unspecified
Rheumatic endocarditis (chronic)
Rheumatic valvulitis (chronic)
EXCLUDES 1   *endocarditis, valve unspecified (I38)*

I09.2   Chronic rheumatic pericarditis   `CC`
Adherent pericardium, rheumatic
Chronic rheumatic mediastinopericarditis
Chronic rheumatic myopericarditis
EXCLUDES 1   *chronic pericarditis not specified as rheumatic (I31.-)*
CC Excl: PDX collection 188

✓5ᵗʰ **I09.8   Other specified rheumatic heart diseases**

    I09.81   Rheumatic heart failure   `CC` `HCC`
Use additional code to identify type of heart failure (I50.-)
DEF: Decreased cardiac output, edema, and hypertension due to rheumatic heart disease.
CC Excl: PDX collection 648

    I09.89   Other specified rheumatic heart diseases
Rheumatic disease of pulmonary valve

I09.9   Rheumatic heart disease, unspecified
Rheumatic carditis
EXCLUDES 1   *rheumatoid carditis (M05.31)*

Hypertensive diseases (I10-I16)

Use additional code to identify:
exposure to environmental tobacco smoke (Z77.22)
history of tobacco dependence (Z87.891)
occupational exposure to environmental tobacco smoke (Z57.31)
tobacco dependence (F17.-)
tobacco use (Z72.0)
EXCLUDES 1   *neonatal hypertension (P29.2)*
           primary pulmonary hypertension (I27.0)
EXCLUDES 2   *hypertensive disease complicating pregnancy, childbirth and the puerperium (O10-O11, O13-O16)*

I10   Essential (primary) hypertension
INCLUDES   high blood pressure
hypertension (arterial) (benign) (essential) (malignant) (primary) (systemic)
EXCLUDES 1   *hypertensive disease complicating pregnancy, childbirth and the puerperium (O10-O11, O13-O16)*
EXCLUDES 2   *essential (primary) hypertension involving vessels of brain (I60-I69)*
           essential (primary) hypertension involving vessels of eye (H35.0-)
AHA: 2018,2Q,9; 2016,4Q,27

✓4ᵗʰ **I11   Hypertensive heart disease**
INCLUDES   any condition in I50.-, I51.4-I51.9 due to hypertension
AHA: 2018,2Q,9
TIP: Do not assign a code from this category when provider documentation indicates the heart disease is attributable to another cause.

    I11.0   Hypertensive heart disease with heart failure   `HCC`
Hypertensive heart failure
Use additional code to identify type of heart failure (I50.-)
AHA: 2017,1Q,47

    I11.9   Hypertensive heart disease without heart failure
Hypertensive heart disease NOS

✓4ᵗʰ **I12   Hypertensive chronic kidney disease**
INCLUDES   any condition in N18 and N26 — due to hypertension
arteriosclerosis of kidney
arteriosclerotic nephritis (chronic) (interstitial)
hypertensive nephropathy
nephrosclerosis
EXCLUDES 1   *hypertension due to kidney disease (I15.0, I15.1)*
           renovascular hypertension (I15.0)
           secondary hypertension (I15.-)
EXCLUDES 2   *acute kidney failure (N17.-)*
AHA: 2018,4Q,88; 2016,3Q,22
TIP: Do not assign a code from this category when provider documentation indicates the chronic kidney disease (CKD) is attributable to another cause.

    I12.0   Hypertensive chronic kidney disease with stage 5 chronic kidney disease or end stage renal disease   `CC` `HCC`
Use additional code to identify the stage of chronic kidney disease (N18.5, N18.6)
CC Excl: PDX collection 649

    I12.9   Hypertensive chronic kidney disease with stage 1 through stage 4 chronic kidney disease, or unspecified chronic kidney disease
Hypertensive chronic kidney disease NOS
Hypertensive renal disease NOS
Use additional code to identify the stage of chronic kidney disease (N18.1-N18.4, N18.9)

✓4ᵗʰ **I13   Hypertensive heart and chronic kidney disease**
INCLUDES   any condition in I11.- with any condition in I12.-
cardiorenal disease
cardiovascular renal disease
TIP: Do not assign a code from this category when provider documentation indicates the heart and/or chronic kidney disease is attributable to another cause.
CC Excl: For CC codes in category I13: PDX collection 650

    I13.0   Hypertensive heart and chronic kidney disease with heart failure and stage 1 through stage 4 chronic kidney disease, or unspecified chronic kidney disease   `CC` `HCC`
Use additional code to identify type of heart failure (I50.-)
Use additional code to identify stage of chronic kidney disease (N18.1-N18.4, N18.9)

✓5ᵗʰ **I13.1   Hypertensive heart and chronic kidney disease without heart failure**

       I13.10   Hypertensive heart and chronic kidney disease without heart failure, with stage 1 through stage 4 chronic kidney disease, or unspecified chronic kidney disease
Hypertensive heart disease and hypertensive chronic kidney disease NOS
Use additional code to identify the stage of chronic kidney disease (N18.1-N18.4, N18.9)

       I13.11   Hypertensive heart and chronic kidney disease without heart failure, with stage 5 chronic kidney disease, or end stage renal disease   `CC` `HCC`
Use additional code to identify the stage of chronic kidney disease (N18.5, N18.6)

    I13.2   Hypertensive heart and chronic kidney disease with heart failure and with stage 5 chronic kidney disease, or end stage renal disease   `CC` `HCC`
Use additional code to identify type of heart failure (I50.-)
Use additional code to identify the stage of chronic kidney disease (N18.5, N18.6)

✓4ᵗʰ **I15   Secondary hypertension**
Code also underlying condition
EXCLUDES 1   *postprocedural hypertension (I97.3)*
EXCLUDES 2   *secondary hypertension involving vessels of brain (I60-I69)*
           secondary hypertension involving vessels of eye (H35.0-)

    I15.0   Renovascular hypertension

    I15.1   Hypertension secondary to other renal disorders
AHA: 2016,3Q,22

    I15.2   Hypertension secondary to endocrine disorders

    I15.8   Other secondary hypertension

    I15.9   Secondary hypertension, unspecified

✓4ᵗʰ **I16   Hypertensive crisis**
Code also any identified hypertensive disease (I10-I15)
AHA: 2016,4Q,26-28

    I16.0   Hypertensive urgency

    I16.1   Hypertensive emergency   `CC`
CC Excl: No Excl

    I16.9   Hypertensive crisis, unspecified   `CC`
CC Excl: No Excl

Ischemic heart diseases (I20-I25)

Use additional code to identify presence of hypertension (I10-I16)

✓4ᵗʰ I20 Angina pectoris

Use additional code to identify:
    exposure to environmental tobacco smoke (Z77.22)
    history of tobacco dependence (Z87.891)
    occupational exposure to environmental tobacco smoke (Z57.31)
    tobacco dependence (F17.-)
    tobacco use (Z72.0)

EXCLUDES 1   *angina pectoris with atherosclerotic heart disease of native coronary arteries (I25.1-)*
        atherosclerosis of coronary artery bypass graft(s) and coronary artery of transplanted heart with angina pectoris (I25.7-)
        postinfarction angina (I23.7)

DEF: Chest pain due to reduced blood flow resulting in a lack of oxygen to the heart muscles.

I20.0 Unstable angina   `CC` `HCC`

Accelerated angina
Crescendo angina
De novo effort angina
Intermediate coronary syndrome
Preinfarction syndrome
Worsening effort angina
DEF: Condition representing an intermediate stage between angina of effort and acute myocardial infarction.
CC Excl: PDX collection 651

I20.1 Angina pectoris with documented spasm   `CC` `HCC`

Angiospastic angina
Prinzmetal angina
Spasm-induced angina
Variant angina
CC Excl: PDX collection 652

I20.8 Other forms of angina pectoris   `HCC`

Angina equivalent
Angina of effort
Coronary slow flow syndrome
Stable angina
Stenocardia
Use additional code(s) for symptoms associated with angina equivalent

I20.9 Angina pectoris, unspecified   `HCC`

Angina NOS
Anginal syndrome
Cardiac angina
Ischemic chest pain

✓4ᵗʰ I21 Acute myocardial infarction

INCLUDES   cardiac infarction
       coronary (artery) embolism
       coronary (artery) occlusion
       coronary (artery) rupture
       coronary (artery) thrombosis
       infarction of heart, myocardium, or ventricle
       myocardial infarction specified as acute or with a stated duration of 4 weeks (28 days) or less from onset

Use additional code, if applicable, to identify:
    exposure to environmental tobacco smoke (Z77.22)
    history of tobacco dependence (Z87.891)
    occupational exposure to environmental tobacco smoke (Z57.31)
    status post administration of tPA (rtPA) in a different facility within the last 24 hours prior to admission to current facility (Z92.82)
    tobacco dependence (F17.-)
    tobacco use (Z72.0)

EXCLUDES 2   *old myocardial infarction (I25.2)*
        postmyocardial infarction syndrome (I24.1)
        subsequent type 1 myocardial infarction (I22.-)

AHA: 2019,2Q,5; 2018,4Q,68; 2018,3Q,5; 2017,4Q,12-14; 2017,1Q,44-45; 2016,4Q,140; 2015,2Q,16; 2013,1Q,25; 2012,4Q,96,102-103
TIP: When chronic total occlusion and myocardial infarction are documented as being in different vessels, assign code I25.82 Chronic total occlusion of coronary artery, in addition to the myocardial infarction code.
CC Excl: For MCC codes in category I21: PDX collection 653

✓5ᵗʰ I21.0 ST elevation (STEMI) myocardial infarction of anterior wall

Type 1 ST elevation myocardial infarction of anterior wall
DEF: ST elevation myocardial infarction: Complete obstruction of one or more coronary arteries causing decreased blood flow (ischemia) and necrosis of myocardial muscle cells.

I21.01 ST elevation (STEMI) myocardial infarction involving left main coronary artery   `CC` `HCC`

I21.02 ST elevation (STEMI) myocardial infarction involving left anterior descending coronary artery   `CC` `HCC`

ST elevation (STEMI) myocardial infarction involving diagonal coronary artery
AHA: 2013,1Q,25

I21.09 ST elevation (STEMI) myocardial infarction involving other coronary artery of anterior wall   `CC` `HCC`

Acute transmural myocardial infarction of anterior wall
Anteroapical transmural (Q wave) infarction (acute)
Anterolateral transmural (Q wave) infarction (acute)
Anteroseptal transmural (Q wave) infarction (acute)
Transmural (Q wave) infarction (acute) (of) anterior (wall) NOS
AHA: 2012,4Q,102-103

✓5ᵗʰ I21.1 ST elevation (STEMI) myocardial infarction of inferior wall

Type 1 ST elevation myocardial infarction of inferior wall
DEF: ST elevation myocardial infarction: Complete obstruction of one or more coronary arteries causing decreased blood flow (ischemia) and necrosis of myocardial muscle cells.

I21.11 ST elevation (STEMI) myocardial infarction involving right coronary artery   `CC` `HCC`

Inferoposterior transmural (Q wave) infarction (acute)

I21.19 ST elevation (STEMI) myocardial infarction involving other coronary artery of inferior wall   `CC` `HCC`

Acute transmural myocardial infarction of inferior wall
Inferolateral transmural (Q wave) infarction (acute)
Transmural (Q wave) infarction (acute) (of) diaphragmatic wall
Transmural (Q wave) infarction (acute) (of) inferior (wall) NOS

EXCLUDES 2   *ST elevation (STEMI) myocardial infarction involving left circumflex coronary artery (I21.21)*

AHA: 2012,4Q,96

√5ᵗʰ **I21.2**   **ST elevation (STEMI) myocardial infarction of other sites**

Type 1 ST elevation myocardial infarction of other sites
DEF: ST elevation myocardial infarction: Complete obstruction of one or more coronary arteries causing decreased blood flow (ischemia) and necrosis of myocardial muscle cells.

     I21.21   **ST elevation (STEMI) myocardial infarction involving left circumflex coronary artery**   CC HCC

ST elevation (STEMI) myocardial infarction involving oblique marginal coronary artery

     I21.29   **ST elevation (STEMI) myocardial infarction involving other sites**   CC HCC

Acute transmural myocardial infarction of other sites
Apical-lateral transmural (Q wave) infarction (acute)
Basal-lateral transmural (Q wave) infarction (acute)
High lateral transmural (Q wave) infarction (acute)
Lateral (wall) NOS transmural (Q wave) infarction (acute)
Posterior (true) transmural (Q wave) infarction (acute)
Posterobasal transmural (Q wave) infarction (acute)
Posterolateral transmural (Q wave) infarction (acute)
Posteroseptal transmural (Q wave) infarction (acute)
Septal transmural (Q wave) infarction (acute) NOS

I21.3   **ST elevation (STEMI) myocardial infarction of unspecified site**   CC HCC

Acute transmural myocardial infarction of unspecified site
Transmural (Q wave) myocardial infarction NOS
Type 1 ST elevation myocardial infarction of unspecified site
DEF: ST elevation myocardial infarction: Complete obstruction of one or more coronary arteries causing decreased blood flow (ischemia) and necrosis of myocardial muscle cells.

I21.4   **Non-ST elevation (NSTEMI) myocardial infarction**   MCC HCC

Acute subendocardial myocardial infarction
Non-Q wave myocardial infarction NOS
Nontransmural myocardial infarction NOS
Type 1 non-ST elevation myocardial infarction
AHA: 2019,2Q,33; 2017,1Q,44-45
DEF: Partial obstruction of one or more coronary arteries that causes decreased blood flow (ischemia) and may cause partial thickness necrosis of myocardial muscle cells.

I21.9   **Acute myocardial infarction, unspecified**   MCC HCC

Myocardial infarction (acute) NOS

√5ᵗʰ **I21.A**   **Other type of myocardial infarction**

AHA: 2019,2Q,5

     I21.A1   **Myocardial infarction type 2**   MCC HCC

Myocardial infarction due to demand ischemia
Myocardial infarction secondary to ischemic imbalance
►Code first the underlying cause, such as:◄
►anemia (D50.0-D64.9)◄
►chronic obstructive pulmonary disease (J44.-)◄
►paroxysmal tachycardia (I47.0-I47.9)◄
►shock (R57.0-R57.9)◄
~~Code also the underlying cause, if known and applicable, such as:~~
~~anemia (D50.0-D64.9)~~
~~chronic obstructive pulmonary disease (J44.-)~~
~~heart failure (I50.-)~~
~~paroxysmal tachycardia (I47.0-I47.9)~~
~~renal failure (N17.0-N19)~~
~~shock (R57.0-R57.9)~~
AHA: 2017,4Q,13-14
DEF: Often referred to as due to demand ischemia, myocardial infarction (MI) type 2 refers to an MI due to ischemia and necrosis resulting from an oxygen imbalance to the heart. This mismatch between oxygen decreased supply and increased demand is caused by conditions other than coronary artery disease such as vasospasm, embolism, anemia, hypertension, hypotension, or arrhythmias.

I21.A9   **Other myocardial infarction type**   MCC HCC

Myocardial infarction associated with revascularization procedure
Myocardial infarction type 3
Myocardial infarction type 4a
Myocardial infarction type 4b
Myocardial infarction type 4c
Myocardial infarction type 5
Code first, if applicable, postprocedural myocardial infarction following cardiac surgery (I97.190), or postprocedural myocardial infarction during cardiac surgery (I97.790)
Code also complication, if known and applicable, such as:
(acute) stent occlusion (T82.897-)
(acute) stent stenosis ►(T82.855-)◄
(acute) stent thrombosis (T82.867-)
cardiac arrest due to underlying cardiac condition (I46.2)
complication of percutaneous coronary intervention (PCI) (I97.89)
occlusion of coronary artery bypass graft (T82.218-)
AHA: 2019,2Q,33

√4ᵗʰ **I22**   **Subsequent ST elevation (STEMI) and non-ST elevation (NSTEMI) myocardial infarction**

INCLUDES   acute myocardial infarction occurring within four weeks (28 days) of a previous acute myocardial infarction, regardless of site
cardiac infarction
coronary (artery) embolism
coronary (artery) occlusion
coronary (artery) rupture
coronary (artery) thrombosis
infarction of heart, myocardium, or ventricle
recurrent myocardial infarction
reinfarction of myocardium
rupture of heart, myocardium, or ventricle
subsequent type 1 myocardial infarction

Use additional code, if applicable, to identify:
exposure to environmental tobacco smoke (Z77.22)
history of tobacco dependence (Z87.891)
occupational exposure to environmental tobacco smoke (Z57.31)
status post administration of tPA (rtPA) in a different facility within the last 24 hours prior to admission to current facility (Z92.82)
tobacco dependence (F17.-)
tobacco use (Z72.0)

EXCLUDES 1   subsequent myocardial infarction, type 2 (I21.A1)
subsequent myocardial infarction of other type (type 3) (type 4) (type 5) (I21.A9)

AHA: 2018,4Q,68; 2018,3Q,5; 2017,4Q,12-13; 2017,2Q,11; 2013,1Q,25; 2012,4Q,97,102-103
DEF: Non-ST elevation myocardial infarction: Partial obstruction of one or more coronary arteries that causes decreased blood flow (ischemia) and may cause partial thickness necrosis of myocardial muscle cells.
DEF: ST elevation myocardial infarction: Complete obstruction of one or more coronary arteries causing decreased blood flow (ischemia) and necrosis of myocardial muscle cells.
TIP: When chronic total occlusion and myocardial infarction are documented as being in different vessels, assign code I25.82 Chronic total occlusion of coronary artery, in addition to the myocardial infarction code.

I22.0   **Subsequent ST elevation (STEMI) myocardial infarction of anterior wall**   CC HCC

Subsequent acute transmural myocardial infarction of anterior wall
Subsequent transmural (Q wave) infarction (acute)(of) anterior (wall) NOS
Subsequent anteroapical transmural (Q wave) infarction (acute)
Subsequent anterolateral transmural (Q wave) infarction (acute)
Subsequent anteroseptal transmural (Q wave) infarction (acute)

I22.1 Subsequent ST elevation (STEMI) myocardial infarction of inferior wall `CC` `HCC`

Subsequent acute transmural myocardial infarction of inferior wall

Subsequent transmural (Q wave) infarction (acute)(of) diaphragmatic wall

Subsequent transmural (Q wave) infarction (acute)(of) inferior (wall) NOS

Subsequent inferolateral transmural (Q wave) infarction (acute)

Subsequent inferoposterior transmural (Q wave) infarction (acute)

AHA: 2012,4Q,102

I22.2 Subsequent non-ST elevation (NSTEMI) myocardial infarction `CC` `HCC`

Subsequent acute subendocardial myocardial infarction

Subsequent non-Q wave myocardial infarction NOS

Subsequent nontransmural myocardial infarction NOS

I22.8 Subsequent ST elevation (STEMI) myocardial infarction of other sites `CC` `HCC`

Subsequent acute transmural myocardial infarction of other sites

Subsequent apical-lateral transmural (Q wave) myocardial infarction (acute)

Subsequent basal-lateral transmural (Q wave) myocardial infarction (acute)

Subsequent high lateral transmural (Q wave) myocardial infarction (acute)

Subsequent transmural (Q wave) myocardial infarction (acute)(of) lateral (wall) NOS

Subsequent posterior (true) transmural (Q wave) myocardial infarction (acute)

Subsequent posterobasal transmural (Q wave) myocardial infarction (acute)

Subsequent posterolateral transmural (Q wave) myocardial infarction (acute)

Subsequent posteroseptal transmural (Q wave) myocardial infarction (acute)

Subsequent septal NOS transmural (Q wave) myocardial infarction (acute)

I22.9 Subsequent ST elevation (STEMI) myocardial infarction of unspecified site `CC` `HCC`

Subsequent acute myocardial infarction of unspecified site

Subsequent myocardial infarction (acute) NOS

√4ᵗʰ **I23 Certain current complications following ST elevation (STEMI) and non-ST elevation (NSTEMI) myocardial infarction (within the 28 day period)**

AHA: 2017,2Q,11

DEF: ST elevation myocardial infarction: Complete obstruction of one or more coronary arteries causing decreased blood flow (ischemia) and necrosis of myocardial muscle cells.

DEF: Non-ST elevation myocardial infarction: Partial obstruction of one or more coronary arteries that causes decreased blood flow (ischemia) and may cause partial thickness necrosis of myocardial muscle cells.

CC Excl: For CC codes in category I23: PDX collection 654

I23.0 Hemopericardium as current complication following acute myocardial infarction `CC` `HCC` `A`

EXCLUDES 1   hemopericardium not specified as current complication following acute myocardial infarction (I31.2)

I23.1 Atrial septal defect as current complication following acute myocardial infarction `CC` `HCC` `A`

EXCLUDES 1   acquired atrial septal defect not specified as current complication following acute myocardial infarction (I51.0)

I23.2 Ventricular septal defect as current complication following acute myocardial infarction `CC` `HCC` `A`

EXCLUDES 1   acquired ventricular septal defect not specified as current complication following acute myocardial infarction (I51.0)

I23.3 Rupture of cardiac wall without hemopericardium as current complication following acute myocardial infarction `CC` `HCC` `A`

I23.4 Rupture of chordae tendineae as current complication following acute myocardial infarction `MCC` `HCC`

EXCLUDES 1   rupture of chordae tendineae not specified as current complication following acute myocardial infarction (I51.1)

CC Excl: PDX collection 655

I23.5 Rupture of papillary muscle as current complication following acute myocardial infarction `MCC` `HCC`

EXCLUDES 1   rupture of papillary muscle not specified as current complication following acute myocardial infarction (I51.2)

CC Excl: PDX collection 656

I23.6 Thrombosis of atrium, auricular appendage, and ventricle as current complications following acute myocardial infarction `CC` `HCC` `A`

EXCLUDES 1   thrombosis of atrium, auricular appendage, and ventricle not specified as current complication following acute myocardial infarction (I51.3)

I23.7 Postinfarction angina `CC` `HCC` `A`

AHA: 2015,2Q,16

TIP: When postinfarction angina occurs with atherosclerotic coronary artery disease, code both I23.7 and I25.118 for atherosclerotic disease with other forms of angina pectoris.

I23.8 Other current complications following acute myocardial infarction `CC` `HCC` `A`

√4ᵗʰ **I24 Other acute ischemic heart diseases**

EXCLUDES 1   angina pectoris (I20.-)

transient myocardial ischemia in newborn (P29.4)

CC Excl: For CC codes in category I24, unless otherwise noted: PDX collection 657

I24.0 Acute coronary thrombosis not resulting in myocardial infarction `CC` `HCC`

Acute coronary (artery) (vein) embolism not resulting in myocardial infarction

Acute coronary (artery) (vein) occlusion not resulting in myocardial infarction

Acute coronary (artery) (vein) thromboembolism not resulting in myocardial infarction

EXCLUDES 1   atherosclerotic heart disease (I25.1-)

AHA: 2013,1Q,24

I24.1 Dressler's syndrome `CC` `HCC`

Postmyocardial infarction syndrome

EXCLUDES 1   postinfarction angina (I23.7)

DEF: Fever, leukocytosis, chest pain, evidence of pericarditis, pleurisy, and pneumonia occurring days or weeks after a myocardial infarction.

CC Excl: PDX collection 658

I24.8 Other forms of acute ischemic heart disease `CC` `HCC`

EXCLUDES 1   myocardial infarction due to demand ischemia (I21.A1)

AHA: 2017,4Q,13

I24.9 Acute ischemic heart disease, unspecified `CC` `HCC`

EXCLUDES 1   ischemic heart disease (chronic) NOS (I25.9)

✓4ᵗʰ **I25 Chronic ischemic heart disease**
Use additional code to identify:
chronic total occlusion of coronary artery (I25.82)
exposure to environmental tobacco smoke (Z77.22)
history of tobacco dependence (Z87.891)
occupational exposure to environmental tobacco smoke (Z57.31)
tobacco dependence (F17.-)
tobacco use (Z72.0)

✓5ᵗʰ **I25.1 Atherosclerotic heart disease of native coronary artery**
Atherosclerotic cardiovascular disease
Coronary (artery) atheroma
Coronary (artery) atherosclerosis
Coronary (artery) disease
Coronary (artery) sclerosis
Use additional code, if applicable, to identify:
coronary atherosclerosis due to calcified coronary lesion (I25.84)
coronary atherosclerosis due to lipid rich plaque (I25.83)
EXCLUDES 2   atheroembolism (I75.-)
atherosclerosis of coronary artery bypass graft(s) and transplanted heart (I25.7-)

Atheromas

Atheromas (fatty tissue and/or plaque)   Lumen

I25.10 Atherosclerotic heart disease of native coronary artery without angina pectoris   Ⓐ
Atherosclerotic heart disease NOS
AHA: 2015,2Q,16; 2012,4Q,92

✓6ᵗʰ **I25.11 Atherosclerotic heart disease of native coronary artery with angina pectoris**

I25.110 Atherosclerotic heart disease of native coronary artery with unstable angina pectoris   CC HCC Ⓐ
EXCLUDES 1   unstable angina without atherosclerotic heart disease (I20.0)
CC Excl: PDX collection 651

I25.111 Atherosclerotic heart disease of native coronary artery with angina pectoris with documented spasm   HCC Ⓐ
EXCLUDES 1   angina pectoris with documented spasm without atherosclerotic heart disease (I20.1)

I25.118 Atherosclerotic heart disease of native coronary artery with other forms of angina pectoris   HCC Ⓐ
EXCLUDES 1   other forms of angina pectoris without atherosclerotic heart disease (I20.8)
AHA: 2015,2Q,16
TIP: When postinfarction angina occurs with atherosclerotic coronary artery disease, code both I23.7 and I25.118 for atherosclerotic disease with other forms of angina pectoris.

I25.119 Atherosclerotic heart disease of native coronary artery with unspecified angina pectoris   HCC Ⓐ
Atherosclerotic heart disease with angina NOS
Atherosclerotic heart disease with ischemic chest pain
EXCLUDES 1   unspecified angina pectoris without atherosclerotic heart disease (I20.9)

I25.2 Old myocardial infarction
Healed myocardial infarction
Past myocardial infarction diagnosed by ECG or other investigation, but currently presenting no symptoms

I25.3 Aneurysm of heart   CC
Mural aneurysm
Ventricular aneurysm
CC Excl: PDX collection 659

✓5ᵗʰ **I25.4 Coronary artery aneurysm and dissection**

I25.41 Coronary artery aneurysm
Coronary arteriovenous fistula, acquired
EXCLUDES 1   congenital coronary (artery) aneurysm (Q24.5)

I25.42 Coronary artery dissection   MCC
DEF: Tear in the intimal arterial wall of a coronary artery resulting in the sudden intrusion of blood within the layers of the wall.
CC Excl: PDX collection 660

I25.5 Ischemic cardiomyopathy
EXCLUDES 2   coronary atherosclerosis (I25.1-, I25.7-)

I25.6 Silent myocardial ischemia

✓5ᵗʰ **I25.7 Atherosclerosis of coronary artery bypass graft(s) and coronary artery of transplanted heart with angina pectoris**
Use additional code, if applicable, to identify:
coronary atherosclerosis due to calcified coronary lesion (I25.84)
coronary atherosclerosis due to lipid rich plaque (I25.83)
EXCLUDES 1   atherosclerosis of bypass graft(s) of transplanted heart without angina pectoris (I25.812)
atherosclerosis of coronary artery bypass graft(s) without angina pectoris (I25.810)
atherosclerosis of native coronary artery of transplanted heart without angina pectoris (I25.811)

✓6ᵗʰ **I25.70 Atherosclerosis of coronary artery bypass graft(s), unspecified, with angina pectoris**

I25.700 Atherosclerosis of coronary artery bypass graft(s), unspecified, with unstable angina pectoris   CC HCC Ⓐ
EXCLUDES 1   unstable angina pectoris without atherosclerosis of coronary artery bypass graft (I20.0)
CC Excl: PDX collection 651

I25.701 Atherosclerosis of coronary artery bypass graft(s), unspecified, with angina pectoris with documented spasm   HCC Ⓐ
EXCLUDES 1   angina pectoris with documented spasm without atherosclerosis of coronary artery bypass graft (I20.1)

I25.708 Atherosclerosis of coronary artery bypass graft(s), unspecified, with other forms of angina pectoris   HCC Ⓐ
EXCLUDES 1   other forms of angina pectoris without atherosclerosis of coronary artery bypass graft (I20.8)

I25.709 Atherosclerosis of coronary artery bypass graft(s), unspecified, with unspecified angina pectoris   HCC Ⓐ
EXCLUDES 1   unspecified angina pectoris without atherosclerosis of coronary artery bypass graft (I20.9)

√6ᵗʰ **I25.71 Atherosclerosis of autologous vein coronary artery bypass graft(s) with angina pectoris**
CC Excl: For CC codes in subcategory I25.71, unless otherwise noted: PDX collection 662

I25.710 Atherosclerosis of autologous `CC` `HCC` `A` **vein coronary artery bypass graft(s) with unstable angina pectoris**
EXCLUDES 1   unstable angina without atherosclerosis of autologous vein coronary artery bypass graft(s) (I20.0)
EXCLUDES 2   embolism or thrombus of coronary artery bypass graft(s) (T82.8-)
CC Excl: PDX collection 661

I25.711 Atherosclerosis of autologous `CC` `HCC` `A` **vein coronary artery bypass graft(s) with angina pectoris with documented spasm**
EXCLUDES 1   angina pectoris with documented spasm without atherosclerosis of autologous vein coronary artery bypass graft(s) (I20.1)

I25.718 Atherosclerosis of autologous `CC` `HCC` `A` **vein coronary artery bypass graft(s) with other forms of angina pectoris**
EXCLUDES 1   other forms of angina pectoris without atherosclerosis of autologous vein coronary artery bypass graft(s) (I20.8)

I25.719 Atherosclerosis of autologous `CC` `HCC` `A` **vein coronary artery bypass graft(s) with unspecified angina pectoris**
EXCLUDES 1   unspecified angina pectoris without atherosclerosis of autologous vein coronary artery bypass graft(s) (I20.9)

√6ᵗʰ **I25.72 Atherosclerosis of autologous artery coronary artery bypass graft(s) with angina pectoris**
Atherosclerosis of internal mammary artery graft with angina pectoris
CC Excl: For CC codes in subcategories I25.72, unless otherwise noted: PDX collection 662

I25.720 Atherosclerosis of autologous `CC` `HCC` `A` **artery coronary artery bypass graft(s) with unstable angina pectoris**
EXCLUDES 1   unstable angina without atherosclerosis of autologous artery coronary artery bypass graft(s) (I20.0)
CC Excl: PDX collection 661

I25.721 Atherosclerosis of autologous `CC` `HCC` `A` **artery coronary artery bypass graft(s) with angina pectoris with documented spasm**
EXCLUDES 1   angina pectoris with documented spasm without atherosclerosis of autologous artery coronary artery bypass graft(s) (I20.1)

I25.728 Atherosclerosis of autologous `CC` `HCC` `A` **artery coronary artery bypass graft(s) with other forms of angina pectoris**
EXCLUDES 1   other forms of angina pectoris without atherosclerosis of autologous artery coronary artery bypass graft(s) (I20.8)

I25.729 Atherosclerosis of autologous `CC` `HCC` `A` **artery coronary artery bypass graft(s) with unspecified angina pectoris**
EXCLUDES 1   unspecified angina pectoris without atherosclerosis of autologous artery coronary artery bypass graft(s) (I20.9)

√6ᵗʰ **I25.73 Atherosclerosis of nonautologous biological coronary artery bypass graft(s) with angina pectoris**
CC Excl: For CC codes in subcategories I25.73, unless otherwise noted: PDX collection 662

I25.730 Atherosclerosis of `CC` `HCC` `A` **nonautologous biological coronary artery bypass graft(s) with unstable angina pectoris**
EXCLUDES 1   unstable angina without atherosclerosis of nonautologous biological coronary artery bypass graft(s) (I20.0)
CC Excl: PDX collection 661

I25.731 Atherosclerosis of `CC` `HCC` `A` **nonautologous biological coronary artery bypass graft(s) with angina pectoris with documented spasm**
EXCLUDES 1   angina pectoris with documented spasm without atherosclerosis of nonautologous biological coronary artery bypass graft(s) (I20.1)

I25.738 Atherosclerosis of `CC` `HCC` `A` **nonautologous biological coronary artery bypass graft(s) with other forms of angina pectoris**
EXCLUDES 1   other forms of angina pectoris without atherosclerosis of nonautologous biological coronary artery bypass graft(s) (I20.8)

I25.739 Atherosclerosis of `CC` `HCC` `A` **nonautologous biological coronary artery bypass graft(s) with unspecified angina pectoris**
EXCLUDES 1   unspecified angina pectoris without atherosclerosis of nonautologous biological coronary artery bypass graft(s) (I20.9)

√6ᵗʰ **I25.75 Atherosclerosis of native coronary artery of transplanted heart with angina pectoris**
EXCLUDES 1   atherosclerosis of native coronary artery of transplanted heart without angina pectoris (I25.811)
CC Excl: For CC codes in subcategory I25.75, unless otherwise noted: PDX collection 664

I25.750 Atherosclerosis of native `CC` `HCC` **coronary artery of transplanted heart with unstable angina**
CC Excl: PDX collection 663

I25.751 Atherosclerosis of native `CC` `HCC` **coronary artery of transplanted heart with angina pectoris with documented spasm**

I25.758 Atherosclerosis of native `CC` `HCC` **coronary artery of transplanted heart with other forms of angina pectoris**

I25.759 Atherosclerosis of native `CC` `HCC` **coronary artery of transplanted heart with unspecified angina pectoris**

√6ᵗʰ **I25.76** **Atherosclerosis of bypass graft of coronary artery of transplanted heart with angina pectoris**

> *EXCLUDES 1*   atherosclerosis of bypass graft of coronary artery of transplanted heart without angina pectoris (I25.812)

> **CC Excl:** For CC codes in subcategory I25.76, unless otherwise noted: PDX collection 666

I25.760 **Atherosclerosis of bypass graft** `CC` `HCC` `A` **of coronary artery of transplanted heart with unstable angina**

> **CC Excl:** PDX collection 665

I25.761 **Atherosclerosis of bypass graft** `CC` `HCC` `A` **of coronary artery of transplanted heart with angina pectoris with documented spasm**

I25.768 **Atherosclerosis of bypass graft** `CC` `HCC` `A` **of coronary artery of transplanted heart with other forms of angina pectoris**

I25.769 **Atherosclerosis of bypass graft** `CC` `HCC` `A` **of coronary artery of transplanted heart with unspecified angina pectoris**

√6ᵗʰ **I25.79** **Atherosclerosis of other coronary artery bypass graft(s) with angina pectoris**

> **CC Excl:** For CC codes in subcategory I25.79, unless otherwise noted: No Excl

I25.790 **Atherosclerosis of other** `CC` `HCC` `A` **coronary artery bypass graft(s) with unstable angina pectoris**

> *EXCLUDES 1*   unstable angina without atherosclerosis of other coronary artery bypass graft(s) (I20.0)

> **CC Excl:** PDX collection 651

I25.791 **Atherosclerosis of other** `CC` `HCC` `A` **coronary artery bypass graft(s) with angina pectoris with documented spasm**

> *EXCLUDES 1*   angina pectoris with documented spasm without atherosclerosis of other coronary artery bypass graft(s) (I20.1)

I25.798 **Atherosclerosis of other** `CC` `HCC` `A` **coronary artery bypass graft(s) with other forms of angina pectoris**

> *EXCLUDES 1*   other forms of angina pectoris without atherosclerosis of other coronary artery bypass graft(s) (I20.8)

I25.799 **Atherosclerosis of other** `CC` `HCC` `A` **coronary artery bypass graft(s) with unspecified angina pectoris**

> *EXCLUDES 1*   unspecified angina pectoris without atherosclerosis of other coronary artery bypass graft(s) (I20.9)

√5ᵗʰ **I25.8** **Other forms of chronic ischemic heart disease**

√6ᵗʰ **I25.81** **Atherosclerosis of other coronary vessels without angina pectoris**

> Use additional code, if applicable, to identify:
> coronary atherosclerosis due to calcified coronary lesion (I25.84)
> coronary atherosclerosis due to lipid rich plaque (I25.83)

> *EXCLUDES 1*   ~~atherosclerotic heart disease of native coronary artery without angina pectoris (I25.10)~~

> *EXCLUDES 2*   ▶atherosclerotic heart disease of native coronary artery without angina pectoris (I25.10)◀

I25.810 **Atherosclerosis of coronary** `CC` `A` **artery bypass graft(s) without angina pectoris**

> Atherosclerosis of coronary artery bypass graft NOS

> *EXCLUDES 1*   atherosclerosis of coronary bypass graft(s) with angina pectoris (I25.70-I25.73-, I25.79-)

> **CC Excl:** No Excl

I25.811 **Atherosclerosis of native** `CC` **coronary artery of transplanted heart without angina pectoris**

> Atherosclerosis of native coronary artery of transplanted heart NOS

> *EXCLUDES 1*   atherosclerosis of native coronary artery of transplanted heart with angina pectoris (I25.75-)

> **CC Excl:** PDX collection 664

I25.812 **Atherosclerosis of bypass graft** `CC` `A` **of coronary artery of transplanted heart without angina pectoris**

> Atherosclerosis of bypass graft of transplanted heart NOS

> *EXCLUDES 1*   atherosclerosis of bypass graft of transplanted heart with angina pectoris (I25.76)

> **CC Excl:** PDX collection 666

I25.82 **Chronic total occlusion of coronary artery**

> Complete occlusion of coronary artery
> Total occlusion of coronary artery
> Code first coronary atherosclerosis (I25.1-, I25.7-, I25.81-)

> *EXCLUDES 1*   acute coronary occlusion with myocardial infarction (I21.0-I21.9, I22.-)
> acute coronary occlusion without myocardial infarction (I24.0)

> **AHA:** 2018,3Q,5
> **DEF:** Complete blockage of the coronary artery due to plaque accumulation over an extended period of time, resulting in substantial reduction of blood flow. Symptoms include angina or chest pain.
> **TIP:** Report this code in addition to a code from category I21 or I22 when the chronic total occlusion and the myocardial infarction are documented as being in different vessels.

I25.83 **Coronary atherosclerosis due to lipid rich plaque** `A`

> Code first coronary atherosclerosis (I25.1-, I25.7-, I25.81-)

I25.84 **Coronary atherosclerosis due to calcified coronary lesion**

> Coronary atherosclerosis due to severely calcified coronary lesion
> Code first coronary atherosclerosis (I25.1-, I25.7-, I25.81-)

I25.89 **Other forms of chronic ischemic heart disease**

I25.9 **Chronic ischemic heart disease, unspecified**

> Ischemic heart disease (chronic) NOS

`N` Newborn: 0   `P` Pediatric: 0-17   `M` Maternity: 9-64   `A` Adult: 15-124   `MCC` Major Complication/Comorbidity   `CC` Complication/Comorbidity   `SW` Severe Wound Dx

652   ICD-10-CM 2020

Pulmonary heart disease and diseases of pulmonary circulation (I26-I28)

✓4ᵗʰ I26 Pulmonary embolism

INCLUDES   pulmonary (acute)(artery)(vein) infarction
pulmonary (acute) (artery)(vein) thromboembolism
pulmonary (acute)(artery)(vein) thrombosis

EXCLUDES 2   chronic pulmonary embolism (I27.82)
personal history of pulmonary embolism (Z86.711)
pulmonary embolism complicating abortion, ectopic or molar pregnancy (O00-O07, O08.2)
pulmonary embolism complicating pregnancy, childbirth and the puerperium (O88.-)
pulmonary embolism due to trauma (T79.0, T79.1)
pulmonary embolism due to complications of surgical and medical care (T80.0, T81.7-, T82.8-)
septic (non-pulmonary) arterial embolism (I76)

✓5ᵗʰ I26.0 Pulmonary embolism with acute cor pulmonale

DEF: Cor pulmonale: Heart-lung disease appearing in identifiable forms as chronic or acute. The chronic form of this heart-lung disease is marked by dilation, hypertrophy and failure of the right ventricle due to a disease that has affected the function of the lungs, excluding congenital or left heart diseases and is also called chronic cardiopulmonary disease. The acute form is an overload of the right ventricle from a rapid onset of pulmonary hypertension, usually arising from a pulmonary embolism.

CC Excl: For MCC codes in subcategory I26.0: PDX collection 667

I26.01   **Septic pulmonary embolism with acute cor pulmonale**   MCC HCC
Code first underlying infection

I26.02   **Saddle embolus of pulmonary artery with acute cor pulmonale**   MCC H10 HCC

I26.09   **Other pulmonary embolism with acute cor pulmonale**   MCC H10 HCC
Acute cor pulmonale NOS
AHA: 2014,4Q,21

✓5ᵗʰ I26.9 Pulmonary embolism without acute cor pulmonale

I26.90   **Septic pulmonary embolism without acute cor pulmonale**   MCC HCC
Code first underlying infection
CC Excl: PDX collection 668

I26.92   **Saddle embolus of pulmonary artery without acute cor pulmonale**   MCC H10 HCC
CC Excl: PDX collection 669

I26.93   **Single subsegmental pulmonary embolism without acute cor pulmonale**   MCC
Subsegmental pulmonary embolism NOS

I26.94   **Multiple subsegmental pulmonary emboli without acute cor pulmonale**   MCC

I26.99   **Other pulmonary embolism without acute cor pulmonale**   MCC H10 HCC
Acute pulmonary embolism NOS
Pulmonary embolism NOS
AHA: 2019,2Q,22
CC Excl: PDX collection 670

✓4ᵗʰ I27 Other pulmonary heart diseases

I27.0   **Primary pulmonary hypertension**   CC HCC
Heritable pulmonary arterial hypertension
Idiopathic pulmonary arterial hypertension
Primary group 1 pulmonary hypertension
Primary pulmonary arterial hypertension

EXCLUDES 1   persistent pulmonary hypertension of newborn (P29.30)
pulmonary hypertension NOS (I27.20)
secondary pulmonary arterial hypertension (I27.21)
secondary pulmonary hypertension (I27.29)

DEF: Condition that occurs when pressure within the pulmonary artery is elevated and vascular resistance is observed in the lungs.
CC Excl: PDX collection 671

I27.1   **Kyphoscoliotic heart disease**   CC HCC
CC Excl: PDX collection 533

✓5ᵗʰ I27.2 Other secondary pulmonary hypertension

Code also associated underlying condition
EXCLUDES 1   Eisenmenger's syndrome (I27.83)
AHA: 2017,4Q,14-15; 2014,4Q,21
DEF: Condition that occurs when pressure within the pulmonary artery is elevated and vascular resistance is observed in the lungs.

I27.20   **Pulmonary hypertension, unspecified**   HCC
Pulmonary hypertension NOS

I27.21   **Secondary pulmonary arterial hypertension**   HCC
(Associated) (drug-induced) (toxin-induced) pulmonary arterial hypertension NOS
(Associated) (drug-induced) (toxin-induced) (secondary) group 1 pulmonary hypertension
Code also associated conditions if applicable, or adverse effects of drugs or toxins, such as:
adverse effect of appetite depressants (T50.5X5)
congenital heart disease (Q20-Q28)
human immunodeficiency virus [HIV] disease (B20)
polymyositis (M33.2-)
portal hypertension (K76.6)
rheumatoid arthritis (M05.-)
schistosomiasis (B65.-)
Sjögren syndrome (M35.0-)
systemic sclerosis (M34.-)

I27.22   **Pulmonary hypertension due to left heart disease**   HCC
Group 2 pulmonary hypertension
Code also associated left heart disease, if known, such as:
multiple valve disease (I08.-)
rheumatic aortic valve diseases (I06.-)
rheumatic mitral valve diseases (I05.-)

I27.23   **Pulmonary hypertension due to lung diseases and hypoxia**   HCC
Group 3 pulmonary hypertension
Code also associated lung disease, if known, such as:
bronchiectasis (J47.-)
cystic fibrosis with pulmonary manifestations (E84.0)
interstitial lung disease (J84.-)
pleural effusion (J90)
sleep apnea (G47.3-)

I27.24   **Chronic thromboembolic pulmonary hypertension**   HCC
Group 4 pulmonary hypertension
Code also associated pulmonary embolism, if applicable (I26.-, I27.82)

I27.29   **Other secondary pulmonary hypertension**   HCC
Group 5 pulmonary hypertension
Pulmonary hypertension with unclear multifactorial mechanisms
Pulmonary hypertension due to hematologic disorders
Pulmonary hypertension due to metabolic disorders
Pulmonary hypertension due to other systemic disorders
Code also other associated disorders, if known, such as:
chronic myeloid leukemia (C92.10- C92.22)
essential thrombocythemia (D47.3)
Gaucher disease (E75.22)
hypertensive chronic kidney disease with end stage renal disease (I12.0, I13.11, I13.2)
hyperthyroidism (E05.-)
hypothyroidism (E00-E03)
polycythemia vera (D45)
sarcoidosis (D86.-)
AHA: 2016,2Q,8

Chapter 9. Diseases of the Circulatory System

I27.8–I31.4

√5th **I27.8 Other specified pulmonary heart diseases**

I27.81 Cor pulmonale (chronic) CC HCC

Cor pulmonale NOS

EXCLUDES 1 *acute cor pulmonale (I26.0-)*

AHA: 2014,4Q,21

DEF: Heart-lung disease appearing in identifiable forms as chronic or acute. The chronic form of this heart-lung disease is marked by dilation, hypertrophy and failure of the right ventricle due to a disease that has affected the function of the lungs, excluding congenital or left heart diseases and is also called chronic cardiopulmonary disease. The acute form is an overload of the right ventricle from a rapid onset of pulmonary hypertension, usually arising from a pulmonary embolism.

I27.82 Chronic pulmonary embolism CC HCC

Use additional code, if applicable, for associated long-term (current) use of anticoagulants (Z79.01)

EXCLUDES 1 *personal history of pulmonary embolism (Z86.711)*

DEF: Long-standing condition commonly associated with pulmonary hypertension in which small blood clots travel to the lungs repeatedly over many weeks, months, or years, requiring continuation of established anticoagulant or thrombolytic therapy.

CC Excl: PDX collection 669

I27.83 Eisenmenger's syndrome HCC

Eisenmenger's complex

(Irreversible) Eisenmenger's disease

Pulmonary hypertension with right to left shunt related to congenital heart disease

Code also underlying heart defect, if known, such as:
atrial septal defect (Q21.1)
Eisenmenger's defect (Q21.8)
patent ductus arteriosus (Q25.0)
ventricular septal defect (Q21.0)

DEF: Pulmonary hypertension with congenital communication between two circulations resulting in a right to left shunt. This causes reduced oxygen saturation in the arterial blood, leading to cyanosis and organ damage. Once it develops, this life-threating condition is irreversible.

I27.89 Other specified pulmonary heart diseases HCC

I27.9 Pulmonary heart disease, unspecified HCC

Chronic cardiopulmonary disease

√4th **I28 Other diseases of pulmonary vessels**

I28.0 Arteriovenous fistula of pulmonary vessels CC HCC

EXCLUDES 1 *congenital arteriovenous fistula (Q25.72)*

CC Excl: PDX collection 672

I28.1 Aneurysm of pulmonary artery CC HCC

EXCLUDES 1 *congenital aneurysm (Q25.79)*
congenital arteriovenous aneurysm (Q25.72)

CC Excl: PDX collection 672

I28.8 Other diseases of pulmonary vessels HCC

Pulmonary arteritis
Pulmonary endarteritis
Rupture of pulmonary vessels
Stenosis of pulmonary vessels
Stricture of pulmonary vessels

I28.9 Disease of pulmonary vessels, unspecified HCC

Other forms of heart disease (I30-I52)

√4th **I30 Acute pericarditis**

INCLUDES acute mediastinopericarditis
acute myopericarditis
acute pericardial effusion
acute pleuropericarditis
acute pneumopericarditis

EXCLUDES 1 *Dressler's syndrome (I24.1)*
rheumatic pericarditis (acute) (I01.0)
viral pericarditis due to Coxsakie virus (B33.23)

DEF: Pericarditis: Inflammation affecting the pericardium, the fibroserous membrane that surrounds the heart.

CC Excl: For CC codes in category I30: PDX collection 673

I30.0 Acute nonspecific idiopathic pericarditis CC

I30.1 Infective pericarditis CC

Pneumococcal pericarditis
Pneumopyopericardium
Purulent pericarditis
Pyopericarditis
Pyopericardium
Pyopneumopericardium
Staphylococcal pericarditis
Streptococcal pericarditis
Suppurative pericarditis
Viral pericarditis

Use additional code (B95-B97) to identify infectious agent

I30.8 Other forms of acute pericarditis CC

I30.9 Acute pericarditis, unspecified CC

√4th **I31 Other diseases of pericardium**

EXCLUDES 1 *diseases of pericardium specified as rheumatic (I09.2)*
postcardiotomy syndrome (I97.0)
traumatic injury to pericardium (S26.-)

I31.0 Chronic adhesive pericarditis CC

Accretio cordis
Adherent pericardium
Adhesive mediastinopericarditis

CC Excl: PDX collection 674

I31.1 Chronic constrictive pericarditis CC

Concretio cordis
Pericardial calcification

CC Excl: PDX collection 674

I31.2 Hemopericardium, not elsewhere classified CC

EXCLUDES 1 *hemopericardium as current complication following acute myocardial infarction (I23.0)*

DEF: Presence of blood in the pericardial sac (pericardium). It can lead to potentially fatal cardiac tamponade if enough blood enters the pericardial cavity.

CC Excl: PDX collection 674

I31.3 Pericardial effusion (noninflammatory) CC

Chylopericardium

EXCLUDES 1 *acute pericardial effusion (I30.9)*

AHA: 2019,1Q,16

TIP: Assign this code for documented malignant pericardial effusion. If the sole reason for admission is to treat the effusion with no treatment rendered for the associated malignancy, this code may be sequenced first.

CC Excl: PDX collection 188

I31.4 Cardiac tamponade CC

Code first underlying cause

DEF: Life-threatening condition in which fluid or blood accumulates in the space between the muscle of the heart (myocardium) and the outer sac that covers the heart (pericardium), resulting in compression of the heart.

CC Excl: PDX collection 188

Cardiac Tamponade

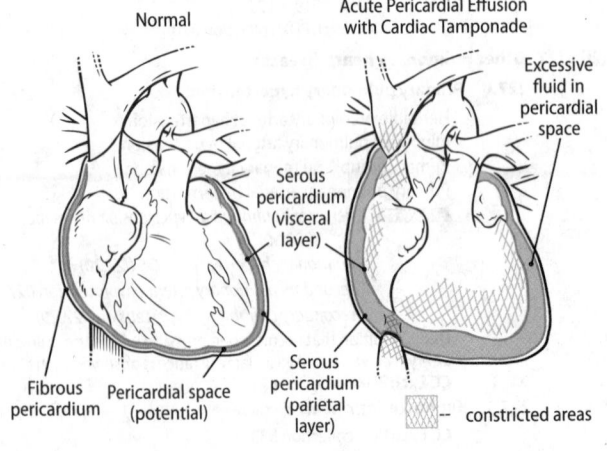

Normal

Acute Pericardial Effusion with Cardiac Tamponade

Excessive fluid in pericardial space

Serous pericardium (visceral layer)

Fibrous pericardium

Pericardial space (potential)

Serous pericardium (parietal layer)

constricted areas

N Newborn: 0   P Pediatric: 0-17   M Maternity: 9-64   A Adult: 15-124   MCC Major Complication/Comorbidity   CC Complication/Comorbidity   SW Severe Wound Dx

654   ICD-10-CM 2020

I31.8   **Other specified diseases of pericardium**   `CC`

     Epicardial plaques

     Focal pericardial adhesions

     CC Excl: PDX collection 188

I31.9   **Disease of pericardium, unspecified**   `CC`

     Pericarditis (chronic) NOS

     CC Excl: PDX collection 188

I32   *Pericarditis in diseases classified elsewhere*   `CC`

     Code first underlying disease

     `EXCLUDES 1`   *pericarditis (in):*

         coxsackie (virus) (B33.23)

         gonococcal (A54.83)

         meningococcal (A39.53)

         rheumatoid (arthritis) (M05.31)

         syphilitic (A52.06)

         systemic lupus erythematosus (M32.12)

         tuberculosis (A18.84)

     DEF: Pericarditis: Inflammation affecting the pericardium, the fibroserous membrane that surrounds the heart.

     CC Excl: PDX collection 673

√4ᵗʰ I33   **Acute and subacute endocarditis**

     `EXCLUDES 1`   *acute rheumatic endocarditis (I01.1)*

         endocarditis NOS (I38)

     DEF: Endocarditis: Inflammatory disease of the interior lining of the heart chamber and heart valves.

I33.0   **Acute and subacute infective endocarditis**   `HIV` `MCC`

     Bacterial endocarditis (acute) (subacute)

     Infective endocarditis (acute) (subacute) NOS

     Endocarditis lenta (acute) (subacute)

     Malignant endocarditis (acute) (subacute)

     Purulent endocarditis (acute) (subacute)

     Septic endocarditis (acute) (subacute)

     Ulcerative endocarditis (acute) (subacute)

     Vegetative endocarditis (acute) (subacute)

     Use additional code (B95-B97) to identify infectious agent

     CC Excl: PDX collection 675

I33.9   **Acute and subacute endocarditis, unspecified**   `HIV` `MCC`

     Acute endocarditis NOS

     Acute myoendocarditis NOS

     Acute periendocarditis NOS

     Subacute endocarditis NOS

     Subacute myoendocarditis NOS

     Subacute periendocarditis NOS

     CC Excl: PDX collection 675

√4ᵗʰ I34   **Nonrheumatic mitral valve disorders**

     `EXCLUDES 1`   *mitral valve disease (I05.9)*

         mitral valve failure (I05.8)

         mitral valve stenosis (I05.0)

         mitral valve disorder of unspecified cause with diseases of aortic and/or tricuspid valve(s) (I08.-)

         mitral valve disorder of unspecified cause with mitral stenosis or obstruction (I05.0)

         mitral valve disorder specified as congenital (Q23.2, Q23.9)

         mitral valve disorder specified as rheumatic (I05.-)

I34.0   **Nonrheumatic mitral (valve) insufficiency**

     Nonrheumatic mitral (valve) incompetence NOS

     Nonrheumatic mitral (valve) regurgitation NOS

I34.1   **Nonrheumatic mitral (valve) prolapse**

     Floppy nonrheumatic mitral valve syndrome

     `EXCLUDES 1`   *Marfan's syndrome (Q87.4-)*

I34.2   **Nonrheumatic mitral (valve) stenosis**

I34.8   **Other nonrheumatic mitral valve disorders**

I34.9   **Nonrheumatic mitral valve disorder, unspecified**

√4ᵗʰ I35   **Nonrheumatic aortic valve disorders**

     `EXCLUDES 1`   *aortic valve disorder of unspecified cause but with diseases of mitral and/or tricuspid valve(s) (I08.-)*

         aortic valve disorder specified as congenital (Q23.0, Q23.1)

         aortic valve disorder specified as rheumatic (I06.-)

         hypertrophic subaortic stenosis (I42.1)

I35.0   **Nonrheumatic aortic (valve) stenosis**

I35.1   **Nonrheumatic aortic (valve) insufficiency**

     Nonrheumatic aortic (valve) incompetence NOS

     Nonrheumatic aortic (valve) regurgitation NOS

I35.2   **Nonrheumatic aortic (valve) stenosis with insufficiency**

I35.8   **Other nonrheumatic aortic valve disorders**

I35.9   **Nonrheumatic aortic valve disorder, unspecified**

√4ᵗʰ I36   **Nonrheumatic tricuspid valve disorders**

     `EXCLUDES 1`   *tricuspid valve disorders of unspecified cause (I07.-)*

         tricuspid valve disorders specified as congenital (Q22.4, Q22.8, Q22.9)

         tricuspid valve disorders specified as rheumatic (I07.-)

         tricuspid valve disorders with aortic and/or mitral valve involvement (I08.-)

I36.0   **Nonrheumatic tricuspid (valve) stenosis**

I36.1   **Nonrheumatic tricuspid (valve) insufficiency**

     Nonrheumatic tricuspid (valve) incompetence

     Nonrheumatic tricuspid (valve) regurgitation

I36.2   **Nonrheumatic tricuspid (valve) stenosis with insufficiency**

I36.8   **Other nonrheumatic tricuspid valve disorders**

I36.9   **Nonrheumatic tricuspid valve disorder, unspecified**

√4ᵗʰ I37   **Nonrheumatic pulmonary valve disorders**

     `EXCLUDES 1`   *pulmonary valve disorder specified as congenital (Q22.1, Q22.2, Q22.3)*

         pulmonary valve disorder specified as rheumatic (I09.89)

I37.0   **Nonrheumatic pulmonary valve stenosis**

I37.1   **Nonrheumatic pulmonary valve insufficiency**

     Nonrheumatic pulmonary valve incompetence

     Nonrheumatic pulmonary valve regurgitation

I37.2   **Nonrheumatic pulmonary valve stenosis with insufficiency**

I37.8   **Other nonrheumatic pulmonary valve disorders**

I37.9   **Nonrheumatic pulmonary valve disorder, unspecified**

I38   **Endocarditis, valve unspecified**   `CC`

     `INCLUDES`   endocarditis (chronic) NOS

         valvular incompetence NOS

         valvular insufficiency NOS

         valvular regurgitation NOS

         valvular stenosis NOS

         valvulitis (chronic) NOS

     `EXCLUDES 1`   *congenital insufficiency of cardiac valve NOS (Q24.8)*

         congenital stenosis of cardiac valve NOS (Q24.8)

         endocardial fibroelastosis (I42.4)

         endocarditis specified as rheumatic (I09.1)

     DEF: Endocarditis: Inflammatory disease of the interior lining of the heart chamber and heart valves.

     CC Excl: PDX collection 676

I39   *Endocarditis and heart valve disorders in diseases classified elsewhere*   `CC`

     Code first underlying disease, such as:

     Q fever (A78)

     `EXCLUDES 1`   *endocardial involvement in:*

         candidiasis (B37.6)

         gonococcal infection (A54.83)

         Libman-Sacks disease (M32.11)

         listerosis (A32.82)

         meningococcal infection (A39.51)

         rheumatoid arthritis (M05.31)

         syphilis (A52.03)

         tuberculosis (A18.84)

         typhoid fever (A01.02)

     DEF: Endocarditis: Inflammatory disease of the interior lining of the heart chamber and heart valves.

     CC Excl: PDX collection 676

√4ᵗʰ I40   **Acute myocarditis**

     `INCLUDES`   subacute myocarditis

     `EXCLUDES 1`   *acute rheumatic myocarditis (I01.2)*

     DEF: Myocarditis: Inflammation of the middle layer of the heart, which is composed of muscle tissue.

     CC Excl: For MCC codes in category I40: PDX collection 677

I40.0   **Infective myocarditis**   `HIV` `MCC`

     Septic myocarditis

     Use additional code (B95-B97) to identify infectious agent

I40.1   **Isolated myocarditis**   `HIV` `MCC`

     Fiedler's myocarditis

     Giant cell myocarditis

     Idiopathic myocarditis

I40.8   **Other acute myocarditis**   `HIV` `MCC`

I40.9   **Acute myocarditis, unspecified**   `HIV` `MCC`

☑ Additional Character Required   ✓ˣ⁷ᵗʰ Placeholder   Unacceptable PDx   Questionable PDx   Manifestation   Unspecified Dx   `H1`-`H14` HAC   `HCC` CMS-HCC Dx   `HIV` HIV Dx

ICD-10-CM 2020   655

I41   Myocarditis in diseases classified elsewhere   `MCC`

Code first underlying disease, such as:
typhus (A75.Ø-A75.9)

> `EXCLUDES 1`   myocarditis (in):
> Chagas' disease (chronic) (B57.2)
> acute (B57.Ø)
> coxsackie (virus) infection (B33.22)
> diphtheritic (A36.81)
> gonococcal (A54.83)
> influenzal (JØ9.X9, J1Ø.82, J11.82)
> meningococcal (A39.52)
> mumps (B26.82)
> rheumatoid arthritis (MØ5.31)
> sarcoid (D86.85)
> syphilis (A52.Ø6)
> toxoplasmosis (B58.81)
> tuberculous (A18.84)

DEF: Myocarditis: Inflammation of the middle layer of the heart, which is composed of muscle tissue.
CC Excl: PDX collection 677

✓4ᵗʰ   I42   Cardiomyopathy

> `INCLUDES`   myocardiopathy

Code first pre-existing cardiomyopathy complicating pregnancy and puerperium (O99.4)

> `EXCLUDES 2`   ischemic cardiomyopathy (I25.5)
> peripartum cardiomyopathy (O9Ø.3)
> ventricular hypertrophy (I51.7)

CC Excl: For CC codes in category I42: PDX collection 678

I42.Ø   **Dilated cardiomyopathy**   `CC` `HCC`
Congestive cardiomyopathy

I42.1   **Obstructive hypertrophic cardiomyopathy**   `HCC`
Hypertrophic subaortic stenosis (idiopathic)
DEF: Cardiomyopathy marked by left ventricle hypertrophy and an enlarged septum that result in obstructed blood flow, arrhythmias, mitral regurgitation, and sudden cardiac death.
TIP: When this condition is described as inherited, assign code Q24.8.

I42.2   **Other hypertrophic cardiomyopathy**   `HCC`
Nonobstructive hypertrophic cardiomyopathy

I42.3   **Endomyocardial (eosinophilic) disease**   `HCC`
Endomyocardial (tropical) fibrosis
Löffler's endocarditis

I42.4   **Endocardial fibroelastosis**   `HCC`
Congenital cardiomyopathy
Elastomyofibrosis

I42.5   **Other restrictive cardiomyopathy**   `HCC`
Constrictive cardiomyopathy NOS

I42.6   **Alcoholic cardiomyopathy**   `CC` `HCC`
Code also presence of alcoholism (F1Ø.-)

I42.7   **Cardiomyopathy due to drug and external agent**   `CC` `HCC`
Code first poisoning due to drug or toxin, if applicable (T36-T65 with fifth or sixth character 1-4 or 6)
Use additional code for adverse effect, if applicable, to identify drug (T36-T5Ø with fifth or sixth character 5)

I42.8   **Other cardiomyopathies**   `CC` `HCC`

I42.9   **Cardiomyopathy, unspecified**   `CC` `HCC`
Cardiomyopathy (primary) (secondary) NOS

I43   Cardiomyopathy in diseases classified elsewhere   `CC` `HCC`

Code first underlying disease, such as:
amyloidosis (E85.-)
glycogen storage disease (E74.Ø)
gout (M1Ø.Ø-)
thyrotoxicosis (EØ5.Ø-EØ5.9-)

> `EXCLUDES 1`   cardiomyopathy (in):
> coxsackie (virus) (B33.24)
> diphtheria (A36.81)
> sarcoidosis (D86.85)
> tuberculosis (A18.84)

CC Excl: PDX collection 678

✓4ᵗʰ   I44   Atrioventricular and left bundle-branch block

I44.Ø   **Atrioventricular block, first degree**

I44.1   **Atrioventricular block, second degree**
Atrioventricular block, type I and II
Möbitz block, type I and II
Second degree block, type I and II
Wenckebach's block

I44.2   **Atrioventricular block, complete**   `CC` `HCC`
Complete heart block NOS
Third degree block
AHA: 2019,2Q,4
CC Excl: PDX collection 679

✓5ᵗʰ   I44.3   **Other and unspecified atrioventricular block**
Atrioventricular block NOS

> **I44.3Ø**   **Unspecified atrioventricular block**
> **I44.39**   **Other atrioventricular block**

I44.4   **Left anterior fascicular block**

I44.5   **Left posterior fascicular block**

✓5ᵗʰ   I44.6   **Other and unspecified fascicular block**

> **I44.6Ø**   **Unspecified fascicular block**
> Left bundle-branch hemiblock NOS
> **I44.69**   **Other fascicular block**

I44.7   **Left bundle-branch block, unspecified**

Conduction Disorders

✓4ᵗʰ   I45   Other conduction disorders

CC Excl: For CC codes in category I45: PDX collection 679

I45.Ø   **Right fascicular block**

✓5ᵗʰ   I45.1   **Other and unspecified right bundle-branch block**

> **I45.1Ø**   **Unspecified right bundle-branch block**
> Right bundle-branch block NOS
> **I45.19**   **Other right bundle-branch block**

I45.2   **Bifascicular block**   `CC`

I45.3   **Trifascicular block**   `CC`

I45.4   **Nonspecific intraventricular block**
Bundle-branch block NOS

I45.5   **Other specified heart block**
Sinoatrial block
Sinoauricular block
> `EXCLUDES 1`   heart block NOS (I45.9)

I45.6   **Pre-excitation syndrome**
Accelerated atrioventricular conduction
Accessory atrioventricular conduction
Anomalous atrioventricular excitation
Lown-Ganong-Levine syndrome
Pre-excitation atrioventricular conduction
Wolff-Parkinson-White syndrome

`N` Newborn: 0   `P` Pediatric: 0-17   `M` Maternity: 9-64   `A` Adult: 15-124   `MCC` Major Complication/Comorbidity   `CC` Complication/Comorbidity   `SW` Severe Wound Dx

656   ICD-10-CM 2020

√5ᵗʰ **I45.8** **Other specified conduction disorders**

I45.81 **Long QT syndrome**
DEF: Condition characterized by recurrent syncope, malignant arrhythmias, and sudden death. This syndrome has a characteristic prolonged Q-T interval on an electrocardiogram.

I45.89 **Other specified conduction disorders**
Atrioventricular [AV] dissociation
Interference dissociation
Isorhythmic dissociation
Nonparoxysmal AV nodal tachycardia
AHA: 2013,2Q,31

I45.9 **Conduction disorder, unspecified**
Heart block NOS
Stokes-Adams syndrome

√4ᵗʰ **I46 Cardiac arrest**
EXCLUDES 1 cardiogenic shock (R57.0)
AHA: 2019,2Q,4-5

I46.2 **Cardiac arrest due to underlying cardiac condition** HCC
Code first underlying cardiac condition

I46.8 **Cardiac arrest due to other underlying condition** HCC
Code first underlying condition

I46.9 **Cardiac arrest, cause unspecified** HCC

√4ᵗʰ **I47 Paroxysmal tachycardia**
Code first tachycardia complicating:
abortion or ectopic or molar pregnancy (O00-O07, O08.8)
obstetric surgery and procedures (O75.4)
EXCLUDES 1 tachycardia NOS (R00.0)
sinoauricular tachycardia NOS (R00.0)
sinus [sinusal] tachycardia NOS (R00.0)
CC Excl: For CC codes in category I47: PDX collection 679

I47.0 **Re-entry ventricular arrhythmia** CC HCC

I47.1 **Supraventricular tachycardia** CC HCC
Atrial (paroxysmal) tachycardia
Atrioventricular [AV] (paroxysmal) tachycardia
Atrioventricular re-entrant (nodal) tachycardia [AVNRT] [AVRT]
Junctional (paroxysmal) tachycardia
Nodal (paroxysmal) tachycardia

I47.2 **Ventricular tachycardia** CC HCC
AHA: 2013,3Q,23

I47.9 **Paroxysmal tachycardia, unspecified** HCC
Bouveret (-Hoffman) syndrome

√4ᵗʰ **I48 Atrial fibrillation and flutter**
CC Excl: For CC codes in category I48: PDX collection 679

I48.0 **Paroxysmal atrial fibrillation** HCC
AHA: 2018,3Q,6

▲ √5ᵗʰ **I48.1** **Persistent atrial fibrillation**
EXCLUDES 1 ▶permanent atrial fibrillation (I48.21)◀
AHA: 2019,2Q,3; 2018,3Q,6

● **I48.11** **Longstanding persistent atrial fibrillation** CC

● **I48.19** **Other persistent atrial fibrillation** CC
Chronic persistent atrial fibrillation
Persistent atrial fibrillation, NOS

▲ √5ᵗʰ **I48.2** **Chronic atrial fibrillation**
~~Permanent atrial fibrillation~~
AHA: 2019,2Q,3; 2018,3Q,6

● **I48.20** **Chronic atrial fibrillation, unspecified** CC
EXCLUDES 1 chronic persistent atrial fibrillation (I48.19)

● **I48.21** **Permanent atrial fibrillation** CC

I48.3 **Typical atrial flutter** CC HCC
Type I atrial flutter

I48.4 **Atypical atrial flutter** CC HCC
Type II atrial flutter

√5ᵗʰ **I48.9** **Unspecified atrial fibrillation and atrial flutter**

I48.91 **Unspecified atrial fibrillation** HCC

I48.92 **Unspecified atrial flutter** CC HCC

√4ᵗʰ **I49 Other cardiac arrhythmias**
Code first cardiac arrhythmia complicating:
abortion or ectopic or molar pregnancy (O00-O07, O08.8)
obstetric surgery and procedures (O75.4)
EXCLUDES 1 neonatal dysrhythmia (P29.1-)
sinoatrial bradycardia (R00.1)
sinus bradycardia (R00.1)
vagal bradycardia (R00.1)
EXCLUDES 2 bradycardia NOS (R00.1)
CC Excl: For CC codes in category I49: PDX collection 679

√5ᵗʰ **I49.0** **Ventricular fibrillation and flutter**

I49.01 **Ventricular fibrillation** CC HCC

I49.02 **Ventricular flutter** CC HCC

I49.1 **Atrial premature depolarization**
Atrial premature beats

I49.2 **Junctional premature depolarization** CC HCC

I49.3 **Ventricular premature depolarization**

√5ᵗʰ **I49.4** **Other and unspecified premature depolarization**

I49.40 **Unspecified premature depolarization**
Premature beats NOS

I49.49 **Other premature depolarization**
Ectopic beats
Extrasystoles
Extrasystolic arrhythmias
Premature contractions

I49.5 **Sick sinus syndrome** HCC
Tachycardia-bradycardia syndrome
AHA: 2019,1Q,33
TIP: The presence of a pacemaker controls but does not cure sick sinus syndrome and therefore is considered a reportable chronic condition. When a pacemaker is evaluated by a provider, this code and code Z95.0 Presence of cardiac pacemaker, should be reported, even in the absence of any notable changes or management.

I49.8 **Other specified cardiac arrhythmias**
Brugada syndrome
Coronary sinus rhythm disorder
Ectopic rhythm disorder
Nodal rhythm disorder

I49.9 **Cardiac arrhythmia, unspecified**
Arrhythmia (cardiac) NOS

√4ᵗʰ **I50 Heart failure**
Code first:
heart failure complicating abortion or ectopic or molar pregnancy (O00-O07, O08.8)
heart failure due to hypertension (I11.0)
heart failure due to hypertension with chronic kidney disease (I13.-)
heart failure following surgery (I97.13-)
obstetric surgery and procedures (O75.4)
rheumatic heart failure (I09.81)
EXCLUDES 1 neonatal cardiac failure (P29.0)
EXCLUDES 2 cardiac arrest (I46.-)
AHA: 2018,4Q,67; 2018,2Q,9; 2017,1Q,47; 2014,1Q,25; 2013,2Q,33
CC Excl: For CC/MCC codes in category I50, unless otherwise noted: PDX collection 682

I50.1 **Left ventricular failure, unspecified** CC HCC
Cardiac asthma
Edema of lung with heart disease NOS
Edema of lung with heart failure
Left heart failure
Pulmonary edema with heart disease NOS
Pulmonary edema with heart failure
EXCLUDES 1 edema of lung without heart disease or heart failure (J81.-)
pulmonary edema without heart disease or failure (J81.-)
CC Excl: PDX collection 681

✓5ᵗʰ **I50.2 Systolic (congestive) heart failure**

Heart failure with reduced ejection fraction [HFrEF]
Systolic left ventricular heart failure
Code also end stage heart failure, if applicable (I50.84)

    EXCLUDES 1   combined systolic (congestive) and diastolic (congestive) heart failure (I50.4-)

AHA: 2017,1Q,46; 2016,1Q,10

   I50.20 Unspecified systolic (congestive) heart failure   CC   HCC

   I50.21 Acute systolic (congestive) heart failure   MCC   HCC
       CC Excl: PDX collection 2025

   I50.22 Chronic systolic (congestive) heart failure   HCC

   I50.23 Acute on chronic systolic (congestive) heart failure   MCC   HCC

✓5ᵗʰ **I50.3 Diastolic (congestive) heart failure**

Diastolic left ventricular heart failure
Heart failure with normal ejection fraction
Heart failure with preserved ejection fraction [HFpEF]
Code also end stage heart failure, if applicable (I50.84)

    EXCLUDES 1   combined systolic (congestive) and diastolic (congestive) heart failure (I50.4-)

AHA: 2017,1Q,46; 2016,1Q,10

   I50.30 Unspecified diastolic (congestive) heart failure   CC   HCC

   I50.31 Acute diastolic (congestive) heart failure   MCC   HCC
       CC Excl: PDX collection 2025

   I50.32 Chronic diastolic (congestive) heart failure   HCC

   I50.33 Acute on chronic diastolic (congestive) heart failure   MCC   HCC

✓5ᵗʰ **I50.4 Combined systolic (congestive) and diastolic (congestive) heart failure**

Combined systolic and diastolic left ventricular heart failure
Heart failure with reduced ejection fraction and diastolic dysfunction
Code also end stage heart failure, if applicable (I50.84)

AHA: 2017,1Q,46; 2016,1Q,10

   I50.40 Unspecified combined systolic (congestive) and diastolic (congestive) heart failure   CC   HCC

   I50.41 Acute combined systolic (congestive) and diastolic (congestive) heart failure   MCC   HCC

   I50.42 Chronic combined systolic (congestive) and diastolic (congestive) heart failure   HCC

   I50.43 Acute on chronic combined systolic (congestive) and diastolic (congestive) heart failure   MCC   HCC

✓5ᵗʰ **I50.8 Other heart failure**

AHA: 2017,4Q,15-16

   ✓6ᵗʰ **I50.81 Right heart failure**

Right ventricular failure

     I50.810 Right heart failure, unspecified   HCC

Right heart failure without mention of left heart failure
Right ventricular failure NOS

     I50.811 Acute right heart failure   HCC

Acute isolated right heart failure
Acute (isolated) right ventricular failure

     I50.812 Chronic right heart failure   HCC

Chronic isolated right heart failure
Chronic (isolated) right ventricular failure

     I50.813 Acute on chronic right heart failure   HCC

Acute on chronic isolated right heart failure
Acute on chronic (isolated) right ventricular failure
Acute decompensation of chronic (isolated) right ventricular failure
Acute exacerbation of chronic (isolated) right ventricular failure

     I50.814 Right heart failure due to left heart failure   HCC

Right ventricular failure secondary to left ventricular failure
Code also the type of left ventricular failure, if known (I50.2-I50.43)

      EXCLUDES 1   right heart failure with but not due to left heart failure (I50.82)

   I50.82 Biventricular heart failure   HCC

Code also the type of left ventricular failure as systolic, diastolic, or combined, if known (I50.2-I50.43)

   I50.83 High output heart failure   HCC

DEF: Occurs when the high demand for blood exceeds the capacity of a normally functioning heart to meet the demand.

   I50.84 End stage heart failure   HCC

Stage D heart failure
Code also the type of heart failure as systolic, diastolic, or combined, if known (I50.2-I50.43)

   I50.89 Other heart failure   HCC

I50.9 Heart failure, unspecified   HCC

Cardiac, heart or myocardial failure NOS
Congestive heart disease
Congestive heart failure NOS

    EXCLUDES 2   ▶fluid overload unrelated to congestive heart failure◀ (E87.70)

AHA: 2017,4Q,15-16; 2017,1Q,45-46; 2014,4Q,21; 2012,4Q,92

✓4ᵗʰ **I51 Complications and ill-defined descriptions of heart disease**

    EXCLUDES 1   any condition in I51.4-I51.9 due to hypertension (I11.-)
              any condition in I51.4-I51.9 due to hypertension and chronic kidney disease (I13.-)
              heart disease specified as rheumatic (I00-I09)

I51.0 Cardiac septal defect, acquired   CC   A

Acquired septal atrial defect (old)
Acquired septal auricular defect (old)
Acquired septal ventricular defect (old)

    EXCLUDES 1   cardiac septal defect as current complication following acute myocardial infarction (I23.1, I23.2)

DEF: Abnormal communication between opposite heart chambers due to a defect of the septum. It is not present at birth.
CC Excl: PDX collection 654

I51.1 Rupture of chordae tendineae, not elsewhere classified   CC   HCC

    EXCLUDES 1   rupture of chordae tendineae as current complication following acute myocardial infarction (I23.4)

I51.2 Rupture of papillary muscle, not elsewhere classified   CC   HCC

    EXCLUDES 1   rupture of papillary muscle as current complication following acute myocardial infarction (I23.5)

I51.3 Intracardiac thrombosis, not elsewhere classified   CC

Apical thrombosis (old)
Atrial thrombosis (old)
Auricular thrombosis (old)
Mural thrombosis (old)
Ventricular thrombosis (old)

    EXCLUDES 1   intracardiac thrombosis as current complication following acute myocardial infarction (I23.6)

AHA: 2013,1Q,24

I51.4 Myocarditis, unspecified   HCC

Chronic (interstitial) myocarditis
Myocardial fibrosis
Myocarditis NOS

    EXCLUDES 1   acute or subacute myocarditis (I40.-)

AHA: 2018,4Q,67; 2018,2Q,9

I51.5 Myocardial degeneration   HCC

Fatty degeneration of heart or myocardium
Myocardial disease
Senile degeneration of heart or myocardium

AHA: 2018,4Q,67; 2018,2Q,9

I51.7   **Cardiomegaly**
Cardiac dilatation
Cardiac hypertrophy
Ventricular dilatation
AHA: 2018,4Q,67; 2018,2Q,9

✓5ᵗʰ **I51.8**   **Other ill-defined heart diseases**
AHA: 2018,2Q,9

    I51.81   **Takotsubo syndrome**   `CC`
Reversible left ventricular dysfunction following
    sudden emotional stress
Stress induced cardiomyopathy
Takotsubo cardiomyopathy
Transient left ventricular apical ballooning syndrome
DEF: Complex of symptoms mimicking myocardial
infarct in absence of heart disease, with the majority
of cases occurring in postmenopausal women. Heart
muscles are temporarily weakened, and a sudden,
massive surge of adrenalin stuns the heart, greatly
reducing the ability to pump blood.
CC Excl: PDX collection 683

    I51.89   **Other ill-defined heart diseases**
Carditis (acute)(chronic)
Pancarditis (acute)(chronic)
AHA: 2019,2Q,5; 2018,4Q,67

   I51.9   **Heart disease, unspecified**
AHA: 2018,4Q,67; 2018,2Q,9

I52   ***Other heart disorders in diseases classified elsewhere***
Code first underlying disease, such as:
congenital syphilis (A50.5)
mucopolysaccharidosis (E76.3)
schistosomiasis (B65.0-B65.9)
   EXCLUDES 1   *heart disease (in):*
       gonococcal infection (A54.83)
       meningococcal infection (A39.50)
       rheumatoid arthritis (M05.31)
       syphilis (A52.06)

Cerebrovascular diseases (I60-I69)

Use additional code to identify presence of:
alcohol abuse and dependence (F10.-)
exposure to environmental tobacco smoke (Z77.22)
history of tobacco dependence (Z87.891)
hypertension (I10-I16)
occupational exposure to environmental tobacco smoke (Z57.31)
tobacco dependence (F17.-)
tobacco use (Z72.0)
   EXCLUDES 1   *traumatic intracranial hemorrhage (S06.-)*
AHA: 2014,3Q,5; 2012,4Q,91-92

✓4ᵗʰ **I60**   **Nontraumatic subarachnoid hemorrhage**
   EXCLUDES 1   *syphilitic ruptured cerebral aneurysm (A52.05)*
   EXCLUDES 2   *sequelae of subarachnoid hemorrhage (I69.0-)*
CC Excl: For MCC codes in category I60: PDX collection 684

✓5ᵗʰ **I60.0**   **Nontraumatic subarachnoid hemorrhage from carotid siphon and bifurcation**
   I60.00   **Nontraumatic subarachnoid hemorrhage**   `MCC` `HCC`
from unspecified carotid siphon and bifurcation
   I60.01   **Nontraumatic subarachnoid hemorrhage**   `MCC` `HCC`
from right carotid siphon and bifurcation
   I60.02   **Nontraumatic subarachnoid hemorrhage**   `MCC` `HCC`
from left carotid siphon and bifurcation

✓5ᵗʰ **I60.1**   **Nontraumatic subarachnoid hemorrhage from middle cerebral artery**
   I60.10   **Nontraumatic subarachnoid hemorrhage**   `MCC` `HCC`
from unspecified middle cerebral artery
   I60.11   **Nontraumatic subarachnoid hemorrhage**   `MCC` `HCC`
from right middle cerebral artery
   I60.12   **Nontraumatic subarachnoid hemorrhage**   `MCC` `HCC`
from left middle cerebral artery

   I60.2   **Nontraumatic subarachnoid hemorrhage from**   `MCC` `HCC`
anterior communicating artery

✓5ᵗʰ **I60.3**   **Nontraumatic subarachnoid hemorrhage from posterior communicating artery**
   I60.30   **Nontraumatic subarachnoid hemorrhage**   `MCC` `HCC`
from unspecified posterior communicating artery
   I60.31   **Nontraumatic subarachnoid hemorrhage**   `MCC` `HCC`
from right posterior communicating artery

   I60.32   **Nontraumatic subarachnoid hemorrhage**   `MCC` `HCC`
from left posterior communicating artery

   I60.4   **Nontraumatic subarachnoid hemorrhage from**   `MCC` `HCC`
basilar artery

✓5ᵗʰ **I60.5**   **Nontraumatic subarachnoid hemorrhage from vertebral artery**
   I60.50   **Nontraumatic subarachnoid hemorrhage**   `MCC` `HCC`
from unspecified vertebral artery
   I60.51   **Nontraumatic subarachnoid hemorrhage**   `MCC` `HCC`
from right vertebral artery
   I60.52   **Nontraumatic subarachnoid hemorrhage**   `MCC` `HCC`
from left vertebral artery

   I60.6   **Nontraumatic subarachnoid hemorrhage from**   `MCC` `HCC`
other intracranial arteries

   I60.7   **Nontraumatic subarachnoid hemorrhage from**   `MCC` `HCC`
unspecified intracranial artery
Ruptured (congenital) berry aneurysm
Ruptured (congenital) cerebral aneurysm
Subarachnoid hemorrhage (nontraumatic) from cerebral artery
  NOS
Subarachnoid hemorrhage (nontraumatic) from communicating
  artery NOS
   EXCLUDES 1   *berry aneurysm, nonruptured (I67.1)*

   I60.8   **Other nontraumatic subarachnoid hemorrhage**   `MCC` `HCC`
Meningeal hemorrhage
Rupture of cerebral arteriovenous malformation

   I60.9   **Nontraumatic subarachnoid hemorrhage,**   `MCC` `HCC`
unspecified

✓4ᵗʰ **I61**   **Nontraumatic intracerebral hemorrhage**
   EXCLUDES 2   *sequelae of intracerebral hemorrhage (I69.1-)*
AHA: 2017,2Q,9-10
CC Excl: For MCC codes in category I61: PDX collection 684

   I61.0   **Nontraumatic intracerebral hemorrhage in**   `MCC` `HCC`
hemisphere, subcortical
Deep intracerebral hemorrhage (nontraumatic)
AHA: 2016,4Q,27

   I61.1   **Nontraumatic intracerebral hemorrhage in**   `MCC` `HCC`
hemisphere, cortical
Cerebral lobe hemorrhage (nontraumatic)
Superficial intracerebral hemorrhage (nontraumatic)

   I61.2   **Nontraumatic intracerebral hemorrhage in**   `MCC` `HCC`
hemisphere, unspecified

   I61.3   **Nontraumatic intracerebral hemorrhage in brain**   `MCC` `HCC`
stem

   I61.4   **Nontraumatic intracerebral hemorrhage in**   `MCC` `HCC`
cerebellum

   I61.5   **Nontraumatic intracerebral hemorrhage,**   `MCC` `HCC`
intraventricular

   I61.6   **Nontraumatic intracerebral hemorrhage, multiple**   `MCC` `HCC`
localized

   I61.8   **Other nontraumatic intracerebral hemorrhage**   `MCC` `HCC`

   I61.9   **Nontraumatic intracerebral hemorrhage,**   `MCC` `HCC`
unspecified

✓4ᵗʰ **I62**   **Other and unspecified nontraumatic intracranial hemorrhage**
   EXCLUDES 2   *sequelae of intracranial hemorrhage (I69.2)*
CC Excl: For CC/MCC codes in category I62: PDX collection 684

✓5ᵗʰ **I62.0**   **Nontraumatic subdural hemorrhage**
   I62.00   **Nontraumatic subdural hemorrhage,**   `MCC` `HCC`
unspecified
   I62.01   **Nontraumatic acute subdural**   `MCC` `HCC`
hemorrhage
   I62.02   **Nontraumatic subacute subdural**   `MCC` `HCC`
hemorrhage
   I62.03   **Nontraumatic chronic subdural**   `CC` `HCC`
hemorrhage

   I62.1   **Nontraumatic extradural hemorrhage**   `MCC` `HCC`
Nontraumatic epidural hemorrhage

   I62.9   **Nontraumatic intracranial hemorrhage,**   `CC` `HCC`
unspecified

√4th **I63 Cerebral infarction**

> INCLUDES   occlusion and stenosis of cerebral and precerebral arteries, resulting in cerebral infarction
>
> Use additional code, if applicable, to identify status post administration of tPA (rtPA) in a different facility within the last 24 hours prior to admission to current facility (Z92.82)
>
> Use additional code, if known, to indicate National Institutes of Health Stroke Scale (NIHSS) score (R29.7-)
>
> EXCLUDES 2   *sequelae of cerebral infarction (I69.3-)*
>
> **AHA:** 2017,2Q,9-10; 2016,4Q,28,61-62; 2014,1Q,23
>
> **TIP:** Weakness on one side of the body documented as secondary to stroke is synonymous with hemiparesis/hemiplegia (G81.-). Weakness of one limb documented as secondary to stroke is synonymous with monoplegia (G83.1-, G83.2-, G83.3-).

√5th **I63.0 Cerebral infarction due to thrombosis of precerebral arteries**

     I63.00 Cerebral infarction due to thrombosis of unspecified precerebral artery MCC HCC
> **CC Excl:** PDX collection 685

     √6th **I63.01 Cerebral infarction due to thrombosis of vertebral artery**
> **CC Excl: For MCC codes in subcategory I63.01:** PDX collection 686

         I63.011 Cerebral infarction due to thrombosis of right vertebral artery MCC HCC

         I63.012 Cerebral infarction due to thrombosis of left vertebral artery MCC HCC

         I63.013 Cerebral infarction due to thrombosis of bilateral vertebral arteries MCC HCC

         I63.019 Cerebral infarction due to thrombosis of unspecified vertebral artery MCC HCC

     I63.02 Cerebral infarction due to thrombosis of basilar artery MCC HCC
> **CC Excl:** PDX collection 685

     √6th **I63.03 Cerebral infarction due to thrombosis of carotid artery**
> **CC Excl: For MCC codes in subcategory I63.03:** PDX collection 687

         I63.031 Cerebral infarction due to thrombosis of right carotid artery MCC HCC

         I63.032 Cerebral infarction due to thrombosis of left carotid artery MCC HCC

         I63.033 Cerebral infarction due to thrombosis of bilateral carotid arteries MCC HCC

         I63.039 Cerebral infarction due to thrombosis of unspecified carotid artery MCC HCC

     I63.09 Cerebral infarction due to thrombosis of other precerebral artery MCC HCC
> **CC Excl:** PDX collection 685

√5th **I63.1 Cerebral infarction due to embolism of precerebral arteries**

     I63.10 Cerebral infarction due to embolism of unspecified precerebral artery MCC HCC
> **CC Excl:** PDX collection 685

     √6th **I63.11 Cerebral infarction due to embolism of vertebral artery**
> **CC Excl: For MCC codes in subcategory I63.13:** PDX collection 686

         I63.111 Cerebral infarction due to embolism of right vertebral artery MCC HCC

         I63.112 Cerebral infarction due to embolism of left vertebral artery MCC HCC

         I63.113 Cerebral infarction due to embolism of bilateral vertebral arteries MCC HCC

         I63.119 Cerebral infarction due to embolism of unspecified vertebral artery MCC HCC

     I63.12 Cerebral infarction due to embolism of basilar artery MCC HCC
> **CC Excl:** PDX collection 685

     √6th **I63.13 Cerebral infarction due to embolism of carotid artery**
> **CC Excl: For MCC codes in subcategory I63.13:** PDX collection 687

         I63.131 Cerebral infarction due to embolism of right carotid artery MCC HCC

         I63.132 Cerebral infarction due to embolism of left carotid artery MCC HCC

         I63.133 Cerebral infarction due to embolism of bilateral carotid arteries MCC HCC

         I63.139 Cerebral infarction due to embolism of unspecified carotid artery MCC HCC

     I63.19 Cerebral infarction due to embolism of other precerebral artery MCC HCC
> **CC Excl:** PDX collection 685

√5th **I63.2 Cerebral infarction due to unspecified occlusion or stenosis of precerebral arteries**

     I63.20 Cerebral infarction due to unspecified occlusion or stenosis of unspecified precerebral arteries MCC HCC
> **CC Excl:** PDX collection 685

     √6th **I63.21 Cerebral infarction due to unspecified occlusion or stenosis of vertebral arteries**
> **CC Excl: For MCC codes in subcategory I63.21:** PDX collection 686

         I63.211 Cerebral infarction due to unspecified occlusion or stenosis of right vertebral artery MCC HCC

         I63.212 Cerebral infarction due to unspecified occlusion or stenosis of left vertebral artery MCC HCC

         I63.213 Cerebral infarction due to unspecified occlusion or stenosis of bilateral vertebral arteries MCC HCC

         I63.219 Cerebral infarction due to unspecified occlusion or stenosis of unspecified vertebral artery MCC HCC

     I63.22 Cerebral infarction due to unspecified occlusion or stenosis of basilar artery MCC HCC
> **CC Excl:** PDX collection 685

     √6th **I63.23 Cerebral infarction due to unspecified occlusion or stenosis of carotid arteries**
> **CC Excl: For MCC codes in subcategory I63.23:** PDX collection 687

         I63.231 Cerebral infarction due to unspecified occlusion or stenosis of right carotid arteries MCC HCC

         I63.232 Cerebral infarction due to unspecified occlusion or stenosis of left carotid arteries MCC HCC

         I63.233 Cerebral infarction due to unspecified occlusion or stenosis of bilateral carotid arteries MCC HCC

         I63.239 Cerebral infarction due to unspecified occlusion or stenosis of unspecified carotid artery MCC HCC

     I63.29 Cerebral infarction due to unspecified occlusion or stenosis of other precerebral arteries MCC HCC
> **CC Excl:** PDX collection 685

√5th **I63.3 Cerebral infarction due to thrombosis of cerebral arteries**
> **CC Excl: For MCC codes in subcategory I63.3:** PDX collection 688

     I63.30 Cerebral infarction due to thrombosis of unspecified cerebral artery MCC HCC

     √6th **I63.31 Cerebral infarction due to thrombosis of middle cerebral artery**

         I63.311 Cerebral infarction due to thrombosis of right middle cerebral artery MCC HCC

         I63.312 Cerebral infarction due to thrombosis of left middle cerebral artery MCC HCC

N Newborn: 0   P Pediatric: 0-17   M Maternity: 9-64   A Adult: 15-124   MCC Major Complication/Comorbidity   CC Complication/Comorbidity   SW Severe Wound Dx

660   ICD-10-CM 2020

I63.313   Cerebral infarction due to thrombosis of bilateral middle cerebral arteries   `MCC` `HCC`

I63.319   Cerebral infarction due to thrombosis of unspecified middle cerebral artery   `MCC` `HCC`

√6ᵗʰ **I63.32**   Cerebral infarction due to thrombosis of anterior cerebral artery

I63.321   Cerebral infarction due to thrombosis of right anterior cerebral artery   `MCC` `HCC`

I63.322   Cerebral infarction due to thrombosis of left anterior cerebral artery   `MCC` `HCC`

I63.323   Cerebral infarction due to thrombosis of bilateral anterior cerebral arteries   `MCC` `HCC`

I63.329   Cerebral infarction due to thrombosis of unspecified anterior cerebral artery   `MCC` `HCC`

√6ᵗʰ **I63.33**   Cerebral infarction due to thrombosis of posterior cerebral artery

I63.331   Cerebral infarction due to thrombosis of right posterior cerebral artery   `MCC` `HCC`

I63.332   Cerebral infarction due to thrombosis of left posterior cerebral artery   `MCC` `HCC`

I63.333   Cerebral infarction due to thrombosis of bilateral posterior cerebral arteries   `MCC` `HCC`

I63.339   Cerebral infarction due to thrombosis of unspecified posterior cerebral artery   `MCC` `HCC`

√6ᵗʰ **I63.34**   Cerebral infarction due to thrombosis of cerebellar artery

I63.341   Cerebral infarction due to thrombosis of right cerebellar artery   `MCC` `HCC`

I63.342   Cerebral infarction due to thrombosis of left cerebellar artery   `MCC` `HCC`

I63.343   Cerebral infarction due to thrombosis of bilateral cerebellar arteries   `MCC` `HCC`

I63.349   Cerebral infarction due to thrombosis of unspecified cerebellar artery   `MCC` `HCC`

I63.39   Cerebral infarction due to thrombosis of other cerebral artery   `MCC` `HCC`

√5ᵗʰ **I63.4**   Cerebral infarction due to embolism of cerebral arteries

> **CC Excl: For MCC codes in subcategory I63.4:** PDX collection 688

I63.40   Cerebral infarction due to embolism of unspecified cerebral artery   `MCC` `HCC`

√6ᵗʰ **I63.41**   Cerebral infarction due to embolism of middle cerebral artery

I63.411   Cerebral infarction due to embolism of right middle cerebral artery   `MCC` `HCC`

I63.412   Cerebral infarction due to embolism of left middle cerebral artery   `MCC` `HCC`

I63.413   Cerebral infarction due to embolism of bilateral middle cerebral arteries   `MCC` `HCC`

I63.419   Cerebral infarction due to embolism of unspecified middle cerebral artery   `MCC` `HCC`

√6ᵗʰ **I63.42**   Cerebral infarction due to embolism of anterior cerebral artery

I63.421   Cerebral infarction due to embolism of right anterior cerebral artery   `MCC` `HCC`

I63.422   Cerebral infarction due to embolism of left anterior cerebral artery   `MCC` `HCC`

I63.423   Cerebral infarction due to embolism of bilateral anterior cerebral arteries   `MCC` `HCC`

I63.429   Cerebral infarction due to embolism of unspecified anterior cerebral artery   `MCC` `HCC`

√6ᵗʰ **I63.43**   Cerebral infarction due to embolism of posterior cerebral artery

I63.431   Cerebral infarction due to embolism of right posterior cerebral artery   `MCC` `HCC`

I63.432   Cerebral infarction due to embolism of left posterior cerebral artery   `MCC` `HCC`

I63.433   Cerebral infarction due to embolism of bilateral posterior cerebral arteries   `MCC` `HCC`

I63.439   Cerebral infarction due to embolism of unspecified posterior cerebral artery   `MCC` `HCC`

√6ᵗʰ **I63.44**   Cerebral infarction due to embolism of cerebellar artery

I63.441   Cerebral infarction due to embolism of right cerebellar artery   `MCC` `HCC`

I63.442   Cerebral infarction due to embolism of left cerebellar artery   `MCC` `HCC`

I63.443   Cerebral infarction due to embolism of bilateral cerebellar arteries   `MCC` `HCC`

I63.449   Cerebral infarction due to embolism of unspecified cerebellar artery   `MCC` `HCC`

I63.49   Cerebral infarction due to embolism of other cerebral artery   `MCC` `HCC`

√5ᵗʰ **I63.5**   Cerebral infarction due to unspecified occlusion or stenosis of cerebral arteries

> **CC Excl: For MCC codes in subcategory I63.5:** PDX collection 688

I63.50   Cerebral infarction due to unspecified occlusion or stenosis of unspecified cerebral artery   `MCC` `HCC`

√6ᵗʰ **I63.51**   Cerebral infarction due to unspecified occlusion or stenosis of middle cerebral artery

I63.511   Cerebral infarction due to unspecified occlusion or stenosis of right middle cerebral artery   `MCC` `HCC`

I63.512   Cerebral infarction due to unspecified occlusion or stenosis of left middle cerebral artery   `MCC` `HCC`

I63.513   Cerebral infarction due to unspecified occlusion or stenosis of bilateral middle cerebral arteries   `MCC` `HCC`

I63.519   Cerebral infarction due to unspecified occlusion or stenosis of unspecified middle cerebral artery   `MCC` `HCC`

√6ᵗʰ **I63.52**   Cerebral infarction due to unspecified occlusion or stenosis of anterior cerebral artery

I63.521   Cerebral infarction due to unspecified occlusion or stenosis of right anterior cerebral artery   `MCC` `HCC`

I63.522   Cerebral infarction due to unspecified occlusion or stenosis of left anterior cerebral artery   `MCC` `HCC`

I63.523   Cerebral infarction due to unspecified occlusion or stenosis of bilateral anterior cerebral arteries   `MCC` `HCC`

I63.529   Cerebral infarction due to unspecified occlusion or stenosis of unspecified anterior cerebral artery   `MCC` `HCC`

√6ᵗʰ **I63.53**   Cerebral infarction due to unspecified occlusion or stenosis of posterior cerebral artery

I63.531   Cerebral infarction due to unspecified occlusion or stenosis of right posterior cerebral artery   `MCC` `HCC`

I63.532   Cerebral infarction due to unspecified occlusion or stenosis of left posterior cerebral artery   `MCC` `HCC`

✔ Additional Character Required   ✔x7ᵗʰ Placeholder   Unacceptable PDx   Questionable PDx   Manifestation   Unspecified Dx   `H1`-`H14` HAC   `HCC` CMS-HCC Dx   `HIV` HIV Dx

ICD-10-CM 2020

661

Chapter 9. Diseases of the Circulatory System

I63.533 Cerebral infarction due to unspecified occlusion or stenosis of bilateral posterior cerebral arteries `MCC` `HCC`

I63.539 Cerebral infarction due to unspecified occlusion or stenosis of unspecified posterior cerebral artery `MCC` `HCC`

√6ᵗʰ **I63.54** Cerebral infarction due to unspecified occlusion or stenosis of cerebellar artery

I63.541 Cerebral infarction due to unspecified occlusion or stenosis of right cerebellar artery `MCC` `HCC`

I63.542 Cerebral infarction due to unspecified occlusion or stenosis of left cerebellar artery `MCC` `HCC`

I63.543 Cerebral infarction due to unspecified occlusion or stenosis of bilateral cerebellar arteries `MCC` `HCC`

I63.549 Cerebral infarction due to unspecified occlusion or stenosis of unspecified cerebellar artery `MCC` `HCC`

I63.59 Cerebral infarction due to unspecified occlusion or stenosis of other cerebral artery `MCC` `HCC`

I63.6 Cerebral infarction due to cerebral venous thrombosis, nonpyogenic `MCC` `HCC`
CC Excl: PDX collection 688

√5ᵗʰ **I63.8** Other cerebral infarction
AHA: 2018,4Q,16

I63.81 Other cerebral infarction due to occlusion or stenosis of small artery `MCC` `HCC`
Lacunar infarction
CC Excl: PDX collection 688

I63.89 Other cerebral infarction `MCC` `HCC`
CC Excl: PDX collection 688

I63.9 Cerebral infarction, unspecified `MCC` `HCC`
Stroke NOS
EXCLUDES 2   transient cerebral ischemic attacks and related syndromes (G45.-)
AHA: 2015,1Q,25
TIP: When provider documentation does not identify the location of an infarction, imaging reports can be used to pinpoint the location and lead to a more specific infarction code.
CC Excl: PDX collection 688

√4ᵗʰ **I65 Occlusion and stenosis of precerebral arteries, not resulting in cerebral infarction**
INCLUDES   embolism of precerebral artery
narrowing of precerebral artery
obstruction (complete) (partial) of precerebral artery
thrombosis of precerebral artery
EXCLUDES 1   insufficiency, NOS, of precerebral artery (G45.-)
insufficiency of precerebral arteries causing cerebral infarction (I63.0-I63.2)
AHA: 2018,2Q,9

√5ᵗʰ **I65.0** Occlusion and stenosis of vertebral artery
I65.01 Occlusion and stenosis of right vertebral artery
I65.02 Occlusion and stenosis of left vertebral artery
I65.03 Occlusion and stenosis of bilateral vertebral arteries `CC`
I65.09 Occlusion and stenosis of unspecified vertebral artery

I65.1 Occlusion and stenosis of basilar artery

√5ᵗʰ **I65.2** Occlusion and stenosis of carotid artery
I65.21 Occlusion and stenosis of right carotid artery
I65.22 Occlusion and stenosis of left carotid artery
I65.23 Occlusion and stenosis of bilateral carotid arteries
I65.29 Occlusion and stenosis of unspecified carotid artery

I65.8 Occlusion and stenosis of other precerebral arteries

I65.9 Occlusion and stenosis of unspecified precerebral artery
Occlusion and stenosis of precerebral artery NOS

√4ᵗʰ **I66 Occlusion and stenosis of cerebral arteries, not resulting in cerebral infarction**
INCLUDES   embolism of cerebral artery
narrowing of cerebral artery
obstruction (complete) (partial) of cerebral artery
thrombosis of cerebral artery
EXCLUDES 1   occlusion and stenosis of cerebral artery causing cerebral infarction (I63.3-I63.5)

√5ᵗʰ **I66.0** Occlusion and stenosis of middle cerebral artery
I66.01 Occlusion and stenosis of right middle cerebral artery
I66.02 Occlusion and stenosis of left middle cerebral artery
I66.03 Occlusion and stenosis of bilateral middle cerebral arteries
I66.09 Occlusion and stenosis of unspecified middle cerebral artery

√5ᵗʰ **I66.1** Occlusion and stenosis of anterior cerebral artery
I66.11 Occlusion and stenosis of right anterior cerebral artery
I66.12 Occlusion and stenosis of left anterior cerebral artery
I66.13 Occlusion and stenosis of bilateral anterior cerebral arteries
I66.19 Occlusion and stenosis of unspecified anterior cerebral artery

√5ᵗʰ **I66.2** Occlusion and stenosis of posterior cerebral artery
I66.21 Occlusion and stenosis of right posterior cerebral artery
I66.22 Occlusion and stenosis of left posterior cerebral artery
I66.23 Occlusion and stenosis of bilateral posterior cerebral arteries
I66.29 Occlusion and stenosis of unspecified posterior cerebral artery

I66.3 Occlusion and stenosis of cerebellar arteries

I66.8 Occlusion and stenosis of other cerebral arteries
Occlusion and stenosis of perforating arteries

I66.9 Occlusion and stenosis of unspecified cerebral artery

√4ᵗʰ **I67 Other cerebrovascular diseases**
EXCLUDES 2   sequelae of the listed conditions (I69.8)

I67.0 Dissection of cerebral arteries, nonruptured `MCC` `HCC`
EXCLUDES 1   ruptured cerebral arteries (I60.7)
CC Excl: PDX collection 689

I67.1 Cerebral aneurysm, nonruptured
Cerebral aneurysm NOS
Cerebral arteriovenous fistula, acquired
Internal carotid artery aneurysm, intracranial portion
Internal carotid artery aneurysm, NOS
> **EXCLUDES 1** congenital cerebral aneurysm, nonruptured (Q28.-)
> ruptured cerebral aneurysm (I60.7)

Berry Aneurysm

Berry aneurysms form at the site of a weakness in an arterial wall, often at a junction

Berry aneurysm

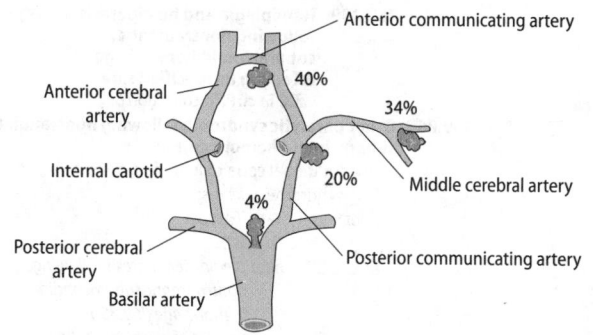

Anterior communicating artery

Anterior cerebral artery — 40%

Internal carotid — 34%

20% — Middle cerebral artery

4%

Posterior cerebral artery — Posterior communicating artery

Basilar artery

Common sites of berry aneurysms in the circle of Willis arteries

I67.2 Cerebral atherosclerosis   `A`
Atheroma of cerebral and precerebral arteries

I67.3 Progressive vascular leukoencephalopathy   `HIV` `CC` `HCC`
Binswanger's disease
CC Excl: PDX collection 133

I67.4 Hypertensive encephalopathy   `CC`
> **EXCLUDES 2** insufficiency, NOS, of precerebral arteries (G45.2)
CC Excl: PDX collection 690

I67.5 Moyamoya disease   `CC`
DEF: Cerebrovascular ischemia. Vessels occlude and rupture, causing tiny hemorrhages at the base of brain. It affects predominantly Japanese people.
CC Excl: PDX collection 691

I67.6 Nonpyogenic thrombosis of intracranial venous system   `CC`
Nonpyogenic thrombosis of cerebral vein
Nonpyogenic thrombosis of intracranial venous sinus
> **EXCLUDES 1** nonpyogenic thrombosis of intracranial venous system causing infarction (I63.6)
CC Excl: PDX collection 692

I67.7 Cerebral arteritis, not elsewhere classified   `CC`
Granulomatous angiitis of the nervous system
> **EXCLUDES 1** allergic granulomatous angiitis (M30.1)
CC Excl: PDX collection 693

√5ᵗʰ **I67.8 Other specified cerebrovascular diseases**
CC Excl: For CC codes in subcategory I67.8, unless otherwise noted: PDX collection 694

I67.81 Acute cerebrovascular insufficiency   `CC`
Acute cerebrovascular insufficiency unspecified as to location or reversibility

I67.82 Cerebral ischemia   `CC`
Chronic cerebral ischemia

I67.83 Posterior reversible encephalopathy syndrome   `HIV` `MCC`
PRES
CC Excl: PDX collection 610

√6ᵗʰ **I67.84 Cerebral vasospasm and vasoconstriction**

I67.841 Reversible cerebrovascular vasoconstriction syndrome   `CC`
Call-Fleming syndrome
Code first underlying condition, if applicable, such as eclampsia (O15.00-O15.9)
CC Excl: PDX collection 586

I67.848 Other cerebrovascular vasospasm and vasoconstriction   `CC`
CC Excl: PDX collection 586

√6ᵗʰ **I67.85 Hereditary cerebrovascular diseases**
AHA: 2018,4Q,17

I67.850 Cerebral autosomal dominant arteriopathy with subcortical infarcts and leukoencephalopathy   `CC`
CADASIL
Code also any associated diagnoses, such as:
epilepsy (G40.-)
stroke (I63.-)
vascular dementia (F01.-)

I67.858 Other hereditary cerebrovascular disease   `CC`

I67.89 Other cerebrovascular disease

I67.9 Cerebrovascular disease, unspecified

√4ᵗʰ **I68 Cerebrovascular disorders in diseases classified elsewhere**

I68.0 Cerebral amyloid angiopathy
Code first underlying amyloidosis (E85.-)

I68.2 Cerebral arteritis in other diseases classified elsewhere   `CC`
Code first underlying disease
> **EXCLUDES 1** cerebral arteritis (in):
> listerosis (A32.89)
> syphilis (A52.04)
> systemic lupus erythematosus (M32.19)
> tuberculosis (A18.89)
CC Excl: PDX collection 693

I68.8 Other cerebrovascular disorders in diseases classified elsewhere
Code first underlying disease
> **EXCLUDES 1** syphilitic cerebral aneurysm (A52.05)

√4ᵗʰ **I69 Sequelae of cerebrovascular disease**

> **NOTE** Category I69 is to be used to indicate conditions in I60-I67 as the cause of sequelae. The "sequelae" include conditions specified as such or as residuals which may occur at any time after the onset of the causal condition

> **EXCLUDES 1** personal history of cerebral infarction without residual deficit (Z86.73)
> personal history of prolonged reversible ischemic neurologic deficit (PRIND) (Z86.73)
> personal history of reversible ischemic neurologcial deficit (RIND) (Z86.73)
> sequelae of traumatic intracranial injury (S06.-)

AHA: 2017,1Q,47; 2016,4Q,28; 2015,1Q,25; 2012,4Q,106
TIP: Weakness on one side of the body (unilateral weakness) documented as secondary to old cerebrovascular disease is synonymous with hemiparesis/hemiplegia. Weakness of one limb documented as secondary to old cerebrovascular disease is synonymous with monoplegia.
TIP: For codes describing hemiplegia, hemiparesis, and monoplegia; if the documentation identifies the affected side but not whether it is the dominant or nondominant side, the default is as follows: for ambidextrous patients, the default is dominant; when the left side is affected, the default is nondominant; and when the right side is affected, the default is dominant.

√5ᵗʰ **I69.0 Sequelae of nontraumatic subarachnoid hemorrhage**

I69.00 Unspecified sequelae of nontraumatic subarachnoid hemorrhage

√6ᵗʰ **I69.01 Cognitive deficits following nontraumatic subarachnoid hemorrhage**

I69.010 Attention and concentration deficit following nontraumatic subarachnoid hemorrhage

I69.011 Memory deficit following nontraumatic subarachnoid hemorrhage

---

I69.012 Visuospatial deficit and spatial neglect following nontraumatic subarachnoid hemorrhage

I69.013 Psychomotor deficit following nontraumatic subarachnoid hemorrhage

I69.014 Frontal lobe and executive function deficit following nontraumatic subarachnoid hemorrhage

I69.015 Cognitive social or emotional deficit following nontraumatic subarachnoid hemorrhage

I69.018 Other symptoms and signs involving cognitive functions following nontraumatic subarachnoid hemorrhage

I69.019 Unspecified symptoms and signs involving cognitive functions following nontraumatic subarachnoid hemorrhage

✓6ᵗʰ **I69.02** Speech and language deficits following nontraumatic subarachnoid hemorrhage

I69.020 Aphasia following nontraumatic subarachnoid hemorrhage

I69.021 Dysphasia following nontraumatic subarachnoid hemorrhage

I69.022 Dysarthria following nontraumatic subarachnoid hemorrhage

I69.023 Fluency disorder following nontraumatic subarachnoid hemorrhage
Stuttering following nontraumatic subarachnoid hemorrhage

I69.028 Other speech and language deficits following nontraumatic subarachnoid hemorrhage

✓6ᵗʰ **I69.03** Monoplegia of upper limb following nontraumatic subarachnoid hemorrhage
AHA: 2017,1Q,47

I69.031 Monoplegia of upper limb following nontraumatic subarachnoid hemorrhage affecting right dominant side [HCC]

I69.032 Monoplegia of upper limb following nontraumatic subarachnoid hemorrhage affecting left dominant side [HCC]

I69.033 Monoplegia of upper limb following nontraumatic subarachnoid hemorrhage affecting right non-dominant side [HCC]

I69.034 Monoplegia of upper limb following nontraumatic subarachnoid hemorrhage affecting left non-dominant side [HCC]

I69.039 Monoplegia of upper limb following nontraumatic subarachnoid hemorrhage affecting unspecified side [HCC]

✓6ᵗʰ **I69.04** Monoplegia of lower limb following nontraumatic subarachnoid hemorrhage
AHA: 2017,1Q,47

I69.041 Monoplegia of lower limb following nontraumatic subarachnoid hemorrhage affecting right dominant side [HCC]

I69.042 Monoplegia of lower limb following nontraumatic subarachnoid hemorrhage affecting left dominant side [HCC]

I69.043 Monoplegia of lower limb following nontraumatic subarachnoid hemorrhage affecting right non-dominant side [HCC]

I69.044 Monoplegia of lower limb following nontraumatic subarachnoid hemorrhage affecting left non-dominant side [HCC]

I69.049 Monoplegia of lower limb following nontraumatic subarachnoid hemorrhage affecting unspecified side [HCC]

✓6ᵗʰ **I69.05** Hemiplegia and hemiparesis following nontraumatic subarachnoid hemorrhage
AHA: 2015,1Q,25

I69.051 Hemiplegia and hemiparesis following nontraumatic subarachnoid hemorrhage affecting right dominant side [CC] [HCC]
CC Excl: PDX collection 695

I69.052 Hemiplegia and hemiparesis following nontraumatic subarachnoid hemorrhage affecting left dominant side [CC] [HCC]
CC Excl: PDX collection 695

I69.053 Hemiplegia and hemiparesis following nontraumatic subarachnoid hemorrhage affecting right non-dominant side [CC] [HCC]
CC Excl: PDX collection 696

I69.054 Hemiplegia and hemiparesis following nontraumatic subarachnoid hemorrhage affecting left non-dominant side [CC] [HCC]
CC Excl: PDX collection 696

I69.059 Hemiplegia and hemiparesis following nontraumatic subarachnoid hemorrhage affecting unspecified side [CC] [HCC]
CC Excl: PDX collection 697

✓6ᵗʰ **I69.06** Other paralytic syndrome following nontraumatic subarachnoid hemorrhage
Use additional code to identify type of paralytic syndrome, such as:
locked-in state (G83.5)
quadriplegia (G82.5-)
EXCLUDES 1 hemiplegia/hemiparesis following nontraumatic subarachnoid hemorrhage (I69.05-)
monoplegia of lower limb following nontraumatic subarachnoid hemorrhage (I69.04-)
monoplegia of upper limb following nontraumatic subarachnoid hemorrhage (I69.03-)

I69.061 Other paralytic syndrome following nontraumatic subarachnoid hemorrhage affecting right dominant side [HCC]

I69.062 Other paralytic syndrome following nontraumatic subarachnoid hemorrhage affecting left dominant side [HCC]

I69.063 Other paralytic syndrome following nontraumatic subarachnoid hemorrhage affecting right non-dominant side [HCC]

I69.064 Other paralytic syndrome following nontraumatic subarachnoid hemorrhage affecting left non-dominant side [HCC]

I69.065 Other paralytic syndrome following nontraumatic subarachnoid hemorrhage, bilateral [HCC]

I69.069 Other paralytic syndrome following nontraumatic subarachnoid hemorrhage affecting unspecified side [HCC]

✓6ᵗʰ **I69.09** Other sequelae of nontraumatic subarachnoid hemorrhage

I69.090 Apraxia following nontraumatic subarachnoid hemorrhage

I69.091 Dysphagia following nontraumatic subarachnoid hemorrhage
Use additional code to identify the type of dysphagia, if known (R13.1-)

I69.092 Facial weakness following nontraumatic subarachnoid hemorrhage
Facial droop following nontraumatic subarachnoid hemorrhage

I69.093 Ataxia following nontraumatic subarachnoid hemorrhage

I69.098 Other sequelae following nontraumatic subarachnoid hemorrhage

Alterations of sensation following nontraumatic subarachnoid hemorrhage

Disturbance of vision following nontraumatic subarachnoid hemorrhage

Use additional code to identify the sequelae

√5ᵗʰ **I69.1 Sequelae of nontraumatic intracerebral hemorrhage**

I69.10 Unspecified sequelae of nontraumatic intracerebral hemorrhage

√6ᵗʰ **I69.11 Cognitive deficits** following nontraumatic intracerebral hemorrhage

I69.110 Attention and concentration deficit following nontraumatic intracerebral hemorrhage

I69.111 Memory deficit following nontraumatic intracerebral hemorrhage

I69.112 Visuospatial deficit and spatial neglect following nontraumatic intracerebral hemorrhage

I69.113 Psychomotor deficit following nontraumatic intracerebral hemorrhage

I69.114 Frontal lobe and executive function deficit following nontraumatic intracerebral hemorrhage

I69.115 Cognitive social or emotional deficit following nontraumatic intracerebral hemorrhage

I69.118 Other symptoms and signs involving cognitive functions following nontraumatic intracerebral hemorrhage

I69.119 Unspecified symptoms and signs involving cognitive functions following nontraumatic intracerebral hemorrhage

√6ᵗʰ **I69.12 Speech and language deficits** following nontraumatic intracerebral hemorrhage

I69.120 Aphasia following nontraumatic intracerebral hemorrhage

I69.121 Dysphasia following nontraumatic intracerebral hemorrhage

I69.122 Dysarthria following nontraumatic intracerebral hemorrhage

I69.123 Fluency disorder following nontraumatic intracerebral hemorrhage

Stuttering following nontraumatic intracerebral hemorrhage

I69.128 Other speech and language deficits following nontraumatic intracerebral hemorrhage

√6ᵗʰ **I69.13 Monoplegia of upper limb** following nontraumatic intracerebral hemorrhage

AHA: 2017,1Q,47

I69.131 Monoplegia of upper limb following nontraumatic intracerebral hemorrhage affecting **right dominant** side   HCC

I69.132 Monoplegia of upper limb following nontraumatic intracerebral hemorrhage affecting **left dominant** side   HCC

I69.133 Monoplegia of upper limb following nontraumatic intracerebral hemorrhage affecting **right non-dominant** side   HCC

I69.134 Monoplegia of upper limb following nontraumatic intracerebral hemorrhage affecting **left non-dominant** side   HCC

I69.139 Monoplegia of upper limb following nontraumatic intracerebral hemorrhage affecting **unspecified** side   HCC

√6ᵗʰ **I69.14 Monoplegia of lower limb** following nontraumatic intracerebral hemorrhage

AHA: 2017,1Q,47

I69.141 Monoplegia of lower limb following nontraumatic intracerebral hemorrhage affecting **right dominant side**   HCC

I69.142 Monoplegia of lower limb following nontraumatic intracerebral hemorrhage affecting **left dominant** side   HCC

I69.143 Monoplegia of lower limb following nontraumatic intracerebral hemorrhage affecting **right non-dominant** side   HCC

I69.144 Monoplegia of lower limb following nontraumatic intracerebral hemorrhage affecting **left non-dominant** side   HCC

I69.149 Monoplegia of lower limb following nontraumatic intracerebral hemorrhage affecting **unspecified** side   HCC

√6ᵗʰ **I69.15 Hemiplegia and hemiparesis** following nontraumatic intracerebral hemorrhage

AHA: 2015,1Q,25

I69.151 Hemiplegia and hemiparesis following nontraumatic intracerebral hemorrhage affecting **right dominant side**   CC HCC
CC Excl: PDX collection 695

I69.152 Hemiplegia and hemiparesis following nontraumatic intracerebral hemorrhage affecting **left dominant side**   CC HCC
CC Excl: PDX collection 695

I69.153 Hemiplegia and hemiparesis following nontraumatic intracerebral hemorrhage affecting **right non-dominant side**   CC HCC
CC Excl: PDX collection 696

I69.154 Hemiplegia and hemiparesis following nontraumatic intracerebral hemorrhage affecting **left non-dominant side**   CC HCC
CC Excl: PDX collection 696

I69.159 Hemiplegia and hemiparesis following nontraumatic intracerebral hemorrhage affecting **unspecified side**   CC HCC
CC Excl: PDX collection 697

√6ᵗʰ **I69.16 Other paralytic syndrome** following nontraumatic intracerebral hemorrhage

Use additional code to identify type of paralytic syndrome, such as:
locked-in state (G83.5)
quadriplegia (G82.5-)

EXCLUDES 1   hemiplegia/hemiparesis following nontraumatic intracerebral hemorrhage (I69.15-)
monoplegia of lower limb following nontraumatic intracerebral hemorrhage (I69.14-)
monoplegia of upper limb following nontraumatic intracerebral hemorrhage (I69.13-)

I69.161 Other paralytic syndrome following nontraumatic intracerebral hemorrhage affecting **right dominant side**   HCC

I69.162 Other paralytic syndrome following nontraumatic intracerebral hemorrhage affecting **left dominant side**   HCC

I69.163 Other paralytic syndrome following nontraumatic intracerebral hemorrhage affecting **right non-dominant** side   HCC

Chapter 9. Diseases of the Circulatory System

I69.164–I69.259

I69.164 Other paralytic syndrome following nontraumatic intracerebral hemorrhage affecting left non-dominant side `HCC`

I69.165 Other paralytic syndrome following nontraumatic intracerebral hemorrhage, bilateral `HCC`

I69.169 Other paralytic syndrome following nontraumatic intracerebral hemorrhage affecting unspecified side `HCC`

✓6ᵗʰ **I69.19** Other sequelae of nontraumatic intracerebral hemorrhage

I69.190 Apraxia following nontraumatic intracerebral hemorrhage

I69.191 Dysphagia following nontraumatic intracerebral hemorrhage
Use additional code to identify the type of dysphagia, if known (R13.1-)

I69.192 Facial weakness following nontraumatic intracerebral hemorrhage
Facial droop following nontraumatic intracerebral hemorrhage

I69.193 Ataxia following nontraumatic intracerebral hemorrhage

I69.198 Other sequelae of nontraumatic intracerebral hemorrhage
Alteration of sensations following nontraumatic intracerebral hemorrhage
Disturbance of vision following nontraumatic intracerebral hemorrhage
Use additional code to identify the sequelae

✓5ᵗʰ **I69.2** Sequelae of other nontraumatic intracranial hemorrhage

I69.20 Unspecified sequelae of other nontraumatic intracranial hemorrhage

✓6ᵗʰ **!I69.21** Cognitive deficits following other nontraumatic intracranial hemorrhage

I69.210 Attention and concentration deficit following other nontraumatic intracranial hemorrhage

I69.211 Memory deficit following other nontraumatic intracranial hemorrhage

I69.212 Visuospatial deficit and spatial neglect following other nontraumatic intracranial hemorrhage

I69.213 Psychomotor deficit following other nontraumatic intracranial hemorrhage

I69.214 Frontal lobe and executive function deficit following other nontraumatic intracranial hemorrhage

I69.215 Cognitive social or emotional deficit following other nontraumatic intracranial hemorrhage

I69.218 Other symptoms and signs involving cognitive functions following other nontraumatic intracranial hemorrhage

I69.219 Unspecified symptoms and signs involving cognitive functions following other nontraumatic intracranial hemorrhage

✓6ᵗʰ **I69.22** Speech and language deficits following other nontraumatic intracranial hemorrhage

I69.220 Aphasia following other nontraumatic intracranial hemorrhage

I69.221 Dysphasia following other nontraumatic intracranial hemorrhage

I69.222 Dysarthria following other nontraumatic intracranial hemorrhage

I69.223 Fluency disorder following other nontraumatic intracranial hemorrhage
Stuttering following other nontraumatic intracranial hemorrhage

I69.228 Other speech and language deficits following other nontraumatic intracranial hemorrhage

✓6ᵗʰ **I69.23** Monoplegia of upper limb following other nontraumatic intracranial hemorrhage
AHA: 2017,1Q,47

I69.231 Monoplegia of upper limb following other nontraumatic intracranial hemorrhage affecting right dominant side `HCC`

I69.232 Monoplegia of upper limb following other nontraumatic intracranial hemorrhage affecting left dominant side `HCC`

I69.233 Monoplegia of upper limb following other nontraumatic intracranial hemorrhage affecting right non-dominant side `HCC`

I69.234 Monoplegia of upper limb following other nontraumatic intracranial hemorrhage affecting left non-dominant side `HCC`

I69.239 Monoplegia of upper limb following other nontraumatic intracranial hemorrhage affecting unspecified side `HCC`

✓6ᵗʰ **I69.24** Monoplegia of lower limb following other nontraumatic intracranial hemorrhage
AHA: 2017,1Q,47

I69.241 Monoplegia of lower limb following other nontraumatic intracranial hemorrhage affecting right dominant side `HCC`

I69.242 Monoplegia of lower limb following other nontraumatic intracranial hemorrhage affecting left dominant side `HCC`

I69.243 Monoplegia of lower limb following other nontraumatic intracranial hemorrhage affecting right non-dominant side `HCC`

I69.244 Monoplegia of lower limb following other nontraumatic intracranial hemorrhage affecting left non-dominant side `HCC`

I69.249 Monoplegia of lower limb following other nontraumatic intracranial hemorrhage affecting unspecified side `HCC`

✓6ᵗʰ **I69.25** Hemiplegia and hemiparesis following other nontraumatic intracranial hemorrhage
AHA: 2015,1Q,25

I69.251 Hemiplegia and hemiparesis following other nontraumatic intracranial hemorrhage affecting right dominant side `CC` `HCC`
CC Excl: PDX collection 695

I69.252 Hemiplegia and hemiparesis following other nontraumatic intracranial hemorrhage affecting left dominant side `CC` `HCC`
CC Excl: PDX collection 695

I69.253 Hemiplegia and hemiparesis following other nontraumatic intracranial hemorrhage affecting right non-dominant side `CC` `HCC`
CC Excl: PDX collection 696

I69.254 Hemiplegia and hemiparesis following other nontraumatic intracranial hemorrhage affecting left non-dominant side `CC` `HCC`
CC Excl: PDX collection 696

I69.259 Hemiplegia and hemiparesis following other nontraumatic intracranial hemorrhage affecting unspecified side `CC` `HCC`
CC Excl: PDX collection 697

`N` Newborn: 0   `P` Pediatric: 0-17   `M` Maternity: 9-64   `A` Adult: 15-124   `MCC` Major Complication/Comorbidity   `CC` Complication/Comorbidity   `SW` Severe Wound Dx

666   ICD-10-CM 2020

✓6ᵗʰ **I69.26** **Other paralytic syndrome following other nontraumatic intracranial hemorrhage**
Use additional code to identify type of paralytic syndrome, such as:
locked-in state (G83.5)
quadriplegia (G82.5-)
EXCLUDES 1   *hemiplegia/hemiparesis following other nontraumatic intracranial hemorrhage (I69.25-)*
monoplegia of lower limb following other nontraumatic intracranial hemorrhage (I69.24-)
monoplegia of upper limb following other nontraumatic intracranial hemorrhage (I69.23-)

I69.261 **Other paralytic syndrome following other nontraumatic intracranial hemorrhage affecting right dominant side**   HCC

I69.262 **Other paralytic syndrome following other nontraumatic intracranial hemorrhage affecting left dominant side**   HCC

I69.263 **Other paralytic syndrome following other nontraumatic intracranial hemorrhage affecting right non-dominant side**   HCC

I69.264 **Other paralytic syndrome following other nontraumatic intracranial hemorrhage affecting left non-dominant side**   HCC

I69.265 **Other paralytic syndrome following other nontraumatic intracranial hemorrhage, bilateral**   HCC

I69.269 **Other paralytic syndrome following other nontraumatic intracranial hemorrhage affecting unspecified side**   HCC

✓6ᵗʰ **I69.29** **Other sequelae of other nontraumatic intracranial hemorrhage**

I69.290 **Apraxia following other nontraumatic intracranial hemorrhage**

I69.291 **Dysphagia following other nontraumatic intracranial hemorrhage**
Use additional code to identify the type of dysphagia, if known (R13.1-)

I69.292 **Facial weakness following other nontraumatic intracranial hemorrhage**
Facial droop following other nontraumatic intracranial hemorrhage

I69.293 **Ataxia following other nontraumatic intracranial hemorrhage**

I69.298 **Other sequelae of other nontraumatic intracranial hemorrhage**
Alteration of sensation following other nontraumatic intracranial hemorrhage
Disturbance of vision following other nontraumatic intracranial hemorrhage
Use additional code to identify the sequelae

✓5ᵗʰ **I69.3** **Sequelae of cerebral infarction**
Sequelae of stroke NOS
AHA: 2013,4Q,127-128; 2012,4Q,92,94

I69.30 **Unspecified sequelae of cerebral infarction**

✓6ᵗʰ **I69.31** **Cognitive deficits following cerebral infarction**

I69.310 **Attention and concentration deficit following cerebral infarction**

I69.311 **Memory deficit following cerebral infarction**

I69.312 **Visuospatial deficit and spatial neglect following cerebral infarction**

I69.313 **Psychomotor deficit following cerebral infarction**

I69.314 **Frontal lobe and executive function deficit following cerebral infarction**

I69.315 **Cognitive social or emotional deficit following cerebral infarction**

I69.318 **Other symptoms and signs involving cognitive functions following cerebral infarction**

I69.319 **Unspecified symptoms and signs involving cognitive functions following cerebral infarction**

✓6ᵗʰ **I69.32** **Speech and language deficits following cerebral infarction**

I69.320 **Aphasia following cerebral infarction**

I69.321 **Dysphasia following cerebral infarction**
AHA: 2012,4Q,91

I69.322 **Dysarthria following cerebral infarction**
EXCLUDES 2   *transient ischemic attack (TIA) (G45.9)*

I69.323 **Fluency disorder following cerebral infarction**
Stuttering following cerebral infarction

I69.328 **Other speech and language deficits following cerebral infarction**

✓6ᵗʰ **I69.33** **Monoplegia of upper limb following cerebral infarction**
AHA: 2017,1Q,47

I69.331 **Monoplegia of upper limb following cerebral infarction affecting right dominant side**   HCC

I69.332 **Monoplegia of upper limb following cerebral infarction affecting left dominant side**   HCC

I69.333 **Monoplegia of upper limb following cerebral infarction affecting right non-dominant side**   HCC

I69.334 **Monoplegia of upper limb following cerebral infarction affecting left non-dominant side**   HCC

I69.339 **Monoplegia of upper limb following cerebral infarction affecting unspecified side**   HCC

✓6ᵗʰ **I69.34** **Monoplegia of lower limb following cerebral infarction**
AHA: 2017,1Q,47

I69.341 **Monoplegia of lower limb following cerebral infarction affecting right dominant side**   HCC

I69.342 **Monoplegia of lower limb following cerebral infarction affecting left dominant side**   HCC

I69.343 **Monoplegia of lower limb following cerebral infarction affecting right non-dominant side**   HCC

I69.344 **Monoplegia of lower limb following cerebral infarction affecting left non-dominant side**   HCC

I69.349 **Monoplegia of lower limb following cerebral infarction affecting unspecified side**   HCC

✓6ᵗʰ **I69.35** **Hemiplegia and hemiparesis following cerebral infarction**
AHA: 2015,1Q,25

I69.351 **Hemiplegia and hemiparesis following cerebral infarction affecting right dominant side**   CC HCC
EXCLUDES 2   *transient ischemic attack (TIA) (G45.9)*
CC Excl: PDX collection 695

I69.352 **Hemiplegia and hemiparesis following cerebral infarction affecting left dominant side**   CC HCC
CC Excl: PDX collection 695

I69.353 **Hemiplegia and hemiparesis following cerebral infarction affecting right non-dominant side**   CC HCC
CC Excl: PDX collection 696

I69.354 **Hemiplegia and hemiparesis following cerebral infarction affecting left non-dominant side**   CC HCC
AHA: 2012,4Q,91
CC Excl: PDX collection 696

Chapter 9. Diseases of the Circulatory System

I69.359–I69.853

I69.359 **Hemiplegia and hemiparesis following cerebral infarction affecting unspecified side** `CC` `HCC`
    CC Excl: PDX collection 697

√6th **I69.36** **Other paralytic syndrome following cerebral infarction**
    Use additional code to identify type of paralytic syndrome, such as:
    locked-in state (G83.5)
    quadriplegia (G82.5-)

    EXCLUDES 1   *hemiplegia/hemiparesis following cerebral infarction (I69.35-)*
             monoplegia of lower limb following cerebral infarction (I69.34-)
             monoplegia of upper limb following cerebral infarction (I69.33-)

    I69.361 **Other paralytic syndrome following cerebral infarction affecting right dominant side** `HCC`

    I69.362 **Other paralytic syndrome following cerebral infarction affecting left dominant side** `HCC`

    I69.363 **Other paralytic syndrome following cerebral infarction affecting right non-dominant side** `HCC`

    I69.364 **Other paralytic syndrome following cerebral infarction affecting left non-dominant side** `HCC`

    I69.365 **Other paralytic syndrome following cerebral infarction, bilateral** `HCC`

    I69.369 **Other paralytic syndrome following cerebral infarction affecting unspecified side** `HCC`

√6th **I69.39** **Other sequelae of cerebral infarction**

    I69.390 **Apraxia following cerebral infarction**

    I69.391 **Dysphagia following cerebral infarction**
        Use additional code to identify the type of dysphagia, if known (R13.1-)

    I69.392 **Facial weakness following cerebral infarction**
        Facial droop following cerebral infarction

    I69.393 **Ataxia following cerebral infarction**

    I69.398 **Other sequelae of cerebral infarction**
        Alteration of sensation following cerebral infarction
        Disturbance of vision following cerebral infarction
        Use additional code to identify the sequelae

√5th **I69.8** **Sequelae of other cerebrovascular diseases**
    EXCLUDES 1   *sequelae of traumatic intracranial injury (S06.-)*

I69.80 **Unspecified sequelae of other cerebrovascular disease**

√6th **I69.81** **Cognitive deficits following other cerebrovascular disease**

    I69.810 **Attention and concentration deficit following other cerebrovascular disease**

    I69.811 **Memory deficit following other cerebrovascular disease**

    I69.812 **Visuospatial deficit and spatial neglect following other cerebrovascular disease**

    I69.813 **Psychomotor deficit following other cerebrovascular disease**

    I69.814 **Frontal lobe and executive function deficit following other cerebrovascular disease**

    I69.815 **Cognitive social or emotional deficit following other cerebrovascular disease**

    I69.818 **Other symptoms and signs involving cognitive functions following other cerebrovascular disease**

    I69.819 **Unspecified symptoms and signs involving cognitive functions following other cerebrovascular disease**

√6th **I69.82** **Speech and language deficits following other cerebrovascular disease**

    I69.820 **Aphasia following other cerebrovascular disease**

    I69.821 **Dysphasia following other cerebrovascular disease**

    I69.822 **Dysarthria following other cerebrovascular disease**

    I69.823 **Fluency disorder following other cerebrovascular disease**
        Stuttering following other cerebrovascular disease

    I69.828 **Other speech and language deficits following other cerebrovascular disease**

√6th **I69.83** **Monoplegia of upper limb following other cerebrovascular disease**
    AHA: 2017,1Q,47

    I69.831 **Monoplegia of upper limb following other cerebrovascular disease affecting right dominant side** `HCC`

    I69.832 **Monoplegia of upper limb following other cerebrovascular disease affecting left dominant side** `HCC`

    I69.833 **Monoplegia of upper limb following other cerebrovascular disease affecting right non-dominant side** `HCC`

    I69.834 **Monoplegia of upper limb following other cerebrovascular disease affecting left non-dominant side** `HCC`

    I69.839 **Monoplegia of upper limb following other cerebrovascular disease affecting unspecified side** `HCC`

√6th **I69.84** **Monoplegia of lower limb following other cerebrovascular disease**
    AHA: 2017,1Q,47

    I69.841 **Monoplegia of lower limb following other cerebrovascular disease affecting right dominant side** `HCC`

    I69.842 **Monoplegia of lower limb following other cerebrovascular disease affecting left dominant side** `HCC`

    I69.843 **Monoplegia of lower limb following other cerebrovascular disease affecting right non-dominant side** `HCC`

    I69.844 **Monoplegia of lower limb following other cerebrovascular disease affecting left non-dominant side** `HCC`

    I69.849 **Monoplegia of lower limb following other cerebrovascular disease affecting unspecified side** `HCC`

√6th **I69.85** **Hemiplegia and hemiparesis following other cerebrovascular disease**
    AHA: 2015,1Q,25

    I69.851 **Hemiplegia and hemiparesis following other cerebrovascular disease affecting right dominant side** `CC` `HCC`
        CC Excl: PDX collection 695

    I69.852 **Hemiplegia and hemiparesis following other cerebrovascular disease affecting left dominant side** `CC` `HCC`
        CC Excl: PDX collection 695

    I69.853 **Hemiplegia and hemiparesis following other cerebrovascular disease affecting right non-dominant side** `CC` `HCC`
        CC Excl: PDX collection 696

N Newborn: 0   P Pediatric: 0-17   M Maternity: 9-64   A Adult: 15-124   MCC Major Complication/Comorbidity   CC Complication/Comorbidity   SW Severe Wound Dx

668   ICD-10-CM 2020

I69.854 Hemiplegia and hemiparesis following other cerebrovascular disease affecting left non-dominant side `CC` `HCC`
    CC Excl: PDX collection 696

I69.859 Hemiplegia and hemiparesis following other cerebrovascular disease affecting unspecified side `CC` `HCC`
    CC Excl: PDX collection 697

√6ᵗʰ **I69.86 Other paralytic syndrome following other cerebrovascular disease**
Use additional code to identify type of paralytic syndrome, such as:
locked-in state (G83.5)
quadriplegia (G82.5-)
    EXCLUDES 1   *hemiplegia/hemiparesis following other cerebrovascular disease (I69.85-)*
        monoplegia of lower limb following other cerebrovascular disease (I69.84-)
        monoplegia of upper limb following other cerebrovascular disease (I69.83-)

I69.861 Other paralytic syndrome following other cerebrovascular disease affecting right dominant side `HCC`

I69.862 Other paralytic syndrome following other cerebrovascular disease affecting left dominant side `HCC`

I69.863 Other paralytic syndrome following other cerebrovascular disease affecting right non-dominant side `HCC`

I69.864 Other paralytic syndrome following other cerebrovascular disease affecting left non-dominant side `HCC`

I69.865 Other paralytic syndrome following other cerebrovascular disease, bilateral `HCC`

I69.869 Other paralytic syndrome following other cerebrovascular disease affecting unspecified side `HCC`

√6ᵗʰ **I69.89 Other sequelae of other cerebrovascular disease**

I69.890 Apraxia following other cerebrovascular disease

I69.891 Dysphagia following other cerebrovascular disease
    Use additional code to identify the type of dysphagia, if known (R13.1-)

I69.892 Facial weakness following other cerebrovascular disease
    Facial droop following other cerebrovascular disease

I69.893 Ataxia following other cerebrovascular disease

I69.898 Other sequelae of other cerebrovascular disease
    Alteration of sensation following other cerebrovascular disease
    Disturbance of vision following other cerebrovascular disease
    Use additional code to identify the sequelae

√5ᵗʰ **I69.9 Sequelae of unspecified cerebrovascular diseases**
    EXCLUDES 1   *sequelae of stroke (I69.3)*
        sequelae of traumatic intracranial injury (S06.-)

I69.90 Unspecified sequelae of unspecified cerebrovascular disease

√6ᵗʰ **I69.91 Cognitive deficits following unspecified cerebrovascular disease**

I69.910 Attention and concentration deficit following unspecified cerebrovascular disease

I69.911 Memory deficit following unspecified cerebrovascular disease

I69.912 Visuospatial deficit and spatial neglect following unspecified cerebrovascular disease

I69.913 Psychomotor deficit following unspecified cerebrovascular disease

I69.914 Frontal lobe and executive function deficit following unspecified cerebrovascular disease

I69.915 Cognitive social or emotional deficit following unspecified cerebrovascular disease

I69.918 Other symptoms and signs involving cognitive functions following unspecified cerebrovascular disease

I69.919 Unspecified symptoms and signs involving cognitive functions following unspecified cerebrovascular disease

√6ᵗʰ **I69.92 Speech and language deficits following unspecified cerebrovascular disease**

I69.920 Aphasia following unspecified cerebrovascular disease

I69.921 Dysphasia following unspecified cerebrovascular disease

I69.922 Dysarthria following unspecified cerebrovascular disease

I69.923 Fluency disorder following unspecified cerebrovascular disease
    Stuttering following unspecified cerebrovascular disease

I69.928 Other speech and language deficits following unspecified cerebrovascular disease

√6ᵗʰ **I69.93 Monoplegia of upper limb following unspecified cerebrovascular disease**
    AHA: 2017,1Q,47

I69.931 Monoplegia of upper limb following unspecified cerebrovascular disease affecting right dominant side `HCC`

I69.932 Monoplegia of upper limb following unspecified cerebrovascular disease affecting left dominant side `HCC`

I69.933 Monoplegia of upper limb following unspecified cerebrovascular disease affecting right non-dominant side `HCC`

I69.934 Monoplegia of upper limb following unspecified cerebrovascular disease affecting left non-dominant side `HCC`

I69.939 Monoplegia of upper limb following unspecified cerebrovascular disease affecting unspecified side `HCC`

√6ᵗʰ **I69.94 Monoplegia of lower limb following unspecified cerebrovascular disease**
    AHA: 2017,1Q,47

I69.941 Monoplegia of lower limb following unspecified cerebrovascular disease affecting right dominant side `HCC`

I69.942 Monoplegia of lower limb following unspecified cerebrovascular disease affecting left dominant side `HCC`

I69.943 Monoplegia of lower limb following unspecified cerebrovascular disease affecting right non-dominant side `HCC`

I69.944 Monoplegia of lower limb following unspecified cerebrovascular disease affecting left non-dominant side `HCC`

I69.949 Monoplegia of lower limb following unspecified cerebrovascular disease affecting unspecified side `HCC`

√6ᵗʰ **I69.95** **Hemiplegia and hemiparesis following unspecified cerebrovascular disease**
AHA: 2015,1Q,25

     I69.951 **Hemiplegia and hemiparesis following unspecified cerebrovascular disease affecting right dominant side** `CC` `HCC`
CC Excl: PDX collection 695

     I69.952 **Hemiplegia and hemiparesis following unspecified cerebrovascular disease affecting left dominant side** `CC` `HCC`
CC Excl: PDX collection 695

     I69.953 **Hemiplegia and hemiparesis following unspecified cerebrovascular disease affecting right non-dominant side** `CC` `HCC`
CC Excl: PDX collection 696

     I69.954 **Hemiplegia and hemiparesis following unspecified cerebrovascular disease affecting left non-dominant side** `CC` `HCC`
CC Excl: PDX collection 696

     I69.959 **Hemiplegia and hemiparesis following unspecified cerebrovascular disease affecting unspecified side** `CC` `HCC`
CC Excl: PDX collection 697

√6ᵗʰ **I69.96** **Other paralytic syndrome following unspecified cerebrovascular disease**
Use additional code to identify type of paralytic syndrome, such as:
locked-in state (G83.5)
quadriplegia (G82.5-)

EXCLUDES 1   *hemiplegia/hemiparesis following unspecified cerebrovascular disease (I69.95-)*
monoplegia of lower limb following unspecified cerebrovascular disease (I69.94-)
monoplegia of upper limb following unspecified cerebrovascular disease (I69.93-)

     I69.961 **Other paralytic syndrome following unspecified cerebrovascular disease affecting right dominant side** `HCC`

     I69.962 **Other paralytic syndrome following unspecified cerebrovascular disease affecting left dominant side** `HCC`

     I69.963 **Other paralytic syndrome following unspecified cerebrovascular disease affecting right non-dominant side** `HCC`

     I69.964 **Other paralytic syndrome following unspecified cerebrovascular disease affecting left non-dominant side** `HCC`

     I69.965 **Other paralytic syndrome following unspecified cerebrovascular disease, bilateral** `HCC`

     I69.969 **Other paralytic syndrome following unspecified cerebrovascular disease affecting unspecified side** `HCC`

√6ᵗʰ **I69.99** **Other sequelae of unspecified cerebrovascular disease**

     I69.990 **Apraxia following unspecified cerebrovascular disease**

     I69.991 **Dysphagia following unspecified cerebrovascular disease**
Use additional code to identify the type of dysphagia, if known (R13.1-)

     I69.992 **Facial weakness following unspecified cerebrovascular disease**
Facial droop following unspecified cerebrovascular disease

     I69.993 **Ataxia following unspecified cerebrovascular disease**

     I69.998 **Other sequelae following unspecified cerebrovascular disease**
Alteration in sensation following unspecified cerebrovascular disease
Disturbance of vision following unspecified cerebrovascular disease
Use additional code to identify the sequelae

Diseases of arteries, arterioles and capillaries (I70-I79)

√4ᵗʰ **I70** **Atherosclerosis**

INCLUDES   arterial degeneration
arteriolosclerosis
arteriosclerosis
arteriosclerotic vascular disease
arteriovascular degeneration
atheroma
endarteritis deformans or obliterans
senile arteritis
senile endarteritis
vascular degeneration

Use additional code to identify:
exposure to environmental tobacco smoke (Z77.22)
history of tobacco dependence (Z87.891)
occupational exposure to environmental tobacco smoke (Z57.31)
tobacco dependence (F17.-)
tobacco use (Z72.0)

EXCLUDES 2   *arteriosclerotic cardiovascular disease (I25.1-)*
arteriosclerotic heart disease (I25.1-)
atheroembolism (I75.-)
cerebral atherosclerosis (I67.2)
coronary atherosclerosis (I25.1-)
mesenteric atherosclerosis (K55.1)
precerebral atherosclerosis (I67.2)
primary pulmonary atherosclerosis (I27.0)

I70.0 **Atherosclerosis of aorta** `HCC` `A`

I70.1 **Atherosclerosis of renal artery** `HCC` `A`
Goldblatt's kidney
EXCLUDES 2   *atherosclerosis of renal arterioles (I12.-)*

√5ᵗʰ **I70.2** **Atherosclerosis of native arteries of the extremities**
Mönckeberg's (medial) sclerosis
Use additional code, if applicable, to identify chronic total occlusion of artery of extremity (I70.92)
EXCLUDES 2   *atherosclerosis of bypass graft of extremities (I70.30-I70.79)*
AHA: 2018,3Q,4; 2018,2Q,7

√6ᵗʰ **I70.20** **Unspecified atherosclerosis of native arteries of extremities**

     I70.201 **Unspecified atherosclerosis of native arteries of extremities, right leg** `HCC` `A`

     I70.202 **Unspecified atherosclerosis of native arteries of extremities, left leg** `HCC` `A`

     I70.203 **Unspecified atherosclerosis of native arteries of extremities, bilateral legs** `HCC` `A`

     I70.208 **Unspecified atherosclerosis of native arteries of extremities, other extremity** `HCC` `A`

     I70.209 **Unspecified atherosclerosis of native arteries of extremities, unspecified extremity** `HCC` `A`

√6ᵗʰ **I70.21** **Atherosclerosis of native arteries of extremities with intermittent claudication**

     I70.211 **Atherosclerosis of native arteries of extremities with intermittent claudication, right leg** `HCC` `A`

     I70.212 **Atherosclerosis of native arteries of extremities with intermittent claudication, left leg** `HCC` `A`

     I70.213 **Atherosclerosis of native arteries of extremities with intermittent claudication, bilateral legs** `HCC` `A`

N Newborn: 0   **P** Pediatric: 0-17   **M** Maternity: 9-64   **A** Adult: 15-124   **MCC** Major Complication/Comorbidity   **CC** Complication/Comorbidity   **SW** Severe Wound Dx

670   ICD-10-CM 2020

I70.218 Atherosclerosis of native arteries of extremities with intermittent claudication, other extremity   HCC A

I70.219 Atherosclerosis of native arteries of extremities with intermittent claudication, unspecified extremity   HCC A

√6ᵗʰ **I70.22** Atherosclerosis of native arteries of extremities with rest pain

> INCLUDES   any condition classifiable to I70.21-

I70.221 Atherosclerosis of native arteries of extremities with rest pain, right leg   HCC A

I70.222 Atherosclerosis of native arteries of extremities with rest pain, left leg   HCC A

I70.223 Atherosclerosis of native arteries of extremities with rest pain, bilateral legs   HCC A

I70.228 Atherosclerosis of native arteries of extremities with rest pain, other extremity   HCC A

I70.229 Atherosclerosis of native arteries of extremities with rest pain, unspecified extremity   HCC A

√6ᵗʰ **I70.23** Atherosclerosis of native arteries of right leg with ulceration

> INCLUDES   any condition classifiable to I70.211 and I70.221

Use additional code to identify severity of ulcer (L97.-)

I70.231 Atherosclerosis of native arteries of right leg with ulceration of thigh   HCC A

I70.232 Atherosclerosis of native arteries of right leg with ulceration of calf   HCC A

I70.233 Atherosclerosis of native arteries of right leg with ulceration of ankle   HCC A

I70.234 Atherosclerosis of native arteries of right leg with ulceration of heel and midfoot   HCC A

> Atherosclerosis of native arteries of right leg with ulceration of plantar surface of midfoot

I70.235 Atherosclerosis of native arteries of right leg with ulceration of other part of foot   HCC A

> Atherosclerosis of native arteries of right leg extremities with ulceration of toe

I70.238 Atherosclerosis of native arteries of right leg with ulceration of other part of lower leg   HCC A

I70.239 Atherosclerosis of native arteries of right leg with ulceration of unspecified site   HCC A

√6ᵗʰ **I70.24** Atherosclerosis of native arteries of left leg with ulceration

> INCLUDES   any condition classifiable to I70.212 and I70.222

Use additional code to identify severity of ulcer (L97.-)

I70.241 Atherosclerosis of native arteries of left leg with ulceration of thigh   HCC A

I70.242 Atherosclerosis of native arteries of left leg with ulceration of calf   HCC A

I70.243 Atherosclerosis of native arteries of left leg with ulceration of ankle   HCC A

I70.244 Atherosclerosis of native arteries of left leg with ulceration of heel and midfoot   HCC A

> Atherosclerosis of native arteries of left leg with ulceration of plantar surface of midfoot

I70.245 Atherosclerosis of native arteries of left leg with ulceration of other part of foot   HCC A

> Atherosclerosis of native arteries of left leg extremities with ulceration of toe

I70.248 Atherosclerosis of native arteries of left leg with ulceration of other part of lower leg   HCC A

I70.249 Atherosclerosis of native arteries of left leg with ulceration of unspecified site   HCC A

I70.25 Atherosclerosis of native arteries of other extremities with ulceration   HCC A

> INCLUDES   any condition classifiable to I70.218 and I70.228

Use additional code to identify the severity of the ulcer (L98.49-)

√6ᵗʰ **I70.26** Atherosclerosis of native arteries of extremities with gangrene

> INCLUDES   any condition classifiable to I70.21-, I70.22-, I70.23-, I70.24-, and I70.25-

Use additional code to identify the severity of any ulcer (L97.-, L98.49-), if applicable

CC Excl: For CC codes in subcategory I70.26: PDX collection 519

I70.261 Atherosclerosis of native arteries of extremities with gangrene, right leg   CC HCC A

I70.262 Atherosclerosis of native arteries of extremities with gangrene, left leg   CC HCC A

I70.263 Atherosclerosis of native arteries of extremities with gangrene, bilateral legs   CC HCC A

I70.268 Atherosclerosis of native arteries of extremities with gangrene, other extremity   CC HCC A

I70.269 Atherosclerosis of native arteries of extremities with gangrene, unspecified extremity   CC HCC A

√6ᵗʰ **I70.29** Other atherosclerosis of native arteries of extremities

I70.291 Other atherosclerosis of native arteries of extremities, right leg   HCC A

I70.292 Other atherosclerosis of native arteries of extremities, left leg   HCC A

I70.293 Other atherosclerosis of native arteries of extremities, bilateral legs   HCC A

I70.298 Other atherosclerosis of native arteries of extremities, other extremity   HCC A

I70.299 Other atherosclerosis of native arteries of extremities, unspecified extremity   HCC A

√5ᵗʰ **I70.3** Atherosclerosis of unspecified type of bypass graft(s) of the extremities

> Use additional code, if applicable, to identify chronic total occlusion of artery of extremity (I70.92)
>
> EXCLUDES 1   embolism or thrombus of bypass graft(s) of extremities (T82.8-)

√6ᵗʰ **I70.30** Unspecified atherosclerosis of unspecified type of bypass graft(s) of the extremities

I70.301 Unspecified atherosclerosis of unspecified type of bypass graft(s) of the extremities, right leg   HCC A

I70.302 Unspecified atherosclerosis of unspecified type of bypass graft(s) of the extremities, left leg   HCC A

I70.303 Unspecified atherosclerosis of unspecified type of bypass graft(s) of the extremities, bilateral legs   HCC A

I70.308 Unspecified atherosclerosis of unspecified type of bypass graft(s) of the extremities, other extremity   HCC A

✔ Additional Character Required   √x7ᵗʰ Placeholder   Unacceptable PDx   Questionable PDx   Manifestation   Unspecified Dx   H1-H14 HAC   HCC CMS-HCC Dx   HIV HIV Dx

ICD-10-CM 2020

671

I70.309 Unspecified atherosclerosis of unspecified type of bypass graft(s) of the extremities, unspecified extremity   HCC   A

√6th **I70.31** Atherosclerosis of unspecified type of bypass graft(s) of the extremities with intermittent claudication

   I70.311 Atherosclerosis of unspecified type of bypass graft(s) of the extremities with intermittent claudication, right leg   HCC   A

   I70.312 Atherosclerosis of unspecified type of bypass graft(s) of the extremities with intermittent claudication, left leg   HCC   A

   I70.313 Atherosclerosis of unspecified type of bypass graft(s) of the extremities with intermittent claudication, bilateral legs   HCC   A

   I70.318 Atherosclerosis of unspecified type of bypass graft(s) of the extremities with intermittent claudication, other extremity   HCC   A

   I70.319 Atherosclerosis of unspecified type of bypass graft(s) of the extremities with intermittent claudication, unspecified extremity   HCC   A

√6th **I70.32** Atherosclerosis of unspecified type of bypass graft(s) of the extremities with rest pain
   INCLUDES   any condition classifiable to I70.31-

   I70.321 Atherosclerosis of unspecified type of bypass graft(s) of the extremities with rest pain, right leg   HCC   A

   I70.322 Atherosclerosis of unspecified type of bypass graft(s) of the extremities with rest pain, left leg   HCC   A

   I70.323 Atherosclerosis of unspecified type of bypass graft(s) of the extremities with rest pain, bilateral legs   HCC   A

   I70.328 Atherosclerosis of unspecified type of bypass graft(s) of the extremities with rest pain, other extremity   HCC   A

   I70.329 Atherosclerosis of unspecified type of bypass graft(s) of the extremities with rest pain, unspecified extremity   HCC   A

√6th **I70.33** Atherosclerosis of unspecified type of bypass graft(s) of the right leg with ulceration
   INCLUDES   any condition classifiable to I70.311 and I70.321
   Use additional code to identify severity of ulcer (L97.-)
   CC Excl: For CC codes in subcategory I70.33: PDX collection 698

   I70.331 Atherosclerosis of unspecified type of bypass graft(s) of the right leg with ulceration of thigh   CC   HCC   A

   I70.332 Atherosclerosis of unspecified type of bypass graft(s) of the right leg with ulceration of calf   CC   HCC   A

   I70.333 Atherosclerosis of unspecified type of bypass graft(s) of the right leg with ulceration of ankle   CC   HCC   A

   I70.334 Atherosclerosis of unspecified type of bypass graft(s) of the right leg with ulceration of heel and midfoot   CC   HCC   A
      Atherosclerosis of unspecified type of bypass graft(s) of right leg with ulceration of plantar surface of midfoot

I70.335 Atherosclerosis of unspecified type of bypass graft(s) of the right leg with ulceration of other part of foot   HCC   A
      Atherosclerosis of unspecified type of bypass graft(s) of the right leg with ulceration of toe

I70.338 Atherosclerosis of unspecified type of bypass graft(s) of the right leg with ulceration of other part of lower leg   CC   HCC   A

I70.339 Atherosclerosis of unspecified type of bypass graft(s) of the right leg with ulceration of unspecified site   CC   HCC   A

√6th **I70.34** Atherosclerosis of unspecified type of bypass graft(s) of the left leg with ulceration
   INCLUDES   any condition classifiable to I70.312 and I70.322
   Use additional code to identify severity of ulcer (L97.-)
   CC Excl: For CC codes in subcategory I70.34: PDX collection 698

   I70.341 Atherosclerosis of unspecified type of bypass graft(s) of the left leg with ulceration of thigh   CC   HCC   A

   I70.342 Atherosclerosis of unspecified type of bypass graft(s) of the left leg with ulceration of calf   CC   HCC   A

   I70.343 Atherosclerosis of unspecified type of bypass graft(s) of the left leg with ulceration of ankle   CC   HCC   A

   I70.344 Atherosclerosis of unspecified type of bypass graft(s) of the left leg with ulceration of heel and midfoot   CC   HCC   A
      Atherosclerosis of unspecified type of bypass graft(s) of left leg with ulceration of plantar surface of midfoot

   I70.345 Atherosclerosis of unspecified type of bypass graft(s) of the left leg with ulceration of other part of foot   HCC   A
      Atherosclerosis of unspecified type of bypass graft(s) of the left leg with ulceration of toe

   I70.348 Atherosclerosis of unspecified type of bypass graft(s) of the left leg with ulceration of other part of lower leg   CC   HCC   A

   I70.349 Atherosclerosis of unspecified type of bypass graft(s) of the left leg with ulceration of unspecified site   CC   HCC   A

I70.35 Atherosclerosis of unspecified type of bypass graft(s) of other extremity with ulceration   HCC   A
   INCLUDES   any condition classifiable to I70.318 and I70.328
   Use additional code to identify severity of ulcer (L98.49-)

√6th **I70.36** Atherosclerosis of unspecified type of bypass graft(s) of the extremities with gangrene
   INCLUDES   any condition classifiable to I70.31-, I70.32-, I70.33-, I70.34-, I70.35
   Use additional code to identify the severity of any ulcer (L97.-, L98.49-), if applicable
   CC Excl: For CC codes in subcategory I70.36: PDX collection 519

   I70.361 Atherosclerosis of unspecified type of bypass graft(s) of the extremities with gangrene, right leg   CC   HCC   A

   I70.362 Atherosclerosis of unspecified type of bypass graft(s) of the extremities with gangrene, left leg   CC   HCC   A

   I70.363 Atherosclerosis of unspecified type of bypass graft(s) of the extremities with gangrene, bilateral legs   CC   HCC   A

N Newborn: 0   P Pediatric: 0-17   M Maternity: 9-64   A Adult: 15-124   MCC Major Complication/Comorbidity   CC Complication/Comorbidity   SW Severe Wound Dx

672   ICD-10-CM 2020

I70.368 Atherosclerosis of unspecified `CC` `HCC` `A` type of bypass graft(s) of the extremities with gangrene, other extremity

I70.369 Atherosclerosis of unspecified `CC` `HCC` `A` type of bypass graft(s) of the extremities with gangrene, unspecified extremity

√6ᵗʰ **I70.39** Other atherosclerosis of unspecified type of bypass graft(s) of the extremities

I70.391 Other atherosclerosis of `HCC` `A` unspecified type of bypass graft(s) of the extremities, right leg

I70.392 Other atherosclerosis of `HCC` `A` unspecified type of bypass graft(s) of the extremities, left leg

I70.393 Other atherosclerosis of `HCC` `A` unspecified type of bypass graft(s) of the extremities, bilateral legs

I70.398 Other atherosclerosis of `HCC` `A` unspecified type of bypass graft(s) of the extremities, other extremity

I70.399 Other atherosclerosis of `HCC` `A` unspecified type of bypass graft(s) of the extremities, unspecified extremity

√5ᵗʰ **I70.4** Atherosclerosis of autologous vein bypass graft(s) of the extremities

Use additional code, if applicable, to identify chronic total occlusion of artery of extremity (I70.92)

√6ᵗʰ **I70.40** Unspecified atherosclerosis of autologous vein bypass graft(s) of the extremities

I70.401 Unspecified atherosclerosis of `HCC` `A` autologous vein bypass graft(s) of the extremities, right leg

I70.402 Unspecified atherosclerosis of `HCC` `A` autologous vein bypass graft(s) of the extremities, left leg

I70.403 Unspecified atherosclerosis of `HCC` `A` autologous vein bypass graft(s) of the extremities, bilateral legs

I70.408 Unspecified atherosclerosis of `HCC` `A` autologous vein bypass graft(s) of the extremities, other extremity

I70.409 Unspecified atherosclerosis of `HCC` `A` autologous vein bypass graft(s) of the extremities, unspecified extremity

√6ᵗʰ **I70.41** Atherosclerosis of autologous vein bypass graft(s) of the extremities with intermittent claudication

I70.411 Atherosclerosis of autologous `HCC` `A` vein bypass graft(s) of the extremities with intermittent claudication, right leg

I70.412 Atherosclerosis of autologous `HCC` `A` vein bypass graft(s) of the extremities with intermittent claudication, left leg

I70.413 Atherosclerosis of autologous `HCC` `A` vein bypass graft(s) of the extremities with intermittent claudication, bilateral legs

I70.418 Atherosclerosis of autologous `HCC` `A` vein bypass graft(s) of the extremities with intermittent claudication, other extremity

I70.419 Atherosclerosis of autologous `HCC` `A` vein bypass graft(s) of the extremities with intermittent claudication, unspecified extremity

√6ᵗʰ **I70.42** Atherosclerosis of autologous vein bypass graft(s) of the extremities with rest pain

`INCLUDES` any condition classifiable to I70.41-

I70.421 Atherosclerosis of autologous `HCC` `A` vein bypass graft(s) of the extremities with rest pain, right leg

I70.422 Atherosclerosis of autologous `HCC` `A` vein bypass graft(s) of the extremities with rest pain, left leg

I70.423 Atherosclerosis of autologous `HCC` `A` vein bypass graft(s) of the extremities with rest pain, bilateral legs

I70.428 Atherosclerosis of autologous `HCC` `A` vein bypass graft(s) of the extremities with rest pain, other extremity

I70.429 Atherosclerosis of autologous `HCC` `A` vein bypass graft(s) of the extremities with rest pain, unspecified extremity

√6ᵗʰ **I70.43** Atherosclerosis of autologous vein bypass graft(s) of the right leg with ulceration

`INCLUDES` any condition classifiable to I70.411 and I70.421

Use additional code to identify severity of ulcer (L97.-)

CC Excl: For CC codes in subcategory I70.43: PDX collection 698

I70.431 Atherosclerosis of autologous `CC` `HCC` `A` vein bypass graft(s) of the right leg with ulceration of thigh

I70.432 Atherosclerosis of autologous `CC` `HCC` `A` vein bypass graft(s) of the right leg with ulceration of calf

I70.433 Atherosclerosis of autologous `CC` `HCC` `A` vein bypass graft(s) of the right leg with ulceration of ankle

I70.434 Atherosclerosis of autologous `CC` `HCC` `A` vein bypass graft(s) of the right leg with ulceration of heel and midfoot

Atherosclerosis of autologous vein bypass graft(s) of right leg with ulceration of plantar surface of midfoot

I70.435 Atherosclerosis of autologous `HCC` `A` vein bypass graft(s) of the right leg with ulceration of other part of foot

Atherosclerosis of autologous vein bypass graft(s) of right leg with ulceration of toe

I70.438 Atherosclerosis of autologous `CC` `HCC` `A` vein bypass graft(s) of the right leg with ulceration of other part of lower leg

I70.439 Atherosclerosis of autologous `CC` `HCC` `A` vein bypass graft(s) of the right leg with ulceration of unspecified site

√6ᵗʰ **I70.44** Atherosclerosis of autologous vein bypass graft(s) of the left leg with ulceration

`INCLUDES` any condition classifiable to I70.412 and I70.422

Use additional code to identify severity of ulcer (L97.-)

CC Excl: For CC codes in subcategory I70.44: PDX collection 698

I70.441 Atherosclerosis of autologous `CC` `HCC` `A` vein bypass graft(s) of the left leg with ulceration of thigh

I70.442 Atherosclerosis of autologous `CC` `HCC` `A` vein bypass graft(s) of the left leg with ulceration of calf

I70.443 Atherosclerosis of autologous `CC` `HCC` `A` vein bypass graft(s) of the left leg with ulceration of ankle

✔ Additional Character Required   √x7ᵗʰ Placeholder   Unacceptable PDx   Questionable PDx   Manifestation   Unspecified Dx   H1 - H14 HAC   `HCC` CMS-HCC Dx   `HIV` HIV Dx

ICD-10-CM 2020   673

Chapter 9. Diseases of the Circulatory System *(side margin)*

I70.444–I70.529 *(side margin)*

I70.444   **Atherosclerosis of autologous** `CC` `HCC` `A`
**vein bypass graft(s) of the left
leg with ulceration of heel and
midfoot**
> Atherosclerosis of autologous vein bypass
> graft(s) of left leg with ulceration of
> plantar surface of midfoot

I70.445   **Atherosclerosis of autologous** `HCC` `A`
**vein bypass graft(s) of the left
leg with ulceration of other
part of foot**
> Atherosclerosis of autologous vein bypass
> graft(s) of left leg with ulceration of
> toe

I70.448   **Atherosclerosis of autologous** `CC` `HCC` `A`
**vein bypass graft(s) of the left
leg with ulceration of other
part of lower leg**

I70.449   **Atherosclerosis of autologous** `CC` `HCC` `A`
**vein bypass graft(s) of the left
leg with ulceration of
unspecified site**

I70.45   **Atherosclerosis of autologous vein** `HCC` `A`
**bypass graft(s) of other extremity with
ulceration**
> **INCLUDES**   any condition classifiable to I70.418,
> I70.428, and I70.438
> Use additional code to identify severity of ulcer
> (L98.49)

√6ᵗʰ **I70.46**   **Atherosclerosis of autologous vein bypass graft(s)
of the extremities with gangrene**
> **INCLUDES**   any condition classifiable to I70.41-,
> I70.42-, and I70.43-, I70.44-, I70.45
> Use additional code to identify the severity of any
> ulcer (L97.-, L98.49-), if applicable
> **CC Excl: For CC codes in subcategory I70.46:** PDX
> collection 519

I70.461   **Atherosclerosis of autologous** `CC` `HCC` `A`
**vein bypass graft(s) of the
extremities with gangrene,
right leg**

I70.462   **Atherosclerosis of autologous** `CC` `HCC` `A`
**vein bypass graft(s) of the
extremities with gangrene, left
leg**

I70.463   **Atherosclerosis of autologous** `CC` `HCC` `A`
**vein bypass graft(s) of the
extremities with gangrene,
bilateral legs**

I70.468   **Atherosclerosis of autologous** `CC` `HCC` `A`
**vein bypass graft(s) of the
extremities with gangrene,
other extremity**

I70.469   **Atherosclerosis of autologous** `CC` `HCC` `A`
**vein bypass graft(s) of the
extremities with gangrene,
unspecified extremity**

√6ᵗʰ **I70.49**   **Other atherosclerosis of autologous vein bypass
graft(s) of the extremities**

I70.491   **Other atherosclerosis of** `HCC` `A`
**autologous vein bypass
graft(s) of the extremities,
right leg**

I70.492   **Other atherosclerosis of** `HCC` `A`
**autologous vein bypass
graft(s) of the extremities, left
leg**

I70.493   **Other atherosclerosis of** `HCC` `A`
**autologous vein bypass
graft(s) of the extremities,
bilateral legs**

I70.498   **Other atherosclerosis of** `HCC` `A`
**autologous vein bypass
graft(s) of the extremities,
other extremity**

I70.499   **Other atherosclerosis of** `HCC` `A`
**autologous vein bypass
graft(s) of the extremities,
unspecified extremity**

√5ᵗʰ **I70.5**   **Atherosclerosis of nonautologous biological bypass graft(s)
of the extremities**
> Use additional code, if applicable, to identify chronic total
> occlusion of artery of extremity (I70.92)

√6ᵗʰ **I70.50**   **Unspecified atherosclerosis of nonautologous
biological bypass graft(s) of the extremities**

I70.501   **Unspecified atherosclerosis of** `HCC` `A`
**nonautologous biological
bypass graft(s) of the
extremities, right leg**

I70.502   **Unspecified atherosclerosis of** `HCC` `A`
**nonautologous biological
bypass graft(s) of the
extremities, left leg**

I70.503   **Unspecified atherosclerosis of** `HCC` `A`
**nonautologous biological
bypass graft(s) of the
extremities, bilateral legs**

I70.508   **Unspecified atherosclerosis of** `HCC` `A`
**nonautologous biological
bypass graft(s) of the
extremities, other extremity**

I70.509   **Unspecified atherosclerosis of** `HCC` `A`
**nonautologous biological
bypass graft(s) of the
extremities, unspecified
extremity**

√6ᵗʰ **I70.51**   **Atherosclerosis of nonautologous biological bypass
graft(s) of the extremities intermittent claudication**

I70.511   **Atherosclerosis of** `HCC` `A`
**nonautologous biological
bypass graft(s) of the
extremities with intermittent
claudication, right leg**

I70.512   **Atherosclerosis of** `HCC` `A`
**nonautologous biological
bypass graft(s) of the
extremities with intermittent
claudication, left leg**

I70.513   **Atherosclerosis of** `HCC` `A`
**nonautologous biological
bypass graft(s) of the
extremities with intermittent
claudication, bilateral legs**

I70.518   **Atherosclerosis of** `HCC` `A`
**nonautologous biological
bypass graft(s) of the
extremities with intermittent
claudication, other extremity**

I70.519   **Atherosclerosis of** `HCC` `A`
**nonautologous biological
bypass graft(s) of the
extremities with intermittent
claudication, unspecified
extremity**

√6ᵗʰ **I70.52**   **Atherosclerosis of nonautologous biological bypass
graft(s) of the extremities with rest pain**
> **INCLUDES**   any condition classifiable to I70.51-

I70.521   **Atherosclerosis of** `HCC` `A`
**nonautologous biological
bypass graft(s) of the
extremities with rest pain,
right leg**

I70.522   **Atherosclerosis of** `HCC` `A`
**nonautologous biological
bypass graft(s) of the
extremities with rest pain, left
leg**

I70.523   **Atherosclerosis of** `HCC` `A`
**nonautologous biological
bypass graft(s) of the
extremities with rest pain,
bilateral legs**

I70.528   **Atherosclerosis of** `HCC` `A`
**nonautologous biological
bypass graft(s) of the
extremities with rest pain,
other extremity**

I70.529   **Atherosclerosis of** `HCC` `A`
**nonautologous biological
bypass graft(s) of the
extremities with rest pain,
unspecified extremity**

`N` Newborn: 0   `P` Pediatric: 0-17   `M` Maternity: 9-64   `A` Adult: 15-124   `MCC` Major Complication/Comorbidity   `CC` Complication/Comorbidity   `SW` Severe Wound Dx

674

ICD-10-CM 2020

√6ᵗʰ **I70.53 Atherosclerosis of nonautologous biological bypass graft(s) of the right leg with ulceration**

INCLUDES any condition classifiable to I70.511 and I70.521

Use additional code to identify severity of ulcer (L97.-)

CC Excl: For CC codes in subcategory I70.53: PDX collection 698

I70.531 Atherosclerosis of nonautologous biological bypass graft(s) of the right leg with ulceration of **thigh** `CC` `HCC` `A`

I70.532 Atherosclerosis of nonautologous biological bypass graft(s) of the right leg with ulceration of **calf** `CC` `HCC` `A`

I70.533 Atherosclerosis of nonautologous biological bypass graft(s) of the right leg with ulceration of **ankle** `CC` `HCC` `A`

I70.534 Atherosclerosis of nonautologous biological bypass graft(s) of the right leg with ulceration of **heel and midfoot** `CC` `HCC` `A`
Atherosclerosis of nonautologous biological bypass graft(s) of right leg with ulceration of plantar surface of midfoot

I70.535 Atherosclerosis of nonautologous biological bypass graft(s) of the right leg with ulceration of other part of foot `HCC` `A`
Atherosclerosis of nonautologous biological bypass graft(s) of the right leg with ulceration of toe

I70.538 Atherosclerosis of nonautologous biological bypass graft(s) of the right leg with ulceration of other part of lower leg `CC` `HCC` `A`

I70.539 Atherosclerosis of nonautologous biological bypass graft(s) of the right leg with ulceration of unspecified site `CC` `HCC` `A`

√6ᵗʰ **I70.54 Atherosclerosis of nonautologous biological bypass graft(s) of the left leg with ulceration**

INCLUDES any condition classifiable to I70.512 and I70.522

Use additional code to identify severity of ulcer (L97.-)

CC Excl: For CC codes in subcategory I70.54: PDX collection 698

I70.541 Atherosclerosis of nonautologous biological bypass graft(s) of the left leg with ulceration of **thigh** `CC` `HCC` `A`

I70.542 Atherosclerosis of nonautologous biological bypass graft(s) of the left leg with ulceration of **calf** `CC` `HCC` `A`

I70.543 Atherosclerosis of nonautologous biological bypass graft(s) of the left leg with ulceration of **ankle** `CC` `HCC` `A`

I70.544 Atherosclerosis of nonautologous biological bypass graft(s) of the left leg with ulceration of **heel and midfoot** `CC` `HCC` `A`
Atherosclerosis of nonautologous biological bypass graft(s) of left leg with ulceration of plantar surface of midfoot

I70.545 Atherosclerosis of nonautologous biological bypass graft(s) of the left leg with ulceration of other part of foot `HCC` `A`
Atherosclerosis of nonautologous biological bypass graft(s) of the left leg with ulceration of toe

I70.548 Atherosclerosis of nonautologous biological bypass graft(s) of the left leg with ulceration of other part of lower leg `CC` `HCC` `A`

I70.549 Atherosclerosis of nonautologous biological bypass graft(s) of the left leg with ulceration of unspecified site `CC` `HCC` `A`

I70.55 Atherosclerosis of nonautologous biological bypass graft(s) of other extremity with ulceration `HCC` `A`

INCLUDES any condition classifiable to I70.518, I70.528, and I70.538

Use additional code to identify severity of ulcer (L98.49)

√6ᵗʰ **I70.56 Atherosclerosis of nonautologous biological bypass graft(s) of the extremities with gangrene**

INCLUDES any condition classifiable to I70.51-, I70.52-, and I70.53-, I70.54-, I70.55

Use additional code to identify the severity of any ulcer (L97.-, L98.49-), if applicable

CC Excl: For CC codes in subcategory I70.56: PDX collection 519

I70.561 Atherosclerosis of nonautologous biological bypass graft(s) of the extremities with gangrene, **right leg** `CC` `HCC` `A`

I70.562 Atherosclerosis of nonautologous biological bypass graft(s) of the extremities with gangrene, **left leg** `CC` `HCC` `A`

I70.563 Atherosclerosis of nonautologous biological bypass graft(s) of the extremities with gangrene, **bilateral legs** `CC` `HCC` `A`

I70.568 Atherosclerosis of nonautologous biological bypass graft(s) of the extremities with gangrene, other extremity `CC` `HCC` `A`

I70.569 Atherosclerosis of nonautologous biological bypass graft(s) of the extremities with gangrene, unspecified extremity `CC` `HCC` `A`

√6ᵗʰ **I70.59 Other atherosclerosis of nonautologous biological bypass graft(s) of the extremities**

I70.591 Other atherosclerosis of nonautologous biological bypass graft(s) of the extremities, **right leg** `HCC` `A`

I70.592 Other atherosclerosis of nonautologous biological bypass graft(s) of the extremities, **left leg** `HCC` `A`

I70.593 Other atherosclerosis of nonautologous biological bypass graft(s) of the extremities, **bilateral legs** `HCC` `A`

I70.598 Other atherosclerosis of nonautologous biological bypass graft(s) of the extremities, other extremity `HCC` `A`

I70.599 Other atherosclerosis of nonautologous biological bypass graft(s) of the extremities, unspecified extremity `HCC` `A`

√5ᵗʰ **I70.6 Atherosclerosis of nonbiological bypass graft(s) of the extremities**

Use additional code, if applicable, to identify chronic total occlusion of artery of extremity (I70.92)

√6ᵗʰ **I70.60 Unspecified atherosclerosis of nonbiological bypass graft(s) of the extremities**

I70.601 Unspecified atherosclerosis of nonbiological bypass graft(s) of the extremities, **right leg** `HCC` `A`

I70.602 Unspecified atherosclerosis of nonbiological bypass graft(s) of the extremities, **left leg** `HCC` `A`

√ Additional Character Required   √x7ᵗʰ Placeholder   Unacceptable PDx   Questionable PDx   Manifestation   Unspecified Dx   H1-H14 HAC   HCC CMS-HCC Dx   HIV HIV Dx

ICD-10-CM 2020   675

Chapter 9. Diseases of the Circulatory System

I70.603 Unspecified atherosclerosis of nonbiological bypass graft(s) of the extremities, **bilateral legs** `HCC` `A`

I70.608 Unspecified atherosclerosis of nonbiological bypass graft(s) of the extremities, **other extremity** `HCC` `A`

I70.609 Unspecified atherosclerosis of nonbiological bypass graft(s) of the extremities, **unspecified extremity** `HCC` `A`

✓6ᵗʰ **I70.61** Atherosclerosis of nonbiological bypass graft(s) of the extremities with **intermittent claudication**

I70.611 Atherosclerosis of nonbiological bypass graft(s) of the extremities with intermittent claudication, **right leg** `HCC` `A`

I70.612 Atherosclerosis of nonbiological bypass graft(s) of the extremities with intermittent claudication, **left leg** `HCC` `A`

I70.613 Atherosclerosis of nonbiological bypass graft(s) of the extremities with intermittent claudication, **bilateral legs** `HCC` `A`

I70.618 Atherosclerosis of nonbiological bypass graft(s) of the extremities with intermittent claudication, **other extremity** `HCC` `A`

I70.619 Atherosclerosis of nonbiological bypass graft(s) of the extremities with intermittent claudication, **unspecified extremity** `HCC` `A`

✓6ᵗʰ **I70.62** Atherosclerosis of nonbiological bypass graft(s) of the extremities with **rest pain**

     `INCLUDES` any condition classifiable to I70.61-

I70.621 Atherosclerosis of nonbiological bypass graft(s) of the extremities with rest pain, **right leg** `HCC` `A`

I70.622 Atherosclerosis of nonbiological bypass graft(s) of the extremities with rest pain, **left leg** `HCC` `A`

I70.623 Atherosclerosis of nonbiological bypass graft(s) of the extremities with rest pain, **bilateral legs** `HCC` `A`

I70.628 Atherosclerosis of nonbiological bypass graft(s) of the extremities with rest pain, **other extremity** `HCC` `A`

I70.629 Atherosclerosis of nonbiological bypass graft(s) of the extremities with rest pain, **unspecified extremity** `HCC` `A`

✓6ᵗʰ **I70.63** Atherosclerosis of nonbiological bypass graft(s) of the **right leg** with **ulceration**

     `INCLUDES` any condition classifiable to I70.611 and I70.621

     Use additional code to identify severity of ulcer (L97.-)

     CC Excl: For CC codes in subcategory I70.63: PDX collection 698

I70.631 Atherosclerosis of nonbiological bypass graft(s) of the right leg with ulceration **of thigh** `CC` `HCC` `A`

I70.632 Atherosclerosis of nonbiological bypass graft(s) of the right leg with ulceration **of calf** `CC` `HCC` `A`

I70.633 Atherosclerosis of nonbiological bypass graft(s) of the right leg with ulceration **of ankle** `CC` `HCC` `A`

I70.634 Atherosclerosis of nonbiological bypass graft(s) of the right leg with ulceration **of heel and midfoot** `CC` `HCC` `A`

     Atherosclerosis of nonbiological bypass graft(s) of right leg with ulceration of plantar surface of midfoot

I70.635 Atherosclerosis of nonbiological bypass graft(s) of the right leg with ulceration **of other part of foot** `HCC` `A`

     Atherosclerosis of nonbiological bypass graft(s) of the right leg with ulceration of toe

I70.638 Atherosclerosis of nonbiological bypass graft(s) of the right leg with ulceration **of other part of lower leg** `CC` `HCC` `A`

I70.639 Atherosclerosis of nonbiological bypass graft(s) of the right leg with ulceration **of unspecified site** `CC` `HCC` `A`

✓6ᵗʰ **I70.64** Atherosclerosis of nonbiological bypass graft(s) of the **left leg** with **ulceration**

     `INCLUDES` any condition classifiable to I70.612 and I70.622

     Use additional code to identify severity of ulcer (L97.-)

     CC Excl: For CC codes in subcategory I70.64: PDX collection 698

I70.641 Atherosclerosis of nonbiological bypass graft(s) of the left leg with ulceration **of thigh** `CC` `HCC` `A`

I70.642 Atherosclerosis of nonbiological bypass graft(s) of the left leg with ulceration **of calf** `CC` `HCC` `A`

I70.643 Atherosclerosis of nonbiological bypass graft(s) of the left leg with ulceration **of ankle** `CC` `HCC` `A`

I70.644 Atherosclerosis of nonbiological bypass graft(s) of the left leg with ulceration **of heel and midfoot** `CC` `HCC` `A`

     Atherosclerosis of nonbiological bypass graft(s) of left leg with ulceration of plantar surface of midfoot

I70.645 Atherosclerosis of nonbiological bypass graft(s) of the left leg with ulceration **of other part of foot** `HCC` `A`

     Atherosclerosis of nonbiological bypass graft(s) of the left leg with ulceration of toe

I70.648 Atherosclerosis of nonbiological bypass graft(s) of the left leg with ulceration **of other part of lower leg** `CC` `HCC` `A`

I70.649 Atherosclerosis of nonbiological bypass graft(s) of the left leg with ulceration **of unspecified site** `CC` `HCC` `A`

I70.65 Atherosclerosis of nonbiological bypass graft(s) of other extremity with ulceration `HCC` `A`

     `INCLUDES` any condition classifiable to I70.618 and I70.628

     Use additional code to identify severity of ulcer (L98.49)

✓6ᵗʰ **I70.66** Atherosclerosis of nonbiological bypass graft(s) of the extremities with **gangrene**

     `INCLUDES` any condition classifiable to I70.61-, I70.62-, I70.63-, I70.64-, I70.65

     Use additional code to identify the severity of any ulcer (L97.-, L98.49-), if applicable

     CC Excl: For CC codes in subcategory I70.66: PDX collection 519

I70.661 Atherosclerosis of nonbiological bypass graft(s) of the extremities with **gangrene, right leg** `CC` `HCC` `A`

Ⓝ Newborn: 0   Ⓟ Pediatric: 0-17   Ⓜ Maternity: 9-64   Ⓐ Adult: 15-124   `MCC` Major Complication/Comorbidity   `CC` Complication/Comorbidity   `SW` Severe Wound Dx

676

ICD-10-CM 2020

Chapter 9. Diseases of the Circulatory System

I70.662 Atherosclerosis of nonbiological bypass graft(s) of the extremities with gangrene, left leg   `CC` `HCC` `A`

I70.663 Atherosclerosis of nonbiological bypass graft(s) of the extremities with gangrene, bilateral legs   `CC` `HCC` `A`

I70.668 Atherosclerosis of nonbiological bypass graft(s) of the extremities with gangrene, other extremity   `CC` `HCC` `A`

I70.669 Atherosclerosis of nonbiological bypass graft(s) of the extremities with gangrene, unspecified extremity   `CC` `HCC` `A`

✓6th **I70.69** Other atherosclerosis of nonbiological bypass graft(s) of the extremities

I70.691 Other atherosclerosis of nonbiological bypass graft(s) of the extremities, right leg   `HCC` `A`

I70.692 Other atherosclerosis of nonbiological bypass graft(s) of the extremities, left leg   `HCC` `A`

I70.693 Other atherosclerosis of nonbiological bypass graft(s) of the extremities, bilateral legs   `HCC` `A`

I70.698 Other atherosclerosis of nonbiological bypass graft(s) of the extremities, other extremity   `HCC` `A`

I70.699 Other atherosclerosis of nonbiological bypass graft(s) of the extremities, unspecified extremity   `HCC` `A`

✓5th **I70.7** Atherosclerosis of other type of bypass graft(s) of the extremities

Use additional code, if applicable, to identify chronic total occlusion of artery of extremity (I70.92)

✓6th **I70.70** Unspecified atherosclerosis of other type of bypass graft(s) of the extremities

I70.701 Unspecified atherosclerosis of other type of bypass graft(s) of the extremities, right leg   `HCC` `A`

I70.702 Unspecified atherosclerosis of other type of bypass graft(s) of the extremities, left leg   `HCC` `A`

I70.703 Unspecified atherosclerosis of other type of bypass graft(s) of the extremities, bilateral legs   `HCC` `A`

I70.708 Unspecified atherosclerosis of other type of bypass graft(s) of the extremities, other extremity   `HCC` `A`

I70.709 Unspecified atherosclerosis of other type of bypass graft(s) of the extremities, unspecified extremity   `HCC` `A`

✓6th **I70.71** Atherosclerosis of other type of bypass graft(s) of the extremities with intermittent claudication

I70.711 Atherosclerosis of other type of bypass graft(s) of the extremities with intermittent claudication, right leg   `HCC` `A`

I70.712 Atherosclerosis of other type of bypass graft(s) of the extremities with intermittent claudication, left leg   `HCC` `A`

I70.713 Atherosclerosis of other type of bypass graft(s) of the extremities with intermittent claudication, bilateral legs   `HCC` `A`

I70.718 Atherosclerosis of other type of bypass graft(s) of the extremities with intermittent claudication, other extremity   `HCC` `A`

I70.719 Atherosclerosis of other type of bypass graft(s) of the extremities with intermittent claudication, unspecified extremity   `HCC` `A`

✓6th **I70.72** Atherosclerosis of other type of bypass graft(s) of the extremities with rest pain

INCLUDES   any condition classifiable to I70.71-

I70.721 Atherosclerosis of other type of bypass graft(s) of the extremities with rest pain, right leg   `HCC` `A`

I70.722 Atherosclerosis of other type of bypass graft(s) of the extremities with rest pain, left leg   `HCC` `A`

I70.723 Atherosclerosis of other type of bypass graft(s) of the extremities with rest pain, bilateral legs   `HCC` `A`

I70.728 Atherosclerosis of other type of bypass graft(s) of the extremities with rest pain, other extremity   `HCC` `A`

I70.729 Atherosclerosis of other type of bypass graft(s) of the extremities with rest pain, unspecified extremity   `HCC` `A`

✓6th **I70.73** Atherosclerosis of other type of bypass graft(s) of the right leg with ulceration

INCLUDES   any condition classifiable to I70.711 and I70.721

Use additional code to identify severity of ulcer (L97.-)

CC Excl: For CC codes in subcategory I70.73: PDX collection 698

I70.731 Atherosclerosis of other type of bypass graft(s) of the right leg with ulceration of thigh   `CC` `HCC` `A`

I70.732 Atherosclerosis of other type of bypass graft(s) of the right leg with ulceration of calf   `CC` `HCC` `A`

I70.733 Atherosclerosis of other type of bypass graft(s) of the right leg with ulceration of ankle   `CC` `HCC` `A`

I70.734 Atherosclerosis of other type of bypass graft(s) of the right leg with ulceration of heel and midfoot   `CC` `HCC` `A`

Atherosclerosis of other type of bypass graft(s) of right leg with ulceration of plantar surface of midfoot

I70.735 Atherosclerosis of other type of bypass graft(s) of the right leg with ulceration of other part of foot   `HCC` `A`

Atherosclerosis of other type of bypass graft(s) of right leg with ulceration of toe

I70.738 Atherosclerosis of other type of bypass graft(s) of the right leg with ulceration of other part of lower leg   `CC` `HCC` `A`

I70.739 Atherosclerosis of other type of bypass graft(s) of the right leg with ulceration of unspecified site   `CC` `HCC` `A`

✓6th **I70.74** Atherosclerosis of other type of bypass graft(s) of the left leg with ulceration

INCLUDES   any condition classifiable to I70.712 and I70.722

Use additional code to identify severity of ulcer (L97.-)

CC Excl: For CC codes in subcategory I70.74: PDX collection 698

I70.741 Atherosclerosis of other type of bypass graft(s) of the left leg with ulceration of thigh   `CC` `HCC` `A`

I70.742 Atherosclerosis of other type of bypass graft(s) of the left leg with ulceration of calf   `CC` `HCC` `A`

I70.743 Atherosclerosis of other type of bypass graft(s) of the left leg with ulceration of ankle   `CC` `HCC` `A`

☑ Additional Character Required   ✓x7th Placeholder   Unacceptable PDx   Questionable PDx   Manifestation   Unspecified Dx   H1-H14 HAC   HCC CMS-HCC Dx   HIV HIV Dx

ICD-10-CM 2020   **677**

I70.744 **Atherosclerosis of other type of bypass graft(s) of the left leg with ulceration of heel and midfoot** `CC` `HCC` `A`

Atherosclerosis of other type of bypass graft(s) of left leg with ulceration of plantar surface of midfoot

I70.745 **Atherosclerosis of other type of bypass graft(s) of the left leg with ulceration of other part of foot** `HCC` `A`

Atherosclerosis of other type of bypass graft(s) of left leg with ulceration of toe

I70.748 **Atherosclerosis of other type of bypass graft(s) of the left leg with ulceration of other part of lower leg** `CC` `HCC` `A`

I70.749 **Atherosclerosis of other type of bypass graft(s) of the left leg with ulceration of unspecified site** `CC` `HCC` `A`

I70.75 **Atherosclerosis of other type of bypass graft(s) of other extremity with ulceration** `HCC` `A`

> **INCLUDES** any condition classifiable to I70.718 and I70.728
>
> Use additional code to identify severity of ulcer (L98.49)

✓6ᵗʰ **I70.76** **Atherosclerosis of other type of bypass graft(s) of the extremities with gangrene**

> **INCLUDES** any condition classifiable to I70.71-, I70.72-, I70.73-, I70.74-, I70.75
>
> Use additional code to identify the severity of any ulcer (L97.-, L98.49-), if applicable
>
> **CC Excl: For CC codes in subcategory I70.76:** PDX collection 519

I70.761 **Atherosclerosis of other type of bypass graft(s) of the extremities with gangrene, right leg** `CC` `HCC` `A`

I70.762 **Atherosclerosis of other type of bypass graft(s) of the extremities with gangrene, left leg** `CC` `HCC` `A`

I70.763 **Atherosclerosis of other type of bypass graft(s) of the extremities with gangrene, bilateral legs** `CC` `HCC` `A`

I70.768 **Atherosclerosis of other type of bypass graft(s) of the extremities with gangrene, other extremity** `CC` `HCC` `A`

I70.769 **Atherosclerosis of other type of bypass graft(s) of the extremities with gangrene, unspecified extremity** `CC` `HCC` `A`

✓6ᵗʰ **I70.79** **Other atherosclerosis of other type of bypass graft(s) of the extremities**

I70.791 **Other atherosclerosis of other type of bypass graft(s) of the extremities, right leg** `HCC` `A`

I70.792 **Other atherosclerosis of other type of bypass graft(s) of the extremities, left leg** `HCC` `A`

I70.793 **Other atherosclerosis of other type of bypass graft(s) of the extremities, bilateral legs** `HCC` `A`

I70.798 **Other atherosclerosis of other type of bypass graft(s) of the extremities, other extremity** `HCC` `A`

I70.799 **Other atherosclerosis of other type of bypass graft(s) of the extremities, unspecified extremity** `HCC` `A`

I70.8 **Atherosclerosis of other arteries** `A`

> **TIP:** Arteriosclerosis of the iliac arteries is coded here.

✓5ᵗʰ **I70.9** **Other and unspecified atherosclerosis**

I70.90 **Unspecified atherosclerosis** `A`

I70.91 **Generalized atherosclerosis** `A`

I70.92 **Chronic total occlusion of artery of the extremities** `CC` `HCC` `A`

Complete occlusion of artery of the extremities
Total occlusion of artery of the extremities
Code first atherosclerosis of arteries of the extremities (I70.2-, I70.3-, I70.4-, I70.5-, I70.6-, I70.7-)
CC Excl: PDX collection 699

✓4ᵗʰ **I71** **Aortic aneurysm and dissection**

> **EXCLUDES 1** aortic ectasia (I77.81-)
> syphilitic aortic aneurysm (A52.01)
> traumatic aortic aneurysm (S25.09, S35.09)
>
> **CC Excl: For MCC codes in category I71:** PDX collection 700

✓5ᵗʰ **I71.0** **Dissection of aorta**

I71.00 **Dissection of unspecified site of aorta** `CC` `HCC`

I71.01 **Dissection of thoracic aorta** `MCC` `HCC`

I71.02 **Dissection of abdominal aorta** `MCC` `HCC`

I71.03 **Dissection of thoracoabdominal aorta** `MCC` `HCC`

I71.1 **Thoracic aortic aneurysm, ruptured** `MCC` `HCC`

I71.2 **Thoracic aortic aneurysm, without rupture** `HCC`

I71.3 **Abdominal aortic aneurysm, ruptured** `MCC` `HCC`

I71.4 **Abdominal aortic aneurysm, without rupture** `HCC`

I71.5 **Thoracoabdominal aortic aneurysm, ruptured** `MCC` `HCC`

I71.6 **Thoracoabdominal aortic aneurysm, without rupture** `HCC`

I71.8 **Aortic aneurysm of unspecified site, ruptured** `MCC` `HCC`

Rupture of aorta NOS

I71.9 **Aortic aneurysm of unspecified site, without rupture** `HCC`

Aneurysm of aorta
Dilatation of aorta
Hyaline necrosis of aorta

✓4ᵗʰ **I72** **Other aneurysm**

> **INCLUDES** aneurysm (cirsoid) (false) (ruptured)
> **EXCLUDES 2** acquired aneurysm (I77.0)
> aneurysm (of) aorta (I71.-)
> aneurysm (of) arteriovenous NOS (Q27.3-)
> carotid artery dissection (I77.71)
> cerebral (nonruptured) aneurysm (I67.1)
> coronary aneurysm (I25.4)
> coronary artery dissection (I25.42)
> dissection of artery NEC (I77.79)
> dissection of precerebral artery, congenital (nonruptured) (Q28.1)
> heart aneurysm (I25.3)
> iliac artery dissection (I77.72)
> precerebral artery, congential (nonruptured) (Q28.1)
> pulmonary artery aneurysm (I28.1)
> renal artery dissection (I77.73)
> retinal aneurysm (H35.0)
> ruptured cerebral aneurysm (I60.7)
> varicose aneurysm (I77.0)
> vertebral artery dissection (I77.74)
>
> **AHA:** 2016,4Q,28-29

I72.0 **Aneurysm of carotid artery** `HCC`

Aneurysm of common carotid artery
Aneurysm of external carotid artery
Aneurysm of internal carotid artery, extracranial portion

> **EXCLUDES 1** aneurysm of internal carotid artery, intracranial portion (I67.1)
> aneurysm of internal carotid artery NOS (I67.1)

I72.1 **Aneurysm of artery of upper extremity** `HCC`

I72.2 **Aneurysm of renal artery** `HCC`

I72.3 **Aneurysm of iliac artery** `HCC`

I72.4 **Aneurysm of artery of lower extremity** `HCC`

> **AHA:** 2019,2Q,21

`N` Newborn: 0   `P` Pediatric: 0-17   `M` Maternity: 9-64   `A` Adult: 15-124   `MCC` Major Complication/Comorbidity   `CC` Complication/Comorbidity   `SW` Severe Wound Dx

I72.5   **Aneurysm of other precerebral arteries**   `HCC`

Aneurysm of basilar artery (trunk)

   `EXCLUDES 2`   *aneurysm of carotid artery (I72.Ø)*
              aneurysm of vertebral artery (I72.6)
              dissection of carotid artery (I77.71)
              dissection of other precerebral arteries (I77.75)
              dissection of vertebral artery (I77.74)

I72.6   **Aneurysm of vertebral artery**   `HCC`

   `EXCLUDES 2`   *dissection of vertebral artery (I77.74)*

I72.8   **Aneurysm of other specified arteries**   `HCC`

I72.9   **Aneurysm of unspecified site**   `HCC`

Aneurysm

Outer layer

Layers of muscular and elastic tissue

Inner layer

Aneurysm

`✓4ᵗʰ` **I73**   **Other peripheral vascular diseases**

   `EXCLUDES 2`   *chilblains (T69.1)*
              frostbite (T33-T34)
              immersion hand or foot (T69.Ø-)
              spasm of cerebral artery (G45.9)

   AHA: 2018,4Q,87

`✓5ᵗʰ` **I73.Ø**   **Raynaud's syndrome**

Raynaud's disease
Raynaud's phenomenon (secondary)
DEF: Constriction of the arteries of the digits caused by cold or by nerve or arterial damage and can be prompted by stress or emotion. Blood cannot reach the skin and soft tissues and the skin turns white with blue mottling.

   I73.ØØ   **Raynaud's syndrome without gangrene**
   I73.Ø1   **Raynaud's syndrome with gangrene**   `CC` `HCC`
         CC Excl: PDX collection 519

I73.1   **Thromboangiitis obliterans [Buerger's disease]**   `HCC`

DEF: Inflammatory disease of the extremity blood vessels, mainly the lower blood vessels. This disease is associated with heavy tobacco use. The arteries are more affected than veins. It occurs primarily in young men and leads to tissue ischemia and gangrene.

`✓5ᵗʰ` **I73.8**   **Other specified peripheral vascular diseases**

   `EXCLUDES 1`   *diabetic (peripheral) angiopathy (EØ8-E13 with .51-.52)*

   I73.81   **Erythromelalgia**   `HCC`
   I73.89   **Other specified peripheral vascular diseases**   `HCC`

Acrocyanosis
Erythrocyanosis
Simple acroparesthesia [Schultze's type]
Vasomotor acroparesthesia [Nothnagel's type]

I73.9   **Peripheral vascular disease, unspecified**   `HCC`

Intermittent claudication
Peripheral angiopathy NOS
Spasm of artery

   `EXCLUDES 1`   *atherosclerosis of the extremities (I70.2-I70.7-)*

   AHA: 2018,2Q,7

`✓4ᵗʰ` **I74**   **Arterial embolism and thrombosis**

   `INCLUDES`   embolic infarction
             embolic occlusion
             thrombotic infarction
             thrombotic occlusion

Code first:
   embolism and thrombosis complicating abortion or ectopic or molar pregnancy (OØØ-OØ7, OØ8.2)
   embolism and thrombosis complicating pregnancy, childbirth and the puerperium (O88.-)

   `EXCLUDES 2`   *atheroembolism (I75.-)*
              basilar embolism and thrombosis (I63.Ø-I63.2, I65.1)
              carotid embolism and thrombosis (I63.Ø-I63.2, I65.2)
              cerebral embolism and thrombosis (I63.3-I63.5, I66.-)
              coronary embolism and thrombosis (I21-I25)
              mesenteric embolism and thrombosis (K55.Ø-)
              ophthalmic embolism and thrombosis (H34.-)
              precerebral embolism and thrombosis NOS (I63.Ø-I63.2, I65.9)
              pulmonary embolism and thrombosis (I26.-)
              renal embolism and thrombosis (N28.Ø)
              retinal embolism and thrombosis (H34.-)
              septic embolism and thrombosis (I76)
              vertebral embolism and thrombosis (I63.Ø-I63.2, I65.Ø)

`✓5ᵗʰ` **I74.Ø**   **Embolism and thrombosis of abdominal aorta**

   I74.Ø1   **Saddle embolus of abdominal aorta**   `MCC` `HCC`
         CC Excl: PDX collection 669
   I74.Ø9   **Other arterial embolism and thrombosis of abdominal aorta**   `CC` `HCC`
         Aortic bifurcation syndrome
         Aortoiliac obstruction
         Leriche's syndrome
         CC Excl: PDX collection 669

`✓5ᵗʰ` **I74.1**   **Embolism and thrombosis of other and unspecified parts of aorta**

   I74.1Ø   **Embolism and thrombosis of unspecified parts of aorta**   `CC` `HCC`
         CC Excl: PDX collection 669
   I74.11   **Embolism and thrombosis of thoracic aorta**   `CC` `HCC`
         CC Excl: PDX collection 701
   I74.19   **Embolism and thrombosis of other parts of aorta**   `CC` `HCC`
         CC Excl: PDX collection 669

I74.2   **Embolism and thrombosis of arteries of the upper extremities**   `CC` `HCC`
   CC Excl: PDX collection 702

I74.3   **Embolism and thrombosis of arteries of the lower extremities**   `CC` `HCC`
   CC Excl: PDX collection 703

I74.4   **Embolism and thrombosis of arteries of extremities, unspecified**   `CC` `HCC`
   Peripheral arterial embolism NOS
   CC Excl: PDX collection 703

I74.5   **Embolism and thrombosis of iliac artery**   `CC` `HCC`
   CC Excl: PDX collection 704

I74.8   **Embolism and thrombosis of other arteries**   `CC` `HCC`
   CC Excl: PDX collection 705

I74.9   **Embolism and thrombosis of unspecified artery**   `CC` `HCC`
   CC Excl: PDX collection 705

`✓4ᵗʰ` **I75**   **Atheroembolism**

   `INCLUDES`   atherothrombotic microembolism
             cholesterol embolism

`✓5ᵗʰ` **I75.Ø**   **Atheroembolism of extremities**

   `✓6ᵗʰ` **I75.Ø1**   **Atheroembolism of upper extremity**
         CC Excl: For CC codes in subcategory I75.Ø1: PDX collection 706

       I75.Ø11   **Atheroembolism of right upper extremity**   `CC` `HCC`
       I75.Ø12   **Atheroembolism of left upper extremity**   `CC` `HCC`
       I75.Ø13   **Atheroembolism of bilateral upper extremities**   `CC` `HCC`
       I75.Ø19   **Atheroembolism of unspecified upper extremity**   `CC` `HCC`

`✓` Additional Character Required   `✓x7ᵗʰ` Placeholder   Unacceptable PDx   Questionable PDx   Manifestation   Unspecified Dx   `H1`-`H14` HAC   `HCC` CMS-HCC Dx   `HIV` HIV Dx

ICD-10-CM 2020   679

✓6ᵗʰ **I75.02 Atheroembolism of lower extremity**

    CC Excl: For CC codes in subcategory I75.02: PDX collection 707

      I75.021 Atheroembolism of right lower extremity `CC` `HCC`

      I75.022 Atheroembolism of left lower extremity `CC` `HCC`

      I75.023 Atheroembolism of bilateral lower extremities `CC` `HCC`

      I75.029 Atheroembolism of unspecified lower extremity `CC` `HCC`

✓5ᵗʰ **I75.8 Atheroembolism of other sites**

    I75.81 Atheroembolism of kidney `CC` `HCC`

      Use additional code for any associated acute kidney failure and chronic kidney disease (N17.-, N18.-)

      CC Excl: PDX collection 708

    I75.89 Atheroembolism of other site `CC` `HCC`

      CC Excl: PDX collection 709

I76 Septic arterial embolism `CC` `HCC`

    Code first underlying infection, such as:

      infective endocarditis (I33.0)

      lung abscess (J85.-)

    Use additional code to identify the site of the embolism (I74.-)

    EXCLUDES 2   septic pulmonary embolism (I26.01, I26.90)

    CC Excl: PDX collection 705

✓4ᵗʰ **I77 Other disorders of arteries and arterioles**

    EXCLUDES 2   collagen (vascular) diseases (M30-M36)

       hypersensitivity angiitis (M31.0)

       pulmonary artery (I28.-)

    I77.0 Arteriovenous fistula, acquired `HCC`

      Aneurysmal varix

      Arteriovenous aneurysm, acquired

      EXCLUDES 1   arteriovenous aneurysm NOS (Q27.3-)

        presence of arteriovenous shunt (fistula) for dialysis (Z99.2)

        traumatic — see injury of blood vessel by body region

      EXCLUDES 2   cerebral (I67.1)

        coronary (I25.4)

      DEF: Communication between an artery and vein caused by trauma or invasive procedures.

    I77.1 Stricture of artery `HCC`

      Narrowing of artery

    I77.2 Rupture of artery `CC` `HCC`

      Erosion of artery

      Fistula of artery

      Ulcer of artery

      EXCLUDES 1   traumatic rupture of artery — see injury of blood vessel by body region

      CC Excl: PDX collection 710

    I77.3 Arterial fibromuscular dysplasia `HCC`

      Fibromuscular hyperplasia (of) carotid artery

      Fibromuscular hyperplasia (of) renal artery

    I77.4 Celiac artery compression syndrome `CC` `HCC`

      CC Excl: PDX collection 711

    I77.5 Necrosis of artery `CC` `HCC`

      CC Excl: PDX collection 712

    I77.6 Arteritis, unspecified `HCC`

      Aortitis NOS

      Endarteritis NOS

      EXCLUDES 1   arteritis or endarteritis:

        aortic arch (M31.4)

        cerebral NEC (I67.7)

        coronary (I25.89)

        deformans (I70.-)

        giant cell (M31.5, M31.6)

        obliterans (I70.-)

        senile (I70.-)

✓5ᵗʰ **I77.7 Other arterial dissection**

    EXCLUDES 2   dissection of aorta (I71.0-)

       dissection of coronary artery (I25.42)

    AHA: 2016,4Q,28-29

    CC Excl: For MCC codes in subcategory I77.7: PDX collection 689

    I77.70 Dissection of unspecified artery `MCC` `HCC`

    I77.71 Dissection of carotid artery `MCC` `HCC`

    I77.72 Dissection of iliac artery `MCC` `HCC`

    I77.73 Dissection of renal artery `MCC` `HCC`

    I77.74 Dissection of vertebral artery `MCC` `HCC`

      EXCLUDES 2   aneurysm of vertebral artery (I72.6)

    I77.75 Dissection of other precerebral arteries `MCC` `HCC`

      Dissection of basilar artery (trunk)

      EXCLUDES 2   aneurysm of carotid artery (I72.0)

        aneurysm of other precerebral arteries (I72.5)

        aneurysm of vertebral artery (I72.6)

        dissection of carotid artery (I77.71)

        dissection of vertebral artery (I77.74)

    I77.76 Dissection of artery of upper extremity `MCC` `HCC`

    I77.77 Dissection of artery of lower extremity `MCC` `HCC`

    I77.79 Dissection of other specified artery `MCC` `HCC`

✓5ᵗʰ **I77.8 Other specified disorders of arteries and arterioles**

    ✓6ᵗʰ **I77.81 Aortic ectasia**

      Ectasis aorta

      EXCLUDES 1   aortic aneurysm and dissection (I71.0-)

       I77.810 Thoracic aortic ectasia `HCC`

       I77.811 Abdominal aortic ectasia `HCC`

       I77.812 Thoracoabdominal aortic ectasia `HCC`

       I77.819 Aortic ectasia, unspecified site `HCC`

    I77.89 Other specified disorders of arteries and arterioles `HCC`

    I77.9 Disorder of arteries and arterioles, unspecified `HCC`

      AHA: 2018,2Q,7

✓4ᵗʰ **I78 Diseases of capillaries**

    I78.0 Hereditary hemorrhagic telangiectasia `HCC`

      Rendu-Osler-Weber disease

    I78.1 Nevus, non-neoplastic

      Araneus nevus

      Senile nevus

      Spider nevus

      Stellar nevus

      EXCLUDES 1   nevus NOS (D22.-)

       vascular NOS (Q82.5)

      EXCLUDES 2   blue nevus (D22.-)

       flammeus nevus (Q82.5)

       hairy nevus (D22.-)

       melanocytic nevus (D22.-)

       pigmented nevus (D22.-)

       portwine nevus (Q82.5)

       sanguineous nevus (Q82.5)

       strawberry nevus (Q82.5)

       verrucous nevus (Q82.5)

      AHA: 2019,1Q,21

    I78.8 Other diseases of capillaries

    I78.9 Disease of capillaries, unspecified

✓4ᵗʰ **I79 Disorders of arteries, arterioles and capillaries in diseases classified elsewhere**

    I79.0 Aneurysm of aorta in diseases classified elsewhere `HCC`

      Code first underlying disease

      EXCLUDES 1   syphilitic aneurysm (A52.01)

    I79.1 Aortitis in diseases classified elsewhere `HCC`

      Code first underlying disease

      EXCLUDES 1   syphilitic aortitis (A52.02)

    I79.8 Other disorders of arteries, arterioles and capillaries in diseases classified elsewhere `HCC`

      Code first underlying disease, such as:

       amyloidosis (E85.-)

      EXCLUDES 1   diabetic (peripheral) angiopathy (E08-E13 with .51-.52)

       syphilitic endarteritis (A52.09)

       tuberculous endarteritis (A18.89)

`N` Newborn: 0   `P` Pediatric: 0-17   `M` Maternity: 9-64   `A` Adult: 15-124   `MCC` Major Complication/Comorbidity   `CC` Complication/Comorbidity   `SW` Severe Wound Dx

680   ICD-10-CM 2020

Diseases of veins, lymphatic vessels and lymph nodes, not elsewhere classified (I80-I89)

✓4ᵗʰ **I80　Phlebitis and thrombophlebitis**

INCLUDES　endophlebitis
inflammation, vein
periphlebitis
suppurative phlebitis

Code first:
phlebitis and thrombophlebitis complicating abortion, ectopic or molar pregnancy (O00-O07, O08.7)
phlebitis and thrombophlebitis complicating pregnancy, childbirth and the puerperium (O22.-, O87.-)

EXCLUDES 1　*venous embolism and thrombosis of lower extremities (I82.4-, I82.5-, I82.81-)*

CC Excl: For CC codes in category I80: PDX collection 713

✓5ᵗʰ **I80.0　Phlebitis and thrombophlebitis of superficial vessels of lower extremities**
Phlebitis and thrombophlebitis of femoropopliteal vein

　　I80.00　Phlebitis and thrombophlebitis of superficial vessels of unspecified lower extremity

　　I80.01　Phlebitis and thrombophlebitis of superficial vessels of right lower extremity

　　I80.02　Phlebitis and thrombophlebitis of superficial vessels of left lower extremity

　　I80.03　Phlebitis and thrombophlebitis of superficial vessels of lower extremities, bilateral

✓5ᵗʰ **I80.1　Phlebitis and thrombophlebitis of femoral vein**
►Phlebitis and thrombophlebitis of common femoral vein◄
►Phlebitis and thrombophlebitis of deep femoral vein◄

　　I80.10　Phlebitis and thrombophlebitis of unspecified femoral vein　CC HCC

　　I80.11　Phlebitis and thrombophlebitis of right femoral vein　CC HCC

　　I80.12　Phlebitis and thrombophlebitis of left femoral vein　CC HCC

　　I80.13　Phlebitis and thrombophlebitis of femoral vein, bilateral

✓5ᵗʰ **I80.2　Phlebitis and thrombophlebitis of other and unspecified deep vessels of lower extremities**

✓6ᵗʰ **I80.20**　Phlebitis and thrombophlebitis of unspecified deep vessels of lower extremities

　　　　I80.201　Phlebitis and thrombophlebitis of unspecified deep vessels of right lower extremity　CC HCC

　　　　I80.202　Phlebitis and thrombophlebitis of unspecified deep vessels of left lower extremity　CC HCC

　　　　I80.203　Phlebitis and thrombophlebitis of unspecified deep vessels of lower extremities, bilateral　CC HCC

　　　　I80.209　Phlebitis and thrombophlebitis of unspecified deep vessels of unspecified lower extremity　CC HCC

✓6ᵗʰ **I80.21**　Phlebitis and thrombophlebitis of iliac vein
►Phlebitis and thrombophlebitis of common iliac vein◄
►Phlebitis and thrombophlebitis of external iliac vein◄
►Phlebitis and thrombophlebitis of internal iliac vein◄

　　　　I80.211　Phlebitis and thrombophlebitis of right iliac vein　CC HCC

　　　　I80.212　Phlebitis and thrombophlebitis of left iliac vein　CC HCC

　　　　I80.213　Phlebitis and thrombophlebitis of iliac vein, bilateral　CC HCC

　　　　I80.219　Phlebitis and thrombophlebitis of unspecified iliac vein　CC HCC

✓6ᵗʰ **I80.22**　Phlebitis and thrombophlebitis of popliteal vein

　　　　I80.221　Phlebitis and thrombophlebitis of right popliteal vein　CC HCC

　　　　I80.222　Phlebitis and thrombophlebitis of left popliteal vein　CC HCC

　　　　I80.223　Phlebitis and thrombophlebitis of popliteal vein, bilateral　CC HCC

　　　　I80.229　Phlebitis and thrombophlebitis of unspecified popliteal vein　CC HCC

✓6ᵗʰ **I80.23**　Phlebitis and thrombophlebitis of tibial vein
►Phlebitis and thrombophlebitis of anterior tibial vein◄
►Phlebitis and thrombophlebitis of posterior tibial vein◄

　　　　I80.231　Phlebitis and thrombophlebitis of right tibial vein　CC HCC

　　　　I80.232　Phlebitis and thrombophlebitis of left tibial vein　CC HCC

　　　　I80.233　Phlebitis and thrombophlebitis of tibial vein, bilateral　CC HCC

　　　　I80.239　Phlebitis and thrombophlebitis of unspecified tibial vein　CC HCC

✓6ᵗʰ **I80.24**　Phlebitis and thrombophlebitis of peroneal vein

　　　　I80.241　Phlebitis and thrombophlebitis of right peroneal vein　CC

　　　　I80.242　Phlebitis and thrombophlebitis of left peroneal vein　CC

　　　　I80.243　Phlebitis and thrombophlebitis of peroneal vein, bilateral　CC

　　　　I80.249　Phlebitis and thrombophlebitis of unspecified peroneal vein　CC

✓6ᵗʰ **I80.25**　Phlebitis and thrombophlebitis of calf muscular vein
Phlebitis and thrombophlebitis of calf muscular vein, NOS
Phlebitis and thrombophlebitis of gastrocnemial vein
Phlebitis and thrombophlebitis of soleal vein

　　　　I80.251　Phlebitis and thrombophlebitis of right calf muscular vein

　　　　I80.252　Phlebitis and thrombophlebitis of left calf muscular vein

　　　　I80.253　Phlebitis and thrombophlebitis of calf muscular vein, bilateral

　　　　I80.259　Phlebitis and thrombophlebitis of unspecified calf muscular vein

✓6ᵗʰ **I80.29**　Phlebitis and thrombophlebitis of other deep vessels of lower extremities

　　　　I80.291　Phlebitis and thrombophlebitis of other deep vessels of right lower extremity　CC HCC

　　　　I80.292　Phlebitis and thrombophlebitis of other deep vessels of left lower extremity　CC HCC

　　　　I80.293　Phlebitis and thrombophlebitis of other deep vessels of lower extremity, bilateral　CC HCC

　　　　I80.299　Phlebitis and thrombophlebitis of other deep vessels of unspecified lower extremity　CC HCC

I80.3　Phlebitis and thrombophlebitis of lower extremities, unspecified

I80.8　Phlebitis and thrombophlebitis of other sites

I80.9　Phlebitis and thrombophlebitis of unspecified site

I81　Portal vein thrombosis　MCC

Portal (vein) obstruction

EXCLUDES 2　*hepatic vein thrombosis (I82.0)*
phlebitis of portal vein (K75.1)

CC Excl: PDX collection 714

Chapter 9. Diseases of the Circulatory System

I82–I82.459

√4ᵗʰ **I82 Other venous embolism and thrombosis**

Code first venous embolism and thrombosis complicating:
abortion, ectopic or molar pregnancy (O00-O07, O08.7)
pregnancy, childbirth and the puerperium (O22.-, O87.-)

EXCLUDES 2   venous embolism and thrombosis (of):
cerebral (I63.6, I67.6)
coronary (I21-I25)
intracranial and intraspinal, septic or NOS (G08)
intracranial, nonpyogenic (I67.6)
intraspinal, nonpyogenic (G95.1)
mesenteric (K55.0-)
portal (I81)
pulmonary (I26.-)

CC Excl: For CC codes in category I82, unless otherwise noted: PDX collection 717

I82.0 Budd-Chiari syndrome   MCC HCC
Hepatic vein thrombosis
DEF: Thrombosis or other obstruction of the hepatic veins. Symptoms include an enlarged liver, extensive collateral vessels, intractable ascites, and severe portal hypertension.
CC Excl: PDX collection 715

I82.1 Thrombophlebitis migrans   CC
CC Excl: PDX collection 716

√5ᵗʰ **I82.2 Embolism and thrombosis of vena cava and other thoracic veins**

   √6ᵗʰ **I82.21 Embolism and thrombosis of superior vena cava**

     I82.210 Acute embolism and thrombosis of superior vena cava   CC HCC
Embolism and thrombosis of superior vena cava NOS

     I82.211 Chronic embolism and thrombosis of superior vena cava   CC HCC

   √6ᵗʰ **I82.22 Embolism and thrombosis of inferior vena cava**

     I82.220 Acute embolism and thrombosis of inferior vena cava   MCC HCC
Embolism and thrombosis of inferior vena cava NOS
CC Excl: PDX collection 718

     I82.221 Chronic embolism and thrombosis of inferior vena cava   MCC HCC
CC Excl: PDX collection 718

   √6ᵗʰ **I82.29 Embolism and thrombosis of other thoracic veins**
Embolism and thrombosis of brachiocephalic (innominate) vein

     I82.290 Acute embolism and thrombosis of other thoracic veins   CC HCC

     I82.291 Chronic embolism and thrombosis of other thoracic veins   CC HCC

I82.3 Embolism and thrombosis of renal vein   CC HCC
CC Excl: PDX collection 719

√5ᵗʰ **I82.4 Acute embolism and thrombosis of deep veins of lower extremity**

   √6ᵗʰ **I82.40 Acute embolism and thrombosis of unspecified deep veins of lower extremity**
Deep vein thrombosis NOS
DVT NOS

     EXCLUDES 1   acute embolism and thrombosis of unspecified deep veins of distal lower extremity (I82.4Z-)
acute embolism and thrombosis of unspecified deep veins of proximal lower extremity (I82.4Y-)

     I82.401 Acute embolism and thrombosis of unspecified deep veins of right lower extremity   CC H10 HCC

     I82.402 Acute embolism and thrombosis of unspecified deep veins of left lower extremity   CC H10 HCC

     I82.403 Acute embolism and thrombosis of unspecified deep veins of lower extremity, bilateral   CC H10 HCC

     I82.409 Acute embolism and thrombosis of unspecified deep veins of unspecified lower extremity   CC H10 HCC

   √6ᵗʰ **I82.41 Acute embolism and thrombosis of femoral vein**
▶Acute embolism and thrombosis of common femoral vein◀
▶Acute embolism and thrombosis of deep femoral vein◀

     I82.411 Acute embolism and thrombosis of right femoral vein   CC H10 HCC

     I82.412 Acute embolism and thrombosis of left femoral vein   CC H10 HCC

     I82.413 Acute embolism and thrombosis of femoral vein, bilateral   CC H10 HCC

     I82.419 Acute embolism and thrombosis of unspecified femoral vein   CC H10 HCC

   √6ᵗʰ **I82.42 Acute embolism and thrombosis of iliac vein**
▶Acute embolism and thrombosis of common iliac vein◀
▶Acute embolism and thrombosis of external iliac vein◀
▶Acute embolism and thrombosis of internal iliac vein◀

     I82.421 Acute embolism and thrombosis of right iliac vein   CC H10 HCC

     I82.422 Acute embolism and thrombosis of left iliac vein   CC H10 HCC

     I82.423 Acute embolism and thrombosis of iliac vein, bilateral   CC H10 HCC

     I82.429 Acute embolism and thrombosis of unspecified iliac vein   CC H10 HCC

   √6ᵗʰ **I82.43 Acute embolism and thrombosis of popliteal vein**

     I82.431 Acute embolism and thrombosis of right popliteal vein   CC H10 HCC

     I82.432 Acute embolism and thrombosis of left popliteal vein   CC H10 HCC

     I82.433 Acute embolism and thrombosis of popliteal vein, bilateral   CC H10 HCC

     I82.439 Acute embolism and thrombosis of unspecified popliteal vein   CC H10 HCC

   √6ᵗʰ **I82.44 Acute embolism and thrombosis of tibial vein**
▶Acute embolism and thrombosis of anterior tibial vein◀
▶Acute embolism and thrombosis of posterior tibial vein◀

     I82.441 Acute embolism and thrombosis of right tibial vein   CC H10 HCC

     I82.442 Acute embolism and thrombosis of left tibial vein   CC H10 HCC

     I82.443 Acute embolism and thrombosis of tibial vein, bilateral   CC H10 HCC

     I82.449 Acute embolism and thrombosis of unspecified tibial vein   CC H10 HCC

   √6ᵗʰ **I82.45 Acute embolism and thrombosis of peroneal vein**

     I82.451 Acute embolism and thrombosis of right peroneal vein   CC

     I82.452 Acute embolism and thrombosis of left peroneal vein   CC

     I82.453 Acute embolism and thrombosis of peroneal vein, bilateral   CC

     I82.459 Acute embolism and thrombosis of unspecified peroneal vein   CC

Ⓝ Newborn: 0   Ⓟ Pediatric: 0-17   Ⓜ Maternity: 9-64   Ⓐ Adult: 15-124   MCC Major Complication/Comorbidity   CC Complication/Comorbidity   SW Severe Wound Dx

√6ᵗʰ **I82.46** **Acute embolism and thrombosis of calf muscular vein**

Acute embolism and thrombosis of calf muscular vein, NOS

Acute embolism and thrombosis of gastrocnemial vein

Acute embolism and thrombosis of soleal vein

I82.461 **Acute embolism and thrombosis of right calf muscular vein**

I82.462 **Acute embolism and thrombosis of left calf muscular vein**

I82.463 **Acute embolism and thrombosis of calf muscular vein, bilateral**

I82.469 **Acute embolism and thrombosis of unspecified calf muscular vein**

√6ᵗʰ **I82.49** **Acute embolism and thrombosis of other specified deep vein of lower extremity**

I82.491 **Acute embolism and thrombosis of other specified deep vein of right lower extremity** `CC` `H10` `HCC`

I82.492 **Acute embolism and thrombosis of other specified deep vein of left lower extremity** `CC` `H10` `HCC`

I82.493 **Acute embolism and thrombosis of other specified deep vein of lower extremity, bilateral** `CC` `H10` `HCC`

I82.499 **Acute embolism and thrombosis of other specified deep vein of unspecified lower extremity** `CC` `H10` `HCC`

√6ᵗʰ **I82.4Y** **Acute embolism and thrombosis of unspecified deep veins of proximal lower extremity**

Acute embolism and thrombosis of deep vein of thigh NOS

Acute embolism and thrombosis of deep vein of upper leg NOS

I82.4Y1 **Acute embolism and thrombosis of unspecified deep veins of right proximal lower extremity** `CC` `H10` `HCC`

I82.4Y2 **Acute embolism and thrombosis of unspecified deep veins of left proximal lower extremity** `CC` `H10` `HCC`

I82.4Y3 **Acute embolism and thrombosis of unspecified deep veins of proximal lower extremity, bilateral** `CC` `H10` `HCC`

I82.4Y9 **Acute embolism and thrombosis of unspecified deep veins of unspecified proximal lower extremity** `CC` `H10` `HCC`

√6ᵗʰ **I82.4Z** **Acute embolism and thrombosis of unspecified deep veins of distal lower extremity**

Acute embolism and thrombosis of deep vein of calf NOS

Acute embolism and thrombosis of deep vein of lower leg NOS

I82.4Z1 **Acute embolism and thrombosis of unspecified deep veins of right distal lower extremity** `CC` `H10` `HCC`

I82.4Z2 **Acute embolism and thrombosis of unspecified deep veins of left distal lower extremity** `CC` `H10` `HCC`

I82.4Z3 **Acute embolism and thrombosis of unspecified deep veins of distal lower extremity, bilateral** `CC` `H10` `HCC`

I82.4Z9 **Acute embolism and thrombosis of unspecified deep veins of unspecified distal lower extremity** `CC` `H10` `HCC`

√5ᵗʰ **I82.5** **Chronic embolism and thrombosis of deep veins of lower extremity**

Use additional code, if applicable, for associated long-term (current) use of anticoagulants (Z79.01)

EXCLUDES 1   *personal history of venous embolism and thrombosis (Z86.718)*

√6ᵗʰ **I82.50** **Chronic embolism and thrombosis of unspecified deep veins of lower extremity**

EXCLUDES 1   *chronic embolism and thrombosis of unspecified deep veins of distal lower extremity (I82.5Z-)*

chronic embolism and thrombosis of unspecified deep veins of proximal lower extremity (I82.5Y-)

I82.501 **Chronic embolism and thrombosis of unspecified deep veins of right lower extremity** `CC` `HCC`

I82.502 **Chronic embolism and thrombosis of unspecified deep veins of left lower extremity** `CC` `HCC`

I82.503 **Chronic embolism and thrombosis of unspecified deep veins of lower extremity, bilateral** `CC` `HCC`

I82.509 **Chronic embolism and thrombosis of unspecified deep veins of unspecified lower extremity** `CC` `HCC`

√6ᵗʰ **I82.51** **Chronic embolism and thrombosis of femoral vein**

►Chronic embolism and thrombosis of common femoral vein◄

►Chronic embolism and thrombosis of deep femoral vein◄

I82.511 **Chronic embolism and thrombosis of right femoral vein** `CC` `HCC`

I82.512 **Chronic embolism and thrombosis of left femoral vein** `CC` `HCC`

I82.513 **Chronic embolism and thrombosis of femoral vein, bilateral** `CC` `HCC`

I82.519 **Chronic embolism and thrombosis of unspecified femoral vein** `CC` `HCC`

√6ᵗʰ **I82.52** **Chronic embolism and thrombosis of iliac vein**

►Chronic embolism and thrombosis of common iliac vein◄

►Chronic embolism and thrombosis of external iliac vein◄

►Chronic embolism and thrombosis of internal iliac vein◄

I82.521 **Chronic embolism and thrombosis of right iliac vein** `CC` `HCC`

I82.522 **Chronic embolism and thrombosis of left iliac vein** `CC` `HCC`

I82.523 **Chronic embolism and thrombosis of iliac vein, bilateral** `CC` `HCC`

I82.529 **Chronic embolism and thrombosis of unspecified iliac vein** `CC` `HCC`

√6ᵗʰ **I82.53** **Chronic embolism and thrombosis of popliteal vein**

I82.531 **Chronic embolism and thrombosis of right popliteal vein** `CC` `HCC`

I82.532 **Chronic embolism and thrombosis of left popliteal vein** `CC` `HCC`

I82.533 **Chronic embolism and thrombosis of popliteal vein, bilateral** `CC` `HCC`

I82.539 **Chronic embolism and thrombosis of unspecified popliteal vein** `CC` `HCC`

☑ Additional Character Required   √x7ᵗʰ Placeholder   Unacceptable PDx   Questionable PDx   Manifestation   Unspecified Dx   `H1`-`H14` HAC   `HCC` CMS-HCC Dx   `HIV` HIV Dx

ICD-10-CM 2020   **683**

√6ᵗʰ **I82.54 Chronic embolism and thrombosis of tibial vein**
▶Chronic embolism and thrombosis of anterior tibial vein◀
▶Chronic embolism and thrombosis of posterior tibial vein◀

I82.541 Chronic embolism and thrombosis of right tibial vein `CC` `HCC`

I82.542 Chronic embolism and thrombosis of left tibial vein `CC` `HCC`

I82.543 Chronic embolism and thrombosis of tibial vein, bilateral `CC` `HCC`

I82.549 Chronic embolism and thrombosis of unspecified tibial vein `CC` `HCC`

√6ᵗʰ **I82.55 Chronic embolism and thrombosis of peroneal vein**

I82.551 Chronic embolism and thrombosis of right peroneal vein `CC`

I82.552 Chronic embolism and thrombosis of left peroneal vein `CC`

I82.553 Chronic embolism and thrombosis of peroneal vein, bilateral `CC`

I82.559 Chronic embolism and thrombosis of unspecified peroneal vein `CC`

√6ᵗʰ **I82.56 Chronic embolism and thrombosis of calf muscular vein**
Chronic embolism and thrombosis of calf muscular vein NOS
Chronic embolism and thrombosis of gastrocnemial vein
Chronic embolism and thrombosis of soleal vein

I82.561 Chronic embolism and thrombosis of right calf muscular vein

I82.562 Chronic embolism and thrombosis of left calf muscular vein

I82.563 Chronic embolism and thrombosis of calf muscular vein, bilateral

I82.569 Chronic embolism and thrombosis of unspecified calf muscular vein

√6ᵗʰ **I82.59 Chronic embolism and thrombosis of other specified deep vein of lower extremity**

I82.591 Chronic embolism and thrombosis of other specified deep vein of right lower extremity `CC` `HCC`

I82.592 Chronic embolism and thrombosis of other specified deep vein of left lower extremity `CC` `HCC`

I82.593 Chronic embolism and thrombosis of other specified deep vein of lower extremity, bilateral `CC` `HCC`

I82.599 Chronic embolism and thrombosis of other specified deep vein of unspecified lower extremity `CC` `HCC`

√6ᵗʰ **I82.5Y Chronic embolism and thrombosis of unspecified deep veins of proximal lower extremity**
Chronic embolism and thrombosis of deep veins of thigh NOS
Chronic embolism and thrombosis of deep veins of upper leg NOS

I82.5Y1 Chronic embolism and thrombosis of unspecified deep veins of right proximal lower extremity `CC` `HCC`

I82.5Y2 Chronic embolism and thrombosis of unspecified deep veins of left proximal lower extremity `CC` `HCC`

I82.5Y3 Chronic embolism and thrombosis of unspecified deep veins of proximal lower extremity, bilateral `CC` `HCC`

I82.5Y9 Chronic embolism and thrombosis of unspecified deep veins of unspecified proximal lower extremity `CC` `HCC`

√6ᵗʰ **I82.5Z Chronic embolism and thrombosis of unspecified deep veins of distal lower extremity**
Chronic embolism and thrombosis of deep veins of calf NOS
Chronic embolism and thrombosis of deep veins of lower leg NOS

I82.5Z1 Chronic embolism and thrombosis of unspecified deep veins of right distal lower extremity `CC` `HCC`

I82.5Z2 Chronic embolism and thrombosis of unspecified deep veins of left distal lower extremity `CC` `HCC`

I82.5Z3 Chronic embolism and thrombosis of unspecified deep veins of distal lower extremity, bilateral `CC` `HCC`

I82.5Z9 Chronic embolism and thrombosis of unspecified deep veins of unspecified distal lower extremity `CC` `HCC`

√5ᵗʰ **I82.6 Acute embolism and thrombosis of veins of upper extremity**

√6ᵗʰ **I82.60 Acute embolism and thrombosis of unspecified veins of upper extremity**

I82.601 Acute embolism and thrombosis of unspecified veins of right upper extremity `CC`

I82.602 Acute embolism and thrombosis of unspecified veins of left upper extremity `CC`

I82.603 Acute embolism and thrombosis of unspecified veins of upper extremity, bilateral `CC`

I82.609 Acute embolism and thrombosis of unspecified veins of unspecified upper extremity `CC`

√6ᵗʰ **I82.61 Acute embolism and thrombosis of superficial veins of upper extremity**
Acute embolism and thrombosis of antecubital vein
Acute embolism and thrombosis of basilic vein
Acute embolism and thrombosis of cephalic vein

I82.611 Acute embolism and thrombosis of superficial veins of right upper extremity `CC`

I82.612 Acute embolism and thrombosis of superficial veins of left upper extremity `CC`

I82.613 Acute embolism and thrombosis of superficial veins of upper extremity, bilateral `CC`

I82.619 Acute embolism and thrombosis of superficial veins of unspecified upper extremity `CC`

√6ᵗʰ **I82.62 Acute embolism and thrombosis of deep veins of upper extremity**
Acute embolism and thrombosis of brachial vein
Acute embolism and thrombosis of radial vein
Acute embolism and thrombosis of ulnar vein

I82.621 Acute embolism and thrombosis of deep veins of right upper extremity `CC` `HCC`

I82.622 Acute embolism and thrombosis of deep veins of left upper extremity `CC` `HCC`

I82.623 Acute embolism and thrombosis of deep veins of upper extremity, bilateral `CC` `HCC`

I82.629 Acute embolism and thrombosis of deep veins of unspecified upper extremity `CC` `HCC`

√5ᵗʰ **I82.7 Chronic embolism and thrombosis of veins of upper extremity**
Use additional code, if applicable, for associated long-term (current) use of anticoagulants (Z79.01)

`EXCLUDES 1`   personal history of venous embolism and thrombosis (Z86.718)

√6ᵗʰ **I82.70 Chronic embolism and thrombosis of unspecified veins of upper extremity**

I82.701 Chronic embolism and thrombosis of unspecified veins of right upper extremity `CC`

Ⓝ Newborn: 0   Ⓟ Pediatric: 0-17   Ⓜ Maternity: 9-64   Ⓐ Adult: 15-124   `MCC` Major Complication/Comorbidity   `CC` Complication/Comorbidity   `SW` Severe Wound Dx

684
ICD-10-CM 2020

I82.702 Chronic embolism and thrombosis of unspecified veins of left upper extremity `CC`

I82.703 Chronic embolism and thrombosis of unspecified veins of upper extremity, bilateral `CC`

I82.709 Chronic embolism and thrombosis of unspecified veins of unspecified upper extremity `CC`

√6ᵗʰ **I82.71** Chronic embolism and thrombosis of superficial veins of upper extremity

  Chronic embolism and thrombosis of antecubital vein
  Chronic embolism and thrombosis of basilic vein
  Chronic embolism and thrombosis of cephalic vein

I82.711 Chronic embolism and thrombosis of superficial veins of right upper extremity `CC`

I82.712 Chronic embolism and thrombosis of superficial veins of left upper extremity `CC`

I82.713 Chronic embolism and thrombosis of superficial veins of upper extremity, bilateral `CC`

I82.719 Chronic embolism and thrombosis of superficial veins of unspecified upper extremity `CC`

√6ᵗʰ **I82.72** Chronic embolism and thrombosis of deep veins of upper extremity

  Chronic embolism and thrombosis of brachial vein
  Chronic embolism and thrombosis of radial vein
  Chronic embolism and thrombosis of ulnar vein

I82.721 Chronic embolism and thrombosis of deep veins of right upper extremity `CC` `HCC`

I82.722 Chronic embolism and thrombosis of deep veins of left upper extremity `CC` `HCC`

I82.723 Chronic embolism and thrombosis of deep veins of upper extremity, bilateral `CC` `HCC`

I82.729 Chronic embolism and thrombosis of deep veins of unspecified upper extremity `CC` `HCC`

√5ᵗʰ **I82.A** Embolism and thrombosis of axillary vein

√6ᵗʰ **I82.A1** Acute embolism and thrombosis of axillary vein

I82.A11 Acute embolism and thrombosis of right axillary vein `CC` `HCC`

I82.A12 Acute embolism and thrombosis of left axillary vein `CC` `HCC`

I82.A13 Acute embolism and thrombosis of axillary vein, bilateral `CC` `HCC`

I82.A19 Acute embolism and thrombosis of unspecified axillary vein `CC` `HCC`

√6ᵗʰ **I82.A2** Chronic embolism and thrombosis of axillary vein

I82.A21 Chronic embolism and thrombosis of right axillary vein `CC` `HCC`

I82.A22 Chronic embolism and thrombosis of left axillary vein `CC` `HCC`

I82.A23 Chronic embolism and thrombosis of axillary vein, bilateral `CC` `HCC`

I82.A29 Chronic embolism and thrombosis of unspecified axillary vein `CC` `HCC`

√5ᵗʰ **I82.B** Embolism and thrombosis of subclavian vein

√6ᵗʰ **I82.B1** Acute embolism and thrombosis of subclavian vein

I82.B11 Acute embolism and thrombosis of right subclavian vein `CC` `HCC`

I82.B12 Acute embolism and thrombosis of left subclavian vein `CC` `HCC`

I82.B13 Acute embolism and thrombosis of subclavian vein, bilateral `CC` `HCC`

I82.B19 Acute embolism and thrombosis of unspecified subclavian vein `CC` `HCC`

√6ᵗʰ **I82.B2** Chronic embolism and thrombosis of subclavian vein

I82.B21 Chronic embolism and thrombosis of right subclavian vein `CC` `HCC`

I82.B22 Chronic embolism and thrombosis of left subclavian vein `CC` `HCC`

I82.B23 Chronic embolism and thrombosis of subclavian vein, bilateral `CC` `HCC`

I82.B29 Chronic embolism and thrombosis of unspecified subclavian vein `CC` `HCC`

√5ᵗʰ **I82.C** Embolism and thrombosis of internal jugular vein

√6ᵗʰ **I82.C1** Acute embolism and thrombosis of internal jugular vein

I82.C11 Acute embolism and thrombosis of right internal jugular vein `CC` `HCC`

I82.C12 Acute embolism and thrombosis of left internal jugular vein `CC` `HCC`

I82.C13 Acute embolism and thrombosis of internal jugular vein, bilateral `CC` `HCC`

I82.C19 Acute embolism and thrombosis of unspecified internal jugular vein `CC` `HCC`

√6ᵗʰ **I82.C2** Chronic embolism and thrombosis of internal jugular vein

I82.C21 Chronic embolism and thrombosis of right internal jugular vein `CC` `HCC`

I82.C22 Chronic embolism and thrombosis of left internal jugular vein `CC` `HCC`

I82.C23 Chronic embolism and thrombosis of internal jugular vein, bilateral `CC` `HCC`

I82.C29 Chronic embolism and thrombosis of unspecified internal jugular vein `CC` `HCC`

√5ᵗʰ **I82.8** Embolism and thrombosis of other specified veins

  Use additional code, if applicable, for associated long-term (current) use of anticoagulants (Z79.01)

√6ᵗʰ **I82.81** Embolism and thrombosis of superficial veins of lower extremities

  Embolism and thrombosis of saphenous vein (greater) (lesser)

I82.811 Embolism and thrombosis of superficial veins of right lower extremity `CC`

I82.812 Embolism and thrombosis of superficial veins of left lower extremity `CC`

I82.813 Embolism and thrombosis of superficial veins of lower extremities, bilateral `CC`

I82.819 Embolism and thrombosis of superficial veins of unspecified lower extremity `CC`

√6ᵗʰ **I82.89** Embolism and thrombosis of other specified veins

I82.890 Acute embolism and thrombosis of other specified veins `CC`

I82.891 Chronic embolism and thrombosis of other specified veins `CC`

√5ᵗʰ **I82.9** Embolism and thrombosis of unspecified vein

I82.90 Acute embolism and thrombosis of unspecified vein `CC`

  Embolism of vein NOS
  Thrombosis (vein) NOS

I82.91 Chronic embolism and thrombosis of unspecified vein `CC`

✔ Additional Character Required   √x7ᵗʰ Placeholder   Unacceptable PDx   Questionable PDx   Manifestation   Unspecified Dx   `H1`-`H14` HAC   `HCC` CMS-HCC Dx   `HIV` HIV Dx

Chapter 9. Diseases of the Circulatory System

✓4ᵗʰ **I83   Varicose veins of lower extremities**

EXCLUDES 1   *varicose veins complicating pregnancy (O22.0-)*
                varicose veins complicating the puerperium (O87.4)

✓5ᵗʰ **I83.0   Varicose veins of lower extremities with ulcer**

Use additional code to identify severity of ulcer (L97.-)

✓6ᵗʰ **I83.00   Varicose veins of unspecified lower extremity with ulcer**

     I83.001   Varicose veins of unspecified lower extremity with ulcer of thigh   HCC A

     I83.002   Varicose veins of unspecified lower extremity with ulcer of calf   HCC A

     I83.003   Varicose veins of unspecified lower extremity with ulcer of ankle   HCC A

     I83.004   Varicose veins of unspecified lower extremity with ulcer of heel and midfoot   HCC A

       Varicose veins of unspecified lower extremity with ulcer of plantar surface of midfoot

     I83.005   Varicose veins of unspecified lower extremity with ulcer other part of foot   HCC A

       Varicose veins of unspecified lower extremity with ulcer of toe

     I83.008   Varicose veins of unspecified lower extremity with ulcer other part of lower leg   HCC A

     I83.009   Varicose veins of unspecified lower extremity with ulcer of unspecified site   HCC A

✓6ᵗʰ **I83.01   Varicose veins of right lower extremity with ulcer**

     I83.011   Varicose veins of right lower extremity with ulcer of thigh   HCC A

     I83.012   Varicose veins of right lower extremity with ulcer of calf   HCC A

     I83.013   Varicose veins of right lower extremity with ulcer of ankle   HCC A

     I83.014   Varicose veins of right lower extremity with ulcer of heel and midfoot   HCC A

       Varicose veins of right lower extremity with ulcer of plantar surface of midfoot

     I83.015   Varicose veins of right lower extremity with ulcer other part of foot   HCC A

       Varicose veins of right lower extremity with ulcer of toe

     I83.018   Varicose veins of right lower extremity with ulcer other part of lower leg   HCC A

     I83.019   Varicose veins of right lower extremity with ulcer of unspecified site   HCC A

✓6ᵗʰ **I83.02   Varicose veins of left lower extremity with ulcer**

     I83.021   Varicose veins of left lower extremity with ulcer of thigh   HCC A

     I83.022   Varicose veins of left lower extremity with ulcer of calf   HCC A

     I83.023   Varicose veins of left lower extremity with ulcer of ankle   HCC A

     I83.024   Varicose veins of left lower extremity with ulcer of heel and midfoot   HCC A

       Varicose veins of left lower extremity with ulcer of plantar surface of midfoot

     I83.025   Varicose veins of left lower extremity with ulcer other part of foot   HCC A

       Varicose veins of left lower extremity with ulcer of toe

     I83.028   Varicose veins of left lower extremity with ulcer other part of lower leg   HCC A

     I83.029   Varicose veins of left lower extremity with ulcer of unspecified site   HCC A

✓5ᵗʰ **I83.1   Varicose veins of lower extremities with inflammation**

     I83.10   Varicose veins of unspecified lower extremity with inflammation   A

     I83.11   Varicose veins of right lower extremity with inflammation   A

     I83.12   Varicose veins of left lower extremity with inflammation   A

✓5ᵗʰ **I83.2   Varicose veins of lower extremities with both ulcer and inflammation**

Use additional code to identify severity of ulcer (L97.-)

CC Excl: For CC codes in subcategory I83.2: PDX collection 720

✓6ᵗʰ **I83.20   Varicose veins of unspecified lower extremity with both ulcer and inflammation**

     I83.201   Varicose veins of unspecified lower extremity with both ulcer of thigh and inflammation   CC HCC A

     I83.202   Varicose veins of unspecified lower extremity with both ulcer of calf and inflammation   CC HCC A

     I83.203   Varicose veins of unspecified lower extremity with both ulcer of ankle and inflammation   CC HCC A

     I83.204   Varicose veins of unspecified lower extremity with both ulcer of heel and midfoot and inflammation   CC HCC A

       Varicose veins of unspecified lower extremity with both ulcer of plantar surface of midfoot and inflammation

     I83.205   Varicose veins of unspecified lower extremity with both ulcer of other part of foot and inflammation   CC HCC A

       Varicose veins of unspecified lower extremity with both ulcer of toe and inflammation

     I83.208   Varicose veins of unspecified lower extremity with both ulcer of other part of lower extremity and inflammation   CC HCC A

     I83.209   Varicose veins of unspecified lower extremity with both ulcer of unspecified site and inflammation   CC HCC A

✓6ᵗʰ **I83.21   Varicose veins of right lower extremity with both ulcer and inflammation**

     I83.211   Varicose veins of right lower extremity with both ulcer of thigh and inflammation   CC HCC A

     I83.212   Varicose veins of right lower extremity with both ulcer of calf and inflammation   CC HCC A

     I83.213   Varicose veins of right lower extremity with both ulcer of ankle and inflammation   CC HCC A

     I83.214   Varicose veins of right lower extremity with both ulcer of heel and midfoot and inflammation   CC HCC A

       Varicose veins of right lower extremity with both ulcer of plantar surface of midfoot and inflammation

     I83.215   Varicose veins of right lower extremity with both ulcer other part of foot and inflammation   CC HCC A

       Varicose veins of right lower extremity with both ulcer of toe and inflammation

     I83.218   Varicose veins of right lower extremity with both ulcer of other part of lower extremity and inflammation   CC HCC A

     I83.219   Varicose veins of right lower extremity with both ulcer of unspecified site and inflammation   CC HCC A

✓6ᵗʰ **I83.22   Varicose veins of left lower extremity with both ulcer and inflammation**

     I83.221   Varicose veins of left lower extremity with both ulcer of thigh and inflammation   CC HCC A

     I83.222   Varicose veins of left lower extremity with both ulcer of calf and inflammation   CC HCC A

N Newborn: 0   P Pediatric: 0-17   M Maternity: 9-64   A Adult: 15-124   MCC Major Complication/Comorbidity   CC Complication/Comorbidity   SW Severe Wound Dx

686   ICD-10-CM 2020

I83.223   **Varicose veins of left lower** `CC` `HCC` `A`
    extremity with both ulcer of ankle and inflammation

I83.224   **Varicose veins of left lower** `CC` `HCC` `A`
    extremity with both ulcer of heel and midfoot and inflammation
       Varicose veins of left lower extremity with both ulcer of plantar surface of midfoot and inflammation

I83.225   **Varicose veins of left lower** `CC` `HCC` `A`
    extremity with both ulcer other part of foot and inflammation
       Varicose veins of left lower extremity with both ulcer of toe and inflammation

I83.228   **Varicose veins of left lower** `CC` `HCC` `A`
    extremity with both ulcer of other part of lower extremity and inflammation

I83.229   **Varicose veins of left lower** `CC` `HCC` `A`
    extremity with both ulcer of unspecified site and inflammation

√5th **I83.8**   **Varicose veins of lower extremities with other complications**

√6th **I83.81**   **Varicose veins of lower extremities with pain**

I83.811   **Varicose veins of right lower** `A`
    extremity with pain

I83.812   **Varicose veins of left lower** `A`
    extremity with pain

I83.813   **Varicose veins of bilateral** `A`
    lower extremities with pain

I83.819   **Varicose veins of unspecified** `A`
    lower extremity with pain

√6th **I83.89**   **Varicose veins of lower extremities with other complications**
     Varicose veins of lower extremities with edema
     Varicose veins of lower extremities with swelling

I83.891   **Varicose veins of right lower** `A`
    extremity with other complications

I83.892   **Varicose veins of left lower** `A`
    extremity with other complications

I83.893   **Varicose veins of bilateral** `A`
    lower extremities with other complications

I83.899   **Varicose veins of unspecified** `A`
    lower extremity with other complications

√5th **I83.9**   **Asymptomatic varicose veins of lower extremities**
     Phlebectasia of lower extremities
     Varicose veins of lower extremities
     Varix of lower extremities

I83.90   **Asymptomatic varicose veins of** `A`
    unspecified lower extremity
       Varicose veins NOS

I83.91   **Asymptomatic varicose veins of right** `A`
    lower extremity

I83.92   **Asymptomatic varicose veins of left** `A`
    lower extremity

I83.93   **Asymptomatic varicose veins of bilateral** `A`
    lower extremities

√4th **I85**   **Esophageal varices**
     Use additional code to identify:
       alcohol abuse and dependence (F10.-)

√5th **I85.0**   **Esophageal varices**
     Idiopathic esophageal varices
     Primary esophageal varices

I85.00   **Esophageal varices without bleeding** `CC` `HCC`
     Esophageal varices NOS
     CC Excl: PDX collection 721

I85.01   **Esophageal varices with bleeding** `MCC` `HCC`
     CC Excl: PDX collection 722

√5th **I85.1**   **Secondary esophageal varices**
     Esophageal varices secondary to alcoholic liver disease
     Esophageal varices secondary to cirrhosis of liver
     Esophageal varices secondary to schistosomiasis
     Esophageal varices secondary to toxic liver disease
     Code first underlying disease

I85.10   **Secondary esophageal varices without** `CC` `HCC`
    bleeding
     CC Excl: PDX collection 723

I85.11   **Secondary esophageal varices with** `MCC` `HCC`
    bleeding
     CC Excl: PDX collection 724

√4th **I86**   **Varicose veins of other sites**
     EXCLUDES 1   *varicose veins of unspecified site (I83.9-)*
     EXCLUDES 2   *retinal varices (H35.0-)*

I86.0   **Sublingual varices**
     DEF: Distended, tortuous veins beneath the tongue.

I86.1   **Scrotal varices**   ♂
     Varicocele

I86.2   **Pelvic varices**

I86.3   **Vulval varices**   ♀
     EXCLUDES 1   *vulval varices complicating childbirth and the puerperium (O87.8)*
          vulval varices complicating pregnancy (O22.1-)

I86.4   **Gastric varices**

I86.8   **Varicose veins of other specified sites** `A`
     Varicose ulcer of nasal septum

√4th **I87**   **Other disorders of veins**

√5th **I87.0**   **Postthrombotic syndrome**
     Chronic venous hypertension due to deep vein thrombosis
     Postphlebitic syndrome
     EXCLUDES 1   *chronic venous hypertension without deep vein thrombosis (I87.3-)*
     CC Excl: For CC codes in subcategory I87.0: PDX collection 725

√6th **I87.00**   **Postthrombotic syndrome without complications**
     Asymptomatic postthrombotic syndrome

I87.001   **Postthrombotic syndrome without complications of right lower extremity**

I87.002   **Postthrombotic syndrome without complications of left lower extremity**

I87.003   **Postthrombotic syndrome without complications of bilateral lower extremity**

I87.009   **Postthrombotic syndrome without complications of unspecified extremity**
     Postthrombotic syndrome NOS

√6th **I87.01**   **Postthrombotic syndrome with ulcer**
     Use additional code to specify site and severity of ulcer (L97.-)

I87.011   **Postthrombotic syndrome with** `CC` `HCC`
    ulcer of right lower extremity

I87.012   **Postthrombotic syndrome with** `CC` `HCC`
    ulcer of left lower extremity

I87.013   **Postthrombotic syndrome with** `CC` `HCC`
    ulcer of bilateral lower extremity

I87.019   **Postthrombotic syndrome with** `CC` `HCC`
    ulcer of unspecified lower extremity

√6th **I87.02**   **Postthrombotic syndrome with inflammation**

I87.021   **Postthrombotic syndrome with inflammation of right lower extremity**

I87.022   **Postthrombotic syndrome with inflammation of left lower extremity**

I87.023   **Postthrombotic syndrome with inflammation of bilateral lower extremity**

I87.029   **Postthrombotic syndrome with inflammation of unspecified lower extremity**

√6th **I87.03**   **Postthrombotic syndrome with ulcer and inflammation**
     Use additional code to specify site and severity of ulcer (L97.-)

I87.031   **Postthrombotic syndrome with** `CC` `HCC`
    ulcer and inflammation of right lower extremity

I87.032   **Postthrombotic syndrome with** `CC` `HCC`
    ulcer and inflammation of left lower extremity

✓ Additional Character Required   ✓x7th Placeholder   Unacceptable PDx   Questionable PDx   Manifestation   Unspecified Dx   H1-H14 HAC   HCC CMS-HCC Dx   HIV HIV Dx

ICD-10-CM 2020   687

Chapter 9. Diseases of the Circulatory System

I87.033–I89.8

    I87.033   **Postthrombotic syndrome with** `CC` `HCC`
              ulcer and inflammation of
              bilateral lower extremity

    I87.039   **Postthrombotic syndrome with** `CC` `HCC`
              ulcer and inflammation of
              unspecified lower extremity

 √6ᵗʰ **I87.09** **Postthrombotic syndrome with other complications**

    I87.091   **Postthrombotic syndrome with other complications of right lower extremity**

    I87.092   **Postthrombotic syndrome with other complications of left lower extremity**

    I87.093   **Postthrombotic syndrome with other complications of bilateral lower extremity**

    I87.099   **Postthrombotic syndrome with other complications of unspecified lower extremity**

I87.1   **Compression of vein** `CC`

    Stricture of vein

    Vena cava syndrome (inferior) (superior)

    EXCLUDES 2   *compression of pulmonary vein (I28.8)*

    CC Excl: PDX collection 726

I87.2   **Venous insufficiency (chronic) (peripheral)**

    Stasis dermatitis

    EXCLUDES 1   *stasis dermatitis with varicose veins of lower extremities (I83.1-, I83.2-)*

    DEF: Insufficient drainage of venous blood in any part of the body that results in edema or dermatosis.

√5ᵗʰ **I87.3**   **Chronic venous hypertension (idiopathic)**

    Stasis edema

    EXCLUDES 1   *chronic venous hypertension due to deep vein thrombosis (I87.0-)*

              varicose veins of lower extremities (I83.-)

    CC Excl: For CC codes in subcategory I87.3: PDX collection 727

 √6ᵗʰ **I87.30** **Chronic venous hypertension (idiopathic) without complications**

    Asymptomatic chronic venous hypertension (idiopathic)

    I87.301   **Chronic venous hypertension (idiopathic) without complications of right lower extremity**

    I87.302   **Chronic venous hypertension (idiopathic) without complications of left lower extremity**

    I87.303   **Chronic venous hypertension (idiopathic) without complications of bilateral lower extremity**

    I87.309   **Chronic venous hypertension (idiopathic) without complications of unspecified lower extremity**

              Chronic venous hypertension NOS

 √6ᵗʰ **I87.31** **Chronic venous hypertension (idiopathic) with ulcer**

    Use additional code to specify site and severity of ulcer (L97.-)

    I87.311   **Chronic venous hypertension** `CC` `HCC`
              (idiopathic) with ulcer of right lower extremity

    I87.312   **Chronic venous hypertension** `CC` `HCC`
              (idiopathic) with ulcer of left lower extremity

    I87.313   **Chronic venous hypertension** `CC` `HCC`
               (idiopathic) with ulcer of bilateral lower extremity

    I87.319   **Chronic venous hypertension** `CC` `HCC`
               (idiopathic) with ulcer of unspecified lower extremity

 √6ᵗʰ **I87.32** **Chronic venous hypertension (idiopathic) with inflammation**

    I87.321   **Chronic venous hypertension (idiopathic) with inflammation of right lower extremity**

    I87.322   **Chronic venous hypertension (idiopathic) with inflammation of left lower extremity**

    I87.323   **Chronic venous hypertension (idiopathic) with inflammation of bilateral lower extremity**

    I87.329   **Chronic venous hypertension (idiopathic) with inflammation of unspecified lower extremity**

 √6ᵗʰ **I87.33** **Chronic venous hypertension (idiopathic) with ulcer and inflammation**

    Use additional code to specify site and severity of ulcer (L97.-)

    I87.331   **Chronic venous hypertension** `CC` `HCC`
              (idiopathic) with ulcer and inflammation of right lower extremity

    I87.332   **Chronic venous hypertension** `CC` `HCC`
              (idiopathic) with ulcer and inflammation of left lower extremity

    I87.333   **Chronic venous hypertension** `CC` `HCC`
              (idiopathic) with ulcer and inflammation of bilateral lower extremity

    I87.339   **Chronic venous hypertension** `CC` `HCC`
              (idiopathic) with ulcer and inflammation of unspecified lower extremity

 √6ᵗʰ **I87.39** **Chronic venous hypertension (idiopathic) with other complications**

    I87.391   **Chronic venous hypertension (idiopathic) with other complications of right lower extremity**

    I87.392   **Chronic venous hypertension (idiopathic) with other complications of left lower extremity**

    I87.393   **Chronic venous hypertension (idiopathic) with other complications of bilateral lower extremity**

    I87.399   **Chronic venous hypertension (idiopathic) with other complications of unspecified lower extremity**

I87.8   **Other specified disorders of veins**

    Phlebosclerosis

    Venofibrosis

I87.9   **Disorder of vein, unspecified**

√4ᵗʰ **I88** **Nonspecific lymphadenitis**

    EXCLUDES 1   *acute lymphadenitis, except mesenteric (L04.-)*

              enlarged lymph nodes NOS (R59.-)

              human immunodeficiency virus [HIV] disease resulting in generalized lymphadenopathy (B20)

I88.0   **Nonspecific mesenteric lymphadenitis**

    Mesenteric lymphadenitis (acute)(chronic)

I88.1   **Chronic lymphadenitis, except mesenteric**

    Adenitis

    Lymphadenitis

I88.8   **Other nonspecific lymphadenitis**

I88.9   **Nonspecific lymphadenitis, unspecified**

    Lymphadenitis NOS

√4ᵗʰ **I89** **Other noninfective disorders of lymphatic vessels and lymph nodes**

    EXCLUDES 1   *chylocele, tunica vaginalis (nonfilarial) NOS (N50.89)*

              enlarged lymph nodes NOS (R59.-)

              filarial chylocele (B74.-)

              hereditary lymphedema (Q82.0)

I89.0   **Lymphedema, not elsewhere classified**

    Elephantiasis (nonfilarial) NOS

    Lymphangiectasis

    Obliteration, lymphatic vessel

    Praecox lymphedema

    Secondary lymphedema

    EXCLUDES 1   *postmastectomy lymphedema (I97.2)*

I89.1   **Lymphangitis**

    Chronic lymphangitis

    Lymphangitis NOS

    Subacute lymphangitis

    EXCLUDES 1   *acute lymphangitis (L03.-)*

I89.8   **Other specified noninfective disorders of lymphatic vessels and lymph nodes**

    Chylocele (nonfilarial)

    Chylous ascites

    Chylous cyst

    Lipomelanotic reticulosis

    Lymph node or vessel fistula

    Lymph node or vessel infarction

    Lymph node or vessel rupture

N Newborn: 0   **P** Pediatric: 0-17   **M** Maternity: 9-64   **A** Adult: 15-124   `MCC` Major Complication/Comorbidity   `CC` Complication/Comorbidity   `SW` Severe Wound Dx

688   ICD-10-CM 2020

I89.9　**Noninfective disorder of lymphatic vessels and lymph nodes, unspecified**
Disease of lymphatic vessels NOS

Other and unspecified disorders of the circulatory system (I95-I99)

✓4ᵗʰ I95　Hotension
EXCLUDES 1　cardiovascular collapse (R57.9) (~R57.9)
maternal hypotension syndrome (O26.5-)
nonspecific low blood pressure reading NOS (R03.1)

I95.0　**Idiopathic hypotension**

I95.1　**Orthostatic hypotension**
Hypotension, postural
EXCLUDES 1　neurogenic orthostatic hypotension [Shy-Drager] (G90.3)
orthostatic hypotension due to drugs (I95.2)

I95.2　**Hypotension due to drugs**
Orthostatic hypotension due to drugs
Use additional code for adverse effect, if applicable, to identify drug (T36-T50 with fifth or sixth character 5)

I95.3　**Hypotension of hemodialysis**
Intra-dialytic hypotension

✓5ᵗʰ I95.8　**Other hypotension**
　　I95.81　**Postprocedural hypotension**
　　I95.89　**Other hypotension**
　　　　Chronic hypotension

I95.9　**Hypotension, unspecified**

I96　Gangrene, not elsewhere classified　`CC` `HCC`
Gangrenous cellulitis
EXCLUDES 1　gangrene in atherosclerosis of native arteries of the extremities (I70.26)
gangrene in hernia (K40.1, K40.4, K41.1, K41.4, K42.1, K43.1-, K44.1, K45.1, K46.1)
gangrene in other peripheral vascular diseases (I73.-)
gangrene of certain specified sites — see Alphabetical Index
gas gangrene (A48.0)
pyoderma gangrenosum (L88)
EXCLUDES 2　gangrene in diabetes mellitus (E08-E13 with .52)
AHA: 2018,4Q,87; 2018,3Q,3; 2017,3Q,6; 2013,2Q,34
CC Excl: PDX collection 519

✓4ᵗʰ I97　Intraoperative and postprocedural complications and disorders of circulatory system, not elsewhere classified
EXCLUDES 2　postprocedural shock (T81.1-)
AHA: 2019,2Q,21

I97.0　**Postcardiotomy syndrome**

✓5ᵗʰ I97.1　**Other postprocedural cardiac functional disturbances**
EXCLUDES 2　acute pulmonary insufficiency following thoracic surgery (J95.1)
intraoperative cardiac functional disturbances (I97.7-)
CC Excl: For CC codes in subcategory I97.1: PDX collection 728

✓6ᵗʰ I97.11　**Postprocedural cardiac insufficiency**
　　I97.110　**Postprocedural cardiac insufficiency following cardiac surgery**
　　I97.111　**Postprocedural cardiac insufficiency following other surgery**

✓6ᵗʰ I97.12　**Postprocedural cardiac arrest**
　　I97.120　**Postprocedural cardiac arrest following cardiac surgery**　`CC`
　　I97.121　**Postprocedural cardiac arrest following other surgery**　`CC`

✓6ᵗʰ I97.13　**Postprocedural heart failure**
Use additional code to identify the heart failure (I50.-)
　　I97.130　**Postprocedural heart failure following cardiac surgery**　`CC`
　　I97.131　**Postprocedural heart failure following other surgery**　`CC`

✓6ᵗʰ I97.19　**Other postprocedural cardiac functional disturbances**
Use additional code, if applicable, to further specify disorder
　　I97.190　**Other postprocedural cardiac functional disturbances following cardiac surgery**　`CC`
　　　　Use additional code, if applicable, for type 4 or type 5 myocardial infarction, to further specify disorder
　　　　AHA: 2019,2Q,33
　　I97.191　**Other postprocedural cardiac functional disturbances following other surgery**　`CC`

I97.2　**Postmastectomy lymphedema syndrome**　`A`
Elephantiasis due to mastectomy
Obliteration of lymphatic vessels

I97.3　**Postprocedural hypertension**

✓5ᵗʰ I97.4　**Intraoperative hemorrhage and hematoma of a circulatory system organ or structure complicating a procedure**
EXCLUDES 1　intraoperative hemorrhage and hematoma of a circulatory system organ or structure due to accidental puncture and laceration during a procedure (I97.5-)
EXCLUDES 2　intraoperative cerebrovascular hemorrhage complicating a procedure (G97.3-)
CC Excl: For CC codes in subcategory I97.4: PDX collection 729

✓6ᵗʰ I97.41　**Intraoperative hemorrhage and hematoma of a circulatory system organ or structure complicating a circulatory system procedure**
　　I97.410　**Intraoperative hemorrhage and hematoma of a circulatory system organ or structure complicating a cardiac catheterization**　`CC`
　　I97.411　**Intraoperative hemorrhage and hematoma of a circulatory system organ or structure complicating a cardiac bypass**　`CC`
　　I97.418　**Intraoperative hemorrhage and hematoma of a circulatory system organ or structure complicating other circulatory system procedure**　`CC`

I97.42　**Intraoperative hemorrhage and hematoma of a circulatory system organ or structure complicating other procedure**　`CC`

✓5ᵗʰ I97.5　**Accidental puncture and laceration of a circulatory system organ or structure during a procedure**
EXCLUDES 2　accidental puncture and laceration of brain during a procedure (G97.4-)

I97.51　**Accidental puncture and laceration of a circulatory system organ or structure during a circulatory system procedure**　`CC`
AHA: 2019,2Q,24
CC Excl: PDX collection 509

I97.52　**Accidental puncture and laceration of a circulatory system organ or structure during other procedure**　`CC`
CC Excl: PDX collection 509

✓5ᵗʰ I97.6　**Postprocedural hemorrhage, hematoma and seroma of a circulatory system organ or structure following a procedure**
EXCLUDES 2　postprocedural cerebrovascular hemorrhage complicating a procedure (G97.5-)
AHA: 2016,4Q,9-10
CC Excl: For CC codes in subcategory I97.6: PDX collection 729

✓6ᵗʰ I97.61　**Postprocedural hemorrhage of a circulatory system organ or structure following a circulatory system procedure**
　　I97.610　**Postprocedural hemorrhage of a circulatory system organ or structure following a cardiac catheterization**　`CC`
　　I97.611　**Postprocedural hemorrhage of a circulatory system organ or structure following cardiac bypass**　`CC`
　　I97.618　**Postprocedural hemorrhage of a circulatory system organ or structure following other circulatory system procedure**　`CC`

Chapter 9. Diseases of the Circulatory System

I97.62–I99.9

√6ᵗʰ **I97.62 Postprocedural hemorrhage, hematoma and seroma** of a circulatory system organ or structure following **other procedure**

     I97.620 Postprocedural hemorrhage of a circulatory system organ or structure following other procedure   `CC`

     I97.621 Postprocedural hematoma of a circulatory system organ or structure following other procedure   `CC`

     I97.622 Postprocedural seroma of a circulatory system organ or structure following other procedure   `CC`

√6ᵗʰ **I97.63 Postprocedural hematoma** of a circulatory system organ or structure following a **circulatory system procedure**

     I97.630 Postprocedural hematoma of a circulatory system organ or structure following a cardiac catheterization   `CC`

     I97.631 Postprocedural hematoma of a circulatory system organ or structure following cardiac bypass   `CC`

     I97.638 Postprocedural hematoma of a circulatory system organ or structure following other circulatory system procedure   `CC`

√6ᵗʰ **I97.64 Postprocedural seroma** of a circulatory system organ or structure following a circulatory system procedure

     I97.640 Postprocedural seroma of a circulatory system organ or structure following a cardiac catheterization   `CC`

     I97.641 Postprocedural seroma of a circulatory system organ or structure following cardiac bypass   `CC`

     I97.648 Postprocedural seroma of a circulatory system organ or structure following other circulatory system procedure   `CC`

√5ᵗʰ **I97.7 Intraoperative cardiac functional disturbances**

     EXCLUDES 2   acute pulmonary insufficiency following thoracic surgery (J95.1)
             postprocedural cardiac functional disturbances (I97.1-)

     CC Excl: For CC codes in subcategory I97.7: PDX collection 728

√6ᵗʰ **I97.71 Intraoperative cardiac arrest**

     I97.710 Intraoperative cardiac arrest during cardiac surgery   `CC`

     I97.711 Intraoperative cardiac arrest during other surgery   `CC`

√6ᵗʰ **I97.79 Other intraoperative cardiac functional disturbances**

     Use additional code, if applicable, to further specify disorder

     I97.790 Other intraoperative cardiac functional disturbances during cardiac surgery   `CC`

     I97.791 Other intraoperative cardiac functional disturbances during other surgery   `CC`

√6ᵗʰ **I97.8 Other intraoperative and postprocedural complications and disorders of the circulatory system, not elsewhere classified**

     Use additional code, if applicable, to further specify disorder

     CC Excl: For CC codes in subcatgory I97.8, unless otherwise noted: PDX collection 617

√6ᵗʰ **I97.81 Intraoperative cerebrovascular infarction**

     I97.810 Intraoperative cerebrovascular infarction during cardiac surgery   `CC` `HCC`

     I97.811 Intraoperative cerebrovascular infarction during other surgery   `CC` `HCC`

√6ᵗʰ **I97.82 Postprocedural cerebrovascular infarction**

     I97.820 Postprocedural cerebrovascular infarction following cardiac surgery   `CC` `HCC`

     I97.821 Postprocedural cerebrovascular infarction following other surgery   `CC` `HCC`

     I97.88 Other intraoperative complications of the circulatory system, not elsewhere classified   `CC`

         CC Excl: PDX collection 728

     I97.89 Other postprocedural complications and disorders of the circulatory system, not elsewhere classified   `CC`

         AHA: 2019,2Q,33

         CC Excl: PDX collection 728

√4ᵗʰ **I99 Other and unspecified disorders of circulatory system**

     I99.8 Other disorder of circulatory system

     I99.9 Unspecified disorder of circulatory system

`N` Newborn: 0   `P` Pediatric: 0-17   `M` Maternity: 9-64   `A` Adult: 15-124   `MCC` Major Complication/Comorbidity   `CC` Complication/Comorbidity   `SW` Severe Wound Dx

690

ICD-10-CM 2020

Chapter 10. Diseases of the Respiratory System (J00–J99)

Chapter-specific Guidelines with Coding Examples

The chapter-specific guidelines from the ICD-10-CM Official Guidelines for Coding and Reporting have been provided below. Along with these guidelines are coding examples, contained in the shaded boxes, that have been developed to help illustrate the coding and/or sequencing guidance found in these guidelines.

a. Chronic obstructive pulmonary disease [COPD] and asthma

1) Acute exacerbation of chronic obstructive bronchitis and asthma

The codes in categories J44 and J45 distinguish between uncomplicated cases and those in acute exacerbation. An acute exacerbation is a worsening or a decompensation of a chronic condition. An acute exacerbation is not equivalent to an infection superimposed on a chronic condition, though an exacerbation may be triggered by an infection.

> Vancomycin IV was started to treat a patient with acute pneumonia due to *Streptococcus pneumoniae*. Patient also with acute exacerbation of COPD continued on home meds.
>
> **J13**   **Pneumonia due to Streptococcus pneumoniae**
>
> **J44.0**   **Chronic obstructive pulmonary disease with (acute) lower respiratory infection**
>
> **J44.1**   **Chronic obstructive pulmonary disease with (acute) exacerbation**
>
> *Explanation*: ICD-10-CM uses combination codes to create organism-specific classifications for acute pneumonia. Category J44 codes include combination codes with severity components, which differentiate between COPD with acute lower respiratory infection (acute pneumonia), COPD with acute exacerbation, and COPD without mention of a complication (unspecified).
>
> An acute exacerbation is a worsening or a decompensation of a chronic condition. An acute exacerbation is not equivalent to an infection superimposed on a chronic condition, though an exacerbation may be triggered by an infection, as in this example. Treatment of the pneumonia necessitated the inpatient admission. Instructional notes at J44.0 say to "code also to identify the infection," which informs the coder that another code must be assigned if applicable. Sequencing of the pneumonia and COPD exacerbation are governed by the Section II, "Selection of Principal Diagnosis," guidelines. In this case it was the pneumonia that was "chiefly responsible for occasioning the admission" with the IV vancomycin treatment.

> Exacerbation of moderate persistent asthma with status asthmaticus
>
> **J45.42**   **Moderate persistent asthma with status asthmaticus**
>
> *Explanation*: Category J45 Asthma includes severity-specific subcategories and fifth-character codes to distinguish between uncomplicated cases, those in acute exacerbation, and those with status asthmaticus.

b. Acute respiratory failure

1) Acute respiratory failure as principal diagnosis

A code from subcategory J96.0, Acute respiratory failure, or subcategory J96.2, Acute and chronic respiratory failure, may be assigned as a principal diagnosis when it is the condition established after study to be chiefly responsible for occasioning the admission to the hospital, and the selection is supported by the Alphabetic Index and Tabular List. However, chapter-specific coding guidelines (such as obstetrics, poisoning, HIV, newborn) that provide sequencing direction take precedence.

> Acute hypoxic respiratory failure due to COPD exacerbation
>
> **J96.01**   **Acute respiratory failure with hypoxia**
>
> **J44.1**   **Chronic obstructive pulmonary disease with (acute) exacerbation**
>
> *Explanation*: Category J96 classifies respiratory failure with combination codes that designate the severity and the presence of hypoxia and hypercapnia. Code J96.01 is sequenced as the first-listed diagnosis, as the reason for the admission. Respiratory failure may be assigned as a principal diagnosis when it is the condition established after study to be chiefly responsible for occasioning the admission to the hospital and the selection is supported by the Alphabetic Index and Tabular List.

2) Acute respiratory failure as secondary diagnosis

Respiratory failure may be listed as a secondary diagnosis if it occurs after admission, or if it is present on admission, but does not meet the definition of principal diagnosis.

> Acute respiratory failure due to accidental oxycodone overdose
>
> **T40.2X1A**   **Poisoning by other opioids, accidental (unintentional), initial encounter**
>
> **J96.00**   **Acute respiratory failure, unspecified whether with hypoxia or hypercapnia**
>
> *Explanation*: Respiratory failure may be assigned as a principal diagnosis when it is the condition established after study to be chiefly responsible for occasioning the admission to the hospital, and the selection is supported by the Alphabetic Index and Tabular List. However, chapter-specific coding guidelines, such as poisoning, that provide sequencing direction take precedence. When coding a poisoning or reaction to the improper use of a medication (e.g. overdose, wrong substance given or taken in error, wrong route of administration), first assign the appropriate code from categories T36–T50. Use additional code(s) for all manifestations of the poisoning. In this instance, the respiratory failure is a manifestation of the poisoning and is sequenced as a secondary diagnosis.

> Acute pneumococcal pneumonia with subsequent development of acute respiratory failure
>
> **J13**   **Pneumonia due to Streptococcus pneumoniae**
>
> **J96.00**   **Acute respiratory failure, unspecified whether with hypoxia or hypercapnia**
>
> *Explanation*: Acute respiratory failure may be listed as a secondary diagnosis if it occurs after admission, or if it is present on admission but does not meet the definition of principal diagnosis.

3) Sequencing of acute respiratory failure and another acute condition

When a patient is admitted with respiratory failure and another acute condition, (e.g., myocardial infarction, cerebrovascular accident, aspiration pneumonia), the principal diagnosis will not be the same in every situation. This applies whether the other acute condition is a respiratory or nonrespiratory condition. Selection of the principal diagnosis will be dependent on the circumstances of admission. If both the respiratory failure and the other acute condition are equally responsible for occasioning the admission to the hospital, and there are no chapter-specific sequencing rules, the guideline regarding two or more diagnoses that equally meet the definition for principal diagnosis (*Section II, C.*) may be applied in these situations.

If the documentation is not clear as to whether acute respiratory failure and another condition are equally responsible for occasioning the admission, query the provider for clarification.

> Acute pneumococcal pneumonia and acute respiratory failure, both present on admission
>
> **J96.00**   **Acute respiratory failure, unspecified whether with hypoxia or hypercapnia**
>
> **J13**   **Pneumonia due to Streptococcus pneumoniae**
>
> *Explanation*: When a patient is admitted with respiratory failure and another acute condition, such as a bacterial pneumonia, the principal diagnosis is not the same in every situation. This applies whether the other acute condition is a respiratory or nonrespiratory condition. The principal diagnosis depends on the circumstances of admission.

c. Influenza due to certain identified influenza viruses

Code only confirmed cases of influenza due to certain identified influenza viruses (category J09), and due to other identified influenza virus (category J10). This is an exception to the hospital inpatient guideline Section II, H. (Uncertain Diagnosis).

In this context, "confirmation" does not require documentation of positive laboratory testing specific for avian or other novel influenza A or other identified influenza virus. However, coding should be based on the provider's diagnostic statement that the patient has avian influenza, or other novel influenza A, for category J09, or has another particular identified strain of influenza, such as H1N1 or H3N2, but not identified as novel or variant, for category J10.

If the provider records "suspected" or "possible" or "probable" avian influenza, or novel influenza, or other identified influenza, then the appropriate influenza code from category J11, Influenza due to unidentified influenza virus, should be assigned. A code from category J09, Influenza due to certain identified influenza viruses, should not be assigned nor should a code from category J10, Influenza due to other identified influenza virus.

> Influenza due to avian influenza virus with pneumonia
>
> **J09.X1   Influenza due to identified novel influenza A virus with pneumonia**
>
> *Explanation*: Codes in category J09 Influenza due to certain identified influenza viruses should be assigned only for confirmed cases. "Confirmation" does not require positive laboratory testing of a specific influenza virus but does need to be based on the provider's diagnostic statement, which should not include terms such as "possible," "probable," or "suspected."

d. Ventilator associated pneumonia

1) Documentation of ventilator associated pneumonia

As with all procedural or postprocedural complications, code assignment is based on the provider's documentation of the relationship between the condition and the procedure.

Code J95.851, Ventilator associated pneumonia, should be assigned only when the provider has documented ventilator associated pneumonia (VAP). An additional code to identify the organism (e.g., Pseudomonas aeruginosa, code B96.5) should also be assigned. Do not assign an additional code from categories J12-J18 to identify the type of pneumonia.

Code J95.851 should not be assigned for cases where the patient has pneumonia and is on a mechanical ventilator and the provider has not specifically stated that the pneumonia is ventilator-associated pneumonia. If the documentation is unclear as to whether the patient has a pneumonia that is a complication attributable to the mechanical ventilator, query the provider.

2) Ventilator associated pneumonia develops after admission

A patient may be admitted with one type of pneumonia (e.g., code J13, Pneumonia due to Streptococcus pneumonia) and subsequently develop VAP. In this instance, the principal diagnosis would be the appropriate code from categories J12-J18 for the pneumonia diagnosed at the time of admission. Code J95.851, Ventilator associated pneumonia, would be assigned as an additional diagnosis when the provider has also documented the presence of ventilator associated pneumonia.

> Patient with pneumonia due to *Klebsiella pneumoniae* develops superimposed MRSA ventilator-associated pneumonia
>
> **J15.0   Pneumonia due to Klebsiella pneumoniae**
>
> **J95.851   Ventilator associated pneumonia**
>
> **B95.62   Methicillin resistant Staphylococcus aureus infection as the cause of diseases classified elsewhere**
>
> *Explanation*: Code assignment for ventilator-associated pneumonia is based on the provider's documentation of the relationship between the condition and the procedure and is reported only when the provider has documented ventilator-associated pneumonia (VAP).
>
> A patient may be admitted with one type of pneumonia and subsequently develop VAP. In this example, the principal diagnosis code describes the pneumonia diagnosed at the time of admission, with code J95.851 Ventilator associated pneumonia, assigned as secondary.

Chapter 10. Diseases of the Respiratory System (J00-J99)

> **NOTE** When a respiratory condition is described as occurring in more than one site and is not specifically indexed, it should be classified to the lower anatomic site (e.g., tracheobronchitis to bronchitis in J40).

Use additional code, where applicable, to identify:
exposure to environmental tobacco smoke (Z77.22)
exposure to tobacco smoke in the perinatal period (P96.81)
history of tobacco dependence (Z87.891)
occupational exposure to environmental tobacco smoke (Z57.31)
tobacco dependence (F17.-)
tobacco use (Z72.0)

> **EXCLUDES 2** *certain conditions originating in the perinatal period (P04-P96)*
> *certain infectious and parasitic diseases (A00-B99)*
> *complications of pregnancy, childbirth and the puerperium (O00-O9A)*
> *congenital malformations, deformations and chromosomal abnormalities (Q00-Q99)*
> *endocrine, nutritional and metabolic diseases (E00-E88)*
> *injury, poisoning and certain other consequences of external causes (S00-T88)*
> *neoplasms (C00-D49)*
> *smoke inhalation (T59.81-)*
> *symptoms, signs and abnormal clinical and laboratory findings, not elsewhere classified (R00-R94)*

This chapter contains the following blocks:
J00-J06   Acute upper respiratory infections
J09-J18   Influenza and pneumonia
J20-J22   Other acute lower respiratory infections
J30-J39   Other diseases of upper respiratory tract
J40-J47   Chronic lower respiratory diseases
J60-J70   Lung diseases due to external agents
J80-J84   Other respiratory diseases principally affecting the interstitium
J85-J86   Suppurative and necrotic conditions of the lower respiratory tract
J90-J94   Other diseases of the pleura
J95   Intraoperative and postprocedural complications and disorders of respiratory system, not elsewhere classified
J96-J99   Other diseases of the respiratory system

Acute upper respiratory infections (J00-J06)

> **EXCLUDES 1** *chronic obstructive pulmonary disease with acute lower respiratory infection (J44.0)*
> *influenza virus with other respiratory manifestations (J09.X2, J10.1, J11.1)*

J00   Acute nasopharyngitis [common cold]
Acute rhinitis
Coryza (acute)
Infective nasopharyngitis NOS
Infective rhinitis
Nasal catarrh, acute
Nasopharyngitis NOS

> **EXCLUDES 1** *acute pharyngitis (J02.-)*
> *acute sore throat NOS (J02.9)*
> *pharyngitis NOS (J02.9)*
> *rhinitis NOS (J31.0)*
> *sore throat NOS (J02.9)*

> **EXCLUDES 2** *allergic rhinitis (J30.1-J30.9)*
> *chronic pharyngitis (J31.2)*
> *chronic rhinitis (J31.0)*
> *chronic sore throat (J31.2)*
> *nasopharyngitis, chronic (J31.1)*
> *vasomotor rhinitis (J30.0)*

DEF: Acute inflammation of the mucous membranes that extends from the nares to the pharynx. It is characterized by nasal obstruction, sneezing, runny nose, and sore throat.

☑4ᵗʰ **J01   Acute sinusitis**
> **INCLUDES**   acute abscess of sinus
> acute empyema of sinus
> acute infection of sinus
> acute inflammation of sinus
> acute suppuration of sinus

Use additional code (B95-B97) to identify infectious agent
> **EXCLUDES 1** *sinusitis NOS (J32.9)*
> **EXCLUDES 2** *chronic sinusitis (J32.0-J32.8)*

☑5ᵗʰ   **J01.0   Acute maxillary sinusitis**
Acute antritis
    J01.00   Acute maxillary sinusitis, unspecified
    J01.01   Acute recurrent maxillary sinusitis

☑5ᵗʰ   **J01.1   Acute frontal sinusitis**
    J01.10   Acute frontal sinusitis, unspecified
    J01.11   Acute recurrent frontal sinusitis

☑5ᵗʰ   **J01.2   Acute ethmoidal sinusitis**
    J01.20   Acute ethmoidal sinusitis, unspecified
    J01.21   Acute recurrent ethmoidal sinusitis

☑5ᵗʰ   **J01.3   Acute sphenoidal sinusitis**
    J01.30   Acute sphenoidal sinusitis, unspecified
    J01.31   Acute recurrent sphenoidal sinusitis

☑5ᵗʰ   **J01.4   Acute pansinusitis**
    J01.40   Acute pansinusitis, unspecified
    J01.41   Acute recurrent pansinusitis

☑5ᵗʰ   **J01.8   Other acute sinusitis**
    J01.80   Other acute sinusitis
       Acute sinusitis involving more than one sinus but not pansinusitis
    J01.81   Other acute recurrent sinusitis
       Acute recurrent sinusitis involving more than one sinus but not pansinusitis

☑5ᵗʰ   **J01.9   Acute sinusitis, unspecified**
    J01.90   Acute sinusitis, unspecified
    J01.91   Acute recurrent sinusitis, unspecified

☑4ᵗʰ **J02   Acute pharyngitis**
> **INCLUDES**   acute sore throat
> **EXCLUDES 1** *acute laryngopharyngitis (J06.0)*
> *peritonsillar abscess (J36)*
> *pharyngeal abscess (J39.1)*
> *retropharyngeal abscess (J39.0)*
> **EXCLUDES 2** *chronic pharyngitis (J31.2)*

    J02.0   Streptococcal pharyngitis
Septic pharyngitis
Streptococcal sore throat
> **EXCLUDES 2** *scarlet fever (A38.-)*

    J02.8   Acute pharyngitis due to other specified organisms
Use additional code (B95-B97) to identify infectious agent
> **EXCLUDES 1** *acute pharyngitis due to coxsackie virus (B08.5)*
> *acute pharyngitis due to gonococcus (A54.5)*
> *acute pharyngitis due to herpes [simplex] virus (B00.2)*
> *acute pharyngitis due to infectious mononucleosis (B27.-)*
> *enteroviral vesicular pharyngitis (B08.5)*

    J02.9   Acute pharyngitis, unspecified
Gangrenous pharyngitis (acute)
Infective pharyngitis (acute) NOS
Pharyngitis (acute) NOS
Sore throat (acute) NOS
Suppurative pharyngitis (acute)
Ulcerative pharyngitis (acute)

☑4ᵗʰ **J03   Acute tonsillitis**
> **EXCLUDES 1** *acute sore throat (J02.-)*
> *hypertrophy of tonsils (J35.1)*
> *peritonsillar abscess (J36)*
> *sore throat NOS (J02.9)*
> *streptococcal sore throat (J02.0)*
> **EXCLUDES 2** *chronic tonsillitis (J35.0)*

☑5ᵗʰ   **J03.0   Streptococcal tonsillitis**
    J03.00   Acute streptococcal tonsillitis, unspecified
    J03.01   Acute recurrent streptococcal tonsillitis

☑5ᵗʰ   **J03.8   Acute tonsillitis due to other specified organisms**
Use additional code (B95-B97) to identify infectious agent
> **EXCLUDES 1** *diphtheritic tonsillitis (A36.0)*
> *herpesviral pharyngotonsillitis (B00.2)*
> *streptococcal tonsillitis (J03.0)*
> *tuberculous tonsillitis (A15.8)*
> *Vincent's tonsillitis (A69.1)*

    J03.80   Acute tonsillitis due to other specified organisms
    J03.81   Acute recurrent tonsillitis due to other specified organisms

✓5ᵗʰ **J03.9** **Acute tonsillitis, unspecified**
Follicular tonsillitis (acute)
Gangrenous tonsillitis (acute)
Infective tonsillitis (acute)
Tonsillitis (acute) NOS
Ulcerative tonsillitis (acute)

    J03.90 **Acute tonsillitis, unspecified**
    J03.91 **Acute recurrent tonsillitis, unspecified**

✓4ᵗʰ **J04** **Acute laryngitis and tracheitis**
Use additional code (B95-B97) to identify infectious agent
    EXCLUDES 1   *acute obstructive laryngitis [croup] and epiglottitis (J05.-)*
    EXCLUDES 2   *laryngismus (stridulus) (J38.5)*

J04.0 **Acute laryngitis**
Edematous laryngitis (acute)
Laryngitis (acute) NOS
Subglottic laryngitis (acute)
Suppurative laryngitis (acute)
Ulcerative laryngitis (acute)
    EXCLUDES 1   *acute obstructive laryngitis (J05.0)*
    EXCLUDES 2   *chronic laryngitis (J37.0)*

✓5ᵗʰ **J04.1** **Acute tracheitis**
Acute viral tracheitis
Catarrhal tracheitis (acute)
Tracheitis (acute) NOS
    EXCLUDES 2   *chronic tracheitis (J42)*

J04.10 **Acute tracheitis without obstruction**
J04.11 **Acute tracheitis with obstruction**   MCC
    CC Excl: PDX collection 730

J04.2 **Acute laryngotracheitis**
Laryngotracheitis NOS
Tracheitis (acute) with laryngitis (acute)
    EXCLUDES 1   *acute obstructive laryngotracheitis (J05.0)*
    EXCLUDES 2   *chronic laryngotracheitis (J37.1)*

✓5ᵗʰ **J04.3** **Supraglottitis, unspecified**

    J04.30 **Supraglottitis, unspecified, without obstruction**
    J04.31 **Supraglottitis, unspecified, with obstruction**   MCC
       CC Excl: PDX collection 731

✓4ᵗʰ **J05** **Acute obstructive laryngitis [croup] and epiglottitis**
Use additional code (B95-B97) to identify infectious agent

J05.0 **Acute obstructive laryngitis [croup]**
Obstructive laryngitis (acute) NOS
Obstructive laryngotracheitis NOS
    DEF: Acute laryngeal obstruction due to allergies, foreign bodies, or in the majority of cases a viral infection. Symptoms include a harsh, barking cough, hoarseness, and a persistent, high-pitched respiratory sound (stridor).

✓5ᵗʰ **J05.1** **Acute epiglottitis**
    EXCLUDES 2   *epiglottitis, chronic (J37.0)*

J05.10 **Acute epiglottitis without obstruction**   CC
Epiglottitis NOS
    CC Excl: PDX collection 732

J05.11 **Acute epiglottitis with obstruction**   MCC
    CC Excl: PDX collection 730

✓4ᵗʰ **J06** **Acute upper respiratory infections of multiple and unspecified sites**
    EXCLUDES 1   *acute respiratory infection NOS (J22)*
           streptococcal pharyngitis (J02.0)

J06.0 **Acute laryngopharyngitis**
J06.9 **Acute upper respiratory infection, unspecified**
Upper respiratory disease, acute
Upper respiratory infection NOS
▶Use additional code (B95-B97) to identify infectious agent, if known, such as:◀
▶respiratory syncytial virus (RSV) (B97.4)◀

Influenza and pneumonia (J09-J18)

    EXCLUDES 2   *allergic or eosinophilic pneumonia (J82)*
           aspiration pneumonia NOS (J69.0)
           meconium pneumonia (P24.01)
           neonatal aspiration pneumonia (P24.-)
           pneumonia due to solids and liquids (J69.-)
           congenital pneumonia (P23.9)
           lipid pneumonia (J69.1)
           rheumatic pneumonia (I00)
           ventilator associated pneumonia (J95.851)

AHA: 2017,4Q,96
TIP: Documentation of lobar pneumonia or multilobar pneumonia should be coded to J18.1 when the specific organism causing the pneumonia is not identified. When the organism is documented, lobar pneumonia or multilobar pneumonia should be coded using categories J12-J16, depending on the organism that is present.
TIP: Hemoptysis (R04.2) is not customarily associated with pneumonia and may be reported separately.
CC Excl: For MCC codes in categories J09-J18, unless otherwise noted: PDX collection 110

✓4ᵗʰ **J09** **Influenza due to certain identified influenza viruses**
    EXCLUDES 1   *influenza A/H1N1 (J10.-)*
           influenza due to other identified influenza virus (J10.-)
           influenza due to unidentified influenza virus (J11.-)
           seasonal influenza due to other identified influenza virus (J10.-)
           seasonal influenza due to unidentified influenza virus (J11.-)

✓5ᵗʰ **J09.X** **Influenza due to identified novel influenza A virus**
Avian influenza
Bird influenza
Influenza A/H5N1
Influenza of other animal origin, not bird or swine
Swine influenza virus (viruses that normally cause infections in pigs)
AHA: 2016,3Q,10

J09.X1 **Influenza due to identified novel influenza A virus with pneumonia**   HIV MCC
Code also, if applicable, associated:
    lung abscess (J85.1)
    other specified type of pneumonia

J09.X2 **Influenza due to identified novel influenza A virus with other respiratory manifestations**
Influenza due to identified novel influenza A virus NOS
Influenza due to identified novel influenza A virus with laryngitis
Influenza due to identified novel influenza A virus with pharyngitis
Influenza due to identified novel influenza A virus with upper respiratory symptoms
Use additional code, if applicable, for associated:
    pleural effusion (J91.8)
    sinusitis (J01.-)

J09.X3 **Influenza due to identified novel influenza A virus with gastrointestinal manifestations**
Influenza due to identified novel influenza A virus gastroenteritis
    EXCLUDES 1   *'intestinal flu' [viral gastroenteritis] (A08.-)*

J09.X9 **Influenza due to identified novel influenza A virus with other manifestations**
Influenza due to identified novel influenza A virus with encephalopathy
Influenza due to identified novel influenza A virus with myocarditis
Influenza due to identified novel influenza A virus with otitis media
Use additional code to identify manifestation

✓4ᵗʰ **J10** **Influenza due to other identified influenza virus**
    EXCLUDES 1   *influenza due to avian influenza virus (J09.X-)*
           influenza due to swine flu (J09.X-)
           influenza due to unidentifed influenza virus (J11.-)

✓5ᵗʰ **J10.0** **Influenza due to other identified influenza virus with pneumonia**
Code also associated lung abscess, if applicable (J85.1)

    J10.00 **Influenza due to other identified influenza virus with unspecified type of pneumonia**   MCC

J10.Ø1   Influenza due to other identified influenza virus with the same other identified influenza virus pneumonia   `MCC`

J10.Ø8   Influenza due to other identified influenza virus with other specified pneumonia   `HIV` `MCC`
> Code also other specified type of pneumonia
> **CC Excl:** PDX collection 733

J10.1   Influenza due to other identified influenza virus with other respiratory manifestations   `CC`
> Influenza due to other identified influenza virus NOS
> Influenza due to other identified influenza virus with laryngitis
> Influenza due to other identified influenza virus with pharyngitis
> Influenza due to other identified influenza virus with upper respiratory symptoms
> Use additional code for associated pleural effusion, if applicable (J91.8)
> Use additional code for associated sinusitis, if applicable (J01.-)
> **AHA:** 2016,3Q,10-11

J10.2   Influenza due to other identified influenza virus with gastrointestinal manifestations
> Influenza due to other identified influenza virus gastroenteritis
> **EXCLUDES 1**   "intestinal flu" [viral gastroenteritis] (A08.-)

✓5ᵗʰ **J10.8**   Influenza due to other identified influenza virus with other manifestations

     J10.81   Influenza due to other identified influenza virus with encephalopathy

     J10.82   Influenza due to other identified influenza virus with myocarditis

     J10.83   Influenza due to other identified influenza virus with otitis media
> > Use additional code for any associated perforated tympanic membrane (H72.-)

     J10.89   Influenza due to other identified influenza virus with other manifestations
> > Use additional codes to identify the manifestations

✓4ᵗʰ **J11**   **Influenza due to unidentified influenza virus**

     ✓5ᵗʰ **J11.Ø**   Influenza due to unidentified influenza virus with pneumonia
> > Code also associated lung abscess, if applicable (J85.1)
> > **AHA:** 2016,3Q,11

         J11.ØØ   Influenza due to unidentified influenza virus with unspecified type of pneumonia   `MCC`
> > > Influenza with pneumonia NOS

         J11.Ø8   Influenza due to unidentified influenza virus with specified pneumonia   `MCC`
> > > Code also other specified type of pneumonia

     J11.1   Influenza due to unidentified influenza virus with other respiratory manifestations
> > Influenza NOS
> > Influenzal laryngitis NOS
> > Influenzal pharyngitis NOS
> > Influenza with upper respiratory symptoms NOS
> > Use additional code for associated pleural effusion, if applicable (J91.8)
> > Use additional code for associated sinusitis, if applicable (J01.-)

     J11.2   Influenza due to unidentified influenza virus with gastrointestinal manifestations
> > Influenza gastroenteritis NOS
> > **EXCLUDES 1**   "intestinal flu" [viral gastroenteritis] (A08.-)

     ✓5ᵗʰ **J11.8**   Influenza due to unidentified influenza virus with other manifestations

         J11.81   Influenza due to unidentified influenza virus with encephalopathy
> > > Influenzal encephalopathy NOS

         J11.82   Influenza due to unidentified influenza virus with myocarditis
> > > Influenzal myocarditis NOS

         J11.83   Influenza due to unidentified influenza virus with otitis media
> > > Influenzal otitis media NOS
> > > Use additional code for any associated perforated tympanic membrane (H72.-)

         J11.89   Influenza due to unidentified influenza virus with other manifestations
> > > Use additional codes to identify the manifestations

✓4ᵗʰ **J12**   **Viral pneumonia, not elsewhere classified**
> **INCLUDES**   bronchopneumonia due to viruses other than influenza viruses
> Code first associated influenza, if applicable (J09.X1, J10.0-, J11.0-)
> Code also associated abscess, if applicable (J85.1)
> **EXCLUDES 1**   aspiration pneumonia due to anesthesia during labor and delivery (O74.0)
> > aspiration pneumonia due to anesthesia during pregnancy (O29)
> > aspiration pneumonia due to anesthesia during puerperium (O89.0)
> > aspiration pneumonia due to solids and liquids (J69.-)
> > aspiration pneumonia NOS (J69.0)
> > congenital pneumonia (P23.0)
> > congenital rubella pneumonitis (P35.0)
> > interstitial pneumonia NOS (J84.9)
> > lipid pneumonia (J69.1)
> > neonatal aspiration pneumonia (P24.-)
> **AHA:** 2019,1Q,35; 2018,3Q,24; 2016,3Q,15; 2013,4Q,118
> **CC Excl: For MCC codes in category J12, unless otherwise noted:** PDX collection 734

     J12.Ø   Adenoviral pneumonia   `MCC`

     J12.1   Respiratory syncytial virus pneumonia   `MCC`
> > ▶RSV pneumonia◀

     J12.2   Parainfluenza virus pneumonia   `MCC`

     J12.3   Human metapneumovirus pneumonia   `HIV` `MCC`

     ✓5ᵗʰ **J12.8**   Other viral pneumonia

         J12.81   Pneumonia due to SARS-associated coronavirus   `HIV` `MCC`
> > > Severe acute respiratory syndrome NOS
> > > **DEF:** Severe adult respiratory syndrome caused by the coronavirus, specified as inflammation of the lungs with consolidation.
> > > **CC Excl:** PDX collection 735

         J12.89   Other viral pneumonia   `HIV` `MCC`

     J12.9   Viral pneumonia, unspecified   `HIV` `MCC`

J13   **Pneumonia due to Streptococcus pneumoniae**   `HIV` `MCC` `HCC`
> Bronchopneumonia due to S. pneumoniae
> Code first associated influenza, if applicable (J09.X1, J10.0-, J11.0-)
> Code also associated abscess, if applicable (J85.1)
> **EXCLUDES 1**   congenital pneumonia due to S. pneumoniae (P23.6)
> > lobar pneumonia, unspecified organism (J18.1)
> > pneumonia due to other streptococci (J15.3-J15.4)
> **AHA:** 2019,1Q,35; 2018,3Q,24; 2016,3Q,15; 2013,4Q,118

J14   **Pneumonia due to Hemophilus influenzae**   `HIV` `MCC` `HCC`
> Bronchopneumonia due to H. influenzae
> Code first associated influenza, if applicable (J09.X1, J10.0-, J11.0-)
> Code also associated abscess, if applicable (J85.1)
> **EXCLUDES 1**   congenital pneumonia due to H. influenzae (P23.6)
> **AHA:** 2019,1Q,35; 2018,3Q,24; 2016,3Q,15; 2013,4Q,118

✓4ᵗʰ **J15**   **Bacterial pneumonia, not elsewhere classified**
> **INCLUDES**   Bronchopneumonia due to bacteria other than S. pneumoniae and H. influenzae
> Code first associated influenza, if applicable (J09.X1, J10.0-, -J11.0-)
> Code also associated abscess, if applicable (J85.1)
> **EXCLUDES 1**   chlamydial pneumonia (J16.0)
> > congenital pneumonia (P23.-)
> > Legionnaires' disease (A48.1)
> > spirochetal pneumonia (A69.8)
> **AHA:** 2019,1Q,35; 2018,3Q,24; 2016,3Q,15; 2013,4Q,118

     J15.Ø   Pneumonia due to Klebsiella pneumoniae   `HIV` `MCC` `HCC`

     J15.1   Pneumonia due to Pseudomonas   `HIV` `MCC` `HCC`

     ✓5ᵗʰ **J15.2**   Pneumonia due to staphylococcus

         J15.2Ø   Pneumonia due to staphylococcus, unspecified   `HIV` `MCC` `HCC`

         ✓6ᵗʰ **J15.21**   Pneumonia due to Staphylococcus aureus

             J15.211   Pneumonia due to methicillin susceptible Staphylococcus aureus   `HIV` `MCC` `HCC`
> > > > MSSA pneumonia
> > > > Pneumonia due to Staphylococcus aureus NOS

☑ Additional Character Required   ✓x7ᵗʰ Placeholder   Unacceptable PDx   Questionable PDx   Manifestation   Unspecified Dx   `H1`-`H14` HAC   `HCC` CMS-HCC Dx   `HIV` HIV Dx

ICD-10-CM 2020   **695**

| | J15.212 | **Pneumonia due to methicillin resistant Staphylococcus aureus** | HIV MCC HCC |
| | J15.29 | **Pneumonia due to other staphylococcus** | HIV MCC HCC |

J15.3 **Pneumonia due to streptococcus, group B** HIV MCC HCC

J15.4 **Pneumonia due to other streptococci** HIV MCC HCC

> EXCLUDES 1 pneumonia due to streptococcus, group B (J15.3)
> pneumonia due to Streptococcus pneumoniae (J13)

J15.5 **Pneumonia due to Escherichia coli** HIV MCC HCC

J15.6 **Pneumonia due to other Gram-negative bacteria** HIV MCC HCC

Pneumonia due to other aerobic Gram-negative bacteria
Pneumonia due to Serratia marcescens

J15.7 **Pneumonia due to Mycoplasma pneumoniae** MCC

J15.8 **Pneumonia due to other specified bacteria** HIV MCC HCC

J15.9 **Unspecified bacterial pneumonia** HIV MCC

Pneumonia due to gram-positive bacteria

✓4th **J16** **Pneumonia due to other infectious organisms, not elsewhere classified**

Code first associated influenza, if applicable (J09.X1, J10.0-, J11.0-)
Code also associated abscess, if applicable (J85.1)

> EXCLUDES 1 congenital pneumonia (P23.-)
> ornithosis (A70)
> pneumocystosis (B59)
> pneumonia NOS (J18.9)

AHA: 2019,1Q,35; 2018,3Q,24; 2016,3Q,15; 2013,4Q,118

J16.0 **Chlamydial pneumonia** MCC

J16.8 **Pneumonia due to other specified infectious organisms** MCC

J17 *Pneumonia in diseases classified elsewhere* MCC

Code first underlying disease, such as:
Q fever (A78)
rheumatic fever (I00)
schistosomiasis (B65.0-B65.9)

> EXCLUDES 1 candidial pneumonia (B37.1)
> chlamydial pneumonia (J16.0)
> gonorrheal pneumonia (A54.84)
> histoplasmosis pneumonia (B39.0-B39.2)
> measles pneumonia (B05.2)
> nocardiosis pneumonia (A43.0)
> pneumocystosis (B59)
> pneumonia due to Pneumocystis carinii (B59)
> pneumonia due to Pneumocystis jiroveci (B59)
> pneumonia in actinomycosis (A42.0)
> pneumonia in anthrax (A22.1)
> pneumonia in ascariasis (B77.81)
> pneumonia in aspergillosis (B44.0-B44.1)
> pneumonia in coccidioidomycosis (B38.0-B38.2)
> pneumonia in cytomegalovirus disease (B25.0)
> pneumonia in toxoplasmosis (B58.3)
> rubella pneumonia (B06.81)
> salmonella pneumonia (A02.22)
> spirochetal infection NEC with pneumonia (A69.8)
> tularemia (A21.2)
> typhoid fever with pneumonia (A01.03)
> varicella pneumonia (B01.2)
> whooping cough with pneumonia (A37 with fifth character 1)

AHA: 2019,1Q,35; 2016,3Q,15; 2013,4Q,118

✓4th **J18** **Pneumonia, unspecified organism**

Code first associated influenza, if applicable (J09.X1, J10.0-, J11.0-)

> EXCLUDES 1 abscess of lung with pneumonia (J85.1)
> aspiration pneumonia due to anesthesia during labor and delivery (O74.0)
> aspiration pneumonia due to anesthesia during pregnancy (O29)
> aspiration pneumonia due to anesthesia during puerperium (O89.0)
> aspiration pneumonia due to solids and liquids (J69.-)
> aspiration pneumonia NOS (J69.0)
> congenital pneumonia (P23.0)
> drug-induced interstitial lung disorder (J70.2-J70.4)
> interstitial pneumonia NOS (J84.9)
> lipid pneumonia (J69.1)
> neonatal aspiration pneumonia (P24.-)
> pneumonitis due to external agents (J67-J70)
> pneumonitis due to fumes and vapors (J68.0)
> usual interstitial pneumonia (J84.17)

AHA: 2019,1Q,35; 2016,3Q,15; 2013,4Q,118

J18.0 **Bronchopneumonia, unspecified organism** MCC

> EXCLUDES 1 hypostatic bronchopneumonia (J18.2)
> lipid pneumonia (J69.1)
> EXCLUDES 2 acute bronchiolitis (J21.-)
> chronic bronchiolitis (J44.9)

J18.1 **Lobar pneumonia, unspecified organism** HIV MCC HCC

AHA: 2018,3Q,24

TIP: Use this code for documented lobar pneumonia or multilobar pneumonia when the causal organism is not identified. If the causal organism is identified, codes from categories J12-J16 should be used, depending on the organism that is present.

J18.2 **Hypostatic pneumonia, unspecified organism** CC

Hypostatic bronchopneumonia
Passive pneumonia
CC Excl: PDX collection 736

J18.8 **Other pneumonia, unspecified organism** HIV MCC

J18.9 **Pneumonia, unspecified organism** HIV MCC

AHA: 2019,2Q,28; 2014,3Q,4; 2013,4Q,119; 2012,4Q,94

Other acute lower respiratory infections (J20-J22)

> EXCLUDES 2 chronic obstructive pulmonary disease with acute lower respiratory infection (J44.0)

✓4th **J20** **Acute bronchitis**

> INCLUDES acute and subacute bronchitis (with) bronchospasm
> acute and subacute bronchitis (with) tracheitis
> acute and subacute bronchitis (with) tracheobronchitis, acute
> acute and subacute fibrinous bronchitis
> acute and subacute membranous bronchitis
> acute and subacute purulent bronchitis
> acute and subacute septic bronchitis
> EXCLUDES 1 bronchitis NOS (J40)
> tracheobronchitis NOS (J40)
> EXCLUDES 2 acute bronchitis with bronchiectasis (J47.0)
> acute bronchitis with chronic obstructive asthma (J44.0)
> acute bronchitis with chronic obstructive pulmonary disease (J44.0)
> allergic bronchitis NOS (J45.909-)
> bronchitis due to chemicals, fumes and vapors (J68.0)
> chronic bronchitis NOS (J42)
> chronic mucopurulent bronchitis (J41.1)
> chronic obstructive bronchitis (J44.-)
> chronic obstructive tracheobronchitis (J44.-)
> chronic simple bronchitis (J41.0)
> chronic tracheobronchitis (J42)

AHA: 2019,1Q,35; 2016,3Q,10,16

DEF: Acute inflammation of the main branches of the bronchial tree due to infectious or irritant agents. Symptoms include cough with a varied production of sputum, fever, substernal soreness, and lung rales. Bronchitis usually lasts three to 10 days.

J20.0 **Acute bronchitis due to Mycoplasma pneumoniae**

J20.1 **Acute bronchitis due to Hemophilus influenzae**

J20.2 **Acute bronchitis due to streptococcus**

J20.3 **Acute bronchitis due to coxsackievirus**

J20.4 **Acute bronchitis due to parainfluenza virus**

J20.5   **Acute bronchitis due to** respiratory syncytial virus
▶Acute bronchitis due to RSV◀

J20.6   **Acute bronchitis due to** rhinovirus

J20.7   **Acute bronchitis due to** echovirus

J20.8   **Acute bronchitis due to other specified organisms**

J20.9   **Acute bronchitis, unspecified**

✓4ᵗʰ **J21   Acute bronchiolitis**

     INCLUDES   acute bronchiolitis with bronchospasm

     EXCLUDES 2   *respiratory bronchiolitis interstitial lung disease (J84.115)*

     CC Excl: For CC codes in category J21, unless otherwise noted: PDX collection 738

J21.0   **Acute bronchiolitis due to** respiratory syncytial virus   CC
▶Acute bronchiolitis due to RSV◀
     CC Excl: PDX collection 737

J21.1   **Acute bronchiolitis due to** human metapneumovirus   CC

J21.8   **Acute bronchiolitis due to other specified organisms**   CC

J21.9   **Acute bronchiolitis, unspecified**   CC
Bronchiolitis (acute)
     EXCLUDES 1   *chronic bronchiolitis (J44.-)*

J22   Unspecified acute lower respiratory infection
Acute (lower) respiratory (tract) infection NOS
     EXCLUDES 1   *upper respiratory infection (acute) (J06.9)*

Other diseases of upper respiratory tract (J30-J39)

✓4ᵗʰ **J30   Vasomotor and allergic rhinitis**

     INCLUDES   spasmodic rhinorrhea

     EXCLUDES 1   *allergic rhinitis with asthma (bronchial) (J45.909)*
                 rhinitis NOS (J31.0)

J30.0   **Vasomotor** rhinitis
     DEF: Noninfectious and nonallergic type of rhinitis for which the cause is often unknown. Symptoms often mimic those of allergic rhinitis with a diagnosis of vasomotor rhinitis typically made after ruling out allergens as the cause.

J30.1   **Allergic** rhinitis **due to pollen**
Allergy NOS due to pollen
Hay fever
Pollinosis

J30.2   **Other** seasonal allergic rhinitis

J30.5   **Allergic** rhinitis **due to food**

✓5ᵗʰ **J30.8**   **Other allergic rhinitis**

     J30.81   **Allergic rhinitis due to** animal (cat) (dog) hair and dander

     J30.89   **Other allergic rhinitis**
              Perennial allergic rhinitis

J30.9   **Allergic rhinitis, unspecified**

✓4ᵗʰ **J31   Chronic rhinitis, nasopharyngitis and pharyngitis**
Use additional code to identify:
     exposure to environmental tobacco smoke (Z77.22)
     exposure to tobacco smoke in the perinatal period (P96.81)
     history of tobacco dependence (Z87.891)
     occupational exposure to environmental tobacco smoke (Z57.31)
     tobacco dependence (F17.-)
     tobacco use (Z72.0)

J31.0   **Chronic rhinitis**
Atrophic rhinitis (chronic)
Granulomatous rhinitis (chronic)
Hypertrophic rhinitis (chronic)
Obstructive rhinitis (chronic)
Ozena
Purulent rhinitis (chronic)
Rhinitis (chronic) NOS
Ulcerative rhinitis (chronic)
     EXCLUDES 1   *allergic rhinitis (J30.1-J30.9)*
                 vasomotor rhinitis (J30.0)
     DEF: Persistent inflammation of the mucous membranes of the nose, characterized by a postnasal drip.

J31.1   **Chronic nasopharyngitis**
     EXCLUDES 2   *acute nasopharyngitis (J00)*
     DEF: Persistent inflammation of the mucous membranes extending from the nares to the pharynx. It is characterized by constant irritation in the nasopharynx and postnasal drip.

J31.2   **Chronic pharyngitis**
Atrophic pharyngitis (chronic)
Chronic sore throat
Granular pharyngitis (chronic)
Hypertrophic pharyngitis (chronic)
     EXCLUDES 2   *acute pharyngitis (J02.9)*

✓4ᵗʰ **J32   Chronic sinusitis**

     INCLUDES   sinus abscess
               sinus empyema
               sinus infection
               sinus suppuration
Use additional code to identify:
     exposure to environmental tobacco smoke (Z77.22)
     exposure to tobacco smoke in the perinatal period (P96.81)
     history of tobacco dependence (Z87.891)
     infectious agent (B95-B97)
     occupational exposure to environmental tobacco smoke (Z57.31)
     tobacco dependence (F17.-)
     tobacco use (Z72.0)
     EXCLUDES 2   *acute sinusitis (J01.-)*

J32.0   **Chronic** maxillary **sinusitis**
Antritis (chronic)
Maxillary sinusitis NOS

J32.1   **Chronic** frontal **sinusitis**
Frontal sinusitis NOS

J32.2   **Chronic** ethmoidal **sinusitis**
Ethmoidal sinusitis NOS
     EXCLUDES 1   *Woakes' ethmoiditis (J33.1)*

J32.3   **Chronic** sphenoidal **sinusitis**
Sphenoidal sinusitis NOS

J32.4   **Chronic** pansinusitis
Pansinusitis NOS

J32.8   **Other chronic sinusitis**
Sinusitis (chronic) involving more than one sinus but not pansinusitis

J32.9   **Chronic sinusitis, unspecified**
Sinusitis (chronic) NOS

✓4ᵗʰ **J33   Nasal polyp**
Use additional code to identify:
     exposure to environmental tobacco smoke (Z77.22)
     exposure to tobacco smoke in the perinatal period (P96.81)
     history of tobacco dependence (Z87.891)
     occupational exposure to environmental tobacco smoke (Z57.31)
     tobacco dependence (F17.-)
     tobacco use (Z72.0)
     EXCLUDES 1   *adenomatous polyps (D14.0)*

J33.0   **Polyp of nasal cavity**
Choanal polyp
Nasopharyngeal polyp

J33.1   **Polypoid sinus degeneration**
Woakes' syndrome or ethmoiditis

J33.8   **Other polyp of sinus**
Accessory polyp of sinus
Ethmoidal polyp of sinus
Maxillary polyp of sinus
Sphenoidal polyp of sinus

J33.9   **Nasal polyp, unspecified**

✓4ᵗʰ **J34   Other and unspecified disorders of nose and nasal sinuses**
     EXCLUDES 2   *varicose ulcer of nasal septum (I86.8)*

J34.0   **Abscess, furuncle and carbuncle of nose**
Cellulitis of nose
Necrosis of nose
Ulceration of nose

J34.1   **Cyst and mucocele of nose and nasal sinus**

J34.2   **Deviated nasal septum**
Deflection or deviation of septum (nasal) (acquired)
     EXCLUDES 1   *congenital deviated nasal septum (Q67.4)*
     DEF: Condition in which the nasal septum, a thin wall composed of cartilage and bone that separates the two nostrils, is crooked or displaced from the midline.

J34.3   **Hypertrophy of nasal turbinates**
     DEF: Overgrowth of bones within the nasal turbinate, which are ridges of bone and soft tissue that project from the sidewalls of the nasal passages. Hypertrophy can cause obstruction of the nasal passages.

√5ᵗʰ **J34.8 Other specified disorders of nose and nasal sinuses**

J34.81 Nasal mucositis (ulcerative)
Code also type of associated therapy, such as:
antineoplastic and immunosuppressive drugs (T45.1X-)
radiological procedure and radiotherapy (Y84.2)
EXCLUDES 2 *gastrointestinal mucositis (ulcerative) (K92.81)*
mucositis (ulcerative) of vagina and vulva (N76.81)
oral mucositis (ulcerative) (K12.3-)

J34.89 Other specified disorders of nose and nasal sinuses
Perforation of nasal septum NOS
Rhinolith

J34.9 Unspecified disorder of nose and nasal sinuses

√4ᵗʰ **J35 Chronic diseases of tonsils and adenoids**
Use additional code to identify:
exposure to environmental tobacco smoke (Z77.22)
exposure to tobacco smoke in the perinatal period (P96.81)
history of tobacco dependence (Z87.891)
occupational exposure to environmental tobacco smoke (Z57.31)
tobacco dependence (F17.-)
tobacco use (Z72.0)

√5ᵗʰ **J35.0 Chronic tonsillitis and adenoiditis**
EXCLUDES 2 *acute tonsillitis (J03.-)*

J35.01 Chronic tonsillitis
J35.02 Chronic adenoiditis
J35.03 Chronic tonsillitis and adenoiditis

J35.1 Hypertrophy of tonsils
Enlargement of tonsils
EXCLUDES 1 *hypertrophy of tonsils with tonsillitis (J35.0-)*

J35.2 Hypertrophy of adenoids
Enlargement of adenoids
EXCLUDES 1 *hypertrophy of adenoids with adenoiditis (J35.0-)*

J35.3 Hypertrophy of tonsils with hypertrophy of adenoids
EXCLUDES 1 *hypertrophy of tonsils and adenoids with tonsillitis and adenoiditis (J35.03)*

J35.8 Other chronic diseases of tonsils and adenoids
Adenoid vegetations
Amygdalolith
Calculus, tonsil
Cicatrix of tonsil (and adenoid)
Tonsillar tag
Ulcer of tonsil

J35.9 Chronic disease of tonsils and adenoids, unspecified
Disease (chronic) of tonsils and adenoids NOS

J36 Peritonsillar abscess CC
INCLUDES abscess of tonsil
peritonsillar cellulitis
quinsy
Use additional code (B95-B97) to identify infectious agent
EXCLUDES 1 *acute tonsillitis (J03.-)*
chronic tonsillitis (J35.0)
retropharyngeal abscess (J39.0)
tonsillitis NOS (J03.9-)
CC Excl: PDX collection 739

√4ᵗʰ **J37 Chronic laryngitis and laryngotracheitis**
Use additional code to identify:
exposure to environmental tobacco smoke (Z77.22)
exposure to tobacco smoke in the perinatal period (P96.81)
history of tobacco dependence (Z87.891)
infectious agent (B95-B97)
occupational exposure to environmental tobacco smoke (Z57.31)
tobacco dependence (F17.-)
tobacco use (Z72.0)

J37.0 Chronic laryngitis
Catarrhal laryngitis
Hypertrophic laryngitis
Sicca laryngitis
EXCLUDES 2 *acute laryngitis (J04.0)*
obstructive (acute) laryngitis (J05.0)

J37.1 Chronic laryngotracheitis
Laryngitis, chronic, with tracheitis (chronic)
Tracheitis, chronic, with laryngitis
EXCLUDES 1 *chronic tracheitis (J42)*
EXCLUDES 2 *acute laryngotracheitis (J04.2)*
acute tracheitis (J04.1)

√4ᵗʰ **J38 Diseases of vocal cords and larynx, not elsewhere classified**
Use additional code to identify:
exposure to environmental tobacco smoke (Z77.22)
exposure to tobacco smoke in the perinatal period (P96.81)
history of tobacco dependence (Z87.891)
occupational exposure to environmental tobacco smoke (Z57.31)
tobacco dependence (F17.-)
tobacco use (Z72.0)
EXCLUDES 1 *congenital laryngeal stridor (P28.89)*
obstructive laryngitis (acute) (J05.0)
postprocedural subglottic stenosis (J95.5)
stridor (R06.1)
ulcerative laryngitis (J04.0)

√5ᵗʰ **J38.0 Paralysis of vocal cords and larynx**
Laryngoplegia
Paralysis of glottis

J38.00 Paralysis of vocal cords and larynx, unspecified
J38.01 Paralysis of vocal cords and larynx, unilateral
J38.02 Paralysis of vocal cords and larynx, bilateral

J38.1 Polyp of vocal cord and larynx
EXCLUDES 1 *adenomatous polyps (D14.1)*

J38.2 Nodules of vocal cords
Chorditis (fibrinous)(nodosa)(tuberosa)
Singer's nodes
Teacher's nodes

J38.3 Other diseases of vocal cords
Abscess of vocal cords
Cellulitis of vocal cords
Granuloma of vocal cords
Leukokeratosis of vocal cords
Leukoplakia of vocal cords

J38.4 Edema of larynx
Edema (of) glottis
Subglottic edema
Supraglottic edema
EXCLUDES 1 *acute obstructive laryngitis [croup] (J05.0)*
edematous laryngitis (J04.0)

J38.5 Laryngeal spasm
Laryngismus (stridulus)

J38.6 Stenosis of larynx

J38.7 Other diseases of larynx
Abscess of larynx
Cellulitis of larynx
Disease of larynx NOS
Necrosis of larynx
Pachyderma of larynx
Perichondritis of larynx
Ulcer of larynx

√4ᵗʰ **J39 Other diseases of upper respiratory tract**
EXCLUDES 1 *acute respiratory infection NOS (J22)*
acute upper respiratory infection (J06.9)
upper respiratory inflammation due to chemicals, gases, fumes or vapors (J68.2)

J39.0 Retropharyngeal and parapharyngeal abscess CC
Peripharyngeal abscess
EXCLUDES 1 *peritonsillar abscess (J36)*
DEF: Purulent infection behind the pharynx and the front of the precerebral fascia, characterized by neck stiffness, cervical lymphadenopathy, sore throat, fever, and stridor.
CC Excl: PDX collection 740

J39.1 Other abscess of pharynx CC
Cellulitis of pharynx
Nasopharyngeal abscess
CC Excl: PDX collection 740

J39.2 Other diseases of pharynx
Cyst of pharynx
Edema of pharynx
> EXCLUDES 2   *chronic pharyngitis (J31.2)*
> *ulcerative pharyngitis (J02.9)*

J39.3 Upper respiratory tract hypersensitivity reaction, site unspecified
> EXCLUDES 1   *hypersensitivity reaction of upper respiratory tract, such as:*
> *extrinsic allergic alveolitis (J67.9)*
> *pneumoconiosis (J60-J67.9)*

J39.8 Other specified diseases of upper respiratory tract
J39.9 Disease of upper respiratory tract, unspecified

Chronic lower respiratory diseases (J40-J47)

> EXCLUDES 1   *bronchitis due to chemicals, gases, fumes and vapors (J68.0)*
> EXCLUDES 2   *cystic fibrosis (E84.-)*

J40 Bronchitis, not specified as acute or chronic
Bronchitis NOS
Bronchitis with tracheitis NOS
Catarrhal bronchitis
Tracheobronchitis NOS
Use additional code to identify:
  exposure to environmental tobacco smoke (Z77.22)
  exposure to tobacco smoke in the perinatal period (P96.81)
  history of tobacco dependence (Z87.891)
  occupational exposure to environmental tobacco smoke (Z57.31)
  tobacco dependence (F17.-)
  tobacco use (Z72.0)
> EXCLUDES 1   *acute bronchitis (J20.-)*
> *allergic bronchitis NOS (J45.909-)*
> *asthmatic bronchitis NOS (J45.9-)*
> *bronchitis due to chemicals, gases, fumes and vapors (J68.0)*

✓4ᵗʰ J41 Simple and mucopurulent chronic bronchitis
Use additional code to identify:
  exposure to environmental tobacco smoke (Z77.22)
  exposure to tobacco smoke in the perinatal period (P96.81)
  history of tobacco dependence (Z87.891)
  occupational exposure to environmental tobacco smoke (Z57.31)
  tobacco dependence (F17.-)
  tobacco use (Z72.0)
> EXCLUDES 1   *chronic bronchitis NOS (J42)*
> *chronic obstructive bronchitis (J44.-)*

J41.0 Simple chronic bronchitis   HCC
J41.1 Mucopurulent chronic bronchitis   HCC
J41.8 Mixed simple and mucopurulent chronic bronchitis   HCC

J42 Unspecified chronic bronchitis   HCC
Chronic bronchitis NOS
Chronic tracheitis
Chronic tracheobronchitis
Use additional code to identify:
  exposure to environmental tobacco smoke (Z77.22)
  exposure to tobacco smoke in the perinatal period (P96.81)
  history of tobacco dependence (Z87.891)
  occupational exposure to environmental tobacco smoke (Z57.31)
  tobacco dependence (F17.-)
  tobacco use (Z72.0)
> EXCLUDES 1   *chronic asthmatic bronchitis (J44.-)*
> *chronic bronchitis with airways obstruction (J44.-)*
> *chronic emphysematous bronchitis (J44.-)*
> *chronic obstructive pulmonary disease NOS (J44.9)*
> *simple and mucopurulent chronic bronchitis (J41.-)*

✓4ᵗʰ J43 Emphysema
Use additional code to identify:
  exposure to environmental tobacco smoke (Z77.22)
  history of tobacco dependence (Z87.891)
  occupational exposure to environmental tobacco smoke (Z57.31)
  tobacco dependence (F17.-)
  tobacco use (Z72.0)
> EXCLUDES 1   *compensatory emphysema (J98.3)*
> *emphysema due to inhalation of chemicals, gases, fumes or vapors (J68.4)*
> *emphysema with chronic (obstructive) bronchitis (J44.-)*
> *emphysematous (obstructive) bronchitis (J44.-)*
> *interstitial emphysema (J98.2)*
> *mediastinal emphysema (J98.2)*
> *neonatal interstitial emphysema (P25.0)*
> *surgical (subcutaneous) emphysema (T81.82)*
> *traumatic subcutaneous emphysema (T79.7)*

DEF: Pathological condition in which there is destructive enlargement of the air sacs in the lungs resulting in damage and lack of elasticity to the alveolar walls, commonly seen in long-term smokers.

Emphysema

Healthy alveoli — Patent bronchiole — Well-vascularized — Dilated alveoli — Excess mucus

Alveoli w/ Emphysema — Collapsed bronchiole — Enlarged alveoli — Broken/fewer capillaries — Alveolar membranes break down

J43.0 Unilateral pulmonary emphysema [MacLeod's syndrome]   HCC
Swyer-James syndrome
Unilateral emphysema
Unilateral hyperlucent lung
Unilateral pulmonary artery functional hypoplasia
Unilateral transparency of lung

J43.1 Panlobular emphysema   HCC
Panacinar emphysema

J43.2 Centrilobular emphysema   HCC
J43.8 Other emphysema   HCC
J43.9 Emphysema, unspecified   HCC
Bullous emphysema (lung)(pulmonary)
Emphysema (lung)(pulmonary) NOS
Emphysematous bleb
Vesicular emphysema (lung)(pulmonary)
AHA: 2019,1Q,34-36; 2017,4Q,97-98

☑ Additional Character Required   ✓x7ᵗʰ Placeholder   Unacceptable PDx   Questionable PDx   Manifestation   Unspecified Dx   H1-H14 HAC   HCC CMS-HCC Dx   HIV HIV Dx
ICD-10-CM 2020   **699**

J39.2–J43.9

✓4ᵗʰ **J44 Other chronic obstructive pulmonary disease**

> **INCLUDES** asthma with chronic obstructive pulmonary disease
> chronic asthmatic (obstructive) bronchitis
> chronic bronchitis with airways obstruction
> chronic bronchitis with emphysema
> chronic emphysematous bronchitis
> chronic obstructive asthma
> chronic obstructive bronchitis
> chronic obstructive tracheobronchitis

Code also type of asthma, if applicable (J45.-)
Use additional code to identify:
  exposure to environmental tobacco smoke (Z77.22)
  history of tobacco dependence (Z87.891)
  occupational exposure to environmental tobacco smoke (Z57.31)
  tobacco dependence (F17.-)
  tobacco use (Z72.0)

> **EXCLUDES 1** bronchiectasis (J47.-)
> chronic bronchitis NOS (J42)
> chronic simple and mucopurulent bronchitis (J41.-)
> chronic tracheitis (J42)
> chronic tracheobronchitis (J42)
> emphysema without chronic bronchitis (J43.-)

AHA: 2019,1Q,34-36; 2017,4Q,97-98; 2017,1Q,25-26; 2016,3Q,15-16; 2013,4Q,109

▲ **J44.0 Chronic obstructive pulmonary disease with**   CC HCC
(acute) lower respiratory infection
  Code also to identify the infection
  AHA: 2019,1Q,35; 2017,4Q,96; 2017,1Q,24-25
  TIP: Do not assign when only aspiration pneumonia is present. Aspiration pneumonis is not classified as a respiratory infection.

J44.1 Chronic obstructive pulmonary disease with   CC HCC
(acute) exacerbation
  Decompensated COPD
  Decompensated COPD with (acute) exacerbation
  > **EXCLUDES 2** chronic obstructive pulmonary disease [COPD] with acute bronchitis (J44.0)
  > lung diseases due to external agents (J60-J70)
  AHA: 2019,1Q,34; 2017,4Q,96; 2017,1Q,26; 2016,1Q,36
  TIP: Exacerbation of COPD should not be assumed based upon worsening of a concomitant respiratory disease or when COPD is described as end-stage.
  CC Excl: PDX collection 741

J44.9 Chronic obstructive pulmonary disease,   HCC
unspecified
  Chronic obstructive airway disease NOS
  Chronic obstructive lung disease NOS
  > **EXCLUDES 2** lung diseases due to external agents (J60-J70)
  AHA: 2019,1Q,36; 2017,4Q,96-97; 2016,1Q,36; 2014,4Q,21; 2013,4Q,109

✓4ᵗʰ **J45 Asthma**

> **INCLUDES** allergic (predominantly) asthma
> allergic bronchitis NOS
> allergic rhinitis with asthma
> atopic asthma
> extrinsic allergic asthma
> hay fever with asthma
> idiosyncratic asthma
> intrinsic nonallergic asthma
> nonallergic asthma

Use additional code to identify:
  exposure to environmental tobacco smoke (Z77.22)
  exposure to tobacco smoke in the perinatal period (P96.81)
  history of tobacco dependence (Z87.891)
  occupational exposure to environmental tobacco smoke (Z57.31)
  tobacco dependence (F17.-)
  tobacco use (Z72.0)

> **EXCLUDES 1** detergent asthma (J69.8)
> eosinophilic asthma (J82)
> miner's asthma (J60)
> wheezing NOS (R06.2)
> wood asthma (J67.8)

> **EXCLUDES 2** asthma with chronic obstructive pulmonary disease (J44.9)
> chronic asthmatic (obstructive) bronchitis (J44.9)
> chronic obstructive asthma (J44.9)

AHA: 2019,1Q,36; 2017,1Q,25-26; 2012,4Q,99
DEF: Status asthmaticus: Severe, intractable episode of asthma that is unresponsive to normal therapeutic measures.
CC Excl: For CC codes in category J45: PDX collection 742

Asthma

Smooth muscle fibers
Contraction of smooth muscle fibers
Respiratory bronchiole
Mucus lining bronchial tubes
Alveoli
Extra mucus secretion in inflamed bronchial tubes
Air trapped within alveoli

Normal alveoli   Asthmatic alveoli

✓5ᵗʰ **J45.2 Mild intermittent asthma**

J45.20 Mild intermittent asthma, uncomplicated
  Mild intermittent asthma NOS

J45.21 Mild intermittent asthma with   CC
(acute) exacerbation

J45.22 Mild intermittent asthma with status   CC
asthmaticus

✓5ᵗʰ **J45.3 Mild persistent asthma**

J45.30 Mild persistent asthma, uncomplicated
  Mild persistent asthma NOS

J45.31 Mild persistent asthma with (acute)   CC
exacerbation
  AHA: 2016,1Q,35

J45.32 Mild persistent asthma with status   CC
asthmaticus

✓5ᵗʰ **J45.4 Moderate persistent asthma**

J45.40 Moderate persistent asthma, uncomplicated
  Moderate persistent asthma NOS

J45.41 Moderate persistent asthma with   CC
(acute) exacerbation
  AHA: 2017,1Q,26

J45.42 Moderate persistent asthma with   CC
status asthmaticus

✓5ᵗʰ **J45.5 Severe persistent asthma**

     J45.50 Severe persistent asthma, uncomplicated
         Severe persistent asthma NOS

     J45.51 Severe persistent asthma with (acute) exacerbation `MCC`

     J45.52 Severe persistent asthma with status asthmaticus `CC`

✓5ᵗʰ **J45.9 Other and unspecified asthma**

     ✓6ᵗʰ **J45.90 Unspecified asthma**
         Asthmatic bronchitis NOS
         Childhood asthma NOS
         Late onset asthma
         AHA: 2017,4Q,96; 2017,1Q,25

         J45.901 Unspecified asthma with (acute) exacerbation `CC`

         J45.902 Unspecified asthma with status asthmaticus `CC`

         J45.909 Unspecified asthma, uncomplicated
            Asthma NOS
            EXCLUDES 2   lung diseases due to external agents (J60-J70)
            AHA: 2017,1Q,25

     ✓6ᵗʰ **J45.99 Other asthma**

         J45.990 Exercise induced bronchospasm
         J45.991 Cough variant asthma
         J45.998 Other asthma

✓4ᵗʰ **J47 Bronchiectasis**

     `INCLUDES`   bronchiolectasis

     Use additional code to identify:
       exposure to environmental tobacco smoke (Z77.22)
       exposure to tobacco smoke in the perinatal period (P96.81)
       history of tobacco dependence (Z87.891)
       occupational exposure to environmental tobacco smoke (Z57.31)
       tobacco dependence (F17.-)
       tobacco use (Z72.0)

     EXCLUDES 1   congenital bronchiectasis (Q33.4)
              tuberculous bronchiectasis (current disease) (A15.0)

     DEF: Dilation of the bronchi with mucus production and persistent cough due to infection or chronic conditions that causes diminished lung capacity and frequent infections of the lung.

     J47.0 Bronchiectasis with acute lower respiratory infection `CC` `HCC`
         Bronchiectasis with acute bronchitis
         Use additional code to identify the infection
         CC Excl: PDX collection 743

     J47.1 Bronchiectasis with (acute) exacerbation `CC` `HCC`
         CC Excl: PDX collection 743

     J47.9 Bronchiectasis, uncomplicated `HCC`
         Bronchiectasis NOS

Lung diseases due to external agents (J60-J70)

EXCLUDES 2   asthma (J45.-)
            malignant neoplasm of bronchus and lung (C34.-)

DEF: Pneumoconiosis: Condition caused by inhaling inorganic dust particles, typically associated with occupations that require regular exposure to mineral dusts. A form of interstitial lung disease that contributes to the inflammation of the air sacs, causing the lung tissue to harden.

CC Excl: For CC/MCC codes in categories J60-J70: PDX collection 110

J60 Coalworker's pneumoconiosis `HCC` `A`

     Anthracosilicosis
     Anthracosis
     Black lung disease
     Coalworker's lung

     EXCLUDES 1   coalworker pneumoconiosis with tuberculosis, any type in A15 (J65)

J61 Pneumoconiosis due to asbestos and other mineral fibers `HCC` `A`

     Asbestosis

     EXCLUDES 1   pleural plaque with asbestosis (J92.0)
              pneumoconiosis with tuberculosis, any type in A15 (J65)

✓4ᵗʰ **J62 Pneumoconiosis due to dust containing silica**

     `INCLUDES`   silicotic fibrosis (massive) of lung
     EXCLUDES 1   pneumoconiosis with tuberculosis, any type in A15 (J65)

     J62.0 Pneumoconiosis due to talc dust `HCC`

     J62.8 Pneumoconiosis due to other dust containing silica
         Silicosis NOS

✓4ᵗʰ **J63 Pneumoconiosis due to other inorganic dusts**

     EXCLUDES 1   pneumoconiosis with tuberculosis, any type in A15 (J65)

     J63.0 Aluminosis (of lung) `HCC`
     J63.1 Bauxite fibrosis (of lung) `HCC`
     J63.2 Berylliosis `HCC`
     J63.3 Graphite fibrosis (of lung) `HCC`
     J63.4 Siderosis `HCC`
     J63.5 Stannosis `HCC`
     J63.6 Pneumoconiosis due to other specified inorganic dusts `HCC`

J64 Unspecified pneumoconiosis `HCC`

     EXCLUDES 1   pneumonoconiosis with tuberculosis, any type in A15 (J65)

J65 Pneumoconiosis associated with tuberculosis `HCC`

     Any condition in J60-J64 with tuberculosis, any type in A15
     Silicotuberculosis

✓4ᵗʰ **J66 Airway disease due to specific organic dust**

     EXCLUDES 2   allergic alveolitis (J67.-)
              asbestosis (J61)
              bagassosis (J67.1)
              farmer's lung (J67.0)
              hypersensitivity pneumonitis due to organic dust (J67.-)
              reactive airways dysfunction syndrome (J68.3)

     J66.0 Byssinosis `HCC`
         Airway disease due to cotton dust

     J66.1 Flax-dressers' disease `HCC`

     J66.2 Cannabinosis `HCC`

     J66.8 Airway disease due to other specific organic dusts `HCC`

✓4ᵗʰ **J67 Hypersensitivity pneumonitis due to organic dust**

     `INCLUDES`   allergic alveolitis and pneumonitis due to inhaled organic dust and particles of fungal, actinomycetic or other origin

     EXCLUDES 1   pneumonitis due to inhalation of chemicals, gases, fumes or vapors (J68.0)

     J67.0 Farmer's lung `HCC`
         Harvester's lung
         Haymaker's lung
         Moldy hay disease

     J67.1 Bagassosis `HCC`
         Bagasse disease
         Bagasse pneumonitis

     J67.2 Bird fancier's lung `HCC`
         Budgerigar fancier's disease or lung
         Pigeon fancier's disease or lung

     J67.3 Suberosis `HCC`
         Corkhandler's disease or lung
         Corkworker's disease or lung

     J67.4 Maltworker's lung `HCC`
         Alveolitis due to Aspergillus clavatus

     J67.5 Mushroom-worker's lung `HCC`

     J67.6 Maple-bark-stripper's lung `HCC`
         Alveolitis due to Cryptostroma corticale
         Cryptostromosis

     J67.7 Air conditioner and humidifier lung `CC` `HCC`
         Allergic alveolitis due to fungal, thermophilic actinomycetes and other organisms growing in ventilation [air conditioning] systems

     J67.8 Hypersensitivity pneumonitis due to other organic dusts `CC` `HCC`
         Cheese-washer's lung
         Coffee-worker's lung
         Fish-meal worker's lung
         Furrier's lung
         Sequoiosis

✔ Additional Character Required   ✗x7ᵗʰ Placeholder   Unacceptable PDx   Questionable PDx   Manifestation   Unspecified Dx   H1-H14 HAC   HCC CMS-HCC Dx   HIV HIV Dx

ICD-10-CM 2020   701

J67.9 **Hypersensitivity pneumonitis due to unspecified organic dust** `CC` `HCC`
> Allergic alveolitis (extrinsic) NOS
> Hypersensitivity pneumonitis NOS

`√4ᵗʰ` **J68** **Respiratory conditions due to inhalation of chemicals, gases, fumes and vapors**
> Code first (T51-T65) to identify cause
> Use additional code to identify associated respiratory conditions, such as:
> acute respiratory failure (J96.0-)

     J68.0 **Bronchitis and pneumonitis due to chemicals, gases, fumes and vapors** `CC` `HCC`
> Chemical bronchitis (acute)
> **AHA:** 2019,2Q,31

     J68.1 **Pulmonary edema due to chemicals, gases, fumes and vapors** `MCC` `HCC`
> Chemical pulmonary edema (acute) (chronic)
> *EXCLUDES 1*   *pulmonary edema (acute) (chronic) NOS (J81.-)*

     J68.2 **Upper respiratory inflammation due to chemicals, gases, fumes and vapors, not elsewhere classified** `HCC`

     J68.3 **Other acute and subacute respiratory conditions due to chemicals, gases, fumes and vapors** `HCC`
> Reactive airways dysfunction syndrome

     J68.4 **Chronic respiratory conditions due to chemicals, gases, fumes and vapors** `HCC`
> Emphysema (diffuse) (chronic) due to inhalation of chemicals, gases, fumes and vapors
> Obliterative bronchiolitis (chronic) (subacute) due to inhalation of chemicals, gases, fumes and vapors
> Pulmonary fibrosis (chronic) due to inhalation of chemicals, gases, fumes and vapors
> *EXCLUDES 1*   *chronic pulmonary edema due to chemicals, gases, fumes and vapors (J68.1)*

     J68.8 **Other respiratory conditions due to chemicals, gases, fumes and vapors** `HCC`

     J68.9 **Unspecified respiratory condition due to chemicals, gases, fumes and vapors** `HCC`

`√4ᵗʰ` **J69** **Pneumonitis due to solids and liquids**
> *EXCLUDES 1*   *neonatal aspiration syndromes (P24.-)*
>   *postprocedural pneumonitis (J95.4)*
>
> **AHA:** 2017,1Q,24
> **DEF:** Pneumonitis: Noninfectious inflammation of the walls of the alveoli in the lung tissue due to inhalation of food, vomit, oils, essences, or other solids or liquids.

     J69.0 **Pneumonitis due to inhalation of food and vomit** `MCC` `HCC`
> Aspiration pneumonia NOS
> Aspiration pneumonia (due to) food (regurgitated)
> Aspiration pneumonia (due to) gastric secretions
> Aspiration pneumonia (due to) milk
> Aspiration pneumonia (due to) vomit
> Code also any associated foreign body in respiratory tract (T17.-)
> *EXCLUDES 1*   *chemical pneumonitis due to anesthesia (J95.4)*
>   *obstetric aspiration pneumonitis (O74.0)*
>
> **AHA:** 2019,2Q,6,31

     J69.1 **Pneumonitis due to inhalation of oils and essences** `MCC` `HCC`
> Exogenous lipoid pneumonia
> Lipid pneumonia NOS
> Code first (T51-T65) to identify substance
> *EXCLUDES 1*   *endogenous lipoid pneumonia (J84.89)*

     J69.8 **Pneumonitis due to inhalation of other solids and liquids** `MCC` `HCC`
> Pneumonitis due to aspiration of blood
> Pneumonitis due to aspiration of detergent
> Code first (T51-T65) to identify substance

`√4ᵗʰ` **J70** **Respiratory conditions due to other external agents**

     J70.0 **Acute pulmonary manifestations due to radiation** `CC` `HCC`
> Radiation pneumonitis
> Use additional code (W88-W90, X39.0-) to identify the external cause

     J70.1 **Chronic and other pulmonary manifestations due to radiation** `CC` `HCC`
> Fibrosis of lung following radiation
> Use additional code (W88-W90, X39.0-) to identify the external cause

     J70.2 **Acute drug-induced interstitial lung disorders** `HCC`
> Use additional code for adverse effect, if applicable, to identify drug (T36-T50 with fifth or sixth character 5)
> *EXCLUDES 1*   *interstitial pneumonia NOS (J84.9)*
>   *lymphoid interstitial pneumonia (J84.2)*
>
> **AHA:** 2019,2Q,28

     J70.3 **Chronic drug-induced interstitial lung disorders** `HCC`
> Use additional code for adverse effect, if applicable, to identify drug (T36-T50 with fifth or sixth character 5)
> *EXCLUDES 1*   *interstitial pneumonia NOS (J84.9)*
>   *lymphoid interstitial pneumonia (J84.2)*

     J70.4 **Drug-induced interstitial lung disorders, unspecified** `HCC`
> Use additional code for adverse effect, if applicable, to identify drug (T36-T50 with fifth or sixth character 5)
> *EXCLUDES 1*   *interstitial pneumonia NOS (J84.9)*
>   *lymphoid interstitial pneumonia (J84.2)*
>
> **AHA:** 2019,2Q,28

     J70.5 **Respiratory conditions due to smoke inhalation** `HCC`
> Smoke inhalation NOS
> *EXCLUDES 1*   *smoke inhalation due to chemicals, gases, fumes and vapors (J68.9)*
>
> **AHA:** 2013,4Q,121

     J70.8 **Respiratory conditions due to other specified external agents** `HCC`
> Code first (T51-T65) to identify the external agent

     J70.9 **Respiratory conditions due to unspecified external agent** `HCC`
> Code first (T51-T65) to identify the external agent

Other respiratory diseases principally affecting the interstitium (J80-J84)

J80 **Acute respiratory distress syndrome** `MCC` `HCC`
> Acute respiratory distress syndrome in adult or child
> Adult hyaline membrane disease
> *EXCLUDES 1*   *respiratory distress syndrome in newborn (perinatal) (P22.0)*
>
> **AHA:** 2017,1Q,26
> **DEF:** Lung inflammation or injury resulting in a build-up of fluid in the air sacs, preventing the passage of oxygen from the air into the bloodstream.
> **CC Excl:** PDX collection 744

`√4ᵗʰ` **J81** **Pulmonary edema**
> Use additional code to identify:
> exposure to environmental tobacco smoke (Z77.22)
> history of tobacco dependence (Z87.891)
> occupational exposure to environmental tobacco smoke (Z57.31)
> tobacco dependence (F17.-)
> tobacco use (Z72.0)
> *EXCLUDES 1*   *chemical (acute) pulmonary edema (J68.1)*
>   *hypostatic pneumonia (J18.2)*
>   *passive pneumonia (J18.2)*
>   *pulmonary edema due to external agents (J60-J70)*
>   *pulmonary edema with heart disease NOS (I50.1)*
>   *pulmonary edema with heart failure (I50.1)*
>
> **DEF:** Accumulation of fluid in the air sacs of the lungs, making it difficult to breath.

     J81.0 **Acute pulmonary edema** `MCC` `HCC`
> Acute edema of lung
> **CC Excl:** PDX collection 745

     J81.1 **Chronic pulmonary edema** `CC`
> Pulmonary congestion (chronic) (passive)
> Pulmonary edema NOS
> **CC Excl:** PDX collection 736

`N` Newborn: 0   `P` Pediatric: 0-17   `M` Maternity: 9-64   `A` Adult: 15-124   `MCC` Major Complication/Comorbidity   `CC` Complication/Comorbidity   `SW` Severe Wound Dx

702   ICD-10-CM 2020

J82 Pulmonary eosinophilia, not elsewhere classified `CC` `HCC`

Allergic pneumonia
Eosinophilic asthma
Eosinophilic pneumonia
Löffler's pneumonia
Tropical (pulmonary) eosinophilia NOS

> `EXCLUDES 1`   *pulmonary eosinophilia due to aspergillosis (B44.-)*
> *pulmonary eosinophilia due to drugs (J70.2-J70.4)*
> *pulmonary eosinophilia due to specified parasitic infection (B50-B83)*
> *pulmonary eosinophilia due to systemic connective tissue disorders (M30-M36)*
> *pulmonary infiltrate NOS (R91.8)*

DEF: Infiltration of eosinophils (white blood cells of the immune system) into the parenchyma of the lungs, resulting in cough, fever, and dyspnea.
CC Excl: PDX collection 746

`✓4th` **J84 Other interstitial pulmonary diseases**

> `EXCLUDES 1`   *drug-induced interstitial lung disorders (J70.2-J70.4)*
> *interstitial emphysema (J98.2)*
> `EXCLUDES 2`   *lung diseases due to external agents (J60-J70)*

DEF: Interstitial: Within the small spaces or gaps occurring in tissue or organs.
CC Excl: For CC/MCC codes in category J84, unless otherwise noted: PDX collection 747

`✓5th` **J84.0 Alveolar and parieto-alveolar conditions**

     J84.01 Alveolar proteinosis `CC` `HCC`

         DEF: Reduced ventilation due to proteinaceous deposits on alveoli. Symptoms include dyspnea, cough, chest pain, weakness, weight loss, and hemoptysis.

     J84.02 Pulmonary alveolar microlithiasis `CC` `HCC`

     J84.03 *Idiopathic pulmonary hemosiderosis* `CC` `HCC`

         Essential brown induration of lung
         Code first underlying disease, such as:
         disorders of iron metabolism (E83.1-)

>   `EXCLUDES 1`   *acute idiopathic pulmonary hemorrhage in infants [AIPHI] (R04.81)*

         DEF: Fibrosis of the alveolar walls marked by abnormal accumulation of iron as hemosiderin in the lungs. It primarily affects children and symptoms include anemia, fluid in the lungs, and blood in the sputum. Etiology is unknown.

     J84.09 Other alveolar and parieto-alveolar conditions `CC` `HCC`

`✓5th` **J84.1 Other interstitial pulmonary diseases with fibrosis**

> `EXCLUDES 1`   *pulmonary fibrosis (chronic) due to inhalation of chemicals, gases, fumes or vapors (J68.4)*
> *pulmonary fibrosis (chronic) following radiation (J70.1)*

     J84.10 Pulmonary fibrosis, unspecified `HCC`

         Capillary fibrosis of lung
         Cirrhosis of lung (chronic) NOS
         Fibrosis of lung (atrophic) (chronic) (confluent) (massive) (perialveolar) (peribronchial) NOS
         Induration of lung (chronic) NOS
         Postinflammatory pulmonary fibrosis

`✓6th`   **J84.11 Idiopathic interstitial pneumonia**

>   `EXCLUDES 1`   *lymphoid interstitial pneumonia (J84.2)*
> *pneumocystis pneumonia (B59)*

     J84.111 Idiopathic interstitial pneumonia, not otherwise specified `HCC`

     J84.112 Idiopathic pulmonary fibrosis `HCC`

         Cryptogenic fibrosing alveolitis
         Idiopathic fibrosing alveolitis

     J84.113 Idiopathic non-specific interstitial pneumonitis `HCC`

>   `EXCLUDES 1`   *non-specific interstitial pneumonia NOS, or due to known underlying cause (J84.89)*

     J84.114 Acute interstitial pneumonitis `CC` `HCC`

         Hamman-Rich syndrome

>   `EXCLUDES 1`   *pneumocystis pneumonia (B59)*

     J84.115 Respiratory bronchiolitis interstitial lung disease `HCC`

     J84.116 Cryptogenic organizing pneumonia `CC` `HCC`

>   `EXCLUDES 1`   *organizing pneumonia NOS, or due to known underlying cause (J84.89)*

     J84.117 Desquamative interstitial pneumonia `CC` `HCC`

`J84.17`   ***Other interstitial pulmonary diseases with fibrosis in diseases classified elsewhere*** `HCC`

     Interstitial pneumonia (nonspecific) (usual) due to collagen vascular disease
     Interstitial pneumonia (nonspecific) (usual) in diseases classified elsewhere
     Organizing pneumonia due to collagen vascular disease
     Organizing pneumonia in diseases classified elsewhere
     Code first underlying disease, such as:
         progressive systemic sclerosis (M34.0)
         rheumatoid arthritis (M05.00-M06.9)
         systemic lupus erythematosis (M32.0-M32.9)

J84.2 Lymphoid interstitial pneumonia `CC` `HCC`

Lymphoid interstitial pneumonitis

`✓5th` **J84.8 Other specified interstitial pulmonary diseases**

> `EXCLUDES 1`   *exogenous lipoid pneumonia (J69.1)*
> *unspecified lipoid pneumonia (J69.1)*

     J84.81 Lymphangioleiomyomatosis `MCC` `HCC`

         Lymphangiomyomatosis

     J84.82 Adult pulmonary Langerhans cell histiocytosis `CC` `HCC` `A`

         Adult PLCH

     J84.83 Surfactant mutations of the lung `MCC` `HCC`

         DEF: Genetic disorder resulting in insufficient secretion of a complex mixture of phospholipids and proteins that reduce surface tension in the alveoli following the onset of breathing to facilitate lung expansion in the newborn. It is the leading indication for pediatric lung transplantation.
         CC Excl: PDX collection 748

`✓6th`   **J84.84 Other interstitial lung diseases of childhood**

     CC Excl: For MCC codes in subcategory J84.84: PDX collection 748

     J84.841 Neuroendocrine cell hyperplasia of infancy `MCC` `HCC`

     J84.842 Pulmonary interstitial glycogenosis `MCC` `HCC`

     J84.843 Alveolar capillary dysplasia with vein misalignment `MCC` `HCC`

     J84.848 Other interstitial lung diseases of childhood `MCC` `HCC`

     J84.89 Other specified interstitial pulmonary diseases `HCC`

         Endogenous lipoid pneumonia
         Interstitial pneumonitis
         Non-specific interstitial pneumonitis NOS
         Organizing pneumonia NOS
         Code first, if applicable:
         poisoning due to drug or toxin (T51-T65 with fifth or sixth character to indicate intent), for toxic pneumonopathy
         underlying cause of pneumonopathy, if known
         Use additional code, for adverse effect, to identify drug (T36-T50 with fifth or sixth character 5), if drug-induced

>   `EXCLUDES 1`   *cryptogenic organizing pneumonia (J84.116)*
> *idiopathic non-specific interstitial pneumonitis (J84.113)*
> *lymphoid interstitial pneumonia (J84.2)*
> *lipoid pneumonia, exogenous or unspecified (J69.1)*

         AHA: 2019,2Q,28

J84.9   **Interstitial pulmonary disease, unspecified**   `HCC`

Interstitial pneumonia NOS

Suppurative and necrotic conditions of the lower respiratory tract (J85-J86)

✓4ᵗʰ   **J85**   **Abscess of lung and mediastinum**

Use additional code (B95-B97) to identify infectious agent

CC Excl: For MCC codes in category J85, unless otherwise noted: PDX collection 749

J85.0   **Gangrene and necrosis of lung**   `MCC` `HCC`

J85.1   **Abscess of lung with pneumonia**   `MCC` `HCC`

Code also the type of pneumonia

J85.2   **Abscess of lung without pneumonia**   `MCC` `HCC`

Abscess of lung NOS

J85.3   **Abscess of mediastinum**   `MCC` `HCC`

CC Excl: PDX collection 750

✓4ᵗʰ   **J86**   **Pyothorax**

Use additional code (B95-B97) to identify infectious agent

EXCLUDES 1   abscess of lung (J85.-)

pyothorax due to tuberculosis (A15.6)

DEF: Collection of pus in the pleural space that is commonly caused by an infection that spreads from the lung, such as bacterial pneumonia or a lung abscess.

J86.0   **Pyothorax with fistula**   `MCC` `HCC` `SW`

Bronchocutaneous fistula

Bronchopleural fistula

Hepatopleural fistula

Mediastinal fistula

Pleural fistula

Thoracic fistula

Any condition classifiable to J86.9 with fistula

DEF: Purulent infection of the respiratory cavity, with communication from a cavity to another structure.

CC Excl: PDX collection 751

J86.9   **Pyothorax without fistula**   `MCC` `HCC`

Abscess of pleura

Abscess of thorax

Empyema (chest) (lung) (pleura)

Fibrinopurulent pleurisy

Purulent pleurisy

Pyopneumothorax

Septic pleurisy

Seropurulent pleurisy

Suppurative pleurisy

CC Excl: PDX collection 751

Other diseases of the pleura (J90-J94)

J90   **Pleural effusion, not elsewhere classified**   `CC`

Encysted pleurisy

Pleural effusion NOS

Pleurisy with effusion (exudative) (serous)

EXCLUDES 1   chylous (pleural) effusion (J94.0)

malignant pleural effusion (J91.0))

pleurisy NOS (R09.1)

tuberculous pleural effusion (A15.6)

DEF: Collection of lymph and other fluid within the pleural space.

CC Excl: PDX collection 752

✓4ᵗʰ   **J91**   **Pleural effusion in conditions classified elsewhere**

EXCLUDES 2   pleural effusion in heart failure (I50.-)

pleural effusion in systemic lupus erythematosus (M32.13)

DEF: Collection of lymph and other fluid within the pleural space.

J91.0   *Malignant pleural effusion*   `CC`

Code first underlying neoplasm

CC Excl: PDX collection 753

J91.8   *Pleural effusion in other conditions classified elsewhere*   `CC`

Code first underlying disease, such as:

filariasis (B74.0-B74.9)

influenza (J09.X2, J10.1, J11.1)

AHA: 2015,2Q,15

TIP: Assign this code as a secondary diagnosis to congestive heart failure (I50.-) only if pleural effusion is specifically evaluated or treated.

CC Excl: PDX collection 752

Pleural Effusion

✓4ᵗʰ   **J92**   **Pleural plaque**

INCLUDES   pleural thickening

DEF: Areas of fibrous thickening that form on the parietal or visceral pleura, the membranes that line the ribs and lungs.

J92.0   **Pleural plaque with presence of asbestos**

J92.9   **Pleural plaque without asbestos**

Pleural plaque NOS

✓4ᵗʰ   **J93**   **Pneumothorax and air leak**

EXCLUDES 1   congenital or perinatal pneumothorax (P25.1)

postprocedural air leak (J95.812)

postprocedural pneumothorax (J95.811)

pyopneumothorax (J86.-)

traumatic pneumothorax (S27.0)

tuberculous (current disease) pneumothorax (A15.-)

DEF: Pneumothorax: Lung displacement due to abnormal leakage of air or gas that is trapped in the pleural space formed by the membrane that encloses the lungs and lines the thoracic cavity.

CC Excl: For CC/MCC codes in category J93: PDX collection 754

J93.0   **Spontaneous tension pneumothorax**   `MCC`

DEF: Leaking air from the lung into the lining, causing collapse.

✓5ᵗʰ   **J93.1**   **Other spontaneous pneumothorax**

J93.11   **Primary spontaneous pneumothorax**   `CC`

J93.12   **Secondary spontaneous pneumothorax**   `CC`

Code first underlying condition, such as:

catamenial pneumothorax due to endometriosis (N80.8)

cystic fibrosis (E84.-)

eosinophilic pneumonia (J82)

lymphangioleiomyomatosis (J84.81)

malignant neoplasm of bronchus and lung (C34.-)

Marfan's syndrome (Q87.4)

pneumonia due to Pneumocystis carinii (B59)

secondary malignant neoplasm of lung (C78.0-)

spontaneous rupture of the esophagus (K22.3)

✓5ᵗʰ   **J93.8**   **Other pneumothorax and air leak**

J93.81   **Chronic pneumothorax**   `CC`

J93.82   **Other air leak**   `CC`

Persistent air leak

N Newborn: 0   P Pediatric: 0-17   M Maternity: 9-64   A Adult: 15-124   MCC Major Complication/Comorbidity   CC Complication/Comorbidity   SW Severe Wound Dx

704   ICD-10-CM 2020

J93.83   **Other pneumothorax**   `CC`

Acute pneumothorax

Spontaneous pneumothorax NOS

J93.9   **Pneumothorax, unspecified**   `CC`

Pneumothorax NOS

`√4ᵗʰ` **J94**   **Other pleural conditions**

> `EXCLUDES 1`   *pleurisy NOS (R09.1)*
> *traumatic hemopneumothorax (S27.2)*
> *traumatic hemothorax (S27.1)*
> *tuberculous pleural conditions (current disease) (A15.-)*

J94.0   **Chylous effusion**   `CC`

Chyliform effusion

DEF: Fluid within the pleural space due to the leaking of lymph contents into the space, usually as a result of thoracic duct damage or injury or mediastinal lymphoma.

CC Excl: PDX collection 752

J94.1   **Fibrothorax**

DEF: Fibrosis within the pleural lining of the lungs commonly seen as a stiff layer surrounding the lung typically attributed to traumatic hemothorax or pleural effusion.

J94.2   **Hemothorax**   `CC`

Hemopneumothorax

CC Excl: PDX collection 752

J94.8   **Other specified pleural conditions**   `CC`

Hydropneumothorax

Hydrothorax

CC Excl: No Excl

J94.9   **Pleural condition, unspecified**

Intraoperative and postprocedural complications and disorders of respiratory system, not elsewhere classified (J95)

`√4ᵗʰ` **J95**   **Intraoperative and postprocedural complications and disorders of respiratory system, not elsewhere classified**

> `EXCLUDES 2`   *aspiration pneumonia (J69.-)*
> *emphysema (subcutaneous) resulting from a procedure (T81.82)*
> *hypostatic pneumonia (J18.2)*
> *pulmonary manifestations due to radiation (J70.0-J70.1)*

`√5ᵗʰ` **J95.0**   **Tracheostomy complications**

DEF: Tracheostomy: Formation of a tracheal opening on the neck surface with tube insertion to allow for respiration in cases of obstruction or decreased patency. A tracheostomy may be planned or performed on an emergency basis for temporary or long-term use.

CC Excl: For CC codes in subcategory J95.0: PDX collection 755

Tracheostomy

Tracheostomy in place

Incision in trachea

Trachea

Tracheostomy tube

J95.00   **Unspecified tracheostomy complication**   `CC` `HCC`

J95.01   **Hemorrhage from tracheostomy stoma**   `CC` `HCC`

J95.02   **Infection of tracheostomy stoma**   `CC` `HCC`

Use additional code to identify type of infection, such as:

cellulitis of neck (L03.221)

sepsis (A40, A41.-)

J95.03   **Malfunction of tracheostomy stoma**   `CC` `HCC`

Mechanical complication of tracheostomy stoma

Obstruction of tracheostomy airway

Tracheal stenosis due to tracheostomy

J95.04   **Tracheo-esophageal fistula following tracheostomy**   `CC` `HCC`

J95.09   **Other tracheostomy complication**   `CC` `HCC`

J95.1   **Acute pulmonary insufficiency following thoracic surgery**   `CC` `HCC`

> `EXCLUDES 2`   *functional disturbances following cardiac surgery (I97.0, I97.1-)*

J95.2   **Acute pulmonary insufficiency following nonthoracic surgery**   `MCC` `HCC`

> `EXCLUDES 2`   *functional disturbances following cardiac surgery (I97.0, I97.1-)*

CC Excl: PDX collection 756

J95.3   **Chronic pulmonary insufficiency following surgery**   `MCC` `HCC`

> `EXCLUDES 2`   *functional disturbances following cardiac surgery (I97.0, I97.1-)*

CC Excl: PDX collection 756

J95.4   **Chemical pneumonitis due to anesthesia**   `CC`

Mendelson's syndrome

Postprocedural aspiration pneumonia

Use additional code for adverse effect, if applicable, to identify drug (T41.- with fifth or sixth character 5)

> `EXCLUDES 1`   *aspiration pneumonitis due to anesthesia complicating labor and delivery (O74.0)*
> *aspiration pneumonitis due to anesthesia complicating pregnancy (O29)*
> *aspiration pneumonitis due to anesthesia complicating the puerperium (O89.01)*

CC Excl: PDX collection 757

J95.5   **Postprocedural subglottic stenosis**   `CC`

CC Excl: PDX collection 757

`√5ᵗʰ` **J95.6**   **Intraoperative hemorrhage and hematoma of a respiratory system organ or structure complicating a procedure**

> `EXCLUDES 1`   *intraoperative hemorrhage and hematoma of a respiratory system organ or structure due to accidental puncture and laceration during procedure (J95.7-)*

J95.61   **Intraoperative hemorrhage and hematoma of a respiratory system organ or structure complicating a respiratory system procedure**   `CC`

CC Excl: PDX collection 758

J95.62   **Intraoperative hemorrhage and hematoma of a respiratory system organ or structure complicating other procedure**   `CC`

CC Excl: PDX collection 758

`√5ᵗʰ` **J95.7**   **Accidental puncture and laceration of a respiratory system organ or structure during a procedure**

> `EXCLUDES 2`   *postprocedural pneumothorax (J95.811)*

J95.71   **Accidental puncture and laceration of a respiratory system organ or structure during a respiratory system procedure**   `CC`

CC Excl: PDX collection 509

J95.72   **Accidental puncture and laceration of a respiratory system organ or structure during other procedure**   `CC`

CC Excl: PDX collection 509

`√5ᵗʰ` **J95.8**   **Other intraoperative and postprocedural complications and disorders of respiratory system, not elsewhere classified**

AHA: 2016,4Q,9-10

`√6ᵗʰ` **J95.81**   **Postprocedural pneumothorax and air leak**

J95.811   **Postprocedural pneumothorax**   `CC` `H14`

CC Excl: PDX collection 754

☑ Additional Character Required   `√x7ᵗʰ` Placeholder   Unacceptable PDx   Questionable PDx   Manifestation   Unspecified Dx   `H1`-`H14` HAC   `HCC` CMS-HCC Dx   `HIV` HIV Dx

ICD-10-CM 2020   705

J95.812 Postprocedural air leak `CC`
    CC Excl: PDX collection 754

√6ᵗʰ **J95.82 Postprocedural respiratory failure**
    EXCLUDES 1 respiratory failure in other conditions
        (J96.-)

J95.821 Acute postprocedural `CC` `HCC`
    respiratory failure
    Postprocedural respiratory failure NOS

J95.822 Acute and chronic `MCC` `HCC`
    postprocedural
    respiratory failure
    CC Excl: PDX collection 756

√6ᵗʰ **J95.83 Postprocedural hemorrhage of a respiratory system organ or structure following a procedure**

J95.830 Postprocedural `CC`
    hemorrhage of a
    respiratory system organ
    or structure following a
    respiratory system
    procedure
    CC Excl: PDX collection 758

J95.831 Postprocedural `CC`
    hemorrhage of a
    respiratory system organ
    or structure following
    other procedure
    CC Excl: PDX collection 758

J95.84 Transfusion-related acute lung `CC`
injury (TRALI)
    DEF: Relatively rare, but serious, pulmonary
    complication of blood transfusion, with acute
    respiratory distress, noncardiogenic pulmonary edema,
    cyanosis, hypoxemia, hypotension, fever, and chills.
    CC Excl: PDX collection 757

√6ᵗʰ **J95.85 Complication of respirator [ventilator]**

J95.850 Mechanical complication `CC` `HCC`
    of respirator
    EXCLUDES 1 encounter for respirator
        [ventilator] dependence
        during power failure
        (Z99.12)
    CC Excl: PDX collection 759

J95.851 Ventilator associated `CC` `HCC`
    pneumonia
    Ventilator associated pneumonitis
    Use additional code to identify the
        organism, if known (B95.-, B96.-,
        B97.-)
    EXCLUDES 1 ventilator lung in newborn
        (P27.8)
    AHA: 2017,1Q,25
    CC Excl: PDX collection 757

J95.859 Other complication of `CC` `HCC`
    respirator [ventilator]
    CC Excl: PDX collection 757

√6ᵗʰ **J95.86 Postprocedural hematoma and seroma of a respiratory system organ or structure following a procedure**
    CC Excl: For CC codes in subcategory J95.86: PDX
    collection 758

J95.860 Postprocedural hematoma `CC`
    of a respiratory system
    organ or structure
    following a respiratory
    system procedure

J95.861 Postprocedural hematoma `CC`
    of a respiratory system
    organ or structure
    following other procedure

J95.862 Postprocedural seroma of `CC`
    a respiratory system organ
    or structure following a
    respiratory system
    procedure

J95.863 Postprocedural seroma of `CC`
    a respiratory system organ
    or structure following
    other procedure

J95.88 Other intraoperative complications `CC`
of respiratory system, not elsewhere
classified
    CC Excl: PDX collection 757

J95.89 Other postprocedural complications `CC`
and disorders of respiratory system,
not elsewhere classified
    Use additional code to identify disorder, such as:
        aspiration pneumonia (J69.-)
        bacterial or viral pneumonia (J12-J18)
    EXCLUDES 2 acute pulmonary insufficiency following
        thoracic surgery (J95.1)
        postprocedural subglottic stenosis (J95.5)
    CC Excl: PDX collection 757

Other diseases of the respiratory system (J96-J99)

√4ᵗʰ **J96 Respiratory failure, not elsewhere classified**
    EXCLUDES 1 acute respiratory distress syndrome (J80)
        cardiorespiratory failure (R09.2)
        newborn respiratory distress syndrome (P22.0)
        postprocedural respiratory failure (J95.82-)
        respiratory arrest (R09.2)
        respiratory arrest of newborn (P28.81)
        respiratory failure of newborn (P28.5)
    CC Excl: For CC/MCC codes in category J96: PDX collection 744

√5ᵗʰ **J96.0 Acute respiratory failure**

J96.00 Acute respiratory failure, `MCC` `HCC`
    unspecified whether with hypoxia
    or hypercapnia
    AHA: 2016,3Q,14; 2013,4Q,121

J96.01 Acute respiratory failure with `MCC` `HCC`
    hypoxia

J96.02 Acute respiratory failure with `MCC` `HCC`
    hypercapnia

√5ᵗʰ **J96.1 Chronic respiratory failure**

J96.10 Chronic respiratory failure, `CC` `HCC`
    unspecified whether with hypoxia
    or hypercapnia
    AHA: 2016,1Q,38; 2015,1Q,21

J96.11 Chronic respiratory failure with `CC` `HCC`
    hypoxia
    AHA: 2013,4Q,129

J96.12 Chronic respiratory failure with `CC` `HCC`
    hypercapnia

√5ᵗʰ **J96.2 Acute and chronic respiratory failure**
    Acute on chronic respiratory failure

J96.20 Acute and chronic respiratory `MCC` `HCC`
    failure, unspecified whether with
    hypoxia or hypercapnia

J96.21 Acute and chronic respiratory failure `MCC` `HCC`
    with hypoxia

J96.22 Acute and chronic respiratory failure `MCC` `HCC`
    with hypercapnia

√5ᵗʰ **J96.9 Respiratory failure, unspecified**

J96.90 Respiratory failure, unspecified, `MCC` `HCC`
    unspecified whether with hypoxia
    or hypercapnia

J96.91 Respiratory failure, unspecified with `MCC` `HCC`
    hypoxia

J96.92 Respiratory failure, unspecified with `MCC` `HCC`
    hypercapnia

✅4ᵗʰ **J98 Other respiratory disorders**

Use additional code to identify:
exposure to environmental tobacco smoke (Z77.22)
exposure to tobacco smoke in the perinatal period (P96.81)
history of tobacco dependence (Z87.891)
occupational exposure to environmental tobacco smoke (Z57.31)
tobacco dependence (F17.-)
tobacco use (Z72.0)

EXCLUDES 1   *newborn apnea (P28.4)*
newborn sleep apnea (P28.3)

EXCLUDES 2   *apnea NOS (R06.81)*
sleep apnea (G47.3-)

✅5ᵗʰ **J98.0 Diseases of bronchus, not elsewhere classified**

J98.01 Acute bronchospasm   CC

EXCLUDES 1   *acute bronchiolitis with bronchospasm (J21.-)*
acute bronchitis with bronchospasm (J20.-)
asthma (J45.-)
exercise induced bronchospasm (J45.990)

J98.09 Other diseases of bronchus, not elsewhere classified
Broncholithiasis
Calcification of bronchus
Stenosis of bronchus
Tracheobronchial collapse
Tracheobronchial dyskinesia
Ulcer of bronchus

✅5ᵗʰ **J98.1 Pulmonary collapse**

EXCLUDES 1   *therapeutic collapse of lung status (Z98.3)*

J98.11 Atelectasis   CC

EXCLUDES 1   *newborn atelectasis*
tuberculous atelectasis (current disease) (A15)

DEF: Collapse of lung tissue affecting part or all of one lung, preventing normal oxygen absorption to healthy tissues.
CC Excl: PDX collection 760

J98.19 Other pulmonary collapse   CC
CC Excl: PDX collection 760

J98.2 Interstitial emphysema   HCC
Mediastinal emphysema

EXCLUDES 1   *emphysema NOS (J43.9)*
emphysema in newborn (P25.0)
surgical emphysema (subcutaneous) (T81.82)
traumatic subcutaneous emphysema (T79.7)

J98.3 Compensatory emphysema   HCC
DEF: Distention of all or part of the lung caused by disease processes or surgical intervention that decreased volume in another part of the lung, causing an overcompensation reaction. Compensatory emphysema occurs in association with pneumonias, pleural effusions, atelectasis, empyema, and pneumothorax.

J98.4 Other disorders of lung
Calcification of lung
Cystic lung disease (acquired)
Lung disease NOS
Pulmolithiasis

EXCLUDES 1   *acute interstitial pneumonitis (J84.114)*
pulmonary insufficiency following surgery (J95.1-J95.2)

✅5ᵗʰ **J98.5 Diseases of mediastinum, not elsewhere classified**

EXCLUDES 2   *abscess of mediastinum (J85.3)*

AHA: 2016,4Q,29

J98.51 Mediastinitis   MCC   H8
Code first underlying condition, if applicable, such as postoperative mediastinitis (T81.-)
CC Excl: No Excl

J98.59 Other diseases of mediastinum, not elsewhere classified   MCC   H8
Fibrosis of mediastinum
Hernia of mediastinum
Retraction of mediastinum
CC Excl: No Excl

J98.6 Disorders of diaphragm
Diaphragmatitis
Paralysis of diaphragm
Relaxation of diaphragm

EXCLUDES 1   *congenital malformation of diaphragm NEC (Q79.1)*
congenital diaphragmatic hernia (Q79.0)

EXCLUDES 2   *diaphragmatic hernia (K44.-)*

J98.8 Other specified respiratory disorders

J98.9 Respiratory disorder, unspecified
Respiratory disease (chronic) NOS

J99 Respiratory disorders in diseases classified elsewhere   HCC
Code first underlying disease, such as:
amyloidosis (E85.-)
ankylosing spondylitis (M45)
congenital syphilis (A50.5)
cryoglobulinemia (D89.1)
early congenital syphilis (A50.0)
plasminogen deficiency (E88.02)
schistosomiasis (B65.0-B65.9)

EXCLUDES 1   *respiratory disorders in:*
amebiasis (A06.5)
blastomycosis (B40.0-B40.2)
candidiasis (B37.1)
coccidioidomycosis (B38.0-B38.2)
cystic fibrosis with pulmonary manifestations (E84.0)
dermatomyositis (M33.01, M33.11)
histoplasmosis (B39.0-B39.2)
late syphilis (A52.72, A52.73)
polymyositis (M33.21)
sicca syndrome (M35.02)
systemic lupus erythematosus (M32.13)
systemic sclerosis (M34.81)
Wegener's granulomatosis (M31.30-M31.31)

 Additional Character Required   ✔x7ᵗʰ Placeholder   Unacceptable PDx   Questionable PDx   Manifestation   Unspecified Dx   H1- H14 HAC   HCC CMS-HCC Dx   HIV HIV Dx

ICD-10-CM 2020   **707**

Chapter 11. Diseases of the Digestive System (KØØ–K95)

Chapter-specific Guidelines with Coding Examples
Reserved for future guideline expansion.

Chapter 11. Diseases of the Digestive System (K00-K95)

EXCLUDES 2   *certain conditions originating in the perinatal period (P04-P96)*
certain infectious and parasitic diseases (A00-B99)
complications of pregnancy, childbirth and the puerperium (O00-O9A)
congenital malformations, deformations and chromosomal abnormalities (Q00-Q99)
endocrine, nutritional and metabolic diseases (E00-E88)
injury, poisoning and certain other consequences of external causes (S00-T88)
neoplasms (C00-D49)
symptoms, signs and abnormal clinical and laboratory findings, not elsewhere classified (R00-R94)

This chapter contains the following blocks:

K00-K14   Diseases of oral cavity and salivary glands
K20-K31   Diseases of esophagus, stomach and duodenum
K35-K38   Diseases of appendix
K40-K46   Hernia
K50-K52   Noninfective enteritis and colitis
K55-K64   Other diseases of intestines
K65-K68   Diseases of peritoneum and retroperitoneum
K70-K77   Diseases of liver
K80-K87   Disorders of gallbladder, biliary tract and pancreas
K90-K95   Other diseases of the digestive system

Diseases of oral cavity and salivary glands (K00-K14)

√4ᵗʰ **K00   Disorders of tooth development and eruption**

> EXCLUDES 2   *embedded and impacted teeth (K01.-)*

K00.0   Anodontia
Hypodontia
Oligodontia
> EXCLUDES 1   *acquired absence of teeth (K08.1-)*

DEF: Partial or complete absence of teeth due to a congenital defect involving the tooth bud.

K00.1   Supernumerary teeth
Distomolar
Fourth molar
Mesiodens
Paramolar
Supplementary teeth
> EXCLUDES 2   *supernumerary roots (K00.2)*

K00.2   Abnormalities of size and form of teeth
Concrescence of teeth
Dens evaginatus
Dens in dente
Dens invaginatus
Enamel pearls
Fusion of teeth
Gemination of teeth
Macrodontia
Microdontia
Peg-shaped [conical] teeth
Supernumerary roots
Taurodontism
Tuberculum paramolare
> EXCLUDES 1   *abnormalities of teeth due to congenital syphilis (A50.5)*
> *tuberculum Carabelli, which is regarded as a normal variation and should not be coded*

K00.3   Mottled teeth
Dental fluorosis
Mottling of enamel
Nonfluoride enamel opacities
> EXCLUDES 2   *deposits [accretions] on teeth (K03.6)*

K00.4   Disturbances in tooth formation
Aplasia and hypoplasia of cementum
Dilaceration of tooth
Enamel hypoplasia (neonatal) (postnatal) (prenatal)
Regional odontodysplasia
Turner's tooth
> EXCLUDES 1   *Hutchinson's teeth and mulberry molars in congenital syphilis (A50.5)*
> EXCLUDES 2   *mottled teeth (K00.3)*

K00.5   Hereditary disturbances in tooth structure, not elsewhere classified
Amelogenesis imperfecta
Dentinogenesis imperfecta
Odontogenesis imperfecta
Dentinal dysplasia
Shell teeth

K00.6   Disturbances in tooth eruption
Dentia praecox
Natal tooth
Neonatal tooth
Premature eruption of tooth
Premature shedding of primary [deciduous] tooth
Prenatal teeth
Retained [persistent] primary tooth
> EXCLUDES 2   *embedded and impacted teeth (K01.-)*

K00.7   Teething syndrome

K00.8   Other disorders of tooth development
Color changes during tooth formation
Intrinsic staining of teeth NOS
> EXCLUDES 2   *posteruptive color changes (K03.7)*

K00.9   Disorder of tooth development, unspecified
Disorder of odontogenesis NOS

√4ᵗʰ **K01   Embedded and impacted teeth**

> EXCLUDES 1   *abnormal position of fully erupted teeth (M26.3-)*

K01.0   Embedded teeth

K01.1   Impacted teeth

√4ᵗʰ **K02   Dental caries**

> INCLUDES   caries of dentine
> dental cavities
> early childhood caries
> pre-eruptive caries
> recurrent caries (dentino enamel junction) (enamel) (to the pulp)
> tooth decay

DEF: Localized section of tooth decay that begins on the tooth surface with destruction of the calcified enamel, allowing bacterial destruction to continue and form cavities and may extend to the dentin and pulp.

Tooth Anatomy

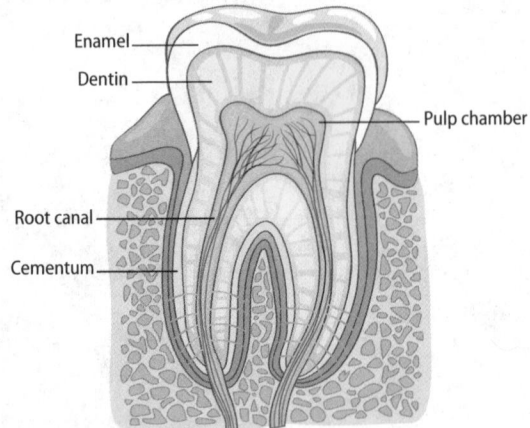

Enamel
Dentin
Pulp chamber
Root canal
Cementum

K02.3   Arrested dental caries
Arrested coronal and root caries

√5ᵗʰ **K02.5   Dental caries on pit and fissure surface**
Dental caries on chewing surface of tooth

K02.51   Dental caries on pit and fissure surface limited to enamel
White spot lesions [initial caries] on pit and fissure surface of tooth

K02.52   Dental caries on pit and fissure surface penetrating into dentin
Primary dental caries, cervical origin

K02.53   Dental caries on pit and fissure surface penetrating into pulp

N Newborn: 0   P Pediatric: 0-17   M Maternity: 9-64   A Adult: 15-124   MCC Major Complication/Comorbidity   CC Complication/Comorbidity   SW Severe Wound Dx

710   ICD-10-CM 2020

√5ᵗʰ K02.6 Dental caries on smooth surface

    K02.61 Dental caries on smooth surface limited to enamel
        White spot lesions [initial caries] on smooth surface of tooth

    K02.62 Dental caries on smooth surface penetrating into dentin

    K02.63 Dental caries on smooth surface penetrating into pulp

K02.7 Dental root caries

K02.9 Dental caries, unspecified

√4ᵗʰ K03 Other diseases of hard tissues of teeth

    EXCLUDES 2   *bruxism (F45.8)*
        dental caries (K02.-)
        teeth-grinding NOS (F45.8)

K03.0 Excessive attrition of teeth
    Approximal wear of teeth
    Occlusal wear of teeth
    DEF: Attrition: In dentistry, wearing away or erosion of tooth surface from abrasive food or grinding teeth.

K03.1 Abrasion of teeth
    Dentifrice abrasion of teeth
    Habitual abrasion of teeth
    Occupational abrasion of teeth
    Ritual abrasion of teeth
    Traditional abrasion of teeth
    Wedge defect NOS

K03.2 Erosion of teeth
    Erosion of teeth due to diet
    Erosion of teeth due to drugs and medicaments
    Erosion of teeth due to persistent vomiting
    Erosion of teeth NOS
    Idiopathic erosion of teeth
    Occupational erosion of teeth

K03.3 Pathological resorption of teeth
    Internal granuloma of pulp
    Resorption of teeth (external)

K03.4 Hypercementosis
    Cementation hyperplasia

K03.5 Ankylosis of teeth

K03.6 Deposits [accretions] on teeth
    Betel deposits [accretions] on teeth
    Black deposits [accretions] on teeth
    Extrinsic staining of teeth NOS
    Green deposits [accretions] on teeth
    Materia alba deposits [accretions] on teeth
    Orange deposits [accretions] on teeth
    Staining of teeth NOS
    Subgingival dental calculus
    Supragingival dental calculus
    Tobacco deposits [accretions] on teeth

K03.7 Posteruptive color changes of dental hard tissues
    EXCLUDES 2   *deposits [accretions] on teeth (K03.6)*

√5ᵗʰ K03.8 Other specified diseases of hard tissues of teeth

    K03.81 Cracked tooth
        EXCLUDES 1   *asymptomatic craze lines in enamel - omit code*
            broken or fractured tooth due to trauma (S02.5)

    K03.89 Other specified diseases of hard tissues of teeth

K03.9 Disease of hard tissues of teeth, unspecified

√4ᵗʰ K04 Diseases of pulp and periapical tissues

    AHA: 2016,4Q,29-30

√5ᵗʰ K04.0 Pulpitis
    Acute pulpitis
    Chronic (hyperplastic) (ulcerative) pulpitis

    K04.01 Reversible pulpitis

    K04.02 Irreversible pulpitis   **CC**
        CC Excl: PDX collection 761

K04.1 Necrosis of pulp
    Pulpal gangrene

K04.2 Pulp degeneration
    Denticles
    Pulpal calcifications
    Pulpal stones

K04.3 Abnormal hard tissue formation in pulp
    Secondary or irregular dentine

K04.4 Acute apical periodontitis of pulpal origin
    Acute apical periodontitis NOS
    EXCLUDES 1   *acute periodontitis (K05.2-)*
    DEF: Severe inflammation of the area surrounding the tip of a tooth's root that is often secondary to infection or trauma.

K04.5 Chronic apical periodontitis
    Apical or periapical granuloma
    Apical periodontitis NOS
    EXCLUDES 1   *chronic periodontitis (K05.3-)*

K04.6 Periapical abscess with sinus   **SW**
    Dental abscess with sinus
    Dentoalveolar abscess with sinus

K04.7 Periapical abscess without sinus
    Dental abscess without sinus
    Dentoalveolar abscess without sinus

K04.8 Radicular cyst
    Apical (periodontal) cyst
    Periapical cyst
    Residual radicular cyst
    EXCLUDES 2   *lateral periodontal cyst (K09.0)*
    DEF: Most common odontogenic cyst in tissue around the tooth apex due to chronic inflammation of dental pulp.

√5ᵗʰ K04.9 Other and unspecified diseases of pulp and periapical tissues

    K04.90 Unspecified diseases of pulp and periapical tissues

    K04.99 Other diseases of pulp and periapical tissues

√4ᵗʰ K05 Gingivitis and periodontal diseases

    Use additional code to identify:
    alcohol abuse and dependence (F10.-)
    exposure to environmental tobacco smoke (Z77.22)
    exposure to tobacco smoke in the perinatal period (P96.81)
    history of tobacco dependence (Z87.891)
    occupational exposure to environmental tobacco smoke (Z57.31)
    tobacco dependence (F17.-)
    tobacco use (Z72.0)
    AHA: 2016,4Q,29-30

√5ᵗʰ K05.0 Acute gingivitis

    EXCLUDES 1   *acute necrotizing ulcerative gingivitis (A69.1)*
            herpesviral [herpes simplex] gingivostomatitis (B00.2)

    K05.00 Acute gingivitis, plaque induced
        Acute gingivitis NOS
        Plaque induced gingival disease

    K05.01 Acute gingivitis, non-plaque induced

√5ᵗʰ K05.1 Chronic gingivitis

    Desquamative gingivitis (chronic)
    Gingivitis (chronic) NOS
    Hyperplastic gingivitis (chronic)
    Pregnancy associated gingivitis
    Simple marginal gingivitis (chronic)
    Ulcerative gingivitis (chronic)
    Code first, if applicable, diseases of the digestive system complicating pregnacy (O99.61-)

    K05.10 Chronic gingivitis, plaque induced
        Chronic gingivitis NOS
        Gingivitis NOS

    K05.11 Chronic gingivitis, non-plaque induced

√5ᵗʰ K05.2 Aggressive periodontitis

    Acute pericoronitis
    EXCLUDES 1   *acute apical periodontitis (K04.4)*
            periapical abscess (K04.7)
            periapical abscess with sinus (K04.6)

    K05.20 Aggressive periodontitis, unspecified

    √6ᵗʰ K05.21 Aggressive periodontitis, localized
        Periodontal abscess

        K05.211 Aggressive periodontitis, localized, slight

        K05.212 Aggressive periodontitis, localized, moderate

        K05.213 Aggressive periodontitis, localized, severe

        K05.219 Aggressive periodontitis, localized, unspecified severity

    √6ᵗʰ K05.22 Aggressive periodontitis, generalized

        K05.221 Aggressive periodontitis, generalized, slight

K05.222 Aggressive periodontitis, generalized, moderate

K05.223 Aggressive periodontitis, generalized, severe

K05.229 Aggressive periodontitis, generalized, unspecified severity

√5ᵗʰ **K05.3 Chronic periodontitis**

Chronic pericoronitis

Complex periodontitis

Periodontitis NOS

Simplex periodontitis

EXCLUDES 1   *chronic apical periodontitis (K04.5)*

K05.30 Chronic periodontitis, unspecified

√6ᵗʰ **K05.31 Chronic periodontitis, localized**

K05.311 Chronic periodontitis, localized, slight

K05.312 Chronic periodontitis, localized, moderate

K05.313 Chronic periodontitis, localized, severe

K05.319 Chronic periodontitis, localized, unspecified severity

√6ᵗʰ **K05.32 Chronic periodontitis, generalized**

K05.321 Chronic periodontitis, generalized, slight

K05.322 Chronic periodontitis, generalized, moderate

K05.323 Chronic periodontitis, generalized, severe

K05.329 Chronic periodontitis, generalized, unspecified

K05.4 Periodontosis

Juvenile periodontosis

K05.5 Other periodontal diseases

Combined periodontic-endodontic lesion

Narrow gingival width (of periodontal soft tissue)

EXCLUDES 2   *leukoplakia of gingiva (K13.21)*

K05.6 Periodontal disease, unspecified

√4ᵗʰ **K06 Other disorders of gingiva and edentulous alveolar ridge**

EXCLUDES 2   *acute gingivitis (K05.0)*

atrophy of edentulous alveolar ridge (K08.2)

chronic gingivitis (K05.1)

gingivitis NOS (K05.1)

AHA: 2016,4Q,29-30

√5ᵗʰ **K06.0 Gingival recession**

Gingival recession (postinfective) (postprocedural)

AHA: 2017,4Q,16

√6ᵗʰ **K06.01 Gingival recession, localized**

K06.010 Localized gingival recession, unspecified

Localized gingival recession, NOS

K06.011 Localized gingival recession, minimal

K06.012 Localized gingival recession, moderate

K06.013 Localized gingival recession, severe

√6ᵗʰ **K06.02 Gingival recession, generalized**

K06.020 Generalized gingival recession, unspecified

Generalized gingival recession, NOS

K06.021 Generalized gingival recession, minimal

K06.022 Generalized gingival recession, moderate

K06.023 Generalized gingival recession, severe

K06.1 Gingival enlargement

Gingival fibromatosis

K06.2 Gingival and edentulous alveolar ridge lesions associated with trauma

Irritative hyperplasia of edentulous ridge [denture hyperplasia]

Use additional code (Chapter 20) to identify external cause or denture status (Z97.2)

K06.3 Horizontal alveolar bone loss

K06.8 Other specified disorders of gingiva and edentulous alveolar ridge

Fibrous epulis

Flabby alveolar ridge

Giant cell epulis

Peripheral giant cell granuloma of gingiva

Pyogenic granuloma of gingiva

Vertical ridge deficiency

EXCLUDES 2   *gingival cyst (K09.0)*

K06.9 Disorder of gingiva and edentulous alveolar ridge, unspecified

√4ᵗʰ **K08 Other disorders of teeth and supporting structures**

EXCLUDES 2   *dentofacial anomalies [including malocclusion] (M26.-)*

disorders of jaw (M27.-)

AHA: 2016,4Q,29-30

K08.0 Exfoliation of teeth due to systemic causes

Code also underlying systemic condition

√5ᵗʰ **K08.1 Complete loss of teeth**

Acquired loss of teeth, complete

EXCLUDES 1   *congenital absence of teeth (K00.0)*

exfoliation of teeth due to systemic causes (K08.0)

partial loss of teeth (K08.4-)

DEF: Loss of all teeth as a result of caries, trauma, extraction, periodontal disease, or other specified or unspecified causes.

Synonym(s): *complete edentulism*

√6ᵗʰ **K08.10 Complete loss of teeth, unspecified cause**

K08.101 Complete loss of teeth, unspecified cause, class I

K08.102 Complete loss of teeth, unspecified cause, class II

K08.103 Complete loss of teeth, unspecified cause, class III

K08.104 Complete loss of teeth, unspecified cause, class IV

K08.109 Complete loss of teeth, unspecified cause, unspecified class

Edentulism NOS

√6ᵗʰ **K08.11 Complete loss of teeth due to trauma**

K08.111 Complete loss of teeth due to trauma, class I

K08.112 Complete loss of teeth due to trauma, class II

K08.113 Complete loss of teeth due to trauma, class III

K08.114 Complete loss of teeth due to trauma, class IV

K08.119 Complete loss of teeth due to trauma, unspecified class

√6ᵗʰ **K08.12 Complete loss of teeth due to periodontal diseases**

K08.121 Complete loss of teeth due to periodontal diseases, class I

K08.122 Complete loss of teeth due to periodontal diseases, class II

K08.123 Complete loss of teeth due to periodontal diseases, class III

K08.124 Complete loss of teeth due to periodontal diseases, class IV

K08.129 Complete loss of teeth due to periodontal diseases, unspecified class

√6ᵗʰ **K08.13 Complete loss of teeth due to caries**

K08.131 Complete loss of teeth due to caries, class I

K08.132 Complete loss of teeth due to caries, class II

K08.133 Complete loss of teeth due to caries, class III

K08.134 Complete loss of teeth due to caries, class IV

K08.139 Complete loss of teeth due to caries, unspecified class

√6ᵗʰ **K08.19 Complete loss of teeth due to other specified cause**

K08.191 Complete loss of teeth due to other specified cause, class I

K08.192 Complete loss of teeth due to other specified cause, class II

K08.193 Complete loss of teeth due to other specified cause, class III

K08.194 Complete loss of teeth due to other specified cause, class IV

K08.199 Complete loss of teeth due to other specified cause, unspecified class

√5ᵗʰ **K08.2 Atrophy of edentulous alveolar ridge**

K08.20 Unspecified atrophy of edentulous alveolar ridge

Atrophy of the mandible NOS

Atrophy of the maxilla NOS

K08.21 Minimal atrophy of the mandible

Minimal atrophy of the edentulous mandible

K08.22 Moderate atrophy of the mandible

Moderate atrophy of the edentulous mandible

N Newborn: 0   P Pediatric: 0-17   M Maternity: 9-64   A Adult: 15-124   MCC Major Complication/Comorbidity   CC Complication/Comorbidity   SW Severe Wound Dx

712   ICD-10-CM 2020

KØ8.23   Severe **atrophy of the** mandible
> Severe atrophy of the edentulous mandible

KØ8.24   Minimal **atrophy of** maxilla
> Minimal atrophy of the edentulous maxilla

KØ8.25   Moderate **atrophy of the** maxilla
> Moderate atrophy of the edentulous maxilla

KØ8.26   Severe **atrophy of the** maxilla
> Severe atrophy of the edentulous maxilla

KØ8.3   **Retained dental root**

☑5ᵗʰ **KØ8.4**   **Partial loss of teeth**
> Acquired loss of teeth, partial
> > EXCLUDES 1   *complete loss of teeth (KØ8.1-)*
> > *congenital absence of teeth (KØØ.Ø)*
> > EXCLUDES 2   *exfoliation of teeth due to systemic causes (KØ8.Ø)*

    ☑6ᵗʰ **KØ8.40**   **Partial loss of teeth, unspecified cause**

      KØ8.401   **Partial loss of teeth, unspecified cause, class I**

      KØ8.402   **Partial loss of teeth, unspecified cause, class II**

      KØ8.403   **Partial loss of teeth, unspecified cause, class III**

      KØ8.404   **Partial loss of teeth, unspecified cause, class IV**

      KØ8.409   **Partial loss of teeth, unspecified cause, unspecified class**
> > Tooth extraction status NOS

    ☑6ᵗʰ **KØ8.41**   **Partial loss of teeth due to** trauma

      KØ8.411   **Partial loss of teeth due to trauma,** class I

      KØ8.412   **Partial loss of teeth due to trauma,** class II

      KØ8.413   **Partial loss of teeth due to trauma,** class III

      KØ8.414   **Partial loss of teeth due to trauma,** class IV

      KØ8.419   **Partial loss of teeth due to trauma, unspecified class**

    ☑6ᵗʰ **KØ8.42**   **Partial loss of teeth due to** periodontal diseases

      KØ8.421   **Partial loss of teeth due to periodontal diseases,** class I

      KØ8.422   **Partial loss of teeth due to periodontal diseases,** class II

      KØ8.423   **Partial loss of teeth due to periodontal diseases,** class III

      KØ8.424   **Partial loss of teeth due to periodontal diseases,** class IV

      KØ8.429   **Partial loss of teeth due to periodontal diseases, unspecified class**

    ☑6ᵗʰ **KØ8.43**   **Partial loss of teeth due to** caries

      KØ8.431   **Partial loss of teeth due to caries,** class I

      KØ8.432   **Partial loss of teeth due to caries,** class II

      KØ8.433   **Partial loss of teeth due to caries,** class III

      KØ8.434   **Partial loss of teeth due to caries,** class IV

      KØ8.439   **Partial loss of teeth due to caries, unspecified class**

    ☑6ᵗʰ **KØ8.49**   **Partial loss of teeth due to other specified cause**

      KØ8.491   **Partial loss of teeth due to other specified cause,** class I

      KØ8.492   **Partial loss of teeth due to other specified cause,** class II

      KØ8.493   **Partial loss of teeth due to other specified cause,** class III

      KØ8.494   **Partial loss of teeth due to other specified cause,** class IV

      KØ8.499   **Partial loss of teeth due to other specified cause, unspecified class**

☑5ᵗʰ **KØ8.5**   **Unsatisfactory restoration of tooth**
> Defective bridge, crown, filling
> Defective dental restoration
> > EXCLUDES 1   *dental restoration status (Z98.811)*
> > EXCLUDES 2   *endosseous dental implant failure (M27.6-)*
> > *unsatisfactory endodontic treatment (M27.5-)*

    KØ8.50   **Unsatisfactory restoration of tooth, unspecified**
> > Defective dental restoration NOS

    KØ8.51   **Open restoration margins of tooth**
> > Dental restoration failure of marginal integrity
> > Open margin on tooth restoration
> > Poor gingival margin to tooth restoration

KØ8.52   **Unrepairable overhanging of dental restorative materials**
> Overhanging of tooth restoration

☑6ᵗʰ **KØ8.53**   **Fractured dental restorative material**
> > EXCLUDES 1   *cracked tooth (KØ3.81)*
> > *traumatic fracture of tooth (SØ2.5)*

    KØ8.530   **Fractured dental restorative material without loss of material**

    KØ8.531   **Fractured dental restorative material with loss of material**

    KØ8.539   **Fractured dental restorative material, unspecified**

KØ8.54   **Contour of existing restoration of tooth biologically incompatible with oral health**
> Dental restoration failure of periodontal anatomical integrity
> Unacceptable contours of existing restoration of tooth
> Unacceptable morphology of existing restoration of tooth

KØ8.55   **Allergy to existing dental restorative material**
> Use additional code to identify the specific type of allergy

KØ8.56   **Poor aesthetic of existing restoration of tooth**
> Dental restoration aesthetically inadequate or displeasing

KØ8.59   **Other unsatisfactory restoration of tooth**
> Other defective dental restoration

☑5ᵗʰ **KØ8.8**   **Other specified disorders of teeth and supporting structures**

    KØ8.81   **Primary occlusal trauma**

    KØ8.82   **Secondary occlusal trauma**

    KØ8.89   **Other specified disorders of teeth and supporting structures**
> > Enlargement of alveolar ridge NOS
> > Insufficient anatomic crown height
> > Insufficient clinical crown length
> > Irregular alveolar process
> > Toothache NOS

KØ8.9   **Disorder of teeth and supporting structures, unspecified**

☑4ᵗʰ **K09**   **Cysts of oral region, not elsewhere classified**
> INCLUDES   lesions showing histological features both of aneurysmal cyst and of another fibro-osseous lesion
> > EXCLUDES 2   *cysts of jaw (M27.Ø-, M27.4-)*
> > *radicular cyst (KØ4.8)*

K09.Ø   **Developmental odontogenic cysts**
> Dentigerous cyst
> Eruption cyst
> Follicular cyst
> Gingival cyst
> Lateral periodontal cyst
> Primordial cyst
> > EXCLUDES 2   *keratocysts (D16.4, D16.5)*
> > *odontogenic keratocystic tumors (D16.4, D16.5)*

K09.1   **Developmental (nonodontogenic) cysts of oral region**
> Cyst (of) incisive canal
> Cyst (of) palatine of papilla
> Globulomaxillary cyst
> Median palatal cyst
> Nasoalveolar cyst
> Nasolabial cyst
> Nasopalatine duct cyst

K09.8   **Other cysts of oral region, not elsewhere classified**
> Dermoid cyst
> Epidermoid cyst
> Lymphoepithelial cyst
> Epstein's pearl

K09.9   **Cyst of oral region, unspecified**

☑4ᵗʰ **K11**   **Diseases of salivary glands**
> Use additional code to identify:
> alcohol abuse and dependence (F10.-)
> exposure to environmental tobacco smoke (Z77.22)
> exposure to tobacco smoke in the perinatal period (P96.81)
> history of tobacco dependence (Z87.891)
> occupational exposure to environmental tobacco smoke (Z57.31)
> tobacco dependence (F17.-)
> tobacco use (Z72.Ø)

K11.Ø   **Atrophy of salivary gland**

☑ Additional Character Required   ☑7ᵗʰ Placeholder   Unacceptable PDx   Questionable PDx   Manifestation   Unspecified Dx   **H1**-**H14** HAC   **HCC** CMS-HCC Dx   **HIV** HIV Dx

ICD-10-CM 2020   **713**

Chapter 11. Diseases of the Digestive System

K11.1   **Hypertrophy of salivary gland**
DEF: Overgrowth of or enlarged salivary gland tissue caused by infection, salivary duct blockage, autoimmune diseases, and benign and malignant tumors.

✓5ᵗʰ **K11.2**   **Sialoadenitis**
Parotitis
EXCLUDES 1   *epidemic parotitis (B26.-)*
      mumps (B26.-)
      uveoparotid fever [Heerfordt] (D86.89)
DEF: Inflammation of the salivary gland.

   K11.20   **Sialoadenitis, unspecified**
   K11.21   **Acute sialoadenitis**
      EXCLUDES 1   *acute recurrent sialoadenitis (K11.22)*
   K11.22   **Acute recurrent sialoadenitis**
   K11.23   **Chronic sialoadenitis**

K11.3   **Abscess of salivary gland**

K11.4   **Fistula of salivary gland**   SW
EXCLUDES 1   *congenital fistula of salivary gland (Q38.4)*

K11.5   **Sialolithiasis**
Calculus of salivary gland or duct
Stone of salivary gland or duct

K11.6   **Mucocele of salivary gland**
Mucous extravasation cyst of salivary gland
Mucous retention cyst of salivary gland
Ranula

K11.7   **Disturbances of salivary secretion**
Hypoptyalism
Ptyalism
Xerostomia
EXCLUDES 2   *dry mouth NOS (R68.2)*

K11.8   **Other diseases of salivary glands**
Benign lymphoepithelial lesion of salivary gland
Mikulicz' disease
Necrotizing sialometaplasia
Sialectasia
Stenosis of salivary duct
Stricture of salivary duct
EXCLUDES 1   *sicca syndrome [Sjögren] (M35.0-)*

K11.9   **Disease of salivary gland, unspecified**
Sialoadenopathy NOS

✓4ᵗʰ **K12**   **Stomatitis and related lesions**
Use additional code to identify:
   alcohol abuse and dependence (F10.-)
   exposure to environmental tobacco smoke (Z77.22)
   exposure to tobacco smoke in the perinatal period (P96.81)
   history of tobacco dependence (Z87.891)
   occupational exposure to environmental tobacco smoke (Z57.31)
   tobacco dependence (F17.-)
   tobacco use (Z72.0)
EXCLUDES 1   *cancrum oris (A69.0)*
      cheilitis (K13.0)
      gangrenous stomatitis (A69.0)
      herpesviral [herpes simplex] gingivostomatitis (B00.2)
      noma (A69.0)

K12.0   **Recurrent oral aphthae**
Aphthous stomatitis (major) (minor)
Bednar's aphthae
Periadenitis mucosa necrotica recurrens
Recurrent aphthous ulcer
Stomatitis herpetiformis
DEF: Disorder of unknown etiology with small oval or round painful ulcers of the mouth marked by a grayish exudate and a red halo effect.

K12.1   **Other forms of stomatitis**
Stomatitis NOS
Denture stomatitis
Ulcerative stomatitis
Vesicular stomatitis
EXCLUDES 1   *acute necrotizing ulcerative stomatitis (A69.1)*
      Vincent's stomatitis (A69.1)

K12.2   **Cellulitis and abscess of mouth**   CC
Cellulitis of mouth (floor)
Submandibular abscess
EXCLUDES 2   *abscess of salivary gland (K11.3)*
      abscess of tongue (K14.0)
      periapical abscess (K04.6-K04.7)
      periodontal abscess (K05.21)
      peritonsillar abscess (J36)
CC Excl: PDX collection 763

✓5ᵗʰ **K12.3**   **Oral mucositis (ulcerative)**
Mucositis (oral) (oropharyneal)
EXCLUDES 2   *gastrointestinal mucositis (ulcerative) (K92.81)*
      mucositis (ulcerative) of vagina and vulva (N76.81)
      nasal mucositis (ulcerative) (J34.81)

   K12.30   **Oral mucositis (ulcerative), unspecified**
   K12.31   **Oral mucositis (ulcerative) due to antineoplastic therapy**
     Use additional code for adverse effect, if applicable, to identify antineoplastic and immunosuppressive drugs (T45.1X5)
     Use additional code for other antineoplastic therapy, such as:
       radiological procedure and radiotherapy (Y84.2)
   K12.32   **Oral mucositis (ulcerative) due to other drugs**
     Use additional code for adverse effect, if applicable, to identify drug (T36-T50 with fifth or sixth character 5)
   K12.33   **Oral mucositis (ulcerative) due to radiation**
     Use additional external cause code (W88-W90, X39.0-) to identify cause
   K12.39   **Other oral mucositis (ulcerative)**
     Viral oral mucositis (ulcerative)

✓4ᵗʰ **K13**   **Other diseases of lip and oral mucosa**
INCLUDES   epithelial disturbances of tongue
Use additional code to identify:
   alcohol abuse and dependence (F10.-)
   exposure to environmental tobacco smoke (Z77.22)
   exposure to tobacco smoke in the perinatal period (P96.81)
   history of tobacco dependence (Z87.891)
   occupational exposure to environmental tobacco smoke (Z57.31)
   tobacco dependence (F17.-)
   tobacco use (Z72.0)
EXCLUDES 2   *certain disorders of gingiva and edentulous alveolar ridge (K05-K06)*
      cysts of oral region (K09.-)
      diseases of tongue (K14.-)
      stomatitis and related lesions (K12.-)

K13.0   **Diseases of lips**
Abscess of lips
Angular cheilitis
Cellulitis of lips
Cheilitis NOS
Cheilodynia
Cheilosis
Exfoliative cheilitis
Fistula of lips
Glandular cheilitis
Hypertrophy of lips
Perlèche NEC
EXCLUDES 1   *ariboflavinosis (E53.0)*
      cheilitis due to radiation-related disorders (L55-L59)
      congenital fistula of lips (Q38.0)
      congenital hypertrophy of lips (Q18.6)
      perlèche due to candidiasis (B37.83)
      perlèche due to riboflavin deficiency (E53.0)

K13.1   **Cheek and lip biting**

N Newborn: 0   P Pediatric: 0-17   M Maternity: 9-64   A Adult: 15-124   **MCC** Major Complication/Comorbidity   **CC** Complication/Comorbidity   **SW** Severe Wound Dx

714   ICD-10-CM 2020

K11.1–K13.1

✓5ᵗʰ **K13.2** **Leukoplakia and other disturbances of oral epithelium, including tongue**
     EXCLUDES 1   *carcinoma in situ of oral epithelium (D00.0-)*
                  hairy leukoplakia (K13.3)
     DEF: Leukoplakia: Thickened white patches or lesions appearing on a mucous membrane, such as oral mucosa or tongue.

     K13.21 **Leukoplakia of oral mucosa, including tongue**
          Leukokeratosis of oral mucosa
          Leukoplakia of gingiva, lips, tongue
          EXCLUDES 1   *hairy leukoplakia (K13.3)*
                      leukokeratosis nicotina palati (K13.24)

     K13.22 **Minimal keratinized residual ridge mucosa**
          Minimal keratinization of alveolar ridge mucosa

     K13.23 **Excessive keratinized residual ridge mucosa**
          Excessive keratinization of alveolar ridge mucosa

     K13.24 **Leukokeratosis nicotina palati**
          Smoker's palate

     K13.29 **Other disturbances of oral epithelium, including tongue**
          Erythroplakia of mouth or tongue
          Focal epithelial hyperplasia of mouth or tongue
          Leukoedema of mouth or tongue
          Other oral epithelium disturbances

K13.3 **Hairy leukoplakia**

K13.4 **Granuloma and granuloma-like lesions of oral mucosa**
     Eosinophilic granuloma
     Granuloma pyogenicum
     Verrucous xanthoma

K13.5 **Oral submucous fibrosis**
     Submucous fibrosis of tongue

K13.6 **Irritative hyperplasia of oral mucosa**
     EXCLUDES 2   *irritative hyperplasia of edentulous ridge [denture hyperplasia] (K06.2)*

✓5ᵗʰ **K13.7** **Other and unspecified lesions of oral mucosa**
     K13.70 **Unspecified lesions of oral mucosa**
     K13.79 **Other lesions of oral mucosa**
          Focal oral mucinosis

✓4ᵗʰ **K14** **Diseases of tongue**
     Use additional code to identify:
       alcohol abuse and dependence (F10.-)
       exposure to environmental tobacco smoke (Z77.22)
       history of tobacco dependence (Z87.891)
       occupational exposure to environmental tobacco smoke (Z57.31)
       tobacco dependence (F17.-)
       tobacco use (Z72.0)
     EXCLUDES 2   *erythroplakia (K13.29)*
                  focal epithelial hyperplasia (K13.29)
                  leukedema of tongue (K13.29)
                  leukoplakia of tongue (K13.21)
                  hairy leukoplakia (K13.3)
                  macroglossia (congenital) (Q38.2)
                  submucous fibrosis of tongue (K13.5)

     K14.0 **Glossitis**
          Abscess of tongue
          Ulceration (traumatic) of tongue
          EXCLUDES 1   *atrophic glossitis (K14.4)*
          DEF: Inflammation and swelling of the tongue that may be associated with infection, adverse drug reactions, smoking, or injury.

     K14.1 **Geographic tongue**
          Benign migratory glossitis
          Glossitis areata exfoliativa

     K14.2 **Median rhomboid glossitis**

     K14.3 **Hypertrophy of tongue papillae**
          Black hairy tongue
          Coated tongue
          Hypertrophy of foliate papillae
          Lingua villosa nigra

     K14.4 **Atrophy of tongue papillae**
          Atrophic glossitis

     K14.5 **Plicated tongue**
          Fissured tongue
          Furrowed tongue
          Scrotal tongue
          EXCLUDES 1   *fissured tongue, congenital (Q38.3)*

     K14.6 **Glossodynia**
          Glossopyrosis
          Painful tongue

     K14.8 **Other diseases of tongue**
          Atrophy of tongue
          Crenated tongue
          Enlargement of tongue
          Glossocele
          Glossoptosis
          Hypertrophy of tongue

     K14.9 **Disease of tongue, unspecified**
          Glossopathy NOS

Diseases of esophagus, stomach and duodenum (K20-K31)

     EXCLUDES 2   *hiatus hernia (K44.-)*

✓4ᵗʰ **K20** **Esophagitis**
     Use additional code to identify:
       alcohol abuse and dependence (F10.-)
     EXCLUDES 1   *erosion of esophagus (K22.1-)*
                  esophagitis with gastro-esophageal reflux disease (K21.0)
                  reflux esophagitis (K21.0)
                  ulcerative esophagitis (K22.1-)
     EXCLUDES 2   *eosinophilic gastritis or gastroenteritis (K52.81)*

     K20.0 **Eosinophilic esophagitis**

     K20.8 **Other esophagitis**
          Abscess of esophagus

     K20.9 **Esophagitis, unspecified**
          Esophagitis NOS

✓4ᵗʰ **K21** **Gastro-esophageal reflux disease**
     EXCLUDES 1   *newborn esophageal reflux (P78.83)*

     K21.0 **Gastro-esophageal reflux disease with esophagitis**
          Reflux esophagitis

     K21.9 **Gastro-esophageal reflux disease without esophagitis**
          Esophageal reflux NOS
          AHA: 2016,1Q,18

✓4ᵗʰ **K22** **Other diseases of esophagus**
     EXCLUDES 2   *esophageal varices (I85.-)*

     K22.0 **Achalasia of cardia**
          Achalasia NOS
          Cardiospasm
          EXCLUDES 1   *congenital cardiospasm (Q39.5)*
          DEF: Esophageal motility disorder that is caused by absence of the esophageal peristalsis and impaired relaxation of the lower esophageal sphincter. It is characterized by dysphagia, regurgitation, and heartburn.

✓5ᵗʰ   **K22.1** **Ulcer of esophagus**
          Barrett's ulcer
          Erosion of esophagus
          Fungal ulcer of esophagus
          Peptic ulcer of esophagus
          Ulcer of esophagus due to ingestion of chemicals
          Ulcer of esophagus due to ingestion of drugs and medicaments
          Ulcerative esophagitis
          Code first poisoning due to drug or toxin, if applicable (T36-T65 with fifth or sixth character 1-4 or 6)
          Use additional code for adverse effect, if applicable, to identify drug (T36-T50 with fifth or sixth character 5)
          EXCLUDES 1   *Barrett's esophagus (K22.7-)*
          AHA: 2018,3Q,22; 2017,3Q,27
          TIP: Assign a code for "with bleeding" when an esophageal ulcer and bleeding (hematemesis) are documented. The ICD-10-CM classification assumes the two are related without the provider linking the two conditions. Evidence of bleeding during a procedure is not required.
          TIP: For bleeding ulcers resulting from anticoagulant therapy, code D68.32 Hemorrhagic disorder due to extrinsic circulating anticoagulant, and an adverse-effect code from subcategory T45.5- should also be assigned. Either the bleeding ulcer code or code D68.32 may be sequenced first, depending on the circumstances of admission.

          K22.10 **Ulcer of esophagus without bleeding**   **CC**
               Ulcer of esophagus NOS
               CC Excl: PDX collection 764

K22.11   **Ulcer of esophagus with bleeding**   `MCC`

    EXCLUDES 2   bleeding esophageal varices (I85.01, I85.11)

    CC Excl: PDX collection 765

K22.2   **Esophageal obstruction**

   Compression of esophagus
   Constriction of esophagus
   Stenosis of esophagus
   Stricture of esophagus

    EXCLUDES 1   congenital stenosis or stricture of esophagus (Q39.3)

K22.3   **Perforation of esophagus**   `MCC`

   Rupture of esophagus

    EXCLUDES 1   traumatic perforation of (thoracic) esophagus (S27.8-)

    CC Excl: PDX collection 766

K22.4   **Dyskinesia of esophagus**

   Corkscrew esophagus
   Diffuse esophageal spasm
   Spasm of esophagus

    EXCLUDES 1   cardiospasm (K22.0)

K22.5   **Diverticulum of esophagus, acquired**

   Esophageal pouch, acquired

    EXCLUDES 1   diverticulum of esophagus (congenital) (Q39.6)

K22.6   **Gastro-esophageal laceration-hemorrhage syndrome**   `MCC`

   Mallory-Weiss syndrome

    CC Excl: PDX collection 767

√5ᵗʰ **K22.7**   **Barrett's esophagus**

   Barrett's disease
   Barrett's syndrome

    EXCLUDES 1   Barrett's ulcer (K22.1)

           malignant neoplasm of esophagus (C15.-)

    DEF: Metaplastic disorder in which specialized columnar epithelial cells replace the normal squamous epithelial cells. Secondary to chronic gastroesophageal reflux damage to the mucosa, this disorder increases the risk of developing adenocarcinoma.

   K22.70   **Barrett's esophagus without dysplasia**

    Barrett's esophagus NOS

√6ᵗʰ **K22.71**   **Barrett's esophagus with dysplasia**

     K22.710   **Barrett's esophagus with low grade dysplasia**

     K22.711   **Barrett's esophagus with high grade dysplasia**

     K22.719   **Barrett's esophagus with dysplasia, unspecified**

K22.8   **Other specified diseases of esophagus**

   Hemorrhage of esophagus NOS

    EXCLUDES 2   esophageal varices (I85.-)

           Paterson-Kelly syndrome (D50.1)

K22.9   **Disease of esophagus, unspecified**

K23   **Disorders of esophagus in diseases classified elsewhere**

   Code first underlying disease, such as:
    congenital syphilis (A50.5)

    EXCLUDES 1   late syphilis (A52.79)

           megaesophagus due to Chagas' disease (B57.31)

           tuberculosis (A18.83)

√4ᵗʰ **K25**   **Gastric ulcer**

    `INCLUDES`   erosion (acute) of stomach
           pylorus ulcer (peptic)
           stomach ulcer (peptic)

   Use additional code to identify:
    alcohol abuse and dependence (F10.-)

    EXCLUDES 1   acute gastritis (K29.0-)

           peptic ulcer NOS (K27.-)

    AHA: 2017,3Q,27

    TIP: Assign a code for "with hemorrhage" when a gastric ulcer and GI bleeding are documented. The ICD-10-CM classification assumes the two are related without the provider linking the two conditions. Evidence of bleeding during a procedure is not required.

    TIP: For bleeding ulcers resulting from anticoagulant therapy, code D68.32 Hemorrhagic disorder due to extrinsic circulating anticoagulant, and an adverse-effect code from subcategory T45.5- should also be assigned. Either the bleeding ulcer code or code D68.32 may be sequenced first, depending on the circumstances of admission.

    CC Excl: For MCC codes in category K25: PDX collection 765

K25.0   **Acute gastric ulcer with hemorrhage**   `MCC`

K25.1   **Acute gastric ulcer with perforation**   `MCC` `HCC`

K25.2   **Acute gastric ulcer with both hemorrhage and perforation**   `MCC` `HCC`

K25.3   **Acute gastric ulcer without hemorrhage or perforation**   `CC`

    CC Excl: PDX collection 765

K25.4   **Chronic or unspecified gastric ulcer with hemorrhage**   `MCC`

K25.5   **Chronic or unspecified gastric ulcer with perforation**   `MCC` `HCC`

K25.6   **Chronic or unspecified gastric ulcer with both hemorrhage and perforation**   `MCC` `HCC`

K25.7   **Chronic gastric ulcer without hemorrhage or perforation**   `CC`

K25.9   **Gastric ulcer, unspecified as acute or chronic, without hemorrhage or perforation**   `CC`

Gastrointestinal Ulcers

Esophagus
Esophageal ulcer
Stomach
Duodenal ulcer
Gastric ulcer
Small intestine

√4ᵗʰ **K26**   **Duodenal ulcer**

    `INCLUDES`   erosion (acute) of duodenum
           duodenum ulcer (peptic)
           postpyloric ulcer (peptic)

   Use additional code to identify:
    alcohol abuse and dependence (F10.-)

    EXCLUDES 1   peptic ulcer NOS (K27.-)

    AHA: 2017,3Q,27

    TIP: Assign a code for "with hemorrhage" when a duodenal ulcer and GI bleeding are documented. The ICD-10-CM classification assumes the two are related without the provider linking the two conditions. Evidence of bleeding during a procedure is not required.

    TIP: For bleeding ulcers resulting from anticoagulant therapy, code D68.32 Hemorrhagic disorder due to extrinsic circulating anticoagulant, and an adverse-effect code from subcategory T45.5- should also be assigned. Either the bleeding ulcer code or code D68.32 may be sequenced first, depending on the circumstances of admission.

    CC Excl: For MCC codes in category K26: PDX collection 768

K26.0   **Acute duodenal ulcer with hemorrhage**   `MCC`

K26.1   **Acute duodenal ulcer with perforation**   `MCC` `HCC`

K26.2   **Acute duodenal ulcer with both hemorrhage and perforation**   `MCC` `HCC`

K26.3   **Acute duodenal ulcer without hemorrhage or perforation**   `CC`

    CC Excl: PDX collection 769

K26.4   **Chronic or unspecified duodenal ulcer with hemorrhage**   `MCC`

    AHA: 2016,1Q,14

K26.5   **Chronic or unspecified duodenal ulcer with perforation**   `MCC` `HCC`

K26.6   **Chronic or unspecified duodenal ulcer with both hemorrhage and perforation**   `MCC` `HCC`

K26.7   **Chronic duodenal ulcer without hemorrhage or perforation**

K26.9   **Duodenal ulcer, unspecified as acute or chronic, without hemorrhage or perforation**

N Newborn: 0   **P** Pediatric: 0-17   **M** Maternity: 9-64   **A** Adult: 15-124   `MCC` Major Complication/Comorbidity   `CC` Complication/Comorbidity   `SW` Severe Wound Dx

716   ICD-10-CM 2020

✓4ᵗʰ K27 Peptic ulcer, site unspecified

> **INCLUDES**   gastroduodenal ulcer NOS
>   peptic ulcer NOS
>
> Use additional code to identify:
>   alcohol abuse and dependence (F10.-)
>
> **EXCLUDES 1**   peptic ulcer of newborn (P78.82)
>
> **AHA:** 2017,3Q,27
>
> **TIP:** Assign a code for "with hemorrhage" when a peptic ulcer and GI bleeding are documented. The ICD-10-CM classification assumes the two are related without the provider linking the two conditions. Evidence of bleeding during a procedure is not required.
>
> **TIP:** For bleeding ulcers resulting from anticoagulant therapy, code D68.32 Hemorrhagic disorder due to extrinsic circulating anticoagulant, and an adverse-effect code from subcategory T45.5- should also be assigned. Either the bleeding ulcer code or code D68.32 may be sequenced first, depending on the circumstances of admission.
>
> **CC Excl: For CC/MCC codes in category K27:** PDX collection 768

K27.0   Acute **peptic ulcer, site unspecified, with hemorrhage**   `MCC`

K27.1   Acute **peptic ulcer, site unspecified, with perforation**   `MCC` `HCC`

K27.2   Acute **peptic ulcer, site unspecified, with both hemorrhage and perforation**   `MCC` `HCC`

K27.3   Acute **peptic ulcer, site unspecified, without hemorrhage or perforation**   `CC`

K27.4   Chronic **or unspecified peptic ulcer, site unspecified, with hemorrhage**   `MCC`

K27.5   Chronic **or unspecified peptic ulcer, site unspecified, with perforation**   `MCC` `HCC`

K27.6   Chronic **or unspecified peptic ulcer, site unspecified, with both hemorrhage and perforation**   `MCC` `HCC`

K27.7   Chronic **peptic ulcer, site unspecified, without hemorrhage or perforation**

K27.9   Peptic ulcer, site unspecified, unspecified as acute or chronic, without hemorrhage or perforation

✓4ᵗʰ K28 Gastrojejunal ulcer

> **INCLUDES**   anastomotic ulcer (peptic) or erosion
>   gastrocolic ulcer (peptic) or erosion
>   gastrointestinal ulcer (peptic) or erosion
>   gastrojejunal ulcer (peptic) or erosion
>   jejunal ulcer (peptic) or erosion
>   marginal ulcer (peptic) or erosion
>   stomal ulcer (peptic) or erosion
>
> Use additional code to identify:
>   alcohol abuse and dependence (F10.-)
>
> **EXCLUDES 1**   primary ulcer of small intestine (K63.3)
>
> **AHA:** 2017,3Q,27
>
> **TIP:** Assign a code for "with hemorrhage" when a gastrojejunal ulcer and GI bleeding are documented. The ICD-10-CM classification assumes the two are related without the provider linking the two conditions. Evidence of bleeding during a procedure is not required.
>
> **TIP:** For bleeding ulcers resulting from anticoagulant therapy, code D68.32 Hemorrhagic disorder due to extrinsic circulating anticoagulant, and an adverse-effect code from subcategory T45.5- should also be assigned. Either the bleeding ulcer code or code D68.32 may be sequenced first, depending on the circumstances of admission.
>
> **CC Excl: For CC/MCC codes in category K28:** PDX collection 765

K28.0   Acute **gastrojejunal ulcer with hemorrhage**   `MCC`

K28.1   Acute **gastrojejunal ulcer with perforation**   `MCC` `HCC`

K28.2   Acute **gastrojejunal ulcer with both hemorrhage and perforation**   `MCC` `HCC`

K28.3   Acute **gastrojejunal ulcer without hemorrhage or perforation**   `CC`

K28.4   Chronic **or unspecified gastrojejunal ulcer with hemorrhage**   `MCC`

K28.5   Chronic **or unspecified gastrojejunal ulcer with perforation**   `MCC` `HCC`

K28.6   Chronic **or unspecified gastrojejunal ulcer with both hemorrhage and perforation**   `MCC` `HCC`

K28.7   Chronic **gastrojejunal ulcer without hemorrhage or perforation**

K28.9   Gastrojejunal ulcer, unspecified as acute or chronic, without hemorrhage or perforation

✓4ᵗʰ K29 Gastritis and duodenitis

> **EXCLUDES 1**   eosinophilic gastritis or gastroenteritis (K52.81)
>   Zollinger-Ellison syndrome (E16.4)
>
> **AHA:** 2018,3Q,22
>
> **TIP:** Assign a code for "with bleeding" when gastritis or duodenitis and GI bleeding are documented. The ICD-10-CM classification assumes the two are related without the provider linking the two conditions. Evidence of bleeding during a procedure is not required.
>
> **TIP:** For bleeding resulting from anticoagulant therapy, code D68.32 Hemorrhagic disorder due to extrinsic circulating anticoagulant, and an adverse-effect code from subcategory T45.5- should also be assigned. Either code K29 or code D68.32 may be sequenced first, depending on the circumstances of admission.
>
> **CC Excl: For MCC codes in category K29:** PDX collection 770

✓5ᵗʰ K29.0 Acute gastritis

> Use additional code to identify:
>   alcohol abuse and dependence (F10.-)
>
> **EXCLUDES 1**   erosion (acute) of stomach (K25.-)

K29.00   **Acute gastritis without bleeding**   `CC`

K29.01   **Acute gastritis with bleeding**   `MCC`

✓5ᵗʰ K29.2 Alcoholic gastritis

> Use additional code to identify:
>   alcohol abuse and dependence (F10.-)

K29.20   **Alcoholic gastritis without bleeding**

K29.21   **Alcoholic gastritis with bleeding**   `MCC`

✓5ᵗʰ K29.3 Chronic superficial gastritis

K29.30   **Chronic superficial gastritis without bleeding**

K29.31   **Chronic superficial gastritis with bleeding**   `MCC`

✓5ᵗʰ K29.4 Chronic atrophic gastritis

> Gastric atrophy

K29.40   **Chronic atrophic gastritis without bleeding**

K29.41   **Chronic atrophic gastritis with bleeding**   `MCC`

✓5ᵗʰ K29.5 Unspecified chronic gastritis

> Chronic antral gastritis
> Chronic fundal gastritis

K29.50   **Unspecified chronic gastritis without bleeding**

K29.51   **Unspecified chronic gastritis with bleeding**   `MCC`

✓5ᵗʰ K29.6 Other gastritis

> Giant hypertrophic gastritis
> Granulomatous gastritis
> Ménétrier's disease

K29.60   **Other gastritis without bleeding**

K29.61   **Other gastritis with bleeding**   `MCC`

✓5ᵗʰ K29.7 Gastritis, unspecified

K29.70   **Gastritis, unspecified, without bleeding**

K29.71   **Gastritis, unspecified, with bleeding**   `MCC`

✓5ᵗʰ K29.8 Duodenitis

K29.80   **Duodenitis without bleeding**

K29.81   **Duodenitis with bleeding**   `MCC`

✓5ᵗʰ K29.9 Gastroduodenitis, unspecified

K29.90   **Gastroduodenitis, unspecified, without bleeding**

K29.91   **Gastroduodenitis, unspecified, with bleeding**   `MCC`

K30 Functional dyspepsia

> Indigestion
>
> **EXCLUDES 1**   dyspepsia NOS (R10.13)
>   heartburn (R12)
>   nervous dyspepsia (F45.8)
>   neurotic dyspepsia (F45.8)
>   psychogenic dyspepsia (F45.8)

✓4ᵗʰ K31 Other diseases of stomach and duodenum

> **INCLUDES**   functional disorders of stomach
>
> **EXCLUDES 2**   diabetic gastroparesis (E08.43, E09.43, E10.43, E11.43, E13.43)
>   diverticulum of duodenum (K57.00-K57.13)

K31.0   **Acute dilatation of stomach**   `CC`

> Acute distention of stomach
> **CC Excl:** PDX collection 771

☑ Additional Character Required   ✓×7ᵗʰ Placeholder   Unacceptable PDx   Questionable PDx   Manifestation   Unspecified Dx   H1-H14 HAC   HCC CMS-HCC Dx   HIV HIV Dx

ICD-10-CM 2020   **717**

Chapter 11. Diseases of the Digestive System

K31.1–K40.01

K31.1 Adult hypertrophic pyloric stenosis `CC` `A`
Pyloric stenosis NOS
EXCLUDES 1   *congenital or infantile pyloric stenosis (Q40.0)*
CC Excl: PDX collection 772

K31.2 Hourglass stricture and stenosis of stomach
EXCLUDES 1   *congenital hourglass stomach (Q40.2)*
        hourglass contraction of stomach (K31.89)

K31.3 Pylorospasm, not elsewhere classified
EXCLUDES 1   *congenital or infantile pylorospasm (Q40.0)*
        neurotic pylorospasm (F45.8)
        psychogenic pylorospasm (F45.8)

K31.4 Gastric diverticulum
EXCLUDES 1   *congenital diverticulum of stomach (Q40.2)*

K31.5 Obstruction of duodenum `CC`
Constriction of duodenum
Duodenal ileus (chronic)
Stenosis of duodenum
Stricture of duodenum
Volvulus of duodenum
EXCLUDES 1   *congenital stenosis of duodenum (Q41.0)*
CC Excl: PDX collection 773

K31.6 Fistula of stomach and duodenum `CC` `SW`
Gastrocolic fistula
Gastrojejunocolic fistula
CC Excl: PDX collection 774

K31.7 Polyp of stomach and duodenum `CC`
EXCLUDES 1   *adenomatous polyp of stomach (D13.1)*

√5ᵗʰ **K31.8 Other specified diseases of stomach and duodenum**

√6ᵗʰ **K31.81 Angiodysplasia of stomach and duodenum**
TIP: Assign a code for "with bleeding" when angiodysplasia of the stomach or the duodenum and GI bleeding are documented. The ICD-10-CM classification assumes the two are related without the provider linking the two conditions. Evidence of bleeding during a procedure is not required.

K31.811 Angiodysplasia of stomach and duodenum with bleeding `CC`

K31.819 Angiodysplasia of stomach and duodenum without bleeding
Angiodysplasia of stomach and duodenum NOS

K31.82 Dieulafoy lesion (hemorrhagic) of stomach and duodenum `MCC`
EXCLUDES 2   *Dieulafoy lesion of intestine (K63.81)*
DEF: Abnormally large submucosal artery protruding through a defect in the stomach mucosa or intestines that can cause massive and life-threatening hemorrhaging.
CC Excl: PDX collection 775

K31.83 Achlorhydria
DEF: Absence of hydrochloric acid in gastric secretions due to gastric mucosa atrophy. Achlorhydria is unresponsive to histamines.

K31.84 Gastroparesis
Gastroparalysis
Code first underlying disease, if known, such as:
anorexia nervosa (F50.0-)
diabetes mellitus (E08.43, E09.43, E10.43, E11.43, E13.43)
scleroderma (M34.-)
AHA: 2013,4Q,114

K31.89 Other diseases of stomach and duodenum
AHA: 2017,1Q,28

K31.9 Disease of stomach and duodenum, unspecified

Diseases of appendix (K35-K38)

√4ᵗʰ **K35 Acute appendicitis**
AHA: 2018,4Q,17-18

√5ᵗʰ **K35.2 Acute appendicitis with generalized peritonitis**
Appendicitis (acute) with generalized (diffuse) peritonitis following rupture or perforation of appendix

K35.20 Acute appendicitis with generalized peritonitis, without abscess
(Acute) appendicitis with generalized peritonitis NOS

K35.21 Acute appendicitis with generalized peritonitis, with abscess

√5ᵗʰ **K35.3 Acute appendicitis with localized peritonitis**

K35.30 Acute appendicitis with localized peritonitis, without perforation or gangrene
Acute appendicitis with localized peritonitis NOS

K35.31 Acute appendicitis with localized peritonitis and gangrene, without perforation

K35.32 Acute appendicitis with perforation and localized peritonitis, without abscess
(Acute) appendicitis with perforation NOS
Perforated appendix NOS
Ruptured appendix (with localized peritonitis) NOS

K35.33 Acute appendicitis with perforation and localized peritonitis, with abscess
(Acute) appendicitis with (peritoneal) abscess NOS
Ruptured appendix with localized peritonitis and abscess

√5ᵗʰ **K35.8 Other and unspecified acute appendicitis**
CC Excl: For CC codes in subcategory K35.8: PDX collection 776

K35.80 Unspecified acute appendicitis `CC`
Acute appendicitis NOS
Acute appendicitis without (localized) (generalized) peritonitis

√6ᵗʰ **K35.89 Other acute appendicitis**

K35.890 Other acute appendicitis without perforation or gangrene `CC`

K35.891 Other acute appendicitis without perforation, with gangrene `CC`
(Acute) appendicitis with gangrene NOS

K36 Other appendicitis
Chronic appendicitis
Recurrent appendicitis

K37 Unspecified appendicitis
EXCLUDES 1   *unspecified appendicitis with peritonitis (K35.2-, K35.3-)*

√4ᵗʰ **K38 Other diseases of appendix**

K38.0 Hyperplasia of appendix

K38.1 Appendicular concretions
Fecalith of appendix
Stercolith of appendix

K38.2 Diverticulum of appendix

K38.3 Fistula of appendix

K38.8 Other specified diseases of appendix
Intussusception of appendix

K38.9 Disease of appendix, unspecified

Hernia (K40-K46)

`NOTE`   Hernia with both gangrene and obstruction is classified to hernia with gangrene.

`INCLUDES`   acquired hernia
congenital [except diaphragmatic or hiatus] hernia
recurrent hernia

√4ᵗʰ **K40 Inguinal hernia**
`INCLUDES`   bubonocele
direct inguinal hernia
double inguinal hernia
indirect inguinal hernia
inguinal hernia NOS
oblique inguinal hernia
scrotal hernia
DEF: Within the groin region.
CC Excl: For CC/MCC codes in category K40: PDX collection 777

√5ᵗʰ **K40.0 Bilateral inguinal hernia, with obstruction, without gangrene**
Inguinal hernia (bilateral) causing obstruction without gangrene
Incarcerated inguinal hernia (bilateral) without gangrene
Irreducible inguinal hernia (bilateral) without gangrene
Strangulated inguinal hernia (bilateral) without gangrene

K40.00 Bilateral inguinal hernia, with obstruction, without gangrene, not specified as recurrent `CC`
Bilateral inguinal hernia, with obstruction, without gangrene NOS

K40.01 Bilateral inguinal hernia, with obstruction, without gangrene, recurrent `CC`

`N` Newborn: 0   `P` Pediatric: 0-17   `M` Maternity: 9-64   `A` Adult: 15-124   `MCC` Major Complication/Comorbidity   `CC` Complication/Comorbidity   `SW` Severe Wound Dx

✓5ᵗʰ **K40.1** **Bilateral inguinal hernia, with gangrene**

     K40.10 **Bilateral inguinal hernia, with**   `MCC`
         gangrene, not specified as recurrent
         Bilateral inguinal hernia, with gangrene NOS

     K40.11 **Bilateral inguinal hernia, with**   `MCC`
         gangrene, recurrent

✓5ᵗʰ **K40.2** **Bilateral inguinal hernia, without obstruction or gangrene**

     K40.20 **Bilateral inguinal hernia, without obstruction or**
         gangrene, not specified as recurrent
         Bilateral inguinal hernia NOS

     K40.21 **Bilateral inguinal hernia, without obstruction or**
         gangrene, recurrent

✓5ᵗʰ **K40.3** **Unilateral inguinal hernia, with obstruction, without gangrene**

     Inguinal hernia (unilateral) causing obstruction without gangrene
     Incarcerated inguinal hernia (unilateral) without gangrene
     Irreducible inguinal hernia (unilateral) without gangrene
     Strangulated inguinal hernia (unilateral) without gangrene

     K40.30 **Unilateral inguinal hernia, with**   `CC`
         obstruction, without gangrene, not
         specified as recurrent
         Inguinal hernia, with obstruction NOS
         Unilateral inguinal hernia, with obstruction, without gangrene NOS

     K40.31 **Unilateral inguinal hernia, with**   `CC`
         obstruction, without gangrene, recurrent

✓5ᵗʰ **K40.4** **Unilateral inguinal hernia, with gangrene**

     K40.40 **Unilateral inguinal hernia, with**   `MCC`
         gangrene, not specified as recurrent
         Inguinal hernia with gangrene NOS
         Unilateral inguinal hernia with gangrene NOS

     K40.41 **Unilateral inguinal hernia, with**   `MCC`
         gangrene, recurrent

✓5ᵗʰ **K40.9** **Unilateral inguinal hernia, without obstruction or gangrene**

     K40.90 **Unilateral inguinal hernia, without obstruction or**
         gangrene, not specified as recurrent
         Inguinal hernia NOS
         Unilateral inguinal hernia NOS

     K40.91 **Unilateral inguinal hernia, without obstruction or**
         gangrene, recurrent

Hernia Sites

✓4ᵗʰ **K41** **Femoral hernia**

CC Excl: For codes in category K41:
For MCC codes: PDX collection 779
For CC codes: PDX collection 778

✓5ᵗʰ **K41.0** **Bilateral femoral hernia, with obstruction, without gangrene**

     Femoral hernia (bilateral) causing obstruction, without gangrene
     Incarcerated femoral hernia (bilateral), without gangrene
     Irreducible femoral hernia (bilateral), without gangrene
     Strangulated femoral hernia (bilateral), without gangrene

     K41.00 **Bilateral femoral hernia, with**   `CC`
         obstruction, without gangrene, not
         specified as recurrent
         Bilateral femoral hernia, with obstruction, without gangrene NOS

     K41.01 **Bilateral femoral hernia, with**   `CC`
         obstruction, without gangrene, recurrent

✓5ᵗʰ **K41.1** **Bilateral femoral hernia, with gangrene**

     K41.10 **Bilateral femoral hernia, with**   `MCC`
         gangrene, not specified as recurrent
         Bilateral femoral hernia, with gangrene NOS

     K41.11 **Bilateral femoral hernia, with**   `MCC`
         gangrene, recurrent

✓5ᵗʰ **K41.2** **Bilateral femoral hernia, without obstruction or gangrene**

     K41.20 **Bilateral femoral hernia, without obstruction or**
         gangrene, not specified as recurrent
         Bilateral femoral hernia NOS

     K41.21 **Bilateral femoral hernia, without obstruction or**
         gangrene, recurrent

✓5ᵗʰ **K41.3** **Unilateral femoral hernia, with obstruction, without gangrene**

     Femoral hernia (unilateral) causing obstruction, without gangrene
     Incarcerated femoral hernia (unilateral), without gangrene
     Irreducible femoral hernia (unilateral), without gangrene
     Strangulated femoral hernia (unilateral), without gangrene

     K41.30 **Unilateral femoral hernia, with**   `CC`
         obstruction, without gangrene, not
         specified as recurrent
         Femoral hernia, with obstruction NOS
         Unilateral femoral hernia, with obstruction NOS

     K41.31 **Unilateral femoral hernia, with**   `CC`
         obstruction, without gangrene, recurrent

✓5ᵗʰ **K41.4** **Unilateral femoral hernia, with gangrene**

     K41.40 **Unilateral femoral hernia, with**   `MCC`
         gangrene, not specified as recurrent
         Femoral hernia, with gangrene NOS
         Unilateral femoral hernia, with gangrene NOS

     K41.41 **Unilateral femoral hernia, with**   `MCC`
         gangrene, recurrent

✓5ᵗʰ **K41.9** **Unilateral femoral hernia, without obstruction or gangrene**

     K41.90 **Unilateral femoral hernia, without obstruction or**
         gangrene, not specified as recurrent
         Femoral hernia NOS
         Unilateral femoral hernia NOS

     K41.91 **Unilateral femoral hernia, without obstruction or**
         gangrene, recurrent

✓4ᵗʰ **K42** **Umbilical hernia**

     `INCLUDES` paraumbilical hernia
     `EXCLUDES 1` omphalocele (Q79.2)

     K42.0 **Umbilical hernia with obstruction, without**   `CC`
         gangrene
         Umbilical hernia causing obstruction, without gangrene
         Incarcerated umbilical hernia, without gangrene
         Irreducible umbilical hernia, without gangrene
         Strangulated umbilical hernia, without gangrene
         CC Excl: PDX collection 780

     K42.1 **Umbilical hernia with gangrene**   `MCC`
         Gangrenous umbilical hernia
         CC Excl: PDX collection 781

     K42.9 **Umbilical hernia without obstruction or gangrene**
         Umbilical hernia NOS

✓4ᵗʰ **K43** **Ventral hernia**

     DEF: Condition in which a loop of bowel protrudes through a weakness in the abdominal wall muscles that may occur as a birth defect, past surgical site (incisional), or form at a stomal site (parastomal).
     CC Excl: For codes in category K43:
     For MCC codes: PDX collection 781
     For CC codes: PDX collection 780

     K43.0 **Incisional hernia with obstruction, without**   `CC`
         gangrene
         Incisional hernia causing obstruction, without gangrene
         Incarcerated incisional hernia, without gangrene
         Irreducible incisional hernia, without gangrene
         Strangulated incisional hernia, without gangrene

     K43.1 **Incisional hernia with gangrene**   `MCC`
         Gangrenous incisional hernia

     K43.2 **Incisional hernia without obstruction or gangrene**
         Incisional hernia NOS

☑ Additional Character Required   ✓ₓ7ᵗʰ Placeholder   Unacceptable PDx   Questionable PDx   Manifestation   Unspecified Dx   `H1`-`H14` HAC   `HCC` CMS-HCC Dx   `HIV` HIV Dx

ICD-10-CM 2020   719

K43.3 Parastomal hernia with obstruction, without gangrene `CC`
Incarcerated parastomal hernia, without gangrene
Irreducible parastomal hernia, without gangrene
Parastomal hernia causing obstruction, without gangrene
Strangulated parastomal hernia, without gangrene

K43.4 Parastomal hernia with gangrene `MCC`
Gangrenous parastomal hernia

K43.5 Parastomal hernia without obstruction or gangrene
Parastomal hernia NOS

K43.6 Other and unspecified ventral hernia with obstruction, without gangrene `CC`
Epigastric hernia causing obstruction, without gangrene
Hypogastric hernia causing obstruction, without gangrene
Incarcerated epigastric hernia without gangrene
Incarcerated hypogastric hernia without gangrene
Incarcerated midline hernia without gangrene
Incarcerated spigelian hernia without gangrene
Incarcerated subxiphoid hernia without gangrene
Irreducible epigastric hernia without gangrene
Irreducible hypogastric hernia without gangrene
Irreducible midline hernia without gangrene
Irreducible spigelian hernia without gangrene
Irreducible subxiphoid hernia without gangrene
Midline hernia causing obstruction, without gangrene
Spigelian hernia causing obstruction, without gangrene
Strangulated epigastric hernia without gangrene
Strangulated hypogastric hernia without gangrene
Strangulated midline hernia without gangrene
Strangulated spigelian hernia without gangrene
Strangulated subxiphoid hernia without gangrene
Subxiphoid hernia causing obstruction, without gangrene

K43.7 Other and unspecified ventral hernia with gangrene `MCC`
Any condition listed under K43.6 specified as gangrenous

K43.9 Ventral hernia without obstruction or gangrene
Epigastric hernia
Ventral hernia NOS

✓4ᵗʰ K44 Diaphragmatic hernia
[INCLUDES]   hiatus hernia (esophageal) (sliding)
paraesophageal hernia
[EXCLUDES 1]   congenital diaphragmatic hernia (Q79.0)
congenital hiatus hernia (Q40.1)
DEF: Protrusion of an abdominal organ, usually the stomach, through the esophageal opening within the diaphragm and occurring in two types: the sliding hiatal hernia and the paraesophageal hernia.

Hiatal Hernia

Sliding hiatal hernia

Gastroesophageal junction (slides up and down)

Gastroesophageal junction (remains in place)

Esophagus

Stomach

Diaphragm

Paraesophageal hiatal hernia

K44.0 Diaphragmatic hernia with obstruction, without gangrene `CC`
Diaphragmatic hernia causing obstruction
Incarcerated diaphragmatic hernia
Irreducible diaphragmatic hernia
Strangulated diaphragmatic hernia
CC Excl: PDX collection 782

K44.1 Diaphragmatic hernia with gangrene `MCC`
Gangrenous diaphragmatic hernia
CC Excl: PDX collection 782

K44.9 Diaphragmatic hernia without obstruction or gangrene
Diaphragmatic hernia NOS

✓4ᵗʰ K45 Other abdominal hernia
[INCLUDES]   abdominal hernia, specified site NEC
lumbar hernia
obturator hernia
pudendal hernia
retroperitoneal hernia
sciatic hernia

K45.0 Other specified abdominal hernia with obstruction, without gangrene `CC`
Other specified abdominal hernia causing obstruction
Other specified incarcerated abdominal hernia
Other specified irreducible abdominal hernia
Other specified strangulated abdominal hernia
CC Excl: PDX collection 783

K45.1 Other specified abdominal hernia with gangrene `MCC`
Any condition listed under K45 specified as gangrenous
CC Excl: PDX collection 784

K45.8 Other specified abdominal hernia without obstruction or gangrene

✓4ᵗʰ K46 Unspecified abdominal hernia
[INCLUDES]   enterocele
epiplocele
hernia NOS
interstitial hernia
intestinal hernia
intra-abdominal hernia
[EXCLUDES 1]   vaginal enterocele (N81.5)

K46.0 Unspecified abdominal hernia with obstruction, without gangrene `CC`
Unspecified abdominal hernia causing obstruction
Unspecified incarcerated abdominal hernia
Unspecified irreducible abdominal hernia
Unspecified strangulated abdominal hernia
CC Excl: PDX collection 783

K46.1 Unspecified abdominal hernia with gangrene `MCC`
Any condition listed under K46 specified as gangrenous
CC Excl: PDX collection 784

K46.9 Unspecified abdominal hernia without obstruction or gangrene
Abdominal hernia NOS

Noninfective enteritis and colitis (K50-K52)

[INCLUDES]   noninfective inflammatory bowel disease
[EXCLUDES 1]   irritable bowel syndrome (K58.-)
megacolon (K59.3-)

✓4ᵗʰ K50 Crohn's disease [regional enteritis]
[INCLUDES]   granulomatous enteritis
Use additional code to identify manifestations, such as:
pyoderma gangrenosum (L88)
[EXCLUDES 1]   ulcerative colitis (K51.-)
AHA: 2012,4Q,104
DEF: Chronic inflammation of the gastrointestinal tract characterized by chronic granulomatous disease, most commonly affecting the intestines and the terminal ileum.

✓5ᵗʰ K50.0 Crohn's disease of small intestine
Crohn's disease [regional enteritis] of duodenum
Crohn's disease [regional enteritis] of ileum
Crohn's disease [regional enteritis] of jejunum
Regional ileitis
Terminal ileitis
[EXCLUDES 1]   Crohn's disease of both small and large intestine (K50.8-)

K50.00 Crohn's disease of small intestine without complications `HCC`

✓6ᵗʰ K50.01 Crohn's disease of small intestine with complications

K50.011 Crohn's disease of small intestine with rectal bleeding `HCC`

`N` Newborn: 0   `P` Pediatric: 0-17   `M` Maternity: 9-64   `A` Adult: 15-124   `MCC` Major Complication/Comorbidity   `CC` Complication/Comorbidity   `SW` Severe Wound Dx

K50.012 **Crohn's disease of small intestine with intestinal obstruction** `HCC`

K50.013 **Crohn's disease of small intestine with fistula** `HCC` `SW`

K50.014 **Crohn's disease of small intestine with abscess** `HCC`
    AHA: 2012,4Q,104

K50.018 **Crohn's disease of small intestine with other complication** `HCC`

K50.019 **Crohn's disease of small intestine with unspecified complications** `HCC`

√5ᵗʰ **K50.1** **Crohn's disease of large intestine**
    Crohn's disease [regional enteritis] of colon
    Crohn's disease [regional enteritis] of large bowel
    Crohn's disease [regional enteritis] of rectum
    Granulomatous colitis
    Regional colitis
    EXCLUDES 1   *Crohn's disease of both small and large intestine (K50.8)*

K50.10 **Crohn's disease of large intestine without complications** `HCC`

√6ᵗʰ **K50.11** **Crohn's disease of large intestine with complications**

K50.111 **Crohn's disease of large intestine with rectal bleeding** `HCC`

K50.112 **Crohn's disease of large intestine with intestinal obstruction** `HCC`

K50.113 **Crohn's disease of large intestine with fistula** `HCC` `SW`

K50.114 **Crohn's disease of large intestine with abscess** `HCC`

K50.118 **Crohn's disease of large intestine with other complication** `HCC`

K50.119 **Crohn's disease of large intestine with unspecified complications** `HCC`

√5ᵗʰ **K50.8** **Crohn's disease of both small and large intestine**

K50.80 **Crohn's disease of both small and large intestine without complications** `HCC`

√6ᵗʰ **K50.81·** **Crohn's disease of both small and large intestine with complications**

K50.811 **Crohn's disease of both small and large intestine with rectal bleeding** `HCC`

K50.812 **Crohn's disease of both small and large intestine with intestinal obstruction** `HCC`

K50.813 **Crohn's disease of both small and large intestine with fistula** `HCC` `SW`

K50.814 **Crohn's disease of both small and large intestine with abscess** `HCC`

K50.818 **Crohn's disease of both small and large intestine with other complication** `HCC`

K50.819 **Crohn's disease of both small and large intestine with unspecified complications** `HCC`

√5ᵗʰ **K50.9** **Crohn's disease, unspecified**

K50.90 **Crohn's disease, unspecified, without complications** `HCC`
    Crohn's disease NOS
    Regional enteritis NOS

√6ᵗʰ **K50.91** **Crohn's disease, unspecified, with complications**

K50.911 **Crohn's disease, unspecified, with rectal bleeding** `HCC`

K50.912 **Crohn's disease, unspecified, with intestinal obstruction** `HCC`

K50.913 **Crohn's disease, unspecified, with fistula** `HCC` `SW`

K50.914 **Crohn's disease, unspecified, with abscess** `HCC`

K50.918 **Crohn's disease, unspecified, with other complication** `HCC`

K50.919 **Crohn's disease, unspecified, with unspecified complications** `HCC`

√4ᵗʰ **K51** **Ulcerative colitis**
    Use additional code to identify manifestations, such as:
    pyoderma gangrenosum (L88)
    EXCLUDES 1   *Crohn's disease [regional enteritis] (K50.-)*

√5ᵗʰ **K51.0** **Ulcerative (chronic) pancolitis**
    Backwash ileitis

K51.00 **Ulcerative (chronic) pancolitis without complications** `HCC`
    Ulcerative (chronic) pancolitis NOS

√6ᵗʰ **K51.01** **Ulcerative (chronic) pancolitis with complications**

K51.011 **Ulcerative (chronic) pancolitis with rectal bleeding** `HCC`

K51.012 **Ulcerative (chronic) pancolitis with intestinal obstruction** `HCC`

K51.013 **Ulcerative (chronic) pancolitis with fistula** `HCC` `SW`

K51.014 **Ulcerative (chronic) pancolitis with abscess** `HCC`

K51.018 **Ulcerative (chronic) pancolitis with other complication** `HCC`

K51.019 **Ulcerative (chronic) pancolitis with unspecified complications** `HCC`

√5ᵗʰ **K51.2** **Ulcerative (chronic) proctitis**

K51.20 **Ulcerative (chronic) proctitis without complications** `HCC`
    Ulcerative (chronic) proctitis NOS

√6ᵗʰ **K51.21** **Ulcerative (chronic) proctitis with complications**

K51.211 **Ulcerative (chronic) proctitis with rectal bleeding** `HCC`

K51.212 **Ulcerative (chronic) proctitis with intestinal obstruction** `CC` `HCC`
    CC Excl: PDX collection 785

K51.213 **Ulcerative (chronic) proctitis with fistula** `HCC` `SW`

K51.214 **Ulcerative (chronic) proctitis with abscess** `HCC`

K51.218 **Ulcerative (chronic) proctitis with other complication** `HCC`

K51.219 **Ulcerative (chronic) proctitis with unspecified complications** `HCC`

√5ᵗʰ **K51.3** **Ulcerative (chronic) rectosigmoiditis**

K51.30 **Ulcerative (chronic) rectosigmoiditis without complications** `HCC`
    Ulcerative (chronic) rectosigmoiditis NOS

√6ᵗʰ **K51.31** **Ulcerative (chronic) rectosigmoiditis with complications**

K51.311 **Ulcerative (chronic) rectosigmoiditis with rectal bleeding** `HCC`

K51.312 **Ulcerative (chronic) rectosigmoiditis with intestinal obstruction** `HCC`

K51.313 **Ulcerative (chronic) rectosigmoiditis with fistula** `HCC` `SW`

K51.314 **Ulcerative (chronic) rectosigmoiditis with abscess** `HCC`

K51.318 **Ulcerative (chronic) rectosigmoiditis with other complication** `HCC`

K51.319 **Ulcerative (chronic) rectosigmoiditis with unspecified complications** `HCC`

☑ Additional Character Required   √x7ᵗʰ Placeholder   Unacceptable PDx   Questionable PDx   Manifestation   Unspecified Dx   `H1`-`H14` HAC   `HCC` CMS-HCC Dx   `HIV` HIV Dx

ICD-10-CM 2020   721

Chapter 11. Diseases of the Digestive System

K51.4–K52.89

✓5th K51.4   Inflammatory polyps of colon

> **EXCLUDES 1**   adenomatous polyp of colon (D12.6)
> polyposis of colon (D12.6)
> polyps of colon NOS (K63.5)

K51.40   **Inflammatory polyps of colon** without complications   HCC
Inflammatory polyps of colon NOS

✓6th **K51.41**   **Inflammatory polyps of colon** with complications

     K51.411   **Inflammatory polyps of colon with** rectal bleeding   HCC

     K51.412   **Inflammatory polyps of colon with** intestinal obstruction   HCC

     K51.413   **Inflammatory polyps of colon with** fistula   CC HCC SW
        CC Excl: PDX collection 785

     K51.414   **Inflammatory polyps of colon with** abscess   HCC

     K51.418   **Inflammatory polyps of colon with other** complication   HCC

     K51.419   **Inflammatory polyps of colon with unspecified** complications   HCC

✓5th K51.5   Left sided colitis

Left hemicolitis

K51.50   **Left sided colitis** without complications   HCC
Left sided colitis NOS

✓6th **K51.51**   **Left sided colitis** with complications

     K51.511   **Left sided colitis with** rectal bleeding   HCC

     K51.512   **Left sided colitis with** intestinal obstruction   HCC

     K51.513   **Left sided colitis with** fistula   HCC SW

     K51.514   **Left sided colitis with** abscess   HCC

     K51.518   **Left sided colitis with other** complication   HCC

     K51.519   **Left sided colitis with** unspecified complications   HCC

✓5th K51.8   Other ulcerative colitis

> **CC Excl: For CC codes in subcategory K51.8:** PDX collection 785

K51.80   **Other ulcerative colitis** without complications   HCC

✓6th **K51.81**   **Other ulcerative colitis** with complications

     K51.811   **Other ulcerative colitis with** rectal bleeding   CC HCC

     K51.812   **Other ulcerative colitis with** intestinal obstruction   CC HCC

     K51.813   **Other ulcerative colitis with** fistula   CC HCC SW

     K51.814   **Other ulcerative colitis with** abscess   CC HCC

     K51.818   **Other ulcerative colitis with other complication**   CC HCC

     K51.819   **Other ulcerative colitis with unspecified complications**   CC HCC

✓5th K51.9   Ulcerative colitis, unspecified

> **CC Excl: For CC codes in subcategory K51.9:** PDX collection 787

K51.90   **Ulcerative colitis, unspecified, without complications**   HCC

✓6th **K51.91**   **Ulcerative colitis, unspecified, with complications**

     K51.911   **Ulcerative colitis, unspecified with** rectal bleeding   CC HCC

     K51.912   **Ulcerative colitis, unspecified with** intestinal obstruction   CC HCC

     K51.913   **Ulcerative colitis, unspecified with** fistula   CC HCC SW

     K51.914   **Ulcerative colitis, unspecified with** abscess   CC HCC

     K51.918   **Ulcerative colitis, unspecified with other complication**   CC HCC

     K51.919   **Ulcerative colitis, unspecified with unspecified complications**   CC HCC

✓4th K52   Other and unspecified noninfective gastroenteritis and colitis

AHA: 2016,4Q,30-31

K52.0   **Gastroenteritis and colitis due to** radiation   CC
     CC Excl: PDX collection 788

K52.1   **Toxic** gastroenteritis and colitis   CC
Drug-induced gastroenteritis and colitis
Code first (T51-T65) to identify toxic agent
Use additional code for adverse effect, if applicable, to identify drug (T36-T50 with fifth or sixth character 5)
AHA: 2019,1Q,17
CC Excl: PDX collection 789

✓5th K52.2   Allergic and dietetic gastroenteritis and colitis

Food hypersensitivity gastroenteritis or colitis
Use additional code to identify type of food allergy (Z91.01-, Z91.02-)

> **EXCLUDES 2**   allergic eosinophilic colitis (K52.82)
> allergic eosinophilic esophagitis (K20.0)
> allergic eosinophilic gastritis (K52.81)
> allergic eosinophilic gastroenteritis (K52.81)
> food protein-induced proctocolitis (K52.82)

DEF: True immunoglobulin E (IgE)-mediated allergic reaction of the lining of the stomach, intestines, or colon to food proteins. It causes nausea, vomiting, diarrhea, and abdominal cramping.
TIP: Assign a code for "with hemorrhage" when angiodysplasia and GI bleeding are documented. The ICD-10-CM classification assumes the two are related without the provider linking the two conditions. Evidence of bleeding during a procedure is not required.

K52.21   **Food protein-induced** enterocolitis syndrome
FPIES
Use additional code for hypovolemic shock, if present (R57.1)

K52.22   **Food protein-induced** enteropathy

K52.29   **Other allergic and dietetic gastroenteritis and colitis**
Food hypersensitivity gastroenteritis or colitis
Immediate gastrointestinal hypersensitivity

K52.3   **Indeterminate** colitis
Colonic inflammatory bowel disease unclassified (IBDU)
> **EXCLUDES 1**   unspecified colitis (K52.9)

✓5th K52.8   Other specified noninfective gastroenteritis and colitis

K52.81   **Eosinophilic gastritis or gastroenteritis**
Eosinophilic enteritis
> **EXCLUDES 2**   eosinophilic esophagitis (K20.0)

DEF: Disorder involving the accumulation of eosinophil in the lining of the stomach or multiple levels of the gastrointestinal tract, but without a known cause such as connective tissue disease, drug reaction, malignancy, or parasitic infection.

K52.82   **Eosinophilic colitis**
Allergic proctocolitis
Food-induced eosinophilic proctocolitis
Food protein-induced proctocolitis
Milk protein-induced proctocolitis
DEF: Disorder involving the accumulation of eosinophil in the tissues lining the colon, but without a known cause such as connective tissue disease, drug reaction, malignancy, or parasitic infection. The resultant inflammation may cause extreme abdominal pain, diarrhea, or bloody stool.

✓6th **K52.83**   **Microscopic colitis**

     K52.831   **Collagenous** colitis
     K52.832   **Lymphocytic** colitis
     K52.838   **Other microscopic colitis**
     K52.839   **Microscopic colitis, unspecified**

K52.89   **Other specified noninfective gastroenteritis and colitis**
AHA: 2019,1Q,20

N Newborn: 0   P Pediatric: 0-17   M Maternity: 9-64   A Adult: 15-124   MCC Major Complication/Comorbidity   CC Complication/Comorbidity   SW Severe Wound Dx

K52.9   **Noninfective gastroenteritis and colitis, unspecified**
Colitis NOS
Enteritis NOS
Gastroenteritis NOS
Ileitis NOS
Jejunitis NOS
Sigmoiditis NOS
> *EXCLUDES 1*   diarrhea NOS (R19.7)
> functional diarrhea (K59.1)
> infectious gastroenteritis and colitis NOS (A09)
> neonatal diarrhea (noninfective) (P78.3)
> psychogenic diarrhea (F45.8)

Other diseases of intestines (K55-K64)

☑4ᵗʰ K55   **Vascular disorders of intestine**
> *EXCLUDES 1*   necrotizing enterocolitis of newborn (P77.-)
AHA: 2016,4Q,32
CC Excl: For MCC codes in category K55, unless otherwise noted: PDX collection 790

☑5ᵗʰ K55.0   **Acute vascular disorders of intestine**
Infarction of appendices epiploicae
Mesenteric (artery) (vein) embolism
Mesenteric (artery) (vein) infarction
Mesenteric (artery) (vein) thrombosis

☑6ᵗʰ K55.01   **Acute (reversible) ischemia of small intestine**
> **K55.011**   **Focal (segmental) acute**   `MCC` `HCC`
> **(reversible) ischemia of small intestine**
> **K55.012**   **Diffuse acute (reversible)**   `MCC` `HCC`
> **ischemia of small intestine**
> **K55.019**   **Acute (reversible)**   `MCC` `HCC`
> **ischemia of small intestine, extent unspecified**

☑6ᵗʰ K55.02   **Acute infarction of small intestine**
Gangrene of small intestine
Necrosis of small intestine
> **K55.021**   **Focal (segmental) acute**   `MCC` `HCC`
> **infarction of small intestine**
> **K55.022**   **Diffuse acute infarction of**   `MCC` `HCC`
> **small intestine**
> **K55.029**   **Acute infarction of small**   `MCC` `HCC`
> **intestine, extent unspecified**

☑6ᵗʰ K55.03   **Acute (reversible) ischemia of large intestine**
Acute fulminant ischemic colitis
Subacute ischemic colitis
> **K55.031**   **Focal (segmental) acute**   `MCC` `HCC`
> **(reversible) ischemia of large intestine**
> **K55.032**   **Diffuse acute (reversible)**   `MCC` `HCC`
> **ischemia of large intestine**
> **K55.039**   **Acute (reversible)**   `MCC` `HCC`
> **ischemia of large intestine, extent unspecified**

☑6ᵗʰ K55.04   **Acute infarction of large intestine**
Gangrene of large intestine
Necrosis of large intestine
> **K55.041**   **Focal (segmental) acute**   `MCC` `HCC`
> **infarction of large intestine**
> **K55.042**   **Diffuse acute infarction of**   `MCC` `HCC`
> **large intestine**
> **K55.049**   **Acute infarction of large**   `MCC` `HCC`
> **intestine, extent unspecified**

☑6ᵗʰ K55.05   **Acute (reversible) ischemia of intestine, part unspecified**
> **K55.051**   **Focal (segmental) acute**   `MCC` `HCC`
> **(reversible) ischemia of intestine, part unspecified**
> **K55.052**   **Diffuse acute (reversible)**   `MCC` `HCC`
> **ischemia of intestine, part unspecified**
> **K55.059**   **Acute (reversible)**   `MCC` `HCC`
> **ischemia of intestine, part and extent unspecified**

☑6ᵗʰ K55.06   **Acute infarction of intestine, part unspecified**
Acute intestinal infarction
Gangrene of intestine
Necrosis of intestine
> **K55.061**   **Focal (segmental) acute**   `MCC` `HCC`
> **infarction of intestine, part unspecified**
> **K55.062**   **Diffuse acute infarction of**   `MCC` `HCC`
> **intestine, part unspecified**
> **K55.069**   **Acute infarction of**   `MCC` `HCC`
> **intestine, part and extent unspecified**

K55.1   **Chronic vascular disorders of intestine**   `HCC`
Chronic ischemic colitis
Chronic ischemic enteritis
Chronic ischemic enterocolitis
Ischemic stricture of intestine
Mesenteric atherosclerosis
Mesenteric vascular insufficiency

☑5ᵗʰ K55.2   **Angiodysplasia of colon**
AHA: 2018,3Q,21
TIP: Assign a code for "with hemorrhage" when angiodysplasia and GI bleeding are documented. The ICD-10-CM classification assumes the two are related without the provider linking the two conditions. Evidence of bleeding during a procedure is not required.
K55.20   **Angiodysplasia of colon without hemorrhage**
K55.21   **Angiodysplasia of colon with**   `MCC`
hemorrhage
> **DEF:** Small vascular abnormalities due to fragile blood vessels in the colon, resulting in blood loss from the gastrointestinal (GI) tract.
> **CC Excl:** PDX collection 770

☑5ᵗʰ K55.3   **Necrotizing enterocolitis**
> *EXCLUDES 1*   necrotizing enterocolitis of newborn (P77.-)
> *EXCLUDES 2*   necrotizing enterocolitis due to Clostridium difficile (A04.7-)
K55.30   **Necrotizing enterocolitis,**   `MCC` `HCC`
unspecified
Necrotizing enterocolitis, NOS
K55.31   **Stage 1 necrotizing enterocolitis**   `MCC` `HCC`
Necrotizing enterocolitis without pneumatosis, without perforation
K55.32   **Stage 2 necrotizing enterocolitis**   `MCC` `HCC`
Necrotizing enterocolitis with pneumatosis, without perforation
K55.33   **Stage 3 necrotizing enterocolitis**   `MCC` `HCC`
Necrotizing enterocolitis with perforation
Necrotizing enterocolitis with pneumatosis and perforation

K55.8   **Other vascular disorders of intestine**   `HCC`

K55.9   **Vascular disorder of intestine, unspecified**   `HCC`
Ischemic colitis
Ischemic enteritis
Ischemic enterocolitis

☑4ᵗʰ K56   **Paralytic ileus and intestinal obstruction without hernia**
> *EXCLUDES 1*   congenital stricture or stenosis of intestine (Q41-Q42)
> cystic fibrosis with meconium ileus (E84.11)
> ischemic stricture of intestine (K55.1)
> meconium ileus NOS (P76.0)
> neonatal intestinal obstructions classifiable to P76.-
> obstruction of duodenum (K31.5)
> postprocedural intestinal obstruction (K91.3-)
> stenosis of anus or rectum (K62.4)
CC Excl: For CC codes in category K56: PDX collection 792

K56.0   **Paralytic ileus**   `CC` `HCC`
Paralysis of bowel
Paralysis of colon
Paralysis of intestine
> *EXCLUDES 1*   gallstone ileus (K56.3)
> ileus NOS (K56.7)
> obstructive ileus NOS (K56.69-)
DEF: Intestinal obstruction due to paralysis of bowel motility or peristalsis.

K56.1 Intussusception `CC` `HCC`

Intussusception or invagination of bowel
Intussusception or invagination of colon
Intussusception or invagination of intestine
Intussusception or invagination of rectum
> *EXCLUDES 2*   *intussusception of appendix (K38.8)*

DEF: Intestinal obstruction due to prolapse of a bowel section into an adjacent section. It occurs primarily in children and symptoms include acute abdominal pain, vomiting, and passage of blood and mucus from the rectum.

K56.2 Volvulus `CC` `HCC`

Strangulation of colon or intestine
Torsion of colon or intestine
Twist of colon or intestine
> *EXCLUDES 2*   *volvulus of duodenum (K31.5)*

DEF: Twisting, knotting, or entanglement of the bowel on itself that may quickly compromise oxygen supply to the intestinal tissues. A volvulus usually occurs at the sigmoid and ileocecal areas of the intestines.

Volvulus

Knotted intestine (volvulus)

K56.3 Gallstone ileus `CC` `HCC`

Obstruction of intestine by gallstone

✓5ᵗʰ K56.4 Other impaction of intestine

K56.41 Fecal impaction `CC` `HCC`
> *EXCLUDES 1*   *constipation (K59.0-)*
> *incomplete defecation (R15.0)*

K56.49 Other impaction of intestine `CC` `HCC`

✓5ᵗʰ K56.5 Intestinal adhesions [bands] with obstruction (postinfection)

Abdominal hernia due to adhesions with obstruction
Peritoneal adhesions [bands] with intestinal obstruction (postinfection)
AHA: 2017,4Q,16-17

K56.50 Intestinal adhesions [bands], unspecified as to partial versus complete obstruction `CC` `HCC`

Intestinal adhesions with obstruction NOS

K56.51 Intestinal adhesions [bands], with partial obstruction `CC` `HCC`

Intestinal adhesions with incomplete obstruction

K56.52 Intestinal adhesions [bands] with complete obstruction `CC` `HCC`

✓5ᵗʰ K56.6 Other and unspecified intestinal obstruction

AHA: 2017,4Q,16-17; 2017,2Q,12

✓6ᵗʰ K56.60 Unspecified intestinal obstruction
> *EXCLUDES 1*   *intestinal obstruction due to specified condition - code to condition*

K56.600 Partial intestinal obstruction, unspecified as to cause `CC` `HCC`

Incomplete intestinal obstruction, NOS

K56.601 Complete intestinal obstruction, unspecified as to cause `CC` `HCC`

K56.609 Unspecified intestinal obstruction, unspecified as to partial versus complete obstruction `CC` `HCC`

Intestinal obstruction NOS

✓6ᵗʰ K56.69 Other intestinal obstruction

Enterostenosis NOS
Obstructive ileus NOS
Occlusion of colon or intestine NOS
Stenosis of colon or intestine NOS
Stricture of colon or intestine NOS
> *EXCLUDES 1*   *intestinal obstruction due to specified condition - code to condition*

K56.690 Other partial intestinal obstruction `CC` `HCC`

Other incomplete intestinal obstruction

K56.691 Other complete intestinal obstruction `CC` `HCC`

K56.699 Other intestinal obstruction unspecified as to partial versus complete obstruction `CC` `HCC`

Other intestinal obstruction, NEC

K56.7 Ileus, unspecified `CC` `HCC`
> *EXCLUDES 1*   *obstructive ileus (K56.69-)*
> *EXCLUDES 2*   *intestinal obstruction with hernia (K40-K46)*

AHA: 2017,1Q,40

✓4ᵗʰ K57 Diverticular disease of intestine

Code also if applicable peritonitis K65.-
> *EXCLUDES 1*   *congenital diverticulum of intestine (Q43.8)*
> *Meckel's diverticulum (Q43.0)*
> *EXCLUDES 2*   *diverticulum of appendix (K38.2)*

AHA: 2018,3Q,21

TIP: Assign a code for "with bleeding" when diverticular disease of the intestine and GI bleeding are documented. The ICD-10-CM classification assumes the two are related without the provider linking the two conditions. Evidence of bleeding during a procedure is not required.

CC Excl: For codes in category K57:
For MCC codes: PDX collection 770
For CC codes, unless otherwise noted: PDX collection 794

✓5ᵗʰ K57.0 Diverticulitis of small intestine with perforation and abscess

Diverticulitis of small intestine with peritonitis
> *EXCLUDES 1*   *diverticulitis of both small and large intestine with perforation and abscess (K57.4-)*

K57.00 Diverticulitis of small intestine with perforation and abscess without bleeding `CC`

CC Excl: PDX collection 793

K57.01 Diverticulitis of small intestine with perforation and abscess with bleeding `MCC`

✓5ᵗʰ K57.1 Diverticular disease of small intestine without perforation or abscess
> *EXCLUDES 1*   *diverticular disease of both small and large intestine without perforation or abscess (K57.5-)*

K57.10 Diverticulosis of small intestine without perforation or abscess without bleeding

Diverticular disease of small intestine NOS

K57.11 Diverticulosis of small intestine without perforation or abscess with bleeding `MCC`

K57.12 Diverticulitis of small intestine without perforation or abscess without bleeding

K57.13 Diverticulitis of small intestine without perforation or abscess with bleeding `MCC`

✓5ᵗʰ K57.2 Diverticulitis of large intestine with perforation and abscess

Diverticulitis of colon with peritonitis
> *EXCLUDES 1*   *diverticulitis of both small and large intestine with perforation and abscess (K57.4-)*

K57.20 Diverticulitis of large intestine with perforation and abscess without bleeding `CC`

K57.21 Diverticulitis of large intestine with perforation and abscess with bleeding `MCC`

🅝 Newborn: 0   🅟 Pediatric: 0-17   🅜 Maternity: 9-64   🅐 Adult: 15-124   `MCC` Major Complication/Comorbidity   `CC` Complication/Comorbidity   `SW` Severe Wound Dx

724   ICD-10-CM 2020

√5ᵗʰ **K57.3** **Diverticular disease of** large intestine without perforation or abscess

> EXCLUDES 1   *diverticular disease of both small and large intestine without perforation or abscess (K57.5-)*

     K57.30 **Diverticulosis of** large intestine without perforation or abscess **without bleeding**
Diverticular disease of colon NOS

     K57.31 **Diverticulosis** of large intestine without perforation or abscess **with bleeding**   `CC`

     K57.32 **Diverticulitis** of large intestine without perforation or abscess **without bleeding**   `CC`

     K57.33 **Diverticulitis** of large intestine without perforation or abscess **with bleeding**   `CC`

√5ᵗʰ **K57.4** **Diverticulitis of both** small and large intestine with perforation and abscess

Diverticulitis of both small and large intestine with peritonitis

     K57.40 **Diverticulitis of both small and large intestine with perforation and abscess without bleeding**   `CC`

     K57.41 **Diverticulitis of both small and large intestine with perforation and abscess with bleeding**   `MCC`

√5ᵗʰ **K57.5** **Diverticular disease of** both small and large intestine without perforation or abscess

     K57.50 **Diverticulosis of both small and large intestine without perforation or abscess without bleeding**
Diverticular disease of both small and large intestine NOS

     K57.51 **Diverticulosis** of both small and large intestine without perforation or abscess **with bleeding**   `MCC`

     K57.52 **Diverticulitis** of both small and large intestine without perforation or abscess **without bleeding**   `CC`

     K57.53 **Diverticulitis** of both small and large intestine without perforation or abscess **with bleeding**   `MCC`

√5ᵗʰ **K57.8** **Diverticulitis of intestine, part unspecified,** with perforation and abscess

Diverticulitis of intestine NOS with peritonitis

     K57.80 **Diverticulitis of intestine, part unspecified, with perforation and abscess without bleeding**   `CC`

     K57.81 **Diverticulitis of intestine, part unspecified, with perforation and abscess with bleeding**   `MCC`

√5ᵗʰ **K57.9** **Diverticular disease of intestine, part unspecified,** without perforation or abscess

     K57.90 **Diverticulosis of intestine, part unspecified, without perforation or abscess without bleeding**
Diverticular disease of intestine NOS

     K57.91 **Diverticulosis of intestine, part unspecified, without perforation or abscess with bleeding**   `MCC`

     K57.92 **Diverticulitis of intestine, part unspecified, without perforation or abscess without bleeding**   `CC`

     K57.93 **Diverticulitis of intestine, part unspecified, without perforation or abscess with bleeding**   `MCC`

√4ᵗʰ **K58** **Irritable bowel syndrome**

> INCLUDES   irritable colon
> spastic colon

AHA: 2016,4Q,32-33

K58.0 **Irritable bowel syndrome** with diarrhea

K58.1 **Irritable bowel syndrome** with constipation

K58.2 **Mixed irritable bowel syndrome**

K58.8 **Other irritable bowel syndrome**

K58.9 **Irritable bowel syndrome** without diarrhea
Irritable bowel syndrome NOS

√4ᵗʰ **K59** **Other functional intestinal disorders**

> EXCLUDES 1   *change in bowel habit NOS (R19.4)*
> *intestinal malabsorption (K90.-)*
> *psychogenic intestinal disorders (F45.8)*
> EXCLUDES 2   *functional disorders of stomach (K31.-)*

√5ᵗʰ **K59.0** **Constipation**

~~Use additional code for adverse effect, if applicable, to identify drug (T36-T50 with fifth or sixth character 5)~~

> EXCLUDES 1   *fecal impaction (K56.41)*
> *incomplete defecation (R15.0)*

AHA: 2016,4Q,33

     K59.00 **Constipation, unspecified**

     K59.01 **Slow transit constipation**
DEF: Delay in the transit of fecal material through the colon secondary to smooth muscle dysfunction or decreased peristaltic contractions along the colon.

     K59.02 **Outlet dysfunction constipation**

     K59.03 **Drug induced constipation**
Use additional code for adverse effect, if applicable, to identify drug (T36-T50 with fifth or sixth character 5)

     K59.04 **Chronic idiopathic constipation**
Functional constipation

     K59.09 **Other constipation**
Chronic constipation

K59.1 **Functional diarrhea**

> EXCLUDES 1   *diarrhea NOS (R19.7)*
> *irritable bowel syndrome with diarrhea (K58.0)*

K59.2 **Neurogenic bowel, not elsewhere classified**   `CC`
DEF: Disorder of bowel due to a spinal cord lesion due to injury or as a complication of conditions such as multiple sclerosis (MS) or spina bifida. Loss of bowel control is the primary symptom, manifested as constipation or bowel incontinence.
CC Excl: PDX collection 795

√5ᵗʰ **K59.3** **Megacolon, not elsewhere classified**
Dilatation of colon
Code first, if applicable (T51-T65) to identify toxic agent

> EXCLUDES 1   *congenital megacolon (aganglionic) (Q43.1)*
> *megacolon (due to) (in) Chagas' disease (B57.32)*
> *megacolon (due to) (in) Clostridium difficile (A04.7-)*
> *megacolon (due to) (in) Hirschsprung's disease (Q43.1)*

AHA: 2016,4Q,33-34

     K59.31 **Toxic megacolon**   `CC` `HCC`
CC Excl: PDX collection 795

     K59.39 **Other megacolon**   `CC`
Megacolon NOS
CC Excl: PDX collection 795

K59.4 **Anal spasm**
Proctalgia fugax

K59.8 **Other specified functional intestinal disorders**
Atony of colon
Pseudo-obstruction (acute) (chronic) of intestine

K59.9 **Functional intestinal disorder, unspecified**

√4ᵗʰ **K60** **Fissure and fistula of anal and rectal regions**

> EXCLUDES 1   *fissure and fistula of anal and rectal regions with abscess or cellulitis (K61.-)*
> EXCLUDES 2   *anal sphincter tear (healed) (nontraumatic) (old) (K62.81)*

K60.0 **Acute anal fissure**

K60.1 **Chronic anal fissure**

K60.2 **Anal fissure, unspecified**

K60.3 **Anal fistula**   `SW`

K60.4 **Rectal fistula**   `SW`

Fistula of rectum to skin

> EXCLUDES 1   *rectovaginal fistula (N82.3)*
> *vesicorectal fistual (N32.1)*

K60.5 **Anorectal fistula**   `SW`

√4ᵗʰ **K61** **Abscess of anal and rectal regions**

> INCLUDES   abscess of anal and rectal regions
> cellulitis of anal and rectal regions

K61.0 **Anal abscess**
Perianal abscess

> EXCLUDES 2   *intrasphincteric abscess (K61.4)*

☑ Additional Character Required   √x 7ᵗʰ Placeholder   <u>Unacceptable PDx</u>   Questionable PDx   Manifestation   Unspecified Dx   `H1`-`H14` HAC   `HCC` CMS-HCC Dx   `HIV` HIV Dx

K61.1 **Rectal abscess**
Perirectal abscess
> *EXCLUDES 1*   ischiorectal abscess (K61.39)

AHA: 2012,4Q,104

K61.2 **Anorectal abscess**

✓5ᵗʰ **K61.3** **Ischiorectal abscess**
AHA: 2018,4Q,19

     K61.31 **Horseshoe abscess**

     K61.39 **Other ischiorectal abscess**
       Abscess of ischiorectal fossa
       Ischiorectal abscess, NOS

K61.4 **Intrasphincteric abscess**
Intersphincteric abscess

K61.5 **Supralevator abscess**
AHA: 2018,4Q,19

✓4ᵗʰ **K62** **Other diseases of anus and rectum**
> *INCLUDES*   anal canal
> *EXCLUDES 2*   colostomy and enterostomy malfunction (K94.0-, K94.1-)
>   fecal incontinence (R15.-)
>   hemorrhoids (K64.-)

K62.0 **Anal polyp**

K62.1 **Rectal polyp**
> *EXCLUDES 1*   adenomatous polyp (D12.8)

AHA: 2018,1Q,6

K62.2 **Anal prolapse**
Prolapse of anal canal

K62.3 **Rectal prolapse**
Prolapse of rectal mucosa

K62.4 **Stenosis of anus and rectum**
Stricture of anus (sphincter)
AHA: 2019,2Q,13

K62.5 **Hemorrhage of anus and rectum**
> *EXCLUDES 1*   gastrointestinal bleeding NOS (K92.2)
>   melena (K92.1)
>   neonatal rectal hemorrhage (P54.2)

AHA: 2019,1Q,21

K62.6 **Ulcer of anus and rectum**
Solitary ulcer of anus and rectum
Stercoral ulcer of anus and rectum
> *EXCLUDES 1*   fissure and fistula of anus and rectum (K60.-)
>   ulcerative colitis (K51.-)

K62.7 **Radiation proctitis**
Use additional code to identify the type of radiation (W90.-)
AHA: 2019,1Q,21

✓5ᵗʰ **K62.8** **Other specified diseases of anus and rectum**
> *EXCLUDES 2*   ulcerative proctitis (K51.2)

     K62.81 **Anal sphincter tear (healed) (nontraumatic) (old)**
       Tear of anus, nontraumatic
       Use additional code for any associated fecal
       incontinence (R15.-)
>   *EXCLUDES 2*   anal fissure (K60.-)
>   anal sphincter tear (healed) (old)
>   complicating delivery (O34.7-)
>   traumatic tear of anal sphincter (S31.831)

     K62.82 **Dysplasia of anus**
       Anal intraepithelial neoplasia I and II (AIN I and II)
       (histologically confirmed)
       Dysplasia of anus NOS
       Mild and moderate dysplasia of anus (histologically
       confirmed)
>   *EXCLUDES 1*   abnormal results from anal cytologic
>   examination without histologic
>   confirmation (R85.61-)
>   anal intraepithelial neoplasia III (D01.3)
>   carcinoma in situ of anus (D01.3)
>   HGSIL of anus (R85.613)
>   severe dysplasia of anus (D01.3)

     K62.89 **Other specified diseases of anus and rectum**
       Proctitis NOS
       Use additional code for any associated fecal
       incontinence (R15.-)

K62.9 **Disease of anus and rectum, unspecified**

✓4ᵗʰ **K63** **Other diseases of intestine**

K63.0 **Abscess of intestine**   `CC`
> *EXCLUDES 1*   abscess of intestine with Crohn's disease (K50.014,
>   K50.114, K50.814, K50.914)
>   abscess of intestine with diverticular disease (K57.0,
>   K57.2, K57.4, K57.8)
>   abscess of intestine with ulcerative colitis (K51.014,
>   K51.214, K51.314, K51.414, K51.514, K51.814,
>   K51.914)
> *EXCLUDES 2*   abscess of anal and rectal regions (K61.-)
>   abscess of appendix (K35.3-)

CC Excl: PDX collection 798

K63.1 **Perforation of intestine (nontraumatic)**   `CC` `HCC`
Perforation (nontraumatic) of rectum
> *EXCLUDES 1*   perforation (nontraumatic) of duodenum (K26.-)
>   perforation (nontraumatic) of intestine with
>   diverticular disease (K57.0, K57.2, K57.4, K57.8)
> *EXCLUDES 2*   perforation (nontraumatic) of appendix (K35.2-,
>   K35.3-)

K63.2 **Fistula of intestine**   `CC` `SW`
> *EXCLUDES 1*   fistula of duodenum (K31.6)
>   fistula of intestine with Crohn's disease (K50.013,
>   K50.113, K50.813, K50.913)
>   fistula of intestine with ulcerative colitis (K51.013,
>   K51.213, K51.313, K51.413, K51.513, K51.813,
>   K51.913)
> *EXCLUDES 2*   fistula of anal and rectal regions (K60.-)
>   fistula of appendix (K38.3)
>   intestinal-genital fistula, female (N82.2-N82.4)
>   vesicointestinal fistula (N32.1)

AHA: 2017,3Q,4
CC Excl: PDX collection 800

K63.3 **Ulcer of intestine**   `CC`
Primary ulcer of small intestine
> *EXCLUDES 1*   duodenal ulcer (K26.-)
>   gastrointestinal ulcer (K28.-)
>   gastrojejunal ulcer (K28.-)
>   jejunal ulcer (K28.-)
>   peptic ulcer, site unspecified (K27.-)
>   ulcer of intestine with perforation (K63.1)
>   ulcer of anus or rectum (K62.6)
>   ulcerative colitis (K51.-)

CC Excl: PDX collection 801

K63.4 **Enteroptosis**

K63.5 **Polyp of colon**
> *EXCLUDES 1*   adenomatous polyp of colon ▶(D12.-)◀
>   inflammatory polyp of colon (K51.4-)
>   polyposis of colon (D12.6)

AHA: 2019,1Q,33; 2018,2Q,14; 2017,1Q,15; 2015,2Q,14
TIP: Assign this code when documentation states hyperplastic
colon polyp regardless of the site in the colon. Slow-growing,
hyperplastic polyps are not precancerous and are classified
differently from benign or adenomatous polyps.

✓5ᵗʰ **K63.8** **Other specified diseases of intestine**

     K63.81 **Dieulafoy lesion of intestine**   `MCC`
>   *EXCLUDES 2*   Dieulafoy lesion of stomach and
>   duodenum (K31.82)

       DEF: Abnormally large submucosal artery protruding
       through a defect in the stomach mucosa or intestines
       that can cause massive and life-threatening
       hemorrhaging.
       CC Excl: PDX collection 802

     K63.89 **Other specified diseases of intestine**
       AHA: 2013,2Q,31

K63.9 **Disease of intestine, unspecified**

`N` Newborn: 0   `P` Pediatric: 0-17   `M` Maternity: 9-64   `A` Adult: 15-124   `MCC` Major Complication/Comorbidity   `CC` Complication/Comorbidity   `SW` Severe Wound Dx

726   ICD-10-CM 2020

✓4ᵗʰ K64 Hemorrhoids and perianal venous thrombosis

     INCLUDES   piles

     EXCLUDES 1   hemorrhoids complicating childbirth and the puerperium (O87.2)

           hemorrhoids complicating pregnancy (O22.4)

Hemorrhoids

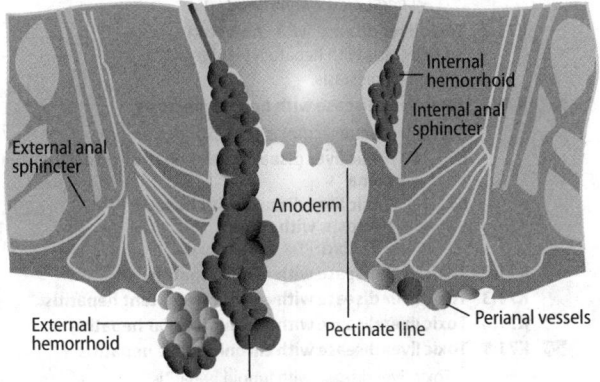

K64.Ø   First degree hemorrhoids

Grade/stage I hemorrhoids

Hemorrhoids (bleeding) without prolapse outside of anal canal

K64.1   Second degree hemorrhoids

Grade/stage II hemorrhoids

Hemorrhoids (bleeding) that prolapse with straining, but retract spontaneously

K64.2   Third degree hemorrhoids

Grade/stage III hemorrhoids

Hemorrhoids (bleeding) that prolapse with straining and require manual replacement back inside anal canal

K64.3   Fourth degree hemorrhoids

Grade/stage IV hemorrhoids

Hemorrhoids (bleeding) with prolapsed tissue that cannot be manually replaced

K64.4   Residual hemorrhoidal skin tags

External hemorrhoids, NOS

Skin tags of anus

K64.5   Perianal venous thrombosis

External hemorrhoids with thrombosis

Perianal hematoma

Thrombosed hemorrhoids NOS

K64.8   Other hemorrhoids

Internal hemorrhoids, without mention of degree

Prolapsed hemorrhoids, degree not specified

K64.9   Unspecified hemorrhoids

Hemorrhoids (bleeding) NOS

Hemorrhoids (bleeding) without mention of degree

Diseases of peritoneum and retroperitoneum (K65-K68)

CC Excl: For CC/MCC codes in categories K65-K68, unless otherwise noted: PDX collection 803

✓4ᵗʰ K65   Peritonitis

Use additional code (B95-B97), to identify infectious agent, if known

Code also if applicable diverticular disease of intestine (K57.-)

     EXCLUDES 1   acute appendicitis with generalized peritonitis (K35.2-)

           aseptic peritonitis (T81.6)

           benign paroxysmal peritonitis (E85.Ø)

           chemical peritonitis (T81.6)

           gonococcal peritonitis (A54.85)

           neonatal peritonitis (P78.Ø-P78.1)

           pelvic peritonitis, female (N73.3-N73.5)

           periodic familial peritonitis (E85.Ø)

           peritonitis due to talc or other foreign substance (T81.6)

           peritonitis in chlamydia (A74.81)

           peritonitis in diphtheria (A36.89)

           peritonitis in syphilis (late) (A52.74)

           peritonitis in tuberculosis (A18.31)

           peritonitis with or following abortion or ectopic or molar pregnancy (OØØ-OØ7, OØ8.Ø)

           peritonitis with or following appendicitis (K35.-)

           puerperal peritonitis (O85)

           retroperitoneal infections (K68.-)

K65.Ø   Generalized (acute) peritonitis   MCC   HCC

Pelvic peritonitis (acute), male

Subphrenic peritonitis (acute)

Suppurative peritonitis (acute)

K65.1   Peritoneal abscess   MCC   HCC

Abdominopelvic abscess

Abscess (of) omentum

Abscess (of) peritoneum

Mesenteric abscess

Retrocecal abscess

Subdiaphragmatic abscess

Subhepatic abscess

Subphrenic abscess

AHA: 2019,1Q,15

K65.2   Spontaneous bacterial peritonitis   MCC   HCC

     EXCLUDES 1   bacterial peritonitis NOS (K65.9)

K65.3   Choleperitonitis   MCC   HCC

Peritonitis due to bile

DEF: Inflammation of the peritoneum due to leakage of bile into the peritoneal cavity resulting from rupture of the bile passages or gallbladder.

K65.4   Sclerosing mesenteritis   CC   HCC

Fat necrosis of peritoneum

(Idiopathic) sclerosing mesenteric fibrosis

Mesenteric lipodystrophy

Mesenteric panniculitis

Retractile mesenteritis

K65.8   Other peritonitis   MCC   HCC

Chronic proliferative peritonitis

Peritonitis due to urine

K65.9   Peritonitis, unspecified   MCC   HCC

Bacterial peritonitis NOS

AHA: 2013,2Q,31

✓4ᵗʰ K66   Other disorders of peritoneum

     EXCLUDES 2   ascites (R18.-)

           peritoneal effusion (chronic) (R18.8)

K66.Ø   Peritoneal adhesions (postprocedural) (postinfection)

Adhesions (of) abdominal (wall)

Adhesions (of) diaphragm

Adhesions (of) intestine

Adhesions (of) male pelvis

Adhesions (of) omentum

Adhesions (of) stomach

Adhesive bands

Mesenteric adhesions

     EXCLUDES 1   female pelvic adhesions [bands] (N73.6)

           peritoneal adhesions with intestinal obstruction (K56.5-)

✓ Additional Character Required   ✓x7ᵗʰ Placeholder   Unacceptable PDx   Questionable PDx   Manifestation   Unspecified Dx   H1 - H14 HAC   HCC CMS-HCC Dx   HIV HIV Dx

ICD-10-CM 2020   727

Chapter 11. Diseases of the Digestive System

K66.1   **Hemoperitoneum**   `MCC`
> `EXCLUDES 1`   *traumatic hemoperitoneum (S36.8-)*
> **CC Excl:** PDX collection 804

K66.8   **Other specified disorders of peritoneum**

K66.9   **Disorder of peritoneum, unspecified**

K67   *Disorders of peritoneum in infectious diseases*   `MCC` `HCC`
classified elsewhere
> Code first underlying disease, such as:
>   congenital syphilis (A50.0)
>   helminthiasis (B65.0-B83.9)
> `EXCLUDES 1`   *peritonitis in chlamydia (A74.81)*
>   *peritonitis in diphtheria (A36.89)*
>   *peritonitis in gonococcal (A54.85)*
>   *peritonitis in syphilis (late) (A52.74)*
>   *peritonitis in tuberculosis (A18.31)*

✓4ᵗʰ **K68**   **Disorders of retroperitoneum**

✓5ᵗʰ **K68.1**   **Retroperitoneal abscess**

   K68.11   **Postprocedural retroperitoneal**   `CC` `H11` `H12` `H13`
      abscess
> `EXCLUDES 2`   *infection following procedure (T81.4-)*
> **CC Excl:** PDX collection 805

   K68.12   **Psoas muscle abscess**   `MCC` `HCC`
> **CC Excl:** PDX collection 806

   K68.19   **Other retroperitoneal abscess**   `MCC` `HCC`
> **AHA:** 2019,1Q,15
> **TIP:** This code should be used for a diagnosis of internal presacral abscess. If an intra-abdominal abscess is also present, code K65.1 can also be assigned; sequencing depends on the circumstances of admission.

K68.9   **Other disorders of retroperitoneum**   `MCC`

Diseases of liver (K70-K77)

`EXCLUDES 1`   *jaundice NOS (R17)*
`EXCLUDES 2`   *hemochromatosis (E83.11-)*
     Reye's syndrome (G93.7)
     viral hepatitis (B15-B19)
     Wilson's disease (E83.0)

✓4ᵗʰ **K70**   **Alcoholic liver disease**
> Use additional code to identify:
>   alcohol abuse and dependence (F10.-)

K70.0   **Alcoholic fatty liver**   `A`

✓5ᵗʰ **K70.1**   **Alcoholic hepatitis**

   K70.10   **Alcoholic hepatitis without ascites**   `A`

   K70.11   **Alcoholic hepatitis with ascites**   `A`

K70.2   **Alcoholic fibrosis and sclerosis of liver**   `A`

✓5ᵗʰ **K70.3**   **Alcoholic cirrhosis of liver**
> Alcoholic cirrhosis NOS

   K70.30   **Alcoholic cirrhosis of liver without**   `HCC` `A`
      ascites

   K70.31   **Alcoholic cirrhosis of liver with**   `HCC` `A`
      ascites
> **AHA:** 2018,1Q,4

✓5ᵗʰ **K70.4**   **Alcoholic hepatic failure**
> Acute alcoholic hepatic failure
> Alcoholic hepatic failure NOS
> Chronic alcoholic hepatic failure
> Subacute alcoholic hepatic failure

   K70.40   **Alcoholic hepatic failure without**   `HCC` `A`
      coma

   K70.41   **Alcoholic hepatic failure with coma**   `MCC` `HCC` `A`
> **CC Excl:** PDX collection 807

K70.9   **Alcoholic liver disease, unspecified**   `HCC` `A`

✓4ᵗʰ **K71**   **Toxic liver disease**
> `INCLUDES`   drug-induced idiosyncratic (unpredictable) liver disease
>   drug-induced toxic (predictable) liver disease
> Code first poisoning due to drug or toxin, if applicable (T36-T65 with fifth or sixth character 1-4 or 6)
> Use additional code for adverse effect, if applicable, to identify drug (T36-T50 with fifth or sixth character 5)
> `EXCLUDES 2`   *alcoholic liver disease (K70.-)*
>   *Budd-Chiari syndrome (I82.0)*

K71.0   **Toxic liver disease with cholestasis**
> Cholestasis with hepatocyte injury
> "Pure" cholestasis

✓5ᵗʰ **K71.1**   **Toxic liver disease with hepatic necrosis**
> Hepatic failure (acute) (chronic) due to drugs

   K71.10   **Toxic liver disease with hepatic necrosis, without coma**

   K71.11   **Toxic liver disease with hepatic**   `MCC` `HCC`
      necrosis, with coma
> **CC Excl:** PDX collection 807

K71.2   **Toxic liver disease with acute hepatitis**

K71.3   **Toxic liver disease with chronic persistent hepatitis**

K71.4   **Toxic liver disease with chronic lobular hepatitis**

✓5ᵗʰ **K71.5**   **Toxic liver disease with chronic active hepatitis**
> Toxic liver disease with lupoid hepatitis

   K71.50   **Toxic liver disease with chronic active hepatitis without ascites**

   K71.51   **Toxic liver disease with chronic active hepatitis with ascites**
> **AHA:** 2018,1Q,4

K71.6   **Toxic liver disease with hepatitis, not elsewhere classified**

K71.7   **Toxic liver disease with fibrosis and cirrhosis of liver**

K71.8   **Toxic liver disease with other disorders of liver**
> Toxic liver disease with focal nodular hyperplasia
> Toxic liver disease with hepatic granulomas
> Toxic liver disease with peliosis hepatis
> Toxic liver disease with veno-occlusive disease of liver

K71.9   **Toxic liver disease, unspecified**

✓4ᵗʰ **K72**   **Hepatic failure, not elsewhere classified**
> `INCLUDES`   fulminant hepatitis NEC, with hepatic failure
>   hepatic encephalopathy NOS
>   liver (cell) necrosis with hepatic failure
>   malignant hepatitis NEC, with hepatic failure
>   yellow liver atrophy or dystrophy
> `EXCLUDES 1`   *alcoholic hepatic failure (K70.4)*
>   *hepatic failure with toxic liver disease (K71.1-)*
>   *icterus of newborn (P55-P59)*
>   *postprocedural hepatic failure (K91.82)*
> `EXCLUDES 2`   *hepatic failure complicating abortion or ectopic or molar pregnancy (O00-O07, O08.8)*
>   *hepatic failure complicating pregnancy, childbirth and the puerperium (O26.6-)*
>   *viral hepatitis with hepatic coma (B15-B19)*
> **AHA:** 2017,1Q,41

✓5ᵗʰ **K72.0**   **Acute and subacute hepatic failure**
> Acute non-viral hepatitis NOS
> **AHA:** 2015,2Q,17; 2014,2Q,13

   K72.00   **Acute and subacute hepatic failure**   `MCC`
      without coma
> **CC Excl:** PDX collection 808

   K72.01   **Acute and subacute hepatic failure**   `MCC` `HCC`
      with coma
> **CC Excl:** PDX collection 808

✓5ᵗʰ **K72.1**   **Chronic hepatic failure**

   K72.10   **Chronic hepatic failure without coma**   `HCC`

   K72.11   **Chronic hepatic failure with coma**   `MCC` `HCC`
> **CC Excl:** PDX collection 807

✓5ᵗʰ **K72.9**   **Hepatic failure, unspecified**

   K72.90   **Hepatic failure, unspecified without**   `HCC`
      coma
> **AHA:** 2018,4Q,20; 2016,2Q,35

   K72.91   **Hepatic failure, unspecified with**   `MCC` `HCC`
      coma
> Hepatic coma NOS
> **CC Excl:** PDX collection 807

`N` Newborn: 0   `P` Pediatric: 0-17   `M` Maternity: 9-64   `A` Adult: 15-124   `MCC` Major Complication/Comorbidity   `CC` Complication/Comorbidity   `SW` Severe Wound Dx

728   ICD-10-CM 2020

✓4ᵗʰ **K73** **Chronic hepatitis, not elsewhere classified**

    EXCLUDES 1   alcoholic hepatitis (chronic) (K70.1-)

              drug-induced hepatitis (chronic) (K71.-)

              granulomatous hepatitis (chronic) NEC (K75.3)

              reactive, nonspecific hepatitis (chronic) (K75.2)

              viral hepatitis (chronic) (B15-B19)

     K73.0 **Chronic persistent hepatitis, not elsewhere classified** `HCC`

     K73.1 **Chronic lobular hepatitis, not elsewhere classified** `HCC`

     K73.2 **Chronic active hepatitis, not elsewhere classified** `HCC`

     K73.8 **Other chronic hepatitis, not elsewhere classified** `HCC`

     K73.9 **Chronic hepatitis, unspecified** `HCC`

✓4ᵗʰ **K74** **Fibrosis and cirrhosis of liver**

     Code also, if applicable, viral hepatitis (acute) (chronic) (B15-B19)

    EXCLUDES 1   alcoholic cirrhosis (of liver) (K70.3)

              alcoholic fibrosis of liver (K70.2)

              cardiac sclerosis of liver (K76.1)

              cirrhosis (of liver) with toxic liver disease (K71.7)

              congenital cirrhosis (of liver) (P78.81)

              pigmentary cirrhosis (of liver) (E83.110)

     K74.0 **Hepatic fibrosis**

     K74.1 **Hepatic sclerosis**

     K74.2 **Hepatic fibrosis with hepatic sclerosis**

     K74.3 **Primary biliary cirrhosis** `HCC`

         Chronic nonsuppurative destructive cholangitis

         Primary biliary cholangitis

        EXCLUDES 2 ▶primary sclerosing cholangitis◀ (K83.01)

     K74.4 **Secondary biliary cirrhosis** `HCC`

     K74.5 **Biliary cirrhosis, unspecified** `HCC`

    ✓5ᵗʰ **K74.6** **Other and unspecified cirrhosis of liver**

         K74.60 **Unspecified cirrhosis of liver** `HCC`

             Cirrhosis (of liver) NOS

             AHA: 2018,1Q,4

         K74.69 **Other cirrhosis of liver** `HCC`

             Cryptogenic cirrhosis (of liver)

             Macronodular cirrhosis (of liver)

             Micronodular cirrhosis (of liver)

             Mixed type cirrhosis (of liver)

             Portal cirrhosis (of liver)

             Postnecrotic cirrhosis (of liver)

✓4ᵗʰ **K75** **Other inflammatory liver diseases**

    EXCLUDES 2   toxic liver disease (K71.-)

     K75.0 **Abscess of liver** `MCC`

         Cholangitic hepatic abscess

         Hematogenic hepatic abscess

         Hepatic abscess NOS

         Lymphogenic hepatic abscess

         Pylephlebitic hepatic abscess

        EXCLUDES 1   amebic liver abscess (A06.4)

              cholangitis without liver abscess (K83.09)

              pylephlebitis without liver abscess (K75.1)

        EXCLUDES 2   acute or subacute hepatitis NOS (B17.9)

              acute or subacute non-viral hepatitis (K72.0)

              chronic hepatitis NEC (K73.8)

         CC Excl: PDX collection 809

     K75.1 **Phlebitis of portal vein** `MCC`

         Pylephlebitis

        EXCLUDES 1   pylephlebitic liver abscess (K75.0)

         DEF: Inflammation of the portal vein or branches due to diverticulitis, perforated appendicitis, or peritonitis. Symptoms include fever, chills, jaundice, sweating, and abscess in various body parts.

         CC Excl: PDX collection 809

     K75.2 **Nonspecific reactive hepatitis**

        EXCLUDES 1   acute or subacute hepatitis (K72.0-)

              chronic hepatitis NEC (K73.-)

              viral hepatitis (B15-B19)

     K75.3 **Granulomatous hepatitis, not elsewhere classified**

        EXCLUDES 1   acute or subacute hepatitis (K72.0-)

              chronic hepatitis NEC (K73.-)

              viral hepatitis (B15-B19)

     K75.4 **Autoimmune hepatitis** `HCC`

         Lupoid hepatitis NEC

    ✓5ᵗʰ **K75.8** **Other specified inflammatory liver diseases**

         K75.81 **Nonalcoholic steatohepatitis (NASH)**

         K75.89 **Other specified inflammatory liver diseases**

     K75.9 **Inflammatory liver disease, unspecified**

         Hepatitis NOS

        EXCLUDES 1   acute or subacute hepatitis (K72.0-)

              chronic hepatitis NEC (K73.-)

              viral hepatitis (B15-B19)

         AHA: 2015,2Q,17

✓4ᵗʰ **K76** **Other diseases of liver**

    EXCLUDES 2   alcoholic liver disease (K70.-)

              amyloid degeneration of liver (E85.-)

              cystic disease of liver (congenital) (Q44.6)

              hepatic vein thrombosis (I82.0)

              hepatomegaly NOS (R16.0)

              pigmentary cirrhosis (of liver) (E83.110)

              portal vein thrombosis (I81)

              toxic liver disease (K71.-)

     K76.0 **Fatty (change of) liver, not elsewhere classified**

         Nonalcoholic fatty liver disease (NAFLD)

        EXCLUDES 1   nonalcoholic steatohepatitis (NASH) (K75.81)

     K76.1 **Chronic passive congestion of liver** `CC`

         Cardiac cirrhosis

         Cardiac sclerosis

     K76.2 **Central hemorrhagic necrosis of liver** `MCC`

        EXCLUDES 1   liver necrosis with hepatic failure (K72.-)

         CC Excl: PDX collection 808

     K76.3 **Infarction of liver** `MCC`

         CC Excl: PDX collection 808

     K76.4 **Peliosis hepatis**

         Hepatic angiomatosis

     K76.5 **Hepatic veno-occlusive disease**

        EXCLUDES 1   Budd-Chiari syndrome (I82.0)

     K76.6 **Portal hypertension** `CC` `HCC`

         Use additional code for any associated complications, such as:

           portal hypertensive gastropathy (K31.89)

         CC Excl: PDX collection 810

     K76.7 **Hepatorenal syndrome** `MCC` `HCC`

        EXCLUDES 1   hepatorenal syndrome following labor and delivery (O90.4)

              postprocedural hepatorenal syndrome (K91.83)

         CC Excl: PDX collection 811

    ✓5ᵗʰ **K76.8** **Other specified diseases of liver**

         K76.81 **Hepatopulmonary syndrome** `HCC`

             Code first underlying liver disease, such as:

               alcoholic cirrhosis of liver (K70.3-)

               cirrhosis of liver without mention of alcohol (K74.6-)

         K76.89 **Other specified diseases of liver**

             Cyst (simple) of liver

             Focal nodular hyperplasia of liver

             Hepatoptosis

     K76.9 **Liver disease, unspecified**

K77 Liver disorders in diseases classified elsewhere   `CC`

Code first underlying disease, such as:
amyloidosis (E85.-)
congenital syphilis (A50.0, A50.5)
congenital toxoplasmosis (P37.1)
schistosomiasis (B65.0-B65.9)

EXCLUDES 1   alcoholic hepatitis (K70.1-)
alcoholic liver disease (K70.-)
cytomegaloviral hepatitis (B25.1)
herpesviral [herpes simplex] hepatitis (B00.81)
infectious mononucleosis with liver disease (B27.0-B27.9 with .9)
mumps hepatitis (B26.81)
sarcoidosis with liver disease (D86.89)
secondary syphilis with liver disease (A51.45)
syphilis (late) with liver disease (A52.74)
toxoplasmosis (acquired) hepatitis (B58.1)
tuberculosis with liver disease (A18.83)

CC Excl: No Excl

Disorders of gallbladder, biliary tract and pancreas (K80-K87)

✓⁴ᵗʰ K80 Cholelithiasis

EXCLUDES 1   retained cholelithiasis following cholecystectomy (K91.86)

AHA: 2018,4Q,20

DEF: Presence or formation of concretions (calculi or "gallstones") in the gallbladder. The stones contain cholesterol, calcium carbonate, or calcium bilirubinate in pure forms or in various combinations.

Cholelithiasis

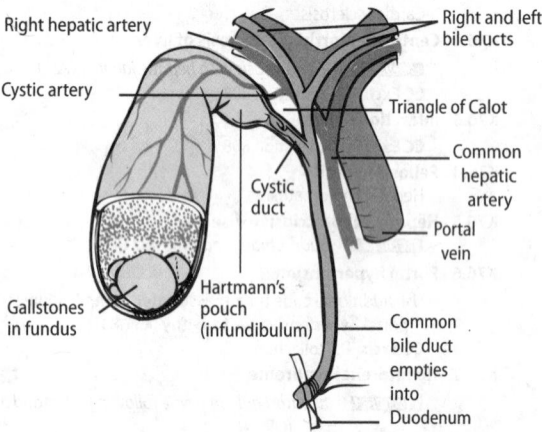

Right hepatic artery — Right and left bile ducts
Cystic artery — Triangle of Calot
Cystic duct — Common hepatic artery
— Portal vein
Gallstones in fundus — Hartmann's pouch (infundibulum)
— Common bile duct empties into Duodenum

✓⁵ᵗʰ K80.0 Calculus of gallbladder with acute cholecystitis

Any condition listed in K80.2 with acute cholecystitis
Use additional code if applicable for associated gangrene of gallbladder (K82.A1), or perforation of gallbladder (K82.A2)

K80.00 Calculus of gallbladder with acute cholecystitis without obstruction

K80.01 Calculus of gallbladder with acute cholecystitis with obstruction   `CC`
     CC Excl: PDX collection 813

✓⁵ᵗʰ K80.1 Calculus of gallbladder with other cholecystitis

Use additional code if applicable for associated gangrene of gallbladder (K82.A1), or perforation of gallbladder (K82.A2)

CC Excl: For CC codes in subcategory K80.1: PDX collection 813

K80.10 Calculus of gallbladder with chronic cholecystitis without obstruction
     Cholelithiasis with cholecystitis NOS

K80.11 Calculus of gallbladder with chronic cholecystitis with obstruction   `CC`

K80.12 Calculus of gallbladder with acute and chronic cholecystitis without obstruction

K80.13 Calculus of gallbladder with acute and chronic cholecystitis with obstruction   `CC`

K80.18 Calculus of gallbladder with other cholecystitis without obstruction

K80.19 Calculus of gallbladder with other cholecystitis with obstruction   `CC`

✓⁵ᵗʰ K80.2 Calculus of gallbladder without cholecystitis

Cholecystolithiasis without cholecystitis
Cholelithiasis (without cholecystitis)
Colic (recurrent) of gallbladder (without cholecystitis)
Gallstone (impacted) of cystic duct (without cholecystitis)
Gallstone (impacted) of gallbladder (without cholecystitis)

K80.20 Calculus of gallbladder without cholecystitis without obstruction

K80.21 Calculus of gallbladder without cholecystitis with obstruction   `CC`
     CC Excl: PDX collection 813

✓⁵ᵗʰ K80.3 Calculus of bile duct with cholangitis

Any condition listed in K80.5 with cholangitis
DEF: Cholangitis: Inflammation of the bile ducts.
CC Excl: For CC codes in subcategory K80.3, unless otherwise noted: PDX collection 814

K80.30 Calculus of bile duct with cholangitis, unspecified, without obstruction   `CC`

K80.31 Calculus of bile duct with cholangitis, unspecified, with obstruction
     CC Excl: PDX collection 815

K80.32 Calculus of bile duct with acute cholangitis without obstruction   `CC`

K80.33 Calculus of bile duct with acute cholangitis with obstruction   `CC`
     CC Excl: PDX collection 815

K80.34 Calculus of bile duct with chronic cholangitis without obstruction   `CC`

K80.35 Calculus of bile duct with chronic cholangitis with obstruction   `CC`
     CC Excl: PDX collection 815

K80.36 Calculus of bile duct with acute and chronic cholangitis without obstruction   `CC`

K80.37 Calculus of bile duct with acute and chronic cholangitis with obstruction   `CC`
     CC Excl: PDX collection 815

✓⁵ᵗʰ K80.4 Calculus of bile duct with cholecystitis

Any condition listed in K80.5 with cholecystitis (with cholangitis)
Use additional code if applicable for associated gangrene of gallbladder (K82.A1), or perforation of gallbladder (K82.A2)
AHA: 2019,1Q,17
CC Excl: For CC codes in subcategory K80.4: PDX collection 815

K80.40 Calculus of bile duct with cholecystitis, unspecified, without obstruction   `CC`

K80.41 Calculus of bile duct with cholecystitis, unspecified, with obstruction   `CC`
     AHA: 2019,1Q,17

K80.42 Calculus of bile duct with acute cholecystitis without obstruction   `CC`

K80.43 Calculus of bile duct with acute cholecystitis with obstruction   `CC`

K80.44 Calculus of bile duct with chronic cholecystitis without obstruction   `CC`

K80.45 Calculus of bile duct with chronic cholecystitis with obstruction   `CC`

K80.46 Calculus of bile duct with acute and chronic cholecystitis without obstruction   `CC`

K80.47 Calculus of bile duct with acute and chronic cholecystitis with obstruction   `CC`

✓⁵ᵗʰ K80.5 Calculus of bile duct without cholangitis or cholecystitis

Choledocholithiasis (without cholangitis or cholecystitis)
Gallstone (impacted) of bile duct NOS (without cholangitis or cholecystitis)
Gallstone (impacted) of common duct (without cholangitis or cholecystitis)
Gallstone (impacted) of hepatic duct (without cholangitis or cholecystitis)
Hepatic cholelithiasis (without cholangitis or cholecystitis)
Hepatic colic (recurrent) (without cholangitis or cholecystitis)
DEF: Cholangitis: Inflammation of the bile ducts.

K80.50 Calculus of bile duct without cholangitis or cholecystitis without obstruction   `CC`

`N` Newborn: 0   `P` Pediatric: 0-17   `M` Maternity: 9-64   `A` Adult: 15-124   `MCC` Major Complication/Comorbidity   `CC` Complication/Comorbidity   `SW` Severe Wound Dx

730   ICD-10-CM 2020

K80.51 **Calculus of bile duct without cholangitis or cholecystitis with obstruction** `CC`
  CC Excl: PDX collection 815

✓5ᵗʰ **K80.6** **Calculus of gallbladder and bile duct with cholecystitis**
  Use additional code if applicable for associated gangrene of gallbladder (K82.A1), or perforation of gallbladder (K82.A2)
  CC Excl: For CC codes in subcategory K80.6, unless otherwise noted: PDX collection 815

  K80.60 **Calculus of gallbladder and bile duct with cholecystitis, unspecified, without obstruction** `CC`

  K80.61 **Calculus of gallbladder and bile duct with cholecystitis, unspecified, with obstruction** `CC`

  K80.62 **Calculus of gallbladder and bile duct with acute cholecystitis without obstruction** `CC`
    CC Excl: PDX collection 816

  K80.63 **Calculus of gallbladder and bile duct with acute cholecystitis with obstruction** `CC`
    CC Excl: PDX collection 816

  K80.64 **Calculus of gallbladder and bile duct with chronic cholecystitis without obstruction** `CC`

  K80.65 **Calculus of gallbladder and bile duct with chronic cholecystitis with obstruction** `CC`

  K80.66 **Calculus of gallbladder and bile duct with acute and chronic cholecystitis without obstruction** `CC`
    CC Excl: PDX collection 817

  K80.67 **Calculus of gallbladder and bile duct with acute and chronic cholecystitis with obstruction** `CC`

✓5ᵗʰ **K80.7** **Calculus of gallbladder and bile duct without cholecystitis**

  K80.70 **Calculus of gallbladder and bile duct without cholecystitis without obstruction** `CC`

  K80.71 **Calculus of gallbladder and bile duct without cholecystitis with obstruction** `CC`
    CC Excl: PDX collection 815

✓5ᵗʰ **K80.8** **Other cholelithiasis**

  K80.80 **Other cholelithiasis without obstruction**

  K80.81 **Other cholelithiasis with obstruction** `CC`
    CC Excl: PDX collection 815

✓4ᵗʰ **K81** **Cholecystitis**
  Use additional code if applicable for associated gangrene of gallbladder (K82.A1), or perforation of gallbladder (K82.A2)
  EXCLUDES 1 cholecystitis with cholelithiasis (K80.-)
  AHA: 2018,4Q,20

  K81.0 **Acute cholecystitis** `CC`
    Abscess of gallbladder
    Angiocholecystitis
    Emphysematous (acute) cholecystitis
    Empyema of gallbladder
    Gangrene of gallbladder
    Gangrenous cholecystitis
    Suppurative cholecystitis
    CC Excl: PDX collection 818

  K81.1 **Chronic cholecystitis**

  K81.2 **Acute cholecystitis with chronic cholecystitis** `CC`
    CC Excl: PDX collection 819

  K81.9 **Cholecystitis, unspecified**

✓4ᵗʰ **K82** **Other diseases of gallbladder**
  EXCLUDES 1 nonvisualization of gallbladder (R93.2)
    postcholecystectomy syndrome (K91.5)
  CC Excl: For CC codes in category K82: PDX collection 820

  K82.0 **Obstruction of gallbladder** `CC`
    Occlusion of cystic duct or gallbladder without cholelithiasis
    Stenosis of cystic duct or gallbladder without cholelithiasis
    Stricture of cystic duct or gallbladder without cholelithiasis
    EXCLUDES 1 obstruction of gallbladder with cholelithiasis (K80.-)

  K82.1 **Hydrops of gallbladder**
    Mucocele of gallbladder

K82.2 **Perforation of gallbladder** `CC`
  Rupture of cystic duct or gallbladder
  EXCLUDES 1 perforation of gallbladder in cholecystitis (K82.A2)

K82.3 **Fistula of gallbladder** `CC`
  Cholecystocolic fistula
  Cholecystoduodenal fistula

K82.4 **Cholesterolosis of gallbladder**
  Strawberry gallbladder
  EXCLUDES 1 cholesterolosis of gallbladder with cholecystitis (K81.-)
    cholesterolosis of gallbladder with cholelithiasis (K80.-)

K82.8 **Other specified diseases of gallbladder**
  Adhesions of cystic duct or gallbladder
  Atrophy of cystic duct or gallbladder
  Cyst of cystic duct or gallbladder
  Dyskinesia of cystic duct or gallbladder
  Hypertrophy of cystic duct or gallbladder
  Nonfunctioning of cystic duct or gallbladder
  Ulcer of cystic duct or gallbladder

K82.9 **Disease of gallbladder, unspecified**

✓5ᵗʰ **K82.A** **Disorders of gallbladder in diseases classified elsewhere**
  Code first the type of cholecystitis (K81.-), or cholelithiasis with cholecystitis (K80.00-K80.19, K80.40-K80.47, K80.60-K80.67)
  AHA: 2018,4Q,19-20

  K82.A1 *Gangrene of gallbladder in cholecystitis*

  K82.A2 *Perforation of gallbladder in cholecystitis* `CC`

✓4ᵗʰ **K83** **Other diseases of biliary tract**
  EXCLUDES 1 postcholecystectomy syndrome (K91.5)
  EXCLUDES 2 conditions involving the gallbladder (K81-K82)
    conditions involving the cystic duct (K81-K82)

✓5ᵗʰ **K83.0** **Cholangitis**
  EXCLUDES 1 cholangitic liver abscess (K75.0)
    cholangitis with choledocholithiasis (K80.3-, K80.4-)
  EXCLUDES 2 chronic nonsuppurative destructive cholangitis (K74.3)
    primary biliary cholangitis (K74.3)
    primary biliary cirrhosis (K74.3)
  AHA: 2018,4Q,20

  K83.01 **Primary sclerosing cholangitis** `CC`
    CC Excl: PDX collection 814

  K83.09 **Other cholangitis** `CC`
    Ascending cholangitis
    Cholangitis NOS
    Primary cholangitis
    Recurrent cholangitis
    Sclerosing cholangitis
    Secondary cholangitis
    Stenosing cholangitis
    Suppurative cholangitis
    CC Excl: PDX collection 814

K83.1 **Obstruction of bile duct** `MCC`
  Occlusion of bile duct without cholelithiasis
  Stenosis of bile duct without cholelithiasis
  Stricture of bile duct without cholelithiasis
  EXCLUDES 1 congenital obstruction of bile duct (Q44.3)
    obstruction of bile duct with cholelithiasis (K80.-)
  AHA: 2016,1Q,18
  CC Excl: PDX collection 821

K83.2 **Perforation of bile duct** `MCC`
  Rupture of bile duct
  CC Excl: PDX collection 822

K83.3 **Fistula of bile duct** `CC`
  Choledochoduodenal fistula
  AHA: 2019,1Q,17
  CC Excl: PDX collection 822

K83.4 **Spasm of sphincter of Oddi**

K83.5 **Biliary cyst**

K83.8 **Other specified diseases of biliary tract**
  Adhesions of biliary tract
  Atrophy of biliary tract
  Hypertrophy of biliary tract
  Ulcer of biliary tract

K83.9 **Disease of biliary tract, unspecified**

Chapter 11. Diseases of the Digestive System

K85-K91.0

√4ᵗʰ K85 Acute pancreatitis

INCLUDES   acute (recurrent) pancreatitis
    subacute pancreatitis

AHA: 2016,4Q,34

CC Excl: For MCC codes in category K85: PDX collection 177

√5ᵗʰ K85.0 Idiopathic acute pancreatitis

K85.00 Idiopathic acute pancreatitis without necrosis or infection   MCC

K85.01 Idiopathic acute pancreatitis with uninfected necrosis   MCC

K85.02 Idiopathic acute pancreatitis with infected necrosis   MCC

√5ᵗʰ K85.1 Biliary acute pancreatitis

Gallstone pancreatitis

K85.10 Biliary acute pancreatitis without necrosis or infection   MCC

K85.11 Biliary acute pancreatitis with uninfected necrosis   MCC

K85.12 Biliary acute pancreatitis with infected necrosis   MCC

√5ᵗʰ K85.2 Alcohol induced acute pancreatitis

EXCLUDES 2   alcohol induced chronic pancreatitis (K86.0)

K85.20 Alcohol induced acute pancreatitis without necrosis or infection   MCC

K85.21 Alcohol induced acute pancreatitis with uninfected necrosis   MCC

K85.22 Alcohol induced acute pancreatitis with infected necrosis   MCC

√5ᵗʰ K85.3 Drug induced acute pancreatitis

Use additional code for adverse effect, if applicable, to identify drug (T36-T50 with fifth or sixth character 5)
Use additional code to identify drug abuse and dependence (F11.- F17.-)

K85.30 Drug induced acute pancreatitis without necrosis or infection   MCC

K85.31 Drug induced acute pancreatitis with uninfected necrosis   MCC

K85.32 Drug induced acute pancreatitis with infected necrosis   MCC

√5ᵗʰ K85.8 Other acute pancreatitis

K85.80 Other acute pancreatitis without necrosis or infection   MCC

K85.81 Other acute pancreatitis with uninfected necrosis   MCC

K85.82 Other acute pancreatitis with infected necrosis   MCC

√5ᵗʰ K85.9 Acute pancreatitis, unspecified

Pancreatitis NOS

K85.90 Acute pancreatitis without necrosis or infection, unspecified   MCC

K85.91 Acute pancreatitis with uninfected necrosis, unspecified   MCC

K85.92 Acute pancreatitis with infected necrosis, unspecified   MCC

√4ᵗʰ K86 Other diseases of pancreas

EXCLUDES 2   fibrocystic disease of pancreas (E84.-)
    islet cell tumor (of pancreas) (D13.7)
    pancreatic steatorrhea (K90.3)

K86.0 Alcohol-induced chronic pancreatitis   HCC

Use additional code to identify:
    alcohol abuse and dependence (F10.-)
Code also exocrine pancreatic insufficiency (K86.81)
EXCLUDES 2   alcohol induced acute pancreatitis (K85.2-)

K86.1 Other chronic pancreatitis   HCC

Chronic pancreatitis NOS
Infectious chronic pancreatitis
Recurrent chronic pancreatitis
Relapsing chronic pancreatitis
Code also exocrine pancreatic insufficiency (K86.81)

K86.2 Cyst of pancreas

K86.3 Pseudocyst of pancreas

√5ᵗʰ K86.8 Other specified diseases of pancreas

AHA: 2016,4Q,34-35

K86.81 Exocrine pancreatic insufficiency

K86.89 Other specified diseases of pancreas

Aseptic pancreatic necrosis, unrelated to acute pancreatitis
Atrophy of pancreas
Calculus of pancreas
Cirrhosis of pancreas
Fibrosis of pancreas
Pancreatic fat necrosis, unrelated to acute pancreatitis
Pancreatic infantilism
Pancreatic necrosis NOS, unrelated to acute pancreatitis

K86.9 Disease of pancreas, unspecified

K87 Disorders of gallbladder, biliary tract and pancreas in diseases classified elsewhere

Code first underlying disease
EXCLUDES 1   cytomegaloviral pancreatitis (B25.2)
    mumps pancreatitis (B26.3)
    syphilitic gallbladder (A52.74)
    syphilitic pancreas (A52.74)
    tuberculosis of gallbladder (A18.83)
    tuberculosis of pancreas (A18.83)

Other diseases of the digestive system (K90-K95)

√4ᵗʰ K90 Intestinal malabsorption

EXCLUDES 1   intestinal malabsorption following gastrointestinal surgery (K91.2)

AHA: 2017,4Q,108

K90.0 Celiac disease

Celiac disease with steatorrhea
Celiac gluten-sensitive enteropathy
Nontropical sprue
Use additional code for associated disorders including:
    dermatitis herpetiformis (L13.0)
    gluten ataxia (G32.81)
Code also exocrine pancreatic insufficiency (K86.81)
DEF: Malabsorption syndrome due to gluten consumption. Symptoms include fetid, bulky, frothy, oily stools; a distended abdomen; gas; asthenia; electrolyte depletion; and vitamin B, D, and K deficiency.

K90.1 Tropical sprue

Sprue NOS
Tropical steatorrhea

K90.2 Blind loop syndrome, not elsewhere classified

Blind loop syndrome NOS
EXCLUDES 1   congenital blind loop syndrome (Q43.8)
    postsurgical blind loop syndrome (K91.2)

K90.3 Pancreatic steatorrhea

√5ᵗʰ K90.4 Other malabsorption due to intolerance

EXCLUDES 2   celiac gluten-sensitive enteropathy (K90.0)
    lactose intolerance (E73.-)

AHA: 2016,4Q,35-36

K90.41 Non-celiac gluten sensitivity

Gluten sensitivity NOS
Non-celiac gluten sensitive enteropathy

K90.49 Malabsorption due to intolerance, not elsewhere classified

Malabsorption due to intolerance to carbohydrate
Malabsorption due to intolerance to fat
Malabsorption due to intolerance to protein
Malabsorption due to intolerance to starch

√5ᵗʰ K90.8 Other intestinal malabsorption

K90.81 Whipple's disease

K90.89 Other intestinal malabsorption

K90.9 Intestinal malabsorption, unspecified

√4ᵗʰ K91 Intraoperative and postprocedural complications and disorders of digestive system, not elsewhere classified

EXCLUDES 2   complications of artificial opening of digestive system (K94.-)
    complications of bariatric procedures (K95.-)
    gastrojejunal ulcer (K28.-)
    postprocedural (radiation) retroperitoneal abscess (K68.11)
    radiation colitis (K52.0)
    radiation gastroenteritis (K52.0)
    radiation proctitis (K62.7)

AHA: 2016,4Q,9-10

K91.0 Vomiting following gastrointestinal surgery

N Newborn: 0   P Pediatric: 0-17   M Maternity: 9-64   A Adult: 15-124   MCC Major Complication/Comorbidity   CC Complication/Comorbidity   SW Severe Wound Dx

732   ICD-10-CM 2020

K91.1   **Postgastric surgery syndromes**
Dumping syndrome
Postgastrectomy syndrome
Postvagotomy syndrome

K91.2   **Postsurgical malabsorption, not elsewhere classified**
Postsurgical blind loop syndrome
> EXCLUDES 1   *malabsorption osteomalacia in adults (M83.2)*
> *malabsorption osteoporosis, postsurgical (M80.8-,
> M81.8)*

✓5ᵗʰ **K91.3**   **Postprocedural intestinal obstruction**
AHA: 2017,4Q,16-17; 2017,1Q,40
CC Excl: For CC codes in subcategory K91.3: PDX collection 792

    K91.30   **Postprocedural intestinal**   CC
**obstruction, unspecified as to partial
versus complete**
Postprocedural intestinal obstruction NOS

    K91.31   **Postprocedural partial intestinal**   CC
obstruction
Postprocedural incomplete intestinal obstruction

    K91.32   **Postprocedural complete intestinal**   MCC
obstruction

K91.5   **Postcholecystectomy syndrome**

✓5ᵗʰ **K91.6**   **Intraoperative hemorrhage and hematoma of a digestive
system organ or structure complicating a procedure**
> EXCLUDES 1   *intraoperative hemorrhage and hematoma of a
> digestive system organ or structure due to
> accidental puncture and laceration during a
> procedure (K91.7-)*

    K91.61   **Intraoperative hemorrhage and**   CC
**hematoma of a digestive system
organ or structure complicating a
digestive system procedure**
CC Excl: PDX collection 829

    K91.62   **Intraoperative hemorrhage and**   CC
**hematoma of a digestive system
organ or structure complicating
other procedure**
CC Excl: PDX collection 829

✓5ᵗʰ **K91.7**   **Accidental puncture and laceration of a digestive system
organ or structure during a procedure**

    K91.71   **Accidental puncture and laceration**   CC
**of a digestive system organ or
structure during a digestive system
procedure**
CC Excl: PDX collection 509

    K91.72   **Accidental puncture and laceration**   CC
**of a digestive system organ or
structure during other procedure**
AHA: 2019,2Q,23
CC Excl: PDX collection 509

✓5ᵗʰ **K91.8**   **Other intraoperative and postprocedural complications and
disorders of digestive system**
**CC Excl: For CC codes in subcategory K91.8, unless otherwise
noted:** PDX collection 828

    K91.81   **Other intraoperative complications**   CC
of digestive system

    K91.82   **Postprocedural hepatic failure**   CC

    K91.83   **Postprocedural hepatorenal**   CC
syndrome

   ✓6ᵗʰ **K91.84**   **Postprocedural hemorrhage of a digestive system
organ or structure following a procedure**

      K91.840   **Postprocedural**   CC
**hemorrhage of a digestive
system organ or structure
following a digestive
system procedure**
AHA: 2016,1Q,15
CC Excl: PDX collection 829

      K91.841   **Postprocedural**   CC
**hemorrhage of a digestive
system organ or structure
following other procedure**
CC Excl: PDX collection 829

   ✓6ᵗʰ **K91.85**   **Complications of intestinal pouch**

      K91.850   **Pouchitis**   CC   HCC
Inflammation of internal ileoanal pouch
DEF: Inflammatory complication of an
existing surgically created ileoanal pouch,
resulting in multiple GI complaints,
including diarrhea, abdominal pain, rectal
bleeding, fecal urgency, or incontinence.

      K91.858   **Other complications of**   CC   HCC
intestinal pouch
AHA: 2019,2Q,13

    K91.86   **Retained cholelithiasis following**   CC
cholecystectomy

   ✓6ᵗʰ **K91.87**   **Postprocedural hematoma and seroma of a
digestive system organ or structure following a
procedure**
CC Excl: For CC codes in subcategory K91.87: PDX
collection 829

      K91.870   **Postprocedural hematoma**   CC
**of a digestive system
organ or structure
following a digestive
system procedure**

      K91.871   **Postprocedural hematoma**   CC
**of a digestive system
organ or structure
following other procedure**

      K91.872   **Postprocedural seroma of**   CC
**a digestive system organ
or structure following a
digestive system
procedure**

      K91.873   **Postprocedural seroma of**   CC
**a digestive system organ
or structure following
other procedure**

    K91.89   **Other postprocedural complications**   CC
and disorders of digestive system
Use additional code, if applicable, to further specify
disorder
> EXCLUDES 2   *postprocedural retroperitoneal abscess
> (K68.11)*

AHA: 2017,1Q,40

✓4ᵗʰ **K92**   **Other diseases of digestive system**
> EXCLUDES 1   *neonatal gastrointestinal hemorrhage (P54.0-P54.3)*

CC Excl: For CC codes in category K92, unless otherwise noted: PDX
collection 770

K92.0   **Hematemesis**   CC

K92.1   **Melena**   CC
> EXCLUDES 1   *occult blood in feces (R19.5)*

K92.2   **Gastrointestinal hemorrhage, unspecified**   CC
Gastric hemorrhage NOS
Intestinal hemorrhage NOS
> EXCLUDES 1   *acute hemorrhagic gastritis (K29.01)*
> *hemorrhage of anus and rectum (K62.5)*
> *angiodysplasia of stomach with hemorrhage
> (K31.811)*
> *diverticular disease with hemorrhage (K57.-)*
> *gastritis and duodenitis with hemorrhage (K29.-)*
> *peptic ulcer with hemorrhage (K25-K28)*

✓5ᵗʰ **K92.8**   **Other specified diseases of the digestive system**

    K92.81   **Gastrointestinal mucositis**   CC
(ulcerative)
Code also type of associated therapy, such as:
antineoplastic and immunosuppressive drugs
(T45.1X-)
radiological procedure and radiotherapy (Y84.2)
> EXCLUDES 2   *mucositis (ulcerative) of vagina and vulva
> (N76.81)*
> *nasal mucositis (ulcerative) (J34.81)*
> *oral mucositis (ulcerative) (K12.3-)*

CC Excl: PDX collection 765

    K92.89   **Other specified diseases of the digestive system**

K92.9   **Disease of digestive system, unspecified**

✓4ᵗʰ K94 Complications of artificial openings of the digestive system

CC Excl: For CC codes in category K94, unless otherwise noted: PDX collection 830

✓5ᵗʰ K94.0 Colostomy complications

- **K94.00 Colostomy complication, unspecified** `HCC`
- **K94.01 Colostomy hemorrhage** `CC` `HCC`
- **K94.02 Colostomy infection** `CC` `HCC`

  Use additional code to specify type of infection, such as:

  cellulitis of abdominal wall (L03.311)

  sepsis (A40.-, A41.-)

- **K94.03 Colostomy malfunction** `CC` `HCC`

  Mechanical complication of colostomy

  CC Excl: PDX collection 831

- **K94.09 Other complications of colostomy** `CC` `HCC`

✓5ᵗʰ K94.1 Enterostomy complications

- **K94.10 Enterostomy complication, unspecified** `HCC`
- **K94.11 Enterostomy hemorrhage** `CC` `HCC`
- **K94.12 Enterostomy infection** `CC` `HCC`

  Use additional code to specify type of infection, such as:

  cellulitis of abdominal wall (L03.311)

  sepsis (A40.-, A41.-)

- **K94.13 Enterostomy malfunction** `CC` `HCC`

  Mechanical complication of enterostomy

  CC Excl: PDX collection 831

- **K94.19 Other complications of enterostomy** `CC` `HCC`

✓5ᵗʰ K94.2 Gastrostomy complications

- **K94.20 Gastrostomy complication, unspecified** `HCC`
- **K94.21 Gastrostomy hemorrhage** `HCC`
- **K94.22 Gastrostomy infection** `CC` `HCC`

  Use additional code to specify type of infection, such as:

  cellulitis of abdominal wall (L03.311)

  sepsis (A40.-, A41.-)

  CC Excl: PDX collection 828

- **K94.23 Gastrostomy malfunction** `CC` `HCC`

  Mechanical complication of gastrostomy

  AHA: 2019,1Q,26

  CC Excl: PDX collection 828

- **K94.29 Other complications of gastrostomy** `HCC`

✓5ᵗʰ K94.3 Esophagostomy complications

CC Excl: For CC codes in subcategory K94.3: PDX collection 828

- **K94.30 Esophagostomy complications, unspecified** `CC` `HCC`
- **K94.31 Esophagostomy hemorrhage** `CC` `HCC`
- **K94.32 Esophagostomy infection** `CC` `HCC`

  Use additional code to identify the infection

- **K94.33 Esophagostomy malfunction** `CC` `HCC`

  Mechanical complication of esophagostomy

- **K94.39 Other complications of esophagostomy** `CC` `HCC`

✓4ᵗʰ K95 Complications of bariatric procedures

CC Excl: For CC codes in category K95: PDX collection 828

✓5ᵗʰ K95.0 Complications of gastric band procedure

- **K95.01 Infection due to gastric band procedure** `CC` `H11`

  Use additional code to specify type of infection or organism, such as:

  bacterial and viral infectious agents (B95.-, B96.-)

  cellulitis of abdominal wall (L03.311)

  sepsis (A40.-, A41.-)

- **K95.09 Other complications of gastric band procedure** `CC`

  Use additional code, if applicable, to further specify complication

✓5ᵗʰ K95.8 Complications of other bariatric procedure

EXCLUDES 1   complications of gastric band surgery (K95.0-)

- **K95.81 Infection due to other bariatric procedure** `CC` `H11`

  Use additional code to specify type of infection or organism, such as:

  bacterial and viral infectious agents (B95.-, B96.-)

  cellulitis of abdominal wall (L03.311)

  sepsis (A40.-, A41.-)

- **K95.89 Other complications of other bariatric procedure** `CC`

  Use additional code, if applicable, to further specify complication

---

N Newborn: 0   P Pediatric: 0-17   M Maternity: 9-64   A Adult: 15-124   `MCC` Major Complication/Comorbidity   `CC` Complication/Comorbidity   `SW` Severe Wound Dx

Chapter 12. Diseases of the Skin and Subcutaneous Tissue (L00–L99)

Chapter-specific Guidelines with Coding Examples

The chapter-specific guidelines from the ICD-10-CM Official Guidelines for Coding and Reporting have been provided below. Along with these guidelines are coding examples, contained in the shaded boxes, that have been developed to help illustrate the coding and/or sequencing guidance found in these guidelines.

a. Pressure ulcer stage codes

1) Pressure ulcer stages

Codes in category L89, Pressure ulcer, identify the site **and stage** of the pressure ulcer.

The ICD-10-CM classifies pressure ulcer stages based on severity, which is designated by stages 1-4, **deep tissue pressure injury,** unspecified stage, and unstageable.

Assign as many codes from category L89 as needed to identify all the pressure ulcers the patient has, if applicable.

See Section I.B.14 for pressure ulcer stage documentation by clinicians other than patient's provider

> Nursing notes: Dressings changed daily on stage 4 ulcer on heel and stage 2 ulcer on elbow
>
> Discharge summary: Pressure ulcers on right heel and left elbow
>
> **L89.614   Pressure ulcer of right heel, stage 4**
>
> **L89.022   Pressure ulcer of left elbow, stage 2**
>
> *Explanation:* Right heel and left elbow pressure ulcers were documented by the patient's provider in the discharge summary. Although the stage of these ulcers was not included in the provider's diagnostic statement, it is appropriate to code the stage from documentation from other clinicians involved in the patient's care, such as the nurse's notes, according to section I.B.14. Combination codes from category L89 Pressure ulcer, identify the site of the pressure ulcer as well as the stage. Assign as many codes from category L89 as needed to identify all the pressure ulcers the patient has.

2) Unstageable pressure ulcers

Assignment of the code for unstageable pressure ulcer (L89.--0) should be based on the clinical documentation. These codes are used for pressure ulcers whose stage cannot be clinically determined (e.g., the ulcer is covered by eschar or has been treated with a skin or muscle graft). This code should not be confused with the codes for unspecified stage (L89.--9). When there is no documentation regarding the stage of the pressure ulcer, assign the appropriate code for unspecified stage (L89.--9).

> Pressure ulcer of the right lower back documented as unstageable due to the presence of thick eschar covering the ulcer
>
> **L89.130   Pressure ulcer of right lower back, unstageable**
>
> *Explanation:* Codes for unstageable pressure ulcers are assigned when the stage cannot be clinically determined (e.g., the ulcer is covered by eschar or has been treated with a skin or muscle graft).

3) Documented pressure ulcer stage

Assignment of the pressure ulcer stage code should be guided by clinical documentation of the stage or documentation of the terms found in the Alphabetic Index. For clinical terms describing the stage that are not found in the Alphabetic Index, and there is no documentation of the stage, the provider should be queried.

> Left heel pressure ulcer with partial thickness skin loss involving the dermis
>
> **L89.622   Pressure ulcer of left heel, stage 2**
>
> *Explanation:* Code assignment for the pressure ulcer stage should be guided by either the clinical documentation of the stage or the documentation of terms found in the Alphabetic Index. The clinical documentation describing the left heel pressure ulcer "partial thickness skin loss involving the dermis" matches the ICD-10-CM index parenthetical description for stage 2 "(abrasion, blister, partial thickness skin loss involving epidermis and/or dermis)."

4) Patients admitted with pressure ulcers documented as healed

No code is assigned if the documentation states that the pressure ulcer is completely healed **at the time of admission**.

5) Pressure ulcers documented as healing

Pressure ulcers described as healing should be assigned the appropriate pressure ulcer stage code based on the documentation in the medical record. If the documentation does not provide information about the stage of the healing pressure ulcer, assign the appropriate code for unspecified stage.

If the documentation is unclear as to whether the patient has a current (new) pressure ulcer or if the patient is being treated for a healing pressure ulcer, query the provider.

For ulcers that were present on admission but healed at the time of discharge, assign the code for the site and stage of the pressure ulcer at the time of admission.

> H & P noted healing stage 2 sacral pressure ulcer. Resolved at time of discharge summary.
>
> **L89.152   Pressure ulcer of sacral region, stage 2**
>
> *Explanation:* Although completely healed upon discharge, the pressure ulcer required observation and/or treatment and should be coded based on the site and stage upon admission.

6) Patient admitted with pressure ulcer evolving into another stage during the admission

If a patient is admitted to an inpatient hospital with a pressure ulcer at one stage and it progresses to a higher stage, two separate codes should be assigned: one code for the site and stage of the ulcer on admission and a second code for the same ulcer site and the highest stage reported during the stay.

> Stage 3 right hip pressure ulcer worsened during admission to a stage 4
>
> **L89.213   Pressure ulcer of right hip, stage 3**
>
> **L89.214   Pressure ulcer of right hip, stage 4**
>
> *Explanation:* A pressure ulcer that progresses from a lower stage to a higher stage is assigned two codes, one for the documented stage upon admission and one for the documented stage at discharge.

7) Pressure-induced deep tissue damage

For pressure-induced deep tissue damage or deep tissue pressure injury, assign only the appropriate code for pressure-induced deep tissue damage (L89.--6).

b. Non-pressure chronic ulcers

1) Patients admitted with non-pressure ulcers documented as healed

No code is assigned if the documentation states that the non-pressure ulcer is completely healed **at the time of admission**.

2) Non-pressure ulcers documented as healing

Non-pressure ulcers described as healing should be assigned the appropriate non-pressure ulcer code based on the documentation in the medical record. If the documentation does not provide information about the severity of the healing non-pressure ulcer, assign the appropriate code for unspecified severity.

If the documentation is unclear as to whether the patient has a current (new) non-pressure ulcer or if the patient is being treated for a healing non-pressure ulcer, query the provider.

For ulcers that were present on admission but healed at the time of discharge, assign the code for the site and severity of the non-pressure ulcer at the time of admission.

> Admission diagnosis: Chronic ulcer, fat layer exposed, on left ankle
>
> Discharge diagnosis: Resolution of ulcer on the left ankle
>
> **L97.322   Non-pressure chronic ulcer of left ankle with fat layer exposed**
>
> *Explanation:* Although the ulcer was documented as resolved (healed) at discharge, a code representing the site and severity of the ulcer upon admission should be appended.

3) Patient admitted with non-pressure ulcer that progresses to another severity level during the admission

If a patient is admitted to an inpatient hospital with a non-pressure ulcer at one severity level and it progresses to a higher severity level, two separate codes should be assigned: one code for the site and severity level of the ulcer on admission and a second code for the same ulcer site and the highest severity level reported during the stay.

See Section I.B.14 for pressure ulcer stage documentation by clinicians other than patient's provider

Chapter 12. Diseases of the Skin and Subcutaneous Tissue (L00-L99)

EXCLUDES 2   certain conditions originating in the perinatal period (P04-P96)
certain infectious and parasitic diseases (A00-B99)
complications of pregnancy, childbirth and the puerperium (O00-O9A)
congenital malformations, deformations, and chromosomal abnormalities (Q00-Q99)
endocrine, nutritional and metabolic diseases (E00-E88)
lipomelanotic reticulosis (I89.8)
neoplasms (C00-D49)
symptoms, signs and abnormal clinical and laboratory findings, not elsewhere classified (R00-R94)
systemic connective tissue disorders (M30-M36)
viral warts (B07.-)

This chapter contains the following blocks:
L00-L08   Infections of the skin and subcutaneous tissue
L10-L14   Bullous disorders
L20-L30   Dermatitis and eczema
L40-L45   Papulosquamous disorders
L49-L54   Urticaria and erythema
L55-L59   Radiation-related disorders of the skin and subcutaneous tissue
L60-L75   Disorders of skin appendages
L76   Intraoperative and postprocedural complications of skin and subcutaneous tissue
L80-L99   Other disorders of the skin and subcutaneous tissue

Infections of the skin and subcutaneous tissue (L00-L08)

Use additional code (B95-B97) to identify infectious agent
EXCLUDES 2   hordeolum (H00.0)
infective dermatitis (L30.3)
local infections of skin classified in Chapter 1
lupus panniculitis (L93.2)
panniculitis NOS (M79.3)
panniculitis of neck and back (M54.0-)
perlèche NOS (K13.0)
perlèche due to candidiasis (B37.0)
perlèche due to riboflavin deficiency (E53.0)
pyogenic granuloma (L98.0)
relapsing panniculitis [Weber-Christian] (M35.6)
viral warts (B07.-)
zoster (B02.-)

L00   **Staphylococcal scalded skin syndrome**
Ritter's disease
Use additional code to identify percentage of skin exfoliation (L49.-)
EXCLUDES 1   bullous impetigo (L01.03)
pemphigus neonatorum (L01.03)
toxic epidermal necrolysis [Lyell] (L51.2)
DEF: Infectious skin disease of children younger than 5 years marked by eruptions ranging from a few localized blisters to widespread, easily ruptured, fine vesicles and bullae affecting almost the entire body. It results in exfoliation of large planes of skin and leaves raw areas.

✓4ᵗʰ **L01**   **Impetigo**
EXCLUDES 1   impetigo herpetiformis (L40.1)
DEF: Acute, superficial, highly contagious skin infection commonly occurring in children. Skin lesions usually appear on the face and consist of vesicles and bullae that burst and form yellow crusts.

✓5ᵗʰ **L01.0**   **Impetigo**
     Impetigo contagiosa
     Impetigo vulgaris
     L01.00   **Impetigo, unspecified**
         Impetigo NOS
     L01.01   **Non-bullous impetigo**
     L01.02   **Bockhart's impetigo**
         Impetigo follicularis
         Perifolliculitis NOS
         Superficial pustular perifolliculitis
         DEF: Superficial inflammation of the hair follicles most commonly caused by staph aureus that manifests as rounded, sphere-shaped, pustular eruptions in the areas of the scalp, beard, underarms, extremities, and buttocks.
     L01.03   **Bullous impetigo**
         Impetigo neonatorum
         Pemphigus neonatorum
     L01.09   **Other impetigo**
         Ulcerative impetigo
   L01.1   **Impetiginization of other dermatoses**

✓4ᵗʰ **L02**   **Cutaneous abscess, furuncle and carbuncle**
Use additional code to identify organism (B95-B96)
EXCLUDES 2   abscess of anus and rectal regions (K61.-)
abscess of female genital organs (external) (N76.4)
abscess of male genital organs (external) (N48.2, N49.-)
DEF: Carbuncle: Infection of the skin that arises from a collection of interconnected infected boils or furuncles, usually from hair follicles infected by *Staphylococcus*. This condition can produce pus and form drainage cavities.
DEF: Furuncle: Inflamed, painful abscess, cyst, or nodule on the skin caused by bacteria, often *Staphylococcus,* entering along the hair follicle.

✓5ᵗʰ **L02.0**   **Cutaneous abscess, furuncle and carbuncle of face**
EXCLUDES 2   abscess of ear, external (H60.0)
abscess of eyelid (H00.0)
abscess of head [any part, except face] (L02.8)
abscess of lacrimal gland (H04.0)
abscess of lacrimal passages (H04.3)
abscess of mouth (K12.2)
abscess of nose (J34.0)
abscess of orbit (H05.0)
submandibular abscess (K12.2)
     L02.01   **Cutaneous abscess of face**
     L02.02   **Furuncle of face**
         Boil of face
         Folliculitis of face
     L02.03   **Carbuncle of face**

✓5ᵗʰ **L02.1**   **Cutaneous abscess, furuncle and carbuncle of neck**
     L02.11   **Cutaneous abscess of neck**
     L02.12   **Furuncle of neck**
         Boil of neck
         Folliculitis of neck
     L02.13   **Carbuncle of neck**

✓5ᵗʰ **L02.2**   **Cutaneous abscess, furuncle and carbuncle of trunk**
EXCLUDES 1   non-newborn omphalitis (L08.82)
omphalitis of newborn (P38.-)
EXCLUDES 2   abscess of breast (N61.1)
abscess of buttocks (L02.3)
abscess of female external genital organs (N76.4)
abscess of hip (L02.4)
abscess of male external genital organs (N48.2, N49.-)
CC Excl: For CC codes in subcategory L02.2: PDX collection 833

✓6ᵗʰ   **L02.21**   **Cutaneous abscess of trunk**
     L02.211   **Cutaneous abscess of abdominal wall**   CC
     L02.212   **Cutaneous abscess of back [any part, except buttock]**   CC
     L02.213   **Cutaneous abscess of chest wall**   CC
     L02.214   **Cutaneous abscess of groin**   CC
     L02.215   **Cutaneous abscess of perineum**   CC
     L02.216   **Cutaneous abscess of umbilicus**   CC
     L02.219   **Cutaneous abscess of trunk, unspecified**

✓6ᵗʰ   **L02.22**   **Furuncle of trunk**
     Boil of trunk
     Folliculitis of trunk
     L02.221   **Furuncle of abdominal wall**
     L02.222   **Furuncle of back [any part, except buttock]**
     L02.223   **Furuncle of chest wall**
     L02.224   **Furuncle of groin**
     L02.225   **Furuncle of perineum**
     L02.226   **Furuncle of umbilicus**
     L02.229   **Furuncle of trunk, unspecified**

✓6ᵗʰ   **L02.23**   **Carbuncle of trunk**
     L02.231   **Carbuncle of abdominal wall**
     L02.232   **Carbuncle of back [any part, except buttock]**
     L02.233   **Carbuncle of chest wall**
     L02.234   **Carbuncle of groin**
     L02.235   **Carbuncle of perineum**
     L02.236   **Carbuncle of umbilicus**
     L02.239   **Carbuncle of trunk, unspecified**

✓5th **L02.3** **Cutaneous abscess, furuncle and carbuncle of buttock**

> *EXCLUDES 1*   pilonidal cyst with abscess (L05.01)

L02.31   **Cutaneous abscess of buttock**   `CC`

> Cutaneous abscess of gluteal region
> **CC Excl:** PDX collection 834

L02.32   **Furuncle of buttock**

> Boil of buttock
> Folliculitis of buttock
> Furuncle of gluteal region

L02.33   **Carbuncle of buttock**

> Carbuncle of gluteal region

✓5th **L02.4** **Cutaneous abscess, furuncle and carbuncle of limb**

> *EXCLUDES 2*   cutaneous abscess, furuncle and carbuncle of groin
> (L02.214, L02.224, L02.234)
> cutaneous abscess, furuncle and carbuncle of hand
> (L02.5-)
> cutaneous abscess, furuncle and carbuncle of foot
> (L02.6-)

CC Excl: For CC codes in subcategory L02.4: PDX collection 835

✓6th **L02.41**   **Cutaneous abscess of limb**

L02.411   **Cutaneous abscess of right axilla**   `CC`

L02.412   **Cutaneous abscess of left axilla**   `CC`

L02.413   **Cutaneous abscess of right upper limb**

L02.414   **Cutaneous abscess of left upper limb**

L02.415   **Cutaneous abscess of right lower limb**

L02.416   **Cutaneous abscess of left lower limb**

L02.419   **Cutaneous abscess of limb, unspecified**

✓6th **L02.42**   **Furuncle of limb**

> Boil of limb
> Folliculitis of limb

L02.421   **Furuncle of right axilla**

L02.422   **Furuncle of left axilla**

L02.423   **Furuncle of right upper limb**

L02.424   **Furuncle of left upper limb**

L02.425   **Furuncle of right lower limb**

L02.426   **Furuncle of left lower limb**

L02.429   **Furuncle of limb, unspecified**

✓6th **L02.43**   **Carbuncle of limb**

L02.431   **Carbuncle of right axilla**

L02.432   **Carbuncle of left axilla**

L02.433   **Carbuncle of right upper limb**

L02.434   **Carbuncle of left upper limb**

L02.435   **Carbuncle of right lower limb**

L02.436   **Carbuncle of left lower limb**

L02.439   **Carbuncle of limb, unspecified**

✓5th **L02.5** **Cutaneous abscess, furuncle and carbuncle of hand**

✓6th **L02.51**   **Cutaneous abscess of hand**

L02.511   **Cutaneous abscess of right hand**

L02.512   **Cutaneous abscess of left hand**

L02.519   **Cutaneous abscess of unspecified hand**

✓6th **L02.52**   **Furuncle hand**

> Boil of hand
> Folliculitis of hand

L02.521   **Furuncle right hand**

L02.522   **Furuncle left hand**

L02.529   **Furuncle unspecified hand**

✓6th **L02.53**   **Carbuncle of hand**

L02.531   **Carbuncle of right hand**

L02.532   **Carbuncle of left hand**

L02.539   **Carbuncle of unspecified hand**

✓5th **L02.6** **Cutaneous abscess, furuncle and carbuncle of foot**

CC Excl: For CC codes in subcategory L02.6: PDX collection 838

✓6th **L02.61**   **Cutaneous abscess of foot**

L02.611   **Cutaneous abscess of right foot**   `CC`

L02.612   **Cutaneous abscess of left foot**   `CC`

L02.619   **Cutaneous abscess of unspecified foot**   `CC`

✓6th **L02.62**   **Furuncle of foot**

> Boil of foot
> Folliculitis of foot

L02.621   **Furuncle of right foot**

L02.622   **Furuncle of left foot**

L02.629   **Furuncle of unspecified foot**

✓6th **L02.63**   **Carbuncle of foot**

L02.631   **Carbuncle of right foot**

L02.632   **Carbuncle of left foot**

L02.639   **Carbuncle of unspecified foot**

✓5th **L02.8** **Cutaneous abscess, furuncle and carbuncle of other sites**

✓6th **L02.81**   **Cutaneous abscess of other sites**

L02.811   **Cutaneous abscess of head [any part, except face]**

L02.818   **Cutaneous abscess of other sites**

✓6th **L02.82**   **Furuncle of other sites**

> Boil of other sites
> Folliculitis of other sites

L02.821   **Furuncle of head [any part, except face]**

L02.828   **Furuncle of other sites**

✓6th **L02.83**   **Carbuncle of other sites**

L02.831   **Carbuncle of head [any part, except face]**

L02.838   **Carbuncle of other sites**

✓5th **L02.9** **Cutaneous abscess, furuncle and carbuncle, unspecified**

L02.91   **Cutaneous abscess, unspecified**

L02.92   **Furuncle, unspecified**

> Boil NOS
> Furunculosis NOS

L02.93   **Carbuncle, unspecified**

✓4th **L03** **Cellulitis and acute lymphangitis**

> *EXCLUDES 2*   cellulitis of anal and rectal region (K61.-)
> cellulitis of external auditory canal (H60.1)
> cellulitis of eyelid (H00.0)
> cellulitis of female external genital organs (N76.4)
> cellulitis of lacrimal apparatus (H04.3)
> cellulitis of male external genital organs (N48.2, N49.-)
> cellulitis of mouth (K12.2)
> cellulitis of nose (J34.0)
> eosinophilic cellulitis [Wells] (L98.3)
> febrile neutrophilic dermatosis [Sweet] (L98.2)
> lymphangitis (chronic) (subacute) (I89.1)

AHA: 2017,4Q,100

DEF: Cellulitis: Infection of the skin and subcutaneous tissues, most often caused by *Staphylococcus* or *Streptococcus* bacteria secondary to a cutaneous lesion. Progression of the inflammation may lead to abscess and tissue death, or even systemic infection-like bacteremia.

DEF: Lymphangitis: Inflammation of the lymph channels most often caused by *Streptococcus*.

✓5th **L03.0** **Cellulitis and acute lymphangitis of finger and toe**

> Infection of nail
> Onychia
> Paronychia
> Perionychia

✓6th **L03.01**   **Cellulitis of finger**

> Felon
> Whitlow
> *EXCLUDES 1*   herpetic whitlow (B00.89)
> **DEF:** Felon: Superficial bacterial skin infection at the tip of the finger.

L03.011   **Cellulitis of right finger**

L03.012   **Cellulitis of left finger**

L03.019   **Cellulitis of unspecified finger**

✓6th **L03.02**   **Acute lymphangitis of finger**

> Hangnail with lymphangitis of finger

L03.021   **Acute lymphangitis of right finger**

L03.022   **Acute lymphangitis of left finger**

L03.029   **Acute lymphangitis of unspecified finger**

✓6th **L03.03**   **Cellulitis of toe**

L03.031   **Cellulitis of right toe**

L03.032   **Cellulitis of left toe**

L03.039   **Cellulitis of unspecified toe**

✓6th **L03.04**   **Acute lymphangitis of toe**

> Hangnail with lymphangitis of toe

L03.041   **Acute lymphangitis of right toe**

L03.042   **Acute lymphangitis of left toe**

L03.049   **Acute lymphangitis of unspecified toe**

☑ Additional Character Required   ✓x7th Placeholder   Unacceptable PDx   Questionable PDx   Manifestation   Unspecified Dx   H1-H14 HAC   HCC CMS-HCC Dx   HIV HIV Dx

ICD-10-CM 2020   737

Chapter 12. Diseases of the Skin and Subcutaneous Tissue

L03.1–L04.0

√5ᵗʰ **L03.1**   **Cellulitis and acute lymphangitis of other parts of limb**

> **CC Excl: For CC codes in subcategory L03.1, unless otherwise noted:** PDX collection 835

   √6ᵗʰ **L03.11**   **Cellulitis of other parts of limb**

> EXCLUDES 2   cellulitis of fingers (L03.01-)
> cellulitis of toes (L03.03-)
> groin (L03.314)

     L03.111   **Cellulitis of right axilla**   CC

     L03.112   **Cellulitis of left axilla**   CC

     L03.113   **Cellulitis of right upper limb**   CC

     L03.114   **Cellulitis of left upper limb**   CC

     L03.115   **Cellulitis of right lower limb**   CC

> **CC Excl:** PDX collection 836

     L03.116   **Cellulitis of left lower limb**   CC

> **CC Excl:** PDX collection 836

     L03.119   **Cellulitis of unspecified part of limb**   CC

> **CC Excl:** PDX collection 836

   √6ᵗʰ **L03.12**   **Acute lymphangitis of other parts of limb**

> EXCLUDES 2   acute lymphangitis of fingers (L03.2-)
> acute lymphangitis of groin (L03.324)
> acute lymphangitis of toes (L03.04-)

     L03.121   **Acute lymphangitis of right axilla**   CC

     L03.122   **Acute lymphangitis of left axilla**   CC

     L03.123   **Acute lymphangitis of right upper limb**   CC

     L03.124   **Acute lymphangitis of left upper limb**   CC

     L03.125   **Acute lymphangitis of right lower limb**   CC

> **CC Excl:** PDX collection 836

     L03.126   **Acute lymphangitis of left lower limb**   CC

> **CC Excl:** PDX collection 836

     L03.129   **Acute lymphangitis of unspecified part of limb**   CC

> **CC Excl:** PDX collection 836

√5ᵗʰ **L03.2**   **Cellulitis and acute lymphangitis of face and neck**

   √6ᵗʰ **L03.21**   **Cellulitis and acute lymphangitis of face**

     L03.211   **Cellulitis of face**   CC

> EXCLUDES 2   abscess of orbit (H05.01-)
> cellulitis of ear (H60.1-)
> cellulitis of eyelid (H00.0-)
> cellulitis of head (L03.81)
> cellulitis of lacrimal apparatus (H04.3)
> cellulitis of lip (K13.0)
> cellulitis of mouth (K12.2)
> cellulitis of nose (internal) (J34.0)
> cellulitis of orbit (H05.01-)
> cellulitis of scalp (L03.81)

> **AHA:** 2013,4Q,123
> **CC Excl:** PDX collection 840

     L03.212   **Acute lymphangitis of face**   CC

> **CC Excl:** No Excl

     L03.213   **Periorbital cellulitis**   CC

> Preseptal cellulitis
> **AHA:** 2016,4Q,36
> **CC Excl:** PDX collection 840

   √6ᵗʰ **L03.22**   **Cellulitis and acute lymphangitis of neck**

     L03.221   **Cellulitis of neck**   CC

> **CC Excl:** PDX collection 832

     L03.222   **Acute lymphangitis of neck**   CC

> **CC Excl:** PDX collection 832

√5ᵗʰ **L03.3**   **Cellulitis and acute lymphangitis of trunk**

> **CC Excl: For CC codes in subcategory L03.3, unless otherwise noted:** PDX collection 833

   √6ᵗʰ **L03.31**   **Cellulitis of trunk**

> EXCLUDES 2   cellulitis of anal and rectal regions (K61.-)
> cellulitis of breast NOS (N61.0)
> cellulitis of female external genital organs (N76.4)
> cellulitis of male external genital organs (N48.2, N49.-)
> omphalitis of newborn (P38.-)
> puerperal cellulitis of breast (O91.2)

     L03.311   **Cellulitis of abdominal wall**   CC

> EXCLUDES 2   cellulitis of umbilicus (L03.316)
> cellulitis of groin (L03.314)

     L03.312   **Cellulitis of back [any part except buttock]**   CC

     L03.313   **Cellulitis of chest wall**   CC

     L03.314   **Cellulitis of groin**   CC

     L03.315   **Cellulitis of perineum**   CC

     L03.316   **Cellulitis of umbilicus**   CC

     L03.317   **Cellulitis of buttock**   CC

> **CC Excl:** PDX collection 834

     L03.319   **Cellulitis of trunk, unspecified**   CC

   √6ᵗʰ **L03.32**   **Acute lymphangitis of trunk**

     L03.321   **Acute lymphangitis of abdominal wall**   CC

     L03.322   **Acute lymphangitis of back [any part except buttock]**   CC

     L03.323   **Acute lymphangitis of chest wall**   CC

     L03.324   **Acute lymphangitis of groin**   CC

     L03.325   **Acute lymphangitis of perineum**   CC

     L03.326   **Acute lymphangitis of umbilicus**   CC

     L03.327   **Acute lymphangitis of buttock**   CC

> **CC Excl:** PDX collection 834

     L03.329   **Acute lymphangitis of trunk, unspecified**   CC

√5ᵗʰ **L03.8**   **Cellulitis and acute lymphangitis of other sites**

> **CC Excl: For CC codes in subcategory L03.8:** PDX collection 839

   √6ᵗʰ **L03.81**   **Cellulitis of other sites**

     L03.811   **Cellulitis of head [any part, except face]**   CC

> Cellulitis of scalp
> EXCLUDES 2   cellulitis of face (L03.211)

     L03.818   **Cellulitis of other sites**   CC

   √6ᵗʰ **L03.89**   **Acute lymphangitis of other sites**

     L03.891   **Acute lymphangitis of head [any part, except face]**   CC

     L03.898   **Acute lymphangitis of other sites**   CC

√5ᵗʰ **L03.9**   **Cellulitis and acute lymphangitis, unspecified**

     L03.90   **Cellulitis, unspecified**   CC

> **CC Excl:** PDX collection 839

     L03.91   **Acute lymphangitis, unspecified**   CC

> EXCLUDES 1   lymphangitis NOS (I89.1)
> **CC Excl:** PDX collection 839

√4ᵗʰ **L04**   **Acute lymphadenitis**

> INCLUDES   abscess (acute) of lymph nodes, except mesenteric
> acute lymphadenitis, except mesenteric
> EXCLUDES 1   chronic or subacute lymphadenitis, except mesenteric (I88.1)
> enlarged lymph nodes (R59.-)
> human immunodeficiency virus [HIV] disease resulting in generalized lymphadenopathy (B20)
> lymphadenitis NOS (I88.9)
> nonspecific mesenteric lymphadenitis (I88.0)

> **DEF:** Inflammation or enlargement of the lymph nodes.

L04.0   **Acute lymphadenitis of face, head and neck**

N Newborn: 0   P Pediatric: 0-17   M Maternity: 9-64   A Adult: 15-124   MCC Major Complication/Comorbidity   CC Complication/Comorbidity   SW Severe Wound Dx

738   ICD-10-CM 2020

L04.1 **Acute lymphadenitis of** trunk

L04.2 **Acute lymphadenitis of** upper limb

    Acute lymphadenitis of axilla

    Acute lymphadenitis of shoulder

L04.3 **Acute lymphadenitis of** lower limb

    Acute lymphadenitis of hip

    EXCLUDES 2   *acute lymphadenitis of groin (L04.1)*

L04.8 **Acute lymphadenitis of other sites**

L04.9 **Acute lymphadenitis, unspecified**

✓4th **L05 Pilonidal cyst and sinus**

    DEF: Pilonidal cyst: Sac or sinus cavity of trapped epithelial tissues in the sacrococcygeal region, usually associated with ingrown hair.

    DEF: Pilonidal sinus: Fistula, tract, or channel that extends from an infected area of ingrown hair to another site within the skin or out to the skin surface.

Pilonidal Cyst

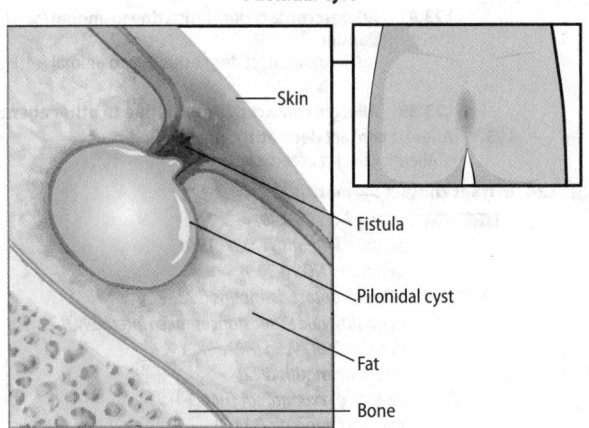

    — Skin

    — Fistula

    — Pilonidal cyst

    — Fat

    — Bone

✓5th **L05.0 Pilonidal cyst and sinus with abscess**

    L05.01 Pilonidal cyst with abscess   `CC` `SW`

        Pilonidal abscess

        Pilonidal dimple with abscess

        Postanal dimple with abscess

        EXCLUDES 2   *congenital sacral dimple (Q82.6)*

                   parasacral dimple (Q82.6)

        CC Excl: PDX collection 841

    L05.02 Pilonidal sinus with abscess   `CC` `SW`

        Coccygeal fistula with abscess

        Coccygeal sinus with abscess

        Pilonidal fistula with abscess

        CC Excl: PDX collection 841

✓5th **L05.9 Pilonidal cyst and sinus without abscess**

    L05.91 Pilonidal cyst without abscess

        Pilonidal dimple

        Postanal dimple

        Pilonidal cyst NOS

        EXCLUDES 2   *congenital sacral dimple (Q82.6)*

                   parasacral dimple (Q82.6)

    L05.92 Pilonidal sinus without abscess   `SW`

        Coccygeal fistula

        Coccygeal sinus without abscess

        Pilonidal fistula

✓4th **L08 Other local infections of skin and subcutaneous tissue**

    L08.0 Pyoderma

        Dermatitis gangrenosa

        Purulent dermatitis

        Septic dermatitis

        Suppurative dermatitis

        EXCLUDES 1   *pyoderma gangrenosum (L88)*

                   pyoderma vegetans (L08.81)

        DEF: Any superficial skin disease commonly characterized by the discharging of pus not attributed to another condition.

    L08.1 Erythrasma   `HIV` `CC`

        DEF: Chronic, superficial skin infection of brown scaly patches, commonly found in skin folds most prevalent in the overweight or diabetic population.

        CC Excl: PDX collection 107

✓5th **L08.8 Other specified local infections of the skin and subcutaneous tissue**

    L08.81 Pyoderma vegetans

        EXCLUDES 1   *pyoderma gangrenosum (L88)*

                   pyoderma NOS (L08.0)

    L08.82 Omphalitis not of newborn

        EXCLUDES 1   *omphalitis of newborn (P38.-)*

    L08.89 Other specified local infections of the skin and subcutaneous tissue

    L08.9 Local infection of the skin and subcutaneous tissue, unspecified

Bullous disorders (L10-L14)

    EXCLUDES 1   *benign familial pemphigus [Hailey-Hailey] (Q82.8)*

               staphylococcal scalded skin syndrome (L00)

               toxic epidermal necrolysis [Lyell] (L51.2)

CC Excl: For CC codes in categories L10-L14, unless otherwise noted: PDX collection 842

✓4th **L10 Pemphigus**

    EXCLUDES 1   *pemphigus neonatorum (L01.03)*

    L10.0 Pemphigus vulgaris   `CC`

    L10.1 Pemphigus vegetans   `CC`

    L10.2 Pemphigus foliaceous   `CC`

    L10.3 Brazilian pemphigus [fogo selvagem]   `CC`

    L10.4 Pemphigus erythematosus   `CC`

        Senear-Usher syndrome

    L10.5 Drug-induced pemphigus   `CC`

        Use additional code for adverse effect, if applicable, to identify drug (T36-T50 with fifth or sixth character 5)

✓5th **L10.8 Other pemphigus**

    L10.81 Paraneoplastic pemphigus   `CC`

    L10.89 Other pemphigus   `CC`

    L10.9 Pemphigus, unspecified   `CC`

✓4th **L11 Other acantholytic disorders**

    L11.0 Acquired keratosis follicularis

        EXCLUDES 1   *keratosis follicularis (congenital) [Darier-White] (Q82.8)*

    L11.1 Transient acantholytic dermatosis [Grover]

    L11.8 Other specified acantholytic disorders

    L11.9 Acantholytic disorder, unspecified

✓4th **L12 Pemphigoid**

    EXCLUDES 1   *herpes gestationis (O26.4-)*

               impetigo herpetiformis (L40.1)

    L12.0 Bullous pemphigoid   `CC`

    L12.1 Cicatricial pemphigoid

        Benign mucous membrane pemphigoid

        DEF: Chronic autoimmune disease characterized by subepidermal blistering lesions of the mucosa, including the conjunctiva. It is seen predominantly in the elderly and produces adhesions and scarring.

    L12.2 Chronic bullous disease of childhood   `P`

        Juvenile dermatitis herpetiformis

✓5th **L12.3 Acquired epidermolysis bullosa**

        EXCLUDES 1   *epidermolysis bullosa (congenital) (Q81.-)*

        CC Excl: For CC codes in subcategory L12.3: PDX collection 843

    L12.30 Acquired epidermolysis bullosa, unspecified   `CC` `HCC`

    L12.31 Epidermolysis bullosa due to drug   `CC` `HCC`

        Use additional code for adverse effect, if applicable, to identify drug (T36-T50 with fifth or sixth character 5)

    L12.35 Other acquired epidermolysis bullosa   `CC` `HCC`

    L12.8 Other pemphigoid   `CC`

    L12.9 Pemphigoid, unspecified   `CC`

☑ Additional Character Required   ✓x7th Placeholder   <u>Unacceptable PDx</u>   <u>Questionable PDx</u>   <u>Manifestation</u>   <u>Unspecified Dx</u>   `H1`-`H14` HAC   `HCC` CMS-HCC Dx   `HIV` HIV Dx

ICD-10-CM 2020   **739**

✓4ᵗʰ L13   Other bullous disorders

    L13.0   Dermatitis herpetiformis
        Duhring's disease
        Hydroa herpetiformis
        EXCLUDES 1   *juvenile dermatitis herpetiformis (L12.2)*
                      senile dermatitis herpetiformis (L12.0)
        DEF: Skin disease to which people are genetically predisposed resulting from an immunological response to gluten. Dermatitis herpetiformis is an extremely pruritic eruption of various lesions that frequently heal, leaving hyperpigmentation or hypopigmentation and occasionally scarring. It is usually associated with asymptomatic gluten-sensitive enteropathy.

    L13.1   Subcorneal pustular dermatitis
        Sneddon-Wilkinson disease

    L13.8   Other specified bullous disorders

    L13.9   Bullous disorder, unspecified

L14   *Bullous disorders in diseases classified elsewhere*
    Code first underlying disease

Dermatitis and eczema (L20-L30)

NOTE   In this block the terms dermatitis and eczema are used synonymously and interchangeably.

EXCLUDES 2   *chronic (childhood) granulomatous disease (D71)*
        dermatitis gangrenosa (L08.0)
        dermatitis herpetiformis (L13.0)
        dry skin dermatitis (L85.3)
        factitial dermatitis (L98.1)
        perioral dermatitis (L71.0)
        radiation-related disorders of the skin and subcutaneous tissue (L55-L59)
        stasis dermatitis (I87.2)

✓4ᵗʰ L20   Atopic dermatitis

    L20.0   Besnier's prurigo

    ✓5ᵗʰ L20.8   Other atopic dermatitis
        EXCLUDES 2   *circumscribed neurodermatitis (L28.0)*

        L20.81   Atopic neurodermatitis
            Diffuse neurodermatitis

        L20.82   Flexural eczema

        L20.83   Infantile (acute) (chronic) eczema   P

        L20.84   Intrinsic (allergic) eczema

        L20.89   Other atopic dermatitis

    L20.9   Atopic dermatitis, unspecified

✓4ᵗʰ L21   Seborrheic dermatitis

    EXCLUDES 2   *infective dermatitis (L30.3)*
                seborrheic keratosis (L82.-)

    L21.0   Seborrhea capitis
        Cradle cap
        AHA: 2018,1Q,6
        TIP: Assign for dandruff in an adult patient.

    L21.1   Seborrheic infantile dermatitis   P

    L21.8   Other seborrheic dermatitis

    L21.9   Seborrheic dermatitis, unspecified
        Seborrhea NOS

L22   Diaper dermatitis
    Diaper erythema
    Diaper rash
    Psoriasiform diaper rash

✓4ᵗʰ L23   Allergic contact dermatitis

    EXCLUDES 1   *allergy NOS (T78.40)*
                contact dermatitis NOS (L25.9)
                dermatitis NOS (L30.9)
    EXCLUDES 2   *dermatitis due to substances taken internally (L27.-)*
                dermatitis of eyelid (H01.1-)
                diaper dermatitis (L22)
                eczema of external ear (H60.5-)
                irritant contact dermatitis (L24.-)
                perioral dermatitis (L71.0)
                radiation-related disorders of the skin and subcutaneous tissue (L55-L59)

    L23.0   Allergic contact dermatitis due to metals
        Allergic contact dermatitis due to chromium
        Allergic contact dermatitis due to nickel

    L23.1   Allergic contact dermatitis due to adhesives

    L23.2   Allergic contact dermatitis due to cosmetics

    L23.3   Allergic contact dermatitis due to drugs in contact with skin
        Use additional code for adverse effect, if applicable, to identify drug (T36-T50 with fifth or sixth character 5)
        EXCLUDES 2   *dermatitis due to ingested drugs and medicaments (L27.0-L27.1)*

    L23.4   Allergic contact dermatitis due to dyes

    L23.5   Allergic contact dermatitis due to other chemical products
        Allergic contact dermatitis due to cement
        Allergic contact dermatitis due to insecticide
        Allergic contact dermatitis due to plastic
        Allergic contact dermatitis due to rubber

    L23.6   Allergic contact dermatitis due to food in contact with the skin
        EXCLUDES 2   *dermatitis due to ingested food (L27.2)*

    L23.7   Allergic contact dermatitis due to plants, except food
        EXCLUDES 2   *allergy NOS due to pollen (J30.1)*

    ✓5ᵗʰ L23.8   Allergic contact dermatitis due to other agents

        L23.81   Allergic contact dermatitis due to animal (cat) (dog) dander
            Allergic contact dermatitis due to animal (cat) (dog) hair

        L23.89   Allergic contact dermatitis due to other agents

    L23.9   Allergic contact dermatitis, unspecified cause
        Allergic contact eczema NOS

✓4ᵗʰ L24   Irritant contact dermatitis

    EXCLUDES 1   *allergy NOS (T78.40)*
                contact dermatitis NOS (L25.9)
                dermatitis NOS (L30.9)
    EXCLUDES 2   *allergic contact dermatitis (L23.-)*
                dermatitis due to substances taken internally (L27.-)
                dermatitis of eyelid (H01.1-)
                diaper dermatitis (L22)
                eczema of external ear (H60.5-)
                perioral dermatitis (L71.0)
                radiation-related disorders of the skin and subcutaneous tissue (L55-L59)

    L24.0   Irritant contact dermatitis due to detergents

    L24.1   Irritant contact dermatitis due to oils and greases

    L24.2   Irritant contact dermatitis due to solvents
        Irritant contact dermatitis due to chlorocompound
        Irritant contact dermatitis due to cyclohexane
        Irritant contact dermatitis due to ester
        Irritant contact dermatitis due to glycol
        Irritant contact dermatitis due to hydrocarbon
        Irritant contact dermatitis due to ketone

    L24.3   Irritant contact dermatitis due to cosmetics

    L24.4   Irritant contact dermatitis due to drugs in contact with skin
        Use additional code for adverse effect, if applicable, to identify drug (T36-T50 with fifth or sixth character 5)

    L24.5   Irritant contact dermatitis due to other chemical products
        Irritant contact dermatitis due to cement
        Irritant contact dermatitis due to insecticide
        Irritant contact dermatitis due to plastic
        Irritant contact dermatitis due to rubber

    L24.6   Irritant contact dermatitis due to food in contact with skin
        EXCLUDES 2   *dermatitis due to ingested food (L27.2)*

    L24.7   Irritant contact dermatitis due to plants, except food
        EXCLUDES 2   *allergy NOS to pollen (J30.1)*

    ✓5ᵗʰ L24.8   Irritant contact dermatitis due to other agents

        L24.81   Irritant contact dermatitis due to metals
            Irritant contact dermatitis due to chromium
            Irritant contact dermatitis due to nickel

        L24.89   Irritant contact dermatitis due to other agents
            Irritant contact dermatitis due to dyes

    L24.9   Irritant contact dermatitis, unspecified cause
        Irritant contact eczema NOS

✓4ᵗʰ L25 Unspecified contact dermatitis

> EXCLUDES 1   allergic contact dermatitis (L23.-)
> allergy NOS (T78.40)
> dermatitis NOS (L30.9)
> irritant contact dermatitis (L24.-)
>
> EXCLUDES 2   dermatitis due to ingested substances (L27.-)
> dermatitis of eyelid (H01.1-)
> eczema of external ear (H60.5-)
> perioral dermatitis (L71.0)
> radiation-related disorders of the skin and subcutaneous tissue (L55-L59)

L25.0 Unspecified contact dermatitis due to cosmetics

L25.1 Unspecified contact dermatitis due to drugs in contact with skin

> Use additional code for adverse effect, if applicable, to identify drug (T36-T50 with fifth or sixth character 5)
>
> EXCLUDES 2   dermatitis due to ingested drugs and medicaments (L27.0-L27.1)

L25.2 Unspecified contact dermatitis due to dyes

L25.3 Unspecified contact dermatitis due to other chemical products

> Unspecified contact dermatitis due to cement
> Unspecified contact dermatitis due to insecticide

L25.4 Unspecified contact dermatitis due to food in contact with skin

> EXCLUDES 2   dermatitis due to ingested food (L27.2)

L25.5 Unspecified contact dermatitis due to plants, except food

> EXCLUDES 1   nettle rash (L50.9)
> EXCLUDES 2   allergy NOS due to pollen (J30.1)

L25.8 Unspecified contact dermatitis due to other agents

L25.9 Unspecified contact dermatitis, unspecified cause

> Contact dermatitis (occupational) NOS
> Contact eczema (occupational) NOS

L26 Exfoliative dermatitis

> Hebra's pityriasis
>
> EXCLUDES 1   Ritter's disease (L00)

✓4ᵗʰ L27 Dermatitis due to substances taken internally

> EXCLUDES 1   allergy NOS (T78.40)
>
> EXCLUDES 2   adverse food reaction, except dermatitis (T78.0-T78.1)
> contact dermatitis (L23-L25)
> drug photoallergic response (L56.1)
> drug phototoxic response (L56.0)
> urticaria (L50.-)

L27.0 Generalized skin eruption due to drugs and medicaments taken internally   `CC`

> Use additional code for adverse effect, if applicable, to identify drug (T36-T50 with fifth or sixth character 5)

L27.1 Localized skin eruption due to drugs and medicaments taken internally   `CC`

> Use additional code for adverse effect, if applicable, to identify drug (T36-T50 with fifth or sixth character 5)

L27.2 Dermatitis due to ingested food

> EXCLUDES 2   dermatitis due to food in contact with skin (L23.6, L24.6, L25.4)

L27.8 Dermatitis due to other substances taken internally

L27.9 Dermatitis due to unspecified substance taken internally

✓4ᵗʰ L28 Lichen simplex chronicus and prurigo

L28.0 Lichen simplex chronicus
> Circumscribed neurodermatitis
> Lichen NOS

L28.1 Prurigo nodularis

L28.2 Other prurigo
> Prurigo NOS
> Prurigo Hebra
> Prurigo mitis
> Urticaria papulosa

✓4ᵗʰ L29 Pruritus

> EXCLUDES 1   neurotic excoriation (L98.1)
> psychogenic pruritus (F45.8)

L29.0 Pruritus ani

L29.1 Pruritus scroti   ♂

L29.2 Pruritus vulvae   ♀

L29.3 Anogenital pruritus, unspecified

L29.8 Other pruritus

L29.9 Pruritus, unspecified
> Itch NOS

✓4ᵗʰ L30 Other and unspecified dermatitis

> EXCLUDES 2   contact dermatitis (L23-L25)
> dry skin dermatitis (L85.3)
> small plaque parapsoriasis (L41.3)
> stasis dermatitis (I87.2)

L30.0 Nummular dermatitis

L30.1 Dyshidrosis [pompholyx]

L30.2 Cutaneous autosensitization
> Candidid [levurid]
> Dermatophytid
> Eczematid

L30.3 Infective dermatitis
> Infectious eczematoid dermatitis

L30.4 Erythema intertrigo

L30.5 Pityriasis alba
> AHA: 2018,1Q,6

L30.8 Other specified dermatitis

L30.9 Dermatitis, unspecified
> Eczema NOS

Papulosquamous disorders (L40-L45)

✓4ᵗʰ L40 Psoriasis

> DEF: Chronic autoimmune condition that speeds up skin cell growth, causing excessive immature skin cells to form raised, rounded erythematous lesions covered by dry, silvery scaling patches. Most commonly found on the scalp, elbows, knees, hands, feet, and genitals, it can also affect the joints with stiffness and swelling.

L40.0 Psoriasis vulgaris
> Nummular psoriasis
> Plaque psoriasis

L40.1 Generalized pustular psoriasis
> Impetigo herpetiformis
> Von Zumbusch's disease

L40.2 Acrodermatitis continua

L40.3 Pustulosis palmaris et plantaris

L40.4 Guttate psoriasis

✓5ᵗʰ L40.5 Arthropathic psoriasis

> **L40.50 Arthropathic psoriasis, unspecified**   `HCC`
>
> **L40.51 Distal interphalangeal psoriatic arthropathy**   `HCC`
>
> **L40.52 Psoriatic arthritis mutilans**   `HCC`
>
> **L40.53 Psoriatic spondylitis**   `HCC`
>
> **L40.54 Psoriatic juvenile arthropathy**   `HCC`
>
> **L40.59 Other psoriatic arthropathy**   `HCC`

L40.8 Other psoriasis
> Flexural psoriasis

L40.9 Psoriasis, unspecified

✓4ᵗʰ L41 Parapsoriasis

> EXCLUDES 1   poikiloderma vasculare atrophicans (L94.5)

L41.0 Pityriasis lichenoides et varioliformis acuta
> Mucha-Habermann disease

L41.1 Pityriasis lichenoides chronica

L41.3 Small plaque parapsoriasis

L41.4 Large plaque parapsoriasis

L41.5 Retiform parapsoriasis

L41.8 Other parapsoriasis

L41.9 Parapsoriasis, unspecified

L42 Pityriasis rosea

✓4ᵗʰ L43 Lichen planus

> EXCLUDES 1   lichen planopilaris (L66.1)

L43.0 Hypertrophic lichen planus

L43.1 Bullous lichen planus

L43.2 Lichenoid drug reaction
> Use additional code for adverse effect, if applicable, to identify drug (T36-T50 with fifth or sixth character 5)

L43.3 Subacute (active) lichen planus
> Lichen planus tropicus

L43.8 Other lichen planus

L43.9 Lichen planus, unspecified

✓4ᵗʰ L44 Other papulosquamous disorders

L44.0 Pityriasis rubra pilaris

✓ Additional Character Required   ✓x7ᵗʰ Placeholder   Unacceptable PDx   Questionable PDx   Manifestation   Unspecified Dx   H1-H14 HAC   HCC CMS-HCC Dx   HIV HIV Dx

ICD-10-CM 2020   741

Chapter 12. Diseases of the Skin and Subcutaneous Tissue

L44.1 Lichen nitidus
> **DEF:** Chronic, inflammatory, asymptomatic skin disorder, characterized by numerous glistening, flat-topped, discrete, skin-colored micropapules, most often on the penis, lower abdomen, inner thighs, wrists, forearms, breasts, and buttocks.

L44.2 Lichen striatus

L44.3 Lichen ruber moniliformis

L44.4 Infantile papular acrodermatitis [P]
[Gianotti-Crosti]

L44.8 Other specified papulosquamous disorders

L44.9 Papulosquamous disorder, unspecified

L45 Papulosquamous disorders in diseases classified elsewhere
> Code first underlying disease

Urticaria and erythema (L49-L54)

EXCLUDES 1 Lyme disease (A69.2-)
rosacea (L71.-)

✓4ᵗʰ L49 Exfoliation due to erythematous conditions according to extent of body surface involved
> Code first erythematous condition causing exfoliation, such as:
> Ritter's disease (L00)
> ►(Staphylococcal) scalded skin syndrome◄ (L00)
> Stevens-Johnson syndrome (L51.1)
> Stevens-Johnson syndrome-toxic epidermal necrolysis overlap syndrome (L51.3)
> toxic epidermal necrolysis (L51.2)
> **DEF:** Exfoliation: Falling or sloughing off skin in layers.

L49.0 Exfoliation due to erythematous condition involving less than 10 percent of body surface
> Exfoliation due to erythematous condition NOS

L49.1 Exfoliation due to erythematous condition involving 10-19 percent of body surface

L49.2 Exfoliation due to erythematous condition involving 20-29 percent of body surface

L49.3 Exfoliation due to erythematous condition involving 30-39 percent of body surface [CC]
> **CC Excl:** PDX collection 844

L49.4 Exfoliation due to erythematous condition involving 40-49 percent of body surface [CC]
> **CC Excl:** PDX collection 845

L49.5 Exfoliation due to erythematous condition involving 50-59 percent of body surface [CC]
> **CC Excl:** PDX collection 846

L49.6 Exfoliation due to erythematous condition involving 60-69 percent of body surface [CC]
> **CC Excl:** PDX collection 847

L49.7 Exfoliation due to erythematous condition involving 70-79 percent of body surface [CC]
> **CC Excl:** PDX collection 848

L49.8 Exfoliation due to erythematous condition involving 80-89 percent of body surface [CC]
> **CC Excl:** PDX collection 849

L49.9 Exfoliation due to erythematous condition involving 90 or more percent of body surface [CC]
> **CC Excl:** PDX collection 850

✓4ᵗʰ L50 Urticaria

EXCLUDES 1 allergic contact dermatitis (L23.-)
angioneurotic edema (T78.3)
giant urticaria (T78.3)
hereditary angio-edema (D84.1)
Quincke's edema (T78.3)
serum urticaria (T80.6-)
solar urticaria (L56.3)
urticaria neonatorum (P83.8)
urticaria papulosa (L28.2)
urticaria pigmentosa ►(D47.01)◄

> **DEF:** Eruption of itching edema of the skin. **Synonym(s):** hives.

L50.0 Allergic urticaria

L50.1 Idiopathic urticaria

L50.2 Urticaria due to cold and heat
EXCLUDES 2 familial cold urticaria (M04.2)

L50.3 Dermatographic urticaria

L50.4 Vibratory urticaria

L50.5 Cholinergic urticaria

L50.6 Contact urticaria

L50.8 Other urticaria
> Chronic urticaria
> Recurrent periodic urticaria

L50.9 Urticaria, unspecified

✓4ᵗʰ L51 Erythema multiforme
> Use additional code for adverse effect, if applicable, to identify drug (T36-T50 with fifth or sixth character 5)
> Use additional code to identify associated manifestations, such as:
> arthropathy associated with dermatological disorders (M14.8-)
> conjunctival edema (H11.42)
> conjunctivitis (H10.22-)
> corneal scars and opacities (H17.-)
> corneal ulcer (H16.0-)
> edema of eyelid (H02.84-)
> inflammation of eyelid (H01.8)
> keratoconjunctivitis sicca (H16.22-)
> mechanical lagophthalmos (H02.22-)
> stomatitis (K12.-)
> symblepharon (H11.23-)
> Use additional code to identify percentage of skin exfoliation (L49.-)
> **EXCLUDES 1** staphylococcal scalded skin syndrome (L00)
> Ritter's disease (L00)
> **DEF:** Acute complex of symptoms with a varied pattern of skin eruptions, such as macular, bullous, popular, nodose, or vesicular lesions on the neck, face, and legs. Erythema (redness of skin and mucous membranes) multiforme (multiple forms) is a hypersensitivity (allergic) reaction that can occur at any age but primarily affects children or young adults.
> **CC Excl: For CC codes in category L51:** PDX collection 843

L51.0 Nonbullous erythema multiforme

L51.1 Stevens-Johnson syndrome [CC] [HCC]

L51.2 Toxic epidermal necrolysis [Lyell] [CC] [HCC]

L51.3 Stevens-Johnson syndrome-toxic epidermal [CC] [HCC]
necrolysis overlap syndrome
> SJS-TEN overlap syndrome

L51.8 Other erythema multiforme

L51.9 Erythema multiforme, unspecified
> Erythema iris
> Erythema multiforme major NOS
> Erythema multiforme minor NOS
> Herpes iris

L52 Erythema nodosum
> **EXCLUDES 1** tuberculous erythema nodosum (A18.4)
> **DEF:** Form of panniculitis (inflammation of the fat layer beneath the skin) most often occurring in women. Commonly seen as a hypersensitivity reaction to infections, drugs, sarcoidosis, and specific enteropathies. The acute stage is associated with fever, malaise, and arthralgia. The lesions are pink to blue in color as tender nodules and are found on the front of the legs below the knees.

✓4ᵗʰ L53 Other erythematous conditions
> **EXCLUDES 1** erythema ab igne (L59.0)
> erythema due to external agents in contact with skin (L23-L25)
> erythema intertrigo (L30.4)
> **CC Excl: For CC codes in category L53:** PDX collection 851

L53.0 Toxic erythema [CC]
> Code first poisoning due to drug or toxin, if applicable (T36-T65 with fifth or sixth character 1-4 or 6)
> Use additional code for adverse effect, if applicable, to identify drug (T36-T50 with fifth or sixth character 5)
> **EXCLUDES 1** neonatal erythema toxicum (P83.1)

L53.1 Erythema annulare centrifugum [CC]

L53.2 Erythema marginatum [CC]

L53.3 Other chronic figurate erythema [CC]

L53.8 Other specified erythematous conditions

L53.9 Erythematous condition, unspecified
> Erythema NOS
> Erythroderma NOS

L54 Erythema in diseases classified elsewhere
> Code first underlying disease

Radiation-related disorders of the skin and subcutaneous tissue (L55-L59)

✓4ᵗʰ L55 Sunburn

L55.0 Sunburn of first degree

L55.1 Sunburn of second degree

[N] Newborn: 0 [P] Pediatric: 0-17 [M] Maternity: 9-64 [A] Adult: 15-124 [MCC] Major Complication/Comorbidity [CC] Complication/Comorbidity [SW] Severe Wound Dx

742 ICD-10-CM 2020

L55.2 **Sunburn of** third degree
L55.9 **Sunburn, unspecified**

√4ᵗʰ **L56 Other acute skin changes due to ultraviolet radiation**
Use additional code to identify the source of the ultraviolet radiation (W89, X32)

L56.0 **Drug phototoxic response**
Use additional code for adverse effect, if applicable, to identify drug (T36-T50 with fifth or sixth character 5)

L56.1 **Drug photoallergic response**
Use additional code for adverse effect, if applicable, to identify drug (T36-T50 with fifth or sixth character 5)

L56.2 **Photocontact dermatitis [berloque dermatitis]**
L56.3 **Solar urticaria**
L56.4 **Polymorphous light eruption**
L56.5 **Disseminated superficial actinic porokeratosis (DSAP)**
DEF: Autosomal dominant skin condition occurring in sun-exposed areas of the skin (particularly the arms and legs), characterized by superficial annular, keratotic, brownish-red spots or thickenings with depressed centers and sharp, ridged borders. It may evolve into squamous cell carcinoma.

L56.8 **Other specified acute skin changes due to ultraviolet radiation**
L56.9 **Acute skin change due to ultraviolet radiation, unspecified**

√4ᵗʰ **L57 Skin changes due to chronic exposure to nonionizing radiation**
Use additional code to identify the source of the ultraviolet radiation (W89)

L57.0 **Actinic keratosis**
Keratosis NOS
Senile keratosis
Solar keratosis

L57.1 **Actinic reticuloid**
L57.2 **Cutis rhomboidalis nuchae**
L57.3 **Poikiloderma of Civatte**
L57.4 **Cutis laxa senilis**
Elastosis senilis

L57.5 **Actinic granuloma**
L57.8 **Other skin changes due to chronic exposure to nonionizing radiation**
Farmer's skin
Sailor's skin
Solar dermatitis

L57.9 **Skin changes due to chronic exposure to nonionizing radiation, unspecified**

√4ᵗʰ **L58 Radiodermatitis**
Use additional code to identify the source of the radiation (W88, W90)

L58.0 **Acute radiodermatitis**
L58.1 **Chronic radiodermatitis**
L58.9 **Radiodermatitis, unspecified**

√4ᵗʰ **L59 Other disorders of skin and subcutaneous tissue related to radiation**
L59.0 **Erythema ab igne [dermatitis ab igne]**
L59.8 **Other specified disorders of the skin and subcutaneous tissue related to radiation**
AHA: 2017,1Q,33

L59.9 **Disorder of the skin and subcutaneous tissue related to radiation, unspecified**

Disorders of skin appendages (L60-L75)

EXCLUDES 1   congenital malformations of integument (Q84.-)

√4ᵗʰ **L60 Nail disorders**
EXCLUDES 2   clubbing of nails (R68.3)
onychia and paronychia (L03.0-)

Nail Disorders

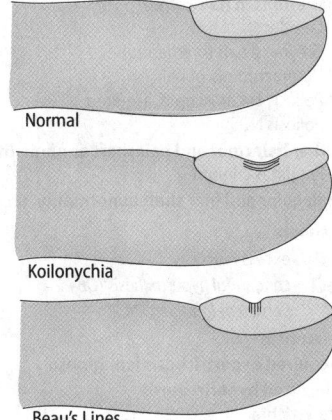

Normal

Koilonychia

Beau's Lines

L60.0 **Ingrowing nail**
L60.1 **Onycholysis**
L60.2 **Onychogryphosis**
L60.3 **Nail dystrophy**
L60.4 **Beau's lines**
L60.5 **Yellow nail syndrome**
L60.8 **Other nail disorders**
L60.9 **Nail disorder, unspecified**

L62 Nail disorders in diseases classified elsewhere
Code first underlying disease, such as:
pachydermoperiostosis (M89.4-)

√4ᵗʰ **L63 Alopecia areata**
L63.0 **Alopecia (capitis)** totalis
L63.1 **Alopecia** universalis
L63.2 **Ophiasis**
L63.8 **Other alopecia areata**
L63.9 **Alopecia areata, unspecified**

√4ᵗʰ **L64 Androgenic alopecia**
INCLUDES   male-pattern baldness

L64.0 **Drug-induced androgenic alopecia**
Use additional code for adverse effect, if applicable, to identify drug (T36-T50 with fifth or sixth character 5)

L64.8 **Other androgenic alopecia**
L64.9 **Androgenic alopecia, unspecified**

√4ᵗʰ **L65 Other nonscarring hair loss**
Use additional code for adverse effect, if applicable, to identify drug (T36-T50 with fifth or sixth character 5)
EXCLUDES 1   trichotillomania (F63.3)

L65.0 **Telogen effluvium**
DEF: Form of nonscarring alopecia characterized by shedding of hair from premature telogen development in follicles due to stress, including shock, childbirth, surgery, drugs, or weight loss.

L65.1 **Anagen effluvium**
L65.2 **Alopecia mucinosa**
L65.8 **Other specified nonscarring hair loss**
L65.9 **Nonscarring hair loss, unspecified**
Alopecia NOS

√4ᵗʰ **L66 Cicatricial alopecia [scarring hair loss]**
L66.0 **Pseudopelade**
L66.1 **Lichen planopilaris**
Follicular lichen planus

L66.2 **Folliculitis decalvans**
L66.3 **Perifolliculitis capitis abscedens**
L66.4 **Folliculitis ulerythematosa reticulata**

L66.8 Other cicatricial alopecia
     AHA: 2015,1Q,19

L66.9 Cicatricial alopecia, unspecified

√4ᵗʰ **L67 Hair color and hair shaft abnormalities**
     EXCLUDES 1   monilethrix (Q84.1)
                pili annulati (Q84.1)
                telogen effluvium (L65.0)

L67.0 Trichorrhexis nodosa

L67.1 Variations in hair color
     Canities
     Greyness, hair (premature)
     Heterochromia of hair
     Poliosis circumscripta, acquired
     Poliosis NOS

L67.8 Other hair color and hair shaft abnormalities
     Fragilitas crinium

L67.9 Hair color and hair shaft abnormality, unspecified

√4ᵗʰ **L68 Hypertrichosis**
     INCLUDES   excess hair
     EXCLUDES 1   congenital hypertrichosis (Q84.2)
                persistent lanugo (Q84.2)

L68.0 Hirsutism

L68.1 Acquired hypertrichosis lanuginosa

L68.2 Localized hypertrichosis

L68.3 Polytrichia

L68.8 Other hypertrichosis

L68.9 Hypertrichosis, unspecified

√4ᵗʰ **L70 Acne**
     EXCLUDES 2   acne keloid (L73.0)

L70.0 Acne vulgaris

L70.1 Acne conglobata

L70.2 Acne varioliformis
     Acne necrotica miliaris
     DEF: Rare form of acne characterized by development of persistent brown papulopustules followed by scar formation. This type of acne usually presents on the brow and temporoparietal part of the scalp.

L70.3 Acne tropica

L70.4 Infantile acne   P

L70.5 Acné excoriée
     Acné excoriée des jeunes filles
     Picker's acne

L70.8 Other acne

L70.9 Acne, unspecified

√4ᵗʰ **L71 Rosacea**
     Use additional code for adverse effect, if applicable, to identify drug (T36-T50 with fifth or sixth character 5)

L71.0 Perioral dermatitis

L71.1 Rhinophyma

L71.8 Other rosacea
     AHA: 2018,4Q,15

L71.9 Rosacea, unspecified

√4ᵗʰ **L72 Follicular cysts of skin and subcutaneous tissue**

L72.0 Epidermal cyst

√5ᵗʰ **L72.1 Pilar and trichodermal cyst**

     L72.11 Pilar cyst

     L72.12 Trichodermal cyst
         Trichilemmal (proliferating) cyst

L72.2 Steatocystoma multiplex

L72.3 Sebaceous cyst
     EXCLUDES 2   pilar cyst (L72.11)
                trichilemmal (proliferating) cyst (L72.12)

L72.8 Other follicular cysts of the skin and subcutaneous tissue

L72.9 Follicular cyst of the skin and subcutaneous tissue, unspecified

√4ᵗʰ **L73 Other follicular disorders**

L73.0 Acne keloid

L73.1 Pseudofolliculitis barbae

L73.2 Hidradenitis suppurativa

L73.8 Other specified follicular disorders
     Sycosis barbae

L73.9 Follicular disorder, unspecified

√4ᵗʰ **L74 Eccrine sweat disorders**
     EXCLUDES 2   generalized hyperhidrosis (R61)
     DEF: Eccrine sweat glands: Glands found in the dermal and hypodermal layer of the skin throughout the body, particularly on the forehead, scalp, axillae, palms, and soles. These glands produce watery and neutral or slightly acidic sweat.

L74.0 Miliaria rubra

L74.1 Miliaria crystallina

L74.2 Miliaria profunda
     Miliaria tropicalis

L74.3 Miliaria, unspecified

L74.4 Anhidrosis
     Hypohidrosis
     DEF: Inability to sweat normally. When the body can't cool itself through perspiration it can lead to heatstroke, a life-threatening condition.

√5ᵗʰ **L74.5 Focal hyperhidrosis**

√6ᵗʰ **L74.51 Primary focal hyperhidrosis**

     L74.510 Primary focal hyperhidrosis, axilla
     L74.511 Primary focal hyperhidrosis, face
     L74.512 Primary focal hyperhidrosis, palms
     L74.513 Primary focal hyperhidrosis, soles
     L74.519 Primary focal hyperhidrosis, unspecified

     L74.52 Secondary focal hyperhidrosis
         Frey's syndrome

L74.8 Other eccrine sweat disorders

L74.9 Eccrine sweat disorder, unspecified
     Sweat gland disorder NOS

√4ᵗʰ **L75 Apocrine sweat disorders**
     EXCLUDES 1   dyshidrosis (L30.1)
                hidradenitis suppurativa (L73.2)
     DEF: Apocrine sweat glands: Found in the axilla, areola, and circumanal region, these glands begin to function in puberty and produce viscid milky secretions in response to external stimuli.

L75.0 Bromhidrosis

L75.1 Chromhidrosis

L75.2 Apocrine miliaria
     Fox-Fordyce disease
     DEF: Chronic, usually pruritic disease evidenced by small follicular papular eruptions, especially in the axillary and pubic areas. Apocrine miliaria develops from the closure and rupture of the affected apocrine glands' intraepidermal portion of the ducts.

L75.8 Other apocrine sweat disorders

L75.9 Apocrine sweat disorder, unspecified

Intraoperative and postprocedural complications of skin and subcutaneous tissue (L76)

√4ᵗʰ **L76 Intraoperative and postprocedural complications of skin and subcutaneous tissue**
     AHA: 2016,4Q,9-10
     CC Excl: For CC codes in category L76, unless otheerwise noted: PDX collection 852

√5ᵗʰ **L76.0 Intraoperative hemorrhage and hematoma of skin and subcutaneous tissue complicating a procedure**
     EXCLUDES 1   intraoperative hemorrhage and hematoma of skin and subcutaneous tissue due to accidental puncture and laceration during a procedure (L76.1-)

     L76.01 Intraoperative hemorrhage and hematoma of skin and subcutaneous tissue complicating a dermatologic procedure   CC

     L76.02 Intraoperative hemorrhage and hematoma of skin and subcutaneous tissue complicating other procedure   CC

√5ᵗʰ **L76.1 Accidental puncture and laceration of skin and subcutaneous tissue during a procedure**

     L76.11 Accidental puncture and laceration of skin and subcutaneous tissue during a dermatologic procedure   CC
         CC Excl: PDX collection 509

     L76.12 Accidental puncture and laceration of skin and subcutaneous tissue during other procedure   CC
         CC Excl: PDX collection 509

N Newborn: 0   P Pediatric: 0-17   M Maternity: 9-64   A Adult: 15-124   MCC Major Complication/Comorbidity   CC Complication/Comorbidity   SW Severe Wound Dx

744   ICD-10-CM 2020

✓5ᵗʰ **L76.2** **Postprocedural hemorrhage** of skin and subcutaneous tissue following a procedure

L76.21 **Postprocedural hemorrhage of skin and subcutaneous tissue following a dermatologic procedure** CC

L76.22 **Postprocedural hemorrhage of skin and subcutaneous tissue following other procedure** CC

✓5ᵗʰ **L76.3** **Postprocedural hematoma and seroma** of skin and subcutaneous tissue following a procedure

L76.31 **Postprocedural hematoma of skin and subcutaneous tissue following a dermatologic procedure** CC

L76.32 **Postprocedural hematoma of skin and subcutaneous tissue following other procedure** CC

L76.33 **Postprocedural seroma of skin and subcutaneous tissue following a dermatologic procedure** CC

L76.34 **Postprocedural seroma of skin and subcutaneous tissue following other procedure** CC

✓5ᵗʰ **L76.8** **Other intraoperative and postprocedural complications of skin and subcutaneous tissue**
Use additional code, if applicable, to further specify disorder

L76.81 **Other intraoperative complications of skin and subcutaneous tissue**

L76.82 **Other postprocedural complications of skin and subcutaneous tissue**
AHA: 2017,3Q,6

Other disorders of the skin and subcutaneous tissue (L80-L99)

L80 **Vitiligo**
EXCLUDES 2   *vitiligo of eyelids (H02.73-)*
vitiligo of vulva (N90.89)
DEF: Persistent, progressive development of nonpigmented white patches on otherwise normal skin.

✓4ᵗʰ **L81** **Other disorders of pigmentation**
EXCLUDES 1   *birthmark NOS (Q82.5)*
Peutz-Jeghers syndrome (Q85.8)
EXCLUDES 2   *nevus — see Alphabetical Index*

L81.0 **Postinflammatory hyperpigmentation**
L81.1 **Chloasma**
L81.2 **Freckles**
L81.3 **Café au lait spots**
L81.4 **Other melanin hyperpigmentation**
Lentigo
L81.5 **Leukoderma, not elsewhere classified**
L81.6 **Other disorders of diminished melanin formation**
L81.7 **Pigmented purpuric dermatosis**
Angioma serpiginosum
L81.8 **Other specified disorders of pigmentation**
Iron pigmentation
Tattoo pigmentation
L81.9 **Disorder of pigmentation, unspecified**

✓4ᵗʰ **L82** **Seborrheic keratosis**
INCLUDES   basal cell papilloma
dermatosis papulosa nigra
Leser-Trélat disease
EXCLUDES 2   *seborrheic dermatitis (L21.-)*
DEF: Common, benign, noninvasive, lightly pigmented, warty growth composed of basaloid cells that usually appear at middle age as soft, easily crumbling plaques on the face, trunk, and extremities.
L82.0 **Inflamed seborrheic keratosis**
L82.1 **Other seborrheic keratosis**
Seborrheic keratosis NOS

L83 **Acanthosis nigricans**
Confluent and reticulated papillomatosis
DEF: Diffuse, velvety hyperplasia of the spinous skin layer of the axilla and other body folds marked by gray, brown, or black pigmentation. In adult form, it is often associated with malignant acanthosis nigricans in a benign, nevoid form relatively generalized.

L84 **Corns and callosities**
Callus
Clavus

✓4ᵗʰ **L85** **Other epidermal thickening**
EXCLUDES 2   *hypertrophic disorders of the skin (L91.-)*

L85.0 **Acquired ichthyosis**
EXCLUDES 1   *congenital ichthyosis (Q80.-)*

L85.1 **Acquired keratosis [keratoderma] palmaris et plantaris**
EXCLUDES 1   *inherited keratosis palmaris et plantaris (Q82.8)*

L85.2 **Keratosis punctata (palmaris et plantaris)**
L85.3 **Xerosis cutis**
Dry skin dermatitis
L85.8 **Other specified epidermal thickening**
Cutaneous horn
L85.9 **Epidermal thickening, unspecified**

L86 *Keratoderma in diseases classified elsewhere*
Code first underlying disease, such as:
Reiter's disease (M02.3-)
EXCLUDES 1   *gonococcal keratoderma (A54.89)*
gonococcal keratosis (A54.89)
keratoderma due to vitamin A deficiency (E50.8)
keratosis due to vitamin A deficiency (E50.8)
xeroderma due to vitamin A deficiency (E50.8)

✓4ᵗʰ **L87** **Transepidermal elimination disorders**
EXCLUDES 1   *granuloma annulare (perforating) (L92.0)*

L87.0 **Keratosis follicularis et parafollicularis in cutem penetrans**
Hyperkeratosis follicularis penetrans
Kyrle disease
L87.1 **Reactive perforating collagenosis**
L87.2 **Elastosis perforans serpiginosa**
L87.8 **Other transepidermal elimination disorders**
L87.9 **Transepidermal elimination disorder, unspecified**

L88 **Pyoderma gangrenosum** CC
Phagedenic pyoderma
EXCLUDES 1   *dermatitis gangrenosa (L08.0)*
DEF: Persistent debilitating skin disease characterized by irregular, boggy, blue-red ulcerations, with central healing and undermined edges.
CC Excl: PDX collection 853

✓4ᵗʰ L89 Pressure ulcer

INCLUDES
- bed sore
- decubitus ulcer
- plaster ulcer
- pressure area
- pressure sore

Code first any associated gangrene (I96)

EXCLUDES 2
- decubitus (trophic) ulcer of cervix (uteri) (N86)
- diabetic ulcers (E08.621, E08.622, E09.621, E09.622, E10.621, E10.622, E11.621, E11.622, E13.621, E13.622)
- non-pressure chronic ulcer of skin (L97.-)
- skin infections (L00-L08)
- varicose ulcer (I83.0, I83.2)

AHA: 2018,4Q,69; 2018,3Q,3; 2018,2Q,21; 2017,4Q,109; 2017,1Q,49; 2016,4Q,143

TIP: The stage of a diagnosed pressure ulcer can be based on documentation from clinicians who are not the patient's provider.

Four Stages of Pressure Ulcer

Epidermis
Dermis

Stage 1
Persistent focal edema

Subcutaneous tissue

Stage 2
Abrasion, blister, partial thickness skin loss involving epidermis and/or dermis

Superficial fascia
Muscle

Stage 3
Full thickness skin loss involving damage or necrosis of subcutaneous tissue

Deep fascia
Bone

Stage 4
Necrosis of soft tissues through to underlying muscle, tendon, or bone

✓5ᵗʰ L89.0 Pressure ulcer of elbow

    ✓6ᵗʰ L89.00 Pressure ulcer of unspecified elbow

        L89.000 Pressure ulcer of unspecified elbow, unstageable `CC` `HCC` `SW`

        L89.001 Pressure ulcer of unspecified elbow, stage 1 `CC`
          Healing pressure ulcer of unspecified elbow, stage 1
          Pressure pre-ulcer skin changes limited to persistent focal edema, unspecified elbow

        L89.002 Pressure ulcer of unspecified elbow, stage 2 `CC` `HCC`
          Healing pressure ulcer of unspecified elbow, stage 2
          Pressure ulcer with abrasion, blister, partial thickness skin loss involving epidermis and/or dermis, unspecified elbow

        L89.003 Pressure ulcer of unspecified elbow, stage 3 `CC` `H4` `HCC` `SW`
          Healing pressure ulcer of unspecified elbow, stage 3
          Pressure ulcer with full thickness skin loss involving damage or necrosis of subcutaneous tissue, unspecified elbow

L89.004 Pressure ulcer of unspecified elbow, stage 4 `CC` `H4` `HCC` `SW`
    Healing pressure ulcer of unspecified elbow, stage 4
    Pressure ulcer with necrosis of soft tissues through to underlying muscle, tendon, or bone, unspecified elbow

L89.006 Pressure-induced deep tissue damage of unspecified elbow `CC`

L89.009 Pressure ulcer of unspecified elbow, unspecified stage `CC`
    Healing pressure ulcer of elbow NOS
    Healing pressure ulcer of unspecified elbow, unspecified stage

✓6ᵗʰ L89.01 Pressure ulcer of right elbow

    L89.010 Pressure ulcer of right elbow, unstageable `CC` `HCC` `SW`

    L89.011 Pressure ulcer of right elbow, stage 1 `CC`
      Healing pressure ulcer of right elbow, stage 1
      Pressure pre-ulcer skin changes limited to persistent focal edema, right elbow

    L89.012 Pressure ulcer of right elbow, stage 2 `CC` `HCC`
      Healing pressure ulcer of right elbow, stage 2
      Pressure ulcer with abrasion, blister, partial thickness skin loss involving epidermis and/or dermis, right elbow

    L89.013 Pressure ulcer of right elbow, stage 3 `CC` `H4` `HCC` `SW`
      Healing pressure ulcer of right elbow, stage 3
      Pressure ulcer with full thickness skin loss involving damage or necrosis of subcutaneous tissue, right elbow

    L89.014 Pressure ulcer of right elbow, stage 4 `CC` `H4` `HCC` `SW`
      Healing pressure ulcer of right elbow, stage 4
      Pressure ulcer with necrosis of soft tissues through to underlying muscle, tendon, or bone, right elbow

L89.016 Pressure-induced deep tissue damage of right elbow `CC`

L89.019 Pressure ulcer of right elbow, unspecified stage `CC`
    Healing pressure right of elbow NOS
    Healing pressure ulcer of right elbow, unspecified stage

✓6ᵗʰ L89.02 Pressure ulcer of left elbow

    L89.020 Pressure ulcer of left elbow, unstageable `CC` `HCC` `SW`

    L89.021 Pressure ulcer of left elbow, stage 1 `CC`
      Healing pressure ulcer of left elbow, stage 1
      Pressure pre-ulcer skin changes limited to persistent focal edema, left elbow

    L89.022 Pressure ulcer of left elbow, stage 2 `CC` `HCC`
      Healing pressure ulcer of left elbow, stage 2
      Pressure ulcer with abrasion, blister, partial thickness skin loss involving epidermis and/or dermis, left elbow

    L89.023 Pressure ulcer of left elbow, stage 3 `CC` `H4` `HCC` `SW`
      Healing pressure ulcer of left elbow, stage 3
      Pressure ulcer with full thickness skin loss involving damage or necrosis of subcutaneous tissue, left elbow

L89.024   **Pressure ulcer of left**   `CC` `H4` `HCC` `SW`
elbow, stage 4
    Healing pressure ulcer of left elbow, stage 4
    Pressure ulcer with necrosis of soft tissues through to underlying muscle, tendon, or bone, left elbow

L89.026   **Pressure-induced deep**   `CC`
tissue damage of left elbow

L89.029   **Pressure ulcer of left**   `CC`
elbow, unspecified stage
    Healing pressure ulcer of left of elbow NOS
    Healing pressure ulcer of left elbow, unspecified stage

√5th **L89.1**   **Pressure ulcer of back**

√6th   **L89.10**   **Pressure ulcer of unspecified part of back**

L89.100   **Pressure ulcer of**   `CC` `HCC` `SW`
unspecified part of back, unstageable

L89.101   **Pressure ulcer of**   `CC`
unspecified part of back, stage 1
    Healing pressure ulcer of unspecified part of back, stage 1
    Pressure pre-ulcer skin changes limited to persistent focal edema, unspecified part of back

L89.102   **Pressure ulcer of**   `CC` `HCC`
unspecified part of back, stage 2
    Healing pressure ulcer of unspecified part of back, stage 2
    Pressure ulcer with abrasion, blister, partial thickness skin loss involving epidermis and/or dermis, unspecified part of back

L89.103   **Pressure ulcer of**   `CC` `H4` `HCC` `SW`
unspecified part of back, stage 3
    Healing pressure ulcer of unspecified part of back, stage 3
    Pressure ulcer with full thickness skin loss involving damage or necrosis of subcutaneous tissue, unspecified part of back

L89.104   **Pressure ulcer of**   `CC` `H4` `HCC` `SW`
unspecified part of back, stage 4
    Healing pressure ulcer of unspecified part of back, stage 4
    Pressure ulcer with necrosis of soft tissues through to underlying muscle, tendon, or bone, unspecified part of back

L89.106   **Pressure-induced deep**   `CC`
tissue damage of unspecified part of back

L89.109   **Pressure ulcer of**   `CC`
unspecified part of back, unspecified stage
    Healing pressure ulcer of unspecified part of back NOS
    Healing pressure ulcer of unspecified part of back, unspecified stage

√6th   **L89.11**   **Pressure ulcer of right upper back**
    Pressure ulcer of right shoulder blade

L89.110   **Pressure ulcer of right**   `CC` `HCC` `SW`
upper back, unstageable

L89.111   **Pressure ulcer of right**   `CC`
upper back, stage 1
    Healing pressure ulcer of right upper back, stage 1
    Pressure pre-ulcer skin changes limited to persistent focal edema, right upper back

L89.112   **Pressure ulcer of right**   `CC` `HCC`
upper back, stage 2
    Healing pressure ulcer of right upper back, stage 2
    Pressure ulcer with abrasion, blister, partial thickness skin loss involving epidermis and/or dermis, right upper back

L89.113   **Pressure ulcer of right**   `CC` `H4` `HCC` `SW`
upper back, stage 3
    Healing pressure ulcer of right upper back, stage 3
    Pressure ulcer with full thickness skin loss involving damage or necrosis of subcutaneous tissue, right upper back

L89.114   **Pressure ulcer of right**   `CC` `H4` `HCC` `SW`
upper back, stage 4
    Healing pressure ulcer of right upper back, stage 4
    Pressure ulcer with necrosis of soft tissues through to underlying muscle, tendon, or bone, right upper back

L89.116   **Pressure-induced deep**   `CC`
tissue damage of right upper back

L89.119   **Pressure ulcer of right**   `CC`
upper back, unspecified stage
    Healing pressure ulcer of right upper back NOS
    Healing pressure ulcer of right upper back, unspecified stage

√6th   **L89.12**   **Pressure ulcer of left upper back**
    Pressure ulcer of left shoulder blade

L89.120   **Pressure ulcer of left**   `CC` `HCC` `SW`
upper back, unstageable

L89.121   **Pressure ulcer of left**   `CC`
upper back, stage 1
    Healing pressure ulcer of left upper back, stage 1
    Pressure pre-ulcer skin changes limited to persistent focal edema, left upper back

L89.122   **Pressure ulcer of left**   `CC` `HCC`
upper back, stage 2
    Healing pressure ulcer of left upper back, stage 2
    Pressure ulcer with abrasion, blister, partial thickness skin loss involving epidermis and/or dermis, left upper back

L89.123   **Pressure ulcer of left**   `CC` `H4` `HCC` `SW`
upper back, stage 3
    Healing pressure ulcer of left upper back, stage 3
    Pressure ulcer with full thickness skin loss involving damage or necrosis of subcutaneous tissue, left upper back

L89.124   **Pressure ulcer of left**   `CC` `H4` `HCC` `SW`
upper back, stage 4
    Healing pressure ulcer of left upper back, stage 4
    Pressure ulcer with necrosis of soft tissues through to underlying muscle, tendon, or bone, left upper back

L89.126   **Pressure-induced deep**   `CC`
tissue damage of left upper back

L89.129   **Pressure ulcer of left**   `CC`
upper back, unspecified stage
    Healing pressure ulcer of left upper back NOS
    Healing pressure ulcer of left upper back, unspecified stage

√6th   **L89.13**   **Pressure ulcer of right lower back**

L89.130   **Pressure ulcer of right**   `CC` `HCC` `SW`
lower back, unstageable

✓ Additional Character Required   √x7th Placeholder   Unacceptable PDx   Questionable PDx   Manifestation   Unspecified Dx   `H1`-`H14` HAC   `HCC` CMS-HCC Dx   `HIV` HIV Dx

ICD-10-CM 2020   747

L89.131   **Pressure ulcer of right** `cc`
    lower back, stage 1
      Healing pressure ulcer of right lower back, stage 1
      Pressure pre-ulcer skin changes limited to persistent focal edema, right lower back

L89.132   **Pressure ulcer of right** `cc` `HCC`
    lower back, stage 2
      Healing pressure ulcer of right lower back, stage 2
      Pressure ulcer with abrasion, blister, partial thickness skin loss involving epidermis and/or dermis, right lower back

L89.133   **Pressure ulcer of right** `cc` `H4` `HCC` `SW`
    lower back, stage 3
      Healing pressure ulcer of right lower back, stage 3
      Pressure ulcer with full thickness skin loss involving damage or necrosis of subcutaneous tissue, right lower back

L89.134   **Pressure ulcer of right** `cc` `H4` `HCC` `SW`
    lower back, stage 4
      Healing pressure ulcer of right lower back, stage 4
      Pressure ulcer with necrosis of soft tissues through to underlying muscle, tendon, or bone, right lower back

L89.136   **Pressure-induced deep** `cc`
    tissue damage of right
    lower back

L89.139   **Pressure ulcer of right** `cc`
    lower back, unspecified
    stage
      Healing pressure ulcer of right lower back NOS
      Healing pressure ulcer of right lower back, unspecified stage

√6ᵗʰ **L89.14**   **Pressure ulcer of left lower back**

L89.140   **Pressure ulcer of left lower** `cc` `HCC` `SW`
    back, unstageable

L89.141   **Pressure ulcer of left lower** `cc`
    back, stage 1
      Healing pressure ulcer of left lower back, stage 1
      Pressure pre-ulcer skin changes limited to persistent focal edema, left lower back

L89.142   **Pressure ulcer of left lower** `cc` `HCC`
    back, stage 2
      Healing pressure ulcer of left lower back, stage 2
      Pressure ulcer with abrasion, blister, partial thickness skin loss involving epidermis and/or dermis, left lower back

L89.143   **Pressure ulcer of left lower** `cc` `H4` `HCC` `SW`
    back, stage 3
      Healing pressure ulcer of left lower back, stage 3
      Pressure ulcer with full thickness skin loss involving damage or necrosis of subcutaneous tissue, left lower back

L89.144   **Pressure ulcer of left lower** `cc` `H4` `HCC` `SW`
    back, stage 4
      Healing pressure ulcer of left lower back, stage 4
      Pressure ulcer with necrosis of soft tissues through to underlying muscle, tendon, or bone, left lower back

L89.146   **Pressure-induced deep** `cc`
    tissue damage of left
    lower back

L89.149   **Pressure ulcer of left lower** `cc`
    back, unspecified stage
      Healing pressure ulcer of left lower back NOS
      Healing pressure ulcer of left lower back, unspecified stage

√6ᵗʰ **L89.15**   **Pressure ulcer of sacral region**
      Pressure ulcer of coccyx
      Pressure ulcer of tailbone

L89.150   **Pressure ulcer of sacral** `cc` `HCC` `SW`
    region, unstageable

L89.151   **Pressure ulcer of sacral** `cc`
    region, stage 1
      Healing pressure ulcer of sacral region, stage 1
      Pressure pre-ulcer skin changes limited to persistent focal edema, sacral region

L89.152   **Pressure ulcer of sacral** `cc` `HCC`
    region, stage 2
      Healing pressure ulcer of sacral region, stage 2
      Pressure ulcer with abrasion, blister, partial thickness skin loss involving epidermis and/or dermis, sacral region

L89.153   **Pressure ulcer of sacral** `cc` `H4` `HCC` `SW`
    region, stage 3
      Healing pressure ulcer of sacral region, stage 3
      Pressure ulcer with full thickness skin loss involving damage or necrosis of subcutaneous tissue, sacral region

L89.154   **Pressure ulcer of sacral** `cc` `H4` `HCC` `SW`
    region, stage 4
      Healing pressure ulcer of sacral region, stage 4
      Pressure ulcer with necrosis of soft tissues through to underlying muscle, tendon, or bone, sacral region

L89.156   **Pressure-induced deep** `cc`
    tissue damage of sacral
    region

L89.159   **Pressure ulcer of sacral** `cc`
    region, unspecified stage
      Healing pressure ulcer of sacral region NOS
      Healing pressure ulcer of sacral region, unspecified stage

√5ᵗʰ **L89.2**   **Pressure ulcer of hip**

√6ᵗʰ **L89.20**   **Pressure ulcer of unspecified hip**

L89.200   **Pressure ulcer of** `cc` `HCC` `SW`
    unspecified hip,
    unstageable

L89.201   **Pressure ulcer of** `cc`
    unspecified hip, stage 1
      Healing pressure ulcer of unspecified hip back, stage 1
      Pressure pre-ulcer skin changes limited to persistent focal edema, unspecified hip

L89.202   **Pressure ulcer of** `cc` `HCC`
    unspecified hip, stage 2
      Healing pressure ulcer of unspecified hip, stage 2
      Pressure ulcer with abrasion, blister, partial thickness skin loss involving epidermis and/or dermis, unspecified hip

L89.203   **Pressure ulcer of** `cc` `H4` `HCC` `SW`
    unspecified hip, stage 3
      Healing pressure ulcer of unspecified hip, stage 3
      Pressure ulcer with full thickness skin loss involving damage or necrosis of subcutaneous tissue, unspecified hip

Ⓝ Newborn: 0   Ⓟ Pediatric: 0-17   Ⓜ Maternity: 9-64   Ⓐ Adult: 15-124   `MCC` Major Complication/Comorbidity   `CC` Complication/Comorbidity   `SW` Severe Wound Dx

748   ICD-10-CM 2020

L89.204 Pressure ulcer of unspecified hip, stage 4 `CC` `H4` `HCC` `SW`
Healing pressure ulcer of unspecified hip, stage 4
Pressure ulcer with necrosis of soft tissues through to underlying muscle, tendon, or bone, unspecified hip

● **L89.206 Pressure-induced deep tissue damage of unspecified hip** `CC`

L89.209 Pressure ulcer of unspecified hip, unspecified stage `CC`
Healing pressure ulcer of unspecified hip NOS
Healing pressure ulcer of unspecified hip, unspecified stage

√6th **L89.21 Pressure ulcer of right hip**

L89.210 Pressure ulcer of right hip, unstageable `CC` `HCC` `SW`

L89.211 Pressure ulcer of right hip, stage 1 `CC`
Healing pressure ulcer of right hip back, stage 1
Pressure pre-ulcer skin changes limited to persistent focal edema, right hip

L89.212 Pressure ulcer of right hip, stage 2 `CC` `HCC`
Healing pressure ulcer of right hip, stage 2
Pressure ulcer with abrasion, blister, partial thickness skin loss involving epidermis and/or dermis, right hip

L89.213 Pressure ulcer of right hip, stage 3 `CC` `H4` `HCC` `SW`
Healing pressure ulcer of right hip, stage 3
Pressure ulcer with full thickness skin loss involving damage or necrosis of subcutaneous tissue, right hip

L89.214 Pressure ulcer of right hip, stage 4 `CC` `H4` `HCC` `SW`
Healing pressure ulcer of right hip, stage 4
Pressure ulcer with necrosis of soft tissues through to underlying muscle, tendon, or bone, right hip

● **L89.216 Pressure-induced deep tissue damage of right hip** `CC`

L89.219 Pressure ulcer of right hip, unspecified stage `CC`
Healing pressure ulcer of right hip NOS
Healing pressure ulcer of right hip, unspecified stage

√6th **L89.22 Pressure ulcer of left hip**

L89.220 Pressure ulcer of left hip, unstageable `CC` `HCC` `SW`

L89.221 Pressure ulcer of left hip, stage 1 `CC`
Healing pressure ulcer of left hip back, stage 1
Pressure pre-ulcer skin changes limited to persistent focal edema, left hip

L89.222 Pressure ulcer of left hip, stage 2 `CC` `HCC`
Healing pressure ulcer of left hip, stage 2
Pressure ulcer with abrasion, blister, partial thickness skin loss involving epidermis and/or dermis, left hip

L89.223 Pressure ulcer of left hip, stage 3 `CC` `H4` `HCC` `SW`
Healing pressure ulcer of left hip, stage 3
Pressure ulcer with full thickness skin loss involving damage or necrosis of subcutaneous tissue, left hip

L89.224 Pressure ulcer of left hip, stage 4 `CC` `H4` `HCC` `SW`
Healing pressure ulcer of left hip, stage 4
Pressure ulcer with necrosis of soft tissues through to underlying muscle, tendon, or bone, left hip

● **L89.226 Pressure-induced deep tissue damage of left hip** `CC`

L89.229 Pressure ulcer of left hip, unspecified stage `CC`
Healing pressure ulcer of left hip NOS
Healing pressure ulcer of left hip, unspecified stage

√5th **L89.3 Pressure ulcer of buttock**

√6th **L89.30 Pressure ulcer of unspecified buttock**

L89.300 Pressure ulcer of unspecified buttock, unstageable `CC` `HCC` `SW`

L89.301 Pressure ulcer of unspecified buttock, stage 1 `CC`
Healing pressure ulcer of unspecified buttock, stage 1
Pressure pre-ulcer skin changes limited to persistent focal edema, unspecified buttock

L89.302 Pressure ulcer of unspecified buttock, stage 2 `CC` `HCC`
Healing pressure ulcer of unspecified buttock, stage 2
Pressure ulcer with abrasion, blister, partial thickness skin loss involving epidermis and/or dermis, unspecified buttock

L89.303 Pressure ulcer of unspecified buttock, stage 3 `CC` `H4` `HCC` `SW`
Healing pressure ulcer of unspecified buttock, stage 3
Pressure ulcer with full thickness skin loss involving damage or necrosis of subcutaneous tissue, unspecified buttock

L89.304 Pressure ulcer of unspecified buttock, stage 4 `CC` `H4` `HCC` `SW`
Healing pressure ulcer of unspecified buttock, stage 4
Pressure ulcer with necrosis of soft tissues through to underlying muscle, tendon, or bone, unspecified buttock

● **L89.306 Pressure-induced deep tissue damage of unspecified buttock** `CC`

L89.309 Pressure ulcer of unspecified buttock, unspecified stage `CC`
Healing pressure ulcer of unspecified buttock NOS
Healing pressure ulcer of unspecified buttock, unspecified stage

√6th **L89.31 Pressure ulcer of right buttock**

L89.310 Pressure ulcer of right buttock, unstageable `CC` `HCC` `SW`

L89.311 Pressure ulcer of right buttock, stage 1 `CC`
Healing pressure ulcer of right buttock, stage 1
Pressure pre-ulcer skin changes limited to persistent focal edema, right buttock

L89.312 Pressure ulcer of right buttock, stage 2 `CC` `HCC`
Healing pressure ulcer of right buttock, stage 2
Pressure ulcer with abrasion, blister, partial thickness skin loss involving epidermis and/or dermis, right buttock

L89.313 Pressure ulcer of right buttock, stage 3 `CC` `H4` `HCC` `SW`
Healing pressure ulcer of right buttock, stage 3
Pressure ulcer with full thickness skin loss involving damage or necrosis of subcutaneous tissue, right buttock

L89.314 Pressure ulcer of right buttock, stage 4 `CC` `H4` `HCC` `SW`
    Healing pressure ulcer of right buttock, stage 4
    Pressure ulcer with necrosis of soft tissues through to underlying muscle, tendon, or bone, right buttock

● **L89.316 Pressure-induced deep tissue damage of right buttock** `CC`

L89.319 Pressure ulcer of right buttock, unspecified stage `CC`
    Healing pressure ulcer of right buttock NOS
    Healing pressure ulcer of right buttock, unspecified stage

✓6ᵗʰ **L89.32 Pressure ulcer of left buttock**

L89.320 Pressure ulcer of left buttock, unstageable `CC` `HCC` `SW`

L89.321 Pressure ulcer of left buttock, stage 1 `CC`
    Healing pressure ulcer of left buttock, stage 1
    Pressure pre-ulcer skin changes limited to persistent focal edema, left buttock

L89.322 Pressure ulcer of left buttock, stage 2 `CC` `HCC`
    Healing pressure ulcer of left buttock, stage 2
    Pressure ulcer with abrasion, blister, partial thickness skin loss involving epidermis and/or dermis, left buttock

L89.323 Pressure ulcer of left buttock, stage 3 `CC` `H4` `HCC` `SW`
    Healing pressure ulcer of left buttock, stage 3
    Pressure ulcer with full thickness skin loss involving damage or necrosis of subcutaneous tissue, left buttock

L89.324 Pressure ulcer of left buttock, stage 4 `CC` `H4` `HCC` `SW`
    Healing pressure ulcer of left buttock, stage 4
    Pressure ulcer with necrosis of soft tissues through to underlying muscle, tendon, or bone, left buttock

● **L89.326 Pressure-induced deep tissue damage of left buttock** `CC`

L89.329 Pressure ulcer of left buttock, unspecified stage `CC`
    Healing pressure ulcer of left buttock NOS
    Healing pressure ulcer of left buttock, unspecified stage

✓5ᵗʰ **L89.4 Pressure ulcer of contiguous site of back, buttock and hip**

L89.40 Pressure ulcer of contiguous site of back, buttock and hip, unspecified stage `CC`
    Healing pressure ulcer of contiguous site of back, buttock and hip NOS
    Healing pressure ulcer of contiguous site of back, buttock and hip, unspecified stage

L89.41 Pressure ulcer of contiguous site of back, buttock and hip, stage 1 `CC`
    Healing pressure ulcer of contiguous site of back, buttock and hip, stage 1
    Pressure pre-ulcer skin changes limited to persistent focal edema, contiguous site of back, buttock and hip

L89.42 Pressure ulcer of contiguous site of back, buttock and hip, stage 2 `CC` `HCC`
    Healing pressure ulcer of contiguous site of back, buttock and hip, stage 2
    Pressure ulcer with abrasion, blister, partial thickness skin loss involving epidermis and/or dermis, contiguous site of back, buttock and hip

L89.43 Pressure ulcer of contiguous site of back, buttock and hip, stage 3 `CC` `H4` `HCC` `SW`
    Healing pressure ulcer of contiguous site of back, buttock and hip, stage 3
    Pressure ulcer with full thickness skin loss involving damage or necrosis of subcutaneous tissue, contiguous site of back, buttock and hip

L89.44 Pressure ulcer of contiguous site of back, buttock and hip, stage 4 `CC` `H4` `HCC` `SW`
    Healing pressure ulcer of contiguous site of back, buttock and hip, stage 4
    Pressure ulcer with necrosis of soft tissues through to underlying muscle, tendon, or bone, contiguous site of back, buttock and hip

L89.45 Pressure ulcer of contiguous site of back, buttock and hip, unstageable `CC` `HCC` `SW`

● **L89.46 Pressure-induced deep tissue damage of contiguous site of back, buttock and hip** `CC`

✓5ᵗʰ **L89.5 Pressure ulcer of ankle**

✓6ᵗʰ **L89.50 Pressure ulcer of unspecified ankle**

L89.500 Pressure ulcer of unspecified ankle, unstageable `CC` `HCC` `SW`

L89.501 Pressure ulcer of unspecified ankle, stage 1 `CC`
    Healing pressure ulcer of unspecified ankle, stage 1
    Pressure pre-ulcer skin changes limited to persistent focal edema, unspecified ankle

L89.502 Pressure ulcer of unspecified ankle, stage 2 `CC` `HCC`
    Healing pressure ulcer of unspecified ankle, stage 2
    Pressure ulcer with abrasion, blister, partial thickness skin loss involving epidermis and/or dermis, unspecified ankle

L89.503 Pressure ulcer of unspecified ankle, stage 3 `CC` `H4` `HCC` `SW`
    Healing pressure ulcer of unspecified ankle, stage 3
    Pressure ulcer with full thickness skin loss involving damage or necrosis of subcutaneous tissue, unspecified ankle

L89.504 Pressure ulcer of unspecified ankle, stage 4 `CC` `H4` `HCC` `SW`
    Healing pressure ulcer of unspecified ankle, stage 4
    Pressure ulcer with necrosis of soft tissues through to underlying muscle, tendon, or bone, unspecified ankle

● **L89.506 Pressure-induced deep tissue damage of unspecified ankle** `CC`

L89.509 Pressure ulcer of unspecified ankle, unspecified stage `CC`
    Healing pressure ulcer of unspecified ankle NOS
    Healing pressure ulcer of unspecified ankle, unspecified stage

✓6ᵗʰ **L89.51 Pressure ulcer of right ankle**

L89.510 Pressure ulcer of right ankle, unstageable `CC` `HCC` `SW`

L89.511 Pressure ulcer of right ankle, stage 1 `CC`
    Healing pressure ulcer of right ankle, stage 1
    Pressure pre-ulcer skin changes limited to persistent focal edema, right ankle

L89.512 Pressure ulcer of right ankle, stage 2 `CC` `HCC`
: Healing pressure ulcer of right ankle, stage 2
: Pressure ulcer with abrasion, blister, partial thickness skin loss involving epidermis and/or dermis, right ankle

L89.513 Pressure ulcer of right ankle, stage 3 `CC` `H4` `HCC` `SW`
: Healing pressure ulcer of right ankle, stage 3
: Pressure ulcer with full thickness skin loss involving damage or necrosis of subcutaneous tissue, right ankle

L89.514 Pressure ulcer of right ankle, stage 4 `CC` `H4` `HCC` `SW`
: Healing pressure ulcer of right ankle, stage 4
: Pressure ulcer with necrosis of soft tissues through to underlying muscle, tendon, or bone, right ankle

L89.516 Pressure-induced deep tissue damage of right ankle `CC`

L89.519 Pressure ulcer of right ankle, unspecified stage `CC`
: Healing pressure ulcer of right ankle NOS
: Healing pressure ulcer of right ankle, unspecified stage

√6ᵗʰ **L89.52 Pressure ulcer of left ankle**

L89.520 Pressure ulcer of left ankle, unstageable `CC` `HCC` `SW`

L89.521 Pressure ulcer of left ankle, stage 1 `CC`
: Healing pressure ulcer of left ankle, stage 1
: Pressure pre-ulcer skin changes limited to persistent focal edema, left ankle

L89.522 Pressure ulcer of left ankle, stage 2 `CC` `HCC`
: Healing pressure ulcer of left ankle, stage 2
: Pressure ulcer with abrasion, blister, partial thickness skin loss involving epidermis and/or dermis, left ankle

L89.523 Pressure ulcer of left ankle, stage 3 `CC` `H4` `HCC` `SW`
: Healing pressure ulcer of left ankle, stage 3
: Pressure ulcer with full thickness skin loss involving damage or necrosis of subcutaneous tissue, left ankle

L89.524 Pressure ulcer of left ankle, stage 4 `CC` `H4` `HCC` `SW`
: Healing pressure ulcer of left ankle, stage 4
: Pressure ulcer with necrosis of soft tissues through to underlying muscle, tendon, or bone, left ankle

L89.526 Pressure-induced deep tissue damage of left ankle `CC`

L89.529 Pressure ulcer of left ankle, unspecified stage `CC`
: Healing pressure ulcer of left ankle NOS
: Healing pressure ulcer of left ankle, unspecified stage

√5ᵗʰ **L89.6 Pressure ulcer of heel**

√6ᵗʰ **L89.60 Pressure ulcer of unspecified heel**

L89.600 Pressure ulcer of unspecified heel, unstageable `CC` `HCC` `SW`

L89.601 Pressure ulcer of unspecified heel, stage 1 `CC`
: Healing pressure ulcer of unspecified heel, stage 1
: Pressure pre-ulcer skin changes limited to persistent focal edema, unspecified heel

L89.602 Pressure ulcer of unspecified heel, stage 2 `CC` `HCC`
: Healing pressure ulcer of unspecified heel, stage 2
: Pressure ulcer with abrasion, blister, partial thickness skin loss involving epidermis and/or dermis, unspecified heel

L89.603 Pressure ulcer of unspecified heel, stage 3 `CC` `H4` `HCC` `SW`
: Healing pressure ulcer of unspecified heel, stage 3
: Pressure ulcer with full thickness skin loss involving damage or necrosis of subcutaneous tissue, unspecified heel

L89.604 Pressure ulcer of unspecified heel, stage 4 `CC` `H4` `HCC` `SW`
: Healing pressure ulcer of unspecified heel, stage 4
: Pressure ulcer with necrosis of soft tissues through to underlying muscle, tendon, or bone, unspecified heel

L89.606 Pressure-induced deep tissue damage of unspecified heel `CC`

L89.609 Pressure ulcer of unspecified heel, unspecified stage `CC`
: Healing pressure ulcer of unspecified heel NOS
: Healing pressure ulcer of unspecified heel, unspecified stage

√6ᵗʰ **L89.61 Pressure ulcer of right heel**

L89.610 Pressure ulcer of right heel, unstageable `CC` `HCC` `SW`

L89.611 Pressure ulcer of right heel, stage 1 `CC`
: Healing pressure ulcer of right heel, stage 1
: Pressure pre-ulcer skin changes limited to persistent focal edema, right heel

L89.612 Pressure ulcer of right heel, stage 2 `CC` `HCC`
: Healing pressure ulcer of right heel, stage 2
: Pressure ulcer with abrasion, blister, partial thickness skin loss involving epidermis and/or dermis, right heel

L89.613 Pressure ulcer of right heel, stage 3 `CC` `H4` `HCC` `SW`
: Healing pressure ulcer of right heel, stage 3
: Pressure ulcer with full thickness skin loss involving damage or necrosis of subcutaneous tissue, right heel

L89.614 Pressure ulcer of right heel, stage 4 `CC` `H4` `HCC` `SW`
: Healing pressure ulcer of right heel, stage 4
: Pressure ulcer with necrosis of soft tissues through to underlying muscle, tendon, or bone, right heel

L89.616 Pressure-induced deep tissue damage of right heel `CC`

L89.619 Pressure ulcer of right heel, unspecified stage `CC`
: Healing pressure ulcer of right heel NOS
: Healing pressure ulcer of right heel, unspecified stage

√6ᵗʰ **L89.62 Pressure ulcer of left heel**

L89.620 Pressure ulcer of left heel, unstageable `CC` `HCC` `SW`

L89.621 Pressure ulcer of left heel, stage 1 `CC`
: Healing pressure ulcer of left heel, stage 1
: Pressure pre-ulcer skin changes limited to persistent focal edema, left heel

L89.622   **Pressure ulcer of left heel,** `CC` `HCC`
stage 2
> Healing pressure ulcer of left heel, stage 2
> Pressure ulcer with abrasion, blister, partial thickness skin loss involving epidermis and/or dermis, left heel

L89.623   **Pressure ulcer of left heel,** `CC` `H4` `HCC` `SW`
stage 3
> Healing pressure ulcer of left heel, stage 3
> Pressure ulcer with full thickness skin loss involving damage or necrosis of subcutaneous tissue, left heel

L89.624   **Pressure ulcer of left heel,** `CC` `H4` `HCC` `SW`
stage 4
> Healing pressure ulcer of left heel, stage 4
> Pressure ulcer with necrosis of soft tissues through to underlying muscle, tendon, or bone, left heel

●   **L89.626**   **Pressure-induced deep** `CC`
tissue damage of left heel

L89.629   **Pressure ulcer of left heel,** `CC`
unspecified stage
> Healing pressure ulcer of left heel NOS
> Healing pressure ulcer of left heel, unspecified stage

√5ᵗʰ **L89.8**   **Pressure ulcer of other site**

√6ᵗʰ   **L89.81**   **Pressure ulcer of head**
> Pressure ulcer of face

L89.810   **Pressure ulcer of head,** `CC` `HCC` `SW`
unstageable

L89.811   **Pressure ulcer of head,** `CC`
stage 1
> Healing pressure ulcer of head, stage 1
> Pressure pre-ulcer skin changes limited to persistent focal edema, head

L89.812   **Pressure ulcer of head,** `CC` `HCC`
stage 2
> Healing pressure ulcer of head, stage 2
> Pressure ulcer with abrasion, blister, partial thickness skin loss involving epidermis and/or dermis, head

L89.813   **Pressure ulcer of head,** `CC` `H4` `HCC` `SW`
stage 3
> Healing pressure ulcer of head, stage 3
> Pressure ulcer with full thickness skin loss involving damage or necrosis of subcutaneous tissue, head

L89.814   **Pressure ulcer of head,** `CC` `H4` `HCC` `SW`
stage 4
> Healing pressure ulcer of head, stage 4
> Pressure ulcer with necrosis of soft tissues through to underlying muscle, tendon, or bone, head

●   **L89.816**   **Pressure-induced deep** `CC`
tissue damage of head

L89.819   **Pressure ulcer of head,** `CC`
unspecified stage
> Healing pressure ulcer of head NOS
> Healing pressure ulcer of head, unspecified stage

√6ᵗʰ   **L89.89**   **Pressure ulcer of other site**

L89.890   **Pressure ulcer of other** `CC` `HCC` `SW`
site, unstageable

L89.891   **Pressure ulcer of other** `CC`
site, stage 1
> Healing pressure ulcer of other site, stage 1
> Pressure pre-ulcer skin changes limited to persistent focal edema, other site

L89.892   **Pressure ulcer of other** `CC` `HCC`
site, stage 2
> Healing pressure ulcer of other site, stage 2
> Pressure ulcer with abrasion, blister, partial thickness skin loss involving epidermis and/or dermis, other site

L89.893   **Pressure ulcer of other** `CC` `H4` `HCC` `SW`
site, stage 3
> Healing pressure ulcer of other site, stage 3
> Pressure ulcer with full thickness skin loss involving damage or necrosis of subcutaneous tissue, other site

L89.894   **Pressure ulcer of other** `CC` `H4` `HCC` `SW`
site, stage 4
> Healing pressure ulcer of other site, stage 4
> Pressure ulcer with necrosis of soft tissues through to underlying muscle, tendon, or bone, other site

●   **L89.896**   **Pressure-induced deep** `CC`
tissue damage of other
site

L89.899   **Pressure ulcer of other** `CC`
site, unspecified stage
> Healing pressure ulcer of other site NOS
> Healing pressure ulcer of other site, unspecified stage

√5ᵗʰ **L89.9**   **Pressure ulcer of unspecified site**

L89.90   **Pressure ulcer of unspecified site,** `CC`
unspecified stage
> Healing pressure ulcer of unspecified site NOS
> Healing pressure ulcer of unspecified site, unspecified stage

L89.91   **Pressure ulcer of unspecified site,** `CC`
stage 1
> Healing pressure ulcer of unspecified site, stage 1
> Pressure pre-ulcer skin changes limited to persistent focal edema, unspecified site

L89.92   **Pressure ulcer of unspecified site,** `CC` `HCC`
stage 2
> Healing pressure ulcer of unspecified site, stage 2
> Pressure ulcer with abrasion, blister, partial thickness skin loss involving epidermis and/or dermis, unspecified site

L89.93   **Pressure ulcer of unspecified site,** `CC` `H4` `HCC` `SW`
stage 3
> Healing pressure ulcer of unspecified site, stage 3
> Pressure ulcer with full thickness skin loss involving damage or necrosis of subcutaneous tissue, unspecified site

L89.94   **Pressure ulcer of unspecified site,** `CC` `H4` `HCC` `SW`
stage 4
> Healing pressure ulcer of unspecified site, stage 4
> Pressure ulcer with necrosis of soft tissues through to underlying muscle, tendon, or bone, unspecified site

L89.95   **Pressure ulcer of unspecified site,** `CC` `HCC` `SW`
unstageable

●   **L89.96**   **Pressure-induced deep tissue** `CC`
damage of unspecified site

√4ᵗʰ **L90**   **Atrophic disorders of skin**

L90.0   **Lichen sclerosus et atrophicus**
> *EXCLUDES 2*   *lichen sclerosus of external female genital organs (N90.4)*
> *lichen sclerosus of external male genital organs (N48.0)*

L90.1   **Anetoderma of Schweninger-Buzzi**

L90.2   **Anetoderma of Jadassohn-Pellizzari**

L90.3   **Atrophoderma of Pasini and Pierini**

L90.4   **Acrodermatitis chronica atrophicans**

L90.5   **Scar conditions and fibrosis of skin**
> Adherent scar (skin)
> Cicatrix
> Disfigurement of skin due to scar
> Fibrosis of skin NOS
> Scar NOS
> *EXCLUDES 2*   *hypertrophic scar (L91.0)*
> *keloid scar (L91.0)*
> **AHA:** 2016,2Q,5; 2015,1Q,19

L90.6   **Striae atrophicae**

L90.8   **Other atrophic disorders of skin**

L90.9   **Atrophic disorder of skin, unspecified**

Ⓝ Newborn: 0   Ⓟ Pediatric: 0-17   Ⓜ Maternity: 9-64   Ⓐ Adult: 15-124   `MCC` Major Complication/Comorbidity   `CC` Complication/Comorbidity   `SW` Severe Wound Dx

752   **ICD-10-CM 2020**

✓4ᵗʰ **L91 Hypertrophic disorders of skin**

L91.0 Hypertrophic scar
Keloid
Keloid scar
EXCLUDES 2   acne keloid (L73.0)
scar NOS (L90.5)
DEF: Overgrowth of scar tissue due to excess amounts of collagen during connective tissue repair, occurring mainly on the upper trunk and face.

L91.8 Other hypertrophic disorders of the skin

L91.9 Hypertrophic disorder of the skin, unspecified

✓4ᵗʰ **L92 Granulomatous disorders of skin and subcutaneous tissue**
EXCLUDES 2   actinic granuloma (L57.5)

L92.0 Granuloma annulare
Perforating granuloma annulare

L92.1 Necrobiosis lipoidica, not elsewhere classified
EXCLUDES 1   necrobiosis lipoidica associated with diabetes mellitus (E08-E13 with .620)

L92.2 Granuloma faciale [eosinophilic granuloma of skin]

L92.3 Foreign body granuloma of the skin and subcutaneous tissue
Use additional code to identify the type of retained foreign body (Z18.-)

L92.8 Other granulomatous disorders of the skin and subcutaneous tissue

L92.9 Granulomatous disorder of the skin and subcutaneous tissue, unspecified
EXCLUDES 2   umbilical granuloma (P83.81)
AHA: 2017,4Q,21-22

✓4ᵗʰ **L93 Lupus erythematosus**
Use additional code for adverse effect, if applicable, to identify drug (T36-T50 with fifth or sixth character 5)
EXCLUDES 1   lupus exedens (A18.4)
lupus vulgaris (A18.4)
scleroderma (M34.-)
systemic lupus erythematosus (M32.-)
DEF: Inflammatory, autoimmune skin condition in which the body's autoimmune system attacks healthy tissue of the integumentary system.

L93.0 Discoid lupus erythematosus
Lupus erythematosus NOS

L93.1 Subacute cutaneous lupus erythematosus

L93.2 Other local lupus erythematosus
Lupus erythematosus profundus
Lupus panniculitis

✓4ᵗʰ **L94 Other localized connective tissue disorders**
EXCLUDES 1   systemic connective tissue disorders (M30-M36)

L94.0 Localized scleroderma [morphea]
Circumscribed scleroderma

L94.1 Linear scleroderma
En coup de sabre lesion

L94.2 Calcinosis cutis

L94.3 Sclerodactyly

L94.4 Gottron's papules

L94.5 Poikiloderma vasculare atrophicans

L94.6 Ainhum

L94.8 Other specified localized connective tissue disorders

L94.9 Localized connective tissue disorder, unspecified

✓4ᵗʰ **L95 Vasculitis limited to skin, not elsewhere classified**
EXCLUDES 1   angioma serpiginosum (L81.7)
Henoch(-Schönlein) purpura (D69.0)
hypersensitivity angiitis (M31.0)
lupus panniculitis (L93.2)
panniculitis NOS (M79.3)
panniculitis of neck and back (M54.0-)
polyarteritis nodosa (M30.0)
relapsing panniculitis (M35.6)
rheumatoid vasculitis (M05.2)
serum sickness (T80.6-)
urticaria (L50.-)
Wegener's granulomatosis (M31.3-)

L95.0 Livedoid vasculitis
Atrophie blanche (en plaque)

L95.1 Erythema elevatum diutinum

L95.8 Other vasculitis limited to the skin

L95.9 Vasculitis limited to the skin, unspecified

✓4ᵗʰ **L97 Non-pressure chronic ulcer of lower limb, not elsewhere classified**
INCLUDES   chronic ulcer of skin of lower limb NOS
non-healing ulcer of skin
non-infected sinus of skin
trophic ulcer NOS
tropical ulcer NOS
ulcer of skin of lower limb NOS
Code first any associated underlying condition, such as:
any associated gangrene (I96)
atherosclerosis of the lower extremities (I70.23-, I70.24-, I70.33-, I70.34-, I70.43-, I70.44-, I70.53-, I70.54-, I70.63-, I70.64-, I70.73-, I70.74-)
chronic venous hypertension (I87.31-, I87.33-)
diabetic ulcers (E08.621, E08.622, E09.621, E09.622, E10.621, E10.622, E11.621, E11.622, E13.621, E13.622)
postphlebitic syndrome (I87.01-, I87.03-)
postthrombotic syndrome (I87.01-, I87.03-)
varicose ulcer (I83.0-, I83.2-)
EXCLUDES 2   pressure ulcer (pressure area) (L89.-)
skin infections (L00-L08)
specific infections classified to A00-B99
AHA: 2018,4Q,69; 2017,4Q,17
TIP: The depth and/or severity of a diagnosed nonpressure ulcer can be determined based on medical record documentation from clinicians who are not the patient's provider.
TIP: Assign a code from this category/subcategory for nonpressure ulcers documented as acute.
CC Excl: For CC codes in category L97: PDX collection 698

✓5ᵗʰ **L97.1 Non-pressure chronic ulcer of thigh**

✓6ᵗʰ **L97.10 Non-pressure chronic ulcer of unspecified thigh**

L97.101 Non-pressure chronic ulcer of unspecified thigh limited to breakdown of skin   CC HCC

L97.102 Non-pressure chronic ulcer of unspecified thigh with fat layer exposed   CC HCC SW

L97.103 Non-pressure chronic ulcer of unspecified thigh with necrosis of muscle   CC HCC SW

L97.104 Non-pressure chronic ulcer of unspecified thigh with necrosis of bone   CC HCC SW

L97.105 Non-pressure chronic ulcer of unspecified thigh with muscle involvement without evidence of necrosis   CC HCC

L97.106 Non-pressure chronic ulcer of unspecified thigh with bone involvement without evidence of necrosis   CC HCC

L97.108 Non-pressure chronic ulcer of unspecified thigh with other specified severity   CC HCC

L97.109 Non-pressure chronic ulcer of unspecified thigh with unspecified severity   CC HCC

✓6ᵗʰ **L97.11 Non-pressure chronic ulcer of right thigh**

L97.111 Non-pressure chronic ulcer of right thigh limited to breakdown of skin   CC HCC

L97.112 Non-pressure chronic ulcer of right thigh with fat layer exposed   CC HCC SW

L97.113 Non-pressure chronic ulcer of right thigh with necrosis of muscle   CC HCC SW

L97.114 Non-pressure chronic ulcer of right thigh with necrosis of bone   CC HCC SW

L97.115 Non-pressure chronic ulcer of right thigh with muscle involvement without evidence of necrosis   CC HCC

L97.116 Non-pressure chronic ulcer of right thigh with bone involvement without evidence of necrosis   CC HCC

L97.118 Non-pressure chronic ulcer of right thigh with other specified severity   CC HCC

L97.119 Non-pressure chronic ulcer of right thigh with unspecified severity   `CC` `HCC`

√6th **L97.12** Non-pressure chronic ulcer of left thigh

L97.121 Non-pressure chronic ulcer of left thigh limited to breakdown of skin   `CC` `HCC`

L97.122 Non-pressure chronic ulcer of left thigh with fat layer exposed   `CC` `HCC` `SW`

L97.123 Non-pressure chronic ulcer of left thigh with necrosis of muscle   `CC` `HCC` `SW`

L97.124 Non-pressure chronic ulcer of left thigh with necrosis of bone   `CC` `HCC` `SW`

L97.125 Non-pressure chronic ulcer of left thigh with muscle involvement without evidence of necrosis   `CC` `HCC`

L97.126 Non-pressure chronic ulcer of left thigh with bone involvement without evidence of necrosis   `CC` `HCC`

L97.128 Non-pressure chronic ulcer of left thigh with other specified severity   `CC` `HCC`

L97.129 Non-pressure chronic ulcer of left thigh with unspecified severity   `CC` `HCC`

√5th **L97.2** Non-pressure chronic ulcer of calf

√6th **L97.20** Non-pressure chronic ulcer of unspecified calf

L97.201 Non-pressure chronic ulcer of unspecified calf limited to breakdown of skin   `CC` `HCC`

L97.202 Non-pressure chronic ulcer of unspecified calf with fat layer exposed   `CC` `HCC` `SW`

L97.203 Non-pressure chronic ulcer of unspecified calf with necrosis of muscle   `CC` `HCC` `SW`

L97.204 Non-pressure chronic ulcer of unspecified calf with necrosis of bone   `CC` `HCC` `SW`

L97.205 Non-pressure chronic ulcer of unspecified calf with muscle involvement without evidence of necrosis   `CC` `HCC`

L97.206 Non-pressure chronic ulcer of unspecified calf with bone involvement without evidence of necrosis   `CC` `HCC`

L97.208 Non-pressure chronic ulcer of unspecified calf with other specified severity   `CC` `HCC`

L97.209 Non-pressure chronic ulcer of unspecified calf with unspecified severity   `CC` `HCC`

√6th **L97.21** Non-pressure chronic ulcer of right calf

L97.211 Non-pressure chronic ulcer of right calf limited to breakdown of skin   `CC` `HCC`

L97.212 Non-pressure chronic ulcer of right calf with fat layer exposed   `CC` `HCC` `SW`

L97.213 Non-pressure chronic ulcer of right calf with necrosis of muscle   `CC` `HCC` `SW`

L97.214 Non-pressure chronic ulcer of right calf with necrosis of bone   `CC` `HCC` `SW`

L97.215 Non-pressure chronic ulcer of right calf with muscle involvement without evidence of necrosis   `CC` `HCC`

L97.216 Non-pressure chronic ulcer of right calf with bone involvement without evidence of necrosis   `CC` `HCC`

L97.218 Non-pressure chronic ulcer of right calf with other specified severity   `CC` `HCC`

L97.219 Non-pressure chronic ulcer of right calf with unspecified severity   `CC` `HCC`

√6th **L97.22** Non-pressure chronic ulcer of left calf

L97.221 Non-pressure chronic ulcer of left calf limited to breakdown of skin   `CC` `HCC`

L97.222 Non-pressure chronic ulcer of left calf with fat layer exposed   `CC` `HCC` `SW`

L97.223 Non-pressure chronic ulcer of left calf with necrosis of muscle   `CC` `HCC` `SW`

L97.224 Non-pressure chronic ulcer of left calf with necrosis of bone   `CC` `HCC` `SW`

L97.225 Non-pressure chronic ulcer of left calf with muscle involvement without evidence of necrosis   `CC` `HCC`

L97.226 Non-pressure chronic ulcer of left calf with bone involvement without evidence of necrosis   `CC` `HCC`

L97.228 Non-pressure chronic ulcer of left calf with other specified severity   `CC` `HCC`

L97.229 Non-pressure chronic ulcer of left calf with unspecified severity   `CC` `HCC`

√5th **L97.3** Non-pressure chronic ulcer of ankle

√6th **L97.30** Non-pressure chronic ulcer of unspecified ankle

L97.301 Non-pressure chronic ulcer of unspecified ankle limited to breakdown of skin   `CC` `HCC`

L97.302 Non-pressure chronic ulcer of unspecified ankle with fat layer exposed   `CC` `HCC` `SW`

L97.303 Non-pressure chronic ulcer of unspecified ankle with necrosis of muscle   `CC` `HCC` `SW`

L97.304 Non-pressure chronic ulcer of unspecified ankle with necrosis of bone   `CC` `HCC` `SW`

L97.305 Non-pressure chronic ulcer of unspecified ankle with muscle involvement without evidence of necrosis   `CC` `HCC`

L97.306 Non-pressure chronic ulcer of unspecified ankle with bone involvement without evidence of necrosis   `CC` `HCC`

L97.308 Non-pressure chronic ulcer of unspecified ankle with other specified severity   `CC` `HCC`

L97.309 Non-pressure chronic ulcer of unspecified ankle with unspecified severity   `CC` `HCC`

√6th **L97.31** Non-pressure chronic ulcer of right ankle

L97.311 Non-pressure chronic ulcer of right ankle limited to breakdown of skin   `CC` `HCC`

L97.312 Non-pressure chronic ulcer of right ankle with fat layer exposed   `CC` `HCC` `SW`

L97.313 Non-pressure chronic ulcer of right ankle with necrosis of muscle   `CC` `HCC` `SW`

L97.314 Non-pressure chronic ulcer of right ankle with necrosis of bone   `CC` `HCC` `SW`

L97.315 Non-pressure chronic ulcer of right ankle with muscle involvement without evidence of necrosis   `CC` `HCC`

L97.316 Non-pressure chronic ulcer of right ankle with bone involvement without evidence of necrosis   `CC` `HCC`

L97.318 Non-pressure chronic ulcer of right ankle with other specified severity   `CC` `HCC`

N Newborn: 0   P Pediatric: 0-17   M Maternity: 9-64   A Adult: 15-124   MCC Major Complication/Comorbidity   CC Complication/Comorbidity   SW Severe Wound Dx

754   ICD-10-CM 2020

L97.319 Non-pressure chronic ulcer of right ankle with unspecified severity `CC` `HCC`

✓6ᵗʰ **L97.32 Non-pressure chronic ulcer of left ankle**

L97.321 Non-pressure chronic ulcer of left ankle limited to breakdown of skin `CC` `HCC`

L97.322 Non-pressure chronic ulcer of left ankle with fat layer exposed `CC` `HCC` `SW`

L97.323 Non-pressure chronic ulcer of left ankle with necrosis of muscle `CC` `HCC` `SW`

L97.324 Non-pressure chronic ulcer of left ankle with necrosis of bone `CC` `HCC` `SW`

L97.325 Non-pressure chronic ulcer of left ankle with muscle involvement without evidence of necrosis `CC` `HCC`

L97.326 Non-pressure chronic ulcer of left ankle with bone involvement without evidence of necrosis `CC` `HCC`

L97.328 Non-pressure chronic ulcer of left ankle with other specified severity `CC` `HCC`

L97.329 Non-pressure chronic ulcer of left ankle with unspecified severity `CC` `HCC`

✓5ᵗʰ **L97.4 Non-pressure chronic ulcer of heel and midfoot**

Non-pressure chronic ulcer of plantar surface of midfoot

✓6ᵗʰ **L97.40 Non-pressure chronic ulcer of unspecified heel and midfoot**

L97.401 Non-pressure chronic ulcer of unspecified heel and midfoot limited to breakdown of skin `CC` `HCC`

L97.402 Non-pressure chronic ulcer of unspecified heel and midfoot with fat layer exposed `CC` `HCC` `SW`

L97.403 Non-pressure chronic ulcer of unspecified heel and midfoot with necrosis of muscle `CC` `HCC` `SW`

L97.404 Non-pressure chronic ulcer of unspecified heel and midfoot with necrosis of bone `CC` `HCC` `SW`

L97.405 Non-pressure chronic ulcer of unspecified heel and midfoot with muscle involvement without evidence of necrosis `CC` `HCC`

L97.406 Non-pressure chronic ulcer of unspecified heel and midfoot with bone involvement without evidence of necrosis `CC` `HCC`

L97.408 Non-pressure chronic ulcer of unspecified heel and midfoot with other specified severity `CC` `HCC`

L97.409 Non-pressure chronic ulcer of unspecified heel and midfoot with unspecified severity `CC` `HCC`

✓6ᵗʰ **L97.41 Non-pressure chronic ulcer of right heel and midfoot**

L97.411 Non-pressure chronic ulcer of right heel and midfoot limited to breakdown of skin `CC` `HCC`

L97.412 Non-pressure chronic ulcer of right heel and midfoot with fat layer exposed `CC` `HCC` `SW`

L97.413 Non-pressure chronic ulcer of right heel and midfoot with necrosis of muscle `CC` `HCC` `SW`

L97.414 Non-pressure chronic ulcer of right heel and midfoot with necrosis of bone `CC` `HCC` `SW`

L97.415 Non-pressure chronic ulcer of right heel and midfoot with muscle involvement without evidence of necrosis `CC` `HCC`

L97.416 Non-pressure chronic ulcer of right heel and midfoot with bone involvement without evidence of necrosis `CC` `HCC`

L97.418 Non-pressure chronic ulcer of right heel and midfoot with other specified severity `CC` `HCC`

L97.419 Non-pressure chronic ulcer of right heel and midfoot with unspecified severity `CC` `HCC`

✓6ᵗʰ **L97.42 Non-pressure chronic ulcer of left heel and midfoot**

L97.421 Non-pressure chronic ulcer of left heel and midfoot limited to breakdown of skin `CC` `HCC`

AHA: 2016,1Q,12

L97.422 Non-pressure chronic ulcer of left heel and midfoot with fat layer exposed `CC` `HCC` `SW`

L97.423 Non-pressure chronic ulcer of left heel and midfoot with necrosis of muscle `CC` `HCC` `SW`

L97.424 Non-pressure chronic ulcer of left heel and midfoot with necrosis of bone `CC` `HCC` `SW`

L97.425 Non-pressure chronic ulcer of left heel and midfoot with muscle involvement without evidence of necrosis `CC` `HCC`

L97.426 Non-pressure chronic ulcer of left heel and midfoot with bone involvement without evidence of necrosis `CC` `HCC`

L97.428 Non-pressure chronic ulcer of left heel and midfoot with other specified severity `CC` `HCC`

L97.429 Non-pressure chronic ulcer of left heel and midfoot with unspecified severity `CC` `HCC`

✓5ᵗʰ **L97.5 Non-pressure chronic ulcer of other part of foot**

Non-pressure chronic ulcer of toe

✓6ᵗʰ **L97.50 Non-pressure chronic ulcer of other part of unspecified foot**

L97.501 Non-pressure chronic ulcer of other part of unspecified foot limited to breakdown of skin `HCC`

L97.502 Non-pressure chronic ulcer of other part of unspecified foot with fat layer exposed `HCC` `SW`

L97.503 Non-pressure chronic ulcer of other part of unspecified foot with necrosis of muscle `HCC` `SW`

L97.504 Non-pressure chronic ulcer of other part of unspecified foot with necrosis of bone `HCC` `SW`

L97.505 Non-pressure chronic ulcer of other part of unspecified foot with muscle involvement without evidence of necrosis `CC` `HCC`

L97.506 Non-pressure chronic ulcer of other part of unspecified foot with bone involvement without evidence of necrosis `CC` `HCC`

L97.508 Non-pressure chronic ulcer of other part of unspecified foot with other specified severity `CC` `HCC`

L97.509 Non-pressure chronic ulcer of other part of unspecified foot with unspecified severity `HCC`

√6ᵗʰ L97.51 Non-pressure chronic ulcer of other part of right foot

L97.511 Non-pressure chronic ulcer of other part of right foot limited to breakdown of skin `HCC`

L97.512 Non-pressure chronic ulcer of other part of right foot with fat layer exposed `HCC` `SW`

L97.513 Non-pressure chronic ulcer of other part of right foot with necrosis of muscle `HCC` `SW`

L97.514 Non-pressure chronic ulcer of other part of right foot with necrosis of bone `HCC` `SW`

L97.515 Non-pressure chronic ulcer of other part of right foot with muscle involvement without evidence of necrosis `CC` `HCC`

L97.516 Non-pressure chronic ulcer of other part of right foot with bone involvement without evidence of necrosis `CC` `HCC`

L97.518 Non-pressure chronic ulcer of other part of right foot with other specified severity `CC` `HCC`

L97.519 Non-pressure chronic ulcer of other part of right foot with unspecified severity `HCC`

√6ᵗʰ L97.52 Non-pressure chronic ulcer of other part of left foot

L97.521 Non-pressure chronic ulcer of other part of left foot limited to breakdown of skin `HCC`

L97.522 Non-pressure chronic ulcer of other part of left foot with fat layer exposed `HCC` `SW`

L97.523 Non-pressure chronic ulcer of other part of left foot with necrosis of muscle `HCC` `SW`

L97.524 Non-pressure chronic ulcer of other part of left foot with necrosis of bone `HCC` `SW`

L97.525 Non-pressure chronic ulcer of other part of left foot with muscle involvement without evidence of necrosis `CC` `HCC`

L97.526 Non-pressure chronic ulcer of other part of left foot with bone involvement without evidence of necrosis `CC` `HCC`

L97.528 Non-pressure chronic ulcer of other part of left foot with other specified severity `CC` `HCC`

L97.529 Non-pressure chronic ulcer of other part of left foot with unspecified severity `HCC`

√6ᵗʰ L97.8 Non-pressure chronic ulcer of other part of lower leg

√6ᵗʰ L97.80 Non-pressure chronic ulcer of other part of unspecified lower leg

L97.801 Non-pressure chronic ulcer of other part of unspecified lower leg limited to breakdown of skin `CC` `HCC`

L97.802 Non-pressure chronic ulcer of other part of unspecified lower leg with fat layer exposed `CC` `HCC` `SW`

L97.803 Non-pressure chronic ulcer of other part of unspecified lower leg with necrosis of muscle `CC` `HCC` `SW`

L97.804 Non-pressure chronic ulcer of other part of unspecified lower leg with necrosis of bone `CC` `HCC` `SW`

L97.805 Non-pressure chronic ulcer of other part of unspecified lower leg with muscle involvement without evidence of necrosis `CC` `HCC`

L97.806 Non-pressure chronic ulcer of other part of unspecified lower leg with bone involvement without evidence of necrosis `CC` `HCC`

L97.808 Non-pressure chronic ulcer of other part of unspecified lower leg with other specified severity `CC` `HCC`

L97.809 Non-pressure chronic ulcer of other part of unspecified lower leg with unspecified severity `CC` `HCC`

√6ᵗʰ L97.81 Non-pressure chronic ulcer of other part of right lower leg

L97.811 Non-pressure chronic ulcer of other part of right lower leg limited to breakdown of skin `CC` `HCC`

L97.812 Non-pressure chronic ulcer of other part of right lower leg with fat layer exposed `CC` `HCC` `SW`

L97.813 Non-pressure chronic ulcer of other part of right lower leg with necrosis of muscle `CC` `HCC` `SW`

L97.814 Non-pressure chronic ulcer of other part of right lower leg with necrosis of bone `CC` `HCC` `SW`

L97.815 Non-pressure chronic ulcer of other part of right lower leg with muscle involvement without evidence of necrosis `CC` `HCC`

L97.816 Non-pressure chronic ulcer of other part of right lower leg with bone involvement without evidence of necrosis `CC` `HCC`

L97.818 Non-pressure chronic ulcer of other part of right lower leg with other specified severity `CC` `HCC`

L97.819 Non-pressure chronic ulcer of other part of right lower leg with unspecified severity `CC` `HCC`

√6ᵗʰ L97.82 Non-pressure chronic ulcer of other part of left lower leg

L97.821 Non-pressure chronic ulcer of other part of left lower leg limited to breakdown of skin `CC` `HCC`

L97.822 Non-pressure chronic ulcer of other part of left lower leg with fat layer exposed `CC` `HCC` `SW`

L97.823 Non-pressure chronic ulcer of other part of left lower leg with necrosis of muscle `CC` `HCC` `SW`

L97.824 Non-pressure chronic ulcer of other part of left lower leg with necrosis of bone `CC` `HCC` `SW`

L97.825 Non-pressure chronic ulcer of other part of left lower leg with muscle involvement without evidence of necrosis `CC` `HCC`

L97.826 Non-pressure chronic ulcer of other part of left lower leg with bone involvement without evidence of necrosis `CC` `HCC`

L97.828 Non-pressure chronic ulcer of other part of left lower leg with other specified severity `CC` `HCC`

N Newborn: 0   **P** Pediatric: 0-17   **M** Maternity: 9-64   **A** Adult: 15-124   **MCC** Major Complication/Comorbidity   **CC** Complication/Comorbidity   **SW** Severe Wound Dx

756

ICD-10-CM 2020

        L97.829 Non-pressure chronic ulcer of other part of left lower leg with unspecified severity   `CC` `HCC`

√5th **L97.9** Non-pressure chronic ulcer of unspecified part of lower leg

  √6th **L97.90** Non-pressure chronic ulcer of unspecified part of unspecified lower leg

        L97.901 Non-pressure chronic ulcer of unspecified part of unspecified lower leg limited to breakdown of skin   `CC` `HCC`

        L97.902 Non-pressure chronic ulcer of unspecified part of unspecified lower leg with fat layer exposed   `CC` `HCC` `SW`

        L97.903 Non-pressure chronic ulcer of unspecified part of unspecified lower leg with necrosis of muscle   `CC` `HCC` `SW`

        L97.904 Non-pressure chronic ulcer of unspecified part of unspecified lower leg with necrosis of bone   `CC` `HCC` `SW`

        L97.905 Non-pressure chronic ulcer of unspecified part of unspecified lower leg with muscle involvement without evidence of necrosis   `CC` `HCC`

        L97.906 Non-pressure chronic ulcer of unspecified part of unspecified lower leg with bone involvement without evidence of necrosis   `CC` `HCC`

        L97.908 Non-pressure chronic ulcer of unspecified part of unspecified lower leg with other specified severity   `CC` `HCC`

        L97.909 Non-pressure chronic ulcer of unspecified part of unspecified lower leg with unspecified severity   `CC` `HCC`

  √6th **L97.91** Non-pressure chronic ulcer of unspecified part of right lower leg

        L97.911 Non-pressure chronic ulcer of unspecified part of right lower leg limited to breakdown of skin   `CC` `HCC`

        L97.912 Non-pressure chronic ulcer of unspecified part of right lower leg with fat layer exposed   `CC` `HCC` `SW`

        L97.913 Non-pressure chronic ulcer of unspecified part of right lower leg with necrosis of muscle   `CC` `HCC` `SW`

        L97.914 Non-pressure chronic ulcer of unspecified part of right lower leg with necrosis of bone   `CC` `HCC` `SW`

        L97.915 Non-pressure chronic ulcer of unspecified part of right lower leg with muscle involvement without evidence of necrosis   `CC` `HCC`

        L97.916 Non-pressure chronic ulcer of unspecified part of right lower leg with bone involvement without evidence of necrosis   `CC` `HCC`

        L97.918 Non-pressure chronic ulcer of unspecified part of right lower leg with other specified severity   `CC` `HCC`

        L97.919 Non-pressure chronic ulcer of unspecified part of right lower leg with unspecified severity   `CC` `HCC`

  √6th **L97.92** Non-pressure chronic ulcer of unspecified part of left lower leg

        L97.921 Non-pressure chronic ulcer of unspecified part of left lower leg limited to breakdown of skin   `CC` `HCC` `SW`

        L97.922 Non-pressure chronic ulcer of unspecified part of left lower leg with fat layer exposed   `CC` `HCC` `SW`

        L97.923 Non-pressure chronic ulcer of unspecified part of left lower leg with necrosis of muscle   `CC` `HCC` `SW`

        L97.924 Non-pressure chronic ulcer of unspecified part of left lower leg with necrosis of bone   `CC` `HCC` `SW`

        L97.925 Non-pressure chronic ulcer of unspecified part of left lower leg with muscle involvement without evidence of necrosis   `CC` `HCC`

        L97.926 Non-pressure chronic ulcer of unspecified part of left lower leg with bone involvement without evidence of necrosis   `CC` `HCC`

        L97.928 Non-pressure chronic ulcer of unspecified part of left lower leg with other specified severity   `CC` `HCC`

        L97.929 Non-pressure chronic ulcer of unspecified part of left lower leg with unspecified severity   `CC` `HCC`

√4th **L98** Other disorders of skin and subcutaneous tissue, not elsewhere classified

  L98.0 Pyogenic granuloma

    EXCLUDES 2   pyogenic granuloma of gingiva (K06.8)

         pyogenic granuloma of maxillary alveolar ridge (K04.5)

         pyogenic granuloma of oral mucosa (K13.4)

    DEF: Solitary polypoid capillary hemangioma often associated with local irritation, trauma, and superimposed inflammation. Located on the skin and gingival or oral mucosa, they bleed easily and may ulcerate and form crusted sores.

  L98.1 Factitial dermatitis

    Neurotic excoriation

    EXCLUDES 1   excoriation (skin-picking) disorder (F42.4)

    AHA: 2016,4Q,15

    DEF: Self-inflicted skin lesions to satisfy an unconscious psychological or emotional need. Methods used to injure the skin include deep excoriations with a sharp instrument, scarification with a knife, or the application of caustic chemicals and burning, sometimes with a cigarette.

  L98.2 Febrile neutrophilic dermatosis [Sweet]

  L98.3 Eosinophilic cellulitis [Wells]   `CC`

    CC Excl: PDX collection 839

√5th **L98.4** Non-pressure chronic ulcer of skin, not elsewhere classified

    Chronic ulcer of skin NOS

    Tropical ulcer NOS

    Ulcer of skin NOS

    EXCLUDES 2   gangrene (I96)

         pressure ulcer (pressure area) (L89.-)

         skin infections (L00-L08)

         specific infections classified to A00-B99

         ulcer of lower limb NEC (L97.-)

         varicose ulcer (I83.0-I82.2)

    AHA: 2017,4Q,17

    TIP: The depth and/or severity of a diagnosed nonpressure ulcer can be determined based on medical record documentation from clinicians who are not the patient's provider.

    TIP: Assign a code from this category/subcategory for nonpressure ulcers documented as acute.

    CC Excl: For CC codes in subcategory L98.4: PDX collection 698

  √6th **L98.41** Non-pressure chronic ulcer of buttock

        L98.411 Non-pressure chronic ulcer of buttock limited to breakdown of skin   `HCC`

        L98.412 Non-pressure chronic ulcer of buttock with fat layer exposed   `HCC` `SW`

        L98.413 Non-pressure chronic ulcer of buttock with necrosis of muscle   `HCC` `SW`

☑ Additional Character Required   √x7th Placeholder   Unacceptable PDx   Questionable PDx   Manifestation   Unspecified Dx   `H1`-`H14` HAC   `HCC` CMS-HCC Dx   `HIV` HIV Dx

L98.414 Non-pressure chronic ulcer of buttock with necrosis of bone `HCC` `SW`

L98.415 Non-pressure chronic ulcer of buttock with muscle involvement without evidence of necrosis `CC` `HCC`

L98.416 Non-pressure chronic ulcer of buttock with bone involvement without evidence of necrosis `CC` `HCC`

L98.418 Non-pressure chronic ulcer of buttock with other specified severity `CC` `HCC`

L98.419 Non-pressure chronic ulcer of buttock with unspecified severity `HCC`

√6ᵗʰ **L98.42** Non-pressure chronic ulcer of back

L98.421 Non-pressure chronic ulcer of back limited to breakdown of skin `HCC`

L98.422 Non-pressure chronic ulcer of back with fat layer exposed `HCC` `SW`

L98.423 Non-pressure chronic ulcer of back with necrosis of muscle `HCC` `SW`

L98.424 Non-pressure chronic ulcer of back with necrosis of bone `HCC` `SW`

L98.425 Non-pressure chronic ulcer of back with muscle involvement without evidence of necrosis `CC` `HCC`

L98.426 Non-pressure chronic ulcer of back with bone involvement without evidence of necrosis `CC` `HCC`

L98.428 Non-pressure chronic ulcer of back with other specified severity `CC` `HCC`

L98.429 Non-pressure chronic ulcer of back with unspecified severity `HCC`

√6ᵗʰ **L98.49** Non-pressure chronic ulcer of skin of other sites

Non-pressure chronic ulcer of skin NOS

L98.491 Non-pressure chronic ulcer of skin of other sites limited to breakdown of skin `HCC`

L98.492 Non-pressure chronic ulcer of skin of other sites with fat layer exposed `HCC` `SW`

L98.493 Non-pressure chronic ulcer of skin of other sites with necrosis of muscle `HCC` `SW`

L98.494 Non-pressure chronic ulcer of skin of other sites with necrosis of bone `HCC` `SW`

L98.495 Non-pressure chronic ulcer of skin of other sites with muscle involvement without evidence of necrosis `CC` `HCC`

L98.496 Non-pressure chronic ulcer of skin of other sites with bone involvement without evidence of necrosis `CC` `HCC`

L98.498 Non-pressure chronic ulcer of skin of other sites with other specified severity `CC` `HCC`

L98.499 Non-pressure chronic ulcer of skin of other sites with unspecified severity `HCC`

L98.5 Mucinosis of the skin

Focal mucinosis

Lichen myxedematosus

Reticular erythematous mucinosis

EXCLUDES 1   *focal oral mucinosis (K13.79)*
        myxedema (E03.9)

L98.6 Other infiltrative disorders of the skin and subcutaneous tissue

EXCLUDES 1   *hyalinosis cutis et mucosae (E78.89)*

L98.7 Excessive and redundant skin and subcutaneous tissue

Loose or sagging skin, following bariatric surgery weight loss

Loose or sagging skin following dietary weight loss

Loose or sagging skin, NOS

EXCLUDES 2   *acquired excess or redundant skin of eyelid (H02.3-)*
        congenital excess or redundant skin of eyelid (Q10.3)
        skin changes due to chronic exposure to nonionizing radiation (L57.-)

AHA: 2016,4Q,36

L98.8 Other specified disorders of the skin and subcutaneous tissue

AHA: 2013,2Q,32

L98.9 Disorder of the skin and subcutaneous tissue, unspecified

L99 *Other disorders of skin and subcutaneous tissue in diseases classified elsewhere*

Code first underlying disease, such as:

amyloidosis (E85.-)

EXCLUDES 1   *skin disorders in diabetes (E08-E13 with .62)*
        skin disorders in gonorrhea (A54.89)
        skin disorders in syphilis (A51.31, A52.79)

`N` Newborn: 0   `P` Pediatric: 0-17   `M` Maternity: 9-64   `A` Adult: 15-124   `MCC` Major Complication/Comorbidity   `CC` Complication/Comorbidity   `SW` Severe Wound Dx

Chapter 13. Diseases of the Musculoskeletal System and Connective Tissue (M00–M99)

Chapter-specific Guidelines with Coding Examples

The chapter-specific guidelines from the ICD-10-CM Official Guidelines for Coding and Reporting have been provided below. Along with these guidelines are coding examples, contained in the shaded boxes, that have been developed to help illustrate the coding and/or sequencing guidance found in these guidelines.

a. Site and laterality

Most of the codes within Chapter 13 have site and laterality designations. The site represents the bone, joint or the muscle involved. For some conditions where more than one bone, joint or muscle is usually involved, such as osteoarthritis, there is a "multiple sites" code available. For categories where no multiple site code is provided and more than one bone, joint or muscle is involved, multiple codes should be used to indicate the different sites involved.

Rheumatoid arthritis of multiple sites without rheumatoid factor

M06.09   Rheumatoid arthritis without rheumatoid factor, multiple sites

Explanation: For some conditions where more than one bone, joint or muscle is usually involved, such as rheumatoid arthritis, there is a "multiple sites" code available.

Osteomyelitis of the fourth thoracic and second lumbar vertebrae

M46.24   Osteomyelitis of vertebra, thoracic region

M46.26   Osteomyelitis of vertebra, lumbar region

Explanation: For categories without a multiple site code and more than one bone, joint, or muscle is involved, multiple codes should be used to indicate the different sites involved.

1) Bone versus joint

For certain conditions, the bone may be affected at the upper or lower end, (e.g., avascular necrosis of bone, M87, Osteoporosis, M80, M81). Though the portion of the bone affected may be at the joint, the site designation will be the bone, not the joint.

Idiopathic avascular necrosis of the femoral head of the left hip joint

M87.052   Idiopathic aseptic necrosis of left femur

Explanation: For certain conditions such as avascular necrosis, the bone may be affected at the joint, but the site designation is the bone, not the joint.

b. Acute traumatic versus chronic or recurrent musculoskeletal conditions

Many musculoskeletal conditions are a result of previous injury or trauma to a site, or are recurrent conditions. Bone, joint or muscle conditions that are the result of a healed injury are usually found in chapter 13. Recurrent bone, joint or muscle conditions are also usually found in chapter 13. Any current, acute injury should be coded to the appropriate injury code from chapter 19. Chronic or recurrent conditions should generally be coded with a code from chapter 13. If it is difficult to determine from the documentation in the record which code is best to describe a condition, query the provider.

Acute traumatic bucket-handle tear of right medial meniscus

S83.211A   Bucket-handle tear of medial meniscus, current injury, right knee, initial encounter

Explanation: Any current, acute injury is not coded in chapter 13. It should instead be coded to the appropriate injury code from chapter 19.

Old bucket-handle tear of right medial meniscus

M23.203   Derangement of unspecified medial meniscus due to old tear or injury, right knee

Explanation: Chronic or recurrent conditions should generally be coded with a code from chapter 13.

c. Coding of pathologic fractures

7th character A is for use as long as the patient is receiving active treatment for the fracture. Examples of active treatment are: surgical treatment, emergency department encounter, evaluation and continuing treatment by the same or a different physician. While the patient may be seen by a new or different provider over the course of treatment for a pathological fracture,

assignment of the 7th character is based on whether the patient is undergoing active treatment and not whether the provider is seeing the patient for the first time.

Patient admitted for repair of pathologic fracture of left foot, unknown cause. The surgery will be performed by his orthopedic specialist who he has been seeing for this fracture for the past month.

M84.475A   Pathological fracture, left foot, initial encounter for fracture

Explanation: Seventh character A is for use as long as the patient is receiving active treatment for a pathologic fracture. Examples of active treatment are surgical treatment, emergency department encounter, evaluation, and continuing treatment by the same or a different physician.

The seventh character is based on whether the patient is undergoing active treatment such as surgery, and not whether the provider is seeing the patient for the first time.

7th character D is to be used for encounters after the patient has completed active treatment for the fracture and is receiving routine care for the fracture during the healing or recovery phase. The other 7th characters, listed under each subcategory in the Tabular List, are to be used for subsequent encounters for treatment of problems associated with the healing, such as malunions, nonunions, and sequelae.

Care for complications of surgical treatment for fracture repairs during the healing or recovery phase should be coded with the appropriate complication codes.

See Section I.C.19. Coding of traumatic fractures.

d. Osteoporosis

Osteoporosis is a systemic condition, meaning that all bones of the musculoskeletal system are affected. Therefore, site is not a component of the codes under category M81, Osteoporosis without current pathological fracture. The site codes under category M80, Osteoporosis with current pathological fracture, identify the site of the fracture, not the osteoporosis.

1) Osteoporosis without pathological fracture

Category M81, Osteoporosis without current pathological fracture, is for use for patients with osteoporosis who do not currently have a pathologic fracture due to the osteoporosis, even if they have had a fracture in the past. For patients with a history of osteoporosis fractures, status code Z87.310, Personal history of (healed) osteoporosis fracture, should follow the code from M81.

Age-related osteoporosis with healed osteoporotic fracture of the lumbar vertebra

M81.0   Age-related osteoporosis without current pathological fracture

Z87.310   Personal history of (healed) osteoporosis fracture

Explanation: Category M81 is used for patients with osteoporosis who do not currently have a pathologic fracture due to the osteoporosis. To report a previous (healed) fracture, status code Z87.310 Personal history of (healed) osteoporosis fracture, should follow the code from M81.

2) Osteoporosis with current pathological fracture

Category M80, Osteoporosis with current pathological fracture, is for patients who have a current pathologic fracture at the time of an encounter. The codes under M80 identify the site of the fracture. A code from category M80, not a traumatic fracture, should be used for any patient with known osteoporosis who suffers a fracture, even if the patient had a minor fall or trauma, if that fall or trauma would not usually break a normal, healthy bone.

Disuse osteoporosis with current fracture of right shoulder sustained lifting a grocery bag, initial encounter

M80.811A   Other osteoporosis with current pathological fracture, right shoulder, initial encounter for fracture

Explanation: A code from category M80, not a traumatic fracture code, should be used for any patient with known osteoporosis who suffers a fracture, even if the patient had a minor fall or trauma, if that fall or trauma would not usually break a normal, healthy bone.

Muscle/Tendon Table

ICD-10-CM categorizes certain muscles and tendons in the upper and lower extremities by their action (e.g., extension, flexion), their anatomical location (e.g., posterior, anterior), and/or whether they are intrinsic or extrinsic to a certain anatomical area. The Muscle/Tendon Table is provided at the beginning of chapters 13 and 19 as a resource to help users when code selection depends on one or more of these characteristics. Please note that this table is not all-inclusive, and proper code assignment should be based on the provider's documentation.

Body Region	Muscle	Extensor Tendon	Flexor Tendon	Other Tendon
Shoulder				
	Deltoid	Posterior deltoid	Anterior deltoid	
	Rotator cuff			
	Infraspinatus			Infraspinatus
	Subscapularis			Subscapularis
	Supraspinatus			Supraspinatus
	Teres minor			Teres minor
	Teres major	Teres major		
Upper arm				
	Anterior muscles			
	Biceps brachii — long head		Biceps brachii — long head	
	Biceps brachii — short head		Biceps brachii — short head	
	Brachialis		Brachialis	
	Coracobrachialis		Coracobrachialis	
	Posterior muscles			
	Triceps brachii	Triceps brachii		
Forearm				
	Anterior muscles			
	Flexors			
	Deep			
	Flexor digitorum profundus		Flexor digitorum profundus	
	Flexor pollicis longus		Flexor pollicis longus	
	Intermediate			
	Flexor digitorum superficialis		Flexor digitorum superficialis	
	Superficial			
	Flexor carpi radialis		Flexor carpi radialis	
	Flexor carpi ulnaris		Flexor carpi ulnaris	
	Palmaris longus		Palmaris longus	
	Pronators			
	Pronator quadratus			Pronator quadratus
	Pronator teres			Pronator teres
	Posterior muscles			
	Extensors			
	Deep			
	Abductor pollicis longus			Abductor pollicis longus
	Extensor indicis	Extensor indicis		
	Extensor pollicis brevis	Extensor pollicis brevis		
	Extensor pollicis longus	Extensor pollicis longus		
	Superficial			
	Brachioradialis			Brachioradialis
	Extensor carpi radialis brevis	Extensor carpi radialis brevis		
	Extensor carpi radialis longus	Extensor carpi radialis longus		
	Extensor carpi ulnaris	Extensor carpi ulnaris		
	Extensor digiti minimi	Extensor digiti minimi		
	Extensor digitorum	Extensor digitorum		
	Anconeus	Anconeus		
	Supinator			Supinator

Body Region	Muscle	Extensor Tendon	Flexor Tendon	Other Tendon
Hand				
Extrinsic — attach to a site in the forearm as well as a site in the hand with action related to hand movement at the wrist				
	Extensor carpi radialis brevis	Extensor carpi radialis brevis		
	Extensor carpi radialis longus	Extensor carpie radialis longus		
	Extensor carpi ulnaris	Extensor carpi ulnaris		
	Flexor carpi radialis		Flexor carpi radialis	
	Flexor carpi ulnaris		Flexor carpi ulnaris	
	Flexor digitorum superficialis		Flexor digitorum superficialis	
	Palmaris longus		Palmaris longus	
Extrinsic — attach to a site in the forearm as well as a site in the hand with action in the hand related to finger movement				
	Adductor pollicis longus			Adductor pollicis longus
	Extensor digiti minimi	Extensor digiti minimi		
	Extensor digitorum	Extensor digitorum		
	Extensor indicis	Extensor indicis		
	Flexor digitorum profundus		Flexor digitorum profundus	
	Flexor digitorum superficialis		Flexor digitorum superficialis	
Extrinsic — attach to a site in the forearm as well as a site in the hand with action in the hand related to thumb movement				
	Extensor pollicis brevis	Extensor pollicis brevis		
	Extensor pollicis longus	Extensor pollicis longus		
	Flexor pollicis longus		Flexor pollicis longus	
Intrinsic — found within the hand only				
	Adductor pollicis			Adductor pollicis
	Dorsal interossei	Dorsal interossei	Dorsal interossei	
	Lumbricals	Lumbricals	Lumbricals	
	Palmaris brevis			Palmaris brevis
	Palmar interossei	Palmar interossei	Palmar interossei	
	Hypothenar muscles			
	Abductor digiti minimi			Abductor digiti minimi
	Flexor digiti minimi brevis		Flexor digiti minimi brevis	
	Oppenens digiti minimi		Oppenens digiti minimi	
	Thenar muscles			
	Abductor pollicis brevis			Abductor pollicis brevis
	Flexor pollicis brevis		Flexor pollicis brevis	
	Oppenens pollicis		Oppenens pollicis	
Thigh				
	Anterior muscles			
	Iliopsoas		Iliopsoas	
	Pectineus		Pectineus	
	Quadriceps	Quadriceps		
	Rectus femoris	Rectus femoris — Extends knee	Rectus femoris — Flexes hip	
	Vastus intermedius	Vastus intermedius		
	Vastus lateralis	Vastus lateralis		
	Vastus medialis	Vastus medialis		
	Sartorius		Sartorius	
	Medial muscles			
	Adductor brevis			Adductor brevis
	Adductor longus			Adductor longus
	Adductor magnus			Adductor magnus
	Gracilis			Gracilis
	Obturator externus			Obturator externus
	Posterior muscles			
	Hamstring	Hamstring — Extends hip	Hamstring — Flexes knee	
	Biceps femoris	Biceps femoris	Biceps femoris	
	Semimembranosus	Semimembranosus	Semimembranosus	
	Semitendinosus	Semitendinosus	Semitendinosus	

Chapter 13. Diseases of the Musculoskeletal System and Connective Tissue

Body Region	Muscle	Extensor Tendon	Flexor Tendon	Other Tendon
Lower leg				
	Anterior muscles			
	Extensor digitorum longus	Extensor digitorum longus		
	Extensor hallucis longus	Extensor hallucis longus		
	Fibularis (peroneus) tertius	Fibularis (peroneus) tertius		
	Tibialis anterior	Tibialis anterior		Tibialis anterior
	Lateral muscles			
	Fibularis (peroneus) brevis		Fibularis (peroneus) brevis	
	Fibularis (peroneus) longus		Fibularis (peroneus) longus	
	Posterior muscles			
	Deep			
	Flexor digitorum longus		Flexor digitorum longus	
	Flexor hallucis longus		Flexor hallucis longus	
	Popliteus		Popliteus	
	Tibialis posterior		Tibialis posterior	
	Superficial			
	Gastrocnemius		Gastrocnemius	
	Plantaris		Plantaris	
	Soleus		Soleus	
				Calcaneal (Achilles)
Ankle/Foot				
Extrinsic — attach to a site in the lower leg as well as a site in the foot with action related to foot movement at the ankle				
	Plantaris		Plantaris	
	Soleus		Soleus	
	Tibialis anterior	Tibialis anterior		
	Tibialis posterior		Tibialis posterior	
Extrinsic — attach to a site in the lower leg as well as a site in the foot with action in the foot related to toe movement				
	Extensor digitorum longus	Extensor digitorum longus		
	Extensor hallicus longus	Extensor hallicus longus		
	Flexor digitorum longus		Flexor digitorum longus	
	Flexor hallucis longus		Flexor hallucis longus	
Intrinsic — found within the ankle/foot only				
	Dorsal muscles			
	Extensor digitorum brevis	Extensor digitorum brevis		
	Extensor hallucis brevis	Extensor hallucis brevis		
	Plantar muscles			
	Abductor digiti minimi		Abductor digiti minimi	
	Abductor hallucis		Abductor hallucis	
	Dorsal interossei	Dorsal interossei	Dorsal interossei	
	Flexor digiti minimi brevis		Flexor digiti minimi brevis	
	Flexor digitorum brevis		Flexor digitorum brevis	
	Flexor hallucis brevis		Flexor hallucis brevis	
	Lumbricals	Lumbricals	Lumbricals	
	Quadratus plantae		Quadratus plantae	
	Plantar interossei	Plantar interossei	Plantar interossei	

Chapter 13. Diseases of the Musculoskeletal System and Connective Tissue (M00-M99)

NOTE Use an external cause code following the code for the musculoskeletal condition, if applicable, to identify the cause of the musculoskeletal condition

EXCLUDES 2 arthropathic psoriasis (L40.5-)
certain conditions originating in the perinatal period (P04-P96)
certain infectious and parasitic diseases (A00-B99)
compartment syndrome (traumatic) (T79.A-)
complications of pregnancy, childbirth and the puerperium (O00-O9A)
congenital malformations, deformations, and chromosomal abnormalities (Q00-Q99)
endocrine, nutritional and metabolic diseases (E00-E88)
injury, poisoning and certain other consequences of external causes (S00-T88)
neoplasms (C00-D49)
symptoms, signs and abnormal clinical and laboratory findings, not elsewhere classified (R00-R94)

This chapter contains the following blocks:

M00-M02   Infectious arthropathies
M04   Autoinflammatory syndromes
M05-M14   Inflammatory polyarthropathies
M15-M19   Osteoarthritis
M20-M25   Other joint disorders
M26-M27   Dentofacial anomalies [including malocclusion] and other disorders of jaw
M30-M36   Systemic connective tissue disorders
M40-M43   Deforming dorsopathies
M45-M49   Spondylopathies
M50-M54   Other dorsopathies
M60-M63   Disorders of muscles
M65-M67   Disorders of synovium and tendon
M70-M79   Other soft tissue disorders
M80-M85   Disorders of bone density and structure
M86-M90   Other osteopathies
M91-M94   Chondropathies
M95   Other disorders of the musculoskeletal system and connective tissue
M96   Intraoperative and postprocedural complications and disorders of musculoskeletal system, not elsewhere classified
M97   Periprosthetic fracture around internal prosthetic joint
M99   Biomechanical lesions, not elsewhere classified

ARTHROPATHIES (M00-M25)

INCLUDES disorders affecting predominantly peripheral (limb) joints

Infectious arthropathies (M00-M02)

NOTE This block comprises arthropathies due to microbiological agents. Distinction is made between the following types of etiological relationship:

a) direct infection of joint, where organisms invade synovial tissue and microbial antigen is present in the joint;

b) indirect infection, which may be of two types: a reactive arthropathy, where microbial infection of the body is established but neither organisms nor antigens can be identified in the joint, and a postinfective arthropathy, where microbial antigen is present but recovery of an organism is inconstant and evidence of local multiplication is lacking.

√4th M00 Pyogenic arthritis

DEF: Pyogenic: Relating to or involving pus production, often referred to as suppurative or purulent.

√5th M00.0 Staphylococcal arthritis and polyarthritis

Use additional code (B95.61-B95.8) to identify bacterial agent

EXCLUDES 2 infection and inflammatory reaction due to internal joint prosthesis (T84.5-)

M00.00 Staphylococcal arthritis, unspecified joint   CC HCC
     CC Excl: PDX collection 855

√6th M00.01 Staphylococcal arthritis, shoulder
     CC Excl: For CC codes in subcategory M00.01: PDX collection 856

     M00.011 Staphylococcal arthritis, right shoulder   CC HCC

     M00.012 Staphylococcal arthritis, left shoulder   CC HCC

     M00.019 Staphylococcal arthritis, unspecified shoulder   CC HCC

√6th M00.02 Staphylococcal arthritis, elbow
     CC Excl: For CC codes in subcategory M00.02: PDX collection 857

     M00.021 Staphylococcal arthritis, right elbow   CC HCC

     M00.022 Staphylococcal arthritis, left elbow   CC HCC

     M00.029 Staphylococcal arthritis, unspecified elbow   CC HCC

√6th M00.03 Staphylococcal arthritis, wrist
     Staphylococcal arthritis of carpal bones
     CC Excl: For CC codes in subcategory M00.03: PDX collection 858

     M00.031 Staphylococcal arthritis, right wrist   CC HCC

     M00.032 Staphylococcal arthritis, left wrist   CC HCC

     M00.039 Staphylococcal arthritis, unspecified wrist   CC HCC

√6th M00.04 Staphylococcal arthritis, hand
     Staphylococcal arthritis of metacarpus and phalanges
     CC Excl: For CC codes in subcategory M00.04: PDX collection 859

     M00.041 Staphylococcal arthritis, right hand   CC HCC

     M00.042 Staphylococcal arthritis, left hand   CC HCC

     M00.049 Staphylococcal arthritis, unspecified hand   CC HCC

√6th M00.05 Staphylococcal arthritis, hip
     CC Excl: For CC codes in subcategory M00.05: PDX collection 860

     M00.051 Staphylococcal arthritis, right hip   CC HCC

     M00.052 Staphylococcal arthritis, left hip   CC HCC

     M00.059 Staphylococcal arthritis, unspecified hip   CC HCC

√6th M00.06 Staphylococcal arthritis, knee
     CC Excl: For CC codes in subcategory M00.06: PDX collection 861

     M00.061 Staphylococcal arthritis, right knee   CC HCC

     M00.062 Staphylococcal arthritis, left knee   CC HCC

     M00.069 Staphylococcal arthritis, unspecified knee   CC HCC

√6th M00.07 Staphylococcal arthritis, ankle and foot
     Staphylococcal arthritis, tarsus, metatarsus and phalanges
     CC Excl: For CC codes in subcategory M00.07: PDX collection 862

     M00.071 Staphylococcal arthritis, right ankle and foot   CC HCC

     M00.072 Staphylococcal arthritis, left ankle and foot   CC HCC

     M00.079 Staphylococcal arthritis, unspecified ankle and foot   CC HCC

M00.08 Staphylococcal arthritis, vertebrae   CC HCC
     CC Excl: PDX collection 855

M00.09 Staphylococcal polyarthritis   CC HCC
     CC Excl: PDX collection 855

√5th M00.1 Pneumococcal arthritis and polyarthritis

M00.10 Pneumococcal arthritis, unspecified joint   CC HCC
     CC Excl: PDX collection 855

√6th M00.11 Pneumococcal arthritis, shoulder
     CC Excl: For CC codes in subcategory M00.11: PDX collection 856

     M00.111 Pneumococcal arthritis, right shoulder   CC HCC

     M00.112 Pneumococcal arthritis, left shoulder   CC HCC

     M00.119 Pneumococcal arthritis, unspecified shoulder   CC HCC

✓ Additional Character Required   ✓x7th Placeholder   Unacceptable PDx   Questionable PDx   Manifestation   Unspecified Dx   H1-H14 HAC   HCC CMS-HCC Dx   HIV HIV Dx

ICD-10-CM 2020

763

Chapter 13. Diseases of the Musculoskeletal System and Connective Tissue

M00.12–M00.811

✓6ᵗʰ **M00.12 Pneumococcal arthritis, elbow**

CC Excl: For CC codes in subcategory M00.12: PDX collection 857

   M00.121 Pneumococcal arthritis, right elbow CC HCC

   M00.122 Pneumococcal arthritis, left elbow CC HCC

   M00.129 Pneumococcal arthritis, unspecified elbow CC HCC

✓6ᵗʰ **M00.13 Pneumococcal arthritis, wrist**

Pneumococcal arthritis of carpal bones

CC Excl: For CC codes in subcategory M00.13: PDX collection 858

   M00.131 Pneumococcal arthritis, right wrist CC HCC

   M00.132 Pneumococcal arthritis, left wrist CC HCC

   M00.139 Pneumococcal arthritis, unspecified wrist CC HCC

✓6ᵗʰ **M00.14 Pneumococcal arthritis, hand**

Pneumococcal arthritis of metacarpus and phalanges

CC Excl: For CC codes in subcategory M00.14: PDX collection 859

   M00.141 Pneumococcal arthritis, right hand CC HCC

   M00.142 Pneumococcal arthritis, left hand CC HCC

   M00.149 Pneumococcal arthritis, unspecified hand CC HCC

✓6ᵗʰ **M00.15 Pneumococcal arthritis, hip**

CC Excl: For CC codes in subcategory M00.15: PDX collection 860

   M00.151 Pneumococcal arthritis, right hip CC HCC

   M00.152 Pneumococcal arthritis, left hip CC HCC

   M00.159 Pneumococcal arthritis, unspecified hip CC HCC

✓6ᵗʰ **M00.16 Pneumococcal arthritis, knee**

CC Excl: For CC codes in subcategory M00.16: PDX collection 861

   M00.161 Pneumococcal arthritis, right knee CC HCC

   M00.162 Pneumococcal arthritis, left knee CC HCC

   M00.169 Pneumococcal arthritis, unspecified knee CC HCC

✓6ᵗʰ **M00.17 Pneumococcal arthritis, ankle and foot**

Pneumococcal arthritis, tarsus, metatarsus and phalanges

CC Excl: For CC codes in subcategory M00.17: PDX collection 862

   M00.171 Pneumococcal arthritis, right ankle and foot CC HCC

   M00.172 Pneumococcal arthritis, left ankle and foot CC HCC

   M00.179 Pneumococcal arthritis, unspecified ankle and foot CC HCC

   M00.18 Pneumococcal arthritis, vertebrae CC HCC

CC Excl: PDX collection 855

   M00.19 Pneumococcal polyarthritis CC HCC

CC Excl: PDX collection 855

✓5ᵗʰ **M00.2 Other streptococcal arthritis and polyarthritis**

Use additional code (B95.0-B95.2, B95.4-B95.5) to identify bacterial agent

   M00.20 Other streptococcal arthritis, unspecified joint CC HCC

CC Excl: PDX collection 855

✓6ᵗʰ **M00.21 Other streptococcal arthritis, shoulder**

CC Excl: For CC codes in subcategory M00.21: PDX collection 856

   M00.211 Other streptococcal arthritis, right shoulder CC HCC

   M00.212 Other streptococcal arthritis, left shoulder CC HCC

   M00.219 Other streptococcal arthritis, unspecified shoulder CC HCC

✓6ᵗʰ **M00.22 Other streptococcal arthritis, elbow**

CC Excl: For CC codes in subcategory M00.22: PDX collection 857

   M00.221 Other streptococcal arthritis, right elbow CC HCC

   M00.222 Other streptococcal arthritis, left elbow CC HCC

   M00.229 Other streptococcal arthritis, unspecified elbow CC HCC

✓6ᵗʰ **M00.23 Other streptococcal arthritis, wrist**

Other streptococcal arthritis of carpal bones

CC Excl: For CC codes in subcategory M00.23: PDX collection 858

   M00.231 Other streptococcal arthritis, right wrist CC HCC

   M00.232 Other streptococcal arthritis, left wrist CC HCC

   M00.239 Other streptococcal arthritis, unspecified wrist CC HCC

✓6ᵗʰ **M00.24 Other streptococcal arthritis, hand**

Other streptococcal arthritis metacarpus and phalanges

CC Excl: For CC codes in subcategory M00.24: PDX collection 859

   M00.241 Other streptococcal arthritis, right hand CC HCC

   M00.242 Other streptococcal arthritis, left hand CC HCC

   M00.249 Other streptococcal arthritis, unspecified hand CC HCC

✓6ᵗʰ **M00.25 Other streptococcal arthritis, hip**

CC Excl: For CC codes in subcategory M00.25: PDX collection 860

   M00.251 Other streptococcal arthritis, right hip CC HCC

   M00.252 Other streptococcal arthritis, left hip CC HCC

   M00.259 Other streptococcal arthritis, unspecified hip CC HCC

✓6ᵗʰ **M00.26 Other streptococcal arthritis, knee**

CC Excl: For CC codes in subcategory M00.26: PDX collection 861

   M00.261 Other streptococcal arthritis, right knee CC HCC

   M00.262 Other streptococcal arthritis, left knee CC HCC

   M00.269 Other streptococcal arthritis, unspecified knee CC HCC

✓6ᵗʰ **M00.27 Other streptococcal arthritis, ankle and foot**

Other streptococcal arthritis, tarsus, metatarsus and phalanges

CC Excl: For CC codes in subcategory M00.27: PDX collection 862

   M00.271 Other streptococcal arthritis, right ankle and foot CC HCC

   M00.272 Other streptococcal arthritis, left ankle and foot CC HCC

   M00.279 Other streptococcal arthritis, unspecified ankle and foot CC HCC

   M00.28 Other streptococcal arthritis, vertebrae CC HCC

CC Excl: PDX collection 855

   M00.29 Other streptococcal polyarthritis CC HCC

CC Excl: PDX collection 855

✓5ᵗʰ **M00.8 Arthritis and polyarthritis due to other bacteria**

Use additional code (B96) to identify bacteria

   M00.80 Arthritis due to other bacteria, unspecified joint CC HCC

CC Excl: PDX collection 855

✓6ᵗʰ **M00.81 Arthritis due to other bacteria, shoulder**

CC Excl: For CC codes in subcategory M00.81: PDX collection 856

   M00.811 Arthritis due to other bacteria, right shoulder CC HCC

N Newborn: 0   P Pediatric: 0-17   M Maternity: 9-64   A Adult: 15-124   HCC Major Complication/Comorbidity   CC Complication/Comorbidity   SW Severe Wound Dx

764   ICD-10-CM 2020

M00.812	**Arthritis due to other bacteria, left shoulder**	`CC` `HCC`
M00.819	**Arthritis due to other bacteria, unspecified shoulder**	`CC` `HCC`

✓6ᵗʰ M00.82 Arthritis due to other bacteria, elbow

> **CC Excl: For CC codes in subcategory M00.82:** PDX collection 857

M00.821	**Arthritis due to other bacteria, right elbow**	`CC` `HCC`
M00.822	**Arthritis due to other bacteria, left elbow**	`CC` `HCC`
M00.829	**Arthritis due to other bacteria, unspecified elbow**	`CC` `HCC`

✓6ᵗʰ M00.83 Arthritis due to other bacteria, wrist

Arthritis due to other bacteria, carpal bones

> **CC Excl: For CC codes in subcategory M00.83:** PDX collection 858

M00.831	**Arthritis due to other bacteria, right wrist**	`CC` `HCC`
M00.832	**Arthritis due to other bacteria, left wrist**	`CC` `HCC`
M00.839	**Arthritis due to other bacteria, unspecified wrist**	`CC` `HCC`

✓6ᵗʰ M00.84 Arthritis due to other bacteria, hand

Arthritis due to other bacteria, metacarpus and phalanges

> **CC Excl: For CC codes in subcategory M00.84:** PDX collection 859

M00.841	**Arthritis due to other bacteria, right hand**	`CC` `HCC`
M00.842	**Arthritis due to other bacteria, left hand**	`CC` `HCC`
M00.849	**Arthritis due to other bacteria, unspecified hand**	`CC` `HCC`

✓6ᵗʰ M00.85 Arthritis due to other bacteria, hip

> **CC Excl: For CC codes in subcategory M00.85:** PDX collection 860

M00.851	**Arthritis due to other bacteria, right hip**	`CC` `HCC`
M00.852	**Arthritis due to other bacteria, left hip**	`CC` `HCC`
M00.859	**Arthritis due to other bacteria, unspecified hip**	`CC` `HCC`

✓6ᵗʰ M00.86 Arthritis due to other bacteria, knee

> **CC Excl: For CC codes in subcategory M00.86:** PDX collection 861

M00.861	**Arthritis due to other bacteria, right knee**	`CC` `HCC`
M00.862	**Arthritis due to other bacteria, left knee**	`CC` `HCC`
M00.869	**Arthritis due to other bacteria, unspecified knee**	`CC` `HCC`

✓6ᵗʰ M00.87 Arthritis due to other bacteria, ankle and foot

Arthritis due to other bacteria, tarsus, metatarsus, and phalanges

> **CC Excl: For CC codes in subcategory M00.87:** PDX collection 862

M00.871	**Arthritis due to other bacteria, right ankle and foot**	`CC` `HCC`
M00.872	**Arthritis due to other bacteria, left ankle and foot**	`CC` `HCC`
M00.879	**Arthritis due to other bacteria, unspecified ankle and foot**	`CC` `HCC`
M00.88	**Arthritis due to other bacteria, vertebrae**	`CC` `HCC`

> **CC Excl:** PDX collection 855

M00.89	**Polyarthritis due to other bacteria**	`CC` `HCC`

> **CC Excl:** PDX collection 855

M00.9	**Pyogenic arthritis, unspecified**	`CC` `HCC`

Infective arthritis NOS

> **CC Excl:** PDX collection 855

✓4ᵗʰ M01 Direct infections of joint in infectious and parasitic diseases classified elsewhere

Code first underlying disease, such as:
leprosy [Hansen's disease] (A30.-)
mycoses (B35-B49)
O'nyong-nyong fever (A92.1)
paratyphoid fever (A01.1-A01.4)

> **EXCLUDES 1**   *arthropathy in Lyme disease (A69.23)*
> *gonococcal arthritis (A54.42)*
> *meningococcal arthritis (A39.83)*
> *mumps arthritis (B26.85)*
> *postinfective arthropathy (M02.-)*
> *postmeningococcal arthritis (A39.84)*
> *reactive arthritis (M02.3)*
> *rubella arthritis (B06.82)*
> *sarcoidosis arthritis (D86.86)*
> *typhoid fever arthritis (A01.04)*
> *tuberculosis arthritis (A18.01-A18.02)*

CC Excl: For CC codes in category M01, unless otherwise noted: PDX collection 863

✓5ᵗʰ M01.X Direct infection of joint in infectious and parasitic diseases classified elsewhere

M01.X0	**Direct infection of unspecified joint in infectious and parasitic diseases classified elsewhere**	`CC` `HCC`

✓6ᵗʰ M01.X1 Direct infection of shoulder joint in infectious and parasitic diseases classified elsewhere

> **CC Excl: For CC codes in subcategory M01.X1:** PDX collection 864

M01.X11	**Direct infection of right shoulder in infectious and parasitic diseases classified elsewhere**	`CC` `HCC`
M01.X12	**Direct infection of left shoulder in infectious and parasitic diseases classified elsewhere**	`CC` `HCC`
M01.X19	**Direct infection of unspecified shoulder in infectious and parasitic diseases classified elsewhere**	`CC` `HCC`

✓6ᵗʰ M01.X2 Direct infection of elbow in infectious and parasitic diseases classified elsewhere

M01.X21	**Direct infection of right elbow in infectious and parasitic diseases classified elsewhere**	`CC` `HCC`
M01.X22	**Direct infection of left elbow in infectious and parasitic diseases classified elsewhere**	`CC` `HCC`
M01.X29	**Direct infection of unspecified elbow in infectious and parasitic diseases classified elsewhere**	`CC` `HCC`

✓6ᵗʰ M01.X3 Direct infection of wrist in infectious and parasitic diseases classified elsewhere

Direct infection of carpal bones in infectious and parasitic diseases classified elsewhere

M01.X31	**Direct infection of right wrist in infectious and parasitic diseases classified elsewhere**	`CC` `HCC`
M01.X32	**Direct infection of left wrist in infectious and parasitic diseases classified elsewhere**	`CC` `HCC`
M01.X39	**Direct infection of unspecified wrist in infectious and parasitic diseases classified elsewhere**	`CC` `HCC`

✓ Additional Character Required   ✓x7ᵗʰ Placeholder   Unacceptable PDx   Questionable PDx   Manifestation   Unspecified Dx   H1-H14 HAC   HCC CMS-HCC Dx   HIV HIV Dx

ICD-10-CM 2020   765

√6ᵗʰ **M01.X4** **Direct infection of hand in infectious and parasitic diseases classified elsewhere**
> Direct infection of metacarpus and phalanges in infectious and parasitic diseases classified elsewhere

     M01.X41 ***Direct infection of right hand in infectious and parasitic diseases classified elsewhere***   `CC` `HCC`

     M01.X42 ***Direct infection of left hand in infectious and parasitic diseases classified elsewhere***   `CC` `HCC`

     M01.X49 ***Direct infection of unspecified hand in infectious and parasitic diseases classified elsewhere***   `CC` `HCC`

√6ᵗʰ **M01.X5** **Direct infection of hip in infectious and parasitic diseases classified elsewhere**

     M01.X51 ***Direct infection of right hip in infectious and parasitic diseases classified elsewhere***   `CC` `HCC`

     M01.X52 ***Direct infection of left hip in infectious and parasitic diseases classified elsewhere***   `CC` `HCC`

     M01.X59 ***Direct infection of unspecified hip in infectious and parasitic diseases classified elsewhere***   `CC` `HCC`

√6ᵗʰ **M01.X6** **Direct infection of knee in infectious and parasitic diseases classified elsewhere**

     M01.X61 ***Direct infection of right knee in infectious and parasitic diseases classified elsewhere***   `CC` `HCC`

     M01.X62 ***Direct infection of left knee in infectious and parasitic diseases classified elsewhere***   `CC` `HCC`

     M01.X69 ***Direct infection of unspecified knee in infectious and parasitic diseases classified elsewhere***   `CC` `HCC`

√6ᵗʰ **M01.X7** **Direct infection of ankle and foot in infectious and parasitic diseases classified elsewhere**
> Direct infection of tarsus, metatarsus and phalanges in infectious and parasitic diseases classified elsewhere

     M01.X71 ***Direct infection of right ankle and foot in infectious and parasitic diseases classified elsewhere***   `CC` `HCC`

     M01.X72 ***Direct infection of left ankle and foot in infectious and parasitic diseases classified elsewhere***   `CC` `HCC`

     M01.X79 ***Direct infection of unspecified ankle and foot in infectious and parasitic diseases classified elsewhere***   `CC` `HCC`

     M01.X8 ***Direct infection of vertebrae in infectious and parasitic diseases classified elsewhere***   `CC` `HCC`

     M01.X9 ***Direct infection of multiple joints in infectious and parasitic diseases classified elsewhere***   `CC` `HCC`

√4ᵗʰ **M02** **Postinfective and reactive arthropathies**
> Code first underlying disease, such as:
> congenital syphilis [Clutton's joints] (A50.5)
> enteritis due to Yersinia enterocolitica (A04.6)
> infective endocarditis (I33.0)
> viral hepatitis (B15-B19)

> **EXCLUDES 1**   Behçet's disease (M35.2)
> direct infections of joint in infectious and parasitic diseases classified elsewhere (M01.-)
> mumps arthritis (B26.85)
> postmeningococcal arthritis (A39.84)
> rheumatic fever (I00)
> rubella arthritis (B06.82)
> syphilis arthritis (late) (A52.77)
> tabetic arthropathy [Charcôt's] (A52.16)

√5ᵗʰ **M02.0** **Arthropathy following intestinal bypass**

     M02.00 **Arthropathy following intestinal bypass, unspecified site**

     √6ᵗʰ **M02.01** **Arthropathy following intestinal bypass, shoulder**

       M02.011 **Arthropathy following intestinal bypass, right shoulder**

       M02.012 **Arthropathy following intestinal bypass, left shoulder**

       M02.019 **Arthropathy following intestinal bypass, unspecified shoulder**

     √6ᵗʰ **M02.02** **Arthropathy following intestinal bypass, elbow**

       M02.021 **Arthropathy following intestinal bypass, right elbow**

       M02.022 **Arthropathy following intestinal bypass, left elbow**

       M02.029 **Arthropathy following intestinal bypass, unspecified elbow**

     √6ᵗʰ **M02.03** **Arthropathy following intestinal bypass, wrist**
> Arthropathy following intestinal bypass, carpal bones

       M02.031 **Arthropathy following intestinal bypass, right wrist**

       M02.032 **Arthropathy following intestinal bypass, left wrist**

       M02.039 **Arthropathy following intestinal bypass, unspecified wrist**

     √6ᵗʰ **M02.04** **Arthropathy following intestinal bypass, hand**
> Arthropathy following intestinal bypass, metacarpals and phalanges

       M02.041 **Arthropathy following intestinal bypass, right hand**

       M02.042 **Arthropathy following intestinal bypass, left hand**

       M02.049 **Arthropathy following intestinal bypass, unspecified hand**

     √6ᵗʰ **M02.05** **Arthropathy following intestinal bypass, hip**

       M02.051 **Arthropathy following intestinal bypass, right hip**

       M02.052 **Arthropathy following intestinal bypass, left hip**

       M02.059 **Arthropathy following intestinal bypass, unspecified hip**

     √6ᵗʰ **M02.06** **Arthropathy following intestinal bypass, knee**

       M02.061 **Arthropathy following intestinal bypass, right knee**

       M02.062 **Arthropathy following intestinal bypass, left knee**

       M02.069 **Arthropathy following intestinal bypass, unspecified knee**

     √6ᵗʰ **M02.07** **Arthropathy following intestinal bypass, ankle and foot**
> Arthropathy following intestinal bypass, tarsus, metatarsus and phalanges

       M02.071 **Arthropathy following intestinal bypass, right ankle and foot**

       M02.072 **Arthropathy following intestinal bypass, left ankle and foot**

       M02.079 **Arthropathy following intestinal bypass, unspecified ankle and foot**

     M02.08 **Arthropathy following intestinal bypass, vertebrae**

     M02.09 **Arthropathy following intestinal bypass, multiple sites**

√5ᵗʰ **M02.1** **Postdysenteric arthropathy**

     M02.10 **Postdysenteric arthropathy, unspecified site**   `HCC`

Ⓝ Newborn: 0   Ⓟ Pediatric: 0-17   Ⓜ Maternity: 9-64   Ⓐ Adult: 15-124   `MCC` Major Complication/Comorbidity   `CC` Complication/Comorbidity   `SW` Severe Wound Dx

766   ICD-10-CM 2020

✓6ᵗʰ **M02.11 Postdysenteric arthropathy, shoulder**
- M02.111 Postdysenteric arthropathy, right shoulder `HCC`
- M02.112 Postdysenteric arthropathy, left shoulder `HCC`
- M02.119 Postdysenteric arthropathy, unspecified shoulder `HCC`

✓6ᵗʰ **M02.12 Postdysenteric arthropathy, elbow**
- M02.121 Postdysenteric arthropathy, right elbow `HCC`
- M02.122 Postdysenteric arthropathy, left elbow `HCC`
- M02.129 Postdysenteric arthropathy, unspecified elbow `HCC`

✓6ᵗʰ **M02.13 Postdysenteric arthropathy, wrist**
  Postdysenteric arthropathy, carpal bones
- M02.131 Postdysenteric arthropathy, right wrist `HCC`
- M02.132 Postdysenteric arthropathy, left wrist `HCC`
- M02.139 Postdysenteric arthropathy, unspecified wrist `HCC`

✓6ᵗʰ **M02.14 Postdysenteric arthropathy, hand**
  Postdysenteric arthropathy, metacarpus and phalanges
- M02.141 Postdysenteric arthropathy, right hand `HCC`
- M02.142 Postdysenteric arthropathy, left hand `HCC`
- M02.149 Postdysenteric arthropathy, unspecified hand `HCC`

✓6ᵗʰ **M02.15 Postdysenteric arthropathy, hip**
- M02.151 Postdysenteric arthropathy, right hip `HCC`
- M02.152 Postdysenteric arthropathy, left hip `HCC`
- M02.159 Postdysenteric arthropathy, unspecified hip `HCC`

✓6ᵗʰ **M02.16 Postdysenteric arthropathy, knee**
- M02.161 Postdysenteric arthropathy, right knee `HCC`
- M02.162 Postdysenteric arthropathy, left knee `HCC`
- M02.169 Postdysenteric arthropathy, unspecified knee `HCC`

✓6ᵗʰ **M02.17 Postdysenteric arthropathy, ankle and foot**
  Postdysenteric arthropathy, tarsus, metatarsus and phalanges
- M02.171 Postdysenteric arthropathy, right ankle and foot `HCC`
- M02.172 Postdysenteric arthropathy, left ankle and foot `HCC`
- M02.179 Postdysenteric arthropathy, unspecified ankle and foot `HCC`

- M02.18 Postdysenteric arthropathy, vertebrae `HCC`
- M02.19 Postdysenteric arthropathy, multiple sites `HCC`

✓5ᵗʰ **M02.2 Postimmunization arthropathy**
- M02.20 Postimmunization arthropathy, unspecified site

✓6ᵗʰ **M02.21 Postimmunization arthropathy, shoulder**
- M02.211 Postimmunization arthropathy, right shoulder
- M02.212 Postimmunization arthropathy, left shoulder
- M02.219 Postimmunization arthropathy, unspecified shoulder

✓6ᵗʰ **M02.22 Postimmunization arthropathy, elbow**
- M02.221 Postimmunization arthropathy, right elbow
- M02.222 Postimmunization arthropathy, left elbow
- M02.229 Postimmunization arthropathy, unspecified elbow

✓6ᵗʰ **M02.23 Postimmunization arthropathy, wrist**
  Postimmunization arthropathy, carpal bones
- M02.231 Postimmunization arthropathy, right wrist
- M02.232 Postimmunization arthropathy, left wrist
- M02.239 Postimmunization arthropathy, unspecified wrist

✓6ᵗʰ **M02.24 Postimmunization arthropathy, hand**
  Postimmunization arthropathy, metacarpus and phalanges
- M02.241 Postimmunization arthropathy, right hand
- M02.242 Postimmunization arthropathy, left hand
- M02.249 Postimmunization arthropathy, unspecified hand

✓6ᵗʰ **M02.25 Postimmunization arthropathy, hip**
- M02.251 Postimmunization arthropathy, right hip
- M02.252 Postimmunization arthropathy, left hip
- M02.259 Postimmunization arthropathy, unspecified hip

✓6ᵗʰ **M02.26 Postimmunization arthropathy, knee**
- M02.261 Postimmunization arthropathy, right knee
- M02.262 Postimmunization arthropathy, left knee
- M02.269 Postimmunization arthropathy, unspecified knee

✓6ᵗʰ **M02.27 Postimmunization arthropathy, ankle and foot**
  Postimmunization arthropathy, tarsus, metatarsus and phalanges
- M02.271 Postimmunization arthropathy, right ankle and foot
- M02.272 Postimmunization arthropathy, left ankle and foot
- M02.279 Postimmunization arthropathy, unspecified ankle and foot

- M02.28 Postimmunization arthropathy, vertebrae
- M02.29 Postimmunization arthropathy, multiple sites

✓5ᵗʰ **M02.3 Reiter's disease**
  Reactive arthritis
  DEF: Arthritis, iridocyclitis, and urethritis, sometimes with diarrhea. While symptoms may recur, arthritis is constant.
- M02.30 Reiter's disease, unspecified site `HCC`

✓6ᵗʰ **M02.31 Reiter's disease, shoulder**
- M02.311 Reiter's disease, right shoulder `HCC`
- M02.312 Reiter's disease, left shoulder `HCC`
- M02.319 Reiter's disease, unspecified shoulder `HCC`

✓6ᵗʰ **M02.32 Reiter's disease, elbow**
- M02.321 Reiter's disease, right elbow `HCC`
- M02.322 Reiter's disease, left elbow `HCC`
- M02.329 Reiter's disease, unspecified elbow `HCC`

✓6ᵗʰ **M02.33 Reiter's disease, wrist**
  Reiter's disease, carpal bones
- M02.331 Reiter's disease, right wrist `HCC`
- M02.332 Reiter's disease, left wrist `HCC`
- M02.339 Reiter's disease, unspecified wrist `HCC`

✓6ᵗʰ **M02.34 Reiter's disease, hand**
  Reiter's disease, metacarpus and phalanges
- M02.341 Reiter's disease, right hand `HCC`
- M02.342 Reiter's disease, left hand `HCC`
- M02.349 Reiter's disease, unspecified hand `HCC`

✓6ᵗʰ **M02.35 Reiter's disease, hip**
- M02.351 Reiter's disease, right hip `HCC`
- M02.352 Reiter's disease, left hip `HCC`
- M02.359 Reiter's disease, unspecified hip `HCC`

✓6ᵗʰ **M02.36** Reiter's disease, knee

     M02.361 Reiter's disease, right knee   HCC

     M02.362 Reiter's disease, left knee   HCC

     M02.369 Reiter's disease, unspecified knee   HCC

✓6ᵗʰ **M02.37** Reiter's disease, ankle and foot

     Reiter's disease, tarsus, metatarsus and phalanges

     M02.371 Reiter's disease, right ankle and foot   HCC

     M02.372 Reiter's disease, left ankle and foot   HCC

     M02.379 Reiter's disease, unspecified ankle and foot   HCC

   M02.38 Reiter's disease, vertebrae   HCC

   M02.39 Reiter's disease, multiple sites   HCC

✓5ᵗʰ **M02.8** Other reactive arthropathies

   M02.80 Other reactive arthropathies, unspecified site   HCC

✓6ᵗʰ **M02.81** Other reactive arthropathies, shoulder

     M02.811 Other reactive arthropathies, right shoulder   HCC

     M02.812 Other reactive arthropathies, left shoulder   HCC

     M02.819 Other reactive arthropathies, unspecified shoulder   HCC

✓6ᵗʰ **M02.82** Other reactive arthropathies, elbow

     M02.821 Other reactive arthropathies, right elbow   HCC

     M02.822 Other reactive arthropathies, left elbow   HCC

     M02.829 Other reactive arthropathies, unspecified elbow   HCC

✓6ᵗʰ **M02.83** Other reactive arthropathies, wrist

     Other reactive arthropathies, carpal bones

     M02.831 Other reactive arthropathies, right wrist   HCC

     M02.832 Other reactive arthropathies, left wrist   HCC

     M02.839 Other reactive arthropathies, unspecified wrist   HCC

✓6ᵗʰ **M02.84** Other reactive arthropathies, hand

     Other reactive arthropathies, metacarpus and phalanges

     M02.841 Other reactive arthropathies, right hand   HCC

     M02.842 Other reactive arthropathies, left hand   HCC

     M02.849 Other reactive arthropathies, unspecified hand   HCC

✓6ᵗʰ **M02.85** Other reactive arthropathies, hip

     M02.851 Other reactive arthropathies, right hip   HCC

     M02.852 Other reactive arthropathies, left hip   HCC

     M02.859 Other reactive arthropathies, unspecified hip   HCC

✓6ᵗʰ **M02.86** Other reactive arthropathies, knee

     M02.861 Other reactive arthropathies, right knee   HCC

     M02.862 Other reactive arthropathies, left knee   HCC

     M02.869 Other reactive arthropathies, unspecified knee   HCC

✓6ᵗʰ **M02.87** Other reactive arthropathies, ankle and foot

     Other reactive arthropathies, tarsus, metatarsus and phalanges

     M02.871 Other reactive arthropathies, right ankle and foot   HCC

     M02.872 Other reactive arthropathies, left ankle and foot   HCC

     M02.879 Other reactive arthropathies, unspecified ankle and foot   HCC

   M02.88 Other reactive arthropathies, vertebrae   HCC

   M02.89 Other reactive arthropathies, multiple sites   HCC

M02.9 Reactive arthropathy, unspecified   HCC

Autoinflammatory syndromes (M04)

✓4ᵗʰ **M04** Autoinflammatory syndromes

   EXCLUDES 2   Crohn's disease (K50.-)

   AHA: 2016,4Q,37

  M04.1 Periodic fever syndromes   HCC

     Familial Mediterranean fever

     Hyperimmunoglobin D syndrome

     Mevalonate kinase deficiency

     Tumor necrosis factor receptor associated periodic syndrome [TRAPS]

  M04.2 Cryopyrin-associated periodic syndromes   HCC

     Chronic infantile neurological, cutaneous and articular syndrome [CINCA]

     Familial cold autoinflammatory syndrome

     Familial cold urticaria

     Muckle-Wells syndrome

     Neonatal onset multisystemic inflammatory disorder [NOMID]

  M04.8 Other autoinflammatory syndromes   HCC

     Blau syndrome

     Deficiency of interleukin 1 receptor antagonist [DIRA]

     Majeed syndrome

     Periodic fever, aphthous stomatitis, pharyngitis, and adenopathy syndrome [PFAPA]

     Pyogenic arthritis, pyoderma gangrenosum, and acne syndrome [PAPA]

  M04.9 Autoinflammatory syndrome, unspecified   HCC

Inflammatory polyarthropathies (M05-M14)

✓4ᵗʰ **M05** Rheumatoid arthritis with rheumatoid factor

   EXCLUDES 1   rheumatic fever (I00)

        juvenile rheumatoid arthritis (M08.-)

        rheumatoid arthritis of spine (M45.-)

   DEF: Rheumatoid arthritis: Autoimmune systemic disease that causes chronic inflammation of the joints and other areas of the body, manifested by inflammatory changes in articular structures and synovial membranes, atrophy, and loss in bone density.

✓5ᵗʰ **M05.0** Felty's syndrome

     Rheumatoid arthritis with splenoadenomegaly and leukopenia

   M05.00 Felty's syndrome, unspecified site   HCC

✓6ᵗʰ **M05.01** Felty's syndrome, shoulder

     M05.011 Felty's syndrome, right shoulder   HCC

     M05.012 Felty's syndrome, left shoulder   HCC

     M05.019 Felty's syndrome, unspecified shoulder   HCC

✓6ᵗʰ **M05.02** Felty's syndrome, elbow

     M05.021 Felty's syndrome, right elbow   HCC

     M05.022 Felty's syndrome, left elbow   HCC

     M05.029 Felty's syndrome, unspecified elbow   HCC

✓6ᵗʰ **M05.03** Felty's syndrome, wrist

     Felty's syndrome, carpal bones

     M05.031 Felty's syndrome, right wrist   HCC

     M05.032 Felty's syndrome, left wrist   HCC

     M05.039 Felty's syndrome, unspecified wrist   HCC

✓6ᵗʰ **M05.04** Felty's syndrome, hand

     Felty's syndrome, metacarpus and phalanges

     M05.041 Felty's syndrome, right hand   HCC

     M05.042 Felty's syndrome, left hand   HCC

N Newborn: 0   P Pediatric: 0-17   M Maternity: 9-64   A Adult: 15-124   MCC Major Complication/Comorbidity   CC Complication/Comorbidity   SW Severe Wound Dx

768   ICD-10-CM 2020

M05.049 Felty's syndrome, unspecified hand HCC

√6ᵗʰ **M05.05** Felty's syndrome, hip

    M05.051 Felty's syndrome, right hip HCC

    M05.052 Felty's syndrome, left hip HCC

    M05.059 Felty's syndrome, unspecified hip HCC

√6ᵗʰ **M05.06** Felty's syndrome, knee

    M05.061 Felty's syndrome, right knee HCC

    M05.062 Felty's syndrome, left knee HCC

    M05.069 Felty's syndrome, unspecified knee HCC

√6ᵗʰ **M05.07** Felty's syndrome, ankle and foot

    Felty's syndrome, tarsus, metatarsus and phalanges

    M05.071 Felty's syndrome, right ankle and foot HCC

    M05.072 Felty's syndrome, left ankle and foot HCC

    M05.079 Felty's syndrome, unspecified ankle and foot HCC

    M05.09 Felty's syndrome, multiple sites HCC

√5ᵗʰ **M05.1** Rheumatoid lung disease with rheumatoid arthritis

    DEF: Lung disorders associated with rheumatoid arthritis.

    M05.10 Rheumatoid lung disease with rheumatoid arthritis of unspecified site HCC

√6ᵗʰ **M05.11** Rheumatoid lung disease with rheumatoid arthritis of shoulder

    M05.111 Rheumatoid lung disease with rheumatoid arthritis of right shoulder HCC

    M05.112 Rheumatoid lung disease with rheumatoid arthritis of left shoulder HCC

    M05.119 Rheumatoid lung disease with rheumatoid arthritis of unspecified shoulder HCC

√6ᵗʰ **M05.12** Rheumatoid lung disease with rheumatoid arthritis of elbow

    M05.121 Rheumatoid lung disease with rheumatoid arthritis of right elbow HCC

    M05.122 Rheumatoid lung disease with rheumatoid arthritis of left elbow HCC

    M05.129 Rheumatoid lung disease with rheumatoid arthritis of unspecified elbow HCC

√6ᵗʰ **M05.13** Rheumatoid lung disease with rheumatoid arthritis of wrist

    Rheumatoid lung disease with rheumatoid arthritis, carpal bones

    M05.131 Rheumatoid lung disease with rheumatoid arthritis of right wrist HCC

    M05.132 Rheumatoid lung disease with rheumatoid arthritis of left wrist HCC

    M05.139 Rheumatoid lung disease with rheumatoid arthritis of unspecified wrist HCC

√6ᵗʰ **M05.14** Rheumatoid lung disease with rheumatoid arthritis of hand

    Rheumatoid lung disease with rheumatoid arthritis, metacarpus and phalanges

    M05.141 Rheumatoid lung disease with rheumatoid arthritis of right hand HCC

    M05.142 Rheumatoid lung disease with rheumatoid arthritis of left hand HCC

    M05.149 Rheumatoid lung disease with rheumatoid arthritis of unspecified hand HCC

√6ᵗʰ **M05.15** Rheumatoid lung disease with rheumatoid arthritis of hip

    M05.151 Rheumatoid lung disease with rheumatoid arthritis of right hip HCC

    M05.152 Rheumatoid lung disease with rheumatoid arthritis of left hip HCC

    M05.159 Rheumatoid lung disease with rheumatoid arthritis of unspecified hip HCC

√6ᵗʰ **M05.16** Rheumatoid lung disease with rheumatoid arthritis of knee

    M05.161 Rheumatoid lung disease with rheumatoid arthritis of right knee HCC

    M05.162 Rheumatoid lung disease with rheumatoid arthritis of left knee HCC

    M05.169 Rheumatoid lung disease with rheumatoid arthritis of unspecified knee HCC

√6ᵗʰ **M05.17** Rheumatoid lung disease with rheumatoid arthritis of ankle and foot

    Rheumatoid lung disease with rheumatoid arthritis, tarsus, metatarsus and phalanges

    M05.171 Rheumatoid lung disease with rheumatoid arthritis of right ankle and foot HCC

    M05.172 Rheumatoid lung disease with rheumatoid arthritis of left ankle and foot HCC

    M05.179 Rheumatoid lung disease with rheumatoid arthritis of unspecified ankle and foot HCC

    M05.19 Rheumatoid lung disease with rheumatoid arthritis of multiple sites HCC

√5ᵗʰ **M05.2** Rheumatoid vasculitis with rheumatoid arthritis

    M05.20 Rheumatoid vasculitis with rheumatoid arthritis of unspecified site HCC

√6ᵗʰ **M05.21** Rheumatoid vasculitis with rheumatoid arthritis of shoulder

    M05.211 Rheumatoid vasculitis with rheumatoid arthritis of right shoulder HCC

    M05.212 Rheumatoid vasculitis with rheumatoid arthritis of left shoulder HCC

    M05.219 Rheumatoid vasculitis with rheumatoid arthritis of unspecified shoulder HCC

√6ᵗʰ **M05.22** Rheumatoid vasculitis with rheumatoid arthritis of elbow

    M05.221 Rheumatoid vasculitis with rheumatoid arthritis of right elbow HCC

    M05.222 Rheumatoid vasculitis with rheumatoid arthritis of left elbow HCC

    M05.229 Rheumatoid vasculitis with rheumatoid arthritis of unspecified elbow HCC

√6ᵗʰ **M05.23** Rheumatoid vasculitis with rheumatoid arthritis of wrist

    Rheumatoid vasculitis with rheumatoid arthritis, carpal bones

    M05.231 Rheumatoid vasculitis with rheumatoid arthritis of right wrist HCC

    M05.232 Rheumatoid vasculitis with rheumatoid arthritis of left wrist HCC

    M05.239 Rheumatoid vasculitis with rheumatoid arthritis of unspecified wrist HCC

√6ᵗʰ **M05.24** Rheumatoid vasculitis with rheumatoid arthritis of hand

    Rheumatoid vasculitis with rheumatoid arthritis, metacarpus and phalanges

    M05.241 Rheumatoid vasculitis with rheumatoid arthritis of right hand HCC

    M05.242 Rheumatoid vasculitis with rheumatoid arthritis of left hand HCC

☑ Additional Character Required   √x7ᵗʰ Placeholder   Unacceptable PDx   Questionable PDx   Manifestation   Unspecified Dx   H1-H4 HAC   HCC CMS-HCC Dx   HIV HIV Dx

ICD-10-CM 2020   **769**

  M05.249   Rheumatoid vasculitis with rheumatoid arthritis of unspecified hand   HCC

✓6th   **M05.25**   Rheumatoid vasculitis with rheumatoid arthritis of hip

  M05.251   Rheumatoid vasculitis with rheumatoid arthritis of right hip   HCC

  M05.252   Rheumatoid vasculitis with rheumatoid arthritis of left hip   HCC

  M05.259   Rheumatoid vasculitis with rheumatoid arthritis of unspecified hip   HCC

✓6th   **M05.26**   Rheumatoid vasculitis with rheumatoid arthritis of knee

  M05.261   Rheumatoid vasculitis with rheumatoid arthritis of right knee   HCC

  M05.262   Rheumatoid vasculitis with rheumatoid arthritis of left knee   HCC

  M05.269   Rheumatoid vasculitis with rheumatoid arthritis of unspecified knee   HCC

✓6th   **M05.27**   Rheumatoid vasculitis with rheumatoid arthritis of ankle and foot

  Rheumatoid vasculitis with rheumatoid arthritis, tarsus, metatarsus and phalanges

  M05.271   Rheumatoid vasculitis with rheumatoid arthritis of right ankle and foot   HCC

  M05.272   Rheumatoid vasculitis with rheumatoid arthritis of left ankle and foot   HCC

  M05.279   Rheumatoid vasculitis with rheumatoid arthritis of unspecified ankle and foot   HCC

  M05.29   Rheumatoid vasculitis with rheumatoid arthritis of multiple sites   HCC

✓5th   **M05.3**   Rheumatoid heart disease with rheumatoid arthritis

  Rheumatoid carditis

  Rheumatoid endocarditis

  Rheumatoid myocarditis

  Rheumatoid pericarditis

  M05.30   Rheumatoid heart disease with rheumatoid arthritis of unspecified site   HCC

✓6th   **M05.31**   Rheumatoid heart disease with rheumatoid arthritis of shoulder

  M05.311   Rheumatoid heart disease with rheumatoid arthritis of right shoulder   HCC

  M05.312   Rheumatoid heart disease with rheumatoid arthritis of left shoulder   HCC

  M05.319   Rheumatoid heart disease with rheumatoid arthritis of unspecified shoulder   HCC

✓6th   **M05.32**   Rheumatoid heart disease with rheumatoid arthritis of elbow

  M05.321   Rheumatoid heart disease with rheumatoid arthritis of right elbow   HCC

  M05.322   Rheumatoid heart disease with rheumatoid arthritis of left elbow   HCC

  M05.329   Rheumatoid heart disease with rheumatoid arthritis of unspecified elbow   HCC

✓6th   **M05.33**   Rheumatoid heart disease with rheumatoid arthritis of wrist

  Rheumatoid heart disease with rheumatoid arthritis, carpal bones

  M05.331   Rheumatoid heart disease with rheumatoid arthritis of right wrist   HCC

  M05.332   Rheumatoid heart disease with rheumatoid arthritis of left wrist   HCC

  M05.339   Rheumatoid heart disease with rheumatoid arthritis of unspecified wrist   HCC

✓6th   **M05.34**   Rheumatoid heart disease with rheumatoid arthritis of hand

  Rheumatoid heart disease with rheumatoid arthritis, metacarpus and phalanges

  M05.341   Rheumatoid heart disease with rheumatoid arthritis of right hand   HCC

  M05.342   Rheumatoid heart disease with rheumatoid arthritis of left hand   HCC

  M05.349   Rheumatoid heart disease with rheumatoid arthritis of unspecified hand   HCC

✓6th   **M05.35**   Rheumatoid heart disease with rheumatoid arthritis of hip

  M05.351   Rheumatoid heart disease with rheumatoid arthritis of right hip   HCC

  M05.352   Rheumatoid heart disease with rheumatoid arthritis of left hip   HCC

  M05.359   Rheumatoid heart disease with rheumatoid arthritis of unspecified hip   HCC

✓6th   **M05.36**   Rheumatoid heart disease with rheumatoid arthritis of knee

  M05.361   Rheumatoid heart disease with rheumatoid arthritis of right knee   HCC

  M05.362   Rheumatoid heart disease with rheumatoid arthritis of left knee   HCC

  M05.369   Rheumatoid heart disease with rheumatoid arthritis of unspecified knee   HCC

✓6th   **M05.37**   Rheumatoid heart disease with rheumatoid arthritis of ankle and foot

  Rheumatoid heart disease with rheumatoid arthritis, tarsus, metatarsus and phalanges

  M05.371   Rheumatoid heart disease with rheumatoid arthritis of right ankle and foot   HCC

  M05.372   Rheumatoid heart disease with rheumatoid arthritis of left ankle and foot   HCC

  M05.379   Rheumatoid heart disease with rheumatoid arthritis of unspecified ankle and foot   HCC

  M05.39   Rheumatoid heart disease with rheumatoid arthritis of multiple sites   HCC

✓5th   **M05.4**   Rheumatoid myopathy with rheumatoid arthritis

  M05.40   Rheumatoid myopathy with rheumatoid arthritis of unspecified site   HCC

✓6th   **M05.41**   Rheumatoid myopathy with rheumatoid arthritis of shoulder

  M05.411   Rheumatoid myopathy with rheumatoid arthritis of right shoulder   HCC

  M05.412   Rheumatoid myopathy with rheumatoid arthritis of left shoulder   HCC

  M05.419   Rheumatoid myopathy with rheumatoid arthritis of unspecified shoulder   HCC

✓6th   **M05.42**   Rheumatoid myopathy with rheumatoid arthritis of elbow

  M05.421   Rheumatoid myopathy with rheumatoid arthritis of right elbow   HCC

  M05.422   Rheumatoid myopathy with rheumatoid arthritis of left elbow   HCC

  M05.429   Rheumatoid myopathy with rheumatoid arthritis of unspecified elbow   HCC

✓6th   **M05.43**   Rheumatoid myopathy with rheumatoid arthritis of wrist

  Rheumatoid myopathy with rheumatoid arthritis, carpal bones

  M05.431   Rheumatoid myopathy with rheumatoid arthritis of right wrist   HCC

N Newborn: 0   P Pediatric: 0-17   M Maternity: 9-64   A Adult: 15-124   MCC Major Complication/Comorbidity   CC Complication/Comorbidity   SW Severe Wound Dx

770   ICD-10-CM 2020

        M05.432 **Rheumatoid myopathy** `HCC`
              with rheumatoid arthritis
              of left wrist

        M05.439 **Rheumatoid myopathy** `HCC`
              with rheumatoid arthritis
              of unspecified wrist

√6ᵗʰ **M05.44** **Rheumatoid myopathy with rheumatoid arthritis of hand**
         Rheumatoid myopathy with rheumatoid arthritis, metacarpus and phalanges

        M05.441 **Rheumatoid myopathy** `HCC`
              with rheumatoid arthritis
              of right hand

        M05.442 **Rheumatoid myopathy** `HCC`
              with rheumatoid arthritis
              of left hand

        M05.449 **Rheumatoid myopathy** `HCC`
              with rheumatoid arthritis
              of unspecified hand

√6ᵗʰ **M05.45** **Rheumatoid myopathy with rheumatoid arthritis of hip**

        M05.451 **Rheumatoid myopathy** `HCC`
              with rheumatoid arthritis
              of right hip

        M05.452 **Rheumatoid myopathy** `HCC`
              with rheumatoid arthritis
              of left hip

        M05.459 **Rheumatoid myopathy** `HCC`
              with rheumatoid arthritis
              of unspecified hip

√6ᵗʰ **M05.46** **Rheumatoid myopathy with rheumatoid arthritis of knee**

        M05.461 **Rheumatoid myopathy** `HCC`
              with rheumatoid arthritis
              of right knee

        M05.462 **Rheumatoid myopathy** `HCC`
              with rheumatoid arthritis
              of left knee

        M05.469 **Rheumatoid myopathy** `HCC`
              with rheumatoid arthritis
              of unspecified knee

√6ᵗʰ **M05.47** **Rheumatoid myopathy with rheumatoid arthritis of ankle and foot**
         Rheumatoid myopathy with rheumatoid arthritis, tarsus, metatarsus and phalanges

        M05.471 **Rheumatoid myopathy** `HCC`
              with rheumatoid arthritis
              of right ankle and foot

        M05.472 **Rheumatoid myopathy** `HCC`
              with rheumatoid arthritis
              of left ankle and foot

        M05.479 **Rheumatoid myopathy** `HCC`
              with rheumatoid arthritis
              of unspecified ankle and foot

        M05.49 **Rheumatoid myopathy with** `HCC`
              rheumatoid arthritis of multiple sites

√5ᵗʰ **M05.5** **Rheumatoid polyneuropathy with rheumatoid arthritis**

      M05.50 **Rheumatoid polyneuropathy with** `HCC`
           rheumatoid arthritis of unspecified site

√6ᵗʰ **M05.51** **Rheumatoid polyneuropathy with rheumatoid arthritis of shoulder**

        M05.511 **Rheumatoid** `HCC`
              polyneuropathy with
              rheumatoid arthritis of
              right shoulder

        M05.512 **Rheumatoid** `HCC`
              polyneuropathy with
              rheumatoid arthritis of
              left shoulder

        M05.519 **Rheumatoid** `HCC`
              polyneuropathy with
              rheumatoid arthritis of
              unspecified shoulder

√6ᵗʰ **M05.52** **Rheumatoid polyneuropathy with rheumatoid arthritis of elbow**

        M05.521 **Rheumatoid** `HCC`
              polyneuropathy with
              rheumatoid arthritis of
              right elbow

        M05.522 **Rheumatoid** `HCC`
              polyneuropathy with
              rheumatoid arthritis of
              left elbow

        M05.529 **Rheumatoid** `HCC`
              polyneuropathy with
              rheumatoid arthritis of
              unspecified elbow

√6ᵗʰ **M05.53** **Rheumatoid polyneuropathy with rheumatoid arthritis of wrist**
         Rheumatoid polyneuropathy with rheumatoid arthritis, carpal bones

        M05.531 **Rheumatoid** `HCC`
              polyneuropathy with
              rheumatoid arthritis of
              right wrist

        M05.532 **Rheumatoid** `HCC`
              polyneuropathy with
              rheumatoid arthritis of
              left wrist

        M05.539 **Rheumatoid** `HCC`
              polyneuropathy with
              rheumatoid arthritis of
              unspecified wrist

√6ᵗʰ **M05.54** **Rheumatoid polyneuropathy with rheumatoid arthritis of hand**
         Rheumatoid polyneuropathy with rheumatoid arthritis, metacarpus and phalanges

        M05.541 **Rheumatoid** `HCC`
              polyneuropathy with
              rheumatoid arthritis of
              right hand

        M05.542 **Rheumatoid** `HCC`
              polyneuropathy with
              rheumatoid arthritis of
              left hand

        M05.549 **Rheumatoid** `HCC`
              polyneuropathy with
              rheumatoid arthritis of
              unspecified hand

√6ᵗʰ **M05.55** **Rheumatoid polyneuropathy with rheumatoid arthritis of hip**

        M05.551 **Rheumatoid** `HCC`
              polyneuropathy with
              rheumatoid arthritis of
              right hip

        M05.552 **Rheumatoid** `HCC`
              polyneuropathy with
              rheumatoid arthritis of
              left hip

        M05.559 **Rheumatoid** `HCC`
              polyneuropathy with
              rheumatoid arthritis of
              unspecified hip

√6ᵗʰ **M05.56** **Rheumatoid polyneuropathy with rheumatoid arthritis of knee**

        M05.561 **Rheumatoid** `HCC`
              polyneuropathy with
              rheumatoid arthritis of
              right knee

        M05.562 **Rheumatoid** `HCC`
              polyneuropathy with
              rheumatoid arthritis of
              left knee

        M05.569 **Rheumatoid** `HCC`
              polyneuropathy with
              rheumatoid arthritis of
              unspecified knee

√6ᵗʰ **M05.57** **Rheumatoid polyneuropathy with rheumatoid arthritis of ankle and foot**
         Rheumatoid polyneuropathy with rheumatoid arthritis, tarsus, metatarsus and phalanges

        M05.571 **Rheumatoid** `HCC`
              polyneuropathy with
              rheumatoid arthritis of
              right ankle and foot

        M05.572 **Rheumatoid** `HCC`
              polyneuropathy with
              rheumatoid arthritis of
              left ankle and foot

        M05.579 **Rheumatoid** `HCC`
              polyneuropathy with
              rheumatoid arthritis of
              unspecified ankle and foot

☑ Additional Character Required   √x7ᵗʰ Placeholder   Unacceptable PDx   Questionable PDx   Manifestation   Unspecified Dx   H1-H14 HAC   HCC CMS-HCC Dx   HIV HIV Dx

ICD-10-CM 2020   771

M05.59 Rheumatoid polyneuropathy with rheumatoid arthritis of multiple sites `HCC`

✓5ᵗʰ **M05.6** Rheumatoid arthritis with involvement of other organs and systems

    M05.60 Rheumatoid arthritis of unspecified site with involvement of other organs and systems `HCC`

✓6ᵗʰ **M05.61** Rheumatoid arthritis of shoulder with involvement of other organs and systems

    M05.611 Rheumatoid arthritis of right shoulder with involvement of other organs and systems `HCC`

    M05.612 Rheumatoid arthritis of left shoulder with involvement of other organs and systems `HCC`

    M05.619 Rheumatoid arthritis of unspecified shoulder with involvement of other organs and systems `HCC`

✓6ᵗʰ **M05.62** Rheumatoid arthritis of elbow with involvement of other organs and systems

    M05.621 Rheumatoid arthritis of right elbow with involvement of other organs and systems `HCC`

    M05.622 Rheumatoid arthritis of left elbow with involvement of other organs and systems `HCC`

    M05.629 Rheumatoid arthritis of unspecified elbow with involvement of other organs and systems `HCC`

✓6ᵗʰ **M05.63** Rheumatoid arthritis of wrist with involvement of other organs and systems

Rheumatoid arthritis of carpal bones with involvement of other organs and systems

    M05.631 Rheumatoid arthritis of right wrist with involvement of other organs and systems `HCC`

    M05.632 Rheumatoid arthritis of left wrist with involvement of other organs and systems `HCC`

    M05.639 Rheumatoid arthritis of unspecified wrist with involvement of other organs and systems `HCC`

✓6ᵗʰ **M05.64** Rheumatoid arthritis of hand with involvement of other organs and systems

Rheumatoid arthritis of metacarpus and phalanges with involvement of other organs and systems

    M05.641 Rheumatoid arthritis of right hand with involvement of other organs and systems `HCC`

    M05.642 Rheumatoid arthritis of left hand with involvement of other organs and systems `HCC`

    M05.649 Rheumatoid arthritis of unspecified hand with involvement of other organs and systems `HCC`

✓6ᵗʰ **M05.65** Rheumatoid arthritis of hip with involvement of other organs and systems

    M05.651 Rheumatoid arthritis of right hip with involvement of other organs and systems `HCC`

    M05.652 Rheumatoid arthritis of left hip with involvement of other organs and systems `HCC`

    M05.659 Rheumatoid arthritis of unspecified hip with involvement of other organs and systems `HCC`

✓6ᵗʰ **M05.66** Rheumatoid arthritis of knee with involvement of other organs and systems

    M05.661 Rheumatoid arthritis of right knee with involvement of other organs and systems `HCC`

    M05.662 Rheumatoid arthritis of left knee with involvement of other organs and systems `HCC`

    M05.669 Rheumatoid arthritis of unspecified knee with involvement of other organs and systems `HCC`

✓6ᵗʰ **M05.67** Rheumatoid arthritis of ankle and foot with involvement of other organs and systems

Rheumatoid arthritis of tarsus, metatarsus and phalanges with involvement of other organs and systems

    M05.671 Rheumatoid arthritis of right ankle and foot with involvement of other organs and systems `HCC`

    M05.672 Rheumatoid arthritis of left ankle and foot with involvement of other organs and systems `HCC`

    M05.679 Rheumatoid arthritis of unspecified ankle and foot with involvement of other organs and systems `HCC`

M05.69 Rheumatoid arthritis of multiple sites with involvement of other organs and systems `HCC`

✓5ᵗʰ **M05.7** Rheumatoid arthritis with rheumatoid factor without organ or systems involvement

    M05.70 Rheumatoid arthritis with rheumatoid factor of unspecified site without organ or systems involvement `HCC`

✓6ᵗʰ **M05.71** Rheumatoid arthritis with rheumatoid factor of shoulder without organ or systems involvement

    M05.711 Rheumatoid arthritis with rheumatoid factor of right shoulder without organ or systems involvement `HCC`

    M05.712 Rheumatoid arthritis with rheumatoid factor of left shoulder without organ or systems involvement `HCC`

    M05.719 Rheumatoid arthritis with rheumatoid factor of unspecified shoulder without organ or systems involvement `HCC`

✓6ᵗʰ **M05.72** Rheumatoid arthritis with rheumatoid factor of elbow without organ or systems involvement

    M05.721 Rheumatoid arthritis with rheumatoid factor of right elbow without organ or systems involvement `HCC`

    M05.722 Rheumatoid arthritis with rheumatoid factor of left elbow without organ or systems involvement `HCC`

    M05.729 Rheumatoid arthritis with rheumatoid factor of unspecified elbow without organ or systems involvement `HCC`

✓6ᵗʰ **M05.73** Rheumatoid arthritis with rheumatoid factor of wrist without organ or systems involvement

    M05.731 Rheumatoid arthritis with rheumatoid factor of right wrist without organ or systems involvement `HCC`

    M05.732 Rheumatoid arthritis with rheumatoid factor of left wrist without organ or systems involvement `HCC`

    M05.739 Rheumatoid arthritis with rheumatoid factor of unspecified wrist without organ or systems involvement `HCC`

Ⓝ Newborn: 0   Ⓟ Pediatric: 0-17   Ⓜ Maternity: 9-64   Ⓐ Adult: 15-124   `MCC` Major Complication/Comorbidity   `CC` Complication/Comorbidity   `SW` Severe Wound Dx

772   ICD-10-CM 2020

√6ᵗʰ **M05.74** **Rheumatoid arthritis with rheumatoid factor of hand without organ or systems involvement**

    M05.741 Rheumatoid arthritis with rheumatoid factor of right hand without organ or systems involvement   `HCC`

    M05.742 Rheumatoid arthritis with rheumatoid factor of left hand without organ or systems involvement   `HCC`

    M05.749 Rheumatoid arthritis with rheumatoid factor of unspecified hand without organ or systems involvement   `HCC`

√6ᵗʰ **M05.75** **Rheumatoid arthritis with rheumatoid factor of hip without organ or systems involvement**

    M05.751 Rheumatoid arthritis with rheumatoid factor of right hip without organ or systems involvement   `HCC`

    M05.752 Rheumatoid arthritis with rheumatoid factor of left hip without organ or systems involvement   `HCC`

    M05.759 Rheumatoid arthritis with rheumatoid factor of unspecified hip without organ or systems involvement   `HCC`

√6ᵗʰ **M05.76** **Rheumatoid arthritis with rheumatoid factor of knee without organ or systems involvement**

    M05.761 Rheumatoid arthritis with rheumatoid factor of right knee without organ or systems involvement   `HCC`

    M05.762 Rheumatoid arthritis with rheumatoid factor of left knee without organ or systems involvement   `HCC`

    M05.769 Rheumatoid arthritis with rheumatoid factor of unspecified knee without organ or systems involvement   `HCC`

√6ᵗʰ **M05.77** **Rheumatoid arthritis with rheumatoid factor of ankle and foot without organ or systems involvement**

    M05.771 Rheumatoid arthritis with rheumatoid factor of right ankle and foot without organ or systems involvement   `HCC`

    M05.772 Rheumatoid arthritis with rheumatoid factor of left ankle and foot without organ or systems involvement   `HCC`

    M05.779 Rheumatoid arthritis with rheumatoid factor of unspecified ankle and foot without organ or systems involvement   `HCC`

    M05.79 Rheumatoid arthritis with rheumatoid factor of multiple sites without organ or systems involvement   `HCC`

√5ᵗʰ **M05.8** **Other rheumatoid arthritis with rheumatoid factor**

    M05.80 Other rheumatoid arthritis with rheumatoid factor of unspecified site   `HCC`

√6ᵗʰ **M05.81** **Other rheumatoid arthritis with rheumatoid factor of shoulder**

    M05.811 Other rheumatoid arthritis with rheumatoid factor of right shoulder   `HCC`

    M05.812 Other rheumatoid arthritis with rheumatoid factor of left shoulder   `HCC`

    M05.819 Other rheumatoid arthritis with rheumatoid factor of unspecified shoulder   `HCC`

√6ᵗʰ **M05.82** **Other rheumatoid arthritis with rheumatoid factor of elbow**

    M05.821 Other rheumatoid arthritis with rheumatoid factor of right elbow   `HCC`

    M05.822 Other rheumatoid arthritis with rheumatoid factor of left elbow   `HCC`

    M05.829 Other rheumatoid arthritis with rheumatoid factor of unspecified elbow   `HCC`

√6ᵗʰ **M05.83** **Other rheumatoid arthritis with rheumatoid factor of wrist**

    M05.831 Other rheumatoid arthritis with rheumatoid factor of right wrist   `HCC`

    M05.832 Other rheumatoid arthritis with rheumatoid factor of left wrist   `HCC`

    M05.839 Other rheumatoid arthritis with rheumatoid factor of unspecified wrist   `HCC`

√6ᵗʰ **M05.84** **Other rheumatoid arthritis with rheumatoid factor of hand**

    M05.841 Other rheumatoid arthritis with rheumatoid factor of right hand   `HCC`

    M05.842 Other rheumatoid arthritis with rheumatoid factor of left hand   `HCC`

    M05.849 Other rheumatoid arthritis with rheumatoid factor of unspecified hand   `HCC`

√6ᵗʰ **M05.85** **Other rheumatoid arthritis with rheumatoid factor of hip**

    M05.851 Other rheumatoid arthritis with rheumatoid factor of right hip   `HCC`

    M05.852 Other rheumatoid arthritis with rheumatoid factor of left hip   `HCC`

    M05.859 Other rheumatoid arthritis with rheumatoid factor of unspecified hip   `HCC`

√6ᵗʰ **M05.86** **Other rheumatoid arthritis with rheumatoid factor of knee**

    M05.861 Other rheumatoid arthritis with rheumatoid factor of right knee   `HCC`

    M05.862 Other rheumatoid arthritis with rheumatoid factor of left knee   `HCC`

    M05.869 Other rheumatoid arthritis with rheumatoid factor of unspecified knee   `HCC`

√6ᵗʰ **M05.87** **Other rheumatoid arthritis with rheumatoid factor of ankle and foot**

    M05.871 Other rheumatoid arthritis with rheumatoid factor of right ankle and foot   `HCC`

    M05.872 Other rheumatoid arthritis with rheumatoid factor of left ankle and foot   `HCC`

    M05.879 Other rheumatoid arthritis with rheumatoid factor of unspecified ankle and foot   `HCC`

    M05.89 Other rheumatoid arthritis with rheumatoid factor of multiple sites   `HCC`

    M05.9 Rheumatoid arthritis with rheumatoid factor, unspecified   `HCC`

√4ᵗʰ **M06** **Other rheumatoid arthritis**

DEF: Rheumatoid arthritis: Autoimmune systemic disease that causes chronic inflammation of the joints and other areas of the body, manifested by inflammatory changes in articular structures and synovial membranes, atrophy, and loss in bone density.

√5ᵗʰ **M06.0** **Rheumatoid arthritis without rheumatoid factor**

    M06.00 Rheumatoid arthritis without rheumatoid factor, unspecified site   `HCC`

√6ᵗʰ **M06.01** **Rheumatoid arthritis without rheumatoid factor, shoulder**

    M06.011 Rheumatoid arthritis without rheumatoid factor, right shoulder   `HCC`

✔ Additional Character Required   √x7ᵗʰ Placeholder   Unacceptable PDx   Questionable PDx   Manifestation   Unspecified Dx   H1-H14 HAC   HCC CMS-HCC Dx   HIV HIV Dx

ICD-10-CM 2020   773

           M06.012 **Rheumatoid arthritis without rheumatoid factor, left shoulder** `HCC`

           M06.019 **Rheumatoid arthritis without rheumatoid factor, unspecified shoulder** `HCC`

✓6ᵗʰ **M06.02** **Rheumatoid arthritis without rheumatoid factor, elbow**

           M06.021 **Rheumatoid arthritis without rheumatoid factor, right elbow** `HCC`

           M06.022 **Rheumatoid arthritis without rheumatoid factor, left elbow** `HCC`

           M06.029 **Rheumatoid arthritis without rheumatoid factor, unspecified elbow** `HCC`

✓6ᵗʰ **M06.03** **Rheumatoid arthritis without rheumatoid factor, wrist**

           M06.031 **Rheumatoid arthritis without rheumatoid factor, right wrist** `HCC`

           M06.032 **Rheumatoid arthritis without rheumatoid factor, left wrist** `HCC`

           M06.039 **Rheumatoid arthritis without rheumatoid factor, unspecified wrist** `HCC`

✓6ᵗʰ **M06.04** **Rheumatoid arthritis without rheumatoid factor, hand**

           M06.041 **Rheumatoid arthritis without rheumatoid factor, right hand** `HCC`

           M06.042 **Rheumatoid arthritis without rheumatoid factor, left hand** `HCC`

           M06.049 **Rheumatoid arthritis without rheumatoid factor, unspecified hand** `HCC`

✓6ᵗʰ **M06.05** **Rheumatoid arthritis without rheumatoid factor, hip**

           M06.051 **Rheumatoid arthritis without rheumatoid factor, right hip** `HCC`

           M06.052 **Rheumatoid arthritis without rheumatoid factor, left hip** `HCC`

           M06.059 **Rheumatoid arthritis without rheumatoid factor, unspecified hip** `HCC`

✓6ᵗʰ **M06.06** **Rheumatoid arthritis without rheumatoid factor, knee**

           M06.061 **Rheumatoid arthritis without rheumatoid factor, right knee** `HCC`

           M06.062 **Rheumatoid arthritis without rheumatoid factor, left knee** `HCC`

           M06.069 **Rheumatoid arthritis without rheumatoid factor, unspecified knee** `HCC`

✓6ᵗʰ **M06.07** **Rheumatoid arthritis without rheumatoid factor, ankle and foot**

           M06.071 **Rheumatoid arthritis without rheumatoid factor, right ankle and foot** `HCC`

           M06.072 **Rheumatoid arthritis without rheumatoid factor, left ankle and foot** `HCC`

           M06.079 **Rheumatoid arthritis without rheumatoid factor, unspecified ankle and foot** `HCC`

    M06.08 **Rheumatoid arthritis without rheumatoid factor, vertebrae** `HCC`

    M06.09 **Rheumatoid arthritis without rheumatoid factor, multiple sites** `HCC`

M06.1 **Adult-onset Still's disease** `HCC` `A`

    EXCLUDES 1   *Still's disease NOS (M08.2-)*

    DEF: Type of systemic arthritis characterized by a transient rash and spiking fevers. This condition may resolve or develop into a chronic condition and may affect internal organs, as well as joints.

    Synonym(s): AOSD

✓5ᵗʰ **M06.2** **Rheumatoid bursitis**

    M06.20 **Rheumatoid bursitis, unspecified site** `HCC`

✓6ᵗʰ **M06.21** **Rheumatoid bursitis, shoulder**

           M06.211 **Rheumatoid bursitis, right shoulder** `HCC`

           M06.212 **Rheumatoid bursitis, left shoulder** `HCC`

           M06.219 **Rheumatoid bursitis, unspecified shoulder** `HCC`

✓6ᵗʰ **M06.22** **Rheumatoid bursitis, elbow**

           M06.221 **Rheumatoid bursitis, right elbow** `HCC`

           M06.222 **Rheumatoid bursitis, left elbow** `HCC`

           M06.229 **Rheumatoid bursitis, unspecified elbow** `HCC`

✓6ᵗʰ **M06.23** **Rheumatoid bursitis, wrist**

           M06.231 **Rheumatoid bursitis, right wrist** `HCC`

           M06.232 **Rheumatoid bursitis, left wrist** `HCC`

           M06.239 **Rheumatoid bursitis, unspecified wrist** `HCC`

✓6ᵗʰ **M06.24** **Rheumatoid bursitis, hand**

           M06.241 **Rheumatoid bursitis, right hand** `HCC`

           M06.242 **Rheumatoid bursitis, left hand** `HCC`

           M06.249 **Rheumatoid bursitis, unspecified hand** `HCC`

✓6ᵗʰ **M06.25** **Rheumatoid bursitis, hip**

           M06.251 **Rheumatoid bursitis, right hip** `HCC`

           M06.252 **Rheumatoid bursitis, left hip** `HCC`

           M06.259 **Rheumatoid bursitis, unspecified hip** `HCC`

✓6ᵗʰ **M06.26** **Rheumatoid bursitis, knee**

           M06.261 **Rheumatoid bursitis, right knee** `HCC`

           M06.262 **Rheumatoid bursitis, left knee** `HCC`

           M06.269 **Rheumatoid bursitis, unspecified knee** `HCC`

✓6ᵗʰ **M06.27** **Rheumatoid bursitis, ankle and foot**

           M06.271 **Rheumatoid bursitis, right ankle and foot** `HCC`

           M06.272 **Rheumatoid bursitis, left ankle and foot** `HCC`

           M06.279 **Rheumatoid bursitis, unspecified ankle and foot** `HCC`

    M06.28 **Rheumatoid bursitis, vertebrae** `HCC`

    M06.29 **Rheumatoid bursitis, multiple sites** `HCC`

✓5ᵗʰ **M06.3** **Rheumatoid nodule**

    M06.30 **Rheumatoid nodule, unspecified site** `HCC`

✓6ᵗʰ **M06.31** **Rheumatoid nodule, shoulder**

           M06.311 **Rheumatoid nodule, right shoulder** `HCC`

           M06.312 **Rheumatoid nodule, left shoulder** `HCC`

           M06.319 **Rheumatoid nodule, unspecified shoulder** `HCC`

✓6ᵗʰ **M06.32** **Rheumatoid nodule, elbow**

           M06.321 **Rheumatoid nodule, right elbow** `HCC`

           M06.322 **Rheumatoid nodule, left elbow** `HCC`

           M06.329 **Rheumatoid nodule, unspecified elbow** `HCC`

✓6ᵗʰ **M06.33** **Rheumatoid nodule, wrist**

           M06.331 **Rheumatoid nodule, right wrist** `HCC`

`N` Newborn: 0   `P` Pediatric: 0-17   `M` Maternity: 9-64   `A` Adult: 15-124   `MCC` Major Complication/Comorbidity   `CC` Complication/Comorbidity   `SW` Severe Wound Dx

774   ICD-10-CM 2020

M06.332 **Rheumatoid nodule, left wrist** `HCC`

M06.339 **Rheumatoid nodule, unspecified wrist** `HCC`

√6ᵗʰ M06.34 **Rheumatoid nodule, hand**

M06.341 **Rheumatoid nodule, right hand** `HCC`

M06.342 **Rheumatoid nodule, left hand** `HCC`

M06.349 **Rheumatoid nodule, unspecified hand** `HCC`

√6ᵗʰ M06.35 **Rheumatoid nodule, hip**

M06.351 **Rheumatoid nodule, right hip** `HCC`

M06.352 **Rheumatoid nodule, left hip** `HCC`

M06.359 **Rheumatoid nodule, unspecified hip** `HCC`

√6ᵗʰ M06.36 **Rheumatoid nodule, knee**

M06.361 **Rheumatoid nodule, right knee** `HCC`

M06.362 **Rheumatoid nodule, left knee** `HCC`

M06.369 **Rheumatoid nodule, unspecified knee** `HCC`

√6ᵗʰ M06.37 **Rheumatoid nodule, ankle and foot**

M06.371 **Rheumatoid nodule, right ankle and foot** `HCC`

M06.372 **Rheumatoid nodule, left ankle and foot** `HCC`

M06.379 **Rheumatoid nodule, unspecified ankle and foot** `HCC`

M06.38 **Rheumatoid nodule, vertebrae** `HCC`

M06.39 **Rheumatoid nodule, multiple sites** `HCC`

M06.4 **Inflammatory polyarthropathy** `HCC`

EXCLUDES 1 *polyarthritis NOS (M13.0)*

√5ᵗʰ M06.8 **Other specified rheumatoid arthritis**

M06.80 **Other specified rheumatoid arthritis, unspecified site** `HCC`

√6ᵗʰ M06.81 **Other specified rheumatoid arthritis, shoulder**

M06.811 **Other specified rheumatoid arthritis, right shoulder** `HCC`

M06.812 **Other specified rheumatoid arthritis, left shoulder** `HCC`

M06.819 **Other specified rheumatoid arthritis, unspecified shoulder** `HCC`

√6ᵗʰ M06.82 **Other specified rheumatoid arthritis, elbow**

M06.821 **Other specified rheumatoid arthritis, right elbow** `HCC`

M06.822 **Other specified rheumatoid arthritis, left elbow** `HCC`

M06.829 **Other specified rheumatoid arthritis, unspecified elbow** `HCC`

√6ᵗʰ M06.83 **Other specified rheumatoid arthritis, wrist**

M06.831 **Other specified rheumatoid arthritis, right wrist** `HCC`

M06.832 **Other specified rheumatoid arthritis, left wrist** `HCC`

M06.839 **Other specified rheumatoid arthritis, unspecified wrist** `HCC`

√6ᵗʰ M06.84 **Other specified rheumatoid arthritis, hand**

M06.841 **Other specified rheumatoid arthritis, right hand** `HCC`

M06.842 **Other specified rheumatoid arthritis, left hand** `HCC`

M06.849 **Other specified rheumatoid arthritis, unspecified hand** `HCC`

√6ᵗʰ M06.85 **Other specified rheumatoid arthritis, hip**

M06.851 **Other specified rheumatoid arthritis, right hip** `HCC`

M06.852 **Other specified rheumatoid arthritis, left hip** `HCC`

M06.859 **Other specified rheumatoid arthritis, unspecified hip** `HCC`

√6ᵗʰ M06.86 **Other specified rheumatoid arthritis, knee**

M06.861 **Other specified rheumatoid arthritis, right knee** `HCC`

M06.862 **Other specified rheumatoid arthritis, left knee** `HCC`

M06.869 **Other specified rheumatoid arthritis, unspecified knee** `HCC`

√6ᵗʰ M06.87 **Other specified rheumatoid arthritis, ankle and foot**

M06.871 **Other specified rheumatoid arthritis, right ankle and foot** `HCC`

M06.872 **Other specified rheumatoid arthritis, left ankle and foot** `HCC`

M06.879 **Other specified rheumatoid arthritis, unspecified ankle and foot** `HCC`

M06.88 **Other specified rheumatoid arthritis, vertebrae** `HCC`

M06.89 **Other specified rheumatoid arthritis, multiple sites** `HCC`

M06.9 **Rheumatoid arthritis, unspecified** `HCC`

√4ᵗʰ **M07 Enteropathic arthropathies**

Code also associated enteropathy, such as:
regional enteritis [Crohn's disease] (K50.-)
ulcerative colitis (K51.-)

EXCLUDES 1 *psoriatic arthropathies (L40.5-)*

√5ᵗʰ M07.6 **Enteropathic arthropathies**

M07.60 **Enteropathic arthropathies, unspecified site**

√6ᵗʰ M07.61 **Enteropathic arthropathies, shoulder**

M07.611 **Enteropathic arthropathies, right shoulder**

M07.612 **Enteropathic arthropathies, left shoulder**

M07.619 **Enteropathic arthropathies, unspecified shoulder**

√6ᵗʰ M07.62 **Enteropathic arthropathies, elbow**

M07.621 **Enteropathic arthropathies, right elbow**

M07.622 **Enteropathic arthropathies, left elbow**

M07.629 **Enteropathic arthropathies, unspecified elbow**

√6ᵗʰ M07.63 **Enteropathic arthropathies, wrist**

M07.631 **Enteropathic arthropathies, right wrist**

M07.632 **Enteropathic arthropathies, left wrist**

M07.639 **Enteropathic arthropathies, unspecified wrist**

√6ᵗʰ M07.64 **Enteropathic arthropathies, hand**

M07.641 **Enteropathic arthropathies, right hand**

M07.642 **Enteropathic arthropathies, left hand**

M07.649 **Enteropathic arthropathies, unspecified hand**

√6ᵗʰ M07.65 **Enteropathic arthropathies, hip**

M07.651 **Enteropathic arthropathies, right hip**

M07.652 **Enteropathic arthropathies, left hip**

M07.659 **Enteropathic arthropathies, unspecified hip**

√6ᵗʰ M07.66 **Enteropathic arthropathies, knee**

M07.661 **Enteropathic arthropathies, right knee**

M07.662 **Enteropathic arthropathies, left knee**

M07.669 **Enteropathic arthropathies, unspecified knee**

√6ᵗʰ M07.67 **Enteropathic arthropathies, ankle and foot**

M07.671 **Enteropathic arthropathies, right ankle and foot**

M07.672 **Enteropathic arthropathies, left ankle and foot**

✔ Additional Character Required   √x7ᵗʰ Placeholder   Unacceptable PDx   Questionable PDx   Manifestation   Unspecified Dx   H1 -H14 HAC   HCC CMS-HCC Dx   HIV HIV Dx

ICD-10-CM 2020 775

M07.679	Enteropathic arthropathies, unspecified ankle and foot
M07.68	Enteropathic arthropathies, **vertebrae**
M07.69	Enteropathic arthropathies, **multiple sites**

✓4ᵗʰ M08 Juvenile arthritis

Code also any associated underlying condition, such as:
regional enteritis [Crohn's disease] (K50.-)
ulcerative colitis (K51.-)

EXCLUDES 1   arthropathy in Whipple's disease (M14.8)
Felty's syndrome (M05.0)
juvenile dermatomyositis (M33.0-)
psoriatic juvenile arthropathy (L40.54)

✓5ᵗʰ M08.0 Unspecified juvenile rheumatoid arthritis

Juvenile rheumatoid arthritis with or without rheumatoid factor

M08.00	Unspecified juvenile rheumatoid arthritis of unspecified site	HCC
✓6ᵗʰ M08.01	Unspecified juvenile rheumatoid arthritis, **shoulder**	
	M08.011 Unspecified juvenile rheumatoid arthritis, **right** shoulder	HCC
	M08.012 Unspecified juvenile rheumatoid arthritis, **left** shoulder	HCC
	M08.019 Unspecified juvenile rheumatoid arthritis, unspecified shoulder	HCC
✓6ᵗʰ M08.02	Unspecified juvenile rheumatoid arthritis of **elbow**	
	M08.021 Unspecified juvenile rheumatoid arthritis, **right** elbow	HCC
	M08.022 Unspecified juvenile rheumatoid arthritis, **left** elbow	HCC
	M08.029 Unspecified juvenile rheumatoid arthritis, unspecified elbow	HCC
✓6ᵗʰ M08.03	Unspecified juvenile rheumatoid arthritis, **wrist**	
	M08.031 Unspecified juvenile rheumatoid arthritis, **right** wrist	HCC
	M08.032 Unspecified juvenile rheumatoid arthritis, **left** wrist	HCC
	M08.039 Unspecified juvenile rheumatoid arthritis, unspecified wrist	HCC
✓6ᵗʰ M08.04	Unspecified juvenile rheumatoid arthritis, **hand**	
	M08.041 Unspecified juvenile rheumatoid arthritis, **right** hand	HCC
	M08.042 Unspecified juvenile rheumatoid arthritis, **left** hand	HCC
	M08.049 Unspecified juvenile rheumatoid arthritis, unspecified hand	HCC
✓6ᵗʰ M08.05	Unspecified juvenile rheumatoid arthritis, **hip**	
	M08.051 Unspecified juvenile rheumatoid arthritis, **right** hip	HCC
	M08.052 Unspecified juvenile rheumatoid arthritis, **left** hip	HCC
	M08.059 Unspecified juvenile rheumatoid arthritis, unspecified hip	HCC
✓6ᵗʰ M08.06	Unspecified juvenile rheumatoid arthritis, **knee**	
	M08.061 Unspecified juvenile rheumatoid arthritis, **right** knee	HCC
	M08.062 Unspecified juvenile rheumatoid arthritis, **left** knee	HCC
	M08.069 Unspecified juvenile rheumatoid arthritis, unspecified knee	HCC
✓6ᵗʰ M08.07	Unspecified juvenile rheumatoid arthritis, **ankle and foot**	
	M08.071 Unspecified juvenile rheumatoid arthritis, **right** ankle and foot	HCC

M08.072	Unspecified juvenile rheumatoid arthritis, **left** ankle and foot	HCC
M08.079	Unspecified juvenile rheumatoid arthritis, unspecified ankle and foot	HCC
M08.08	Unspecified juvenile rheumatoid arthritis, **vertebrae**	HCC
M08.09	Unspecified juvenile rheumatoid arthritis, **multiple sites**	HCC

M08.1 Juvenile ankylosing spondylitis   HCC

EXCLUDES 1   ankylosing spondylitis in adults (M45.0-)

✓5ᵗʰ M08.2 Juvenile rheumatoid arthritis with systemic onset

Still's disease NOS

EXCLUDES 1   adult-onset Still's disease (M06.1-)

DEF: Systemic juvenile rheumatoid arthritis characterized by a transient rash and spiking fevers that may affect internal organs, as well as joints.

M08.20	Juvenile rheumatoid arthritis with systemic onset, unspecified site	HCC
✓6ᵗʰ M08.21	Juvenile rheumatoid arthritis with systemic onset, **shoulder**	
	M08.211 Juvenile rheumatoid arthritis with systemic onset, **right shoulder**	HCC
	M08.212 Juvenile rheumatoid arthritis with systemic onset, **left shoulder**	HCC
	M08.219 Juvenile rheumatoid arthritis with systemic onset, unspecified shoulder	HCC
✓6ᵗʰ M08.22	Juvenile rheumatoid arthritis with systemic onset, **elbow**	
	M08.221 Juvenile rheumatoid arthritis with systemic onset, **right elbow**	HCC
	M08.222 Juvenile rheumatoid arthritis with systemic onset, **left elbow**	HCC
	M08.229 Juvenile rheumatoid arthritis with systemic onset, unspecified elbow	HCC
✓6ᵗʰ M08.23	Juvenile rheumatoid arthritis with systemic onset, **wrist**	
	M08.231 Juvenile rheumatoid arthritis with systemic onset, **right wrist**	HCC
	M08.232 Juvenile rheumatoid arthritis with systemic onset, **left wrist**	HCC
	M08.239 Juvenile rheumatoid arthritis with systemic onset, unspecified wrist	HCC
✓6ᵗʰ M08.24	Juvenile rheumatoid arthritis with systemic onset, **hand**	
	M08.241 Juvenile rheumatoid arthritis with systemic onset, **right hand**	HCC
	M08.242 Juvenile rheumatoid arthritis with systemic onset, **left hand**	HCC
	M08.249 Juvenile rheumatoid arthritis with systemic onset, unspecified hand	HCC
✓6ᵗʰ M08.25	Juvenile rheumatoid arthritis with systemic onset, **hip**	
	M08.251 Juvenile rheumatoid arthritis with systemic onset, **right hip**	HCC
	M08.252 Juvenile rheumatoid arthritis with systemic onset, **left hip**	HCC
	M08.259 Juvenile rheumatoid arthritis with systemic onset, unspecified hip	HCC
✓6ᵗʰ M08.26	Juvenile rheumatoid arthritis with systemic onset, **knee**	
	M08.261 Juvenile rheumatoid arthritis with systemic onset, **right knee**	HCC
	M08.262 Juvenile rheumatoid arthritis with systemic onset, **left knee**	HCC

Ⓝ Newborn: 0   Ⓟ Pediatric: 0-17   Ⓜ Maternity: 9-64   Ⓐ Adult: 15-124   **MCC** Major Complication/Comorbidity   **CC** Complication/Comorbidity   **SW** Severe Wound Dx

776   ICD-10-CM 2020

M08.269   **Juvenile rheumatoid arthritis with systemic onset, unspecified knee**   HCC

√6ᵗʰ   **M08.27**   **Juvenile rheumatoid arthritis with systemic onset, ankle and foot**

M08.271   **Juvenile rheumatoid arthritis with systemic onset, right ankle and foot**   HCC

M08.272   **Juvenile rheumatoid arthritis with systemic onset, left ankle and foot**   HCC

M08.279   **Juvenile rheumatoid arthritis with systemic onset, unspecified ankle and foot**   HCC

M08.28   **Juvenile rheumatoid arthritis with systemic onset, vertebrae**   HCC

M08.29   **Juvenile rheumatoid arthritis with systemic onset, multiple sites**   HCC

M08.3   **Juvenile rheumatoid polyarthritis (seronegative)**   HCC

√5ᵗʰ   **M08.4**   **Pauciarticular juvenile rheumatoid arthritis**

M08.40   **Pauciarticular juvenile rheumatoid arthritis, unspecified site**   HCC

√6ᵗʰ   **M08.41**   **Pauciarticular juvenile rheumatoid arthritis, shoulder**

M08.411   **Pauciarticular juvenile rheumatoid arthritis, right shoulder**   HCC

M08.412   **Pauciarticular juvenile rheumatoid arthritis, left shoulder**   HCC

M08.419   **Pauciarticular juvenile rheumatoid arthritis, unspecified shoulder**   HCC

√6ᵗʰ   **M08.42**   **Pauciarticular juvenile rheumatoid arthritis, elbow**

M08.421   **Pauciarticular juvenile rheumatoid arthritis, right elbow**   HCC

M08.422   **Pauciarticular juvenile rheumatoid arthritis, left elbow**   HCC

M08.429   **Pauciarticular juvenile rheumatoid arthritis, unspecified elbow**   HCC

√6ᵗʰ   **M08.43**   **Pauciarticular juvenile rheumatoid arthritis, wrist**

M08.431   **Pauciarticular juvenile rheumatoid arthritis, right wrist**   HCC

M08.432   **Pauciarticular juvenile rheumatoid arthritis, left wrist**   HCC

M08.439   **Pauciarticular juvenile rheumatoid arthritis, unspecified wrist**   HCC

√6ᵗʰ   **M08.44**   **Pauciarticular juvenile rheumatoid arthritis, hand**

M08.441   **Pauciarticular juvenile rheumatoid arthritis, right hand**   HCC

M08.442   **Pauciarticular juvenile rheumatoid arthritis, left hand**   HCC

M08.449   **Pauciarticular juvenile rheumatoid arthritis, unspecified hand**   HCC

√6ᵗʰ   **M08.45**   **Pauciarticular juvenile rheumatoid arthritis, hip**

M08.451   **Pauciarticular juvenile rheumatoid arthritis, right hip**   HCC

M08.452   **Pauciarticular juvenile rheumatoid arthritis, left hip**   HCC

M08.459   **Pauciarticular juvenile rheumatoid arthritis, unspecified hip**   HCC

√6ᵗʰ   **M08.46**   **Pauciarticular juvenile rheumatoid arthritis, knee**

M08.461   **Pauciarticular juvenile rheumatoid arthritis, right knee**   HCC

M08.462   **Pauciarticular juvenile rheumatoid arthritis, left knee**   HCC

M08.469   **Pauciarticular juvenile rheumatoid arthritis, unspecified knee**   HCC

√6ᵗʰ   **M08.47**   **Pauciarticular juvenile rheumatoid arthritis, ankle and foot**

M08.471   **Pauciarticular juvenile rheumatoid arthritis, right ankle and foot**   HCC

M08.472   **Pauciarticular juvenile rheumatoid arthritis, left ankle and foot**   HCC

M08.479   **Pauciarticular juvenile rheumatoid arthritis, unspecified ankle and foot**   HCC

M08.48   **Pauciarticular juvenile rheumatoid arthritis, vertebrae**   HCC

√5ᵗʰ   **M08.8**   **Other juvenile arthritis**

M08.80   **Other juvenile arthritis, unspecified site**   HCC

√6ᵗʰ   **M08.81**   **Other juvenile arthritis, shoulder**

M08.811   **Other juvenile arthritis, right shoulder**   HCC

M08.812   **Other juvenile arthritis, left shoulder**   HCC

M08.819   **Other juvenile arthritis, unspecified shoulder**   HCC

√6ᵗʰ   **M08.82**   **Other juvenile arthritis, elbow**

M08.821   **Other juvenile arthritis, right elbow**   HCC

M08.822   **Other juvenile arthritis, left elbow**   HCC

M08.829   **Other juvenile arthritis, unspecified elbow**   HCC

√6ᵗʰ   **M08.83**   **Other juvenile arthritis, wrist**

M08.831   **Other juvenile arthritis, right wrist**   HCC

M08.832   **Other juvenile arthritis, left wrist**   HCC

M08.839   **Other juvenile arthritis, unspecified wrist**   HCC

√6ᵗʰ   **M08.84**   **Other juvenile arthritis, hand**

M08.841   **Other juvenile arthritis, right hand**   HCC

M08.842   **Other juvenile arthritis, left hand**   HCC

M08.849   **Other juvenile arthritis, unspecified hand**   HCC

√6ᵗʰ   **M08.85**   **Other juvenile arthritis, hip**

M08.851   **Other juvenile arthritis, right hip**   HCC

M08.852   **Other juvenile arthritis, left hip**   HCC

M08.859   **Other juvenile arthritis, unspecified hip**   HCC

√6ᵗʰ   **M08.86**   **Other juvenile arthritis, knee**

M08.861   **Other juvenile arthritis, right knee**   HCC

M08.862   **Other juvenile arthritis, left knee**   HCC

M08.869   **Other juvenile arthritis, unspecified knee**   HCC

√6ᵗʰ   **M08.87**   **Other juvenile arthritis, ankle and foot**

M08.871   **Other juvenile arthritis, right ankle and foot**   HCC

M08.872   **Other juvenile arthritis, left ankle and foot**   HCC

M08.879   **Other juvenile arthritis, unspecified ankle and foot**   HCC

M08.88   **Other juvenile arthritis, other specified site**   HCC

Other juvenile arthritis, vertebrae

M08.89   **Other juvenile arthritis, multiple sites**   HCC

√5ᵗʰ   **M08.9**   **Juvenile arthritis, unspecified**

> EXCLUDES 1   *juvenile rheumatoid arthritis, unspecified (M08.0-)*

M08.90   **Juvenile arthritis, unspecified, unspecified site**   HCC

☑ Additional Character Required   √x7ᵗʰ Placeholder   Unacceptable PDx   Questionable PDx   Manifestation   Unspecified Dx   H1-H14 HAC   HCC CMS-HCC Dx   HIV HIV Dx

ICD-10-CM 2020   777

Chapter 13. Diseases of the Musculoskeletal System and Connective Tissue

√6ᵗʰ **M08.91** **Juvenile arthritis, unspecified, shoulder**

     M08.911 Juvenile arthritis, unspecified, **right** shoulder   `HCC`

     M08.912 Juvenile arthritis, unspecified, **left** shoulder   `HCC`

     M08.919 Juvenile arthritis, unspecified, unspecified shoulder   `HCC`

√6ᵗʰ **M08.92** **Juvenile arthritis, unspecified, elbow**

     M08.921 Juvenile arthritis, unspecified, **right** elbow   `HCC`

     M08.922 Juvenile arthritis, unspecified, **left** elbow   `HCC`

     M08.929 Juvenile arthritis, unspecified, unspecified elbow   `HCC`

√6ᵗʰ **M08.93** **Juvenile arthritis, unspecified, wrist**

     M08.931 Juvenile arthritis, unspecified, **right** wrist   `HCC`

     M08.932 Juvenile arthritis, unspecified, **left** wrist   `HCC`

     M08.939 Juvenile arthritis, unspecified, unspecified wrist   `HCC`

√6ᵗʰ **M08.94** **Juvenile arthritis, unspecified, hand**

     M08.941 Juvenile arthritis, unspecified, **right** hand   `HCC`

     M08.942 Juvenile arthritis, unspecified, **left** hand   `HCC`

     M08.949 Juvenile arthritis, unspecified, unspecified hand   `HCC`

√6ᵗʰ **M08.95** **Juvenile arthritis, unspecified, hip**

     M08.951 Juvenile arthritis, unspecified, **right** hip   `HCC`

     M08.952 Juvenile arthritis, unspecified, **left** hip   `HCC`

     M08.959 Juvenile arthritis, unspecified, unspecified hip   `HCC`

√6ᵗʰ **M08.96** **Juvenile arthritis, unspecified, knee**

     M08.961 Juvenile arthritis, unspecified, **right** knee   `HCC`

     M08.962 Juvenile arthritis, unspecified, **left** knee   `HCC`

     M08.969 Juvenile arthritis, unspecified, unspecified knee   `HCC`

√6ᵗʰ **M08.97** **Juvenile arthritis, unspecified, ankle and foot**

     M08.971 Juvenile arthritis, unspecified, **right** ankle and foot   `HCC`

     M08.972 Juvenile arthritis, unspecified, **left** ankle and foot   `HCC`

     M08.979 Juvenile arthritis, unspecified, unspecified ankle and foot   `HCC`

M08.98 **Juvenile arthritis, unspecified, vertebrae**   `HCC`

M08.99 **Juvenile arthritis, unspecified, multiple sites**   `HCC`

√4ᵗʰ **M1A** **Chronic gout**

Use additional code to identify:

     autonomic neuropathy in diseases classified elsewhere (G99.0)

     calculus of urinary tract in diseases classified elsewhere (N22)

     cardiomyopathy in diseases classified elsewhere (I43)

     disorders of external ear in diseases classified elsewhere (H61.1-, H62.8-)

     disorders of iris and ciliary body in diseases classified elsewhere (H22)

     glomerular disorders in diseases classified elsewhere (N08)

   EXCLUDES 1   gout NOS (M10.-)

   EXCLUDES 2   acute gout (M10.-)

The appropriate 7th character is to be added to each code from category M1A.

   0   without tophus (tophi)

   1   with tophus (tophi)

√5ᵗʰ **M1A.0** **Idiopathic chronic gout**

     Chronic gouty bursitis

     Primary chronic gout

√x7ᵗʰ **M1A.00** Idiopathic chronic gout, unspecified site

√6ᵗʰ **M1A.01** Idiopathic chronic gout, **shoulder**

     √7ᵗʰ **M1A.011** Idiopathic chronic gout, **right** shoulder

     √7ᵗʰ **M1A.012** Idiopathic chronic gout, **left** shoulder

     √7ᵗʰ **M1A.019** Idiopathic chronic gout, unspecified shoulder

√6ᵗʰ **M1A.02** Idiopathic chronic gout, **elbow**

     √7ᵗʰ **M1A.021** Idiopathic chronic gout, **right** elbow

     √7ᵗʰ **M1A.022** Idiopathic chronic gout, **left** elbow

     √7ᵗʰ **M1A.029** Idiopathic chronic gout, unspecified elbow

√6ᵗʰ **M1A.03** Idiopathic chronic gout, **wrist**

     √7ᵗʰ **M1A.031** Idiopathic chronic gout, **right** wrist

     √7ᵗʰ **M1A.032** Idiopathic chronic gout, **left** wrist

     √7ᵗʰ **M1A.039** Idiopathic chronic gout, unspecified wrist

√6ᵗʰ **M1A.04** Idiopathic chronic gout, **hand**

     √7ᵗʰ **M1A.041** Idiopathic chronic gout, **right** hand

     √7ᵗʰ **M1A.042** Idiopathic chronic gout, **left** hand

     √7ᵗʰ **M1A.049** Idiopathic chronic gout, unspecified hand

√6ᵗʰ **M1A.05** Idiopathic chronic gout, **hip**

     √7ᵗʰ **M1A.051** Idiopathic chronic gout, **right** hip

     √7ᵗʰ **M1A.052** Idiopathic chronic gout, **left** hip

     √7ᵗʰ **M1A.059** Idiopathic chronic gout, unspecified hip

√6ᵗʰ **M1A.06** Idiopathic chronic gout, **knee**

     √7ᵗʰ **M1A.061** Idiopathic chronic gout, **right** knee

     √7ᵗʰ **M1A.062** Idiopathic chronic gout, **left** knee

     √7ᵗʰ **M1A.069** Idiopathic chronic gout, unspecified knee

√6ᵗʰ **M1A.07** Idiopathic chronic gout, **ankle and foot**

     √7ᵗʰ **M1A.071** Idiopathic chronic gout, **right** ankle and foot

     √7ᵗʰ **M1A.072** Idiopathic chronic gout, **left** ankle and foot

     √7ᵗʰ **M1A.079** Idiopathic chronic gout, unspecified ankle and foot

√x7ᵗʰ **M1A.08** Idiopathic chronic gout, **vertebrae**

√x7ᵗʰ **M1A.09** Idiopathic chronic gout, **multiple sites**

√5ᵗʰ **M1A.1** **Lead-induced chronic gout**

     Code first toxic effects of lead and its compounds (T56.0-)

√x7ᵗʰ **M1A.10** Lead-induced chronic gout, unspecified site

√6ᵗʰ **M1A.11** Lead-induced chronic gout, **shoulder**

     √7ᵗʰ **M1A.111** Lead-induced chronic gout, **right** shoulder

     √7ᵗʰ **M1A.112** Lead-induced chronic gout, **left** shoulder

     √7ᵗʰ **M1A.119** Lead-induced chronic gout, unspecified shoulder

√6ᵗʰ **M1A.12** Lead-induced chronic gout, **elbow**

     √7ᵗʰ **M1A.121** Lead-induced chronic gout, **right** elbow

     √7ᵗʰ **M1A.122** Lead-induced chronic gout, **left** elbow

     √7ᵗʰ **M1A.129** Lead-induced chronic gout, unspecified elbow

√6ᵗʰ **M1A.13** Lead-induced chronic gout, **wrist**

     √7ᵗʰ **M1A.131** Lead-induced chronic gout, **right** wrist

     √7ᵗʰ **M1A.132** Lead-induced chronic gout, **left** wrist

Ⓝ Newborn: 0   Ⓟ Pediatric: 0-17   Ⓜ Maternity: 9-64   Ⓐ Adult: 15-124   `MCC` Major Complication/Comorbidity   `CC` Complication/Comorbidity   `SW` Severe Wound Dx

778   ICD-10-CM 2020

√7ᵗʰ **M1A.139 Lead-induced chronic gout, unspecified wrist**

√6ᵗʰ **M1A.14 Lead-induced chronic gout, hand**

    √7ᵗʰ **M1A.141 Lead-induced chronic gout, right hand**

    √7ᵗʰ **M1A.142 Lead-induced chronic gout, left hand**

    √7ᵗʰ **M1A.149 Lead-induced chronic gout, unspecified hand**

√6ᵗʰ **M1A.15 Lead-induced chronic gout, hip**

    √7ᵗʰ **M1A.151 Lead-induced chronic gout, right hip**

    √7ᵗʰ **M1A.152 Lead-induced chronic gout, left hip**

    √7ᵗʰ **M1A.159 Lead-induced chronic gout, unspecified hip**

√6ᵗʰ **M1A.16 Lead-induced chronic gout, knee**

    √7ᵗʰ **M1A.161 Lead-induced chronic gout, right knee**

    √7ᵗʰ **M1A.162 Lead-induced chronic gout, left knee**

    √7ᵗʰ **M1A.169 Lead-induced chronic gout, unspecified knee**

√6ᵗʰ **M1A.17 Lead-induced chronic gout, ankle and foot**

    √7ᵗʰ **M1A.171 Lead-induced chronic gout, right ankle and foot**

    √7ᵗʰ **M1A.172 Lead-induced chronic gout, left ankle and foot**

    √7ᵗʰ **M1A.179 Lead-induced chronic gout, unspecified ankle and foot**

√x7ᵗʰ **M1A.18 Lead-induced chronic gout, vertebrae**

√x7ᵗʰ **M1A.19 Lead-induced chronic gout, multiple sites**

√5ᵗʰ **M1A.2 Drug-induced chronic gout**

Use additional code for adverse effect, if applicable, to identify drug (T36-T50 with fifth or sixth character 5)

√x7ᵗʰ **M1A.20 Drug-induced chronic gout, unspecified site**

√6ᵗʰ **M1A.21 Drug-induced chronic gout, shoulder**

    √7ᵗʰ **M1A.211 Drug-induced chronic gout, right shoulder**

    √7ᵗʰ **M1A.212 Drug-induced chronic gout, left shoulder**

    √7ᵗʰ **M1A.219 Drug-induced chronic gout, unspecified shoulder**

√6ᵗʰ **M1A.22 Drug-induced chronic gout, elbow**

    √7ᵗʰ **M1A.221 Drug-induced chronic gout, right elbow**

    √7ᵗʰ **M1A.222 Drug-induced chronic gout, left elbow**

    √7ᵗʰ **M1A.229 Drug-induced chronic gout, unspecified elbow**

√6ᵗʰ **M1A.23 Drug-induced chronic gout, wrist**

    √7ᵗʰ **M1A.231 Drug-induced chronic gout, right wrist**

    √7ᵗʰ **M1A.232 Drug-induced chronic gout, left wrist**

    √7ᵗʰ **M1A.239 Drug-induced chronic gout, unspecified wrist**

√6ᵗʰ **M1A.24 Drug-induced chronic gout, hand**

    √7ᵗʰ **M1A.241 Drug-induced chronic gout, right hand**

    √7ᵗʰ **M1A.242 Drug-induced chronic gout, left hand**

    √7ᵗʰ **M1A.249 Drug-induced chronic gout, unspecified hand**

√6ᵗʰ **M1A.25 Drug-induced chronic gout, hip**

    √7ᵗʰ **M1A.251 Drug-induced chronic gout, right hip**

    √7ᵗʰ **M1A.252 Drug-induced chronic gout, left hip**

    √7ᵗʰ **M1A.259 Drug-induced chronic gout, unspecified hip**

√6ᵗʰ **M1A.26 Drug-induced chronic gout, knee**

    √7ᵗʰ **M1A.261 Drug-induced chronic gout, right knee**

    √7ᵗʰ **M1A.262 Drug-induced chronic gout, left knee**

    √7ᵗʰ **M1A.269 Drug-induced chronic gout, unspecified knee**

√6ᵗʰ **M1A.27 Drug-induced chronic gout, ankle and foot**

    √7ᵗʰ **M1A.271 Drug-induced chronic gout, right ankle and foot**

    √7ᵗʰ **M1A.272 Drug-induced chronic gout, left ankle and foot**

    √7ᵗʰ **M1A.279 Drug-induced chronic gout, unspecified ankle and foot**

√x7ᵗʰ **M1A.28 Drug-induced chronic gout, vertebrae**

√x7ᵗʰ **M1A.29 Drug-induced chronic gout, multiple sites**

√5ᵗʰ **M1A.3 Chronic gout due to renal impairment**

Code first associated renal disease

√x7ᵗʰ **M1A.30 Chronic gout due to renal impairment, unspecified site**

√6ᵗʰ **M1A.31 Chronic gout due to renal impairment, shoulder**

    √7ᵗʰ **M1A.311 Chronic gout due to renal impairment, right shoulder**

    √7ᵗʰ **M1A.312 Chronic gout due to renal impairment, left shoulder**

    √7ᵗʰ **M1A.319 Chronic gout due to renal impairment, unspecified shoulder**

√6ᵗʰ **M1A.32 Chronic gout due to renal impairment, elbow**

    √7ᵗʰ **M1A.321 Chronic gout due to renal impairment, right elbow**

    √7ᵗʰ **M1A.322 Chronic gout due to renal impairment, left elbow**

    √7ᵗʰ **M1A.329 Chronic gout due to renal impairment, unspecified elbow**

√6ᵗʰ **M1A.33 Chronic gout due to renal impairment, wrist**

    √7ᵗʰ **M1A.331 Chronic gout due to renal impairment, right wrist**

    √7ᵗʰ **M1A.332 Chronic gout due to renal impairment, left wrist**

    √7ᵗʰ **M1A.339 Chronic gout due to renal impairment, unspecified wrist**

√6ᵗʰ **M1A.34 Chronic gout due to renal impairment, hand**

    √7ᵗʰ **M1A.341 Chronic gout due to renal impairment, right hand**

    √7ᵗʰ **M1A.342 Chronic gout due to renal impairment, left hand**

    √7ᵗʰ **M1A.349 Chronic gout due to renal impairment, unspecified hand**

√6ᵗʰ **M1A.35 Chronic gout due to renal impairment, hip**

    √7ᵗʰ **M1A.351 Chronic gout due to renal impairment, right hip**

    √7ᵗʰ **M1A.352 Chronic gout due to renal impairment, left hip**

    √7ᵗʰ **M1A.359 Chronic gout due to renal impairment, unspecified hip**

√6ᵗʰ **M1A.36 Chronic gout due to renal impairment, knee**

    √7ᵗʰ **M1A.361 Chronic gout due to renal impairment, right knee**

    √7ᵗʰ **M1A.362 Chronic gout due to renal impairment, left knee**

    √7ᵗʰ **M1A.369 Chronic gout due to renal impairment, unspecified knee**

√6ᵗʰ **M1A.37 Chronic gout due to renal impairment, ankle and foot**

    √7ᵗʰ **M1A.371 Chronic gout due to renal impairment, right ankle and foot**

    √7ᵗʰ **M1A.372 Chronic gout due to renal impairment, left ankle and foot**

    √7ᵗʰ **M1A.379 Chronic gout due to renal impairment, unspecified ankle and foot**

√x7ᵗʰ **M1A.38 Chronic gout due to renal impairment, vertebrae**

√x7ᵗʰ **M1A.39 Chronic gout due to renal impairment, multiple sites**

√5ᵗʰ **M1A.4 Other secondary chronic gout**

Code first associated condition

√x7ᵗʰ **M1A.40 Other secondary chronic gout, unspecified site**

√6ᵗʰ **M1A.41 Other secondary chronic gout, shoulder**

    √7ᵗʰ **M1A.411 Other secondary chronic gout, right shoulder**

    √7ᵗʰ **M1A.412 Other secondary chronic gout, left shoulder**

    √7ᵗʰ **M1A.419 Other secondary chronic gout, unspecified shoulder**

√6ᵗʰ **M1A.42 Other secondary chronic gout, elbow**

    √7ᵗʰ **M1A.421 Other secondary chronic gout, right elbow**

    √7ᵗʰ **M1A.422 Other secondary chronic gout, left elbow**

    √7ᵗʰ **M1A.429 Other secondary chronic gout, unspecified elbow**

√6ᵗʰ **M1A.43 Other secondary chronic gout, wrist**

    √7ᵗʰ **M1A.431 Other secondary chronic gout, right wrist**

    √7ᵗʰ **M1A.432 Other secondary chronic gout, left wrist**

    √7ᵗʰ **M1A.439 Other secondary chronic gout, unspecified wrist**

✔ Additional Character Required   √x7ᵗʰ Placeholder   Unacceptable PDx   Questionable PDx   Manifestation   Unspecified Dx   H1 - H14 HAC   HCC CMS-HCC Dx   HIV HIV Dx

ICD-10-CM 2020   779

✓6ᵗʰ **M1A.44** Other secondary chronic gout, hand

  ✓7ᵗʰ **M1A.441** Other secondary chronic gout, right hand

  ✓7ᵗʰ **M1A.442** Other secondary chronic gout, left hand

  ✓7ᵗʰ **M1A.449** Other secondary chronic gout, unspecified hand

✓6ᵗʰ **M1A.45** Other secondary chronic gout, hip

  ✓7ᵗʰ **M1A.451** Other secondary chronic gout, right hip

  ✓7ᵗʰ **M1A.452** Other secondary chronic gout, left hip

  ✓7ᵗʰ **M1A.459** Other secondary chronic gout, unspecified hip

✓6ᵗʰ **M1A.46** Other secondary chronic gout, knee

  ✓7ᵗʰ **M1A.461** Other secondary chronic gout, right knee

  ✓7ᵗʰ **M1A.462** Other secondary chronic gout, left knee

  ✓7ᵗʰ **M1A.469** Other secondary chronic gout, unspecified knee

✓6ᵗʰ **M1A.47** Other secondary chronic gout, ankle and foot

  ✓7ᵗʰ **M1A.471** Other secondary chronic gout, right ankle and foot

  ✓7ᵗʰ **M1A.472** Other secondary chronic gout, left ankle and foot

  ✓7ᵗʰ **M1A.479** Other secondary chronic gout, unspecified ankle and foot

✓x7ᵗʰ **M1A.48** Other secondary chronic gout, vertebrae

✓x7ᵗʰ **M1A.49** Other secondary chronic gout, multiple sites

✓x7ᵗʰ **M1A.9** Chronic gout, unspecified

✓4ᵗʰ **M10 Gout**

Acute gout

Gout attack

Gout flare

Podagra

Use additional code to identify:

  autonomic neuropathy in diseases classified elsewhere (G99.0)

  calculus of urinary tract in diseases classified elsewhere (N22)

  cardiomyopathy in diseases classified elsewhere (I43)

  disorders of external ear in diseases classified elsewhere (H61.1-, H62.8-)

  disorders of iris and ciliary body in diseases classified elsewhere (H22)

  glomerular disorders in diseases classified elsewhere (N08)

EXCLUDES 2   chronic gout (M1A.-)

DEF: Purine and pyrimidine metabolic disorders, manifested by hyperuricemia and recurrent acute inflammatory arthritis. Monosodium urate or monohydrate crystals may be deposited in and around the joints, leading to joint destruction and severe crippling.

✓5ᵗʰ **M10.0 Idiopathic gout**

Gouty bursitis

Primary gout

M10.00 Idiopathic gout, unspecified site

✓6ᵗʰ **M10.01** Idiopathic gout, shoulder

  M10.011 Idiopathic gout, right shoulder

  M10.012 Idiopathic gout, left shoulder

  M10.019 Idiopathic gout, unspecified shoulder

✓6ᵗʰ **M10.02** Idiopathic gout, elbow

  M10.021 Idiopathic gout, right elbow

  M10.022 Idiopathic gout, left elbow

  M10.029 Idiopathic gout, unspecified elbow

✓6ᵗʰ **M10.03** Idiopathic gout, wrist

  M10.031 Idiopathic gout, right wrist

  M10.032 Idiopathic gout, left wrist

  M10.039 Idiopathic gout, unspecified wrist

✓6ᵗʰ **M10.04** Idiopathic gout, hand

  M10.041 Idiopathic gout, right hand

  M10.042 Idiopathic gout, left hand

  M10.049 Idiopathic gout, unspecified hand

✓6ᵗʰ **M10.05** Idiopathic gout, hip

  M10.051 Idiopathic gout, right hip

  M10.052 Idiopathic gout, left hip

  M10.059 Idiopathic gout, unspecified hip

✓6ᵗʰ **M10.06** Idiopathic gout, knee

  M10.061 Idiopathic gout, right knee

  M10.062 Idiopathic gout, left knee

  M10.069 Idiopathic gout, unspecified knee

✓6ᵗʰ **M10.07** Idiopathic gout, ankle and foot

  M10.071 Idiopathic gout, right ankle and foot

  M10.072 Idiopathic gout, left ankle and foot

  M10.079 Idiopathic gout, unspecified ankle and foot

M10.08 Idiopathic gout, vertebrae

M10.09 Idiopathic gout, multiple sites

✓5ᵗʰ **M10.1 Lead-induced gout**

Code first toxic effects of lead and its compounds (T56.0-)

M10.10 Lead-induced gout, unspecified site

✓6ᵗʰ **M10.11** Lead-induced gout, shoulder

  M10.111 Lead-induced gout, right shoulder

  M10.112 Lead-induced gout, left shoulder

  M10.119 Lead-induced gout, unspecified shoulder

✓6ᵗʰ **M10.12** Lead-induced gout, elbow

  M10.121 Lead-induced gout, right elbow

  M10.122 Lead-induced gout, left elbow

  M10.129 Lead-induced gout, unspecified elbow

✓6ᵗʰ **M10.13** Lead-induced gout, wrist

  M10.131 Lead-induced gout, right wrist

  M10.132 Lead-induced gout, left wrist

  M10.139 Lead-induced gout, unspecified wrist

✓6ᵗʰ **M10.14** Lead-induced gout, hand

  M10.141 Lead-induced gout, right hand

  M10.142 Lead-induced gout, left hand

  M10.149 Lead-induced gout, unspecified hand

✓6ᵗʰ **M10.15** Lead-induced gout, hip

  M10.151 Lead-induced gout, right hip

  M10.152 Lead-induced gout, left hip

  M10.159 Lead-induced gout, unspecified hip

✓6ᵗʰ **M10.16** Lead-induced gout, knee

  M10.161 Lead-induced gout, right knee

  M10.162 Lead-induced gout, left knee

  M10.169 Lead-induced gout, unspecified knee

✓6ᵗʰ **M10.17** Lead-induced gout, ankle and foot

  M10.171 Lead-induced gout, right ankle and foot

  M10.172 Lead-induced gout, left ankle and foot

  M10.179 Lead-induced gout, unspecified ankle and foot

M10.18 Lead-induced gout, vertebrae

M10.19 Lead-induced gout, multiple sites

✓5ᵗʰ **M10.2 Drug-induced gout**

Use additional code for adverse effect, if applicable, to identify drug (T36-T50 with fifth or sixth character 5)

M10.20 Drug-induced gout, unspecified site

✓6ᵗʰ **M10.21** Drug-induced gout, shoulder

  M10.211 Drug-induced gout, right shoulder

  M10.212 Drug-induced gout, left shoulder

  M10.219 Drug-induced gout, unspecified shoulder

✓6ᵗʰ **M10.22** Drug-induced gout, elbow

  M10.221 Drug-induced gout, right elbow

  M10.222 Drug-induced gout, left elbow

  M10.229 Drug-induced gout, unspecified elbow

✓6ᵗʰ **M10.23** Drug-induced gout, wrist

  M10.231 Drug-induced gout, right wrist

  M10.232 Drug-induced gout, left wrist

  M10.239 Drug-induced gout, unspecified wrist

✓6ᵗʰ **M10.24** Drug-induced gout, hand

  M10.241 Drug-induced gout, right hand

  M10.242 Drug-induced gout, left hand

  M10.249 Drug-induced gout, unspecified hand

✓6ᵗʰ **M10.25** Drug-induced gout, hip

  M10.251 Drug-induced gout, right hip

  M10.252 Drug-induced gout, left hip

  M10.259 Drug-induced gout, unspecified hip

✓6ᵗʰ **M10.26** Drug-induced gout, knee

  M10.261 Drug-induced gout, right knee

  M10.262 Drug-induced gout, left knee

  M10.269 Drug-induced gout, unspecified knee

✓6ᵗʰ **M10.27** Drug-induced gout, ankle and foot

  M10.271 Drug-induced gout, right ankle and foot

  M10.272 Drug-induced gout, left ankle and foot

  M10.279 Drug-induced gout, unspecified ankle and foot

M10.28 Drug-induced gout, vertebrae

M10.29 Drug-induced gout, multiple sites

Ⓝ Newborn: 0   Ⓟ Pediatric: 0-17   Ⓜ Maternity: 9-64   Ⓐ Adult: 15-124   MCC Major Complication/Comorbidity   CC Complication/Comorbidity   SW Severe Wound Dx

780   ICD-10-CM 2020

M10.3 Gout due to renal impairment
Code first associated renal disease

- **M10.30** Gout due to renal impairment, unspecified site
- **M10.31** Gout due to renal impairment, shoulder
  - M10.311 Gout due to renal impairment, right shoulder
  - M10.312 Gout due to renal impairment, left shoulder
  - **M10.319** Gout due to renal impairment, unspecified shoulder
- **M10.32** Gout due to renal impairment, elbow
  - M10.321 Gout due to renal impairment, right elbow
  - M10.322 Gout due to renal impairment, left elbow
  - **M10.329** Gout due to renal impairment, unspecified elbow
- **M10.33** Gout due to renal impairment, wrist
  - M10.331 Gout due to renal impairment, right wrist
  - M10.332 Gout due to renal impairment, left wrist
  - **M10.339** Gout due to renal impairment, unspecified wrist
- **M10.34** Gout due to renal impairment, hand
  - M10.341 Gout due to renal impairment, right hand
  - M10.342 Gout due to renal impairment, left hand
  - **M10.349** Gout due to renal impairment, unspecified hand
- **M10.35** Gout due to renal impairment, hip
  - M10.351 Gout due to renal impairment, right hip
  - M10.352 Gout due to renal impairment, left hip
  - **M10.359** Gout due to renal impairment, unspecified hip
- **M10.36** Gout due to renal impairment, knee
  - M10.361 Gout due to renal impairment, right knee
  - M10.362 Gout due to renal impairment, left knee
  - **M10.369** Gout due to renal impairment, unspecified knee
- **M10.37** Gout due to renal impairment, ankle and foot
  - M10.371 Gout due to renal impairment, right ankle and foot
  - M10.372 Gout due to renal impairment, left ankle and foot
  - **M10.379** Gout due to renal impairment, unspecified ankle and foot
- **M10.38** Gout due to renal impairment, vertebrae
- **M10.39** Gout due to renal impairment, multiple sites

M10.4 Other secondary gout
Code first associated condition

- **M10.40** Other secondary gout, unspecified site
- **M10.41** Other secondary gout, shoulder
  - M10.411 Other secondary gout, right shoulder
  - M10.412 Other secondary gout, left shoulder
  - **M10.419** Other secondary gout, unspecified shoulder
- **M10.42** Other secondary gout, elbow
  - M10.421 Other secondary gout, right elbow
  - M10.422 Other secondary gout, left elbow
  - **M10.429** Other secondary gout, unspecified elbow
- **M10.43** Other secondary gout, wrist
  - M10.431 Other secondary gout, right wrist
  - M10.432 Other secondary gout, left wrist
  - **M10.439** Other secondary gout, unspecified wrist
- **M10.44** Other secondary gout, hand
  - M10.441 Other secondary gout, right hand
  - M10.442 Other secondary gout, left hand
  - **M10.449** Other secondary gout, unspecified hand
- **M10.45** Other secondary gout, hip
  - M10.451 Other secondary gout, right hip
  - M10.452 Other secondary gout, left hip
  - **M10.459** Other secondary gout, unspecified hip
- **M10.46** Other secondary gout, knee
  - M10.461 Other secondary gout, right knee
  - M10.462 Other secondary gout, left knee
  - **M10.469** Other secondary gout, unspecified knee
- **M10.47** Other secondary gout, ankle and foot
  - M10.471 Other secondary gout, right ankle and foot
  - M10.472 Other secondary gout, left ankle and foot
  - **M10.479** Other secondary gout, unspecified ankle and foot
- **M10.48** Other secondary gout, vertebrae
- **M10.49** Other secondary gout, multiple sites

M10.9 Gout, unspecified
Gout NOS

M11 Other crystal arthropathies

M11.0 Hydroxyapatite deposition disease
DEF: Disease caused by deposits of calcium phosphate crystals in the soft tissues close to the joint (especially tendons) or in the joints. These calcifications can be mono or polyarticular and can cause destruction of the joint involved.

- **M11.00** Hydroxyapatite deposition disease, unspecified site
- **M11.01** Hydroxyapatite deposition disease, shoulder
  - M11.011 Hydroxyapatite deposition disease, right shoulder
  - M11.012 Hydroxyapatite deposition disease, left shoulder
  - **M11.019** Hydroxyapatite deposition disease, unspecified shoulder
- **M11.02** Hydroxyapatite deposition disease, elbow
  - M11.021 Hydroxyapatite deposition disease, right elbow
  - M11.022 Hydroxyapatite deposition disease, left elbow
  - **M11.029** Hydroxyapatite deposition disease, unspecified elbow
- **M11.03** Hydroxyapatite deposition disease, wrist
  - M11.031 Hydroxyapatite deposition disease, right wrist
  - M11.032 Hydroxyapatite deposition disease, left wrist
  - **M11.039** Hydroxyapatite deposition disease, unspecified wrist
- **M11.04** Hydroxyapatite deposition disease, hand
  - M11.041 Hydroxyapatite deposition disease, right hand
  - M11.042 Hydroxyapatite deposition disease, left hand
  - **M11.049** Hydroxyapatite deposition disease, unspecified hand
- **M11.05** Hydroxyapatite deposition disease, hip
  - M11.051 Hydroxyapatite deposition disease, right hip
  - M11.052 Hydroxyapatite deposition disease, left hip
  - **M11.059** Hydroxyapatite deposition disease, unspecified hip
- **M11.06** Hydroxyapatite deposition disease, knee
  - M11.061 Hydroxyapatite deposition disease, right knee
  - M11.062 Hydroxyapatite deposition disease, left knee
  - **M11.069** Hydroxyapatite deposition disease, unspecified knee
- **M11.07** Hydroxyapatite deposition disease, ankle and foot
  - M11.071 Hydroxyapatite deposition disease, right ankle and foot
  - M11.072 Hydroxyapatite deposition disease, left ankle and foot
  - **M11.079** Hydroxyapatite deposition disease, unspecified ankle and foot
- **M11.08** Hydroxyapatite deposition disease, vertebrae
- **M11.09** Hydroxyapatite deposition disease, multiple sites

M11.1 Familial chondrocalcinosis

- **M11.10** Familial chondrocalcinosis, unspecified site
- **M11.11** Familial chondrocalcinosis, shoulder
  - M11.111 Familial chondrocalcinosis, right shoulder
  - M11.112 Familial chondrocalcinosis, left shoulder
  - **M11.119** Familial chondrocalcinosis, unspecified shoulder
- **M11.12** Familial chondrocalcinosis, elbow
  - M11.121 Familial chondrocalcinosis, right elbow
  - M11.122 Familial chondrocalcinosis, left elbow
  - **M11.129** Familial chondrocalcinosis, unspecified elbow
- **M11.13** Familial chondrocalcinosis, wrist
  - M11.131 Familial chondrocalcinosis, right wrist

M11.132 Familial chondrocalcinosis, left wrist
M11.139 Familial chondrocalcinosis, unspecified wrist

√6ᵗʰ M11.14 Familial chondrocalcinosis, hand
M11.141 Familial chondrocalcinosis, right hand
M11.142 Familial chondrocalcinosis, left hand
M11.149 Familial chondrocalcinosis, unspecified hand

√6ᵗʰ M11.15 Familial chondrocalcinosis, hip
M11.151 Familial chondrocalcinosis, right hip
M11.152 Familial chondrocalcinosis, left hip
M11.159 Familial chondrocalcinosis, unspecified hip

√6ᵗʰ M11.16 Familial chondrocalcinosis, knee
M11.161 Familial chondrocalcinosis, right knee
M11.162 Familial chondrocalcinosis, left knee
M11.169 Familial chondrocalcinosis, unspecified knee

√6ᵗʰ M11.17 Familial chondrocalcinosis, ankle and foot
M11.171 Familial chondrocalcinosis, right ankle and foot
M11.172 Familial chondrocalcinosis, left ankle and foot
M11.179 Familial chondrocalcinosis, unspecified ankle and foot

M11.18 Familial chondrocalcinosis, vertebrae
M11.19 Familial chondrocalcinosis, multiple sites

√5ᵗʰ M11.2 Other chondrocalcinosis
Chondrocalcinosis NOS
AHA: 2018,3Q,20
TIP: Pseudogout is captured with codes in this subcategory.

M11.20 Other chondrocalcinosis, unspecified site

√6ᵗʰ M11.21 Other chondrocalcinosis, shoulder
M11.211 Other chondrocalcinosis, right shoulder
M11.212 Other chondrocalcinosis, left shoulder
M11.219 Other chondrocalcinosis, unspecified shoulder

√6ᵗʰ M11.22 Other chondrocalcinosis, elbow
M11.221 Other chondrocalcinosis, right elbow
M11.222 Other chondrocalcinosis, left elbow
M11.229 Other chondrocalcinosis, unspecified elbow

√6ᵗʰ M11.23 Other chondrocalcinosis, wrist
M11.231 Other chondrocalcinosis, right wrist
M11.232 Other chondrocalcinosis, left wrist
M11.239 Other chondrocalcinosis, unspecified wrist

√6ᵗʰ M11.24 Other chondrocalcinosis, hand
M11.241 Other chondrocalcinosis, right hand
M11.242 Other chondrocalcinosis, left hand
M11.249 Other chondrocalcinosis, unspecified hand

√6ᵗʰ M11.25 Other chondrocalcinosis, hip
M11.251 Other chondrocalcinosis, right hip
M11.252 Other chondrocalcinosis, left hip
M11.259 Other chondrocalcinosis, unspecified hip

√6ᵗʰ M11.26 Other chondrocalcinosis, knee
M11.261 Other chondrocalcinosis, right knee
M11.262 Other chondrocalcinosis, left knee
M11.269 Other chondrocalcinosis, unspecified knee

√6ᵗʰ M11.27 Other chondrocalcinosis, ankle and foot
M11.271 Other chondrocalcinosis, right ankle and foot
M11.272 Other chondrocalcinosis, left ankle and foot
M11.279 Other chondrocalcinosis, unspecified ankle and foot

M11.28 Other chondrocalcinosis, vertebrae
M11.29 Other chondrocalcinosis, multiple sites

√5ᵗʰ M11.8 Other specified crystal arthropathies
M11.80 Other specified crystal arthropathies, unspecified site

√6ᵗʰ M11.81 Other specified crystal arthropathies, shoulder
M11.811 Other specified crystal arthropathies, right shoulder
M11.812 Other specified crystal arthropathies, left shoulder

M11.819 Other specified crystal arthropathies, unspecified shoulder

√6ᵗʰ M11.82 Other specified crystal arthropathies, elbow
M11.821 Other specified crystal arthropathies, right elbow
M11.822 Other specified crystal arthropathies, left elbow
M11.829 Other specified crystal arthropathies, unspecified elbow

√6ᵗʰ M11.83 Other specified crystal arthropathies, wrist
M11.831 Other specified crystal arthropathies, right wrist
M11.832 Other specified crystal arthropathies, left wrist
M11.839 Other specified crystal arthropathies, unspecified wrist

√6ᵗʰ M11.84 Other specified crystal arthropathies, hand
M11.841 Other specified crystal arthropathies, right hand
M11.842 Other specified crystal arthropathies, left hand
M11.849 Other specified crystal arthropathies, unspecified hand

√6ᵗʰ M11.85 Other specified crystal arthropathies, hip
M11.851 Other specified crystal arthropathies, right hip
M11.852 Other specified crystal arthropathies, left hip
M11.859 Other specified crystal arthropathies, unspecified hip

√6ᵗʰ M11.86 Other specified crystal arthropathies, knee
M11.861 Other specified crystal arthropathies, right knee
M11.862 Other specified crystal arthropathies, left knee
M11.869 Other specified crystal arthropathies, unspecified knee

√6ᵗʰ M11.87 Other specified crystal arthropathies, ankle and foot
M11.871 Other specified crystal arthropathies, right ankle and foot
M11.872 Other specified crystal arthropathies, left ankle and foot
M11.879 Other specified crystal arthropathies, unspecified ankle and foot

M11.88 Other specified crystal arthropathies, vertebrae
M11.89 Other specified crystal arthropathies, multiple sites
M11.9 Crystal arthropathy, unspecified

√4ᵗʰ M12 Other and unspecified arthropathy
EXCLUDES 1   arthrosis (M15-M19)
              cricoarytenoid arthropathy (J38.7)

√5ᵗʰ M12.0 Chronic postrheumatic arthropathy [Jaccoud]

M12.00 Chronic postrheumatic arthropathy [Jaccoud], unspecified site   HCC

√6ᵗʰ M12.01 Chronic postrheumatic arthropathy [Jaccoud], shoulder
M12.011 Chronic postrheumatic arthropathy [Jaccoud], right shoulder   HCC
M12.012 Chronic postrheumatic arthropathy [Jaccoud], left shoulder   HCC
M12.019 Chronic postrheumatic arthropathy [Jaccoud], unspecified shoulder   HCC

√6ᵗʰ M12.02 Chronic postrheumatic arthropathy [Jaccoud], elbow
M12.021 Chronic postrheumatic arthropathy [Jaccoud], right elbow   HCC
M12.022 Chronic postrheumatic arthropathy [Jaccoud], left elbow   HCC
M12.029 Chronic postrheumatic arthropathy [Jaccoud], unspecified elbow   HCC

√6ᵗʰ M12.03 Chronic postrheumatic arthropathy [Jaccoud], wrist
M12.031 Chronic postrheumatic arthropathy [Jaccoud], right wrist   HCC

M12.032   Chronic postrheumatic arthropathy [Jaccoud], left wrist   `HCC`

M12.039   Chronic postrheumatic arthropathy [Jaccoud], unspecified wrist   `HCC`

√6ᵗʰ   **M12.04**   Chronic postrheumatic arthropathy [Jaccoud], hand

M12.041   Chronic postrheumatic arthropathy [Jaccoud], right hand   `HCC`

M12.042   Chronic postrheumatic arthropathy [Jaccoud], left hand   `HCC`

M12.049   Chronic postrheumatic arthropathy [Jaccoud], unspecified hand   `HCC`

√6ᵗʰ   **M12.05**   Chronic postrheumatic arthropathy [Jaccoud], hip

M12.051   Chronic postrheumatic arthropathy [Jaccoud], right hip   `HCC`

M12.052   Chronic postrheumatic arthropathy [Jaccoud], left hip   `HCC`

M12.059   Chronic postrheumatic arthropathy [Jaccoud], unspecified hip   `HCC`

√6ᵗʰ   **M12.06**   Chronic postrheumatic arthropathy [Jaccoud], knee

M12.061   Chronic postrheumatic arthropathy [Jaccoud], right knee   `HCC`

M12.062   Chronic postrheumatic arthropathy [Jaccoud], left knee   `HCC`

M12.069   Chronic postrheumatic arthropathy [Jaccoud], unspecified knee   `HCC`

√6ᵗʰ   **M12.07**   Chronic postrheumatic arthropathy [Jaccoud], ankle and foot

M12.071   Chronic postrheumatic arthropathy [Jaccoud], right ankle and foot   `HCC`

M12.072   Chronic postrheumatic arthropathy [Jaccoud], left ankle and foot   `HCC`

M12.079   Chronic postrheumatic arthropathy [Jaccoud], unspecified ankle and foot   `HCC`

M12.08   Chronic postrheumatic arthropathy [Jaccoud], other specified site   `HCC`

    Chronic postrheumatic arthropathy [Jaccoud], vertebrae

M12.09   Chronic postrheumatic arthropathy [Jaccoud], multiple sites   `HCC`

√5ᵗʰ   **M12.1**   **Kaschin-Beck disease**

    Osteochondroarthrosis deformans endemica

M12.10   Kaschin-Beck disease, unspecified site

√6ᵗʰ   **M12.11**   Kaschin-Beck disease, shoulder

M12.111   Kaschin-Beck disease, right shoulder

M12.112   Kaschin-Beck disease, left shoulder

M12.119   Kaschin-Beck disease, unspecified shoulder

√6ᵗʰ   **M12.12**   Kaschin-Beck disease, elbow

M12.121   Kaschin-Beck disease, right elbow

M12.122   Kaschin-Beck disease, left elbow

M12.129   Kaschin-Beck disease, unspecified elbow

√6ᵗʰ   **M12.13**   Kaschin-Beck disease, wrist

M12.131   Kaschin-Beck disease, right wrist

M12.132   Kaschin-Beck disease, left wrist

M12.139   Kaschin-Beck disease, unspecified wrist

√6ᵗʰ   **M12.14**   Kaschin-Beck disease, hand

M12.141   Kaschin-Beck disease, right hand

M12.142   Kaschin-Beck disease, left hand

M12.149   Kaschin-Beck disease, unspecified hand

√6ᵗʰ   **M12.15**   Kaschin-Beck disease, hip

M12.151   Kaschin-Beck disease, right hip

M12.152   Kaschin-Beck disease, left hip

M12.159   Kaschin-Beck disease, unspecified hip

√6ᵗʰ   **M12.16**   Kaschin-Beck disease, knee

M12.161   Kaschin-Beck disease, right knee

M12.162   Kaschin-Beck disease, left knee

M12.169   Kaschin-Beck disease, unspecified knee

√6ᵗʰ   **M12.17**   Kaschin-Beck disease, ankle and foot

M12.171   Kaschin-Beck disease, right ankle and foot

M12.172   Kaschin-Beck disease, left ankle and foot

M12.179   Kaschin-Beck disease, unspecified ankle and foot

M12.18   Kaschin-Beck disease, vertebrae

M12.19   Kaschin-Beck disease, multiple sites

√5ᵗʰ   **M12.2**   **Villonodular synovitis (pigmented)**

M12.20   Villonodular synovitis (pigmented), unspecified site

√6ᵗʰ   **M12.21**   Villonodular synovitis (pigmented), shoulder

M12.211   Villonodular synovitis (pigmented), right shoulder

M12.212   Villonodular synovitis (pigmented), left shoulder

M12.219   Villonodular synovitis (pigmented), unspecified shoulder

√6ᵗʰ   **M12.22**   Villonodular synovitis (pigmented), elbow

M12.221   Villonodular synovitis (pigmented), right elbow

M12.222   Villonodular synovitis (pigmented), left elbow

M12.229   Villonodular synovitis (pigmented), unspecified elbow

√6ᵗʰ   **M12.23**   Villonodular synovitis (pigmented), wrist

M12.231   Villonodular synovitis (pigmented), right wrist

M12.232   Villonodular synovitis (pigmented), left wrist

M12.239   Villonodular synovitis (pigmented), unspecified wrist

√6ᵗʰ   **M12.24**   Villonodular synovitis (pigmented), hand

M12.241   Villonodular synovitis (pigmented), right hand

M12.242   Villonodular synovitis (pigmented), left hand

M12.249   Villonodular synovitis (pigmented), unspecified hand

√6ᵗʰ   **M12.25**   Villonodular synovitis (pigmented), hip

M12.251   Villonodular synovitis (pigmented), right hip

M12.252   Villonodular synovitis (pigmented), left hip

M12.259   Villonodular synovitis (pigmented), unspecified hip

√6ᵗʰ   **M12.26**   Villonodular synovitis (pigmented), knee

M12.261   Villonodular synovitis (pigmented), right knee

M12.262   Villonodular synovitis (pigmented), left knee

M12.269   Villonodular synovitis (pigmented), unspecified knee

√6ᵗʰ   **M12.27**   Villonodular synovitis (pigmented), ankle and foot

M12.271   Villonodular synovitis (pigmented), right ankle and foot

M12.272   Villonodular synovitis (pigmented), left ankle and foot

M12.279   Villonodular synovitis (pigmented), unspecified ankle and foot

M12.28   Villonodular synovitis (pigmented), other specified site

    Villonodular synovitis (pigmented), vertebrae

M12.29   Villonodular synovitis (pigmented), multiple sites

√5ᵗʰ   **M12.3**   **Palindromic rheumatism**

    DEF: Sudden and recurring attacks of moderate to severe joint pain and swelling generally occurring in the hands or feet of unknown etiology. After the attack subsides, the joints appear normal again.

M12.30   Palindromic rheumatism, unspecified site

√6ᵗʰ   **M12.31**   Palindromic rheumatism, shoulder

M12.311   Palindromic rheumatism, right shoulder

M12.312   Palindromic rheumatism, left shoulder

M12.319   Palindromic rheumatism, unspecified shoulder

√6ᵗʰ   **M12.32**   Palindromic rheumatism, elbow

M12.321   Palindromic rheumatism, right elbow

M12.322   Palindromic rheumatism, left elbow

☑ Additional Character Required   √x7ᵗʰ Placeholder   Unacceptable PDx   Questionable PDx   Manifestation   Unspecified Dx   `H1`-`H14` HAC   `HCC` CMS-HCC Dx   `HIV` HIV Dx

M12.329 **Palindromic rheumatism, unspecified elbow**

✓6ᵗʰ M12.33 **Palindromic rheumatism, wrist**

M12.331 **Palindromic rheumatism, right wrist**
M12.332 **Palindromic rheumatism, left wrist**
M12.339 **Palindromic rheumatism, unspecified wrist**

✓6ᵗʰ M12.34 **Palindromic rheumatism, hand**

M12.341 **Palindromic rheumatism, right hand**
M12.342 **Palindromic rheumatism, left hand**
M12.349 **Palindromic rheumatism, unspecified hand**

✓6ᵗʰ M12.35 **Palindromic rheumatism, hip**

M12.351 **Palindromic rheumatism, right hip**
M12.352 **Palindromic rheumatism, left hip**
M12.359 **Palindromic rheumatism, unspecified hip**

✓6ᵗʰ M12.36 **Palindromic rheumatism, knee**

M12.361 **Palindromic rheumatism, right knee**
M12.362 **Palindromic rheumatism, left knee**
M12.369 **Palindromic rheumatism, unspecified knee**

✓6ᵗʰ M12.37 **Palindromic rheumatism, ankle and foot**

M12.371 **Palindromic rheumatism, right ankle and foot**
M12.372 **Palindromic rheumatism, left ankle and foot**
M12.379 **Palindromic rheumatism, unspecified ankle and foot**

M12.38 **Palindromic rheumatism, other specified site**
Palindromic rheumatism, vertebrae

M12.39 **Palindromic rheumatism, multiple sites**

✓5ᵗʰ M12.4 **Intermittent hydrarthrosis**

M12.40 **Intermittent hydrarthrosis, unspecified site**

✓6ᵗʰ M12.41 **Intermittent hydrarthrosis, shoulder**

M12.411 **Intermittent hydrarthrosis, right shoulder**
M12.412 **Intermittent hydrarthrosis, left shoulder**
M12.419 **Intermittent hydrarthrosis, unspecified shoulder**

✓6ᵗʰ M12.42 **Intermittent hydrarthrosis, elbow**

M12.421 **Intermittent hydrarthrosis, right elbow**
M12.422 **Intermittent hydrarthrosis, left elbow**
M12.429 **Intermittent hydrarthrosis, unspecified elbow**

✓6ᵗʰ M12.43 **Intermittent hydrarthrosis, wrist**

M12.431 **Intermittent hydrarthrosis, right wrist**
M12.432 **Intermittent hydrarthrosis, left wrist**
M12.439 **Intermittent hydrarthrosis, unspecified wrist**

✓6ᵗʰ M12.44 **Intermittent hydrarthrosis, hand**

M12.441 **Intermittent hydrarthrosis, right hand**
M12.442 **Intermittent hydrarthrosis, left hand**
M12.449 **Intermittent hydrarthrosis, unspecified hand**

✓6ᵗʰ M12.45 **Intermittent hydrarthrosis, hip**

M12.451 **Intermittent hydrarthrosis, right hip**
M12.452 **Intermittent hydrarthrosis, left hip**
M12.459 **Intermittent hydrarthrosis, unspecified hip**

✓6ᵗʰ M12.46 **Intermittent hydrarthrosis, knee**

M12.461 **Intermittent hydrarthrosis, right knee**
M12.462 **Intermittent hydrarthrosis, left knee**
M12.469 **Intermittent hydrarthrosis, unspecified knee**

✓6ᵗʰ M12.47 **Intermittent hydrarthrosis, ankle and foot**

M12.471 **Intermittent hydrarthrosis, right ankle and foot**
M12.472 **Intermittent hydrarthrosis, left ankle and foot**
M12.479 **Intermittent hydrarthrosis, unspecified ankle and foot**

M12.48 **Intermittent hydrarthrosis, other site**

M12.49 **Intermittent hydrarthrosis, multiple sites**

✓5ᵗʰ M12.5 **Traumatic arthropathy**

EXCLUDES 1   *current injury–see Alphabetic Index*
post-traumatic osteoarthritis of first carpometacarpal joint (M18.2-M18.3)
post-traumatic osteoarthritis of hip (M16.4-M16.5)
post-traumatic osteoarthritis of knee (M17.2-M17.3)
post-traumatic osteoarthritis NOS (M19.1-)
post-traumatic osteoarthritis of other single joints (M19.1-)

AHA: 2015,1Q,17

M12.50 **Traumatic arthropathy, unspecified site**

✓6ᵗʰ M12.51 **Traumatic arthropathy, shoulder**

M12.511 **Traumatic arthropathy, right shoulder**
M12.512 **Traumatic arthropathy, left shoulder**
M12.519 **Traumatic arthropathy, unspecified shoulder**

✓6ᵗʰ M12.52 **Traumatic arthropathy, elbow**

M12.521 **Traumatic arthropathy, right elbow**
M12.522 **Traumatic arthropathy, left elbow**
M12.529 **Traumatic arthropathy, unspecified elbow**

✓6ᵗʰ M12.53 **Traumatic arthropathy, wrist**

M12.531 **Traumatic arthropathy, right wrist**
M12.532 **Traumatic arthropathy, left wrist**
M12.539 **Traumatic arthropathy, unspecified wrist**

✓6ᵗʰ M12.54 **Traumatic arthropathy, hand**

M12.541 **Traumatic arthropathy, right hand**
M12.542 **Traumatic arthropathy, left hand**
M12.549 **Traumatic arthropathy, unspecified hand**

✓6ᵗʰ M12.55 **Traumatic arthropathy, hip**

M12.551 **Traumatic arthropathy, right hip**
M12.552 **Traumatic arthropathy, left hip**
M12.559 **Traumatic arthropathy, unspecified hip**

✓6ᵗʰ M12.56 **Traumatic arthropathy, knee**

M12.561 **Traumatic arthropathy, right knee**
M12.562 **Traumatic arthropathy, left knee**
M12.569 **Traumatic arthropathy, unspecified knee**

✓6ᵗʰ M12.57 **Traumatic arthropathy, ankle and foot**

M12.571 **Traumatic arthropathy, right ankle and foot**
M12.572 **Traumatic arthropathy, left ankle and foot**
M12.579 **Traumatic arthropathy, unspecified ankle and foot**

M12.58 **Traumatic arthropathy, other specified site**
Traumatic arthropathy, vertebrae

M12.59 **Traumatic arthropathy, multiple sites**

✓5ᵗʰ M12.8 **Other specific arthropathies, not elsewhere classified**
Transient arthropathy

M12.80 **Other specific arthropathies, not elsewhere classified, unspecified site**

✓6ᵗʰ M12.81 **Other specific arthropathies, not elsewhere classified, shoulder**

M12.811 **Other specific arthropathies, not elsewhere classified, right shoulder**
M12.812 **Other specific arthropathies, not elsewhere classified, left shoulder**
M12.819 **Other specific arthropathies, not elsewhere classified, unspecified shoulder**

✓6ᵗʰ M12.82 **Other specific arthropathies, not elsewhere classified, elbow**

M12.821 **Other specific arthropathies, not elsewhere classified, right elbow**
M12.822 **Other specific arthropathies, not elsewhere classified, left elbow**
M12.829 **Other specific arthropathies, not elsewhere classified, unspecified elbow**

✓6ᵗʰ M12.83 **Other specific arthropathies, not elsewhere classified, wrist**

M12.831 **Other specific arthropathies, not elsewhere classified, right wrist**
M12.832 **Other specific arthropathies, not elsewhere classified, left wrist**
M12.839 **Other specific arthropathies, not elsewhere classified, unspecified wrist**

N Newborn: 0   P Pediatric: 0-17   M Maternity: 9-64   A Adult: 15-124   MCC Major Complication/Comorbidity   CC Complication/Comorbidity   SW Severe Wound Dx

784   ICD-10-CM 2020

√6ᵗʰ **M12.84** Other specific arthropathies, not elsewhere classified, hand

    M12.841 Other specific arthropathies, not elsewhere classified, right hand

    M12.842 Other specific arthropathies, not elsewhere classified, left hand

    M12.849 Other specific arthropathies, not elsewhere classified, unspecified hand

√6ᵗʰ **M12.85** Other specific arthropathies, not elsewhere classified, hip

    M12.851 Other specific arthropathies, not elsewhere classified, right hip

    M12.852 Other specific arthropathies, not elsewhere classified, left hip

    M12.859 Other specific arthropathies, not elsewhere classified, unspecified hip

√6ᵗʰ **M12.86** Other specific arthropathies, not elsewhere classified, knee

    M12.861 Other specific arthropathies, not elsewhere classified, right knee

    M12.862 Other specific arthropathies, not elsewhere classified, left knee

    M12.869 Other specific arthropathies, not elsewhere classified, unspecified knee

√6ᵗʰ **M12.87** Other specific arthropathies, not elsewhere classified, ankle and foot

    M12.871 Other specific arthropathies, not elsewhere classified, right ankle and foot

    M12.872 Other specific arthropathies, not elsewhere classified, left ankle and foot

    M12.879 Other specific arthropathies, not elsewhere classified, unspecified ankle and foot

M12.88 Other specific arthropathies, not elsewhere classified, other specified site

    Other specific arthropathies, not elsewhere classified, vertebrae

M12.89 Other specific arthropathies, not elsewhere classified, multiple sites

M12.9 Arthropathy, unspecified

√4ᵗʰ **M13** Other arthritis

  EXCLUDES 1   arthrosis (M15-M19)

        osteoarthritis (M15-M19)

M13.0 Polyarthritis, unspecified

√5ᵗʰ **M13.1** Monoarthritis, not elsewhere classified

  M13.10 Monoarthritis, not elsewhere classified, unspecified site

√6ᵗʰ **M13.11** Monoarthritis, not elsewhere classified, shoulder

    M13.111 Monoarthritis, not elsewhere classified, right shoulder

    M13.112 Monoarthritis, not elsewhere classified, left shoulder

    M13.119 Monoarthritis, not elsewhere classified, unspecified shoulder

√6ᵗʰ **M13.12** Monoarthritis, not elsewhere classified, elbow

    M13.121 Monoarthritis, not elsewhere classified, right elbow

    M13.122 Monoarthritis, not elsewhere classified, left elbow

    M13.129 Monoarthritis, not elsewhere classified, unspecified elbow

√6ᵗʰ **M13.13** Monoarthritis, not elsewhere classified, wrist

    M13.131 Monoarthritis, not elsewhere classified, right wrist

    M13.132 Monoarthritis, not elsewhere classified, left wrist

    M13.139 Monoarthritis, not elsewhere classified, unspecified wrist

√6ᵗʰ **M13.14** Monoarthritis, not elsewhere classified, hand

    M13.141 Monoarthritis, not elsewhere classified, right hand

    M13.142 Monoarthritis, not elsewhere classified, left hand

    M13.149 Monoarthritis, not elsewhere classified, unspecified hand

√6ᵗʰ **M13.15** Monoarthritis, not elsewhere classified, hip

    M13.151 Monoarthritis, not elsewhere classified, right hip

    M13.152 Monoarthritis, not elsewhere classified, left hip

    M13.159 Monoarthritis, not elsewhere classified, unspecified hip

√6ᵗʰ **M13.16** Monoarthritis, not elsewhere classified, knee

    M13.161 Monoarthritis, not elsewhere classified, right knee

    M13.162 Monoarthritis, not elsewhere classified, left knee

    M13.169 Monoarthritis, not elsewhere classified, unspecified knee

√6ᵗʰ **M13.17** Monoarthritis, not elsewhere classified, ankle and foot

    M13.171 Monoarthritis, not elsewhere classified, right ankle and foot

    M13.172 Monoarthritis, not elsewhere classified, left ankle and foot

    M13.179 Monoarthritis, not elsewhere classified, unspecified ankle and foot

√5ᵗʰ **M13.8** Other specified arthritis

  Allergic arthritis

  EXCLUDES 1   osteoarthritis (M15-M19)

  M13.80 Other specified arthritis, unspecified site

√6ᵗʰ **M13.81** Other specified arthritis, shoulder

    M13.811 Other specified arthritis, right shoulder

    M13.812 Other specified arthritis, left shoulder

    M13.819 Other specified arthritis, unspecified shoulder

√6ᵗʰ **M13.82** Other specified arthritis, elbow

    M13.821 Other specified arthritis, right elbow

    M13.822 Other specified arthritis, left elbow

    M13.829 Other specified arthritis, unspecified elbow

√6ᵗʰ **M13.83** Other specified arthritis, wrist

    M13.831 Other specified arthritis, right wrist

    M13.832 Other specified arthritis, left wrist

    M13.839 Other specified arthritis, unspecified wrist

√6ᵗʰ **M13.84** Other specified arthritis, hand

    M13.841 Other specified arthritis, right hand

    M13.842 Other specified arthritis, left hand

    M13.849 Other specified arthritis, unspecified hand

√6ᵗʰ **M13.85** Other specified arthritis, hip

    M13.851 Other specified arthritis, right hip

    M13.852 Other specified arthritis, left hip

    M13.859 Other specified arthritis, unspecified hip

√6ᵗʰ **M13.86** Other specified arthritis, knee

    M13.861 Other specified arthritis, right knee

    M13.862 Other specified arthritis, left knee

    M13.869 Other specified arthritis, unspecified knee

√6ᵗʰ **M13.87** Other specified arthritis, ankle and foot

    M13.871 Other specified arthritis, right ankle and foot

    M13.872 Other specified arthritis, left ankle and foot

    M13.879 Other specified arthritis, unspecified ankle and foot

M13.88 Other specified arthritis, other site

M13.89 Other specified arthritis, multiple sites

☑ Additional Character Required   √x7ᵗʰ Placeholder   Unacceptable PDx   Questionable PDx   Manifestation   Unspecified Dx   H1-H14 HAC   HCC CMS-HCC Dx   HIV HIV Dx

ICD-10-CM 2020   **785**

Chapter 13. Diseases of the Musculoskeletal System and Connective Tissue

M14–M16.0

✓4ᵗʰ **M14 Arthropathies in other diseases classified elsewhere**

> **EXCLUDES 1**   arthropathy in:
> > diabetes mellitus (E08-E13 with .61-)
> > hematological disorders (M36.2-M36.3)
> > hypersensitivity reactions (M36.4)
> > neoplastic disease (M36.1)
> > neurosyphillis (A52.16)
> > sarcoidosis (D86.86)
> > enteropathic arthropathies (M07.-)
> > juvenile psoriatic arthropathy (L40.54)
> > lipoid dermatoarthritis (E78.81)

✓5ᵗʰ **M14.6 Charcôt's joint**

> Neuropathic arthropathy
>
> **EXCLUDES 1**   Charcôt's joint in diabetes mellitus (E08-E13 with .610)
> > Charcôt's joint in tabes dorsalis (A52.16)
>
> **DEF:** Progressive neurologic arthropathy in which chronic degeneration of joints in the weight-bearing areas with peripheral hypertrophy occurs as a complication of a neuropathy disorder. Supporting structures relax from a loss of sensation resulting in chronic joint instability.

   M14.60 Charcôt's joint, unspecified site

✓6ᵗʰ **M14.61 Charcôt's joint, shoulder**

     M14.611 Charcôt's joint, right shoulder
     M14.612 Charcôt's joint, left shoulder
     M14.619 Charcôt's joint, unspecified shoulder

✓6ᵗʰ **M14.62 Charcôt's joint, elbow**

     M14.621 Charcôt's joint, right elbow
     M14.622 Charcôt's joint, left elbow
     M14.629 Charcôt's joint, unspecified elbow

✓6ᵗʰ **M14.63 Charcôt's joint, wrist**

     M14.631 Charcôt's joint, right wrist
     M14.632 Charcôt's joint, left wrist
     M14.639 Charcôt's joint, unspecified wrist

✓6ᵗʰ **M14.64 Charcôt's joint, hand**

     M14.641 Charcôt's joint, right hand
     M14.642 Charcôt's joint, left hand
     M14.649 Charcôt's joint, unspecified hand

✓6ᵗʰ **M14.65 Charcôt's joint, hip**

     M14.651 Charcôt's joint, right hip
     M14.652 Charcôt's joint, left hip
     M14.659 Charcôt's joint, unspecified hip

✓6ᵗʰ **M14.66 Charcôt's joint, knee**

     M14.661 Charcôt's joint, right knee
     M14.662 Charcôt's joint, left knee
     M14.669 Charcôt's joint, unspecified knee

✓6ᵗʰ **M14.67 Charcôt's joint, ankle and foot**

     M14.671 Charcôt's joint, right ankle and foot
     M14.672 Charcôt's joint, left ankle and foot
     M14.679 Charcôt's joint, unspecified ankle and foot

   M14.68 Charcôt's joint, vertebrae

   M14.69 Charcôt's joint, multiple sites

✓5ᵗʰ **M14.8 Arthropathies in other specified diseases classified elsewhere**

> Code first underlying disease, such as:
> > amyloidosis (E85.-)
> > erythema multiforme (L51.-)
> > erythema nodosum (L52)
> > hemochromatosis (E83.11-)
> > hyperparathyroidism (E21.-)
> > hypothyroidism (E00-E03)
> > sickle-cell disorders (D57.-)
> > thyrotoxicosis [hyperthyroidism] (E05.-)
> > Whipple's disease (K90.81)

   M14.80 Arthropathies in other specified diseases classified elsewhere, unspecified site

✓6ᵗʰ *M14.81 Arthropathies in other specified diseases classified elsewhere, shoulder*

     M14.811 Arthropathies in other specified diseases classified elsewhere, right shoulder
     M14.812 Arthropathies in other specified diseases classified elsewhere, left shoulder
     M14.819 Arthropathies in other specified diseases classified elsewhere, unspecified shoulder

✓6ᵗʰ *M14.82 Arthropathies in other specified diseases classified elsewhere, elbow*

     M14.821 Arthropathies in other specified diseases classified elsewhere, right elbow
     M14.822 Arthropathies in other specified diseases classified elsewhere, left elbow
     M14.829 Arthropathies in other specified diseases classified elsewhere, unspecified elbow

✓6ᵗʰ *M14.83 Arthropathies in other specified diseases classified elsewhere, wrist*

     M14.831 Arthropathies in other specified diseases classified elsewhere, right wrist
     M14.832 Arthropathies in other specified diseases classified elsewhere, left wrist
     M14.839 Arthropathies in other specified diseases classified elsewhere, unspecified wrist

✓6ᵗʰ *M14.84 Arthropathies in other specified diseases classified elsewhere, hand*

     M14.841 Arthropathies in other specified diseases classified elsewhere, right hand
     M14.842 Arthropathies in other specified diseases classified elsewhere, left hand
     M14.849 Arthropathies in other specified diseases classified elsewhere, unspecified hand

✓6ᵗʰ *M14.85 Arthropathies in other specified diseases classified elsewhere, hip*

     M14.851 Arthropathies in other specified diseases classified elsewhere, right hip
     M14.852 Arthropathies in other specified diseases classified elsewhere, left hip
     M14.859 Arthropathies in other specified diseases classified elsewhere, unspecified hip

✓6ᵗʰ *M14.86 Arthropathies in other specified diseases classified elsewhere, knee*

     M14.861 Arthropathies in other specified diseases classified elsewhere, right knee
     M14.862 Arthropathies in other specified diseases classified elsewhere, left knee
     M14.869 Arthropathies in other specified diseases classified elsewhere, unspecified knee

✓6ᵗʰ *M14.87 Arthropathies in other specified diseases classified elsewhere, ankle and foot*

     M14.871 Arthropathies in other specified diseases classified elsewhere, right ankle and foot
     M14.872 Arthropathies in other specified diseases classified elsewhere, left ankle and foot
     M14.879 Arthropathies in other specified diseases classified elsewhere, unspecified ankle and foot

   M14.88 Arthropathies in other specified diseases classified elsewhere, vertebrae

   M14.89 Arthropathies in other specified diseases classified elsewhere, multiple sites

Osteoarthritis (M15-M19)

> **EXCLUDES 2**   osteoarthritis of spine (M47.-)
>
> **TIP:** Assign a primary osteoarthritis code when the type of osteoarthritis—primary, secondary, or generalized—is not specified in the documentation. Primary is considered the default.

✓4ᵗʰ **M15 Polyosteoarthritis**

> **INCLUDES**   arthritis of multiple sites
> **EXCLUDES 1**   bilateral involvement of single joint (M16-M19)

   M15.0 Primary generalized (osteo)arthritis

   M15.1 Heberden's nodes (with arthropathy)
     Interphalangeal distal osteoarthritis

   M15.2 Bouchard's nodes (with arthropathy)
     Juxtaphalangeal distal osteoarthritis

   M15.3 Secondary multiple arthritis
     Post-traumatic polyosteoarthritis

   M15.4 Erosive (osteo)arthritis

   M15.8 Other polyosteoarthritis

   M15.9 Polyosteoarthritis, unspecified
     Generalized osteoarthritis NOS

✓4ᵗʰ **M16 Osteoarthritis of hip**

> **AHA:** 2016,4Q,146

   M16.0 Bilateral primary osteoarthritis of hip
     AHA: 2018,2Q,15

N Newborn: 0   **P** Pediatric: 0-17   **M** Maternity: 9-64   **A** Adult: 15-124   **MCC** Major Complication/Comorbidity   **CC** Complication/Comorbidity   **SW** Severe Wound Dx

786   ICD-10-CM 2020

✓5ᵗʰ **M16.1** **Unilateral primary osteoarthritis of hip**
> Primary osteoarthritis of hip NOS
> **AHA:** 2018,2Q,15

> **M16.10** **Unilateral primary osteoarthritis, unspecified hip**
> **M16.11** **Unilateral primary osteoarthritis, right hip**
> **M16.12** **Unilateral primary osteoarthritis, left hip**

M16.2 **Bilateral osteoarthritis resulting from hip dysplasia**

✓5ᵗʰ **M16.3** **Unilateral osteoarthritis resulting from hip dysplasia**
> Dysplastic osteoarthritis of hip NOS

> **M16.30** **Unilateral osteoarthritis resulting from hip dysplasia, unspecified hip**
> **M16.31** **Unilateral osteoarthritis resulting from hip dysplasia, right hip**
> **M16.32** **Unilateral osteoarthritis resulting from hip dysplasia, left hip**

M16.4 **Bilateral post-traumatic osteoarthritis of hip**

✓5ᵗʰ **M16.5** **Unilateral post-traumatic osteoarthritis of hip**
> Post-traumatic osteoarthritis of hip NOS

> **M16.50** **Unilateral post-traumatic osteoarthritis, unspecified hip**
> **M16.51** **Unilateral post-traumatic osteoarthritis, right hip**
> **M16.52** **Unilateral post-traumatic osteoarthritis, left hip**

M16.6 **Other bilateral secondary osteoarthritis of hip**

M16.7 **Other unilateral secondary osteoarthritis of hip**
> Secondary osteoarthritis of hip NOS

M16.9 **Osteoarthritis of hip, unspecified**

✓4ᵗʰ **M17** **Osteoarthritis of knee**
> **AHA:** 2016,4Q,146-147

M17.0 **Bilateral primary osteoarthritis of knee**
> **AHA:** 2018,2Q,15

✓5ᵗʰ **M17.1** **Unilateral primary osteoarthritis of knee**
> Primary osteoarthritis of knee NOS
> **AHA:** 2018,2Q,15

> **M17.10** **Unilateral primary osteoarthritis, unspecified knee**
> **M17.11** **Unilateral primary osteoarthritis, right knee**
> **M17.12** **Unilateral primary osteoarthritis, left knee**

M17.2 **Bilateral post-traumatic osteoarthritis of knee**

✓5ᵗʰ **M17.3** **Unilateral post-traumatic osteoarthritis of knee**
> Post-traumatic osteoarthritis of knee NOS

> **M17.30** **Unilateral post-traumatic osteoarthritis, unspecified knee**
> **M17.31** **Unilateral post-traumatic osteoarthritis, right knee**
> **M17.32** **Unilateral post-traumatic osteoarthritis, left knee**

M17.4 **Other bilateral secondary osteoarthritis of knee**

M17.5 **Other unilateral secondary osteoarthritis of knee**
> Secondary osteoarthritis of knee NOS

M17.9 **Osteoarthritis of knee, unspecified**

✓4ᵗʰ **M18** **Osteoarthritis of first carpometacarpal joint**

M18.0 **Bilateral primary osteoarthritis of first carpometacarpal joints**

✓5ᵗʰ **M18.1** **Unilateral primary osteoarthritis of first carpometacarpal joint**
> Primary osteoarthritis of first carpometacarpal joint NOS

> **M18.10** **Unilateral primary osteoarthritis of first carpometacarpal joint, unspecified hand**
> **M18.11** **Unilateral primary osteoarthritis of first carpometacarpal joint, right hand**
> **M18.12** **Unilateral primary osteoarthritis of first carpometacarpal joint, left hand**

M18.2 **Bilateral post-traumatic osteoarthritis of first carpometacarpal joints**

✓5ᵗʰ **M18.3** **Unilateral post-traumatic osteoarthritis of first carpometacarpal joint**
> Post-traumatic osteoarthritis of first carpometacarpal joint NOS

> **M18.30** **Unilateral post-traumatic osteoarthritis of first carpometacarpal joint, unspecified hand**
> **M18.31** **Unilateral post-traumatic osteoarthritis of first carpometacarpal joint, right hand**
> **M18.32** **Unilateral post-traumatic osteoarthritis of first carpometacarpal joint, left hand**

M18.4 **Other bilateral secondary osteoarthritis of first carpometacarpal joints**

✓5ᵗʰ **M18.5** **Other unilateral secondary osteoarthritis of first carpometacarpal joint**
> Secondary osteoarthritis of first carpometacarpal joint NOS

> **M18.50** **Other unilateral secondary osteoarthritis of first carpometacarpal joint, unspecified hand**

M18.51 **Other unilateral secondary osteoarthritis of first carpometacarpal joint, right hand**

M18.52 **Other unilateral secondary osteoarthritis of first carpometacarpal joint, left hand**

M18.9 **Osteoarthritis of first carpometacarpal joint, unspecified**

✓4ᵗʰ **M19** **Other and unspecified osteoarthritis**

> *EXCLUDES 1*   polyarthritis (M15.-)
> *EXCLUDES 2*   arthrosis of spine (M47.-)
>   hallux rigidus (M20.2)
>   osteoarthritis of spine (M47.-)

✓5ᵗʰ **M19.0** **Primary osteoarthritis of other joints**
> **AHA:** 2018,2Q,15; 2016,4Q,145

✓6ᵗʰ **M19.01** **Primary osteoarthritis, shoulder**

> **M19.011** **Primary osteoarthritis, right shoulder**
> **M19.012** **Primary osteoarthritis, left shoulder**
> **M19.019** **Primary osteoarthritis, unspecified shoulder**

✓6ᵗʰ **M19.02** **Primary osteoarthritis, elbow**

> **M19.021** **Primary osteoarthritis, right elbow**
> **M19.022** **Primary osteoarthritis, left elbow**
> **M19.029** **Primary osteoarthritis, unspecified elbow**

✓6ᵗʰ **M19.03** **Primary osteoarthritis, wrist**

> **M19.031** **Primary osteoarthritis, right wrist**
> **M19.032** **Primary osteoarthritis, left wrist**
> **M19.039** **Primary osteoarthritis, unspecified wrist**

✓6ᵗʰ **M19.04** **Primary osteoarthritis, hand**

> *EXCLUDES 2*   primary osteoarthritis of first carpometacarpal joint (M18.0-, M18.1-)

> **M19.041** **Primary osteoarthritis, right hand**
> **M19.042** **Primary osteoarthritis, left hand**
> **M19.049** **Primary osteoarthritis, unspecified hand**

✓6ᵗʰ **M19.07** **Primary osteoarthritis ankle and foot**

> **M19.071** **Primary osteoarthritis, right ankle and foot**
> **M19.072** **Primary osteoarthritis, left ankle and foot**
> **M19.079** **Primary osteoarthritis, unspecified ankle and foot**

✓5ᵗʰ **M19.1** **Post-traumatic osteoarthritis of other joints**

✓6ᵗʰ **M19.11** **Post-traumatic osteoarthritis, shoulder**

> **M19.111** **Post-traumatic osteoarthritis, right shoulder**
> **M19.112** **Post-traumatic osteoarthritis, left shoulder**
> **M19.119** **Post-traumatic osteoarthritis, unspecified shoulder**

✓6ᵗʰ **M19.12** **Post-traumatic osteoarthritis, elbow**

> **M19.121** **Post-traumatic osteoarthritis, right elbow**
> **M19.122** **Post-traumatic osteoarthritis, left elbow**
> **M19.129** **Post-traumatic osteoarthritis, unspecified elbow**

✓6ᵗʰ **M19.13** **Post-traumatic osteoarthritis, wrist**

> **M19.131** **Post-traumatic osteoarthritis, right wrist**
> **M19.132** **Post-traumatic osteoarthritis, left wrist**
> **M19.139** **Post-traumatic osteoarthritis, unspecified wrist**

✓6ᵗʰ **M19.14** **Post-traumatic osteoarthritis, hand**

> *EXCLUDES 2*   post-traumatic osteoarthritis of first carpometacarpal joint (M18.2-, M18.3-)

> **M19.141** **Post-traumatic osteoarthritis, right hand**
> **M19.142** **Post-traumatic osteoarthritis, left hand**
> **M19.149** **Post-traumatic osteoarthritis, unspecified hand**

✓6ᵗʰ **M19.17** **Post-traumatic osteoarthritis, ankle and foot**

> **M19.171** **Post-traumatic osteoarthritis, right ankle and foot**
> **M19.172** **Post-traumatic osteoarthritis, left ankle and foot**
> **M19.179** **Post-traumatic osteoarthritis, unspecified ankle and foot**

✓5ᵗʰ **M19.2** **Secondary osteoarthritis of other joints**

✓6ᵗʰ **M19.21** **Secondary osteoarthritis, shoulder**

> **M19.211** **Secondary osteoarthritis, right shoulder**
> **M19.212** **Secondary osteoarthritis, left shoulder**

✓ Additional Character Required   ✓x7ᵗʰ Placeholder   Unacceptable PDx   Questionable PDx   Manifestation   Unspecified Dx   H1-H14 HAC   HCC CMS-HCC Dx   HIV HIV Dx

ICD-10-CM 2020   787

Chapter 13. Diseases of the Musculoskeletal System and Connective Tissue

M19.219–M21.00

M19.219 Secondary osteoarthritis, unspecified shoulder

✓6ᵗʰ **M19.22 Secondary osteoarthritis, elbow**

M19.221 Secondary osteoarthritis, right elbow
M19.222 Secondary osteoarthritis, left elbow
M19.229 Secondary osteoarthritis, unspecified elbow

✓6ᵗʰ **M19.23 Secondary osteoarthritis, wrist**

M19.231 Secondary osteoarthritis, right wrist
M19.232 Secondary osteoarthritis, left wrist
M19.239 Secondary osteoarthritis, unspecified wrist

✓6ᵗʰ **M19.24 Secondary osteoarthritis, hand**

M19.241 Secondary osteoarthritis, right hand
M19.242 Secondary osteoarthritis, left hand
M19.249 Secondary osteoarthritis, unspecified hand

✓6ᵗʰ **M19.27 Secondary osteoarthritis, ankle and foot**

M19.271 Secondary osteoarthritis, right ankle and foot
M19.272 Secondary osteoarthritis, left ankle and foot
M19.279 Secondary osteoarthritis, unspecified ankle and foot

✓5ᵗʰ **M19.9 Osteoarthritis, unspecified site**

M19.90 **Unspecified osteoarthritis, unspecified site**
Arthrosis NOS
Arthritis NOS
Osteoarthritis NOS
AHA: 2016,4Q,147

M19.91 **Primary osteoarthritis, unspecified site**
Primary osteoarthritis NOS

M19.92 **Post-traumatic osteoarthritis, unspecified site**
Post-traumatic osteoarthritis NOS

M19.93 **Secondary osteoarthritis, unspecified site**
Secondary osteoarthritis NOS

Other joint disorders (M20-M25)

EXCLUDES 2   joints of the spine (M40-M54)

✓4ᵗʰ **M20 Acquired deformities of fingers and toes**

EXCLUDES 1   acquired absence of fingers and toes (Z89.-)
congenital absence of fingers and toes (Q71.3-, Q72.3-)
congenital deformities and malformations of fingers and toes (Q66.-, Q68-Q70, Q74.-)

✓5ᵗʰ **M20.0 Deformity of finger(s)**

EXCLUDES 1   clubbing of fingers (R68.3)
palmar fascial fibromatosis [Dupuytren] (M72.0)
trigger finger (M65.3)

✓6ᵗʰ **M20.00 Unspecified deformity of finger(s)**

M20.001 Unspecified deformity of right finger(s)
M20.002 Unspecified deformity of left finger(s)
M20.009 Unspecified deformity of unspecified finger(s)

✓6ᵗʰ **M20.01 Mallet finger**

M20.011 Mallet finger of right finger(s)
M20.012 Mallet finger of left finger(s)
M20.019 Mallet finger of unspecified finger(s)

✓6ᵗʰ **M20.02 Boutonnière deformity**

DEF: Deformity of the finger caused by flexion of the proximal interphalangeal joint and hyperextension of the distal joint. The deformity results from rheumatoid arthritis, osteoarthritis, or injury.

M20.021 Boutonnière deformity of right finger(s)
M20.022 Boutonnière deformity of left finger(s)
M20.029 Boutonnière deformity of unspecified finger(s)

✓6ᵗʰ **M20.03 Swan-neck deformity**

DEF: Flexed distal and hyperextended proximal interphalangeal joint most commonly caused by rheumatoid arthritis.

M20.031 Swan-neck deformity of right finger(s)
M20.032 Swan-neck deformity of left finger(s)
M20.039 Swan-neck deformity of unspecified finger(s)

✓6ᵗʰ **M20.09 Other deformity of finger(s)**

M20.091 Other deformity of right finger(s)
M20.092 Other deformity of left finger(s)

M20.099 Other deformity of finger(s), unspecified finger(s)

✓5ᵗʰ **M20.1 Hallux valgus (acquired)**

EXCLUDES 2   bunion (M21.6-)

AHA: 2016,4Q,38
DEF: Deformity in which the great toe deviates toward the other toes and may even be positioned over or under the second toe.

Hallux Valgus

Hallux valgus

Medial eminence of metatarsal bone

Right foot

M20.10 Hallux valgus (acquired), unspecified foot
M20.11 Hallux valgus (acquired), right foot
M20.12 Hallux valgus (acquired), left foot

✓5ᵗʰ **M20.2 Hallux rigidus**

M20.20 Hallux rigidus, unspecified foot
M20.21 Hallux rigidus, right foot
M20.22 Hallux rigidus, left foot

✓5ᵗʰ **M20.3 Hallux varus (acquired)**

DEF: Deformity in which the great toe deviates away from the other toes.

M20.30 Hallux varus (acquired), unspecified foot
M20.31 Hallux varus (acquired), right foot
M20.32 Hallux varus (acquired), left foot

✓5ᵗʰ **M20.4 Other hammer toe(s) (acquired)**

M20.40 Other hammer toe(s) (acquired), unspecified foot
M20.41 Other hammer toe(s) (acquired), right foot
M20.42 Other hammer toe(s) (acquired), left foot

✓5ᵗʰ **M20.5 Other deformities of toe(s) (acquired)**

✓6ᵗʰ **M20.5X Other deformities of toe(s) (acquired)**

M20.5X1 Other deformities of toe(s) (acquired), right foot
M20.5X2 Other deformities of toe(s) (acquired), left foot
M20.5X9 Other deformities of toe(s) (acquired), unspecified foot

✓5ᵗʰ **M20.6 Acquired deformities of toe(s), unspecified**

M20.60 **Acquired deformities of toe(s), unspecified, unspecified foot**
M20.61 **Acquired deformities of toe(s), unspecified, right foot**
M20.62 **Acquired deformities of toe(s), unspecified, left foot**

✓4ᵗʰ **M21 Other acquired deformities of limbs**

EXCLUDES 1   acquired absence of limb (Z89.-)
congenital absence of limbs (Q71-Q73)
congenital deformities and malformations of limbs (Q65-Q66, Q68-Q74)

EXCLUDES 2   acquired deformities of fingers or toes (M20.-)
coxa plana (M91.2)

✓5ᵗʰ **M21.0 Valgus deformity, not elsewhere classified**

EXCLUDES 1   metatarsus valgus (Q66.6)
talipes calcaneovalgus ▶(Q66.4-)◄

M21.00 **Valgus deformity, not elsewhere classified, unspecified site**

√6ᵗʰ **M21.02 Valgus deformity, not elsewhere classified, elbow**
Cubitus valgus

M21.021 Valgus deformity, not elsewhere classified, right elbow

M21.022 Valgus deformity, not elsewhere classified, left elbow

M21.029 Valgus deformity, not elsewhere classified, unspecified elbow

√6ᵗʰ **M21.05 Valgus deformity, not elsewhere classified, hip**

M21.051 Valgus deformity, not elsewhere classified, right hip

M21.052 Valgus deformity, not elsewhere classified, left hip

M21.059 Valgus deformity, not elsewhere classified, unspecified hip

√6ᵗʰ **M21.06 Valgus deformity, not elsewhere classified, knee**
Genu valgum
Knock knee
DEF: Genu valga/valgum: Condition in which the thighs slant inward, causing the knees to be angled abnormally close together, leaving the space between the ankles wider than normal.

Genu Valga (knock-knee)

M21.061 Valgus deformity, not elsewhere classified, right knee

M21.062 Valgus deformity, not elsewhere classified, left knee

M21.069 Valgus deformity, not elsewhere classified, unspecified knee

√6ᵗʰ **M21.07 Valgus deformity, not elsewhere classified, ankle**

M21.071 Valgus deformity, not elsewhere classified, right ankle

M21.072 Valgus deformity, not elsewhere classified, left ankle

M21.079 Valgus deformity, not elsewhere classified, unspecified ankle

√5ᵗʰ **M21.1 Varus deformity, not elsewhere classified**

EXCLUDES 1   metatarsus varus ▶(Q66.22-)◀
tibia vara (M92.5)

M21.10 Varus deformity, not elsewhere classified, unspecified site

√6ᵗʰ **M21.12 Varus deformity, not elsewhere classified, elbow**
Cubitus varus, elbow

M21.121 Varus deformity, not elsewhere classified, right elbow

M21.122 Varus deformity, not elsewhere classified, left elbow

M21.129 Varus deformity, not elsewhere classified, unspecified elbow

√6ᵗʰ **M21.15 Varus deformity, not elsewhere classified, hip**

M21.151 Varus deformity, not elsewhere classified, right hip

M21.152 Varus deformity, not elsewhere classified, left hip

M21.159 Varus deformity, not elsewhere classified, unspecified

√6ᵗʰ **M21.16 Varus deformity, not elsewhere classified, knee**
Bow leg
Genu varum
DEF: Genu varus/varum: Condition in which the thighs and/or legs are bowed in an outward curve with an abnormally increased space between the knees.

Genu Varus (bowleg)

M21.161 Varus deformity, not elsewhere classified, right knee

M21.162 Varus deformity, not elsewhere classified, left knee

M21.169 Varus deformity, not elsewhere classified, unspecified knee

√6ᵗʰ **M21.17 Varus deformity, not elsewhere classified, ankle**

M21.171 Varus deformity, not elsewhere classified, right ankle

M21.172 Varus deformity, not elsewhere classified, left ankle

M21.179 Varus deformity, not elsewhere classified, unspecified ankle

√5ᵗʰ **M21.2 Flexion deformity**

M21.20 Flexion deformity, unspecified site

√6ᵗʰ **M21.21 Flexion deformity, shoulder**

M21.211 Flexion deformity, right shoulder
M21.212 Flexion deformity, left shoulder
M21.219 Flexion deformity, unspecified shoulder

√6ᵗʰ **M21.22 Flexion deformity, elbow**

M21.221 Flexion deformity, right elbow
M21.222 Flexion deformity, left elbow
M21.229 Flexion deformity, unspecified elbow

√6ᵗʰ **M21.23 Flexion deformity, wrist**

M21.231 Flexion deformity, right wrist
M21.232 Flexion deformity, left wrist
M21.239 Flexion deformity, unspecified wrist

√6ᵗʰ **M21.24 Flexion deformity, finger joints**

M21.241 Flexion deformity, right finger joints
M21.242 Flexion deformity, left finger joints
M21.249 Flexion deformity, unspecified finger joints

√6ᵗʰ **M21.25 Flexion deformity, hip**

M21.251 Flexion deformity, right hip
M21.252 Flexion deformity, left hip
M21.259 Flexion deformity, unspecified hip

√6ᵗʰ **M21.26 Flexion deformity, knee**

M21.261 Flexion deformity, right knee
M21.262 Flexion deformity, left knee
M21.269 Flexion deformity, unspecified knee

√6ᵗʰ **M21.27 Flexion deformity, ankle and toes**

M21.271 Flexion deformity, right ankle and toes
M21.272 Flexion deformity, left ankle and toes

M21.279 Flexion deformity, unspecified ankle and toes

✓5ᵗʰ **M21.3** Wrist or foot drop (acquired)

  ✓6ᵗʰ **M21.33** Wrist drop (acquired)

    M21.331 Wrist drop, right wrist

    M21.332 Wrist drop, left wrist

    M21.339 Wrist drop, unspecified wrist

  ✓6ᵗʰ **M21.37** Foot drop (acquired)

    M21.371 Foot drop, right foot

    M21.372 Foot drop, left foot

    M21.379 Foot drop, unspecified foot

✓5ᵗʰ **M21.4** Flat foot [pes planus] (acquired)

    EXCLUDES 1   congenital pes planus (Q66.5-)

  M21.40 Flat foot [pes planus] (acquired), unspecified foot

  M21.41 Flat foot [pes planus] (acquired), right foot

  M21.42 Flat foot [pes planus] (acquired), left foot

✓5ᵗʰ **M21.5** Acquired clawhand, clubhand, clawfoot and clubfoot

    EXCLUDES 1   clubfoot, not specified as acquired (Q66.89)

  ✓6ᵗʰ **M21.51** Acquired clawhand

    M21.511 Acquired clawhand, right hand

    M21.512 Acquired clawhand, left hand

    M21.519 Acquired clawhand, unspecified hand

  ✓6ᵗʰ **M21.52** Acquired clubhand

    M21.521 Acquired clubhand, right hand

    M21.522 Acquired clubhand, left hand

    M21.529 Acquired clubhand, unspecified hand

  ✓6ᵗʰ **M21.53** Acquired clawfoot

    DEF: High foot arch with hyperextended toes at the metatarsophalangeal joint and flexed toes at the distal joints.

    M21.531 Acquired clawfoot, right foot

    M21.532 Acquired clawfoot, left foot

    M21.539 Acquired clawfoot, unspecified foot

  ✓6ᵗʰ **M21.54** Acquired clubfoot

    DEF: Acquired anomaly of the foot with the heel elevated and rotated outward and the toes pointing inward.

    M21.541 Acquired clubfoot, right foot

    M21.542 Acquired clubfoot, left foot

    M21.549 Acquired clubfoot, unspecified foot

✓5ᵗʰ **M21.6** Other acquired deformities of foot

    EXCLUDES 2   deformities of toe (acquired) (M20.1-M20.6-)

    AHA: 2016,4Q,38

  ✓6ᵗʰ **M21.61** Bunion

    M21.611 Bunion of right foot

    M21.612 Bunion of left foot

    M21.619 Bunion of unspecified foot

  ✓6ᵗʰ **M21.62** Bunionette

    M21.621 Bunionette of right foot

    M21.622 Bunionette of left foot

    M21.629 Bunionette of unspecified foot

  ✓6ᵗʰ **M21.6X** Other acquired deformities of foot

    M21.6X1 Other acquired deformities of right foot

    M21.6X2 Other acquired deformities of left foot

    M21.6X9 Other acquired deformities of unspecified foot

✓5ᵗʰ **M21.7** Unequal limb length (acquired)

    NOTE   The site used should correspond to the shorter limb

  M21.70 Unequal limb length (acquired), unspecified site

  ✓6ᵗʰ **M21.72** Unequal limb length (acquired), humerus

    M21.721 Unequal limb length (acquired), right humerus

    M21.722 Unequal limb length (acquired), left humerus

    M21.729 Unequal limb length (acquired), unspecified humerus

  ✓6ᵗʰ **M21.73** Unequal limb length (acquired), ulna and radius

    M21.731 Unequal limb length (acquired), right ulna

    M21.732 Unequal limb length (acquired), left ulna

    M21.733 Unequal limb length (acquired), right radius

    M21.734 Unequal limb length (acquired), left radius

    M21.739 Unequal limb length (acquired), unspecified ulna and radius

  ✓6ᵗʰ **M21.75** Unequal limb length (acquired), femur

    M21.751 Unequal limb length (acquired), right femur

    M21.752 Unequal limb length (acquired), left femur

    M21.759 Unequal limb length (acquired), unspecified femur

  ✓6ᵗʰ **M21.76** Unequal limb length (acquired), tibia and fibula

    M21.761 Unequal limb length (acquired), right tibia

    M21.762 Unequal limb length (acquired), left tibia

    M21.763 Unequal limb length (acquired), right fibula

    M21.764 Unequal limb length (acquired), left fibula

    M21.769 Unequal limb length (acquired), unspecified tibia and fibula

✓5ᵗʰ **M21.8** Other specified acquired deformities of limbs

    EXCLUDES 2   coxa plana (M91.2)

  M21.80 Other specified acquired deformities of unspecified limb

  ✓6ᵗʰ **M21.82** Other specified acquired deformities of upper arm

    M21.821 Other specified acquired deformities of right upper arm

    M21.822 Other specified acquired deformities of left upper arm

    M21.829 Other specified acquired deformities of unspecified upper arm

  ✓6ᵗʰ **M21.83** Other specified acquired deformities of forearm

    M21.831 Other specified acquired deformities of right forearm

    M21.832 Other specified acquired deformities of left forearm

    M21.839 Other specified acquired deformities of unspecified forearm

  ✓6ᵗʰ **M21.85** Other specified acquired deformities of thigh

    M21.851 Other specified acquired deformities of right thigh

    M21.852 Other specified acquired deformities of left thigh

    M21.859 Other specified acquired deformities of unspecified thigh

  ✓6ᵗʰ **M21.86** Other specified acquired deformities of lower leg

    M21.861 Other specified acquired deformities of right lower leg

    M21.862 Other specified acquired deformities of left lower leg

    M21.869 Other specified acquired deformities of unspecified lower leg

✓5ᵗʰ **M21.9** Unspecified acquired deformity of limb and hand

  M21.90 Unspecified acquired deformity of unspecified limb

  ✓6ᵗʰ **M21.92** Unspecified acquired deformity of upper arm

    M21.921 Unspecified acquired deformity of right upper arm

    M21.922 Unspecified acquired deformity of left upper arm

    M21.929 Unspecified acquired deformity of unspecified upper arm

  ✓6ᵗʰ **M21.93** Unspecified acquired deformity of forearm

    M21.931 Unspecified acquired deformity of right forearm

    M21.932 Unspecified acquired deformity of left forearm

    M21.939 Unspecified acquired deformity of unspecified forearm

  ✓6ᵗʰ **M21.94** Unspecified acquired deformity of hand

    M21.941 Unspecified acquired deformity of hand, right hand

    M21.942 Unspecified acquired deformity of hand, left hand

    M21.949 Unspecified acquired deformity of hand, unspecified hand

  ✓6ᵗʰ **M21.95** Unspecified acquired deformity of thigh

    M21.951 Unspecified acquired deformity of right thigh

    M21.952 Unspecified acquired deformity of left thigh

    M21.959 Unspecified acquired deformity of unspecified thigh

N Newborn: 0 **P** Pediatric: 0-17 **M** Maternity: 9-64 **A** Adult: 15-124 **MCC** Major Complication/Comorbidity **CC** Complication/Comorbidity **SW** Severe Wound Dx

790 ICD-10-CM 2020

√6ᵗʰ **M21.96** Unspecified acquired deformity of lower leg

    M21.961 Unspecified acquired deformity of right lower leg

    M21.962 Unspecified acquired deformity of left lower leg

    M21.969 Unspecified acquired deformity of unspecified lower leg

√4ᵗʰ **M22** Disorder of patella

    EXCLUDES 1   traumatic dislocation of patella (S83.0-)

  √5ᵗʰ **M22.0** Recurrent dislocation of patella

    M22.00 Recurrent dislocation of patella, unspecified knee

    M22.01 Recurrent dislocation of patella, right knee

    M22.02 Recurrent dislocation of patella, left knee

  √5ᵗʰ **M22.1** Recurrent subluxation of patella

    Incomplete dislocation of patella

    M22.10 Recurrent subluxation of patella, unspecified knee

    M22.11 Recurrent subluxation of patella, right knee

    M22.12 Recurrent subluxation of patella, left knee

  √5ᵗʰ **M22.2** Patellofemoral disorders

    √6ᵗʰ **M22.2X** Patellofemoral disorders

      M22.2X1 Patellofemoral disorders, right knee

      M22.2X2 Patellofemoral disorders, left knee

      M22.2X9 Patellofemoral disorders, unspecified knee

  √5ᵗʰ **M22.3** Other derangements of patella

    √6ᵗʰ **M22.3X** Other derangements of patella

      M22.3X1 Other derangements of patella, right knee

      M22.3X2 Other derangements of patella, left knee

      M22.3X9 Other derangements of patella, unspecified knee

  √5ᵗʰ **M22.4** Chondromalacia patellae

    M22.40 Chondromalacia patellae, unspecified knee

    M22.41 Chondromalacia patellae, right knee

    M22.42 Chondromalacia patellae, left knee

  √5ᵗʰ **M22.8** Other disorders of patella

    √6ᵗʰ **M22.8X** Other disorders of patella

      M22.8X1 Other disorders of patella, right knee

      M22.8X2 Other disorders of patella, left knee

      M22.8X9 Other disorders of patella, unspecified knee

  √5ᵗʰ **M22.9** Unspecified disorder of patella

    M22.90 Unspecified disorder of patella, unspecified knee

    M22.91 Unspecified disorder of patella, right knee

    M22.92 Unspecified disorder of patella, left knee

√4ᵗʰ **M23** Internal derangement of knee

    EXCLUDES 1   ankylosis (M24.66)

        current injury — see injury of knee and lower leg (S80-S89)

        deformity of knee (M21.-)

        osteochondritis dissecans (M93.2)

        recurrent dislocation or subluxation of joints (M24.4)

        recurrent dislocation or subluxation of patella (M22.0-M22.1)

  √5ᵗʰ **M23.0** Cystic meniscus

    √6ᵗʰ **M23.00** Cystic meniscus, unspecified meniscus

      Cystic meniscus, unspecified lateral meniscus

      Cystic meniscus, unspecified medial meniscus

      M23.000 Cystic meniscus, unspecified lateral meniscus, right knee

      M23.001 Cystic meniscus, unspecified lateral meniscus, left knee

      M23.002 Cystic meniscus, unspecified lateral meniscus, unspecified knee

      M23.003 Cystic meniscus, unspecified medial meniscus, right knee

      M23.004 Cystic meniscus, unspecified medial meniscus, left knee

      M23.005 Cystic meniscus, unspecified medial meniscus, unspecified knee

      M23.006 Cystic meniscus, unspecified meniscus, right knee

      M23.007 Cystic meniscus, unspecified meniscus, left knee

      M23.009 Cystic meniscus, unspecified meniscus, unspecified knee

---

    √6ᵗʰ **M23.01** Cystic meniscus, anterior horn of medial meniscus

      M23.011 Cystic meniscus, anterior horn of medial meniscus, right knee

      M23.012 Cystic meniscus, anterior horn of medial meniscus, left knee

      M23.019 Cystic meniscus, anterior horn of medial meniscus, unspecified knee

    √6ᵗʰ **M23.02** Cystic meniscus, posterior horn of medial meniscus

      M23.021 Cystic meniscus, posterior horn of medial meniscus, right knee

      M23.022 Cystic meniscus, posterior horn of medial meniscus, left knee

      M23.029 Cystic meniscus, posterior horn of medial meniscus, unspecified knee

    √6ᵗʰ **M23.03** Cystic meniscus, other medial meniscus

      M23.031 Cystic meniscus, other medial meniscus, right knee

      M23.032 Cystic meniscus, other medial meniscus, left knee

      M23.039 Cystic meniscus, other medial meniscus, unspecified knee

    √6ᵗʰ **M23.04** Cystic meniscus, anterior horn of lateral meniscus

      M23.041 Cystic meniscus, anterior horn of lateral meniscus, right knee

      M23.042 Cystic meniscus, anterior horn of lateral meniscus, left knee

      M23.049 Cystic meniscus, anterior horn of lateral meniscus, unspecified knee

    √6ᵗʰ **M23.05** Cystic meniscus, posterior horn of lateral meniscus

      M23.051 Cystic meniscus, posterior horn of lateral meniscus, right knee

      M23.052 Cystic meniscus, posterior horn of lateral meniscus, left knee

      M23.059 Cystic meniscus, posterior horn of lateral meniscus, unspecified knee

    √6ᵗʰ **M23.06** Cystic meniscus, other lateral meniscus

      M23.061 Cystic meniscus, other lateral meniscus, right knee

      M23.062 Cystic meniscus, other lateral meniscus, left knee

      M23.069 Cystic meniscus, other lateral meniscus, unspecified knee

  √5ᵗʰ **M23.2** Derangement of meniscus due to old tear or injury

    Old bucket-handle tear

    AHA: 2019,2Q,26

Derangement of Meniscus

Bucket handle tear

Radial tear

Meniscus

Lateral meniscus

Posterior cruciate ligament

Medial meniscus

Anterior horns

Patellar ligament

Anterior cruciate ligament

Posterior horns

Overhead view of right knee

    √6ᵗʰ **M23.20** Derangement of unspecified meniscus due to old tear or injury

      Derangement of unspecified lateral meniscus due to old tear or injury

      Derangement of unspecified medial meniscus due to old tear or injury

      M23.200 Derangement of unspecified lateral meniscus due to old tear or injury, right knee

✔ Additional Character Required   √x7ᵗʰ Placeholder   Unacceptable PDx   Questionable PDx   Manifestation   Unspecified Dx   H1-H14 HAC   HCC CMS-HCC Dx   HIV HIV Dx

ICD-10-CM 2020   791

M23.201 Derangement of unspecified lateral meniscus due to old tear or injury, left knee

M23.202 Derangement of unspecified lateral meniscus due to old tear or injury, unspecified knee

M23.203 Derangement of unspecified medial meniscus due to old tear or injury, right knee

M23.204 Derangement of unspecified medial meniscus due to old tear or injury, left knee

M23.205 Derangement of unspecified medial meniscus due to old tear or injury, unspecified knee

M23.206 Derangement of unspecified meniscus due to old tear or injury, right knee

M23.207 Derangement of unspecified meniscus due to old tear or injury, left knee

M23.209 Derangement of unspecified meniscus due to old tear or injury, unspecified knee

✓6ᵗʰ **M23.21** Derangement of anterior horn of medial meniscus due to old tear or injury

M23.211 Derangement of anterior horn of medial meniscus due to old tear or injury, right knee

M23.212 Derangement of anterior horn of medial meniscus due to old tear or injury, left knee

M23.219 Derangement of anterior horn of medial meniscus due to old tear or injury, unspecified knee

✓6ᵗʰ **M23.22** Derangement of posterior horn of medial meniscus due to old tear or injury

M23.221 Derangement of posterior horn of medial meniscus due to old tear or injury, right knee

M23.222 Derangement of posterior horn of medial meniscus due to old tear or injury, left knee

M23.229 Derangement of posterior horn of medial meniscus due to old tear or injury, unspecified knee

✓6ᵗʰ **M23.23** Derangement of other medial meniscus due to old tear or injury

M23.231 Derangement of other medial meniscus due to old tear or injury, right knee

M23.232 Derangement of other medial meniscus due to old tear or injury, left knee

M23.239 Derangement of other medial meniscus due to old tear or injury, unspecified knee

✓6ᵗʰ **M23.24** Derangement of anterior horn of lateral meniscus due to old tear or injury

M23.241 Derangement of anterior horn of lateral meniscus due to old tear or injury, right knee

M23.242 Derangement of anterior horn of lateral meniscus due to old tear or injury, left knee

M23.249 Derangement of anterior horn of lateral meniscus due to old tear or injury, unspecified knee

✓6ᵗʰ **M23.25** Derangement of posterior horn of lateral meniscus due to old tear or injury

M23.251 Derangement of posterior horn of lateral meniscus due to old tear or injury, right knee

M23.252 Derangement of posterior horn of lateral meniscus due to old tear or injury, left knee

M23.259 Derangement of posterior horn of lateral meniscus due to old tear or injury, unspecified knee

✓6ᵗʰ **M23.26** Derangement of other lateral meniscus due to old tear or injury

M23.261 Derangement of other lateral meniscus due to old tear or injury, right knee

M23.262 Derangement of other lateral meniscus due to old tear or injury, left knee

M23.269 Derangement of other lateral meniscus due to old tear or injury, unspecified knee

✓5ᵗʰ **M23.3** Other meniscus derangements

Degenerate meniscus

Detached meniscus

Retained meniscus

✓6ᵗʰ **M23.30** Other meniscus derangements, unspecified meniscus

Other meniscus derangements, unspecified lateral meniscus

Other meniscus derangements, unspecified medial meniscus

M23.300 Other meniscus derangements, unspecified lateral meniscus, right knee

M23.301 Other meniscus derangements, unspecified lateral meniscus, left knee

M23.302 Other meniscus derangements, unspecified lateral meniscus, unspecified knee

M23.303 Other meniscus derangements, unspecified medial meniscus, right knee

M23.304 Other meniscus derangements, unspecified medial meniscus, left knee

M23.305 Other meniscus derangements, unspecified medial meniscus, unspecified knee

M23.306 Other meniscus derangements, unspecified meniscus, right knee

M23.307 Other meniscus derangements, unspecified meniscus, left knee

M23.309 Other meniscus derangements, unspecified meniscus, unspecified knee

✓6ᵗʰ **M23.31** Other meniscus derangements, anterior horn of medial meniscus

M23.311 Other meniscus derangements, anterior horn of medial meniscus, right knee

M23.312 Other meniscus derangements, anterior horn of medial meniscus, left knee

M23.319 Other meniscus derangements, anterior horn of medial meniscus, unspecified knee

✓6ᵗʰ **M23.32** Other meniscus derangements, posterior horn of medial meniscus

M23.321 Other meniscus derangements, posterior horn of medial meniscus, right knee

M23.322 Other meniscus derangements, posterior horn of medial meniscus, left knee

M23.329 Other meniscus derangements, posterior horn of medial meniscus, unspecified knee

✓6ᵗʰ **M23.33** Other meniscus derangements, other medial meniscus

M23.331 Other meniscus derangements, other medial meniscus, right knee

M23.332 Other meniscus derangements, other medial meniscus, left knee

M23.339 Other meniscus derangements, other medial meniscus, unspecified knee

✓6ᵗʰ **M23.34** Other meniscus derangements, anterior horn of lateral meniscus

M23.341 Other meniscus derangements, anterior horn of lateral meniscus, right knee

M23.342 Other meniscus derangements, anterior horn of lateral meniscus, left knee

M23.349 Other meniscus derangements, anterior horn of lateral meniscus, unspecified knee

✓6ᵗʰ **M23.35** Other meniscus derangements, posterior horn of lateral meniscus

M23.351 Other meniscus derangements, posterior horn of lateral meniscus, right knee

M23.352 Other meniscus derangements, posterior horn of lateral meniscus, left knee

M23.359 Other meniscus derangements, posterior horn of lateral meniscus, unspecified knee

✓6ᵗʰ **M23.36** Other meniscus derangements, other lateral meniscus

M23.361 Other meniscus derangements, other lateral meniscus, right knee

M23.362 Other meniscus derangements, other lateral meniscus, left knee

M23.369 Other meniscus derangements, other lateral meniscus, unspecified knee

N Newborn: 0   P Pediatric: 0-17   M Maternity: 9-64   A Adult: 15-124   MCC Major Complication/Comorbidity   CC Complication/Comorbidity   SW Severe Wound Dx

792

ICD-10-CM 2020

√5ᵗʰ **M23.4 Loose body in knee**

M23.40 Loose body in knee, unspecified knee
M23.41 Loose body in knee, right knee
M23.42 Loose body in knee, left knee

√5ᵗʰ **M23.5 Chronic instability of knee**

M23.50 Chronic instability of knee, unspecified knee
M23.51 Chronic instability of knee, right knee
M23.52 Chronic instability of knee, left knee

√5ᵗʰ **M23.6 Other spontaneous disruption of ligament(s) of knee**

√6ᵗʰ   **M23.60** Other spontaneous disruption of unspecified ligament of knee
     M23.601 Other spontaneous disruption of unspecified ligament of right knee
     M23.602 Other spontaneous disruption of unspecified ligament of left knee
     M23.609 Other spontaneous disruption of unspecified ligament of unspecified knee

√6ᵗʰ   **M23.61** Other spontaneous disruption of anterior cruciate ligament of knee
     M23.611 Other spontaneous disruption of anterior cruciate ligament of right knee
     M23.612 Other spontaneous disruption of anterior cruciate ligament of left knee
     M23.619 Other spontaneous disruption of anterior cruciate ligament of unspecified knee

√6ᵗʰ   **M23.62** Other spontaneous disruption of posterior cruciate ligament of knee
     M23.621 Other spontaneous disruption of posterior cruciate ligament of right knee
     M23.622 Other spontaneous disruption of posterior cruciate ligament of left knee
     M23.629 Other spontaneous disruption of posterior cruciate ligament of unspecified knee

√6ᵗʰ   **M23.63** Other spontaneous disruption of medial collateral ligament of knee
     M23.631 Other spontaneous disruption of medial collateral ligament of right knee
     M23.632 Other spontaneous disruption of medial collateral ligament of left knee
     M23.639 Other spontaneous disruption of medial collateral ligament of unspecified knee

√6ᵗʰ   **M23.64** Other spontaneous disruption of lateral collateral ligament of knee
     M23.641 Other spontaneous disruption of lateral collateral ligament of right knee
     M23.642 Other spontaneous disruption of lateral collateral ligament of left knee
     M23.649 Other spontaneous disruption of lateral collateral ligament of unspecified knee

√6ᵗʰ   **M23.67** Other spontaneous disruption of capsular ligament of knee
     M23.671 Other spontaneous disruption of capsular ligament of right knee
     M23.672 Other spontaneous disruption of capsular ligament of left knee
     M23.679 Other spontaneous disruption of capsular ligament of unspecified knee

√5ᵗʰ **M23.8 Other internal derangements of knee**

Laxity of ligament of knee
Snapping knee

√6ᵗʰ   **M23.8X** Other internal derangements of knee
     M23.8X1 Other internal derangements of right knee
     M23.8X2 Other internal derangements of left knee
     M23.8X9 Other internal derangements of unspecified knee

√5ᵗʰ **M23.9 Unspecified internal derangement of knee**

M23.90 Unspecified internal derangement of unspecified knee
M23.91 Unspecified internal derangement of right knee
M23.92 Unspecified internal derangement of left knee

√4ᵗʰ **M24 Other specific joint derangements**

EXCLUDES 1   current injury — see injury of joint by body region
EXCLUDES 2   ganglion (M67.4)
     snapping knee (M23.8-)
     temporomandibular joint disorders (M26.6-)

√5ᵗʰ **M24.0 Loose body in joint**

EXCLUDES 2   loose body in knee (M23.4)

M24.00 Loose body in unspecified joint

√6ᵗʰ   **M24.01** Loose body in shoulder
     M24.011 Loose body in right shoulder
     M24.012 Loose body in left shoulder
     M24.019 Loose body in unspecified shoulder

√6ᵗʰ   **M24.02** Loose body in elbow
     M24.021 Loose body in right elbow
     M24.022 Loose body in left elbow
     M24.029 Loose body in unspecified elbow

√6ᵗʰ   **M24.03** Loose body in wrist
     M24.031 Loose body in right wrist
     M24.032 Loose body in left wrist
     M24.039 Loose body in unspecified wrist

√6ᵗʰ   **M24.04** Loose body in finger joints
     M24.041 Loose body in right finger joint(s)
     M24.042 Loose body in left finger joint(s)
     M24.049 Loose body in unspecified finger joint(s)

√6ᵗʰ   **M24.05** Loose body in hip
     M24.051 Loose body in right hip
     M24.052 Loose body in left hip
     M24.059 Loose body in unspecified hip

√6ᵗʰ   **M24.07** Loose body in ankle and toe joints
     M24.071 Loose body in right ankle
     M24.072 Loose body in left ankle
     M24.073 Loose body in unspecified ankle
     M24.074 Loose body in right toe joint(s)
     M24.075 Loose body in left toe joint(s)
     M24.076 Loose body in unspecified toe joints

M24.08 Loose body, other site

√5ᵗʰ **M24.1 Other articular cartilage disorders**

EXCLUDES 2   chondrocalcinosis (M11.1, M11.2-)
     internal derangement of knee (M23.-)
     metastatic calcification (E83.5)
     ochronosis (E70.2)

M24.10 Other articular cartilage disorders, unspecified site

√6ᵗʰ   **M24.11** Other articular cartilage disorders, shoulder
     M24.111 Other articular cartilage disorders, right shoulder
     M24.112 Other articular cartilage disorders, left shoulder
     M24.119 Other articular cartilage disorders, unspecified shoulder

√6ᵗʰ   **M24.12** Other articular cartilage disorders, elbow
     M24.121 Other articular cartilage disorders, right elbow
     M24.122 Other articular cartilage disorders, left elbow
     M24.129 Other articular cartilage disorders, unspecified elbow

√6ᵗʰ   **M24.13** Other articular cartilage disorders, wrist
     M24.131 Other articular cartilage disorders, right wrist
     M24.132 Other articular cartilage disorders, left wrist
     M24.139 Other articular cartilage disorders, unspecified wrist

√6ᵗʰ   **M24.14** Other articular cartilage disorders, hand
     M24.141 Other articular cartilage disorders, right hand
     M24.142 Other articular cartilage disorders, left hand
     M24.149 Other articular cartilage disorders, unspecified hand

√6ᵗʰ   **M24.15** Other articular cartilage disorders, hip
     M24.151 Other articular cartilage disorders, right hip
     M24.152 Other articular cartilage disorders, left hip
     M24.159 Other articular cartilage disorders, unspecified hip

Chapter 13. Diseases of the Musculoskeletal System and Connective Tissue

M24.17–M24.474

√6ᵗʰ **M24.17 Other articular cartilage disorders, ankle and foot**

    M24.171 Other articular cartilage disorders, right ankle

    M24.172 Other articular cartilage disorders, left ankle

    M24.173 Other articular cartilage disorders, unspecified ankle

    M24.174 Other articular cartilage disorders, right foot

    M24.175 Other articular cartilage disorders, left foot

    M24.176 Other articular cartilage disorders, unspecified foot

√5ᵗʰ **M24.2 Disorder of ligament**

    Instability secondary to old ligament injury

    Ligamentous laxity NOS

    EXCLUDES 1 *familial ligamentous laxity (M35.7)*

    EXCLUDES 2 *internal derangement of knee ▶(M23.5-M23.8X9)◀*

    M24.20 Disorder of ligament, unspecified site

√6ᵗʰ **M24.21 Disorder of ligament, shoulder**

    M24.211 Disorder of ligament, right shoulder

    M24.212 Disorder of ligament, left shoulder

    M24.219 Disorder of ligament, unspecified shoulder

√6ᵗʰ **M24.22 Disorder of ligament, elbow**

    M24.221 Disorder of ligament, right elbow

    M24.222 Disorder of ligament, left elbow

    M24.229 Disorder of ligament, unspecified elbow

√6ᵗʰ **M24.23 Disorder of ligament, wrist**

    M24.231 Disorder of ligament, right wrist

    M24.232 Disorder of ligament, left wrist

    M24.239 Disorder of ligament, unspecified wrist

√6ᵗʰ **M24.24 Disorder of ligament, hand**

    M24.241 Disorder of ligament, right hand

    M24.242 Disorder of ligament, left hand

    M24.249 Disorder of ligament, unspecified hand

√6ᵗʰ **M24.25 Disorder of ligament, hip**

    M24.251 Disorder of ligament, right hip

    M24.252 Disorder of ligament, left hip

    M24.259 Disorder of ligament, unspecified hip

√6ᵗʰ **M24.27 Disorder of ligament, ankle and foot**

    M24.271 Disorder of ligament, right ankle

    M24.272 Disorder of ligament, left ankle

    M24.273 Disorder of ligament, unspecified ankle

    M24.274 Disorder of ligament, right foot

    M24.275 Disorder of ligament, left foot

    M24.276 Disorder of ligament, unspecified foot

    M24.28 Disorder of ligament, vertebrae

√5ᵗʰ **M24.3 Pathological dislocation of joint, not elsewhere classified**

    EXCLUDES 1 *congenital dislocation or displacement of joint — see congenital malformations and deformations of the musculoskeletal system (Q65-Q79)*

    current injury — see injury of joints and ligaments by body region

    recurrent dislocation of joint (M24.4-)

    M24.30 Pathological dislocation of unspecified joint, not elsewhere classified

√6ᵗʰ **M24.31 Pathological dislocation of shoulder, not elsewhere classified**

    M24.311 Pathological dislocation of right shoulder, not elsewhere classified

    M24.312 Pathological dislocation of left shoulder, not elsewhere classified

    M24.319 Pathological dislocation of unspecified shoulder, not elsewhere classified

√6ᵗʰ **M24.32 Pathological dislocation of elbow, not elsewhere classified**

    M24.321 Pathological dislocation of right elbow, not elsewhere classified

    M24.322 Pathological dislocation of left elbow, not elsewhere classified

    M24.329 Pathological dislocation of unspecified elbow, not elsewhere classified

√6ᵗʰ **M24.33 Pathological dislocation of wrist, not elsewhere classified**

    M24.331 Pathological dislocation of right wrist, not elsewhere classified

    M24.332 Pathological dislocation of left wrist, not elsewhere classified

    M24.339 Pathological dislocation of unspecified wrist, not elsewhere classified

√6ᵗʰ **M24.34 Pathological dislocation of hand, not elsewhere classified**

    M24.341 Pathological dislocation of right hand, not elsewhere classified

    M24.342 Pathological dislocation of left hand, not elsewhere classified

    M24.349 Pathological dislocation of unspecified hand, not elsewhere classified

√6ᵗʰ **M24.35 Pathological dislocation of hip, not elsewhere classified**

    M24.351 Pathological dislocation of right hip, not elsewhere classified

    M24.352 Pathological dislocation of left hip, not elsewhere classified

    M24.359 Pathological dislocation of unspecified hip, not elsewhere classified

√6ᵗʰ **M24.36 Pathological dislocation of knee, not elsewhere classified**

    M24.361 Pathological dislocation of right knee, not elsewhere classified

    M24.362 Pathological dislocation of left knee, not elsewhere classified

    M24.369 Pathological dislocation of unspecified knee, not elsewhere classified

√6ᵗʰ **M24.37 Pathological dislocation of ankle and foot, not elsewhere classified**

    M24.371 Pathological dislocation of right ankle, not elsewhere classified

    M24.372 Pathological dislocation of left ankle, not elsewhere classified

    M24.373 Pathological dislocation of unspecified ankle, not elsewhere classified

    M24.374 Pathological dislocation of right foot, not elsewhere classified

    M24.375 Pathological dislocation of left foot, not elsewhere classified

    M24.376 Pathological dislocation of unspecified foot, not elsewhere classified

√5ᵗʰ **M24.4 Recurrent dislocation of joint**

    Recurrent subluxation of joint

    EXCLUDES 2 *recurrent dislocation of patella (M22.0-M22.1)*

    recurrent vertebral dislocation (M43.3-, M43.4, M43.5-)

    M24.40 Recurrent dislocation, unspecified joint

√6ᵗʰ **M24.41 Recurrent dislocation, shoulder**

    M24.411 Recurrent dislocation, right shoulder

    M24.412 Recurrent dislocation, left shoulder

    M24.419 Recurrent dislocation, unspecified shoulder

√6ᵗʰ **M24.42 Recurrent dislocation, elbow**

    M24.421 Recurrent dislocation, right elbow

    M24.422 Recurrent dislocation, left elbow

    M24.429 Recurrent dislocation, unspecified elbow

√6ᵗʰ **M24.43 Recurrent dislocation, wrist**

    M24.431 Recurrent dislocation, right wrist

    M24.432 Recurrent dislocation, left wrist

    M24.439 Recurrent dislocation, unspecified wrist

√6ᵗʰ **M24.44 Recurrent dislocation, hand and finger(s)**

    M24.441 Recurrent dislocation, right hand

    M24.442 Recurrent dislocation, left hand

    M24.443 Recurrent dislocation, unspecified hand

    M24.444 Recurrent dislocation, right finger

    M24.445 Recurrent dislocation, left finger

    M24.446 Recurrent dislocation, unspecified finger

√6ᵗʰ **M24.45 Recurrent dislocation, hip**

    M24.451 Recurrent dislocation, right hip

    M24.452 Recurrent dislocation, left hip

    M24.459 Recurrent dislocation, unspecified hip

√6ᵗʰ **M24.46 Recurrent dislocation, knee**

    M24.461 Recurrent dislocation, right knee

    M24.462 Recurrent dislocation, left knee

    M24.469 Recurrent dislocation, unspecified knee

√6ᵗʰ **M24.47 Recurrent dislocation, ankle, foot and toes**

    M24.471 Recurrent dislocation, right ankle

    M24.472 Recurrent dislocation, left ankle

    M24.473 Recurrent dislocation, unspecified ankle

    M24.474 Recurrent dislocation, right foot

Ⓝ Newborn: 0   Ⓟ Pediatric: 0-17   Ⓜ Maternity: 9-64   Ⓐ Adult: 15-124   **MCC** Major Complication/Comorbidity   **CC** Complication/Comorbidity   **SW** Severe Wound Dx

794   ICD-10-CM 2020

M24.475 **Recurrent dislocation, left foot**
M24.476 **Recurrent dislocation, unspecified foot**
M24.477 **Recurrent dislocation, right toe(s)**
M24.478 **Recurrent dislocation, left toe(s)**
M24.479 **Recurrent dislocation, unspecified toe(s)**

✓5ᵗʰ **M24.5 Contracture of joint**
　EXCLUDES 1　contracture of muscle without contracture of joint (M62.4-)
　　　　contracture of tendon (sheath) without contracture of joint (M62.4-)
　　　　Dupuytren's contracture (M72.0)
　EXCLUDES 2　acquired deformities of limbs (M20-M21)
　AHA: 2016,2Q,6

M24.50 Contracture, unspecified joint
✓6ᵗʰ **M24.51 Contracture, shoulder**
M24.511 **Contracture, right shoulder**
M24.512 **Contracture, left shoulder**
M24.519 **Contracture, unspecified shoulder**
✓6ᵗʰ **M24.52 Contracture, elbow**
M24.521 **Contracture, right elbow**
M24.522 **Contracture, left elbow**
M24.529 **Contracture, unspecified elbow**
✓6ᵗʰ **M24.53 Contracture, wrist**
M24.531 **Contracture, right wrist**
M24.532 **Contracture, left wrist**
M24.539 **Contracture, unspecified wrist**
✓6ᵗʰ **M24.54 Contracture, hand**
M24.541 **Contracture, right hand**
M24.542 **Contracture, left hand**
M24.549 **Contracture, unspecified hand**
✓6ᵗʰ **M24.55 Contracture, hip**
M24.551 **Contracture, right hip**
M24.552 **Contracture, left hip**
M24.559 **Contracture, unspecified hip**
✓6ᵗʰ **M24.56 Contracture, knee**
M24.561 **Contracture, right knee**
M24.562 **Contracture, left knee**
M24.569 **Contracture, unspecified knee**
✓6ᵗʰ **M24.57 Contracture, ankle and foot**
M24.571 **Contracture, right ankle**
M24.572 **Contracture, left ankle**
M24.573 **Contracture, unspecified ankle**
M24.574 **Contracture, right foot**
M24.575 **Contracture, left foot**
M24.576 **Contracture, unspecified foot**

✓5ᵗʰ **M24.6 Ankylosis of joint**
　EXCLUDES 1　stiffness of joint without ankylosis (M25.6-)
　EXCLUDES 2　spine (M43.2-)
　DEF: Ankylosis: Abnormal union or fusion of bones in a joint, which is normally moveable.

M24.60 Ankylosis, unspecified joint
✓6ᵗʰ **M24.61 Ankylosis, shoulder**
M24.611 **Ankylosis, right shoulder**
M24.612 **Ankylosis, left shoulder**
M24.619 **Ankylosis, unspecified shoulder**
✓6ᵗʰ **M24.62 Ankylosis, elbow**
M24.621 **Ankylosis, right elbow**
M24.622 **Ankylosis, left elbow**
M24.629 **Ankylosis, unspecified elbow**
✓6ᵗʰ **M24.63 Ankylosis, wrist**
M24.631 **Ankylosis, right wrist**
M24.632 **Ankylosis, left wrist**
M24.639 **Ankylosis, unspecified wrist**
✓6ᵗʰ **M24.64 Ankylosis, hand**
M24.641 **Ankylosis, right hand**
M24.642 **Ankylosis, left hand**
M24.649 **Ankylosis, unspecified hand**
✓6ᵗʰ **M24.65 Ankylosis, hip**
M24.651 **Ankylosis, right hip**
M24.652 **Ankylosis, left hip**
M24.659 **Ankylosis, unspecified hip**
✓6ᵗʰ **M24.66 Ankylosis, knee**
M24.661 **Ankylosis, right knee**
M24.662 **Ankylosis, left knee**
M24.669 **Ankylosis, unspecified knee**

✓6ᵗʰ **M24.67 Ankylosis, ankle and foot**
M24.671 **Ankylosis, right ankle**
M24.672 **Ankylosis, left ankle**
M24.673 **Ankylosis, unspecified ankle**
M24.674 **Ankylosis, right foot**
M24.675 **Ankylosis, left foot**
M24.676 **Ankylosis, unspecified foot**

M24.7 Protrusio acetabuli
　DEF: Intrapelvic protrusion of the acetabulum characterized by the sinking of the floor of the acetabulum, causing the femoral head to protrude. It limits hip movement and is of unknown etiology. **Synonym(s):** Otto's pelvis.

✓5ᵗʰ **M24.8 Other specific joint derangements, not elsewhere classified**
　EXCLUDES 2　iliotibial band syndrome (M76.3)

M24.80 Other specific joint derangements of unspecified joint, not elsewhere classified
✓6ᵗʰ **M24.81 Other specific joint derangements of shoulder, not elsewhere classified**
M24.811 **Other specific joint derangements of right shoulder, not elsewhere classified**
M24.812 **Other specific joint derangements of left shoulder, not elsewhere classified**
M24.819 **Other specific joint derangements of unspecified shoulder, not elsewhere classified**
✓6ᵗʰ **M24.82 Other specific joint derangements of elbow, not elsewhere classified**
M24.821 **Other specific joint derangements of right elbow, not elsewhere classified**
M24.822 **Other specific joint derangements of left elbow, not elsewhere classified**
M24.829 **Other specific joint derangements of unspecified elbow, not elsewhere classified**
✓6ᵗʰ **M24.83 Other specific joint derangements of wrist, not elsewhere classified**
M24.831 **Other specific joint derangements of right wrist, not elsewhere classified**
M24.832 **Other specific joint derangements of left wrist, not elsewhere classified**
M24.839 **Other specific joint derangements of unspecified wrist, not elsewhere classified**
✓6ᵗʰ **M24.84 Other specific joint derangements of hand, not elsewhere classified**
M24.841 **Other specific joint derangements of right hand, not elsewhere classified**
M24.842 **Other specific joint derangements of left hand, not elsewhere classified**
M24.849 **Other specific joint derangements of unspecified hand, not elsewhere classified**
✓6ᵗʰ **M24.85 Other specific joint derangements of hip, not elsewhere classified**
　Irritable hip
M24.851 **Other specific joint derangements of right hip, not elsewhere classified**
M24.852 **Other specific joint derangements of left hip, not elsewhere classified**
M24.859 **Other specific joint derangements of unspecified hip, not elsewhere classified**
✓6ᵗʰ **M24.87 Other specific joint derangements of ankle and foot, not elsewhere classified**
M24.871 **Other specific joint derangements of right ankle, not elsewhere classified**
M24.872 **Other specific joint derangements of left ankle, not elsewhere classified**
M24.873 **Other specific joint derangements of unspecified ankle, not elsewhere classified**
M24.874 **Other specific joint derangements of right foot, not elsewhere classified**
M24.875 **Other specific joint derangements of left foot, not elsewhere classified**
M24.876 **Other specific joint derangements of unspecified foot, not elsewhere classified**

M24.9 Joint derangement, unspecified

Chapter 13. Diseases of the Musculoskeletal System and Connective Tissue

M25–M25.28

√4th **M25** **Other joint disorder, not elsewhere classified**

EXCLUDES 2   abnormality of gait and mobility (R26.-)
acquired deformities of limb (M20-M21)
calcification of bursa (M71.4-)
calcification of shoulder (joint) (M75.3)
calcification of tendon (M65.2-)
difficulty in walking (R26.2)
temporomandibular joint disorder (M26.6-)

√5th **M25.0** **Hemarthrosis**

EXCLUDES 1   current injury — see injury of joint by body region
hemophilic arthropathy (M36.2)

M25.00 **Hemarthrosis, unspecified joint**   CC
CC Excl: PDX collection 868

√6th **M25.01** **Hemarthrosis, shoulder**
CC Excl: For CC codes in subcategory M25.01: PDX collection 869

M25.011 **Hemarthrosis, right shoulder**   CC

M25.012 **Hemarthrosis, left shoulder**   CC

M25.019 **Hemarthrosis, unspecified shoulder**   CC

√6th **M25.02** **Hemarthrosis, elbow**
CC Excl: For CC codes in subcategory M25.02: PDX collection 870

M25.021 **Hemarthrosis, right elbow**   CC

M25.022 **Hemarthrosis, left elbow**   CC

M25.029 **Hemarthrosis, unspecified elbow**   CC

√6th **M25.03** **Hemarthrosis, wrist**
CC Excl: For CC codes in subcategory M25.03: PDX collection 871

M25.031 **Hemarthrosis, right wrist**   CC

M25.032 **Hemarthrosis, left wrist**   CC

M25.039 **Hemarthrosis, unspecified wrist**   CC

√6th **M25.04** **Hemarthrosis, hand**
CC Excl: For CC codes in subcategory M25.04: PDX collection 872

M25.041 **Hemarthrosis, right hand**   CC

M25.042 **Hemarthrosis, left hand**   CC

M25.049 **Hemarthrosis, unspecified hand**   CC

√6th **M25.05** **Hemarthrosis, hip**
CC Excl: For CC codes in subcategory M25.05: PDX collection 868

M25.051 **Hemarthrosis, right hip**   CC

M25.052 **Hemarthrosis, left hip**   CC

M25.059 **Hemarthrosis, unspecified hip**   CC

√6th **M25.06** **Hemarthrosis, knee**
CC Excl: For CC codes in subcategory M25.06: PDX collection 873

M25.061 **Hemarthrosis, right knee**   CC

M25.062 **Hemarthrosis, left knee**   CC

M25.069 **Hemarthrosis, unspecified knee**   CC

√6th **M25.07** **Hemarthrosis, ankle and foot**
CC Excl: For CC codes in subcategory M25.07: PDX collection 873

M25.071 **Hemarthrosis, right ankle**   CC

M25.072 **Hemarthrosis, left ankle**   CC

M25.073 **Hemarthrosis, unspecified ankle**   CC

M25.074 **Hemarthrosis, right foot**   CC

M25.075 **Hemarthrosis, left foot**   CC

M25.076 **Hemarthrosis, unspecified foot**   CC

M25.08 **Hemarthrosis, other specified site**   CC
Hemarthrosis, vertebrae
CC Excl: PDX collection 868

√5th **M25.1** **Fistula of joint**

M25.10 **Fistula, unspecified joint**   SW

√6th **M25.11** **Fistula, shoulder**

M25.111 **Fistula, right shoulder**   SW

M25.112 **Fistula, left shoulder**   SW

M25.119 **Fistula, unspecified shoulder**   SW

√6th **M25.12** **Fistula, elbow**

M25.121 **Fistula, right elbow**   SW

M25.122 **Fistula, left elbow**   SW

M25.129 **Fistula, unspecified elbow**   SW

√6th **M25.13** **Fistula, wrist**

M25.131 **Fistula, right wrist**   SW

M25.132 **Fistula, left wrist**   SW

M25.139 **Fistula, unspecified wrist**   SW

√6th **M25.14** **Fistula, hand**

M25.141 **Fistula, right hand**   SW

M25.142 **Fistula, left hand**   SW

M25.149 **Fistula, unspecified hand**   SW

√6th **M25.15** **Fistula, hip**

M25.151 **Fistula, right hip**   SW

M25.152 **Fistula, left hip**   SW

M25.159 **Fistula, unspecified hip**   SW

√6th **M25.16** **Fistula, knee**

M25.161 **Fistula, right knee**   SW

M25.162 **Fistula, left knee**   SW

M25.169 **Fistula, unspecified knee**   SW

√6th **M25.17** **Fistula, ankle and foot**

M25.171 **Fistula, right ankle**   SW

M25.172 **Fistula, left ankle**   SW

M25.173 **Fistula, unspecified ankle**   SW

M25.174 **Fistula, right foot**   SW

M25.175 **Fistula, left foot**   SW

M25.176 **Fistula, unspecified foot**   SW

M25.18 **Fistula, other specified site**   SW
Fistula, vertebrae

√5th **M25.2** **Flail joint**
DEF: Hinged joint that exhibits an abnormal or excessive degree of range and mobility.

M25.20 **Flail joint, unspecified joint**

√6th **M25.21** **Flail joint, shoulder**

M25.211 **Flail joint, right shoulder**

M25.212 **Flail joint, left shoulder**

M25.219 **Flail joint, unspecified shoulder**

√6th **M25.22** **Flail joint, elbow**

M25.221 **Flail joint, right elbow**

M25.222 **Flail joint, left elbow**

M25.229 **Flail joint, unspecified elbow**

√6th **M25.23** **Flail joint, wrist**

M25.231 **Flail joint, right wrist**

M25.232 **Flail joint, left wrist**

M25.239 **Flail joint, unspecified wrist**

√6th **M25.24** **Flail joint, hand**

M25.241 **Flail joint, right hand**

M25.242 **Flail joint, left hand**

M25.249 **Flail joint, unspecified hand**

√6th **M25.25** **Flail joint, hip**

M25.251 **Flail joint, right hip**

M25.252 **Flail joint, left hip**

M25.259 **Flail joint, unspecified hip**

√6th **M25.26** **Flail joint, knee**

M25.261 **Flail joint, right knee**

M25.262 **Flail joint, left knee**

M25.269 **Flail joint, unspecified knee**

√6th **M25.27** **Flail joint, ankle and foot**

M25.271 **Flail joint, right ankle and foot**

M25.272 **Flail joint, left ankle and foot**

M25.279 **Flail joint, unspecified ankle and foot**

M25.28 **Flail joint, other site**

N Newborn: 0   P Pediatric: 0-17   M Maternity: 9-64   A Adult: 15-124   MCC Major Complication/Comorbidity   CC Complication/Comorbidity   SW Severe Wound Dx

796   ICD-10-CM 2020

√5ᵗʰ **M25.3 Other instability of joint**

     EXCLUDES 1   *instability of joint secondary to old ligament injury (M24.2-)*

                instability of joint secondary to removal of joint prosthesis (M96.8-)

     EXCLUDES 2   *spinal instabilities (M53.2-)*

     M25.30 Other instability, unspecified joint

√6ᵗʰ **M25.31 Other instability, shoulder**

     M25.311 Other instability, right shoulder
     M25.312 Other instability, left shoulder
     M25.319 Other instability, unspecified shoulder

√6ᵗʰ **M25.32 Other instability, elbow**

     M25.321 Other instability, right elbow
     M25.322 Other instability, left elbow
     M25.329 Other instability, unspecified elbow

√6ᵗʰ **M25.33 Other instability, wrist**

     M25.331 Other instability, right wrist
     M25.332 Other instability, left wrist
     M25.339 Other instability, unspecified wrist

√6ᵗʰ **M25.34 Other instability, hand**

     M25.341 Other instability, right hand
     M25.342 Other instability, left hand
     M25.349 Other instability, unspecified hand

√6ᵗʰ **M25.35 Other instability, hip**

     M25.351 Other instability, right hip
     M25.352 Other instability, left hip
     M25.359 Other instability, unspecified hip

√6ᵗʰ **M25.36 Other instability, knee**

     M25.361 Other instability, right knee
     M25.362 Other instability, left knee
     M25.369 Other instability, unspecified knee

√6ᵗʰ **M25.37 Other instability, ankle and foot**

     M25.371 Other instability, right ankle
     M25.372 Other instability, left ankle
     M25.373 Other instability, unspecified ankle
     M25.374 Other instability, right foot
     M25.375 Other instability, left foot
     M25.376 Other instability, unspecified foot

√5ᵗʰ **M25.4 Effusion of joint**

     EXCLUDES 1   *hydrarthrosis in yaws (A66.6)*

                intermittent hydrarthrosis (M12.4-)

                other infective (teno)synovitis (M65.1-)

     M25.40 Effusion, unspecified joint

√6ᵗʰ **M25.41 Effusion, shoulder**

     M25.411 Effusion, right shoulder
     M25.412 Effusion, left shoulder
     M25.419 Effusion, unspecified shoulder

√6ᵗʰ **M25.42 Effusion, elbow**

     M25.421 Effusion, right elbow
     M25.422 Effusion, left elbow
     M25.429 Effusion, unspecified elbow

√6ᵗʰ **M25.43 Effusion, wrist**

     M25.431 Effusion, right wrist
     M25.432 Effusion, left wrist
     M25.439 Effusion, unspecified wrist

√6ᵗʰ **M25.44 Effusion, hand**

     M25.441 Effusion, right hand
     M25.442 Effusion, left hand
     M25.449 Effusion, unspecified hand

√6ᵗʰ **M25.45 Effusion, hip**

     M25.451 Effusion, right hip
     M25.452 Effusion, left hip
     M25.459 Effusion, unspecified hip

√6ᵗʰ **M25.46 Effusion, knee**

     M25.461 Effusion, right knee
     M25.462 Effusion, left knee
     M25.469 Effusion, unspecified knee

√6ᵗʰ **M25.47 Effusion, ankle and foot**

     M25.471 Effusion, right ankle
     M25.472 Effusion, left ankle
     M25.473 Effusion, unspecified ankle
     M25.474 Effusion, right foot
     M25.475 Effusion, left foot
     M25.476 Effusion, unspecified foot

     M25.48 Effusion, other site

√5ᵗʰ **M25.5 Pain in joint**

     EXCLUDES 2   *pain in hand (M79.64-)*

                pain in fingers (M79.64-)

                pain in foot (M79.67-)

                pain in limb (M79.6-)

                pain in toes (M79.67-)

     M25.50 Pain in unspecified joint

√6ᵗʰ **M25.51 Pain in shoulder**

     M25.511 Pain in right shoulder
     M25.512 Pain in left shoulder
     M25.519 Pain in unspecified shoulder

√6ᵗʰ **M25.52 Pain in elbow**

     M25.521 Pain in right elbow
     M25.522 Pain in left elbow
     M25.529 Pain in unspecified elbow

√6ᵗʰ **M25.53 Pain in wrist**

     M25.531 Pain in right wrist
     M25.532 Pain in left wrist
     M25.539 Pain in unspecified wrist

√6ᵗʰ **M25.54 Pain in joints of hand**

     AHA: 2016,4Q,38
     M25.541 Pain in joints of right hand
     M25.542 Pain in joints of left hand
     M25.549 Pain in joints of unspecified hand
             Pain in joints of hand NOS

√6ᵗʰ **M25.55 Pain in hip**

     M25.551 Pain in right hip
     M25.552 Pain in left hip
     M25.559 Pain in unspecified hip

√6ᵗʰ **M25.56 Pain in knee**

     M25.561 Pain in right knee
     M25.562 Pain in left knee
     M25.569 Pain in unspecified knee

√6ᵗʰ **M25.57 Pain in ankle and joints of foot**

     M25.571 Pain in right ankle and joints of right foot
     M25.572 Pain in left ankle and joints of left foot
     M25.579 Pain in unspecified ankle and joints of unspecified foot

√5ᵗʰ **M25.6 Stiffness of joint, not elsewhere classified**

     EXCLUDES 1   *ankylosis of joint (M24.6-)*

                contracture of joint (M24.5-)

     M25.60 Stiffness of unspecified joint, not elsewhere classified

√6ᵗʰ **M25.61 Stiffness of shoulder, not elsewhere classified**

     M25.611 Stiffness of right shoulder, not elsewhere classified
     M25.612 Stiffness of left shoulder, not elsewhere classified
     M25.619 Stiffness of unspecified shoulder, not elsewhere classified

√6ᵗʰ **M25.62 Stiffness of elbow, not elsewhere classified**

     M25.621 Stiffness of right elbow, not elsewhere classified
     M25.622 Stiffness of left elbow, not elsewhere classified
     M25.629 Stiffness of unspecified elbow, not elsewhere classified

√6ᵗʰ **M25.63 Stiffness of wrist, not elsewhere classified**

     M25.631 Stiffness of right wrist, not elsewhere classified
     M25.632 Stiffness of left wrist, not elsewhere classified
     M25.639 Stiffness of unspecified wrist, not elsewhere classified

√6ᵗʰ **M25.64 Stiffness of hand, not elsewhere classified**

     M25.641 Stiffness of right hand, not elsewhere classified
     M25.642 Stiffness of left hand, not elsewhere classified
     M25.649 Stiffness of unspecified hand, not elsewhere classified

√6ᵗʰ **M25.65 Stiffness of hip, not elsewhere classified**

     M25.651 Stiffness of right hip, not elsewhere classified
     M25.652 Stiffness of left hip, not elsewhere classified

☑ Additional Character Required   √x7ᵗʰ Placeholder   Unacceptable PDx   Questionable PDx   Manifestation   Unspecified Dx   **H1**-**H14** HAC   **HCC** CMS-HCC Dx   **HIV** HIV Dx

ICD-10-CM 2020   **797**

M25.659 Stiffness of unspecified hip, not elsewhere classified

√6ᵗʰ M25.66 Stiffness of knee, not elsewhere classified

M25.661 Stiffness of right knee, not elsewhere classified

M25.662 Stiffness of left knee, not elsewhere classified

M25.669 Stiffness of unspecified knee, not elsewhere classified

√6ᵗʰ M25.67 Stiffness of ankle and foot, not elsewhere classified

M25.671 Stiffness of right ankle, not elsewhere classified

M25.672 Stiffness of left ankle, not elsewhere classified

M25.673 Stiffness of unspecified ankle, not elsewhere classified

M25.674 Stiffness of right foot, not elsewhere classified

M25.675 Stiffness of left foot, not elsewhere classified

M25.676 Stiffness of unspecified foot, not elsewhere classified

√5ᵗʰ M25.7 Osteophyte

M25.70 Osteophyte, unspecified joint

√6ᵗʰ M25.71 Osteophyte, shoulder

M25.711 Osteophyte, right shoulder
M25.712 Osteophyte, left shoulder
M25.719 Osteophyte, unspecified shoulder

√6ᵗʰ M25.72 Osteophyte, elbow

M25.721 Osteophyte, right elbow
M25.722 Osteophyte, left elbow
M25.729 Osteophyte, unspecified elbow

√6ᵗʰ M25.73 Osteophyte, wrist

M25.731 Osteophyte, right wrist
M25.732 Osteophyte, left wrist
M25.739 Osteophyte, unspecified wrist

√6ᵗʰ M25.74 Osteophyte, hand

M25.741 Osteophyte, right hand
M25.742 Osteophyte, left hand
M25.749 Osteophyte, unspecified hand

√6ᵗʰ M25.75 Osteophyte, hip

M25.751 Osteophyte, right hip
M25.752 Osteophyte, left hip
M25.759 Osteophyte, unspecified hip

√6ᵗʰ M25.76 Osteophyte, knee

M25.761 Osteophyte, right knee
M25.762 Osteophyte, left knee
M25.769 Osteophyte, unspecified knee

√6ᵗʰ M25.77 Osteophyte, ankle and foot

M25.771 Osteophyte, right ankle
M25.772 Osteophyte, left ankle
M25.773 Osteophyte, unspecified ankle
M25.774 Osteophyte, right foot
M25.775 Osteophyte, left foot
M25.776 Osteophyte, unspecified foot

M25.78 Osteophyte, vertebrae

√5ᵗʰ M25.8 Other specified joint disorders

M25.80 Other specified joint disorders, unspecified joint

√6ᵗʰ M25.81 Other specified joint disorders, shoulder

M25.811 Other specified joint disorders, right shoulder
M25.812 Other specified joint disorders, left shoulder
M25.819 Other specified joint disorders, unspecified shoulder

√6ᵗʰ M25.82 Other specified joint disorders, elbow

M25.821 Other specified joint disorders, right elbow
M25.822 Other specified joint disorders, left elbow
M25.829 Other specified joint disorders, unspecified elbow

√6ᵗʰ M25.83 Other specified joint disorders, wrist

M25.831 Other specified joint disorders, right wrist
M25.832 Other specified joint disorders, left wrist
M25.839 Other specified joint disorders, unspecified wrist

√6ᵗʰ M25.84 Other specified joint disorders, hand

M25.841 Other specified joint disorders, right hand
M25.842 Other specified joint disorders, left hand
M25.849 Other specified joint disorders, unspecified hand

√6ᵗʰ M25.85 Other specified joint disorders, hip

AHA: 2014,4Q,25

M25.851 Other specified joint disorders, right hip
M25.852 Other specified joint disorders, left hip
M25.859 Other specified joint disorders, unspecified hip

√6ᵗʰ M25.86 Other specified joint disorders, knee

M25.861 Other specified joint disorders, right knee
M25.862 Other specified joint disorders, left knee
M25.869 Other specified joint disorders, unspecified knee

√6ᵗʰ M25.87 Other specified joint disorders, ankle and foot

M25.871 Other specified joint disorders, right ankle and foot
M25.872 Other specified joint disorders, left ankle and foot
M25.879 Other specified joint disorders, unspecified ankle and foot

M25.9 Joint disorder, unspecified

Dentofacial anomalies [including malocclusion] and other disorders of jaw (M26-M27)

EXCLUDES 1 hemifacial atrophy or hypertrophy (Q67.4)
unilateral condylar hyperplasia or hypoplasia (M27.8)

√4ᵗʰ M26 Dentofacial anomalies [including malocclusion]

√5ᵗʰ M26.0 Major anomalies of jaw size

EXCLUDES 1 acromegaly (E22.0)
Robin's syndrome (Q87.0)

M26.00 Unspecified anomaly of jaw size
M26.01 Maxillary hyperplasia
M26.02 Maxillary hypoplasia
AHA: 2014,3Q,23
M26.03 Mandibular hyperplasia
M26.04 Mandibular hypoplasia
M26.05 Macrogenia
M26.06 Microgenia
M26.07 Excessive tuberosity of jaw
Entire maxillary tuberosity
M26.09 Other specified anomalies of jaw size

√5ᵗʰ M26.1 Anomalies of jaw-cranial base relationship

M26.10 Unspecified anomaly of jaw-cranial base relationship
M26.11 Maxillary asymmetry
M26.12 Other jaw asymmetry
M26.19 Other specified anomalies of jaw-cranial base relationship

√5ᵗʰ M26.2 Anomalies of dental arch relationship

M26.20 Unspecified anomaly of dental arch relationship

√6ᵗʰ M26.21 Malocclusion, Angle's class

M26.211 Malocclusion, Angle's class I
Neutro-occlusion
M26.212 Malocclusion, Angle's class II
Disto-occlusion Division I
Disto-occlusion Division II
M26.213 Malocclusion, Angle's class III
Mesio-occlusion
M26.219 Malocclusion, Angle's class, unspecified

√6ᵗʰ M26.22 Open occlusal relationship

M26.220 Open anterior occlusal relationship
Anterior open bite
M26.221 Open posterior occlusal relationship
Posterior open bite

M26.23 Excessive horizontal overlap
Excessive horizontal overjet
M26.24 Reverse articulation
Crossbite (anterior) (posterior)
M26.25 Anomalies of interarch distance

N Newborn: 0   P Pediatric: 0-17   M Maternity: 9-64   A Adult: 15-124   MCC Major Complication/Comorbidity   CC Complication/Comorbidity   SW Severe Wound Dx

798   ICD-10-CM 2020

M26.29 **Other anomalies of dental arch relationship**
Midline deviation of dental arch
Overbite (excessive) deep
Overbite (excessive) horizontal
Overbite (excessive) vertical
Posterior lingual occlusion of mandibular teeth

√5ᵗʰ **M26.3** **Anomalies of tooth position of fully erupted tooth or teeth**
EXCLUDES 2   *embedded and impacted teeth (K01.-)*

M26.30 **Unspecified anomaly of tooth position of fully erupted tooth or teeth**
Abnormal spacing of fully erupted tooth or teeth NOS
Displacement of fully erupted tooth or teeth NOS
Transposition of fully erupted tooth or teeth NOS

M26.31 **Crowding of fully erupted teeth**

M26.32 **Excessive spacing of fully erupted teeth**
Diastema of fully erupted tooth or teeth NOS

M26.33 **Horizontal displacement of fully erupted tooth or teeth**
Tipped tooth or teeth
Tipping of fully erupted tooth

M26.34 **Vertical displacement of fully erupted tooth or teeth**
Extruded tooth
Infraeruption of tooth or teeth
Supraeruption of tooth or teeth

M26.35 **Rotation of fully erupted tooth or teeth**

M26.36 **Insufficient interocclusal distance of fully erupted teeth (ridge)**
Lack of adequate intermaxillary vertical dimension of fully erupted teeth

M26.37 **Excessive interocclusal distance of fully erupted teeth**
Excessive intermaxillary vertical dimension of fully erupted teeth
Loss of occlusal vertical dimension of fully erupted teeth

M26.39 **Other anomalies of tooth position of fully erupted tooth or teeth**

M26.4 **Malocclusion, unspecified**

√5ᵗʰ **M26.5** **Dentofacial functional abnormalities**
EXCLUDES 1   *bruxism (F45.8)*
            teeth-grinding NOS (F45.8)

M26.50 **Dentofacial functional abnormalities, unspecified**

M26.51 **Abnormal jaw closure**

M26.52 **Limited mandibular range of motion**

M26.53 **Deviation in opening and closing of the mandible**

M26.54 **Insufficient anterior guidance**
Insufficient anterior occlusal guidance

M26.55 **Centric occlusion maximum intercuspation discrepancy**
EXCLUDES 1   *centric occlusion NOS (M26.59)*

M26.56 **Non-working side interference**
Balancing side interference

M26.57 **Lack of posterior occlusal support**

M26.59 **Other dentofacial functional abnormalities**
Centric occlusion (of teeth) NOS
Malocclusion due to abnormal swallowing
Malocclusion due to mouth breathing
Malocclusion due to tongue, lip or finger habits

√5ᵗʰ **M26.6** **Temporomandibular joint disorders**
EXCLUDES 2   *current temporomandibular joint dislocation (S03.0)*
            current temporomandibular joint sprain (S03.4)
AHA: 2016,4Q,38-39

Temporomandibular Joint

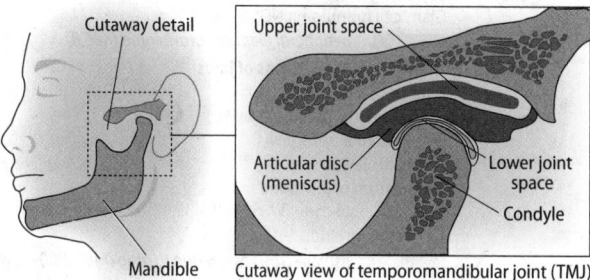

Cutaway detail
Upper joint space
Articular disc (meniscus)
Lower joint space
Condyle
Mandible
Cutaway view of temporomandibular joint (TMJ)

√6ᵗʰ **M26.60** **Temporomandibular joint disorder, unspecified**

M26.601 **Right temporomandibular joint disorder, unspecified**

M26.602 **Left temporomandibular joint disorder, unspecified**

M26.603 **Bilateral temporomandibular joint disorder, unspecified**

M26.609 **Unspecified temporomandibular joint disorder, unspecified side**
Temporomandibular joint disorder NOS

√6ᵗʰ **M26.61** **Adhesions and ankylosis of temporomandibular joint**

M26.611 **Adhesions and ankylosis of right temporomandibular joint**

M26.612 **Adhesions and ankylosis of left temporomandibular joint**

M26.613 **Adhesions and ankylosis of bilateral temporomandibular joint**

M26.619 **Adhesions and ankylosis of temporomandibular joint, unspecified side**

√6ᵗʰ **M26.62** **Arthralgia of temporomandibular joint**

M26.621 **Arthralgia of right temporomandibular joint**

M26.622 **Arthralgia of left temporomandibular joint**

M26.623 **Arthralgia of bilateral temporomandibular joint**

M26.629 **Arthralgia of temporomandibular joint, unspecified side**

√6ᵗʰ **M26.63** **Articular disc disorder of temporomandibular joint**

M26.631 **Articular disc disorder of right temporomandibular joint**

M26.632 **Articular disc disorder of left temporomandibular joint**

M26.633 **Articular disc disorder of bilateral temporomandibular joint**

M26.639 **Articular disc disorder of temporomandibular joint, unspecified side**

M26.69 **Other specified disorders of temporomandibular joint**

√5ᵗʰ **M26.7** **Dental alveolar anomalies**

M26.70 **Unspecified alveolar anomaly**

M26.71 **Alveolar maxillary hyperplasia**

M26.72 **Alveolar mandibular hyperplasia**

M26.73 **Alveolar maxillary hypoplasia**

M26.74 **Alveolar mandibular hypoplasia**

M26.79 **Other specified alveolar anomalies**

√5ᵗʰ **M26.8** **Other dentofacial anomalies**

M26.81 **Anterior soft tissue impingement**
Anterior soft tissue impingement on teeth

M26.82 **Posterior soft tissue impingement**
Posterior soft tissue impingement on teeth

M26.89 **Other dentofacial anomalies**

M26.9 **Dentofacial anomaly, unspecified**

✓4ᵗʰ **M27   Other diseases of jaws**

M27.0   Developmental disorders of jaws
Latent bone cyst of jaw
Stafne's cyst
Torus mandibularis
Torus palatinus

M27.1   Giant cell granuloma, central
Giant cell granuloma NOS
EXCLUDES 1   *peripheral giant cell granuloma (K06.8)*

M27.2   Inflammatory conditions of jaws
Osteitis of jaw(s)
Osteomyelitis (neonatal) jaw(s)
Osteoradionecrosis jaw(s)
Periostitis jaw(s)
Sequestrum of jaw bone
Use additional code (W88-W90, X39.0) to identify radiation, if
     radiation-induced
EXCLUDES 2   *osteonecrosis of jaw due to drug (M87.180)*

M27.3   Alveolitis of jaws
Alveolar osteitis
Dry socket

✓5ᵗʰ **M27.4   Other and unspecified cysts of jaw**
EXCLUDES 1   *cysts of oral region (K09.-)*
            latent bone cyst of jaw (M27.0)
            Stafne's cyst (M27.0)

     M27.40   Unspecified cyst of jaw
            Cyst of jaw NOS

     M27.49   Other cysts of jaw
            Aneurysmal cyst of jaw
            Hemorrhagic cyst of jaw
            Traumatic cyst of jaw

✓5ᵗʰ **M27.5   Periradicular pathology associated with previous endodontic treatment**
     M27.51   Perforation of root canal space due to endodontic treatment
     M27.52   Endodontic overfill
     M27.53   Endodontic underfill
     M27.59   Other periradicular pathology associated with previous endodontic treatment

✓5ᵗʰ **M27.6   Endosseous dental implant failure**
     M27.61   Osseointegration failure of dental implant
            Hemorrhagic complications of dental implant placement
            Iatrogenic osseointegration failure of dental implant
            Osseointegration failure of dental implant due to complications of systemic disease
            Osseointegration failure of dental implant due to poor bone quality
            Pre-integration failure of dental implant NOS
            Pre-osseointegration failure of dental implant

     M27.62   Post-osseointegration biological failure of dental implant
            Failure of dental implant due to lack of attached gingiva
            Failure of dental implant due to occlusal trauma (caused by poor prosthetic design)
            Failure of dental implant due to parafunctional habits
            Failure of dental implant due to periodontal infection (peri-implantitis)
            Failure of dental implant due to poor oral hygiene
            Iatrogenic post-osseointegration failure of dental implant
            Post-osseointegration failure of dental implant due to complications of systemic disease

     M27.63   Post-osseointegration mechanical failure of dental implant
            Failure of dental prosthesis causing loss of dental implant
            Fracture of dental implant
            EXCLUDES 2   *cracked tooth (K03.81)*
                     fractured dental restorative material with loss of material (K08.531)
                     fractured dental restorative material without loss of material (K08.530)
                     fractured tooth (S02.5)

M27.69   Other endosseous dental implant failure
Dental implant failure NOS

M27.8   Other specified diseases of jaws
Cherubism
Exostosis
Fibrous dysplasia
Unilateral condylar hyperplasia
Unilateral condylar hypoplasia
EXCLUDES 1   *jaw pain (R68.84)*

M27.9   Disease of jaws, unspecified

Systemic connective tissue disorders (M30-M36)

INCLUDES   autoimmune disease NOS
            collagen (vascular) disease NOS
            systemic autoimmune disease
            systemic collagen (vascular) disease
EXCLUDES 1   *autoimmune disease, single organ or single cell-type-code to relevant condition category*

✓4ᵗʰ **M30   Polyarteritis nodosa and related conditions**
EXCLUDES 1   *microscopic polyarteritis (M31.7)*
CC Excl: For CC codes in category M30, unless otherwise noted: PDX collection 874

M30.0   Polyarteritis nodosa   CC   HCC

M30.1   Polyarteritis with lung involvement [Churg-Strauss]   CC   HCC
Allergic granulomatous angiitis

M30.2   Juvenile polyarteritis   CC   HCC

M30.3   Mucocutaneous lymph node syndrome [Kawasaki]   CC   HCC
CC Excl: PDX collection 875

M30.8   Other conditions related to polyarteritis nodosa   CC   HCC
Polyangiitis overlap syndrome

✓4ᵗʰ **M31   Other necrotizing vasculopathies**
CC Excl: For CC/MCC codes in category M31, unless otherwise noted: PDX collection 874

M31.0   Hypersensitivity angiitis   CC   HCC
Goodpasture's syndrome

M31.1   Thrombotic microangiopathy   MCC   HCC
Thrombotic thrombocytopenic purpura

M31.2   Lethal midline granuloma   CC   HCC

✓5ᵗʰ **M31.3   Wegener's granulomatosis**
Necrotizing respiratory granulomatosis

     M31.30   Wegener's granulomatosis without renal involvement   HCC
            Wegener's granulomatosis NOS

     M31.31   Wegener's granulomatosis with renal involvement   CC   HCC

M31.4   Aortic arch syndrome [Takayasu]   CC   HCC

M31.5   Giant cell arteritis with polymyalgia rheumatica   HCC

M31.6   Other giant cell arteritis   HCC

M31.7   Microscopic polyangiitis   CC   HCC
Microscopic polyarteritis
EXCLUDES 1   *polyarteritis nodosa (M30.0)*

M31.8   Other specified necrotizing vasculopathies   CC   HCC
Hypocomplementemic vasculitis
Septic vasculitis
CC Excl: PDX collection 712

M31.9   Necrotizing vasculopathy, unspecified   CC   HCC
CC Excl: PDX collection 712

✓4ᵗʰ **M32   Systemic lupus erythematosus (SLE)**
EXCLUDES 1   *lupus erythematosus (discoid) (NOS) (L93.0)*
AHA: 2018,3Q,14
TIP: There is no default code for "lupus NOS." Query the provider for the specific type of lupus in order to assign the appropriate code.

M32.0   Drug-induced systemic lupus erythematosus   HCC
Use additional code for adverse effect, if applicable, to identify drug (T36-T50 with fifth or sixth character 5)

✓6ᵗʰ **M32.1   Systemic lupus erythematosus with organ or system involvement**
     M32.10   Systemic lupus erythematosus, organ or system involvement unspecified   HCC

M32.11 Endocarditis in systemic lupus erythematosus `CC` `HCC`
Libman-Sacks disease
CC Excl: PDX collection 676

M32.12 Pericarditis in systemic lupus erythematosus `CC` `HCC`
Lupus pericarditis
CC Excl: PDX collection 673

M32.13 Lung involvement in systemic lupus erythematosus `HCC`
Pleural effusion due to systemic lupus erythematosus

M32.14 Glomerular disease in systemic lupus erythematosus `HCC`
Lupus renal disease NOS
AHA: 2013,4Q,125

M32.15 Tubulo-interstitial nephropathy in systemic lupus erythematosus `HCC`

M32.19 Other organ or system involvement in systemic lupus erythematosus `HCC`

M32.8 Other forms of systemic lupus erythematosus `HCC`

M32.9 Systemic lupus erythematosus, unspecified `HCC`
SLE NOS
Systemic lupus erythematosus NOS
Systemic lupus erythematosus without organ involvement

✓4ᵗʰ **M33 Dermatopolymyositis**
AHA: 2017,4Q,18
CC Excl: For CC codes in category M33, unless otherwise noted: PDX collection 876

✓5ᵗʰ **M33.0 Juvenile dermatomyositis**

M33.00 Juvenile dermatomyositis, organ involvement unspecified `CC` `HCC`

M33.01 Juvenile dermatomyositis with respiratory involvement `CC` `HCC`

M33.02 Juvenile dermatomyositis with myopathy `CC` `HCC`
CC Excl: PDX collection 877

M33.03 Juvenile dermatomyositis without myopathy `CC` `HCC`

M33.09 Juvenile dermatomyositis with other organ involvement `CC` `HCC`

✓5ᵗʰ **M33.1 Other dermatomyositis**
Adult dermatomyositis

M33.10 Other dermatomyositis, organ involvement unspecified `CC` `HCC`

M33.11 Other dermatomyositis with respiratory involvement `CC` `HCC`

M33.12 Other dermatomyositis with myopathy `CC` `HCC`
CC Excl: PDX collection 877

M33.13 Other dermatomyositis without myopathy `CC` `HCC`
Dermatomyositis NOS

M33.19 Other dermatomyositis with other organ involvement `CC` `HCC`

✓5ᵗʰ **M33.2 Polymyositis**

M33.20 Polymyositis, organ involvement unspecified `CC` `HCC`
CC Excl: PDX collection 878

M33.21 Polymyositis with respiratory involvement `CC` `HCC`
CC Excl: PDX collection 878

M33.22 Polymyositis with myopathy `CC` `HCC`
CC Excl: PDX collection 879

M33.29 Polymyositis with other organ involvement `CC` `HCC`
CC Excl: PDX collection 878

✓5ᵗʰ **M33.9 Dermatopolymyositis, unspecified**

M33.90 Dermatopolymyositis, unspecified, organ involvement unspecified `CC` `HCC`

M33.91 Dermatopolymyositis, unspecified with respiratory involvement `CC` `HCC`

M33.92 Dermatopolymyositis, unspecified with myopathy `CC` `HCC`
CC Excl: PDX collection 877

M33.93 Dermatopolymyositis, unspecified without myopathy `CC` `HCC`

M33.99 Dermatopolymyositis, unspecified with other organ involvement `CC` `HCC`

✓4ᵗʰ **M34 Systemic sclerosis [scleroderma]**
EXCLUDES 1   circumscribed scleroderma (L94.0)
    neonatal scleroderma ▶(P83.88)◀

M34.0 Progressive systemic sclerosis `HCC`

M34.1 CR(E)ST syndrome `HCC`
Combination of calcinosis, Raynaud's phenomenon, esophageal dysfunction, sclerodactyly, telangiectasia

M34.2 Systemic sclerosis induced by drug and chemical `HCC`
Code first poisoning due to drug or toxin, if applicable (T36-T65 with fifth or sixth character 1-4 or 6)
Use additional code for adverse effect, if applicable, to identify drug (T36-T50 with fifth or sixth character 5)

✓5ᵗʰ **M34.8 Other forms of systemic sclerosis**

M34.81 Systemic sclerosis with lung involvement `CC` `HCC`
CC Excl: No Excl

M34.82 Systemic sclerosis with myopathy `CC` `HCC`
CC Excl: PDX collection 867

M34.83 Systemic sclerosis with polyneuropathy `HCC`

M34.89 Other systemic sclerosis `HCC`

M34.9 Systemic sclerosis, unspecified `HCC`

✓4ᵗʰ **M35 Other systemic involvement of connective tissue**
EXCLUDES 1   reactive perforating collagenosis (L87.1)

✓5ᵗʰ **M35.0 Sicca syndrome [Sjögren]**
DEF: Autoimmune disease associated with keratoconjunctivitis, laryngopharyngitis, rhinitis, dry mouth, enlarged parotid gland, and chronic polyarthritis.

M35.00 Sicca syndrome, unspecified `HCC`

M35.01 Sicca syndrome with keratoconjunctivitis `HCC`

M35.02 Sicca syndrome with lung involvement `HCC`

M35.03 Sicca syndrome with myopathy `CC` `HCC`
CC Excl: PDX collection 867

M35.04 Sicca syndrome with tubulo-interstitial nephropathy `HCC`
Renal tubular acidosis in sicca syndrome

M35.09 Sicca syndrome with other organ involvement `HCC`

M35.1 Other overlap syndromes `CC` `HCC`
Mixed connective tissue disease
EXCLUDES 1   polyangiitis overlap syndrome (M30.8)
CC Excl: PDX collection 880

M35.2 Behçet's disease `CC` `HCC`
CC Excl: PDX collection 863

M35.3 Polymyalgia rheumatica `HCC`
EXCLUDES 1   polymyalgia rheumatica with giant cell arteritis (M31.5)

M35.4 Diffuse (eosinophilic) fasciitis

M35.5 Multifocal fibrosclerosis `CC` `HCC`
CC Excl: PDX collection 880

M35.6 Relapsing panniculitis [Weber-Christian]
EXCLUDES 1   lupus panniculitis (L93.2)
    panniculitis NOS (M79.3-)

M35.7 Hypermobility syndrome
Familial ligamentous laxity
EXCLUDES 1   Ehlers-Danlos syndrome ▶(Q79.6-)◀
    ligamentous laxity, NOS (M24.2-)

M35.8 Other specified systemic involvement of connective tissue `CC` `HCC`
CC Excl: PDX collection 880

M35.9 Systemic involvement of connective tissue, unspecified `HCC`
Autoimmune disease (systemic) NOS
Collagen (vascular) disease NOS

✓4ᵗʰ **M36 Systemic disorders of connective tissue in diseases classified elsewhere**
EXCLUDES 2   arthropathies in diseases classified elsewhere (M14.-)

M36.0 Dermato(poly)myositis in neoplastic disease `CC` `HCC`
Code first underlying neoplasm (C00-D49)
CC Excl: PDX collection 876

M36.1 *Arthropathy in neoplastic disease*
Code first underlying neoplasm, such as:
leukemia (C91-C95)
malignant histiocytosis (C96.A)
multiple myeloma (C90.0)

M36.2 *Hemophilic arthropathy*
Hemarthrosis in hemophilic arthropathy
Code first underlying disease, such as:
factor VIII deficiency (D66)
with vascular defect (D68.0)
factor IX deficiency (D67)
hemophilia (classical) (D66)
hemophilia B (D67)
hemophilia C (D68.1)

M36.3 *Arthropathy in other blood disorders*

M36.4 *Arthropathy in hypersensitivity reactions classified elsewhere*
Code first underlying disease, such as:
Henoch (-Schönlein) purpura (D69.0)
serum sickness (T80.6-)

M36.8 *Systemic disorders of connective tissue in other* `HCC`
diseases classified elsewhere
Code first underlying disease, such as:
alkaptonuria (E70.2)
hypogammaglobulinemia (D80.-)
ochronosis (E70.2)

DORSOPATHIES (M40-M54)

Deforming dorsopathies (M40-M43)

✓4ᵗʰ **M40** **Kyphosis and lordosis**
`EXCLUDES 1` *congenital kyphosis and lordosis (Q76.4)*
kyphoscoliosis (M41.-)
postprocedural kyphosis and lordosis (M96.-)

Kyphosis and Lordosis

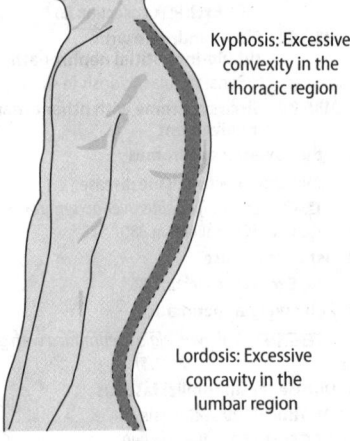

Kyphosis: Excessive convexity in the thoracic region

Lordosis: Excessive concavity in the lumbar region

✓5ᵗʰ **M40.0** **Postural kyphosis**
`EXCLUDES 1` *osteochondrosis of spine (M42.-)*
M40.00 Postural kyphosis, site unspecified
M40.03 Postural kyphosis, cervicothoracic **region**
M40.04 Postural kyphosis, thoracic **region**
M40.05 Postural kyphosis, thoracolumbar **region**

✓5ᵗʰ **M40.1** **Other secondary kyphosis**
M40.10 Other secondary kyphosis, site unspecified
M40.12 Other secondary kyphosis, cervical **region**
M40.13 Other secondary kyphosis, cervicothoracic **region**
M40.14 Other secondary kyphosis, thoracic **region**
M40.15 Other secondary kyphosis, thoracolumbar **region**

✓5ᵗʰ **M40.2** **Other and unspecified kyphosis**
✓6ᵗʰ **M40.20** **Unspecified kyphosis**
M40.202 Unspecified kyphosis, cervical **region**
M40.203 Unspecified kyphosis, cervicothoracic **region**
M40.204 Unspecified kyphosis, thoracic **region**
M40.205 Unspecified kyphosis, thoracolumbar **region**
M40.209 Unspecified kyphosis, site unspecified

✓6ᵗʰ **M40.29** **Other kyphosis**
M40.292 Other kyphosis, cervical **region**
M40.293 Other kyphosis, cervicothoracic **region**
M40.294 Other kyphosis, thoracic **region**
M40.295 Other kyphosis, thoracolumbar **region**
M40.299 Other kyphosis, site unspecified

✓5ᵗʰ **M40.3** **Flatback syndrome**
M40.30 Flatback syndrome, site unspecified
M40.35 Flatback syndrome, thoracolumbar **region**
M40.36 Flatback syndrome, lumbar **region**
M40.37 Flatback syndrome, lumbosacral **region**

✓5ᵗʰ **M40.4** **Postural lordosis**
Acquired lordosis
M40.40 Postural lordosis, site unspecified
M40.45 Postural lordosis, thoracolumbar **region**
M40.46 Postural lordosis, lumbar **region**
M40.47 Postural lordosis, lumbosacral **region**

✓5ᵗʰ **M40.5** **Lordosis, unspecified**
M40.50 Lordosis, unspecified, site unspecified
M40.55 Lordosis, unspecified, thoracolumbar **region**
M40.56 Lordosis, unspecified, lumbar **region**
M40.57 Lordosis, unspecified, lumbosacral **region**

✓4ᵗʰ **M41** **Scoliosis**
`INCLUDES` kyphoscoliosis
`EXCLUDES 1` *congenital scoliosis due to bony malformation (Q76.3)*
congenital scoliosis NOS (Q67.5)
kyphoscoliotic heart disease (I27.1)
postprocedural scoliosis (M96.-)
postural congenital scoliosis (Q67.5)

Scoliosis

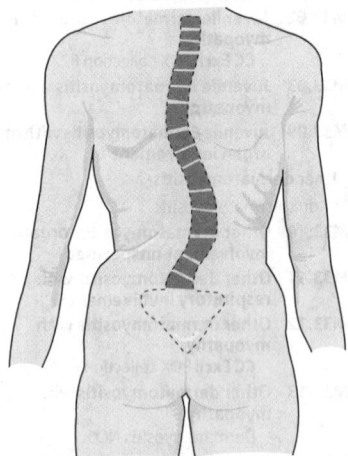

Lateral curvature of spine

✓5ᵗʰ **M41.0** **Infantile idiopathic scoliosis**
AHA: 2014,4Q,26
M41.00 Infantile idiopathic scoliosis, site unspecified
M41.02 Infantile idiopathic scoliosis, cervical **region**
M41.03 Infantile idiopathic scoliosis, cervicothoracic **region**
M41.04 Infantile idiopathic scoliosis, thoracic **region**
M41.05 Infantile idiopathic scoliosis, thoracolumbar **region**
M41.06 Infantile idiopathic scoliosis, lumbar **region**
M41.07 Infantile idiopathic scoliosis, lumbosacral **region**
M41.08 Infantile idiopathic scoliosis, sacral and sacrococcygeal **region**

✓5ᵗʰ **M41.1** **Juvenile and adolescent idiopathic scoliosis**
✓6ᵗʰ **M41.11** **Juvenile idiopathic scoliosis**
AHA: 2014,4Q,28
M41.112 Juvenile idiopathic scoliosis, cervical **region**
M41.113 Juvenile idiopathic scoliosis, cervicothoracic **region**
M41.114 Juvenile idiopathic scoliosis, thoracic **region**
M41.115 Juvenile idiopathic scoliosis, thoracolumbar **region**

M41.116   **Juvenile idiopathic scoliosis, lumbar region**

M41.117   **Juvenile idiopathic scoliosis, lumbosacral region**

M41.119   **Juvenile idiopathic scoliosis, site unspecified**

√6ᵗʰ **M41.12**   **Adolescent scoliosis**

M41.122   **Adolescent idiopathic scoliosis, cervical region**

M41.123   **Adolescent idiopathic scoliosis, cervicothoracic region**

M41.124   **Adolescent idiopathic scoliosis, thoracic region**

M41.125   **Adolescent idiopathic scoliosis, thoracolumbar region**

M41.126   **Adolescent idiopathic scoliosis, lumbar region**

M41.127   **Adolescent idiopathic scoliosis, lumbosacral region**

M41.129   **Adolescent idiopathic scoliosis, site unspecified**

√5ᵗʰ **M41.2**   **Other idiopathic scoliosis**

M41.20   **Other idiopathic scoliosis, site unspecified**

M41.22   **Other idiopathic scoliosis, cervical region**

M41.23   **Other idiopathic scoliosis, cervicothoracic region**

M41.24   **Other idiopathic scoliosis, thoracic region**

M41.25   **Other idiopathic scoliosis, thoracolumbar region**

M41.26   **Other idiopathic scoliosis, lumbar region**

M41.27   **Other idiopathic scoliosis, lumbosacral region**

√5ᵗʰ **M41.3**   **Thoracogenic scoliosis**

M41.30   **Thoracogenic scoliosis, site unspecified**

M41.34   **Thoracogenic scoliosis, thoracic region**

M41.35   **Thoracogenic scoliosis, thoracolumbar region**

√5ᵗʰ **M41.4**   **Neuromuscular scoliosis**

Scoliosis secondary to cerebral palsy, Friedreich's ataxia, poliomyelitis and other neuromuscular disorders

Code also underlying condition

AHA: 2014,4Q,27

M41.40   **Neuromuscular scoliosis, site unspecified**

M41.41   **Neuromuscular scoliosis, occipito-atlanto-axial region**

M41.42   **Neuromuscular scoliosis, cervical region**

M41.43   **Neuromuscular scoliosis, cervicothoracic region**

M41.44   **Neuromuscular scoliosis, thoracic region**

M41.45   **Neuromuscular scoliosis, thoracolumbar region**

M41.46   **Neuromuscular scoliosis, lumbar region**

M41.47   **Neuromuscular scoliosis, lumbosacral region**

√5ᵗʰ **M41.5**   **Other secondary scoliosis**

AHA: 2019,1Q,19

M41.50   **Other secondary scoliosis, site unspecified**

M41.52   **Other secondary scoliosis, cervical region**

M41.53   **Other secondary scoliosis, cervicothoracic region**

M41.54   **Other secondary scoliosis, thoracic region**

M41.55   **Other secondary scoliosis, thoracolumbar region**

M41.56   **Other secondary scoliosis, lumbar region**

M41.57   **Other secondary scoliosis, lumbosacral region**

√5ᵗʰ **M41.8**   **Other forms of scoliosis**

M41.80   **Other forms of scoliosis, site unspecified**

M41.82   **Other forms of scoliosis, cervical region**

M41.83   **Other forms of scoliosis, cervicothoracic region**

M41.84   **Other forms of scoliosis, thoracic region**

M41.85   **Other forms of scoliosis, thoracolumbar region**

M41.86   **Other forms of scoliosis, lumbar region**

M41.87   **Other forms of scoliosis, lumbosacral region**

M41.9   **Scoliosis, unspecified**

√4ᵗʰ **M42**   **Spinal osteochondrosis**

√5ᵗʰ **M42.0**   **Juvenile osteochondrosis of spine**

Calvé's disease

Scheuermann's disease

EXCLUDES 1   *postural kyphosis (M40.0)*

M42.00   **Juvenile osteochondrosis of spine, site unspecified**

M42.01   **Juvenile osteochondrosis of spine, occipito-atlanto-axial region**

M42.02   **Juvenile osteochondrosis of spine, cervical region**

M42.03   **Juvenile osteochondrosis of spine, cervicothoracic region**

M42.04   **Juvenile osteochondrosis of spine, thoracic region**

M42.05   **Juvenile osteochondrosis of spine, thoracolumbar region**

M42.06   **Juvenile osteochondrosis of spine, lumbar region**

M42.07   **Juvenile osteochondrosis of spine, lumbosacral region**

M42.08   **Juvenile osteochondrosis of spine, sacral and sacrococcygeal region**

M42.09   **Juvenile osteochondrosis of spine, multiple sites in spine**

√5ᵗʰ **M42.1**   **Adult osteochondrosis of spine**

M42.10   **Adult osteochondrosis of spine, site unspecified**   Ⓐ

M42.11   **Adult osteochondrosis of spine, occipito-atlanto-axial region**   Ⓐ

M42.12   **Adult osteochondrosis of spine, cervical region**   Ⓐ

M42.13   **Adult osteochondrosis of spine, cervicothoracic region**   Ⓐ

M42.14   **Adult osteochondrosis of spine, thoracic region**   Ⓐ

M42.15   **Adult osteochondrosis of spine, thoracolumbar region**   Ⓐ

M42.16   **Adult osteochondrosis of spine, lumbar region**   Ⓐ

M42.17   **Adult osteochondrosis of spine, lumbosacral region**   Ⓐ

M42.18   **Adult osteochondrosis of spine, sacral and sacrococcygeal region**   Ⓐ

M42.19   **Adult osteochondrosis of spine, multiple sites in spine**   Ⓐ

M42.9   **Spinal osteochondrosis, unspecified**

√4ᵗʰ **M43**   **Other deforming dorsopathies**

EXCLUDES 1   *congenital spondylolysis and spondylolisthesis (Q76.2)*

hemivertebra (Q76.3-Q76.4)

Klippel-Feil syndrome (Q76.1)

lumbarization and sacralization (Q76.4)

platyspondylisis (Q76.4)

spina bifida occulta (Q76.0)

spinal curvature in osteoporosis (M80.-)

spinal curvature in Paget's disease of bone [osteitis deformans] (M88.-)

√5ᵗʰ **M43.0**   **Spondylolysis**

EXCLUDES 1   *congenital spondylolysis (Q76.2)*

spondylolisthesis (M43.1)

M43.00   **Spondylolysis, site unspecified**

M43.01   **Spondylolysis, occipito-atlanto-axial region**

M43.02   **Spondylolysis, cervical region**

M43.03   **Spondylolysis, cervicothoracic region**

M43.04   **Spondylolysis, thoracic region**

M43.05   **Spondylolysis, thoracolumbar region**

M43.06   **Spondylolysis, lumbar region**

M43.07   **Spondylolysis, lumbosacral region**

M43.08   **Spondylolysis, sacral and sacrococcygeal region**

M43.09   **Spondylolysis, multiple sites in spine**

√5ᵗʰ **M43.1**   **Spondylolisthesis**

EXCLUDES 1   *acute traumatic of lumbosacral region (S33.1)*

acute traumatic of sites other than lumbosacral — code to Fracture, vertebra, by region

congenital spondylolisthesis (Q76.2)

AHA: 2018,3Q,18

TIP: Code also any associated radiculopathy (M54.1-) and/or myelopathy (G99.2).

M43.10   **Spondylolisthesis, site unspecified**

M43.11   **Spondylolisthesis, occipito-atlanto-axial region**

M43.12   **Spondylolisthesis, cervical region**

M43.13   **Spondylolisthesis, cervicothoracic region**

M43.14   **Spondylolisthesis, thoracic region**

M43.15   **Spondylolisthesis, thoracolumbar region**

M43.16   **Spondylolisthesis, lumbar region**

M43.17   **Spondylolisthesis, lumbosacral region**

M43.18   **Spondylolisthesis, sacral and sacrococcygeal region**

M43.19   **Spondylolisthesis, multiple sites in spine**

☑ Additional Character Required   √x7ᵗʰ Placeholder   Unacceptable PDx   Questionable PDx   Manifestation   Unspecified Dx   H1-H14 HAC   HCC CMS-HCC Dx   HIV HIV Dx

ICD-10-CM 2020   **803**

Chapter 13. Diseases of the Musculoskeletal System and Connective Tissue

M43.2–M46.30

✓5th **M43.2** **Fusion of spine**

Ankylosis of spinal joint

EXCLUDES 1 *ankylosing spondylitis (M45.0-)*
congenital fusion of spine (Q76.4)

EXCLUDES 2 *arthrodesis status (Z98.1)*
pseudoarthrosis after fusion or arthrodesis (M96.0)

M43.20 **Fusion of spine, site unspecified**
M43.21 **Fusion of spine, occipito-atlanto-axial region**
M43.22 **Fusion of spine, cervical region**
M43.23 **Fusion of spine, cervicothoracic region**
M43.24 **Fusion of spine, thoracic region**
M43.25 **Fusion of spine, thoracolumbar region**
M43.26 **Fusion of spine, lumbar region**
M43.27 **Fusion of spine, lumbosacral region**
M43.28 **Fusion of spine, sacral and sacrococcygeal region**

M43.3 **Recurrent atlantoaxial dislocation with myelopathy**

M43.4 **Other recurrent atlantoaxial dislocation**

✓5th **M43.5** **Other recurrent vertebral dislocation**

EXCLUDES 1 *biomechanical lesions NEC (M99.-)*

✓6th **M43.5X** **Other recurrent vertebral dislocation**

M43.5X2 **Other recurrent vertebral dislocation, cervical region**
M43.5X3 **Other recurrent vertebral dislocation, cervicothoracic region**
M43.5X4 **Other recurrent vertebral dislocation, thoracic region**
M43.5X5 **Other recurrent vertebral dislocation, thoracolumbar region**
M43.5X6 **Other recurrent vertebral dislocation, lumbar region**
M43.5X7 **Other recurrent vertebral dislocation, lumbosacral region**
M43.5X8 **Other recurrent vertebral dislocation, sacral and sacrococcygeal region**
M43.5X9 **Other recurrent vertebral dislocation, site unspecified**

M43.6 **Torticollis**

EXCLUDES 1 *congenital (sternomastoid) torticollis (Q68.0)*
current injury — see Injury, of spine, by body region
ocular torticollis (R29.891)
psychogenic torticollis (F45.8)
spasmodic torticollis (G24.3)
torticollis due to birth injury (P15.2)

DEF: Twisted, unnatural position of the neck due to contracted cervical muscles that pull the head to one side.

✓5th **M43.8** **Other specified deforming dorsopathies**

EXCLUDES 2 *kyphosis and lordosis (M40.-)*
scoliosis (M41.-)

✓6th **M43.8X** **Other specified deforming dorsopathies**

M43.8X1 **Other specified deforming dorsopathies, occipito-atlanto-axial region**
M43.8X2 **Other specified deforming dorsopathies, cervical region**
M43.8X3 **Other specified deforming dorsopathies, cervicothoracic region**
M43.8X4 **Other specified deforming dorsopathies, thoracic region**
M43.8X5 **Other specified deforming dorsopathies, thoracolumbar region**
M43.8X6 **Other specified deforming dorsopathies, lumbar region**
M43.8X7 **Other specified deforming dorsopathies, lumbosacral region**
M43.8X8 **Other specified deforming dorsopathies, sacral and sacrococcygeal region**
M43.8X9 **Other specified deforming dorsopathies, site unspecified**

M43.9 **Deforming dorsopathy, unspecified**

Curvature of spine NOS

Spondylopathies (M45-M49)

✓4th **M45** **Ankylosing spondylitis**

Rheumatoid arthritis of spine

EXCLUDES 1 *arthropathy in Reiter's disease (M02.3-)*
juvenile (ankylosing) spondylitis (M08.1)

EXCLUDES 2 *Behçet's disease (M35.2)*

M45.0 **Ankylosing spondylitis of multiple sites in spine** HCC
M45.1 **Ankylosing spondylitis of occipito-atlanto-axial region** HCC
M45.2 **Ankylosing spondylitis of cervical region** HCC
M45.3 **Ankylosing spondylitis of cervicothoracic region** HCC
M45.4 **Ankylosing spondylitis of thoracic region** HCC
M45.5 **Ankylosing spondylitis of thoracolumbar region** HCC
M45.6 **Ankylosing spondylitis lumbar region** HCC
M45.7 **Ankylosing spondylitis of lumbosacral region** HCC
M45.8 **Ankylosing spondylitis sacral and sacrococcygeal region** HCC
M45.9 **Ankylosing spondylitis of unspecified sites in spine** HCC

✓4th **M46** **Other inflammatory spondylopathies**

✓5th **M46.0** **Spinal enthesopathy**

Disorder of ligamentous or muscular attachments of spine

M46.00 **Spinal enthesopathy, site unspecified** HCC
M46.01 **Spinal enthesopathy, occipito-atlanto-axial region** HCC
M46.02 **Spinal enthesopathy, cervical region** HCC
M46.03 **Spinal enthesopathy, cervicothoracic region** HCC
M46.04 **Spinal enthesopathy, thoracic region** HCC
M46.05 **Spinal enthesopathy, thoracolumbar region** HCC
M46.06 **Spinal enthesopathy, lumbar region** HCC
M46.07 **Spinal enthesopathy, lumbosacral region** HCC
M46.08 **Spinal enthesopathy, sacral and sacrococcygeal region** HCC
M46.09 **Spinal enthesopathy, multiple sites in spine** HCC

M46.1 **Sacroiliitis, not elsewhere classified** HCC

DEF: Inflammation of the sacroiliac joint (situated at the juncture of the sacrum and hip). Symptoms include pain in the buttocks or lower back that can extend down one or both legs.

✓5th **M46.2** **Osteomyelitis of vertebra**

CC Excl: For CC codes in subcategory M46.2: PDX collection 881

M46.20 **Osteomyelitis of vertebra, site unspecified** CC HCC
M46.21 **Osteomyelitis of vertebra, occipito-atlanto-axial region** CC HCC
M46.22 **Osteomyelitis of vertebra, cervical region** CC HCC
M46.23 **Osteomyelitis of vertebra, cervicothoracic region** CC HCC
M46.24 **Osteomyelitis of vertebra, thoracic region** CC HCC
M46.25 **Osteomyelitis of vertebra, thoracolumbar region** CC HCC
M46.26 **Osteomyelitis of vertebra, lumbar region** CC HCC
M46.27 **Osteomyelitis of vertebra, lumbosacral region** CC HCC
M46.28 **Osteomyelitis of vertebra, sacral and sacrococcygeal region** CC HCC

✓5th **M46.3** **Infection of intervertebral disc (pyogenic)**

Use additional code (B95-B97) to identify infectious agent

CC Excl: For CC codes in subcategory M46.3: PDX collection 882

M46.30 **Infection of intervertebral disc (pyogenic), site unspecified** CC HCC

N Newborn: 0 P Pediatric: 0-17 M Maternity: 9-64 A Adult: 15-124 MCC Major Complication/Comorbidity CC Complication/Comorbidity SW Severe Wound Dx

804 ICD-10-CM 2020

M46.31 Infection of intervertebral disc (pyogenic), **occipito-atlanto-axial** region `CC` `HCC`

M46.32 Infection of intervertebral disc (pyogenic), **cervical** region `CC` `HCC`

M46.33 Infection of intervertebral disc (pyogenic), **cervicothoracic** region `CC` `HCC`

M46.34 Infection of intervertebral disc (pyogenic), **thoracic** region `CC` `HCC`

M46.35 Infection of intervertebral disc (pyogenic), **thoracolumbar** region `CC` `HCC`

M46.36 Infection of intervertebral disc (pyogenic), **lumbar** region `CC` `HCC`

M46.37 Infection of intervertebral disc (pyogenic), **lumbosacral** region `CC` `HCC`

M46.38 Infection of intervertebral disc (pyogenic), **sacral and sacrococcygeal** region `CC` `HCC`

M46.39 Infection of intervertebral disc (pyogenic), **multiple sites** in spine `CC` `HCC`

✓5ᵗʰ **M46.4** Discitis, unspecified

M46.40 Discitis, unspecified, site unspecified

M46.41 Discitis, unspecified, occipito-atlanto-axial region

M46.42 Discitis, unspecified, cervical region

M46.43 Discitis, unspecified, cervicothoracic region

M46.44 Discitis, unspecified, thoracic region

M46.45 Discitis, unspecified, thoracolumbar region

M46.46 Discitis, unspecified, lumbar region

M46.47 Discitis, unspecified, lumbosacral region

M46.48 Discitis, unspecified, sacral and sacrococcygeal region

M46.49 Discitis, unspecified, multiple sites in spine

✓5ᵗʰ **M46.5** Other infective spondylopathies

M46.50 Other infective spondylopathies, site unspecified `HCC`

M46.51 Other infective spondylopathies, **occipito-atlanto-axial** region `HCC`

M46.52 Other infective spondylopathies, **cervical** region `HCC`

M46.53 Other infective spondylopathies, **cervicothoracic** region `HCC`

M46.54 Other infective spondylopathies, **thoracic** region `HCC`

M46.55 Other infective spondylopathies, **thoracolumbar** region `HCC`

M46.56 Other infective spondylopathies, **lumbar** region `HCC`

M46.57 Other infective spondylopathies, **lumbosacral** region `HCC`

M46.58 Other infective spondylopathies, **sacral and sacrococcygeal** region `HCC`

M46.59 Other infective spondylopathies, **multiple sites** in spine `HCC`

✓5ᵗʰ **M46.8** Other specified inflammatory spondylopathies

M46.80 Other specified inflammatory spondylopathies, site unspecified `HCC`

M46.81 Other specified inflammatory spondylopathies, **occipito-atlanto-axial** region `HCC`

M46.82 Other specified inflammatory spondylopathies, **cervical** region `HCC`

M46.83 Other specified inflammatory spondylopathies, **cervicothoracic** region `HCC`

M46.84 Other specified inflammatory spondylopathies, **thoracic** region `HCC`

M46.85 Other specified inflammatory spondylopathies, **thoracolumbar** region `HCC`

M46.86 Other specified inflammatory spondylopathies, **lumbar** region `HCC`

M46.87 Other specified inflammatory spondylopathies, **lumbosacral** region `HCC`

M46.88 Other specified inflammatory spondylopathies, **sacral and sacrococcygeal** region `HCC`

M46.89 Other specified inflammatory spondylopathies, **multiple sites** in spine `HCC`

✓5ᵗʰ **M46.9** Unspecified inflammatory spondylopathy

M46.90 Unspecified inflammatory spondylopathy, site unspecified `HCC`

M46.91 Unspecified inflammatory spondylopathy, **occipito-atlanto-axial** region `HCC`

M46.92 Unspecified inflammatory spondylopathy, **cervical** region `HCC`

M46.93 Unspecified inflammatory spondylopathy, **cervicothoracic** region `HCC`

M46.94 Unspecified inflammatory spondylopathy, **thoracic** region `HCC`

M46.95 Unspecified inflammatory spondylopathy, **thoracolumbar** region `HCC`

M46.96 Unspecified inflammatory spondylopathy, **lumbar** region `HCC`

M46.97 Unspecified inflammatory spondylopathy, **lumbosacral** region `HCC`

M46.98 Unspecified inflammatory spondylopathy, **sacral and sacrococcygeal** region `HCC`

M46.99 Unspecified inflammatory spondylopathy, **multiple sites** in spine `HCC`

✓4ᵗʰ **M47** Spondylosis

INCLUDES arthrosis or osteoarthritis of spine
degeneration of facet joints

CC Excl: For CC codes in category M47, unless otherwise noted: PDX collection 883

✓5ᵗʰ **M47.0** Anterior spinal and vertebral artery **compression syndromes**

✓6ᵗʰ **M47.01** Anterior spinal artery **compression syndromes**

M47.011 Anterior spinal artery compression syndromes, **occipito-atlanto-axial** region `CC`

M47.012 Anterior spinal artery compression syndromes, **cervical** region `CC`

M47.013 Anterior spinal artery compression syndromes, **cervicothoracic** region `CC`

M47.014 Anterior spinal artery compression syndromes, **thoracic** region `CC`

M47.015 Anterior spinal artery compression syndromes, **thoracolumbar** region `CC`

M47.016 Anterior spinal artery compression syndromes, **lumbar** region `CC`

M47.019 Anterior spinal artery compression syndromes, **site unspecified** `CC`

✓6ᵗʰ **M47.02** Vertebral artery **compression syndromes**

M47.021 Vertebral artery compression syndromes, **occipito-atlanto-axial** region `CC`

M47.022 Vertebral artery compression syndromes, **cervical** region `CC`

M47.029 Vertebral artery compression syndromes, **site unspecified** `CC`

✓5ᵗʰ **M47.1** Other spondylosis **with myelopathy**

Spondylogenic compression of spinal cord

EXCLUDES 1   vertebral subluxation ▶*(M43.3-M43.5X9)*◀

M47.10 Other spondylosis with myelopathy, site unspecified `CC`

CC Excl: PDX collection 884

M47.11 Other spondylosis with myelopathy, **occipito-atlanto-axial** region `CC`

M47.12 Other spondylosis with myelopathy, **cervical** region `CC`

M47.13 Other spondylosis with myelopathy, **cervicothoracic** region `CC`

Chapter 13. Diseases of the Musculoskeletal System and Connective Tissue

M47.14 Other spondylosis with myelopathy, thoracic region   `CC`
     CC Excl: PDX collection 885

M47.15 Other spondylosis with myelopathy, thoracolumbar region   `CC`
     CC Excl: PDX collection 885

M47.16 Other spondylosis with myelopathy, lumbar region   `CC`
     CC Excl: PDX collection 886

✓5ᵗʰ **M47.2** Other spondylosis with radiculopathy

M47.20 Other spondylosis with radiculopathy, site unspecified

M47.21 Other spondylosis with radiculopathy, occipito-atlanto-axial region

M47.22 Other spondylosis with radiculopathy, cervical region

M47.23 Other spondylosis with radiculopathy, cervicothoracic region

M47.24 Other spondylosis with radiculopathy, thoracic region

M47.25 Other spondylosis with radiculopathy, thoracolumbar region

M47.26 Other spondylosis with radiculopathy, lumbar region

M47.27 Other spondylosis with radiculopathy, lumbosacral region

M47.28 Other spondylosis with radiculopathy, sacral and sacrococcygeal region

✓5ᵗʰ **M47.8** Other spondylosis

✓6ᵗʰ **M47.81** Spondylosis without myelopathy or radiculopathy
     AHA: 2018,2Q,14

M47.811 Spondylosis without myelopathy or radiculopathy, occipito-atlanto-axial region

M47.812 Spondylosis without myelopathy or radiculopathy, cervical region

M47.813 Spondylosis without myelopathy or radiculopathy, cervicothoracic region

M47.814 Spondylosis without myelopathy or radiculopathy, thoracic region

M47.815 Spondylosis without myelopathy or radiculopathy, thoracolumbar region

M47.816 Spondylosis without myelopathy or radiculopathy, lumbar region

M47.817 Spondylosis without myelopathy or radiculopathy, lumbosacral region

M47.818 Spondylosis without myelopathy or radiculopathy, sacral and sacrococcygeal region

M47.819 Spondylosis without myelopathy or radiculopathy, site unspecified

✓6ᵗʰ **M47.89** Other spondylosis

M47.891 Other spondylosis, occipito-atlanto-axial region

M47.892 Other spondylosis, cervical region

M47.893 Other spondylosis, cervicothoracic region

M47.894 Other spondylosis, thoracic region

M47.895 Other spondylosis, thoracolumbar region

M47.896 Other spondylosis, lumbar region

M47.897 Other spondylosis, lumbosacral region

M47.898 Other spondylosis, sacral and sacrococcygeal region

M47.899 Other spondylosis, site unspecified

M47.9 Spondylosis, unspecified

✓4ᵗʰ **M48** Other spondylopathies

✓5ᵗʰ **M48.0** Spinal stenosis
     Caudal stenosis
     AHA: 2018,3Q,18-19
     TIP: Code also any associated radiculopathy (M54.1-) and/or myelopathy (G99.2).

M48.00 Spinal stenosis, site unspecified

M48.01 Spinal stenosis, occipito-atlanto-axial region

M48.02 Spinal stenosis, cervical region

M48.03 Spinal stenosis, cervicothoracic region

M48.04 Spinal stenosis, thoracic region

M48.05 Spinal stenosis, thoracolumbar region

✓6ᵗʰ **M48.06** Spinal stenosis, lumbar region
     AHA: 2018,3Q,19; 2017,4Q,18-19
     DEF: Spinal canal narrowing in the lumbar area with nerve root compression, causing muscle pain, fatigue, and weakness during extension of the lumbar spine. Pain is relieved by sitting or bending.

M48.061 Spinal stenosis, lumbar region without neurogenic claudication
     Spinal stenosis, lumbar region NOS

M48.062 Spinal stenosis, lumbar region with neurogenic claudication

M48.07 Spinal stenosis, lumbosacral region

M48.08 Spinal stenosis, sacral and sacrococcygeal region

✓5ᵗʰ **M48.1** Ankylosing hyperostosis [Forestier]
     Diffuse idiopathic skeletal hyperostosis [DISH]

M48.10 Ankylosing hyperostosis [Forestier], site unspecified

M48.11 Ankylosing hyperostosis [Forestier], occipito-atlanto-axial region

M48.12 Ankylosing hyperostosis [Forestier], cervical region

M48.13 Ankylosing hyperostosis [Forestier], cervicothoracic region

M48.14 Ankylosing hyperostosis [Forestier], thoracic region

M48.15 Ankylosing hyperostosis [Forestier], thoracolumbar region

M48.16 Ankylosing hyperostosis [Forestier], lumbar region

M48.17 Ankylosing hyperostosis [Forestier], lumbosacral region

M48.18 Ankylosing hyperostosis [Forestier], sacral and sacrococcygeal region

M48.19 Ankylosing hyperostosis [Forestier], multiple sites in spine

✓5ᵗʰ **M48.2** Kissing spine

M48.20 Kissing spine, site unspecified

M48.21 Kissing spine, occipito-atlanto-axial region

M48.22 Kissing spine, cervical region

M48.23 Kissing spine, cervicothoracic region

M48.24 Kissing spine, thoracic region

M48.25 Kissing spine, thoracolumbar region

M48.26 Kissing spine, lumbar region

M48.27 Kissing spine, lumbosacral region

✓5ᵗʰ **M48.3** Traumatic spondylopathy

     CC Excl: For CC codes in subcategory M48.3: PDX collection 887

M48.30 Traumatic spondylopathy, site unspecified   `CC`

M48.31 Traumatic spondylopathy, occipito-atlanto-axial region   `CC`

M48.32 Traumatic spondylopathy, cervical region   `CC`

M48.33 Traumatic spondylopathy, cervicothoracic region   `CC`

M48.34 Traumatic spondylopathy, thoracic region   `CC`

M48.35 Traumatic spondylopathy, thoracolumbar region   `CC`

M48.36 Traumatic spondylopathy, lumbar region   `CC`

M48.37 Traumatic spondylopathy, lumbosacral region   `CC`

M48.38 Traumatic spondylopathy, sacral and sacrococcygeal region   `CC`

N Newborn: 0   P Pediatric: 0-17   M Maternity: 9-64   A Adult: 15-124   `MCC` Major Complication/Comorbidity   `CC` Complication/Comorbidity   `SW` Severe Wound Dx

806   ICD-10-CM 2020

√5ᵗʰ **M48.4 Fatigue fracture of vertebra**

Stress fracture of vertebra

EXCLUDES 1   *pathological fracture NOS (M84.4-)*

pathological fracture of vertebra due to neoplasm (M84.58)

pathological fracture of vertebra due to osteoporosis (M80.-)

pathological fracture of vertebra due to other diagnosis (M84.68)

traumatic fracture of vertebrae (S12.0-S12.3-, S22.0-, S32.0-)

> The appropriate 7th character is to be added to each code from subcategory M48.4.
> A   initial encounter for fracture
> D   subsequent encounter for fracture with routine healing
> G   subsequent encounter for fracture with delayed healing
> S   sequela of fracture

√x7ᵗʰ **M48.40 Fatigue fracture of vertebra, site unspecified**

√x7ᵗʰ **M48.41 Fatigue fracture of vertebra, occipito-atlanto-axial region**

√x7ᵗʰ **M48.42 Fatigue fracture of vertebra, cervical region**

√x7ᵗʰ **M48.43 Fatigue fracture of vertebra, cervicothoracic region**

√x7ᵗʰ **M48.44 Fatigue fracture of vertebra, thoracic region**

√x7ᵗʰ **M48.45 Fatigue fracture of vertebra, thoracolumbar region**

√x7ᵗʰ **M48.46 Fatigue fracture of vertebra, lumbar region**

√x7ᵗʰ **M48.47 Fatigue fracture of vertebra, lumbosacral region**

√x7ᵗʰ **M48.48 Fatigue fracture of vertebra, sacral and sacrococcygeal region**

√5ᵗʰ **M48.5 Collapsed vertebra, not elsewhere classified**

Collapsed vertebra NOS

Compression fracture of vertebra NOS

Wedging of vertebra NOS

EXCLUDES 1   *current injury — see Injury of spine, by body region*

fatigue fracture of vertebra (M48.4)

pathological fracture NOS (M84.4-)

pathological fracture of vertebra due to neoplasm (M84.58)

pathological fracture of vertebra due to osteoporosis (M80.-)

pathological fracture of vertebra due to other diagnosis (M84.68)

stress fracture of vertebra (M48.4-)

traumatic fracture of vertebra (S12.-, S22.-, S32.-)

> The appropriate 7th character is to be added to each code from subcategory M48.5.
> A   initial encounter for fracture
> D   subsequent encounter for fracture with routine healing
> G   subsequent encounter for fracture with delayed healing
> S   sequela of fracture

CC Excl: For CC codes in subcategory M48.5: PDX collection 888

6 √x7ᵗʰ **M48.50 Collapsed vertebra, not elsewhere classified, site unspecified**   CC HCC

6 √x7ᵗʰ **M48.51 Collapsed vertebra, not elsewhere classified, occipito-atlanto-axial region**   CC HCC

6 √x7ᵗʰ **M48.52 Collapsed vertebra, not elsewhere classified, cervical region**   CC HCC

6 √x7ᵗʰ **M48.53 Collapsed vertebra, not elsewhere classified, cervicothoracic region**   CC HCC

6 √x7ᵗʰ **M48.54 Collapsed vertebra, not elsewhere classified, thoracic region**   CC HCC

6 √x7ᵗʰ **M48.55 Collapsed vertebra, not elsewhere classified, thoracolumbar region**   CC HCC

6 √x7ᵗʰ **M48.56 Collapsed vertebra, not elsewhere classified, lumbar region**   CC HCC

6 √x7ᵗʰ **M48.57 Collapsed vertebra, not elsewhere classified, lumbosacral region**   CC HCC

6 √x7ᵗʰ **M48.58 Collapsed vertebra, not elsewhere classified, sacral and sacrococcygeal region**   CC HCC

√5ᵗʰ **M48.8 Other specified spondylopathies**

Ossification of posterior longitudinal ligament

√6ᵗʰ **M48.8X Other specified spondylopathies**

M48.8X1 Other specified spondylopathies, occipito-atlanto-axial region   HCC

M48.8X2 Other specified spondylopathies, cervical region   HCC

M48.8X3 Other specified spondylopathies, cervicothoracic region   HCC

M48.8X4 Other specified spondylopathies, thoracic region   HCC

M48.8X5 Other specified spondylopathies, thoracolumbar region   HCC

M48.8X6 Other specified spondylopathies, lumbar region   HCC

M48.8X7 Other specified spondylopathies, lumbosacral region   HCC

M48.8X8 Other specified spondylopathies, sacral and sacrococcygeal region   HCC

M48.8X9 Other specified spondylopathies, site unspecified   HCC

M48.9 Spondylopathy, unspecified

√4ᵗʰ **M49 Spondylopathies in diseases classified elsewhere**

INCLUDES   curvature of spine in diseases classified elsewhere

deformity of spine in diseases classified elsewhere

kyphosis in diseases classified elsewhere

scoliosis in diseases classified elsewhere

spondylopathy in diseases classified elsewhere

Code first underlying disease, such as:

brucellosis (A23.-)

Charcôt-Marie-Tooth disease (G60.0)

enterobacterial infections (A01-A04)

osteitis fibrosa cystica (E21.0)

EXCLUDES 1   *curvature of spine in tuberculosis [Pott's] (A18.01)*

enteropathic arthropathies (M07.-)

gonococcal spondylitis (A54.41)

neuropathic spondylopathy in syringomyelia (G95.0)

neuropathic spondylopathy in tabes dorsalis (A52.11)

neuropathic [tabes dorsalis] spondylitis (A52.11)

nonsyphilitic neuropathic spondylopathy NEC (G98.0)

spondylitis in syphilis (acquired) (A52.77)

tuberculous spondylitis (A18.01)

typhoid fever spondylitis (A01.05)

√5ᵗʰ **M49.8 Spondylopathy in diseases classified elsewhere**

M49.80 *Spondylopathy in diseases classified elsewhere, site unspecified*   HCC

M49.81 *Spondylopathy in diseases classified elsewhere, occipito-atlanto-axial region*   HCC

M49.82 *Spondylopathy in diseases classified elsewhere, cervical region*   HCC

M49.83 *Spondylopathy in diseases classified elsewhere, cervicothoracic region*   HCC

M49.84 *Spondylopathy in diseases classified elsewhere, thoracic region*   HCC

M49.85 *Spondylopathy in diseases classified elsewhere, thoracolumbar region*   HCC

M49.86 *Spondylopathy in diseases classified elsewhere, lumbar region*   HCC

M49.87 *Spondylopathy in diseases classified elsewhere, lumbosacral region*   HCC

M49.88 *Spondylopathy in diseases classified elsewhere, sacral and sacrococcygeal region*   HCC

M49.89 *Spondylopathy in diseases classified elsewhere, multiple sites in spine*   HCC

Chapter 13. Diseases of the Musculoskeletal System and Connective Tissue

M50–M50.923

Other dorsopathies (M50-M54)

EXCLUDES 1   current injury — see injury of spine by body region
discitis NOS (M46.4-)

√4ᵗʰ **M50 Cervical disc disorders**

> NOTE   Code to the most superior level of disorder
>
> INCLUDES   cervicothoracic disc disorders
> cervicothoracic disc disorders with cervicalgia
>
> AHA: 2016,4Q,39-40; 2016,1Q,17

√5ᵗʰ **M50.0 Cervical disc disorder with myelopathy**

> AHA: 2018,3Q,19
>
> CC Excl: For CC codes in subcategory M50.0: PDX collection 889

    M50.00 Cervical disc disorder with myelopathy, unspecified cervical region   CC

    M50.01 Cervical disc disorder with myelopathy, high cervical region   CC
C2-C3 disc disorder with myelopathy
C3-C4 disc disorder with myelopathy

√6ᵗʰ   **M50.02 Cervical disc disorder with myelopathy, mid-cervical region**

    M50.020 Cervical disc disorder with myelopathy, mid-cervical region, unspecified level   CC

    M50.021 Cervical disc disorder at C4-C5 level with myelopathy   CC
C4-C5 disc disorder with myelopathy

    M50.022 Cervical disc disorder at C5-C6 level with myelopathy   CC
C5-C6 disc disorder with myelopathy

    M50.023 Cervical disc disorder at C6-C7 level with myelopathy   CC
C6-C7 disc disorder with myelopathy

    M50.03 Cervical disc disorder with myelopathy, cervicothoracic region   CC
C7-T1 disc disorder with myelopathy

√5ᵗʰ **M50.1 Cervical disc disorder with radiculopathy**

> EXCLUDES 2   brachial radiculitis NOS (M54.13)
>
> AHA: 2018,3Q,19

    M50.10 Cervical disc disorder with radiculopathy, unspecified cervical region

    M50.11 Cervical disc disorder with radiculopathy, high cervical region
C2-C3 disc disorder with radiculopathy
C3 radiculopathy due to disc disorder
C3-C4 disc disorder with radiculopathy
C4 radiculopathy due to disc disorder

√6ᵗʰ   **M50.12 Cervical disc disorder with radiculopathy, mid-cervical region**

    M50.120 Mid-cervical disc disorder, unspecified level

    M50.121 Cervical disc disorder at C4-C5 level with radiculopathy
C4-C5 disc disorder with radiculopathy
C5 radiculopathy due to disc disorder

    M50.122 Cervical disc disorder at C5-C6 level with radiculopathy
C5-C6 disc disorder with radiculopathy
C6 radiculopathy due to disc disorder

    M50.123 Cervical disc disorder at C6-C7 level with radiculopathy
C6-C7 disc disorder with radiculopathy
C7 radiculopathy due to disc disorder

    M50.13 Cervical disc disorder with radiculopathy, cervicothoracic region
C7-T1 disc disorder with radiculopathy
C8 radiculopathy due to disc disorder

√5ᵗʰ **M50.2 Other cervical disc displacement**

    M50.20 Other cervical disc displacement, unspecified cervical region

    M50.21 Other cervical disc displacement, high cervical region
Other C2-C3 cervical disc displacement
Other C3-C4 cervical disc displacement

√6ᵗʰ   **M50.22 Other cervical disc displacement, mid-cervical region**

    M50.220 Other cervical disc displacement, mid-cervical region, unspecified level

    M50.221 Other cervical disc displacement at C4-C5 level
Other C4-C5 cervical disc displacement

    M50.222 Other cervical disc displacement at C5-C6 level
Other C5-C6 cervical disc displacement

    M50.223 Other cervical disc displacement at C6-C7 level
Other C6-C7 cervical disc displacement

    M50.23 Other cervical disc displacement, cervicothoracic region
Other C7-T1 cervical disc displacement

√5ᵗʰ **M50.3 Other cervical disc degeneration**

    M50.30 Other cervical disc degeneration, unspecified cervical region

    M50.31 Other cervical disc degeneration, high cervical region
Other C2-C3 cervical disc degeneration
Other C3-C4 cervical disc degeneration

√6ᵗʰ   **M50.32 Other cervical disc degeneration, mid-cervical region**

    M50.320 Other cervical disc degeneration, mid-cervical region, unspecified level

    M50.321 Other cervical disc degeneration at C4-C5 level
Other C4-C5 cervical disc degeneration

    M50.322 Other cervical disc degeneration at C5-C6 level
Other C5-C6 cervical disc degeneration

    M50.323 Other cervical disc degeneration at C6-C7 level
Other C6-C7 cervical disc degeneration

    M50.33 Other cervical disc degeneration, cervicothoracic region
Other C7-T1 cervical disc degeneration

√5ᵗʰ **M50.8 Other cervical disc disorders**

    M50.80 Other cervical disc disorders, unspecified cervical region

    M50.81 Other cervical disc disorders, high cervical region
Other C2-C3 cervical disc disorders
Other C3-C4 cervical disc disorders

√6ᵗʰ   **M50.82 Other cervical disc disorders, mid-cervical region**

    M50.820 Other cervical disc disorders, mid-cervical region, unspecified level

    M50.821 Other cervical disc disorders at C4-C5 level
Other C4-C5 cervical disc disorders

    M50.822 Other cervical disc disorders at C5-C6 level
Other C5-C6 cervical disc disorders

    M50.823 Other cervical disc disorders at C6-C7 level
Other C6-C7 cervical disc disorders

    M50.83 Other cervical disc disorders, cervicothoracic region
Other C7-T1 cervical disc disorders

√5ᵗʰ **M50.9 Cervical disc disorder, unspecified**

    M50.90 Cervical disc disorder, unspecified, unspecified cervical region

    M50.91 Cervical disc disorder, unspecified, high cervical region
C2-C3 cervical disc disorder, unspecified
C3-C4 cervical disc disorder, unspecified

√6ᵗʰ   **M50.92 Cervical disc disorder, unspecified, mid-cervical region**

    M50.920 Unspecified cervical disc disorder, mid-cervical region, unspecified level

    M50.921 Unspecified cervical disc disorder at C4-C5 level
Unspecified C4-C5 cervical disc disorder

    M50.922 Unspecified cervical disc disorder at C5-C6 level
Unspecified C5-C6 cervical disc disorder

    M50.923 Unspecified cervical disc disorder at C6-C7 level
Unspecified C6-C7 cervical disc disorder

M50.93 Cervical disc disorder, unspecified, cervicothoracic region
C7-T1 cervical disc disorder, unspecified

√4ᵗʰ **M51 Thoracic, thoracolumbar, and lumbosacral intervertebral disc disorders**
EXCLUDES 2   *cervical and cervicothoracic disc disorders (M50.-)*
sacral and sacrococcygeal disorders (M53.3)

√5ᵗʰ **M51.0 Thoracic, thoracolumbar and lumbosacral intervertebral disc disorders with myelopathy**

M51.04 Intervertebral disc disorders with myelopathy, thoracic region   CC
CC Excl: PDX collection 890

M51.05 Intervertebral disc disorders with myelopathy, thoracolumbar region   CC
CC Excl: PDX collection 890

M51.06 Intervertebral disc disorders with myelopathy, lumbar region   CC
CC Excl: PDX collection 891

√5ᵗʰ **M51.1 Thoracic, thoracolumbar and lumbosacral intervertebral disc disorders with radiculopathy**
Sciatica due to intervertebral disc disorder
EXCLUDES 1   *lumbar radiculitis NOS (M54.16)*
sciatica NOS (M54.3)
AHA: 2018,3Q,18

M51.14 Intervertebral disc disorders with radiculopathy, thoracic region

M51.15 Intervertebral disc disorders with radiculopathy, thoracolumbar region

M51.16 Intervertebral disc disorders with radiculopathy, lumbar region

M51.17 Intervertebral disc disorders with radiculopathy, lumbosacral region

√5ᵗʰ **M51.2 Other thoracic, thoracolumbar and lumbosacral intervertebral disc displacement**
Lumbago due to displacement of intervertebral disc

Displacement Intervertebral Disc

Normal Top View   Herniated Top View
Lamina
Ligamentum flavum
Nucleus pulposus
Disc annulus
Nucleus pulposus
Spinal cord
Herniates through annulus
Spinal nerve

M51.24 Other intervertebral disc displacement, thoracic region

M51.25 Other intervertebral disc displacement, thoracolumbar region

M51.26 Other intervertebral disc displacement, lumbar region

M51.27 Other intervertebral disc displacement, lumbosacral region

√5ᵗʰ **M51.3 Other thoracic, thoracolumbar and lumbosacral intervertebral disc degeneration**
AHA: 2018,2Q,15; 2013,3Q,22

M51.34 Other intervertebral disc degeneration, thoracic region

M51.35 Other intervertebral disc degeneration, thoracolumbar region

M51.36 Other intervertebral disc degeneration, lumbar region

M51.37 Other intervertebral disc degeneration, lumbosacral region

√5ᵗʰ **M51.4 Schmorl's nodes**
DEF: Irregular bone defect in the margin of the vertebral body that causes herniation into the end plate of the vertebral body.

M51.44 Schmorl's nodes, thoracic region

M51.45 Schmorl's nodes, thoracolumbar region

M51.46 Schmorl's nodes, lumbar region

M51.47 Schmorl's nodes, lumbosacral region

√5ᵗʰ **M51.8 Other thoracic, thoracolumbar and lumbosacral intervertebral disc disorders**

M51.84 Other intervertebral disc disorders, thoracic region

M51.85 Other intervertebral disc disorders, thoracolumbar region

M51.86 Other intervertebral disc disorders, lumbar region

M51.87 Other intervertebral disc disorders, lumbosacral region

M51.9 Unspecified thoracic, thoracolumbar and lumbosacral intervertebral disc disorder

√4ᵗʰ **M53 Other and unspecified dorsopathies, not elsewhere classified**

M53.0 Cervicocranial syndrome
Posterior cervical sympathetic syndrome

M53.1 Cervicobrachial syndrome
EXCLUDES 2   *cervical disc disorder (M50.-)*
thoracic outlet syndrome (G54.0)

√5ᵗʰ **M53.2 Spinal instabilities**

√6ᵗʰ **M53.2X Spinal instabilities**

M53.2X1 Spinal instabilities, occipito-atlanto-axial region

M53.2X2 Spinal instabilities, cervical region

M53.2X3 Spinal instabilities, cervicothoracic region

M53.2X4 Spinal instabilities, thoracic region

M53.2X5 Spinal instabilities, thoracolumbar region

M53.2X6 Spinal instabilities, lumbar region

M53.2X7 Spinal instabilities, lumbosacral region

M53.2X8 Spinal instabilities, sacral and sacrococcygeal region

M53.2X9 Spinal instabilities, site unspecified

M53.3 Sacrococcygeal disorders, not elsewhere classified
Coccygodynia

√5ᵗʰ **M53.8 Other specified dorsopathies**

M53.80 Other specified dorsopathies, site unspecified

M53.81 Other specified dorsopathies, occipito-atlanto-axial region

M53.82 Other specified dorsopathies, cervical region

M53.83 Other specified dorsopathies, cervicothoracic region

M53.84 Other specified dorsopathies, thoracic region

M53.85 Other specified dorsopathies, thoracolumbar region

M53.86 Other specified dorsopathies, lumbar region

M53.87 Other specified dorsopathies, lumbosacral region

M53.88 Other specified dorsopathies, sacral and sacrococcygeal region

M53.9 Dorsopathy, unspecified

√4ᵗʰ **M54 Dorsalgia**
EXCLUDES 1   *psychogenic dorsalgia (F45.41)*

√5ᵗʰ **M54.0 Panniculitis affecting regions of neck and back**
EXCLUDES 1   *lupus panniculitis (L93.2)*
panniculitis NOS (M79.3)
relapsing [Weber-Christian] panniculitis (M35.6)

M54.00 Panniculitis affecting regions of neck and back, site unspecified

M54.01 Panniculitis affecting regions of neck and back, occipito-atlanto-axial region

M54.02 Panniculitis affecting regions of neck and back, cervical region

M54.03 Panniculitis affecting regions of neck and back, cervicothoracic region

M54.04 Panniculitis affecting regions of neck and back, thoracic region

M54.05 Panniculitis affecting regions of neck and back, thoracolumbar region

M54.06 Panniculitis affecting regions of neck and back, lumbar region

M54.07 Panniculitis affecting regions of neck and back, lumbosacral region

M54.08 Panniculitis affecting regions of neck and back, sacral and sacrococcygeal region

M54.09 Panniculitis affecting regions, neck and back, multiple sites in spine

✓5ᵗʰ **M54.1 Radiculopathy**

Brachial neuritis or radiculitis NOS
Lumbar neuritis or radiculitis NOS
Lumbosacral neuritis or radiculitis NOS
Thoracic neuritis or radiculitis NOS
Radiculitis NOS

> *EXCLUDES 1*   neuralgia and neuritis NOS (M79.2)
> radiculopathy with cervical disc disorder (M50.1)
> radiculopathy with lumbar and other intervertebral disc disorder (M51.1-)
> radiculopathy with spondylosis (M47.2-)

AHA: 2018,3Q,18

TIP: A code from this subcategory can be used in addition to a spondylolisthesis code (M43.1-) or a spinal stenosis code (M48.0-) when either condition is documented as the cause of the radiculopathy.

    M54.10 Radiculopathy, site unspecified
    M54.11 Radiculopathy, occipito-atlanto-axial region
    M54.12 Radiculopathy, cervical region
    M54.13 Radiculopathy, cervicothoracic region
    M54.14 Radiculopathy, thoracic region
    M54.15 Radiculopathy, thoracolumbar region
    M54.16 Radiculopathy, lumbar region
    M54.17 Radiculopathy, lumbosacral region
    M54.18 Radiculopathy, sacral and sacrococcygeal region

M54.2 Cervicalgia

> *EXCLUDES 1*   cervicalgia due to intervertebral cervical disc disorder (M50.-)

✓5ᵗʰ **M54.3 Sciatica**

> *EXCLUDES 1*   lesion of sciatic nerve (G57.0)
> sciatica due to intervertebral disc disorder (M51.1-)
> sciatica with lumbago (M54.4-)

    M54.30 Sciatica, unspecified side
    M54.31 Sciatica, right side
    M54.32 Sciatica, left side

✓5ᵗʰ **M54.4 Lumbago with sciatica**

> *EXCLUDES 1*   lumbago with sciatica due to intervertebral disc disorder (M51.1-)

AHA: 2016,2Q,7

    M54.40 Lumbago with sciatica, unspecified side
    M54.41 Lumbago with sciatica, right side
    M54.42 Lumbago with sciatica, left side

M54.5 Low back pain

Loin pain
Lumbago NOS

> *EXCLUDES 1*   low back strain (S39.012)
> lumbago due to intervertebral disc displacement (M51.2-)
> lumbago with sciatica (M54.4-)

M54.6 Pain in thoracic spine

> *EXCLUDES 1*   pain in thoracic spine due to intervertebral disc disorder (M51.-)

✓5ᵗʰ **M54.8 Other dorsalgia**

> *EXCLUDES 1*   dorsalgia in thoracic region (M54.6)
> low back pain (M54.5)

    M54.81 Occipital neuralgia
    M54.89 Other dorsalgia

M54.9 Dorsalgia, unspecified

Backache NOS
Back pain NOS

SOFT TISSUE DISORDERS (M60-M79)

Disorders of muscles (M60-M63)

> *EXCLUDES 1*   dermatopolymyositis (M33.-)
> muscular dystrophies and myopathies (G71-G72)
> myopathy in amyloidosis (E85.-)
> myopathy in polyarteritis nodosa (M30.0)
> myopathy in rheumatoid arthritis (M05.32)
> myopathy in scleroderma (M34.-)
> myopathy in Sjögren's syndrome (M35.03)
> myopathy in systemic lupus erythematosus (M32.-)

✓4ᵗʰ **M60 Myositis**

> *EXCLUDES 2*   inclusion body myositis [IBM] (G72.41)

✓5ᵗʰ **M60.0 Infective myositis**

Tropical pyomyositis
Use additional code (B95-B97) to identify infectious agent

CC Excl: For CC codes in subcategory M60.0: PDX collection 806

✓6ᵗʰ **M60.00 Infective myositis, unspecified site**

    M60.000 Infective myositis, unspecified right arm `CC`
      Infective myositis, right upper limb NOS

    M60.001 Infective myositis, unspecified left arm `CC`
      Infective myositis, left upper limb NOS

    M60.002 Infective myositis, unspecified arm `CC`
      Infective myositis, upper limb NOS

    M60.003 Infective myositis, unspecified right leg `CC`
      Infective myositis, right lower limb NOS

    M60.004 Infective myositis, unspecified left leg `CC`
      Infective myositis, left lower limb NOS

    M60.005 Infective myositis, unspecified leg `CC`
      Infective myositis, lower limb NOS

    M60.009 Infective myositis, unspecified site `CC`

✓6ᵗʰ **M60.01 Infective myositis, shoulder**

    M60.011 Infective myositis, right shoulder `CC`
    M60.012 Infective myositis, left shoulder `CC`
    M60.019 Infective myositis, unspecified shoulder `CC`

✓6ᵗʰ **M60.02 Infective myositis, upper arm**

    M60.021 Infective myositis, right upper arm `CC`
    M60.022 Infective myositis, left upper arm `CC`
    M60.029 Infective myositis, unspecified upper arm `CC`

✓6ᵗʰ **M60.03 Infective myositis, forearm**

    M60.031 Infective myositis, right forearm `CC`
    M60.032 Infective myositis, left forearm `CC`
    M60.039 Infective myositis, unspecified forearm `CC`

✓6ᵗʰ **M60.04 Infective myositis, hand and fingers**

    M60.041 Infective myositis, right hand `CC`
    M60.042 Infective myositis, left hand `CC`
    M60.043 Infective myositis, unspecified hand `CC`
    M60.044 Infective myositis, right finger(s) `CC`
    M60.045 Infective myositis, left finger(s) `CC`
    M60.046 Infective myositis, unspecified finger(s) `CC`

✓6ᵗʰ **M60.05 Infective myositis, thigh**

    M60.051 Infective myositis, right thigh `CC`
    M60.052 Infective myositis, left thigh `CC`

N Newborn: 0   P Pediatric: 0-17   M Maternity: 9-64   A Adult: 15-124   MCC Major Complication/Comorbidity   CC Complication/Comorbidity   SW Severe Wound Dx

810   ICD-10-CM 2020

M60.059 Infective myositis, unspecified thigh `CC`

✓6ᵗʰ M60.06 Infective myositis, lower leg

M60.061 Infective myositis, right lower leg `CC`

M60.062 Infective myositis, left lower leg `CC`

M60.069 Infective myositis, unspecified lower leg `CC`

✓6ᵗʰ M60.07 Infective myositis, ankle, foot and toes

M60.070 Infective myositis, right ankle `CC`

M60.071 Infective myositis, left ankle `CC`

M60.072 Infective myositis, unspecified ankle `CC`

M60.073 Infective myositis, right foot `CC`

M60.074 Infective myositis, left foot `CC`

M60.075 Infective myositis, unspecified foot `CC`

M60.076 Infective myositis, right toe(s) `CC`

M60.077 Infective myositis, left toe(s) `CC`

M60.078 Infective myositis, unspecified toe(s) `CC`

M60.08 Infective myositis, other site `CC`

M60.09 Infective myositis, multiple sites `CC`

✓5ᵗʰ M60.1 Interstitial myositis

M60.10 Interstitial myositis of unspecified site

✓6ᵗʰ M60.11 Interstitial myositis, shoulder

M60.111 Interstitial myositis, right shoulder

M60.112 Interstitial myositis, left shoulder

M60.119 Interstitial myositis, unspecified shoulder

✓6ᵗʰ M60.12 Interstitial myositis, upper arm

M60.121 Interstitial myositis, right upper arm

M60.122 Interstitial myositis, left upper arm

M60.129 Interstitial myositis, unspecified upper arm

✓6ᵗʰ M60.13 Interstitial myositis, forearm

M60.131 Interstitial myositis, right forearm

M60.132 Interstitial myositis, left forearm

M60.139 Interstitial myositis, unspecified forearm

✓6ᵗʰ M60.14 Interstitial myositis, hand

M60.141 Interstitial myositis, right hand

M60.142 Interstitial myositis, left hand

M60.149 Interstitial myositis, unspecified hand

✓6ᵗʰ M60.15 Interstitial myositis, thigh

M60.151 Interstitial myositis, right thigh

M60.152 Interstitial myositis, left thigh

M60.159 Interstitial myositis, unspecified thigh

✓6ᵗʰ M60.16 Interstitial myositis, lower leg

M60.161 Interstitial myositis, right lower leg

M60.162 Interstitial myositis, left lower leg

M60.169 Interstitial myositis, unspecified lower leg

✓6ᵗʰ M60.17 Interstitial myositis, ankle and foot

M60.171 Interstitial myositis, right ankle and foot

M60.172 Interstitial myositis, left ankle and foot

M60.179 Interstitial myositis, unspecified ankle and foot

M60.18 Interstitial myositis, other site

M60.19 Interstitial myositis, multiple sites

✓5ᵗʰ M60.2 Foreign body granuloma of soft tissue, not elsewhere classified

Use additional code to identify the type of retained foreign body (Z18.-)

EXCLUDES 1   foreign body granuloma of skin and subcutaneous tissue (L92.3)

M60.20 Foreign body granuloma of soft tissue, not elsewhere classified, unspecified site

✓6ᵗʰ M60.21 Foreign body granuloma of soft tissue, not elsewhere classified, shoulder

M60.211 Foreign body granuloma of soft tissue, not elsewhere classified, right shoulder

M60.212 Foreign body granuloma of soft tissue, not elsewhere classified, left shoulder

M60.219 Foreign body granuloma of soft tissue, not elsewhere classified, unspecified shoulder

✓6ᵗʰ M60.22 Foreign body granuloma of soft tissue, not elsewhere classified, upper arm

M60.221 Foreign body granuloma of soft tissue, not elsewhere classified, right upper arm

M60.222 Foreign body granuloma of soft tissue, not elsewhere classified, left upper arm

M60.229 Foreign body granuloma of soft tissue, not elsewhere classified, unspecified upper arm

✓6ᵗʰ M60.23 Foreign body granuloma of soft tissue, not elsewhere classified, forearm

M60.231 Foreign body granuloma of soft tissue, not elsewhere classified, right forearm

M60.232 Foreign body granuloma of soft tissue, not elsewhere classified, left forearm

M60.239 Foreign body granuloma of soft tissue, not elsewhere classified, unspecified forearm

✓6ᵗʰ M60.24 Foreign body granuloma of soft tissue, not elsewhere classified, hand

M60.241 Foreign body granuloma of soft tissue, not elsewhere classified, right hand

M60.242 Foreign body granuloma of soft tissue, not elsewhere classified, left hand

M60.249 Foreign body granuloma of soft tissue, not elsewhere classified, unspecified hand

✓6ᵗʰ M60.25 Foreign body granuloma of soft tissue, not elsewhere classified, thigh

M60.251 Foreign body granuloma of soft tissue, not elsewhere classified, right thigh

M60.252 Foreign body granuloma of soft tissue, not elsewhere classified, left thigh

M60.259 Foreign body granuloma of soft tissue, not elsewhere classified, unspecified thigh

✓6ᵗʰ M60.26 Foreign body granuloma of soft tissue, not elsewhere classified, lower leg

M60.261 Foreign body granuloma of soft tissue, not elsewhere classified, right lower leg

M60.262 Foreign body granuloma of soft tissue, not elsewhere classified, left lower leg

M60.269 Foreign body granuloma of soft tissue, not elsewhere classified, unspecified lower leg

✓6ᵗʰ M60.27 Foreign body granuloma of soft tissue, not elsewhere classified, ankle and foot

M60.271 Foreign body granuloma of soft tissue, not elsewhere classified, right ankle and foot

M60.272 Foreign body granuloma of soft tissue, not elsewhere classified, left ankle and foot

M60.279 Foreign body granuloma of soft tissue, not elsewhere classified, unspecified ankle and foot

M60.28 Foreign body granuloma of soft tissue, not elsewhere classified, other site

✓5ᵗʰ M60.8 Other myositis

M60.80 Other myositis, unspecified site

✓6ᵗʰ M60.81 Other myositis shoulder

M60.811 Other myositis, right shoulder

M60.812 Other myositis, left shoulder

M60.819 Other myositis, unspecified shoulder

✓6ᵗʰ M60.82 Other myositis, upper arm

M60.821 Other myositis, right upper arm

M60.822 Other myositis, left upper arm

M60.829 Other myositis, unspecified upper arm

✓6ᵗʰ M60.83 Other myositis, forearm

M60.831 Other myositis, right forearm

M60.832 Other myositis, left forearm

M60.839 Other myositis, unspecified forearm

✓6ᵗʰ M60.84 Other myositis, hand

M60.841 Other myositis, right hand

M60.842 Other myositis, left hand

M60.849 Other myositis, unspecified hand

✓6ᵗʰ M60.85 Other myositis, thigh

M60.851 Other myositis, right thigh

✓ Additional Character Required   ✓x7ᵗʰ Placeholder   Unacceptable PDx   Questionable PDx   Manifestation   Unspecified Dx   H1-H14 HAC   HCC CMS-HCC Dx   HIV HIV Dx

ICD-10-CM 2020   811

M60.852   Other myositis, left thigh
M60.859   Other myositis, unspecified thigh

√6ᵗʰ   M60.86   Other myositis, lower leg
M60.861   Other myositis, right lower leg
M60.862   Other myositis, left lower leg
M60.869   Other myositis, unspecified lower leg

√6ᵗʰ   M60.87   Other myositis, ankle and foot
M60.871   Other myositis, right ankle and foot
M60.872   Other myositis, left ankle and foot
M60.879   Other myositis, unspecified ankle and foot

M60.88   Other myositis, other site
M60.89   Other myositis, multiple sites

M60.9   Myositis, unspecified

√4ᵗʰ   **M61**   **Calcification and ossification of muscle**

√5ᵗʰ   **M61.0**   Myositis ossificans traumatica

M61.00   Myositis ossificans traumatica, unspecified site

√6ᵗʰ   **M61.01**   Myositis ossificans traumatica, shoulder
M61.011   Myositis ossificans traumatica, right shoulder
M61.012   Myositis ossificans traumatica, left shoulder
M61.019   Myositis ossificans traumatica, unspecified shoulder

√6ᵗʰ   **M61.02**   Myositis ossificans traumatica, upper arm
M61.021   Myositis ossificans traumatica, right upper arm
M61.022   Myositis ossificans traumatica, left upper arm
M61.029   Myositis ossificans traumatica, unspecified upper arm

√6ᵗʰ   **M61.03**   Myositis ossificans traumatica, forearm
M61.031   Myositis ossificans traumatica, right forearm
M61.032   Myositis ossificans traumatica, left forearm
M61.039   Myositis ossificans traumatica, unspecified forearm

√6ᵗʰ   **M61.04**   Myositis ossificans traumatica, hand
M61.041   Myositis ossificans traumatica, right hand
M61.042   Myositis ossificans traumatica, left hand
M61.049   Myositis ossificans traumatica, unspecified hand

√6ᵗʰ   **M61.05**   Myositis ossificans traumatica, thigh
M61.051   Myositis ossificans traumatica, right thigh
M61.052   Myositis ossificans traumatica, left thigh
M61.059   Myositis ossificans traumatica, unspecified thigh

√6ᵗʰ   **M61.06**   Myositis ossificans traumatica, lower leg
M61.061   Myositis ossificans traumatica, right lower leg
M61.062   Myositis ossificans traumatica, left lower leg
M61.069   Myositis ossificans traumatica, unspecified lower leg

√6ᵗʰ   **M61.07**   Myositis ossificans traumatica, ankle and foot
M61.071   Myositis ossificans traumatica, right ankle and foot
M61.072   Myositis ossificans traumatica, left ankle and foot
M61.079   Myositis ossificans traumatica, unspecified ankle and foot

M61.08   Myositis ossificans traumatica, other site
M61.09   Myositis ossificans traumatica, multiple sites

√5ᵗʰ   **M61.1**   Myositis ossificans progressiva
Fibrodysplasia ossificans progressiva

M61.10   Myositis ossificans progressiva, unspecified site

√6ᵗʰ   **M61.11**   Myositis ossificans progressiva, shoulder
M61.111   Myositis ossificans progressiva, right shoulder
M61.112   Myositis ossificans progressiva, left shoulder
M61.119   Myositis ossificans progressiva, unspecified shoulder

√6ᵗʰ   **M61.12**   Myositis ossificans progressiva, upper arm
M61.121   Myositis ossificans progressiva, right upper arm

M61.122   Myositis ossificans progressiva, left upper arm
M61.129   Myositis ossificans progressiva, unspecified arm

√6ᵗʰ   **M61.13**   Myositis ossificans progressiva, forearm
M61.131   Myositis ossificans progressiva, right forearm
M61.132   Myositis ossificans progressiva, left forearm
M61.139   Myositis ossificans progressiva, unspecified forearm

√6ᵗʰ   **M61.14**   Myositis ossificans progressiva, hand and finger(s)
M61.141   Myositis ossificans progressiva, right hand
M61.142   Myositis ossificans progressiva, left hand
M61.143   Myositis ossificans progressiva, unspecified hand
M61.144   Myositis ossificans progressiva, right finger(s)
M61.145   Myositis ossificans progressiva, left finger(s)
M61.146   Myositis ossificans progressiva, unspecified finger(s)

√6ᵗʰ   **M61.15**   Myositis ossificans progressiva, thigh
M61.151   Myositis ossificans progressiva, right thigh
M61.152   Myositis ossificans progressiva, left thigh
M61.159   Myositis ossificans progressiva, unspecified thigh

√6ᵗʰ   **M61.16**   Myositis ossificans progressiva, lower leg
M61.161   Myositis ossificans progressiva, right lower leg
M61.162   Myositis ossificans progressiva, left lower leg
M61.169   Myositis ossificans progressiva, unspecified lower leg

√6ᵗʰ   **M61.17**   Myositis ossificans progressiva, ankle, foot and toe(s)
M61.171   Myositis ossificans progressiva, right ankle
M61.172   Myositis ossificans progressiva, left ankle
M61.173   Myositis ossificans progressiva, unspecified ankle
M61.174   Myositis ossificans progressiva, right foot
M61.175   Myositis ossificans progressiva, left foot
M61.176   Myositis ossificans progressiva, unspecified foot
M61.177   Myositis ossificans progressiva, right toe(s)
M61.178   Myositis ossificans progressiva, left toe(s)
M61.179   Myositis ossificans progressiva, unspecified toe(s)

M61.18   Myositis ossificans progressiva, other site
M61.19   Myositis ossificans progressiva, multiple sites

√5ᵗʰ   **M61.2**   Paralytic calcification and ossification of muscle
Myositis ossificans associated with quadriplegia or paraplegia

M61.20   Paralytic calcification and ossification of muscle, unspecified site

√6ᵗʰ   **M61.21**   Paralytic calcification and ossification of muscle, shoulder
M61.211   Paralytic calcification and ossification of muscle, right shoulder
M61.212   Paralytic calcification and ossification of muscle, left shoulder
M61.219   Paralytic calcification and ossification of muscle, unspecified shoulder

√6ᵗʰ   **M61.22**   Paralytic calcification and ossification of muscle, upper arm
M61.221   Paralytic calcification and ossification of muscle, right upper arm
M61.222   Paralytic calcification and ossification of muscle, left upper arm
M61.229   Paralytic calcification and ossification of muscle, unspecified upper arm

√6ᵗʰ   **M61.23**   Paralytic calcification and ossification of muscle, forearm
M61.231   Paralytic calcification and ossification of muscle, right forearm
M61.232   Paralytic calcification and ossification of muscle, left forearm

M61.239   Paralytic calcification and ossification of muscle, unspecified forearm

✓6ᵗʰ   **M61.24**   **Paralytic calcification and ossification of muscle, hand**

M61.241   Paralytic calcification and ossification of muscle, right hand

M61.242   Paralytic calcification and ossification of muscle, left hand

M61.249   Paralytic calcification and ossification of muscle, unspecified hand

✓6ᵗʰ   **M61.25**   **Paralytic calcification and ossification of muscle, thigh**

M61.251   Paralytic calcification and ossification of muscle, right thigh

M61.252   Paralytic calcification and ossification of muscle, left thigh

M61.259   Paralytic calcification and ossification of muscle, unspecified thigh

✓6ᵗʰ   **M61.26**   **Paralytic calcification and ossification of muscle, lower leg**

M61.261   Paralytic calcification and ossification of muscle, right lower leg

M61.262   Paralytic calcification and ossification of muscle, left lower leg

M61.269   Paralytic calcification and ossification of muscle, unspecified lower leg

✓6ᵗʰ   **M61.27**   **Paralytic calcification and ossification of muscle, ankle and foot**

M61.271   Paralytic calcification and ossification of muscle, right ankle and foot

M61.272   Paralytic calcification and ossification of muscle, left ankle and foot

M61.279   Paralytic calcification and ossification of muscle, unspecified ankle and foot

M61.28   Paralytic calcification and ossification of muscle, other site

M61.29   Paralytic calcification and ossification of muscle, multiple sites

✓5ᵗʰ   **M61.3**   **Calcification and ossification of muscles associated with burns**

Myositis ossificans associated with burns

M61.30   Calcification and ossification of muscles associated with burns, unspecified site

✓6ᵗʰ   **M61.31**   **Calcification and ossification of muscles associated with burns, shoulder**

M61.311   Calcification and ossification of muscles associated with burns, right shoulder

M61.312   Calcification and ossification of muscles associated with burns, left shoulder

M61.319   Calcification and ossification of muscles associated with burns, unspecified shoulder

✓6ᵗʰ   **M61.32**   **Calcification and ossification of muscles associated with burns, upper arm**

M61.321   Calcification and ossification of muscles associated with burns, right upper arm

M61.322   Calcification and ossification of muscles associated with burns, left upper arm

M61.329   Calcification and ossification of muscles associated with burns, unspecified upper arm

✓6ᵗʰ   **M61.33**   **Calcification and ossification of muscles associated with burns, forearm**

M61.331   Calcification and ossification of muscles associated with burns, right forearm

M61.332   Calcification and ossification of muscles associated with burns, left forearm

M61.339   Calcification and ossification of muscles associated with burns, unspecified forearm

✓6ᵗʰ   **M61.34**   **Calcification and ossification of muscles associated with burns, hand**

M61.341   Calcification and ossification of muscles associated with burns, right hand

M61.342   Calcification and ossification of muscles associated with burns, left hand

M61.349   Calcification and ossification of muscles associated with burns, unspecified hand

✓6ᵗʰ   **M61.35**   **Calcification and ossification of muscles associated with burns, thigh**

M61.351   Calcification and ossification of muscles associated with burns, right thigh

M61.352   Calcification and ossification of muscles associated with burns, left thigh

M61.359   Calcification and ossification of muscles associated with burns, unspecified thigh

✓6ᵗʰ   **M61.36**   **Calcification and ossification of muscles associated with burns, lower leg**

M61.361   Calcification and ossification of muscles associated with burns, right lower leg

M61.362   Calcification and ossification of muscles associated with burns, left lower leg

M61.369   Calcification and ossification of muscles associated with burns, unspecified lower leg

✓6ᵗʰ   **M61.37**   **Calcification and ossification of muscles associated with burns, ankle and foot**

M61.371   Calcification and ossification of muscles associated with burns, right ankle and foot

M61.372   Calcification and ossification of muscles associated with burns, left ankle and foot

M61.379   Calcification and ossification of muscles associated with burns, unspecified ankle and foot

M61.38   Calcification and ossification of muscles associated with burns, other site

M61.39   Calcification and ossification of muscles associated with burns, multiple sites

✓5ᵗʰ   **M61.4**   **Other calcification of muscle**

> EXCLUDES 1   calcific tendinitis NOS (M65.2-)
> calcific tendinitis of shoulder (M75.3)

M61.40   Other calcification of muscle, unspecified site

✓6ᵗʰ   **M61.41**   **Other calcification of muscle, shoulder**

M61.411   Other calcification of muscle, right shoulder

M61.412   Other calcification of muscle, left shoulder

M61.419   Other calcification of muscle, unspecified shoulder

✓6ᵗʰ   **M61.42**   **Other calcification of muscle, upper arm**

M61.421   Other calcification of muscle, right upper arm

M61.422   Other calcification of muscle, left upper arm

M61.429   Other calcification of muscle, unspecified upper arm

✓6ᵗʰ   **M61.43**   **Other calcification of muscle, forearm**

M61.431   Other calcification of muscle, right forearm

M61.432   Other calcification of muscle, left forearm

M61.439   Other calcification of muscle, unspecified forearm

✓6ᵗʰ   **M61.44**   **Other calcification of muscle, hand**

M61.441   Other calcification of muscle, right hand

M61.442   Other calcification of muscle, left hand

M61.449   Other calcification of muscle, unspecified hand

✓6ᵗʰ   **M61.45**   **Other calcification of muscle, thigh**

M61.451   Other calcification of muscle, right thigh

M61.452   Other calcification of muscle, left thigh

M61.459   Other calcification of muscle, unspecified thigh

✓6ᵗʰ   **M61.46**   **Other calcification of muscle, lower leg**

M61.461   Other calcification of muscle, right lower leg

M61.462   Other calcification of muscle, left lower leg

M61.469   Other calcification of muscle, unspecified lower leg

✓6ᵗʰ   **M61.47**   **Other calcification of muscle, ankle and foot**

M61.471   Other calcification of muscle, right ankle and foot

M61.472   Other calcification of muscle, left ankle and foot

M61.479   Other calcification of muscle, unspecified ankle and foot

M61.48   Other calcification of muscle, other site

M61.49   Other calcification of muscle, multiple sites

✓5ᵗʰ   **M61.5**   **Other ossification of muscle**

M61.50   Other ossification of muscle, unspecified site

☑ Additional Character Required   ✓x7ᵗʰ Placeholder   Unacceptable PDx   Questionable PDx   Manifestation   Unspecified Dx   H1-H14 HAC   HCC CMS-HCC Dx   HIV HIV Dx

ICD-10-CM 2020

813

√6ᵗʰ **M61.51** Other ossification of muscle, shoulder

     M61.511 Other ossification of muscle, right shoulder

     M61.512 Other ossification of muscle, left shoulder

     M61.519 Other ossification of muscle, unspecified shoulder

√6ᵗʰ **M61.52** Other ossification of muscle, upper arm

     M61.521 Other ossification of muscle, right upper arm

     M61.522 Other ossification of muscle, left upper arm

     M61.529 Other ossification of muscle, unspecified upper arm

√6ᵗʰ **M61.53** Other ossification of muscle, forearm

     M61.531 Other ossification of muscle, right forearm

     M61.532 Other ossification of muscle, left forearm

     M61.539 Other ossification of muscle, unspecified forearm

√6ᵗʰ **M61.54** Other ossification of muscle, hand

     M61.541 Other ossification of muscle, right hand

     M61.542 Other ossification of muscle, left hand

     M61.549 Other ossification of muscle, unspecified hand

√6ᵗʰ **M61.55** Other ossification of muscle, thigh

     M61.551 Other ossification of muscle, right thigh

     M61.552 Other ossification of muscle, left thigh

     M61.559 Other ossification of muscle, unspecified thigh

√6ᵗʰ **M61.56** Other ossification of muscle, lower leg

     M61.561 Other ossification of muscle, right lower leg

     M61.562 Other ossification of muscle, left lower leg

     M61.569 Other ossification of muscle, unspecified lower leg

√6ᵗʰ **M61.57** Other ossification of muscle, ankle and foot

     M61.571 Other ossification of muscle, right ankle and foot

     M61.572 Other ossification of muscle, left ankle and foot

     M61.579 Other ossification of muscle, unspecified ankle and foot

     M61.58 Other ossification of muscle, other site

     M61.59 Other ossification of muscle, multiple sites

M61.9 Calcification and ossification of muscle, unspecified

√4ᵗʰ **M62** Other disorders of muscle

     EXCLUDES 1   alcoholic myopathy (G72.1)

             cramp and spasm (R25.2)

             drug-induced myopathy (G72.0)

             myalgia (M79.1-)

             stiff-man syndrome (G25.82)

     EXCLUDES 2   nontraumatic hematoma of muscle (M79.81)

√5ᵗʰ **M62.0** Separation of muscle (nontraumatic)

     Diastasis of muscle

     EXCLUDES 1   diastasis recti complicating pregnancy, labor and delivery (O71.8)

             traumatic separation of muscle — see strain of muscle by body region

     M62.00 Separation of muscle (nontraumatic), unspecified site

√6ᵗʰ **M62.01** Separation of muscle (nontraumatic), shoulder

     M62.011 Separation of muscle (nontraumatic), right shoulder

     M62.012 Separation of muscle (nontraumatic), left shoulder

     M62.019 Separation of muscle (nontraumatic), unspecified shoulder

√6ᵗʰ **M62.02** Separation of muscle (nontraumatic), upper arm

     M62.021 Separation of muscle (nontraumatic), right upper arm

     M62.022 Separation of muscle (nontraumatic), left upper arm

     M62.029 Separation of muscle (nontraumatic), unspecified upper arm

√6ᵗʰ **M62.03** Separation of muscle (nontraumatic), forearm

     M62.031 Separation of muscle (nontraumatic), right forearm

     M62.032 Separation of muscle (nontraumatic), left forearm

     M62.039 Separation of muscle (nontraumatic), unspecified forearm

√6ᵗʰ **M62.04** Separation of muscle (nontraumatic), hand

     M62.041 Separation of muscle (nontraumatic), right hand

     M62.042 Separation of muscle (nontraumatic), left hand

     M62.049 Separation of muscle (nontraumatic), unspecified hand

√6ᵗʰ **M62.05** Separation of muscle (nontraumatic), thigh

     M62.051 Separation of muscle (nontraumatic), right thigh

     M62.052 Separation of muscle (nontraumatic), left thigh

     M62.059 Separation of muscle (nontraumatic), unspecified thigh

√6ᵗʰ **M62.06** Separation of muscle (nontraumatic), lower leg

     M62.061 Separation of muscle (nontraumatic), right lower leg

     M62.062 Separation of muscle (nontraumatic), left lower leg

     M62.069 Separation of muscle (nontraumatic), unspecified lower leg

√6ᵗʰ **M62.07** Separation of muscle (nontraumatic), ankle and foot

     M62.071 Separation of muscle (nontraumatic), right ankle and foot

     M62.072 Separation of muscle (nontraumatic), left ankle and foot

     M62.079 Separation of muscle (nontraumatic), unspecified ankle and foot

     M62.08 Separation of muscle (nontraumatic), other site

√5ᵗʰ **M62.1** Other rupture of muscle (nontraumatic)

     EXCLUDES 1   traumatic rupture of muscle — see strain of muscle by body region

     EXCLUDES 2   rupture of tendon (M66.-)

     M62.10 Other rupture of muscle (nontraumatic), unspecified site

√6ᵗʰ **M62.11** Other rupture of muscle (nontraumatic), shoulder

     M62.111 Other rupture of muscle (nontraumatic), right shoulder

     M62.112 Other rupture of muscle (nontraumatic), left shoulder

     M62.119 Other rupture of muscle (nontraumatic), unspecified shoulder

√6ᵗʰ **M62.12** Other rupture of muscle (nontraumatic), upper arm

     M62.121 Other rupture of muscle (nontraumatic), right upper arm

     M62.122 Other rupture of muscle (nontraumatic), left upper arm

     M62.129 Other rupture of muscle (nontraumatic), unspecified upper arm

√6ᵗʰ **M62.13** Other rupture of muscle (nontraumatic), forearm

     M62.131 Other rupture of muscle (nontraumatic), right forearm

     M62.132 Other rupture of muscle (nontraumatic), left forearm

     M62.139 Other rupture of muscle (nontraumatic), unspecified forearm

√6ᵗʰ **M62.14** Other rupture of muscle (nontraumatic), hand

     M62.141 Other rupture of muscle (nontraumatic), right hand

     M62.142 Other rupture of muscle (nontraumatic), left hand

     M62.149 Other rupture of muscle (nontraumatic), unspecified hand

√6ᵗʰ **M62.15** Other rupture of muscle (nontraumatic), thigh

     M62.151 Other rupture of muscle (nontraumatic), right thigh

     M62.152 Other rupture of muscle (nontraumatic), left thigh

     M62.159 Other rupture of muscle (nontraumatic), unspecified thigh

√6ᵗʰ **M62.16** Other rupture of muscle (nontraumatic), lower leg

     M62.161 Other rupture of muscle (nontraumatic), right lower leg

     M62.162 Other rupture of muscle (nontraumatic), left lower leg

Ⓝ Newborn: 0   Ⓟ Pediatric: 0-17   Ⓜ Maternity: 9-64   Ⓐ Adult: 15-124   ᴹᶜᶜ Major Complication/Comorbidity   ᶜᶜ Complication/Comorbidity   ˢʷ Severe Wound Dx

814   ICD-10-CM 2020

M62.169 Other rupture of muscle (nontraumatic), unspecified lower leg

√6ᵗʰ **M62.17** Other rupture of muscle (nontraumatic), **ankle and foot**

    M62.171 Other rupture of muscle (nontraumatic), **right ankle and foot**

    M62.172 Other rupture of muscle (nontraumatic), **left ankle and foot**

    M62.179 Other rupture of muscle (nontraumatic), unspecified ankle and foot

  M62.18 Other rupture of muscle (nontraumatic), other site

√5ᵗʰ **M62.2** Nontraumatic ischemic infarction of muscle

    EXCLUDES 1   compartment syndrome (traumatic) (T79.A-)
           nontraumatic compartment syndrome (M79.A-)
           rhabdomyolysis (M62.82)
           traumatic ischemia of muscle (T79.6)
           Volkmann's ischemic contracture (T79.6)

  M62.20 Nontraumatic ischemic infarction of muscle, unspecified site

√6ᵗʰ **M62.21** Nontraumatic ischemic infarction of muscle, shoulder

    M62.211 Nontraumatic ischemic infarction of muscle, right shoulder

    M62.212 Nontraumatic ischemic infarction of muscle, left shoulder

    M62.219 Nontraumatic ischemic infarction of muscle, unspecified shoulder

√6ᵗʰ **M62.22** Nontraumatic ischemic infarction of muscle, **upper arm**

    M62.221 Nontraumatic ischemic infarction of muscle, right upper arm

    M62.222 Nontraumatic ischemic infarction of muscle, left upper arm

    M62.229 Nontraumatic ischemic infarction of muscle, unspecified upper arm

√6ᵗʰ **M62.23** Nontraumatic ischemic infarction of muscle, **forearm**

    M62.231 Nontraumatic ischemic infarction of muscle, right forearm

    M62.232 Nontraumatic ischemic infarction of muscle, left forearm

    M62.239 Nontraumatic ischemic infarction of muscle, unspecified forearm

√6ᵗʰ **M62.24** Nontraumatic ischemic infarction of muscle, **hand**

    M62.241 Nontraumatic ischemic infarction of muscle, right hand

    M62.242 Nontraumatic ischemic infarction of muscle, left hand

    M62.249 Nontraumatic ischemic infarction of muscle, unspecified hand

√6ᵗʰ **M62.25** Nontraumatic ischemic infarction of muscle, **thigh**

    M62.251 Nontraumatic ischemic infarction of muscle, right thigh

    M62.252 Nontraumatic ischemic infarction of muscle, left thigh

    M62.259 Nontraumatic ischemic infarction of muscle, unspecified thigh

√6ᵗʰ **M62.26** Nontraumatic ischemic infarction of muscle, **lower leg**

    M62.261 Nontraumatic ischemic infarction of muscle, right lower leg

    M62.262 Nontraumatic ischemic infarction of muscle, left lower leg

    M62.269 Nontraumatic ischemic infarction of muscle, unspecified lower leg

√6ᵗʰ **M62.27** Nontraumatic ischemic infarction of muscle, **ankle and foot**

    M62.271 Nontraumatic ischemic infarction of muscle, right ankle and foot

    M62.272 Nontraumatic ischemic infarction of muscle, left ankle and foot

    M62.279 Nontraumatic ischemic infarction of muscle, unspecified ankle and foot

  M62.28 Nontraumatic ischemic infarction of muscle, other site

  M62.3 Immobility syndrome (paraplegic)   **CC**

√5ᵗʰ **M62.4** Contracture of muscle

    Contracture of tendon (sheath)
    EXCLUDES 1   contracture of joint (M24.5-)

  M62.40 Contracture of muscle, unspecified site

√6ᵗʰ **M62.41** Contracture of muscle, **shoulder**

    M62.411 Contracture of muscle, **right shoulder**

    M62.412 Contracture of muscle, **left shoulder**

    M62.419 Contracture of muscle, unspecified shoulder

√6ᵗʰ **M62.42** Contracture of muscle, **upper arm**

    M62.421 Contracture of muscle, **right upper arm**

    M62.422 Contracture of muscle, **left upper arm**

    M62.429 Contracture of muscle, unspecified upper arm

√6ᵗʰ **M62.43** Contracture of muscle, **forearm**

    M62.431 Contracture of muscle, **right forearm**

    M62.432 Contracture of muscle, **left forearm**

    M62.439 Contracture of muscle, unspecified forearm

√6ᵗʰ **M62.44** Contracture of muscle, **hand**

    M62.441 Contracture of muscle, **right hand**

    M62.442 Contracture of muscle, **left hand**

    M62.449 Contracture of muscle, unspecified hand

√6ᵗʰ **M62.45** Contracture of muscle, **thigh**

    M62.451 Contracture of muscle, **right thigh**

    M62.452 Contracture of muscle, **left thigh**

    M62.459 Contracture of muscle, unspecified thigh

√6ᵗʰ **M62.46** Contracture of muscle, **lower leg**

    M62.461 Contracture of muscle, **right lower leg**

    M62.462 Contracture of muscle, **left lower leg**

    M62.469 Contracture of muscle, unspecified lower leg

√6ᵗʰ **M62.47** Contracture of muscle, **ankle and foot**

    M62.471 Contracture of muscle, **right ankle and foot**

    M62.472 Contracture of muscle, **left ankle and foot**

    M62.479 Contracture of muscle, unspecified ankle and foot

  M62.48 Contracture of muscle, other site

  M62.49 Contracture of muscle, **multiple sites**

√5ᵗʰ **M62.5** Muscle wasting and atrophy, not elsewhere classified

    Disuse atrophy NEC
    EXCLUDES 1   neuralgic amyotrophy (G54.5)
           progressive muscular atrophy (G12.21)
           sarcopenia (M62.84)
    EXCLUDES 2   pelvic muscle wasting (N81.84)

  M62.50 Muscle wasting and atrophy, not elsewhere classified, unspecified site

√6ᵗʰ **M62.51** Muscle wasting and atrophy, not elsewhere classified, **shoulder**

    M62.511 Muscle wasting and atrophy, not elsewhere classified, **right shoulder**

    M62.512 Muscle wasting and atrophy, not elsewhere classified, **left shoulder**

    M62.519 Muscle wasting and atrophy, not elsewhere classified, unspecified shoulder

√6ᵗʰ **M62.52** Muscle wasting and atrophy, not elsewhere classified, **upper arm**

    M62.521 Muscle wasting and atrophy, not elsewhere classified, **right upper arm**

    M62.522 Muscle wasting and atrophy, not elsewhere classified, **left upper arm**

    M62.529 Muscle wasting and atrophy, not elsewhere classified, unspecified upper arm

√6ᵗʰ **M62.53** Muscle wasting and atrophy, not elsewhere classified, **forearm**

    M62.531 Muscle wasting and atrophy, not elsewhere classified, **right forearm**

    M62.532 Muscle wasting and atrophy, not elsewhere classified, **left forearm**

    M62.539 Muscle wasting and atrophy, not elsewhere classified, unspecified forearm

√6ᵗʰ **M62.54** Muscle wasting and atrophy, not elsewhere classified, **hand**

    M62.541 Muscle wasting and atrophy, not elsewhere classified, **right hand**

    M62.542 Muscle wasting and atrophy, not elsewhere classified, **left hand**

    M62.549 Muscle wasting and atrophy, not elsewhere classified, unspecified hand

☑ Additional Character Required   √x7ᵗʰ Placeholder   Unacceptable PDx   Questionable PDx   Manifestation   Unspecified Dx   **H1–H14** HAC   **HCC** CMS-HCC Dx   **HIV** HIV Dx

ICD-10-CM 2020   815

√6ᵗʰ **M62.55 Muscle wasting and atrophy, not elsewhere classified, thigh**

    M62.551 Muscle wasting and atrophy, not elsewhere classified, **right thigh**

    M62.552 Muscle wasting and atrophy, not elsewhere classified, **left thigh**

    M62.559 Muscle wasting and atrophy, not elsewhere classified, **unspecified thigh**

√6ᵗʰ **M62.56 Muscle wasting and atrophy, not elsewhere classified, lower leg**

    M62.561 Muscle wasting and atrophy, not elsewhere classified, **right lower leg**

    M62.562 Muscle wasting and atrophy, not elsewhere classified, **left lower leg**

    M62.569 Muscle wasting and atrophy, not elsewhere classified, **unspecified lower leg**

√6ᵗʰ **M62.57 Muscle wasting and atrophy, not elsewhere classified, ankle and foot**

    M62.571 Muscle wasting and atrophy, not elsewhere classified, **right ankle and foot**

    M62.572 Muscle wasting and atrophy, not elsewhere classified, **left ankle and foot**

    M62.579 Muscle wasting and atrophy, not elsewhere classified, **unspecified ankle and foot**

  M62.58 Muscle wasting and atrophy, not elsewhere classified, other site

  M62.59 Muscle wasting and atrophy, not elsewhere classified, multiple sites

√5ᵗʰ **M62.8 Other specified disorders of muscle**

    EXCLUDES 2   *nontraumatic hematoma of muscle (M79.81)*

  M62.81 Muscle weakness (generalized)

    EXCLUDES 1   *muscle weakness in sarcopenia (M62.84)*

  M62.82 Rhabdomyolysis   CC

    EXCLUDES 1   *traumatic rhabdomyolysis (T79.6)*

    AHA: 2019,2Q,12

    DEF: Rapid disintegration or destruction of skeletal muscle caused by direct or indirect injury, resulting in the excretion of muscle protein myoglobin into the urine.

    CC Excl: PDX collection 892

√6ᵗʰ **M62.83 Muscle spasm**

    M62.83Ø Muscle spasm of **back**

    M62.831 Muscle spasm of **calf**

        Charley-horse

    M62.838 Other muscle spasm

  M62.84 Sarcopenia

    Age-related sarcopenia

    Code first underlying disease, if applicable, such as:

      disorders of myoneural junction and muscle disease in diseases classified elsewhere (G73.-)

      other and unspecified myopathies (G72.-)

      primary disorders of muscles (G71.-)

    AHA: 2016,4Q,41

  M62.89 Other specified disorders of muscle

    Muscle (sheath) hernia

  M62.9 Disorder of muscle, unspecified

√4ᵗʰ **M63 Disorders of muscle in diseases classified elsewhere**

  Code first underlying disease, such as:

    leprosy (A3Ø.-)

    neoplasm (C49.-, C79.89, D21.-, D48.1)

    schistosomiasis (B65.-)

    trichinellosis (B75)

    EXCLUDES 1   *myopathy in cysticercosis (B69.81)*

        myopathy in endocrine diseases (G73.7)

        myopathy in metabolic diseases (G73.7)

        myopathy in sarcoidosis (D86.87)

        myopathy in secondary syphilis (A51.49)

        myopathy in syphilis (late) (A52.78)

        myopathy in toxoplasmosis (B58.82)

        myopathy in tuberculosis (A18.Ø9)

√5ᵗʰ **M63.8 Disorders of muscle in diseases classified elsewhere**

  M63.8Ø Disorders of muscle in diseases classified elsewhere, unspecified site

√6ᵗʰ **M63.81 Disorders of muscle in diseases classified elsewhere, shoulder**

    M63.811 Disorders of muscle in diseases classified elsewhere, right shoulder

    M63.812 Disorders of muscle in diseases classified elsewhere, left shoulder

    M63.819 Disorders of muscle in diseases classified elsewhere, unspecified shoulder

√6ᵗʰ **M63.82 Disorders of muscle in diseases classified elsewhere, upper arm**

    M63.821 Disorders of muscle in diseases classified elsewhere, right upper arm

    M63.822 Disorders of muscle in diseases classified elsewhere, left upper arm

    M63.829 Disorders of muscle in diseases classified elsewhere, unspecified upper arm

√6ᵗʰ **M63.83 Disorders of muscle in diseases classified elsewhere, forearm**

    M63.831 Disorders of muscle in diseases classified elsewhere, right forearm

    M63.832 Disorders of muscle in diseases classified elsewhere, left forearm

    M63.839 Disorders of muscle in diseases classified elsewhere, unspecified forearm

√6ᵗʰ **M63.84 Disorders of muscle in diseases classified elsewhere, hand**

    M63.841 Disorders of muscle in diseases classified elsewhere, right hand

    M63.842 Disorders of muscle in diseases classified elsewhere, left hand

    M63.849 Disorders of muscle in diseases classified elsewhere, unspecified hand

√6ᵗʰ **M63.85 Disorders of muscle in diseases classified elsewhere, thigh**

    M63.851 Disorders of muscle in diseases classified elsewhere, right thigh

    M63.852 Disorders of muscle in diseases classified elsewhere, left thigh

    M63.859 Disorders of muscle in diseases classified elsewhere, unspecified thigh

√6ᵗʰ **M63.86 Disorders of muscle in diseases classified elsewhere, lower leg**

    M63.861 Disorders of muscle in diseases classified elsewhere, right lower leg

    M63.862 Disorders of muscle in diseases classified elsewhere, left lower leg

    M63.869 Disorders of muscle in diseases classified elsewhere, unspecified lower leg

√6ᵗʰ **M63.87 Disorders of muscle in diseases classified elsewhere, ankle and foot**

    M63.871 Disorders of muscle in diseases classified elsewhere, right ankle and foot

    M63.872 Disorders of muscle in diseases classified elsewhere, left ankle and foot

    M63.879 Disorders of muscle in diseases classified elsewhere, unspecified ankle and foot

  M63.88 Disorders of muscle in diseases classified elsewhere, other site

  M63.89 Disorders of muscle in diseases classified elsewhere, multiple sites

Disorders of synovium and tendon (M65-M67)

√4ᵗʰ **M65 Synovitis and tenosynovitis**

  EXCLUDES 1   *chronic crepitant synovitis of hand and wrist (M7Ø.Ø-)*

    current injury — see injury of ligament or tendon by body region

    soft tissue disorders related to use, overuse and pressure (M7Ø.-)

√5ᵗʰ **M65.Ø Abscess of tendon sheath**

  Use additional code (B95-B96) to identify bacterial agent.

  M65.ØØ Abscess of tendon sheath, unspecified site

√6ᵗʰ **M65.Ø1 Abscess of tendon sheath, shoulder**

    M65.Ø11 Abscess of tendon sheath, **right shoulder**

    M65.Ø12 Abscess of tendon sheath, **left shoulder**

    M65.Ø19 Abscess of tendon sheath, **unspecified shoulder**

√6ᵗʰ **M65.Ø2 Abscess of tendon sheath, upper arm**

    M65.Ø21 Abscess of tendon sheath, **right upper arm**

    M65.Ø22 Abscess of tendon sheath, **left upper arm**

    M65.Ø29 Abscess of tendon sheath, **unspecified upper arm**

√6ᵗʰ **M65.Ø3 Abscess of tendon sheath, forearm**

    M65.Ø31 Abscess of tendon sheath, **right forearm**

N Newborn: 0   P Pediatric: 0-17   M Maternity: 9-64   A Adult: 15-124   MCC Major Complication/Comorbidity   CC Complication/Comorbidity   SW Severe Wound Dx

816   ICD-10-CM 2020

M65.032 Abscess of tendon sheath, left forearm
M65.039 Abscess of tendon sheath, unspecified forearm

√6ᵗʰ **M65.04** Abscess of tendon sheath, hand
M65.041 Abscess of tendon sheath, right hand
M65.042 Abscess of tendon sheath, left hand
M65.049 Abscess of tendon sheath, unspecified hand

√6ᵗʰ **M65.05** Abscess of tendon sheath, thigh
M65.051 Abscess of tendon sheath, right thigh
M65.052 Abscess of tendon sheath, left thigh
M65.059 Abscess of tendon sheath, unspecified thigh

√6ᵗʰ **M65.06** Abscess of tendon sheath, lower leg
M65.061 Abscess of tendon sheath, right lower leg
M65.062 Abscess of tendon sheath, left lower leg
M65.069 Abscess of tendon sheath, unspecified lower leg

√6ᵗʰ **M65.07** Abscess of tendon sheath, ankle and foot
M65.071 Abscess of tendon sheath, right ankle and foot
M65.072 Abscess of tendon sheath, left ankle and foot
M65.079 Abscess of tendon sheath, unspecified ankle and foot

M65.08 Abscess of tendon sheath, other site

√5ᵗʰ **M65.1** Other infective (teno)synovitis
M65.10 Other infective (teno)synovitis, unspecified site

√6ᵗʰ **M65.11** Other infective (teno)synovitis, shoulder
M65.111 Other infective (teno)synovitis, right shoulder
M65.112 Other infective (teno)synovitis, left shoulder
M65.119 Other infective (teno)synovitis, unspecified shoulder

√6ᵗʰ **M65.12** Other infective (teno)synovitis, elbow
M65.121 Other infective (teno)synovitis, right elbow
M65.122 Other infective (teno)synovitis, left elbow
M65.129 Other infective (teno)synovitis, unspecified elbow

√6ᵗʰ **M65.13** Other infective (teno)synovitis, wrist
M65.131 Other infective (teno)synovitis, right wrist
M65.132 Other infective (teno)synovitis, left wrist
M65.139 Other infective (teno)synovitis, unspecified wrist

√6ᵗʰ **M65.14** Other infective (teno)synovitis, hand
M65.141 Other infective (teno)synovitis, right hand
M65.142 Other infective (teno)synovitis, left hand
M65.149 Other infective (teno)synovitis, unspecified hand

√6ᵗʰ **M65.15** Other infective (teno)synovitis, hip
M65.151 Other infective (teno)synovitis, right hip
M65.152 Other infective (teno)synovitis, left hip
M65.159 Other infective (teno)synovitis, unspecified hip

√6ᵗʰ **M65.16** Other infective (teno)synovitis, knee
M65.161 Other infective (teno)synovitis, right knee
M65.162 Other infective (teno)synovitis, left knee
M65.169 Other infective (teno)synovitis, unspecified knee

√6ᵗʰ **M65.17** Other infective (teno)synovitis, ankle and foot
M65.171 Other infective (teno)synovitis, right ankle and foot
M65.172 Other infective (teno)synovitis, left ankle and foot
M65.179 Other infective (teno)synovitis, unspecified ankle and foot

M65.18 Other infective (teno)synovitis, other site
M65.19 Other infective (teno)synovitis, multiple sites

√5ᵗʰ **M65.2** Calcific tendinitis
EXCLUDES 1   tendinitis as classified in M75-M77
calcified tendinitis of shoulder (M75.3)

M65.20 Calcific tendinitis, unspecified site
√6ᵗʰ **M65.22** Calcific tendinitis, upper arm
M65.221 Calcific tendinitis, right upper arm
M65.222 Calcific tendinitis, left upper arm

M65.229 Calcific tendinitis, unspecified upper arm

√6ᵗʰ **M65.23** Calcific tendinitis, forearm
M65.231 Calcific tendinitis, right forearm
M65.232 Calcific tendinitis, left forearm
M65.239 Calcific tendinitis, unspecified forearm

√6ᵗʰ **M65.24** Calcific tendinitis, hand
M65.241 Calcific tendinitis, right hand
M65.242 Calcific tendinitis, left hand
M65.249 Calcific tendinitis, unspecified hand

√6ᵗʰ **M65.25** Calcific tendinitis, thigh
M65.251 Calcific tendinitis, right thigh
M65.252 Calcific tendinitis, left thigh
M65.259 Calcific tendinitis, unspecified thigh

√6ᵗʰ **M65.26** Calcific tendinitis, lower leg
M65.261 Calcific tendinitis, right lower leg
M65.262 Calcific tendinitis, left lower leg
M65.269 Calcific tendinitis, unspecified lower leg

√6ᵗʰ **M65.27** Calcific tendinitis, ankle and foot
M65.271 Calcific tendinitis, right ankle and foot
M65.272 Calcific tendinitis, left ankle and foot
M65.279 Calcific tendinitis, unspecified ankle and foot

M65.28 Calcific tendinitis, other site
M65.29 Calcific tendinitis, multiple sites

√5ᵗʰ **M65.3** Trigger finger
Nodular tendinous disease

M65.30 Trigger finger, unspecified finger
√6ᵗʰ **M65.31** Trigger thumb
M65.311 Trigger thumb, right thumb
M65.312 Trigger thumb, left thumb
M65.319 Trigger thumb, unspecified thumb

√6ᵗʰ **M65.32** Trigger finger, index finger
M65.321 Trigger finger, right index finger
M65.322 Trigger finger, left index finger
M65.329 Trigger finger, unspecified index finger

√6ᵗʰ **M65.33** Trigger finger, middle finger
M65.331 Trigger finger, right middle finger
M65.332 Trigger finger, left middle finger
M65.339 Trigger finger, unspecified middle finger

√6ᵗʰ **M65.34** Trigger finger, ring finger
M65.341 Trigger finger, right ring finger
M65.342 Trigger finger, left ring finger
M65.349 Trigger finger, unspecified ring finger

√6ᵗʰ **M65.35** Trigger finger, little finger
M65.351 Trigger finger, right little finger
M65.352 Trigger finger, left little finger
M65.359 Trigger finger, unspecified little finger

M65.4 Radial styloid tenosynovitis [de Quervain]

√5ᵗʰ **M65.8** Other synovitis and tenosynovitis
M65.80 Other synovitis and tenosynovitis, unspecified site
√6ᵗʰ **M65.81** Other synovitis and tenosynovitis, shoulder
M65.811 Other synovitis and tenosynovitis, right shoulder
M65.812 Other synovitis and tenosynovitis, left shoulder
M65.819 Other synovitis and tenosynovitis, unspecified shoulder

√6ᵗʰ **M65.82** Other synovitis and tenosynovitis, upper arm
M65.821 Other synovitis and tenosynovitis, right upper arm
M65.822 Other synovitis and tenosynovitis, left upper arm
M65.829 Other synovitis and tenosynovitis, unspecified upper arm

√6ᵗʰ **M65.83** Other synovitis and tenosynovitis, forearm
M65.831 Other synovitis and tenosynovitis, right forearm
M65.832 Other synovitis and tenosynovitis, left forearm
M65.839 Other synovitis and tenosynovitis, unspecified forearm

√6ᵗʰ **M65.84** Other synovitis and tenosynovitis, hand
M65.841 Other synovitis and tenosynovitis, right hand
M65.842 Other synovitis and tenosynovitis, left hand

M65.849 Other synovitis and tenosynovitis, unspecified hand

✓6ᵗʰ **M65.85** Other synovitis and tenosynovitis, **thigh**

　M65.851 Other synovitis and tenosynovitis, **right thigh**

　M65.852 Other synovitis and tenosynovitis, **left thigh**

　M65.859 Other synovitis and tenosynovitis, unspecified thigh

✓6ᵗʰ **M65.86** Other synovitis and tenosynovitis, **lower leg**

　M65.861 Other synovitis and tenosynovitis, **right lower leg**

　M65.862 Other synovitis and tenosynovitis, **left lower leg**

　M65.869 Other synovitis and tenosynovitis, unspecified lower leg

✓6ᵗʰ **M65.87** Other synovitis and tenosynovitis, **ankle and foot**

　M65.871 Other synovitis and tenosynovitis, **right ankle and foot**

　M65.872 Other synovitis and tenosynovitis, **left ankle and foot**

　M65.879 Other synovitis and tenosynovitis, unspecified ankle and foot

　M65.88 Other synovitis and tenosynovitis, other site

　M65.89 Other synovitis and tenosynovitis, multiple sites

M65.9 Synovitis and tenosynovitis, unspecified

✓4ᵗʰ **M66** **Spontaneous rupture of synovium and tendon**

　INCLUDES rupture that occurs when a normal force is applied to tissues that are inferred to have less than normal strength

　EXCLUDES 2 rotator cuff syndrome (M75.1-)

　rupture where an abnormal force is applied to normal tissue — see injury of tendon by body region

M66.0 Rupture of popliteal cyst

✓5ᵗʰ **M66.1** Rupture of synovium

　Rupture of synovial cyst

　EXCLUDES 2 rupture of popliteal cyst (M66.0)

　M66.10 Rupture of synovium, unspecified joint

✓6ᵗʰ **M66.11** Rupture of synovium, **shoulder**

　M66.111 Rupture of synovium, **right shoulder**
　M66.112 Rupture of synovium, **left shoulder**
　M66.119 Rupture of synovium, unspecified shoulder

✓6ᵗʰ **M66.12** Rupture of synovium, **elbow**

　M66.121 Rupture of synovium, **right elbow**
　M66.122 Rupture of synovium, **left elbow**
　M66.129 Rupture of synovium, unspecified elbow

✓6ᵗʰ **M66.13** Rupture of synovium, **wrist**

　M66.131 Rupture of synovium, **right wrist**
　M66.132 Rupture of synovium, **left wrist**
　M66.139 Rupture of synovium, unspecified wrist

✓6ᵗʰ **M66.14** Rupture of synovium, **hand and fingers**

　M66.141 Rupture of synovium, **right hand**
　M66.142 Rupture of synovium, **left hand**
　M66.143 Rupture of synovium, unspecified hand
　M66.144 Rupture of synovium, **right finger(s)**
　M66.145 Rupture of synovium, **left finger(s)**
　M66.146 Rupture of synovium, unspecified finger(s)

✓6ᵗʰ **M66.15** Rupture of synovium, **hip**

　M66.151 Rupture of synovium, **right hip**
　M66.152 Rupture of synovium, **left hip**
　M66.159 Rupture of synovium, unspecified hip

✓6ᵗʰ **M66.17** Rupture of synovium, **ankle, foot and toes**

　M66.171 Rupture of synovium, **right ankle**
　M66.172 Rupture of synovium, **left ankle**
　M66.173 Rupture of synovium, unspecified ankle
　M66.174 Rupture of synovium, **right foot**
　M66.175 Rupture of synovium, **left foot**
　M66.176 Rupture of synovium, unspecified foot
　M66.177 Rupture of synovium, **right toe(s)**
　M66.178 Rupture of synovium, **left toe(s)**
　M66.179 Rupture of synovium, unspecified toe(s)

　M66.18 Rupture of synovium, other site

✓5ᵗʰ **M66.2** **Spontaneous rupture of extensor tendons**

　TIP: Refer to the Muscle/Tendon table at the beginning of this chapter.

　M66.20 Spontaneous rupture of extensor tendons, unspecified site

✓6ᵗʰ **M66.21** Spontaneous rupture of extensor tendons, **shoulder**

　M66.211 Spontaneous rupture of extensor tendons, **right shoulder**
　M66.212 Spontaneous rupture of extensor tendons, **left shoulder**
　M66.219 Spontaneous rupture of extensor tendons, unspecified shoulder

✓6ᵗʰ **M66.22** Spontaneous rupture of extensor tendons, **upper arm**

　M66.221 Spontaneous rupture of extensor tendons, **right upper arm**
　M66.222 Spontaneous rupture of extensor tendons, **left upper arm**
　M66.229 Spontaneous rupture of extensor tendons, unspecified upper arm

✓6ᵗʰ **M66.23** Spontaneous rupture of extensor tendons, **forearm**

　M66.231 Spontaneous rupture of extensor tendons, **right forearm**
　M66.232 Spontaneous rupture of extensor tendons, **left forearm**
　M66.239 Spontaneous rupture of extensor tendons, unspecified forearm

✓6ᵗʰ **M66.24** Spontaneous rupture of extensor tendons, **hand**

　M66.241 Spontaneous rupture of extensor tendons, **right hand**
　M66.242 Spontaneous rupture of extensor tendons, **left hand**
　M66.249 Spontaneous rupture of extensor tendons, unspecified hand

✓6ᵗʰ **M66.25** Spontaneous rupture of extensor tendons, **thigh**

　M66.251 Spontaneous rupture of extensor tendons, **right thigh**
　M66.252 Spontaneous rupture of extensor tendons, **left thigh**
　M66.259 Spontaneous rupture of extensor tendons, unspecified thigh

✓6ᵗʰ **M66.26** Spontaneous rupture of extensor tendons, **lower leg**

　M66.261 Spontaneous rupture of extensor tendons, **right lower leg**
　M66.262 Spontaneous rupture of extensor tendons, **left lower leg**
　M66.269 Spontaneous rupture of extensor tendons, unspecified lower leg

✓6ᵗʰ **M66.27** Spontaneous rupture of extensor tendons, **ankle and foot**

　M66.271 Spontaneous rupture of extensor tendons, **right ankle and foot**
　M66.272 Spontaneous rupture of extensor tendons, **left ankle and foot**
　M66.279 Spontaneous rupture of extensor tendons, unspecified ankle and foot

　M66.28 Spontaneous rupture of extensor tendons, other site

　M66.29 Spontaneous rupture of extensor tendons, **multiple sites**

✓5ᵗʰ **M66.3** **Spontaneous rupture of flexor tendons**

　TIP: Refer to the Muscle/Tendon table at the beginning of this chapter.

　M66.30 Spontaneous rupture of flexor tendons, unspecified site

✓6ᵗʰ **M66.31** Spontaneous rupture of flexor tendons, **shoulder**

　M66.311 Spontaneous rupture of flexor tendons, **right shoulder**
　M66.312 Spontaneous rupture of flexor tendons, **left shoulder**
　M66.319 Spontaneous rupture of flexor tendons, unspecified shoulder

✓6ᵗʰ **M66.32** Spontaneous rupture of flexor tendons, **upper arm**

　M66.321 Spontaneous rupture of flexor tendons, **right upper arm**
　M66.322 Spontaneous rupture of flexor tendons, **left upper arm**
　M66.329 Spontaneous rupture of flexor tendons, unspecified upper arm

N Newborn: 0　**P** Pediatric: 0-17　**M** Maternity: 9-64　**A** Adult: 15-124　**MCC** Major Complication/Comorbidity　**CC** Complication/Comorbidity　**SW** Severe Wound Dx

818　ICD-10-CM 2020

✓6ᵗʰ **M66.33** Spontaneous rupture of flexor tendons, forearm

     M66.331 Spontaneous rupture of flexor tendons, right forearm

     M66.332 Spontaneous rupture of flexor tendons, left forearm

     M66.339 Spontaneous rupture of flexor tendons, unspecified forearm

✓6ᵗʰ **M66.34** Spontaneous rupture of flexor tendons, hand

     M66.341 Spontaneous rupture of flexor tendons, right hand

     M66.342 Spontaneous rupture of flexor tendons, left hand

     M66.349 Spontaneous rupture of flexor tendons, unspecified hand

✓6ᵗʰ **M66.35** Spontaneous rupture of flexor tendons, thigh

     M66.351 Spontaneous rupture of flexor tendons, right thigh

     M66.352 Spontaneous rupture of flexor tendons, left thigh

     M66.359 Spontaneous rupture of flexor tendons, unspecified thigh

✓6ᵗʰ **M66.36** Spontaneous rupture of flexor tendons, lower leg

     M66.361 Spontaneous rupture of flexor tendons, right lower leg

     M66.362 Spontaneous rupture of flexor tendons, left lower leg

     M66.369 Spontaneous rupture of flexor tendons, unspecified lower leg

✓6ᵗʰ **M66.37** Spontaneous rupture of flexor tendons, ankle and foot

     M66.371 Spontaneous rupture of flexor tendons, right ankle and foot

     M66.372 Spontaneous rupture of flexor tendons, left ankle and foot

     M66.379 Spontaneous rupture of flexor tendons, unspecified ankle and foot

     M66.38 Spontaneous rupture of flexor tendons, other site

     M66.39 Spontaneous rupture of flexor tendons, multiple sites

✓5ᵗʰ **M66.8** Spontaneous rupture of other tendons

     TIP: Refer to the Muscle/Tendon table at the beginning of this chapter.

     M66.80 Spontaneous rupture of other tendons, unspecified site

✓6ᵗʰ **M66.81** Spontaneous rupture of other tendons, shoulder

     M66.811 Spontaneous rupture of other tendons, right shoulder

     M66.812 Spontaneous rupture of other tendons, left shoulder

     M66.819 Spontaneous rupture of other tendons, unspecified shoulder

✓6ᵗʰ **M66.82** Spontaneous rupture of other tendons, upper arm

     M66.821 Spontaneous rupture of other tendons, right upper arm

     M66.822 Spontaneous rupture of other tendons, left upper arm

     M66.829 Spontaneous rupture of other tendons, unspecified upper arm

✓6ᵗʰ **M66.83** Spontaneous rupture of other tendons, forearm

     M66.831 Spontaneous rupture of other tendons, right forearm

     M66.832 Spontaneous rupture of other tendons, left forearm

     M66.839 Spontaneous rupture of other tendons, unspecified forearm

✓6ᵗʰ **M66.84** Spontaneous rupture of other tendons, hand

     M66.841 Spontaneous rupture of other tendons, right hand

     M66.842 Spontaneous rupture of other tendons, left hand

     M66.849 Spontaneous rupture of other tendons, unspecified hand

✓6ᵗʰ **M66.85** Spontaneous rupture of other tendons, thigh

     M66.851 Spontaneous rupture of other tendons, right thigh

     M66.852 Spontaneous rupture of other tendons, left thigh

     M66.859 Spontaneous rupture of other tendons, unspecified thigh

✓6ᵗʰ **M66.86** Spontaneous rupture of other tendons, lower leg

     M66.861 Spontaneous rupture of other tendons, right lower leg

     M66.862 Spontaneous rupture of other tendons, left lower leg

     M66.869 Spontaneous rupture of other tendons, unspecified lower leg

✓6ᵗʰ **M66.87** Spontaneous rupture of other tendons, ankle and foot

     M66.871 Spontaneous rupture of other tendons, right ankle and foot

     M66.872 Spontaneous rupture of other tendons, left ankle and foot

     M66.879 Spontaneous rupture of other tendons, unspecified ankle and foot

     M66.88 Spontaneous rupture of other tendons, other sites

     M66.89 Spontaneous rupture of other tendons, multiple sites

     M66.9 Spontaneous rupture of unspecified tendon

         Rupture at musculotendinous junction, nontraumatic

✓4ᵗʰ **M67** Other disorders of synovium and tendon

     EXCLUDES 1   palmar fascial fibromatosis [Dupuytren] (M72.0)

         tendinitis NOS (M77.9-)

         xanthomatosis localized to tendons (E78.2)

✓5ᵗʰ **M67.0** Short Achilles tendon (acquired)

     M67.00 Short Achilles tendon (acquired), unspecified ankle

     M67.01 Short Achilles tendon (acquired), right ankle

     M67.02 Short Achilles tendon (acquired), left ankle

✓5ᵗʰ **M67.2** Synovial hypertrophy, not elsewhere classified

     EXCLUDES 1   villonodular synovitis (pigmented) (M12.2-)

     M67.20 Synovial hypertrophy, not elsewhere classified, unspecified site

✓6ᵗʰ **M67.21** Synovial hypertrophy, not elsewhere classified, shoulder

     M67.211 Synovial hypertrophy, not elsewhere classified, right shoulder

     M67.212 Synovial hypertrophy, not elsewhere classified, left shoulder

     M67.219 Synovial hypertrophy, not elsewhere classified, unspecified shoulder

✓6ᵗʰ **M67.22** Synovial hypertrophy, not elsewhere classified, upper arm

     M67.221 Synovial hypertrophy, not elsewhere classified, right upper arm

     M67.222 Synovial hypertrophy, not elsewhere classified, left upper arm

     M67.229 Synovial hypertrophy, not elsewhere classified, unspecified upper arm

✓6ᵗʰ **M67.23** Synovial hypertrophy, not elsewhere classified, forearm

     M67.231 Synovial hypertrophy, not elsewhere classified, right forearm

     M67.232 Synovial hypertrophy, not elsewhere classified, left forearm

     M67.239 Synovial hypertrophy, not elsewhere classified, unspecified forearm

✓6ᵗʰ **M67.24** Synovial hypertrophy, not elsewhere classified, hand

     M67.241 Synovial hypertrophy, not elsewhere classified, right hand

     M67.242 Synovial hypertrophy, not elsewhere classified, left hand

     M67.249 Synovial hypertrophy, not elsewhere classified, unspecified hand

✓6ᵗʰ **M67.25** Synovial hypertrophy, not elsewhere classified, thigh

     M67.251 Synovial hypertrophy, not elsewhere classified, right thigh

     M67.252 Synovial hypertrophy, not elsewhere classified, left thigh

     M67.259 Synovial hypertrophy, not elsewhere classified, unspecified thigh

✓6ᵗʰ **M67.26** Synovial hypertrophy, not elsewhere classified, lower leg

     M67.261 Synovial hypertrophy, not elsewhere classified, right lower leg

     M67.262 Synovial hypertrophy, not elsewhere classified, left lower leg

     M67.269 Synovial hypertrophy, not elsewhere classified, unspecified lower leg

✓ Additional Character Required   ✓x7ᵗʰ Placeholder   Unacceptable PDx   Questionable PDx   Manifestation   Unspecified Dx   H1-H14 HAC   HCC CMS-HCC Dx   HIV HIV Dx

ICD-10-CM 2020   819

✓6th **M67.27** **Synovial hypertrophy, not elsewhere classified, ankle and foot**
  M67.271 Synovial hypertrophy, not elsewhere classified, right ankle and foot
  M67.272 Synovial hypertrophy, not elsewhere classified, left ankle and foot
  M67.279 Synovial hypertrophy, not elsewhere classified, unspecified ankle and foot
M67.28 **Synovial hypertrophy, not elsewhere classified, other site**
M67.29 **Synovial hypertrophy, not elsewhere classified, multiple sites**

✓5th **M67.3** **Transient synovitis**
  Toxic synovitis
  EXCLUDES 1   palindromic rheumatism (M12.3-)
  M67.30 **Transient synovitis, unspecified site**
  ✓6th **M67.31** **Transient synovitis, shoulder**
    M67.311 Transient synovitis, right shoulder
    M67.312 Transient synovitis, left shoulder
    M67.319 Transient synovitis, unspecified shoulder
  ✓6th **M67.32** **Transient synovitis, elbow**
    M67.321 Transient synovitis, right elbow
    M67.322 Transient synovitis, left elbow
    M67.329 Transient synovitis, unspecified elbow
  ✓6th **M67.33** **Transient synovitis, wrist**
    M67.331 Transient synovitis, right wrist
    M67.332 Transient synovitis, left wrist
    M67.339 Transient synovitis, unspecified wrist
  ✓6th **M67.34** **Transient synovitis, hand**
    M67.341 Transient synovitis, right hand
    M67.342 Transient synovitis, left hand
    M67.349 Transient synovitis, unspecified hand
  ✓6th **M67.35** **Transient synovitis, hip**
    M67.351 Transient synovitis, right hip
    M67.352 Transient synovitis, left hip
    M67.359 Transient synovitis, unspecified hip
  ✓6th **M67.36** **Transient synovitis, knee**
    M67.361 Transient synovitis, right knee
    M67.362 Transient synovitis, left knee
    M67.369 Transient synovitis, unspecified knee
  ✓6th **M67.37** **Transient synovitis, ankle and foot**
    M67.371 Transient synovitis, right ankle and foot
    M67.372 Transient synovitis, left ankle and foot
    M67.379 Transient synovitis, unspecified ankle and foot
  M67.38 **Transient synovitis, other site**
  M67.39 **Transient synovitis, multiple sites**

✓5th **M67.4** **Ganglion**
  Ganglion of joint or tendon (sheath)
  EXCLUDES 1   ganglion in yaws (A66.6)
  EXCLUDES 2   cyst of bursa (M71.2-M71.3)
              cyst of synovium (M71.2-M71.3)
  DEF: Fluid-filled, benign cyst appearing on a tendon sheath or aponeurosis, frequently connecting to an underlying joint.
  M67.40 **Ganglion, unspecified site**
  ✓6th **M67.41** **Ganglion, shoulder**
    M67.411 Ganglion, right shoulder
    M67.412 Ganglion, left shoulder
    M67.419 Ganglion, unspecified shoulder
  ✓6th **M67.42** **Ganglion, elbow**
    M67.421 Ganglion, right elbow
    M67.422 Ganglion, left elbow
    M67.429 Ganglion, unspecified elbow

✓6th **M67.43** **Ganglion, wrist**

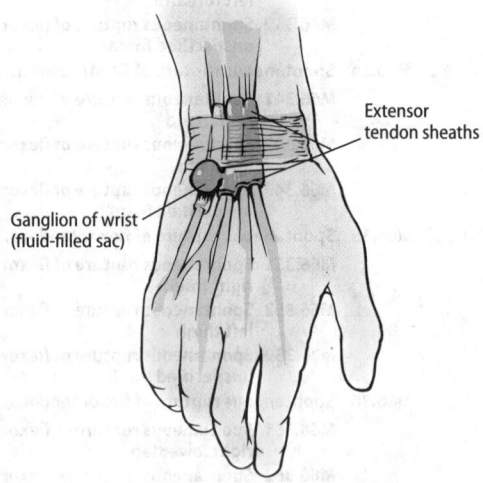

Ganglion of Wrist

Extensor tendon sheaths

Ganglion of wrist (fluid-filled sac)

    M67.431 Ganglion, right wrist
    M67.432 Ganglion, left wrist
    M67.439 Ganglion, unspecified wrist
  ✓6th **M67.44** **Ganglion, hand**
    M67.441 Ganglion, right hand
    M67.442 Ganglion, left hand
    M67.449 Ganglion, unspecified hand
  ✓6th **M67.45** **Ganglion, hip**
    M67.451 Ganglion, right hip
    M67.452 Ganglion, left hip
    M67.459 Ganglion, unspecified hip
  ✓6th **M67.46** **Ganglion, knee**
    M67.461 Ganglion, right knee
    M67.462 Ganglion, left knee
    M67.469 Ganglion, unspecified knee
  ✓6th **M67.47** **Ganglion, ankle and foot**
    M67.471 Ganglion, right ankle and foot
    M67.472 Ganglion, left ankle and foot
    M67.479 Ganglion, unspecified ankle and foot
  M67.48 **Ganglion, other site**
  M67.49 **Ganglion, multiple sites**

✓5th **M67.5** **Plica syndrome**
  Plica knee
  M67.50 **Plica syndrome, unspecified knee**
  M67.51 **Plica syndrome, right knee**
  M67.52 **Plica syndrome, left knee**

✓5th **M67.8** **Other specified disorders of synovium and tendon**
  M67.80 **Other specified disorders of synovium and tendon, unspecified site**
  ✓6th **M67.81** **Other specified disorders of synovium and tendon, shoulder**
    M67.811 Other specified disorders of synovium, right shoulder
    M67.812 Other specified disorders of synovium, left shoulder
    M67.813 Other specified disorders of tendon, right shoulder
    M67.814 Other specified disorders of tendon, left shoulder
    M67.819 Other specified disorders of synovium and tendon, unspecified shoulder
  ✓6th **M67.82** **Other specified disorders of synovium and tendon, elbow**
    M67.821 Other specified disorders of synovium, right elbow
    M67.822 Other specified disorders of synovium, left elbow
    M67.823 Other specified disorders of tendon, right elbow
    M67.824 Other specified disorders of tendon, left elbow

M67.829   Other specified disorders of synovium and tendon, unspecified elbow

√6ᵗʰ M67.83   **Other specified disorders of synovium and tendon, wrist**

M67.831   Other specified disorders of synovium, right wrist

M67.832   Other specified disorders of synovium, left wrist

M67.833   Other specified disorders of tendon, right wrist

M67.834   Other specified disorders of tendon, left wrist

▲   M67.839   Other specified disorders of synovium and tendon, unspecified wrist

√6ᵗʰ M67.84   **Other specified disorders of synovium and tendon, hand**

M67.841   Other specified disorders of synovium, right hand

M67.842   Other specified disorders of synovium, left hand

M67.843   Other specified disorders of tendon, right hand

M67.844   Other specified disorders of tendon, left hand

M67.849   Other specified disorders of synovium and tendon, unspecified hand

√6ᵗʰ M67.85   **Other specified disorders of synovium and tendon, hip**

M67.851   Other specified disorders of synovium, right hip

M67.852   Other specified disorders of synovium, left hip

M67.853   Other specified disorders of tendon, right hip

M67.854   Other specified disorders of tendon, left hip

M67.859   Other specified disorders of synovium and tendon, unspecified hip

√6ᵗʰ M67.86   **Other specified disorders of synovium and tendon, knee**

M67.861   Other specified disorders of synovium, right knee

M67.862   Other specified disorders of synovium, left knee

M67.863   Other specified disorders of tendon, right knee

M67.864   Other specified disorders of tendon, left knee

M67.869   Other specified disorders of synovium and tendon, unspecified knee

√6ᵗʰ M67.87   **Other specified disorders of synovium and tendon, ankle and foot**

M67.871   Other specified disorders of synovium, right ankle and foot

M67.872   Other specified disorders of synovium, left ankle and foot

M67.873   Other specified disorders of tendon, right ankle and foot

M67.874   Other specified disorders of tendon, left ankle and foot

M67.879   Other specified disorders of synovium and tendon, unspecified ankle and foot

M67.88   Other specified disorders of synovium and tendon, other site

M67.89   Other specified disorders of synovium and tendon, multiple sites

√5ᵗʰ M67.9   **Unspecified disorder of synovium and tendon**

M67.90   Unspecified disorder of synovium and tendon, unspecified site

√6ᵗʰ M67.91   Unspecified disorder of synovium and tendon, shoulder

M67.911   Unspecified disorder of synovium and tendon, right shoulder

M67.912   Unspecified disorder of synovium and tendon, left shoulder

M67.919   Unspecified disorder of synovium and tendon, unspecified shoulder

√6ᵗʰ M67.92   Unspecified disorder of synovium and tendon, upper arm

M67.921   Unspecified disorder of synovium and tendon, right upper arm

M67.922   Unspecified disorder of synovium and tendon, left upper arm

M67.929   Unspecified disorder of synovium and tendon, unspecified upper arm

√6ᵗʰ M67.93   Unspecified disorder of synovium and tendon, forearm

M67.931   Unspecified disorder of synovium and tendon, right forearm

M67.932   Unspecified disorder of synovium and tendon, left forearm

M67.939   Unspecified disorder of synovium and tendon, unspecified forearm

√6ᵗʰ M67.94   Unspecified disorder of synovium and tendon, hand

M67.941   Unspecified disorder of synovium and tendon, right hand

M67.942   Unspecified disorder of synovium and tendon, left hand

M67.949   Unspecified disorder of synovium and tendon, unspecified hand

√6ᵗʰ M67.95   Unspecified disorder of synovium and tendon, thigh

M67.951   Unspecified disorder of synovium and tendon, right thigh

M67.952   Unspecified disorder of synovium and tendon, left thigh

M67.959   Unspecified disorder of synovium and tendon, unspecified thigh

√6ᵗʰ M67.96   Unspecified disorder of synovium and tendon, lower leg

M67.961   Unspecified disorder of synovium and tendon, right lower leg

M67.962   Unspecified disorder of synovium and tendon, left lower leg

M67.969   Unspecified disorder of synovium and tendon, unspecified lower leg

√6ᵗʰ M67.97   Unspecified disorder of synovium and tendon, ankle and foot

M67.971   Unspecified disorder of synovium and tendon, right ankle and foot

M67.972   Unspecified disorder of synovium and tendon, left ankle and foot

M67.979   Unspecified disorder of synovium and tendon, unspecified ankle and foot

M67.98   Unspecified disorder of synovium and tendon, other site

M67.99   Unspecified disorder of synovium and tendon, multiple sites

Other soft tissue disorders (M70-M79)

√4ᵗʰ **M70**   **Soft tissue disorders related to use, overuse and pressure**

INCLUDES   soft tissue disorders of occupational origin

Use additional external cause code to identify activity causing disorder (Y93.-)

EXCLUDES 1   bursitis NOS (M71.9-)

EXCLUDES 2   bursitis of shoulder (M75.5)

            enthesopathies (M76-M77)

            pressure ulcer (pressure area) (L89.-)

√5ᵗʰ M70.0   **Crepitant synovitis (acute) (chronic) of hand and wrist**

√6ᵗʰ M70.03   Crepitant synovitis (acute) (chronic), wrist

M70.031   Crepitant synovitis (acute) (chronic), right wrist

M70.032   Crepitant synovitis (acute) (chronic), left wrist

M70.039   Crepitant synovitis (acute) (chronic), unspecified wrist

√6ᵗʰ M70.04   Crepitant synovitis (acute) (chronic), hand

M70.041   Crepitant synovitis (acute) (chronic), right hand

M70.042   Crepitant synovitis (acute) (chronic), left hand

M70.049   Crepitant synovitis (acute) (chronic), unspecified hand

√5ᵗʰ M70.1   **Bursitis of hand**

M70.10   Bursitis, unspecified hand

M70.11   Bursitis, right hand

M70.12   Bursitis, left hand

√5ᵗʰ M70.2   **Olecranon bursitis**

M70.20   Olecranon bursitis, unspecified elbow

M70.21   Olecranon bursitis, right elbow

M70.22   Olecranon bursitis, left elbow

✔ Additional Character Required   √x7ᵗʰ Placeholder   Unacceptable PDx   Questionable PDx   Manifestation   Unspecified Dx   H1-H14 HAC   HCC CMS-HCC Dx   HIV HIV Dx

ICD-10-CM 2020   821

Chapter 13. Diseases of the Musculoskeletal System and Connective Tissue

M70.3–M70.949

✓5ᵗʰ **M70.3 Other bursitis of elbow**

    M70.30 Other bursitis of elbow, unspecified elbow

    M70.31 Other bursitis of elbow, right elbow

    M70.32 Other bursitis of elbow, left elbow

✓5ᵗʰ **M70.4 Prepatellar bursitis**

    M70.40 Prepatellar bursitis, unspecified knee

    M70.41 Prepatellar bursitis, right knee

    M70.42 Prepatellar bursitis, left knee

Knee Bursae

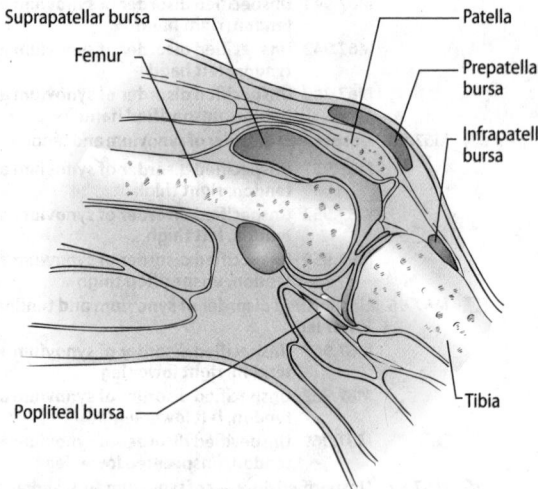

Suprapatellar bursa — Femur — Patella — Prepatellar bursa — Infrapatellar bursa — Popliteal bursa — Tibia

✓5ᵗʰ **M70.5 Other bursitis of knee**

    M70.50 Other bursitis of knee, unspecified knee

    M70.51 Other bursitis of knee, right knee

    M70.52 Other bursitis of knee, left knee

✓5ᵗʰ **M70.6 Trochanteric bursitis**

    Trochanteric tendinitis

    M70.60 Trochanteric bursitis, unspecified hip

    M70.61 Trochanteric bursitis, right hip

    M70.62 Trochanteric bursitis, left hip

✓5ᵗʰ **M70.7 Other bursitis of hip**

    Ischial bursitis

    M70.70 Other bursitis of hip, unspecified hip

    M70.71 Other bursitis of hip, right hip

    M70.72 Other bursitis of hip, left hip

✓5ᵗʰ **M70.8 Other soft tissue disorders related to use, overuse and pressure**

    M70.80 Other soft tissue disorders related to use, overuse and pressure of unspecified site

    ✓6ᵗʰ **M70.81** Other soft tissue disorders related to use, overuse and pressure of shoulder

        M70.811 Other soft tissue disorders related to use, overuse and pressure, right shoulder

        M70.812 Other soft tissue disorders related to use, overuse and pressure, left shoulder

        M70.819 Other soft tissue disorders related to use, overuse and pressure, unspecified shoulder

    ✓6ᵗʰ **M70.82** Other soft tissue disorders related to use, overuse and pressure of upper arm

        M70.821 Other soft tissue disorders related to use, overuse and pressure, right upper arm

        M70.822 Other soft tissue disorders related to use, overuse and pressure, left upper arm

        M70.829 Other soft tissue disorders related to use, overuse and pressure, unspecified upper arms

    ✓6ᵗʰ **M70.83** Other soft tissue disorders related to use, overuse and pressure of forearm

        M70.831 Other soft tissue disorders related to use, overuse and pressure, right forearm

        M70.832 Other soft tissue disorders related to use, overuse and pressure, left forearm

        M70.839 Other soft tissue disorders related to use, overuse and pressure, unspecified forearm

✓6ᵗʰ **M70.84** Other soft tissue disorders related to use, overuse and pressure of hand

    M70.841 Other soft tissue disorders related to use, overuse and pressure, right hand

    M70.842 Other soft tissue disorders related to use, overuse and pressure, left hand

    M70.849 Other soft tissue disorders related to use, overuse and pressure, unspecified hand

✓6ᵗʰ **M70.85** Other soft tissue disorders related to use, overuse and pressure of thigh

    M70.851 Other soft tissue disorders related to use, overuse and pressure, right thigh

    M70.852 Other soft tissue disorders related to use, overuse and pressure, left thigh

    M70.859 Other soft tissue disorders related to use, overuse and pressure, unspecified thigh

✓6ᵗʰ **M70.86** Other soft tissue disorders related to use, overuse and pressure lower leg

    M70.861 Other soft tissue disorders related to use, overuse and pressure, right lower leg

    M70.862 Other soft tissue disorders related to use, overuse and pressure, left lower leg

    M70.869 Other soft tissue disorders related to use, overuse and pressure, unspecified leg

✓6ᵗʰ **M70.87** Other soft tissue disorders related to use, overuse and pressure of ankle and foot

    M70.871 Other soft tissue disorders related to use, overuse and pressure, right ankle and foot

    M70.872 Other soft tissue disorders related to use, overuse and pressure, left ankle and foot

    M70.879 Other soft tissue disorders related to use, overuse and pressure, unspecified ankle and foot

M70.88 Other soft tissue disorders related to use, overuse and pressure other site

M70.89 Other soft tissue disorders related to use, overuse and pressure multiple sites

✓5ᵗʰ **M70.9 Unspecified soft tissue disorder related to use, overuse and pressure**

    M70.90 Unspecified soft tissue disorder related to use, overuse and pressure of unspecified site

    ✓6ᵗʰ **M70.91** Unspecified soft tissue disorder related to use, overuse and pressure of shoulder

        M70.911 Unspecified soft tissue disorder related to use, overuse and pressure, right shoulder

        M70.912 Unspecified soft tissue disorder related to use, overuse and pressure, left shoulder

        M70.919 Unspecified soft tissue disorder related to use, overuse and pressure, unspecified shoulder

    ✓6ᵗʰ **M70.92** Unspecified soft tissue disorder related to use, overuse and pressure of upper arm

        M70.921 Unspecified soft tissue disorder related to use, overuse and pressure, right upper arm

        M70.922 Unspecified soft tissue disorder related to use, overuse and pressure, left upper arm

        M70.929 Unspecified soft tissue disorder related to use, overuse and pressure, unspecified upper arm

    ✓6ᵗʰ **M70.93** Unspecified soft tissue disorder related to use, overuse and pressure of forearm

        M70.931 Unspecified soft tissue disorder related to use, overuse and pressure, right forearm

        M70.932 Unspecified soft tissue disorder related to use, overuse and pressure, left forearm

        M70.939 Unspecified soft tissue disorder related to use, overuse and pressure, unspecified forearm

    ✓6ᵗʰ **M70.94** Unspecified soft tissue disorder related to use, overuse and pressure of hand

        M70.941 Unspecified soft tissue disorder related to use, overuse and pressure, right hand

        M70.942 Unspecified soft tissue disorder related to use, overuse and pressure, left hand

        M70.949 Unspecified soft tissue disorder related to use, overuse and pressure, unspecified hand

N Newborn: 0   P Pediatric: 0-17   M Maternity: 9-64   A Adult: 15-124   MCC Major Complication/Comorbidity   CC Complication/Comorbidity   SW Severe Wound Dx

822   ICD-10-CM 2020

√6ᵗʰ **M70.95 Unspecified soft tissue disorder related to use, overuse and pressure of** thigh

M70.951 Unspecified soft tissue disorder related to use, overuse and pressure, right **thigh**

M70.952 Unspecified soft tissue disorder related to use, overuse and pressure, left **thigh**

M70.959 Unspecified soft tissue disorder related to use, overuse and pressure, unspecified thigh

√6ᵗʰ **M70.96 Unspecified soft tissue disorder related to use, overuse and pressure** lower leg

M70.961 Unspecified soft tissue disorder related to use, overuse and pressure, right **lower leg**

M70.962 Unspecified soft tissue disorder related to use, overuse and pressure, left **lower leg**

M70.969 Unspecified soft tissue disorder related to use, overuse and pressure, unspecified lower leg

√6ᵗʰ **M70.97 Unspecified soft tissue disorder related to use, overuse and pressure of** ankle and foot

M70.971 Unspecified soft tissue disorder related to use, overuse and pressure, right **ankle and foot**

M70.972 Unspecified soft tissue disorder related to use, overuse and pressure, left **ankle and foot**

M70.979 Unspecified soft tissue disorder related to use, overuse and pressure, unspecified ankle and foot

M70.98 Unspecified soft tissue disorder related to use, overuse and pressure other

M70.99 Unspecified soft tissue disorder related to use, overuse and pressure multiple sites

√4ᵗʰ **M71 Other bursopathies**

EXCLUDES 1   *bunion (M20.1)*
bursitis related to use, overuse or pressure (M70.-)
enthesopathies (M76-M77)

√5ᵗʰ **M71.0 Abscess of bursa**

Use additional code (B95.-, B96.-) to identify causative organism

M71.00 Abscess of bursa, unspecified site

√6ᵗʰ **M71.01 Abscess of bursa,** shoulder

M71.011 Abscess of bursa, right **shoulder**
M71.012 Abscess of bursa, left **shoulder**
M71.019 Abscess of bursa, unspecified shoulder

√6ᵗʰ **M71.02 Abscess of bursa,** elbow

M71.021 Abscess of bursa, right **elbow**
M71.022 Abscess of bursa, left **elbow**
M71.029 Abscess of bursa, unspecified elbow

√6ᵗʰ **M71.03 Abscess of bursa,** wrist

M71.031 Abscess of bursa, right **wrist**
M71.032 Abscess of bursa, left **wrist**
M71.039 Abscess of bursa, unspecified wrist

√6ᵗʰ **M71.04 Abscess of bursa,** hand

M71.041 Abscess of bursa, right **hand**
M71.042 Abscess of bursa, left **hand**
M71.049 Abscess of bursa, unspecified hand

√6ᵗʰ **M71.05 Abscess of bursa,** hip

M71.051 Abscess of bursa, right **hip**
M71.052 Abscess of bursa, left **hip**
M71.059 Abscess of bursa, unspecified hip

√6ᵗʰ **M71.06 Abscess of bursa,** knee

M71.061 Abscess of bursa, right **knee**
M71.062 Abscess of bursa, left **knee**
M71.069 Abscess of bursa, unspecified knee

√6ᵗʰ **M71.07 Abscess of bursa,** ankle and foot

M71.071 Abscess of bursa, right **ankle and foot**
M71.072 Abscess of bursa, left **ankle and foot**
M71.079 Abscess of bursa, unspecified ankle and foot

M71.08 Abscess of bursa, other site

M71.09 Abscess of bursa, multiple sites

√5ᵗʰ **M71.1 Other infective bursitis**

Use additional code (B95.-, B96.-) to identify causative organism

M71.10 Other infective bursitis, unspecified site

√6ᵗʰ **M71.11 Other infective bursitis,** shoulder

M71.111 Other infective bursitis, right **shoulder**
M71.112 Other infective bursitis, left **shoulder**
M71.119 Other infective bursitis, unspecified shoulder

√6ᵗʰ **M71.12 Other infective bursitis,** elbow

M71.121 Other infective bursitis, right **elbow**
M71.122 Other infective bursitis, left **elbow**
M71.129 Other infective bursitis, unspecified elbow

√6ᵗʰ **M71.13 Other infective bursitis,** wrist

M71.131 Other infective bursitis, right **wrist**
M71.132 Other infective bursitis, left **wrist**
M71.139 Other infective bursitis, unspecified wrist

√6ᵗʰ **M71.14 Other infective bursitis,** hand

M71.141 Other infective bursitis, right **hand**
M71.142 Other infective bursitis, left **hand**
M71.149 Other infective bursitis, unspecified hand

√6ᵗʰ **M71.15 Other infective bursitis,** hip

M71.151 Other infective bursitis, right **hip**
M71.152 Other infective bursitis, left **hip**
M71.159 Other infective bursitis, unspecified hip

√6ᵗʰ **M71.16 Other infective bursitis,** knee

M71.161 Other infective bursitis, right **knee**
M71.162 Other infective bursitis, left **knee**
M71.169 Other infective bursitis, unspecified knee

√6ᵗʰ **M71.17 Other infective bursitis,** ankle and foot

M71.171 Other infective bursitis, right **ankle and foot**
M71.172 Other infective bursitis, left **ankle and foot**
M71.179 Other infective bursitis, unspecified ankle and foot

M71.18 Other infective bursitis, other site

M71.19 Other infective bursitis, multiple sites

√5ᵗʰ **M71.2 Synovial cyst of popliteal space [Baker]**

EXCLUDES 1   *synovial cyst of popliteal space with rupture (M66.0)*

DEF: Sac filled with clear synovial fluid in adults, usually secondary to disease inside the joint, located on the back of the knee in the popliteal fossa area. In children, the cyst usually represents a ganglion of one of the tendons in the knee.

Baker's Cyst

Baker's cyst connected to knee joint synovial cavity

M71.20 Synovial cyst of popliteal space [Baker], unspecified knee

M71.21 Synovial cyst of popliteal space [Baker], right **knee**

M71.22 Synovial cyst of popliteal space [Baker], left **knee**

√5ᵗʰ **M71.3 Other bursal cyst**

Synovial cyst NOS

EXCLUDES 1   *synovial cyst with rupture (M66.1-)*

M71.30 Other bursal cyst, unspecified site

√6ᵗʰ **M71.31 Other bursal cyst,** shoulder

M71.311 Other bursal cyst, right **shoulder**
M71.312 Other bursal cyst, left **shoulder**
M71.319 Other bursal cyst, unspecified shoulder

√6ᵗʰ **M71.32 Other bursal cyst,** elbow

M71.321 Other bursal cyst, right **elbow**

        M71.322   Other bursal cyst, left elbow
        M71.329   Other bursal cyst, unspecified elbow

√6ᵗʰ   M71.33   **Other bursal cyst, wrist**

        M71.331   Other bursal cyst, right wrist
        M71.332   Other bursal cyst, left wrist
        M71.339   Other bursal cyst, unspecified wrist

√6ᵗʰ   M71.34   **Other bursal cyst, hand**

        M71.341   Other bursal cyst, right hand
        M71.342   Other bursal cyst, left hand
        M71.349   Other bursal cyst, unspecified hand

√6ᵗʰ   M71.35   **Other bursal cyst, hip**

        M71.351   Other bursal cyst, right hip
        M71.352   Other bursal cyst, left hip
        M71.359   Other bursal cyst, unspecified hip

√6ᵗʰ   M71.37   **Other bursal cyst, ankle and foot**

        M71.371   Other bursal cyst, right ankle and foot
        M71.372   Other bursal cyst, left ankle and foot
        M71.379   Other bursal cyst, unspecified ankle and foot

       M71.38   **Other bursal cyst, other site**

       M71.39   **Other bursal cyst, multiple sites**

√5ᵗʰ   **M71.4   Calcium deposit in bursa**

         EXCLUDES 2   *calcium deposit in bursa of shoulder (M75.3)*

       M71.40   **Calcium deposit in bursa, unspecified site**

√6ᵗʰ   M71.42   **Calcium deposit in bursa, elbow**

        M71.421   Calcium deposit in bursa, right elbow
        M71.422   Calcium deposit in bursa, left elbow
        M71.429   Calcium deposit in bursa, unspecified elbow

√6ᵗʰ   M71.43   **Calcium deposit in bursa, wrist**

        M71.431   Calcium deposit in bursa, right wrist
        M71.432   Calcium deposit in bursa, left wrist
        M71.439   Calcium deposit in bursa, unspecified wrist

√6ᵗʰ   M71.44   **Calcium deposit in bursa, hand**

        M71.441   Calcium deposit in bursa, right hand
        M71.442   Calcium deposit in bursa, left hand
        M71.449   Calcium deposit in bursa, unspecified hand

√6ᵗʰ   M71.45   **Calcium deposit in bursa, hip**

        M71.451   Calcium deposit in bursa, right hip
        M71.452   Calcium deposit in bursa, left hip
        M71.459   Calcium deposit in bursa, unspecified hip

√6ᵗʰ   M71.46   **Calcium deposit in bursa, knee**

        M71.461   Calcium deposit in bursa, right knee
        M71.462   Calcium deposit in bursa, left knee
        M71.469   Calcium deposit in bursa, unspecified knee

√6ᵗʰ   M71.47   **Calcium deposit in bursa, ankle and foot**

        M71.471   Calcium deposit in bursa, right ankle and foot
        M71.472   Calcium deposit in bursa, left ankle and foot
        M71.479   Calcium deposit in bursa, unspecified ankle and foot

       M71.48   **Calcium deposit in bursa, other site**

       M71.49   **Calcium deposit in bursa, multiple sites**

√5ᵗʰ   **M71.5   Other bursitis, not elsewhere classified**

         EXCLUDES 1   *bursitis NOS (M71.9-)*
         EXCLUDES 2   *bursitis of shoulder (M75.5)*
                 bursitis of tibial collateral [Pellegrini-Stieda] (M76.4-)

       M71.50   **Other bursitis, not elsewhere classified, unspecified site**

√6ᵗʰ   M71.52   **Other bursitis, not elsewhere classified, elbow**

        M71.521   Other bursitis, not elsewhere classified, right elbow
        M71.522   Other bursitis, not elsewhere classified, left elbow
        M71.529   Other bursitis, not elsewhere classified, unspecified elbow

√6ᵗʰ   M71.53   **Other bursitis, not elsewhere classified, wrist**

        M71.531   Other bursitis, not elsewhere classified, right wrist
        M71.532   Other bursitis, not elsewhere classified, left wrist
        M71.539   Other bursitis, not elsewhere classified, unspecified wrist

√6ᵗʰ   M71.54   **Other bursitis, not elsewhere classified, hand**

        M71.541   Other bursitis, not elsewhere classified, right hand
        M71.542   Other bursitis, not elsewhere classified, left hand
        M71.549   Other bursitis, not elsewhere classified, unspecified hand

√6ᵗʰ   M71.55   **Other bursitis, not elsewhere classified, hip**

        M71.551   Other bursitis, not elsewhere classified, right hip
        M71.552   Other bursitis, not elsewhere classified, left hip
        M71.559   Other bursitis, not elsewhere classified, unspecified hip

√6ᵗʰ   M71.56   **Other bursitis, not elsewhere classified, knee**

        M71.561   Other bursitis, not elsewhere classified, right knee
        M71.562   Other bursitis, not elsewhere classified, left knee
        M71.569   Other bursitis, not elsewhere classified, unspecified knee

√6ᵗʰ   M71.57   **Other bursitis, not elsewhere classified, ankle and foot**

        M71.571   Other bursitis, not elsewhere classified, right ankle and foot
        M71.572   Other bursitis, not elsewhere classified, left ankle and foot
        M71.579   Other bursitis, not elsewhere classified, unspecified ankle and foot

       M71.58   **Other bursitis, not elsewhere classified, other site**

√5ᵗʰ   **M71.8   Other specified bursopathies**

       M71.80   **Other specified bursopathies, unspecified site**

√6ᵗʰ   M71.81   **Other specified bursopathies, shoulder**

        M71.811   Other specified bursopathies, right shoulder
        M71.812   Other specified bursopathies, left shoulder
        M71.819   Other specified bursopathies, unspecified shoulder

√6ᵗʰ   M71.82   **Other specified bursopathies, elbow**

        M71.821   Other specified bursopathies, right elbow
        M71.822   Other specified bursopathies, left elbow
        M71.829   Other specified bursopathies, unspecified elbow

√6ᵗʰ   M71.83   **Other specified bursopathies, wrist**

        M71.831   Other specified bursopathies, right wrist
        M71.832   Other specified bursopathies, left wrist
        M71.839   Other specified bursopathies, unspecified wrist

√6ᵗʰ   M71.84   **Other specified bursopathies, hand**

        M71.841   Other specified bursopathies, right hand
        M71.842   Other specified bursopathies, left hand
        M71.849   Other specified bursopathies, unspecified hand

√6ᵗʰ   M71.85   **Other specified bursopathies, hip**

        M71.851   Other specified bursopathies, right hip
        M71.852   Other specified bursopathies, left hip
        M71.859   Other specified bursopathies, unspecified hip

√6ᵗʰ   M71.86   **Other specified bursopathies, knee**

        M71.861   Other specified bursopathies, right knee
        M71.862   Other specified bursopathies, left knee
        M71.869   Other specified bursopathies, unspecified knee

√6ᵗʰ   M71.87   **Other specified bursopathies, ankle and foot**

        M71.871   Other specified bursopathies, right ankle and foot
        M71.872   Other specified bursopathies, left ankle and foot
        M71.879   Other specified bursopathies, unspecified ankle and foot

       M71.88   **Other specified bursopathies, other site**

       M71.89   **Other specified bursopathies, multiple sites**

    M71.9   Bursopathy, unspecified
         Bursitis NOS

N Newborn: 0   P Pediatric: 0-17   M Maternity: 9-64   A Adult: 15-124   **MCC** Major Complication/Comorbidity   **CC** Complication/Comorbidity   **SW** Severe Wound Dx

824   ICD-10-CM 2020

✓4ᵗʰ **M72　Fibroblastic disorders**

　　EXCLUDES 2　*retroperitoneal fibromatosis (D48.3)*

M72.0　Palmar fascial fibromatosis [Dupuytren]　　A

　　DEF: Dupuytren's contracture: Flexion deformity of a finger, due to shortened, thickened fibrosing of palmar fascia. The cause is unknown, but it is associated with long-standing epilepsy.

M72.1　Knuckle pads

M72.2　Plantar fascial fibromatosis
　　Plantar fasciitis
　　DEF: Rapid-growing and multiplanar nodular swellings and pain in the foot that is not associated with contractures.

M72.4　Pseudosarcomatous fibromatosis
　　Nodular fasciitis

M72.6　Necrotizing fasciitis　　MCC HCC
　　Use additional code (B95.-, B96.-) to identify causative organism
　　CC Excl: PDX collection 806

M72.8　Other fibroblastic disorders
　　Abscess of fascia
　　Fasciitis NEC
　　Other infective fasciitis
　　Use additional code to (B95.-, B96.-) identify causative organism
　　　EXCLUDES 1　*diffuse (eosinophilic) fasciitis (M35.4)*
　　　　　necrotizing fasciitis (M72.6)
　　　　　nodular fasciitis (M72.4)
　　　　　perirenal fasciitis NOS (N13.5)
　　　　　perirenal fasciitis with infection (N13.6)
　　　　　plantar fasciitis (M72.2)

M72.9　Fibroblastic disorder, unspecified
　　Fasciitis NOS
　　Fibromatosis NOS

✓4ᵗʰ **M75　Shoulder lesions**

　　EXCLUDES 2　*shoulder-hand syndrome (M89.0-)*

✓5ᵗʰ **M75.0　Adhesive capsulitis of shoulder**
　　Frozen shoulder
　　Periarthritis of shoulder
　　AHA: 2015,2Q,23
　　M75.00　Adhesive capsulitis of unspecified shoulder
　　M75.01　Adhesive capsulitis of right shoulder
　　M75.02　Adhesive capsulitis of left shoulder

✓5ᵗʰ **M75.1　Rotator cuff tear or rupture, not specified as traumatic**
　　Rotator cuff syndrome
　　Supraspinatus syndrome
　　Supraspinatus tear or rupture, not specified as traumatic
　　　EXCLUDES 1　*tear of rotator cuff, traumatic (S46.01-)*

✓6ᵗʰ **M75.10**　**Unspecified rotator cuff tear or rupture, not specified as traumatic**
　　M75.100　Unspecified rotator cuff tear or rupture of unspecified shoulder, not specified as traumatic
　　M75.101　Unspecified rotator cuff tear or rupture of right shoulder, not specified as traumatic
　　M75.102　Unspecified rotator cuff tear or rupture of left shoulder, not specified as traumatic

✓6ᵗʰ **M75.11**　**Incomplete rotator cuff tear or rupture not specified as traumatic**
　　M75.110　Incomplete rotator cuff tear or rupture of unspecified shoulder, not specified as traumatic
　　M75.111　Incomplete rotator cuff tear or rupture of right shoulder, not specified as traumatic
　　M75.112　Incomplete rotator cuff tear or rupture of left shoulder, not specified as traumatic

✓6ᵗʰ **M75.12**　**Complete rotator cuff tear or rupture not specified as traumatic**
　　M75.120　Complete rotator cuff tear or rupture of unspecified shoulder, not specified as traumatic
　　M75.121　Complete rotator cuff tear or rupture of right shoulder, not specified as traumatic　　CC
　　M75.122　Complete rotator cuff tear or rupture of left shoulder, not specified as traumatic　　CC

✓5ᵗʰ **M75.2　Bicipital tendinitis**
　　M75.20　Bicipital tendinitis, unspecified shoulder
　　M75.21　Bicipital tendinitis, right shoulder
　　M75.22　Bicipital tendinitis, left shoulder

✓5ᵗʰ **M75.3　Calcific tendinitis of shoulder**
　　Calcified bursa of shoulder
　　M75.30　Calcific tendinitis of unspecified shoulder
　　M75.31　Calcific tendinitis of right shoulder
　　M75.32　Calcific tendinitis of left shoulder

✓5ᵗʰ **M75.4　Impingement syndrome of shoulder**
　　M75.40　Impingement syndrome of unspecified shoulder
　　M75.41　Impingement syndrome of right shoulder
　　M75.42　Impingement syndrome of left shoulder

✓5ᵗʰ **M75.5　Bursitis of shoulder**
　　M75.50　Bursitis of unspecified shoulder
　　M75.51　Bursitis of right shoulder
　　M75.52　Bursitis of left shoulder

✓5ᵗʰ **M75.8　Other shoulder lesions**
　　M75.80　Other shoulder lesions, unspecified shoulder
　　M75.81　Other shoulder lesions, right shoulder
　　M75.82　Other shoulder lesions, left shoulder

✓5ᵗʰ **M75.9　Shoulder lesion, unspecified**
　　M75.90　Shoulder lesion, unspecified, unspecified shoulder
　　M75.91　Shoulder lesion, unspecified, right shoulder
　　M75.92　Shoulder lesion, unspecified, left shoulder

✓4ᵗʰ **M76　Enthesopathies, lower limb, excluding foot**

　　EXCLUDES 2　*bursitis due to use, overuse and pressure (M70.-)*
　　　　　enthesopathies of ankle and foot (M77.5-)

✓5ᵗʰ **M76.0　Gluteal tendinitis**
　　M76.00　Gluteal tendinitis, unspecified hip
　　M76.01　Gluteal tendinitis, right hip
　　M76.02　Gluteal tendinitis, left hip

✓5ᵗʰ **M76.1　Psoas tendinitis**
　　M76.10　Psoas tendinitis, unspecified hip
　　M76.11　Psoas tendinitis, right hip
　　M76.12　Psoas tendinitis, left hip

✓5ᵗʰ **M76.2　Iliac crest spur**
　　M76.20　Iliac crest spur, unspecified hip
　　M76.21　Iliac crest spur, right hip
　　M76.22　Iliac crest spur, left hip

✓5ᵗʰ **M76.3　Iliotibial band syndrome**
　　M76.30　Iliotibial band syndrome, unspecified leg
　　M76.31　Iliotibial band syndrome, right leg
　　M76.32　Iliotibial band syndrome, left leg

✓5ᵗʰ **M76.4　Tibial collateral bursitis [Pellegrini-Stieda]**
　　M76.40　Tibial collateral bursitis [Pellegrini-Stieda], unspecified leg
　　M76.41　Tibial collateral bursitis [Pellegrini-Stieda], right leg
　　M76.42　Tibial collateral bursitis [Pellegrini-Stieda], left leg

✓5ᵗʰ **M76.5　Patellar tendinitis**
　　M76.50　Patellar tendinitis, unspecified knee
　　M76.51　Patellar tendinitis, right knee
　　M76.52　Patellar tendinitis, left knee

✓5ᵗʰ **M76.6　Achilles tendinitis**
　　Achilles bursitis
　　M76.60　Achilles tendinitis, unspecified leg
　　M76.61　Achilles tendinitis, right leg
　　M76.62　Achilles tendinitis, left leg

✓5ᵗʰ **M76.7　Peroneal tendinitis**
　　M76.70　Peroneal tendinitis, unspecified leg
　　M76.71　Peroneal tendinitis, right leg
　　M76.72　Peroneal tendinitis, left leg

✓5ᵗʰ **M76.8　Other specified enthesopathies of lower limb, excluding foot**
　　✓6ᵗʰ **M76.81**　**Anterior tibial syndrome**
　　　M76.811　Anterior tibial syndrome, right leg
　　　M76.812　Anterior tibial syndrome, left leg
　　　M76.819　Anterior tibial syndrome, unspecified leg
　　✓6ᵗʰ **M76.82**　**Posterior tibial tendinitis**
　　　M76.821　Posterior tibial tendinitis, right leg
　　　M76.822　Posterior tibial tendinitis, left leg
　　　M76.829　Posterior tibial tendinitis, unspecified leg

√6ᵗʰ **M76.89 Other specified enthesopathies of lower limb, excluding foot**
    M76.891 Other specified enthesopathies of right lower limb, excluding foot
    M76.892 Other specified enthesopathies of left lower limb, excluding foot
    M76.899 Other specified enthesopathies of unspecified lower limb, excluding foot
M76.9 Unspecified enthesopathy, lower limb, excluding foot

√4ᵗʰ **M77 Other enthesopathies**
    EXCLUDES 1 *bursitis NOS (M71.9-)*
    EXCLUDES 2 *bursitis due to use, overuse and pressure (M70.-)*
        osteophyte (M25.7)
        spinal enthesopathy (M46.0-)

√5ᵗʰ **M77.0 Medial epicondylitis**
    M77.00 Medial epicondylitis, unspecified elbow
    M77.01 Medial epicondylitis, right elbow
    M77.02 Medial epicondylitis, left elbow

√5ᵗʰ **M77.1 Lateral epicondylitis**
    Tennis elbow
    M77.10 Lateral epicondylitis, unspecified elbow
    M77.11 Lateral epicondylitis, right elbow
    M77.12 Lateral epicondylitis, left elbow

√5ᵗʰ **M77.2 Periarthritis of wrist**
    M77.20 Periarthritis, unspecified wrist
    M77.21 Periarthritis, right wrist
    M77.22 Periarthritis, left wrist

√5ᵗʰ **M77.3 Calcaneal spur**
    DEF: Overgrowth of calcaneus bone on the underside of the heel that causes pain on walking. Calcaneal spur is due to a chronic avulsion injury of the plantar fascia from the calcaneus.
    M77.30 Calcaneal spur, unspecified foot
    M77.31 Calcaneal spur, right foot
    M77.32 Calcaneal spur, left foot

√5ᵗʰ **M77.4 Metatarsalgia**
    EXCLUDES 1 *Morton's metatarsalgia (G57.6)*
    M77.40 Metatarsalgia, unspecified foot
    M77.41 Metatarsalgia, right foot
    M77.42 Metatarsalgia, left foot

▲ √5ᵗʰ **M77.5 Other enthesopathy of foot and ankle**
▲   **M77.50 Other enthesopathy of unspecified foot and ankle**
▲   **M77.51 Other enthesopathy of right foot and ankle**
▲   **M77.52 Other enthesopathy of left foot and ankle**

M77.8 Other enthesopathies, not elsewhere classified
M77.9 Enthesopathy, unspecified
    Bone spur NOS
    Capsulitis NOS
    Periarthritis NOS
    Tendinitis NOS

√4ᵗʰ **M79 Other and unspecified soft tissue disorders, not elsewhere classified**
    EXCLUDES 1 *psychogenic rheumatism (F45.8)*
        soft tissue pain, psychogenic (F45.41)

M79.0 Rheumatism, unspecified
    EXCLUDES 1 *fibromyalgia (M79.7)*
        palindromic rheumatism (M12.3-)

√5ᵗʰ **M79.1 Myalgia**
    Myofascial pain syndrome
    EXCLUDES 1 *fibromyalgia (M79.7)*
        myositis (M60.-)
    AHA: 2018,4Q,21
    M79.10 Myalgia, unspecified site
    M79.11 Myalgia of mastication muscle
    M79.12 Myalgia of auxiliary muscles, head and neck
    M79.18 Myalgia, other site

M79.2 Neuralgia and neuritis, unspecified
    EXCLUDES 1 *brachial radiculitis NOS (M54.1)*
        lumbosacral radiculitis NOS (M54.1)
        mononeuropathies (G56-G58)
        radiculitis NOS (M54.1)
        sciatica (M54.3-M54.4)
    TIP: Assign for documented neuropathic pain.

M79.3 Panniculitis, unspecified CC
    EXCLUDES 1 *lupus panniculitis (L93.2)*
        neck and back panniculitis (M54.0-)
        relapsing [Weber-Christian] panniculitis (M35.6)

M79.4 Hypertrophy of (infrapatellar) fat pad
M79.5 Residual foreign body in soft tissue
    EXCLUDES 1 *foreign body granuloma of skin and subcutaneous tissue (L92.3)*
        foreign body granuloma of soft tissue (M60.2-)

√5ᵗʰ **M79.6 Pain in limb, hand, foot, fingers and toes**
    EXCLUDES 2 *pain in joint (M25.5-)*

√6ᵗʰ **M79.60 Pain in limb, unspecified**
    M79.601 Pain in right arm
        Pain in right upper limb NOS
    M79.602 Pain in left arm
        Pain in left upper limb NOS
    M79.603 Pain in arm, unspecified
        Pain in upper limb NOS
    M79.604 Pain in right leg
        Pain in right lower limb NOS
    M79.605 Pain in left leg
        Pain in left lower limb NOS
    M79.606 Pain in leg, unspecified
        Pain in lower limb NOS
    M79.609 Pain in unspecified limb
        Pain in limb NOS

√6ᵗʰ **M79.62 Pain in upper arm**
    Pain in axillary region
    M79.621 Pain in right upper arm
    M79.622 Pain in left upper arm
    M79.629 Pain in unspecified upper arm

√6ᵗʰ **M79.63 Pain in forearm**
    M79.631 Pain in right forearm
    M79.632 Pain in left forearm
    M79.639 Pain in unspecified forearm

√6ᵗʰ **M79.64 Pain in hand and fingers**
    M79.641 Pain in right hand
    M79.642 Pain in left hand
    M79.643 Pain in unspecified hand
    M79.644 Pain in right finger(s)
    M79.645 Pain in left finger(s)
    M79.646 Pain in unspecified finger(s)

√6ᵗʰ **M79.65 Pain in thigh**
    M79.651 Pain in right thigh
    M79.652 Pain in left thigh
    M79.659 Pain in unspecified thigh

√6ᵗʰ **M79.66 Pain in lower leg**
    M79.661 Pain in right lower leg
    M79.662 Pain in left lower leg
    M79.669 Pain in unspecified lower leg

√6ᵗʰ **M79.67 Pain in foot and toes**
    M79.671 Pain in right foot
    M79.672 Pain in left foot
    M79.673 Pain in unspecified foot
    M79.674 Pain in right toe(s)
    M79.675 Pain in left toe(s)
    M79.676 Pain in unspecified toe(s)

M79.7 Fibromyalgia
    Fibromyositis
    Fibrositis
    Myofibrositis

√5ᵗʰ **M79.A Nontraumatic compartment syndrome**
    Code first, if applicable, associated postprocedural complication
    EXCLUDES 1 *compartment syndrome NOS (T79.A-)*
        fibromyalgia (M79.7)
        nontraumatic ischemic infarction of muscle (M62.2-)
        traumatic compartment syndrome (T79.A-)

√6ᵗʰ **M79.A1 Nontraumatic compartment syndrome of upper extremity**
    Nontraumatic compartment syndrome of shoulder, arm, forearm, wrist, hand, and fingers
    CC Excl: For CC codes in subcategory M79.A1: PDX collection 893

    M79.A11 Nontraumatic compartment syndrome of right upper extremity CC

N Newborn: 0   P Pediatric: 0-17   M Maternity: 9-64   A Adult: 15-124   MCC Major Complication/Comorbidity   CC Complication/Comorbidity   SW Severe Wound Dx

826

ICD-10-CM 2020

M79.A12 Nontraumatic compartment syndrome of **left upper extremity** `CC`

M79.A19 Nontraumatic compartment syndrome of **unspecified upper extremity** `CC`

√6ᵗʰ **M79.A2** Nontraumatic compartment syndrome of **lower extremity**

Nontraumatic compartment syndrome of hip, buttock, thigh, leg, foot, and toes

CC Excl: For CC codes in subcategory M79.A2: PDX collection 894

M79.A21 Nontraumatic compartment syndrome of **right lower extremity** `CC`

M79.A22 Nontraumatic compartment syndrome of **left lower extremity** `CC`

M79.A29 Nontraumatic compartment syndrome of **unspecified lower extremity** `CC`

M79.A3 Nontraumatic compartment syndrome of **abdomen** `CC`

CC Excl: PDX collection 895

M79.A9 Nontraumatic compartment syndrome of **other sites** `CC`

CC Excl: PDX collection 896

√5ᵗʰ **M79.8** Other specified soft tissue disorders

M79.81 Nontraumatic hematoma of soft tissue

Nontraumatic hematoma of muscle
Nontraumatic seroma of muscle and soft tissue

M79.89 Other specified soft tissue disorders

Polyalgia

M79.9 Soft tissue disorder, unspecified

OSTEOPATHIES AND CHONDROPATHIES (M80-M94)

Disorders of bone density and structure (M80-M85)

√4ᵗʰ **M80** **Osteoporosis** with current pathological fracture

`INCLUDES` osteoporosis with current fragility fracture

Use additional code to identify major osseous defect, if applicable (M89.7-)

`EXCLUDES 1` collapsed vertebra NOS (M48.5)
pathological fracture NOS (M84.4)
wedging of vertebra NOS (M48.5)

`EXCLUDES 2` personal history of (healed) osteoporosis fracture (Z87.310)

AHA: 2018,2Q,12

TIP: The site codes in this category identify the site of the fracture, not the site of the osteoporosis.

The appropriate 7th character is to be added to each code from category M80:

A   initial encounter for fracture
D   subsequent encounter for fracture with routine healing
G   subsequent encounter for fracture with delayed healing
K   subsequent encounter for fracture with nonunion
P   subsequent encounter for fracture with malunion
S   sequela

CC Excl: For codes in category M80:
CC with 7th character A: PDX collection 888
CC with 7th character K or P: PDX collection 897

√5ᵗʰ **M80.0** **Age-related** osteoporosis with current pathological fracture

Involutional osteoporosis with current pathological fracture
Osteoporosis NOS with current pathological fracture
Postmenopausal osteoporosis with current pathological fracture
Senile osteoporosis with current pathological fracture

³ √x7ᵗʰ **M80.00** Age-related osteoporosis with current pathological fracture, unspecified site `CC` `A`

√6ᵗʰ **M80.01** Age-related osteoporosis with current pathological fracture, **shoulder**

³ √7ᵗʰ **M80.011** Age-related osteoporosis with current pathological fracture, **right shoulder** `CC` `A`

³ √7ᵗʰ **M80.012** Age-related osteoporosis with current pathological fracture, **left shoulder** `CC` `A`

³ √7ᵗʰ **M80.019** Age-related osteoporosis with current pathological fracture, unspecified **shoulder** `CC` `A`

√6ᵗʰ **M80.02** Age-related osteoporosis with current pathological fracture, **humerus**

³ √7ᵗʰ **M80.021** Age-related osteoporosis with current pathological fracture, **right humerus** `CC` `A`

³ √7ᵗʰ **M80.022** Age-related osteoporosis with current pathological fracture, **left humerus** `CC` `A`

³ √7ᵗʰ **M80.029** Age-related osteoporosis with current pathological fracture, unspecified **humerus** `CC` `A`

√6ᵗʰ **M80.03** Age-related osteoporosis with current pathological fracture, **forearm**

Age-related osteoporosis with current pathological fracture of wrist

³ √7ᵗʰ **M80.031** Age-related osteoporosis with current pathological fracture, **right forearm** `CC` `A`

³ √7ᵗʰ **M80.032** Age-related osteoporosis with current pathological fracture, **left forearm** `CC` `A`

³ √7ᵗʰ **M80.039** Age-related osteoporosis with current pathological fracture, unspecified **forearm** `CC` `A`

√6ᵗʰ **M80.04** Age-related osteoporosis with current pathological fracture, **hand**

³ √7ᵗʰ **M80.041** Age-related osteoporosis with current pathological fracture, **right hand** `CC` `A`

³ √7ᵗʰ **M80.042** Age-related osteoporosis with current pathological fracture, **left hand** `CC` `A`

³ √7ᵗʰ **M80.049** Age-related osteoporosis with current pathological fracture, unspecified **hand** `CC` `A`

√6ᵗʰ **M80.05** Age-related osteoporosis with current pathological fracture, **femur**

Age-related osteoporosis with current pathological fracture of hip

³,⁶ √7ᵗʰ **M80.051** Age-related osteoporosis with current pathological fracture, **right femur** `CC` `HCC` `A`

³,⁶ √7ᵗʰ **M80.052** Age-related osteoporosis with current pathological fracture, **left femur** `CC` `HCC` `A`

³,⁶ √7ᵗʰ **M80.059** Age-related osteoporosis with current pathological fracture, unspecified **femur** `CC` `HCC` `A`

√6ᵗʰ **M80.06** Age-related osteoporosis with current pathological fracture, **lower leg**

³ √7ᵗʰ **M80.061** Age-related osteoporosis with current pathological fracture, **right lower leg** `CC` `A`

³ √7ᵗʰ **M80.062** Age-related osteoporosis with current pathological fracture, **left lower leg** `CC` `A`

³ √7ᵗʰ **M80.069** Age-related osteoporosis with current pathological fracture, unspecified **lower leg** `CC` `A`

√6ᵗʰ **M80.07** Age-related osteoporosis with current pathological fracture, **ankle and foot**

³ √7ᵗʰ **M80.071** Age-related osteoporosis with current pathological fracture, **right ankle and foot** `CC` `A`

³ √7ᵗʰ **M80.072** Age-related osteoporosis with current pathological fracture, **left ankle and foot** `CC` `A`

³ √7ᵗʰ **M80.079** Age-related osteoporosis with current pathological fracture, unspecified **ankle and foot** `CC` `A`

³,⁶ √x7ᵗʰ **M80.08** Age-related osteoporosis with current pathological fracture, **vertebra(e)** `CC` `HCC` `A`

√5ᵗʰ **M80.8** **Other osteoporosis with current pathological fracture**

Drug-induced osteoporosis with current pathological fracture

Idiopathic osteoporosis with current pathological fracture

Osteoporosis of disuse with current pathological fracture

Postoophorectomy osteoporosis with current pathological fracture

Postsurgical malabsorption osteoporosis with current pathological fracture

Post-traumatic osteoporosis with current pathological fracture

Use additional code for adverse effect, if applicable, to identify drug (T36–T50 with fifth or sixth character 5)

3 √x7ᵗʰ **M80.80** **Other osteoporosis with current pathological fracture, unspecified site**   CC

√6ᵗʰ **M80.81** **Other osteoporosis with pathological fracture, shoulder**

    3 √7ᵗʰ **M80.811** **Other osteoporosis with current pathological fracture, right shoulder**   CC

    3 √7ᵗʰ **M80.812** **Other osteoporosis with current pathological fracture, left shoulder**   CC

    3 √7ᵗʰ **M80.819** **Other osteoporosis with current pathological fracture, unspecified shoulder**   CC

√6ᵗʰ **M80.82** **Other osteoporosis with current pathological fracture, humerus**

    3 √7ᵗʰ **M80.821** **Other osteoporosis with current pathological fracture, right humerus**   CC

    3 √7ᵗʰ **M80.822** **Other osteoporosis with current pathological fracture, left humerus**   CC

    3 √7ᵗʰ **M80.829** **Other osteoporosis with current pathological fracture, unspecified humerus**   CC

√6ᵗʰ **M80.83** **Other osteoporosis with current pathological fracture, forearm**

Other osteoporosis with current pathological fracture of wrist

    3 √7ᵗʰ **M80.831** **Other osteoporosis with current pathological fracture, right forearm**   CC

    3 √7ᵗʰ **M80.832** **Other osteoporosis with current pathological fracture, left forearm**   CC

    3 √7ᵗʰ **M80.839** **Other osteoporosis with current pathological fracture, unspecified forearm**   CC

√6ᵗʰ **M80.84** **Other osteoporosis with current pathological fracture, hand**

    3 √7ᵗʰ **M80.841** **Other osteoporosis with current pathological fracture, right hand**   CC

    3 √7ᵗʰ **M80.842** **Other osteoporosis with current pathological fracture, left hand**   CC

    3 √7ᵗʰ **M80.849** **Other osteoporosis with current pathological fracture, unspecified hand**   CC

√6ᵗʰ **M80.85** **Other osteoporosis with current pathological fracture, femur**

Other osteoporosis with current pathological fracture of hip

    3,6 √7ᵗʰ **M80.851** **Other osteoporosis with current pathological fracture, right femur**   CC HCC

    3,6 √7ᵗʰ **M80.852** **Other osteoporosis with current pathological fracture, left femur**   CC HCC

    3,6 √7ᵗʰ **M80.859** **Other osteoporosis with current pathological fracture, unspecified femur**   CC HCC

√6ᵗʰ **M80.86** **Other osteoporosis with current pathological fracture, lower leg**

    3 √7ᵗʰ **M80.861** **Other osteoporosis with current pathological fracture, right lower leg**   CC

    3 √7ᵗʰ **M80.862** **Other osteoporosis with current pathological fracture, left lower leg**   CC

    3 √7ᵗʰ **M80.869** **Other osteoporosis with current pathological fracture, unspecified lower leg**   CC

√6ᵗʰ **M80.87** **Other osteoporosis with current pathological fracture, ankle and foot**

    3 √7ᵗʰ **M80.871** **Other osteoporosis with current pathological fracture, right ankle and foot**   CC

    3 √7ᵗʰ **M80.872** **Other osteoporosis with current pathological fracture, left ankle and foot**   CC

    3 √7ᵗʰ **M80.879** **Other osteoporosis with current pathological fracture, unspecified ankle and foot**   CC

3,6 √x7ᵗʰ **M80.88** **Other osteoporosis with current pathological fracture, vertebra(e)**   CC HCC

√4ᵗʰ **M81** **Osteoporosis without current pathological fracture**

Use additional code to identify:

major osseous defect, if applicable (M89.7-)

personal history of (healed) osteoporosis fracture, if applicable (Z87.310)

    EXCLUDES 1   osteoporosis with current pathological fracture (M80.-)

               Sudeck's atrophy (M89.0)

M81.0 **Age-related osteoporosis without current pathological fracture**   A

Involutional osteoporosis without current pathological fracture

Osteoporosis NOS

Postmenopausal osteoporosis without current pathological fracture

Senile osteoporosis without current pathological fracture

M81.6 **Localized osteoporosis [Lequesne]**

    EXCLUDES 1   Sudeck's atrophy (M89.0)

M81.8 **Other osteoporosis without current pathological fracture**

Drug-induced osteoporosis without current pathological fracture

Idiopathic osteoporosis without current pathological fracture

Osteoporosis of disuse without current pathological fracture

Postoophorectomy osteoporosis without current pathological fracture

Postsurgical malabsorption osteoporosis without current pathological fracture

Post-traumatic osteoporosis without current pathological fracture

Use additional code for adverse effect, if applicable, to identify drug (T36–T50 with fifth or sixth character 5)

√4ᵗʰ **M83** **Adult osteomalacia**

    EXCLUDES 1   infantile and juvenile osteomalacia (E55.0)

               renal osteodystrophy (N25.0)

               rickets (active) (E55.0)

               rickets (active) sequelae (E64.3)

               vitamin D-resistant osteomalacia (E83.3)

               vitamin D-resistant rickets (active) (E83.3)

M83.0 **Puerperal osteomalacia**   M ♀

M83.1 **Senile osteomalacia**   A

M83.2 **Adult osteomalacia due to malabsorption**   A

Postsurgical malabsorption osteomalacia in adults

M83.3 **Adult osteomalacia due to malnutrition**   A

M83.4 **Aluminum bone disease**

M83.5 **Other drug-induced osteomalacia in adults**   A

Use additional code for adverse effect, if applicable, to identify drug (T36–T50 with fifth or sixth character 5)

M83.8 **Other adult osteomalacia**   A

M83.9 **Adult osteomalacia, unspecified**   A

N Newborn: 0   P Pediatric: 0-17   M Maternity: 9-64   A Adult: 15-124   MCC Major Complication/Comorbidity   CC Complication/Comorbidity   SW Severe Wound Dx

828   ICD-10-CM 2020

√4ʰ **M84 Disorder of continuity of bone**

     EXCLUDES 2   *traumatic fracture of bone-see fracture, by site*

   √5ʰ **M84.3 Stress fracture**

     Fatigue fracture
     March fracture
     Stress fracture NOS
     Stress reaction
     Use additional external cause code(s) to identify the cause of the stress fracture

     EXCLUDES 1   *pathological fracture due to osteoporosis (M80.-)*
             pathological fracture NOS (M84.4.-)
             traumatic fracture (S12.-, S22.-, S32.-, S42.-, S52.-, S62.-, S72.-, S82.-, S92.-)

     EXCLUDES 2   *personal history of (healed) stress (fatigue) fracture (Z87.312)*
             stress fracture of vertebra (M48.4-)

> The appropriate 7th character is to be added to each code from subcategory M84.3.
> A   initial encounter for fracture
> D   subsequent encounter for fracture with routine healing
> G   subsequent encounter for fracture with delayed healing
> K   subsequent encounter for fracture with nonunion
> P   subsequent encounter for fracture with malunion
> S   sequela

> **CC Excl: For codes in subcategory M84.3:**
> **CC with 7th character K or P:** PDX collection 897

4 √x7ʰ   **M84.30**   **Stress fracture, unspecified site**   cc

   √6ʰ   **M84.31**   **Stress fracture, shoulder**

     4 √7ʰ   **M84.311**   **Stress fracture, right shoulder**   cc

     4 √7ʰ   **M84.312**   **Stress fracture, left shoulder**   cc

     4 √7ʰ   **M84.319**   **Stress fracture, unspecified shoulder**   cc

   √6ʰ   **M84.32**   **Stress fracture, humerus**

     4 √7ʰ   **M84.321**   **Stress fracture, right humerus**   cc

     4 √7ʰ   **M84.322**   **Stress fracture, left humerus**   cc

     4 √7ʰ   **M84.329**   **Stress fracture, unspecified humerus**   cc

   √6ʰ   **M84.33**   **Stress fracture, ulna and radius**

     4 √7ʰ   **M84.331**   **Stress fracture, right ulna**   cc

     4 √7ʰ   **M84.332**   **Stress fracture, left ulna**   cc

     4 √7ʰ   **M84.333**   **Stress fracture, right radius**   cc

     4 √7ʰ   **M84.334**   **Stress fracture, left radius**   cc

     4 √7ʰ   **M84.339**   **Stress fracture, unspecified ulna and radius**   cc

   √6ʰ   **M84.34**   **Stress fracture, hand and fingers**

     4 √7ʰ   **M84.341**   **Stress fracture, right hand**   cc

     4 √7ʰ   **M84.342**   **Stress fracture, left hand**   cc

     4 √7ʰ   **M84.343**   **Stress fracture, unspecified hand**   cc

     4 √7ʰ   **M84.344**   **Stress fracture, right finger(s)**

     4 √7ʰ   **M84.345**   **Stress fracture, left finger(s)**

     4 √7ʰ   **M84.346**   **Stress fracture, unspecified finger(s)**   cc

   √6ʰ   **M84.35**   **Stress fracture, pelvis and femur**

     Stress fracture, hip

     4 √7ʰ   **M84.350**   **Stress fracture, pelvis**   cc

     4 √7ʰ   **M84.351**   **Stress fracture, right femur**   cc

     4 √7ʰ   **M84.352**   **Stress fracture, left femur**   cc

     4 √7ʰ   **M84.353**   **Stress fracture, unspecified femur**   cc

     4 √7ʰ   **M84.359**   **Stress fracture, hip, unspecified**   cc

   √6ʰ   **M84.36**   **Stress fracture, tibia and fibula**

     4 √7ʰ   **M84.361**   **Stress fracture, right tibia**   cc

     4 √7ʰ   **M84.362**   **Stress fracture, left tibia**   cc

     4 √7ʰ   **M84.363**   **Stress fracture, right fibula**

     4 √7ʰ   **M84.364**   **Stress fracture, left fibula**   cc

     4 √7ʰ   **M84.369**   **Stress fracture, unspecified tibia and fibula**   cc

   √6ʰ   **M84.37**   **Stress fracture, ankle, foot and toes**

     4 √7ʰ   **M84.371**   **Stress fracture, right ankle**   cc

     4 √7ʰ   **M84.372**   **Stress fracture, left ankle**   cc

     4 √7ʰ   **M84.373**   **Stress fracture, unspecified ankle**   cc

     4 √7ʰ   **M84.374**   **Stress fracture, right foot**   cc

     4 √7ʰ   **M84.375**   **Stress fracture, left foot**   cc

     4 √7ʰ   **M84.376**   **Stress fracture, unspecified foot**   cc

     4 √7ʰ   **M84.377**   **Stress fracture, right toe(s)**   cc

     4 √7ʰ   **M84.378**   **Stress fracture, left toe(s)**   cc

     4 √7ʰ   **M84.379**   **Stress fracture, unspecified toe(s)**   cc

4 √x7ʰ   **M84.38**   **Stress fracture, other site**   cc

     EXCLUDES 2   *stress fracture of vertebra (M48.4-)*

   √5ʰ **M84.4 Pathological fracture, not elsewhere classified**

     Chronic fracture
     Pathological fracture NOS

     EXCLUDES 1   *collapsed vertebra NEC (M48.5)*
             pathological fracture in neoplastic disease (M84.5-)
             pathological fracture in osteoporosis (M80.-)
             pathological fracture in other disease (M84.6-)
             stress fracture (M84.3-)
             traumatic fracture (S12.-, S22.-, S32.-, S42.-, S52.-, S62.-, S72.-, S82.-, S92.-)

     EXCLUDES 2   *personal history of (healed) pathological fracture (Z87.311)*

> The appropriate 7th character is to be added to each code from subcategory M84.4.
> A   initial encounter for fracture
> D   subsequent encounter for fracture with routine healing
> G   subsequent encounter for fracture with delayed healing
> K   subsequent encounter for fracture with nonunion
> P   subsequent encounter for fracture with malunion
> S   sequela

> **CC Excl: For codes in subcategory M84.4:**
> **CC with 7th character A:** PDX collection 888
> **CC with 7th character K or P:** PDX collection 897

3 √x7ʰ   **M84.40**   **Pathological fracture, unspecified site**   cc

   √6ʰ   **M84.41**   **Pathological fracture, shoulder**

     3 √7ʰ   **M84.411**   **Pathological fracture, right shoulder**   cc

     3 √7ʰ   **M84.412**   **Pathological fracture, left shoulder**   cc

     3 √7ʰ   **M84.419**   **Pathological fracture, unspecified shoulder**   cc

   √6ʰ   **M84.42**   **Pathological fracture, humerus**

     3 √7ʰ   **M84.421**   **Pathological fracture, right humerus**   cc

     3 √7ʰ   **M84.422**   **Pathological fracture, left humerus**   cc

     3 √7ʰ   **M84.429**   **Pathological fracture, unspecified humerus**   cc

   √6ʰ   **M84.43**   **Pathological fracture, ulna and radius**

     3 √7ʰ   **M84.431**   **Pathological fracture, right ulna**   cc

     3 √7ʰ   **M84.432**   **Pathological fracture, left ulna**   cc

     3 √7ʰ   **M84.433**   **Pathological fracture, right radius**

     3 √7ʰ   **M84.434**   **Pathological fracture, left radius**   cc

     3 √7ʰ   **M84.439**   **Pathological fracture, unspecified ulna and radius**   cc

   √6ʰ   **M84.44**   **Pathological fracture, hand and fingers**

     3 √7ʰ   **M84.441**   **Pathological fracture, right hand**   cc

     3 √7ʰ   **M84.442**   **Pathological fracture, left hand**   cc

     3 √7ʰ   **M84.443**   **Pathological fracture, unspecified hand**   cc

3 ✓7ᵗʰ **M84.444 Pathological fracture, right finger(s)** CC

3 ✓7ᵗʰ **M84.445 Pathological fracture, left finger(s)** CC

3 ✓7ᵗʰ **M84.446 Pathological fracture, unspecified finger(s)** CC

✓6ᵗʰ **M84.45 Pathological fracture, femur and pelvis**
AHA: 2016,4Q,43

3,6 ✓7ᵗʰ **M84.451 Pathological fracture, right femur** CC HCC

3,6 ✓7ᵗʰ **M84.452 Pathological fracture, left femur** CC HCC

3,6 ✓7ᵗʰ **M84.453 Pathological fracture, unspecified femur** CC HCC

3 ✓7ᵗʰ **M84.454 Pathological fracture, pelvis** CC

3,6 ✓7ᵗʰ **M84.459 Pathological fracture, hip, unspecified** CC HCC

✓6ᵗʰ **M84.46 Pathological fracture, tibia and fibula**

3 ✓7ᵗʰ **M84.461 Pathological fracture, right tibia** CC

3 ✓7ᵗʰ **M84.462 Pathological fracture, left tibia** CC

3 ✓7ᵗʰ **M84.463 Pathological fracture, right fibula** CC

3 ✓7ᵗʰ **M84.464 Pathological fracture, left fibula** CC

3 ✓7ᵗʰ **M84.469 Pathological fracture, unspecified tibia and fibula** CC

✓6ᵗʰ **M84.47 Pathological fracture, ankle, foot and toes**

3 ✓7ᵗʰ **M84.471 Pathological fracture, right ankle** CC

3 ✓7ᵗʰ **M84.472 Pathological fracture, left ankle** CC

3 ✓7ᵗʰ **M84.473 Pathological fracture, unspecified ankle** CC

3 ✓7ᵗʰ **M84.474 Pathological fracture, right foot** CC

3 ✓7ᵗʰ **M84.475 Pathological fracture, left foot** CC

3 ✓7ᵗʰ **M84.476 Pathological fracture, unspecified foot** CC

3 ✓7ᵗʰ **M84.477 Pathological fracture, right toe(s)** CC

3 ✓7ᵗʰ **M84.478 Pathological fracture, left toe(s)** CC

3 ✓7ᵗʰ **M84.479 Pathological fracture, unspecified toe(s)** CC

3 ✓x7ᵗʰ **M84.48 Pathological fracture, other site** CC

✓5ᵗʰ **M84.5 Pathological fracture in neoplastic disease**

Code also underlying neoplasm

The appropriate 7th character is to be added to each code from subcategory M84.5.
A   initial encounter for fracture
D   subsequent encounter for fracture with routine healing
G   subsequent encounter for fracture with delayed healing
K   subsequent encounter for fracture with nonunion
P   subsequent encounter for fracture with malunion
S   sequela

CC Excl: For codes in subcategory M84.5:
CC with 7th character A: PDX collection 888
CC with 7th character K or P: PDX collection 897

3 ✓x7ᵗʰ **M84.50 Pathological fracture in neoplastic disease, unspecified site** CC

✓6ᵗʰ **M84.51 Pathological fracture in neoplastic disease, shoulder**

3 ✓7ᵗʰ **M84.511 Pathological fracture in neoplastic disease, right shoulder** CC

3 ✓7ᵗʰ **M84.512 Pathological fracture in neoplastic disease, left shoulder** CC

3 ✓7ᵗʰ **M84.519 Pathological fracture in neoplastic disease, unspecified shoulder** CC

✓6ᵗʰ **M84.52 Pathological fracture in neoplastic disease, humerus**

3 ✓7ᵗʰ **M84.521 Pathological fracture in neoplastic disease, right humerus** CC

3 ✓7ᵗʰ **M84.522 Pathological fracture in neoplastic disease, left humerus** CC

3 ✓7ᵗʰ **M84.529 Pathological fracture in neoplastic disease, unspecified humerus** CC

✓6ᵗʰ **M84.53 Pathological fracture in neoplastic disease, ulna and radius**

3 ✓7ᵗʰ **M84.531 Pathological fracture in neoplastic disease, right ulna** CC

3 ✓7ᵗʰ **M84.532 Pathological fracture in neoplastic disease, left ulna** CC

3 ✓7ᵗʰ **M84.533 Pathological fracture in neoplastic disease, right radius** CC

3 ✓7ᵗʰ **M84.534 Pathological fracture in neoplastic disease, left radius** CC

3 ✓7ᵗʰ **M84.539 Pathological fracture in neoplastic disease, unspecified ulna and radius** CC

✓6ᵗʰ **M84.54 Pathological fracture in neoplastic disease, hand**

3 ✓7ᵗʰ **M84.541 Pathological fracture in neoplastic disease, right hand** CC

3 ✓7ᵗʰ **M84.542 Pathological fracture in neoplastic disease, left hand** CC

3 ✓7ᵗʰ **M84.549 Pathological fracture in neoplastic disease, unspecified hand** CC

✓6ᵗʰ **M84.55 Pathological fracture in neoplastic disease, pelvis and femur**

3 ✓7ᵗʰ **M84.550 Pathological fracture in neoplastic disease, pelvis** CC

3,6 ✓7ᵗʰ **M84.551 Pathological fracture in neoplastic disease, right femur** CC HCC

3,6 ✓7ᵗʰ **M84.552 Pathological fracture in neoplastic disease, left femur** CC HCC

3,6 ✓7ᵗʰ **M84.553 Pathological fracture in neoplastic disease, unspecified femur** CC HCC

3,6 ✓7ᵗʰ **M84.559 Pathological fracture in neoplastic disease, hip, unspecified** CC HCC

✓6ᵗʰ **M84.56 Pathological fracture in neoplastic disease, tibia and fibula**

3 ✓7ᵗʰ **M84.561 Pathological fracture in neoplastic disease, right tibia** CC

3 ✓7ᵗʰ **M84.562 Pathological fracture in neoplastic disease, left tibia** CC

3 ✓7ᵗʰ **M84.563 Pathological fracture in neoplastic disease, right fibula** CC

3 ✓7ᵗʰ **M84.564 Pathological fracture in neoplastic disease, left fibula** CC

3 ✓7ᵗʰ **M84.569 Pathological fracture in neoplastic disease, unspecified tibia and fibula** CC

✓6ᵗʰ **M84.57 Pathological fracture in neoplastic disease, ankle and foot**

3 ✓7ᵗʰ **M84.571 Pathological fracture in neoplastic disease, right ankle** CC

3 ✓7ᵗʰ **M84.572 Pathological fracture in neoplastic disease, left ankle** CC

3 ✓7ᵗʰ **M84.573 Pathological fracture in neoplastic disease, unspecified ankle** CC

3 ✓7ᵗʰ **M84.574 Pathological fracture in neoplastic disease, right foot** CC

3 ✓7ᵗʰ **M84.575 Pathological fracture in neoplastic disease, left foot** CC

3 √7ᵗʰ **M84.576 Pathological fracture in neoplastic disease, unspecified foot** CC

3 √x7ᵗʰ **M84.58 Pathological fracture in neoplastic disease, other specified site** CC

Pathological fracture in neoplastic disease, vertebrae

√5ᵗʰ **M84.6 Pathological fracture in other disease**

Code also underlying condition

EXCLUDES 1 *pathological fracture in osteoporosis (M80.-)*

The appropriate 7th character is to be added to each code from subcategory M84.6.
A   initial encounter for fracture
D   subsequent encounter for fracture with routine healing
G   subsequent encounter for fracture with delayed healing
K   subsequent encounter for fracture with nonunion
P   subsequent encounter for fracture with malunion
S   sequela

CC Excl: For codes in subcategory M84.6:
CC with 7th character A: PDX collection 888
CC with 7th character K or P: PDX collection 897

3 √x7ᵗʰ **M84.60 Pathological fracture in other disease, unspecified site** CC

√6ᵗʰ **M84.61 Pathological fracture in other disease, shoulder**

3 √7ᵗʰ **M84.611 Pathological fracture in other disease, right shoulder** CC

3 √7ᵗʰ **M84.612 Pathological fracture in other disease, left shoulder** CC

3 √7ᵗʰ **M84.619 Pathological fracture in other disease, unspecified shoulder** CC

√6ᵗʰ **M84.62 Pathological fracture in other disease, humerus**

3 √7ᵗʰ **M84.621 Pathological fracture in other disease, right humerus** CC

3 √7ᵗʰ **M84.622 Pathological fracture in other disease, left humerus** CC

3 √7ᵗʰ **M84.629 Pathological fracture in other disease, unspecified humerus** CC

√6ᵗʰ **M84.63 Pathological fracture in other disease, ulna and radius**

3 √7ᵗʰ **M84.631 Pathological fracture in other disease, right ulna** CC

3 √7ᵗʰ **M84.632 Pathological fracture in other disease, left ulna** CC

3 √7ᵗʰ **M84.633 Pathological fracture in other disease, right radius** CC

3 √7ᵗʰ **M84.634 Pathological fracture in other disease, left radius** CC

3 √7ᵗʰ **M84.639 Pathological fracture in other disease, unspecified ulna and radius** CC

√6ᵗʰ **M84.64 Pathological fracture in other disease, hand**

3 √7ᵗʰ **M84.641 Pathological fracture in other disease, right hand** CC

3 √7ᵗʰ **M84.642 Pathological fracture in other disease, left hand** CC

3 √7ᵗʰ **M84.649 Pathological fracture in other disease, unspecified hand** CC

√6ᵗʰ **M84.65 Pathological fracture in other disease, pelvis and femur**

3 √7ᵗʰ **M84.650 Pathological fracture in other disease, pelvis** CC

3,6 √7ᵗʰ **M84.651 Pathological fracture in other disease, right femur** CC HCC

3,6 √7ᵗʰ **M84.652 Pathological fracture in other disease, left femur** CC HCC

3,6 √7ᵗʰ **M84.653 Pathological fracture in other disease, unspecified femur** CC HCC

3,6 √7ᵗʰ **M84.659 Pathological fracture in other disease, hip, unspecified** CC HCC

√6ᵗʰ **M84.66 Pathological fracture in other disease, tibia and fibula**

3 √7ᵗʰ **M84.661 Pathological fracture in other disease, right tibia** CC

3 √7ᵗʰ **M84.662 Pathological fracture in other disease, left tibia** CC

3 √7ᵗʰ **M84.663 Pathological fracture in other disease, right fibula** CC

3 √7ᵗʰ **M84.664 Pathological fracture in other disease, left fibula** CC

3 √7ᵗʰ **M84.669 Pathological fracture in other disease, unspecified tibia and fibula** CC

√6ᵗʰ **M84.67 Pathological fracture in other disease, ankle and foot**

3 √7ᵗʰ **M84.671 Pathological fracture in other disease, right ankle** CC

3 √7ᵗʰ **M84.672 Pathological fracture in other disease, left ankle** CC

3 √7ᵗʰ **M84.673 Pathological fracture in other disease, unspecified ankle** CC

3 √7ᵗʰ **M84.674 Pathological fracture in other disease, right foot** CC

3 √7ᵗʰ **M84.675 Pathological fracture in other disease, left foot** CC

3 √7ᵗʰ **M84.676 Pathological fracture in other disease, unspecified foot** CC

3 √x7ᵗʰ **M84.68 Pathological fracture in other disease, other site** CC

√5ᵗʰ **M84.7 Nontraumatic fracture, not elsewhere classified**

√6ᵗʰ **M84.75 Atypical femoral fracture**

AHA: 2016,4Q,41-42

The appropriate 7th character is to be added to each code from M84.75.
A   initial encounter for fracture
D   subsequent encounter for fracture with routine healing
G   subsequent encounter for fracture with delayed healing
K   subsequent encounter for fracture with nonunion
P   subsequent encounter for fracture with malunion
S   sequela

CC Excl: For codes in subcategory M84.75:
CC with 7th character A: PDX collection 888
CC with 7th character K or P: PDX collection 897

3 √7ᵗʰ **M84.750 Atypical femoral fracture, unspecified** CC

3 √7ᵗʰ **M84.751 Incomplete atypical femoral fracture, right leg** CC

3 √7ᵗʰ **M84.752 Incomplete atypical femoral fracture, left leg** CC

3 √7ᵗʰ **M84.753 Incomplete atypical femoral fracture, unspecified leg** CC

3,6 √7ᵗʰ **M84.754 Complete transverse atypical femoral fracture, right leg** CC HCC

3,6 √7ᵗʰ **M84.755 Complete transverse atypical femoral fracture, left leg** CC HCC

3,6 √7ᵗʰ **M84.756 Complete transverse atypical femoral fracture, unspecified leg** CC HCC

3,6 √7ᵗʰ **M84.757 Complete oblique atypical femoral fracture, right leg** CC HCC

3,6 √7ᵗʰ **M84.758 Complete oblique atypical femoral fracture, left leg** CC HCC

3,6 √7ᵗʰ **M84.759 Complete oblique atypical femoral fracture, unspecified leg** CC HCC

√5ᵗʰ **M84.8 Other disorders of continuity of bone**

M84.80 Other disorders of continuity of bone, unspecified site

√6ᵗʰ **M84.81 Other disorders of continuity of bone, shoulder**

M84.811 Other disorders of continuity of bone, right shoulder

M84.812 Other disorders of continuity of bone, left shoulder

M84.819 Other disorders of continuity of bone, unspecified shoulder

√6ᵗʰ **M84.82** **Other disorders of continuity of bone, humerus**
  M84.821 Other disorders of continuity of bone, right humerus
  M84.822 Other disorders of continuity of bone, left humerus
  M84.829 Other disorders of continuity of bone, unspecified humerus

√6ᵗʰ **M84.83** **Other disorders of continuity of bone, ulna and radius**
  M84.831 Other disorders of continuity of bone, right ulna
  M84.832 Other disorders of continuity of bone, left ulna
  M84.833 Other disorders of continuity of bone, right radius
  M84.834 Other disorders of continuity of bone, left radius
  M84.839 Other disorders of continuity of bone, unspecified ulna and radius

√6ᵗʰ **M84.84** **Other disorders of continuity of bone, hand** .
  M84.841 Other disorders of continuity of bone, right hand
  M84.842 Other disorders of continuity of bone, left hand
  M84.849 Other disorders of continuity of bone, unspecified hand

√6ᵗʰ **M84.85** **Other disorders of continuity of bone, pelvic region and thigh**
  M84.851 Other disorders of continuity of bone, right pelvic region and thigh
  M84.852 Other disorders of continuity of bone, left pelvic region and thigh
  M84.859 Other disorders of continuity of bone, unspecified pelvic region and thigh

√6ᵗʰ **M84.86** **Other disorders of continuity of bone, tibia and fibula**
  M84.861 Other disorders of continuity of bone, right tibia
  M84.862 Other disorders of continuity of bone, left tibia
  M84.863 Other disorders of continuity of bone, right fibula
  M84.864 Other disorders of continuity of bone, left fibula
  M84.869 Other disorders of continuity of bone, unspecified tibia and fibula

√6ᵗʰ **M84.87** **Other disorders of continuity of bone, ankle and foot**
  M84.871 Other disorders of continuity of bone, right ankle and foot
  M84.872 Other disorders of continuity of bone, left ankle and foot
  M84.879 Other disorders of continuity of bone, unspecified ankle and foot

  M84.88 **Other disorders of continuity of bone, other site**

  M84.9 **Disorder of continuity of bone, unspecified**

√4ᵗʰ **M85** **Other disorders of bone density and structure**
  EXCLUDES 1 osteogenesis imperfecta (Q78.0)
       osteopetrosis (Q78.2)
       osteopoikilosis (Q78.8)
       polyostotic fibrous dysplasia (Q78.1)

√5ᵗʰ **M85.0** **Fibrous dysplasia (monostotic)**
  EXCLUDES 2 fibrous dysplasia of jaw (M27.8)
  M85.00 **Fibrous dysplasia (monostotic), unspecified site**

√6ᵗʰ **M85.01** **Fibrous dysplasia (monostotic), shoulder**
  M85.011 Fibrous dysplasia (monostotic), right shoulder
  M85.012 Fibrous dysplasia (monostotic), left shoulder
  M85.019 Fibrous dysplasia (monostotic), unspecified shoulder

√6ᵗʰ **M85.02** **Fibrous dysplasia (monostotic), upper arm**
  M85.021 Fibrous dysplasia (monostotic), right upper arm
  M85.022 Fibrous dysplasia (monostotic), left upper arm
  M85.029 Fibrous dysplasia (monostotic), unspecified upper arm

√6ᵗʰ **M85.03** **Fibrous dysplasia (monostotic), forearm**
  M85.031 Fibrous dysplasia (monostotic), right forearm
  M85.032 Fibrous dysplasia (monostotic), left forearm
  M85.039 Fibrous dysplasia (monostotic), unspecified forearm

√6ᵗʰ **M85.04** **Fibrous dysplasia (monostotic), hand**
  M85.041 Fibrous dysplasia (monostotic), right hand
  M85.042 Fibrous dysplasia (monostotic), left hand
  M85.049 Fibrous dysplasia (monostotic), unspecified hand

√6ᵗʰ **M85.05** **Fibrous dysplasia (monostotic), thigh**
  M85.051 Fibrous dysplasia (monostotic), right thigh
  M85.052 Fibrous dysplasia (monostotic), left thigh
  M85.059 Fibrous dysplasia (monostotic), unspecified thigh

√6ᵗʰ **M85.06** **Fibrous dysplasia (monostotic), lower leg**
  M85.061 Fibrous dysplasia (monostotic), right lower leg
  M85.062 Fibrous dysplasia (monostotic), left lower leg
  M85.069 Fibrous dysplasia (monostotic), unspecified lower leg

√6ᵗʰ **M85.07** **Fibrous dysplasia (monostotic), ankle and foot**
  M85.071 Fibrous dysplasia (monostotic), right ankle and foot
  M85.072 Fibrous dysplasia (monostotic), left ankle and foot
  M85.079 Fibrous dysplasia (monostotic), unspecified ankle and foot

  M85.08 **Fibrous dysplasia (monostotic), other site**
  M85.09 **Fibrous dysplasia (monostotic), multiple sites**

√5ᵗʰ **M85.1** **Skeletal fluorosis**
  M85.10 **Skeletal fluorosis, unspecified site**

√6ᵗʰ **M85.11** **Skeletal fluorosis, shoulder**
  M85.111 Skeletal fluorosis, right shoulder
  M85.112 Skeletal fluorosis, left shoulder
  M85.119 Skeletal fluorosis, unspecified shoulder

√6ᵗʰ **M85.12** **Skeletal fluorosis, upper arm**
  M85.121 Skeletal fluorosis, right upper arm
  M85.122 Skeletal fluorosis, left upper arm
  M85.129 Skeletal fluorosis, unspecified upper arm

√6ᵗʰ **M85.13** **Skeletal fluorosis, forearm**
  M85.131 Skeletal fluorosis, right forearm
  M85.132 Skeletal fluorosis, left forearm
  M85.139 Skeletal fluorosis, unspecified forearm

√6ᵗʰ **M85.14** **Skeletal fluorosis, hand**
  M85.141 Skeletal fluorosis, right hand
  M85.142 Skeletal fluorosis, left hand
  M85.149 Skeletal fluorosis, unspecified hand

√6ᵗʰ **M85.15** **Skeletal fluorosis, thigh**
  M85.151 Skeletal fluorosis, right thigh
  M85.152 Skeletal fluorosis, left thigh
  M85.159 Skeletal fluorosis, unspecified thigh

√6ᵗʰ **M85.16** **Skeletal fluorosis, lower leg**
  M85.161 Skeletal fluorosis, right lower leg
  M85.162 Skeletal fluorosis, left lower leg
  M85.169 Skeletal fluorosis, unspecified lower leg

√6ᵗʰ **M85.17** **Skeletal fluorosis, ankle and foot**
  M85.171 Skeletal fluorosis, right ankle and foot
  M85.172 Skeletal fluorosis, left ankle and foot
  M85.179 Skeletal fluorosis, unspecified ankle and foot

  M85.18 **Skeletal fluorosis, other site**
  M85.19 **Skeletal fluorosis, multiple sites**

  M85.2 **Hyperostosis of skull**
    DEF: Abnormal bone growth on the inner aspect of the cranial bones.

√5ᵗʰ **M85.3** **Osteitis condensans**
  M85.30 **Osteitis condensans, unspecified site**
√6ᵗʰ **M85.31** **Osteitis condensans, shoulder**
  M85.311 Osteitis condensans, right shoulder
  M85.312 Osteitis condensans, left shoulder

M85.319   Osteitis condensans, unspecified shoulder

√6ᵗʰ M85.32   **Osteitis condensans, upper arm**

    M85.321   Osteitis condensans, **right upper arm**

    M85.322   Osteitis condensans, **left upper arm**

    M85.329   Osteitis condensans, unspecified upper arm

√6ᵗʰ M85.33   **Osteitis condensans, forearm**

    M85.331   Osteitis condensans, **right forearm**

    M85.332   Osteitis condensans, **left forearm**

    M85.339   Osteitis condensans, unspecified forearm

√6ᵗʰ M85.34   **Osteitis condensans, hand**

    M85.341   Osteitis condensans, **right hand**

    M85.342   Osteitis condensans, **left hand**

    M85.349   Osteitis condensans, unspecified hand

√6ᵗʰ M85.35   **Osteitis condensans, thigh**

    M85.351   Osteitis condensans, **right thigh**

    M85.352   Osteitis condensans, **left thigh**

    M85.359   Osteitis condensans, unspecified thigh

√6ᵗʰ M85.36   **Osteitis condensans, lower leg**

    M85.361   Osteitis condensans, **right lower leg**

    M85.362   Osteitis condensans, **left lower leg**

    M85.369   Osteitis condensans, unspecified lower leg

√6ᵗʰ M85.37   **Osteitis condensans, ankle and foot**

    M85.371   Osteitis condensans, **right ankle and foot**

    M85.372   Osteitis condensans, **left ankle and foot**

    M85.379   Osteitis condensans, unspecified ankle and foot

    M85.38   **Osteitis condensans, other site**

    M85.39   **Osteitis condensans, multiple sites**

√5ᵗʰ M85.4   **Solitary bone cyst**

    EXCLUDES 2   solitary cyst of jaw (M27.4)

    M85.40   **Solitary bone cyst, unspecified site**

√6ᵗʰ M85.41   **Solitary bone cyst, shoulder**

    M85.411   Solitary bone cyst, **right shoulder**

    M85.412   Solitary bone cyst, **left shoulder**

    M85.419   Solitary bone cyst, unspecified shoulder

√6ᵗʰ M85.42   **Solitary bone cyst, humerus**

    M85.421   Solitary bone cyst, **right humerus**

    M85.422   Solitary bone cyst, **left humerus**

    M85.429   Solitary bone cyst, unspecified humerus

√6ᵗʰ M85.43   **Solitary bone cyst, ulna and radius**

    M85.431   Solitary bone cyst, **right ulna and radius**

    M85.432   Solitary bone cyst, **left ulna and radius**

    M85.439   Solitary bone cyst, unspecified ulna and radius

√6ᵗʰ M85.44   **Solitary bone cyst, hand**

    M85.441   Solitary bone cyst, **right hand**

    M85.442   Solitary bone cyst, **left hand**

    M85.449   Solitary bone cyst, unspecified hand

√6ᵗʰ M85.45   **Solitary bone cyst, pelvis**

    M85.451   Solitary bone cyst, **right pelvis**

    M85.452   Solitary bone cyst, **left pelvis**

    M85.459   Solitary bone cyst, unspecified pelvis

√6ᵗʰ M85.46   **Solitary bone cyst, tibia and fibula**

    M85.461   Solitary bone cyst, **right tibia and fibula**

    M85.462   Solitary bone cyst, **left tibia and fibula**

    M85.469   Solitary bone cyst, unspecified tibia and fibula

√6ᵗʰ M85.47   **Solitary bone cyst, ankle and foot**

    M85.471   Solitary bone cyst, **right ankle and foot**

    M85.472   Solitary bone cyst, **left ankle and foot**

    M85.479   Solitary bone cyst, unspecified ankle and foot

    M85.48   **Solitary bone cyst, other site**

√5ᵗʰ M85.5   **Aneurysmal bone cyst**

    EXCLUDES 2   aneurysmal cyst of jaw (M27.4)

    DEF: Solitary bone lesion that bulges into the periosteum and is marked by a calcified rim.

    M85.50   **Aneurysmal bone cyst, unspecified site**

√6ᵗʰ M85.51   **Aneurysmal bone cyst, shoulder**

    M85.511   Aneurysmal bone cyst, **right shoulder**

    M85.512   Aneurysmal bone cyst, **left shoulder**

    M85.519   Aneurysmal bone cyst, unspecified shoulder

√6ᵗʰ M85.52   **Aneurysmal bone cyst, upper arm**

    M85.521   Aneurysmal bone cyst, **right upper arm**

    M85.522   Aneurysmal bone cyst, **left upper arm**

    M85.529   Aneurysmal bone cyst, unspecified upper arm

√6ᵗʰ M85.53   **Aneurysmal bone cyst, forearm**

    M85.531   Aneurysmal bone cyst, **right forearm**

    M85.532   Aneurysmal bone cyst, **left forearm**

    M85.539   Aneurysmal bone cyst, unspecified forearm

√6ᵗʰ M85.54   **Aneurysmal bone cyst, hand**

    M85.541   Aneurysmal bone cyst, **right hand**

    M85.542   Aneurysmal bone cyst, **left hand**

    M85.549   Aneurysmal bone cyst, unspecified hand

√6ᵗʰ M85.55   **Aneurysmal bone cyst, thigh**

    M85.551   Aneurysmal bone cyst, **right thigh**

    M85.552   Aneurysmal bone cyst, **left thigh**

    M85.559   Aneurysmal bone cyst, unspecified thigh

√6ᵗʰ M85.56   **Aneurysmal bone cyst, lower leg**

    M85.561   Aneurysmal bone cyst, **right lower leg**

    M85.562   Aneurysmal bone cyst, **left lower leg**

    M85.569   Aneurysmal bone cyst, unspecified lower leg

√6ᵗʰ M85.57   **Aneurysmal bone cyst, ankle and foot**

    M85.571   Aneurysmal bone cyst, **right ankle and foot**

    M85.572   Aneurysmal bone cyst, **left ankle and foot**

    M85.579   Aneurysmal bone cyst, unspecified ankle and foot

    M85.58   **Aneurysmal bone cyst, other site**

    M85.59   **Aneurysmal bone cyst, multiple sites**

√5ᵗʰ M85.6   **Other cyst of bone**

    EXCLUDES 1   cyst of jaw NEC (M27.4)

            osteitis fibrosa cystica generalisata [von Recklinghausen's disease of bone] (E21.Ø)

    M85.60   **Other cyst of bone, unspecified site**

√6ᵗʰ M85.61   **Other cyst of bone, shoulder**

    M85.611   Other cyst of bone, **right shoulder**

    M85.612   Other cyst of bone, **left shoulder**

    M85.619   Other cyst of bone, unspecified shoulder

√6ᵗʰ M85.62   **Other cyst of bone, upper arm**

    M85.621   Other cyst of bone, **right upper arm**

    M85.622   Other cyst of bone, **left upper arm**

    M85.629   Other cyst of bone, unspecified upper arm

√6ᵗʰ M85.63   **Other cyst of bone, forearm**

    M85.631   Other cyst of bone, **right forearm**

    M85.632   Other cyst of bone, **left forearm**

    M85.639   Other cyst of bone, unspecified forearm

√6ᵗʰ M85.64   **Other cyst of bone, hand**

    M85.641   Other cyst of bone, **right hand**

    M85.642   Other cyst of bone, **left hand**

    M85.649   Other cyst of bone, unspecified hand

√6ᵗʰ M85.65   **Other cyst of bone, thigh**

    M85.651   Other cyst of bone, **right thigh**

    M85.652   Other cyst of bone, **left thigh**

    M85.659   Other cyst of bone, unspecified thigh

√6ᵗʰ M85.66   **Other cyst of bone, lower leg**

    M85.661   Other cyst of bone, **right lower leg**

    M85.662   Other cyst of bone, **left lower leg**

    M85.669   Other cyst of bone, unspecified lower leg

√6ᵗʰ M85.67   **Other cyst of bone, ankle and foot**

    M85.671   Other cyst of bone, **right ankle and foot**

    M85.672   Other cyst of bone, **left ankle and foot**

    M85.679   Other cyst of bone, unspecified ankle and foot

    M85.68   **Other cyst of bone, other site**

    M85.69   **Other cyst of bone, multiple sites**

√5ᵗʰ M85.8   **Other specified disorders of bone density and structure**

    Hyperostosis of bones, except skull

    Osteosclerosis, acquired

    EXCLUDES 1   diffuse idiopathic skeletal hyperostosis [DISH] (M48.1)

            osteosclerosis congenita (Q77.4)

            osteosclerosis fragilitas (generalista) (Q78.2)

            osteosclerosis myelofibrosis (D75.81)

    M85.80   **Other specified disorders of bone density and structure, unspecified site**

✔ Additional Character Required   √x7ᵗʰ Placeholder   Unacceptable PDx   Questionable PDx   Manifestation   Unspecified Dx   H1-H14 HAC   HCC CMS-HCC Dx   HIV HIV Dx

ICD-10-CM 2020   833

√6ᵗʰ **M85.81** Other specified disorders of bone density and structure, **shoulder**

M85.811 Other specified disorders of bone density and structure, **right shoulder**

M85.812 Other specified disorders of bone density and structure, **left shoulder**

M85.819 Other specified disorders of bone density and structure, **unspecified shoulder**

√6ᵗʰ **M85.82** Other specified disorders of bone density and structure, **upper arm**

M85.821 Other specified disorders of bone density and structure, **right upper arm**

M85.822 Other specified disorders of bone density and structure, **left upper arm**

M85.829 Other specified disorders of bone density and structure, **unspecified upper arm**

√6ᵗʰ **M85.83** Other specified disorders of bone density and structure, **forearm**

M85.831 Other specified disorders of bone density and structure, **right forearm**

M85.832 Other specified disorders of bone density and structure, **left forearm**

M85.839 Other specified disorders of bone density and structure, **unspecified forearm**

√6ᵗʰ **M85.84** Other specified disorders of bone density and structure, **hand**

M85.841 Other specified disorders of bone density and structure, **right hand**

M85.842 Other specified disorders of bone density and structure, **left hand**

M85.849 Other specified disorders of bone density and structure, **unspecified hand**

√6ᵗʰ **M85.85** Other specified disorders of bone density and structure, **thigh**

M85.851 Other specified disorders of bone density and structure, **right thigh**

M85.852 Other specified disorders of bone density and structure, **left thigh**

M85.859 Other specified disorders of bone density and structure, **unspecified thigh**

√6ᵗʰ **M85.86** Other specified disorders of bone density and structure, **lower leg**

M85.861 Other specified disorders of bone density and structure, **right lower leg**

M85.862 Other specified disorders of bone density and structure, **left lower leg**

M85.869 Other specified disorders of bone density and structure, **unspecified lower leg**

√6ᵗʰ **M85.87** Other specified disorders of bone density and structure, **ankle and foot**

M85.871 Other specified disorders of bone density and structure, **right ankle and foot**

M85.872 Other specified disorders of bone density and structure, **left ankle and foot**

M85.879 Other specified disorders of bone density and structure, **unspecified ankle and foot**

M85.88 Other specified disorders of bone density and structure, **other site**

M85.89 Other specified disorders of bone density and structure, **multiple sites**

M85.9 Disorder of bone density and structure, unspecified

Other osteopathies (M86-M90)

EXCLUDES 1 | postprocedural osteopathies (M96.-)

√4ᵗʰ **M86 Osteomyelitis**

Use additional code (B95-B97) to identify infectious agent

Use additional code to identify major osseous defect, if applicable (M89.7-)

EXCLUDES 1 | osteomyelitis due to:
echinococcus (B67.2)
gonococcus (A54.43)
salmonella (A02.24)

EXCLUDES 2 | osteomyelitis of:
orbit (H05.0-)
petrous bone (H70.2-)
vertebra (M46.2-)

√5ᵗʰ **M86.0** Acute hematogenous **osteomyelitis**

M86.00 Acute hematogenous osteomyelitis, unspecified site   CC HCC
CC Excl: PDX collection 898

√6ᵗʰ **M86.01** Acute hematogenous osteomyelitis, **shoulder**

CC Excl: For CC codes in subcategory M86.01: PDX collection 899

M86.011 Acute hematogenous osteomyelitis, **right shoulder**   CC HCC

M86.012 Acute hematogenous osteomyelitis, **left shoulder**   CC HCC

M86.019 Acute hematogenous osteomyelitis, unspecified **shoulder**   CC HCC

√6ᵗʰ **M86.02** Acute hematogenous osteomyelitis, **humerus**

CC Excl: For CC codes in subcategory M86.02: PDX collection 900

M86.021 Acute hematogenous osteomyelitis, **right humerus**   CC HCC

M86.022 Acute hematogenous osteomyelitis, **left humerus**   CC HCC

M86.029 Acute hematogenous osteomyelitis, unspecified **humerus**   CC HCC

√6ᵗʰ **M86.03** Acute hematogenous osteomyelitis, **radius and ulna**

CC Excl: For CC codes in subcategory M86.03: PDX collection 901

M86.031 Acute hematogenous osteomyelitis, **right radius and ulna**   CC HCC

M86.032 Acute hematogenous osteomyelitis, **left radius and ulna**   CC HCC

M86.039 Acute hematogenous osteomyelitis, unspecified **radius and ulna**   CC HCC

√6ᵗʰ **M86.04** Acute hematogenous osteomyelitis, **hand**

CC Excl: For CC codes in subcategory M86.04: PDX collection 902

M86.041 Acute hematogenous osteomyelitis, **right hand**   CC HCC

M86.042 Acute hematogenous osteomyelitis, **left hand**   CC HCC

M86.049 Acute hematogenous osteomyelitis, unspecified **hand**   CC HCC

√6ᵗʰ **M86.05** Acute hematogenous osteomyelitis, **femur**

CC Excl: For CC codes in subcategory M86.05: PDX collection 903

M86.051 Acute hematogenous osteomyelitis, **right femur**   CC HCC

M86.052 Acute hematogenous osteomyelitis, **left femur**   CC HCC

M86.059 Acute hematogenous osteomyelitis, unspecified **femur**   CC HCC

√6ᵗʰ **M86.06** Acute hematogenous osteomyelitis, **tibia and fibula**

CC Excl: For CC codes in subcategory M86.06: PDX collection 904

M86.061 Acute hematogenous osteomyelitis, **right tibia and fibula**   CC HCC

M86.062 Acute hematogenous osteomyelitis, **left tibia and fibula**   CC HCC

M86.069 Acute hematogenous osteomyelitis, unspecified **tibia and fibula**   CC HCC

√6ᵗʰ **M86.07** Acute hematogenous osteomyelitis, **ankle and foot**

CC Excl: For CC codes in subcategory M86.07: PDX collection 905

M86.071 Acute hematogenous osteomyelitis, **right ankle and foot**   CC HCC

M86.072 Acute hematogenous osteomyelitis, **left ankle and foot**   CC HCC

M86.079 Acute hematogenous osteomyelitis, unspecified **ankle and foot**   CC HCC

N Newborn: 0 | P Pediatric: 0-17 | M Maternity: 9-64 | A Adult: 15-124 | MCC Major Complication/Comorbidity | CC Complication/Comorbidity | SW Severe Wound Dx

M86.08 **Acute hematogenous osteomyelitis, other sites** `CC` `HCC`
CC Excl: PDX collection 882

M86.09 **Acute hematogenous osteomyelitis, multiple sites** `CC` `HCC`
CC Excl: PDX collection 898

√5ᵗʰ **M86.1** **Other acute osteomyelitis**

     M86.10 **Other acute osteomyelitis, unspecified site** `CC` `HCC`
CC Excl: PDX collection 898

     √6ᵗʰ **M86.11** **Other acute osteomyelitis, shoulder**
CC Excl: For CC codes in subcategory M86.11: PDX collection 899

         M86.111 **Other acute osteomyelitis, right shoulder** `CC` `HCC`

         M86.112 **Other acute osteomyelitis, left shoulder** `CC` `HCC`

         M86.119 **Other acute osteomyelitis, unspecified shoulder** `CC` `HCC`

     √6ᵗʰ **M86.12** **Other acute osteomyelitis, humerus**
CC Excl: For CC codes in subcategory M86.12: PDX collection 900

         M86.121 **Other acute osteomyelitis, right humerus** `CC` `HCC`

         M86.122 **Other acute osteomyelitis, left humerus** `CC` `HCC`

         M86.129 **Other acute osteomyelitis, unspecified humerus** `CC` `HCC`

     √6ᵗʰ **M86.13** **Other acute osteomyelitis, radius and ulna**
CC Excl: For CC codes in subcategory M86.13: PDX collection 901

         M86.131 **Other acute osteomyelitis, right radius and ulna** `CC` `HCC`

         M86.132 **Other acute osteomyelitis, left radius and ulna** `CC` `HCC`

         M86.139 **Other acute osteomyelitis, unspecified radius and ulna** `CC` `HCC`

     √6ᵗʰ **M86.14** **Other acute osteomyelitis, hand**
CC Excl: For CC codes in subcategory M86.14: PDX collection 902

         M86.141 **Other acute osteomyelitis, right hand** `CC` `HCC`

         M86.142 **Other acute osteomyelitis, left hand** `CC` `HCC`

         M86.149 **Other acute osteomyelitis, unspecified hand** `CC` `HCC`

     √6ᵗʰ **M86.15** **Other acute osteomyelitis, femur**
CC Excl: For CC codes in subcategory M86.15: PDX collection 903

         M86.151 **Other acute osteomyelitis, right femur** `CC` `HCC`

         M86.152 **Other acute osteomyelitis, left femur** `CC` `HCC`

         M86.159 **Other acute osteomyelitis, unspecified femur** `CC` `HCC`

     √6ᵗʰ **M86.16** **Other acute osteomyelitis, tibia and fibula**
CC Excl: For CC codes in subcategory M86.16: PDX collection 904

         M86.161 **Other acute osteomyelitis, right tibia and fibula** `CC` `HCC`

         M86.162 **Other acute osteomyelitis, left tibia and fibula** `CC` `HCC`

         M86.169 **Other acute osteomyelitis, unspecified tibia and fibula** `CC` `HCC`

     √6ᵗʰ **M86.17** **Other acute osteomyelitis, ankle and foot**
CC Excl: For CC codes in subcategory M86.17: PDX collection 905

         M86.171 **Other acute osteomyelitis, right ankle and foot** `CC` `HCC`

         M86.172 **Other acute osteomyelitis, left ankle and foot** `CC` `HCC`

         M86.179 **Other acute osteomyelitis, unspecified ankle and foot** `CC` `HCC`

     M86.18 **Other acute osteomyelitis, other site** `CC` `HCC`
CC Excl: PDX collection 882

     M86.19 **Other acute osteomyelitis, multiple sites** `CC` `HCC`
CC Excl: PDX collection 898

√5ᵗʰ **M86.2** **Subacute osteomyelitis**

     M86.20 **Subacute osteomyelitis, unspecified site** `CC` `HCC`
CC Excl: PDX collection 898

     √6ᵗʰ **M86.21** **Subacute osteomyelitis, shoulder**
CC Excl: For CC codes in subcategory M86.21: PDX collection 899

         M86.211 **Subacute osteomyelitis, right shoulder** `CC` `HCC`

         M86.212 **Subacute osteomyelitis, left shoulder** `CC` `HCC`

         M86.219 **Subacute osteomyelitis, unspecified shoulder** `CC` `HCC`

     √6ᵗʰ **M86.22** **Subacute osteomyelitis, humerus**
CC Excl: For CC codes in subcategory M86.22: PDX collection 900

         M86.221 **Subacute osteomyelitis, right humerus** `CC` `HCC`

         M86.222 **Subacute osteomyelitis, left humerus** `CC` `HCC`

         M86.229 **Subacute osteomyelitis, unspecified humerus** `CC` `HCC`

     √6ᵗʰ **M86.23** **Subacute osteomyelitis, radius and ulna**
CC Excl: For CC codes in subcategory M86.23: PDX collection 901

         M86.231 **Subacute osteomyelitis, right radius and ulna** `CC` `HCC`

         M86.232 **Subacute osteomyelitis, left radius and ulna** `CC` `HCC`

         M86.239 **Subacute osteomyelitis, unspecified radius and ulna** `CC` `HCC`

     √6ᵗʰ **M86.24** **Subacute osteomyelitis, hand**
CC Excl: For CC codes in subcategory M86.24: PDX collection 902

         M86.241 **Subacute osteomyelitis, right hand** `CC` `HCC`

         M86.242 **Subacute osteomyelitis, left hand** `CC` `HCC`

         M86.249 **Subacute osteomyelitis, unspecified hand** `CC` `HCC`

     √6ᵗʰ **M86.25** **Subacute osteomyelitis, femur**
CC Excl: For CC codes in subcategory M86.25: PDX collection 903

         M86.251 **Subacute osteomyelitis, right femur** `CC` `HCC`

         M86.252 **Subacute osteomyelitis, left femur** `CC` `HCC`

         M86.259 **Subacute osteomyelitis, unspecified femur** `CC` `HCC`

     √6ᵗʰ **M86.26** **Subacute osteomyelitis, tibia and fibula**
CC Excl: For CC codes in subcategory M86.26: PDX collection 904

         M86.261 **Subacute osteomyelitis, right tibia and fibula** `CC` `HCC`

         M86.262 **Subacute osteomyelitis, left tibia and fibula** `CC` `HCC`

         M86.269 **Subacute osteomyelitis, unspecified tibia and fibula** `CC` `HCC`

     √6ᵗʰ **M86.27** **Subacute osteomyelitis, ankle and foot**
CC Excl: For CC codes in subcategory M86.27: PDX collection 905

         M86.271 **Subacute osteomyelitis, right ankle and foot** `CC` `HCC`

         M86.272 **Subacute osteomyelitis, left ankle and foot** `CC` `HCC`

         M86.279 **Subacute osteomyelitis, unspecified ankle and foot** `CC` `HCC`

     M86.28 **Subacute osteomyelitis, other site** `CC` `HCC`
CC Excl: PDX collection 882

     M86.29 **Subacute osteomyelitis, multiple sites** `CC` `HCC`
CC Excl: PDX collection 898

Chapter 13. Diseases of the Musculoskeletal System and Connective Tissue

M86.3–M86.49

√5th **M86.3** Chronic multifocal **osteomyelitis**

     CC Excl: For CC codes in subcategory M86.3, unless otherwise noted: PDX collection 881

     M86.30 Chronic multifocal osteomyelitis, unspecified site   `CC` `HCC`

         CC Excl: PDX collection 906

     √6th **M86.31** Chronic multifocal osteomyelitis, **shoulder**

         M86.311 Chronic multifocal osteomyelitis, **right** shoulder   `CC` `HCC`

         M86.312 Chronic multifocal osteomyelitis, **left** shoulder   `CC` `HCC`

         M86.319 Chronic multifocal osteomyelitis, unspecified shoulder   `CC` `HCC`

     √6th **M86.32** Chronic multifocal osteomyelitis, **humerus**

         M86.321 Chronic multifocal osteomyelitis, **right** humerus   `CC` `HCC`

         M86.322 Chronic multifocal osteomyelitis, **left** humerus   `CC` `HCC`

         M86.329 Chronic multifocal osteomyelitis, unspecified humerus   `CC` `HCC`

     √6th **M86.33** Chronic multifocal osteomyelitis, **radius and ulna**

         M86.331 Chronic multifocal osteomyelitis, **right** radius and ulna   `CC` `HCC`

         M86.332 Chronic multifocal osteomyelitis, **left** radius and ulna   `CC` `HCC`

         M86.339 Chronic multifocal osteomyelitis, unspecified radius and ulna   `CC` `HCC`

     √6th **M86.34** Chronic multifocal osteomyelitis, **hand**

         M86.341 Chronic multifocal osteomyelitis, **right** hand   `CC` `HCC`

         M86.342 Chronic multifocal osteomyelitis, **left** hand   `CC` `HCC`

         M86.349 Chronic multifocal osteomyelitis, unspecified hand   `CC` `HCC`

     √6th **M86.35** Chronic multifocal osteomyelitis, **femur**

         M86.351 Chronic multifocal osteomyelitis, **right** femur   `CC` `HCC`

         M86.352 Chronic multifocal osteomyelitis, **left** femur   `CC` `HCC`

         M86.359 Chronic multifocal osteomyelitis, unspecified femur   `CC` `HCC`

     √6th **M86.36** Chronic multifocal osteomyelitis, **tibia and fibula**

         M86.361 Chronic multifocal osteomyelitis, **right** tibia and fibula   `CC` `HCC`

         M86.362 Chronic multifocal osteomyelitis, **left** tibia and fibula   `CC` `HCC`

         M86.369 Chronic multifocal osteomyelitis, unspecified tibia and fibula   `CC` `HCC`

     √6th **M86.37** Chronic multifocal osteomyelitis, **ankle and foot**

         M86.371 Chronic multifocal osteomyelitis, **right** ankle and foot   `CC` `HCC`

         M86.372 Chronic multifocal osteomyelitis, **left** ankle and foot   `CC` `HCC`

         M86.379 Chronic multifocal osteomyelitis, unspecified ankle and foot   `CC` `HCC`

     M86.38 Chronic multifocal osteomyelitis, other site   `CC` `HCC`

     M86.39 Chronic multifocal osteomyelitis, multiple sites   `CC` `HCC`

√5th **M86.4** Chronic **osteomyelitis** with draining sinus

     CC Excl: For CC codes in subcategory M86.4, unless otherwise noted: PDX collection 881

     M86.40 Chronic osteomyelitis with draining sinus, unspecified site   `CC` `HCC`

         CC Excl: PDX collection 906

     √6th **M86.41** Chronic osteomyelitis with draining sinus, **shoulder**

         M86.411 Chronic osteomyelitis with draining sinus, **right** shoulder   `CC` `HCC`

         M86.412 Chronic osteomyelitis with draining sinus, **left** shoulder   `CC` `HCC`

         M86.419 Chronic osteomyelitis with draining sinus, unspecified shoulder   `CC` `HCC`

     √6th **M86.42** Chronic osteomyelitis with draining sinus, **humerus**

         M86.421 Chronic osteomyelitis with draining sinus, **right** humerus   `CC` `HCC`

         M86.422 Chronic osteomyelitis with draining sinus, **left** humerus   `CC` `HCC`

         M86.429 Chronic osteomyelitis with draining sinus, unspecified humerus   `CC` `HCC`

     √6th **M86.43** Chronic osteomyelitis with draining sinus, **radius and ulna**

         M86.431 Chronic osteomyelitis with draining sinus, **right** radius and ulna   `CC` `HCC`

         M86.432 Chronic osteomyelitis with draining sinus, **left** radius and ulna   `CC` `HCC`

         M86.439 Chronic osteomyelitis with draining sinus, unspecified radius and ulna   `CC` `HCC`

     √6th **M86.44** Chronic osteomyelitis with draining sinus, **hand**

         M86.441 Chronic osteomyelitis with draining sinus, **right** hand   `CC` `HCC`

         M86.442 Chronic osteomyelitis with draining sinus, **left** hand   `CC` `HCC`

         M86.449 Chronic osteomyelitis with draining sinus, unspecified hand   `CC` `HCC`

     √6th **M86.45** Chronic osteomyelitis with draining sinus, **femur**

         M86.451 Chronic osteomyelitis with draining sinus, **right** femur   `CC` `HCC`

         M86.452 Chronic osteomyelitis with draining sinus, **left** femur   `CC` `HCC`

         M86.459 Chronic osteomyelitis with draining sinus, unspecified femur   `CC` `HCC`

     √6th **M86.46** Chronic osteomyelitis with draining sinus, **tibia and fibula**

         M86.461 Chronic osteomyelitis with draining sinus, **right** tibia and fibula   `CC` `HCC`

         M86.462 Chronic osteomyelitis with draining sinus, **left** tibia and fibula   `CC` `HCC`

         M86.469 Chronic osteomyelitis with draining sinus, unspecified tibia and fibula   `CC` `HCC`

     √6th **M86.47** Chronic osteomyelitis with draining sinus, **ankle and foot**

         M86.471 Chronic osteomyelitis with draining sinus, **right** ankle and foot   `CC` `HCC`

         M86.472 Chronic osteomyelitis with draining sinus, **left** ankle and foot   `CC` `HCC`

         M86.479 Chronic osteomyelitis with draining sinus, unspecified ankle and foot   `CC` `HCC`

     M86.48 Chronic osteomyelitis with draining sinus, other site   `CC` `HCC`

     M86.49 Chronic osteomyelitis with draining sinus, multiple sites   `CC` `HCC`

N Newborn: 0   P Pediatric: 0-17   M Maternity: 9-64   A Adult: 15-124   **MCC** Major Complication/Comorbidity   **CC** Complication/Comorbidity   **SW** Severe Wound Dx

836   ICD-10-CM 2020

✓5ᵗʰ M86.5   Other chronic hematogenous osteomyelitis

CC Excl: For CC codes in subcategory M86.5, unless otherwise noted: PDX collection 881

    M86.50   Other chronic hematogenous osteomyelitis, unspecified site   `CC` `HCC`
       CC Excl: PDX collection 906

   ✓6ᵗʰ M86.51   Other chronic hematogenous osteomyelitis, shoulder

       M86.511   Other chronic hematogenous osteomyelitis, right shoulder   `CC` `HCC`

       M86.512   Other chronic hematogenous osteomyelitis, left shoulder   `CC` `HCC`

       M86.519   Other chronic hematogenous osteomyelitis, unspecified shoulder   `CC` `HCC`

   ✓6ᵗʰ M86.52   Other chronic hematogenous osteomyelitis, humerus

       M86.521   Other chronic hematogenous osteomyelitis, right humerus   `CC` `HCC`

       M86.522   Other chronic hematogenous osteomyelitis, left humerus   `CC` `HCC`

       M86.529   Other chronic hematogenous osteomyelitis, unspecified humerus   `CC` `HCC`

   ✓6ᵗʰ M86.53   Other chronic hematogenous osteomyelitis, radius and ulna

       M86.531   Other chronic hematogenous osteomyelitis, right radius and ulna   `CC` `HCC`

       M86.532   Other chronic hematogenous osteomyelitis, left radius and ulna   `CC` `HCC`

       M86.539   Other chronic hematogenous osteomyelitis, unspecified radius and ulna   `CC` `HCC`

   ✓6ᵗʰ M86.54   Other chronic hematogenous osteomyelitis, hand

       M86.541   Other chronic hematogenous osteomyelitis, right hand   `CC` `HCC`

       M86.542   Other chronic hematogenous osteomyelitis, left hand   `CC` `HCC`

       M86.549   Other chronic hematogenous osteomyelitis, unspecified hand   `CC` `HCC`

   ✓6ᵗʰ M86.55   Other chronic hematogenous osteomyelitis, femur

       M86.551   Other chronic hematogenous osteomyelitis, right femur   `CC` `HCC`

       M86.552   Other chronic hematogenous osteomyelitis, left femur   `CC` `HCC`

       M86.559   Other chronic hematogenous osteomyelitis, unspecified femur   `CC` `HCC`

   ✓6ᵗʰ M86.56   Other chronic hematogenous osteomyelitis, tibia and fibula

       M86.561   Other chronic hematogenous osteomyelitis, right tibia and fibula   `CC` `HCC`

       M86.562   Other chronic hematogenous osteomyelitis, left tibia and fibula   `CC` `HCC`

       M86.569   Other chronic hematogenous osteomyelitis, unspecified tibia and fibula   `CC` `HCC`

   ✓6ᵗʰ M86.57   Other chronic hematogenous osteomyelitis, ankle and foot

       M86.571   Other chronic hematogenous osteomyelitis, right ankle and foot   `CC` `HCC`

       M86.572   Other chronic hematogenous osteomyelitis, left ankle and foot   `CC` `HCC`

       M86.579   Other chronic hematogenous osteomyelitis, unspecified ankle and foot   `CC` `HCC`

     M86.58   Other chronic hematogenous osteomyelitis, other site   `CC` `HCC`

     M86.59   Other chronic hematogenous osteomyelitis, multiple sites   `CC` `HCC`

✓5ᵗʰ M86.6   Other chronic osteomyelitis

CC Excl: For CC codes in subcategory M86.6, unless otherwise noted: PDX collection 881

    M86.60   Other chronic osteomyelitis, unspecified site   `CC` `HCC`
       CC Excl: PDX collection 906

   ✓6ᵗʰ M86.61   Other chronic osteomyelitis, shoulder

       M86.611   Other chronic osteomyelitis, right shoulder   `CC` `HCC`

       M86.612   Other chronic osteomyelitis, left shoulder   `CC` `HCC`

       M86.619   Other chronic osteomyelitis, unspecified shoulder   `CC` `HCC`

   ✓6ᵗʰ M86.62   Other chronic osteomyelitis, humerus

       M86.621   Other chronic osteomyelitis, right humerus   `CC` `HCC`

       M86.622   Other chronic osteomyelitis, left humerus   `CC` `HCC`

       M86.629   Other chronic osteomyelitis, unspecified humerus   `CC` `HCC`

   ✓6ᵗʰ M86.63   Other chronic osteomyelitis, radius and ulna

       M86.631   Other chronic osteomyelitis, right radius and ulna   `CC` `HCC`

       M86.632   Other chronic osteomyelitis, left radius and ulna   `CC` `HCC`

       M86.639   Other chronic osteomyelitis, unspecified radius and ulna   `CC` `HCC`

   ✓6ᵗʰ M86.64   Other chronic osteomyelitis, hand

       M86.641   Other chronic osteomyelitis, right hand   `CC` `HCC`

       M86.642   Other chronic osteomyelitis, left hand   `CC` `HCC`

       M86.649   Other chronic osteomyelitis, unspecified hand   `CC` `HCC`

   ✓6ᵗʰ M86.65   Other chronic osteomyelitis, thigh

       M86.651   Other chronic osteomyelitis, right thigh   `CC` `HCC`

       M86.652   Other chronic osteomyelitis, left thigh   `CC` `HCC`

       M86.659   Other chronic osteomyelitis, unspecified thigh   `CC` `HCC`

   ✓6ᵗʰ M86.66   Other chronic osteomyelitis, tibia and fibula

       M86.661   Other chronic osteomyelitis, right tibia and fibula   `CC` `HCC`

       M86.662   Other chronic osteomyelitis, left tibia and fibula   `CC` `HCC`

       M86.669   Other chronic osteomyelitis, unspecified tibia and fibula   `CC` `HCC`

☑ Additional Character Required   ✓x7ᵗʰ Placeholder   Unacceptable PDx   Questionable PDx   Manifestation   Unspecified Dx   `H1`-`H14` HAC   `HCC` CMS-HCC Dx   `HIV` HIV Dx

ICD-10-CM 2020   837

√6ᵗʰ **M86.67** **Other chronic osteomyelitis, ankle and foot**

    M86.671 **Other chronic** `CC` `HCC`
       osteomyelitis, right ankle
       and foot
         AHA: 2016,1Q,13

    M86.672 **Other chronic** `CC` `HCC`
       osteomyelitis, left ankle
       and foot

    M86.679 **Other chronic** `CC` `HCC`
       osteomyelitis, unspecified
       ankle and foot

M86.68 **Other chronic osteomyelitis, other** `CC` `HCC`
    site

M86.69 **Other chronic osteomyelitis,** `CC` `HCC`
    multiple sites

√5ᵗʰ **M86.8** **Other osteomyelitis**

    Brodie's abscess

    CC Excl: For CC codes in subcategory M86.8, unless otherwise noted: PDX collection 881

√6ᵗʰ **M86.8X** **Other osteomyelitis**

    M86.8X0 **Other osteomyelitis,** `CC` `HCC`
       multiple sites

    M86.8X1 **Other osteomyelitis,** `CC` `HCC`
       shoulder

    M86.8X2 **Other osteomyelitis,** `CC` `HCC`
       upper arm

    M86.8X3 **Other osteomyelitis,** `CC` `HCC`
       forearm

    M86.8X4 **Other osteomyelitis, hand** `CC` `HCC`

    M86.8X5 **Other osteomyelitis, thigh** `CC` `HCC`

    M86.8X6 **Other osteomyelitis, lower** `CC` `HCC`
       leg

    M86.8X7 **Other osteomyelitis, ankle** `CC` `HCC`
       and foot

    M86.8X8 **Other osteomyelitis, other** `CC` `HCC`
       site

    M86.8X9 **Other osteomyelitis,** `CC` `HCC`
       unspecified sites
         CC Excl: PDX collection 906

M86.9 **Osteomyelitis, unspecified** `CC` `HCC`

    Infection of bone NOS

    Periostitis without osteomyelitis

    CC Excl: PDX collection 906

√4ᵗʰ **M87** **Osteonecrosis**

    INCLUDES   avascular necrosis of bone

    Use additional code to identify major osseous defect, if applicable (M89.7-)

    EXCLUDES 1   juvenile osteonecrosis (M91-M92)
                osteochondropathies (M90-M93)

    CC Excl: For CC codes in category M87, unless otherwise noted: PDX collection 907

√5ᵗʰ **M87.0** **Idiopathic aseptic necrosis of bone**

    M87.00 **Idiopathic aseptic necrosis of** `CC` `HCC`
       unspecified bone

√6ᵗʰ **M87.01** **Idiopathic aseptic necrosis of shoulder**

    Idiopathic aseptic necrosis of clavicle and scapula

    CC Excl: For CC codes in subcategory M87.01: PDX collection 908

    M87.011 **Idiopathic aseptic necrosis** `CC` `HCC`
       of right shoulder

    M87.012 **Idiopathic aseptic necrosis** `CC` `HCC`
       of left shoulder

    M87.019 **Idiopathic aseptic necrosis** `CC` `HCC`
       of unspecified shoulder

√6ᵗʰ **M87.02** **Idiopathic aseptic necrosis of humerus**

    CC Excl: For CC codes in subcategory M87.02: PDX collection 908

    M87.021 **Idiopathic aseptic necrosis** `CC` `HCC`
       of right humerus

    M87.022 **Idiopathic aseptic necrosis** `CC` `HCC`
       of left humerus

    M87.029 **Idiopathic aseptic necrosis** `CC` `HCC`
       of unspecified humerus

√6ᵗʰ **M87.03** **Idiopathic aseptic necrosis of radius, ulna and carpus**

    M87.031 **Idiopathic aseptic necrosis** `CC` `HCC`
       of right radius

    M87.032 **Idiopathic aseptic necrosis** `CC` `HCC`
       of left radius

    M87.033 **Idiopathic aseptic necrosis** `CC` `HCC`
       of unspecified radius

    M87.034 **Idiopathic aseptic necrosis** `CC` `HCC`
       of right ulna

    M87.035 **Idiopathic aseptic necrosis** `CC` `HCC`
       of left ulna

    M87.036 **Idiopathic aseptic necrosis** `CC` `HCC`
       of unspecified ulna

    M87.037 **Idiopathic aseptic necrosis** `CC` `HCC`
       of right carpus

    M87.038 **Idiopathic aseptic necrosis** `CC` `HCC`
       of left carpus

    M87.039 **Idiopathic aseptic necrosis** `CC` `HCC`
       of unspecified carpus

√6ᵗʰ **M87.04** **Idiopathic aseptic necrosis of hand and fingers**

    Idiopathic aseptic necrosis of metacarpals and phalanges of hands

    M87.041 **Idiopathic aseptic necrosis** `CC` `HCC`
       of right hand

    M87.042 **Idiopathic aseptic necrosis** `CC` `HCC`
       of left hand

    M87.043 **Idiopathic aseptic necrosis** `CC` `HCC`
       of unspecified hand

    M87.044 **Idiopathic aseptic necrosis** `CC` `HCC`
       of right finger(s)

    M87.045 **Idiopathic aseptic necrosis** `CC` `HCC`
       of left finger(s)

    M87.046 **Idiopathic aseptic necrosis** `CC` `HCC`
       of unspecified finger(s)

√6ᵗʰ **M87.05** **Idiopathic aseptic necrosis of pelvis and femur**

    M87.050 **Idiopathic aseptic necrosis** `CC` `HCC`
       of pelvis

    M87.051 **Idiopathic aseptic necrosis** `CC` `HCC`
       of right femur
         CC Excl: PDX collection 909

    M87.052 **Idiopathic aseptic necrosis** `CC` `HCC`
       of left femur
         CC Excl: PDX collection 909

    M87.059 **Idiopathic aseptic necrosis** `CC` `HCC`
       of unspecified femur
         CC Excl: PDX collection 909

√6ᵗʰ **M87.06** **Idiopathic aseptic necrosis of tibia and fibula**

    M87.061 **Idiopathic aseptic necrosis** `CC` `HCC`
       of right tibia

    M87.062 **Idiopathic aseptic necrosis** `CC` `HCC`
       of left tibia

    M87.063 **Idiopathic aseptic necrosis** `CC` `HCC`
       of unspecified tibia

    M87.064 **Idiopathic aseptic necrosis** `CC` `HCC`
       of right fibula

    M87.065 **Idiopathic aseptic necrosis** `CC` `HCC`
       of left fibula

    M87.066 **Idiopathic aseptic necrosis** `CC` `HCC`
       of unspecified fibula

√6ᵗʰ **M87.07** **Idiopathic aseptic necrosis of ankle, foot and toes**

    Idiopathic aseptic necrosis of metatarsus, tarsus, and phalanges of toes

    M87.071 **Idiopathic aseptic necrosis** `CC` `HCC`
       of right ankle

    M87.072 **Idiopathic aseptic necrosis** `CC` `HCC`
       of left ankle

    M87.073 **Idiopathic aseptic necrosis** `CC` `HCC`
       of unspecified ankle

    M87.074 **Idiopathic aseptic necrosis** `CC` `HCC`
       of right foot
         CC Excl: PDX collection 910

    M87.075 **Idiopathic aseptic necrosis** `CC` `HCC`
       of left foot
         CC Excl: PDX collection 910

    M87.076 **Idiopathic aseptic necrosis** `CC` `HCC`
       of unspecified foot
         CC Excl: PDX collection 910

    M87.077 **Idiopathic aseptic necrosis** `CC` `HCC`
       of right toe(s)

    M87.078 **Idiopathic aseptic necrosis** `CC` `HCC`
       of left toe(s)

    M87.079 **Idiopathic aseptic necrosis** `CC` `HCC`
       of unspecified toe(s)

M87.08 **Idiopathic aseptic necrosis of bone,** `CC` `HCC`
    other site

M87.09 **Idiopathic aseptic necrosis of bone,** `CC` `HCC`
    multiple sites

N Newborn: 0   P Pediatric: 0-17   M Maternity: 9-64   A Adult: 15-124   **MCC** Major Complication/Comorbidity   **CC** Complication/Comorbidity   **SW** Severe Wound Dx

838   ICD-10-CM 2020

√5ᵗʰ M87.1 Osteonecrosis due to drugs

Use additional code for adverse effect, if applicable, to identify drug (T36-T50 with fifth or sixth character 5)

M87.10 Osteonecrosis due to drugs, unspecified bone `CC` `HCC`

√6ᵗʰ M87.11 Osteonecrosis due to drugs, shoulder

    M87.111 Osteonecrosis due to drugs, right shoulder `CC` `HCC`

    M87.112 Osteonecrosis due to drugs, left shoulder `CC` `HCC`

    M87.119 Osteonecrosis due to drugs, unspecified shoulder `CC` `HCC`

√6ᵗʰ M87.12 Osteonecrosis due to drugs, humerus

    CC Excl: For CC codes in subcategory M87.12: PDX collection 908

    M87.121 Osteonecrosis due to drugs, right humerus `CC` `HCC`

    M87.122 Osteonecrosis due to drugs, left humerus `CC` `HCC`

    M87.129 Osteonecrosis due to drugs, unspecified humerus `CC` `HCC`

√6ᵗʰ M87.13 Osteonecrosis due to drugs of radius, ulna and carpus

    M87.131 Osteonecrosis due to drugs of right radius `CC` `HCC`

    M87.132 Osteonecrosis due to drugs of left radius `CC` `HCC`

    M87.133 Osteonecrosis due to drugs of unspecified radius `CC` `HCC`

    M87.134 Osteonecrosis due to drugs of right ulna `CC` `HCC`

    M87.135 Osteonecrosis due to drugs of left ulna `CC` `HCC`

    M87.136 Osteonecrosis due to drugs of unspecified ulna `CC` `HCC`

    M87.137 Osteonecrosis due to drugs of right carpus `CC` `HCC`

    M87.138 Osteonecrosis due to drugs of left carpus `CC` `HCC`

    M87.139 Osteonecrosis due to drugs of unspecified carpus `CC` `HCC`

√6ᵗʰ M87.14 Osteonecrosis due to drugs, hand and fingers

    M87.141 Osteonecrosis due to drugs, right hand `CC` `HCC`

    M87.142 Osteonecrosis due to drugs, left hand `CC` `HCC`

    M87.143 Osteonecrosis due to drugs, unspecified hand `CC` `HCC`

    M87.144 Osteonecrosis due to drugs, right finger(s) `CC` `HCC`

    M87.145 Osteonecrosis due to drugs, left finger(s) `CC` `HCC`

    M87.146 Osteonecrosis due to drugs, unspecified finger(s) `CC` `HCC`

√6ᵗʰ M87.15 Osteonecrosis due to drugs, pelvis and femur

    CC Excl: For CC codes in subcategory M87.15: PDX collection 909

    M87.150 Osteonecrosis due to drugs, pelvis `CC` `HCC`

    M87.151 Osteonecrosis due to drugs, right femur `CC` `HCC`

    M87.152 Osteonecrosis due to drugs, left femur `CC` `HCC`

    M87.159 Osteonecrosis due to drugs, unspecified femur `CC` `HCC`

√6ᵗʰ M87.16 Osteonecrosis due to drugs, tibia and fibula

    M87.161 Osteonecrosis due to drugs, right tibia `CC` `HCC`

    M87.162 Osteonecrosis due to drugs, left tibia `CC` `HCC`

    M87.163 Osteonecrosis due to drugs, unspecified tibia `CC` `HCC`

    M87.164 Osteonecrosis due to drugs, right fibula `CC` `HCC`

    M87.165 Osteonecrosis due to drugs, left fibula `CC` `HCC`

    M87.166 Osteonecrosis due to drugs, unspecified fibula `CC` `HCC`

√6ᵗʰ M87.17 Osteonecrosis due to drugs, ankle, foot and toes

    M87.171 Osteonecrosis due to drugs, right ankle `CC` `HCC`

    M87.172 Osteonecrosis due to drugs, left ankle `CC` `HCC`

    M87.173 Osteonecrosis due to drugs, unspecified ankle `CC` `HCC`

    M87.174 Osteonecrosis due to drugs, right foot `CC` `HCC`
        CC Excl: PDX collection 910

    M87.175 Osteonecrosis due to drugs, left foot `CC` `HCC`
        CC Excl: PDX collection 910

    M87.176 Osteonecrosis due to drugs, unspecified foot `CC` `HCC`
        CC Excl: PDX collection 910

    M87.177 Osteonecrosis due to drugs, right toe(s) `CC` `HCC`

    M87.178 Osteonecrosis due to drugs, left toe(s) `CC` `HCC`

    M87.179 Osteonecrosis due to drugs, unspecified toe(s) `CC` `HCC`

√6ᵗʰ M87.18 Osteonecrosis due to drugs, other site

    M87.180 Osteonecrosis due to drugs, jaw `CC` `HCC`

    M87.188 Osteonecrosis due to drugs, other site `CC` `HCC`

M87.19 Osteonecrosis due to drugs, multiple sites `CC` `HCC`

√5ᵗʰ M87.2 Osteonecrosis due to previous trauma

M87.20 Osteonecrosis due to previous trauma, unspecified bone `CC` `HCC`

√6ᵗʰ M87.21 Osteonecrosis due to previous trauma, shoulder

    M87.211 Osteonecrosis due to previous trauma, right shoulder `CC` `HCC`

    M87.212 Osteonecrosis due to previous trauma, left shoulder `CC` `HCC`

    M87.219 Osteonecrosis due to previous trauma, unspecified shoulder `CC` `HCC`

√6ᵗʰ M87.22 Osteonecrosis due to previous trauma, humerus

    CC Excl: For CC codes in subcategory M87.22: PDX collection 908

    M87.221 Osteonecrosis due to previous trauma, right humerus `CC` `HCC`

    M87.222 Osteonecrosis due to previous trauma, left humerus `CC` `HCC`

    M87.229 Osteonecrosis due to previous trauma, unspecified humerus `CC` `HCC`

√6ᵗʰ M87.23 Osteonecrosis due to previous trauma of radius, ulna and carpus

    M87.231 Osteonecrosis due to previous trauma of right radius `CC` `HCC`

    M87.232 Osteonecrosis due to previous trauma of left radius `CC` `HCC`

    M87.233 Osteonecrosis due to previous trauma of unspecified radius `CC` `HCC`

    M87.234 Osteonecrosis due to previous trauma of right ulna `CC` `HCC`

    M87.235 Osteonecrosis due to previous trauma of left ulna `CC` `HCC`

    M87.236 Osteonecrosis due to previous trauma of unspecified ulna `CC` `HCC`

    M87.237 Osteonecrosis due to previous trauma of right carpus `CC` `HCC`

    M87.238 Osteonecrosis due to previous trauma of left carpus `CC` `HCC`

M87.239	Osteonecrosis due to previous trauma of unspecified carpus	CC HCC

✓6ᵗʰ **M87.24** Osteonecrosis due to previous trauma, **hand and fingers**

M87.241	Osteonecrosis due to previous trauma, **right hand**	CC HCC
M87.242	Osteonecrosis due to previous trauma, **left hand**	CC HCC
M87.243	Osteonecrosis due to previous trauma, **unspecified hand**	CC HCC
M87.244	Osteonecrosis due to previous trauma, **right finger(s)**	CC HCC
M87.245	Osteonecrosis due to previous trauma, **left finger(s)**	CC HCC
M87.246	Osteonecrosis due to previous trauma, **unspecified finger(s)**	CC HCC

✓6ᵗʰ **M87.25** Osteonecrosis due to previous trauma, **pelvis and femur**

M87.250	Osteonecrosis due to previous trauma, **pelvis**	CC HCC
M87.251	Osteonecrosis due to previous trauma, **right femur**	CC HCC
	CC Excl: PDX collection 909	
M87.252	Osteonecrosis due to previous trauma, **left femur**	CC HCC
	CC Excl: PDX collection 909	
M87.256	Osteonecrosis due to previous trauma, **unspecified femur**	CC HCC
	CC Excl: PDX collection 909	

✓6ᵗʰ **M87.26** Osteonecrosis due to previous trauma, **tibia and fibula**

M87.261	Osteonecrosis due to previous trauma, **right tibia**	CC HCC
M87.262	Osteonecrosis due to previous trauma, **left tibia**	CC HCC
M87.263	Osteonecrosis due to previous trauma, **unspecified tibia**	CC HCC
M87.264	Osteonecrosis due to previous trauma, **right fibula**	CC HCC
M87.265	Osteonecrosis due to previous trauma, **left fibula**	CC HCC
M87.266	Osteonecrosis due to previous trauma, **unspecified fibula**	CC HCC

✓6ᵗʰ **M87.27** Osteonecrosis due to previous trauma, **ankle, foot and toes**

M87.271	Osteonecrosis due to previous trauma, **right ankle**	CC HCC
M87.272	Osteonecrosis due to previous trauma, **left ankle**	CC HCC
M87.273	Osteonecrosis due to previous trauma, **unspecified ankle**	CC HCC
M87.274	Osteonecrosis due to previous trauma, **right foot**	CC HCC
	CC Excl: PDX collection 910	
M87.275	Osteonecrosis due to previous trauma, **left foot**	CC HCC
	CC Excl: PDX collection 910	
M87.276	Osteonecrosis due to previous trauma, **unspecified foot**	CC HCC
	CC Excl: PDX collection 910	
M87.277	Osteonecrosis due to previous trauma, **right toe(s)**	CC HCC
M87.278	Osteonecrosis due to previous trauma, **left toe(s)**	CC HCC

M87.279	Osteonecrosis due to previous trauma, **unspecified toe(s)**	CC HCC
M87.28	Osteonecrosis due to previous trauma, **other site**	CC HCC
M87.29	Osteonecrosis due to previous trauma, **multiple sites**	CC HCC

✓5ᵗʰ **M87.3** Other **secondary osteonecrosis**

M87.30	Other secondary osteonecrosis, **unspecified bone**	CC HCC

✓6ᵗʰ **M87.31** Other secondary osteonecrosis, **shoulder**

M87.311	Other secondary osteonecrosis, **right shoulder**	CC HCC
M87.312	Other secondary osteonecrosis, **left shoulder**	CC HCC
M87.319	Other secondary osteonecrosis, **unspecified shoulder**	CC HCC

✓6ᵗʰ **M87.32** Other secondary osteonecrosis, **humerus**

CC Excl: For CC codes in subcategory M87.32: PDX collection 908

M87.321	Other secondary osteonecrosis, **right humerus**	CC HCC
M87.322	Other secondary osteonecrosis, **left humerus**	CC HCC
M87.329	Other secondary osteonecrosis, **unspecified humerus**	CC HCC

✓6ᵗʰ **M87.33** Other secondary osteonecrosis of **radius, ulna and carpus**

M87.331	Other secondary osteonecrosis of **right radius**	CC HCC
M87.332	Other secondary osteonecrosis of **left radius**	CC HCC
M87.333	Other secondary osteonecrosis of **unspecified radius**	CC HCC
M87.334	Other secondary osteonecrosis of **right ulna**	CC HCC
M87.335	Other secondary osteonecrosis of **left ulna**	CC HCC
M87.336	Other secondary osteonecrosis of **unspecified ulna**	CC HCC
M87.337	Other secondary osteonecrosis of **right carpus**	CC HCC
M87.338	Other secondary osteonecrosis of **left carpus**	CC HCC
M87.339	Other secondary osteonecrosis of **unspecified carpus**	CC HCC

✓6ᵗʰ **M87.34** Other secondary osteonecrosis, **hand and fingers**

M87.341	Other secondary osteonecrosis, **right hand**	CC HCC
M87.342	Other secondary osteonecrosis, **left hand**	CC HCC
M87.343	Other secondary osteonecrosis, **unspecified hand**	CC HCC
M87.344	Other secondary osteonecrosis, **right finger(s)**	CC HCC
M87.345	Other secondary osteonecrosis, **left finger(s)**	CC HCC
M87.346	Other secondary osteonecrosis, **unspecified finger(s)**	CC HCC

✓6ᵗʰ **M87.35** Other secondary osteonecrosis, **pelvis and femur**

CC Excl: For CC codes in subcategory M87.35: PDX collection 909

M87.350	Other secondary osteonecrosis, **pelvis**	CC HCC
M87.351	Other secondary osteonecrosis, **right femur**	CC HCC

Ⓝ Newborn: 0   Ⓟ Pediatric: 0-17   Ⓜ Maternity: 9-64   Ⓐ Adult: 15-124   **MCC** Major Complication/Comorbidity   **CC** Complication/Comorbidity   **SW** Severe Wound Dx

840   ICD-10-CM 2020

M87.352   Other secondary osteonecrosis, left femur   `CC` `HCC`

M87.353   Other secondary osteonecrosis, unspecified femur   `CC` `HCC`

✓6th   **M87.36   Other secondary osteonecrosis, tibia and fibula**

M87.361   Other secondary osteonecrosis, right tibia   `CC` `HCC`

M87.362   Other secondary osteonecrosis, left tibia   `CC` `HCC`

M87.363   Other secondary osteonecrosis, unspecified tibia   `CC` `HCC`

M87.364   Other secondary osteonecrosis, right fibula   `CC` `HCC`

M87.365   Other secondary osteonecrosis, left fibula   `CC` `HCC`

M87.366   Other secondary osteonecrosis, unspecified fibula   `CC` `HCC`

✓6th   **M87.37   Other secondary osteonecrosis, ankle and foot**

M87.371   Other secondary osteonecrosis, right ankle   `CC` `HCC`

M87.372   Other secondary osteonecrosis, left ankle   `CC` `HCC`

M87.373   Other secondary osteonecrosis, unspecified ankle   `CC` `HCC`

M87.374   Other secondary osteonecrosis, right foot   `CC` `HCC`
    CC Excl: PDX collection 910

M87.375   Other secondary osteonecrosis, left foot   `CC` `HCC`
    CC Excl: PDX collection 910

M87.376   Other secondary osteonecrosis, unspecified foot   `CC` `HCC`
    CC Excl: PDX collection 910

M87.377   Other secondary osteonecrosis, right toe(s)   `CC` `HCC`

M87.378   Other secondary osteonecrosis, left toe(s)   `CC` `HCC`

M87.379   Other secondary osteonecrosis, unspecified toe(s)   `CC` `HCC`

M87.38   Other secondary osteonecrosis, other site   `CC` `HCC`

M87.39   Other secondary osteonecrosis, multiple sites   `CC` `HCC`

✓5th   **M87.8   Other osteonecrosis**

M87.80   Other osteonecrosis, unspecified bone   `CC` `HCC`

✓6th   **M87.81   Other osteonecrosis, shoulder**

M87.811   Other osteonecrosis, right shoulder   `CC` `HCC`

M87.812   Other osteonecrosis, left shoulder   `CC` `HCC`

M87.819   Other osteonecrosis, unspecified shoulder   `CC` `HCC`

✓6th   **M87.82   Other osteonecrosis, humerus**

    CC Excl: For CC codes in subcategory M87.82: PDX collection 908

M87.821   Other osteonecrosis, right humerus   `CC` `HCC`

M87.822   Other osteonecrosis, left humerus   `CC` `HCC`

M87.829   Other osteonecrosis, unspecified humerus   `CC` `HCC`

✓6th   **M87.83   Other osteonecrosis of radius, ulna and carpus**

M87.831   Other osteonecrosis of right radius   `CC` `HCC`

M87.832   Other osteonecrosis of left radius   `CC` `HCC`

M87.833   Other osteonecrosis of unspecified radius   `CC` `HCC`

M87.834   Other osteonecrosis of right ulna   `CC` `HCC`

M87.835   Other osteonecrosis of left ulna   `CC` `HCC`

M87.836   Other osteonecrosis of unspecified ulna   `CC` `HCC`

M87.837   Other osteonecrosis of right carpus   `CC` `HCC`

M87.838   Other osteonecrosis of left carpus   `CC` `HCC`

M87.839   Other osteonecrosis of unspecified carpus   `CC` `HCC`

✓6th   **M87.84   Other osteonecrosis, hand and fingers**

M87.841   Other osteonecrosis, right hand   `CC` `HCC`

M87.842   Other osteonecrosis, left hand   `CC` `HCC`

M87.843   Other osteonecrosis, unspecified hand   `CC` `HCC`

M87.844   Other osteonecrosis, right finger(s)   `CC` `HCC`

M87.845   Other osteonecrosis, left finger(s)   `CC` `HCC`

M87.849   Other osteonecrosis, unspecified finger(s)   `CC` `HCC`

✓6th   **M87.85   Other osteonecrosis, pelvis and femur**

    CC Excl: For CC codes in subcategory M87.85: PDX collection 909

M87.850   Other osteonecrosis, pelvis   `CC` `HCC`

M87.851   Other osteonecrosis, right femur   `CC` `HCC`

M87.852   Other osteonecrosis, left femur   `CC` `HCC`

M87.859   Other osteonecrosis, unspecified femur   `CC` `HCC`

✓6th   **M87.86   Other osteonecrosis, tibia and fibula**

M87.861   Other osteonecrosis, right tibia   `CC` `HCC`

M87.862   Other osteonecrosis, left tibia   `CC` `HCC`

M87.863   Other osteonecrosis, unspecified tibia   `CC` `HCC`

M87.864   Other osteonecrosis, right fibula   `CC` `HCC`

M87.865   Other osteonecrosis, left fibula   `CC` `HCC`

M87.869   Other osteonecrosis, unspecified fibula   `CC` `HCC`

✓6th   **M87.87   Other osteonecrosis, ankle, foot and toes**

M87.871   Other osteonecrosis, right ankle   `CC` `HCC`

M87.872   Other osteonecrosis, left ankle   `CC` `HCC`

M87.873   Other osteonecrosis, unspecified ankle   `CC` `HCC`

M87.874   Other osteonecrosis, right foot   `CC` `HCC`
    CC Excl: PDX collection 910

M87.875   Other osteonecrosis, left foot   `CC` `HCC`
    CC Excl: PDX collection 910

M87.876   Other osteonecrosis, unspecified foot   `CC` `HCC`
    CC Excl: PDX collection 910

M87.877   Other osteonecrosis, right toe(s)   `CC` `HCC`

M87.878   Other osteonecrosis, left toe(s)   `CC` `HCC`

M87.879   Other osteonecrosis, unspecified toe(s)   `CC` `HCC`

M87.88   Other osteonecrosis, other site   `CC` `HCC`

M87.89   Other osteonecrosis, multiple sites   `CC` `HCC`

M87.9   Osteonecrosis, unspecified   `CC` `HCC`

    Necrosis of bone NOS

✓4th   **M88   Osteitis deformans [Paget's disease of bone]**

    EXCLUDES 1   osteitis deformans in neoplastic disease (M90.6)

    DEF: Bone disease characterized by numerous cycles of bone resorption by the body. Resorption is followed by accelerated repair attempts, causing bone deformities and bowing, with associated fractures and pain.

M88.0   Osteitis deformans of skull

M88.1   Osteitis deformans of vertebrae

✓5th   **M88.8   Osteitis deformans of other bones**

✓6th   **M88.81   Osteitis deformans of shoulder**

M88.811   Osteitis deformans of right shoulder

M88.812   Osteitis deformans of left shoulder

Chapter 13. Diseases of the Musculoskeletal System and Connective Tissue

M88.819 Osteitis deformans of unspecified shoulder

√6ᵗʰ **M88.82** Osteitis deformans of upper arm

M88.821 Osteitis deformans of right upper arm
M88.822 Osteitis deformans of left upper arm
M88.829 Osteitis deformans of unspecified upper arm

√6ᵗʰ **M88.83** Osteitis deformans of forearm

M88.831 Osteitis deformans of right forearm
M88.832 Osteitis deformans of left forearm
M88.839 Osteitis deformans of unspecified forearm

√6ᵗʰ **M88.84** Osteitis deformans of hand

M88.841 Osteitis deformans of right hand
M88.842 Osteitis deformans of left hand
M88.849 Osteitis deformans of unspecified hand

√6ᵗʰ **M88.85** Osteitis deformans of thigh

M88.851 Osteitis deformans of right thigh
M88.852 Osteitis deformans of left thigh
M88.859 Osteitis deformans of unspecified thigh

√6ᵗʰ **M88.86** Osteitis deformans of lower leg

M88.861 Osteitis deformans of right lower leg
M88.862 Osteitis deformans of left lower leg
M88.869 Osteitis deformans of unspecified lower leg

√6ᵗʰ **M88.87** Osteitis deformans of ankle and foot

M88.871 Osteitis deformans of right ankle and foot
M88.872 Osteitis deformans of left ankle and foot
M88.879 Osteitis deformans of unspecified ankle and foot

M88.88 Osteitis deformans of other bones
EXCLUDES 2 osteitis deformans of skull (M88.0)
osteitis deformans of vertebrae (M88.1)

M88.89 Osteitis deformans of multiple sites

M88.9 Osteitis deformans of unspecified bone

√4ᵗʰ **M89** Other disorders of bone

√5ᵗʰ **M89.0** Algoneurodystrophy

Shoulder-hand syndrome
Sudeck's atrophy
EXCLUDES 1 causalgia, lower limb (G57.7-)
causalgia, upper limb (G56.4-)
complex regional pain syndrome II, lower limb (G57.7-)
complex regional pain syndrome II, upper limb (G56.4-)
reflex sympathetic dystrophy (G90.5-)

M89.00 Algoneurodystrophy, unspecified site

√6ᵗʰ **M89.01** Algoneurodystrophy, shoulder

M89.011 Algoneurodystrophy, right shoulder
M89.012 Algoneurodystrophy, left shoulder
M89.019 Algoneurodystrophy, unspecified shoulder

√6ᵗʰ **M89.02** Algoneurodystrophy, upper arm

M89.021 Algoneurodystrophy, right upper arm
M89.022 Algoneurodystrophy, left upper arm
M89.029 Algoneurodystrophy, unspecified upper arm

√6ᵗʰ **M89.03** Algoneurodystrophy, forearm

M89.031 Algoneurodystrophy, right forearm
M89.032 Algoneurodystrophy, left forearm
M89.039 Algoneurodystrophy, unspecified forearm

√6ᵗʰ **M89.04** Algoneurodystrophy, hand

M89.041 Algoneurodystrophy, right hand
M89.042 Algoneurodystrophy, left hand
M89.049 Algoneurodystrophy, unspecified hand

√6ᵗʰ **M89.05** Algoneurodystrophy, thigh

M89.051 Algoneurodystrophy, right thigh
M89.052 Algoneurodystrophy, left thigh
M89.059 Algoneurodystrophy, unspecified thigh

√6ᵗʰ **M89.06** Algoneurodystrophy, lower leg

M89.061 Algoneurodystrophy, right lower leg
M89.062 Algoneurodystrophy, left lower leg
M89.069 Algoneurodystrophy, unspecified lower leg

√6ᵗʰ **M89.07** Algoneurodystrophy, ankle and foot

M89.071 Algoneurodystrophy, right ankle and foot
M89.072 Algoneurodystrophy, left ankle and foot
M89.079 Algoneurodystrophy, unspecified ankle and foot

M89.08 Algoneurodystrophy, other site
M89.09 Algoneurodystrophy, multiple sites

√5ᵗʰ **M89.1** Physeal arrest

Arrest of growth plate
Epiphyseal arrest
Growth plate arrest

√6ᵗʰ **M89.12** Physeal arrest, humerus

M89.121 Complete physeal arrest, right proximal humerus
M89.122 Complete physeal arrest, left proximal humerus
M89.123 Partial physeal arrest, right proximal humerus
M89.124 Partial physeal arrest, left proximal humerus
M89.125 Complete physeal arrest, right distal humerus
M89.126 Complete physeal arrest, left distal humerus
M89.127 Partial physeal arrest, right distal humerus
M89.128 Partial physeal arrest, left distal humerus
M89.129 Physeal arrest, humerus, unspecified

√6ᵗʰ **M89.13** Physeal arrest, forearm

M89.131 Complete physeal arrest, right distal radius
M89.132 Complete physeal arrest, left distal radius
M89.133 Partial physeal arrest, right distal radius
M89.134 Partial physeal arrest, left distal radius
M89.138 Other physeal arrest of forearm
M89.139 Physeal arrest, forearm, unspecified

√6ᵗʰ **M89.15** Physeal arrest, femur

M89.151 Complete physeal arrest, right proximal femur
M89.152 Complete physeal arrest, left proximal femur
M89.153 Partial physeal arrest, right proximal femur
M89.154 Partial physeal arrest, left proximal femur
M89.155 Complete physeal arrest, right distal femur
M89.156 Complete physeal arrest, left distal femur
M89.157 Partial physeal arrest, right distal femur
M89.158 Partial physeal arrest, left distal femur
M89.159 Physeal arrest, femur, unspecified

√6ᵗʰ **M89.16** Physeal arrest, lower leg

M89.160 Complete physeal arrest, right proximal tibia
M89.161 Complete physeal arrest, left proximal tibia
M89.162 Partial physeal arrest, right proximal tibia
M89.163 Partial physeal arrest, left proximal tibia
M89.164 Complete physeal arrest, right distal tibia
M89.165 Complete physeal arrest, left distal tibia
M89.166 Partial physeal arrest, right distal tibia
M89.167 Partial physeal arrest, left distal tibia
M89.168 Other physeal arrest of lower leg
M89.169 Physeal arrest, lower leg, unspecified

M89.18 Physeal arrest, other site

√5ᵗʰ **M89.2** Other disorders of bone development and growth

M89.20 Other disorders of bone development and growth, unspecified site

√6ᵗʰ **M89.21** Other disorders of bone development and growth, shoulder

M89.211 Other disorders of bone development and growth, right shoulder
M89.212 Other disorders of bone development and growth, left shoulder
M89.219 Other disorders of bone development and growth, unspecified shoulder

√6ᵗʰ **M89.22** Other disorders of bone development and growth, humerus

M89.221 Other disorders of bone development and growth, right humerus

N Newborn: 0   **P** Pediatric: 0-17   **M** Maternity: 9-64   **A** Adult: 15-124   **MCC** Major Complication/Comorbidity   **CC** Complication/Comorbidity   **SW** Severe Wound Dx

842

ICD-10-CM 2020

M89.222   Other disorders of bone development and growth, left humerus

M89.229   Other disorders of bone development and growth, unspecified humerus

✓6th M89.23   Other disorders of bone development and growth, ulna and radius

M89.231   Other disorders of bone development and growth, right ulna

M89.232   Other disorders of bone development and growth, left ulna

M89.233   Other disorders of bone development and growth, right radius

M89.234   Other disorders of bone development and growth, left radius

M89.239   Other disorders of bone development and growth, unspecified ulna and radius

✓6th M89.24   Other disorders of bone development and growth, hand

M89.241   Other disorders of bone development and growth, right hand

M89.242   Other disorders of bone development and growth, left hand

M89.249   Other disorders of bone development and growth, unspecified hand

✓6th M89.25   Other disorders of bone development and growth, femur

M89.251   Other disorders of bone development and growth, right femur

M89.252   Other disorders of bone development and growth, left femur

M89.259   Other disorders of bone development and growth, unspecified femur

✓6th M89.26   Other disorders of bone development and growth, tibia and fibula

M89.261   Other disorders of bone development and growth, right tibia

M89.262   Other disorders of bone development and growth, left tibia

M89.263   Other disorders of bone development and growth, right fibula

M89.264   Other disorders of bone development and growth, left fibula

M89.269   Other disorders of bone development and growth, unspecified lower leg

✓6th M89.27   Other disorders of bone development and growth, ankle and foot

M89.271   Other disorders of bone development and growth, right ankle and foot

M89.272   Other disorders of bone development and growth, left ankle and foot

M89.279   Other disorders of bone development and growth, unspecified ankle and foot

M89.28   Other disorders of bone development and growth, other site

M89.29   Other disorders of bone development and growth, multiple sites

✓5th M89.3   Hypertrophy of bone

M89.30   Hypertrophy of bone, unspecified site

✓6th M89.31   Hypertrophy of bone, shoulder

M89.311   Hypertrophy of bone, right shoulder

M89.312   Hypertrophy of bone, left shoulder

M89.319   Hypertrophy of bone, unspecified shoulder

✓6th M89.32   Hypertrophy of bone, humerus

M89.321   Hypertrophy of bone, right humerus

M89.322   Hypertrophy of bone, left humerus

M89.329   Hypertrophy of bone, unspecified humerus

✓6th M89.33   Hypertrophy of bone, ulna and radius

M89.331   Hypertrophy of bone, right ulna

M89.332   Hypertrophy of bone, left ulna

M89.333   Hypertrophy of bone, right radius

M89.334   Hypertrophy of bone, left radius

M89.339   Hypertrophy of bone, unspecified ulna and radius

✓6th M89.34   Hypertrophy of bone, hand

M89.341   Hypertrophy of bone, right hand

M89.342   Hypertrophy of bone, left hand

M89.349   Hypertrophy of bone, unspecified hand

✓6th M89.35   Hypertrophy of bone, femur

M89.351   Hypertrophy of bone, right femur

M89.352   Hypertrophy of bone, left femur

M89.359   Hypertrophy of bone, unspecified femur

✓6th M89.36   Hypertrophy of bone, tibia and fibula

M89.361   Hypertrophy of bone, right tibia

M89.362   Hypertrophy of bone, left tibia

M89.363   Hypertrophy of bone, right fibula

M89.364   Hypertrophy of bone, left fibula

M89.369   Hypertrophy of bone, unspecified tibia and fibula

✓6th M89.37   Hypertrophy of bone, ankle and foot

M89.371   Hypertrophy of bone, right ankle and foot

M89.372   Hypertrophy of bone, left ankle and foot

M89.379   Hypertrophy of bone, unspecified ankle and foot

M89.38   Hypertrophy of bone, other site

M89.39   Hypertrophy of bone, multiple sites

✓5th M89.4   Other hypertrophic osteoarthropathy

Marie-Bamberger disease
Pachydermoperiostosis

M89.40   Other hypertrophic osteoarthropathy, unspecified site

✓6th M89.41   Other hypertrophic osteoarthropathy, shoulder

M89.411   Other hypertrophic osteoarthropathy, right shoulder

M89.412   Other hypertrophic osteoarthropathy, left shoulder

M89.419   Other hypertrophic osteoarthropathy, unspecified shoulder

✓6th M89.42   Other hypertrophic osteoarthropathy, upper arm

M89.421   Other hypertrophic osteoarthropathy, right upper arm

M89.422   Other hypertrophic osteoarthropathy, left upper arm

M89.429   Other hypertrophic osteoarthropathy, unspecified upper arm

✓6th M89.43   Other hypertrophic osteoarthropathy, forearm

M89.431   Other hypertrophic osteoarthropathy, right forearm

M89.432   Other hypertrophic osteoarthropathy, left forearm

M89.439   Other hypertrophic osteoarthropathy, unspecified forearm

✓6th M89.44   Other hypertrophic osteoarthropathy, hand

M89.441   Other hypertrophic osteoarthropathy, right hand

M89.442   Other hypertrophic osteoarthropathy, left hand

M89.449   Other hypertrophic osteoarthropathy, unspecified hand

✓6th M89.45   Other hypertrophic osteoarthropathy, thigh

M89.451   Other hypertrophic osteoarthropathy, right thigh

M89.452   Other hypertrophic osteoarthropathy, left thigh

M89.459   Other hypertrophic osteoarthropathy, unspecified thigh

✓6th M89.46   Other hypertrophic osteoarthropathy, lower leg

M89.461   Other hypertrophic osteoarthropathy, right lower leg

M89.462   Other hypertrophic osteoarthropathy, left lower leg

M89.469   Other hypertrophic osteoarthropathy, unspecified lower leg

✓6th M89.47   Other hypertrophic osteoarthropathy, ankle and foot

M89.471   Other hypertrophic osteoarthropathy, right ankle and foot

M89.472   Other hypertrophic osteoarthropathy, left ankle and foot

M89.479   Other hypertrophic osteoarthropathy, unspecified ankle and foot

M89.48   Other hypertrophic osteoarthropathy, other site

M89.49   Other hypertrophic osteoarthropathy, multiple sites

☑ Additional Character Required   ✓x7th Placeholder   Unacceptable PDx   Questionable PDx   Manifestation   Unspecified Dx   H1 - H14 HAC   HCC CMS-HCC Dx   HIV HIV Dx

ICD-10-CM 2020   843

✓5ᵗʰ **M89.5** **Osteolysis**

> Use additional code to identify major osseous defect, if applicable (M89.7-)
>
> EXCLUDES 2   *periprosthetic osteolysis of internal prosthetic joint (T84.Ø5-)*

     M89.5Ø **Osteolysis, unspecified site**

✓6ᵗʰ **M89.51** **Osteolysis,** shoulder

     M89.511 **Osteolysis, right shoulder**
     M89.512 **Osteolysis, left shoulder**
     M89.519 **Osteolysis, unspecified shoulder**

✓6ᵗʰ **M89.52** **Osteolysis,** upper arm

     M89.521 **Osteolysis, right upper arm**
     M89.522 **Osteolysis, left upper arm**
     M89.529 **Osteolysis, unspecified upper arm**

✓6ᵗʰ **M89.53** **Osteolysis,** forearm

     M89.531 **Osteolysis, right forearm**
     M89.532 **Osteolysis, left forearm**
     M89.539 **Osteolysis, unspecified forearm**

✓6ᵗʰ **M89.54** **Osteolysis,** hand

     M89.541 **Osteolysis, right hand**
     M89.542 **Osteolysis, left hand**
     M89.549 **Osteolysis, unspecified hand**

✓6ᵗʰ **M89.55** **Osteolysis,** thigh

     M89.551 **Osteolysis, right thigh**
     M89.552 **Osteolysis, left thigh**
     M89.559 **Osteolysis, unspecified thigh**

✓6ᵗʰ **M89.56** **Osteolysis,** lower leg

     M89.561 **Osteolysis, right lower leg**
     M89.562 **Osteolysis, left lower leg**
     M89.569 **Osteolysis, unspecified lower leg**

✓6ᵗʰ **M89.57** **Osteolysis,** ankle and foot

     M89.571 **Osteolysis, right ankle and foot**
     M89.572 **Osteolysis, left ankle and foot**
     M89.579 **Osteolysis, unspecified ankle and foot**

     M89.58 **Osteolysis, other site**
     M89.59 **Osteolysis, multiple sites**

✓5ᵗʰ **M89.6** **Osteopathy after poliomyelitis**

> Use additional code (B91) to identify previous poliomyelitis
>
> EXCLUDES 1   *postpolio syndrome (G14)*

     M89.6Ø **Osteopathy after poliomyelitis, unspecified site**   HCC

✓6ᵗʰ **M89.61** **Osteopathy after poliomyelitis,** shoulder

     M89.611 **Osteopathy after poliomyelitis, right shoulder**   HCC
     M89.612 **Osteopathy after poliomyelitis, left shoulder**   HCC
     M89.619 **Osteopathy after poliomyelitis, unspecified shoulder**   HCC

✓6ᵗʰ **M89.62** **Osteopathy after poliomyelitis,** upper arm

     M89.621 **Osteopathy after poliomyelitis, right upper arm**   HCC
     M89.622 **Osteopathy after poliomyelitis, left upper arm**   HCC
     M89.629 **Osteopathy after poliomyelitis, unspecified upper arm**   HCC

✓6ᵗʰ **M89.63** **Osteopathy after poliomyelitis,** forearm

     M89.631 **Osteopathy after poliomyelitis, right forearm**   HCC
     M89.632 **Osteopathy after poliomyelitis, left forearm**   HCC
     M89.639 **Osteopathy after poliomyelitis, unspecified forearm**   HCC

✓6ᵗʰ **M89.64** **Osteopathy after poliomyelitis,** hand

     M89.641 **Osteopathy after poliomyelitis, right hand**   HCC
     M89.642 **Osteopathy after poliomyelitis, left hand**   HCC
     M89.649 **Osteopathy after poliomyelitis, unspecified hand**   HCC

✓6ᵗʰ **M89.65** **Osteopathy after poliomyelitis,** thigh

     M89.651 **Osteopathy after poliomyelitis, right thigh**   HCC
     M89.652 **Osteopathy after poliomyelitis, left thigh**   HCC
     M89.659 **Osteopathy after poliomyelitis, unspecified thigh**   HCC

✓6ᵗʰ **M89.66** **Osteopathy after poliomyelitis,** lower leg

     M89.661 **Osteopathy after poliomyelitis, right lower leg**   HCC
     M89.662 **Osteopathy after poliomyelitis, left lower leg**   HCC
     M89.669 **Osteopathy after poliomyelitis, unspecified lower leg**   HCC

✓6ᵗʰ **M89.67** **Osteopathy after poliomyelitis,** ankle and foot

     M89.671 **Osteopathy after poliomyelitis, right ankle and foot**   HCC
     M89.672 **Osteopathy after poliomyelitis, left ankle and foot**   HCC
     M89.679 **Osteopathy after poliomyelitis, unspecified ankle and foot**   HCC

     M89.68 **Osteopathy after poliomyelitis, other site**   HCC
     M89.69 **Osteopathy after poliomyelitis, multiple sites**   HCC

✓5ᵗʰ **M89.7** **Major osseous defect**

> Code first underlying disease, if known, such as:
> aseptic necrosis of bone (M87.-)
> malignant neoplasm of bone (C4Ø.-)
> osteolysis (M89.5)
> osteomyelitis (M86.-)
> osteonecrosis (M87.-)
> osteoporosis (M8Ø.-, M81.-)
> periprosthetic osteolysis (T84.Ø5-)

     M89.7Ø **Major osseous defect, unspecified site**

✓6ᵗʰ **M89.71** **Major osseous defect,** shoulder region

> Major osseous defect clavicle or scapula

     M89.711 **Major osseous defect, right shoulder region**
     M89.712 **Major osseous defect, left shoulder region**
     M89.719 **Major osseous defect, unspecified shoulder region**

✓6ᵗʰ **M89.72** **Major osseous defect,** humerus

     M89.721 **Major osseous defect, right humerus**
     M89.722 **Major osseous defect, left humerus**
     M89.729 **Major osseous defect, unspecified humerus**

✓6ᵗʰ **M89.73** **Major osseous defect,** forearm

> Major osseous defect of radius and ulna

     M89.731 **Major osseous defect, right forearm**
     M89.732 **Major osseous defect, left forearm**
     M89.739 **Major osseous defect, unspecified forearm**

✓6ᵗʰ **M89.74** **Major osseous defect,** hand

> Major osseous defect of carpus, fingers, metacarpus

     M89.741 **Major osseous defect, right hand**
     M89.742 **Major osseous defect, left hand**
     M89.749 **Major osseous defect, unspecified hand**

✓6ᵗʰ **M89.75** **Major osseous defect,** pelvic region and thigh

> Major osseous defect of femur and pelvis

     M89.751 **Major osseous defect, right pelvic region and thigh**
     M89.752 **Major osseous defect, left pelvic region and thigh**
     M89.759 **Major osseous defect, unspecified pelvic region and thigh**

✓6ᵗʰ **M89.76** **Major osseous defect,** lower leg

> Major osseous defect of fibula and tibia

     M89.761 **Major osseous defect, right lower leg**
     M89.762 **Major osseous defect, left lower leg**
     M89.769 **Major osseous defect, unspecified lower leg**

N Newborn: 0   P Pediatric: 0-17   M Maternity: 9-64   A Adult: 15-124   MCC Major Complication/Comorbidity   CC Complication/Comorbidity   SW Severe Wound Dx

844   ICD-10-CM 2020

√6ᵗʰ **M89.77** **Major osseous defect,** ankle and foot

      Major osseous defect of metatarsus, tarsus, toes

      M89.771 **Major osseous defect,** right **ankle and foot**

      M89.772 **Major osseous defect,** left **ankle and foot**

      M89.779 **Major osseous defect, unspecified ankle and foot**

    M89.78 **Major osseous defect, other site**

    M89.79 **Major osseous defect,** multiple sites

√5ᵗʰ **M89.8** **Other specified disorders of bone**

      Infantile cortical hyperostoses

      Post-traumatic subperiosteal ossification

√6ᵗʰ **M89.8X** **Other specified disorders of bone**

      M89.8X0 **Other specified disorders of bone, multiple sites**

      M89.8X1 **Other specified disorders of bone, shoulder**

      M89.8X2 **Other specified disorders of bone,** upper arm

      M89.8X3 **Other specified disorders of bone, forearm**

      M89.8X4 **Other specified disorders of bone, hand**

      M89.8X5 **Other specified disorders of bone, thigh**

      M89.8X6 **Other specified disorders of bone, lower leg**

      M89.8X7 **Other specified disorders of bone, ankle and foot**

      M89.8X8 **Other specified disorders of bone, other site**

      M89.8X9 **Other specified disorders of bone, unspecified site**

    M89.9 **Disorder of bone, unspecified**

√4ᵗʰ **M90** **Osteopathies in diseases classified elsewhere**

      EXCLUDES 1   osteochondritis, osteomyelitis, and osteopathy (in):

         cryptococcosis (B45.3)

         diabetes mellitus (E08-E13 with .69-)

         gonococcal (A54.43)

         neurogenic syphilis (A52.11)

         renal osteodystrophy (N25.0)

         salmonellosis (A02.24)

         secondary syphilis (A51.46)

         syphilis (late) (A52.77)

√5ᵗʰ **M90.5** **Osteonecrosis in diseases classified elsewhere**

      Code first underlying disease, such as:

         caisson disease (T70.3)

         hemoglobinopathy (D50-D64)

      CC Excl: For CC codes in subcategory M90.5, unless otherwise noted: PDX collection 907

    M90.50 **Osteonecrosis in diseases classified elsewhere, unspecified site**   CC HCC

√6ᵗʰ **M90.51** **Osteonecrosis in diseases classified elsewhere, shoulder**

      CC Excl: For CC codes in subcategory M90.51: PDX collection 908

      M90.511 **Osteonecrosis in diseases classified elsewhere,** right **shoulder**   CC HCC

      M90.512 **Osteonecrosis in diseases classified elsewhere,** left **shoulder**   CC HCC

      M90.519 **Osteonecrosis in diseases classified elsewhere, unspecified shoulder**   CC HCC

√6ᵗʰ **M90.52** **Osteonecrosis in diseases classified elsewhere, upper arm**

      M90.521 **Osteonecrosis in diseases classified elsewhere,** right **upper arm**   CC HCC

      M90.522 **Osteonecrosis in diseases classified elsewhere,** left **upper arm**   CC HCC

      M90.529 **Osteonecrosis in diseases classified elsewhere, unspecified upper arm**   CC HCC

√6ᵗʰ **M90.53** **Osteonecrosis in diseases classified elsewhere, forearm**

      M90.531 **Osteonecrosis in diseases classified elsewhere,** right **forearm**   CC HCC

      M90.532 **Osteonecrosis in diseases classified elsewhere,** left **forearm**   CC HCC

      M90.539 **Osteonecrosis in diseases classified elsewhere, unspecified forearm**   CC HCC

√6ᵗʰ **M90.54** **Osteonecrosis in diseases classified elsewhere,** hand

      M90.541 **Osteonecrosis in diseases classified elsewhere,** right **hand**   CC HCC

      M90.542 **Osteonecrosis in diseases classified elsewhere,** left **hand**   CC HCC

      M90.549 **Osteonecrosis in diseases classified elsewhere, unspecified hand**   CC HCC

√6ᵗʰ **M90.55** **Osteonecrosis in diseases classified elsewhere, thigh**

      CC Excl: For CC codes in subcategory M90.55: PDX collection 909

      M90.551 **Osteonecrosis in diseases classified elsewhere,** right **thigh**   CC HCC

      M90.552 **Osteonecrosis in diseases classified elsewhere,** left **thigh**   CC HCC

      M90.559 **Osteonecrosis in diseases classified elsewhere, unspecified thigh**   CC HCC

√6ᵗʰ **M90.56** **Osteonecrosis in diseases classified elsewhere, lower leg**

      M90.561 **Osteonecrosis in diseases classified elsewhere,** right **lower leg**   CC HCC

      M90.562 **Osteonecrosis in diseases classified elsewhere,** left **lower leg**   CC HCC

      M90.569 **Osteonecrosis in diseases classified elsewhere, unspecified lower leg**   CC HCC

√6ᵗʰ **M90.57** **Osteonecrosis in diseases classified elsewhere, ankle and foot**

      M90.571 **Osteonecrosis in diseases classified elsewhere,** right **ankle and foot**   CC HCC

      M90.572 **Osteonecrosis in diseases classified elsewhere,** left **ankle and foot**   CC HCC

      M90.579 **Osteonecrosis in diseases classified elsewhere, unspecified ankle and foot**   CC HCC

    M90.58 **Osteonecrosis in diseases classified elsewhere, other site**   CC HCC

    M90.59 **Osteonecrosis in diseases classified elsewhere,** multiple sites   CC HCC

√5ᵗʰ **M90.6** **Osteitis deformans in neoplastic diseases**

      Osteitis deformans in malignant neoplasm of bone

      Code first the neoplasm (C40.-, C41.-)

      EXCLUDES 1   osteitis deformans [Paget's disease of bone] (M88.-)

    M90.60 **Osteitis deformans in neoplastic diseases, unspecified site**

√6ᵗʰ **M90.61** **Osteitis deformans in neoplastic diseases,** shoulder

      M90.611 **Osteitis deformans in neoplastic diseases,** right **shoulder**

      M90.612 **Osteitis deformans in neoplastic diseases,** left **shoulder**

      M90.619 **Osteitis deformans in neoplastic diseases, unspecified shoulder**

√6ᵗʰ **M90.62** **Osteitis deformans in neoplastic diseases,** upper arm

      M90.621 **Osteitis deformans in neoplastic diseases,** right **upper arm**

      M90.622 **Osteitis deformans in neoplastic diseases,** left **upper arm**

      M90.629 **Osteitis deformans in neoplastic diseases, unspecified upper arm**

√6ᵗʰ **M90.63** **Osteitis deformans in neoplastic diseases,** forearm

      M90.631 **Osteitis deformans in neoplastic diseases,** right **forearm**

      M90.632 **Osteitis deformans in neoplastic diseases,** left **forearm**

      M90.639 **Osteitis deformans in neoplastic diseases, unspecified forearm**

☑ Additional Character Required   √x7ᵗʰ Placeholder   Unacceptable PDx   Questionable PDx   Manifestation   Unspecified Dx   H1-H14 HAC   HCC CMS-HCC Dx   HIV HIV Dx

ICD-10-CM 2020   **845**

M90.64–M92.10

Chapter 13. Diseases of the Musculoskeletal System and Connective Tissue

√6ᵗʰ **M90.64** Osteitis deformans in neoplastic diseases, hand

     M90.641 *Osteitis deformans in neoplastic diseases, right hand*

     M90.642 *Osteitis deformans in neoplastic diseases, left hand*

     M90.649 *Osteitis deformans in neoplastic diseases, unspecified hand*

√6ᵗʰ **M90.65** Osteitis deformans in neoplastic diseases, thigh

     M90.651 *Osteitis deformans in neoplastic diseases, right thigh*

     M90.652 *Osteitis deformans in neoplastic diseases, left thigh*

     M90.659 *Osteitis deformans in neoplastic diseases, unspecified thigh*

√6ᵗʰ **M90.66** Osteitis deformans in neoplastic diseases, lower leg

     M90.661 *Osteitis deformans in neoplastic diseases, right lower leg*

     M90.662 *Osteitis deformans in neoplastic diseases, left lower leg*

     M90.669 *Osteitis deformans in neoplastic diseases, unspecified lower leg*

√6ᵗʰ **M90.67** Osteitis deformans in neoplastic diseases, ankle and foot

     M90.671 *Osteitis deformans in neoplastic diseases, right ankle and foot*

     M90.672 *Osteitis deformans in neoplastic diseases, left ankle and foot*

     M90.679 *Osteitis deformans in neoplastic diseases, unspecified ankle and foot*

   M90.68 Osteitis deformans in neoplastic diseases, other site

   M90.69 *Osteitis deformans in neoplastic diseases, multiple sites*

√5ᵗʰ **M90.8** Osteopathy in diseases classified elsewhere

     Code first underlying disease, such as:
     rickets (E55.0)
     vitamin-D-resistant rickets (E83.3)

     M90.80 *Osteopathy in diseases classified elsewhere, unspecified site*

√6ᵗʰ **M90.81** Osteopathy in diseases classified elsewhere, shoulder

     M90.811 *Osteopathy in diseases classified elsewhere, right shoulder*

     M90.812 *Osteopathy in diseases classified elsewhere, left shoulder*

     M90.819 *Osteopathy in diseases classified elsewhere, unspecified shoulder*

√6ᵗʰ **M90.82** Osteopathy in diseases classified elsewhere, upper arm

     M90.821 *Osteopathy in diseases classified elsewhere, right upper arm*

     M90.822 *Osteopathy in diseases classified elsewhere, left upper arm*

     M90.829 *Osteopathy in diseases classified elsewhere, unspecified upper arm*

√6ᵗʰ **M90.83** Osteopathy in diseases classified elsewhere, forearm

     M90.831 *Osteopathy in diseases classified elsewhere, right forearm*

     M90.832 *Osteopathy in diseases classified elsewhere, left forearm*

     M90.839 *Osteopathy in diseases classified elsewhere, unspecified forearm*

√6ᵗʰ **M90.84** Osteopathy in diseases classified elsewhere, hand

     M90.841 *Osteopathy in diseases classified elsewhere, right hand*

     M90.842 *Osteopathy in diseases classified elsewhere, left hand*

     M90.849 *Osteopathy in diseases classified elsewhere, unspecified hand*

√6ᵗʰ **M90.85** Osteopathy in diseases classified elsewhere, thigh

     M90.851 *Osteopathy in diseases classified elsewhere, right thigh*

     M90.852 *Osteopathy in diseases classified elsewhere, left thigh*

     M90.859 *Osteopathy in diseases classified elsewhere, unspecified thigh*

√6ᵗʰ **M90.86** Osteopathy in diseases classified elsewhere, lower leg

     M90.861 *Osteopathy in diseases classified elsewhere, right lower leg*

     M90.862 *Osteopathy in diseases classified elsewhere, left lower leg*

     M90.869 *Osteopathy in diseases classified elsewhere, unspecified lower leg*

√6ᵗʰ **M90.87** Osteopathy in diseases classified elsewhere, ankle and foot

     M90.871 *Osteopathy in diseases classified elsewhere, right ankle and foot*

     M90.872 *Osteopathy in diseases classified elsewhere, left ankle and foot*

     M90.879 *Osteopathy in diseases classified elsewhere, unspecified ankle and foot*

   M90.88 Osteopathy in diseases classified elsewhere, other site

   M90.89 Osteopathy in diseases classified elsewhere, *multiple sites*

Chondropathies (M91-M94)

EXCLUDES 1   *postprocedural chondropathies (M96.-)*

√4ᵗʰ **M91** Juvenile osteochondrosis of hip and pelvis

     EXCLUDES 1   *slipped upper femoral epiphysis (nontraumatic) (M93.0)*

   M91.0 Juvenile osteochondrosis of pelvis

     Osteochondrosis (juvenile) of acetabulum

     Osteochondrosis (juvenile) of iliac crest [Buchanan]

     Osteochondrosis (juvenile) of ischiopubic synchondrosis [van Neck]

     Osteochondrosis (juvenile) of symphysis pubis [Pierson]

√5ᵗʰ **M91.1** Juvenile osteochondrosis of head of femur [Legg-Calvé-Perthes]

     M91.10 Juvenile osteochondrosis of head of femur [Legg-Calvé-Perthes], unspecified leg

     M91.11 Juvenile osteochondrosis of head of femur [Legg-Calvé-Perthes], right leg

     M91.12 Juvenile osteochondrosis of head of femur [Legg-Calvé-Perthes], left leg

√5ᵗʰ **M91.2** Coxa plana

     Hip deformity due to previous juvenile osteochondrosis

     M91.20 Coxa plana, unspecified hip

     M91.21 Coxa plana, right hip

     M91.22 Coxa plana, left hip

√5ᵗʰ **M91.3** Pseudocoxalgia

     M91.30 Pseudocoxalgia, unspecified hip

     M91.31 Pseudocoxalgia, right hip

     M91.32 Pseudocoxalgia, left hip

√5ᵗʰ **M91.4** Coxa magna

     M91.40 Coxa magna, unspecified hip

     M91.41 Coxa magna, right hip

     M91.42 Coxa magna, left hip

√5ᵗʰ **M91.8** Other juvenile osteochondrosis of hip and pelvis

     Juvenile osteochondrosis after reduction of congenital dislocation of hip

     M91.80 Other juvenile osteochondrosis of hip and pelvis, unspecified leg

     M91.81 Other juvenile osteochondrosis of hip and pelvis, right leg

     M91.82 Other juvenile osteochondrosis of hip and pelvis, left leg

√5ᵗʰ **M91.9** Juvenile osteochondrosis of hip and pelvis, unspecified

     M91.90 Juvenile osteochondrosis of hip and pelvis, unspecified, unspecified leg

     M91.91 Juvenile osteochondrosis of hip and pelvis, unspecified, right leg

     M91.92 Juvenile osteochondrosis of hip and pelvis, unspecified, left leg

√4ᵗʰ **M92** Other juvenile osteochondrosis

√5ᵗʰ **M92.0** Juvenile osteochondrosis of humerus

     Osteochondrosis (juvenile) of capitulum of humerus [Panner]

     Osteochondrosis (juvenile) of head of humerus [Haas]

     M92.00 Juvenile osteochondrosis of humerus, unspecified arm

     M92.01 Juvenile osteochondrosis of humerus, right arm

     M92.02 Juvenile osteochondrosis of humerus, left arm

√5ᵗʰ **M92.1** Juvenile osteochondrosis of radius and ulna

     Osteochondrosis (juvenile) of lower ulna [Burns]

     Osteochondrosis (juvenile) of radial head [Brailsford]

     M92.10 Juvenile osteochondrosis of radius and ulna, unspecified arm

N Newborn: 0   **P** Pediatric: 0-17   **M** Maternity: 9-64   **A** Adult: 15-124   **MCC** Major Complication/Comorbidity   **CC** Complication/Comorbidity   **SW** Severe Wound Dx

846   ICD-10-CM 2020

M92.11   **Juvenile osteochondrosis of radius and ulna, right arm**

M92.12   **Juvenile osteochondrosis of radius and ulna, left arm**

√5ᵗʰ **M92.2**   **Juvenile osteochondrosis, hand**

    √6ᵗʰ **M92.20**   **Unspecified juvenile osteochondrosis, hand**

      M92.201   **Unspecified juvenile osteochondrosis, right hand**

      M92.202   **Unspecified juvenile osteochondrosis, left hand**

      M92.209   **Unspecified juvenile osteochondrosis, unspecified hand**

    √6ᵗʰ **M92.21**   **Osteochondrosis (juvenile) of carpal lunate [Kienböck]**

      M92.211   **Osteochondrosis (juvenile) of carpal lunate [Kienböck], right hand**

      M92.212   **Osteochondrosis (juvenile) of carpal lunate [Kienböck], left hand**

      M92.219   **Osteochondrosis (juvenile) of carpal lunate [Kienböck], unspecified hand**

    √6ᵗʰ **M92.22**   **Osteochondrosis (juvenile) of metacarpal heads [Mauclaire]**

      M92.221   **Osteochondrosis (juvenile) of metacarpal heads [Mauclaire], right hand**

      M92.222   **Osteochondrosis (juvenile) of metacarpal heads [Mauclaire], left hand**

      M92.229   **Osteochondrosis (juvenile) of metacarpal heads [Mauclaire], unspecified hand**

    √6ᵗʰ **M92.29**   **Other juvenile osteochondrosis, hand**

      M92.291   **Other juvenile osteochondrosis, right hand**

      M92.292   **Other juvenile osteochondrosis, left hand**

      M92.299   **Other juvenile osteochondrosis, unspecified hand**

√5ᵗʰ **M92.3**   **Other juvenile osteochondrosis, upper limb**

    M92.30   **Other juvenile osteochondrosis, unspecified upper limb**

    M92.31   **Other juvenile osteochondrosis, right upper limb**

    M92.32   **Other juvenile osteochondrosis, left upper limb**

√5ᵗʰ **M92.4**   **Juvenile osteochondrosis of patella**

    Osteochondrosis (juvenile) of primary patellar center [Köhler]

    Osteochondrosis (juvenile) of secondary patellar centre [Sinding Larsen]

    M92.40   **Juvenile osteochondrosis of patella, unspecified knee**

    M92.41   **Juvenile osteochondrosis of patella, right knee**

    M92.42   **Juvenile osteochondrosis of patella, left knee**

√5ᵗʰ **M92.5**   **Juvenile osteochondrosis of tibia and fibula**

    Osteochondrosis (juvenile) of proximal tibia [Blount]

    Osteochondrosis (juvenile) of tibial tubercle [Osgood-Schlatter]

    Tibia vara

    M92.50   **Juvenile osteochondrosis of tibia and fibula, unspecified leg**

    M92.51   **Juvenile osteochondrosis of tibia and fibula, right leg**

    M92.52   **Juvenile osteochondrosis of tibia and fibula, left leg**

√5ᵗʰ **M92.6**   **Juvenile osteochondrosis of tarsus**

    Osteochondrosis (juvenile) of calcaneum [Sever]

    Osteochondrosis (juvenile) of os tibiale externum [Haglund]

    Osteochondrosis (juvenile) of talus [Diaz]

    Osteochondrosis (juvenile) of tarsal navicular [Köhler]

    M92.60   **Juvenile osteochondrosis of tarsus, unspecified ankle**

    M92.61   **Juvenile osteochondrosis of tarsus, right ankle**

    M92.62   **Juvenile osteochondrosis of tarsus, left ankle**

√5ᵗʰ **M92.7**   **Juvenile osteochondrosis of metatarsus**

    Osteochondrosis (juvenile) of fifth metatarsus [Iselin]

    Osteochondrosis (juvenile) of second metatarsus [Freiberg]

    M92.70   **Juvenile osteochondrosis of metatarsus, unspecified foot**

    M92.71   **Juvenile osteochondrosis of metatarsus, right foot**

    M92.72   **Juvenile osteochondrosis of metatarsus, left foot**

M92.8   **Other specified juvenile osteochondrosis**

    Calcaneal apophysitis

    DEF: Calcaneal apophysitis: Inflammation of the calcaneus at the point of Achilles tendon insertion usually occurring in boys ages 8 to 14. Pain, tenderness, and localized swelling are present.

M92.9   **Juvenile osteochondrosis, unspecified**

    Juvenile apophysitis NOS

    Juvenile epiphysitis NOS

    Juvenile osteochondritis NOS

    Juvenile osteochondrosis NOS

√4ᵗʰ **M93**   **Other osteochondropathies**

    EXCLUDES 2   osteochondrosis of spine (M42.-)

√5ᵗʰ **M93.0**   **Slipped upper femoral epiphysis (nontraumatic)**

    Use additional code for associated chondrolysis (M94.3)

    √6ᵗʰ **M93.00**   **Unspecified slipped upper femoral epiphysis (nontraumatic)**

      M93.001   **Unspecified slipped upper femoral epiphysis (nontraumatic), right hip**

      M93.002   **Unspecified slipped upper femoral epiphysis (nontraumatic), left hip**

      M93.003   **Unspecified slipped upper femoral epiphysis (nontraumatic), unspecified hip**

    √6ᵗʰ **M93.01**   **Acute slipped upper femoral epiphysis (nontraumatic)**

      M93.011   **Acute slipped upper femoral epiphysis (nontraumatic), right hip**

      M93.012   **Acute slipped upper femoral epiphysis (nontraumatic), left hip**

      M93.013   **Acute slipped upper femoral epiphysis (nontraumatic), unspecified hip**

    √6ᵗʰ **M93.02**   **Chronic slipped upper femoral epiphysis (nontraumatic)**

      M93.021   **Chronic slipped upper femoral epiphysis (nontraumatic), right hip**

      M93.022   **Chronic slipped upper femoral epiphysis (nontraumatic), left hip**

      M93.023   **Chronic slipped upper femoral epiphysis (nontraumatic), unspecified hip**

    √6ᵗʰ **M93.03**   **Acute on chronic slipped upper femoral epiphysis (nontraumatic)**

      M93.031   **Acute on chronic slipped upper femoral epiphysis (nontraumatic), right hip**

      M93.032   **Acute on chronic slipped upper femoral epiphysis (nontraumatic), left hip**

      M93.033   **Acute on chronic slipped upper femoral epiphysis (nontraumatic), unspecified hip**

M93.1   **Kienböck's disease of adults**   Ⓐ

    Adult osteochondrosis of carpal lunates

√5ᵗʰ **M93.2**   **Osteochondritis dissecans**

    DEF: Avascular necrosis caused by lack of blood flow to the bone and cartilage of a joint causing the bone to die. This can result in splinters or pieces of cartilage breaking off in the joint.

    M93.20   **Osteochondritis dissecans of unspecified site**

    √6ᵗʰ **M93.21**   **Osteochondritis dissecans of shoulder**

      M93.211   **Osteochondritis dissecans, right shoulder**

      M93.212   **Osteochondritis dissecans, left shoulder**

      M93.219   **Osteochondritis dissecans, unspecified shoulder**

    √6ᵗʰ **M93.22**   **Osteochondritis dissecans of elbow**

      M93.221   **Osteochondritis dissecans, right elbow**

      M93.222   **Osteochondritis dissecans, left elbow**

      M93.229   **Osteochondritis dissecans, unspecified elbow**

    √6ᵗʰ **M93.23**   **Osteochondritis dissecans of wrist**

      M93.231   **Osteochondritis dissecans, right wrist**

      M93.232   **Osteochondritis dissecans, left wrist**

      M93.239   **Osteochondritis dissecans, unspecified wrist**

    √6ᵗʰ **M93.24**   **Osteochondritis dissecans of joints of hand**

      M93.241   **Osteochondritis dissecans, joints of right hand**

      M93.242   **Osteochondritis dissecans, joints of left hand**

      M93.249   **Osteochondritis dissecans, joints of unspecified hand**

    √6ᵗʰ **M93.25**   **Osteochondritis dissecans of hip**

      M93.251   **Osteochondritis dissecans, right hip**

      M93.252   **Osteochondritis dissecans, left hip**

      M93.259   **Osteochondritis dissecans, unspecified hip**

    √6ᵗʰ **M93.26**   **Osteochondritis dissecans knee**

      M93.261   **Osteochondritis dissecans, right knee**

      M93.262   **Osteochondritis dissecans, left knee**

✔ Additional Character Required   ✔x7ᵗʰ Placeholder   Unacceptable PDx   Questionable PDx   Manifestation   Unspecified Dx   H1-H14 HAC   HCC CMS-HCC Dx   HIV HIV Dx

ICD-10-CM 2020   **847**

M93.269 Osteochondritis dissecans, unspecified knee

✓6ᵗʰ M93.27 Osteochondritis dissecans of ankle and joints of foot

M93.271 Osteochondritis dissecans, right ankle and joints of right foot

M93.272 Osteochondritis dissecans, left ankle and joints of left foot

M93.279 Osteochondritis dissecans, unspecified ankle and joints of foot

M93.28 Osteochondritis dissecans other site

M93.29 Osteochondritis dissecans multiple sites

✓5ᵗʰ M93.8 Other specified osteochondropathies

M93.80 Other specified osteochondropathies of unspecified site

✓6ᵗʰ M93.81 Other specified osteochondropathies of shoulder

M93.811 Other specified osteochondropathies, right shoulder

M93.812 Other specified osteochondropathies, left shoulder

M93.819 Other specified osteochondropathies, unspecified shoulder

✓6ᵗʰ M93.82 Other specified osteochondropathies of upper arm

M93.821 Other specified osteochondropathies, right upper arm

M93.822 Other specified osteochondropathies, left upper arm

M93.829 Other specified osteochondropathies, unspecified upper arm

✓6ᵗʰ M93.83 Other specified osteochondropathies of forearm

M93.831 Other specified osteochondropathies, right forearm

M93.832 Other specified osteochondropathies, left forearm

M93.839 Other specified osteochondropathies, unspecified forearm

✓6ᵗʰ M93.84 Other specified osteochondropathies of hand

M93.841 Other specified osteochondropathies, right hand

M93.842 Other specified osteochondropathies, left hand

M93.849 Other specified osteochondropathies, unspecified hand

✓6ᵗʰ M93.85 Other specified osteochondropathies of thigh

M93.851 Other specified osteochondropathies, right thigh

M93.852 Other specified osteochondropathies, left thigh

M93.859 Other specified osteochondropathies, unspecified thigh

✓6ᵗʰ M93.86 Other specified osteochondropathies lower leg

M93.861 Other specified osteochondropathies, right lower leg

M93.862 Other specified osteochondropathies, left lower leg

M93.869 Other specified osteochondropathies, unspecified lower leg

✓6ᵗʰ M93.87 Other specified osteochondropathies of ankle and foot

M93.871 Other specified osteochondropathies, right ankle and foot

M93.872 Other specified osteochondropathies, left ankle and foot

M93.879 Other specified osteochondropathies, unspecified ankle and foot

M93.88 Other specified osteochondropathies other site

M93.89 Other specified osteochondropathies multiple sites

✓5ᵗʰ M93.9 Osteochondropathy, unspecified

Apophysitis NOS

Epiphysitis NOS

Osteochondritis NOS

Osteochondrosis NOS

M93.90 Osteochondropathy, unspecified of unspecified site

✓6ᵗʰ M93.91 Osteochondropathy, unspecified of shoulder

M93.911 Osteochondropathy, unspecified, right shoulder

M93.912 Osteochondropathy, unspecified, left shoulder

M93.919 Osteochondropathy, unspecified, unspecified shoulder

✓6ᵗʰ M93.92 Osteochondropathy, unspecified of upper arm

M93.921 Osteochondropathy, unspecified, right upper arm

M93.922 Osteochondropathy, unspecified, left upper arm

M93.929 Osteochondropathy, unspecified, unspecified upper arm

✓6ᵗʰ M93.93 Osteochondropathy, unspecified of forearm

M93.931 Osteochondropathy, unspecified, right forearm

M93.932 Osteochondropathy, unspecified, left forearm

M93.939 Osteochondropathy, unspecified, unspecified forearm

✓6ᵗʰ M93.94 Osteochondropathy, unspecified of hand

M93.941 Osteochondropathy, unspecified, right hand

M93.942 Osteochondropathy, unspecified, left hand

M93.949 Osteochondropathy, unspecified, unspecified hand

✓6ᵗʰ M93.95 Osteochondropathy, unspecified of thigh

M93.951 Osteochondropathy, unspecified, right thigh

M93.952 Osteochondropathy, unspecified, left thigh

M93.959 Osteochondropathy, unspecified, unspecified thigh

✓6ᵗʰ M93.96 Osteochondropathy, unspecified lower leg

M93.961 Osteochondropathy, unspecified, right lower leg

M93.962 Osteochondropathy, unspecified, left lower leg

M93.969 Osteochondropathy, unspecified, unspecified lower leg

✓6ᵗʰ M93.97 Osteochondropathy, unspecified of ankle and foot

M93.971 Osteochondropathy, unspecified, right ankle and foot

M93.972 Osteochondropathy, unspecified, left ankle and foot

M93.979 Osteochondropathy, unspecified, unspecified ankle and foot

M93.98 Osteochondropathy, unspecified other site

M93.99 Osteochondropathy, unspecified multiple sites

✓4ᵗʰ M94 Other disorders of cartilage

M94.0 Chondrocostal junction syndrome [Tietze]

Costochondritis

M94.1 Relapsing polychondritis

✓5ᵗʰ M94.2 Chondromalacia

EXCLUDES 1   chondromalacia patellae (M22.4)

M94.20 Chondromalacia, unspecified site

✓6ᵗʰ M94.21 Chondromalacia, shoulder

M94.211 Chondromalacia, right shoulder

M94.212 Chondromalacia, left shoulder

M94.219 Chondromalacia, unspecified shoulder

✓6ᵗʰ M94.22 Chondromalacia, elbow

M94.221 Chondromalacia, right elbow

M94.222 Chondromalacia, left elbow

M94.229 Chondromalacia, unspecified elbow

✓6ᵗʰ M94.23 Chondromalacia, wrist

M94.231 Chondromalacia, right wrist

M94.232 Chondromalacia, left wrist

M94.239 Chondromalacia, unspecified wrist

✓6ᵗʰ M94.24 Chondromalacia, joints of hand

M94.241 Chondromalacia, joints of right hand

M94.242 Chondromalacia, joints of left hand

M94.249 Chondromalacia, joints of unspecified hand

✓6ᵗʰ M94.25 Chondromalacia, hip

M94.251 Chondromalacia, right hip

M94.252 Chondromalacia, left hip

M94.259 Chondromalacia, unspecified hip

✓6ᵗʰ M94.26 Chondromalacia, knee

M94.261 Chondromalacia, right knee

M94.262 Chondromalacia, left knee

N Newborn: 0   P Pediatric: 0-17   M Maternity: 9-64   A Adult: 15-124   MCC Major Complication/Comorbidity   CC Complication/Comorbidity   SW Severe Wound Dx

848   ICD-10-CM 2020

          M94.269 Chondromalacia, unspecified knee

✓6th **M94.27** Chondromalacia, ankle and joints of foot

          M94.271 Chondromalacia, right ankle and joints of right foot

          M94.272 Chondromalacia, left ankle and joints of left foot

          M94.279 Chondromalacia, unspecified ankle and joints of foot

     M94.28 Chondromalacia, other site

     M94.29 Chondromalacia, multiple sites

✓5th **M94.3** Chondrolysis

       Code first any associated slipped upper femoral epiphysis (nontraumatic) (M93.0-)

   ✓6th **M94.35** Chondrolysis, hip

          M94.351 Chondrolysis, right hip

          M94.352 Chondrolysis, left hip

          M94.359 Chondrolysis, unspecified hip

✓5th **M94.8** Other specified disorders of cartilage

   ✓6th **M94.8X** Other specified disorders of cartilage

          M94.8X0 Other specified disorders of cartilage, multiple sites

          M94.8X1 Other specified disorders of cartilage, shoulder

          M94.8X2 Other specified disorders of cartilage, upper arm

          M94.8X3 Other specified disorders of cartilage, forearm

          M94.8X4 Other specified disorders of cartilage, hand

          M94.8X5 Other specified disorders of cartilage, thigh

          M94.8X6 Other specified disorders of cartilage, lower leg

          M94.8X7 Other specified disorders of cartilage, ankle and foot

          M94.8X8 Other specified disorders of cartilage, other site

          M94.8X9 Other specified disorders of cartilage, unspecified sites

   M94.9 Disorder of cartilage, unspecified

Other disorders of the musculoskeletal system and connective tissue (M95)

✓4th **M95** Other acquired deformities of musculoskeletal system and connective tissue

     EXCLUDES 2   acquired absence of limbs and organs (Z89-Z90)

           acquired deformities of limbs (M20-M21)

           congenital malformations and deformations of the musculoskeletal system (Q65-Q79)

           deforming dorsopathies (M40-M43)

           dentofacial anomalies [including malocclusion] (M26.-)

           postprocedural musculoskeletal disorders (M96.-)

   M95.0 Acquired deformity of nose

     EXCLUDES 2   deviated nasal septum (J34.2)

✓5th **M95.1** Cauliflower ear

     EXCLUDES 2   other acquired deformities of ear (H61.1)

     DEF: Acquired deformity of the external ear due to injury or subsequent perichondritis.

     M95.10 Cauliflower ear, unspecified ear

     M95.11 Cauliflower ear, right ear

     M95.12 Cauliflower ear, left ear

   M95.2 Other acquired deformity of head

   M95.3 Acquired deformity of neck

   M95.4 Acquired deformity of chest and rib

     AHA: 2014,4Q,26-27

   M95.5 Acquired deformity of pelvis

     EXCLUDES 1   maternal care for known or suspected disproportion (O33.-)

   M95.8 Other specified acquired deformities of musculoskeletal system

   M95.9 Acquired deformity of musculoskeletal system, unspecified

Intraoperative and postprocedural complications and disorders of musculoskeletal system, not elsewhere classified (M96)

✓4th **M96** Intraoperative and postprocedural complications and disorders of musculoskeletal system, not elsewhere classified

     EXCLUDES 2   arthropathy following intestinal bypass (M02.0-)

           complications of internal orthopedic prosthetic devices, implants and grafts (T84.-)

           disorders associated with osteoporosis (M80)

           periprosthetic fracture around internal prosthetic joint (M97.-)

           presence of functional implants and other devices (Z96-Z97)

   M96.0 Pseudarthrosis after fusion or arthrodesis   CC

     CC Excl: No Excl

   M96.1 Postlaminectomy syndrome, not elsewhere classified

   M96.2 Postradiation kyphosis

   M96.3 Postlaminectomy kyphosis

   M96.4 Postsurgical lordosis

   M96.5 Postradiation scoliosis

✓5th **M96.6** Fracture of bone following insertion of orthopedic implant, joint prosthesis, or bone plate

     Intraoperative fracture of bone during insertion of orthopedic implant, joint prosthesis, or bone plate

     EXCLUDES 2   complication of internal orthopedic devices, implants or grafts (T84.-)

     CC Excl: For CC codes in subcategory M96.6: PDX collection 911

   ✓6th **M96.62** Fracture of humerus following insertion of orthopedic implant, joint prosthesis, or bone plate

          M96.621 Fracture of humerus following insertion of orthopedic implant, joint prosthesis, or bone plate, right arm   CC HCC

          M96.622 Fracture of humerus following insertion of orthopedic implant, joint prosthesis, or bone plate, left arm   CC HCC

          M96.629 Fracture of humerus following insertion of orthopedic implant, joint prosthesis, or bone plate, unspecified arm   CC HCC

   ✓6th **M96.63** Fracture of radius or ulna following insertion of orthopedic implant, joint prosthesis, or bone plate

          M96.631 Fracture of radius or ulna following insertion of orthopedic implant, joint prosthesis, or bone plate, right arm   CC HCC

          M96.632 Fracture of radius or ulna following insertion of orthopedic implant, joint prosthesis, or bone plate, left arm   CC HCC

          M96.639 Fracture of radius or ulna following insertion of orthopedic implant, joint prosthesis, or bone plate, unspecified arm   CC HCC

     M96.65 Fracture of pelvis following insertion of orthopedic implant, joint prosthesis, or bone plate   CC HCC

   ✓6th **M96.66** Fracture of femur following insertion of orthopedic implant, joint prosthesis, or bone plate

          M96.661 Fracture of femur following insertion of orthopedic implant, joint prosthesis, or bone plate, right leg   CC HCC

          M96.662 Fracture of femur following insertion of orthopedic implant, joint prosthesis, or bone plate, left leg   CC HCC

          M96.669 Fracture of femur following insertion of orthopedic implant, joint prosthesis, or bone plate, unspecified leg   CC HCC

Chapter 13. Diseases of the Musculoskeletal System and Connective Tissue

√6ᵗʰ **M96.67** **Fracture of tibia or fibula following insertion of orthopedic implant, joint prosthesis, or bone plate**

     M96.671 **Fracture of tibia or fibula following insertion of orthopedic implant, joint prosthesis, or bone plate, right leg** `CC` `HCC`

     M96.672 **Fracture of tibia or fibula following insertion of orthopedic implant, joint prosthesis, or bone plate, left leg** `CC` `HCC`

     M96.679 **Fracture of tibia or fibula following insertion of orthopedic implant, joint prosthesis, or bone plate, unspecified leg** `CC` `HCC`

     M96.69 **Fracture of other bone following insertion of orthopedic implant, joint prosthesis, or bone plate** `CC` `HCC`

√5ᵗʰ **M96.8** **Other intraoperative and postprocedural complications and disorders of musculoskeletal system, not elsewhere classified**

     AHA: 2016,4Q,9-10

     CC Excl: For CC codes in subcategory M96.8, unless otherwise noted: PDX collection 912

√6ᵗʰ **M96.81** **Intraoperative hemorrhage and hematoma of a musculoskeletal structure complicating a procedure**

     EXCLUDES 1   intraoperative hemorrhage and hematoma of a musculoskeletal structure due to accidental puncture and laceration during a procedure (M96.82-)

     M96.810 **Intraoperative hemorrhage and hematoma of a musculoskeletal structure complicating a musculoskeletal system procedure** `CC`

     M96.811 **Intraoperative hemorrhage and hematoma of a musculoskeletal structure complicating other procedure** `CC`

√6ᵗʰ **M96.82** **Accidental puncture and laceration of a musculoskeletal structure during a procedure**

     M96.820 **Accidental puncture and laceration of a musculoskeletal structure during a musculoskeletal system procedure** `CC`

         CC Excl: PDX collection 509

     M96.821 **Accidental puncture and laceration of a musculoskeletal structure during other procedure** `CC`

         CC Excl: PDX collection 509

√6ᵗʰ **M96.83** **Postprocedural hemorrhage of a musculoskeletal structure following a procedure**

     M96.830 **Postprocedural hemorrhage of a musculoskeletal structure following a musculoskeletal system procedure** `CC`

     M96.831 **Postprocedural hemorrhage of a musculoskeletal structure following other procedure** `CC`

√6ᵗʰ **M96.84** **Postprocedural hematoma and seroma of a musculoskeletal structure following a procedure**

     M96.840 **Postprocedural hematoma of a musculoskeletal structure following a musculoskeletal system procedure** `CC`

     M96.841 **Postprocedural hematoma of a musculoskeletal structure following other procedure** `CC`

         AHA: 2016,4Q,10

     M96.842 **Postprocedural seroma of a musculoskeletal structure following a musculoskeletal system procedure** `CC`

     M96.843 **Postprocedural seroma of a musculoskeletal structure following other procedure** `CC`

         AHA: 2018,3Q,6

     M96.89 **Other intraoperative and postprocedural complications and disorders of the musculoskeletal system** `CC`

         Instability of joint secondary to removal of joint prosthesis

         Use additional code, if applicable, to further specify disorder

         CC Excl: PDX collection 643

Periprosthetic fractures around internal prosthetic joint (M97)

√4ᵗʰ **M97** **Periprosthetic fracture around internal prosthetic joint**

     EXCLUDES 2   breakage (fracture) of prosthetic joint (T84.01-)
            fracture of bone following insertion of orthopedic implant, joint prosthesis or bone plate (M96.6-)

     AHA: 2016,4Q,42-43

     The appropriate 7th character is to be added to each code from category M97.
     A   initial encounter
     D   subsequent encounter
     S   sequela

     CC Excl: For CC codes in category M97: PDX collection 911

√5ᵗʰ **M97.0** **Periprosthetic fracture around internal prosthetic hip joint**

     AHA: 2018,1Q,21; 2016,4Q,42

     √x7ᵗʰ **M97.01** **Periprosthetic fracture around internal prosthetic right hip joint** `CC` `HCC`

     √x7ᵗʰ **M97.02** **Periprosthetic fracture around internal prosthetic left hip joint** `CC` `HCC`

√5ᵗʰ **M97.1** **Periprosthetic fracture around internal prosthetic knee joint**

     √x7ᵗʰ **M97.11** **Periprosthetic fracture around internal prosthetic right knee joint** `CC`

     √x7ᵗʰ **M97.12** **Periprosthetic fracture around internal prosthetic left knee joint** `CC`

√5ᵗʰ **M97.2** **Periprosthetic fracture around internal prosthetic ankle joint**

     √x7ᵗʰ **M97.21** **Periprosthetic fracture around internal prosthetic right ankle joint** `CC`

     √x7ᵗʰ **M97.22** **Periprosthetic fracture around internal prosthetic left ankle joint** `CC`

√5ᵗʰ **M97.3** **Periprosthetic fracture around internal prosthetic shoulder joint**

     √x7ᵗʰ **M97.31** **Periprosthetic fracture around internal prosthetic right shoulder joint** `CC`

     √x7ᵗʰ **M97.32** **Periprosthetic fracture around internal prosthetic left shoulder joint** `CC`

√5ᵗʰ **M97.4** **Periprosthetic fracture around internal prosthetic elbow joint**

     √x7ᵗʰ **M97.41** **Periprosthetic fracture around internal prosthetic right elbow joint** `CC`

     √x7ᵗʰ **M97.42** **Periprosthetic fracture around internal prosthetic left elbow joint** `CC`

√x7ᵗʰ **M97.8** **Periprosthetic fracture around other internal prosthetic joint** `CC`

     Periprosthetic fracture around internal prosthetic finger joint
     Periprosthetic fracture around internal prosthetic spinal joint
     Periprosthetic fracture around internal prosthetic toe joint
     Periprosthetic fracture around internal prosthetic wrist joint
     Use additional code to identify the joint (Z96.6-)

√x7ᵗʰ **M97.9** **Periprosthetic fracture around unspecified internal prosthetic joint** `CC`

N Newborn: 0   P Pediatric: 0-17   M Maternity: 9-64   A Adult: 15-124   `MCC` Major Complication/Comorbidity   `CC` Complication/Comorbidity   `SW` Severe Wound Dx

850   ICD-10-CM 2020

Biomechanical lesions, not elsewhere classified (M99)

✓4ᵗʰ M99 Biomechanical lesions, not elsewhere classified

> **NOTE**   This category should not be used if the condition can be classified elsewhere.
>
> **DEF:** Biomechanical lesion: Term used by osteopathic and chiropractic physicians to describe musculoskeletal conditions treated that are not more appropriately classified elsewhere.

  ✓6ᵗʰ M99.0 Segmental and somatic dysfunction

    M99.00 Segmental and somatic dysfunction of head region
    M99.01 Segmental and somatic dysfunction of cervical region
    M99.02 Segmental and somatic dysfunction of thoracic region
    M99.03 Segmental and somatic dysfunction of lumbar region
    M99.04 Segmental and somatic dysfunction of sacral region
    M99.05 Segmental and somatic dysfunction of pelvic region
    M99.06 Segmental and somatic dysfunction of lower extremity
    M99.07 Segmental and somatic dysfunction of upper extremity
    M99.08 Segmental and somatic dysfunction of rib cage
    M99.09 Segmental and somatic dysfunction of abdomen and other regions

  ✓5ᵗʰ M99.1 Subluxation complex (vertebral)

    M99.10 Subluxation complex (vertebral) of head region   CC H5
        CC Excl: PDX collection 913
    M99.11 Subluxation complex (vertebral) of cervical region   CC H5
        CC Excl: PDX collection 913
    M99.12 Subluxation complex (vertebral) of thoracic region
    M99.13 Subluxation complex (vertebral) of lumbar region
    M99.14 Subluxation complex (vertebral) of sacral region
    M99.15 Subluxation complex (vertebral) of pelvic region
    M99.16 Subluxation complex (vertebral) of lower extremity
    M99.17 Subluxation complex (vertebral) of upper extremity
    M99.18 Subluxation complex (vertebral) of rib cage   CC H5
        CC Excl: PDX collection 914
    M99.19 Subluxation complex (vertebral) of abdomen and other regions

  ✓5ᵗʰ M99.2 Subluxation stenosis of neural canal

    M99.20 Subluxation stenosis of neural canal of head region
    M99.21 Subluxation stenosis of neural canal of cervical region
    M99.22 Subluxation stenosis of neural canal of thoracic region
    M99.23 Subluxation stenosis of neural canal of lumbar region
    M99.24 Subluxation stenosis of neural canal of sacral region
    M99.25 Subluxation stenosis of neural canal of pelvic region
    M99.26 Subluxation stenosis of neural canal of lower extremity
    M99.27 Subluxation stenosis of neural canal of upper extremity
    M99.28 Subluxation stenosis of neural canal of rib cage
    M99.29 Subluxation stenosis of neural canal of abdomen and other regions

  ✓5ᵗʰ M99.3 Osseous stenosis of neural canal

    M99.30 Osseous stenosis of neural canal of head region
    M99.31 Osseous stenosis of neural canal of cervical region
    M99.32 Osseous stenosis of neural canal of thoracic region
    M99.33 Osseous stenosis of neural canal of lumbar region
    M99.34 Osseous stenosis of neural canal of sacral region
    M99.35 Osseous stenosis of neural canal of pelvic region
    M99.36 Osseous stenosis of neural canal of lower extremity
    M99.37 Osseous stenosis of neural canal of upper extremity
    M99.38 Osseous stenosis of neural canal of rib cage
    M99.39 Osseous stenosis of neural canal of abdomen and other regions

  ✓5ᵗʰ M99.4 Connective tissue stenosis of neural canal

    M99.40 Connective tissue stenosis of neural canal of head region
    M99.41 Connective tissue stenosis of neural canal of cervical region

    M99.42 Connective tissue stenosis of neural canal of thoracic region
    M99.43 Connective tissue stenosis of neural canal of lumbar region
    M99.44 Connective tissue stenosis of neural canal of sacral region
    M99.45 Connective tissue stenosis of neural canal of pelvic region
    M99.46 Connective tissue stenosis of neural canal of lower extremity
    M99.47 Connective tissue stenosis of neural canal of upper extremity
    M99.48 Connective tissue stenosis of neural canal of rib cage
    M99.49 Connective tissue stenosis of neural canal of abdomen and other regions

  ✓5ᵗʰ M99.5 Intervertebral disc stenosis of neural canal

    M99.50 Intervertebral disc stenosis of neural canal of head region
    M99.51 Intervertebral disc stenosis of neural canal of cervical region
    M99.52 Intervertebral disc stenosis of neural canal of thoracic region
    M99.53 Intervertebral disc stenosis of neural canal of lumbar region
    M99.54 Intervertebral disc stenosis of neural canal of sacral region
    M99.55 Intervertebral disc stenosis of neural canal of pelvic region
    M99.56 Intervertebral disc stenosis of neural canal of lower extremity
    M99.57 Intervertebral disc stenosis of neural canal of upper extremity
    M99.58 Intervertebral disc stenosis of neural canal of rib cage
    M99.59 Intervertebral disc stenosis of neural canal of abdomen and other regions

  ✓5ᵗʰ M99.6 Osseous and subluxation stenosis of intervertebral foramina

    M99.60 Osseous and subluxation stenosis of intervertebral foramina of head region
    M99.61 Osseous and subluxation stenosis of intervertebral foramina of cervical region
    M99.62 Osseous and subluxation stenosis of intervertebral foramina of thoracic region
    M99.63 Osseous and subluxation stenosis of intervertebral foramina of lumbar region
    M99.64 Osseous and subluxation stenosis of intervertebral foramina of sacral region
    M99.65 Osseous and subluxation stenosis of intervertebral foramina of pelvic region
    M99.66 Osseous and subluxation stenosis of intervertebral foramina of lower extremity
    M99.67 Osseous and subluxation stenosis of intervertebral foramina of upper extremity
    M99.68 Osseous and subluxation stenosis of intervertebral foramina of rib cage
    M99.69 Osseous and subluxation stenosis of intervertebral foramina of abdomen and other regions

  ✓5ᵗʰ M99.7 Connective tissue and disc stenosis of intervertebral foramina

    M99.70 Connective tissue and disc stenosis of intervertebral foramina of head region
    M99.71 Connective tissue and disc stenosis of intervertebral foramina of cervical region
    M99.72 Connective tissue and disc stenosis of intervertebral foramina of thoracic region
    M99.73 Connective tissue and disc stenosis of intervertebral foramina of lumbar region
    M99.74 Connective tissue and disc stenosis of intervertebral foramina of sacral region
    M99.75 Connective tissue and disc stenosis of intervertebral foramina of pelvic region
    M99.76 Connective tissue and disc stenosis of intervertebral foramina of lower extremity
    M99.77 Connective tissue and disc stenosis of intervertebral foramina of upper extremity
    M99.78 Connective tissue and disc stenosis of intervertebral foramina of rib cage
    M99.79 Connective tissue and disc stenosis of intervertebral foramina of abdomen and other regions

  ✓5ᵗʰ M99.8 Other biomechanical lesions

    M99.80 Other biomechanical lesions of head region

☑ Additional Character Required   ✓x7ᵗʰ Placeholder   Unacceptable PDx   • Questionable PDx   Manifestation   Unspecified Dx   H1–H14 HAC   HCC CMS-HCC Dx   HIV HIV Dx

M99.81	**Other biomechanical lesions of cervical region**
M99.82	**Other biomechanical lesions of thoracic region**
M99.83	**Other biomechanical lesions of lumbar region**
M99.84	**Other biomechanical lesions of sacral region**
M99.85	**Other biomechanical lesions of pelvic region**
M99.86	**Other biomechanical lesions of lower extremity**
M99.87	**Other biomechanical lesions of upper extremity**
M99.88	**Other biomechanical lesions of rib cage**
M99.89	**Other biomechanical lesions of abdomen and other regions**

M99.9 **Biomechanical lesion, unspecified**

Ⓝ Newborn: 0   Ⓟ Pediatric: 0-17   Ⓜ Maternity: 9-64   Ⓐ Adult: 15-124   **MCC** Major Complication/Comorbidity   **CC** Complication/Comorbidity   **SW** Severe Wound Dx

852

ICD-10-CM 2020

Chapter 14. Diseases of Genitourinary System (NØØ–N99)

Chapter-specific Guidelines with Coding Examples

The chapter-specific guidelines from the ICD-10-CM Official Guidelines for Coding and Reporting have been provided below. Along with these guidelines are coding examples, contained in the shaded boxes, that have been developed to help illustrate the coding and/or sequencing guidance found in these guidelines.

a. Chronic kidney disease

1) Stages of chronic kidney disease (CKD)

The ICD-10-CM classifies CKD based on severity. The severity of CKD is designated by stages 1-5. Stage 2, code N18.2, equates to mild CKD; stage 3, code N18.3, equates to moderate CKD; and stage 4, code N18.4, equates to severe CKD. Code N18.6, End stage renal disease (ESRD), is assigned when the provider has documented end-stage renal disease (ESRD).

If both a stage of CKD and ESRD are documented, assign code N18.6 only.

> Stage 5 chronic kidney disease with ESRD requiring chronic dialysis
>
> **N18.6**   **End stage renal disease**
>
> **Z99.2**   **Dependence on renal dialysis**
>
> *Explanation:* The diagnostic statement indicates the patient has chronic kidney disease, documented both as stage 5 and as ESRD requiring chronic dialysis. Code N18.6 End stage renal disease (ESRD), is assigned when the provider has documented end-stage-renal disease (ESRD). If both a stage of CKD and ESRD are documented, assign code N18.6 only.

2) Chronic kidney disease and kidney transplant status

Patients who have undergone kidney transplant may still have some form of chronic kidney disease (CKD) because the kidney transplant may not fully restore kidney function. Therefore, the presence of CKD alone does not constitute a transplant complication. Assign the appropriate N18 code for the patient's stage of CKD and code Z94.0, Kidney transplant status. If a transplant complication such as failure or rejection or other transplant complication is documented, see section I.C.19.g for information on coding complications of a kidney transplant. If the documentation is unclear as to whether the patient has a complication of the transplant, query the provider.

> Patient with residual chronic kidney disease stage 1 after kidney transplant
>
> **N18.1**   **Chronic kidney disease, stage 1**
>
> **Z94.Ø**   **Kidney transplant status**
>
> *Explanation:* Patients who have undergone kidney transplant may still have some form of chronic kidney disease (CKD) because the kidney transplant may not fully restore kidney function. The presence of CKD alone does not constitute a transplant complication. Assign the appropriate N18 code for the patient's stage of CKD and code Z94.0 Kidney transplant status.

3) Chronic kidney disease with other conditions

Patients with CKD may also suffer from other serious conditions, most commonly diabetes mellitus and hypertension. The sequencing of the CKD code in relationship to codes for other contributing conditions is based on the conventions in the Tabular List.

See I.C.9. Hypertensive chronic kidney disease.

See I.C.19. Chronic kidney disease and kidney transplant complications.

> Type 1 diabetic chronic kidney disease, stage 2
>
> **E10.22**   **Type 1 diabetes mellitus with diabetic chronic kidney disease**
>
> **N18.2**   **Chronic kidney disease, stage 2 (mild)**
>
> *Explanation:* Patients with CKD may also suffer from other serious conditions such as diabetes mellitus. The sequencing of the CKD code in relationship to codes for other contributing conditions is based on the conventions in the Tabular List. Diabetic CKD code E10.22 includes an instructional note to "Use additional code to identify stage of chronic kidney disease (N18.1–N18.6)," thus providing sequencing direction.

Chapter 14. Diseases of the Genitourinary System (N00-N99)

EXCLUDES 2   certain conditions originating in the perinatal period (P04-P96)
certain infectious and parasitic diseases (A00-B99)
complications of pregnancy, childbirth and the puerperium (O00-O9A)
congenital malformations, deformations and chromosomal abnormalities (Q00-Q99)
endocrine, nutritional and metabolic diseases (E00-E88)
injury, poisoning and certain other consequences of external causes (S00-T88)
neoplasms (C00-D49)
symptoms, signs and abnormal clinical and laboratory findings, not elsewhere classified (R00-R94)

This chapter contains the following blocks:
N00-N08   Glomerular diseases
N10-N16   Renal tubulo-interstitial diseases
N17-N19   Acute kidney failure and chronic kidney disease
N20-N23   Urolithiasis
N25-N29   Other disorders of kidney and ureter
N30-N39   Other diseases of the urinary system
N40-N53   Diseases of male genital organs
N60-N65   Disorders of breast
N70-N77   Inflammatory diseases of female pelvic organs
N80-N98   Noninflammatory disorders of female genital tract
N99   Intraoperative and postprocedural complications and disorders of genitourinary system, not elsewhere classified

Glomerular diseases (N00-N08)

Code also any associated kidney failure (N17-N19).
EXCLUDES 1   hypertensive chronic kidney disease (I12.-)
DEF: Glomeruli: Clusters of microscopic blood vessels located within the kidneys containing small pores through which waste products are filtered from the blood and urine is formed.
DEF: Glomerulonephritis: Disease of the kidney with diffuse inflammation of the capillary loops of the glomeruli.

✓4ᵗʰ N00 Acute nephritic syndrome

INCLUDES   acute glomerular disease
acute glomerulonephritis
acute nephritis
EXCLUDES 1   acute tubulo-interstitial nephritis (N10)
nephritic syndrome NOS (N05.-)

CC Excl: For MCC codes in category N00, unless otherwise noted: PDX collection 915

N00.0 Acute nephritic syndrome with minor glomerular abnormality   MCC
Acute nephritic syndrome with minimal change lesion

N00.1 Acute nephritic syndrome with focal and segmental glomerular lesions   MCC
Acute nephritic syndrome with focal and segmental hyalinosis
Acute nephritic syndrome with focal and segmental sclerosis
Acute nephritic syndrome with focal glomerulonephritis

N00.2 Acute nephritic syndrome with diffuse membranous glomerulonephritis   MCC

N00.3 Acute nephritic syndrome with diffuse mesangial proliferative glomerulonephritis   MCC

N00.4 Acute nephritic syndrome with diffuse endocapillary proliferative glomerulonephritis   MCC

N00.5 Acute nephritic syndrome with diffuse mesangiocapillary glomerulonephritis   MCC
Acute nephritic syndrome with membranoproliferative glomerulonephritis, types 1 and 3, or NOS

N00.6 Acute nephritic syndrome with dense deposit disease   MCC
Acute nephritic syndrome with membranoproliferative glomerulonephritis, type 2

N00.7 Acute nephritic syndrome with diffuse crescentic glomerulonephritis   MCC
Acute nephritic syndrome with extracapillary glomerulonephritis

N00.8 Acute nephritic syndrome with other morphologic changes   MCC
Acute nephritic syndrome with proliferative glomerulonephritis NOS
CC Excl: PDX collection 916

N00.9 Acute nephritic syndrome with unspecified morphologic changes   MCC

✓4ᵗʰ N01 Rapidly progressive nephritic syndrome

INCLUDES   rapidly progressive glomerular disease
rapidly progressive glomerulonephritis
rapidly progressive nephritis
EXCLUDES 1   nephritic syndrome NOS (N05.-)

CC Excl: For MCC codes in category N01: PDX collection 915

N01.0 Rapidly progressive nephritic syndrome with minor glomerular abnormality   MCC
Rapidly progressive nephritic syndrome with minimal change lesion

N01.1 Rapidly progressive nephritic syndrome with focal and segmental glomerular lesions   MCC
Rapidly progressive nephritic syndrome with focal and segmental hyalinosis
Rapidly progressive nephritic syndrome with focal and segmental sclerosis
Rapidly progressive nephritic syndrome with focal glomerulonephritis

N01.2 Rapidly progressive nephritic syndrome with diffuse membranous glomerulonephritis   MCC

N01.3 Rapidly progressive nephritic syndrome with diffuse mesangial proliferative glomerulonephritis   MCC

N01.4 Rapidly progressive nephritic syndrome with diffuse endocapillary proliferative glomerulonephritis   MCC

N01.5 Rapidly progressive nephritic syndrome with diffuse mesangiocapillary glomerulonephritis   MCC
Rapidly progressive nephritic syndrome with membranoproliferative glomerulonephritis, types 1 and 3, or NOS

N01.6 Rapidly progressive nephritic syndrome with dense deposit disease   MCC
Rapidly progressive nephritic syndrome with membranoproliferative glomerulonephritis, type 2

N01.7 Rapidly progressive nephritic syndrome with diffuse crescentic glomerulonephritis   MCC
Rapidly progressive nephritic syndrome with extracapillary glomerulonephritis

N01.8 Rapidly progressive nephritic syndrome with other morphologic changes   MCC
Rapidly progressive nephritic syndrome with proliferative glomerulonephritis NOS

N01.9 Rapidly progressive nephritic syndrome with unspecified morphologic changes   MCC

✓4ᵗʰ N02 Recurrent and persistent hematuria

EXCLUDES 1   acute cystitis with hematuria (N30.01)
hematuria NOS (R31.9)
hematuria not associated with specified morphologic lesions (R31.-)

CC Excl: For CC codes in category N02, unless otherwise noted: PDX collection 917

N02.0 Recurrent and persistent hematuria with minor glomerular abnormality   CC
Recurrent and persistent hematuria with minimal change lesion

N02.1 Recurrent and persistent hematuria with focal and segmental glomerular lesions   CC
Recurrent and persistent hematuria with focal and segmental hyalinosis
Recurrent and persistent hematuria with focal and segmental sclerosis
Recurrent and persistent hematuria with focal glomerulonephritis

N02.2 Recurrent and persistent hematuria with diffuse membranous glomerulonephritis   CC

N02.3 Recurrent and persistent hematuria with diffuse mesangial proliferative glomerulonephritis   CC

N02.4 Recurrent and persistent hematuria with diffuse endocapillary proliferative glomerulonephritis   CC

N02.5 Recurrent and persistent hematuria with diffuse mesangiocapillary glomerulonephritis   CC
Recurrent and persistent hematuria with membranoproliferative glomerulonephritis, types 1 and 3, or NOS

N Newborn: 0   P Pediatric: 0-17   M Maternity: 9-64   A Adult: 15-124   MCC Major Complication/Comorbidity   CC Complication/Comorbidity   SW Severe Wound Dx

N02.6 **Recurrent and persistent hematuria with dense deposit disease** `CC`
Recurrent and persistent hematuria with membranoproliferative glomerulonephritis, type 2

N02.7 **Recurrent and persistent hematuria with diffuse crescentic glomerulonephritis** `CC`
Recurrent and persistent hematuria with extracapillary glomerulonephritis

N02.8 **Recurrent and persistent hematuria with other morphologic changes** `CC`
Recurrent and persistent hematuria with proliferative glomerulonephritis NOS
CC Excl: PDX collection 915

N02.9 **Recurrent and persistent hematuria with unspecified morphologic changes** `CC`
AHA: 2017,2Q,5
CC Excl: PDX collection 915

☑4ᵗʰ **N03** **Chronic nephritic syndrome**
    INCLUDES chronic glomerular disease
            chronic glomerulonephritis
            chronic nephritis
    EXCLUDES 1 *chronic tubulo-interstitial nephritis (N11.-)*
             diffuse sclerosing glomerulonephritis (N05.8-)
             nephritic syndrome NOS (N05.-)
DEF: Slow, progressive type of nephritis characterized by inflammation of the capillary loops in the glomeruli of the kidney, which leads to renal failure.
CC Excl: For CC codes in category N03: PDX collection 918

N03.0 **Chronic nephritic syndrome with minor glomerular abnormality** `CC`
Chronic nephritic syndrome with minimal change lesion

N03.1 **Chronic nephritic syndrome with focal and segmental glomerular lesions** `CC`
Chronic nephritic syndrome with focal and segmental hyalinosis
Chronic nephritic syndrome with focal and segmental sclerosis
Chronic nephritic syndrome with focal glomerulonephritis

N03.2 **Chronic nephritic syndrome with diffuse membranous glomerulonephritis** `CC`

N03.3 **Chronic nephritic syndrome with diffuse mesangial proliferative glomerulonephritis** `CC`

N03.4 **Chronic nephritic syndrome with diffuse endocapillary proliferative glomerulonephritis** `CC`

N03.5 **Chronic nephritic syndrome with diffuse mesangiocapillary glomerulonephritis** `CC`
Chronic nephritic syndrome with membranoproliferative glomerulonephritis, types 1 and 3, or NOS

N03.6 **Chronic nephritic syndrome with dense deposit disease** `CC`
Chronic nephritic syndrome with membranoproliferative glomerulonephritis, type 2

N03.7 **Chronic nephritic syndrome with diffuse crescentic glomerulonephritis** `CC`
Chronic nephritic syndrome with extracapillary glomerulonephritis

N03.8 **Chronic nephritic syndrome with other morphologic changes** `CC`
Chronic nephritic syndrome with proliferative glomerulonephritis NOS

N03.9 **Chronic nephritic syndrome with unspecified morphologic changes** `CC`

☑4ᵗʰ **N04** **Nephrotic syndrome**
    INCLUDES congenital nephrotic syndrome
            lipoid nephrosis
CC Excl: For CC codes in category N04, unless otherwise noted: PDX collection 917

N04.0 **Nephrotic syndrome with minor glomerular abnormality** `CC`
Nephrotic syndrome with minimal change lesion

N04.1 **Nephrotic syndrome with focal and segmental glomerular lesions** `CC`
Nephrotic syndrome with focal and segmental hyalinosis
Nephrotic syndrome with focal and segmental sclerosis
Nephrotic syndrome with focal glomerulonephritis

N04.2 **Nephrotic syndrome with diffuse membranous glomerulonephritis** `CC`

N04.3 **Nephrotic syndrome with diffuse mesangial proliferative glomerulonephritis** `CC`

N04.4 **Nephrotic syndrome with diffuse endocapillary proliferative glomerulonephritis** `CC`

N04.5 **Nephrotic syndrome with diffuse mesangiocapillary glomerulonephritis** `CC`
Nephrotic syndrome with membranoproliferative glomerulonephritis, types 1 and 3, or NOS

N04.6 **Nephrotic syndrome with dense deposit disease** `CC`
Nephrotic syndrome with membranoproliferative glomerulonephritis, type 2

N04.7 **Nephrotic syndrome with diffuse crescentic glomerulonephritis** `CC`
Nephrotic syndrome with extracapillary glomerulonephritis
CC Excl: PDX collection 915

N04.8 **Nephrotic syndrome with other morphologic changes** `CC`
Nephrotic syndrome with proliferative glomerulonephritis NOS
CC Excl: PDX collection 915

N04.9 **Nephrotic syndrome with unspecified morphologic changes** `CC`
CC Excl: PDX collection 915

☑4ᵗʰ **N05** **Unspecified nephritic syndrome**
    INCLUDES glomerular disease NOS
            glomerulonephritis NOS
            nephritis NOS
            nephropathy NOS and renal disease NOS with morphological lesion specified in .0-.8
    EXCLUDES 1 *nephropathy NOS with no stated morphological lesion (N28.9)*
             renal disease NOS with no stated morphological lesion (N28.9)
             tubulo-interstitial nephritis NOS (N12)
CC Excl: For CC codes in category N05: PDX collection 918

N05.0 **Unspecified nephritic syndrome with minor glomerular abnormality**
Unspecified nephritic syndrome with minimal change lesion

N05.1 **Unspecified nephritic syndrome with focal and segmental glomerular lesions**
Unspecified nephritic syndrome with focal and segmental hyalinosis
Unspecified nephritic syndrome with focal and segmental sclerosis
Unspecified nephritic syndrome with focal glomerulonephritis

N05.2 **Unspecified nephritic syndrome with diffuse membranous glomerulonephritis** `CC`

N05.3 **Unspecified nephritic syndrome with diffuse mesangial proliferative glomerulonephritis** `CC`

N05.4 **Unspecified nephritic syndrome with diffuse endocapillary proliferative glomerulonephritis** `CC`

N05.5 **Unspecified nephritic syndrome with diffuse mesangiocapillary glomerulonephritis** `CC`
Unspecified nephritic syndrome with membranoproliferative glomerulonephritis, types 1 and 3, or NOS

N05.6 **Unspecified nephritic syndrome with dense deposit disease**
Unspecified nephritic syndrome with membranoproliferative glomerulonephritis, type 2

N05.7 **Unspecified nephritic syndrome with diffuse crescentic glomerulonephritis**
Unspecified nephritic syndrome with extracapillary glomerulonephritis

N05.8 **Unspecified nephritic syndrome with other morphologic changes**
Unspecified nephritic syndrome with proliferative glomerulonephritis NOS

N05.9 **Unspecified nephritic syndrome with unspecified morphologic changes**

☑4ᵗʰ **N06** **Isolated proteinuria with specified morphological lesion**
    EXCLUDES 1 *proteinuria not associated with specific morphologic lesions (R80.0)*
CC Excl: For CC codes in category N06: PDX collection 918

N06.0 **Isolated proteinuria with minor glomerular abnormality**
Isolated proteinuria with minimal change lesion

N06.1 **Isolated proteinuria with focal and segmental glomerular lesions**
Isolated proteinuria with focal and segmental hyalinosis
Isolated proteinuria with focal and segmental sclerosis
Isolated proteinuria with focal glomerulonephritis

N06.2 **Isolated proteinuria with diffuse membranous glomerulonephritis** `CC`

N06.3 **Isolated proteinuria with** diffuse mesangial proliferative glomerulonephritis   `CC`

N06.4 **Isolated proteinuria with** diffuse endocapillary proliferative glomerulonephritis   `CC`

N06.5 **Isolated proteinuria with** diffuse mesangiocapillary glomerulonephritis   `CC`
Isolated proteinuria with membranoproliferative glomerulonephritis, types 1 and 3, or NOS

N06.6 **Isolated proteinuria with** dense deposit disease
Isolated proteinuria with membranoproliferative glomerulonephritis, type 2

N06.7 **Isolated proteinuria with** diffuse crescentic glomerulonephritis
Isolated proteinuria with extracapillary glomerulonephritis

N06.8 **Isolated proteinuria with other morphologic lesion**
Isolated proteinuria with proliferative glomerulonephritis NOS

N06.9 **Isolated proteinuria with unspecified morphologic lesion**

`√4th` **N07** **Hereditary nephropathy, not elsewhere classified**
    `EXCLUDES 2`   Alport's syndrome (Q87.81-)
       hereditary amyloid nephropathy (E85.-)
       nail patella syndrome (Q87.2)
       non-neuropathic heredofamilial amyloidosis (E85.-)
    CC Excl: For CC codes in category N07: PDX collection 918

N07.0 **Hereditary nephropathy, not elsewhere classified with minor glomerular abnormality**
Hereditary nephropathy, not elsewhere classified with minimal change lesion

N07.1 **Hereditary nephropathy, not elsewhere classified with focal and segmental glomerular lesions**
Hereditary nephropathy, not elsewhere classified with focal and segmental hyalinosis
Hereditary nephropathy, not elsewhere classified with focal and segmental sclerosis
Hereditary nephropathy, not elsewhere classified with focal glomerulonephritis

N07.2 **Hereditary nephropathy, not elsewhere classified with** diffuse membranous glomerulonephritis   `CC`

N07.3 **Hereditary nephropathy, not elsewhere classified with** diffuse mesangial proliferative glomerulonephritis   `CC`

N07.4 **Hereditary nephropathy, not elsewhere classified with** diffuse endocapillary proliferative glomerulonephritis   `CC`

N07.5 **Hereditary nephropathy, not elsewhere classified with** diffuse mesangiocapillary glomerulonephritis   `CC`
Hereditary nephropathy, not elsewhere classified with membranoproliferative glomerulonephritis, types 1 and 3, or NOS

N07.6 **Hereditary nephropathy, not elsewhere classified with** dense deposit disease
Hereditary nephropathy, not elsewhere classified with membranoproliferative glomerulonephritis, type 2

N07.7 **Hereditary nephropathy, not elsewhere classified with** diffuse crescentic glomerulonephritis
Hereditary nephropathy, not elsewhere classified with extracapillary glomerulonephritis

N07.8 **Hereditary nephropathy, not elsewhere classified with other morphologic lesions**
Hereditary nephropathy, not elsewhere classified with proliferative glomerulonephritis NOS

N07.9 **Hereditary nephropathy, not elsewhere classified with unspecified morphologic lesions**

N08 *Glomerular disorders in diseases classified elsewhere*
Glomerulonephritis
Nephritis
Nephropathy
Code first underlying disease, such as:
    amyloidosis (E85.-)
    congenital syphilis (A50.5)
    cryoglobulinemia (D89.1)
    disseminated intravascular coagulation (D65)
    gout (M1A.-, M10.-)
    microscopic polyangiitis (M31.7)
    multiple myeloma (C90.0-)
    sepsis (A40.0-A41.9)
    sickle-cell disease (D57.0-D57.8)
    `EXCLUDES 1`   glomerulonephritis, nephritis and nephropathy (in):
         antiglomerular basement membrane disease (M31.0)
         diabetes (E08-E13 with .21)
         gonococcal (A54.21)
         Goodpasture's syndrome (M31.0)
         hemolytic-uremic syndrome (D59.3)
         lupus (M32.14)
         mumps (B26.83)
         syphilis (A52.75)
         systemic lupus erythematosus (M32.14)
         Wegener's granulomatosis (M31.31)
       pyelonephritis in diseases classified elsewhere (N16)
       renal tubulo-interstitial disorders classified elsewhere (N16)

Renal tubulo-interstitial diseases (N10-N16)

`INCLUDES`   pyelonephritis
`EXCLUDES 1`   pyeloureteritis cystica (N28.85)

N10 **Acute pyelonephritis**   `H6`
Acute infectious interstitial nephritis
Acute pyelitis
Acute tubulo-interstitial nephritis
Hemoglobin nephrosis
Myoglobin nephrosis
Use additional code (B95-B97), to identify infectious agent

`√4th` **N11** **Chronic tubulo-interstitial nephritis**
    `INCLUDES`   chronic infectious interstitial nephritis
         chronic pyelitis
         chronic pyelonephritis
Use additional code (B95-B97), to identify infectious agent

N11.0 **Nonobstructive reflux-associated chronic pyelonephritis**
Pyelonephritis (chronic) associated with (vesicoureteral) reflux
    `EXCLUDES 1`   vesicoureteral reflux NOS (N13.70)

N11.1 **Chronic obstructive pyelonephritis**   `CC`
Pyelonephritis (chronic) associated with anomaly of pelviureteric junction
Pyelonephritis (chronic) associated with anomaly of pyeloureteric junction
Pyelonephritis (chronic) associated with crossing of vessel
Pyelonephritis (chronic) associated with kinking of ureter
Pyelonephritis (chronic) associated with obstruction of ureter
Pyelonephritis (chronic) associated with stricture of pelviureteric junction
Pyelonephritis (chronic) associated with stricture of ureter
    `EXCLUDES 1`   calculous pyelonephritis (N20.9)
         obstructive uropathy (N13.-)
    CC Excl: PDX collection 920

N11.8 **Other chronic tubulo-interstitial nephritis**   `CC`
Nonobstructive chronic pyelonephritis NOS
    CC Excl: PDX collection 921

N11.9 **Chronic tubulo-interstitial nephritis, unspecified**   `CC` `H6`
Chronic interstitial nephritis NOS
Chronic pyelitis NOS
Chronic pyelonephritis NOS
    CC Excl: PDX collection 922

`N` Newborn: 0   `P` Pediatric: 0-17   `M` Maternity: 9-64   `A` Adult: 15-124   `MCC` Major Complication/Comorbidity   `CC` Complication/Comorbidity   `SW` Severe Wound Dx

856   **ICD-10-CM 2020**

N12 Tubulo-interstitial nephritis, not specified as acute or chronic `CC` `H6`
Interstitial nephritis NOS
Pyelitis NOS
Pyelonephritis NOS
EXCLUDES 1   *calculous pyelonephritis (N20.9)*
CC Excl: PDX collection 922

✓4ᵗʰ **N13 Obstructive and reflux uropathy**
EXCLUDES 2   *calculus of kidney and ureter without hydronephrosis (N20.-)*
congenital obstructive defects of renal pelvis and ureter (Q62.0-Q62.3)
hydronephrosis with ureteropelvic junction obstruction (Q62.11)
obstructive pyelonephritis (N11.1)
DEF: Hydronephrosis: Distension of the kidney caused by an accumulation of urine that cannot flow out due to an obstruction that may be caused by conditions such as kidney stones or vesicoureteral reflux.
CC Excl: For CC codes in category N13, unless otherwise noted: PDX collection 922

N13.0 Hydronephrosis with ureteropelvic junction obstruction `CC`
Hydronephrosis due to acquired occlusion of ureteropelvic junction
EXCLUDES 2   *hydronephrosis with ureteropelvic junction obstruction due to calculus (N13.2)*
AHA: 2016,4Q,43

Hydronephrosis/UPJ Obstruction

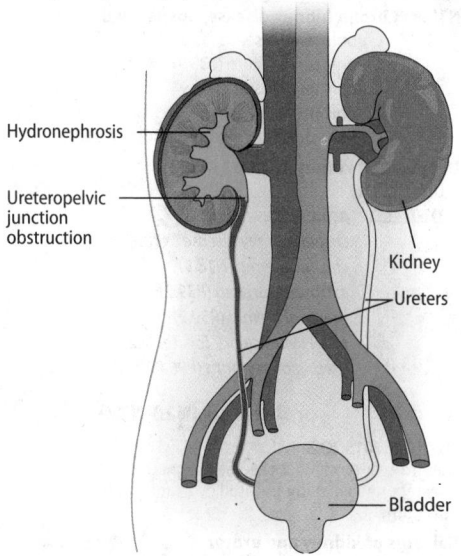

N13.1 Hydronephrosis with ureteral stricture, not elsewhere classified `CC`
EXCLUDES 1   *hydronephrosis with ureteral stricture with infection (N13.6)*

N13.2 Hydronephrosis with renal and ureteral calculous obstruction `CC`
EXCLUDES 1   *hydronephrosis with renal and ureteral calculous obstruction with infection (N13.6)*

✓5ᵗʰ **N13.3 Other and unspecified hydronephrosis**
EXCLUDES 1   *hydronephrosis with infection (N13.6)*
    N13.30 Unspecified hydronephrosis `CC`
    N13.39 Other hydronephrosis `CC`

N13.4 Hydroureter `CC`
EXCLUDES 1   *congenital hydroureter (Q62.3-)*
hydroureter with infection (N13.6)
vesicoureteral-reflux with hydroureter (N13.73-)
DEF: Abnormal enlargement or distension of the ureter with water or urine caused by an obstruction.
CC Excl: PDX collection 923

N13.5 Crossing vessel and stricture of ureter without hydronephrosis
Kinking and stricture of ureter without hydronephrosis
EXCLUDES 1   *crossing vessel and stricture of ureter without hydronephrosis with infection (N13.6)*

N13.6 Pyonephrosis `CC` `H6`
Conditions in N13.0-N13.5 with infection
Obstructive uropathy with infection
Use additional code (B95-B97), to identify infectious agent
AHA: 2018,2Q,21

✓5ᵗʰ **N13.7 Vesicoureteral-reflux**
EXCLUDES 1   *reflux-associated pyelonephritis (N11.0)*
DEF: Urine passage from the bladder flows backward up into the ureter and kidneys that can lead to bacterial infection and an increase in hydrostatic pressure, causing kidney damage.

Vesicoureteral Reflux

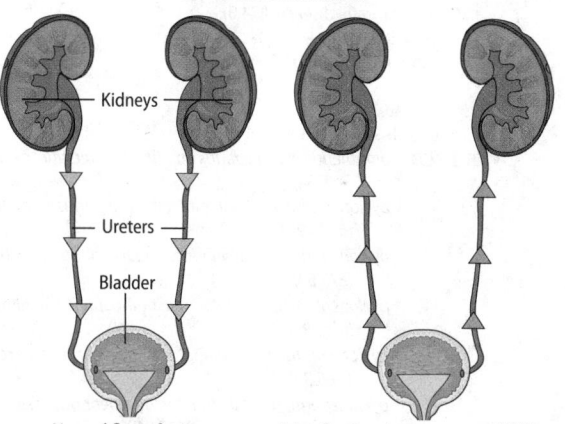

Normal flow of urine   Urine flowing the wrong way (VUR)

N13.70 Vesicoureteral-reflux, unspecified
Vesicoureteral-reflux NOS
N13.71 Vesicoureteral-reflux without reflux nephropathy
✓6ᵗʰ **N13.72 Vesicoureteral-reflux with reflux nephropathy without hydroureter**
    N13.721 Vesicoureteral-reflux with reflux nephropathy without hydroureter, unilateral
    N13.722 Vesicoureteral-reflux with reflux nephropathy without hydroureter, bilateral
    N13.729 Vesicoureteral-reflux with reflux nephropathy without hydroureter, unspecified
✓6ᵗʰ **N13.73 Vesicoureteral-reflux with reflux nephropathy with hydroureter**
    N13.731 Vesicoureteral-reflux with reflux nephropathy with hydroureter, unilateral
    N13.732 Vesicoureteral-reflux with reflux nephropathy with hydroureter, bilateral
    N13.739 Vesicoureteral-reflux with reflux nephropathy with hydroureter, unspecified

N13.8 Other obstructive and reflux uropathy `CC`
Urinary tract obstruction due to specified cause
Code first, if applicable, any causal condition, such as:
enlarged prostate (N40.1)
CC Excl: PDX collection 920

N13.9 Obstructive and reflux uropathy, unspecified
Urinary tract obstruction NOS

✓4ᵗʰ **N14 Drug- and heavy-metal-induced tubulo-interstitial and tubular conditions**
Code first poisoning due to drug or toxin, if applicable (T36-T65 with fifth or sixth character 1-4 or 6)
Use additional code for adverse effect, if applicable, to identify drug (T36-T50 with fifth or sixth character 5)

N14.0 Analgesic nephropathy
N14.1 Nephropathy induced by other drugs, medicaments and biological substances
N14.2 Nephropathy induced by unspecified drug, medicament or biological substance
N14.3 Nephropathy induced by heavy metals
N14.4 Toxic nephropathy, not elsewhere classified

✓4ᵗʰ **N15 Other renal tubulo-interstitial diseases**

N15.0 Balkan nephropathy
Balkan endemic nephropathy

N15.1 Renal and perinephric abscess `MCC` `H6`
  CC Excl: PDX collection 919

N15.8 Other specified renal tubulo-interstitial diseases

N15.9 Renal tubulo-interstitial disease, unspecified
  Infection of kidney NOS
    EXCLUDES 1 *urinary tract infection NOS (N39.0)*

N16 Renal tubulo-interstitial disorders in diseases classified elsewhere
  Pyelonephritis
  Tubulo-interstitial nephritis
  Code first underlying disease, such as:
    brucellosis (A23.0-A23.9)
    cryoglobulinemia (D89.1)
    glycogen storage disease (E74.0)
    leukemia (C91-C95)
    lymphoma (C81.0-C85.9, C96.0-C96.9)
    multiple myeloma (C90.0-)
    sepsis (A40.0-A41.9)
    Wilson's disease (E83.0)
    EXCLUDES 1 *diphtheritic pyelonephritis and tubulo-interstitial nephritis (A36.84)*
      pyelonephritis and tubulo-interstitial nephritis in candidiasis (B37.49)
      pyelonephritis and tubulo-interstitial nephritis in cystinosis (E72.04)
      pyelonephritis and tubulo-interstitial nephritis in salmonella infection (A02.25)
      pyelonephritis and tubulo-interstitial nephritis in sarcoidosis (D86.84)
      pyelonephritis and tubulo-interstitial nephritis in sicca syndrome [Sjogren's] (M35.04)
      pyelonephritis and tubulo-interstitial nephritis in systemic lupus erythematosus (M32.15)
      pyelonephritis and tubulo-interstitial nephritis in toxoplasmosis (B58.83)
      renal tubular degeneration in diabetes (E08-E13 with .29)
      syphilitic pyelonephritis and tubulo-interstitial nephritis (A52.75)

Acute kidney failure and chronic kidney disease (N17-N19)

EXCLUDES 2 *congenital renal failure (P96.0)*
  drug- and heavy-metal-induced tubulo-interstitial and tubular conditions (N14.-)
  extrarenal uremia (R39.2)
  hemolytic-uremic syndrome (D59.3)
  hepatorenal syndrome (K76.7)
  postpartum hepatorenal syndrome (O90.4)
  posttraumatic renal failure (T79.5)
  prerenal uremia (R39.2)
  renal failure complicating abortion or ectopic or molar pregnancy (O00-O07, O08.4)
  renal failure following labor and delivery (O90.4)
  renal failure postprocedural (N99.0)

N17 Acute kidney failure `√4th`
  Code also associated underlying condition
    EXCLUDES 1 *posttraumatic renal failure (T79.5)*
  AHA: 2019,2Q,7; 2019,1Q,12; 2013,4Q,124
  CC Excl: For CC/MCC codes in category N17, unless otherwise noted:
  PDX collection 924

  N17.0 Acute kidney failure with tubular necrosis `MCC` `HCC`
    Acute tubular necrosis
    Renal tubular necrosis
    Tubular necrosis NOS

  N17.1 Acute kidney failure with acute cortical necrosis `MCC` `HCC`
    Acute cortical necrosis
    Cortical necrosis NOS
    Renal cortical necrosis

  N17.2 Acute kidney failure with medullary necrosis `MCC` `HCC`
    Medullary [papillary] necrosis NOS
    Acute medullary [papillary] necrosis
    Renal medullary [papillary] necrosis

  N17.8 Other acute kidney failure `CC` `HCC`
    CC Excl: PDX collection 925

N17.9 Acute kidney failure, unspecified `CC` `HCC`
  Acute kidney injury (nontraumatic)
    EXCLUDES 2 *traumatic kidney injury (S37.0-)*

N18 Chronic kidney disease (CKD) `√4th`
  Code first any associated:
    diabetic chronic kidney disease (E08.22, E09.22, E10.22, E11.22, E13.22)
    hypertensive chronic kidney disease (I12.-, I13.-)
  Use additional code to identify kidney transplant status, if applicable, (Z94.0)
  AHA: 2013,1Q,24

  N18.1 Chronic kidney disease, stage 1

  N18.2 Chronic kidney disease, stage 2 (mild)

  N18.3 Chronic kidney disease, stage 3 (moderate) `HCC`

  N18.4 Chronic kidney disease, stage 4 (severe) `HCC`

  N18.5 Chronic kidney disease, stage 5 `HCC`
    EXCLUDES 1 *chronic kidney disease, stage 5 requiring chronic dialysis (N18.6)*
    DEF: End-stage renal disease (ESRD) with a GFR value of 15 ml/min or less not yet requiring chronic dialysis.
    TIP: When both ESRD and CKD 5 are documented, code only for ESRD.

  N18.6 End stage renal disease `CC` `HCC`
    Chronic kidney disease requiring chronic dialysis
    Use additional code to identify dialysis status (Z99.2)
    AHA: 2016,3Q,22; 2016,1Q,12; 2013,4Q,124-125
    TIP: When both ESRD and CKD 5 are documented, code only for ESRD.

  N18.9 Chronic kidney disease, unspecified
    Chronic renal disease
    Chronic renal failure NOS
    Chronic renal insufficiency
    Chronic uremia NOS
    Diffuse sclerosing glomerulonephritis NOS

N19 Unspecified kidney failure
  Uremia NOS
    EXCLUDES 1 *acute kidney failure (N17.-)*
      chronic kidney disease (N18.-)
      chronic uremia (N18.9)
      extrarenal uremia (R39.2)
      prerenal uremia (R39.2)
      renal insufficiency (acute) (N28.9)
      uremia of newborn (P96.0)

Urolithiasis (N20-N23)

AHA: 2017,1Q,5; 2015,2Q,8
TIP: Codes from this code block can be assigned based on the diagnosis listed in a radiology report when authenticated by a radiologist and available at the time of code assignment.

N20 Calculus of kidney and ureter `√4th`
  Calculous pyelonephritis
    EXCLUDES 1 *nephrocalcinosis (E83.5)*
      that with hydronephrosis (N13.2)

  N20.0 Calculus of kidney
    Nephrolithiasis NOS
    Renal calculus
    Renal stone
    Staghorn calculus
    Stone in kidney

  N20.1 Calculus of ureter `CC`
    Ureteric stone
    AHA: 2016,3Q,22
    CC Excl: PDX collection 928

  N20.2 Calculus of kidney with calculus of ureter `CC`
    CC Excl: PDX collection 928

  N20.9 Urinary calculus, unspecified

N21 Calculus of lower urinary tract `√4th`
  INCLUDES calculus of lower urinary tract with cystitis and urethritis

  N21.0 Calculus in bladder
    Calculus in diverticulum of bladder
    Urinary bladder stone
    EXCLUDES 2 *staghorn calculus (N20.0)*

  N21.1 Calculus in urethra
    EXCLUDES 2 *calculus of prostate (N42.0)*

  N21.8 Other lower urinary tract calculus

`N` Newborn: 0   `P` Pediatric: 0-17   `M` Maternity: 9-64   `A` Adult: 15-124   `MCC` Major Complication/Comorbidity   `CC` Complication/Comorbidity   `SW` Severe Wound Dx

N21.9　Calculus of lower urinary tract, unspecified
> EXCLUDES 1　*calculus of urinary tract NOS (N20.9)*

N22　*Calculus of urinary tract in diseases classified elsewhere*
> Code first underlying disease, such as:
> gout (M1A.-, M10.-)
> schistosomiasis (B65.0-B65.9)

N23　Unspecified renal colic

Other disorders of kidney and ureter (N25-N29)

> EXCLUDES 2　*disorders of kidney and ureter with urolithiasis (N20-N23)*

✓4ᵗʰ　N25　Disorders resulting from impaired renal tubular function

N25.0　Renal osteodystrophy
> Azotemic osteodystrophy
> Phosphate-losing tubular disorders
> Renal rickets
> Renal short stature
> EXCLUDES 2　*metabolic disorders classifiable to E70-E88*
> **DEF:** Various bone diseases occurring when kidney function is impaired or fails. Abnormal levels of phosphorous and calcium can lead to osteomalacia, osteoporosis, or osteosclerosis.

N25.1　Nephrogenic diabetes insipidus　　CC HCC
> EXCLUDES 1　*diabetes insipidus NOS (E23.2)*
> **DEF:** Type of diabetes due to the inability of renal tubules to reabsorb water back into the body. It is not responsive to vasopressin (antidiuretic hormone) and it is characterized by excessive thirst and excessive urine production. It may develop into chronic renal insufficiency.
> **CC Excl:** PDX collection 929

✓5ᵗʰ　N25.8　Other disorders resulting from impaired renal tubular function

N25.81　Secondary hyperparathyroidism of renal origin　　CC HCC
> EXCLUDES 1　*secondary hyperparathyroidism, non-renal (E21.1)*
> EXCLUDES 2　*metabolic disorders classifiable to E70-E88*
> **DEF:** Parathyroid dysfunction caused by chronic renal failure. Phosphate clearance and vitamin D production is impaired resulting in lowered calcium blood levels and an excessive production of parathyroid hormone.
> **CC Excl:** PDX collection 930

N25.89　Other disorders resulting from impaired renal tubular function
> Hypokalemic nephropathy
> Lightwood-Albright syndrome
> Renal tubular acidosis NOS

N25.9　Disorder resulting from impaired renal tubular function, unspecified

✓4ᵗʰ　N26　Unspecified contracted kidney
> EXCLUDES 1　*contracted kidney due to hypertension (I12.-)*
> *diffuse sclerosing glomerulonephritis (N05.8.-)*
> *hypertensive nephrosclerosis (arteriolar) (arteriosclerotic) (I12.-)*
> *small kidney of unknown cause (N27.-)*

N26.1　Atrophy of kidney (terminal)

N26.2　Page kidney

N26.9　Renal sclerosis, unspecified

✓4ᵗʰ　N27　Small kidney of unknown cause
> INCLUDES　oligonephronia

N27.0　Small kidney, unilateral

N27.1　Small kidney, bilateral

N27.9　Small kidney, unspecified

✓4ᵗʰ　N28　Other disorders of kidney and ureter, not elsewhere classified

N28.0　Ischemia and infarction of kidney　　CC HCC
> Renal artery embolism
> Renal artery obstruction
> Renal artery occlusion
> Renal artery thrombosis
> Renal infarct
> EXCLUDES 1　*atherosclerosis of renal artery (extrarenal part) (I70.1)*
> *congenital stenosis of renal artery (Q27.1)*
> *Goldblatt's kidney (I70.1)*
> **CC Excl:** PDX collection 931

N28.1　Cyst of kidney, acquired
> Cyst (multiple) (solitary) of kidney (acquired)
> EXCLUDES 1　*cystic kidney disease (congenital) (Q61.-)*

✓5ᵗʰ　N28.8　Other specified disorders of kidney and ureter
> EXCLUDES 1　*hydroureter (N13.4)*
> *ureteric stricture with hydronephrosis (N13.1)*
> *ureteric stricture without hydronephrosis (N13.5)*
> **CC Excl:** For CC codes in subcategory N28.8: PDX collection 922

N28.81　Hypertrophy of kidney

N28.82　Megaloureter

N28.83　Nephroptosis

N28.84　Pyelitis cystica　　CC H6

N28.85　Pyeloureteritis cystica　　CC H6

N28.86　Ureteritis cystica　　CC H6

N28.89　Other specified disorders of kidney and ureter

N28.9　Disorder of kidney and ureter, unspecified
> Nephropathy NOS
> Renal disease (acute) NOS
> Renal insufficiency (acute)
> EXCLUDES 1　*chronic renal insufficiency (N18.9)*
> *unspecified nephritic syndrome (N05.-)*
> **AHA:** 2016,1Q,13

N29　*Other disorders of kidney and ureter in diseases classified elsewhere*
> Code first underlying disease, such as:
> amyloidosis (E85.-)
> nephrocalcinosis (E83.5)
> schistosomiasis (B65.0-B65.9)
> EXCLUDES 1　*disorders of kidney and ureter in:*
> *cystinosis (E72.0)*
> *gonorrhea (A54.21)*
> *syphilis (A52.75)*
> *tuberculosis (A18.11)*

Other diseases of the urinary system (N30-N39)

> EXCLUDES 1　*urinary infection (complicating):*
> *abortion or ectopic or molar pregnancy (O00-O07, O08.8)*
> *pregnancy, childbirth and the puerperium (O23.-, O75.3, O86.2-)*

✓4ᵗʰ　N30　Cystitis
> Use additional code to identify infectious agent (B95-B97)
> EXCLUDES 1　*prostatocystitis (N41.3)*
> **AHA:** 2017,1Q,6
> **DEF:** Inflammation of the urinary bladder. Symptoms include dysuria, frequency of urination, urgency, and hematuria.
> **CC Excl:** For CC codes in category N30: PDX collection 932

✓5ᵗʰ　N30.0　Acute cystitis
> EXCLUDES 1　*irradiation cystitis (N30.4-)*
> *trigonitis (N30.3-)*

N30.00　Acute cystitis without hematuria　　H6

N30.01　Acute cystitis with hematuria　　H6

✓5ᵗʰ　N30.1　Interstitial cystitis (chronic)

N30.10　Interstitial cystitis (chronic) without hematuria

N30.11　Interstitial cystitis (chronic) with hematuria

✓5ᵗʰ　N30.2　Other chronic cystitis

N30.20　Other chronic cystitis without hematuria

N30.21　Other chronic cystitis with hematuria

✓5ᵗʰ　N30.3　Trigonitis
> Urethrotrigonitis

N30.30　Trigonitis without hematuria

N30.31　Trigonitis with hematuria

✓5ᵗʰ　N30.4　Irradiation cystitis

N30.40　Irradiation cystitis without hematuria　　CC

N30.41　Irradiation cystitis with hematuria　　CC

✓5ᵗʰ　N30.8　Other cystitis
> Abscess of bladder

N30.80　Other cystitis without hematuria

N30.81　Other cystitis with hematuria

✓5ᵗʰ　N30.9　Cystitis, unspecified

N30.90　Cystitis, unspecified without hematuria

N30.91　Cystitis, unspecified with hematuria

✓4ᵗʰ N31 Neuromuscular dysfunction of bladder, not elsewhere classified

Use additional code to identify any associated urinary incontinence (N39.3-N39.4-)

> EXCLUDES 1   cord bladder NOS (G95.89)
> neurogenic bladder due to cauda equina syndrome (G83.4)
> neuromuscular dysfunction due to spinal cord lesion (G95.89)

N31.0 Uninhibited neuropathic bladder, not elsewhere classified

N31.1 Reflex neuropathic bladder, not elsewhere classified

N31.2 Flaccid neuropathic bladder, not elsewhere classified
Atonic (motor) (sensory) neuropathic bladder
Autonomous neuropathic bladder
Nonreflex neuropathic bladder

N31.8 Other neuromuscular dysfunction of bladder

N31.9 Neuromuscular dysfunction of bladder, unspecified
Neurogenic bladder dysfunction NOS

✓4ᵗʰ N32 Other disorders of bladder

> EXCLUDES 2   calculus of bladder (N21.0)
> cystocele (N81.1-)
> hernia or prolapse of bladder, female (N81.1-)

N32.0 Bladder-neck obstruction
Bladder-neck stenosis (acquired)
> EXCLUDES 1   congenital bladder-neck obstruction (Q64.3-)

DEF: Bladder outlet and vesicourethral obstruction that occurs as a consequence of benign prostatic hypertrophy or prostatic cancer. It may also occur in either sex due to strictures, radiation, cystoscopy, catheterization, injury, infection, blood clots, bladder cancer, impaction, or other disease that compresses the bladder neck.

N32.1 Vesicointestinal fistula   `CC`
Vesicorectal fistula
CC Excl: PDX collection 933

N32.2 Vesical fistula, not elsewhere classified   `CC`
> EXCLUDES 1   fistula between bladder and female genital tract (N82.0-N82.1)

CC Excl: PDX collection 933

N32.3 Diverticulum of bladder
> EXCLUDES 1   congenital diverticulum of bladder (Q64.6)
> diverticulitis of bladder (N30.8-)

✓5ᵗʰ N32.8 Other specified disorders of bladder

N32.81 Overactive bladder
Detrusor muscle hyperactivity
> EXCLUDES 1   frequent urination due to specified bladder condition — code to condition

DEF: Sudden involuntary contractions of the muscular wall of the bladder that results in a sudden, strong urge to urinate.

N32.89 Other specified disorders of bladder
Bladder hemorrhage
Bladder hypertrophy
Calcified bladder
Contracted bladder

N32.9 Bladder disorder, unspecified

N33 Bladder disorders in diseases classified elsewhere

Code first underlying disease, such as:
schistosomiasis (B65.0-B65.9)

> EXCLUDES 1   bladder disorder in syphilis (A52.76)
> bladder disorder in tuberculosis (A18.12)
> candidal cystitis (B37.41)
> chlamydial cystitis (A56.01)
> cystitis in gonorrhea (A54.01)
> cystitis in neurogenic bladder (N31.-)
> diphtheritic cystitis (A36.85)
> neurogenic bladder (N31.-)
> syphilitic cystitis (A52.76)
> trichomonal cystitis (A59.03)

✓4ᵗʰ N34 Urethritis and urethral syndrome

Use additional code (B95-B97), to identify infectious agent

> EXCLUDES 2   Reiter's disease (M02.3-)
> urethritis in diseases with a predominantly sexual mode of transmission (A50-A64)
> urethrotrigonitis (N30.3-)

AHA: 2017,1Q,6

N34.0 Urethral abscess   `CC` `H6`
Abscess (of) Cowper's gland
Abscess (of) Littré's gland
Abscess (of) urethral (gland)
Periurethral abscess
> EXCLUDES 1   urethral caruncle (N36.2)

CC Excl: PDX collection 934

N34.1 Nonspecific urethritis
Nongonococcal urethritis
Nonvenereal urethritis

N34.2 Other urethritis
Meatitis, urethral
Postmenopausal urethritis
Ulcer of urethra (meatus)
Urethritis NOS

N34.3 Urethral syndrome, unspecified

✓4ᵗʰ N35 Urethral stricture

> EXCLUDES 1   congenital urethral stricture (Q64.3-)
> postprocedural urethral stricture (N99.1-)

AHA: 2018,4Q,21-22

✓5ᵗʰ N35.0 Post-traumatic urethral stricture

Urethral stricture due to injury
> EXCLUDES 1   postprocedural urethral stricture (N99.1-)

✓6ᵗʰ N35.01 Post-traumatic urethral stricture, male

N35.010 Post-traumatic urethral stricture, male, meatal	♂
N35.011 Post-traumatic bulbous urethral stricture	♂
N35.012 Post-traumatic membranous urethral stricture	♂
N35.013 Post-traumatic anterior urethral stricture	♂
N35.014 Post-traumatic urethral stricture, male, unspecified	♂
N35.016 Post-traumatic urethral stricture, male, overlapping sites	♂

✓6ᵗʰ N35.02 Post-traumatic urethral stricture, female

N35.021 Urethral stricture due to childbirth	♀
N35.028 Other post-traumatic urethral stricture, female	♀

✓5ᵗʰ N35.1 Postinfective urethral stricture, not elsewhere classified

> EXCLUDES 1   gonococcal urethral stricture (A54.01)
> syphilitic urethral stricture (A52.76)
> urethral stricture associated with schistosomiasis (B65.-, N29)

✓6ᵗʰ N35.11 Postinfective urethral stricture, not elsewhere classified, male

N35.111 Postinfective urethral stricture, not elsewhere classified, male, meatal	♂
N35.112 Postinfective bulbous urethral stricture, not elsewhere classified, male	♂
N35.113 Postinfective membranous urethral stricture, not elsewhere classified, male	♂
N35.114 Postinfective anterior urethral stricture, not elsewhere classified, male	♂
N35.116 Postinfective urethral stricture, not elsewhere classified, male, overlapping sites	♂
N35.119 Postinfective urethral stricture, not elsewhere classified, male, unspecified	♂

`N` Newborn: 0   `P` Pediatric: 0-17   `M` Maternity: 9-64   `A` Adult: 15-124   `MCC` Major Complication/Comorbidity   `CC` Complication/Comorbidity   `SW` Severe Wound Dx

N35.12 Postinfective urethral stricture, not elsewhere classified, female ♀

✓5ᵗʰ **N35.8** Other urethral stricture
> **EXCLUDES 1**   postprocedural urethral stricture (N99.1-)

  ✓6ᵗʰ **N35.81** Other urethral stricture, male ♂

N35.811 Other urethral stricture, male, meatal ♂

N35.812 Other urethral bulbous stricture, male ♂

N35.813 Other membranous urethral stricture, male ♂

N35.814 Other anterior urethral stricture, male ♂

N35.816 Other urethral stricture, male, overlapping sites ♂

N35.819 Other urethral stricture, male, unspecified site ♂

N35.82 Other urethral stricture, female ♀

✓5ᵗʰ **N35.9** Urethral stricture, unspecified

  ✓6ᵗʰ **N35.91** Urethral stricture, unspecified, male ♂

N35.911 Unspecified urethral stricture, male, meatal ♂

N35.912 Unspecified bulbous urethral stricture, male ♂

N35.913 Unspecified membranous urethral stricture, male ♂

N35.914 Unspecified anterior urethral stricture, male ♂

N35.916 Unspecified urethral stricture, male, overlapping sites ♂

N35.919 Unspecified urethral stricture, male, unspecified site ♂
> Pinhole meatus NOS
> Urethral stricture NOS

N35.92 Unspecified urethral stricture, female ♀

✓4ᵗʰ **N36** Other disorders of urethra

N36.0 Urethral fistula   CC
> Urethroperineal fistula
> Urethrorectal fistula
> Urinary fistula NOS
> **EXCLUDES 1**   urethroscrotal fistula (N50.89)
>   urethrovaginal fistula (N82.1)
>   urethrovesicovaginal fistula (N82.1)
>
> **CC Excl:** PDX collection 935

N36.1 Urethral diverticulum

N36.2 Urethral caruncle

✓5ᵗʰ **N36.4** Urethral functional and muscular disorders
> Use additional code to identify associated urinary stress incontinence (N39.3)

N36.41 Hypermobility of urethra

N36.42 Intrinsic sphincter deficiency (ISD)

N36.43 Combined hypermobility of urethra and intrinsic sphincter deficiency

N36.44 Muscular disorders of urethra
> Bladder sphincter dyssynergy

N36.5 Urethral false passage

N36.8 Other specified disorders of urethra
> **EXCLUDES 1**   congenital urethrocele (Q64.7)
>   female urethrocele (N81.0)

N36.9 Urethral disorder, unspecified

N37 *Urethral disorders in diseases classified elsewhere*
> Code first underlying disease
> **EXCLUDES 1**   urethritis (in):
>   candidal infection (B37.41)
>   chlamydial (A56.01)
>   gonorrhea (A54.01)
>   syphilis (A52.76)
>   trichomonal infection (A59.03)
>   tuberculosis (A18.13)

✓4ᵗʰ **N39** Other disorders of urinary system
> **EXCLUDES 2**   hematuria NOS (R31.-)
>   recurrent or persistent hematuria (N02.-)
>   recurrent or persistent hematuria with specified morphological lesion (N02.-)
>   proteinuria NOS (R80.-)

N39.0 Urinary tract infection, site not specified   CC H6
> Use additional code (B95-B97), to identify infectious agent
> **EXCLUDES 1**   candidiasis of urinary tract (B37.4-)
>   neonatal urinary tract infection (P39.3)
>   ▶pyuria (R82.81)◀
>   urinary tract infection of specified site, such as:
>   cystitis (N30.-)
>   urethritis (N34.-)
>
> **AHA:** 2018,2Q,21,22; 2018,1Q,16; 2017,1Q,6; 2012,4Q,94
> **CC Excl:** PDX collection 936

N39.3 Stress incontinence (female) (male)
> Code also any associated overactive bladder (N32.81)
> **EXCLUDES 1**   mixed incontinence (N39.46)

✓5ᵗʰ **N39.4** Other specified urinary incontinence
> Code also any associated overactive bladder (N32.81)
> **EXCLUDES 1**   enuresis NOS (R32)
>   functional urinary incontinence (R39.81)
>   urinary incontinence associated with cognitive impairment (R39.81)
>   urinary incontinence NOS (R32)
>   urinary incontinence of nonorganic origin (F98.0)

N39.41 Urge incontinence
> **EXCLUDES 1**   mixed incontinence (N39.46)

N39.42 Incontinence without sensory awareness
> Insensible (urinary) incontinence

N39.43 Post-void dribbling

N39.44 Nocturnal enuresis

N39.45 Continuous leakage

N39.46 Mixed incontinence
> Urge and stress incontinence

✓6ᵗʰ **N39.49** Other specified urinary incontinence
> **AHA:** 2016,4Q,44

N39.490 Overflow incontinence

N39.491 Coital incontinence

N39.492 Postural (urinary) incontinence

N39.498 Other specified urinary incontinence
> Reflex incontinence
> Total incontinence

N39.8 Other specified disorders of urinary system

N39.9 Disorder of urinary system, unspecified

Diseases of male genital organs (N40-N53)

✓4ᵗʰ **N40** Benign prostatic hyperplasia
> **INCLUDES**   adenofibromatous hypertrophy of prostate
>   benign hypertrophy of the prostate
>   benign prostatic hypertrophy
>   BPH
>   enlarged prostate
>   nodular prostate
>   polyp of prostate
> **EXCLUDES 1**   benign neoplasms of prostate (adenoma, benign) (fibroadenoma) (fibroma) (myoma) (D29.1)
> **EXCLUDES 2**   malignant neoplasm of prostate (C61)
>
> **DEF:** Enlargement of the prostate gland due to an abnormal proliferation of fibrostromal tissue in the paraurethral glands. This condition causes impingement of the urethra resulting in obstructed urinary flow.

N40.0 Benign prostatic hyperplasia without lower urinary tract symptoms   A ♂
> Enlarged prostate NOS
> Enlarged prostate without LUTS

✓ Additional Character Required   ✓x7ᵗʰ Placeholder   Unacceptable PDx   Questionable PDx   Manifestation   Unspecified Dx   H1-H14 HAC   HCC CMS-HCC Dx   HIV HIV Dx

ICD-10-CM 2020   861

N4Ø.1　Benign prostatic hyperplasia with lower urinary tract symptoms　Ⓐ ♂

Enlarged prostate with LUTS

Use additional code for associated symptoms, when specified:
incomplete bladder emptying (R39.14)
nocturia (R35.1)
straining on urination (R39.16)
urinary frequency (R35.Ø)
urinary hesitancy (R39.11)
urinary incontinence (N39.4-)
urinary obstruction (N13.8)
urinary retention (R33.8)
urinary urgency (R39.15)
weak urinary stream (R39.12)

AHA: 2018,4Q,55

N4Ø.2　Nodular prostate without lower urinary tract symptoms　Ⓐ ♂

Nodular prostate without LUTS

N4Ø.3　Nodular prostate with lower urinary tract symptoms　Ⓐ ♂

Use additional code for associated symptoms, when specified:
incomplete bladder emptying (R39.14)
nocturia (R35.1)
straining on urination (R39.16)
urinary frequency (R35.Ø)
urinary hesitancy (R39.11)
urinary incontinence (N39.4-)
urinary obstruction (N13.8)
urinary retention (R33.8)
urinary urgency (R39.15)
weak urinary stream (R39.12)

✓4ᵗʰ **N41　Inflammatory diseases of prostate**

Use additional code (B95-B97), to identify infectious agent

N41.Ø　Acute prostatitis　Ⓐ ♂

N41.1　Chronic prostatitis　Ⓐ ♂

N41.2　Abscess of prostate　ᴄᴄ Ⓐ ♂

CC Excl: PDX collection 937

N41.3　Prostatocystitis　Ⓐ ♂

N41.4　Granulomatous prostatitis　Ⓐ ♂

N41.8　Other inflammatory diseases of prostate　Ⓐ ♂

N41.9　Inflammatory disease of prostate, unspecified　Ⓐ ♂

Prostatitis NOS

✓4ᵗʰ **N42　Other and unspecified disorders of prostate**

N42.Ø　Calculus of prostate　Ⓐ ♂

Prostatic stone

DEF: Formation of a small, solid stone often composed of calcium carbonate or calcium phosphate in the prostate gland.

N42.1　Congestion and hemorrhage of prostate　Ⓐ ♂

EXCLUDES 1　enlarged prostate (N4Ø.-)
hematuria (R31.-)
hyperplasia of prostate (N4Ø.-)
inflammatory diseases of prostate (N41.-)

✓5ᵗʰ **N42.3　Dysplasia of prostate**

AHA: 2016,4Q,44

N42.3Ø　Unspecified dysplasia of prostate　♂

N42.31　Prostatic intraepithelial neoplasia　♂

PIN
Prostatic intraepithelial neoplasia I (PIN I)
Prostatic intraepithelial neoplasia II (PIN II)

EXCLUDES 1　prostatic intraepithelial neoplasia III (PIN III) (DØ7.5)

DEF: Abnormality of shape and size of the intraepithelial tissues of the prostate. It is a premalignant condition characterized by stalks and absence of a basilar cell layer.

N42.32　Atypical small acinar proliferation of prostate　♂

N42.39　Other dysplasia of prostate　♂

✓5ᵗʰ **N42.8　Other specified disorders of prostate**

N42.81　Prostatodynia syndrome　Ⓐ ♂

Painful prostate syndrome

N42.82　Prostatosis syndrome　Ⓐ ♂

N42.83　Cyst of prostate　Ⓐ ♂

N42.89　Other specified disorders of prostate　Ⓐ ♂

N42.9　Disorder of prostate, unspecified　Ⓐ ♂

✓4ᵗʰ **N43　Hydrocele and spermatocele**

INCLUDES　hydrocele of spermatic cord, testis or tunica vaginalis

EXCLUDES 1　congenital hydrocele (P83.5)

DEF: Hydrocele: Serous fluid that collects in the tunica vaginalis of the scrotum along the spermatic cord in males.

N43.Ø　Encysted hydrocele　♂

N43.1　Infected hydrocele　ᴄᴄ ♂

Use additional code (B95-B97), to identify infectious agent

CC Excl: PDX collection 938

N43.2　Other hydrocele　♂

Hydrocele

Normal　Noncommunicating hydrocele　Communicating hydrocele　Hydrocele of the cord

(labels: Testicle, Scrotum)

N43.3　Hydrocele, unspecified　♂

✓5ᵗʰ **N43.4　Spermatocele of epididymis**

Spermatic cyst

DEF: Spermatocele: Noncancerous accumulation of fluid and dead sperm cells normally located at the head of the epididymis that exhibits itself as a hard, smooth scrotal mass and do not normally require treatment unless they become enlarged or cause pain.

N43.4Ø　Spermatocele of epididymis, unspecified　♂

N43.41　Spermatocele of epididymis, single　♂

N43.42　Spermatocele of epididymis, multiple　♂

✓4ᵗʰ **N44　Noninflammatory disorders of testis**

CC Excl: For CC codes in category N44: PDX collection 939

✓5ᵗʰ **N44.Ø　Torsion of testis**

N44.ØØ　Torsion of testis, unspecified　ᴄᴄ ♂

N44.Ø1　Extravaginal torsion of spermatic cord　ᴄᴄ ♂

DEF: Torsion of the spermatic cord just below the tunica vaginalis attachments.

N44.Ø2　Intravaginal torsion of spermatic cord　ᴄᴄ ♂

Torsion of spermatic cord NOS

N44.Ø3　Torsion of appendix testis　ᴄᴄ ♂

N44.Ø4　Torsion of appendix epididymis　ᴄᴄ ♂

N44.1　Cyst of tunica albuginea testis　♂

N44.2　Benign cyst of testis　♂

N44.8　Other noninflammatory disorders of the testis　♂

✓4ᵗʰ **N45　Orchitis and epididymitis**

Use additional code (B95-B97), to identify infectious agent

N45.1　Epididymitis　♂

N45.2　Orchitis　♂

N45.3　Epididymo-orchitis　♂

N45.4　Abscess of epididymis or testis　ᴄᴄ ♂

CC Excl: PDX collection 940

Ⓝ Newborn: 0　Ⓟ Pediatric: 0-17　Ⓜ Maternity: 9-64　Ⓐ Adult: 15-124　ᴹᶜᶜ Major Complication/Comorbidity　ᴄᴄ Complication/Comorbidity　ˢʷ Severe Wound Dx

✓4ᵗʰ N46   Male infertility

> EXCLUDES 1   vasectomy status (Z98.52)

✓5ᵗʰ N46.0   Azoospermia

Absolute male infertility
Male infertility due to germinal (cell) aplasia
Male infertility due to spermatogenic arrest (complete)
DEF: Failure of the development of sperm or the absence of sperm in semen.

N46.01   Organic azoospermia   🄰 ♂

Azoospermia NOS

✓6ᵗʰ N46.02   Azoospermia due to extratesticular causes

Code also associated cause

- N46.021   Azoospermia due to drug therapy   🄰 ♂
- N46.022   Azoospermia due to infection   🄰 ♂
- N46.023   Azoospermia due to obstruction of efferent ducts   🄰 ♂
- N46.024   Azoospermia due to radiation   🄰 ♂
- N46.025   Azoospermia due to systemic disease   🄰 ♂
- N46.029   Azoospermia due to other extratesticular causes   🄰 ♂

✓5ᵗʰ N46.1   Oligospermia

Male infertility due to germinal cell desquamation
Male infertility due to hypospermatogenesis
Male infertility due to incomplete spermatogenic arrest
DEF: Insufficient production of sperm in semen.

N46.11   Organic oligospermia   🄰 ♂

Oligospermia NOS

✓6ᵗʰ N46.12   Oligospermia due to extratesticular causes

Code also associated cause

- N46.121   Oligospermia due to drug therapy   🄰 ♂
- N46.122   Oligospermia due to infection   🄰 ♂
- N46.123   Oligospermia due to obstruction of efferent ducts   🄰 ♂
- N46.124   Oligospermia due to radiation   🄰 ♂
- N46.125   Oligospermia due to systemic disease   🄰 ♂
- N46.129   Oligospermia due to other extratesticular causes   🄰 ♂

N46.8   Other male infertility   🄰 ♂

N46.9   Male infertility, unspecified   🄰 ♂

✓4ᵗʰ N47   Disorders of prepuce

N47.0   Adherent prepuce, newborn   Ⓝ ♂

N47.1   Phimosis   ♂

DEF: Condition in which the foreskin is contracted and cannot be drawn back behind the glans penis.

N47.2   Paraphimosis   ♂

N47.3   Deficient foreskin   ♂

N47.4   Benign cyst of prepuce   ♂

N47.5   Adhesions of prepuce and glans penis   ♂

N47.6   Balanoposthitis   ♂

Use additional code (B95-B97), to identify infectious agent
> EXCLUDES 1   balanitis (N48.1)

N47.7   Other inflammatory diseases of prepuce   ♂

Use additional code (B95-B97), to identify infectious agent

N47.8   Other disorders of prepuce   ♂

✓4ᵗʰ N48   Other disorders of penis

N48.0   Leukoplakia of penis   ♂

Balanitis xerotica obliterans
Kraurosis of penis
Lichen sclerosus of external male genital organs
> EXCLUDES 1   carcinoma in situ of penis (D07.4)

N48.1   Balanitis   ♂

Use additional code (B95-B97), to identify infectious agent
> EXCLUDES 1   amebic balanitis (A06.8)
> balanitis xerotica obliterans (N48.0)
> candidal balanitis (B37.42)
> gonococcal balanitis (A54.23)
> herpesviral [herpes simplex] balanitis (A60.01)

DEF: Inflammation of the glans penis, most often affecting uncircumcised males.

✓5ᵗʰ N48.2   Other inflammatory disorders of penis

Use additional code (B95-B97), to identify infectious agent
> EXCLUDES 1   balanitis (N48.1)
> balanitis xerotica obliterans (N48.0)
> balanoposthitis (N47.6)

- N48.21   Abscess of corpus cavernosum and penis   ♂
- N48.22   Cellulitis of corpus cavernosum and penis   ♂
- N48.29   Other inflammatory disorders of penis   ♂

✓5ᵗʰ N48.3   Priapism

Painful erection
Code first underlying cause
CC Excl: For CC codes in subcategory N48.3: PDX collection 941

- N48.30   Priapism, unspecified   🄲🄲 ♂
- N48.31   Priapism due to trauma   🄲🄲 ♂
- N48.32   *Priapism due to disease classified elsewhere*   🄲🄲 ♂
- N48.33   Priapism, drug-induced   🄲🄲 ♂
- N48.39   Other priapism   🄲🄲 ♂

N48.5   Ulcer of penis   ♂

N48.6   Induration penis plastica   ♂

Peyronie's disease
Plastic induration of penis

✓5ᵗʰ N48.8   Other specified disorders of penis

- N48.81   Thrombosis of superficial vein of penis   ♂
- N48.82   Acquired torsion of penis   ♂
  Acquired torsion of penis NOS
  > EXCLUDES 1   congenital torsion of penis (Q55.63)
- N48.83   Acquired buried penis   ♂
  > EXCLUDES 1   congenital hidden penis (Q55.64)
- N48.89   Other specified disorders of penis   ♂

N48.9   Disorder of penis, unspecified   ♂

✓4ᵗʰ N49   Inflammatory disorders of male genital organs, not elsewhere classified

Use additional code (B95-B97), to identify infectious agent
> EXCLUDES 1   inflammation of penis (N48.1, N48.2-)
> orchitis and epididymitis (N45.-)

N49.0   Inflammatory disorders of seminal vesicle   ♂

Vesiculitis NOS

N49.1   Inflammatory disorders of spermatic cord, tunica vaginalis and vas deferens   ♂

Vasitis

N49.2   Inflammatory disorders of scrotum   ♂

N49.3   Fournier gangrene   ♂

N49.8   Inflammatory disorders of other specified male genital organs   ♂

Inflammation of multiple sites in male genital organs

N49.9   Inflammatory disorder of unspecified male genital organ   ♂

Abscess of unspecified male genital organ
Boil of unspecified male genital organ
Carbuncle of unspecified male genital organ
Cellulitis of unspecified male genital organ

✓4ᵗʰ N50   Other and unspecified disorders of male genital organs

> EXCLUDES 2   torsion of testis (N44.0-)

N50.0   Atrophy of testis   ♂

✓ Additional Character Required   ✓x7ᵗʰ Placeholder   Unacceptable PDx   Questionable PDx   Manifestation   Unspecified Dx   🄷🄷 HAC   🄷🄲🄲 CMS-HCC Dx   🄷🄸🅅 HIV Dx

ICD-10-CM 2020   863

Chapter 14. Diseases of the Genitourinary System

N50.1 Vascular disorders of male genital organs ♂

Hematocele, NOS, of male genital organs
Hemorrhage of male genital organs
Thrombosis of male genital organs

N50.3 Cyst of epididymis ♂

√5ᵗʰ **N50.8 Other specified disorders of male genital organs**

AHA: 2016,4Q,45

√6ᵗʰ **N50.81 Testicular pain**

N50.811 Right testicular pain ♂

N50.812 Left testicular pain ♂

N50.819 Testicular pain, unspecified ♂

N50.82 Scrotal pain ♂

N50.89 Other specified disorders of the male genital organs ♂

Atrophy of scrotum, seminal vesicle, spermatic cord, tunica vaginalis and vas deferens
Chylocele, tunica vaginalis (nonfilarial) NOS
Edema of scrotum, seminal vesicle, spermatic cord, tunica vaginalis and vas deferens
Hypertrophy of scrotum, seminal vesicle, spermatic cord, tunica vaginalis and vas deferens
Stricture of spermatic cord, tunica vaginalis, and vas deferens
Ulcer of scrotum, seminal vesicle, spermatic cord, testis, tunica vaginalis and vas deferens
Urethroscrotal fistula

N50.9 Disorder of male genital organs, unspecified ♂

N51 Disorders of male genital organs in diseases classified elsewhere ♂

Code first underlying disease, such as:
filariasis (B74.0-B74.9)

EXCLUDES 1   amebic balanitis (A06.8)
candidal balanitis (B37.42)
gonococcal balanitis (A54.23)
gonococcal prostatitis (A54.22)
herpesviral [herpes simplex] balanitis (A60.01)
trichomonal prostatitis (A59.02)
tuberculous prostatitis (A18.14)

√4ᵗʰ **N52 Male erectile dysfunction**

EXCLUDES 1   psychogenic impotence (F52.21)

√5ᵗʰ **N52.0 Vasculogenic erectile dysfunction**

N52.01 Erectile dysfunction due to arterial insufficiency A ♂

N52.02 Corporo-venous occlusive erectile dysfunction A ♂

N52.03 Combined arterial insufficiency and corporo-venous occlusive erectile dysfunction A ♂

N52.1 Erectile dysfunction due to diseases classified elsewhere A ♂

Code first underlying disease

N52.2 Drug-induced erectile dysfunction A ♂

√5ᵗʰ **N52.3 Postprocedural erectile dysfunction**

AHA: 2016,4Q,45

N52.31 Erectile dysfunction following radical prostatectomy A ♂

N52.32 Erectile dysfunction following radical cystectomy A ♂

N52.33 Erectile dysfunction following urethral surgery A ♂

N52.34 Erectile dysfunction following simple prostatectomy A ♂

N52.35 Erectile dysfunction following radiation therapy A ♂

N52.36 Erectile dysfunction following interstitial seed therapy A ♂

N52.37 Erectile dysfunction following prostate ablative therapy A ♂

Erectile dysfunction following cryotherapy
Erectile dysfunction following other prostate ablative therapies
Erectile dysfunction following ultrasound ablative therapies

N52.39 Other and unspecified postprocedural erectile dysfunction A ♂

N52.8 Other male erectile dysfunction A ♂

N52.9 Male erectile dysfunction, unspecified A ♂

Impotence NOS

√4ᵗʰ **N53 Other male sexual dysfunction**

EXCLUDES 1   psychogenic sexual dysfunction (F52.-)

√5ᵗʰ **N53.1 Ejaculatory dysfunction**

EXCLUDES 1   premature ejaculation (F52.4)

N53.11 Retarded ejaculation ♂

N53.12 Painful ejaculation ♂

N53.13 Anejaculatory orgasm ♂

N53.14 Retrograde ejaculation ♂

DEF: Form of male sexual dysfunction in which the semen enters the bladder instead of going out through the urethra during ejaculation.

N53.19 Other ejaculatory dysfunction ♂

Ejaculatory dysfunction NOS

N53.8 Other male sexual dysfunction ♂

N53.9 Unspecified male sexual dysfunction ♂

Disorders of breast (N60-N65)

EXCLUDES 1   disorders of breast associated with childbirth (O91-O92)

√4ᵗʰ **N60 Benign mammary dysplasia**

INCLUDES   fibrocystic mastopathy

√5ᵗʰ **N60.0 Solitary cyst of breast**

Cyst of breast

N60.01 Solitary cyst of right breast
N60.02 Solitary cyst of left breast
N60.09 Solitary cyst of unspecified breast

√5ᵗʰ **N60.1 Diffuse cystic mastopathy**

Cystic breast
Fibrocystic disease of breast

EXCLUDES 1   diffuse cystic mastopathy with epithelial proliferation (N60.3-)

N60.11 Diffuse cystic mastopathy of right breast A

N60.12 Diffuse cystic mastopathy of left breast A

N60.19 Diffuse cystic mastopathy of unspecified breast A

√5ᵗʰ **N60.2 Fibroadenosis of breast**

Adenofibrosis of breast

EXCLUDES 2   fibroadenoma of breast (D24.-)

N60.21 Fibroadenosis of right breast
N60.22 Fibroadenosis of left breast
N60.29 Fibroadenosis of unspecified breast

√5ᵗʰ **N60.3 Fibrosclerosis of breast**

Cystic mastopathy with epithelial proliferation

N60.31 Fibrosclerosis of right breast
N60.32 Fibrosclerosis of left breast
N60.39 Fibrosclerosis of unspecified breast

√5ᵗʰ **N60.4 Mammary duct ectasia**

N60.41 Mammary duct ectasia of right breast
N60.42 Mammary duct ectasia of left breast
N60.49 Mammary duct ectasia of unspecified breast

√5ᵗʰ **N60.8 Other benign mammary dysplasias**

N60.81 Other benign mammary dysplasias of right breast
N60.82 Other benign mammary dysplasias of left breast
N60.89 Other benign mammary dysplasias of unspecified breast

√5ᵗʰ **N60.9 Unspecified benign mammary dysplasia**

N60.91 Unspecified benign mammary dysplasia of right breast
N60.92 Unspecified benign mammary dysplasia of left breast
N60.99 Unspecified benign mammary dysplasia of unspecified breast

N Newborn: 0   P Pediatric: 0-17   M Maternity: 9-64   A Adult: 15-124   MCC Major Complication/Comorbidity   CC Complication/Comorbidity   SW Severe Wound Dx

864   ICD-10-CM 2020

N61 Inflammatory disorders of breast

EXCLUDES 1   inflammatory carcinoma of breast (C50.9)
inflammatory disorder of breast associated with childbirth (O91.-)
neonatal infective mastitis (P39.0)
thrombophlebitis of breast [Mondor's disease] (I80.8)

N61.0 Mastitis without abscess
Infective mastitis (acute) (nonpuerperal) (subacute)
Mastitis (acute) (nonpuerperal) (subacute) NOS
Cellulitis (acute) (nonpuerperal) (subacute) of breast NOS
Cellulitis (acute) (nonpuerperal) (subacute) of nipple NOS

N61.1 Abscess of the breast and nipple
Abscess (acute) (chronic) (nonpuerperal) of areola
Abscess (acute) (chronic) (nonpuerperal) of breast
Carbuncle of breast
Mastitis with abscess

N62 Hypertrophy of breast
Gynecomastia
Hypertrophy of breast NOS
Massive pubertal hypertrophy of breast
EXCLUDES 1   breast engorgement of newborn (P83.4)
disproportion of reconstructed breast (N65.1)

N63 Unspecified lump in breast
Nodule(s) NOS in breast
AHA: 2017,4Q,19

N63.0 Unspecified lump in unspecified breast

N63.1 Unspecified lump in the right breast

  N63.10 Unspecified lump in the right breast, unspecified quadrant
  N63.11 Unspecified lump in the right breast, upper outer quadrant
  N63.12 Unspecified lump in the right breast, upper inner quadrant
  N63.13 Unspecified lump in the right breast, lower outer quadrant
  N63.14 Unspecified lump in the right breast, lower inner quadrant
  N63.15 Unspecified lump in the right breast, overlapping quadrants

N63.2 Unspecified lump in the left breast

  N63.20 Unspecified lump in the left breast, unspecified quadrant
  N63.21 Unspecified lump in the left breast, upper outer quadrant
  N63.22 Unspecified lump in the left breast, upper inner quadrant
  N63.23 Unspecified lump in the left breast, lower outer quadrant
  N63.24 Unspecified lump in the left breast, lower inner quadrant
  N63.25 Unspecified lump in the left breast, overlapping quadrants

N63.3 Unspecified lump in axillary tail
  N63.31 Unspecified lump in axillary tail of the right breast
  N63.32 Unspecified lump in axillary tail of the left breast

N63.4 Unspecified lump in breast, subareolar
  N63.41 Unspecified lump in right breast, subareolar
  N63.42 Unspecified lump in left breast, subareolar

N64 Other disorders of breast
EXCLUDES 2   mechanical complication of breast prosthesis and implant (T85.4-)

N64.0 Fissure and fistula of nipple
N64.1 Fat necrosis of breast
Fat necrosis (segmental) of breast
Code first breast necrosis due to breast graft (T85.898)
N64.2 Atrophy of breast
N64.3 Galactorrhea not associated with childbirth
N64.4 Mastodynia
N64.5 Other signs and symptoms in breast
EXCLUDES 2   abnormal findings on diagnostic imaging of breast (R92.-)
  N64.51 Induration of breast
  N64.52 Nipple discharge
  EXCLUDES 1   abnormal findings in nipple discharge (R89.-)
  N64.53 Retraction of nipple

  N64.59 Other signs and symptoms in breast
N64.8 Other specified disorders of breast
  N64.81 Ptosis of breast   ▲
  EXCLUDES 1   ptosis of native breast in relation to reconstructed breast (N65.1)
  N64.82 Hypoplasia of breast   ▲
  Micromastia
  EXCLUDES 1   congenital absence of breast (Q83.0)
  hypoplasia of native breast in relation to reconstructed breast (N65.1)
  N64.89 Other specified disorders of breast
  Galactocele
  Subinvolution of breast (postlactational)
  AHA: 2019,1Q,32; 2018,1Q,3
N64.9 Disorder of breast, unspecified

N65 Deformity and disproportion of reconstructed breast

N65.0 Deformity of reconstructed breast   ▲
Contour irregularity in reconstructed breast
Excess tissue in reconstructed breast
Misshapen reconstructed breast

N65.1 Disproportion of reconstructed breast   ▲
Breast asymmetry between native breast and reconstructed breast
Disproportion between native breast and reconstructed breast

Inflammatory diseases of female pelvic organs (N70-N77)

EXCLUDES 1   inflammatory diseases of female pelvic organs complicating:
abortion or ectopic or molar pregnancy (O00-O07, O08.0)
pregnancy, childbirth and the puerperium (O23.-, O75.3, O85, O86.-)
CC Excl: For CC/MCC codes in categories N70-N77, unless otherwise noted: PDX collection 942

N70 Salpingitis and oophoritis

INCLUDES   abscess (of) fallopian tube
abscess (of) ovary
pyosalpinx
salpingo-oophoritis
tubo-ovarian abscess
tubo-ovarian inflammatory disease
Use additional code (B95-B97), to identify infectious agent
EXCLUDES 1   gonococcal infection (A54.24)
tuberculous infection (A18.17)

N70.0 Acute salpingitis and oophoritis
  N70.01 Acute salpingitis   CC ♀
  N70.02 Acute oophoritis   CC ♀
  N70.03 Acute salpingitis and oophoritis   CC ♀
N70.1 Chronic salpingitis and oophoritis
  Hydrosalpinx
  N70.11 Chronic salpingitis   ♀
  N70.12 Chronic oophoritis   ♀
  N70.13 Chronic salpingitis and oophoritis   ♀
N70.9 Salpingitis and oophoritis, unspecified
  N70.91 Salpingitis, unspecified   ♀
  N70.92 Oophoritis, unspecified   ♀
  N70.93 Salpingitis and oophoritis, unspecified

N71 Inflammatory disease of uterus, except cervix

INCLUDES   endo (myo) metritis
metritis
myometritis
pyometra
uterine abscess
Use additional code (B95-B97), to identify infectious agent
EXCLUDES 1   hyperplastic endometritis (N85.0-)
infection of uterus following delivery (O85, O86.-)

N71.0 Acute inflammatory disease of uterus   CC ♀
  CC Excl: PDX collection 943
N71.1 Chronic inflammatory disease of uterus   ♀
N71.9 Inflammatory disease of uterus, unspecified   ♀

Chapter 14. Diseases of the Genitourinary System

N72   Inflammatory disease of cervix uteri ♀

> **INCLUDES**   cervicitis (with or without erosion or ectropion)
> endocervicitis (with or without erosion or ectropion)
> exocervicitis (with or without erosion or ectropion)
> Use additional code (B95-B97), to identify infectious agent
> **EXCLUDES 1**   erosion and ectropion of cervix without cervicitis (N86)

✓4ᵗʰ N73   Other female pelvic inflammatory diseases

> Use additional code (B95-B97), to identify infectious agent

N73.0   Acute parametritis and pelvic cellulitis CC ♀

> Abscess of broad ligament
> Abscess of parametrium
> Pelvic cellulitis, female
> **DEF:** Parametritis: Inflammation of the parametrium.

N73.1   Chronic parametritis and pelvic cellulitis ♀

> Any condition in N73.0 specified as chronic
> **EXCLUDES 1**   tuberculous parametritis and pelvic cellultis (A18.17)

N73.2   Unspecified parametritis and pelvic cellulitis ♀

> Any condition in N73.0 unspecified whether acute or chronic

N73.3   Female acute pelvic peritonitis MCC ♀

N73.4   Female chronic pelvic peritonitis CC ♀

> **EXCLUDES 1**   tuberculous pelvic (female) peritonitis (A18.17)

N73.5   Female pelvic peritonitis, unspecified ♀

N73.6   Female pelvic peritoneal adhesions (postinfective) ♀

> **EXCLUDES 2**   postprocedural pelvic peritoneal adhesions (N99.4)
> **AHA:** 2014,1Q,6

N73.8   Other specified female pelvic inflammatory diseases ♀

N73.9   Female pelvic inflammatory disease, unspecified ♀

> Female pelvic infection or inflammation NOS

N74   Female pelvic inflammatory disorders in diseases classified elsewhere ♀

> Code first underlying disease
> **EXCLUDES 1**   chlamydial cervicitis (A56.02)
> chlamydial pelvic inflammatory disease (A56.11)
> gonococcal cervicitis (A54.03)
> gonococcal pelvic inflammatory disease (A54.24)
> herpesviral [herpes simplex] cervicitis (A60.03)
> herpesviral [herpes simplex] pelvic inflammatory disease (A60.09)
> syphilitic cervicitis (A52.76)
> syphilitic pelvic inflammatory disease (A52.76)
> trichomonal cervicitis (A59.09)
> tuberculous cervicitis (A18.16)
> tuberculous pelvic inflammatory disease (A18.17)

✓4ᵗʰ N75   Diseases of Bartholin's gland

> **DEF:** Bartholin's gland: Mucous-producing gland found in the vestibular bulbs on either side of the vaginal orifice and connected to the mucosal membrane at the opening by a duct.

N75.0   Cyst of Bartholin's gland ♀

N75.1   Abscess of Bartholin's gland CC ♀

> **CC Excl:** PDX collection 944

N75.8   Other diseases of Bartholin's gland ♀

> Bartholinitis

N75.9   Disease of Bartholin's gland, unspecified ♀

✓4ᵗʰ N76   Other inflammation of vagina and vulva

> Use additional code (B95-B97), to identify infectious agent
> **EXCLUDES 2**   senile (atrophic) vaginitis (N95.2)
> vulvar vestibulitis (N94.810)

N76.0   Acute vaginitis ♀

> Acute vulvovaginitis
> Vaginitis NOS
> Vulvovaginitis NOS

N76.1   Subacute and chronic vaginitis ♀

> Chronic vulvovaginitis
> Subacute vulvovaginitis

N76.2   Acute vulvitis ♀

> Vulvitis NOS

N76.3   Subacute and chronic vulvitis ♀

N76.4   Abscess of vulva ♀

> Furuncle of vulva

N76.5   Ulceration of vagina ♀

N76.6   Ulceration of vulva ♀

✓5ᵗʰ N76.8   Other specified inflammation of vagina and vulva

N76.81   Mucositis (ulcerative) of vagina and vulva CC ♀

> Code also type of associated therapy, such as:
> antineoplastic and immunosuppressive drugs (T45.1X-)
> radiological procedure and radiotherapy (Y84.2)
> **EXCLUDES 2**   gastrointestinal mucositis (ulcerative) (K92.81)
> nasal mucositis (ulcerative) (J34.81)
> oral mucositis (ulcerative) (K12.3-)
> **CC Excl:** PDX collection 945

N76.89   Other specified inflammation of vagina and vulva ♀

✓4ᵗʰ N77   Vulvovaginal ulceration and inflammation in diseases classified elsewhere

N77.0   Ulceration of vulva in diseases classified elsewhere ♀

> Code first underlying disease, such as:
> Behçet's disease (M35.2)
> **EXCLUDES 1**   ulceration of vulva in gonococcal infection (A54.02)
> ulceration of vulva in herpesviral [herpes simplex] infection (A60.04)
> ulceration of vulva in syphilis (A51.0)
> ulceration of vulva in tuberculosis (A18.18)

N77.1   Vaginitis, vulvitis and vulvovaginitis in diseases classified elsewhere ♀

> Code first underlying disease, such as:
> pinworm (B80)
> **EXCLUDES 1**   candidal vulvovaginitis (B37.3)
> chlamydial vulvovaginitis (A56.02)
> gonococcal vulvovaginitis (A54.02)
> herpesviral [herpes simplex] vulvovaginitis (A60.04)
> trichomonal vulvovaginitis (A59.01)
> tuberculous vulvovaginitis (A18.18)
> vulvovaginitis in early syphilis (A51.0)
> vulvovaginitis in late syphilis (A52.76)

Noninflammatory disorders of female genital tract (N80-N98)

✓4ᵗʰ N80   Endometriosis

> **DEF:** Aberrant uterine mucosal tissue appearing in areas of the pelvic cavity outside of its normal location, lining the uterus, and inflaming surrounding tissues often resulting in infertility or spontaneous abortion.

N80.0   Endometriosis of uterus ♀

> Adenomyosis
> **EXCLUDES 1**   stromal endometriosis (D39.0)

N80.1   Endometriosis of ovary ♀

N80.2   Endometriosis of fallopian tube ♀

N80.3   Endometriosis of pelvic peritoneum ♀

N80.4   Endometriosis of rectovaginal septum and vagina ♀

N80.5   Endometriosis of intestine ♀

N80.6   Endometriosis in cutaneous scar ♀

N80.8   Other endometriosis ♀

> Endometriosis of thorax

N80.9   Endometriosis, unspecified ♀

N Newborn: 0   P Pediatric: 0-17   M Maternity: 9-64   A Adult: 15-124   MCC Major Complication/Comorbidity   CC Complication/Comorbidity   SW Severe Wound Dx

866   ICD-10-CM 2020

✓4ᵗʰ N81 Female genital prolapse

> EXCLUDES 1   *genital prolapse complicating pregnancy, labor or delivery (O34.5-)*
> *prolapse and hernia of ovary and fallopian tube (N83.4-)*
> *prolapse of vaginal vault after hysterectomy (N99.3)*

Types of Pelvic Organ Prolapse

Urethrocele
Bladder
Uterus
Rectum
Urethra
Vaginal canal
Urethrocele

Cystocele
Bladder
Uterus
Rectum
Urethra
Vaginal canal
Cystocele

Rectocele
Bladder
Uterus
Rectum
Urethra
Vaginal canal
Rectocele

Enterocele
Bladder
Uterus
Rectum
Enterocele
Urethra
Vaginal canal
Terminal ileum

N81.Ø Urethrocele ♀

> EXCLUDES 1   *urethrocele with cystocele (N81.1-)*
> *urethrocele with prolapse of uterus (N81.2-N81.4)*

✓5ᵗʰ N81.1 Cystocele
Cystocele with urethrocele
Cystourethrocele

> EXCLUDES 1   *cystocele with prolapse of uterus (N81.2-N81.4)*

    N81.1Ø Cystocele, unspecified ♀
       Prolapse of (anterior) vaginal wall NOS

    N81.11 Cystocele, midline ♀

    N81.12 Cystocele, lateral ♀
       Paravaginal cystocele
       DEF: Detachment of the lateral support connections of the vagina at the arcus tendineus fasciae pelvis (ATFP) that results in bladder drop. The bladder herniates into the vagina laterally.

N81.2 Incomplete uterovaginal prolapse ♀
First degree uterine prolapse
Prolapse of cervix NOS
Second degree uterine prolapse

> EXCLUDES 1   *cervical stump prolapse (N81.85)*

N81.3 Complete uterovaginal prolapse ♀
Procidentia (uteri) NOS
Third degree uterine prolapse

N81.4 Uterovaginal prolapse, unspecified ♀
Prolapse of uterus NOS

N81.5 Vaginal enterocele ♀

> EXCLUDES 1   *enterocele with prolapse of uterus (N81.2-N81.4)*

N81.6 Rectocele ♀
Prolapse of posterior vaginal wall
Use additional code for any associated fecal incontinence, if applicable (R15.-)

> EXCLUDES 2   *perineocele (N81.81)*
> *rectal prolapse (K62.3)*
> *rectocele with prolapse of uterus (N81.2-N81.4)*

✓5ᵗʰ N81.8 Other female genital prolapse

    N81.81 Perineocele ♀

    N81.82 Incompetence or weakening of pubocervical tissue ♀

    N81.83 Incompetence or weakening of rectovaginal tissue ♀

    N81.84 Pelvic muscle wasting ♀
       Disuse atrophy of pelvic muscles and anal sphincter

    N81.85 Cervical stump prolapse ♀

    N81.89 Other female genital prolapse ♀
       Deficient perineum
       Old laceration of muscles of pelvic floor

N81.9 Female genital prolapse, unspecified ♀

✓4ᵗʰ N82 Fistulae involving female genital tract

> EXCLUDES 1   *vesicointestinal fistulae (N32.1)*

CC Excl: For CC codes in category N82: PDX collection 946

N82.Ø Vesicovaginal fistula   CC SW ♀

N82.1 Other female urinary-genital tract fistulae   CC ♀
Cervicovesical fistula
Ureterovaginal fistula
Urethrovaginal fistula
Uteroureteric fistula
Uterovesical fistula
AHA: 2017,3Q,3

N82.2 Fistula of vagina to small intestine   CC SW ♀

N82.3 Fistula of vagina to large intestine   CC SW ♀
Rectovaginal fistula

N82.4 Other female intestinal-genital tract fistulae   CC SW ♀
Intestinouterine fistula

N82.5 Female genital tract-skin fistulae   CC SW ♀
Uterus to abdominal wall fistula
Vaginoperineal fistula

N82.8 Other female genital tract fistulae   CC ♀

N82.9 Female genital tract fistula, unspecified   CC ♀

✓4ᵗʰ N83 Noninflammatory disorders of ovary, fallopian tube and broad ligament

> EXCLUDES 2   *hydrosalpinx (N70.1-)*

AHA: 2016,4Q,46

✓5ᵗʰ N83.Ø Follicular cyst of ovary
Cyst of graafian follicle
Hemorrhagic follicular cyst (of ovary)

    N83.ØØ Follicular cyst of ovary, unspecified side ♀

    N83.Ø1 Follicular cyst of right ovary ♀

    N83.Ø2 Follicular cyst of left ovary ♀

✓5ᵗʰ N83.1 Corpus luteum cyst
Hemorrhagic corpus luteum cyst

    N83.1Ø Corpus luteum cyst of ovary, unspecified side ♀

    N83.11 Corpus luteum cyst of right ovary ♀

    N83.12 Corpus luteum cyst of left ovary ♀

✓5ᵗʰ N83.2 Other and unspecified ovarian cysts

> EXCLUDES 1   *developmental ovarian cyst (Q5Ø.1)*
> *neoplastic ovarian cyst (D27.-)*
> *polycystic ovarian syndrome (E28.2)*
> *Stein-Leventhal syndrome (E28.2)*

    ✓6ᵗʰ N83.2Ø Unspecified ovarian cysts

       N83.2Ø1 Unspecified ovarian cyst, right side ♀

       N83.2Ø2 Unspecified ovarian cyst, left side ♀

       N83.2Ø9 Unspecified ovarian cyst, unspecified side ♀
          Ovarian cyst, NOS

    ✓6ᵗʰ N83.29 Other ovarian cysts
       Retention cyst of ovary
       Simple cyst of ovary

       N83.291 Other ovarian cyst, right side ♀

       N83.292 Other ovarian cyst, left side ♀

       N83.299 Other ovarian cyst, unspecified side ♀

✓5ᵗʰ N83.3 Acquired atrophy of ovary and fallopian tube

    ✓6ᵗʰ N83.31 Acquired atrophy of ovary

       N83.311 Acquired atrophy of right ovary ♀

       N83.312 Acquired atrophy of left ovary ♀

Chapter 14. Diseases of the Genitourinary System

N83.319   **Acquired atrophy of ovary, unspecified side**   ♀
     Acquired atrophy of ovary, NOS

☑6ᵗʰ **N83.32**   **Acquired atrophy of fallopian tube**

     N83.321   **Acquired atrophy of right fallopian tube**   ♀

     N83.322   **Acquired atrophy of left fallopian tube**   ♀

     N83.329   **Acquired atrophy of fallopian tube, unspecified side**   ♀
       Acquired atrophy of fallopian tube, NOS

☑6ᵗʰ **N83.33**   **Acquired atrophy of ovary and fallopian tube**

     N83.331   **Acquired atrophy of right ovary and fallopian tube**   ♀

     N83.332   **Acquired atrophy of left ovary and fallopian tube**   ♀

     N83.339   **Acquired atrophy of ovary and fallopian tube, unspecified side**   ♀
       Acquired atrophy of ovary and fallopian tube, NOS

☑5ᵗʰ **N83.4**   **Prolapse and hernia of ovary and fallopian tube**

     N83.40   **Prolapse and hernia of ovary and fallopian tube, unspecified side**   ♀
       Prolapse and hernia of ovary and fallopian tube, NOS

     N83.41   **Prolapse and hernia of right ovary and fallopian tube**   ♀

     N83.42   **Prolapse and hernia of left ovary and fallopian tube**   ♀

☑5ᵗʰ **N83.5**   **Torsion of ovary, ovarian pedicle and fallopian tube**
     Torsion of accessory tube
     CC Excl: For CC codes in subcategory N83.5: PDX collection 947

     ☑6ᵗʰ **N83.51**   **Torsion of ovary and ovarian pedicle**

       N83.511   **Torsion of right ovary and ovarian pedicle**   CC ♀

       N83.512   **Torsion of left ovary and ovarian pedicle**   CC ♀

       N83.519   **Torsion of ovary and ovarian pedicle, unspecified side**   CC ♀
         Torsion of ovary and ovarian pedicle, NOS

     ☑6ᵗʰ **N83.52**   **Torsion of fallopian tube**
       Torsion of hydatid of Morgagni

       N83.521   **Torsion of right fallopian tube**   CC ♀

       N83.522   **Torsion of left fallopian tube**   CC ♀

       N83.529   **Torsion of fallopian tube, unspecified side**   CC ♀
         Torsion of fallopian tube, NOS

     N83.53   **Torsion of ovary, ovarian pedicle and fallopian tube**   CC ♀

N83.6   **Hematosalpinx**   ♀
     EXCLUDES 1   *hematosalpinx (with) (in):*
       hematocolpos (N89.7)
       hematometra (N85.7)
       tubal pregnancy (O00.1-)

N83.7   **Hematoma of broad ligament**   ♀

N83.8   **Other noninflammatory disorders of ovary, fallopian tube and broad ligament**   ♀
     Broad ligament laceration syndrome [Allen-Masters]

N83.9   **Noninflammatory disorder of ovary, fallopian tube and broad ligament, unspecified**   ♀

☑4ᵗʰ **N84**   **Polyp of female genital tract**
     EXCLUDES 1   *adenomatous polyp (D28.-)*
       placental polyp (O90.89)

N84.0   **Polyp of corpus uteri**   ♀
     Polyp of endometrium
     Polyp of uterus NOS
     EXCLUDES 1   *polypoid endometrial hyperplasia (N85.0-)*

N84.1   **Polyp of cervix uteri**   ♀
     Mucous polyp of cervix

N84.2   **Polyp of vagina**   ♀

N84.3   **Polyp of vulva**   ♀
     Polyp of labia

N84.8   **Polyp of other parts of female genital tract**   ♀

N84.9   **Polyp of female genital tract, unspecified**   ♀

☑4ᵗʰ **N85**   **Other noninflammatory disorders of uterus, except cervix**
     EXCLUDES 1   *endometriosis (N80.-)*
       inflammatory diseases of uterus (N71.-)
       noninflammatory disorders of cervix, except malposition (N86-N88)
       polyp of corpus uteri (N84.0)
       uterine prolapse (N81.-)

☑5ᵗʰ **N85.0**   **Endometrial hyperplasia**

     N85.00   **Endometrial hyperplasia, unspecified**   ♀
       Hyperplasia (adenomatous) (cystic) (glandular) of endometrium
       Hyperplastic endometritis

     N85.01   **Benign endometrial hyperplasia**   ♀
       Endometrial hyperplasia (complex) (simple) without atypia

     N85.02   **Endometrial intraepithelial neoplasia [EIN]**   ♀
       Endometrial hyperplasia with atypia
       EXCLUDES 1   *malignant neoplasm of endometrium (with endometrial intraepithelial neoplasia [EIN]) (C54.1)*

N85.2   **Hypertrophy of uterus**   ♀
     Bulky or enlarged uterus
     EXCLUDES 1   *puerperal hypertrophy of uterus (O90.89)*

N85.3   **Subinvolution of uterus**   ♀
     EXCLUDES 1   *puerperal subinvolution of uterus (O90.89)*

N85.4   **Malposition of uterus**   ♀
     Anteversion of uterus
     Retroflexion of uterus
     Retroversion of uterus
     EXCLUDES 1   *malposition of uterus complicating pregnancy, labor or delivery (O34.5-, O65.5)*

N85.5   **Inversion of uterus**   ♀
     EXCLUDES 1   *current obstetric trauma (O71.2)*
       postpartum inversion of uterus (O71.2)
     DEF: Abnormality in which the uterus turns inside out.

Inversion of Uterus

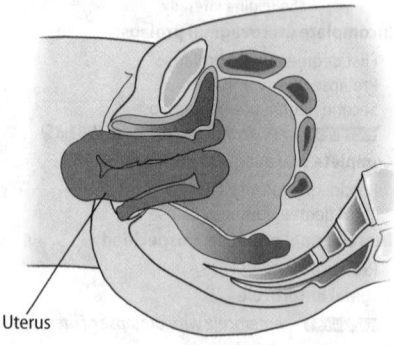

Uterus

N85.6   **Intrauterine synechiae**   ♀

N85.7   **Hematometra**   ♀
     Hematosalpinx with hematometra
     EXCLUDES 1   *hematometra with hematocolpos (N89.7)*
     DEF: Accumulation of blood within the uterus.

N85.8   **Other specified noninflammatory disorders of uterus**   ♀
     Atrophy of uterus, acquired
     Fibrosis of uterus NOS

N85.9   **Noninflammatory disorder of uterus, unspecified**   ♀
     Disorder of uterus NOS

Ⓝ Newborn: 0   Ⓟ Pediatric: 0-17   Ⓜ Maternity: 9-64   Ⓐ Adult: 15-124   MCC Major Complication/Comorbidity   CC Complication/Comorbidity   SW Severe Wound Dx

868   ICD-10-CM 2020

N86   Erosion and ectropion of cervix uteri ♀

     Decubitus (trophic) ulcer of cervix
     Eversion of cervix
     EXCLUDES 1   erosion and ectropion of cervix with cervicitis (N72)

✓4ᵗʰ **N87   Dysplasia of cervix uteri**

     EXCLUDES 1   abnormal results from cervical cytologic examination without
                histologic confirmation (R87.61-)
                carcinoma in situ of cervix uteri (D06.-)
                cervical intraepithelial neoplasia III [CIN III] (D06.-)
                HGSIL of cervix (R87.613)
                severe dysplasia of cervix uteri (D06.-)

     N87.0   Mild cervical dysplasia ♀

         Cervical intraepithelial neoplasia I [CIN I]

     N87.1   Moderate cervical dysplasia ♀

         Cervical intraepithelial neoplasia II [CIN II]

     N87.9   Dysplasia of cervix uteri, unspecified ♀

         Anaplasia of cervix
         Cervical atypism
         Cervical dysplasia NOS

✓4ᵗʰ **N88   Other noninflammatory disorders of cervix uteri**

     EXCLUDES 2   inflammatory disease of cervix (N72)
                polyp of cervix (N84.1)

     N88.0   Leukoplakia of cervix uteri ♀

     N88.1   Old laceration of cervix uteri ♀

         Adhesions of cervix
         EXCLUDES 1   current obstetric trauma (O71.3)

     N88.2   Stricture and stenosis of cervix uteri ♀

         EXCLUDES 1   stricture and stenosis of cervix uteri complicating
                labor (O65.5)

     N88.3   Incompetence of cervix uteri ♀

         Investigation and management of (suspected) cervical
            incompetence in a nonpregnant woman
         EXCLUDES 1   cervical incompetence complicating pregnancy
                (O34.3-)
         DEF: Inadequate functioning of the cervix marked by abnormal
         widening during pregnancy and causing premature birth or
         miscarriage.

     N88.4   Hypertrophic elongation of cervix uteri ♀

     **N88.8   Other specified noninflammatory disorders
              of cervix uteri** ♀

         EXCLUDES 1   current obstetric trauma (O71.3)

     **N88.9   Noninflammatory disorder of cervix uteri,
              unspecified** ♀

✓4ᵗʰ **N89   Other noninflammatory disorders of vagina**

     EXCLUDES 1   abnormal results from vaginal cytologic examination without
                histologic confirmation (R87.62-)
                carcinoma in situ of vagina (D07.2)
                HGSIL of vagina (R87.623)
                inflammation of vagina (N76.-)
                senile (atrophic) vaginitis (N95.2)
                severe dysplasia of vagina (D07.2)
                trichomonal leukorrhea (A59.00)
                vaginal intraepithelial neoplasia [VAIN], grade III (D07.2)

     N89.0   Mild vaginal dysplasia ♀

         Vaginal intraepithelial neoplasia [VAIN], grade I

     N89.1   Moderate vaginal dysplasia ♀

         Vaginal intraepithelial neoplasia [VAIN], grade II

     N89.3   Dysplasia of vagina, unspecified ♀

     N89.4   Leukoplakia of vagina ♀

     N89.5   Stricture and atresia of vagina ♀

         Vaginal adhesions
         Vaginal stenosis
         EXCLUDES 1   congenital atresia or stricture (Q52.4)
                postprocedural adhesions of vagina (N99.2)

     N89.6   Tight hymenal ring ♀

         Rigid hymen
         Tight introitus
         EXCLUDES 1   imperforate hymen (Q52.3)

     N89.7   Hematocolpos ♀

         Hematocolpos with hematometra or hematosalpinx
         AHA: 2016,4Q,58

     **N89.8   Other specified noninflammatory disorders
              of vagina** ♀

         Leukorrhea NOS
         Old vaginal laceration
         Pessary ulcer of vagina
         EXCLUDES 1   current obstetric trauma (O70.-, O71.4, O71.7-O71.8)
                old laceration involving muscles of pelvic floor
                (N81.8)

     **N89.9   Noninflammatory disorder of vagina,
              unspecified** ♀

✓4ᵗʰ **N90   Other noninflammatory disorders of vulva and perineum**

     EXCLUDES 1   anogenital (venereal) warts (A63.0)
                carcinoma in situ of vulva (D07.1)
                condyloma acuminatum (A63.0)
                current obstetric trauma (O70.-, O71.7-O71.8)
                inflammation of vulva (N76.-)
                severe dysplasia of vulva (D07.1)
                vulvar intraepithelial neoplasm III [VIN III] (D07.1)

     N90.0   Mild vulvar dysplasia ♀

         Vulvar intraepithelial neoplasia [VIN], grade I

     N90.1   Moderate vulvar dysplasia ♀

         Vulvar intraepithelial neoplasia [VIN], grade II

     N90.3   Dysplasia of vulva, unspecified ♀

     N90.4   Leukoplakia of vulva ♀

         Dystrophy of vulva
         Kraurosis of vulva
         Lichen sclerosus of external female genital organs

     N90.5   Atrophy of vulva ♀

         Stenosis of vulva

✓5ᵗʰ   **N90.6   Hypertrophy of vulva**

         AHA: 2016,4Q,46

         N90.60   Unspecified hypertrophy of vulva ♀

             Unspecified hypertrophy of labia

         **N90.61   Childhood asymmetric labium majus
                 enlargement** ♀

             CALME

         N90.69   Other specified hypertrophy of vulva ♀

             Other specified hypertrophy of labia

     N90.7   Vulvar cyst ♀

✓5ᵗʰ   **N90.8   Other specified noninflammatory disorders of vulva and
              perineum**

     ✓6ᵗʰ   **N90.81   Female genital mutilation status**

             Female genital cutting status

             **N90.810   Female genital mutilation
                    status, unspecified** ♀

                  Female genital cutting status, unspecified
                  Female genital mutilation status NOS

             **N90.811   Female genital mutilation
                    Type I status** ♀

                  Clitorectomy status
                  Female genital cutting Type I status

             **N90.812   Female genital mutilation
                    Type II status** ♀

                  Clitorectomy with excision of labia minora
                    status
                  Female genital cutting Type II status

             **N90.813   Female genital mutilation
                    Type III status** ♀

                  Female genital cutting Type III status
                  Infibulation status

             **N90.818   Other female genital
                    mutilation status** ♀

                  Female genital cutting Type IV status
                  Female genital mutilation Type IV status
                  Other female genital cutting status

         **N90.89   Other specified noninflammatory
                 disorders of vulva and perineum** ♀

             Adhesions of vulva
             Hypertrophy of clitoris

     **N90.9   Noninflammatory disorder of vulva and
              perineum, unspecified** ♀

✓4ᵗʰ **N91   Absent, scanty and rare menstruation**

     EXCLUDES 1   ovarian dysfunction (E28.-)

     N91.0   Primary amenorrhea ♀

     N91.1   Secondary amenorrhea ♀

N91.2   **Amenorrhea, unspecified** ♀

N91.3   **Primary oligomenorrhea** ♀

N91.4   **Secondary oligomenorrhea** ♀

N91.5   **Oligomenorrhea, unspecified** ♀

     Hypomenorrhea NOS

✓4ᵗʰ **N92**   **Excessive, frequent and irregular menstruation**

     EXCLUDES 1   *postmenopausal bleeding (N95.0)*

           precocious puberty (menstruation) (E30.1)

N92.0   **Excessive and frequent menstruation with regular cycle** ♀

     Heavy periods NOS

     Menorrhagia NOS

     Polymenorrhea

N92.1   **Excessive and frequent menstruation with irregular cycle** ♀

     Irregular intermenstrual bleeding

     Irregular, shortened intervals between menstrual bleeding

     Menometrorrhagia

     Metrorrhagia

N92.2   **Excessive menstruation at puberty** P ♀

     Excessive bleeding associated with onset of menstrual periods

     Pubertal menorrhagia

     Puberty bleeding

N92.3   **Ovulation bleeding** ♀

     Regular intermenstrual bleeding

N92.4   **Excessive bleeding in the premenopausal period** ♀

     Climacteric menorrhagia or metrorrhagia

     Menopausal menorrhagia or metrorrhagia

     ▶Perimenopausal bleeding◀

     ▶Perimenopausal menorrhagia or metrorrhagia◀

     Preclimacteric menorrhagia or metrorrhagia

     Premenopausal menorrhagia or metrorrhagia

N92.5   **Other specified irregular menstruation** ♀

N92.6   **Irregular menstruation, unspecified** ♀

     Irregular bleeding NOS

     Irregular periods NOS

     EXCLUDES 1   *irregular menstruation with:*

           lengthened intervals or scanty bleeding (N91.3-N91.5)

           shortened intervals or excessive bleeding (N92.1)

✓4ᵗʰ **N93**   **Other abnormal uterine and vaginal bleeding**

     EXCLUDES 1   *neonatal vaginal hemorrhage (P54.6)*

           precocious puberty (menstruation) (E30.1)

           pseudomenses (P54.6)

N93.0   **Postcoital and contact bleeding** ♀

N93.1   **Pre-pubertal vaginal bleeding** ♀

     AHA: 2016,4Q,47

N93.8   **Other specified abnormal uterine and vaginal bleeding** ♀

     Dysfunctional or functional uterine or vaginal bleeding NOS

N93.9   **Abnormal uterine and vaginal bleeding, unspecified** ♀

✓4ᵗʰ **N94**   **Pain and other conditions associated with female genital organs and menstrual cycle**

N94.0   **Mittelschmerz** ♀

     DEF: One-sided, lower abdominal pain occurring between menstrual periods that is associated with ovulation.

✓5ᵗʰ **N94.1**   **Dyspareunia**

     EXCLUDES 1   *psychogenic dyspareunia (F52.6)*

     AHA: 2016,4Q,47

     N94.10   **Unspecified dyspareunia** ♀

     N94.11   **Superficial (introital) dyspareunia** ♀

     N94.12   **Deep dyspareunia** ♀

     N94.19   **Other specified dyspareunia** ♀

N94.2   **Vaginismus** ♀

     EXCLUDES 1   *psychogenic vaginismus (F52.5)*

     DEF: Spontaneous contractions of the muscles surrounding the vagina, causing it to constrict or close.

N94.3   **Premenstrual tension syndrome** ♀

     Code also associated menstrual migraine (G43.82-, G43.83-)

     EXCLUDES 1   *premenstrual dysphoric disorder (F32.81)*

N94.4   **Primary dysmenorrhea** ♀

N94.5   **Secondary dysmenorrhea** ♀

N94.6   **Dysmenorrhea, unspecified** ♀

     EXCLUDES 1   *psychogenic dysmenorrhea (F45.8)*

✓5ᵗʰ **N94.8**   **Other specified conditions associated with female genital organs and menstrual cycle**

     ✓6ᵗʰ **N94.81**   **Vulvodynia**

         N94.810   **Vulvar vestibulitis** ♀

         N94.818   **Other vulvodynia** ♀

         N94.819   **Vulvodynia, unspecified** ♀

           Vulvodynia NOS

     N94.89   **Other specified conditions associated with female genital organs and menstrual cycle** ♀

         DEF: Hydrocele: Serous fluid that collects in the canal of Nuck in females.

N94.9   **Unspecified condition associated with female genital organs and menstrual cycle**

✓4ᵗʰ **N95**   **Menopausal and other perimenopausal disorders**

     Menopausal and other perimenopausal disorders due to naturally occurring (age-related) menopause and perimenopause

     EXCLUDES 1   *excessive bleeding in the premenopausal period (N92.4)*

           menopausal and perimenopausal disorders due to artificial or premature menopause (E89.4-, E28.31-)

           premature menopause (E28.31-)

     EXCLUDES 2   *postmenopausal osteoporosis (M81.0-)*

           postmenopausal osteoporosis with current pathological fracture (M80.0-)

           postmenopausal urethritis (N34.2)

N95.0   **Postmenopausal bleeding** ♀

N95.1   **Menopausal and female climacteric states** ♀

     Symptoms such as flushing, sleeplessness, headache, lack of concentration, associated with natural (age-related) menopause

     Use additional code for associated symptoms

     EXCLUDES 1   *asymptomatic menopausal state (Z78.0)*

           symptoms associated with artificial menopause (E89.41)

           symptoms associated with premature menopause (E28.310)

N95.2   **Postmenopausal atrophic vaginitis** ♀

     Senile (atrophic) vaginitis

N95.8   **Other specified menopausal and perimenopausal disorders** ♀

N95.9   **Unspecified menopausal and perimenopausal disorder** ♀

N96   **Recurrent pregnancy loss** ♀

     Investigation or care in a nonpregnant woman with history of recurrent pregnancy loss

     EXCLUDES 1   *recurrent pregnancy loss with current pregnancy (O26.2-)*

✓4ᵗʰ **N97**   **Female infertility**

     INCLUDES   inability to achieve a pregnancy

           sterility, female NOS

     EXCLUDES 1   *female infertility associated with:*

           hypopituitarism (E23.0)

           Stein-Leventhal syndrome (E28.2)

     EXCLUDES 2   *incompetence of cervix uteri (N88.3)*

     DEF: Infertility: Inability to conceive for at least one year with regular intercourse.

     DEF: Primary infertility: Infertility occurring in patients who have never conceived.

     DEF: Secondary infertility: Infertility occurring in patients who have previously conceived.

N97.0   **Female infertility associated with anovulation** ♀

N97.1   **Female infertility of tubal origin** ♀

     Female infertility associated with congenital anomaly of tube

     Female infertility due to tubal block

     Female infertility due to tubal occlusion

     Female infertility due to tubal stenosis

N97.2   **Female infertility of** uterine origin   ♀

Female infertility associated with congenital anomaly of uterus

Female infertility due to nonimplantation of ovum

N97.8   **Female infertility of** other origin   ♀

N97.9   **Female infertility, unspecified**   ♀

☑4th **N98**   **Complications associated with artificial fertilization**

CC Excl: For CC codes in category N98, unless otherwise noted: PDX collection 643

N98.0   **Infection associated with artificial insemination**   CC ♀

CC Excl: PDX collection 948

N98.1   **Hyperstimulation of ovaries**   CC ♀

Hyperstimulation of ovaries NOS

Hyperstimulation of ovaries associated with induced ovulation

N98.2   **Complications of attempted introduction of fertilized ovum following in vitro fertilization**   CC ♀

N98.3   **Complications of attempted introduction of embryo in embryo transfer**   CC ♀

N98.8   **Other complications associated with artificial fertilization**   CC ♀

N98.9   **Complication associated with artificial fertilization, unspecified**   CC ♀

Intraoperative and postprocedural complications and disorders of genitourinary system, not elsewhere classified (N99)

CC Excl: For CC codes in category N99, unless otherwise noted: PDX collection 952

☑4th **N99**   **Intraoperative and postprocedural complications and disorders of genitourinary system, not elsewhere classified**

   EXCLUDES 2   irradiation cystitis (N30.4-)

     postoophorectomy osteoporosis with current pathological fracture (M80.8-)

     postoophorectomy osteoporosis without current pathological fracture (M81.8)

N99.0   **Postprocedural (acute) (chronic) kidney failure**

Use additional code to type of kidney disease

☑5th **N99.1**   **Postprocedural urethral stricture**

Postcatheterization urethral stricture

   ☑6th **N99.11**   **Postprocedural urethral stricture, male**

     AHA: 2016,4Q,47-48

     N99.110   **Postprocedural urethral stricture, male,** meatal   ♂

     N99.111   **Postprocedural** bulbous **urethral stricture, male**   ♂

     N99.112   **Postprocedural** membranous **urethral stricture, male**   ♂

     N99.113   **Postprocedural** anterior bulbous **urethral stricture, male**   ♂

     N99.114   **Postprocedural urethral stricture, male, unspecified**   ♂

     N99.115   **Postprocedural** fossa navicularis **urethral stricture**   ♂

     N99.116   **Postprocedural urethral stricture, male,** overlapping **sites**   ♂

   N99.12   **Postprocedural urethral stricture, female**   ♀

N99.2   **Postprocedural** adhesions of vagina   ♀

N99.3   **Prolapse of vaginal vault** after hysterectomy   ♀

N99.4   **Postprocedural** pelvic peritoneal adhesions

   EXCLUDES 2   pelvic peritoneal adhesions NOS (N73.6)

     postinfective pelvic peritoneal adhesions (N73.6)

☑5th **N99.5**   **Complications of stoma of urinary tract**

   EXCLUDES 2   mechanical complication of urinary catheter (T83.0-)

   AHA: 2016,4Q,48

   ☑6th **N99.51**   **Complication of** cystostomy

     N99.510   **Cystostomy** hemorrhage   CC HCC

       CC Excl: PDX collection 949

     N99.511   **Cystostomy infection**   CC HCC

       CC Excl: PDX collection 950

     N99.512   **Cystostomy malfunction**   CC HCC

       CC Excl: PDX collection 951

     N99.518   **Other cystostomy complication**   CC HCC

       CC Excl: PDX collection 949

   ☑6th **N99.52**   **Complication of** incontinent external stoma **of urinary tract**

     N99.520   **Hemorrhage of incontinent external stoma of urinary tract**   HCC

     N99.521   **Infection of incontinent external stoma of urinary tract**   HCC

     N99.522   **Malfunction of incontinent external stoma of urinary tract**   HCC

     N99.523   **Herniation of incontinent stoma of urinary tract**   HCC

     N99.524   **Stenosis of incontinent stoma of urinary tract**   HCC

     N99.528   **Other complication of incontinent external stoma of urinary tract**   HCC

   ☑6th **N99.53**   **Complication of** continent stoma **of urinary tract**

     N99.530   **Hemorrhage of continent stoma of urinary tract**   HCC

     N99.531   **Infection of continent stoma of urinary tract**   HCC

     N99.532   **Malfunction of continent stoma of urinary tract**   HCC

     N99.533   **Herniation of continent stoma of urinary tract**   HCC

     N99.534   **Stenosis of continent stoma of urinary tract**   HCC

     N99.538   **Other complication of continent stoma of urinary tract**   HCC

☑5th **N99.6**   **Intraoperative hemorrhage and hematoma of a genitourinary system organ or structure complicating a procedure**

   EXCLUDES 1   intraoperative hemorrhage and hematoma of a genitourinary system organ or structure due to accidental puncture or laceration during a procedure (N99.7-)

   N99.61   **Intraoperative hemorrhage and hematoma of a genitourinary system organ or structure complicating a genitourinary system procedure**   CC

   N99.62   **Intraoperative hemorrhage and hematoma of a genitourinary system organ or structure complicating other procedure**   CC

☑5th **N99.7**   **Accidental puncture and laceration of a genitourinary system organ or structure during a procedure**

   N99.71   **Accidental puncture and laceration of a genitourinary system organ or structure during a genitourinary system procedure**   CC

     CC Excl: PDX collection 509

   N99.72   **Accidental puncture and laceration of a genitourinary system organ or structure during other procedure**   CC

     CC Excl: PDX collection 509

☑5th **N99.8**   **Other intraoperative and postprocedural complications and disorders of genitourinary system**

   AHA: 2016,4Q,9-10

   N99.81   **Other** intraoperative complications **of genitourinary system**

   ☑6th **N99.82**   **Postprocedural hemorrhage of a genitourinary system organ or structure following a procedure**

     N99.820   **Postprocedural hemorrhage of a genitourinary system organ or structure following a genitourinary system procedure**   CC

     N99.821   **Postprocedural hemorrhage of a genitourinary system organ or structure following other procedure**   CC

   N99.83   **Residual ovary syndrome**   ♀

☑ Additional Character Required   ☑x7th Placeholder   Unacceptable PDx   Questionable PDx   Manifestation   Unspecified Dx   H1-H14 HAC   HCC CMS-HCC Dx   HIV HIV Dx

ICD-10-CM 2020   871

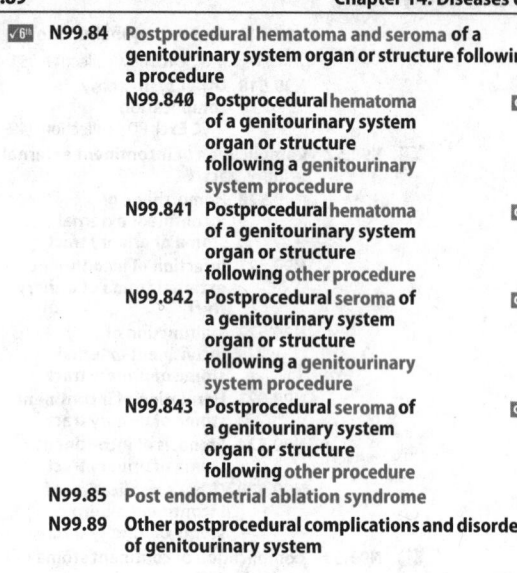

√6ᵗ   **N99.84**   **Postprocedural hematoma and seroma of a genitourinary system organ or structure following a procedure**

     N99.840   **Postprocedural hematoma of a genitourinary system organ or structure following a genitourinary system procedure**   `CC`

     N99.841   **Postprocedural hematoma of a genitourinary system organ or structure following other procedure**   `CC`

     N99.842   **Postprocedural seroma of a genitourinary system organ or structure following a genitourinary system procedure**   `CC`

     N99.843   **Postprocedural seroma of a genitourinary system organ or structure following other procedure**   `CC`

   N99.85   **Post endometrial ablation syndrome**

   N99.89   **Other postprocedural complications and disorders of genitourinary system**

N Newborn: 0   **P** Pediatric: 0-17   **M** Maternity: 9-64   **A** Adult: 15-124   **MCC** Major Complication/Comorbidity   **CC** Complication/Comorbidity   **SW** Severe Wound Dx

872

ICD-10-CM 2020

Chapter 15. Pregnancy, Childbirth and the Puerperium (O00–O9A)

Chapter-specific Guidelines with Coding Examples

The chapter-specific guidelines from the ICD-10-CM Official Guidelines for Coding and Reporting have been provided below. Along with these guidelines are coding examples, contained in the shaded boxes, that have been developed to help illustrate the coding and/or sequencing guidance found in these guidelines.

a. General rules for obstetric cases

1) Codes from Chapter 15 and sequencing priority

Obstetric cases require codes from chapter 15, codes in the range O00-O9A, Pregnancy, Childbirth, and the Puerperium. Chapter 15 codes have sequencing priority over codes from other chapters. Additional codes from other chapters may be used in conjunction with chapter 15 codes to further specify conditions. Should the provider document that the pregnancy is incidental to the encounter, then code Z33.1, Pregnant state, incidental, should be used in place of any chapter 15 codes. It is the provider's responsibility to state that the condition being treated is not affecting the pregnancy.

> Pregnant patient at 25 weeks' gestation admitted for bladder abscess
>
> **O23.12**   **Infections of bladder in pregnancy, second trimester**
>
> **N30.80**   **Other cystitis without hematuria**
>
> **Z3A.25**   **25 weeks gestation of pregnancy**
>
> *Explanation:* The documentation does not indicate that the pregnancy is incidental or in any way unaffected by the bladder abscess; therefore, an obstetrics code should be sequenced first. An additional code was provided to identify the specific bladder condition as this information is not called out specifically in the obstetrics code.

2) Chapter 15 codes used only on the maternal record

Chapter 15 codes are to be used only on the maternal record, never on the record of the newborn.

3) Final character for trimester

The majority of codes in Chapter 15 have a final character indicating the trimester of pregnancy. The timeframes for the trimesters are indicated at the beginning of the chapter. If trimester is not a component of a code, it is because the condition always occurs in a specific trimester, or the concept of trimester of pregnancy is not applicable. Certain codes have characters for only certain trimesters because the condition does not occur in all trimesters, but it may occur in more than just one.

Assignment of the final character for trimester should be based on the provider's documentation of the trimester (or number of weeks) for the current admission/encounter. This applies to the assignment of trimester for pre-existing conditions as well as those that develop during or are due to the pregnancy. The provider's documentation of the number of weeks may be used to assign the appropriate code identifying the trimester.

Whenever delivery occurs during the current admission, and there is an "in childbirth" option for the obstetric complication being coded, the "in childbirth" code should be assigned.

> Pregnant patient at 21 weeks' gestation admitted with excessive vomiting
>
> **O21.2**   **Late vomiting of pregnancy**
>
> **Z3A.21**   **21 weeks gestation of pregnancy**
>
> *Explanation:* Category O21 classifies vomiting in pregnancy. Although code selection is based on whether the vomiting is before or after 20 completed weeks, these codes are not further classified by trimester. If vomiting only in the second trimester was documented, the provider should be queried for the specific week of gestation, as this will affect code selection.

4) Selection of trimester for inpatient admissions that encompass more than one trimester

In instances when a patient is admitted to a hospital for complications of pregnancy during one trimester and remains in the hospital into a subsequent trimester, the trimester character for the antepartum complication code should be assigned on the basis of the trimester when the complication developed, not the trimester of the discharge. If the condition developed prior to the current admission/encounter or represents a pre-existing condition, the trimester character for the trimester at the time of the admission/encounter should be assigned.

> Patient admitted at 27 6/7 weeks' gestation for hemorrhaging from partial placenta previa; three days after admission at 28 1/7 weeks' gestation, she developed gestational hypertension
>
> **O44.32**   **Partial placenta previa with hemorrhage, second trimester**
>
> **O13.3**   **Gestational [pregnancy-induced] hypertension without significant proteinuria, third trimester**
>
> **Z3A.27**   **27 weeks gestation of pregnancy**
>
> *Explanation:* The patient presented with hemorrhaging from partial placenta previa while still in her 27th week, which falls within the second trimester. The gestational hypertension did not occur until three days after admission, putting the patient in her 28th week of pregnancy or what is considered to be the third trimester. The weeks of gestation captured by a code from category Z3A should represent only the gestational weeks upon admission.

5) Unspecified trimester

Each category that includes codes for trimester has a code for "unspecified trimester." The "unspecified trimester" code should rarely be used, such as when the documentation in the record is insufficient to determine the trimester and it is not possible to obtain clarification.

6) 7th character for fetus identification

Where applicable, a 7th character is to be assigned for certain categories (O31, O32, O33.3 - O33.6, O35, O36, O40, O41, O60.1, O60.2, O64, and O69) to identify the fetus for which the complication code applies.

Assign 7th character "0":

- For single gestations
- When the documentation in the record is insufficient to determine the fetus affected and it is not possible to obtain clarification.
- When it is not possible to clinically determine which fetus is affected.

> Maternal patient with twin gestations is seen after ultrasound identifies fetus B to be in breech presentation
>
> **O32.1XX2**   **Maternal care for breech presentation, fetus 2**
>
> *Explanation:* The documentation indicates that although there are two fetuses, only one fetus is determined to be in breech presentation. Whether fetus 2 or fetus B is used, the coder can assign the seventh character of 2 to identify the second fetus as the one in breech.

b. Selection of OB principal or first-listed diagnosis

1) Routine outpatient prenatal visits

For routine outpatient prenatal visits when no complications are present, a code from category Z34, Encounter for supervision of normal pregnancy, should be used as the first-listed diagnosis. These codes should not be used in conjunction with chapter 15 codes.

2) Supervision of high-risk pregnancy

Codes from category O09, Supervision of high-risk pregnancy, are intended for use only during the prenatal period. For complications during the labor or delivery episode as a result of a high-risk pregnancy, assign the applicable complication codes from Chapter 15. If there are no complications during the labor or delivery episode, assign code O80, Encounter for full-term uncomplicated delivery.

For routine prenatal outpatient visits for patients with high-risk pregnancies, a code from category O09, Supervision of high-risk pregnancy, should be used as the first-listed diagnosis. Secondary chapter 15 codes may be used in conjunction with these codes if appropriate.

> 36-year-old with history of preterm labor admitted in labor with second child at 39 weeks' gestation, delivered healthy baby without complications
>
> **O80**   **Encounter for full-term uncomplicated delivery**
>
> **Z3A.39**   **39 weeks gestation of pregnancy**
>
> **Z37.0**   **Single live birth**
>
> *Explanation:* Although this patient is over 35 and having her second child (elderly multigravida) and has a history of preterm labor with her first child, no codes from category O09.- should be appended. In the absence of any other complications noted during the encounter, code O80 is the most appropriate code to describe the principal diagnosis.

Chapter 15. Pregnancy, Childbirth and the Puerperium

3) Episodes when no delivery occurs

In episodes when no delivery occurs, the principal diagnosis should correspond to the principal complication of the pregnancy which necessitated the encounter. Should more than one complication exist, all of which are treated or monitored, any of the complication codes may be sequenced first.

4) When a delivery occurs

When an obstetric patient is admitted and delivers during that admission, the condition that prompted the admission should be sequenced as the principal diagnosis. If multiple conditions prompted the admission, sequence the one most related to the delivery as the principal diagnosis. A code for any complication of the delivery should be assigned as an additional diagnosis. In cases of cesarean delivery, if the patient was admitted with a condition that resulted in the performance of a cesarean procedure, that condition should be selected as the principal diagnosis. If the reason for the admission was unrelated to the condition resulting in the cesarean delivery, the condition related to the reason for the admission should be selected as the principal diagnosis.

> Maternal patient with diet-controlled gestational diabetes was admitted at 38 weeks' gestation in obstructed labor due to footling presentation; cesarean performed for the malpresentation
>
> | O64.8XX0 | Obstructed labor due to other malposition and malpresentation, not applicable or unspecified |
> |---|---|
> | O24.420 | Gestational diabetes mellitus in childbirth, diet controlled |
> | Z3A.38 | 38 weeks gestation of pregnancy |
> | Z37.0 | Single live birth |
>
> *Explanation:* The obstructed labor necessitated the cesarean procedure.

> At 39 weeks' gestation, a maternal patient presents with hemorrhage with coagulation defect; the next day the patient goes into labor and eventually delivers via cesarean section due to arrested active phase of labor
>
> | O46.003 | Antepartum hemorrhage with coagulation defect, unspecified, third trimester |
> |---|---|
> | O62.1 | Secondary uterine inertia |
> | Z3A.39 | 39 weeks gestation of pregnancy |
> | Z37.0 | Single live birth |
>
> *Explanation:* The patient was admitted because of the antepartum hemorrhage with coagulation defect. The arrested active phase, although the reason for the cesarean delivery, did not develop until later into the stay.

5) Outcome of delivery

A code from category Z37, Outcome of delivery, should be included on every maternal record when a delivery has occurred. These codes are not to be used on subsequent records or on the newborn record.

c. Pre-existing conditions versus conditions due to the pregnancy

Certain categories in Chapter 15 distinguish between conditions of the mother that existed prior to pregnancy (pre-existing) and those that are a direct result of pregnancy. When assigning codes from Chapter 15, it is important to assess if a condition was pre-existing prior to pregnancy or developed during or due to the pregnancy in order to assign the correct code.

Categories that do not distinguish between pre-existing and pregnancy-related conditions may be used for either. It is acceptable to use codes specifically for the puerperium with codes complicating pregnancy and childbirth if a condition arises postpartum during the delivery encounter.

d. Pre-existing hypertension in pregnancy

Category O10, Pre-existing hypertension complicating pregnancy, childbirth and the puerperium, includes codes for hypertensive heart and hypertensive chronic kidney disease. When assigning one of the O10 codes that includes hypertensive heart disease or hypertensive chronic kidney disease, it is necessary to add a secondary code from the appropriate hypertension category to specify the type of heart failure or chronic kidney disease.

See Section I.C.9. Hypertension.

e. Fetal conditions affecting the management of the mother

1) Codes from categories O35 and O36

Codes from categories O35, Maternal care for known or suspected fetal abnormality and damage, and O36, Maternal care for other fetal problems, are assigned only when the fetal condition is actually responsible for modifying the management of the mother, i.e., by requiring diagnostic studies, additional observation, special care, or termination of pregnancy. The fact that the fetal condition exists does not justify assigning a code from this series to the mother's record.

> A patient is seen in ED for spotting 15 weeks into her pregnancy; the doctors also suspect fetal hydrocephalus.
>
> | O26.852 | Spotting complicating pregnancy, second trimester |
> |---|---|
> | Z3A.15 | 15 weeks gestation of pregnancy |
>
> *Explanation:* Whether the fetal hydrocephalus was suspected or confirmed, an additional code is not warranted for this condition as the documentation does not indicate that this fetal condition is in any way altering the management of the mother or complicating her pregnancy.

2) In utero surgery

In cases when surgery is performed on the fetus, a diagnosis code from category O35, Maternal care for known or suspected fetal abnormality and damage, should be assigned identifying the fetal condition. Assign the appropriate procedure code for the procedure performed.

No code from Chapter 16, the perinatal codes, should be used on the mother's record to identify fetal conditions. Surgery performed in utero on a fetus is still to be coded as an obstetric encounter.

f. HIV infection in pregnancy, childbirth and the puerperium

During pregnancy, childbirth or the puerperium, a patient admitted because of an HIV-related illness should receive a principal diagnosis from subcategory O98.7-, Human immunodeficiency [HIV] disease complicating pregnancy, childbirth and the puerperium, followed by the code(s) for the HIV-related illness(es).

Patients with asymptomatic HIV infection status admitted during pregnancy, childbirth, or the puerperium should receive codes of O98.7- and Z21, Asymptomatic human immunodeficiency virus [HIV] infection status.

> A previously asymptomatic HIV patient who is 13 weeks pregnant is admitted with oral thrush.
>
> | O98.711 | Human immunodeficiency virus [HIV] disease complicating pregnancy, first trimester |
> |---|---|
> | B20 | Human immunodeficiency virus [HIV] disease |
> | B37.0 | Candidal stomatitis |
> | Z3A.13 | 13 weeks gestation of pregnancy |
>
> *Explanation:* Because oral thrush is an HIV-related condition, this patient is now considered to have HIV disease. An obstetrics code indicating that HIV is complicating the pregnancy is coded first, followed by B20 for HIV disease as well as a code for the oral thrush.

g. Diabetes mellitus in pregnancy

Diabetes mellitus is a significant complicating factor in pregnancy. Pregnant women who are diabetic should be assigned a code from category O24, Diabetes mellitus in pregnancy, childbirth, and the puerperium, first, followed by the appropriate diabetes code(s) (E08-E13) from Chapter 4.

h. Long term use of insulin and oral hypoglycemics

See section I.C.4.a.3 for information on the long term use of insulin and oral hypoglycemic.

i. Gestational (pregnancy induced) diabetes

Gestational (pregnancy induced) diabetes can occur during the second and third trimester of pregnancy in women who were not diabetic prior to pregnancy. Gestational diabetes can cause complications in the pregnancy similar to those of pre-existing diabetes mellitus. It also puts the woman at greater risk of developing diabetes after the pregnancy. Codes for gestational diabetes are in subcategory O24.4, Gestational diabetes mellitus. No other code from category O24, Diabetes mellitus in pregnancy, childbirth, and the puerperium, should be used with a code from O24.4.

The codes under subcategory O24.4 include diet controlled, insulin controlled, and controlled by oral hypoglycemic drugs. If a patient with gestational diabetes is treated with both diet and insulin, only the code for insulin-controlled is required. If a patient with gestational diabetes is treated with both diet and oral hypoglycemic medications, only the code for "controlled by oral hypoglycemic drugs" is required. Code Z79.4, Long-term (current) use of insulin or code Z79.84, Long-term (current) use of oral hypoglycemic drugs, should not be assigned with codes from subcategory O24.4.

An abnormal glucose tolerance in pregnancy is assigned a code from subcategory O99.81, Abnormal glucose complicating pregnancy, childbirth, and the puerperium.

> Patient at 39 weeks term pregnancy with gestational diabetes was admitted in labor and delivered a healthy newborn. Patient is on a diabetic diet with daily metformin.
>
> | O24.425 | Gestational diabetes mellitus in childbirth, controlled by oral hypoglycemic drugs |
> |---|---|
> | Z3A.39 | 39 weeks gestation of pregnancy |
> | Z37.0 | Single live birth |
>
> *Explanation:* When the patient is admitted for delivery and the patient's gestational diabetes is controlled by both diet and oral hypoglycemic medications, only the combination code in subcategory O24.4-Gestational diabetes mellitus, is reported. No code is added for diet controlled diabetes, and no Z code for long-term use of oral hypoglycemics is reported with the O24.4 combination codes.

j. Sepsis and septic shock complicating abortion, pregnancy, childbirth and the puerperium

When assigning a chapter 15 code for sepsis complicating abortion, pregnancy, childbirth, and the puerperium, a code for the specific type of infection should be assigned as an additional diagnosis. If severe sepsis is present, a code from subcategory R65.2, Severe sepsis, and code(s) for associated organ dysfunction(s) should also be assigned as additional diagnoses.

> Patient is seen several days after a miscarriage with sepsis; cultures return MSSA
>
> | O03.87 | Sepsis following complete or unspecified spontaneous abortion |
> |---|---|
> | B95.61 | Methicillin susceptible Staphylococcus aureus infection as the cause of diseases classified elsewhere |
>
> *Explanation:* The type of infection that caused this patient to become septic was methicillin susceptible *Staphylococcus aureus* (MSSA), which as a secondary code helps capture all aspects related to this patient's septic condition.

k. Puerperal sepsis

Code O85, Puerperal sepsis, should be assigned with a secondary code to identify the causal organism (e.g., for a bacterial infection, assign a code from category B95-B96, Bacterial infections in conditions classified elsewhere). A code from category A40, Streptococcal sepsis, or A41, Other sepsis, should not be used for puerperal sepsis. If applicable, use additional codes to identify severe sepsis (R65.2-) and any associated acute organ dysfunction.

l. Alcohol, tobacco *and drug* use during pregnancy, childbirth and the puerperium

1) Alcohol use during pregnancy, childbirth and the puerperium

Codes under subcategory O99.31, Alcohol use complicating pregnancy, childbirth, and the puerperium, should be assigned for any pregnancy case when a mother uses alcohol during the pregnancy or postpartum. A secondary code from category F10, Alcohol related disorders, should also be assigned to identify manifestations of the alcohol use.

2) Tobacco use during pregnancy, childbirth and the puerperium

Codes under subcategory O99.33, Smoking (tobacco) complicating pregnancy, childbirth, and the puerperium, should be assigned for any pregnancy case when a mother uses any type of tobacco product during the pregnancy or postpartum. A secondary code from category F17, Nicotine dependence, should also be assigned to identify the type of nicotine dependence.

3) Drug use during pregnancy, childbirth and the puerperium

Codes under subcategory O99.32, Drug use complicating pregnancy, childbirth, and the puerperium, should be assigned for any pregnancy case when a mother uses drugs during the pregnancy or postpartum. This can involve illegal drugs, or inappropriate use or abuse of prescription drugs. Secondary code(s) from categories F11-F16 and F18-F19 should also be assigned to identify manifestations of the drug use.

m. Poisoning, toxic effects, adverse effects and underdosing in a pregnant patient

A code from subcategory O9A.2, Injury, poisoning and certain other consequences of external causes complicating pregnancy, childbirth, and the puerperium, should be sequenced first, followed by the appropriate injury, poisoning, toxic effect, adverse effect or underdosing code, and then the additional code(s) that specifies the condition caused by the poisoning, toxic effect, adverse effect or underdosing.

See Section I.C.19. Adverse effects, poisoning, underdosing and toxic effects.

> Patient admitted with accidental carbon monoxide poisoning from a gas heating implement; the patient is 18 weeks' pregnant
>
> | O9A.212 | Injury, poisoning and certain other consequences of external causes complicating pregnancy, second trimester |
> |---|---|
> | T58.11XA | Toxic effect of carbon monoxide from utility gas, accidental (unintentional), initial encounter |
> | Z3A.18 | 18 weeks gestation of pregnancy |
>
> *Explanation:* Although the carbon monoxide poisoning is the reason the patient was admitted, a code from the obstetrics chapter must be sequenced first. Chapter 15 codes have sequencing priority over codes from other chapters.

n. Normal delivery, code O80

1) Encounter for full term uncomplicated delivery

Code O80 should be assigned when a woman is admitted for a full-term normal delivery and delivers a single, healthy infant without any complications antepartum, during the delivery, or postpartum during the delivery episode. Code O80 is always a principal diagnosis. It is not to be used if any other code from chapter 15 is needed to describe a current complication of the antenatal, delivery, or **postnatal** period. Additional codes from other chapters may be used with code O80 if they are not related to or are in any way complicating the pregnancy.

2) Uncomplicated delivery with resolved antepartum complication

Code O80 may be used if the patient had a complication at some point during the pregnancy, but the complication is not present at the time of the admission for delivery.

> Patient presents in labor at 39 weeks' gestation and delivers a healthy newborn; patient had abnormal glucose levels in her first trimester, which have since resolved
>
> | O80 | Encounter for full-term uncomplicated delivery |
> |---|---|
> | Z37.0 | Single live birth |
>
> *Explanation:* The abnormal glucose levels during the first trimester cannot be coded if they are not affecting the patient's current trimester. Without additional complications associated with the pregnancy, fetus, or mother, code O80 is appropriate.

3) Outcome of delivery for O80

Z37.0, Single live birth, is the only outcome of delivery code appropriate for use with O80.

o. The peripartum and postpartum periods

1) Peripartum and postpartum periods

The postpartum period begins immediately after delivery and continues for six weeks following delivery. The peripartum period is defined as the last month of pregnancy to five months postpartum.

2) Peripartum and postpartum complication

A postpartum complication is any complication occurring within the six-week period.

3) Pregnancy-related complications after 6 week period

Chapter 15 codes may also be used to describe pregnancy-related complications after the peripartum or postpartum period if the provider documents that a condition is pregnancy related.

Patient admitted for varicose veins. She had a baby boy three months ago; the varicose veins started to appear one month ago. The doctor attributes the patient's pregnancy as the cause of the varicose veins, which continue to be painful and bother the patient. She is seeking surgical relief.

O87.4   Varicose veins of the lower extremity in the puerperium

Explanation: Although the varicose veins occurred several months after the delivery of the newborn, the doctor attributed the varicose veins to pregnancy and therefore a code from chapter 15 is appropriate.

4) Admission for routine postpartum care following delivery outside hospital

When the mother delivers outside the hospital prior to admission and is admitted for routine postpartum care and no complications are noted, code Z39.0, Encounter for care and examination of mother immediately after delivery, should be assigned as the principal diagnosis.

5) Pregnancy associated cardiomyopathy

Pregnancy associated cardiomyopathy, code O90.3, is unique in that it may be diagnosed in the third trimester of pregnancy but may continue to progress months after delivery. For this reason, it is referred to as peripartum cardiomyopathy. Code O90.3 is only for use when the cardiomyopathy develops as a result of pregnancy in a woman who did not have pre-existing heart disease.

p. Code O94, Sequelae of complication of pregnancy, childbirth, and the puerperium

1) Code O94

Code O94, Sequelae of complication of pregnancy, childbirth, and the puerperium, is for use in those cases when an initial complication of a pregnancy develops a sequelae requiring care or treatment at a future date.

2) After the initial postpartum period

This code may be used at any time after the initial postpartum period.

3) Sequencing of code O94

This code, like all sequela codes, is to be sequenced following the code describing the sequelae of the complication.

q. Termination of pregnancy and spontaneous abortions

1) Abortion with liveborn fetus

When an attempted termination of pregnancy results in a liveborn fetus, assign code Z33.2, Encounter for elective termination of pregnancy and a code from category Z37, Outcome of Delivery.

2) Retained products of conception following an abortion

Subsequent encounters for retained products of conception following a spontaneous abortion or elective termination of pregnancy, without complications are assigned O03.4, Incomplete spontaneous, abortion without complication, or code O07.4, Failed attempted termination of pregnancy without complication. This advice is appropriate even when the patient was discharged previously with a discharge diagnosis of complete abortion. If the patient has a specific complication associated with the spontaneous abortion or elective termination of pregnancy in addition to retained products of conception, assign the appropriate complication **code (e.g., O03.-, O04.-, O07.-)** instead of code O03.4 or O07.4.

Patient was seen two days ago for complete spontaneous abortion but returns today for urinary tract infection (UTI) with ultrasound showing retained products of conception

O03.38   Urinary tract infection following incomplete spontaneous abortion

Explanation: Although the diagnosis from the patient's previous stay indicated that the patient had a complete abortion, it is now determined that there were actually retained products of conception (POC). An abortion with retained POC is considered incomplete and in this case resulted in the patient developing a UTI.

3) Complications leading to abortion

Codes from Chapter 15 may be used as additional codes to identify any documented complications of the pregnancy in conjunction with codes in categories in O04, O07 and O08.

r. Abuse in a pregnant patient

For suspected or confirmed cases of abuse of a pregnant patient, a code(s) from subcategories O9A.3, Physical abuse complicating pregnancy, childbirth, and the puerperium, O9A.4, Sexual abuse complicating pregnancy, childbirth, and the puerperium, and O9A.5, Psychological abuse complicating pregnancy, childbirth, and the puerperium, should be sequenced first, followed by the appropriate codes (if applicable) to identify any associated current injury due to physical abuse, sexual abuse, and the perpetrator of abuse.

See Section I.C.19. Adult and child abuse, neglect and other maltreatment.

Chapter 15. Pregnancy, Childbirth and the Puerperium (O00–O9A)

NOTE CODES FROM THIS CHAPTER ARE FOR USE ONLY ON MATERNAL RECORDS, NEVER ON NEWBORN RECORDS

Codes from this chapter are for use for conditions related to or aggravated by the pregnancy, childbirth, or by the puerperium (maternal causes or obstetric causes)

NOTE Trimesters are counted from the first day of the last menstrual period. They are defined as follows:

1st trimester- less than 14 weeks 0 days

2nd trimester- 14 weeks 0 days to less than 28 weeks 0 days

3rd trimester- 28 weeks 0 days until delivery

Use additional code from category Z3A, Weeks of gestation, to identify the specific week of the pregnancy, if known.

EXCLUDES 1 *supervision of normal pregnancy (Z34.-)*

EXCLUDES 2 *mental and behavioral disorders associated with the puerperium (F53.-)*
obstetrical tetanus (A34)
postpartum necrosis of pituitary gland (E23.0)
puerperal osteomalacia (M83.0)

AHA: 2016,1Q,3-5; 2014,3Q,17

This chapter contains the following blocks:

O00-O08   Pregnancy with abortive outcome
O09   Supervision of high risk pregnancy
O10-O16   Edema, proteinuria and hypertensive disorders in pregnancy, childbirth and the puerperium
O20-O29   Other maternal disorders predominantly related to pregnancy
O30-O48   Maternal care related to the fetus and amniotic cavity and possible delivery problems
O60-O77   Complications of labor and delivery
O80-O82   Encounter for delivery
O85-O92   Complications predominantly related to the puerperium
O94-O9A   Other obstetric conditions, not elsewhere classified

Pregnancy with abortive outcome (O00-O08)

EXCLUDES 1 *continuing pregnancy in multiple gestation after abortion of one fetus or more (O31.1-, O31.3-)*

TIP: Do not assign a code from category Z3A with codes in this code block.

√4ᵗʰ **O00 Ectopic pregnancy**

INCLUDES ruptured ectopic pregnancy

Use additional code from category O08 to identify any associated complication

AHA: 2016,4Q,48-50; 2014,3Q,17

DEF: Implantation of a fertilized egg outside the uterus, usually in the fallopian tube or abdomen that requires emergency treatment.

CC Excl: For CC codes in category O00: PDX collection 953

Ectopic Pregnancy

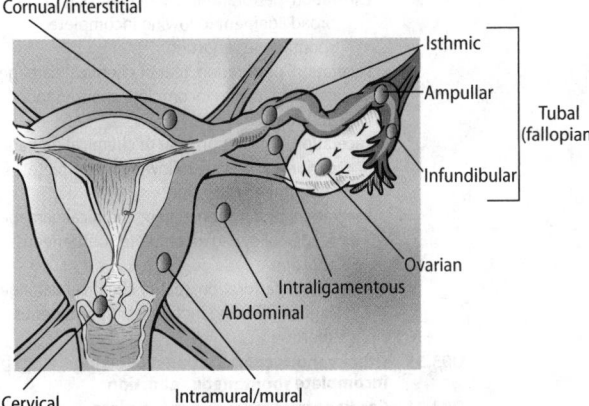

Cornual/interstitial
Isthmic
Ampullar
Tubal (fallopian)
Infundibular
Ovarian
Intraligamentous
Abdominal
Cervical
Intramural/mural

√5ᵗʰ **O00.0 Abdominal pregnancy**

EXCLUDES 1 *maternal care for viable fetus in abdominal pregnancy (O36.7-)*

O00.00 Abdominal pregnancy without intrauterine pregnancy   cc M ♀
Abdominal pregnancy NOS

O00.01 Abdominal pregnancy with intrauterine pregnancy   cc M ♀

√5ᵗʰ **O00.1 Tubal pregnancy**
Fallopian pregnancy
Rupture of (fallopian) tube due to pregnancy
Tubal abortion
AHA: 2017,4Q,20

√6ᵗʰ **O00.10 Tubal pregnancy without intrauterine pregnancy**
Tubal pregnancy NOS

O00.101 Right tubal pregnancy without intrauterine pregnancy   cc M ♀

O00.102 Left tubal pregnancy without intrauterine pregnancy   cc M ♀

O00.109 Unspecified tubal pregnancy without intrauterine pregnancy   cc M ♀

√6ᵗʰ **O00.11 Tubal pregnancy with intrauterine pregnancy**

O00.111 Right tubal pregnancy with intrauterine pregnancy   cc M ♀

O00.112 Left tubal pregnancy with intrauterine pregnancy   cc M ♀

O00.119 Unspecified tubal pregnancy with intrauterine pregnancy   cc M ♀

√5ᵗʰ **O00.2 Ovarian pregnancy**
AHA: 2017,4Q,20

√6ᵗʰ **O00.20 Ovarian pregnancy without intrauterine pregnancy**
Ovarian pregnancy NOS

O00.201 Right ovarian pregnancy without intrauterine pregnancy   cc M ♀

O00.202 Left ovarian pregnancy without intrauterine pregnancy   cc M ♀

O00.209 Unspecified ovarian pregnancy without intrauterine pregnancy   cc M ♀

√6ᵗʰ **O00.21 Ovarian pregnancy with intrauterine pregnancy**

O00.211 Right ovarian pregnancy with intrauterine pregnancy   cc M ♀

O00.212 Left ovarian pregnancy with intrauterine pregnancy   cc M ♀

O00.219 Unspecified ovarian pregnancy with intrauterine pregnancy   cc M ♀

√5ᵗʰ **O00.8 Other ectopic pregnancy**
Cervical pregnancy
Cornual pregnancy
Intraligamentous pregnancy
Mural pregnancy

O00.80 Other ectopic pregnancy without intrauterine pregnancy   cc M ♀
Other ectopic pregnancy NOS

O00.81 Other ectopic pregnancy with intrauterine pregnancy   cc M ♀

√5ᵗʰ **O00.9 Ectopic pregnancy, unspecified**

O00.90 Unspecified ectopic pregnancy without intrauterine pregnancy   cc M ♀
Ectopic pregnancy NOS

O00.91 Unspecified ectopic pregnancy with intrauterine pregnancy   cc M ♀

√4ᵗʰ **O01 Hydatidiform mole**

Use additional code from category O08 to identify any associated complication

EXCLUDES 1 *chorioadenoma (destruens) (D39.2)*
malignant hydatidiform mole (D39.2)

AHA: 2014,3Q,17

DEF: Abnormal product of pregnancy, marked by a mass of cysts resembling a bunch of grapes due to chorionic villi proliferation and dissolution. It must be surgically removed.

O01.0 Classical hydatidiform mole   M ♀
Complete hydatidiform mole

O01.1 Incomplete and partial hydatidiform mole   M ♀

O01.9 Hydatidiform mole, unspecified   M ♀
Trophoblastic disease NOS
Vesicular mole NOS

☑ Additional Character Required   √x7ᵗʰ Placeholder   Unacceptable PDx   Questionable PDx   Manifestation   Unspecified Dx   H1 - H14 HAC   HCC CMS-HCC Dx   HIV HIV Dx

ICD-10-CM 2020   **877**

☑4ᵗʰ **O02 Other abnormal products of conception**

Use additional code from category O08 to identify any associated complication

EXCLUDES 1   *papyraceous fetus (O31.0-)*

AHA: 2014,3Q,17

O02.0 Blighted ovum and nonhydatidiform mole   M ♀

Carneous mole
Fleshy mole
Intrauterine mole NOS
Molar pregnancy NEC
Pathological ovum

O02.1 Missed abortion   M ♀

Early fetal death, before completion of 20 weeks of gestation, with retention of dead fetus

EXCLUDES 1   *failed induced abortion (O07.-)*
fetal death (intrauterine) (late) (O36.4)
missed abortion with blighted ovum (O02.0)
missed abortion with hydatidiform mole (O01.-)
missed abortion with nonhydatidiform (O02.0)
missed abortion with other abnormal products of conception (O02.8-)
missed delivery (O36.4)
stillbirth (P95)

☑5ᵗʰ **O02.8 Other specified abnormal products of conception**

EXCLUDES 1   *abnormal products of conception with blighted ovum (O02.0)*
abnormal products of conception with hydatidiform mole (O01.-)
abnormal products of conception with nonhydatidiform mole (O02.0)

O02.81 Inappropriate change in quantitative human chorionic gonadotropin (hCG) in early pregnancy   M ♀

Biochemical pregnancy
Chemical pregnancy
Inappropriate level of quantitative human chorionic gonadotropin (hCG) for gestational age in early pregnancy

O02.89 Other abnormal products of conception   M ♀

O02.9 Abnormal product of conception, unspecified   M ♀

☑4ᵗʰ **O03 Spontaneous abortion**

NOTE   Incomplete abortion includes retained products of conception following spontaneous abortion

INCLUDES   miscarriage

CC Excl: For CC/MCC codes in category O03: PDX collection 954

O03.0 Genital tract and pelvic infection following incomplete spontaneous abortion   CC M ♀

Endometritis following incomplete spontaneous abortion
Oophoritis following incomplete spontaneous abortion
Parametritis following incomplete spontaneous abortion
Pelvic peritonitis following incomplete spontaneous abortion
Salpingitis following incomplete spontaneous abortion
Salpingo-oophoritis following incomplete spontaneous abortion

EXCLUDES 1   *sepsis following incomplete spontaneous abortion (O03.37)*
urinary tract infection following incomplete spontaneous abortion (O03.38)

O03.1 Delayed or excessive hemorrhage following incomplete spontaneous abortion   M ♀

Afibrinogenemia following incomplete spontaneous abortion
Defibrination syndrome following incomplete spontaneous abortion
Hemolysis following incomplete spontaneous abortion
Intravascular coagulation following incomplete spontaneous abortion

O03.2 Embolism following incomplete spontaneous abortion   MCC M ♀

Air embolism following incomplete spontaneous abortion
Amniotic fluid embolism following incomplete spontaneous abortion
Blood-clot embolism following incomplete spontaneous abortion
Embolism NOS following incomplete spontaneous abortion
Fat embolism following incomplete spontaneous abortion
Pulmonary embolism following incomplete spontaneous abortion
Pyemic embolism following incomplete spontaneous abortion
Septic or septicopyemic embolism following incomplete spontaneous abortion
Soap embolism following incomplete spontaneous abortion

☑5ᵗʰ **O03.3 Other and unspecified complications following incomplete spontaneous abortion**

O03.30 Unspecified complication following incomplete spontaneous abortion   CC M ♀

O03.31 Shock following incomplete spontaneous abortion   MCC M ♀

Circulatory collapse following incomplete spontaneous abortion
Shock (postprocedural) following incomplete spontaneous abortion

EXCLUDES 1   *shock due to infection following incomplete spontaneous abortion (O03.37)*

O03.32 Renal failure following incomplete spontaneous abortion   MCC M ♀

Kidney failure (acute) following incomplete spontaneous abortion
Oliguria following incomplete spontaneous abortion
Renal shutdown following incomplete spontaneous abortion
Renal tubular necrosis following incomplete spontaneous abortion
Uremia following incomplete spontaneous abortion

O03.33 Metabolic disorder following incomplete spontaneous abortion   CC M ♀

O03.34 Damage to pelvic organs following incomplete spontaneous abortion   CC M ♀

Laceration, perforation, tear or chemical damage of bladder following incomplete spontaneous abortion
Laceration, perforation, tear or chemical damage of bowel following incomplete spontaneous abortion
Laceration, perforation, tear or chemical damage of broad ligament following incomplete spontaneous abortion
Laceration, perforation, tear or chemical damage of cervix following incomplete spontaneous abortion
Laceration, perforation, tear or chemical damage of periurethral tissue following incomplete spontaneous abortion
Laceration, perforation, tear or chemical damage of uterus following incomplete spontaneous abortion
Laceration, perforation, tear or chemical damage of vagina following incomplete spontaneous abortion

O03.35 Other venous complications following incomplete spontaneous abortion   CC M ♀

O03.36 Cardiac arrest following incomplete spontaneous abortion   CC M ♀

O03.37 Sepsis following incomplete spontaneous abortion   CC M ♀

Use additional code to identify infectious agent (B95-B97)
Use additional code to identify severe sepsis, if applicable (R65.2-)

EXCLUDES 1   *septic or septicopyemic embolism following incomplete spontaneous abortion (O03.2)*

N Newborn: 0   P Pediatric: 0-17   M Maternity: 9-64   A Adult: 15-124   MCC Major Complication/Comorbidity   CC Complication/Comorbidity   SW Severe Wound Dx

878   ICD-10-CM 2020

O03.38 **Urinary tract infection following** **incomplete spontaneous abortion** `cc` `M` ♀
    Cystitis following incomplete spontaneous abortion

O03.39 **Incomplete spontaneous abortion with** **other complications** `cc` `M` ♀

O03.4 **Incomplete spontaneous abortion without** **complication** `M` ♀

O03.5 **Genital tract and pelvic infection following** **complete or unspecified spontaneous abortion** `cc` `M` ♀
    Endometritis following complete or unspecified spontaneous abortion
    Oophoritis following complete or unspecified spontaneous abortion
    Parametritis following complete or unspecified spontaneous abortion
    Pelvic peritonitis following complete or unspecified spontaneous abortion
    Salpingitis following complete or unspecified spontaneous abortion
    Salpingo-oophoritis following complete or unspecified spontaneous abortion

    EXCLUDES 1   *sepsis following complete or unspecified spontaneous abortion (O03.87)*
        urinary tract infection following complete or unspecified spontaneous abortion (O03.88)

O03.6 **Delayed or excessive hemorrhage following** **complete or unspecified spontaneous abortion** `M` ♀
    Afibrinogenemia following complete or unspecified spontaneous abortion
    Defibrination syndrome following complete or unspecified spontaneous abortion
    Hemolysis following complete or unspecified spontaneous abortion
    Intravascular coagulation following complete or unspecified spontaneous abortion

O03.7 **Embolism following complete or unspecified** **spontaneous abortion** `cc` `M` ♀
    Air embolism following complete or unspecified spontaneous abortion
    Amniotic fluid embolism following complete or unspecified spontaneous abortion
    Blood-clot embolism following complete or unspecified spontaneous abortion
    Embolism NOS following complete or unspecified spontaneous abortion
    Fat embolism following complete or unspecified spontaneous abortion
    Pulmonary embolism following complete or unspecified spontaneous abortion
    Pyemic embolism following complete or unspecified spontaneous abortion
    Septic or septicopyemic embolism following complete or unspecified spontaneous abortion
    Soap embolism following complete or unspecified spontaneous abortion

√5ᵗʰ **O03.8** **Other and unspecified complications following complete or** **unspecified spontaneous abortion**

    O03.80 **Unspecified complication following** **complete or unspecified spontaneous abortion** `cc` `M` ♀

    O03.81 **Shock following complete or unspecified** **spontaneous abortion** `mcc` `M` ♀
        Circulatory collapse following complete or unspecified spontaneous abortion
        Shock (postprocedural) following complete or unspecified spontaneous abortion
        EXCLUDES 1 *shock due to infection following complete or unspecified spontaneous abortion (O03.87)*

O03.82 **Renal failure following complete or** **unspecified spontaneous abortion** `mcc` `M` ♀
    Kidney failure (acute) following complete or unspecified spontaneous abortion
    Oliguria following complete or unspecified spontaneous abortion
    Renal shutdown following complete or unspecified spontaneous abortion
    Renal tubular necrosis following complete or unspecified spontaneous abortion
    Uremia following complete or unspecified spontaneous abortion

O03.83 **Metabolic disorder following complete** **or unspecified spontaneous abortion** `cc` `M` ♀

O03.84 **Damage to pelvic organs following** **complete or unspecified spontaneous abortion** `cc` `M` ♀
    Laceration, perforation, tear or chemical damage of bladder following complete or unspecified spontaneous abortion
    Laceration, perforation, tear or chemical damage of bowel following complete or unspecified spontaneous abortion
    Laceration, perforation, tear or chemical damage of broad ligament following complete or unspecified spontaneous abortion
    Laceration, perforation, tear or chemical damage of cervix following complete or unspecified spontaneous abortion
    Laceration, perforation, tear or chemical damage of periurethral tissue following complete or unspecified spontaneous abortion
    Laceration, perforation, tear or chemical damage of uterus following complete or unspecified spontaneous abortion
    Laceration, perforation, tear or chemical damage of vagina following complete or unspecified spontaneous abortion

O03.85 **Other venous complications following** **complete or unspecified spontaneous abortion** `cc` `M` ♀

O03.86 **Cardiac arrest following complete or** **unspecified spontaneous abortion** `cc` `M` ♀

O03.87 **Sepsis following complete or unspecified** **spontaneous abortion** `cc` `M` ♀
    Use additional code to identify infectious agent (B95-B97)
    Use additional code to identify severe sepsis, if applicable (R65.2-)
    EXCLUDES 1 *septic or septicopyemic embolism following complete or unspecified spontaneous abortion (O03.7)*

O03.88 **Urinary tract infection following** **complete or unspecified spontaneous abortion** `cc` `M` ♀
    Cystitis following complete or unspecified spontaneous abortion

O03.89 **Complete or unspecified spontaneous** **abortion with other complications** `cc` `M` ♀

O03.9 **Complete or unspecified spontaneous abortion** **without complication** `M` ♀
    Miscarriage NOS
    Spontaneous abortion NOS

✓4ᵗʰ O04 Complications following (induced) termination of pregnancy

INCLUDES   complications following (induced) termination of pregnancy

EXCLUDES 1   encounter for elective termination of pregnancy, uncomplicated (Z33.2)

failed attempted termination of pregnancy (O07.-)

CC Excl: For CC/MCC codes in category O04, unless otherwise noted: PDX collection 954

O04.5 Genital tract and pelvic infection following (induced) termination of pregnancy   CC M ♀

Endometritis following (induced) termination of pregnancy

Oophoritis following (induced) termination of pregnancy

Parametritis following (induced) termination of pregnancy

Pelvic peritonitis following (induced) termination of pregnancy

Salpingitis following (induced) termination of pregnancy

Salpingo-oophoritis following (induced) termination of pregnancy

EXCLUDES 1   sepsis following (induced) termination of pregnancy (O04.87)

urinary tract infection following (induced) termination of pregnancy (O04.88)

O04.6 Delayed or excessive hemorrhage following (induced) termination of pregnancy   M ♀

Afibrinogenemia following (induced) termination of pregnancy

Defibrination syndrome following (induced) termination of pregnancy

Hemolysis following (induced) termination of pregnancy

Intravascular coagulation following (induced) termination of pregnancy

O04.7 Embolism following (induced) termination of pregnancy   MCC M ♀

Air embolism following (induced) termination of pregnancy

Amniotic fluid embolism following (induced) termination of pregnancy

Blood-clot embolism following (induced) termination of pregnancy

Embolism NOS following (induced) termination of pregnancy

Fat embolism following (induced) termination of pregnancy

Pulmonary embolism following (induced) termination of pregnancy

Pyemic embolism following (induced) termination of pregnancy

Septic or septicopyemic embolism following (induced) termination of pregnancy

Soap embolism following (induced) termination of pregnancy

✓5ᵗʰ O04.8 (Induced) termination of pregnancy with other and unspecified complications

O04.80 (Induced) termination of pregnancy with unspecified complications   CC M ♀

O04.81 Shock following (induced) termination of pregnancy   MCC M ♀

Circulatory collapse following (induced) termination of pregnancy

Shock (postprocedural) following (induced) termination of pregnancy

EXCLUDES 1   shock due to infection following (induced) termination of pregnancy (O04.87)

O04.82 Renal failure following (induced) termination of pregnancy   MCC M ♀

Kidney failure (acute) following (induced) termination of pregnancy

Oliguria following (induced) termination of pregnancy

Renal shutdown following (induced) termination of pregnancy

Renal tubular necrosis following (induced) termination of pregnancy

Uremia following (induced) termination of pregnancy

O04.83 Metabolic disorder following (induced) termination of pregnancy   CC M ♀

O04.84 Damage to pelvic organs following (induced) termination of pregnancy   CC M ♀

Laceration, perforation, tear or chemical damage of bladder following (induced) termination of pregnancy

Laceration, perforation, tear or chemical damage of bowel following (induced) termination of pregnancy

Laceration, perforation, tear or chemical damage of broad ligament following (induced) termination of pregnancy

Laceration, perforation, tear or chemical damage of cervix following (induced) termination of pregnancy

Laceration, perforation, tear or chemical damage of periurethral tissue following (induced) termination of pregnancy

Laceration, perforation, tear or chemical damage of uterus following (induced) termination of pregnancy

Laceration, perforation, tear or chemical damage of vagina following (induced) termination of pregnancy

O04.85 Other venous complications following (induced) termination of pregnancy   CC M ♀

O04.86 Cardiac arrest following (induced) termination of pregnancy   CC M ♀

O04.87 Sepsis following (induced) termination of pregnancy   CC M ♀

Use additional code to identify infectious agent (B95-B97)

Use additional code to identify severe sepsis, if applicable (R65.2-)

EXCLUDES 1   septic or septicopyemic embolism following (induced) termination of pregnancy (O04.7)

CC Excl: PDX collection 955

O04.88 Urinary tract infection following (induced) termination of pregnancy   CC M ♀

Cystitis following (induced) termination of pregnancy

O04.89 (Induced) termination of pregnancy with other complications   CC M ♀

✓4ᵗʰ O07 Failed attempted termination of pregnancy

INCLUDES   failure of attempted induction of termination of pregnancy

incomplete elective abortion

EXCLUDES 1   incomplete spontaneous abortion (O03.0-)

O07.0 Genital tract and pelvic infection following failed attempted termination of pregnancy   CC M ♀

Endometritis following failed attempted termination of pregnancy

Oophoritis following failed attempted termination of pregnancy

Parametritis following failed attempted termination of pregnancy

Pelvic peritonitis following failed attempted termination of pregnancy

Salpingitis following failed attempted termination of pregnancy

Salpingo-oophoritis following failed attempted termination of pregnancy

EXCLUDES 1   sepsis following failed attempted termination of pregnancy (O07.37)

urinary tract infection following failed attempted termination of pregnancy (O07.38)

CC Excl: PDX collection 956

O07.1 Delayed or excessive hemorrhage following failed attempted termination of pregnancy   CC M ♀

Afibrinogenemia following failed attempted termination of pregnancy

Defibrination syndrome following failed attempted termination of pregnancy

Hemolysis following failed attempted termination of pregnancy

Intravascular coagulation following failed attempted termination of pregnancy

CC Excl: PDX collection 957

N Newborn: 0   P Pediatric: 0-17   M Maternity: 9-64   A Adult: 15-124   MCC Major Complication/Comorbidity   CC Complication/Comorbidity   SW Severe Wound Dx

O07.2 Embolism following failed attempted termination `MCC` `♀`
of pregnancy
  Air embolism following failed attempted termination of
    pregnancy
  Amniotic fluid embolism following failed attempted termination
    of pregnancy
  Blood-clot embolism following failed attempted termination
    of pregnancy
  Embolism NOS following failed attempted termination of
    pregnancy
  Fat embolism following failed attempted termination of
    pregnancy
  Pulmonary embolism following failed attempted termination
    of pregnancy
  Pyemic embolism following failed attempted termination of
    pregnancy
  Septic or septicopyemic embolism following failed attempted
    termination of pregnancy
  Soap embolism following failed attempted termination of
    pregnancy
  CC Excl: PDX collection 958

☑5ᵗʰ O07.3 Failed attempted termination of pregnancy with other and
unspecified complications
  CC Excl: For CC codes in subcategory O07.3, unless otherwise
  noted: PDX collection 954

  O07.30 Failed attempted termination of `cc` `M` `♀`
    pregnancy with unspecified
    complications

  O07.31 Shock following failed attempted `MCC` `M` `♀`
    termination of pregnancy
    Circulatory collapse following failed attempted
      termination of pregnancy
    Shock (postprocedural) following failed attempted
      termination of pregnancy
    EXCLUDES 1 shock due to infection following failed
        attempted termination of pregnancy
        (O07.37)
    CC Excl: PDX collection 959

  O07.32 Renal failure following failed attempted `MCC` `M` `♀`
    termination of pregnancy
    Kidney failure (acute) following failed attempted
      termination of pregnancy
    Oliguria following failed attempted termination of
      pregnancy
    Renal shutdown following failed attempted
      termination of pregnancy
    Renal tubular necrosis following failed attempted
      termination of pregnancy
    Uremia following failed attempted termination of
      pregnancy
    CC Excl: PDX collection 960

  O07.33 Metabolic disorder following failed `cc` `♀`
    attempted termination of pregnancy

  O07.34 Damage to pelvic organs following failed `cc` `M` `♀`
    attempted termination of pregnancy
    Laceration, perforation, tear or chemical damage of
      bladder following failed attempted termination
      of pregnancy
    Laceration, perforation, tear or chemical damage of
      bowel following failed attempted termination
      of pregnancy
    Laceration, perforation, tear or chemical damage of
      broad ligament following failed attempted
      termination of pregnancy
    Laceration, perforation, tear or chemical damage of
      cervix following failed attempted termination
      of pregnancy
    Laceration, perforation, tear or chemical damage of
      periurethral tissue following failed attempted
      termination of pregnancy
    Laceration, perforation, tear or chemical damage of
      uterus following failed attempted termination
      of pregnancy
    Laceration, perforation, tear or chemical damage of
      vagina following failed attempted termination
      of pregnancy
    CC Excl: PDX collection 961

  O07.35 Other venous complications following `cc` `M` `♀`
    failed attempted termination of
    pregnancy

O07.36 Cardiac arrest following failed attempted `cc` `M` `♀`
termination of pregnancy

O07.37 Sepsis following failed attempted `cc` `M` `♀`
termination of pregnancy
  Use additional code (B95-B97), to identify infectious
    agent
  Use additional code (R65.2-) to identify severe sepsis,
    if applicable
  EXCLUDES 1 septic or septicopyemic embolism
        following failed attempted
        termination of pregnancy (O07.2)
  CC Excl: PDX collection 956

O07.38 Urinary tract infection following failed `cc` `M` `♀`
attempted termination of pregnancy
  Cystitis following failed attempted termination of
    pregnancy

O07.39 Failed attempted termination of `cc` `M` `♀`
pregnancy with other complications

O07.4 Failed attempted termination of pregnancy `M` `♀`
without complication

☑4ᵗʰ O08 Complications following ectopic and molar pregnancy
  This category is for use with categories O00-O02 to identify any
    associated complications
  CC Excl: For CC/MCC codes in category O08, unless otherwise noted:
  PDX collection 963

O08.0 Genital tract and pelvic infection following ectopic `cc` `M` `♀`
and molar pregnancy
  Endometritis following ectopic and molar pregnancy
  Oophoritis following ectopic and molar pregnancy
  Parametritis following ectopic and molar pregnancy
  Pelvic peritonitis following ectopic and molar pregnancy
  Salpingitis following ectopic and molar pregnancy
  Salpingo-oophoritis following ectopic and molar pregnancy
  EXCLUDES 1 sepsis following ectopic and molar pregnancy
        (O08.82)
        urinary tract infection (O08.83)
  CC Excl: PDX collection 85

O08.1 Delayed or excessive hemorrhage following `cc` `M` `♀`
ectopic and molar pregnancy
  Afibrinogenemia following ectopic and molar pregnancy
  Defibrination syndrome following ectopic and molar pregnancy
  Hemolysis following ectopic and molar pregnancy
  Intravascular coagulation following ectopic and molar
    pregnancy
  EXCLUDES 1 delayed or excessive hemorrhage due to incomplete
        abortion (O03.1)
  CC Excl: PDX collection 962

O08.2 Embolism following ectopic and molar pregnancy `MCC` `M` `♀`
  Air embolism following ectopic and molar pregnancy
  Amniotic fluid embolism following ectopic and molar pregnancy
  Blood-clot embolism following ectopic and molar pregnancy
  Embolism NOS following ectopic and molar pregnancy
  Fat embolism following ectopic and molar pregnancy
  Pulmonary embolism following ectopic and molar pregnancy
  Pyemic embolism following ectopic and molar pregnancy
  Septic or septicopyemic embolism following ectopic and molar
    pregnancy
  Soap embolism following ectopic and molar pregnancy

O08.3 Shock following ectopic and molar pregnancy `MCC` `M` `♀`
  Circulatory collapse following ectopic and molar pregnancy
  Shock (postprocedural) following ectopic and molar pregnancy
  EXCLUDES 1 shock due to infection following ectopic and molar
        pregnancy (O08.82)

O08.4 Renal failure following ectopic and molar `MCC` `M` `♀`
pregnancy
  Kidney failure (acute) following ectopic and molar pregnancy
  Oliguria following ectopic and molar pregnancy
  Renal shutdown following ectopic and molar pregnancy
  Renal tubular necrosis following ectopic and molar pregnancy
  Uremia following ectopic and molar pregnancy

O08.5 Metabolic disorders following an ectopic and `cc` `M` `♀`
molar pregnancy

O08.6 **Damage to pelvic organs and tissues following an** ☐cc ☐M ♀
ectopic and molar pregnancy
    Laceration, perforation, tear or chemical damage of bladder
      following an ectopic and molar pregnancy
    Laceration, perforation, tear or chemical damage of bowel
      following an ectopic and molar pregnancy
    Laceration, perforation, tear or chemical damage of broad
      ligament following an ectopic and molar pregnancy
    Laceration, perforation, tear or chemical damage of cervix
      following an ectopic and molar pregnancy
    Laceration, perforation, tear or chemical damage of periurethral
      tissue following an ectopic and molar pregnancy
    Laceration, perforation, tear or chemical damage of uterus
      following an ectopic and molar pregnancy
    Laceration, perforation, tear or chemical damage of vagina
      following an ectopic and molar pregnancy

O08.7 **Other venous complications following an ectopic** ☐cc ☐M ♀
and molar pregnancy

√5ᵗʰ **O08.8** **Other complications following an ectopic and molar**
pregnancy

    O08.81 **Cardiac arrest following an ectopic and** ☐cc ☐M ♀
      molar pregnancy

    O08.82 **Sepsis following ectopic and molar** ☐cc ☐M ♀
      pregnancy
        Use additional code (B95-B97), to identify infectious
          agent
        Use additional code (R65.2-) to identify severe sepsis,
          if applicable
        EXCLUDES 1 *septic or septicopyemic embolism*
            following ectopic and molar
            pregnancy (O08.2)
        CC Excl: PDX collection 85

    O08.83 **Urinary tract infection following an** ☐cc ☐M ♀
      ectopic and molar pregnancy
        Cystitis following an ectopic and molar pregnancy

    O08.89 **Other complications following an ectopic** ☐cc ☐M ♀
      and molar pregnancy

O08.9 **Unspecified complication following an ectopic and** ☐cc ☐M ♀
molar pregnancy

Supervision of high risk pregnancy (O09)

√4ᵗʰ **O09** **Supervision of high risk pregnancy**
    AHA: 2016,4Q,48-50,150

√5ᵗʰ **O09.0** **Supervision of pregnancy with history of infertility**
    DEF: Infertility: Inability to conceive for at least one year with
      regular intercourse.

    O09.00 **Supervision of pregnancy with history of** ☐M ♀
      infertility, unspecified trimester

    O09.01 **Supervision of pregnancy with history of** ☐M ♀
      infertility, first trimester

    O09.02 **Supervision of pregnancy with history of** ☐M ♀
      infertility, second trimester

    O09.03 **Supervision of pregnancy with history of** ☐M ♀
      infertility, third trimester

√5ᵗʰ **O09.1** **Supervision of pregnancy with history of ectopic pregnancy**
    DEF: Ectopic pregnancy: Implantation of a fertilized egg outside
      the uterus, usually in the fallopian tube or abdomen that requires
      emergency treatment.

    O09.10 **Supervision of pregnancy with history of** ☐M ♀
      ectopic pregnancy, unspecified trimester

    O09.11 **Supervision of pregnancy with history of** ☐M ♀
      ectopic pregnancy, first trimester

    O09.12 **Supervision of pregnancy with history of** ☐M ♀
      ectopic pregnancy, second trimester

    O09.13 **Supervision of pregnancy with history of** ☐M ♀
      ectopic pregnancy, third trimester

√5ᵗʰ **O09.A** **Supervision of pregnancy with history of molar pregnancy**
    DEF: Molar pregnancy: Trophoblastic neoplasm that mimics
      pregnancy by proliferating from a pathologic ovum and resulting
      only in a mass of cysts resembling grapes, 80 percent of which
      are benign, but require surgical removal.

    O09.A0 **Supervision of pregnancy with history of** ☐M ♀
      molar pregnancy, unspecified trimester

    O09.A1 **Supervision of pregnancy with history of** ☐M ♀
      molar pregnancy, first trimester

    O09.A2 **Supervision of pregnancy with history of** ☐M ♀
      molar pregnancy, second trimester

    O09.A3 **Supervision of pregnancy with history of** ☐M ♀
      molar pregnancy, third trimester

√5ᵗʰ **O09.2** **Supervision of pregnancy with other poor reproductive or**
obstetric history
    EXCLUDES 2 *pregnancy care for patient with history of recurrent*
            pregnancy loss (O26.2-)

  √6ᵗʰ **O09.21** **Supervision of pregnancy with history of pre-term**
      labor

      O09.211 **Supervision of pregnancy with** ☐M ♀
        history of pre-term labor, first
        trimester

      O09.212 **Supervision of pregnancy with** ☐M ♀
        history of pre-term labor,
        second trimester

      O09.213 **Supervision of pregnancy with** ☐M ♀
        history of pre-term labor, third
        trimester

      O09.219 **Supervision of pregnancy with** ☐M ♀
        history of pre-term labor,
        unspecified trimester

  √6ᵗʰ **O09.29** **Supervision of pregnancy with other poor**
      reproductive or obstetric history
        Supervision of pregnancy with history of neonatal
          death
        Supervision of pregnancy with history of stillbirth

      O09.291 **Supervision of pregnancy with** ☐M ♀
        other poor reproductive or
        obstetric history, first trimester

      O09.292 **Supervision of pregnancy with** ☐M ♀
        other poor reproductive or
        obstetric history, second
        trimester

      O09.293 **Supervision of pregnancy with** ☐M ♀
        other poor reproductive or
        obstetric history, third
        trimester

      O09.299 **Supervision of pregnancy with** ☐M ♀
        other poor reproductive or
        obstetric history, unspecified
        trimester

√5ᵗʰ **O09.3** **Supervision of pregnancy with insufficient antenatal care**
    Supervision of concealed pregnancy
    Supervision of hidden pregnancy

    O09.30 **Supervision of pregnancy with** ☐M ♀
      insufficient antenatal care, unspecified
      trimester

    O09.31 **Supervision of pregnancy with** ☐M ♀
      insufficient antenatal care, first trimester

    O09.32 **Supervision of pregnancy with** ☐M ♀
      insufficient antenatal care, second
      trimester

    O09.33 **Supervision of pregnancy with** ☐M ♀
      insufficient antenatal care, third
      trimester

√5ᵗʰ **O09.4** **Supervision of pregnancy with grand multiparity**

    O09.40 **Supervision of pregnancy with grand** ☐M ♀
      multiparity, unspecified trimester

    O09.41 **Supervision of pregnancy with grand** ☐M ♀
      multiparity, first trimester

    O09.42 **Supervision of pregnancy with grand** ☐M ♀
      multiparity, second trimester

    O09.43 **Supervision of pregnancy with grand** ☐M ♀
      multiparity, third trimester

√5ᵗʰ **O09.5** **Supervision of elderly primigravida and multigravida**
    Pregnancy for a female 35 years and older at expected date of
      delivery

  √6ᵗʰ **O09.51** **Supervision of elderly primigravida**

      O09.511 **Supervision of elderly** ☐M ♀
        primigravida, first trimester

      O09.512 **Supervision of elderly** ☐M ♀
        primigravida, second trimester

      O09.513 **Supervision of elderly** ☐M ♀
        primigravida, third trimester

      O09.519 **Supervision of elderly** ☐M ♀
        primigravida, unspecified
        trimester

  √6ᵗʰ **O09.52** **Supervision of elderly multigravida**

      O09.521 **Supervision of elderly** ☐M ♀
        multigravida, first trimester

      O09.522 **Supervision of elderly** ☐M ♀
        multigravida, second trimester

      O09.523 **Supervision of elderly** ☐M ♀
        multigravida, third trimester

N Newborn: 0   **P** Pediatric: 0-17   **M** Maternity: 9-64   **A** Adult: 15-124   **MCC** Major Complication/Comorbidity   **CC** Complication/Comorbidity   **SW** Severe Wound Dx

882   ICD-10-CM 2020

O09.529 **Supervision of elderly multigravida, unspecified trimester** M ♀

√6th **O09.6 Supervision of young primigravida and multigravida**
Supervision of pregnancy for a female less than 16 years old at expected date of delivery

√6th **O09.61 Supervision of young primigravida**

O09.611 **Supervision of young primigravida, first trimester** M ♀

O09.612 **Supervision of young primigravida, second trimester** M ♀

O09.613 **Supervision of young primigravida, third trimester** M ♀

O09.619 **Supervision of young primigravida, unspecified trimester** M ♀

√6th **O09.62 Supervision of young multigravida**

O09.621 **Supervision of young multigravida, first trimester** M ♀

O09.622 **Supervision of young multigravida, second trimester** M ♀

O09.623 **Supervision of young multigravida, third trimester** M ♀

O09.629 **Supervision of young multigravida, unspecified trimester** M ♀

√5th **O09.7 Supervision of high risk pregnancy due to social problems**

O09.70 **Supervision of high risk pregnancy due to social problems, unspecified trimester** M ♀

O09.71 **Supervision of high risk pregnancy due to social problems, first trimester** M ♀

O09.72 **Supervision of high risk pregnancy due to social problems, second trimester** M ♀

O09.73 **Supervision of high risk pregnancy due to social problems, third trimester** M ♀

√5th **O09.8 Supervision of other high risk pregnancies**

√6th **O09.81 Supervision of pregnancy resulting from assisted reproductive technology**
Supervision of pregnancy resulting from in-vitro fertilization
EXCLUDES 2   gestational carrier status (Z33.3)

O09.811 **Supervision of pregnancy resulting from assisted reproductive technology, first trimester** M ♀

O09.812 **Supervision of pregnancy resulting from assisted reproductive technology, second trimester** M ♀

O09.813 **Supervision of pregnancy resulting from assisted reproductive technology, third trimester** M ♀

O09.819 **Supervision of pregnancy resulting from assisted reproductive technology, unspecified trimester** M ♀

√6th **O09.82 Supervision of pregnancy with history of in utero procedure during previous pregnancy**

O09.821 **Supervision of pregnancy with history of in utero procedure during previous pregnancy, first trimester** M ♀

O09.822 **Supervision of pregnancy with history of in utero procedure during previous pregnancy, second trimester** M ♀

O09.823 **Supervision of pregnancy with history of in utero procedure during previous pregnancy, third trimester** M ♀

O09.829 **Supervision of pregnancy with history of in utero procedure during previous pregnancy, unspecified trimester** M ♀
EXCLUDES 1   supervision of pregnancy affected by in utero procedure during current pregnancy (O35.7)

√6th **O09.89 Supervision of other high risk pregnancies**

O09.891 **Supervision of other high risk pregnancies, first trimester** M ♀

O09.892 **Supervision of other high risk pregnancies, second trimester** M ♀

O09.893 **Supervision of other high risk pregnancies, third trimester** M ♀

O09.899 **Supervision of other high risk pregnancies, unspecified trimester** M ♀

√5th **O09.9 Supervision of high risk pregnancy, unspecified**

O09.90 **Supervision of high risk pregnancy, unspecified, unspecified trimester** M ♀

O09.91 **Supervision of high risk pregnancy, unspecified, first trimester** M ♀

O09.92 **Supervision of high risk pregnancy, unspecified, second trimester** M ♀

O09.93 **Supervision of high risk pregnancy, unspecified, third trimester** M ♀

Edema, proteinuria and hypertensive disorders in pregnancy, childbirth and the puerperium (O10-O16)

AHA: 2016,4Q,50
CC Excl: For CC/MCC codes in categories O10-O16, unless otherwise noted: PDX collection 964

√4th **O10 Pre-existing hypertension complicating pregnancy, childbirth and the puerperium**
INCLUDES   pre-existing hypertension with pre-existing proteinuria complicating pregnancy, childbirth and the puerperium
EXCLUDES 2   pre-existing hypertension with superimposed pre-eclampsia complicating pregnancy, childbirth and the puerperium (O11.-)

√5th **O10.0 Pre-existing essential hypertension complicating pregnancy, childbirth and the puerperium**
Any condition in I10 specified as a reason for obstetric care during pregnancy, childbirth or the puerperium

√6th **O10.01 Pre-existing essential hypertension complicating pregnancy**

O10.011 **Pre-existing essential hypertension complicating pregnancy, first trimester** CC M ♀

O10.012 **Pre-existing essential hypertension complicating pregnancy, second trimester** CC M ♀

O10.013 **Pre-existing essential hypertension complicating pregnancy, third trimester** CC M ♀

O10.019 **Pre-existing essential hypertension complicating pregnancy, unspecified trimester** M ♀

O10.02 **Pre-existing essential hypertension complicating childbirth** CC M ♀

O10.03 **Pre-existing essential hypertension complicating the puerperium** M ♀

√5th **O10.1 Pre-existing hypertensive heart disease complicating pregnancy, childbirth and the puerperium**
Any condition in I11 specified as a reason for obstetric care during pregnancy, childbirth or the puerperium
Use additional code from I11 to identify the type of hypertensive heart disease

√6th **O10.11 Pre-existing hypertensive heart disease complicating pregnancy**

O10.111 **Pre-existing hypertensive heart disease complicating pregnancy, first trimester** M ♀

O10.112 **Pre-existing hypertensive heart disease complicating pregnancy, second trimester** M ♀

O10.113 **Pre-existing hypertensive heart disease complicating pregnancy, third trimester** M ♀

O10.119 **Pre-existing hypertensive heart disease complicating pregnancy, unspecified trimester** M ♀

O10.12 **Pre-existing hypertensive heart disease complicating childbirth** M ♀

O10.13 **Pre-existing hypertensive heart disease complicating the puerperium** M ♀

√5ᵗʰ **O1Ø.2** **Pre-existing hypertensive chronic kidney disease complicating pregnancy, childbirth and the puerperium**
Any condition in I12 specified as a reason for obstetric care during pregnancy, childbirth or the puerperium
Use additional code from I12 to identify the type of hypertensive chronic kidney disease

√6ᵗʰ **O1Ø.21** **Pre-existing hypertensive chronic kidney disease complicating pregnancy**

O1Ø.211 Pre-existing hypertensive chronic kidney disease complicating pregnancy, first trimester   M ♀

O1Ø.212 Pre-existing hypertensive chronic kidney disease complicating pregnancy, second trimester   M ♀

O1Ø.213 Pre-existing hypertensive chronic kidney disease complicating pregnancy, third trimester   M ♀

O1Ø.219 Pre-existing hypertensive chronic kidney disease complicating pregnancy, unspecified trimester   M ♀

O1Ø.22 **Pre-existing hypertensive chronic kidney disease complicating childbirth**   M ♀

O1Ø.23 **Pre-existing hypertensive chronic kidney disease complicating the puerperium**   M ♀

√5ᵗʰ **O1Ø.3** **Pre-existing hypertensive heart and chronic kidney disease complicating pregnancy, childbirth and the puerperium**
Any condition in I13 specified as a reason for obstetric care during pregnancy, childbirth or the puerperium
Use additional code from I13 to identify the type of hypertensive heart and chronic kidney disease

√6ᵗʰ **O1Ø.31** **Pre-existing hypertensive heart and chronic kidney disease complicating pregnancy**

O1Ø.311 Pre-existing hypertensive heart and chronic kidney disease complicating pregnancy, first trimester   M ♀

O1Ø.312 Pre-existing hypertensive heart and chronic kidney disease complicating pregnancy, second trimester   M ♀

O1Ø.313 Pre-existing hypertensive heart and chronic kidney disease complicating pregnancy, third trimester   M ♀

O1Ø.319 Pre-existing hypertensive heart and chronic kidney disease complicating pregnancy, unspecified trimester   M ♀

O1Ø.32 **Pre-existing hypertensive heart and chronic kidney disease complicating childbirth**   M ♀

O1Ø.33 **Pre-existing hypertensive heart and chronic kidney disease complicating the puerperium**   M ♀

√5ᵗʰ **O1Ø.4** **Pre-existing secondary hypertension complicating pregnancy, childbirth and the puerperium**
Any condition in I15 specified as a reason for obstetric care during pregnancy, childbirth or the puerperium
Use additional code from I15 to identify the type of secondary hypertension

√6ᵗʰ **O1Ø.41** **Pre-existing secondary hypertension complicating pregnancy**

O1Ø.411 Pre-existing secondary hypertension complicating pregnancy, first trimester   CC M ♀

O1Ø.412 Pre-existing secondary hypertension complicating pregnancy, second trimester   CC M ♀

O1Ø.413 Pre-existing secondary hypertension complicating pregnancy, third trimester   CC M ♀

O1Ø.419 Pre-existing secondary hypertension complicating pregnancy, unspecified trimester   M ♀

O1Ø.42 **Pre-existing secondary hypertension complicating childbirth**   MCC M ♀

O1Ø.43 **Pre-existing secondary hypertension complicating the puerperium**   CC M ♀

√5ᵗʰ **O1Ø.9** **Unspecified pre-existing hypertension complicating pregnancy, childbirth and the puerperium**

√6ᵗʰ **O1Ø.91** **Unspecified pre-existing hypertension complicating pregnancy**

O1Ø.911 Unspecified pre-existing hypertension complicating pregnancy, first trimester   CC M ♀

O1Ø.912 Unspecified pre-existing hypertension complicating pregnancy, second trimester   CC M ♀

O1Ø.913 Unspecified pre-existing hypertension complicating pregnancy, third trimester   CC M ♀

O1Ø.919 Unspecified pre-existing hypertension complicating pregnancy, unspecified trimester   M ♀

O1Ø.92 **Unspecified pre-existing hypertension complicating childbirth**   CC M ♀

O1Ø.93 **Unspecified pre-existing hypertension complicating the puerperium**   M ♀

√4ᵗʰ **O11** **Pre-existing hypertension with pre-eclampsia**
INCLUDES conditions in O1Ø complicated by pre-eclampsia
pre-eclampsia superimposed pre-existing in hypertension
Use additional code from O1Ø to identify the type of hypertension
DEF: Complication of pregnancy manifesting in the development of borderline hypertension, protein in the urine, and unresponsive swelling between the 20th week of pregnancy and the end of the first week following birth in mild to moderate cases. Severe preeclampsia presents with hypertension, associated with marked swelling, proteinuria, abdominal pain, and/or visual changes.

O11.1 **Pre-existing hypertension with pre-eclampsia, first trimester**   MCC M ♀

O11.2 **Pre-existing hypertension with pre-eclampsia, second trimester**   MCC M ♀

O11.3 **Pre-existing hypertension with pre-eclampsia, third trimester**   MCC M ♀

O11.4 **Pre-existing hypertension with pre-eclampsia, complicating childbirth**   M ♀

O11.5 **Pre-existing hypertension with pre-eclampsia, complicating the puerperium**   M ♀

O11.9 **Pre-existing hypertension with pre-eclampsia, unspecified trimester**   M ♀

√4ᵗʰ **O12** **Gestational [pregnancy-induced] edema and proteinuria without hypertension**
CC Excl: For CC codes in category O12: PDX collection 965

√5ᵗʰ **O12.Ø** **Gestational edema**

O12.ØØ Gestational edema, unspecified trimester   M ♀

O12.Ø1 Gestational edema, first trimester   M ♀

O12.Ø2 Gestational edema, second trimester   M ♀

O12.Ø3 Gestational edema, third trimester   M ♀

O12.Ø4 Gestational edema, complicating childbirth   M ♀

O12.Ø5 Gestational edema, complicating the puerperium   M ♀

√5ᵗʰ **O12.1** **Gestational proteinuria**

O12.1Ø Gestational proteinuria, unspecified trimester   M ♀

O12.11 Gestational proteinuria, first trimester   CC M ♀

O12.12 Gestational proteinuria, second trimester   CC M ♀

O12.13 Gestational proteinuria, third trimester   CC M ♀

O12.14 Gestational proteinuria, complicating childbirth   M ♀

O12.15 Gestational proteinuria, complicating the puerperium   M ♀

√5ᵗʰ **O12.2** **Gestational edema with proteinuria**

O12.2Ø Gestational edema with proteinuria, unspecified trimester   M ♀

O12.21 Gestational edema with proteinuria, first trimester   CC M ♀

O12.22 Gestational edema with proteinuria, second trimester   CC M ♀

O12.23 Gestational edema with proteinuria, third trimester   CC M ♀

O12.24 Gestational edema with proteinuria, complicating childbirth   M ♀

O12.25 Gestational edema with proteinuria, complicating the puerperium   M ♀

✓4ᵗʰ **O13** **Gestational [pregnancy-induced] hypertension without significant proteinuria**

INCLUDES　gestational hypertension NOS
transient hypertension of pregnancy
AHA: 2016,1Q,5

O13.1 **Gestational [pregnancy-induced] hypertension without significant proteinuria, first trimester**　M ♀

O13.2 **Gestational [pregnancy-induced] hypertension without significant proteinuria, second trimester**　M ♀

O13.3 **Gestational [pregnancy-induced] hypertension without significant proteinuria, third trimester**　M ♀

O13.4 **Gestational [pregnancy-induced] hypertension without significant proteinuria, complicating childbirth**

O13.5 **Gestational [pregnancy-induced] hypertension without significant proteinuria, complicating the puerperium**

O13.9 **Gestational [pregnancy-induced] hypertension without significant proteinuria, unspecified trimester**　M ♀

✓4ᵗʰ **O14** **Pre-eclampsia**

EXCLUDES 1　pre-existing hypertension with pre-eclampsia (O11)
DEF: Complication of pregnancy manifesting in the development of borderline hypertension, protein in the urine, and unresponsive swelling between the 20th week of pregnancy and the end of the first week following birth in mild to moderate cases. Severe preeclampsia presents with hypertension, associated with marked swelling, proteinuria, abdominal pain, and/or visual changes.

✓5ᵗʰ **O14.0** **Mild to moderate pre-eclampsia**

AHA: 2019,2Q,8

O14.00 **Mild to moderate pre-eclampsia, unspecified trimester**　M ♀

O14.02 **Mild to moderate pre-eclampsia, second trimester**　CC M ♀

O14.03 **Mild to moderate pre-eclampsia, third trimester**　CC M ♀

O14.04 **Mild to moderate pre-eclampsia, complicating childbirth**　M ♀

AHA: 2019,2Q,8

O14.05 **Mild to moderate pre-eclampsia, complicating the puerperium**　M ♀

✓5ᵗʰ **O14.1** **Severe pre-eclampsia**

EXCLUDES 1　HELLP syndrome (O14.2-)

O14.10 **Severe pre-eclampsia, unspecified trimester**　M ♀

O14.12 **Severe pre-eclampsia, second trimester**　MCC M ♀

O14.13 **Severe pre-eclampsia, third trimester**　MCC M ♀

O14.14 **Severe pre-eclampsia complicating childbirth**　M ♀

O14.15 **Severe pre-eclampsia, complicating the puerperium**　M ♀

✓5ᵗʰ **O14.2** **HELLP syndrome**

Severe pre-eclampsia with hemolysis, elevated liver enzymes and low platelet count (HELLP)

O14.20 **HELLP syndrome (HELLP), unspecified trimester**　M ♀

O14.22 **HELLP syndrome (HELLP), second trimester**　MCC M ♀

O14.23 **HELLP syndrome (HELLP), third trimester**　MCC M ♀

O14.24 **HELLP syndrome, complicating childbirth**　M ♀

O14.25 **HELLP syndrome, complicating the puerperium**　M ♀

✓5ᵗʰ **O14.9** **Unspecified pre-eclampsia**

O14.90 **Unspecified pre-eclampsia, unspecified trimester**　M ♀

O14.92 **Unspecified pre-eclampsia, second trimester**　CC M ♀

O14.93 **Unspecified pre-eclampsia, third trimester**　CC M ♀

O14.94 **Unspecified pre-eclampsia, complicating childbirth**　M ♀

O14.95 **Unspecified pre-eclampsia, complicating the puerperium**　M ♀

✓4ᵗʰ **O15** **Eclampsia**

INCLUDES　convulsions following conditions in O10-O14 and O16
DEF: Tetany and toxemia producing seizure activity or coma in a pregnant patient who most often has presented with prior preeclampsia (i.e., hypertension, albuminuria, and edema).

✓5ᵗʰ **O15.0** **Eclampsia complicating pregnancy**

O15.00 **Eclampsia complicating pregnancy, unspecified trimester**　M ♀

O15.02 **Eclampsia complicating pregnancy, second trimester**　MCC M ♀

O15.03 **Eclampsia complicating pregnancy, third trimester**　MCC M ♀

O15.1 **Eclampsia complicating labor**　MCC M ♀

O15.2 **Eclampsia complicating the puerperium**　MCC M ♀

O15.9 **Eclampsia, unspecified as to time period**　M ♀

Eclampsia NOS

✓4ᵗʰ **O16** **Unspecified maternal hypertension**

O16.1 **Unspecified maternal hypertension, first trimester**　CC M ♀

O16.2 **Unspecified maternal hypertension, second trimester**　CC M ♀

O16.3 **Unspecified maternal hypertension, third trimester**　CC M ♀

O16.4 **Unspecified maternal hypertension, complicating childbirth**　M ♀

O16.5 **Unspecified maternal hypertension, complicating the puerperium**　M ♀

O16.9 **Unspecified maternal hypertension, unspecified trimester**　M ♀

Other maternal disorders predominantly related to pregnancy (O20–O29)

EXCLUDES 2　maternal care related to the fetus and amniotic cavity and possible delivery problems (O30-O48)
maternal diseases classifiable elsewhere but complicating pregnancy, labor and delivery, and the puerperium (O98-O99)

✓4ᵗʰ **O20** **Hemorrhage in early pregnancy**

INCLUDES　hemorrhage before completion of 20 weeks gestation
EXCLUDES 1　pregnancy with abortive outcome (O00-O08)

O20.0 **Threatened abortion**　CC M ♀

Hemorrhage specified as due to threatened abortion
DEF: Bloody discharge during pregnancy. The cervix may be dilated and pregnancy threatened, but the pregnancy is not terminated.
CC Excl: PDX collection 966

O20.8 **Other hemorrhage in early pregnancy**　M ♀

O20.9 **Hemorrhage in early pregnancy, unspecified**　CC M ♀

CC Excl: PDX collection 966

✓4ᵗʰ **O21** **Excessive vomiting in pregnancy**

O21.0 **Mild hyperemesis gravidarum**　M ♀

Hyperemesis gravidarum, mild or unspecified, starting before the end of the 20th week of gestation

O21.1 **Hyperemesis gravidarum with metabolic disturbance**　M ♀

Hyperemesis gravidarum, starting before the end of the 20th week of gestation, with metabolic disturbance such as carbohydrate depletion
Hyperemesis gravidarum, starting before the end of the 20th week of gestation, with metabolic disturbance such as dehydration
Hyperemesis gravidarum, starting before the end of the 20th week of gestation, with metabolic disturbance such as electrolyte imbalance

O21.2 **Late vomiting of pregnancy**　M ♀

Excessive vomiting starting after 20 completed weeks of gestation

O21.8 **Other vomiting complicating pregnancy**　M ♀

Vomiting due to diseases classified elsewhere, complicating pregnancy
Use additional code, to identify cause

O21.9 **Vomiting of pregnancy, unspecified**　M ♀

Chapter 15. Pregnancy, Childbirth and the Puerperium

O22–O23.33

√4ᵗʰ **O22 Venous complications and hemorrhoids in pregnancy**

EXCLUDES 1   venous complications of:
- abortion NOS (O03.9)
- ectopic or molar pregnancy (O08.7)
- failed attempted abortion (O07.35)
- induced abortion (O04.85)
- spontaneous abortion (O03.89)

EXCLUDES 2   obstetric pulmonary embolism (O88.-)
venous complications and hemorrhoids of childbirth and the puerperium (O87.-)

CC Excl: For CC/MCC codes in category O22: PDX collection 967

√5ᵗʰ **O22.0 Varicose veins of lower extremity in pregnancy**

Varicose veins NOS in pregnancy
DEF: Distended, tortuous veins of the lower extremities associated with pregnancy.

O22.00 Varicose veins of lower extremity in pregnancy, unspecified trimester   M ♀

O22.01 Varicose veins of lower extremity in pregnancy, first trimester   M ♀

O22.02 Varicose veins of lower extremity in pregnancy, second trimester   M ♀

O22.03 Varicose veins of lower extremity in pregnancy, third trimester   M ♀

√5ᵗʰ **O22.1 Genital varices in pregnancy**

Perineal varices in pregnancy
Vaginal varices in pregnancy
Vulval varices in pregnancy

O22.10 Genital varices in pregnancy, unspecified trimester   M ♀

O22.11 Genital varices in pregnancy, first trimester   M ♀

O22.12 Genital varices in pregnancy, second trimester   M ♀

O22.13 Genital varices in pregnancy, third trimester   M ♀

√5ᵗʰ **O22.2 Superficial thrombophlebitis in pregnancy**

Phlebitis in pregnancy NOS
Thrombophlebitis of legs in pregnancy
Thrombosis in pregnancy NOS
Use additional code to identify the superficial thrombophlebitis (I80.0-)

O22.20 Superficial thrombophlebitis in pregnancy, unspecified trimester   CC M ♀

O22.21 Superficial thrombophlebitis in pregnancy, first trimester   CC M ♀

O22.22 Superficial thrombophlebitis in pregnancy, second trimester   CC M ♀

O22.23 Superficial thrombophlebitis in pregnancy, third trimester   CC M ♀

√5ᵗʰ **O22.3 Deep phlebothrombosis in pregnancy**

Deep vein thrombosis, antepartum
Use additional code to identify the deep vein thrombosis (I82.4-, I82.5-, I82.62-, I82.72-)
Use additional code, if applicable, for associated long-term (current) use of anticoagulants (Z79.01)

O22.30 Deep phlebothrombosis in pregnancy, unspecified trimester   CC M ♀

O22.31 Deep phlebothrombosis in pregnancy, first trimester   MCC M ♀

O22.32 Deep phlebothrombosis in pregnancy, second trimester   MCC M ♀

O22.33 Deep phlebothrombosis in pregnancy, third trimester   MCC M ♀

√5ᵗʰ **O22.4 Hemorrhoids in pregnancy**

O22.40 Hemorrhoids in pregnancy, unspecified trimester   CC M ♀

O22.41 Hemorrhoids in pregnancy, first trimester   CC M ♀

O22.42 Hemorrhoids in pregnancy, second trimester   CC M ♀

O22.43 Hemorrhoids in pregnancy, third trimester   CC M ♀

√5ᵗʰ **O22.5 Cerebral venous thrombosis in pregnancy**

Cerebrovenous sinus thrombosis in pregnancy

O22.50 Cerebral venous thrombosis in pregnancy, unspecified trimester   CC M ♀

O22.51 Cerebral venous thrombosis in pregnancy, first trimester   CC M ♀

O22.52 Cerebral venous thrombosis in pregnancy, second trimester   CC M ♀

O22.53 Cerebral venous thrombosis in pregnancy, third trimester   CC M ♀

√5ᵗʰ **O22.8 Other venous complications in pregnancy**

√6ᵗʰ **O22.8X Other venous complications in pregnancy**

O22.8X1 Other venous complications in pregnancy, first trimester   CC M ♀

O22.8X2 Other venous complications in pregnancy, second trimester   CC M ♀

O22.8X3 Other venous complications in pregnancy, third trimester   CC M ♀

O22.8X9 Other venous complications in pregnancy, unspecified trimester   CC M ♀

√5ᵗʰ **O22.9 Venous complication in pregnancy, unspecified**

Gestational phlebitis NOS
Gestational phlebopathy NOS
Gestational thrombosis NOS

O22.90 Venous complication in pregnancy, unspecified, unspecified trimester   CC M ♀

O22.91 Venous complication in pregnancy, unspecified, first trimester   M ♀

O22.92 Venous complication in pregnancy, unspecified, second trimester   M ♀

O22.93 Venous complication in pregnancy, unspecified, third trimester   M ♀

√4ᵗʰ **O23 Infections of genitourinary tract in pregnancy**

Use additional code to identify organism (B95.-, B96.-)

EXCLUDES 2   gonococcal infections complicating pregnancy, childbirth and the puerperium (O98.2)
infections with a predominantly sexual mode of transmission NOS complicating pregnancy, childbirth and the puerperium (O98.3)
syphilis complicating pregnancy, childbirth and the puerperium (O98.1)
tuberculosis of genitourinary system complicating pregnancy, childbirth and the puerperium (O98.0)
venereal disease NOS complicating pregnancy, childbirth and the puerperium (O98.3)

AHA: 2018,2Q,20

CC Excl: For CC codes in category O23: PDX collection 968

√5ᵗʰ **O23.0 Infections of kidney in pregnancy**

Pyelonephritis in pregnancy

O23.00 Infections of kidney in pregnancy, unspecified trimester   M ♀

O23.01 Infections of kidney in pregnancy, first trimester   CC M ♀

O23.02 Infections of kidney in pregnancy, second trimester   CC M ♀

O23.03 Infections of kidney in pregnancy, third trimester   CC M ♀

√5ᵗʰ **O23.1 Infections of bladder in pregnancy**

O23.10 Infections of bladder in pregnancy, unspecified trimester   M ♀

O23.11 Infections of bladder in pregnancy, first trimester   CC M ♀

O23.12 Infections of bladder in pregnancy, second trimester   CC M ♀

O23.13 Infections of bladder in pregnancy, third trimester   CC M ♀

√5ᵗʰ **O23.2 Infections of urethra in pregnancy**

O23.20 Infections of urethra in pregnancy, unspecified trimester   M ♀

O23.21 Infections of urethra in pregnancy, first trimester   CC M ♀

O23.22 Infections of urethra in pregnancy, second trimester   CC M ♀

O23.23 Infections of urethra in pregnancy, third trimester   CC M ♀

√5ᵗʰ **O23.3 Infections of other parts of urinary tract in pregnancy**

O23.30 Infections of other parts of urinary tract in pregnancy, unspecified trimester   M ♀

O23.31 Infections of other parts of urinary tract in pregnancy, first trimester   CC M ♀

O23.32 Infections of other parts of urinary tract in pregnancy, second trimester   CC M ♀

O23.33 Infections of other parts of urinary tract in pregnancy, third trimester   CC M ♀

N Newborn: 0   P Pediatric: 0-17   M Maternity: 9-64   A Adult: 15-124   MCC Major Complication/Comorbidity   CC Complication/Comorbidity   SW Severe Wound Dx

886   ICD-10-CM 2020

√5ᵗʰ **O23.4** **Unspecified infection of urinary tract in pregnancy**

     O23.40 **Unspecified infection of urinary tract in pregnancy, unspecified trimester**   M ♀

     O23.41 **Unspecified infection of urinary tract in pregnancy, first trimester**   CC M ♀

     O23.42 **Unspecified infection of urinary tract in pregnancy, second trimester**   CC M ♀

     O23.43 **Unspecified infection of urinary tract in pregnancy, third trimester**   CC M ♀

√5ᵗʰ **O23.5** **Infections of the genital tract in pregnancy**

     √6ᵗʰ **O23.51** **Infection of cervix in pregnancy**

         O23.511 **Infections of cervix in pregnancy, first trimester**   CC M ♀

         O23.512 **Infections of cervix in pregnancy, second trimester**   CC M ♀

         O23.513 **Infections of cervix in pregnancy, third trimester**   CC M ♀

         O23.519 **Infections of cervix in pregnancy, unspecified trimester**   M ♀

     √6ᵗʰ **O23.52** **Salpingo-oophoritis in pregnancy**

         Oophoritis in pregnancy
         Salpingitis in pregnancy

         O23.521 **Salpingo-oophoritis in pregnancy, first trimester**   CC M ♀

         O23.522 **Salpingo-oophoritis in pregnancy, second trimester**   CC M ♀

         O23.523 **Salpingo-oophoritis in pregnancy, third trimester**   CC M ♀

         O23.529 **Salpingo-oophoritis in pregnancy, unspecified trimester**   M ♀

     √6ᵗʰ **O23.59** **Infection of other part of genital tract in pregnancy**

         O23.591 **Infection of other part of genital tract in pregnancy, first trimester**   CC M ♀

         O23.592 **Infection of other part of genital tract in pregnancy, second trimester**   CC M ♀

         O23.593 **Infection of other part of genital tract in pregnancy, third trimester**   CC M ♀

         O23.599 **Infection of other part of genital tract in pregnancy, unspecified trimester**   M ♀

√5ᵗʰ **O23.9** **Unspecified genitourinary tract infection in pregnancy**

     Genitourinary tract infection in pregnancy NOS

     O23.90 **Unspecified genitourinary tract infection in pregnancy, unspecified trimester**   M ♀

     O23.91 **Unspecified genitourinary tract infection in pregnancy, first trimester**   CC M ♀

     O23.92 **Unspecified genitourinary tract infection in pregnancy, second trimester**   CC M ♀

     O23.93 **Unspecified genitourinary tract infection in pregnancy, third trimester**   CC M ♀

√4ᵗʰ **O24** **Diabetes mellitus in pregnancy, childbirth and the puerperium**

     CC Excl: For CC codes in category O24: PDX collection 969

     √5ᵗʰ **O24.0** **Pre-existing type 1 diabetes mellitus, in pregnancy, childbirth and the puerperium**

         Juvenile onset diabetes mellitus, in pregnancy, childbirth and the puerperium
         Ketosis-prone diabetes mellitus in pregnancy, childbirth and the puerperium
         Use additional code from category E10 to further identify any manifestations

         √6ᵗʰ **O24.01** **Pre-existing type 1 diabetes mellitus, in pregnancy**

             O24.011 **Pre-existing type 1 diabetes mellitus, in pregnancy, first trimester**   CC M ♀

             O24.012 **Pre-existing type 1 diabetes mellitus, in pregnancy, second trimester**   CC M ♀

             O24.013 **Pre-existing type 1 diabetes mellitus, in pregnancy, third trimester**   CC M ♀

             O24.019 **Pre-existing type 1 diabetes mellitus, in pregnancy, unspecified trimester**   CC M ♀

         O24.02 **Pre-existing type 1 diabetes mellitus, in childbirth**   CC M ♀

         O24.03 **Pre-existing type 1 diabetes mellitus, in the puerperium**   CC M ♀

     √5ᵗʰ **O24.1** **Pre-existing type 2 diabetes mellitus, in pregnancy, childbirth and the puerperium**

         Insulin-resistant diabetes mellitus in pregnancy, childbirth and the puerperium
         Use additional code (for):
         from category E11 to further identify any manifestations
         long-term (current) use of insulin (Z79.4)

         √6ᵗʰ **O24.11** **Pre-existing type 2 diabetes mellitus, in pregnancy**

             O24.111 **Pre-existing type 2 diabetes mellitus, in pregnancy, first trimester**   CC M ♀

             O24.112 **Pre-existing type 2 diabetes mellitus, in pregnancy, second trimester**   CC M ♀

             O24.113 **Pre-existing type 2 diabetes mellitus, in pregnancy, third trimester**   CC M ♀

             O24.119 **Pre-existing type 2 diabetes mellitus, in pregnancy, unspecified trimester**   CC M ♀

         O24.12 **Pre-existing type 2 diabetes mellitus, in childbirth**   CC M ♀

         O24.13 **Pre-existing type 2 diabetes mellitus, in the puerperium**   CC M ♀

     √5ᵗʰ **O24.3** **Unspecified pre-existing diabetes mellitus in pregnancy, childbirth and the puerperium**

         Use additional code (for):
         from category E11 to further identify any manifestation
         long-term (current) use of insulin (Z79.4)

         √6ᵗʰ **O24.31** **Unspecified pre-existing diabetes mellitus in pregnancy**

             O24.311 **Unspecified pre-existing diabetes mellitus in pregnancy, first trimester**   CC M ♀

             O24.312 **Unspecified pre-existing diabetes mellitus in pregnancy, second trimester**   CC M ♀

             O24.313 **Unspecified pre-existing diabetes mellitus in pregnancy, third trimester**   CC M ♀

             O24.319 **Unspecified pre-existing diabetes mellitus in pregnancy, unspecified trimester**   CC M ♀

         O24.32 **Unspecified pre-existing diabetes mellitus in childbirth**   CC M ♀

         O24.33 **Unspecified pre-existing diabetes mellitus in the puerperium**   CC M ♀

     √5ᵗʰ **O24.4** **Gestational diabetes mellitus**

         Diabetes mellitus arising in pregnancy
         Gestational diabetes mellitus NOS
         AHA: 2016,4Q,50; 2015,4Q,34

         √6ᵗʰ **O24.41** **Gestational diabetes mellitus in pregnancy**

             O24.410 **Gestational diabetes mellitus in pregnancy, diet controlled**   M ♀

             O24.414 **Gestational diabetes mellitus in pregnancy, insulin controlled**   CC M ♀

             O24.415 **Gestational diabetes mellitus in pregnancy, controlled by oral hypoglycemic drugs**   CC M ♀

                 Gestational diabetes mellitus in pregnancy, controlled by oral antidiabetic drugs

             O24.419 **Gestational diabetes mellitus in pregnancy, unspecified control**   M ♀

         √6ᵗʰ **O24.42** **Gestational diabetes mellitus in childbirth**

             AHA: 2016,1Q,5

             O24.420 **Gestational diabetes mellitus in childbirth, diet controlled**   M ♀

             O24.424 **Gestational diabetes mellitus in childbirth, insulin controlled**   CC M ♀

             O24.425 **Gestational diabetes mellitus in childbirth, controlled by oral hypoglycemic drugs**   CC M ♀

                 Gestational diabetes mellitus in childbirth, controlled by oral antidiabetic drugs

             O24.429 **Gestational diabetes mellitus in childbirth, unspecified control**   M ♀

✓ Additional Character Required   ✓7ᵗʰ Placeholder   Unacceptable PDx   Questionable PDx   Manifestation   Unspecified Dx   H1-H4 HAC   HCC CMS-HCC Dx   HIV HIV Dx

ICD-10-CM 2020   **887**

Chapter 15. Pregnancy, Childbirth and the Puerperium

O24.43–O26.712

√6th **O24.43**   Gestational diabetes mellitus in the **puerperium**

    O24.430   Gestational diabetes mellitus in the puerperium, **diet controlled**   M ♀

    O24.434   Gestational diabetes mellitus in the puerperium, **insulin controlled**   CC M ♀

    O24.435   Gestational diabetes mellitus in puerperium, **controlled by oral hypoglycemic drugs**   CC M ♀
       Gestational diabetes mellitus in puerperium, controlled by oral antidiabetic drugs

    O24.439   Gestational diabetes mellitus in the puerperium, unspecified control   M ♀

√5th **O24.8**   **Other pre-existing diabetes mellitus in pregnancy, childbirth, and the puerperium**
    Use additional code (for):
       from categories E08, E09 and E13 to further identify any manifestation
       long-term (current) use of insulin (Z79.4)

   √6th **O24.81**   Other pre-existing diabetes mellitus in **pregnancy**

    O24.811   Other pre-existing diabetes mellitus in pregnancy, **first trimester**   CC M ♀

    O24.812   Other pre-existing diabetes mellitus in pregnancy, **second trimester**   CC M ♀

    O24.813   Other pre-existing diabetes mellitus in pregnancy, **third trimester**   CC M ♀

    O24.819   Other pre-existing diabetes mellitus in pregnancy, **unspecified trimester**   CC M ♀

   O24.82   Other pre-existing diabetes mellitus in **childbirth**   CC M ♀

   O24.83   Other pre-existing diabetes mellitus in the **puerperium**   CC M ♀

√5th **O24.9**   **Unspecified diabetes mellitus in pregnancy, childbirth and the puerperium**
    Use additional code for long-term (current) use of insulin (Z79.4)

   √6th **O24.91**   Unspecified diabetes mellitus in **pregnancy**

    O24.911   Unspecified diabetes mellitus in pregnancy, **first trimester**   CC M ♀

    O24.912   Unspecified diabetes mellitus in pregnancy, **second trimester**   CC M ♀

    O24.913   Unspecified diabetes mellitus in pregnancy, **third trimester**   CC M ♀

    O24.919   Unspecified diabetes mellitus in pregnancy, **unspecified trimester**   CC M ♀

   O24.92   Unspecified diabetes mellitus in **childbirth**   CC M ♀

   O24.93   Unspecified diabetes mellitus in the **puerperium**   CC M ♀

√4th **O25**   **Malnutrition in pregnancy, childbirth and the puerperium**

   √5th **O25.1**   **Malnutrition in pregnancy**

    O25.10   Malnutrition in pregnancy, unspecified trimester   M ♀

    O25.11   Malnutrition in pregnancy, **first trimester**   M ♀

    O25.12   Malnutrition in pregnancy, **second trimester**   M ♀

    O25.13   Malnutrition in pregnancy, **third trimester**   M ♀

   O25.2   Malnutrition in **childbirth**   M ♀

   O25.3   Malnutrition in the **puerperium**   M ♀

√4th **O26**   **Maternal care for other conditions predominantly related to pregnancy**

   √5th **O26.0**   **Excessive weight gain in pregnancy**
     EXCLUDES 2   gestational edema (O12.0, O12.2)

    O26.00   Excessive weight gain in pregnancy, unspecified trimester   M ♀

    O26.01   Excessive weight gain in pregnancy, **first trimester**   M ♀

    O26.02   Excessive weight gain in pregnancy, **second trimester**   M ♀

    O26.03   Excessive weight gain in pregnancy, **third trimester**   M ♀

√5th **O26.1**   **Low weight gain in pregnancy**

    O26.10   Low weight gain in pregnancy, unspecified trimester   M ♀

    O26.11   Low weight gain in pregnancy, **first trimester**   M ♀

    O26.12   Low weight gain in pregnancy, **second trimester**   M ♀

    O26.13   Low weight gain in pregnancy, **third trimester**   M ♀

√5th **O26.2**   **Pregnancy care for patient with recurrent pregnancy loss**

    O26.20   Pregnancy care for patient with recurrent pregnancy loss, unspecified trimester   M ♀

    O26.21   Pregnancy care for patient with recurrent pregnancy loss, **first trimester**   M ♀

    O26.22   Pregnancy care for patient with recurrent pregnancy loss, **second trimester**   M ♀

    O26.23   Pregnancy care for patient with recurrent pregnancy loss, **third trimester**   M ♀

√5th **O26.3**   **Retained intrauterine contraceptive device in pregnancy**

    O26.30   Retained intrauterine contraceptive device in pregnancy, unspecified trimester   M ♀

    O26.31   Retained intrauterine contraceptive device in pregnancy, **first trimester**   M ♀

    O26.32   Retained intrauterine contraceptive device in pregnancy, **second trimester**   M ♀

    O26.33   Retained intrauterine contraceptive device in pregnancy, **third trimester**   M ♀

√5th **O26.4**   **Herpes gestationis**
    DEF: Rare skin disorder of unknown origin that appears on the abdomen in the second and third trimester as intensely itchy blisters that spread to other sites.

    O26.40   Herpes gestationis, unspecified trimester   M ♀

    O26.41   Herpes gestationis, **first trimester**   M ♀

    O26.42   Herpes gestationis, **second trimester**   M ♀

    O26.43   Herpes gestationis, **third trimester**   M ♀

√5th **O26.5**   **Maternal hypotension syndrome**
    Supine hypotensive syndrome

    O26.50   Maternal hypotension syndrome, unspecified trimester   M ♀

    O26.51   Maternal hypotension syndrome, **first trimester**   M ♀

    O26.52   Maternal hypotension syndrome, **second trimester**   M ♀

    O26.53   Maternal hypotension syndrome, **third trimester**   M ♀

√5th **O26.6**   **Liver and biliary tract disorders in pregnancy, childbirth and the puerperium**
    Use additional code to identify the specific disorder
     EXCLUDES 2   hepatorenal syndrome following labor and delivery (O90.4)

    CC Excl: For CC codes in subcategory O26.6: PDX collection 972

   √6th **O26.61**   Liver and biliary tract disorders in **pregnancy**

    O26.611   Liver and biliary tract disorders in pregnancy, **first trimester**   CC M ♀

    O26.612   Liver and biliary tract disorders in pregnancy, **second trimester**   CC M ♀

    O26.613   Liver and biliary tract disorders in pregnancy, **third trimester**   CC M ♀

    O26.619   Liver and biliary tract disorders in pregnancy, unspecified trimester   M ♀

   O26.62   Liver and biliary tract disorders in **childbirth**   CC M ♀

   O26.63   Liver and biliary tract disorders in the **puerperium**   M ♀

√5th **O26.7**   **Subluxation of symphysis (pubis) in pregnancy, childbirth and the puerperium**
     EXCLUDES 1   traumatic separation of symphysis (pubis) during childbirth (O71.6)

   √6th **O26.71**   Subluxation of symphysis (pubis) in **pregnancy**

    O26.711   Subluxation of symphysis (pubis) in pregnancy, **first trimester**   M ♀

    O26.712   Subluxation of symphysis (pubis) in pregnancy, **second trimester**   M ♀

N Newborn: 0   P Pediatric: 0-17   M Maternity: 9-64   A Adult: 15-124   MCC Major Complication/Comorbidity   CC Complication/Comorbidity   SW Severe Wound Dx

888   ICD-10-CM 2020

O26.713 Subluxation of symphysis (pubis) in pregnancy, **third trimester**   M ♀

O26.719 Subluxation of symphysis (pubis) in pregnancy, **unspecified trimester**   M ♀

O26.72 Subluxation of symphysis (pubis) in childbirth   M ♀

O26.73 Subluxation of symphysis (pubis) in the puerperium   M ♀

✓5ᵗʰ **O26.8** Other specified pregnancy related conditions

   ✓6ᵗʰ **O26.81** Pregnancy related exhaustion and fatigue

     O26.811 Pregnancy related exhaustion and fatigue, **first trimester**   M ♀

     O26.812 Pregnancy related exhaustion and fatigue, **second trimester**   M ♀

     O26.813 Pregnancy related exhaustion and fatigue, **third trimester**   M ♀

     O26.819 Pregnancy related exhaustion and fatigue, **unspecified trimester**   M ♀

   ✓6ᵗʰ **O26.82** Pregnancy related peripheral neuritis

     O26.821 Pregnancy related peripheral neuritis, **first trimester**   M ♀

     O26.822 Pregnancy related peripheral neuritis, **second trimester**   M ♀

     O26.823 Pregnancy related peripheral neuritis, **third trimester**   M ♀

     O26.829 Pregnancy related peripheral neuritis, **unspecified trimester**   M ♀

   ✓6ᵗʰ **O26.83** Pregnancy related renal disease

     Use additional code to identify the specific disorder

     CC Excl: For CC codes in subcategory O26.83: PDX collection 965

     O26.831 Pregnancy related renal disease, **first trimester**   cc M ♀

     O26.832 Pregnancy related renal disease, **second trimester**   cc M ♀

     O26.833 Pregnancy related renal disease, **third trimester**   cc M ♀

     O26.839 Pregnancy related renal disease, **unspecified trimester**   M ♀

   ✓6ᵗʰ **O26.84** Uterine size-date discrepancy complicating pregnancy

     EXCLUDES 1   encounter for suspected problem with fetal growth ruled out (Z03.74)

     O26.841 Uterine size-date discrepancy, **first trimester**   M ♀

     O26.842 Uterine size-date discrepancy, **second trimester**   M ♀

     O26.843 Uterine size-date discrepancy, **third trimester**   M ♀

     O26.849 Uterine size-date discrepancy, **unspecified trimester**   M ♀

   ✓6ᵗʰ **O26.85** Spotting complicating pregnancy

     O26.851 Spotting complicating pregnancy, **first trimester**   M ♀

     O26.852 Spotting complicating pregnancy, **second trimester**   M ♀

     O26.853 Spotting complicating pregnancy, **third trimester**   M ♀

     O26.859 Spotting complicating pregnancy, **unspecified trimester**   M ♀

   O26.86 Pruritic urticarial papules and plaques of pregnancy (PUPPP)   M ♀

     Polymorphic eruption of pregnancy

   ✓6ᵗʰ **O26.87** Cervical shortening

     EXCLUDES 1   encounter for suspected cervical shortening ruled out (Z03.75)

     DEF: Cervix that has shortened to less than 25 mm before the 24th week of pregnancy. A shortened cervix is a warning sign for impending premature delivery and is treated by cervical cerclage placement or progesterone.

     CC Excl: For CC codes in subcategory O26.87: PDX collection 973

     O26.872 Cervical shortening, **second trimester**   cc M ♀

     O26.873 Cervical shortening, **third trimester**   cc M ♀

     O26.879 Cervical shortening, **unspecified trimester**   cc M ♀

   ✓6ᵗʰ **O26.89** Other specified pregnancy related conditions

     AHA: 2015,3Q,40

     O26.891 Other specified pregnancy related conditions, **first trimester**   M ♀

     O26.892 Other specified pregnancy related conditions, **second trimester**   M ♀

     O26.893 Other specified pregnancy related conditions, **third trimester**   M ♀

     O26.899 Other specified pregnancy related conditions, **unspecified trimester**   M ♀

   ✓5ᵗʰ **O26.9** Pregnancy related conditions, unspecified

     O26.90 Pregnancy related conditions, unspecified, **unspecified trimester**   M ♀

     O26.91 Pregnancy related conditions, unspecified, **first trimester**   M ♀

     O26.92 Pregnancy related conditions, unspecified, **second trimester**   M ♀

     O26.93 Pregnancy related conditions, unspecified, **third trimester**   M ♀

✓4ᵗʰ **O28** Abnormal findings on antenatal screening of mother

   EXCLUDES 1   diagnostic findings classified elsewhere — see Alphabetical Index

   O28.0 Abnormal **hematological** finding on antenatal screening of mother   M ♀

   O28.1 Abnormal **biochemical** finding on antenatal screening of mother   M ♀

   O28.2 Abnormal **cytological** finding on antenatal screening of mother   M ♀

   O28.3 Abnormal **ultrasonic** finding on antenatal screening of mother   M ♀

   O28.4 Abnormal **radiological** finding on antenatal screening of mother   M ♀

   O28.5 Abnormal **chromosomal and genetic** finding on antenatal screening of mother   M ♀

   O28.8 Other abnormal findings on antenatal screening of mother   M ♀

   O28.9 Unspecified abnormal findings on antenatal screening of mother   M ♀

✓4ᵗʰ **O29** Complications of anesthesia during pregnancy

   INCLUDES   maternal complications arising from the administration of a general, regional or local anesthetic, analgesic or other sedation during pregnancy

   Use additional code, if necessary, to identify the complication

   EXCLUDES 2   complications of anesthesia during labor and delivery (O74.-)
       complications of anesthesia during the puerperium (O89.-)

   ✓5ᵗʰ **O29.0** Pulmonary complications of anesthesia during pregnancy

     ✓6ᵗʰ **O29.01** Aspiration pneumonitis due to anesthesia during pregnancy

       Inhalation of stomach contents or secretions NOS due to anesthesia during pregnancy

       Mendelson's syndrome due to anesthesia during pregnancy

       O29.011 Aspiration pneumonitis due to anesthesia during pregnancy, **first trimester**   M ♀

       O29.012 Aspiration pneumonitis due to anesthesia during pregnancy, **second trimester**   M ♀

       O29.013 Aspiration pneumonitis due to anesthesia during pregnancy, **third trimester**   M ♀

       O29.019 Aspiration pneumonitis due to anesthesia during pregnancy, **unspecified trimester**   M ♀

     ✓6ᵗʰ **O29.02** Pressure collapse of lung due to anesthesia during pregnancy

       O29.021 Pressure collapse of lung due to anesthesia during pregnancy, **first trimester**   M ♀

       O29.022 Pressure collapse of lung due to anesthesia during pregnancy, **second trimester**   M ♀

☑ Additional Character Required   ✓x7ᵗʰ Placeholder   Unacceptable PDx   Questionable PDx   Manifestation   Unspecified Dx   H1-H14 HAC   HCC CMS-HCC Dx   HIV HIV Dx

ICD-10-CM 2020   **889**

O29.023 Pressure collapse of lung due to anesthesia during pregnancy, third trimester M ♀

O29.029 Pressure collapse of lung due to anesthesia during pregnancy, unspecified trimester M ♀

✓6th **O29.09** Other pulmonary complications of anesthesia during pregnancy

O29.091 Other pulmonary complications of anesthesia during pregnancy, first trimester M ♀

O29.092 Other pulmonary complications of anesthesia during pregnancy, second trimester M ♀

O29.093 Other pulmonary complications of anesthesia during pregnancy, third trimester M ♀

O29.099 Other pulmonary complications of anesthesia during pregnancy, unspecified trimester M ♀

✓5th **O29.1** Cardiac complications of anesthesia during pregnancy

✓6th **O29.11** Cardiac arrest due to anesthesia during pregnancy

O29.111 Cardiac arrest due to anesthesia during pregnancy, first trimester M ♀

O29.112 Cardiac arrest due to anesthesia during pregnancy, second trimester M ♀

O29.113 Cardiac arrest due to anesthesia during pregnancy, third trimester M ♀

O29.119 Cardiac arrest due to anesthesia during pregnancy, unspecified trimester M ♀

✓6th **O29.12** Cardiac failure due to anesthesia during pregnancy

O29.121 Cardiac failure due to anesthesia during pregnancy, first trimester M ♀

O29.122 Cardiac failure due to anesthesia during pregnancy, second trimester M ♀

O29.123 Cardiac failure due to anesthesia during pregnancy, third trimester M ♀

O29.129 Cardiac failure due to anesthesia during pregnancy, unspecified trimester M ♀

✓6th **O29.19** Other cardiac complications of anesthesia during pregnancy

O29.191 Other cardiac complications of anesthesia during pregnancy, first trimester M ♀

O29.192 Other cardiac complications of anesthesia during pregnancy, second trimester M ♀

O29.193 Other cardiac complications of anesthesia during pregnancy, third trimester M ♀

O29.199 Other cardiac complications of anesthesia during pregnancy, unspecified trimester M ♀

✓5th **O29.2** Central nervous system complications of anesthesia during pregnancy

✓6th **O29.21** Cerebral anoxia due to anesthesia during pregnancy

O29.211 Cerebral anoxia due to anesthesia during pregnancy, first trimester M ♀

O29.212 Cerebral anoxia due to anesthesia during pregnancy, second trimester M ♀

O29.213 Cerebral anoxia due to anesthesia during pregnancy, third trimester M ♀

O29.219 Cerebral anoxia due to anesthesia during pregnancy, unspecified trimester M ♀

✓6th **O29.29** Other central nervous system complications of anesthesia during pregnancy

O29.291 Other central nervous system complications of anesthesia during pregnancy, first trimester M ♀

O29.292 Other central nervous system complications of anesthesia during pregnancy, second trimester M ♀

O29.293 Other central nervous system complications of anesthesia during pregnancy, third trimester M ♀

O29.299 Other central nervous system complications of anesthesia during pregnancy, unspecified trimester M ♀

✓5th **O29.3** Toxic reaction to local anesthesia during pregnancy

✓6th **O29.3X** Toxic reaction to local anesthesia during pregnancy

O29.3X1 Toxic reaction to local anesthesia during pregnancy, first trimester M ♀

O29.3X2 Toxic reaction to local anesthesia during pregnancy, second trimester M ♀

O29.3X3 Toxic reaction to local anesthesia during pregnancy, third trimester M ♀

O29.3X9 Toxic reaction to local anesthesia during pregnancy, unspecified trimester M ♀

✓5th **O29.4** Spinal and epidural anesthesia induced headache during pregnancy

O29.40 Spinal and epidural anesthesia induced headache during pregnancy, unspecified trimester M ♀

O29.41 Spinal and epidural anesthesia induced headache during pregnancy, first trimester M ♀

O29.42 Spinal and epidural anesthesia induced headache during pregnancy, second trimester M ♀

O29.43 Spinal and epidural anesthesia induced headache during pregnancy, third trimester M ♀

✓5th **O29.5** Other complications of spinal and epidural anesthesia during pregnancy

✓6th **O29.5X** Other complications of spinal and epidural anesthesia during pregnancy

O29.5X1 Other complications of spinal and epidural anesthesia during pregnancy, first trimester M ♀

O29.5X2 Other complications of spinal and epidural anesthesia during pregnancy, second trimester M ♀

O29.5X3 Other complications of spinal and epidural anesthesia during pregnancy, third trimester M ♀

O29.5X9 Other complications of spinal and epidural anesthesia during pregnancy, unspecified trimester M ♀

✓5th **O29.6** Failed or difficult intubation for anesthesia during pregnancy

O29.60 Failed or difficult intubation for anesthesia during pregnancy, unspecified trimester M ♀

O29.61 Failed or difficult intubation for anesthesia during pregnancy, first trimester M ♀

O29.62 Failed or difficult intubation for anesthesia during pregnancy, second trimester M ♀

O29.63 Failed or difficult intubation for anesthesia during pregnancy, third trimester M ♀

✓5th **O29.8** Other complications of anesthesia during pregnancy

✓6th **O29.8X** Other complications of anesthesia during pregnancy

O29.8X1 Other complications of anesthesia during pregnancy, first trimester M ♀

      O29.8X2 **Other complications of**   Ⓜ♀
anesthesia during pregnancy, **second trimester**

      O29.8X3 **Other complications of**   Ⓜ♀
anesthesia during pregnancy, **third trimester**

      O29.8X9 **Other complications of**   Ⓜ♀
anesthesia during pregnancy, **unspecified trimester**

✓⁵ᵗʰ **O29.9 Unspecified complication of anesthesia during pregnancy**

    O29.90 **Unspecified complication of anesthesia** Ⓜ♀
during pregnancy, **unspecified trimester**

    O29.91 **Unspecified complication of anesthesia** Ⓜ♀
during pregnancy, **first trimester**

    O29.92 **Unspecified complication of anesthesia** Ⓜ♀
during pregnancy, **second trimester**

    O29.93 **Unspecified complication of anesthesia** Ⓜ♀
during pregnancy, **third trimester**

Maternal care related to the fetus and amniotic cavity and possible delivery problems (O30-O48)

✓⁴ᵗʰ **O30 Multiple gestation**

Code also any complications specific to multiple gestation
AHA: 2016,4Q,51
CC Excl: For CC codes in category O30: PDX collection 976

✓⁵ᵗʰ **O30.0 Twin pregnancy**

  ✓⁶ᵗʰ **O30.00** **Twin pregnancy, unspecified number of placenta and unspecified number of amniotic sacs**

      O30.001 **Twin pregnancy, unspecified** Ⓜ♀
number of placenta and unspecified number of amniotic sacs, **first trimester**

      O30.002 **Twin pregnancy, unspecified** Ⓜ♀
number of placenta and unspecified number of amniotic sacs, **second trimester**

      O30.003 **Twin pregnancy, unspecified** Ⓜ♀
number of placenta and unspecified number of amniotic sacs, **third trimester**

      O30.009 **Twin pregnancy, unspecified** Ⓜ♀
number of placenta and unspecified number of amniotic sacs, **unspecified trimester**

  ✓⁶ᵗʰ **O30.01** **Twin pregnancy, monochorionic/monoamniotic**

Twin pregnancy, one placenta, one amniotic sac
EXCLUDES 1 conjoined twins (O30.02-)

Twin Gestation – Monochorionic/Monoamniotic

- 1 Chorionic sac
- 1 Amniotic sac
- 2 Fetuses
- 2 Umbilical cords
- 1 Placenta

    O30.011 **Twin pregnancy,** Ⓜ♀
monochorionic/monoamniotic, **first trimester**

    O30.012 **Twin pregnancy,** Ⓜ♀
monochorionic/monoamniotic, **second trimester**

    O30.013 **Twin pregnancy,** Ⓜ♀
monochorionic/monoamniotic, **third trimester**

    O30.019 **Twin pregnancy,** Ⓜ♀
monochorionic/monoamniotic, **unspecified trimester**

  ✓⁶ᵗʰ **O30.02** **Conjoined twin pregnancy**

    O30.021 **Conjoined twin pregnancy,** Ⓜ♀
first trimester

    O30.022 **Conjoined twin pregnancy,** Ⓜ♀
second trimester

    O30.023 **Conjoined twin pregnancy,** CC Ⓜ♀
third trimester

    O30.029 **Conjoined twin pregnancy,** Ⓜ♀
unspecified trimester

  ✓⁶ᵗʰ **O30.03** **Twin pregnancy, monochorionic/diamniotic**

Twin pregnancy, one placenta, two amniotic sacs

Twin Gestation – Monochorionic/Diamniotic

- 1 Chorionic sac
- 2 Amniotic sacs
- 2 Fetuses
- 2 Umbilical cords
- 1 Placenta

    O30.031 **Twin pregnancy,** Ⓜ♀
monochorionic/diamniotic, **first trimester**

    O30.032 **Twin pregnancy,** Ⓜ♀
monochorionic/diamniotic, **second trimester**

    O30.033 **Twin pregnancy,** Ⓜ♀
monochorionic/diamniotic, **third trimester**

    O30.039 **Twin pregnancy,** Ⓜ♀
monochorionic/diamniotic, **unspecified trimester**

  ✓⁶ᵗʰ **O30.04** **Twin pregnancy, dichorionic/diamniotic**

Twin pregnancy, two placentae, two amniotic sacs

Twin Gestation – Dichorionic/Diamniotic

- 2 Chorionic sacs
- 2 Amniotic sacs
- 2 Fetuses
- 2 Umbilical cords
- 2 Placentas

    O30.041 **Twin pregnancy,** Ⓜ♀
dichorionic/diamniotic, **first trimester**

    O30.042 **Twin pregnancy,** Ⓝ♀
dichorionic/diamniotic, **second trimester**

    O30.043 **Twin pregnancy,** Ⓜ♀
dichorionic/diamniotic, **third trimester**

    O30.049 **Twin pregnancy,** Ⓜ♀
dichorionic/diamniotic, **unspecified trimester**

Chapter 15. Pregnancy, Childbirth and the Puerperium

O30.09–O30.239

√6ᵗʰ **O30.09** Twin pregnancy, unable to determine number of placenta and number of amniotic sacs

    O30.091 Twin pregnancy, unable to determine number of placenta and number of amniotic sacs, first trimester   M ♀

    O30.092 Twin pregnancy, unable to determine number of placenta and number of amniotic sacs, second trimester   M ♀

    O30.093 Twin pregnancy, unable to determine number of placenta and number of amniotic sacs, third trimester   M ♀

    O30.099 Twin pregnancy, unable to determine number of placenta and number of amniotic sacs, unspecified trimester   M ♀

√5ᵗʰ **O30.1** Triplet pregnancy

  √6ᵗʰ **O30.10** Triplet pregnancy, unspecified number of placenta and unspecified number of amniotic sacs

    AHA: 2016,2Q,8

    O30.101 Triplet pregnancy, unspecified number of placenta and unspecified number of amniotic sacs, first trimester   CC M ♀

    O30.102 Triplet pregnancy, unspecified number of placenta and unspecified number of amniotic sacs, second trimester   CC M ♀

    O30.103 Triplet pregnancy, unspecified number of placenta and unspecified number of amniotic sacs, third trimester   CC M ♀

    O30.109 Triplet pregnancy, unspecified number of placenta and unspecified number of amniotic sacs, unspecified trimester   M ♀

  √6ᵗʰ **O30.11** Triplet pregnancy with two or more monochorionic fetuses

    O30.111 Triplet pregnancy with two or more monochorionic fetuses, first trimester   CC M ♀

    O30.112 Triplet pregnancy with two or more monochorionic fetuses, second trimester   CC M ♀

    O30.113 Triplet pregnancy with two or more monochorionic fetuses, third trimester   CC M ♀

    O30.119 Triplet pregnancy with two or more monochorionic fetuses, unspecified trimester   M ♀

  √6ᵗʰ **O30.12** Triplet pregnancy with two or more monoamniotic fetuses

    O30.121 Triplet pregnancy with two or more monoamniotic fetuses, first trimester   CC M ♀

    O30.122 Triplet pregnancy with two or more monoamniotic fetuses, second trimester   CC M ♀

    O30.123 Triplet pregnancy with two or more monoamniotic fetuses, third trimester   CC M ♀

    O30.129 Triplet pregnancy with two or more monoamniotic fetuses, unspecified trimester   M ♀

  √6ᵗʰ **O30.13** Triplet pregnancy, trichorionic/triamniotic

    AHA: 2018,4Q,22

    O30.131 Triplet pregnancy, trichorionic/triamniotic, first trimester   CC M ♀

    O30.132 Triplet pregnancy, trichorionic/triamniotic, second trimester   CC M ♀

    O30.133 Triplet pregnancy, trichorionic/triamniotic, third trimester   CC M ♀

    O30.139 Triplet pregnancy, trichorionic/triamniotic, unspecified trimester   M ♀

√6ᵗʰ **O30.19** Triplet pregnancy, unable to determine number of placenta and number of amniotic sacs

    O30.191 Triplet pregnancy, unable to determine number of placenta and number of amniotic sacs, first trimester   CC M ♀

    O30.192 Triplet pregnancy, unable to determine number of placenta and number of amniotic sacs, second trimester   CC M ♀

    O30.193 Triplet pregnancy, unable to determine number of placenta and number of amniotic sacs, third trimester   CC M ♀

    O30.199 Triplet pregnancy, unable to determine number of placenta and number of amniotic sacs, unspecified trimester   M ♀

√5ᵗʰ **O30.2** Quadruplet pregnancy

  √6ᵗʰ **O30.20** Quadruplet pregnancy, unspecified number of placenta and unspecified number of amniotic sacs

    O30.201 Quadruplet pregnancy, unspecified number of placenta and unspecified number of amniotic sacs, first trimester   CC M ♀

    O30.202 Quadruplet pregnancy, unspecified number of placenta and unspecified number of amniotic sacs, second trimester   CC M ♀

    O30.203 Quadruplet pregnancy, unspecified number of placenta and unspecified number of amniotic sacs, third trimester   CC M ♀

    O30.209 Quadruplet pregnancy, unspecified number of placenta and unspecified number of amniotic sacs, unspecified trimester   M ♀

  √6ᵗʰ **O30.21** Quadruplet pregnancy with two or more monochorionic fetuses

    O30.211 Quadruplet pregnancy with two or more monochorionic fetuses, first trimester   CC M ♀

    O30.212 Quadruplet pregnancy with two or more monochorionic fetuses, second trimester   CC M ♀

    O30.213 Quadruplet pregnancy with two or more monochorionic fetuses, third trimester   CC M ♀

    O30.219 Quadruplet pregnancy with two or more monochorionic fetuses, unspecified trimester   M ♀

  √6ᵗʰ **O30.22** Quadruplet pregnancy with two or more monoamniotic fetuses

    O30.221 Quadruplet pregnancy with two or more monoamniotic fetuses, first trimester   CC M ♀

    O30.222 Quadruplet pregnancy with two or more monoamniotic fetuses, second trimester   CC M ♀

    O30.223 Quadruplet pregnancy with two or more monoamniotic fetuses, third trimester   CC M ♀

    O30.229 Quadruplet pregnancy with two or more monoamniotic fetuses, unspecified trimester   M ♀

  √6ᵗʰ **O30.23** Quadruplet pregnancy, quadrachorionic/quadra-amniotic

    AHA: 2018,4Q,22

    O30.231 Quadruplet pregnancy, quadrachorionic/quadra-amniotic, first trimester   CC M ♀

    O30.232 Quadruplet pregnancy, quadrachorionic/quadra-amniotic, second trimester   CC M ♀

    O30.233 Quadruplet pregnancy, quadrachorionic/quadra-amniotic, third trimester   CC M ♀

    O30.239 Quadruplet pregnancy, quadrachorionic/quadra-amniotic, unspecified trimester   M ♀

N Newborn: 0   P Pediatric: 0-17   M Maternity: 9-64   A Adult: 15-124   MCC Major Complication/Comorbidity   CC Complication/Comorbidity   SW Severe Wound Dx

892   ICD-10-CM 2020

✓6ᵗʰ **O30.29 Quadruplet pregnancy,** unable to determine number of placenta and number of amniotic sacs

     O30.291 Quadruplet pregnancy, unable **cc M ♀**
         to determine number of
         placenta and number of
         amniotic sacs, first trimester

     O30.292 Quadruplet pregnancy, unable **cc M ♀**
         to determine number of
         placenta and number of
         amniotic sacs, second trimester

     O30.293 Quadruplet pregnancy, unable **cc M ♀**
         to determine number of
         placenta and number of
         amniotic sacs, third trimester

     O30.299 Quadruplet pregnancy, unable **M ♀**
         to determine number of
         placenta and number of
         amniotic sacs, unspecified
         trimester

✓5ᵗʰ **O30.8 Other specified multiple gestation**

     Multiple gestation pregnancy greater then quadruplets

✓6ᵗʰ **O30.80 Other specified multiple gestation, unspecified number of placenta and unspecified number of amniotic sacs**

     O30.801 Other specified multiple **cc M ♀**
         gestation, unspecified number
         of placenta and unspecified
         number of amniotic sacs, first
         trimester

     O30.802 Other specified multiple **cc M ♀**
         gestation, unspecified number
         of placenta and unspecified
         number of amniotic sacs,
         second trimester

     O30.803 Other specified multiple **cc M ♀**
         gestation, unspecified number
         of placenta and unspecified
         number of amniotic sacs, third
         trimester

     O30.809 Other specified multiple **M ♀**
         gestation, unspecified number
         of placenta and unspecified
         number of amniotic sacs,
         unspecified trimester

✓6ᵗʰ **O30.81 Other specified multiple gestation with** two or more monochorionic fetuses

     O30.811 Other specified multiple **cc ♀**
         gestation with two or more
         monochorionic fetuses, first
         trimester

     O30.812 Other specified multiple **cc ♀**
         gestation with two or more
         monochorionic fetuses, second
         trimester

     O30.813 Other specified multiple **cc ♀**
         gestation with two or more
         monochorionic fetuses, third
         trimester

     O30.819 Other specified multiple **M ♀**
         gestation with two or more
         monochorionic fetuses,
         unspecified trimester

✓6ᵗʰ **O30.82 Other specified multiple gestation with** two or more monoamniotic fetuses

     O30.821 Other specified multiple **cc ♀**
         gestation with two or more
         monoamniotic fetuses, first
         trimester

     O30.822 Other specified multiple **cc ♀**
         gestation with two or more
         monoamniotic fetuses, second
         trimester

     O30.823 Other specified multiple **cc ♀**
         gestation with two or more
         monoamniotic fetuses, third
         trimester

     O30.829 Other specified multiple **M ♀**
         gestation with two or more
         monoamniotic fetuses,
         unspecified trimester

✓6ᵗʰ **O30.83 Other specified multiple gestation,** number of chorions and amnions are both equal to the number of fetuses

     Pentachorionic, penta-amniotic pregnancy (quintuplets)
     Hexachorionic, hexa-amniotic pregnancy (sextuplets)
     Heptachorionic, hepta-amniotic pregnancy (septuplets)
     AHA: 2018,4Q,22

     O30.831 Other specified multiple **cc M ♀**
         gestation, number of chorions
         and amnions are both equal to
         the number of fetuses, first
         trimester

     O30.832 Other specified multiple **cc M ♀**
         gestation, number of chorions
         and amnions are both equal to
         the number of fetuses, second
         trimester

     O30.833 Other specified multiple **cc M ♀**
         gestation, number of chorions
         and amnions are both equal to
         the number of fetuses, third
         trimester

     O30.839 Other specified multiple **M ♀**
         gestation, number of chorions
         and amnions are both equal to
         the number of fetuses,
         unspecified trimester

✓6ᵗʰ **O30.89 Other specified multiple gestation,** unable to determine number of placenta and number of amniotic sacs

     O30.891 Other specified multiple **cc M ♀**
         gestation, unable to determine
         number of placenta and
         number of amniotic sacs, first
         trimester

     O30.892 Other specified multiple **cc M ♀**
         gestation, unable to determine
         number of placenta and
         number of amniotic sacs,
         second trimester

     O30.893 Other specified multiple **cc M ♀**
         gestation, unable to determine
         number of placenta and
         number of amniotic sacs, third
         trimester

     O30.899 Other specified multiple **M ♀**
         gestation, unable to determine
         number of placenta and
         number of amniotic sacs,
         unspecified trimester

✓5ᵗʰ **O30.9 Multiple gestation, unspecified**

     Multiple pregnancy NOS

     O30.90 Multiple gestation, unspecified, **M ♀**
         unspecified trimester

     O30.91 Multiple gestation, unspecified, first **M ♀**
         trimester

     O30.92 Multiple gestation, unspecified, second **M ♀**
         trimester

     O30.93 Multiple gestation, unspecified, third **M ♀**
         trimester

☑ Additional Character Required   ✓x7ᵗʰ Placeholder   Unacceptable PDx   Questionable PDx   Manifestation   Unspecified Dx   H1-H14 HAC   HCC CMS-HCC Dx   HIV HIV Dx

ICD-10-CM 2020   893

✓4ᵗʰ O31 Complications specific to multiple gestation

> EXCLUDES 2   delayed delivery of second twin, triplet, etc. (O63.2)
> malpresentation of one fetus or more (O32.9)
> placental transfusion syndromes (O43.0-)

AHA: 2012,4Q,107

> One of the following 7th characters is to be assigned to each code under category O31. 7th character Ø is for single gestations and multiple gestations where the fetus is unspecified. 7th characters 1 through 9 are for cases of multiple gestations to identify the fetus for which the code applies. The appropriate code from category O3Ø, Multiple gestation, must also be assigned when assigning a code from category O31 that has a 7th character of 1 through 9.
> Ø   not applicable or unspecified
> 1   fetus 1
> 2   fetus 2
> 3   fetus 3
> 4   fetus 4
> 5   fetus 5
> 9   other fetus

✓5ᵗʰ O31.Ø Papyraceous fetus

Fetus compressus

DEF: Fetus that has died, but remains in utero for weeks before delivery, becoming compacted and mummified in appearance, with skin resembling parchment. Occurs most commonly in multigestational pregnancies. *Synonym(s):* paper doll fetus.

✓7ᵗʰ **O31.ØØ** Papyraceous fetus, unspecified trimester   M ♀
✓7ᵗʰ **O31.Ø1** Papyraceous fetus, first trimester   M ♀
✓7ᵗʰ **O31.Ø2** Papyraceous fetus, second trimester   M ♀
✓7ᵗʰ **O31.Ø3** Papyraceous fetus, third trimester   M ♀

✓5ᵗʰ O31.1 Continuing pregnancy after spontaneous abortion of one fetus or more

✓7ᵗʰ **O31.1Ø** Continuing pregnancy after spontaneous abortion of one fetus or more, unspecified trimester   M ♀
✓7ᵗʰ **O31.11** Continuing pregnancy after spontaneous abortion of one fetus or more, first trimester   M ♀
✓7ᵗʰ **O31.12** Continuing pregnancy after spontaneous abortion of one fetus or more, second trimester   M ♀
✓7ᵗʰ **O31.13** Continuing pregnancy after spontaneous abortion of one fetus or more, third trimester   M ♀

✓5ᵗʰ O31.2 Continuing pregnancy after intrauterine death of one fetus or more

✓7ᵗʰ **O31.2Ø** Continuing pregnancy after intrauterine death of one fetus or more, unspecified trimester   M ♀
✓7ᵗʰ **O31.21** Continuing pregnancy after intrauterine death of one fetus or more, first trimester   M ♀
✓7ᵗʰ **O31.22** Continuing pregnancy after intrauterine death of one fetus or more, second trimester   M ♀
✓7ᵗʰ **O31.23** Continuing pregnancy after intrauterine death of one fetus or more, third trimester   M ♀

✓5ᵗʰ O31.3 Continuing pregnancy after elective fetal reduction of one fetus or more

Continuing pregnancy after selective termination of one fetus or more

✓7ᵗʰ **O31.3Ø** Continuing pregnancy after elective fetal reduction of one fetus or more, unspecified trimester   M ♀
✓7ᵗʰ **O31.31** Continuing pregnancy after elective fetal reduction of one fetus or more, first trimester   M ♀
✓7ᵗʰ **O31.32** Continuing pregnancy after elective fetal reduction of one fetus or more, second trimester   M ♀
✓7ᵗʰ **O31.33** Continuing pregnancy after elective fetal reduction of one fetus or more, third trimester   M ♀

✓5ᵗʰ O31.8 Other complications specific to multiple gestation

✓6ᵗʰ O31.8X Other complications specific to multiple gestation

CC Excl: For CC codes in subcategory O31.8X: PDX collection 976

✓7ᵗʰ **O31.8X1** Other complications specific to multiple gestation, first trimester   CC ♀

✓7ᵗʰ **O31.8X2** Other complications specific to multiple gestation, second trimester   CC M ♀
✓7ᵗʰ **O31.8X3** Other complications specific to multiple gestation, third trimester   CC M ♀
✓7ᵗʰ **O31.8X9** Other complications specific to multiple gestation, unspecified trimester   CC M ♀

✓4ᵗʰ O32 Maternal care for malpresentation of fetus

> INCLUDES   the listed conditions as a reason for observation, hospitalization or other obstetric care of the mother, or for cesarean delivery before onset of labor

> EXCLUDES 1   malpresentation of fetus with obstructed labor (O64.-)

AHA: 2012,4Q,107

> One of the following 7th characters is to be assigned to each code under category O32. 7th character Ø is for single gestations and multiple gestations where the fetus is unspecified. 7th characters 1 through 9 are for cases of multiple gestations to identify the fetus for which the code applies. The appropriate code from category O3Ø, Multiple gestation, must also be assigned when assigning a code from category O32 that has a 7th character of 1 through 9.
> Ø   not applicable or unspecified
> 1   fetus 1
> 2   fetus 2
> 3   fetus 3
> 4   fetus 4
> 5   fetus 5
> 9   other fetus

✓7ᵗʰ **O32.Ø** Maternal care for unstable lie   M ♀

✓7ᵗʰ **O32.1** Maternal care for breech presentation   M ♀

Maternal care for buttocks presentation
Maternal care for complete breech
Maternal care for frank breech

> EXCLUDES 1   footling presentation (O32.8)
> incomplete breech (O32.8)

DEF: Fetus presentation in a longitudinal lie with the buttocks or feet closest to birth canal that may require external cephalic version or cesarean delivery.

✓7ᵗʰ **O32.2** Maternal care for transverse and oblique lie   M ♀

Maternal care for oblique presentation
Maternal care for transverse presentation

✓7ᵗʰ **O32.3** Maternal care for face, brow and chin presentation   M ♀
✓7ᵗʰ **O32.4** Maternal care for high head at term   M ♀

Maternal care for failure of head to enter pelvic brim

✓7ᵗʰ **O32.6** Maternal care for compound presentation   M ♀
✓7ᵗʰ **O32.8** Maternal care for other malpresentation of fetus   M ♀

Maternal care for footling presentation
Maternal care for incomplete breech

✓7ᵗʰ **O32.9** Maternal care for malpresentation of fetus, unspecified   M ♀

Fetal Malpresentation

Breech
Mother's pelvis
Face (mentum)
Shoulder (arm prolapse)
Compound (extremity together with head)
Oblique

N Newborn: 0   P Pediatric: 0-17   M Maternity: 9-64   A Adult: 15-124   MCC Major Complication/Comorbidity   CC Complication/Comorbidity   SW Severe Wound Dx

894   ICD-10-CM 2020

✓4ᵗʰ O33 Maternal care for disproportion

> **INCLUDES**   the listed conditions as a reason for observation, hospitalization or other obstetric care of the mother, or for cesarean delivery before onset of labor
>
> **EXCLUDES 1**   *disproportion with obstructed labor (O65-O66)*

O33.0 Maternal care for disproportion due to deformity of maternal pelvic bones   **CC M ♀**

> Maternal care for disproportion due to pelvic deformity causing disproportion NOS
>
> **CC Excl:** PDX collection 977

O33.1 Maternal care for disproportion due to generally contracted pelvis   **M ♀**

> Maternal care for disproportion due to contracted pelvis NOS causing disproportion

O33.2 Maternal care for disproportion due to inlet contraction of pelvis   **M ♀**

> Maternal care for disproportion due to inlet contraction (pelvis) causing disproportion

✓x7ᵗʰ O33.3 Maternal care for disproportion due to outlet contraction of pelvis   **M ♀**

> Maternal care for disproportion due to mid-cavity contraction (pelvis)
>
> Maternal care for disproportion due to outlet contraction (pelvis)
>
> One of the following 7th characters is to be assigned to code O33.3. 7th character 0 is for single gestations and multiple gestations where the fetus is unspecified. 7th characters 1 through 9 are for cases of multiple gestations to identify the fetus for which the code applies. The appropriate code from category O30, Multiple gestation, must also be assigned when assigning code O33.3 with a 7th character of 1 through 9.
>
> 0   not applicable or unspecified
> 1   fetus 1
> 2   fetus 2
> 3   fetus 3
> 4   fetus 4
> 5   fetus 5
> 9   other fetus

✓x7ᵗʰ O33.4 Maternal care for disproportion of mixed maternal and fetal origin   **M ♀**

> One of the following 7th characters is to be assigned to code O33.4. 7th character 0 is for single gestations and multiple gestations where the fetus is unspecified. 7th characters 1 through 9 are for cases of multiple gestations to identify the fetus for which the code applies. The appropriate code from category O30, Multiple gestation, must also be assigned when assigning code O33.4 with a 7th character of 1 through 9.
>
> 0   not applicable or unspecified
> 1   fetus 1
> 2   fetus 2
> 3   fetus 3
> 4   fetus 4
> 5   fetus 5
> 9   other fetus

✓x7ᵗʰ O33.5 Maternal care for disproportion due to unusually large fetus   **M ♀**

> Maternal care for disproportion due to disproportion of fetal origin with normally formed fetus
>
> Maternal care for disproportion due to fetal disproportion NOS
>
> One of the following 7th characters is to be assigned to code O33.5. 7th character 0 is for single gestations and multiple gestations where the fetus is unspecified. 7th characters 1 through 9 are for cases of multiple gestations to identify the fetus for which the code applies. The appropriate code from category O30, Multiple gestation, must also be assigned when assigning code O33.5 with a 7th character of 1 through 9.
>
> 0   not applicable or unspecified
> 1   fetus 1
> 2   fetus 2
> 3   fetus 3
> 4   fetus 4
> 5   fetus 5
> 9   other fetus

✓x7ᵗʰ O33.6 Maternal care for disproportion due to hydrocephalic fetus   **M ♀**

> One of the following 7th characters is to be assigned to code O33.6. 7th character 0 is for single gestations and multiple gestations where the fetus is unspecified. 7th characters 1 through 9 are for cases of multiple gestations to identify the fetus for which the code applies. The appropriate code from category O30, Multiple gestation, must also be assigned when assigning code O33.6 with a 7th character of 1 through 9.
>
> 0   not applicable or unspecified
> 1   fetus 1
> 2   fetus 2
> 3   fetus 3
> 4   fetus 4
> 5   fetus 5
> 9   other fetus

✓x7ᵗʰ O33.7 Maternal care for disproportion due to other fetal deformities   **M ♀**

> Maternal care for disproportion due to fetal ascites
> Maternal care for disproportion due to fetal hydrops
> Maternal care for disproportion due to fetal meningomyelocele
> Maternal care for disproportion due to fetal sacral teratoma
> Maternal care for disproportion due to fetal tumor
>
> **EXCLUDES 1**   *obstructed labor due to other fetal deformities (O66.3)*
>
> **AHA:** 2016,4Q,51
>
> One of the following 7th characters is to be assigned to code O33.7. 7th character 0 is for single gestations and multiple gestations where the fetus is unspecified. 7th characters 1 through 9 are for cases of multiple gestations to identify the fetus for which the code applies. The appropriate code from category O30, Multiple gestation, must also be assigned when assigning code O33.7 with a 7th character of 1 through 9.
>
> 0   not applicable or unspecified
> 1   fetus 1
> 2   fetus 2
> 3   fetus 3
> 4   fetus 4
> 5   fetus 5
> 9   other fetus

O33.8 Maternal care for disproportion of other origin   **M ♀**

O33.9 Maternal care for disproportion, unspecified   **M ♀**

> Maternal care for disproportion due to cephalopelvic disproportion NOS
>
> Maternal care for disproportion due to fetopelvic disproportion NOS

✓4ᵗʰ O34 Maternal care for abnormality of pelvic organs

> **INCLUDES**   the listed conditions as a reason for hospitalization or other obstetric care of the mother, or for cesarean delivery before onset of labor
>
> Code first any associated obstructed labor (O65.5)
> Use additional code for specific condition

✓5ᵗʰ O34.0 Maternal care for congenital malformation of uterus

> Maternal care for double uterus
> Maternal care for uterus bicornis

O34.00 Maternal care for unspecified congenital malformation of uterus, unspecified trimester   **M ♀**

O34.01 Maternal care for unspecified congenital malformation of uterus, first trimester   **M ♀**

O34.02 Maternal care for unspecified congenital malformation of uterus, second trimester   **M ♀**

O34.03 Maternal care for unspecified congenital malformation of uterus, third trimester   **M ♀**

✓5ᵗʰ O34.1 Maternal care for benign tumor of corpus uteri

> **EXCLUDES 2**   *maternal care for benign tumor of cervix (O34.4-)*
>
> *maternal care for malignant neoplasm of uterus (O9A.1-)*

O34.10 Maternal care for benign tumor of corpus uteri, unspecified trimester   **M ♀**

O34.11 Maternal care for benign tumor of corpus uteri, first trimester   **M ♀**

O34.12 Maternal care for benign tumor of corpus uteri, second trimester   **M ♀**

O34.13 Maternal care for benign tumor of corpus uteri, third trimester   **M ♀**

√5ᵗʰ **O34.2** **Maternal care due to** uterine scar from previous surgery
    AHA: 2016,4Q,76

  √6ᵗʰ **O34.21** **Maternal care for scar** from previous cesarean delivery
      AHA: 2018,3Q,23; 2016,4Q,51-52

     O34.211 **Maternal care for** low transverse scar from previous cesarean delivery   Ⓜ ♀

     O34.212 **Maternal care for** vertical scar from previous cesarean delivery   Ⓜ ♀

        Maternal care for classical scar from previous cesarean delivery

     O34.219 **Maternal care for unspecified type scar from previous cesarean delivery**   Ⓜ ♀

  O34.29 **Maternal care due to** uterine scar from other previous surgery   Ⓜ ♀

     Maternal care due to uterine scar from other transmural uterine incision

√5ᵗʰ **O34.3** **Maternal care for** cervical incompetence

  Maternal care for cerclage with or without cervical incompetence

  Maternal care for Shirodkar suture with or without cervical incompetence

  DEF: Inadequate functioning of the cervix marked by abnormal widening during pregnancy and causing premature birth or miscarriage.

  CC Excl: For MCC codes in subcategory O34.3: PDX collection 973

  O34.30 **Maternal care for cervical incompetence, unspecified trimester**   Ⓜ ♀

  O34.31 **Maternal care for cervical incompetence,** first trimester   ᴹᶜᶜ Ⓜ ♀

  O34.32 **Maternal care for cervical incompetence,** second trimester   ᴹᶜᶜ Ⓜ ♀

  O34.33 **Maternal care for cervical incompetence,** third trimester   ᴹᶜᶜ Ⓜ ♀

√5ᵗʰ **O34.4** **Maternal care for** other abnormalities of cervix

  O34.40 **Maternal care for other abnormalities of cervix, unspecified trimester**   Ⓜ ♀

  O34.41 **Maternal care for other abnormalities of cervix,** first trimester   Ⓜ ♀

  O34.42 **Maternal care for other abnormalities of cervix,** second trimester   Ⓜ ♀

  O34.43 **Maternal care for other abnormalities of cervix,** third trimester   Ⓜ ♀

√5ᵗʰ **O34.5** **Maternal care for** other abnormalities of gravid uterus

  √6ᵗʰ **O34.51** **Maternal care for** incarceration of gravid uterus

     O34.511 **Maternal care for incarceration of gravid uterus,** first trimester   Ⓜ ♀

     O34.512 **Maternal care for incarceration of gravid uterus,** second trimester   Ⓜ ♀

     O34.513 **Maternal care for incarceration of gravid uterus,** third trimester   Ⓜ ♀

     O34.519 **Maternal care for incarceration of gravid uterus, unspecified trimester**   Ⓜ ♀

  √6ᵗʰ **O34.52** **Maternal care for** prolapse of gravid uterus

     O34.521 **Maternal care for prolapse of gravid uterus,** first trimester   Ⓜ ♀

     O34.522 **Maternal care for prolapse of gravid uterus,** second trimester   Ⓜ ♀

     O34.523 **Maternal care for prolapse of gravid uterus,** third trimester   Ⓜ ♀

     O34.529 **Maternal care for prolapse of gravid uterus, unspecified trimester**   Ⓜ ♀

  √6ᵗʰ **O34.53** **Maternal care for** retroversion of gravid uterus

     O34.531 **Maternal care for retroversion of gravid uterus,** first trimester   Ⓜ ♀

     O34.532 **Maternal care for retroversion of gravid uterus,** second trimester   Ⓜ ♀

     O34.533 **Maternal care for retroversion of gravid uterus,** third trimester   Ⓜ ♀

     O34.539 **Maternal care for retroversion of gravid uterus, unspecified trimester**   Ⓜ ♀

  √6ᵗʰ **O34.59** **Maternal care for other abnormalities of gravid uterus**

     O34.591 **Maternal care for other abnormalities of gravid uterus, first trimester**   Ⓜ ♀

     O34.592 **Maternal care for other abnormalities of gravid uterus, second trimester**   Ⓜ ♀

     O34.593 **Maternal care for other abnormalities of gravid uterus, third trimester**   Ⓜ ♀

     O34.599 **Maternal care for other abnormalities of gravid uterus, unspecified trimester**   Ⓜ ♀

√5ᵗʰ **O34.6** **Maternal care for** abnormality of vagina

  EXCLUDES 2   maternal care for vaginal varices in pregnancy (O22.1-)

  O34.60 **Maternal care for abnormality of vagina, unspecified trimester**   Ⓜ ♀

  O34.61 **Maternal care for abnormality of vagina,** first trimester   Ⓜ ♀

  O34.62 **Maternal care for abnormality of vagina,** second trimester   Ⓜ ♀

  O34.63 **Maternal care for abnormality of vagina,** third trimester   Ⓜ ♀

√5ᵗʰ **O34.7** **Maternal care for** abnormality of vulva and perineum

  EXCLUDES 2   maternal care for perineal and vulval varices in pregnancy (O22.1-)

  O34.70 **Maternal care for abnormality of vulva and perineum, unspecified trimester**   Ⓜ ♀

  O34.71 **Maternal care for abnormality of vulva and perineum,** first trimester   Ⓜ ♀

  O34.72 **Maternal care for abnormality of vulva and perineum,** second trimester   Ⓜ ♀

  O34.73 **Maternal care for abnormality of vulva and perineum,** third trimester   Ⓜ ♀

√5ᵗʰ **O34.8** **Maternal care for** other abnormalities of pelvic organs

  O34.80 **Maternal care for other abnormalities of pelvic organs, unspecified trimester**   Ⓜ ♀

  O34.81 **Maternal care for other abnormalities of pelvic organs, first trimester**   Ⓜ ♀

  O34.82 **Maternal care for other abnormalities of pelvic organs, second trimester**   Ⓜ ♀

  O34.83 **Maternal care for other abnormalities of pelvic organs, third trimester**   Ⓜ ♀

√5ᵗʰ **O34.9** **Maternal care for abnormality of pelvic organ, unspecified**

  O34.90 **Maternal care for abnormality of pelvic organ, unspecified, unspecified trimester**   Ⓜ ♀

  O34.91 **Maternal care for abnormality of pelvic organ, unspecified,** first trimester   Ⓜ ♀

  O34.92 **Maternal care for abnormality of pelvic organ, unspecified,** second trimester   Ⓜ ♀

  O34.93 **Maternal care for abnormality of pelvic organ, unspecified,** third trimester   Ⓜ ♀

✓4th O35 Maternal care for known or suspected fetal abnormality and damage

INCLUDES the listed conditions in the fetus as a reason for hospitalization or other obstetric care to the mother, or for termination of pregnancy

Code also any associated maternal condition

EXCLUDES 1 *encounter for suspected maternal and fetal conditions ruled out (Z03.7-)*

One of the following 7th characters is to be assigned to each code under category O35. 7th character 0 is for single gestations and multiple gestations where the fetus is unspecified. 7th characters 1 through 9 are for cases of multiple gestations to identify the fetus for which the code applies. The appropriate code from category O30, Multiple gestation, must also be assigned when assigning a code from category O35 that has a 7th character of 1 through 9.

- 0   not applicable or unspecified
- 1   fetus 1
- 2   fetus 2
- 3   fetus 3
- 4   fetus 4
- 5   fetus 5
- 9   other fetus

✓x7th O35.0 Maternal care for (suspected) central nervous system malformation in fetus   M ♀
- Maternal care for fetal anencephaly
- Maternal care for fetal hydrocephalus
- Maternal care for fetal spina bifida
- **EXCLUDES 2** *chromosomal abnormality in fetus (O35.1)*

✓x7th O35.1 Maternal care for (suspected) chromosomal abnormality in fetus   M ♀

✓x7th O35.2 Maternal care for (suspected) hereditary disease in fetus   M ♀
- **EXCLUDES 2** *chromosomal abnormality in fetus (O35.1)*

✓x7th O35.3 Maternal care for (suspected) damage to fetus from viral disease in mother   M ♀
- Maternal care for damage to fetus from maternal cytomegalovirus infection
- Maternal care for damage to fetus from maternal rubella

✓x7th O35.4 Maternal care for (suspected) damage to fetus from alcohol   M ♀

✓x7th O35.5 Maternal care for (suspected) damage to fetus by drugs   M ♀
- Maternal care for damage to fetus from drug addiction

✓x7th O35.6 Maternal care for (suspected) damage to fetus by radiation   M ♀

✓x7th O35.7 Maternal care for (suspected) damage to fetus by other medical procedures   M ♀
- Maternal care for damage to fetus by amniocentesis
- Maternal care for damage to fetus by biopsy procedures
- Maternal care for damage to fetus by hematological investigation
- Maternal care for damage to fetus by intrauterine contraceptive device
- Maternal care for damage to fetus by intrauterine surgery

✓x7th O35.8 Maternal care for other (suspected) fetal abnormality and damage   M ♀
- Maternal care for damage to fetus from maternal listeriosis
- Maternal care for damage to fetus from maternal toxoplasmosis

✓x7th O35.9 Maternal care for (suspected) fetal abnormality and damage, unspecified   M ♀

✓4th O36 Maternal care for other fetal problems

INCLUDES the listed conditions in the fetus as a reason for hospitalization or other obstetric care of the mother, or for termination of pregnancy

EXCLUDES 1 *encounter for suspected maternal and fetal conditions ruled out (Z03.7-)*
placental transfusion syndromes (O43.0-)

EXCLUDES 2 *labor and delivery complicated by fetal stress (O77.-)*

AHA: 2015,3Q,40

One of the following 7th characters is to be assigned to each code under category O36. 7th character 0 is for single gestations and multiple gestations where the fetus is unspecified. 7th characters 1 through 9 are for cases of multiple gestations to identify the fetus for which the code applies. The appropriate code from category O30, Multiple gestation, must also be assigned when assigning a code from category O36 that has a 7th character of 1 through 9.

- 0   not applicable or unspecified
- 1   fetus 1
- 2   fetus 2
- 3   fetus 3
- 4   fetus 4
- 5   fetus 5
- 9   other fetus

✓5th O36.0 Maternal care for rhesus isoimmunization
- Maternal care for Rh incompatibility (with hydrops fetalis)
- **CC Excl: For CC codes in subcategory O36.0:** PDX collection 978

    ✓6th O36.01 Maternal care for anti-D [Rh] antibodies
       AHA: 2014,4Q,17

       ✓7th O36.011 Maternal care for anti-D [Rh] antibodies, first trimester   CC M ♀

       ✓7th O36.012 Maternal care for anti-D [Rh] antibodies, second trimester   CC M ♀

       ✓7th O36.013 Maternal care for anti-D [Rh] antibodies, third trimester   CC M ♀

       ✓7th O36.019 Maternal care for anti-D [Rh] antibodies, unspecified trimester   M ♀

    ✓6th O36.09 Maternal care for other rhesus isoimmunization

       ✓7th O36.091 Maternal care for other rhesus isoimmunization, first trimester   CC M ♀

       ✓7th O36.092 Maternal care for other rhesus isoimmunization, second trimester   CC M ♀

       ✓7th O36.093 Maternal care for other rhesus isoimmunization, third trimester   CC M ♀

       ✓7th O36.099 Maternal care for other rhesus isoimmunization, unspecified trimester   M ♀

✓5th O36.1 Maternal care for other isoimmunization
- Maternal care for ABO isoimmunization

    ✓6th O36.11 Maternal care for Anti-A sensitization
       Maternal care for isoimmunization NOS (with hydrops fetalis)

       ✓7th O36.111 Maternal care for Anti-A sensitization, first trimester   M ♀

       ✓7th O36.112 Maternal care for Anti-A sensitization, second trimester   M ♀

       ✓7th O36.113 Maternal care for Anti-A sensitization, third trimester   M ♀

       ✓7th O36.119 Maternal care for Anti-A sensitization, unspecified trimester   M ♀

    ✓6th O36.19 Maternal care for other isoimmunization
       Maternal care for Anti-B sensitization

       ✓7th O36.191 Maternal care for other isoimmunization, first trimester   CC M ♀

       ✓7th O36.192 Maternal care for other isoimmunization, second trimester   M ♀

       ✓7th O36.193 Maternal care for other isoimmunization, third trimester   M ♀

       ✓7th O36.199 Maternal care for other isoimmunization, unspecified trimester   M ♀

✔ Additional Character Required   ✓x7th Placeholder   Unacceptable PDx   Questionable PDx   Manifestation   Unspecified Dx   H1-H14 HAC   HCC CMS-HCC Dx   HIV HIV Dx

ICD-10-CM 2020   897

✓5ᵗʰ O36.2 Maternal care for hydrops fetalis

Maternal care for hydrops fetalis NOS

Maternal care for hydrops fetalis not associated with isoimmunization

> **EXCLUDES 1**   *hydrops fetalis associated with ABO isoimmunization (O36.1-)*
> *hydrops fetalis associated with rhesus isoimmunization (O36.0-)*

DEF: Hydrops fetalis: Abnormal fluid buildup in at least two of the following fetal organ spaces: the skin (edema), abdomen (ascites), around the heart (pericardia effusion), and around the lung (pleural effusion). Fluid accumulation may also occur in the mother as polyhydramnios and edema of the placenta.

   ✓x7ᵗʰ O36.20 Maternal care for hydrops fetalis, unspecified trimester   Ⓜ ♀

   ✓x7ᵗʰ O36.21 Maternal care for hydrops fetalis, first trimester   Ⓜ ♀

   ✓x7ᵗʰ O36.22 Maternal care for hydrops fetalis, second trimester   Ⓜ ♀

   ✓x7ᵗʰ O36.23 Maternal care for hydrops fetalis, third trimester   Ⓜ ♀

✓x7ᵗʰ O36.4 Maternal care for intrauterine death   ⒸⒸ Ⓜ ♀

Maternal care for intrauterine fetal death NOS

Maternal care for intrauterine fetal death after completion of 20 weeks of gestation

Maternal care for late fetal death

Maternal care for missed delivery

> **EXCLUDES 1**   *missed abortion (O02.1)*
> *stillbirth (P95)*

CC Excl: PDX collection 979

✓5ᵗʰ O36.5 Maternal care for known or suspected poor fetal growth

   ✓6ᵗʰ O36.51 Maternal care for known or suspected placental insufficiency

     ✓7ᵗʰ O36.511 Maternal care for known or suspected placental insufficiency, first trimester   Ⓜ ♀

     ✓7ᵗʰ O36.512 Maternal care for known or suspected placental insufficiency, second trimester   Ⓜ ♀

     ✓7ᵗʰ O36.513 Maternal care for known or suspected placental insufficiency, third trimester   Ⓜ ♀

     ✓7ᵗʰ O36.519 Maternal care for known or suspected placental insufficiency, unspecified trimester   Ⓜ ♀

   ✓6ᵗʰ O36.59 Maternal care for other known or suspected poor fetal growth

Maternal care for known or suspected light-for-dates NOS

Maternal care for known or suspected small-for-dates NOS

     ✓7ᵗʰ O36.591 Maternal care for other known or suspected poor fetal growth, first trimester   Ⓜ ♀

     ✓7ᵗʰ O36.592 Maternal care for other known or suspected poor fetal growth, second trimester   Ⓜ ♀

     ✓7ᵗʰ O36.593 Maternal care for other known or suspected poor fetal growth, third trimester   Ⓜ ♀

     ✓7ᵗʰ O36.599 Maternal care for other known or suspected poor fetal growth, unspecified trimester   Ⓜ ♀

✓5ᵗʰ O36.6 Maternal care for excessive fetal growth

Maternal care for known or suspected large-for-dates

   ✓x7ᵗʰ O36.60 Maternal care for excessive fetal growth, unspecified trimester   Ⓜ ♀

   ✓x7ᵗʰ O36.61 Maternal care for excessive fetal growth, first trimester   Ⓜ ♀

   ✓x7ᵗʰ O36.62 Maternal care for excessive fetal growth, second trimester   Ⓜ ♀

   ✓x7ᵗʰ O36.63 Maternal care for excessive fetal growth, third trimester   Ⓜ ♀

✓5ᵗʰ O36.7 Maternal care for viable fetus in abdominal pregnancy

   ✓x7ᵗʰ O36.70 Maternal care for viable fetus in abdominal pregnancy, unspecified trimester   Ⓜ ♀

   ✓x7ᵗʰ O36.71 Maternal care for viable fetus in abdominal pregnancy, first trimester   Ⓜ ♀

   ✓x7ᵗʰ O36.72 Maternal care for viable fetus in abdominal pregnancy, second trimester   Ⓜ ♀

   ✓x7ᵗʰ O36.73 Maternal care for viable fetus in abdominal pregnancy, third trimester   Ⓜ ♀

✓5ᵗʰ O36.8 Maternal care for other specified fetal problems

   ✓x7ᵗʰ O36.80 Pregnancy with inconclusive fetal viability   Ⓜ ♀

Encounter to determine fetal viability of pregnancy

AHA: 2019,2Q,29

   ✓6ᵗʰ O36.81 Decreased fetal movements

     ✓7ᵗʰ O36.812 Decreased fetal movements, second trimester   Ⓜ ♀

     ✓7ᵗʰ O36.813 Decreased fetal movements, third trimester   Ⓜ ♀

     ✓7ᵗʰ O36.819 Decreased fetal movements, unspecified trimester   Ⓜ ♀

   ✓6ᵗʰ O36.82 Fetal anemia and thrombocytopenia

     ✓7ᵗʰ O36.821 Fetal anemia and thrombocytopenia, first trimester   Ⓜ ♀

     ✓7ᵗʰ O36.822 Fetal anemia and thrombocytopenia, second trimester   Ⓜ ♀

     ✓7ᵗʰ O36.823 Fetal anemia and thrombocytopenia, third trimester   Ⓜ ♀

     ✓7ᵗʰ O36.829 Fetal anemia and thrombocytopenia, unspecified trimester   Ⓜ ♀

   ✓6ᵗʰ O36.83 Maternal care for abnormalities of the fetal heart rate or rhythm

▶Maternal care for depressed fetal heart rate tones◀

▶Maternal care for fetal bradycardia◀

▶Maternal care for fetal heart rate abnormal variability◀

▶Maternal care for fetal heart rate decelerations◀

▶Maternal care for fetal heart rate irregularity◀

▶Maternal care for fetal tachycardia◀

▶Maternal care for non-reassuring fetal heart rate or rhythm◀

AHA: 2017,4Q,20

TIP: Assign for documented fetal tachycardia, bradycardia, decelerations, or loss of variability detected during antenatal testing.

     ✓7ᵗʰ O36.831 Maternal care for abnormalities of the fetal heart rate or rhythm, first trimester   Ⓜ ♀

     ✓7ᵗʰ O36.832 Maternal care for abnormalities of the fetal heart rate or rhythm, second trimester   Ⓜ ♀

     ✓7ᵗʰ O36.833 Maternal care for abnormalities of the fetal heart rate or rhythm, third trimester   Ⓜ ♀

     ✓7ᵗʰ O36.839 Maternal care for abnormalities of the fetal heart rate or rhythm, unspecified trimester   Ⓜ ♀

   ✓6ᵗʰ O36.89 Maternal care for other specified fetal problems

     ✓7ᵗʰ O36.891 Maternal care for other specified fetal problems, first trimester   Ⓜ ♀

     ✓7ᵗʰ O36.892 Maternal care for other specified fetal problems, second trimester   Ⓜ ♀

     ✓7ᵗʰ O36.893 Maternal care for other specified fetal problems, third trimester   Ⓜ ♀

     ✓7ᵗʰ O36.899 Maternal care for other specified fetal problems, unspecified trimester   Ⓜ ♀

✓5ᵗʰ O36.9 Maternal care for fetal problem, unspecified

   ✓x7ᵗʰ O36.90 Maternal care for fetal problem, unspecified, unspecified trimester   Ⓜ ♀

   ✓x7ᵗʰ O36.91 Maternal care for fetal problem, unspecified, first trimester   Ⓜ ♀

   ✓x7ᵗʰ O36.92 Maternal care for fetal problem, unspecified, second trimester   Ⓜ ♀

   ✓x7ᵗʰ O36.93 Maternal care for fetal problem, unspecified, third trimester   Ⓜ ♀

Ⓝ Newborn: 0   Ⓟ Pediatric: 0-17   Ⓜ Maternity: 9-64   Ⓐ Adult: 15-124   ⓂⒸⒸ Major Complication/Comorbidity   ⒸⒸ Complication/Comorbidity   ⓈⓌ Severe Wound Dx

898   ICD-10-CM 2020

Chapter 15. Pregnancy, Childbirth and the Puerperium

O40–O42.111

✓4ᵗʰ O40 Polyhydramnios

INCLUDES   hydramnios

EXCLUDES 1   *encounter for suspected maternal and fetal conditions ruled out (Z03.7-)*

AHA: 2016,1Q,4

DEF: Excess amniotic fluid surrounding the fetus, typically defined as a total fluid volume of greater than 24.0 cc.

One of the following 7th characters is to be assigned to each code under category O40. 7th character Ø is for single gestations and multiple gestations where the fetus is unspecified. 7th characters 1 through 9 are for cases of multiple gestations to identify the fetus for which the code applies. The appropriate code from category O30, Multiple gestation, must also be assigned when assigning a code from category O40 that has a 7th character of 1 through 9.

- Ø   not applicable or unspecified
- 1   fetus 1
- 2   fetus 2
- 3   fetus 3
- 4   fetus 4
- 5   fetus 5
- 9   other fetus

✓x7ᵗʰ	**O40.1**	**Polyhydramnios, first trimester**	Ⓜ ♀
✓x7ᵗʰ	**O40.2**	**Polyhydramnios, second trimester**	Ⓜ ♀
✓x7ᵗʰ	**O40.3**	**Polyhydramnios, third trimester**	Ⓜ ♀
✓x7ᵗʰ	**O40.9**	**Polyhydramnios, unspecified trimester**	Ⓜ ♀

✓4ᵗʰ O41 Other disorders of amniotic fluid and membranes

EXCLUDES 1   *encounter for suspected maternal and fetal conditions ruled out (Z03.7-)*

One of the following 7th characters is to be assigned to each code under category O41. 7th character Ø is for single gestations and multiple gestations where the fetus is unspecified. 7th characters 1 through 9 are for cases of multiple gestations to identify the fetus for which the code applies. The appropriate code from category O30, Multiple gestation, must also be assigned when assigning a code from category O41 that has a 7th character of 1 through 9.

- Ø   not applicable or unspecified
- 1   fetus 1
- 2   fetus 2
- 3   fetus 3
- 4   fetus 4
- 5   fetus 5
- 9   other fetus

✓5ᵗʰ O41.0 Oligohydramnios

Oligohydramnios without rupture of membranes

DEF: Low amniotic fluid, occurring most frequently in the last trimester.

CC Excl: For CC codes in category O41.0: PDX collection 982

✓x7ᵗʰ	**O41.00**	**Oligohydramnios, unspecified trimester**	Ⓜ ♀
✓x7ᵗʰ	**O41.01**	**Oligohydramnios, first trimester**	CC Ⓜ ♀
✓x7ᵗʰ	**O41.02**	**Oligohydramnios, second trimester**	CC Ⓜ ♀
✓x7ᵗʰ	**O41.03**	**Oligohydramnios, third trimester**	CC Ⓜ ♀

✓5ᵗʰ O41.1 Infection of amniotic sac and membranes

CC Excl: For MCC codes in subcategory O41.1: PDX collection 983

✓6ᵗʰ O41.10 Infection of amniotic sac and membranes, unspecified

✓7ᵗʰ	**O41.101**	**Infection of amniotic sac and membranes, unspecified, first trimester**	MCC Ⓜ ♀
✓7ᵗʰ	**O41.102**	**Infection of amniotic sac and membranes, unspecified, second trimester**	MCC Ⓜ ♀
✓7ᵗʰ	**O41.103**	**Infection of amniotic sac and membranes, unspecified, third trimester**	MCC Ⓜ ♀
✓7ᵗʰ	**O41.109**	**Infection of amniotic sac and membranes, unspecified, unspecified trimester**	Ⓜ ♀

✓6ᵗʰ O41.12 Chorioamnionitis

AHA: 2019,2Q,34

✓7ᵗʰ	**O41.121**	**Chorioamnionitis, first trimester**	MCC Ⓜ ♀
✓7ᵗʰ	**O41.122**	**Chorioamnionitis, second trimester**	MCC Ⓜ ♀
✓7ᵗʰ	**O41.123**	**Chorioamnionitis, third trimester**	MCC Ⓜ ♀
✓7ᵗʰ	**O41.129**	**Chorioamnionitis, unspecified trimester**	Ⓜ ♀

✓6ᵗʰ O41.14 Placentitis

✓7ᵗʰ	**O41.141**	**Placentitis, first trimester**	MCC Ⓜ ♀
✓7ᵗʰ	**O41.142**	**Placentitis, second trimester**	MCC Ⓜ ♀
✓7ᵗʰ	**O41.143**	**Placentitis, third trimester**	MCC Ⓜ ♀
✓7ᵗʰ	**O41.149**	**Placentitis, unspecified trimester**	Ⓜ ♀

✓5ᵗʰ O41.8 Other specified disorders of amniotic fluid and membranes

✓6ᵗʰ O41.8X Other specified disorders of amniotic fluid and membranes

✓7ᵗʰ	**O41.8X1**	**Other specified disorders of amniotic fluid and membranes, first trimester**	Ⓜ ♀
✓7ᵗʰ	**O41.8X2**	**Other specified disorders of amniotic fluid and membranes, second trimester**	Ⓜ ♀
✓7ᵗʰ	**O41.8X3**	**Other specified disorders of amniotic fluid and membranes, third trimester**	Ⓜ ♀
✓7ᵗʰ	**O41.8X9**	**Other specified disorders of amniotic fluid and membranes, unspecified trimester**	Ⓜ ♀

✓5ᵗʰ O41.9 Disorder of amniotic fluid and membranes, unspecified

✓x7ᵗʰ	**O41.90**	**Disorder of amniotic fluid and membranes, unspecified, unspecified trimester**	Ⓜ ♀
✓x7ᵗʰ	**O41.91**	**Disorder of amniotic fluid and membranes, unspecified, first trimester**	Ⓜ ♀
✓x7ᵗʰ	**O41.92**	**Disorder of amniotic fluid and membranes, unspecified, second trimester**	Ⓜ ♀
✓x7ᵗʰ	**O41.93**	**Disorder of amniotic fluid and membranes, unspecified, third trimester**	Ⓜ ♀

✓4ᵗʰ O42 Premature rupture of membranes

AHA: 2016,1Q,3

✓5ᵗʰ O42.0 Premature rupture of membranes, onset of labor within 24 hours of rupture

O42.00   **Premature rupture of membranes, onset of labor within 24 hours of rupture, unspecified weeks of gestation**   Ⓜ ♀

✓6ᵗʰ O42.01 Preterm premature rupture of membranes, onset of labor within 24 hours of rupture

Premature rupture of membranes before 37 completed weeks of gestation

	O42.011	**Preterm premature rupture of membranes, onset of labor within 24 hours of rupture, first trimester**	Ⓜ ♀
	O42.012	**Preterm premature rupture of membranes, onset of labor within 24 hours of rupture, second trimester**	Ⓜ ♀
	O42.013	**Preterm premature rupture of membranes, onset of labor within 24 hours of rupture, third trimester**	Ⓜ ♀
	O42.019	**Preterm premature rupture of membranes, onset of labor within 24 hours of rupture, unspecified trimester**	Ⓜ ♀

O42.02   **Full-term premature rupture of membranes, onset of labor within 24 hours of rupture**   Ⓜ ♀

Premature rupture of membranes at or after 37 completed weeks of gestation, onset of labor within 24 hours of rupture

✓5ᵗʰ O42.1 Premature rupture of membranes, onset of labor more than 24 hours following rupture

AHA: 2016,1Q,5

O42.10   **Premature rupture of membranes, onset of labor more than 24 hours following rupture, unspecified weeks of gestation**   Ⓜ ♀

✓6ᵗʰ O42.11 Preterm premature rupture of membranes, onset of labor more than 24 hours following rupture

Premature rupture of membranes before 37 completed weeks of gestation

| | **O42.111** | **Preterm premature rupture of membranes, onset of labor more than 24 hours following rupture, first trimester** | Ⓜ ♀ |

☑ Additional Character Required   ✓x7ᵗʰ Placeholder   Unacceptable PDx   Questionable PDx   Manifestation   Unspecified Dx   H1-H14 HAC   HCC CMS-HCC Dx   HIV HIV Dx

ICD-10-CM 2020

899

Chapter 15. Pregnancy, Childbirth and the Puerperium

O42.112   **Preterm premature rupture of membranes, onset of labor more than 24 hours following rupture, second trimester** Ⓜ♀

O42.113   **Preterm premature rupture of membranes, onset of labor more than 24 hours following rupture, third trimester** Ⓜ♀

O42.119   **Preterm premature rupture of membranes, onset of labor more than 24 hours following rupture, unspecified trimester** Ⓜ♀

O42.12   **Full-term premature rupture of membranes, onset of labor more than 24 hours following rupture** Ⓜ♀
Premature rupture of membranes at or after 37 completed weeks of gestation, onset of labor more than 24 hours following rupture

✓5th **O42.9**   **Premature rupture of membranes, unspecified as to length of time between rupture and onset of labor**

O42.90   **Premature rupture of membranes, unspecified as to length of time between rupture and onset of labor, unspecified weeks of gestation** Ⓜ♀

✓6th **O42.91**   **Preterm premature rupture of membranes, unspecified as to length of time between rupture and onset of labor**
Premature rupture of membranes before 37 completed weeks of gestation

O42.911   **Preterm premature rupture of membranes, unspecified as to length of time between rupture and onset of labor, first trimester** Ⓜ♀

O42.912   **Preterm premature rupture of membranes, unspecified as to length of time between rupture and onset of labor, second trimester** Ⓜ♀

O42.913   **Preterm premature rupture of membranes, unspecified as to length of time between rupture and onset of labor, third trimester** Ⓜ♀

O42.919   **Preterm premature rupture of membranes, unspecified as to length of time between rupture and onset of labor, unspecified trimester** Ⓜ♀

O42.92   **Full-term premature rupture of membranes, unspecified as to length of time between rupture and onset of labor** Ⓜ♀
Premature rupture of membranes at or after 37 completed weeks of gestation, unspecified as to length of time between rupture and onset of labor

✓4th **O43**   **Placental disorders**
EXCLUDES 2   maternal care for poor fetal growth due to placental insufficiency (O36.5-)
placenta previa (O44.-)
placental polyp (O90.89)
placentitis (O41.14-)
premature separation of placenta [abruptio placentae] (O45.-)

✓5th **O43.0**   **Placental transfusion syndromes**

✓6th **O43.01**   **Fetomaternal placental transfusion syndrome**
Maternofetal placental transfusion syndrome

O43.011   **Fetomaternal placental transfusion syndrome, first trimester** Ⓜ♀

O43.012   **Fetomaternal placental transfusion syndrome, second trimester** Ⓜ♀

O43.013   **Fetomaternal placental transfusion syndrome, third trimester** Ⓜ♀

O43.019   **Fetomaternal placental transfusion syndrome, unspecified trimester** Ⓜ♀

✓6th **O43.02**   **Fetus-to-fetus placental transfusion syndrome**
DEF: Condition in which an imbalance in amniotic fluid occurs due to uneven blood flow between twins sharing a placenta.

Twin to Twin Transfusion Syndrome (TTTS)

Healthy twins   Twins with TTTS

O43.021   **Fetus-to-fetus placental transfusion syndrome, first trimester** Ⓜ♀

O43.022   **Fetus-to-fetus placental transfusion syndrome, second trimester** Ⓜ♀

O43.023   **Fetus-to-fetus placental transfusion syndrome, third trimester** Ⓜ♀

O43.029   **Fetus-to-fetus placental transfusion syndrome, unspecified trimester** Ⓜ♀

✓5th **O43.1**   **Malformation of placenta**

✓6th **O43.10**   **Malformation of placenta, unspecified**
Abnormal placenta NOS

O43.101   **Malformation of placenta, unspecified, first trimester** Ⓜ♀

O43.102   **Malformation of placenta, unspecified, second trimester** Ⓜ♀

O43.103   **Malformation of placenta, unspecified, third trimester** Ⓜ♀

O43.109   **Malformation of placenta, unspecified, unspecified trimester** Ⓜ♀

✓6th **O43.11**   **Circumvallate placenta**

O43.111   **Circumvallate placenta, first trimester** Ⓜ♀

O43.112   **Circumvallate placenta, second trimester** Ⓜ♀

O43.113   **Circumvallate placenta, third trimester** Ⓜ♀

O43.119   **Circumvallate placenta, unspecified trimester** Ⓜ♀

✓6th **O43.12**   **Velamentous insertion of umbilical cord**

O43.121   **Velamentous insertion of umbilical cord, first trimester** Ⓜ♀

O43.122   **Velamentous insertion of umbilical cord, second trimester** Ⓜ♀

O43.123   **Velamentous insertion of umbilical cord, third trimester** Ⓜ♀

O43.129   **Velamentous insertion of umbilical cord, unspecified trimester** Ⓜ♀

✓6th **O43.19**   **Other malformation of placenta**

O43.191   **Other malformation of placenta, first trimester** Ⓜ♀

O43.192   **Other malformation of placenta, second trimester** Ⓜ♀

O43.193   **Other malformation of placenta, third trimester** Ⓜ♀

O43.199   **Other malformation of placenta, unspecified trimester** Ⓜ♀

Ⓝ Newborn: 0   Ⓟ Pediatric: 0-17   Ⓜ Maternity: 9-64   Ⓐ Adult: 15-124   MCC Major Complication/Comorbidity   CC Complication/Comorbidity   SW Severe Wound Dx

900   ICD-10-CM 2020

O42.112–O43.199

√5ᵗʰ **O43.2 Morbidly adherent placenta**

Code also associated third stage postpartum hemorrhage, if applicable (O72.0)

EXCLUDES 1   *retained placenta (O73.-)*

√6ᵗʰ **O43.21 Placenta** accreta

DEF: Condition where the placenta adheres too deeply to the uterine wall; often associated with placenta previa.

O43.211 Placenta accreta, first trimester   M ♀

O43.212 Placenta accreta, second trimester   M ♀

O43.213 Placenta accreta, third trimester   M ♀

O43.219 Placenta accreta, unspecified trimester   M ♀

√6ᵗʰ **O43.22 Placenta** increta

DEF: Condition where the placenta adheres too deeply to the uterine wall and penetrates the muscle; often associated with placenta previa.

O43.221 Placenta increta, first trimester   M ♀

O43.222 Placenta increta, second trimester   M ♀

O43.223 Placenta increta, third trimester   M ♀

O43.229 Placenta increta, unspecified trimester   M ♀

√6ᵗʰ **O43.23 Placenta** percreta

DEF: Condition where the placenta attaches through the uterine muscle and may invade other organs, resulting in antenatal complications, premature delivery, retention of all or a portion of the placenta, or postpartum bleeding.

O43.231 Placenta percreta, first trimester   M ♀

O43.232 Placenta percreta, second trimester   M ♀

O43.233 Placenta percreta, third trimester   M ♀

O43.239 Placenta percreta, unspecified trimester   M ♀

√5ᵗʰ **O43.8 Other placental disorders**

√6ᵗʰ **O43.81 Placental infarction**

O43.811 Placental infarction, first trimester   M ♀

O43.812 Placental infarction, second trimester   M ♀

O43.813 Placental infarction, third trimester   M ♀

O43.819 Placental infarction, unspecified trimester   M ♀

√6ᵗʰ **O43.89 Other placental disorders**

Placental dysfunction

O43.891 Other placental disorders, first trimester   M ♀

O43.892 Other placental disorders, second trimester   M ♀

O43.893 Other placental disorders, third trimester   M ♀

O43.899 Other placental disorders, unspecified trimester   M ♀

√5ᵗʰ **O43.9 Unspecified placental disorder**

O43.90 Unspecified placental disorder, unspecified trimester   M ♀

O43.91 Unspecified placental disorder, first trimester   M ♀

O43.92 Unspecified placental disorder, second trimester   M ♀

O43.93 Unspecified placental disorder, third trimester   M ♀

√4ᵗʰ **O44 Placenta previa**

AHA: 2016,4Q,52-53

DEF: Placenta implanted in the lower segment of the uterus, which commonly causes hemorrhage in the last trimester of pregnancy.

CC Excl: For CC/MCC codes in category O44: PDX collection 966

√5ᵗʰ **O44.0 Complete placenta previa NOS or without hemorrhage**

Placenta previa NOS

O44.00 Complete placenta previa NOS or without hemorrhage, unspecified trimester   M ♀

O44.01 Complete placenta previa NOS or without hemorrhage, first trimester   CC M ♀

O44.02 Complete placenta previa NOS or without hemorrhage, second trimester   CC M ♀

O44.03 Complete placenta previa NOS or without hemorrhage, third trimester   CC M ♀

√5ᵗʰ **O44.1 Complete placenta previa with hemorrhage**

EXCLUDES 1   *labor and delivery complicated by hemorrhage from vasa previa (O69.4)*

O44.10 Complete placenta previa with hemorrhage, unspecified trimester   M ♀

O44.11 Complete placenta previa with hemorrhage, first trimester   MCC M ♀

O44.12 Complete placenta previa with hemorrhage, second trimester   MCC M ♀

O44.13 Complete placenta previa with hemorrhage, third trimester   MCC M ♀

√5ᵗʰ **O44.2 Partial placenta previa without hemorrhage**

Marginal placenta previa, NOS or without hemorrhage

O44.20 Partial placenta previa NOS or without hemorrhage, unspecified trimester   M ♀

O44.21 Partial placenta previa NOS or without hemorrhage, first trimester   CC M ♀

O44.22 Partial placenta previa NOS or without hemorrhage, second trimester   CC M ♀

O44.23 Partial placenta previa NOS or without hemorrhage, third trimester   CC ♀

√5ᵗʰ **O44.3 Partial placenta previa with hemorrhage**

Marginal placenta previa with hemorrhage

O44.30 Partial placenta previa with hemorrhage, unspecified trimester   M ♀

O44.31 Partial placenta previa with hemorrhage, first trimester   MCC M ♀

O44.32 Partial placenta previa with hemorrhage, second trimester   MCC M ♀

O44.33 Partial placenta previa with hemorrhage, third trimester   MCC M ♀

√5ᵗʰ **O44.4 Low lying placenta NOS or without hemorrhage**

Low implantation of placenta NOS or without hemorrhage

O44.40 Low lying placenta NOS or without hemorrhage, unspecified trimester   M ♀

O44.41 Low lying placenta NOS or without hemorrhage, first trimester   CC M ♀

O44.42 Low lying placenta NOS or without hemorrhage, second trimester   CC M ♀

O44.43 Low lying placenta NOS or without hemorrhage, third trimester   CC M ♀

√5ᵗʰ **O44.5 Low lying placenta with hemorrhage**

Low implantation of placenta with hemorrhage

O44.50 Low lying placenta with hemorrhage, unspecified trimester   M ♀

O44.51 Low lying placenta with hemorrhage, first trimester   MCC M ♀

O44.52 Low lying placenta with hemorrhage, second trimester   MCC M ♀

O44.53 Low lying placenta with hemorrhage, third trimester   MCC M ♀

√4ᵗʰ **O45 Premature separation of placenta [abruptio placentae]**

√5ᵗʰ **O45.0 Premature separation of placenta with coagulation defect**

CC Excl: For MCC codes in subcategory O45.0: PDX collection 985

√6ᵗʰ **O45.00 Premature separation of placenta with coagulation defect, unspecified**

O45.001 Premature separation of placenta with coagulation defect, unspecified, first trimester   MCC M ♀

O45.002 Premature separation of placenta with coagulation defect, unspecified, second trimester   MCC M ♀

O45.003 Premature separation of placenta with coagulation defect, unspecified, third trimester   MCC M ♀

O45.009 Premature separation of placenta with coagulation defect, unspecified, unspecified trimester   M ♀

✔ Additional Character Required   √ˣ7ᵗʰ Placeholder   Unacceptable PDx   Questionable PDx   Manifestation   Unspecified Dx   H1-H4 HAC   HCC CMS-HCC Dx   HIV HIV Dx

ICD-10-CM 2020   901

✓6ᵗʰ **O45.01** **Premature separation of placenta with afibrinogenemia**
Premature separation of placenta with hypofibrinogenemia

     O45.011 **Premature separation of placenta with afibrinogenemia, first trimester**   MCC M ♀

     O45.012 **Premature separation of placenta with afibrinogenemia, second trimester**   MCC M ♀

     O45.013 **Premature separation of placenta with afibrinogenemia, third trimester**   MCC M ♀

     O45.019 **Premature separation of placenta with afibrinogenemia, unspecified trimester**   M ♀

✓6ᵗʰ **O45.02** **Premature separation of placenta with disseminated intravascular coagulation**

     O45.021 **Premature separation of placenta with disseminated intravascular coagulation, first trimester**   MCC M ♀

     O45.022 **Premature separation of placenta with disseminated intravascular coagulation, second trimester**   MCC M ♀

     O45.023 **Premature separation of placenta with disseminated intravascular coagulation, third trimester**   MCC M ♀

     O45.029 **Premature separation of placenta with disseminated intravascular coagulation, unspecified trimester**   M ♀

✓6ᵗʰ **O45.09** **Premature separation of placenta with other coagulation defect**

     O45.091 **Premature separation of placenta with other coagulation defect, first trimester**   MCC M ♀

     O45.092 **Premature separation of placenta with other coagulation defect, second trimester**   MCC M ♀

     O45.093 **Premature separation of placenta with other coagulation defect, third trimester**   MCC M ♀

     O45.099 **Premature separation of placenta with other coagulation defect, unspecified trimester**   M ♀

✓5ᵗʰ **O45.8** **Other premature separation of placenta**

> **CC Excl: For MCC codes in subcategory O45.8:** PDX collection 986

✓6ᵗʰ **O45.8X** **Other premature separation of placenta**

     O45.8X1 **Other premature separation of placenta, first trimester**   MCC M ♀

     O45.8X2 **Other premature separation of placenta, second trimester**   MCC M ♀

     O45.8X3 **Other premature separation of placenta, third trimester**   MCC M ♀

     O45.8X9 **Other premature separation of placenta, unspecified trimester**   M ♀

✓5ᵗʰ **O45.9** **Premature separation of placenta, unspecified**
Abruptio placentae NOS

> **CC Excl: For MCC codes in subcategory O45.9:** PDX collection 986

     O45.90 **Premature separation of placenta, unspecified, unspecified trimester**   M ♀

     O45.91 **Premature separation of placenta, unspecified, first trimester**   MCC M ♀

     O45.92 **Premature separation of placenta, unspecified, second trimester**   MCC M ♀

     O45.93 **Premature separation of placenta, unspecified, third trimester**   MCC M ♀

✓4ᵗʰ **O46** **Antepartum hemorrhage, not elsewhere classified**

> EXCLUDES 1   *hemorrhage in early pregnancy (O20.-)*
> *intrapartum hemorrhage NEC (O67.-)*
> *placenta previa (O44.-)*
> *premature separation of placenta [abruptio placentae] (O45.-)*

DEF: Uterine hemorrhage prior to delivery that is not related to placenta previa or abruptio placentae.

✓5ᵗʰ **O46.0** **Antepartum hemorrhage with coagulation defect**

> **CC Excl: For MCC codes in subcategory O46.0:** PDX collection 985

✓6ᵗʰ **O46.00** **Antepartum hemorrhage with coagulation defect, unspecified**

     O46.001 **Antepartum hemorrhage with coagulation defect, unspecified, first trimester**   MCC M ♀

     O46.002 **Antepartum hemorrhage with coagulation defect, unspecified, second trimester**   MCC M ♀

     O46.003 **Antepartum hemorrhage with coagulation defect, unspecified, third trimester**   MCC M ♀

     O46.009 **Antepartum hemorrhage with coagulation defect, unspecified, unspecified trimester**   M ♀

✓6ᵗʰ **O46.01** **Antepartum hemorrhage with afibrinogenemia**
Antepartum hemorrhage with hypofibrinogenemia

     O46.011 **Antepartum hemorrhage with afibrinogenemia, first trimester**   MCC M ♀

     O46.012 **Antepartum hemorrhage with afibrinogenemia, second trimester**   MCC M ♀

     O46.013 **Antepartum hemorrhage with afibrinogenemia, third trimester**   MCC M ♀

     O46.019 **Antepartum hemorrhage with afibrinogenemia, unspecified trimester**   M ♀

✓6ᵗʰ **O46.02** **Antepartum hemorrhage with disseminated intravascular coagulation**

     O46.021 **Antepartum hemorrhage with disseminated intravascular coagulation, first trimester**   MCC M ♀

     O46.022 **Antepartum hemorrhage with disseminated intravascular coagulation, second trimester**   MCC M ♀

     O46.023 **Antepartum hemorrhage with disseminated intravascular coagulation, third trimester**   MCC M ♀

     O46.029 **Antepartum hemorrhage with disseminated intravascular coagulation, unspecified trimester**   M ♀

✓6ᵗʰ **O46.09** **Antepartum hemorrhage with other coagulation defect**

     O46.091 **Antepartum hemorrhage with other coagulation defect, first trimester**   MCC M ♀

     O46.092 **Antepartum hemorrhage with other coagulation defect, second trimester**   MCC M ♀

     O46.093 **Antepartum hemorrhage with other coagulation defect, third trimester**   MCC M ♀

     O46.099 **Antepartum hemorrhage with other coagulation defect, unspecified trimester**   M ♀

✓5ᵗʰ **O46.8** **Other antepartum hemorrhage**

✓6ᵗʰ **O46.8X** **Other antepartum hemorrhage**

     O46.8X1 **Other antepartum hemorrhage, first trimester**   M ♀

     O46.8X2 **Other antepartum hemorrhage, second trimester**   M ♀

     O46.8X3 **Other antepartum hemorrhage, third trimester**   M ♀

     O46.8X9 **Other antepartum hemorrhage, unspecified trimester**   M ♀

✓5ᵗʰ **O46.9** **Antepartum hemorrhage, unspecified**

     O46.90 **Antepartum hemorrhage, unspecified, unspecified trimester**   M ♀

N Newborn: 0   P Pediatric: 0-17   M Maternity: 9-64   A Adult: 15-124   MCC Major Complication/Comorbidity   CC Complication/Comorbidity   SW Severe Wound Dx

902   ICD-10-CM 2020

O46.91   **Antepartum hemorrhage, unspecified, first trimester**   M ♀

O46.92   **Antepartum hemorrhage, unspecified, second trimester**   M ♀

O46.93   **Antepartum hemorrhage, unspecified, third trimester**   M ♀

√4ᵗʰ **O47**   **False labor**

INCLUDES   Braxton Hicks contractions
threatened labor

EXCLUDES 1   *preterm labor (O60.-)*

CC Excl: For CC codes in category O47: PDX collection 987

√5ᵗʰ **O47.0**   **False labor** before 37 completed weeks of gestation

O47.00   **False labor before 37 completed weeks of gestation, unspecified trimester**   M ♀

O47.02   **False labor before 37 completed weeks of gestation, second trimester**   CC M ♀

O47.03   **False labor before 37 completed weeks of gestation, third trimester**   CC M ♀

O47.1   **False labor** at or after 37 completed weeks of gestation   CC M ♀

O47.9   **False labor, unspecified**   M ♀

√4ᵗʰ **O48**   **Late pregnancy**

O48.0   **Post-term pregnancy**   M ♀

Pregnancy over 40 completed weeks to 42 completed weeks gestation

O48.1   **Prolonged pregnancy**   M ♀

Pregnancy which has advanced beyond 42 completed weeks gestation

AHA: 2016,1Q,5

Complications of labor and delivery (O60-O77)

√4ᵗʰ **O60**   **Preterm labor**

INCLUDES   onset (spontaneous) of labor before 37 completed weeks of gestation

EXCLUDES 1   *false labor (O47.0-)*
threatened labor NOS (O47.0-)

CC Excl: For CC/MCC codes in category O60: PDX collection 987

√5ᵗʰ **O60.0**   **Preterm labor** without delivery

O60.00   **Preterm labor without delivery, unspecified trimester**   M ♀

O60.02   **Preterm labor without delivery, second trimester**   MCC M ♀

O60.03   **Preterm labor without delivery, third trimester**   MCC M ♀

√5ᵗʰ **O60.1**   **Preterm labor** with preterm delivery

AHA: 2016,2Q,10

One of the following 7th characters is to be assigned to each code under subcategory O60.1. 7th character 0 is for single gestations and multiple gestations where the fetus is unspecified. 7th characters 1 through 9 are for cases of multiple gestations to identify the fetus for which the code applies. The appropriate code from category O30, Multiple gestation, must also be assigned when assigning a code from subcategory O60.1 that has a 7th character of 1 through 9.

0   not applicable or unspecified
1   fetus 1
2   fetus 2
3   fetus 3
4   fetus 4
5   fetus 5
9   other fetus

√x7ᵗʰ **O60.10**   **Preterm labor with preterm delivery, unspecified trimester**   CC M ♀

Preterm labor with delivery NOS

√x7ᵗʰ **O60.12**   **Preterm labor** second trimester **with preterm delivery** second trimester   MCC M ♀

√x7ᵗʰ **O60.13**   **Preterm labor** second trimester **with preterm delivery** third trimester   MCC M ♀

√x7ᵗʰ **O60.14**   **Preterm labor** third trimester **with preterm delivery** third trimester   MCC M ♀

√5ᵗʰ **O60.2**   **Term delivery with preterm labor**

One of the following 7th characters is to be assigned to each code under subcategory O60.2. 7th character 0 is for single gestations and multiple gestations where the fetus is unspecified. 7th characters 1 through 9 are for cases of multiple gestations to identify the fetus for which the code applies. The appropriate code from category O30, Multiple gestation, must also be assigned when assigning a code from subcategory O60.2 that has a 7th character of 1 through 9.

0   not applicable or unspecified
1   fetus 1
2   fetus 2
3   fetus 3
4   fetus 4
5   fetus 5
9   other fetus

√x7ᵗʰ **O60.20**   **Term delivery with preterm labor, unspecified trimester**   CC M ♀

√x7ᵗʰ **O60.22**   **Term delivery with preterm labor, second trimester**   MCC M ♀

√x7ᵗʰ **O60.23**   **Term delivery with preterm labor, third trimester**   MCC M ♀

√4ᵗʰ **O61**   **Failed induction of labor**

O61.0   **Failed** medical **induction of labor**   M ♀

Failed induction (of labor) by oxytocin
Failed induction (of labor) by prostaglandins

O61.1   **Failed** instrumental **induction of labor**   M ♀

Failed mechanical induction (of labor)
Failed surgical induction (of labor)

O61.8   **Other failed induction of labor**   M ♀

O61.9   **Failed induction of labor, unspecified**   M ♀

√4ᵗʰ **O62**   **Abnormalities of forces of labor**

DEF: Uterine inertia: Weak or poorly coordinated contractions of the uterus during labor.

O62.0   **Primary inadequate contractions**   M ♀

Failure of cervical dilatation
Primary hypotonic uterine dysfunction
Uterine inertia during latent phase of labor

O62.1   **Secondary uterine inertia**   M ♀

Arrested active phase of labor
Secondary hypotonic uterine dysfunction

O62.2   **Other uterine inertia**   M ♀

Atony of uterus without hemorrhage
Atony of uterus NOS
Desultory labor
Hypotonic uterine dysfunction NOS
Irregular labor
Poor contractions
Slow slope active phase of labor
Uterine inertia NOS

EXCLUDES 1   *atony of uterus with hemorrhage (postpartum) (O72.1)*
postpartum atony of uterus without hemorrhage (O75.89)

DEF: Uterine atony: Failure of the uterine muscles to contract after the fetus and placenta are delivered.

O62.3   **Precipitate labor**   M ♀

DEF: Rapid labor with delivery occurring in three hours or less from the onset of contractions.

O62.4   **Hypertonic, incoordinate, and prolonged uterine contractions**   M ♀

Cervical spasm
Contraction ring dystocia
Dyscoordinate labor
Hour-glass contraction of uterus
Hypertonic uterine dysfunction
Incoordinate uterine action
Tetanic contractions
Uterine dystocia NOS
Uterine spasm

EXCLUDES 1   *dystocia (fetal) (maternal) NOS (O66.9)*

O62.8   **Other abnormalities of forces of labor**   M ♀

O62.9   **Abnormality of forces of labor, unspecified**   M ♀

☑ Additional Character Required   √x7ᵗʰ Placeholder   Unacceptable PDx   Questionable PDx   Manifestation   Unspecified Dx   H1-H14 HAC   HCC CMS-HCC Dx   HIV HIV Dx

ICD-10-CM 2020   **903**

✓4ᵗʰ **O63 Long labor**

    O63.0 Prolonged first stage (of labor)   Ⓜ♀

    O63.1 Prolonged second stage (of labor)   Ⓜ♀

    O63.2 Delayed delivery of second twin, triplet, etc.   Ⓜ♀

    O63.9 Long labor, unspecified   ⒸⒸ♀

        Prolonged labor NOS
        CC Excl: PDX collection 988

✓4ᵗʰ **O64 Obstructed labor due to malposition and malpresentation of fetus**

> One of the following 7th characters is to be assigned to each code under category O64. 7th character Ø is for single gestations and multiple gestations where the fetus is unspecified. 7th characters 1 through 9 are for cases of multiple gestations to identify the fetus for which the code applies. The appropriate code from category O30, Multiple gestation, must also be assigned when assigning a code from category O64 that has a 7th character of 1 through 9.
>
> Ø not applicable or unspecified
> 1 fetus 1
> 2 fetus 2
> 3 fetus 3
> 4 fetus 4
> 5 fetus 5
> 9 other fetus

Fetal Malposition

Breech

Shoulder (arm prolapse)

Mother's pelvis

Compound (extremity together with head)

Face (mentum)

Oblique

✓x7ᵗʰ **O64.0 Obstructed labor due to incomplete rotation of fetal head**   Ⓜ♀

    Deep transverse arrest
    Obstructed labor due to persistent occipitoiliac (position)
    Obstructed labor due to persistent occipitoposterior (position)
    Obstructed labor due to persistent occipitosacral (position)
    Obstructed labor due to persistent occipitotransverse (position)

✓x7ᵗʰ **O64.1 Obstructed labor due to breech presentation**   Ⓜ♀

    Obstructed labor due to buttocks presentation
    Obstructed labor due to complete breech presentation
    Obstructed labor due to frank breech presentation

✓x7ᵗʰ **O64.2 Obstructed labor due to face presentation**   Ⓜ♀

    Obstructed labor due to chin presentation

✓x7ᵗʰ **O64.3 Obstructed labor due to brow presentation**   Ⓜ♀

✓x7ᵗʰ **O64.4 Obstructed labor due to shoulder presentation**   Ⓜ♀

    Prolapsed arm
    EXCLUDES 1   impacted shoulders (O66.0)
              shoulder dystocia (O66.0)

✓x7ᵗʰ **O64.5 Obstructed labor due to compound presentation**   Ⓜ♀

✓x7ᵗʰ **O64.8 Obstructed labor due to other malposition and malpresentation**   Ⓜ♀

    Obstructed labor due to footling presentation
    Obstructed labor due to incomplete breech presentation

✓x7ᵗʰ **O64.9 Obstructed labor due to malposition and malpresentation, unspecified**   Ⓜ♀

✓4ᵗʰ **O65 Obstructed labor due to maternal pelvic abnormality**

    O65.0 Obstructed labor due to deformed pelvis   Ⓜ♀

    O65.1 Obstructed labor due to generally contracted pelvis   Ⓜ♀

    O65.2 Obstructed labor due to pelvic inlet contraction   Ⓜ♀

    O65.3 Obstructed labor due to pelvic outlet and mid-cavity contraction   Ⓜ♀

    O65.4 Obstructed labor due to fetopelvic disproportion, unspecified   Ⓜ♀

        EXCLUDES 1   dystocia due to abnormality of fetus (O66.2-O66.3)

    O65.5 Obstructed labor due to abnormality of maternal pelvic organs   Ⓜ♀

        Obstructed labor due to conditions listed in O34.-
        Use additional code to identify abnormality of pelvic organs O34.-

    O65.8 Obstructed labor due to other maternal pelvic abnormalities   Ⓜ♀

    O65.9 Obstructed labor due to maternal pelvic abnormality, unspecified   Ⓜ♀

✓4ᵗʰ **O66 Other obstructed labor**

    O66.0 Obstructed labor due to shoulder dystocia   Ⓜ♀

        Impacted shoulders
        DEF: Obstructed labor due to impacted fetal shoulders. It is an emergency condition that may require cesarean section, forceps delivery, vacuum extraction, or symphysiotomy.

    O66.1 Obstructed labor due to locked twins   Ⓜ♀

    O66.2 Obstructed labor due to unusually large fetus   Ⓜ♀

    O66.3 Obstructed labor due to other abnormalities of fetus   Ⓜ♀

        Dystocia due to fetal ascites
        Dystocia due to fetal hydrops
        Dystocia due to fetal meningomyelocele
        Dystocia due to fetal sacral teratoma
        Dystocia due to fetal tumor
        Dystocia due to hydrocephalic fetus
        Use additional code to identify cause of obstruction

✓5ᵗʰ **O66.4 Failed trial of labor**

    O66.40 Failed trial of labor, unspecified   Ⓜ♀

    O66.41 Failed attempted vaginal birth after previous cesarean delivery   Ⓜ♀

        Code first rupture of uterus, if applicable (O71.0-, O71.1)

    O66.5 Attempted application of vacuum extractor and forceps   Ⓜ♀

        Attempted application of vacuum or forceps, with subsequent delivery by forceps or cesarean delivery

    O66.6 Obstructed labor due to other multiple fetuses   Ⓜ♀

    O66.8 Other specified obstructed labor   Ⓜ♀

        Use additional code to identify cause of obstruction

    O66.9 Obstructed labor, unspecified   Ⓜ♀

        Dystocia NOS
        Fetal dystocia NOS
        Maternal dystocia NOS

✓4ᵗʰ **O67 Labor and delivery complicated by intrapartum hemorrhage, not elsewhere classified**

    EXCLUDES 1   antepartum hemorrhage NEC (O46.-)
              placenta previa (O44.-)
              premature separation of placenta [abruptio placentae] (O45.-)
    EXCLUDES 2   postpartum hemorrhage (O72.-)

    O67.0 Intrapartum hemorrhage with coagulation defect   ⓂⒸⒸⓂ♀

        Intrapartum hemorrhage (excessive) associated with afibrinogenemia
        Intrapartum hemorrhage (excessive) associated with disseminated intravascular coagulation
        Intrapartum hemorrhage (excessive) associated with hyperfibrinolysis
        Intrapartum hemorrhage (excessive) associated with hypofibrinogenemia
        CC Excl: PDX collection 985

    O67.8 Other intrapartum hemorrhage   Ⓜ♀

        Excessive intrapartum hemorrhage

    O67.9 Intrapartum hemorrhage, unspecified   Ⓜ♀

Ⓝ Newborn: 0   Ⓟ Pediatric: 0-17   Ⓜ Maternity: 9-64   Ⓐ Adult: 15-124   ⓂⒸⒸ Major Complication/Comorbidity   ⒸⒸ Complication/Comorbidity   ⓈⓌ Severe Wound Dx

904   ICD-10-CM 2020

O68 Labor and delivery complicated by abnormality of fetal acid-base balance `CC` `M` ♀

Fetal acidemia complicating labor and delivery
Fetal acidosis complicating labor and delivery
Fetal alkalosis complicating labor and delivery
Fetal metabolic acidemia complicating labor and delivery

EXCLUDES 1   *fetal stress NOS (O77.9)*
labor and delivery complicated by electrocardiographic evidence of fetal stress (O77.8)
labor and delivery complicated by ultrasonic evidence of fetal stress (O77.8)

EXCLUDES 2   *abnormality in fetal heart rate or rhythm (O76)*
labor and delivery complicated by meconium in amniotic fluid (O77.0)

CC Excl: PDX collection 989

✓4ᵗʰ **O69 Labor and delivery complicated by umbilical cord complications**

AHA: 2016,1Q,5

One of the following 7th characters is to be assigned to each code under category O69. 7th character 0 is for single gestations and multiple gestations where the fetus is unspecified. 7th characters 1 through 9 are for cases of multiple gestations to identify the fetus for which the code applies. The appropriate code from category O30, Multiple gestation, must also be assigned when assigning a code from category O69 that has a 7th character of 1 through 9.

0   not applicable or unspecified
1   fetus 1
2   fetus 2
3   fetus 3
4   fetus 4
5   fetus 5
9   other fetus

✓x7ᵗʰ **O69.0 Labor and delivery complicated by prolapse of cord** `M` ♀
DEF: Abnormal presentation of the fetus marked by a protruding umbilical cord during labor. It can cause fetal death.

✓x7ᵗʰ **O69.1 Labor and delivery complicated by cord around neck, with compression** `M` ♀
EXCLUDES 1   *labor and delivery complicated by cord around neck, without compression (O69.81)*

✓x7ᵗʰ **O69.2 Labor and delivery complicated by other cord entanglement, with compression** `M` ♀
Labor and delivery complicated by compression of cord NOS
Labor and delivery complicated by entanglement of cords of twins in monoamniotic sac
Labor and delivery complicated by knot in cord
EXCLUDES 1   *labor and delivery complicated by other cord entanglement, without compression (O69.82)*

✓x7ᵗʰ **O69.3 Labor and delivery complicated by short cord** `M` ♀

✓x7ᵗʰ **O69.4 Labor and delivery complicated by vasa previa** `M` ♀
Labor and delivery complicated by hemorrhage from vasa previa

✓x7ᵗʰ **O69.5 Labor and delivery complicated by vascular lesion of cord** `M` ♀
Labor and delivery complicated by cord bruising
Labor and delivery complicated by cord hematoma
Labor and delivery complicated by thrombosis of umbilical vessels

✓5ᵗʰ **O69.8 Labor and delivery complicated by other cord complications**

✓x7ᵗʰ **O69.81 Labor and delivery complicated by cord around neck, without compression** `M` ♀
AHA: 2016,1Q,5

✓x7ᵗʰ **O69.82 Labor and delivery complicated by other cord entanglement, without compression** `M` ♀

✓x7ᵗʰ **O69.89 Labor and delivery complicated by other cord complications** `M` ♀

✓x7ᵗʰ **O69.9 Labor and delivery complicated by cord complication, unspecified** `M` ♀

✓4ᵗʰ **O70 Perineal laceration during delivery**

INCLUDES   episiotomy extended by laceration
EXCLUDES 1   *obstetric high vaginal laceration alone (O71.4)*

AHA: 2016,2Q,34; 2016,1Q,3-4,5

O70.0 First degree perineal laceration during delivery `M` ♀
Perineal laceration, rupture or tear involving fourchette during delivery
Perineal laceration, rupture or tear involving labia during delivery
Perineal laceration, rupture or tear involving skin during delivery
Perineal laceration, rupture or tear involving vagina during delivery
Perineal laceration, rupture or tear involving vulva during delivery
Slight perineal laceration, rupture or tear during delivery

O70.1 Second degree perineal laceration during delivery `M` ♀
Perineal laceration, rupture or tear during delivery as in O70.0, also involving pelvic floor
Perineal laceration, rupture or tear during delivery as in O70.0, also involving perineal muscles
Perineal laceration, rupture or tear during delivery as in O70.0, also involving vaginal muscles
EXCLUDES 1   *perineal laceration involving anal sphincter (O70.2)*

✓5ᵗʰ **O70.2 Third degree perineal laceration during delivery**
Perineal laceration, rupture or tear during delivery as in O70.1, also involving anal sphincter
Perineal laceration, rupture or tear during delivery as in O70.1, also involving rectovaginal septum
Perineal laceration, rupture or tear during delivery as in O70.1, also involving sphincter NOS
EXCLUDES 1   *anal sphincter tear during delivery without third degree perineal laceration (O70.4)*
perineal laceration involving anal or rectal mucosa (O70.3)

AHA: 2016,4Q,53-54

CC Excl: For CC codes in subcategory O70.2: PDX collection 990

O70.20 Third degree perineal laceration during delivery, unspecified `CC` `M` ♀

O70.21 Third degree perineal laceration during delivery, IIIa `CC` `M` ♀
Third degree perineal laceration during delivery with less than 50% of external anal sphincter (EAS) thickness torn

O70.22 Third degree perineal laceration during delivery, IIIb `CC` `M` ♀
Third degree perineal laceration during delivery with more than 50% external anal sphincter (EAS) thickness torn

O70.23 Third degree perineal laceration during delivery, IIIc `CC` `M` ♀
Third degree perineal laceration during delivery with both external anal sphincter (EAS) and internal anal sphincter (IAS) torn

O70.3 Fourth degree perineal laceration during delivery `CC` `M` ♀
Perineal laceration, rupture or tear during delivery as in O70.2, also involving anal mucosa
Perineal laceration, rupture or tear during delivery as in O70.2, also involving rectal mucosa
CC Excl: PDX collection 991

O70.4 Anal sphincter tear complicating delivery, not associated with third degree laceration `CC` `M` ♀
EXCLUDES 1   *anal sphincter tear with third degree perineal laceration (O70.2)*
CC Excl: PDX collection 992

O70.9 Perineal laceration during delivery, unspecified `M` ♀

✓4ᵗʰ **O71 Other obstetric trauma**

INCLUDES   obstetric damage from instruments

✓5ᵗʰ **O71.0 Rupture of uterus (spontaneous) before onset of labor**
EXCLUDES 1   *disruption of (current) cesarean delivery wound (O90.0)*
laceration of uterus, NEC (O71.81)

O71.00 Rupture of uterus before onset of labor, unspecified trimester `M` ♀

✅ Additional Character Required   ✓x7ᵗʰ Placeholder   Unacceptable PDx   Questionable PDx   Manifestation   Unspecified Dx   `H1`-`H14` HAC   `HCC` CMS-HCC Dx   `HIV` HIV Dx

ICD-10-CM 2020   905

Chapter 15. Pregnancy, Childbirth and the Puerperium

O71.02   **Rupture of uterus before onset of labor, second trimester**   MCC M ♀
     CC Excl: PDX collection 993

O71.03   **Rupture of uterus before onset of labor, third trimester**   MCC M ♀
     CC Excl: PDX collection 993

O71.1   **Rupture of uterus during labor**   MCC M ♀
    Rupture of uterus not stated as occurring before onset of labor
     EXCLUDES 1   disruption of cesarean delivery wound (O90.0)
         laceration of uterus, NEC (O71.81)
     CC Excl: PDX collection 993

O71.2   **Postpartum inversion of uterus**   CC M ♀
     CC Excl: PDX collection 994

O71.3   **Obstetric laceration of cervix**   CC M ♀
    Annular detachment of cervix
     CC Excl: PDX collection 995

O71.4   **Obstetric high vaginal laceration alone**   CC M ♀
    Laceration of vaginal wall without perineal laceration
     EXCLUDES 1   obstetric high vaginal laceration with perineal laceration (O70.-)
     AHA: 2016,1Q,5
     CC Excl: PDX collection 996

O71.5   **Other obstetric injury to pelvic organs**   CC M ♀
    Obstetric injury to bladder
    Obstetric injury to urethra
     EXCLUDES 2   obstetric periurethral trauma (O71.82)
     AHA: 2014,4Q,18
     CC Excl: PDX collection 993

O71.6   **Obstetric damage to pelvic joints and ligaments**   CC M ♀
    Obstetric avulsion of inner symphyseal cartilage
    Obstetric damage to coccyx
    Obstetric traumatic separation of symphysis (pubis)
     CC Excl: PDX collection 997

O71.7   **Obstetric hematoma of pelvis**   CC M ♀
    Obstetric hematoma of perineum
    Obstetric hematoma of vagina
    Obstetric hematoma of vulva
     CC Excl: PDX collection 998

✓5ᵗʰ **O71.8**   **Other specified obstetric trauma**

    O71.81   **Laceration of uterus, not elsewhere classified**   M ♀

    O71.82   **Other specified trauma to perineum and vulva**   M ♀
       Obstetric periurethral trauma
       AHA: 2016,1Q,4; 2014,4Q,18

    O71.89   **Other specified obstetric trauma**   M ♀

    O71.9   **Obstetric trauma, unspecified**   M ♀

✓4ᵗʰ **O72**   **Postpartum hemorrhage**
    INCLUDES   hemorrhage after delivery of fetus or infant

    O72.0   **Third-stage hemorrhage**   CC M ♀
       Hemorrhage associated with retained, trapped or adherent placenta
       Retained placenta NOS
       Code also type of adherent placenta (O43.2-)
       CC Excl: PDX collection 999

    O72.1   **Other immediate postpartum hemorrhage**   CC M ♀
       Hemorrhage following delivery of placenta
       Postpartum hemorrhage (atonic) NOS
       Uterine atony with hemorrhage
        EXCLUDES 1   uterine atony NOS (O62.2)
           uterine atony without hemorrhage (O62.2)
           postpartum atony of uterus without hemorrhage (O75.89)
       AHA: 2016,1Q,4
       DEF: Uterine atony: Failure of the uterine muscles to contract after the fetus and placenta are delivered.
       CC Excl: PDX collection 1000

    O72.2   **Delayed and secondary postpartum hemorrhage**   CC M ♀
       Hemorrhage associated with retained portions of placenta or membranes after the first 24 hours following delivery of placenta
       Retained products of conception NOS, following delivery
       CC Excl: PDX collection 1001

    O72.3   **Postpartum coagulation defects**   M ♀
       Postpartum afibrinogenemia
       Postpartum fibrinolysis

✓4ᵗʰ **O73**   **Retained placenta and membranes, without hemorrhage**
     EXCLUDES 1   placenta accreta (O43.21-)
         placenta increta (O43.22-)
         placenta percreta (O43.23-)
    DEF: Postpartum condition resulting from failure to expel placental membrane tissues due to failed contractions of the uterine wall.

    O73.0   **Retained placenta without hemorrhage**   M ♀
       Adherent placenta, without hemorrhage
       Trapped placenta without hemorrhage

    O73.1   **Retained portions of placenta and membranes, without hemorrhage**   M ♀
       Retained products of conception following delivery, without hemorrhage

✓4ᵗʰ **O74**   **Complications of anesthesia during labor and delivery**
    INCLUDES   maternal complications arising from the administration of a general, regional or local anesthetic, analgesic or other sedation during labor and delivery
    Use additional code, if applicable, to identify specific complication

    O74.0   **Aspiration pneumonitis due to anesthesia during labor and delivery**   M ♀
       Inhalation of stomach contents or secretions NOS due to anesthesia during labor and delivery
       Mendelson's syndrome due to anesthesia during labor and delivery

    O74.1   **Other pulmonary complications of anesthesia during labor and delivery**   M ♀

    O74.2   **Cardiac complications of anesthesia during labor and delivery**   M ♀

    O74.3   **Central nervous system complications of anesthesia during labor and delivery**   M ♀

    O74.4   **Toxic reaction to local anesthesia during labor and delivery**   M ♀

    O74.5   **Spinal and epidural anesthesia-induced headache during labor and delivery**   M ♀

    O74.6   **Other complications of spinal and epidural anesthesia during labor and delivery**   M ♀

    O74.7   **Failed or difficult intubation for anesthesia during labor and delivery**   M ♀

    O74.8   **Other complications of anesthesia during labor and delivery**   M ♀

    O74.9   **Complication of anesthesia during labor and delivery, unspecified**   M ♀

✓4ᵗʰ **O75**   **Other complications of labor and delivery, not elsewhere classified**
     EXCLUDES 2   puerperal (postpartum) infection (O86.-)
         puerperal (postpartum) sepsis (O85)

    O75.0   **Maternal distress during labor and delivery**   M ♀

    O75.1   **Shock during or following labor and delivery**   MCC M ♀
       Obstetric shock following labor and delivery
       CC Excl: PDX collection 1002

    O75.2   **Pyrexia during labor, not elsewhere classified**   CC M ♀
       CC Excl: PDX collection 1003

    O75.3   **Other infection during labor**   MCC M ♀
       Sepsis during labor
       Use additional code (B95-B97), to identify infectious agent
       CC Excl: PDX collection 1004

    O75.4   **Other complications of obstetric surgery and procedures**   M ♀
       Cardiac arrest following obstetric surgery or procedures
       Cardiac failure following obstetric surgery or procedures
       Cerebral anoxia following obstetric surgery or procedures
       Pulmonary edema following obstetric surgery or procedures
       Use additional code to identify specific complication
        EXCLUDES 2   complications of anesthesia during labor and delivery (O74.-)
           disruption of obstetrical (surgical) wound (O90.0-O90.1)
           hematoma of obstetrical (surgical) wound (O90.2)
           infection of obstetrical (surgical) wound (O86.0-)

    O75.5   **Delayed delivery after artificial rupture of membranes**   M ♀

✓5ᵗʰ **O75.8**   **Other specified complications of labor and delivery**

    O75.81   **Maternal exhaustion complicating labor and delivery**   M ♀

N Newborn: 0   P Pediatric: 0-17   M Maternity: 9-64   A Adult: 15-124   MCC Major Complication/Comorbidity   CC Complication/Comorbidity   SW Severe Wound Dx

906   ICD-10-CM 2020

O75.82 **Onset (spontaneous) of labor after 37 completed weeks of gestation but before 39 completed weeks gestation, with delivery by (planned) cesarean section**   M ♀

Delivery by (planned) cesarean section occurring after 37 completed weeks of gestation but before 39 completed weeks gestation due to (spontaneous) onset of labor

Code first to specify reason for planned cesarean section such as:

cephalopelvic disproportion (normally formed fetus) (O33.9)

previous cesarean delivery (O34.21)

O75.89 **Other specified complications of labor and delivery**   M ♀

O75.9 **Complication of labor and delivery, unspecified**   M ♀

O76 **Abnormality in fetal heart rate and rhythm complicating labor and delivery**   CC M ♀

Depressed fetal heart rate tones complicating labor and delivery

Fetal bradycardia complicating labor and delivery

Fetal heart rate decelerations complicating labor and delivery

Fetal heart rate irregularity complicating labor and delivery

Fetal heart rate abnormal variability complicating labor and delivery

Fetal tachycardia complicating labor and delivery

Non-reassuring fetal heart rate or rhythm complicating labor and delivery

> EXCLUDES 1   fetal stress NOS (O77.9)
>
> labor and delivery complicated by electrocardiographic evidence of fetal stress (O77.8)
>
> labor and delivery complicated by ultrasonic evidence of fetal stress (O77.8)
>
> EXCLUDES 2   fetal metabolic acidemia (O68)
>
> other fetal stress (O77.0-O77.1)

AHA: 2013,4Q,118

O77 **Other fetal stress complicating labor and delivery** ✓4th

O77.0 **Labor and delivery complicated by meconium in amniotic fluid**   M ♀

AHA: 2013,4Q,117-118

O77.1 **Fetal stress in labor or delivery due to drug administration**   M ♀

O77.8 **Labor and delivery complicated by other evidence of fetal stress**   M ♀

Labor and delivery complicated by electrocardiographic evidence of fetal stress

Labor and delivery complicated by ultrasonic evidence of fetal stress

> EXCLUDES 1   abnormality of fetal acid-base balance (O68)
>
> abnormality in fetal heart rate or rhythm (O76)
>
> fetal metabolic acidemia (O68)

O77.9 **Labor and delivery complicated by fetal stress, unspecified**   M ♀

> EXCLUDES 1   abnormality of fetal acid-base balance (O68)
>
> abnormality in fetal heart rate or rhythm (O76)
>
> fetal metabolic acidemia (O68)

Encounter for delivery (O80-O82)

O80 **Encounter for full-term uncomplicated delivery**   M ♀

> NOTE   Delivery requiring minimal or no assistance, with or without episiotomy, without fetal manipulation [e.g., rotation version] or instrumentation [forceps] of a spontaneous, cephalic, vaginal, full-term, single, live-born infant. This code is for use as a single diagnosis code and is not to be used with any other code from chapter 15.

Use additional code to indicate outcome of delivery (Z37.0)

AHA: 2016,4Q,150; 2014,2Q,9

O82 **Encounter for cesarean delivery without indication**   M ♀

Use additional code to indicate outcome of delivery (Z37.0)

Complications predominantly related to the puerperium (O85-O92)

> EXCLUDES 2   mental and behavioral disorders associated with the puerperium (F53.-)
>
> obstetrical tetanus (A34)
>
> puerperal osteomalacia (M83.0)

O85 **Puerperal sepsis**   MCC M ♀

Postpartum sepsis

Puerperal peritonitis

Puerperal pyemia

Use additional code (B95-B97), to identify infectious agent

Use additional code (R65.2-) to identify severe sepsis, if applicable

> EXCLUDES 1   fever of unknown origin following delivery (O86.4)
>
> genital tract infection following delivery (O86.1-)
>
> obstetric pyemic and septic embolism (O88.3-)
>
> puerperal septic thrombophlebitis (O86.81)
>
> urinary tract infection following delivery (O86.2-)
>
> EXCLUDES 2   sepsis during labor (O75.3)

AHA: 2018,4Q,23

CC Excl: PDX collection 1005

O86 **Other puerperal infections** ✓4th

Use additional code (B95-B97), to identify infectious agent

> EXCLUDES 2   infection during labor (O75.3)
>
> obstetrical tetanus (A34)

CC Excl: For codes in category O86:

For MCC codes: PDX collection 1005

For CC codes, unless otherwise noted: PDX collection 968

O86.0 **Infection of obstetric surgical wound** ✓5th

Infected cesarean delivery wound following delivery

Infected perineal repair following delivery

> EXCLUDES 1   complications of procedures, not elsewhere classified (T81.4-)
>
> postprocedural fever NOS (R50.82)
>
> postprocedural retroperitoneal abscess (K68.11)

AHA: 2018,4Q,22-23,62

O86.00 **Infection of obstetric surgical wound, unspecified**   M ♀

O86.01 **Infection of obstetric surgical wound, superficial incisional site**   M ♀

Subcutaneous abscess following an obstetrical procedure

Stitch abscess following an obstetrical procedure

O86.02 **Infection of obstetric surgical wound, deep incisional site**   M ♀

Intramuscular abscess following an obstetrical procedure

▶Sub-fascial abscess following an obstetrical procedure◀

O86.03 **Infection of obstetric surgical wound, organ and space site**   M ♀

Intraabdominal abscess following an obstetrical procedure

Subphrenic abscess following an obstetrical procedure

O86.04 **Sepsis following an obstetrical procedure**   MCC M ♀

Use additional code to identify the sepsis

AHA: 2019,2Q,39

O86.09 **Infection of obstetric surgical wound, other surgical site**   M ♀

O86.1 **Other infection of genital tract following delivery** ✓5th

O86.11 **Cervicitis following delivery**   CC M ♀

O86.12 **Endometritis following delivery**   CC M ♀

CC Excl: PDX collection 1005

O86.13 **Vaginitis following delivery**   CC M ♀

O86.19 **Other infection of genital tract following delivery**   CC M ♀

O86.2 **Urinary tract infection following delivery** ✓5th

O86.20 **Urinary tract infection following delivery, unspecified**   CC M ♀

Puerperal urinary tract infection NOS

O86.21 **Infection of kidney following delivery**   CC M ♀

O86.22 **Infection of bladder following delivery**   CC M ♀

Infection of urethra following delivery

O86.29 **Other urinary tract infection following delivery**   CC M ♀

✓ Additional Character Required   ✓x7th Placeholder   Unacceptable PDx   Questionable PDx   Manifestation   Unspecified Dx   H1-H14 HAC   HCC CMS-HCC Dx   HIV HIV Dx

ICD-10-CM 2020

907

Chapter 15. Pregnancy, Childbirth and the Puerperium

O86.4   **Pyrexia of unknown origin following delivery**   CC M ♀

Puerperal infection NOS following delivery

Puerperal pyrexia NOS following delivery

EXCLUDES 2   *pyrexia during labor (O75.2)*

DEF: Fever of unknown origin experienced by the mother after childbirth.

CC Excl: PDX collection 1006

√5ᵗʰ O86.8   **Other specified puerperal infections**

O86.81   **Puerperal septic thrombophlebitis**   MCC M ♀

O86.89   **Other specified puerperal infections**   MCC M ♀

√4ᵗʰ O87   **Venous complications and hemorrhoids in the puerperium**

INCLUDES   venous complications in labor, delivery and the puerperium

EXCLUDES 2   *obstetric embolism (O88.-)*

puerperal septic thrombophlebitis (O86.81)

venous complications in pregnancy (O22.-)

CC Excl: For CC/MCC codes in category O87: PDX collection 967

O87.0   **Superficial thrombophlebitis in the puerperium**   CC M ♀

Puerperal phlebitis NOS

Puerperal thrombosis NOS

O87.1   **Deep phlebothrombosis in the puerperium**   MCC M ♀

Deep vein thrombosis, postpartum

Pelvic thrombophlebitis, postpartum

Use additional code to identify the deep vein thrombosis (I82.4-, I82.5-, I82.62-. I82.72-)

Use additional code, if applicable, for associated long-term (current) use of anticoagulants (Z79.01)

O87.2   **Hemorrhoids in the puerperium**   CC M ♀

O87.3   **Cerebral venous thrombosis in the puerperium**   CC M ♀

Cerebrovenous sinus thrombosis in the puerperium

O87.4   **Varicose veins of lower extremity in the puerperium**   M ♀

O87.8   **Other venous complications in the puerperium**   CC M ♀

Genital varices in the puerperium

O87.9   **Venous complication in the puerperium, unspecified**   M ♀

Puerperal phlebopathy NOS

√4ᵗʰ O88   **Obstetric embolism**

EXCLUDES 1   *embolism complicating abortion NOS (O03.2)*

embolism complicating ectopic or molar pregnancy (O08.2)

embolism complicating failed attempted abortion (O07.2)

embolism complicating induced abortion (O04.7)

embolism complicating spontaneous abortion (O03.2, O03.7)

CC Excl: For CC/MCC codes in category O88: PDX collection 1007

√5ᵗʰ O88.0   **Obstetric air embolism**

DEF: Sudden blocking of the pulmonary artery or right ventricle with air or nitrogen bubbles.

√6ᵗʰ O88.01   **Obstetric air embolism in pregnancy**

O88.011   **Air embolism in pregnancy, first trimester**   MCC M ♀

O88.012   **Air embolism in pregnancy, second trimester**   MCC M ♀

O88.013   **Air embolism in pregnancy, third trimester**   MCC M ♀

O88.019   **Air embolism in pregnancy, unspecified trimester**   M ♀

O88.02   **Air embolism in childbirth**   MCC M ♀

O88.03   **Air embolism in the puerperium**   MCC M ♀

√5ᵗʰ O88.1   **Amniotic fluid embolism**

Anaphylactoid syndrome in pregnancy

√6ᵗʰ O88.11   **Amniotic fluid embolism in pregnancy**

O88.111   **Amniotic fluid embolism in pregnancy, first trimester**   MCC M ♀

O88.112   **Amniotic fluid embolism in pregnancy, second trimester**   MCC M ♀

O88.113   **Amniotic fluid embolism in pregnancy, third trimester**   MCC M ♀

O88.119   **Amniotic fluid embolism in pregnancy, unspecified trimester**   M ♀

O88.12   **Amniotic fluid embolism in childbirth**   MCC M ♀

O88.13   **Amniotic fluid embolism in the puerperium**   MCC M ♀

√5ᵗʰ O88.2   **Obstetric thromboembolism**

√6ᵗʰ O88.21   **Thromboembolism in pregnancy**

Obstetric (pulmonary) embolism NOS

O88.211   **Thromboembolism in pregnancy, first trimester**   MCC M ♀

O88.212   **Thromboembolism in pregnancy, second trimester**   MCC M ♀

O88.213   **Thromboembolism in pregnancy, third trimester**   MCC M ♀

O88.219   **Thromboembolism in pregnancy, unspecified trimester**   M ♀

O88.22   **Thromboembolism in childbirth**   MCC M ♀

O88.23   **Thromboembolism in the puerperium**   MCC M ♀

Puerperal (pulmonary) embolism NOS

√5ᵗʰ O88.3   **Obstetric pyemic and septic embolism**

√6ᵗʰ O88.31   **Pyemic and septic embolism in pregnancy**

O88.311   **Pyemic and septic embolism in pregnancy, first trimester**   MCC M ♀

O88.312   **Pyemic and septic embolism in pregnancy, second trimester**   MCC M ♀

O88.313   **Pyemic and septic embolism in pregnancy, third trimester**   MCC M ♀

O88.319   **Pyemic and septic embolism in pregnancy, unspecified trimester**   CC M ♀

O88.32   **Pyemic and septic embolism in childbirth**   MCC M ♀

O88.33   **Pyemic and septic embolism in the puerperium**   MCC M ♀

√5ᵗʰ O88.8   **Other obstetric embolism**

Obstetric fat embolism

√6ᵗʰ O88.81   **Other embolism in pregnancy**

O88.811   **Other embolism in pregnancy, first trimester**   MCC M ♀

O88.812   **Other embolism in pregnancy, second trimester**   MCC M ♀

O88.813   **Other embolism in pregnancy, third trimester**   MCC M ♀

O88.819   **Other embolism in pregnancy, unspecified trimester**   M ♀

O88.82   **Other embolism in childbirth**   MCC M ♀

O88.83   **Other embolism in the puerperium**   MCC M ♀

√4ᵗʰ O89   **Complications of anesthesia during the puerperium**

INCLUDES   maternal complications arising from the administration of a general, regional or local anesthetic, analgesic or other sedation during the puerperium

Use additional code, if applicable, to identify specific complication

√5ᵗʰ O89.0   **Pulmonary complications of anesthesia during the puerperium**

O89.01   **Aspiration pneumonitis due to anesthesia during the puerperium**   M ♀

Inhalation of stomach contents or secretions NOS due to anesthesia during the puerperium

Mendelson's syndrome due to anesthesia during the puerperium

O89.09   **Other pulmonary complications of anesthesia during the puerperium**   M ♀

O89.1   **Cardiac complications of anesthesia during the puerperium**   M ♀

O89.2   **Central nervous system complications of anesthesia during the puerperium**   M ♀

O89.3   **Toxic reaction to local anesthesia during the puerperium**   M ♀

O89.4   **Spinal and epidural anesthesia-induced headache during the puerperium**   M ♀

O89.5   **Other complications of spinal and epidural anesthesia during the puerperium**   M ♀

O89.6   **Failed or difficult intubation for anesthesia during the puerperium**   M ♀

O89.8   **Other complications of anesthesia during the puerperium**   M ♀

O89.9   **Complication of anesthesia during the puerperium, unspecified**   M ♀

N Newborn: 0   P Pediatric: 0-17   M Maternity: 9-64   A Adult: 15-124   MCC Major Complication/Comorbidity   CC Complication/Comorbidity   SW Severe Wound Dx

908   ICD-10-CM 2020

✓4ᵗʰ **O90 Complications of the puerperium, not elsewhere classified**

O90.0 Disruption of cesarean delivery wound   Ⓜ♀

Dehiscence of cesarean delivery wound

> EXCLUDES 1   *rupture of uterus (spontaneous) before onset of labor (O71.0-)*
> *rupture of uterus during labor (O71.1)*

O90.1 Disruption of perineal obstetric wound   Ⓜ♀

Disruption of wound of episiotomy
Disruption of wound of perineal laceration
Secondary perineal tear

O90.2 Hematoma of obstetric wound   Ⓜ♀

O90.3 Peripartum cardiomyopathy   MCC Ⓜ♀

Conditions in I42- arising during pregnancy and the puerperium

> EXCLUDES 1   *pre-existing heart disease complicating pregnancy and the puerperium (O99.4-)*

DEF: Any structural or functional abnormality of the ventricular myocardium. It is a noninflammatory disease of obscure or unknown etiology with onset during the postpartum period.
CC Excl: PDX collection 1008

O90.4 Postpartum acute kidney failure   MCC Ⓜ♀

Hepatorenal syndrome following labor and delivery
CC Excl: PDX collection 1009

O90.5 Postpartum thyroiditis   Ⓜ♀

O90.6 Postpartum mood disturbance   Ⓜ♀

Postpartum blues
Postpartum dysphoria
Postpartum sadness

> EXCLUDES 1   *postpartum depression (F53.0)*
> *puerperal psychosis (F53.1)*

✓5ᵗʰ **O90.8 Other complications of the puerperium, not elsewhere classified**

O90.81 Anemia of the puerperium   Ⓜ♀

Postpartum anemia NOS

> EXCLUDES 1   *pre-existing anemia complicating the puerperium (O99.03)*

O90.89 Other complications of the puerperium, not elsewhere classified   Ⓜ♀

Placental polyp

O90.9 Complication of the puerperium, unspecified   Ⓜ♀

✓4ᵗʰ **O91 Infections of breast associated with pregnancy, the puerperium and lactation**

Use additional code to identify infection

✓5ᵗʰ **O91.0 Infection of nipple associated with pregnancy, the puerperium and lactation**

✓6ᵗʰ **O91.01 Infection of nipple associated with pregnancy**

Gestational abscess of nipple

O91.011 Infection of nipple associated with pregnancy, first trimester   Ⓜ♀

O91.012 Infection of nipple associated with pregnancy, second trimester   Ⓜ♀

O91.013 Infection of nipple associated with pregnancy, third trimester   Ⓜ♀

O91.019 Infection of nipple associated with pregnancy, unspecified trimester   Ⓜ♀

O91.02 Infection of nipple associated with the puerperium   Ⓜ♀

Puerperal abscess of nipple

O91.03 Infection of nipple associated with lactation   Ⓜ♀

Abscess of nipple associated with lactation

✓5ᵗʰ **O91.1 Abscess of breast associated with pregnancy, the puerperium and lactation**

✓6ᵗʰ **O91.11 Abscess of breast associated with pregnancy**

Gestational mammary abscess
Gestational purulent mastitis
Gestational subareolar abscess

O91.111 Abscess of breast associated with pregnancy, first trimester   Ⓜ♀

O91.112 Abscess of breast associated with pregnancy, second trimester   Ⓜ♀

O91.113 Abscess of breast associated with pregnancy, third trimester   Ⓜ♀

O91.119 Abscess of breast associated with pregnancy, unspecified trimester   Ⓜ♀

O91.12 Abscess of breast associated with the puerperium   Ⓜ♀

Puerperal mammary abscess
Puerperal purulent mastitis
Puerperal subareolar abscess

O91.13 Abscess of breast associated with lactation   Ⓜ♀

Mammary abscess associated with lactation
Purulent mastitis associated with lactation
Subareolar abscess associated with lactation

✓5ᵗʰ **O91.2 Nonpurulent mastitis associated with pregnancy, the puerperium and lactation**

✓6ᵗʰ **O91.21 Nonpurulent mastitis associated with pregnancy**

Gestational interstitial mastitis
Gestational lymphangitis of breast
Gestational mastitis NOS
Gestational parenchymatous mastitis

O91.211 Nonpurulent mastitis associated with pregnancy, first trimester   Ⓜ♀

O91.212 Nonpurulent mastitis associated with pregnancy, second trimester   Ⓜ♀

O91.213 Nonpurulent mastitis associated with pregnancy, third trimester   Ⓜ♀

O91.219 Nonpurulent mastitis associated with pregnancy, unspecified trimester   Ⓜ♀

O91.22 Nonpurulent mastitis associated with the puerperium   Ⓜ♀

Puerperal interstitial mastitis
Puerperal lymphangitis of breast
Puerperal mastitis NOS
Puerperal parenchymatous mastitis

O91.23 Nonpurulent mastitis associated with lactation   Ⓜ♀

Interstitial mastitis associated with lactation
Lymphangitis of breast associated with lactation
Mastitis NOS associated with lactation
Parenchymatous mastitis associated with lactation

✓4ᵗʰ **O92 Other disorders of breast and disorders of lactation associated with pregnancy and the puerperium**

✓5ᵗʰ **O92.0 Retracted nipple associated with pregnancy, the puerperium, and lactation**

✓6ᵗʰ **O92.01 Retracted nipple associated with pregnancy**

O92.011 Retracted nipple associated with pregnancy, first trimester   Ⓜ♀

O92.012 Retracted nipple associated with pregnancy, second trimester   Ⓜ♀

O92.013 Retracted nipple associated with pregnancy, third trimester   Ⓜ♀

O92.019 Retracted nipple associated with pregnancy, unspecified trimester   Ⓜ♀

O92.02 Retracted nipple associated with the puerperium   Ⓜ♀

O92.03 Retracted nipple associated with lactation   Ⓜ♀

✓5ᵗʰ **O92.1 Cracked nipple associated with pregnancy, the puerperium, and lactation**

Fissure of nipple, gestational or puerperal

✓6ᵗʰ **O92.11 Cracked nipple associated with pregnancy**

O92.111 Cracked nipple associated with pregnancy, first trimester   Ⓜ♀

O92.112 Cracked nipple associated with pregnancy, second trimester   Ⓜ♀

O92.113 Cracked nipple associated with pregnancy, third trimester   Ⓜ♀

O92.119 Cracked nipple associated with pregnancy, unspecified trimester   Ⓜ♀

O92.12 Cracked nipple associated with the puerperium   Ⓜ♀

O92.13 Cracked nipple associated with lactation   Ⓜ♀

√5ᵗʰ O92.2 Other and unspecified disorders of breast associated with pregnancy and the puerperium

    O92.20 Unspecified disorder of breast associated M ♀
        with pregnancy and the puerperium

    O92.29 Other disorders of breast associated with M ♀
        pregnancy and the puerperium

O92.3 Agalactia   M ♀

    Primary agalactia

    EXCLUDES 1   *elective agalactia (O92.5)*
              secondary agalactia (O92.5)
              therapeutic agalactia (O92.5)

    DEF: Absence of milk secretion in a female after delivery.

O92.4 Hypogalactia   M ♀

O92.5 Suppressed lactation   M ♀

    Elective agalactia
    Secondary agalactia
    Therapeutic agalactia

    EXCLUDES 1   *primary agalactia (O92.3)*

O92.6 Galactorrhea   M ♀

    DEF: Excessive or persistent milk secretion by the breast that may occur in the absence of nursing.

√5ᵗʰ O92.7 Other and unspecified disorders of lactation

    O92.70 Unspecified disorders of lactation   M ♀

    O92.79 Other disorders of lactation   M ♀

        Puerperal galactocele

Other obstetric conditions, not elsewhere classified (O94-O9A)

O94 Sequelae of complication of pregnancy, childbirth, and M ♀
the puerperium

    NOTE   This category is to be used to indicate conditions in O00-O77.-, O85-O94 and O98-O9A.- as the cause of late effects. The sequelae include conditions specified as such, or as late effects, which may occur at any time after the puerperium

    Code first condition resulting from (sequela) of complication of pregnancy, childbirth, and the puerperium

√4ᵗʰ O98 Maternal infectious and parasitic diseases classifiable elsewhere but complicating pregnancy, childbirth and the puerperium

    INCLUDES   the listed conditions when complicating the pregnant state, when aggravated by the pregnancy, or as a reason for obstetric care

    Use additional code (Chapter 1), to identify specific infectious or parasitic disease

    EXCLUDES 2   *herpes gestationis (O26.4-)*
             infectious carrier state (O99.82-, O99.83-)
             obstetrical tetanus (A34)
             puerperal infection (O86.-)
             puerperal sepsis (O85)
             when the reason for maternal care is that the disease is known or suspected to have affected the fetus (O35-O36)

√5ᵗʰ O98.0 Tuberculosis complicating pregnancy, childbirth and the puerperium

    Conditions in A15-A19

    CC Excl: For CC codes in subcategory O98.0: PDX collection 1011

    √6ᵗʰ O98.01 Tuberculosis complicating pregnancy

        O98.011 Tuberculosis complicating CC M ♀
            pregnancy, first trimester

        O98.012 Tuberculosis complicating CC M ♀
            pregnancy, second trimester

        O98.013 Tuberculosis complicating CC M ♀
            pregnancy, third trimester

        O98.019 Tuberculosis complicating M ♀
            pregnancy, unspecified trimester

    O98.02 Tuberculosis complicating childbirth CC M ♀

    O98.03 Tuberculosis complicating the CC M ♀
        puerperium

√5ᵗʰ O98.1 Syphilis complicating pregnancy, childbirth, and the puerperium

    Conditions in A50-A53

    CC Excl: For CC codes in subcategory O98.1: PDX collection 1012

    √6ᵗʰ O98.11 Syphilis complicating pregnancy

        O98.111 Syphilis complicating CC M ♀
            pregnancy, first trimester

        O98.112 Syphilis complicating CC M ♀
            pregnancy, second trimester

        O98.113 Syphilis complicating CC M ♀
            pregnancy, third trimester

        O98.119 Syphilis complicating M ♀
            pregnancy, unspecified trimester

    O98.12 Syphilis complicating childbirth CC M ♀

    O98.13 Syphilis complicating the puerperium CC M ♀

√5ᵗʰ O98.2 Gonorrhea complicating pregnancy, childbirth and the puerperium

    Conditions in A54.-

    CC Excl: For CC codes in subcategory O98.2: PDX collection 1012

    √6ᵗʰ O98.21 Gonorrhea complicating pregnancy

        O98.211 Gonorrhea complicating CC M ♀
            pregnancy, first trimester

        O98.212 Gonorrhea complicating CC M ♀
            pregnancy, second trimester

        O98.213 Gonorrhea complicating CC M ♀
            pregnancy, third trimester

        O98.219 Gonorrhea complicating M ♀
            pregnancy, unspecified trimester

    O98.22 Gonorrhea complicating childbirth CC M ♀

    O98.23 Gonorrhea complicating the puerperium CC M ♀

√5ᵗʰ O98.3 Other infections with a predominantly sexual mode of transmission complicating pregnancy, childbirth and the puerperium

    Conditions in A55-A64

    √6ᵗʰ O98.31 Other infections with a predominantly sexual mode of transmission complicating pregnancy

        O98.311 Other infections with a M ♀
            predominantly sexual mode of transmission complicating pregnancy, first trimester

        O98.312 Other infections with a M ♀
            predominantly sexual mode of transmission complicating pregnancy, second trimester

        O98.313 Other infections with a M ♀
            predominantly sexual mode of transmission complicating pregnancy, third trimester

        O98.319 Other infections with a M ♀
            predominantly sexual mode of transmission complicating pregnancy, unspecified trimester

    O98.32 Other infections with a predominantly M ♀
        sexual mode of transmission complicating childbirth

    O98.33 Other infections with a predominantly M ♀
        sexual mode of transmission complicating the puerperium

√5ᵗʰ O98.4 Viral hepatitis complicating pregnancy, childbirth and the puerperium

    Conditions in B15-B19

    CC Excl: For CC codes in subcategory O98.4: PDX collection 1013

    √6ᵗʰ O98.41 Viral hepatitis complicating pregnancy

        O98.411 Viral hepatitis complicating CC M ♀
            pregnancy, first trimester

        O98.412 Viral hepatitis complicating CC M ♀
            pregnancy, second trimester

        O98.413 Viral hepatitis complicating CC M ♀
            pregnancy, third trimester

        O98.419 Viral hepatitis complicating M ♀
            pregnancy, unspecified trimester

    O98.42 Viral hepatitis complicating childbirth CC M ♀

    O98.43 Viral hepatitis complicating the CC M ♀
        puerperium

N Newborn: 0   P Pediatric: 0-17   M Maternity: 9-64   A Adult: 15-124   MCC Major Complication/Comorbidity   CC Complication/Comorbidity   SW Severe Wound Dx

910   ICD-10-CM 2020

√5ᵗʰ **O98.5 Other viral diseases complicating pregnancy, childbirth and the puerperium**
Conditions in A80-B09, B25-B34, R87.81-, R87.82-
  EXCLUDES 1 *human immunodeficiency virus [HIV] disease complicating pregnancy, childbirth and the puerperium (O98.7-)*
CC Excl: For CC codes in subcategory O98.5: PDX collection 1013

√6ᵗʰ **O98.51 Other viral diseases complicating pregnancy**
- **O98.511 Other viral diseases complicating pregnancy, first trimester** cc M ♀
- **O98.512 Other viral diseases complicating pregnancy, second trimester** cc M ♀
- **O98.513 Other viral diseases complicating pregnancy, third trimester** cc M ♀
- **O98.519 Other viral diseases complicating pregnancy, unspecified trimester** M ♀
O98.52 Other viral diseases complicating childbirth M ♀
O98.53 Other viral diseases complicating the puerperium cc M ♀

√5ᵗʰ **O98.6 Protozoal diseases complicating pregnancy, childbirth and the puerperium**
Conditions in B50-B64
CC Excl: For CC codes in subcategory O98.6, unless otherwise noted: PDX collection 1014

√6ᵗʰ **O98.61 Protozoal diseases complicating pregnancy**
- **O98.611 Protozoal diseases complicating pregnancy, first trimester** cc M ♀
- **O98.612 Protozoal diseases complicating pregnancy, second trimester** cc M ♀
- **O98.613 Protozoal diseases complicating pregnancy, third trimester** cc M ♀
- **O98.619 Protozoal diseases complicating pregnancy, unspecified trimester** M ♀
O98.62 Protozoal diseases complicating childbirth cc M ♀
  CC Excl: PDX collection 1015
O98.63 Protozoal diseases complicating the puerperium cc M ♀
  CC Excl: PDX collection 1015

√5ᵗʰ **O98.7 Human immunodeficiency virus [HIV] disease complicating pregnancy, childbirth and the puerperium**
Use additional code to identify the type of HIV disease:
  acquired immune deficiency syndrome (AIDS) (B20)
  asymptomatic HIV status (Z21)
  HIV positive NOS (Z21)
  symptomatic HIV disease (B20)
CC Excl: For CC codes in subcategory O98.7: PDX collection 1013

√6ᵗʰ **O98.71 Human immunodeficiency virus [HIV] disease complicating pregnancy**
- **O98.711 Human immunodeficiency virus [HIV] disease complicating pregnancy, first trimester** cc M ♀
- **O98.712 Human immunodeficiency virus [HIV] disease complicating pregnancy, second trimester** cc M ♀
- **O98.713 Human immunodeficiency virus [HIV] disease complicating pregnancy, third trimester** cc M ♀
- **O98.719 Human immunodeficiency virus [HIV] disease complicating pregnancy, unspecified trimester** M ♀
O98.72 Human immunodeficiency virus [HIV] disease complicating childbirth cc M ♀
O98.73 Human immunodeficiency virus [HIV] disease complicating the puerperium cc M ♀

√5ᵗʰ **O98.8 Other maternal infectious and parasitic diseases complicating pregnancy, childbirth and the puerperium**
CC Excl: For CC codes in subcategory O98.8: PDX collection 1013

√6ᵗʰ **O98.81 Other maternal infectious and parasitic diseases complicating pregnancy**
- **O98.811 Other maternal infectious and parasitic diseases complicating pregnancy, first trimester** cc M ♀
- **O98.812 Other maternal infectious and parasitic diseases complicating pregnancy, second trimester** cc M ♀
- **O98.813 Other maternal infectious and parasitic diseases complicating pregnancy, third trimester** cc M ♀
- **O98.819 Other maternal infectious and parasitic diseases complicating pregnancy, unspecified trimester** M ♀
O98.82 Other maternal infectious and parasitic diseases complicating childbirth cc M ♀
O98.83 Other maternal infectious and parasitic diseases complicating the puerperium cc M ♀

√5ᵗʰ **O98.9 Unspecified maternal infectious and parasitic disease complicating pregnancy, childbirth and the puerperium**
CC Excl: For CC codes in subcategory O98.9: PDX collection 1013

√6ᵗʰ **O98.91 Unspecified maternal infectious and parasitic disease complicating pregnancy**
- **O98.911 Unspecified maternal infectious and parasitic disease complicating pregnancy, first trimester** cc M ♀
- **O98.912 Unspecified maternal infectious and parasitic disease complicating pregnancy, second trimester** cc M ♀
- **O98.913 Unspecified maternal infectious and parasitic disease complicating pregnancy, third trimester** cc M ♀
- **O98.919 Unspecified maternal infectious and parasitic disease complicating pregnancy, unspecified trimester** M ♀
O98.92 Unspecified maternal infectious and parasitic disease complicating childbirth cc M ♀
O98.93 Unspecified maternal infectious and parasitic disease complicating the puerperium cc M ♀

√4ᵗʰ **O99 Other maternal diseases classifiable elsewhere but complicating pregnancy, childbirth and the puerperium**
  INCLUDES conditions which complicate the pregnant state, are aggravated by the pregnancy or are a main reason for obstetric care
Use additional code to identify specific condition
  EXCLUDES 2 *when the reason for maternal care is that the condition is known or suspected to have affected the fetus (O35-O36)*

√5ᵗʰ **O99.0 Anemia complicating pregnancy, childbirth and the puerperium**
Conditions in D50-D64
  EXCLUDES 1 *anemia arising in the puerperium (O90.81)*
    postpartum anemia NOS (O90.81)

√6ᵗʰ **O99.01 Anemia complicating pregnancy**
  AHA: 2016,1Q,4
- **O99.011 Anemia complicating pregnancy, first trimester** M ♀
- **O99.012 Anemia complicating pregnancy, second trimester** M ♀
- **O99.013 Anemia complicating pregnancy, third trimester** M ♀
- **O99.019 Anemia complicating pregnancy, unspecified trimester** M ♀
O99.02 Anemia complicating childbirth M ♀
O99.03 Anemia complicating the puerperium M ♀
  EXCLUDES 1 *postpartum anemia not pre-existing prior to delivery (O90.81)*

√5ᵗʰ **O99.1** **Other diseases of the blood and blood-forming organs and certain disorders involving the immune mechanism complicating pregnancy, childbirth and the puerperium**
Conditions in D65-D89
EXCLUDES 1 *hemorrhage with coagulation defects (O45.-, O46.0-, O67.0, O72.3)*
CC Excl: For CC codes in subcategory O99.1, unless otherwise noted: PDX collection 1016

√6ᵗʰ **O99.11** **Other diseases of the blood and blood-forming organs and certain disorders involving the immune mechanism complicating** pregnancy

O99.111 Other diseases of the blood and blood-forming organs and certain disorders involving the immune mechanism complicating pregnancy, **first trimester**   CC M ♀

O99.112 Other diseases of the blood and blood-forming organs and certain disorders involving the immune mechanism complicating pregnancy, **second trimester**   CC M ♀

O99.113 Other diseases of the blood and blood-forming organs and certain disorders involving the immune mechanism complicating pregnancy, **third trimester**   CC M ♀

O99.119 Other diseases of the blood and blood-forming organs and certain disorders involving the immune mechanism complicating pregnancy, **unspecified trimester**   CC M ♀
CC Excl: PDX collection 1017

O99.12 Other diseases of the blood and blood-forming organs and certain disorders involving the immune mechanism complicating **childbirth**   CC M ♀

O99.13 Other diseases of the blood and blood-forming organs and certain disorders involving the immune mechanism complicating the **puerperium**   CC M ♀

√5ᵗʰ **O99.2** **Endocrine, nutritional and metabolic diseases complicating pregnancy, childbirth and the puerperium**
Conditions in E00-E88
EXCLUDES 2 *diabetes mellitus (O24.-)*
malnutrition (O25.-)
postpartum thyroiditis (O90.5)

√6ᵗʰ **O99.21** **Obesity complicating pregnancy, childbirth, and the puerperium**
Use additional code to identify the type of obesity (E66.-)
AHA: 2018,4Q,80
TIP: Do not assign a BMI code (Z68.-) for obese or overweight patients who are pregnant.

O99.210 Obesity complicating pregnancy, unspecified trimester   M ♀

O99.211 Obesity complicating pregnancy, **first trimester**   M ♀

O99.212 Obesity complicating pregnancy, **second trimester**   M ♀

O99.213 Obesity complicating pregnancy, **third trimester**   M ♀

O99.214 Obesity complicating **childbirth**   M ♀

O99.215 Obesity complicating the **puerperium**   M ♀

√6ᵗʰ **O99.28** **Other endocrine, nutritional and metabolic diseases complicating pregnancy, childbirth and the puerperium**

O99.280 Endocrine, nutritional and metabolic diseases complicating pregnancy, unspecified trimester   M ♀

O99.281 Endocrine, nutritional and metabolic diseases complicating pregnancy, **first trimester**   M ♀

O99.282 Endocrine, nutritional and metabolic diseases complicating pregnancy, **second trimester**   M ♀

O99.283 Endocrine, nutritional and metabolic diseases complicating pregnancy, **third trimester**   M ♀

O99.284 Endocrine, nutritional and metabolic diseases complicating **childbirth**   M ♀

O99.285 Endocrine, nutritional and metabolic diseases complicating the **puerperium**   M ♀

√5ᵗʰ **O99.3** **Mental disorders and diseases of the nervous system complicating pregnancy, childbirth and the puerperium**
CC Excl: For CC codes in subcategory O99.3, unless otherwise noted: PDX collection 1018

√6ᵗʰ **O99.31** **Alcohol use complicating pregnancy, childbirth, and the puerperium**
Use additional code(s) from F10 to identify manifestations of the alcohol use

O99.310 Alcohol use complicating pregnancy, unspecified trimester   M ♀

O99.311 Alcohol use complicating pregnancy, **first trimester**   M ♀

O99.312 Alcohol use complicating pregnancy, **second trimester**   M ♀

O99.313 Alcohol use complicating pregnancy, **third trimester**   M ♀

O99.314 Alcohol use complicating **childbirth**   M ♀

O99.315 Alcohol use complicating the **puerperium**   M ♀

√6ᵗʰ **O99.32** **Drug use complicating pregnancy, childbirth, and the puerperium**
Use additional code(s) from F11-F16 and F18-F19 to identify manifestations of the drug use
AHA: 2018,4Q,69-70; 2018,2Q,10
TIP: When drug use is documented during pregnancy, assign first a code from this subcategory followed by an additional code from F11-F16 and F18-F19 identifying the specific drug use even if not documented as associated with a physical, mental, or behavioral disorder. According to chapter 15 guidelines, it is the provider's responsibility to state that the condition being treated is *not* affecting the pregnancy.

O99.320 Drug use complicating pregnancy, unspecified trimester   M ♀

O99.321 Drug use complicating pregnancy, **first trimester**   CC M ♀

O99.322 Drug use complicating pregnancy, **second trimester**   CC M ♀

O99.323 Drug use complicating pregnancy, **third trimester**   CC M ♀

O99.324 Drug use complicating **childbirth**   CC M ♀

O99.325 Drug use complicating the **puerperium**   CC M ♀

√6ᵗʰ **O99.33** **Tobacco use disorder complicating pregnancy, childbirth, and the puerperium**
Smoking complicating pregnancy, childbirth, and the puerperium
Use additional code from category F17 to identify type of tobacco nicotine dependence

O99.330 Smoking (tobacco) complicating pregnancy, unspecified trimester   M ♀

O99.331 Smoking (tobacco) complicating pregnancy, **first trimester**   M ♀

O99.332 Smoking (tobacco) complicating pregnancy, **second trimester**   M ♀

O99.333 Smoking (tobacco) complicating pregnancy, **third trimester**   M ♀

O99.334 Smoking (tobacco) complicating **childbirth**   M ♀

O99.335 Smoking (tobacco) complicating the **puerperium**   M ♀

✓6ᵗʰ **O99.34** **Other mental disorders complicating pregnancy, childbirth, and the puerperium**
▶Conditions in F01-F09, F20-F99 and F54-F99◀
EXCLUDES 2 *postpartum mood disturbance (O90.6)*
postnatal psychosis (F53.1)
puerperal psychosis (F53.1)

O99.340 Other mental disorders complicating pregnancy, unspecified trimester M ♀

O99.341 Other mental disorders complicating pregnancy, first trimester M ♀

O99.342 Other mental disorders complicating pregnancy, second trimester M ♀

O99.343 Other mental disorders complicating pregnancy, third trimester M ♀

O99.344 Other mental disorders complicating childbirth M ♀

O99.345 Other mental disorders complicating the puerperium M ♀
AHA: 2018,4Q,8

✓6ᵗʰ **O99.35** **Diseases of the nervous system complicating pregnancy, childbirth, and the puerperium**
Conditions in G00-G99
EXCLUDES 2 *pregnancy related peripheral neuritis (O26.8-)*

O99.350 Diseases of the nervous system complicating pregnancy, unspecified trimester M ♀

O99.351 Diseases of the nervous system complicating pregnancy, first trimester M ♀

O99.352 Diseases of the nervous system complicating pregnancy, second trimester M ♀

O99.353 Diseases of the nervous system complicating pregnancy, third trimester M ♀

O99.354 Diseases of the nervous system complicating childbirth CC M ♀
CC Excl: PDX collection 1016

O99.355 Diseases of the nervous system complicating the puerperium CC M ♀
CC Excl: PDX collection 1016

✓5ᵗʰ **O99.4** **Diseases of the circulatory system complicating pregnancy, childbirth and the puerperium**
Conditions in I00-I99
EXCLUDES 1 *peripartum cardiomyopathy (O90.3)*
EXCLUDES 2 *hypertensive disorders (O10-O16)*
obstetric embolism (O88.-)
venous complications and cerebrovenous sinus thrombosis in labor, childbirth and the puerperium (O87.-)
venous complications and cerebrovenous sinus thrombosis in pregnancy (O22.-)
AHA: 2016,2Q,8
CC Excl: For CC codes in subcategory O99.4, unless otherwise noted: PDX collection 1019

✓6ᵗʰ **O99.41** **Diseases of the circulatory system complicating pregnancy**

O99.411 Diseases of the circulatory system complicating pregnancy, first trimester CC M ♀

O99.412 Diseases of the circulatory system complicating pregnancy, second trimester CC M ♀

O99.413 Diseases of the circulatory system complicating pregnancy, third trimester CC M ♀

O99.419 Diseases of the circulatory system complicating pregnancy, unspecified trimester M ♀

O99.42 Diseases of the circulatory system complicating childbirth MCC M ♀
CC Excl: PDX collection 1008

O99.43 Diseases of the circulatory system complicating the puerperium CC M ♀

✓5ᵗʰ **O99.5** **Diseases of the respiratory system complicating pregnancy, childbirth and the puerperium**
Conditions in J00-J99

✓6ᵗʰ **O99.51** **Diseases of the respiratory system complicating pregnancy**

O99.511 Diseases of the respiratory system complicating pregnancy, first trimester M ♀

O99.512 Diseases of the respiratory system complicating pregnancy, second trimester M ♀

O99.513 Diseases of the respiratory system complicating pregnancy, third trimester M ♀

O99.519 Diseases of the respiratory system complicating pregnancy, unspecified trimester M ♀

O99.52 Diseases of the respiratory system complicating childbirth M ♀

O99.53 Diseases of the respiratory system complicating the puerperium M ♀

✓5ᵗʰ **O99.6** **Diseases of the digestive system complicating pregnancy, childbirth and the puerperium**
Conditions in K00-K93
EXCLUDES 2 *hemorrhoids in pregnancy (O22.4-)*
liver and biliary tract disorders in pregnancy, childbirth and the puerperium (O26.6-)

✓6ᵗʰ **O99.61** **Diseases of the digestive system complicating pregnancy**
AHA: 2016,1Q,4

O99.611 Diseases of the digestive system complicating pregnancy, first trimester M ♀

O99.612 Diseases of the digestive system complicating pregnancy, second trimester M ♀

O99.613 Diseases of the digestive system complicating pregnancy, third trimester M ♀

O99.619 Diseases of the digestive system complicating pregnancy, unspecified trimester M ♀

O99.62 Diseases of the digestive system complicating childbirth M ♀

O99.63 Diseases of the digestive system complicating the puerperium M ♀

✓5ᵗʰ **O99.7** **Diseases of the skin and subcutaneous tissue complicating pregnancy, childbirth and the puerperium**
Conditions in L00-L99
EXCLUDES 2 *herpes gestationis (O26.4)*
pruritic urticarial papules and plaques of pregnancy (PUPPP) (O26.86)

✓6ᵗʰ **O99.71** **Diseases of the skin and subcutaneous tissue complicating pregnancy**

O99.711 Diseases of the skin and subcutaneous tissue complicating pregnancy, first trimester M ♀

O99.712 Diseases of the skin and subcutaneous tissue complicating pregnancy, second trimester M ♀

O99.713 Diseases of the skin and subcutaneous tissue complicating pregnancy, third trimester M ♀

O99.719 Diseases of the skin and subcutaneous tissue complicating pregnancy, unspecified trimester M ♀

O99.72 Diseases of the skin and subcutaneous tissue complicating childbirth M ♀

O99.73 Diseases of the skin and subcutaneous tissue complicating the puerperium M ♀

✓5ᵗʰ O99.8 Other specified diseases and conditions complicating pregnancy, childbirth and the puerperium
Conditions in D00-D48, H00-H95, M00-N99, and Q00-Q99
Use additional code to identify condition
    EXCLUDES 2   genitourinary infections in pregnancy (O23.-)
         infection of genitourinary tract following delivery
           ▶(O86.1-O86.4)◀
         malignant neoplasm complicating pregnancy,
           childbirth and the puerperium (O9A.1-)
         maternal care for known or suspected abnormality
           of maternal pelvic organs (O34.-)
         postpartum acute kidney failure (O90.4)
         traumatic injuries in pregnancy (O9A.2-)
    CC Excl: For CC codes in subcategory O99.8: PDX collection 1013

✓6ᵗʰ O99.81 Abnormal glucose complicating pregnancy, childbirth and the puerperium
    EXCLUDES 1   gestational diabetes (O24.4-)
    O99.810 Abnormal glucose complicating pregnancy Ⓜ ♀
    O99.814 Abnormal glucose complicating childbirth Ⓜ ♀
    O99.815 Abnormal glucose complicating the puerperium Ⓜ ♀

✓6ᵗʰ O99.82 Streptococcus B carrier state complicating pregnancy, childbirth and the puerperium
    EXCLUDES 1   carrier of streptococcus group B (GBS) in a nonpregnant woman (Z22.330)
    DEF: *Streptococcus* group B colonization: Bacteria normally found in the vagina or lower intestine of many healthy adult women that may infect the fetus during childbirth, causing mental or physical handicaps or death. Women who test positive for *streptococcus* Group B during pregnancy are considered a "colonized" status and are treated with IV antibiotics at the time of delivery and may also be treated with oral antibiotics during the pregnancy.
    O99.820 Streptococcus B carrier state complicating pregnancy Ⓜ ♀
    O99.824 Streptococcus B carrier state complicating childbirth Ⓜ ♀
          AHA: 2019,2Q,8
    O99.825 Streptococcus B carrier state complicating the puerperium Ⓜ ♀

✓6ᵗʰ O99.83 Other infection carrier state complicating pregnancy, childbirth and the puerperium
    Use additional code to identify the carrier state (Z22.-)
    O99.830 Other infection carrier state complicating pregnancy ᴄᴄ Ⓜ ♀
    O99.834 Other infection carrier state complicating childbirth ᴄᴄ Ⓜ ♀
    O99.835 Other infection carrier state complicating the puerperium ᴄᴄ Ⓜ ♀

✓6ᵗʰ O99.84 Bariatric surgery status complicating pregnancy, childbirth and the puerperium
    Gastric banding status complicating pregnancy, childbirth and the puerperium
    Gastric bypass status for obesity complicating pregnancy, childbirth and the puerperium
    Obesity surgery status complicating pregnancy, childbirth and the puerperium
    O99.840 Bariatric surgery status complicating pregnancy, unspecified trimester Ⓜ ♀
    O99.841 Bariatric surgery status complicating pregnancy, first trimester Ⓜ ♀
    O99.842 Bariatric surgery status complicating pregnancy, second trimester Ⓜ ♀
    O99.843 Bariatric surgery status complicating pregnancy, third trimester Ⓜ ♀
    O99.844 Bariatric surgery status complicating childbirth Ⓜ ♀
    O99.845 Bariatric surgery status complicating the puerperium Ⓜ ♀

O99.89 Other specified diseases and conditions complicating pregnancy, childbirth and the puerperium Ⓜ ♀

✓4ᵗʰ O9A Maternal malignant neoplasms, traumatic injuries and abuse classifiable elsewhere but complicating pregnancy, childbirth and the puerperium

✓5ᵗʰ O9A.1 Malignant neoplasm complicating pregnancy, childbirth and the puerperium
Conditions in C00-C96
Use additional code to identify neoplasm
    EXCLUDES 2   maternal care for benign tumor of corpus uteri (O34.1-)
         maternal care for benign tumor of cervix (O34.4-)
    AHA: 2015,3Q,19

✓6ᵗʰ O9A.11 Malignant neoplasm complicating pregnancy
    O9A.111 Malignant neoplasm complicating pregnancy, first trimester Ⓜ ♀
    O9A.112 Malignant neoplasm complicating pregnancy, second trimester Ⓜ ♀
    O9A.113 Malignant neoplasm complicating pregnancy, third trimester Ⓜ ♀
    O9A.119 Malignant neoplasm complicating pregnancy, unspecified trimester Ⓜ ♀

O9A.12 Malignant neoplasm complicating childbirth Ⓜ ♀

O9A.13 Malignant neoplasm complicating the puerperium Ⓜ ♀

✓5ᵗʰ O9A.2 Injury, poisoning and certain other consequences of external causes complicating pregnancy, childbirth and the puerperium
Conditions in S00-T88, except T74 and T76
Use additional code(s) to identify the injury or poisoning
    EXCLUDES 2   physical, sexual and psychological abuse complicating pregnancy, childbirth and the puerperium (O9A.3-, O9A.4-, O9A.5-)

✓6ᵗʰ O9A.21 Injury, poisoning and certain other consequences of external causes complicating pregnancy
    O9A.211 Injury, poisoning and certain other consequences of external causes complicating pregnancy, first trimester Ⓜ ♀
    O9A.212 Injury, poisoning and certain other consequences of external causes complicating pregnancy, second trimester Ⓜ ♀
    O9A.213 Injury, poisoning and certain other consequences of external causes complicating pregnancy, third trimester Ⓜ ♀
    O9A.219 Injury, poisoning and certain other consequences of external causes complicating pregnancy, unspecified trimester Ⓜ ♀

O9A.22 Injury, poisoning and certain other consequences of external causes complicating childbirth Ⓜ ♀

O9A.23 Injury, poisoning and certain other consequences of external causes complicating the puerperium Ⓜ ♀

✓5ᵗʰ O9A.3 Physical abuse complicating pregnancy, childbirth and the puerperium
Conditions in T74.11 or T76.11
Use additional code (if applicable):
    to identify any associated current injury due to physical abuse
    to identify the perpetrator of abuse (Y07.-)
    EXCLUDES 2   sexual abuse complicating pregnancy, childbirth and the puerperium (O9A.4)

✓6ᵗʰ O9A.31 Physical abuse complicating pregnancy
    O9A.311 Physical abuse complicating pregnancy, first trimester Ⓜ ♀
    O9A.312 Physical abuse complicating pregnancy, second trimester Ⓜ ♀
    O9A.313 Physical abuse complicating pregnancy, third trimester Ⓜ ♀
    O9A.319 Physical abuse complicating pregnancy, unspecified trimester Ⓜ ♀

O9A.32 Physical abuse complicating childbirth Ⓜ ♀

O9A.33 Physical abuse complicating the puerperium Ⓜ ♀

√5ᵗʰ **O9A.4** **Sexual abuse** complicating pregnancy, childbirth and the puerperium
Conditions in T74.21 or T76.21
Use additional code (if applicable):
to identify any associated current injury due to sexual abuse
to identify the perpetrator of abuse (Y07.-)

√6ᵗʰ **O9A.41** **Sexual abuse complicating** pregnancy

O9A.411 **Sexual abuse complicating pregnancy, first trimester** Ⓜ ♀

O9A.412 **Sexual abuse complicating pregnancy, second trimester** Ⓜ ♀

O9A.413 **Sexual abuse complicating pregnancy, third trimester** Ⓜ ♀

O9A.419 **Sexual abuse complicating pregnancy, unspecified trimester** Ⓜ ♀

O9A.42 **Sexual abuse complicating** childbirth Ⓜ ♀

O9A.43 **Sexual abuse complicating the puerperium** Ⓜ ♀

√5ᵗʰ **O9A.5** **Psychological abuse** complicating pregnancy, childbirth and the puerperium
Conditions in T74.31 or T76.31
Use additional code to identify the perpetrator of abuse (Y07.-)

√6ᵗʰ **O9A.51** **Psychological abuse complicating** pregnancy

O9A.511 **Psychological abuse complicating pregnancy, first trimester** Ⓜ ♀

O9A.512 **Psychological abuse complicating pregnancy, second trimester** Ⓜ ♀

O9A.513 **Psychological abuse complicating pregnancy, third trimester** Ⓜ ♀

O9A.519 **Psychological abuse complicating pregnancy, unspecified trimester** Ⓜ ♀

O9A.52 **Psychological abuse complicating childbirth** Ⓜ ♀

O9A.53 **Psychological abuse complicating the puerperium** Ⓜ ♀

Chapter 16. Certain Conditions Originating in the Perinatal Period (P00–P96)

Chapter-specific Guidelines with Coding Examples

The chapter-specific guidelines from the ICD-10-CM Official Guidelines for Coding and Reporting have been provided below. Along with these guidelines are coding examples, contained in the shaded boxes, that have been developed to help illustrate the coding and/or sequencing guidance found in these guidelines.

For coding and reporting purposes the perinatal period is defined as before birth through the 28th day following birth. The following guidelines are provided for reporting purposes

a. General perinatal rules

1) Use of Chapter 16 codes

Codes in this chapter are <u>never</u> for use on the maternal record. Codes from Chapter 15, the obstetric chapter, are never permitted on the newborn record. Chapter 16 codes may be used throughout the life of the patient if the condition is still present.

2) Principal diagnosis for birth record

When coding the birth episode in a newborn record, assign a code from category Z38, Liveborn infants according to place of birth and type of delivery, as the principal diagnosis. A code from category Z38 is assigned only once, to a newborn at the time of birth. If a newborn is transferred to another institution, a code from category Z38 should not be used at the receiving hospital.

A code from category Z38 is used only on the newborn record, not on the mother's record.

> Newborn delivered via vaginal delivery in Rural Hospital A, experienced meconium aspiration resulting in pneumonia. Rural Hospital A is not equipped to handle the extensive respiratory therapy this baby needs and transfers the patient to Metropolis Hospital B, where the pneumonia resolves and the newborn is eventually discharged.
>
> *Rural Hospital A*
>
> **Z38.00**   **Single liveborn infant, delivered vaginally**
>
> **P24.01**   **Meconium aspiration with respiratory symptoms**
>
> *Metropolis Hospital B*
>
> **P24.01**   **Meconium aspiration with respiratory symptoms**
>
> *Explanation:* A code from category Z38 is a one-time use only code. The hospital that actually delivered the newborn, in this case Rural Hospital A, can append a code from category Z38 but for the delivery admission only. Once the patient is transferred or discharged, the Z38 category no longer applies for that patient.
>
> The reason for the transfer to Metropolis Hospital B was for the respiratory symptoms (pneumonia) the newborn was exhibiting secondary to aspirating meconium.

3) Use of codes from other chapters with codes from Chapter 16

Codes from other chapters may be used with codes from chapter 16 if the codes from the other chapters provide more specific detail. Codes for signs and symptoms may be assigned when a definitive diagnosis has not been established. If the reason for the encounter is a perinatal condition, the code from chapter 16 should be sequenced first.

4) Use of Chapter 16 codes after the perinatal period

Should a condition originate in the perinatal period, and continue throughout the life of the patient, the perinatal code should continue to be used regardless of the patient's age.

> A 7-year-old patient with history of birth injury that resulted in Erb's palsy is seen for subscapularis release
>
> **P14.0**   **Erb's paralysis due to birth injury**
>
> *Explanation:* Although in this instance Erb's palsy is specifically related to a birth injury, it has not resolved and continues to be a health concern. A perinatal code is appropriate even though this patient is beyond the perinatal period.

5) Birth process or community acquired conditions

If a newborn has a condition that may be either due to the birth process or community acquired and the documentation does not indicate which it is, the default is due to the birth process and the code from Chapter 16 should be used. If the condition is community-acquired, a code from Chapter 16 should not be assigned.

6) Code all clinically significant conditions

All clinically significant conditions noted on routine newborn examination should be coded. A condition is clinically significant if it requires:

clinical evaluation; or

therapeutic treatment; or

diagnostic procedures; or

extended length of hospital stay; or

increased nursing care and/or monitoring; or

has implications for future health care needs

Note: The perinatal guidelines listed above are the same as the general coding guidelines for "additional diagnoses", except for the final point regarding implications for future health care needs. Codes should be assigned for conditions that have been specified by the provider as having implications for future health care needs.

b. Observation and evaluation of newborns for suspected conditions not found

1) Use of Z05 codes

Assign a code from category Z05, Observation and evaluation of newborns and infants for suspected conditions ruled out, to identify those instances when a healthy newborn is evaluated for a suspected condition that is determined after study not to be present. Do not use a code from category Z05 when the patient has identified signs or symptoms of a suspected problem; in such cases code the sign or symptom.

2) Z05 on Other than the birth record

A code from category Z05 may also be assigned as a principal or first-listed code for readmissions or encounters when the code from category Z38 code no longer applies. Codes from category Z05 are for use only for healthy newborns and infants for which no condition after study is found to be present.

3) Z05 on a birth record

A code from category Z05 is to be used as a secondary code after the code from category Z38, Liveborn infants according to place of birth and type of delivery.

> Newborn delivered via vaginal delivery; previous ultrasounds showed what appeared to be an abnormality of the right kidney. Kidney function tests were performed and ultrasounds taken and any genitourinary conditions ruled out.
>
> **Z38.00**   **Single liveborn infant, delivered vaginally**
>
> **Z05.6**   **Observation and evaluation of newborn for suspected genitourinary condition ruled out**
>
> Explanation: The newborn had no signs or symptoms of kidney or other genitourinary condition but was evaluated after delivery due to the abnormal prenatal ultrasound findings. A Z code describing the type and place of birth should be coded first, followed by a Z05 category code for the work performed to rule out a suspected genitourinary condition.

c. Coding additional perinatal diagnoses

1) Assigning codes for conditions that require treatment

Assign codes for conditions that require treatment or further investigation, prolong the length of stay, or require resource utilization.

Chapter 16. Certain Conditions Originating in the Perinatal Period

2) Codes for conditions specified as having implications for future health care needs

Assign codes for conditions that have been specified by the provider as having implications for future health care needs.

Note: This guideline should not be used for adult patients.

> An abnormal noise was heard in the left hip of a post-term newborn during a physical examination. The pediatrician would like to follow the patient after discharge as a hip click can be an early sign of hip dysplasia. The newborn was delivered via cesarean at 41 weeks.
>
> **Z38.01** **Single liveborn infant, delivered by cesarean**
>
> **P08.21** **Post-term newborn**
>
> **R29.4** **Clicking hip**
>
> *Explanation:* The abnormal hip noise or click is appended as a secondary diagnosis not only because it is an abnormal finding upon examination, but also due to its potential to be part of a bigger health issue. The hip dysplasia has not yet been diagnosed and does not warrant a code at this time.

d. Prematurity and fetal growth retardation

Providers utilize different criteria in determining prematurity. A code for prematurity should not be assigned unless it is documented. Assignment of codes in categories P05, Disorders of newborn related to slow fetal growth and fetal malnutrition, and P07, Disorders of newborn related to short gestation and low birth weight, not elsewhere classified, should be based on the recorded birth weight and estimated gestational age.

When both birth weight and gestational age are available, two codes from category P07 should be assigned, with the code for birth weight sequenced before the code for gestational age.

e. Low birth weight and immaturity status

Codes from category P07, Disorders of newborn related to short gestation and low birth weight, not elsewhere classified, are for use for a child or adult who was premature or had a low birth weight as a newborn and this is affecting the patient's current health status.

See Section I.C.21. Factors influencing health status and contact with health services, Status.

> A 35-year-old patient, who weighed 659 grams at birth, is seen for heart disease documented as being a consequence of the low birth weight
>
> **I51.9** **Heart disease, unspecified**
>
> **P07.02** **Extremely low birth weight newborn, 500–749 grams**
>
> *Explanation:* A code from subcategories P07.0- and P07.1- is appropriate, regardless of the age of the patient, as long as the documentation provides a clear link between the patient's current illness and the low birth weight.

f. Bacterial sepsis of newborn

Category P36, Bacterial sepsis of newborn, includes congenital sepsis. If a perinate is documented as having sepsis without documentation of congenital or community acquired, the default is congenital and a code from category P36 should be assigned. If the P36 code includes the causal organism, an additional code from category B95, Streptococcus, Staphylococcus, and Enterococcus as the cause of diseases classified elsewhere, or B96, Other bacterial agents as the cause of diseases classified elsewhere, should not be assigned. If the P36 code does not include the causal organism, assign an additional code from category B96. If applicable, use additional codes to identify severe sepsis (R65.2-) and any associated acute organ dysfunction.

> A full-term infant develops severe sepsis 24 hours after discharge from the hospital and is readmitted; cultures identified *E. coli* as the infective agent
>
> **P36.4** **Sepsis of newborn due to Escherichia coli**
>
> **R65.20** **Severe sepsis without septic shock**
>
> *Explanation:* Even though this newborn was discharged and could have acquired *E. coli* from his/her external environment, due to the lack of documentation specifying specifically how this pathogen was acquired, the default is to code the *E. coli* sepsis as congenital. A code from chapter 1, "Certain Infectious and Parasitic Diseases," is not required because the perinatal sepsis code identifies both the sepsis and the bacteria causing the sepsis.

g. Stillbirth

Code P95, Stillbirth, is only for use in institutions that maintain separate records for stillbirths. No other code should be used with P95. Code P95 should not be used on the mother's record.

Chapter 16. Certain Conditions Originating in the Perinatal Period (P00–P96)

NOTE Codes from this chapter are for use on newborn records only, never on maternal records

INCLUDES conditions that have their origin in the fetal or perinatal period (before birth through the first 28 days after birth) even if morbidity occurs later

EXCLUDES 2 congenital malformations, deformations and chromosomal abnormalities (Q00-Q99)

endocrine, nutritional and metabolic diseases (E00-E88)

injury, poisoning and certain other consequences of external causes (S00-T88)

neoplasms (C00-D49)

tetanus neonatorum (A33)

This chapter contains the following blocks:

P00-P04	Newborn affected by maternal factors and by complications of pregnancy, labor, and delivery
P05-P08	Disorders of newborn related to length of gestation and fetal growth
P09	Abnormal findings on neonatal screening
P10-P15	Birth trauma
P19-P29	Respiratory and cardiovascular disorders specific to the perinatal period
P35-P39	Infections specific to the perinatal period
P50-P61	Hemorrhagic and hematological disorders of newborn
P70-P74	Transitory endocrine and metabolic disorders specific to newborn
P76-P78	Digestive system disorders of newborn
P80-P83	Conditions involving the integument and temperature regulation of newborn
P84	Other problems with newborn
P90-P96	Other disorders originating in the perinatal period

Newborn affected by maternal factors and by complications of pregnancy, labor, and delivery (P00-P04)

NOTE These codes are for use when the listed maternal conditions are specified as the cause of confirmed morbidity or potential morbidity which have their origin in the perinatal period (before birth through the first 28 days after birth).

AHA: 2016,4Q,54-55

✓4ᵗʰ P00 Newborn affected by maternal conditions that may be unrelated to present pregnancy

Code first any current condition in newborn

EXCLUDES 2 encounter for observation of newborn for suspected diseases and conditions ruled out (Z05.-)

newborn affected by maternal complications of pregnancy (P01.-)

newborn affected by maternal endocrine and metabolic disorders (P70-P74)

newborn affected by noxious substances transmitted via placenta or breast milk (P04.-)

P00.0 Newborn affected by maternal hypertensive disorders

Newborn affected by maternal conditions classifiable to O10-O11, O13-O16

P00.1 Newborn affected by maternal renal and urinary tract diseases

Newborn affected by maternal conditions classifiable to N00-N39

P00.2 Newborn affected by maternal infectious and parasitic diseases

Newborn affected by maternal infectious disease classifiable to A00-B99, J09 and J10

EXCLUDES 1 maternal genital tract or other localized infections (P00.8)

EXCLUDES 2 infections specific to the perinatal period (P35-P39)

AHA: 2019,2Q,10; 2015,3Q,20

P00.3 Newborn affected by other maternal circulatory and respiratory diseases

Newborn affected by maternal conditions classifiable to I00-I99, J00-J99, Q20-Q34 and not included in P00.0, P00.2

P00.4 Newborn affected by maternal nutritional disorders

Newborn affected by maternal disorders classifiable to E40-E64

Maternal malnutrition NOS

P00.5 Newborn affected by maternal injury

Newborn affected by maternal conditions classifiable to O9A.2-

P00.6 Newborn affected by surgical procedure on mother

Newborn affected by amniocentesis

EXCLUDES 1 Cesarean delivery for present delivery (P03.4)

damage to placenta from amniocentesis, Cesarean delivery or surgical induction (P02.1)

previous surgery to uterus or pelvic organs (P03.89)

EXCLUDES 2 newborn affected by complication of (fetal) intrauterine procedure (P96.5)

P00.7 Newborn affected by other medical procedures on mother, not elsewhere classified

Newborn affected by radiation to mother

EXCLUDES 1 damage to placenta from amniocentesis, cesarean delivery or surgical induction (P02.1)

newborn affected by other complications of labor and delivery (P03.-)

✓5ᵗʰ P00.8 Newborn affected by other maternal conditions

P00.81 Newborn affected by periodontal disease in mother

P00.89 Newborn affected by other maternal conditions

Newborn affected by conditions classifiable to T80-T88

Newborn affected by maternal genital tract or other localized infections

Newborn affected by maternal systemic lupus erythematosus

AHA: 2019,2Q,9

P00.9 Newborn affected by unspecified maternal condition

✓4ᵗʰ P01 Newborn affected by maternal complications of pregnancy

Code first any current condition in newborn

EXCLUDES 2 encounter for observation of newborn for suspected diseases and conditions ruled out (Z05.-)

P01.0 Newborn affected by incompetent cervix

P01.1 Newborn affected by premature rupture of membranes

P01.2 Newborn affected by oligohydramnios

EXCLUDES 1 oligohydramnios due to premature rupture of membranes (P01.1)

DEF: Oligohydramnios: Low amniotic fluid level, resulting in underdeveloped organs in the fetus.

P01.3 Newborn affected by polyhydramnios

Newborn affected by hydramnios

DEF: Polyhydramnios: Excess amniotic fluid surrounding the fetus, typically defined as a total fluid volume of greater than 24.0 cc.

P01.4 Newborn affected by ectopic pregnancy

Newborn affected by abdominal pregnancy

P01.5 Newborn affected by multiple pregnancy

Newborn affected by triplet (pregnancy)

Newborn affected by twin (pregnancy)

P01.6 Newborn affected by maternal death

P01.7 Newborn affected by malpresentation before labor

Newborn affected by breech presentation before labor

Newborn affected by external version before labor

Newborn affected by face presentation before labor

Newborn affected by transverse lie before labor

Newborn affected by unstable lie before labor

P01.8 Newborn affected by other maternal complications of pregnancy

P01.9 Newborn affected by maternal complication of pregnancy, unspecified

✓4ᵗʰ P02 Newborn affected by complications of placenta, cord and membranes

Code first any current condition in newborn

EXCLUDES 2 encounter for observation of newborn for suspected diseases and conditions ruled out (Z05.-)

P02.0 Newborn affected by placenta previa

DEF: Placenta developed in the lower segment of the uterus that can cause hemorrhaging leading to preterm delivery.

P02.1 Newborn affected by other forms of placental separation and hemorrhage

Newborn affected by abruptio placenta

Newborn affected by accidental hemorrhage

Newborn affected by antepartum hemorrhage

Newborn affected by damage to placenta from amniocentesis, cesarean delivery or surgical induction

Newborn affected by maternal blood loss

Newborn affected by premature separation of placenta

✓5ᵗʰ P02.2 Newborn affected by other and unspecified morphological and functional abnormalities of placenta

P02.20 Newborn affected by unspecified morphological and functional abnormalities of placenta

✓ Additional Character Required   **✓x7ᵗʰ** Placeholder   Unacceptable PDx   Questionable PDx   Manifestation   Unspecified Dx   **H1-H14** HAC   **HCC** CMS-HCC Dx   **HIV** HIV Dx

ICD-10-CM 2020   **919**

P02.29   **Newborn affected by other morphological and functional abnormalities of placenta**
Newborn affected by placental dysfunction
Newborn affected by placental infarction
Newborn affected by placental insufficiency

P02.3   **Newborn affected by placental transfusion syndromes**
Newborn affected by placental and cord abnormalities resulting in twin-to-twin or other transplacental transfusion

P02.4   **Newborn affected by prolapsed cord**

P02.5   **Newborn affected by other compression of umbilical cord**
Newborn affected by umbilical cord (tightly) around neck
Newborn affected by entanglement of umbilical cord
Newborn affected by knot in umbilical cord

✓5ᵗʰ **P02.6**   **Newborn affected by other and unspecified conditions of umbilical cord**

    P02.60   **Newborn affected by unspecified conditions of umbilical cord**

    P02.69   **Newborn affected by other conditions of umbilical cord**
Newborn affected by short umbilical cord
Newborn affected by vasa previa
EXCLUDES 1   *newborn affected by single umbilical artery (Q27.0)*

✓5ᵗʰ **P02.7**   **Newborn affected by chorioamnionitis**
AHA: 2018,4Q,23-24
DEF: Inflammation of the fetal membranes due to maternal infection characterized by fetal tachycardia, respiratory distress, apnea, weak cries, and poor sucking.

    P02.70   **Newborn affected by fetal inflammatory response syndrome**   HCC
Newborn affected by FIRS

    P02.78   **Newborn affected by other conditions from chorioamnionitis**
Newborn affected by amnionitis
Newborn affected by membranitis
Newborn affected by placentitis

P02.8   **Newborn affected by other abnormalities of membranes**

P02.9   **Newborn affected by abnormality of membranes, unspecified**

✓4ᵗʰ **P03**   **Newborn affected by other complications of labor and delivery**
Code first any current condition in newborn
EXCLUDES 2   *encounter for observation of newborn for suspected diseases and conditions ruled out (Z05.-)*

P03.0   **Newborn affected by breech delivery and extraction**

P03.1   **Newborn affected by other malpresentation, malposition and disproportion during labor and delivery**
Newborn affected by contracted pelvis
Newborn affected by conditions classifiable to O64-O66
Newborn affected by persistent occipitoposterior
Newborn affected by transverse lie

P03.2   **Newborn affected by forceps delivery**

Forceps Assisted Birth

Forceps extractor

P03.3   **Newborn affected by delivery by vacuum extractor [ventouse]**

Vacuum Assisted Birth

Vacuum extractor

P03.4   **Newborn affected by Cesarean delivery**

P03.5   **Newborn affected by precipitate delivery**
Newborn affected by rapid second stage

P03.6   **Newborn affected by abnormal uterine contractions**
Newborn affected by conditions classifiable to O62.-, except O62.3
Newborn affected by hypertonic labor
Newborn affected by uterine inertia

✓5ᵗʰ **P03.8**   **Newborn affected by other specified complications of labor and delivery**

   ✓6ᵗʰ **P03.81**   **Newborn affected by abnormality in fetal (intrauterine) heart rate or rhythm**
EXCLUDES 1   *neonatal cardiac dysrhythmia (P29.1-)*

    P03.810   **Newborn affected by abnormality in fetal (intrauterine) heart rate or rhythm before the onset of labor**

    P03.811   **Newborn affected by abnormality in fetal (intrauterine) heart rate or rhythm during labor**

    P03.819   **Newborn affected by abnormality in fetal (intrauterine) heart rate or rhythm, unspecified as to time of onset**

   P03.82   **Meconium passage during delivery**
EXCLUDES 1   *meconium aspiration (P24.00, P24.01)*
meconium staining (P96.83)
DEF: Fetal intestinal activity that increases in response to a fetomaternal distressed state during delivery. The anal sphincter relaxes and meconium is passed into the amniotic fluid.

   P03.89   **Newborn affected by other specified complications of labor and delivery**
Newborn affected by abnormality of maternal soft tissues
Newborn affected by conditions classifiable to O60-O75 and by procedures used in labor and delivery not included in P02.- and P03.0-P03.6
Newborn affected by induction of labor

P03.9   **Newborn affected by complication of labor and delivery, unspecified**

✓4ᵗʰ **P04**   **Newborn affected by noxious substances transmitted via placenta or breast milk**
INCLUDES   nonteratogenic effects of substances transmitted via placenta
EXCLUDES 2   *congenital malformations (Q00-Q99)*
encounter for observation of newborn for suspected diseases and conditions ruled out (Z05.-)
neonatal jaundice from excessive hemolysis due to drugs or toxins transmitted from mother (P58.4)
newborn in contact with and (suspected) exposures hazardous to health not transmitted via placenta or breast milk (Z77.-)

P04.0   **Newborn affected by maternal anesthesia and analgesia in pregnancy, labor and delivery**
Newborn affected by reactions and intoxications from maternal opiates and tranquilizers administered for procedures during pregnancy or labor and delivery
EXCLUDES 2   *newborn affected by other maternal medication (P04.1-)*

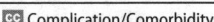

Ⓝ Newborn: 0   Ⓟ Pediatric: 0-17   Ⓜ Maternity: 9-64   Ⓐ Adult: 15-124   **MCC** Major Complication/Comorbidity   **CC** Complication/Comorbidity   **SW** Severe Wound Dx

920   ICD-10-CM 2020

✓5ᵗʰ **P04.1 Newborn affected by other maternal medication**

Code first withdrawal symptoms from maternal use of drugs of addiction, if applicable (P96.1)

> EXCLUDES 1   dysmorphism due to warfarin (Q86.2)
> fetal hydantoin syndrome (Q86.1)

> EXCLUDES 2   maternal anesthesia and analgesia in pregnancy, labor and delivery (P04.0)
> maternal use of drugs of addiction (P04.4-)

AHA: 2018,4Q,24-25

P04.11 Newborn affected by maternal antineoplastic chemotherapy

P04.12 Newborn affected by maternal cytotoxic drugs

P04.13 Newborn affected by maternal use of anticonvulsants

P04.14 Newborn affected by maternal use of opiates

P04.15 Newborn affected by maternal use of antidepressants

P04.16 Newborn affected by maternal use of amphetamines

P04.17 Newborn affected by maternal use of sedative-hypnotics

P04.1A Newborn affected by maternal use of anxiolytics

P04.18 Newborn affected by other maternal medication

P04.19 Newborn affected by maternal use of unspecified medication

P04.2 Newborn affected by maternal use of tobacco

Newborn affected by exposure in utero to tobacco smoke

> EXCLUDES 2   newborn exposure to environmental tobacco smoke (P96.81)

P04.3 Newborn affected by maternal use of alcohol

> EXCLUDES 1   fetal alcohol syndrome (Q86.0)

✓5ᵗʰ **P04.4 Newborn affected by maternal use of drugs of addiction**

AHA: 2018,4Q,25

P04.40 Newborn affected by maternal use of unspecified drugs of addiction

P04.41 Newborn affected by maternal use of cocaine
"Crack baby"

P04.42 Newborn affected by maternal use of hallucinogens

> EXCLUDES 2   newborn affected by other maternal medication (P04.1-)

P04.49 Newborn affected by maternal use of other drugs of addiction

> EXCLUDES 2   newborn affected by maternal anesthesia and analgesia (P04.0)
> withdrawal symptoms from maternal use of drugs of addiction (P96.1)

P04.5 Newborn affected by maternal use of nutritional chemical substances

P04.6 Newborn affected by maternal exposure to environmental chemical substances

✓5ᵗʰ **P04.8 Newborn affected by other maternal noxious substances**

AHA: 2018,4Q,25

P04.81 Newborn affected by maternal use of cannabis

P04.89 Newborn affected by other maternal noxious substances

P04.9 Newborn affected by maternal noxious substance, unspecified

Disorders of newborn related to length of gestation and fetal growth (P05-P08)

✓4ᵗʰ **P05 Disorders of newborn related to slow fetal growth and fetal malnutrition**

AHA: 2016,4Q,55-56

✓5ᵗʰ **P05.0 Newborn light for gestational age**

Newborn light-for-dates

Weight below but length above 10th percentile for gestational age

P05.00 Newborn light for gestational age, unspecified weight

P05.01 Newborn light for gestational age, less than 500 grams

P05.02 Newborn light for gestational age, 500-749 grams

P05.03 Newborn light for gestational age, 750-999 grams

P05.04 Newborn light for gestational age, 1000-1249 grams

P05.05 Newborn light for gestational age, 1250-1499 grams

P05.06 Newborn light for gestational age, 1500-1749 grams

P05.07 Newborn light for gestational age, 1750-1999 grams

P05.08 Newborn light for gestational age, 2000-2499 grams

P05.09 Newborn light for gestational age, 2500 grams and over

Newborn light for gestational age, other

✓5ᵗʰ **P05.1 Newborn small for gestational age**

Newborn small-and-light-for-dates

Newborn small-for-dates

Weight and length below 10th percentile for gestational age

P05.10 Newborn small for gestational age, unspecified weight

P05.11 Newborn small for gestational age, less than 500 grams

P05.12 Newborn small for gestational age, 500-749 grams

P05.13 Newborn small for gestational age, 750-999 grams

P05.14 Newborn small for gestational age, 1000-1249 grams

P05.15 Newborn small for gestational age, 1250-1499 grams

P05.16 Newborn small for gestational age, 1500-1749 grams

P05.17 Newborn small for gestational age, 1750-1999 grams

P05.18 Newborn small for gestational age, 2000-2499 grams

P05.19 Newborn small for gestational age, other

Newborn small for gestational age, 2500 grams and over

P05.2 Newborn affected by fetal (intrauterine) malnutrition not light or small for gestational age

Infant, not light or small for gestational age, showing signs of fetal malnutrition, such as dry, peeling skin and loss of subcutaneous tissue

> EXCLUDES 1   newborn affected by fetal malnutrition with light for gestational age (P05.0-)
> newborn affected by fetal malnutrition with small for gestational age (P05.1-)

P05.9 Newborn affected by slow intrauterine growth, unspecified

Newborn affected by fetal growth retardation NOS

✓4ᵗʰ **P07 Disorders of newborn related to short gestation and low birth weight, not elsewhere classified**

> NOTE   When both birth weight and gestational age of the newborn are available, both should be coded with birth weight sequenced before gestational age

> INCLUDES   the listed conditions, without further specification, as the cause of morbidity or additional care, in newborn

✓5ᵗʰ **P07.0 Extremely low birth weight newborn**

Newborn birth weight 999 g. or less

> EXCLUDES 1   low birth weight due to slow fetal growth and fetal malnutrition (P05.-)

P07.00 Extremely low birth weight newborn, unspecified weight

P07.01 Extremely low birth weight newborn, less than 500 grams

P07.02 Extremely low birth weight newborn, 500-749 grams

P07.03 Extremely low birth weight newborn, 750-999 grams

✓5ᵗʰ **P07.1 Other low birth weight newborn**

Newborn birth weight 1000-2499 g.

> EXCLUDES 1   low birth weight due to slow fetal growth and fetal malnutrition (P05.-)

P07.10 Other low birth weight newborn, unspecified weight

P07.14 Other low birth weight newborn, 1000-1249 grams

P07.15 Other low birth weight newborn, 1250-1499 grams

P07.16 Other low birth weight newborn, 1500-1749 grams

P07.17 Other low birth weight newborn, 1750-1999 grams

P07.18 Other low birth weight newborn, 2000-2499 grams

✔ Additional Character Required   ✓x7ᵗʰ Placeholder   Unacceptable PDx   Questionable PDx   Manifestation   Unspecified Dx   H1 - H14 HAC   HCC CMS-HCC Dx   HIV HIV Dx

ICD-10-CM 2020   **921**

Chapter 16. Certain Conditions Originating in the Perinatal Period

✓5ᵗʰ **P07.2 Extreme immaturity of newborn**

Less than 28 completed weeks (less than 196 completed days) of gestation.

P07.20 Extreme immaturity of newborn, unspecified weeks of gestation

Gestational age less than 28 completed weeks NOS

P07.21 Extreme immaturity of newborn, gestational age less than 23 completed weeks

Extreme immaturity of newborn, gestational age less than 23 weeks, 0 days

P07.22 Extreme immaturity of newborn, gestational age 23 completed weeks

Extreme immaturity of newborn, gestational age 23 weeks, 0 days through 23 weeks, 6 days

P07.23 Extreme immaturity of newborn, gestational age 24 completed weeks

Extreme immaturity of newborn, gestational age 24 weeks, 0 days through 24 weeks, 6 days

P07.24 Extreme immaturity of newborn, gestational age 25 completed weeks

Extreme immaturity of newborn, gestational age 25 weeks, 0 days through 25 weeks, 6 days

P07.25 Extreme immaturity of newborn, gestational age 26 completed weeks

Extreme immaturity of newborn, gestational age 26 weeks, 0 days through 26 weeks, 6 days

P07.26 Extreme immaturity of newborn, gestational age 27 completed weeks

Extreme immaturity of newborn, gestational age 27 weeks, 0 days through 27 weeks, 6 days

✓5ᵗʰ **P07.3 Preterm [premature] newborn [other]**

28 completed weeks or more but less than 37 completed weeks (196 completed days but less than 259 completed days) of gestation

Prematurity NOS

AHA: 2017,3Q,26

P07.30 Preterm newborn, unspecified weeks of gestation

P07.31 Preterm newborn, gestational age 28 completed weeks

Preterm newborn, gestational age 28 weeks, 0 days through 28 weeks, 6 days

P07.32 Preterm newborn, gestational age 29 completed weeks

Preterm newborn, gestational age 29 weeks, 0 days through 29 weeks, 6 days

P07.33 Preterm newborn, gestational age 30 completed weeks

Preterm newborn, gestational age 30 weeks, 0 days through 30 weeks, 6 days

P07.34 Preterm newborn, gestational age 31 completed weeks

Preterm newborn, gestational age 31 weeks, 0 days through 31 weeks, 6 days

P07.35 Preterm newborn, gestational age 32 completed weeks

Preterm newborn, gestational age 32 weeks, 0 days through 32 weeks, 6 days

P07.36 Preterm newborn, gestational age 33 completed weeks

Preterm newborn, gestational age 33 weeks, 0 days through 33 weeks, 6 days

P07.37 Preterm newborn, gestational age 34 completed weeks

Preterm newborn, gestational age 34 weeks, 0 days through 34 weeks, 6 days

P07.38 Preterm newborn, gestational age 35 completed weeks

Preterm newborn, gestational age 35 weeks, 0 days through 35 weeks, 6 days

P07.39 Preterm newborn, gestational age 36 completed weeks

Preterm newborn, gestational age 36 weeks, 0 days through 36 weeks, 6 days

✓4ᵗʰ **P08 Disorders of newborn related to long gestation and high birth weight**

NOTE When both birth weight and gestational age of the newborn are available, priority of assignment should be given to birth weight

INCLUDES the listed conditions, without further specification, as causes of morbidity or additional care, in newborn

P08.0 Exceptionally large newborn baby

Usually implies a birth weight of 4500 g. or more

EXCLUDES 1 syndrome of infant of diabetic mother (P70.1)

syndrome of infant of mother with gestational diabetes (P70.0)

P08.1 Other heavy for gestational age newborn

Other newborn heavy- or large-for-dates regardless of period of gestation

Usually implies a birth weight of 4000 g. to 4499 g.

EXCLUDES 1 newborn with a birth weight of 4500 or more (P08.0)

syndrome of infant of diabetic mother (P70.1)

syndrome of infant of mother with gestational diabetes (P70.0).

✓5ᵗʰ **P08.2 Late newborn, not heavy for gestational age**

AHA: 2014,1Q,14

P08.21 Post-term newborn

Newborn with gestation period over 40 completed weeks to 42 completed weeks

P08.22 Prolonged gestation of newborn

Newborn with gestation period over 42 completed weeks (294 days or more), not heavy- or large-for-dates.

Postmaturity NOS

Abnormal findings on neonatal screening (P09)

P09 Abnormal findings on neonatal screening

Use additional code to identify signs, symptoms and conditions associated with the screening

EXCLUDES 2 nonspecific serologic evidence of human immunodeficiency virus [HIV] (R75)

Birth trauma (P10-P15)

CC Excl: For MCC codes in categories P10-P15, unless otherwise noted: PDX collection 1020

✓4ᵗʰ **P10 Intracranial laceration and hemorrhage due to birth injury**

EXCLUDES 1 intracranial hemorrhage of newborn NOS (P52.9)

intracranial hemorrhage of newborn due to anoxia or hypoxia (P52.-)

nontraumatic intracranial hemorrhage of newborn (P52.-)

P10.0 Subdural hemorrhage due to birth injury `MCC`

Subdural hematoma (localized) due to birth injury

EXCLUDES 1 subdural hemorrhage accompanying tentorial tear (P10.4)

P10.1 Cerebral hemorrhage due to birth injury `MCC`

P10.2 Intraventricular hemorrhage due to birth injury `CC`

CC Excl: PDX collection 1021

P10.3 Subarachnoid hemorrhage due to birth injury `MCC`

CC Excl: PDX collection 1022

P10.4 Tentorial tear due to birth injury `MCC`

P10.8 Other intracranial lacerations and hemorrhages due to birth injury `MCC`

P10.9 Unspecified intracranial laceration and hemorrhage due to birth injury `MCC`

✓4ᵗʰ **P11 Other birth injuries to central nervous system**

P11.0 Cerebral edema due to birth injury `MCC`

P11.1 Other specified brain damage due to birth injury

P11.2 Unspecified brain damage due to birth injury `MCC`

P11.3 Birth injury to facial nerve

Facial palsy due to birth injury

P11.4 Birth injury to other cranial nerves

P11.5 Birth injury to spine and spinal cord

Fracture of spine due to birth injury

P11.9 Birth injury to central nervous system, unspecified `MCC`

Ⓝ Newborn: 0   Ⓟ Pediatric: 0-17   Ⓜ Maternity: 9-64   Ⓐ Adult: 15-124   `MCC` Major Complication/Comorbidity   `CC` Complication/Comorbidity   `SW` Severe Wound Dx

922   ICD-10-CM 2020

P07.2–P11.9

✓4ᵗʰ **P12 Birth injury to** scalp

Birth Injuries to Scalp

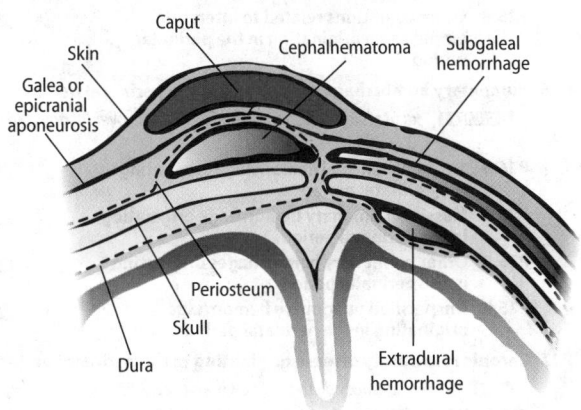

P12.0 Cephalhematoma due to birth injury
DEF: Condition that occurs in a neonate when blood vessels between the skull and periosteum rupture and blood collects in the subperiosteal space (below the periosteum). It is typically caused by prolonged labor or trauma due to instrument-assisted delivery (e.g., forceps, vacuum extraction), although in rare circumstances, it may indicate a linear skull fracture with intracranial hemorrhage.

P12.1 Chignon (from vacuum extraction) due to birth injury
DEF: Artificial swelling of the scalp that occurs when a collection of interstitial fluid and blood forms in the area of the scalp where the suction cup was applied during a vacuum-assisted delivery.

P12.2 Epicranial subaponeurotic hemorrhage due CC **to birth injury**
Subgaleal hemorrhage
CC Excl: PDX collection 1023

P12.3 Bruising of scalp due to birth injury

P12.4 Injury of scalp of newborn due to monitoring equipment
Sampling incision of scalp of newborn
Scalp clip (electrode) injury of newborn

✓5ᵗʰ **P12.8 Other birth injuries to scalp**

P12.81 Caput succedaneum
DEF: Swelling of the scalp as a result of pressure being exerted on the head from the vaginal walls, uterus, or instrumentation used in assisting a delivery (e.g., vacuum).

P12.89 Other birth injuries to scalp

P12.9 Birth injury to scalp, unspecified

✓4ᵗʰ **P13 Birth injury to skeleton**
EXCLUDES 2   birth injury to spine (P11.5)

P13.0 Fracture of skull due to birth injury

P13.1 Other birth injuries to skull
EXCLUDES 1   cephalhematoma (P12.0)

P13.2 Birth injury to femur

P13.3 Birth injury to other long bones

P13.4 Fracture of clavicle due to birth injury

P13.8 Birth injuries to other parts of skeleton

P13.9 Birth injury to skeleton, unspecified

✓4ᵗʰ **P14 Birth injury to peripheral nervous system**

P14.0 Erb's paralysis due to birth injury
DEF: Erb's paralysis: Most common type of brachial plexus (peripheral nerve) injury in a neonate that involves nerve damage at the level of C5-C6. **Synonym(s):** Erb's palsy

P14.1 Klumpke's paralysis due to birth injury

P14.2 Phrenic nerve paralysis due to birth injury

P14.3 Other brachial plexus birth injuries

P14.8 Birth injuries to other parts of peripheral nervous system

P14.9 Birth injury to peripheral nervous system, unspecified

✓4ᵗʰ **P15 Other birth injuries**

P15.0 Birth injury to liver
Rupture of liver due to birth injury

P15.1 Birth injury to spleen
Rupture of spleen due to birth injury

P15.2 Sternomastoid injury due to birth injury

P15.3 Birth injury to eye
Subconjunctival hemorrhage due to birth injury
Traumatic glaucoma due to birth injury

P15.4 Birth injury to face
Facial congestion due to birth injury

P15.5 Birth injury to external genitalia

P15.6 Subcutaneous fat necrosis due to birth injury

P15.8 Other specified birth injuries
TIP: Use for any injury of newborn from scalpel.

P15.9 Birth injury, unspecified

Respiratory and cardiovascular disorders specific to the perinatal period (P19-P29)

CC Excl: For MCC codes in categories P19-P29, unless otherwise noted: PDX collection 748

✓4ᵗʰ **P19 Metabolic acidemia in newborn**
INCLUDES   metabolic acidemia in newborn

P19.0 Metabolic acidemia in newborn first noted before onset of labor

P19.1 Metabolic acidemia in newborn first noted during labor

P19.2 Metabolic acidemia noted at birth

P19.9 Metabolic acidemia, unspecified

✓4ᵗʰ **P22 Respiratory distress of newborn**
EXCLUDES 1   *respiratory arrest of newborn (P28.81)*
           respiratory failure of newborn NOS (P28.5)
AHA: 2019,2Q,29

P22.0 Respiratory distress syndrome of newborn MCC
Cardiorespiratory distress syndrome of newborn
Hyaline membrane disease
Idiopathic respiratory distress syndrome [IRDS or RDS] of newborn
Pulmonary hypoperfusion syndrome
Respiratory distress syndrome, type I
EXCLUDES 2 ▶respiratory arrest of newborn (P28.81)◀
         ▶respiratory failure of newborn NOS (P28.5)◀
AHA: 2019,2Q,29
DEF: Severe chest contractions upon air intake and expiratory grunting. The infant appears blue due to oxygen deficiency and has a rapid respiratory rate, formerly called hyaline membrane disease.

P22.1 Transient tachypnea of newborn
Idiopathic tachypnea of newborn
Respiratory distress syndrome, type II
Wet lung syndrome
DEF: Rapid, labored breathing of a newborn. It is a short-term problem that begins after birth and lasts about three days.

P22.8 Other respiratory distress of newborn
EXCLUDES 1 ▶respiratory arrest of newborn (P28.81)◀
         ▶respiratory failure of newborn NOS (P28.5)◀

P22.9 Respiratory distress of newborn, unspecified
EXCLUDES 1 ▶respiratory arrest of newborn (P28.81)◀
         ▶respiratory failure of newborn NOS (P28.5)◀

✓4ᵗʰ **P23 Congenital pneumonia**
INCLUDES   infective pneumonia acquired in utero or during birth
EXCLUDES 1   neonatal pneumonia resulting from aspiration (P24.-)

P23.0 Congenital pneumonia due to viral agent MCC
Use additional code (B97) to identify organism
EXCLUDES 1   congenital rubella pneumonitis (P35.0)

P23.1 Congenital pneumonia due to Chlamydia MCC

P23.2 Congenital pneumonia due to staphylococcus MCC

P23.3 Congenital pneumonia due to streptococcus, group B MCC

P23.4 Congenital pneumonia due to Escherichia coli MCC

P23.5 Congenital pneumonia due to Pseudomonas MCC

P23.6 Congenital pneumonia due to other bacterial agents MCC
Congenital pneumonia due to Hemophilus influenzae
Congenital pneumonia due to Klebsiella pneumoniae
Congenital pneumonia due to Mycoplasma
Congenital pneumonia due to Streptococcus, except group B
Use additional code (B95-B96) to identify organism

P23.8 Congenital pneumonia due to other organisms MCC

P23.9 Congenital pneumonia, unspecified MCC

✓4ᵗʰ **P24 Neonatal aspiration**

INCLUDES   aspiration in utero and during delivery

✓5ᵗʰ **P24.0 Meconium aspiration**

EXCLUDES 1   meconium passage (without aspiration) during delivery (P03.82)

meconium staining (P96.83)

DEF: Meconium in the trachea or seen on chest x-ray after birth.

P24.00 Meconium aspiration without respiratory symptoms

Meconium aspiration NOS

P24.01 Meconium aspiration with respiratory symptoms   MCC

Meconium aspiration pneumonia

Meconium aspiration pneumonitis

Meconium aspiration syndrome NOS

Use additional code to identify any secondary pulmonary hypertension, if applicable (I27.2-)

DEF: Aspiration of fetal intestinal material during or prior to delivery. If is usually a complication of placental insufficiency, causing pneumonitis and bronchial obstruction (inflammatory reaction of lungs).

✓5ᵗʰ **P24.1 Neonatal aspiration of (clear) amniotic fluid and mucus**

Neonatal aspiration of liquor (amnii)

P24.10 Neonatal aspiration of (clear) amniotic fluid and mucus without respiratory symptoms

Neonatal aspiration of amniotic fluid and mucus NOS

P24.11 Neonatal aspiration of (clear) amniotic fluid and mucus with respiratory symptoms   MCC

Neonatal aspiration of amniotic fluid and mucus with pneumonia

Neonatal aspiration of amniotic fluid and mucus with pneumonitis

Use additional code to identify any secondary pulmonary hypertension, if applicable (I27.2-)

✓5ᵗʰ **P24.2 Neonatal aspiration of blood**

P24.20 Neonatal aspiration of blood without respiratory symptoms

Neonatal aspiration of blood NOS

P24.21 Neonatal aspiration of blood with respiratory symptoms   MCC

Neonatal aspiration of blood with pneumonia

Neonatal aspiration of blood with pneumonitis

Use additional code to identify any secondary pulmonary hypertension, if applicable (I27.2-)

✓5ᵗʰ **P24.3 Neonatal aspiration of milk and regurgitated food**

Neonatal aspiration of stomach contents

P24.30 Neonatal aspiration of milk and regurgitated food without respiratory symptoms

Neonatal aspiration of milk and regurgitated food NOS

P24.31 Neonatal aspiration of milk and regurgitated food with respiratory symptoms   MCC

Neonatal aspiration of milk and regurgitated food with pneumonia

Neonatal aspiration of milk and regurgitated food with pneumonitis

Use additional code to identify any secondary pulmonary hypertension, if applicable (I27.2-)

✓5ᵗʰ **P24.8 Other neonatal aspiration**

P24.80 Other neonatal aspiration without respiratory symptoms

Neonatal aspiration NEC

P24.81 Other neonatal aspiration with respiratory symptoms   MCC

Neonatal aspiration pneumonia NEC

Neonatal aspiration with pneumonitis NEC

Neonatal aspiration with pneumonia NOS

Neonatal aspiration with pneumonitis NOS

Use additional code to identify any secondary pulmonary hypertension, if applicable (I27.2-)

P24.9 Neonatal aspiration, unspecified

✓4ᵗʰ **P25 Interstitial emphysema and related conditions originating in the perinatal period**

P25.0 Interstitial emphysema originating in the perinatal period   MCC

P25.1 Pneumothorax originating in the perinatal period   MCC

P25.2 Pneumomediastinum originating in the perinatal period   MCC

P25.3 Pneumopericardium originating in the perinatal period   MCC

P25.8 Other conditions related to interstitial emphysema originating in the perinatal period   MCC

✓4ᵗʰ **P26 Pulmonary hemorrhage originating in the perinatal period**

EXCLUDES 1   acute idiopathic hemorrhage in infants over 28 days old (R04.81)

P26.0 Tracheobronchial hemorrhage originating in the perinatal period   MCC

P26.1 Massive pulmonary hemorrhage originating in the perinatal period   MCC

P26.8 Other pulmonary hemorrhages originating in the perinatal period   MCC

P26.9 Unspecified pulmonary hemorrhage originating in the perinatal period   MCC

✓4ᵗʰ **P27 Chronic respiratory disease originating in the perinatal period**

EXCLUDES 2   respiratory distress of newborn (P22.0-P22.9)

P27.0 Wilson-Mikity syndrome   MCC

Pulmonary dysmaturity

DEF: Pulmonary insufficiency in newborn babies, especially those with low birth weight. Rapid onset of hypercapnia and cyanosis occur during the first month of life frequently resulting in death.

P27.1 Bronchopulmonary dysplasia originating in the perinatal period   MCC

P27.8 Other chronic respiratory diseases originating in the perinatal period   MCC

Congenital pulmonary fibrosis

Ventilator lung in newborn

P27.9 Unspecified chronic respiratory disease originating in the perinatal period   MCC

✓4ᵗʰ **P28 Other respiratory conditions originating in the perinatal period**

EXCLUDES 1   congenital malformations of the respiratory system (Q30-Q34)

P28.0 Primary atelectasis of newborn   CC

Primary failure to expand terminal respiratory units

Pulmonary hypoplasia associated with short gestation

Pulmonary immaturity NOS

✓5ᵗʰ **P28.1 Other and unspecified atelectasis of newborn**

P28.10 Unspecified atelectasis of newborn   CC

Atelectasis of newborn NOS

P28.11 Resorption atelectasis without respiratory distress syndrome   CC

EXCLUDES 1   resorption atelectasis with respiratory distress syndrome (P22.0)

P28.19 Other atelectasis of newborn   CC

Partial atelectasis of newborn

Secondary atelectasis of newborn

P28.2 Cyanotic attacks of newborn   CC

EXCLUDES 1   apnea of newborn (P28.3-P28.4)

CC Excl: PDX collection 1024

P28.3 Primary sleep apnea of newborn   CC

Central sleep apnea of newborn

Obstructive sleep apnea of newborn

Sleep apnea of newborn NOS

DEF: Unexplained cessation of breathing when a neonate makes no respiratory effort for 20 seconds or longer or when a neonate's breathing cessation is accompanied by cyanosis, bradycardia, or hypotonia.

CC Excl: PDX collection 1025

P28.4 Other apnea of newborn   CC

Apnea of prematurity

Obstructive apnea of newborn

EXCLUDES 1   obstructive sleep apnea of newborn (P28.3)

CC Excl: PDX collection 1026

P28.5 Respiratory failure of newborn   MCC

EXCLUDES 1   respiratory arrest of newborn (P28.81)

respiratory distress of newborn (P22.0-)

AHA: 2019,2Q,29

✓5ᵗʰ **P28.8 Other specified respiratory conditions of newborn**

P28.81 Respiratory arrest of newborn   MCC

CC Excl: PDX collection 1027

N Newborn: 0   P Pediatric: 0-17   M Maternity: 9-64   A Adult: 15-124   MCC Major Complication/Comorbidity   CC Complication/Comorbidity   SW Severe Wound Dx

924   ICD-10-CM 2020

P28.89 **Other specified respiratory conditions of newborn**
Congenital laryngeal stridor
Sniffles in newborn
Snuffles in newborn
EXCLUDES 1 *early congenital syphilitic rhinitis (A50.05)*

P28.9 **Respiratory condition of newborn, unspecified**
Respiratory depression in newborn

✓4ᵗʰ **P29** **Cardiovascular disorders originating in the perinatal period**
EXCLUDES 1 *congenital malformations of the circulatory system (Q20-Q28)*

P29.0 **Neonatal cardiac failure**

✓5ᵗʰ **P29.1** **Neonatal cardiac dysrhythmia**

P29.11 **Neonatal tachycardia**
P29.12 **Neonatal bradycardia**

P29.2 **Neonatal hypertension**

✓5ᵗʰ **P29.3** **Persistent fetal circulation**
AHA: 2017,4Q,20-21

P29.30 **Pulmonary hypertension of newborn** `MCC`
Persistent pulmonary hypertension of newborn
DEF: Condition that occurs when pressure within the pulmonary artery is elevated and vascular resistance is observed in the lungs.
CC Excl: PDX collection 1028

P29.38 **Other persistent fetal circulation** `MCC`
Delayed closure of ductus arteriosus
CC Excl: PDX collection 1028

P29.4 **Transient myocardial ischemia in newborn**

✓5ᵗʰ **P29.8** **Other cardiovascular disorders originating in the perinatal period**

P29.81 **Cardiac arrest of newborn** `MCC`
CC Excl: PDX collection 1029

P29.89 **Other cardiovascular disorders originating in the perinatal period**
AHA: 2014,4Q,23

P29.9 **Cardiovascular disorder originating in the perinatal period, unspecified**

Infections specific to the perinatal period (P35-P39)

Infections acquired in utero, during birth via the umbilicus, or during the first 28 days after birth

EXCLUDES 2 *asymptomatic human immunodeficiency virus [HIV] infection status (Z21)*
congenital gonococcal infection (A54.-)
congenital pneumonia (P23.-)
congenital syphilis (A50.-)
human immunodeficiency virus [HIV] disease (B20)
infant botulism (A48.51)
infectious diseases not specific to the perinatal period (A00-B99, J09, J10.-)
intestinal infectious disease (A00-A09)
laboratory evidence of human immunodeficiency virus [HIV] (R75)
tetanus neonatorum (A33)

✓4ᵗʰ **P35** **Congenital viral diseases**
`INCLUDES` infections acquired in utero or during birth
CC Excl: For MCC codes in category P35, unless otherwise noted: PDX collection 562

P35.0 **Congenital rubella syndrome** `CC`
Congenital rubella pneumonitis
CC Excl: PDX collection 1030

P35.1 **Congenital cytomegalovirus infection** `MCC`
CC Excl: PDX collection 1030

P35.2 **Congenital herpesviral [herpes simplex] infection** `MCC`

P35.3 **Congenital viral hepatitis** `MCC`

P35.4 **Congenital Zika virus disease** `MCC`
Use additional code to identify manifestations of congenital Zika virus disease
AHA: 2018,4Q,25-26

P35.8 **Other congenital viral diseases** `MCC`
Congenital varicella [chickenpox]

P35.9 **Congenital viral disease, unspecified** `MCC`

✓4ᵗʰ **P36** **Bacterial sepsis of newborn**
`INCLUDES` congenital sepsis
Use additional code(s), if applicable, to identify severe sepsis (R65.2-) and associated acute organ dysfunction(s)
CC Excl: For MCC codes in category P36: PDX collection 1031

P36.0 **Sepsis of newborn due to streptococcus, group B** `MCC` `HCC`

✓5ᵗʰ **P36.1** **Sepsis of newborn due to other and unspecified streptococci**

P36.10 **Sepsis of newborn due to unspecified streptococci** `MCC` `HCC`

P36.19 **Sepsis of newborn due to other streptococci** `MCC` `HCC`

P36.2 **Sepsis of newborn due to Staphylococcus aureus** `MCC` `HCC`

✓5ᵗʰ **P36.3** **Sepsis of newborn due to other and unspecified staphylococci**

P36.30 **Sepsis of newborn due to unspecified staphylococci** `MCC` `HCC`

P36.39 **Sepsis of newborn due to other staphylococci** `MCC` `HCC`

P36.4 **Sepsis of newborn due to Escherichia coli** `MCC` `HCC`

P36.5 **Sepsis of newborn due to anaerobes** `MCC` `HCC`

P36.8 **Other bacterial sepsis of newborn** `MCC` `HCC`
Use additional code from category B96 to identify organism

P36.9 **Bacterial sepsis of newborn, unspecified** `MCC` `HCC`

✓4ᵗʰ **P37** **Other congenital infectious and parasitic diseases**
EXCLUDES 2 *congenital syphilis (A50.-)*
infectious neonatal diarrhea (A00-A09)
necrotizing enterocolitis in newborn (P77.-)
noninfectious neonatal diarrhea (P78.3)
ophthalmia neonatorum due to gonococcus (A54.31)
tetanus neonatorum (A33)
CC Excl: For MCC codes in category P37: PDX collection 562

P37.0 **Congenital tuberculosis** `MCC`

P37.1 **Congenital toxoplasmosis** `MCC`
Hydrocephalus due to congenital toxoplasmosis

P37.2 **Neonatal (disseminated) listeriosis** `MCC`

P37.3 **Congenital falciparum malaria** `MCC`

P37.4 **Other congenital malaria** `MCC`

P37.5 **Neonatal candidiasis**

P37.8 **Other specified congenital infectious and parasitic diseases** `MCC`

P37.9 **Congenital infectious or parasitic disease, unspecified** `MCC`

✓4ᵗʰ **P38** **Omphalitis of newborn**
EXCLUDES 1 *omphalitis not of newborn (L08.82)*
tetanus omphalitis (A33)
umbilical hemorrhage of newborn (P51.-)
DEF: Omphalitis: Infection and inflammation of the umbilical stump, often due to bacteria that can spread beyond the umbilical stump to the fascia, muscle, or even the umbilical vessels.

P38.1 **Omphalitis with mild hemorrhage** `CC`
CC Excl: PDX collection 1032

P38.9 **Omphalitis without hemorrhage** `CC`
Omphalitis of newborn NOS
CC Excl: PDX collection 1032

✓4ᵗʰ **P39** **Other infections specific to the perinatal period**
Use additional code to identify organism or specific infection
CC Excl: For CC codes in category P39, unless otherwise noted: PDX collection 1033

P39.0 **Neonatal infective mastitis** `CC`
EXCLUDES 1 *breast engorgement of newborn (P83.4)*
noninfective mastitis of newborn (P83.4)
CC Excl: PDX collection 1032

P39.1 **Neonatal conjunctivitis and dacryocystitis**
Neonatal chlamydial conjunctivitis
Ophthalmia neonatorum NOS
EXCLUDES 1 *gonococcal conjunctivitis (A54.31)*

P39.2 **Intra-amniotic infection affecting newborn, not elsewhere classified** `CC`

P39.3 **Neonatal urinary tract infection** `CC`
CC Excl: PDX collection 1034

Chapter 16. Certain Conditions Originating in the Perinatal Period

P39.4–P58.2

P39.4 **Neonatal skin infection** `CC`

Neonatal pyoderma

> **EXCLUDES 1**   *pemphigus neonatorum (L00)*
>
>   *staphylococcal scalded skin syndrome (L00)*

P39.8 **Other specified infections specific to the perinatal period** `CC`

P39.9 **Infection specific to the perinatal period, unspecified** `CC`

Hemorrhagic and hematological disorders of newborn (P50-P61)

> **EXCLUDES 1**   *congenital stenosis and stricture of bile ducts (Q44.3)*
>
>   *Crigler-Najjar syndrome (E80.5)*
>
>   *Dubin-Johnson syndrome (E80.6)*
>
>   *Gilbert syndrome (E80.4)*
>
>   *hereditary hemolytic anemias (D55-D58)*

✓4ᵗʰ **P50** **Newborn affected by intrauterine (fetal) blood loss**

> **EXCLUDES 1**   *congenital anemia from intrauterine (fetal) blood loss (P61.3)*

P50.0 **Newborn affected by intrauterine (fetal) blood loss from vasa previa**

P50.1 **Newborn affected by intrauterine (fetal) blood loss from ruptured cord**

P50.2 **Newborn affected by intrauterine (fetal) blood loss from placenta**

P50.3 **Newborn affected by hemorrhage into co-twin**

P50.4 **Newborn affected by hemorrhage into maternal circulation**

P50.5 **Newborn affected by intrauterine (fetal) blood loss from cut end of co-twin's cord**

P50.8 **Newborn affected by other intrauterine (fetal) blood loss**

P50.9 **Newborn affected by intrauterine (fetal) blood loss, unspecified**

Newborn affected by fetal hemorrhage NOS

✓4ᵗʰ **P51** **Umbilical hemorrhage of newborn**

> **EXCLUDES 1**   *omphalitis with mild hemorrhage (P38.1)*
>
>   *umbilical hemorrhage from cut end of co-twins cord (P50.5)*

P51.0 **Massive umbilical hemorrhage of newborn**

P51.8 **Other umbilical hemorrhages of newborn**

Slipped umbilical ligature NOS

P51.9 **Umbilical hemorrhage of newborn, unspecified**

✓4ᵗʰ **P52** **Intracranial nontraumatic hemorrhage of newborn**

> **INCLUDES**   intracranial hemorrhage due to anoxia or hypoxia
>
> **EXCLUDES 1**   *intracranial hemorrhage due to birth injury (P10.-)*
>
>   *intracranial hemorrhage due to other injury (S06.-)*

CC Excl: For codes in category P52:
For MCC codes, unless otherwise noted: PDX collection 1020
For CC codes: PDX collection 1021

P52.0 **Intraventricular (nontraumatic) hemorrhage, grade 1, of newborn** `CC`

Subependymal hemorrhage (without intraventricular extension)

Bleeding into germinal matrix

P52.1 **Intraventricular (nontraumatic) hemorrhage, grade 2, of newborn** `CC`

Subependymal hemorrhage with intraventricular extension

Bleeding into ventricle

✓5ᵗʰ **P52.2** **Intraventricular (nontraumatic) hemorrhage, grade 3 and grade 4, of newborn**

   P52.21 **Intraventricular (nontraumatic) hemorrhage, grade 3, of newborn** `MCC`

     Subependymal hemorrhage with intraventricular extension with enlargement of ventricle

     CC Excl: PDX collection 1021

   P52.22 **Intraventricular (nontraumatic) hemorrhage, grade 4, of newborn** `MCC`

     Bleeding into cerebral cortex

     Subependymal hemorrhage with intracerebral extension

     CC Excl: PDX collection 1021

P52.3 **Unspecified intraventricular (nontraumatic) hemorrhage of newborn** `CC`

P52.4 **Intracerebral (nontraumatic) hemorrhage of newborn** `MCC`

P52.5 **Subarachnoid (nontraumatic) hemorrhage of newborn** `MCC`

   CC Excl: PDX collection 1022

P52.6 **Cerebellar (nontraumatic) and posterior fossa hemorrhage of newborn** `MCC`

P52.8 **Other intracranial (nontraumatic) hemorrhages of newborn** `MCC`

P52.9 **Intracranial (nontraumatic) hemorrhage of newborn, unspecified** `MCC`

P53 **Hemorrhagic disease of newborn** `CC`

Vitamin K deficiency of newborn
CC Excl: PDX collection 1035

✓4ᵗʰ **P54** **Other neonatal hemorrhages**

> **EXCLUDES 1**   *newborn affected by (intrauterine) blood loss (P50.-)*
>
>   *pulmonary hemorrhage originating in the perinatal period (P26.-)*

CC Excl: For CC/MCC codes in category P54: PDX collection 1036

P54.0 **Neonatal hematemesis**

> **EXCLUDES 1**   *neonatal hematemesis due to swallowed maternal blood (P78.2)*

P54.1 **Neonatal melena** `MCC`

> **EXCLUDES 1**   *neonatal melena due to swallowed maternal blood (P78.2)*

P54.2 **Neonatal rectal hemorrhage** `MCC`

P54.3 **Other neonatal gastrointestinal hemorrhage** `MCC`

P54.4 **Neonatal adrenal hemorrhage** `CC`

P54.5 **Neonatal cutaneous hemorrhage**

Neonatal bruising

Neonatal ecchymoses

Neonatal petechiae

Neonatal superficial hematomata

> **EXCLUDES 2**   *bruising of scalp due to birth injury (P12.3)*
>
>   *cephalhematoma due to birth injury (P12.0)*

P54.6 **Neonatal vaginal hemorrhage** ♀

Neonatal pseudomenses

P54.8 **Other specified neonatal hemorrhages**

P54.9 **Neonatal hemorrhage, unspecified**

✓4ᵗʰ **P55** **Hemolytic disease of newborn**

P55.0 **Rh isoimmunization of newborn**

   DEF: Incompatible Rh fetal-maternal blood grouping that prematurely destroys red blood cells. Symptoms include jaundice, asphyxia, pulmonary hypertension, edema, respiratory distress, kernicterus, and coagulopathies. It is detected by a Coombs test.

   TIP: A positive Coombs test without documentation of associated Rh isoimmunization should be coded to R79.89 Other specified abnormal findings of blood chemistry.

P55.1 **ABO isoimmunization of newborn**
   AHA: 2015,3Q,20

P55.8 **Other hemolytic diseases of newborn**
   AHA: 2018,3Q,24

P55.9 **Hemolytic disease of newborn, unspecified**

✓4ᵗʰ **P56** **Hydrops fetalis due to hemolytic disease**

> **EXCLUDES 1**   *hydrops fetalis NOS (P83.2)*

CC Excl: For MCC codes in category P56: PDX collection 1037

P56.0 **Hydrops fetalis due to isoimmunization** `MCC`

✓5ᵗʰ **P56.9** **Hydrops fetalis due to other and unspecified hemolytic disease**

   P56.90 **Hydrops fetalis due to unspecified hemolytic disease** `MCC`

   P56.99 **Hydrops fetalis due to other hemolytic disease** `MCC`

✓4ᵗʰ **P57** **Kernicterus**

P57.0 **Kernicterus due to isoimmunization** `MCC`

   DEF: Complication of erythroblastosis fetalis associated with severe neural symptoms, high blood bilirubin levels, and nerve cell destruction. It results in bilirubin-pigmented gray matter of the central nervous system.

   CC Excl: PDX collection 1037

P57.8 **Other specified kernicterus** `MCC`

> **EXCLUDES 1**   *Crigler-Najjar syndrome (E80.5)*

   CC Excl: PDX collection 1038

P57.9 **Kernicterus, unspecified** `MCC`

   CC Excl: PDX collection 1038

✓4ᵗʰ **P58** **Neonatal jaundice due to other excessive hemolysis**

> **EXCLUDES 1**   *jaundice due to isoimmunization (P55-P57)*

P58.0 **Neonatal jaundice due to bruising**

P58.1 **Neonatal jaundice due to bleeding**

P58.2 **Neonatal jaundice due to infection**

N Newborn: 0   P Pediatric: 0-17   M Maternity: 9-64   A Adult: 15-124   MCC Major Complication/Comorbidity   CC Complication/Comorbidity   SW Severe Wound Dx

926   ICD-10-CM 2020

P58.3 **Neonatal jaundice due to** polycythemia

√5ᵗʰ P58.4 **Neonatal jaundice due to** drugs or toxins transmitted from mother or given to newborn

    Code first poisoning due to drug or toxin, if applicable (T36-T65 with fifth or sixth character 1-4 or 6)

    Use additional code for adverse effect, if applicable, to identify drug (T36-T50 with fifth or sixth character 5)

    P58.41 **Neonatal jaundice due to drugs or toxins transmitted from mother**

    P58.42 **Neonatal jaundice due to drugs or toxins** given to **newborn**

P58.5 **Neonatal jaundice due to** swallowed maternal blood

P58.8 **Neonatal jaundice due to other specified excessive hemolysis**

P58.9 **Neonatal jaundice due to excessive hemolysis, unspecified**

√4ᵗʰ P59 **Neonatal jaundice from other and unspecified causes**

    EXCLUDES 1   *jaundice due to inborn errors of metabolism (E70-E88)*

          kernicterus (P57.-)

    CC Excl: For MCC codes in category P59: PDX collection 1038

P59.0 **Neonatal jaundice associated with** preterm delivery

    Hyperbilirubinemia of prematurity

    Jaundice due to delayed conjugation associated with preterm delivery

P59.1 **Inspissated bile syndrome**   `MCC`

    DEF: Biliary obstruction in newborn resulting from obstruction of outflow tract.

√5ᵗʰ P59.2 **Neonatal jaundice from other and unspecified** hepatocellular damage

    EXCLUDES 1   *congenital viral hepatitis (P35.3)*

    P59.20 **Neonatal jaundice from unspecified hepatocellular damage**   `MCC`

    P59.29 **Neonatal jaundice from other hepatocellular damage**   `MCC`

        Neonatal giant cell hepatitis

        Neonatal (idiopathic) hepatitis

P59.3 **Neonatal jaundice from** breast milk inhibitor

P59.8 **Neonatal jaundice from other specified causes**

P59.9 **Neonatal jaundice, unspecified**

    Neonatal physiological jaundice (intense)(prolonged) NOS

    AHA: 2015,3Q,20

P60 **Disseminated intravascular coagulation of newborn**   `MCC`

    Defibrination syndrome of newborn

    CC Excl: PDX collection 1035

√4ᵗʰ P61 **Other perinatal hematological disorders**

    EXCLUDES 1   *transient hypogammaglobulinemia of infancy (D80.7)*

P61.0 **Transient neonatal thrombocytopenia**   `MCC`

    Neonatal thrombocytopenia due to exchange transfusion

    Neonatal thrombocytopenia due to idiopathic maternal thrombocytopenia

    Neonatal thrombocytopenia due to isoimmunization

    DEF: Temporary decrease in blood platelets of a newborn that is secondary to placental insufficiency.

    CC Excl: PDX collection 1035

P61.1 **Polycythemia neonatorum**

    DEF: Abnormal increase of total red blood cells of a newborn that results in hyperviscosity, which slows the flow of blood through small blood vessels.

P61.2 **Anemia of prematurity**   `CC`

    CC Excl: PDX collection 1039

P61.3 **Congenital anemia from fetal blood loss**   `CC`

    CC Excl: PDX collection 1039

P61.4 **Other congenital anemias, not elsewhere classified**   `CC`

    Congenital anemia NOS

    CC Excl: PDX collection 1039

P61.5 **Transient neonatal neutropenia**   `MCC`

    EXCLUDES 1   *congenital neutropenia (nontransient) (D70.0)*

    DEF: Low blood neutrophil counts of newborn that occurs due to maternal hypertension, sepsis, twin-twin transfusion, alloimmunization, and hemolytic disease.

    CC Excl: PDX collection 1040

P61.6 **Other transient neonatal disorders of coagulation**   `CC`

    CC Excl: PDX collection 1035

P61.8 **Other specified perinatal hematological disorders**

P61.9 **Perinatal hematological disorder, unspecified**

Transitory endocrine and metabolic disorders specific to newborn (P70-P74)

INCLUDES   transitory endocrine and metabolic disturbances caused by the infant's response to maternal endocrine and metabolic factors, or its adjustment to extrauterine environment

AHA: 2018,2Q,6

√4ᵗʰ P70 **Transitory disorders of** carbohydrate metabolism **specific to newborn**

P70.0 **Syndrome of infant of mother with** gestational diabetes

    Newborn (with hypoglycemia) affected by maternal gestational diabetes

    EXCLUDES 1   *newborn (with hypoglycemia) affected by maternal (pre-existing) diabetes mellitus (P70.1)*

          syndrome of infant of a diabetic mother (P70.1)

P70.1 **Syndrome of infant of a** diabetic mother

    Newborn (with hypoglycemia) affected by maternal (pre-existing) diabetes mellitus

    EXCLUDES 1   *newborn (with hypoglycemia) affected by maternal gestational diabetes (P70.0)*

          syndrome of infant of mother with gestational diabetes (P70.0)

P70.2 **Neonatal diabetes mellitus**   `CC`

    CC Excl: PDX collection 1041

P70.3 **Iatrogenic** neonatal hypoglycemia

P70.4 **Other neonatal hypoglycemia**

    Transitory neonatal hypoglycemia

P70.8 **Other transitory disorders of carbohydrate metabolism of newborn**   `CC`

    CC Excl: PDX collection 1042

P70.9 **Transitory disorder of carbohydrate metabolism of newborn, unspecified**

√4ᵗʰ P71 **Transitory neonatal disorders of** calcium and magnesium **metabolism**

    CC Excl: For CC codes in category P71: PDX collection 1041

P71.0 **Cow's milk hypocalcemia in newborn**   `CC`

P71.1 **Other neonatal hypocalcemia**   `CC`

    EXCLUDES 1   *neonatal hypoparathyroidism (P71.4)*

P71.2 **Neonatal hypomagnesemia**   `CC`

P71.3 **Neonatal tetany without calcium or magnesium deficiency**   `CC`

    Neonatal tetany NOS

P71.4 **Transitory neonatal** hypoparathyroidism   `CC`

P71.8 **Other transitory neonatal disorders of calcium and magnesium metabolism**   `CC`

    AHA: 2016,4Q,54

P71.9 **Transitory neonatal disorder of calcium and magnesium metabolism, unspecified**   `CC`

√4ᵗʰ P72 **Other transitory neonatal** endocrine disorders.

    EXCLUDES 1   *congenital hypothyroidism with or without goiter (E03.0-E03.1)*

          dyshormogenetic goiter (E07.1)

          Pendred's syndrome (E07.1)

    CC Excl: For CC codes in category P72, unless otherwise noted: PDX collection 1042 .

P72.0 **Neonatal goiter, not elsewhere classified**   `CC`

    Transitory congenital goiter with normal functioning

P72.1 **Transitory** neonatal hyperthyroidism   `CC`

    Neonatal thyrotoxicosis

    CC Excl: PDX collection 1041

P72.2 **Other transitory neonatal disorders of thyroid function, not elsewhere classified**   `CC`

    Transitory neonatal hypothyroidism

P72.8 **Other specified transitory neonatal endocrine disorders**   `CC`

P72.9 **Transitory neonatal endocrine disorder, unspecified**

√4ᵗʰ P74 **Other transitory neonatal** electrolyte and metabolic **disturbances**

    AHA: 2018,4Q,26-27

    CC Excl: For CC codes in category P74: PDX collection 1042

P74.0 **Late metabolic acidosis of newborn**   `MCC`

    EXCLUDES 1   *(fetal) metabolic acidosis of newborn (P19)*

    CC Excl: PDX collection 1041

P74.1 **Dehydration of newborn**

☑ Additional Character Required   √x7ᵗʰ Placeholder   <u>Unacceptable PDx</u>   Questionable PDx   Manifestation   Unspecified Dx   `H1`-`H14` HAC   `HCC` CMS-HCC Dx   `HIV` HIV Dx

ICD-10-CM 2020   **927**

P58.3–P74.1

√5ᵗʰ **P74.2 Disturbances of sodium balance of newborn**

     P74.21 Hypernatremia of newborn
     P74.22 Hyponatremia of newborn

√5ᵗʰ **P74.3 Disturbances of potassium balance of newborn**

     P74.31 Hyperkalemia of newborn
     P74.32 Hypokalemia of newborn

√5ᵗʰ **P74.4 Other transitory electrolyte disturbances of newborn**

     P74.41 Alkalosis of newborn   `CC`

         Hyperbicarbonatemia

√6ᵗʰ   **P74.42 Disturbances of chlorine balance of newborn**

         P74.421 Hyperchloremia of newborn

            Hyperchloremic metabolic acidosis

            EXCLUDES 2   *late metabolic acidosis of the newborn ▶(P74.0)◀*

         P74.422 Hypochloremia of newborn

     P74.49 Other transitory electrolyte disturbance of newborn

P74.5 Transitory tyrosinemia of newborn   `CC`

P74.6 Transitory hyperammonemia of newborn   `CC`

P74.8 Other transitory metabolic disturbances of newborn   `CC`

     Amino-acid metabolic disorders described as transitory

P74.9 Transitory metabolic disturbance of newborn, unspecified

Digestive system disorders of newborn (P76-P78)

√4ᵗʰ **P76 Other intestinal obstruction of newborn**

     P76.0 Meconium plug syndrome

         Meconium ileus NOS

         EXCLUDES 1   *meconium ileus in cystic fibrosis (E84.11)*

         DEF: Meconium obstruction of a newborn's intestines, resulting from unusually thick or hard meconium.

     P76.1 Transitory ileus of newborn   `CC`

         EXCLUDES 1   *Hirschsprung's disease (Q43.1)*

         CC Excl: PDX collection 1043

     P76.2 Intestinal obstruction due to inspissated milk

     P76.8 Other specified intestinal obstruction of newborn

         EXCLUDES 1   *intestinal obstruction classifiable to K56.-*

     P76.9 Intestinal obstruction of newborn, unspecified

√4ᵗʰ **P77 Necrotizing enterocolitis of newborn**

     DEF: Serious intestinal infection and inflammation in preterm infants. Severity is measured by stages and may progress to life-threatening perforation or peritonitis. Resection surgical treatment may be necessary.

     CC Excl: For MCC codes in category P77: PDX collection 1044

     P77.1 Stage 1 necrotizing enterocolitis in newborn   `MCC`

         Necrotizing enterocolitis without pneumatosis, without perforation

         DEF: Broad-spectrum symptoms with nonspecific signs, including feeding intolerance, abdominal distention, bradycardia, and metabolic abnormalities.

     P77.2 Stage 2 necrotizing enterocolitis in newborn   `MCC`

         Necrotizing enterocolitis with pneumatosis, without perforation

         DEF: Radiographic confirmation of necrotizing enterocolitis showing intestinal dilatation, fixed loops of bowels, pneumatosis intestinalis, metabolic acidosis, and thrombocytopenia.

     P77.3 Stage 3 necrotizing enterocolitis in newborn   `MCC`

         Necrotizing enterocolitis with perforation

         Necrotizing enterocolitis with pneumatosis and perforation

         DEF: Advanced stage in which an infant demonstrates signs of bowel perforation, septic shock, metabolic acidosis, ascites, disseminated intravascular coagulopathy, and neutropenia.

     P77.9 Necrotizing enterocolitis in newborn, unspecified   `MCC`

         Necrotizing enterocolitis in newborn, NOS

√4ᵗʰ **P78 Other perinatal digestive system disorders**

     EXCLUDES 1   *cystic fibrosis (E84.0-E84.9)*

            neonatal gastrointestinal hemorrhages (P54.0-P54.3)

     P78.0 Perinatal intestinal perforation   `MCC`

         Meconium peritonitis

         CC Excl: PDX collection 1044

     P78.1 Other neonatal peritonitis

         Neonatal peritonitis NOS

     P78.2 Neonatal hematemesis and melena due to swallowed maternal blood

---

P78.3 Noninfective neonatal diarrhea

     Neonatal diarrhea NOS

√5ᵗʰ **P78.8 Other specified perinatal digestive system disorders**

     P78.81 Congenital cirrhosis (of liver)

     P78.82 Peptic ulcer of newborn

     P78.83 Newborn esophageal reflux

         Neonatal esophageal reflux

     P78.84 Gestational alloimmune liver disease

         GALD

         Neonatal hemochromatosis

         EXCLUDES 1   *hemochromatosis (E83.11-)*

         AHA: 2017,4Q,21

         DEF: Severe hepatic injury with onset during fetal development with manifestations beginning during fetal life. It is due to maternal antibodies to fetal hepatic cells (hepatocytes) that cross the placenta into the fetal circulation, causing hepatic cell necrosis.

     P78.89 Other specified perinatal digestive system disorders

P78.9 Perinatal digestive system disorder, unspecified

Conditions involving the integument and temperature regulation of newborn (P80-P83)

√4ᵗʰ **P80 Hypothermia of newborn**

     DEF: Decrease in newborn body temperature due to their larger ratio of surface area to body weight, thin skin with blood vessels close to the surface, and a limited amount of subcutaneous fat.

     P80.0 Cold injury syndrome

         Severe and usually chronic hypothermia associated with a pink flushed appearance, edema and neurological and biochemical abnormalities.

         EXCLUDES 1   *mild hypothermia of newborn (P80.8)*

     P80.8 Other hypothermia of newborn

         Mild hypothermia of newborn

     P80.9 Hypothermia of newborn, unspecified

√4ᵗʰ **P81 Other disturbances of temperature regulation of newborn**

     P81.0 Environmental hyperthermia of newborn

     P81.8 Other specified disturbances of temperature regulation of newborn

     P81.9 Disturbance of temperature regulation of newborn, unspecified

         Fever of newborn NOS

√4ᵗʰ **P83 Other conditions of integument specific to newborn**

     EXCLUDES 1   *congenital malformations of skin and integument (Q80-Q84)*

            hydrops fetalis due to hemolytic disease (P56.-)

            neonatal skin infection (P39.4)

            staphylococcal scalded skin syndrome (L00)

     EXCLUDES 2   *cradle cap (L21.0)*

            diaper [napkin] dermatitis (L22)

     P83.0 Sclerema neonatorum   `CC`

         DEF: Diffuse, rapidly progressing white, waxy, nonpitting hardening of tissue, usually of legs and feet that is life-threatening. It is found in preterm or debilitated infants. Etiology is unknown.

         CC Excl: PDX collection 1045

     P83.1 Neonatal erythema toxicum

     P83.2 Hydrops fetalis not due to hemolytic disease   `MCC`

         Hydrops fetalis NOS

         DEF: Severe, life-threatening problem of a newborn characterized by severe edema of the entire body. It is unrelated to immune response.

         CC Excl: PDX collection 1046

√5ᵗʰ **P83.3 Other and unspecified edema specific to newborn**

     P83.30 Unspecified edema specific to newborn   `CC`

         CC Excl: PDX collection 1047

     P83.39 Other edema specific to newborn   `CC`

         CC Excl: PDX collection 1047

     P83.4 Breast engorgement of newborn

         Noninfective mastitis of newborn

     P83.5 Congenital hydrocele   ♂

         DEF: Hydrocele: Serous fluid that collects in the tunica vaginalis of the scrotum along the spermatic cord in males.

     P83.6 Umbilical polyp of newborn

Ⓝ Newborn: 0   Ⓟ Pediatric: 0-17   Ⓜ Maternity: 9-64   Ⓐ Adult: 15-124   `MCC` Major Complication/Comorbidity   `CC` Complication/Comorbidity   `SW` Severe Wound Dx

928   ICD-10-CM 2020

✓5ᵗʰ **P83.8 Other specified conditions of integument specific to newborn**
AHA: 2017,4Q,21-22

P83.81 Umbilical granuloma
EXCLUDES 2 *granulomatous disorder of the skin and subcutaneous tissue, unspecified (L92.9)*

P83.88 Other specified conditions of integument specific to newborn
Bronze baby syndrome
Neonatal scleroderma
Urticaria neonatorum

P83.9 Condition of the integument specific to newborn, unspecified

Other problems with newborn (P84)

P84 Other problems with newborn
Acidemia of newborn
Acidosis of newborn
Anoxia of newborn NOS
Asphyxia of newborn NOS
Hypercapnia of newborn
Hypoxemia of newborn
Hypoxia of newborn NOS
Mixed metabolic and respiratory acidosis of newborn
EXCLUDES 1 *intracranial hemorrhage due to anoxia or hypoxia (P52.-)*
hypoxic ischemic encephalopathy [HIE] (P91.6-)
late metabolic acidosis of newborn (P74.0)

Other disorders originating in the perinatal period (P90-P96)

P90 Convulsions of newborn   MCC
EXCLUDES 1 *benign myoclonic epilepsy in infancy (G40.3-)*
benign neonatal convulsions (familial) (G40.3-)
CC Excl: PDX collection 1048

✓4ᵗʰ **P91 Other disturbances of cerebral status of newborn**
CC Excl: For MCC codes in category P91, unless otherwise noted: PDX collection 1049

P91.0 Neonatal cerebral ischemia   MCC

P91.1 Acquired periventricular cysts of newborn   MCC

P91.2 Neonatal cerebral leukomalacia   MCC
Periventricular leukomalacia
CC Excl: PDX collection 1022

P91.3 Neonatal cerebral irritability   MCC

P91.4 Neonatal cerebral depression   MCC

P91.5 Neonatal coma   MCC

✓5ᵗʰ **P91.6 Hypoxic ischemic encephalopathy [HIE]**
EXCLUDES 1 *neonatal cerebral depression (P91.4)*
neonatal cerebral irritability (P91.3)
neonatal coma (P91.5)
AHA: 2017,4Q,22
CC Excl: For CC/MCC codes in subcategory P91.6: PDX collection 1050

P91.60 Hypoxic ischemic encephalopathy [HIE], unspecified   CC

P91.61 Mild hypoxic ischemic encephalopathy [HIE]   CC

P91.62 Moderate hypoxic ischemic encephalopathy [HIE]   CC

P91.63 Severe hypoxic ischemic encephalopathy [HIE]   MCC

✓5ᵗʰ **P91.8 Other specified disturbances of cerebral status of newborn**
AHA: 2017,4Q,22

✓6ᵗʰ **P91.81 Neonatal encephalopathy**

P91.811 Neonatal encephalopathy in diseases classified elsewhere
Code first underlying condition, if known, such as:
congenital cirrhosis (of liver) (P78.81)
intracranial nontraumatic hemorrhage of newborn (P52.-)
kernicterus (P57.-)

P91.819 Neonatal encephalopathy, unspecified

P91.88 Other specified disturbances of cerebral status of newborn

P91.9 Disturbance of cerebral status of newborn, unspecified

✓4ᵗʰ **P92 Feeding problems of newborn**
EXCLUDES 1 *eating disorders (F50.-)*
feeding problems in child over 28 days old (R63.3)
AHA: 2016,3Q,19
TIP: Continue to assign a code from this category for feeding problems in a patient greater than 28 days old when that feeding problem was initially diagnosed between day 0 and day 28. Do not assign code R63.3.

✓5ᵗʰ **P92.0 Vomiting of newborn**
EXCLUDES 1 *vomiting of child over 28 days old (R11.-)*

P92.01 Bilious vomiting of newborn   MCC
EXCLUDES 1 *bilious vomiting in child over 28 days old (R11.14)*
CC Excl: PDX collection 1051

P92.09 Other vomiting of newborn
EXCLUDES 1 *regurgitation of food in newborn (P92.1)*

P92.1 Regurgitation and rumination of newborn

P92.2 Slow feeding of newborn

P92.3 Underfeeding of newborn

P92.4 Overfeeding of newborn

P92.5 Neonatal difficulty in feeding at breast
AHA: 2017,1Q,28

P92.6 Failure to thrive in newborn
EXCLUDES 1 *failure to thrive in child over 28 days old (R62.51)*

P92.8 Other feeding problems of newborn

P92.9 Feeding problem of newborn, unspecified

✓4ᵗʰ **P93 Reactions and intoxications due to drugs administered to newborn**
INCLUDES reactions and intoxications due to drugs administered to fetus affecting newborn
EXCLUDES 1 *jaundice due to drugs or toxins transmitted from mother or given to newborn (P58.4-)*
reactions and intoxications from maternal opiates, tranquilizers and other medication (P04.0-P04.1, P04.4-)
withdrawal symptoms from maternal use of drugs of addiction (P96.1)
withdrawal symptoms from therapeutic use of drugs in newborn (P96.2)

P93.0 Grey baby syndrome   CC
Grey syndrome from chloramphenicol administration in newborn
CC Excl: PDX collection 1052

P93.8 Other reactions and intoxications due to drugs administered to newborn   CC
Use additional code for adverse effect, if applicable, to identify drug (T36-T50 with fifth or sixth character 5)
CC Excl: PDX collection 1052

✓4ᵗʰ **P94 Disorders of muscle tone of newborn**

P94.0 Transient neonatal myasthenia gravis   CC
EXCLUDES 1 *myasthenia gravis (G70.0)*
CC Excl: PDX collection 1041

P94.1 Congenital hypertonia

P94.2 Congenital hypotonia
Floppy baby syndrome, unspecified

P94.8 Other disorders of muscle tone of newborn

P94.9 Disorder of muscle tone of newborn, unspecified

P95 Stillbirth
Deadborn fetus NOS
Fetal death of unspecified cause
Stillbirth NOS
EXCLUDES 1 *maternal care for intrauterine death (O36.4)*
missed abortion (O02.1)
outcome of delivery, stillbirth (Z37.1, Z37.3, Z37.4, Z37.7)

✓4ᵗʰ **P96 Other conditions originating in the perinatal period**

P96.0 Congenital renal failure
Uremia of newborn

P96.1 Neonatal withdrawal symptoms from maternal use of drugs of addiction   CC
Drug withdrawal syndrome in infant of dependent mother
Neonatal abstinence syndrome
EXCLUDES 1 *reactions and intoxications from maternal opiates and tranquilizers administered during labor and delivery (P04.0)*
AHA: 2018,4Q,24-25
CC Excl: PDX collection 1052

P96.2 **Withdrawal symptoms from therapeutic use of drugs in newborn** `CC`
　　　CC Excl: PDX collection 1052

P96.3 **Wide cranial sutures of newborn**
　　　Neonatal craniotabes

P96.5 **Complication to newborn due to (fetal) intrauterine procedure**
　　　EXCLUDES 2 newborn affected by amniocentesis (P00.6)

√5ᵗʰ **P96.8** **Other specified conditions originating in the perinatal period**

　　P96.81 **Exposure to (parental) (environmental) tobacco smoke in the perinatal period**
　　　　EXCLUDES 2 newborn affected by in utero exposure to tobacco (P04.2)
　　　　　　exposure to environmental tobacco smoke after the perinatal period (Z77.22)

　　P96.82 **Delayed separation of umbilical cord**
　　P96.83 **Meconium staining**
　　　　EXCLUDES 1 meconium aspiration (P24.00, P24.01)
　　　　　　meconium passage during delivery (P03.82)

　　　　DEF: Meconium passed in utero causing discoloration on the fetal skin and nails or on the umbilicus. This staining may be incidental or may be an indicator of significant fetal stress that could affect outcomes.

　　P96.89 **Other specified conditions originating in the perinatal period**
　　　　Use additional code to specify condition

P96.9 **Condition originating in the perinatal period, unspecified**
　　　Congenital debility NOS

Chapter 17. Congenital Malformations, Deformations and Chromosomal Abnormalities (Q00–Q99)

Chapter-specific Guidelines with Coding Examples

The chapter-specific guidelines from the ICD-10-CM Official Guidelines for Coding and Reporting have been provided below. Along with these guidelines are coding examples, contained in the shaded boxes, that have been developed to help illustrate the coding and/or sequencing guidance found in these guidelines.

Assign an appropriate code(s) from categories Q00-Q99, Congenital malformations, deformations, and chromosomal abnormalities when a malformation/deformation or chromosomal abnormality is documented. A malformation/deformation/or chromosomal abnormality may be the principal/first-listed diagnosis on a record or a secondary diagnosis.

When a malformation/deformation/or chromosomal abnormality does not have a unique code assignment, assign additional code(s) for any manifestations that may be present.

When the code assignment specifically identifies the malformation/deformation/or chromosomal abnormality, manifestations that are an inherent component of the anomaly should not be coded separately. Additional codes should be assigned for manifestations that are not an inherent component.

8-day-old infant with tetralogy of Fallot and pulmonary stenosis

Q21.3   **Tetralogy of Fallot**

Explanation: Pulmonary stenosis is inherent in the disease process of tetralogy of Fallot. When the code assignment specifically identifies the malformation/deformation/or chromosomal abnormality, manifestations that are inherent components of the anomaly should not be coded separately.

7-month-old infant with Down syndrome and common atrioventricular canal

Q90.9   **Down syndrome, unspecified**

Q21.2   **Atrioventricular septal defect**

Explanation: While a common atrioventricular canal is often associated with patients with Down syndrome, this manifestation is not an inherent component and may be reported separately. When the code assignment specifically identifies the anomaly, manifestations that are inherent components of the condition should not be coded separately. Additional codes should be assigned for manifestations that are not inherent components.

Codes from Chapter 17 may be used throughout the life of the patient. If a congenital malformation or deformity has been corrected, a personal history code should be used to identify the history of the malformation or deformity. Although present at birth, **a** malformation/deformation/or chromosomal abnormality may not be identified until later in life. Whenever the condition is diagnosed by the **provider**, it is appropriate to assign a code from codes Q00-Q99. For the birth admission, the appropriate code from category Z38, Liveborn infants, according to place of birth and type of delivery, should be sequenced as the principal diagnosis, followed by any congenital anomaly codes, Q00- Q99.

Three-year-old with history of corrected ventricular septal defect

Z87.74   **Personal history of (corrected) congenital malformations of heart and circulatory system**

Explanation: If a congenital malformation or deformity has been corrected, a personal history code should be used to identify the history of the malformation or deformity.

Forty-year-old man with headaches diagnosed with congenital arteriovenous malformation of cerebral vessels by brain scan

Q28.2   **Arteriovenous malformation of cerebral vessels**

Explanation: Although present at birth, malformations may not be identified until later in life. Whenever a congenital condition is diagnosed by the physician, it is appropriate to assign a code from the range Q00–Q99.

Newborn with anencephaly delivered vaginally in hospital

Z38.00   **Single liveborn infant, delivered vaginally**

Q00.0   **Anencephaly**

Explanation: For the birth admission, the appropriate code from category Z38 Liveborn infants, according to place of birth and type of delivery, should be sequenced as the principal diagnosis, followed by any congenital anomaly codes, Q00–Q99.

Chapter 17. Congenital Malformations, Deformations and Chromosomal Abnormalities

Chapter 17. Congenital Malformations, Deformations and Chromosomal Abnormalities (Q00–Q99)

| NOTE | Codes from this chapter are not for use on maternal records |

EXCLUDES 2   inborn errors of metabolism (E70-E88)

This chapter contains the following blocks:

Q00-Q07   Congenital malformations of the nervous system
Q10-Q18   Congenital malformations of eye, ear, face and neck
Q20-Q28   Congenital malformations of the circulatory system
Q30-Q34   Congenital malformations of the respiratory system
Q35-Q37   Cleft lip and cleft palate
Q38-Q45   Other congenital malformations of the digestive system
Q50-Q56   Congenital malformations of genital organs
Q60-Q64   Congenital malformations of the urinary system
Q65-Q79   Congenital malformations and deformations of the musculoskeletal system
Q80-Q89   Other congenital malformations
Q90-Q99   Chromosomal abnormalities, not elsewhere classified

Congenital malformations of the nervous system (Q00-Q07)

✓4ᵗʰ **Q00   Anencephaly and similar malformations**

CC Excl: For MCC codes in category Q00, unless otherwise noted: PDX collection 1053

Q00.0   Anencephaly   `MCC` `HCC`

Acephaly
Acrania
Amyelencephaly
Hemianencephaly
Hemicephaly

Q00.1   Craniorachischisis   `MCC` `HCC`

Q00.2   Iniencephaly   `MCC` `HCC`

✓4ᵗʰ **Q01   Encephalocele**

| INCLUDES | Arnold-Chiari syndrome, type III |

encephalocystocele
encephalomyelocele
hydroencephalocele
hydromeningocele, cranial
meningocele, cerebral
meningoencephalocele

EXCLUDES 1   Meckel-Gruber syndrome (Q61.9)

DEF: Congenital protrusion of brain tissue through a defect in the skull.
CC Excl: For CC codes in category Q01: PDX collection 1054

Q01.0   Frontal encephalocele   `CC` `HCC`

Q01.1   Nasofrontal encephalocele   `CC` `HCC`

Q01.2   Occipital encephalocele   `CC` `HCC`

Q01.8   Encephalocele of other sites   `CC` `HCC`

Q01.9   Encephalocele, unspecified   `CC` `HCC`

Q02   Microcephaly   `HCC`

| INCLUDES | hydromicrocephaly |

micrencephalon

▶Code first, if applicable, congenital Zika virus disease◀
~~Use additional code, if applicable, to identify congenital Zika virus disease~~

EXCLUDES 1   Meckel-Gruber syndrome (Q61.9)

AHA: 2018,4Q,26
DEF: Congenital disorder in which the head circumference is more than two standard deviations below the mean for age, sex, race, and gestation and associated with a decreased life expectancy.

✓4ᵗʰ **Q03   Congenital hydrocephalus**

| INCLUDES | hydrocephalus in newborn |

EXCLUDES 1   Arnold-Chiari syndrome, type II (Q07.0-)
acquired hydrocephalus (G91.-)
hydrocephalus due to congenital toxoplasmosis (P37.1)
hydrocephalus with spina bifida (Q05.0-Q05.4)

DEF: Hydrocephalus: Abnormal buildup of cerebrospinal fluid in the brain causing dilation of the ventricles.

Congenital Hydrocephalus

Pressure

Normal ventricles   Hydrocephalic ventricles

Q03.0   Malformations of aqueduct of Sylvius   `HCC`

Anomaly of aqueduct of Sylvius
Obstruction of aqueduct of Sylvius, congenital
Stenosis of aqueduct of Sylvius

Q03.1   Atresia of foramina of Magendie and Luschka   `HCC`

Dandy-Walker syndrome

Q03.8   Other congenital hydrocephalus   `HCC`

Q03.9   Congenital hydrocephalus, unspecified   `HCC`

✓4ᵗʰ **Q04   Other congenital malformations of brain**

EXCLUDES 1   cyclopia (Q87.0)
macrocephaly (Q75.3)

CC Excl: For codes in category Q04:
For MCC codes: PDX collection 1054
For CC codes: PDX collection 1055

Q04.0   Congenital malformations of corpus callosum   `MCC` `HCC`

Agenesis of corpus callosum

Q04.1   Arhinencephaly   `MCC` `HCC`

Q04.2   Holoprosencephaly   `MCC` `HCC`

Q04.3   Other reduction deformities of brain   `MCC` `HCC`

Absence of part of brain
Agenesis of part of brain
Agyria
Aplasia of part of brain
Hydranencephaly
Hypoplasia of part of brain
Lissencephaly
Microgyria
Pachygyria

EXCLUDES 1   congenital malformations of corpus callosum (Q04.0)

Q04.4   Septo-optic dysplasia of brain   `CC` `HCC`

Q04.5   Megalencephaly   `CC` `HCC`

Q04.6   Congenital cerebral cysts   `CC` `HCC`

Porencephaly
Schizencephaly

EXCLUDES 1   acquired porencephalic cyst (G93.0)

Q04.8   Other specified congenital malformations of brain   `CC` `HCC`

Arnold-Chiari syndrome, type IV
Macrogyria

Q04.9   Congenital malformation of brain, unspecified   `HCC`

Congenital anomaly NOS of brain
Congenital deformity NOS of brain
Congenital disease or lesion NOS of brain
Multiple anomalies NOS of brain, congenital

N Newborn: 0   P Pediatric: 0-17   M Maternity: 9-64   A Adult: 15-124   MCC Major Complication/Comorbidity   CC Complication/Comorbidity   SW Severe Wound Dx

932   ICD-10-CM 2020

✓4ᵗʰ Q05   Spina bifida

INCLUDES   hydromeningocele (spinal)
meningocele (spinal)
meningomyelocele
myelocele
myelomeningocele
rachischisis
spina bifida (aperta)(cystica)
syringomyelocele

Use additional code for any associated paraplegia (paraparesis) (G82.2-)

EXCLUDES 1   Arnold-Chiari syndrome, type II (Q07.0-)
spina bifida occulta (Q76.0)

DEF: Lack of closure in the vertebral column with protrusion of the spinal cord through the defect, often in the lumbosacral area. This condition can be recognized by the presence of alpha-fetoproteins in the amniotic fluid.

CC Excl: For CC codes in category Q05: PDX collection 1056

Spina Bifida

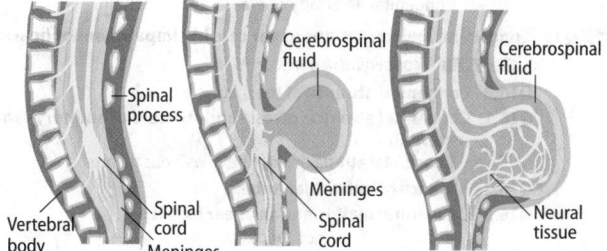

Spina bifida occulta   Meningocele   Myelomeningocele

Q05.0	**Cervical spina bifida with hydrocephalus**	CC HCC
Q05.1	**Thoracic spina bifida with hydrocephalus**	CC HCC
	Dorsal spina bifida with hydrocephalus	
	Thoracolumbar spina bifida with hydrocephalus	
Q05.2	**Lumbar spina bifida with hydrocephalus**	CC HCC
	Lumbosacral spina bifida with hydrocephalus	
Q05.3	**Sacral spina bifida with hydrocephalus**	CC HCC
Q05.4	**Unspecified spina bifida with hydrocephalus**	CC HCC
Q05.5	**Cervical spina bifida without hydrocephalus**	HCC
Q05.6	**Thoracic spina bifida without hydrocephalus**	HCC
	Dorsal spina bifida NOS	
	Thoracolumbar spina bifida NOS	
Q05.7	**Lumbar spina bifida without hydrocephalus**	HCC
	Lumbosacral spina bifida NOS	
Q05.8	**Sacral spina bifida without hydrocephalus**	HCC
Q05.9	**Spina bifida, unspecified**	HCC

✓4ᵗʰ Q06   Other congenital malformations of spinal cord

Q06.0	**Amyelia**	HCC
Q06.1	**Hypoplasia and dysplasia of spinal cord**	HCC
	Atelomyelia	
	Myelatelia	
	Myelodysplasia of spinal cord	
Q06.2	**Diastematomyelia**	HCC

DEF: Rare congenital anomaly often associated with spina bifida. The spinal cord is separated into longitudinal halves by a bony, cartilaginous or fibrous septum, each half surrounded by a dural sac.

Q06.3	**Other congenital cauda equina malformations**	HCC
Q06.4	**Hydromyelia**	HCC
	Hydrorachis	
Q06.8	**Other specified congenital malformations of spinal cord**	
Q06.9	**Congenital malformation of spinal cord, unspecified**	HCC
	Congenital anomaly NOS of spinal cord	
	Congenital deformity NOS of spinal cord	
	Congenital disease or lesion NOS of spinal cord	

✓4ᵗʰ Q07   Other congenital malformations of nervous system

EXCLUDES 2   congenital central alveolar hypoventilation syndrome (G47.35)
familial dysautonomia [Riley-Day] (G90.1)
neurofibromatosis (nonmalignant) (Q85.0-)

CC Excl: For CC codes in category Q07: PDX collection 1056

✓5ᵗʰ Q07.0   Arnold-Chiari syndrome

Arnold-Chiari syndrome, type II

EXCLUDES 1   Arnold-Chiari syndrome, type III (Q01.-)
Arnold-Chiari syndrome, type IV (Q04.8)

DEF: Congenital malformation of the brain in which the cerebellum protrudes through the foramen magnum into the spinal canal.

Q07.00	**Arnold-Chiari syndrome without spina bifida or hydrocephalus**	HCC
Q07.01	**Arnold-Chiari syndrome with spina bifida**	HCC
Q07.02	**Arnold-Chiari syndrome with hydrocephalus**	CC HCC
Q07.03	**Arnold-Chiari syndrome with spina bifida and hydrocephalus**	CC HCC
Q07.8	**Other specified congenital malformations of nervous system**	HCC
	Agenesis of nerve	
	Displacement of brachial plexus	
	Jaw-winking syndrome	
	Marcus Gunn's syndrome	
Q07.9	**Congenital malformation of nervous system, unspecified**	HCC
	Congenital anomaly NOS of nervous system	
	Congenital deformity NOS of nervous system	
	Congenital disease or lesion NOS of nervous system	

Congenital malformations of eye, ear, face and neck (Q10-Q18)

EXCLUDES 2   cleft lip and cleft palate (Q35-Q37)
congenital malformation of cervical spine (Q05.0, Q05.5, Q67.5, Q76.0-Q76.4)
congenital malformation of larynx (Q31.-)
congenital malformation of lip NEC (Q38.0)
congenital malformation of nose (Q30.-)
congenital malformation of parathyroid gland (Q89.2)
congenital malformation of thyroid gland (Q89.2)

✓4ᵗʰ Q10   Congenital malformations of eyelid, lacrimal apparatus and orbit

EXCLUDES 1   cryptophthalmos NOS (Q11.2)
cryptophthalmos syndrome (Q87.0)

Q10.0 **Congenital ptosis**
DEF: Congenital drooping of the eyelid. Ptosis is mostly idiopathic, but may occur genetically.

Q10.1 **Congenital ectropion**

Q10.2 **Congenital entropion**

Q10.3 **Other congenital malformations of eyelid**
Ablepharon
Blepharophimosis, congenital
Coloboma of eyelid
Congenital absence or agenesis of cilia
Congenital absence or agenesis of eyelid
Congenital accessory eyelid
Congenital accessory eye muscle
Congenital malformation of eyelid NOS

Q10.4 **Absence and agenesis of lacrimal apparatus**
Congenital absence of punctum lacrimale

Q10.5 **Congenital stenosis and stricture of lacrimal duct**

Q10.6 **Other congenital malformations of lacrimal apparatus**
Congenital malformation of lacrimal apparatus NOS

Q10.7 **Congenital malformation of orbit**

✓4ᵗʰ Q11   Anophthalmos, microphthalmos and macrophthalmos

Q11.0 **Cystic eyeball**

Q11.1 **Other anophthalmos**
Anophthalmos NOS
Agenesis of eye
Aplasia of eye

✓ Additional Character Required   ✓x7ᵗʰ Placeholder   Unacceptable PDx   Questionable PDx   Manifestation   Unspecified Dx   H1-H14 HAC   HCC CMS-HCC Dx   HIV HIV Dx

ICD-10-CM 2020   933

Q11.2 Microphthalmos
Cryptophthalmos NOS
Dysplasia of eye
Hypoplasia of eye
Rudimentary eye
EXCLUDES 1 cryptophthalmos syndrome (Q87.0)

Q11.3 Macrophthalmos
EXCLUDES 1 macrophthalmos in congenital glaucoma (Q15.0)

✓4ᵗʰ **Q12 Congenital lens malformations**

Q12.0 Congenital cataract

Q12.1 Congenital displaced lens

Q12.2 Coloboma of lens

Coloboma of Lens

Coloboma

Q12.3 Congenital aphakia

Q12.4 Spherophakia

Q12.8 Other congenital lens malformations
Microphakia

Q12.9 Congenital lens malformation, unspecified

✓4ᵗʰ **Q13 Congenital malformations of anterior segment of eye**

Q13.0 Coloboma of iris
Coloboma NOS
DEF: Defective or absent section of ocular tissue that may present as mild cupping or a small pit in the ocular disc due to extensive defects in the iris, ciliary body, choroids, and retina.

Q13.1 Absence of iris
Aniridia
Use additional code for associated glaucoma (H42)
DEF: Incompletely formed or absent iris. It affects both eyes and is a dominant trait.

Q13.2 Other congenital malformations of iris
Anisocoria, congenital
Atresia of pupil
Congenital malformation of iris NOS
Corectopia

Q13.3 Congenital corneal opacity

Q13.4 Other congenital corneal malformations
Congenital malformation of cornea NOS
Microcornea
Peter's anomaly

Q13.5 Blue sclera

✓5ᵗʰ **Q13.8 Other congenital malformations of anterior segment of eye**

Q13.81 Rieger's anomaly
Use additional code for associated glaucoma (H42)

Q13.89 Other congenital malformations of anterior segment of eye

Q13.9 Congenital malformation of anterior segment of eye, unspecified

✓4ᵗʰ **Q14 Congenital malformations of posterior segment of eye**
EXCLUDES 2 optic nerve hypoplasia (H47.03-)

Q14.0 Congenital malformation of vitreous humor
Congenital vitreous opacity

Q14.1 Congenital malformation of retina
Congenital retinal aneurysm

Q14.2 Congenital malformation of optic disc
Coloboma of optic disc

Q14.3 Congenital malformation of choroid

Q14.8 Other congenital malformations of posterior segment of eye
Coloboma of the fundus

Q14.9 Congenital malformation of posterior segment of eye, unspecified

✓4ᵗʰ **Q15 Other congenital malformations of eye**
EXCLUDES 1 congenital nystagmus (H55.01)
ocular albinism (E70.31-)
optic nerve hypoplasia (H47.03-)
retinitis pigmentosa (H35.52)

Q15.0 Congenital glaucoma
Axenfeld's anomaly
Buphthalmos
Glaucoma of childhood
Glaucoma of newborn
Hydrophthalmos
Keratoglobus, congenital, with glaucoma
Macrocornea with glaucoma
Macrophthalmos in congenital glaucoma
Megalocornea with glaucoma

Q15.8 Other specified congenital malformations of eye

Q15.9 Congenital malformation of eye, unspecified
Congenital anomaly of eye
Congenital deformity of eye

✓4ᵗʰ **Q16 Congenital malformations of ear causing impairment of hearing**
EXCLUDES 1 congenital deafness (H90.-)

Q16.0 Congenital absence of (ear) auricle

Q16.1 Congenital absence, atresia and stricture of auditory canal (external)
Congenital atresia or stricture of osseous meatus

Q16.2 Absence of eustachian tube

Q16.3 Congenital malformation of ear ossicles
Congenital fusion of ear ossicles

Q16.4 Other congenital malformations of middle ear
Congenital malformation of middle ear NOS

Q16.5 Congenital malformation of inner ear
Congenital anomaly of membranous labyrinth
Congenital anomaly of organ of Corti

Q16.9 Congenital malformation of ear causing impairment of hearing, unspecified
Congenital absence of ear NOS

✓4ᵗʰ **Q17 Other congenital malformations of ear**
EXCLUDES 1 congenital malformations of ear with impairment of hearing (Q16.0-Q16.9)
preauricular sinus (Q18.1)

Q17.0 Accessory auricle
Accessory tragus
Polyotia
Preauricular appendage or tag
Supernumerary ear
Supernumerary lobule

Q17.1 Macrotia
DEF: Birth defect characterized by abnormal enlargement of the pinna of the ear.

Q17.2 Microtia

Q17.3 Other misshapen ear
Pointed ear

Q17.4 Misplaced ear
Low-set ears
EXCLUDES 1 cervical auricle (Q18.2)

Q17.5 Prominent ear
Bat ear

Q17.8 Other specified congenital malformations of ear
Congenital absence of lobe of ear

Q17.9 Congenital malformation of ear, unspecified
Congenital anomaly of ear NOS

✓4ᵗʰ **Q18 Other congenital malformations of face and neck**
EXCLUDES 1 cleft lip and cleft palate (Q35-Q37)
conditions classified to Q67.0-Q67.4
congenital malformations of skull and face bones (Q75.-)
cyclopia (Q87.0)
dentofacial anomalies [including malocclusion] (M26.-)
malformation syndromes affecting facial appearance (Q87.0)
persistent thyroglossal duct (Q89.2)

Q18.0 Sinus, fistula and cyst of branchial cleft
Branchial vestige

Q18.1 Preauricular sinus and cyst SW
Fistula of auricle, congenital
Cervicoaural fistula

Q18.2 **Other branchial cleft malformations**
    Branchial cleft malformation NOS
    Cervical auricle
    Otocephaly

Q18.3 **Webbing of neck**
    Pterygium colli
    DEF: Congenital malformation characterized by a thick, triangular skinfold that stretches from the lateral side of the neck across the shoulder. It is associated with genetic conditions such as Turner's and Noonan's syndromes.

Q18.4 **Macrostomia**
    DEF: Rare congenital craniofacial bilateral or unilateral anomaly of the mouth due to malformed maxillary and mandibular processes. It results in an abnormally large mouth extending toward the ear.

Q18.5 **Microstomia**

Q18.6 **Macrocheilia**
    Hypertrophy of lip, congenital

Q18.7 **Microcheilia**

Q18.8 **Other specified congenital malformations of face and neck**
    Medial cyst of face and neck
    Medial fistula of face and neck
    Medial sinus of face and neck

Q18.9 **Congenital malformation of face and neck, unspecified**
    Congenital anomaly NOS of face and neck

Congenital malformations of the circulatory system (Q20-Q28)

✓4ᵗʰ **Q20** **Congenital malformations of cardiac chambers and connections**
    EXCLUDES 1   *dextrocardia with situs inversus (Q89.3)*
                 mirror-image atrial arrangement with situs inversus (Q89.3)
    CC Excl: For CC/MCC codes in category Q20: PDX collection 1057

    Q20.0 **Common arterial trunk**   `MCC`
        Persistent truncus arteriosus
        EXCLUDES 1   *aortic septal defect (Q21.4)*

    Q20.1 **Double outlet right ventricle**   `MCC`
        Taussig-Bing syndrome

    Q20.2 **Double outlet left ventricle**   `MCC`

    Q20.3 **Discordant ventriculoarterial connection**   `MCC`
        Dextrotransposition of aorta
        Transposition of great vessels (complete)

    Q20.4 **Double inlet ventricle**   `MCC`
        Common ventricle
        Cor triloculare biatriatum
        Single ventricle

    Q20.5 **Discordant atrioventricular connection**   `CC`
        Corrected transposition
        Levotransposition
        Ventricular inversion

    Q20.6 **Isomerism of atrial appendages**
        Isomerism of atrial appendages with asplenia or polysplenia

    Q20.8 **Other congenital malformations of cardiac chambers and connections**
        Cor binoculare

    Q20.9 **Congenital malformation of cardiac chambers and connections, unspecified**

✓4ᵗʰ **Q21** **Congenital malformations of cardiac septa**
    EXCLUDES 1   *acquired cardiac septal defect (I51.0)*

    Q21.0 **Ventricular septal defect**
        Roger's disease

Ventricular Septal Defect

    Q21.1 **Atrial septal defect**
        Coronary sinus defect
        Patent or persistent foramen ovale
        Patent or persistent ostium secundum defect (type II)
        Patent or persistent sinus venosus defect

Atrial Septal Defect

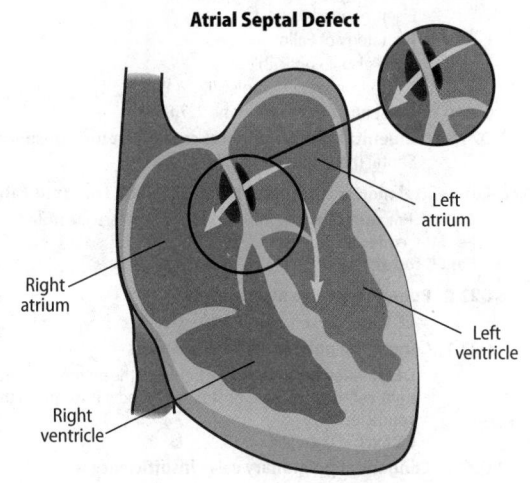

Right atrium

Left atrium

Right ventricle

Left ventricle

✔ Additional Character Required   ✓x7ᵗʰ Placeholder   Unacceptable PDx   Questionable PDx   Manifestation   Unspecified Dx   H1 - H14 HAC   HCC CMS-HCC Dx   HIV HIV Dx

ICD-10-CM 2020   **935**

Q21.2 Atrioventricular septal defect
Common atrioventricular canal
Endocardial cushion defect
Ostium primum atrial septal defect (type I)

Atrioventricular Septal Defect

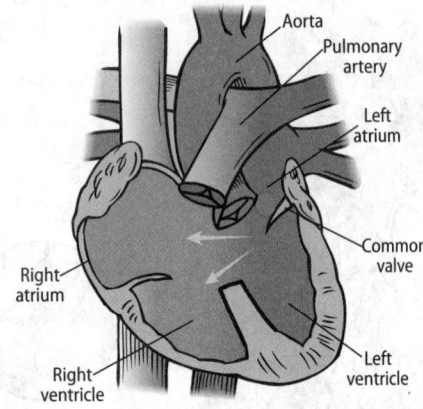

Labels: Aorta, Pulmonary artery, Left atrium, Common valve, Left ventricle, Right atrium, Right ventricle

Q21.3 Tetralogy of Fallot   `MCC`
Ventricular septal defect with pulmonary stenosis or atresia, dextroposition of aorta and hypertrophy of right ventricle.
AHA: 2014,3Q,16
CC Excl: PDX collection 1057

Q21.4 Aortopulmonary septal defect
Aortic septal defect
Aortopulmonary window

Q21.8 Other congenital malformations of cardiac septa
Eisenmenger's defect
Pentalogy of Fallot
Code also if applicable:
    Eisenmenger's complex (I27.83)
    Eisenmenger's syndrome (I27.83)

Q21.9 Congenital malformation of cardiac septum, unspecified
Septal (heart) defect NOS

✓4ᵗʰ Q22 Congenital malformations of pulmonary and tricuspid valves
CC Excl: For codes in category Q22, unless otherwise noted:
For MCC codes: PDX collection 1061
For CC codes: PDX collection 1060

Q22.0 Pulmonary valve atresia   `MCC`
CC Excl: PDX collection 1059

Q22.1 Congenital pulmonary valve stenosis   `CC`
DEF: Stenosis of the opening between the pulmonary artery and right ventricle, causing obstructed blood outflow from the right ventricle.
CC Excl: PDX collection 1059

Q22.2 Congenital pulmonary valve insufficiency   `CC`
Congenital pulmonary valve regurgitation

Q22.3 Other congenital malformations of pulmonary valve   `CC`
Congenital malformation of pulmonary valve NOS
Supernumerary cusps of pulmonary valve

Q22.4 Congenital tricuspid stenosis   `MCC`
Congenital tricuspid atresia

Q22.5 Ebstein's anomaly   `MCC`
DEF: Malformation of the tricuspid valve characterized by septal and posterior leaflets attaching to the wall of the right ventricle. Ebstein's anomaly causes the right ventricle to fuse with the atrium into a large right atrium and a small ventricle and leads to heart failure and abnormal cardiac rhythm.

Q22.6 Hypoplastic right heart syndrome   `MCC`

Q22.8 Other congenital malformations of tricuspid valve   `MCC`

Q22.9 Congenital malformation of tricuspid valve, unspecified   `MCC`

✓4ᵗʰ Q23 Congenital malformations of aortic and mitral valves

Q23.0 Congenital stenosis of aortic valve
Congenital aortic atresia
Congenital aortic stenosis NOS
EXCLUDES 1 *congenital stenosis of aortic valve in hypoplastic left heart syndrome (Q23.4)*
congenital subaortic stenosis (Q24.4)
supravalvular aortic stenosis (congenital) (Q25.3)

Q23.1 Congenital insufficiency of aortic valve
Bicuspid aortic valve
Congenital aortic insufficiency

Q23.2 Congenital mitral stenosis
Congenital mitral atresia
DEF: Congenital stenosis of the mitral valve orifice between the left atrium and ventricle, at the supravalvular, valvular, or subvalvular levels, causing obstruction to left ventricular filling.

Q23.3 Congenital mitral insufficiency

Q23.4 Hypoplastic left heart syndrome   `MCC`
CC Excl: PDX collection 1061

Q23.8 Other congenital malformations of aortic and mitral valves

Q23.9 Congenital malformation of aortic and mitral valves, unspecified

✓4ᵗʰ Q24 Other congenital malformations of heart
EXCLUDES 1 *endocardial fibroelastosis (I42.4)*

Q24.0 Dextrocardia   `CC`
EXCLUDES 1 *dextrocardia with situs inversus (Q89.3)*
isomerism of atrial appendages (with asplenia or polysplenia) (Q20.6)
mirror-image atrial arrangement with situs inversus (Q89.3)
DEF: Congenital condition in which the heart is located on the right side of the chest rather than in its normal position on the left.
CC Excl: PDX collection 1062

Q24.1 Levocardia   `CC`
CC Excl: PDX collection 1062

Q24.2 Cor triatriatum   `MCC`
CC Excl: PDX collection 1063

Q24.3 Pulmonary infundibular stenosis   `CC`
Subvalvular pulmonic stenosis
CC Excl: PDX collection 1063

Q24.4 Congenital subaortic stenosis   `MCC`
DEF: Congenital heart defect characterized by stenosis of the left ventricular outflow tract due to a fibrous tissue ring or septal hypertrophy below the aortic valve.
CC Excl: PDX collection 1063

Q24.5 Malformation of coronary vessels
Congenital coronary (artery) aneurysm

Q24.6 Congenital heart block   `MCC`
CC Excl: PDX collection 1065

Q24.8 Other specified congenital malformations of heart
Congenital diverticulum of left ventricle
Congenital malformation of myocardium
Congenital malformation of pericardium
Malposition of heart
Uhl's disease

Q24.9 Congenital malformation of heart, unspecified
Congenital anomaly of heart
Congenital disease of heart

N Newborn: 0   **P** Pediatric: 0-17   **M** Maternity: 9-64   **A** Adult: 15-124   `MCC` Major Complication/Comorbidity   `CC` Complication/Comorbidity   `SW` Severe Wound Dx

936   ICD-10-CM 2020

✓4ᵗʰ Q25 Congenital malformations of great arteries

Q25.0 Patent ductus arteriosus `CC`

Patent ductus Botallo
Persistent ductus arteriosus
DEF: Condition in which the normal channel between the pulmonary artery and the aorta fails to close at birth, causing arterial blood to recirculate in the lungs and inhibiting the blood supply to the aorta. ***Synonym(s):*** *PDA.*
CC Excl: PDX collection 1066

Patent Ductus Arteriosus

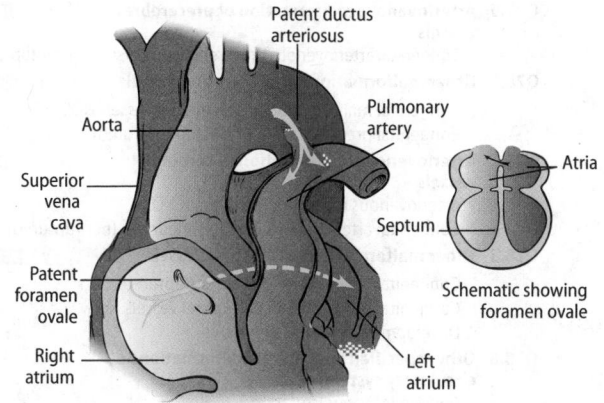

Schematic showing foramen ovale

Q25.1 Coarctation of aorta `CC`

Coarctation of aorta (preductal) (postductal)
Stenosis of aorta
AHA: 2016,4Q,56-57
CC Excl: PDX collection 1067

✓5ᵗʰ Q25.2 Atresia of aorta

AHA: 2016,4Q,56-57

Q25.21 Interruption of aortic arch `CC`

Atresia of aortic arch
CC Excl: PDX collection 1068

Q25.29 Other atresia of aorta `CC`

Atresia of aorta
CC Excl: PDX collection 1068

Q25.3 Supravalvular aortic stenosis `CC`

`EXCLUDES 1` *congenital aortic stenosis NOS (Q23.0)*
congenital stenosis of aortic valve (Q23.0)
CC Excl: PDX collection 1068

✓5ᵗʰ Q25.4 Other congenital malformations of aorta

`EXCLUDES 1` *hypoplasia of aorta in hypoplastic left heart syndrome (Q23.4)*
AHA: 2016,4Q,57
CC Excl: For CC codes in subcategory Q25.4: PDX collection 1069

Q25.40 Congenital malformation of aorta unspecified `CC`

Q25.41 Absence and aplasia of aorta `CC`

Q25.42 Hypoplasia of aorta `CC`

Q25.43 Congenital aneurysm of aorta `CC`

Congenital aneurysm of aortic root
Congenital aneurysm of aortic sinus

Q25.44 Congenital dilation of aorta `CC`

Q25.45 Double aortic arch `CC`

Vascular ring of aorta

Aortic Arch Anomalies

Aortic arch — Esophagus
— Trachea

Normal aortic arch

Double aortic arch   Right aortic arch

Q25.46 Tortuous aortic arch `CC`

Persistent convolutions of aortic arch

Q25.47 Right aortic arch `CC`

Persistent right aortic arch

Q25.48 Anomalous origin of subclavian artery `CC`

Q25.49 Other congenital malformations of aorta `CC`

Aortic arch
Bovine arch

Q25.5 Atresia of pulmonary artery `MCC`

CC Excl: PDX collection 1070

Q25.6 Stenosis of pulmonary artery `MCC`

Supravalvular pulmonary stenosis
CC Excl: PDX collection 1070

✓5ᵗʰ Q25.7 Other congenital malformations of pulmonary artery

CC Excl: For MCC codes in subcategory Q25.7: PDX collection 1070

Q25.71 Coarctation of pulmonary artery `MCC`

Q25.72 Congenital pulmonary arteriovenous malformation `MCC`

Congenital pulmonary arteriovenous aneurysm

Q25.79 Other congenital malformations of pulmonary artery `MCC`

Aberrant pulmonary artery
Agenesis of pulmonary artery
Congenital aneurysm of pulmonary artery
Congenital anomaly of pulmonary artery
Hypoplasia of pulmonary artery

Q25.8 Other congenital malformations of other great arteries `CC`

CC Excl: PDX collection 1069

Q25.9 Congenital malformation of great arteries, unspecified `CC`

CC Excl: PDX collection 1069

✓4ᵗʰ Q26 Congenital malformations of great veins

Q26.0 Congenital stenosis of vena cava `CC`

Congenital stenosis of vena cava (inferior)(superior)
CC Excl: PDX collection 1071

Q26.1 Persistent left superior vena cava `CC`

CC Excl: PDX collection 1071

Chapter 17. Congenital Malformations, Deformations and Chromosomal Abnormalities

Q26.2 **Total anomalous pulmonary venous connection** `CC`
Total anomalous pulmonary venous return [TAPVR], subdiaphragmatic
Total anomalous pulmonary venous return [TAPVR], supradiaphragmatic
CC Excl: PDX collection 1072

Q26.3 **Partial anomalous pulmonary venous connection** `CC`
Partial anomalous pulmonary venous return
CC Excl: PDX collection 1073

Q26.4 **Anomalous pulmonary venous connection, unspecified** `CC`
CC Excl: PDX collection 1073

Q26.5 **Anomalous portal venous connection**

Q26.6 **Portal vein-hepatic artery fistula**

Q26.8 **Other congenital malformations of great veins** `CC`
Absence of vena cava (inferior) (superior)
Azygos continuation of inferior vena cava
Persistent left posterior cardinal vein
Scimitar syndrome
CC Excl: PDX collection 1071

Q26.9 **Congenital malformation of great vein, unspecified** `CC`
Congenital anomaly of vena cava (inferior) (superior) NOS
CC Excl: PDX collection 1074

✓4ᵗʰ **Q27** **Other congenital malformations of peripheral vascular system**
EXCLUDES 2   anomalies of cerebral and precerebral vessels (Q28.0-Q28.3)
anomalies of coronary vessels (Q24.5)
anomalies of pulmonary artery (Q25.5-Q25.7)
congenital retinal aneurysm (Q14.1)
hemangioma and lymphangioma (D18.-)

Q27.0 **Congenital absence and hypoplasia of umbilical artery**
Single umbilical artery

Q27.1 **Congenital renal artery stenosis**

Q27.2 **Other congenital malformations of renal artery**
Congenital malformation of renal artery NOS
Multiple renal arteries

✓5ᵗʰ **Q27.3** **Arteriovenous malformation (peripheral)**
Arteriovenous aneurysm
EXCLUDES 1   acquired arteriovenous aneurysm (I77.0)
EXCLUDES 2   arteriovenous malformation of cerebral vessels (Q28.2)
arteriovenous malformation of precerebral vessels (Q28.0)
DEF: Arteriovenous malformation: Connecting passage between an artery and a vein.

     Q27.30 **Arteriovenous malformation, site unspecified** `CC`
CC Excl: PDX collection 1075

     Q27.31 **Arteriovenous malformation of vessel of upper limb**

     Q27.32 **Arteriovenous malformation of vessel of lower limb**

     Q27.33 **Arteriovenous malformation of digestive system vessel**
AHA: 2018,3Q,21

     Q27.34 **Arteriovenous malformation of renal vessel**

     Q27.39 **Arteriovenous malformation, other site**

Q27.4 **Congenital phlebectasia** `CC`
CC Excl: PDX collection 1075

Q27.8 **Other specified congenital malformations of peripheral vascular system**
Absence of peripheral vascular system
Atresia of peripheral vascular system
Congenital aneurysm (peripheral)
Congenital stricture, artery
Congenital varix
EXCLUDES 1   arteriovenous malformation (Q27.3-)

Q27.9 **Congenital malformation of peripheral vascular system, unspecified**
Anomaly of artery or vein NOS

✓4ᵗʰ **Q28** **Other congenital malformations of circulatory system**
EXCLUDES 1   congenital aneurysm NOS (Q27.8)
congenital coronary aneurysm (Q24.5)
ruptured cerebral arteriovenous malformation (I60.8)
ruptured malformation of precerebral vessels (I72.0)
EXCLUDES 2   congenital peripheral aneurysm (Q27.8)
congenital pulmonary aneurysm (Q25.79)
congenital retinal aneurysm (Q14.1)
CC Excl: For codes in category Q28:
For MCC codes: PDX collection 1076
For CC codes, unless otherwise noted: PDX collection 1075

Q28.0 **Arteriovenous malformation of precerebral vessels** `CC`
Congenital arteriovenous precerebral aneurysm (nonruptured)

Q28.1 **Other malformations of precerebral vessels** `CC`
Congenital malformation of precerebral vessels NOS
Congenital precerebral aneurysm (nonruptured)

Q28.2 **Arteriovenous malformation of cerebral vessels** `MCC`
Arteriovenous malformation of brain NOS
Congenital arteriovenous cerebral aneurysm (nonruptured)

Q28.3 **Other malformations of cerebral vessels** `MCC`
Congenital cerebral aneurysm (nonruptured)
Congenital malformation of cerebral vessels NOS
Developmental venous anomaly

Q28.8 **Other specified congenital malformations of circulatory system** `CC`
Congenital aneurysm, specified site NEC
Spinal vessel anomaly

Q28.9 **Congenital malformation of circulatory system, unspecified** `CC`
CC Excl: PDX collection 1077

Congenital malformations of the respiratory system (Q30-Q34)

✓4ᵗʰ **Q30** **Congenital malformations of nose**
EXCLUDES 1   congenital deviation of nasal septum (Q67.4)

Q30.0 **Choanal atresia**
Atresia of nares (anterior) (posterior)
Congenital stenosis of nares (anterior) (posterior)

Q30.1 **Agenesis and underdevelopment of nose**
Congenital absent of nose

Q30.2 **Fissured, notched and cleft nose**

Q30.3 **Congenital perforated nasal septum**

Q30.8 **Other congenital malformations of nose**
Accessory nose
Congenital anomaly of nasal sinus wall

Q30.9 **Congenital malformation of nose, unspecified**

✓4ᵗʰ **Q31** **Congenital malformations of larynx**
EXCLUDES 1   congenital laryngeal stridor NOS (P28.89)
CC Excl: For CC codes in category Q31: PDX collection 1078

Q31.0 **Web of larynx**
Glottic web of larynx
Subglottic web of larynx
Web of larynx NOS
DEF: Congenital malformation of the larynx marked by thin, translucent, or thick fibrotic membrane-like structure between the vocal folds. It is characterized by shortness of breath and stridor.

Q31.1 **Congenital subglottic stenosis** `CC`

Q31.2 **Laryngeal hypoplasia** `CC`

Q31.3 **Laryngocele** `CC`

Q31.5 **Congenital laryngomalacia** `CC`

Q31.8 **Other congenital malformations of larynx** `CC`
Absence of larynx
Agenesis of larynx
Atresia of larynx
Congenital cleft thyroid cartilage
Congenital fissure of epiglottis
Congenital stenosis of larynx NEC
Posterior cleft of cricoid cartilage

Q31.9 **Congenital malformation of larynx, unspecified** `CC`

✓4ᵗʰ **Q32　Congenital malformations of trachea and bronchus**

　　　EXCLUDES 1　congenital bronchiectasis (Q33.4)

　　CC Excl: For CC codes in category Q32: PDX collection 1078

　　Q32.Ø　Congenital tracheomalacia　　　　`CC`

　　Q32.1　Other congenital malformations of trachea　　`CC`

　　　　Atresia of trachea
　　　　Congenital anomaly of tracheal cartilage
　　　　Congenital dilatation of trachea
　　　　Congenital malformation of trachea
　　　　Congenital stenosis of trachea
　　　　Congenital tracheocele

　　Q32.2　Congenital bronchomalacia　　　　`CC`

　　Q32.3　Congenital stenosis of bronchus　　`CC`

　　Q32.4　Other congenital malformations of bronchus　`CC`

　　　　Absence of bronchus
　　　　Agenesis of bronchus
　　　　Atresia of bronchus
　　　　Congenital diverticulum of bronchus
　　　　Congenital malformation of bronchus NOS

✓4ᵗʰ **Q33　Congenital malformations of lung**

　　CC Excl: For MCC codes in category Q33: PDX collection 1079

　　Q33.Ø　Congenital cystic lung　　　　`CC`

　　　　Congenital cystic lung disease
　　　　Congenital honeycomb lung
　　　　Congenital polycystic lung disease
　　　　EXCLUDES 1　cystic fibrosis (E84.Ø)
　　　　　　　　cystic lung disease, acquired or unspecified (J98.4)
　　　　CC Excl: PDX collection 1079

　　Q33.1　Accessory lobe of lung
　　　　Azygos lobe (fissured), lung

　　Q33.2　Sequestration of lung　　　　`MCC`

　　Q33.3　Agenesis of lung　　　　`MCC`
　　　　Congenital absence of lung (lobe)

　　Q33.4　Congenital bronchiectasis　　　　`CC`
　　　　CC Excl: PDX collection 1080

　　Q33.5　Ectopic tissue in lung

　　Q33.6　Congenital hypoplasia and dysplasia of lung　`MCC`
　　　　EXCLUDES 1　pulmonary hypoplasia associated with short
　　　　　　　　gestation (P28.Ø)

　　Q33.8　Other congenital malformations of lung

　　Q33.9　Congenital malformation of lung, unspecified

✓4ᵗʰ **Q34　Other congenital malformations of respiratory system**

　　　EXCLUDES 2　congenital central alveolar hypoventilation syndrome
　　　　　　　(G47.35)

　　Q34.Ø　Anomaly of pleura

　　Q34.1　Congenital cyst of mediastinum

　　Q34.8　Other specified congenital malformations of respiratory system
　　　　Atresia of nasopharynx

　　Q34.9　Congenital malformation of respiratory system, unspecified
　　　　Congenital absence of respiratory system
　　　　Congenital anomaly of respiratory system NOS

Cleft lip and cleft palate (Q35-Q37)

Use additional code to identify associated malformation of the nose (Q3Ø.2)

EXCLUDES 1　Robin's syndrome (Q87.Ø)

✓4ᵗʰ **Q35　Cleft palate**

　　INCLUDES　fissure of palate
　　　　　palatoschisis

　　EXCLUDES 1　cleft palate with cleft lip (Q37.-)

　　DEF: Congenital fissure or defect of the roof of the mouth opening to the
　　nasal cavity due to failure of embryonic cells to fuse completely.

Cleft Palate

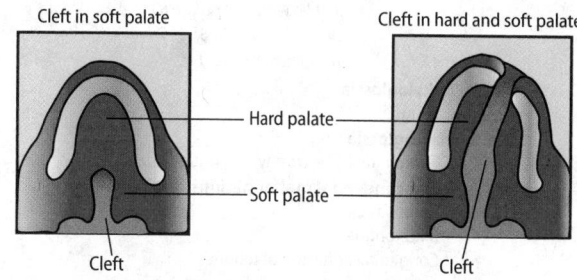

Cleft in soft palate　　　　　　　　　　Cleft in hard and soft palate

Hard palate

Soft palate

Cleft　　　　　　　　　　　　　　　Cleft

　　Q35.1　Cleft hard palate

　　Q35.3　Cleft soft palate

　　Q35.5　Cleft hard palate with cleft soft palate

　　Q35.7　Cleft uvula

　　Q35.9　Cleft palate, unspecified
　　　　Cleft palate NOS

✓4ᵗʰ **Q36　Cleft lip**

　　INCLUDES　cheiloschisis
　　　　　congenital fissure of lip
　　　　　harelip
　　　　　labium leporinum

　　EXCLUDES 1　cleft lip with cleft palate (Q37.-)

　　DEF: Congenital fissure or opening in the upper lip due to failure of
　　embryonic cells to fuse completely.

Cleft Lip

Unilateral incomplete　　　Unilateral complete　　　Bilateral complete

　　Q36.Ø　Cleft lip, bilateral

　　Q36.1　Cleft lip, median

　　Q36.9　Cleft lip, unilateral
　　　　Cleft lip NOS

✓4ᵗʰ **Q37　Cleft palate with cleft lip**

　　INCLUDES　cheilopalatoschisis

　　Q37.Ø　Cleft hard palate with bilateral cleft lip

　　Q37.1　Cleft hard palate with unilateral cleft lip
　　　　Cleft hard palate with cleft lip NOS

　　Q37.2　Cleft soft palate with bilateral cleft lip

　　Q37.3　Cleft soft palate with unilateral cleft lip
　　　　Cleft soft palate with cleft lip NOS

　　Q37.4　Cleft hard and soft palate with bilateral cleft lip

　　Q37.5　Cleft hard and soft palate with unilateral cleft lip
　　　　Cleft hard and soft palate with cleft lip NOS

　　Q37.8　Unspecified cleft palate with bilateral cleft lip

　　Q37.9　Unspecified cleft palate with unilateral cleft lip
　　　　Cleft palate with cleft lip NOS

☑ Additional Character Required　　✓x7ᵗʰ Placeholder　　Unacceptable PDx　　Questionable PDx　　Manifestation　　Unspecified Dx　　**H1**-**H14** HAC　　**HCC** CMS-HCC Dx　　**HIV** HIV Dx

ICD-10-CM 2020　　　　　　　　　　　　　　　　　　　　　　　　　　　　　**939**

Other congenital malformations of the digestive system (Q38-Q45)

☑4ᵗʰ **Q38 Other congenital malformations of tongue, mouth and pharynx**

> **EXCLUDES 1**   *dentofacial anomalies (M26.-)*
> *macrostomia (Q18.4)*
> *microstomia (Q18.5)*

Q38.0 Congenital malformations of lips, not elsewhere classified
Congenital fistula of lip
Congenital malformation of lip NOS
Van der Woude's syndrome
> **EXCLUDES 1**   *cleft lip (Q36.-)*
> *cleft lip with cleft palate (Q37.-)*
> *macrocheilia (Q18.6)*
> *microcheilia (Q18.7)*

Q38.1 Ankyloglossia
Tongue tie

Q38.2 Macroglossia
Congenital hypertrophy of tongue

Q38.3 Other congenital malformations of tongue
Aglossia
Bifid tongue
Congenital adhesion of tongue
Congenital fissure of tongue
Congenital malformation of tongue NOS
Double tongue
Hypoglossia
Hypoplasia of tongue
Microglossia

Q38.4 Congenital malformations of salivary glands and ducts
Atresia of salivary glands and ducts
Congenital absence of salivary glands and ducts
Congenital accessory salivary glands and ducts
Congenital fistula of salivary gland

Q38.5 Congenital malformations of palate, not elsewhere classified
Congenital absence of uvula
Congenital malformation of palate NOS
Congenital high arched palate
> **EXCLUDES 1**   *cleft palate (Q35.-)*
> *cleft palate with cleft lip (Q37.-)*

Q38.6 Other congenital malformations of mouth
Congenital malformation of mouth NOS

Q38.7 Congenital pharyngeal pouch
Congenital diverticulum of pharynx
> **EXCLUDES 1**   *pharyngeal pouch syndrome (D82.1)*

Q38.8 Other congenital malformations of pharynx
Congenital malformation of pharynx NOS
Imperforate pharynx

☑4ᵗʰ **Q39 Congenital malformations of esophagus**

> **CC Excl: For codes in category Q39:**
> **For MCC codes:** PDX collection 1081
> **For CC codes:** PDX collection 1082

Q39.0 Atresia of esophagus without fistula   `MCC`
Atresia of esophagus NOS

Q39.1 Atresia of esophagus with tracheo-esophageal fistula   `MCC`
Atresia of esophagus with broncho-esophageal fistula

Q39.2 Congenital tracheo-esophageal fistula without atresia   `MCC`
Congenital tracheo-esophageal fistula NOS

Q39.3 Congenital stenosis and stricture of esophagus   `MCC`

Q39.4 Esophageal web   `CC`

Q39.5 Congenital dilatation of esophagus   `CC`
Congenital cardiospasm

Q39.6 Congenital diverticulum of esophagus   `CC`
Congenital esophageal pouch

Q39.8 Other congenital malformations of esophagus   `CC`
Congenital absence of esophagus
Congenital displacement of esophagus
Congenital duplication of esophagus

Q39.9 Congenital malformation of esophagus, unspecified   `CC`

☑4ᵗʰ **Q40 Other congenital malformations of upper alimentary tract**

Q40.0 Congenital hypertrophic pyloric stenosis
Congenital or infantile constriction
Congenital or infantile hypertromphy
Congenital or infantile spasm
Congenital or infantile stenosis
Congenital or infantile stricture

Q40.1 Congenital hiatus hernia
Congenital displacement of cardia through esophageal hiatus
> **EXCLUDES 1**   *congenital diaphragmatic hernia (Q79.0)*

Q40.2 Other specified congenital malformations of stomach
Congenital displacement of stomach
Congenital diverticulum of stomach
Congenital hourglass stomach
Congenital duplication of stomach
Megalogastria
Microgastria

Q40.3 Congenital malformation of stomach, unspecified

Q40.8 Other specified congenital malformations of upper alimentary tract

Q40.9 Congenital malformation of upper alimentary tract, unspecified
Congenital anomaly of upper alimentary tract
Congenital deformity of upper alimentary tract

☑4ᵗʰ **Q41 Congenital absence, atresia and stenosis of small intestine**

> **INCLUDES**   congenital obstruction, occlusion or stricture of small intestine or intestine NOS
> **EXCLUDES 1**   *cystic fibrosis with intestinal manifestation (E84.11)*
> *meconium ileus NOS (without cystic fibrosis) (P76.0)*

> **CC Excl: For CC codes in category Q41:** PDX collection 1083

Q41.0 Congenital absence, atresia and stenosis of duodenum   `CC`

Q41.1 Congenital absence, atresia and stenosis of jejunum   `CC`
Apple peel syndrome
Imperforate jejunum

Q41.2 Congenital absence, atresia and stenosis of ileum   `CC`

Q41.8 Congenital absence, atresia and stenosis of other specified parts of small intestine   `CC`

Q41.9 Congenital absence, atresia and stenosis of small intestine, part unspecified   `CC`
Congenital absence, atresia and stenosis of intestine NOS

☑4ᵗʰ **Q42 Congenital absence, atresia and stenosis of large intestine**

> **INCLUDES**   congenital obstruction, occlusion and stricture of large intestine

> **CC Excl: For CC codes in category Q42:** PDX collection 1084

Q42.0 Congenital absence, atresia and stenosis of rectum with fistula   `CC`

Q42.1 Congenital absence, atresia and stenosis of rectum without fistula   `CC`
Imperforate rectum

Q42.2 Congenital absence, atresia and stenosis of anus with fistula   `CC`

Q42.3 Congenital absence, atresia and stenosis of anus without fistula   `CC`
Imperforate anus

Q42.8 Congenital absence, atresia and stenosis of other parts of large intestine   `CC`

Q42.9 Congenital absence, atresia and stenosis of large intestine, part unspecified   `CC`

☑4ᵗʰ **Q43 Other congenital malformations of intestine**

> **CC Excl: For CC codes in category Q43, unless otherwise noted:** PDX collection 1087

Q43.0 Meckel's diverticulum (displaced) (hypertrophic)
Persistent omphalomesenteric duct
Persistent vitelline duct
DEF: Congenital, abnormal remnant of embryonic digestive system development that leaves a sacculation or outpouching from the wall of the small intestine near the terminal part of the ileum made of acid-secreting tissue as in the stomach.

N Newborn: 0   P Pediatric: 0-17   M Maternity: 9-64   A Adult: 15-124   `MCC` Major Complication/Comorbidity   `CC` Complication/Comorbidity   `SW` Severe Wound Dx

940   ICD-10-CM 2020

Q43.1 Hirschsprung's disease `CC`

Aganglionosis
Congenital (aganglionic) megacolon
DEF: Congenital enlargement or dilation of the colon, with the absence of nerve cells in a segment of colon distally that causes the inability to defecate.
CC Excl: PDX collection 1085

Q43.2 Other congenital functional disorders of colon `CC`

Congenital dilatation of colon
CC Excl: PDX collection 1085

Q43.3 Congenital malformations of intestinal fixation `CC`

Congenital omental, anomalous adhesions [bands]
Congenital peritoneal adhesions [bands]
Incomplete rotation of cecum and colon
Insufficient rotation of cecum and colon
Jackson's membrane
Malrotation of colon
Rotation failure of cecum and colon
Universal mesentery
CC Excl: PDX collection 1086

Q43.4 Duplication of intestine `CC`

Q43.5 Ectopic anus `CC`

Q43.6 Congenital fistula of rectum and anus `CC`

EXCLUDES 1   congenital fistula of anus with absence, atresia and stenosis (Q42.2)
congenital fistula of rectum with absence, atresia and stenosis (Q42.0)
congenital rectovaginal fistula (Q52.2)
congenital urethrorectal fistula (Q64.73)
pilonidal fistula or sinus (L05.-)

Q43.7 Persistent cloaca `CC`

Cloaca NOS

Q43.8 Other specified congenital malformations of intestine `CC`

Congenital blind loop syndrome
Congenital diverticulitis, colon
Congenital diverticulum, intestine
Dolichocolon
Megaloappendix
Megaloduodenum
Microcolon
Transposition of appendix
Transposition of colon
Transposition of intestine
AHA: 2013,2Q,31

Q43.9 Congenital malformation of intestine, unspecified `CC`

✓4ᵗʰ **Q44 Congenital malformations of gallbladder, bile ducts and liver**

CC Excl: For codes in category Q44:
For MCC codes: PDX collection 1089
For CC codes, unless otherwise noted: PDX collection 1088

Q44.0 Agenesis, aplasia and hypoplasia of gallbladder `CC`

Congenital absence of gallbladder

Q44.1 Other congenital malformations of gallbladder `CC`

Congenital malformation of gallbladder NOS
Intrahepatic gallbladder

Q44.2 Atresia of bile ducts `MCC`

Q44.3 Congenital stenosis and stricture of bile ducts `MCC`

Q44.4 Choledochal cyst `CC`

Q44.5 Other congenital malformations of bile ducts `CC`

Accessory hepatic duct
Biliary duct duplication
Congenital malformation of bile duct NOS
Cystic duct duplication

Q44.6 Cystic disease of liver `CC`

Fibrocystic disease of liver
CC Excl: PDX collection 1090

Q44.7 Other congenital malformations of liver `CC`

Accessory liver
Alagille's syndrome
Congenital absence of liver
Congenital hepatomegaly
Congenital malformation of liver NOS

✓4ᵗʰ **Q45 Other congenital malformations of digestive system**

EXCLUDES 2   congenital diaphragmatic hernia (Q79.0)
congenital hiatus hernia (Q40.1)

CC Excl: For CC codes in category Q45: PDX collection 1091

Q45.0 Agenesis, aplasia and hypoplasia of pancreas `CC`

Congenital absence of pancreas

Q45.1 Annular pancreas `CC`

Q45.2 Congenital pancreatic cyst `CC`

Q45.3 Other congenital malformations of pancreas and pancreatic duct `CC`

Accessory pancreas
Congenital malformation of pancreas or pancreatic duct NOS
EXCLUDES 1   congenital diabetes mellitus (E10.-)
cystic fibrosis (E84.0-E84.9)
fibrocystic disease of pancreas (E84.-)
neonatal diabetes mellitus (P70.2)

Q45.8 Other specified congenital malformations of digestive system

Absence (complete) (partial) of alimentary tract NOS
Duplication of digestive system
Malposition, congenital of digestive system

Q45.9 Congenital malformation of digestive system, unspecified

Congenital anomaly of digestive system
Congenital deformity of digestive system

Congenital malformations of genital organs (Q50-Q56)

EXCLUDES 1   androgen insensitivity syndrome (E34.5-)
syndromes associated with anomalies in the number and form of chromosomes (Q90-Q99)

✓4ᵗʰ **Q50 Congenital malformations of ovaries, fallopian tubes and broad ligaments**

✓5ᵗʰ **Q50.0 Congenital absence of ovary**

EXCLUDES 1   Turner's syndrome (Q96.-)

Q50.01 Congenital absence of ovary, unilateral ♀

Q50.02 Congenital absence of ovary, bilateral ♀

Q50.1 Developmental ovarian cyst ♀

Q50.2 Congenital torsion of ovary ♀

✓5ᵗʰ **Q50.3 Other congenital malformations of ovary**

Q50.31 Accessory ovary ♀

Q50.32 Ovarian streak ♀

46, XX with streak gonads

Q50.39 Other congenital malformation of ovary ♀

Congenital malformation of ovary NOS

Q50.4 Embryonic cyst of fallopian tube ♀

Fimbrial cyst

Q50.5 Embryonic cyst of broad ligament ♀

Epoophoron cyst
Parovarian cyst

Q50.6 Other congenital malformations of fallopian tube and broad ligament ♀

Absence of fallopian tube and broad ligament
Accessory fallopian tube and broad ligament
Atresia of fallopian tube and broad ligament
Congenital malformation of fallopian tube or broad ligament NOS

✓4ᵗʰ **Q51 Congenital malformations of uterus and cervix**

Q51.0 Agenesis and aplasia of uterus ♀

Congenital absence of uterus

✓5ᵗʰ **Q51.1 Doubling of uterus with doubling of cervix and vagina**

Q51.10 Doubling of uterus with doubling of cervix and vagina without obstruction ♀

Doubling of uterus with doubling of cervix and vagina NOS

Q51.11 Doubling of uterus with doubling of cervix and vagina with obstruction ♀

✓5th **Q51.2 Other doubling of uterus**
Doubling of uterus NOS
Septate uterus
AHA: 2018,4Q,27

     Q51.20 Other doubling of uterus, unspecified ♀
         Septate uterus, unspecified

     Q51.21 Other complete doubling of uterus ♀
         Complete septate uterus

     Q51.22 Other partial doubling of uterus ♀
         Partial septate uterus

     Q51.28 Other doubling of uterus, other specified ♀
         Septate uterus, other specified

Q51.3 Bicornate uterus ♀
Bicornate uterus, complete or partial

Q51.4 Unicornate uterus ♀
Unicornate uterus with or without a separate uterine horn
Uterus with only one functioning horn

Q51.5 Agenesis and aplasia of cervix ♀
Congenital absence of cervix

Q51.6 Embryonic cyst of cervix ♀

Q51.7 Congenital fistulae between uterus and digestive and urinary tracts ♀

✓5th **Q51.8 Other congenital malformations of uterus and cervix**

   ✓6th **Q51.81 Other congenital malformations of uterus**

     Q51.810 Arcuate uterus ♀
         Arcuatus uterus

     Q51.811 Hypoplasia of uterus ♀

     Q51.818 Other congenital malformations of uterus ♀
         Müllerian anomaly of uterus NEC

   ✓6th **Q51.82 Other congenital malformations of cervix**

     Q51.820 Cervical duplication ♀

     Q51.821 Hypoplasia of cervix ♀

     Q51.828 Other congenital malformations of cervix ♀

Q51.9 Congenital malformation of uterus and cervix, unspecified ♀

✓4th **Q52 Other congenital malformations of female genitalia**

Q52.0 Congenital absence of vagina ♀
Vaginal agenesis, total or partial

✓5th **Q52.1 Doubling of vagina**

     EXCLUDES 1 *doubling of vagina with doubling of uterus and cervix (Q51.1-)*

     Q52.10 Doubling of vagina, unspecified ♀
         Septate vagina NOS

     Q52.11 Transverse vaginal septum ♀

   ✓6th **Q52.12 Longitudinal vaginal septum**
     AHA: 2016,4Q,58-59

     Q52.120 Longitudinal vaginal septum, nonobstructing ♀

     Q52.121 Longitudinal vaginal septum, obstructing, right side ♀

     Q52.122 Longitudinal vaginal septum, obstructing, left side ♀

     Q52.123 Longitudinal vaginal septum, microperforate, right side ♀

     Q52.124 Longitudinal vaginal septum, microperforate, left side ♀

     Q52.129 Other and unspecified longitudinal vaginal septum ♀

Q52.2 Congenital rectovaginal fistula ♀
     EXCLUDES 1 *cloaca (Q43.7)*

Q52.3 Imperforate hymen ♀
     DEF: Obstructive anomaly of vagina, characterized by complete closure of the membranous fold around the external opening of the vagina, obstructing the vaginal introitus.

Q52.4 Other congenital malformations of vagina ♀
Canal of Nuck cyst, congenital
Congenital malformation of vagina NOS
Embryonic vaginal cyst
Gartner's duct cyst

Q52.5 Fusion of labia ♀

Q52.6 Congenital malformation of clitoris ♀

✓5th **Q52.7 Other and unspecified congenital malformations of vulva**

     Q52.70 Unspecified congenital malformations of vulva ♀
         Congenital malformation of vulva NOS

     Q52.71 Congenital absence of vulva ♀

     Q52.79 Other congenital malformations of vulva ♀
         Congenital cyst of vulva

Q52.8 Other specified congenital malformations of female genitalia ♀

Q52.9 Congenital malformation of female genitalia, unspecified ♀

✓4th **Q53 Undescended and ectopic testicle**

✓5th **Q53.0 Ectopic testis**

     Q53.00 Ectopic testis, unspecified ♂

     Q53.01 Ectopic testis, unilateral ♂

     Q53.02 Ectopic testes, bilateral ♂

✓5th **Q53.1 Undescended testicle, unilateral**
     AHA: 2017,4Q,22-23

     Q53.10 Unspecified undescended testicle, unilateral ♂

   ✓6th **Q53.11 Abdominal testis, unilateral**

     Q53.111 Unilateral intraabdominal testis ♂

     Q53.112 Unilateral inguinal testis ♂

     Q53.12 Ectopic perineal testis, unilateral ♂

     Q53.13 Unilateral high scrotal testis ♂

✓5th **Q53.2 Undescended testicle, bilateral**
     AHA: 2017,4Q,22-23

     Q53.20 Undescended testicle, unspecified, bilateral ♂

   ✓6th **Q53.21 Abdominal testis, bilateral**

     Q53.211 Bilateral intraabdominal testes ♂

     Q53.212 Bilateral inguinal testes ♂

     Q53.22 Ectopic perineal testis, bilateral ♂

     Q53.23 Bilateral high scrotal testes ♂

Q53.9 Undescended testicle, unspecified ♂
Cryptorchism NOS

✓4th **Q54 Hypospadias**
     EXCLUDES 1 *epispadias (Q64.0)*
     DEF: Abnormal opening of the urethra on the ventral (underside) surface of the penis.

Hypospadias

- Balanic (glanular, coronal) hypospadias
- Subcoronal hypospadias
- Penile hypospadias
- Penile raphe
- Scrotal hypospadias
- Penoscrotal hypospadias
- Scrotum
- Scrotal raphe
- Perineal hypospadias

Hypospadias (ventral view)

Q54.0 Hypospadias, balanic ♂
Hypospadias, coronal
Hypospadias, glandular

Q54.1 Hypospadias, penile ♂

Q54.2 **Hypospadias, penoscrotal** ♂

Q54.3 **Hypospadias, perineal** ♂

Q54.4 **Congenital chordee** ♂
Chordee without hypospadias

Q54.8 **Other hypospadias** ♂
Hypospadias with intersex state

Q54.9 **Hypospadias, unspecified** ♂

✓4ᵗʰ **Q55 Other congenital malformations of male genital organs**
EXCLUDES 1   congenital hydrocele (P83.5)
hypospadias (Q54.-)

Q55.0 **Absence and aplasia of testis** ♂
Monorchism

Q55.1 **Hypoplasia of testis and scrotum** ♂
Fusion of testes

✓5ᵗʰ Q55.2 **Other and unspecified congenital malformations of testis and scrotum**

Q55.20 **Unspecified congenital malformations of testis and scrotum** ♂
Congenital malformation of testis or scrotum NOS

Q55.21 **Polyorchism** ♂
DEF: Congenital anomaly in which there are more than two testes.

Q55.22 **Retractile testis** ♂

Q55.23 **Scrotal transposition** ♂

Q55.29 **Other congenital malformations of testis and scrotum** ♂

Q55.3 **Atresia of vas deferens** ♂
Code first any associated cystic fibrosis (E84.-)

Q55.4 **Other congenital malformations of vas deferens, epididymis, seminal vesicles and prostate** ♂
Absence or aplasia of prostate
Absence or aplasia of spermatic cord
Congenital malformation of vas deferens, epididymis, seminal vesicles or prostate NOS

Q55.5 **Congenital absence and aplasia of penis** ♂

✓5ᵗʰ Q55.6 **Other congenital malformations of penis**

Q55.61 **Curvature of penis (lateral)** ♂

Q55.62 **Hypoplasia of penis** ♂
Micropenis

Q55.63 **Congenital torsion of penis** ♂
EXCLUDES 1   acquired torsion of penis (N48.82)

Q55.64 **Hidden penis** ♂
Buried penis
Concealed penis
EXCLUDES 1   acquired buried penis (N48.83)

Q55.69 **Other congenital malformation of penis**
Congenital malformation of penis NOS

Q55.7 **Congenital vasocutaneous fistula** ♂

Q55.8 **Other specified congenital malformations of male genital organs** ♂

Q55.9 **Congenital malformation of male genital organ, unspecified** ♂
Congenital anomaly of male genital organ
Congenital deformity of male genital organ

✓4ᵗʰ **Q56 Indeterminate sex and pseudohermaphroditism**
EXCLUDES 1   46, XX true hermaphrodite (Q99.1)
androgen insensitivity syndrome (E34.5-)
chimera 46, XX/46, XY true hermaphrodite (Q99.0)
female pseudohermaphroditism with adrenocortical disorder (E25.-)
pseudohermaphroditism with specified chromosomal anomaly (Q96-Q99)
pure gonadal dysgenesis (Q99.1)
DEF: Indeterminate sex: External genitalia that is nondescript, lacking the physical appearance specific to either sex.
DEF: Pseudohermaphroditism: Presence of gonads of one sex and external genitalia of another sex.

Q56.0 **Hermaphroditism, not elsewhere classified**
Ovotestis

Q56.1 **Male pseudohermaphroditism, not elsewhere classified** ♂
46, XY with streak gonads
Male pseudohermaphroditism NOS

Q56.2 **Female pseudohermaphroditism, not elsewhere classified** ♀
Female pseudohermaphroditism NOS

Q56.3 **Pseudohermaphroditism, unspecified**

Q56.4 **Indeterminate sex, unspecified**
Ambiguous genitalia

Congenital malformations of the urinary system (Q60-Q64)

✓4ᵗʰ **Q60 Renal agenesis and other reduction defects of kidney**
INCLUDES   congenital absence of kidney
congenital atrophy of kidney
infantile atrophy of kidney

Q60.0 **Renal agenesis, unilateral**

Q60.1 **Renal agenesis, bilateral**

Q60.2 **Renal agenesis, unspecified**

Q60.3 **Renal hypoplasia, unilateral**

Q60.4 **Renal hypoplasia, bilateral**

Q60.5 **Renal hypoplasia, unspecified**

Q60.6 **Potter's syndrome**

✓4ᵗʰ **Q61 Cystic kidney disease**
EXCLUDES 1   acquired cyst of kidney (N28.1)
Potter's syndrome (Q60.6)

✓5ᵗʰ Q61.0 **Congenital renal cyst**

Q61.00 **Congenital renal cyst, unspecified**
Cyst of kidney NOS (congenital)

Q61.01 **Congenital single renal cyst**

Q61.02 **Congenital multiple renal cysts**

✓5ᵗʰ Q61.1 **Polycystic kidney, infantile type**
Polycystic kidney, autosomal recessive

Q61.11 **Cystic dilatation of collecting ducts**

Q61.19 **Other polycystic kidney, infantile type**

Q61.2 **Polycystic kidney, adult type**
Polycystic kidney, autosomal dominant

Q61.3 **Polycystic kidney, unspecified**
AHA: 2016,3Q,22

Q61.4 **Renal dysplasia**
Multicystic dysplastic kidney
Multicystic kidney (development)
Multicystic kidney disease
Multicystic renal dysplasia
EXCLUDES 1   polycystic kidney disease (Q61.11-Q61.3)

Q61.5 **Medullary cystic kidney**
Nephronopthisis
Sponge kidney NOS
DEF: Sponge kidney: Dilated collecting tubules that are usually asymptomatic. Calcinosis in tubules may cause renal insufficiency.

Q61.8 **Other cystic kidney diseases** CC
Fibrocystic kidney
Fibrocystic renal degeneration or disease
CC Excl: PDX collection 1095

Q61.9 **Cystic kidney disease, unspecified** CC
Meckel-Gruber syndrome
CC Excl: PDX collection 1093

✓4ᵗʰ **Q62 Congenital obstructive defects of renal pelvis and congenital malformations of ureter**
CC Excl: For CC codes in category Q62: PDX collection 1098

Q62.0 **Congenital hydronephrosis** CC

✓5ᵗʰ Q62.1 **Congenital occlusion of ureter**
Atresia and stenosis of ureter

Q62.10 **Congenital occlusion of ureter, unspecified** CC

Q62.11 **Congenital occlusion of ureteropelvic junction** CC

Q62.12 **Congenital occlusion of ureterovesical orifice** CC

Q62.2 **Congenital megaureter** CC
Congenital dilatation of ureter

✓5ᵗʰ Q62.3 **Other obstructive defects of renal pelvis and ureter**

Q62.31 **Congenital ureterocele, orthotopic** CC

Q62.32　Cecoureterocele CC
　Ectopic ureterocele

Q62.39　Other obstructive defects of renal pelvis and ureter CC
　Ureteropelvic junction obstruction NOS

Q62.4　Agenesis of ureter
　Congenital absence ureter

Q62.5　Duplication of ureter
　Accessory ureter
　Double ureter

✓5ᵗʰ **Q62.6　Malposition of ureter**

　Q62.60　Malposition of ureter, unspecified

　Q62.61　Deviation of ureter

　Q62.62　Displacement of ureter

　Q62.63　Anomalous implantation of ureter
　　Ectopia of ureter
　　Ectopic ureter

　Q62.69　Other malposition of ureter

Q62.7　Congenital vesico-uretero-renal reflux

Q62.8　Other congenital malformations of ureter
　Anomaly of ureter NOS

✓4ᵗʰ **Q63　Other congenital malformations of kidney**

　EXCLUDES 1　congenital nephrotic syndrome (N04.-)

Q63.0　Accessory kidney

Q63.1　Lobulated, fused and horseshoe kidney

Q63.2　Ectopic kidney
　Congenital displaced kidney
　Malrotation of kidney

Q63.3　Hyperplastic and giant kidney
　Compensatory hypertrophy of kidney

Q63.8　Other specified congenital malformations of kidney
　Congenital renal calculi

Q63.9　Congenital malformation of kidney, unspecified

✓4ᵗʰ **Q64　Other congenital malformations of urinary system**

Q64.0　Epispadias

　EXCLUDES 1　hypospadias (Q54.-)

Epispadias

Epispadias (dorsal view)

✓5ᵗʰ **Q64.1　Exstrophy of urinary bladder**

　CC Excl: For CC codes in subcategory Q64.1: PDX collection 1099

　Q64.10　Exstrophy of urinary bladder, unspecified CC
　　Ectopia vesicae

　Q64.11　Supravesical fissure of urinary bladder CC

　Q64.12　Cloacal exstrophy of urinary bladder CC

　Q64.19　Other exstrophy of urinary bladder CC
　　Extroversion of bladder

Q64.2　Congenital posterior urethral valves CC

　CC Excl: PDX collection 1100

✓5ᵗʰ **Q64.3　Other atresia and stenosis of urethra and bladder neck**

　CC Excl: For CC codes in subcategory Q64.3: PDX collection 1100

　Q64.31　Congenital bladder neck obstruction CC
　　Congenital obstruction of vesicourethral orifice

　Q64.32　Congenital stricture of urethra CC

　Q64.33　Congenital stricture of urinary meatus CC

Q64.39　Other atresia and stenosis of urethra and bladder neck CC
　Atresia and stenosis of urethra and bladder neck NOS

Q64.4　Malformation of urachus
　Cyst of urachus
　Patent urachus
　Prolapse of urachus

Q64.5　Congenital absence of bladder and urethra

Q64.6　Congenital diverticulum of bladder

✓5ᵗʰ **Q64.7　Other and unspecified congenital malformations of bladder and urethra**

　EXCLUDES 1　congenital prolapse of bladder (mucosa) (Q79.4)

　Q64.70　Unspecified congenital malformation of bladder and urethra
　　Malformation of bladder or urethra NOS

　Q64.71　Congenital prolapse of urethra

　Q64.72　Congenital prolapse of urinary meatus

　Q64.73　Congenital urethrorectal fistula

　Q64.74　Double urethra

　Q64.75　Double urinary meatus

　Q64.79　Other congenital malformations of bladder and urethra

Q64.8　Other specified congenital malformations of urinary system

Q64.9　Congenital malformation of urinary system, unspecified
　Congenital anomaly NOS of urinary system
　Congenital deformity NOS of urinary system

Congenital malformations and deformations of the musculoskeletal system (Q65-Q79)

✓4ᵗʰ **Q65　Congenital deformities of hip**

　EXCLUDES 1　clicking hip (R29.4)

✓5ᵗʰ **Q65.0　Congenital dislocation of hip, unilateral**

　Q65.00　Congenital dislocation of unspecified hip, unilateral

　Q65.01　Congenital dislocation of right hip, unilateral

　Q65.02　Congenital dislocation of left hip, unilateral

Q65.1　Congenital dislocation of hip, bilateral

Q65.2　Congenital dislocation of hip, unspecified

✓5ᵗʰ **Q65.3　Congenital partial dislocation of hip, unilateral**

　Q65.30　Congenital partial dislocation of unspecified hip, unilateral

　Q65.31　Congenital partial dislocation of right hip, unilateral

　Q65.32　Congenital partial dislocation of left hip, unilateral

Q65.4　Congenital partial dislocation of hip, bilateral

Q65.5　Congenital partial dislocation of hip, unspecified

Q65.6　Congenital unstable hip
　Congenital dislocatable hip

✓5ᵗʰ **Q65.8　Other congenital deformities of hip**

　Q65.81　Congenital coxa valga

　Q65.82　Congenital coxa vara

　Q65.89　Other specified congenital deformities of hip
　　Anteversion of femoral neck
　　Congenital acetabular dysplasia

Q65.9　Congenital deformity of hip, unspecified

✓4ᵗʰ **Q66　Congenital deformities of feet**

　EXCLUDES 1　reduction defects of feet (Q72.-)
　　valgus deformities (acquired) (M21.0-)
　　varus deformities (acquired) (M21.1-)

▲ ✓5ᵗʰ **Q66.0　Congenital talipes equinovarus**

　● **Q66.00　Congenital talipes equinovarus, unspecified foot**

　● **Q66.01　Congenital talipes equinovarus, right foot**

　● **Q66.02　Congenital talipes equinovarus, left foot**

▲ ✓5ᵗʰ **Q66.1　Congenital talipes calcaneovarus**

　● **Q66.10　Congenital talipes calcaneovarus, unspecified foot**

　● **Q66.11　Congenital talipes calcaneovarus, right foot**

　● **Q66.12　Congenital talipes calcaneovarus, left foot**

✓5ᵗʰ **Q66.2　Congenital metatarsus (primus) varus**
　AHA: 2016,4Q,59

▲ ✓6ᵗʰ **Q66.21　Congenital metatarsus primus varus**

　● **Q66.211　Congenital metatarsus primus varus, right foot**

　● **Q66.212　Congenital metatarsus primus varus, left foot**

Q66.219 Congenital metatarsus primus varus, unspecified foot

▲ ☑6ᵗʰ **Q66.22 Congenital metatarsus adductus**

    Congenital metatarsus varus

Q66.221 Congenital metatarsus adductus, right foot

Q66.222 Congenital metatarsus adductus, left foot

Q66.229 Congenital metatarsus adductus, unspecified foot

▲ ☑5ᵗʰ **Q66.3 Other congenital varus deformities of feet**

    Hallux varus, congenital

Q66.30 Other congenital varus deformities of feet, unspecified foot

Q66.31 Other congenital varus deformities of feet, right foot

Q66.32 Other congenital varus deformities of feet, left foot

▲ ☑5ᵗʰ **Q66.4 Congenital talipes calcaneovalgus**

Q66.40 Congenital talipes calcaneovalgus, unspecified foot

Q66.41 Congenital talipes calcaneovalgus, right foot

Q66.42 Congenital talipes calcaneovalgus, left foot

☑5ᵗʰ **Q66.5 Congenital pes planus**

    Congenital flat foot

    Congenital rigid flat foot

    Congenital spastic (everted) flat foot

    EXCLUDES 1   pes planus, acquired (M21.4)

Q66.50 Congenital pes planus, unspecified foot

Q66.51 Congenital pes planus, right foot

Q66.52 Congenital pes planus, left foot

Q66.6 Other congenital valgus deformities of feet

    Congenital metatarsus valgus

▲ ☑5ᵗʰ **Q66.7 Congenital pes cavus**

Q66.70 Congenital pes cavus, unspecified foot

Q66.71 Congenital pes cavus, right foot

Q66.72 Congenital pes cavus, left foot

☑5ᵗʰ **Q66.8 Other congenital deformities of feet**

Q66.80 Congenital vertical talus deformity, unspecified foot

Q66.81 Congenital vertical talus deformity, right foot

Q66.82 Congenital vertical talus deformity, left foot

Q66.89 Other specified congenital deformities of feet

    Congenital asymmetric talipes

    Congenital clubfoot NOS

    Congenital talipes NOS

    Congenital tarsal coalition

    Hammer toe, congenital

    DEF: Clubfoot: Congenital anomaly of the foot with the heel elevated and rotated outward and the toes pointing inward.

▲ ☑5ᵗʰ **Q66.9 Congenital deformity of feet, unspecified**

Q66.90 Congenital deformity of feet, unspecified, unspecified foot

Q66.91 Congenital deformity of feet, unspecified, right foot

Q66.92 Congenital deformity of feet, unspecified, left foot

☑4ᵗʰ **Q67 Congenital musculoskeletal deformities of head, face, spine and chest**

    EXCLUDES 1   congenital malformation syndromes classified to Q87.-

            Potter's syndrome (Q60.6)

Q67.0 Congenital facial asymmetry

Q67.1 Congenital compression facies

Q67.2 Dolichocephaly

Q67.3 Plagiocephaly

Q67.4 Other congenital deformities of skull, face and jaw

    Congenital depressions in skull

    Congenital hemifacial atrophy or hypertrophy

    Deviation of nasal septum, congenital

    Squashed or bent nose, congenital

    EXCLUDES 1   dentofacial anomalies [including malocclusion] (M26.-)

            syphilitic saddle nose (A50.5)

    DEF: Deviated septum: Condition in which the nasal septum, a thin wall composed of cartilage and bone that separates the two nostrils, is crooked or displaced from the midline.

Q67.5 Congenital deformity of spine   cc

    Congenital postural scoliosis

    Congenital scoliosis NOS

    EXCLUDES 1   infantile idiopathic scoliosis (M41.0)

            scoliosis due to congenital bony malformation (Q76.3)

    AHA: 2014,4Q,26

    CC Excl: PDX collection 1101

Q67.6 Pectus excavatum

    Congenital funnel chest

Q67.7 Pectus carinatum

    Congenital pigeon chest

Q67.8 Other congenital deformities of chest   cc

    Congenital deformity of chest wall NOS

    CC Excl: PDX collection 1102

☑4ᵗʰ **Q68 Other congenital musculoskeletal deformities**

    EXCLUDES 1   reduction defects of limb(s) (Q71-Q73)

    EXCLUDES 2   congenital myotonic chondrodystrophy (G71.13)

Q68.0 Congenital deformity of sternocleidomastoid muscle

    Congenital contracture of sternocleidomastoid (muscle)

    Congenital (sternomastoid) torticollis

    Sternomastoid tumor (congenital)

Q68.1 Congenital deformity of finger(s) and hand   cc

    Congenital clubfinger

    Spade-like hand (congenital)

    CC Excl: PDX collection 1102

Q68.2 Congenital deformity of knee

    Congenital dislocation of knee

    Congenital genu recurvatum

Q68.3 Congenital bowing of femur

    EXCLUDES 1   anteversion of femur (neck) (Q65.89)

Q68.4 Congenital bowing of tibia and fibula

Q68.5 Congenital bowing of long bones of leg, unspecified

Q68.6 Discoid meniscus

Q68.8 Other specified congenital musculoskeletal deformities

    Congenital deformity of clavicle

    Congenital deformity of elbow

    Congenital deformity of forearm

    Congenital deformity of scapula

    Congenital deformity of wrist

    Congenital dislocation of elbow

    Congenital dislocation of shoulder

    Congenital dislocation of wrist

☑4ᵗʰ **Q69 Polydactyly**

Q69.0 Accessory finger(s)

Q69.1 Accessory thumb(s)

Q69.2 Accessory toe(s)

    Accessory hallux

Q69.9 Polydactyly, unspecified

    Supernumerary digit(s) NOS

☑4ᵗʰ **Q70 Syndactyly**

☑5ᵗʰ **Q70.0 Fused fingers**

    Complex syndactyly of fingers with synostosis

Q70.00 Fused fingers, unspecified hand

Q70.01 Fused fingers, right hand

Q70.02 Fused fingers, left hand

Q70.03 Fused fingers, bilateral

☑5ᵗʰ **Q70.1 Webbed fingers**

    Simple syndactyly of fingers without synostosis

Q70.10 Webbed fingers, unspecified hand

Q70.11 Webbed fingers, right hand

Q70.12 Webbed fingers, left hand

Q70.13 Webbed fingers, bilateral

☑6ᵗʰ **Q70.2 Fused toes**

    Complex syndactyly of toes with synostosis

Q70.20 Fused toes, unspecified foot

Q70.21 Fused toes, right foot

Q70.22 Fused toes, left foot

Q70.23 Fused toes, bilateral

☑5ᵗʰ **Q70.3 Webbed toes**

    Simple syndactyly of toes without synostosis

Q70.30 Webbed toes, unspecified foot

Q70.31 Webbed toes, right foot

Q70.32 Webbed toes, left foot

☑ Additional Character Required   ☑7ᵗʰ Placeholder   Unacceptable PDx   Questionable PDx   Manifestation   Unspecified Dx   H1-H14 HAC   HCC CMS-HCC Dx   HIV HIV Dx

ICD-10-CM 2020   945

Q70.33 Webbed toes, bilateral

Q70.4 Polysyndactyly, unspecified
> EXCLUDES 1   *specified syndactyly of hand and feet — code to specified conditions (Q70.0-Q70.3-)*

Q70.9 Syndactyly, unspecified
Symphalangy NOS

✓4ᵗʰ **Q71 Reduction defects of upper limb**

  ✓5ᵗʰ **Q71.0 Congenital complete absence of upper limb**

    Q71.00 Congenital complete absence of unspecified upper limb
    Q71.01 Congenital complete absence of right upper limb
    Q71.02 Congenital complete absence of left upper limb
    Q71.03 Congenital complete absence of upper limb, bilateral

  ✓5ᵗʰ **Q71.1 Congenital absence of upper arm and forearm with hand present**

    Q71.10 Congenital absence of unspecified upper arm and forearm with hand present
    Q71.11 Congenital absence of right upper arm and forearm with hand present
    Q71.12 Congenital absence of left upper arm and forearm with hand present
    Q71.13 Congenital absence of upper arm and forearm with hand present, bilateral

  ✓5ᵗʰ **Q71.2 Congenital absence of both forearm and hand**

    Q71.20 Congenital absence of both forearm and hand, unspecified upper limb
    Q71.21 Congenital absence of both forearm and hand, right upper limb
    Q71.22 Congenital absence of both forearm and hand, left upper limb
    Q71.23 Congenital absence of both forearm and hand, bilateral

  ✓5ᵗʰ **Q71.3 Congenital absence of hand and finger**

    Q71.30 Congenital absence of unspecified hand and finger
    Q71.31 Congenital absence of right hand and finger
    Q71.32 Congenital absence of left hand and finger
    Q71.33 Congenital absence of hand and finger, bilateral

  ✓5ᵗʰ **Q71.4 Longitudinal reduction defect of radius**

    Clubhand (congenital)
    Radial clubhand
    Q71.40 Longitudinal reduction defect of unspecified radius
    Q71.41 Longitudinal reduction defect of right radius
    Q71.42 Longitudinal reduction defect of left radius
    Q71.43 Longitudinal reduction defect of radius, bilateral

  ✓5ᵗʰ **Q71.5 Longitudinal reduction defect of ulna**

    Q71.50 Longitudinal reduction defect of unspecified ulna
    Q71.51 Longitudinal reduction defect of right ulna
    Q71.52 Longitudinal reduction defect of left ulna
    Q71.53 Longitudinal reduction defect of ulna, bilateral

  ✓5ᵗʰ **Q71.6 Lobster-claw hand**

    Q71.60 Lobster-claw hand, unspecified hand
    Q71.61 Lobster-claw right hand
    Q71.62 Lobster-claw left hand
    Q71.63 Lobster-claw hand, bilateral

  ✓5ᵗʰ **Q71.8 Other reduction defects of upper limb**

    ✓6ᵗʰ **Q71.81 Congenital shortening of upper limb**
      Q71.811 Congenital shortening of right upper limb
      Q71.812 Congenital shortening of left upper limb
      Q71.813 Congenital shortening of upper limb, bilateral
      Q71.819 Congenital shortening of unspecified upper limb

    ✓6ᵗʰ **Q71.89 Other reduction defects of upper limb**
      Q71.891 Other reduction defects of right upper limb
      Q71.892 Other reduction defects of left upper limb
      Q71.893 Other reduction defects of upper limb, bilateral
      Q71.899 Other reduction defects of unspecified upper limb

  ✓5ᵗʰ **Q71.9 Unspecified reduction defect of upper limb**

    Q71.90 Unspecified reduction defect of unspecified upper limb
    Q71.91 Unspecified reduction defect of right upper limb
    Q71.92 Unspecified reduction defect of left upper limb
    Q71.93 Unspecified reduction defect of upper limb, bilateral

✓4ᵗʰ **Q72 Reduction defects of lower limb**

  ✓5ᵗʰ **Q72.0 Congenital complete absence of lower limb**

    Q72.00 Congenital complete absence of unspecified lower limb
    Q72.01 Congenital complete absence of right lower limb
    Q72.02 Congenital complete absence of left lower limb
    Q72.03 Congenital complete absence of lower limb, bilateral

  ✓5ᵗʰ **Q72.1 Congenital absence of thigh and lower leg with foot present**

    Q72.10 Congenital absence of unspecified thigh and lower leg with foot present
    Q72.11 Congenital absence of right thigh and lower leg with foot present
    Q72.12 Congenital absence of left thigh and lower leg with foot present
    Q72.13 Congenital absence of thigh and lower leg with foot present, bilateral

  ✓5ᵗʰ **Q72.2 Congenital absence of both lower leg and foot**

    Q72.20 Congenital absence of both lower leg and foot, unspecified lower limb
    Q72.21 Congenital absence of both lower leg and foot, right lower limb
    Q72.22 Congenital absence of both lower leg and foot, left lower limb
    Q72.23 Congenital absence of both lower leg and foot, bilateral

  ✓5ᵗʰ **Q72.3 Congenital absence of foot and toe(s)**

    Q72.30 Congenital absence of unspecified foot and toe(s)
    Q72.31 Congenital absence of right foot and toe(s)
    Q72.32 Congenital absence of left foot and toe(s)
    Q72.33 Congenital absence of foot and toe(s), bilateral

  ✓5ᵗʰ **Q72.4 Longitudinal reduction defect of femur**

    Proximal femoral focal deficiency
    Q72.40 Longitudinal reduction defect of unspecified femur
    Q72.41 Longitudinal reduction defect of right femur
    Q72.42 Longitudinal reduction defect of left femur
    Q72.43 Longitudinal reduction defect of femur, bilateral

  ✓5ᵗʰ **Q72.5 Longitudinal reduction defect of tibia**

    Q72.50 Longitudinal reduction defect of unspecified tibia
    Q72.51 Longitudinal reduction defect of right tibia
    Q72.52 Longitudinal reduction defect of left tibia
    Q72.53 Longitudinal reduction defect of tibia, bilateral

  ✓5ᵗʰ **Q72.6 Longitudinal reduction defect of fibula**

    Q72.60 Longitudinal reduction defect of unspecified fibula
    Q72.61 Longitudinal reduction defect of right fibula
    Q72.62 Longitudinal reduction defect of left fibula
    Q72.63 Longitudinal reduction defect of fibula, bilateral

  ✓5ᵗʰ **Q72.7 Split foot**

    Q72.70 Split foot, unspecified lower limb
    Q72.71 Split foot, right lower limb
    Q72.72 Split foot, left lower limb
    Q72.73 Split foot, bilateral

  ✓5ᵗʰ **Q72.8 Other reduction defects of lower limb**

    ✓6ᵗʰ **Q72.81 Congenital shortening of lower limb**
      Q72.811 Congenital shortening of right lower limb
      Q72.812 Congenital shortening of left lower limb
      Q72.813 Congenital shortening of lower limb, bilateral
      Q72.819 Congenital shortening of unspecified lower limb

    ✓6ᵗʰ **Q72.89 Other reduction defects of lower limb**
      Q72.891 Other reduction defects of right lower limb
      Q72.892 Other reduction defects of left lower limb
      Q72.893 Other reduction defects of lower limb, bilateral
      Q72.899 Other reduction defects of unspecified lower limb

  ✓5ᵗʰ **Q72.9 Unspecified reduction defect of lower limb**

    Q72.90 Unspecified reduction defect of unspecified lower limb
    Q72.91 Unspecified reduction defect of right lower limb
    Q72.92 Unspecified reduction defect of left lower limb
    Q72.93 Unspecified reduction defect of lower limb, bilateral

N Newborn: 0   P Pediatric: 0-17   M Maternity: 9-64   A Adult: 15-124   MCC Major Complication/Comorbidity   CC Complication/Comorbidity   SW Severe Wound Dx

946   ICD-10-CM 2020

✓4ᵗʰ Q73 Reduction defects of unspecified limb

Q73.0 Congenital absence of unspecified limb(s)
Amelia NOS

Q73.1 Phocomelia, unspecified limb(s)
Phocomelia NOS

Q73.8 Other reduction defects of unspecified limb(s)
Longitudinal reduction deformity of unspecified limb(s)
Ectromelia of limb NOS
Hemimelia of limb NOS
Reduction defect of limb NOS

✓4ᵗʰ Q74 Other congenital malformations of limb(s)

EXCLUDES 1   polydactyly (Q69.-)
reduction defect of limb (Q71-Q73)
syndactyly (Q70.-)

Q74.0 Other congenital malformations of upper limb(s), including shoulder girdle
Accessory carpal bones
Cleidocranial dysostosis
Congenital pseudarthrosis of clavicle
Macrodactylia (fingers)
Madelung's deformity
Radioulnar synostosis
Sprengel's deformity
Triphalangeal thumb

Q74.1 Congenital malformation of knee
Congenital absence of patella
Congenital dislocation of patella
Congenital genu valgum
Congenital genu varum
Rudimentary patella
EXCLUDES 1   congenital dislocation of knee (Q68.2)
congenital genu recurvatum (Q68.2)
nail patella syndrome (Q87.2)

Q74.2 Other congenital malformations of lower limb(s), including pelvic girdle
Congenital fusion of sacroiliac joint
Congenital malformation of ankle joint
Congenital malformation of sacroiliac joint
EXCLUDES 1   anteversion of femur (neck) (Q65.89)

Q74.3 Arthrogryposis multiplex congenita   CC
CC Excl: PDX collection 1102

Q74.8 Other specified congenital malformations of limb(s)

Q74.9 Unspecified congenital malformation of limb(s)
Congenital anomaly of limb(s) NOS

✓4ᵗʰ Q75 Other congenital malformations of skull and face bones

EXCLUDES 1   congenital malformation of face NOS (Q18.-)
congenital malformation syndromes classified to Q87.-
dentofacial anomalies [including malocclusion] (M26.-)
musculoskeletal deformities of head and face (Q67.0-Q67.4)
skull defects associated with congenital anomalies of brain
such as:
anencephaly (Q00.0)
encephalocele (Q01.-)
hydrocephalus (Q03.-)
microcephaly (Q02)

Q75.0 Craniosynostosis
Acrocephaly
Imperfect fusion of skull
Oxycephaly
Trigonocephaly
DEF: Congenital condition in which one or more of the cranial sutures fuse prematurely, creating a deformed or aberrant head shape.

Q75.1 Craniofacial dysostosis
Crouzon's disease

Q75.2 Hypertelorism

Q75.3 Macrocephaly

Q75.4 Mandibulofacial dysostosis
Franceschetti syndrome
Treacher Collins syndrome

Q75.5 Oculomandibular dysostosis

Q75.8 Other specified congenital malformations of skull and face bones
Absence of skull bone, congenital
Congenital deformity of forehead
Platybasia

Q75.9 Congenital malformation of skull and face bones, unspecified
Congenital anomaly of face bones NOS
Congenital anomaly of skull NOS

✓4ᵗʰ Q76 Congenital malformations of spine and bony thorax

EXCLUDES 1   congenital musculoskeletal deformities of spine and chest (Q67.5-Q67.8)

Q76.0 Spina bifida occulta
EXCLUDES 1   meningocele (spinal) (Q05.-)
spina bifida (aperta) (cystica) (Q05.-)

Q76.1 Klippel-Feil syndrome
Cervical fusion syndrome

Q76.2 Congenital spondylolisthesis
Congenital spondylolysis
EXCLUDES 1   spondylolisthesis (acquired) (M43.1-)
spondylolysis (acquired) (M43.0-)

Q76.3 Congenital scoliosis due to congenital bony malformation   CC
Hemivertebra fusion or failure of segmentation with scoliosis
CC Excl: PDX collection 1101

✓5ᵗʰ Q76.4 Other congenital malformations of spine, not associated with scoliosis
CC Excl: For CC codes in subcategory Q76.4: PDX collection 1101

✓6ᵗʰ Q76.41 Congenital kyphosis
Q76.411 Congenital kyphosis, occipito-atlanto-axial region
Q76.412 Congenital kyphosis, cervical region
Q76.413 Congenital kyphosis, cervicothoracic region
Q76.414 Congenital kyphosis, thoracic region
Q76.415 Congenital kyphosis, thoracolumbar region
Q76.419 Congenital kyphosis, unspecified region

✓6ᵗʰ Q76.42 Congenital lordosis
Q76.425 Congenital lordosis, thoracolumbar region   CC
Q76.426 Congenital lordosis, lumbar region   CC
Q76.427 Congenital lordosis, lumbosacral region   CC
Q76.428 Congenital lordosis, sacral and sacrococcygeal region   CC
Q76.429 Congenital lordosis, unspecified region   CC

Q76.49 Other congenital malformations of spine, not associated with scoliosis
Congenital absence of vertebra NOS
Congenital fusion of spine NOS
Congenital malformation of lumbosacral (joint) (region) NOS
Congenital malformation of spine NOS
Hemivertebra NOS
Malformation of spine NOS
Platyspondylisis NOS
Supernumerary vertebra NOS

Q76.5 Cervical rib
Supernumerary rib in cervical region

Q76.6 Other congenital malformations of ribs   CC
Accessory rib
Congenital absence of rib
Congenital fusion of ribs
Congenital malformation of ribs NOS
EXCLUDES 1   short rib syndrome (Q77.2)
CC Excl: PDX collection 1103

Q76.7 Congenital malformation of sternum   CC
Congenital absence of sternum
Sternum bifidum
CC Excl: PDX collection 1103

Q76.8 Other congenital malformations of bony thorax   CC
CC Excl: PDX collection 1103

Chapter 17. Congenital Malformations, Deformations and Chromosomal Abnormalities

Q73–Q76.8

Q76.9 **Congenital malformation of bony thorax, unspecified** `CC`
 CC Excl: PDX collection 1103

✓4ᵗʰ **Q77** **Osteochondrodysplasia with defects of growth of tubular bones and spine**
 EXCLUDES 1 *mucopolysaccharidosis (E76.0-E76.3)*
 EXCLUDES 2 *congenital myotonic chondrodystrophy (G71.13)*

 Q77.0 **Achondrogenesis**
  Hypochondrogenesis

 Q77.1 **Thanatophoric short stature**

 Q77.2 **Short rib syndrome** `CC`
  Asphyxiating thoracic dysplasia [Jeune]
  CC Excl: PDX collection 1103

 Q77.3 **Chondrodysplasia punctata**
  EXCLUDES 1 *Rhizomelic chondrodysplasia punctata (E71.43)*

 Q77.4 **Achondroplasia**
  Hypochondroplasia
  Osteosclerosis congenita

 Q77.5 **Diastrophic dysplasia**

 Q77.6 **Chondroectodermal dysplasia**
  Ellis-van Creveld syndrome

 Q77.7 **Spondyloepiphyseal dysplasia**

 Q77.8 **Other osteochondrodysplasia with defects of growth of tubular bones and spine**

 Q77.9 **Osteochondrodysplasia with defects of growth of tubular bones and spine, unspecified**

✓4ᵗʰ **Q78** **Other osteochondrodysplasias**
 EXCLUDES 2 *congenital myotonic chondrodystrophy (G71.13)*

 Q78.0 **Osteogenesis imperfecta** `CC`
  Fragilitas ossium
  Osteopsathyrosis
  CC Excl: PDX collection 1104

 Q78.1 **Polyostotic fibrous dysplasia**
  Albright(-McCune)(-Sternberg) syndrome

 Q78.2 **Osteopetrosis** `CC`
  Albers-Schönberg syndrome
  Osteosclerosis NOS
  DEF: Rare congenital condition in which the bones are excessively dense, resulting from a discrepancy in the formation and breakdown of bone.
  CC Excl: PDX collection 1104

 Q78.3 **Progressive diaphyseal dysplasia**
  Camurati-Engelmann syndrome

 Q78.4 **Enchondromatosis**
  Maffucci's syndrome
  Ollier's disease

 Q78.5 **Metaphyseal dysplasia**
  Pyle's syndrome

 Q78.6 **Multiple congenital exostoses**
  Diaphyseal aclasis

 Q78.8 **Other specified osteochondrodysplasias**
  Osteopoikilosis

 Q78.9 **Osteochondrodysplasia, unspecified**
  Chondrodystrophy NOS
  Osteodystrophy NOS

✓4ᵗʰ **Q79** **Congenital malformations of musculoskeletal system, not elsewhere classified**
 EXCLUDES 2 *congenital (sternomastoid) torticollis (Q68.0)*
 CC Excl: For MCC codes in category Q79, unless otherwise noted: PDX collection 1106

 Q79.0 **Congenital diaphragmatic hernia** `MCC`
  EXCLUDES 1 *congenital hiatus hernia (Q40.1)*
  CC Excl: PDX collection 1105

 Q79.1 **Other congenital malformations of diaphragm** `MCC`
  Absence of diaphragm
  Congenital malformation of diaphragm NOS
  Eventration of diaphragm
  CC Excl: PDX collection 1105

 Q79.2 **Exomphalos** `MCC`
  Omphalocele
  EXCLUDES 1 *umbilical hernia (K42.-)*

 Q79.3 **Gastroschisis** `MCC`

Gastroschisis

Herniated small bowel (gastroschisis)
Rectus abdominus m.
Umbilicus
distal
skin
proximal
Defect

 Q79.4 **Prune belly syndrome** `CC`
  Congenital prolapse of bladder mucosa
  Eagle-Barrett syndrome

✓5ᵗʰ **Q79.5** **Other congenital malformations of abdominal wall**
  EXCLUDES 1 *umbilical hernia (K42.-)*

  Q79.51 **Congenital hernia of bladder** `CC`

  Q79.59 **Other congenital malformations of abdominal wall** `CC`

▲ ✓5ᵗʰ **Q79.6** **Ehlers-Danlos syndromes**
  DEF: Connective tissue disorder that causes hyperextended skin and joints and results in fragile blood vessels with bleeding, poor wound healing, and subcutaneous pseudotumors.

  Q79.60 **Ehlers-Danlos syndrome, unspecified**

  Q79.61 **Classical Ehlers-Danlos syndrome**
   Classical EDS (cEDS)

  Q79.62 **Hypermobile Ehlers-Danlos syndrome**
   Hypermobile EDS (hEDS)

  Q79.63 **Vascular Ehlers-Danlos syndrome**
   Vascular EDS (vEDS)

  Q79.69 **Other Ehlers-Danlos syndromes**

 Q79.8 **Other congenital malformations of musculoskeletal system**
  Absence of muscle
  Absence of tendon
  Accessory muscle
  Amyotrophia congenita
  Congenital constricting bands
  Congenital shortening of tendon
  Poland syndrome

 Q79.9 **Congenital malformation of musculoskeletal system, unspecified**
  Congenital anomaly of musculoskeletal system NOS
  Congenital deformity of musculoskeletal system NOS

Other congenital malformations (Q80-Q89)

✓4ᵗʰ **Q80** **Congenital ichthyosis**
 EXCLUDES 1 *Refsum's disease (G60.1)*
 DEF: Excessive production of skin cells resulting in red, dry, scaly skin.

 Q80.0 **Ichthyosis vulgaris**

 Q80.1 **X-linked ichthyosis**

 Q80.2 **Lamellar ichthyosis**
  Collodion baby

 Q80.3 **Congenital bullous ichthyosiform erythroderma**

 Q80.4 **Harlequin fetus**

 Q80.8 **Other congenital ichthyosis**

 Q80.9 **Congenital ichthyosis, unspecified**

✓4ᵗʰ **Q81** **Epidermolysis bullosa**

 Q81.0 **Epidermolysis bullosa simplex**
  EXCLUDES 1 *Cockayne's syndrome ▶(Q87.19)◀*

 Q81.1 **Epidermolysis bullosa letalis**
  Herlitz' syndrome

 Q81.2 **Epidermolysis bullosa dystrophica**

 Q81.8 **Other epidermolysis bullosa**

 Q81.9 **Epidermolysis bullosa, unspecified**

N Newborn: 0 P Pediatric: 0-17 M Maternity: 9-64 A Adult: 15-124 `MCC` Major Complication/Comorbidity `CC` Complication/Comorbidity `SW` Severe Wound Dx

948 ICD-10-CM 2020

☑4ᵗʰ **Q82 Other congenital malformations of skin**
> EXCLUDES 1   *acrodermatitis enteropathica (E83.2)*
> *congenital erythropoietic porphyria (E80.0)*
> *pilonidal cyst or sinus (L05.-)*
> *Sturge-Weber (-Dimitri) syndrome (Q85.8)*

Q82.0 Hereditary lymphedema

Q82.1 Xeroderma pigmentosum

Q82.2 Congenital cutaneous mastocytosis
Congenital diffuse cutaneous mastocytosis
Congenital maculopapular cutaneous mastocytosis
Congenital urticaria pigmentosa
> EXCLUDES 1   *cutaneous mastocytosis NOS (D47.01)*
> *diffuse cutaneous mastocytosis (with onset after newborn period) (D47.01)*
> *malignant mastocytosis (C96.2-)*
> *systemic mastocytosis (D47.02)*
> *urticaria pigmentosa (non-congenital) (with onset after newborn period) (D47.01)*

AHA: 2017,4Q,5

Q82.3 Incontinentia pigmenti

Q82.4 Ectodermal dysplasia (anhidrotic)
> EXCLUDES 1   *Ellis-van Creveld syndrome (Q77.6)*

Q82.5 Congenital non-neoplastic nevus
Birthmark NOS
Flammeus Nevus
Portwine Nevus
Sanguineous Nevus
Strawberry Nevus
Vascular Nevus NOS
Verrucous Nevus
> EXCLUDES 2   *araneus nevus (I78.1)*
> *Café au lait spots (L81.3)*
> *lentigo (L81.4)*
> *melanocytic nevus (D22.-)*
> *nevus NOS (D22.-)*
> *pigmented nevus (D22.-)*
> *spider nevus (I78.1)*
> *stellar nevus (I78.1)*

Q82.6 Congenital sacral dimple
Parasacral dimple
> EXCLUDES 2   *pilonidal cyst with abscess (L05.01)*
> *pilonidal cyst without abscess (L05.91)*

AHA: 2016,4Q,60

Q82.8 Other specified congenital malformations of skin
Abnormal palmar creases
Accessory skin tags
Benign familial pemphigus [Hailey-Hailey]
Congenital poikiloderma
Cutis laxa (hyperelastica)
Dermatoglyphic anomalies
Inherited keratosis palmaris et plantaris
Keratosis follicularis [Darier-White]
> EXCLUDES 1   *Ehlers-Danlos syndrome ▶(Q79.6-)◀*

AHA: 2016,1Q,17

Q82.9 Congenital malformation of skin, unspecified

☑4ᵗʰ **Q83 Congenital malformations of breast**
> EXCLUDES 2   *absence of pectoral muscle (Q79.8)*
> *hypoplasia of breast (N64.82)*
> *micromastia (N64.82)*

Q83.0 Congenital absence of breast with absent nipple

Q83.1 Accessory breast
Supernumerary breast

Q83.2 Absent nipple

Q83.3 Accessory nipple
Supernumerary nipple

Q83.8 Other congenital malformations of breast

Q83.9 Congenital malformation of breast, unspecified

☑4ᵗʰ **Q84 Other congenital malformations of integument**

Q84.0 Congenital alopecia
Congenital atrichosis

Q84.1 Congenital morphological disturbances of hair, not elsewhere classified
Beaded hair
Monilethrix
Pili annulati
> EXCLUDES 1   *Menkes' kinky hair syndrome (E83.0)*

Q84.2 Other congenital malformations of hair
Congenital hypertrichosis
Congenital malformation of hair NOS
Persistent lanugo

Q84.3 Anonychia
> EXCLUDES 1   *nail patella syndrome (Q87.2)*

Q84.4 Congenital leukonychia

Q84.5 Enlarged and hypertrophic nails
Congenital onychauxis
Pachyonychia

Q84.6 Other congenital malformations of nails
Congenital clubnail
Congenital koilonychia
Congenital malformation of nail NOS

Q84.8 Other specified congenital malformations of integument
Aplasia cutis congenita

Q84.9 Congenital malformation of integument, unspecified
Congenital anomaly of integument NOS
Congenital deformity of integument NOS

☑4ᵗʰ **Q85 Phakomatoses, not elsewhere classified**
> EXCLUDES 1   *ataxia telangiectasia [Louis-Bar] (G11.3)*
> *familial dysautonomia [Riley-Day] (G90.1)*

☑5ᵗʰ **Q85.0 Neurofibromatosis (nonmalignant)**

Q85.00 Neurofibromatosis, unspecified   HCC

Q85.01 Neurofibromatosis, type 1   HCC
Von Recklinghausen disease

Q85.02 Neurofibromatosis, type 2   HCC
Acoustic neurofibromatosis
DEF: Inherited condition with cutaneous lesions, benign tumors of peripheral nerves, and bilateral 8th nerve masses.

Q85.03 Schwannomatosis   HCC
DEF: Genetic mutation (SMARCB1/INI1) causing multiple benign tumors along the nerve pathways, except on the 8th cranial (vestibular) nerve.

Q85.09 Other neurofibromatosis   HCC

Q85.1 Tuberous sclerosis   CC HCC
Bourneville's disease
Epiloia
CC Excl: PDX collection 1108

Q85.8 Other phakomatoses, not elsewhere classified   CC HCC
Peutz-Jeghers Syndrome
Sturge-Weber(-Dimitri) syndrome
von Hippel-Lindau syndrome
> EXCLUDES 1   *Meckel-Gruber syndrome (Q61.9)*

CC Excl: PDX collection 1109

Q85.9 Phakomatosis, unspecified   CC HCC
Hamartosis NOS
CC Excl: PDX collection 1109

☑4ᵗʰ **Q86 Congenital malformation syndromes due to known exogenous causes, not elsewhere classified**
> EXCLUDES 2   *iodine-deficiency-related hypothyroidism (E00-E02)*
> *nonteratogenic effects of substances transmitted via placenta or breast milk (P04.-)*

Q86.0 Fetal alcohol syndrome (dysmorphic)

Q86.1 Fetal hydantoin syndrome
Meadow's syndrome

Q86.2 Dysmorphism due to warfarin

Q86.8 Other congenital malformation syndromes due to known exogenous causes

✓4ᵗʰ **Q87** **Other specified congenital malformation syndromes affecting multiple systems**

Use additional code(s) to identify all associated manifestations

Q87.0 **Congenital malformation syndromes predominantly affecting facial appearance**

Acrocephalopolysyndactyly
Acrocephalosyndactyly [Apert]
Cryptophthalmos syndrome
Cyclopia
Goldenhar syndrome
Moebius syndrome
Oro-facial-digital syndrome
Robin syndrome
Whistling face

▲ ✓5ᵗʰ **Q87.1** **Congenital malformation syndromes predominantly associated with short stature**

~~Aarskog syndrome~~
~~Cockayne syndrome~~
~~De Lange syndrome~~
~~Dubowitz syndrome~~
~~Noonan syndrome~~
~~Prader-Willi syndrome~~
~~Robinow-Silverman-Smith syndrome~~
~~Russell-Silver syndrome~~
~~Seckel syndrome~~

EXCLUDES 1   *Ellis-van Creveld syndrome (Q77.6)*
                Smith-Lemli-Opitz syndrome (E78.72)

● **Q87.11** **Prader-Willi syndrome**

● **Q87.19** **Other congenital malformation syndromes predominantly associated with short stature**

Aarskog syndrome
Cockayne syndrome
De Lange syndrome
Dubowitz syndrome
Noonan syndrome
Robinow-Silverman-Smith syndrome
Russell-Silver syndrome
Seckel syndrome

Q87.2 **Congenital malformation syndromes predominantly involving limbs**

Holt-Oram syndrome
Klippel-Trenaunay-Weber syndrome
Nail patella syndrome
Rubinstein-Taybi syndrome
Sirenomelia syndrome
Thrombocytopenia with absent radius [TAR] syndrome
VATER syndrome

Q87.3 **Congenital malformation syndromes involving early overgrowth**

Beckwith-Wiedemann syndrome
Sotos syndrome
Weaver syndrome

✓5ᵗʰ **Q87.4** **Marfan's syndrome**

DEF: Disorder that affects the connective tissue of multiple systems, including disproportionally long or abnormal bone structure and eye and cardiovascular complications.
CC Excl: For CC codes in subcategory Q87.4: PDX collection 1110

Q87.40 **Marfan's syndrome, unspecified**   CC

✓6ᵗʰ **Q87.41** **Marfan's syndrome with cardiovascular manifestations**

Q87.410 **Marfan's syndrome with aortic dilation**   CC

Q87.418 **Marfan's syndrome with other cardiovascular manifestations**   CC

Q87.42 **Marfan's syndrome with ocular manifestations**   CC

Q87.43 **Marfan's syndrome with skeletal manifestation**   CC

Q87.5 **Other congenital malformation syndromes with other skeletal changes**   CC

CC Excl: PDX collection 540

✓5ᵗʰ **Q87.8** **Other specified congenital malformation syndromes, not elsewhere classified**

EXCLUDES 1   *Zellweger syndrome (E71.510)*

Q87.81 **Alport syndrome**

Use additional code to identify stage of chronic kidney disease (N18.1-N18.6)

Q87.82 **Arterial tortuosity syndrome**

.**AHA:** 2016,4Q,60-61

Q87.89 **Other specified congenital malformation syndromes, not elsewhere classified**

Laurence-Moon (-Bardet)-Biedl syndrome

✓4ᵗʰ **Q89** **Other congenital malformations, not elsewhere classified**

✓5ᵗʰ **Q89.0** **Congenital absence and malformations of spleen**

EXCLUDES 1   *isomerism of atrial appendages (with asplenia or polysplenia) (Q20.6)*

Q89.01 **Asplenia (congenital)**

Q89.09 **Congenital malformations of spleen**

Congenital splenomegaly

Q89.1 **Congenital malformations of adrenal gland**

EXCLUDES 1   *adrenogenital disorders (E25.-)*
                congenital adrenal hyperplasia (E25.0)

Q89.2 **Congenital malformations of other endocrine glands**

Congenital malformation of parathyroid or thyroid gland
Persistent thyroglossal duct
Thyroglossal cyst

EXCLUDES 1   *congenital goiter (E03.0)*
                congenital hypothyroidism (E03.1)

Q89.3 **Situs inversus**

Dextrocardia with situs inversus
Mirror-image atrial arrangement with situs inversus
Situs inversus or transversus abdominalis
Situs inversus or transversus thoracis
Transposition of abdominal viscera
Transposition of thoracic viscera

EXCLUDES 1   *dextrocardia NOS (Q24.0)*

DEF: Congenital anomaly in which the internal thoracic and abdominal organs are transposed laterally and found on the opposite side from the normal position.

Q89.4 **Conjoined twins**   MCC

Craniopagus
Dicephaly
Pygopagus
Thoracopagus

CC Excl: PDX collection 1113

Q89.7 **Multiple congenital malformations, not elsewhere classified**

Multiple congenital anomalies NOS
Multiple congenital deformities NOS

EXCLUDES 1   *congenital malformation syndromes affecting multiple systems (Q87.-)*

Q89.8 **Other specified congenital malformations**

Use additional code(s) to identify all associated manifestations

Q89.9 **Congenital malformation, unspecified**

Congenital anomaly NOS
Congenital deformity NOS

Chromosomal abnormalities, not elsewhere classified (Q90-Q99)

EXCLUDES 2   *mitochondrial metabolic disorders (E88.4-)*

✓4ᵗʰ **Q90** **Down syndrome**

Use additional code(s) to identify any associated physical conditions and degree of intellectual disabilities (F70-F79)

Q90.0 **Trisomy 21, nonmosaicism (meiotic nondisjunction)**

Q90.1 **Trisomy 21, mosaicism (mitotic nondisjunction)**

Q90.2 **Trisomy 21, translocation**

Q90.9 **Down syndrome, unspecified**

Trisomy 21 NOS

✓4ᵗʰ **Q91** **Trisomy 18 and Trisomy 13**

Q91.0 **Trisomy 18, nonmosaicism (meiotic nondisjunction)**

Q91.1 **Trisomy 18, mosaicism (mitotic nondisjunction)**

Q91.2 **Trisomy 18, translocation**

Q91.3 **Trisomy 18, unspecified**

Q91.4 **Trisomy 13, nonmosaicism (meiotic nondisjunction)**

Q91.5 **Trisomy 13, mosaicism (mitotic nondisjunction)**

Q91.6 **Trisomy 13, translocation**

Q91.7 **Trisomy 13, unspecified**

N Newborn: 0   P Pediatric: 0-17   M Maternity: 9-64   A Adult: 15-124   MCC Major Complication/Comorbidity   CC Complication/Comorbidity   SW Severe Wound Dx

950   ICD-10-CM 2020

✓4ᵗʰ **Q92 Other trisomies and partial trisomies of the autosomes, not elsewhere classified**

INCLUDES unbalanced translocations and insertions

EXCLUDES 1 *trisomies of chromosomes 13, 18, 21 (Q90–Q91)*

Q92.0 Whole chromosome trisomy, nonmosaicism (meiotic nondisjunction)

Q92.1 Whole chromosome trisomy, mosaicism (mitotic nondisjunction)

Q92.2 Partial trisomy

Less than whole arm duplicated

Whole arm or more duplicated

EXCLUDES 1 *partial trisomy due to unbalanced translocation (Q92.5)*

Q92.5 Duplications with other complex rearrangements

Partial trisomy due to unbalanced translocations

Code also any associated deletions due to unbalanced translocations, inversions and insertions (Q93.7)

✓5ᵗʰ **Q92.6 Marker chromosomes**

Trisomies due to dicentrics

Trisomies due to extra rings

Trisomies due to isochromosomes

Individual with marker heterochromatin

Q92.61 Marker chromosomes in normal individual

Q92.62 Marker chromosomes in abnormal individual

Q92.7 Triploidy and polyploidy

Q92.8 Other specified trisomies and partial trisomies of autosomes

Duplications identified by fluorescence in situ hybridization (FISH)

Duplications identified by in situ hybridization (ISH)

Duplications seen only at prometaphase

Q92.9 Trisomy and partial trisomy of autosomes, unspecified

✓4ᵗʰ **Q93 Monosomies and deletions from the autosomes, not elsewhere classified**

Q93.0 Whole chromosome monosomy, nonmosaicism (meiotic nondisjunction)

Q93.1 Whole chromosome monosomy, mosaicism (mitotic nondisjunction)

Q93.2 Chromosome replaced with ring, dicentric or isochromosome

Q93.3 Deletion of short arm of chromosome 4

Wolff-Hirschorn syndrome

Q93.4 Deletion of short arm of chromosome 5

Cri-du-chat syndrome

✓5ᵗʰ **Q93.5 Other deletions of part of a chromosome**

AHA: 2018,4Q,28

Q93.51 Angelman syndrome CC

CC Excl: PDX collection 1114

Q93.59 Other deletions of part of a chromosome CC

CC Excl: PDX collection 1114

Q93.7 Deletions with other complex rearrangements

Deletions due to unbalanced translocations, inversions and insertions

Code also any associated duplications due to unbalanced translocations, inversions and insertions (Q92.5)

✓5ᵗʰ **Q93.8 Other deletions from the autosomes**

Q93.81 Velo-cardio-facial syndrome CC

Deletion 22q11.2

DEF: Microdeletion syndrome affecting multiple organs characterized by a cleft palate, heart defects, an elongated face with almond-shaped eyes, wide nose, small ears, weak immune system, weak musculature, hypothyroidism, short stature, and scoliosis. The deletion occurs at q11.2 on the long arm of the chromosome 22.

Q93.82 Williams syndrome CC

AHA: 2018,4Q,28-29

CC Excl: PDX collection 1114

Q93.88 Other microdeletions CC

Miller-Dieker syndrome

Smith-Magenis syndrome

CC Excl: PDX collection 1118

Q93.89 Other deletions from the autosomes CC

Deletions identified by fluorescence in situ hybridization (FISH)

Deletions identified by in situ hybridization (ISH)

Deletions seen only at prometaphase

CC Excl: PDX collection 1115

Q93.9 Deletion from autosomes, unspecified CC

CC Excl: PDX collection 1115

✓4ᵗʰ **Q95 Balanced rearrangements and structural markers, not elsewhere classified**

INCLUDES Robertsonian and balanced reciprocal translocations and insertions

Q95.0 Balanced translocation and insertion in normal individual

Q95.1 Chromosome inversion in normal individual

Q95.2 Balanced autosomal rearrangement in abnormal individual

Q95.3 Balanced sex/autosomal rearrangement in abnormal individual

Q95.5 Individual with autosomal fragile site

Q95.8 Other balanced rearrangements and structural markers

Q95.9 Balanced rearrangement and structural marker, unspecified

✓4ᵗʰ **Q96 Turner's syndrome**

EXCLUDES 1 *Noonan syndrome ▶(Q87.19)◀*

Q96.0 Karyotype 45, X ♀

Q96.1 Karyotype 46, X iso (Xq) ♀

Karyotype 46, isochromosome Xq

Q96.2 Karyotype 46, X with abnormal sex chromosome, except iso (Xq) ♀

Karyotype 46, X with abnormal sex chromosome, except isochromosome Xq

Q96.3 Mosaicism, 45, X/46, XX or XY ♀

Q96.4 Mosaicism, 45, X/other cell line(s) with abnormal sex chromosome ♀

Q96.8 Other variants of Turner's syndrome ♀

Q96.9 Turner's syndrome, unspecified ♀

✓4ᵗʰ **Q97 Other sex chromosome abnormalities, female phenotype, not elsewhere classified**

EXCLUDES 1 *Turner's syndrome (Q96.-)*

Q97.0 Karyotype 47, XXX ♀

Q97.1 Female with more than three X chromosomes ♀

Q97.2 Mosaicism, lines with various numbers of X chromosomes ♀

Q97.3 Female with 46, XY karyotype ♀

Q97.8 Other specified sex chromosome abnormalities, female phenotype

Q97.9 Sex chromosome abnormality, female phenotype, unspecified ♀

✓4ᵗʰ **Q98 Other sex chromosome abnormalities, male phenotype, not elsewhere classified**

Q98.0 Klinefelter syndrome karyotype 47, XXY ♂

Q98.1 Klinefelter syndrome, male with more than two X chromosomes ♂

Q98.3 Other male with 46, XX karyotype ♂

Q98.4 Klinefelter syndrome, unspecified ♂

Q98.5 Karyotype 47, XYY ♂

Q98.6 Male with structurally abnormal sex chromosome ♂

Q98.7 Male with sex chromosome mosaicism ♂

Q98.8 Other specified sex chromosome abnormalities, male phenotype ♂

Q98.9 Sex chromosome abnormality, male phenotype, unspecified ♂

✓4ᵗʰ **Q99 Other chromosome abnormalities, not elsewhere classified**

Q99.0 Chimera 46, XX/46, XY

Chimera 46, XX/46, XY true hermaphrodite

Q99.1 46, XX true hermaphrodite

46, XX with streak gonads

46, XY with streak gonads

Pure gonadal dysgenesis

Q99.2 Fragile X chromosome

Fragile X syndrome

Q99.8 Other specified chromosome abnormalities

Q99.9 Chromosomal abnormality, unspecified

✓ Additional Character Required ✓x7ᵗʰ Placeholder Unacceptable PDx Questionable PDx Manifestation Unspecified Dx H1 - H4 HAC HCC CMS-HCC Dx HIV HIV Dx

ICD-10-CM 2020

951

Chapter 18. Symptoms, Signs and Abnormal Clinical and Laboratory Findings, Not Elsewhere Classified (RØØ–R99)

Chapter-specific Guidelines with Coding Examples

The chapter-specific guidelines from the ICD-10-CM Official Guidelines for Coding and Reporting have been provided below. Along with these guidelines are coding examples, contained in the shaded boxes, that have been developed to help illustrate the coding and/or sequencing guidance found in these guidelines.

Chapter 18 includes symptoms, signs, abnormal results of clinical or other investigative procedures, and ill-defined conditions regarding which no diagnosis classifiable elsewhere is recorded. Signs and symptoms that point to a specific diagnosis have been assigned to a category in other chapters of the classification.

a. Use of symptom codes

Codes that describe symptoms and signs are acceptable for reporting purposes when a related definitive diagnosis has not been established (confirmed) by the provider.

Chest pain of unknown origin

RØ7.9   Chest pain, unspecified

Explanation: Codes that describe symptoms such as chest pain are acceptable for reporting purposes when the provider has not established (confirmed) a related definitive diagnosis.

b. Use of a symptom code with a definitive diagnosis code

Codes for signs and symptoms may be reported in addition to a related definitive diagnosis when the sign or symptom is not routinely associated with that diagnosis, such as the various signs and symptoms associated with complex syndromes. The definitive diagnosis code should be sequenced before the symptom code.

Signs or symptoms that are associated routinely with a disease process should not be assigned as additional codes, unless otherwise instructed by the classification.

Pneumonia with hemoptysis

J18.9   Pneumonia, unspecified organism

RØ4.2   Hemoptysis

Explanation: Codes for signs and symptoms may be reported in addition to a related definitive diagnosis when the sign or symptom is not routinely associated with that diagnosis.

Abdominal pain due to acute appendicitis

K35.8Ø   Unspecified acute appendicitis

Explanation: Codes for signs or symptoms routinely associated with a disease process should not be assigned unless the classification instructs otherwise.

c. Combination codes that include symptoms

ICD-10-CM contains a number of combination codes that identify both the definitive diagnosis and common symptoms of that diagnosis. When using one of these combination codes, an additional code should not be assigned for the symptom.

Acute gastritis with hemorrhage

K29.Ø1   Acute gastritis with bleeding

Explanation: When a combination code identifies both the definitive diagnosis and the symptom, an additional code should not be assigned for the symptom.

d. Repeated falls

Code R29.6, Repeated falls, is for use for encounters when a patient has recently fallen and the reason for the fall is being investigated.

Code Z91.81, History of falling, is for use when a patient has fallen in the past and is at risk for future falls. When appropriate, both codes R29.6 and Z91.81 may be assigned together.

e. Coma scale

The coma scale codes (R40.2-) can be used in conjunction with traumatic brain injury codes, acute cerebrovascular disease or sequelae of cerebrovascular disease codes. These codes are primarily for use by trauma registries, but they may be used in any setting where this information is collected. The coma scale may also be used to assess the status of the central nervous system for other non-trauma conditions, such as monitoring patients in the intensive care unit regardless of medical condition. The coma scale codes should be sequenced after the diagnosis code(s).

These codes, one from each subcategory, are needed to complete the scale. The 7th character indicates when the scale was recorded. The 7th character should match for all three codes.

At a minimum, report the initial score documented on presentation at your facility. This may be a score from the emergency medicine technician (EMT) or in the emergency department. If desired, a facility may choose to capture multiple coma scale scores.

Assign code R40.24, Glasgow coma scale, total score, when only the total score is documented in the medical record and not the individual score(s).

Do not report codes for individual or total Glasgow coma scale scores for a patient with a medically induced coma or a sedated patient.

See Section I.B.14 for coma scale documentation by clinicians other than patient's provider

23-year-old man found down after unknown injury with skull fracture and with concussion and loss of consciousness of unknown duration. EMS evaluated the patient in the field and reported the individual Glasgow coma scores:

Eye opening response—3: eyes open to speech

Verbal response—4: confused but coherent speech

Motor response—6: obeys commands fully

SØ2.ØXXA   Fracture of vault of skull, initial encounter for closed fracture

SØ6.ØX9A   Concussion with loss of consciousness of unspecified duration, initial encounter

R4Ø.2131   Coma scale, eyes open, to sound, in the field [EMT or ambulance]

R4Ø.2241   Coma scale, best verbal response, confused conversation, in the field [EMT or ambulance]

R4Ø.2361   Coma scale, best motor response, obeys commands, in the field [EMT or ambulance]

Explanation: When individual scores for the Glasgow coma scale are documented, one code from each category is needed to complete the scale. The seventh character indicates when the scale was recorded and should match for all three codes. Assign a code from subcategory R40.24- Glasgow coma scale, total score, when only the total and not the individual score(s) is documented.

Patient with intractable epilepsy with status epilepticus arrives to ED with alteration of consciousness. Coma scale performed en route by EMT documented total coma score as 11. Another coma score was performed upon hospital admission that was documented as 14.

G4Ø.911   Epilepsy, unspecified, intractable, with status epilepticus

R4Ø.2421   Glasgow coma scale score 9-12, in the field [EMT or ambulance]

R4Ø.2413   Glasgow coma scale score 13-15, at hospital admission

Explanation: Coma scores may be used to assess mental status in non-trauma conditions. Use only code R40.24- Glasgow coma scale, total scores when individual scores are unavailable. Multiple scores may be reported with the seventh character representing where or when the assessment was made.

f. Functional quadriplegia

GUIDELINE HAS BEEN DELETED EFFECTIVE OCTOBER 1, 2Ø17

Chapter 18. Symptoms, Signs and Abnormal Clinical and Laboratory Findings, Not Elsewhere Classified

g. SIRS due to non-infectious process

The systemic inflammatory response syndrome (SIRS) can develop as a result of certain non-infectious disease processes, such as trauma, malignant neoplasm, or pancreatitis. When SIRS is documented with a noninfectious condition, and no subsequent infection is documented, the code for the underlying condition, such as an injury, should be assigned, followed by code R65.10, Systemic inflammatory response syndrome (SIRS) of non-infectious origin without acute organ dysfunction, or code R65.11, Systemic inflammatory response syndrome (SIRS) of non-infectious origin with acute organ dysfunction. If an associated acute organ dysfunction is documented, the appropriate code(s) for the specific type of organ dysfunction(s) should be assigned in addition to code R65.11. If acute organ dysfunction is documented, but it cannot be determined if the acute organ dysfunction is associated with SIRS or due to another condition (e.g., directly due to the trauma), the provider should be queried.

Systemic inflammatory response syndrome (SIRS) due to acute gallstone pancreatitis

K85.10   **Biliary acute pancreatitis without necrosis or infection**

R65.10   **Systemic inflammatory response syndrome [SIRS] of non-infectious origin without acute organ dysfunction**

Explanation: When SIRS is documented with a non-infectious condition without subsequent infection documented, the code for the underlying condition such as pancreatitis should be assigned followed by the appropriate code for SIRS of noninfectious origin, either with or without associated organ dysfunction.

h. Death NOS

Code R99, Ill-defined and unknown cause of mortality, is only for use in the very limited circumstance when a patient who has already died is brought into an emergency department or other healthcare facility and is pronounced dead upon arrival. It does not represent the discharge disposition of death.

i. NIHSS stroke scale

The NIH stroke scale (NIHSS) codes (R29.7- -) can be used in conjunction with acute stroke codes (I63) to identify the patient's neurological status and the severity of the stroke. The stroke scale codes should be sequenced after the acute stroke diagnosis code(s).

At a minimum, report the initial score documented. If desired, a facility may choose to capture multiple stroke scale scores.

See Section I.B.14 for NIHSS stroke scale documentation by clinicians other than patient's provider

Patient admitted with CVA seen by neurology consult who documents moderate to severe stroke, 17 on NIHSS stroke scale.

I63.9   **Cerebral infarction, unspecified**

R29.717   **NIHSS score 17**

Explanation: Unspecified cerebral vascular accident (CVA) is sequenced before the NIHSS stroke scale score code. The stroke scale is an assessment tool to help measure stroke-related neurological deficits. Fifteen items are evaluated by trained observers and include such conditions as levels of consciousness, language, dysarthria, ataxia, and sensory loss. A facility may report multiple stroke scale scores if it wants to.

Chapter 18. Symptoms, Signs and Abnormal Clinical and Laboratory Findings, Not Elsewhere Classified (R00-R99)

NOTE This chapter includes symptoms, signs, abnormal results of clinical or other investigative procedures, and ill-defined conditions regarding which no diagnosis classifiable elsewhere is recorded.

Signs and symptoms that point rather definitely to a given diagnosis have been assigned to a category in other chapters of the classification. In general, categories in this chapter include the less well-defined conditions and symptoms that, without the necessary study of the case to establish a final diagnosis, point perhaps equally to two or more diseases or to two or more systems of the body. Practically all categories in the chapter could be designated 'not otherwise specified', 'unknown etiology' or 'transient'. The Alphabetical Index should be consulted to determine which symptoms and signs are to be allocated here and which to other chapters. The residual subcategories, numbered .8, are generally provided for other relevant symptoms that cannot be allocated elsewhere in the classification.

The conditions and signs or symptoms included in categories R00-R94 consist of:

(a) cases for which no more specific diagnosis can be made even after all the facts bearing on the case have been investigated;

(b) signs or symptoms existing at the time of initial encounter that proved to be transient and whose causes could not be determined;

(c) provisional diagnosis in a patient who failed to return for further investigation or care;

(d) cases referred elsewhere for investigation or treatment before the diagnosis was made;

(e) cases in which a more precise diagnosis was not available for any other reason;

(f) certain symptoms, for which supplementary information is provided, that represent important problems in medical care in their own right.

EXCLUDES 2 *abnormal findings on antenatal screening of mother (O28.-)*
certain conditions originating in the perinatal period (P04-P96)
signs and symptoms classified in the body system chapters
signs and symptoms of breast (N63, N64.5)

AHA: 2017,1Q,6,7

This chapter contains the following blocks:

R00-R09 Symptoms and signs involving the circulatory and respiratory systems
R10-R19 Symptoms and signs involving the digestive system and abdomen
R20-R23 Symptoms and signs involving the skin and subcutaneous tissue
R25-R29 Symptoms and signs involving the nervous and musculoskeletal systems
R30-R39 Symptoms and signs involving the genitourinary system
R40-R46 Symptoms and signs involving cognition, perception, emotional state and behavior
R47-R49 Symptoms and signs involving speech and voice
R50-R69 General symptoms and signs
R70-R79 Abnormal findings on examination of blood, without diagnosis
R80-R82 Abnormal findings on examination of urine, without diagnosis
R83-R89 Abnormal findings on examination of other body fluids, substances and tissues, without diagnosis
R90-R94 Abnormal findings on diagnostic imaging and in function studies, without diagnosis
R97 Abnormal tumor markers
R99 Ill-defined and unknown cause of mortality

Symptoms and signs involving the circulatory and respiratory systems (R00-R09)

✓4ᵗʰ **R00 Abnormalities of heart beat**

EXCLUDES 1 *abnormalities originating in the perinatal period (P29.1-)*
EXCLUDES 2 *specified arrhythmias (I47-I49)*

R00.0 Tachycardia, unspecified
Rapid heart beat
Sinoauricular tachycardia NOS
Sinus [sinusal] tachycardia NOS
EXCLUDES 1 *neonatal tachycardia (P29.11)*
paroxysmal tachycardia (I47.-)
DEF: Excessively rapid heart rate of more than 100 beats per minute.

R00.1 Bradycardia, unspecified
Sinoatrial bradycardia
Sinus bradycardia
Slow heart beat
Vagal bradycardia
Use additional code for adverse effect, if applicable, to identify drug (T36-T50 with fifth or sixth character 5)
EXCLUDES 1 *neonatal bradycardia (P29.12)*
DEF: Slowed heartbeat, usually defined as a rate fewer than 60 beats per minute. Heart rhythm may be slow as a result of a congenital defect or an acquired problem.

R00.2 Palpitations
Awareness of heart beat

R00.8 Other abnormalities of heart beat

R00.9 Unspecified abnormalities of heart beat

✓4ᵗʰ **R01 Cardiac murmurs and other cardiac sounds**

EXCLUDES 1 *cardiac murmurs and sounds originating in the perinatal period (P29.8)*

R01.0 Benign and innocent cardiac murmurs
Functional cardiac murmur

R01.1 Cardiac murmur, unspecified
Cardiac bruit NOS
Heart murmur NOS
Systolic murmur NOS

R01.2 Other cardiac sounds
Cardiac dullness, increased or decreased
Precordial friction

✓4ᵗʰ **R03 Abnormal blood-pressure reading, without diagnosis**

R03.0 Elevated blood-pressure reading, without diagnosis of hypertension

NOTE This category is to be used to record an episode of elevated blood pressure in a patient in whom no formal diagnosis of hypertension has been made, or as an isolated incidental finding.

R03.1 Nonspecific low blood-pressure reading
EXCLUDES 1 *hypotension (I95.-)*
maternal hypotension syndrome (O26.5-)
neurogenic orthostatic hypotension (G90.3)

✓4ᵗʰ **R04 Hemorrhage from respiratory passages**

CC Excl: For CC codes in category R04: PDX collection 1119

R04.0 Epistaxis   CC
Hemorrhage from nose
Nosebleed

R04.1 Hemorrhage from throat   CC
EXCLUDES 2 *hemoptysis (R04.2)*

R04.2 Hemoptysis   CC
Blood-stained sputum
Cough with hemorrhage
AHA: 2013,4Q,118

✓5ᵗʰ **R04.8 Hemorrhage from other sites in respiratory passages**

R04.81 Acute idiopathic pulmonary hemorrhage in infants   CC P
AIPHI
Acute idiopathic hemorrhage in infants over 28 days old
EXCLUDES 1 *perinatal pulmonary hemorrhage (P26.-)*
von Willebrand's disease (D68.0)

R04.89 Hemorrhage from other sites in respiratory passages   CC
Pulmonary hemorrhage NOS

R04.9 Hemorrhage from respiratory passages, unspecified   CC

R05 Cough
EXCLUDES 1 *cough with hemorrhage (R04.2)*
smoker's cough (J41.0)
AHA: 2016,2Q,33

☑ Additional Character Required   ✓x7ᵗʰ Placeholder   Unacceptable PDx   Questionable PDx   Manifestation   Unspecified Dx   H1-H14 HAC   HCC CMS-HCC Dx   HIV HIV Dx

ICD-10-CM 2020

955

R00–R05

✓4ᵗʰ **R06   Abnormalities of breathing**

> *EXCLUDES 1*   acute respiratory distress syndrome (J80)
> respiratory arrest (R09.2)
> respiratory arrest of newborn (P28.81)
> respiratory distress syndrome of newborn (P22.-)
> respiratory failure (J96.-)
> respiratory failure of newborn (P28.5)

✓5ᵗʰ **R06.0   Dyspnea**

> *EXCLUDES 1*   tachypnea NOS (R06.82)
> transient tachypnea of newborn (P22.1)

R06.00   Dyspnea, unspecified
AHA: 2017,1Q,26

R06.01   Orthopnea

R06.02   Shortness of breath

R06.03   Acute respiratory distress
AHA: 2017,4Q,23

R06.09   Other forms of dyspnea

R06.1   Stridor

> *EXCLUDES 1*   congenital laryngeal stridor (P28.89)
> laryngismus (stridulus) (J38.5)

DEF: Certain type of wheezing described as a loud, constant, musical sound produced when breathing with an obstructed airway, like the inspiratory sound heard when laryngeal or esophageal obstruction is present.

R06.2   Wheezing

> *EXCLUDES 1*   asthma (J45.-)

AHA: 2016,2Q,33
DEF: High-pitched whistling sound during breathing due to stenosis of the respiratory passageway. Wheezing is associated with asthma, sleep apnea, bronchiectasis, bronchiolitis, COPD, and pleural effusion.

R06.3   Periodic breathing   CC

Cheyne-Stokes breathing
CC Excl: PDX collection 1120

R06.4   Hyperventilation

> *EXCLUDES 1*   psychogenic hyperventilation (F45.8)

R06.5   Mouth breathing

> *EXCLUDES 2*   dry mouth NOS (R68.2)

R06.6   Hiccough

> *EXCLUDES 1*   psychogenic hiccough (F45.8)

R06.7   Sneezing

✓5ᵗʰ **R06.8   Other abnormalities of breathing**

R06.81   Apnea, not elsewhere classified
Apnea NOS

> *EXCLUDES 1*   apnea (of) newborn (P28.4)
> sleep apnea (G47.3-)
> sleep apnea of newborn (primary) (P28.3)

R06.82   Tachypnea, not elsewhere classified
Tachypnea NOS

> *EXCLUDES 1*   transitory tachypnea of newborn (P22.1)

R06.83   Snoring

R06.89   Other abnormalities of breathing
Breath-holding (spells)
Sighing

R06.9   Unspecified abnormalities of breathing

✓4ᵗʰ **R07   Pain in throat and chest**

> *EXCLUDES 1*   epidemic myalgia (B33.0)
> *EXCLUDES 2*   jaw pain R68.84
> pain in breast (N64.4)

R07.0   Pain in throat

> *EXCLUDES 1*   chronic sore throat (J31.2)
> sore throat (acute) NOS (J02.9)
> *EXCLUDES 2*   dysphagia (R13.1-)
> pain in neck (M54.2)

R07.1   Chest pain on breathing
Painful respiration

R07.2   Precordial pain
DEF: Pain felt in the anterior (front) chest wall over the region of the heart. This type of pain is generally felt slightly to the left of the sternum, but may also extend into the surrounding chest wall region.

R07.8   Other chest pain   ✓5ᵗʰ

R07.81   Pleurodynia
Pleurodynia NOS

> *EXCLUDES 1*   epidemic pleurodynia (B33.0)

R07.82   Intercostal pain

R07.89   Other chest pain
Anterior chest-wall pain NOS

R07.9   Chest pain, unspecified

✓4ᵗʰ **R09   Other symptoms and signs involving the circulatory and respiratory system**

> *EXCLUDES 1*   acute respiratory distress syndrome (J80)
> respiratory arrest of newborn (P28.81)
> respiratory distress syndrome of newborn (P22.0)
> respiratory failure (J96.-)
> respiratory failure of newborn (P28.5)

✓5ᵗʰ **R09.0   Asphyxia and hypoxemia**

> *EXCLUDES 1*   asphyxia due to carbon monoxide (T58.-)
> asphyxia due to foreign body in respiratory tract (T17.-)
> birth (intrauterine) asphyxia (P84)
> hyperventilation (R06.4)
> traumatic asphyxia (T71.-)
> *EXCLUDES 2*   hypercapnia (R06.89)

R09.01   Asphyxia   CC
DEF: Interference of oxygen intake due to obstruction or injury of airways resulting in a lack of oxygen perfusion to the tissues or excessive carbon dioxide in the blood. Can cause unconsciousness or death.
CC Excl: PDX collection 1121

R09.02   Hypoxemia
DEF: Insufficient oxygen in the arterial blood resulting in inadequate delivery of oxygen to the body tissues.

R09.1   Pleurisy

> *EXCLUDES 1*   pleurisy with effusion (J90)

¹ **R09.2   Respiratory arrest**   MCC   HCC
Cardiorespiratory failure

> *EXCLUDES 1*   cardiac arrest (I46.-)
> respiratory arrest of newborn (P28.81)
> respiratory distress of newborn (P22.0)
> respiratory failure (J96.-)
> respiratory failure of newborn (P28.5)
> respiratory insufficiency (R06.89)
> respiratory insufficiency of newborn (P28.5)

CC Excl: PDX collection 1121

R09.3   Abnormal sputum
Abnormal amount of sputum
Abnormal color of sputum
Abnormal odor of sputum
Excessive sputum

> *EXCLUDES 1*   blood-stained sputum (R04.2)

✓5ᵗʰ **R09.8   Other specified symptoms and signs involving the circulatory and respiratory systems**

R09.81   Nasal congestion

R09.82   Postnasal drip

R09.89   Other specified symptoms and signs involving the circulatory and respiratory systems
Abnormal chest percussion
Bruit (arterial)
Chest tympany
Choking sensation
Feeling of foreign body in throat
Friction sounds in chest
Rales
Weak pulse

> *EXCLUDES 2*   foreign body in throat (T17.2-)
> wheezing (R06.2)

Ⓝ Newborn: 0   Ⓟ Pediatric: 0-17   Ⓜ Maternity: 9-64   Ⓐ Adult: 15-124   MCC Major Complication/Comorbidity   CC Complication/Comorbidity   SW Severe Wound Dx

956   ICD-10-CM 2020

Symptoms and signs involving the digestive system and abdomen (R10-R19)

> **EXCLUDES 2**   congenital or infantile pylorospasm (Q40.0)
> gastrointestinal hemorrhage (K92.0-K92.2)
> intestinal obstruction (K56.-)
> newborn gastrointestinal hemorrhage (P54.0-P54.3)
> newborn intestinal obstruction (P76.-)
> pylorospasm (K31.3)
> signs and symptoms involving the urinary system (R30-R39)
> symptoms referable to female genital organs (N94.-)
> symptoms referable to male genital organs (N48-N50)

✓4ᵗʰ **R10 Abdominal and pelvic pain**

> **EXCLUDES 1**   renal colic (N23)
> **EXCLUDES 2**   dorsalgia (M54.-)
> flatulence and related conditions (R14.-)

R10.0 Acute abdomen

Severe abdominal pain (generalized) (with abdominal rigidity)

> **EXCLUDES 1**   abdominal rigidity NOS (R19.3)
> generalized abdominal pain NOS (R10.84)
> localized abdominal pain (R10.1-R10.3-)

✓5ᵗʰ **R10.1 Pain localized to upper abdomen**

R10.10 Upper abdominal pain, unspecified
R10.11 Right upper quadrant pain
R10.12 Left upper quadrant pain
R10.13 Epigastric pain
Dyspepsia

> **EXCLUDES 1**   functional dyspepsia (K30)

Abdominal Pain

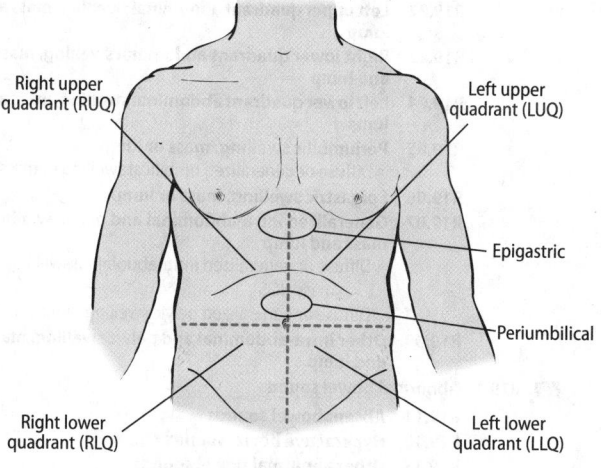

Right upper quadrant (RUQ)

Left upper quadrant (LUQ)

Epigastric

Periumbilical

Right lower quadrant (RLQ)

Left lower quadrant (LLQ)

R10.2 Pelvic and perineal pain

> **EXCLUDES 1**   vulvodynia (N94.81)

✓5ᵗʰ **R10.3 Pain localized to other parts of lower abdomen**

R10.30 Lower abdominal pain, unspecified
R10.31 Right lower quadrant pain
R10.32 Left lower quadrant pain
R10.33 Periumbilical pain

✓5ᵗʰ **R10.8 Other abdominal pain**

✓6ᵗʰ **R10.81 Abdominal tenderness**
Abdominal tenderness NOS

R10.811 Right upper quadrant abdominal tenderness
R10.812 Left upper quadrant abdominal tenderness
R10.813 Right lower quadrant abdominal tenderness
R10.814 Left lower quadrant abdominal tenderness
R10.815 Periumbilic abdominal tenderness
R10.816 Epigastric abdominal tenderness
R10.817 Generalized abdominal tenderness
R10.819 Abdominal tenderness, unspecified site

✓6ᵗʰ **R10.82 Rebound abdominal tenderness**

R10.821 Right upper quadrant rebound abdominal tenderness

R10.822 Left upper quadrant rebound abdominal tenderness
R10.823 Right lower quadrant rebound abdominal tenderness
R10.824 Left lower quadrant rebound abdominal tenderness
R10.825 Periumbilic rebound abdominal tenderness
R10.826 Epigastric rebound abdominal tenderness
R10.827 Generalized rebound abdominal tenderness
R10.829 Rebound abdominal tenderness, unspecified site

R10.83 Colic   P
Colic NOS
Infantile colic

> **EXCLUDES 1**   colic in adult and child over 12 months old (R10.84)

DEF: Inconsolable crying in an otherwise well-fed and healthy infant for more than three hours a day, three days a week, for more than three weeks.

R10.84 Generalized abdominal pain

> **EXCLUDES 1**   generalized abdominal pain associated with acute abdomen (R10.0)

R10.9 Unspecified abdominal pain

✓4ᵗʰ **R11 Nausea and vomiting**

> **EXCLUDES 1**   cyclical vomiting associated with migraine (G43.A-)
> excessive vomiting in pregnancy (O21.-)
> hematemesis (K92.0)
> neonatal hematemesis (P54.0)
> newborn vomiting (P92.0-)
> psychogenic vomiting (F50.89)
> vomiting associated with bulimia nervosa (F50.2)
> vomiting following gastrointestinal surgery (K91.0)

AHA: 2017,1Q,28

TIP: Assign a code from this category along with K31.89 Other diseases of stomach and duodenum, to describe cyclical vomiting not due to migraine.

R11.0 Nausea
Nausea NOS
Nausea without vomiting

✓5ᵗʰ **R11.1 Vomiting**

R11.10 Vomiting, unspecified
Vomiting NOS

R11.11 Vomiting without nausea
R11.12 Projectile vomiting
R11.13 Vomiting of fecal matter
R11.14 Bilious vomiting
Bilious emesis

R11.15 Cyclical vomiting syndrome unrelated to migraine
Cyclic vomiting syndrome NOS
Persistent vomiting

> **EXCLUDES 1**   cyclical vomiting in migraine (G43.A-)
> **EXCLUDES 2**   bulimia nervosa (F50.2)
> diabetes mellitus due to underlying condition (E08.-)

R11.2 Nausea with vomiting, unspecified
Persistent nausea with vomiting NOS

R12 Heartburn

> **EXCLUDES 1**   dyspepsia NOS (R10.13)
> functional dyspepsia (K30)

✓4ᵗʰ **R13 Aphagia and dysphagia**

R13.0 Aphagia   CC
Inability to swallow

> **EXCLUDES 1**   psychogenic aphagia (F50.9)

☑ Additional Character Required   ✓x7ᵗʰ Placeholder   Unacceptable PDx   Questionable PDx   Manifestation   Unspecified Dx   H1-H14 HAC   HCC CMS-HCC Dx   HIV HIV Dx

ICD-10-CM 2020   **957**

Chapter 18. Symptoms, Signs and Abnormal Clinical and Laboratory Findings

R13.1–R19.4

✓5ᵗʰ R13.1 Dysphagia

Code first, if applicable, dysphagia following cerebrovascular disease (I69. with final characters -91)

EXCLUDES 1 *psychogenic dysphagia (F45.8)*

Swallowing Function

Oral phase

Oropharyngeal phase

Pharyngeal phase

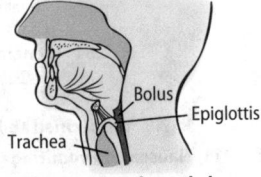

Pharyngoesophageal phase

R13.10	**Dysphagia, unspecified** Difficulty in swallowing NOS
R13.11	**Dysphagia, oral phase**
R13.12	**Dysphagia, oropharyngeal phase**
R13.13	**Dysphagia, pharyngeal phase**
R13.14	**Dysphagia, pharyngoesophageal phase**
R13.19	**Other dysphagia** Cervical dysphagia Neurogenic dysphagia

✓4ᵗʰ R14 Flatulence and related conditions

EXCLUDES 1 *psychogenic aerophagy (F45.8)*

R14.0 Abdominal distension (gaseous)
Bloating
Tympanites (abdominal) (intestinal)

R14.1 Gas pain

R14.2 Eructation

R14.3 Flatulence

✓4ᵗʰ R15 Fecal incontinence

INCLUDES encopresis NOS

EXCLUDES 1 *fecal incontinence of nonorganic origin (F98.1)*

R15.0 Incomplete defecation
EXCLUDES 1 *constipation (K59.0-)*
fecal impaction (K56.41)

R15.1 Fecal smearing
Fecal soiling

R15.2 Fecal urgency

R15.9 Full incontinence of feces
Fecal incontinence NOS

✓4ᵗʰ R16 Hepatomegaly and splenomegaly, not elsewhere classified

R16.0 Hepatomegaly, not elsewhere classified
Hepatomegaly NOS

R16.1 Splenomegaly, not elsewhere classified
Splenomegaly NOS

R16.2 Hepatomegaly with splenomegaly, not elsewhere classified
Hepatosplenomegaly NOS

R17 Unspecified jaundice   **CC**

EXCLUDES 1 *neonatal jaundice (P55, P57-P59)*
CC Excl: PDX collection 1122

✓4ᵗʰ R18 Ascites

INCLUDES fluid in peritoneal cavity

EXCLUDES 1 *ascites in alcoholic cirrhosis (K70.31)*
ascites in alcoholic hepatitis (K70.11)
ascites in toxic liver disease with chronic active hepatitis (K71.51)

DEF: Abnormal accumulation of free fluid in the abdominal cavity, causing distention and tightness in addition to shortness of breath as the fluid accumulates. Ascites is usually an underlying disorder and can be a manifestation of any number of diseases.

R18.0 Malignant ascites   **CC**

Code first malignancy, such as:
malignant neoplasm of ovary (C56.-)
secondary malignant neoplasm of retroperitoneum and peritoneum (C78.6)
CC Excl: PDX collection 1123

R18.8 Other ascites   **CC**

Ascites NOS
Peritoneal effusion (chronic)
AHA: 2018,1Q,4
CC Excl: PDX collection 1123

✓4ᵗʰ R19 Other symptoms and signs involving the digestive system and abdomen

EXCLUDES 1 *acute abdomen (R10.0)*

✓5ᵗʰ R19.0 Intra-abdominal and pelvic swelling, mass and lump

EXCLUDES 1 *abdominal distension (gaseous) (R14.-)*
ascites (R18.-)

R19.00	**Intra-abdominal and pelvic swelling, mass and lump, unspecified site**
R19.01	**Right upper quadrant abdominal swelling, mass and lump**
R19.02	**Left upper quadrant abdominal swelling, mass and lump**
R19.03	**Right lower quadrant abdominal swelling, mass and lump**
R19.04	**Left lower quadrant abdominal swelling, mass and lump**
R19.05	**Periumbilic swelling, mass or lump** Diffuse or generalized umbilical swelling or mass
R19.06	**Epigastric swelling, mass or lump**
R19.07	**Generalized intra-abdominal and pelvic swelling, mass and lump** Diffuse or generalized intra-abdominal swelling or mass NOS Diffuse or generalized pelvic swelling or mass NOS
R19.09	**Other intra-abdominal and pelvic swelling, mass and lump**

✓5ᵗʰ R19.1 Abnormal bowel sounds

R19.11 Absent bowel sounds

R19.12 Hyperactive bowel sounds

R19.15 Other abnormal bowel sounds
Abnormal bowel sounds NOS

R19.2 Visible peristalsis

Hyperperistalsis
DEF: Visible movements of muscular attempts to move food through the digestive tract due to pyloric obstruction, stomach obstruction, or intestinal obstruction.

✓5ᵗʰ R19.3 Abdominal rigidity

EXCLUDES 1 *abdominal rigidity with severe abdominal pain (R10.0)*

R19.30	**Abdominal rigidity, unspecified site**
R19.31	**Right upper quadrant abdominal rigidity**
R19.32	**Left upper quadrant abdominal rigidity**
R19.33	**Right lower quadrant abdominal rigidity**
R19.34	**Left lower quadrant abdominal rigidity**
R19.35	**Periumbilic abdominal rigidity**
R19.36	**Epigastric abdominal rigidity**
R19.37	**Generalized abdominal rigidity**

R19.4 Change in bowel habit

EXCLUDES 1 *constipation (K59.0-)*
functional diarrhea (K59.1)

N Newborn: 0   **P** Pediatric: 0-17   **M** Maternity: 9-64   **A** Adult: 15-124   **MCC** Major Complication/Comorbidity   **CC** Complication/Comorbidity   **SW** Severe Wound Dx

958   ICD-10-CM 2020

R19.5 Other fecal abnormalities
Abnormal stool color
Bulky stools
Mucus in stools
Occult blood in feces
Occult blood in stools
> EXCLUDES 1   melena (K92.1)
>   neonatal melena (P54.1)
AHA: 2019,1Q,32

R19.6 Halitosis

R19.7 Diarrhea, unspecified
Diarrhea NOS
> EXCLUDES 1   functional diarrhea (K59.1)
>   neonatal diarrhea (P78.3)
>   psychogenic diarrhea (F45.8)

R19.8 Other specified symptoms and signs involving the digestive system and abdomen

Symptoms and signs involving the skin and subcutaneous tissue (R20-R23)

> EXCLUDES 2   symptoms relating to breast (N64.4-N64.5)

✓4th **R20 Disturbances of skin sensation**
> EXCLUDES 1   dissociative anesthesia and sensory loss (F44.6)
>   psychogenic disturbances (F45.8)

R20.0 Anesthesia of skin

R20.1 Hypoesthesia of skin

R20.2 Paresthesia of skin
Formication
Pins and needles
Tingling skin
> EXCLUDES 1   acroparesthesia (I73.8)

R20.3 Hyperesthesia

R20.8 Other disturbances of skin sensation

R20.9 Unspecified disturbances of skin sensation

R21 Rash and other nonspecific skin eruption
> INCLUDES   rash NOS
> EXCLUDES 1   specified type of rash — code to condition
>   vesicular eruption (R23.8)

✓4th **R22 Localized swelling, mass and lump of skin and subcutaneous tissue**
> INCLUDES   subcutaneous nodules (localized)(superficial)
> EXCLUDES 1   abnormal findings on diagnostic imaging (R90-R93)
>   edema (R60.-)
>   enlarged lymph nodes (R59.-)
>   localized adiposity (E65)
>   swelling of joint (M25.4-)

R22.0 Localized swelling, mass and lump, head

R22.1 Localized swelling, mass and lump, neck

R22.2 Localized swelling, mass and lump, trunk
> EXCLUDES 1   intra-abdominal or pelvic mass and lump (R19.0-)
>   intra-abdominal or pelvic swelling (R19.0-)
> EXCLUDES 2   breast mass and lump (N63)

✓5th **R22.3 Localized swelling, mass and lump, upper limb**

R22.30 Localized swelling, mass and lump, unspecified upper limb

R22.31 Localized swelling, mass and lump, right upper limb

R22.32 Localized swelling, mass and lump, left upper limb

R22.33 Localized swelling, mass and lump, upper limb, bilateral

✓5th **R22.4 Localized swelling, mass and lump, lower limb**

R22.40 Localized swelling, mass and lump, unspecified lower limb

R22.41 Localized swelling, mass and lump, right lower limb

R22.42 Localized swelling, mass and lump, left lower limb

R22.43 Localized swelling, mass and lump, lower limb, bilateral

R22.9 Localized swelling, mass and lump, unspecified

✓4th **R23 Other skin changes**

R23.0 Cyanosis
> EXCLUDES 1   acrocyanosis (I73.8)
>   cyanotic attacks of newborn (P28.2)
DEF: Bluish or purplish discoloration of the skin due to an inadequate oxygen blood level.

R23.1 Pallor
Clammy skin

R23.2 Flushing
Excessive blushing
Code first, if applicable, menopausal and female climacteric states (N95.1)

R23.3 Spontaneous ecchymoses
Petechiae
> EXCLUDES 1   ecchymoses of newborn (P54.5)
>   purpura (D69.-)

R23.4 Changes in skin texture
Desquamation of skin
Induration of skin
Scaling of skin
> EXCLUDES 1   epidermal thickening NOS (L85.9)

R23.8 Other skin changes

R23.9 Unspecified skin changes

Symptoms and signs involving the nervous and musculoskeletal systems (R25-R29)

✓4th **R25 Abnormal involuntary movements**
> EXCLUDES 1   specific movement disorders (G20-G26)
>   stereotyped movement disorders (F98.4)
>   tic disorders (F95.-)

R25.0 Abnormal head movements

R25.1 Tremor, unspecified
> EXCLUDES 1   chorea NOS (G25.5)
>   essential tremor (G25.0)
>   hysterical tremor (F44.4)
>   intention tremor (G25.2)

R25.2 Cramp and spasm
> EXCLUDES 2   carpopedal spasm (R29.0)
>   charley-horse (M62.831)
>   infantile spasms (G40.4-)
>   muscle spasm of back (M62.830)
>   muscle spasm of calf (M62.831)

R25.3 Fasciculation
Twitching NOS

R25.8 Other abnormal involuntary movements

R25.9 Unspecified abnormal involuntary movements

✓4th **R26 Abnormalities of gait and mobility**
> EXCLUDES 1   ataxia NOS (R27.0)
>   hereditary ataxia (G11.-)
>   locomotor (syphilitic) ataxia (A52.11)
>   immobility syndrome (paraplegic) (M62.3)

R26.0 Ataxic gait
Staggering gait

R26.1 Paralytic gait
Spastic gait

R26.2 Difficulty in walking, not elsewhere classified
> EXCLUDES 1   falling (R29.6)
>   unsteadiness on feet (R26.81)
AHA: 2016,2Q,7

✓5th **R26.8 Other abnormalities of gait and mobility**

R26.81 Unsteadiness on feet

R26.89 Other abnormalities of gait and mobility

R26.9 Unspecified abnormalities of gait and mobility

✓4th **R27 Other lack of coordination**
> EXCLUDES 1   ataxic gait (R26.0)
>   hereditary ataxia (G11.-)
>   vertigo NOS (R42)

R27.0 Ataxia, unspecified
> EXCLUDES 1   ataxia following cerebrovascular disease (I69. with final characters -93)

R27.8 Other lack of coordination

R27.9 Unspecified lack of coordination

Chapter 18. Symptoms, Signs and Abnormal Clinical and Laboratory Findings

R19.5–R27.9

√4ᵗʰ **R29 Other symptoms and signs involving the nervous and musculoskeletal systems**

R29.0 Tetany   CC

Carpopedal spasm

EXCLUDES 1   *hysterical tetany (F44.5)*

neonatal tetany (P71.3)

parathyroid tetany (E20.9)

post-thyroidectomy tetany (E89.2)

DEF: Calcium or other mineral imbalance causing voluntary muscles such as hands, feet, or larynx to spasm rhythmically.

CC Excl: PDX collection 1124

R29.1 Meningismus   CC

CC Excl: PDX collection 1125

R29.2 Abnormal reflex

EXCLUDES 2   *abnormal pupillary reflex (H57.0)*

hyperactive gag reflex (J39.2)

vasovagal reaction or syncope (R55)

R29.3 Abnormal posture

R29.4 Clicking hip

EXCLUDES 1   *congenital deformities of hip (Q65.-)*

R29.5 Transient paralysis   CC

Code first any associated spinal cord injury (S14.0, S14.1-, S24.0, S24.1-, S34.0-, S34.1-)

EXCLUDES 1   *transient ischemic attack (G45.9)*

CC Excl: PDX collection 1126

R29.6 Repeated falls

Falling

Tendency to fall

EXCLUDES 2   *at risk for falling (Z91.81)*

history of falling (Z91.81)

AHA: 2016,2Q,6

TIP: Code in addition to Parkinson's disease (G20), when documented.

√5ᵗʰ **R29.7 National Institutes of Health Stroke Scale (NIHSS) score**

Code first the type of cerebral infarction (I63.-)

AHA: 2016,4Q,61-62

TIP: Codes from this subcategory may be assigned based on medical record documentation from clinicians who are not the patient's provider.

√6ᵗʰ **R29.70 NIHSS score 0-9**

R29.700 **NIHSS score 0**

R29.701 **NIHSS score 1**

R29.702 **NIHSS score 2**

R29.703 **NIHSS score 3**

R29.704 **NIHSS score 4**

R29.705 **NIHSS score 5**

R29.706 **NIHSS score 6**

R29.707 **NIHSS score 7**

R29.708 **NIHSS score 8**

R29.709 **NIHSS score 9**

√6ᵗʰ **R29.71 NIHSS score 10-19**

R29.710 **NIHSS score 10**

R29.711 **NIHSS score 11**

R29.712 **NIHSS score 12**

R29.713 **NIHSS score 13**

R29.714 **NIHSS score 14**

R29.715 **NIHSS score 15**

R29.716 **NIHSS score 16**

R29.717 **NIHSS score 17**

R29.718 **NIHSS score 18**

R29.719 **NIHSS score 19**

√6ᵗʰ **R29.72 NIHSS score 20-29**

R29.720 **NIHSS score 20**

R29.721 **NIHSS score 21**

R29.722 **NIHSS score 22**

R29.723 **NIHSS score 23**

R29.724 **NIHSS score 24**

R29.725 **NIHSS score 25**

R29.726 **NIHSS score 26**

R29.727 **NIHSS score 27**

R29.728 **NIHSS score 28**

R29.729 **NIHSS score 29**

√6ᵗʰ **R29.73 NIHSS score 30-39**

R29.730 **NIHSS score 30**

R29.731 **NIHSS score 31**

R29.732 **NIHSS score 32**

R29.733 **NIHSS score 33**

R29.734 **NIHSS score 34**

R29.735 **NIHSS score 35**

R29.736 **NIHSS score 36**

R29.737 **NIHSS score 37**

R29.738 **NIHSS score 38**

R29.739 **NIHSS score 39**

√6ᵗʰ **R29.74 NIHSS score 40-42**

R29.740 **NIHSS score 40**

R29.741 **NIHSS score 41**

R29.742 **NIHSS score 42**

√5ᵗʰ **R29.8 Other symptoms and signs involving the nervous and musculoskeletal systems**

√6ᵗʰ **R29.81 Other symptoms and signs involving the nervous system**

R29.810 Facial weakness

Facial droop

EXCLUDES 1   *Bell's palsy (G51.0)*

facial weakness following cerebrovascular disease (I69. with final characters -92)

R29.818 Other symptoms and signs involving the nervous system

√6ᵗʰ **R29.89 Other symptoms and signs involving the musculoskeletal system**

EXCLUDES 2   *pain in limb (M79.6-)*

R29.890 Loss of height

EXCLUDES 1   *osteoporosis (M80-M81)*

R29.891 Ocular torticollis

EXCLUDES 1   *congenital (sternomastoid) torticollis Q68.0*

psychogenic torticollis (F45.8)

spasmodic torticollis (G24.3)

torticollis due to birth injury (P15.8)

torticollis NOS M43.6

DEF: Abnormal head posture as a result of a contracted state of cervical muscles to correct a visual disturbance, either double vision or a visual field defect.

R29.898 Other symptoms and signs involving the musculoskeletal system

√5ᵗʰ **R29.9 Unspecified symptoms and signs involving the nervous and musculoskeletal systems**

R29.90 Unspecified symptoms and signs involving the nervous system

R29.91 Unspecified symptoms and signs involving the musculoskeletal system

Symptoms and signs involving the genitourinary system (R30-R39)

√4ᵗʰ **R30 Pain associated with micturition**

EXCLUDES 1   *psychogenic pain associated with micturition (F45.8)*

R30.0 Dysuria

Strangury

R30.1 Vesical tenesmus

DEF: Feeling of a full bladder even when there is little or no urine in the bladder.

R30.9 Painful micturition, unspecified

Painful urination NOS

√4ᵗʰ **R31 Hematuria**

EXCLUDES 1   *hematuria included with underlying conditions, such as:*

acute cystitis with hematuria (N30.01)

recurrent and persistent hematuria in glomerular diseases (N02.-)

AHA: 2017,1Q,17

R31.0 Gross hematuria

R31.1 Benign essential microscopic hematuria

√5ᵗʰ **R31.2 Other microscopic hematuria**

AHA: 2016,4Q,62

R31.21 Asymptomatic microscopic hematuria

AMH

R31.29 Other microscopic hematuria

R31.9 Hematuria, unspecified

N Newborn: 0   P Pediatric: 0-17   M Maternity: 9-64   A Adult: 15-124   MCC Major Complication/Comorbidity   CC Complication/Comorbidity   SW Severe Wound Dx

960   ICD-10-CM 2020

R32 Unspecified urinary incontinence
Enuresis NOS
> *EXCLUDES 1* *functional urinary incontinence (R39.81)*
> *nonorganic enuresis (F98.0)*
> *stress incontinence and other specified urinary incontinence (N39.3-N39.4-)*
> *urinary incontinence associated with cognitive impairment (R39.81)*

√4ᵗʰ R33 Retention of urine
> *EXCLUDES 1* *psychogenic retention of urine (F45.8)*

R33.0 Drug induced retention of urine
Use additional code for adverse effect, if applicable, to identify drug (T36-T50 with fifth or sixth character 5)

R33.8 Other retention of urine
Code first, if applicable, any causal condition, such as:
enlarged prostate (N40.1)
AHA: 2018,4Q,55

R33.9 Retention of urine, unspecified

R34 Anuria and oliguria
> *EXCLUDES 1* *anuria and oliguria complicating abortion or ectopic or molar pregnancy (O00-O07, O08.4)*
> *anuria and oliguria complicating pregnancy (O26.83-)*
> *anuria and oliguria complicating the puerperium (O90.4)*

√4ᵗʰ R35 Polyuria
Code first, if applicable, any causal condition, such as:
enlarged prostate (N40.1)
> *EXCLUDES 1* *psychogenic polyuria (F45.8)*

R35.0 Frequency of micturition
R35.1 Nocturia
R35.8 Other polyuria
Polyuria NOS

√4ᵗʰ R36 Urethral discharge
R36.0 Urethral discharge without blood
R36.1 Hematospermia   ♂
R36.9 Urethral discharge, unspecified
Penile discharge NOS
Urethrorrhea

R37 Sexual dysfunction, unspecified

√4ᵗʰ R39 Other and unspecified symptoms and signs involving the genitourinary system
R39.0 Extravasation of urine   CC
CC Excl: PDX collection 1127

√5ᵗʰ R39.1 Other difficulties with micturition
Code first, if applicable, any causal condition, such as:
enlarged prostate (N40.1)
R39.11 Hesitancy of micturition
R39.12 Poor urinary stream
Weak urinary steam
R39.13 Splitting of urinary stream
R39.14 Feeling of incomplete bladder emptying
R39.15 Urgency of urination
> *EXCLUDES 1* *urge incontinence (N39.41, N39.46)*
R39.16 Straining to void
√6ᵗʰ R39.19 Other difficulties with micturition
AHA: 2016,4Q,63
R39.191 Need to immediately re-void
R39.192 Position dependent micturition
R39.198 Other difficulties with micturition

R39.2 Extrarenal uremia
Prerenal uremia
> *EXCLUDES 1* *uremia NOS (N19)*

√5ᵗʰ R39.8 Other symptoms and signs involving the genitourinary system
AHA: 2017,4Q,22-23
R39.81 Functional urinary incontinence
Urinary incontinence due to cognitive impairment, or severe physical disability or immobility
> *EXCLUDES 1* *stress incontinence and other specified urinary incontinence (N39.3-N39.4-)*
> *urinary incontinence NOS (R32)*
R39.82 Chronic bladder pain
AHA: 2016,4Q,64
R39.83 Unilateral non-palpable testicle   ♂
R39.84 Bilateral non-palpable testicles   ♂

R39.89 Other symptoms and signs involving the genitourinary system
R39.9 Unspecified symptoms and signs involving the genitourinary system

Symptoms and signs involving cognition, perception, emotional state and behavior (R40-R46)

> *EXCLUDES 2* *symptoms and signs constituting part of a pattern of mental disorder (F01-F99)*

√4ᵗʰ R40 Somnolence, stupor and coma
> *EXCLUDES 1* *neonatal coma (P91.5)*
> *somnolence, stupor and coma in diabetes (E08-E13)*
> *somnolence, stupor and coma in hepatic failure (K72.-)*
> *somnolence, stupor and coma in hypoglycemia (nondiabetic) (E15)*

R40.0 Somnolence
Drowsiness
> *EXCLUDES 1* *coma (R40.2-)*

R40.1 Stupor
Catatonic stupor
Semicoma
> *EXCLUDES 1* *catatonic schizophrenia (F20.2)*
> *coma (R40.2-)*
> *depressive stupor (F31-F33)*
> *dissociative stupor (F44.2)*
> *manic stupor (F30.2)*

√5ᵗʰ R40.2 Coma
Code first any associated:
fracture of skull (S02.-)
intracranial injury (S06.-)
> **NOTE** One code from each subcategory, R40.21-R40.23, is required to complete the coma scale

AHA: 2019,2Q,12; 2018,4Q,70; 2017,4Q,23-25,95; 2015,2Q,17; 2014,1Q,19
TIP: Codes for individual (R40.21-, R40.22, R40.23-) or total (R40.24-) coma scale scores may be assigned based on medical record documentation from clinicians who are not the patient's provider.
TIP: It is not appropriate to assign individual (R40.21-, R40.22-, R40.23-) or total (R40.24-) coma scale score codes for patients who are sedated or in medically induced comas.
CC Excl: For MCC codes in subcategory R40.2: PDX collection 515

R40.20 Unspecified coma   MCC HCC
Coma NOS
Unconsciousness NOS

√6ᵗʰ R40.21 Coma scale, eyes open

> The following appropriate 7th character is to be added to subcategory R40.21-, R40.22-, R40.23-, and R40.24-.
> 0 unspecified time
> 1 in the field [EMT or ambulance]
> 2 at arrival to emergency department
> 3 at hospital admission
> 4 24 hours or more after hospital admission

√7ᵗʰ R40.211 Coma scale, eyes open, never   MCC HCC
Coma scale eye opening score of 1
√7ᵗʰ R40.212 Coma scale, eyes open, to pain   MCC HCC
Coma scale eye opening score of 2
√7ᵗʰ R40.213 Coma scale, eyes open, to sound
Coma scale eye opening score of 3
√7ᵗʰ R40.214 Coma scale, eyes open, spontaneous
Coma scale eye opening score of 4

√6ᵗʰ R40.22 Coma scale, best verbal response

√7ᵗʰ R40.221 Coma scale, best verbal response, none   MCC HCC
Coma scale verbal score of 1

√7ᵗʰ **R40.222 Coma scale, best verbal response, incomprehensible words** `MCC` `HCC`
Coma scale verbal score of 2
Incomprehensible sounds (2-5 years of age)
Moans/grunts to pain; restless (< 2 years old)

√7ᵗʰ **R40.223 Coma scale, best verbal response, inappropriate words**
Coma scale verbal score of 3
Inappropriate crying or screaming (< 2 years of age)
Screaming (2-5 years of age)

√7ᵗʰ **R40.224 Coma scale, best verbal response, confused conversation**
Coma scale verbal score of 4
Inappropriate words (2-5 years of age)
Irritable cries (< 2 years of age)

√7ᵗʰ **R40.225 Coma scale, best verbal response, oriented**
Coma scale verbal score of 5
Cooing or babbling or crying appropriately (< 2 years of age)
Uses appropriate words (2-5 years of age)

√6ᵗʰ **R40.23 Coma scale, best motor response**

√7ᵗʰ **R40.231 Coma scale, best motor response, none** `MCC` `HCC`
Coma scale motor score of 1

√7ᵗʰ **R40.232 Coma scale, best motor response, extension** `MCC` `HCC`
Abnormal extensor posturing to pain or noxious stimuli (< 2 years of age)
Coma scale motor score of 2
Extensor posturing to pain or noxious stimuli (2-5 years of age)

√7ᵗʰ **R40.233 Coma scale, best motor response, abnormal flexion**
Abnormal flexure posturing to pain or noxious stimuli (2-5 years of age)
Coma scale motor score of 3
Flexion/decorticate posturing (< 2 years of age)

√7ᵗʰ **R40.234 Coma scale, best motor response, flexion withdrawal** `MCC` `HCC`
Coma scale motor score of 4
Withdraws from pain or noxious stimuli (2-5 years of age)

√7ᵗʰ **R40.235 Coma scale, best motor response, localizes pain**
Coma scale motor score of 5
Localizes pain (2-5 years of age)
Withdraws to touch (< 2 years of age)

√7ᵗʰ **R40.236 Coma scale, best motor response, obeys commands**
Coma scale motor score of 6
Normal or spontaneous movement (< 2 years of age)
Obeys commands (2-5 years of age)

√6ᵗʰ **R40.24 Glasgow coma scale, total score**
> `NOTE` Assign a code from subcategory R40.24, when only the total coma score is documented

AHA: 2016,4Q,64-65

√7ᵗʰ **R40.241 Glasgow coma scale score 13-15**

√7ᵗʰ **R40.242 Glasgow coma scale score 9-12**

√7ᵗʰ **R40.243 Glasgow coma scale score 3-8** `HCC`

√7ᵗʰ **R40.244 Other coma, without documented Glasgow coma scale score, or with partial score reported** `HCC`

R40.3 Persistent vegetative state `CC` `HCC`
DEF: Persistent wakefulness without consciousness due to a nonfunctioning cerebral cortex.
CC Excl: PDX collection 515

R40.4 Transient alteration of awareness

√4ᵗʰ **R41 Other symptoms and signs involving cognitive functions and awareness**
> `EXCLUDES 1` dissociative [conversion] disorders (F44.-)
> mild cognitive impairment, so stated (G31.84)

R41.0 Disorientation, unspecified
Confusion NOS
Delirium NOS
AHA: 2019,2Q,34

R41.1 Anterograde amnesia

R41.2 Retrograde amnesia

R41.3 Other amnesia
Amnesia NOS
Memory loss NOS
> `EXCLUDES 1` amnestic disorder due to known physiologic condition (F04)
> amnestic syndrome due to psychoactive substance use (F10-F19 with 5th character .6)
> mild memory disturbance due to known physiological condition (F06.8)
> transient global amnesia (G45.4)

R41.4 Neurologic neglect syndrome `CC`
Asomatognosia
Hemi-akinesia
Hemi-inattention
Hemispatial neglect
Left-sided neglect
Sensory neglect
Visuospatial neglect
> `EXCLUDES 1` visuospatial deficit (R41.842)
CC Excl: PDX collection 1128

√5ᵗʰ **R41.8 Other symptoms and signs involving cognitive functions and awareness**

R41.81 Age-related cognitive decline `A`
Senility NOS

R41.82 Altered mental status, unspecified
Change in mental status NOS
> `EXCLUDES 1` altered level of consciousness (R40.-)
> altered mental status due to known condition — code to condition
> delirium NOS (R41.0)
AHA: 2012,4Q,97

R41.83 Borderline intellectual functioning
IQ level 71 to 84
> `EXCLUDES 1` intellectual disabilities (F70-F79)

√6ᵗʰ **R41.84 Other specified cognitive deficit**
> `EXCLUDES 1` cognitive deficits as sequelae of cerebrovascular disease (I69.01-, I69.11-, I69.21-, I69.31-, I69.81-, I69.91-)

R41.840 Attention and concentration deficit
> `EXCLUDES 1` attention-deficit hyperactivity disorders (F90.-)

R41.841 Cognitive communication deficit

R41.842 Visuospatial deficit

R41.843 Psychomotor deficit

R41.844 Frontal lobe and executive function deficit

R41.89 Other symptoms and signs involving cognitive functions and awareness
Anosognosia

R41.9 Unspecified symptoms and signs involving cognitive functions and awareness
Unspecified neurocognitive disorder

R42 Dizziness and giddiness
Light-headedness
Vertigo NOS
> `EXCLUDES 1` vertiginous syndromes (H81.-)
> vertigo from infrasound (T75.23)

√4ᵗʰ **R43 Disturbances of smell and taste**

R43.0 Anosmia
DEF: Permanent or transient absence of smell that may be congenital or acquired.

R43.1 Parosmia
DEF: Abnormal perception of smell usually triggered by environmental odors.

R43.2 Parageusia
    DEF: Abnormal perception of taste.

R43.8 Other disturbances of smell and taste
    Mixed disturbance of smell and taste

R43.9 Unspecified disturbances of smell and taste

☑4ᵗʰ **R44 Other symptoms and signs involving general sensations and perceptions**
    EXCLUDES 1   alcoholic hallucinations (F1.5)
          hallucinations in drug psychosis (F11-F19 with .5)
          hallucinations in mood disorders with psychotic symptoms (F30.2, F31.5, F32.3, F33.3)
          hallucinations in schizophrenia, schizotypal and delusional disorders (F20-F29)
    EXCLUDES 2   disturbances of skin sensation (R20.-)
    CC Excl: For CC codes in category R44: PDX collection 1129

R44.0 Auditory hallucinations   CC

R44.1 Visual hallucinations

R44.2 Other hallucinations   CC

R44.3 Hallucinations, unspecified   CC

R44.8 Other symptoms and signs involving general sensations and perceptions

R44.9 Unspecified symptoms and signs involving general sensations and perceptions

☑4ᵗʰ **R45 Symptoms and signs involving emotional state**

R45.0 Nervousness
    Nervous tension

R45.1 Restlessness and agitation

R45.2 Unhappiness

R45.3 Demoralization and apathy
    EXCLUDES 1   anhedonia (R45.84)

R45.4 Irritability and anger

R45.5 Hostility

R45.6 Violent behavior

R45.7 State of emotional shock and stress, unspecified

☑5ᵗʰ **R45.8 Other symptoms and signs involving emotional state**

    R45.81 Low self-esteem

    R45.82 Worries

    R45.83 Excessive crying of child, adolescent or adult
         EXCLUDES 1   excessive crying of infant (baby) R68.11

    R45.84 Anhedonia

    ☑6ᵗʰ **R45.85 Homicidal and suicidal ideations**
         EXCLUDES 1   suicide attempt (T14.91)

         R45.850 Homicidal ideations

         R45.851 Suicidal ideations   CC
             DEF: Thoughts of committing suicide but no actual attempt of suicide has been made.
             CC Excl: PDX collection 1130

    R45.86 Emotional lability

    R45.87 Impulsiveness

    R45.89 Other symptoms and signs involving emotional state

☑4ᵗʰ **R46 Symptoms and signs involving appearance and behavior**
    EXCLUDES 1   appearance and behavior in schizophrenia, schizotypal and delusional disorders (F20-F29)
          mental and behavioral disorders (F01-F99)

R46.0 Very low level of personal hygiene

R46.1 Bizarre personal appearance

R46.2 Strange and inexplicable behavior

R46.3 Overactivity

R46.4 Slowness and poor responsiveness
    EXCLUDES 1   stupor (R40.1)

R46.5 Suspiciousness and marked evasiveness

R46.6 Undue concern and preoccupation with stressful events

R46.7 Verbosity and circumstantial detail obscuring reason for contact

☑5ᵗʰ **R46.8 Other symptoms and signs involving appearance and behavior**

    R46.81 Obsessive-compulsive behavior
         EXCLUDES 1   obsessive-compulsive disorder (F42-)

    R46.89 Other symptoms and signs involving appearance and behavior

Symptoms and signs involving speech and voice (R47-R49)

☑4ᵗʰ **R47 Speech disturbances, not elsewhere classified**
    EXCLUDES 1   autism (F84.0)
          cluttering (F80.81)
          specific developmental disorders of speech and language (F80.-)
          stuttering (F80.81)

☑5ᵗʰ **R47.0 Dysphasia and aphasia**

    R47.01 Aphasia   CC
         EXCLUDES 1   aphasia following cerebrovascular disease (I69. with final characters -20)
              progressive isolated aphasia (G31.01)
         CC Excl: PDX collection 1131

    R47.02 Dysphasia
         EXCLUDES 1   dysphasia following cerebrovascular disease (I69. with final characters -21)

R47.1 Dysarthria and anarthria
    EXCLUDES 1   dysarthria following cerebrovascular disease (I69. with final characters -22)

☑5ᵗʰ **R47.8 Other speech disturbances**
    EXCLUDES 1   dysarthria following cerebrovascular disease (I69. with final characters -28)

    R47.81 Slurred speech

    R47.82 Fluency disorder in conditions classified elsewhere
         Stuttering in conditions classified elsewhere
         Code first underlying disease or condition, such as:
         Parkinson's disease (G20)
         EXCLUDES 1   adult onset fluency disorder (F98.5)
              childhood onset fluency disorder (F80.81)
              fluency disorder (stuttering) following cerebrovascular disease (I69. with final characters -23)

    R47.89 Other speech disturbances

R47.9 Unspecified speech disturbances

☑4ᵗʰ **R48 Dyslexia and other symbolic dysfunctions, not elsewhere classified**
    EXCLUDES 1   specific developmental disorders of scholastic skills (F81.-)

R48.0 Dyslexia and alexia

R48.1 Agnosia
    Astereognosia (astereognosis)
    Autotopagnosia
    EXCLUDES 1   visual object agnosia (R48.3)
    DEF: Inability to recognize common things such as faces, objects, smells, or voices.

R48.2 Apraxia
    EXCLUDES 1   apraxia following cerebrovascular disease (I69. with final characters -90)

R48.3 Visual agnosia
    Prosopagnosia
    Simultanagnosia (asimultagnosia)

R48.8 Other symbolic dysfunctions
    Acalculia
    Agraphia
    AHA: 2017,1Q,27

R48.9 Unspecified symbolic dysfunctions

☑4ᵗʰ **R49 Voice and resonance disorders**
    EXCLUDES 1   psychogenic voice and resonance disorders (F44.4)

R49.0 Dysphonia
    Hoarseness

R49.1 Aphonia
    Loss of voice

☑5ᵗʰ **R49.2 Hypernasality and hyponasality**

    R49.21 Hypernasality

    R49.22 Hyponasality

R49.8 Other voice and resonance disorders

R49.9 Unspecified voice and resonance disorder
    Change in voice NOS
    Resonance disorder NOS

☑ Additional Character Required   ☑x7ᵗʰ Placeholder   Unacceptable PDx   Questionable PDx   Manifestation   Unspecified Dx   H1-H14 HAC   HCC CMS-HCC Dx   HIV HIV Dx

ICD-10-CM 2020   963

Chapter 18. Symptoms, Signs and Abnormal Clinical and Laboratory Findings

R50–R54

General symptoms and signs (R50-R69)

✓4th R50　Fever of other and unknown origin

> **EXCLUDES 1**　chills without fever (R68.83)
> febrile convulsions (R56.0-)
> fever of unknown origin during labor (O75.2)
> fever of unknown origin in newborn (P81.9)
> hypothermia due to illness (R68.0)
> malignant hyperthermia due to anesthesia (T88.3)
> puerperal pyrexia NOS (O86.4)

R50.2　Drug induced fever　　　　CC

> Use additional code for adverse effect, if applicable, to identify drug (T36-T50 with fifth or sixth character 5)
> **EXCLUDES 1**　postvaccination (postimmunization) fever (R50.83)

✓5th R50.8　Other specified fever

> **R50.81　Fever presenting with conditions classified elsewhere**
> Code first underlying condition when associated fever is present, such as with:
> leukemia (C91-C95)
> neutropenia (D70.-)
> sickle-cell disease (D57.-)
> **AHA:** 2014,4Q,22

> **R50.82　Postprocedural fever**　　　　CC
> **EXCLUDES 1**　postprocedural infection (T81.4-)
> posttransfusion fever (R50.84)
> postvaccination (postimmunization) fever (R50.83)

> **R50.83　Postvaccination fever**
> Postimmunization fever

> **R50.84　Febrile nonhemolytic transfusion reaction**
> FNHTR
> Posttransfusion fever

R50.9　Fever, unspecified
> Fever NOS
> Fever of unknown origin [FUO]
> Fever with chills
> Fever with rigors
> Hyperpyrexia NOS
> Persistent fever
> Pyrexia NOS

R51　Headache
> Facial pain NOS
> **EXCLUDES 1**　atypical face pain (G50.1)
> migraine and other headache syndromes (G43-G44)
> trigeminal neuralgia (G50.0)

R52　Pain, unspecified
> Acute pain NOS
> Generalized pain NOS
> Pain NOS
> **EXCLUDES 1**　acute and chronic pain, not elsewhere classified (G89.-)
> localized pain, unspecified type — code to pain by site, such as:
> abdomen pain (R10.-)
> back pain (M54.9)
> breast pain (N64.4)
> chest pain (R07.1-R07.9)
> ear pain (H92.0-)
> eye pain (H57.1)
> headache (R51)
> joint pain (M25.5-)
> limb pain (M79.6-)
> lumbar region pain (M54.5)
> pelvic and perineal pain (R10.2)
> renal colic (N23)
> shoulder pain (M25.51-)
> spine pain (M54.-)
> throat pain (R07.0)
> tongue pain (K14.6)
> tooth pain (K08.8)
> pain disorders exclusively related to psychological factors (F45.41)

✓4th R53　Malaise and fatigue

R53.0　Neoplastic (malignant) related fatigue
> Code first associated neoplasm

R53.1　Weakness
> Asthenia NOS
> **EXCLUDES 1**　age-related weakness (R54)
> muscle weakness (M62.8-)
> sarcopenia (M62.84)
> senile asthenia (R54)
> **AHA:** 2017,1Q,7; 2015,1Q,25

R53.2　Functional quadriplegia　　　　MCC　HCC
> Complete immobility due to severe physical disability or frailty
> **EXCLUDES 1**　frailty NOS (R54)
> hysterical paralysis (F44.4)
> immobility syndrome (M62.3)
> neurologic quadriplegia (G82.5-)
> quadriplegia (G82.50)
> **AHA:** 2016,2Q,6
> **DEF:** Inability to move due to a nonphysiological condition, such as dementia. The patient has no mental ability to move independently.
> **CC Excl:** PDX collection 595

✓5th R53.8　Other malaise and fatigue
> **EXCLUDES 1**　combat exhaustion and fatigue (F43.0)
> congenital debility (P96.9)
> exhaustion and fatigue due to excessive exertion (T73.3)
> exhaustion and fatigue due to exposure (T73.2)
> exhaustion and fatigue due to heat (T67.-)
> exhaustion and fatigue due to pregnancy (O26.8-)
> exhaustion and fatigue due to recurrent depressive episode (F33)
> exhaustion and fatigue due to senile debility (R54)

> **R53.81　Other malaise**
> Chronic debility
> Debility NOS
> General physical deterioration
> Malaise NOS
> Nervous debility
> **EXCLUDES 1**　age-related physical debility (R54)

> **R53.82　Chronic fatigue, unspecified**
> Chronic fatigue syndrome NOS
> **EXCLUDES 1**　postviral fatigue syndrome (G93.3)

> **R53.83　Other fatigue**
> Fatigue NOS
> Lack of energy
> Lethargy
> Tiredness
> **EXCLUDES 2**　exhaustion and fatigue due to depressive episode (F32.-)

R54　Age-related physical debility　　　　A
> Frailty
> Old age
> Senescence
> Senile asthenia
> Senile debility
> **EXCLUDES 1**　age-related cognitive decline (R41.81)
> sarcopenia (M62.84)
> senile psychosis (F03)
> senility NOS (R41.81)

N Newborn: 0　　**P** Pediatric: 0-17　　**M** Maternity: 9-64　　**A** Adult: 15-124　　**MCC** Major Complication/Comorbidity　　**CC** Complication/Comorbidity　　**SW** Severe Wound Dx

964　　　　ICD-10-CM 2020

R55 Syncope and collapse
Blackout
Fainting
Vasovagal attack
> *EXCLUDES 1*   *cardiogenic shock (R57.0)*
> *carotid sinus syncope (G90.01)*
> *heat syncope (T67.1)*
> *neurocirculatory asthenia (F45.8)*
> *neurogenic orthostatic hypotension (G90.3)*
> *orthostatic hypotension (I95.1)*
> *postprocedural shock (T81.1-)*
> *psychogenic syncope (F48.8)*
> *shock NOS (R57.9)*
> *shock complicating or following abortion or ectopic or molar*
>   *pregnancy (O00–O07, O08.3)*
> *shock complicating or following labor and delivery (O75.1)*
> *Stokes-Adams attack (I45.9)*
> *unconsciousness NOS (R40.2-)*

✓4ᵗʰ R56 Convulsions, not elsewhere classified
> *EXCLUDES 1*   *dissociative convulsions and seizures (F44.5)*
> *epileptic convulsions and seizures (G40.-)*
> *newborn convulsions and seizures (P90)*

✓5ᵗʰ R56.0 Febrile convulsions

   R56.00 Simple febrile convulsions   `CC` `HCC`

     Febrile convulsion NOS
     Febrile seizure NOS
     CC Excl: PDX collection 1132

   R56.01 Complex febrile convulsions   `CC` `HCC`

     Atypical febrile seizure
     Complex febrile seizure
     Complicated febrile seizure
> *EXCLUDES 1*   *status epilepticus (G40.901)*
     CC Excl: PDX collection 1132

R56.1 Post traumatic seizures   `CC` `HCC`
> *EXCLUDES 1*   *post traumatic epilepsy (G40.-)*
CC Excl: PDX collection 582

R56.9 Unspecified convulsions   `HCC`

Convulsion disorder
Fit NOS
Recurrent convulsions
Seizure(s) (convulsive) NOS
AHA: 2019,1Q,19

✓4ᵗʰ R57 Shock, not elsewhere classified
> *EXCLUDES 1*   *anaphylactic shock NOS (T78.2)*
> *anaphylactic reaction or shock due to adverse food reaction*
>   *(T78.0-)*
> *anaphylactic shock due to adverse effect of correct drug or*
>   *medicament properly administered (T88.6)*
> *anaphylactic shock due to serum (T80.5-)*
> *anesthetic shock (T88.3)*
> *electric shock (T75.4)*
> *obstetric shock (O75.1)*
> *postprocedural shock (T81.1-)*
> *psychic shock (F43.0)*
> *shock complicating or following ectopic or molar pregnancy*
>   *(O00–O07, O08.3)*
> *shock due to lightning (T75.01)*
> *traumatic shock (T79.4)*
> *toxic shock syndrome (A48.3)*

CC Excl: For CC/MCC codes in category R57: PDX collection 1133

¹ **R57.0 Cardiogenic shock**   `MCC` `HCC`
> *EXCLUDES 2*   *septic shock (R65.21)*
DEF: Associated with myocardial infarction, cardiac tamponade, and massive pulmonary embolism. Symptoms include mental confusion, reduced blood pressure, tachycardia, pallor, and cold, clammy skin.

¹ **R57.1 Hypovolemic shock**   `MCC` `HCC`
AHA: 2019,2Q,7

¹ **R57.8 Other shock**   `MCC` `HCC`

R57.9 Shock, unspecified   `CC` `HCC`
Failure of peripheral circulation NOS

R58 Hemorrhage, not elsewhere classified   `CC`
Hemorrhage NOS
> *EXCLUDES 1*   *hemorrhage included with underlying conditions, such as:*
> *acute duodenal ulcer with hemorrhage (K26.0)*
> *acute gastritis with bleeding (K29.01)*
> *ulcerative enterocolitis with rectal bleeding (K51.01)*

✓4ᵗʰ R59 Enlarged lymph nodes
> `INCLUDES`   swollen glands
> *EXCLUDES 1*   *acute lymphadenitis (L04.-)*
> *chronic lymphadenitis (I88.1)*
> *lymphadenitis NOS (I88.9)*
> *mesenteric (acute) (chronic) lymphadenitis (I88.0)*

R59.0 Localized enlarged lymph nodes
R59.1 Generalized enlarged lymph nodes
Lymphadenopathy NOS
R59.9 Enlarged lymph nodes, unspecified

✓4ᵗʰ R60 Edema, not elsewhere classified
> *EXCLUDES 1*   *angioneurotic edema (T78.3)*
> *ascites (R18.-)*
> *cerebral edema (G93.6)*
> *cerebral edema due to birth injury (P11.0)*
> *edema of larynx (J38.4)*
> *edema of nasopharynx (J39.2)*
> *edema of pharynx (J39.2)*
> *gestational edema (O12.0-)*
> *hereditary edema (Q82.0)*
> *hydrops fetalis NOS (P83.2)*
> *hydrothorax (J94.8)*
> *hydrops fetalis NOS (P83.2)*
> *newborn edema (P83.3)*
> *pulmonary edema (J81.-)*

R60.0 Localized edema
R60.1 Generalized edema   `CC`
> *EXCLUDES 2*   *nutritional edema (E40-E46)*

R60.9 Edema, unspecified
Fluid retention NOS

R61 Generalized hyperhidrosis
Excessive sweating
Night sweats
Secondary hyperhidrosis
Code first, if applicable, menopausal and female climacteric states (N95.1)
> *EXCLUDES 1*   *focal (primary) (secondary) hyperhidrosis (L74.5-)*
> *Frey's syndrome (L74.52)*
> *localized (primary) (secondary) hyperhidrosis (L74.5-)*

✓4ᵗʰ R62 Lack of expected normal physiological development in childhood and adults
> *EXCLUDES 1*   *delayed puberty (E30.0)*
> *gonadal dysgenesis (Q99.1)*
> *hypopituitarism (E23.0)*

R62.0 Delayed milestone in childhood   `P`

Delayed attainment of expected physiological developmental stage
Late talker
Late walker

✓5ᵗʰ R62.5 Other and unspecified lack of expected normal physiological development in childhood
> *EXCLUDES 1*   *HIV disease resulting in failure to thrive (B20)*
> *physical retardation due to malnutrition (E45)*

   R62.50 Unspecified lack of expected normal physiological development in childhood
     Infantilism NOS

   R62.51 Failure to thrive (child)   `P`

     Failure to gain weight
> *EXCLUDES 1*   *failure to thrive in child under 28 days old*
>   *(P92.6)*

     AHA: 2018,4Q,82
     DEF: Organic failure to thrive (FTT): Acute or chronic illness that interferes with nutritional intake, absorption, metabolism excretion, and energy requirements.
     DEF: Nonorganic failure to thrive (FTT): Symptom of neglect or abuse.

✓ Additional Character Required   ✓x 7ᵗʰ Placeholder   Unacceptable PDx   Questionable PDx   Manifestation   Unspecified Dx   `H1`-`H14` HAC   `HCC` CMS-HCC Dx   `HIV` HIV Dx

ICD-10-CM 2020   **965**

Chapter 18. Symptoms, Signs and Abnormal Clinical and Laboratory Findings

R62.52   **Short stature (child)**
Lack of growth
Physical retardation
Short stature NOS
> EXCLUDES 1   *short stature due to endocrine disorder (E34.3)*

R62.59   **Other lack of expected normal physiological development in childhood**

R62.7   **Adult failure to thrive**   CC A

✓4ᵗʰ **R63**   **Symptoms and signs concerning food and fluid intake**
> EXCLUDES 1   *bulimia NOS (F50.2)*
> *eating disorders of nonorganic origin (F50.-)*
> *malnutrition (E40-E46)*

R63.0   **Anorexia**
Loss of appetite
> EXCLUDES 1   *anorexia nervosa (F50.0-)*
> *loss of appetite of nonorganic origin (F50.89)*

AHA: 2018,4Q,82
TIP: Assign an additional code from category Z68 when BMI is documented. BMI can be based on documentation from clinicians who are not the patient's provider.

R63.1   **Polydipsia**
Excessive thirst

R63.2   **Polyphagia**
Excessive eating
Hyperalimentation NOS

R63.3   **Feeding difficulties**   CC
Feeding problem (elderly) (infant) NOS
Picky eater
> EXCLUDES 1   *eating disorders (F50.-)*
> *feeding problems of newborn (P92.-)*
> *infant feeding disorder of nonorganic origin (F98.2-)*

AHA: 2017,1Q,28; 2016,3Q,19
TIP: Do not assign for feeding problems in a patient greater than 28 days old if the feeding problem was initially diagnosed between day 0 and day 28; use a code from category P92 instead.

R63.4   **Abnormal weight loss**
AHA: 2018,4Q,82
TIP: Assign an additional code from category Z68 when BMI is documented. BMI can be based on documentation from clinicians who are not the patient's provider.

R63.5   **Abnormal weight gain**
> EXCLUDES 1   *excessive weight gain in pregnancy (O26.0-)*
> *obesity (E66.-)*

AHA: 2018,4Q,82
TIP: Assign an additional code from category Z68 when BMI is documented. BMI can be based on documentation from clinicians who are not the patient's provider.

R63.6   **Underweight**
Use additional code to identify body mass index (BMI), if known (Z68.-)
> EXCLUDES 1   *abnormal weight loss (R63.4)*
> *anorexia nervosa (F50.0-)*
> *malnutrition (E40-E46)*

AHA: 2018,4Q,82

R63.8   **Other symptoms and signs concerning food and fluid intake**

R64   **Cachexia**   CC HCC
Wasting syndrome
Code first underlying condition, if known
> EXCLUDES 1   *abnormal weight loss (R63.4)*
> *nutritional marasmus (E41)*

AHA: 2018,4Q,82; 2017,3Q,24
CC Excl: PDX collection 1134

✓4ᵗʰ **R65**   **Symptoms and signs specifically associated with systemic inflammation and infection**
AHA: 2019,2Q,38
TIP: When documentation states SIRS with an infection, assign only a code for the infection. ICD-10-CM does not offer a code for SIRS due to infectious process. If sepsis is suspected, query the provider.
CC Excl: For CC/MCC codes in category R65, unless otherwise noted: PDX collection 71

✓5ᵗʰ **R65.1**   **Systemic inflammatory response syndrome [SIRS] of non-infectious origin**
Code first underlying condition, such as:
heatstroke ▶(T67.0-)◄
injury and trauma (S00-T88)
> EXCLUDES 1   *sepsis — code to infection*
> *severe sepsis (R65.2)*

R65.10   **Systemic inflammatory response syndrome [SIRS] of non-infectious origin without acute organ dysfunction**   CC HCC
Systemic inflammatory response syndrome (SIRS) NOS
AHA: 2019,2Q,24

R65.11   **Systemic inflammatory response syndrome [SIRS] of non-infectious origin with acute organ dysfunction**   CC HCC
Use additional code to identify specific acute organ dysfunction, such as:
acute kidney failure (N17.-)
acute respiratory failure (J96.0-)
critical illness myopathy (G72.81)
critical illness polyneuropathy (G62.81)
disseminated intravascular coagulopathy [DIC] (D65)
encephalopathy (metabolic) (septic) (G93.41)
hepatic failure (K72.0-)

✓5ᵗʰ **R65.2**   **Severe sepsis**
Infection with associated acute organ dysfunction
Sepsis with acute organ dysfunction
Sepsis with multiple organ dysfunction
Systemic inflammatory response syndrome due to infectious process with acute organ dysfunction
Code first underlying infection, such as:
infection following a procedure (T81.4-)
infections following infusion, transfusion and therapeutic injection (T80.2-)
puerperal sepsis (O85)
sepsis following complete or unspecified spontaneous abortion (O03.87)
sepsis following ectopic and molar pregnancy (O08.82)
sepsis following incomplete spontaneous abortion (O03.37)
sepsis following (induced) termination of pregnancy (O04.87)
sepsis NOS (A41.9)
Use additional code to identify specific acute organ dysfunction, such as:
acute kidney failure (N17.-)
acute respiratory failure (J96.0-)
critical illness myopathy (G72.81)
critical illness polyneuropathy (G62.81)
disseminated intravascular coagulopathy [DIC] (D65)
encephalopathy (metabolic) (septic) (G93.41)
hepatic failure (K72.0-)
AHA: 2018,4Q,62-63; 2017,4Q,98-99; 2016,3Q,8

R65.20   **Severe sepsis without septic shock**   MCC HCC
Severe sepsis NOS
AHA: 2016,3Q,14; 2013,4Q,119

R65.21   **Severe sepsis with septic shock**   MCC HCC
AHA: 2018,4Q,63
CC Excl: PDX collection 1133

✓4ᵗʰ **R68**   **Other general symptoms and signs**

R68.0   **Hypothermia, not associated with low environmental temperature**
> EXCLUDES 1   *hypothermia NOS (accidental) (T68)*
> *hypothermia due to anesthesia (T88.51)*
> *hypothermia due to low environmental temperature (T68)*
> *newborn hypothermia (P80.-)*

✓5ᵗʰ **R68.1 Nonspecific symptoms peculiar to infancy**

    EXCLUDES 1   colic, infantile (R10.83)

           neonatal cerebral irritability (P91.3)

           teething syndrome (K00.7)

    R68.11 Excessive crying of infant (baby)   P

          EXCLUDES 1   excessive crying of child, adolescent, or adult (R45.83)

    R68.12 Fussy infant (baby)   P

           Irritable infant

    R68.13 Apparent life threatening event in infant (ALTE)   P

           Apparent life threatening event in newborn

           Brief resolved unexplained event (BRUE)

           Code first confirmed diagnosis, if known

           Use additional code(s) for associated signs and symptoms if no confirmed diagnosis established, or if signs and symptoms are not associated routinely with confirmed diagnosis, or provide additional information for cause of ALTE

    R68.19 Other nonspecific symptoms peculiar to infancy   P

R68.2 Dry mouth, unspecified

    EXCLUDES 1   dry mouth due to dehydration (E86.0)

           dry mouth due to sicca syndrome [Sjögren] (M35.0-)

           salivary gland hyposecretion (K11.7)

R68.3 Clubbing of fingers

     Clubbing of nails

    EXCLUDES 1   congenital clubfinger (Q68.1)

    DEF: Enlarged soft tissue of the distal fingers that usually occurs in heart and lung diseases.

✓5ᵗʰ **R68.8 Other general symptoms and signs**

    R68.81 Early satiety

          DEF: Premature feeling of being full after eating only a small amount of food. The mechanism of satiety is multifactorial.

    R68.82 Decreased libido   A

           Decreased sexual desire

    R68.83 Chills (without fever)

           Chills NOS

          EXCLUDES 1   chills with fever (R50.9)

    R68.84 Jaw pain

           Mandibular pain

           Maxilla pain

          EXCLUDES 1   temporomandibular joint arthralgia (M26.62-)

    R68.89 Other general symptoms and signs

R69 Illness, unspecified

     Unknown and unspecified cases of morbidity

Abnormal findings on examination of blood, without diagnosis (R70-R79)

EXCLUDES 2   abnormal findings on antenatal screening of mother (O28.-)

           abnormalities of lipids (E78.-)

           abnormalities of platelets and thrombocytes (D69.-)

           abnormalities of white blood cells classified elsewhere (D70-D72)

           coagulation hemorrhagic disorders (D65-D68)

           diagnostic abnormal findings classified elsewhere — see Alphabetical Index

           hemorrhagic and hematological disorders of newborn (P50-P61)

✓4ᵗʰ **R70 Elevated erythrocyte sedimentation rate and abnormality of plasma viscosity**

    R70.0 Elevated erythrocyte sedimentation rate

    R70.1 Abnormal plasma viscosity

✓4ᵗʰ **R71 Abnormality of red blood cells**

    EXCLUDES 1   anemias (D50-D64)

           anemia of premature infant (P61.2)

           benign (familial) polycythemia (D75.0)

           congenital anemias (P61.2-P61.4)

           newborn anemia due to isoimmunization (P55.-)

           polycythemia neonatorum (P61.1)

           polycythemia NOS (D75.1)

           polycythemia vera (D45)

           secondary polycythemia (D75.1)

    R71.0 Precipitous drop in hematocrit   CC

           Drop (precipitous) in hemoglobin

           Drop in hematocrit

          CC Excl: PDX collection 1135

    R71.8 Other abnormality of red blood cells

           Abnormal red-cell morphology NOS

           Abnormal red-cell volume NOS

           Anisocytosis

           Poikilocytosis

✓4ᵗʰ **R73 Elevated blood glucose level**

    EXCLUDES 1   diabetes mellitus (E08-E13)

           diabetes mellitus in pregnancy, childbirth and the puerperium (O24.-)

           neonatal disorders (P70.0-P70.2)

           postsurgical hypoinsulinemia (E89.1)

    ✓5ᵗʰ **R73.0 Abnormal glucose**

          EXCLUDES 1   abnormal glucose in pregnancy (O99.81-)

                 diabetes mellitus (E08-E13)

                 dysmetabolic syndrome X (E88.81)

                 gestational diabetes (O24.4-)

                 glycosuria (R81)

                 hypoglycemia (E16.2)

        R73.01 Impaired fasting glucose

              Elevated fasting glucose

        R73.02 Impaired glucose tolerance (oral)

              Elevated glucose tolerance

        R73.03 Prediabetes

              Latent diabetes

             AHA: 2016,4Q,65

        R73.09 Other abnormal glucose

              Abnormal glucose NOS

              Abnormal non-fasting glucose tolerance

    R73.9 Hyperglycemia, unspecified

✓4ᵗʰ **R74 Abnormal serum enzyme levels**

    R74.0 Nonspecific elevation of levels of transaminase and lactic acid dehydrogenase [LDH]

    R74.8 Abnormal levels of other serum enzymes

           Abnormal level of acid phosphatase

           Abnormal level of alkaline phosphatase

           Abnormal level of amylase

           Abnormal level of lipase [triacylglycerol lipase]

          AHA: 2019,2Q,6

    R74.9 Abnormal serum enzyme level, unspecified

R75 Inconclusive laboratory evidence of human immunodeficiency virus [HIV]

     Nonconclusive HIV-test finding in infants

    EXCLUDES 1   asymptomatic human immunodeficiency virus [HIV] infection status (Z21)

           human immunodeficiency virus [HIV] disease (B20)

    TIP: Do not assign for patients previously diagnosed with an HIV-related illness; assign code B20 instead.

✓4ᵗʰ **R76 Other abnormal immunological findings in serum**

    R76.0 Raised antibody titer

          EXCLUDES 1   isoimmunization in pregnancy (O36.0-O36.1)

                 isoimmunization affecting newborn (P55.-)

☑ Additional Character Required   ✓ₓ7ᵗʰ Placeholder   Unacceptable PDx   Questionable PDx   Manifestation   Unspecified Dx   H1-H14 HAC   HCC CMS-HCC Dx   HIV HIV Dx

ICD-10-CM 2020   967

√5ᵗʰ R76.1 Nonspecific reaction to test for tuberculosis

R76.11 Nonspecific reaction to tuberculin skin test without active tuberculosis
Abnormal result of Mantoux test
PPD positive
Tuberculin (skin test) positive
Tuberculin (skin test) reactor
EXCLUDES 1   *nonspecific reaction to cell mediated immunity measurement of gamma interferon antigen response without active tuberculosis (R76.12)*

R76.12 Nonspecific reaction to cell mediated immunity measurement of gamma interferon antigen response without active tuberculosis
Nonspecific reaction to QuantiFERON-TB test (QFT) without active tuberculosis
EXCLUDES 1   *nonspecific reaction to tuberculin skin test without active tuberculosis (R76.11)*
positive tuberculin skin test (R76.11)

R76.8 Other specified abnormal immunological findings in serum
Raised level of immunoglobulins NOS

R76.9 Abnormal immunological finding in serum, unspecified

√4ᵗʰ R77 Other abnormalities of plasma proteins
EXCLUDES 1   *disorders of plasma-protein metabolism (E88.0-)*

R77.0 Abnormality of albumin

R77.1 Abnormality of globulin
Hyperglobulinemia NOS

R77.2 Abnormality of alphafetoprotein

R77.8 Other specified abnormalities of plasma proteins

R77.9 Abnormality of plasma protein, unspecified
AHA: 2019,2Q,6

√4ᵗʰ R78 Findings of drugs and other substances, not normally found in blood
Use additional code to identify the any retained foreign body, if applicable (Z18.-)
EXCLUDES 1   *mental or behavioral disorders due to psychoactive substance use (F10-F19)*

R78.0 Finding of alcohol in blood
Use additional external cause code (Y90.-), for detail regarding alcohol level

R78.1 Finding of opiate drug in blood

R78.2 Finding of cocaine in blood

R78.3 Finding of hallucinogen in blood

R78.4 Finding of other drugs of addictive potential in blood

R78.5 Finding of other psychotropic drug in blood

R78.6 Finding of steroid agent in blood

√5ᵗʰ R78.7 Finding of abnormal level of heavy metals in blood

R78.71 Abnormal lead level in blood
EXCLUDES 1   *lead poisoning (T56.0-)*

R78.79 Finding of abnormal level of heavy metals in blood

√5ᵗʰ R78.8 Finding of other specified substances, not normally found in blood

R78.81 Bacteremia   MCC
EXCLUDES 1   *sepsis — code to specified infection*
DEF: Laboratory finding of bacteria in the blood in the absence of two or more signs of sepsis. Transient in nature, it can progress to septicemia with a severe infectious process.

R78.89 Finding of other specified substances, not normally found in blood
Finding of abnormal level of lithium in blood

R78.9 Finding of unspecified substance, not normally found in blood

√4ᵗʰ R79 Other abnormal findings of blood chemistry
Use additional code to identify any retained foreign body, if applicable (Z18.-)
EXCLUDES 1   *asymptomatic hyperuricemia (E79.0)*
hyperglycemia NOS (R73.9)
hypoglycemia NOS (E16.2)
neonatal hypoglycemia (P70.3-P70.4)
specific findings indicating disorder of amino-acid metabolism (E70-E72)
specific findings indicating disorder of carbohydrate metabolism (E73-E74)
specific findings indicating disorder of lipid metabolism (E75.-)

R79.0 Abnormal level of blood mineral
Abnormal blood level of cobalt
Abnormal blood level of copper
Abnormal blood level of iron
Abnormal blood level of magnesium
Abnormal blood level of mineral NEC
Abnormal blood level of zinc
EXCLUDES 1   *abnormal level of lithium (R78.89)*
disorders of mineral metabolism (E83.-)
neonatal hypomagnesemia (P71.2)
nutritional mineral deficiency (E58-E61)

R79.1 Abnormal coagulation profile
Abnormal or prolonged bleeding time
Abnormal or prolonged coagulation time
Abnormal or prolonged partial thromboplastin time [PTT]
Abnormal or prolonged prothrombin time [PT]
EXCLUDES 1   *coagulation defects (D68.-)*
EXCLUDES 2   *abnormality of fluid, electrolyte or acid-base balance (E86-E87)*

√5ᵗʰ R79.8 Other specified abnormal findings of blood chemistry

R79.81 Abnormal blood-gas level

R79.82 Elevated C-reactive protein [CRP]

R79.89 Other specified abnormal findings of blood chemistry
AHA: 2019,2Q,6
TIP: Assign for documented abnormal or elevated troponin level when a definitive diagnosis has not been established.
TIP: Assign for positive Coombs test when not further clarified in the documentation.

R79.9 Abnormal finding of blood chemistry, unspecified

Abnormal findings on examination of urine, without diagnosis (R80-R82)

EXCLUDES 1   *abnormal findings on antenatal screening of mother (O28.-)*
diagnostic abnormal findings classified elsewhere — see Alphabetical Index
specific findings indicating disorder of amino-acid metabolism (E70-E72)
specific findings indicating disorder of carbohydrate metabolism (E73-E74)

√4ᵗʰ R80 Proteinuria
EXCLUDES 1   *gestational proteinuria (O12.1-)*

R80.0 Isolated proteinuria
Idiopathic proteinuria
EXCLUDES 1   *isolated proteinuria with specific morphological lesion (N06.-)*

R80.1 Persistent proteinuria, unspecified

R80.2 Orthostatic proteinuria, unspecified
Postural proteinuria

R80.3 Bence Jones proteinuria

R80.8 Other proteinuria

R80.9 Proteinuria, unspecified
Albuminuria NOS

R81 Glycosuria
EXCLUDES 1   *renal glycosuria (E74.8)*

✓4ᵗʰ **R82 Other and unspecified abnormal findings in urine**

    INCLUDES   chromoabnormalities in urine

    Use additional code to identify any retained foreign body, if applicable (Z18.-)

    EXCLUDES 2   hematuria (R31.-)

  R82.0 Chyluria   CC
    EXCLUDES 1   filarial chyluria (B74.-)
    CC Excl: PDX collection 1137

  R82.1 Myoglobinuria   CC
    CC Excl: PDX collection 1138

  R82.2 Biliuria

  R82.3 Hemoglobinuria
    EXCLUDES 1   hemoglobinuria due to hemolysis from external causes NEC (D59.6)
        hemoglobinuria due to paroxysmal nocturnal [Marchiafava-Micheli] (D59.5)
    DEF: Free hemoglobin in blood due to rapid hemolysis of red blood cells. Causes include burns, crushed injury, sickle cell anemia, thalassemia, parasitic infections, or kidney infections.

  R82.4 Acetonuria
    Ketonuria
    DEF: Excessive excretion of acetone in urine that commonly occurs in diabetic acidosis.

  R82.5 Elevated urine levels of drugs, medicaments and biological substances
    Elevated urine levels of catecholamines
    Elevated urine levels of indoleacetic acid
    Elevated urine levels of 17-ketosteroids
    Elevated urine levels of steroids

  R82.6 Abnormal urine levels of substances chiefly nonmedicinal as to source
    Abnormal urine level of heavy metals

✓5ᵗʰ **R82.7 Abnormal findings on microbiological examination of urine**
    EXCLUDES 1   colonization status (Z22.-)
    AHA: 2016,4Q,65

    R82.71 Bacteriuria

    R82.79 Other abnormal findings on microbiological examination of urine
        Positive culture findings of urine

▲ ✓5ᵗʰ **R82.8 Abnormal findings on cytological and histological examination of urine**

●   **R82.81 Pyuria**
        Sterile pyuria

●   **R82.89 Other abnormal findings on cytological and histological examination of urine**

✓5ᵗʰ **R82.9 Other and unspecified abnormal findings in urine**

    R82.90 Unspecified abnormal findings in urine

    R82.91 Other chromoabnormalities of urine
        Chromoconversion (dipstick)
        Idiopathic dipstick converts positive for blood with no cellular forms in sediment
        EXCLUDES 1   hemoglobinuria (R82.3)
            myoglobinuria (R82.1)

    ✓6ᵗʰ **R82.99 Other abnormal findings in urine**
        AHA: 2018,4Q,29-30

        R82.991 Hypocitraturia

        R82.992 Hyperoxaluria
            EXCLUDES 1   primary hyperoxaluria (E72.53)

▲   **R82.993 Hyperuricosuria**

        R82.994 Hypercalciuria
            Idiopathic hypercalciuria

        R82.998 Other abnormal findings in urine
            Cells and casts in urine
            Crystalluria
            Melanuria

Abnormal findings on examination of other body fluids, substances and tissues, without diagnosis (R83-R89)

  EXCLUDES 1   abnormal findings on antenatal screening of mother (O28.-)
    diagnostic abnormal findings classified elsewhere — see Alphabetical Index

  EXCLUDES 2   abnormal findings on examination of blood, without diagnosis (R70-R79)
    abnormal findings on examination of urine, without diagnosis (R80-R82)
    abnormal tumor markers (R97.-)

✓4ᵗʰ **R83 Abnormal findings in cerebrospinal fluid**

Cerebrospinal Fluid

Ventricles

Cerebrospinal fluid

Spinal cord

  R83.0 Abnormal level of enzymes in cerebrospinal fluid

  R83.1 Abnormal level of hormones in cerebrospinal fluid

  R83.2 Abnormal level of other drugs, medicaments and biological substances in cerebrospinal fluid

  R83.3 Abnormal level of substances chiefly nonmedicinal as to source in cerebrospinal fluid

  R83.4 Abnormal immunological findings in cerebrospinal fluid

  R83.5 Abnormal microbiological findings in cerebrospinal fluid
    Positive culture findings in cerebrospinal fluid
    EXCLUDES 1   colonization status (Z22.-)

  R83.6 Abnormal cytological findings in cerebrospinal fluid

  R83.8 Other abnormal findings in cerebrospinal fluid
    Abnormal chromosomal findings in cerebrospinal fluid

  R83.9 Unspecified abnormal finding in cerebrospinal fluid

✓4ᵗʰ **R84 Abnormal findings in specimens from respiratory organs and thorax**
    INCLUDES   abnormal findings in bronchial washings
        abnormal findings in nasal secretions
        abnormal findings in pleural fluid
        abnormal findings in sputum
        abnormal findings in throat scrapings
    EXCLUDES 1   blood-stained sputum (R04.2)

  R84.0 Abnormal level of enzymes in specimens from respiratory organs and thorax

  R84.1 Abnormal level of hormones in specimens from respiratory organs and thorax

  R84.2 Abnormal level of other drugs, medicaments and biological substances in specimens from respiratory organs and thorax

  R84.3 Abnormal level of substances chiefly nonmedicinal as to source in specimens from respiratory organs and thorax

  R84.4 Abnormal immunological findings in specimens from respiratory organs and thorax

✔ Additional Character Required   ✓x7ᵗʰ Placeholder   Unacceptable PDx   Questionable PDx   Manifestation   Unspecified Dx   H1-H14 HAC   HCC CMS-HCC Dx   HIV HIV Dx

ICD-10-CM 2020   969

R84.5 **Abnormal microbiological findings in specimens from respiratory organs and thorax**
  Positive culture findings in specimens from respiratory organs and thorax
  EXCLUDES 1 colonization status (Z22.-)

R84.6 **Abnormal cytological findings in specimens from respiratory organs and thorax**

R84.7 **Abnormal histological findings in specimens from respiratory organs and thorax**

R84.8 **Other abnormal findings in specimens from respiratory organs and thorax**
  Abnormal chromosomal findings in specimens from respiratory organs and thorax

R84.9 **Unspecified abnormal finding in specimens from respiratory organs and thorax**

√4ᵗʰ **R85** **Abnormal findings in specimens from digestive organs and abdominal cavity**
  INCLUDES abnormal findings in peritoneal fluid
    abnormal findings in saliva
  EXCLUDES 1 cloudy peritoneal dialysis effluent (R88.0)
    fecal abnormalities (R19.5)

R85.0 **Abnormal level of enzymes in specimens from digestive organs and abdominal cavity**

R85.1 **Abnormal level of hormones in specimens from digestive organs and abdominal cavity**

R85.2 **Abnormal level of other drugs, medicaments and biological substances in specimens from digestive organs and abdominal cavity**

R85.3 **Abnormal level of substances chiefly nonmedicinal as to source in specimens from digestive organs and abdominal cavity**

R85.4 **Abnormal immunological findings in specimens from digestive organs and abdominal cavity**

R85.5 **Abnormal microbiological findings in specimens from digestive organs and abdominal cavity**
  Positive culture findings in specimens from digestive organs and abdominal cavity
  EXCLUDES 1 colonization status (Z22.-)

√5ᵗʰ **R85.6** **Abnormal cytological findings in specimens from digestive organs and abdominal cavity**

√6ᵗʰ **R85.61** **Abnormal cytologic smear of anus**
  EXCLUDES 1 abnormal cytological findings in specimens from other digestive organs and abdominal cavity (R85.69)
    anal intraepithelial neoplasia I [AIN I] (K62.82)
    anal intraepithelial neoplasia II [AIN II] (K62.82)
    anal intraepithelial neoplasia III [AIN III] (D01.3)
    carcinoma in situ of anus (histologically confirmed) (D01.3)
    dysplasia (mild) (moderate) of anus (histologically confirmed) (K62.82)
    severe dysplasia of anus (histologically confirmed) (D01.3)
  EXCLUDES 2 anal high risk human papillomavirus (HPV) DNA test positive (R85.81)
    anal low risk human papillomavirus (HPV) DNA test positive (R85.82)

R85.610 **Atypical squamous cells of undetermined significance on cytologic smear of anus [ASC-US]**

R85.611 **Atypical squamous cells cannot exclude high grade squamous intraepithelial lesion on cytologic smear of anus [ASC-H]**

R85.612 **Low grade squamous intraepithelial lesion on cytologic smear of anus [LGSIL]**

R85.613 **High grade squamous intraepithelial lesion on cytologic smear of anus [HGSIL]**

R85.614 **Cytologic evidence of malignancy on smear of anus**

R85.615 **Unsatisfactory cytologic smear of anus**
  Inadequate sample of cytologic smear of anus

R85.616 **Satisfactory anal smear but lacking transformation zone**

R85.618 **Other abnormal cytological findings on specimens from anus**

R85.619 **Unspecified abnormal cytological findings in specimens from anus**
  Abnormal anal cytology NOS
  Atypical glandular cells of anus NOS

R85.69 **Abnormal cytological findings in specimens from other digestive organs and abdominal cavity**

R85.7 **Abnormal histological findings in specimens from digestive organs and abdominal cavity**

√5ᵗʰ **R85.8** **Other abnormal findings in specimens from digestive organs and abdominal cavity**

R85.81 **Anal high risk human papillomavirus [HPV] DNA test positive**
  EXCLUDES 1 anogenital warts due to human papillomavirus (HPV) (A63.0)
    condyloma acuminatum (A63.0)

R85.82 **Anal low risk human papillomavirus [HPV] DNA test positive**
  Use additional code for associated human papillomavirus (B97.7)

R85.89 **Other abnormal findings in specimens from digestive organs and abdominal cavity**
  Abnormal chromosomal findings in specimens from digestive organs and abdominal cavity

R85.9 **Unspecified abnormal finding in specimens from digestive organs and abdominal cavity**

√4ᵗʰ **R86** **Abnormal findings in specimens from male genital organs**
  INCLUDES abnormal findings in prostatic secretions
    abnormal findings in semen, seminal fluid
    abnormal spermatozoa
  EXCLUDES 1 azoospermia (N46.0-)
    oligospermia (N46.1-)

R86.0 **Abnormal level of enzymes in specimens from male genital organs** ♂

R86.1 **Abnormal level of hormones in specimens from male genital organs** ♂

R86.2 **Abnormal level of other drugs, medicaments and biological substances in specimens from male genital organs** ♂

R86.3 **Abnormal level of substances chiefly nonmedicinal as to source in specimens from male genital organs** ♂

R86.4 **Abnormal immunological findings in specimens from male genital organs** ♂

R86.5 **Abnormal microbiological findings in specimens from male genital organs** ♂
  Positive culture findings in specimens from male genital organs
  EXCLUDES 1 colonization status (Z22.-)

R86.6 **Abnormal cytological findings in specimens from male genital organs** ♂

R86.7 **Abnormal histological findings in specimens from male genital organs** ♂

R86.8 **Other abnormal findings in specimens from male genital organs** ♂
  Abnormal chromosomal findings in specimens from male genital organs

R86.9 **Unspecified abnormal finding in specimens from male genital organs** ♂

√4ᵗʰ **R87** **Abnormal findings in specimens from female genital organs**
  INCLUDES abnormal findings in secretion and smears from cervix uteri
    abnormal findings in secretion and smears from vagina
    abnormal findings in secretion and smears from vulva

R87.0 **Abnormal level of enzymes from female genital organs** ♀

R87.1 **Abnormal level of hormones in specimens from female genital organs** ♀

R87.2 **Abnormal level of other drugs, medicaments and biological substances in specimens from female genital organs** ♀

R87.3 **Abnormal level of substances chiefly nonmedicinal as to source in specimens from female genital organs** ♀

R87.4 **Abnormal immunological findings in specimens from female genital organs** ♀

R87.5 **Abnormal microbiological findings in specimens from female genital organs** ♀
  Positive culture findings in specimens from female genital organs
  EXCLUDES 1 colonization status (Z22.-)

√5ᵗʰ **R87.6** **Abnormal** cytological **findings in specimens from female genital organs**

√6ᵗʰ **R87.61** **Abnormal cytological findings in specimens from cervix uteri**

EXCLUDES 1   *abnormal cytological findings in specimens from other female genital organs (R87.69)*

abnormal cytological findings in specimens from vagina (R87.62-)

carcinoma in situ of cervix uteri (histologically confirmed) (D06.-)

cervical intraepithelial neoplasia I [CIN I] (N87.0)

cervical intraepithelial neoplasia II [CIN II] (N87.1)

cervical intraepithelial neoplasia III [CIN III] (D06.-)

dysplasia (mild) (moderate) of cervix uteri (histologically confirmed) (N87.-)

severe dysplasia of cervix uteri (histologically confirmed) (D06.-)

EXCLUDES 2   *cervical high risk human papillomavirus (HPV) DNA test positive (R87.810)*

cervical low risk human papillomavirus (HPV) DNA test positive (R87.820)

R87.610 **Atypical squamous cells of undetermined significance on cytologic smear of cervix [ASC-US]** ♀

R87.611 **Atypical squamous cells cannot exclude high grade squamous intraepithelial lesion on cytologic smear of cervix [ASC-H]** ♀

R87.612 **Low grade squamous intraepithelial lesion on cytologic smear of cervix [LGSIL]** ♀

R87.613 **High grade squamous intraepithelial lesion on cytologic smear of cervix [HGSIL]** ♀

R87.614 **Cytologic evidence of malignancy on smear of cervix** ♀

R87.615 **Unsatisfactory cytologic smear of cervix** ♀

Inadequate sample of cytologic smear of cervix

R87.616 **Satisfactory cervical smear but lacking transformation zone** ♀

R87.618 **Other abnormal cytological findings on specimens from cervix uteri** ♀

R87.619 **Unspecified abnormal cytological findings in specimens from cervix uteri** ♀

Abnormal cervical cytology NOS

Abnormal Papanicolaou smear of cervix NOS

Abnormal thin preparation smear of cervix NOS

Atypical endocervial cells of cervix NOS

Atypical endometrial cells of cervix NOS

Atypical glandular cells of cervix NOS

√6ᵗʰ **R87.62** **Abnormal cytological findings in specimens from vagina**

Use additional code to identify acquired absence of uterus and cervix, if applicable (Z90.71-)

EXCLUDES 1   *abnormal cytological findings in specimens from cervix uteri (R87.61-)*

abnormal cytological findings in specimens from other female genital organs (R87.69)

carcinoma in situ of vagina (histologically confirmed) (D07.2)

dysplasia (mild) (moderate) of vagina (histologically confirmed) (N89.-)

severe dysplasia of vagina (histologically confirmed) (D07.2)

vaginal intraepithelial neoplasia I [VAIN I] (N89.0)

vaginal intraepithelial neoplasia II [VAIN II] (N89.1)

vaginal intraepithelial neoplasia III [VAIN III] (D07.2)

EXCLUDES 2   *vaginal high risk human papillomavirus (HPV) DNA test positive (R87.811)*

vaginal low risk human papillomavirus (HPV) DNA test positive (R87.821)

R87.620 **Atypical squamous cells of undetermined significance on cytologic smear of vagina [ASC-US]** ♀

R87.621 **Atypical squamous cells cannot exclude high grade squamous intraepithelial lesion on cytologic smear of vagina [ASC-H]** ♀

R87.622 **Low grade squamous intraepithelial lesion on cytologic smear of vagina [LGSIL]** ♀

R87.623 **High grade squamous intraepithelial lesion on cytologic smear of vagina [HGSIL]** ♀

R87.624 **Cytologic evidence of malignancy on smear of vagina** ♀

R87.625 **Unsatisfactory cytologic smear of vagina** ♀

Inadequate sample of cytologic smear of vagina

R87.628 **Other abnormal cytological findings on specimens from vagina** ♀

R87.629 **Unspecified abnormal cytological findings in specimens from vagina** ♀

Abnormal Papanicolaou smear of vagina NOS

Abnormal thin preparation smear of vagina NOS

Abnormal vaginal cytology NOS

Atypical endocervical cells of vagina NOS

Atypical endometrial cells of vagina NOS

Atypical glandular cells of vagina NOS

R87.69 **Abnormal cytological findings in specimens from other female genital organs** ♀

Abnormal cytological findings in specimens from female genital organs NOS

EXCLUDES 1   *dysplasia of vulva (histologically confirmed) (N90.0-N90.3)*

✔ Additional Character Required   √x7ᵗʰ Placeholder   Unacceptable PDx   Questionable PDx   Manifestation   Unspecified Dx   H1-H14 HAC   HCC CMS-HCC Dx   HIV HIV Dx

ICD-10-CM 2020   971

R87.7 **Abnormal histological findings in specimens from female genital organs** ♀

EXCLUDES 1   *carcinoma in situ (histologically confirmed) of female genital organs (D06-D07.3)*
cervical intraepithelial neoplasia I [CIN I] (N87.0)
cervical intraepithelial neoplasia II [CIN II] (N87.1)
cervical intraepithelial neoplasia III [CIN III] (D06.-)
dysplasia (mild) (moderate) of cervix uteri (histologically confirmed) (N87.-)
dysplasia (mild) (moderate) of vagina (histologically confirmed) (N89.-)
severe dysplasia of cervix uteri (histologically confirmed) (D06.-)
severe dysplasia of vagina (histologically confirmed) (D07.2)
vaginal intraepithelial neoplasia I [VAIN I] (N89.0)
vaginal intraepithelial neoplasia II [VAIN II] (N89.1)
vaginal intraepithelial neoplasia III [VAIN III] (D07.2)

√5ᵗʰ **R87.8** **Other abnormal findings in specimens from female genital organs**

√6ᵗʰ **R87.81** **High risk human papillomavirus [HPV] DNA test positive from female genital organs**

EXCLUDES 1   *anogenital warts due to human papillomavirus (HPV) (A63.0)*
condyloma acuminatum (A63.0)

  R87.810 **Cervical high risk human papillomavirus [HPV] DNA test positive** ♀

  R87.811 **Vaginal high risk human papillomavirus [HPV] DNA test positive** ♀

√6ᵗʰ **R87.82** **Low risk human papillomavirus [HPV] DNA test positive from female genital organs**

Use additional code for associated human papillomavirus (B97.7)

  R87.820 **Cervical low risk human papillomavirus [HPV] DNA test positive** ♀

  R87.821 **Vaginal low risk human papillomavirus [HPV] DNA test positive** ♀

  R87.89 **Other abnormal findings in specimens from female genital organs** ♀

Abnormal chromosomal findings in specimens from female genital organs

R87.9 **Unspecified abnormal finding in specimens from female genital organs** ♀

√4ᵗʰ **R88** **Abnormal findings in other body fluids and substances**

  R88.0 **Cloudy (hemodialysis) (peritoneal) dialysis effluent**

  R88.8 **Abnormal findings in other body fluids and substances**

√4ᵗʰ **R89** **Abnormal findings in specimens from other organs, systems and tissues**

INCLUDES   abnormal findings in nipple discharge
abnormal findings in synovial fluid
abnormal findings in wound secretions

  R89.0 **Abnormal level of enzymes in specimens from other organs, systems and tissues**

  R89.1 **Abnormal level of hormones in specimens from other organs, systems and tissues**

  R89.2 **Abnormal level of other drugs, medicaments and biological substances in specimens from other organs, systems and tissues**

  R89.3 **Abnormal level of substances chiefly nonmedicinal as to source in specimens from other organs, systems and tissues**

  R89.4 **Abnormal immunological findings in specimens from other organs, systems and tissues**

  R89.5 **Abnormal microbiological findings in specimens from other organs, systems and tissues**

Positive culture findings in specimens from other organs, systems and tissues

EXCLUDES 1   *colonization status (Z22.-)*

  R89.6 **Abnormal cytological findings in specimens from other organs, systems and tissues**

  R89.7 **Abnormal histological findings in specimens from other organs, systems and tissues**

  R89.8 **Other abnormal findings in specimens from other organs, systems and tissues**

Abnormal chromosomal findings in specimens from other organs, systems and tissues

  R89.9 **Unspecified abnormal finding in specimens from other organs, systems and tissues**

Abnormal findings on diagnostic imaging and in function studies, without diagnosis (R90-R94)

INCLUDES   nonspecific abnormal findings on diagnostic imaging by computerized axial tomography [CAT scan]
nonspecific abnormal findings on diagnostic imaging by magnetic resonance imaging [MRI][NMR]
nonspecific abnormal findings on diagnostic imaging by positron emission tomography [PET scan]
nonspecific abnormal findings on diagnostic imaging by thermography
nonspecific abnormal findings on diagnostic imaging by ultrasound [echogram]
nonspecific abnormal findings on diagnostic imaging by X-ray examination

EXCLUDES 1   *abnormal findings on antenatal screening of mother (O28.-)*
diagnostic abnormal findings classified elsewhere — see Alphabetical Index

√4ᵗʰ **R90** **Abnormal findings on diagnostic imaging of central nervous system**

  R90.0 **Intracranial space-occupying lesion found on diagnostic imaging of central nervous system**

√6ᵗʰ **R90.8** **Other abnormal findings on diagnostic imaging of central nervous system**

  R90.81 **Abnormal echoencephalogram**

  R90.82 **White matter disease, unspecified**

  R90.89 **Other abnormal findings on diagnostic imaging of central nervous system**

Other cerebrovascular abnormality found on diagnostic imaging of central nervous system

√4ᵗʰ **R91** **Abnormal findings on diagnostic imaging of lung**

  R91.1 **Solitary pulmonary nodule**

Coin lesion lung
Solitary pulmonary nodule, subsegmental branch of the bronchial tree

  R91.8 **Other nonspecific abnormal finding of lung field**

Lung mass NOS found on diagnostic imaging of lung
Pulmonary infiltrate NOS
Shadow, lung

√4ᵗʰ **R92** **Abnormal and inconclusive findings on diagnostic imaging of breast**

  R92.0 **Mammographic microcalcification found on diagnostic imaging of breast**

EXCLUDES 2   *mammographic calcification (calculus) found on diagnostic imaging of breast (R92.1)*

DEF: Calcium and cellular debris deposits in the breast that cannot be felt but can be detected on a mammogram. The deposits can be a sign of cancer, benign conditions, or changes in the breast tissue as a result of inflammation, injury, or an obstructed duct.

  R92.1 **Mammographic calcification found on diagnostic imaging of breast**

Mammographic calculus found on diagnostic imaging of breast

  R92.2 **Inconclusive mammogram**

Dense breasts NOS
Inconclusive mammogram NEC
Inconclusive mammography due to dense breasts
Inconclusive mammography NEC
AHA: 2015,1Q,24

  R92.8 **Other abnormal and inconclusive findings on diagnostic imaging of breast**

√4ᵗʰ **R93** **Abnormal findings on diagnostic imaging of other body structures**

  R93.0 **Abnormal findings on diagnostic imaging of skull and head, not elsewhere classified**

EXCLUDES 1   *intracranial space-occupying lesion found on diagnostic imaging (R90.0)*

  R93.1 **Abnormal findings on diagnostic imaging of heart and coronary circulation**

Abnormal echocardiogram NOS
Abnormal heart shadow

  R93.2 **Abnormal findings on diagnostic imaging of liver and biliary tract**

Nonvisualization of gallbladder

R93.3   **Abnormal findings on diagnostic imaging of other parts of digestive tract**

✓5ᵗʰ **R93.4**   **Abnormal findings on diagnostic imaging of urinary organs**
     EXCLUDES 2   hypertrophy of kidney (N28.81)
     AHA: 2016,4Q,66

     R93.41   **Abnormal radiologic findings on diagnostic imaging of renal pelvis, ureter, or bladder**
         Filling defect of bladder found on diagnostic imaging
         Filling defect of renal pelvis found on diagnostic imaging
         Filling defect of ureter found on diagnostic imaging

     ✓6ᵗʰ **R93.42**   **Abnormal radiologic findings on diagnostic imaging of kidney**
         R93.421   **Abnormal radiologic findings on diagnostic imaging of right kidney**
         R93.422   **Abnormal radiologic findings on diagnostic imaging of left kidney**
         R93.429   **Abnormal radiologic findings on diagnostic imaging of unspecified kidney**

     R93.49   **Abnormal radiologic findings on diagnostic imaging of other urinary organs**

R93.5   **Abnormal findings on diagnostic imaging of other abdominal regions, including retroperitoneum**

R93.6   **Abnormal findings on diagnostic imaging of limbs**
     EXCLUDES 2   abnormal finding in skin and subcutaneous tissue (R93.8-)

R93.7   **Abnormal findings on diagnostic imaging of other parts of musculoskeletal system**
     EXCLUDES 2   abnormal findings on diagnostic imaging of skull (R93.0)

✓5ᵗʰ **R93.8**   **Abnormal findings on diagnostic imaging of other specified body structures**
     AHA: 2018,4Q,30

     ✓6ᵗʰ **R93.81**   **Abnormal radiologic findings on diagnostic imaging of testis**
         R93.811   **Abnormal radiologic findings on diagnostic imaging of right testicle**   ♂
         R93.812   **Abnormal radiologic findings on diagnostic imaging of left testicle**   ♂
         R93.813   **Abnormal radiologic findings on diagnostic imaging of testicles, bilateral**   ♂
         R93.819   **Abnormal radiologic findings on diagnostic imaging of unspecified testicle**   ♂

     R93.89   **Abnormal findings on diagnostic imaging of other specified body structures**
         Abnormal finding by radioisotope localization of placenta
         Abnormal radiological finding in skin and subcutaneous tissue
         Mediastinal shift

R93.9   **Diagnostic imaging inconclusive due to excess body fat of patient**

✓4ᵗʰ **R94**   **Abnormal results of function studies**
     INCLUDES   abnormal results of radionuclide [radioisotope] uptake studies
                abnormal results of scintigraphy

✓5ᵗʰ **R94.0**   **Abnormal results of function studies of central nervous system**
     R94.01   **Abnormal electroencephalogram [EEG]**
     R94.02   **Abnormal brain scan**
     R94.09   **Abnormal results of other function studies of central nervous system**

✓5ᵗʰ **R94.1**   **Abnormal results of function studies of peripheral nervous system and special senses**
     ✓6ᵗʰ **R94.11**   **Abnormal results of function studies of eye**
         R94.110   **Abnormal electro-oculogram [EOG]**
         R94.111   **Abnormal electroretinogram [ERG]**
             Abnormal retinal function study
         R94.112   **Abnormal visually evoked potential [VEP]**
         R94.113   **Abnormal oculomotor study**
         R94.118   **Abnormal results of other function studies of eye**

     ✓6ᵗʰ **R94.12**   **Abnormal results of function studies of ear and other special senses**
         AHA: 2016,3Q,17
         R94.120   **Abnormal auditory function study**
         R94.121   **Abnormal vestibular function study**
         R94.128   **Abnormal results of other function studies of ear and other special senses**

     ✓6ᵗʰ **R94.13**   **Abnormal results of function studies of peripheral nervous system**
         R94.130   **Abnormal response to nerve stimulation, unspecified**
         R94.131   **Abnormal electromyogram [EMG]**
            EXCLUDES 1   electromyogram of eye (R94.113)
         R94.138   **Abnormal results of other function studies of peripheral nervous system**

R94.2   **Abnormal results of pulmonary function studies**
     Reduced ventilatory capacity
     Reduced vital capacity

✓5ᵗʰ **R94.3**   **Abnormal results of cardiovascular function studies**
     R94.30   **Abnormal result of cardiovascular function study, unspecified**
     R94.31   **Abnormal electrocardiogram [ECG] [EKG]**
         EXCLUDES 1   long QT syndrome (I45.81)
     R94.39   **Abnormal result of other cardiovascular function study**
         Abnormal electrophysiological intracardiac studies
         Abnormal phonocardiogram
         Abnormal vectorcardiogram

R94.4   **Abnormal results of kidney function studies**
     Abnormal renal function test

R94.5   **Abnormal results of liver function studies**

R94.6   **Abnormal results of thyroid function studies**

R94.7   **Abnormal results of other endocrine function studies**
     EXCLUDES 2   abnormal glucose (R73.0-)

R94.8   **Abnormal results of function studies of other organs and systems**
     Abnormal basal metabolic rate [BMR]
     Abnormal bladder function test
     Abnormal splenic function test

Abnormal tumor markers (R97)

✓4ᵗʰ **R97**   **Abnormal tumor markers**
     Elevated tumor associated antigens [TAA]
     Elevated tumor specific antigens [TSA]

R97.0   **Elevated carcinoembryonic antigen [CEA]**

R97.1   **Elevated cancer antigen 125 [CA 125]**

✓5ᵗʰ **R97.2**   **Elevated prostate specific antigen [PSA]**
     AHA: 2016,4Q,66
     R97.20   **Elevated prostate specific antigen [PSA]**   Ⓐ♂
     R97.21   **Rising PSA following treatment for malignant neoplasm of prostate**   Ⓐ♂

R97.8   **Other abnormal tumor markers**

Ill-defined and unknown cause of mortality (R99)

R99   **Ill-defined and unknown cause of mortality**
     Death (unexplained) NOS
     Unspecified cause of mortality

Chapter 19. Injury, Poisoning and Certain Other Consequences of External Causes (SØØ–T88)

Chapter-specific Guidelines with Coding Examples

The chapter-specific guidelines from the ICD-10-CM Official Guidelines for Coding and Reporting have been provided below. Along with these guidelines are coding examples, contained in the shaded boxes, that have been developed to help illustrate the coding and/or sequencing guidance found in these guidelines.

a. Application of 7th characters in Chapter 19

Most categories in chapter 19 have a 7th character requirement for each applicable code. Most categories in this chapter have three 7th character values (with the exception of fractures): A, initial encounter, D, subsequent encounter and S, sequela. Categories for traumatic fractures have additional 7th character values. While the patient may be seen by a new or different provider over the course of treatment for an injury, assignment of the 7th character is based on whether the patient is undergoing active treatment and not whether the provider is seeing the patient for the first time.

For complication codes, active treatment refers to treatment for the condition described by the code, even though it may be related to an earlier precipitating problem. For example, code T84.50XA, Infection and inflammatory reaction due to unspecified internal joint prosthesis, initial encounter, is used when active treatment is provided for the infection, even though the condition relates to the prosthetic device, implant or graft that was placed at a previous encounter.

7th character "A", initial encounter is used for each encounter where the patient is receiving active treatment for the condition.

> Patient admitted after fall from a skateboard onto the sidewalk, x-rays identify a nondisplaced fracture to the distal pole of the right scaphoid bone. The patient is placed in a cast.
>
> **S62.Ø14A**   **Nondisplaced fracture of distal pole of navicular [scaphoid] bone of right wrist, initial encounter for closed fracture**
>
> **VØØ.131A**   **Fall from skateboard, initial encounter**
>
> **Y92.48Ø**   **Sidewalk as the place of occurrence of the external cause**
>
> **Y93.51**   **Activity, roller skating (inline) and skateboarding**
>
> **Y99.8**   **Other external cause status**
>
> *Explanation:* This fracture would be coded with a seventh character A for initial encounter because the patient received x-rays to identify the site of the fracture and treatment was rendered; this would be considered active treatment.

7th character "D" subsequent encounter is used for encounters after the patient has completed active treatment of the condition and is receiving routine care for the condition during the healing or recovery phase.

> Patient admitted after fall from a skateboard onto the sidewalk resulted in casting of the right arm. X-rays are taken to evaluate how well the nondisplaced fracture to the distal pole of the right scaphoid bone is healing. The physician feels the fracture is healing appropriately; no adjustments to the cast are made.
>
> **S62.Ø14D**   **Nondisplaced fracture of distal pole of navicular [scaphoid] bone of right wrist, subsequent encounter for fracture with routine healing**
>
> **VØØ.131D**   **Fall from skateboard, subsequent encounter**
>
> *Explanation:* This fracture would be coded with a seventh character D for subsequent encounter, whether the same physician who provided the initial cast application or a different physician is now seeing the patient. Although the patient received x-rays, the intent of the x-rays was to assess how the fracture was healing. There was no active treatment rendered and the visit is therefore considered a subsequent encounter.

The aftercare Z codes should not be used for aftercare for conditions such as injuries or poisonings, where 7th characters are provided to identify subsequent care. For example, for aftercare of an injury, assign the acute injury code with the 7th character "D" (subsequent encounter).

7th character "S", sequela, is for use for complications or conditions that arise as a direct result of a condition, such as scar formation after a burn. The scars are sequelae of the burn. When using 7th character "S", it is

necessary to use both the injury code that precipitated the sequela and the code for the sequela itself. The "S" is added only to the injury code, not the sequela code. The 7th character "S" identifies the injury responsible for the sequela. The specific type of sequela (e.g. scar) is sequenced first, followed by the injury code.

See Section I.B.1Ø Sequelae, (Late Effects)

> Patient with a history of a nondisplaced fracture to the distal pole of the right scaphoid bone due to a fall from a skateboard is admitted for evaluation of arthritis to the right wrist that has developed as a consequence of the traumatic fracture.
>
> **M12.531**   **Traumatic arthropathy, right wrist**
>
> **S62.Ø14S**   **Nondisplaced fracture of distal pole of navicular [scaphoid] bone of right wrist, sequela**
>
> **VØØ.131S**   **Fall from skateboard, sequela**
>
> *Explanation:* The code identifying the specific sequela condition (traumatic arthritis) should be coded first followed by the injury that instigated the development of the sequela (fracture). The scaphoid fracture injury code is given a 7th character S for sequela to represent its role as the inciting injury. The fracture has healed and is not being managed or treated on this admit and therefore is not applicable as a first listed or principal diagnosis. However, it is directly related to the development of the arthritis and should be appended as a secondary code to signify this cause and effect relationship.

b. Coding of injuries

When coding injuries, assign separate codes for each injury unless a combination code is provided, in which case the combination code is assigned. Codes from category TØ7, Unspecified multiple injuries should not be assigned in the inpatient setting unless information for a more specific code is not available. Traumatic injury codes (SØØ-T14.9) are not to be used for normal, healing surgical wounds or to identify complications of surgical wounds.

The code for the most serious injury, as determined by the provider and the focus of treatment, is sequenced first.

1) Superficial injuries

Superficial injuries such as abrasions or contusions are not coded when associated with more severe injuries of the same site.

2) Primary injury with damage to nerves/blood vessels

When a primary injury results in minor damage to peripheral nerves or blood vessels, the primary injury is sequenced first with additional code(s) for injuries to nerves and spinal cord (such as category SØ4), and/or injury to blood vessels (such as category S15). When the primary injury is to the blood vessels or nerves, that injury should be sequenced first.

3) Iatrogenic injuries

Injury codes from Chapter 19 should not be assigned for injuries that occur during, or as a result of, a medical intervention. Assign the appropriate complication code(s).

c. Coding of traumatic fractures

The principles of multiple coding of injuries should be followed in coding fractures. Fractures of specified sites are coded individually by site in accordance with both the provisions within categories SØ2, S12, S22, S32, S42, S49, S52, S59, S62, S72, S79, S82, S89, S92 and the level of detail furnished by medical record content.

A fracture not indicated as open or closed should be coded to closed. A fracture not indicated whether displaced or not displaced should be coded to displaced.

More specific guidelines are as follows:

1) Initial vs. subsequent encounter for fractures

Traumatic fractures are coded using the appropriate 7th character for initial encounter (A, B, C) for each encounter where the patient is receiving active treatment for the fracture. The appropriate 7th character for initial encounter should also be assigned for a patient who delayed seeking treatment for the fracture or nonunion. Fractures are coded using the appropriate 7th character for subsequent care for encounters after the patient has completed active treatment of the fracture and is receiving routine care for the fracture during the healing or recovery phase.

Care for complications of surgical treatment for fracture repairs during the healing or recovery phase should be coded with the appropriate complication codes.

Care of complications of fractures, such as malunion and nonunion, should be reported with the appropriate 7th character for subsequent care with nonunion (K, M, N,) or subsequent care with malunion (P, Q, R).

Malunion/nonunion: The appropriate 7th character for initial encounter should also be assigned for a patient who delayed seeking treatment for the fracture or nonunion.

Female patient fell during a forest hiking excursion almost six months ago and until recently did not feel she needed to seek medical attention for her left ankle pain; x-rays show nonunion of lateral malleolus and surgery has been scheduled	
S82.62XA	Displaced fracture of lateral malleolus of left fibula, initial encounter for closed fracture
W01.0XXA	Fall on same level from slipping, tripping and stumbling without subsequent striking against object, initial encounter
Y92.821	Forest as place of occurrence of the external cause
Y93.01	Activity, walking, marching and hiking
Y99.8	Other external cause status

Explanation: A seventh character of A is used for the lateral malleolus nonunion fracture to signify that the fracture is receiving active treatment. The delayed care for the fracture has resulted in a nonunion, but capturing the nonunion in the seventh character is trumped by the provision of active care.

The open fracture designations in the assignment of the 7th character for fractures of the forearm, femur and lower leg, including ankle are based on the Gustilo open fracture classification. When the Gustilo classification type is not specified for an open fracture, the 7th character for open fracture type I or II should be assigned (B, E, H, M, Q).

A 17-year-old arrives at the trauma center with open, displaced right forearm fracture with extensive soft tissue damage. He fell while being tackled playing football for his high school team. On-call orthopaedic specialist documents segmental type IIIA fracture of radial shaft with no need for plastic consult.	
S52.361C	Displaced segmental fracture of shaft of radius, right arm, initial encounter for open fracture type IIIA, IIIB, or IIIC
W03.XXXA	Other fall on same level due to collision with another person, initial encounter
Y92.321	Football field as the place of occurrence of the external cause
Y93.61	Activity, American tackle football

Explanation: The seventh character for forearm fractures capture the type of encounter and whether the fracture is open or closed; open fractures are broken down further by the type of fracture based on the Gustilo classification. The Gustilo classification describes the severity of open fracture and soft tissue injury. Type IIIA describes an open fracture with extensive soft tissue injury but adequate soft tissue remaining for wound coverage. A segmental fracture means that the bone is broken in two places, leaving at least one segment unattached to the bone. There is no need to report an additional code for the soft tissue injury as it is captured in the fracture code.

A code from category M80, not a traumatic fracture code, should be used for any patient with known osteoporosis who suffers a fracture, even if the patient had a minor fall or trauma, if that fall or trauma would not usually break a normal, healthy bone.

See Section I.C.13. Osteoporosis.

The aftercare Z codes should not be used for aftercare for traumatic fractures. For aftercare of a traumatic fracture, assign the acute fracture code with the appropriate 7th character.

2) Multiple fractures sequencing

Multiple fractures are sequenced in accordance with the severity of the fracture.

3) Physeal fractures

For physeal fractures, assign only the code identifying the type of physeal fracture. Do not assign a separate code to identify the specific bone that is fractured.

d. Coding of burns and corrosions

The ICD-10-CM makes a distinction between burns and corrosions. The burn codes are for thermal burns, except sunburns, that come from a heat source, such as a fire or hot appliance. The burn codes are also for burns resulting from electricity and radiation. Corrosions are burns due to chemicals. The guidelines are the same for burns and corrosions.

Current burns (T20-T25) are classified by depth, extent and by agent (X code). Burns are classified by depth as first degree (erythema), second degree (blistering), and third degree (full-thickness involvement). Burns of the eye and internal organs (T26-T28) are classified by site, but not by degree.

1) Sequencing of burn and related condition codes

Sequence first the code that reflects the highest degree of burn when more than one burn is present.

a. When the reason for the admission or encounter is for treatment of external multiple burns, sequence first the code that reflects the burn of the highest degree.

b. When a patient has both internal and external burns, the circumstances of admission govern the selection of the principal diagnosis or first-listed diagnosis.

c. When a patient is admitted for burn injuries and other related conditions such as smoke inhalation and/or respiratory failure, the circumstances of admission govern the selection of the principal or first-listed diagnosis.

Patient admitted with minor first-degree burns to multiple sites of her right and left hands as well as severe smoke inhalation. While she was sleeping at home, a candle on her dresser lit the bedroom curtains on fire.	
T59.811A	Toxic effect of smoke, accidental (unintentional), initial encounter
J70.5	Respiratory conditions due to smoke inhalation
T23.191A	Burn of first degree of multiple sites of right wrist and hand, initial encounter
T23.192A	Burn of first degree of multiple sites of left wrist and hand, initial encounter
X08.8XXA	Exposure to other specified smoke, fire and flames, initial encounter
Y92.003	Bedroom of unspecified non-institutional (private) residence as the place of occurrence of the external cause
Y93.84	Activity, sleeping

Explanation: Based on the documentation, the inhalation injury is more severe than the first-degree burns and is sequenced first. The burns to the hands are appended as secondary diagnoses.

2) Burns of the same anatomic site

Classify burns of the same anatomic site and on the same side but of different degrees to the subcategory identifying the highest degree recorded in the diagnosis (e.g., for second and third degree burns of right thigh, assign only code T24.311-).

3) Non-healing burns

Non-healing burns are coded as acute burns.

Necrosis of burned skin should be coded as a non-healed burn.

4) Infected burn

For any documented infected burn site, use an additional code for the infection.

5) Assign separate codes for each burn site

When coding burns, assign separate codes for each burn site. Category T30, Burn and corrosion, body region unspecified is extremely vague and should rarely be used.

Codes for burns of "multiple sites" should only be assigned when the medical record documentation does not specify the individual sites.

Patient is admitted with third-degree burns of the scalp as well as second-degree burns to the back of the right hand

T20.35XA | **Burn of third degree of scalp [any part], initial encounter**

T23.261A | **Burn of second degree of back of right hand, initial encounter**

Explanation: Two codes may be reported as the hand and face represent distinct burn sites.

---

6) **Burns and corrosions classified according to extent of body surface involved**

Assign codes from category T31, Burns classified according to extent of body surface involved, or T32, Corrosions classified according to extent of body surface involved, when the site of the burn is not specified or when there is a need for additional data. It is advisable to use category T31 as additional coding when needed to provide data for evaluating burn mortality, such as that needed by burn units. It is also advisable to use category T31 as an additional code for reporting purposes when there is mention of a third-degree burn involving 20 percent or more of the body surface.

Categories T31 and T32 are based on the classic "rule of nines" in estimating body surface involved: head and neck are assigned nine percent, each arm nine percent, each leg 18 percent, the anterior trunk 18 percent, posterior trunk 18 percent, and genitalia one percent. Providers may change these percentage assignments where necessary to accommodate infants and children who have proportionally larger heads than adults, and patients who have large buttocks, thighs, or abdomen that involve burns.

Patient seen in burn unit for dressing change after he accidentally spilled acetic acid on himself two days ago. The second-degree burns to his right thigh, covering about 3 percent of his body surface, are healing appropriately.

T54.2X1D | **Toxic effect of corrosive acids and acid-like substances, accidental (unintentional), subsequent encounter**

T24.611D | **Corrosion of second degree of right thigh, subsequent encounter**

T32.0 | **Corrosions involving less than 10% of body surface**

Explanation: Code T32.0 provides additional information as to how much of the patient's body was affected by the corrosive substance.

---

7) **Encounters for treatment of sequela of burns**

Encounters for the treatment of the late effects of burns or corrosions (i.e., scars or joint contractures) should be coded with a burn or corrosion code with the 7th character "S" for sequela.

8) **Sequelae with a late effect code and current burn**

When appropriate, both a code for a current burn or corrosion with 7th character "A" or "D" and a burn or corrosion code with 7th character "S" may be assigned on the same record (when both a current burn and sequelae of an old burn exist). Burns and corrosions do not heal at the same rate and a current healing wound may still exist with sequela of a healed burn or corrosion.

See Section I.B.10 Sequela (Late Effects)

Female patient seen in ED for second-degree burn to the left ear; she also has significant scarring on her left elbow from a third-degree burn from childhood

T20.212A | **Burn of second degree of left ear [any part, except ear drum], initial encounter**

L90.5 | **Scar conditions and fibrosis of skin**

T22.322S | **Burn of third degree of left elbow, sequela**

Explanation: The patient is being seen for management of a current second-degree burn, which is reflected in the code by appending the seventh character of A, indicating active treatment or management of this burn. The elbow scarring is a sequela of a previous third-degree burn. The sequela condition precedes the original burn injury, which is appended with a seventh character of S.

---

9) **Use of an external cause code with burns and corrosions**

An external cause code should be used with burns and corrosions to identify the source and intent of the burn, as well as the place where it occurred.

e. **Adverse effects, poisoning, underdosing and toxic effects**

Codes in categories T36-T65 are combination codes that include the substance that was taken as well as the intent. No additional external cause code is required for poisonings, toxic effects, adverse effects and underdosing codes.

1) **Do not code directly from the Table of Drugs**

Do not code directly from the Table of Drugs and Chemicals. Always refer back to the Tabular List.

2) **Use as many codes as necessary to describe**

Use as many codes as necessary to describe completely all drugs, medicinal or biological substances.

3) **If the same code would describe the causative agent**

If the same code would describe the causative agent for more than one adverse reaction, poisoning, toxic effect or underdosing, assign the code only once.

4) **If two or more drugs, medicinal or biological substances**

If two or more drugs, medicinal or biological substances are **taken**, code each individually unless a combination code is listed in the Table of Drugs and Chemicals.

If multiple unspecified drugs, medicinal or biological substances were taken, assign the appropriate code from subcategory T50.91, Poisoning by, adverse effect of and underdosing of multiple unspecified drugs, medicaments and biological substances.

5) **The occurrence of drug toxicity is classified in ICD-10-CM as follows:**
(a) **Adverse effect**

When coding an adverse effect of a drug that has been correctly prescribed and properly administered, assign the appropriate code for the nature of the adverse effect followed by the appropriate code for the adverse effect of the drug (T36-T50). The code for the drug should have a 5th or 6th character "5" (for example T36.0X5-) Examples of the nature of an adverse effect are tachycardia, delirium, gastrointestinal hemorrhaging, vomiting, hypokalemia, hepatitis, renal failure, or respiratory failure.

Patient admitted for stomach pain and jaundice, indicated by physician as possible side-effects of Inderal, recently started for hypertension. Inderal was discontinued and the patient switched to Atenolol instead.

R10.9 | **Unspecified abdominal pain**

R17 | **Unspecified jaundice**

T44.7X5A | **Adverse effect of beta-adrenoreceptor antagonists, initial encounter**

I10 | **Essential (primary) hypertension**

Explanation: The side-effects caused by the drug are listed first, followed by the code for the adverse effect of the drug to capture the specific drug that was used.

(b) **Poisoning**

When coding a poisoning or reaction to the improper use of a medication (e.g., overdose, wrong substance given or taken in error, wrong route of administration), first assign the appropriate code from categories T36-T50. The poisoning codes have an associated intent as their 5th or 6th character (accidental, intentional self-harm, assault and undetermined. If the intent of the poisoning is unknown or unspecified, code the intent as accidental intent. The undetermined intent is only for use if the documentation in the record specifies that the intent cannot be determined. Use additional code(s) for all manifestations of poisonings.

A 55-year-old female status post recent left knee replacement is admitted due to confusion, dizziness, and nausea. Her spouse brought in her prescribed Xanax, Ambien, and Percocet bottles but has no idea how many she took. It is suspected that her symptoms are due to an overdose of these medications.

T42.4X1A	**Poisoning by benzodiazepines, accidental (unintentional), initial encounter**
T42.6X1A	**Poisoning by other antiepileptic and sedative-hypnotic drugs, accidental (unintentional), initial encounter**
T40.2X1A	**Poisoning by other opioids, accidental (unintentional), initial encounter**
R41.0	**Disorientation, unspecified**
R42	**Dizziness and giddiness**
R11.0	**Nausea**

Explanation: It was not documented whether the overdose of the drugs was accidental or intentional; therefore the correct reporting of the poisoning codes is accidental intent. The poisoning codes are sequenced first, followed by manifestations of the poisoning.

If there is also a diagnosis of abuse or dependence of the substance, the abuse or dependence is assigned as an additional code.

Examples of poisoning include:

  (i)   Error was made in drug prescription

       Errors made in drug prescription or in the administration of the drug by provider, nurse, patient, or other person.

  (ii) Overdose of a drug intentionally taken

       If an overdose of a drug was intentionally taken or administered and resulted in drug toxicity, it would be coded as a poisoning.

  (iii) Nonprescribed drug taken with correctly prescribed and properly administered drug

       If a nonprescribed drug or medicinal agent was taken in combination with a correctly prescribed and properly administered drug, any drug toxicity or other reaction resulting from the interaction of the two drugs would be classified as a poisoning.

  (iv) Interaction of drug(s) and alcohol

       When a reaction results from the interaction of a drug(s) and alcohol, this would be classified as poisoning.

       See Section I.C.4. if poisoning is the result of insulin pump malfunctions.

(c) Underdosing

Underdosing refers to taking less of a medication than is prescribed by a provider or a manufacturer's instruction. Discontinuing the use of a prescribed medication on the patient's own initiative (not directed by the patient's provider) is also classified as an underdosing. For underdosing, assign the code from categories T36-T50 (fifth or sixth character "6").

Codes for underdosing should never be assigned as principal or first-listed codes. If a patient has a relapse or exacerbation of the medical condition for which the drug is prescribed because of the reduction in dose, then the medical condition itself should be coded.

Noncompliance (Z91.12-, Z91.13- and Z91.14-) or complication of care (Y63.6-Y63.9) codes are to be used with an underdosing code to indicate intent, if known.

Patient admitted for atrial fibrillation with history of chronic atrial fibrillation for which she is prescribed amiodarone. Financial concerns have left the patient unable to pay for her prescriptions and she has been skipping her amiodarone dose every other day to offset the cost.

I48.20	**Chronic atrial fibrillation, unspecified**
T46.2X6A	**Underdosing of other antidysrhythmic drugs, initial encounter**
Z91.120	**Patient's intentional underdosing of medication regimen due to financial hardship**

Explanation: By skipping her amiodarone pill every other day, the patient's atrial fibrillation returned. The condition for which the drug was being taken is reported first, followed by an underdosing code to show that the patient was not adhering to her prescription regimen. The Z code helps elaborate on the patient's social and/or economic circumstances that led to the patient taking less then what she was prescribed.

(d) Toxic effects

When a harmful substance is ingested or comes in contact with a person, this is classified as a toxic effect. The toxic effect codes are in categories T51-T65.

Toxic effect codes have an associated intent: accidental, intentional self-harm, assault and undetermined.

f. Adult and child abuse, neglect and other maltreatment

Sequence first the appropriate code from categories T74.- (Adult and child abuse, neglect and other maltreatment, confirmed) or T76.- (Adult and child abuse, neglect and other maltreatment, suspected) for abuse, neglect and other maltreatment, followed by any accompanying mental health or injury code(s).

If the documentation in the medical record states abuse or neglect it is coded as confirmed (T74.-). It is coded as suspected if it is documented as suspected (T76.-).

For cases of confirmed abuse or neglect an external cause code from the assault section (X92-Y09) should be added to identify the cause of any physical injuries. A perpetrator code (Y07) should be added when the perpetrator of the abuse is known. For suspected cases of abuse or neglect, do not report external cause or perpetrator code.

If a suspected case of abuse, neglect or mistreatment is ruled out during an encounter code Z04.71, Encounter for examination and observation following alleged physical adult abuse, ruled out, or code Z04.72, Encounter for examination and observation following alleged child physical abuse, ruled out, should be used, not a code from T76.

If a suspected case of alleged rape or sexual abuse is ruled out during an encounter code Z04.41, Encounter for examination and observation following alleged adult rape or code Z04.42, Encounter for examination and observation following alleged child rape, should be used, not a code from T76.

If a suspected case of forced sexual exploitation or forced labor exploitation is ruled out during an encounter, code Z04.81, Encounter for examination and observation of victim following forced sexual exploitation, or code Z04.82, Encounter for examination and observation of victim following forced labor exploitation, should be used, not a code from T76.

See Section I.C.15. Abuse in a pregnant patient.

g. Complications of care

1) General guidelines for complications of care

(a) Documentation of complications of care

     See Section I.B.16. for information on documentation of complications of care.

2) Pain due to medical devices

Pain associated with devices, implants or grafts left in a surgical site (for example painful hip prosthesis) is assigned to the appropriate code(s) found in Chapter 19, Injury, poisoning, and certain other consequences of external causes. Specific codes for pain due to medical devices are found in the T code section of the ICD-10-CM. Use additional code(s) from category G89 to identify acute or chronic pain due to presence of the device, implant or graft (G89.18 or G89.28).

Chronic left breast pain secondary to breast implant

T85.848A	**Pain due to other internal prosthetic devices, implants and grafts, initial encounter**
N64.4	**Mastodynia**
G89.28	**Other chronic postprocedural pain**

Explanation: As the pain is a complication related to the breast implant, the complication code is sequenced first. The T code does not describe the site or type of pain, so additional codes may be appended to indicate that the patient is experiencing chronic pain in the breast.

3) Transplant complications

(a) Transplant complications other than kidney

Codes under category T86, Complications of transplanted organs and tissues, are for use for both complications and rejection of transplanted organs. A transplant complication code is only assigned if the complication affects the function of the transplanted organ. Two codes are required to fully describe a transplant complication: the appropriate code from category T86 and a secondary code that identifies the complication.

Pre-existing conditions or conditions that develop after the transplant are not coded as complications unless they affect the function of the transplanted organs.

See I.C.21. for transplant organ removal status

See I.C.2. for malignant neoplasm associated with transplanted organ.

(b) Kidney transplant complications

Patients who have undergone kidney transplant may still have some form of chronic kidney disease (CKD) because the kidney transplant may not fully restore kidney function. Code T86.1- should be assigned for documented complications of a kidney transplant, such as transplant failure or rejection or other transplant complication. Code T86.1- should not be assigned for post kidney transplant patients who have chronic kidney (CKD) unless a transplant complication such as transplant failure or rejection is documented. If the documentation is unclear as to whether the patient has a complication of the transplant, query the provider.

Conditions that affect the function of the transplanted kidney, other than CKD, should be assigned a code from subcategory T86.1, Complications of transplanted organ, Kidney, and a secondary code that identifies the complication.

For patients with CKD following a kidney transplant, but who do not have a complication such as failure or rejection, *see section I.C.14. Chronic kidney disease and kidney transplant status.*

Patient with chronic kidney disease stage 2; history of successful kidney transplant with no complications identified

N18.2	**Chronic kidney disease, stage 2 (mild)**
Z94.0	**Kidney transplant status**

Explanation: This patient's stage 2 CKD is not indicated as being due to the transplanted kidney but instead is just the residual disease the patient had prior to the transplant.

4) Complication codes that include the external cause

As with certain other T codes, some of the complications of care codes have the external cause included in the code. The code includes the nature of the complication as well as the type of procedure that caused the complication. No external cause code indicating the type of procedure is necessary for these codes.

5) Complications of care codes within the body system chapters

Intraoperative and postprocedural complication codes are found within the body system chapters with codes specific to the organs and structures of that body system. These codes should be sequenced first, followed by a code(s) for the specific complication, if applicable.

Complication codes from the body system chapters should be assigned for intraoperative and postprocedural complications (e.g., the appropriate complication code from chapter 9 would be assigned for a vascular intraoperative or postprocedural complication) unless the complication is specifically indexed to a T code in chapter 19.

During a spinal fusion procedure, the surgeon inadvertently punctured the dura. The midline durotomy was repaired, and the fusion procedure was completed.

G97.41	**Accidental puncture or laceration of dura during a procedure**

Explanation: The accidental durotomy is not coded to an injury code in chapter 19 but instead is categorized to the nervous system chapter.

Muscle/Tendon Table

ICD-10-CM categorizes certain muscles and tendons in the upper and lower extremities by their action (e.g., extension, flexion), their anatomical location (e.g., posterior, anterior), and/or whether they are intrinsic or extrinsic to a certain anatomical area. The Muscle/Tendon Table is provided at the beginning of chapters 13 and 19 as a resource to help users when code selection depends on one or more of these characteristics. Please note that this table is not all-inclusive, and proper code assignment should be based on the provider's documentation.

Body Region	Muscle	Extensor Tendon	Flexor Tendon	Other Tendon
Shoulder				
	Deltoid	Posterior deltoid	Anterior deltoid	
	Rotator cuff			
	Infraspinatus			Infraspinatus
	Subscapularis			Subscapularis
	Supraspinatus			Supraspinatus
	Teres minor			Teres minor
	Teres major	Teres major		
Upper arm				
	Anterior muscles			
	Biceps brachii — long head		Biceps brachii — long head	
	Biceps brachii — short head		Biceps brachii — short head	
	Brachialis		Brachialis	
	Coracobrachialis		Coracobrachialis	
	Posterior muscles			
	Triceps brachii	Triceps brachii		
Forearm				
	Anterior muscles			
	Flexors			
	Deep			
	Flexor digitorum profundus		Flexor digitorum profundus	
	Flexor pollicis longus		Flexor pollicis longus	
	Intermediate			
	Flexor digitorum superficialis		Flexor digitorum superficialis	
	Superficial			
	Flexor carpi radialis		Flexor carpi radialis	
	Flexor carpi ulnaris		Flexor carpi ulnaris	
	Palmaris longus		Palmaris longus	
	Pronators			
	Pronator quadratus			Pronator quadratus
	Pronator teres			Pronator teres
	Posterior muscles			
	Extensors			
	Deep			
	Abductor pollicis longus			Abductor pollicis longus
	Extensor indicis	Extensor indicis		
	Extensor pollicis brevis	Extensor pollicis brevis		
	Extensor pollicis longus	Extensor pollicis longus		
	Superficial			
	Brachioradialis			Brachioradialis
	Extensor carpi radialis brevis	Extensor carpi radialis brevis		
	Extensor carpi radialis longus	Extensor carpi radialis longus		
	Extensor carpi ulnaris	Extensor carpi ulnaris		
	Extensor digiti minimi	Extensor digiti minimi		
	Extensor digitorum	Extensor digitorum		
	Anconeus	Anconeus		
	Supinator			Supinator

Body Region	Muscle	Extensor Tendon	Flexor Tendon	Other Tendon
Hand				
Extrinsic — attach to a site in the forearm as well as a site in the hand with action related to hand movement at the wrist				
	Extensor carpi radialis brevis	Extensor carpi radialis brevis		
	Extensor carpi radialis longus	Extensor carpie radialis longus		
	Extensor carpi ulnaris	Extensor carpi ulnaris		
	Flexor carpi radialis		Flexor carpi radialis	
	Flexor carpi ulnaris		Flexor carpi ulnaris	
	Flexor digitorum superficialis		Flexor digitorum superficialis	
	Palmaris longus		Palmaris longus	
Extrinsic — attach to a site in the forearm as well as a site in the hand with action in the hand related to finger movement				
	Adductor pollicis longus			Adductor pollicis longus
	Extensor digiti minimi	Extensor digiti minimi		
	Extensor digitorum	Extensor digitorum		
	Extensor indicis	Extensor indicis		
	Flexor digitorum profundus		Flexor digitorum profundus	
	Flexor digitorum superficialis		Flexor digitorum superficialis	
Extrinsic — attach to a site in the forearm as well as a site in the hand with action in the hand related to thumb movement				
	Extensor pollicis brevis	Extensor pollicis brevis		
	Extensor pollicis longus	Extensor pollicis longus		
	Flexor pollicis longus		Flexor pollicis longus	
Intrinsic — found within the hand only				
	Adductor pollicis			Adductor pollicis
	Dorsal interossei	Dorsal interossei	Dorsal interossei	
	Lumbricals	Lumbricals	Lumbricals	
	Palmaris brevis			Palmaris brevis
	Palmar interossei	Palmar interossei	Palmar interossei	
	Hypothenar muscles			
	Abductor digiti minimi			Abductor digiti minimi
	Flexor digiti minimi brevis		Flexor digiti minimi brevis	
	Oppenens digiti minimi		Oppenens digiti minimi	
	Thenar muscles			
	Abductor pollicis brevis			Abductor pollicis brevis
	Flexor pollicis brevis		Flexor pollicis brevis	
	Oppenens pollicis		Oppenens pollicis	
Thigh				
	Anterior muscles			
	Iliopsoas		Iliopsoas	
	Pectineus		Pectineus	
	Quadriceps	Quadriceps		
	Rectus femoris	Rectus femoris — Extends knee	Rectus femoris — Flexes hip	
	Vastus intermedius	Vastus intermedius		
	Vastus lateralis	Vastus lateralis		
	Vastus medialis	Vastus medialis		
	Sartorius		Sartorius	
	Medial muscles			
	Adductor brevis			Adductor brevis
	Adductor longus			Adductor longus
	Adductor magnus			Adductor magnus
	Gracilis			Gracilis
	Obturator externus			Obturator externus
	Posterior muscles			
	Hamstring	Hamstring — Extends hip	Hamstring — Flexes knee	
	Biceps femoris	Biceps femoris	Biceps femoris	
	Semimembranosus	Semimembranosus	Semimembranosus	
	Semitendinosus	Semitendinosus	Semitendinosus	

Chapter 19. Injury, Poisoning and Certain Other Consequences of External Causes

Body Region	Muscle	Extensor Tendon	Flexor Tendon	Other Tendon
Lower leg				
	Anterior muscles			
	Extensor digitorum longus	Extensor digitorum longus		
	Extensor hallucis longus	Extensor hallucis longus		
	Fibularis (peroneus) tertius	Fibularis (peroneus) tertius		
	Tibialis anterior	Tibialis anterior		Tibialis anterior
	Lateral muscles			
	Fibularis (peroneus) brevis		Fibularis (peroneus) brevis	
	Fibularis (peroneus) longus		Fibularis (peroneus) longus	
	Posterior muscles			
	Deep			
	Flexor digitorum longus		Flexor digitorum longus	
	Flexor hallucis longus		Flexor hallucis longus	
	Popliteus		Popliteus	
	Tibialis posterior		Tibialis posterior	
	Superficial			
	Gastrocnemius		Gastrocnemius	
	Plantaris		Plantaris	
	Soleus		Soleus	
				Calcaneal (Achilles)
Ankle/Foot				
Extrinsic — attach to a site in the lower leg as well as a site in the foot with action related to foot movement at the ankle				
	Plantaris		Plantaris	
	Soleus		Soleus	
	Tibialis anterior	Tibialis anterior		
	Tibialis posterior		Tibialis posterior	
Extrinsic — attach to a site in the lower leg as well as a site in the foot with action in the foot related to toe movement				
	Extensor digitorum longus	Extensor digitorum longus		
	Extensor hallicus longus	Extensor hallicus longus		
	Flexor digitorum longus		Flexor digitorum longus	
	Flexor hallucis longus		Flexor hallucis longus	
Intrinsic — found within the ankle/foot only				
	Dorsal muscles			
	Extensor digitorum brevis	Extensor digitorum brevis		
	Extensor hallucis brevis	Extensor hallucis brevis		
	Plantar muscles			
	Abductor digiti minimi		Abductor digiti minimi	
	Abductor hallucis		Abductor hallucis	
	Dorsal interossei	Dorsal interossei	Dorsal interossei	
	Flexor digiti minimi brevis		Flexor digiti minimi brevis	
	Flexor digitorum brevis		Flexor digitorum brevis	
	Flexor hallucis brevis		Flexor hallucis brevis	
	Lumbricals	Lumbricals	Lumbricals	
	Quadratus plantae		Quadratus plantae	
	Plantar interossei	Plantar interossei	Plantar interossei	

Chapter 19. Injury, Poisoning and Certain Other Consequences of External Causes

Chapter 19. Injury, Poisoning and Certain Other Consequences of External Causes (S00-T88)

NOTE   Use secondary code(s) from Chapter 20, External causes of morbidity, to indicate cause of injury. Codes within the T section that include the external cause do not require an additional external cause code.

Use additional code to identify any retained foreign body, if applicable (Z18.-)

EXCLUDES 1   birth trauma (P10-P15)
       obstetric trauma (O70-O71)

NOTE   The chapter uses the S-section for coding different types of injuries related to single body regions and the T-section to cover injuries to unspecified body regions as well as poisoning and certain other consequences of external causes.

AHA: 2016,2Q,3-7; 2015,4Q,35-38; 2015,3Q,37-39,40; 2015,2Q,6; 2015,1Q,3-21
TIP: The specific site of an injury can be determined from the radiology report when authenticated by a radiologist and available at the time of code assignment.

This chapter contains the following blocks:

S00-S09   Injuries to the head
S10-S19   Injuries to the neck
S20-S29   Injuries to the thorax
S30-S39   Injuries to the abdomen, lower back, lumbar spine, pelvis and external genitals
S40-S49   Injuries to the shoulder and upper arm
S50-S59   Injuries to the elbow and forearm
S60-S69   Injuries to the wrist, hand and fingers
S70-S79   Injuries to the hip and thigh
S80-S89   Injuries to the knee and lower leg
S90-S99   Injuries to the ankle and foot
T07   Injuries involving multiple body regions
T14   Injury of unspecified body region
T15-T19   Effects of foreign body entering through natural orifice
T20-T25   Burns and corrosions of external body surface, specified by site
T26-T28   Burns and corrosions confined to eye and internal organs
T30-T32   Burns and corrosions of multiple and unspecified body regions
T33-T34   Frostbite
T36-T50   Poisoning by, adverse effect of and underdosing of drugs, medicaments and biological substances
T51-T65   Toxic effects of substances chiefly nonmedicinal as to source
T66-T78   Other and unspecified effects of external causes
T79   Certain early complications of trauma
T80-T88   Complications of surgical and medical care, not elsewhere classified

Injuries to the head (S00-S09)

INCLUDES   injuries of ear
       injuries of eye
       injuries of face [any part]
       injuries of gum
       injuries of jaw
       injuries of oral cavity
       injuries of palate
       injuries of periocular area
       injuries of scalp
       injuries of temporomandibular joint area
       injuries of tongue
       injuries of tooth

Code also for any associated infection

EXCLUDES 2   burns and corrosions (T20-T32)
       effects of foreign body in ear (T16)
       effects of foreign body in larynx (T17.3)
       effects of foreign body in mouth NOS (T18.0)
       effects of foreign body in nose (T17.0-T17.1)
       effects of foreign body in pharynx (T17.2)
       effects of foreign body on external eye (T15.-)
       frostbite (T33-T34)
       insect bite or sting, venomous (T63.4)

✓4ᵗʰ S00   Superficial injury of head

EXCLUDES 1   diffuse cerebral contusion (S06.2-)
       focal cerebral contusion (S06.3-)
       injury of eye and orbit (S05.-)
       open wound of head (S01.-)

The appropriate 7th character is to be added to each code from category S00.
A   initial encounter
D   subsequent encounter
S   sequela

   ✓5ᵗʰ S00.0   Superficial injury of scalp

     ✓x 7ᵗʰ   **S00.00   Unspecified superficial injury of scalp**

     ✓x 7ᵗʰ   **S00.01   Abrasion of scalp**

     ✓x 7ᵗʰ   **S00.02   Blister (nonthermal) of scalp**

     ✓x 7ᵗʰ   **S00.03   Contusion of scalp**
         Bruise of scalp
         Hematoma of scalp

     ✓x 7ᵗʰ   **S00.04   External constriction of part of scalp**

     ✓x 7ᵗʰ   **S00.05   Superficial foreign body of scalp**
         Splinter in the scalp

     ✓x 7ᵗʰ   **S00.06   Insect bite (nonvenomous) of scalp**

     ✓x 7ᵗʰ   **S00.07   Other superficial bite of scalp**
         EXCLUDES 1   open bite of scalp (S01.05)

   ✓5ᵗʰ S00.1   Contusion of eyelid and periocular area
       Black eye
       EXCLUDES 2   contusion of eyeball and orbital tissues (S05.1)

     ✓x 7ᵗʰ   **S00.10   Contusion of unspecified eyelid and periocular area**

     ✓x 7ᵗʰ   **S00.11   Contusion of right eyelid and periocular area**

     ✓x 7ᵗʰ   **S00.12   Contusion of left eyelid and periocular area**

   ✓5ᵗʰ S00.2   Other and unspecified superficial injuries of eyelid and periocular area
       EXCLUDES 2   superficial injury of conjunctiva and cornea (S05.0-)

     ✓6ᵗʰ   **S00.20   Unspecified superficial injury of eyelid and periocular area**

       ✓7ᵗʰ   **S00.201   Unspecified superficial injury of right eyelid and periocular area**

       ✓7ᵗʰ   **S00.202   Unspecified superficial injury of left eyelid and periocular area**

       ✓7ᵗʰ   **S00.209   Unspecified superficial injury of unspecified eyelid and periocular area**

     ✓6ᵗʰ   **S00.21   Abrasion of eyelid and periocular area**

       ✓7ᵗʰ   **S00.211   Abrasion of right eyelid and periocular area**

       ✓7ᵗʰ   **S00.212   Abrasion of left eyelid and periocular area**

       ✓7ᵗʰ   **S00.219   Abrasion of unspecified eyelid and periocular area**

     ✓6ᵗʰ   **S00.22   Blister (nonthermal) of eyelid and periocular area**

       ✓7ᵗʰ   **S00.221   Blister (nonthermal) of right eyelid and periocular area**

       ✓7ᵗʰ   **S00.222   Blister (nonthermal) of left eyelid and periocular area**

       ✓7ᵗʰ   **S00.229   Blister (nonthermal) of unspecified eyelid and periocular area**

     ✓6ᵗʰ   **S00.24   External constriction of eyelid and periocular area**

       ✓7ᵗʰ   **S00.241   External constriction of right eyelid and periocular area**

       ✓7ᵗʰ   **S00.242   External constriction of left eyelid and periocular area**

       ✓7ᵗʰ   **S00.249   External constriction of unspecified eyelid and periocular area**

     ✓6ᵗʰ   **S00.25   Superficial foreign body of eyelid and periocular area**
       Splinter of eyelid and periocular area
       EXCLUDES 2   retained foreign body in eyelid (H02.81-)

       ✓7ᵗʰ   **S00.251   Superficial foreign body of right eyelid and periocular area**

       ✓7ᵗʰ   **S00.252   Superficial foreign body of left eyelid and periocular area**

       ✓7ᵗʰ   **S00.259   Superficial foreign body of unspecified eyelid and periocular area**

     ✓6ᵗʰ   **S00.26   Insect bite (nonvenomous) of eyelid and periocular area**

       ✓7ᵗʰ   **S00.261   Insect bite (nonvenomous) of right eyelid and periocular area**

       ✓7ᵗʰ   **S00.262   Insect bite (nonvenomous) of left eyelid and periocular area**

       ✓7ᵗʰ   **S00.269   Insect bite (nonvenomous) of unspecified eyelid and periocular area**

     ✓6ᵗʰ   **S00.27   Other superficial bite of eyelid and periocular area**
       EXCLUDES 1   open bite of eyelid and periocular area (S01.15)

       ✓7ᵗʰ   **S00.271   Other superficial bite of right eyelid and periocular area**

       ✓7ᵗʰ   **S00.272   Other superficial bite of left eyelid and periocular area**

       ✓7ᵗʰ   **S00.279   Other superficial bite of unspecified eyelid and periocular area**

   ✓5ᵗʰ S00.3   Superficial injury of nose

     ✓x 7ᵗʰ   **S00.30   Unspecified superficial injury of nose**

     ✓x 7ᵗʰ   **S00.31   Abrasion of nose**

     ✓x 7ᵗʰ   **S00.32   Blister (nonthermal) of nose**

☑ Additional Character Required   ✓x7ᵗʰ Placeholder   Unacceptable PDx   Questionable PDx   Manifestation   Unspecified Dx   H1-H14 HAC   HCC CMS-HCC Dx   HIV HIV Dx

ICD-10-CM 2020   983

√x7ᵗʰ **S00.33** **Contusion** of nose
     Bruise of nose
     Hematoma of nose

√x7ᵗʰ **S00.34** **External constriction** of nose

√x7ᵗʰ **S00.35** **Superficial** foreign body of nose
     Splinter in the nose

√x7ᵗʰ **S00.36** **Insect bite (nonvenomous)** of nose

√x7ᵗʰ **S00.37** **Other superficial** bite of nose
     EXCLUDES 1   *open bite of nose (S01.25)*

√5ᵗʰ **S00.4** **Superficial injury** of ear

   √6ᵗʰ **S00.40** **Unspecified superficial injury of ear**

     √7ᵗʰ **S00.401** **Unspecified superficial injury of** right **ear**

     √7ᵗʰ **S00.402** **Unspecified superficial injury of** left **ear**

     √7ᵗʰ **S00.409** **Unspecified superficial injury of unspecified ear**

   √6ᵗʰ **S00.41** **Abrasion** of ear

     √7ᵗʰ **S00.411** **Abrasion of** right **ear**

     √7ᵗʰ **S00.412** **Abrasion of** left **ear**

     √7ᵗʰ **S00.419** **Abrasion of unspecified ear**

   √6ᵗʰ **S00.42** **Blister (nonthermal)** of ear

     √7ᵗʰ **S00.421** **Blister (nonthermal) of** right **ear**

     √7ᵗʰ **S00.422** **Blister (nonthermal) of** left **ear**

     √7ᵗʰ **S00.429** **Blister (nonthermal) of unspecified ear**

   √6ᵗʰ **S00.43** **Contusion** of ear
     Bruise of ear
     Hematoma of ear

     √7ᵗʰ **S00.431** **Contusion of** right **ear**

     √7ᵗʰ **S00.432** **Contusion of** left **ear**

     √7ᵗʰ **S00.439** **Contusion of unspecified ear**

   √6ᵗʰ **S00.44** **External constriction** of ear

     √7ᵗʰ **S00.441** **External constriction of** right **ear**

     √7ᵗʰ **S00.442** **External constriction of** left **ear**

     √7ᵗʰ **S00.449** **External constriction of unspecified ear**

   √6ᵗʰ **S00.45** **Superficial** foreign body of ear
     Splinter in the ear

     √7ᵗʰ **S00.451** **Superficial foreign body of** right **ear**

     √7ᵗʰ **S00.452** **Superficial foreign body of** left **ear**

     √7ᵗʰ **S00.459** **Superficial foreign body of unspecified ear**

   √6ᵗʰ **S00.46** **Insect bite (nonvenomous)** of ear

     √7ᵗʰ **S00.461** **Insect bite (nonvenomous) of** right **ear**

     √7ᵗʰ **S00.462** **Insect bite (nonvenomous) of** left **ear**

     √7ᵗʰ **S00.469** **Insect bite (nonvenomous) of unspecified ear**

   √6ᵗʰ **S00.47** **Other superficial** bite of ear
     EXCLUDES 1   *open bite of ear (S01.35)*

     √7ᵗʰ **S00.471** **Other superficial bite of** right **ear**

     √7ᵗʰ **S00.472** **Other superficial bite of** left **ear**

     √7ᵗʰ **S00.479** **Other superficial bite of unspecified ear**

√5ᵗʰ **S00.5** **Superficial injury** of lip and oral cavity

   √6ᵗʰ **S00.50** **Unspecified superficial injury of lip and oral cavity**

     √7ᵗʰ **S00.501** **Unspecified superficial injury of** lip

     √7ᵗʰ **S00.502** **Unspecified superficial injury of** oral cavity

   √6ᵗʰ **S00.51** **Abrasion** of lip and oral cavity

     √7ᵗʰ **S00.511** **Abrasion of** lip

     √7ᵗʰ **S00.512** **Abrasion of** oral cavity

   √6ᵗʰ **S00.52** **Blister (nonthermal)** of lip and oral cavity

     √7ᵗʰ **S00.521** **Blister (nonthermal) of** lip

     √7ᵗʰ **S00.522** **Blister (nonthermal) of** oral cavity

   √6ᵗʰ **S00.53** **Contusion** of lip and oral cavity

     √7ᵗʰ **S00.531** **Contusion of** lip
       Bruise of lip
       Hematoma of lip

     √7ᵗʰ **S00.532** **Contusion of** oral cavity
       Bruise of oral cavity
       Hematoma of oral cavity

   √6ᵗʰ **S00.54** **External constriction** of lip and oral cavity

     √7ᵗʰ **S00.541** **External constriction of** lip

√7ᵗʰ **S00.542** **External constriction** of oral cavity

   √6ᵗʰ **S00.55** **Superficial** foreign body of lip and oral cavity

     √7ᵗʰ **S00.551** **Superficial foreign body of** lip
       Splinter of lip and oral cavity

     √7ᵗʰ **S00.552** **Superficial foreign body of** oral cavity
       Splinter of lip and oral cavity

   √6ᵗʰ **S00.56** **Insect bite (nonvenomous)** of lip and oral cavity

     √7ᵗʰ **S00.561** **Insect bite (nonvenomous) of** lip

     √7ᵗʰ **S00.562** **Insect bite (nonvenomous) of** oral cavity

   √6ᵗʰ **S00.57** **Other superficial** bite of lip and oral cavity

     √7ᵗʰ **S00.571** **Other superficial bite of** lip
       EXCLUDES 1   *open bite of lip (S01.551)*

     √7ᵗʰ **S00.572** **Other superficial bite of** oral cavity
       EXCLUDES 1   *open bite of oral cavity (S01.552)*

√5ᵗʰ **S00.8** **Superficial injury** of other parts of head
     Superficial injuries of face [any part]

   √x7ᵗʰ **S00.80** **Unspecified superficial injury of other part of head**

   √x7ᵗʰ **S00.81** **Abrasion of other part of head**

   √x7ᵗʰ **S00.82** **Blister (nonthermal) of other part of head**

   √x7ᵗʰ **S00.83** **Contusion of other part of head**
     Bruise of other part of head
     Hematoma of other part of head

   √x7ᵗʰ **S00.84** **External constriction** of other part of head

   √x7ᵗʰ **S00.85** **Superficial** foreign body of other part of head
     Splinter in other part of head

   √x7ᵗʰ **S00.86** **Insect bite (nonvenomous) of other part of head**

   √x7ᵗʰ **S00.87** **Other superficial** bite of other part of head
     EXCLUDES 1   *open bite of other part of head (S01.85)*

√5ᵗʰ **S00.9** **Superficial injury** of unspecified part of head

   √x7ᵗʰ **S00.90** **Unspecified superficial injury of unspecified part of head**

   √x7ᵗʰ **S00.91** **Abrasion of unspecified part of head**

   √x7ᵗʰ **S00.92** **Blister (nonthermal) of unspecified part of head**

   √x7ᵗʰ **S00.93** **Contusion of unspecified part of head**
     Bruise of head
     Hematoma of head

   √x7ᵗʰ **S00.94** **External constriction** of unspecified part of head

   √x7ᵗʰ **S00.95** **Superficial** foreign body of unspecified part of head
     Splinter of head

   √x7ᵗʰ **S00.96** **Insect bite (nonvenomous) of unspecified part of head**

   √x7ᵗʰ **S00.97** **Other superficial** bite of unspecified part of head
     EXCLUDES 1   *open bite of head (S01.95)*

√4ᵗʰ **S01** **Open wound of head**
     Code also any associated:
       injury of cranial nerve (S04.-)
       injury of muscle and tendon of head (S09.1-)
       intracranial injury (S06.-)
       wound infection
     EXCLUDES 1   *open skull fracture (S02.- with 7th character B)*
     EXCLUDES 2   *injury of eye and orbit (S05.-)*
                 traumatic amputation of part of head (S08.-)

> The appropriate 7th character is to be added to each code from category S01.
> A   initial encounter
> D   subsequent encounter
> S   sequela

√5ᵗʰ **S01.0** **Open wound of scalp**
     EXCLUDES 1   *avulsion of scalp (S08.0)*

   √x7ᵗʰ **S01.00** **Unspecified open wound of scalp**

   √x7ᵗʰ **S01.01** **Laceration without foreign body of scalp**

   √x7ᵗʰ **S01.02** **Laceration with foreign body of scalp**

   √x7ᵗʰ **S01.03** **Puncture wound without foreign body of scalp**

   √x7ᵗʰ **S01.04** **Puncture wound with foreign body of scalp**

   √x7ᵗʰ **S01.05** **Open bite of scalp**
     Bite of scalp NOS
     EXCLUDES 1   *superficial bite of scalp (S00.06, S00.07-)*

Ⓝ Newborn: 0   Ⓟ Pediatric: 0-17   Ⓜ Maternity: 9-64   Ⓐ Adult: 15-124   **MCC** Major Complication/Comorbidity   **CC** Complication/Comorbidity   **SW** Severe Wound Dx

984   ICD-10-CM 2020

✓5th **S01.1** **Open wound of eyelid and periocular area**

Open wound of eyelid and periocular area with or without involvement of lacrimal passages

  ✓6th **S01.10** **Unspecified open wound of eyelid and periocular area**

       CC Excl: For CC codes in subcategory S01.10: PDX collection 1139

    ✓7th **S01.101** Unspecified open wound of right eyelid and periocular area   **CC**

    ✓7th **S01.102** Unspecified open wound of left eyelid and periocular area   **CC**

    ✓7th **S01.109** Unspecified open wound of unspecified eyelid and periocular area   **CC**

  ✓6th **S01.11** Laceration without foreign body of eyelid and periocular area

    ✓7th **S01.111** Laceration without foreign body of right eyelid and periocular area

    ✓7th **S01.112** Laceration without foreign body of left eyelid and periocular area

    ✓7th **S01.119** Laceration without foreign body of unspecified eyelid and periocular area

  ✓6th **S01.12** Laceration with foreign body of eyelid and periocular area

    ✓7th **S01.121** Laceration with foreign body of right eyelid and periocular area

    ✓7th **S01.122** Laceration with foreign body of left eyelid and periocular area

    ✓7th **S01.129** Laceration with foreign body of unspecified eyelid and periocular area

  ✓6th **S01.13** Puncture wound without foreign body of eyelid and periocular area

    ✓7th **S01.131** Puncture wound without foreign body of right eyelid and periocular area

    ✓7th **S01.132** Puncture wound without foreign body of left eyelid and periocular area

    ✓7th **S01.139** Puncture wound without foreign body of unspecified eyelid and periocular area

  ✓6th **S01.14** Puncture wound with foreign body of eyelid and periocular area

    ✓7th **S01.141** Puncture wound with foreign body of right eyelid and periocular area

    ✓7th **S01.142** Puncture wound with foreign body of left eyelid and periocular area

    ✓7th **S01.149** Puncture wound with foreign body of unspecified eyelid and periocular area

  ✓6th **S01.15** Open bite of eyelid and periocular area

Bite of eyelid and periocular area NOS

     EXCLUDES 1   *superficial bite of eyelid and periocular area (S00.26, S00.27)*

    ✓7th **S01.151** Open bite of right eyelid and periocular area

    ✓7th **S01.152** Open bite of left eyelid and periocular area

    ✓7th **S01.159** Open bite of unspecified eyelid and periocular area

✓5th **S01.2** **Open wound of nose**

  ✓x7th **S01.20** **Unspecified open wound of nose**

  ✓x7th **S01.21** Laceration without foreign body of nose

  ✓x7th **S01.22** Laceration with foreign body of nose

  ✓x7th **S01.23** Puncture wound without foreign body of nose

  ✓x7th **S01.24** Puncture wound with foreign body of nose

  ✓x7th **S01.25** Open bite of nose

Bite of nose NOS

     EXCLUDES 1   *superficial bite of nose (S00.36, S00.37)*

✓5th **S01.3** **Open wound of ear**

  ✓6th **S01.30** **Unspecified open wound of ear**

    ✓7th **S01.301** Unspecified open wound of right ear

    ✓7th **S01.302** Unspecified open wound of left ear

    ✓7th **S01.309** Unspecified open wound of unspecified ear

  ✓6th **S01.31** Laceration without foreign body of ear

    ✓7th **S01.311** Laceration without foreign body of right ear

    ✓7th **S01.312** Laceration without foreign body of left ear

    ✓7th **S01.319** Laceration without foreign body of unspecified ear

  ✓6th **S01.32** Laceration with foreign body of ear

    ✓7th **S01.321** Laceration with foreign body of right ear

    ✓7th **S01.322** Laceration with foreign body of left ear

    ✓7th **S01.329** Laceration with foreign body of unspecified ear

  ✓6th **S01.33** Puncture wound without foreign body of ear

    ✓7th **S01.331** Puncture wound without foreign body of right ear

    ✓7th **S01.332** Puncture wound without foreign body of left ear

    ✓7th **S01.339** Puncture wound without foreign body of unspecified ear

  ✓6th **S01.34** Puncture wound with foreign body of ear

    ✓7th **S01.341** Puncture wound with foreign body of right ear

    ✓7th **S01.342** Puncture wound with foreign body of left ear

    ✓7th **S01.349** Puncture wound with foreign body of unspecified ear

  ✓6th **S01.35** Open bite of ear

Bite of ear NOS

     EXCLUDES 1   *superficial bite of ear (S00.46, S00.47)*

    ✓7th **S01.351** Open bite of right ear

    ✓7th **S01.352** Open bite of left ear

    ✓7th **S01.359** Open bite of unspecified ear

✓5th **S01.4** **Open wound of cheek and temporomandibular area**

  ✓6th **S01.40** **Unspecified open wound of cheek and temporomandibular area**

    ✓7th **S01.401** Unspecified open wound of right cheek and temporomandibular area

    ✓7th **S01.402** Unspecified open wound of left cheek and temporomandibular area

    ✓7th **S01.409** Unspecified open wound of unspecified cheek and temporomandibular area

  ✓6th **S01.41** Laceration without foreign body of cheek and temporomandibular area

    ✓7th **S01.411** Laceration without foreign body of right cheek and temporomandibular area

    ✓7th **S01.412** Laceration without foreign body of left cheek and temporomandibular area

    ✓7th **S01.419** Laceration without foreign body of unspecified cheek and temporomandibular area

  ✓6th **S01.42** Laceration with foreign body of cheek and temporomandibular area

    ✓7th **S01.421** Laceration with foreign body of right cheek and temporomandibular area

    ✓7th **S01.422** Laceration with foreign body of left cheek and temporomandibular area

    ✓7th **S01.429** Laceration with foreign body of unspecified cheek and temporomandibular area

  ✓6th **S01.43** Puncture wound without foreign body of cheek and temporomandibular area

    ✓7th **S01.431** Puncture wound without foreign body of right cheek and temporomandibular area

    ✓7th **S01.432** Puncture wound without foreign body of left cheek and temporomandibular area

    ✓7th **S01.439** Puncture wound without foreign body of unspecified cheek and temporomandibular area

  ✓6th **S01.44** Puncture wound with foreign body of cheek and temporomandibular area

    ✓7th **S01.441** Puncture wound with foreign body of right cheek and temporomandibular area

    ✓7th **S01.442** Puncture wound with foreign body of left cheek and temporomandibular area

    ✓7th **S01.449** Puncture wound with foreign body of unspecified cheek and temporomandibular area

  ✓6th **S01.45** Open bite of cheek and temporomandibular area

Bite of cheek and temporomandibular area NOS

     EXCLUDES 2   *superficial bite of cheek and temporomandibular area (S00.86, S00.87)*

    ✓7th **S01.451** Open bite of right cheek and temporomandibular area

---

☑ Additional Character Required   ✓x7th Placeholder   Unacceptable PDx   Questionable PDx   Manifestation   Unspecified Dx   **H1–H14** HAC   **HCC** CMS-HCC Dx   **HIV** HIV Dx

ICD-10-CM 2020   **985**

√7ᵗʰ **S01.452** **Open bite of** left **cheek and temporomandibular area**

√7ᵗʰ **S01.459** **Open bite of unspecified cheek and temporomandibular area**

√5ᵗʰ **S01.5** **Open wound of** lip and oral cavity

EXCLUDES 2   *tooth dislocation (S03.2)*
           tooth fracture (S02.5)

√6ᵗʰ **S01.50** **Unspecified open wound of lip and oral cavity**

√7ᵗʰ **S01.501** **Unspecified open wound of lip**

√7ᵗʰ **S01.502** **Unspecified open wound of oral cavity**

√6ᵗʰ **S01.51** **Laceration of lip and oral cavity** without foreign **body**

√7ᵗʰ **S01.511** **Laceration without foreign body of lip**

√7ᵗʰ **S01.512** **Laceration without foreign body of oral cavity**

√6ᵗʰ **S01.52** **Laceration of lip and oral cavity** with foreign **body**

√7ᵗʰ **S01.521** **Laceration with foreign body of lip**

√7ᵗʰ **S01.522** **Laceration with foreign body of oral cavity**

√6ᵗʰ **S01.53** **Puncture wound of lip and oral cavity** without **foreign body**

√7ᵗʰ **S01.531** **Puncture wound without foreign body of lip**

√7ᵗʰ **S01.532** **Puncture wound without foreign body of oral cavity**

√6ᵗʰ **S01.54** **Puncture wound of lip and oral cavity** with foreign **body**

√7ᵗʰ **S01.541** **Puncture wound with foreign body of lip**

√7ᵗʰ **S01.542** **Puncture wound with foreign body of oral cavity**

√6ᵗʰ **S01.55** **Open bite of lip and oral cavity**

√7ᵗʰ **S01.551** **Open bite of lip**

Bite of lip NOS

EXCLUDES 1   *superficial bite of lip (S00.571)*

√7ᵗʰ **S01.552** **Open bite of oral cavity**

Bite of oral cavity NOS

EXCLUDES 1   *superficial bite of oral cavity (S00.572)*

√5ᵗʰ **S01.8** **Open wound of other parts of head**

√x7ᵗʰ **S01.80** **Unspecified open wound of other part of head**

√x7ᵗʰ **S01.81** **Laceration without foreign body of other part of head**

√x7ᵗʰ **S01.82** **Laceration with foreign body of other part of head**

√x7ᵗʰ **S01.83** **Puncture wound without foreign body of other part of head**

√x7ᵗʰ **S01.84** **Puncture wound with foreign body of other part of head**

√x7ᵗʰ **S01.85** **Open bite of other part of head**

Bite of other part of head NOS

EXCLUDES 1   *superficial bite of other part of head (S00.87)*

√5ᵗʰ **S01.9** **Open wound of unspecified part of head**

√x7ᵗʰ **S01.90** **Unspecified open wound of unspecified part of head**

√x7ᵗʰ **S01.91** **Laceration without foreign body of unspecified part of head**

√x7ᵗʰ **S01.92** **Laceration with foreign body of unspecified part of head**

√x7ᵗʰ **S01.93** **Puncture wound without foreign body of unspecified part of head**

√x7ᵗʰ **S01.94** **Puncture wound with foreign body of unspecified part of head**

√x7ᵗʰ **S01.95** **Open bite of unspecified part of head**

Bite of head NOS

EXCLUDES 1   *superficial bite of head NOS (S00.97)*

√4ᵗʰ **S02** **Fracture of skull and facial bones**

NOTE   A fracture not indicated as open or closed should be coded to closed.

Code also any associated intracranial injury (S06.-)

AHA: 2017,1Q,42; 2016,4Q,66-67

The appropriate 7th character is to be added to each code from category S02.
A   initial encounter for closed fracture
B   initial encounter for open fracture
D   subsequent encounter for fracture with routine healing
G   subsequent encounter for fracture with delayed healing
K   subsequent encounter for fracture with nonunion
S   sequela

2,3,7 √x7ᵗʰ **S02.0** **Fracture of vault of skull**   MCC CC H5 HCC

Fracture of frontal bone
Fracture of parietal bone

CC Excl: For codes in subcategory S02.0:
CC with 7th character A or MCC with 7th character B: PDX collection 1140
CC with 7th character K: PDX collection 897

√5ᵗʰ **S02.1** **Fracture of base of skull**

EXCLUDES 1   *orbit NOS (S02.8)*
EXCLUDES 2   ▶*lateral orbital wall (S02.84-)*◀
           ▶*medial orbital wall (S02.83-)*◀
           orbital floor (S02.3-)

CC Excl: For codes in subcategory S02.1:
CC with 7th character A or MCC with 7th character B: PDX collection 1140
CC with 7th character K: PDX collection 897

√6ᵗʰ **S02.10** **Unspecified fracture of base of skull**

2,3,7 √7ᵗʰ **S02.101** **Fracture of base of skull, right side**   MCC CC H5 HCC

2,3,7 √7ᵗʰ **S02.102** **Fracture of base of skull, left side**   MCC CC H5 HCC

2,3,7 √7ᵗʰ **S02.109** **Fracture of base of skull, unspecified side**   MCC CC H5 HCC

√6ᵗʰ **S02.11** **Fracture of occiput**

2,3,7 √7ᵗʰ **S02.110** **Type I occipital condyle fracture, unspecified side**   MCC CC H5 HCC

2,3,7 √7ᵗʰ **S02.111** **Type II occipital condyle fracture, unspecified side**   MCC CC H5 HCC

2,3,7 √7ᵗʰ **S02.112** **Type III occipital condyle fracture, unspecified side**   MCC CC H5 HCC

2,3,7 √7ᵗʰ **S02.113** **Unspecified occipital condyle fracture**   MCC CC H5 HCC

2,3,7 √7ᵗʰ **S02.118** **Other fracture of occiput, unspecified side**   MCC CC H5 HCC

2,3,7 √7ᵗʰ **S02.119** **Unspecified fracture of occiput**   MCC CC H5 HCC

2,3,7 √7ᵗʰ **S02.11A** **Type I occipital condyle fracture, right side**   MCC CC H5 HCC

2,3,7 √7ᵗʰ **S02.11B** **Type I occipital condyle fracture, left side**   MCC CC H5 HCC

2,3,7 √7ᵗʰ **S02.11C** **Type II occipital condyle fracture, right side**   MCC CC H5 HCC

2,3,7 √7ᵗʰ **S02.11D** **Type II occipital condyle fracture, left side**   MCC CC H5 HCC

2,3,7 √7ᵗʰ **S02.11E** **Type III occipital condyle fracture, right side**   MCC CC H5 HCC

2,3,7 √7ᵗʰ **S02.11F** **Type III occipital condyle fracture, left side**   MCC CC H5 HCC

2,3,7 √7ᵗʰ **S02.11G** **Other fracture of occiput, right side**   MCC CC H5 HCC

2,3,7 √7ᵗʰ **S02.11H** **Other fracture of occiput, left side**   MCC CC H5 HCC

√6ᵗʰ **S02.12** **Fracture of orbital roof**

2,3 √7ᵗʰ **S02.121** **Fracture of orbital roof, right side**   MCC CC

2,3 √7ᵗʰ **S02.122** **Fracture of orbital roof, left side**   MCC CC

2,3 √7ᵗʰ **S02.129** **Fracture of orbital roof, unspecified side**   MCC CC

2,3,7 √x7th **S02.19   Other fracture of base of skull**   MCC CC H5 HCC

Fracture of anterior fossa of base of skull
Fracture of ethmoid sinus
Fracture of frontal sinus
Fracture of middle fossa of base of skull
~~Fracture of orbital roof~~
Fracture of posterior fossa of base of skull
Fracture of sphenoid
Fracture of temporal bone

3 √x7th **S02.2   Fracture of nasal bones**   CC H5

CC Excl: CC with 7th character B: PDX collection 1141
CC Excl: CC with 7th character K: PDX collection 897

√5th **S02.3   Fracture of orbital floor**

▶Fracture of inferior orbital wall◀

EXCLUDES 1   orbit NOS ▶(S02.85)◀
EXCLUDES 2   ▶lateral orbital wall (S02.84-)◀
▶medial orbital wall (S02.83-) ◀
orbital roof (S02.1-)

CC Excl: For codes in subcategory S02.3:
CC with 7th character A or B: PDX collection 1142
CC with 7th character K: PDX collection 897

3,7 √x7th **S02.30   Fracture of orbital floor, unspecified side**   CC H5 HCC

3,7 √x7th **S02.31   Fracture of orbital floor, right side**   CC H5 HCC

3,7 √x7th **S02.32   Fracture of orbital floor, left side**   CC H5 HCC

√5th **S02.4   Fracture of malar, maxillary and zygoma bones**

Fracture of superior maxilla
Fracture of upper jaw (bone)
Fracture of zygomatic process of temporal bone

CC Excl: For codes in subcategory S02.4, unless otherwise noted:
CC with 7th character A or B: PDX collection 1143
CC with 7th character K: PDX collection 897

√6th **S02.40   Fracture of malar, maxillary and zygoma bones, unspecified**

3,7 √7th **S02.400   Malar fracture, unspecified side**   CC H5 HCC

3,7 √7th **S02.401   Maxillary fracture, unspecified side**   CC H5 HCC

3,7 √7th **S02.402   Zygomatic fracture, unspecified side**   CC H5 HCC

3,7 √7th **S02.40A   Malar fracture, right side**   CC H5 HCC

3,7 √7th **S02.40B   Malar fracture, left side**   CC H5 HCC

3,7 √7th **S02.40C   Maxillary fracture, right side**   CC H5 HCC

3,7 √7th **S02.40D   Maxillary fracture, left side**   CC H5 HCC

3,7 √7th **S02.40E   Zygomatic fracture, right side**   CC H5 HCC

3,7 √7th **S02.40F   Zygomatic fracture, left side**   CC H5 HCC

√6th **S02.41   LeFort fracture**

DEF: Named for Rene Le Fort, these fractures describe different combinations of multiple fractures that occur from significant force to the midface. A common denominator in all three types of LeFort fractures is fracture of the pterygoid processes, which are two bony plates resembling wings that extend downward from the sphenoid bone.

LeFort Fracture Types

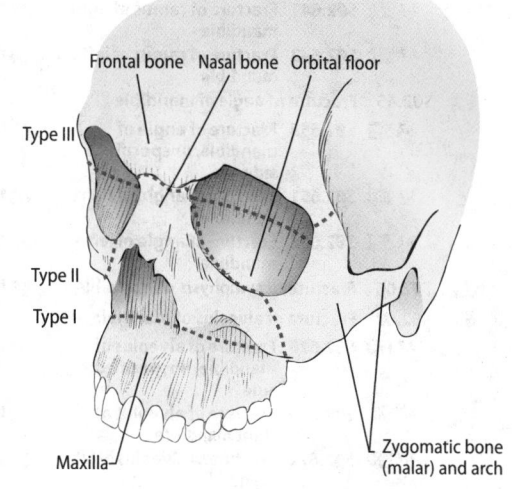

Frontal bone   Nasal bone   Orbital floor

Type III

Type II

Type I

Maxilla

Zygomatic bone (malar) and arch

3,7 √7th **S02.411   LeFort I fracture**   CC H5 HCC

3,7 √7th **S02.412   LeFort II fracture**   CC H5 HCC

3,7 √7th **S02.413   LeFort III fracture**   CC H5 HCC

3,7 √x7th **S02.42   Fracture of alveolus of maxilla**   CC H5 HCC

CC Excl: CC with 7th character B: PDX collection 1141
CC Excl: CC with 7th character K: PDX collection 897

4 √x7th **S02.5   Fracture of tooth (traumatic)**   CC

Broken tooth
EXCLUDES 1   cracked tooth (nontraumatic) (K03.81)
CC Excl: CC with 7th character K: PDX collection 897

√5th **S02.6   Fracture of mandible**

Fracture of lower jaw (bone)
CC Excl: For codes in subcategory S02.6:
CC with 7th character A or B: PDX collection 1143
CC with 7th character K: PDX collection 897

√6th **S02.60   Fracture of mandible, unspecified**

3,7 √7th **S02.600   Fracture of unspecified part of body of mandible, unspecified side**   CC H5 HCC

3,7 √7th **S02.601   Fracture of unspecified part of body of right mandible**   CC H5 HCC

3,7 √7th **S02.602   Fracture of unspecified part of body of left mandible**   CC H5 HCC

3,7 √7th **S02.609   Fracture of mandible, unspecified**   CC H5 HCC

√6th **S02.61   Fracture of condylar process of mandible**

3,7 √7th **S02.610   Fracture of condylar process of mandible, unspecified side**   CC H5 HCC

3,7 √7th **S02.611   Fracture of condylar process of right mandible**   CC H5 HCC

3,7 √7th **S02.612   Fracture of condylar process of left mandible**   CC H5 HCC

√6th **S02.62   Fracture of subcondylar process of mandible**

3,7 √7th **S02.620   Fracture of subcondylar process of mandible, unspecified side**   CC H5 HCC

3,7 √7th **S02.621   Fracture of subcondylar process of right mandible**   CC H5 HCC

3,7 √7th **S02.622   Fracture of subcondylar process of left mandible**   CC H5 HCC

√6ᵗʰ **S02.63** Fracture of **coronoid process of mandible**

3,7 √7ᵗʰ **S02.630** Fracture of coronoid process of mandible, unspecified side   CC H5 HCC

3,7 √7ᵗʰ **S02.631** Fracture of coronoid process of **right** mandible   CC H5 HCC

3,7 √7ᵗʰ **S02.632** Fracture of coronoid process of **left** mandible   CC H5 HCC

√6ᵗʰ **S02.64** Fracture of **ramus of mandible**

3,7 √7ᵗʰ **S02.640** Fracture of ramus of mandible, unspecified side   CC H5 HCC

3,7 √7ᵗʰ **S02.641** Fracture of ramus of **right** mandible   CC H5 HCC

3,7 √7ᵗʰ **S02.642** Fracture of ramus of **left** mandible   CC H5 HCC

√6ᵗʰ **S02.65** Fracture of **angle of mandible**

3,7 √7ᵗʰ **S02.650** Fracture of angle of mandible, unspecified side   CC H5 HCC

3,7 √7ᵗʰ **S02.651** Fracture of angle of **right** mandible   CC H5 HCC

3,7 √7ᵗʰ **S02.652** Fracture of angle of **left** mandible   CC H5 HCC

3,7 √x7ᵗʰ **S02.66** Fracture of **symphysis of mandible**   CC H5 HCC

√6ᵗʰ **S02.67** Fracture of **alveolus of mandible**

3,7 √7ᵗʰ **S02.670** Fracture of alveolus of mandible, unspecified side   CC H5 HCC

3,7 √7ᵗʰ **S02.671** Fracture of alveolus of **right** mandible   CC H5 HCC

3,7 √7ᵗʰ **S02.672** Fracture of alveolus of **left** mandible   CC H5 HCC

3,7 √x7ᵗʰ **S02.69** Fracture of **mandible of other specified site**   CC H5 HCC

√5ᵗʰ **S02.8** Fractures of other specified skull and facial bones

Fracture of orbit NOS

Fracture of palate

EXCLUDES 1   *fracture of orbital floor (S02.3-)*

fracture of orbital roof (S02.1-)

EXCLUDES 2   ▶*fracture of orbital floor (S02.3-)*◀

▶*fracture of orbital roof (S02.12-)*◀

CC Excl: For codes in subcategory S02.8:

CC with 7th character A or B: PDX collection 1142

CC with 7th character K: PDX collection 897

3,7 √x7ᵗʰ **S02.80** Fracture of other specified skull and facial bones, unspecified side   CC H5 HCC

3,7 √x7ᵗʰ **S02.81** Fracture of other specified skull and facial bones, **right** side   CC H5 HCC

3,7 √x7ᵗʰ **S02.82** Fracture of other specified skull and facial bones, **left** side   CC H5 HCC

√6ᵗʰ **S02.83** Fracture of **medial orbital wall**

EXCLUDES 2   *orbital floor (S02.3-)*

orbital roof (S02.12-)

3 √7ᵗʰ **S02.831** Fracture of medial orbital wall, **right** side   CC

3 √7ᵗʰ **S02.832** Fracture of medial orbital wall, **left** side   CC

3 √7ᵗʰ **S02.839** Fracture of medial orbital wall, **unspecified** side   CC

√6ᵗʰ **S02.84** Fracture of **lateral orbital wall**

EXCLUDES 2   *orbital floor (S02.3-)*

orbital roof (S02.12-)

3 √7ᵗʰ **S02.841** Fracture of lateral orbital wall, **right** side   CC

3 √7ᵗʰ **S02.842** Fracture of lateral orbital wall, **left** side   CC

3 √7ᵗʰ **S02.849** Fracture of lateral orbital wall, **unspecified** side   CC

3 √x7ᵗʰ **S02.85** Fracture of orbit, unspecified   CC

Fracture of orbit NOS

Fracture of orbit wall NOS

EXCLUDES 1   *lateral orbital wall (S02.84-)*

medial orbital wall (S02.83-)

orbital floor (S02.3-)

orbital roof (S02.12-)

√5ᵗʰ **S02.9** Fracture of unspecified skull and facial bones

2,3,7 √x7ᵗʰ **S02.91** Unspecified fracture of **skull**   MCC CC H5 HCC

CC Excl: CC with 7th character A or MCC with 7th character B: PDX collection 1140

CC Excl: CC with 7th character K: PDX collection 897

3,7 √x7ᵗʰ **S02.92** Unspecified fracture of **facial bones**   CC H5 HCC

CC Excl: CC with 7th character A or B: PDX collection 1142

CC Excl: CC with 7th character K: PDX collection 897

√4ᵗʰ **S03** Dislocation and sprain of joints and ligaments of head

INCLUDES   avulsion of joint (capsule) or ligament of head

laceration of cartilage, joint (capsule) or ligament of head

sprain of cartilage, joint (capsule) or ligament of head

traumatic hemarthrosis of joint or ligament of head

traumatic rupture of joint or ligament of head

traumatic subluxation of joint or ligament of head

traumatic tear of joint or ligament of head

Code also any associated open wound

EXCLUDES 2   *strain of muscle or tendon of head (S09.1)*

The appropriate 7th character is to be added to each code from category S03.

A   initial encounter

D   subsequent encounter

S   sequela

√5ᵗʰ **S03.0** Dislocation of jaw

Dislocation of jaw (cartilage) (meniscus)

Dislocation of mandible

Dislocation of temporomandibular (joint)

AHA: 2016,4Q,67

√x7ᵗʰ **S03.00** Dislocation of jaw, unspecified side

√x7ᵗʰ **S03.01** Dislocation of jaw, **right** side

√x7ᵗʰ **S03.02** Dislocation of jaw, **left** side

√x7ᵗʰ **S03.03** Dislocation of jaw, **bilateral**

√x7ᵗʰ **S03.1** Dislocation of septal cartilage of nose

√x7ᵗʰ **S03.2** Dislocation of tooth

√5ᵗʰ **S03.4** Sprain of jaw

Sprain of temporomandibular (joint) (ligament)

AHA: 2016,4Q,67

√x7ᵗʰ **S03.40** Sprain of jaw, unspecified side

√x7ᵗʰ **S03.41** Sprain of jaw, **right** side

√x7ᵗʰ **S03.42** Sprain of jaw, **left** side

√x7ᵗʰ **S03.43** Sprain of jaw, **bilateral**

√x7ᵗʰ **S03.8** Sprain of joints and ligaments of other parts of head

√x7ᵗʰ **S03.9** Sprain of joints and ligaments of unspecified parts of head

√4ᵗʰ **S04** Injury of cranial nerve

The selection of side should be based on the side of the body being affected

Code first any associated intracranial injury (S06.-)

Code also any associated:

open wound of head (S01.-)

skull fracture (S02.-)

The appropriate 7th character is to be added to each code from category S04.

A   initial encounter

D   subsequent encounter

S   sequela

√5ᵗʰ **S04.0** Injury of optic nerve and pathways

Use additional code to identify any visual field defect or blindness (H53.4-, H54.-)

CC Excl: For CC codes in subcategory S04.0: PDX collection 1144

√6ᵗʰ **S04.01** Injury of **optic nerve**

Injury of 2nd cranial nerve

√7ᵗʰ **S04.011** Injury of optic nerve, **right** eye   CC

√7ᵗʰ **S04.012** Injury of optic nerve, **left** eye   CC

√7ᵗʰ **S04.019** Injury of optic nerve, **unspecified** eye   CC

Injury of optic nerve NOS

√x7ᵗʰ **S04.02** Injury of optic **chiasm**   CC

N Newborn: 0   P Pediatric: 0-17   M Maternity: 9-64   A Adult: 15-124   MCC Major Complication/Comorbidity   CC Complication/Comorbidity   SW Severe Wound Dx

988   ICD-10-CM 2020

√6ᵗʰ **S04.03 Injury of optic tract and pathways**
Injury of optic radiation

√7ᵗʰ **S04.031 Injury of optic tract and pathways, right side** cc

√7ᵗʰ **S04.032 Injury of optic tract and pathways, left side** cc

√7ᵗʰ **S04.039 Injury of optic tract and pathways, unspecified side**
Injury of optic tract and pathways NOS

√6ᵗʰ **S04.04 Injury of visual cortex**

√7ᵗʰ **S04.041 Injury of visual cortex, right side** cc

√7ᵗʰ **S04.042 Injury of visual cortex, left side** cc

√7ᵗʰ **S04.049 Injury of visual cortex, unspecified side**
Injury of visual cortex NOS

√5ᵗʰ **S04.1 Injury of oculomotor nerve**
Injury of 3rd cranial nerve
CC Excl: For CC codes in subcategory S04.1: PDX collection 1145

√7ᵗʰ **S04.10 Injury of oculomotor nerve, unspecified side** cc

√x7ᵗʰ **S04.11 Injury of oculomotor nerve, right side** cc

√x7ᵗʰ **S04.12 Injury of oculomotor nerve, left side** cc

√5ᵗʰ **S04.2 Injury of trochlear nerve**
Injury of 4th cranial nerve
CC Excl: For CC codes in subcategory S04.2: PDX collection 1146

√x7ᵗʰ **S04.20 Injury of trochlear nerve, unspecified side** cc

√x7ᵗʰ **S04.21 Injury of trochlear nerve, right side** cc

√x7ᵗʰ **S04.22 Injury of trochlear nerve, left side** cc

√5ᵗʰ **S04.3 Injury of trigeminal nerve**
Injury of 5th cranial nerve
CC Excl: For CC codes in subcategory S04.3: PDX collection 1147

√x7ᵗʰ **S04.30 Injury of trigeminal nerve, unspecified side** cc

√x7ᵗʰ **S04.31 Injury of trigeminal nerve, right side** cc

√x7ᵗʰ **S04.32 Injury of trigeminal nerve, left side** cc

√5ᵗʰ **S04.4 Injury of abducent nerve**
Injury of 6th cranial nerve
CC Excl: For CC codes in subcategory S04.4: PDX collection 1148

√x7ᵗʰ **S04.40 Injury of abducent nerve, unspecified side** cc

√x7ᵗʰ **S04.41 Injury of abducent nerve, right side** cc

√x7ᵗʰ **S04.42 Injury of abducent nerve, left side** cc

√5ᵗʰ **S04.5 Injury of facial nerve**
Injury of 7th cranial nerve
CC Excl: For CC codes in subcategory S04.5: PDX collection 1149

√x7ᵗʰ **S04.50 Injury of facial nerve, unspecified side** cc

√x7ᵗʰ **S04.51 Injury of facial nerve, right side** cc

√x7ᵗʰ **S04.52 Injury of facial nerve, left side** cc

√5ᵗʰ **S04.6 Injury of acoustic nerve**
Injury of auditory nerve
Injury of 8th cranial nerve
CC Excl: For CC codes in subcategory S04.6: PDX collection 1150

√x7ᵗʰ **S04.60 Injury of acoustic nerve, unspecified side** cc

√x7ᵗʰ **S04.61 Injury of acoustic nerve, right side** cc

√x7ᵗʰ **S04.62 Injury of acoustic nerve, left side** cc

√5ᵗʰ **S04.7 Injury of accessory nerve**
Injury of 11th cranial nerve
CC Excl: For CC codes in subcategory S04.7: PDX collection 1151

√x7ᵗʰ **S04.70 Injury of accessory nerve, unspecified side** cc

√x7ᵗʰ **S04.71 Injury of accessory nerve, right side** cc

√x7ᵗʰ **S04.72 Injury of accessory nerve, left side** cc

√5ᵗʰ **S04.8 Injury of other cranial nerves**
CC Excl: For CC codes in subcategory S04.8: PDX collection 1152

√6ᵗʰ **S04.81 Injury of olfactory [1st] nerve**

√7ᵗʰ **S04.811 Injury of olfactory [1st] nerve, right side** cc

√7ᵗʰ **S04.812 Injury of olfactory [1st] nerve, left side** cc

√7ᵗʰ **S04.819 Injury of olfactory [1st] nerve, unspecified side** cc

√6ᵗʰ **S04.89 Injury of other cranial nerves**
Injury of vagus [10th] nerve

√7ᵗʰ **S04.891 Injury of other cranial nerves, right side** cc

√7ᵗʰ **S04.892 Injury of other cranial nerves, left side** cc

√7ᵗʰ **S04.899 Injury of other cranial nerves, unspecified side** cc

√x7ᵗʰ **S04.9 Injury of unspecified cranial nerve** cc
CC Excl: PDX collection 1152

√4ᵗʰ **S05 Injury of eye and orbit**
INCLUDES open wound of eye and orbit
EXCLUDES 2 *2nd cranial [optic] nerve injury (S04.0-)*
3rd cranial [oculomotor] nerve injury (S04.1-)
open wound of eyelid and periocular area (S01.1-)
orbital bone fracture (S02.1-, S02.3-, S02.8-)
superficial injury of eyelid (S00.1-S00.2)

The appropriate 7th character is to be added to each code from category S05.
A   initial encounter
D   subsequent encounter
S   sequela

CC Excl: For CC codes in category S05, unless otherwise noted: PDX collection 1139

√5ᵗʰ **S05.0 Injury of conjunctiva and corneal abrasion without foreign body**
EXCLUDES 1 *foreign body in conjunctival sac (T15.1)*
foreign body in cornea (T15.0)

√x7ᵗʰ **S05.00 Injury of conjunctiva and corneal abrasion without foreign body, unspecified eye**

√x7ᵗʰ **S05.01 Injury of conjunctiva and corneal abrasion without foreign body, right eye**

√x7ᵗʰ **S05.02 Injury of conjunctiva and corneal abrasion without foreign body, left eye**

√5ᵗʰ **S05.1 Contusion of eyeball and orbital tissues**
Traumatic hyphema
EXCLUDES 2 *black eye NOS (S00.1)*
contusion of eyelid and periocular area (S00.1)

√x7ᵗʰ **S05.10 Contusion of eyeball and orbital tissues, unspecified eye**

√x7ᵗʰ **S05.11 Contusion of eyeball and orbital tissues, right eye**

√x7ᵗʰ **S05.12 Contusion of eyeball and orbital tissues, left eye**

√5ᵗʰ **S05.2 Ocular laceration and rupture with prolapse or loss of intraocular tissue**

√x7ᵗʰ **S05.20 Ocular laceration and rupture with prolapse or loss of intraocular tissue, unspecified eye** cc

√x7ᵗʰ **S05.21 Ocular laceration and rupture with prolapse or loss of intraocular tissue, right eye** cc

√x7ᵗʰ **S05.22 Ocular laceration and rupture with prolapse or loss of intraocular tissue, left eye** cc

√5ᵗʰ **S05.3 Ocular laceration without prolapse or loss of intraocular tissue**
Laceration of eye NOS
DEF: Tear in ocular tissue without displacing structures that is due to blunt trauma. It is characterized by pain, redness, and decreased vision.

√x7ᵗʰ **S05.30 Ocular laceration without prolapse or loss of intraocular tissue, unspecified eye** cc

√x7ᵗʰ **S05.31 Ocular laceration without prolapse or loss of intraocular tissue, right eye** cc

√x7ᵗʰ **S05.32 Ocular laceration without prolapse or loss of intraocular tissue, left eye** cc

Chapter 19. Injury, Poisoning and Certain Other Consequences of External Causes

✓5ᵗʰ **S05.4 Penetrating wound** of orbit with or without foreign body

> EXCLUDES 2   *retained (old) foreign body following penetrating wound in orbit (H05.5-)*

    ✓x7ᵗʰ **S05.40 Penetrating wound of orbit with or without foreign body, unspecified eye**   CC

    ✓x7ᵗʰ **S05.41 Penetrating wound of orbit with or without foreign body, right eye**   CC

    ✓x7ᵗʰ **S05.42 Penetrating wound of orbit with or without foreign body, left eye**   CC

✓5ᵗʰ **S05.5 Penetrating wound with foreign body** of eyeball

> EXCLUDES 2   *retained (old) intraocular foreign body (H44.6-, H44.7)*

> **CC Excl:** For CC Codes in subcategory S05.5: PDX collection 1153

    ✓x7ᵗʰ **S05.50 Penetrating wound with foreign body of unspecified eyeball**   CC

    ✓x7ᵗʰ **S05.51 Penetrating wound with foreign body of right eyeball**   CC

    ✓x7ᵗʰ **S05.52 Penetrating wound with foreign body of left eyeball**   CC

✓5ᵗʰ **S05.6 Penetrating wound without foreign body** of eyeball

    Ocular penetration NOS

    ✓x7ᵗʰ **S05.60 Penetrating wound without foreign body of unspecified eyeball**

    ✓x7ᵗʰ **S05.61 Penetrating wound without foreign body of right eyeball**

    ✓x7ᵗʰ **S05.62 Penetrating wound without foreign body of left eyeball**

✓5ᵗʰ **S05.7 Avulsion of eye**

    Traumatic enucleation

    ✓x7ᵗʰ **S05.70 Avulsion of unspecified eye**   CC

    ✓x7ᵗʰ **S05.71 Avulsion of right eye**   CC

    ✓x7ᵗʰ **S05.72 Avulsion of left eye**   CC

✓5ᵗʰ **S05.8 Other injuries of eye and orbit**

    Lacrimal duct injury

    ✓6ᵗʰ **S05.8X Other injuries of eye and orbit**

      ✓7ᵗʰ **S05.8X1 Other injuries of right eye and orbit**   CC

      ✓7ᵗʰ **S05.8X2 Other injuries of left eye and orbit**   CC

      ✓7ᵗʰ **S05.8X9 Other injuries of unspecified eye and orbit**   CC

✓5ᵗʰ **S05.9 Unspecified injury of eye and orbit**

    Injury of eye NOS

    ✓x7ᵗʰ **S05.90 Unspecified injury of unspecified eye and orbit**

    ✓x7ᵗʰ **S05.91 Unspecified injury of right eye and orbit**   CC

    ✓x7ᵗʰ **S05.92 Unspecified injury of left eye and orbit**   CC

✓4ᵗʰ **S06 Intracranial injury**

> **NOTE**   7th characters D and S do not apply to codes in category S06 with 6th character 7 – death due to brain injury prior to regaining consciousness, or 8 – death due to other cause prior to regaining consciousness.

> **INCLUDES**   traumatic brain injury

Code also any associated:
   open wound of head (S01.-)
   skull fracture (S02.-)

> EXCLUDES 1   *head injury NOS (S09.90)*

AHA: 2017,4Q,25; 2017,1Q,42; 2015,3Q,37

TIP: Do not assign Z87.820 Personal history of traumatic brain injury, when residual conditions persist after an intracranial injury. The codes for the residual conditions should be first listed, followed by a code from category S06 using seventh character S to identify sequelae.

> The appropriate 7th character is to be added to each code from category S06.
> A   initial encounter
> D   subsequent encounter
> S   sequela

> **CC Excl:** For CC/MCC codes in category S06, unless otherwise noted: PDX collection 1154

✓5ᵗʰ **S06.0 Concussion**

    Commotio cerebri

> EXCLUDES 1   *concussion with other intracranial injuries classified in subcategories S06.1- to S06.6- , S06.81- and S06.82- — code to specified intracranial injury*

    AHA: 2016,4Q,67-68

    ✓6ᵗʰ **S06.0X Concussion**

      8 ✓7ᵗʰ **S06.0X0 Concussion** without loss of consciousness   CC HCC

      8 ✓7ᵗʰ **S06.0X1 Concussion with loss of consciousness of 30 minutes or less**   CC H5 HCC

      8 ✓7ᵗʰ **S06.0X9 Concussion with loss of consciousness of unspecified duration**   CC H5 HCC
       Concussion NOS

✓5ᵗʰ **S06.1 Traumatic cerebral edema**

    Diffuse traumatic cerebral edema
    Focal traumatic cerebral edema

> **CC Excl:** For MCC codes in category S06.1, unless otherwise noted: PDX collection 1155

    ✓6ᵗʰ **S06.1X Traumatic** cerebral edema

      7 ✓7ᵗʰ **S06.1X0 Traumatic cerebral edema without loss of consciousness**   MCC HCC
       CC Excl: PDX collection 612

      7 ✓7ᵗʰ **S06.1X1 Traumatic cerebral edema with loss of consciousness of 30 minutes or less**   MCC H5 HCC

      7 ✓7ᵗʰ **S06.1X2 Traumatic cerebral edema with loss of consciousness of 31 minutes to 59 minutes**   MCC H5 HCC

      7 ✓7ᵗʰ **S06.1X3 Traumatic cerebral edema with loss of consciousness of 1 hour to 5 hours 59 minutes**   MCC H5 HCC

      7 ✓7ᵗʰ **S06.1X4 Traumatic cerebral edema with loss of consciousness of 6 hours to 24 hours**   MCC H5 HCC

      7 ✓7ᵗʰ **S06.1X5 Traumatic cerebral edema with loss of consciousness greater than 24 hours with return to pre-existing conscious level**   MCC H5 HCC

      7 ✓7ᵗʰ **S06.1X6 Traumatic cerebral edema with loss of consciousness greater than 24 hours without return to pre-existing conscious level with patient surviving**   MCC H5 HCC
       CC Excl: PDX collection 1154

N Newborn: 0   P Pediatric: 0-17   M Maternity: 9-64   A Adult: 15-124   MCC Major Complication/Comorbidity   CC Complication/Comorbidity   SW Severe Wound Dx

990   ICD-10-CM 2020

S05.4–S06.1X6

√7ᵗʰ **S06.1X7 Traumatic cerebral edema with loss of consciousness of** any duration with death due to brain injury prior to regaining consciousness   `MCC` `H5`
    CC Excl: PDX collection 1154

√7ᵗʰ **S06.1X8 Traumatic cerebral edema with loss of consciousness of** any duration with death due to **other** cause prior to regaining consciousness   `MCC` `H5`
    CC Excl: PDX collection 1154

7 √7ᵗʰ **S06.1X9 Traumatic cerebral edema with loss of consciousness of unspecified duration**   `MCC` `H5` `HCC`
    Traumatic cerebral edema NOS

√5ᵗʰ **S06.2 Diffuse traumatic brain injury**
    Diffuse axonal brain injury
    EXCLUDES 1   traumatic diffuse cerebral edema (S06.1X-)

√6ᵗʰ **S06.2X Diffuse traumatic brain injury**

7 √7ᵗʰ **S06.2X0 Diffuse traumatic brain injury** without loss of consciousness   `HCC`

7 √7ᵗʰ **S06.2X1 Diffuse traumatic brain injury with loss of consciousness of** 30 minutes or less   `CC` `H5` `HCC`

7 √7ᵗʰ **S06.2X2 Diffuse traumatic brain injury with loss of consciousness of** 31 minutes to 59 minutes   `CC` `H5` `HCC`

7 √7ᵗʰ **S06.2X3 Diffuse traumatic brain injury with loss of consciousness of** 1 hour to 5 hours 59 minutes   `CC` `H5` `HCC`

7 √7ᵗʰ **S06.2X4 Diffuse traumatic brain injury with loss of consciousness of** 6 hours to 24 hours   `CC` `H5` `HCC`

7 √7ᵗʰ **S06.2X5 Diffuse traumatic brain injury with loss of consciousness** greater than 24 hours with return to pre-existing conscious levels   `CC` `H5` `HCC`

7 √7ᵗʰ **S06.2X6 Diffuse traumatic brain injury with loss of consciousness** greater than 24 hours without return to pre-existing conscious level with patient surviving   `MCC` `H5` `HCC`

√7ᵗʰ **S06.2X7 Diffuse traumatic brain injury with loss of consciousness of** any duration with death due to brain injury prior to regaining consciousness   `MCC` `H5`

√7ᵗʰ **S06.2X8 Diffuse traumatic brain injury with loss of consciousness of** any duration with death due to **other** cause prior to regaining consciousness   `MCC` `H5`

7 √7ᵗʰ **S06.2X9 Diffuse traumatic brain injury with loss of consciousness of unspecified duration**   `CC` `H5` `HCC`
    Diffuse traumatic brain injury NOS

√5ᵗʰ **S06.3 Focal traumatic brain injury**
    EXCLUDES 1   any condition classifiable to S06.4-S06.6
            focal cerebral edema (S06.1)

√6ᵗʰ **S06.30 Unspecified focal traumatic brain injury**

7 √7ᵗʰ **S06.300 Unspecified focal traumatic brain injury** without loss of consciousness   `HCC`

7 √7ᵗʰ **S06.301 Unspecified focal traumatic brain injury with loss of consciousness of** 30 minutes or less   `CC` `H5` `HCC`

7 √7ᵗʰ **S06.302 Unspecified focal traumatic brain injury with loss of consciousness of** 31 minutes to 59 minutes   `CC` `H5` `HCC`

7 √7ᵗʰ **S06.303 Unspecified focal traumatic brain injury with loss of consciousness of** 1 hour to 5 hours 59 minutes   `CC` `H5` `HCC`

7 √7ᵗʰ **S06.304 Unspecified focal traumatic brain injury with loss of consciousness of** 6 hours to 24 hours   `CC` `H5` `HCC`

7 √7ᵗʰ **S06.305 Unspecified focal traumatic brain injury with loss of consciousness** greater than 24 hours with return to pre-existing conscious level   `CC` `H5` `HCC`

7 √7ᵗʰ **S06.306 Unspecified focal traumatic brain injury with loss of consciousness** greater than 24 hours without return to pre-existing conscious level with patient surviving   `MCC` `H5` `HCC`

√7ᵗʰ **S06.307 Unspecified focal traumatic brain injury with loss of consciousness of** any duration with death due to brain injury prior to regaining consciousness   `MCC` `H5`

√7ᵗʰ **S06.308 Unspecified focal traumatic brain injury with loss of consciousness of** any duration with death due to **other** cause prior to regaining consciousness   `MCC` `H5`

7 √7ᵗʰ **S06.309 Unspecified focal traumatic brain injury with loss of consciousness of unspecified duration**   `CC` `H5` `HCC`
    Unspecified focal traumatic brain injury NOS

√6ᵗʰ **S06.31 Contusion and laceration of** right cerebrum

7 √7ᵗʰ **S06.310 Contusion and laceration of right cerebrum** without loss of consciousness   `MCC` `H5` `HCC`

7 √7ᵗʰ **S06.311 Contusion and laceration of right cerebrum with loss of consciousness of** 30 minutes or less   `MCC` `H5` `HCC`

7 √7ᵗʰ **S06.312 Contusion and laceration of right cerebrum with loss of consciousness of** 31 minutes to 59 minutes   `MCC` `H5` `HCC`

7 √7ᵗʰ **S06.313 Contusion and laceration of right cerebrum with loss of consciousness of** 1 hour to 5 hours 59 minutes   `MCC` `H5` `HCC`

7 √7ᵗʰ **S06.314 Contusion and laceration of right cerebrum with loss of consciousness of** 6 hours to 24 hours   `MCC` `H5` `HCC`

7 √7ᵗʰ **S06.315 Contusion and laceration of right cerebrum with loss of consciousness** greater than 24 hours with return to pre-existing conscious level   `MCC` `H5` `HCC`

7 √7ᵗʰ **S06.316 Contusion and laceration of right cerebrum with loss of consciousness** greater than 24 hours without return to pre-existing conscious level with patient surviving   `MCC` `H5` `HCC`

√7ᵗʰ **S06.317** **Contusion and laceration of right cerebrum with loss of consciousness of any duration with death due to brain injury prior to regaining consciousness** MCC H5

√7ᵗʰ **S06.318** **Contusion and laceration of right cerebrum with loss of consciousness of any duration with death due to other cause prior to regaining consciousness** MCC H5

7 √7ᵗʰ **S06.319** **Contusion and laceration of right cerebrum with loss of consciousness of unspecified duration** MCC H5 HCC

Contusion and laceration of right cerebrum NOS

√6ᵗʰ **S06.32** **Contusion and laceration of left cerebrum**

7 √7ᵗʰ **S06.320** **Contusion and laceration of left cerebrum without loss of consciousness** MCC H5 HCC

7 √7ᵗʰ **S06.321** **Contusion and laceration of left cerebrum with loss of consciousness of 30 minutes or less** MCC H5 HCC

7 √7ᵗʰ **S06.322** **Contusion and laceration of left cerebrum with loss of consciousness of 31 minutes to 59 minutes** MCC H5 HCC

7 √7ᵗʰ **S06.323** **Contusion and laceration of left cerebrum with loss of consciousness of 1 hour to 5 hours 59 minutes** MCC H5 HCC

7 √7ᵗʰ **S06.324** **Contusion and laceration of left cerebrum with loss of consciousness of 6 hours to 24 hours** MCC H5 HCC

7 √7ᵗʰ **S06.325** **Contusion and laceration of left cerebrum with loss of consciousness greater than 24 hours with return to pre-existing conscious level** MCC H5 HCC

7 √7ᵗʰ **S06.326** **Contusion and laceration of left cerebrum with loss of consciousness greater than 24 hours without return to pre-existing conscious level with patient surviving** MCC H5 HCC

√7ᵗʰ **S06.327** **Contusion and laceration of left cerebrum with loss of consciousness of any duration with death due to brain injury prior to regaining consciousness** MCC H5

√7ᵗʰ **S06.328** **Contusion and laceration of left cerebrum with loss of consciousness of any duration with death due to other cause prior to regaining consciousness** MCC H5

7 √7ᵗʰ **S06.329** **Contusion and laceration of left cerebrum with loss of consciousness of unspecified duration** MCC H5 HCC

Contusion and laceration of left cerebrum NOS

√6ᵗʰ **S06.33** **Contusion and laceration of cerebrum, unspecified**

7 √7ᵗʰ **S06.330** **Contusion and laceration of cerebrum, unspecified, without loss of consciousness** MCC H5 HCC

7 √7ᵗʰ **S06.331** **Contusion and laceration of cerebrum, unspecified, with loss of consciousness of 30 minutes or less** MCC H5 HCC

7 √7ᵗʰ **S06.332** **Contusion and laceration of cerebrum, unspecified, with loss of consciousness of 31 minutes to 59 minutes** MCC H5 HCC

7 √7ᵗʰ **S06.333** **Contusion and laceration of cerebrum, unspecified, with loss of consciousness of 1 hour to 5 hours 59 minutes** MCC H5 HCC

7 √7ᵗʰ **S06.334** **Contusion and laceration of cerebrum, unspecified, with loss of consciousness of 6 hours to 24 hours** MCC H5 HCC

7 √7ᵗʰ **S06.335** **Contusion and laceration of cerebrum, unspecified, with loss of consciousness greater than 24 hours with return to pre-existing conscious level** MCC H5 HCC

7 √7ᵗʰ **S06.336** **Contusion and laceration of cerebrum, unspecified, with loss of consciousness greater than 24 hours without return to pre-existing conscious level with patient surviving** MCC H5 HCC

√7ᵗʰ **S06.337** **Contusion and laceration of cerebrum, unspecified, with loss of consciousness of any duration with death due to brain injury prior to regaining consciousness** MCC H5

√7ᵗʰ **S06.338** **Contusion and laceration of cerebrum, unspecified, with loss of consciousness of any duration with death due to other cause prior to regaining consciousness** MCC H5

7 √7ᵗʰ **S06.339** **Contusion and laceration of cerebrum, unspecified, with loss of consciousness of unspecified duration** MCC H5 HCC

Contusion and laceration of cerebrum NOS

√6ᵗʰ **S06.34** **Traumatic hemorrhage of right cerebrum**

Traumatic intracerebral hemorrhage and hematoma of right cerebrum

7 √7ᵗʰ **S06.340** **Traumatic hemorrhage of right cerebrum without loss of consciousness** MCC H5 HCC

7 √7ᵗʰ **S06.341** **Traumatic hemorrhage of right cerebrum with loss of consciousness of 30 minutes or less** MCC H5 HCC

7 √7ᵗʰ **S06.342** **Traumatic hemorrhage of right cerebrum with loss of consciousness of 31 minutes to 59 minutes** MCC H5 HCC

7 √7ᵗʰ **S06.343** **Traumatic hemorrhage of right cerebrum with loss of consciousness of 1 hours to 5 hours 59 minutes** MCC H5 HCC

7 √7ᵗʰ **S06.344** **Traumatic hemorrhage of right cerebrum with loss of consciousness of 6 hours to 24 hours** MCC H5 HCC

7 √7ᵗʰ **S06.345** **Traumatic hemorrhage of right cerebrum with loss of consciousness greater than 24 hours with return to pre-existing conscious level** MCC H5 HCC

7 √7ᵗʰ **S06.346** **Traumatic hemorrhage of right cerebrum with loss of consciousness greater than 24 hours without return to pre-existing conscious level with patient surviving** MCC H5 HCC

√7ᵗʰ **S06.347** **Traumatic hemorrhage of right cerebrum with loss of consciousness of any duration with death due to brain injury prior to regaining consciousness** MCC H5

N Newborn: 0   P Pediatric: 0-17   M Maternity: 9-64   A Adult: 15-124   **MCC** Major Complication/Comorbidity   **CC** Complication/Comorbidity   **SW** Severe Wound Dx

992   ICD-10-CM 2020

7 ✓7ʰ **S06.348** **Traumatic hemorrhage of right cerebrum with loss of consciousness of any duration with death due to other cause prior to regaining consciousness** `MCC` `H5`

7 ✓7ʰ **S06.349** **Traumatic hemorrhage of right cerebrum with loss of consciousness of unspecified duration** `MCC` `H5` `HCC`
Traumatic hemorrhage of right cerebrum NOS

✓6ʰ **S06.35** **Traumatic hemorrhage of left cerebrum**
Traumatic intracerebral hemorrhage and hematoma of left cerebrum

7 ✓7ʰ **S06.350** **Traumatic hemorrhage of left cerebrum without loss of consciousness** `MCC` `H5` `HCC`

7 ✓7ʰ **S06.351** **Traumatic hemorrhage of left cerebrum with loss of consciousness of 30 minutes or less** `MCC` `H5` `HCC`

7 ✓7ʰ **S06.352** **Traumatic hemorrhage of left cerebrum with loss of consciousness of 31 minutes to 59 minutes** `MCC` `H5` `HCC`

7 ✓7ʰ **S06.353** **Traumatic hemorrhage of left cerebrum with loss of consciousness of 1 hours to 5 hours 59 minutes** `MCC` `H5` `HCC`

7 ✓7ʰ **S06.354** **Traumatic hemorrhage of left cerebrum with loss of consciousness of 6 hours to 24 hours** `MCC` `H5` `HCC`

7 ✓7ʰ **S06.355** **Traumatic hemorrhage of left cerebrum with loss of consciousness greater than 24 hours with return to pre-existing conscious level** `MCC` `H5` `HCC`

7 ✓7ʰ **S06.356** **Traumatic hemorrhage of left cerebrum with loss of consciousness greater than 24 hours without return to pre-existing conscious level with patient surviving** `MCC` `H5` `HCC`

✓7ʰ **S06.357** **Traumatic hemorrhage of left cerebrum with loss of consciousness of any duration with death due to brain injury prior to regaining consciousness** `MCC` `H5`

✓7ʰ **S06.358** **Traumatic hemorrhage of left cerebrum with loss of consciousness of any duration with death due to other cause prior to regaining consciousness** `MCC` `H5`

7 ✓7ʰ **S06.359** **Traumatic hemorrhage of left cerebrum with loss of consciousness of unspecified duration** `MCC` `H5` `HCC`
Traumatic hemorrhage of left cerebrum NOS

✓6ʰ **S06.36** **Traumatic hemorrhage of cerebrum, unspecified**
Traumatic intracerebral hemorrhage and hematoma, unspecified

7 ✓7ʰ **S06.360** **Traumatic hemorrhage of cerebrum, unspecified, without loss of consciousness** `MCC` `H5` `HCC`

7 ✓7ʰ **S06.361** **Traumatic hemorrhage of cerebrum, unspecified, with loss of consciousness of 30 minutes or less** `MCC` `H5` `HCC`

7 ✓7ʰ **S06.362** **Traumatic hemorrhage of cerebrum, unspecified, with loss of consciousness of 31 minutes to 59 minutes** `MCC` `H5` `HCC`

7 ✓7ʰ **S06.363** **Traumatic hemorrhage of cerebrum, unspecified, with loss of consciousness of 1 hours to 5 hours 59 minutes** `MCC` `H5` `HCC`

7 ✓7ʰ **S06.364** **Traumatic hemorrhage of cerebrum, unspecified, with loss of consciousness of 6 hours to 24 hours** `MCC` `H5` `HCC`

7 ✓7ʰ **S06.365** **Traumatic hemorrhage of cerebrum, unspecified, with loss of consciousness greater than 24 hours with return to pre-existing conscious level** `MCC` `H5` `HCC`

7 ✓7ʰ **S06.366** **Traumatic hemorrhage of cerebrum, unspecified, with loss of consciousness greater than 24 hours without return to pre-existing conscious level with patient surviving** `MCC` `H5` `HCC`

✓7ʰ **S06.367** **Traumatic hemorrhage of cerebrum, unspecified, with loss of consciousness of any duration with death due to brain injury prior to regaining consciousness** `MCC` `H5`

✓7ʰ **S06.368** **Traumatic hemorrhage of cerebrum, unspecified, with loss of consciousness of any duration with death due to other cause prior to regaining consciousness** `MCC` `H5`

7 ✓7ʰ **S06.369** **Traumatic hemorrhage of cerebrum, unspecified, with loss of consciousness of unspecified duration** `MCC` `H5` `HCC`
Traumatic hemorrhage of cerebrum NOS

✓6ʰ **S06.37** **Contusion, laceration, and hemorrhage of cerebellum**

7 ✓7ʰ **S06.370** **Contusion, laceration, and hemorrhage of cerebellum without loss of consciousness** `MCC` `H5` `HCC`
CC Excl: No Excl

7 ✓7ʰ **S06.371** **Contusion, laceration, and hemorrhage of cerebellum with loss of consciousness of 30 minutes or less** `CC` `H5` `HCC`

7 ✓7ʰ **S06.372** **Contusion, laceration, and hemorrhage of cerebellum with loss of consciousness of 31 minutes to 59 minutes** `CC` `H5` `HCC`

7 ✓7ʰ **S06.373** **Contusion, laceration, and hemorrhage of cerebellum with loss of consciousness of 1 hour to 5 hours 59 minutes** `CC` `H5` `HCC`

7 ✓7ʰ **S06.374** **Contusion, laceration, and hemorrhage of cerebellum with loss of consciousness of 6 hours to 24 hours** `CC` `H5` `HCC`

7 ✓7ʰ **S06.375** **Contusion, laceration, and hemorrhage of cerebellum with loss of consciousness greater than 24 hours with return to pre-existing conscious level** `CC` `H5` `HCC`

7 ✓7ʰ **S06.376** **Contusion, laceration, and hemorrhage of cerebellum with loss of consciousness greater than 24 hours without return to pre-existing conscious level with patient surviving** `MCC` `H5` `HCC`

✓7ʰ **S06.377** **Contusion, laceration, and hemorrhage of cerebellum with loss of consciousness of any duration with death due to brain injury prior to regaining consciousness** `MCC` `H5`

√7ᵗʰ **S06.378** **Contusion, laceration, and hemorrhage of cerebellum with loss of consciousness of any duration with death due to other cause prior to regaining consciousness**   MCC H5

7 √7ᵗʰ **S06.379** **Contusion, laceration, and hemorrhage of cerebellum with loss of consciousness of unspecified duration**   CC H5 HCC
Contusion, laceration, and hemorrhage of cerebellum NOS

√6ᵗʰ **S06.38** **Contusion, laceration, and hemorrhage of brainstem**

7 √7ᵗʰ **S06.380** **Contusion, laceration, and hemorrhage of brainstem without loss of consciousness**   MCC H5 HCC
CC Excl: No Excl

7 √7ᵗʰ **S06.381** **Contusion, laceration, and hemorrhage of brainstem with loss of consciousness of 30 minutes or less**   CC H5 HCC

7 √7ᵗʰ **S06.382** **Contusion, laceration, and hemorrhage of brainstem with loss of consciousness of 31 minutes to 59 minutes**   CC H5 HCC

7 √7ᵗʰ **S06.383** **Contusion, laceration, and hemorrhage of brainstem with loss of consciousness of 1 hour to 5 hours 59 minutes**   CC H5 HCC

7 √7ᵗʰ **S06.384** **Contusion, laceration, and hemorrhage of brainstem with loss of consciousness of 6 hours to 24 hours**   CC H5 HCC

7 √7ᵗʰ **S06.385** **Contusion, laceration, and hemorrhage of brainstem with loss of consciousness greater than 24 hours with return to pre-existing conscious level**   CC H5 HCC

7 √7ᵗʰ **S06.386** **Contusion, laceration, and hemorrhage of brainstem with loss of consciousness greater than 24 hours without return to pre-existing conscious level with patient surviving**   MCC H5 HCC

√7ᵗʰ **S06.387** **Contusion, laceration, and hemorrhage of brainstem with loss of consciousness of any duration with death due to brain injury prior to regaining consciousness**   MCC H5

√7ᵗʰ **S06.388** **Contusion, laceration, and hemorrhage of brainstem with loss of consciousness of any duration with death due to other cause prior to regaining consciousness**   MCC H5

7 √7ᵗʰ **S06.389** **Contusion, laceration, and hemorrhage of brainstem with loss of consciousness of unspecified duration**   CC H5 HCC
Contusion, laceration, and hemorrhage of brainstem NOS

√5ᵗʰ **S06.4** **Epidural hemorrhage**
Extradural hemorrhage NOS
Extradural hemorrhage (traumatic)
DEF: Epidural space: Space between the endosteum of the cranium (skull) and the dura mater, the outermost layer of a three-layer membrane that covers the brain.

√6ᵗʰ **S06.4X** **Epidural hemorrhage**

7 √7ᵗʰ **S06.4X0** **Epidural hemorrhage without loss of consciousness**   MCC H5 HCC

7 √7ᵗʰ **S06.4X1** **Epidural hemorrhage with loss of consciousness of 30 minutes or less**   MCC H5 HCC

7 √7ᵗʰ **S06.4X2** **Epidural hemorrhage with loss of consciousness of 31 minutes to 59 minutes**   MCC H5 HCC

7 √7ᵗʰ **S06.4X3** **Epidural hemorrhage with loss of consciousness of 1 hour to 5 hours 59 minutes**   MCC H5 HCC

7 √7ᵗʰ **S06.4X4** **Epidural hemorrhage with loss of consciousness of 6 hours to 24 hours**   MCC H5 HCC

7 √7ᵗʰ **S06.4X5** **Epidural hemorrhage with loss of consciousness greater than 24 hours with return to pre-existing conscious level**   MCC H5 HCC

7 √7ᵗʰ **S06.4X6** **Epidural hemorrhage with loss of consciousness greater than 24 hours without return to pre-existing conscious level with patient surviving**   MCC H5 HCC

√7ᵗʰ **S06.4X7** **Epidural hemorrhage with loss of consciousness of any duration with death due to brain injury prior to regaining consciousness**   MCC H5

√7ᵗʰ **S06.4X8** **Epidural hemorrhage with loss of consciousness of any duration with death due to other causes prior to regaining consciousness**   MCC H5

7 √7ᵗʰ **S06.4X9** **Epidural hemorrhage with loss of consciousness of unspecified duration**   MCC H5 HCC
Epidural hemorrhage NOS

√5ᵗʰ **S06.5** **Traumatic subdural hemorrhage**
DEF: Subdural: Potential space between the dura mater and arachnoid membrane around the brain.

√6ᵗʰ **S06.5X** **Traumatic subdural hemorrhage**

7 √7ᵗʰ **S06.5X0** **Traumatic subdural hemorrhage without loss of consciousness**   MCC H5 HCC

7 √7ᵗʰ **S06.5X1** **Traumatic subdural hemorrhage with loss of consciousness of 30 minutes or less**   MCC H5 HCC

7 √7ᵗʰ **S06.5X2** **Traumatic subdural hemorrhage with loss of consciousness of 31 minutes to 59 minutes**   MCC H5 HCC

7 √7ᵗʰ **S06.5X3** **Traumatic subdural hemorrhage with loss of consciousness of 1 hour to 5 hours 59 minutes**   MCC H5 HCC

7 √7ᵗʰ **S06.5X4** **Traumatic subdural hemorrhage with loss of consciousness of 6 hours to 24 hours**   MCC H5 HCC

7 √7ᵗʰ **S06.5X5** **Traumatic subdural hemorrhage with loss of consciousness greater than 24 hours with return to pre-existing conscious level**   MCC H5 HCC

7 √7ᵗʰ **S06.5X6** **Traumatic subdural hemorrhage with loss of consciousness greater than 24 hours without return to pre-existing conscious level with patient surviving**   MCC H5 HCC

√7ᵗʰ **S06.5X7** **Traumatic subdural hemorrhage with loss of consciousness of any duration with death due to brain injury before regaining consciousness**   MCC H5

√7ᵗʰ **S06.5X8** **Traumatic subdural hemorrhage with loss of consciousness of any duration with death due to other cause before regaining consciousness**   MCC H5

7 ✓7th **S06.5X9** **Traumatic subdural hemorrhage with loss of consciousness of unspecified duration** `MCC` `H5` `HCC`
Traumatic subdural hemorrhage NOS

✓5th **S06.6** **Traumatic subarachnoid hemorrhage**
DEF: Subarachnoid: Space located between the arachnoid membrane and the pia mater that contains cerebrospinal fluid.

✓6th **S06.6X** **Traumatic subarachnoid hemorrhage**

7 ✓7th **S06.6X0** **Traumatic subarachnoid hemorrhage without loss of consciousness** `MCC` `H5` `HCC`

7 ✓7th **S06.6X1** **Traumatic subarachnoid hemorrhage with loss of consciousness of 30 minutes or less** `MCC` `H5` `HCC`

7 ✓7th **S06.6X2** **Traumatic subarachnoid hemorrhage with loss of consciousness of 31 minutes to 59 minutes** `MCC` `H5` `HCC`

7 ✓7th **S06.6X3** **Traumatic subarachnoid hemorrhage with loss of consciousness of 1 hour to 5 hours 59 minutes** `MCC` `H5` `HCC`

7 ✓7th **S06.6X4** **Traumatic subarachnoid hemorrhage with loss of consciousness of 6 hours to 24 hours** `MCC` `H5` `HCC`

7 ✓7th **S06.6X5** **Traumatic subarachnoid hemorrhage with loss of consciousness greater than 24 hours with return to pre-existing conscious level** `MCC` `H5` `HCC`

7 ✓7th **S06.6X6** **Traumatic subarachnoid hemorrhage with loss of consciousness greater than 24 hours without return to pre-existing conscious level with patient surviving** `MCC` `H5` `HCC`

✓7th **S06.6X7** **Traumatic subarachnoid hemorrhage with loss of consciousness of any duration with death due to brain injury prior to regaining consciousness** `MCC` `H5`

✓7th **S06.6X8** **Traumatic subarachnoid hemorrhage with loss of consciousness of any duration with death due to other cause prior to regaining consciousness** `MCC` `H5`

7 ✓7th **S06.6X9** **Traumatic subarachnoid hemorrhage with loss of consciousness of unspecified duration** `MCC` `H5` `HCC`
Traumatic subarachnoid hemorrhage NOS

✓5th **S06.8** **Other specified intracranial injuries**

✓6th **S06.81** **Injury of right internal carotid artery, intracranial portion, not elsewhere classified**

7 ✓7th **S06.810** **Injury of right internal carotid artery, intracranial portion, not elsewhere classified without loss of consciousness** `HCC`

7 ✓7th **S06.811** **Injury of right internal carotid artery, intracranial portion, not elsewhere classified with loss of consciousness of 30 minutes or less** `CC` `H5` `HCC`

7 ✓7th **S06.812** **Injury of right internal carotid artery, intracranial portion, not elsewhere classified with loss of consciousness of 31 minutes to 59 minutes** `CC` `H5` `HCC`

7 ✓7th **S06.813** **Injury of right internal carotid artery, intracranial portion, not elsewhere classified with loss of consciousness of 1 hour to 5 hours 59 minutes** `CC` `H5` `HCC`

7 ✓7th **S06.814** **Injury of right internal carotid artery, intracranial portion, not elsewhere classified with loss of consciousness of 6 hours to 24 hours** `CC` `H5` `HCC`

7 ✓7th **S06.815** **Injury of right internal carotid artery, intracranial portion, not elsewhere classified with loss of consciousness greater than 24 hours with return to pre-existing conscious level** `CC` `H5` `HCC`

7 ✓7th **S06.816** **Injury of right internal carotid artery, intracranial portion, not elsewhere classified with loss of consciousness greater than 24 hours without return to pre-existing conscious level with patient surviving** `MCC` `H5` `HCC`

✓7th **S06.817** **Injury of right internal carotid artery, intracranial portion, not elsewhere classified with loss of consciousness of any duration with death due to brain injury prior to regaining consciousness** `MCC` `H5`

✓7th **S06.818** **Injury of right internal carotid artery, intracranial portion, not elsewhere classified with loss of consciousness of any duration with death due to other cause prior to regaining consciousness** `MCC` `H5`

7 ✓7th **S06.819** **Injury of right internal carotid artery, intracranial portion, not elsewhere classified with loss of consciousness of unspecified duration** `CC` `H5` `HCC`
Injury of right internal carotid artery, intracranial portion, not elsewhere classified NOS

✓6th **S06.82** **Injury of left internal carotid artery, intracranial portion, not elsewhere classified**

7 ✓7th **S06.820** **Injury of left internal carotid artery, intracranial portion, not elsewhere classified without loss of consciousness** `HCC`

7 ✓7th **S06.821** **Injury of left internal carotid artery, intracranial portion, not elsewhere classified with loss of consciousness of 30 minutes or less** `CC` `H5` `HCC`

7 ✓7th **S06.822** **Injury of left internal carotid artery, intracranial portion, not elsewhere classified with loss of consciousness of 31 minutes to 59 minutes** `CC` `H5` `HCC`

7 ✓7th **S06.823** **Injury of left internal carotid artery, intracranial portion, not elsewhere classified with loss of consciousness of 1 hour to 5 hours 59 minutes** `CC` `H5` `HCC`

7 ✓7th **S06.824** **Injury of left internal carotid artery, intracranial portion, not elsewhere classified with loss of consciousness of 6 hours to 24 hours** `CC` `H5` `HCC`

7 ✓7th **S06.825** **Injury of left internal carotid artery, intracranial portion, not elsewhere classified with loss of consciousness greater than 24 hours with return to pre-existing conscious level** `CC` `H5` `HCC`

7 √7ᵗʰ **S06.826** **Injury of left internal carotid artery, intracranial portion, not elsewhere classified with loss of consciousness** greater than 24 hours without return to pre-existing conscious level with patient surviving   `MCC` `H5` `HCC`

√7ᵗʰ **S06.827** **Injury of left internal carotid artery, intracranial portion, not elsewhere classified with loss of consciousness** of any duration with death due to brain injury prior to regaining consciousness   `MCC` `H5`

√7ᵗʰ **S06.828** **Injury of left internal carotid artery, intracranial portion, not elsewhere classified with loss of consciousness** of any duration with death due to other cause prior to regaining consciousness   `MCC` `H5`

7 √7ᵗʰ **S06.829** **Injury of left internal carotid artery, intracranial portion, not elsewhere classified with loss of consciousness** of unspecified duration   `CC` `H5` `HCC`

Injury of left internal carotid artery, intracranial portion, not elsewhere classified NOS

√6ᵗʰ **S06.89** **Other specified intracranial injury**

EXCLUDES 1   concussion (S06.0X-)

7 √7ᵗʰ **S06.890** **Other specified intracranial injury** without loss of consciousness   `HCC`

7 √7ᵗʰ **S06.891** **Other specified intracranial injury with loss of consciousness of** 30 minutes or less   `CC` `H5` `HCC`

7 √7ᵗʰ **S06.892** **Other specified intracranial injury with loss of consciousness of** 31 minutes to 59 minutes   `CC` `H5` `HCC`

7 √7ᵗʰ **S06.893** **Other specified intracranial injury with loss of consciousness of** 1 hour to 5 hours 59 minutes   `CC` `H5` `HCC`

7 √7ᵗʰ **S06.894** **Other specified intracranial injury with loss of consciousness of** 6 hours to 24 hours   `CC` `H5` `HCC`

7 √7ᵗʰ **S06.895** **Other specified intracranial injury with loss of consciousness** greater than 24 hours with return to pre-existing conscious level   `CC` `H5` `HCC`

7 √7ᵗʰ **S06.896** **Other specified intracranial injury with loss of consciousness** greater than 24 hours without return to pre-existing conscious level with patient surviving   `MCC` `H5` `HCC`

√7ᵗʰ **S06.897** **Other specified intracranial injury with loss of consciousness of** any duration with death due to brain injury prior to regaining consciousness   `MCC` `H5`

√7ᵗʰ **S06.898** **Other specified intracranial injury with loss of consciousness of** any duration with death due to other cause prior to regaining consciousness   `MCC` `H5`

7 √7ᵗʰ **S06.899** **Other specified intracranial injury with loss of consciousness of** unspecified duration   `CC` `H5` `HCC`

√5ᵗʰ **S06.9** **Unspecified intracranial injury**

Brain injury NOS

Head injury NOS with loss of consciousness

Traumatic brain injury NOS

EXCLUDES 1   conditions classifiable to S06.0- to S06.8- code to specified intracranial injury

head injury NOS (S09.90)

√6ᵗʰ **S06.9X** **Unspecified intracranial injury**

7 √7ᵗʰ **S06.9X0** **Unspecified intracranial injury** without loss of consciousness   `HCC`

7 √7ᵗʰ **S06.9X1** **Unspecified intracranial injury with loss of consciousness of** 30 minutes or less   `CC` `H5` `HCC`

7 √7ᵗʰ **S06.9X2** **Unspecified intracranial injury with loss of consciousness of** 31 minutes to 59 minutes   `CC` `H5` `HCC`

7 √7ᵗʰ **S06.9X3** **Unspecified intracranial injury with loss of consciousness of** 1 hour to 5 hours 59 minutes   `CC` `H5` `HCC`

7 √7ᵗʰ **S06.9X4** **Unspecified intracranial injury with loss of consciousness of** 6 hours to 24 hours   `CC` `H5` `HCC`

7 √7ᵗʰ **S06.9X5** **Unspecified intracranial injury with loss of consciousness** greater than 24 hours with return to pre-existing conscious level   `CC` `H5` `HCC`

7 √7ᵗʰ **S06.9X6** **Unspecified intracranial injury with loss of consciousness** greater than 24 hours without return to pre-existing conscious level with patient surviving   `MCC` `H5` `HCC`

√7ᵗʰ **S06.9X7** **Unspecified intracranial injury with loss of consciousness of** any duration with death due to brain injury prior to regaining consciousness   `MCC` `H5`

√7ᵗʰ **S06.9X8** **Unspecified intracranial injury with loss of consciousness of** any duration with death due to other cause prior to regaining consciousness   `MCC` `H5`

7 √7ᵗʰ **S06.9X9** **Unspecified intracranial injury with loss of consciousness of** unspecified duration   `CC` `H5` `HCC`

√4ᵗʰ **S07** **Crushing injury of head**

Use additional code for all associated injuries, such as:

intracranial injuries (S06.-)

skull fractures (S02.-)

The appropriate 7th character is to be added to each code from category S07.

A   initial encounter

D   subsequent encounter

S   sequela

CC Excl: For CC codes in category S07: PDX collection 1156

√x7ᵗʰ **S07.0** **Crushing injury of face**   `CC` `H5`

√x7ᵗʰ **S07.1** **Crushing injury of skull**   `CC` `H5`

√x7ᵗʰ **S07.8** **Crushing injury of other parts of head**   `CC` `H5`

√x7ᵗʰ **S07.9** **Crushing injury of head, part unspecified**   `CC` `H5`

√4ᵗʰ **S08** **Avulsion and traumatic amputation of part of head**

An amputation not identified as partial or complete should be coded to complete

The appropriate 7th character is to be added to each code from category S08.

A   initial encounter

D   subsequent encounter

S   sequela

√x7ᵗʰ **S08.0** **Avulsion of scalp**

N Newborn: 0   P Pediatric: 0-17   M Maternity: 9-64   A Adult: 15-124   MCC Major Complication/Comorbidity   CC Complication/Comorbidity   SW Severe Wound Dx

996   ICD-10-CM 2020

√5ᵗʰ **S08.1** **Traumatic amputation of** ear
  √6ᵗʰ **S08.11** **Complete** traumatic amputation of ear
    √7ᵗʰ **S08.111** **Complete** traumatic amputation of **right** ear
    √7ᵗʰ **S08.112** **Complete** traumatic amputation of **left** ear
    √7ᵗʰ **S08.119** **Complete** traumatic amputation of **unspecified ear**
  √6ᵗʰ **S08.12** **Partial** traumatic amputation of ear
    √7ᵗʰ **S08.121** **Partial** traumatic amputation of **right** ear
    √7ᵗʰ **S08.122** **Partial** traumatic amputation of **left** ear
    √7ᵗʰ **S08.129** **Partial** traumatic amputation of **unspecified ear**
√5ᵗʰ **S08.8** **Traumatic amputation of other parts of head**
  √6ᵗʰ **S08.81** **Traumatic amputation of** nose
    √7ᵗʰ **S08.811** **Complete** traumatic amputation of nose
    √7ᵗʰ **S08.812** **Partial** traumatic amputation of nose
  √7ᵗʰ **S08.89** **Traumatic amputation of other parts of head**

√4ᵗʰ **S09** **Other and unspecified injuries of head**

> The appropriate 7th character is to be added to each code from category S09.
> A   initial encounter
> D   subsequent encounter
> S   sequela

CC Excl: For CC codes in category S09, unless otherwise noted: PDX collection 1158

√x7ᵗʰ **S09.0** **Injury of** blood vessels **of head, not elsewhere classified**   **cc**
  EXCLUDES 1 injury of cerebral blood vessels (S06.-)
  injury of precerebral blood vessels (S15.-)
  CC Excl: PDX collection 1157
√5ᵗʰ **S09.1** **Injury of** muscle and tendon **of head**
  Code also any associated open wound (S01.-)
  EXCLUDES 2 sprain to joints and ligament of head (S03.9)
  √7ᵗʰ **S09.10** **Unspecified injury of muscle and tendon of head**
    Injury of muscle and tendon of head NOS
  √x7ᵗʰ **S09.11** **Strain of muscle and tendon of head**
  √x7ᵗʰ **S09.12** **Laceration of muscle and tendon of head**
  √x7ᵗʰ **S09.19** **Other specified injury of muscle and tendon of head**
√5ᵗʰ **S09.2** **Traumatic rupture of** ear drum
  EXCLUDES 1 traumatic rupture of ear drum due to blast injury (S09.31-)
  √x7ᵗʰ **S09.20** **Traumatic rupture of unspecified ear drum**   **cc**
  √x7ᵗʰ **S09.21** **Traumatic rupture of right ear drum**   **cc**
  √x7ᵗʰ **S09.22** **Traumatic rupture of left ear drum**   **cc**
√5ᵗʰ **S09.3** **Other specified and unspecified injury of middle and inner ear**
  EXCLUDES 1 injury to ear NOS (S09.91-)
  EXCLUDES 2 injury to external ear (S00.4-, S01.3-, S08.1-)
  √6ᵗʰ **S09.30** **Unspecified injury of** middle and inner ear
    √7ᵗʰ **S09.301** **Unspecified injury of** right middle and inner ear   **cc**
    √7ᵗʰ **S09.302** **Unspecified injury of** left middle and inner ear   **cc**
    √7ᵗʰ **S09.309** **Unspecified injury of unspecified middle and inner ear**   **cc**
  √6ᵗʰ **S09.31** **Primary** blast injury **of ear**
    Blast injury of ear NOS
    √7ᵗʰ **S09.311** **Primary blast injury of right ear**   **cc**
    √7ᵗʰ **S09.312** **Primary blast injury of left ear**   **cc**
    √7ᵗʰ **S09.313** **Primary blast injury of ear, bilateral**   **cc**
    √7ᵗʰ **S09.319** **Primary blast injury of unspecified ear**   **cc**
  √6ᵗʰ **S09.39** **Other specified injury of middle and inner ear**
    Secondary blast injury to ear
    √7ᵗʰ **S09.391** **Other specified injury of right middle and inner ear**   **cc**
    √7ᵗʰ **S09.392** **Other specified injury of left middle and inner ear**   **cc**

√7ᵗʰ **S09.399** **Other specified injury of unspecified middle and inner ear**   **cc**
√x7ᵗʰ **S09.8** **Other specified injuries of head**
√5ᵗʰ **S09.9** **Unspecified injury of face and head**
  √x7ᵗʰ **S09.90** **Unspecified injury of** head
    Head injury NOS
    EXCLUDES 1 brain injury NOS (S06.9-)
    head injury NOS with loss of consciousness (S06.9-)
    intracranial injury NOS (S06.9-)
  √x7ᵗʰ **S09.91** **Unspecified injury of** ear
    Injury of ear NOS
  √x7ᵗʰ **S09.92** **Unspecified injury of** nose
    Injury of nose NOS
  √x7ᵗʰ **S09.93** **Unspecified injury of** face
    Injury of face NOS
    AHA: 2019,2Q,23

Injuries to the neck (S10-S19)

INCLUDES injuries of nape
  injuries of supraclavicular region
  injuries of throat
EXCLUDES 2 burns and corrosions (T20-T32)
  effects of foreign body in esophagus (T18.1)
  effects of foreign body in larynx (T17.3)
  effects of foreign body in pharynx (T17.2)
  effects of foreign body in trachea (T17.4)
  frostbite (T33-T34)
  insect bite or sting, venomous (T63.4)

√4ᵗʰ **S10** **Superficial injury of neck**

> The appropriate 7th character is to be added to each code from category S10.
> A   initial encounter
> D   subsequent encounter
> S   sequela

√x7ᵗʰ **S10.0** **Contusion of throat**
  Contusion of cervical esophagus
  Contusion of larynx
  Contusion of pharynx
  Contusion of trachea
√5ᵗʰ **S10.1** **Other and unspecified superficial injuries of throat**
  √x7ᵗʰ **S10.10** **Unspecified superficial injuries of throat**
  √x7ᵗʰ **S10.11** **Abrasion of throat**
  √x7ᵗʰ **S10.12** **Blister (nonthermal) of throat**
  √x7ᵗʰ **S10.14** **External constriction of part of throat**
  √x7ᵗʰ **S10.15** **Superficial foreign body of throat**
    Splinter in the throat
  √x7ᵗʰ **S10.16** **Insect bite (nonvenomous) of throat**
  √x7ᵗʰ **S10.17** **Other superficial bite of throat**
    EXCLUDES 1 open bite of throat (S11.85)
√5ᵗʰ **S10.8** **Superficial injury of other specified parts of neck**
  √x7ᵗʰ **S10.80** **Unspecified superficial injury of other specified part of neck**
  √x7ᵗʰ **S10.81** **Abrasion of other specified part of neck**
  √x7ᵗʰ **S10.82** **Blister (nonthermal) of other specified part of neck**
  √x7ᵗʰ **S10.83** **Contusion of other specified part of neck**
  √x7ᵗʰ **S10.84** **External constriction of other specified part of neck**
  √x7ᵗʰ **S10.85** **Superficial foreign body of other specified part of neck**
    Splinter in other specified part of neck
  √x7ᵗʰ **S10.86** **Insect bite of other specified part of neck**
  √x7ᵗʰ **S10.87** **Other superficial bite of other specified part of neck**
    EXCLUDES 1 open bite of other specified parts of neck (S11.85)
√5ᵗʰ **S10.9** **Superficial injury of unspecified part of neck**
  √x7ᵗʰ **S10.90** **Unspecified superficial injury of unspecified part of neck**
  √x7ᵗʰ **S10.91** **Abrasion of unspecified part of neck**
  √x7ᵗʰ **S10.92** **Blister (nonthermal) of unspecified part of neck**
  √x7ᵗʰ **S10.93** **Contusion of unspecified part of neck**
  √x7ᵗʰ **S10.94** **External constriction of unspecified part of neck**

√x7ᵗʰ **S10.95**   Superficial **foreign body of unspecified part of neck**

√x7ᵗʰ **S10.96**   Insect bite **of unspecified part of neck**

√x7ᵗʰ **S10.97**   Other superficial **bite of unspecified part of neck**

√4ᵗʰ **S11   Open wound of neck**

Code also any associated:
    spinal cord injury (S14.0, S14.1-)
    wound infection
EXCLUDES 2   *open fracture of vertebra (S12.- with 7th character B)*

The appropriate 7th character is to be added to each code from category S11.
A   initial encounter
D   subsequent encounter
S   sequela

√5ᵗʰ **S11.0   Open wound of larynx and trachea**

CC Excl: For MCC codes in subcategory S11.0: PDX collection 1159

√6ᵗʰ **S11.01   Open wound of larynx**

EXCLUDES 2   *open wound of vocal cord (S11.03)*

√7ᵗʰ **S11.011   Laceration without foreign body of larynx**   MCC

√7ᵗʰ **S11.012   Laceration with foreign body of larynx**   MCC

√7ᵗʰ **S11.013   Puncture wound without foreign body of larynx**   MCC

√7ᵗʰ **S11.014   Puncture wound with foreign body of larynx**   MCC

√7ᵗʰ **S11.015   Open bite of larynx**   MCC

Bite of larynx NOS

√7ᵗʰ **S11.019   Unspecified open wound of larynx**   MCC

√6ᵗʰ **S11.02   Open wound of trachea**

Open wound of cervical trachea
Open wound of trachea NOS
EXCLUDES 2   *open wound of thoracic trachea (S27.5-)*

√7ᵗʰ **S11.021   Laceration without foreign body of trachea**   MCC

√7ᵗʰ **S11.022   Laceration with foreign body of trachea**   MCC

√7ᵗʰ **S11.023   Puncture wound without foreign body of trachea**   MCC

√7ᵗʰ **S11.024   Puncture wound with foreign body of trachea**   MCC

√7ᵗʰ **S11.025   Open bite of trachea**   MCC

Bite of trachea NOS

√7ᵗʰ **S11.029   Unspecified open wound of trachea**   MCC

√6ᵗʰ **S11.03   Open wound of vocal cord**

√7ᵗʰ **S11.031   Laceration without foreign body of vocal cord**   MCC

√7ᵗʰ **S11.032   Laceration with foreign body of vocal cord**   MCC

√7ᵗʰ **S11.033   Puncture wound without foreign body of vocal cord**   MCC

√7ᵗʰ **S11.034   Puncture wound with foreign body of vocal cord**   MCC

√7ᵗʰ **S11.035   Open bite of vocal cord**   MCC

Bite of vocal cord NOS

√7ᵗʰ **S11.039   Unspecified open wound of vocal cord**   MCC

√5ᵗʰ **S11.1   Open wound of thyroid gland**

CC Excl: For CC codes in subcategory S11.1, unless otherwise noted: PDX collection 1160

√x7ᵗʰ **S11.10   Unspecified open wound of thyroid gland**   CC

√x7ᵗʰ **S11.11   Laceration without foreign body of thyroid gland**   CC

√x7ᵗʰ **S11.12   Laceration with foreign body of thyroid gland**   CC

CC Excl: PDX collection 1161

√x7ᵗʰ **S11.13   Puncture wound without foreign body of thyroid gland**   CC

√x7ᵗʰ **S11.14   Puncture wound with foreign body of thyroid gland**   CC

CC Excl: PDX collection 1161

√x7ᵗʰ **S11.15   Open bite of thyroid gland**   CC

Bite of thyroid gland NOS

√5ᵗʰ **S11.2   Open wound of pharynx and cervical esophagus**

EXCLUDES 1   *open wound of esophagus NOS (S27.8-)*

CC Excl: For CC codes in subcategory S11.2, unless otherwise noted: PDX collection 1162

√x7ᵗʰ **S11.20   Unspecified open wound of pharynx and cervical esophagus**   CC

√x7ᵗʰ **S11.21   Laceration without foreign body of pharynx and cervical esophagus**   CC

√x7ᵗʰ **S11.22   Laceration with foreign body of pharynx and cervical esophagus**   CC

CC Excl: PDX collection 1163

√x7ᵗʰ **S11.23   Puncture wound without foreign body of pharynx and cervical esophagus**   CC

√x7ᵗʰ **S11.24   Puncture wound with foreign body of pharynx and cervical esophagus**   CC

CC Excl: PDX collection 1163

√x7ᵗʰ **S11.25   Open bite of pharynx and cervical esophagus**   CC

Bite of pharynx and cervical esophagus NOS

√5ᵗʰ **S11.8   Open wound of other specified parts of neck**

√x7ᵗʰ **S11.80   Unspecified open wound of other specified part of neck**

√x7ᵗʰ **S11.81   Laceration without foreign body of other specified part of neck**

√x7ᵗʰ **S11.82   Laceration with foreign body of other specified part of neck**

√x7ᵗʰ **S11.83   Puncture wound without foreign body of other specified part of neck**

√x7ᵗʰ **S11.84   Puncture wound with foreign body of other specified part of neck**

√x7ᵗʰ **S11.85   Open bite of other specified part of neck**

Bite of other specified part of neck NOS
EXCLUDES 1   *superficial bite of other specified part of neck (S10.87)*

√x7ᵗʰ **S11.89   Other open wound of other specified part of neck**

√5ᵗʰ **S11.9   Open wound of unspecified part of neck**

√x7ᵗʰ **S11.90   Unspecified open wound of unspecified part of neck**

√x7ᵗʰ **S11.91   Laceration without foreign body of unspecified part of neck**

√x7ᵗʰ **S11.92   Laceration with foreign body of unspecified part of neck**

√x7ᵗʰ **S11.93   Puncture wound without foreign body of unspecified part of neck**

√x7ᵗʰ **S11.94   Puncture wound with foreign body of unspecified part of neck**

√x7ᵗʰ **S11.95   Open bite of unspecified part of neck**

Bite of neck NOS
EXCLUDES 1   *superficial bite of neck (S10.97)*

√4ᵗʰ **S12 Fracture of cervical vertebra and other parts of neck**

NOTE A fracture not indicated as displaced or nondisplaced should be coded to displaced.

A fracture not indicated as open or closed should be coded to closed.

INCLUDES fracture of cervical neural arch
fracture of cervical spine
fracture of cervical spinous process
fracture of cervical transverse process
fracture of cervical vertebral arch
fracture of neck

Code first any associated cervical spinal cord injury (S14.0, S14.1-)

AHA: 2018,2Q,12; 2015,3Q,37-39

The appropriate 7th character is to be added to all codes from subcategories S12.0-S12.6.
A initial encounter for closed fracture
B initial encounter for open fracture
D subsequent encounter for fracture with routine healing
G subsequent encounter for fracture with delayed healing
K subsequent encounter for fracture with nonunion
S sequela

CC Excl: For codes in category S12, unless otherwise noted:
CC with 7th character A or MCC with 7th character B: PDX collection 1164
CC with 7th character K: PDX collection 897

√5ᵗʰ **S12.0 Fracture of first cervical vertebra**
Atlas

√6ᵗʰ **S12.00 Unspecified fracture of first cervical vertebra**

2,3,6 √7ᵗʰ **S12.000 Unspecified displaced fracture of first cervical vertebra** MCC CC H5 HCC

2,3,6 √7ᵗʰ **S12.001 Unspecified nondisplaced fracture of first cervical vertebra** MCC CC H5 HCC

2,3,6 √x7ᵗʰ **S12.01 Stable burst fracture of first cervical vertebra** MCC CC H5 HCC

2,3,6 √x7ᵗʰ **S12.02 Unstable burst fracture of first cervical vertebra** MCC CC H5 HCC

√6ᵗʰ **S12.03 Posterior arch fracture of first cervical vertebra**

2,3,6 √7ᵗʰ **S12.030 Displaced posterior arch fracture of first cervical vertebra** MCC CC H5 HCC

2,3,6 √7ᵗʰ **S12.031 Nondisplaced posterior arch fracture of first cervical vertebra** MCC CC H5 HCC

√6ᵗʰ **S12.04 Lateral mass fracture of first cervical vertebra**

2,3,6 √7ᵗʰ **S12.040 Displaced lateral mass fracture of first cervical vertebra** MCC CC H5 HCC

2,3,6 √7ᵗʰ **S12.041 Nondisplaced lateral mass fracture of first cervical vertebra** MCC CC H5 HCC

√6ᵗʰ **S12.09 Other fracture of first cervical vertebra**

2,3,6 √7ᵗʰ **S12.090 Other displaced fracture of first cervical vertebra** MCC CC H5 HCC

2,3,6 √7ᵗʰ **S12.091 Other nondisplaced fracture of first cervical vertebra** MCC CC H5 HCC

√5ᵗʰ **S12.1 Fracture of second cervical vertebra**
Axis

√6ᵗʰ **S12.10 Unspecified fracture of second cervical vertebra**

2,3,6 √7ᵗʰ **S12.100 Unspecified displaced fracture of second cervical vertebra** MCC CC H5 HCC

2,3,6 √7ᵗʰ **S12.101 Unspecified nondisplaced fracture of second cervical vertebra** MCC CC H5 HCC

√6ᵗʰ **S12.11 Type II dens fracture**

2,3,6 √7ᵗʰ **S12.110 Anterior displaced Type II dens fracture** MCC CC H5 HCC

2,3,6 √7ᵗʰ **S12.111 Posterior displaced Type II dens fracture** MCC CC H5 HCC

2,3,6 √7ᵗʰ **S12.112 Nondisplaced Type II dens fracture** MCC CC H5 HCC

√6ᵗʰ **S12.12 Other dens fracture**

2,3,6 √7ᵗʰ **S12.120 Other displaced dens fracture** MCC CC H5 HCC

2,3,6 √7ᵗʰ **S12.121 Other nondisplaced dens fracture** MCC CC H5 HCC

√6ᵗʰ **S12.13 Unspecified traumatic spondylolisthesis of second cervical vertebra**

2,3,6 √7ᵗʰ **S12.130 Unspecified traumatic displaced spondylolisthesis of second cervical vertebra** MCC CC H5 HCC

2,3,6 √7ᵗʰ **S12.131 Unspecified traumatic nondisplaced spondylolisthesis of second cervical vertebra** MCC CC H5 HCC

2,3,6 √x7ᵗʰ **S12.14 Type III traumatic spondylolisthesis of second cervical vertebra** MCC CC H5 HCC

√6ᵗʰ **S12.15 Other traumatic spondylolisthesis of second cervical vertebra**

2,3,6 √7ᵗʰ **S12.150 Other traumatic displaced spondylolisthesis of second cervical vertebra** MCC CC H5 HCC

2,3,6 √7ᵗʰ **S12.151 Other traumatic nondisplaced spondylolisthesis of second cervical vertebra** MCC CC H5 HCC

√6ᵗʰ **S12.19 Other fracture of second cervical vertebra**

2,3,6 √7ᵗʰ **S12.190 Other displaced fracture of second cervical vertebra** MCC CC H5 HCC

2,3,6 √7ᵗʰ **S12.191 Other nondisplaced fracture of second cervical vertebra** MCC CC H5 HCC

√5ᵗʰ **S12.2 Fracture of third cervical vertebra**

√6ᵗʰ **S12.20 Unspecified fracture of third cervical vertebra**

2,3,6 √7ᵗʰ **S12.200 Unspecified displaced fracture of third cervical vertebra** MCC CC H5 HCC

2,3,6 √7ᵗʰ **S12.201 Unspecified nondisplaced fracture of third cervical vertebra** MCC CC H5 HCC

√6ᵗʰ **S12.23 Unspecified traumatic spondylolisthesis of third cervical vertebra**

2,3,6 √7ᵗʰ **S12.230 Unspecified traumatic displaced spondylolisthesis of third cervical vertebra** MCC CC H5 HCC

2,3,6 √7ᵗʰ **S12.231 Unspecified traumatic nondisplaced spondylolisthesis of third cervical vertebra** MCC CC H5 HCC

2,3,6 √x7ᵗʰ **S12.24 Type III traumatic spondylolisthesis of third cervical vertebra** MCC CC H5 HCC

√6ᵗʰ **S12.25 Other traumatic spondylolisthesis of third cervical vertebra**

2,3,6 √7ᵗʰ **S12.250 Other traumatic displaced spondylolisthesis of third cervical vertebra** MCC CC H5 HCC

2,3,6 √7ᵗʰ **S12.251 Other traumatic nondisplaced spondylolisthesis of third cervical vertebra** MCC CC H5 HCC

√6ᵗʰ **S12.29 Other fracture of third cervical vertebra**

2,3,6 √7ᵗʰ **S12.290 Other displaced fracture of third cervical vertebra** MCC CC H5 HCC

2,3,6 √7ᵗʰ **S12.291 Other nondisplaced fracture of third cervical vertebra** MCC CC H5 HCC

√5ᵗʰ **S12.3 Fracture of fourth cervical vertebra**

√6ᵗʰ **S12.30 Unspecified fracture of fourth cervical vertebra**

2,3,6 √7ᵗʰ **S12.300 Unspecified displaced fracture of fourth cervical vertebra** MCC CC H5 HCC

2,3,6 √7ᵗʰ **S12.301 Unspecified nondisplaced fracture of fourth cervical vertebra** MCC CC H5 HCC

√6ᵗʰ **S12.33 Unspecified traumatic spondylolisthesis of fourth cervical vertebra**

2,3,6 √7ᵗʰ **S12.330 Unspecified traumatic displaced spondylolisthesis of fourth cervical vertebra** MCC CC H5 HCC

2,3,6 √7ᵗʰ **S12.331 Unspecified traumatic nondisplaced spondylolisthesis of fourth cervical vertebra** MCC CC H5 HCC

2,3,6 √x7ᵗʰ **S12.34** Type III traumatic spondylolisthesis `MCC` `CC` `HS` `HCC`
of fourth cervical vertebra

√6ᵗʰ **S12.35** Other traumatic spondylolisthesis of fourth cervical
vertebra

2,3,6 √7ᵗʰ **S12.350** Other traumatic displaced `MCC` `CC` `HS` `HCC`
spondylolisthesis of fourth
cervical vertebra

2,3,6 √7ᵗʰ **S12.351** Other traumatic `MCC` `CC` `HS` `HCC`
nondisplaced
spondylolisthesis of fourth
cervical vertebra

√6ᵗʰ **S12.39** Other fracture of fourth cervical vertebra

2,3,6 √7ᵗʰ **S12.390** Other displaced fracture `MCC` `CC` `HS` `HCC`
of fourth cervical vertebra

2,3,6 √7ᵗʰ **S12.391** Other nondisplaced `MCC` `CC` `HS` `HCC`
fracture of fourth cervical
vertebra

√5ᵗʰ **S12.4** Fracture of fifth cervical vertebra

√6ᵗʰ **S12.40** Unspecified fracture of fifth cervical vertebra

2,3,6 √7ᵗʰ **S12.400** Unspecified displaced `MCC` `CC` `HS` `HCC`
fracture of fifth cervical
vertebra

2,3,6 √7ᵗʰ **S12.401** Unspecified nondisplaced `MCC` `CC` `HS` `HCC`
fracture of fifth cervical
vertebra

√6ᵗʰ **S12.43** Unspecified traumatic spondylolisthesis of fifth
cervical vertebra

2,3,6 √7ᵗʰ **S12.430** Unspecified traumatic `MCC` `CC` `HS` `HCC`
displaced
spondylolisthesis of fifth
cervical vertebra

2,3,6 √7ᵗʰ **S12.431** Unspecified traumatic `MCC` `CC` `HS` `HCC`
nondisplaced
spondylolisthesis of fifth
cervical vertebra

2,3,6 √x7ᵗʰ **S12.44** Type III traumatic spondylolisthesis `MCC` `CC` `HS` `HCC`
of fifth cervical vertebra

√6ᵗʰ **S12.45** Other traumatic spondylolisthesis of fifth cervical
vertebra

2,3,6 √7ᵗʰ **S12.450** Other traumatic displaced `MCC` `CC` `HS` `HCC`
spondylolisthesis of fifth
cervical vertebra

2,3,6 √7ᵗʰ **S12.451** Other traumatic `MCC` `CC` `HS` `HCC`
nondisplaced
spondylolisthesis of fifth
cervical vertebra

√6ᵗʰ **S12.49** Other fracture of fifth cervical vertebra

2,3,6 √7ᵗʰ **S12.490** Other displaced fracture `MCC` `CC` `HS` `HCC`
of fifth cervical vertebra

2,3,6 √7ᵗʰ **S12.491** Other nondisplaced `MCC` `CC` `HS` `HCC`
fracture of fifth cervical
vertebra

√5ᵗʰ **S12.5** Fracture of sixth cervical vertebra

√6ᵗʰ **S12.50** Unspecified fracture of sixth cervical vertebra

2,3,6 √7ᵗʰ **S12.500** Unspecified displaced `MCC` `CC` `HS` `HCC`
fracture of sixth cervical
vertebra

2,3,6 √7ᵗʰ **S12.501** Unspecified nondisplaced `MCC` `CC` `HS` `HCC`
fracture of sixth cervical
vertebra

√6ᵗʰ **S12.53** Unspecified traumatic spondylolisthesis of sixth
cervical vertebra

2,3,6 √7ᵗʰ **S12.530** Unspecified traumatic `MCC` `CC` `HS` `HCC`
displaced
spondylolisthesis of sixth
cervical vertebra

2,3,6 √7ᵗʰ **S12.531** Unspecified traumatic `MCC` `CC` `HS` `HCC`
nondisplaced
spondylolisthesis of sixth
cervical vertebra

2,3,6 √x7ᵗʰ **S12.54** Type III traumatic spondylolisthesis `MCC` `CC` `HS` `HCC`
of sixth cervical vertebra

√6ᵗʰ **S12.55** Other traumatic spondylolisthesis of sixth cervical
vertebra

2,3,6 √7ᵗʰ **S12.550** Other traumatic displaced `MCC` `CC` `HS` `HCC`
spondylolisthesis of sixth
cervical vertebra

2,3,6 √7ᵗʰ **S12.551** Other traumatic `MCC` `CC` `HS` `HCC`
nondisplaced
spondylolisthesis of sixth
cervical vertebra

√6ᵗʰ **S12.59** Other fracture of sixth cervical vertebra

2,3,6 √7ᵗʰ **S12.590** Other displaced fracture `MCC` `CC` `HS` `HCC`
of sixth cervical vertebra

2,3,6 √7ᵗʰ **S12.591** Other nondisplaced `MCC` `CC` `HS` `HCC`
fracture of sixth cervical
vertebra

√5ᵗʰ **S12.6** Fracture of seventh cervical vertebra

√6ᵗʰ **S12.60** Unspecified fracture of seventh cervical vertebra

2,3,6 √7ᵗʰ **S12.600** Unspecified displaced `MCC` `CC` `HS` `HCC`
fracture of seventh
cervical vertebra

2,3,6 √7ᵗʰ **S12.601** Unspecified nondisplaced `MCC` `CC` `HS` `HCC`
fracture of seventh
cervical vertebra

√6ᵗʰ **S12.63** Unspecified traumatic spondylolisthesis of seventh
cervical vertebra

2,3,6 √7ᵗʰ **S12.630** Unspecified traumatic `MCC` `CC` `HS` `HCC`
displaced
spondylolisthesis of
seventh cervical vertebra

2,3,6 √7ᵗʰ **S12.631** Unspecified traumatic `MCC` `CC` `HS` `HCC`
nondisplaced
spondylolisthesis of
seventh cervical vertebra

2,3,6 √x7ᵗʰ **S12.64** Type III traumatic spondylolisthesis `MCC` `CC` `HS` `HCC`
of seventh cervical vertebra

√6ᵗʰ **S12.65** Other traumatic spondylolisthesis of seventh
cervical vertebra

2,3,6 √7ᵗʰ **S12.650** Other traumatic displaced `MCC` `CC` `HS` `HCC`
spondylolisthesis of
seventh cervical vertebra

2,3,6 √7ᵗʰ **S12.651** Other traumatic `MCC` `CC` `HS` `HCC`
nondisplaced
spondylolisthesis of
seventh cervical vertebra

√6ᵗʰ **S12.69** Other fracture of seventh cervical vertebra

2,3,6 √7ᵗʰ **S12.690** Other displaced fracture `MCC` `CC` `HS` `HCC`
of seventh cervical
vertebra

2,3,6 √7ᵗʰ **S12.691** Other nondisplaced `MCC` `CC` `HS` `HCC`
fracture of seventh
cervical vertebra

6 √x7ᵗʰ **S12.8** Fracture of other parts of neck `MCC` `HS` `HCC`

Hyoid bone
Larynx
Thyroid cartilage
Trachea

> The appropriate 7th character is to be added to code S12.8.
> A   initial encounter
> D   subsequent encounter
> S   sequela

CC Excl: PDX collection 1165

6 √x7ᵗʰ **S12.9** Fracture of neck, unspecified `CC` `HS` `HCC`

Fracture of neck NOS
Fracture of cervical spine NOS
Fracture of cervical vertebra NOS

> The appropriate 7th character is to be added to code S12.9.
> A   initial encounter
> D   subsequent encounter
> S   sequela

CC Excl: PDX collection 1164

N Newborn: 0 — P Pediatric: 0-17 — M Maternity: 9-64 — A Adult: 15-124 — `MCC` Major Complication/Comorbidity — `CC` Complication/Comorbidity — `SW` Severe Wound Dx

1000

ICD-10-CM 2020

√4th **S13** **Dislocation and sprain of joints and ligaments at neck level**

INCLUDES   avulsion of joint or ligament at neck level
laceration of cartilage, joint or ligament at neck level
sprain of cartilage, joint or ligament at neck level
traumatic hemarthrosis of joint or ligament at neck level
traumatic rupture of joint or ligament at neck level
traumatic subluxation of joint or ligament at neck level
traumatic tear of joint or ligament at neck level

Code also any associated open wound
EXCLUDES 2   *strain of muscle or tendon at neck level (S16.1)*

The appropriate 7th character is to be added to each code from category S13.
A   initial encounter
D   subsequent encounter
S   sequela

CC Excl: For CC codes in category S13: PDX collection 913

√x7th **S13.Ø** **Traumatic rupture of cervical intervertebral disc**   CC H5
EXCLUDES 1   *rupture or displacement (nontraumatic) of cervical intervertebral disc NOS (M5Ø.-)*

√5th **S13.1** **Subluxation and dislocation of cervical vertebrae**
Code also any associated:
open wound of neck (S11.-)
spinal cord injury (S14.1-)
EXCLUDES 2   *fracture of cervical vertebrae (S12.Ø-S12.3-)*

√6th **S13.10** **Subluxation and dislocation of unspecified cervical vertebrae**
√7th **S13.100** **Subluxation of unspecified cervical vertebrae**   CC H5
√7th **S13.101** **Dislocation of unspecified cervical vertebrae**   CC H5

√6th **S13.11** **Subluxation and dislocation of CØ/C1 cervical vertebrae**
Subluxation and dislocation of atlantooccipital joint
Subluxation and dislocation of atloidooccipital joint
Subluxation and dislocation of occipitoatloid joint
√7th **S13.110** **Subluxation of CØ/C1 cervical vertebrae**   CC H5
√7th **S13.111** **Dislocation of CØ/C1 cervical vertebrae**   CC H5

√6th **S13.12** **Subluxation and dislocation of C1/C2 cervical vertebrae**
Subluxation and dislocation of atlantoaxial joint
√7th **S13.120** **Subluxation of C1/C2 cervical vertebrae**   CC H5
√7th **S13.121** **Dislocation of C1/C2 cervical vertebrae**   CC H5

√6th **S13.13** **Subluxation and dislocation of C2/C3 cervical vertebrae**
√7th **S13.130** **Subluxation of C2/C3 cervical vertebrae**   CC H5
√7th **S13.131** **Dislocation of C2/C3 cervical vertebrae**   CC H5

√6th **S13.14** **Subluxation and dislocation of C3/C4 cervical vertebrae**
√7th **S13.140** **Subluxation of C3/C4 cervical vertebrae**   CC H5
√7th **S13.141** **Dislocation of C3/C4 cervical vertebrae**   CC H5

√6th **S13.15** **Subluxation and dislocation of C4/C5 cervical vertebrae**
√7th **S13.150** **Subluxation of C4/C5 cervical vertebrae**   CC H5
√7th **S13.151** **Dislocation of C4/C5 cervical vertebrae**   CC H5

√6th **S13.16** **Subluxation and dislocation of C5/C6 cervical vertebrae**
√7th **S13.160** **Subluxation of C5/C6 cervical vertebrae**   CC H5
√7th **S13.161** **Dislocation of C5/C6 cervical vertebrae**   CC H5

√6th **S13.17** **Subluxation and dislocation of C6/C7 cervical vertebrae**
√7th **S13.170** **Subluxation of C6/C7 cervical vertebrae**   CC H5
√7th **S13.171** **Dislocation of C6/C7 cervical vertebrae**   CC H5

√6th **S13.18** **Subluxation and dislocation of C7/T1 cervical vertebrae**
√7th **S13.180** **Subluxation of C7/T1 cervical vertebrae**   CC H5
√7th **S13.181** **Dislocation of C7/T1 cervical vertebrae**   CC H5

√5th **S13.2** **Dislocation of other and unspecified parts of neck**
√x7th **S13.20** **Dislocation of unspecified parts of neck**   CC H5
√x7th **S13.29** **Dislocation of other parts of neck**   CC H5

√x7th **S13.4** **Sprain of ligaments of cervical spine**
Sprain of anterior longitudinal (ligament), cervical
Sprain of atlanto-axial (joints)
Sprain of atlanto-occipital (joints)
Whiplash injury of cervical spine

√x7th **S13.5** **Sprain of thyroid region**
Sprain of cricoarytenoid (joint) (ligament)
Sprain of cricothyroid (joint) (ligament)
Sprain of thyroid cartilage

√x7th **S13.8** **Sprain of joints and ligaments of other parts of neck**

√x7th **S13.9** **Sprain of joints and ligaments of unspecified parts of neck**

√4th **S14** **Injury of nerves and spinal cord at neck level**

NOTE   Code to highest level of cervical cord injury

Code also any associated:
fracture of cervical vertebra (S12.Ø- — S12.6.-)
open wound of neck (S11.-)
transient paralysis (R29.5)

The appropriate 7th character is to be added to each code from category S14.
A   initial encounter
D   subsequent encounter
S   sequela

CC Excl: For MCC codes in category S14: PDX collection 1166

√x7th **S14.Ø** **Concussion and edema of cervical spinal cord**   MCC HCC

√5th **S14.1** **Other and unspecified injuries of cervical spinal cord**
√6th **S14.10** **Unspecified injury of cervical spinal cord**
√7th **S14.101** **Unspecified injury at C1 level of cervical spinal cord**   MCC H5 HCC
√7th **S14.102** **Unspecified injury at C2 level of cervical spinal cord**   MCC H5 HCC
√7th **S14.103** **Unspecified injury at C3 level of cervical spinal cord**   MCC H5 HCC
√7th **S14.104** **Unspecified injury at C4 level of cervical spinal cord**   MCC H5 HCC
√7th **S14.105** **Unspecified injury at C5 level of cervical spinal cord**   MCC H5 HCC
√7th **S14.106** **Unspecified injury at C6 level of cervical spinal cord**   MCC H5 HCC
√7th **S14.107** **Unspecified injury at C7 level of cervical spinal cord**   MCC H5 HCC
√7th **S14.108** **Unspecified injury at C8 level of cervical spinal cord**   MCC HCC
√7th **S14.109** **Unspecified injury at unspecified level of cervical spinal cord**   HCC
Injury of cervical spinal cord NOS

√6th **S14.11** **Complete lesion of cervical spinal cord**
√7th **S14.111** **Complete lesion at C1 level of cervical spinal cord**   MCC H5 HCC
√7th **S14.112** **Complete lesion at C2 level of cervical spinal cord**   MCC H5 HCC
√7th **S14.113** **Complete lesion at C3 level of cervical spinal cord**   MCC H5 HCC
√7th **S14.114** **Complete lesion at C4 level of cervical spinal cord**   MCC H5 HCC

√7ᵗʰ **S14.115** Complete lesion at C5 level of cervical spinal cord `MCC` `H5` `HCC`

√7ᵗʰ **S14.116** Complete lesion at C6 level of cervical spinal cord `MCC` `H5` `HCC`

√7ᵗʰ **S14.117** Complete lesion at C7 level of cervical spinal cord `MCC` `H5` `HCC`

√7ᵗʰ **S14.118** Complete lesion at C8 level of cervical spinal cord `MCC` `HCC`

√7ᵗʰ **S14.119** Complete lesion at unspecified level of cervical spinal cord `HCC`

√6ᵗʰ **S14.12** Central cord syndrome of cervical spinal cord

√7ᵗʰ **S14.121** Central cord syndrome at C1 level of cervical spinal cord `MCC` `H5` `HCC`

√7ᵗʰ **S14.122** Central cord syndrome at C2 level of cervical spinal cord `MCC` `H5` `HCC`

√7ᵗʰ **S14.123** Central cord syndrome at C3 level of cervical spinal cord `MCC` `H5` `HCC`

√7ᵗʰ **S14.124** Central cord syndrome at C4 level of cervical spinal cord `MCC` `H5` `HCC`

√7ᵗʰ **S14.125** Central cord syndrome at C5 level of cervical spinal cord `MCC` `H5` `HCC`

√7ᵗʰ **S14.126** Central cord syndrome at C6 level of cervical spinal cord `MCC` `H5` `HCC`

√7ᵗʰ **S14.127** Central cord syndrome at C7 level of cervical spinal cord `MCC` `H5` `HCC`

√7ᵗʰ **S14.128** Central cord syndrome at C8 level of cervical spinal cord `MCC` `HCC`

√7ᵗʰ **S14.129** Central cord syndrome at unspecified level of cervical spinal cord `HCC`

√6ᵗʰ **S14.13** Anterior cord syndrome of cervical spinal cord

√7ᵗʰ **S14.131** Anterior cord syndrome at C1 level of cervical spinal cord `MCC` `H5` `HCC`

√7ᵗʰ **S14.132** Anterior cord syndrome at C2 level of cervical spinal cord `MCC` `H5` `HCC`

√7ᵗʰ **S14.133** Anterior cord syndrome at C3 level of cervical spinal cord `MCC` `H5` `HCC`

√7ᵗʰ **S14.134** Anterior cord syndrome at C4 level of cervical spinal cord `MCC` `H5` `HCC`

√7ᵗʰ **S14.135** Anterior cord syndrome at C5 level of cervical spinal cord `MCC` `H5` `HCC`

√7ᵗʰ **S14.136** Anterior cord syndrome at C6 level of cervical spinal cord `MCC` `H5` `HCC`

√7ᵗʰ **S14.137** Anterior cord syndrome at C7 level of cervical spinal cord `MCC` `H5` `HCC`

√7ᵗʰ **S14.138** Anterior cord syndrome at C8 level of cervical spinal cord `MCC` `HCC`

√7ᵗʰ **S14.139** Anterior cord syndrome at unspecified level of cervical spinal cord `HCC`

√6ᵗʰ **S14.14** Brown-Séquard syndrome of cervical spinal cord

√7ᵗʰ **S14.141** Brown-Séquard syndrome at C1 level of cervical spinal cord `MCC` `HCC`

√7ᵗʰ **S14.142** Brown-Séquard syndrome at C2 level of cervical spinal cord `MCC` `HCC`

√7ᵗʰ **S14.143** Brown-Séquard syndrome at C3 level of cervical spinal cord `MCC` `HCC`

√7ᵗʰ **S14.144** Brown-Séquard syndrome at C4 level of cervical spinal cord `MCC` `HCC`

√7ᵗʰ **S14.145** Brown-Séquard syndrome at C5 level of cervical spinal cord `MCC` `HCC`

√7ᵗʰ **S14.146** Brown-Séquard syndrome at C6 level of cervical spinal cord `MCC` `HCC`

√7ᵗʰ **S14.147** Brown-Séquard syndrome at C7 level of cervical spinal cord `MCC` `HCC`

√7ᵗʰ **S14.148** Brown-Séquard syndrome at C8 level of cervical spinal cord `MCC` `HCC`

√7ᵗʰ **S14.149** Brown-Séquard syndrome at unspecified level of cervical spinal cord `HCC`

√6ᵗʰ **S14.15** Other incomplete lesions of cervical spinal cord

Incomplete lesion of cervical spinal cord NOS
Posterior cord syndrome of cervical spinal cord

√7ᵗʰ **S14.151** Other incomplete lesion at C1 level of cervical spinal cord `MCC` `H5` `HCC`

√7ᵗʰ **S14.152** Other incomplete lesion at C2 level of cervical spinal cord `MCC` `H5` `HCC`

√7ᵗʰ **S14.153** Other incomplete lesion at C3 level of cervical spinal cord `MCC` `H5` `HCC`

√7ᵗʰ **S14.154** Other incomplete lesion at C4 level of cervical spinal cord `MCC` `H5` `HCC`

√7ᵗʰ **S14.155** Other incomplete lesion at C5 level of cervical spinal cord `MCC` `H5` `HCC`

√7ᵗʰ **S14.156** Other incomplete lesion at C6 level of cervical spinal cord `MCC` `H5` `HCC`

√7ᵗʰ **S14.157** Other incomplete lesion at C7 level of cervical spinal cord `MCC` `H5` `HCC`

√7ᵗʰ **S14.158** Other incomplete lesion at C8 level of cervical spinal cord `MCC` `HCC`

√7ᵗʰ **S14.159** Other incomplete lesion at unspecified level of cervical spinal cord `HCC`

√x7ᵗʰ **S14.2** Injury of nerve root of cervical spine

√x7ᵗʰ **S14.3** Injury of brachial plexus

√x7ᵗʰ **S14.4** Injury of peripheral nerves of neck

√x7ᵗʰ **S14.5** Injury of cervical sympathetic nerves

√x7ᵗʰ **S14.8** Injury of other specified nerves of neck

√x7ᵗʰ **S14.9** Injury of unspecified nerves of neck

√4ᵗʰ **S15** Injury of blood vessels at neck level

Code also any associated open wound (S11.-)

The appropriate 7th character is to be added to each code from category S15.
A initial encounter
D subsequent encounter
S sequela

CC Excl: For CC codes in category S15, unless otherwise noted: PDX collection 1157

√5ᵗʰ **S15.0** Injury of carotid artery of neck

Injury of carotid artery (common) (external) (internal, extracranial portion)
Injury of carotid artery NOS

EXCLUDES 1 injury of internal carotid artery, intracranial portion (S06.8)

CC Excl: For CC codes in subcategory S15.0: PDX collection 1167

√6ᵗʰ **S15.00** Unspecified injury of carotid artery

√7ᵗʰ **S15.001** Unspecified injury of right carotid artery `CC`

√7ᵗʰ **S15.002** Unspecified injury of left carotid artery `CC`

√7ᵗʰ **S15.009** Unspecified injury of unspecified carotid artery `CC`

N Newborn: 0 **P** Pediatric: 0-17 **M** Maternity: 9-64 **A** Adult: 15-124 `MCC` Major Complication/Comorbidity `CC` Complication/Comorbidity `SW` Severe Wound Dx

1002 ICD-10-CM 2020

√6ᵗʰ **S15.01** **Minor laceration of carotid artery**

Incomplete transection of carotid artery
Laceration of carotid artery NOS
Superficial laceration of carotid artery

  √7ᵗʰ **S15.011** **Minor laceration of right carotid artery** `cc`

  √7ᵗʰ **S15.012** **Minor laceration of left carotid artery**

  √7ᵗʰ **S15.019** **Minor laceration of unspecified carotid artery** `cc`

√6ᵗʰ **S15.02** **Major laceration of carotid artery**

Complete transection of carotid artery
Traumatic rupture of carotid artery

  √7ᵗʰ **S15.021** **Major laceration of right carotid artery**

  √7ᵗʰ **S15.022** **Major laceration of left carotid artery** `cc`

  √7ᵗʰ **S15.029** **Major laceration of unspecified carotid artery**

√6ᵗʰ **S15.09** **Other specified injury of carotid artery**

  √7ᵗʰ **S15.091** **Other specified injury of right carotid artery** `cc`

  √7ᵗʰ **S15.092** **Other specified injury of left carotid artery** `cc`

  √7ᵗʰ **S15.099** **Other specified injury of unspecified carotid artery** `cc`

√5ᵗʰ **S15.1** **Injury of vertebral artery**

√6ᵗʰ **S15.10** **Unspecified injury of vertebral artery**

  √7ᵗʰ **S15.101** **Unspecified injury of right vertebral artery** `cc`

  √7ᵗʰ **S15.102** **Unspecified injury of left vertebral artery** `cc`

  √7ᵗʰ **S15.109** **Unspecified injury of unspecified vertebral artery** `cc`

√6ᵗʰ **S15.11** **Minor laceration of vertebral artery**

Incomplete transection of vertebral artery
Laceration of vertebral artery NOS
Superficial laceration of vertebral artery

  √7ᵗʰ **S15.111** **Minor laceration of right vertebral artery** `cc`

  √7ᵗʰ **S15.112** **Minor laceration of left vertebral artery** `cc`

  √7ᵗʰ **S15.119** **Minor laceration of unspecified vertebral artery** `cc`

√6ᵗʰ **S15.12** **Major laceration of vertebral artery**

Complete transection of vertebral artery
Traumatic rupture of vertebral artery

  √7ᵗʰ **S15.121** **Major laceration of right vertebral artery** `cc`

  √7ᵗʰ **S15.122** **Major laceration of left vertebral artery** `cc`

  √7ᵗʰ **S15.129** **Major laceration of unspecified vertebral artery** `cc`

√6ᵗʰ **S15.19** **Other specified injury of vertebral artery**

  √7ᵗʰ **S15.191** **Other specified injury of right vertebral artery** `cc`

  √7ᵗʰ **S15.192** **Other specified injury of left vertebral artery** `cc`

  √7ᵗʰ **S15.199** **Other specified injury of unspecified vertebral artery** `cc`

√5ᵗʰ **S15.2** **Injury of external jugular vein**

√6ᵗʰ **S15.20** **Unspecified injury of external jugular vein**

  √7ᵗʰ **S15.201** **Unspecified injury of right external jugular vein** `cc`

  √7ᵗʰ **S15.202** **Unspecified injury of left external jugular vein** `cc`

  √7ᵗʰ **S15.209** **Unspecified injury of unspecified external jugular vein** `cc`

√6ᵗʰ **S15.21** **Minor laceration of external jugular vein**

Incomplete transection of external jugular vein
Laceration of external jugular vein NOS
Superficial laceration of external jugular vein

  √7ᵗʰ **S15.211** **Minor laceration of right external jugular vein** `cc`

  √7ᵗʰ **S15.212** **Minor laceration of left external jugular vein** `cc`

  √7ᵗʰ **S15.219** **Minor laceration of unspecified external jugular vein** `cc`

√6ᵗʰ **S15.22** **Major laceration of external jugular vein**

Complete transection of external jugular vein
Traumatic rupture of external jugular vein

  √7ᵗʰ **S15.221** **Major laceration of right external jugular vein** `cc`

  √7ᵗʰ **S15.222** **Major laceration of left external jugular vein** `cc`

  √7ᵗʰ **S15.229** **Major laceration of unspecified external jugular vein** `cc`

√6ᵗʰ **S15.29** **Other specified injury of external jugular vein**

  √7ᵗʰ **S15.291** **Other specified injury of right external jugular vein** `cc`

  √7ᵗʰ **S15.292** **Other specified injury of left external jugular vein**

  √7ᵗʰ **S15.299** **Other specified injury of unspecified external jugular vein** `cc`

√5ᵗʰ **S15.3** **Injury of internal jugular vein**

√6ᵗʰ **S15.30** **Unspecified injury of internal jugular vein**

  √7ᵗʰ **S15.301** **Unspecified injury of right internal jugular vein** `cc`

  √7ᵗʰ **S15.302** **Unspecified injury of left internal jugular vein** `cc`

  √7ᵗʰ **S15.309** **Unspecified injury of unspecified internal jugular vein** `cc`

√6ᵗʰ **S15.31** **Minor laceration of internal jugular vein**

Incomplete transection of internal jugular vein
Laceration of internal jugular vein NOS
Superficial laceration of internal jugular vein

  √7ᵗʰ **S15.311** **Minor laceration of right internal jugular vein** `cc`

  √7ᵗʰ **S15.312** **Minor laceration of left internal jugular vein** `cc`

  √7ᵗʰ **S15.319** **Minor laceration of unspecified internal jugular vein** `cc`

√6ᵗʰ **S15.32** **Major laceration of internal jugular vein**

Complete transection of internal jugular vein
Traumatic rupture of internal jugular vein

  √7ᵗʰ **S15.321** **Major laceration of right internal jugular vein** `cc`

  √7ᵗʰ **S15.322** **Major laceration of left internal jugular vein** `cc`

  √7ᵗʰ **S15.329** **Major laceration of unspecified internal jugular vein** `cc`

√6ᵗʰ **S15.39** **Other specified injury of internal jugular vein**

  √7ᵗʰ **S15.391** **Other specified injury of right internal jugular vein** `cc`

  √7ᵗʰ **S15.392** **Other specified injury of left internal jugular vein** `cc`

  √7ᵗʰ **S15.399** **Other specified injury of unspecified internal jugular vein** `cc`

√x7ᵗʰ **S15.8** **Injury of other specified blood vessels at neck level** `cc`

√x7ᵗʰ **S15.9** **Injury of unspecified blood vessel at neck level** `cc`

√4ᵗʰ **S16** **Injury of muscle, fascia and tendon at neck level**

Code also any associated open wound (S11.-)

EXCLUDES 2   sprain of joint or ligament at neck level (S13.9)

The appropriate 7th character is to be added to each code from category S16.
A initial encounter
D subsequent encounter
S sequela

√x7ᵗʰ **S16.1** **Strain of muscle, fascia and tendon at neck level**

√x7ᵗʰ **S16.2** **Laceration of muscle, fascia and tendon at neck level**

√x7ᵗʰ **S16.8** **Other specified injury of muscle, fascia and tendon at neck level**

√x7ᵗʰ **S16.9** **Unspecified injury of muscle, fascia and tendon at neck level**

✔ Additional Character Required   √x7ᵗʰ Placeholder   Unacceptable PDx   Questionable PDx   Manifestation   Unspecified Dx   **H1**-**H14** HAC   **HCC** CMS-HCC Dx   **HIV** HIV Dx

ICD-10-CM 2020

1003

Chapter 19. Injury, Poisoning and Certain Other Consequences of External Causes

S15.01–S16.9

√4ᵗʰ S17 Crushing injury of neck

Use additional code for all associated injuries, such as:
injury of blood vessels (S15.-)
open wound of neck (S11.-)
spinal cord injury (S14.0, S14.1-)
vertebral fracture (S12.0- — S12.3-)

The appropriate 7th character is to be added to each code from category S17.
A   initial encounter
D   subsequent encounter
S   sequela

CC Excl: For CC codes in category S17: PDX collection 1156

√x7ᵗʰ **S17.0 Crushing injury of larynx and trachea** `CC` `H5`

√x7ᵗʰ **S17.8 Crushing injury of other specified parts of neck** `CC` `H5`

√x7ᵗʰ **S17.9 Crushing injury of neck, part unspecified** `CC` `H5`

√4ᵗʰ S19 Other specified and unspecified injuries of neck

The appropriate 7th character is to be added to each code from category S19.
A   initial encounter
D   subsequent encounter
S   sequela

√5ᵗʰ **S19.8 Other specified injuries of neck**

√x7ᵗʰ **S19.80 Other specified injuries of unspecified part of neck**

√x7ᵗʰ **S19.81 Other specified injuries of larynx**

√x7ᵗʰ **S19.82 Other specified injuries of cervical trachea**

EXCLUDES 2   other specified injury of thoracic trachea (S27.5-)

√x7ᵗʰ **S19.83 Other specified injuries of vocal cord**

√x7ᵗʰ **S19.84 Other specified injuries of thyroid gland**

√x7ᵗʰ **S19.85 Other specified injuries of pharynx and cervical esophagus**

√x7ᵗʰ **S19.89 Other specified injuries of other specified part of neck**

√x7ᵗʰ **S19.9 Unspecified injury of neck**

Injuries to the thorax (S20-S29)

INCLUDES   injuries of breast
injuries of chest (wall)
injuries of interscapular area

EXCLUDES 2   burns and corrosions (T20-T32)
effects of foreign body in bronchus (T17.5)
effects of foreign body in esophagus (T18.1)
effects of foreign body in lung (T17.8)
effects of foreign body in trachea (T17.4)
frostbite (T33-T34)
injuries of axilla
injuries of clavicle
injuries of scapular region
injuries of shoulder
insect bite or sting, venomous (T63.4)

√4ᵗʰ S20 Superficial injury of thorax

The appropriate 7th character is to be added to each code from category S20.
A   initial encounter
D   subsequent encounter
S   sequela

√5ᵗʰ **S20.0 Contusion of breast**

√x7ᵗʰ **S20.00 Contusion of breast, unspecified breast**

√x7ᵗʰ **S20.01 Contusion of right breast**

√x7ᵗʰ **S20.02 Contusion of left breast**

√5ᵗʰ **S20.1 Other and unspecified superficial injuries of breast**

√6ᵗʰ **S20.10 Unspecified superficial injuries of breast**

√7ᵗʰ **S20.101 Unspecified superficial injuries of breast, right breast**

√7ᵗʰ **S20.102 Unspecified superficial injuries of breast, left breast**

√7ᵗʰ **S20.109 Unspecified superficial injuries of breast, unspecified breast**

√6ᵗʰ **S20.11 Abrasion of breast**

√7ᵗʰ **S20.111 Abrasion of breast, right breast**

√7ᵗʰ **S20.112 Abrasion of breast, left breast**

√7ᵗʰ **S20.119 Abrasion of breast, unspecified breast**

√6ᵗʰ **S20.12 Blister (nonthermal) of breast**

√7ᵗʰ **S20.121 Blister (nonthermal) of breast, right breast**

√7ᵗʰ **S20.122 Blister (nonthermal) of breast, left breast**

√7ᵗʰ **S20.129 Blister (nonthermal) of breast, unspecified breast**

√6ᵗʰ **S20.14 External constriction of part of breast**

√7ᵗʰ **S20.141 External constriction of part of breast, right breast**

√7ᵗʰ **S20.142 External constriction of part of breast, left breast**

√7ᵗʰ **S20.149 External constriction of part of breast, unspecified breast**

√6ᵗʰ **S20.15 Superficial foreign body of breast**

Splinter in the breast

√7ᵗʰ **S20.151 Superficial foreign body of breast, right breast**

√7ᵗʰ **S20.152 Superficial foreign body of breast, left breast**

√7ᵗʰ **S20.159 Superficial foreign body of breast, unspecified breast**

√6ᵗʰ **S20.16 Insect bite (nonvenomous) of breast**

√7ᵗʰ **S20.161 Insect bite (nonvenomous) of breast, right breast**

√7ᵗʰ **S20.162 Insect bite (nonvenomous) of breast, left breast**

√7ᵗʰ **S20.169 Insect bite (nonvenomous) of breast, unspecified breast**

√6ᵗʰ **S20.17 Other superficial bite of breast**

EXCLUDES 1   open bite of breast (S21.05-)

√7ᵗʰ **S20.171 Other superficial bite of breast, right breast**

√7ᵗʰ **S20.172 Other superficial bite of breast, left breast**

√7ᵗʰ **S20.179 Other superficial bite of breast, unspecified breast**

√5ᵗʰ **S20.2 Contusion of thorax**

√x7ᵗʰ **S20.20 Contusion of thorax, unspecified**

√6ᵗʰ **S20.21 Contusion of front wall of thorax**

√7ᵗʰ **S20.211 Contusion of right front wall of thorax**

√7ᵗʰ **S20.212 Contusion of left front wall of thorax**

√7ᵗʰ **S20.219 Contusion of unspecified front wall of thorax**

√6ᵗʰ **S20.22 Contusion of back wall of thorax**

√7ᵗʰ **S20.221 Contusion of right back wall of thorax**

√7ᵗʰ **S20.222 Contusion of left back wall of thorax**

√7ᵗʰ **S20.229 Contusion of unspecified back wall of thorax**

√5ᵗʰ **S20.3 Other and unspecified superficial injuries of front wall of thorax**

√6ᵗʰ **S20.30 Unspecified superficial injuries of front wall of thorax**

√7ᵗʰ **S20.301 Unspecified superficial injuries of right front wall of thorax**

√7ᵗʰ **S20.302 Unspecified superficial injuries of left front wall of thorax**

√7ᵗʰ **S20.309 Unspecified superficial injuries of unspecified front wall of thorax**

√6ᵗʰ **S20.31 Abrasion of front wall of thorax**

√7ᵗʰ **S20.311 Abrasion of right front wall of thorax**

√7ᵗʰ **S20.312 Abrasion of left front wall of thorax**

√7ᵗʰ **S20.319 Abrasion of unspecified front wall of thorax**

√6ᵗʰ **S20.32 Blister (nonthermal) of front wall of thorax**

√7ᵗʰ **S20.321 Blister (nonthermal) of right front wall of thorax**

√7ᵗʰ **S20.322 Blister (nonthermal) of left front wall of thorax**

√7ᵗʰ **S20.329 Blister (nonthermal) of unspecified front wall of thorax**

√6ᵗʰ **S20.34 External constriction of front wall of thorax**

√7ᵗʰ **S20.341 External constriction of right front wall of thorax**

√7ᵗʰ **S20.342 External constriction of left front wall of thorax**

√7ᵗʰ **S20.349 External constriction of unspecified front wall of thorax**

`N` Newborn: 0   `P` Pediatric: 0-17   `M` Maternity: 9-64   `A` Adult: 15-124   `MCC` Major Complication/Comorbidity   `CC` Complication/Comorbidity   `SW` Severe Wound Dx

1004   ICD-10-CM 2020

✓6ᵗʰ **S20.35** **Superficial** foreign body **of front wall of thorax**
     Splinter in front wall of thorax

     ✓7ᵗʰ **S20.351** **Superficial foreign body of** right **front wall of thorax**

     ✓7ᵗʰ **S20.352** **Superficial foreign body of** left **front wall of thorax**

     ✓7ᵗʰ **S20.359** **Superficial foreign body of unspecified front wall of thorax**

✓6ᵗʰ **S20.36** **Insect bite (nonvenomous) of front wall of thorax**

     ✓7ᵗʰ **S20.361** **Insect bite (nonvenomous) of** right **front wall of thorax**

     ✓7ᵗʰ **S20.362** **Insect bite (nonvenomous) of** left **front wall of thorax**

     ✓7ᵗʰ **S20.369** **Insect bite (nonvenomous) of unspecified front wall of thorax**

✓6ᵗʰ **S20.37** **Other superficial** bite **of front wall of thorax**
     EXCLUDES 1   *open bite of front wall of thorax (S21.15)*

     ✓7ᵗʰ **S20.371** **Other superficial bite of** right **front wall of thorax**

     ✓7ᵗʰ **S20.372** **Other superficial bite of** left **front wall of thorax**

     ✓7ᵗʰ **S20.379** **Other superficial bite of unspecified front wall of thorax**

✓5ᵗʰ **S20.4** **Other and unspecified superficial injuries of** back wall of thorax

     ✓6ᵗʰ **S20.40** **Unspecified superficial injuries of back wall of thorax**

         ✓7ᵗʰ **S20.401** **Unspecified superficial injuries of** right **back wall of thorax**

         ✓7ᵗʰ **S20.402** **Unspecified superficial injuries of** left **back wall of thorax**

         ✓7ᵗʰ **S20.409** **Unspecified superficial injuries of unspecified back wall of thorax**

     ✓6ᵗʰ **S20.41** **Abrasion of back wall of thorax**

         ✓7ᵗʰ **S20.411** **Abrasion of** right **back wall of thorax**

         ✓7ᵗʰ **S20.412** **Abrasion of** left **back wall of thorax**

         ✓7ᵗʰ **S20.419** **Abrasion of unspecified back wall of thorax**

     ✓6ᵗʰ **S20.42** **Blister (nonthermal) of back wall of thorax**

         ✓7ᵗʰ **S20.421** **Blister (nonthermal) of** right **back wall of thorax**

         ✓7ᵗʰ **S20.422** **Blister (nonthermal) of** left **back wall of thorax**

         ✓7ᵗʰ **S20.429** **Blister (nonthermal) of unspecified back wall of thorax**

     ✓6ᵗʰ **S20.44** **External constriction of back wall of thorax**

         ✓7ᵗʰ **S20.441** **External constriction of** right **back wall of thorax**

         ✓7ᵗʰ **S20.442** **External constriction of** left **back wall of thorax**

         ✓7ᵗʰ **S20.449** **External constriction of unspecified back wall of thorax**

     ✓6ᵗʰ **S20.45** **Superficial** foreign body **of back wall of thorax**
         Splinter of back wall of thorax

         ✓7ᵗʰ **S20.451** **Superficial foreign body of** right **back wall of thorax**

         ✓7ᵗʰ **S20.452** **Superficial foreign body of** left **back wall of thorax**

         ✓7ᵗʰ **S20.459** **Superficial foreign body of unspecified back wall of thorax**

     ✓6ᵗʰ **S20.46** **Insect bite (nonvenomous) of back wall of thorax**

         ✓7ᵗʰ **S20.461** **Insect bite (nonvenomous) of** right **back wall of thorax**

         ✓7ᵗʰ **S20.462** **Insect bite (nonvenomous) of** left **back wall of thorax**

         ✓7ᵗʰ **S20.469** **Insect bite (nonvenomous) of unspecified back wall of thorax**

     ✓6ᵗʰ **S20.47** **Other superficial** bite **of back wall of thorax**
         EXCLUDES 1   *open bite of back wall of thorax (S21.25)*

         ✓7ᵗʰ **S20.471** **Other superficial bite of** right **back wall of thorax**

         ✓7ᵗʰ **S20.472** **Other superficial bite of** left **back wall of thorax**

         ✓7ᵗʰ **S20.479** **Other superficial bite of unspecified back wall of thorax**

✓5ᵗʰ **S20.9** **Superficial injury of unspecified parts of thorax**
     EXCLUDES 1   *contusion of thorax NOS (S20.20)*

     ✓x7ᵗʰ **S20.90** **Unspecified superficial injury of unspecified parts of thorax**
         Superficial injury of thoracic wall NOS

     ✓x7ᵗʰ **S20.91** **Abrasion of unspecified parts of thorax**

     ✓x7ᵗʰ **S20.92** **Blister (nonthermal) of unspecified parts of thorax**

     ✓x7ᵗʰ **S20.94** **External constriction of unspecified parts of thorax**

     ✓x7ᵗʰ **S20.95** **Superficial** foreign body **of unspecified parts of thorax**
         Splinter in thorax NOS

     ✓x7ᵗʰ **S20.96** **Insect bite (nonvenomous) of unspecified parts of thorax**

     ✓x7ᵗʰ **S20.97** **Other superficial bite of unspecified parts of thorax**
         EXCLUDES 1   *open bite of thorax NOS (S21.95)*

✓4ᵗʰ **S21** **Open wound of thorax**

Code also any associated injury, such as:
     injury of heart (S26.-)
     injury of intrathoracic organs (S27.-)
     rib fracture (S22.3-, S22.4-)
     spinal cord injury (S24.0-, S24.1-)
     traumatic hemopneumothorax (S27.3)
     traumatic hemothorax (S27.1)
     traumatic pneumothorax (S27.0)
     wound infection

     EXCLUDES 1   *traumatic amputation (partial) of thorax (S28.1)*

The appropriate 7th character is to be added to each code from category S21.
A   initial encounter
D   subsequent encounter
S   sequela

CC Excl: For codes in category S21:
For MCC codes, unless otherwise noted: PDX collection 1169
For CC codes: PDX collection 1168

✓5ᵗʰ **S21.0** **Open wound of breast**

     ✓6ᵗʰ **S21.00** **Unspecified open wound of breast**

         ✓7ᵗʰ **S21.001** **Unspecified open wound of** right **breast**

         ✓7ᵗʰ **S21.002** **Unspecified open wound of** left **breast**

         ✓7ᵗʰ **S21.009** **Unspecified open wound of unspecified breast**

     ✓6ᵗʰ **S21.01** **Laceration without foreign body of breast**

         ✓7ᵗʰ **S21.011** **Laceration without foreign body of** right **breast**

         ✓7ᵗʰ **S21.012** **Laceration without foreign body of** left **breast**

         ✓7ᵗʰ **S21.019** **Laceration without foreign body of unspecified breast**

     ✓6ᵗʰ **S21.02** **Laceration with foreign body of breast**

         ✓7ᵗʰ **S21.021** **Laceration with foreign body of** right **breast**

         ✓7ᵗʰ **S21.022** **Laceration with foreign body of** left **breast**

         ✓7ᵗʰ **S21.029** **Laceration with foreign body of unspecified breast**

     ✓6ᵗʰ **S21.03** **Puncture wound without foreign body of breast**

         ✓7ᵗʰ **S21.031** **Puncture wound without foreign body of** right **breast**

         ✓7ᵗʰ **S21.032** **Puncture wound without foreign body of** left **breast**

         ✓7ᵗʰ **S21.039** **Puncture wound without foreign body of unspecified breast**

     ✓6ᵗʰ **S21.04** **Puncture wound with foreign body of breast**

         ✓7ᵗʰ **S21.041** **Puncture wound with foreign body of** right **breast**

         ✓7ᵗʰ **S21.042** **Puncture wound with foreign body of** left **breast**

         ✓7ᵗʰ **S21.049** **Puncture wound with foreign body of unspecified breast**

     ✓6ᵗʰ **S21.05** **Open bite of breast**
         Bite of breast NOS
         EXCLUDES 1   *superficial bite of breast (S20.17)*

         ✓7ᵗʰ **S21.051** **Open bite of** right **breast**

         ✓7ᵗʰ **S21.052** **Open bite of** left **breast**

         ✓7ᵗʰ **S21.059** **Open bite of unspecified breast**

✓ Additional Character Required   ✓x7ᵗʰ Placeholder   Unacceptable PDx   Questionable PDx   Manifestation   Unspecified Dx   H1-H14 HAC   HCC CMS-HCC Dx   HIV HIV Dx

ICD-10-CM 2020   1005

√5ᵗʰ **S21.1** **Open wound of** front wall of thorax **without penetration into thoracic cavity**

Open wound of chest without penetration into thoracic cavity

   √6ᵗʰ **S21.10** **Unspecified open wound of front wall of thorax without penetration into thoracic cavity**

      √7ᵗʰ **S21.101** **Unspecified open wound of** right **front wall of thorax without penetration into thoracic cavity**   `CC`

      √7ᵗʰ **S21.102** **Unspecified open wound of** left **front wall of thorax without penetration into thoracic cavity**   `CC`

      √7ᵗʰ **S21.109** **Unspecified open wound of unspecified front wall of thorax without penetration into thoracic cavity**   `CC`

   √6ᵗʰ **S21.11** **Laceration without foreign body of front wall of thorax without penetration into thoracic cavity**

      √7ᵗʰ **S21.111** **Laceration without foreign body of** right **front wall of thorax without penetration into thoracic cavity**   `CC`

      √7ᵗʰ **S21.112** **Laceration without foreign body of** left **front wall of thorax without penetration into thoracic cavity**   `CC`

      √7ᵗʰ **S21.119** **Laceration without foreign body of unspecified front wall of thorax without penetration into thoracic cavity**   `CC`

   √6ᵗʰ **S21.12** **Laceration with foreign body** of front wall of thorax **without penetration into thoracic cavity**

      √7ᵗʰ **S21.121** **Laceration with foreign body of** right **front wall of thorax without penetration into thoracic cavity**   `CC`

      √7ᵗʰ **S21.122** **Laceration with foreign body of** left **front wall of thorax without penetration into thoracic cavity**   `CC`

      √7ᵗʰ **S21.129** **Laceration with foreign body of unspecified front wall of thorax without penetration into thoracic cavity**   `CC`

   √6ᵗʰ **S21.13** **Puncture wound without foreign body of front wall of thorax without penetration into thoracic cavity**

      √7ᵗʰ **S21.131** **Puncture wound without foreign body of** right **front wall of thorax without penetration into thoracic cavity**   `CC`

      √7ᵗʰ **S21.132** **Puncture wound without foreign body of** left **front wall of thorax without penetration into thoracic cavity**   `CC`

      √7ᵗʰ **S21.139** **Puncture wound without foreign body of unspecified front wall of thorax without penetration into thoracic cavity**   `CC`

   √6ᵗʰ **S21.14** **Puncture wound with foreign body** of front wall of thorax **without penetration into thoracic cavity**

      √7ᵗʰ **S21.141** **Puncture wound with foreign body of** right **front wall of thorax without penetration into thoracic cavity**   `CC`

      √7ᵗʰ **S21.142** **Puncture wound with foreign body of** left **front wall of thorax without penetration into thoracic cavity**   `CC`

      √7ᵗʰ **S21.149** **Puncture wound with foreign body of unspecified front wall of thorax without penetration into thoracic cavity**   `CC`

   √6ᵗʰ **S21.15** **Open bite** of front wall of thorax **without penetration into thoracic cavity**

Bite of front wall of thorax NOS

EXCLUDES 1   *superficial bite of front wall of thorax (S20.37)*

      √7ᵗʰ **S21.151** **Open bite of** right **front wall of thorax without penetration into thoracic cavity**   `CC`

      √7ᵗʰ **S21.152** **Open bite of** left **front wall of thorax without penetration into thoracic cavity**   `CC`

      √7ᵗʰ **S21.159** **Open bite of unspecified front wall of thorax without penetration into thoracic cavity**   `CC`

√5ᵗʰ **S21.2** **Open wound of** back wall of thorax **without penetration into thoracic cavity**

   √6ᵗʰ **S21.20** **Unspecified open wound of back wall of thorax without penetration into thoracic cavity**

      √7ᵗʰ **S21.201** **Unspecified open wound of** right **back wall of thorax without penetration into thoracic cavity**

      √7ᵗʰ **S21.202** **Unspecified open wound of** left **back wall of thorax without penetration into thoracic cavity**

      √7ᵗʰ **S21.209** **Unspecified open wound of unspecified back wall of thorax without penetration into thoracic cavity**

   √6ᵗʰ **S21.21** **Laceration without foreign body** of back wall of **thorax without penetration into thoracic cavity**

      √7ᵗʰ **S21.211** **Laceration without foreign body of** right **back wall of thorax without penetration into thoracic cavity**

      √7ᵗʰ **S21.212** **Laceration without foreign body of** left **back wall of thorax without penetration into thoracic cavity**

      √7ᵗʰ **S21.219** **Laceration without foreign body of unspecified back wall of thorax without penetration into thoracic cavity**

   √6ᵗʰ **S21.22** **Laceration with foreign body** of back wall of thorax **without penetration into thoracic cavity**

      √7ᵗʰ **S21.221** **Laceration with foreign body of** right **back wall of thorax without penetration into thoracic cavity**

      √7ᵗʰ **S21.222** **Laceration with foreign body of** left **back wall of thorax without penetration into thoracic cavity**

      √7ᵗʰ **S21.229** **Laceration with foreign body of unspecified back wall of thorax without penetration into thoracic cavity**

   √6ᵗʰ **S21.23** **Puncture wound without foreign body** of back wall **of thorax without penetration into thoracic cavity**

      √7ᵗʰ **S21.231** **Puncture wound without foreign body of** right **back wall of thorax without penetration into thoracic cavity**

      √7ᵗʰ **S21.232** **Puncture wound without foreign body of** left **back wall of thorax without penetration into thoracic cavity**

      √7ᵗʰ **S21.239** **Puncture wound without foreign body of unspecified back wall of thorax without penetration into thoracic cavity**

   √6ᵗʰ **S21.24** **Puncture wound with foreign body** of back wall of **thorax without penetration into thoracic cavity**

      √7ᵗʰ **S21.241** **Puncture wound with foreign body of** right **back wall of thorax without penetration into thoracic cavity**

      √7ᵗʰ **S21.242** **Puncture wound with foreign body of** left **back wall of thorax without penetration into thoracic cavity**

      √7ᵗʰ **S21.249** **Puncture wound with foreign body of unspecified back wall of thorax without penetration into thoracic cavity**

`N` Newborn: 0   `P` Pediatric: 0-17   `M` Maternity: 9-64   `A` Adult: 15-124   `MCC` Major Complication/Comorbidity   `CC` Complication/Comorbidity   `SW` Severe Wound Dx

1006   ICD–10-CM 2020

√6ᵗʰ **S21.25** Open bite of back wall of thorax without penetration into thoracic cavity

Bite of back wall of thorax NOS

> EXCLUDES 1   superficial bite of back wall of thorax (S20.47)

√7ᵗʰ **S21.251** Open bite of right back wall of thorax without penetration into thoracic cavity

√7ᵗʰ **S21.252** Open bite of left back wall of thorax without penetration into thoracic cavity

√7ᵗʰ **S21.259** Open bite of unspecified back wall of thorax without penetration into thoracic cavity

√5ᵗʰ **S21.3** Open wound of front wall of thorax with penetration into thoracic cavity

Open wound of chest with penetration into thoracic cavity

√6ᵗʰ **S21.30** Unspecified open wound of front wall of thorax with penetration into thoracic cavity

√7ᵗʰ **S21.301** Unspecified open wound of right front wall of thorax with penetration into thoracic cavity   `MCC`

√7ᵗʰ **S21.302** Unspecified open wound of left front wall of thorax with penetration into thoracic cavity   `MCC`

√7ᵗʰ **S21.309** Unspecified open wound of unspecified front wall of thorax with penetration into thoracic cavity   `MCC`

CC Excl: PDX collection 1170

√6ᵗʰ **S21.31** Laceration without foreign body of front wall of thorax with penetration into thoracic cavity

√7ᵗʰ **S21.311** Laceration without foreign body of right front wall of thorax with penetration into thoracic cavity   `MCC`

√7ᵗʰ **S21.312** Laceration without foreign body of left front wall of thorax with penetration into thoracic cavity   `MCC`

√7ᵗʰ **S21.319** Laceration without foreign body of unspecified front wall of thorax with penetration into thoracic cavity   `MCC`

√6ᵗʰ **S21.32** Laceration with foreign body of front wall of thorax with penetration into thoracic cavity

√7ᵗʰ **S21.321** Laceration with foreign body of right front wall of thorax with penetration into thoracic cavity   `MCC`

√7ᵗʰ **S21.322** Laceration with foreign body of left front wall of thorax with penetration into thoracic cavity   `MCC`

√7ᵗʰ **S21.329** Laceration with foreign body of unspecified front wall of thorax with penetration into thoracic cavity   `MCC`

√6ᵗʰ **S21.33** Puncture wound without foreign body of front wall of thorax with penetration into thoracic cavity

√7ᵗʰ **S21.331** Puncture wound without foreign body of right front wall of thorax with penetration into thoracic cavity   `MCC`

√7ᵗʰ **S21.332** Puncture wound without foreign body of left front wall of thorax with penetration into thoracic cavity   `MCC`

√7ᵗʰ **S21.339** Puncture wound without foreign body of unspecified front wall of thorax with penetration into thoracic cavity   `MCC`

√6ᵗʰ **S21.34** Puncture wound with foreign body of front wall of thorax with penetration into thoracic cavity

√7ᵗʰ **S21.341** Puncture wound with foreign body of right front wall of thorax with penetration into thoracic cavity   `MCC`

√7ᵗʰ **S21.342** Puncture wound with foreign body of left front wall of thorax with penetration into thoracic cavity   `MCC`

√7ᵗʰ **S21.349** Puncture wound with foreign body of unspecified front wall of thorax with penetration into thoracic cavity   `MCC`

√6ᵗʰ **S21.35** Open bite of front wall of thorax with penetration into thoracic cavity

> EXCLUDES 1   superficial bite of front wall of thorax (S20.37)

√7ᵗʰ **S21.351** Open bite of right front wall of thorax with penetration into thoracic cavity   `MCC`

√7ᵗʰ **S21.352** Open bite of left front wall of thorax with penetration into thoracic cavity   `MCC`

√7ᵗʰ **S21.359** Open bite of unspecified front wall of thorax with penetration into thoracic cavity   `MCC`

√5ᵗʰ **S21.4** Open wound of back wall of thorax with penetration into thoracic cavity

√6ᵗʰ **S21.40** Unspecified open wound of back wall of thorax with penetration into thoracic cavity

√7ᵗʰ **S21.401** Unspecified open wound of right back wall of thorax with penetration into thoracic cavity   `MCC`

√7ᵗʰ **S21.402** Unspecified open wound of left back wall of thorax with penetration into thoracic cavity   `MCC`

√7ᵗʰ **S21.409** Unspecified open wound of unspecified back wall of thorax with penetration into thoracic cavity   `MCC`

√6ᵗʰ **S21.41** Laceration without foreign body of back wall of thorax with penetration into thoracic cavity

√7ᵗʰ **S21.411** Laceration without foreign body of right back wall of thorax with penetration into thoracic cavity   `MCC`

√7ᵗʰ **S21.412** Laceration without foreign body of left back wall of thorax with penetration into thoracic cavity   `MCC`

√7ᵗʰ **S21.419** Laceration without foreign body of unspecified back wall of thorax with penetration into thoracic cavity   `MCC`

√6ᵗʰ **S21.42** Laceration with foreign body of back wall of thorax with penetration into thoracic cavity

√7ᵗʰ **S21.421** Laceration with foreign body of right back wall of thorax with penetration into thoracic cavity   `MCC`

√7ᵗʰ **S21.422** Laceration with foreign body of left back wall of thorax with penetration into thoracic cavity   `MCC`

√7ᵗʰ **S21.429** Laceration with foreign body of unspecified back wall of thorax with penetration into thoracic cavity   `MCC`

☑ Additional Character Required   √x7ᵗʰ Placeholder   Unacceptable PDx   Questionable PDx   Manifestation   Unspecified Dx   H1-H14 HAC   HCC CMS-HCC Dx   HIV HIV Dx

ICD-10-CM 2020   1007

√6ᵗʰ **S21.43** Puncture wound without foreign body of back wall of thorax with penetration into thoracic cavity

√7ᵗʰ **S21.431** Puncture wound without foreign body of right back wall of thorax with penetration into thoracic cavity `MCC`

√7ᵗʰ **S21.432** Puncture wound without foreign body of left back wall of thorax with penetration into thoracic cavity `MCC`

√7ᵗʰ **S21.439** Puncture wound without foreign body of unspecified back wall of thorax with penetration into thoracic cavity `MCC`

√6ᵗʰ **S21.44** Puncture wound with foreign body of back wall of thorax with penetration into thoracic cavity

√7ᵗʰ **S21.441** Puncture wound with foreign body of right back wall of thorax with penetration into thoracic cavity `MCC`

√7ᵗʰ **S21.442** Puncture wound with foreign body of left back wall of thorax with penetration into thoracic cavity `MCC`

√7ᵗʰ **S21.449** Puncture wound with foreign body of unspecified back wall of thorax with penetration into thoracic cavity `MCC`

√6ᵗʰ **S21.45** Open bite of back wall of thorax with penetration into thoracic cavity

Bite of back wall of thorax NOS

EXCLUDES 1 superficial bite of back wall of thorax (S20.47)

√7ᵗʰ **S21.451** Open bite of right back wall of thorax with penetration into thoracic cavity `MCC`

√7ᵗʰ **S21.452** Open bite of left back wall of thorax with penetration into thoracic cavity `MCC`

√7ᵗʰ **S21.459** Open bite of unspecified back wall of thorax with penetration into thoracic cavity `MCC`

√5ᵗʰ **S21.9** Open wound of unspecified part of thorax

Open wound of thoracic wall NOS

√x7ᵗʰ **S21.90** Unspecified open wound of unspecified part of thorax `CC`

√x7ᵗʰ **S21.91** Laceration without foreign body of unspecified part of thorax `CC`

√x7ᵗʰ **S21.92** Laceration with foreign body of unspecified part of thorax `CC`

√x7ᵗʰ **S21.93** Puncture wound without foreign body of unspecified part of thorax `CC`

√x7ᵗʰ **S21.94** Puncture wound with foreign body of unspecified part of thorax `CC`

√x7ᵗʰ **S21.95** Open bite of unspecified part of thorax `CC`

EXCLUDES 1 superficial bite of thorax (S20.97)

√4ᵗʰ **S22 Fracture of rib(s), sternum and thoracic spine**

`NOTE` A fracture not indicated as displaced or nondisplaced should be coded to displaced

A fracture not indicated as open or closed should be coded to closed

`INCLUDES` fracture of thoracic neural arch
fracture of thoracic spinous process
fracture of thoracic transverse process
fracture of thoracic vertebra
fracture of thoracic vertebral arch

Code first any associated:
injury of intrathoracic organ (S27.-)
spinal cord injury (S24.0-, S24.1-)

EXCLUDES 1 transection of thorax (S28.1)

EXCLUDES 2 fracture of clavicle (S42.0-)
fracture of scapula (S42.1-)

AHA: 2018,2Q,12; 2015,3Q,37-39

The appropriate 7th character is to be added to each code from category S22.
A initial encounter for closed fracture
B initial encounter for open fracture
D subsequent encounter for fracture with routine healing
G subsequent encounter for fracture with delayed healing
K subsequent encounter for fracture with nonunion
S sequela

√5ᵗʰ **S22.0 Fracture of thoracic vertebra**

CC Excl: For codes in subcategory S22.0:
CC with 7th character A or MCC with 7th character B: PDX collection 1171
CC with 7th character K: PDX collection 897

√6ᵗʰ **S22.00** Fracture of unspecified thoracic vertebra

2,3,6 √7ᵗʰ **S22.000** Wedge compression fracture of unspecified thoracic vertebra `MCC` `CC` `H5` `HCC`

2,3,6 √7ᵗʰ **S22.001** Stable burst fracture of unspecified thoracic vertebra `MCC` `CC` `H5` `HCC`

2,3,6 √7ᵗʰ **S22.002** Unstable burst fracture of unspecified thoracic vertebra `MCC` `CC` `H5` `HCC`

2,3,6 √7ᵗʰ **S22.008** Other fracture of unspecified thoracic vertebra `MCC` `CC` `H5` `HCC`

2,3,6 √7ᵗʰ **S22.009** Unspecified fracture of unspecified thoracic vertebra `MCC` `CC` `H5` `HCC`

√6ᵗʰ **S22.01** Fracture of first thoracic vertebra

2,3,6 √7ᵗʰ **S22.010** Wedge compression fracture of first thoracic vertebra `MCC` `CC` `H5` `HCC`

2,3,6 √7ᵗʰ **S22.011** Stable burst fracture of first thoracic vertebra `MCC` `CC` `H5` `HCC`

2,3,6 √7ᵗʰ **S22.012** Unstable burst fracture of first thoracic vertebra `MCC` `CC` `H5` `HCC`

2,3,6 √7ᵗʰ **S22.018** Other fracture of first thoracic vertebra `MCC` `CC` `H5` `HCC`

2,3,6 √7ᵗʰ **S22.019** Unspecified fracture of first thoracic vertebra `MCC` `CC` `H5` `HCC`

√6ᵗʰ **S22.02** Fracture of second thoracic vertebra

2,3,6 √7ᵗʰ **S22.020** Wedge compression fracture of second thoracic vertebra `MCC` `CC` `H5` `HCC`

2,3,6 √7ᵗʰ **S22.021** Stable burst fracture of second thoracic vertebra `MCC` `CC` `H5` `HCC`

2,3,6 √7ᵗʰ **S22.022** Unstable burst fracture of second thoracic vertebra `MCC` `CC` `H5` `HCC`

2,3,6 √7ᵗʰ **S22.028** Other fracture of second thoracic vertebra `MCC` `CC` `H5` `HCC`

2,3,6 √7ᵗʰ **S22.029** Unspecified fracture of second thoracic vertebra `MCC` `CC` `H5` `HCC`

√6ᵗʰ **S22.03** Fracture of third thoracic vertebra

2,3,6 √7ᵗʰ **S22.030** Wedge compression fracture of third thoracic vertebra `MCC` `CC` `H5` `HCC`

2,3,6 √7ᵗʰ **S22.031** Stable burst fracture of third thoracic vertebra `MCC` `CC` `H5` `HCC`

2,3,6 √7ᵗʰ **S22.032** Unstable burst fracture of third thoracic vertebra `MCC` `CC` `H5` `HCC`

N Newborn: 0 **P** Pediatric: 0-17 **M** Maternity: 9-64 **A** Adult: 15-124 `MCC` Major Complication/Comorbidity `CC` Complication/Comorbidity `SW` Severe Wound Dx

1008 ICD-10-CM 2020

2,3,6 √7th **S22.038 Other fracture of third thoracic vertebra** `MCC` `CC` `H5` `HCC`

2,3,6 √7th **S22.039 Unspecified fracture of third thoracic vertebra** `MCC` `CC` `H5` `HCC`

√6th **S22.04 Fracture of fourth thoracic vertebra**

2,3,6 √7th **S22.040 Wedge compression fracture of fourth thoracic vertebra** `MCC` `CC` `H5` `HCC`

2,3,6 √7th **S22.041 Stable burst fracture of fourth thoracic vertebra** `MCC` `CC` `H5` `HCC`

2,3,6 √7th **S22.042 Unstable burst fracture of fourth thoracic vertebra** `MCC` `CC` `H5` `HCC`

2,3,6 √7th **S22.048 Other fracture of fourth thoracic vertebra** `MCC` `CC` `H5` `HCC`

2,3,6 √7th **S22.049 Unspecified fracture of fourth thoracic vertebra** `MCC` `CC` `H5` `HCC`

√6th **S22.05 Fracture of T5-T6 vertebra**

2,3,6 √7th **S22.050 Wedge compression fracture of T5-T6 vertebra** `MCC` `CC` `H5` `HCC`

2,3,6 √7th **S22.051 Stable burst fracture of T5-T6 vertebra** `MCC` `CC` `H5` `HCC`

2,3,6 √7th **S22.052 Unstable burst fracture of T5-T6 vertebra** `MCC` `CC` `H5` `HCC`

2,3,6 √7th **S22.058 Other fracture of T5-T6 vertebra** `MCC` `CC` `H5` `HCC`

2,3,6 √7th **S22.059 Unspecified fracture of T5-T6 vertebra** `MCC` `CC` `H5` `HCC`

√6th **S22.06 Fracture of T7-T8 vertebra**

2,3,6 √7th **S22.060 Wedge compression fracture of T7-T8 vertebra** `MCC` `CC` `H5` `HCC`

2,3,6 √7th **S22.061 Stable burst fracture of T7-T8 vertebra** `MCC` `CC` `H5` `HCC`

2,3,6 √7th **S22.062 Unstable burst fracture of T7-T8 vertebra** `MCC` `CC` `H5` `HCC`

2,3,6 √7th **S22.068 Other fracture of T7-T8 thoracic vertebra** `MCC` `CC` `H5` `HCC`

2,3,6 √7th **S22.069 Unspecified fracture of T7-T8 vertebra** `MCC` `CC` `H5` `HCC`

√6th **S22.07 Fracture of T9-T10 vertebra**

2,3,6 √7th **S22.070 Wedge compression fracture of T9-T10 vertebra** `MCC` `CC` `H5` `HCC`

2,3,6 √7th **S22.071 Stable burst fracture of T9-T10 vertebra** `MCC` `CC` `H5` `HCC`

2,3,6 √7th **S22.072 Unstable burst fracture of T9-T10 vertebra** `MCC` `CC` `H5` `HCC`

2,3,6 √7th **S22.078 Other fracture of T9-T10 vertebra** `MCC` `CC` `H5` `HCC`

2,3,6 √7th **S22.079 Unspecified fracture of T9-T10 vertebra** `MCC` `CC` `H5` `HCC`

√6th **S22.08 Fracture of T11-T12 vertebra**

2,3,6 √7th **S22.080 Wedge compression fracture of T11-T12 vertebra** `MCC` `CC` `H5` `HCC`

2,3,6 √7th **S22.081 Stable burst fracture of T11-T12 vertebra** `MCC` `CC` `H5` `HCC`

2,3,6 √7th **S22.082 Unstable burst fracture of T11-T12 vertebra** `MCC` `CC` `H5` `HCC`

2,3,6 √7th **S22.088 Other fracture of T11-T12 vertebra** `MCC` `CC` `H5` `HCC`

2,3,6 √7th **S22.089 Unspecified fracture of T11-T12 vertebra** `MCC` `CC` `H5` `HCC`

√5th **S22.2 Fracture of sternum**

DEF: Break in flat bone (breast bone) in the anterior thorax caused by blunt trauma to the anterior chest.
CC Excl: For codes in subcategory S22.2:
CC with 7th character A or MCC with 7th character B: PDX collection 1172
CC with 7th character K: PDX collection 897

2,4 √x7th **S22.20 Unspecified fracture of sternum** `MCC` `CC` `H5`

2,3 √x7th **S22.21 Fracture of manubrium** `MCC` `CC` `H5`

2,3 √x7th **S22.22 Fracture of body of sternum** `MCC` `CC` `H5`

2,3 √x7th **S22.23 Sternal manubrial dissociation** `MCC` `CC` `H5`

2,3 √x7th **S22.24 Fracture of xiphoid process** `MCC` `CC` `H5`

√5th **S22.3 Fracture of one rib**

CC Excl: For codes in subcategory S22.3:
CC with 7th character A: PDX collection 1173
MCC with 7th character B: PDX collection 1174
CC with 7th character K: PDX collection 897

2,3 √x7th **S22.31 Fracture of one rib, right side** `MCC` `CC` `H5`

2,3 √x7th **S22.32 Fracture of one rib, left side** `MCC` `CC` `H5`

2,3 √x7th **S22.39 Fracture of one rib, unspecified side** `MCC` `CC` `H5`

√5th **S22.4 Multiple fractures of ribs**

Fractures of two or more ribs
EXCLUDES 1 flail chest (S22.5-)
CC Excl: For codes in subcategory S22.4, unless otherwise noted:
CC with 7th character A or or MCC with 7th character B: PDX collection 1174
CC with 7th character K: PDX collection 897

2,3 √x7th **S22.41 Multiple fractures of ribs, right side** `MCC` `CC` `H5`

2,3 √x7th **S22.42 Multiple fractures of ribs, left side** `MCC` `CC` `H5`

2,3 √x7th **S22.43 Multiple fractures of ribs, bilateral** `MCC` `CC` `H5`

2,3 √x7th **S22.49 Multiple fractures of ribs, unspecified side** `MCC` `CC` `H5`
CC Excl: CC with 7th character A: PDX collection 1174
CC Excl: MCC with 7th character B: No Excl
CC Excl: CC with 7th character K: PDX collection 897

4 √x7th **S22.5 Flail chest** `MCC` `CC` `H5`
CC Excl: MCC with 7th character A or B: PDX collection 1175
CC Excl: CC with 7th character K: PDX collection 897

2,3 √x7th **S22.9 Fracture of bony thorax, part unspecified** `MCC` `CC` `H5`
CC Excl: CC with 7th character A or MCC with 7th character B: PDX collection 1176
CC Excl: CC with 7th character K: PDX collection 897

√4th **S23 Dislocation and sprain of joints and ligaments of thorax**

INCLUDES   avulsion of joint or ligament of thorax
laceration of cartilage, joint or ligament of thorax
sprain of cartilage, joint or ligament of thorax
traumatic hemarthrosis of joint or ligament of thorax
traumatic rupture of joint or ligament of thorax
traumatic subluxation of joint or ligament of thorax
traumatic tear of joint or ligament of thorax
Code also any associated open wound
EXCLUDES 2 dislocation, sprain of sternoclavicular joint (S43.2, S43.6)
strain of muscle or tendon of thorax (S29.01-)

The appropriate 7th character is to be added to each code from category S23.
A   initial encounter
D   subsequent encounter
S   sequela

√x7th **S23.0 Traumatic rupture of thoracic intervertebral disc**
EXCLUDES 1 rupture or displacement (nontraumatic) of thoracic intervertebral disc NOS (M51.- with fifth character 4)

√5th **S23.1 Subluxation and dislocation of thoracic vertebra**
Code also any associated:
open wound of thorax (S21.-)
spinal cord injury (S24.0-, S24.1-)
EXCLUDES 2 fracture of thoracic vertebrae (S22.0-)

√6th **S23.10 Subluxation and dislocation of unspecified thoracic vertebra**

√7th **S23.100 Subluxation of unspecified thoracic vertebra**

√7th **S23.101 Dislocation of unspecified thoracic vertebra**

√6th **S23.11 Subluxation and dislocation of T1/T2 thoracic vertebra**

√7th **S23.110 Subluxation of T1/T2 thoracic vertebra**

√7th **S23.111 Dislocation of T1/T2 thoracic vertebra**

√6th **S23.12 Subluxation and dislocation of T2/T3-T3/T4 thoracic vertebra**

√7th **S23.120 Subluxation of T2/T3 thoracic vertebra**

√7th **S23.121 Dislocation of T2/T3 thoracic vertebra**

√7th **S23.122 Subluxation of T3/T4 thoracic vertebra**

√7th **S23.123 Dislocation of T3/T4 thoracic vertebra**

√6ᵗʰ **S23.13** **Subluxation and dislocation of** T4/T5-T5/T6 **thoracic vertebra**
- √7ᵗʰ **S23.130** Subluxation of T4/T5 thoracic vertebra
- √7ᵗʰ **S23.131** Dislocation of T4/T5 thoracic vertebra
- √7ᵗʰ **S23.132** Subluxation of T5/T6 thoracic vertebra
- √7ᵗʰ **S23.133** Dislocation of T5/T6 thoracic vertebra

√6ᵗʰ **S23.14** **Subluxation and dislocation of** T6/T7-T7/T8 **thoracic vertebra**
- √7ᵗʰ **S23.140** Subluxation of T6/T7 thoracic vertebra
- √7ᵗʰ **S23.141** Dislocation of T6/T7 thoracic vertebra
- √7ᵗʰ **S23.142** Subluxation of T7/T8 thoracic vertebra
- √7ᵗʰ **S23.143** Dislocation of T7/T8 thoracic vertebra

√6ᵗʰ **S23.15** **Subluxation and dislocation of** T8/T9-T9/T10 **thoracic vertebra**
- √7ᵗʰ **S23.150** Subluxation of T8/T9 thoracic vertebra
- √7ᵗʰ **S23.151** Dislocation of T8/T9 thoracic vertebra
- √7ᵗʰ **S23.152** Subluxation of T9/T10 thoracic vertebra
- √7ᵗʰ **S23.153** Dislocation of T9/T10 thoracic vertebra

√6ᵗʰ **S23.16** **Subluxation and dislocation of** T10/T11-T11/T12 **thoracic vertebra**
- √7ᵗʰ **S23.160** Subluxation of T10/T11 thoracic vertebra
- √7ᵗʰ **S23.161** Dislocation of T10/T11 thoracic vertebra
- √7ᵗʰ **S23.162** Subluxation of T11/T12 thoracic vertebra
- √7ᵗʰ **S23.163** Dislocation of T11/T12 thoracic vertebra

√6ᵗʰ **S23.17** **Subluxation and dislocation of** T12/L1 **thoracic vertebra**
- √7ᵗʰ **S23.170** Subluxation of T12/L1 thoracic vertebra
- √7ᵗʰ **S23.171** Dislocation of T12/L1 thoracic vertebra

√5ᵗʰ **S23.2** **Dislocation of other and unspecified parts of thorax**
- √x7ᵗʰ **S23.20** **Dislocation of unspecified part of thorax**
- √x7ᵗʰ **S23.29** **Dislocation of other parts of thorax**

√x7ᵗʰ **S23.3** **Sprain of ligaments of thoracic spine**

√5ᵗʰ **S23.4** **Sprain of ribs and sternum**
- √x7ᵗʰ **S23.41** **Sprain of ribs**
- √6ᵗʰ **S23.42** **Sprain of sternum**
  - √7ᵗʰ **S23.420** Sprain of sternoclavicular (joint) (ligament)
  - √7ᵗʰ **S23.421** Sprain of chondrosternal joint
  - √7ᵗʰ **S23.428** Other sprain of sternum
  - √7ᵗʰ **S23.429** Unspecified sprain of sternum

√x7ᵗʰ **S23.8** **Sprain of other specified parts of thorax**

√x7ᵗʰ **S23.9** **Sprain of unspecified parts of thorax**

√4ᵗʰ **S24** **Injury of nerves and spinal cord at thorax level**

NOTE Code to highest level of thoracic spinal cord injury.

Injuries to the spinal cord (S24.0 and S24.1) refer to the cord level and not bone level injury, and can affect nerve roots at and below the level given.

Code also any associated:
 fracture of thoracic vertebra (S22.0-)
 open wound of thorax (S21.-)
 transient paralysis (R29.5)

EXCLUDES 2 injury of brachial plexus (S14.3)

The appropriate 7th character is to be added to each code from category S24.
- A   initial encounter
- D   subsequent encounter
- S   sequela

CC Excl: For MCC codes in category S24: PDX collection 1177

√x7ᵗʰ **S24.0** **Concussion and edema of thoracic spinal cord** MCC HCC

√5ᵗʰ **S24.1** **Other and unspecified injuries of thoracic spinal cord**
- √6ᵗʰ **S24.10** **Unspecified injury of thoracic spinal cord**
  - √7ᵗʰ **S24.101** Unspecified injury at T1 level of thoracic spinal cord   MCC H5 HCC
  - √7ᵗʰ **S24.102** Unspecified injury at T2-T6 level of thoracic spinal cord   MCC H5 HCC
  - √7ᵗʰ **S24.103** Unspecified injury at T7-T10 level of thoracic spinal cord   MCC H5 HCC
  - √7ᵗʰ **S24.104** Unspecified injury at T11-T12 level of thoracic spinal cord   MCC H5 HCC
  - √7ᵗʰ **S24.109** Unspecified injury at unspecified level of thoracic spinal cord   HCC
    Injury of thoracic spinal cord NOS
- √6ᵗʰ **S24.11** **Complete lesion of thoracic spinal cord**
  - √7ᵗʰ **S24.111** Complete lesion at T1 level of thoracic spinal cord   MCC H5 HCC
  - √7ᵗʰ **S24.112** Complete lesion at T2-T6 level of thoracic spinal cord   MCC H5 HCC
  - √7ᵗʰ **S24.113** Complete lesion at T7-T10 level of thoracic spinal cord   MCC H5 HCC
  - √7ᵗʰ **S24.114** Complete lesion at T11-T12 level of thoracic spinal cord   MCC H5 HCC
  - √7ᵗʰ **S24.119** Complete lesion at unspecified level of thoracic spinal cord   HCC
- √6ᵗʰ **S24.13** **Anterior cord syndrome of thoracic spinal cord**
  - √7ᵗʰ **S24.131** Anterior cord syndrome at T1 level of thoracic spinal cord   MCC H5 HCC
  - √7ᵗʰ **S24.132** Anterior cord syndrome at T2-T6 level of thoracic spinal cord   MCC H5 HCC
  - √7ᵗʰ **S24.133** Anterior cord syndrome at T7-T10 level of thoracic spinal cord   MCC H5 HCC
  - √7ᵗʰ **S24.134** Anterior cord syndrome at T11-T12 level of thoracic spinal cord   MCC H5 HCC
  - √7ᵗʰ **S24.139** Anterior cord syndrome at unspecified level of thoracic spinal cord   HCC
- √6ᵗʰ **S24.14** **Brown-Séquard syndrome of thoracic spinal cord**
  - √7ᵗʰ **S24.141** Brown-Séquard syndrome at T1 level of thoracic spinal cord   MCC HCC
  - √7ᵗʰ **S24.142** Brown-Séquard syndrome at T2-T6 level of thoracic spinal cord   MCC HCC
  - √7ᵗʰ **S24.143** Brown-Séquard syndrome at T7-T10 level of thoracic spinal cord   MCC HCC
  - √7ᵗʰ **S24.144** Brown-Séquard syndrome at T11-T12 level of thoracic spinal cord   MCC HCC
  - √7ᵗʰ **S24.149** Brown-Séquard syndrome at unspecified level of thoracic spinal cord   HCC
- √6ᵗʰ **S24.15** **Other incomplete lesions of thoracic spinal cord**
    Incomplete lesion of thoracic spinal cord NOS
    Posterior cord syndrome of thoracic spinal cord
  - √7ᵗʰ **S24.151** Other incomplete lesion at T1 level of thoracic spinal cord   MCC H5 HCC
  - √7ᵗʰ **S24.152** Other incomplete lesion at T2-T6 level of thoracic spinal cord   MCC H5 HCC
  - √7ᵗʰ **S24.153** Other incomplete lesion at T7-T10 level of thoracic spinal cord   MCC H5 HCC
  - √7ᵗʰ **S24.154** Other incomplete lesion at T11-T12 level of thoracic spinal cord   MCC H5 HCC
  - √7ᵗʰ **S24.159** Other incomplete lesion at unspecified level of thoracic spinal cord   HCC

√x7ᵗʰ **S24.2** **Injury of nerve root of thoracic spine**

√x7ᵗʰ **S24.3** **Injury of peripheral nerves of thorax**

√x7ᵗʰ **S24.4** **Injury of thoracic sympathetic nervous system**
    Injury of cardiac plexus
    Injury of esophageal plexus
    Injury of pulmonary plexus
    Injury of stellate ganglion
    Injury of thoracic sympathetic ganglion

√x7ᵗʰ **S24.8** **Injury of other specified nerves of thorax**

√x7ᵗʰ **S24.9** **Injury of unspecified nerve of thorax**

√4ᵗʰ **S25** **Injury of blood vessels of thorax**

Code also any associated open wound (S21.-)

The appropriate 7th character is to be added to each code from category S25.
A initial encounter
D subsequent encounter
S sequela

√5ᵗʰ **S25.0** **Injury of thoracic aorta**

Injury of aorta NOS
CC Excl: For MCC codes in subcategory S25.0: PDX collection 1178

√x7ᵗʰ **S25.00** **Unspecified injury of thoracic aorta**   `MCC`

√x7ᵗʰ **S25.01** **Minor laceration of thoracic aorta**   `MCC`

Incomplete transection of thoracic aorta
Laceration of thoracic aorta NOS
Superficial laceration of thoracic aorta

√x7ᵗʰ **S25.02** **Major laceration of thoracic aorta**   `MCC`

Complete transection of thoracic aorta
Traumatic rupture of thoracic aorta

√x7ᵗʰ **S25.09** **Other specified injury of thoracic aorta**   `MCC`

√5ᵗʰ **S25.1** **Injury of innominate or subclavian artery**

CC Excl: For MCC codes in subcategory S25.1: PDX collection 1179

√6ᵗʰ **S25.10** **Unspecified injury of innominate or subclavian artery**

√7ᵗʰ **S25.101** **Unspecified injury of right innominate or subclavian artery**   `MCC`

√7ᵗʰ **S25.102** **Unspecified injury of left innominate or subclavian artery**   `MCC`

√7ᵗʰ **S25.109** **Unspecified injury of unspecified innominate or subclavian artery**   `MCC`

√6ᵗʰ **S25.11** **Minor laceration of innominate or subclavian artery**

Incomplete transection of innominate or subclavian artery
Laceration of innominate or subclavian artery NOS
Superficial laceration of innominate or subclavian artery

√7ᵗʰ **S25.111** **Minor laceration of right innominate or subclavian artery**   `MCC`

√7ᵗʰ **S25.112** **Minor laceration of left innominate or subclavian artery**   `MCC`

√7ᵗʰ **S25.119** **Minor laceration of unspecified innominate or subclavian artery**   `MCC`

√6ᵗʰ **S25.12** **Major laceration of innominate or subclavian artery**

Complete transection of innominate or subclavian artery
Traumatic rupture of innominate or subclavian artery

√7ᵗʰ **S25.121** **Major laceration of right innominate or subclavian artery**   `MCC`

√7ᵗʰ **S25.122** **Major laceration of left innominate or subclavian artery**   `MCC`

√7ᵗʰ **S25.129** **Major laceration of unspecified innominate or subclavian artery**   `MCC`

√6ᵗʰ **S25.19** **Other specified injury of innominate or subclavian artery**

√7ᵗʰ **S25.191** **Other specified injury of right innominate or subclavian artery**   `MCC`

√7ᵗʰ **S25.192** **Other specified injury of left innominate or subclavian artery**   `MCC`

√7ᵗʰ **S25.199** **Other specified injury of unspecified innominate or subclavian artery**   `MCC`

√5ᵗʰ **S25.2** **Injury of superior vena cava**

Injury of vena cava NOS
CC Excl: For MCC codes in subcategory S25.2: PDX collection 1180

√x7ᵗʰ **S25.20** **Unspecified injury of superior vena cava**   `MCC`

√x7ᵗʰ **S25.21** **Minor laceration of superior vena cava**   `MCC`

Incomplete transection of superior vena cava
Laceration of superior vena cava NOS
Superficial laceration of superior vena cava

√x7ᵗʰ **S25.22** **Major laceration of superior vena cava**   `MCC`

Complete transection of superior vena cava
Traumatic rupture of superior vena cava

√x7ᵗʰ **S25.29** **Other specified injury of superior vena cava**   `MCC`

√5ᵗʰ **S25.3** **Injury of innominate or subclavian vein**

CC Excl: For MCC codes in subcategory S25.3: PDX collection 1181

√6ᵗʰ **S25.30** **Unspecified injury of innominate or subclavian vein**

√7ᵗʰ **S25.301** **Unspecified injury of right innominate or subclavian vein**   `MCC`

√7ᵗʰ **S25.302** **Unspecified injury of left innominate or subclavian vein**   `MCC`

√7ᵗʰ **S25.309** **Unspecified injury of unspecified innominate or subclavian vein**   `MCC`

√6ᵗʰ **S25.31** **Minor laceration of innominate or subclavian vein**

Incomplete transection of innominate or subclavian vein
Laceration of innominate or subclavian vein NOS
Superficial laceration of innominate or subclavian vein

√7ᵗʰ **S25.311** **Minor laceration of right innominate or subclavian vein**   `MCC`

√7ᵗʰ **S25.312** **Minor laceration of left innominate or subclavian vein**   `MCC`

√7ᵗʰ **S25.319** **Minor laceration of unspecified innominate or subclavian vein**   `MCC`

√6ᵗʰ **S25.32** **Major laceration of innominate or subclavian vein**

Complete transection of innominate or subclavian vein
Traumatic rupture of innominate or subclavian vein

√7ᵗʰ **S25.321** **Major laceration of right innominate or subclavian vein**   `MCC`

√7ᵗʰ **S25.322** **Major laceration of left innominate or subclavian vein**   `MCC`

√7ᵗʰ **S25.329** **Major laceration of unspecified innominate or subclavian vein**   `MCC`

√6ᵗʰ **S25.39** **Other specified injury of innominate or subclavian vein**

√7ᵗʰ **S25.391** **Other specified injury of right innominate or subclavian vein**   `MCC`

√7ᵗʰ **S25.392** **Other specified injury of left innominate or subclavian vein**   `MCC`

√7ᵗʰ **S25.399** **Other specified injury of unspecified innominate or subclavian vein**   `MCC`

√5ᵗʰ **S25.4** **Injury of pulmonary blood vessels**

CC Excl: For MCC codes in subcategory S25.4, unless otherwise noted: PDX collection 1182

√6ᵗʰ **S25.40** **Unspecified injury of pulmonary blood vessels**

√7ᵗʰ **S25.401** **Unspecified injury of right pulmonary blood vessels**   `MCC`

√7ᵗʰ **S25.402** **Unspecified injury of left pulmonary blood vessels**   `MCC`

√7ᵗʰ **S25.409** **Unspecified injury of unspecified pulmonary blood vessels**   `MCC`

☑ Additional Character Required   √x7ᵗʰ Placeholder   Unacceptable PDx   Questionable PDx   Manifestation   Unspecified Dx   `H1`-`H14` HAC   `HCC` CMS-HCC Dx   `HIV` HIV Dx

ICD-10-CM 2020   **1011**

√6th **S25.41 Minor laceration of pulmonary blood vessels**

    Incomplete transection of pulmonary blood vessels
    Laceration of pulmonary blood vessels NOS
    Superficial laceration of pulmonary blood vessels

    √7th **S25.411 Minor laceration of right pulmonary blood vessels** `MCC`

    √7th **S25.412 Minor laceration of left pulmonary blood vessels** `MCC`

    √7th **S25.419 Minor laceration of unspecified pulmonary blood vessels** `MCC`

√6th **S25.42 Major laceration of pulmonary blood vessels**

    Complete transection of pulmonary blood vessels
    Traumatic rupture of pulmonary blood vessels

    √7th **S25.421 Major laceration of right pulmonary blood vessels** `MCC`
        CC Excl: PDX collection 1183

    √7th **S25.422 Major laceration of left pulmonary blood vessels** `MCC`

    √7th **S25.429 Major laceration of unspecified pulmonary blood vessels** `MCC`

√6th **S25.49 Other specified injury of pulmonary blood vessels**

    √7th **S25.491 Other specified injury of right pulmonary blood vessels** `MCC`

    √7th **S25.492 Other specified injury of left pulmonary blood vessels** `MCC`

    √7th **S25.499 Other specified injury of unspecified pulmonary blood vessels** `MCC`

√5th **S25.5 Injury of intercostal blood vessels**

    CC Excl: For CC codes in subcategory S25.5: PDX collection 1184

√6th **S25.50 Unspecified injury of intercostal blood vessels**

    √7th **S25.501 Unspecified injury of intercostal blood vessels, right side** `CC`

    √7th **S25.502 Unspecified injury of intercostal blood vessels, left side** `CC`

    √7th **S25.509 Unspecified injury of intercostal blood vessels, unspecified side** `CC`

√6th **S25.51 Laceration of intercostal blood vessels**

    √7th **S25.511 Laceration of intercostal blood vessels, right side** `CC`

    √7th **S25.512 Laceration of intercostal blood vessels, left side** `CC`

    √7th **S25.519 Laceration of intercostal blood vessels, unspecified side** `CC`

√6th **S25.59 Other specified injury of intercostal blood vessels**

    √7th **S25.591 Other specified injury of intercostal blood vessels, right side** `CC`

    √7th **S25.592 Other specified injury of intercostal blood vessels, left side** `CC`

    √7th **S25.599 Other specified injury of intercostal blood vessels, unspecified side** `CC`

√5th **S25.8 Injury of other blood vessels of thorax**

    Injury of azygos vein
    Injury of mammary artery or vein
    CC Excl: For CC codes in subcategory S25.8: PDX collection 1185

√6th **S25.80 Unspecified injury of other blood vessels of thorax**

    √7th **S25.801 Unspecified injury of other blood vessels of thorax, right side** `CC`

    √7th **S25.802 Unspecified injury of other blood vessels of thorax, left side** `CC`

    √7th **S25.809 Unspecified injury of other blood vessels of thorax, unspecified side** `CC`

√6th **S25.81 Laceration of other blood vessels of thorax**

    √7th **S25.811 Laceration of other blood vessels of thorax, right side** `CC`

    √7th **S25.812 Laceration of other blood vessels of thorax, left side** `CC`

    √7th **S25.819 Laceration of other blood vessels of thorax, unspecified side** `CC`

√6th **S25.89 Other specified injury of other blood vessels of thorax**

    √7th **S25.891 Other specified injury of other blood vessels of thorax, right side** `CC`

    √7th **S25.892 Other specified injury of other blood vessels of thorax, left side** `CC`

    √7th **S25.899 Other specified injury of other blood vessels of thorax, unspecified side** `CC`

√5th **S25.9 Injury of unspecified blood vessel of thorax**

    CC Excl: For CC codes in subcategory S25.9: PDX collection 1185

√x7th **S25.90 Unspecified injury of unspecified blood vessel of thorax** `CC`

√x7th **S25.91 Laceration of unspecified blood vessel of thorax** `CC`

√x7th **S25.99 Other specified injury of unspecified blood vessel of thorax** `CC`

√4th **S26 Injury of heart**

    Code also any associated:
      open wound of thorax (S21.-)
      traumatic hemopneumothorax (S27.2)
      traumatic hemothorax (S27.1)
      traumatic pneumothorax (S27.0)

    The appropriate 7th character is to be added to each code from category S26.
    A   initial encounter
    D   subsequent encounter
    S   sequela

    CC Excl: For codes in category S26:
    For MCC codes: PDX collection 1187
    For CC codes, unless otherwise noted: PDX collection 1186

√5th **S26.0 Injury of heart with hemopericardium**

    √x7th **S26.00 Unspecified injury of heart with hemopericardium** `CC`

    √x7th **S26.01 Contusion of heart with hemopericardium** `CC`
        CC Excl: PDX collection 1187

    √6th **S26.02 Laceration of heart with hemopericardium**

        √7th **S26.020 Mild laceration of heart with hemopericardium** `MCC`
            Laceration of heart without penetration of heart chamber

        √7th **S26.021 Moderate laceration of heart with hemopericardium** `MCC`
            Laceration of heart with penetration of heart chamber

        √7th **S26.022 Major laceration of heart with hemopericardium** `MCC`
            Laceration of heart with penetration of multiple heart chambers

    √x7th **S26.09 Other injury of heart with hemopericardium** `CC`

√5th **S26.1 Injury of heart without hemopericardium**

    √x7th **S26.10 Unspecified injury of heart without hemopericardium** `CC`

    √x7th **S26.11 Contusion of heart without hemopericardium** `CC`

    √x7th **S26.12 Laceration of heart without hemopericardium** `MCC`

    √x7th **S26.19 Other injury of heart without hemopericardium** `CC`

√5th **S26.9 Injury of heart, unspecified with or without hemopericardium**

    √x7th **S26.90 Unspecified injury of heart, unspecified with or without hemopericardium** `CC`

N Newborn: 0   P Pediatric: 0-17   M Maternity: 9-64   A Adult: 15-124   MCC Major Complication/Comorbidity   CC Complication/Comorbidity   SW Severe Wound Dx

1012   ICD-10-CM 2020

√x7ᵗʰ **S26.91** **Contusion** of heart, unspecified with or without hemopericardium   `CC`
> **DEF:** Bruising within the heart muscle, with no mention of an open wound, usually caused by blunt chest trauma in motor vehicle accidents, falling from great heights, or receiving CPR.

√x7ᵗʰ **S26.92** **Laceration** of heart, unspecified with or without hemopericardium   `MCC`
> Laceration of heart NOS
> **AHA:** 2019,2Q,24

√x7ᵗʰ **S26.99** **Other injury** of heart, unspecified with or without hemopericardium   `CC`

√4ᵗʰ **S27** **Injury of other and unspecified intrathoracic organs**
> Code also any associated open wound of thorax (S21.-)
> *EXCLUDES 2*   injury of cervical esophagus (S10–S19)
>   injury of trachea (cervical) (S10–S19)

> The appropriate 7th character is to be added to each code from category S27.
> A   initial encounter
> D   subsequent encounter
> S   sequela

√x7ᵗʰ **S27.0** **Traumatic pneumothorax**   `CC`
> *EXCLUDES 1*   spontaneous pneumothorax (J93.-)
> **CC Excl:** PDX collection 1188

√x7ᵗʰ **S27.1** **Traumatic hemothorax**   `MCC`
> **CC Excl:** PDX collection 1188

√x7ᵗʰ **S27.2** **Traumatic hemopneumothorax**   `MCC`
> **CC Excl:** PDX collection 1188

√5ᵗʰ **S27.3** **Other and unspecified injuries of lung**
> **CC Excl: For codes in subcategory S27.3:**
> **MCC codes:** PDX collection 1190
> **CC codes:** PDX collection 1189

√6ᵗʰ   **S27.30** **Unspecified injury of lung**
> √7ᵗʰ   **S27.301** **Unspecified injury of lung,** unilateral   `CC`
> √7ᵗʰ   **S27.302** **Unspecified injury of lung,** bilateral   `CC`
> √7ᵗʰ   **S27.309** **Unspecified injury of lung,** unspecified   `CC`

√6ᵗʰ   **S27.31** **Primary blast injury of lung**
> Blast injury of lung NOS
> √7ᵗʰ   **S27.311** **Primary blast injury of lung,** unilateral   `CC`
> √7ᵗʰ   **S27.312** **Primary blast injury of lung,** bilateral   `CC`
> √7ᵗʰ   **S27.319** **Primary blast injury of lung,** unspecified   `CC`

√6ᵗʰ   **S27.32** **Contusion of lung**
> **DEF:** Bruising of the lung without mention of an open wound.
> √7ᵗʰ   **S27.321** **Contusion of lung,** unilateral   `CC`
> √7ᵗʰ   **S27.322** **Contusion of lung,** bilateral   `CC`
> √7ᵗʰ   **S27.329** **Contusion of lung,** unspecified   `CC`

√6ᵗʰ   **S27.33** **Laceration of lung**
> √7ᵗʰ   **S27.331** **Laceration of lung,** unilateral   `MCC`
> √7ᵗʰ   **S27.332** **Laceration of lung,** bilateral   `MCC`
> √7ᵗʰ   **S27.339** **Laceration of lung,** unspecified   `MCC`

√6ᵗʰ   **S27.39** **Other injuries of lung**
> Secondary blast injury of lung
> √7ᵗʰ   **S27.391** **Other injuries of lung,** unilateral   `CC`
> √7ᵗʰ   **S27.392** **Other injuries of lung,** bilateral   `CC`
> √7ᵗʰ   **S27.399** **Other injuries of lung,** unspecified   `CC`

√5ᵗʰ **S27.4** **Injury of bronchus**
> **CC Excl: For MCC codes in subcategory S27.4:** PDX collection 1191

√6ᵗʰ   **S27.40** **Unspecified injury of bronchus**
> √7ᵗʰ   **S27.401** **Unspecified injury of bronchus, unilateral**   `MCC`
> √7ᵗʰ   **S27.402** **Unspecified injury of bronchus, bilateral**   `MCC`
> √7ᵗʰ   **S27.409** **Unspecified injury of bronchus, unspecified**   `MCC`

√6ᵗʰ   **S27.41** **Primary blast injury of bronchus**
> Blast injury of bronchus NOS
> √7ᵗʰ   **S27.411** **Primary blast injury of bronchus, unilateral**   `MCC`
> √7ᵗʰ   **S27.412** **Primary blast injury of bronchus, bilateral**   `MCC`
> √7ᵗʰ   **S27.419** **Primary blast injury of bronchus, unspecified**   `MCC`

√6ᵗʰ   **S27.42** **Contusion of bronchus**
> √7ᵗʰ   **S27.421** **Contusion of bronchus, unilateral**   `MCC`
> √7ᵗʰ   **S27.422** **Contusion of bronchus, bilateral**   `MCC`
> √7ᵗʰ   **S27.429** **Contusion of bronchus, unspecified**   `MCC`

√6ᵗʰ   **S27.43** **Laceration of bronchus**
> √7ᵗʰ   **S27.431** **Laceration of bronchus, unilateral**   `MCC`
> √7ᵗʰ   **S27.432** **Laceration of bronchus, bilateral**   `MCC`
> √7ᵗʰ   **S27.439** **Laceration of bronchus, unspecified**   `MCC`

√6ᵗʰ   **S27.49** **Other injury of bronchus**
> Secondary blast injury of bronchus
> √7ᵗʰ   **S27.491** **Other injury of bronchus, unilateral**   `MCC`
> √7ᵗʰ   **S27.492** **Other injury of bronchus, bilateral**   `MCC`
> √7ᵗʰ   **S27.499** **Other injury of bronchus, unspecified**   `MCC`

√5ᵗʰ **S27.5** **Injury of thoracic trachea**
> **CC Excl: For CC codes in subcategory S27.5:** PDX collection 1169

√x7ᵗʰ   **S27.50** **Unspecified injury of thoracic trachea**   `CC`
√x7ᵗʰ   **S27.51** **Primary blast injury of thoracic trachea**   `CC`
> Blast injury of thoracic trachea NOS
√x7ᵗʰ   **S27.52** **Contusion of thoracic trachea**   `CC`
√x7ᵗʰ   **S27.53** **Laceration of thoracic trachea**   `CC`
√x7ᵗʰ   **S27.59** **Other injury of thoracic trachea**   `CC`
> Secondary blast injury of thoracic trachea

√5ᵗʰ **S27.6** **Injury of pleura**
> **CC Excl: For CC codes in subcategory S27.6:** PDX collection 1169

√x7ᵗʰ   **S27.60** **Unspecified injury of pleura**   `CC`
√x7ᵗʰ   **S27.63** **Laceration of pleura**   `CC`
√x7ᵗʰ   **S27.69** **Other injury of pleura**   `CC`

√5ᵗʰ **S27.8** **Injury of other specified intrathoracic organs**

√6ᵗʰ   **S27.80** **Injury of diaphragm**
> **CC Excl: For CC codes in subcategory S27.80:** PDX collection 1192
> √7ᵗʰ   **S27.802** **Contusion of diaphragm**   `CC`
> √7ᵗʰ   **S27.803** **Laceration of diaphragm**   `CC`
> √7ᵗʰ   **S27.808** **Other injury of diaphragm**   `CC`
> √7ᵗʰ   **S27.809** **Unspecified injury of diaphragm**   `CC`

√6ᵗʰ   **S27.81** **Injury of esophagus (thoracic part)**
> **CC Excl: For MCC codes in subcategory S27.81:** PDX collection 1193
> √7ᵗʰ   **S27.812** **Contusion of esophagus (thoracic part)**   `MCC`
> √7ᵗʰ   **S27.813** **Laceration of esophagus (thoracic part)**   `MCC`
> √7ᵗʰ   **S27.818** **Other injury of esophagus (thoracic part)**   `MCC`
> √7ᵗʰ   **S27.819** **Unspecified injury of esophagus (thoracic part)**   `MCC`

✔ Additional Character Required   √x7ᵗʰ Placeholder   Unacceptable PDx   Questionable PDx   Manifestation   Unspecified Dx   H1-H14 HAC   HCC CMS-HCC Dx   HIV HIV Dx

ICD-10-CM 2020   **1013**

√6ᵗʰ **S27.89 Injury of other specified intrathoracic organs**

Injury of lymphatic thoracic duct

Injury of thymus gland

CC Excl: For CC codes in subcategory S27.89: PDX collection 1169

√7ᵗʰ **S27.892 Contusion of other specified intrathoracic organs** `CC`

√7ᵗʰ **S27.893 Laceration of other specified intrathoracic organs** `CC`

√7ᵗʰ **S27.898 Other injury of other specified intrathoracic organs** `CC`

√7ᵗʰ **S27.899 Unspecified injury of other specified intrathoracic organs** `CC`

√x7ᵗʰ **S27.9 Injury of unspecified intrathoracic organ** `CC`

CC Excl: PDX collection 1194

√4ᵗʰ **S28 Crushing injury of thorax, and traumatic amputation of part of thorax**

The appropriate 7th character is to be added to each code from category S28.
A initial encounter
D subsequent encounter
S sequela

√x7ᵗʰ **S28.0 Crushed chest**

Use additional code for all associated injuries

EXCLUDES 1 flail chest (S22.5)

√x7ᵗʰ **S28.1 Traumatic amputation (partial) of part of thorax, except breast** `CC`

CC Excl: PDX collection 1168

√5ᵗʰ **S28.2 Traumatic amputation of breast**

√6ᵗʰ **S28.21 Complete traumatic amputation of breast**

Traumatic amputation of breast NOS

√7ᵗʰ **S28.211 Complete traumatic amputation of right breast**

√7ᵗʰ **S28.212 Complete traumatic amputation of left breast**

√7ᵗʰ **S28.219 Complete traumatic amputation of unspecified breast**

√6ᵗʰ **S28.22 Partial traumatic amputation of breast**

√7ᵗʰ **S28.221 Partial traumatic amputation of right breast**

√7ᵗʰ **S28.222 Partial traumatic amputation of left breast**

√7ᵗʰ **S28.229 Partial traumatic amputation of unspecified breast**

√4ᵗʰ **S29 Other and unspecified injuries of thorax**

Code also any associated open wound (S21.-)

The appropriate 7th character is to be added to each code from category S29.
A initial encounter
D subsequent encounter
S sequela

√5ᵗʰ **S29.0 Injury of muscle and tendon at thorax level**

√6ᵗʰ **S29.00 Unspecified injury of muscle and tendon of thorax**

√7ᵗʰ **S29.001 Unspecified injury of muscle and tendon of front wall of thorax**

√7ᵗʰ **S29.002 Unspecified injury of muscle and tendon of back wall of thorax**

√7ᵗʰ **S29.009 Unspecified injury of muscle and tendon of unspecified wall of thorax**

√6ᵗʰ **S29.01 Strain of muscle and tendon of thorax**

√7ᵗʰ **S29.011 Strain of muscle and tendon of front wall of thorax**

√7ᵗʰ **S29.012 Strain of muscle and tendon of back wall of thorax**

√7ᵗʰ **S29.019 Strain of muscle and tendon of unspecified wall of thorax**

√6ᵗʰ **S29.02 Laceration of muscle and tendon of thorax**

√7ᵗʰ **S29.021 Laceration of muscle and tendon of front wall of thorax** `CC`

CC Excl: PDX collection 1168

√7ᵗʰ **S29.022 Laceration of muscle and tendon of back wall of thorax**

√7ᵗʰ **S29.029 Laceration of muscle and tendon of unspecified wall of thorax** `CC`

CC Excl: PDX collection 1168

√6ᵗʰ **S29.09 Other injury of muscle and tendon of thorax**

√7ᵗʰ **S29.091 Other injury of muscle and tendon of front wall of thorax**

√7ᵗʰ **S29.092 Other injury of muscle and tendon of back wall of thorax**

√7ᵗʰ **S29.099 Other injury of muscle and tendon of unspecified wall of thorax**

√x7ᵗʰ **S29.8 Other specified injuries of thorax**

√x7ᵗʰ **S29.9 Unspecified injury of thorax**

Injuries to the abdomen, lower back, lumbar spine, pelvis and external genitals (S30-S39)

INCLUDES injuries to the abdominal wall
injuries to the anus
injuries to the buttock
injuries to the external genitalia
injuries to the flank
injuries to the groin

EXCLUDES 2 burns and corrosions (T20-T32)
effects of foreign body in anus and rectum (T18.5)
effects of foreign body in genitourinary tract (T19.-)
effects of foreign body in stomach, small intestine and colon (T18.2-T18.4)
frostbite (T33-T34)
insect bite or sting, venomous (T63.4)

√4ᵗʰ **S30 Superficial injury of abdomen, lower back, pelvis and external genitals**

EXCLUDES 2 superficial injury of hip (S70.-)

The appropriate 7th character is to be added to each code from category S30.
A initial encounter
D subsequent encounter
S sequela

√x7ᵗʰ **S30.0 Contusion of lower back and pelvis**

Contusion of buttock

√x7ᵗʰ **S30.1 Contusion of abdominal wall**

Contusion of flank

Contusion of groin

√5ᵗʰ **S30.2 Contusion of external genital organs**

√6ᵗʰ **S30.20 Contusion of unspecified external genital organ**

√7ᵗʰ **S30.201 Contusion of unspecified external genital organ, male** ♂

√7ᵗʰ **S30.202 Contusion of unspecified external genital organ, female** ♀

√x7ᵗʰ **S30.21 Contusion of penis** ♂

√x7ᵗʰ **S30.22 Contusion of scrotum and testes** ♂

√x7ᵗʰ **S30.23 Contusion of vagina and vulva** ♀

√x7ᵗʰ **S30.3 Contusion of anus**

√5ᵗʰ **S30.8 Other superficial injuries of abdomen, lower back, pelvis and external genitals**

√6ᵗʰ **S30.81 Abrasion of abdomen, lower back, pelvis and external genitals**

√7ᵗʰ **S30.810 Abrasion of lower back and pelvis**

√7ᵗʰ **S30.811 Abrasion of abdominal wall**

√7ᵗʰ **S30.812 Abrasion of penis** ♂

√7ᵗʰ **S30.813 Abrasion of scrotum and testes** ♂

√7ᵗʰ **S30.814 Abrasion of vagina and vulva** ♀

√7ᵗʰ **S30.815 Abrasion of unspecified external genital organs, male** ♂

√7ᵗʰ **S30.816 Abrasion of unspecified external genital organs, female** ♀

√7ᵗʰ **S30.817 Abrasion of anus**

√6ᵗʰ **S30.82 Blister (nonthermal) of abdomen, lower back, pelvis and external genitals**

√7ᵗʰ **S30.820 Blister (nonthermal) of lower back and pelvis**

√7ᵗʰ **S30.821 Blister (nonthermal) of abdominal wall**

Ⓝ Newborn: 0 Ⓟ Pediatric: 0-17 Ⓜ Maternity: 9-64 Ⓐ Adult: 15-124 **MCC** Major Complication/Comorbidity **CC** Complication/Comorbidity **SW** Severe Wound Dx

1014

ICD-10-CM 2020

√7ᵗʰ **S30.822** Blister (nonthermal) of penis ♂

√7ᵗʰ **S30.823** Blister (nonthermal) of scrotum and testes ♂

√7ᵗʰ **S30.824** Blister (nonthermal) of vagina and vulva ♀

√7ᵗʰ **S30.825** Blister (nonthermal) of unspecified external genital organs, male ♂

√7ᵗʰ **S30.826** Blister (nonthermal) of unspecified external genital organs, female ♀

√7ᵗʰ **S30.827** Blister (nonthermal) of anus

√6ᵗʰ **S30.84** External constriction of abdomen, lower back, pelvis and external genitals

√7ᵗʰ **S30.840** External constriction of lower back and pelvis

√7ᵗʰ **S30.841** External constriction of abdominal wall

√7ᵗʰ **S30.842** External constriction of penis ♂

     Hair tourniquet syndrome of penis
     Use additional cause code to identify the constricting item (W49.0-)

√7ᵗʰ **S30.843** External constriction of scrotum and testes ♂

√7ᵗʰ **S30.844** External constriction of vagina and vulva ♀

√7ᵗʰ **S30.845** External constriction of unspecified external genital organs, male ♂

√7ᵗʰ **S30.846** External constriction of unspecified external genital organs, female ♀

√6ᵗʰ **S30.85** Superficial foreign body of abdomen, lower back, pelvis and external genitals

     Splinter in the abdomen, lower back, pelvis and external genitals

√7ᵗʰ **S30.850** Superficial foreign body of lower back and pelvis

√7ᵗʰ **S30.851** Superficial foreign body of abdominal wall

√7ᵗʰ **S30.852** Superficial foreign body of penis ♂

√7ᵗʰ **S30.853** Superficial foreign body of scrotum and testes ♂

√7ᵗʰ **S30.854** Superficial foreign body of vagina and vulva ♀

√7ᵗʰ **S30.855** Superficial foreign body of unspecified external genital organs, male ♂

√7ᵗʰ **S30.856** Superficial foreign body of unspecified external genital organs, female ♀

√7ᵗʰ **S30.857** Superficial foreign body of anus

√6ᵗʰ **S30.86** Insect bite (nonvenomous) of abdomen, lower back, pelvis and external genitals

√7ᵗʰ **S30.860** Insect bite (nonvenomous) of lower back and pelvis

√7ᵗʰ **S30.861** Insect bite (nonvenomous) of abdominal wall

√7ᵗʰ **S30.862** Insect bite (nonvenomous) of penis ♂

√7ᵗʰ **S30.863** Insect bite (nonvenomous) of scrotum and testes ♂

√7ᵗʰ **S30.864** Insect bite (nonvenomous) of vagina and vulva ♀

√7ᵗʰ **S30.865** Insect bite (nonvenomous) of unspecified external genital organs, male ♂

√7ᵗʰ **S30.866** Insect bite (nonvenomous) of unspecified external genital organs, female ♀

√7ᵗʰ **S30.867** Insect bite (nonvenomous) of anus

√6ᵗʰ **S30.87** Other superficial bite of abdomen, lower back, pelvis and external genitals

     EXCLUDES 1   open bite of abdomen, lower back, pelvis and external genitals (S31.05, S31.15, S31.25, S31.35, S31.45, S31.55)

√7ᵗʰ **S30.870** Other superficial bite of lower back and pelvis

√7ᵗʰ **S30.871** Other superficial bite of abdominal wall

√7ᵗʰ **S30.872** Other superficial bite of penis ♂

√7ᵗʰ **S30.873** Other superficial bite of scrotum and testes ♂

√7ᵗʰ **S30.874** Other superficial bite of vagina and vulva ♀

√7ᵗʰ **S30.875** Other superficial bite of unspecified external genital organs, male ♂

√7ᵗʰ **S30.876** Other superficial bite of unspecified external genital organs, female ♀

√7ᵗʰ **S30.877** Other superficial bite of anus

√5ᵗʰ **S30.9** Unspecified superficial injury of abdomen, lower back, pelvis and external genitals

√x7ᵗʰ **S30.91** Unspecified superficial injury of lower back and pelvis

√x7ᵗʰ **S30.92** Unspecified superficial injury of abdominal wall

√x7ᵗʰ **S30.93** Unspecified superficial injury of penis ♂

√x7ᵗʰ **S30.94** Unspecified superficial injury of scrotum and testes ♂

√x7ᵗʰ **S30.95** Unspecified superficial injury of vagina and vulva ♀

√x7ᵗʰ **S30.96** Unspecified superficial injury of unspecified external genital organs, male ♂

√x7ᵗʰ **S30.97** Unspecified superficial injury of unspecified external genital organs, female ♀

√x7ᵗʰ **S30.98** Unspecified superficial injury of anus

√4ᵗʰ **S31** Open wound of abdomen, lower back, pelvis and external genitals

     Code also any associated:
         spinal cord injury (S24.0, S24.1-, S34.0-, S34.1-)
         wound infection

     EXCLUDES 1   traumatic amputation of part of abdomen, lower back and pelvis (S38.2-, S38.3)

     EXCLUDES 2   open wound of hip (S71.00-S71.02)
           open fracture of pelvis (S32.1- – S32.9 with 7th character B)

     The appropriate 7th character is to be added to each code from category S31.
     A   initial encounter
     D   subsequent encounter
     S   sequela

     CC Excl: For MCC codes in category S31: PDX collection 1195

√5ᵗʰ **S31.0** Open wound of lower back and pelvis

√6ᵗʰ **S31.00** Unspecified open wound of lower back and pelvis

√7ᵗʰ **S31.000** Unspecified open wound of lower back and pelvis without penetration into retroperitoneum

     Unspecified open wound of lower back and pelvis NOS

√7ᵗʰ **S31.001** Unspecified open wound of lower back and pelvis with penetration into retroperitoneum   MCC

√6ᵗʰ **S31.01** Laceration without foreign body of lower back and pelvis

√7ᵗʰ **S31.010** Laceration without foreign body of lower back and pelvis without penetration into retroperitoneum

     Laceration without foreign body of lower back and pelvis NOS

√7ᵗʰ **S31.011** Laceration without foreign body of lower back and pelvis with penetration into retroperitoneum   MCC

√6ᵗʰ **S31.02** Laceration with foreign body of lower back and pelvis

√7ᵗʰ **S31.020** Laceration with foreign body of lower back and pelvis without penetration into retroperitoneum

     Laceration with foreign body of lower back and pelvis NOS

√7ᵗʰ **S31.021** Laceration with foreign body of lower back and pelvis with penetration into retroperitoneum   MCC

☑ Additional Character Required   √x7ᵗʰ Placeholder   Unacceptable PDx   Questionable PDx   Manifestation   Unspecified Dx   H1-H14 HAC   HCC CMS-HCC Dx   HIV HIV Dx

√6th **S31.Ø3** **Puncture wound without foreign body** of lower back and pelvis

√7th **S31.Ø3Ø** **Puncture wound without foreign body of lower back and pelvis** without penetration into retroperitoneum
Puncture wound without foreign body of lower back and pelvis NOS

√7th **S31.Ø31** **Puncture wound without foreign body of lower back and pelvis** with penetration into retroperitoneum   MCC

√6th **S31.Ø4** **Puncture wound with foreign body** of lower back and pelvis

√7th **S31.Ø4Ø** **Puncture wound with foreign body of lower back and pelvis** without penetration into retroperitoneum
Puncture wound with foreign body of lower back and pelvis NOS

√7th **S31.Ø41** **Puncture wound with foreign body of lower back and pelvis** with penetration into retroperitoneum   MCC

√6th **S31.Ø5** **Open bite** of lower back and pelvis
Bite of lower back and pelvis NOS
EXCLUDES 1   *superficial bite of lower back and pelvis (S3Ø.86Ø, S3Ø.87Ø)*

√7th **S31.Ø5Ø** **Open bite of lower back and pelvis** without penetration into retroperitoneum
Open bite of lower back and pelvis NOS

√7th **S31.Ø51** **Open bite of lower back and pelvis** with penetration into retroperitoneum   MCC

√5th **S31.1** **Open wound of** abdominal wall without penetration into peritoneal cavity
Open wound of abdominal wall NOS
EXCLUDES 2   *open wound of abdominal wall with penetration into peritoneal cavity (S31.6-)*

√6th **S31.1Ø** **Unspecified open wound of abdominal wall without penetration into peritoneal cavity**

√7th **S31.1ØØ** **Unspecified open wound of abdominal wall, right upper quadrant** without penetration into peritoneal cavity

√7th **S31.1Ø1** **Unspecified open wound of abdominal wall, left upper quadrant** without penetration into peritoneal cavity

√7th **S31.1Ø2** **Unspecified open wound of abdominal wall, epigastric region** without penetration into peritoneal cavity

√7th **S31.1Ø3** **Unspecified open wound of abdominal wall, right lower quadrant** without penetration into peritoneal cavity

√7th **S31.1Ø4** **Unspecified open wound of abdominal wall, left lower quadrant** without penetration into peritoneal cavity

√7th **S31.1Ø5** **Unspecified open wound of abdominal wall, periumbilic region** without penetration into peritoneal cavity

√7th **S31.1Ø9** **Unspecified open wound of abdominal wall, unspecified quadrant** without penetration into peritoneal cavity
Unspecified open wound of abdominal wall NOS

√6th **S31.11** **Laceration without foreign body** of abdominal wall without penetration into peritoneal cavity

√7th **S31.11Ø** **Laceration without foreign body of abdominal wall, right upper quadrant** without penetration into peritoneal cavity

√7th **S31.111** **Laceration without foreign body of abdominal wall, left upper quadrant** without penetration into peritoneal cavity

√7th **S31.112** **Laceration without foreign body of abdominal wall, epigastric region** without penetration into peritoneal cavity

√7th **S31.113** **Laceration without foreign body of abdominal wall, right lower quadrant** without penetration into peritoneal cavity

√7th **S31.114** **Laceration without foreign body of abdominal wall, left lower quadrant** without penetration into peritoneal cavity

√7th **S31.115** **Laceration without foreign body of abdominal wall, periumbilic region** without penetration into peritoneal cavity

√7th **S31.119** **Laceration without foreign body of abdominal wall, unspecified quadrant** without penetration into peritoneal cavity

√6th **S31.12** **Laceration with foreign body** of abdominal wall without penetration into peritoneal cavity

√7th **S31.12Ø** **Laceration of abdominal wall with foreign body, right upper quadrant** without penetration into peritoneal cavity

√7th **S31.121** **Laceration of abdominal wall with foreign body, left upper quadrant** without penetration into peritoneal cavity

√7th **S31.122** **Laceration of abdominal wall with foreign body, epigastric region** without penetration into peritoneal cavity

√7th **S31.123** **Laceration of abdominal wall with foreign body, right lower quadrant** without penetration into peritoneal cavity

√7th **S31.124** **Laceration of abdominal wall with foreign body, left lower quadrant** without penetration into peritoneal cavity

√7th **S31.125** **Laceration of abdominal wall with foreign body, periumbilic region** without penetration into peritoneal cavity

√7th **S31.129** **Laceration of abdominal wall with foreign body, unspecified quadrant** without penetration into peritoneal cavity

√6th **S31.13** **Puncture wound of abdominal wall** without foreign body without penetration into peritoneal cavity

√7th **S31.13Ø** **Puncture wound of abdominal wall without foreign body, right upper quadrant** without penetration into peritoneal cavity

√7th **S31.131** **Puncture wound of abdominal wall without foreign body, left upper quadrant** without penetration into peritoneal cavity

√7th **S31.132** **Puncture wound of abdominal wall without foreign body, epigastric region** without penetration into peritoneal cavity

√7th **S31.133** **Puncture wound of abdominal wall without foreign body, right lower quadrant** without penetration into peritoneal cavity

√7th **S31.134** **Puncture wound of abdominal wall without foreign body, left lower quadrant** without penetration into peritoneal cavity

√7th **S31.135** **Puncture wound of abdominal wall without foreign body, periumbilic region** without penetration into peritoneal cavity

√7th **S31.139** **Puncture wound of abdominal wall without foreign body, unspecified quadrant** without penetration into peritoneal cavity

√6th **S31.14** **Puncture wound of abdominal wall with foreign body** without penetration into peritoneal cavity

√7th **S31.14Ø** **Puncture wound of abdominal wall with foreign body, right upper quadrant** without penetration into peritoneal cavity

√7th **S31.141** **Puncture wound of abdominal wall with foreign body, left upper quadrant** without penetration into peritoneal cavity

√7th **S31.142** **Puncture wound of abdominal wall with foreign body, epigastric region** without penetration into peritoneal cavity

√7th **S31.143** **Puncture wound of abdominal wall with foreign body, right lower quadrant** without penetration into peritoneal cavity

√7th **S31.144** **Puncture wound of abdominal wall with foreign body, left lower quadrant** without penetration into peritoneal cavity

√7ᵗʰ **S31.145** **Puncture wound of abdominal wall with foreign body, periumbilic region without penetration into peritoneal cavity**

√7ᵗʰ **S31.149** **Puncture wound of abdominal wall with foreign body, unspecified quadrant without penetration into peritoneal cavity**

√6ᵗʰ **S31.15** **Open bite of abdominal wall without penetration into peritoneal cavity**

Bite of abdominal wall NOS

EXCLUDES 1 *superficial bite of abdominal wall (S30.871)*

√7ᵗʰ **S31.150** **Open bite of abdominal wall, right upper quadrant without penetration into peritoneal cavity**

√7ᵗʰ **S31.151** **Open bite of abdominal wall, left upper quadrant without penetration into peritoneal cavity**

√7ᵗʰ **S31.152** **Open bite of abdominal wall, epigastric region without penetration into peritoneal cavity**

√7ᵗʰ **S31.153** **Open bite of abdominal wall, right lower quadrant without penetration into peritoneal cavity**

√7ᵗʰ **S31.154** **Open bite of abdominal wall, left lower quadrant without penetration into peritoneal cavity**

√7ᵗʰ **S31.155** **Open bite of abdominal wall, periumbilic region without penetration into peritoneal cavity**

√7ᵗʰ **S31.159** **Open bite of abdominal wall, unspecified quadrant without penetration into peritoneal cavity**

√5ᵗʰ **S31.2** **Open wound of penis**

√x7ᵗʰ **S31.20** **Unspecified open wound of penis** ♂

√x7ᵗʰ **S31.21** **Laceration without foreign body of penis** ♂

√x7ᵗʰ **S31.22** **Laceration with foreign body of penis** ♂

√x7ᵗʰ **S31.23** **Puncture wound without foreign body of penis** ♂

√x7ᵗʰ **S31.24** **Puncture wound with foreign body of penis** ♂

√x7ᵗʰ **S31.25** **Open bite of penis** ♂

Bite of penis NOS

EXCLUDES 1 *superficial bite of penis (S30.862, S30.872)*

√6ᵗʰ **S31.3** **Open wound of scrotum and testes**

√x7ᵗʰ **S31.30** **Unspecified open wound of scrotum and testes** ♂

√x7ᵗʰ **S31.31** **Laceration without foreign body of scrotum and testes** ♂

√x7ᵗʰ **S31.32** **Laceration with foreign body of scrotum and testes** ♂

√x7ᵗʰ **S31.33** **Puncture wound without foreign body of scrotum and testes** ♂

√x7ᵗʰ **S31.34** **Puncture wound with foreign body of scrotum and testes** ♂

√x7ᵗʰ **S31.35** **Open bite of scrotum and testes** ♂

Bite of scrotum and testes NOS

EXCLUDES 1 *superficial bite of scrotum and testes (S30.863, S30.873)*

√5ᵗʰ **S31.4** **Open wound of vagina and vulva**

EXCLUDES 1 *injury to vagina and vulva during delivery (O70.-, O71.4)*

√x7ᵗʰ **S31.40** **Unspecified open wound of vagina and vulva** ♀

√x7ᵗʰ **S31.41** **Laceration without foreign body of vagina and vulva** ♀

√x7ᵗʰ **S31.42** **Laceration with foreign body of vagina and vulva** ♀

√x7ᵗʰ **S31.43** **Puncture wound without foreign body of vagina and vulva** ♀

√x7ᵗʰ **S31.44** **Puncture wound with foreign body of vagina and vulva** ♀

√x7ᵗʰ **S31.45** **Open bite of vagina and vulva** ♀

Bite of vagina and vulva NOS

EXCLUDES 1 *superficial bite of vagina and vulva (S30.864, S30.874)*

√5ᵗʰ **S31.5** **Open wound of unspecified external genital organs**

EXCLUDES 1 *traumatic amputation of external genital organs (S38.21, S38.22)*

√6ᵗʰ **S31.50** **Unspecified open wound of unspecified external genital organs**

√7ᵗʰ **S31.501** **Unspecified open wound of unspecified external genital organs, male** ♂

√7ᵗʰ **S31.502** **Unspecified open wound of unspecified external genital organs, female** ♀

√6ᵗʰ **S31.51** **Laceration without foreign body of unspecified external genital organs**

√7ᵗʰ **S31.511** **Laceration without foreign body of unspecified external genital organs, male** ♂

√7ᵗʰ **S31.512** **Laceration without foreign body of unspecified external genital organs, female** ♀

√6ᵗʰ **S31.52** **Laceration with foreign body of unspecified external genital organs**

√7ᵗʰ **S31.521** **Laceration with foreign body of unspecified external genital organs, male** ♂

√7ᵗʰ **S31.522** **Laceration with foreign body of unspecified external genital organs, female** ♀

√6ᵗʰ **S31.53** **Puncture wound without foreign body of unspecified external genital organs**

√7ᵗʰ **S31.531** **Puncture wound without foreign body of unspecified external genital organs, male** ♂

√7ᵗʰ **S31.532** **Puncture wound without foreign body of unspecified external genital organs, female** ♀

√6ᵗʰ **S31.54** **Puncture wound with foreign body of unspecified external genital organs**

√7ᵗʰ **S31.541** **Puncture wound with foreign body of unspecified external genital organs, male** ♂

√7ᵗʰ **S31.542** **Puncture wound with foreign body of unspecified external genital organs, female** ♀

√6ᵗʰ **S31.55** **Open bite of unspecified external genital organs**

Bite of unspecified external genital organs NOS

EXCLUDES 1 *superficial bite of unspecified external genital organs (S30.865, S30.866, S30.875, S30.876)*

√7ᵗʰ **S31.551** **Open bite of unspecified external genital organs, male** ♂

√7ᵗʰ **S31.552** **Open bite of unspecified external genital organs, female** ♀

√5ᵗʰ **S31.6** **Open wound of abdominal wall with penetration into peritoneal cavity**

√6ᵗʰ **S31.60** **Unspecified open wound of abdominal wall with penetration into peritoneal cavity**

√7ᵗʰ **S31.600** **Unspecified open wound of abdominal wall, right upper quadrant with penetration into peritoneal cavity** MCC

√7ᵗʰ **S31.601** **Unspecified open wound of abdominal wall, left upper quadrant with penetration into peritoneal cavity** MCC

√7ᵗʰ **S31.602** **Unspecified open wound of abdominal wall, epigastric region with penetration into peritoneal cavity** MCC

☑ Additional Character Required   √x7ᵗʰ Placeholder   Unacceptable PDx   Questionable PDx   Manifestation   Unspecified Dx   H1-H14 HAC   HCC CMS-HCC Dx   HIV HIV Dx

ICD-10-CM 2020   **1017**

Chapter 19. Injury, Poisoning and Certain Other Consequences of External Causes

S31.145–S31.602

√7ᵗʰ **S31.603** Unspecified open wound of abdominal wall, right lower quadrant with penetration into peritoneal cavity   MCC

√7ᵗʰ **S31.604** Unspecified open wound of abdominal wall, left lower quadrant with penetration into peritoneal cavity   MCC

√7ᵗʰ **S31.605** Unspecified open wound of abdominal wall, periumbilic region with penetration into peritoneal cavity   MCC

√7ᵗʰ **S31.609** Unspecified open wound of abdominal wall, unspecified quadrant with penetration into peritoneal cavity   MCC

√6ᵗʰ **S31.61** Laceration without foreign body of abdominal wall with penetration into peritoneal cavity

√7ᵗʰ **S31.610** Laceration without foreign body of abdominal wall, right upper quadrant with penetration into peritoneal cavity   MCC

√7ᵗʰ **S31.611** Laceration without foreign body of abdominal wall, left upper quadrant with penetration into peritoneal cavity   MCC

√7ᵗʰ **S31.612** Laceration without foreign body of abdominal wall, epigastric region with penetration into peritoneal cavity   MCC

√7ᵗʰ **S31.613** Laceration without foreign body of abdominal wall, right lower quadrant with penetration into peritoneal cavity   MCC

√7ᵗʰ **S31.614** Laceration without foreign body of abdominal wall, left lower quadrant with penetration into peritoneal cavity   MCC

√7ᵗʰ **S31.615** Laceration without foreign body of abdominal wall, periumbilic region with penetration into peritoneal cavity   MCC

√7ᵗʰ **S31.619** Laceration without foreign body of abdominal wall, unspecified quadrant with penetration into peritoneal cavity   MCC

√6ᵗʰ **S31.62** Laceration with foreign body of abdominal wall with penetration into peritoneal cavity

√7ᵗʰ **S31.620** Laceration with foreign body of abdominal wall, right upper quadrant with penetration into peritoneal cavity   MCC

√7ᵗʰ **S31.621** Laceration with foreign body of abdominal wall, left upper quadrant with penetration into peritoneal cavity   MCC

√7ᵗʰ **S31.622** Laceration with foreign body of abdominal wall, epigastric region with penetration into peritoneal cavity   MCC

√7ᵗʰ **S31.623** Laceration with foreign body of abdominal wall, right lower quadrant with penetration into peritoneal cavity   MCC

√7ᵗʰ **S31.624** Laceration with foreign body of abdominal wall, left lower quadrant with penetration into peritoneal cavity   MCC

√7ᵗʰ **S31.625** Laceration with foreign body of abdominal wall, periumbilic region with penetration into peritoneal cavity   MCC

√7ᵗʰ **S31.629** Laceration with foreign body of abdominal wall, unspecified quadrant with penetration into peritoneal cavity   MCC

√6ᵗʰ **S31.63** Puncture wound without foreign body of abdominal wall with penetration into peritoneal cavity

√7ᵗʰ **S31.630** Puncture wound without foreign body of abdominal wall, right upper quadrant with penetration into peritoneal cavity   MCC

√7ᵗʰ **S31.631** Puncture wound without foreign body of abdominal wall, left upper quadrant with penetration into peritoneal cavity   MCC

√7ᵗʰ **S31.632** Puncture wound without foreign body of abdominal wall, epigastric region with penetration into peritoneal cavity   MCC

√7ᵗʰ **S31.633** Puncture wound without foreign body of abdominal wall, right lower quadrant with penetration into peritoneal cavity   MCC

√7ᵗʰ **S31.634** Puncture wound without foreign body of abdominal wall, left lower quadrant with penetration into peritoneal cavity   MCC

√7ᵗʰ **S31.635** Puncture wound without foreign body of abdominal wall, periumbilic region with penetration into peritoneal cavity   MCC

√7ᵗʰ **S31.639** Puncture wound without foreign body of abdominal wall, unspecified quadrant with penetration into peritoneal cavity   MCC

√6ᵗʰ **S31.64** Puncture wound with foreign body of abdominal wall with penetration into peritoneal cavity

√7ᵗʰ **S31.640** Puncture wound with foreign body of abdominal wall, right upper quadrant with penetration into peritoneal cavity   MCC

√7ᵗʰ **S31.641** Puncture wound with foreign body of abdominal wall, left upper quadrant with penetration into peritoneal cavity   MCC

√7ᵗʰ **S31.642** Puncture wound with foreign body of abdominal wall, epigastric region with penetration into peritoneal cavity   MCC

√7ᵗʰ **S31.643** Puncture wound with foreign body of abdominal wall, right lower quadrant with penetration into peritoneal cavity   MCC

√7ᵗʰ **S31.644** Puncture wound with foreign body of abdominal wall, left lower quadrant with penetration into peritoneal cavity   MCC

√7ᵗʰ **S31.645** Puncture wound with foreign body of abdominal wall, periumbilic region with penetration into peritoneal cavity   MCC

√7ᵗʰ **S31.649** Puncture wound with foreign body of abdominal wall, unspecified quadrant with penetration into peritoneal cavity   MCC

Ⓝ Newborn: 0   Ⓟ Pediatric: 0-17   Ⓜ Maternity: 9-64   Ⓐ Adult: 15-124   MCC Major Complication/Comorbidity   CC Complication/Comorbidity   SW Severe Wound Dx

1018   ICD-10-CM 2020

✓6ᵗʰ **S31.65** **Open bite** of abdominal wall with penetration into peritoneal cavity

    EXCLUDES 1   superficial bite of abdominal wall (S30.861, S30.871)

    ✓7ᵗʰ **S31.650** Open bite of abdominal wall, **right upper quadrant** with penetration into peritoneal cavity   MCC

    ✓7ᵗʰ **S31.651** Open bite of abdominal wall, **left upper quadrant** with penetration into peritoneal cavity   MCC

    ✓7ᵗʰ **S31.652** Open bite of abdominal wall, **epigastric region** with penetration into peritoneal cavity   MCC

    ✓7ᵗʰ **S31.653** Open bite of abdominal wall, **right lower quadrant** with penetration into peritoneal cavity   MCC

    ✓7ᵗʰ **S31.654** Open bite of abdominal wall, **left lower quadrant** with penetration into peritoneal cavity   MCC

    ✓7ᵗʰ **S31.655** Open bite of abdominal wall, **periumbilic region** with penetration into peritoneal cavity   MCC

    ✓7ᵗʰ **S31.659** Open bite of abdominal wall, **unspecified quadrant** with penetration into peritoneal cavity   MCC

✓5ᵗʰ **S31.8** **Open wound of other parts of abdomen, lower back and pelvis**

    ✓6ᵗʰ **S31.80** **Open wound of unspecified buttock**

      ✓7ᵗʰ **S31.801** Laceration without foreign body of unspecified buttock

      ✓7ᵗʰ **S31.802** Laceration with foreign body of unspecified buttock

      ✓7ᵗʰ **S31.803** Puncture wound without foreign body of unspecified buttock

      ✓7ᵗʰ **S31.804** Puncture wound with foreign body of unspecified buttock

      ✓7ᵗʰ **S31.805** Open bite of unspecified buttock

        Bite of buttock NOS

        EXCLUDES 1   superficial bite of buttock (S30.870)

      ✓7ᵗʰ **S31.809** Unspecified open wound of unspecified buttock

    ✓6ᵗʰ **S31.81** **Open wound of right buttock**

      ✓7ᵗʰ **S31.811** Laceration without foreign body of right buttock

      ✓7ᵗʰ **S31.812** Laceration with foreign body of right buttock

      ✓7ᵗʰ **S31.813** Puncture wound without foreign body of right buttock

      ✓7ᵗʰ **S31.814** Puncture wound with foreign body of right buttock

      ✓7ᵗʰ **S31.815** Open bite of right buttock

        Bite of right buttock NOS

        EXCLUDES 1   superficial bite of buttock (S30.870)

      ✓7ᵗʰ **S31.819** Unspecified open wound of right buttock

    ✓6ᵗʰ **S31.82** **Open wound of left buttock**

      ✓7ᵗʰ **S31.821** Laceration without foreign body of left buttock

      ✓7ᵗʰ **S31.822** Laceration with foreign body of left buttock

      ✓7ᵗʰ **S31.823** Puncture wound without foreign body of left buttock

      ✓7ᵗʰ **S31.824** Puncture wound with foreign body of left buttock

      ✓7ᵗʰ **S31.825** Open bite of left buttock

        Bite of left buttock NOS

        EXCLUDES 1   superficial bite of buttock (S30.870)

      ✓7ᵗʰ **S31.829** Unspecified open wound of left buttock

    ✓6ᵗʰ **S31.83** **Open wound of anus**

      ✓7ᵗʰ **S31.831** Laceration without foreign body of anus

      ✓7ᵗʰ **S31.832** Laceration with foreign body of anus

      ✓7ᵗʰ **S31.833** Puncture wound without foreign body of anus

      ✓7ᵗʰ **S31.834** Puncture wound with foreign body of anus

      ✓7ᵗʰ **S31.835** Open bite of anus

        Bite of anus NOS

        EXCLUDES 1   superficial bite of anus (S30.877)

      ✓7ᵗʰ **S31.839** Unspecified open wound of anus

✓4ᵗʰ **S32** **Fracture of lumbar spine and pelvis**

    NOTE   A fracture not indicated as displaced or nondisplaced should be coded to displaced.

        A fracture not indicated as opened or closed should be coded to closed.

    INCLUDES   fracture of lumbosacral neural arch

        fracture of lumbosacral spinous process

        fracture of lumbosacral transverse process

        fracture of lumbosacral vertebra

        fracture of lumbosacral vertebral arch

Code first any associated spinal cord and spinal nerve injury (S34.-)

    EXCLUDES 1   transection of abdomen (S38.3)

    EXCLUDES 2   fracture of hip NOS (S72.0-)

AHA: 2018,2Q,12; 2015,3Q,37-39; 2012,4Q,93

The appropriate 7th character is to be added to each code from category S32.
A   initial encounter for closed fracture
B   initial encounter for open fracture
D   subsequent encounter for fracture with routine healing
G   subsequent encounter for fracture with delayed healing
K   subsequent encounter for fracture with nonunion
S   sequela

✓5ᵗʰ **S32.0** **Fracture of lumbar vertebra**

    Fracture of lumbar spine NOS

    CC Excl: For codes in subcategory S32.0:
    CC with 7th character A or MCC with 7th character B: PDX collection 1196
    CC with 7th character K: PDX collection 897

    ✓6ᵗʰ **S32.00** **Fracture of unspecified lumbar vertebra**

      2,3,6 ✓7ᵗʰ **S32.000** Wedge compression fracture of unspecified lumbar vertebra   MCC CC H5 HCC

      2,3,6 ✓7ᵗʰ **S32.001** Stable burst fracture of unspecified lumbar vertebra   MCC CC H5 HCC

      2,3,6 ✓7ᵗʰ **S32.002** Unstable burst fracture of unspecified lumbar vertebra   MCC CC H5 HCC

      2,3,6 ✓7ᵗʰ **S32.008** Other fracture of unspecified lumbar vertebra   MCC CC H5 HCC

      2,3,6 ✓7ᵗʰ **S32.009** Unspecified fracture of unspecified lumbar vertebra   MCC CC H5 HCC

    ✓6ᵗʰ **S32.01** **Fracture of first lumbar vertebra**

      2,3,6 ✓7ᵗʰ **S32.010** Wedge compression fracture of first lumbar vertebra   MCC CC H5 HCC

      2,3,6 ✓7ᵗʰ **S32.011** Stable burst fracture of first lumbar vertebra   MCC CC H5 HCC

      2,3,6 ✓7ᵗʰ **S32.012** Unstable burst fracture of first lumbar vertebra   MCC CC H5 HCC

      2,3,6 ✓7ᵗʰ **S32.018** Other fracture of first lumbar vertebra   MCC CC H5 HCC

      2,3,6 ✓7ᵗʰ **S32.019** Unspecified fracture of first lumbar vertebra   MCC CC H5 HCC

    ✓6ᵗʰ **S32.02** **Fracture of second lumbar vertebra**

      2,3,6 ✓7ᵗʰ **S32.020** Wedge compression fracture of second lumbar vertebra   MCC CC H5 HCC

      2,3,6 ✓7ᵗʰ **S32.021** Stable burst fracture of second lumbar vertebra   MCC CC H5 HCC

      2,3,6 ✓7ᵗʰ **S32.022** Unstable burst fracture of second lumbar vertebra   MCC CC H5 HCC

      2,3,6 ✓7ᵗʰ **S32.028** Other fracture of second lumbar vertebra   MCC CC H5 HCC

      2,3,6 ✓7ᵗʰ **S32.029** Unspecified fracture of second lumbar vertebra   MCC CC H5 HCC

☑ Additional Character Required   ✓x7ᵗʰ Placeholder   Unacceptable PDx   Questionable PDx   Manifestation   Unspecified Dx   H1-H14 HAC   HCC CMS-HCC Dx   HIV HIV Dx

ICD-10-CM 2020   1019

Chapter 19. Injury, Poisoning and Certain Other Consequences of External Causes (side margin)

S32.03–S32.316 (side margin)

√6ᵗʰ **S32.03** **Fracture of third lumbar vertebra**

2,3,6 √7ᵗʰ **S32.030** **Wedge compression fracture of third lumbar vertebra** `MCC` `CC` `H5` `HCC`

2,3,6 √7ᵗʰ **S32.031** **Stable burst fracture of third lumbar vertebra** `MCC` `CC` `H5` `HCC`

2,3,6 √7ᵗʰ **S32.032** **Unstable burst fracture of third lumbar vertebra** `MCC` `CC` `H5` `HCC`

2,3,6 √7ᵗʰ **S32.038** **Other fracture of third lumbar vertebra** `MCC` `CC` `H5` `HCC`

2,3,6 √7ᵗʰ **S32.039** **Unspecified fracture of third lumbar vertebra** `MCC` `CC` `H5` `HCC`

√6ᵗʰ **S32.04** **Fracture of fourth lumbar vertebra**

2,3,6 √7ᵗʰ **S32.040** **Wedge compression fracture of fourth lumbar vertebra** `MCC` `CC` `H5` `HCC`

2,3,6 √7ᵗʰ **S32.041** **Stable burst fracture of fourth lumbar vertebra** `MCC` `CC` `H5` `HCC`

2,3,6 √7ᵗʰ **S32.042** **Unstable burst fracture of fourth lumbar vertebra** `MCC` `CC` `H5` `HCC`

2,3,6 √7ᵗʰ **S32.048** **Other fracture of fourth lumbar vertebra** `MCC` `CC` `H5` `HCC`

2,3,6 √7ᵗʰ **S32.049** **Unspecified fracture of fourth lumbar vertebra** `MCC` `CC` `H5` `HCC`

√6ᵗʰ **S32.05** **Fracture of fifth lumbar vertebra**

2,3,6 √7ᵗʰ **S32.050** **Wedge compression fracture of fifth lumbar vertebra** `MCC` `CC` `H5` `HCC`

2,3,6 √7ᵗʰ **S32.051** **Stable burst fracture of fifth lumbar vertebra** `MCC` `CC` `H5` `HCC`

2,3,6 √7ᵗʰ **S32.052** **Unstable burst fracture of fifth lumbar vertebra** `MCC` `CC` `H5` `HCC`

2,3,6 √7ᵗʰ **S32.058** **Other fracture of fifth lumbar vertebra** `MCC` `CC` `H5` `HCC`

2,3,6 √7ᵗʰ **S32.059** **Unspecified fracture of fifth lumbar vertebra** `MCC` `CC` `H5` `HCC`

√5ᵗʰ **S32.1** **Fracture of sacrum**

> `NOTE` For vertical fractures, code to most medial fracture extension
>
> Use two codes if both a vertical and transverse fracture are present
>
> Code also any associated fracture of pelvic ring (S32.8-)
>
> **CC Excl: For codes in subcategory S32.1:**
> **CC with 7th character A or MCC with 7th character B:** PDX collection 1197
> **CC with 7th character K:** PDX collection 897

2,3,6 √x7ᵗʰ **S32.10** **Unspecified fracture of sacrum** `MCC` `CC` `H5` `HCC`

√6ᵗʰ **S32.11** **Zone I fracture of sacrum**

> Vertical sacral ala fracture of sacrum

Vertical Sacral Fracture Zones

Zones: ① ② ③

2,3,6 √7ᵗʰ **S32.110** **Nondisplaced Zone I fracture of sacrum** `MCC` `CC` `H5` `HCC`

2,3,6 √7ᵗʰ **S32.111** **Minimally displaced Zone I fracture of sacrum** `MCC` `CC` `H5` `HCC`

2,3,6 √7ᵗʰ **S32.112** **Severely displaced Zone I fracture of sacrum** `MCC` `CC` `H5` `HCC`

2,3,6 √7ᵗʰ **S32.119** **Unspecified Zone I fracture of sacrum** `MCC` `CC` `H5` `HCC`

√6ᵗʰ **S32.12** **Zone II fracture of sacrum**

> Vertical foraminal region fracture of sacrum

2,3,6 √7ᵗʰ **S32.120** **Nondisplaced Zone II fracture of sacrum** `MCC` `CC` `H5` `HCC`

2,3,6 √7ᵗʰ **S32.121** **Minimally displaced Zone II fracture of sacrum** `MCC` `CC` `H5` `HCC`

2,3,6 √7ᵗʰ **S32.122** **Severely displaced Zone II fracture of sacrum** `MCC` `CC` `H5` `HCC`

2,3,6 √7ᵗʰ **S32.129** **Unspecified Zone II fracture of sacrum** `MCC` `CC` `H5` `HCC`

√6ᵗʰ **S32.13** **Zone III fracture of sacrum**

> Vertical fracture into spinal canal region of sacrum

2,3,6 √7ᵗʰ **S32.130** **Nondisplaced Zone III fracture of sacrum** `MCC` `CC` `H5` `HCC`

2,3,6 √7ᵗʰ **S32.131** **Minimally displaced Zone III fracture of sacrum** `MCC` `CC` `H5` `HCC`

2,3,6 √7ᵗʰ **S32.132** **Severely displaced Zone III fracture of sacrum** `MCC` `CC` `H5` `HCC`

2,3,6 √7ᵗʰ **S32.139** **Unspecified Zone III fracture of sacrum** `MCC` `CC` `H5` `HCC`

Transverse Sacral Fracture Types

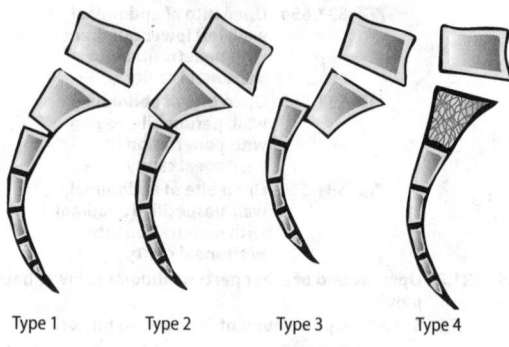

Type 1   Type 2   Type 3   Type 4

2,3,6 √x7ᵗʰ **S32.14** **Type 1 fracture of sacrum** `MCC` `CC` `H5` `HCC`

> Transverse flexion fracture of sacrum without displacement

2,3,6 √x7ᵗʰ **S32.15** **Type 2 fracture of sacrum** `MCC` `CC` `H5` `HCC`

> Transverse flexion fracture of sacrum with posterior displacement

2,3,6 √x7ᵗʰ **S32.16** **Type 3 fracture of sacrum** `MCC` `CC` `H5` `HCC`

> Transverse extension fracture of sacrum with anterior displacement

2,3,6 √x7ᵗʰ **S32.17** **Type 4 fracture of sacrum** `MCC` `CC` `H5` `HCC`

> Transverse segmental comminution of upper sacrum

2,3,6 √x7ᵗʰ **S32.19** **Other fracture of sacrum** `MCC` `CC` `H5` `HCC`

2,3,6 √x7ᵗʰ **S32.2** **Fracture of coccyx** `MCC` `CC` `H5` `HCC`

> **CC Excl:** See code S32.1

√5ᵗʰ **S32.3** **Fracture of ilium**

> *EXCLUDES 1*   *fracture of ilium with associated disruption of pelvic ring (S32.8-)*
>
> **CC Excl: For codes in subcategory S32.3:**
> **CC with 7th character A:** PDX collection 1176
> **MCC with 7th character B:** PDX collection 1198
> **CC with 7th character K:** PDX collection 897

√6ᵗʰ **S32.30** **Unspecified fracture of ilium**

2,3,6 √7ᵗʰ **S32.301** **Unspecified fracture of right ilium** `MCC` `CC` `H5` `HCC`

2,3,6 √7ᵗʰ **S32.302** **Unspecified fracture of left ilium** `MCC` `CC` `H5` `HCC`

2,3,6 √7ᵗʰ **S32.309** **Unspecified fracture of unspecified ilium** `MCC` `CC` `H5` `HCC`

√6ᵗʰ **S32.31** **Avulsion fracture of ilium**

2,3,6 √7ᵗʰ **S32.311** **Displaced avulsion fracture of right ilium** `MCC` `CC` `H5` `HCC`

2,3,6 √7ᵗʰ **S32.312** **Displaced avulsion fracture of left ilium** `MCC` `CC` `H5` `HCC`

2,3,6 √7ᵗʰ **S32.313** **Displaced avulsion fracture of unspecified ilium** `MCC` `CC` `H5` `HCC`

2,3,6 √7ᵗʰ **S32.314** **Nondisplaced avulsion fracture of right ilium** `MCC` `CC` `H5` `HCC`

2,3,6 √7ᵗʰ **S32.315** **Nondisplaced avulsion fracture of left ilium** `MCC` `CC` `H5` `HCC`

2,3,6 √7ᵗʰ **S32.316** **Nondisplaced avulsion fracture of unspecified ilium** `MCC` `CC` `H5` `HCC`

`N` Newborn: 0   `P` Pediatric: 0-17   `M` Maternity: 9-64   `A` Adult: 15-124   `MCC` Major Complication/Comorbidity   `CC` Complication/Comorbidity   `SW` Severe Wound Dx

1020   ICD-10-CM 2020

ICD-10-CM 2020   Chapter 19. Injury, Poisoning and Certain Other Consequences of External Causes   S32.39–S32.474

√6ᵗʰ **S32.39**   **Other fracture of ilium**

2,3,6 √7ᵗʰ   **S32.391**   Other fracture of right ilium   `MCC` `CC` `H5` `HCC`

2,3,6 √7ᵗʰ   **S32.392**   Other fracture of left ilium   `MCC` `CC` `H5` `HCC`

2,3,6 √7ᵗʰ   **S32.399**   Other fracture of unspecified ilium   `MCC` `CC` `H5` `HCC`

√5ᵗʰ **S32.4**   **Fracture of acetabulum**

   Code also any associated fracture of pelvic ring (S32.8-)

   AHA: 2016,3Q,16

   CC Excl: For codes in subcategory S32.4:
   MCC with 7th character A: PDX collection 1199
   MCC with 7th character B: PDX collection 1200
   CC with 7th character K: PDX collection 897

√6ᵗʰ **S32.40**   **Unspecified fracture of acetabulum**

2,3,6 √7ᵗʰ   **S32.401**   Unspecified fracture of right acetabulum   `MCC` `CC` `H5` `HCC`

2,3,6 √7ᵗʰ   **S32.402**   Unspecified fracture of left acetabulum   `MCC` `CC` `H5` `HCC`

2,3,6 √7ᵗʰ   **S32.409**   Unspecified fracture of unspecified acetabulum   `MCC` `CC` `H5` `HCC`

√6ᵗʰ **S32.41**   **Fracture of anterior wall of acetabulum**

4,6 √7ᵗʰ   **S32.411**   Displaced fracture of anterior wall of right acetabulum   `MCC` `CC` `H5` `HCC`

4,6 √7ᵗʰ   **S32.412**   Displaced fracture of anterior wall of left acetabulum   `MCC` `CC` `H5` `HCC`

4,6 √7ᵗʰ   **S32.413**   Displaced fracture of anterior wall of unspecified acetabulum   `MCC` `CC` `H5` `HCC`

4,6 √7ᵗʰ   **S32.414**   Nondisplaced fracture of anterior wall of right acetabulum   `MCC` `CC` `H5` `HCC`

4,6 √7ᵗʰ   **S32.415**   Nondisplaced fracture of anterior wall of left acetabulum   `MCC` `CC` `H5` `HCC`

4,6 √7ᵗʰ   **S32.416**   Nondisplaced fracture of anterior wall of unspecified acetabulum   `MCC` `CC` `H5` `HCC`

√6ᵗʰ **S32.42**   **Fracture of posterior wall of acetabulum**

4,6 √7ᵗʰ   **S32.421**   Displaced fracture of posterior wall of right acetabulum   `MCC` `CC` `H5` `HCC`

4,6 √7ᵗʰ   **S32.422**   Displaced fracture of posterior wall of left acetabulum   `MCC` `CC` `H5` `HCC`

4,6 √7ᵗʰ   **S32.423**   Displaced fracture of posterior wall of unspecified acetabulum   `MCC` `CC` `H5` `HCC`

4,6 √7ᵗʰ   **S32.424**   Nondisplaced fracture of posterior wall of right acetabulum   `MCC` `CC` `H5` `HCC`

4,6 √7ᵗʰ   **S32.425**   Nondisplaced fracture of posterior wall of left acetabulum   `MCC` `CC` `H5` `HCC`

4,6 √7ᵗʰ   **S32.426**   Nondisplaced fracture of posterior wall of unspecified acetabulum   `MCC` `CC` `H5` `HCC`

√6ᵗʰ **S32.43**   **Fracture of anterior column [iliopubic] of acetabulum**

4,6 √7ᵗʰ   **S32.431**   Displaced fracture of anterior column [iliopubic] of right acetabulum   `MCC` `CC` `H5` `HCC`

4,6 √7ᵗʰ   **S32.432**   Displaced fracture of anterior column [iliopubic] of left acetabulum   `MCC` `CC` `H5` `HCC`

4,6 √7ᵗʰ   **S32.433**   Displaced fracture of anterior column [iliopubic] of unspecified acetabulum   `MCC` `CC` `H5` `HCC`

4,6 √7ᵗʰ   **S32.434**   Nondisplaced fracture of anterior column [iliopubic] of right acetabulum   `MCC` `CC` `H5` `HCC`

4,6 √7ᵗʰ   **S32.435**   Nondisplaced fracture of anterior column [iliopubic] of left acetabulum   `MCC` `CC` `H5` `HCC`

4,6 √7ᵗʰ   **S32.436**   Nondisplaced fracture of anterior column [iliopubic] of unspecified acetabulum   `MCC` `CC` `H5` `HCC`

√6ᵗʰ **S32.44**   **Fracture of posterior column [ilioischial] of acetabulum**

4,6 √7ᵗʰ   **S32.441**   Displaced fracture of posterior column [ilioischial] of right acetabulum   `MCC` `CC` `H5` `HCC`

4,6 √7ᵗʰ   **S32.442**   Displaced fracture of posterior column [ilioischial] of left acetabulum   `MCC` `CC` `H5` `HCC`

4,6 √7ᵗʰ   **S32.443**   Displaced fracture of posterior column [ilioischial] of unspecified acetabulum   `MCC` `CC` `H5` `HCC`

4,6 √7ᵗʰ   **S32.444**   Nondisplaced fracture of posterior column [ilioischial] of right acetabulum   `MCC` `CC` `H5` `HCC`

4,6 √7ᵗʰ   **S32.445**   Nondisplaced fracture of posterior column [ilioischial] of left acetabulum   `MCC` `CC` `H5` `HCC`

4,6 √7ᵗʰ   **S32.446**   Nondisplaced fracture of posterior column [ilioischial] of unspecified acetabulum   `MCC` `CC` `H5` `HCC`

√6ᵗʰ **S32.45**   **Transverse fracture of acetabulum**

4,6 √7ᵗʰ   **S32.451**   Displaced transverse fracture of right acetabulum   `MCC` `CC` `H5` `HCC`

4,6 √7ᵗʰ   **S32.452**   Displaced transverse fracture of left acetabulum   `MCC` `CC` `H5` `HCC`

4,6 √7ᵗʰ   **S32.453**   Displaced transverse fracture of unspecified acetabulum   `MCC` `CC` `H5` `HCC`

4,6 √7ᵗʰ   **S32.454**   Nondisplaced transverse fracture of right acetabulum   `MCC` `CC` `H5` `HCC`

4,6 √7ᵗʰ   **S32.455**   Nondisplaced transverse fracture of left acetabulum   `MCC` `CC` `H5` `HCC`

4,6 √7ᵗʰ   **S32.456**   Nondisplaced transverse fracture of unspecified acetabulum   `MCC` `CC` `H5` `HCC`

√6ᵗʰ **S32.46**   **Associated transverse-posterior fracture of acetabulum**

4,6 √7ᵗʰ   **S32.461**   Displaced associated transverse-posterior fracture of right acetabulum   `MCC` `CC` `H5` `HCC`

4,6 √7ᵗʰ   **S32.462**   Displaced associated transverse-posterior fracture of left acetabulum   `MCC` `CC` `H5` `HCC`

4,6 √7ᵗʰ   **S32.463**   Displaced associated transverse-posterior fracture of unspecified acetabulum   `MCC` `CC` `H5` `HCC`

4,6 √7ᵗʰ   **S32.464**   Nondisplaced associated transverse-posterior fracture of right acetabulum   `MCC` `CC` `H5` `HCC`

4,6 √7ᵗʰ   **S32.465**   Nondisplaced associated transverse-posterior fracture of left acetabulum   `MCC` `CC` `H5` `HCC`

4,6 √7ᵗʰ   **S32.466**   Nondisplaced associated transverse-posterior fracture of unspecified acetabulum   `MCC` `CC` `H5` `HCC`

√6ᵗʰ **S32.47**   **Fracture of medial wall of acetabulum**

4,6 √7ᵗʰ   **S32.471**   Displaced fracture of medial wall of right acetabulum   `MCC` `CC` `H5` `HCC`

4,6 √7ᵗʰ   **S32.472**   Displaced fracture of medial wall of left acetabulum   `MCC` `CC` `H5` `HCC`

4,6 √7ᵗʰ   **S32.473**   Displaced fracture of medial wall of unspecified acetabulum   `MCC` `CC` `H5` `HCC`

4,6 √7ᵗʰ   **S32.474**   Nondisplaced fracture of medial wall of right acetabulum   `MCC` `CC` `H5` `HCC`

☑ Additional Character Required   √x7ᵗʰ Placeholder   Unacceptable PDx   Questionable PDx   Manifestation   Unspecified Dx   `H1`-`H14` HAC   `HCC` CMS-HCC Dx   `HIV` HIV Dx

ICD-10-CM 2020   1021

4,6 √7ᵗʰ **S32.475** **Nondisplaced** fracture of `MCC` `CC` `H5` `HCC` **medial wall of left acetabulum**

4,6 √7ᵗʰ **S32.476** **Nondisplaced** fracture of `MCC` `CC` `H5` `HCC` **medial wall of unspecified acetabulum**

√6ᵗʰ **S32.48** **Dome fracture of acetabulum**

4,6 √7ᵗʰ **S32.481** **Displaced dome fracture** `MCC` `CC` `H5` `HCC` **of right acetabulum**

4,6 √7ᵗʰ **S32.482** **Displaced dome fracture** `MCC` `CC` `H5` `HCC` **of left acetabulum**

4,6 √7ᵗʰ **S32.483** **Displaced dome fracture** `MCC` `CC` `H5` `HCC` **of unspecified acetabulum**

4,6 √7ᵗʰ **S32.484** **Nondisplaced dome** `MCC` `CC` `H5` `HCC` **fracture of right acetabulum**

4,6 √7ᵗʰ **S32.485** **Nondisplaced dome** `MCC` `CC` `H5` `HCC` **fracture of left acetabulum**

4,6 √7ᵗʰ **S32.486** **Nondisplaced dome** `MCC` `CC` `H5` `HCC` **fracture of unspecified acetabulum**

√6ᵗʰ **S32.49** **Other specified fracture of acetabulum**

4,6 √7ᵗʰ **S32.491** **Other specified fracture of** `MCC` `CC` `H5` `HCC` **right acetabulum**

4,6 √7ᵗʰ **S32.492** **Other specified fracture of** `MCC` `CC` `H5` `HCC` **left acetabulum**

4,6 √7ᵗʰ **S32.499** **Other specified fracture of** `MCC` `CC` `H5` `HCC` **unspecified acetabulum**

√5ᵗʰ **S32.5** **Fracture of pubis**

> *EXCLUDES 1*   *fracture of pubis with associated disruption of pelvic ring (S32.8-)*

CC Excl: For codes in subcategory S32.5:
MCC with 7th character B: PDX collection 1201

√6ᵗʰ **S32.50** **Unspecified fracture of pubis**

2,6 √7ᵗʰ **S32.501** **Unspecified fracture of** `MCC` `H5` `HCC` **right pubis**

2,6 √7ᵗʰ **S32.502** **Unspecified fracture of left** `MCC` `H5` `HCC` **pubis**

2,6 √7ᵗʰ **S32.509** **Unspecified fracture of** `MCC` `H5` `HCC` **unspecified pubis**

√6ᵗʰ **S32.51** **Fracture of superior rim of pubis**

2,6 √7ᵗʰ **S32.511** **Fracture of superior rim of** `MCC` `H5` `HCC` **right pubis**

2,6 √7ᵗʰ **S32.512** **Fracture of superior rim of** `MCC` `H5` `HCC` **left pubis**

2,6 √7ᵗʰ **S32.519** **Fracture of superior rim of** `MCC` `H5` `HCC` **unspecified pubis**

√6ᵗʰ **S32.59** **Other specified fracture of pubis**

2,6 √7ᵗʰ **S32.591** **Other specified fracture of** `MCC` `H5` `HCC` **right pubis**

2,6 √7ᵗʰ **S32.592** **Other specified fracture of** `MCC` `H5` `HCC` **left pubis**

2,6 √7ᵗʰ **S32.599** **Other specified fracture of** `MCC` `H5` `HCC` **unspecified pubis**

√5ᵗʰ **S32.6** **Fracture of ischium**

> *EXCLUDES 1*   *fracture of ischium with associated disruption of pelvic ring (S32.8-)*

CC Excl: For codes in subcategory S32.6:
CC with 7th character A: PDX collection 1202
MCC with 7th character B: PDX collection 1203
CC with 7th character K: PDX collection 897

√6ᵗʰ **S32.60** **Unspecified fracture of ischium**

2,3,6 √7ᵗʰ **S32.601** **Unspecified fracture of** `MCC` `CC` `H5` `HCC` **right ischium**

2,3,6 √7ᵗʰ **S32.602** **Unspecified fracture of left** `MCC` `CC` `H5` `HCC` **ischium**

2,3,6 √7ᵗʰ **S32.609** **Unspecified fracture of** `MCC` `CC` `H5` `HCC` **unspecified ischium**

√6ᵗʰ **S32.61** **Avulsion fracture of ischium**

2,3,6 √7ᵗʰ **S32.611** **Displaced avulsion** `MCC` `CC` `H5` `HCC` **fracture of right ischium**

2,3,6 √7ᵗʰ **S32.612** **Displaced avulsion** `MCC` `CC` `H5` `HCC` **fracture of left ischium**

2,3,6 √7ᵗʰ **S32.613** **Displaced avulsion** `MCC` `CC` `H5` `HCC` **fracture of unspecified ischium**

2,3,6 √7ᵗʰ **S32.614** **Nondisplaced avulsion** `MCC` `CC` `H5` `HCC` **fracture of right ischium**

2,3,6 √7ᵗʰ **S32.615** **Nondisplaced avulsion** `MCC` `CC` `H5` `HCC` **fracture of left ischium**

2,3,6 √7ᵗʰ **S32.616** **Nondisplaced avulsion** `MCC` `CC` `H5` `HCC` **fracture of unspecified ischium**

√6ᵗʰ **S32.69** **Other specified fracture of ischium**

2,3,6 √7ᵗʰ **S32.691** **Other specified fracture of** `MCC` `CC` `H5` `HCC` **right ischium**

2,3,6 √7ᵗʰ **S32.692** **Other specified fracture of** `MCC` `CC` `H5` `HCC` **left ischium**

2,3,6 √7ᵗʰ **S32.699** **Other specified fracture of** `MCC` `CC` `H5` `HCC` **unspecified ischium**

√5ᵗʰ **S32.8** **Fracture of other parts of pelvis**

> Code also any associated:
> fracture of acetabulum (S32.4-)
> sacral fracture (S32.1-)

Fractures Disrupting Pelvic Circle

√6ᵗʰ **S32.81** **Multiple fractures of pelvis with disruption of pelvic ring**

> Multiple pelvic fractures with disruption of pelvic circle

CC Excl: For codes in subcategory S32.81:
CC with 7th character A or MCC with 7th character B: PDX collection 1204
CC with 7th character K: PDX collection 897

2,3,6 √7ᵗʰ **S32.810** **Multiple fractures of pelvis** `MCC` `CC` `H5` `HCC` **with stable disruption of pelvic ring**

2,3,6 √7ᵗʰ **S32.811** **Multiple fractures of pelvis** `MCC` `CC` `H5` `HCC` **with unstable disruption of pelvic ring**

2,3,6 √x7ᵗʰ **S32.82** **Multiple fractures of pelvis without** `MCC` `CC` `H5` `HCC` **disruption of pelvic ring**

> Multiple pelvic fractures without disruption of pelvic circle

CC Excl: CC with 7th character A or MCC with 7th character B: PDX collection 1205
CC Excl: CC with 7th character K: PDX collection 897

2,3,6 √x7ᵗʰ **S32.89** **Fracture of other parts of pelvis** `MCC` `CC` `H5` `HCC`

CC Excl: CC with 7th character A or MCC with 7th character B: PDX collection 1206
CC Excl: CC with 7th character K: PDX collection 897

2,3,6 √x7ᵗʰ **S32.9** **Fracture of unspecified parts of lumbosacral** `MCC` `CC` `H5` `HCC` **spine and pelvis**

> Fracture of lumbosacral spine NOS
> Fracture of pelvis NOS

AHA: 2012,4Q,93
CC Excl: CC with 7th character A or MCC with 7th character B: PDX collection 1204
CC Excl: CC with 7th character K: PDX collection 897

☑4ᵗʰ **S33 Dislocation and sprain of joints and ligaments of lumbar spine and pelvis**

INCLUDES   avulsion of joint or ligament of lumbar spine and pelvis

laceration of cartilage, joint or ligament of lumbar spine and pelvis

sprain of cartilage, joint or ligament of lumbar spine and pelvis

traumatic hemarthrosis of joint or ligament of lumbar spine and pelvis

traumatic rupture of joint or ligament of lumbar spine and pelvis

traumatic subluxation of joint or ligament of lumbar spine and pelvis

traumatic tear of joint or ligament of lumbar spine and pelvis

Code also any associated open wound

EXCLUDES 1   nontraumatic rupture or displacement of lumbar intervertebral disc NOS (M51.-)

obstetric damage to pelvic joints and ligaments (O71.6)

EXCLUDES 2   dislocation and sprain of joints and ligaments of hip (S73.-)

strain of muscle of lower back and pelvis (S39.01-)

> The appropriate 7th character is to be added to each code from category S33.
> A   initial encounter
> D   subsequent encounter
> S   sequela

☑x7ᵗʰ **S33.0 Traumatic rupture of lumbar intervertebral disc**

EXCLUDES 1   rupture or displacement (nontraumatic) of lumbar intervertebral disc NOS (M51.- with fifth character 6)

☑5ᵗʰ **S33.1 Subluxation and dislocation of lumbar vertebra**

Code also any associated:

open wound of abdomen, lower back and pelvis (S31)

spinal cord injury (S24.0, S24.1-, S34.0-, S34.1-)

EXCLUDES 2   fracture of lumbar vertebrae (S32.0-)

☑6ᵗʰ **S33.10 Subluxation and dislocation of unspecified lumbar vertebra**

☑7ᵗʰ **S33.100 Subluxation** of unspecified lumbar vertebra

☑7ᵗʰ **S33.101 Dislocation** of unspecified lumbar vertebra

☑6ᵗʰ **S33.11 Subluxation and dislocation of L1/L2 lumbar vertebra**

☑7ᵗʰ **S33.110 Subluxation** of L1/L2 lumbar vertebra

☑7ᵗʰ **S33.111 Dislocation** of L1/L2 lumbar vertebra

☑6ᵗʰ **S33.12 Subluxation and dislocation of L2/L3 lumbar vertebra**

☑7ᵗʰ **S33.120 Subluxation** of L2/L3 lumbar vertebra

☑7ᵗʰ **S33.121 Dislocation** of L2/L3 lumbar vertebra

☑6ᵗʰ **S33.13 Subluxation and dislocation of L3/L4 lumbar vertebra**

☑7ᵗʰ **S33.130 Subluxation** of L3/L4 lumbar vertebra

☑7ᵗʰ **S33.131 Dislocation** of L3/L4 lumbar vertebra

☑6ᵗʰ **S33.14 Subluxation and dislocation of L4/L5 lumbar vertebra**

☑7ᵗʰ **S33.140 Subluxation** of L4/L5 lumbar vertebra

☑7ᵗʰ **S33.141 Dislocation** of L4/L5 lumbar vertebra

☑x7ᵗʰ **S33.2 Dislocation of sacroiliac and sacrococcygeal joint**

☑5ᵗʰ **S33.3 Dislocation of other and unspecified parts of lumbar spine and pelvis**

☑x7ᵗʰ **S33.30 Dislocation of unspecified parts of lumbar spine and pelvis**

☑x7ᵗʰ **S33.39 Dislocation of other parts of lumbar spine and pelvis**

☑x7ᵗʰ **S33.4 Traumatic rupture of symphysis pubis**

☑x7ᵗʰ **S33.5 Sprain of ligaments of lumbar spine**

☑x7ᵗʰ **S33.6 Sprain of sacroiliac joint**

☑x7ᵗʰ **S33.8 Sprain of other parts of lumbar spine and pelvis**

☑x7ᵗʰ **S33.9 Sprain of unspecified parts of lumbar spine and pelvis**

☑4ᵗʰ **S34 Injury of lumbar and sacral spinal cord and nerves at abdomen, lower back and pelvis level**

NOTE   Code to highest level of lumbar cord injury.

Injuries to the spinal cord (S34.0 and S34.1) refer to the cord level and not bone level injury, and can affect nerve roots at and below the level given.

Code also any associated:

fracture of vertebra (S22.0-, S32.0-)

open wound of abdomen, lower back and pelvis (S31.-)

transient paralysis (R29.5)

> The appropriate 7th character is to be added to each code from category S34.
> A   initial encounter
> D   subsequent encounter
> S   sequela

CC Excl: For MCC codes in category S34, unless otherwise noted: PDX collection 1207

☑5ᵗʰ **S34.0 Concussion and edema of lumbar and sacral spinal cord**

☑7ᵗʰ **S34.01 Concussion and edema of lumbar spinal cord**   MCC HCC

☑7ᵗʰ **S34.02 Concussion and edema of sacral spinal cord**   MCC HCC

Concussion and edema of conus medullaris

CC Excl: PDX collection 1208

☑5ᵗʰ **S34.1 Other and unspecified injury of lumbar and sacral spinal cord**

☑6ᵗʰ **S34.10 Unspecified injury to lumbar spinal cord**

☑7ᵗʰ **S34.101 Unspecified injury to L1 level of lumbar spinal cord**   MCC H5 HCC

Unspecified injury to lumbar spinal cord level 1

☑7ᵗʰ **S34.102 Unspecified injury to L2 level of lumbar spinal cord**   MCC H5 HCC

Unspecified injury to lumbar spinal cord level 2

☑7ᵗʰ **S34.103 Unspecified injury to L3 level of lumbar spinal cord**   MCC H5 HCC

Unspecified injury to lumbar spinal cord level 3

☑7ᵗʰ **S34.104 Unspecified injury to L4 level of lumbar spinal cord**   MCC H5 HCC

Unspecified injury to lumbar spinal cord level 4

☑7ᵗʰ **S34.105 Unspecified injury to L5 level of lumbar spinal cord**   MCC H5 HCC

Unspecified injury to lumbar spinal cord level 5

☑7ᵗʰ **S34.109 Unspecified injury to unspecified level of lumbar spinal cord**   MCC H5 HCC

☑6ᵗʰ **S34.11 Complete lesion of lumbar spinal cord**

☑7ᵗʰ **S34.111 Complete lesion of L1 level of lumbar spinal cord**   MCC H5 HCC

Complete lesion of lumbar spinal cord level 1

☑7ᵗʰ **S34.112 Complete lesion of L2 level of lumbar spinal cord**   MCC H5 HCC

Complete lesion of lumbar spinal cord level 2

☑7ᵗʰ **S34.113 Complete lesion of L3 level of lumbar spinal cord**   MCC H5 HCC

Complete lesion of lumbar spinal cord level 3

☑7ᵗʰ **S34.114 Complete lesion of L4 level of lumbar spinal cord**   MCC H5 HCC

Complete lesion of lumbar spinal cord level 4

☑7ᵗʰ **S34.115 Complete lesion of L5 level of lumbar spinal cord**   MCC H5 HCC

Complete lesion of lumbar spinal cord level 5

☑7ᵗʰ **S34.119 Complete lesion of unspecified level of lumbar spinal cord**   MCC H5 HCC

Chapter 19. Injury, Poisoning and Certain Other Consequences of External Causes

S34.12–S35.239

√6ᵗʰ **S34.12** **Incomplete lesion of lumbar spinal cord**

√7ᵗʰ **S34.121** **Incomplete lesion of L1 level of lumbar spinal cord** `MCC` `H5` `HCC`
Incomplete lesion of lumbar spinal cord level 1

√7ᵗʰ **S34.122** **Incomplete lesion of L2 level of lumbar spinal cord** `MCC` `H5` `HCC`
Incomplete lesion of lumbar spinal cord level 2

√7ᵗʰ **S34.123** **Incomplete lesion of L3 level of lumbar spinal cord** `MCC` `H5` `HCC`
Incomplete lesion of lumbar spinal cord level 3

√7ᵗʰ **S34.124** **Incomplete lesion of L4 level of lumbar spinal cord** `MCC` `H5` `HCC`
Incomplete lesion of lumbar spinal cord level 4

√7ᵗʰ **S34.125** **Incomplete lesion of L5 level of lumbar spinal cord** `MCC` `H5` `HCC`
Incomplete lesion of lumbar spinal cord level 5

√7ᵗʰ **S34.129** **Incomplete lesion of unspecified level of lumbar spinal cord** `MCC` `H5` `HCC`

√6ᵗʰ **S34.13** **Other and unspecified injury to sacral spinal cord**
Other injury to conus medullaris
CC Excl: For MCC codes in subcategory S34.13: PDX collection 1208

√7ᵗʰ **S34.131** **Complete lesion of sacral spinal cord** `MCC` `H5` `HCC`
Complete lesion of conus medullaris

√7ᵗʰ **S34.132** **Incomplete lesion of sacral spinal cord** `MCC` `H5` `HCC`
Incomplete lesion of conus medullaris

√7ᵗʰ **S34.139** **Unspecified injury to sacral spinal cord** `MCC` `H5` `HCC`
Unspecified injury of conus medullaris

√5ᵗʰ **S34.2** **Injury of nerve root of lumbar and sacral spine**

√x7ᵗʰ **S34.21** **Injury of nerve root of lumbar spine**

√x7ᵗʰ **S34.22** **Injury of nerve root of sacral spine**

⁶ √x7ᵗʰ **S34.3** **Injury of cauda equina** `MCC` `H5` `HCC`
CC Excl: PDX collection 1208

√x7ᵗʰ **S34.4** **Injury of lumbosacral plexus**

√x7ᵗʰ **S34.5** **Injury of lumbar, sacral and pelvic sympathetic nerves**
Injury of celiac ganglion or plexus
Injury of hypogastric plexus
Injury of mesenteric plexus (inferior) (superior)
Injury of splanchnic nerve

√x7ᵗʰ **S34.6** **Injury of peripheral nerve(s) at abdomen, lower back and pelvis level**

√x7ᵗʰ **S34.8** **Injury of other nerves at abdomen, lower back and pelvis level**

√x7ᵗʰ **S34.9** **Injury of unspecified nerves at abdomen, lower back and pelvis level**

√4ᵗʰ **S35** **Injury of blood vessels at abdomen, lower back and pelvis level**
Code also any associated open wound (S31.-)

The appropriate 7th character is to be added to each code from category S35.
A   initial encounter
D   subsequent encounter
S   sequela

√5ᵗʰ **S35.0** **Injury of abdominal aorta**
EXCLUDES 1   injury of aorta NOS (S25.0)
CC Excl: For MCC codes in subcategory S35.0: PDX collection 1209

√x7ᵗʰ **S35.00** **Unspecified injury of abdominal aorta** `MCC`

√x7ᵗʰ **S35.01** **Minor laceration of abdominal aorta** `MCC`
Incomplete transection of abdominal aorta
Laceration of abdominal aorta NOS
Superficial laceration of abdominal aorta

√x7ᵗʰ **S35.02** **Major laceration of abdominal aorta** `MCC`
Complete transection of abdominal aorta
Traumatic rupture of abdominal aorta

√x7ᵗʰ **S35.09** **Other injury of abdominal aorta** `MCC`

√5ᵗʰ **S35.1** **Injury of inferior vena cava**
Injury of hepatic vein
EXCLUDES 1   injury of vena cava NOS (S25.2)
CC Excl: For MCC codes in subcategory S35.1: PDX collection 1210

√x7ᵗʰ **S35.10** **Unspecified injury of inferior vena cava** `MCC`

√x7ᵗʰ **S35.11** **Minor laceration of inferior vena cava** `MCC`
Incomplete transection of inferior vena cava
Laceration of inferior vena cava NOS
Superficial laceration of inferior vena cava

√x7ᵗʰ **S35.12** **Major laceration of inferior vena cava** `MCC`
Complete transection of inferior vena cava
Traumatic rupture of inferior vena cava

√x7ᵗʰ **S35.19** **Other injury of inferior vena cava** `MCC`

√5ᵗʰ **S35.2** **Injury of celiac or mesenteric artery and branches**

√6ᵗʰ **S35.21** **Injury of celiac artery**
CC Excl: For MCC codes in subcategory S35.21: PDX collection 1211

√7ᵗʰ **S35.211** **Minor laceration of celiac artery** `MCC`
Incomplete transection of celiac artery
Laceration of celiac artery NOS
Superficial laceration of celiac artery

√7ᵗʰ **S35.212** **Major laceration of celiac artery** `MCC`
Complete transection of celiac artery
Traumatic rupture of celiac artery

√7ᵗʰ **S35.218** **Other injury of celiac artery** `MCC`

√7ᵗʰ **S35.219** **Unspecified injury of celiac artery** `MCC`

√6ᵗʰ **S35.22** **Injury of superior mesenteric artery**
CC Excl: For MCC codes in subcategory S35.22: PDX collection 1212

√7ᵗʰ **S35.221** **Minor laceration of superior mesenteric artery** `MCC`
Incomplete transection of superior mesenteric artery
Laceration of superior mesenteric artery NOS
Superficial laceration of superior mesenteric artery

√7ᵗʰ **S35.222** **Major laceration of superior mesenteric artery** `MCC`
Complete transection of superior mesenteric artery
Traumatic rupture of superior mesenteric artery

√7ᵗʰ **S35.228** **Other injury of superior mesenteric artery** `MCC`

√7ᵗʰ **S35.229** **Unspecified injury of superior mesenteric artery** `MCC`

√6ᵗʰ **S35.23** **Injury of inferior mesenteric artery**
CC Excl: For MCC codes in subcategory S35.23: PDX collection 1213

√7ᵗʰ **S35.231** **Minor laceration of inferior mesenteric artery** `MCC`
Incomplete transection of inferior mesenteric artery
Laceration of inferior mesenteric artery NOS
Superficial laceration of inferior mesenteric artery

√7ᵗʰ **S35.232** **Major laceration of inferior mesenteric artery** `MCC`
Complete transection of inferior mesenteric artery
Traumatic rupture of inferior mesenteric artery

√7ᵗʰ **S35.238** **Other injury of inferior mesenteric artery** `MCC`

√7ᵗʰ **S35.239** **Unspecified injury of inferior mesenteric artery** `MCC`

✓6ᵗʰ **S35.29** **Injury of branches of celiac and mesenteric artery**
Injury of gastric artery
Injury of gastroduodenal artery
Injury of hepatic artery
Injury of splenic artery

✓7ᵗʰ **S35.291** **Minor laceration of branches of celiac and mesenteric artery**   MCC
Incomplete transection of branches of celiac and mesenteric artery
Laceration of branches of celiac and mesenteric artery NOS
Superficial laceration of branches of celiac and mesenteric artery
CC Excl: PDX collection 1214

✓7ᵗʰ **S35.292** **Major laceration of branches of celiac and mesenteric artery**   MCC
Complete transection of branches of celiac and mesenteric artery
Traumatic rupture of branches of celiac and mesenteric artery
CC Excl: PDX collection 1215

✓7ᵗʰ **S35.298** **Other injury of branches of celiac and mesenteric artery**   MCC
CC Excl: PDX collection 1215

✓7ᵗʰ **S35.299** **Unspecified injury of branches of celiac and mesenteric artery**   MCC
CC Excl: PDX collection 1216

✓5ᵗʰ **S35.3** **Injury of portal or splenic vein and branches**

✓6ᵗʰ **S35.31** **Injury of portal vein**
CC Excl: For MCC codes in subcategory S35.31: PDX collection 1217

✓7ᵗʰ **S35.311** **Laceration of portal vein**   MCC

✓7ᵗʰ **S35.318** **Other specified injury of portal vein**   MCC

✓7ᵗʰ **S35.319** **Unspecified injury of portal vein**   MCC

✓6ᵗʰ **S35.32** **Injury of splenic vein**
CC Excl: For MCC codes in subcategory S35.32: PDX collection 1218

✓7ᵗʰ **S35.321** **Laceration of splenic vein**   MCC

✓7ᵗʰ **S35.328** **Other specified injury of splenic vein**   MCC

✓7ᵗʰ **S35.329** **Unspecified injury of splenic vein**   MCC

✓6ᵗʰ **S35.33** **Injury of superior mesenteric vein**
CC Excl: For MCC codes in subcategory S35.33: PDX collection 1219

✓7ᵗʰ **S35.331** **Laceration of superior mesenteric vein**   MCC

✓7ᵗʰ **S35.338** **Other specified injury of superior mesenteric vein**   MCC

✓7ᵗʰ **S35.339** **Unspecified injury of superior mesenteric vein**   MCC

✓6ᵗʰ **S35.34** **Injury of inferior mesenteric vein**
CC Excl: For MCC codes in subcategory S35.34: PDX collection 1220

✓7ᵗʰ **S35.341** **Laceration of inferior mesenteric vein**   MCC

✓7ᵗʰ **S35.348** **Other specified injury of inferior mesenteric vein**   MCC

✓7ᵗʰ **S35.349** **Unspecified injury of inferior mesenteric vein**   MCC

✓5ᵗʰ **S35.4** **Injury of renal blood vessels**
CC Excl: For MCC codes in subcategory S35.4, unless otherwise noted: PDX collection 1221

✓6ᵗʰ **S35.40** **Unspecified injury of renal blood vessel**

✓7ᵗʰ **S35.401** **Unspecified injury of right renal artery**   MCC

✓7ᵗʰ **S35.402** **Unspecified injury of left renal artery**   MCC

✓7ᵗʰ **S35.403** **Unspecified injury of unspecified renal artery**   MCC

✓7ᵗʰ **S35.404** **Unspecified injury of right renal vein**   MCC
CC Excl: PDX collection 1222

✓7ᵗʰ **S35.405** **Unspecified injury of left renal vein**   MCC
CC Excl: PDX collection 1222

✓7ᵗʰ **S35.406** **Unspecified injury of unspecified renal vein**   MCC
CC Excl: PDX collection 1222

✓6ᵗʰ **S35.41** **Laceration of renal blood vessel**

✓7ᵗʰ **S35.411** **Laceration of right renal artery**   MCC

✓7ᵗʰ **S35.412** **Laceration of left renal artery**   MCC

✓7ᵗʰ **S35.413** **Laceration of unspecified renal artery**   MCC

✓7ᵗʰ **S35.414** **Laceration of right renal vein**   MCC
CC Excl: PDX collection 1222

✓7ᵗʰ **S35.415** **Laceration of left renal vein**   MCC
CC Excl: PDX collection 1222

✓7ᵗʰ **S35.416** **Laceration of unspecified renal vein**   MCC
CC Excl: PDX collection 1222

✓6ᵗʰ **S35.49** **Other specified injury of renal blood vessel**

✓7ᵗʰ **S35.491** **Other specified injury of right renal artery**   MCC

✓7ᵗʰ **S35.492** **Other specified injury of left renal artery**   MCC

✓7ᵗʰ **S35.493** **Other specified injury of unspecified renal artery**   MCC

✓7ᵗʰ **S35.494** **Other specified injury of right renal vein**   MCC
CC Excl: PDX collection 1222

✓7ᵗʰ **S35.495** **Other specified injury of left renal vein**   MCC
CC Excl: PDX collection 1222

✓7ᵗʰ **S35.496** **Other specified injury of unspecified renal vein**   MCC
CC Excl: PDX collection 1222

✓5ᵗʰ **S35.5** **Injury of iliac blood vessels**

✓×7ᵗʰ **S35.50** **Injury of unspecified iliac blood vessel(s)**   MCC
CC Excl: PDX collection 1223

✓6ᵗʰ **S35.51** **Injury of iliac artery or vein**
Injury of hypogastric artery or vein

✓7ᵗʰ **S35.511** **Injury of right iliac artery**   MCC
CC Excl: PDX collection 1224

✓7ᵗʰ **S35.512** **Injury of left iliac artery**   MCC
CC Excl: PDX collection 1224

✓7ᵗʰ **S35.513** **Injury of unspecified iliac artery**   MCC
CC Excl: PDX collection 1224

✓7ᵗʰ **S35.514** **Injury of right iliac vein**   MCC
CC Excl: PDX collection 1225

✓7ᵗʰ **S35.515** **Injury of left iliac vein**   MCC
CC Excl: PDX collection 1225

✓7ᵗʰ **S35.516** **Injury of unspecified iliac vein**   MCC
CC Excl: PDX collection 1225

✓6ᵗʰ **S35.53** **Injury of uterine artery or vein**

✓7ᵗʰ **S35.531** **Injury of right uterine artery**   CC ♀
CC Excl: PDX collection 1226

✓7ᵗʰ **S35.532** **Injury of left uterine artery**   CC ♀
CC Excl: PDX collection 1226

✓7ᵗʰ **S35.533** **Injury of unspecified uterine artery**   CC ♀
CC Excl: PDX collection 1226

✓7ᵗʰ **S35.534** **Injury of right uterine vein**   CC ♀
CC Excl: PDX collection 1227

✓7ᵗʰ **S35.535** **Injury of left uterine vein**   CC ♀
CC Excl: PDX collection 1227

✓7ᵗʰ **S35.536** **Injury of unspecified uterine vein**   CC ♀
CC Excl: PDX collection 1227

✓×7ᵗʰ **S35.59** **Injury of other iliac blood vessels**   MCC
CC Excl: PDX collection 1223

Chapter 19. Injury, Poisoning and Certain Other Consequences of External Causes

S35.8–S36.241

√5ᵗʰ **S35.8**   **Injury of other blood vessels at abdomen, lower back and pelvis level**

Injury of ovarian artery or vein

√6ᵗʰ **S35.8X**   **Injury of other blood vessels at abdomen, lower back and pelvis level**

CC Excl: For CC codes in subcategory S35.8X: PDX collection 1228

√7ᵗʰ **S35.8X1**   **Laceration of other blood vessels at abdomen, lower back and pelvis level**   `CC`

√7ᵗʰ **S35.8X8**   **Other specified injury of other blood vessels at abdomen, lower back and pelvis level**   `CC`

√7ᵗʰ **S35.8X9**   **Unspecified injury of other blood vessels at abdomen, lower back and pelvis level**   `CC`

√5ᵗʰ **S35.9**   **Injury of unspecified blood vessel at abdomen, lower back and pelvis level**

CC Excl: For CC codes in subcategory S35.9: PDX collection 1229

√x7ᵗʰ **S35.90**   **Unspecified injury of unspecified blood vessel at abdomen, lower back and pelvis level**   `CC`

√x7ᵗʰ **S35.91**   **Laceration of unspecified blood vessel at abdomen, lower back and pelvis level**   `CC`

√x7ᵗʰ **S35.99**   **Other specified injury of unspecified blood vessel at abdomen, lower back and pelvis level**   `CC`

√4ᵗʰ **S36**   **Injury of intra-abdominal organs**

Code also any associated open wound (S31.-)

The appropriate 7th character is to be added to each code from category S36.
A   initial encounter
D   subsequent encounter
S   sequela

√5ᵗʰ **S36.0**   **Injury of spleen**

AHA: 2015,2Q,36; 2015,1Q,10
CC Excl: For CC/MCC codes in subcategory S36.0: PDX collection 1230

√x7ᵗʰ **S36.00**   **Unspecified injury of spleen**   `CC`

√6ᵗʰ **S36.02**   **Contusion of spleen**

TIP: When both traumatic splenic laceration and contusion are documented in the same encounter, code only the laceration, as contusions are not coded when they occur with a more severe injury in the same body site.

√7ᵗʰ **S36.020**   **Minor contusion of spleen**   `CC`

Contusion of spleen less than 2 cm

√7ᵗʰ **S36.021**   **Major contusion of spleen**   `CC`

Contusion of spleen greater than 2 cm

√7ᵗʰ **S36.029**   **Unspecified contusion of spleen**   `CC`

√6ᵗʰ **S36.03**   **Laceration of spleen**

TIP: When both traumatic splenic laceration and contusion are documented in the same encounter, code only the laceration, as contusions are not coded when they occur with a more severe injury in the same body site.

√7ᵗʰ **S36.030**   **Superficial (capsular) laceration of spleen**   `CC`

Laceration of spleen less than 1 cm
Minor laceration of spleen

√7ᵗʰ **S36.031**   **Moderate laceration of spleen**   `MCC`

Laceration of spleen 1 to 3 cm

√7ᵗʰ **S36.032**   **Major laceration of spleen**   `MCC`

Avulsion of spleen
Laceration of spleen greater than 3 cm
Massive laceration of spleen
Multiple moderate lacerations of spleen
Stellate laceration of spleen

√7ᵗʰ **S36.039**   **Unspecified laceration of spleen**   `CC`

√x7ᵗʰ **S36.09**   **Other injury of spleen**   `CC`

√5ᵗʰ **S36.1**   **Injury of liver and gallbladder and bile duct**

√6ᵗʰ **S36.11**   **Injury of liver**

CC Excl: For CC/MCC codes in subcategory S36.11: PDX collection 1231

√7ᵗʰ **S36.112**   **Contusion of liver**   `CC`

√7ᵗʰ **S36.113**   **Laceration of liver, unspecified degree**   `CC`

√7ᵗʰ **S36.114**   **Minor laceration of liver**   `CC`

Laceration involving capsule only, or, without significant involvement of hepatic parenchyma [i.e., less than 1 cm deep]

√7ᵗʰ **S36.115**   **Moderate laceration of liver**   `MCC`

Laceration involving parenchyma but without major disruption of parenchyma [i.e., less than 10 cm long and less than 3 cm deep]

√7ᵗʰ **S36.116**   **Major laceration of liver**   `MCC`

Laceration with significant disruption of hepatic parenchyma [i.e., greater than 10 cm long and 3 cm deep]
Multiple moderate lacerations, with or without hematoma
Stellate laceration of liver

√7ᵗʰ **S36.118**   **Other injury of liver**   `CC`

√7ᵗʰ **S36.119**   **Unspecified injury of liver**   `CC`

√6ᵗʰ **S36.12**   **Injury of gallbladder**

CC Excl: For CC codes in subcategory S36.12: PDX collection 1232

√7ᵗʰ **S36.122**   **Contusion of gallbladder**   `CC`

√7ᵗʰ **S36.123**   **Laceration of gallbladder**   `CC`

√7ᵗʰ **S36.128**   **Other injury of gallbladder**   `CC`

√7ᵗʰ **S36.129**   **Unspecified injury of gallbladder**   `CC`

√x7ᵗʰ **S36.13**   **Injury of bile duct**   `CC`

CC Excl: PDX collection 1232

√5ᵗʰ **S36.2**   **Injury of pancreas**

CC Excl: For CC codes in subcategory S36.2: PDX collection 1233

√6ᵗʰ **S36.20**   **Unspecified injury of pancreas**

√7ᵗʰ **S36.200**   **Unspecified injury of head of pancreas**   `CC`

√7ᵗʰ **S36.201**   **Unspecified injury of body of pancreas**   `CC`

√7ᵗʰ **S36.202**   **Unspecified injury of tail of pancreas**   `CC`

√7ᵗʰ **S36.209**   **Unspecified injury of unspecified part of pancreas**   `CC`

√6ᵗʰ **S36.22**   **Contusion of pancreas**

√7ᵗʰ **S36.220**   **Contusion of head of pancreas**   `CC`

√7ᵗʰ **S36.221**   **Contusion of body of pancreas**   `CC`

√7ᵗʰ **S36.222**   **Contusion of tail of pancreas**   `CC`

√7ᵗʰ **S36.229**   **Contusion of unspecified part of pancreas**   `CC`

√6ᵗʰ **S36.23**   **Laceration of pancreas, unspecified degree**

√7ᵗʰ **S36.230**   **Laceration of head of pancreas, unspecified degree**   `CC`

√7ᵗʰ **S36.231**   **Laceration of body of pancreas, unspecified degree**   `CC`

√7ᵗʰ **S36.232**   **Laceration of tail of pancreas, unspecified degree**   `CC`

√7ᵗʰ **S36.239**   **Laceration of unspecified part of pancreas, unspecified degree**   `CC`

√6ᵗʰ **S36.24**   **Minor laceration of pancreas**

√7ᵗʰ **S36.240**   **Minor laceration of head of pancreas**   `CC`

√7ᵗʰ **S36.241**   **Minor laceration of body of pancreas**   `CC`

`N` Newborn: 0   `P` Pediatric: 0-17   `M` Maternity: 9-64   `A` Adult: 15-124   `MCC` Major Complication/Comorbidity   `CC` Complication/Comorbidity   `SW` Severe Wound Dx

1026   ICD-10-CM 2020

√7ᵗʰ **S36.242** Minor laceration of tail of pancreas   CC

√7ᵗʰ **S36.249** Minor laceration of unspecified part of pancreas   CC

√6ᵗʰ **S36.25** Moderate laceration of pancreas

√7ᵗʰ **S36.250** Moderate laceration of head of pancreas   CC

√7ᵗʰ **S36.251** Moderate laceration of body of pancreas   CC

√7ᵗʰ **S36.252** Moderate laceration of tail of pancreas   CC

√7ᵗʰ **S36.259** Moderate laceration of unspecified part of pancreas   CC

√6ᵗʰ **S36.26** Major laceration of pancreas

√7ᵗʰ **S36.260** Major laceration of head of pancreas   CC

√7ᵗʰ **S36.261** Major laceration of body of pancreas   CC

√7ᵗʰ **S36.262** Major laceration of tail of pancreas   CC

√7ᵗʰ **S36.269** Major laceration of unspecified part of pancreas   CC

√6ᵗʰ **S36.29** Other injury of pancreas

√7ᵗʰ **S36.290** Other injury of head of pancreas   CC

√7ᵗʰ **S36.291** Other injury of body of pancreas   CC

√7ᵗʰ **S36.292** Other injury of tail of pancreas   CC

√7ᵗʰ **S36.299** Other injury of unspecified part of pancreas   CC

√5ᵗʰ **S36.3** Injury of stomach

CC Excl: For CC codes in subcategory S36.3: PDX collection 1234

√x7ᵗʰ **S36.30** Unspecified injury of stomach   CC

√x7ᵗʰ **S36.32** Contusion of stomach   CC

√x7ᵗʰ **S36.33** Laceration of stomach   CC

√x7ᵗʰ **S36.39** Other injury of stomach   CC

√5ᵗʰ **S36.4** Injury of small intestine

CC Excl: For CC codes in subcategory S36.4: PDX collection 1235

√6ᵗʰ **S36.40** Unspecified injury of small intestine

√7ᵗʰ **S36.400** Unspecified injury of duodenum   CC

√7ᵗʰ **S36.408** Unspecified injury of other part of small intestine   CC

√7ᵗʰ **S36.409** Unspecified injury of unspecified part of small intestine   CC

√6ᵗʰ **S36.41** Primary blast injury of small intestine

Blast injury of small intestine NOS

√7ᵗʰ **S36.410** Primary blast injury of duodenum   CC

√7ᵗʰ **S36.418** Primary blast injury of other part of small intestine   CC

√7ᵗʰ **S36.419** Primary blast injury of unspecified part of small intestine   CC

√6ᵗʰ **S36.42** Contusion of small intestine

√7ᵗʰ **S36.420** Contusion of duodenum   CC

√7ᵗʰ **S36.428** Contusion of other part of small intestine   CC

√7ᵗʰ **S36.429** Contusion of unspecified part of small intestine   CC

√6ᵗʰ **S36.43** Laceration of small intestine

√7ᵗʰ **S36.430** Laceration of duodenum   CC

√7ᵗʰ **S36.438** Laceration of other part of small intestine   CC

√7ᵗʰ **S36.439** Laceration of unspecified part of small intestine   CC

√6ᵗʰ **S36.49** Other injury of small intestine

√7ᵗʰ **S36.490** Other injury of duodenum   CC

√7ᵗʰ **S36.498** Other injury of other part of small intestine   CC

√7ᵗʰ **S36.499** Other injury of unspecified part of small intestine   CC

√5ᵗʰ **S36.5** Injury of colon

EXCLUDES 2   injury of rectum (S36.6-)

CC Excl: For CC codes in subcategory S36.5: PDX collection 1236

√6ᵗʰ **S36.50** Unspecified injury of colon

√7ᵗʰ **S36.500** Unspecified injury of ascending [right] colon   CC

√7ᵗʰ **S36.501** Unspecified injury of transverse colon   CC

√7ᵗʰ **S36.502** Unspecified injury of descending [left] colon   CC

√7ᵗʰ **S36.503** Unspecified injury of sigmoid colon   CC

√7ᵗʰ **S36.508** Unspecified injury of other part of colon   CC

√7ᵗʰ **S36.509** Unspecified injury of unspecified part of colon   CC

√6ᵗʰ **S36.51** Primary blast injury of colon

Blast injury of colon NOS

√7ᵗʰ **S36.510** Primary blast injury of ascending [right] colon   CC

√7ᵗʰ **S36.511** Primary blast injury of transverse colon   CC

√7ᵗʰ **S36.512** Primary blast injury of descending [left] colon   CC

√7ᵗʰ **S36.513** Primary blast injury of sigmoid colon   CC

√7ᵗʰ **S36.518** Primary blast injury of other part of colon   CC

√7ᵗʰ **S36.519** Primary blast injury of unspecified part of colon   CC

√6ᵗʰ **S36.52** Contusion of colon

√7ᵗʰ **S36.520** Contusion of ascending [right] colon   CC

√7ᵗʰ **S36.521** Contusion of transverse colon   CC

√7ᵗʰ **S36.522** Contusion of descending [left] colon   CC

√7ᵗʰ **S36.523** Contusion of sigmoid colon   CC

√7ᵗʰ **S36.528** Contusion of other part of colon   CC

√7ᵗʰ **S36.529** Contusion of unspecified part of colon   CC

√6ᵗʰ **S36.53** Laceration of colon

√7ᵗʰ **S36.530** Laceration of ascending [right] colon   CC

√7ᵗʰ **S36.531** Laceration of transverse colon   CC

√7ᵗʰ **S36.532** Laceration of descending [left] colon   CC

√7ᵗʰ **S36.533** Laceration of sigmoid colon   CC

√7ᵗʰ **S36.538** Laceration of other part of colon   CC

√7ᵗʰ **S36.539** Laceration of unspecified part of colon   CC

√6ᵗʰ **S36.59** Other injury of colon

Secondary blast injury of colon

√7ᵗʰ **S36.590** Other injury of ascending [right] colon   CC

√7ᵗʰ **S36.591** Other injury of transverse colon   CC

√7ᵗʰ **S36.592** Other injury of descending [left] colon   CC

√7ᵗʰ **S36.593** Other injury of sigmoid colon   CC

√7ᵗʰ **S36.598** Other injury of other part of colon   CC

√7ᵗʰ **S36.599** Other injury of unspecified part of colon   CC

√5ᵗʰ **S36.6** Injury of rectum

CC Excl: For CC codes in subcategory S36.6: PDX collection 1236

√x7ᵗʰ **S36.60** Unspecified injury of rectum   CC

√x7ᵗʰ **S36.61** Primary blast injury of rectum   CC

Blast injury of rectum NOS

√x7ᵗʰ **S36.62** Contusion of rectum   CC

☑ Additional Character Required   √x7ᵗʰ Placeholder   Unacceptable PDx   Questionable PDx   Manifestation   Unspecified Dx   H1-H14 HAC   HCC CMS-HCC Dx   HIV HIV Dx

ICD-10-CM 2020   1027

√x7ᵗʰ **S36.63** **Laceration of rectum** CC

√x7ᵗʰ **S36.69** **Other injury of rectum** CC

Secondary blast injury of rectum

√5ᵗʰ **S36.8** **Injury of other intra-abdominal organs**

CC Excl: For CC codes in subcategory S36.8: PDX collection 1195

√x7ᵗʰ **S36.81** **Injury of peritoneum** CC

√6ᵗʰ **S36.89** **Injury of other intra-abdominal organs**

Injury of retroperitoneum

√7ᵗʰ **S36.892** **Contusion of other intra-abdominal organs** CC

√7ᵗʰ **S36.893** **Laceration of other intra-abdominal organs** CC

√7ᵗʰ **S36.898** **Other injury of other intra-abdominal organs** CC

√7ᵗʰ **S36.899** **Unspecified injury of other intra-abdominal organs** CC

√5ᵗʰ **S36.9** **Injury of unspecified intra-abdominal organ**

CC Excl: For CC codes in subcategory S36.9: PDX collection 1195

√x7ᵗʰ **S36.90** **Unspecified injury of unspecified intra-abdominal organ** CC

√x7ᵗʰ **S36.92** **Contusion of unspecified intra-abdominal organ** CC

√x7ᵗʰ **S36.93** **Laceration of unspecified intra-abdominal organ** CC

√x7ᵗʰ **S36.99** **Other injury of unspecified intra-abdominal organ** CC

√4ᵗʰ **S37** **Injury of urinary and pelvic organs**

BOSS code

Code also any associated open wound (S31.-)

EXCLUDES 1 obstetric trauma to pelvic organs (O71.-)

EXCLUDES 2 injury of peritoneum (S36.81)

injury of retroperitoneum (S36.89-)

The appropriate 7th character is to be added to each code from category S37.

A initial encounter
D subsequent encounter
S sequela

√5ᵗʰ **S37.0** **Injury of kidney**

EXCLUDES 2 acute kidney injury (nontraumatic) (N17.9)

CC Excl: For CC/MCC codes in subcategory S37.0: PDX collection 1237

√6ᵗʰ **S37.00** **Unspecified injury of kidney**

√7ᵗʰ **S37.001** **Unspecified injury of right kidney** CC

√7ᵗʰ **S37.002** **Unspecified injury of left kidney** CC

√7ᵗʰ **S37.009** **Unspecified injury of unspecified kidney** CC

√6ᵗʰ **S37.01** **Minor contusion of kidney**

Contusion of kidney less than 2 cm
Contusion of kidney NOS

√7ᵗʰ **S37.011** **Minor contusion of right kidney** CC

√7ᵗʰ **S37.012** **Minor contusion of left kidney** CC

√7ᵗʰ **S37.019** **Minor contusion of unspecified kidney** CC

√6ᵗʰ **S37.02** **Major contusion of kidney**

Contusion of kidney greater than 2 cm

√7ᵗʰ **S37.021** **Major contusion of right kidney** CC

√7ᵗʰ **S37.022** **Major contusion of left kidney** CC

√7ᵗʰ **S37.029** **Major contusion of unspecified kidney** CC

√6ᵗʰ **S37.03** **Laceration of kidney, unspecified degree**

√7ᵗʰ **S37.031** **Laceration of right kidney, unspecified degree** CC

√7ᵗʰ **S37.032** **Laceration of left kidney, unspecified degree** CC

√7ᵗʰ **S37.039** **Laceration of unspecified kidney, unspecified degree** CC

√6ᵗʰ **S37.04** **Minor laceration of kidney**

Laceration of kidney less than 1 cm

√7ᵗʰ **S37.041** **Minor laceration of right kidney** CC

√7ᵗʰ **S37.042** **Minor laceration of left kidney** CC

√7ᵗʰ **S37.049** **Minor laceration of unspecified kidney** CC

√6ᵗʰ **S37.05** **Moderate laceration of kidney**

Laceration of kidney 1 to 3 cm

√7ᵗʰ **S37.051** **Moderate laceration of right kidney** CC

√7ᵗʰ **S37.052** **Moderate laceration of left kidney** CC

√7ᵗʰ **S37.059** **Moderate laceration of unspecified kidney** CC

√6ᵗʰ **S37.06** **Major laceration of kidney**

Avulsion of kidney
Laceration of kidney greater than 3 cm
Massive laceration of kidney
Multiple moderate lacerations of kidney
Stellate laceration of kidney

√7ᵗʰ **S37.061** **Major laceration of right kidney** MCC

√7ᵗʰ **S37.062** **Major laceration of left kidney** MCC

√7ᵗʰ **S37.069** **Major laceration of unspecified kidney** MCC

√6ᵗʰ **S37.09** **Other injury of kidney**

√7ᵗʰ **S37.091** **Other injury of right kidney** MCC

√7ᵗʰ **S37.092** **Other injury of left kidney** MCC

√7ᵗʰ **S37.099** **Other injury of unspecified kidney** MCC

√5ᵗʰ **S37.1** **Injury of ureter**

CC Excl: For CC codes in subcategory S37.1: PDX collection 1238

√x7ᵗʰ **S37.10** **Unspecified injury of ureter** CC

√x7ᵗʰ **S37.12** **Contusion of ureter** CC

√x7ᵗʰ **S37.13** **Laceration of ureter** CC

√x7ᵗʰ **S37.19** **Other injury of ureter** CC

√5ᵗʰ **S37.2** **Injury of bladder**

CC Excl: For CC codes in subcategory S37.2: PDX collection 1239

√x7ᵗʰ **S37.20** **Unspecified injury of bladder** CC

√x7ᵗʰ **S37.22** **Contusion of bladder** CC

√x7ᵗʰ **S37.23** **Laceration of bladder** CC

√x7ᵗʰ **S37.29** **Other injury of bladder** CC

√5ᵗʰ **S37.3** **Injury of urethra**

CC Excl: For CC codes in subcategory S37.3: PDX collection 1239

√x7ᵗʰ **S37.30** **Unspecified injury of urethra** CC

√x7ᵗʰ **S37.32** **Contusion of urethra** CC

√x7ᵗʰ **S37.33** **Laceration of urethra** CC

√x7ᵗʰ **S37.39** **Other injury of urethra** CC

√5ᵗʰ **S37.4** **Injury of ovary**

√6ᵗʰ **S37.40** **Unspecified injury of ovary**

√7ᵗʰ **S37.401** **Unspecified injury of ovary, unilateral** ♀

√7ᵗʰ **S37.402** **Unspecified injury of ovary, bilateral** ♀

√7ᵗʰ **S37.409** **Unspecified injury of ovary, unspecified** ♀

√6ᵗʰ **S37.42** **Contusion of ovary**

√7ᵗʰ **S37.421** **Contusion of ovary, unilateral** ♀

√7ᵗʰ **S37.422** **Contusion of ovary, bilateral** ♀

√7ᵗʰ **S37.429** **Contusion of ovary, unspecified** ♀

√6ᵗʰ **S37.43** **Laceration of ovary**

√7ᵗʰ **S37.431** **Laceration of ovary, unilateral** ♀

√7ᵗʰ **S37.432** **Laceration of ovary, bilateral** ♀

Ⓝ Newborn: 0 Ⓟ Pediatric: 0-17 Ⓜ Maternity: 9-64 Ⓐ Adult: 15-124 **MCC** Major Complication/Comorbidity **CC** Complication/Comorbidity **SW** Severe Wound Dx

1028

ICD-10-CM 2020

√7ᵗʰ **S37.439** Laceration of ovary, unspecified ♀

√6ᵗʰ **S37.49** Other injury of ovary

√7ᵗʰ **S37.491** Other injury of ovary, unilateral ♀

√7ᵗʰ **S37.492** Other injury of ovary, bilateral ♀

√7ᵗʰ **S37.499** Other injury of ovary, unspecified ♀

√5ᵗʰ **S37.5** Injury of fallopian tube

√6ᵗʰ **S37.50** Unspecified injury of fallopian tube

√7ᵗʰ **S37.501** Unspecified injury of fallopian tube, unilateral ♀

√7ᵗʰ **S37.502** Unspecified injury of fallopian tube, bilateral ♀

√7ᵗʰ **S37.509** Unspecified injury of fallopian tube, unspecified ♀

√6ᵗʰ **S37.51** Primary blast injury of fallopian tube

Blast injury of fallopian tube NOS

√7ᵗʰ **S37.511** Primary blast injury of fallopian tube, unilateral ♀

√7ᵗʰ **S37.512** Primary blast injury of fallopian tube, bilateral ♀

√7ᵗʰ **S37.519** Primary blast injury of fallopian tube, unspecified ♀

√6ᵗʰ **S37.52** Contusion of fallopian tube

√7ᵗʰ **S37.521** Contusion of fallopian tube, unilateral ♀

√7ᵗʰ **S37.522** Contusion of fallopian tube, bilateral ♀

√7ᵗʰ **S37.529** Contusion of fallopian tube, unspecified ♀

√6ᵗʰ **S37.53** Laceration of fallopian tube

√7ᵗʰ **S37.531** Laceration of fallopian tube, unilateral ♀

√7ᵗʰ **S37.532** Laceration of fallopian tube, bilateral ♀

√7ᵗʰ **S37.539** Laceration of fallopian tube, unspecified ♀

√6ᵗʰ **S37.59** Other injury of fallopian tube

Secondary blast injury of fallopian tube

√7ᵗʰ **S37.591** Other injury of fallopian tube, unilateral ♀

√7ᵗʰ **S37.592** Other injury of fallopian tube, bilateral ♀

√7ᵗʰ **S37.599** Other injury of fallopian tube, unspecified ♀

√5ᵗʰ **S37.6** Injury of uterus

EXCLUDES 1   injury to gravid uterus (O9A.2-)

injury to uterus during delivery (O71.-)

CC Excl: For CC codes in subcategory S37.6: PDX collection 1240

√x7ᵗʰ **S37.60** Unspecified injury of uterus cc ♀

√x7ᵗʰ **S37.62** Contusion of uterus cc ♀

√x7ᵗʰ **S37.63** Laceration of uterus cc ♀

√x7ᵗʰ **S37.69** Other injury of uterus cc ♀

√5ᵗʰ **S37.8** Injury of other urinary and pelvic organs

√6ᵗʰ **S37.81** Injury of adrenal gland

CC Excl: For CC codes in subcategory S37.81: PDX collection 1241

√7ᵗʰ **S37.812** Contusion of adrenal gland cc

√7ᵗʰ **S37.813** Laceration of adrenal gland cc

√7ᵗʰ **S37.818** Other injury of adrenal gland cc

√7ᵗʰ **S37.819** Unspecified injury of adrenal gland cc

√6ᵗʰ **S37.82** Injury of prostate

√7ᵗʰ **S37.822** Contusion of prostate ♂

√7ᵗʰ **S37.823** Laceration of prostate ♂

√7ᵗʰ **S37.828** Other injury of prostate ♂

√7ᵗʰ **S37.829** Unspecified injury of prostate ♂

√6ᵗʰ **S37.89** Injury of other urinary and pelvic organ

CC Excl: For CC codes in subcategory S37.89: PDX collection 1242

√7ᵗʰ **S37.892** Contusion of other urinary and pelvic organ cc

√7ᵗʰ **S37.893** Laceration of other urinary and pelvic organ cc

√7ᵗʰ **S37.898** Other injury of other urinary and pelvic organ cc

√7ᵗʰ **S37.899** Unspecified injury of other urinary and pelvic organ cc

√5ᵗʰ **S37.9** Injury of unspecified urinary and pelvic organ

CC Excl: For CC codes in subcategory S37.9: PDX collection 1242

√x7ᵗʰ **S37.90** Unspecified injury of unspecified urinary and pelvic organ cc

√x7ᵗʰ **S37.92** Contusion of unspecified urinary and pelvic organ cc

√x7ᵗʰ **S37.93** Laceration of unspecified urinary and pelvic organ cc

√x7ᵗʰ **S37.99** Other injury of unspecified urinary and pelvic organ cc

√4ᵗʰ **S38** Crushing injury and traumatic amputation of abdomen, lower back, pelvis and external genitals

NOTE   An amputation not identified as partial or complete should be coded to complete

The appropriate 7th character is to be added to each code from category S38.
A   initial encounter
D   subsequent encounter
S   sequela

√5ᵗʰ **S38.0** Crushing injury of external genital organs

Use additional code for any associated injuries

√6ᵗʰ **S38.00** Crushing injury of unspecified external genital organs

√7ᵗʰ **S38.001** Crushing injury of unspecified external genital organs, male ♂

√7ᵗʰ **S38.002** Crushing injury of unspecified external genital organs, female ♀

√x7ᵗʰ **S38.01** Crushing injury of penis ♂

√x7ᵗʰ **S38.02** Crushing injury of scrotum and testis ♂

√x7ᵗʰ **S38.03** Crushing injury of vulva ♀

√x7ᵗʰ **S38.1** Crushing injury of abdomen, lower back, and pelvis

Use additional code for all associated injuries, such as:
fracture of thoracic or lumbar spine and pelvis (S22.0-, S32.-)
injury to intra-abdominal organs (S36.-)
injury to urinary and pelvic organs (S37.-)
open wound of abdominal wall (S31.-)
spinal cord injury (S34.0, S34.1-)

EXCLUDES 2   crushing injury of external genital organs (S38.0-)

√5ᵗʰ **S38.2** Traumatic amputation of external genital organs

√6ᵗʰ **S38.21** Traumatic amputation of female external genital organs

Traumatic amputation of clitoris
Traumatic amputation of labium (majus) (minus)
Traumatic amputation of vulva

√7ᵗʰ **S38.211** Complete traumatic amputation of female external genital organs ♀

√7ᵗʰ **S38.212** Partial traumatic amputation of female external genital organs ♀

√6ᵗʰ **S38.22** Traumatic amputation of penis

√7ᵗʰ **S38.221** Complete traumatic amputation of penis ♂

√7ᵗʰ **S38.222** Partial traumatic amputation of penis ♂

√6ᵗʰ **S38.23** Traumatic amputation of scrotum and testis

√7ᵗʰ **S38.231** Complete traumatic amputation of scrotum and testis ♂

√7ᵗʰ **S38.232** Partial traumatic amputation of scrotum and testis ♂

√x7ᵗʰ **S38.3** Transection (partial) of abdomen

☑ Additional Character Required   √x7ᵗʰ Placeholder   Unacceptable PDx   Questionable PDx   Manifestation   Unspecified Dx   H1-H14 HAC   HCC CMS-HCC Dx   HIV HIV Dx

ICD-10-CM 2020   1029

✓4ᵗʰ **S39** **Other and unspecified injuries of abdomen, lower back, pelvis and external genitals**

> Code also any associated open wound (S31.-)
>
> EXCLUDES 2   *sprain of joints and ligaments of lumbar spine and pelvis (S33.-)*

> The appropriate 7th character is to be added to each code from category S39.
> A   initial encounter
> D   subsequent encounter
> S   sequela

✓5ᵗʰ **S39.0** **Injury of muscle, fascia and tendon of abdomen, lower back and pelvis**

  ✓6ᵗʰ **S39.00** **Unspecified injury of muscle, fascia and tendon of abdomen, lower back and pelvis**

    ✓7ᵗʰ **S39.001** **Unspecified injury of muscle, fascia and tendon of** abdomen

    ✓7ᵗʰ **S39.002** **Unspecified injury of muscle, fascia and tendon of** lower back

    S39.003 **Unspecified injury of muscle, fascia and tendon of** pelvis

  ✓6ᵗʰ **S39.01** **Strain of muscle, fascia and tendon of abdomen, lower back and pelvis**

    ✓7ᵗʰ **S39.011** **Strain of muscle, fascia and tendon of** abdomen

    S39.012 **Strain of muscle, fascia and tendon of** lower back

    S39.013 **Strain of muscle, fascia and tendon of** pelvis

  ✓6ᵗʰ **S39.02** **Laceration of muscle, fascia and tendon of abdomen, lower back and pelvis**

    ✓7ᵗʰ **S39.021** **Laceration of muscle, fascia and tendon of** abdomen

    ✓7ᵗʰ **S39.022** **Laceration of muscle, fascia and tendon of** lower back

    ✓7ᵗʰ **S39.023** **Laceration of muscle, fascia and tendon of** pelvis

  ✓6ᵗʰ **S39.09** **Other injury of muscle, fascia and tendon of abdomen, lower back and pelvis**

    ✓7ᵗʰ **S39.091** **Other injury of muscle, fascia and tendon of** abdomen

    ✓7ᵗʰ **S39.092** **Other injury of muscle, fascia and tendon of** lower back

    ✓7ᵗʰ **S39.093** **Other injury of muscle, fascia and tendon of** pelvis

✓5ᵗʰ **S39.8** **Other specified injuries of abdomen, lower back, pelvis and external genitals**

  ✓×7ᵗʰ **S39.81** **Other specified injuries of** abdomen

  ✓×7ᵗʰ **S39.82** **Other specified injuries of** lower back

  ✓×7ᵗʰ **S39.83** **Other specified injuries of** pelvis

  ✓6ᵗʰ **S39.84** **Other specified injuries of** external genitals

    ✓7ᵗʰ **S39.840** **Fracture of** corpus cavernosum penis ♂

    ✓7ᵗʰ **S39.848** **Other specified injuries of external genitals**

> **TIP:** Assign for traumatic rupture of testis.

✓5ᵗʰ **S39.9** **Unspecified injury of abdomen, lower back, pelvis and external genitals**

  ✓×7ᵗʰ **S39.91** **Unspecified injury of** abdomen

  ✓×7ᵗʰ **S39.92** **Unspecified injury of** lower back

  ✓×7ᵗʰ **S39.93** **Unspecified injury of** pelvis

  ✓×7ᵗʰ **S39.94** **Unspecified injury of** external genitals

Injuries to the shoulder and upper arm (S40-S49)

> INCLUDES   injuries of axilla
>   injuries of scapular region
> EXCLUDES 2   *burns and corrosions (T20-T32)*
>   *frostbite (T33-T34)*
>   *injuries of elbow (S50-S59)*
>   *insect bite or sting, venomous (T63.4)*

✓4ᵗʰ **S40** **Superficial injury of shoulder and upper arm**

> The appropriate 7th character is to be added to each code from category S40.
> A   initial encounter
> D   subsequent encounter
> S   sequela

✓5ᵗʰ **S40.0** **Contusion of shoulder and upper arm**

  ✓6ᵗʰ **S40.01** **Contusion of** shoulder

    ✓7ᵗʰ **S40.011** **Contusion of** right shoulder

    ✓7ᵗʰ **S40.012** **Contusion of** left shoulder

    ✓7ᵗʰ **S40.019** **Contusion of unspecified shoulder**

  ✓6ᵗʰ **S40.02** **Contusion of** upper arm

    ✓7ᵗʰ **S40.021** **Contusion of** right upper arm

    ✓7ᵗʰ **S40.022** **Contusion of** left upper arm

    ✓7ᵗʰ **S40.029** **Contusion of unspecified upper arm**

✓5ᵗʰ **S40.2** **Other superficial injuries of** shoulder

  ✓6ᵗʰ **S40.21** **Abrasion** of shoulder

    ✓7ᵗʰ **S40.211** **Abrasion of** right shoulder

    ✓7ᵗʰ **S40.212** **Abrasion of** left shoulder

    ✓7ᵗʰ **S40.219** **Abrasion of unspecified shoulder**

  ✓6ᵗʰ **S40.22** **Blister (nonthermal) of shoulder**

    ✓7ᵗʰ **S40.221** **Blister (nonthermal) of** right shoulder

    ✓7ᵗʰ **S40.222** **Blister (nonthermal) of** left shoulder

    ✓7ᵗʰ **S40.229** **Blister (nonthermal) of unspecified shoulder**

  ✓6ᵗʰ **S40.24** **External constriction** of shoulder

    ✓7ᵗʰ **S40.241** **External constriction of** right shoulder

    ✓7ᵗʰ **S40.242** **External constriction of** left shoulder

    ✓7ᵗʰ **S40.249** **External constriction of unspecified shoulder**

  ✓6ᵗʰ **S40.25** **Superficial foreign body of shoulder**

    Splinter in the shoulder

    ✓7ᵗʰ **S40.251** **Superficial foreign body of** right shoulder

    ✓7ᵗʰ **S40.252** **Superficial foreign body of** left shoulder

    ✓7ᵗʰ **S40.259** **Superficial foreign body of unspecified shoulder**

  ✓6ᵗʰ **S40.26** **Insect bite (nonvenomous) of shoulder**

    ✓7ᵗʰ **S40.261** **Insect bite (nonvenomous) of** right shoulder

    ✓7ᵗʰ **S40.262** **Insect bite (nonvenomous) of** left shoulder

    ✓7ᵗʰ **S40.269** **Insect bite (nonvenomous) of unspecified shoulder**

  ✓6ᵗʰ **S40.27** **Other superficial bite of shoulder**

    EXCLUDES 1   *open bite of shoulder (S41.05)*

    ✓7ᵗʰ **S40.271** **Other superficial bite of** right shoulder

    ✓7ᵗʰ **S40.272** **Other superficial bite of** left shoulder

    ✓7ᵗʰ **S40.279** **Other superficial bite of unspecified shoulder**

✓5ᵗʰ **S40.8** **Other superficial injuries of** upper arm

  ✓6ᵗʰ **S40.81** **Abrasion** of upper arm

    ✓7ᵗʰ **S40.811** **Abrasion of** right upper arm

    ✓7ᵗʰ **S40.812** **Abrasion of** left upper arm

    ✓7ᵗʰ **S40.819** **Abrasion of unspecified upper arm**

  ✓6ᵗʰ **S40.82** **Blister (nonthermal) of upper arm**

    ✓7ᵗʰ **S40.821** **Blister (nonthermal) of** right upper arm

    ✓7ᵗʰ **S40.822** **Blister (nonthermal) of** left upper arm

    ✓7ᵗʰ **S40.829** **Blister (nonthermal) of unspecified upper arm**

  ✓6ᵗʰ **S40.84** **External constriction** of upper arm

    ✓7ᵗʰ **S40.841** **External constriction of** right upper arm

    ✓7ᵗʰ **S40.842** **External constriction of** left upper arm

N Newborn: 0   P Pediatric: 0-17   M Maternity: 9-64   A Adult: 15-124   MCC Major Complication/Comorbidity   CC Complication/Comorbidity   SW Severe Wound Dx

1030   ICD-10-CM 2020

√7ᵗʰ **S40.849** External constriction of unspecified upper arm

√6ᵗʰ **S40.85** Superficial foreign body of upper arm

    Splinter in the upper arm

√7ᵗʰ **S40.851** Superficial foreign body of right upper arm

√7ᵗʰ **S40.852** Superficial foreign body of left upper arm

√7ᵗʰ **S40.859** Superficial foreign body of unspecified upper arm

√6ᵗʰ **S40.86** Insect bite (nonvenomous) of upper arm

√7ᵗʰ **S40.861** Insect bite (nonvenomous) of right upper arm

√7ᵗʰ **S40.862** Insect bite (nonvenomous) of left upper arm

√7ᵗʰ **S40.869** Insect bite (nonvenomous) of unspecified upper arm

√6ᵗʰ **S40.87** Other superficial bite of upper arm

    EXCLUDES 1   open bite of upper arm (S41.14)

    EXCLUDES 2   other superficial bite of shoulder (S40.27-)

√7ᵗʰ **S40.871** Other superficial bite of right upper arm

√7ᵗʰ **S40.872** Other superficial bite of left upper arm

√7ᵗʰ **S40.879** Other superficial bite of unspecified upper arm

√5ᵗʰ **S40.9** Unspecified superficial injury of shoulder and upper arm

√6ᵗʰ **S40.91** Unspecified superficial injury of shoulder

√7ᵗʰ **S40.911** Unspecified superficial injury of right shoulder

√7ᵗʰ **S40.912** Unspecified superficial injury of left shoulder

√7ᵗʰ **S40.919** Unspecified superficial injury of unspecified shoulder

√6ᵗʰ **S40.92** Unspecified superficial injury of upper arm

√7ᵗʰ **S40.921** Unspecified superficial injury of right upper arm

√7ᵗʰ **S40.922** Unspecified superficial injury of left upper arm

√7ᵗʰ **S40.929** Unspecified superficial injury of unspecified upper arm

√4ᵗʰ **S41** **Open wound of shoulder and upper arm**

    Code also any associated wound infection

    EXCLUDES 1   traumatic amputation of shoulder and upper arm (S48.-)

    EXCLUDES 2   open fracture of shoulder and upper arm (S42.- with 7th character B or C)

> The appropriate 7th character is to be added to each code from category S41.
> A   initial encounter
> D   subsequent encounter
> S   sequela

√5ᵗʰ **S41.0** Open wound of shoulder

√6ᵗʰ **S41.00** Unspecified open wound of shoulder

√7ᵗʰ **S41.001** Unspecified open wound of right shoulder

√7ᵗʰ **S41.002** Unspecified open wound of left shoulder

√7ᵗʰ **S41.009** Unspecified open wound of unspecified shoulder

√6ᵗʰ **S41.01** Laceration without foreign body of shoulder

√7ᵗʰ **S41.011** Laceration without foreign body of right shoulder

√7ᵗʰ **S41.012** Laceration without foreign body of left shoulder

√7ᵗʰ **S41.019** Laceration without foreign body of unspecified shoulder

√6ᵗʰ **S41.02** Laceration with foreign body of shoulder

√7ᵗʰ **S41.021** Laceration with foreign body of right shoulder

√7ᵗʰ **S41.022** Laceration with foreign body of left shoulder

√7ᵗʰ **S41.029** Laceration with foreign body of unspecified shoulder

√6ᵗʰ **S41.03** Puncture wound without foreign body of shoulder

√7ᵗʰ **S41.031** Puncture wound without foreign body of right shoulder

√7ᵗʰ **S41.032** Puncture wound without foreign body of left shoulder

√7ᵗʰ **S41.039** Puncture wound without foreign body of unspecified shoulder

√6ᵗʰ **S41.04** Puncture wound with foreign body of shoulder

√7ᵗʰ **S41.041** Puncture wound with foreign body of right shoulder

√7ᵗʰ **S41.042** Puncture wound with foreign body of left shoulder

√7ᵗʰ **S41.049** Puncture wound with foreign body of unspecified shoulder

√6ᵗʰ **S41.05** Open bite of shoulder

    Bite of shoulder NOS

    EXCLUDES 1   superficial bite of shoulder (S40.27)

√7ᵗʰ **S41.051** Open bite of right shoulder

√7ᵗʰ **S41.052** Open bite of left shoulder

√7ᵗʰ **S41.059** Open bite of unspecified shoulder

√5ᵗʰ **S41.1** Open wound of upper arm

√6ᵗʰ **S41.10** Unspecified open wound of upper arm

    AHA: 2016,3Q,24

√7ᵗʰ **S41.101** Unspecified open wound of right upper arm

√7ᵗʰ **S41.102** Unspecified open wound of left upper arm

√7ᵗʰ **S41.109** Unspecified open wound of unspecified upper arm

√6ᵗʰ **S41.11** Laceration without foreign body of upper arm

√7ᵗʰ **S41.111** Laceration without foreign body of right upper arm

√7ᵗʰ **S41.112** Laceration without foreign body of left upper arm

√7ᵗʰ **S41.119** Laceration without foreign body of unspecified upper arm

√6ᵗʰ **S41.12** Laceration with foreign body of upper arm

√7ᵗʰ **S41.121** Laceration with foreign body of right upper arm

√7ᵗʰ **S41.122** Laceration with foreign body of left upper arm

√7ᵗʰ **S41.129** Laceration with foreign body of unspecified upper arm

√6ᵗʰ **S41.13** Puncture wound without foreign body of upper arm

    AHA: 2016,3Q,24

√7ᵗʰ **S41.131** Puncture wound without foreign body of right upper arm

√7ᵗʰ **S41.132** Puncture wound without foreign body of left upper arm

√7ᵗʰ **S41.139** Puncture wound without foreign body of unspecified upper arm

√6ᵗʰ **S41.14** Puncture wound with foreign body of upper arm

    AHA: 2016,3Q,24

√7ᵗʰ **S41.141** Puncture wound with foreign body of right upper arm

√7ᵗʰ **S41.142** Puncture wound with foreign body of left upper arm

√7ᵗʰ **S41.149** Puncture wound with foreign body of unspecified upper arm

√6ᵗʰ **S41.15** Open bite of upper arm

    Bite of upper arm NOS

    EXCLUDES 1   superficial bite of upper arm (S40.87)

√7ᵗʰ **S41.151** Open bite of right upper arm

√7ᵗʰ **S41.152** Open bite of left upper arm

√7ᵗʰ **S41.159** Open bite of unspecified upper arm

☑ Additional Character Required   ✓x7ᵗʰ Placeholder   Unacceptable PDx   Questionable PDx   Manifestation   Unspecified Dx   H1-H14 HAC   HCC CMS-HCC Dx   HIV HIV Dx

ICD-10-CM 2020   1031

√4th **S42 Fracture of shoulder and upper arm**

> **NOTE** A fracture not indicated as displaced or nondisplaced should be coded to displaced
>
> A fracture not indicated as open or closed should be coded to closed

EXCLUDES 1 *traumatic amputation of shoulder and upper arm (S48.-)*

AHA: 2018,2Q,12; 2015,3Q,37-39
DEF: Diaphysis: Central shaft of a long bone.
DEF: Epiphysis: Proximal and distal rounded ends of a long bone, communicates with the joint.
DEF: Metaphysis: Section of a long bone located between the epiphysis and diaphysis at the proximal and distal ends.
DEF: Physis (growth plate): Narrow zone of cartilaginous tissue between the epiphysis and metaphysis at each end of a long bone. In childhood, proliferation of cells in this zone lengthens the bone. As the bone matures, this area thins, ossification eventually fusing into solid bone and growth stops. *Synonyms: Epiphyseal plate.*

> The appropriate 7th character is to be added to all codes from category S42 [unless otherwise indicated].
> A initial encounter for closed fracture
> B initial encounter for open fracture
> D subsequent encounter for fracture with routine healing
> G subsequent encounter for fracture with delayed healing
> K subsequent encounter for fracture with nonunion
> P subsequent encounter for fracture with malunion
> S sequela

√5th **S42.0 Fracture of clavicle**

> **CC Excl: For codes in subcategory S42.0:**
> **CC with 7th character B:** PDX collection 1243
> **CC with 7th character K or P:** PDX collection 897

√6th **S42.00 Fracture of unspecified part of clavicle**

3 √7th **S42.001 Fracture of unspecified part of right clavicle** `CC` `H5`

3 √7th **S42.002 Fracture of unspecified part of left clavicle** `CC` `H5`

3 √7th **S42.009 Fracture of unspecified part of unspecified clavicle** `CC` `H5`
AHA: 2012,4Q,93

√6th **S42.01 Fracture of sternal end of clavicle**

3 √7th **S42.011 Anterior displaced fracture of sternal end of right clavicle** `CC` `H5`

3 √7th **S42.012 Anterior displaced fracture of sternal end of left clavicle** `CC` `H5`

3 √7th **S42.013 Anterior displaced fracture of sternal end of unspecified clavicle** `CC` `H5`
Displaced fracture of sternal end of clavicle NOS

3 √7th **S42.014 Posterior displaced fracture of sternal end of right clavicle** `CC` `H5`

3 √7th **S42.015 Posterior displaced fracture of sternal end of left clavicle** `CC` `H5`

3 √7th **S42.016 Posterior displaced fracture of sternal end of unspecified clavicle** `CC` `H5`

3 √7th **S42.017 Nondisplaced fracture of sternal end of right clavicle** `CC` `H5`

3 √7th **S42.018 Nondisplaced fracture of sternal end of left clavicle** `CC` `H5`

3 √7th **S42.019 Nondisplaced fracture of sternal end of unspecified clavicle** `CC` `H5`

√6th **S42.02 Fracture of shaft of clavicle**

3 √7th **S42.021 Displaced fracture of shaft of right clavicle** `CC` `H5`

3 √7th **S42.022 Displaced fracture of shaft of left clavicle** `CC` `H5`

3 √7th **S42.023 Displaced fracture of shaft of unspecified clavicle** `CC` `H5`

3 √7th **S42.024 Nondisplaced fracture of shaft of right clavicle** `CC` `H5`

3 √7th **S42.025 Nondisplaced fracture of shaft of left clavicle** `CC` `H5`

3 √7th **S42.026 Nondisplaced fracture of shaft of unspecified clavicle** `CC` `H5`

√6th **S42.03 Fracture of lateral end of clavicle**
Fracture of acromial end of clavicle

3 √7th **S42.031 Displaced fracture of lateral end of right clavicle** `CC` `H5`

3 √7th **S42.032 Displaced fracture of lateral end of left clavicle** `CC` `H5`

3 √7th **S42.033 Displaced fracture of lateral end of unspecified clavicle** `CC` `H5`

3 √7th **S42.034 Nondisplaced fracture of lateral end of right clavicle** `CC` `H5`

3 √7th **S42.035 Nondisplaced fracture of lateral end of left clavicle** `CC` `H5`

3 √7th **S42.036 Nondisplaced fracture of lateral end of unspecified clavicle** `CC` `H5`

√5th **S42.1 Fracture of scapula**

> **CC Excl: For codes in subcategory S42.1:**
> **CC with 7th character B:** PDX collection 1244
> **CC with 7th character K or P:** PDX collection 897

√6th **S42.10 Fracture of unspecified part of scapula**

3 √7th **S42.101 Fracture of unspecified part of scapula, right shoulder** `CC` `H5`

3 √7th **S42.102 Fracture of unspecified part of scapula, left shoulder** `CC` `H5`

3 √7th **S42.109 Fracture of unspecified part of scapula, unspecified shoulder** `CC` `H5`

√6th **S42.11 Fracture of body of scapula**

3 √7th **S42.111 Displaced fracture of body of scapula, right shoulder** `CC` `H5`

3 √7th **S42.112 Displaced fracture of body of scapula, left shoulder** `CC` `H5`

3 √7th **S42.113 Displaced fracture of body of scapula, unspecified shoulder** `CC` `H5`

3 √7th **S42.114 Nondisplaced fracture of body of scapula, right shoulder** `CC` `H5`

3 √7th **S42.115 Nondisplaced fracture of body of scapula, left shoulder** `CC` `H5`

3 √7th **S42.116 Nondisplaced fracture of body of scapula, unspecified shoulder** `CC` `H5`

√6th **S42.12 Fracture of acromial process**

3 √7th **S42.121 Displaced fracture of acromial process, right shoulder** `CC` `H5`

3 √7th **S42.122 Displaced fracture of acromial process, left shoulder** `CC` `H5`

3 √7th **S42.123 Displaced fracture of acromial process, unspecified shoulder** `CC` `H5`

3 √7th **S42.124 Nondisplaced fracture of acromial process, right shoulder** `CC` `H5`

3 √7th **S42.125 Nondisplaced fracture of acromial process, left shoulder** `CC` `H5`

3 √7th **S42.126 Nondisplaced fracture of acromial process, unspecified shoulder** `CC` `H5`

√6th **S42.13 Fracture of coracoid process**

3 √7th **S42.131 Displaced fracture of coracoid process, right shoulder** `CC` `H5`

3 √7th **S42.132 Displaced fracture of coracoid process, left shoulder** `CC` `H5`

3 √7th **S42.133 Displaced fracture of coracoid process, unspecified shoulder** `CC` `H5`

3 √7th **S42.134 Nondisplaced fracture of coracoid process, right shoulder** `CC` `H5`

N Newborn: 0   P Pediatric: 0-17   M Maternity: 9-64   A Adult: 15-124   **MCC** Major Complication/Comorbidity   **CC** Complication/Comorbidity   **SW** Severe Wound Dx

1032

ICD-10-CM 2020

3 √7ᵗʰ **S42.135** Nondisplaced fracture of coracoid process, left shoulder   `CC` `H5`

3 √7ᵗʰ **S42.136** Nondisplaced fracture of coracoid process, unspecified shoulder   `CC` `H5`

√6ᵗʰ **S42.14** Fracture of glenoid cavity of scapula

3 √7ᵗʰ **S42.141** Displaced fracture of glenoid cavity of scapula, right shoulder   `CC` `H5`

3 √7ᵗʰ **S42.142** Displaced fracture of glenoid cavity of scapula, left shoulder   `CC` `H5`

3 √7ᵗʰ **S42.143** Displaced fracture of glenoid cavity of scapula, unspecified shoulder   `CC` `H5`

3 √7ᵗʰ **S42.144** Nondisplaced fracture of glenoid cavity of scapula, right shoulder   `CC` `H5`

3 √7ᵗʰ **S42.145** Nondisplaced fracture of glenoid cavity of scapula, left shoulder   `CC` `H5`

3 √7ᵗʰ **S42.146** Nondisplaced fracture of glenoid cavity of scapula, unspecified shoulder   `CC` `H5`

√6ᵗʰ **S42.15** Fracture of neck of scapula

3 √7ᵗʰ **S42.151** Displaced fracture of neck of scapula, right shoulder   `CC` `H5`

3 √7ᵗʰ **S42.152** Displaced fracture of neck of scapula, left shoulder   `CC` `H5`

3 √7ᵗʰ **S42.153** Displaced fracture of neck of scapula, unspecified shoulder   `CC` `H5`

3 √7ᵗʰ **S42.154** Nondisplaced fracture of neck of scapula, right shoulder   `CC` `H5`

3 √7ᵗʰ **S42.155** Nondisplaced fracture of neck of scapula, left shoulder   `CC` `H5`

3 √7ᵗʰ **S42.156** Nondisplaced fracture of neck of scapula, unspecified shoulder   `CC` `H5`

√6ᵗʰ **S42.19** Fracture of other part of scapula

3 √7ᵗʰ **S42.191** Fracture of other part of scapula, right shoulder   `CC` `H5`

3 √7ᵗʰ **S42.192** Fracture of other part of scapula, left shoulder   `CC` `H5`

3 √7ᵗʰ **S42.199** Fracture of other part of scapula, unspecified shoulder   `CC` `H5`

√5ᵗʰ **S42.2** Fracture of upper end of humerus

Fracture of proximal end of humerus

EXCLUDES 2   fracture of shaft of humerus (S42.3-)

physeal fracture of upper end of humerus (S49.0-)

CC Excl: For CC/MCC codes in subcategory S42.2, unless otherwise noted:
Right side: See code S42.201
Left side: See code S42.202
Unspecified side: See code S42.209

√6ᵗʰ **S42.20** Unspecified fracture of upper end of humerus

2,3 √7ᵗʰ **S42.201** Unspecified fracture of upper end of right humerus   `MCC` `CC` `H5`
    CC Excl: CC with 7th character A: PDX collection 1245
    CC Excl: MCC with 7th character B: PDX collection 1246
    CC Excl: CC with 7th character K or P: PDX collection 897

2,3 √7ᵗʰ **S42.202** Unspecified fracture of upper end of left humerus   `MCC` `CC` `H5`
    CC Excl: CC with 7th character A: PDX collection 1247
    CC Excl: MCC with 7th character B: PDX collection 1246
    CC Excl: CC with 7th character K or P: PDX collection 897

2,3 √7ᵗʰ **S42.209** Unspecified fracture of upper end of unspecified humerus   `MCC` `CC` `H5`
    CC Excl: CC with 7th character A: PDX collection 1248
    CC Excl: MCC with 7th character B: PDX collection 1246
    CC Excl: CC with 7th character K or P: PDX collection 897

√6ᵗʰ **S42.21** Unspecified fracture of surgical neck of humerus

Fracture of neck of humerus NOS

2,3 √7ᵗʰ **S42.211** Unspecified displaced fracture of surgical neck of right humerus   `MCC` `CC` `H5`

2,3 √7ᵗʰ **S42.212** Unspecified displaced fracture of surgical neck of left humerus   `MCC` `CC` `H5`

2,3 √7ᵗʰ **S42.213** Unspecified displaced fracture of surgical neck of unspecified humerus   `MCC` `CC` `H5`

2,3 √7ᵗʰ **S42.214** Unspecified nondisplaced fracture of surgical neck of right humerus   `MCC` `CC` `H5`

2,3 √7ᵗʰ **S42.215** Unspecified nondisplaced fracture of surgical neck of left humerus   `MCC` `CC` `H5`

2,3 √7ᵗʰ **S42.216** Unspecified nondisplaced fracture of surgical neck of unspecified humerus   `MCC` `CC` `H5`

√6ᵗʰ **S42.22** 2-part fracture of surgical neck of humerus

2,3 √7ᵗʰ **S42.221** 2-part displaced fracture of surgical neck of right humerus   `MCC` `CC` `H5`

2,3 √7ᵗʰ **S42.222** 2-part displaced fracture of surgical neck of left humerus   `MCC` `CC` `H5`

2,3 √7ᵗʰ **S42.223** 2-part displaced fracture of surgical neck of unspecified humerus   `MCC` `CC` `H5`

2,3 √7ᵗʰ **S42.224** 2-part nondisplaced fracture of surgical neck of right humerus   `MCC` `CC` `H5`

2,3 √7ᵗʰ **S42.225** 2-part nondisplaced fracture of surgical neck of left humerus   `MCC` `CC` `H5`

2,3 √7ᵗʰ **S42.226** 2-part nondisplaced fracture of surgical neck of unspecified humerus   `MCC` `CC` `H5`

√6ᵗʰ **S42.23** 3-part fracture of surgical neck of humerus

2,3 √7ᵗʰ **S42.231** 3-part fracture of surgical neck of right humerus   `MCC` `CC` `H5`

2,3 √7ᵗʰ **S42.232** 3-part fracture of surgical neck of left humerus   `MCC` `CC` `H5`

2,3 √7ᵗʰ **S42.239** 3-part fracture of surgical neck of unspecified humerus   `MCC` `CC` `H5`

√6ᵗʰ **S42.24** 4-part fracture of surgical neck of humerus

2,3 √7ᵗʰ **S42.241** 4-part fracture of surgical neck of right humerus   `MCC` `CC` `H5`

2,3 √7ᵗʰ **S42.242** 4-part fracture of surgical neck of left humerus   `MCC` `CC` `H5`

2,3 √7ᵗʰ **S42.249** 4-part fracture of surgical neck of unspecified humerus   `MCC` `CC` `H5`

√6ᵗʰ **S42.25** Fracture of greater tuberosity of humerus

2,3 √7ᵗʰ **S42.251** Displaced fracture of greater tuberosity of right humerus   `MCC` `CC` `H5`

2,3 √7ᵗʰ **S42.252** Displaced fracture of greater tuberosity of left humerus   `MCC` `CC` `H5`

2,3 √7ᵗʰ **S42.253** Displaced fracture of greater tuberosity of unspecified humerus   `MCC` `CC` `H5`

2,3 √7ᵗʰ **S42.254** Nondisplaced fracture of greater tuberosity of right humerus   `MCC` `CC` `H5`

2,3 √7ᵗʰ **S42.255** Nondisplaced fracture of greater tuberosity of left humerus   `MCC` `CC` `H5`

2,3 √7ᵗʰ **S42.256** Nondisplaced fracture of greater tuberosity of unspecified humerus   `MCC` `CC` `H5`

√6ᵗʰ **S42.26**   Fracture of lesser tuberosity of humerus

2,3 √7ᵗʰ **S42.261**   Displaced fracture of lesser tuberosity of right humerus   `MCC` `CC` `H5`

2,3 √7ᵗʰ **S42.262**   Displaced fracture of lesser tuberosity of left humerus   `MCC` `CC` `H5`

2,3 √7ᵗʰ **S42.263**   Displaced fracture of lesser tuberosity of unspecified humerus   `MCC` `CC` `H5`

2,3 √7ᵗʰ **S42.264**   Nondisplaced fracture of lesser tuberosity of right humerus   `MCC` `CC` `H5`

2,3 √7ᵗʰ **S42.265**   Nondisplaced fracture of lesser tuberosity of left humerus   `MCC` `CC` `H5`

2,3 √7ᵗʰ **S42.266**   Nondisplaced fracture of lesser tuberosity of unspecified humerus   `MCC` `CC` `H5`

√6ᵗʰ **S42.27**   Torus fracture of upper end of humerus

> The appropriate 7th character is to be added to all codes in subcategory S42.27
> A   initial encounter for closed fracture
> D   subsequent encounter for fracture with routine healing
> G   subsequent encounter for fracture with delayed healing
> K   subsequent encounter for fracture with nonunion
> P   subsequent encounter for fracture with malunion
> S   sequela

3 √7ᵗʰ **S42.271**   Torus fracture of upper end of right humerus   `CC` `H5`
CC Excl: CC with 7th character A: PDX collection 1245
CC Excl: CC with 7th character K or P: PDX collection 897

3 √7ᵗʰ **S42.272**   Torus fracture of upper end of left humerus   `CC` `H5`
CC Excl: CC with 7th character A: PDX collection 1247
CC Excl: CC with 7th character K or P: PDX collection 897

3 √7ᵗʰ **S42.279**   Torus fracture of upper end of unspecified humerus   `CC` `H5`
CC Excl: CC with 7th character A: PDX collection 1248
CC Excl: CC with 7th character K or P: PDX collection 897

√6ᵗʰ **S42.29**   Other fracture of upper end of humerus
Fracture of anatomical neck of humerus
Fracture of articular head of humerus
AHA: 2019,1Q,18

2,3 √7ᵗʰ **S42.291**   Other displaced fracture of upper end of right humerus   `MCC` `CC` `H5`

2,3 √7ᵗʰ **S42.292**   Other displaced fracture of upper end of left humerus   `MCC` `CC` `H5`

2,3 √7ᵗʰ **S42.293**   Other displaced fracture of upper end of unspecified humerus   `MCC` `CC` `H5`

2,3 √7ᵗʰ **S42.294**   Other nondisplaced fracture of upper end of right humerus   `MCC` `CC` `H5`

2,3 √7ᵗʰ **S42.295**   Other nondisplaced fracture of upper end of left humerus   `MCC` `CC` `H5`

2,3 √7ᵗʰ **S42.296**   Other nondisplaced fracture of upper end of unspecified humerus   `MCC` `CC` `H5`

√5ᵗʰ **S42.3**   Fracture of shaft of humerus
Fracture of humerus NOS
Fracture of upper arm NOS
EXCLUDES 2   physeal fractures of upper end of humerus (S49.0-)
physeal fractures of lower end of humerus (S49.1-)
CC Excl: For CC/MCC codes in subcategory S42.3, unless otherwise noted:
Right side: See code S42.321
Left side: See code S42.322
Unspecified side: See code S42.323

√6ᵗʰ **S42.30**   Unspecified fracture of shaft of humerus

2,3 √7ᵗʰ **S42.301**   Unspecified fracture of shaft of humerus, right arm   `MCC` `CC` `H5`

2,3 √7ᵗʰ **S42.302**   Unspecified fracture of shaft of humerus, left arm   `MCC` `CC` `H5`

2,3 √7ᵗʰ **S42.309**   Unspecified fracture of shaft of humerus, unspecified arm   `MCC` `CC` `H5`

√6ᵗʰ **S42.31**   Greenstick fracture of shaft of humerus

> The appropriate 7th character is to be added to all codes in subcategory S42.31
> A   initial encounter for closed fracture
> D   subsequent encounter for fracture with routine healing
> G   subsequent encounter for fracture with delayed healing
> K   subsequent encounter for fracture with nonunion
> P   subsequent encounter for fracture with malunion
> S   sequela

3 √7ᵗʰ **S42.311**   Greenstick fracture of shaft of humerus, right arm   `CC` `H5`
CC Excl: CC with 7th character A: PDX collection 1249
CC Excl: CC with 7th character K or P: PDX collection 897

3 √7ᵗʰ **S42.312**   Greenstick fracture of shaft of humerus, left arm   `CC` `H5`
CC Excl: CC with 7th character A: PDX collection 1250
CC Excl: CC with 7th character K or P: PDX collection 897

3 √7ᵗʰ **S42.319**   Greenstick fracture of shaft of humerus, unspecified arm   `CC` `H5`
CC Excl: CC with 7th character A: PDX collection 1251
CC Excl: CC with 7th character K or P: PDX collection 897

√6ᵗʰ **S42.32**   Transverse fracture of shaft of humerus

2,3 √7ᵗʰ **S42.321**   Displaced transverse fracture of shaft of humerus, right arm   `MCC` `CC` `H5`
CC Excl: CC with 7th character A: PDX collection 1249
CC Excl: MCC with 7th character B: PDX collection 1246
CC Excl: CC with 7th character K or P: PDX collection 897

2,3 √7ᵗʰ **S42.322**   Displaced transverse fracture of shaft of humerus, left arm   `MCC` `CC` `H5`
CC Excl: CC with 7th character A: PDX collection 1250
CC Excl: MCC with 7th character B: PDX collection 1246
CC Excl: CC with 7th character K or P: PDX collection 897

2,3 √7ᵗʰ **S42.323**   Displaced transverse fracture of shaft of humerus, unspecified arm   `MCC` `CC` `H5`
CC Excl: CC with 7th character A: PDX collection 1251
CC Excl: MCC with 7th character B: PDX collection 1246
CC Excl: CC with 7th character K or P: PDX collection 897

2,3 √7ᵗʰ **S42.324** Nondisplaced transverse fracture of shaft of humerus, **right arm**   MCC CC H5

2,3 √7ᵗʰ **S42.325** Nondisplaced transverse fracture of shaft of humerus, **left arm**   MCC CC H5

2,3 √7ᵗʰ **S42.326** Nondisplaced transverse fracture of shaft of humerus, **unspecified arm**   MCC CC H5

√6ᵗʰ **S42.33** Oblique fracture of shaft of humerus

2,3 √7ᵗʰ **S42.331** Displaced oblique fracture of shaft of humerus, **right arm**   MCC CC H5

2,3 √7ᵗʰ **S42.332** Displaced oblique fracture of shaft of humerus, **left arm**   MCC CC H5

2,3 √7ᵗʰ **S42.333** Displaced oblique fracture of shaft of humerus, **unspecified arm**   MCC CC H5

2,3 √7ᵗʰ **S42.334** Nondisplaced oblique fracture of shaft of humerus, **right arm**   MCC CC H5

2,3 √7ᵗʰ **S42.335** Nondisplaced oblique fracture of shaft of humerus, **left arm**   MCC CC H5

2,3 √7ᵗʰ **S42.336** Nondisplaced oblique fracture of shaft of humerus, **unspecified arm**   MCC CC H5

√6ᵗʰ **S42.34** Spiral fracture of shaft of humerus

2,3 √7ᵗʰ **S42.341** Displaced spiral fracture of shaft of humerus, **right arm**   MCC CC H5

2,3 √7ᵗʰ **S42.342** Displaced spiral fracture of shaft of humerus, **left arm**   MCC CC H5

2,3 √7ᵗʰ **S42.343** Displaced spiral fracture of shaft of humerus, **unspecified arm**   MCC CC H5

2,3 √7ᵗʰ **S42.344** Nondisplaced spiral fracture of shaft of humerus, **right arm**   MCC CC H5

2,3 √7ᵗʰ **S42.345** Nondisplaced spiral fracture of shaft of humerus, **left arm**   MCC CC H5

2,3 √7ᵗʰ **S42.346** Nondisplaced spiral fracture of shaft of humerus, **unspecified arm**   MCC CC H5

√6ᵗʰ **S42.35** Comminuted fracture of shaft of humerus

2,3 √7ᵗʰ **S42.351** Displaced comminuted fracture of shaft of humerus, **right arm**   MCC CC H5

2,3 √7ᵗʰ **S42.352** Displaced comminuted fracture of shaft of humerus, **left arm**   MCC CC H5

2,3 √7ᵗʰ **S42.353** Displaced comminuted fracture of shaft of humerus, **unspecified arm**   MCC CC H5

2,3 √7ᵗʰ **S42.354** Nondisplaced comminuted fracture of shaft of humerus, **right arm**   MCC CC H5

2,3 √7ᵗʰ **S42.355** Nondisplaced comminuted fracture of shaft of humerus, **left arm**   MCC CC H5

2,3 √7ᵗʰ **S42.356** Nondisplaced comminuted fracture of shaft of humerus, **unspecified arm**   MCC CC H5

√6ᵗʰ **S42.36** Segmental fracture of shaft of humerus

2,3 √7ᵗʰ **S42.361** Displaced segmental fracture of shaft of humerus, **right arm**   MCC CC H5

2,3 √7ᵗʰ **S42.362** Displaced segmental fracture of shaft of humerus, **left arm**   MCC CC H5

2,3 √7ᵗʰ **S42.363** Displaced segmental fracture of shaft of humerus, **unspecified arm**   MCC CC H5

2,3 √7ᵗʰ **S42.364** Nondisplaced segmental fracture of shaft of humerus, **right arm**   MCC CC H5

2,3 √7ᵗʰ **S42.365** Nondisplaced segmental fracture of shaft of humerus, **left arm**   MCC CC H5

2,3 √7ᵗʰ **S42.366** Nondisplaced segmental fracture of shaft of humerus, **unspecified arm**   MCC CC H5

√6ᵗʰ **S42.39** Other fracture of shaft of humerus

2,3 √7ᵗʰ **S42.391** Other fracture of shaft of **right** humerus   MCC CC H5

2,3 √7ᵗʰ **S42.392** Other fracture of shaft of **left** humerus   MCC CC H5

2,3 √7ᵗʰ **S42.399** Other fracture of shaft of **unspecified** humerus   MCC CC H5

√5ᵗʰ **S42.4** Fracture of lower end of humerus

Fracture of distal end of humerus

EXCLUDES 2   *fracture of shaft of humerus (S42.3-)*
           physeal fracture of lower end of humerus (S49.1-)

CC Excl: For CC/MCC codes in subcategory S42.4, unless otherwise noted:
Right side: See code S42.201
Left side: See code S42.202
Unspecified side: See code S42.209

√6ᵗʰ **S42.40** Unspecified fracture of lower end of humerus

Fracture of elbow NOS

2,3 √7ᵗʰ **S42.401** Unspecified fracture of lower end of **right** humerus   MCC CC H5

2,3 √7ᵗʰ **S42.402** Unspecified fracture of lower end of **left** humerus   MCC CC H5

2,3 √7ᵗʰ **S42.409** Unspecified fracture of lower end of unspecified humerus   MCC CC H5

√6ᵗʰ **S42.41** Simple supracondylar fracture without intercondylar fracture of humerus

2,3 √7ᵗʰ **S42.411** Displaced simple supracondylar fracture without intercondylar fracture of **right** humerus   MCC CC H5

2,3 √7ᵗʰ **S42.412** Displaced simple supracondylar fracture without intercondylar fracture of **left** humerus   MCC CC H5

2,3 √7ᵗʰ **S42.413** Displaced simple supracondylar fracture without intercondylar fracture of unspecified humerus   MCC CC H5

2,3 √7ᵗʰ **S42.414** Nondisplaced simple supracondylar fracture without intercondylar fracture of **right** humerus   MCC CC H5

2,3 √7ᵗʰ **S42.415** Nondisplaced simple supracondylar fracture without intercondylar fracture of **left** humerus   MCC CC H5

2,3 √7ᵗʰ **S42.416** Nondisplaced simple supracondylar fracture without intercondylar fracture of unspecified humerus   MCC CC H5

√6ᵗʰ **S42.42** Comminuted supracondylar fracture without intercondylar fracture of humerus

2,3 √7ᵗʰ **S42.421** Displaced comminuted supracondylar fracture without intercondylar fracture of **right** humerus   MCC CC H5

2,3 √7ᵗʰ **S42.422** Displaced comminuted supracondylar fracture without intercondylar fracture of **left** humerus   MCC CC H5

2,3 √7ᵗʰ **S42.423** Displaced comminuted supracondylar fracture without intercondylar fracture of unspecified humerus   MCC CC H5

2,3 √7ᵗʰ **S42.424** Nondisplaced comminuted supracondylar fracture without intercondylar fracture of **right** humerus   MCC CC H5

2,3 √7ᵗʰ **S42.425** Nondisplaced comminuted supracondylar fracture without intercondylar fracture of **left** humerus   MCC CC H5

2,3 √7ᵗʰ **S42.426** Nondisplaced comminuted supracondylar fracture without intercondylar fracture of unspecified humerus `MCC` `CC` `H5`

√6ᵗʰ **S42.43** Fracture (avulsion) of lateral epicondyle of humerus

2,3 √7ᵗʰ **S42.431** Displaced fracture (avulsion) of lateral epicondyle of right humerus `MCC` `CC` `H5`

2,3 √7ᵗʰ **S42.432** Displaced fracture (avulsion) of lateral epicondyle of left humerus `MCC` `CC` `H5`

2,3 √7ᵗʰ **S42.433** Displaced fracture (avulsion) of lateral epicondyle of unspecified humerus `MCC` `CC` `H5`

2,3 √7ᵗʰ **S42.434** Nondisplaced fracture (avulsion) of lateral epicondyle of right humerus `MCC` `CC` `H5`

2,3 √7ᵗʰ **S42.435** Nondisplaced fracture (avulsion) of lateral epicondyle of left humerus `MCC` `CC` `H5`

2,3 √7ᵗʰ **S42.436** Nondisplaced fracture (avulsion) of lateral epicondyle of unspecified humerus `MCC` `CC` `H5`

√6ᵗʰ **S42.44** Fracture (avulsion) of medial epicondyle of humerus

2,3 √7ᵗʰ **S42.441** Displaced fracture (avulsion) of medial epicondyle of right humerus `MCC` `CC` `H5`

2,3 √7ᵗʰ **S42.442** Displaced fracture (avulsion) of medial epicondyle of left humerus `MCC` `CC` `H5`

2,3 √7ᵗʰ **S42.443** Displaced fracture (avulsion) of medial epicondyle of unspecified humerus `MCC` `CC` `H5`

2,3 √7ᵗʰ **S42.444** Nondisplaced fracture (avulsion) of medial epicondyle of right humerus `MCC` `CC` `H5`

2,3 √7ᵗʰ **S42.445** Nondisplaced fracture (avulsion) of medial epicondyle of left humerus `MCC` `CC` `H5`

2,3 √7ᵗʰ **S42.446** Nondisplaced fracture (avulsion) of medial epicondyle of unspecified humerus `MCC` `CC` `H5`

2,3 √7ᵗʰ **S42.447** Incarcerated fracture (avulsion) of medial epicondyle of right humerus `MCC` `CC` `H5`

2,3 √7ᵗʰ **S42.448** Incarcerated fracture (avulsion) of medial epicondyle of left humerus `MCC` `CC` `H5`

2,3 √7ᵗʰ **S42.449** Incarcerated fracture (avulsion) of medial epicondyle of unspecified humerus `MCC` `CC` `H5`

√6ᵗʰ **S42.45** Fracture of lateral condyle of humerus

Fracture of capitellum of humerus

2,3 √7ᵗʰ **S42.451** Displaced fracture of lateral condyle of right humerus `MCC` `CC` `H5`

2,3 √7ᵗʰ **S42.452** Displaced fracture of lateral condyle of left humerus `MCC` `CC` `H5`

2,3 √7ᵗʰ **S42.453** Displaced fracture of lateral condyle of unspecified humerus `MCC` `CC` `H5`

2,3 √7ᵗʰ **S42.454** Nondisplaced fracture of lateral condyle of right humerus `MCC` `CC` `H5`

2,3 √7ᵗʰ **S42.455** Nondisplaced fracture of lateral condyle of left humerus `MCC` `CC` `H5`

2,3 √7ᵗʰ **S42.456** Nondisplaced fracture of lateral condyle of unspecified humerus `MCC` `CC` `H5`

√6ᵗʰ **S42.46** Fracture of medial condyle of humerus

Trochlea fracture of humerus

2,3 √7ᵗʰ **S42.461** Displaced fracture of medial condyle of right humerus `MCC` `CC` `H5`

2,3 √7ᵗʰ **S42.462** Displaced fracture of medial condyle of left humerus `MCC` `CC` `H5`

2,3 √7ᵗʰ **S42.463** Displaced fracture of medial condyle of unspecified humerus `MCC` `CC` `H5`

2,3 √7ᵗʰ **S42.464** Nondisplaced fracture of medial condyle of right humerus `MCC` `CC` `H5`

2,3 √7ᵗʰ **S42.465** Nondisplaced fracture of medial condyle of left humerus `MCC` `CC` `H5`

2,3 √7ᵗʰ **S42.466** Nondisplaced fracture of medial condyle of unspecified humerus `MCC` `CC` `H5`

√6ᵗʰ **S42.47** Transcondylar fracture of humerus

2,3 √7ᵗʰ **S42.471** Displaced transcondylar fracture of right humerus `MCC` `CC` `H5`

2,3 √7ᵗʰ **S42.472** Displaced transcondylar fracture of left humerus `MCC` `CC` `H5`

2,3 √7ᵗʰ **S42.473** Displaced transcondylar fracture of unspecified humerus `MCC` `CC` `H5`

2,3 √7ᵗʰ **S42.474** Nondisplaced transcondylar fracture of right humerus `MCC` `CC` `H5`

2,3 √7ᵗʰ **S42.475** Nondisplaced transcondylar fracture of left humerus `MCC` `CC` `H5`

2,3 √7ᵗʰ **S42.476** Nondisplaced transcondylar fracture of unspecified humerus `MCC` `CC` `H5`

√6ᵗʰ **S42.48** Torus fracture of lower end of humerus

> The appropriate 7th character is to be added to all codes in subcategory S42.48.
> A initial encounter for closed fracture
> D subsequent encounter for fracture with routine healing
> G subsequent encounter for fracture with delayed healing
> K subsequent encounter for fracture with nonunion
> P subsequent encounter for fracture with malunion
> S sequela

3 √7ᵗʰ **S42.481** Torus fracture of lower end of right humerus `CC` `H5`
CC Excl: CC with 7th character A: PDX collection 1245
CC Excl: CC with 7th character K or P: PDX collection 897

3 √7ᵗʰ **S42.482** Torus fracture of lower end of left humerus `CC` `H5`
CC Excl: CC with 7th character A: PDX collection 1247
CC Excl: CC with 7th character K or P: PDX collection 897

3 √7ᵗʰ **S42.489** Torus fracture of lower end of unspecified humerus `CC` `H5`
CC Excl: CC with 7th character A: PDX collection 1248
CC Excl: CC with 7th character K or P: PDX collection 897

√6ᵗʰ **S42.49** Other fracture of lower end of humerus

2,3 √7ᵗʰ **S42.491** Other displaced fracture of lower end of right humerus `MCC` `CC` `H5`

2,3 √7ᵗʰ **S42.492** Other displaced fracture of lower end of left humerus `MCC` `CC` `H5`

2,3 √7ᵗʰ **S42.493** Other displaced fracture of lower end of unspecified humerus `MCC` `CC` `H5`

`N` Newborn: 0   `P` Pediatric: 0-17   `M` Maternity: 9-64   `A` Adult: 15-124   `MCC` Major Complication/Comorbidity   `CC` Complication/Comorbidity   `SW` Severe Wound Dx

2,3 √7ᵗʰ **S42.494** Other **nondisplaced fracture of lower end of right humerus** `MCC` `CC` `H5`

2,3 √7ᵗʰ **S42.495** Other **nondisplaced fracture of lower end of left humerus** `MCC` `CC` `H5`

2,3 √7ᵗʰ **S42.496** Other **nondisplaced fracture of lower end of unspecified humerus** `MCC` `CC` `H5`

√5ᵗʰ **S42.9** **Fracture of shoulder girdle, part unspecified**

Fracture of shoulder NOS

CC Excl: For CC/MCC codes in subcategory S42.9: See code S42.209

2,3 √x7ᵗʰ **S42.90** **Fracture of unspecified shoulder girdle, part unspecified** `MCC` `CC` `H5`

2,3 √x7ᵗʰ **S42.91** **Fracture of right shoulder girdle, part unspecified** `MCC` `CC` `H5`

2,3 √x7ᵗʰ **S42.92** **Fracture of left shoulder girdle, part unspecified** `MCC` `CC` `H5`

√4ᵗʰ **S43** **Dislocation and sprain of joints and ligaments of shoulder girdle**

`INCLUDES` avulsion of joint or ligament of shoulder girdle

laceration of cartilage, joint or ligament of shoulder girdle

sprain of cartilage, joint or ligament of shoulder girdle

traumatic hemarthrosis of joint or ligament of shoulder girdle

traumatic rupture of joint or ligament of shoulder girdle

traumatic subluxation of joint or ligament of shoulder girdle

traumatic tear of joint or ligament of shoulder girdle

Code also any associated open wound

`EXCLUDES 2` *strain of muscle, fascia and tendon of shoulder and upper arm (S46.-)*

The appropriate 7th character is to be added to each code from category S43.
A   initial encounter
D   subsequent encounter
S   sequela

√5ᵗʰ **S43.0** **Subluxation and dislocation of shoulder joint**

Dislocation of glenohumeral joint

Subluxation of glenohumeral joint

√6ᵗʰ **S43.00** **Unspecified subluxation and dislocation of shoulder joint**

Dislocation of humerus NOS

Subluxation of humerus NOS

√7ᵗʰ **S43.001** **Unspecified subluxation of right shoulder joint**

√7ᵗʰ **S43.002** **Unspecified subluxation of left shoulder joint**

√7ᵗʰ **S43.003** **Unspecified subluxation of unspecified shoulder joint**

√7ᵗʰ **S43.004** **Unspecified dislocation of right shoulder joint**

√7ᵗʰ **S43.005** **Unspecified dislocation of left shoulder joint**

√7ᵗʰ **S43.006** **Unspecified dislocation of unspecified shoulder joint**

√6ᵗʰ **S43.01** **Anterior subluxation and dislocation of humerus**

√7ᵗʰ **S43.011** **Anterior subluxation of right humerus**

√7ᵗʰ **S43.012** **Anterior subluxation of left humerus**

√7ᵗʰ **S43.013** **Anterior subluxation of unspecified humerus**

√7ᵗʰ **S43.014** **Anterior dislocation of right humerus**

√7ᵗʰ **S43.015** **Anterior dislocation of left humerus**

√7ᵗʰ **S43.016** **Anterior dislocation of unspecified humerus**

√6ᵗʰ **S43.02** **Posterior subluxation and dislocation of humerus**

√7ᵗʰ **S43.021** **Posterior subluxation of right humerus**

√7ᵗʰ **S43.022** **Posterior subluxation of left humerus**

√7ᵗʰ **S43.023** **Posterior subluxation of unspecified humerus**

√7ᵗʰ **S43.024** **Posterior dislocation of right humerus**

√7ᵗʰ **S43.025** **Posterior dislocation of left humerus**

√7ᵗʰ **S43.026** **Posterior dislocation of unspecified humerus**

√6ᵗʰ **S43.03** **Inferior subluxation and dislocation of humerus**

√7ᵗʰ **S43.031** **Inferior subluxation of right humerus**

√7ᵗʰ **S43.032** **Inferior subluxation of left humerus**

√7ᵗʰ **S43.033** **Inferior subluxation of unspecified humerus**

√7ᵗʰ **S43.034** **Inferior dislocation of right humerus**

√7ᵗʰ **S43.035** **Inferior dislocation of left humerus**

√7ᵗʰ **S43.036** **Inferior dislocation of unspecified humerus**

√6ᵗʰ **S43.08** **Other subluxation and dislocation of shoulder joint**

√7ᵗʰ **S43.081** **Other subluxation of right shoulder joint**

√7ᵗʰ **S43.082** **Other subluxation of left shoulder joint**

√7ᵗʰ **S43.083** **Other subluxation of unspecified shoulder joint**

√7ᵗʰ **S43.084** **Other dislocation of right shoulder joint**

√7ᵗʰ **S43.085** **Other dislocation of left shoulder joint**

√7ᵗʰ **S43.086** **Other dislocation of unspecified shoulder joint**

√5ᵗʰ **S43.1** **Subluxation and dislocation of acromioclavicular joint**

√6ᵗʰ **S43.10** **Unspecified dislocation of acromioclavicular joint**

√7ᵗʰ **S43.101** **Unspecified dislocation of right acromioclavicular joint**

√7ᵗʰ **S43.102** **Unspecified dislocation of left acromioclavicular joint**

√7ᵗʰ **S43.109** **Unspecified dislocation of unspecified acromioclavicular joint**

√6ᵗʰ **S43.11** **Subluxation of acromioclavicular joint**

√7ᵗʰ **S43.111** **Subluxation of right acromioclavicular joint**

√7ᵗʰ **S43.112** **Subluxation of left acromioclavicular joint**

√7ᵗʰ **S43.119** **Subluxation of unspecified acromioclavicular joint**

√6ᵗʰ **S43.12** **Dislocation of acromioclavicular joint, 100%-200% displacement**

√7ᵗʰ **S43.121** **Dislocation of right acromioclavicular joint, 100%-200% displacement**

√7ᵗʰ **S43.122** **Dislocation of left acromioclavicular joint, 100%-200% displacement**

√7ᵗʰ **S43.129** **Dislocation of unspecified acromioclavicular joint, 100%-200% displacement**

√6ᵗʰ **S43.13** **Dislocation of acromioclavicular joint, greater than 200% displacement**

√7ᵗʰ **S43.131** **Dislocation of right acromioclavicular joint, greater than 200% displacement**

√7ᵗʰ **S43.132** **Dislocation of left acromioclavicular joint, greater than 200% displacement**

√7ᵗʰ **S43.139** **Dislocation of unspecified acromioclavicular joint, greater than 200% displacement**

√6ᵗʰ **S43.14** **Inferior dislocation of acromioclavicular joint**

√7ᵗʰ **S43.141** **Inferior dislocation of right acromioclavicular joint**

√7ᵗʰ **S43.142** **Inferior dislocation of left acromioclavicular joint**

√7ᵗʰ **S43.149** **Inferior dislocation of unspecified acromioclavicular joint**

√6ᵗʰ **S43.15** **Posterior dislocation of acromioclavicular joint**

√7ᵗʰ **S43.151** **Posterior dislocation of right acromioclavicular joint**

√7ᵗʰ **S43.152** **Posterior dislocation of left acromioclavicular joint**

√7ᵗʰ **S43.159** **Posterior dislocation of unspecified acromioclavicular joint**

√5ᵗʰ **S43.2** **Subluxation and dislocation of sternoclavicular joint**

CC Excl: For CC codes in subcategory S43.2:
Right side: PDX collection 1252
Left side: PDX collection 1253
Unspecified side: PDX collection 914

√6ᵗʰ **S43.20** **Unspecified subluxation and dislocation of sternoclavicular joint**

√7ᵗʰ **S43.201** **Unspecified subluxation of right sternoclavicular joint** `CC` `H5`

√7ᵗʰ **S43.202** **Unspecified subluxation of left sternoclavicular joint** `CC` `H5`

√7ᵗʰ **S43.203** **Unspecified subluxation of unspecified sternoclavicular joint** `CC` `H5`

√7ᵗʰ **S43.204** **Unspecified dislocation of right sternoclavicular joint** `CC` `H5`

☑ Additional Character Required   √x7ᵗʰ Placeholder   Unacceptable PDx   Questionable PDx   Manifestation   Unspecified Dx   `H1`-`H14` HAC   `HCC` CMS-HCC Dx   `HIV` HIV Dx

ICD-10-CM 2020   **1037**

√7ᵗʰ **S43.205** Unspecified dislocation of left sternoclavicular joint   CC H5

√7ᵗʰ **S43.206** Unspecified dislocation of unspecified sternoclavicular joint   CC H5

√6ᵗʰ **S43.21** Anterior subluxation and dislocation of sternoclavicular joint

√7ᵗʰ **S43.211** Anterior subluxation of right sternoclavicular joint   CC H5

√7ᵗʰ **S43.212** Anterior subluxation of left sternoclavicular joint   CC H5

√7ᵗʰ **S43.213** Anterior subluxation of unspecified sternoclavicular joint   CC H5

√7ᵗʰ **S43.214** Anterior dislocation of right sternoclavicular joint   CC H5

√7ᵗʰ **S43.215** Anterior dislocation of left sternoclavicular joint   CC H5

√7ᵗʰ **S43.216** Anterior dislocation of unspecified sternoclavicular joint   CC H5

√6ᵗʰ **S43.22** Posterior subluxation and dislocation of sternoclavicular joint

√7ᵗʰ **S43.221** Posterior subluxation of right sternoclavicular joint   CC H5

√7ᵗʰ **S43.222** Posterior subluxation of left sternoclavicular joint   CC H5

√7ᵗʰ **S43.223** Posterior subluxation of unspecified sternoclavicular joint   CC H5

√7ᵗʰ **S43.224** Posterior dislocation of right sternoclavicular joint   CC H5

√7ᵗʰ **S43.225** Posterior dislocation of left sternoclavicular joint   CC H5

√7ᵗʰ **S43.226** Posterior dislocation of unspecified sternoclavicular joint   CC H5

√5ᵗʰ **S43.3** Subluxation and dislocation of other and unspecified parts of shoulder girdle

√6ᵗʰ **S43.30** Subluxation and dislocation of unspecified parts of shoulder girdle

Dislocation of shoulder girdle NOS

Subluxation of shoulder girdle NOS

√7ᵗʰ **S43.301** Subluxation of unspecified parts of right shoulder girdle

√7ᵗʰ **S43.302** Subluxation of unspecified parts of left shoulder girdle

√7ᵗʰ **S43.303** Subluxation of unspecified parts of unspecified shoulder girdle

√7ᵗʰ **S43.304** Dislocation of unspecified parts of right shoulder girdle

√7ᵗʰ **S43.305** Dislocation of unspecified parts of left shoulder girdle

√7ᵗʰ **S43.306** Dislocation of unspecified parts of unspecified shoulder girdle

√6ᵗʰ **S43.31** Subluxation and dislocation of scapula

√7ᵗʰ **S43.311** Subluxation of right scapula

√7ᵗʰ **S43.312** Subluxation of left scapula

√7ᵗʰ **S43.313** Subluxation of unspecified scapula

√7ᵗʰ **S43.314** Dislocation of right scapula

√7ᵗʰ **S43.315** Dislocation of left scapula

√7ᵗʰ **S43.316** Dislocation of unspecified scapula

√6ᵗʰ **S43.39** Subluxation and dislocation of other parts of shoulder girdle

√7ᵗʰ **S43.391** Subluxation of other parts of right shoulder girdle

√7ᵗʰ **S43.392** Subluxation of other parts of left shoulder girdle

√7ᵗʰ **S43.393** Subluxation of other parts of unspecified shoulder girdle

√7ᵗʰ **S43.394** Dislocation of other parts of right shoulder girdle

√7ᵗʰ **S43.395** Dislocation of other parts of left shoulder girdle

√7ᵗʰ **S43.396** Dislocation of other parts of unspecified shoulder girdle

√5ᵗʰ **S43.4** Sprain of shoulder joint

√6ᵗʰ **S43.40** Unspecified sprain of shoulder joint

√7ᵗʰ **S43.401** Unspecified sprain of right shoulder joint

√7ᵗʰ **S43.402** Unspecified sprain of left shoulder joint

√7ᵗʰ **S43.409** Unspecified sprain of unspecified shoulder joint

√6ᵗʰ **S43.41** Sprain of coracohumeral (ligament)

√7ᵗʰ **S43.411** Sprain of right coracohumeral (ligament)

√7ᵗʰ **S43.412** Sprain of left coracohumeral (ligament)

√7ᵗʰ **S43.419** Sprain of unspecified coracohumeral (ligament)

√6ᵗʰ **S43.42** Sprain of rotator cuff capsule

EXCLUDES 1   rotator cuff syndrome (complete) (incomplete), not specified as traumatic (M75.1-)

EXCLUDES 2   injury of tendon of rotator cuff (S46.0-)

√7ᵗʰ **S43.421** Sprain of right rotator cuff capsule

√7ᵗʰ **S43.422** Sprain of left rotator cuff capsule

√7ᵗʰ **S43.429** Sprain of unspecified rotator cuff capsule

√6ᵗʰ **S43.43** Superior glenoid labrum lesion

SLAP lesion

AHA: 2019,2Q,26

DEF: Detachment injury of the superior aspect of the glenoid labrum, which is the ring of fibrocartilage attached to the rim of the glenoid cavity of the scapula.

√7ᵗʰ **S43.431** Superior glenoid labrum lesion of right shoulder

√7ᵗʰ **S43.432** Superior glenoid labrum lesion of left shoulder

√7ᵗʰ **S43.439** Superior glenoid labrum lesion of unspecified shoulder

√6ᵗʰ **S43.49** Other sprain of shoulder joint

√7ᵗʰ **S43.491** Other sprain of right shoulder joint

√7ᵗʰ **S43.492** Other sprain of left shoulder joint

√7ᵗʰ **S43.499** Other sprain of unspecified shoulder joint

√5ᵗʰ **S43.5** Sprain of acromioclavicular joint

Sprain of acromioclavicular ligament

√x7ᵗʰ **S43.50** Sprain of unspecified acromioclavicular joint

√x7ᵗʰ **S43.51** Sprain of right acromioclavicular joint

√x7ᵗʰ **S43.52** Sprain of left acromioclavicular joint

√5ᵗʰ **S43.6** Sprain of sternoclavicular joint

√x7ᵗʰ **S43.60** Sprain of unspecified sternoclavicular joint

√x7ᵗʰ **S43.61** Sprain of right sternoclavicular joint

√x7ᵗʰ **S43.62** Sprain of left sternoclavicular joint

√5ᵗʰ **S43.8** Sprain of other specified parts of shoulder girdle

√x7ᵗʰ **S43.80** Sprain of other specified parts of unspecified shoulder girdle

√x7ᵗʰ **S43.81** Sprain of other specified parts of right shoulder girdle

√x7ᵗʰ **S43.82** Sprain of other specified parts of left shoulder girdle

√5ᵗʰ **S43.9** Sprain of unspecified parts of shoulder girdle

√x7ᵗʰ **S43.90** Sprain of unspecified parts of unspecified shoulder girdle

Sprain of shoulder girdle NOS

√x7ᵗʰ **S43.91** Sprain of unspecified parts of right shoulder girdle

√x7ᵗʰ **S43.92** Sprain of unspecified parts of left shoulder girdle

√4ᵗʰ **S44** Injury of nerves at shoulder and upper arm level

Code also any associated open wound (S41.-)

EXCLUDES 2   injury of brachial plexus (S14.3-)

The appropriate 7th character is to be added to each code from category S44.
A   initial encounter
D   subsequent encounter
S   sequela

√5ᵗʰ **S44.0** Injury of ulnar nerve at upper arm level

EXCLUDES 1   ulnar nerve NOS (S54.0)

√x7ᵗʰ **S44.00** Injury of ulnar nerve at upper arm level, unspecified arm

√x7ᵗʰ **S44.01** Injury of ulnar nerve at upper arm level, right arm

√x7ᵗʰ **S44.02** Injury of ulnar nerve at upper arm level, left arm

√5ᵗʰ **S44.1** Injury of median nerve at upper arm level

EXCLUDES 1   median nerve NOS (S54.1)

√x7ᵗʰ **S44.10** Injury of median nerve at upper arm level, unspecified arm

√x7ᵗʰ **S44.11** Injury of median nerve at upper arm level, right arm

---

N Newborn: 0   P Pediatric: 0-17   M Maternity: 9-64   A Adult: 15-124   MCC Major Complication/Comorbidity   CC Complication/Comorbidity   SW Severe Wound Dx

√x7ᵗʰ **S44.12** Injury of median nerve at upper arm level, left arm

√5ᵗʰ **S44.2** Injury of radial nerve at upper arm level
  EXCLUDES 1   radial nerve NOS (S54.2)
  √x7ᵗʰ **S44.20** Injury of radial nerve at upper arm level, unspecified arm
  √x7ᵗʰ **S44.21** Injury of radial nerve at upper arm level, right arm
  √x7ᵗʰ **S44.22** Injury of radial nerve at upper arm level, left arm

√5ᵗʰ **S44.3** Injury of axillary nerve
  √x7ᵗʰ **S44.30** Injury of axillary nerve, unspecified arm
  √x7ᵗʰ **S44.31** Injury of axillary nerve, right arm
  √x7ᵗʰ **S44.32** Injury of axillary nerve, left arm

√5ᵗʰ **S44.4** Injury of musculocutaneous nerve
  √x7ᵗʰ **S44.40** Injury of musculocutaneous nerve, unspecified arm
  √x7ᵗʰ **S44.41** Injury of musculocutaneous nerve, right arm
  √x7ᵗʰ **S44.42** Injury of musculocutaneous nerve, left arm

√5ᵗʰ **S44.5** Injury of cutaneous sensory nerve at shoulder and upper arm level
  √x7ᵗʰ **S44.50** Injury of cutaneous sensory nerve at shoulder and upper arm level, unspecified arm
  √x7ᵗʰ **S44.51** Injury of cutaneous sensory nerve at shoulder and upper arm level, right arm
  √x7ᵗʰ **S44.52** Injury of cutaneous sensory nerve at shoulder and upper arm level, left arm

√5ᵗʰ **S44.8** Injury of other nerves at shoulder and upper arm level
  √6ᵗʰ **S44.8X** Injury of other nerves at shoulder and upper arm level
    √7ᵗʰ **S44.8X1** Injury of other nerves at shoulder and upper arm level, right arm
    √7ᵗʰ **S44.8X2** Injury of other nerves at shoulder and upper arm level, left arm
    √7ᵗʰ **S44.8X9** Injury of other nerves at shoulder and upper arm level, unspecified arm

√5ᵗʰ **S44.9** Injury of unspecified nerve at shoulder and upper arm level
  √x7ᵗʰ **S44.90** Injury of unspecified nerve at shoulder and upper arm level, unspecified arm
  √x7ᵗʰ **S44.91** Injury of unspecified nerve at shoulder and upper arm level, right arm
  √x7ᵗʰ **S44.92** Injury of unspecified nerve at shoulder and upper arm level, left arm

√4ᵗʰ **S45** Injury of blood vessels at shoulder and upper arm level
  Code also any associated open wound (S41.-)
  EXCLUDES 2   injury of subclavian artery (S25.1)
                injury of subclavian vein (S25.3)

  The appropriate 7th character is to be added to each code from category S45.
  A   initial encounter
  D   subsequent encounter
  S   sequela

  √5ᵗʰ **S45.0** Injury of axillary artery
    CC Excl: For MCC codes in subcategory S45.0:
    Right side: PDX collection 1254
    Left side: PDX collection 1255
    Unspecified side: PDX collection 1256

    √6ᵗʰ **S45.00** Unspecified injury of axillary artery
      √7ᵗʰ **S45.001** Unspecified injury of axillary artery, right side   MCC
      √7ᵗʰ **S45.002** Unspecified injury of axillary artery, left side   MCC
      √7ᵗʰ **S45.009** Unspecified injury of axillary artery, unspecified side   MCC
    √6ᵗʰ **S45.01** Laceration of axillary artery
      √7ᵗʰ **S45.011** Laceration of axillary artery, right side   MCC
      √7ᵗʰ **S45.012** Laceration of axillary artery, left side   MCC
      √7ᵗʰ **S45.019** Laceration of axillary artery, unspecified side   MCC
    √6ᵗʰ **S45.09** Other specified injury of axillary artery
      √7ᵗʰ **S45.091** Other specified injury of axillary artery, right side   MCC
      √7ᵗʰ **S45.092** Other specified injury of axillary artery, left side   MCC
      √7ᵗʰ **S45.099** Other specified injury of axillary artery, unspecified side   MCC

  √5ᵗʰ **S45.1** Injury of brachial artery
    CC Excl: For CC codes in subcategory S45.1:
    Right side: PDX collection 1257
    Left side: PDX collection 1258
    Unspecified side: PDX collection 1259

    √6ᵗʰ **S45.10** Unspecified injury of brachial artery
      √7ᵗʰ **S45.101** Unspecified injury of brachial artery, right side   CC
      √7ᵗʰ **S45.102** Unspecified injury of brachial artery, left side   CC
      √7ᵗʰ **S45.109** Unspecified injury of brachial artery, unspecified side   CC
    √6ᵗʰ **S45.11** Laceration of brachial artery
      √7ᵗʰ **S45.111** Laceration of brachial artery, right side   CC
      √7ᵗʰ **S45.112** Laceration of brachial artery, left side   CC
      √7ᵗʰ **S45.119** Laceration of brachial artery, unspecified side   CC
    √6ᵗʰ **S45.19** Other specified injury of brachial artery
      √7ᵗʰ **S45.191** Other specified injury of brachial artery, right side   CC
      √7ᵗʰ **S45.192** Other specified injury of brachial artery, left side   CC
      √7ᵗʰ **S45.199** Other specified injury of brachial artery, unspecified side   CC

  √5ᵗʰ **S45.2** Injury of axillary or brachial vein
    CC Excl: For CC codes in subcategory S45.2:
    Right side: PDX collection 1257
    Left side: PDX collection 1258
    Unspecified side: PDX collection 1259

    √6ᵗʰ **S45.20** Unspecified injury of axillary or brachial vein
      √7ᵗʰ **S45.201** Unspecified injury of axillary or brachial vein, right side   CC
      √7ᵗʰ **S45.202** Unspecified injury of axillary or brachial vein, left side   CC
      √7ᵗʰ **S45.209** Unspecified injury of axillary or brachial vein, unspecified side   CC
    √6ᵗʰ **S45.21** Laceration of axillary or brachial vein
      √7ᵗʰ **S45.211** Laceration of axillary or brachial vein, right side   CC
      √7ᵗʰ **S45.212** Laceration of axillary or brachial vein, left side   CC
      √7ᵗʰ **S45.219** Laceration of axillary or brachial vein, unspecified side   CC
    √6ᵗʰ **S45.29** Other specified injury of axillary or brachial vein
      √7ᵗʰ **S45.291** Other specified injury of axillary or brachial vein, right side   CC
      √7ᵗʰ **S45.292** Other specified injury of axillary or brachial vein, left side   CC
      √7ᵗʰ **S45.299** Other specified injury of axillary or brachial vein, unspecified side   CC

  √5ᵗʰ **S45.3** Injury of superficial vein at shoulder and upper arm level
    CC Excl: For CC codes in subcategory S45.3:
    Right side: PDX collection 1260
    Left side: PDX collection 1261
    Unspecified side: PDX collection 1262

    √6ᵗʰ **S45.30** Unspecified injury of superficial vein at shoulder and upper arm level
      √7ᵗʰ **S45.301** Unspecified injury of superficial vein at shoulder and upper arm level, right arm   CC
      √7ᵗʰ **S45.302** Unspecified injury of superficial vein at shoulder and upper arm level, left arm   CC
      √7ᵗʰ **S45.309** Unspecified injury of superficial vein at shoulder and upper arm level, unspecified arm   CC

√6ᵗʰ **S45.31** Laceration of superficial vein at shoulder and upper arm level

√7ᵗʰ **S45.311** Laceration of superficial vein at shoulder and upper arm level, right arm `CC`

√7ᵗʰ **S45.312** Laceration of superficial vein at shoulder and upper arm level, left arm `CC`

√7ᵗʰ **S45.319** Laceration of superficial vein at shoulder and upper arm level, unspecified arm `CC`

√6ᵗʰ **S45.39** Other specified injury of superficial vein at shoulder and upper arm level

√7ᵗʰ **S45.391** Other specified injury of superficial vein at shoulder and upper arm level, right arm `CC`

√7ᵗʰ **S45.392** Other specified injury of superficial vein at shoulder and upper arm level, left arm `CC`

√7ᵗʰ **S45.399** Other specified injury of superficial vein at shoulder and upper arm level, unspecified arm `CC`

√5ᵗʰ **S45.8** Injury of other specified blood vessels at shoulder and upper arm level

CC Excl: For CC codes in subcategory S45.8:
Right side: PDX collection 1260
Left side: PDX collection 1261
Unspecified side: PDX collection 1262

√6ᵗʰ **S45.80** Unspecified injury of other specified blood vessels at shoulder and upper arm level

√7ᵗʰ **S45.801** Unspecified injury of other specified blood vessels at shoulder and upper arm level, right arm `CC`

√7ᵗʰ **S45.802** Unspecified injury of other specified blood vessels at shoulder and upper arm level, left arm `CC`

√7ᵗʰ **S45.809** Unspecified injury of other specified blood vessels at shoulder and upper arm level, unspecified arm `CC`

√6ᵗʰ **S45.81** Laceration of other specified blood vessels at shoulder and upper arm level

√7ᵗʰ **S45.811** Laceration of other specified blood vessels at shoulder and upper arm level, right arm `CC`

√7ᵗʰ **S45.812** Laceration of other specified blood vessels at shoulder and upper arm level, left arm `CC`

√7ᵗʰ **S45.819** Laceration of other specified blood vessels at shoulder and upper arm level, unspecified arm `CC`

√6ᵗʰ **S45.89** Other specified injury of other specified blood vessels at shoulder and upper arm level

√7ᵗʰ **S45.891** Other specified injury of other specified blood vessels at shoulder and upper arm level, right arm `CC`

√7ᵗʰ **S45.892** Other specified injury of other specified blood vessels at shoulder and upper arm level, left arm `CC`

√7ᵗʰ **S45.899** Other specified injury of other specified blood vessels at shoulder and upper arm level, unspecified arm `CC`

√5ᵗʰ **S45.9** Injury of unspecified blood vessel at shoulder and upper arm level

CC Excl: For CC codes in subcategory S45.9:
Right side: PDX collection 1260
Left side: PDX collection 1261
Unspecified side: PDX collection 1262

√6ᵗʰ **S45.90** Unspecified injury of unspecified blood vessel at shoulder and upper arm level

√7ᵗʰ **S45.901** Unspecified injury of unspecified blood vessel at shoulder and upper arm level, right arm `CC`

√7ᵗʰ **S45.902** Unspecified injury of unspecified blood vessel at shoulder and upper arm level, left arm `CC`

√7ᵗʰ **S45.909** Unspecified injury of unspecified blood vessel at shoulder and upper arm level, unspecified arm `CC`

√6ᵗʰ **S45.91** Laceration of unspecified blood vessel at shoulder and upper arm level

√7ᵗʰ **S45.911** Laceration of unspecified blood vessel at shoulder and upper arm level, right arm `CC`

√7ᵗʰ **S45.912** Laceration of unspecified blood vessel at shoulder and upper arm level, left arm `CC`

√7ᵗʰ **S45.919** Laceration of unspecified blood vessel at shoulder and upper arm level, unspecified arm `CC`

√6ᵗʰ **S45.99** Other specified injury of unspecified blood vessel at shoulder and upper arm level

√7ᵗʰ **S45.991** Other specified injury of unspecified blood vessel at shoulder and upper arm level, right arm `CC`

√7ᵗʰ **S45.992** Other specified injury of unspecified blood vessel at shoulder and upper arm level, left arm `CC`

√7ᵗʰ **S45.999** Other specified injury of unspecified blood vessel at shoulder and upper arm level, unspecified arm `CC`

√4ᵗʰ **S46** Injury of muscle, fascia and tendon at shoulder and upper arm level

Code also any associated open wound (S41.-)

EXCLUDES 2   injury of muscle, fascia and tendon at elbow (S56.-)
sprain of joints and ligaments of shoulder girdle (S43.9)

TIP: Refer to the Muscle/Tendon table at the beginning of this chapter.

The appropriate 7th character is to be added to each code from category S46.
A   initial encounter
D   subsequent encounter
S   sequela

CC Excl: For CC codes in category S46:
Right side: PDX collection 1263
Left side: PDX collection 1264
Unspecified side: PDX collection 1265

√5ᵗʰ **S46.0** Injury of muscle(s) and tendon(s) of the rotator cuff of shoulder

√6ᵗʰ **S46.00** Unspecified injury of muscle(s) and tendon(s) of the rotator cuff of shoulder

√7ᵗʰ **S46.001** Unspecified injury of muscle(s) and tendon(s) of the rotator cuff of right shoulder

√7ᵗʰ **S46.002** Unspecified injury of muscle(s) and tendon(s) of the rotator cuff of left shoulder

√7ᵗʰ **S46.009** Unspecified injury of muscle(s) and tendon(s) of the rotator cuff of unspecified shoulder

√6ᵗʰ **S46.01** Strain of muscle(s) and tendon(s) of the rotator cuff of shoulder

√7ᵗʰ **S46.011** Strain of muscle(s) and tendon(s) of the rotator cuff of right shoulder

√7ᵗʰ **S46.012** Strain of muscle(s) and tendon(s) of the rotator cuff of left shoulder

     √7ᵗʰ **S46.019** Strain of muscle(s) and tendon(s) of the rotator cuff of unspecified shoulder

√6ᵗʰ **S46.02** Laceration of muscle(s) and tendon(s) of the rotator cuff of shoulder

     √7ᵗʰ **S46.021** Laceration of muscle(s) and tendon(s) of the rotator cuff of right shoulder   `CC`

     √7ᵗʰ **S46.022** Laceration of muscle(s) and tendon(s) of the rotator cuff of left shoulder   `CC`

     √7ᵗʰ **S46.029** Laceration of muscle(s) and tendon(s) of the rotator cuff of unspecified shoulder   `CC`

√6ᵗʰ **S46.09** Other injury of muscle(s) and tendon(s) of the rotator cuff of shoulder

     √7ᵗʰ **S46.091** Other injury of muscle(s) and tendon(s) of the rotator cuff of right shoulder

     √7ᵗʰ **S46.092** Other injury of muscle(s) and tendon(s) of the rotator cuff of left shoulder

     √7ᵗʰ **S46.099** Other injury of muscle(s) and tendon(s) of the rotator cuff of unspecified shoulder

√5ᵗʰ **S46.1** Injury of muscle, fascia and tendon of long head of biceps

√6ᵗʰ **S46.10** Unspecified injury of muscle, fascia and tendon of long head of biceps

     √7ᵗʰ **S46.101** Unspecified injury of muscle, fascia and tendon of long head of biceps, right arm

     √7ᵗʰ **S46.102** Unspecified injury of muscle, fascia and tendon of long head of biceps, left arm

     √7ᵗʰ **S46.109** Unspecified injury of muscle, fascia and tendon of long head of biceps, unspecified arm

√6ᵗʰ **S46.11** Strain of muscle, fascia and tendon of long head of biceps

     AHA: 2019,2Q,27

     √7ᵗʰ **S46.111** Strain of muscle, fascia and tendon of long head of biceps, right arm

     √7ᵗʰ **S46.112** Strain of muscle, fascia and tendon of long head of biceps, left arm

     √7ᵗʰ **S46.119** Strain of muscle, fascia and tendon of long head of biceps, unspecified arm

√6ᵗʰ **S46.12** Laceration of muscle, fascia and tendon of long head of biceps

     √7ᵗʰ **S46.121** Laceration of muscle, fascia and tendon of long head of biceps, right arm   `CC`

     √7ᵗʰ **S46.122** Laceration of muscle, fascia and tendon of long head of biceps, left arm   `CC`

     √7ᵗʰ **S46.129** Laceration of muscle, fascia and tendon of long head of biceps, unspecified arm   `CC`

√6ᵗʰ **S46.19** Other injury of muscle, fascia and tendon of long head of biceps

     √7ᵗʰ **S46.191** Other injury of muscle, fascia and tendon of long head of biceps, right arm

     √7ᵗʰ **S46.192** Other injury of muscle, fascia and tendon of long head of biceps, left arm

     √7ᵗʰ **S46.199** Other injury of muscle, fascia and tendon of long head of biceps, unspecified arm

√5ᵗʰ **S46.2** Injury of muscle, fascia and tendon of other parts of biceps

√6ᵗʰ **S46.20** Unspecified injury of muscle, fascia and tendon of other parts of biceps

     √7ᵗʰ **S46.201** Unspecified injury of muscle, fascia and tendon of other parts of biceps, right arm

     √7ᵗʰ **S46.202** Unspecified injury of muscle, fascia and tendon of other parts of biceps, left arm

     √7ᵗʰ **S46.209** Unspecified injury of muscle, fascia and tendon of other parts of biceps, unspecified arm

√6ᵗʰ **S46.21** Strain of muscle, fascia and tendon of other parts of biceps

     √7ᵗʰ **S46.211** Strain of muscle, fascia and tendon of other parts of biceps, right arm

     √7ᵗʰ **S46.212** Strain of muscle, fascia and tendon of other parts of biceps, left arm

     √7ᵗʰ **S46.219** Strain of muscle, fascia and tendon of other parts of biceps, unspecified arm

√6ᵗʰ **S46.22** Laceration of muscle, fascia and tendon of other parts of biceps

     √7ᵗʰ **S46.221** Laceration of muscle, fascia and tendon of other parts of biceps, right arm   `CC`

     √7ᵗʰ **S46.222** Laceration of muscle, fascia and tendon of other parts of biceps, left arm   `CC`

     √7ᵗʰ **S46.229** Laceration of muscle, fascia and tendon of other parts of biceps, unspecified arm   `CC`

√6ᵗʰ **S46.29** Other injury of muscle, fascia and tendon of other parts of biceps

     √7ᵗʰ **S46.291** Other injury of muscle, fascia and tendon of other parts of biceps, right arm

     √7ᵗʰ **S46.292** Other injury of muscle, fascia and tendon of other parts of biceps, left arm

     √7ᵗʰ **S46.299** Other injury of muscle, fascia and tendon of other parts of biceps, unspecified arm

√5ᵗʰ **S46.3** Injury of muscle, fascia and tendon of triceps

√6ᵗʰ **S46.30** Unspecified injury of muscle, fascia and tendon of triceps

     √7ᵗʰ **S46.301** Unspecified injury of muscle, fascia and tendon of triceps, right arm

     √7ᵗʰ **S46.302** Unspecified injury of muscle, fascia and tendon of triceps, left arm

     √7ᵗʰ **S46.309** Unspecified injury of muscle, fascia and tendon of triceps, unspecified arm

√6ᵗʰ **S46.31** Strain of muscle, fascia and tendon of triceps

     √7ᵗʰ **S46.311** Strain of muscle, fascia and tendon of triceps, right arm

     √7ᵗʰ **S46.312** Strain of muscle, fascia and tendon of triceps, left arm

     √7ᵗʰ **S46.319** Strain of muscle, fascia and tendon of triceps, unspecified arm

√6ᵗʰ **S46.32** Laceration of muscle, fascia and tendon of triceps

     √7ᵗʰ **S46.321** Laceration of muscle, fascia and tendon of triceps, right arm   `CC`

     √7ᵗʰ **S46.322** Laceration of muscle, fascia and tendon of triceps, left arm   `CC`

     √7ᵗʰ **S46.329** Laceration of muscle, fascia and tendon of triceps, unspecified arm   `CC`

√6ᵗʰ **S46.39** Other injury of muscle, fascia and tendon of triceps

     √7ᵗʰ **S46.391** Other injury of muscle, fascia and tendon of triceps, right arm

     √7ᵗʰ **S46.392** Other injury of muscle, fascia and tendon of triceps, left arm

     √7ᵗʰ **S46.399** Other injury of muscle, fascia and tendon of triceps, unspecified arm

√5ᵗʰ **S46.8** Injury of other muscles, fascia and tendons at shoulder and upper arm level

√6ᵗʰ **S46.80** Unspecified injury of other muscles, fascia and tendons at shoulder and upper arm level

     √7ᵗʰ **S46.801** Unspecified injury of other muscles, fascia and tendons at shoulder and upper arm level, right arm

     √7ᵗʰ **S46.802** Unspecified injury of other muscles, fascia and tendons at shoulder and upper arm level, left arm

     √7ᵗʰ **S46.809** Unspecified injury of other muscles, fascia and tendons at shoulder and upper arm level, unspecified arm

√6ᵗʰ **S46.81** Strain of other muscles, fascia and tendons at shoulder and upper arm level

     √7ᵗʰ **S46.811** Strain of other muscles, fascia and tendons at shoulder and upper arm level, right arm

     √7ᵗʰ **S46.812** Strain of other muscles, fascia and tendons at shoulder and upper arm level, left arm

     √7ᵗʰ **S46.819** Strain of other muscles, fascia and tendons at shoulder and upper arm level, unspecified arm

√6ᵗʰ **S46.82** Laceration of other muscles, fascia and tendons at shoulder and upper arm level

     √7ᵗʰ **S46.821** Laceration of other muscles, fascia and tendons at shoulder and upper arm level, right arm   `CC`

☑ Additional Character Required   √x7ᵗʰ Placeholder   Unacceptable PDx   Questionable PDx   Manifestation   Unspecified Dx   `H1`-`H4` HAC   `HCC` CMS-HCC Dx   `HIV` HIV Dx

ICD-10-CM 2020   1041

    √7ᵗʰ **S46.822** **Laceration of other muscles, fascia and tendons at shoulder and upper arm level, left arm**   cc

    √7ᵗʰ **S46.829** **Laceration of other muscles, fascia and tendons at shoulder and upper arm level, unspecified arm**   cc

√6ᵗʰ **S46.89** **Other injury of other muscles, fascia and tendons at shoulder and upper arm level**

    √7ᵗʰ **S46.891** **Other injury of other muscles, fascia and tendons at shoulder and upper arm level, right arm**

    √7ᵗʰ **S46.892** **Other injury of other muscles, fascia and tendons at shoulder and upper arm level, left arm**

    √7ᵗʰ **S46.899** **Other injury of other muscles, fascia and tendons at shoulder and upper arm level, unspecified arm**

√5ᵗʰ **S46.9** **Injury of unspecified muscle, fascia and tendon at shoulder and upper arm level**

√6ᵗʰ **S46.90** **Unspecified injury of unspecified muscle, fascia and tendon at shoulder and upper arm level**

    √7ᵗʰ **S46.901** **Unspecified injury of unspecified muscle, fascia and tendon at shoulder and upper arm level, right arm**

    √7ᵗʰ **S46.902** **Unspecified injury of unspecified muscle, fascia and tendon at shoulder and upper arm level, left arm**

    √7ᵗʰ **S46.909** **Unspecified injury of unspecified muscle, fascia and tendon at shoulder and upper arm level, unspecified arm**

√6ᵗʰ **S46.91** **Strain of unspecified muscle, fascia and tendon at shoulder and upper arm level**

    √7ᵗʰ **S46.911** **Strain of unspecified muscle, fascia and tendon at shoulder and upper arm level, right arm**

    √7ᵗʰ **S46.912** **Strain of unspecified muscle, fascia and tendon at shoulder and upper arm level, left arm**

    √7ᵗʰ **S46.919** **Strain of unspecified muscle, fascia and tendon at shoulder and upper arm level, unspecified arm**

√6ᵗʰ **S46.92** **Laceration of unspecified muscle, fascia and tendon at shoulder and upper arm level**

    √7ᵗʰ **S46.921** **Laceration of unspecified muscle, fascia and tendon at shoulder and upper arm level, right arm**   cc

    √7ᵗʰ **S46.922** **Laceration of unspecified muscle, fascia and tendon at shoulder and upper arm level, left arm**   cc

    √7ᵗʰ **S46.929** **Laceration of unspecified muscle, fascia and tendon at shoulder and upper arm level, unspecified arm**   cc

√6ᵗʰ **S46.99** **Other injury of unspecified muscle, fascia and tendon at shoulder and upper arm level**

    √7ᵗʰ **S46.991** **Other injury of unspecified muscle, fascia and tendon at shoulder and upper arm level, right arm**

    √7ᵗʰ **S46.992** **Other injury of unspecified muscle, fascia and tendon at shoulder and upper arm level, left arm**

    √7ᵗʰ **S46.999** **Other injury of unspecified muscle, fascia and tendon at shoulder and upper arm level, unspecified arm**

√4ᵗʰ **S47** **Crushing injury of shoulder and upper arm**

Use additional code for all associated injuries

EXCLUDES 2   *crushing injury of elbow (S57.0-)*

The appropriate 7th character is to be added to each code from category S47.
A   initial encounter
D   subsequent encounter
S   sequela

√x7ᵗʰ **S47.1** **Crushing injury of right shoulder and upper arm**

√x7ᵗʰ **S47.2** **Crushing injury of left shoulder and upper arm**

√x7ᵗʰ **S47.9** **Crushing injury of shoulder and upper arm, unspecified arm**

√4ᵗʰ **S48** **Traumatic amputation of shoulder and upper arm**

An amputation not identified as partial or complete should be coded to complete

EXCLUDES 1   *traumatic amputation at elbow level (S58.0)*

The appropriate 7th character is to be added to each code from category S48.
A   initial encounter
D   subsequent encounter
S   sequela

CC Excl: For CC codes in category S48:
Right side: PDX collection 1,266
Left side: PDX collection 1,267
Unspecified side: PDX collection 1,268

√5ᵗʰ **S48.0** **Traumatic amputation at shoulder joint**

√6ᵗʰ **S48.01** **Complete traumatic amputation at shoulder joint**

    7 √7ᵗʰ **S48.011** **Complete traumatic amputation at right shoulder joint**   cc HCC

    7 √7ᵗʰ **S48.012** **Complete traumatic amputation at left shoulder joint**   cc HCC

    7 √7ᵗʰ **S48.019** **Complete traumatic amputation at unspecified shoulder joint**   cc HCC

√6ᵗʰ **S48.02** **Partial traumatic amputation at shoulder joint**

    7 √7ᵗʰ **S48.021** **Partial traumatic amputation at right shoulder joint**   cc HCC

    7 √7ᵗʰ **S48.022** **Partial traumatic amputation at left shoulder joint**   cc HCC

    7 √7ᵗʰ **S48.029** **Partial traumatic amputation at unspecified shoulder joint**   cc HCC

√5ᵗʰ **S48.1** **Traumatic amputation at level between shoulder and elbow**

√6ᵗʰ **S48.11** **Complete traumatic amputation at level between shoulder and elbow**

    7 √7ᵗʰ **S48.111** **Complete traumatic amputation at level between right shoulder and elbow**   cc HCC

    7 √7ᵗʰ **S48.112** **Complete traumatic amputation at level between left shoulder and elbow**   cc HCC

    7 √7ᵗʰ **S48.119** **Complete traumatic amputation at level between unspecified shoulder and elbow**   cc HCC

√6ᵗʰ **S48.12** **Partial traumatic amputation at level between shoulder and elbow**

    7 √7ᵗʰ **S48.121** **Partial traumatic amputation at level between right shoulder and elbow**   cc HCC

    7 √7ᵗʰ **S48.122** **Partial traumatic amputation at level between left shoulder and elbow**   cc HCC

    7 √7ᵗʰ **S48.129** **Partial traumatic amputation at level between unspecified shoulder and elbow**   cc HCC

√5ᵗʰ **S48.9** **Traumatic amputation of shoulder and upper arm, level unspecified**

√6ᵗʰ **S48.91** **Complete traumatic amputation of shoulder and upper arm, level unspecified**

    7 √7ᵗʰ **S48.911** **Complete traumatic amputation of right shoulder and upper arm, level unspecified**   cc HCC

    7 √7ᵗʰ **S48.912** **Complete traumatic amputation of left shoulder and upper arm, level unspecified**   cc HCC

    7 √7ᵗʰ **S48.919** **Complete traumatic amputation of unspecified shoulder and upper arm, level unspecified**   cc HCC

√6ᵗʰ **S48.92** **Partial traumatic amputation of shoulder and upper arm, level unspecified**

    7 √7ᵗʰ **S48.921** **Partial traumatic amputation of right shoulder and upper arm, level unspecified**   `CC` `HCC`

    7 √7ᵗʰ **S48.922** **Partial traumatic amputation of left shoulder and upper arm, level unspecified**   `CC` `HCC`

    7 √7ᵗʰ **S48.929** **Partial traumatic amputation of unspecified shoulder and upper arm, level unspecified**   `CC` `HCC`

√4ᵗʰ **S49** **Other and unspecified injuries of shoulder and upper arm**

    AHA: 2018,2Q,12; 2018,1Q,3

> The appropriate 7th character is to be added to each code from subcategories S49.0 and S49.1.
> A   initial encounter for closed fracture
> D   subsequent encounter for fracture with routine healing
> G   subsequent encounter for fracture with delayed healing
> K   subsequent encounter for fracture with nonunion
> P   subsequent encounter for fracture with malunion
> S   sequela

CC Excl: For CC codes in category S49:
Right side: See code S49.001
Left side: See code S49.002
Unspecified side: See code S49.009

√5ᵗʰ **S49.0** **Physeal fracture of upper end of humerus**

    √6ᵗʰ **S49.00** **Unspecified physeal fracture of upper end of humerus**

       3 √7ᵗʰ **S49.001** **Unspecified physeal fracture of upper end of humerus, right arm**   `CC` `H5`
         CC Excl: CC with 7th character A: PDX collection 1245
         CC Excl: CC with 7th character K or P: PDX collection 897

       3 √7ᵗʰ **S49.002** **Unspecified physeal fracture of upper end of humerus, left arm**   `CC` `H5`
         CC Excl: CC with 7th character A: PDX collection 1247
         CC Excl: CC with 7th character K or P: PDX collection 897

       3 √7ᵗʰ **S49.009** **Unspecified physeal fracture of upper end of humerus, unspecified arm**   `CC` `H5`
         CC Excl: CC with 7th character A: PDX collection 1248
         CC Excl: CC with 7th character K or P: PDX collection 897

    √6ᵗʰ **S49.01** **Salter-Harris Type I physeal fracture of upper end of humerus**

       3 √7ᵗʰ **S49.011** **Salter-Harris Type I physeal fracture of upper end of humerus, right arm**   `CC` `H5`

       3 √7ᵗʰ **S49.012** **Salter-Harris Type I physeal fracture of upper end of humerus, left arm**   `CC` `H5`

       3 √7ᵗʰ **S49.019** **Salter-Harris Type I physeal fracture of upper end of humerus, unspecified arm**   `CC` `H5`

    √6ᵗʰ **S49.02** **Salter-Harris Type II physeal fracture of upper end of humerus**

       3 √7ᵗʰ **S49.021** **Salter-Harris Type II physeal fracture of upper end of humerus, right arm**   `CC` `H5`

       3 √7ᵗʰ **S49.022** **Salter-Harris Type II physeal fracture of upper end of humerus, left arm**   `CC` `H5`

       3 √7ᵗʰ **S49.029** **Salter-Harris Type II physeal fracture of upper end of humerus, unspecified arm**   `CC` `H5`

    √6ᵗʰ **S49.03** **Salter-Harris Type III physeal fracture of upper end of humerus**

       3 √7ᵗʰ **S49.031** **Salter-Harris Type III physeal fracture of upper end of humerus, right arm**   `CC` `H5`

       3 √7ᵗʰ **S49.032** **Salter-Harris Type III physeal fracture of upper end of humerus, left arm**   `CC` `H5`

       3 √7ᵗʰ **S49.039** **Salter-Harris Type III physeal fracture of upper end of humerus, unspecified arm**   `CC` `H5`

    √6ᵗʰ **S49.04** **Salter-Harris Type IV physeal fracture of upper end of humerus**

       3 √7ᵗʰ **S49.041** **Salter-Harris Type IV physeal fracture of upper end of humerus, right arm**   `CC` `H5`

       3 √7ᵗʰ **S49.042** **Salter-Harris Type IV physeal fracture of upper end of humerus, left arm**   `CC` `H5`

       3 √7ᵗʰ **S49.049** **Salter-Harris Type IV physeal fracture of upper end of humerus, unspecified arm**   `CC` `H5`

    √6ᵗʰ **S49.09** **Other physeal fracture of upper end of humerus**

       3 √7ᵗʰ **S49.091** **Other physeal fracture of upper end of humerus, right arm**   `CC` `H5`

       3 √7ᵗʰ **S49.092** **Other physeal fracture of upper end of humerus, left arm**   `CC` `H5`

       3 √7ᵗʰ **S49.099** **Other physeal fracture of upper end of humerus, unspecified arm**   `CC` `H5`

√5ᵗʰ **S49.1** **Physeal fracture of lower end of humerus**

    √6ᵗʰ **S49.10** **Unspecified physeal fracture of lower end of humerus**

       3 √7ᵗʰ **S49.101** **Unspecified physeal fracture of lower end of humerus, right arm**   `CC` `H5`

       3 √7ᵗʰ **S49.102** **Unspecified physeal fracture of lower end of humerus, left arm**   `CC` `H5`

       3 √7ᵗʰ **S49.109** **Unspecified physeal fracture of lower end of humerus, unspecified arm**   `CC` `H5`

    √6ᵗʰ **S49.11** **Salter-Harris Type I physeal fracture of lower end of humerus**

       3 √7ᵗʰ **S49.111** **Salter-Harris Type I physeal fracture of lower end of humerus, right arm**   `CC` `H5`

       3 √7ᵗʰ **S49.112** **Salter-Harris Type I physeal fracture of lower end of humerus, left arm**   `CC` `H5`

       3 √7ᵗʰ **S49.119** **Salter-Harris Type I physeal fracture of lower end of humerus, unspecified arm**   `CC` `H5`

    √6ᵗʰ **S49.12** **Salter-Harris Type II physeal fracture of lower end of humerus**

       3 √7ᵗʰ **S49.121** **Salter-Harris Type II physeal fracture of lower end of humerus, right arm**   `CC` `H5`

       3 √7ᵗʰ **S49.122** **Salter-Harris Type II physeal fracture of lower end of humerus, left arm**   `CC` `H5`

       3 √7ᵗʰ **S49.129** **Salter-Harris Type II physeal fracture of lower end of humerus, unspecified arm**   `CC` `H5`

    √6ᵗʰ **S49.13** **Salter-Harris Type III physeal fracture of lower end of humerus**

       3 √7ᵗʰ **S49.131** **Salter-Harris Type III physeal fracture of lower end of humerus, right arm**   `CC` `H5`

       3 √7ᵗʰ **S49.132** **Salter-Harris Type III physeal fracture of lower end of humerus, left arm**   `CC` `H5`

       3 √7ᵗʰ **S49.139** **Salter-Harris Type III physeal fracture of lower end of humerus, unspecified arm**   `CC` `H5`

    √6ᵗʰ **S49.14** **Salter-Harris Type IV physeal fracture of lower end of humerus**

       3 √7ᵗʰ **S49.141** **Salter-Harris Type IV physeal fracture of lower end of humerus, right arm**   `CC` `H5`

3 ✓7ᵗʰ **S49.142 Salter-Harris Type IV physeal fracture of lower end of humerus, left arm** `CC` `H5`

3 ✓7ᵗʰ **S49.149 Salter-Harris Type IV physeal fracture of lower end of humerus, unspecified arm** `CC` `H5`

✓6ᵗʰ **S49.19 Other physeal fracture of lower end of humerus**

    3 ✓7ᵗʰ **S49.191 Other physeal fracture of lower end of humerus, right arm** `CC` `H5`

    3 ✓7ᵗʰ **S49.192 Other physeal fracture of lower end of humerus, left arm** `CC` `H5`

    3 ✓7ᵗʰ **S49.199 Other physeal fracture of lower end of humerus, unspecified arm** `CC` `H5`

✓5ᵗʰ **S49.8 Other specified injuries of shoulder and upper arm**

> The appropriate 7th character is to be added to each code in subcategory S49.8.
> A   initial encounter
> D   subsequent encounter
> S   sequela

✓x7ᵗʰ **S49.80 Other specified injuries of shoulder and upper arm, unspecified arm**

✓x7ᵗʰ **S49.81 Other specified injuries of right shoulder and upper arm**

✓x7ᵗʰ **S49.82 Other specified injuries of left shoulder and upper arm**

✓5ᵗʰ **S49.9 Unspecified injury of shoulder and upper arm**

> The appropriate 7th character is to be added to each code in subcategory S49.9.
> A   initial encounter
> D   subsequent encounter
> S   sequela

✓x7ᵗʰ **S49.90 Unspecified injury of shoulder and upper arm, unspecified arm**

✓x7ᵗʰ **S49.91 Unspecified injury of right shoulder and upper arm**

✓x7ᵗʰ **S49.92 Unspecified injury of left shoulder and upper arm**

Injuries to the elbow and forearm (S50-S59)

EXCLUDES 2   burns and corrosions (T20-T32)
     frostbite (T33-T34)
     injuries of wrist and hand (S60-S69)
     insect bite or sting, venomous (T63.4)

✓4ᵗʰ **S50 Superficial injury of elbow and forearm**

    EXCLUDES 2   superficial injury of wrist and hand (S60.-)

> The appropriate 7th character is to be added to each code from category S50.
> A   initial encounter
> D   subsequent encounter
> S   sequela

✓5ᵗʰ **S50.0 Contusion of elbow**

✓x7ᵗʰ **S50.00 Contusion of unspecified elbow**

✓x7ᵗʰ **S50.01 Contusion of right elbow**

✓x7ᵗʰ **S50.02 Contusion of left elbow**

✓5ᵗʰ **S50.1 Contusion of forearm**

✓x7ᵗʰ **S50.10 Contusion of unspecified forearm**

✓x7ᵗʰ **S50.11 Contusion of right forearm**

✓x7ᵗʰ **S50.12 Contusion of left forearm**

✓5ᵗʰ **S50.3 Other superficial injuries of elbow**

✓6ᵗʰ **S50.31 Abrasion of elbow**

    ✓7ᵗʰ **S50.311 Abrasion of right elbow**

    ✓7ᵗʰ **S50.312 Abrasion of left elbow**

    ✓7ᵗʰ **S50.319 Abrasion of unspecified elbow**

✓6ᵗʰ **S50.32 Blister (nonthermal) of elbow**

    ✓7ᵗʰ **S50.321 Blister (nonthermal) of right elbow**

    ✓7ᵗʰ **S50.322 Blister (nonthermal) of left elbow**

    ✓7ᵗʰ **S50.329 Blister (nonthermal) of unspecified elbow**

✓6ᵗʰ **S50.34 External constriction of elbow**

    ✓7ᵗʰ **S50.341 External constriction of right elbow**

    ✓7ᵗʰ **S50.342 External constriction of left elbow**

    ✓7ᵗʰ **S50.349 External constriction of unspecified elbow**

✓6ᵗʰ **S50.35 Superficial foreign body of elbow**

    Splinter in the elbow

    ✓7ᵗʰ **S50.351 Superficial foreign body of right elbow**

    ✓7ᵗʰ **S50.352 Superficial foreign body of left elbow**

    ✓7ᵗʰ **S50.359 Superficial foreign body of unspecified elbow**

✓6ᵗʰ **S50.36 Insect bite (nonvenomous) of elbow**

    ✓7ᵗʰ **S50.361 Insect bite (nonvenomous) of right elbow**

    ✓7ᵗʰ **S50.362 Insect bite (nonvenomous) of left elbow**

    ✓7ᵗʰ **S50.369 Insect bite (nonvenomous) of unspecified elbow**

✓6ᵗʰ **S50.37 Other superficial bite of elbow**

    EXCLUDES 1   open bite of elbow (S51.05)

    ✓7ᵗʰ **S50.371 Other superficial bite of right elbow**

    ✓7ᵗʰ **S50.372 Other superficial bite of left elbow**

    ✓7ᵗʰ **S50.379 Other superficial bite of unspecified elbow**

✓5ᵗʰ **S50.8 Other superficial injuries of forearm**

✓6ᵗʰ **S50.81 Abrasion of forearm**

    ✓7ᵗʰ **S50.811 Abrasion of right forearm**

    ✓7ᵗʰ **S50.812 Abrasion of left forearm**

    ✓7ᵗʰ **S50.819 Abrasion of unspecified forearm**

✓6ᵗʰ **S50.82 Blister (nonthermal) of forearm**

    ✓7ᵗʰ **S50.821 Blister (nonthermal) of right forearm**

    ✓7ᵗʰ **S50.822 Blister (nonthermal) of left forearm**

    ✓7ᵗʰ **S50.829 Blister (nonthermal) of unspecified forearm**

✓6ᵗʰ **S50.84 External constriction of forearm**

    ✓7ᵗʰ **S50.841 External constriction of right forearm**

    ✓7ᵗʰ **S50.842 External constriction of left forearm**

    ✓7ᵗʰ **S50.849 External constriction of unspecified forearm**

✓6ᵗʰ **S50.85 Superficial foreign body of forearm**

    Splinter in the forearm

    ✓7ᵗʰ **S50.851 Superficial foreign body of right forearm**

    ✓7ᵗʰ **S50.852 Superficial foreign body of left forearm**

    ✓7ᵗʰ **S50.859 Superficial foreign body of unspecified forearm**

✓6ᵗʰ **S50.86 Insect bite (nonvenomous) of forearm**

    ✓7ᵗʰ **S50.861 Insect bite (nonvenomous) of right forearm**

    ✓7ᵗʰ **S50.862 Insect bite (nonvenomous) of left forearm**

    ✓7ᵗʰ **S50.869 Insect bite (nonvenomous) of unspecified forearm**

✓6ᵗʰ **S50.87 Other superficial bite of forearm**

    EXCLUDES 1   open bite of forearm (S51.85)

    ✓7ᵗʰ **S50.871 Other superficial bite of right forearm**

    ✓7ᵗʰ **S50.872 Other superficial bite of left forearm**

    ✓7ᵗʰ **S50.879 Other superficial bite of unspecified forearm**

✓5ᵗʰ **S50.9 Unspecified superficial injury of elbow and forearm**

✓6ᵗʰ **S50.90 Unspecified superficial injury of elbow**

    ✓7ᵗʰ **S50.901 Unspecified superficial injury of right elbow**

    ✓7ᵗʰ **S50.902 Unspecified superficial injury of left elbow**

    ✓7ᵗʰ **S50.909 Unspecified superficial injury of unspecified elbow**

✓6ᵗʰ **S50.91 Unspecified superficial injury of forearm**

    ✓7ᵗʰ **S50.911 Unspecified superficial injury of right forearm**

    ✓7ᵗʰ **S50.912 Unspecified superficial injury of left forearm**

    ✓7ᵗʰ **S50.919 Unspecified superficial injury of unspecified forearm**

√4ᵗʰ **S51 Open wound of elbow and forearm**

Code also any associated wound infection

EXCLUDES 1   *open fracture of elbow and forearm (S52.- with open fracture 7th character)*

traumatic amputation of elbow and forearm (S58.-)

EXCLUDES 2   *open wound of wrist and hand (S61.-)*

The appropriate 7th character is to be added to each code from category S51.

A   initial encounter
D   subsequent encounter
S   sequela

√5ᵗʰ **S51.0 Open wound of elbow**

√6ᵗʰ **S51.00 Unspecified open wound of elbow**

√7ᵗʰ **S51.001 Unspecified open wound of right elbow**

AHA: 2012,4Q,108

√7ᵗʰ **S51.002 Unspecified open wound of left elbow**

√7ᵗʰ **S51.009 Unspecified open wound of unspecified elbow**

Open wound of elbow NOS

√6ᵗʰ **S51.01 Laceration without foreign body of elbow**

√7ᵗʰ **S51.011 Laceration without foreign body of right elbow**

√7ᵗʰ **S51.012 Laceration without foreign body of left elbow**

√7ᵗʰ **S51.019 Laceration without foreign body of unspecified elbow**

√6ᵗʰ **S51.02 Laceration with foreign body of elbow**

√7ᵗʰ **S51.021 Laceration with foreign body of right elbow**

√7ᵗʰ **S51.022 Laceration with foreign body of left elbow**

√7ᵗʰ **S51.029 Laceration with foreign body of unspecified elbow**

√6ᵗʰ **S51.03 Puncture wound without foreign body of elbow**

√7ᵗʰ **S51.031 Puncture wound without foreign body of right elbow**

√7ᵗʰ **S51.032 Puncture wound without foreign body of left elbow**

√7ᵗʰ **S51.039 Puncture wound without foreign body of unspecified elbow**

√6ᵗʰ **S51.04 Puncture wound with foreign body of elbow**

√7ᵗʰ **S51.041 Puncture wound with foreign body of right elbow**

√7ᵗʰ **S51.042 Puncture wound with foreign body of left elbow**

√7ᵗʰ **S51.049 Puncture wound with foreign body of unspecified elbow**

√6ᵗʰ **S51.05 Open bite of elbow**

Bite of elbow NOS

EXCLUDES 1   *superficial bite of elbow (S50.36, S50.37)*

√7ᵗʰ **S51.051 Open bite, right elbow**

√7ᵗʰ **S51.052 Open bite, left elbow**

√7ᵗʰ **S51.059 Open bite, unspecified elbow**

√5ᵗʰ **S51.8 Open wound of forearm**

EXCLUDES 2   *open wound of elbow (S51.0-)*

√6ᵗʰ **S51.80 Unspecified open wound of forearm**

AHA: 2016,3Q,24

√7ᵗʰ **S51.801 Unspecified open wound of right forearm**

√7ᵗʰ **S51.802 Unspecified open wound of left forearm**

√7ᵗʰ **S51.809 Unspecified open wound of unspecified forearm**

Open wound of forearm NOS

√6ᵗʰ **S51.81 Laceration without foreign body of forearm**

√7ᵗʰ **S51.811 Laceration without foreign body of right forearm**

√7ᵗʰ **S51.812 Laceration without foreign body of left forearm**

√7ᵗʰ **S51.819 Laceration without foreign body of unspecified forearm**

√6ᵗʰ **S51.82 Laceration with foreign body of forearm**

√7ᵗʰ **S51.821 Laceration with foreign body of right forearm**

√7ᵗʰ **S51.822 Laceration with foreign body of left forearm**

√7ᵗʰ **S51.829 Laceration with foreign body of unspecified forearm**

√6ᵗʰ **S51.83 Puncture wound without foreign body of forearm**

AHA: 2016,3Q,24

√7ᵗʰ **S51.831 Puncture wound without foreign body of right forearm**

√7ᵗʰ **S51.832 Puncture wound without foreign body of left forearm**

√7ᵗʰ **S51.839 Puncture wound without foreign body of unspecified forearm**

√6ᵗʰ **S51.84 Puncture wound with foreign body of forearm**

AHA: 2016,3Q,24

√7ᵗʰ **S51.841 Puncture wound with foreign body of right forearm**

√7ᵗʰ **S51.842 Puncture wound with foreign body of left forearm**

√7ᵗʰ **S51.849 Puncture wound with foreign body of unspecified forearm**

√6ᵗʰ **S51.85 Open bite of forearm**

Bite of forearm NOS

EXCLUDES 1   *superficial bite of forearm (S50.86, S50.87)*

√7ᵗʰ **S51.851 Open bite of right forearm**

√7ᵗʰ **S51.852 Open bite of left forearm**

√7ᵗʰ **S51.859 Open bite of unspecified forearm**

☑ Additional Character Required   √x7ᵗʰ Placeholder   Unacceptable PDx   Questionable PDx   Manifestation   Unspecified Dx   H1-H14 HAC   HCC CMS-HCC Dx   HIV HIV Dx

ICD-10-CM 2020

1045

√4ᵗʰ **S52 Fracture of forearm**

NOTE A fracture not indicated as displaced or nondisplaced should be coded to displaced.

A fracture not indicated as open or closed should be coded to closed.

The open fracture designations are based on the Gustilo open fracture classification.

EXCLUDES 1 *traumatic amputation of forearm (S58.-)*
EXCLUDES 2 *fracture at wrist and hand level (S62.-)*

AHA: 2018,2Q,12; 2016,1Q,33; 2015,3Q,37-39
DEF: Diaphysis: Central shaft of a long bone.
DEF: Epiphysis: Proximal and distal rounded ends of a long bone, communicates with the joint.
DEF: Metaphysis: Section of a long bone located between the epiphysis and diaphysis at the proximal and distal ends.
DEF: Physis (growth plate): Narrow zone of cartilaginous tissue between the epiphysis and metaphysis at each end of a long bone. In childhood, proliferation of cells in this zone lengthens the bone. As the bone matures, this area thins, ossification eventually fusing into solid bone and growth stops. *Synonyms: Epiphyseal plate.*

The appropriate 7th character is to be added to all codes from category S52 [unless otherwise indicated].
A   initial encounter for closed fracture
B   initial encounter for open fracture type I or II
initial encounter for open fracture NOS
C   initial encounter for open fracture type IIIA, IIIB, or IIIC
D   subsequent encounter for closed fracture with routine healing
E   subsequent encounter for open fracture type I or II with routine healing
F   subsequent encounter for open fracture type IIIA, IIIB, or IIIC with routine healing
G   subsequent encounter for closed fracture with delayed healing
H   subsequent encounter for open fracture type I or II with delayed healing
J   subsequent encounter for open fracture type IIIA, IIIB, or IIIC with delayed healing
K   subsequent encounter for closed fracture with nonunion
M   subsequent encounter for open fracture type I or II with nonunion
N   subsequent encounter for open fracture type IIIA, IIIB, or IIIC with nonunion
P   subsequent encounter for closed fracture with malunion
Q   subsequent encounter for open fracture type I or II with malunion
R   subsequent encounter for open fracture type IIIA, IIIB, or IIIC with malunion
S   sequela

√5ᵗʰ **S52.0 Fracture of upper end of ulna**
Fracture of proximal end of ulna
EXCLUDES 2 *fracture of elbow NOS (S42.40-)*
fractures of shaft of ulna (S52.2-)

√6ᵗʰ **S52.00 Unspecified fracture of upper end of ulna**

CC Excl: For codes in subcategory S52.00:
MCC with 7th character B or C: PDX collection 1296
CC with 7th character K, M, N, P, Q, or R: PDX collection 897

2,4 √7ᵗʰ **S52.001 Unspecified fracture of upper end of right ulna** MCC CC H5

2,4 √7ᵗʰ **S52.002 Unspecified fracture of upper end of left ulna** MCC CC H5

2,4 √7ᵗʰ **S52.009 Unspecified fracture of upper end of unspecified ulna** MCC CC H5

√6ᵗʰ **S52.01 Torus fracture of upper end of ulna**

The appropriate 7th character is to be added to all codes in subcategory S52.01
A   initial encounter for closed fracture
D   subsequent encounter for fracture with routine healing
G   subsequent encounter for fracture with delayed healing
K   subsequent encounter for fracture with nonunion
P   subsequent encounter for fracture with malunion
S   sequela

3 √7ᵗʰ **S52.011 Torus fracture of upper end of right ulna** CC H5
CC Excl: CC with 7th character A: PDX collection 1270
CC Excl: CC with 7th character K or P: PDX collection 897

3 √7ᵗʰ **S52.012 Torus fracture of upper end of left ulna** CC H5
CC Excl: CC with 7th character A: PDX collection 1271
CC Excl: CC with 7th character K or P: PDX collection 897

3 √7ᵗʰ **S52.019 Torus fracture of upper end of unspecified ulna** CC H5
CC Excl: CC with 7th character A: PDX collection 1272
CC Excl: CC with 7th character K or P: PDX collection 897

√6ᵗʰ **S52.02 Fracture of olecranon process without intraarticular extension of ulna**
CC Excl: For codes in subcategory S52.02:
MCC with 7th character B or C: PDX collection 1273
CC with 7th character K, M, N, P, Q, or R: PDX collection 897

2,4 √7ᵗʰ **S52.021 Displaced fracture of olecranon process without intraarticular extension of right ulna** MCC CC H5

2,4 √7ᵗʰ **S52.022 Displaced fracture of olecranon process without intraarticular extension of left ulna** MCC CC H5

2,4 √7ᵗʰ **S52.023 Displaced fracture of olecranon process without intraarticular extension of unspecified ulna** MCC CC H5

2,4 √7ᵗʰ **S52.024 Nondisplaced fracture of olecranon process without intraarticular extension of right ulna** MCC CC H5

2,4 √7ᵗʰ **S52.025 Nondisplaced fracture of olecranon process without intraarticular extension of left ulna** MCC CC H5

2,4 √7ᵗʰ **S52.026 Nondisplaced fracture of olecranon process without intraarticular extension of unspecified ulna** MCC CC H5

√6ᵗʰ **S52.03 Fracture of olecranon process with intraarticular extension of ulna**
CC Excl: For codes in subcategory S52.03:
MCC with 7th character B or C: PDX collection 1273
CC with 7th character K, M, N, P, Q, or R: PDX collection 897

2,4 √7ᵗʰ **S52.031 Displaced fracture of olecranon process with intraarticular extension of right ulna** MCC CC H5

2,4 √7ᵗʰ **S52.032 Displaced fracture of olecranon process with intraarticular extension of left ulna** MCC CC H5

2,4 √7ᵗʰ **S52.033 Displaced fracture of olecranon process with intraarticular extension of unspecified ulna** MCC CC H5

2,4 √7ᵗʰ **S52.034 Nondisplaced fracture of olecranon process with intraarticular extension of right ulna** MCC CC H5

2,4 √7ᵗʰ **S52.035** Nondisplaced fracture of olecranon process with intraarticular extension of left ulna `MCC` `CC` `H5`

2,4 √7ᵗʰ **S52.036** Nondisplaced fracture of olecranon process with intraarticular extension of unspecified ulna `MCC` `CC` `H5`

√6ᵗʰ **S52.04** Fracture of coronoid process of ulna

> **CC Excl: For codes in subcategory S52.04:**
> **MCC with 7th character B or C:** PDX collection 1269
> **CC with 7th character K, M, N, P, Q, or R:** PDX collection 897

2,4 √7ᵗʰ **S52.041** Displaced fracture of coronoid process of right ulna `MCC` `CC` `H5`

2,4 √7ᵗʰ **S52.042** Displaced fracture of coronoid process of left ulna `MCC` `CC` `H5`

2,4 √7ᵗʰ **S52.043** Displaced fracture of coronoid process of unspecified ulna `MCC` `CC` `H5`

2,4 √7ᵗʰ **S52.044** Nondisplaced fracture of coronoid process of right ulna `MCC` `CC` `H5`

2,4 √7ᵗʰ **S52.045** Nondisplaced fracture of coronoid process of left ulna `MCC` `CC` `H5`

2,4 √7ᵗʰ **S52.046** Nondisplaced fracture of coronoid process of unspecified ulna `MCC` `CC` `H5`

√6ᵗʰ **S52.09** Other fracture of upper end of ulna

> **CC Excl: For codes in subcategory S52.09:**
> **MCC with 7th character B or C:** PDX collection 1269
> **CC with 7th character K, M, N, P, Q, or R:** PDX collection 897

2,4 √7ᵗʰ **S52.091** Other fracture of upper end of right ulna `MCC` `CC` `H5`

2,4 √7ᵗʰ **S52.092** Other fracture of upper end of left ulna `MCC` `CC` `H5`

2,4 √7ᵗʰ **S52.099** Other fracture of upper end of unspecified ulna `MCC` `CC` `H5`

√5ᵗʰ **S52.1** Fracture of upper end of radius

Fracture of proximal end of radius

> **EXCLUDES 2**   physeal fractures of upper end of radius (S59.2-)
> fracture of shaft of radius (S52.3-)

> **CC Excl: For codes in subcategory S52.1, unless otherwise noted:**
> **MCC with 7th character B or C:** PDX collection 1269
> **CC with 7th character K, M, N, P, Q, or R:** PDX collection 897

√6ᵗʰ **S52.10** Unspecified fracture of upper end of radius

2,4 √7ᵗʰ **S52.101** Unspecified fracture of upper end of right radius `MCC` `CC` `H5`

2,4 √7ᵗʰ **S52.102** Unspecified fracture of upper end of left radius `MCC` `CC` `H5`

2,4 √7ᵗʰ **S52.109** Unspecified fracture of upper end of unspecified radius `MCC` `CC` `H5`

√6ᵗʰ **S52.11** Torus fracture of upper end of radius

> The appropriate 7th character is to be added to all codes in subcategory S52.11
> A   initial encounter for closed fracture
> D   subsequent encounter for fracture with routine healing
> G   subsequent encounter for fracture with delayed healing
> K   subsequent encounter for fracture with nonunion
> P   subsequent encounter for fracture with malunion
> S   sequela

3 √7ᵗʰ **S52.111** Torus fracture of upper end of right radius `CC` `H5`
     CC Excl: CC with 7th character A: PDX collection 1270
     CC Excl: CC with 7th character K or P: PDX collection 897

3 √7ᵗʰ **S52.112** Torus fracture of upper end of left radius `CC` `H5`
     CC Excl: CC with 7th character A: PDX collection 1271
     CC Excl: CC with 7th character K or P: PDX collection 897

3 √7ᵗʰ **S52.119** Torus fracture of upper end of unspecified radius `CC` `H5`
     CC Excl: CC with 7th character A: PDX collection 1272
     CC Excl: CC with 7th character K or P: PDX collection 897

√6ᵗʰ **S52.12** Fracture of head of radius

2,4 √7ᵗʰ **S52.121** Displaced fracture of head of right radius `MCC` `CC` `H5`

2,4 √7ᵗʰ **S52.122** Displaced fracture of head of left radius `MCC` `CC` `H5`

2,4 √7ᵗʰ **S52.123** Displaced fracture of head of unspecified radius `MCC` `CC` `H5`

2,4 √7ᵗʰ **S52.124** Nondisplaced fracture of head of right radius `MCC` `CC` `H5`

2,4 √7ᵗʰ **S52.125** Nondisplaced fracture of head of left radius `MCC` `CC` `H5`

2,4 √7ᵗʰ **S52.126** Nondisplaced fracture of head of unspecified radius `MCC` `CC` `H5`

√6ᵗʰ **S52.13** Fracture of neck of radius

2,4 √7ᵗʰ **S52.131** Displaced fracture of neck of right radius `MCC` `CC` `H5`

2,4 √7ᵗʰ **S52.132** Displaced fracture of neck of left radius `MCC` `CC` `H5`

2,4 √7ᵗʰ **S52.133** Displaced fracture of neck of unspecified radius `MCC` `CC` `H5`

2,4 √7ᵗʰ **S52.134** Nondisplaced fracture of neck of right radius `MCC` `CC` `H5`

2,4 √7ᵗʰ **S52.135** Nondisplaced fracture of neck of left radius `MCC` `CC` `H5`

2,4 √7ᵗʰ **S52.136** Nondisplaced fracture of neck of unspecified radius `MCC` `CC` `H5`

√6ᵗʰ **S52.18** Other fracture of upper end of radius

2,4 √7ᵗʰ **S52.181** Other fracture of upper end of right radius `MCC` `CC` `H5`

2,4 √7ᵗʰ **S52.182** Other fracture of upper end of left radius `MCC` `CC` `H5`

2,4 √7ᵗʰ **S52.189** Other fracture of upper end of unspecified radius `MCC` `CC` `H5`

√5ᵗʰ **S52.2** Fracture of shaft of ulna

> **CC Excl: For CC/MCC codes in subcategory S52.2, unless otherwise noted:**
> **Right side:** See code S52.201
> **Left side:** See code S52.202
> **Unspecified side:** See code S52.209

√6ᵗʰ **S52.20** Unspecified fracture of shaft of ulna

Fracture of ulna NOS

2,3 √7ᵗʰ **S52.201** Unspecified fracture of shaft of right ulna `MCC` `CC` `H5`
     CC Excl: CC with 7th character A: PDX collection 1270
     CC Excl: MCC with 7th character B or C: PDX collection 1269
     CC Excl: CC with 7th character K, M, N, P, Q, or R: PDX collection 897

2,3 √7ᵗʰ **S52.202** Unspecified fracture of shaft of left ulna `MCC` `CC` `H5`
     CC Excl: CC with 7th character A: PDX collection 1271
     CC Excl: MCC with 7th character B or C: PDX collection 1269
     CC Excl: CC with 7th character K, M, N, P, Q, or R: PDX collection 897

2,3 √7ᵗʰ **S52.209** Unspecified fracture of shaft of unspecified ulna `MCC` `CC` `H5`
     CC Excl: CC with 7th character A: PDX collection 1272
     CC Excl: MCC with 7th character B or C: PDX collection 1269
     CC Excl: CC with 7th character K, M, N, P, Q, or R: PDX collection 897

☑ Additional Character Required   √x7ᵗʰ Placeholder   Unacceptable PDx   Questionable PDx   Manifestation   Unspecified Dx   `H1`-`H14` HAC   `HCC` CMS-HCC Dx   `HIV` HIV Dx

ICD-10-CM 2020   **1047**

√6ᵗʰ **S52.21**   **Greenstick fracture of shaft of ulna**

> The appropriate 7th character is to be added to all codes in subcategory S52.21
> A   initial encounter for closed fracture
> D   subsequent encounter for fracture with routine healing
> G   subsequent encounter for fracture with delayed healing
> K   subsequent encounter for fracture with nonunion
> P   subsequent encounter for fracture with malunion
> S   sequela

3 √7ᵗʰ **S52.211**   **Greenstick fracture of shaft of right ulna**   CC H5
> **CC Excl: CC with 7th character A:** PDX collection 1270
> **CC Excl: CC with 7th character K or P:** PDX collection 897

3 √7ᵗʰ **S52.212**   **Greenstick fracture of shaft of left ulna**   CC H5
> **CC Excl: CC with 7th character A:** PDX collection 1271
> **CC Excl: CC with 7th character K or P:** PDX collection 897

3 √7ᵗʰ **S52.219**   **Greenstick fracture of shaft of unspecified ulna**   CC H5
> **CC Excl: CC with 7th character A:** PDX collection 1272
> **CC Excl: CC with 7th character K or P:** PDX collection 897

√6ᵗʰ **S52.22**   **Transverse fracture of shaft of ulna**

2,3 √7ᵗʰ **S52.221**   **Displaced transverse fracture of shaft of right ulna**   MCC CC H5

2,3 √7ᵗʰ **S52.222**   **Displaced transverse fracture of shaft of left ulna**   MCC CC H5

2,3 √7ᵗʰ **S52.223**   **Displaced transverse fracture of shaft of unspecified ulna**   MCC CC H5

2,3 √7ᵗʰ **S52.224**   **Nondisplaced transverse fracture of shaft of right ulna**   MCC CC H5

2,3 √7ᵗʰ **S52.225**   **Nondisplaced transverse fracture of shaft of left ulna**   MCC CC H5

2,3 √7ᵗʰ **S52.226**   **Nondisplaced transverse fracture of shaft of unspecified ulna**   MCC CC H5

√6ᵗʰ **S52.23**   **Oblique fracture of shaft of ulna**

2,3 √7ᵗʰ **S52.231**   **Displaced oblique fracture of shaft of right ulna**   MCC CC H5

2,3 √7ᵗʰ **S52.232**   **Displaced oblique fracture of shaft of left ulna**   MCC CC H5

2,3 √7ᵗʰ **S52.233**   **Displaced oblique fracture of shaft of unspecified ulna**   MCC CC H5

2,3 √7ᵗʰ **S52.234**   **Nondisplaced oblique fracture of shaft of right ulna**   MCC CC H5

2,3 √7ᵗʰ **S52.235**   **Nondisplaced oblique fracture of shaft of left ulna**   MCC CC H5

2,3 √7ᵗʰ **S52.236**   **Nondisplaced oblique fracture of shaft of unspecified ulna**   MCC CC H5

√6ᵗʰ **S52.24**   **Spiral fracture of shaft of ulna**

2,3 √7ᵗʰ **S52.241**   **Displaced spiral fracture of shaft of ulna, right arm**   MCC CC H5

2,3 √7ᵗʰ **S52.242**   **Displaced spiral fracture of shaft of ulna, left arm**   MCC CC H5

2,3 √7ᵗʰ **S52.243**   **Displaced spiral fracture of shaft of ulna, unspecified arm**   MCC CC H5

2,3 √7ᵗʰ **S52.244**   **Nondisplaced spiral fracture of shaft of ulna, right arm**   MCC CC H5

2,3 √7ᵗʰ **S52.245**   **Nondisplaced spiral fracture of shaft of ulna, left arm**   MCC CC H5

2,3 √7ᵗʰ **S52.246**   **Nondisplaced spiral fracture of shaft of ulna, unspecified arm**   MCC CC H5

√6ᵗʰ **S52.25**   **Comminuted fracture of shaft of ulna**

2,3 √7ᵗʰ **S52.251**   **Displaced comminuted fracture of shaft of ulna, right arm**   MCC CC H5

2,3 √7ᵗʰ **S52.252**   **Displaced comminuted fracture of shaft of ulna, left arm**   MCC CC H5

2,3 √7ᵗʰ **S52.253**   **Displaced comminuted fracture of shaft of ulna, unspecified arm**   MCC CC H5

2,3 √7ᵗʰ **S52.254**   **Nondisplaced comminuted fracture of shaft of ulna, right arm**   MCC CC H5

2,3 √7ᵗʰ **S52.255**   **Nondisplaced comminuted fracture of shaft of ulna, left arm**   MCC CC H5

2,3 √7ᵗʰ **S52.256**   **Nondisplaced comminuted fracture of shaft of ulna, unspecified arm**   MCC CC H5

√6ᵗʰ **S52.26**   **Segmental fracture of shaft of ulna**

2,3 √7ᵗʰ **S52.261**   **Displaced segmental fracture of shaft of ulna, right arm**   MCC CC H5

2,3 √7ᵗʰ **S52.262**   **Displaced segmental fracture of shaft of ulna, left arm**   MCC CC H5

2,3 √7ᵗʰ **S52.263**   **Displaced segmental fracture of shaft of ulna, unspecified arm**   MCC CC H5

2,3 √7ᵗʰ **S52.264**   **Nondisplaced segmental fracture of shaft of ulna, right arm**   MCC CC H5

2,3 √7ᵗʰ **S52.265**   **Nondisplaced segmental fracture of shaft of ulna, left arm**   MCC CC H5

2,3 √7ᵗʰ **S52.266**   **Nondisplaced segmental fracture of shaft of ulna, unspecified arm**   MCC CC H5

√6ᵗʰ **S52.27**   **Monteggia's fracture of ulna**

> Fracture of upper shaft of ulna with dislocation of radial head
> **CC Excl: For codes in subcategory S52.27:**
> **MCC with 7th character B or C:** PDX collection 1269
> **CC with 7th character K, M, N, P, Q, or R:** PDX collection 897

2,4 √7ᵗʰ **S52.271**   **Monteggia's fracture of right ulna**   MCC CC H5

2,4 √7ᵗʰ **S52.272**   **Monteggia's fracture of left ulna**   MCC CC H5

2,4 √7ᵗʰ **S52.279**   **Monteggia's fracture of unspecified ulna**   MCC CC H5

√6ᵗʰ **S52.28**   **Bent bone of ulna**

2,3 √7ᵗʰ **S52.281**   **Bent bone of right ulna**   MCC CC H5

2,3 √7ᵗʰ **S52.282**   **Bent bone of left ulna**   MCC CC H5

2,3 √7ᵗʰ **S52.283**   **Bent bone of unspecified ulna**   MCC CC H5

√6ᵗʰ **S52.29**   **Other fracture of shaft of ulna**

2,3 √7ᵗʰ **S52.291**   **Other fracture of shaft of right ulna**   MCC CC H5

2,3 √7ᵗʰ **S52.292**   **Other fracture of shaft of left ulna**   MCC CC H5

2,3 √7ᵗʰ **S52.299**   **Other fracture of shaft of unspecified ulna**   MCC CC H5

√5ᵗʰ **S52.3**   **Fracture of shaft of radius**

> **CC Excl: For CC/MCC codes in subcategory S52.3, unless otherwise noted:**
> **Right side:** See code S52.201
> **Left side:** See code S52.202
> **Unspecified side:** See code S52.209

√6ᵗʰ **S52.30**   **Unspecified fracture of shaft of radius**

2,3 √7ᵗʰ **S52.301**   **Unspecified fracture of shaft of right radius**   MCC CC H5

2,3 √7ᵗʰ **S52.302**   **Unspecified fracture of shaft of left radius**   MCC CC H5

2,3 √7ᵗʰ **S52.309**   **Unspecified fracture of shaft of unspecified radius**   MCC CC H5

N Newborn: 0   P Pediatric: 0-17   M Maternity: 9-64   A Adult: 15-124   MCC Major Complication/Comorbidity   CC Complication/Comorbidity   SW Severe Wound Dx

1048   ICD-10-CM 2020

√6th **S52.31**   **Greenstick** fracture of shaft of radius

> The appropriate 7th character is to be added to all codes in subcategory S52.31.
> A   initial encounter for closed fracture
> D   subsequent encounter for fracture with routine healing
> G   subsequent encounter for fracture with delayed healing
> K   subsequent encounter for fracture with nonunion
> P   subsequent encounter for fracture with malunion
> S   sequela

3 √7th **S52.311**   **Greenstick** fracture of shaft of radius, **right arm**   CC H5
    CC Excl: See code S52.211

3 √7th **S52.312**   **Greenstick** fracture of shaft of radius, **left arm**   CC H5
    CC Excl: See code S52.212

3 √7th **S52.319**   **Greenstick** fracture of shaft of radius, **unspecified arm**   CC H5
    CC Excl: See code S52.219

√6th **S52.32**   **Transverse** fracture of shaft of radius

2,3 √7th **S52.321**   **Displaced transverse** fracture of shaft of **right radius**   MCC CC H5

2,3 √7th **S52.322**   **Displaced transverse** fracture of shaft of **left radius**   MCC CC H5

2,3 √7th **S52.323**   **Displaced transverse** fracture of shaft of **unspecified radius**   MCC CC H5

2,3 √7th **S52.324**   **Nondisplaced transverse** fracture of shaft of **right radius**   MCC CC H5

2,3 √7th **S52.325**   **Nondisplaced transverse** fracture of shaft of **left radius**   MCC CC H5

2,3 √7th **S52.326**   **Nondisplaced transverse** fracture of shaft of **unspecified radius**   MCC CC H5

√6th **S52.33**   **Oblique** fracture of shaft of radius

2,3 √7th **S52.331**   **Displaced oblique** fracture of shaft of **right radius**   MCC CC H5

2,3 √7th **S52.332**   **Displaced oblique** fracture of shaft of **left radius**   MCC CC H5

2,3 √7th **S52.333**   **Displaced oblique** fracture of shaft of **unspecified radius**   MCC CC H5

2,3 √7th **S52.334**   **Nondisplaced oblique** fracture of shaft of **right radius**   MCC CC H5

2,3 √7th **S52.335**   **Nondisplaced oblique** fracture of shaft of **left radius**   MCC CC H5

2,3 √7th **S52.336**   **Nondisplaced oblique** fracture of shaft of **unspecified radius**   MCC CC H5

√6th **S52.34**   **Spiral** fracture of shaft of radius

2,3 √7th **S52.341**   **Displaced spiral** fracture of shaft of radius, **right arm**   MCC CC H5

2,3 √7th **S52.342**   **Displaced spiral** fracture of shaft of radius, **left arm**   MCC CC H5

2,3 √7th **S52.343**   **Displaced spiral** fracture of shaft of radius, **unspecified arm**   MCC CC H5

2,3 √7th **S52.344**   **Nondisplaced spiral** fracture of shaft of radius, **right arm**   MCC CC H5

2,3 √7th **S52.345**   **Nondisplaced spiral** fracture of shaft of radius, **left arm**   MCC CC H5

2,3 √7th **S52.346**   **Nondisplaced spiral** fracture of shaft of radius, **unspecified arm**   MCC CC H5

√6th **S52.35**   **Comminuted** fracture of shaft of radius

2,3 √7th **S52.351**   **Displaced comminuted** fracture of shaft of radius, **right arm**   MCC CC H5

2,3 √7th **S52.352**   **Displaced comminuted** fracture of shaft of radius, **left arm**   MCC CC H5

2,3 √7th **S52.353**   **Displaced comminuted** fracture of shaft of radius, **unspecified arm**   MCC CC H5

2,3 √7th **S52.354**   **Nondisplaced comminuted** fracture of shaft of radius, **right arm**   MCC CC H5

2,3 √7th **S52.355**   **Nondisplaced comminuted** fracture of shaft of radius, **left arm**   MCC CC H5

2,3 √7th **S52.356**   **Nondisplaced comminuted** fracture of shaft of radius, **unspecified arm**   MCC CC H5

√6th **S52.36**   **Segmental** fracture of shaft of radius

2,3 √7th **S52.361**   **Displaced segmental** fracture of shaft of radius, **right arm**   MCC CC H5

2,3 √7th **S52.362**   **Displaced segmental** fracture of shaft of radius, **left arm**   MCC CC H5

2,3 √7th **S52.363**   **Displaced segmental** fracture of shaft of radius, **unspecified arm**   MCC CC H5

2,3 √7th **S52.364**   **Nondisplaced segmental** fracture of shaft of radius, **right arm**   MCC CC H5

2,3 √7th **S52.365**   **Nondisplaced segmental** fracture of shaft of radius, **left arm**   MCC CC H5

2,3 √7th **S52.366**   **Nondisplaced segmental** fracture of shaft of radius, **unspecified arm**   MCC CC H5

√6th **S52.37**   **Galeazzi's** fracture

> Fracture of lower shaft of radius with radioulnar joint dislocation

2,3 √7th **S52.371**   **Galeazzi's** fracture of **right radius**   MCC CC H5

2,3 √7th **S52.372**   **Galeazzi's** fracture of **left radius**   MCC CC H5

2,3 √7th **S52.379**   **Galeazzi's** fracture of **unspecified radius**   MCC CC H5

√6th **S52.38**   **Bent bone** of radius

2,3 √7th **S52.381**   **Bent bone** of **right radius**   MCC CC H5

2,3 √7th **S52.382**   **Bent bone** of **left radius**   MCC CC H5

2,3 √7th **S52.389**   **Bent bone** of **unspecified radius**   MCC CC H5

√6th **S52.39**   **Other** fracture of shaft of radius

2,3 √7th **S52.391**   **Other** fracture of shaft of radius, **right arm**   MCC CC H5

2,3 √7th **S52.392**   **Other** fracture of shaft of radius, **left arm**   MCC CC H5

2,3 √7th **S52.399**   **Other** fracture of shaft of radius, **unspecified arm**   MCC CC H5

√5th **S52.5**   Fracture of lower end of radius

> Fracture of distal end of radius
>
> **EXCLUDES 2**   *physeal fractures of lower end of radius (S59.2-)*
>
> **DEF:** Fracture of the distal end of the radius above the wrist, most commonly caused by a fall onto an outstretched hand.
>
> **CC Excl: For CC/MCC codes in subcategory S52.5, unless otherwise noted:**
> **Right side:** See code S52.201
> **Left side:** See code S52.202
> **Unspecified side:** See code S52.209

√6th **S52.50**   **Unspecified** fracture of the lower end of radius

2,3 √7th **S52.501**   **Unspecified** fracture of the lower end of **right radius**   MCC CC H5

2,3 √7th **S52.502**   **Unspecified** fracture of the lower end of **left radius**   MCC CC H5

2,3 √7th **S52.509**   **Unspecified** fracture of the lower end of **unspecified radius**   MCC CC H5

√6th **S52.51**   Fracture of radial styloid process

2,3 √7th **S52.511**   **Displaced** fracture of **right radial styloid process**   MCC CC H5

2,3 √7th **S52.512**   **Displaced** fracture of **left radial styloid process**   MCC CC H5

Chapter 19. Injury, Poisoning and Certain Other Consequences of External Causes

S52.513–S52.92

2,3 √7th **S52.513** **Displaced** fracture of unspecified radial styloid process `MCC` `CC` `H5`

2,3 √7th **S52.514** **Nondisplaced** fracture of right radial styloid process `MCC` `CC` `H5`

2,3 √7th **S52.515** **Nondisplaced** fracture of left radial styloid process `MCC` `CC` `H5`

2,3 √7th **S52.516** **Nondisplaced** fracture of unspecified radial styloid process `MCC` `CC` `H5`

√6th **S52.52** **Torus** fracture of lower end of radius

The appropriate 7th character is to be added to all codes in subcategory S52.52.
A initial encounter for closed fracture
D subsequent encounter for fracture with routine healing
G subsequent encounter for fracture with delayed healing
K subsequent encounter for fracture with nonunion
P subsequent encounter for fracture with malunion
S sequela

3 √7th **S52.521** **Torus fracture of lower end of right radius** `CC` `H5`
CC Excl: See code S52.211

3 √7th **S52.522** **Torus fracture of lower end of left radius** `CC` `H5`
CC Excl: See code S52.212

3 √7th **S52.529** **Torus fracture of lower end of unspecified radius** `CC` `H5`
CC Excl: See code S52.219

√6th **S52.53** **Colles' fracture**
AHA: 2016,2Q,4
DEF: Fracture of the radius at the wrist in which the distal fragment is pushed posteriorly. The dorsal angulation of the fragment results in the wrist cocking up.

2,3 √7th **S52.531** **Colles' fracture of right radius** `MCC` `CC` `H5`

2,3 √7th **S52.532** **Colles' fracture of left radius** `MCC` `CC` `H5`

2,3 √7th **S52.539** **Colles' fracture of unspecified radius** `MCC` `CC` `H5`

√6th **S52.54** **Smith's fracture**

2,3 √7th **S52.541** **Smith's fracture of right radius** `MCC` `CC` `H5`

2,3 √7th **S52.542** **Smith's fracture of left radius** `MCC` `CC` `H5`

2,3 √7th **S52.549** **Smith's fracture of unspecified radius** `MCC` `CC` `H5`

√6th **S52.55** **Other extraarticular** fracture of lower end of radius

2,3 √7th **S52.551** **Other extraarticular fracture of lower end of right radius** `MCC` `CC` `H5`

2,3 √7th **S52.552** **Other extraarticular fracture of lower end of left radius** `MCC` `CC` `H5`

2,3 √7th **S52.559** **Other extraarticular fracture of lower end of unspecified radius** `MCC` `CC` `H5`

√6th **S52.56** **Barton's fracture**

2,3 √7th **S52.561** **Barton's fracture of right radius** `MCC` `CC` `H5`

2,3 √7th **S52.562** **Barton's fracture of left radius** `MCC` `CC` `H5`

2,3 √7th **S52.569** **Barton's fracture of unspecified radius** `MCC` `CC` `H5`

√6th **S52.57** **Other intraarticular** fracture of lower end of radius

2,3 √7th **S52.571** **Other intraarticular fracture of lower end of right radius** `MCC` `CC` `H5`

2,3 √7th **S52.572** **Other intraarticular fracture of lower end of left radius** `MCC` `CC` `H5`

2,3 √7th **S52.579** **Other intraarticular fracture of lower end of unspecified radius** `MCC` `CC` `H5`

√6th **S52.59** **Other fractures of lower end of radius**

2,3 √7th **S52.591** **Other fractures of lower end of right radius** `MCC` `CC` `H5`

2,3 √7th **S52.592** **Other fractures of lower end of left radius** `MCC` `CC` `H5`

2,3 √7th **S52.599** **Other fractures of lower end of unspecified radius** `MCC` `CC` `H5`

√5th **S52.6** **Fracture of lower end of ulna**

CC Excl: For CC/MCC codes in subcategory S52.6, unless otherwise noted:
Right side: See code S52.201
Left side: See code S52.202
Unspecified side: See code S52.209

√6th **S52.60** **Unspecified fracture of lower end of ulna**

2,3 √7th **S52.601** **Unspecified fracture of lower end of right ulna** `MCC` `CC` `H5`

2,3 √7th **S52.602** **Unspecified fracture of lower end of left ulna** `MCC` `CC` `H5`

2,3 √7th **S52.609** **Unspecified fracture of lower end of unspecified ulna** `MCC` `CC` `H5`

√6th **S52.61** **Fracture of ulna styloid process**

2,3 √7th **S52.611** **Displaced fracture of right ulna styloid process** `MCC` `CC` `H5`

2,3 √7th **S52.612** **Displaced fracture of left ulna styloid process** `MCC` `CC` `H5`

2,3 √7th **S52.613** **Displaced fracture of unspecified ulna styloid process** `MCC` `CC` `H5`

2,3 √7th **S52.614** **Nondisplaced fracture of right ulna styloid process** `MCC` `CC` `H5`

2,3 √7th **S52.615** **Nondisplaced fracture of left ulna styloid process** `MCC` `CC` `H5`

2,3 √7th **S52.616** **Nondisplaced fracture of unspecified ulna styloid process** `MCC` `CC` `H5`

√6th **S52.62** **Torus** fracture of lower end of ulna

The appropriate 7th character is to be added to all codes in subcategory S52.62.
A initial encounter for closed fracture
D subsequent encounter for fracture with routine healing
G subsequent encounter for fracture with delayed healing
K subsequent encounter for fracture with nonunion
P subsequent encounter for fracture with malunion
S sequela

3 √7th **S52.621** **Torus fracture of lower end of right ulna** `CC` `H5`
CC Excl: See code S52.211

3 √7th **S52.622** **Torus fracture of lower end of left ulna** `CC` `H5`
CC Excl: See code S52.212

3 √7th **S52.629** **Torus fracture of lower end of unspecified ulna** `CC` `H5`
CC Excl: See code S52.219

√6th **S52.69** **Other fracture of lower end of ulna**

2,3 √7th **S52.691** **Other fracture of lower end of right ulna** `MCC` `CC` `H5`

2,3 √7th **S52.692** **Other fracture of lower end of left ulna** `MCC` `CC` `H5`

2,3 √7th **S52.699** **Other fracture of lower end of unspecified ulna** `MCC` `CC` `H5`

√5th **S52.9** **Unspecified fracture of forearm**

CC Excl: For CC/MCC codes in subcategory S52.9: See code S52.209

2,3 √x7th **S52.90** **Unspecified fracture of unspecified forearm** `MCC` `CC` `H5`

2,3 √x7th **S52.91** **Unspecified fracture of right forearm** `MCC` `CC` `H5`

2,3 √x7th **S52.92** **Unspecified fracture of left forearm** `MCC` `CC` `H5`

√4th S53 Dislocation and sprain of joints and ligaments of elbow

INCLUDES   avulsion of joint or ligament of elbow
laceration of cartilage, joint or ligament of elbow
sprain of cartilage, joint or ligament of elbow
traumatic hemarthrosis of joint or ligament of elbow
traumatic rupture of joint or ligament of elbow
traumatic subluxation of joint or ligament of elbow
traumatic tear of joint or ligament of elbow
Code also any associated open wound
EXCLUDES 2   strain of muscle, fascia and tendon at forearm level (S56.-)

The appropriate 7th character is to be added to each code from category S53.
A   initial encounter
D   subsequent encounter
S   sequela

√5th S53.0   Subluxation and dislocation of radial head
Dislocation of radiohumeral joint
Subluxation of radiohumeral joint
EXCLUDES 1   Monteggia's fracture-dislocation (S52.27-)

√6th S53.00   Unspecified subluxation and dislocation of radial head
√7th **S53.001** Unspecified subluxation of right radial head
√7th **S53.002** Unspecified subluxation of left radial head
√7th **S53.003** Unspecified subluxation of unspecified radial head
√7th **S53.004** Unspecified dislocation of right radial head
√7th **S53.005** Unspecified dislocation of left radial head
√7th **S53.006** Unspecified dislocation of unspecified radial head

√6th S53.01   Anterior subluxation and dislocation of radial head
Anteriomedial subluxation and dislocation of radial head
√7th **S53.011** Anterior subluxation of right radial head
√7th **S53.012** Anterior subluxation of left radial head
√7th **S53.013** Anterior subluxation of unspecified radial head
√7th **S53.014** Anterior dislocation of right radial head
√7th **S53.015** Anterior dislocation of left radial head
√7th **S53.016** Anterior dislocation of unspecified radial head

√6th S53.02   Posterior subluxation and dislocation of radial head
Posteriolateral subluxation and dislocation of radial head
√7th **S53.021** Posterior subluxation of right radial head
√7th **S53.022** Posterior subluxation of left radial head
√7th **S53.023** Posterior subluxation of unspecified radial head
√7th **S53.024** Posterior dislocation of right radial head
√7th **S53.025** Posterior dislocation of left radial head
√7th **S53.026** Posterior dislocation of unspecified radial head

√6th S53.03   Nursemaid's elbow
√7th **S53.031** Nursemaid's elbow, right elbow
√7th **S53.032** Nursemaid's elbow, left elbow
√7th **S53.033** Nursemaid's elbow, unspecified elbow

√6th S53.09   Other subluxation and dislocation of radial head
√7th **S53.091** Other subluxation of right radial head
√7th **S53.092** Other subluxation of left radial head
√7th **S53.093** Other subluxation of unspecified radial head
√7th **S53.094** Other dislocation of right radial head
√7th **S53.095** Other dislocation of left radial head
√7th **S53.096** Other dislocation of unspecified radial head

√5th S53.1   Subluxation and dislocation of ulnohumeral joint
Subluxation and dislocation of elbow NOS
EXCLUDES 1   dislocation of radial head alone (S53.0-)

√6th S53.10   Unspecified subluxation and dislocation of ulnohumeral joint
√7th **S53.101** Unspecified subluxation of right ulnohumeral joint
√7th **S53.102** Unspecified subluxation of left ulnohumeral joint
√7th **S53.103** Unspecified subluxation of unspecified ulnohumeral joint
√7th **S53.104** Unspecified dislocation of right ulnohumeral joint
√7th **S53.105** Unspecified dislocation of left ulnohumeral joint
√7th **S53.106** Unspecified dislocation of unspecified ulnohumeral joint

√6th S53.11   Anterior subluxation and dislocation of ulnohumeral joint
√7th **S53.111** Anterior subluxation of right ulnohumeral joint
√7th **S53.112** Anterior subluxation of left ulnohumeral joint
√7th **S53.113** Anterior subluxation of unspecified ulnohumeral joint
√7th **S53.114** Anterior dislocation of right ulnohumeral joint
AHA: 2012,4Q,108
√7th **S53.115** Anterior dislocation of left ulnohumeral joint
√7th **S53.116** Anterior dislocation of unspecified ulnohumeral joint

√6th S53.12   Posterior subluxation and dislocation of ulnohumeral joint
√7th **S53.121** Posterior subluxation of right ulnohumeral joint
√7th **S53.122** Posterior subluxation of left ulnohumeral joint
√7th **S53.123** Posterior subluxation of unspecified ulnohumeral joint
√7th **S53.124** Posterior dislocation of right ulnohumeral joint
√7th **S53.125** Posterior dislocation of left ulnohumeral joint
√7th **S53.126** Posterior dislocation of unspecified ulnohumeral joint

√6th S53.13   Medial subluxation and dislocation of ulnohumeral joint
√7th **S53.131** Medial subluxation of right ulnohumeral joint
√7th **S53.132** Medial subluxation of left ulnohumeral joint
√7th **S53.133** Medial subluxation of unspecified ulnohumeral joint
√7th **S53.134** Medial dislocation of right ulnohumeral joint
√7th **S53.135** Medial dislocation of left ulnohumeral joint
√7th **S53.136** Medial dislocation of unspecified ulnohumeral joint

√6th S53.14   Lateral subluxation and dislocation of ulnohumeral joint
√7th **S53.141** Lateral subluxation of right ulnohumeral joint
√7th **S53.142** Lateral subluxation of left ulnohumeral joint
√7th **S53.143** Lateral subluxation of unspecified ulnohumeral joint
√7th **S53.144** Lateral dislocation of right ulnohumeral joint
√7th **S53.145** Lateral dislocation of left ulnohumeral joint
√7th **S53.146** Lateral dislocation of unspecified ulnohumeral joint

√6th S53.19   Other subluxation and dislocation of ulnohumeral joint
√7th **S53.191** Other subluxation of right ulnohumeral joint
√7th **S53.192** Other subluxation of left ulnohumeral joint
√7th **S53.193** Other subluxation of unspecified ulnohumeral joint
√7th **S53.194** Other dislocation of right ulnohumeral joint
√7th **S53.195** Other dislocation of left ulnohumeral joint
√7th **S53.196** Other dislocation of unspecified ulnohumeral joint

Chapter 19. Injury, Poisoning and Certain Other Consequences of External Causes

√5ᵗʰ **S53.2** **Traumatic rupture of radial collateral ligament**

     EXCLUDES 1   *sprain of radial collateral ligament NOS (S53.43-)*

    √x7ᵗʰ **S53.20** **Traumatic rupture of unspecified radial collateral ligament**

    √x7ᵗʰ **S53.21** **Traumatic rupture of right radial collateral ligament**

    √x7ᵗʰ **S53.22** **Traumatic rupture of left radial collateral ligament**

√5ᵗʰ **S53.3** **Traumatic rupture of ulnar collateral ligament**

     EXCLUDES 1   *sprain of ulnar collateral ligament (S53.44-)*

    √x7ᵗʰ **S53.30** **Traumatic rupture of unspecified ulnar collateral ligament**

    √x7ᵗʰ **S53.31** **Traumatic rupture of right ulnar collateral ligament**

    √x7ᵗʰ **S53.32** **Traumatic rupture of left ulnar collateral ligament**

√5ᵗʰ **S53.4** **Sprain of elbow**

     EXCLUDES 2   *traumatic rupture of radial collateral ligament (S53.2-)*

          traumatic rupture of ulnar collateral ligament (S53.3-)

   √6ᵗʰ **S53.40** **Unspecified sprain of elbow**

     √7ᵗʰ **S53.401** **Unspecified sprain of right elbow**

     √7ᵗʰ **S53.402** **Unspecified sprain of left elbow**

     √7ᵗʰ **S53.409** **Unspecified sprain of unspecified elbow**

         Sprain of elbow NOS

   √6ᵗʰ **S53.41** **Radiohumeral (joint) sprain**

     √7ᵗʰ **S53.411** **Radiohumeral (joint) sprain of right elbow**

     √7ᵗʰ **S53.412** **Radiohumeral (joint) sprain of left elbow**

     √7ᵗʰ **S53.419** **Radiohumeral (joint) sprain of unspecified elbow**

   √6ᵗʰ **S53.42** **Ulnohumeral (joint) sprain**

     √7ᵗʰ **S53.421** **Ulnohumeral (joint) sprain of right elbow**

     √7ᵗʰ **S53.422** **Ulnohumeral (joint) sprain of left elbow**

     √7ᵗʰ **S53.429** **Ulnohumeral (joint) sprain of unspecified elbow**

   √6ᵗʰ **S53.43** **Radial collateral ligament sprain**

     √7ᵗʰ **S53.431** **Radial collateral ligament sprain of right elbow**

     √7ᵗʰ **S53.432** **Radial collateral ligament sprain of left elbow**

     √7ᵗʰ **S53.439** **Radial collateral ligament sprain of unspecified elbow**

   √6ᵗʰ **S53.44** **Ulnar collateral ligament sprain**

     √7ᵗʰ **S53.441** **Ulnar collateral ligament sprain of right elbow**

     √7ᵗʰ **S53.442** **Ulnar collateral ligament sprain of left elbow**

     √7ᵗʰ **S53.449** **Ulnar collateral ligament sprain of unspecified elbow**

   √6ᵗʰ **S53.49** **Other sprain of elbow**

     √7ᵗʰ **S53.491** **Other sprain of right elbow**

     √7ᵗʰ **S53.492** **Other sprain of left elbow**

     √7ᵗʰ **S53.499** **Other sprain of unspecified elbow**

√4ᵗʰ **S54** **Injury of nerves at forearm level**

    Code also any associated open wound (S51.-)

     EXCLUDES 2   *injury of nerves at wrist and hand level (S64.-)*

    The appropriate 7th character is to be added to each code from category S54.
    A   initial encounter
    D   subsequent encounter
    S   sequela

√5ᵗʰ **S54.0** **Injury of ulnar nerve at forearm level**

     Injury of ulnar nerve NOS

   √x7ᵗʰ **S54.00** **Injury of ulnar nerve at forearm level, unspecified arm**

   √x7ᵗʰ **S54.01** **Injury of ulnar nerve at forearm level, right arm**

   √x7ᵗʰ **S54.02** **Injury of ulnar nerve at forearm level, left arm**

√5ᵗʰ **S54.1** **Injury of median nerve at forearm level**

     Injury of median nerve NOS

   √x7ᵗʰ **S54.10** **Injury of median nerve at forearm level, unspecified arm**

   √x7ᵗʰ **S54.11** **Injury of median nerve at forearm level, right arm**

   √x7ᵗʰ **S54.12** **Injury of median nerve at forearm level, left arm**

√5ᵗʰ **S54.2** **Injury of radial nerve at forearm level**

     Injury of radial nerve NOS

   √x7ᵗʰ **S54.20** **Injury of radial nerve at forearm level, unspecified arm**

   √x7ᵗʰ **S54.21** **Injury of radial nerve at forearm level, right arm**

   √x7ᵗʰ **S54.22** **Injury of radial nerve at forearm level, left arm**

√5ᵗʰ **S54.3** **Injury of cutaneous sensory nerve at forearm level**

   √x7ᵗʰ **S54.30** **Injury of cutaneous sensory nerve at forearm level, unspecified arm**

   √x7ᵗʰ **S54.31** **Injury of cutaneous sensory nerve at forearm level, right arm**

   √x7ᵗʰ **S54.32** **Injury of cutaneous sensory nerve at forearm level, left arm**

√5ᵗʰ **S54.8** **Injury of other nerves at forearm level**

   √6ᵗʰ **S54.8X** **Injury of other nerves at forearm level**

     √7ᵗʰ **S54.8X1** **Injury of other nerves at forearm level, right arm**

     √7ᵗʰ **S54.8X2** **Injury of other nerves at forearm level, left arm**

     √7ᵗʰ **S54.8X9** **Injury of other nerves at forearm level, unspecified arm**

√5ᵗʰ **S54.9** **Injury of unspecified nerve at forearm level**

   √x7ᵗʰ **S54.90** **Injury of unspecified nerve at forearm level, unspecified arm**

   √x7ᵗʰ **S54.91** **Injury of unspecified nerve at forearm level, right arm**

   √x7ᵗʰ **S54.92** **Injury of unspecified nerve at forearm level, left arm**

√4ᵗʰ **S55** **Injury of blood vessels at forearm level**

    Code also any associated open wound (S51.-)

     EXCLUDES 2   *injury of blood vessels at wrist and hand level (S65.-)*

          injury of brachial vessels (S45.1-S45.2)

    The appropriate 7th character is to be added to each code from category S55.
    A   initial encounter
    D   subsequent encounter
    S   sequela

√5ᵗʰ **S55.0** **Injury of ulnar artery at forearm level**

    CC Excl: For CC codes in subcategory S55.0:
    Right side: PDX collection 1274
    Left side: PDX collection 1275
    Unspecified side: PDX collection 1276

   √6ᵗʰ **S55.00** **Unspecified injury of ulnar artery at forearm level**

     √7ᵗʰ **S55.001** **Unspecified injury of ulnar artery at forearm level, right arm**   CC

     √7ᵗʰ **S55.002** **Unspecified injury of ulnar artery at forearm level, left arm**   CC

     √7ᵗʰ **S55.009** **Unspecified injury of ulnar artery at forearm level, unspecified arm**   CC

   √6ᵗʰ **S55.01** **Laceration of ulnar artery at forearm level**

     √7ᵗʰ **S55.011** **Laceration of ulnar artery at forearm level, right arm**   CC

     √7ᵗʰ **S55.012** **Laceration of ulnar artery at forearm level, left arm**   CC

     √7ᵗʰ **S55.019** **Laceration of ulnar artery at forearm level, unspecified arm**   CC

   √6ᵗʰ **S55.09** **Other specified injury of ulnar artery at forearm level**

     √7ᵗʰ **S55.091** **Other specified injury of ulnar artery at forearm level, right arm**   CC

     √7ᵗʰ **S55.092** **Other specified injury of ulnar artery at forearm level, left arm**   CC

     √7ᵗʰ **S55.099** **Other specified injury of ulnar artery at forearm level, unspecified arm**   CC

N Newborn: 0   P Pediatric: 0-17   M Maternity: 9-64   A Adult: 15-124   MCC Major Complication/Comorbidity   CC Complication/Comorbidity   SW Severe Wound Dx

1052   ICD-10-CM 2020

√5ᵗʰ **S55.1** **Injury of radial artery at forearm level**

> **CC Excl: For CC codes in subcategory S55.1:**
> **Right side:** PDX collection 1277
> **Left side:** PDX collection 1278
> **Unspecified side:** PDX collection 1279

√6ᵗʰ **S55.10** **Unspecified injury of radial artery at forearm level**

√7ᵗʰ **S55.101** Unspecified injury of radial artery at forearm level, **right** arm   `CC`

√7ᵗʰ **S55.102** Unspecified injury of radial artery at forearm level, **left** arm   `CC`

√7ᵗʰ **S55.109** Unspecified injury of radial artery at forearm level, unspecified arm   `CC`

√6ᵗʰ **S55.11** **Laceration of radial artery at forearm level**

√7ᵗʰ **S55.111** Laceration of radial artery at forearm level, **right** arm   `CC`

√7ᵗʰ **S55.112** Laceration of radial artery at forearm level, **left** arm   `CC`

√7ᵗʰ **S55.119** Laceration of radial artery at forearm level, unspecified arm   `CC`

√6ᵗʰ **S55.19** **Other specified injury of radial artery at forearm level**

√7ᵗʰ **S55.191** Other specified injury of radial artery at forearm level, **right** arm   `CC`

√7ᵗʰ **S55.192** Other specified injury of radial artery at forearm level, **left** arm   `CC`

√7ᵗʰ **S55.199** Other specified injury of radial artery at forearm level, unspecified arm   `CC`

√5ᵗʰ **S55.2** **Injury of vein at forearm level**

> **CC Excl: For CC codes in subcategory S55.2:**
> **Right side:** PDX collection 1260
> **Left side:** PDX collection 1261
> **Unspecified side:** PDX collection 1262

√6ᵗʰ **S55.20** **Unspecified injury of vein at forearm level**

√7ᵗʰ **S55.201** Unspecified injury of vein at forearm level, **right** arm   `CC`

√7ᵗʰ **S55.202** Unspecified injury of vein at forearm level, **left** arm   `CC`

√7ᵗʰ **S55.209** Unspecified injury of vein at forearm level, unspecified arm   `CC`

√6ᵗʰ **S55.21** **Laceration of vein at forearm level**

√7ᵗʰ **S55.211** Laceration of vein at forearm level, **right** arm   `CC`

√7ᵗʰ **S55.212** Laceration of vein at forearm level, **left** arm   `CC`

√7ᵗʰ **S55.219** Laceration of vein at forearm level, unspecified arm   `CC`

√6ᵗʰ **S55.29** **Other specified injury of vein at forearm level**

√7ᵗʰ **S55.291** Other specified injury of vein at forearm level, **right** arm   `CC`

√7ᵗʰ **S55.292** Other specified injury of vein at forearm level, **left** arm   `CC`

√7ᵗʰ **S55.299** Other specified injury of vein at forearm level, unspecified arm   `CC`

√5ᵗʰ **S55.8** **Injury of other blood vessels at forearm level**

> **CC Excl: For CC codes in subcategory S55.8:**
> **Right side:** PDX collection 1260
> **Left side:** PDX collection 1261
> **Unspecified side:** PDX collection 1262

√6ᵗʰ **S55.80** **Unspecified injury of other blood vessels at forearm level**

√7ᵗʰ **S55.801** Unspecified injury of other blood vessels at forearm level, **right** arm   `CC`

√7ᵗʰ **S55.802** Unspecified injury of other blood vessels at forearm level, **left** arm   `CC`

√7ᵗʰ **S55.809** Unspecified injury of other blood vessels at forearm level, unspecified arm   `CC`

√6ᵗʰ **S55.81** **Laceration of other blood vessels at forearm level**

√7ᵗʰ **S55.811** Laceration of other blood vessels at forearm level, **right** arm   `CC`

√7ᵗʰ **S55.812** Laceration of other blood vessels at forearm level, **left** arm   `CC`

√7ᵗʰ **S55.819** Laceration of other blood vessels at forearm level, unspecified arm   `CC`

√6ᵗʰ **S55.89** **Other specified injury of other blood vessels at forearm level**

√7ᵗʰ **S55.891** Other specified injury of other blood vessels at forearm level, **right** arm   `CC`

√7ᵗʰ **S55.892** Other specified injury of other blood vessels at forearm level, **left** arm   `CC`

√7ᵗʰ **S55.899** Other specified injury of other blood vessels at forearm level, unspecified arm   `CC`

√5ᵗʰ **S55.9** **Injury of unspecified blood vessel at forearm level**

> **CC Excl: For CC codes in subcategory S55.9:**
> **Right side:** PDX collection 1260
> **Left side:** PDX collection 1261
> **Unspecified side:** PDX collection 1262

√6ᵗʰ **S55.90** **Unspecified injury of unspecified blood vessel at forearm level**

√7ᵗʰ **S55.901** Unspecified injury of unspecified blood vessel at forearm level, **right** arm   `CC`

√7ᵗʰ **S55.902** Unspecified injury of unspecified blood vessel at forearm level, **left** arm   `CC`

√7ᵗʰ **S55.909** Unspecified injury of unspecified blood vessel at forearm level, unspecified arm   `CC`

√6ᵗʰ **S55.91** **Laceration of unspecified blood vessel at forearm level**

√7ᵗʰ **S55.911** Laceration of unspecified blood vessel at forearm level, **right** arm   `CC`

√7ᵗʰ **S55.912** Laceration of unspecified blood vessel at forearm level, **left** arm   `CC`

√7ᵗʰ **S55.919** Laceration of unspecified blood vessel at forearm level, unspecified arm   `CC`

√6ᵗʰ **S55.99** **Other specified injury of unspecified blood vessel at forearm level**

√7ᵗʰ **S55.991** Other specified injury of unspecified blood vessel at forearm level, **right** arm   `CC`

√7ᵗʰ **S55.992** Other specified injury of unspecified blood vessel at forearm level, **left** arm   `CC`

√7ᵗʰ **S55.999** Other specified injury of unspecified blood vessel at forearm level, unspecified arm   `CC`

✅ Additional Character Required   √x7ᵗʰ Placeholder   Unacceptable PDx   Questionable PDx   Manifestation   Unspecified Dx   H1-H14 HAC   HCC CMS-HCC Dx   HIV HIV Dx

ICD-10-CM 2020   **1053**

☑4ᵗʰ **S56 Injury of muscle, fascia and tendon at forearm level**

Code also any associated open wound (S51.-)

EXCLUDES 2   *injury of muscle, fascia and tendon at or below wrist (S66.-)*

sprain of joints and ligaments of elbow (S53.4-)

TIP: Refer to the Muscle/Tendon table at the beginning of this chapter

> The appropriate 7th character is to be added to each code from category S56.
> A   initial encounter
> D   subsequent encounter
> S   sequela

CC Excl: For CC codes in category S56:
Right side: PDX collection 1280
Left side: PDX collection 1281
Unspecified side: PDX collection 1282

☑5ᵗʰ **S56.0 Injury of flexor muscle, fascia and tendon of thumb at forearm level**

   ☑6ᵗʰ **S56.00 Unspecified injury of flexor muscle, fascia and tendon of thumb at forearm level**

     ☑7ᵗʰ **S56.001** Unspecified injury of flexor muscle, fascia and tendon of right thumb at forearm level

     ☑7ᵗʰ **S56.002** Unspecified injury of flexor muscle, fascia and tendon of left thumb at forearm level

     ☑7ᵗʰ **S56.009** Unspecified injury of flexor muscle, fascia and tendon of unspecified thumb at forearm level

   ☑6ᵗʰ **S56.01 Strain of flexor muscle, fascia and tendon of thumb at forearm level**

     ☑7ᵗʰ **S56.011** Strain of flexor muscle, fascia and tendon of right thumb at forearm level

     ☑7ᵗʰ **S56.012** Strain of flexor muscle, fascia and tendon of left thumb at forearm level

     ☑7ᵗʰ **S56.019** Strain of flexor muscle, fascia and tendon of unspecified thumb at forearm level

   ☑6ᵗʰ **S56.02 Laceration of flexor muscle, fascia and tendon of thumb at forearm level**

     ☑7ᵗʰ **S56.021** Laceration of flexor muscle, fascia and tendon of right thumb at forearm level   **CC**

     ☑7ᵗʰ **S56.022** Laceration of flexor muscle, fascia and tendon of left thumb at forearm level   **CC**

     ☑7ᵗʰ **S56.029** Laceration of flexor muscle, fascia and tendon of unspecified thumb at forearm level   **CC**

   ☑6ᵗʰ **S56.09 Other injury of flexor muscle, fascia and tendon of thumb at forearm level**

     ☑7ᵗʰ **S56.091** Other injury of flexor muscle, fascia and tendon of right thumb at forearm level

     ☑7ᵗʰ **S56.092** Other injury of flexor muscle, fascia and tendon of left thumb at forearm level

     ☑7ᵗʰ **S56.099** Other injury of flexor muscle, fascia and tendon of unspecified thumb at forearm level

☑5ᵗʰ **S56.1 Injury of flexor muscle, fascia and tendon of other and unspecified finger at forearm level**

   ☑6ᵗʰ **S56.10 Unspecified injury of flexor muscle, fascia and tendon of other and unspecified finger at forearm level**

     ☑7ᵗʰ **S56.101** Unspecified injury of flexor muscle, fascia and tendon of right index finger at forearm level

     ☑7ᵗʰ **S56.102** Unspecified injury of flexor muscle, fascia and tendon of left index finger at forearm level

     ☑7ᵗʰ **S56.103** Unspecified injury of flexor muscle, fascia and tendon of right middle finger at forearm level

     ☑7ᵗʰ **S56.104** Unspecified injury of flexor muscle, fascia and tendon of left middle finger at forearm level

     ☑7ᵗʰ **S56.105** Unspecified injury of flexor muscle, fascia and tendon of right ring finger at forearm level

     ☑7ᵗʰ **S56.106** Unspecified injury of flexor muscle, fascia and tendon of left ring finger at forearm level

     ☑7ᵗʰ **S56.107** Unspecified injury of flexor muscle, fascia and tendon of right little finger at forearm level

     ☑7ᵗʰ **S56.108** Unspecified injury of flexor muscle, fascia and tendon of left little finger at forearm level

     ☑7ᵗʰ **S56.109** Unspecified injury of flexor muscle, fascia and tendon of unspecified finger at forearm level

   ☑6ᵗʰ **S56.11 Strain of flexor muscle, fascia and tendon of other and unspecified finger at forearm level**

     ☑7ᵗʰ **S56.111** Strain of flexor muscle, fascia and tendon of right index finger at forearm level

     ☑7ᵗʰ **S56.112** Strain of flexor muscle, fascia and tendon of left index finger at forearm level

     ☑7ᵗʰ **S56.113** Strain of flexor muscle, fascia and tendon of right middle finger at forearm level

     ☑7ᵗʰ **S56.114** Strain of flexor muscle, fascia and tendon of left middle finger at forearm level

     ☑7ᵗʰ **S56.115** Strain of flexor muscle, fascia and tendon of right ring finger at forearm level

     ☑7ᵗʰ **S56.116** Strain of flexor muscle, fascia and tendon of left ring finger at forearm level

     ☑7ᵗʰ **S56.117** Strain of flexor muscle, fascia and tendon of right little finger at forearm level

     ☑7ᵗʰ **S56.118** Strain of flexor muscle, fascia and tendon of left little finger at forearm level

     ☑7ᵗʰ **S56.119** Strain of flexor muscle, fascia and tendon of finger of unspecified finger at forearm level

   ☑6ᵗʰ **S56.12 Laceration of flexor muscle, fascia and tendon of other and unspecified finger at forearm level**

     ☑7ᵗʰ **S56.121** Laceration of flexor muscle, fascia and tendon of right index finger at forearm level   **CC**

     ☑7ᵗʰ **S56.122** Laceration of flexor muscle, fascia and tendon of left index finger at forearm level   **CC**

     ☑7ᵗʰ **S56.123** Laceration of flexor muscle, fascia and tendon of right middle finger at forearm level   **CC**

     ☑7ᵗʰ **S56.124** Laceration of flexor muscle, fascia and tendon of left middle finger at forearm level   **CC**

     ☑7ᵗʰ **S56.125** Laceration of flexor muscle, fascia and tendon of right ring finger at forearm level   **CC**

     ☑7ᵗʰ **S56.126** Laceration of flexor muscle, fascia and tendon of left ring finger at forearm level   **CC**

     ☑7ᵗʰ **S56.127** Laceration of flexor muscle, fascia and tendon of right little finger at forearm level   **CC**

     ☑7ᵗʰ **S56.128** Laceration of flexor muscle, fascia and tendon of left little finger at forearm level   **CC**

     ☑7ᵗʰ **S56.129** Laceration of flexor muscle, fascia and tendon of unspecified finger at forearm level   **CC**

   ☑6ᵗʰ **S56.19 Other injury of flexor muscle, fascia and tendon of other and unspecified finger at forearm level**

     ☑7ᵗʰ **S56.191** Other injury of flexor muscle, fascia and tendon of right index finger at forearm level

     ☑7ᵗʰ **S56.192** Other injury of flexor muscle, fascia and tendon of left index finger at forearm level

     ☑7ᵗʰ **S56.193** Other injury of flexor muscle, fascia and tendon of right middle finger at forearm level

     ☑7ᵗʰ **S56.194** Other injury of flexor muscle, fascia and tendon of left middle finger at forearm level

     ☑7ᵗʰ **S56.195** Other injury of flexor muscle, fascia and tendon of right ring finger at forearm level

     ☑7ᵗʰ **S56.196** Other injury of flexor muscle, fascia and tendon of left ring finger at forearm level

N Newborn: 0   **P** Pediatric: 0-17   **M** Maternity: 9-64   **A** Adult: 15-124   **MCC** Major Complication/Comorbidity   **CC** Complication/Comorbidity   **SW** Severe Wound Dx

1054   ICD-10-CM 2020

√7ᵗʰ **S56.197** Other injury of flexor muscle, fascia and tendon of right little finger at forearm level

√7ᵗʰ **S56.198** Other injury of flexor muscle, fascia and tendon of left little finger at forearm level

√7ᵗʰ **S56.199** Other injury of flexor muscle, fascia and tendon of unspecified finger at forearm level

√5ᵗʰ **S56.2** Injury of other flexor muscle, fascia and tendon at forearm level

√6ᵗʰ **S56.20** Unspecified injury of other flexor muscle, fascia and tendon at forearm level

√7ᵗʰ **S56.201** Unspecified injury of other flexor muscle, fascia and tendon at forearm level, right arm

√7ᵗʰ **S56.202** Unspecified injury of other flexor muscle, fascia and tendon at forearm level, left arm

√7ᵗʰ **S56.209** Unspecified injury of other flexor muscle, fascia and tendon at forearm level, unspecified arm

√6ᵗʰ **S56.21** Strain of other flexor muscle, fascia and tendon at forearm level

√7ᵗʰ **S56.211** Strain of other flexor muscle, fascia and tendon at forearm level, right arm

√7ᵗʰ **S56.212** Strain of other flexor muscle, fascia and tendon at forearm level, left arm

√7ᵗʰ **S56.219** Strain of other flexor muscle, fascia and tendon at forearm level, unspecified arm

√6ᵗʰ **S56.22** Laceration of other flexor muscle, fascia and tendon at forearm level

√7ᵗʰ **S56.221** Laceration of other flexor muscle, fascia and tendon at forearm level, right arm   `cc`

√7ᵗʰ **S56.222** Laceration of other flexor muscle, fascia and tendon at forearm level, left arm   `cc`

√7ᵗʰ **S56.229** Laceration of other flexor muscle, fascia and tendon at forearm level, unspecified arm   `cc`

√6ᵗʰ **S56.29** Other injury of other flexor muscle, fascia and tendon at forearm level

√7ᵗʰ **S56.291** Other injury of other flexor muscle, fascia and tendon at forearm level, right arm

√7ᵗʰ **S56.292** Other injury of other flexor muscle, fascia and tendon at forearm level, left arm

√7ᵗʰ **S56.299** Other injury of other flexor muscle, fascia and tendon at forearm level, unspecified arm

√5ᵗʰ **S56.3** Injury of extensor or abductor muscles, fascia and tendons of thumb at forearm level

√6ᵗʰ **S56.30** Unspecified injury of extensor or abductor muscles, fascia and tendons of thumb at forearm level

√7ᵗʰ **S56.301** Unspecified injury of extensor or abductor muscles, fascia and tendons of right thumb at forearm level

√7ᵗʰ **S56.302** Unspecified injury of extensor or abductor muscles, fascia and tendons of left thumb at forearm level

√7ᵗʰ **S56.309** Unspecified injury of extensor or abductor muscles, fascia and tendons of unspecified thumb at forearm level

√6ᵗʰ **S56.31** Strain of extensor or abductor muscles, fascia and tendons of thumb at forearm level

√7ᵗʰ **S56.311** Strain of extensor or abductor muscles, fascia and tendons of right thumb at forearm level

√7ᵗʰ **S56.312** Strain of extensor or abductor muscles, fascia and tendons of left thumb at forearm level

√7ᵗʰ **S56.319** Strain of extensor or abductor muscles, fascia and tendons of unspecified thumb at forearm level

√6ᵗʰ **S56.32** Laceration of extensor or abductor muscles, fascia and tendons of thumb at forearm level

√7ᵗʰ **S56.321** Laceration of extensor or abductor muscles, fascia and tendons of right thumb at forearm level   `cc`

√7ᵗʰ **S56.322** Laceration of extensor or abductor muscles, fascia and tendons of left thumb at forearm level   `cc`

√7ᵗʰ **S56.329** Laceration of extensor or abductor muscles, fascia and tendons of unspecified thumb at forearm level   `cc`

√6ᵗʰ **S56.39** Other injury of extensor or abductor muscles, fascia and tendons of thumb at forearm level

√7ᵗʰ **S56.391** Other injury of extensor or abductor muscles, fascia and tendons of right thumb at forearm level

√7ᵗʰ **S56.392** Other injury of extensor or abductor muscles, fascia and tendons of left thumb at forearm level

√7ᵗʰ **S56.399** Other injury of extensor or abductor muscles, fascia and tendons of unspecified thumb at forearm level

√5ᵗʰ **S56.4** Injury of extensor muscle, fascia and tendon of other and unspecified finger at forearm level

√6ᵗʰ **S56.40** Unspecified injury of extensor muscle, fascia and tendon of other and unspecified finger at forearm level

√7ᵗʰ **S56.401** Unspecified injury of extensor muscle, fascia and tendon of right index finger at forearm level

√7ᵗʰ **S56.402** Unspecified injury of extensor muscle, fascia and tendon of left index finger at forearm level

√7ᵗʰ **S56.403** Unspecified injury of extensor muscle, fascia and tendon of right middle finger at forearm level

√7ᵗʰ **S56.404** Unspecified injury of extensor muscle, fascia and tendon of left middle finger at forearm level

√7ᵗʰ **S56.405** Unspecified injury of extensor muscle, fascia and tendon of right ring finger at forearm level

√7ᵗʰ **S56.406** Unspecified injury of extensor muscle, fascia and tendon of left ring finger at forearm level

√7ᵗʰ **S56.407** Unspecified injury of extensor muscle, fascia and tendon of right little finger at forearm level

√7ᵗʰ **S56.408** Unspecified injury of extensor muscle, fascia and tendon of left little finger at forearm level

√7ᵗʰ **S56.409** Unspecified injury of extensor muscle, fascia and tendon of unspecified finger at forearm level

√6ᵗʰ **S56.41** Strain of extensor muscle, fascia and tendon of other and unspecified finger at forearm level

√7ᵗʰ **S56.411** Strain of extensor muscle, fascia and tendon of right index finger at forearm level

√7ᵗʰ **S56.412** Strain of extensor muscle, fascia and tendon of left index finger at forearm level

√7ᵗʰ **S56.413** Strain of extensor muscle, fascia and tendon of right middle finger at forearm level

√7ᵗʰ **S56.414** Strain of extensor muscle, fascia and tendon of left middle finger at forearm level

√7ᵗʰ **S56.415** Strain of extensor muscle, fascia and tendon of right ring finger at forearm level

√7ᵗʰ **S56.416** Strain of extensor muscle, fascia and tendon of left ring finger at forearm level

√7ᵗʰ **S56.417** Strain of extensor muscle, fascia and tendon of right little finger at forearm level

√7ᵗʰ **S56.418** Strain of extensor muscle, fascia and tendon of left little finger at forearm level

√7ᵗʰ **S56.419** Strain of extensor muscle, fascia and tendon of finger, unspecified finger at forearm level

√6ᵗʰ **S56.42** Laceration of extensor muscle, fascia and tendon of other and unspecified finger at forearm level

√7ᵗʰ **S56.421** Laceration of extensor muscle, fascia and tendon of right index finger at forearm level   `cc`

√7ᵗʰ **S56.422** Laceration of extensor muscle, fascia and tendon of left index finger at forearm level   `cc`

√7ᵗʰ **S56.423** Laceration of extensor muscle, fascia and tendon of right middle finger at forearm level   CC

√7ᵗʰ **S56.424** Laceration of extensor muscle, fascia and tendon of left middle finger at forearm level   CC

√7ᵗʰ **S56.425** Laceration of extensor muscle, fascia and tendon of right ring finger at forearm level   CC

√7ᵗʰ **S56.426** Laceration of extensor muscle, fascia and tendon of left ring finger at forearm level   CC

√7ᵗʰ **S56.427** Laceration of extensor muscle, fascia and tendon of right little finger at forearm level   CC

√7ᵗʰ **S56.428** Laceration of extensor muscle, fascia and tendon of left little finger at forearm level   CC

√7ᵗʰ **S56.429** Laceration of extensor muscle, fascia and tendon of unspecified finger at forearm level   CC

√6ᵗʰ **S56.49** Other injury of extensor muscle, fascia and tendon of other and unspecified finger at forearm level

√7ᵗʰ **S56.491** Other injury of extensor muscle, fascia and tendon of right index finger at forearm level

√7ᵗʰ **S56.492** Other injury of extensor muscle, fascia and tendon of left index finger at forearm level

√7ᵗʰ **S56.493** Other injury of extensor muscle, fascia and tendon of right middle finger at forearm level

√7ᵗʰ **S56.494** Other injury of extensor muscle, fascia and tendon of left middle finger at forearm level

√7ᵗʰ **S56.495** Other injury of extensor muscle, fascia and tendon of right ring finger at forearm level

√7ᵗʰ **S56.496** Other injury of extensor muscle, fascia and tendon of left ring finger at forearm level

√7ᵗʰ **S56.497** Other injury of extensor muscle, fascia and tendon of right little finger at forearm level

√7ᵗʰ **S56.498** Other injury of extensor muscle, fascia and tendon of left little finger at forearm level

√7ᵗʰ **S56.499** Other injury of extensor muscle, fascia and tendon of unspecified finger at forearm level

√5ᵗʰ **S56.5** Injury of other extensor muscle, fascia and tendon at forearm level

√6ᵗʰ **S56.50** Unspecified injury of other extensor muscle, fascia and tendon at forearm level

√7ᵗʰ **S56.501** Unspecified injury of other extensor muscle, fascia and tendon at forearm level, right arm

√7ᵗʰ **S56.502** Unspecified injury of other extensor muscle, fascia and tendon at forearm level, left arm

√7ᵗʰ **S56.509** Unspecified injury of other extensor muscle, fascia and tendon at forearm level, unspecified arm

√6ᵗʰ **S56.51** Strain of other extensor muscle, fascia and tendon at forearm level

√7ᵗʰ **S56.511** Strain of other extensor muscle, fascia and tendon at forearm level, right arm

√7ᵗʰ **S56.512** Strain of other extensor muscle, fascia and tendon at forearm level, left arm

√7ᵗʰ **S56.519** Strain of other extensor muscle, fascia and tendon at forearm level, unspecified arm

√6ᵗʰ **S56.52** Laceration of other extensor muscle, fascia and tendon at forearm level

√7ᵗʰ **S56.521** Laceration of other extensor muscle, fascia and tendon at forearm level, right arm   CC

√7ᵗʰ **S56.522** Laceration of other extensor muscle, fascia and tendon at forearm level, left arm   CC

√7ᵗʰ **S56.529** Laceration of other extensor muscle, fascia and tendon at forearm level, unspecified arm   CC

√6ᵗʰ **S56.59** Other injury of other extensor muscle, fascia and tendon at forearm level

√7ᵗʰ **S56.591** Other injury of other extensor muscle, fascia and tendon at forearm level, right arm

√7ᵗʰ **S56.592** Other injury of other extensor muscle, fascia and tendon at forearm level, left arm

√7ᵗʰ **S56.599** Other injury of other extensor muscle, fascia and tendon at forearm level, unspecified arm

√5ᵗʰ **S56.8** Injury of other muscles, fascia and tendons at forearm level

√6ᵗʰ **S56.80** Unspecified injury of other muscles, fascia and tendons at forearm level

√7ᵗʰ **S56.801** Unspecified injury of other muscles, fascia and tendons at forearm level, right arm

√7ᵗʰ **S56.802** Unspecified injury of other muscles, fascia and tendons at forearm level, left arm

√7ᵗʰ **S56.809** Unspecified injury of other muscles, fascia and tendons at forearm level, unspecified arm

√6ᵗʰ **S56.81** Strain of other muscles, fascia and tendons at forearm level

√7ᵗʰ **S56.811** Strain of other muscles, fascia and tendons at forearm level, right arm

√7ᵗʰ **S56.812** Strain of other muscles, fascia and tendons at forearm level, left arm

√7ᵗʰ **S56.819** Strain of other muscles, fascia and tendons at forearm level, unspecified arm

√6ᵗʰ **S56.82** Laceration of other muscles, fascia and tendons at forearm level

√7ᵗʰ **S56.821** Laceration of other muscles, fascia and tendons at forearm level, right arm   CC

√7ᵗʰ **S56.822** Laceration of other muscles, fascia and tendons at forearm level, left arm   CC

√7ᵗʰ **S56.829** Laceration of other muscles, fascia and tendons at forearm level, unspecified arm   CC

√6ᵗʰ **S56.89** Other injury of other muscles, fascia and tendons at forearm level

√7ᵗʰ **S56.891** Other injury of other muscles, fascia and tendons at forearm level, right arm

√7ᵗʰ **S56.892** Other injury of other muscles, fascia and tendons at forearm level, left arm

√7ᵗʰ **S56.899** Other injury of other muscles, fascia and tendons at forearm level, unspecified arm

√5ᵗʰ **S56.9** Injury of unspecified muscles, fascia and tendons at forearm level

√6ᵗʰ **S56.90** Unspecified injury of unspecified muscles, fascia and tendons at forearm level

√7ᵗʰ **S56.901** Unspecified injury of unspecified muscles, fascia and tendons at forearm level, right arm

√7ᵗʰ **S56.902** Unspecified injury of unspecified muscles, fascia and tendons at forearm level, left arm

√7ᵗʰ **S56.909** Unspecified injury of unspecified muscles, fascia and tendons at forearm level, unspecified arm

√6ᵗʰ **S56.91** Strain of unspecified muscles, fascia and tendons at forearm level

√7ᵗʰ **S56.911** Strain of unspecified muscles, fascia and tendons at forearm level, right arm

√7ᵗʰ **S56.912** Strain of unspecified muscles, fascia and tendons at forearm level, left arm

√7ᵗʰ **S56.919** Strain of unspecified muscles, fascia and tendons at forearm level, unspecified arm

N Newborn: 0   P Pediatric: 0-17   M Maternity: 9-64   A Adult: 15-124   MCC Major Complication/Comorbidity   CC Complication/Comorbidity   SW Severe Wound Dx

1056   ICD-10-CM 2020

S56.423–S56.919

√6ᵗʰ **S56.92** **Laceration of unspecified muscles, fascia and tendons at forearm level**

     √7ᵗʰ **S56.921** **Laceration of unspecified muscles, fascia and tendons at forearm level, right arm** `CC`

     √7ᵗʰ **S56.922** **Laceration of unspecified muscles, fascia and tendons at forearm level, left arm** `CC`

     √7ᵗʰ **S56.929** **Laceration of unspecified muscles, fascia and tendons at forearm level, unspecified arm** `CC`

√6ᵗʰ **S56.99** **Other injury of unspecified muscles, fascia and tendons at forearm level**

     √7ᵗʰ **S56.991** **Other injury of unspecified muscles, fascia and tendons at forearm level, right arm**

     √7ᵗʰ **S56.992** **Other injury of unspecified muscles, fascia and tendons at forearm level, left arm**

     √7ᵗʰ **S56.999** **Other injury of unspecified muscles, fascia and tendons at forearm level, unspecified arm**

√4ᵗʰ **S57** **Crushing injury of elbow and forearm**

Use additional code(s) for all associated injuries

EXCLUDES 2   *crushing injury of wrist and hand (S67.-)*

The appropriate 7th character is to be added to each code from category S57.
A   initial encounter
D   subsequent encounter
S   sequela

√5ᵗʰ **S57.0** **Crushing injury of elbow**

   √x7ᵗʰ **S57.00** **Crushing injury of unspecified elbow**

   √x7ᵗʰ **S57.01** **Crushing injury of right elbow**

   √x7ᵗʰ **S57.02** **Crushing injury of left elbow**

√5ᵗʰ **S57.8** **Crushing injury of forearm**

   √x7ᵗʰ **S57.80** **Crushing injury of unspecified forearm**

   √x7ᵗʰ **S57.81** **Crushing injury of right forearm**

   √x7ᵗʰ **S57.82** **Crushing injury of left forearm**

√4ᵗʰ **S58** **Traumatic amputation of elbow and forearm**

An amputation not identified as partial or complete should be coded to complete

EXCLUDES 1   *traumatic amputation of wrist and hand (S68.-)*

The appropriate 7th character is to be added to each code from category S58.
A   initial encounter
D   subsequent encounter
S   sequela

CC Excl: For CC codes in category S58:
Right side: PDX collection 1266
Left side: PDX collection 1267
Unspecified side: PDX collection 1268

√5ᵗʰ **S58.0** **Traumatic amputation at elbow level**

   √6ᵗʰ **S58.01** **Complete traumatic amputation at elbow level**

     7 √7ᵗʰ **S58.011** **Complete traumatic amputation at elbow level, right arm** `CC` `HCC`

     7 √7ᵗʰ **S58.012** **Complete traumatic amputation at elbow level, left arm** `CC` `HCC`

     7 √7ᵗʰ **S58.019** **Complete traumatic amputation at elbow level, unspecified arm** `CC` `HCC`

   √6ᵗʰ **S58.02** **Partial traumatic amputation at elbow level**

     7 √7ᵗʰ **S58.021** **Partial traumatic amputation at elbow level, right arm** `CC` `HCC`

     7 √7ᵗʰ **S58.022** **Partial traumatic amputation at elbow level, left arm** `CC` `HCC`

     7 √7ᵗʰ **S58.029** **Partial traumatic amputation at elbow level, unspecified arm** `CC` `HCC`

√5ᵗʰ **S58.1** **Traumatic amputation at level between elbow and wrist**

   √6ᵗʰ **S58.11** **Complete traumatic amputation at level between elbow and wrist**

     7 √7ᵗʰ **S58.111** **Complete traumatic amputation at level between elbow and wrist, right arm** `CC` `HCC`

     7 √7ᵗʰ **S58.112** **Complete traumatic amputation at level between elbow and wrist, left arm** `CC` `HCC`

     7 √7ᵗʰ **S58.119** **Complete traumatic amputation at level between elbow and wrist, unspecified arm** `CC` `HCC`

   √6ᵗʰ **S58.12** **Partial traumatic amputation at level between elbow and wrist**

     7 √7ᵗʰ **S58.121** **Partial traumatic amputation at level between elbow and wrist, right arm** `CC` `HCC`

     7 √7ᵗʰ **S58.122** **Partial traumatic amputation at level between elbow and wrist, left arm** `CC` `HCC`

     7 √7ᵗʰ **S58.129** **Partial traumatic amputation at level between elbow and wrist, unspecified arm** `CC` `HCC`

√5ᵗʰ **S58.9** **Traumatic amputation of forearm, level unspecified**

EXCLUDES 1   *traumatic amputation of wrist (S68.-)*

   √6ᵗʰ **S58.91** **Complete traumatic amputation of forearm, level unspecified**

     7 √7ᵗʰ **S58.911** **Complete traumatic amputation of right forearm, level unspecified** `CC` `HCC`

     7 √7ᵗʰ **S58.912** **Complete traumatic amputation of left forearm, level unspecified** `CC` `HCC`

     7 √7ᵗʰ **S58.919** **Complete traumatic amputation of unspecified forearm, level unspecified** `CC` `HCC`

   √6ᵗʰ **S58.92** **Partial traumatic amputation of forearm, level unspecified**

     7 √7ᵗʰ **S58.921** **Partial traumatic amputation of right forearm, level unspecified** `CC` `HCC`

     7 √7ᵗʰ **S58.922** **Partial traumatic amputation of left forearm, level unspecified** `CC` `HCC`

     7 √7ᵗʰ **S58.929** **Partial traumatic amputation of unspecified forearm, level unspecified** `CC` `HCC`

√4ᵗʰ **S59** **Other and unspecified injuries of elbow and forearm**

EXCLUDES 2   *other and unspecified injuries of wrist and hand (S69.-)*

AHA: 2018,2Q,12; 2018,1Q,3; 2015,3Q,37-39

The appropriate 7th character is to be added to each code from subcategories S59.0, S59.1, and S59.2.
A   initial encounter for closed fracture
D   subsequent encounter for fracture with routine healing
G   subsequent encounter for fracture with delayed healing
K   subsequent encounter for fracture with nonunion
P   subsequent encounter for fracture with malunion
S   sequela

√5ᵗʰ **S59.0** **Physeal fracture of lower end of ulna**

CC Excl: For CC/MCC codes in subcategory S59.0:
Right side: See code S59.001
Left side: See code S59.002
Unspecified side: See code S59.009

   √6ᵗʰ **S59.00** **Unspecified physeal fracture of lower end of ulna**

     3 √7ᵗʰ **S59.001** **Unspecified physeal fracture of lower end of ulna, right arm** `CC` `H5`

       CC Excl: CC with 7th character A: PDX collection 1270
       CC Excl: CC with 7th character K or P: PDX collection 897

3 √7th **S59.002** Unspecified physeal fracture of lower end of ulna, left arm   CC H5
  CC Excl: CC with 7th character A: PDX collection 1271
  CC Excl: CC with 7th character K or P: PDX collection 897

3 √7th **S59.009** Unspecified physeal fracture of lower end of ulna, unspecified arm   CC H5
  CC Excl: CC with 7th character A: PDX collection 1272
  CC Excl: CC with 7th character K or P: PDX collection 897

√6th **S59.01** Salter-Harris Type I physeal fracture of lower end of ulna

3 √7th **S59.011** Salter-Harris Type I physeal fracture of lower end of ulna, right arm   CC H5

3 √7th **S59.012** Salter-Harris Type I physeal fracture of lower end of ulna, left arm   CC H5

3 √7th **S59.019** Salter-Harris Type I physeal fracture of lower end of ulna, unspecified arm   CC H5

√6th **S59.02** Salter-Harris Type II physeal fracture of lower end of ulna

3 √7th **S59.021** Salter-Harris Type II physeal fracture of lower end of ulna, right arm   CC H5

3 √7th **S59.022** Salter-Harris Type II physeal fracture of lower end of ulna, left arm   CC H5

3 √7th **S59.029** Salter-Harris Type II physeal fracture of lower end of ulna, unspecified arm   CC H5

√6th **S59.03** Salter-Harris Type III physeal fracture of lower end of ulna

3 √7th **S59.031** Salter-Harris Type III physeal fracture of lower end of ulna, right arm   CC H5

3 √7th **S59.032** Salter-Harris Type III physeal fracture of lower end of ulna, left arm   CC H5

3 √7th **S59.039** Salter-Harris Type III physeal fracture of lower end of ulna, unspecified arm   CC H5

√6th **S59.04** Salter-Harris Type IV physeal fracture of lower end of ulna

3 √7th **S59.041** Salter-Harris Type IV physeal fracture of lower end of ulna, right arm   CC H5

3 √7th **S59.042** Salter-Harris Type IV physeal fracture of lower end of ulna, left arm   CC H5

3 √7th **S59.049** Salter-Harris Type IV physeal fracture of lower end of ulna, unspecified arm   CC H5

√6th **S59.09** Other physeal fracture of lower end of ulna

3 √7th **S59.091** Other physeal fracture of lower end of ulna, right arm   CC H5

3 √7th **S59.092** Other physeal fracture of lower end of ulna, left arm   CC H5

3 √7th **S59.099** Other physeal fracture of lower end of ulna, unspecified arm   CC H5

√5th **S59.1** Physeal fracture of upper end of radius
  CC Excl: For CC codes in subcategory S59.1:
  CC with 7th character K or P: PDX collection 897

√6th **S59.10** Unspecified physeal fracture of upper end of radius

4 √7th **S59.101** Unspecified physeal fracture of upper end of radius, right arm   CC

4 √7th **S59.102** Unspecified physeal fracture of upper end of radius, left arm   CC

4 √7th **S59.109** Unspecified physeal fracture of upper end of radius, unspecified arm   CC

√6th **S59.11** Salter-Harris Type I physeal fracture of upper end of radius

4 √7th **S59.111** Salter-Harris Type I physeal fracture of upper end of radius, right arm   CC

4 √7th **S59.112** Salter-Harris Type I physeal fracture of upper end of radius, left arm   CC

4 √7th **S59.119** Salter-Harris Type I physeal fracture of upper end of radius, unspecified arm   CC

√6th **S59.12** Salter-Harris Type II physeal fracture of upper end of radius

4 √7th **S59.121** Salter-Harris Type II physeal fracture of upper end of radius, right arm   CC

4 √7th **S59.122** Salter-Harris Type II physeal fracture of upper end of radius, left arm   CC

4 √7th **S59.129** Salter-Harris Type II physeal fracture of upper end of radius, unspecified arm   CC

√6th **S59.13** Salter-Harris Type III physeal fracture of upper end of radius

4 √7th **S59.131** Salter-Harris Type III physeal fracture of upper end of radius, right arm   CC

4 √7th **S59.132** Salter-Harris Type III physeal fracture of upper end of radius, left arm   CC

4 √7th **S59.139** Salter-Harris Type III physeal fracture of upper end of radius, unspecified arm   CC

√6th **S59.14** Salter-Harris Type IV physeal fracture of upper end of radius

4 √7th **S59.141** Salter-Harris Type IV physeal fracture of upper end of radius, right arm   CC

4 √7th **S59.142** Salter-Harris Type IV physeal fracture of upper end of radius, left arm   CC

4 √7th **S59.149** Salter-Harris Type IV physeal fracture of upper end of radius, unspecified arm   CC

√6th **S59.19** Other physeal fracture of upper end of radius

4 √7th **S59.191** Other physeal fracture of upper end of radius, right arm   CC

4 √7th **S59.192** Other physeal fracture of upper end of radius, left arm   CC

4 √7th **S59.199** Other physeal fracture of upper end of radius, unspecified arm   CC

√5th **S59.2** Physeal fracture of lower end of radius
  CC Excl: For CC codes in subcategory S59.2:
  Right side: See code S59.201
  Left side: See code S59.202
  Unspecified side: See code S59.209

√6th **S59.20** Unspecified physeal fracture of lower end of radius

3 √7th **S59.201** Unspecified physeal fracture of lower end of radius, right arm   CC H5
  CC Excl: CC with 7th character A: PDX collection 1270
  CC Excl: CC with 7th character K or P: PDX collection 897

3 √7th **S59.202** Unspecified physeal fracture of lower end of radius, left arm   CC H5
  CC Excl: CC with 7th character A: PDX collection 1271
  CC Excl: CC with 7th character K or P: PDX collection 897

N Newborn: 0   P Pediatric: 0-17   M Maternity: 9-64   A Adult: 15-124   MCC Major Complication/Comorbidity   CC Complication/Comorbidity   SW Severe Wound Dx

³ √7ᵗʰ S59.209 Unspecified physeal fracture of lower end of radius, unspecified arm   `CC` `H5`
     CC Excl: CC with 7th character A: PDX collection 1272
     CC Excl: CC with 7th character K or P: PDX collection 897

√6ᵗʰ S59.21 Salter-Harris Type I physeal fracture of lower end of radius

    ³ √7ᵗʰ S59.211 Salter-Harris Type I physeal fracture of lower end of radius, right arm   `CC` `H5`

    ³ √7ᵗʰ S59.212 Salter-Harris Type I physeal fracture of lower end of radius, left arm   `CC` `H5`

    ³ √7ᵗʰ S59.219 Salter-Harris Type I physeal fracture of lower end of radius, unspecified arm   `CC` `H5`

√6ᵗʰ S59.22 Salter-Harris Type II physeal fracture of lower end of radius

    ³ √7ᵗʰ S59.221 Salter-Harris Type II physeal fracture of lower end of radius, right arm   `CC` `H5`

    ³ √7ᵗʰ S59.222 Salter-Harris Type II physeal fracture of lower end of radius, left arm   `CC` `H5`

    ³ √7ᵗʰ S59.229 Salter-Harris Type II physeal fracture of lower end of radius, unspecified arm   `CC` `H5`

√6ᵗʰ S59.23 Salter-Harris Type III physeal fracture of lower end of radius

    ³ √7ᵗʰ S59.231 Salter-Harris Type III physeal fracture of lower end of radius, right arm   `CC` `H5`

    ³ √7ᵗʰ S59.232 Salter-Harris Type III physeal fracture of lower end of radius, left arm   `CC` `H5`

    ³ √7ᵗʰ S59.239 Salter-Harris Type III physeal fracture of lower end of radius, unspecified arm   `CC` `H5`

√6ᵗʰ S59.24 Salter-Harris Type IV physeal fracture of lower end of radius

    ³ √7ᵗʰ S59.241 Salter-Harris Type IV physeal fracture of lower end of radius, right arm   `CC` `H5`

    ³ √7ᵗʰ S59.242 Salter-Harris Type IV physeal fracture of lower end of radius, left arm   `CC` `H5`

    ³ √7ᵗʰ S59.249 Salter-Harris Type IV physeal fracture of lower end of radius, unspecified arm   `CC` `H5`

√6ᵗʰ S59.29 Other physeal fracture of lower end of radius

    ³ √7ᵗʰ S59.291 Other physeal fracture of lower end of radius, right arm   `CC` `H5`

    ³ √7ᵗʰ S59.292 Other physeal fracture of lower end of radius, left arm   `CC` `H5`

    ³ √7ᵗʰ S59.299 Other physeal fracture of lower end of radius, unspecified arm   `CC` `H5`

√5ᵗʰ S59.8 Other specified injuries of elbow and forearm

The appropriate 7th character is to be added to each code in subcategory S59.8.
A   initial encounter
D   subsequent encounter
S   sequela

√6ᵗʰ S59.80 Other specified injuries of elbow

    √7ᵗʰ S59.801 Other specified injuries of right elbow

    √7ᵗʰ S59.802 Other specified injuries of left elbow

    √7ᵗʰ S59.809 Other specified injuries of unspecified elbow

√6ᵗʰ S59.81 Other specified injuries of forearm

    √7ᵗʰ S59.811 Other specified injuries right forearm

    √7ᵗʰ S59.812 Other specified injuries left forearm

    √7ᵗʰ S59.819 Other specified injuries unspecified forearm

---

√5ᵗʰ S59.9 Unspecified injury of elbow and forearm

The appropriate 7th character is to be added to each code in subcategory S59.9.
A   initial encounter
D   subsequent encounter
S   sequela

√6ᵗʰ S59.90 Unspecified injury of elbow

    √7ᵗʰ S59.901 Unspecified injury of right elbow

    √7ᵗʰ S59.902 Unspecified injury of left elbow

    √7ᵗʰ S59.909 Unspecified injury of unspecified elbow

√6ᵗʰ S59.91 Unspecified injury of forearm

    √7ᵗʰ S59.911 Unspecified injury of right forearm

    √7ᵗʰ S59.912 Unspecified injury of left forearm

    √7ᵗʰ S59.919 Unspecified injury of unspecified forearm

Injuries to the wrist, hand and fingers (S60-S69)

EXCLUDES 2   burns and corrosions (T20-T32)
     frostbite (T33-T34)
     insect bite or sting, venomous (T63.4)

√4ᵗʰ S60 Superficial injury of wrist, hand and fingers

The appropriate 7th character is to be added to each code from category S60.
A   initial encounter
D   subsequent encounter
S   sequela

√5ᵗʰ S60.0 Contusion of finger without damage to nail

    EXCLUDES 1   contusion involving nail (matrix) (S60.1)

√x7ᵗʰ S60.00 Contusion of unspecified finger without damage to nail
     Contusion of finger(s) NOS

√6ᵗʰ S60.01 Contusion of thumb without damage to nail

    √7ᵗʰ S60.011 Contusion of right thumb without damage to nail

    √7ᵗʰ S60.012 Contusion of left thumb without damage to nail

    √7ᵗʰ S60.019 Contusion of unspecified thumb without damage to nail

√6ᵗʰ S60.02 Contusion of index finger without damage to nail

    √7ᵗʰ S60.021 Contusion of right index finger without damage to nail

    √7ᵗʰ S60.022 Contusion of left index finger without damage to nail

    √7ᵗʰ S60.029 Contusion of unspecified index finger without damage to nail

√6ᵗʰ S60.03 Contusion of middle finger without damage to nail

    √7ᵗʰ S60.031 Contusion of right middle finger without damage to nail

    √7ᵗʰ S60.032 Contusion of left middle finger without damage to nail

    √7ᵗʰ S60.039 Contusion of unspecified middle finger without damage to nail

√6ᵗʰ S60.04 Contusion of ring finger without damage to nail

    √7ᵗʰ S60.041 Contusion of right ring finger without damage to nail

    √7ᵗʰ S60.042 Contusion of left ring finger without damage to nail

    √7ᵗʰ S60.049 Contusion of unspecified ring finger without damage to nail

√6ᵗʰ S60.05 Contusion of little finger without damage to nail

    √7ᵗʰ S60.051 Contusion of right little finger without damage to nail

    √7ᵗʰ S60.052 Contusion of left little finger without damage to nail

    √7ᵗʰ S60.059 Contusion of unspecified little finger without damage to nail

√5ᵗʰ S60.1 Contusion of finger with damage to nail

√x7ᵗʰ S60.10 Contusion of unspecified finger with damage to nail

√6ᵗʰ S60.11 Contusion of thumb with damage to nail

    √7ᵗʰ S60.111 Contusion of right thumb with damage to nail

    √7ᵗʰ S60.112 Contusion of left thumb with damage to nail

    √7ᵗʰ S60.119 Contusion of unspecified thumb with damage to nail

---

√6ᵗʰ **S60.12** Contusion of index finger with damage to nail
- √7ᵗʰ **S60.121** Contusion of right index finger with damage to nail
- √7ᵗʰ **S60.122** Contusion of left index finger with damage to nail
- √7ᵗʰ **S60.129** Contusion of unspecified index finger with damage to nail

√6ᵗʰ **S60.13** Contusion of middle finger with damage to nail
- √7ᵗʰ **S60.131** Contusion of right middle finger with damage to nail
- √7ᵗʰ **S60.132** Contusion of left middle finger with damage to nail
- √7ᵗʰ **S60.139** Contusion of unspecified middle finger with damage to nail

√6ᵗʰ **S60.14** Contusion of ring finger with damage to nail
- √7ᵗʰ **S60.141** Contusion of right ring finger with damage to nail
- √7ᵗʰ **S60.142** Contusion of left ring finger with damage to nail
- √7ᵗʰ **S60.149** Contusion of unspecified ring finger with damage to nail

√6ᵗʰ **S60.15** Contusion of little finger with damage to nail
- √7ᵗʰ **S60.151** Contusion of right little finger with damage to nail
- √7ᵗʰ **S60.152** Contusion of left little finger with damage to nail
- √7ᵗʰ **S60.159** Contusion of unspecified little finger with damage to nail

√5ᵗʰ **S60.2** Contusion of wrist and hand
> EXCLUDES 2   contusion of fingers (S60.0-, S60.1-)

√6ᵗʰ **S60.21** Contusion of wrist
- √7ᵗʰ **S60.211** Contusion of right wrist
- √7ᵗʰ **S60.212** Contusion of left wrist
- √7ᵗʰ **S60.219** Contusion of unspecified wrist

√6ᵗʰ **S60.22** Contusion of hand
- √7ᵗʰ **S60.221** Contusion of right hand
- √7ᵗʰ **S60.222** Contusion of left hand
- √7ᵗʰ **S60.229** Contusion of unspecified hand

√5ᵗʰ **S60.3** Other superficial injuries of thumb

√6ᵗʰ **S60.31** Abrasion of thumb
- √7ᵗʰ **S60.311** Abrasion of right thumb
- √7ᵗʰ **S60.312** Abrasion of left thumb
- √7ᵗʰ **S60.319** Abrasion of unspecified thumb

√6ᵗʰ **S60.32** Blister (nonthermal) of thumb
- √7ᵗʰ **S60.321** Blister (nonthermal) of right thumb
- √7ᵗʰ **S60.322** Blister (nonthermal) of left thumb
- √7ᵗʰ **S60.329** Blister (nonthermal) of unspecified thumb

√6ᵗʰ **S60.34** External constriction of thumb
> Hair tourniquet syndrome of thumb
> Use additional cause code to identify the constricting item (W49.0-)
- √7ᵗʰ **S60.341** External constriction of right thumb
- √7ᵗʰ **S60.342** External constriction of left thumb
- √7ᵗʰ **S60.349** External constriction of unspecified thumb

√6ᵗʰ **S60.35** Superficial foreign body of thumb
> Splinter in the thumb
- √7ᵗʰ **S60.351** Superficial foreign body of right thumb
- √7ᵗʰ **S60.352** Superficial foreign body of left thumb
- √7ᵗʰ **S60.359** Superficial foreign body of unspecified thumb

√6ᵗʰ **S60.36** Insect bite (nonvenomous) of thumb
- √7ᵗʰ **S60.361** Insect bite (nonvenomous) of right thumb
- √7ᵗʰ **S60.362** Insect bite (nonvenomous) of left thumb
- √7ᵗʰ **S60.369** Insect bite (nonvenomous) of unspecified thumb

√6ᵗʰ **S60.37** Other superficial bite of thumb
> EXCLUDES 1   open bite of thumb (S61.05-, S61.15-)
- √7ᵗʰ **S60.371** Other superficial bite of right thumb
- √7ᵗʰ **S60.372** Other superficial bite of left thumb
- √7ᵗʰ **S60.379** Other superficial bite of unspecified thumb

√6ᵗʰ **S60.39** Other superficial injuries of thumb
- √7ᵗʰ **S60.391** Other superficial injuries of right thumb
- √7ᵗʰ **S60.392** Other superficial injuries of left thumb
- √7ᵗʰ **S60.399** Other superficial injuries of unspecified thumb

√5ᵗʰ **S60.4** Other superficial injuries of other fingers

√6ᵗʰ **S60.41** Abrasion of fingers
- √7ᵗʰ **S60.410** Abrasion of right index finger
- √7ᵗʰ **S60.411** Abrasion of left index finger
- √7ᵗʰ **S60.412** Abrasion of right middle finger
- √7ᵗʰ **S60.413** Abrasion of left middle finger
- √7ᵗʰ **S60.414** Abrasion of right ring finger
- √7ᵗʰ **S60.415** Abrasion of left ring finger
- √7ᵗʰ **S60.416** Abrasion of right little finger
- √7ᵗʰ **S60.417** Abrasion of left little finger
- √7ᵗʰ **S60.418** Abrasion of other finger
  > Abrasion of specified finger with unspecified laterality
- √7ᵗʰ **S60.419** Abrasion of unspecified finger

√6ᵗʰ **S60.42** Blister (nonthermal) of fingers
- √7ᵗʰ **S60.420** Blister (nonthermal) of right index finger
- √7ᵗʰ **S60.421** Blister (nonthermal) of left index finger
- √7ᵗʰ **S60.422** Blister (nonthermal) of right middle finger
- √7ᵗʰ **S60.423** Blister (nonthermal) of left middle finger
- √7ᵗʰ **S60.424** Blister (nonthermal) of right ring finger
- √7ᵗʰ **S60.425** Blister (nonthermal) of left ring finger
- √7ᵗʰ **S60.426** Blister (nonthermal) of right little finger
- √7ᵗʰ **S60.427** Blister (nonthermal) of left little finger
- √7ᵗʰ **S60.428** Blister (nonthermal) of other finger
  > Blister (nonthermal) of specified finger with unspecified laterality
- √7ᵗʰ **S60.429** Blister (nonthermal) of unspecified finger

√6ᵗʰ **S60.44** External constriction of fingers
> Hair tourniquet syndrome of finger
> Use additional cause code to identify the constricting item (W49.0-)
- √7ᵗʰ **S60.440** External constriction of right index finger
- √7ᵗʰ **S60.441** External constriction of left index finger
- √7ᵗʰ **S60.442** External constriction of right middle finger
- √7ᵗʰ **S60.443** External constriction of left middle finger
- √7ᵗʰ **S60.444** External constriction of right ring finger
- √7ᵗʰ **S60.445** External constriction of left ring finger
- √7ᵗʰ **S60.446** External constriction of right little finger
- √7ᵗʰ **S60.447** External constriction of left little finger
- √7ᵗʰ **S60.448** External constriction of other finger
  > External constriction of specified finger with unspecified laterality
- √7ᵗʰ **S60.449** External constriction of unspecified finger

√6ᵗʰ **S60.45** Superficial foreign body of fingers
> Splinter in the finger(s)
- √7ᵗʰ **S60.450** Superficial foreign body of right index finger
- √7ᵗʰ **S60.451** Superficial foreign body of left index finger
- √7ᵗʰ **S60.452** Superficial foreign body of right middle finger
- √7ᵗʰ **S60.453** Superficial foreign body of left middle finger
- √7ᵗʰ **S60.454** Superficial foreign body of right ring finger
- √7ᵗʰ **S60.455** Superficial foreign body of left ring finger
- √7ᵗʰ **S60.456** Superficial foreign body of right little finger
- √7ᵗʰ **S60.457** Superficial foreign body of left little finger
- √7ᵗʰ **S60.458** Superficial foreign body of other finger
  > Superficial foreign body of specified finger with unspecified laterality
- √7ᵗʰ **S60.459** Superficial foreign body of unspecified finger

√6ᵗʰ **S60.46   Insect bite (nonvenomous) of fingers**

   √7ᵗʰ **S60.460   Insect bite (nonvenomous) of right index finger**

   √7ᵗʰ **S60.461   Insect bite (nonvenomous) of left index finger**

   √7ᵗʰ **S60.462   Insect bite (nonvenomous) of right middle finger**

   √7ᵗʰ **S60.463   Insect bite (nonvenomous) of left middle finger**

   √7ᵗʰ **S60.464   Insect bite (nonvenomous) of right ring finger**

   √7ᵗʰ **S60.465   Insect bite (nonvenomous) of left ring finger**

   √7ᵗʰ **S60.466   Insect bite (nonvenomous) of right little finger**

   √7ᵗʰ **S60.467   Insect bite (nonvenomous) of left little finger**

   √7ᵗʰ **S60.468   Insect bite (nonvenomous) of other finger**

      Insect bite (nonvenomous) of specified finger with unspecified laterality

   √7ᵗʰ **S60.469   Insect bite (nonvenomous) of unspecified finger**

√6ᵗʰ **S60.47   Other superficial bite of fingers**

   EXCLUDES 1   *open bite of fingers (S61.25-, S61.35-)*

   √7ᵗʰ **S60.470   Other superficial bite of right index finger**

   √7ᵗʰ **S60.471   Other superficial bite of left index finger**

   √7ᵗʰ **S60.472   Other superficial bite of right middle finger**

   √7ᵗʰ **S60.473   Other superficial bite of left middle finger**

   √7ᵗʰ **S60.474   Other superficial bite of right ring finger**

   √7ᵗʰ **S60.475   Other superficial bite of left ring finger**

   √7ᵗʰ **S60.476   Other superficial bite of right little finger**

   √7ᵗʰ **S60.477   Other superficial bite of left little finger**

   √7ᵗʰ **S60.478   Other superficial bite of other finger**

      Other superficial bite of specified finger with unspecified laterality

   √7ᵗʰ **S60.479   Other superficial bite of unspecified finger**

√5ᵗʰ **S60.5   Other superficial injuries of hand**

   EXCLUDES 2   *superficial injuries of fingers (S60.3-, S60.4-)*

√6ᵗʰ **S60.51   Abrasion of hand**

   √7ᵗʰ **S60.511   Abrasion of right hand**

   √7ᵗʰ **S60.512   Abrasion of left hand**

   √7ᵗʰ **S60.519   Abrasion of unspecified hand**

√6ᵗʰ **S60.52   Blister (nonthermal) of hand**

   √7ᵗʰ **S60.521   Blister (nonthermal) of right hand**

   √7ᵗʰ **S60.522   Blister (nonthermal) of left hand**

   √7ᵗʰ **S60.529   Blister (nonthermal) of unspecified hand**

√6ᵗʰ **S60.54   External constriction of hand**

   √7ᵗʰ **S60.541   External constriction of right hand**

   √7ᵗʰ **S60.542   External constriction of left hand**

   √7ᵗʰ **S60.549   External constriction of unspecified hand**

√6ᵗʰ **S60.55   Superficial foreign body of hand**

      Splinter in the hand

   √7ᵗʰ **S60.551   Superficial foreign body of right hand**

   √7ᵗʰ **S60.552   Superficial foreign body of left hand**

   √7ᵗʰ **S60.559   Superficial foreign body of unspecified hand**

√6ᵗʰ **S60.56   Insect bite (nonvenomous) of hand**

   √7ᵗʰ **S60.561   Insect bite (nonvenomous) of right hand**

   √7ᵗʰ **S60.562   Insect bite (nonvenomous) of left hand**

   √7ᵗʰ **S60.569   Insect bite (nonvenomous) of unspecified hand**

√6ᵗʰ **S60.57   Other superficial bite of hand**

   EXCLUDES 1   *open bite of hand (S61.45-)*

   √7ᵗʰ **S60.571   Other superficial bite of hand of right hand**

   √7ᵗʰ **S60.572   Other superficial bite of hand of left hand**

   √7ᵗʰ **S60.579   Other superficial bite of hand of unspecified hand**

√5ᵗʰ **S60.8   Other superficial injuries of wrist**

√6ᵗʰ **S60.81   Abrasion of wrist**

   √7ᵗʰ **S60.811   Abrasion of right wrist**

   √7ᵗʰ **S60.812   Abrasion of left wrist**

   √7ᵗʰ **S60.819   Abrasion of unspecified wrist**

√6ᵗʰ **S60.82   Blister (nonthermal) of wrist**

   √7ᵗʰ **S60.821   Blister (nonthermal) of right wrist**

   √7ᵗʰ **S60.822   Blister (nonthermal) of left wrist**

   √7ᵗʰ **S60.829   Blister (nonthermal) of unspecified wrist**

√6ᵗʰ **S60.84   External constriction of wrist**

   √7ᵗʰ **S60.841   External constriction of right wrist**

   √7ᵗʰ **S60.842   External constriction of left wrist**

   √7ᵗʰ **S60.849   External constriction of unspecified wrist**

√6ᵗʰ **S60.85   Superficial foreign body of wrist**

      Splinter in the wrist

   √7ᵗʰ **S60.851   Superficial foreign body of right wrist**

   √7ᵗʰ **S60.852   Superficial foreign body of left wrist**

   √7ᵗʰ **S60.859   Superficial foreign body of unspecified wrist**

√6ᵗʰ **S60.86   Insect bite (nonvenomous) of wrist**

   √7ᵗʰ **S60.861   Insect bite (nonvenomous) of right wrist**

   √7ᵗʰ **S60.862   Insect bite (nonvenomous) of left wrist**

   √7ᵗʰ **S60.869   Insect bite (nonvenomous) of unspecified wrist**

√6ᵗʰ **S60.87   Other superficial bite of wrist**

   EXCLUDES 1   *open bite of wrist (S61.55)*

   √7ᵗʰ **S60.871   Other superficial bite of right wrist**

   √7ᵗʰ **S60.872   Other superficial bite of left wrist**

   √7ᵗʰ **S60.879   Other superficial bite of unspecified wrist**

√5ᵗʰ **S60.9   Unspecified superficial injury of wrist, hand and fingers**

√6ᵗʰ **S60.91   Unspecified superficial injury of wrist**

   √7ᵗʰ **S60.911   Unspecified superficial injury of right wrist**

   √7ᵗʰ **S60.912   Unspecified superficial injury of left wrist**

   √7ᵗʰ **S60.919   Unspecified superficial injury of unspecified wrist**

√6ᵗʰ **S60.92   Unspecified superficial injury of hand**

   √7ᵗʰ **S60.921   Unspecified superficial injury of right hand**

   √7ᵗʰ **S60.922   Unspecified superficial injury of left hand**

   √7ᵗʰ **S60.929   Unspecified superficial injury of unspecified hand**

√6ᵗʰ **S60.93   Unspecified superficial injury of thumb**

   √7ᵗʰ **S60.931   Unspecified superficial injury of right thumb**

   √7ᵗʰ **S60.932   Unspecified superficial injury of left thumb**

   √7ᵗʰ **S60.939   Unspecified superficial injury of unspecified thumb**

√6ᵗʰ **S60.94   Unspecified superficial injury of other fingers**

   √7ᵗʰ **S60.940   Unspecified superficial injury of right index finger**

   √7ᵗʰ **S60.941   Unspecified superficial injury of left index finger**

   √7ᵗʰ **S60.942   Unspecified superficial injury of right middle finger**

   √7ᵗʰ **S60.943   Unspecified superficial injury of left middle finger**

   √7ᵗʰ **S60.944   Unspecified superficial injury of right ring finger**

   √7ᵗʰ **S60.945   Unspecified superficial injury of left ring finger**

   √7ᵗʰ **S60.946   Unspecified superficial injury of right little finger**

   √7ᵗʰ **S60.947   Unspecified superficial injury of left little finger**

   √7ᵗʰ **S60.948   Unspecified superficial injury of other finger**

      Unspecified superficial injury of specified finger with unspecified laterality

   √7ᵗʰ **S60.949   Unspecified superficial injury of unspecified finger**

☑4ᵗʰ **S61 Open wound of wrist, hand and fingers**

Code also any associated wound infection

EXCLUDES 1 open fracture of wrist, hand and finger (S62.- with 7th character B)

traumatic amputation of wrist and hand (S68.-)

The appropriate 7th character is to be added to each code from category S61.

A initial encounter
D subsequent encounter
S sequela

☑5ᵗʰ **S61.0 Open wound of thumb without damage to nail**

EXCLUDES 1 open wound of thumb with damage to nail (S61.1-)

☑6ᵗʰ **S61.00 Unspecified open wound of thumb without damage to nail**

☑7ᵗʰ **S61.001 Unspecified open wound of right thumb without damage to nail**

☑7ᵗʰ **S61.002 Unspecified open wound of left thumb without damage to nail**

☑7ᵗʰ **S61.009 Unspecified open wound of unspecified thumb without damage to nail**

☑6ᵗʰ **S61.01 Laceration without foreign body of thumb without damage to nail**

☑7ᵗʰ **S61.011 Laceration without foreign body of right thumb without damage to nail**

☑7ᵗʰ **S61.012 Laceration without foreign body of left thumb without damage to nail**

☑7ᵗʰ **S61.019 Laceration without foreign body of unspecified thumb without damage to nail**

☑6ᵗʰ **S61.02 Laceration with foreign body of thumb without damage to nail**

☑7ᵗʰ **S61.021 Laceration with foreign body of right thumb without damage to nail**

☑7ᵗʰ **S61.022 Laceration with foreign body of left thumb without damage to nail**

☑7ᵗʰ **S61.029 Laceration with foreign body of unspecified thumb without damage to nail**

☑6ᵗʰ **S61.03 Puncture wound without foreign body of thumb without damage to nail**

☑7ᵗʰ **S61.031 Puncture wound without foreign body of right thumb without damage to nail**

☑7ᵗʰ **S61.032 Puncture wound without foreign body of left thumb without damage to nail**

☑7ᵗʰ **S61.039 Puncture wound without foreign body of unspecified thumb without damage to nail**

☑6ᵗʰ **S61.04 Puncture wound with foreign body of thumb without damage to nail**

☑7ᵗʰ **S61.041 Puncture wound with foreign body of right thumb without damage to nail**

☑7ᵗʰ **S61.042 Puncture wound with foreign body of left thumb without damage to nail**

☑7ᵗʰ **S61.049 Puncture wound with foreign body of unspecified thumb without damage to nail**

☑6ᵗʰ **S61.05 Open bite of thumb without damage to nail**

Bite of thumb NOS

EXCLUDES 1 superficial bite of thumb (S60.36-, S60.37-)

☑7ᵗʰ **S61.051 Open bite of right thumb without damage to nail**

☑7ᵗʰ **S61.052 Open bite of left thumb without damage to nail**

☑7ᵗʰ **S61.059 Open bite of unspecified thumb without damage to nail**

☑5ᵗʰ **S61.1 Open wound of thumb with damage to nail**

☑6ᵗʰ **S61.10 Unspecified open wound of thumb with damage to nail**

☑7ᵗʰ **S61.101 Unspecified open wound of right thumb with damage to nail**

☑7ᵗʰ **S61.102 Unspecified open wound of left thumb with damage to nail**

☑7ᵗʰ **S61.109 Unspecified open wound of unspecified thumb with damage to nail**

☑6ᵗʰ **S61.11 Laceration without foreign body of thumb with damage to nail**

☑7ᵗʰ **S61.111 Laceration without foreign body of right thumb with damage to nail**

☑7ᵗʰ **S61.112 Laceration without foreign body of left thumb with damage to nail**

☑7ᵗʰ **S61.119 Laceration without foreign body of unspecified thumb with damage to nail**

☑6ᵗʰ **S61.12 Laceration with foreign body of thumb with damage to nail**

☑7ᵗʰ **S61.121 Laceration with foreign body of right thumb with damage to nail**

☑7ᵗʰ **S61.122 Laceration with foreign body of left thumb with damage to nail**

☑7ᵗʰ **S61.129 Laceration with foreign body of unspecified thumb with damage to nail**

☑6ᵗʰ **S61.13 Puncture wound without foreign body of thumb with damage to nail**

☑7ᵗʰ **S61.131 Puncture wound without foreign body of right thumb with damage to nail**

☑7ᵗʰ **S61.132 Puncture wound without foreign body of left thumb with damage to nail**

☑7ᵗʰ **S61.139 Puncture wound without foreign body of unspecified thumb with damage to nail**

☑6ᵗʰ **S61.14 Puncture wound with foreign body of thumb with damage to nail**

☑7ᵗʰ **S61.141 Puncture wound with foreign body of right thumb with damage to nail**

☑7ᵗʰ **S61.142 Puncture wound with foreign body of left thumb with damage to nail**

☑7ᵗʰ **S61.149 Puncture wound with foreign body of unspecified thumb with damage to nail**

☑6ᵗʰ **S61.15 Open bite of thumb with damage to nail**

Bite of thumb with damage to nail NOS

EXCLUDES 1 superficial bite of thumb (S60.36-, S60.37-)

☑7ᵗʰ **S61.151 Open bite of right thumb with damage to nail**

☑7ᵗʰ **S61.152 Open bite of left thumb with damage to nail**

☑7ᵗʰ **S61.159 Open bite of unspecified thumb with damage to nail**

☑5ᵗʰ **S61.2 Open wound of other finger without damage to nail**

EXCLUDES 1 open wound of finger involving nail (matrix) (S61.3-)

EXCLUDES 2 open wound of thumb without damage to nail (S61.0-)

☑6ᵗʰ **S61.20 Unspecified open wound of other finger without damage to nail**

☑7ᵗʰ **S61.200 Unspecified open wound of right index finger without damage to nail**

☑7ᵗʰ **S61.201 Unspecified open wound of left index finger without damage to nail**

☑7ᵗʰ **S61.202 Unspecified open wound of right middle finger without damage to nail**

☑7ᵗʰ **S61.203 Unspecified open wound of left middle finger without damage to nail**

☑7ᵗʰ **S61.204 Unspecified open wound of right ring finger without damage to nail**

☑7ᵗʰ **S61.205 Unspecified open wound of left ring finger without damage to nail**

☑7ᵗʰ **S61.206 Unspecified open wound of right little finger without damage to nail**

☑7ᵗʰ **S61.207 Unspecified open wound of left little finger without damage to nail**

☑7ᵗʰ **S61.208 Unspecified open wound of other finger without damage to nail**

Unspecified open wound of specified finger with unspecified laterality without damage to nail

☑7ᵗʰ **S61.209 Unspecified open wound of unspecified finger without damage to nail**

☑6ᵗʰ **S61.21 Laceration without foreign body of finger without damage to nail**

☑7ᵗʰ **S61.210 Laceration without foreign body of right index finger without damage to nail**

☑7ᵗʰ **S61.211 Laceration without foreign body of left index finger without damage to nail**

☑7ᵗʰ **S61.212 Laceration without foreign body of right middle finger without damage to nail**

☑7ᵗʰ **S61.213 Laceration without foreign body of left middle finger without damage to nail**

☑7ᵗʰ **S61.214 Laceration without foreign body of right ring finger without damage to nail**

☑7ᵗʰ **S61.215 Laceration without foreign body of left ring finger without damage to nail**

☑7ᵗʰ **S61.216 Laceration without foreign body of right little finger without damage to nail**

☑7ᵗʰ **S61.217 Laceration without foreign body of left little finger without damage to nail**

Ⓝ Newborn: 0   Ⓟ Pediatric: 0-17   Ⓜ Maternity: 9-64   Ⓐ Adult: 15-124   **MCC** Major Complication/Comorbidity   **CC** Complication/Comorbidity   **SW** Severe Wound Dx

1062   ICD-10-CM 2020

√7ᵗʰ **S61.218** **Laceration without foreign body of other finger without damage to nail**
Laceration without foreign body of specified finger with unspecified laterality without damage to nail

√7ᵗʰ **S61.219** **Laceration without foreign body of unspecified finger without damage to nail**

√6ᵗʰ **S61.22** **Laceration with foreign body of finger without damage to nail**

√7ᵗʰ **S61.220** **Laceration with foreign body of right index finger without damage to nail**

√7ᵗʰ **S61.221** **Laceration with foreign body of left index finger without damage to nail**

√7ᵗʰ **S61.222** **Laceration with foreign body of right middle finger without damage to nail**

√7ᵗʰ **S61.223** **Laceration with foreign body of left middle finger without damage to nail**

√7ᵗʰ **S61.224** **Laceration with foreign body of right ring finger without damage to nail**

√7ᵗʰ **S61.225** **Laceration with foreign body of left ring finger without damage to nail**

√7ᵗʰ **S61.226** **Laceration with foreign body of right little finger without damage to nail**

√7ᵗʰ **S61.227** **Laceration with foreign body of left little finger without damage to nail**

√7ᵗʰ **S61.228** **Laceration with foreign body of other finger without damage to nail**
Laceration with foreign body of specified finger with unspecified laterality without damage to nail

√7ᵗʰ **S61.229** **Laceration with foreign body of unspecified finger without damage to nail**

√6ᵗʰ **S61.23** **Puncture wound without foreign body of finger without damage to nail**

√7ᵗʰ **S61.230** **Puncture wound without foreign body of right index finger without damage to nail**

√7ᵗʰ **S61.231** **Puncture wound without foreign body of left index finger without damage to nail**

√7ᵗʰ **S61.232** **Puncture wound without foreign body of right middle finger without damage to nail**

√7ᵗʰ **S61.233** **Puncture wound without foreign body of left middle finger without damage to nail**

√7ᵗʰ **S61.234** **Puncture wound without foreign body of right ring finger without damage to nail**

√7ᵗʰ **S61.235** **Puncture wound without foreign body of left ring finger without damage to nail**

√7ᵗʰ **S61.236** **Puncture wound without foreign body of right little finger without damage to nail**

√7ᵗʰ **S61.237** **Puncture wound without foreign body of left little finger without damage to nail**

√7ᵗʰ **S61.238** **Puncture wound without foreign body of other finger without damage to nail**
Puncture wound without foreign body of specified finger with unspecified laterality without damage to nail

√7ᵗʰ **S61.239** **Puncture wound without foreign body of unspecified finger without damage to nail**

√6ᵗʰ **S61.24** **Puncture wound with foreign body of finger without damage to nail**

√7ᵗʰ **S61.240** **Puncture wound with foreign body of right index finger without damage to nail**

√7ᵗʰ **S61.241** **Puncture wound with foreign body of left index finger without damage to nail**

√7ᵗʰ **S61.242** **Puncture wound with foreign body of right middle finger without damage to nail**

√7ᵗʰ **S61.243** **Puncture wound with foreign body of left middle finger without damage to nail**

√7ᵗʰ **S61.244** **Puncture wound with foreign body of right ring finger without damage to nail**

√7ᵗʰ **S61.245** **Puncture wound with foreign body of left ring finger without damage to nail**

√7ᵗʰ **S61.246** **Puncture wound with foreign body of right little finger without damage to nail**

√7ᵗʰ **S61.247** **Puncture wound with foreign body of left little finger without damage to nail**

√7ᵗʰ **S61.248** **Puncture wound with foreign body of other finger without damage to nail**
Puncture wound with foreign body of specified finger with unspecified laterality without damage to nail

√7ᵗʰ **S61.249** **Puncture wound with foreign body of unspecified finger without damage to nail**

√6ᵗʰ **S61.25** **Open bite of finger without damage to nail**
Bite of finger without damage to nail NOS
EXCLUDES 1   superficial bite of finger (S60.46-, S60.47-)

√7ᵗʰ **S61.250** **Open bite of right index finger without damage to nail**

√7ᵗʰ **S61.251** **Open bite of left index finger without damage to nail**

√7ᵗʰ **S61.252** **Open bite of right middle finger without damage to nail**

√7ᵗʰ **S61.253** **Open bite of left middle finger without damage to nail**

√7ᵗʰ **S61.254** **Open bite of right ring finger without damage to nail**

√7ᵗʰ **S61.255** **Open bite of left ring finger without damage to nail**

√7ᵗʰ **S61.256** **Open bite of right little finger without damage to nail**

√7ᵗʰ **S61.257** **Open bite of left little finger without damage to nail**

√7ᵗʰ **S61.258** **Open bite of other finger without damage to nail**
Open bite of specified finger with unspecified laterality without damage to nail

√7ᵗʰ **S61.259** **Open bite of unspecified finger without damage to nail**

√5ᵗʰ **S61.3** **Open wound of other finger with damage to nail**

√6ᵗʰ **S61.30** **Unspecified open wound of finger with damage to nail**

√7ᵗʰ **S61.300** **Unspecified open wound of right index finger with damage to nail**

√7ᵗʰ **S61.301** **Unspecified open wound of left index finger with damage to nail**

√7ᵗʰ **S61.302** **Unspecified open wound of right middle finger with damage to nail**

√7ᵗʰ **S61.303** **Unspecified open wound of left middle finger with damage to nail**

√7ᵗʰ **S61.304** **Unspecified open wound of right ring finger with damage to nail**

√7ᵗʰ **S61.305** **Unspecified open wound of left ring finger with damage to nail**

√7ᵗʰ **S61.306** **Unspecified open wound of right little finger with damage to nail**

√7ᵗʰ **S61.307** **Unspecified open wound of left little finger with damage to nail**

√7ᵗʰ **S61.308** **Unspecified open wound of other finger with damage to nail**
Unspecified open wound of specified finger with unspecified laterality with damage to nail

√7ᵗʰ **S61.309** **Unspecified open wound of unspecified finger with damage to nail**

√6ᵗʰ **S61.31** **Laceration without foreign body of finger with damage to nail**

√7ᵗʰ **S61.310** **Laceration without foreign body of right index finger with damage to nail**

√7ᵗʰ **S61.311** **Laceration without foreign body of left index finger with damage to nail**

√7ᵗʰ **S61.312** **Laceration without foreign body of right middle finger with damage to nail**

√7ᵗʰ **S61.313** **Laceration without foreign body of left middle finger with damage to nail**

√7ᵗʰ **S61.314** **Laceration without foreign body of right ring finger with damage to nail**

√7ᵗʰ **S61.315** **Laceration without foreign body of left ring finger with damage to nail**

√7ᵗʰ **S61.316** **Laceration without foreign body of right little finger with damage to nail**

√7ᵗʰ **S61.317** **Laceration without foreign body of left little finger with damage to nail**

☑ Additional Character Required   √x7ᵗʰ Placeholder   Unacceptable PDx   Questionable PDx   Manifestation   Unspecified Dx   H1-H14 HAC   HCC CMS-HCC Dx   HIV HIV Dx

ICD-10-CM 2020   1063

Chapter 19. Injury, Poisoning and Certain Other Consequences of External Causes

√7ᵗʰ **S61.318 Laceration without foreign body of other finger with damage to nail**
　　Laceration without foreign body of specified finger with unspecified laterality with damage to nail

√7ᵗʰ **S61.319 Laceration without foreign body of unspecified finger with damage to nail**

√6ᵗʰ **S61.32 Laceration with foreign body of finger with damage to nail**

√7ᵗʰ **S61.320 Laceration with foreign body of right index finger with damage to nail**

√7ᵗʰ **S61.321 Laceration with foreign body of left index finger with damage to nail**

√7ᵗʰ **S61.322 Laceration with foreign body of right middle finger with damage to nail**

√7ᵗʰ **S61.323 Laceration with foreign body of left middle finger with damage to nail**

√7ᵗʰ **S61.324 Laceration with foreign body of right ring finger with damage to nail**

√7ᵗʰ **S61.325 Laceration with foreign body of left ring finger with damage to nail**

√7ᵗʰ **S61.326 Laceration with foreign body of right little finger with damage to nail**

√7ᵗʰ **S61.327 Laceration with foreign body of left little finger with damage to nail**

√7ᵗʰ **S61.328 Laceration with foreign body of other finger with damage to nail**
　　Laceration with foreign body of specified finger with unspecified laterality with damage to nail

√7ᵗʰ **S61.329 Laceration with foreign body of unspecified finger with damage to nail**

√6ᵗʰ **S61.33 Puncture wound without foreign body of finger with damage to nail**

√7ᵗʰ **S61.330 Puncture wound without foreign body of right index finger with damage to nail**

√7ᵗʰ **S61.331 Puncture wound without foreign body of left index finger with damage to nail**

√7ᵗʰ **S61.332 Puncture wound without foreign body of right middle finger with damage to nail**

√7ᵗʰ **S61.333 Puncture wound without foreign body of left middle finger with damage to nail**

√7ᵗʰ **S61.334 Puncture wound without foreign body of right ring finger with damage to nail**

√7ᵗʰ **S61.335 Puncture wound without foreign body of left ring finger with damage to nail**

√7ᵗʰ **S61.336 Puncture wound without foreign body of right little finger with damage to nail**

√7ᵗʰ **S61.337 Puncture wound without foreign body of left little finger with damage to nail**

√7ᵗʰ **S61.338 Puncture wound without foreign body of other finger with damage to nail**
　　Puncture wound without foreign body of specified finger with unspecified laterality with damage to nail

√7ᵗʰ **S61.339 Puncture wound without foreign body of unspecified finger with damage to nail**

√6ᵗʰ **S61.34 Puncture wound with foreign body of finger with damage to nail**

√7ᵗʰ **S61.340 Puncture wound with foreign body of right index finger with damage to nail**

√7ᵗʰ **S61.341 Puncture wound with foreign body of left index finger with damage to nail**

√7ᵗʰ **S61.342 Puncture wound with foreign body of right middle finger with damage to nail**

√7ᵗʰ **S61.343 Puncture wound with foreign body of left middle finger with damage to nail**

√7ᵗʰ **S61.344 Puncture wound with foreign body of right ring finger with damage to nail**

√7ᵗʰ **S61.345 Puncture wound with foreign body of left ring finger with damage to nail**

√7ᵗʰ **S61.346 Puncture wound with foreign body of right little finger with damage to nail**

√7ᵗʰ **S61.347 Puncture wound with foreign body of left little finger with damage to nail**

√7ᵗʰ **S61.348 Puncture wound with foreign body of other finger with damage to nail**
　　Puncture wound with foreign body of specified finger with unspecified laterality with damage to nail

√7ᵗʰ **S61.349 Puncture wound with foreign body of unspecified finger with damage to nail**

√6ᵗʰ **S61.35 Open bite of finger with damage to nail**
　　Bite of finger with damage to nail NOS
　　EXCLUDES 1   *superficial bite of finger (S60.46-, S60.47-)*

√7ᵗʰ **S61.350 Open bite of right index finger with damage to nail**

√7ᵗʰ **S61.351 Open bite of left index finger with damage to nail**

√7ᵗʰ **S61.352 Open bite of right middle finger with damage to nail**

√7ᵗʰ **S61.353 Open bite of left middle finger with damage to nail**

√7ᵗʰ **S61.354 Open bite of right ring finger with damage to nail**

√7ᵗʰ **S61.355 Open bite of left ring finger with damage to nail**

√7ᵗʰ **S61.356 Open bite of right little finger with damage to nail**

√7ᵗʰ **S61.357 Open bite of left little finger with damage to nail**

√7ᵗʰ **S61.358 Open bite of other finger with damage to nail**
　　Open bite of specified finger with unspecified laterality with damage to nail

√7ᵗʰ **S61.359 Open bite of unspecified finger with damage to nail**

√5ᵗʰ **S61.4 Open wound of hand**

√6ᵗʰ **S61.40 Unspecified open wound of hand**

√7ᵗʰ **S61.401 Unspecified open wound of right hand**

√7ᵗʰ **S61.402 Unspecified open wound of left hand**

√7ᵗʰ **S61.409 Unspecified open wound of unspecified hand**

√6ᵗʰ **S61.41 Laceration without foreign body of hand**

√7ᵗʰ **S61.411 Laceration without foreign body of right hand**

√7ᵗʰ **S61.412 Laceration without foreign body of left hand**

√7ᵗʰ **S61.419 Laceration without foreign body of unspecified hand**

√6ᵗʰ **S61.42 Laceration with foreign body of hand**

√7ᵗʰ **S61.421 Laceration with foreign body of right hand**

√7ᵗʰ **S61.422 Laceration with foreign body of left hand**

√7ᵗʰ **S61.429 Laceration with foreign body of unspecified hand**

√6ᵗʰ **S61.43 Puncture wound without foreign body of hand**

√7ᵗʰ **S61.431 Puncture wound without foreign body of right hand**

√7ᵗʰ **S61.432 Puncture wound without foreign body of left hand**

√7ᵗʰ **S61.439 Puncture wound without foreign body of unspecified hand**

√6ᵗʰ **S61.44 Puncture wound with foreign body of hand**

√7ᵗʰ **S61.441 Puncture wound with foreign body of right hand**

√7ᵗʰ **S61.442 Puncture wound with foreign body of left hand**

√7ᵗʰ **S61.449 Puncture wound with foreign body of unspecified hand**

√6ᵗʰ **S61.45 Open bite of hand**
　　Bite of hand NOS
　　EXCLUDES 1   *superficial bite of hand (S60.56-, S60.57-)*

√7ᵗʰ **S61.451 Open bite of right hand**

√7ᵗʰ **S61.452 Open bite of left hand**

√7ᵗʰ **S61.459 Open bite of unspecified hand**

√5ᵗʰ **S61.5 Open wound of wrist**

√6ᵗʰ **S61.50 Unspecified open wound of wrist**

√7ᵗʰ **S61.501 Unspecified open wound of right wrist**

√7ᵗʰ **S61.502 Unspecified open wound of left wrist**

√7ᵗʰ **S61.509 Unspecified open wound of unspecified wrist**

√6ᵗʰ **S61.51 Laceration without foreign body of wrist**

√7ᵗʰ **S61.511 Laceration without foreign body of right wrist**

√7ᵗʰ **S61.512 Laceration without foreign body of left wrist**

Ⓝ Newborn: 0   Ⓟ Pediatric: 0-17   Ⓜ Maternity: 9-64   Ⓐ Adult: 15-124   **MCC** Major Complication/Comorbidity   **CC** Complication/Comorbidity   **SW** Severe Wound Dx

1064   ICD-10-CM 2020

√7ᵗʰ **S61.519** Laceration without foreign body of unspecified wrist

√6ᵗʰ **S61.52** Laceration with foreign body of wrist

√7ᵗʰ **S61.521** Laceration with foreign body of right wrist

√7ᵗʰ **S61.522** Laceration with foreign body of left wrist

√7ᵗʰ **S61.529** Laceration with foreign body of unspecified wrist

√6ᵗʰ **S61.53** Puncture wound without foreign body of wrist

√7ᵗʰ **S61.531** Puncture wound without foreign body of right wrist

√7ᵗʰ **S61.532** Puncture wound without foreign body of left wrist

√7ᵗʰ **S61.539** Puncture wound without foreign body of unspecified wrist

√6ᵗʰ **S61.54** Puncture wound with foreign body of wrist

√7ᵗʰ **S61.541** Puncture wound with foreign body of right wrist

√7ᵗʰ **S61.542** Puncture wound with foreign body of left wrist

√7ᵗʰ **S61.549** Puncture wound with foreign body of unspecified wrist

√6ᵗʰ **S61.55** Open bite of wrist

Bite of wrist NOS

EXCLUDES 1   superficial bite of wrist (S60.86-, S60.87-)

√7ᵗʰ **S61.551** Open bite of right wrist

√7ᵗʰ **S61.552** Open bite of left wrist

√7ᵗʰ **S61.559** Open bite of unspecified wrist

√4ᵗʰ **S62 Fracture at wrist and hand level**

NOTE   A fracture not indicated as displaced or nondisplaced should be coded to displaced

A fracture not indicated as open or closed should be coded to closed

EXCLUDES 1   traumatic amputation of wrist and hand (S68.-)

EXCLUDES 2   fracture of distal parts of ulna and radius (S52.-)

AHA: 2018,2Q,12; 2015,3Q,37-39

The appropriate 7th character is to be added to each code from category S62.

A   initial encounter for closed fracture
B   initial encounter for open fracture
D   subsequent encounter for fracture with routine healing
G   subsequent encounter for fracture with delayed healing
K   subsequent encounter for fracture with nonunion
P   subsequent encounter for fracture with malunion
S   sequela

√5ᵗʰ **S62.0 Fracture of navicular [scaphoid] bone of wrist**

CC Excl: For codes in subcategory S62.0:
CC with 7th character B: PDX collection 1283
CC with 7th character K or P: PDX collection 897

√6ᵗʰ **S62.00** Unspecified fracture of navicular [scaphoid] bone of wrist

3 √7ᵗʰ **S62.001** Unspecified fracture of navicular [scaphoid] bone of right wrist   CC H5

3 √7ᵗʰ **S62.002** Unspecified fracture of navicular [scaphoid] bone of left wrist   CC H5

AHA: 2012,4Q,106

3 √7ᵗʰ **S62.009** Unspecified fracture of navicular [scaphoid] bone of unspecified wrist   CC H5

√6ᵗʰ **S62.01** Fracture of distal pole of navicular [scaphoid] bone of wrist

Fracture of volar tuberosity of navicular [scaphoid] bone of wrist

3 √7ᵗʰ **S62.011** Displaced fracture of distal pole of navicular [scaphoid] bone of right wrist   CC H5

3 √7ᵗʰ **S62.012** Displaced fracture of distal pole of navicular [scaphoid] bone of left wrist   CC H5

3 √7ᵗʰ **S62.013** Displaced fracture of distal pole of navicular [scaphoid] bone of unspecified wrist   CC H5

3 √7ᵗʰ **S62.014** Nondisplaced fracture of distal pole of navicular [scaphoid] bone of right wrist   CC H5

3 √7ᵗʰ **S62.015** Nondisplaced fracture of distal pole of navicular [scaphoid] bone of left wrist   CC H5

3 √7ᵗʰ **S62.016** Nondisplaced fracture of distal pole of navicular [scaphoid] bone of unspecified wrist   CC H5

√6ᵗʰ **S62.02** Fracture of middle third of navicular [scaphoid] bone of wrist

3 √7ᵗʰ **S62.021** Displaced fracture of middle third of navicular [scaphoid] bone of right wrist   CC H5

3 √7ᵗʰ **S62.022** Displaced fracture of middle third of navicular [scaphoid] bone of left wrist   CC H5

3 √7ᵗʰ **S62.023** Displaced fracture of middle third of navicular [scaphoid] bone of unspecified wrist   CC H5

3 √7ᵗʰ **S62.024** Nondisplaced fracture of middle third of navicular [scaphoid] bone of right wrist   CC H5

3 √7ᵗʰ **S62.025** Nondisplaced fracture of middle third of navicular [scaphoid] bone of left wrist   CC H5

3 √7ᵗʰ **S62.026** Nondisplaced fracture of middle third of navicular [scaphoid] bone of unspecified wrist   CC H5

√6ᵗʰ **S62.03** Fracture of proximal third of navicular [scaphoid] bone of wrist

3 √7ᵗʰ **S62.031** Displaced fracture of proximal third of navicular [scaphoid] bone of right wrist   CC H5

3 √7ᵗʰ **S62.032** Displaced fracture of proximal third of navicular [scaphoid] bone of left wrist   CC H5

3 √7ᵗʰ **S62.033** Displaced fracture of proximal third of navicular [scaphoid] bone of unspecified wrist   CC H5

3 √7ᵗʰ **S62.034** Nondisplaced fracture of proximal third of navicular [scaphoid] bone of right wrist   CC H5

3 √7ᵗʰ **S62.035** Nondisplaced fracture of proximal third of navicular [scaphoid] bone of left wrist   CC H5

3 √7ᵗʰ **S62.036** Nondisplaced fracture of proximal third of navicular [scaphoid] bone of unspecified wrist   CC H5

√5ᵗʰ **S62.1 Fracture of other and unspecified carpal bone(s)**

EXCLUDES 2   fracture of scaphoid of wrist (S62.0-)

CC Excl: For codes in subcategory S62.1:
CC with 7th character B: PDX collection 1283
CC with 7th character K or P: PDX collection 897

√6ᵗʰ **S62.10** Fracture of unspecified carpal bone

Fracture of wrist NOS

3 √7ᵗʰ **S62.101** Fracture of unspecified carpal bone, right wrist   CC H5

3 √7ᵗʰ **S62.102** Fracture of unspecified carpal bone, left wrist   CC H5

AHA: 2012,4Q,95

3 √7ᵗʰ **S62.109** Fracture of unspecified carpal bone, unspecified wrist   CC H5

√6ᵗʰ **S62.11** Fracture of triquetrum [cuneiform] bone of wrist

3 √7ᵗʰ **S62.111** Displaced fracture of triquetrum [cuneiform] bone, right wrist   CC H5

☑ Additional Character Required   ✔ x 7ᵗʰ Placeholder   Unacceptable PDx   Questionable PDx   Manifestation   Unspecified Dx   H1-H14 HAC   HCC CMS-HCC Dx   HIV HIV Dx

ICD-10-CM 2020   1065

3 √7ᵗʰ **S62.112** Displaced fracture of triquetrum [cuneiform] bone, left wrist   `CC` `H5`

3 √7ᵗʰ **S62.113** Displaced fracture of triquetrum [cuneiform] bone, unspecified wrist   `CC` `H5`

3 √7ᵗʰ **S62.114** Nondisplaced fracture of triquetrum [cuneiform] bone, right wrist   `CC` `H5`

3 √7ᵗʰ **S62.115** Nondisplaced fracture of triquetrum [cuneiform] bone, left wrist   `CC` `H5`

3 √7ᵗʰ **S62.116** Nondisplaced fracture of triquetrum [cuneiform] bone, unspecified wrist   `CC` `H5`

√6ᵗʰ **S62.12** Fracture of lunate [semilunar]

3 √7ᵗʰ **S62.121** Displaced fracture of lunate [semilunar], right wrist   `CC` `H5`

3 √7ᵗʰ **S62.122** Displaced fracture of lunate [semilunar], left wrist   `CC` `H5`

3 √7ᵗʰ **S62.123** Displaced fracture of lunate [semilunar], unspecified wrist   `CC` `H5`

3 √7ᵗʰ **S62.124** Nondisplaced fracture of lunate [semilunar], right wrist   `CC` `H5`

3 √7ᵗʰ **S62.125** Nondisplaced fracture of lunate [semilunar], left wrist   `CC` `H5`

3 √7ᵗʰ **S62.126** Nondisplaced fracture of lunate [semilunar], unspecified wrist   `CC` `H5`

√6ᵗʰ **S62.13** Fracture of capitate [os magnum] bone

3 √7ᵗʰ **S62.131** Displaced fracture of capitate [os magnum] bone, right wrist   `CC` `H5`

3 √7ᵗʰ **S62.132** Displaced fracture of capitate [os magnum] bone, left wrist   `CC` `H5`

3 √7ᵗʰ **S62.133** Displaced fracture of capitate [os magnum] bone, unspecified wrist   `CC` `H5`

3 √7ᵗʰ **S62.134** Nondisplaced fracture of capitate [os magnum] bone, right wrist   `CC` `H5`

3 √7ᵗʰ **S62.135** Nondisplaced fracture of capitate [os magnum] bone, left wrist   `CC` `H5`

3 √7ᵗʰ **S62.136** Nondisplaced fracture of capitate [os magnum] bone, unspecified wrist   `CC` `H5`

√6ᵗʰ **S62.14** Fracture of body of hamate [unciform] bone
Fracture of hamate [unciform] bone NOS

3 √7ᵗʰ **S62.141** Displaced fracture of body of hamate [unciform] bone, right wrist   `CC` `H5`

3 √7ᵗʰ **S62.142** Displaced fracture of body of hamate [unciform] bone, left wrist   `CC` `H5`

3 √7ᵗʰ **S62.143** Displaced fracture of body of hamate [unciform] bone, unspecified wrist   `CC` `H5`

3 √7ᵗʰ **S62.144** Nondisplaced fracture of body of hamate [unciform] bone, right wrist   `CC` `H5`

3 √7ᵗʰ **S62.145** Nondisplaced fracture of body of hamate [unciform] bone, left wrist   `CC` `H5`

3 √7ᵗʰ **S62.146** Nondisplaced fracture of body of hamate [unciform] bone, unspecified wrist   `CC` `H5`

√6ᵗʰ **S62.15** Fracture of hook process of hamate [unciform] bone
Fracture of unciform process of hamate [unciform] bone

3 √7ᵗʰ **S62.151** Displaced fracture of hook process of hamate [unciform] bone, right wrist   `CC` `H5`

3 √7ᵗʰ **S62.152** Displaced fracture of hook process of hamate [unciform] bone, left wrist   `CC` `H5`

3 √7ᵗʰ **S62.153** Displaced fracture of hook process of hamate [unciform] bone, unspecified wrist   `CC` `H5`

3 √7ᵗʰ **S62.154** Nondisplaced fracture of hook process of hamate [unciform] bone, right wrist   `CC` `H5`

3 √7ᵗʰ **S62.155** Nondisplaced fracture of hook process of hamate [unciform] bone, left wrist   `CC` `H5`

3 √7ᵗʰ **S62.156** Nondisplaced fracture of hook process of hamate [unciform] bone, unspecified wrist   `CC` `H5`

√6ᵗʰ **S62.16** Fracture of pisiform

3 √7ᵗʰ **S62.161** Displaced fracture of pisiform, right wrist   `CC` `H5`

3 √7ᵗʰ **S62.162** Displaced fracture of pisiform, left wrist   `CC` `H5`

3 √7ᵗʰ **S62.163** Displaced fracture of pisiform, unspecified wrist   `CC` `H5`

3 √7ᵗʰ **S62.164** Nondisplaced fracture of pisiform, right wrist   `CC` `H5`

3 √7ᵗʰ **S62.165** Nondisplaced fracture of pisiform, left wrist   `CC` `H5`

3 √7ᵗʰ **S62.166** Nondisplaced fracture of pisiform, unspecified wrist   `CC` `H5`

√6ᵗʰ **S62.17** Fracture of trapezium [larger multangular]

3 √7ᵗʰ **S62.171** Displaced fracture of trapezium [larger multangular], right wrist   `CC` `H5`

3 √7ᵗʰ **S62.172** Displaced fracture of trapezium [larger multangular], left wrist   `CC` `H5`

3 √7ᵗʰ **S62.173** Displaced fracture of trapezium [larger multangular], unspecified wrist   `CC` `H5`

3 √7ᵗʰ **S62.174** Nondisplaced fracture of trapezium [larger multangular], right wrist   `CC` `H5`

3 √7ᵗʰ **S62.175** Nondisplaced fracture of trapezium [larger multangular], left wrist   `CC` `H5`

3 √7ᵗʰ **S62.176** Nondisplaced fracture of trapezium [larger multangular], unspecified wrist   `CC` `H5`

√6ᵗʰ **S62.18** Fracture of trapezoid [smaller multangular]

3 √7ᵗʰ **S62.181** Displaced fracture of trapezoid [smaller multangular], right wrist   `CC` `H5`

3 √7ᵗʰ **S62.182** Displaced fracture of trapezoid [smaller multangular], left wrist   `CC` `H5`

3 √7ᵗʰ **S62.183** Displaced fracture of trapezoid [smaller multangular], unspecified wrist   `CC` `H5`

3 √7ᵗʰ **S62.184** Nondisplaced fracture of trapezoid [smaller multangular], right wrist   `CC` `H5`

3 √7ᵗʰ **S62.185** Nondisplaced fracture of trapezoid [smaller multangular], left wrist   `CC` `H5`

3 √7ᵗʰ **S62.186** Nondisplaced fracture of trapezoid [smaller multangular], unspecified wrist   `CC` `H5`

√5ᵗʰ **S62.2** Fracture of first metacarpal bone

CC Excl: For codes in subcategory S62.2:
CC with 7th character B: PDX collection 1284
CC with 7th character K or P: PDX collection 897

√6ᵗʰ **S62.20** Unspecified fracture of first metacarpal bone

3 √7ᵗʰ **S62.201** Unspecified fracture of first metacarpal bone, right hand   `CC` `H5`

3 √7ᵗʰ **S62.202** Unspecified fracture of first metacarpal bone, left hand   `CC` `H5`

`N` Newborn: 0   `P` Pediatric: 0-17   `M` Maternity: 9-64   `A` Adult: 15-124   `MCC` Major Complication/Comorbidity   `CC` Complication/Comorbidity   `SW` Severe Wound Dx

1066   ICD-10-CM 2020

3 √7ᵗʰ **S62.209** Unspecified fracture of first metacarpal bone, unspecified hand   CC H5

√6ᵗʰ **S62.21** Bennett's fracture
> **DEF:** Intra-articular, two-part fracture at the base of the first metacarpal bone (thumb) on the ulnar side at the carpometacarpal (CMC) joint.

3 √7ᵗʰ **S62.211** Bennett's fracture, right hand   CC H5

3 √7ᵗʰ **S62.212** Bennett's fracture, left hand   CC H5

3 √7ᵗʰ **S62.213** Bennett's fracture, unspecified hand   CC H5

√6ᵗʰ **S62.22** Rolando's fracture
> **DEF:** Comminuted, three part intra-articular fracture at the base of the thumb metacarpal.

3 √7ᵗʰ **S62.221** Displaced Rolando's fracture, right hand   CC H5

3 √7ᵗʰ **S62.222** Displaced Rolando's fracture, left hand   CC H5

3 √7ᵗʰ **S62.223** Displaced Rolando's fracture, unspecified hand   CC H5

3 √7ᵗʰ **S62.224** Nondisplaced Rolando's fracture, right hand   CC H5

3 √7ᵗʰ **S62.225** Nondisplaced Rolando's fracture, left hand   CC H5

3 √7ᵗʰ **S62.226** Nondisplaced Rolando's fracture, unspecified hand   CC H5

√6ᵗʰ **S62.23** Other fracture of base of first metacarpal bone

3 √7ᵗʰ **S62.231** Other displaced fracture of base of first metacarpal bone, right hand   CC H5

3 √7ᵗʰ **S62.232** Other displaced fracture of base of first metacarpal bone, left hand   CC H5

3 √7ᵗʰ **S62.233** Other displaced fracture of base of first metacarpal bone, unspecified hand   CC H5

3 √7ᵗʰ **S62.234** Other nondisplaced fracture of base of first metacarpal bone, right hand   CC H5

3 √7ᵗʰ **S62.235** Other nondisplaced fracture of base of first metacarpal bone, left hand   CC H5

3 √7ᵗʰ **S62.236** Other nondisplaced fracture of base of first metacarpal bone, unspecified hand   CC H5

√6ᵗʰ **S62.24** Fracture of shaft of first metacarpal bone

3 √7ᵗʰ **S62.241** Displaced fracture of shaft of first metacarpal bone, right hand   CC H5

3 √7ᵗʰ **S62.242** Displaced fracture of shaft of first metacarpal bone, left hand   CC H5

3 √7ᵗʰ **S62.243** Displaced fracture of shaft of first metacarpal bone, unspecified hand   CC H5

3 √7ᵗʰ **S62.244** Nondisplaced fracture of shaft of first metacarpal bone, right hand   CC H5

3 √7ᵗʰ **S62.245** Nondisplaced fracture of shaft of first metacarpal bone, left hand   CC H5

3 √7ᵗʰ **S62.246** Nondisplaced fracture of shaft of first metacarpal bone, unspecified hand   CC H5

√6ᵗʰ **S62.25** Fracture of neck of first metacarpal bone

3 √7ᵗʰ **S62.251** Displaced fracture of neck of first metacarpal bone, right hand   CC H5

3 √7ᵗʰ **S62.252** Displaced fracture of neck of first metacarpal bone, left hand   CC H5

3 √7ᵗʰ **S62.253** Displaced fracture of neck of first metacarpal bone, unspecified hand   CC H5

3 √7ᵗʰ **S62.254** Nondisplaced fracture of neck of first metacarpal bone, right hand   CC H5

3 √7ᵗʰ **S62.255** Nondisplaced fracture of neck of first metacarpal bone, left hand   CC H5

3 √7ᵗʰ **S62.256** Nondisplaced fracture of neck of first metacarpal bone, unspecified hand   CC H5

√6ᵗʰ **S62.29** Other fracture of first metacarpal bone

3 √7ᵗʰ **S62.291** Other fracture of first metacarpal bone, right hand   CC H5

3 √7ᵗʰ **S62.292** Other fracture of first metacarpal bone, left hand   CC H5

3 √7ᵗʰ **S62.299** Other fracture of first metacarpal bone, unspecified hand   CC H5

√5ᵗʰ **S62.3** Fracture of other and unspecified metacarpal bone
> **EXCLUDES 2**   *fracture of first metacarpal bone (S62.2-)*

CC Excl: For codes in subcategory S62.3:
CC with 7th character B: PDX collection 1284
CC with 7th character K or P: PDX collection 897

√6ᵗʰ **S62.30** Unspecified fracture of other metacarpal bone

3 √7ᵗʰ **S62.300** Unspecified fracture of second metacarpal bone, right hand   CC H5

3 √7ᵗʰ **S62.301** Unspecified fracture of second metacarpal bone, left hand   CC H5

3 √7ᵗʰ **S62.302** Unspecified fracture of third metacarpal bone, right hand   CC H5

3 √7ᵗʰ **S62.303** Unspecified fracture of third metacarpal bone, left hand   CC H5

3 √7ᵗʰ **S62.304** Unspecified fracture of fourth metacarpal bone, right hand   CC H5

3 √7ᵗʰ **S62.305** Unspecified fracture of fourth metacarpal bone, left hand   CC H5

3 √7ᵗʰ **S62.306** Unspecified fracture of fifth metacarpal bone, right hand   CC H5

3 √7ᵗʰ **S62.307** Unspecified fracture of fifth metacarpal bone, left hand   CC H5

3 √7ᵗʰ **S62.308** Unspecified fracture of other metacarpal bone   CC H5
> Unspecified fracture of specified metacarpal bone with unspecified laterality

3 √7ᵗʰ **S62.309** Unspecified fracture of unspecified metacarpal bone   CC H5

√6ᵗʰ **S62.31** Displaced fracture of base of other metacarpal bone

3 √7ᵗʰ **S62.310** Displaced fracture of base of second metacarpal bone, right hand   CC H5

3 √7ᵗʰ **S62.311** Displaced fracture of base of second metacarpal bone, left hand   CC H5

3 √7ᵗʰ **S62.312** Displaced fracture of base of third metacarpal bone, right hand   CC H5

3 √7ᵗʰ **S62.313** Displaced fracture of base of third metacarpal bone, left hand   CC H5

3 √7ᵗʰ **S62.314** Displaced fracture of base of fourth metacarpal bone, right hand   CC H5

3 √7ᵗʰ **S62.315** Displaced fracture of base of fourth metacarpal bone, left hand   CC H5

3 √7ᵗʰ **S62.316** Displaced fracture of base of fifth metacarpal bone, right hand   CC H5

3 √7ᵗʰ **S62.317** Displaced fracture of base of fifth metacarpal bone, left hand   CC H5

3 ✓7ᵗʰ **S62.318** **Displaced fracture of base of other metacarpal bone** `CC` `H5`
         Displaced fracture of base of specified metacarpal bone with unspecified laterality

3 ✓7ᵗʰ **S62.319** **Displaced fracture of base of unspecified metacarpal bone** `CC` `H5`

✓6ᵗʰ **S62.32** **Displaced fracture of shaft of other metacarpal bone**

3 ✓7ᵗʰ **S62.320** **Displaced fracture of shaft of second metacarpal bone, right hand** `CC` `H5`

3 ✓7ᵗʰ **S62.321** **Displaced fracture of shaft of second metacarpal bone, left hand** `CC` `H5`

3 ✓7ᵗʰ **S62.322** **Displaced fracture of shaft of third metacarpal bone, right hand** `CC` `H5`

3 ✓7ᵗʰ **S62.323** **Displaced fracture of shaft of third metacarpal bone, left hand** `CC` `H5`

3 ✓7ᵗʰ **S62.324** **Displaced fracture of shaft of fourth metacarpal bone, right hand** `CC` `H5`

3 ✓7ᵗʰ **S62.325** **Displaced fracture of shaft of fourth metacarpal bone, left hand** `CC` `H5`

3 ✓7ᵗʰ **S62.326** **Displaced fracture of shaft of fifth metacarpal bone, right hand** `CC` `H5`

3 ✓7ᵗʰ **S62.327** **Displaced fracture of shaft of fifth metacarpal bone, left hand** `CC` `H5`

3 ✓7ᵗʰ **S62.328** **Displaced fracture of shaft of other metacarpal bone** `CC` `H5`
         Displaced fracture of shaft of specified metacarpal bone with unspecified laterality

3 ✓7ᵗʰ **S62.329** **Displaced fracture of shaft of unspecified metacarpal bone** `CC` `H5`

✓6ᵗʰ **S62.33** **Displaced fracture of neck of other metacarpal bone**

3 ✓7ᵗʰ **S62.330** **Displaced fracture of neck of second metacarpal bone, right hand** `CC` `H5`

3 ✓7ᵗʰ **S62.331** **Displaced fracture of neck of second metacarpal bone, left hand** `CC` `H5`

3 ✓7ᵗʰ **S62.332** **Displaced fracture of neck of third metacarpal bone, right hand** `CC` `H5`

3 ✓7ᵗʰ **S62.333** **Displaced fracture of neck of third metacarpal bone, left hand** `CC` `H5`

3 ✓7ᵗʰ **S62.334** **Displaced fracture of neck of fourth metacarpal bone, right hand** `CC` `H5`

3 ✓7ᵗʰ **S62.335** **Displaced fracture of neck of fourth metacarpal bone, left hand** `CC` `H5`

3 ✓7ᵗʰ **S62.336** **Displaced fracture of neck of fifth metacarpal bone, right hand** `CC` `H5`

3 ✓7ᵗʰ **S62.337** **Displaced fracture of neck of fifth metacarpal bone, left hand** `CC` `H5`

3 ✓7ᵗʰ **S62.338** **Displaced fracture of neck of other metacarpal bone** `CC` `H5`
         Displaced fracture of neck of specified metacarpal bone with unspecified laterality

3 ✓7ᵗʰ **S62.339** **Displaced fracture of neck of unspecified metacarpal bone** `CC` `H5`

✓6ᵗʰ **S62.34** **Nondisplaced fracture of base of other metacarpal bone**

3 ✓7ᵗʰ **S62.340** **Nondisplaced fracture of base of second metacarpal bone, right hand** `CC` `H5`

3 ✓7ᵗʰ **S62.341** **Nondisplaced fracture of base of second metacarpal bone, left hand** `CC` `H5`

3 ✓7ᵗʰ **S62.342** **Nondisplaced fracture of base of third metacarpal bone, right hand** `CC` `H5`

3 ✓7ᵗʰ **S62.343** **Nondisplaced fracture of base of third metacarpal bone, left hand** `CC` `H5`

3 ✓7ᵗʰ **S62.344** **Nondisplaced fracture of base of fourth metacarpal bone, right hand** `CC` `H5`

3 ✓7ᵗʰ **S62.345** **Nondisplaced fracture of base of fourth metacarpal bone, left hand** `CC` `H5`

3 ✓7ᵗʰ **S62.346** **Nondisplaced fracture of base of fifth metacarpal bone, right hand** `CC` `H5`

3 ✓7ᵗʰ **S62.347** **Nondisplaced fracture of base of fifth metacarpal bone, left hand** `CC` `H5`

3 ✓7ᵗʰ **S62.348** **Nondisplaced fracture of base of other metacarpal bone** `CC` `H5`
         Nondisplaced fracture of base of specified metacarpal bone with unspecified laterality

3 ✓7ᵗʰ **S62.349** **Nondisplaced fracture of base of unspecified metacarpal bone** `CC` `H5`

✓6ᵗʰ **S62.35** **Nondisplaced fracture of shaft of other metacarpal bone**

3 ✓7ᵗʰ **S62.350** **Nondisplaced fracture of shaft of second metacarpal bone, right hand** `CC` `H5`

3 ✓7ᵗʰ **S62.351** **Nondisplaced fracture of shaft of second metacarpal bone, left hand** `CC` `H5`

3 ✓7ᵗʰ **S62.352** **Nondisplaced fracture of shaft of third metacarpal bone, right hand** `CC` `H5`

3 ✓7ᵗʰ **S62.353** **Nondisplaced fracture of shaft of third metacarpal bone, left hand** `CC` `H5`

3 ✓7ᵗʰ **S62.354** **Nondisplaced fracture of shaft of fourth metacarpal bone, right hand** `CC` `H5`

3 ✓7ᵗʰ **S62.355** **Nondisplaced fracture of shaft of fourth metacarpal bone, left hand** `CC` `H5`

3 ✓7ᵗʰ **S62.356** **Nondisplaced fracture of shaft of fifth metacarpal bone, right hand** `CC` `H5`

3 ✓7ᵗʰ **S62.357** **Nondisplaced fracture of shaft of fifth metacarpal bone, left hand** `CC` `H5`

3 ✓7ᵗʰ **S62.358** **Nondisplaced fracture of shaft of other metacarpal bone** `CC` `H5`
         Nondisplaced fracture of shaft of specified metacarpal bone with unspecified laterality

3 ✓7ᵗʰ **S62.359** **Nondisplaced fracture of shaft of unspecified metacarpal bone** `CC` `H5`

✓6ᵗʰ **S62.36** **Nondisplaced fracture of neck of other metacarpal bone**

3 ✓7ᵗʰ **S62.360** **Nondisplaced fracture of neck of second metacarpal bone, right hand** `CC` `H5`

3 ✓7ᵗʰ **S62.361** **Nondisplaced fracture of neck of second metacarpal bone, left hand** `CC` `H5`

3 ✓7ᵗʰ **S62.362** **Nondisplaced fracture of neck of third metacarpal bone, right hand** `CC` `H5`

3 ✓7ᵗʰ **S62.363** **Nondisplaced fracture of neck of third metacarpal bone, left hand** `CC` `H5`

3 ✓7ᵗʰ **S62.364** **Nondisplaced fracture of neck of fourth metacarpal bone, right hand** `CC` `H5`

3 ✓7ᵗʰ **S62.365** **Nondisplaced fracture of neck of fourth metacarpal bone, left hand** `CC` `H5`

Ⓝ Newborn: 0   Ⓟ Pediatric: 0-17   Ⓜ Maternity: 9-64   Ⓐ Adult: 15-124   `MCC` Major Complication/Comorbidity   `CC` Complication/Comorbidity   `SW` Severe Wound Dx

1068   ICD-10-CM 2020

3 √7ᵗʰ	**S62.366**	**Nondisplaced fracture of neck of fifth metacarpal bone, right hand**	CC H5
3 √7ᵗʰ	**S62.367**	**Nondisplaced fracture of neck of fifth metacarpal bone, left hand**	CC H5
3 √7ᵗʰ	**S62.368**	**Nondisplaced fracture of neck of other metacarpal bone**	CC H5
		Nondisplaced fracture of neck of specified metacarpal bone with unspecified laterality	
3 √7ᵗʰ	**S62.369**	**Nondisplaced fracture of neck of unspecified metacarpal bone**	CC H5

√6ᵗʰ **S62.39**   **Other fracture of other metacarpal bone**

3 √7ᵗʰ	**S62.390**	**Other fracture of second metacarpal bone, right hand**	CC H5
3 √7ᵗʰ	**S62.391**	**Other fracture of second metacarpal bone, left hand**	CC H5
3 √7ᵗʰ	**S62.392**	**Other fracture of third metacarpal bone, right hand**	CC H5
3 √7ᵗʰ	**S62.393**	**Other fracture of third metacarpal bone, left hand**	CC H5
3 √7ᵗʰ	**S62.394**	**Other fracture of fourth metacarpal bone, right hand**	CC H5
3 √7ᵗʰ	**S62.395**	**Other fracture of fourth metacarpal bone, left hand**	CC H5
3 √7ᵗʰ	**S62.396**	**Other fracture of fifth metacarpal bone, right hand**	CC H5
3 √7ᵗʰ	**S62.397**	**Other fracture of fifth metacarpal bone, left hand**	CC H5
3 √7ᵗʰ	**S62.398**	**Other fracture of other metacarpal bone**	CC H5
		Other fracture of specified metacarpal bone with unspecified laterality	
3 √7ᵗʰ	**S62.399**	**Other fracture of unspecified metacarpal bone**	CC H5

√5ᵗʰ **S62.5**   **Fracture of thumb**

> **CC Excl:** For codes in subcategory S62.5:
> **CC with 7th character B:** PDX collection 1285
> **CC with 7th character K or P:** PDX collection 897

√6ᵗʰ **S62.50**   **Fracture of unspecified phalanx of thumb**

3 √7ᵗʰ	**S62.501**	**Fracture of unspecified phalanx of right thumb**	CC H5
3 √7ᵗʰ	**S62.502**	**Fracture of unspecified phalanx of left thumb**	CC H5
3 √7ᵗʰ	**S62.509**	**Fracture of unspecified phalanx of unspecified thumb**	CC H5

√6ᵗʰ **S62.51**   **Fracture of proximal phalanx of thumb**

3 √7ᵗʰ	**S62.511**	**Displaced fracture of proximal phalanx of right thumb**	CC H5
3 √7ᵗʰ	**S62.512**	**Displaced fracture of proximal phalanx of left thumb**	CC H5
3 √7ᵗʰ	**S62.513**	**Displaced fracture of proximal phalanx of unspecified thumb**	CC H5
3 √7ᵗʰ	**S62.514**	**Nondisplaced fracture of proximal phalanx of right thumb**	CC H5
3 √7ᵗʰ	**S62.515**	**Nondisplaced fracture of proximal phalanx of left thumb**	CC H5
3 √7ᵗʰ	**S62.516**	**Nondisplaced fracture of proximal phalanx of unspecified thumb**	CC H5

√6ᵗʰ **S62.52**   **Fracture of distal phalanx of thumb**

3 √7ᵗʰ	**S62.521**	**Displaced fracture of distal phalanx of right thumb**	CC H5
3 √7ᵗʰ	**S62.522**	**Displaced fracture of distal phalanx of left thumb**	CC H5
3 √7ᵗʰ	**S62.523**	**Displaced fracture of distal phalanx of unspecified thumb**	CC H5
3 √7ᵗʰ	**S62.524**	**Nondisplaced fracture of distal phalanx of right thumb**	CC H5
3 √7ᵗʰ	**S62.525**	**Nondisplaced fracture of distal phalanx of left thumb**	CC H5
3 √7ᵗʰ	**S62.526**	**Nondisplaced fracture of distal phalanx of unspecified thumb**	CC H5

√5ᵗʰ **S62.6**   **Fracture of other and unspecified finger(s)**

> **EXCLUDES 2**   fracture of thumb (S62.5-)
>
> **CC Excl:** For codes in subcategory S62.6:
> **CC with 7th character B:** PDX collection 1285
> **CC with 7th character K or P:** PDX collection 897

√6ᵗʰ **S62.60**   **Fracture of unspecified phalanx of finger**

3 √7ᵗʰ	**S62.600**	**Fracture of unspecified phalanx of right index finger**	CC H5
3 √7ᵗʰ	**S62.601**	**Fracture of unspecified phalanx of left index finger**	CC H5
3 √7ᵗʰ	**S62.602**	**Fracture of unspecified phalanx of right middle finger**	CC H5
3 √7ᵗʰ	**S62.603**	**Fracture of unspecified phalanx of left middle finger**	CC H5
3 √7ᵗʰ	**S62.604**	**Fracture of unspecified phalanx of right ring finger**	CC H5
3 √7ᵗʰ	**S62.605**	**Fracture of unspecified phalanx of left ring finger**	CC H5
3 √7ᵗʰ	**S62.606**	**Fracture of unspecified phalanx of right little finger**	CC H5
3 √7ᵗʰ	**S62.607**	**Fracture of unspecified phalanx of left little finger**	CC H5
3 √7ᵗʰ	**S62.608**	**Fracture of unspecified phalanx of other finger**	CC H5
		Fracture of unspecified phalanx of specified finger with unspecified laterality	
3 √7ᵗʰ	**S62.609**	**Fracture of unspecified phalanx of unspecified finger**	CC H5

√6ᵗʰ **S62.61**   **Displaced fracture of proximal phalanx of finger**

3 √7ᵗʰ	**S62.610**	**Displaced fracture of proximal phalanx of right index finger**	CC H5
3 √7ᵗʰ	**S62.611**	**Displaced fracture of proximal phalanx of left index finger**	CC H5
3 √7ᵗʰ	**S62.612**	**Displaced fracture of proximal phalanx of right middle finger**	CC H5
3 √7ᵗʰ	**S62.613**	**Displaced fracture of proximal phalanx of left middle finger**	CC H5
3 √7ᵗʰ	**S62.614**	**Displaced fracture of proximal phalanx of right ring finger**	CC H5
3 √7ᵗʰ	**S62.615**	**Displaced fracture of proximal phalanx of left ring finger**	CC H5
3 √7ᵗʰ	**S62.616**	**Displaced fracture of proximal phalanx of right little finger**	CC H5
3 √7ᵗʰ	**S62.617**	**Displaced fracture of proximal phalanx of left little finger**	CC H5
3 √7ᵗʰ	**S62.618**	**Displaced fracture of proximal phalanx of other finger**	CC H5
		Displaced fracture of proximal phalanx of specified finger with unspecified laterality	

3 ✓7ᵗʰ **S62.619** **Displaced fracture of proximal phalanx of unspecified finger** `CC` `H5`

✓6ᵗʰ **S62.62** **Displaced fracture of middle phalanx of finger**

    3 ✓7ᵗʰ **S62.620** **Displaced fracture of middle phalanx of right index finger** `CC` `H5`

    3 ✓7ᵗʰ **S62.621** **Displaced fracture of middle phalanx of left index finger** `CC` `H5`

    3 ✓7ᵗʰ **S62.622** **Displaced fracture of middle phalanx of right middle finger** `CC` `H5`

    3 ✓7ᵗʰ **S62.623** **Displaced fracture of middle phalanx of left middle finger** `CC` `H5`

    3 ✓7ᵗʰ **S62.624** **Displaced fracture of middle phalanx of right ring finger** `CC` `H5`

    3 ✓7ᵗʰ **S62.625** **Displaced fracture of middle phalanx of left ring finger** `CC` `H5`

    3 ✓7ᵗʰ **S62.626** **Displaced fracture of middle phalanx of right little finger** `CC` `H5`

    3 ✓7ᵗʰ **S62.627** **Displaced fracture of middle phalanx of left little finger** `CC` `H5`

    3 ✓7ᵗʰ **S62.628** **Displaced fracture of middle phalanx of other finger** `CC` `H5`

        Displaced fracture of middle phalanx of specified finger with unspecified laterality

    3 ✓7ᵗʰ **S62.629** **Displaced fracture of middle phalanx of unspecified finger** `CC` `H5`

✓6ᵗʰ **S62.63** **Displaced fracture of distal phalanx of finger**

    3 ✓7ᵗʰ **S62.630** **Displaced fracture of distal phalanx of right index finger** `CC` `H5`

    3 ✓7ᵗʰ **S62.631** **Displaced fracture of distal phalanx of left index finger** `CC` `H5`

    3 ✓7ᵗʰ **S62.632** **Displaced fracture of distal phalanx of right middle finger** `CC` `H5`

    3 ✓7ᵗʰ **S62.633** **Displaced fracture of distal phalanx of left middle finger** `CC` `H5`

    3 ✓7ᵗʰ **S62.634** **Displaced fracture of distal phalanx of right ring finger** `CC` `H5`

    3 ✓7ᵗʰ **S62.635** **Displaced fracture of distal phalanx of left ring finger** `CC` `H5`

    3 ✓7ᵗʰ **S62.636** **Displaced fracture of distal phalanx of right little finger** `CC` `H5`

    3 ✓7ᵗʰ **S62.637** **Displaced fracture of distal phalanx of left little finger** `CC` `H5`

    3 ✓7ᵗʰ **S62.638** **Displaced fracture of distal phalanx of other finger** `CC` `H5`

        Displaced fracture of distal phalanx of specified finger with unspecified laterality

    3 ✓7ᵗʰ **S62.639** **Displaced fracture of distal phalanx of unspecified finger** `CC` `H5`

✓6ᵗʰ **S62.64** **Nondisplaced fracture of proximal phalanx of finger**

    3 ✓7ᵗʰ **S62.640** **Nondisplaced fracture of proximal phalanx of right index finger** `CC` `H5`

    3 ✓7ᵗʰ **S62.641** **Nondisplaced fracture of proximal phalanx of left index finger** `CC` `H5`

    3 ✓7ᵗʰ **S62.642** **Nondisplaced fracture of proximal phalanx of right middle finger** `CC` `H5`

    3 ✓7ᵗʰ **S62.643** **Nondisplaced fracture of proximal phalanx of left middle finger** `CC` `H5`

    3 ✓7ᵗʰ **S62.644** **Nondisplaced fracture of proximal phalanx of right ring finger** `CC` `H5`

    3 ✓7ᵗʰ **S62.645** **Nondisplaced fracture of proximal phalanx of left ring finger** `CC` `H5`

    3 ✓7ᵗʰ **S62.646** **Nondisplaced fracture of proximal phalanx of right little finger** `CC` `H5`

    3 ✓7ᵗʰ **S62.647** **Nondisplaced fracture of proximal phalanx of left little finger** `CC` `H5`

    3 ✓7ᵗʰ **S62.648** **Nondisplaced fracture of proximal phalanx of other finger** `CC` `H5`

        Nondisplaced fracture of proximal phalanx of specified finger with unspecified laterality

    3 ✓7ᵗʰ **S62.649** **Nondisplaced fracture of proximal phalanx of unspecified finger** `CC` `H5`

✓6ᵗʰ **S62.65** **Nondisplaced fracture of middle phalanx of finger**

    3 ✓7ᵗʰ **S62.650** **Nondisplaced fracture of middle phalanx of right index finger** `CC` `H5`

    3 ✓7ᵗʰ **S62.651** **Nondisplaced fracture of middle phalanx of left index finger** `CC` `H5`

    3 ✓7ᵗʰ **S62.652** **Nondisplaced fracture of middle phalanx of right middle finger** `CC` `H5`

    3 ✓7ᵗʰ **S62.653** **Nondisplaced fracture of middle phalanx of left middle finger** `CC` `H5`

    3 ✓7ᵗʰ **S62.654** **Nondisplaced fracture of middle phalanx of right ring finger** `CC` `H5`

    3 ✓7ᵗʰ **S62.655** **Nondisplaced fracture of middle phalanx of left ring finger** `CC` `H5`

    3 ✓7ᵗʰ **S62.656** **Nondisplaced fracture of middle phalanx of right little finger** `CC` `H5`

    3 ✓7ᵗʰ **S62.657** **Nondisplaced fracture of middle phalanx of left little finger** `CC` `H5`

    3 ✓7ᵗʰ **S62.658** **Nondisplaced fracture of middle phalanx of other finger** `CC` `H5`

        Nondisplaced fracture of middle phalanx of specified finger with unspecified laterality

    3 ✓7ᵗʰ **S62.659** **Nondisplaced fracture of middle phalanx of unspecified finger** `CC` `H5`

✓6ᵗʰ **S62.66** **Nondisplaced fracture of distal phalanx of finger**

    3 ✓7ᵗʰ **S62.660** **Nondisplaced fracture of distal phalanx of right index finger** `CC` `H5`

    3 ✓7ᵗʰ **S62.661** **Nondisplaced fracture of distal phalanx of left index finger** `CC` `H5`

    3 ✓7ᵗʰ **S62.662** **Nondisplaced fracture of distal phalanx of right middle finger** `CC` `H5`

    3 ✓7ᵗʰ **S62.663** **Nondisplaced fracture of distal phalanx of left middle finger** `CC` `H5`

    3 ✓7ᵗʰ **S62.664** **Nondisplaced fracture of distal phalanx of right ring finger** `CC` `H5`

    3 ✓7ᵗʰ **S62.665** **Nondisplaced fracture of distal phalanx of left ring finger** `CC` `H5`

    3 ✓7ᵗʰ **S62.666** **Nondisplaced fracture of distal phalanx of right little finger** `CC` `H5`

    3 ✓7ᵗʰ **S62.667** **Nondisplaced fracture of distal phalanx of left little finger** `CC` `H5`

N Newborn: 0   **P** Pediatric: 0-17   **M** Maternity: 9-64   **A** Adult: 15-124   **MCC** Major Complication/Comorbidity   **CC** Complication/Comorbidity   **SW** Severe Wound Dx

1070

ICD-10-CM 2020

3 √7ᵗʰ **S62.668 Nondisplaced fracture of distal phalanx of other finger** `CC` `H5`

Nondisplaced fracture of distal phalanx of specified finger with unspecified laterality

3 √7ᵗʰ **S62.669 Nondisplaced fracture of distal phalanx of unspecified finger** `CC` `H5`

√6ᵗʰ **S62.9 Unspecified fracture of wrist and hand**

3 √x7ᵗʰ **S62.90 Unspecified fracture of unspecified wrist and hand** `CC` `H5`

CC Excl: CC with 7th character B: PDX collection 1286
CC Excl: CC with 7th character K or P: PDX collection 897

3 √x7ᵗʰ **S62.91 Unspecified fracture of right wrist and hand** `CC` `H5`

CC Excl: CC with 7th character B: PDX collection 1287
CC Excl: CC with 7th character K or P: PDX collection 897

3 √x7ᵗʰ **S62.92 Unspecified fracture of left wrist and hand** `CC` `H5`

CC Excl: CC with 7th character B: PDX collection 1287
CC Excl: CC with 7th character K or P: PDX collection 897

√4ᵗʰ **S63 Dislocation and sprain of joints and ligaments at wrist and hand level**

`INCLUDES` avulsion of joint or ligament at wrist and hand level
laceration of cartilage, joint or ligament at wrist and hand level
sprain of cartilage, joint or ligament at wrist and hand level
traumatic hemarthrosis of joint or ligament at wrist and hand level
traumatic rupture of joint or ligament at wrist and hand level
traumatic subluxation of joint or ligament at wrist and hand level
traumatic tear of joint or ligament at wrist and hand level

Code also any associated open wound

`EXCLUDES 2` strain of muscle, fascia and tendon of wrist and hand (S66.-)

The appropriate 7th character is to be added to each code from category S63.
A   initial encounter
D   subsequent encounter
S   sequela

√5ᵗʰ **S63.0 Subluxation and dislocation of wrist and hand joints**

√6ᵗʰ **S63.00 Unspecified subluxation and dislocation of wrist and hand**

Dislocation of carpal bone NOS
Dislocation of distal end of radius NOS
Subluxation of carpal bone NOS
Subluxation of distal end of radius NOS

√7ᵗʰ **S63.001 Unspecified subluxation of right wrist and hand**

√7ᵗʰ **S63.002 Unspecified subluxation of left wrist and hand**

√7ᵗʰ **S63.003 Unspecified subluxation of unspecified wrist and hand**

√7ᵗʰ **S63.004 Unspecified dislocation of right wrist and hand**

√7ᵗʰ **S63.005 Unspecified dislocation of left wrist and hand**

√7ᵗʰ **S63.006 Unspecified dislocation of unspecified wrist and hand**

√6ᵗʰ **S63.01 Subluxation and dislocation of distal radioulnar joint**

√7ᵗʰ **S63.011 Subluxation of distal radioulnar joint of right wrist**

√7ᵗʰ **S63.012 Subluxation of distal radioulnar joint of left wrist**

√7ᵗʰ **S63.013 Subluxation of distal radioulnar joint of unspecified wrist**

√7ᵗʰ **S63.014 Dislocation of distal radioulnar joint of right wrist**

√7ᵗʰ **S63.015 Dislocation of distal radioulnar joint of left wrist**

√7ᵗʰ **S63.016 Dislocation of distal radioulnar joint of unspecified wrist**

√6ᵗʰ **S63.02 Subluxation and dislocation of radiocarpal joint**

√7ᵗʰ **S63.021 Subluxation of radiocarpal joint of right wrist**

√7ᵗʰ **S63.022 Subluxation of radiocarpal joint of left wrist**

√7ᵗʰ **S63.023 Subluxation of radiocarpal joint of unspecified wrist**

√7ᵗʰ **S63.024 Dislocation of radiocarpal joint of right wrist**

√7ᵗʰ **S63.025 Dislocation of radiocarpal joint of left wrist**

√7ᵗʰ **S63.026 Dislocation of radiocarpal joint of unspecified wrist**

√6ᵗʰ **S63.03 Subluxation and dislocation of midcarpal joint**

√7ᵗʰ **S63.031 Subluxation of midcarpal joint of right wrist**

√7ᵗʰ **S63.032 Subluxation of midcarpal joint of left wrist**

√7ᵗʰ **S63.033 Subluxation of midcarpal joint of unspecified wrist**

√7ᵗʰ **S63.034 Dislocation of midcarpal joint of right wrist**

√7ᵗʰ **S63.035 Dislocation of midcarpal joint of left wrist**

√7ᵗʰ **S63.036 Dislocation of midcarpal joint of unspecified wrist**

√6ᵗʰ **S63.04 Subluxation and dislocation of carpometacarpal joint of thumb**

`EXCLUDES 2` interphalangeal subluxation and dislocation of thumb (S63.1-)

√7ᵗʰ **S63.041 Subluxation of carpometacarpal joint of right thumb**

√7ᵗʰ **S63.042 Subluxation of carpometacarpal joint of left thumb**

√7ᵗʰ **S63.043 Subluxation of carpometacarpal joint of unspecified thumb**

√7ᵗʰ **S63.044 Dislocation of carpometacarpal joint of right thumb**

√7ᵗʰ **S63.045 Dislocation of carpometacarpal joint of left thumb**

√7ᵗʰ **S63.046 Dislocation of carpometacarpal joint of unspecified thumb**

√6ᵗʰ **S63.05 Subluxation and dislocation of other carpometacarpal joint**

`EXCLUDES 2` subluxation and dislocation of carpometacarpal joint of thumb (S63.04-)

√7ᵗʰ **S63.051 Subluxation of other carpometacarpal joint of right hand**

√7ᵗʰ **S63.052 Subluxation of other carpometacarpal joint of left hand**

√7ᵗʰ **S63.053 Subluxation of other carpometacarpal joint of unspecified hand**

√7ᵗʰ **S63.054 Dislocation of other carpometacarpal joint of right hand**

√7ᵗʰ **S63.055 Dislocation of other carpometacarpal joint of left hand**

√7ᵗʰ **S63.056 Dislocation of other carpometacarpal joint of unspecified hand**

√6ᵗʰ **S63.06 Subluxation and dislocation of metacarpal (bone), proximal end**

√7ᵗʰ **S63.061 Subluxation of metacarpal (bone), proximal end of right hand**

√7ᵗʰ **S63.062 Subluxation of metacarpal (bone), proximal end of left hand**

√7ᵗʰ **S63.063 Subluxation of metacarpal (bone), proximal end of unspecified hand**

√7ᵗʰ **S63.064 Dislocation of metacarpal (bone), proximal end of right hand**

√7ᵗʰ **S63.065 Dislocation of metacarpal (bone), proximal end of left hand**

√7ᵗʰ **S63.066 Dislocation of metacarpal (bone), proximal end of unspecified hand**

√6ᵗʰ **S63.07 Subluxation and dislocation of distal end of ulna**

√7ᵗʰ **S63.071 Subluxation of distal end of right ulna**

√7ᵗʰ **S63.072 Subluxation of distal end of left ulna**

√7ᵗʰ **S63.073 Subluxation of distal end of unspecified ulna**

√7ᵗʰ **S63.074 Dislocation of distal end of right ulna**

√7ᵗʰ **S63.075 Dislocation of distal end of left ulna**

√7ᵗʰ **S63.076 Dislocation of distal end of unspecified ulna**

√6ᵗʰ **S63.09** Other subluxation and dislocation of wrist and hand
- √7ᵗʰ **S63.091** Other subluxation of right wrist and hand
- √7ᵗʰ **S63.092** Other subluxation of left wrist and hand
- √7ᵗʰ **S63.093** Other subluxation of unspecified wrist and hand
- √7ᵗʰ **S63.094** Other dislocation of right wrist and hand
- √7ᵗʰ **S63.095** Other dislocation of left wrist and hand
- √7ᵗʰ **S63.096** Other dislocation of unspecified wrist and hand

√5ᵗʰ **S63.1** Subluxation and dislocation of thumb

√6ᵗʰ **S63.10** Unspecified subluxation and dislocation of thumb
- √7ᵗʰ **S63.101** Unspecified subluxation of right thumb
- √7ᵗʰ **S63.102** Unspecified subluxation of left thumb
- √7ᵗʰ **S63.103** Unspecified subluxation of unspecified thumb
- √7ᵗʰ **S63.104** Unspecified dislocation of right thumb
- √7ᵗʰ **S63.105** Unspecified dislocation of left thumb
- √7ᵗʰ **S63.106** Unspecified dislocation of unspecified thumb

√6ᵗʰ **S63.11** Subluxation and dislocation of metacarpophalangeal joint of thumb
- √7ᵗʰ **S63.111** Subluxation of metacarpophalangeal joint of right thumb
- √7ᵗʰ **S63.112** Subluxation of metacarpophalangeal joint of left thumb
- √7ᵗʰ **S63.113** Subluxation of metacarpophalangeal joint of unspecified thumb
- √7ᵗʰ **S63.114** Dislocation of metacarpophalangeal joint of right thumb
- √7ᵗʰ **S63.115** Dislocation of metacarpophalangeal joint of left thumb
- √7ᵗʰ **S63.116** Dislocation of metacarpophalangeal joint of unspecified thumb

√6ᵗʰ **S63.12** Subluxation and dislocation of interphalangeal joint of thumb
- √7ᵗʰ **S63.121** Subluxation of interphalangeal joint of right thumb
- √7ᵗʰ **S63.122** Subluxation of interphalangeal joint of left thumb
- √7ᵗʰ **S63.123** Subluxation of interphalangeal joint of unspecified thumb
- √7ᵗʰ **S63.124** Dislocation of interphalangeal joint of right thumb
- √7ᵗʰ **S63.125** Dislocation of interphalangeal joint of left thumb
- √7ᵗʰ **S63.126** Dislocation of interphalangeal joint of unspecified thumb

√5ᵗʰ **S63.2** Subluxation and dislocation of other finger(s)

     EXCLUDES 2   subluxation and dislocation of thumb (S63.1-)

√6ᵗʰ **S63.20** Unspecified subluxation of other finger
- √7ᵗʰ **S63.200** Unspecified subluxation of right index finger
- √7ᵗʰ **S63.201** Unspecified subluxation of left index finger
- √7ᵗʰ **S63.202** Unspecified subluxation of right middle finger
- √7ᵗʰ **S63.203** Unspecified subluxation of left middle finger
- √7ᵗʰ **S63.204** Unspecified subluxation of right ring finger
- √7ᵗʰ **S63.205** Unspecified subluxation of left ring finger
- √7ᵗʰ **S63.206** Unspecified subluxation of right little finger
- √7ᵗʰ **S63.207** Unspecified subluxation of left little finger
- √7ᵗʰ **S63.208** Unspecified subluxation of other finger
  Unspecified subluxation of specified finger with unspecified laterality
- √7ᵗʰ **S63.209** Unspecified subluxation of unspecified finger

√6ᵗʰ **S63.21** Subluxation of metacarpophalangeal joint of finger
- √7ᵗʰ **S63.210** Subluxation of metacarpophalangeal joint of right index finger
- √7ᵗʰ **S63.211** Subluxation of metacarpophalangeal joint of left index finger
- √7ᵗʰ **S63.212** Subluxation of metacarpophalangeal joint of right middle finger
- √7ᵗʰ **S63.213** Subluxation of metacarpophalangeal joint of left middle finger
- √7ᵗʰ **S63.214** Subluxation of metacarpophalangeal joint of right ring finger
- √7ᵗʰ **S63.215** Subluxation of metacarpophalangeal joint of left ring finger
- √7ᵗʰ **S63.216** Subluxation of metacarpophalangeal joint of right little finger
- √7ᵗʰ **S63.217** Subluxation of metacarpophalangeal joint of left little finger
- √7ᵗʰ **S63.218** Subluxation of metacarpophalangeal joint of other finger
  Subluxation of metacarpophalangeal joint of specified finger with unspecified laterality
- √7ᵗʰ **S63.219** Subluxation of metacarpophalangeal joint of unspecified finger

√6ᵗʰ **S63.22** Subluxation of unspecified interphalangeal joint of finger
- √7ᵗʰ **S63.220** Subluxation of unspecified interphalangeal joint of right index finger
- √7ᵗʰ **S63.221** Subluxation of unspecified interphalangeal joint of left index finger
- √7ᵗʰ **S63.222** Subluxation of unspecified interphalangeal joint of right middle finger
- √7ᵗʰ **S63.223** Subluxation of unspecified interphalangeal joint of left middle finger
- √7ᵗʰ **S63.224** Subluxation of unspecified interphalangeal joint of right ring finger
- √7ᵗʰ **S63.225** Subluxation of unspecified interphalangeal joint of left ring finger
- √7ᵗʰ **S63.226** Subluxation of unspecified interphalangeal joint of right little finger
- √7ᵗʰ **S63.227** Subluxation of unspecified interphalangeal joint of left little finger
- √7ᵗʰ **S63.228** Subluxation of unspecified interphalangeal joint of other finger
  Subluxation of unspecified interphalangeal joint of specified finger with unspecified laterality
- √7ᵗʰ **S63.229** Subluxation of unspecified interphalangeal joint of unspecified finger

√6ᵗʰ **S63.23** Subluxation of proximal interphalangeal joint of finger
- √7ᵗʰ **S63.230** Subluxation of proximal interphalangeal joint of right index finger
- √7ᵗʰ **S63.231** Subluxation of proximal interphalangeal joint of left index finger
- √7ᵗʰ **S63.232** Subluxation of proximal interphalangeal joint of right middle finger
- √7ᵗʰ **S63.233** Subluxation of proximal interphalangeal joint of left middle finger
- √7ᵗʰ **S63.234** Subluxation of proximal interphalangeal joint of right ring finger
- √7ᵗʰ **S63.235** Subluxation of proximal interphalangeal joint of left ring finger
- √7ᵗʰ **S63.236** Subluxation of proximal interphalangeal joint of right little finger
- √7ᵗʰ **S63.237** Subluxation of proximal interphalangeal joint of left little finger
- √7ᵗʰ **S63.238** Subluxation of proximal interphalangeal joint of other finger
  Subluxation of proximal interphalangeal joint of specified finger with unspecified laterality
- √7ᵗʰ **S63.239** Subluxation of proximal interphalangeal joint of unspecified finger

√6ᵗʰ **S63.24** Subluxation of distal interphalangeal joint of finger
- √7ᵗʰ **S63.240** Subluxation of distal interphalangeal joint of right index finger
- √7ᵗʰ **S63.241** Subluxation of distal interphalangeal joint of left index finger
- √7ᵗʰ **S63.242** Subluxation of distal interphalangeal joint of right middle finger
- √7ᵗʰ **S63.243** Subluxation of distal interphalangeal joint of left middle finger
- √7ᵗʰ **S63.244** Subluxation of distal interphalangeal joint of right ring finger
- √7ᵗʰ **S63.245** Subluxation of distal interphalangeal joint of left ring finger
- √7ᵗʰ **S63.246** Subluxation of distal interphalangeal joint of right little finger

√7ᵗʰ **S63.247** Subluxation of distal interphalangeal joint of left little finger

√7ᵗʰ **S63.248** Subluxation of distal interphalangeal joint of other finger

Subluxation of distal interphalangeal joint of specified finger with unspecified laterality

√7ᵗʰ **S63.249** Subluxation of distal interphalangeal joint of unspecified finger

√6ᵗʰ **S63.25** Unspecified dislocation of other finger

√7ᵗʰ **S63.250** Unspecified dislocation of right index finger

√7ᵗʰ **S63.251** Unspecified dislocation of left index finger

√7ᵗʰ **S63.252** Unspecified dislocation of right middle finger

√7ᵗʰ **S63.253** Unspecified dislocation of left middle finger

√7ᵗʰ **S63.254** Unspecified dislocation of right ring finger

√7ᵗʰ **S63.255** Unspecified dislocation of left ring finger

√7ᵗʰ **S63.256** Unspecified dislocation of right little finger

√7ᵗʰ **S63.257** Unspecified dislocation of left little finger

√7ᵗʰ **S63.258** Unspecified dislocation of other finger

Unspecified dislocation of specified finger with unspecified laterality

√7ᵗʰ **S63.259** Unspecified dislocation of unspecified finger

Unspecified dislocation of unspecified finger with unspecified laterality

√6ᵗʰ **S63.26** Dislocation of metacarpophalangeal joint of finger

√7ᵗʰ **S63.260** Dislocation of metacarpophalangeal joint of right index finger

√7ᵗʰ **S63.261** Dislocation of metacarpophalangeal joint of left index finger

√7ᵗʰ **S63.262** Dislocation of metacarpophalangeal joint of right middle finger

√7ᵗʰ **S63.263** Dislocation of metacarpophalangeal joint of left middle finger

√7ᵗʰ **S63.264** Dislocation of metacarpophalangeal joint of right ring finger

√7ᵗʰ **S63.265** Dislocation of metacarpophalangeal joint of left ring finger

√7ᵗʰ **S63.266** Dislocation of metacarpophalangeal joint of right little finger

√7ᵗʰ **S63.267** Dislocation of metacarpophalangeal joint of left little finger

√7ᵗʰ **S63.268** Dislocation of metacarpophalangeal joint of other finger

Dislocation of metacarpophalangeal joint of specified finger with unspecified laterality

√7ᵗʰ **S63.269** Dislocation of metacarpophalangeal joint of unspecified finger

√6ᵗʰ **S63.27** Dislocation of unspecified interphalangeal joint of finger

√7ᵗʰ **S63.270** Dislocation of unspecified interphalangeal joint of right index finger

√7ᵗʰ **S63.271** Dislocation of unspecified interphalangeal joint of left index finger

√7ᵗʰ **S63.272** Dislocation of unspecified interphalangeal joint of right middle finger

√7ᵗʰ **S63.273** Dislocation of unspecified interphalangeal joint of left middle finger

√7ᵗʰ **S63.274** Dislocation of unspecified interphalangeal joint of right ring finger

√7ᵗʰ **S63.275** Dislocation of unspecified interphalangeal joint of left ring finger

√7ᵗʰ **S63.276** Dislocation of unspecified interphalangeal joint of right little finger

√7ᵗʰ **S63.277** Dislocation of unspecified interphalangeal joint of left little finger

√7ᵗʰ **S63.278** Dislocation of unspecified interphalangeal joint of other finger

Dislocation of unspecified interphalangeal joint of specified finger with unspecified laterality

√7ᵗʰ **S63.279** Dislocation of unspecified interphalangeal joint of unspecified finger

Dislocation of unspecified interphalangeal joint of unspecified finger without specified laterality

√6ᵗʰ **S63.28** Dislocation of proximal interphalangeal joint of finger

√7ᵗʰ **S63.280** Dislocation of proximal interphalangeal joint of right index finger

√7ᵗʰ **S63.281** Dislocation of proximal interphalangeal joint of left index finger

√7ᵗʰ **S63.282** Dislocation of proximal interphalangeal joint of right middle finger

√7ᵗʰ **S63.283** Dislocation of proximal interphalangeal joint of left middle finger

√7ᵗʰ **S63.284** Dislocation of proximal interphalangeal joint of right ring finger

√7ᵗʰ **S63.285** Dislocation of proximal interphalangeal joint of left ring finger

√7ᵗʰ **S63.286** Dislocation of proximal interphalangeal joint of right little finger

√7ᵗʰ **S63.287** Dislocation of proximal interphalangeal joint of left little finger

√7ᵗʰ **S63.288** Dislocation of proximal interphalangeal joint of other finger

Dislocation of proximal interphalangeal joint of specified finger with unspecified laterality

√7ᵗʰ **S63.289** Dislocation of proximal interphalangeal joint of unspecified finger

√6ᵗʰ **S63.29** Dislocation of distal interphalangeal joint of finger

√7ᵗʰ **S63.290** Dislocation of distal interphalangeal joint of right index finger

√7ᵗʰ **S63.291** Dislocation of distal interphalangeal joint of left index finger

√7ᵗʰ **S63.292** Dislocation of distal interphalangeal joint of right middle finger

√7ᵗʰ **S63.293** Dislocation of distal interphalangeal joint of left middle finger

√7ᵗʰ **S63.294** Dislocation of distal interphalangeal joint of right ring finger

√7ᵗʰ **S63.295** Dislocation of distal interphalangeal joint of left ring finger

√7ᵗʰ **S63.296** Dislocation of distal interphalangeal joint of right little finger

√7ᵗʰ **S63.297** Dislocation of distal interphalangeal joint of left little finger

√7ᵗʰ **S63.298** Dislocation of distal interphalangeal joint of other finger

Dislocation of distal interphalangeal joint of specified finger with unspecified laterality

√7ᵗʰ **S63.299** Dislocation of distal interphalangeal joint of unspecified finger

√5ᵗʰ **S63.3** Traumatic rupture of ligament of wrist

√6ᵗʰ **S63.30** Traumatic rupture of unspecified ligament of wrist

√7ᵗʰ **S63.301** Traumatic rupture of unspecified ligament of right wrist

√7ᵗʰ **S63.302** Traumatic rupture of unspecified ligament of left wrist

√7ᵗʰ **S63.309** Traumatic rupture of unspecified ligament of unspecified wrist

√6ᵗʰ **S63.31** Traumatic rupture of collateral ligament of wrist

√7ᵗʰ **S63.311** Traumatic rupture of collateral ligament of right wrist

√7ᵗʰ **S63.312** Traumatic rupture of collateral ligament of left wrist

√7ᵗʰ **S63.319** Traumatic rupture of collateral ligament of unspecified wrist

√6ᵗʰ **S63.32** Traumatic rupture of radiocarpal ligament

√7ᵗʰ **S63.321** Traumatic rupture of right radiocarpal ligament

√7ᵗʰ **S63.322** Traumatic rupture of left radiocarpal ligament

√7ᵗʰ **S63.329** Traumatic rupture of unspecified radiocarpal ligament

√6ᵗʰ **S63.33** Traumatic rupture of ulnocarpal (palmar) ligament

√7ᵗʰ **S63.331** Traumatic rupture of right ulnocarpal (palmar) ligament

√7ᵗʰ **S63.332** Traumatic rupture of left ulnocarpal (palmar) ligament

√7ᵗʰ **S63.339** Traumatic rupture of unspecified ulnocarpal (palmar) ligament

√6ᵗʰ **S63.39** Traumatic rupture of other ligament of wrist

√7ᵗʰ **S63.391** Traumatic rupture of other ligament of right wrist

√7ᵗʰ **S63.392** Traumatic rupture of other ligament of left wrist

√7ᵗʰ **S63.399** Traumatic rupture of other ligament of unspecified wrist

√5ᵗʰ **S63.4** Traumatic rupture of ligament of finger at metacarpophalangeal and interphalangeal joint(s)

√6ᵗʰ **S63.40** Traumatic rupture of unspecified ligament of finger at metacarpophalangeal and interphalangeal joint

√7ᵗʰ **S63.400** Traumatic rupture of unspecified ligament of right index finger at metacarpophalangeal and interphalangeal joint

√7ᵗʰ **S63.401** Traumatic rupture of unspecified ligament of left index finger at metacarpophalangeal and interphalangeal joint

√7ᵗʰ **S63.402** Traumatic rupture of unspecified ligament of right middle finger at metacarpophalangeal and interphalangeal joint

√7ᵗʰ **S63.403** Traumatic rupture of unspecified ligament of left middle finger at metacarpophalangeal and interphalangeal joint

√7ᵗʰ **S63.404** Traumatic rupture of unspecified ligament of right ring finger at metacarpophalangeal and interphalangeal joint

√7ᵗʰ **S63.405** Traumatic rupture of unspecified ligament of left ring finger at metacarpophalangeal and interphalangeal joint

√7ᵗʰ **S63.406** Traumatic rupture of unspecified ligament of right little finger at metacarpophalangeal and interphalangeal joint

√7ᵗʰ **S63.407** Traumatic rupture of unspecified ligament of left little finger at metacarpophalangeal and interphalangeal joint

√7ᵗʰ **S63.408** Traumatic rupture of unspecified ligament of other finger at metacarpophalangeal and interphalangeal joint

Traumatic rupture of unspecified ligament of specified finger with unspecified laterality at metacarpophalangeal and interphalangeal joint

√7ᵗʰ **S63.409** Traumatic rupture of unspecified ligament of unspecified finger at metacarpophalangeal and interphalangeal joint

√6ᵗʰ **S63.41** Traumatic rupture of collateral ligament of finger at metacarpophalangeal and interphalangeal joint

√7ᵗʰ **S63.410** Traumatic rupture of collateral ligament of right index finger at metacarpophalangeal and interphalangeal joint

√7ᵗʰ **S63.411** Traumatic rupture of collateral ligament of left index finger at metacarpophalangeal and interphalangeal joint

√7ᵗʰ **S63.412** Traumatic rupture of collateral ligament of right middle finger at metacarpophalangeal and interphalangeal joint

√7ᵗʰ **S63.413** Traumatic rupture of collateral ligament of left middle finger at metacarpophalangeal and interphalangeal joint

√7ᵗʰ **S63.414** Traumatic rupture of collateral ligament of right ring finger at metacarpophalangeal and interphalangeal joint

√7ᵗʰ **S63.415** Traumatic rupture of collateral ligament of left ring finger at metacarpophalangeal and interphalangeal joint

√7ᵗʰ **S63.416** Traumatic rupture of collateral ligament of right little finger at metacarpophalangeal and interphalangeal joint

√7ᵗʰ **S63.417** Traumatic rupture of collateral ligament of left little finger at metacarpophalangeal and interphalangeal joint

√7ᵗʰ **S63.418** Traumatic rupture of collateral ligament of other finger at metacarpophalangeal and interphalangeal joint

Traumatic rupture of collateral ligament of specified finger with unspecified laterality at metacarpophalangeal and interphalangeal joint

√7ᵗʰ **S63.419** Traumatic rupture of collateral ligament of unspecified finger at metacarpophalangeal and interphalangeal joint

√6ᵗʰ **S63.42** Traumatic rupture of palmar ligament of finger at metacarpophalangeal and interphalangeal joint

√7ᵗʰ **S63.420** Traumatic rupture of palmar ligament of right index finger at metacarpophalangeal and interphalangeal joint

√7ᵗʰ **S63.421** Traumatic rupture of palmar ligament of left index finger at metacarpophalangeal and interphalangeal joint

√7ᵗʰ **S63.422** Traumatic rupture of palmar ligament of right middle finger at metacarpophalangeal and interphalangeal joint

√7ᵗʰ **S63.423** Traumatic rupture of palmar ligament of left middle finger at metacarpophalangeal and interphalangeal joint

√7ᵗʰ **S63.424** Traumatic rupture of palmar ligament of right ring finger at metacarpophalangeal and interphalangeal joint

√7ᵗʰ **S63.425** Traumatic rupture of palmar ligament of left ring finger at metacarpophalangeal and interphalangeal joint

√7ᵗʰ **S63.426** Traumatic rupture of palmar ligament of right little finger at metacarpophalangeal and interphalangeal joint

√7ᵗʰ **S63.427** Traumatic rupture of palmar ligament of left little finger at metacarpophalangeal and interphalangeal joint

√7ᵗʰ **S63.428** Traumatic rupture of palmar ligament of other finger at metacarpophalangeal and interphalangeal joint

Traumatic rupture of palmar ligament of specified finger with unspecified laterality at metacarpophalangeal and interphalangeal joint

√7ᵗʰ **S63.429** Traumatic rupture of palmar ligament of unspecified finger at metacarpophalangeal and interphalangeal joint

√6ᵗʰ **S63.43** Traumatic rupture of volar plate of finger at metacarpophalangeal and interphalangeal joint

√7ᵗʰ **S63.430** Traumatic rupture of volar plate of right index finger at metacarpophalangeal and interphalangeal joint

√7ᵗʰ **S63.431** Traumatic rupture of volar plate of left index finger at metacarpophalangeal and interphalangeal joint

√7ᵗʰ **S63.432** Traumatic rupture of volar plate of right middle finger at metacarpophalangeal and interphalangeal joint

√7ᵗʰ **S63.433** Traumatic rupture of volar plate of left middle finger at metacarpophalangeal and interphalangeal joint

√7ᵗʰ **S63.434** Traumatic rupture of volar plate of right ring finger at metacarpophalangeal and interphalangeal joint

√7ᵗʰ **S63.435** Traumatic rupture of volar plate of left ring finger at metacarpophalangeal and interphalangeal joint

√7ᵗʰ **S63.436** Traumatic rupture of volar plate of right little finger at metacarpophalangeal and interphalangeal joint

√7ᵗʰ **S63.437** Traumatic rupture of volar plate of left little finger at metacarpophalangeal and interphalangeal joint

N Newborn: 0 | P Pediatric: 0-17 | M Maternity: 9-64 | A Adult: 15-124 | MCC Major Complication/Comorbidity | CC Complication/Comorbidity | SW Severe Wound Dx

1074 | ICD-10-CM 2020

√7ᵗʰ **S63.438 Traumatic rupture of volar plate of other finger at metacarpophalangeal and interphalangeal joint**
Traumatic rupture of volar plate of specified finger with unspecified laterality at metacarpophalangeal and interphalangeal joint

√7ᵗʰ **S63.439 Traumatic rupture of volar plate of unspecified finger at metacarpophalangeal and interphalangeal joint**

√6ᵗʰ **S63.49 Traumatic rupture of other ligament of finger at metacarpophalangeal and interphalangeal joint**

√7ᵗʰ **S63.490 Traumatic rupture of other ligament of right index finger at metacarpophalangeal and interphalangeal joint**

√7ᵗʰ **S63.491 Traumatic rupture of other ligament of left index finger at metacarpophalangeal and interphalangeal joint**

√7ᵗʰ **S63.492 Traumatic rupture of other ligament of right middle finger at metacarpophalangeal and interphalangeal joint**

√7ᵗʰ **S63.493 Traumatic rupture of other ligament of left middle finger at metacarpophalangeal and interphalangeal joint**

√7ᵗʰ **S63.494 Traumatic rupture of other ligament of right ring finger at metacarpophalangeal and interphalangeal joint**

√7ᵗʰ **S63.495 Traumatic rupture of other ligament of left ring finger at metacarpophalangeal and interphalangeal joint**

√7ᵗʰ **S63.496 Traumatic rupture of other ligament of right little finger at metacarpophalangeal and interphalangeal joint**

√7ᵗʰ **S63.497 Traumatic rupture of other ligament of left little finger at metacarpophalangeal and interphalangeal joint**

√7ᵗʰ **S63.498 Traumatic rupture of other ligament of other finger at metacarpophalangeal and interphalangeal joint**
Traumatic rupture of ligament of specified finger with unspecified laterality at metacarpophalangeal and interphalangeal joint

√7ᵗʰ **S63.499 Traumatic rupture of other ligament of unspecified finger at metacarpophalangeal and interphalangeal joint**

√5ᵗʰ **S63.5 Other and unspecified sprain of wrist**

√6ᵗʰ **S63.50 Unspecified sprain of wrist**

√7ᵗʰ **S63.501 Unspecified sprain of right wrist**

√7ᵗʰ **S63.502 Unspecified sprain of left wrist**

√7ᵗʰ **S63.509 Unspecified sprain of unspecified wrist**

√6ᵗʰ **S63.51 Sprain of carpal (joint)**

√7ᵗʰ **S63.511 Sprain of carpal joint of right wrist**

√7ᵗʰ **S63.512 Sprain of carpal joint of left wrist**

√7ᵗʰ **S63.519 Sprain of carpal joint of unspecified wrist**

√6ᵗʰ **S63.52 Sprain of radiocarpal joint**

EXCLUDES 1   *traumatic rupture of radiocarpal ligament (S63.32-)*

√7ᵗʰ **S63.521 Sprain of radiocarpal joint of right wrist**

√7ᵗʰ **S63.522 Sprain of radiocarpal joint of left wrist**

√7ᵗʰ **S63.529 Sprain of radiocarpal joint of unspecified wrist**

√6ᵗʰ **S63.59 Other specified sprain of wrist**

√7ᵗʰ **S63.591 Other specified sprain of right wrist**

√7ᵗʰ **S63.592 Other specified sprain of left wrist**

√7ᵗʰ **S63.599 Other specified sprain of unspecified wrist**

√5ᵗʰ **S63.6 Other and unspecified sprain of finger(s)**

EXCLUDES 1   *traumatic rupture of ligament of finger at metacarpophalangeal and interphalangeal joint(s) (S63.4-)*

√6ᵗʰ **S63.60 Unspecified sprain of thumb**

√7ᵗʰ **S63.601 Unspecified sprain of right thumb**

√7ᵗʰ **S63.602 Unspecified sprain of left thumb**

√7ᵗʰ **S63.609 Unspecified sprain of unspecified thumb**

√6ᵗʰ **S63.61 Unspecified sprain of other and unspecified finger(s)**

√7ᵗʰ **S63.610 Unspecified sprain of right index finger**

√7ᵗʰ **S63.611 Unspecified sprain of left index finger**

√7ᵗʰ **S63.612 Unspecified sprain of right middle finger**

√7ᵗʰ **S63.613 Unspecified sprain of left middle finger**

√7ᵗʰ **S63.614 Unspecified sprain of right ring finger**

√7ᵗʰ **S63.615 Unspecified sprain of left ring finger**

√7ᵗʰ **S63.616 Unspecified sprain of right little finger**

√7ᵗʰ **S63.617 Unspecified sprain of left little finger**

√7ᵗʰ **S63.618 Unspecified sprain of other finger**
Unspecified sprain of specified finger with unspecified laterality

√7ᵗʰ **S63.619 Unspecified sprain of unspecified finger**

√6ᵗʰ **S63.62 Sprain of interphalangeal joint of thumb**

√7ᵗʰ **S63.621 Sprain of interphalangeal joint of right thumb**

√7ᵗʰ **S63.622 Sprain of interphalangeal joint of left thumb**

√7ᵗʰ **S63.629 Sprain of interphalangeal joint of unspecified thumb**

√6ᵗʰ **S63.63 Sprain of interphalangeal joint of other and unspecified finger(s)**

√7ᵗʰ **S63.630 Sprain of interphalangeal joint of right index finger**

√7ᵗʰ **S63.631 Sprain of interphalangeal joint of left index finger**

√7ᵗʰ **S63.632 Sprain of interphalangeal joint of right middle finger**

√7ᵗʰ **S63.633 Sprain of interphalangeal joint of left middle finger**

√7ᵗʰ **S63.634 Sprain of interphalangeal joint of right ring finger**

√7ᵗʰ **S63.635 Sprain of interphalangeal joint of left ring finger**

√7ᵗʰ **S63.636 Sprain of interphalangeal joint of right little finger**

√7ᵗʰ **S63.637 Sprain of interphalangeal joint of left little finger**

√7ᵗʰ **S63.638 Sprain of interphalangeal joint of other finger**

√7ᵗʰ **S63.639 Sprain of interphalangeal joint of unspecified finger**

√6ᵗʰ **S63.64 Sprain of metacarpophalangeal joint of thumb**

√7ᵗʰ **S63.641 Sprain of metacarpophalangeal joint of right thumb**

√7ᵗʰ **S63.642 Sprain of metacarpophalangeal joint of left thumb**

√7ᵗʰ **S63.649 Sprain of metacarpophalangeal joint of unspecified thumb**

√6ᵗʰ **S63.65 Sprain of metacarpophalangeal joint of other and unspecified finger(s)**

√7ᵗʰ **S63.650 Sprain of metacarpophalangeal joint of right index finger**

√7ᵗʰ **S63.651 Sprain of metacarpophalangeal joint of left index finger**

√7ᵗʰ **S63.652 Sprain of metacarpophalangeal joint of right middle finger**

√7ᵗʰ **S63.653 Sprain of metacarpophalangeal joint of left middle finger**

√7ᵗʰ **S63.654 Sprain of metacarpophalangeal joint of right ring finger**

√7ᵗʰ **S63.655 Sprain of metacarpophalangeal joint of left ring finger**

√7ᵗʰ **S63.656 Sprain of metacarpophalangeal joint of right little finger**

√7ᵗʰ **S63.657 Sprain of metacarpophalangeal joint of left little finger**

√7ᵗʰ **S63.658 Sprain of metacarpophalangeal joint of other finger**
Sprain of metacarpophalangeal joint of specified finger with unspecified laterality

√7ᵗʰ **S63.659 Sprain of metacarpophalangeal joint of unspecified finger**

√6ᵗʰ **S63.68 Other sprain of thumb**

√7ᵗʰ **S63.681 Other sprain of right thumb**

☑ Additional Character Required   √×7ᵗʰ Placeholder   Unacceptable PDx   Questionable PDx   Manifestation   Unspecified Dx   H1-H14 HAC   HCC CMS-HCC Dx   HIV HIV Dx

ICD-10-CM 2020   1075

√7ᵗʰ **S63.682** Other sprain of left thumb

√7ᵗʰ **S63.689** Other sprain of unspecified thumb

√6ᵗʰ **S63.69** Other sprain of other and unspecified finger(s)

√7ᵗʰ **S63.690** Other sprain of right index finger

√7ᵗʰ **S63.691** Other sprain of left index finger

√7ᵗʰ **S63.692** Other sprain of right middle finger

√7ᵗʰ **S63.693** Other sprain of left middle finger

√7ᵗʰ **S63.694** Other sprain of right ring finger

√7ᵗʰ **S63.695** Other sprain of left ring finger

√7ᵗʰ **S63.696** Other sprain of right little finger

√7ᵗʰ **S63.697** Other sprain of left little finger

√7ᵗʰ **S63.698** Other sprain of other finger

Other sprain of specified finger with unspecified laterality

√7ᵗʰ **S63.699** Other sprain of unspecified finger

√5ᵗʰ **S63.8** Sprain of other part of wrist and hand

√6ᵗʰ **S63.8X** Sprain of other part of wrist and hand

√7ᵗʰ **S63.8X1** Sprain of other part of right wrist and hand

√7ᵗʰ **S63.8X2** Sprain of other part of left wrist and hand

√7ᵗʰ **S63.8X9** Sprain of other part of unspecified wrist and hand

√5ᵗʰ **S63.9** Sprain of unspecified part of wrist and hand

√x7ᵗʰ **S63.90** Sprain of unspecified part of unspecified wrist and hand

√x7ᵗʰ **S63.91** Sprain of unspecified part of right wrist and hand

√x7ᵗʰ **S63.92** Sprain of unspecified part of left wrist and hand

√4ᵗʰ **S64** **Injury of nerves at wrist and hand level**

Code also any associated open wound (S61.-)

The appropriate 7th character is to be added to each code from category S64.
A   initial encounter
D   subsequent encounter
S   sequela

√5ᵗʰ **S64.0** Injury of ulnar nerve at wrist and hand level

√x7ᵗʰ **S64.00** Injury of ulnar nerve at wrist and hand level of unspecified arm

√x7ᵗʰ **S64.01** Injury of ulnar nerve at wrist and hand level of right arm

√x7ᵗʰ **S64.02** Injury of ulnar nerve at wrist and hand level of left arm

√5ᵗʰ **S64.1** Injury of median nerve at wrist and hand level

√x7ᵗʰ **S64.10** Injury of median nerve at wrist and hand level of unspecified arm

√x7ᵗʰ **S64.11** Injury of median nerve at wrist and hand level of right arm

√x7ᵗʰ **S64.12** Injury of median nerve at wrist and hand level of left arm

√5ᵗʰ **S64.2** Injury of radial nerve at wrist and hand level

√x7ᵗʰ **S64.20** Injury of radial nerve at wrist and hand level of unspecified arm

√x7ᵗʰ **S64.21** Injury of radial nerve at wrist and hand level of right arm

√x7ᵗʰ **S64.22** Injury of radial nerve at wrist and hand level of left arm

√5ᵗʰ **S64.3** Injury of digital nerve of thumb

√x7ᵗʰ **S64.30** Injury of digital nerve of unspecified thumb

√x7ᵗʰ **S64.31** Injury of digital nerve of right thumb

√x7ᵗʰ **S64.32** Injury of digital nerve of left thumb

√5ᵗʰ **S64.4** Injury of digital nerve of other and unspecified finger

√x7ᵗʰ **S64.40** Injury of digital nerve of unspecified finger

√6ᵗʰ **S64.49** Injury of digital nerve of other finger

√7ᵗʰ **S64.490** Injury of digital nerve of right index finger

√7ᵗʰ **S64.491** Injury of digital nerve of left index finger

√7ᵗʰ **S64.492** Injury of digital nerve of right middle finger

√7ᵗʰ **S64.493** Injury of digital nerve of left middle finger

√7ᵗʰ **S64.494** Injury of digital nerve of right ring finger

√7ᵗʰ **S64.495** Injury of digital nerve of left ring finger

√7ᵗʰ **S64.496** Injury of digital nerve of right little finger

√7ᵗʰ **S64.497** Injury of digital nerve of left little finger

√7ᵗʰ **S64.498** Injury of digital nerve of other finger

Injury of digital nerve of specified finger with unspecified laterality

√5ᵗʰ **S64.8** Injury of other nerves at wrist and hand level

√6ᵗʰ **S64.8X** Injury of other nerves at wrist and hand level

√7ᵗʰ **S64.8X1** Injury of other nerves at wrist and hand level of right arm

√7ᵗʰ **S64.8X2** Injury of other nerves at wrist and hand level of left arm

√7ᵗʰ **S64.8X9** Injury of other nerves at wrist and hand level of unspecified arm

√5ᵗʰ **S64.9** Injury of unspecified nerve at wrist and hand level

√x7ᵗʰ **S64.90** Injury of unspecified nerve at wrist and hand level of unspecified arm

√x7ᵗʰ **S64.91** Injury of unspecified nerve at wrist and hand level of right arm

√x7ᵗʰ **S64.92** Injury of unspecified nerve at wrist and hand level of left arm

√4ᵗʰ **S65** **Injury of blood vessels at wrist and hand level**

Code also any associated open wound (S61.-)

The appropriate 7th character is to be added to each code from category S65.
A   initial encounter
D   subsequent encounter
S   sequela

√5ᵗʰ **S65.0** Injury of ulnar artery at wrist and hand level

CC Excl: For CC codes in subcategory S65.0:
Right side: PDX collection 1274
Left side: PDX collection 1275
Unspecified side: PDX collection 1276

√6ᵗʰ **S65.00** Unspecified injury of ulnar artery at wrist and hand level

√7ᵗʰ **S65.001** Unspecified injury of ulnar artery at wrist and hand level of right arm   CC

√7ᵗʰ **S65.002** Unspecified injury of ulnar artery at wrist and hand level of left arm   CC

√7ᵗʰ **S65.009** Unspecified injury of ulnar artery at wrist and hand level of unspecified arm   CC

√6ᵗʰ **S65.01** Laceration of ulnar artery at wrist and hand level

√7ᵗʰ **S65.011** Laceration of ulnar artery at wrist and hand level of right arm   CC

√7ᵗʰ **S65.012** Laceration of ulnar artery at wrist and hand level of left arm   CC

√7ᵗʰ **S65.019** Laceration of ulnar artery at wrist and hand level of unspecified arm   CC

√6ᵗʰ **S65.09** Other specified injury of ulnar artery at wrist and hand level

√7ᵗʰ **S65.091** Other specified injury of ulnar artery at wrist and hand level of right arm   CC

√7ᵗʰ **S65.092** Other specified injury of ulnar artery at wrist and hand level of left arm   CC

√7ᵗʰ **S65.099** Other specified injury of ulnar artery at wrist and hand level of unspecified arm   CC

√5ᵗʰ **S65.1** Injury of radial artery at wrist and hand level

CC Excl: For CC codes in subcategory S65.1:
Right side: PDX collection 1277
Left side: PDX collection 1278
Unspecified side: PDX collection 1279

√6ᵗʰ **S65.10** Unspecified injury of radial artery at wrist and hand level

√7ᵗʰ **S65.101** Unspecified injury of radial artery at wrist and hand level of right arm   CC

√7ᵗʰ **S65.102** Unspecified injury of radial artery at wrist and hand level of left arm   CC

N Newborn: 0   **P** Pediatric: 0-17   **M** Maternity: 9-64   **A** Adult: 15-124   **MCC** Major Complication/Comorbidity   **CC** Complication/Comorbidity   **SW** Severe Wound Dx

1076   ICD-10-CM 2020

√7ᵗʰ **S65.109** Unspecified injury of radial artery at wrist and hand level of unspecified arm   `cc`

√6ᵗʰ **S65.11** Laceration of radial artery at wrist and hand level

    √7ᵗʰ **S65.111** Laceration of radial artery at wrist and hand level of right arm   `cc`

    √7ᵗʰ **S65.112** Laceration of radial artery at wrist and hand level of left arm   `cc`

    √7ᵗʰ **S65.119** Laceration of radial artery at wrist and hand level of unspecified arm   `cc`

√6ᵗʰ **S65.19** Other specified injury of radial artery at wrist and hand level

    √7ᵗʰ **S65.191** Other specified injury of radial artery at wrist and hand level of right arm   `cc`

    √7ᵗʰ **S65.192** Other specified injury of radial artery at wrist and hand level of left arm   `cc`

    √7ᵗʰ **S65.199** Other specified injury of radial artery at wrist and hand level of unspecified arm   `cc`

√5ᵗʰ **S65.2** Injury of superficial palmar arch

> **CC Excl: For CC codes in subcategory S65.2:**
> **Right side:** PDX collection 1288
> **Left side:** PDX collection 1289
> **Unspecified side:** PDX collection 1290

√6ᵗʰ **S65.20** Unspecified injury of superficial palmar arch

    √7ᵗʰ **S65.201** Unspecified injury of superficial palmar arch of right hand   `cc`

    √7ᵗʰ **S65.202** Unspecified injury of superficial palmar arch of left hand   `cc`

    √7ᵗʰ **S65.209** Unspecified injury of superficial palmar arch of unspecified hand   `cc`

√6ᵗʰ **S65.21** Laceration of superficial palmar arch

    √7ᵗʰ **S65.211** Laceration of superficial palmar arch of right hand   `cc`

    √7ᵗʰ **S65.212** Laceration of superficial palmar arch of left hand   `cc`

    √7ᵗʰ **S65.219** Laceration of superficial palmar arch of unspecified hand   `cc`

√6ᵗʰ **S65.29** Other specified injury of superficial palmar arch

    √7ᵗʰ **S65.291** Other specified injury of superficial palmar arch of right hand   `cc`

    √7ᵗʰ **S65.292** Other specified injury of superficial palmar arch of left hand   `cc`

    √7ᵗʰ **S65.299** Other specified injury of superficial palmar arch of unspecified hand   `cc`

√5ᵗʰ **S65.3** Injury of deep palmar arch

> **CC Excl: For CC codes in subcategory S65.3:**
> **Right side:** PDX collection 1288
> **Left side:** PDX collection 1289
> **Unspecified side:** PDX collection 1290

√6ᵗʰ **S65.30** Unspecified injury of deep palmar arch

    √7ᵗʰ **S65.301** Unspecified injury of deep palmar arch of right hand   `cc`

    √7ᵗʰ **S65.302** Unspecified injury of deep palmar arch of left hand   `cc`

    √7ᵗʰ **S65.309** Unspecified injury of deep palmar arch of unspecified hand   `cc`

√6ᵗʰ **S65.31** Laceration of deep palmar arch

    √7ᵗʰ **S65.311** Laceration of deep palmar arch of right hand   `cc`

    √7ᵗʰ **S65.312** Laceration of deep palmar arch of left hand   `cc`

    √7ᵗʰ **S65.319** Laceration of deep palmar arch of unspecified hand   `cc`

√6ᵗʰ **S65.39** Other specified injury of deep palmar arch

    √7ᵗʰ **S65.391** Other specified injury of deep palmar arch of right hand   `cc`

    √7ᵗʰ **S65.392** Other specified injury of deep palmar arch of left hand   `cc`

    √7ᵗʰ **S65.399** Other specified injury of deep palmar arch of unspecified hand   `cc`

√5ᵗʰ **S65.4** Injury of blood vessel of thumb

> **CC Excl: For CC codes in subcategory S65.4:**
> **Right side:** PDX collection 1291
> **Left side:** PDX collection 1292
> **Unspecified side:** PDX collection 1293

√6ᵗʰ **S65.40** Unspecified injury of blood vessel of thumb

    √7ᵗʰ **S65.401** Unspecified injury of blood vessel of right thumb   `cc`

    √7ᵗʰ **S65.402** Unspecified injury of blood vessel of left thumb   `cc`

    √7ᵗʰ **S65.409** Unspecified injury of blood vessel of unspecified thumb   `cc`

√6ᵗʰ **S65.41** Laceration of blood vessel of thumb

    √7ᵗʰ **S65.411** Laceration of blood vessel of right thumb   `cc`

    √7ᵗʰ **S65.412** Laceration of blood vessel of left thumb   `cc`

    √7ᵗʰ **S65.419** Laceration of blood vessel of unspecified thumb   `cc`

√6ᵗʰ **S65.49** Other specified injury of blood vessel of thumb

    √7ᵗʰ **S65.491** Other specified injury of blood vessel of right thumb   `cc`

    √7ᵗʰ **S65.492** Other specified injury of blood vessel of left thumb   `cc`

    √7ᵗʰ **S65.499** Other specified injury of blood vessel of unspecified thumb   `cc`

√5ᵗʰ **S65.5** Injury of blood vessel of other and unspecified finger

> **CC Excl: For CC codes in subcategory S65.5:**
> **Right side:** PDX collection 1291
> **Left side:** PDX collection 1292
> **Unspecified side:** PDX collection 1293

√6ᵗʰ **S65.50** Unspecified injury of blood vessel of other and unspecified finger

    √7ᵗʰ **S65.500** Unspecified injury of blood vessel of right index finger   `cc`

    √7ᵗʰ **S65.501** Unspecified injury of blood vessel of left index finger   `cc`

    √7ᵗʰ **S65.502** Unspecified injury of blood vessel of right middle finger   `cc`

    √7ᵗʰ **S65.503** Unspecified injury of blood vessel of left middle finger   `cc`

    √7ᵗʰ **S65.504** Unspecified injury of blood vessel of right ring finger   `cc`

    √7ᵗʰ **S65.505** Unspecified injury of blood vessel of left ring finger   `cc`

    √7ᵗʰ **S65.506** Unspecified injury of blood vessel of right little finger   `cc`

    √7ᵗʰ **S65.507** Unspecified injury of blood vessel of left little finger   `cc`

    √7ᵗʰ **S65.508** Unspecified injury of blood vessel of other finger   `cc`

        Unspecified injury of blood vessel of specified finger with unspecified laterality

    √7ᵗʰ **S65.509** Unspecified injury of blood vessel of unspecified finger   `cc`

☑ Additional Character Required   √ˣ7ᵗʰ Placeholder   Unacceptable PDx   Questionable PDx   Manifestation   Unspecified Dx   H1-H14 HAC   HCC CMS-HCC Dx   HIV HIV Dx

ICD-10-CM 2020   **1077**

Chapter 19. Injury, Poisoning and Certain Other Consequences of External Causes

S65.109–S65.509

√6ᵗʰ **S65.51** **Laceration of blood vessel of other and unspecified finger**

     √7ᵗʰ **S65.510** **Laceration of blood vessel of right index finger** CC

     √7ᵗʰ **S65.511** **Laceration of blood vessel of left index finger** CC

     √7ᵗʰ **S65.512** **Laceration of blood vessel of right middle finger** CC

     √7ᵗʰ **S65.513** **Laceration of blood vessel of left middle finger** CC

     √7ᵗʰ **S65.514** **Laceration of blood vessel of right ring finger** CC

     √7ᵗʰ **S65.515** **Laceration of blood vessel of left ring finger** CC

     √7ᵗʰ **S65.516** **Laceration of blood vessel of right little finger** CC

     √7ᵗʰ **S65.517** **Laceration of blood vessel of left little finger** CC

     √7ᵗʰ **S65.518** **Laceration of blood vessel of other finger** CC
         Laceration of blood vessel of specified finger with unspecified laterality

     √7ᵗʰ **S65.519** **Laceration of blood vessel of unspecified finger** CC

√6ᵗʰ **S65.59** **Other specified injury of blood vessel of other and unspecified finger**

     √7ᵗʰ **S65.590** **Other specified injury of blood vessel of right index finger** CC

     √7ᵗʰ **S65.591** **Other specified injury of blood vessel of left index finger** CC

     √7ᵗʰ **S65.592** **Other specified injury of blood vessel of right middle finger** CC

     √7ᵗʰ **S65.593** **Other specified injury of blood vessel of left middle finger** CC

     √7ᵗʰ **S65.594** **Other specified injury of blood vessel of right ring finger** CC

     √7ᵗʰ **S65.595** **Other specified injury of blood vessel of left ring finger** CC

     √7ᵗʰ **S65.596** **Other specified injury of blood vessel of right little finger** CC

     √7ᵗʰ **S65.597** **Other specified injury of blood vessel of left little finger** CC

     √7ᵗʰ **S65.598** **Other specified injury of blood vessel of other finger** CC
         Other specified injury of blood vessel of specified finger with unspecified laterality

     √7ᵗʰ **S65.599** **Other specified injury of blood vessel of unspecified finger** CC

√5ᵗʰ **S65.8** **Injury of other blood vessels at wrist and hand level**

CC Excl: For CC codes in subcategory S65.8:
Right side: PDX collection 1260
Left side: PDX collection 1261
Unspecified side: PDX collection 1262

√6ᵗʰ **S65.80** **Unspecified injury of other blood vessels at wrist and hand level**

     √7ᵗʰ **S65.801** **Unspecified injury of other blood vessels at wrist and hand level of right arm** CC

     √7ᵗʰ **S65.802** **Unspecified injury of other blood vessels at wrist and hand level of left arm** CC

     √7ᵗʰ **S65.809** **Unspecified injury of other blood vessels at wrist and hand level of unspecified arm** CC

√6ᵗʰ **S65.81** **Laceration of other blood vessels at wrist and hand level**

     √7ᵗʰ **S65.811** **Laceration of other blood vessels at wrist and hand level of right arm** CC

     √7ᵗʰ **S65.812** **Laceration of other blood vessels at wrist and hand level of left arm** CC

     √7ᵗʰ **S65.819** **Laceration of other blood vessels at wrist and hand level of unspecified arm** CC

√6ᵗʰ **S65.89** **Other specified injury of other blood vessels at wrist and hand level**

     √7ᵗʰ **S65.891** **Other specified injury of other blood vessels at wrist and hand level of right arm** CC

     √7ᵗʰ **S65.892** **Other specified injury of other blood vessels at wrist and hand level of left arm** CC

     √7ᵗʰ **S65.899** **Other specified injury of other blood vessels at wrist and hand level of unspecified arm** CC

√5ᵗʰ **S65.9** **Injury of unspecified blood vessel at wrist and hand level**

CC Excl: For CC codes in subcategory S65.9:
Right side: PDX collection 1260
Left side: PDX collection 1261
Unspecified side: PDX collection 1262

√6ᵗʰ **S65.90** **Unspecified injury of unspecified blood vessel at wrist and hand level**

     √7ᵗʰ **S65.901** **Unspecified injury of unspecified blood vessel at wrist and hand level of right arm** CC

     √7ᵗʰ **S65.902** **Unspecified injury of unspecified blood vessel at wrist and hand level of left arm** CC

     √7ᵗʰ **S65.909** **Unspecified injury of unspecified blood vessel at wrist and hand level of unspecified arm** CC

√6ᵗʰ **S65.91** **Laceration of unspecified blood vessel at wrist and hand level**

     √7ᵗʰ **S65.911** **Laceration of unspecified blood vessel at wrist and hand level of right arm** CC

     √7ᵗʰ **S65.912** **Laceration of unspecified blood vessel at wrist and hand level of left arm** CC

     √7ᵗʰ **S65.919** **Laceration of unspecified blood vessel at wrist and hand level of unspecified arm** CC

√6ᵗʰ **S65.99** **Other specified injury of unspecified blood vessel at wrist and hand level**

     √7ᵗʰ **S65.991** **Other specified injury of unspecified blood vessel at wrist and hand of right arm** CC

     √7ᵗʰ **S65.992** **Other specified injury of unspecified blood vessel at wrist and hand of left arm** CC

     √7ᵗʰ **S65.999** **Other specified injury of unspecified blood vessel at wrist and hand of unspecified arm** CC

√4ᵗʰ **S66** **Injury of muscle, fascia and tendon at wrist and hand level**

Code also any associated open wound (S61.-)

EXCLUDES 2   *sprain of joints and ligaments of wrist and hand (S63.-)*

TIP: Refer to the Muscle/Tendon table at the beginning of this chapter.

The appropriate 7th character is to be added to each code from category S66.
A   initial encounter
D   subsequent encounter
S   sequela

CC Excl: For CC codes in category S66:
Right side: PDX collection 1294
Left side: PDX collection 1295
Unspecified side: PDX collection 1296

√5ᵗʰ **S66.0** **Injury of long flexor muscle, fascia and tendon of thumb at wrist and hand level**

√6ᵗʰ **S66.00** **Unspecified injury of long flexor muscle, fascia and tendon of thumb at wrist and hand level**

     √7ᵗʰ **S66.001** **Unspecified injury of long flexor muscle, fascia and tendon of right thumb at wrist and hand level**

√7ᵗʰ **S66.002** **Unspecified injury of long flexor muscle, fascia and tendon of left thumb at wrist and hand level**

√7ᵗʰ **S66.009** **Unspecified injury of long flexor muscle, fascia and tendon of unspecified thumb at wrist and hand level**

√6ᵗʰ **S66.01** **Strain of long flexor muscle, fascia and tendon of thumb at wrist and hand level**

√7ᵗʰ **S66.011** **Strain of long flexor muscle, fascia and tendon of right thumb at wrist and hand level**

√7ᵗʰ **S66.012** **Strain of long flexor muscle, fascia and tendon of left thumb at wrist and hand level**

√7ᵗʰ **S66.019** **Strain of long flexor muscle, fascia and tendon of unspecified thumb at wrist and hand level**

√6ᵗʰ **S66.02** **Laceration of long flexor muscle, fascia and tendon of thumb at wrist and hand level**

√7ᵗʰ **S66.021** **Laceration of long flexor muscle, fascia and tendon of right thumb at wrist and hand level** `CC`

√7ᵗʰ **S66.022** **Laceration of long flexor muscle, fascia and tendon of left thumb at wrist and hand level** `CC`

√7ᵗʰ **S66.029** **Laceration of long flexor muscle, fascia and tendon of unspecified thumb at wrist and hand level** `CC`

√6ᵗʰ **S66.09** **Other specified injury of long flexor muscle, fascia and tendon of thumb at wrist and hand level**

√7ᵗʰ **S66.091** **Other specified injury of long flexor muscle, fascia and tendon of right thumb at wrist and hand level**

√7ᵗʰ **S66.092** **Other specified injury of long flexor muscle, fascia and tendon of left thumb at wrist and hand level**

√7ᵗʰ **S66.099** **Other specified injury of long flexor muscle, fascia and tendon of unspecified thumb at wrist and hand level**

√5ᵗʰ **S66.1** **Injury of flexor muscle, fascia and tendon of other and unspecified finger at wrist and hand level**

> *EXCLUDES 2*   injury of long flexor muscle, fascia and tendon of thumb at wrist and hand level (S66.0-)

√6ᵗʰ **S66.10** **Unspecified injury of flexor muscle, fascia and tendon of other and unspecified finger at wrist and hand level**

√7ᵗʰ **S66.100** **Unspecified injury of flexor muscle, fascia and tendon of right index finger at wrist and hand level**

√7ᵗʰ **S66.101** **Unspecified injury of flexor muscle, fascia and tendon of left index finger at wrist and hand level**

√7ᵗʰ **S66.102** **Unspecified injury of flexor muscle, fascia and tendon of right middle finger at wrist and hand level**

√7ᵗʰ **S66.103** **Unspecified injury of flexor muscle, fascia and tendon of left middle finger at wrist and hand level**

√7ᵗʰ **S66.104** **Unspecified injury of flexor muscle, fascia and tendon of right ring finger at wrist and hand level**

√7ᵗʰ **S66.105** **Unspecified injury of flexor muscle, fascia and tendon of left ring finger at wrist and hand level**

√7ᵗʰ **S66.106** **Unspecified injury of flexor muscle, fascia and tendon of right little finger at wrist and hand level**

√7ᵗʰ **S66.107** **Unspecified injury of flexor muscle, fascia and tendon of left little finger at wrist and hand level**

√7ᵗʰ **S66.108** **Unspecified injury of flexor muscle, fascia and tendon of other finger at wrist and hand level**

> Unspecified injury of flexor muscle, fascia and tendon of specified finger with unspecified laterality at wrist and hand level

√7ᵗʰ **S66.109** **Unspecified injury of flexor muscle, fascia and tendon of unspecified finger at wrist and hand level**

√6ᵗʰ **S66.11** **Strain of flexor muscle, fascia and tendon of other and unspecified finger at wrist and hand level**

√7ᵗʰ **S66.110** **Strain of flexor muscle, fascia and tendon of right index finger at wrist and hand level**

√7ᵗʰ **S66.111** **Strain of flexor muscle, fascia and tendon of left index finger at wrist and hand level**

√7ᵗʰ **S66.112** **Strain of flexor muscle, fascia and tendon of right middle finger at wrist and hand level**

√7ᵗʰ **S66.113** **Strain of flexor muscle, fascia and tendon of left middle finger at wrist and hand level**

√7ᵗʰ **S66.114** **Strain of flexor muscle, fascia and tendon of right ring finger at wrist and hand level**

√7ᵗʰ **S66.115** **Strain of flexor muscle, fascia and tendon of left ring finger at wrist and hand level**

√7ᵗʰ **S66.116** **Strain of flexor muscle, fascia and tendon of right little finger at wrist and hand level**

√7ᵗʰ **S66.117** **Strain of flexor muscle, fascia and tendon of left little finger at wrist and hand level**

√7ᵗʰ **S66.118** **Strain of flexor muscle, fascia and tendon of other finger at wrist and hand level**

> Strain of flexor muscle, fascia and tendon of specified finger with unspecified laterality at wrist and hand level

√7ᵗʰ **S66.119** **Strain of flexor muscle, fascia and tendon of unspecified finger at wrist and hand level**

√6ᵗʰ **S66.12** **Laceration of flexor muscle, fascia and tendon of other and unspecified finger at wrist and hand level**

√7ᵗʰ **S66.120** **Laceration of flexor muscle, fascia and tendon of right index finger at wrist and hand level** `CC`

√7ᵗʰ **S66.121** **Laceration of flexor muscle, fascia and tendon of left index finger at wrist and hand level** `CC`

√7ᵗʰ **S66.122** **Laceration of flexor muscle, fascia and tendon of right middle finger at wrist and hand level** `CC`

√7ᵗʰ **S66.123** **Laceration of flexor muscle, fascia and tendon of left middle finger at wrist and hand level** `CC`

√7ᵗʰ **S66.124** **Laceration of flexor muscle, fascia and tendon of right ring finger at wrist and hand level** `CC`

√7ᵗʰ **S66.125** **Laceration of flexor muscle, fascia and tendon of left ring finger at wrist and hand level** `CC`

√7ᵗʰ **S66.126** **Laceration of flexor muscle, fascia and tendon of right little finger at wrist and hand level** `CC`

√7ᵗʰ **S66.127** **Laceration of flexor muscle, fascia and tendon of left little finger at wrist and hand level** `CC`

√7ᵗʰ **S66.128** **Laceration of flexor muscle, fascia and tendon of other finger at wrist and hand level** `CC`

> Laceration of flexor muscle, fascia and tendon of specified finger with unspecified laterality at wrist and hand level

√7ᵗʰ **S66.129** **Laceration of flexor muscle, fascia and tendon of unspecified finger at wrist and hand level** `CC`

√6ᵗʰ **S66.19** **Other injury of flexor muscle, fascia and tendon of other and unspecified finger at wrist and hand level**

√7ᵗʰ **S66.190** **Other injury of flexor muscle, fascia and tendon of right index finger at wrist and hand level**

√7ᵗʰ **S66.191** **Other injury of flexor muscle, fascia and tendon of left index finger at wrist and hand level**

☑ Additional Character Required   √x7ᵗʰ Placeholder   Unacceptable PDx   Questionable PDx   Manifestation   Unspecified Dx   H1-H14 HAC   HCC CMS-HCC Dx   HIV HIV Dx

ICD-10-CM 2020   1079

√7ᵗʰ **S66.192** Other injury of flexor muscle, fascia and tendon of **right middle** finger at wrist and hand level

√7ᵗʰ **S66.193** Other injury of flexor muscle, fascia and tendon of **left middle** finger at wrist and hand level

√7ᵗʰ **S66.194** Other injury of flexor muscle, fascia and tendon of **right ring** finger at wrist and hand level

√7ᵗʰ **S66.195** Other injury of flexor muscle, fascia and tendon of **left ring** finger at wrist and hand level

√7ᵗʰ **S66.196** Other injury of flexor muscle, fascia and tendon of **right little** finger at wrist and hand level

√7ᵗʰ **S66.197** Other injury of flexor muscle, fascia and tendon of **left little** finger at wrist and hand level

√7ᵗʰ **S66.198** Other injury of flexor muscle, fascia and tendon of other finger at wrist and hand level

Other injury of flexor muscle, fascia and tendon of specified finger with unspecified laterality at wrist and hand level

√7ᵗʰ **S66.199** Other injury of flexor muscle, fascia and tendon of unspecified finger at wrist and hand level

√5ᵗʰ **S66.2** Injury of extensor muscle, fascia and tendon of thumb at wrist and hand level

√6ᵗʰ **S66.20** Unspecified injury of extensor muscle, fascia and tendon of thumb at wrist and hand level

√7ᵗʰ **S66.201** Unspecified injury of extensor muscle, fascia and tendon of right thumb at wrist and hand level

√7ᵗʰ **S66.202** Unspecified injury of extensor muscle, fascia and tendon of left thumb at wrist and hand level

√7ᵗʰ **S66.209** Unspecified injury of extensor muscle, fascia and tendon of unspecified thumb at wrist and hand level

√6ᵗʰ **S66.21** Strain of extensor muscle, fascia and tendon of thumb at wrist and hand level

√7ᵗʰ **S66.211** Strain of extensor muscle, fascia and tendon of right thumb at wrist and hand level

√7ᵗʰ **S66.212** Strain of extensor muscle, fascia and tendon of left thumb at wrist and hand level

√7ᵗʰ **S66.219** Strain of extensor muscle, fascia and tendon of unspecified thumb at wrist and hand level

√6ᵗʰ **S66.22** Laceration of extensor muscle, fascia and tendon of thumb at wrist and hand level

√7ᵗʰ **S66.221** Laceration of extensor muscle, fascia and tendon of right thumb at wrist and hand level `CC`

√7ᵗʰ **S66.222** Laceration of extensor muscle, fascia and tendon of left thumb at wrist and hand level `CC`

√7ᵗʰ **S66.229** Laceration of extensor muscle, fascia and tendon of unspecified thumb at wrist and hand level `CC`

√6ᵗʰ **S66.29** Other specified injury of extensor muscle, fascia and tendon of thumb at wrist and hand level

√7ᵗʰ **S66.291** Other specified injury of extensor muscle, fascia and tendon of right thumb at wrist and hand level

√7ᵗʰ **S66.292** Other specified injury of extensor muscle, fascia and tendon of left thumb at wrist and hand level

√7ᵗʰ **S66.299** Other specified injury of extensor muscle, fascia and tendon of unspecified thumb at wrist and hand level

√5ᵗʰ **S66.3** Injury of extensor muscle, fascia and tendon of other and unspecified finger at wrist and hand level

`EXCLUDES 2` *injury of extensor muscle, fascia and tendon of thumb at wrist and hand level (S66.2-)*

√6ᵗʰ **S66.30** Unspecified injury of extensor muscle, fascia and tendon of other and unspecified finger at wrist and hand level

√7ᵗʰ **S66.300** Unspecified injury of extensor muscle, fascia and tendon of right index finger at wrist and hand level

√7ᵗʰ **S66.301** Unspecified injury of extensor muscle, fascia and tendon of left index finger at wrist and hand level

√7ᵗʰ **S66.302** Unspecified injury of extensor muscle, fascia and tendon of right middle finger at wrist and hand level

√7ᵗʰ **S66.303** Unspecified injury of extensor muscle, fascia and tendon of left middle finger at wrist and hand level

√7ᵗʰ **S66.304** Unspecified injury of extensor muscle, fascia and tendon of right ring finger at wrist and hand level

√7ᵗʰ **S66.305** Unspecified injury of extensor muscle, fascia and tendon of left ring finger at wrist and hand level

√7ᵗʰ **S66.306** Unspecified injury of extensor muscle, fascia and tendon of right little finger at wrist and hand level

√7ᵗʰ **S66.307** Unspecified injury of extensor muscle, fascia and tendon of left little finger at wrist and hand level

√7ᵗʰ **S66.308** Unspecified injury of extensor muscle, fascia and tendon of other finger at wrist and hand level

Unspecified injury of extensor muscle, fascia and tendon of specified finger with unspecified laterality at wrist and hand level

√7ᵗʰ **S66.309** Unspecified injury of extensor muscle, fascia and tendon of unspecified finger at wrist and hand level

√6ᵗʰ **S66.31** Strain of extensor muscle, fascia and tendon of other and unspecified finger at wrist and hand level

√7ᵗʰ **S66.310** Strain of extensor muscle, fascia and tendon of right index finger at wrist and hand level

√7ᵗʰ **S66.311** Strain of extensor muscle, fascia and tendon of left index finger at wrist and hand level

√7ᵗʰ **S66.312** Strain of extensor muscle, fascia and tendon of right middle finger at wrist and hand level

√7ᵗʰ **S66.313** Strain of extensor muscle, fascia and tendon of left middle finger at wrist and hand level

√7ᵗʰ **S66.314** Strain of extensor muscle, fascia and tendon of right ring finger at wrist and hand level

√7ᵗʰ **S66.315** Strain of extensor muscle, fascia and tendon of left ring finger at wrist and hand level

√7ᵗʰ **S66.316** Strain of extensor muscle, fascia and tendon of right little finger at wrist and hand level

√7ᵗʰ **S66.317** Strain of extensor muscle, fascia and tendon of left little finger at wrist and hand level

√7ᵗʰ **S66.318** Strain of extensor muscle, fascia and tendon of other finger at wrist and hand level

Strain of extensor muscle, fascia and tendon of specified finger with unspecified laterality at wrist and hand level

√7ᵗʰ **S66.319** Strain of extensor muscle, fascia and tendon of unspecified finger at wrist and hand level

√6ᵗʰ **S66.32** Laceration of extensor muscle, fascia and tendon of other and unspecified finger at wrist and hand level

√7ᵗʰ **S66.320** Laceration of extensor muscle, fascia and tendon of right index finger at wrist and hand level `CC`

Ⓝ Newborn: 0 Ⓟ Pediatric: 0-17 Ⓜ Maternity: 9-64 Ⓐ Adult: 15-124 `MCC` Major Complication/Comorbidity `CC` Complication/Comorbidity `SW` Severe Wound Dx

1080

ICD-10-CM 2020

√7ᵗʰ **S66.321** **Laceration of extensor muscle, fascia and tendon of left index finger at wrist and hand level** cc

√7ᵗʰ **S66.322** **Laceration of extensor muscle, fascia and tendon of right middle finger at wrist and hand level** cc

√7ᵗʰ **S66.323** **Laceration of extensor muscle, fascia and tendon of left middle finger at wrist and hand level** cc

√7ᵗʰ **S66.324** **Laceration of extensor muscle, fascia and tendon of right ring finger at wrist and hand level** cc

√7ᵗʰ **S66.325** **Laceration of extensor muscle, fascia and tendon of left ring finger at wrist and hand level** cc

√7ᵗʰ **S66.326** **Laceration of extensor muscle, fascia and tendon of right little finger at wrist and hand level** cc

√7ᵗʰ **S66.327** **Laceration of extensor muscle, fascia and tendon of left little finger at wrist and hand level** cc

√7ᵗʰ **S66.328** **Laceration of extensor muscle, fascia and tendon of other finger at wrist and hand level** cc
Laceration of extensor muscle, fascia and tendon of specified finger with unspecified laterality at wrist and hand level

√7ᵗʰ **S66.329** **Laceration of extensor muscle, fascia and tendon of unspecified finger at wrist and hand level** cc

√6ᵗʰ **S66.39** **Other injury of extensor muscle, fascia and tendon of other and unspecified finger at wrist and hand level**

√7ᵗʰ **S66.390** **Other injury of extensor muscle, fascia and tendon of right index finger at wrist and hand level**

√7ᵗʰ **S66.391** **Other injury of extensor muscle, fascia and tendon of left index finger at wrist and hand level**

√7ᵗʰ **S66.392** **Other injury of extensor muscle, fascia and tendon of right middle finger at wrist and hand level**

√7ᵗʰ **S66.393** **Other injury of extensor muscle, fascia and tendon of left middle finger at wrist and hand level**

√7ᵗʰ **S66.394** **Other injury of extensor muscle, fascia and tendon of right ring finger at wrist and hand level**

√7ᵗʰ **S66.395** **Other injury of extensor muscle, fascia and tendon of left ring finger at wrist and hand level**

√7ᵗʰ **S66.396** **Other injury of extensor muscle, fascia and tendon of right little finger at wrist and hand level**

√7ᵗʰ **S66.397** **Other injury of extensor muscle, fascia and tendon of left little finger at wrist and hand level**

√7ᵗʰ **S66.398** **Other injury of extensor muscle, fascia and tendon of other finger at wrist and hand level**
Other injury of extensor muscle, fascia and tendon of specified finger with unspecified laterality at wrist and hand level

√7ᵗʰ **S66.399** **Other injury of extensor muscle, fascia and tendon of unspecified finger at wrist and hand level**

√5ᵗʰ **S66.4** **Injury of intrinsic muscle, fascia and tendon of thumb at wrist and hand level**

√6ᵗʰ **S66.40** **Unspecified injury of intrinsic muscle, fascia and tendon of thumb at wrist and hand level**

√7ᵗʰ **S66.401** **Unspecified injury of intrinsic muscle, fascia and tendon of right thumb at wrist and hand level**

√7ᵗʰ **S66.402** **Unspecified injury of intrinsic muscle, fascia and tendon of left thumb at wrist and hand level**

√7ᵗʰ **S66.409** **Unspecified injury of intrinsic muscle, fascia and tendon of unspecified thumb at wrist and hand level**

√6ᵗʰ **S66.41** **Strain of intrinsic muscle, fascia and tendon of thumb at wrist and hand level**

√7ᵗʰ **S66.411** **Strain of intrinsic muscle, fascia and tendon of right thumb at wrist and hand level**

√7ᵗʰ **S66.412** **Strain of intrinsic muscle, fascia and tendon of left thumb at wrist and hand level**

√7ᵗʰ **S66.419** **Strain of intrinsic muscle, fascia and tendon of unspecified thumb at wrist and hand level**

√6ᵗʰ **S66.42** **Laceration of intrinsic muscle, fascia and tendon of thumb at wrist and hand level**

√7ᵗʰ **S66.421** **Laceration of intrinsic muscle, fascia and tendon of right thumb at wrist and hand level** cc

√7ᵗʰ **S66.422** **Laceration of intrinsic muscle, fascia and tendon of left thumb at wrist and hand level** cc

√7ᵗʰ **S66.429** **Laceration of intrinsic muscle, fascia and tendon of unspecified thumb at wrist and hand level** cc

√6ᵗʰ **S66.49** **Other specified injury of intrinsic muscle, fascia and tendon of thumb at wrist and hand level**

√7ᵗʰ **S66.491** **Other specified injury of intrinsic muscle, fascia and tendon of right thumb at wrist and hand level**

√7ᵗʰ **S66.492** **Other specified injury of intrinsic muscle, fascia and tendon of left thumb at wrist and hand level**

√7ᵗʰ **S66.499** **Other specified injury of intrinsic muscle, fascia and tendon of unspecified thumb at wrist and hand level**

√5ᵗʰ **S66.5** **Injury of intrinsic muscle, fascia and tendon of other and unspecified finger at wrist and hand level**
EXCLUDES 2   injury of intrinsic muscle, fascia and tendon of thumb at wrist and hand level (S66.4-)

√6ᵗʰ **S66.50** **Unspecified injury of intrinsic muscle, fascia and tendon of other and unspecified finger at wrist and hand level**

√7ᵗʰ **S66.500** **Unspecified injury of intrinsic muscle, fascia and tendon of right index finger at wrist and hand level**

√7ᵗʰ **S66.501** **Unspecified injury of intrinsic muscle, fascia and tendon of left index finger at wrist and hand level**

√7ᵗʰ **S66.502** **Unspecified injury of intrinsic muscle, fascia and tendon of right middle finger at wrist and hand level**

√7ᵗʰ **S66.503** **Unspecified injury of intrinsic muscle, fascia and tendon of left middle finger at wrist and hand level**

√7ᵗʰ **S66.504** **Unspecified injury of intrinsic muscle, fascia and tendon of right ring finger at wrist and hand level**

√7ᵗʰ **S66.505** **Unspecified injury of intrinsic muscle, fascia and tendon of left ring finger at wrist and hand level**

√7ᵗʰ **S66.506** **Unspecified injury of intrinsic muscle, fascia and tendon of right little finger at wrist and hand level**

√7ᵗʰ **S66.507** **Unspecified injury of intrinsic muscle, fascia and tendon of left little finger at wrist and hand level**

√7ᵗʰ **S66.508** **Unspecified injury of intrinsic muscle, fascia and tendon of other finger at wrist and hand level**
Unspecified injury of intrinsic muscle, fascia and tendon of specified finger with unspecified laterality at wrist and hand level

√7ᵗʰ **S66.509** **Unspecified injury of intrinsic muscle, fascia and tendon of unspecified finger at wrist and hand level**

✓6ᵗʰ **S66.51** **Strain of intrinsic muscle, fascia and tendon of other and unspecified finger at wrist and hand level**

  ✓7ᵗʰ **S66.510** **Strain of intrinsic muscle, fascia and tendon of right index finger at wrist and hand level**

  ✓7ᵗʰ **S66.511** **Strain of intrinsic muscle, fascia and tendon of left index finger at wrist and hand level**

  ✓7ᵗʰ **S66.512** **Strain of intrinsic muscle, fascia and tendon of right middle finger at wrist and hand level**

  ✓7ᵗʰ **S66.513** **Strain of intrinsic muscle, fascia and tendon of left middle finger at wrist and hand level**

  ✓7ᵗʰ **S66.514** **Strain of intrinsic muscle, fascia and tendon of right ring finger at wrist and hand level**

  ✓7ᵗʰ **S66.515** **Strain of intrinsic muscle, fascia and tendon of left ring finger at wrist and hand level**

  ✓7ᵗʰ **S66.516** **Strain of intrinsic muscle, fascia and tendon of right little finger at wrist and hand level**

  ✓7ᵗʰ **S66.517** **Strain of intrinsic muscle, fascia and tendon of left little finger at wrist and hand level**

  ✓7ᵗʰ **S66.518** **Strain of intrinsic muscle, fascia and tendon of other finger at wrist and hand level**

      Strain of intrinsic muscle, fascia and tendon of specified finger with unspecified laterality at wrist and hand level

  ✓7ᵗʰ **S66.519** **Strain of intrinsic muscle, fascia and tendon of unspecified finger at wrist and hand level**

✓6ᵗʰ **S66.52** **Laceration of intrinsic muscle, fascia and tendon of other and unspecified finger at wrist and hand level**

  ✓7ᵗʰ **S66.520** **Laceration of intrinsic muscle, fascia and tendon of right index finger at wrist and hand level** CC

  ✓7ᵗʰ **S66.521** **Laceration of intrinsic muscle, fascia and tendon of left index finger at wrist and hand level** CC

  ✓7ᵗʰ **S66.522** **Laceration of intrinsic muscle, fascia and tendon of right middle finger at wrist and hand level** CC

  ✓7ᵗʰ **S66.523** **Laceration of intrinsic muscle, fascia and tendon of left middle finger at wrist and hand level** CC

  ✓7ᵗʰ **S66.524** **Laceration of intrinsic muscle, fascia and tendon of right ring finger at wrist and hand level** CC

  ✓7ᵗʰ **S66.525** **Laceration of intrinsic muscle, fascia and tendon of left ring finger at wrist and hand level** CC

  ✓7ᵗʰ **S66.526** **Laceration of intrinsic muscle, fascia and tendon of right little finger at wrist and hand level** CC

  ✓7ᵗʰ **S66.527** **Laceration of intrinsic muscle, fascia and tendon of left little finger at wrist and hand level** CC

  ✓7ᵗʰ **S66.528** **Laceration of intrinsic muscle, fascia and tendon of other finger at wrist and hand level** CC

      Laceration of intrinsic muscle, fascia and tendon of specified finger with unspecified laterality at wrist and hand level

  ✓7ᵗʰ **S66.529** **Laceration of intrinsic muscle, fascia and tendon of unspecified finger at wrist and hand level** CC

✓6ᵗʰ **S66.59** **Other injury of intrinsic muscle, fascia and tendon of other and unspecified finger at wrist and hand level**

  ✓7ᵗʰ **S66.590** **Other injury of intrinsic muscle, fascia and tendon of right index finger at wrist and hand level**

  ✓7ᵗʰ **S66.591** **Other injury of intrinsic muscle, fascia and tendon of left index finger at wrist and hand level**

  ✓7ᵗʰ **S66.592** **Other injury of intrinsic muscle, fascia and tendon of right middle finger at wrist and hand level**

  ✓7ᵗʰ **S66.593** **Other injury of intrinsic muscle, fascia and tendon of left middle finger at wrist and hand level**

  ✓7ᵗʰ **S66.594** **Other injury of intrinsic muscle, fascia and tendon of right ring finger at wrist and hand level**

  ✓7ᵗʰ **S66.595** **Other injury of intrinsic muscle, fascia and tendon of left ring finger at wrist and hand level**

  ✓7ᵗʰ **S66.596** **Other injury of intrinsic muscle, fascia and tendon of right little finger at wrist and hand level**

  ✓7ᵗʰ **S66.597** **Other injury of intrinsic muscle, fascia and tendon of left little finger at wrist and hand level**

  ✓7ᵗʰ **S66.598** **Other injury of intrinsic muscle, fascia and tendon of other finger at wrist and hand level**

      Other injury of intrinsic muscle, fascia and tendon of specified finger with unspecified laterality at wrist and hand level

  ✓7ᵗʰ **S66.599** **Other injury of intrinsic muscle, fascia and tendon of unspecified finger at wrist and hand level**

✓5ᵗʰ **S66.8** **Injury of other specified muscles, fascia and tendons at wrist and hand level**

  ✓6ᵗʰ **S66.80** **Unspecified injury of other specified muscles, fascia and tendons at wrist and hand level**

    ✓7ᵗʰ **S66.801** **Unspecified injury of other specified muscles, fascia and tendons at wrist and hand level, right hand**

    ✓7ᵗʰ **S66.802** **Unspecified injury of other specified muscles, fascia and tendons at wrist and hand level, left hand**

    ✓7ᵗʰ **S66.809** **Unspecified injury of other specified muscles, fascia and tendons at wrist and hand level, unspecified hand**

  ✓6ᵗʰ **S66.81** **Strain of other specified muscles, fascia and tendons at wrist and hand level**

    ✓7ᵗʰ **S66.811** **Strain of other specified muscles, fascia and tendons at wrist and hand level, right hand**

    ✓7ᵗʰ **S66.812** **Strain of other specified muscles, fascia and tendons at wrist and hand level, left hand**

    ✓7ᵗʰ **S66.819** **Strain of other specified muscles, fascia and tendons at wrist and hand level, unspecified hand**

  ✓6ᵗʰ **S66.82** **Laceration of other specified muscles, fascia and tendons at wrist and hand level**

    ✓7ᵗʰ **S66.821** **Laceration of other specified muscles, fascia and tendons at wrist and hand level, right hand** CC

    ✓7ᵗʰ **S66.822** **Laceration of other specified muscles, fascia and tendons at wrist and hand level, left hand** CC

    ✓7ᵗʰ **S66.829** **Laceration of other specified muscles, fascia and tendons at wrist and hand level, unspecified hand** CC

  ✓6ᵗʰ **S66.89** **Other injury of other specified muscles, fascia and tendons at wrist and hand level**

    ✓7ᵗʰ **S66.891** **Other injury of other specified muscles, fascia and tendons at wrist and hand level, right hand**

    ✓7ᵗʰ **S66.892** **Other injury of other specified muscles, fascia and tendons at wrist and hand level, left hand**

N Newborn: 0   P Pediatric: 0-17   M Maternity: 9-64   A Adult: 15-124   MCC Major Complication/Comorbidity   CC Complication/Comorbidity   SW Severe Wound Dx

1082   ICD-10-CM 2020

√7ᵗʰ **S66.899** Other injury of other specified muscles, fascia and tendons at wrist and hand level, unspecified hand

√5ᵗʰ **S66.9** **Injury of unspecified muscle, fascia and tendon at wrist and hand level**

√6ᵗʰ **S66.90** Unspecified injury of unspecified muscle, fascia and tendon at wrist and hand level

  √7ᵗʰ **S66.901** Unspecified injury of unspecified muscle, fascia and tendon at wrist and hand level, right hand

  √7ᵗʰ **S66.902** Unspecified injury of unspecified muscle, fascia and tendon at wrist and hand level, left hand

  √7ᵗʰ **S66.909** Unspecified injury of unspecified muscle, fascia and tendon at wrist and hand level, unspecified hand

√6ᵗʰ **S66.91** Strain of unspecified muscle, fascia and tendon at wrist and hand level

  √7ᵗʰ **S66.911** Strain of unspecified muscle, fascia and tendon at wrist and hand level, right hand

  √7ᵗʰ **S66.912** Strain of unspecified muscle, fascia and tendon at wrist and hand level, left hand

  √7ᵗʰ **S66.919** Strain of unspecified muscle, fascia and tendon at wrist and hand level, unspecified hand

√6ᵗʰ **S66.92** Laceration of unspecified muscle, fascia and tendon at wrist and hand level

  √7ᵗʰ **S66.921** Laceration of unspecified muscle, fascia and tendon at wrist and hand level, right hand   CC

  √7ᵗʰ **S66.922** Laceration of unspecified muscle, fascia and tendon at wrist and hand level, left hand   CC

  √7ᵗʰ **S66.929** Laceration of unspecified muscle, fascia and tendon at wrist and hand level, unspecified hand   CC

√6ᵗʰ **S66.99** Other injury of unspecified muscle, fascia and tendon at wrist and hand level

  √7ᵗʰ **S66.991** Other injury of unspecified muscle, fascia and tendon at wrist and hand level, right hand

  √7ᵗʰ **S66.992** Other injury of unspecified muscle, fascia and tendon at wrist and hand level, left hand

  √7ᵗʰ **S66.999** Other injury of unspecified muscle, fascia and tendon at wrist and hand level, unspecified hand

√4ᵗʰ **S67** **Crushing injury of wrist, hand and fingers**

Use additional code for all associated injuries, such as:
fracture of wrist and hand (S62.-)
open wound of wrist and hand (S61.-)

The appropriate 7th character is to be added to each code from category S67.
A   initial encounter
D   subsequent encounter
S   sequela

√5ᵗʰ **S67.0** **Crushing injury of thumb**

  √x7ᵗʰ **S67.00** Crushing injury of unspecified thumb
  √x7ᵗʰ **S67.01** Crushing injury of right thumb
  √x7ᵗʰ **S67.02** Crushing injury of left thumb

√5ᵗʰ **S67.1** **Crushing injury of other and unspecified finger(s)**

  EXCLUDES 2   crushing injury of thumb (S67.0-)

  √x7ᵗʰ **S67.10** Crushing injury of unspecified finger(s)
  √6ᵗʰ **S67.19** Crushing injury of other finger(s)

    √7ᵗʰ **S67.190** Crushing injury of right index finger
    √7ᵗʰ **S67.191** Crushing injury of left index finger
    √7ᵗʰ **S67.192** Crushing injury of right middle finger
    √7ᵗʰ **S67.193** Crushing injury of left middle finger
    √7ᵗʰ **S67.194** Crushing injury of right ring finger
    √7ᵗʰ **S67.195** Crushing injury of left ring finger
    √7ᵗʰ **S67.196** Crushing injury of right little finger
    √7ᵗʰ **S67.197** Crushing injury of left little finger

  √7ᵗʰ **S67.198** Crushing injury of other finger
Crushing injury of specified finger with unspecified laterality

√5ᵗʰ **S67.2** **Crushing injury of hand**

  EXCLUDES 2   crushing injury of fingers (S67.1-)
             crushing injury of thumb (S67.0-)

  √x7ᵗʰ **S67.20** Crushing injury of unspecified hand
  √x7ᵗʰ **S67.21** Crushing injury of right hand
  √x7ᵗʰ **S67.22** Crushing injury of left hand

√5ᵗʰ **S67.3** **Crushing injury of wrist**

  √x7ᵗʰ **S67.30** Crushing injury of unspecified wrist
  √x7ᵗʰ **S67.31** Crushing injury of right wrist
  √x7ᵗʰ **S67.32** Crushing injury of left wrist

√5ᵗʰ **S67.4** **Crushing injury of wrist and hand**

  EXCLUDES 1   crushing injury of hand alone (S67.2-)
             crushing injury of wrist alone (S67.3-)
  EXCLUDES 2   crushing injury of fingers (S67.1-)
             crushing injury of thumb (S67.0-)

  √x7ᵗʰ **S67.40** Crushing injury of unspecified wrist and hand
  √x7ᵗʰ **S67.41** Crushing injury of right wrist and hand
  √x7ᵗʰ **S67.42** Crushing injury of left wrist and hand

√5ᵗʰ **S67.9** **Crushing injury of unspecified part(s) of wrist, hand and fingers**

  √x7ᵗʰ **S67.90** Crushing injury of unspecified part(s) of unspecified wrist, hand and fingers
  √x7ᵗʰ **S67.91** Crushing injury of unspecified part(s) of right wrist, hand and fingers
  √x7ᵗʰ **S67.92** Crushing injury of unspecified part(s) of left wrist, hand and fingers

√4ᵗʰ **S68** **Traumatic amputation of wrist, hand and fingers**

An amputation not identified as partial or complete should be coded to complete.

The appropriate 7th character is to be added to each code from category S68.
A   initial encounter
D   subsequent encounter
S   sequela

CC Excl: For CC codes in category S68:
Right side: PDX collection 1266
Left side: PDX collection 1267
Unspecified side: PDX collection 1268

√5ᵗʰ **S68.0** **Traumatic metacarpophalangeal amputation of thumb**

Traumatic amputation of thumb NOS

  √6ᵗʰ **S68.01** Complete traumatic metacarpophalangeal amputation of thumb

    8 √7ᵗʰ **S68.011** Complete traumatic metacarpophalangeal amputation of right thumb   HCC

    8 √7ᵗʰ **S68.012** Complete traumatic metacarpophalangeal amputation of left thumb   HCC

    8 √7ᵗʰ **S68.019** Complete traumatic metacarpophalangeal amputation of unspecified thumb   HCC

  √6ᵗʰ **S68.02** Partial traumatic metacarpophalangeal amputation of thumb

    8 √7ᵗʰ **S68.021** Partial traumatic metacarpophalangeal amputation of right thumb   HCC

    8 √7ᵗʰ **S68.022** Partial traumatic metacarpophalangeal amputation of left thumb   HCC

    8 √7ᵗʰ **S68.029** Partial traumatic metacarpophalangeal amputation of unspecified thumb   HCC

√5ᵗʰ **S68.1   Traumatic metacarpophalangeal amputation of other and unspecified finger**

Traumatic amputation of finger NOS

EXCLUDES 2   *traumatic metacarpophalangeal amputation of thumb (S68.0-)*

√6ᵗʰ **S68.11   Complete traumatic metacarpophalangeal amputation of other and unspecified finger**

8 √7ᵗʰ **S68.110   Complete traumatic metacarpophalangeal amputation of right index finger**   HCC

8 √7ᵗʰ **S68.111   Complete traumatic metacarpophalangeal amputation of left index finger**   HCC

8 √7ᵗʰ **S68.112   Complete traumatic metacarpophalangeal amputation of right middle finger**   HCC

8 √7ᵗʰ **S68.113   Complete traumatic metacarpophalangeal amputation of left middle finger**   HCC

8 √7ᵗʰ **S68.114   Complete traumatic metacarpophalangeal amputation of right ring finger**   HCC

8 √7ᵗʰ **S68.115   Complete traumatic metacarpophalangeal amputation of left ring finger**   HCC

8 √7ᵗʰ **S68.116   Complete traumatic metacarpophalangeal amputation of right little finger**   HCC

8 √7ᵗʰ **S68.117   Complete traumatic metacarpophalangeal amputation of left little finger**   HCC

8 √7ᵗʰ **S68.118   Complete traumatic metacarpophalangeal amputation of other finger**   HCC

Complete traumatic metacarpophalangeal amputation of specified finger with unspecified laterality

8 √7ᵗʰ **S68.119   Complete traumatic metacarpophalangeal amputation of unspecified finger**   HCC

√6ᵗʰ **S68.12   Partial traumatic metacarpophalangeal amputation of other and unspecified finger**

8 √7ᵗʰ **S68.120   Partial traumatic metacarpophalangeal amputation of right index finger**   HCC

8 √7ᵗʰ **S68.121   Partial traumatic metacarpophalangeal amputation of left index finger**   HCC

8 √7ᵗʰ **S68.122   Partial traumatic metacarpophalangeal amputation of right middle finger**   HCC

8 √7ᵗʰ **S68.123   Partial traumatic metacarpophalangeal amputation of left middle finger**   HCC

8 √7ᵗʰ **S68.124   Partial traumatic metacarpophalangeal amputation of right ring finger**   HCC

8 √7ᵗʰ **S68.125   Partial traumatic metacarpophalangeal amputation of left ring finger**   HCC

8 √7ᵗʰ **S68.126   Partial traumatic metacarpophalangeal amputation of right little finger**   HCC

8 √7ᵗʰ **S68.127   Partial traumatic metacarpophalangeal amputation of left little finger**   HCC

8 √7ᵗʰ **S68.128   Partial traumatic metacarpophalangeal amputation of other finger**   HCC

Partial traumatic metacarpophalangeal amputation of specified finger with unspecified laterality

8 √7ᵗʰ **S68.129   Partial traumatic metacarpophalangeal amputation of unspecified finger**   HCC

√5ᵗʰ **S68.4   Traumatic amputation of hand at wrist level**

Traumatic amputation of hand NOS

Traumatic amputation of wrist

√6ᵗʰ **S68.41   Complete traumatic amputation of hand at wrist level**

7 √7ᵗʰ **S68.411   Complete traumatic amputation of right hand at wrist level**   CC HCC

7 √7ᵗʰ **S68.412   Complete traumatic amputation of left hand at wrist level**   CC HCC

7 √7ᵗʰ **S68.419   Complete traumatic amputation of unspecified hand at wrist level**   CC HCC

√6ᵗʰ **S68.42   Partial traumatic amputation of hand at wrist level**

7 √7ᵗʰ **S68.421   Partial traumatic amputation of right hand at wrist level**   CC HCC

7 √7ᵗʰ **S68.422   Partial traumatic amputation of left hand at wrist level**   CC HCC

7 √7ᵗʰ **S68.429   Partial traumatic amputation of unspecified hand at wrist level**   CC HCC

√5ᵗʰ **S68.5   Traumatic transphalangeal amputation of thumb**

Traumatic interphalangeal joint amputation of thumb

√6ᵗʰ **S68.51   Complete traumatic transphalangeal amputation of thumb**

8 √7ᵗʰ **S68.511   Complete traumatic transphalangeal amputation of right thumb**   HCC

8 √7ᵗʰ **S68.512   Complete traumatic transphalangeal amputation of left thumb**   HCC

8 √7ᵗʰ **S68.519   Complete traumatic transphalangeal amputation of unspecified thumb**   HCC

√6ᵗʰ **S68.52   Partial traumatic transphalangeal amputation of thumb**

8 √7ᵗʰ **S68.521   Partial traumatic transphalangeal amputation of right thumb**   HCC

8 √7ᵗʰ **S68.522   Partial traumatic transphalangeal amputation of left thumb**   HCC

8 √7ᵗʰ **S68.529   Partial traumatic transphalangeal amputation of unspecified thumb**   HCC

√5ᵗʰ **S68.6   Traumatic transphalangeal amputation of other and unspecified finger**

√6ᵗʰ **S68.61   Complete traumatic transphalangeal amputation of other and unspecified finger(s)**

8 √7ᵗʰ **S68.610   Complete traumatic transphalangeal amputation of right index finger**   HCC

8 √7ᵗʰ **S68.611   Complete traumatic transphalangeal amputation of left index finger**   HCC

8 √7ᵗʰ **S68.612   Complete traumatic transphalangeal amputation of right middle finger**   HCC

8 √7ᵗʰ **S68.613   Complete traumatic transphalangeal amputation of left middle finger**   HCC

N Newborn: 0   P Pediatric: 0-17   M Maternity: 9-64   A Adult: 15-124   MCC Major Complication/Comorbidity   CC Complication/Comorbidity   SW Severe Wound Dx

1084   ICD-10-CM 2020

8 √7ᵗʰ **S68.614** Complete traumatic transphalangeal amputation of right ring finger   `HCC`

8 √7ᵗʰ **S68.615** Complete traumatic transphalangeal amputation of left ring finger   `HCC`

8 √7ᵗʰ **S68.616** Complete traumatic transphalangeal amputation of right little finger   `HCC`

8 √7ᵗʰ **S68.617** Complete traumatic transphalangeal amputation of left little finger   `HCC`

8 √7ᵗʰ **S68.618** Complete traumatic transphalangeal amputation of other finger   `HCC`
> Complete traumatic transphalangeal amputation of specified finger with unspecified laterality

8 √7ᵗʰ **S68.619** Complete traumatic transphalangeal amputation of unspecified finger   `HCC`

√6ᵗʰ **S68.62** Partial traumatic transphalangeal amputation of other and unspecified finger

8 √7ᵗʰ **S68.620** Partial traumatic transphalangeal amputation of right index finger   `HCC`

8 √7ᵗʰ **S68.621** Partial traumatic transphalangeal amputation of left index finger   `HCC`

8 √7ᵗʰ **S68.622** Partial traumatic transphalangeal amputation of right middle finger   `HCC`

8 √7ᵗʰ **S68.623** Partial traumatic transphalangeal amputation of left middle finger   `HCC`

8 √7ᵗʰ **S68.624** Partial traumatic transphalangeal amputation of right ring finger   `HCC`

8 √7ᵗʰ **S68.625** Partial traumatic transphalangeal amputation of left ring finger   `HCC`

8 √7ᵗʰ **S68.626** Partial traumatic transphalangeal amputation of right little finger   `HCC`

8 √7ᵗʰ **S68.627** Partial traumatic transphalangeal amputation of left little finger   `HCC`

8 √7ᵗʰ **S68.628** Partial traumatic transphalangeal amputation of other finger   `HCC`
> Partial traumatic transphalangeal amputation of specified finger with unspecified laterality

8 √7ᵗʰ **S68.629** Partial traumatic transphalangeal amputation of unspecified finger   `HCC`

√5ᵗʰ **S68.7** Traumatic transmetacarpal amputation of hand

√6ᵗʰ **S68.71** Complete traumatic transmetacarpal amputation of hand

7 √7ᵗʰ **S68.711** Complete traumatic transmetacarpal amputation of right hand   `CC` `HCC`

7 √7ᵗʰ **S68.712** Complete traumatic transmetacarpal amputation of left hand   `CC` `HCC`

7 √7ᵗʰ **S68.719** Complete traumatic transmetacarpal amputation of unspecified hand   `CC` `HCC`

√6ᵗʰ **S68.72** Partial traumatic transmetacarpal amputation of hand

7 √7ᵗʰ **S68.721** Partial traumatic transmetacarpal amputation of right hand   `CC` `HCC`

7 √7ᵗʰ **S68.722** Partial traumatic transmetacarpal amputation of left hand   `CC` `HCC`

7 √7ᵗʰ **S68.729** Partial traumatic transmetacarpal amputation of unspecified hand   `CC` `HCC`

√4ᵗʰ **S69** Other and unspecified injuries of wrist, hand and finger(s)

> The appropriate 7th character is to be added to each code from category S69.
> A   initial encounter
> D   subsequent encounter
> S   sequela

√5ᵗʰ **S69.8** Other specified injuries of wrist, hand and finger(s)

√x7ᵗʰ **S69.80** Other specified injuries of unspecified wrist, hand and finger(s)

√x7ᵗʰ **S69.81** Other specified injuries of right wrist, hand and finger(s)

√x7ᵗʰ **S69.82** Other specified injuries of left wrist, hand and finger(s)

√5ᵗʰ **S69.9** Unspecified injury of wrist, hand and finger(s)

√x7ᵗʰ **S69.90** Unspecified injury of unspecified wrist, hand and finger(s)

√x7ᵗʰ **S69.91** Unspecified injury of right wrist, hand and finger(s)

√x7ᵗʰ **S69.92** Unspecified injury of left wrist, hand and finger(s)

Injuries to the hip and thigh (S70-S79)

EXCLUDES 2   burns and corrosions (T20-T32)
> frostbite (T33-T34)
> snake bite (T63.0-)
> venomous insect bite or sting (T63.4-)

√4ᵗʰ **S70** Superficial injury of hip and thigh

> The appropriate 7th character is to be added to each code from category S70.
> A   initial encounter
> D   subsequent encounter
> S   sequela

√5ᵗʰ **S70.0** Contusion of hip

√x7ᵗʰ **S70.00** Contusion of unspecified hip

√x7ᵗʰ **S70.01** Contusion of right hip

√x7ᵗʰ **S70.02** Contusion of left hip

√5ᵗʰ **S70.1** Contusion of thigh

√x7ᵗʰ **S70.10** Contusion of unspecified thigh

√x7ᵗʰ **S70.11** Contusion of right thigh

√x7ᵗʰ **S70.12** Contusion of left thigh

√5ᵗʰ **S70.2** Other superficial injuries of hip

√6ᵗʰ **S70.21** Abrasion of hip

√7ᵗʰ **S70.211** Abrasion, right hip

√7ᵗʰ **S70.212** Abrasion, left hip

√7ᵗʰ **S70.219** Abrasion, unspecified hip

√6ᵗʰ **S70.22** Blister (nonthermal) of hip

√7ᵗʰ **S70.221** Blister (nonthermal), right hip

√7ᵗʰ **S70.222** Blister (nonthermal), left hip

√7ᵗʰ **S70.229** Blister (nonthermal), unspecified hip

√6ᵗʰ **S70.24** External constriction of hip

√7ᵗʰ **S70.241** External constriction, right hip

√7ᵗʰ **S70.242** External constriction, left hip

√7ᵗʰ **S70.249** External constriction, unspecified hip

√6ᵗʰ **S70.25** Superficial foreign body of hip
> Splinter in the hip

√7ᵗʰ **S70.251** Superficial foreign body, right hip

√7ᵗʰ **S70.252** Superficial foreign body, left hip

√7ᵗʰ **S70.259** Superficial foreign body, unspecified hip

√6ᵗʰ **S70.26** Insect bite (nonvenomous) of hip

√7ᵗʰ **S70.261** Insect bite (nonvenomous), right hip

√7ᵗʰ **S70.262** Insect bite (nonvenomous), left hip

☑ Additional Character Required   √x7ᵗʰ Placeholder   Unacceptable PDx   Questionable PDx   Manifestation   Unspecified Dx   H1-H14 HAC   HCC CMS-HCC Dx   HIV HIV Dx

ICD-10-CM 2020   **1085**

     ✓7ᵗʰ **S70.269** Insect bite (nonvenomous), unspecified hip

  ✓6ᵗʰ **S70.27** Other superficial **bite** of hip

         EXCLUDES 1   *open bite of hip (S71.05-)*

     ✓7ᵗʰ **S70.271** Other superficial bite of hip, **right** hip

     ✓7ᵗʰ **S70.272** Other superficial bite of hip, **left** hip

     ✓7ᵗʰ **S70.279** Other superficial bite of hip, unspecified hip

✓5ᵗʰ **S70.3** Other superficial injuries of **thigh**

  ✓6ᵗʰ **S70.31** Abrasion of **thigh**

     ✓7ᵗʰ **S70.311** Abrasion, **right** thigh

     ✓7ᵗʰ **S70.312** Abrasion, **left** thigh

     ✓7ᵗʰ **S70.319** Abrasion, **unspecified** thigh

  ✓6ᵗʰ **S70.32** Blister (nonthermal) of **thigh**

     ✓7ᵗʰ **S70.321** Blister (nonthermal), **right** thigh

     ✓7ᵗʰ **S70.322** Blister (nonthermal), **left** thigh

     ✓7ᵗʰ **S70.329** Blister (nonthermal), **unspecified** thigh

  ✓6ᵗʰ **S70.34** External constriction of **thigh**

     ✓7ᵗʰ **S70.341** External constriction, **right** thigh

     ✓7ᵗʰ **S70.342** External constriction, **left** thigh

     ✓7ᵗʰ **S70.349** External constriction, **unspecified** thigh

  ✓6ᵗʰ **S70.35** Superficial **foreign body** of thigh

       Splinter in the thigh

     ✓7ᵗʰ **S70.351** Superficial foreign body, **right** thigh

     ✓7ᵗʰ **S70.352** Superficial foreign body, **left** thigh

     ✓7ᵗʰ **S70.359** Superficial foreign body, **unspecified** thigh

  ✓6ᵗʰ **S70.36** Insect bite (nonvenomous) of **thigh**

     ✓7ᵗʰ **S70.361** Insect bite (nonvenomous), **right** thigh

     ✓7ᵗʰ **S70.362** Insect bite (nonvenomous), **left** thigh

     ✓7ᵗʰ **S70.369** Insect bite (nonvenomous), **unspecified** thigh

  ✓6ᵗʰ **S70.37** Other superficial **bite** of thigh

         EXCLUDES 1   *open bite of thigh (S71.15)*

     ✓7ᵗʰ **S70.371** Other superficial bite of **right** thigh

     ✓7ᵗʰ **S70.372** Other superficial bite of **left** thigh

     ✓7ᵗʰ **S70.379** Other superficial bite of **unspecified** thigh

✓5ᵗʰ **S70.9** Unspecified superficial injury of **hip and thigh**

  ✓6ᵗʰ **S70.91** Unspecified superficial injury of **hip**

     ✓7ᵗʰ **S70.911** Unspecified superficial injury of **right** hip

     ✓7ᵗʰ **S70.912** Unspecified superficial injury of **left** hip

     ✓7ᵗʰ **S70.919** Unspecified superficial injury of **unspecified** hip

  ✓6ᵗʰ **S70.92** Unspecified superficial injury of **thigh**

     ✓7ᵗʰ **S70.921** Unspecified superficial injury of **right** thigh

     ✓7ᵗʰ **S70.922** Unspecified superficial injury of **left** thigh

     ✓7ᵗʰ **S70.929** Unspecified superficial injury of **unspecified** thigh

✓4ᵗʰ **S71** Open wound of hip and thigh

    Code also any associated wound infection

     EXCLUDES 1   *open fracture of hip and thigh (S72.-)*

                traumatic amputation of hip and thigh (S78.-)

     EXCLUDES 2   *bite of venomous animal (T63.-)*

                open wound of ankle, foot and toes (S91.-)

                open wound of knee and lower leg (S81.-)

> The appropriate 7th character is to be added to each code from category S71.
> A   initial encounter
> D   subsequent encounter
> S   sequela

  ✓5ᵗʰ **S71.0** Open wound of **hip**

    ✓6ᵗʰ **S71.00** Unspecified open wound of **hip**

       ✓7ᵗʰ **S71.001** Unspecified open wound, **right** hip

       ✓7ᵗʰ **S71.002** Unspecified open wound, **left** hip

       ✓7ᵗʰ **S71.009** Unspecified open wound, **unspecified** hip

    ✓6ᵗʰ **S71.01** Laceration without foreign body **of hip**

       ✓7ᵗʰ **S71.011** Laceration without foreign body, **right** hip

       ✓7ᵗʰ **S71.012** Laceration without foreign body, **left** hip

---

       ✓7ᵗʰ **S71.019** Laceration without foreign body, unspecified hip

    ✓6ᵗʰ **S71.02** Laceration with foreign body **of hip**

       ✓7ᵗʰ **S71.021** Laceration with foreign body, **right** hip

       ✓7ᵗʰ **S71.022** Laceration with foreign body, **left** hip

       ✓7ᵗʰ **S71.029** Laceration with foreign body, unspecified hip

    ✓6ᵗʰ **S71.03** Puncture wound without foreign body **of hip**

       ✓7ᵗʰ **S71.031** Puncture wound without foreign body, **right** hip

       ✓7ᵗʰ **S71.032** Puncture wound without foreign body, **left** hip

       ✓7ᵗʰ **S71.039** Puncture wound without foreign body, unspecified hip

    ✓6ᵗʰ **S71.04** Puncture wound with foreign body **of hip**

       ✓7ᵗʰ **S71.041** Puncture wound with foreign body, **right** hip

       ✓7ᵗʰ **S71.042** Puncture wound with foreign body, **left** hip

       ✓7ᵗʰ **S71.049** Puncture wound with foreign body, unspecified hip

    ✓6ᵗʰ **S71.05** Open bite **of hip**

       Bite of hip NOS

        EXCLUDES 1   *superficial bite of hip (S70.26, S70.27)*

       ✓7ᵗʰ **S71.051** Open bite, **right** hip

       ✓7ᵗʰ **S71.052** Open bite, **left** hip

       ✓7ᵗʰ **S71.059** Open bite, **unspecified** hip

  ✓5ᵗʰ **S71.1** Open wound of **thigh**

    ✓6ᵗʰ **S71.10** Unspecified open wound of **thigh**

       AHA: 2016,3Q,24

       ✓7ᵗʰ **S71.101** Unspecified open wound, **right** thigh

       ✓7ᵗʰ **S71.102** Unspecified open wound, **left** thigh

       ✓7ᵗʰ **S71.109** Unspecified open wound, **unspecified** thigh

    ✓6ᵗʰ **S71.11** Laceration without foreign body **of thigh**

       ✓7ᵗʰ **S71.111** Laceration without foreign body, **right** thigh

       ✓7ᵗʰ **S71.112** Laceration without foreign body, **left** thigh

       ✓7ᵗʰ **S71.119** Laceration without foreign body, unspecified thigh

    ✓6ᵗʰ **S71.12** Laceration with foreign body **of thigh**

       ✓7ᵗʰ **S71.121** Laceration with foreign body, **right** thigh

       ✓7ᵗʰ **S71.122** Laceration with foreign body, **left** thigh

       ✓7ᵗʰ **S71.129** Laceration with foreign body, unspecified thigh

    ✓6ᵗʰ **S71.13** Puncture wound without foreign body **of thigh**

       AHA: 2016,3Q,24

       ✓7ᵗʰ **S71.131** Puncture wound without foreign body, **right** thigh

       ✓7ᵗʰ **S71.132** Puncture wound without foreign body, **left** thigh

       ✓7ᵗʰ **S71.139** Puncture wound without foreign body, unspecified thigh

    ✓6ᵗʰ **S71.14** Puncture wound with foreign body **of thigh**

       AHA: 2016,3Q,24

       ✓7ᵗʰ **S71.141** Puncture wound with foreign body, **right** thigh

       ✓7ᵗʰ **S71.142** Puncture wound with foreign body, **left** thigh

       ✓7ᵗʰ **S71.149** Puncture wound with foreign body, unspecified thigh

    ✓6ᵗʰ **S71.15** Open bite **of thigh**

       Bite of thigh NOS

        EXCLUDES 1   *superficial bite of thigh (S70.37-)*

       ✓7ᵗʰ **S71.151** Open bite, **right** thigh

       ✓7ᵗʰ **S71.152** Open bite, **left** thigh

       ✓7ᵗʰ **S71.159** Open bite, **unspecified** thigh

N Newborn: 0   **P** Pediatric: 0-17   **M** Maternity: 9-64   **A** Adult: 15-124   **MCC** Major Complication/Comorbidity   **CC** Complication/Comorbidity   **SW** Severe Wound Dx

1086   ICD-10-CM 2020

√4ᵗʰ **S72   Fracture of femur**

> **NOTE**   A fracture not indicated as displaced or nondisplaced should be coded to displaced.
>
> A fracture not indicated as open or closed should be coded to closed.
>
> The open fracture designations are based on the Gustilo open fracture classification.

> EXCLUDES 1   *traumatic amputation of hip and thigh (S78.-)*
>
> EXCLUDES 2   *fracture of lower leg and ankle (S82.-)*
> *fracture of foot (S92.-)*
> *periprosthetic fracture of prosthetic implant of hip (M97.0-)*

AHA: 2018,2Q,12; 2016,1Q,33; 2015,3Q,37-39; 2015,1Q,17; 2013,4Q,128
DEF: Diaphysis: Central shaft of a long bone.
DEF: Epiphysis: Proximal and distal rounded ends of a long bone communicates with the joint.
DEF: Metaphysis: Section of a long bone located between the epiphysis and diaphysis at the proximal and distal ends.
DEF: Physis (growth plate): Narrow zone of cartilaginous tissue between the epiphysis and metaphysis at each end of a long bone. In childhood, proliferation of cells in this zone lengthens the bone. As the bone matures, this area thins, ossification eventually fusing into solid bone and growth stops. ***Synonyms:*** *Epiphyseal plate.*

> The appropriate 7th character is to be added to all codes from category S72 [unless otherwise indicated].
> A   initial encounter for closed fracture
> B   initial encounter for open fracture type I or II
>   initial encounter for open fracture NOS
> C   initial encounter for open fracture type IIIA, IIIB, or IIIC
> D   subsequent encounter for closed fracture with routine healing
> E   subsequent encounter for open fracture type I or II with routine healing
> F   subsequent encounter for open fracture type IIIA, IIIB, or IIIC with routine healing
> G   subsequent encounter for closed fracture with delayed healing
> H   subsequent encounter for open fracture type I or II with delayed healing
> J   subsequent encounter for open fracture type IIIA, IIIB, or IIIC with delayed healing
> K   subsequent encounter for closed fracture with nonunion
> M   subsequent encounter for open fracture type I or II with nonunion
> N   subsequent encounter for open fracture type IIIA, IIIB, or IIIC with nonunion
> P   subsequent encounter for closed fracture with malunion
> Q   subsequent encounter for open fracture type I or II with malunion
> R   subsequent encounter for open fracture type IIIA, IIIB, or IIIC with malunion
> S   sequela

√5ᵗʰ **S72.0   Fracture of head and neck of femur**

> EXCLUDES 2   *physeal fracture of upper end of femur (S79.0-)*

AHA: 2016,3Q,16
CC Excl: For CC/MCC codes in subcategory S72.0:
Right side: See code S72.001
Left side: See code S72.002
Unspecified side: See code S72.009

√6ᵗʰ **S72.00   Fracture of unspecified part of neck of femur**

Fracture of hip NOS
Fracture of neck of femur NOS

4,6 √7ᵗʰ **S72.001   Fracture of unspecified part of neck of right femur**   MCC CC H5 HCC

> **CC Excl: MCC with 7th character A:** PDX collection 1297
> **CC Excl: MCC with 7th character B or C:** PDX collection 1298
> **CC Excl: CC with 7th character K, M, N, P, Q, or R:** PDX collection 897

4,6 √7ᵗʰ **S72.002   Fracture of unspecified part of neck of left femur**   MCC CC H5 HCC

> **CC Excl: MCC with 7th character A:** PDX collection 1299
> **CC Excl: MCC with 7th character B or C:** PDX collection 1298
> **CC Excl: CC with 7th character K, M, N, P, Q, or R:** PDX collection 897

4,6 √7ᵗʰ **S72.009   Fracture of unspecified part of neck of unspecified femur**   MCC CC H5 HCC

> **CC Excl: MCC with 7th character A, B or C:** PDX collection 1298
> **CC Excl: CC with 7th character K, M, N, P, Q, or R:** PDX collection 897

√6ᵗʰ **S72.01   Unspecified intracapsular fracture of femur**

Subcapital fracture of femur

2,3,6 √7ᵗʰ **S72.011   Unspecified intracapsular fracture of right femur**   MCC CC H5 HCC

2,3,6 √7ᵗʰ **S72.012   Unspecified intracapsular fracture of left femur**   MCC CC H5 HCC

2,3,6 √7ᵗʰ **S72.019   Unspecified intracapsular fracture of unspecified femur**   MCC CC H5 HCC

√6ᵗʰ **S72.02   Fracture of epiphysis (separation) (upper) of femur**

Transepiphyseal fracture of femur

> EXCLUDES 1   *capital femoral epiphyseal fracture (pediatric) of femur (S79.01-)*
> *Salter-Harris Type I physeal fracture of upper end of femur (S79.01-)*

4,6 √7ᵗʰ **S72.021   Displaced fracture of epiphysis (separation) (upper) of right femur**   MCC CC H5 HCC

4,6 √7ᵗʰ **S72.022   Displaced fracture of epiphysis (separation) (upper) of left femur**   MCC CC H5 HCC

4,6 √7ᵗʰ **S72.023   Displaced fracture of epiphysis (separation) (upper) of unspecified femur**   MCC CC H5 HCC

4,6 √7ᵗʰ **S72.024   Nondisplaced fracture of epiphysis (separation) (upper) of right femur**   MCC CC H5 HCC

4,6 √7ᵗʰ **S72.025   Nondisplaced fracture of epiphysis (separation) (upper) of left femur**   MCC CC H5 HCC

4,6 √7ᵗʰ **S72.026   Nondisplaced fracture of epiphysis (separation) (upper) of unspecified femur**   MCC CC H5 HCC

√6ᵗʰ **S72.03   Midcervical fracture of femur**

Transcervical fracture of femur NOS

4,6 √7ᵗʰ **S72.031   Displaced midcervical fracture of right femur**   MCC CC H5 HCC

4,6 √7ᵗʰ **S72.032   Displaced midcervical fracture of left femur**   MCC CC H5 HCC

4,6 √7ᵗʰ **S72.033   Displaced midcervical fracture of unspecified femur**   MCC CC H5 HCC

4,6 √7ᵗʰ **S72.034   Nondisplaced midcervical fracture of right femur**   MCC CC H5 HCC

4,6 √7ᵗʰ **S72.035   Nondisplaced midcervical fracture of left femur**   MCC CC H5 HCC

4,6 √7ᵗʰ **S72.036   Nondisplaced midcervical fracture of unspecified femur**   MCC CC H5 HCC

√6ᵗʰ **S72.04   Fracture of base of neck of femur**

Cervicotrochanteric fracture of femur

4,6 √7ᵗʰ **S72.041   Displaced fracture of base of neck of right femur**   MCC CC H5 HCC

4,6 √7ᵗʰ **S72.042   Displaced fracture of base of neck of left femur**   MCC CC H5 HCC

4,6 √7ᵗʰ **S72.043   Displaced fracture of base of neck of unspecified femur**   MCC CC H5 HCC

4,6 √7ᵗʰ **S72.044   Nondisplaced fracture of base of neck of right femur**   MCC CC H5 HCC

4,6 √7ᵗʰ **S72.045   Nondisplaced fracture of base of neck of left femur**   MCC CC H5 HCC

4,6 √7ᵗʰ **S72.046   Nondisplaced fracture of base of neck of unspecified femur**   MCC CC H5 HCC

√6ᵗʰ **S72.05   Unspecified fracture of head of femur**

Fracture of head of femur NOS

4,6 √7ᵗʰ **S72.051   Unspecified fracture of head of right femur**   MCC CC H5 HCC

4,6 √7ᵗʰ **S72.052   Unspecified fracture of head of left femur**   MCC CC H5 HCC

☑ Additional Character Required   √xᵗʰ Placeholder   Unacceptable PDx   Questionable PDx   Manifestation   Unspecified Dx   H1-H14 HAC   HCC CMS-HCC Dx   HIV HIV Dx

4,6 ✓7th **S72.059** Unspecified fracture of head of unspecified femur   MCC CC H5 HCC

✓6th **S72.06** Articular fracture of head of femur

4,6 ✓7th **S72.061** Displaced articular fracture of head of right femur   MCC CC H5 HCC

4,6 ✓7th **S72.062** Displaced articular fracture of head of left femur   MCC CC H5 HCC

4,6 ✓7th **S72.063** Displaced articular fracture of head of unspecified femur   MCC CC H5 HCC

4,6 ✓7th **S72.064** Nondisplaced articular fracture of head of right femur   MCC CC H5 HCC

4,6 ✓7th **S72.065** Nondisplaced articular fracture of head of left femur   MCC CC H5 HCC

4,6 ✓7th **S72.066** Nondisplaced articular fracture of head of unspecified femur   MCC CC H5 HCC

✓6th **S72.09** Other fracture of head and neck of femur

4,6 ✓7th **S72.091** Other fracture of head and neck of right femur   MCC CC H5 HCC

4,6 ✓7th **S72.092** Other fracture of head and neck of left femur   MCC CC H5 HCC

4,6 ✓7th **S72.099** Other fracture of head and neck of unspecified femur   MCC CC H5 HCC

✓5th **S72.1** Pertrochanteric fracture

AHA: 2016,3Q,16

CC Excl: For CC/MCC codes in subcategory S72.1:
Right side: See code S72.001
Left side: See code S72.002
Unspecified side: See code S72.009

✓6th **S72.10** Unspecified trochanteric fracture of femur

Fracture of trochanter NOS

4,6 ✓7th **S72.101** Unspecified trochanteric fracture of right femur   MCC CC H5 HCC

4,6 ✓7th **S72.102** Unspecified trochanteric fracture of left femur   MCC CC H5 HCC

4,6 ✓7th **S72.109** Unspecified trochanteric fracture of unspecified femur   MCC CC H5 HCC

✓6th **S72.11** Fracture of greater trochanter of femur

2,3,6 ✓7th **S72.111** Displaced fracture of greater trochanter of right femur   MCC CC H5 HCC

2,3,6 ✓7th **S72.112** Displaced fracture of greater trochanter of left femur   MCC CC H5 HCC

2,3,6 ✓7th **S72.113** Displaced fracture of greater trochanter of unspecified femur   MCC CC H5 HCC

2,3,6 ✓7th **S72.114** Nondisplaced fracture of greater trochanter of right femur   MCC CC H5 HCC

2,3,6 ✓7th **S72.115** Nondisplaced fracture of greater trochanter of left femur   MCC CC H5 HCC

2,3,6 ✓7th **S72.116** Nondisplaced fracture of greater trochanter of unspecified femur   MCC CC H5 HCC

✓6th **S72.12** Fracture of lesser trochanter of femur

2,3,6 ✓7th **S72.121** Displaced fracture of lesser trochanter of right femur   MCC CC H5 HCC

2,3,6 ✓7th **S72.122** Displaced fracture of lesser trochanter of left femur   MCC CC H5 HCC

2,3,6 ✓7th **S72.123** Displaced fracture of lesser trochanter of unspecified femur   MCC CC H5 HCC

2,3,6 ✓7th **S72.124** Nondisplaced fracture of lesser trochanter of right femur   MCC CC H5 HCC

2,3,6 ✓7th **S72.125** Nondisplaced fracture of lesser trochanter of left femur   MCC CC H5 HCC

2,3,6 ✓7th **S72.126** Nondisplaced fracture of lesser trochanter of unspecified femur   MCC CC H5 HCC

✓6th **S72.13** Apophyseal fracture of femur

EXCLUDES 1   chronic (nontraumatic) slipped upper femoral epiphysis (M93.0-)

2,3,6 ✓7th **S72.131** Displaced apophyseal fracture of right femur   MCC CC H5 HCC

2,3,6 ✓7th **S72.132** Displaced apophyseal fracture of left femur   MCC CC H5 HCC

2,3,6 ✓7th **S72.133** Displaced apophyseal fracture of unspecified femur   MCC CC H5 HCC

2,3,6 ✓7th **S72.134** Nondisplaced apophyseal fracture of right femur   MCC CC H5 HCC

2,3,6 ✓7th **S72.135** Nondisplaced apophyseal fracture of left femur   MCC CC H5 HCC

2,3,6 ✓7th **S72.136** Nondisplaced apophyseal fracture of unspecified femur   MCC CC H5 HCC

✓6th **S72.14** Intertrochanteric fracture of femur

2,3,6 ✓7th **S72.141** Displaced intertrochanteric fracture of right femur   MCC CC H5 HCC

2,3,6 ✓7th **S72.142** Displaced intertrochanteric fracture of left femur   MCC CC H5 HCC

2,3,6 ✓7th **S72.143** Displaced intertrochanteric fracture of unspecified femur   MCC CC H5 HCC

2,3,6 ✓7th **S72.144** Nondisplaced intertrochanteric fracture of right femur   MCC CC H5 HCC

2,3,6 ✓7th **S72.145** Nondisplaced intertrochanteric fracture of left femur   MCC CC H5 HCC

2,3,6 ✓7th **S72.146** Nondisplaced intertrochanteric fracture of unspecified femur   MCC CC H5 HCC

✓5th **S72.2** Subtrochanteric fracture of femur

CC Excl: For CC/MCC codes in subcategory S72.0: See code S72.009

2,3,6 ✓x7th **S72.21** Displaced subtrochanteric fracture of right femur   MCC CC H5 HCC

2,3,6 ✓x7th **S72.22** Displaced subtrochanteric fracture of left femur   MCC CC H5 HCC

2,3,6 ✓x7th **S72.23** Displaced subtrochanteric fracture of unspecified femur   MCC CC H5 HCC

2,3,6 ✓x7th **S72.24** Nondisplaced subtrochanteric fracture of right femur   MCC CC H5 HCC

2,3,6 ✓x7th **S72.25** Nondisplaced subtrochanteric fracture of left femur   MCC CC H5 HCC

2,3,6 ✓x7th **S72.26** Nondisplaced subtrochanteric fracture of unspecified femur   MCC CC H5 HCC

✓5th **S72.3** Fracture of shaft of femur

CC Excl: For CC/MCC codes in subcategory S72.3:
Right side: See code S72.001
Left side: See code S72.002
Unspecified side: See code S72.009

✓6th **S72.30** Unspecified fracture of shaft of femur

2,3,6 ✓7th **S72.301** Unspecified fracture of shaft of right femur   MCC CC H5 HCC

2,3,6 ✓7th **S72.302** Unspecified fracture of shaft of left femur   MCC CC H5 HCC

2,3,6 ✓7th **S72.309** Unspecified fracture of shaft of unspecified femur   MCC CC H5 HCC

✓6th **S72.32** Transverse fracture of shaft of femur

4,6 ✓7th **S72.321** Displaced transverse fracture of shaft of right femur   MCC CC H5 HCC

4,6 ✓7th **S72.322** Displaced transverse fracture of shaft of left femur   MCC CC H5 HCC

4,6 ✓7th **S72.323** Displaced transverse fracture of shaft of unspecified femur   MCC CC H5 HCC

4,6 ✓7th **S72.324** Nondisplaced transverse fracture of shaft of right femur   MCC CC H5 HCC

4,6 ✓7th **S72.325** Nondisplaced transverse fracture of shaft of left femur   MCC CC H5 HCC

4,6 ✓7th **S72.326** Nondisplaced transverse fracture of shaft of unspecified femur   MCC CC H5 HCC

N Newborn: 0   P Pediatric: 0-17   M Maternity: 9-64   A Adult: 15-124   MCC Major Complication/Comorbidity   CC Complication/Comorbidity   SW Severe Wound Dx

1088   ICD-10-CM 2020

✓6th **S72.33** **Oblique** fracture of shaft of femur

    4,6 ✓7th **S72.331** Displaced **oblique** fracture MCC CC H5 HCC of shaft of **right** femur

    4,6 ✓7th **S72.332** Displaced **oblique** fracture MCC CC H5 HCC of shaft of **left** femur

    4,6 ✓7th **S72.333** Displaced **oblique** fracture MCC CC H5 HCC of shaft of **unspecified** femur

    4,6 ✓7th **S72.334** Nondisplaced **oblique** MCC CC H5 HCC fracture of shaft of **right** femur

    4,6 ✓7th **S72.335** Nondisplaced **oblique** MCC CC H5 HCC fracture of shaft of **left** femur

    4,6 ✓7th **S72.336** Nondisplaced **oblique** MCC CC H5 HCC fracture of shaft of **unspecified** femur

✓6th **S72.34** **Spiral** fracture of shaft of femur

    4,6 ✓7th **S72.341** Displaced **spiral** fracture MCC CC H5 HCC of shaft of **right** femur

    4,6 ✓7th **S72.342** Displaced **spiral** fracture MCC CC H5 HCC of shaft of **left** femur

    4,6 ✓7th **S72.343** Displaced **spiral** fracture MCC CC H5 HCC of shaft of **unspecified** femur

    4,6 ✓7th **S72.344** Nondisplaced **spiral** MCC CC H5 HCC fracture of shaft of **right** femur

    4,6 ✓7th **S72.345** Nondisplaced **spiral** MCC CC H5 HCC fracture of shaft of **left** femur

    4,6 ✓7th **S72.346** Nondisplaced **spiral** MCC CC H5 HCC fracture of shaft of **unspecified** femur

✓6th **S72.35** **Comminuted** fracture of shaft of femur

    4,6 ✓7th **S72.351** Displaced **comminuted** MCC CC H5 HCC fracture of shaft of **right** femur

    4,6 ✓7th **S72.352** Displaced **comminuted** MCC CC H5 HCC fracture of shaft of **left** femur

    4,6 ✓7th **S72.353** Displaced **comminuted** MCC CC H5 HCC fracture of shaft of **unspecified** femur

    4,6 ✓7th **S72.354** Nondisplaced **comminuted** fracture of MCC CC H5 HCC shaft of **right** femur

    4,6 ✓7th **S72.355** Nondisplaced **comminuted** fracture of MCC CC H5 HCC shaft of **left** femur

    4,6 ✓7th **S72.356** Nondisplaced **comminuted** fracture of MCC CC H5 HCC shaft of **unspecified** femur

✓6th **S72.36** **Segmental** fracture of shaft of femur

    4,6 ✓7th **S72.361** Displaced **segmental** MCC CC H5 HCC fracture of shaft or **right** femur

    4,6 ✓7th **S72.362** Displaced **segmental** MCC CC H5 HCC fracture of shaft of **left** femur

    4,6 ✓7th **S72.363** Displaced **segmental** MCC CC H5 HCC fracture of shaft of **unspecified** femur

    4,6 ✓7th **S72.364** Nondisplaced **segmental** MCC CC H5 HCC fracture of shaft of **right** femur

    4,6 ✓7th **S72.365** Nondisplaced **segmental** MCC CC H5 HCC fracture of shaft of **left** femur

    4,6 ✓7th **S72.366** Nondisplaced **segmental** MCC CC H5 HCC fracture of shaft of **unspecified** femur

✓6th **S72.39** Other fracture of shaft of femur

    4,6 ✓7th **S72.391** Other fracture of shaft of MCC CC H5 HCC **right** femur

    4,6 ✓7th **S72.392** Other fracture of shaft of MCC CC H5 HCC **left** femur

    4,6 ✓7th **S72.399** Other fracture of shaft of MCC CC H5 HCC **unspecified** femur

✓5th **S72.4** Fracture of **lower end** of femur

    Fracture of distal end of femur

    EXCLUDES 2   *fracture of shaft of femur (S72.3-)*
           physeal fracture of lower end of femur (S79.1-)

    AHA: 2016,4Q,42

    CC Excl: For CC/MCC codes in subcategory S72.4, unless otherwise noted:
    Right side: See code S72.401
    Left side: See code S72.402
    Unspecified side: See code S72.409

✓6th **S72.40** **Unspecified** fracture of lower end of femur

    AHA: 2018,1Q,21; 2016,4Q,42

    2,3,6 ✓7th **S72.401** **Unspecified** fracture of MCC CC H5 HCC lower end of **right** femur
       CC Excl: CC with 7th character A: PDX collection 1300
       CC Excl: MCC with 7th character B or C: PDX collection 1301
       CC Excl: CC with 7th character K, M, N, P, Q, or R: PDX collection 897

    2,3,6 ✓7th **S72.402** **Unspecified** fracture of MCC CC H5 HCC lower end of **left** femur
       CC Excl: CC with 7th character A: PDX collection 1302
       CC Excl: MCC with 7th character B or C: PDX collection 1301
       CC Excl: CC with 7th character K, M, N, P, Q, or R: PDX collection 897

    2,3,6 ✓7th **S72.409** **Unspecified** fracture of MCC CC H5 HCC lower end of **unspecified** femur
       CC Excl: CC with 7th character A or MCC with 7th character B or C: PDX collection 1301
       CC Excl: CC with 7th character K, M, N, P, Q, or R: PDX collection 897

✓6th **S72.41** **Unspecified condyle** fracture of lower end of femur

    Condyle fracture of femur NOS

    2,3,6 ✓7th **S72.411** Displaced **unspecified** MCC CC H5 HCC condyle fracture of lower end of **right** femur

    2,3,6 ✓7th **S72.412** Displaced **unspecified** MCC CC H5 HCC condyle fracture of lower end of **left** femur

    2,3,6 ✓7th **S72.413** Displaced **unspecified** MCC CC H5 HCC condyle fracture of lower end of **unspecified** femur

    2,3,6 ✓7th **S72.414** Nondisplaced **unspecified** MCC CC H5 HCC condyle fracture of lower end of **right** femur

    2,3,6 ✓7th **S72.415** Nondisplaced **unspecified** MCC CC H5 HCC condyle fracture of lower end of **left** femur

    2,3,6 ✓7th **S72.416** Nondisplaced **unspecified** MCC CC H5 HCC condyle fracture of lower end of **unspecified** femur

✓6th **S72.42** Fracture of **lateral condyle** of femur

    2,3,6 ✓7th **S72.421** Displaced fracture of MCC CC H5 HCC lateral condyle of **right** femur

    2,3,6 ✓7th **S72.422** Displaced fracture of MCC CC H5 HCC lateral condyle of **left** femur

    2,3,6 ✓7th **S72.423** Displaced fracture of MCC CC H5 HCC lateral condyle of **unspecified** femur

    2,3,6 ✓7th **S72.424** Nondisplaced fracture of MCC CC H5 HCC lateral condyle of **right** femur

    2,3,6 ✓7th **S72.425** Nondisplaced fracture of MCC CC H5 HCC lateral condyle of **left** femur

    2,3,6 ✓7th **S72.426** Nondisplaced fracture of MCC CC H5 HCC lateral condyle of **unspecified** femur

✓6th **S72.43** Fracture of **medial condyle** of femur

    2,3,6 ✓7th **S72.431** Displaced fracture of MCC CC H5 HCC medial condyle of **right** femur

    2,3,6 ✓7th **S72.432** Displaced fracture of MCC CC H5 HCC medial condyle of **left** femur

2,3,6 √7ᵗʰ **S72.433** Displaced fracture of `MCC` `CC` `H5` `HCC`
medial condyle of
unspecified femur

2,3,6 √7ᵗʰ **S72.434** Nondisplaced fracture of `MCC` `CC` `H5` `HCC`
medial condyle of right
femur

2,3,6 √7ᵗʰ **S72.435** Nondisplaced fracture of `MCC` `CC` `H5` `HCC`
medial condyle of left
femur

2,3,6 √7ᵗʰ **S72.436** Nondisplaced fracture of `MCC` `CC` `H5` `HCC`
medial condyle of
unspecified femur

√6ᵗʰ **S72.44** Fracture of lower epiphysis (separation) of femur

　　　EXCLUDES 1　*Salter-Harris Type I physeal fracture of
lower end of femur (S79.11-)*

2,3,6 √7ᵗʰ **S72.441** Displaced fracture of `MCC` `CC` `H5` `HCC`
lower epiphysis
(separation) of right femur

2,3,6 √7ᵗʰ **S72.442** Displaced fracture of `MCC` `CC` `H5` `HCC`
lower epiphysis
(separation) of left femur

2,3,6 √7ᵗʰ **S72.443** Displaced fracture of `MCC` `CC` `H5` `HCC`
lower epiphysis
(separation) of
unspecified femur

2,3,6 √7ᵗʰ **S72.444** Nondisplaced fracture of `MCC` `CC` `H5` `HCC`
lower epiphysis
(separation) of right femur

2,3,6 √7ᵗʰ **S72.445** Nondisplaced fracture of `MCC` `CC` `H5` `HCC`
lower epiphysis
(separation) of left femur

2,3,6 √7ᵗʰ **S72.446** Nondisplaced fracture of `MCC` `CC` `H5` `HCC`
lower epiphysis
(separation) of
unspecified femur

√6ᵗʰ **S72.45** Supracondylar fracture without intracondylar
extension of lower end of femur

　　　Supracondylar fracture of lower end of femur NOS

　　　EXCLUDES 1　*supracondylar fracture with intracondylar
extension of lower end of femur
(S72.46-)*

2,3,6 √7ᵗʰ **S72.451** Displaced supracondylar `MCC` `CC` `H5` `HCC`
fracture without
intracondylar extension of
lower end of right femur

2,3,6 √7ᵗʰ **S72.452** Displaced supracondylar `MCC` `CC` `H5` `HCC`
fracture without
intracondylar extension of
lower end of left femur

2,3,6 √7ᵗʰ **S72.453** Displaced supracondylar `MCC` `CC` `H5` `HCC`
fracture without
intracondylar extension of
lower end of unspecified
femur

2,3,6 √7ᵗʰ **S72.454** Nondisplaced `MCC` `CC` `H5` `HCC`
supracondylar fracture
without intracondylar
extension of lower end of
right femur

2,3,6 √7ᵗʰ **S72.455** Nondisplaced `MCC` `CC` `H5` `HCC`
supracondylar fracture
without intracondylar
extension of lower end of
left femur

2,3,6 √7ᵗʰ **S72.456** Nondisplaced `MCC` `CC` `H5` `HCC`
supracondylar fracture
without intracondylar
extension of lower end of
unspecified femur

√6ᵗʰ **S72.46** Supracondylar fracture with intracondylar
extension of lower end of femur

　　　EXCLUDES 1　*supracondylar fracture without
intracondylar extension of lower end
of femur (S72.45-)*

2,3,6 √7ᵗʰ **S72.461** Displaced supracondylar `MCC` `CC` `H5` `HCC`
fracture with
intracondylar extension of
lower end of right femur

2,3,6 √7ᵗʰ **S72.462** Displaced supracondylar `MCC` `CC` `H5` `HCC`
fracture with
intracondylar extension of
lower end of left femur

2,3,6 √7ᵗʰ **S72.463** Displaced supracondylar `MCC` `CC` `H5` `HCC`
fracture with
intracondylar extension of
lower end of unspecified
femur

2,3,6 √7ᵗʰ **S72.464** Nondisplaced `MCC` `CC` `H5` `HCC`
supracondylar fracture
with intracondylar
extension of lower end of
right femur

2,3,6 √7ᵗʰ **S72.465** Nondisplaced `MCC` `CC` `H5` `HCC`
supracondylar fracture
with intracondylar
extension of lower end of
left femur

2,3,6 √7ᵗʰ **S72.466** Nondisplaced `MCC` `CC` `H5` `HCC`
supracondylar fracture
with intracondylar
extension of lower end of
unspecified femur

√6ᵗʰ **S72.47** Torus fracture of lower end of femur

> The appropriate 7th character is to be added to all
> codes in subcategory S72.47.
> A　initial encounter for closed fracture
> D　subsequent encounter for fracture with routine
> 　　healing
> G　subsequent encounter for fracture with delayed
> 　　healing
> K　subsequent encounter for fracture with
> 　　nonunion
> P　subsequent encounter for fracture with
> 　　malunion
> S　sequela

3,6 √7ᵗʰ **S72.471** Torus fracture of lower `CC` `H5` `HCC`
end of right femur
CC Excl: CC with 7th character A: PDX
collection 1300
CC Excl: CC with 7th character K or P: PDX
collection 897

3,6 √7ᵗʰ **S72.472** Torus fracture of lower `CC` `H5` `HCC`
end of left femur
CC Excl: CC with 7th character A: PDX
collection 1302
CC Excl: CC with 7th character K or P: PDX
collection 897

3,6 √7ᵗʰ **S72.479** Torus fracture of lower `CC` `H5` `HCC`
end of unspecified femur
CC Excl: CC with 7th character A: PDX
collection 1301
CC Excl: CC with 7th character K or P: PDX
collection 897

√6ᵗʰ **S72.49** Other fracture of lower end of femur

2,3,6 √7ᵗʰ **S72.491** Other fracture of lower `MCC` `CC` `H5` `HCC`
end of right femur
CC Excl: CC with 7th character A: PDX
collection 1300
CC Excl: MCC with 7th character B or C:
PDX collection 1303
**CC Excl: CC with 7th character K, M, N, P,
Q, or R:** PDX collection 897

2,3,6 √7ᵗʰ **S72.492** Other fracture of lower `MCC` `CC` `H5` `HCC`
end of left femur
CC Excl: CC with 7th character A: PDX
collection 1302
CC Excl: MCC with 7th character B or C:
PDX collection 1303
**CC Excl: CC with 7th character K, M, N, P,
Q, or R:** PDX collection 897

2,3,6 √7ᵗʰ **S72.499** Other fracture of lower `MCC` `CC` `H5` `HCC`
end of unspecified femur
CC Excl: CC with 7th character A: PDX
collection 1301
CC Excl: MCC with 7th character B or C:
PDX collection 1303
**CC Excl: CC with 7th character K, M, N, P,
Q, or R:** PDX collection 897

√5ᵗʰ **S72.8 Other fracture of femur**

√6ᵗʰ **S72.8X Other fracture of femur**

CC Excl: For codes in subcategory S72.8X:
MCC with 7th character A, B or C: PDX collection 1298
CC with 7th character K, M, N, P, Q, or R: PDX collection 897

4,6 √7ᵗʰ **S72.8X1 Other fracture of right femur** `MCC` `CC` `H5` `HCC`

4,6 √7ᵗʰ **S72.8X2 Other fracture of left femur** `MCC` `CC` `H5` `HCC`

4,6 √7ᵗʰ **S72.8X9 Other fracture of unspecified femur** `MCC` `CC` `H5` `HCC`

√5ᵗʰ **S72.9 Unspecified fracture of femur**

Fracture of thigh NOS
Fracture of upper leg NOS

EXCLUDES 1   fracture of hip NOS (S72.00-, S72.01-)

CC Excl: For codes in subcategory S72.9:
MCC with 7th character A, B or C: PDX collection 1298
CC with 7th character K, M, N, P, Q, or R: PDX collection 897

4,6 √x7ᵗʰ **S72.90 Unspecified fracture of unspecified femur** `MCC` `CC` `H5` `HCC`

AHA: 2012,4Q,93

4,6 √x7ᵗʰ **S72.91 Unspecified fracture of right femur** `MCC` `CC` `H5` `HCC`

4,6 √x7ᵗʰ **S72.92 Unspecified fracture of left femur** `MCC` `CC` `H5` `HCC`

√4ᵗʰ **S73 Dislocation and sprain of joint and ligaments of hip**

INCLUDES   avulsion of joint or ligament of hip
laceration of cartilage, joint or ligament of hip
sprain of cartilage, joint or ligament of hip
traumatic hemarthrosis of joint or ligament of hip
traumatic rupture of joint or ligament of hip
traumatic subluxation of joint or ligament of hip
traumatic tear of joint or ligament of hip

Code also any associated open wound

EXCLUDES 2   strain of muscle, fascia and tendon of hip and thigh (S76.-)

The appropriate 7th character is to be added to each code from category S73.
A   initial encounter
D   subsequent encounter
S   sequela

√5ᵗʰ **S73.0 Subluxation and dislocation of hip**

EXCLUDES 2   dislocation and subluxation of hip prosthesis (T84.020, T84.021)

√6ᵗʰ **S73.00 Unspecified subluxation and dislocation of hip**

Dislocation of hip NOS
Subluxation of hip NOS

CC Excl: For CC codes in subcategory S73.00:
Right side: PDX collection 1304
Left side: PDX collection 1305
Unspecified side: PDX collection 1306

6 √7ᵗʰ **S73.001 Unspecified subluxation of right hip** `CC` `H5` `HCC`

6 √7ᵗʰ **S73.002 Unspecified subluxation of left hip** `CC` `H5` `HCC`

6 √7ᵗʰ **S73.003 Unspecified subluxation of unspecified hip** `CC` `H5` `HCC`

6 √7ᵗʰ **S73.004 Unspecified dislocation of right hip** `CC` `H5` `HCC`

6 √7ᵗʰ **S73.005 Unspecified dislocation of left hip** `CC` `H5` `HCC`

6 √7ᵗʰ **S73.006 Unspecified dislocation of unspecified hip** `CC` `H5` `HCC`

√6ᵗʰ **S73.01 Posterior subluxation and dislocation of hip**

CC Excl: For CC codes in subcategory S73.01:
Right side: PDX collection 1307
Left side: PDX collection 1308
Unspecified side: PDX collection 1309

6 √7ᵗʰ **S73.011 Posterior subluxation of right hip** `CC` `H5` `HCC`

6 √7ᵗʰ **S73.012 Posterior subluxation of left hip** `CC` `H5` `HCC`

6 √7ᵗʰ **S73.013 Posterior subluxation of unspecified hip** `CC` `H5` `HCC`

6 √7ᵗʰ **S73.014 Posterior dislocation of right hip** `CC` `H5` `HCC`

6 √7ᵗʰ **S73.015 Posterior dislocation of left hip** `CC` `H5` `HCC`

6 √7ᵗʰ **S73.016 Posterior dislocation of unspecified hip** `CC` `H5` `HCC`

√6ᵗʰ **S73.02 Obturator subluxation and dislocation of hip**

CC Excl: For CC codes in subcategory S73.02:
Right side: PDX collection 1310
Left side: PDX collection 1311
Unspecified side: PDX collection 1312

6 √7ᵗʰ **S73.021 Obturator subluxation of right hip** `CC` `H5` `HCC`

6 √7ᵗʰ **S73.022 Obturator subluxation of left hip** `CC` `H5` `HCC`

6 √7ᵗʰ **S73.023 Obturator subluxation of unspecified hip** `CC` `H5` `HCC`

6 √7ᵗʰ **S73.024 Obturator dislocation of right hip** `CC` `H5` `HCC`

6 √7ᵗʰ **S73.025 Obturator dislocation of left hip** `CC` `H5` `HCC`

6 √7ᵗʰ **S73.026 Obturator dislocation of unspecified hip** `CC` `H5` `HCC`

√6ᵗʰ **S73.03 Other anterior subluxation and dislocation of hip**

CC Excl: For CC codes in subcategory S73.03:
Right side: PDX collection 1313
Left side: PDX collection 1314
Unspecified side: PDX collection 1315

6 √7ᵗʰ **S73.031 Other anterior subluxation of right hip** `CC` `H5` `HCC`

6 √7ᵗʰ **S73.032 Other anterior subluxation of left hip** `CC` `H5` `HCC`

6 √7ᵗʰ **S73.033 Other anterior subluxation of unspecified hip** `CC` `H5` `HCC`

6 √7ᵗʰ **S73.034 Other anterior dislocation of right hip** `CC` `H5` `HCC`

6 √7ᵗʰ **S73.035 Other anterior dislocation of left hip** `CC` `H5` `HCC`

6 √7ᵗʰ **S73.036 Other anterior dislocation of unspecified hip** `CC` `H5` `HCC`

√6ᵗʰ **S73.04 Central subluxation and dislocation of hip**

CC Excl: For CC codes in subcategory S73.04:
Right side: PDX collection 1304
Left side: PDX collection 1305
Unspecified side: PDX collection 1306

6 √7ᵗʰ **S73.041 Central subluxation of right hip** `CC` `H5` `HCC`

6 √7ᵗʰ **S73.042 Central subluxation of left hip** `CC` `H5` `HCC`

6 √7ᵗʰ **S73.043 Central subluxation of unspecified hip** `CC` `H5` `HCC`

6 √7ᵗʰ **S73.044 Central dislocation of right hip** `CC` `H5` `HCC`

6 √7ᵗʰ **S73.045 Central dislocation of left hip** `CC` `H5` `HCC`

6 √7ᵗʰ **S73.046 Central dislocation of unspecified hip** `CC` `H5` `HCC`

√5ᵗʰ **S73.1 Sprain of hip**

AHA: 2014,4Q,25

√6ᵗʰ **S73.10 Unspecified sprain of hip**

√7ᵗʰ **S73.101 Unspecified sprain of right hip**

√7ᵗʰ **S73.102 Unspecified sprain of left hip**

√7ᵗʰ **S73.109 Unspecified sprain of unspecified hip**

√6ᵗʰ **S73.11 Iliofemoral ligament sprain of hip**

√7ᵗʰ **S73.111 Iliofemoral ligament sprain of right hip**

√7ᵗʰ **S73.112 Iliofemoral ligament sprain of left hip**

√7ᵗʰ **S73.119 Iliofemoral ligament sprain of unspecified hip**

√6ᵗʰ **S73.12 Ischiocapsular (ligament) sprain of hip**

√7ᵗʰ **S73.121 Ischiocapsular ligament sprain of right hip**

√7ᵗʰ **S73.122 Ischiocapsular ligament sprain of left hip**

√7ᵗʰ **S73.129 Ischiocapsular ligament sprain of unspecified hip**

√6ᵗʰ **S73.19 Other sprain of hip**

√7ᵗʰ **S73.191 Other sprain of right hip**

√7ᵗʰ **S73.192 Other sprain of left hip**

√7ᵗʰ **S73.199 Other sprain of unspecified hip**

✅ Additional Character Required   √x7ᵗʰ Placeholder   Unacceptable PDx   Questionable PDx   Manifestation   Unspecified Dx   `H1`-`H14` HAC   `HCC` CMS-HCC Dx   `HIV` HIV Dx

Chapter 19. Injury, Poisoning and Certain Other Consequences of External Causes *(left margin)*

S74–S75.199 *(left margin)*

√4ᵗʰ S74 Injury of nerves at hip and thigh level

Code also any associated open wound (S71.-)

EXCLUDES 2 injury of nerves at ankle and foot level (S94.-)

injury of nerves at lower leg level (S84.-)

The appropriate 7th character is to be added to each code from category S74.
A   initial encounter
D   subsequent encounter
S   sequela

√5ᵗʰ S74.0 Injury of sciatic nerve at hip and thigh level

√x7ᵗʰ S74.00 Injury of sciatic nerve at hip and thigh level, unspecified leg

√x7ᵗʰ S74.01 Injury of sciatic nerve at hip and thigh level, right leg

√x7ᵗʰ S74.02 Injury of sciatic nerve at hip and thigh level, left leg

√5ᵗʰ S74.1 Injury of femoral nerve at hip and thigh level

√x7ᵗʰ S74.10 Injury of femoral nerve at hip and thigh level, unspecified leg

√x7ᵗʰ S74.11 Injury of femoral nerve at hip and thigh level, right leg

√x7ᵗʰ S74.12 Injury of femoral nerve at hip and thigh level, left leg

√5ᵗʰ S74.2 Injury of cutaneous sensory nerve at hip and thigh level

√x7ᵗʰ S74.20 Injury of cutaneous sensory nerve at hip and thigh level, unspecified leg

√x7ᵗʰ S74.21 Injury of cutaneous sensory nerve at hip and high level, right leg

√x7ᵗʰ S74.22 Injury of cutaneous sensory nerve at hip and thigh level, left leg

√5ᵗʰ S74.8 Injury of other nerves at hip and thigh level

√6ᵗʰ S74.8X Injury of other nerves at hip and thigh level

√7ᵗʰ S74.8X1 Injury of other nerves at hip and thigh level, right leg

√7ᵗʰ S74.8X2 Injury of other nerves at hip and thigh level, left leg

√7ᵗʰ S74.8X9 Injury of other nerves at hip and thigh level, unspecified leg

√5ᵗʰ S74.9 Injury of unspecified nerve at hip and thigh level

√x7ᵗʰ S74.90 Injury of unspecified nerve at hip and thigh level, unspecified leg

√x7ᵗʰ S74.91 Injury of unspecified nerve at hip and thigh level, right leg

√x7ᵗʰ S74.92 Injury of unspecified nerve at hip and thigh level, left leg

√4ᵗʰ S75 Injury of blood vessels at hip and thigh level

Code also any associated open wound (S71.-)

EXCLUDES 2 injury of blood vessels at lower leg level (S85.-)

injury of popliteal artery (S85.0)

The appropriate 7th character is to be added to each code from category S75.
A   initial encounter
D   subsequent encounter
S   sequela

√5ᵗʰ S75.0 Injury of femoral artery

CC Excl: For MCC codes in subcategory S75.0:
Right side: PDX collection 1316
Left side: PDX collection 1317
Unspecified side: PDX collection 1318

√6ᵗʰ S75.00 Unspecified injury of femoral artery

√7ᵗʰ S75.001 Unspecified injury of femoral artery, right leg `MCC`

√7ᵗʰ S75.002 Unspecified injury of femoral artery, left leg `MCC`

√7ᵗʰ S75.009 Unspecified injury of femoral artery, unspecified leg `MCC`

√6ᵗʰ S75.01 Minor laceration of femoral artery

Incomplete transection of femoral artery
Laceration of femoral artery NOS
Superficial laceration of femoral artery

√7ᵗʰ S75.011 Minor laceration of femoral artery, right leg `MCC`

√7ᵗʰ S75.012 Minor laceration of femoral artery, left leg `MCC`

√7ᵗʰ S75.019 Minor laceration of femoral artery, unspecified leg `MCC`

√6ᵗʰ S75.02 Major laceration of femoral artery

Complete transection of femoral artery
Traumatic rupture of femoral artery

√7ᵗʰ S75.021 Major laceration of femoral artery, right leg `MCC`

√7ᵗʰ S75.022 Major laceration of femoral artery, left leg `MCC`

√7ᵗʰ S75.029 Major laceration of femoral artery, unspecified leg `MCC`

√6ᵗʰ S75.09 Other specified injury of femoral artery

√7ᵗʰ S75.091 Other specified injury of femoral artery, right leg `MCC`

√7ᵗʰ S75.092 Other specified injury of femoral artery, left leg `MCC`

√7ᵗʰ S75.099 Other specified injury of femoral artery, unspecified leg `MCC`

√5ᵗʰ S75.1 Injury of femoral vein at hip and thigh level

CC Excl: For MCC codes in subcategory S75.1:
Right side: PDX collection 1319
Left side: PDX collection 1320
Unspecified side: PDX collection 1321

√6ᵗʰ S75.10 Unspecified injury of femoral vein at hip and thigh level

√7ᵗʰ S75.101 Unspecified injury of femoral vein at hip and thigh level, right leg `MCC`

√7ᵗʰ S75.102 Unspecified injury of femoral vein at hip and thigh level, left leg `MCC`

√7ᵗʰ S75.109 Unspecified injury of femoral vein at hip and thigh level, unspecified leg `MCC`

√6ᵗʰ S75.11 Minor laceration of femoral vein at hip and thigh level

Incomplete transection of femoral vein at hip and thigh level
Laceration of femoral vein at hip and thigh level NOS
Superficial laceration of femoral vein at hip and thigh level

√7ᵗʰ S75.111 Minor laceration of femoral vein at hip and thigh level, right leg `MCC`

√7ᵗʰ S75.112 Minor laceration of femoral vein at hip and thigh level, left leg `MCC`

√7ᵗʰ S75.119 Minor laceration of femoral vein at hip and thigh level, unspecified leg `MCC`

√6ᵗʰ S75.12 Major laceration of femoral vein at hip and thigh level

Complete transection of femoral vein at hip and thigh level
Traumatic rupture of femoral vein at hip and thigh level

√7ᵗʰ S75.121 Major laceration of femoral vein at hip and thigh level, right leg `MCC`

√7ᵗʰ S75.122 Major laceration of femoral vein at hip and thigh level, left leg `MCC`

√7ᵗʰ S75.129 Major laceration of femoral vein at hip and thigh level, unspecified leg `MCC`

√6ᵗʰ S75.19 Other specified injury of femoral vein at hip and thigh level

√7ᵗʰ S75.191 Other specified injury of femoral vein at hip and thigh level, right leg `MCC`

√7ᵗʰ S75.192 Other specified injury of femoral vein at hip and thigh level, left leg `MCC`

√7ᵗʰ S75.199 Other specified injury of femoral vein at hip and thigh level, unspecified leg `MCC`

N Newborn: 0   P Pediatric: 0-17   M Maternity: 9-64   A Adult: 15-124   MCC Major Complication/Comorbidity   CC Complication/Comorbidity   SW Severe Wound Dx

1092 | ICD-10-CM 2020

√5ᵗʰ **S75.2 Injury of greater saphenous vein at hip and thigh level**

> **EXCLUDES 1**   *greater saphenous vein NOS (S85.3)*
>
> **CC Excl: For CC codes in subcategory S75.2:**
> **Right side:** PDX collection 1322
> **Left side:** PDX collection 1323
> **Unspecified side:** PDX collection 1324

√6ᵗʰ **S75.20 Unspecified injury of greater saphenous vein at hip and thigh level**

√7ᵗʰ **S75.201 Unspecified injury of greater saphenous vein at hip and thigh level, right leg**   `CC`

√7ᵗʰ **S75.202 Unspecified injury of greater saphenous vein at hip and thigh level, left leg**   `CC`

√7ᵗʰ **S75.209 Unspecified injury of greater saphenous vein at hip and thigh level, unspecified leg**   `CC`

√6ᵗʰ **S75.21 Minor laceration of greater saphenous vein at hip and thigh level**

Incomplete transection of greater saphenous vein at hip and thigh level

Laceration of greater saphenous vein at hip and thigh level NOS

Superficial laceration of greater saphenous vein at hip and thigh level

√7ᵗʰ **S75.211 Minor laceration of greater saphenous vein at hip and thigh level, right leg**   `CC`

√7ᵗʰ **S75.212 Minor laceration of greater saphenous vein at hip and thigh level, left leg**   `CC`

√7ᵗʰ **S75.219 Minor laceration of greater saphenous vein at hip and thigh level, unspecified leg**   `CC`

√6ᵗʰ **S75.22 Major laceration of greater saphenous vein at hip and thigh level**

Complete transection of greater saphenous vein at hip and thigh level

Traumatic rupture of greater saphenous vein at hip and thigh level

√7ᵗʰ **S75.221 Major laceration of greater saphenous vein at hip and thigh level, right leg**   `CC`

√7ᵗʰ **S75.222 Major laceration of greater saphenous vein at hip and thigh level, left leg**   `CC`

√7ᵗʰ **S75.229 Major laceration of greater saphenous vein at hip and thigh level, unspecified leg**   `CC`

√6ᵗʰ **S75.29 Other specified injury of greater saphenous vein at hip and thigh level**

√7ᵗʰ **S75.291 Other specified injury of greater saphenous vein at hip and thigh level, right leg**   `CC`

√7ᵗʰ **S75.292 Other specified injury of greater saphenous vein at hip and thigh level, left leg**   `CC`

√7ᵗʰ **S75.299 Other specified injury of greater saphenous vein at hip and thigh level, unspecified leg**   `CC`

√5ᵗʰ **S75.8 Injury of other blood vessels at hip and thigh level**

> **CC Excl: For CC codes in subcategory S75.8:**
> **Right side:** PDX collection 1325
> **Left side:** PDX collection 1326
> **Unspecified side:** PDX collection 1327

√6ᵗʰ **S75.80 Unspecified injury of other blood vessels at hip and thigh level**

√7ᵗʰ **S75.801 Unspecified injury of other blood vessels at hip and thigh level, right leg**   `CC`

√7ᵗʰ **S75.802 Unspecified injury of other blood vessels at hip and thigh level, left leg**   `CC`

√7ᵗʰ **S75.809 Unspecified injury of other blood vessels at hip and thigh level, unspecified leg**   `CC`

√6ᵗʰ **S75.81 Laceration of other blood vessels at hip and thigh level**

√7ᵗʰ **S75.811 Laceration of other blood vessels at hip and thigh level, right leg**   `CC`

√7ᵗʰ **S75.812 Laceration of other blood vessels at hip and thigh level, left leg**   `CC`

√7ᵗʰ **S75.819 Laceration of other blood vessels at hip and thigh level, unspecified leg**   `CC`

√6ᵗʰ **S75.89 Other specified injury of other blood vessels at hip and thigh level**

√7ᵗʰ **S75.891 Other specified injury of other blood vessels at hip and thigh level, right leg**   `CC`

√7ᵗʰ **S75.892 Other specified injury of other blood vessels at hip and thigh level, left leg**   `CC`

√7ᵗʰ **S75.899 Other specified injury of other blood vessels at hip and thigh level, unspecified leg**   `CC`

√5ᵗʰ **S75.9 Injury of unspecified blood vessel at hip and thigh level**

> **CC Excl: For CC codes in subcategory S75.9:**
> **Right side:** PDX collection 1325
> **Left side:** PDX collection 1326
> **Unspecified side:** PDX collection 1327

√6ᵗʰ **S75.90 Unspecified injury of unspecified blood vessel at hip and thigh level**

√7ᵗʰ **S75.901 Unspecified injury of unspecified blood vessel at hip and thigh level, right leg**   `CC`

√7ᵗʰ **S75.902 Unspecified injury of unspecified blood vessel at hip and thigh level, left leg**   `CC`

√7ᵗʰ **S75.909 Unspecified injury of unspecified blood vessel at hip and thigh level, unspecified leg**   `CC`

√6ᵗʰ **S75.91 Laceration of unspecified blood vessel at hip and thigh level**

√7ᵗʰ **S75.911 Laceration of unspecified blood vessel at hip and thigh level, right leg**   `CC`

√7ᵗʰ **S75.912 Laceration of unspecified blood vessel at hip and thigh level, left leg**   `CC`

√7ᵗʰ **S75.919 Laceration of unspecified blood vessel at hip and thigh level, unspecified leg**   `CC`

√6ᵗʰ **S75.99 Other specified injury of unspecified blood vessel at hip and thigh level**

√7ᵗʰ **S75.991 Other specified injury of unspecified blood vessel at hip and thigh level, right leg**   `CC`

√7ᵗʰ **S75.992 Other specified injury of unspecified blood vessel at hip and thigh level, left leg**   `CC`

√7ᵗʰ **S75.999 Other specified injury of unspecified blood vessel at hip and thigh level, unspecified leg**   `CC`

✅ Additional Character Required   √x7ᵗʰ Placeholder   Unacceptable PDx   Questionable PDx   Manifestation   Unspecified Dx   **H1**-**H14** HAC   **HCC** CMS-HCC Dx   **HIV** HIV Dx

✓4ᵗʰ S76 Injury of muscle, fascia and tendon at hip and thigh level

Code also any associated open wound (S71.-)

EXCLUDES 2   *injury of muscle, fascia and tendon at lower leg level (S86)*
sprain of joint and ligament of hip (S73.1)

TIP: Refer to the Muscle/Tendon table at the beginning of this chapter.

The appropriate 7th character is to be added to each code from category S76.
A   initial encounter
D   subsequent encounter
S   sequela

CC Excl: For CC codes in category S76:
Right side: PDX collection 1328
Left side: PDX collection 1329
Unspecified side: PDX collection 1330

✓5ᵗʰ S76.0 Injury of muscle, fascia and tendon of hip

    ✓6ᵗʰ S76.00 Unspecified injury of muscle, fascia and tendon of hip

       ✓7ᵗʰ S76.001 Unspecified injury of muscle, fascia and tendon of right hip

       ✓7ᵗʰ S76.002 Unspecified injury of muscle, fascia and tendon of left hip

       ✓7ᵗʰ S76.009 Unspecified injury of muscle, fascia and tendon of unspecified hip

    ✓6ᵗʰ S76.01 Strain of muscle, fascia and tendon of hip

       ✓7ᵗʰ S76.011 Strain of muscle, fascia and tendon of right hip

       ✓7ᵗʰ S76.012 Strain of muscle, fascia and tendon of left hip

       ✓7ᵗʰ S76.019 Strain of muscle, fascia and tendon of unspecified hip

    ✓6ᵗʰ S76.02 Laceration of muscle, fascia and tendon of hip

       ✓7ᵗʰ S76.021 Laceration of muscle, fascia and tendon of right hip `CC`

       ✓7ᵗʰ S76.022 Laceration of muscle, fascia and tendon of left hip `CC`

       ✓7ᵗʰ S76.029 Laceration of muscle, fascia and tendon of unspecified hip `CC`

    ✓6ᵗʰ S76.09 Other specified injury of muscle, fascia and tendon of hip

       ✓7ᵗʰ S76.091 Other specified injury of muscle, fascia and tendon of right hip

       ✓7ᵗʰ S76.092 Other specified injury of muscle, fascia and tendon of left hip

       ✓7ᵗʰ S76.099 Other specified injury of muscle, fascia and tendon of unspecified hip

✓5ᵗʰ S76.1 Injury of quadriceps muscle, fascia and tendon

Injury of patellar ligament (tendon)

    ✓6ᵗʰ S76.10 Unspecified injury of quadriceps muscle, fascia and tendon

       ✓7ᵗʰ S76.101 Unspecified injury of right quadriceps muscle, fascia and tendon

       ✓7ᵗʰ S76.102 Unspecified injury of left quadriceps muscle, fascia and tendon

       ✓7ᵗʰ S76.109 Unspecified injury of unspecified quadriceps muscle, fascia and tendon

    ✓6ᵗʰ S76.11 Strain of quadriceps muscle, fascia and tendon

       ✓7ᵗʰ S76.111 Strain of right quadriceps muscle, fascia and tendon

       ✓7ᵗʰ S76.112 Strain of left quadriceps muscle, fascia and tendon

       ✓7ᵗʰ S76.119 Strain of unspecified quadriceps muscle, fascia and tendon

    ✓6ᵗʰ S76.12 Laceration of quadriceps muscle, fascia and tendon

       ✓7ᵗʰ S76.121 Laceration of right quadriceps muscle, fascia and tendon `CC`

       ✓7ᵗʰ S76.122 Laceration of left quadriceps muscle, fascia and tendon `CC`

       ✓7ᵗʰ S76.129 Laceration of unspecified quadriceps muscle, fascia and tendon `CC`

    ✓6ᵗʰ S76.19 Other specified injury of quadriceps muscle, fascia and tendon

       ✓7ᵗʰ S76.191 Other specified injury of right quadriceps muscle, fascia and tendon

✓7ᵗʰ S76.192 Other specified injury of left quadriceps muscle, fascia and tendon

✓7ᵗʰ S76.199 Other specified injury of unspecified quadriceps muscle, fascia and tendon

✓5ᵗʰ S76.2 Injury of adductor muscle, fascia and tendon of thigh

    ✓6ᵗʰ S76.20 Unspecified injury of adductor muscle, fascia and tendon of thigh

       ✓7ᵗʰ S76.201 Unspecified injury of adductor muscle, fascia and tendon of right thigh

       ✓7ᵗʰ S76.202 Unspecified injury of adductor muscle, fascia and tendon of left thigh

       ✓7ᵗʰ S76.209 Unspecified injury of adductor muscle, fascia and tendon of unspecified thigh

    ✓6ᵗʰ S76.21 Strain of adductor muscle, fascia and tendon of thigh

       ✓7ᵗʰ S76.211 Strain of adductor muscle, fascia and tendon of right thigh

       ✓7ᵗʰ S76.212 Strain of adductor muscle, fascia and tendon of left thigh

       ✓7ᵗʰ S76.219 Strain of adductor muscle, fascia and tendon of unspecified thigh

    ✓6ᵗʰ S76.22 Laceration of adductor muscle, fascia and tendon of thigh

       ✓7ᵗʰ S76.221 Laceration of adductor muscle, fascia and tendon of right thigh `CC`

       ✓7ᵗʰ S76.222 Laceration of adductor muscle, fascia and tendon of left thigh `CC`

       ✓7ᵗʰ S76.229 Laceration of adductor muscle, fascia and tendon of unspecified thigh `CC`

    ✓6ᵗʰ S76.29 Other injury of adductor muscle, fascia and tendon of thigh

       ✓7ᵗʰ S76.291 Other injury of adductor muscle, fascia and tendon of right thigh

       ✓7ᵗʰ S76.292 Other injury of adductor muscle, fascia and tendon of left thigh

       ✓7ᵗʰ S76.299 Other injury of adductor muscle, fascia and tendon of unspecified thigh

✓5ᵗʰ S76.3 Injury of muscle, fascia and tendon of the posterior muscle group at thigh level

    ✓6ᵗʰ S76.30 Unspecified injury of muscle, fascia and tendon of the posterior muscle group at thigh level

       ✓7ᵗʰ S76.301 Unspecified injury of muscle, fascia and tendon of the posterior muscle group at thigh level, right thigh

       ✓7ᵗʰ S76.302 Unspecified injury of muscle, fascia and tendon of the posterior muscle group at thigh level, left thigh

       ✓7ᵗʰ S76.309 Unspecified injury of muscle, fascia and tendon of the posterior muscle group at thigh level, unspecified thigh

    ✓6ᵗʰ S76.31 Strain of muscle, fascia and tendon of the posterior muscle group at thigh level

       ✓7ᵗʰ S76.311 Strain of muscle, fascia and tendon of the posterior muscle group at thigh level, right thigh

       ✓7ᵗʰ S76.312 Strain of muscle, fascia and tendon of the posterior muscle group at thigh level, left thigh

       ✓7ᵗʰ S76.319 Strain of muscle, fascia and tendon of the posterior muscle group at thigh level, unspecified thigh

    ✓6ᵗʰ S76.32 Laceration of muscle, fascia and tendon of the posterior muscle group at thigh level

       ✓7ᵗʰ S76.321 Laceration of muscle, fascia and tendon of the posterior muscle group at thigh level, right thigh `CC`

       ✓7ᵗʰ S76.322 Laceration of muscle, fascia and tendon of the posterior muscle group at thigh level, left thigh `CC`

       ✓7ᵗʰ S76.329 Laceration of muscle, fascia and tendon of the posterior muscle group at thigh level, unspecified thigh `CC`

    ✓6ᵗʰ S76.39 Other specified injury of muscle, fascia and tendon of the posterior muscle group at thigh level

       ✓7ᵗʰ S76.391 Other specified injury of muscle, fascia and tendon of the posterior muscle group at thigh level, right thigh

N Newborn: 0   P Pediatric: 0-17   M Maternity: 9-64   A Adult: 15-124   MCC Major Complication/Comorbidity   CC Complication/Comorbidity   SW Severe Wound Dx

1094   ICD-10-CM 2020

√7ᵗʰ **S76.392** Other specified injury of muscle, fascia and tendon of the posterior muscle group at thigh level, left thigh

√7ᵗʰ **S76.399** Other specified injury of muscle, fascia and tendon of the posterior muscle group at thigh level, unspecified thigh

√5ᵗʰ **S76.8** Injury of other specified muscles, fascia and tendons at thigh level

  √6ᵗʰ **S76.80** Unspecified injury of other specified muscles, fascia and tendons at thigh level

    √7ᵗʰ **S76.801** Unspecified injury of other specified muscles, fascia and tendons at thigh level, right thigh

    √7ᵗʰ **S76.802** Unspecified injury of other specified muscles, fascia and tendons at thigh level, left thigh

    √7ᵗʰ **S76.809** Unspecified injury of other specified muscles, fascia and tendons at thigh level, unspecified thigh

  √6ᵗʰ **S76.81** Strain of other specified muscles, fascia and tendons at thigh level

    √7ᵗʰ **S76.811** Strain of other specified muscles, fascia and tendons at thigh level, right thigh

    √7ᵗʰ **S76.812** Strain of other specified muscles, fascia and tendons at thigh level, left thigh

    √7ᵗʰ **S76.819** Strain of other specified muscles, fascia and tendons at thigh level, unspecified thigh

  √6ᵗʰ **S76.82** Laceration of other specified muscles, fascia and tendons at thigh level

    √7ᵗʰ **S76.821** Laceration of other specified muscles, fascia and tendons at thigh level, right thigh   `CC`

    √7ᵗʰ **S76.822** Laceration of other specified muscles, fascia and tendons at thigh level, left thigh   `CC`

    √7ᵗʰ **S76.829** Laceration of other specified muscles, fascia and tendons at thigh level, unspecified thigh   `CC`

  √6ᵗʰ **S76.89** Other injury of other specified muscles, fascia and tendons at thigh level

    √7ᵗʰ **S76.891** Other injury of other specified muscles, fascia and tendons at thigh level, right thigh

    √7ᵗʰ **S76.892** Other injury of other specified muscles, fascia and tendons at thigh level, left thigh

    √7ᵗʰ **S76.899** Other injury of other specified muscles, fascia and tendons at thigh level, unspecified thigh

√5ᵗʰ **S76.9** Injury of unspecified muscles, fascia and tendons at thigh level

  √6ᵗʰ **S76.90** Unspecified injury of unspecified muscles, fascia and tendons at thigh level

    √7ᵗʰ **S76.901** Unspecified injury of unspecified muscles, fascia and tendons at thigh level, right thigh

    √7ᵗʰ **S76.902** Unspecified injury of unspecified muscles, fascia and tendons at thigh level, left thigh

    √7ᵗʰ **S76.909** Unspecified injury of unspecified muscles, fascia and tendons at thigh level, unspecified thigh

  √6ᵗʰ **S76.91** Strain of unspecified muscles, fascia and tendons at thigh level

    √7ᵗʰ **S76.911** Strain of unspecified muscles, fascia and tendons at thigh level, right thigh

    √7ᵗʰ **S76.912** Strain of unspecified muscles, fascia and tendons at thigh level, left thigh

    √7ᵗʰ **S76.919** Strain of unspecified muscles, fascia and tendons at thigh level, unspecified thigh

  √6ᵗʰ **S76.92** Laceration of unspecified muscles, fascia and tendons at thigh level

    √7ᵗʰ **S76.921** Laceration of unspecified muscles, fascia and tendons at thigh level, right thigh   `CC`

    √7ᵗʰ **S76.922** Laceration of unspecified muscles, fascia and tendons at thigh level, left thigh   `CC`

    √7ᵗʰ **S76.929** Laceration of unspecified muscles, fascia and tendons at thigh level, unspecified thigh   `CC`

  √6ᵗʰ **S76.99** Other specified injury of unspecified muscles, fascia and tendons at thigh level

    √7ᵗʰ **S76.991** Other specified injury of unspecified muscles, fascia and tendons at thigh level, right thigh

    √7ᵗʰ **S76.992** Other specified injury of unspecified muscles, fascia and tendons at thigh level, left thigh

    √7ᵗʰ **S76.999** Other specified injury of unspecified muscles, fascia and tendons at thigh level, unspecified thigh

√4ᵗʰ **S77** **Crushing injury of hip and thigh**

Use additional code(s) for all associated injuries

EXCLUDES 2   crushing injury of ankle and foot (S97.-)
crushing injury of lower leg (S87.-)

The appropriate 7th character is to be added to each code from category S77.
A   initial encounter
D   subsequent encounter
S   sequela

√5ᵗʰ **S77.0** Crushing injury of hip

CC Excl: For CC codes in subcategory S77.0: PDX collection 1331

√x7ᵗʰ **S77.00** Crushing injury of unspecified hip   `CC` `H5`

√x7ᵗʰ **S77.01** Crushing injury of right hip   `CC` `H5`

√x7ᵗʰ **S77.02** Crushing injury of left hip   `CC` `H5`

√5ᵗʰ **S77.1** Crushing injury of thigh

CC Excl: For CC codes in subcategory S77.1: PDX collection 1332

√x7ᵗʰ **S77.10** Crushing injury of unspecified thigh   `CC` `H5`

√x7ᵗʰ **S77.11** Crushing injury of right thigh   `CC` `H5`

√x7ᵗʰ **S77.12** Crushing injury of left thigh   `CC` `H5`

√5ᵗʰ **S77.2** Crushing injury of hip with thigh

√x7ᵗʰ **S77.20** Crushing injury of unspecified hip with thigh

√x7ᵗʰ **S77.21** Crushing injury of right hip with thigh

√x7ᵗʰ **S77.22** Crushing injury of left hip with thigh

√4ᵗʰ **S78** **Traumatic amputation of hip and thigh**

An amputation not identified as partial or complete should be coded to complete

EXCLUDES 1   traumatic amputation of knee (S88.0-)

The appropriate 7th character is to be added to each code from category S78.
A   initial encounter
D   subsequent encounter
S   sequela

CC Excl: For CC codes in category S78:
Right side: PDX collection 1333
Left side: PDX collection 1334
Unspecified side: PDX collection 1335

√5ᵗʰ **S78.0** Traumatic amputation at hip joint

  √6ᵗʰ **S78.01** Complete traumatic amputation at hip joint

    √7ᵗʰ **S78.011** Complete traumatic amputation at right hip joint   `CC` `HCC`

    √7ᵗʰ **S78.012** Complete traumatic amputation at left hip joint   `CC` `HCC`

    √7ᵗʰ **S78.019** Complete traumatic amputation at unspecified hip joint   `CC` `HCC`

  √6ᵗʰ **S78.02** Partial traumatic amputation at hip joint

    √7ᵗʰ **S78.021** Partial traumatic amputation at right hip joint   `CC` `HCC`

    √7ᵗʰ **S78.022** Partial traumatic amputation at left hip joint   `CC` `HCC`

    √7ᵗʰ **S78.029** Partial traumatic amputation at unspecified hip joint   `CC` `HCC`

☑ Additional Character Required   √x7ᵗʰ Placeholder   Unacceptable PDx   Questionable PDx   Manifestation   Unspecified Dx   H1-H14 HAC   HCC CMS-HCC Dx   HIV HIV Dx

ICD-10-CM 2020   1095

✓5ᵗʰ S78.1   Traumatic amputation at level between hip and knee

     EXCLUDES 1   *traumatic amputation of knee (S88.0-)*

   ✓6ᵗʰ S78.11   Complete traumatic amputation at level between hip and knee

     ✓7ᵗʰ S78.111   Complete traumatic amputation at level between right hip and knee   `CC` `HCC`

     ✓7ᵗʰ S78.112   Complete traumatic amputation at level between left hip and knee   `CC` `HCC`

     ✓7ᵗʰ S78.119   Complete traumatic amputation at level between unspecified hip and knee   `CC` `HCC`

   ✓6ᵗʰ S78.12   Partial traumatic amputation at level between hip and knee

     ✓7ᵗʰ S78.121   Partial traumatic amputation at level between right hip and knee   `CC` `HCC`

     ✓7ᵗʰ S78.122   Partial traumatic amputation at level between left hip and knee   `CC` `HCC`

     ✓7ᵗʰ S78.129   Partial traumatic amputation at level between unspecified hip and knee   `CC` `HCC`

✓5ᵗʰ S78.9   Traumatic amputation of hip and thigh, level unspecified

   ✓6ᵗʰ S78.91   Complete traumatic amputation of hip and thigh, level unspecified

     ✓7ᵗʰ S78.911   Complete traumatic amputation of right hip and thigh, level unspecified   `CC` `HCC`

     ✓7ᵗʰ S78.912   Complete traumatic amputation of left hip and thigh, level unspecified   `CC` `HCC`

     ✓7ᵗʰ S78.919   Complete traumatic amputation of unspecified hip and thigh, level unspecified   `CC` `HCC`

   ✓6ᵗʰ S78.92   Partial traumatic amputation of hip and thigh, level unspecified

     ✓7ᵗʰ S78.921   Partial traumatic amputation of right hip and thigh, level unspecified   `CC` `HCC`

     ✓7ᵗʰ S78.922   Partial traumatic amputation of left hip and thigh, level unspecified   `CC` `HCC`

     ✓7ᵗʰ S78.929   Partial traumatic amputation of unspecified hip and thigh, level unspecified   `CC` `HCC`

✓4ᵗʰ S79   Other and unspecified injuries of hip and thigh

   NOTE   A fracture not indicated as open or closed should be coded to closed

AHA: 2018,2Q,12; 2018,1Q,3; 2015,3Q,37-39

The appropriate 7th character is to be added to each code from subcategories S79.0 and S79.1.

A   initial encounter for closed fracture
D   subsequent encounter for fracture with routine healing
G   subsequent encounter for fracture with delayed healing
K   subsequent encounter for fracture with nonunion
P   subsequent encounter for fracture with malunion
S   sequela

✓5ᵗʰ S79.0   Physeal fracture of upper end of femur

     EXCLUDES 1   *apophyseal fracture of upper end of femur (S72.13-)*
           nontraumatic slipped upper femoral epiphysis (M93.0-)

   CC Excl: For CC/MCC codes in subcategory S79.0:
   Right side: See code S79.001
   Left side: See code S79.002
   Unspecified side: See code S79.009

   ✓6ᵗʰ S79.00   Unspecified physeal fracture of upper end of femur

     4,6 **✓7ᵗʰ S79.001   Unspecified physeal fracture of upper end of right femur**   `MCC` `CC` `H5` `HCC`
         CC Excl: MCC with 7th character A: PDX collection 1297
         CC Excl: CC with 7th character K or P: PDX collection 897

     4,6 **✓7ᵗʰ S79.002   Unspecified physeal fracture of upper end of left femur**   `MCC` `CC` `H5` `HCC`
         CC Excl: MCC with 7th character A: PDX collection 1299
         CC Excl: CC with 7th character K or P: PDX collection 897

     4,6 **✓7ᵗʰ S79.009   Unspecified physeal fracture of upper end of unspecified femur**   `MCC` `CC` `H5` `HCC`
         CC Excl: MCC with 7th character A: PDX collection 1298
         CC Excl: CC with 7th character K or P: PDX collection 897

   ✓6ᵗʰ S79.01   Salter-Harris Type I physeal fracture of upper end of femur

     Acute on chronic slipped capital femoral epiphysis (traumatic)
     Acute slipped capital femoral epiphysis (traumatic)
     Capital femoral epiphyseal fracture
     EXCLUDES 1   *chronic slipped upper femoral epiphysis (nontraumatic) (M93.02-)*

     4,6 **✓7ᵗʰ S79.011   Salter-Harris Type I physeal fracture of upper end of right femur**   `MCC` `CC` `H5` `HCC`

     4,6 **✓7ᵗʰ S79.012   Salter-Harris Type I physeal fracture of upper end of left femur**   `MCC` `CC` `H5` `HCC`

     4,6 **✓7ᵗʰ S79.019   Salter-Harris Type I physeal fracture of upper end of unspecified femur**   `MCC` `CC` `H5` `HCC`

   ✓6ᵗʰ S79.09   Other physeal fracture of upper end of femur

     4,6 **✓7ᵗʰ S79.091   Other physeal fracture of upper end of right femur**   `MCC` `CC` `H5` `HCC`

     4,6 **✓7ᵗʰ S79.092   Other physeal fracture of upper end of left femur**   `MCC` `CC` `H5` `HCC`

     4,6 **✓7ᵗʰ S79.099   Other physeal fracture of upper end of unspecified femur**   `MCC` `CC` `H5` `HCC`

N Newborn: 0   **P** Pediatric: 0-17   **M** Maternity: 9-64   **A** Adult: 15-124   `MCC` Major Complication/Comorbidity   `CC` Complication/Comorbidity   `SW` Severe Wound Dx

1096   ICD-10-CM 2020

√5ᵗʰ S79.1 Physeal fracture of lower end of femur

> **CC Excl: For CC/MCC codes in subcategory S79.1:**
> **Right side:** See code S79.101
> **Left side:** See code S79.102
> **Unspecified side:** See code S79.109

    √6ᵗʰ S79.10 Unspecified physeal fracture of lower end of femur

       3,6 √7ᵗʰ S79.101 Unspecified physeal fracture of lower end of right femur   `CC` `H5` `HCC`

> **CC Excl: CC with 7th character A:** PDX collection 1300
> **CC Excl: CC with 7th character K or P:** PDX collection 897

       3,6 √7ᵗʰ S79.102 Unspecified physeal fracture of lower end of left femur   `CC` `H5` `HCC`

> **CC Excl: CC with 7th character A:** PDX collection 1302
> **CC Excl: CC with 7th character K or P:** PDX collection 897

       3,6 √7ᵗʰ S79.109 Unspecified physeal fracture of lower end of unspecified femur   `CC` `H5` `HCC`

> **CC Excl: CC with 7th character A:** PDX collection 1301
> **CC Excl: CC with 7th character K or P:** PDX collection 897

    √6ᵗʰ S79.11 Salter-Harris Type I physeal fracture of lower end of femur

       3,6 √7ᵗʰ S79.111 Salter-Harris Type I physeal fracture of lower end of right femur   `CC` `H5` `HCC`

       3,6 √7ᵗʰ S79.112 Salter-Harris Type I physeal fracture of lower end of left femur   `CC` `H5` `HCC`

       3,6 √7ᵗʰ S79.119 Salter-Harris Type I physeal fracture of lower end of unspecified femur   `CC` `H5` `HCC`

    √6ᵗʰ S79.12 Salter-Harris Type II physeal fracture of lower end of femur

       3,6 √7ᵗʰ S79.121 Salter-Harris Type II physeal fracture of lower end of right femur   `CC` `H5` `HCC`

       3,6 √7ᵗʰ S79.122 Salter-Harris Type II physeal fracture of lower end of left femur   `CC` `H5` `HCC`

       3,6 √7ᵗʰ S79.129 Salter-Harris Type II physeal fracture of lower end of unspecified femur   `CC` `H5` `HCC`

    √6ᵗʰ S79.13 Salter-Harris Type III physeal fracture of lower end of femur

       3,6 √7ᵗʰ S79.131 Salter-Harris Type III physeal fracture of lower end of right femur   `CC` `H5` `HCC`

       3,6 √7ᵗʰ S79.132 Salter-Harris Type III physeal fracture of lower end of left femur   `CC` `H5` `HCC`

       3,6 √7ᵗʰ S79.139 Salter-Harris Type III physeal fracture of lower end of unspecified femur   `CC` `H5` `HCC`

    √6ᵗʰ S79.14 Salter-Harris Type IV physeal fracture of lower end of femur

       3,6 √7ᵗʰ S79.141 Salter-Harris Type IV physeal fracture of lower end of right femur   `CC` `H5` `HCC`

       3,6 √7ᵗʰ S79.142 Salter-Harris Type IV physeal fracture of lower end of left femur   `CC` `H5` `HCC`

       3,6 √7ᵗʰ S79.149 Salter-Harris Type IV physeal fracture of lower end of unspecified femur   `CC` `H5` `HCC`

    √6ᵗʰ S79.19 Other physeal fracture of lower end of femur

       3,6 √7ᵗʰ S79.191 Other physeal fracture of lower end of right femur   `CC` `H5` `HCC`

       3,6 √7ᵗʰ S79.192 Other physeal fracture of lower end of left femur   `CC` `H5` `HCC`

       3,6 √7ᵗʰ S79.199 Other physeal fracture of lower end of unspecified femur   `CC` `H5` `HCC`

√5ᵗʰ S79.8 Other specified injuries of hip and thigh

> The appropriate 7th character is to be added to each code in subcategory S79.8.
> A   initial encounter
> D   subsequent encounter
> S   sequela

    √6ᵗʰ S79.81 Other specified injuries of hip

       √7ᵗʰ S79.811 Other specified injuries of right hip

       √7ᵗʰ S79.812 Other specified injuries of left hip

       √7ᵗʰ S79.819 Other specified injuries of unspecified hip

    √6ᵗʰ S79.82 Other specified injuries of thigh

       √7ᵗʰ S79.821 Other specified injuries of right thigh

       √7ᵗʰ S79.822 Other specified injuries of left thigh

       √7ᵗʰ S79.829 Other specified injuries of unspecified thigh

√5ᵗʰ S79.9 Unspecified injury of hip and thigh

> The appropriate 7th character is to be added to each code in subcategory S79.9.
> A   initial encounter
> D   subsequent encounter
> S   sequela

    √6ᵗʰ S79.91 Unspecified injury of hip

       √7ᵗʰ S79.911 Unspecified injury of right hip

       √7ᵗʰ S79.912 Unspecified injury of left hip

       √7ᵗʰ S79.919 Unspecified injury of unspecified hip

    √6ᵗʰ S79.92 Unspecified injury of thigh

       √7ᵗʰ S79.921 Unspecified injury of right thigh

       √7ᵗʰ S79.922 Unspecified injury of left thigh

       √7ᵗʰ S79.929 Unspecified injury of unspecified thigh

Injuries to the knee and lower leg (S80-S89)

EXCLUDES 2	burns and corrosions (T20-T32)
	frostbite (T33-T34)
	injuries of ankle and foot, except fracture of ankle and malleolus (S90-S99)
	insect bite or sting, venomous (T63.4)

√4ᵗʰ S80 Superficial injury of knee and lower leg

> **EXCLUDES 2**   superficial injury of ankle and foot (S90.-)

> The appropriate 7th character is to be added to each code from category S80.
> A   initial encounter
> D   subsequent encounter
> S   sequela

  √5ᵗʰ S80.0 Contusion of knee

    √x7ᵗʰ S80.00 Contusion of unspecified knee

    √x7ᵗʰ S80.01 Contusion of right knee

    √x7ᵗʰ S80.02 Contusion of left knee

  √5ᵗʰ S80.1 Contusion of lower leg

    √x7ᵗʰ S80.10 Contusion of unspecified lower leg

    √x7ᵗʰ S80.11 Contusion of right lower leg

    √x7ᵗʰ S80.12 Contusion of left lower leg

  √5ᵗʰ S80.2 Other superficial injuries of knee

    √6ᵗʰ S80.21 Abrasion of knee

       √7ᵗʰ S80.211 Abrasion, right knee

       √7ᵗʰ S80.212 Abrasion, left knee

       √7ᵗʰ S80.219 Abrasion, unspecified knee

    √6ᵗʰ S80.22 Blister (nonthermal) of knee

       √7ᵗʰ S80.221 Blister (nonthermal), right knee

       √7ᵗʰ S80.222 Blister (nonthermal), left knee

       √7ᵗʰ S80.229 Blister (nonthermal), unspecified knee

    √6ᵗʰ S80.24 External constriction of knee

       √7ᵗʰ S80.241 External constriction, right knee

       √7ᵗʰ S80.242 External constriction, left knee

       √7ᵗʰ S80.249 External constriction, unspecified knee

    √6ᵗʰ S80.25 Superficial foreign body of knee

       Splinter in the knee

       √7ᵗʰ S80.251 Superficial foreign body, right knee

       √7ᵗʰ S80.252 Superficial foreign body, left knee

✔ Additional Character Required   √x7ᵗʰ Placeholder   Unacceptable PDx   Questionable PDx   Manifestation   Unspecified Dx   H1-H14 HAC   HCC CMS-HCC Dx   HIV HIV Dx

ICD-10-CM 2020   1097

√7ᵗʰ **S80.259** Superficial foreign body, unspecified knee

√6ᵗʰ **S80.26** Insect bite (nonvenomous) of knee

     √7ᵗʰ **S80.261** Insect bite (nonvenomous), right knee

     √7ᵗʰ **S80.262** Insect bite (nonvenomous), left knee

     √7ᵗʰ **S80.269** Insect bite (nonvenomous), unspecified knee

√6ᵗʰ **S80.27** Other superficial bite of knee

     EXCLUDES 1   *open bite of knee (S81.05-)*

     √7ᵗʰ **S80.271** Other superficial bite of right knee

     √7ᵗʰ **S80.272** Other superficial bite of left knee

     √7ᵗʰ **S80.279** Other superficial bite of unspecified knee

√5ᵗʰ **S80.8** Other superficial injuries of lower leg

   √6ᵗʰ **S80.81** Abrasion of lower leg

     √7ᵗʰ **S80.811** Abrasion, right lower leg

     √7ᵗʰ **S80.812** Abrasion, left lower leg

     √7ᵗʰ **S80.819** Abrasion, unspecified lower leg

   √6ᵗʰ **S80.82** Blister (nonthermal) of lower leg

     √7ᵗʰ **S80.821** Blister (nonthermal), right lower leg

     √7ᵗʰ **S80.822** Blister (nonthermal), left lower leg

     √7ᵗʰ **S80.829** Blister (nonthermal), unspecified lower leg

   √6ᵗʰ **S80.84** External constriction of lower leg

     √7ᵗʰ **S80.841** External constriction, right lower leg

     √7ᵗʰ **S80.842** External constriction, left lower leg

     √7ᵗʰ **S80.849** External constriction, unspecified lower leg

   √6ᵗʰ **S80.85** Superficial foreign body of lower leg

     Splinter in the lower leg

     √7ᵗʰ **S80.851** Superficial foreign body, right lower leg

     √7ᵗʰ **S80.852** Superficial foreign body, left lower leg

     √7ᵗʰ **S80.859** Superficial foreign body, unspecified lower leg

   √6ᵗʰ **S80.86** Insect bite (nonvenomous) of lower leg

     √7ᵗʰ **S80.861** Insect bite (nonvenomous), right lower leg

     √7ᵗʰ **S80.862** Insect bite (nonvenomous), left lower leg

     √7ᵗʰ **S80.869** Insect bite (nonvenomous), unspecified lower leg

   √6ᵗʰ **S80.87** Other superficial bite of lower leg

     EXCLUDES 1   *open bite of lower leg (S81.85-)*

     √7ᵗʰ **S80.871** Other superficial bite, right lower leg

     √7ᵗʰ **S80.872** Other superficial bite, left lower leg

     √7ᵗʰ **S80.879** Other superficial bite, unspecified lower leg

√5ᵗʰ **S80.9** Unspecified superficial injury of knee and lower leg

   √6ᵗʰ **S80.91** Unspecified superficial injury of knee

     √7ᵗʰ **S80.911** Unspecified superficial injury of right knee

     √7ᵗʰ **S80.912** Unspecified superficial injury of left knee

     √7ᵗʰ **S80.919** Unspecified superficial injury of unspecified knee

   √6ᵗʰ **S80.92** Unspecified superficial injury of lower leg

     √7ᵗʰ **S80.921** Unspecified superficial injury of right lower leg

     √7ᵗʰ **S80.922** Unspecified superficial injury of left lower leg

     √7ᵗʰ **S80.929** Unspecified superficial injury of unspecified lower leg

√4ᵗʰ **S81** Open wound of knee and lower leg

   Code also any associated wound infection

   EXCLUDES 1   *open fracture of knee and lower leg (S82.-)*

           traumatic amputation of lower leg (S88.-)

   EXCLUDES 2   *open wound of ankle and foot (S91.-)*

   The appropriate 7th character is to be added to each code from category S81.

   A   initial encounter

   D   subsequent encounter

   S   sequela

√5ᵗʰ **S81.0** Open wound of knee

   √6ᵗʰ **S81.00** Unspecified open wound of knee

     √7ᵗʰ **S81.001** Unspecified open wound, right knee

√7ᵗʰ **S81.002** Unspecified open wound, left knee

√7ᵗʰ **S81.009** Unspecified open wound, unspecified knee

√6ᵗʰ **S81.01** Laceration without foreign body of knee

     √7ᵗʰ **S81.011** Laceration without foreign body, right knee

     √7ᵗʰ **S81.012** Laceration without foreign body, left knee

     √7ᵗʰ **S81.019** Laceration without foreign body, unspecified knee

√6ᵗʰ **S81.02** Laceration with foreign body of knee

     √7ᵗʰ **S81.021** Laceration with foreign body, right knee

     √7ᵗʰ **S81.022** Laceration with foreign body, left knee

     √7ᵗʰ **S81.029** Laceration with foreign body, unspecified knee

√6ᵗʰ **S81.03** Puncture wound without foreign body of knee

     √7ᵗʰ **S81.031** Puncture wound without foreign body, right knee

     √7ᵗʰ **S81.032** Puncture wound without foreign body, left knee

     √7ᵗʰ **S81.039** Puncture wound without foreign body, unspecified knee

√6ᵗʰ **S81.04** Puncture wound with foreign body of knee

     √7ᵗʰ **S81.041** Puncture wound with foreign body, right knee

     √7ᵗʰ **S81.042** Puncture wound with foreign body, left knee

     √7ᵗʰ **S81.049** Puncture wound with foreign body, unspecified knee

√6ᵗʰ **S81.05** Open bite of knee

     Bite of knee NOS

     EXCLUDES 1   *superficial bite of knee (S80.27-)*

     √7ᵗʰ **S81.051** Open bite, right knee

     √7ᵗʰ **S81.052** Open bite, left knee

     √7ᵗʰ **S81.059** Open bite, unspecified knee

√5ᵗʰ **S81.8** Open wound of lower leg

   √6ᵗʰ **S81.80** Unspecified open wound of lower leg

     AHA: 2016,3Q,24

     √7ᵗʰ **S81.801** Unspecified open wound, right lower leg

     √7ᵗʰ **S81.802** Unspecified open wound, left lower leg

     √7ᵗʰ **S81.809** Unspecified open wound, unspecified lower leg

   √6ᵗʰ **S81.81** Laceration without foreign body of lower leg

     √7ᵗʰ **S81.811** Laceration without foreign body, right lower leg

     √7ᵗʰ **S81.812** Laceration without foreign body, left lower leg

     √7ᵗʰ **S81.819** Laceration without foreign body, unspecified lower leg

   √6ᵗʰ **S81.82** Laceration with foreign body of lower leg

     √7ᵗʰ **S81.821** Laceration with foreign body, right lower leg

     √7ᵗʰ **S81.822** Laceration with foreign body, left lower leg

     √7ᵗʰ **S81.829** Laceration with foreign body, unspecified lower leg

   √6ᵗʰ **S81.83** Puncture wound without foreign body of lower leg

     AHA: 2016,3Q,24

     √7ᵗʰ **S81.831** Puncture wound without foreign body, right lower leg

     √7ᵗʰ **S81.832** Puncture wound without foreign body, left lower leg

     √7ᵗʰ **S81.839** Puncture wound without foreign body, unspecified lower leg

   √6ᵗʰ **S81.84** Puncture wound with foreign body of lower leg

     AHA: 2016,3Q,24

     √7ᵗʰ **S81.841** Puncture wound with foreign body, right lower leg

     √7ᵗʰ **S81.842** Puncture wound with foreign body, left lower leg

     √7ᵗʰ **S81.849** Puncture wound with foreign body, unspecified lower leg

   √6ᵗʰ **S81.85** Open bite of lower leg

     Bite of lower leg NOS

     EXCLUDES 1   *superficial bite of lower leg (S80.86-, S80.87-)*

     √7ᵗʰ **S81.851** Open bite, right lower leg

N Newborn: 0   P Pediatric: 0-17   M Maternity: 9-64   A Adult: 15-124   **MCC** Major Complication/Comorbidity   **CC** Complication/Comorbidity   **SW** Severe Wound Dx

1098   ICD-10-CM 2020

√7ʰ **S81.852** Open bite, **left lower leg**

√7ʰ **S81.859** Open bite, **unspecified lower leg**

√4ʰ **S82 Fracture of lower leg, including ankle**

> **NOTE** A fracture not indicated as displaced or nondisplaced should be coded to displaced
>
> A fracture not indicated as open or closed should be coded to closed
>
> The open fracture designations are based on the Gustilo open fracture classification.

INCLUDES fracture of malleolus

EXCLUDES 1 *traumatic amputation of lower leg (S88.-)*

EXCLUDES 2 *fracture of foot, except ankle (S92.-)*

periprosthetic fracture of prosthetic implant of knee (M97.0-)

AHA: 2018,2Q,12; 2016,1Q,33; 2015,3Q,37-39

DEF: Diaphysis: Central shaft of a long bone.

DEF: Epiphysis: Proximal and distal rounded ends of a long bone, communicates with the joint.

DEF: Metaphysis: Section of a long bone located between the epiphysis and diaphysis at the proximal and distal ends.

DEF: Physis (growth plate): Narrow zone of cartilaginous tissue between the epiphysis and metaphysis at each end of a long bone. In childhood, proliferation of cells in this zone lengthens the bone. As the bone matures, this area thins, ossification eventually fusing into solid bone and growth stops. *Synonyms: Epiphyseal plate.*

> The appropriate 7th character is to be added to all codes from category S82 [unless otherwise indicated].
>
> A   initial encounter for closed fracture
>
> B   initial encounter for open fracture type I or II
>
>   initial encounter for open fracture NOS
>
> C   initial encounter for open fracture type IIIA, IIIB, or IIIC
>
> D   subsequent encounter for closed fracture with routine healing
>
> E   subsequent encounter for open fracture type I or II with routine healing
>
> F   subsequent encounter for open fracture type IIIA, IIIB, or IIIC with routine healing
>
> G   subsequent encounter for closed fracture with delayed healing
>
> H   subsequent encounter for open fracture type I or II with delayed healing
>
> J   subsequent encounter for open fracture type IIIA, IIIB, or IIIC with delayed healing
>
> K   subsequent encounter for closed fracture with nonunion
>
> M   subsequent encounter for open fracture type I or II with nonunion
>
> N   subsequent encounter for open fracture type IIIA, IIIB, or IIIC with nonunion
>
> P   subsequent encounter for closed fracture with malunion
>
> Q   subsequent encounter for open fracture type I or II with malunion
>
> R   subsequent encounter for open fracture type IIIA, IIIB, or IIIC with malunion
>
> S   sequela

√5ʰ **S82.0 Fracture of patella**

Knee cap

CC Excl: For CC codes in subcategory S82.0:
Right side: See code S82.001
Left side: See code S82.002
Unspecified side: See code S82.009

√6ʰ **S82.00 Unspecified fracture of patella**

3 √7ʰ **S82.001 Unspecified fracture of right patella** CC H5

> CC Excl: CC with 7th character A: PDX collection 1336
> CC Excl: CC with 7th character B or C: PDX collection 1337
> CC Excl: CC with 7th character K, M, N, P, Q, or R: PDX collection 897

3 √7ʰ **S82.002 Unspecified fracture of left patella** CC H5

> CC Excl: CC with 7th character A: PDX collection 1338
> CC Excl: CC with 7th character B or C: PDX collection 1337
> CC Excl: CC with 7th character K, M, N, P, Q, or R: PDX collection 897

3 √7ʰ **S82.009 Unspecified fracture of unspecified patella** CC H5

> CC Excl: CC with 7th character A: PDX collection 1339
> CC Excl: CC with 7th character B or C: PDX collection 1337
> CC Excl: CC with 7th character K, M, N, P, Q, or R: PDX collection 897

√6ʰ **S82.01 Osteochondral fracture of patella**

3 √7ʰ **S82.011 Displaced osteochondral fracture of right patella** CC H5

3 √7ʰ **S82.012 Displaced osteochondral fracture of left patella** CC H5

3 √7ʰ **S82.013 Displaced osteochondral fracture of unspecified patella** CC H5

3 √7ʰ **S82.014 Nondisplaced osteochondral fracture of right patella** CC H5

3 √7ʰ **S82.015 Nondisplaced osteochondral fracture of left patella** CC H5

3 √7ʰ **S82.016 Nondisplaced osteochondral fracture of unspecified patella** CC H5

√6ʰ **S82.02 Longitudinal fracture of patella**

3 √7ʰ **S82.021 Displaced longitudinal fracture of right patella** CC H5

3 √7ʰ **S82.022 Displaced longitudinal fracture of left patella** CC H5

3 √7ʰ **S82.023 Displaced longitudinal fracture of unspecified patella** CC H5

3 √7ʰ **S82.024 Nondisplaced longitudinal fracture of right patella** CC H5

3 √7ʰ **S82.025 Nondisplaced longitudinal fracture of left patella** CC H5

3 √7ʰ **S82.026 Nondisplaced longitudinal fracture of unspecified patella** CC H5

√6ʰ **S82.03 Transverse fracture of patella**

3 √7ʰ **S82.031 Displaced transverse fracture of right patella** CC H5

3 √7ʰ **S82.032 Displaced transverse fracture of left patella** CC H5

3 √7ʰ **S82.033 Displaced transverse fracture of unspecified patella** CC H5

3 √7ʰ **S82.034 Nondisplaced transverse fracture of right patella** CC H5

3 √7ʰ **S82.035 Nondisplaced transverse fracture of left patella** CC H5

3 √7ʰ **S82.036 Nondisplaced transverse fracture of unspecified patella** CC H5

√6ʰ **S82.04 Comminuted fracture of patella**

3 √7ʰ **S82.041 Displaced comminuted fracture of right patella** CC H5

3 √7ʰ **S82.042 Displaced comminuted fracture of left patella** CC H5

3 √7ʰ **S82.043 Displaced comminuted fracture of unspecified patella** CC H5

3 √7ʰ **S82.044 Nondisplaced comminuted fracture of right patella** CC H5

3 √7ʰ **S82.045 Nondisplaced comminuted fracture of left patella** CC H5

3 √7ʰ **S82.046 Nondisplaced comminuted fracture of unspecified patella** CC H5

√6ʰ **S82.09 Other fracture of patella**

3 √7ʰ **S82.091 Other fracture of right patella** CC H5

3 √7ʰ **S82.092 Other fracture of left patella** CC H5

3 √7ʰ **S82.099 Other fracture of unspecified patella** CC H5

☑ Additional Character Required   √x7ʰ Placeholder   Unacceptable PDx   Questionable PDx   Manifestation   Unspecified Dx   H1–H14 HAC   HCC CMS-HCC Dx   HIV HIV Dx

ICD-10-CM 2020   **1099**

√5th **S82.1 Fracture of upper end of tibia**

Fracture of proximal end of tibia

EXCLUDES 2 *fracture of shaft of tibia (S82.2-)*

physeal fracture of upper end of tibia (S89.0-)

CC Excl: For CC/MCC codes in subcategory S82.1:
Right side: See code S82.101
Left side: See code S82.102
Unspecified side: See code S82.109

√6th **S82.10 Unspecified fracture of upper end of tibia**

2,3 √7th **S82.101 Unspecified fracture of upper end of right tibia** `MCC` `CC` `H5`

CC Excl: CC with 7th character A: PDX collection 1340
CC Excl: MCC with 7th character B or C: PDX collection 1341
CC Excl: CC with 7th character K, M, N, P, Q, or R: PDX collection 897

2,3 √7th **S82.102 Unspecified fracture of upper end of left tibia** `MCC` `CC` `H5`

CC Excl: CC with 7th character A: PDX collection 1342
CC Excl: MCC with 7th character B or C: PDX collection 1341
CC Excl: CC with 7th character K, M, N, P, Q, or R: PDX collection 897

2,3 √7th **S82.109 Unspecified fracture of upper end of unspecified tibia** `MCC` `CC` `H5`

CC Excl: CC or MCC with 7th character A, B, or C: PDX collection 1341
CC Excl: CC with 7th character K, M, N, P, Q, or R: PDX collection 897

√6th **S82.11 Fracture of tibial spine**

2,3 √7th **S82.111 Displaced fracture of right tibial spine** `MCC` `CC` `H5`

2,3 √7th **S82.112 Displaced fracture of left tibial spine** `MCC` `CC` `H5`

2,3 √7th **S82.113 Displaced fracture of unspecified tibial spine** `MCC` `CC` `H5`

2,3 √7th **S82.114 Nondisplaced fracture of right tibial spine** `MCC` `CC` `H5`

2,3 √7th **S82.115 Nondisplaced fracture of left tibial spine** `MCC` `CC` `H5`

2,3 √7th **S82.116 Nondisplaced fracture of unspecified tibial spine** `MCC` `CC` `H5`

√6th **S82.12 Fracture of lateral condyle of tibia**

2,3 √7th **S82.121 Displaced fracture of lateral condyle of right tibia** `MCC` `CC` `H5`

2,3 √7th **S82.122 Displaced fracture of lateral condyle of left tibia** `MCC` `CC` `H5`

2,3 √7th **S82.123 Displaced fracture of lateral condyle of unspecified tibia** `MCC` `CC` `H5`

2,3 √7th **S82.124 Nondisplaced fracture of lateral condyle of right tibia** `MCC` `CC` `H5`

2,3 √7th **S82.125 Nondisplaced fracture of lateral condyle of left tibia** `MCC` `CC` `H5`

2,3 √7th **S82.126 Nondisplaced fracture of lateral condyle of unspecified tibia** `MCC` `CC` `H5`

√6th **S82.13 Fracture of medial condyle of tibia**

2,3 √7th **S82.131 Displaced fracture of medial condyle of right tibia** `MCC` `CC` `H5`

2,3 √7th **S82.132 Displaced fracture of medial condyle of left tibia** `MCC` `CC` `H5`

2,3 √7th **S82.133 Displaced fracture of medial condyle of unspecified tibia** `MCC` `CC` `H5`

2,3 √7th **S82.134 Nondisplaced fracture of medial condyle of right tibia** `MCC` `CC` `H5`

2,3 √7th **S82.135 Nondisplaced fracture of medial condyle of left tibia** `MCC` `CC` `H5`

2,3 √7th **S82.136 Nondisplaced fracture of medial condyle of unspecified tibia** `MCC` `CC` `H5`

√6th **S82.14 Bicondylar fracture of tibia**

Fracture of tibial plateau NOS

2,3 √7th **S82.141 Displaced bicondylar fracture of right tibia** `MCC` `CC` `H5`

2,3 √7th **S82.142 Displaced bicondylar fracture of left tibia** `MCC` `CC` `H5`

2,3 √7th **S82.143 Displaced bicondylar fracture of unspecified tibia** `MCC` `CC` `H5`

2,3 √7th **S82.144 Nondisplaced bicondylar fracture of right tibia** `MCC` `CC` `H5`

2,3 √7th **S82.145 Nondisplaced bicondylar fracture of left tibia** `MCC` `CC` `H5`

2,3 √7th **S82.146 Nondisplaced bicondylar fracture of unspecified tibia** `MCC` `CC` `H5`

√6th **S82.15 Fracture of tibial tuberosity**

2,3 √7th **S82.151 Displaced fracture of right tibial tuberosity** `MCC` `CC` `H5`

2,3 √7th **S82.152 Displaced fracture of left tibial tuberosity** `MCC` `CC` `H5`

2,3 √7th **S82.153 Displaced fracture of unspecified tibial tuberosity** `MCC` `CC` `H5`

2,3 √7th **S82.154 Nondisplaced fracture of right tibial tuberosity** `MCC` `CC` `H5`

2,3 √7th **S82.155 Nondisplaced fracture of left tibial tuberosity** `MCC` `CC` `H5`

2,3 √7th **S82.156 Nondisplaced fracture of unspecified tibial tuberosity** `MCC` `CC` `H5`

√6th **S82.16 Torus fracture of upper end of tibia**

The appropriate 7th character is to be added to all codes in subcategory S82.16.
A initial encounter for closed fracture
D subsequent encounter for fracture with routine healing
G subsequent encounter for fracture with delayed healing
K subsequent encounter for fracture with nonunion
P subsequent encounter for fracture with malunion
S sequela

3 √7th **S82.161 Torus fracture of upper end of right tibia** `CC` `H5`

CC Excl: CC with 7th character A: PDX collection 1343
CC Excl: CC with 7th character K or P: PDX collection 897

3 √7th **S82.162 Torus fracture of upper end of left tibia** `CC` `H5`

CC Excl: CC with 7th character A: PDX collection 1344
CC Excl: CC with 7th character K or P: PDX collection 897

3 √7th **S82.169 Torus fracture of upper end of unspecified tibia** `CC` `H5`

CC Excl: CC with 7th character A: PDX collection 1345
CC Excl: CC with 7th character K or P: PDX collection 897

√6th **S82.19 Other fracture of upper end of tibia**

2,3 √7th **S82.191 Other fracture of upper end of right tibia** `MCC` `CC` `H5`

2,3 √7th **S82.192 Other fracture of upper end of left tibia** `MCC` `CC` `H5`

2,3 √7th **S82.199 Other fracture of upper end of unspecified tibia** `MCC` `CC` `H5`

`N` Newborn: 0   `P` Pediatric: 0-17   `M` Maternity: 9-64   `A` Adult: 15-124   `MCC` Major Complication/Comorbidity   `CC` Complication/Comorbidity   `SW` Severe Wound Dx

√5ᵗʰ **S82.2   Fracture of shaft of tibia**

CC Excl: For CC/MCC codes in subcategory S82.2:
Right side: See code S82.101
Left side: See code S82.102
Unspecified side: See code S82.109

√6ᵗʰ **S82.20   Unspecified fracture of shaft of tibia**
Fracture of tibia NOS

2,3 √7ᵗʰ **S82.201   Unspecified fracture of shaft of right tibia**   MCC CC H5
CC Excl: CC with 7th character A: PDX collection 1346
CC Excl: MCC with 7th character B or C: PDX collection 1341
CC Excl: CC with 7th character K, M, N, P, Q, or R: PDX collection 897

2,3 √7ᵗʰ **S82.202   Unspecified fracture of shaft of left tibia**   MCC CC H5
CC Excl: CC with 7th character A: PDX collection 1342
CC Excl: MCC with 7th character B or C: PDX collection 1341
CC Excl: CC with 7th character K, M, N, P, Q, or R: PDX collection 897

2,3 √7ᵗʰ **S82.209   Unspecified fracture of shaft of unspecified tibia**   MCC CC H5
CC Excl: CC or MCC with 7th character A, B, or C: PDX collection 1341
CC Excl: CC with 7th character K, M, N, P, Q, or R: PDX collection 897

√6ᵗʰ **S82.22   Transverse fracture of shaft of tibia**

2,3 √7ᵗʰ **S82.221   Displaced transverse fracture of shaft of right tibia**   MCC CC H5

2,3 √7ᵗʰ **S82.222   Displaced transverse fracture of shaft of left tibia**   MCC CC H5

2,3 √7ᵗʰ **S82.223   Displaced transverse fracture of shaft of unspecified tibia**   MCC CC H5

2,3 √7ᵗʰ **S82.224   Nondisplaced transverse fracture of shaft of right tibia**   MCC CC H5

2,3 √7ᵗʰ **S82.225   Nondisplaced transverse fracture of shaft of left tibia**   MCC CC H5

2,3 √7ᵗʰ **S82.226   Nondisplaced transverse fracture of shaft of unspecified tibia**   MCC CC H5

√6ᵗʰ **S82.23   Oblique fracture of shaft of tibia**

2,3 √7ᵗʰ **S82.231   Displaced oblique fracture of shaft of right tibia**   MCC CC H5

2,3 √7ᵗʰ **S82.232   Displaced oblique fracture of shaft of left tibia**   MCC CC H5

2,3 √7ᵗʰ **S82.233   Displaced oblique fracture of shaft of unspecified tibia**   MCC CC H5

2,3 √7ᵗʰ **S82.234   Nondisplaced oblique fracture of shaft of right tibia**   MCC CC H5

2,3 √7ᵗʰ **S82.235   Nondisplaced oblique fracture of shaft of left tibia**   MCC CC H5

2,3 √7ᵗʰ **S82.236   Nondisplaced oblique fracture of shaft of unspecified tibia**   MCC CC H5

√6ᵗʰ **S82.24   Spiral fracture of shaft of tibia**
Toddler fracture

2,3 √7ᵗʰ **S82.241   Displaced spiral fracture of shaft of right tibia**   MCC CC H5

2,3 √7ᵗʰ **S82.242   Displaced spiral fracture of shaft of left tibia**   MCC CC H5

2,3 √7ᵗʰ **S82.243   Displaced spiral fracture of shaft of unspecified tibia**   MCC CC H5

2,3 √7ᵗʰ **S82.244   Nondisplaced spiral fracture of shaft of right tibia**   MCC CC H5

2,3 √7ᵗʰ **S82.245   Nondisplaced spiral fracture of shaft of left tibia**   MCC CC H5

2,3 √7ᵗʰ **S82.246   Nondisplaced spiral fracture of shaft of unspecified tibia**   MCC CC H5

√6ᵗʰ **S82.25   Comminuted fracture of shaft of tibia**

2,3 √7ᵗʰ **S82.251   Displaced comminuted fracture of shaft of right tibia**   MCC CC H5

2,3 √7ᵗʰ **S82.252   Displaced comminuted fracture of shaft of left tibia**   MCC CC H5

2,3 √7ᵗʰ **S82.253   Displaced comminuted fracture of shaft of unspecified tibia**   MCC CC H5

2,3 √7ᵗʰ **S82.254   Nondisplaced comminuted fracture of shaft of right tibia**   MCC CC H5

2,3 √7ᵗʰ **S82.255   Nondisplaced comminuted fracture of shaft of left tibia**   MCC CC H5

2,3 √7ᵗʰ **S82.256   Nondisplaced comminuted fracture of shaft of unspecified tibia**   MCC CC H5

√6ᵗʰ **S82.26   Segmental fracture of shaft of tibia**

2,3 √7ᵗʰ **S82.261   Displaced segmental fracture of shaft of right tibia**   MCC CC H5

2,3 √7ᵗʰ **S82.262   Displaced segmental fracture of shaft of left tibia**   MCC CC H5

2,3 √7ᵗʰ **S82.263   Displaced segmental fracture of shaft of unspecified tibia**   MCC CC H5

2,3 √7ᵗʰ **S82.264   Nondisplaced segmental fracture of shaft of right tibia**   MCC CC H5

2,3 √7ᵗʰ **S82.265   Nondisplaced segmental fracture of shaft of left tibia**   MCC CC H5

2,3 √7ᵗʰ **S82.266   Nondisplaced segmental fracture of shaft of unspecified tibia**   MCC CC H5

√6ᵗʰ **S82.29   Other fracture of shaft of tibia**

2,3 √7ᵗʰ **S82.291   Other fracture of shaft of right tibia**   MCC CC H5

2,3 √7ᵗʰ **S82.292   Other fracture of shaft of left tibia**   MCC CC H5

2,3 √7ᵗʰ **S82.299   Other fracture of shaft of unspecified tibia**   MCC CC H5

√5ᵗʰ **S82.3   Fracture of lower end of tibia**

EXCLUDES 1   bimalleolar fracture of lower leg (S82.84-)
fracture of medial malleolus alone (S82.5-)
Maisonneuve's fracture (S82.86-)
pilon fracture of distal tibia (S82.87-)
trimalleolar fractures of lower leg (S82.85-)

√6ᵗʰ **S82.30   Unspecified fracture of lower end of tibia**

CC Excl: For codes in subcategory S82.30:
CC with 7th character B or C: PDX collection 1347
CC with 7th character K, M, N, P, Q, or R: PDX collection 897

3 √7ᵗʰ **S82.301   Unspecified fracture of lower end of right tibia**   CC H5

3 √7ᵗʰ **S82.302   Unspecified fracture of lower end of left tibia**   CC H5

3 √7ᵗʰ **S82.309   Unspecified fracture of lower end of unspecified tibia**   CC H5

√6ᵗʰ **S82.31 Torus fracture of lower end of tibia**

The appropriate 7th character is to be added to all codes in subcategory S82.31.
A   initial encounter for closed fracture
D   subsequent encounter for fracture with routine healing
G   subsequent encounter for fracture with delayed healing
K   subsequent encounter for fracture with nonunion
P   subsequent encounter for fracture with malunion
S   sequela

3 √7ᵗʰ **S82.311 Torus fracture of lower end of right tibia**   `CC` `H5`
CC Excl: CC with 7th character A: PDX collection 1343
CC Excl: CC with 7th character K or P: PDX collection 897

3 √7ᵗʰ **S82.312 Torus fracture of lower end of left tibia**   `CC` `H5`
CC Excl: CC with 7th character A: PDX collection 1344
CC Excl: CC with 7th character K or P: PDX collection 897

3 √7ᵗʰ **S82.319 Torus fracture of lower end of unspecified tibia**   `CC` `H5`
CC Excl: CC with 7th character A: PDX collection 1345
CC Excl: CC with 7th character K or P: PDX collection 897

√6ᵗʰ **S82.39 Other fracture of lower end of tibia**
AHA: 2015,1Q,25
CC Excl: For codes in subcategory S82.39:
CC with 7th character B or C: PDX collection 1347
CC with 7th character K, M, N, P, Q, or R: PDX collection 897

3 √7ᵗʰ **S82.391 Other fracture of lower end of right tibia**   `CC` `H5`

3 √7ᵗʰ **S82.392 Other fracture of lower end of left tibia**   `CC` `H5`

3 √7ᵗʰ **S82.399 Other fracture of lower end of unspecified tibia**   `CC` `H5`

√5ᵗʰ **S82.4 Fracture of shaft of fibula**
EXCLUDES 2   fracture of lateral malleolus alone (S82.6-)
CC Excl: For codes in subcategory S82.4:
MCC with 7th character B or C: PDX collection 1341
CC with 7th character K, M, N, P, Q, or R: PDX collection 897

√6ᵗʰ **S82.40 Unspecified fracture of shaft of fibula**

2,4 √7ᵗʰ **S82.401 Unspecified fracture of shaft of right fibula**   `MCC` `CC` `H5`

2,4 √7ᵗʰ **S82.402 Unspecified fracture of shaft of left fibula**   `MCC` `CC` `H5`

2,4 √7ᵗʰ **S82.409 Unspecified fracture of shaft of unspecified fibula**   `MCC` `CC` `H5`

√6ᵗʰ **S82.42 Transverse fracture of shaft of fibula**

2,4 √7ᵗʰ **S82.421 Displaced transverse fracture of shaft of right fibula**   `MCC` `CC` `H5`

2,4 √7ᵗʰ **S82.422 Displaced transverse fracture of shaft of left fibula**   `MCC` `CC` `H5`

2,4 √7ᵗʰ **S82.423 Displaced transverse fracture of shaft of unspecified fibula**   `MCC` `CC` `H5`

2,4 √7ᵗʰ **S82.424 Nondisplaced transverse fracture of shaft of right fibula**   `MCC` `CC` `H5`

2,4 √7ᵗʰ **S82.425 Nondisplaced transverse fracture of shaft of left fibula**   `MCC` `CC` `H5`

2,4 √7ᵗʰ **S82.426 Nondisplaced transverse fracture of shaft of unspecified fibula**   `MCC` `CC` `H5`

√6ᵗʰ **S82.43 Oblique fracture of shaft of fibula**

2,4 √7ᵗʰ **S82.431 Displaced oblique fracture of shaft of right fibula**   `MCC` `CC` `H5`

2,4 √7ᵗʰ **S82.432 Displaced oblique fracture of shaft of left fibula**   `MCC` `CC` `H5`

2,4 √7ᵗʰ **S82.433 Displaced oblique fracture of shaft of unspecified fibula**   `MCC` `CC` `H5`

2,4 √7ᵗʰ **S82.434 Nondisplaced oblique fracture of shaft of right fibula**   `MCC` `CC` `H5`

2,4 √7ᵗʰ **S82.435 Nondisplaced oblique fracture of shaft of left fibula**   `MCC` `CC` `H5`

2,4 √7ᵗʰ **S82.436 Nondisplaced oblique fracture of shaft of unspecified fibula**   `MCC` `CC` `H5`

√6ᵗʰ **S82.44 Spiral fracture of shaft of fibula**

2,4 √7ᵗʰ **S82.441 Displaced spiral fracture of shaft of right fibula**   `MCC` `CC` `H5`

2,4 √7ᵗʰ **S82.442 Displaced spiral fracture of shaft of left fibula**   `MCC` `CC` `H5`

2,4 √7ᵗʰ **S82.443 Displaced spiral fracture of shaft of unspecified fibula**   `MCC` `CC` `H5`

2,4 √7ᵗʰ **S82.444 Nondisplaced spiral fracture of shaft of right fibula**   `MCC` `CC` `H5`

2,4 √7ᵗʰ **S82.445 Nondisplaced spiral fracture of shaft of left fibula**   `MCC` `CC` `H5`

2,4 √7ᵗʰ **S82.446 Nondisplaced spiral fracture of shaft of unspecified fibula**   `MCC` `CC` `H5`

√6ᵗʰ **S82.45 Comminuted fracture of shaft of fibula**

2,4 √7ᵗʰ **S82.451 Displaced comminuted fracture of shaft of right fibula**   `MCC` `CC` `H5`

2,4 √7ᵗʰ **S82.452 Displaced comminuted fracture of shaft of left fibula**   `MCC` `CC` `H5`

2,4 √7ᵗʰ **S82.453 Displaced comminuted fracture of shaft of unspecified fibula**   `MCC` `CC` `H5`

2,4 √7ᵗʰ **S82.454 Nondisplaced comminuted fracture of shaft of right fibula**   `MCC` `CC` `H5`

2,4 √7ᵗʰ **S82.455 Nondisplaced comminuted fracture of shaft of left fibula**   `MCC` `CC` `H5`

2,4 √7ᵗʰ **S82.456 Nondisplaced comminuted fracture of shaft of unspecified fibula**   `MCC` `CC` `H5`

√6ᵗʰ **S82.46 Segmental fracture of shaft of fibula**

2,4 √7ᵗʰ **S82.461 Displaced segmental fracture of shaft of right fibula**   `MCC` `CC` `H5`

2,4 √7ᵗʰ **S82.462 Displaced segmental fracture of shaft of left fibula**   `MCC` `CC` `H5`

2,4 √7ᵗʰ **S82.463 Displaced segmental fracture of shaft of unspecified fibula**   `MCC` `CC` `H5`

2,4 √7ᵗʰ **S82.464 Nondisplaced segmental fracture of shaft of right fibula**   `MCC` `CC` `H5`

2,4 √7ᵗʰ **S82.465 Nondisplaced segmental fracture of shaft of left fibula**   `MCC` `CC` `H5`

2,4 √7ᵗʰ **S82.466 Nondisplaced segmental fracture of shaft of unspecified fibula**   `MCC` `CC` `H5`

√6ᵗʰ **S82.49 Other fracture of shaft of fibula**

2,4 √7ᵗʰ **S82.491 Other fracture of shaft of right fibula**   `MCC` `CC` `H5`

2,4 √7ᵗʰ **S82.492 Other fracture of shaft of left fibula**   `MCC` `CC` `H5`

2,4 √7ᵗʰ **S82.499 Other fracture of shaft of unspecified fibula**   `MCC` `CC` `H5`

√5ᵗʰ **S82.5 Fracture of medial malleolus**
EXCLUDES 1   pilon fracture of distal tibia (S82.87-)
Salter-Harris type III of lower end of tibia (S89.13-)
Salter-Harris type IV of lower end of tibia (S89.14-)
CC Excl: For codes in subcategory S82.5:
CC with 7th character B or C: PDX collection 1347
CC with 7th character K, M, N, P, Q, or R: PDX collection 897

3 √x7ᵗʰ **S82.51 Displaced fracture of medial malleolus of right tibia**   `CC` `H5`

3 √x7th **S82.52** **Displaced fracture of medial malleolus of left tibia**   CC H5

3 √x7th **S82.53** **Displaced fracture of medial malleolus of unspecified tibia**   CC H5

3 √x7th **S82.54** **Nondisplaced fracture of medial malleolus of right tibia**   CC H5

3 √x7th **S82.55** **Nondisplaced fracture of medial malleolus of left tibia**   CC H5

3 √x7th **S82.56** **Nondisplaced fracture of medial malleolus of unspecified tibia**   CC H5

√5th **S82.6** **Fracture of lateral malleolus**

> EXCLUDES 1   pilon fracture of distal tibia (S82.87-)
>
> **CC Excl: For codes in subcategory S82.6:**
> **CC with 7th character B or C:** PDX collection 1347
> **CC with 7th character K, M, N, P, Q, or R:** PDX collection 897

3 √x7th **S82.61** **Displaced fracture of lateral malleolus of right fibula**   CC H5

3 √x7th **S82.62** **Displaced fracture of lateral malleolus of left fibula**   CC H5

3 √x7th **S82.63** **Displaced fracture of lateral malleolus of unspecified fibula**   CC H5

3 √x7th **S82.64** **Nondisplaced fracture of lateral malleolus of right fibula**   CC H5

3 √x7th **S82.65** **Nondisplaced fracture of lateral malleolus of left fibula**   CC H5

3 √x7th **S82.66** **Nondisplaced fracture of lateral malleolus of unspecified fibula**   CC H5

√5th **S82.8** **Other fractures of lower leg**

√6th **S82.81** **Torus fracture of upper end of fibula**

> The appropriate 7th character is to be added to all codes in subcategory S82.81
> A   initial encounter for closed fracture
> D   subsequent encounter for fracture with routine healing
> G   subsequent encounter for fracture with delayed healing
> K   subsequent encounter for fracture with nonunion
> P   subsequent encounter for fracture with malunion
> S   sequela
>
> **CC Excl: For codes in subcategory S82.81:**
> **CC with 7th character K or P:** PDX collection 897

4 √7th **S82.811** **Torus fracture of upper end of right fibula**   CC

4 √7th **S82.812** **Torus fracture of upper end of left fibula**   CC

4 √7th **S82.819** **Torus fracture of upper end of unspecified fibula**   CC

√6th **S82.82** **Torus fracture of lower end of fibula**

> The appropriate 7th character is to be added to all codes in subcategory S82.82.
> A   initial encounter for closed fracture
> D   subsequent encounter for fracture with routine healing
> G   subsequent encounter for fracture with delayed healing
> K   subsequent encounter for fracture with nonunion
> P   subsequent encounter for fracture with malunion
> S   sequela
>
> **CC Excl: For codes in subcategory S82.82:**
> **CC with 7th character K or P:** PDX collection 897

4 √7th **S82.821** **Torus fracture of lower end of right fibula**   CC

4 √7th **S82.822** **Torus fracture of lower end of left fibula**   CC

4 √7th **S82.829** **Torus fracture of lower end of unspecified fibula**   CC

√6th **S82.83** **Other fracture of upper and lower end of fibula**

> **AHA:** 2015,1Q,25
>
> **CC Excl: For codes in subcategory S82.83:**
> **MCC with 7th character B or C:** PDX collection 1341
> **CC with 7th character K, M, N, P, Q, or R:** PDX collection 897

2,4 √7th **S82.831** **Other fracture of upper and lower end of right fibula**   MCC CC H5

2,4 √7th **S82.832** **Other fracture of upper and lower end of left fibula**   MCC CC H5

2,4 √7th **S82.839** **Other fracture of upper and lower end of unspecified fibula**   MCC CC H5

√6th **S82.84** **Bimalleolar fracture of lower leg**

> **CC Excl: For codes in subcategory S82.84:**
> **CC with 7th character B or C:** PDX collection 1347
> **CC with 7th character K, M, N, P, Q, or R:** PDX collection 897

Right Bimalleolar Fracture

- Patella
- Tibial plateau
- Tibial tubercle
- Fibula
- Tibia
- Fracture medial malleolus
- Fracture lateral malleolus
- Talus
- Lateral (fibular) malleolus
- Medial (tibial) malleolus

3 √7th **S82.841** **Displaced bimalleolar fracture of right lower leg**   CC H5

3 √7th **S82.842** **Displaced bimalleolar fracture of left lower leg**   CC H5

3 √7th **S82.843** **Displaced bimalleolar fracture of unspecified lower leg**   CC H5

3 √7th **S82.844** **Nondisplaced bimalleolar fracture of right lower leg**   CC H5

3 √7th **S82.845** **Nondisplaced bimalleolar fracture of left lower leg**   CC H5

3 √7th **S82.846** **Nondisplaced bimalleolar fracture of unspecified lower leg**   CC H5

√6th **S82.85** **Trimalleolar fracture of lower leg**

> **CC Excl: For codes in subcategory S82.85:**
> **CC with 7th character B or C:** PDX collection 1347
> **CC with 7th character K, M, N, P, Q, or R:** PDX collection 897

3 √7th **S82.851** **Displaced trimalleolar fracture of right lower leg**   CC H5

3 √7th **S82.852** **Displaced trimalleolar fracture of left lower leg**   CC H5

3 √7th **S82.853** **Displaced trimalleolar fracture of unspecified lower leg**   CC H5

3 √7th **S82.854** **Nondisplaced trimalleolar fracture of right lower leg**   CC H5

3 √7th **S82.855** **Nondisplaced trimalleolar fracture of left lower leg**   CC H5

☑ Additional Character Required   √x7th Placeholder   Unacceptable PDx   Questionable PDx   Manifestation   Unspecified Dx   H1-H14 HAC   HCC CMS-HCC Dx   HIV HIV Dx

3 √7ᵗʰ **S82.856 Nondisplaced trimalleolar** CC H5
**fracture of unspecified
lower leg**

√6ᵗʰ **S82.86 Maisonneuve's fracture**

CC Excl: For codes in subcategory S82.86:
MCC with 7th character B or C: PDX collection 1341
CC with 7th character K, M, N, P, Q, or R: PDX
collection 897

2,4 √7ᵗʰ **S82.861 Displaced Maisonneuve's** MCC CC H5
fracture of right leg

2,4 √7ᵗʰ **S82.862 Displaced Maisonneuve's** MCC CC H5
fracture of left leg

2,4 √7ᵗʰ **S82.863 Displaced Maisonneuve's** MCC CC H5
fracture of unspecified leg

2,4 √7ᵗʰ **S82.864 Nondisplaced** MCC CC H5
**Maisonneuve's fracture of
right leg**

2,4 √7ᵗʰ **S82.865 Nondisplaced** MCC CC H5
**Maisonneuve's fracture of
left leg**

2,4 √7ᵗʰ **S82.866 Nondisplaced** MCC CC H5
**Maisonneuve's fracture of
unspecified leg**

√6ᵗʰ **S82.87 Pilon fracture of tibia**

CC Excl: For codes in subcategory S82.87:
CC with 7th character B or C: PDX collection 1347
CC with 7th character K, M, N, P, Q, or R: PDX
collection 897

3 √7ᵗʰ **S82.871 Displaced pilon fracture of** CC H5
right tibia

3 √7ᵗʰ **S82.872 Displaced pilon fracture of** CC H5
left tibia

3 √7ᵗʰ **S82.873 Displaced pilon fracture of** CC H5
unspecified tibia

3 √7ᵗʰ **S82.874 Nondisplaced pilon** CC H5
fracture of right tibia

3 √7ᵗʰ **S82.875 Nondisplaced pilon** CC H5
fracture of left tibia

3 √7ᵗʰ **S82.876 Nondisplaced pilon** CC H5
**fracture of unspecified
tibia**

√6ᵗʰ **S82.89 Other fractures of lower leg**

Fracture of ankle NOS

CC Excl: For codes in subcategory S82.89:
CC with 7th character B or C: PDX collection 1347
CC with 7th character K, M, N, P, Q, or R: PDX
collection 897

3 √7ᵗʰ **S82.891 Other fracture of right** CC H5
lower leg

3 √7ᵗʰ **S82.892 Other fracture of left lower** CC H5
leg

3 √7ᵗʰ **S82.899 Other fracture of** CC H5
unspecified lower leg

√5ᵗʰ **S82.9 Unspecified fracture of lower leg**

CC Excl: For codes in subcategory S82.9:
CC with 7th character B or C: PDX collection 1348
CC with 7th character K, M, N, P, Q, or R: PDX collection 897

3 √x7ᵗʰ **S82.90 Unspecified fracture of unspecified** CC H5
lower leg

3 √x7ᵗʰ **S82.91 Unspecified fracture of right lower** CC H5
leg

3 √x7ᵗʰ **S82.92 Unspecified fracture of left lower leg** CC H5

√4ᵗʰ **S83 Dislocation and sprain of joints and ligaments of knee**

INCLUDES avulsion of joint or ligament of knee
laceration of cartilage, joint or ligament of knee
sprain of cartilage, joint or ligament of knee
traumatic hemarthrosis of joint or ligament of knee
traumatic rupture of joint or ligament of knee
traumatic subluxation of joint or ligament of knee
traumatic tear of joint or ligament of knee

Code also any associated open wound

EXCLUDES 1 derangement of patella (M22.0-M22.3)
injury of patellar ligament (tendon) (S76.1-)
internal derangement of knee (M23.-)
old dislocation of knee (M23.8X)
pathological dislocation of knee (M24.36)
recurrent dislocation of knee (M22.0)

EXCLUDES 2 strain of muscle, fascia and tendon of lower leg (S86.-)

The appropriate 7th character is to be added to each code from
category S83.
A initial encounter
D subsequent encounter
S sequela

√5ᵗʰ **S83.0 Subluxation and dislocation of patella**

√6ᵗʰ **S83.00 Unspecified subluxation and dislocation of patella**

√7ᵗʰ **S83.001 Unspecified subluxation of right patella**

√7ᵗʰ **S83.002 Unspecified subluxation of left patella**

√7ᵗʰ **S83.003 Unspecified subluxation of unspecified
patella**

√7ᵗʰ **S83.004 Unspecified dislocation of right patella**

√7ᵗʰ **S83.005 Unspecified dislocation of left patella**

√7ᵗʰ **S83.006 Unspecified dislocation of unspecified
patella**

√6ᵗʰ **S83.01 Lateral subluxation and dislocation of patella**

√7ᵗʰ **S83.011 Lateral subluxation of right patella**

√7ᵗʰ **S83.012 Lateral subluxation of left patella**

√7ᵗʰ **S83.013 Lateral subluxation of unspecified patella**

√7ᵗʰ **S83.014 Lateral dislocation of right patella**

√7ᵗʰ **S83.015 Lateral dislocation of left patella**

√7ᵗʰ **S83.016 Lateral dislocation of unspecified patella**

√6ᵗʰ **S83.09 Other subluxation and dislocation of patella**

√7ᵗʰ **S83.091 Other subluxation of right patella**

√7ᵗʰ **S83.092 Other subluxation of left patella**

√7ᵗʰ **S83.093 Other subluxation of unspecified patella**

√7ᵗʰ **S83.094 Other dislocation of right patella**

√7ᵗʰ **S83.095 Other dislocation of left patella**

√7ᵗʰ **S83.096 Other dislocation of unspecified patella**

√5ᵗʰ **S83.1 Subluxation and dislocation of knee**

EXCLUDES 2 instability of knee prosthesis (T84.022, T84.023)

√6ᵗʰ **S83.10 Unspecified subluxation and dislocation of knee**

√7ᵗʰ **S83.101 Unspecified subluxation of right knee**

√7ᵗʰ **S83.102 Unspecified subluxation of left knee**

√7ᵗʰ **S83.103 Unspecified subluxation of unspecified
knee**

√7ᵗʰ **S83.104 Unspecified dislocation of right knee**

√7ᵗʰ **S83.105 Unspecified dislocation of left knee**

√7ᵗʰ **S83.106 Unspecified dislocation of unspecified
knee**

√6ᵗʰ **S83.11 Anterior subluxation and dislocation of proximal
end of tibia**

Posterior subluxation and dislocation of distal end of
femur

√7ᵗʰ **S83.111 Anterior subluxation of proximal end of
tibia, right knee**

√7ᵗʰ **S83.112 Anterior subluxation of proximal end of
tibia, left knee**

√7ᵗʰ **S83.113 Anterior subluxation of proximal end of
tibia, unspecified knee**

√7ᵗʰ **S83.114 Anterior dislocation of proximal end of
tibia, right knee**

√7ᵗʰ **S83.115 Anterior dislocation of proximal end of
tibia, left knee**

√7ᵗʰ **S83.116 Anterior dislocation of proximal end of
tibia, unspecified knee**

√6ᵗʰ **S83.12** Posterior subluxation and dislocation of proximal end of tibia

Anterior dislocation of distal end of femur

√7ᵗʰ **S83.121** Posterior subluxation of proximal end of tibia, right knee

√7ᵗʰ **S83.122** Posterior subluxation of proximal end of tibia, left knee

√7ᵗʰ **S83.123** Posterior subluxation of proximal end of tibia, unspecified knee

√7ᵗʰ **S83.124** Posterior dislocation of proximal end of tibia, right knee

√7ᵗʰ **S83.125** Posterior dislocation of proximal end of tibia, left knee

√7ᵗʰ **S83.126** Posterior dislocation of proximal end of tibia, unspecified knee

√6ᵗʰ **S83.13** Medial subluxation and dislocation of proximal end of tibia

√7ᵗʰ **S83.131** Medial subluxation of proximal end of tibia, right knee

√7ᵗʰ **S83.132** Medial subluxation of proximal end of tibia, left knee

√7ᵗʰ **S83.133** Medial subluxation of proximal end of tibia, unspecified knee

√7ᵗʰ **S83.134** Medial dislocation of proximal end of tibia, right knee

√7ᵗʰ **S83.135** Medial dislocation of proximal end of tibia, left knee

√7ᵗʰ **S83.136** Medial dislocation of proximal end of tibia, unspecified knee

√6ᵗʰ **S83.14** Lateral subluxation and dislocation of proximal end of tibia

√7ᵗʰ **S83.141** Lateral subluxation of proximal end of tibia, right knee

√7ᵗʰ **S83.142** Lateral subluxation of proximal end of tibia, left knee

√7ᵗʰ **S83.143** Lateral subluxation of proximal end of tibia, unspecified knee

√7ᵗʰ **S83.144** Lateral dislocation of proximal end of tibia, right knee

√7ᵗʰ **S83.145** Lateral dislocation of proximal end of tibia, left knee

√7ᵗʰ **S83.146** Lateral dislocation of proximal end of tibia, unspecified knee

√6ᵗʰ **S83.19** Other subluxation and dislocation of knee

√7ᵗʰ **S83.191** Other subluxation of right knee

√7ᵗʰ **S83.192** Other subluxation of left knee

√7ᵗʰ **S83.193** Other subluxation of unspecified knee

√7ᵗʰ **S83.194** Other dislocation of right knee

√7ᵗʰ **S83.195** Other dislocation of left knee

√7ᵗʰ **S83.196** Other dislocation of unspecified knee

√5ᵗʰ **S83.2** Tear of meniscus, current injury

EXCLUDES 1 *old bucket-handle tear (M23.2)*

AHA: 2019,2Q,26

√6ᵗʰ **S83.20** Tear of unspecified meniscus, current injury

Tear of meniscus of knee NOS

√7ᵗʰ **S83.200** Bucket-handle tear of unspecified meniscus, current injury, right knee

√7ᵗʰ **S83.201** Bucket-handle tear of unspecified meniscus, current injury, left knee

√7ᵗʰ **S83.202** Bucket-handle tear of unspecified meniscus, current injury, unspecified knee

√7ᵗʰ **S83.203** Other tear of unspecified meniscus, current injury, right knee

√7ᵗʰ **S83.204** Other tear of unspecified meniscus, current injury, left knee

√7ᵗʰ **S83.205** Other tear of unspecified meniscus, current injury, unspecified knee

√7ᵗʰ **S83.206** Unspecified tear of unspecified meniscus, current injury, right knee

√7ᵗʰ **S83.207** Unspecified tear of unspecified meniscus, current injury, left knee

√7ᵗʰ **S83.209** Unspecified tear of unspecified meniscus, current injury, unspecified knee

√6ᵗʰ **S83.21** Bucket-handle tear of medial meniscus, current injury

√7ᵗʰ **S83.211** Bucket-handle tear of medial meniscus, current injury, right knee

√7ᵗʰ **S83.212** Bucket-handle tear of medial meniscus, current injury, left knee

√7ᵗʰ **S83.219** Bucket-handle tear of medial meniscus, current injury, unspecified knee

√6ᵗʰ **S83.22** Peripheral tear of medial meniscus, current injury

√7ᵗʰ **S83.221** Peripheral tear of medial meniscus, current injury, right knee

√7ᵗʰ **S83.222** Peripheral tear of medial meniscus, current injury, left knee

√7ᵗʰ **S83.229** Peripheral tear of medial meniscus, current injury, unspecified knee

√6ᵗʰ **S83.23** Complex tear of medial meniscus, current injury

√7ᵗʰ **S83.231** Complex tear of medial meniscus, current injury, right knee

√7ᵗʰ **S83.232** Complex tear of medial meniscus, current injury, left knee

√7ᵗʰ **S83.239** Complex tear of medial meniscus, current injury, unspecified knee

√6ᵗʰ **S83.24** Other tear of medial meniscus, current injury

√7ᵗʰ **S83.241** Other tear of medial meniscus, current injury, right knee

√7ᵗʰ **S83.242** Other tear of medial meniscus, current injury, left knee

√7ᵗʰ **S83.249** Other tear of medial meniscus, current injury, unspecified knee

√6ᵗʰ **S83.25** Bucket-handle tear of lateral meniscus, current injury

√7ᵗʰ **S83.251** Bucket-handle tear of lateral meniscus, current injury, right knee

√7ᵗʰ **S83.252** Bucket-handle tear of lateral meniscus, current injury, left knee

√7ᵗʰ **S83.259** Bucket-handle tear of lateral meniscus, current injury, unspecified knee

√6ᵗʰ **S83.26** Peripheral tear of lateral meniscus, current injury

√7ᵗʰ **S83.261** Peripheral tear of lateral meniscus, current injury, right knee

√7ᵗʰ **S83.262** Peripheral tear of lateral meniscus, current injury, left knee

√7ᵗʰ **S83.269** Peripheral tear of lateral meniscus, current injury, unspecified knee

√6ᵗʰ **S83.27** Complex tear of lateral meniscus, current injury

√7ᵗʰ **S83.271** Complex tear of lateral meniscus, current injury, right knee

√7ᵗʰ **S83.272** Complex tear of lateral meniscus, current injury, left knee

√7ᵗʰ **S83.279** Complex tear of lateral meniscus, current injury, unspecified knee

√6ᵗʰ **S83.28** Other tear of lateral meniscus, current injury

√7ᵗʰ **S83.281** Other tear of lateral meniscus, current injury, right knee

√7ᵗʰ **S83.282** Other tear of lateral meniscus, current injury, left knee

√7ᵗʰ **S83.289** Other tear of lateral meniscus, current injury, unspecified knee

√5ᵗʰ **S83.3** Tear of articular cartilage of knee, current

√x7ᵗʰ **S83.30** Tear of articular cartilage of unspecified knee, current

√x7ᵗʰ **S83.31** Tear of articular cartilage of right knee, current

√x7ᵗʰ **S83.32** Tear of articular cartilage of left knee, current

√5ᵗʰ **S83.4** Sprain of collateral ligament of knee

√6ᵗʰ **S83.40** Sprain of unspecified collateral ligament of knee

√7ᵗʰ **S83.401** Sprain of unspecified collateral ligament of right knee

√7ᵗʰ **S83.402** Sprain of unspecified collateral ligament of left knee

√7ᵗʰ **S83.409** Sprain of unspecified collateral ligament of unspecified knee

√6ᵗʰ **S83.41** Sprain of medial collateral ligament of knee

Sprain of tibial collateral ligament

√7ᵗʰ **S83.411** Sprain of medial collateral ligament of right knee

√7ᵗʰ **S83.412** Sprain of medial collateral ligament of left knee

√7ᵗʰ **S83.419** Sprain of medial collateral ligament of unspecified knee

√6ᵗʰ **S83.42** Sprain of lateral collateral ligament of knee

Sprain of fibular collateral ligament

√7ᵗʰ **S83.421** Sprain of lateral collateral ligament of right knee

√7ᵗʰ **S83.422** Sprain of lateral collateral ligament of left knee

☑ Additional Character Required √x7ᵗʰ Placeholder Unacceptable PDx Questionable PDx Manifestation Unspecified Dx H1–H14 HAC HCC CMS-HCC Dx HIV HIV Dx

ICD-10-CM 2020 **1105**

✓7ᵗʰ **S83.429**   Sprain of lateral collateral ligament of unspecified knee

✓5ᵗʰ **S83.5**   Sprain of cruciate ligament of knee

     AHA: 2016,2Q,3

     ✓6ᵗʰ **S83.50**   Sprain of unspecified cruciate ligament of knee

       ✓7ᵗʰ **S83.501**   Sprain of unspecified cruciate ligament of right knee

       ✓7ᵗʰ **S83.502**   Sprain of unspecified cruciate ligament of left knee

       ✓7ᵗʰ **S83.509**   Sprain of unspecified cruciate ligament of unspecified knee

     ✓6ᵗʰ **S83.51**   Sprain of anterior cruciate ligament of knee

       ✓7ᵗʰ **S83.511**   Sprain of anterior cruciate ligament of right knee

       ✓7ᵗʰ **S83.512**   Sprain of anterior cruciate ligament of left knee

       ✓7ᵗʰ **S83.519**   Sprain of anterior cruciate ligament of unspecified knee

     ✓6ᵗʰ **S83.52**   Sprain of posterior cruciate ligament of knee

       ✓7ᵗʰ **S83.521**   Sprain of posterior cruciate ligament of right knee

       ✓7ᵗʰ **S83.522**   Sprain of posterior cruciate ligament of left knee

       ✓7ᵗʰ **S83.529**   Sprain of posterior cruciate ligament of unspecified knee

✓5ᵗʰ **S83.6**   Sprain of the superior tibiofibular joint and ligament

     ✓x7ᵗʰ **S83.60**   Sprain of the superior tibiofibular joint and ligament, unspecified knee

     ✓x7ᵗʰ **S83.61**   Sprain of the superior tibiofibular joint and ligament, right knee

     ✓x7ᵗʰ **S83.62**   Sprain of the superior tibiofibular joint and ligament, left knee

✓5ᵗʰ **S83.8**   Sprain of other specified parts of knee

     ✓6ᵗʰ **S83.8X**   Sprain of other specified parts of knee

       ✓7ᵗʰ **S83.8X1**   Sprain of other specified parts of right knee

       ✓7ᵗʰ **S83.8X2**   Sprain of other specified parts of left knee

       ✓7ᵗʰ **S83.8X9**   Sprain of other specified parts of unspecified knee

✓5ᵗʰ **S83.9**   Sprain of unspecified site of knee

     ✓x7ᵗʰ **S83.90**   Sprain of unspecified site of unspecified knee

     ✓x7ᵗʰ **S83.91**   Sprain of unspecified site of right knee

     ✓x7ᵗʰ **S83.92**   Sprain of unspecified site of left knee

✓4ᵗʰ **S84**   Injury of nerves at lower leg level

     Code also any associated open wound (S81.-)

     EXCLUDES 2   injury of nerves at ankle and foot level (S94.-)

     The appropriate 7th character is to be added to each code from category S84.
     A   initial encounter
     D   subsequent encounter
     S   sequela

     ✓5ᵗʰ **S84.0**   Injury of tibial nerve at lower leg level

       ✓x7ᵗʰ **S84.00**   Injury of tibial nerve at lower leg level, unspecified leg

       ✓x7ᵗʰ **S84.01**   Injury of tibial nerve at lower leg level, right leg

       ✓x7ᵗʰ **S84.02**   Injury of tibial nerve at lower leg level, left leg

     ✓5ᵗʰ **S84.1**   Injury of peroneal nerve at lower leg level

       ✓x7ᵗʰ **S84.10**   Injury of peroneal nerve at lower leg level, unspecified leg

       ✓x7ᵗʰ **S84.11**   Injury of peroneal nerve at lower leg level, right leg

       ✓x7ᵗʰ **S84.12**   Injury of peroneal nerve at lower leg level, left leg

     ✓5ᵗʰ **S84.2**   Injury of cutaneous sensory nerve at lower leg level

       ✓x7ᵗʰ **S84.20**   Injury of cutaneous sensory nerve at lower leg level, unspecified leg

       ✓x7ᵗʰ **S84.21**   Injury of cutaneous sensory nerve at lower leg level, right leg

       ✓x7ᵗʰ **S84.22**   Injury of cutaneous sensory nerve at lower leg level, left leg

     ✓5ᵗʰ **S84.8**   Injury of other nerves at lower leg level

       ✓6ᵗʰ **S84.80**   Injury of other nerves at lower leg level

         ✓7ᵗʰ **S84.801**   Injury of other nerves at lower leg level, right leg

         ✓7ᵗʰ **S84.802**   Injury of other nerves at lower leg level, left leg

         ✓7ᵗʰ **S84.809**   Injury of other nerves at lower leg level, unspecified leg

     ✓5ᵗʰ **S84.9**   Injury of unspecified nerve at lower leg level

       ✓x7ᵗʰ **S84.90**   Injury of unspecified nerve at lower leg level, unspecified leg

       ✓x7ᵗʰ **S84.91**   Injury of unspecified nerve at lower leg level, right leg

       ✓x7ᵗʰ **S84.92**   Injury of unspecified nerve at lower leg level, left leg

✓4ᵗʰ **S85**   Injury of blood vessels at lower leg level

     Code also any associated open wound (S81.-)

     EXCLUDES 2   injury of blood vessels at ankle and foot level (S95.-)

     The appropriate 7th character is to be added to each code from category S85.
     A   initial encounter
     D   subsequent encounter
     S   sequela

     ✓5ᵗʰ **S85.0**   Injury of popliteal artery

     CC Excl: For MCC codes in subcategory S85.0:
     Right side: PDX collection 1349
     Left side: PDX collection 1350
     Unspecified side: PDX collection 1351

       ✓6ᵗʰ **S85.00**   Unspecified injury of popliteal artery

         ✓7ᵗʰ **S85.001**   Unspecified injury of popliteal artery, right leg   MCC

         ✓7ᵗʰ **S85.002**   Unspecified injury of popliteal artery, left leg   MCC

         ✓7ᵗʰ **S85.009**   Unspecified injury of popliteal artery, unspecified leg   MCC

       ✓6ᵗʰ **S85.01**   Laceration of popliteal artery

         ✓7ᵗʰ **S85.011**   Laceration of popliteal artery, right leg   MCC

         ✓7ᵗʰ **S85.012**   Laceration of popliteal artery, left leg   MCC

         ✓7ᵗʰ **S85.019**   Laceration of popliteal artery, unspecified leg   MCC

       ✓6ᵗʰ **S85.09**   Other specified injury of popliteal artery

         ✓7ᵗʰ **S85.091**   Other specified injury of popliteal artery, right leg   MCC

         ✓7ᵗʰ **S85.092**   Other specified injury of popliteal artery, left leg   MCC

         ✓7ᵗʰ **S85.099**   Other specified injury of popliteal artery, unspecified leg   MCC

     ✓5ᵗʰ **S85.1**   Injury of tibial artery

       ✓6ᵗʰ **S85.10**   Unspecified injury of unspecified tibial artery

         Injury of tibial artery NOS

         ✓7ᵗʰ **S85.101**   Unspecified injury of unspecified tibial artery, right leg   CC
           CC Excl: PDX collection 1352

         ✓7ᵗʰ **S85.102**   Unspecified injury of unspecified tibial artery, left leg   CC
           CC Excl: PDX collection 1353

         ✓7ᵗʰ **S85.109**   Unspecified injury of unspecified tibial artery, unspecified leg   CC
           CC Excl: PDX collection 1354

       ✓6ᵗʰ **S85.11**   Laceration of unspecified tibial artery

         ✓7ᵗʰ **S85.111**   Laceration of unspecified tibial artery, right leg   CC
           CC Excl: PDX collection 1352

         ✓7ᵗʰ **S85.112**   Laceration of unspecified tibial artery, left leg   CC
           CC Excl: PDX collection 1353

         ✓7ᵗʰ **S85.119**   Laceration of unspecified tibial artery, unspecified leg   CC
           CC Excl: PDX collection 1354

       ✓6ᵗʰ **S85.12**   Other specified injury of unspecified tibial artery

         ✓7ᵗʰ **S85.121**   Other specified injury of unspecified tibial artery, right leg   CC
           CC Excl: PDX collection 1352

N Newborn: 0   **P** Pediatric: 0-17   **M** Maternity: 9-64   **A** Adult: 15-124   **MCC** Major Complication/Comorbidity   **CC** Complication/Comorbidity   **SW** Severe Wound Dx

1106   **ICD-10-CM 2020**

√7ᵗʰ **S85.122** Other specified injury of unspecified tibial artery, left leg   `CC`
CC Excl: PDX collection 1353

√7ᵗʰ **S85.129** Other specified injury of unspecified tibial artery, unspecified leg   `CC`
CC Excl: PDX collection 1354

√6ᵗʰ **S85.13** Unspecified injury of anterior tibial artery

√7ᵗʰ **S85.131** Unspecified injury of anterior tibial artery, right leg   `CC`
CC Excl: PDX collection 1355

√7ᵗʰ **S85.132** Unspecified injury of anterior tibial artery, left leg   `CC`
CC Excl: PDX collection 1356

√7ᵗʰ **S85.139** Unspecified injury of anterior tibial artery, unspecified leg   `CC`
CC Excl: PDX collection 1357

√6ᵗʰ **S85.14** Laceration of anterior tibial artery

√7ᵗʰ **S85.141** Laceration of anterior tibial artery, right leg   `CC`
CC Excl: PDX collection 1355

√7ᵗʰ **S85.142** Laceration of anterior tibial artery, left leg   `CC`
CC Excl: PDX collection 1356

√7ᵗʰ **S85.149** Laceration of anterior tibial artery, unspecified leg   `CC`
CC Excl: PDX collection 1357

√6ᵗʰ **S85.15** Other specified injury of anterior tibial artery

√7ᵗʰ **S85.151** Other specified injury of anterior tibial artery, right leg   `CC`
CC Excl: PDX collection 1355

√7ᵗʰ **S85.152** Other specified injury of anterior tibial artery, left leg   `CC`
CC Excl: PDX collection 1356

√7ᵗʰ **S85.159** Other specified injury of anterior tibial artery, unspecified leg   `CC`
CC Excl: PDX collection 1357

√6ᵗʰ **S85.16** Unspecified injury of posterior tibial artery

√7ᵗʰ **S85.161** Unspecified injury of posterior tibial artery, right leg   `CC`
CC Excl: PDX collection 1358

√7ᵗʰ **S85.162** Unspecified injury of posterior tibial artery, left leg   `CC`
CC Excl: PDX collection 1359

√7ᵗʰ **S85.169** Unspecified injury of posterior tibial artery, unspecified leg   `CC`
CC Excl: PDX collection 1360

√6ᵗʰ **S85.17** Laceration of posterior tibial artery

√7ᵗʰ **S85.171** Laceration of posterior tibial artery, right leg   `CC`
CC Excl: PDX collection 1358

√7ᵗʰ **S85.172** Laceration of posterior tibial artery, left leg   `CC`
CC Excl: PDX collection 1359

√7ᵗʰ **S85.179** Laceration of posterior tibial artery, unspecified leg   `CC`
CC Excl: PDX collection 1360

√6ᵗʰ **S85.18** Other specified injury of posterior tibial artery

√7ᵗʰ **S85.181** Other specified injury of posterior tibial artery, right leg   `CC`
CC Excl: PDX collection 1358

√7ᵗʰ **S85.182** Other specified injury of posterior tibial artery, left leg   `CC`
CC Excl: PDX collection 1359

√7ᵗʰ **S85.189** Other specified injury of posterior tibial artery, unspecified leg   `CC`
CC Excl: PDX collection 1360

√5ᵗʰ **S85.2** Injury of peroneal artery

CC Excl: For CC codes in subcategory S85.2:
Right side: PDX collection 1325
Left side: PDX collection 1326
Unspecified side: PDX collection 1327

√6ᵗʰ **S85.20** Unspecified injury of peroneal artery

√7ᵗʰ **S85.201** Unspecified injury of peroneal artery, right leg   `CC`

√7ᵗʰ **S85.202** Unspecified injury of peroneal artery, left leg   `CC`

√7ᵗʰ **S85.209** Unspecified injury of peroneal artery, unspecified leg   `CC`

√6ᵗʰ **S85.21** Laceration of peroneal artery

√7ᵗʰ **S85.211** Laceration of peroneal artery, right leg   `CC`

√7ᵗʰ **S85.212** Laceration of peroneal artery, left leg   `CC`

√7ᵗʰ **S85.219** Laceration of peroneal artery, unspecified leg   `CC`

√6ᵗʰ **S85.29** Other specified injury of peroneal artery

√7ᵗʰ **S85.291** Other specified injury of peroneal artery, right leg   `CC`

√7ᵗʰ **S85.292** Other specified injury of peroneal artery, left leg   `CC`

√7ᵗʰ **S85.299** Other specified injury of peroneal artery, unspecified leg   `CC`

√5ᵗʰ **S85.3** Injury of greater saphenous vein at lower leg level

Injury of greater saphenous vein NOS
Injury of saphenous vein NOS

CC Excl: For CC codes in subcategory S85.3:
Right side: PDX collection 1322
Left side: PDX collection 1323
Unspecified side: PDX collection 1324

√6ᵗʰ **S85.30** Unspecified injury of greater saphenous vein at lower leg level

√7ᵗʰ **S85.301** Unspecified injury of greater saphenous vein at lower leg level, right leg   `CC`

√7ᵗʰ **S85.302** Unspecified injury of greater saphenous vein at lower leg level, left leg   `CC`

√7ᵗʰ **S85.309** Unspecified injury of greater saphenous vein at lower leg level, unspecified leg   `CC`

√6ᵗʰ **S85.31** Laceration of greater saphenous vein at lower leg level

√7ᵗʰ **S85.311** Laceration of greater saphenous vein at lower leg level, right leg   `CC`

√7ᵗʰ **S85.312** Laceration of greater saphenous vein at lower leg level, left leg   `CC`

√7ᵗʰ **S85.319** Laceration of greater saphenous vein at lower leg level, unspecified leg   `CC`

√6ᵗʰ **S85.39** Other specified injury of greater saphenous vein at lower leg level

√7ᵗʰ **S85.391** Other specified injury of greater saphenous vein at lower leg level, right leg   `CC`

√7ᵗʰ **S85.392** Other specified injury of greater saphenous vein at lower leg level, left leg   `CC`

√7ᵗʰ **S85.399** Other specified injury of greater saphenous vein at lower leg level, unspecified leg   `CC`

√5ᵗʰ **S85.4** Injury of lesser saphenous vein at lower leg level

CC Excl: For CC codes in subcategory S85.4:
Right side: PDX collection 1322
Left side: PDX collection 1323
Unspecified side: PDX collection 1324

√6ᵗʰ **S85.40** Unspecified injury of lesser saphenous vein at lower leg level

√7ᵗʰ **S85.401** Unspecified injury of lesser saphenous vein at lower leg level, right leg   `CC`

√7ᵗʰ **S85.402** Unspecified injury of lesser saphenous vein at lower leg level, **left** leg `CC`

√7ᵗʰ **S85.409** Unspecified injury of lesser saphenous vein at lower leg level, unspecified leg `CC`

√6ᵗʰ **S85.41** Laceration of lesser saphenous vein at lower leg level

√7ᵗʰ **S85.411** Laceration of lesser saphenous vein at lower leg level, **right** leg `CC`

√7ᵗʰ **S85.412** Laceration of lesser saphenous vein at lower leg level, **left** leg `CC`

√7ᵗʰ **S85.419** Laceration of lesser saphenous vein at lower leg level, unspecified leg `CC`

√6ᵗʰ **S85.49** Other specified injury of lesser saphenous vein at lower leg level

√7ᵗʰ **S85.491** Other specified injury of lesser saphenous vein at lower leg level, **right** leg `CC`

√7ᵗʰ **S85.492** Other specified injury of lesser saphenous vein at lower leg level, **left** leg `CC`

√7ᵗʰ **S85.499** Other specified injury of lesser saphenous vein at lower leg level, unspecified leg `CC`

√5ᵗʰ **S85.5** Injury of popliteal vein

CC Excl: For MCC codes in subcategory S85.5:
Right side: PDX collection 1361
Left side: PDX collection 1362
Unspecified side: PDX collection 1363

√6ᵗʰ **S85.50** Unspecified injury of popliteal vein

√7ᵗʰ **S85.501** Unspecified injury of popliteal vein, **right** leg `MCC`

√7ᵗʰ **S85.502** Unspecified injury of popliteal vein, **left** leg `MCC`

√7ᵗʰ **S85.509** Unspecified injury of popliteal vein, unspecified leg `MCC`

√6ᵗʰ **S85.51** Laceration of popliteal vein

√7ᵗʰ **S85.511** Laceration of popliteal vein, **right** leg `MCC`

√7ᵗʰ **S85.512** Laceration of popliteal vein, **left** leg `MCC`

√7ᵗʰ **S85.519** Laceration of popliteal vein, unspecified leg `MCC`

√6ᵗʰ **S85.59** Other specified injury of popliteal vein

√7ᵗʰ **S85.591** Other specified injury of popliteal vein, **right** leg `MCC`

√7ᵗʰ **S85.592** Other specified injury of popliteal vein, **left** leg `MCC`

√7ᵗʰ **S85.599** Other specified injury of popliteal vein, unspecified leg `MCC`

√5ᵗʰ **S85.8** Injury of other blood vessels at lower leg level

CC Excl: For CC codes in subcategory S85.8:
Right side: PDX collection 1325
Left side: PDX collection 1326
Unspecified side: PDX collection 1327

√6ᵗʰ **S85.80** Unspecified injury of other blood vessels at lower leg level

√7ᵗʰ **S85.801** Unspecified injury of other blood vessels at lower leg level, **right** leg `CC`

√7ᵗʰ **S85.802** Unspecified injury of other blood vessels at lower leg level, **left** leg `CC`

√7ᵗʰ **S85.809** Unspecified injury of other blood vessels at lower leg level, unspecified leg `CC`

√6ᵗʰ **S85.81** Laceration of other blood vessels at lower leg level

√7ᵗʰ **S85.811** Laceration of other blood vessels at lower leg level, **right** leg `CC`

√7ᵗʰ **S85.812** Laceration of other blood vessels at lower leg level, **left** leg `CC`

√7ᵗʰ **S85.819** Laceration of other blood vessels at lower leg level, unspecified leg `CC`

√6ᵗʰ **S85.89** Other specified injury of other blood vessels at lower leg level

√7ᵗʰ **S85.891** Other specified injury of other blood vessels at lower leg level, **right** leg `CC`

√7ᵗʰ **S85.892** Other specified injury of other blood vessels at lower leg level, **left** leg `CC`

√7ᵗʰ **S85.899** Other specified injury of other blood vessels at lower leg level, unspecified leg `CC`

√5ᵗʰ **S85.9** Injury of unspecified blood vessel at lower leg level

CC Excl: For CC codes in subcategory S85.9:
Right side: PDX collection 1325
Left side: PDX collection 1326
Unspecified side: PDX collection 1327

√6ᵗʰ **S85.90** Unspecified injury of unspecified blood vessel at lower leg level

√7ᵗʰ **S85.901** Unspecified injury of unspecified blood vessel at lower leg level, **right** leg `CC`

√7ᵗʰ **S85.902** Unspecified injury of unspecified blood vessel at lower leg level, **left** leg `CC`

√7ᵗʰ **S85.909** Unspecified injury of unspecified blood vessel at lower leg level, unspecified leg `CC`

√6ᵗʰ **S85.91** Laceration of unspecified blood vessel at lower leg level

√7ᵗʰ **S85.911** Laceration of unspecified blood vessel at lower leg level, **right** leg `CC`

√7ᵗʰ **S85.912** Laceration of unspecified blood vessel at lower leg level, **left** leg `CC`

√7ᵗʰ **S85.919** Laceration of unspecified blood vessel at lower leg level, unspecified leg `CC`

√6ᵗʰ **S85.99** Other specified injury of unspecified blood vessel at lower leg level

√7ᵗʰ **S85.991** Other specified injury of unspecified blood vessel at lower leg level, **right** leg `CC`

√7ᵗʰ **S85.992** Other specified injury of unspecified blood vessel at lower leg level, **left** leg `CC`

√7ᵗʰ **S85.999** Other specified injury of unspecified blood vessel at lower leg level, unspecified leg `CC`

√4ᵗʰ **S86** **Injury of muscle, fascia and tendon at lower leg level**

Code also any associated open wound (S81.-)

EXCLUDES 2 *injury of muscle, fascia and tendon at ankle (S96.-)*
injury of patellar ligament (tendon) (S76.1-)
sprain of joints and ligaments of knee (S83.-)

TIP: Refer to the Muscle/Tendon table at the beginning of this chapter.

The appropriate 7th character is to be added to each code from category S86.
A   initial encounter
D   subsequent encounter
S   sequela

CC Excl: For CC codes in category S86:
Right side: PDX collection 1364
Left side: PDX collection 1365
Unspecified side: PDX collection 1366

√5ᵗʰ **S86.0** Injury of Achilles tendon

√6ᵗʰ **S86.00** Unspecified injury of Achilles tendon

√7ᵗʰ **S86.001** Unspecified injury of **right** Achilles tendon

√7ᵗʰ **S86.002** Unspecified injury of **left** Achilles tendon

√7ᵗʰ **S86.009** Unspecified injury of unspecified Achilles tendon

√6ᵗʰ **S86.01** Strain of Achilles tendon

√7ᵗʰ **S86.011** Strain of **right** Achilles tendon

√7ᵗʰ **S86.012** Strain of **left** Achilles tendon

√7ᵗʰ **S86.019** **Strain of unspecified Achilles tendon**

√6ᵗʰ **S86.02** **Laceration of Achilles tendon**

    √7ᵗʰ **S86.021** **Laceration of** right **Achilles tendon**   CC

    √7ᵗʰ **S86.022** **Laceration of** left **Achilles tendon**   CC

    √7ᵗʰ **S86.029** **Laceration of unspecified Achilles tendon**   CC

√6ᵗʰ **S86.09** **Other specified injury of Achilles tendon·**

    √7ᵗʰ **S86.091** **Other specified injury of** right **Achilles tendon**

    √7ᵗʰ **S86.092** **Other specified injury of** left **Achilles tendon**

    √7ᵗʰ **S86.099** **Other specified injury of unspecified Achilles tendon**

√5ᵗʰ **S86.1** **Injury of other muscle(s) and tendon(s) of** posterior muscle group **at lower leg level**

√6ᵗʰ **S86.10** **Unspecified injury of other muscle(s) and tendon(s) of posterior muscle group at lower leg level**

    √7ᵗʰ **S86.101** **Unspecified injury of other muscle(s) and tendon(s) of posterior muscle group at lower leg level,** right leg

    √7ᵗʰ **S86.102** **Unspecified injury of other muscle(s) and tendon(s) of posterior muscle group at lower leg level,** left leg

    √7ᵗʰ **S86.109** **Unspecified injury of other muscle(s) and tendon(s) of posterior muscle group at lower leg level, unspecified leg**

√6ᵗʰ **S86.11** **Strain of other muscle(s) and tendon(s) of posterior muscle group at lower leg level**

    √7ᵗʰ **S86.111** **Strain of other muscle(s) and tendon(s) of posterior muscle group at lower leg level,** right leg

    √7ᵗʰ **S86.112** **Strain of other muscle(s) and tendon(s) of posterior muscle group at lower leg level,** left leg

    √7ᵗʰ **S86.119** **Strain of other muscle(s) and tendon(s) of posterior muscle group at lower leg level, unspecified leg**

√6ᵗʰ **S86.12** **Laceration of other muscle(s) and tendon(s) of posterior muscle group at lower leg level**

    √7ᵗʰ **S86.121** **Laceration of other muscle(s) and tendon(s) of posterior muscle group at lower leg level,** right leg   CC

    √7ᵗʰ **S86.122** **Laceration of other muscle(s) and tendon(s) of posterior muscle group at lower leg level,** left leg   CC

    √7ᵗʰ **S86.129** **Laceration of other muscle(s) and tendon(s) of posterior muscle group at lower leg level, unspecified leg**   CC

√6ᵗʰ **S86.19** **Other injury of other muscle(s) and tendon(s) of posterior muscle group at lower leg level**

    √7ᵗʰ **S86.191** **Other injury of other muscle(s) and tendon(s) of posterior muscle group at lower leg level,** right leg

    √7ᵗʰ **S86.192** **Other injury of other muscle(s) and tendon(s) of posterior muscle group at lower leg level,** left leg

    √7ᵗʰ **S86.199** **Other injury of other muscle(s) and tendon(s) of posterior muscle group at lower leg level, unspecified leg**

√5ᵗʰ **S86.2** **Injury of muscle(s) and tendon(s) of** anterior muscle group **at lower leg level**

√6ᵗʰ **S86.20** **Unspecified injury of muscle(s) and tendon(s) of anterior muscle group at lower leg level**

    √7ᵗʰ **S86.201** **Unspecified injury of muscle(s) and tendon(s) of anterior muscle group at lower leg level,** right leg

    √7ᵗʰ **S86.202** **Unspecified injury of muscle(s) and tendon(s) of anterior muscle group at lower leg level,** left leg

    √7ᵗʰ **S86.209** **Unspecified injury of muscle(s) and tendon(s) of anterior muscle group at lower leg level, unspecified leg**

√6ᵗʰ **S86.21** **Strain of muscle(s) and tendon(s) of anterior muscle group at lower leg level**

    √7ᵗʰ **S86.211** **Strain of muscle(s) and tendon(s) of anterior muscle group at lower leg level,** right leg

√7ᵗʰ **S86.212** **Strain of muscle(s) and tendon(s) of anterior muscle group at lower leg level,** left leg

√7ᵗʰ **S86.219** **Strain of muscle(s) and tendon(s) of anterior muscle group at lower leg level, unspecified leg**

√6ᵗʰ **S86.22** **Laceration of muscle(s) and tendon(s) of anterior muscle group at lower leg level**

    √7ᵗʰ **S86.221** **Laceration of muscle(s) and tendon(s) of anterior muscle group at lower leg level,** right leg   CC

    √7ᵗʰ **S86.222** **Laceration of muscle(s) and tendon(s) of anterior muscle group at lower leg level,** left leg   CC

    √7ᵗʰ **S86.229** **Laceration of muscle(s) and tendon(s) of anterior muscle group at lower leg level, unspecified leg**   CC

√6ᵗʰ **S86.29** **Other injury of muscle(s) and tendon(s) of anterior muscle group at lower leg level**

    √7ᵗʰ **S86.291** **Other injury of muscle(s) and tendon(s) of anterior muscle group at lower leg level,** right leg

    √7ᵗʰ **S86.292** **Other injury of muscle(s) and tendon(s) of anterior muscle group at lower leg level,** left leg

    √7ᵗʰ **S86.299** **Other injury of muscle(s) and tendon(s) of anterior muscle group at lower leg level, unspecified leg**

√5ᵗʰ **S86.3** **Injury of muscle(s) and tendon(s) of** peroneal muscle group **at lower leg level**

√6ᵗʰ **S86.30** **Unspecified injury of muscle(s) and tendon(s) of peroneal muscle group at lower leg level**

    √7ᵗʰ **S86.301** **Unspecified injury of muscle(s) and tendon(s) of peroneal muscle group at lower leg level,** right leg

    √7ᵗʰ **S86.302** **Unspecified injury of muscle(s) and tendon(s) of peroneal muscle group at lower leg level,** left leg

    √7ᵗʰ **S86.309** **Unspecified injury of muscle(s) and tendon(s) of peroneal muscle group at lower leg level, unspecified leg**

√6ᵗʰ **S86.31** **Strain of muscle(s) and tendon(s) of peroneal muscle group at lower leg level**

    √7ᵗʰ **S86.311** **Strain of muscle(s) and tendon(s) of peroneal muscle group at lower leg level,** right leg

    √7ᵗʰ **S86.312** **Strain of muscle(s) and tendon(s) of peroneal muscle group at lower leg level,** left leg

    √7ᵗʰ **S86.319** **Strain of muscle(s) and tendon(s) of peroneal muscle group at lower leg level, unspecified leg**

√6ᵗʰ **S86.32** **Laceration of muscle(s) and tendon(s) of peroneal muscle group at lower leg level**

    √7ᵗʰ **S86.321** **Laceration of muscle(s) and tendon(s) of peroneal muscle group at lower leg level,** right leg   CC

    √7ᵗʰ **S86.322** **Laceration of muscle(s) and tendon(s) of peroneal muscle group at lower leg level,** left leg   CC

    √7ᵗʰ **S86.329** **Laceration of muscle(s) and tendon(s) of peroneal muscle group at lower leg level, unspecified leg**   CC

√6ᵗʰ **S86.39** **Other injury of muscle(s) and tendon(s) of peroneal muscle group at lower leg level**

    √7ᵗʰ **S86.391** **Other injury of muscle(s) and tendon(s) of peroneal muscle group at lower leg level,** right leg

    √7ᵗʰ **S86.392** **Other injury of muscle(s) and tendon(s) of peroneal muscle group at lower leg level,** left leg

    √7ᵗʰ **S86.399** **Other injury of muscle(s) and tendon(s) of peroneal muscle group at lower leg level, unspecified leg**

√5ᵗʰ **S86.8** **Injury of other muscles and tendons at lower leg level**

√6ᵗʰ **S86.80** **Unspecified injury of other muscles and tendons at lower leg level**

    √7ᵗʰ **S86.801** **Unspecified injury of other muscle(s) and tendon(s) at lower leg level,** right leg

☑ Additional Character Required   √x7ᵗʰ Placeholder   Unacceptable PDx   Questionable PDx   Manifestation   Unspecified Dx   H1–H14 HAC   HCC CMS-HCC Dx   HIV HIV Dx

ICD-10-CM 2020   **1109**

√7ᵗʰ **S86.802** Unspecified injury of other muscle(s) and tendon(s) at lower leg level, **left** leg

√7ᵗʰ **S86.809** Unspecified injury of other muscle(s) and tendon(s) at lower leg level, unspecified leg

√6ᵗʰ **S86.81** Strain of other muscles and tendons at lower leg level

√7ᵗʰ **S86.811** Strain of other muscle(s) and tendon(s) at lower leg level, **right** leg

√7ᵗʰ **S86.812** Strain of other muscle(s) and tendon(s) at lower leg level, **left** leg

√7ᵗʰ **S86.819** Strain of other muscle(s) and tendon(s) at lower leg level, unspecified leg

√6ᵗʰ **S86.82** Laceration of other muscles and tendons at lower leg level

√7ᵗʰ **S86.821** Laceration of other muscle(s) and tendon(s) at lower leg level, **right** leg   `CC`

√7ᵗʰ **S86.822** Laceration of other muscle(s) and tendon(s) at lower leg level, **left** leg   `CC`

√7ᵗʰ **S86.829** Laceration of other muscle(s) and tendon(s) at lower leg level, unspecified leg   `CC`

√6ᵗʰ **S86.89** Other injury of other muscles and tendons at lower leg level

√7ᵗʰ **S86.891** Other injury of other muscle(s) and tendon(s) at lower leg level, **right** leg

√7ᵗʰ **S86.892** Other injury of other muscle(s) and tendon(s) at lower leg level, **left** leg

√7ᵗʰ **S86.899** Other injury of other muscle(s) and tendon(s) at lower leg level, unspecified leg

√5ᵗʰ **S86.9** Injury of unspecified muscle and tendon at lower leg level

√6ᵗʰ **S86.90** Unspecified injury of unspecified muscle and tendon at lower leg level

√7ᵗʰ **S86.901** Unspecified injury of unspecified muscle(s) and tendon(s) at lower leg level, **right** leg

√7ᵗʰ **S86.902** Unspecified injury of unspecified muscle(s) and tendon(s) at lower leg level, **left** leg

√7ᵗʰ **S86.909** Unspecified injury of unspecified muscle(s) and tendon(s) at lower leg level, unspecified leg

√6ᵗʰ **S86.91** Strain of unspecified muscle and tendon at lower leg level

√7ᵗʰ **S86.911** Strain of unspecified muscle(s) and tendon(s) at lower leg level, **right** leg

√7ᵗʰ **S86.912** Strain of unspecified muscle(s) and tendon(s) at lower leg level, **left** leg

√7ᵗʰ **S86.919** Strain of unspecified muscle(s) and tendon(s) at lower leg level, unspecified leg

√6ᵗʰ **S86.92** Laceration of unspecified muscle and tendon at lower leg level

√7ᵗʰ **S86.921** Laceration of unspecified muscle(s) and tendon(s) at lower leg level, **right** leg   `CC`

√7ᵗʰ **S86.922** Laceration of unspecified muscle(s) and tendon(s) at lower leg level, **left** leg   `CC`

√7ᵗʰ **S86.929** Laceration of unspecified muscle(s) and tendon(s) at lower leg level, unspecified leg   `CC`

√6ᵗʰ **S86.99** Other injury of unspecified muscle and tendon at lower leg level

√7ᵗʰ **S86.991** Other injury of unspecified muscle(s) and tendon(s) at lower leg level, **right** leg

√7ᵗʰ **S86.992** Other injury of unspecified muscle(s) and tendon(s) at lower leg level, **left** leg

√7ᵗʰ **S86.999** Other injury of unspecified muscle(s) and tendon(s) at lower leg level, unspecified leg

√4ᵗʰ **S87** Crushing injury of lower leg

Use additional code(s) for all associated injuries

EXCLUDES 2   crushing injury of ankle and foot (S97.-)

The appropriate 7th character is to be added to each code from category S87.
A   initial encounter
D   subsequent encounter
S   sequela

√5ᵗʰ **S87.0** Crushing injury of knee

√x7ᵗʰ **S87.00** Crushing injury of unspecified knee

√x7ᵗʰ **S87.01** Crushing injury of **right** knee

√x7ᵗʰ **S87.02** Crushing injury of **left** knee

√5ᵗʰ **S87.8** Crushing injury of lower leg

√x7ᵗʰ **S87.80** Crushing injury of unspecified lower leg

√x7ᵗʰ **S87.81** Crushing injury of **right** lower leg

√x7ᵗʰ **S87.82** Crushing injury of **left** lower leg

√4ᵗʰ **S88** Traumatic amputation of lower leg

An amputation not identified as partial or complete should be coded to complete

EXCLUDES 1   traumatic amputation of ankle and foot (S98.-)

The appropriate 7th character is to be added to each code from category S88.
A   initial encounter
D   subsequent encounter
S   sequela

CC Excl: For CC codes in category S88:
Right side: PDX collection 1333
Left side: PDX collection 1334
Unspecified side: PDX collection 1335

√5ᵗʰ **S88.0** Traumatic amputation at knee level

√6ᵗʰ **S88.01** Complete traumatic amputation at knee level

√7ᵗʰ **S88.011** Complete traumatic amputation at knee level, **right** lower leg   `CC` `HCC`

√7ᵗʰ **S88.012** Complete traumatic amputation at knee level, **left** lower leg   `CC` `HCC`

√7ᵗʰ **S88.019** Complete traumatic amputation at knee level, unspecified lower leg   `CC` `HCC`

√6ᵗʰ **S88.02** Partial traumatic amputation at knee level

√7ᵗʰ **S88.021** Partial traumatic amputation at knee level, **right** lower leg   `CC` `HCC`

√7ᵗʰ **S88.022** Partial traumatic amputation at knee level, **left** lower leg   `CC` `HCC`

√7ᵗʰ **S88.029** Partial traumatic amputation at knee level, unspecified lower leg   `CC` `HCC`

√5ᵗʰ **S88.1** Traumatic amputation at level between knee and ankle

√6ᵗʰ **S88.11** Complete traumatic amputation at level between knee and ankle

√7ᵗʰ **S88.111** Complete traumatic amputation at level between knee and ankle, **right** lower leg   `CC` `HCC`

√7ᵗʰ **S88.112** Complete traumatic amputation at level between knee and ankle, **left** lower leg   `CC` `HCC`

√7ᵗʰ **S88.119** Complete traumatic amputation at level between knee and ankle, unspecified lower leg   `CC` `HCC`

√6ᵗʰ **S88.12** Partial traumatic amputation at level between knee and ankle

√7ᵗʰ **S88.121** Partial traumatic amputation at level between knee and ankle, **right** lower leg   `CC` `HCC`

√7ᵗʰ **S88.122** Partial traumatic amputation at level between knee and ankle, **left** lower leg   `CC` `HCC`

√7ᵗʰ **S88.129** Partial traumatic amputation at level between knee and ankle, unspecified lower leg `CC` `HCC`

√5ᵗʰ **S88.9** Traumatic amputation of lower leg, level unspecified

  √6ᵗʰ **S88.91** Complete traumatic amputation of lower leg, level unspecified

    √7ᵗʰ **S88.911** Complete traumatic amputation of right lower leg, level unspecified `CC` `HCC`

    √7ᵗʰ **S88.912** Complete traumatic amputation of left lower leg, level unspecified `CC` `HCC`

    √7ᵗʰ **S88.919** Complete traumatic amputation of unspecified lower leg, level unspecified `CC` `HCC`

  √6ᵗʰ **S88.92** Partial traumatic amputation of lower leg, level unspecified

    √7ᵗʰ **S88.921** Partial traumatic amputation of right lower leg, level unspecified `CC` `HCC`

    √7ᵗʰ **S88.922** Partial traumatic amputation of left lower leg, level unspecified `CC` `HCC`

    √7ᵗʰ **S88.929** Partial traumatic amputation of unspecified lower leg, level unspecified `CC` `HCC`

√4ᵗʰ **S89 Other and unspecified injuries of lower leg**

> **NOTE** A fracture not indicated as open or closed should be coded to closed.
>
> *EXCLUDES 2* *other and unspecified injuries of ankle and foot (S99.-)*
>
> **AHA:** 2018,2Q,12; 2018,1Q,3; 2015,3Q,37-39

The appropriate 7th character is to be added to each code from subcategories S89.0, S89.1, S89.2, and S89.3.
A   initial encounter for closed fracture
D   subsequent encounter for fracture with routine healing
G   subsequent encounter for fracture with delayed healing
K   subsequent encounter for fracture with nonunion
P   subsequent encounter for fracture with malunion
S   sequela

√5ᵗʰ **S89.0** Physeal fracture of upper end of tibia

> **CC Excl: For CC codes in subcategory S89.0:**
> **Right side:** See code S89.001
> **Left side:** See code S89.002
> **Unspecified side:** See code S89.009

  √6ᵗʰ **S89.00** Unspecified physeal fracture of upper end of tibia

    3 √7ᵗʰ **S89.001** Unspecified physeal fracture of upper end of right tibia `CC` `H5`
> **CC Excl: CC with 7th character A:** PDX collection 1340
> **CC Excl: CC with 7th character K or P:** PDX collection 897

    3 √7ᵗʰ **S89.002** Unspecified physeal fracture of upper end of left tibia `CC` `H5`
> **CC Excl: CC with 7th character A:** PDX collection 1342
> **CC Excl: CC with 7th character K or P:** PDX collection 897

    3 √7ᵗʰ **S89.009** Unspecified physeal fracture of upper end of unspecified tibia `CC` `H5`
> **CC Excl: CC with 7th character A:** PDX collection 1341
> **CC Excl: CC with 7th character K or P:** PDX collection 897

  √6ᵗʰ **S89.01** Salter-Harris Type I physeal fracture of upper end of tibia

    3 √7ᵗʰ **S89.011** Salter-Harris Type I physeal fracture of upper end of right tibia `CC` `H5`

    3 √7ᵗʰ **S89.012** Salter-Harris Type I physeal fracture of upper end of left tibia `CC` `H5`

    3 √7ᵗʰ **S89.019** Salter-Harris Type I physeal fracture of upper end of unspecified tibia `CC` `H5`

√6ᵗʰ **S89.02** Salter-Harris Type II physeal fracture of upper end of tibia

  3 √7ᵗʰ **S89.021** Salter-Harris Type II physeal fracture of upper end of right tibia `CC` `H5`

  3 √7ᵗʰ **S89.022** Salter-Harris Type II physeal fracture of upper end of left tibia `CC` `H5`

  3 √7ᵗʰ **S89.029** Salter-Harris Type II physeal fracture of upper end of unspecified tibia `CC` `H5`

√6ᵗʰ **S89.03** Salter-Harris Type III physeal fracture of upper end of tibia

  3 √7ᵗʰ **S89.031** Salter-Harris Type III physeal fracture of upper end of right tibia `CC` `H5`

  3 √7ᵗʰ **S89.032** Salter-Harris Type III physeal fracture of upper end of left tibia `CC` `H5`

  3 √7ᵗʰ **S89.039** Salter-Harris Type III physeal fracture of upper end of unspecified tibia `CC` `H5`

√6ᵗʰ **S89.04** Salter-Harris Type IV physeal fracture of upper end of tibia

  3 √7ᵗʰ **S89.041** Salter-Harris Type IV physeal fracture of upper end of right tibia `CC` `H5`

  3 √7ᵗʰ **S89.042** Salter-Harris Type IV physeal fracture of upper end of left tibia `CC` `H5`

  3 √7ᵗʰ **S89.049** Salter-Harris Type IV physeal fracture of upper end of unspecified tibia `CC` `H5`

√6ᵗʰ **S89.09** Other physeal fracture of upper end of tibia

  3 √7ᵗʰ **S89.091** Other physeal fracture of upper end of right tibia `CC` `H5`

  3 √7ᵗʰ **S89.092** Other physeal fracture of upper end of left tibia `CC` `H5`

  3 √7ᵗʰ **S89.099** Other physeal fracture of upper end of unspecified tibia `CC` `H5`

√5ᵗʰ **S89.1** Physeal fracture of lower end of tibia

> **CC Excl: For codes in subcategory S89.1:**
> **CC with 7th character K or P:** PDX collection 897

  √6ᵗʰ **S89.10** Unspecified physeal fracture of lower end of tibia

    4 √7ᵗʰ **S89.101** Unspecified physeal fracture of lower end of right tibia `CC`

    4 √7ᵗʰ **S89.102** Unspecified physeal fracture of lower end of left tibia `CC`

    4 √7ᵗʰ **S89.109** Unspecified physeal fracture of lower end of unspecified tibia `CC`

  √6ᵗʰ **S89.11** Salter-Harris Type I physeal fracture of lower end of tibia

    4 √7ᵗʰ **S89.111** Salter-Harris Type I physeal fracture of lower end of right tibia `CC`

    4 √7ᵗʰ **S89.112** Salter-Harris Type I physeal fracture of lower end of left tibia `CC`

    4 √7ᵗʰ **S89.119** Salter-Harris Type I physeal fracture of lower end of unspecified tibia `CC`

  √6ᵗʰ **S89.12** Salter-Harris Type II physeal fracture of lower end of tibia

    4 √7ᵗʰ **S89.121** Salter-Harris Type II physeal fracture of lower end of right tibia `CC`

    4 √7ᵗʰ **S89.122** Salter-Harris Type II physeal fracture of lower end of left tibia `CC`

    4 √7ᵗʰ **S89.129** Salter-Harris Type II physeal fracture of lower end of unspecified tibia `CC`

  √6ᵗʰ **S89.13** Salter-Harris Type III physeal fracture of lower end of tibia

> *EXCLUDES 1* *fracture of medial malleolus (adult) (S82.5-)*

    4 √7ᵗʰ **S89.131** Salter-Harris Type III physeal fracture of lower end of right tibia `CC`

Chapter 19. Injury, Poisoning and Certain Other Consequences of External Causes

S89.132–S90.119

4 √7ᵗʰ **S89.132** Salter-Harris Type III physeal fracture of lower end of left tibia   CC

4 √7ᵗʰ **S89.139** Salter-Harris Type III physeal fracture of lower end of unspecified tibia   CC

√6ᵗʰ **S89.14** Salter-Harris Type IV physeal fracture of lower end of tibia

> EXCLUDES 1   fracture of medial malleolus (adult) (S82.5-)

4 √7ᵗʰ **S89.141** Salter-Harris Type IV physeal fracture of lower end of right tibia   CC

4 √7ᵗʰ **S89.142** Salter-Harris Type IV physeal fracture of lower end of left tibia   CC

4 √7ᵗʰ **S89.149** Salter-Harris Type IV physeal fracture of lower end of unspecified tibia   CC

√6ᵗʰ **S89.19** Other physeal fracture of lower end of tibia

4 √7ᵗʰ **S89.191** Other physeal fracture of lower end of right tibia   CC

4 √7ᵗʰ **S89.192** Other physeal fracture of lower end of left tibia   CC

4 √7ᵗʰ **S89.199** Other physeal fracture of lower end of unspecified tibia   CC

√5ᵗʰ **S89.2** Physeal fracture of upper end of fibula

> CC Excl: For codes in subcategory S89.2:
> CC with 7th character K or P: PDX collection 897

√6ᵗʰ **S89.20** Unspecified physeal fracture of upper end of fibula

4 √7ᵗʰ **S89.201** Unspecified physeal fracture of upper end of right fibula   CC

4 √7ᵗʰ **S89.202** Unspecified physeal fracture of upper end of left fibula   CC

4 √7ᵗʰ **S89.209** Unspecified physeal fracture of upper end of unspecified fibula   CC

√6ᵗʰ **S89.21** Salter-Harris Type I physeal fracture of upper end of fibula

4 √7ᵗʰ **S89.211** Salter-Harris Type I physeal fracture of upper end of right fibula   CC

4 √7ᵗʰ **S89.212** Salter-Harris Type I physeal fracture of upper end of left fibula   CC

4 √7ᵗʰ **S89.219** Salter-Harris Type I physeal fracture of upper end of unspecified fibula   CC

√6ᵗʰ **S89.22** Salter-Harris Type II physeal fracture of upper end of fibula

4 √7ᵗʰ **S89.221** Salter-Harris Type II physeal fracture of upper end of right fibula   CC

4 √7ᵗʰ **S89.222** Salter-Harris Type II physeal fracture of upper end of left fibula   CC

4 √7ᵗʰ **S89.229** Salter-Harris Type II physeal fracture of upper end of unspecified fibula   CC

√6ᵗʰ **S89.29** Other physeal fracture of upper end of fibula

4 √7ᵗʰ **S89.291** Other physeal fracture of upper end of right fibula   CC

4 √7ᵗʰ **S89.292** Other physeal fracture of upper end of left fibula   CC

4 √7ᵗʰ **S89.299** Other physeal fracture of upper end of unspecified fibula   CC

√5ᵗʰ **S89.3** Physeal fracture of lower end of fibula

> CC Excl: For codes in subcategory S89.3:
> CC with 7th character K or P: PDX collection 897

√6ᵗʰ **S89.30** Unspecified physeal fracture of lower end of fibula

4 √7ᵗʰ **S89.301** Unspecified physeal fracture of lower end of right fibula   CC

4 √7ᵗʰ **S89.302** Unspecified physeal fracture of lower end of left fibula   CC

4 √7ᵗʰ **S89.309** Unspecified physeal fracture of lower end of unspecified fibula   CC

√6ᵗʰ **S89.31** Salter-Harris Type I physeal fracture of lower end of fibula

4 √7ᵗʰ **S89.311** Salter-Harris Type I physeal fracture of lower end of right fibula   CC

4 √7ᵗʰ **S89.312** Salter-Harris Type I physeal fracture of lower end of left fibula   CC

4 √7ᵗʰ **S89.319** Salter-Harris Type I physeal fracture of lower end of unspecified fibula   CC

√6ᵗʰ **S89.32** Salter-Harris Type II physeal fracture of lower end of fibula

4 √7ᵗʰ **S89.321** Salter-Harris Type II physeal fracture of lower end of right fibula   CC

4 √7ᵗʰ **S89.322** Salter-Harris Type II physeal fracture of lower end of left fibula   CC

4 √7ᵗʰ **S89.329** Salter-Harris Type II physeal fracture of lower end of unspecified fibula   CC

√6ᵗʰ **S89.39** Other physeal fracture of lower end of fibula

4 √7ᵗʰ **S89.391** Other physeal fracture of lower end of right fibula   CC

4 √7ᵗʰ **S89.392** Other physeal fracture of lower end of left fibula   CC

4 √7ᵗʰ **S89.399** Other physeal fracture of lower end of unspecified fibula   CC

√5ᵗʰ **S89.8** Other specified injuries of lower leg

> The appropriate 7th character is to be added to each code in subcategory S89.8.
> A   initial encounter
> D   subsequent encounter
> S   sequela

√x7ᵗʰ **S89.80** Other specified injuries of unspecified lower leg

√x7ᵗʰ **S89.81** Other specified injuries of right lower leg

√x7ᵗʰ **S89.82** Other specified injuries of left lower leg

√5ᵗʰ **S89.9** Unspecified injury of lower leg

> The appropriate 7th character is to be added to each code in subcategory S89.9.
> A   initial encounter
> D   subsequent encounter
> S   sequela

√x7ᵗʰ **S89.90** Unspecified injury of unspecified lower leg

√x7ᵗʰ **S89.91** Unspecified injury of right lower leg

√x7ᵗʰ **S89.92** Unspecified injury of left lower leg

Injuries to the ankle and foot (S90-S99)

> EXCLUDES 2   burns and corrosions (T20-T32)
> fracture of ankle and malleolus (S82.-)
> frostbite (T33-T34)
> insect bite or sting, venomous (T63.4)

√4ᵗʰ **S90** Superficial injury of ankle, foot and toes

> The appropriate 7th character is to be added to each code from category S90.
> A   initial encounter
> D   subsequent encounter
> S   sequela

√5ᵗʰ **S90.0** Contusion of ankle

√x7ᵗʰ **S90.00** Contusion of unspecified ankle

√x7ᵗʰ **S90.01** Contusion of right ankle

√x7ᵗʰ **S90.02** Contusion of left ankle

√5ᵗʰ **S90.1** Contusion of toe without damage to nail

√6ᵗʰ **S90.11** Contusion of great toe without damage to nail

√7ᵗʰ **S90.111** Contusion of right great toe without damage to nail

√7ᵗʰ **S90.112** Contusion of left great toe without damage to nail

√7ᵗʰ **S90.119** Contusion of unspecified great toe without damage to nail

N Newborn: 0   P Pediatric: 0-17   M Maternity: 9-64   A Adult: 15-124   MCC Major Complication/Comorbidity   CC Complication/Comorbidity   SW Severe Wound Dx

1112   ICD-10-CM 2020

√6ᵗʰ **S90.12** Contusion of lesser toe without damage to nail
- √7ᵗʰ **S90.121** Contusion of right lesser toe(s) without damage to nail
- √7ᵗʰ **S90.122** Contusion of left lesser toe(s) without damage to nail
- √7ᵗʰ **S90.129** Contusion of unspecified lesser toe(s) without damage to nail
  Contusion of toe NOS

√5ᵗʰ **S90.2** Contusion of toe with damage to nail
- √6ᵗʰ **S90.21** Contusion of great toe with damage to nail
  - √7ᵗʰ **S90.211** Contusion of right great toe with damage to nail
  - √7ᵗʰ **S90.212** Contusion of left great toe with damage to nail
  - √7ᵗʰ **S90.219** Contusion of unspecified great toe with damage to nail
- √6ᵗʰ **S90.22** Contusion of lesser toe with damage to nail
  - √7ᵗʰ **S90.221** Contusion of right lesser toe(s) with damage to nail
  - √7ᵗʰ **S90.222** Contusion of left lesser toe(s) with damage to nail
  - √7ᵗʰ **S90.229** Contusion of unspecified lesser toe(s) with damage to nail

√5ᵗʰ **S90.3** Contusion of foot
  EXCLUDES 2   contusion of toes (S90.1-, S90.2-)
- √×7ᵗʰ **S90.30** Contusion of unspecified foot
  Contusion of foot NOS
- √×7ᵗʰ **S90.31** Contusion of right foot
- √×7ᵗʰ **S90.32** Contusion of left foot

√5ᵗʰ **S90.4** Other superficial injuries of toe
- √6ᵗʰ **S90.41** Abrasion of toe
  - √7ᵗʰ **S90.411** Abrasion, right great toe
  - √7ᵗʰ **S90.412** Abrasion, left great toe
  - √7ᵗʰ **S90.413** Abrasion, unspecified great toe
  - √7ᵗʰ **S90.414** Abrasion, right lesser toe(s)
  - √7ᵗʰ **S90.415** Abrasion, left lesser toe(s)
  - √7ᵗʰ **S90.416** Abrasion, unspecified lesser toe(s)
- √6ᵗʰ **S90.42** Blister (nonthermal) of toe
  - √7ᵗʰ **S90.421** Blister (nonthermal), right great toe
  - √7ᵗʰ **S90.422** Blister (nonthermal), left great toe
  - √7ᵗʰ **S90.423** Blister (nonthermal), unspecified great toe
  - √7ᵗʰ **S90.424** Blister (nonthermal), right lesser toe(s)
  - √7ᵗʰ **S90.425** Blister (nonthermal), left lesser toe(s)
  - √7ᵗʰ **S90.426** Blister (nonthermal), unspecified lesser toe(s)
- √6ᵗʰ **S90.44** External constriction of toe
  Hair tourniquet syndrome of toe
  - √7ᵗʰ **S90.441** External constriction, right great toe
  - √7ᵗʰ **S90.442** External constriction, left great toe
  - √7ᵗʰ **S90.443** External constriction, unspecified great toe
  - √7ᵗʰ **S90.444** External constriction, right lesser toe(s)
  - √7ᵗʰ **S90.445** External constriction, left lesser toe(s)
  - √7ᵗʰ **S90.446** External constriction, unspecified lesser toe(s)
- √6ᵗʰ **S90.45** Superficial foreign body of toe
  Splinter in the toe
  - √7ᵗʰ **S90.451** Superficial foreign body, right great toe
  - √7ᵗʰ **S90.452** Superficial foreign body, left great toe
  - √7ᵗʰ **S90.453** Superficial foreign body, unspecified great toe
  - √7ᵗʰ **S90.454** Superficial foreign body, right lesser toe(s)
  - √7ᵗʰ **S90.455** Superficial foreign body, left lesser toe(s)
  - √7ᵗʰ **S90.456** Superficial foreign body, unspecified lesser toe(s)
- √6ᵗʰ **S90.46** Insect bite (nonvenomous) of toe
  - √7ᵗʰ **S90.461** Insect bite (nonvenomous), right great toe
  - √7ᵗʰ **S90.462** Insect bite (nonvenomous), left great toe
  - √7ᵗʰ **S90.463** Insect bite (nonvenomous), unspecified great toe

- √7ᵗʰ **S90.464** Insect bite (nonvenomous), right lesser toe(s)
- √7ᵗʰ **S90.465** Insect bite (nonvenomous), left lesser toe(s)
- √7ᵗʰ **S90.466** Insect bite (nonvenomous), unspecified lesser toe(s)

√6ᵗʰ **S90.47** Other superficial bite of toe
  EXCLUDES 1   open bite of toe (S91.15-, S91.25-)
- √7ᵗʰ **S90.471** Other superficial bite of right great toe
- √7ᵗʰ **S90.472** Other superficial bite of left great toe
- √7ᵗʰ **S90.473** Other superficial bite of unspecified great toe
- √7ᵗʰ **S90.474** Other superficial bite of right lesser toe(s)
- √7ᵗʰ **S90.475** Other superficial bite of left lesser toe(s)
- √7ᵗʰ **S90.476** Other superficial bite of unspecified lesser toe(s)

√5ᵗʰ **S90.5** Other superficial injuries of ankle
- √6ᵗʰ **S90.51** Abrasion of ankle
  - √7ᵗʰ **S90.511** Abrasion, right ankle
  - √7ᵗʰ **S90.512** Abrasion, left ankle
  - √7ᵗʰ **S90.519** Abrasion, unspecified ankle
- √6ᵗʰ **S90.52** Blister (nonthermal) of ankle
  - √7ᵗʰ **S90.521** Blister (nonthermal), right ankle
  - √7ᵗʰ **S90.522** Blister (nonthermal), left ankle
  - √7ᵗʰ **S90.529** Blister (nonthermal), unspecified ankle
- √6ᵗʰ **S90.54** External constriction of ankle
  - √7ᵗʰ **S90.541** External constriction, right ankle
  - √7ᵗʰ **S90.542** External constriction, left ankle
  - √7ᵗʰ **S90.549** External constriction, unspecified ankle
- √6ᵗʰ **S90.55** Superficial foreign body of ankle
  Splinter in the ankle
  - √7ᵗʰ **S90.551** Superficial foreign body, right ankle
  - √7ᵗʰ **S90.552** Superficial foreign body, left ankle
  - √7ᵗʰ **S90.559** Superficial foreign body, unspecified ankle
- √6ᵗʰ **S90.56** Insect bite (nonvenomous) of ankle
  - √7ᵗʰ **S90.561** Insect bite (nonvenomous), right ankle
  - √7ᵗʰ **S90.562** Insect bite (nonvenomous), left ankle
  - √7ᵗʰ **S90.569** Insect bite (nonvenomous), unspecified ankle
- √6ᵗʰ **S90.57** Other superficial bite of ankle
  EXCLUDES 1   open bite of ankle (S91.05-)
  - √7ᵗʰ **S90.571** Other superficial bite of ankle, right ankle
  - √7ᵗʰ **S90.572** Other superficial bite of ankle, left ankle
  - √7ᵗʰ **S90.579** Other superficial bite of ankle, unspecified ankle

√5ᵗʰ **S90.8** Other superficial injuries of foot
- √6ᵗʰ **S90.81** Abrasion of foot
  - √7ᵗʰ **S90.811** Abrasion, right foot
  - √7ᵗʰ **S90.812** Abrasion, left foot
  - √7ᵗʰ **S90.819** Abrasion, unspecified foot
- √6ᵗʰ **S90.82** Blister (nonthermal) of foot
  - √7ᵗʰ **S90.821** Blister (nonthermal), right foot
  - √7ᵗʰ **S90.822** Blister (nonthermal), left foot
  - √7ᵗʰ **S90.829** Blister (nonthermal), unspecified foot
- √6ᵗʰ **S90.84** External constriction of foot
  - √7ᵗʰ **S90.841** External constriction, right foot
  - √7ᵗʰ **S90.842** External constriction, left foot
  - √7ᵗʰ **S90.849** External constriction, unspecified foot
- √6ᵗʰ **S90.85** Superficial foreign body of foot
  Splinter in the foot
  - √7ᵗʰ **S90.851** Superficial foreign body, right foot
  - √7ᵗʰ **S90.852** Superficial foreign body, left foot
  - √7ᵗʰ **S90.859** Superficial foreign body, unspecified foot
- √6ᵗʰ **S90.86** Insect bite (nonvenomous) of foot
  - √7ᵗʰ **S90.861** Insect bite (nonvenomous), right foot
  - √7ᵗʰ **S90.862** Insect bite (nonvenomous), left foot
  - √7ᵗʰ **S90.869** Insect bite (nonvenomous), unspecified foot

☑ Additional Character Required   √×7ᵗʰ Placeholder   Unacceptable PDx   Questionable PDx   Manifestation   Unspecified Dx   H1-H14 HAC   HCC CMS-HCC Dx   HIV HIV Dx

ICD-10-CM 2020   **1113**

√6th **S90.87   Other superficial bite of foot**
   EXCLUDES 1   *open bite of foot (S91.35-)*
         √7th **S90.871   Other superficial bite of right foot**
         √7th **S90.872   Other superficial bite of left foot**
         √7th **S90.879   Other superficial bite of unspecified foot**

√5th **S90.9   Unspecified superficial injury of ankle, foot and toe**
   √6th **S90.91   Unspecified superficial injury of ankle**
         √7th **S90.911   Unspecified superficial injury of right ankle**
         √7th **S90.912   Unspecified superficial injury of left ankle**
         √7th **S90.919   Unspecified superficial injury of unspecified ankle**
   √6th **S90.92   Unspecified superficial injury of foot**
         √7th **S90.921   Unspecified superficial injury of right foot**
         √7th **S90.922   Unspecified superficial injury of left foot**
         √7th **S90.929   Unspecified superficial injury of unspecified foot**
   √6th **S90.93   Unspecified superficial injury of toes**
         √7th **S90.931   Unspecified superficial injury of right great toe**
         √7th **S90.932   Unspecified superficial injury of left great toe**
         √7th **S90.933   Unspecified superficial injury of unspecified great toe**
         √7th **S90.934   Unspecified superficial injury of right lesser toe(s)**
         √7th **S90.935   Unspecified superficial injury of left lesser toe(s)**
         √7th **S90.936   Unspecified superficial injury of unspecified lesser toe(s)**

√4th **S91   Open wound of ankle, foot and toes**
   Code also any associated wound infection
   EXCLUDES 1   *open fracture of ankle, foot and toes (S92.- with 7th character B)*
            traumatic amputation of ankle and foot (S98.-)

   The appropriate 7th character is to be added to each code from category S91.
   A   initial encounter
   D   subsequent encounter
   S   sequela

   √5th **S91.0   Open wound of ankle**
      √6th **S91.00   Unspecified open wound of ankle**
            √7th **S91.001   Unspecified open wound, right ankle**
            √7th **S91.002   Unspecified open wound, left ankle**
            √7th **S91.009   Unspecified open wound, unspecified ankle**
      √6th **S91.01   Laceration without foreign body of ankle**
            √7th **S91.011   Laceration without foreign body, right ankle**
            √7th **S91.012   Laceration without foreign body, left ankle**
            √7th **S91.019   Laceration without foreign body, unspecified ankle**
      √6th **S91.02   Laceration with foreign body of ankle**
            √7th **S91.021   Laceration with foreign body, right ankle**
            √7th **S91.022   Laceration with foreign body, left ankle**
            √7th **S91.029   Laceration with foreign body, unspecified ankle**
      √6th **S91.03   Puncture wound without foreign body of ankle**
            √7th **S91.031   Puncture wound without foreign body, right ankle**
            √7th **S91.032   Puncture wound without foreign body, left ankle**
            √7th **S91.039   Puncture wound without foreign body, unspecified ankle**
      √6th **S91.04   Puncture wound with foreign body of ankle**
            √7th **S91.041   Puncture wound with foreign body, right ankle**
            √7th **S91.042   Puncture wound with foreign body, left ankle**
            √7th **S91.049   Puncture wound with foreign body, unspecified ankle**
      √6th **S91.05   Open bite of ankle**
            EXCLUDES 1   *superficial bite of ankle (S90.56-, S90.57-)*
            √7th **S91.051   Open bite, right ankle**

         √7th **S91.052   Open bite, left ankle**
         √7th **S91.059   Open bite, unspecified ankle**

√5th **S91.1   Open wound of toe without damage to nail**
   √6th **S91.10   Unspecified open wound of toe without damage to nail**
         √7th **S91.101   Unspecified open wound of right great toe without damage to nail**
         √7th **S91.102   Unspecified open wound of left great toe without damage to nail**
         √7th **S91.103   Unspecified open wound of unspecified great toe without damage to nail**
         √7th **S91.104   Unspecified open wound of right lesser toe(s) without damage to nail**
         √7th **S91.105   Unspecified open wound of left lesser toe(s) without damage to nail**
         √7th **S91.106   Unspecified open wound of unspecified lesser toe(s) without damage to nail**
         √7th **S91.109   Unspecified open wound of unspecified toe(s) without damage to nail**
   √6th **S91.11   Laceration without foreign body of toe without damage to nail**
         √7th **S91.111   Laceration without foreign body of right great toe without damage to nail**
         √7th **S91.112   Laceration without foreign body of left great toe without damage to nail**
         √7th **S91.113   Laceration without foreign body of unspecified great toe without damage to nail**
         √7th **S91.114   Laceration without foreign body of right lesser toe(s) without damage to nail**
         √7th **S91.115   Laceration without foreign body of left lesser toe(s) without damage to nail**
         √7th **S91.116   Laceration without foreign body of unspecified lesser toe(s) without damage to nail**
         √7th **S91.119   Laceration without foreign body of unspecified toe without damage to nail**
   √6th **S91.12   Laceration with foreign body of toe without damage to nail**
         √7th **S91.121   Laceration with foreign body of right great toe without damage to nail**
         √7th **S91.122   Laceration with foreign body of left great toe without damage to nail**
         √7th **S91.123   Laceration with foreign body of unspecified great toe without damage to nail**
         √7th **S91.124   Laceration with foreign body of right lesser toe(s) without damage to nail**
         √7th **S91.125   Laceration with foreign body of left lesser toe(s) without damage to nail**
         √7th **S91.126   Laceration with foreign body of unspecified lesser toe(s) without damage to nail**
         √7th **S91.129   Laceration with foreign body of unspecified toe(s) without damage to nail**
   √6th **S91.13   Puncture wound without foreign body of toe without damage to nail**
         √7th **S91.131   Puncture wound without foreign body of right great toe without damage to nail**
         √7th **S91.132   Puncture wound without foreign body of left great toe without damage to nail**
         √7th **S91.133   Puncture wound without foreign body of unspecified great toe without damage to nail**
         √7th **S91.134   Puncture wound without foreign body of right lesser toe(s) without damage to nail**
         √7th **S91.135   Puncture wound without foreign body of left lesser toe(s) without damage to nail**
         √7th **S91.136   Puncture wound without foreign body of unspecified lesser toe(s) without damage to nail**
         √7th **S91.139   Puncture wound without foreign body of unspecified toe(s) without damage to nail**
   √6th **S91.14   Puncture wound with foreign body of toe without damage to nail**
         √7th **S91.141   Puncture wound with foreign body of right great toe without damage to nail**
         √7th **S91.142   Puncture wound with foreign body of left great toe without damage to nail**
         √7th **S91.143   Puncture wound with foreign body of unspecified great toe without damage to nail**

√7ᵗʰ **S91.144** Puncture wound with foreign body of right lesser toe(s) without damage to nail

√7ᵗʰ **S91.145** Puncture wound with foreign body of left lesser toe(s) without damage to nail

√7ᵗʰ **S91.146** Puncture wound with foreign body of unspecified lesser toe(s) without damage to nail

√7ᵗʰ **S91.149** Puncture wound with foreign body of unspecified toe(s) without damage to nail

√6ᵗʰ **S91.15** Open bite of toe without damage to nail

Bite of toe NOS

EXCLUDES 1   *superficial bite of toe (S90.46-, S90.47-)*

√7ᵗʰ **S91.151** Open bite of right great toe without damage to nail

√7ᵗʰ **S91.152** Open bite of left great toe without damage to nail

√7ᵗʰ **S91.153** Open bite of unspecified great toe without damage to nail

√7ᵗʰ **S91.154** Open bite of right lesser toe(s) without damage to nail

√7ᵗʰ **S91.155** Open bite of left lesser toe(s) without damage to nail

√7ᵗʰ **S91.156** Open bite of unspecified lesser toe(s) without damage to nail

√7ᵗʰ **S91.159** Open bite of unspecified toe(s) without damage to nail

√5ᵗʰ **S91.2** Open wound of toe with damage to nail

√6ᵗʰ **S91.20** Unspecified open wound of toe with damage to nail

√7ᵗʰ **S91.201** Unspecified open wound of right great toe with damage to nail

√7ᵗʰ **S91.202** Unspecified open wound of left great toe with damage to nail

√7ᵗʰ **S91.203** Unspecified open wound of unspecified great toe with damage to nail

√7ᵗʰ **S91.204** Unspecified open wound of right lesser toe(s) with damage to nail

√7ᵗʰ **S91.205** Unspecified open wound of left lesser toe(s) with damage to nail

√7ᵗʰ **S91.206** Unspecified open wound of unspecified lesser toe(s) with damage to nail

√7ᵗʰ **S91.209** Unspecified open wound of unspecified toe(s) with damage to nail

√6ᵗʰ **S91.21** Laceration without foreign body of toe with damage to nail

√7ᵗʰ **S91.211** Laceration without foreign body of right great toe with damage to nail

√7ᵗʰ **S91.212** Laceration without foreign body of left great toe with damage to nail

√7ᵗʰ **S91.213** Laceration without foreign body of unspecified great toe with damage to nail

√7ᵗʰ **S91.214** Laceration without foreign body of right lesser toe(s) with damage to nail

√7ᵗʰ **S91.215** Laceration without foreign body of left lesser toe(s) with damage to nail

√7ᵗʰ **S91.216** Laceration without foreign body of unspecified lesser toe(s) with damage to nail

√7ᵗʰ **S91.219** Laceration without foreign body of unspecified toe(s) with damage to nail

√6ᵗʰ **S91.22** Laceration with foreign body of toe with damage to nail

√7ᵗʰ **S91.221** Laceration with foreign body of right great toe with damage to nail

√7ᵗʰ **S91.222** Laceration with foreign body of left great toe with damage to nail

√7ᵗʰ **S91.223** Laceration with foreign body of unspecified great toe with damage to nail

√7ᵗʰ **S91.224** Laceration with foreign body of right lesser toe(s) with damage to nail

√7ᵗʰ **S91.225** Laceration with foreign body of left lesser toe(s) with damage to nail

√7ᵗʰ **S91.226** Laceration with foreign body of unspecified lesser toe(s) with damage to nail

√7ᵗʰ **S91.229** Laceration with foreign body of unspecified toe(s) with damage to nail

√6ᵗʰ **S91.23** Puncture wound without foreign body of toe with damage to nail

√7ᵗʰ **S91.231** Puncture wound without foreign body of right great toe with damage to nail

√7ᵗʰ **S91.232** Puncture wound without foreign body of left great toe with damage to nail

√7ᵗʰ **S91.233** Puncture wound without foreign body of unspecified great toe with damage to nail

√7ᵗʰ **S91.234** Puncture wound without foreign body of right lesser toe(s) with damage to nail

√7ᵗʰ **S91.235** Puncture wound without foreign body of left lesser toe(s) with damage to nail

√7ᵗʰ **S91.236** Puncture wound without foreign body of unspecified lesser toe(s) with damage to nail

√7ᵗʰ **S91.239** Puncture wound without foreign body of unspecified toe(s) with damage to nail

√6ᵗʰ **S91.24** Puncture wound with foreign body of toe with damage to nail

√7ᵗʰ **S91.241** Puncture wound with foreign body of right great toe with damage to nail

√7ᵗʰ **S91.242** Puncture wound with foreign body of left great toe with damage to nail

√7ᵗʰ **S91.243** Puncture wound with foreign body of unspecified great toe with damage to nail

√7ᵗʰ **S91.244** Puncture wound with foreign body of right lesser toe(s) with damage to nail

√7ᵗʰ **S91.245** Puncture wound with foreign body of left lesser toe(s) with damage to nail

√7ᵗʰ **S91.246** Puncture wound with foreign body of unspecified lesser toe(s) with damage to nail

√7ᵗʰ **S91.249** Puncture wound with foreign body of unspecified toe(s) with damage to nail

√6ᵗʰ **S91.25** Open bite of toe with damage to nail

Bite of toe with damage to nail NOS

EXCLUDES 1   *superficial bite of toe (S90.46-, S90.47-)*

√7ᵗʰ **S91.251** Open bite of right great toe with damage to nail

√7ᵗʰ **S91.252** Open bite of left great toe with damage to nail

√7ᵗʰ **S91.253** Open bite of unspecified great toe with damage to nail

√7ᵗʰ **S91.254** Open bite of right lesser toe(s) with damage to nail

√7ᵗʰ **S91.255** Open bite of left lesser toe(s) with damage to nail

√7ᵗʰ **S91.256** Open bite of unspecified lesser toe(s) with damage to nail

√7ᵗʰ **S91.259** Open bite of unspecified toe(s) with damage to nail

√5ᵗʰ **S91.3** Open wound of foot

√6ᵗʰ **S91.30** Unspecified open wound of foot

√7ᵗʰ **S91.301** Unspecified open wound, right foot

√7ᵗʰ **S91.302** Unspecified open wound, left foot

√7ᵗʰ **S91.309** Unspecified open wound, unspecified foot

√6ᵗʰ **S91.31** Laceration without foreign body of foot

√7ᵗʰ **S91.311** Laceration without foreign body, right foot

√7ᵗʰ **S91.312** Laceration without foreign body, left foot

√7ᵗʰ **S91.319** Laceration without foreign body, unspecified foot

√6ᵗʰ **S91.32** Laceration with foreign body of foot

√7ᵗʰ **S91.321** Laceration with foreign body, right foot

√7ᵗʰ **S91.322** Laceration with foreign body, left foot

√7ᵗʰ **S91.329** Laceration with foreign body, unspecified foot

√6ᵗʰ **S91.33** Puncture wound without foreign body of foot

√7ᵗʰ **S91.331** Puncture wound without foreign body, right foot

√7ᵗʰ **S91.332** Puncture wound without foreign body, left foot

√7ᵗʰ **S91.339** Puncture wound without foreign body, unspecified foot

√6ᵗʰ **S91.34** Puncture wound with foreign body of foot

√7ᵗʰ **S91.341** Puncture wound with foreign body, right foot

√7ᵗʰ **S91.342** Puncture wound with foreign body, left foot

√7ᵗʰ **S91.349** Puncture wound with foreign body, unspecified foot

√6ᵗʰ **S91.35** Open bite of foot

EXCLUDES 1   *superficial bite of foot (S90.86-, S90.87-)*

√7ᵗʰ **S91.351** Open bite, right foot

☑ Additional Character Required   √x7ᵗʰ Placeholder   Unacceptable PDx   Questionable PDx   Manifestation   Unspecified Dx   H1-H14 HAC   HCC CMS-HCC Dx   HIV HIV Dx

ICD-10-CM 2020   1115

√7ᵗʰ **S91.352**   **Open bite, left foot**

√7ᵗʰ **S91.359**   **Open bite, unspecified foot**

√4ᵗʰ **S92**   **Fracture of foot and toe, except ankle**

> **NOTE**   A fracture not indicated as displaced or nondisplaced should be coded to displaced
>
> A fracture not indicated as open or closed should be coded to closed.

EXCLUDES 1   traumatic amputation of ankle and foot (S98.-)

EXCLUDES 2   fracture of ankle (S82.-)

fracture of malleolus (S82.-)

AHA: 2018,2Q,12; 2015,3Q,37-39

The appropriate 7th character is to be added to each code from category S92.
- A   initial encounter for closed fracture
- B   initial encounter for open fracture
- D   subsequent encounter for fracture with routine healing
- G   subsequent encounter for fracture with delayed healing
- K   subsequent encounter for fracture with nonunion
- P   subsequent encounter for fracture with malunion
- S   sequela

√5ᵗʰ **S92.0**   **Fracture of calcaneus**

Heel bone

Os calcis

EXCLUDES 2   physeal fracture of calcaneus (S99.0-)

CC Excl: For codes in subcategory S92.0:
CC with 7th character B: PDX collection 1367
CC with 7th character K or P: PDX collection 897

√6ᵗʰ **S92.00**   **Unspecified fracture of calcaneus**

³ √7ᵗʰ **S92.001**   **Unspecified fracture of right calcaneus**   CC H5

³ √7ᵗʰ **S92.002**   **Unspecified fracture of left calcaneus**   CC H5

³ √7ᵗʰ **S92.009**   **Unspecified fracture of unspecified calcaneus**   CC H5

√6ᵗʰ **S92.01**   **Fracture of body of calcaneus**

³ √7ᵗʰ **S92.011**   **Displaced fracture of body of right calcaneus**   CC H5

³ √7ᵗʰ **S92.012**   **Displaced fracture of body of left calcaneus**   CC H5

³ √7ᵗʰ **S92.013**   **Displaced fracture of body of unspecified calcaneus**   CC H5

³ √7ᵗʰ **S92.014**   **Nondisplaced fracture of body of right calcaneus**   CC H5

³ √7ᵗʰ **S92.015**   **Nondisplaced fracture of body of left calcaneus**   CC H5

³ √7ᵗʰ **S92.016**   **Nondisplaced fracture of body of unspecified calcaneus**   CC H5

√6ᵗʰ **S92.02**   **Fracture of anterior process of calcaneus**

³ √7ᵗʰ **S92.021**   **Displaced fracture of anterior process of right calcaneus**   CC H5

³ √7ᵗʰ **S92.022**   **Displaced fracture of anterior process of left calcaneus**   CC H5

³ √7ᵗʰ **S92.023**   **Displaced fracture of anterior process of unspecified calcaneus**   CC H5

³ √7ᵗʰ **S92.024**   **Nondisplaced fracture of anterior process of right calcaneus**   CC H5

³ √7ᵗʰ **S92.025**   **Nondisplaced fracture of anterior process of left calcaneus**   CC H5

³ √7ᵗʰ **S92.026**   **Nondisplaced fracture of anterior process of unspecified calcaneus**   CC H5

√6ᵗʰ **S92.03**   **Avulsion fracture of tuberosity of calcaneus**

³ √7ᵗʰ **S92.031**   **Displaced avulsion fracture of tuberosity of right calcaneus**   CC H5

³ √7ᵗʰ **S92.032**   **Displaced avulsion fracture of tuberosity of left calcaneus**   CC H5

³ √7ᵗʰ **S92.033**   **Displaced avulsion fracture of tuberosity of unspecified calcaneus**   CC H5

³ **S92.034**   **Nondisplaced avulsion fracture of tuberosity of right calcaneus**   CC H5

³ **S92.035**   **Nondisplaced avulsion fracture of tuberosity of left calcaneus**   CC H5

³ √7ᵗʰ **S92.036**   **Nondisplaced avulsion fracture of tuberosity of unspecified calcaneus**   CC H5

√6ᵗʰ **S92.04**   **Other fracture of tuberosity of calcaneus**

³ √7ᵗʰ **S92.041**   **Displaced other fracture of tuberosity of right calcaneus**   CC H5

³ √7ᵗʰ **S92.042**   **Displaced other fracture of tuberosity of left calcaneus**   CC H5

³ √7ᵗʰ **S92.043**   **Displaced other fracture of tuberosity of unspecified calcaneus**   CC H5

³ √7ᵗʰ **S92.044**   **Nondisplaced other fracture of tuberosity of right calcaneus**   CC H5

³ √7ᵗʰ **S92.045**   **Nondisplaced other fracture of tuberosity of left calcaneus**   CC H5

³ √7ᵗʰ **S92.046**   **Nondisplaced other fracture of tuberosity of unspecified calcaneus**   CC H5

√6ᵗʰ **S92.05**   **Other extraarticular fracture of calcaneus**

³ √7ᵗʰ **S92.051**   **Displaced other extraarticular fracture of right calcaneus**   CC H5

³ √7ᵗʰ **S92.052**   **Displaced other extraarticular fracture of left calcaneus**   CC H5

³ √7ᵗʰ **S92.053**   **Displaced other extraarticular fracture of unspecified calcaneus**   CC H5

³ √7ᵗʰ **S92.054**   **Nondisplaced other extraarticular fracture of right calcaneus**   CC H5

³ √7ᵗʰ **S92.055**   **Nondisplaced other extraarticular fracture of left calcaneus**   CC H5

³ **S92.056**   **Nondisplaced other extraarticular fracture of unspecified calcaneus**   CC H5

√6ᵗʰ **S92.06**   **Intraarticular fracture of calcaneus**

³ √7ᵗʰ **S92.061**   **Displaced intraarticular fracture of right calcaneus**   CC H5

³ √7ᵗʰ **S92.062**   **Displaced intraarticular fracture of left calcaneus**   CC H5

³ √7ᵗʰ **S92.063**   **Displaced intraarticular fracture of unspecified calcaneus**   CC H5

³ √7ᵗʰ **S92.064**   **Nondisplaced intraarticular fracture of right calcaneus**   CC H5

³ √7ᵗʰ **S92.065**   **Nondisplaced intraarticular fracture of left calcaneus**   CC H5

³ √7ᵗʰ **S92.066**   **Nondisplaced intraarticular fracture of unspecified calcaneus**   CC H5

√5ᵗʰ **S92.1**   **Fracture of talus**

Astragalus

CC Excl: For codes in subcategory S92.1:
CC with 7th character B: PDX collection 1368
CC with 7th character K or P: PDX collection 897

√6ᵗʰ **S92.10**   **Unspecified fracture of talus**

³ √7ᵗʰ **S92.101**   **Unspecified fracture of right talus**   CC H5

³ √7ᵗʰ **S92.102**   **Unspecified fracture of left talus**   CC H5

³ √7ᵗʰ **S92.109**   **Unspecified fracture of unspecified talus**   CC H5

√6ᵗʰ **S92.11**   **Fracture of neck of talus**

³ √7ᵗʰ **S92.111**   **Displaced fracture of neck of right talus**   CC H5

³ √7ᵗʰ **S92.112**   **Displaced fracture of neck of left talus**   CC H5

³ √7ᵗʰ **S92.113**   **Displaced fracture of neck of unspecified talus**   CC H5

Ⓝ Newborn: 0   Ⓟ Pediatric: 0-17   Ⓜ Maternity: 9-64   Ⓐ Adult: 15-124   **MCC** Major Complication/Comorbidity   **CC** Complication/Comorbidity   **SW** Severe Wound Dx

1116   ICD-10-CM 2020

3 √7ᵗʰ **S92.114** Nondisplaced fracture of neck of right talus   `CC` `H5`

3 √7ᵗʰ **S92.115** Nondisplaced fracture of neck of left talus   `CC` `H5`

3 √7ᵗʰ **S92.116** Nondisplaced fracture of neck of unspecified talus   `CC` `H5`

√6ᵗʰ **S92.12** Fracture of body of talus

3 √7ᵗʰ **S92.121** Displaced fracture of body of right talus   `CC` `H5`

3 √7ᵗʰ **S92.122** Displaced fracture of body of left talus   `CC` `H5`

3 √7ᵗʰ **S92.123** Displaced fracture of body of unspecified talus   `CC` `H5`

3 √7ᵗʰ **S92.124** Nondisplaced fracture of body of right talus   `CC` `H5`

3 √7ᵗʰ **S92.125** Nondisplaced fracture of body of left talus   `CC` `H5`

3 √7ᵗʰ **S92.126** Nondisplaced fracture of body of unspecified talus   `CC` `H5`

√6ᵗʰ **S92.13** Fracture of posterior process of talus

3 √7ᵗʰ **S92.131** Displaced fracture of posterior process of right talus   `CC` `H5`

3 √7ᵗʰ **S92.132** Displaced fracture of posterior process of left talus   `CC` `H5`

3 √7ᵗʰ **S92.133** Displaced fracture of posterior process of unspecified talus   `CC` `H5`

3 √7ᵗʰ **S92.134** Nondisplaced fracture of posterior process of right talus   `CC` `H5`

3 √7ᵗʰ **S92.135** Nondisplaced fracture of posterior process of left talus   `CC` `H5`

3 √7ᵗʰ **S92.136** Nondisplaced fracture of posterior process of unspecified talus   `CC` `H5`

√6ᵗʰ **S92.14** Dome fracture of talus

EXCLUDES 1   osteochondritis dissecans (M93.2)

3 √7ᵗʰ **S92.141** Displaced dome fracture of right talus   `CC` `H5`

3 √7ᵗʰ **S92.142** Displaced dome fracture of left talus   `CC` `H5`

3 √7ᵗʰ **S92.143** Displaced dome fracture of unspecified talus   `CC` `H5`

3 √7ᵗʰ **S92.144** Nondisplaced dome fracture of right talus   `CC` `H5`

3 √7ᵗʰ **S92.145** Nondisplaced dome fracture of left talus   `CC` `H5`

3 √7ᵗʰ **S92.146** Nondisplaced dome fracture of unspecified talus   `CC` `H5`

√6ᵗʰ **S92.15** Avulsion fracture (chip fracture) of talus

3 √7ᵗʰ **S92.151** Displaced avulsion fracture (chip fracture) of right talus   `CC` `H5`

3 √7ᵗʰ **S92.152** Displaced avulsion fracture (chip fracture) of left talus   `CC` `H5`

3 √7ᵗʰ **S92.153** Displaced avulsion fracture (chip fracture) of unspecified talus   `CC` `H5`

3 √7ᵗʰ **S92.154** Nondisplaced avulsion fracture (chip fracture) of right talus   `CC` `H5`

3 √7ᵗʰ **S92.155** Nondisplaced avulsion fracture (chip fracture) of left talus   `CC` `H5`

3 √7ᵗʰ **S92.156** Nondisplaced avulsion fracture (chip fracture) of unspecified talus   `CC` `H5`

√6ᵗʰ **S92.19** Other fracture of talus

3 √7ᵗʰ **S92.191** Other fracture of right talus   `CC` `H5`

3 √7ᵗʰ **S92.192** Other fracture of left talus   `CC` `H5`

3 √7ᵗʰ **S92.199** Other fracture of unspecified talus   `CC` `H5`

√5ᵗʰ **S92.2** Fracture of other and unspecified tarsal bone(s)

CC Excl: For codes in subcategory S92.2, unless otherwise noted:
CC with 7th character B: PDX collection 1368
CC with 7th character K or P: PDX collection 897

√6ᵗʰ **S92.20** Fracture of unspecified tarsal bone(s)

CC Excl: For codes in subcategory S92.20:
CC with 7th character B: PDX collection 1369

3 √7ᵗʰ **S92.201** Fracture of unspecified tarsal bone(s) of right foot   `CC` `H5`

3 √7ᵗʰ **S92.202** Fracture of unspecified tarsal bone(s) of left foot   `CC` `H5`

3 √7ᵗʰ **S92.209** Fracture of unspecified tarsal bone(s) of unspecified foot   `CC` `H5`

√6ᵗʰ **S92.21** Fracture of cuboid bone

3 √7ᵗʰ **S92.211** Displaced fracture of cuboid bone of right foot   `CC` `H5`

3 √7ᵗʰ **S92.212** Displaced fracture of cuboid bone of left foot   `CC` `H5`

3 √7ᵗʰ **S92.213** Displaced fracture of cuboid bone of unspecified foot   `CC` `H5`

3 √7ᵗʰ **S92.214** Nondisplaced fracture of cuboid bone of right foot   `CC` `H5`

3 √7ᵗʰ **S92.215** Nondisplaced fracture of cuboid bone of left foot   `CC` `H5`

3 √7ᵗʰ **S92.216** Nondisplaced fracture of cuboid bone of unspecified foot   `CC` `H5`

√6ᵗʰ **S92.22** Fracture of lateral cuneiform

3 √7ᵗʰ **S92.221** Displaced fracture of lateral cuneiform of right foot   `CC` `H5`

3 √7ᵗʰ **S92.222** Displaced fracture of lateral cuneiform of left foot   `CC` `H5`

3 √7ᵗʰ **S92.223** Displaced fracture of lateral cuneiform of unspecified foot   `CC` `H5`

3 √7ᵗʰ **S92.224** Nondisplaced fracture of lateral cuneiform of right foot   `CC` `H5`

3 √7ᵗʰ **S92.225** Nondisplaced fracture of lateral cuneiform of left foot   `CC` `H5`

3 √7ᵗʰ **S92.226** Nondisplaced fracture of lateral cuneiform of unspecified foot   `CC` `H5`

√6ᵗʰ **S92.23** Fracture of intermediate cuneiform

3 √7ᵗʰ **S92.231** Displaced fracture of intermediate cuneiform of right foot   `CC` `H5`

3 √7ᵗʰ **S92.232** Displaced fracture of intermediate cuneiform of left foot   `CC` `H5`

3 √7ᵗʰ **S92.233** Displaced fracture of intermediate cuneiform of unspecified foot   `CC` `H5`

3 √7ᵗʰ **S92.234** Nondisplaced fracture of intermediate cuneiform of right foot   `CC` `H5`

3 √7ᵗʰ **S92.235** Nondisplaced fracture of intermediate cuneiform of left foot   `CC` `H5`

3 √7ᵗʰ **S92.236** Nondisplaced fracture of intermediate cuneiform of unspecified foot   `CC` `H5`

√6ᵗʰ **S92.24** Fracture of medial cuneiform

3 √7ᵗʰ **S92.241** Displaced fracture of medial cuneiform of right foot   `CC` `H5`

3 √7ᵗʰ **S92.242** Displaced fracture of medial cuneiform of left foot   `CC` `H5`

3 √7ᵗʰ **S92.243** Displaced fracture of medial cuneiform of unspecified foot   `CC` `H5`

3 √7ᵗʰ **S92.244** Nondisplaced fracture of medial cuneiform of right foot   `CC` `H5`

3 ✓7ᵗʰ **S92.245** Nondisplaced fracture of medial cuneiform of left foot   CC H5

3 ✓7ᵗʰ **S92.246** Nondisplaced fracture of medial cuneiform of unspecified foot   CC H5

✓6ᵗʰ **S92.25** Fracture of navicular [scaphoid] of foot

3 ✓7ᵗʰ **S92.251** Displaced fracture of navicular [scaphoid] of right foot   CC H5

3 ✓7ᵗʰ **S92.252** Displaced fracture of navicular [scaphoid] of left foot   CC H5

3 ✓7ᵗʰ **S92.253** Displaced fracture of navicular [scaphoid] of unspecified foot   CC H5

3 ✓7ᵗʰ **S92.254** Nondisplaced fracture of navicular [scaphoid] of right foot   CC H5

3 ✓7ᵗʰ **S92.255** Nondisplaced fracture of navicular [scaphoid] of left foot   CC H5

3 ✓7ᵗʰ **S92.256** Nondisplaced fracture of navicular [scaphoid] of unspecified foot   CC H5

✓5ᵗʰ **S92.3** Fracture of metatarsal bone(s)

EXCLUDES 2   physeal fracture of metatarsal (S99.1-)

AHA: 2018,1Q,3

CC Excl: For codes in subcategory S92.3:
CC with 7th character B: PDX collection 1368
CC with 7th character K or P: PDX collection 897

✓6ᵗʰ **S92.30** Fracture of unspecified metatarsal bone(s)

3 ✓7ᵗʰ **S92.301** Fracture of unspecified metatarsal bone(s), right foot   CC H5

3 ✓7ᵗʰ **S92.302** Fracture of unspecified metatarsal bone(s), left foot   CC H5

3 ✓7ᵗʰ **S92.309** Fracture of unspecified metatarsal bone(s), unspecified foot   CC H5

✓6ᵗʰ **S92.31** Fracture of first metatarsal bone

3 ✓7ᵗʰ **S92.311** Displaced fracture of first metatarsal bone, right foot   CC H5

3 ✓7ᵗʰ **S92.312** Displaced fracture of first metatarsal bone, left foot   CC H5

3 ✓7ᵗʰ **S92.313** Displaced fracture of first metatarsal bone, unspecified foot   CC H5

3 ✓7ᵗʰ **S92.314** Nondisplaced fracture of first metatarsal bone, right foot   CC H5

3 ✓7ᵗʰ **S92.315** Nondisplaced fracture of first metatarsal bone, left foot   CC H5

3 ✓7ᵗʰ **S92.316** Nondisplaced fracture of first metatarsal bone, unspecified foot   CC H5

✓6ᵗʰ **S92.32** Fracture of second metatarsal bone

3 ✓7ᵗʰ **S92.321** Displaced fracture of second metatarsal bone, right foot   CC H5

3 ✓7ᵗʰ **S92.322** Displaced fracture of second metatarsal bone, left foot   CC H5

3 ✓7ᵗʰ **S92.323** Displaced fracture of second metatarsal bone, unspecified foot   CC H5

3 ✓7ᵗʰ **S92.324** Nondisplaced fracture of second metatarsal bone, right foot   CC H5

3 ✓7ᵗʰ **S92.325** Nondisplaced fracture of second metatarsal bone, left foot   CC H5

3 ✓7ᵗʰ **S92.326** Nondisplaced fracture of second metatarsal bone, unspecified foot   CC H5

✓6ᵗʰ **S92.33** Fracture of third metatarsal bone

3 ✓7ᵗʰ **S92.331** Displaced fracture of third metatarsal bone, right foot   CC H5

3 ✓7ᵗʰ **S92.332** Displaced fracture of third metatarsal bone, left foot   CC H5

3 ✓7ᵗʰ **S92.333** Displaced fracture of third metatarsal bone, unspecified foot   CC H5

3 ✓7ᵗʰ **S92.334** Nondisplaced fracture of third metatarsal bone, right foot   CC H5

3 ✓7ᵗʰ **S92.335** Nondisplaced fracture of third metatarsal bone, left foot   CC H5

3 ✓7ᵗʰ **S92.336** Nondisplaced fracture of third metatarsal bone, unspecified foot   CC H5

✓6ᵗʰ **S92.34** Fracture of fourth metatarsal bone

3 ✓7ᵗʰ **S92.341** Displaced fracture of fourth metatarsal bone, right foot   CC H5

3 ✓7ᵗʰ **S92.342** Displaced fracture of fourth metatarsal bone, left foot   CC H5

3 ✓7ᵗʰ **S92.343** Displaced fracture of fourth metatarsal bone, unspecified foot   CC H5

3 ✓7ᵗʰ **S92.344** Nondisplaced fracture of fourth metatarsal bone, right foot   CC H5

3 ✓7ᵗʰ **S92.345** Nondisplaced fracture of fourth metatarsal bone, left foot   CC H5

3 ✓7ᵗʰ **S92.346** Nondisplaced fracture of fourth metatarsal bone, unspecified foot   CC H5

✓6ᵗʰ **S92.35** Fracture of fifth metatarsal bone

3 ✓7ᵗʰ **S92.351** Displaced fracture of fifth metatarsal bone, right foot   CC H5

3 ✓7ᵗʰ **S92.352** Displaced fracture of fifth metatarsal bone, left foot   CC H5

3 ✓7ᵗʰ **S92.353** Displaced fracture of fifth metatarsal bone, unspecified foot   CC H5

3 ✓7ᵗʰ **S92.354** Nondisplaced fracture of fifth metatarsal bone, right foot   CC H5

3 ✓7ᵗʰ **S92.355** Nondisplaced fracture of fifth metatarsal bone, left foot   CC H5

3 ✓7ᵗʰ **S92.356** Nondisplaced fracture of fifth metatarsal bone, unspecified foot   CC H5

✓5ᵗʰ **S92.4** Fracture of great toe

EXCLUDES 2   physeal fracture of phalanx of toe (S99.2-)

CC Excl: For codes in subcategory S92.4:
CC with 7th character K or P: PDX collection 897

✓6ᵗʰ **S92.40** Unspecified fracture of great toe

4 ✓7ᵗʰ **S92.401** Displaced unspecified fracture of right great toe   CC

4 ✓7ᵗʰ **S92.402** Displaced unspecified fracture of left great toe   CC

4 ✓7ᵗʰ **S92.403** Displaced unspecified fracture of unspecified great toe   CC

4 ✓7ᵗʰ **S92.404** Nondisplaced unspecified fracture of right great toe   CC

4 ✓7ᵗʰ **S92.405** Nondisplaced unspecified fracture of left great toe   CC

4 ✓7ᵗʰ **S92.406** Nondisplaced unspecified fracture of unspecified great toe   CC

✓6ᵗʰ **S92.41** Fracture of proximal phalanx of great toe

4 ✓7ᵗʰ **S92.411** Displaced fracture of proximal phalanx of right great toe   CC

4 ✓7ᵗʰ **S92.412** Displaced fracture of proximal phalanx of left great toe   CC

4 ✓7ᵗʰ **S92.413** Displaced fracture of proximal phalanx of unspecified great toe   CC

4 ✓7ᵗʰ **S92.414** Nondisplaced fracture of proximal phalanx of right great toe   CC

4 √7ᵗʰ **S92.415** Nondisplaced fracture of proximal phalanx of left great toe `CC`

4 √7ᵗʰ **S92.416** Nondisplaced fracture of proximal phalanx of unspecified great toe `CC`

√6ᵗʰ **S92.42** Fracture of distal phalanx of great toe

4 √7ᵗʰ **S92.421** Displaced fracture of distal phalanx of right great toe `CC`

4 √7ᵗʰ **S92.422** Displaced fracture of distal phalanx of left great toe `CC`

4 √7ᵗʰ **S92.423** Displaced fracture of distal phalanx of unspecified great toe `CC`

4 √7ᵗʰ **S92.424** Nondisplaced fracture of distal phalanx of right great toe `CC`

4 √7ᵗʰ **S92.425** Nondisplaced fracture of distal phalanx of left great toe `CC`

4 √7ᵗʰ **S92.426** Nondisplaced fracture of distal phalanx of unspecified great toe `CC`

√6ᵗʰ **S92.49** Other fracture of great toe

4 √7ᵗʰ **S92.491** Other fracture of right great toe `CC`

4 √7ᵗʰ **S92.492** Other fracture of left great toe `CC`

4 √7ᵗʰ **S92.499** Other fracture of unspecified great toe `CC`

√5ᵗʰ **S92.5** Fracture of lesser toe(s)

> *EXCLUDES 2* physeal fracture of phalanx of toe (S99.2-)
>
> **CC Excl: For codes in subcategory S92.5:**
> **CC with 7th character K or P:** PDX collection 897

√6ᵗʰ **S92.50** Unspecified fracture of lesser toe(s)

4 √7ᵗʰ **S92.501** Displaced unspecified fracture of right lesser toe(s) `CC`

4 √7ᵗʰ **S92.502** Displaced unspecified fracture of left lesser toe(s) `CC`

4 √7ᵗʰ **S92.503** Displaced unspecified fracture of unspecified lesser toe(s) `CC`

4 √7ᵗʰ **S92.504** Nondisplaced unspecified fracture of right lesser toe(s) `CC`

4 √7ᵗʰ **S92.505** Nondisplaced unspecified fracture of left lesser toe(s) `CC`

4 √7ᵗʰ **S92.506** Nondisplaced unspecified fracture of unspecified lesser toe(s) `CC`

√6ᵗʰ **S92.51** Fracture of proximal phalanx of lesser toe(s)

4 √7ᵗʰ **S92.511** Displaced fracture of proximal phalanx of right lesser toe(s) `CC`

4 √7ᵗʰ **S92.512** Displaced fracture of proximal phalanx of left lesser toe(s) `CC`

4 √7ᵗʰ **S92.513** Displaced fracture of proximal phalanx of unspecified lesser toe(s) `CC`

4 √7ᵗʰ **S92.514** Nondisplaced fracture of proximal phalanx of right lesser toe(s) `CC`

4 √7ᵗʰ **S92.515** Nondisplaced fracture of proximal phalanx of left lesser toe(s)) `CC`

4 √7ᵗʰ **S92.516** Nondisplaced fracture of proximal phalanx of unspecified lesser toe(s) `CC`

√6ᵗʰ **S92.52** Fracture of middle phalanx of lesser toe(s)

4 √7ᵗʰ **S92.521** Displaced fracture of middle phalanx of right lesser toe(s) `CC`

4 √7ᵗʰ **S92.522** Displaced fracture of middle phalanx of left lesser toe(s) `CC`

4 √7ᵗʰ **S92.523** Displaced fracture of middle phalanx of unspecified lesser toe(s) `CC`

4 √7ᵗʰ **S92.524** Nondisplaced fracture of middle phalanx of right lesser toe(s) `CC`

4 √7ᵗʰ **S92.525** Nondisplaced fracture of middle phalanx of left lesser toe(s) `CC`

4 √7ᵗʰ **S92.526** Nondisplaced fracture of middle phalanx of unspecified lesser toe(s) `CC`

√6ᵗʰ **S92.53** Fracture of distal phalanx of lesser toe(s)

4 √7ᵗʰ **S92.531** Displaced fracture of distal phalanx of right lesser toe(s) `CC`

4 √7ᵗʰ **S92.532** Displaced fracture of distal phalanx of left lesser toe(s) `CC`

4 √7ᵗʰ **S92.533** Displaced fracture of distal phalanx of unspecified lesser toe(s) `CC`

4 √7ᵗʰ **S92.534** Nondisplaced fracture of distal phalanx of right lesser toe(s) `CC`

4 √7ᵗʰ **S92.535** Nondisplaced fracture of distal phalanx of left lesser toe(s) `CC`

4 √7ᵗʰ **S92.536** Nondisplaced fracture of distal phalanx of unspecified lesser toe(s) `CC`

√6ᵗʰ **S92.59** Other fracture of lesser toe(s)

4 √7ᵗʰ **S92.591** Other fracture of right lesser toe(s) `CC`

4 √7ᵗʰ **S92.592** Other fracture of left lesser toe(s) `CC`

4 √7ᵗʰ **S92.599** Other fracture of unspecified lesser toe(s) `CC`

√5ᵗʰ **S92.8** Other fracture of foot, except ankle

√6ᵗʰ **S92.81** Other fracture of foot

> Sesamoid fracture of foot
> **AHA:** 2016,4Q,68
> **CC Excl: For codes in subcategory S92.81:**
> **CC with 7th character B:** PDX collection 1369
> **CC with 7th character K or P:** PDX collection 897

3 √7ᵗʰ **S92.811** Other fracture of right foot `CC` `H5`

3 √7ᵗʰ **S92.812** Other fracture of left foot `CC` `H5`

3 √7ᵗʰ **S92.819** Other fracture of unspecified foot `CC` `H5`

√5ᵗʰ **S92.9** Unspecified fracture of foot and toe

> **CC Excl: For codes in subcategory S92.9, unless otherwise noted:**
> **CC with 7th character K or P:** PDX collection 897

√6ᵗʰ **S92.90** Unspecified fracture of foot

> **CC Excl: For codes in subcategory S92.90:**
> **CC with 7th character B:** PDX collection 1369

3 √7ᵗʰ **S92.901** Unspecified fracture of right foot `CC` `H5`

3 √7ᵗʰ **S92.902** Unspecified fracture of left foot `CC` `H5`

3 √7ᵗʰ **S92.909** Unspecified fracture of unspecified foot `CC` `H5`

√6ᵗʰ **S92.91** Unspecified fracture of toe

4 √7ᵗʰ **S92.911** Unspecified fracture of right toe(s) `CC`

4 √7ᵗʰ **S92.912** Unspecified fracture of left toe(s) `CC`

4 √7ᵗʰ **S92.919** Unspecified fracture of unspecified toe(s) `CC`

✓ Additional Character Required   √x7ᵗʰ Placeholder   Unacceptable PDx   Questionable PDx   Manifestation   Unspecified Dx   H1-H14 HAC   HCC CMS-HCC Dx   HIV HIV Dx

ICD-10-CM 2020   1119

Chapter 19. Injury, Poisoning and Certain Other Consequences of External Causes

S92.415–S92.919

✓4ᵗʰ **S93 Dislocation and sprain of joints and ligaments at ankle, foot and toe level**

INCLUDES   avulsion of joint or ligament of ankle, foot and toe

laceration of cartilage, joint or ligament of ankle, foot and toe

sprain of cartilage, joint or ligament of ankle, foot and toe

traumatic hemarthrosis of joint or ligament of ankle, foot and toe

traumatic rupture of joint or ligament of ankle, foot and toe

traumatic subluxation of joint or ligament of ankle, foot and toe

traumatic tear of joint or ligament of ankle, foot and toe

Code also any associated open wound

EXCLUDES 2   *strain of muscle and tendon of ankle and foot (S96.-)*

The appropriate 7th character is to be added to each code from category S93.
A   initial encounter
D   subsequent encounter
S   sequela

✓5ᵗʰ **S93.0 Subluxation and dislocation of ankle joint**

Subluxation and dislocation of astragalus
Subluxation and dislocation of fibula, lower end
Subluxation and dislocation of talus
Subluxation and dislocation of tibia, lower end

✓x7ᵗʰ **S93.01 Subluxation of right ankle joint**

✓x7ᵗʰ **S93.02 Subluxation of left ankle joint**

✓x7ᵗʰ **S93.03 Subluxation of unspecified ankle joint**

✓x7ᵗʰ **S93.04 Dislocation of right ankle joint**

✓x7ᵗʰ **S93.05 Dislocation of left ankle joint**

✓x7ᵗʰ **S93.06 Dislocation of unspecified ankle joint**

✓5ᵗʰ **S93.1 Subluxation and dislocation of toe**

✓6ᵗʰ **S93.10 Unspecified subluxation and dislocation of toe**

Dislocation of toe NOS
Subluxation of toe NOS

✓7ᵗʰ **S93.101 Unspecified subluxation of right toe(s)**

✓7ᵗʰ **S93.102 Unspecified subluxation of left toe(s)**

✓7ᵗʰ **S93.103 Unspecified subluxation of unspecified toe(s)**

✓7ᵗʰ **S93.104 Unspecified dislocation of right toe(s)**

✓7ᵗʰ **S93.105 Unspecified dislocation of left toe(s)**

✓7ᵗʰ **S93.106 Unspecified dislocation of unspecified toe(s)**

✓6ᵗʰ **S93.11 Dislocation of interphalangeal joint**

✓7ᵗʰ **S93.111 Dislocation of interphalangeal joint of right great toe**

✓7ᵗʰ **S93.112 Dislocation of interphalangeal joint of left great toe**

✓7ᵗʰ **S93.113 Dislocation of interphalangeal joint of unspecified great toe**

✓7ᵗʰ **S93.114 Dislocation of interphalangeal joint of right lesser toe(s)**

✓7ᵗʰ **S93.115 Dislocation of interphalangeal joint of left lesser toe(s)**

✓7ᵗʰ **S93.116 Dislocation of interphalangeal joint of unspecified lesser toe(s)**

✓7ᵗʰ **S93.119 Dislocation of interphalangeal joint of unspecified toe(s)**

✓6ᵗʰ **S93.12 Dislocation of metatarsophalangeal joint**

✓7ᵗʰ **S93.121 Dislocation of metatarsophalangeal joint of right great toe**

✓7ᵗʰ **S93.122 Dislocation of metatarsophalangeal joint of left great toe**

✓7ᵗʰ **S93.123 Dislocation of metatarsophalangeal joint of unspecified great toe**

✓7ᵗʰ **S93.124 Dislocation of metatarsophalangeal joint of right lesser toe(s)**

✓7ᵗʰ **S93.125 Dislocation of metatarsophalangeal joint of left lesser toe(s)**

✓7ᵗʰ **S93.126 Dislocation of metatarsophalangeal joint of unspecified lesser toe(s)**

✓7ᵗʰ **S93.129 Dislocation of metatarsophalangeal joint of unspecified toe(s)**

✓6ᵗʰ **S93.13 Subluxation of interphalangeal joint**

✓7ᵗʰ **S93.131 Subluxation of interphalangeal joint of right great toe**

✓7ᵗʰ **S93.132 Subluxation of interphalangeal joint of left great toe**

✓7ᵗʰ **S93.133 Subluxation of interphalangeal joint of unspecified great toe**

✓7ᵗʰ **S93.134 Subluxation of interphalangeal joint of right lesser toe(s)**

✓7ᵗʰ **S93.135 Subluxation of interphalangeal joint of left lesser toe(s)**

✓7ᵗʰ **S93.136 Subluxation of interphalangeal joint of unspecified lesser toe(s)**

✓7ᵗʰ **S93.139 Subluxation of interphalangeal joint of unspecified toe(s)**

✓6ᵗʰ **S93.14 Subluxation of metatarsophalangeal joint**

✓7ᵗʰ **S93.141 Subluxation of metatarsophalangeal joint of right great toe**

✓7ᵗʰ **S93.142 Subluxation of metatarsophalangeal joint of left great toe**

✓7ᵗʰ **S93.143 Subluxation of metatarsophalangeal joint of unspecified great toe**

✓7ᵗʰ **S93.144 Subluxation of metatarsophalangeal joint of right lesser toe(s)**

✓7ᵗʰ **S93.145 Subluxation of metatarsophalangeal joint of left lesser toe(s)**

✓7ᵗʰ **S93.146 Subluxation of metatarsophalangeal joint of unspecified lesser toe(s)**

✓7ᵗʰ **S93.149 Subluxation of metatarsophalangeal joint of unspecified toe(s)**

✓5ᵗʰ **S93.3 Subluxation and dislocation of foot**

EXCLUDES 2   *dislocation of toe (S93.1-)*

✓6ᵗʰ **S93.30 Unspecified subluxation and dislocation of foot**

Dislocation of foot NOS
Subluxation of foot NOS

✓7ᵗʰ **S93.301 Unspecified subluxation of right foot**

✓7ᵗʰ **S93.302 Unspecified subluxation of left foot**

✓7ᵗʰ **S93.303 Unspecified subluxation of unspecified foot**

✓7ᵗʰ **S93.304 Unspecified dislocation of right foot**

✓7ᵗʰ **S93.305 Unspecified dislocation of left foot**

✓7ᵗʰ **S93.306 Unspecified dislocation of unspecified foot**

✓6ᵗʰ **S93.31 Subluxation and dislocation of tarsal joint**

✓7ᵗʰ **S93.311 Subluxation of tarsal joint of right foot**

✓7ᵗʰ **S93.312 Subluxation of tarsal joint of left foot**

✓7ᵗʰ **S93.313 Subluxation of tarsal joint of unspecified foot**

✓7ᵗʰ **S93.314 Dislocation of tarsal joint of right foot**

✓7ᵗʰ **S93.315 Dislocation of tarsal joint of left foot**

✓7ᵗʰ **S93.316 Dislocation of tarsal joint of unspecified foot**

✓6ᵗʰ **S93.32 Subluxation and dislocation of tarsometatarsal joint**

✓7ᵗʰ **S93.321 Subluxation of tarsometatarsal joint of right foot**

✓7ᵗʰ **S93.322 Subluxation of tarsometatarsal joint of left foot**

✓7ᵗʰ **S93.323 Subluxation of tarsometatarsal joint of unspecified foot**

✓7ᵗʰ **S93.324 Dislocation of tarsometatarsal joint of right foot**

✓7ᵗʰ **S93.325 Dislocation of tarsometatarsal joint of left foot**

✓7ᵗʰ **S93.326 Dislocation of tarsometatarsal joint of unspecified foot**

✓6ᵗʰ **S93.33 Other subluxation and dislocation of foot**

✓7ᵗʰ **S93.331 Other subluxation of right foot**

✓7ᵗʰ **S93.332 Other subluxation of left foot**

✓7ᵗʰ **S93.333 Other subluxation of unspecified foot**

✓7ᵗʰ **S93.334 Other dislocation of right foot**

✓7ᵗʰ **S93.335 Other dislocation of left foot**

✓7ᵗʰ **S93.336 Other dislocation of unspecified foot**

✓5ᵗʰ **S93.4 Sprain of ankle**

EXCLUDES 2   *injury of Achilles tendon (S86.0-)*

✓6ᵗʰ **S93.40 Sprain of unspecified ligament of ankle**

Sprain of ankle NOS
Sprained ankle NOS

✓7ᵗʰ **S93.401 Sprain of unspecified ligament of right ankle**

N Newborn: 0   P Pediatric: 0-17   M Maternity: 9-64   A Adult: 15-124   MCC Major Complication/Comorbidity   CC Complication/Comorbidity   SW Severe Wound Dx

1120   ICD-10-CM 2020

√7ᵗʰ **S93.402** Sprain of unspecified ligament of left ankle

√7ᵗʰ **S93.409** Sprain of unspecified ligament of unspecified ankle

√6ᵗʰ **S93.41** Sprain of calcaneofibular ligament

√7ᵗʰ **S93.411** Sprain of calcaneofibular ligament of right ankle

√7ᵗʰ **S93.412** Sprain of calcaneofibular ligament of left ankle

√7ᵗʰ **S93.419** Sprain of calcaneofibular ligament of unspecified ankle

√6ᵗʰ **S93.42** Sprain of deltoid ligament

√7ᵗʰ **S93.421** Sprain of deltoid ligament of right ankle

√7ᵗʰ **S93.422** Sprain of deltoid ligament of left ankle

√7ᵗʰ **S93.429** Sprain of deltoid ligament of unspecified ankle

√6ᵗʰ **S93.43** Sprain of tibiofibular ligament

√7ᵗʰ **S93.431** Sprain of tibiofibular ligament of right ankle

√7ᵗʰ **S93.432** Sprain of tibiofibular ligament of left ankle

√7ᵗʰ **S93.439** Sprain of tibiofibular ligament of unspecified ankle

√6ᵗʰ **S93.49** Sprain of other ligament of ankle

Sprain of internal collateral ligament
Sprain of talofibular ligament

√7ᵗʰ **S93.491** Sprain of other ligament of right ankle

√7ᵗʰ **S93.492** Sprain of other ligament of left ankle

√7ᵗʰ **S93.499** Sprain of other ligament of unspecified ankle

√5ᵗʰ **S93.5** Sprain of toe

√6ᵗʰ **S93.50** Unspecified sprain of toe

√7ᵗʰ **S93.501** Unspecified sprain of right great toe

√7ᵗʰ **S93.502** Unspecified sprain of left great toe

√7ᵗʰ **S93.503** Unspecified sprain of unspecified great toe

√7ᵗʰ **S93.504** Unspecified sprain of right lesser toe(s)

√7ᵗʰ **S93.505** Unspecified sprain of left lesser toe(s)

√7ᵗʰ **S93.506** Unspecified sprain of unspecified lesser toe(s)

√7ᵗʰ **S93.509** Unspecified sprain of unspecified toe(s)

√6ᵗʰ **S93.51** Sprain of interphalangeal joint of toe

√7ᵗʰ **S93.511** Sprain of interphalangeal joint of right great toe

√7ᵗʰ **S93.512** Sprain of interphalangeal joint of left great toe

√7ᵗʰ **S93.513** Sprain of interphalangeal joint of unspecified great toe

√7ᵗʰ **S93.514** Sprain of interphalangeal joint of right lesser toe(s)

√7ᵗʰ **S93.515** Sprain of interphalangeal joint of left lesser toe(s)

√7ᵗʰ **S93.516** Sprain of interphalangeal joint of unspecified lesser toe(s)

√7ᵗʰ **S93.519** Sprain of interphalangeal joint of unspecified toe(s)

√6ᵗʰ **S93.52** Sprain of metatarsophalangeal joint of toe

√7ᵗʰ **S93.521** Sprain of metatarsophalangeal joint of right great toe

√7ᵗʰ **S93.522** Sprain of metatarsophalangeal joint of left great toe

√7ᵗʰ **S93.523** Sprain of metatarsophalangeal joint of unspecified great toe

√7ᵗʰ **S93.524** Sprain of metatarsophalangeal joint of right lesser toe(s)

√7ᵗʰ **S93.525** Sprain of metatarsophalangeal joint of left lesser toe(s)

√7ᵗʰ **S93.526** Sprain of metatarsophalangeal joint of unspecified lesser toe(s)

√7ᵗʰ **S93.529** Sprain of metatarsophalangeal joint of unspecified toe(s)

√5ᵗʰ **S93.6** Sprain of foot

EXCLUDES 2   sprain of metatarsophalangeal joint of toe (S93.52-)
              sprain of toe (S93.5-)

√6ᵗʰ **S93.60** Unspecified sprain of foot

√7ᵗʰ **S93.601** Unspecified sprain of right foot

√7ᵗʰ **S93.602** Unspecified sprain of left foot

√7ᵗʰ **S93.609** Unspecified sprain of unspecified foot

√6ᵗʰ **S93.61** Sprain of tarsal ligament of foot

√7ᵗʰ **S93.611** Sprain of tarsal ligament of right foot

√7ᵗʰ **S93.612** Sprain of tarsal ligament of left foot

√7ᵗʰ **S93.619** Sprain of tarsal ligament of unspecified foot

√6ᵗʰ **S93.62** Sprain of tarsometatarsal ligament of foot

√7ᵗʰ **S93.621** Sprain of tarsometatarsal ligament of right foot

√7ᵗʰ **S93.622** Sprain of tarsometatarsal ligament of left foot

√7ᵗʰ **S93.629** Sprain of tarsometatarsal ligament of unspecified foot

√6ᵗʰ **S93.69** Other sprain of foot

√7ᵗʰ **S93.691** Other sprain of right foot

√7ᵗʰ **S93.692** Other sprain of left foot

√7ᵗʰ **S93.699** Other sprain of unspecified foot

√4ᵗʰ **S94 Injury of nerves at ankle and foot level**

Code also any associated open wound (S91.-)

The appropriate 7th character is to be added to each code from category S94.
A   initial encounter
D   subsequent encounter
S   sequela

√5ᵗʰ **S94.0** Injury of lateral plantar nerve

√x7ᵗʰ **S94.00** Injury of lateral plantar nerve, unspecified leg

√x7ᵗʰ **S94.01** Injury of lateral plantar nerve, right leg

√x7ᵗʰ **S94.02** Injury of lateral plantar nerve, left leg

√5ᵗʰ **S94.1** Injury of medial plantar nerve

√x7ᵗʰ **S94.10** Injury of medial plantar nerve, unspecified leg

√x7ᵗʰ **S94.11** Injury of medial plantar nerve, right leg

√x7ᵗʰ **S94.12** Injury of medial plantar nerve, left leg

√5ᵗʰ **S94.2** Injury of deep peroneal nerve at ankle and foot level

Injury of terminal, lateral branch of deep peroneal nerve

√x7ᵗʰ **S94.20** Injury of deep peroneal nerve at ankle and foot level, unspecified leg

√x7ᵗʰ **S94.21** Injury of deep peroneal nerve at ankle and foot level, right leg

√x7ᵗʰ **S94.22** Injury of deep peroneal nerve at ankle and foot level, left leg

√5ᵗʰ **S94.3** Injury of cutaneous sensory nerve at ankle and foot level

√x7ᵗʰ **S94.30** Injury of cutaneous sensory nerve at ankle and foot level, unspecified leg

√x7ᵗʰ **S94.31** Injury of cutaneous sensory nerve at ankle and foot level, right leg

√x7ᵗʰ **S94.32** Injury of cutaneous sensory nerve at ankle and foot level, left leg

√5ᵗʰ **S94.8** Injury of other nerves at ankle and foot level

√6ᵗʰ **S94.8X** Injury of other nerves at ankle and foot level

√7ᵗʰ **S94.8X1** Injury of other nerves at ankle and foot level, right leg

√7ᵗʰ **S94.8X2** Injury of other nerves at ankle and foot level, left leg

√7ᵗʰ **S94.8X9** Injury of other nerves at ankle and foot level, unspecified leg

√5ᵗʰ **S94.9** Injury of unspecified nerve at ankle and foot level

√x7ᵗʰ **S94.90** Injury of unspecified nerve at ankle and foot level, unspecified leg

√x7ᵗʰ **S94.91** Injury of unspecified nerve at ankle and foot level, right leg

√x7ᵗʰ **S94.92** Injury of unspecified nerve at ankle and foot level, left leg

✓4ᵗʰ **S95 Injury of blood vessels at ankle and foot level**

Code also any associated open wound (S91.-)

EXCLUDES 2   *injury of posterior tibial artery and vein (S85.1-, S85.8-)*

The appropriate 7th character is to be added to each code from category S95.
A   initial encounter
D   subsequent encounter
S   sequela

CC Excl: For CC codes in category S95, unless otherwise noted:
Right side: PDX collection 1325
Left side: PDX collection 1326
Unspecified side: PDX collection 1327

✓5ᵗʰ **S95.0 Injury of dorsal artery of foot**

✓6ᵗʰ **S95.00   Unspecified injury of dorsal artery of foot**

✓7ᵗʰ **S95.001 Unspecified injury of dorsal artery of right foot** cc

✓7ᵗʰ **S95.002 Unspecified injury of dorsal artery of left foot** cc

✓7ᵗʰ **S95.009 Unspecified injury of dorsal artery of unspecified foot** cc

✓6ᵗʰ **S95.01   Laceration of dorsal artery of foot**

✓7ᵗʰ **S95.011 Laceration of dorsal artery of right foot** cc

✓7ᵗʰ **S95.012 Laceration of dorsal artery of left foot** cc

✓7ᵗʰ **S95.019 Laceration of dorsal artery of unspecified foot** cc

✓6ᵗʰ **S95.09   Other specified injury of dorsal artery of foot**

✓7ᵗʰ **S95.091 Other specified injury of dorsal artery of right foot** cc

✓7ᵗʰ **S95.092 Other specified injury of dorsal artery of left foot** cc

✓7ᵗʰ **S95.099 Other specified injury of dorsal artery of unspecified foot** cc

✓5ᵗʰ **S95.1 Injury of plantar artery of foot**

CC Excl: For CC codes in subcategory S95.1:
Right side: PDX collection 1370
Left side: PDX collection 1371
Unspecified side: PDX collection 1372

✓6ᵗʰ **S95.10   Unspecified injury of plantar artery of foot**

✓7ᵗʰ **S95.101 Unspecified injury of plantar artery of right foot** cc

✓7ᵗʰ **S95.102 Unspecified injury of plantar artery of left foot** cc

✓7ᵗʰ **S95.109 Unspecified injury of plantar artery of unspecified foot** cc

✓6ᵗʰ **S95.11   Laceration of plantar artery of foot**

✓7ᵗʰ **S95.111 Laceration of plantar artery of right foot** cc

✓7ᵗʰ **S95.112 Laceration of plantar artery of left foot** cc

✓7ᵗʰ **S95.119 Laceration of plantar artery of unspecified foot** cc

✓6ᵗʰ **S95.19   Other specified injury of plantar artery of foot**

✓7ᵗʰ **S95.191 Other specified injury of plantar artery of right foot** cc

✓7ᵗʰ **S95.192 Other specified injury of plantar artery of left foot** cc

✓7ᵗʰ **S95.199 Other specified injury of plantar artery of unspecified foot** cc

✓5ᵗʰ **S95.2 Injury of dorsal vein of foot**

✓6ᵗʰ **S95.20   Unspecified injury of dorsal vein of foot**

✓7ᵗʰ **S95.201 Unspecified injury of dorsal vein of right foot** cc

✓7ᵗʰ **S95.202 Unspecified injury of dorsal vein of left foot** cc

✓7ᵗʰ **S95.209 Unspecified injury of dorsal vein of unspecified foot** cc

✓6ᵗʰ **S95.21   Laceration of dorsal vein of foot**

✓7ᵗʰ **S95.211 Laceration of dorsal vein of right foot** cc

✓7ᵗʰ **S95.212 Laceration of dorsal vein of left foot** cc

✓7ᵗʰ **S95.219 Laceration of dorsal vein of unspecified foot** cc

✓6ᵗʰ **S95.29   Other specified injury of dorsal vein of foot**

✓7ᵗʰ **S95.291 Other specified injury of dorsal vein of right foot** cc

✓7ᵗʰ **S95.292 Other specified injury of dorsal vein of left foot** cc

✓7ᵗʰ **S95.299 Other specified injury of dorsal vein of unspecified foot** cc

✓5ᵗʰ **S95.8 Injury of other blood vessels at ankle and foot level**

✓6ᵗʰ **S95.80   Unspecified injury of other blood vessels at ankle and foot level**

✓7ᵗʰ **S95.801 Unspecified injury of other blood vessels at ankle and foot level, right leg** cc

✓7ᵗʰ **S95.802 Unspecified injury of other blood vessels at ankle and foot level, left leg** cc

✓7ᵗʰ **S95.809 Unspecified injury of other blood vessels at ankle and foot level, unspecified leg** cc

✓6ᵗʰ **S95.81   Laceration of other blood vessels at ankle and foot level**

✓7ᵗʰ **S95.811 Laceration of other blood vessels at ankle and foot level, right leg** cc

✓7ᵗʰ **S95.812 Laceration of other blood vessels at ankle and foot level, left leg** cc

✓7ᵗʰ **S95.819 Laceration of other blood vessels at ankle and foot level, unspecified leg** cc

✓6ᵗʰ **S95.89   Other specified injury of other blood vessels at ankle and foot level**

✓7ᵗʰ **S95.891 Other specified injury of other blood vessels at ankle and foot level, right leg** cc

✓7ᵗʰ **S95.892 Other specified injury of other blood vessels at ankle and foot level, left leg** cc

✓7ᵗʰ **S95.899 Other specified injury of other blood vessels at ankle and foot level, unspecified leg** cc

✓5ᵗʰ **S95.9 Injury of unspecified blood vessel at ankle and foot level**

✓6ᵗʰ **S95.90   Unspecified injury of unspecified blood vessel at ankle and foot level**

✓7ᵗʰ **S95.901 Unspecified injury of unspecified blood vessel at ankle and foot level, right leg** cc

✓7ᵗʰ **S95.902 Unspecified injury of unspecified blood vessel at ankle and foot level, left leg** cc

✓7ᵗʰ **S95.909 Unspecified injury of unspecified blood vessel at ankle and foot level, unspecified leg** cc

✓6ᵗʰ **S95.91   Laceration of unspecified blood vessel at ankle and foot level**

✓7ᵗʰ **S95.911 Laceration of unspecified blood vessel at ankle and foot level, right leg** cc

✓7ᵗʰ **S95.912 Laceration of unspecified blood vessel at ankle and foot level, left leg** cc

✓7ᵗʰ **S95.919 Laceration of unspecified blood vessel at ankle and foot level, unspecified leg** cc

✓6ᵗʰ **S95.99   Other specified injury of unspecified blood vessel at ankle and foot level**

✓7ᵗʰ **S95.991 Other specified injury of unspecified blood vessel at ankle and foot level, right leg** cc

✓7ᵗʰ **S95.992 Other specified injury of unspecified blood vessel at ankle and foot level, left leg** cc

☑7ᵗʰ **S95.999 Other specified injury of unspecified blood vessel at ankle and foot level, unspecified leg**   CC

☑4ᵗʰ **S96 Injury of muscle and tendon at ankle and foot level**

    Code also any associated open wound (S91.-)

    EXCLUDES 2   *injury of Achilles tendon (S86.0-)*

                sprain of joints and ligaments of ankle and foot (S93.-)

    TIP: Refer to the Muscle/Tendon table at the beginning of this chapter.

    The appropriate 7th character is to be added to each code from category S96.

    A   initial encounter

    D   subsequent encounter

    S   sequela

    CC Excl: For CC codes in category S96:

    Right side: PDX collection 1364

    Left side: PDX collection 1365

    Unspecified side: PDX collection 1366

☑5ᵗʰ **S96.0 Injury of muscle and tendon of long flexor muscle of toe at ankle and foot level**

   ☑6ᵗʰ **S96.00 Unspecified injury of muscle and tendon of long flexor muscle of toe at ankle and foot level**

     ☑7ᵗʰ **S96.001 Unspecified injury of muscle and tendon of long flexor muscle of toe at ankle and foot level, right foot**

     ☑7ᵗʰ **S96.002 Unspecified injury of muscle and tendon of long flexor muscle of toe at ankle and foot level, left foot**

     ☑7ᵗʰ **S96.009 Unspecified injury of muscle and tendon of long flexor muscle of toe at ankle and foot level, unspecified foot**

   ☑6ᵗʰ **S96.01 Strain of muscle and tendon of long flexor muscle of toe at ankle and foot level**

     ☑7ᵗʰ **S96.011 Strain of muscle and tendon of long flexor muscle of toe at ankle and foot level, right foot**

     ☑7ᵗʰ **S96.012 Strain of muscle and tendon of long flexor muscle of toe at ankle and foot level, left foot**

     ☑7ᵗʰ **S96.019 Strain of muscle and tendon of long flexor muscle of toe at ankle and foot level, unspecified foot**

   ☑6ᵗʰ **S96.02 Laceration of muscle and tendon of long flexor muscle of toe at ankle and foot level**

     ☑7ᵗʰ **S96.021 Laceration of muscle and tendon of long flexor muscle of toe at ankle and foot level, right foot**   CC

     ☑7ᵗʰ **S96.022 Laceration of muscle and tendon of long flexor muscle of toe at ankle and foot level, left foot**   CC

     ☑7ᵗʰ **S96.029 Laceration of muscle and tendon of long flexor muscle of toe at ankle and foot level, unspecified foot**   CC

   ☑6ᵗʰ **S96.09 Other injury of muscle and tendon of long flexor muscle of toe at ankle and foot level**

     ☑7ᵗʰ **S96.091 Other injury of muscle and tendon of long flexor muscle of toe at ankle and foot level, right foot**

     ☑7ᵗʰ **S96.092 Other injury of muscle and tendon of long flexor muscle of toe at ankle and foot level, left foot**

     ☑7ᵗʰ **S96.099 Other injury of muscle and tendon of long flexor muscle of toe at ankle and foot level, unspecified foot**

☑5ᵗʰ **S96.1 Injury of muscle and tendon of long extensor muscle of toe at ankle and foot level**

   ☑6ᵗʰ **S96.10 Unspecified injury of muscle and tendon of long extensor muscle of toe at ankle and foot level**

     ☑7ᵗʰ **S96.101 Unspecified injury of muscle and tendon of long extensor muscle of toe at ankle and foot level, right foot**

     ☑7ᵗʰ **S96.102 Unspecified injury of muscle and tendon of long extensor muscle of toe at ankle and foot level, left foot**

     ☑7ᵗʰ **S96.109 Unspecified injury of muscle and tendon of long extensor muscle of toe at ankle and foot level, unspecified foot**

☑6ᵗʰ **S96.11 Strain of muscle and tendon of long extensor muscle of toe at ankle and foot level**

     ☑7ᵗʰ **S96.111 Strain of muscle and tendon of long extensor muscle of toe at ankle and foot level, right foot**

     ☑7ᵗʰ **S96.112 Strain of muscle and tendon of long extensor muscle of toe at ankle and foot level, left foot**

     ☑7ᵗʰ **S96.119 Strain of muscle and tendon of long extensor muscle of toe at ankle and foot level, unspecified foot**

   ☑6ᵗʰ **S96.12 Laceration of muscle and tendon of long extensor muscle of toe at ankle and foot level**

     ☑7ᵗʰ **S96.121 Laceration of muscle and tendon of long extensor muscle of toe at ankle and foot level, right foot**   CC

     ☑7ᵗʰ **S96.122 Laceration of muscle and tendon of long extensor muscle of toe at ankle and foot level, left foot**   CC

     ☑7ᵗʰ **S96.129 Laceration of muscle and tendon of long extensor muscle of toe at ankle and foot level, unspecified foot**   CC

   ☑6ᵗʰ **S96.19 Other specified injury of muscle and tendon of long extensor muscle of toe at ankle and foot level**

     ☑7ᵗʰ **S96.191 Other specified injury of muscle and tendon of long extensor muscle of toe at ankle and foot level, right foot**

     ☑7ᵗʰ **S96.192 Other specified injury of muscle and tendon of long extensor muscle of toe at ankle and foot level, left foot**

     ☑7ᵗʰ **S96.199 Other specified injury of muscle and tendon of long extensor muscle of toe at ankle and foot level, unspecified foot**

☑5ᵗʰ **S96.2 Injury of intrinsic muscle and tendon at ankle and foot level**

   ☑6ᵗʰ **S96.20 Unspecified injury of intrinsic muscle and tendon at ankle and foot level**

     ☑7ᵗʰ **S96.201 Unspecified injury of intrinsic muscle and tendon at ankle and foot level, right foot**

     ☑7ᵗʰ **S96.202 Unspecified injury of intrinsic muscle and tendon at ankle and foot level, left foot**

     ☑7ᵗʰ **S96.209 Unspecified injury of intrinsic muscle and tendon at ankle and foot level, unspecified foot**

   ☑6ᵗʰ **S96.21 Strain of intrinsic muscle and tendon at ankle and foot level**

     ☑7ᵗʰ **S96.211 Strain of intrinsic muscle and tendon at ankle and foot level, right foot**

     ☑7ᵗʰ **S96.212 Strain of intrinsic muscle and tendon at ankle and foot level, left foot**

     ☑7ᵗʰ **S96.219 Strain of intrinsic muscle and tendon at ankle and foot level, unspecified foot**

   ☑6ᵗʰ **S96.22 Laceration of intrinsic muscle and tendon at ankle and foot level**

     ☑7ᵗʰ **S96.221 Laceration of intrinsic muscle and tendon at ankle and foot level, right foot**   CC

     ☑7ᵗʰ **S96.222 Laceration of intrinsic muscle and tendon at ankle and foot level, left foot**   CC

     ☑7ᵗʰ **S96.229 Laceration of intrinsic muscle and tendon at ankle and foot level, unspecified foot**   CC

   ☑6ᵗʰ **S96.29 Other specified injury of intrinsic muscle and tendon at ankle and foot level**

     ☑7ᵗʰ **S96.291 Other specified injury of intrinsic muscle and tendon at ankle and foot level, right foot**

     ☑7ᵗʰ **S96.292 Other specified injury of intrinsic muscle and tendon at ankle and foot level, left foot**

     ☑7ᵗʰ **S96.299 Other specified injury of intrinsic muscle and tendon at ankle and foot level, unspecified foot**

☑ Additional Character Required   ☑x7ᵗʰ Placeholder   Unacceptable PDx   Questionable PDx   Manifestation   Unspecified Dx   H1-H14 HAC   HCC CMS-HCC Dx   HIV HIV Dx

ICD-10-CM 2020   1123

√5ᵗʰ **S96.8** **Injury of other specified muscles and tendons at ankle and foot level**

√6ᵗʰ **S96.80** **Unspecified injury of other specified muscles and tendons at ankle and foot level**

√7ᵗʰ **S96.801** **Unspecified injury of other specified muscles and tendons at ankle and foot level, right foot**

√7ᵗʰ **S96.802** **Unspecified injury of other specified muscles and tendons at ankle and foot level, left foot**

√7ᵗʰ **S96.809** **Unspecified injury of other specified muscles and tendons at ankle and foot level, unspecified foot**

√6ᵗʰ **S96.81** **Strain of other specified muscles and tendons at ankle and foot level**

√7ᵗʰ **S96.811** **Strain of other specified muscles and tendons at ankle and foot level, right foot**

√7ᵗʰ **S96.812** **Strain of other specified muscles and tendons at ankle and foot level, left foot**

√7ᵗʰ **S96.819** **Strain of other specified muscles and tendons at ankle and foot level, unspecified foot**

√6ᵗʰ **S96.82** **Laceration of other specified muscles and tendons at ankle and foot level**

√7ᵗʰ **S96.821** **Laceration of other specified muscles and tendons at ankle and foot level, right foot** **CC**

√7ᵗʰ **S96.822** **Laceration of other specified muscles and tendons at ankle and foot level, left foot** **CC**

√7ᵗʰ **S96.829** **Laceration of other specified muscles and tendons at ankle and foot level, unspecified foot** **CC**

√6ᵗʰ **S96.89** **Other specified injury of other specified muscles and tendons at ankle and foot level**

√7ᵗʰ **S96.891** **Other specified injury of other specified muscles and tendons at ankle and foot level, right foot**

√7ᵗʰ **S96.892** **Other specified injury of other specified muscles and tendons at ankle and foot level, left foot**

√7ᵗʰ **S96.899** **Other specified injury of other specified muscles and tendons at ankle and foot level, unspecified foot**

√5ᵗʰ **S96.9** **Injury of unspecified muscle and tendon at ankle and foot level**

√6ᵗʰ **S96.90** **Unspecified injury of unspecified muscle and tendon at ankle and foot level**

√7ᵗʰ **S96.901** **Unspecified injury of unspecified muscle and tendon at ankle and foot level, right foot**

√7ᵗʰ **S96.902** **Unspecified injury of unspecified muscle and tendon at ankle and foot level, left foot**

√7ᵗʰ **S96.909** **Unspecified injury of unspecified muscle and tendon at ankle and foot level, unspecified foot**

√6ᵗʰ **S96.91** **Strain of unspecified muscle and tendon at ankle and foot level**

√7ᵗʰ **S96.911** **Strain of unspecified muscle and tendon at ankle and foot level, right foot**

√7ᵗʰ **S96.912** **Strain of unspecified muscle and tendon at ankle and foot level, left foot**

√7ᵗʰ **S96.919** **Strain of unspecified muscle and tendon at ankle and foot level, unspecified foot**

√6ᵗʰ **S96.92** **Laceration of unspecified muscle and tendon at ankle and foot level**

√7ᵗʰ **S96.921** **Laceration of unspecified muscle and tendon at ankle and foot level, right foot** **CC**

√7ᵗʰ **S96.922** **Laceration of unspecified muscle and tendon at ankle and foot level, left foot** **CC**

√7ᵗʰ **S96.929** **Laceration of unspecified muscle and tendon at ankle and foot level, unspecified foot** **CC**

√6ᵗʰ **S96.99** **Other specified injury of unspecified muscle and tendon at ankle and foot level**

√7ᵗʰ **S96.991** **Other specified injury of unspecified muscle and tendon at ankle and foot level, right foot**

√7ᵗʰ **S96.992** **Other specified injury of unspecified muscle and tendon at ankle and foot level, left foot**

√7ᵗʰ **S96.999** **Other specified injury of unspecified muscle and tendon at ankle and foot level, unspecified foot**

√4ᵗʰ **S97** **Crushing injury of ankle and foot**

Use additional code(s) for all associated injuries

The appropriate 7th character is to be added to each code from category S97.
A   initial encounter
D   subsequent encounter
S   sequela

√5ᵗʰ **S97.0** **Crushing injury of ankle**

√x7ᵗʰ **S97.00** **Crushing injury of unspecified ankle**

√x7ᵗʰ **S97.01** **Crushing injury of right ankle**

√x7ᵗʰ **S97.02** **Crushing injury of left ankle**

√5ᵗʰ **S97.1** **Crushing injury of toe**

√6ᵗʰ **S97.10** **Crushing injury of unspecified toe(s)**

√7ᵗʰ **S97.101** **Crushing injury of unspecified right toe(s)**

√7ᵗʰ **S97.102** **Crushing injury of unspecified left toe(s)**

√7ᵗʰ **S97.109** **Crushing injury of unspecified toe(s)**
Crushing injury of toe NOS

√6ᵗʰ **S97.11** **Crushing injury of great toe**

√7ᵗʰ **S97.111** **Crushing injury of right great toe**

√7ᵗʰ **S97.112** **Crushing injury of left great toe**

√7ᵗʰ **S97.119** **Crushing injury of unspecified great toe**

√6ᵗʰ **S97.12** **Crushing injury of lesser toe(s)**

√7ᵗʰ **S97.121** **Crushing injury of right lesser toe(s)**

√7ᵗʰ **S97.122** **Crushing injury of left lesser toe(s)**

√7ᵗʰ **S97.129** **Crushing injury of unspecified lesser toe(s)**

√5ᵗʰ **S97.8** **Crushing injury of foot**

√x7ᵗʰ **S97.80** **Crushing injury of unspecified foot**
Crushing injury of foot NOS

√x7ᵗʰ **S97.81** **Crushing injury of right foot**

√x7ᵗʰ **S97.82** **Crushing injury of left foot**

√4ᵗʰ **S98** **Traumatic amputation of ankle and foot**

An amputation not identified as partial or complete should be coded to complete

The appropriate 7th character is to be added to each code from category S98.
A   initial encounter
D   subsequent encounter
S   sequela

CC Excl: For CC codes in category S98:
Right side: PDX collection 1333
Left side: PDX collection 1334
Unspecified side: PDX collection 1335

√5ᵗʰ **S98.0** **Traumatic amputation of foot at ankle level**

√6ᵗʰ **S98.01** **Complete traumatic amputation of foot at ankle level**

√7ᵗʰ **S98.011** **Complete traumatic amputation of right foot at ankle level** **CC** **HCC**

√7ᵗʰ **S98.012** **Complete traumatic amputation of left foot at ankle level** **CC** **HCC**

√7ᵗʰ **S98.019** **Complete traumatic amputation of unspecified foot at ankle level** **CC** **HCC**

√6ᵗʰ **S98.02** **Partial traumatic amputation of foot at ankle level**

√7ᵗʰ **S98.021** **Partial traumatic amputation of right foot at ankle level** **CC** **HCC**

√7ᵗʰ **S98.022** **Partial traumatic amputation of left foot at ankle level** **CC** **HCC**

√7th **S98.029** Partial traumatic amputation of unspecified foot at ankle level   `CC` `HCC`

√5th **S98.1** **Traumatic amputation of** one toe

√6th **S98.11** **Complete** traumatic amputation of **great** toe

    √7th **S98.111** **Complete traumatic amputation of** right **great toe**   `HCC`

    √7th **S98.112** **Complete traumatic amputation of** left **great toe**   `HCC`

    √7th **S98.119** **Complete traumatic amputation of unspecified great toe**   `HCC`

√6th **S98.12** **Partial** traumatic amputation of **great** toe

    √7th **S98.121** **Partial traumatic amputation of** right **great toe**   `HCC`

    √7th **S98.122** **Partial traumatic amputation of** left **great toe**   `HCC`

    √7th **S98.129** **Partial traumatic amputation of unspecified great toe**   `HCC`

√6th **S98.13** **Complete** traumatic amputation of **one lesser toe**
Traumatic amputation of toe NOS

    √7th **S98.131** **Complete traumatic amputation of one** right **lesser toe**   `HCC`

    √7th **S98.132** **Complete traumatic amputation of one** left **lesser toe**   `HCC`

    √7th **S98.139** **Complete traumatic amputation of one unspecified lesser toe**   `HCC`

√6th **S98.14** **Partial** traumatic amputation of **one lesser toe**

    √7th **S98.141** **Partial traumatic amputation of one** right **lesser toe**   `HCC`

    √7th **S98.142** **Partial traumatic amputation of one** left **lesser toe**   `HCC`

    √7th **S98.149** **Partial traumatic amputation of one unspecified lesser toe**   `HCC`

√5th **S98.2** **Traumatic amputation of** two or more lesser toes

√6th **S98.21** **Complete** traumatic amputation of two or more lesser toes

    √7th **S98.211** **Complete traumatic amputation of two or more** right **lesser toes**   `HCC`

    √7th **S98.212** **Complete traumatic amputation of two or more** left **lesser toes**   `HCC`

    √7th **S98.219** **Complete traumatic amputation of two or more unspecified lesser toes**   `HCC`

√6th **S98.22** **Partial** traumatic amputation of two or more lesser toes

    √7th **S98.221** **Partial traumatic amputation of two or more** right **lesser toes**   `HCC`

    √7th **S98.222** **Partial traumatic amputation of two or more** left **lesser toes**   `HCC`

    √7th **S98.229** **Partial traumatic amputation of two or more unspecified lesser toes**   `HCC`

√5th **S98.3** **Traumatic amputation of** midfoot

√6th **S98.31** **Complete** traumatic amputation of midfoot

    √7th **S98.311** **Complete traumatic amputation of** right **midfoot**   `CC` `HCC`

    √7th **S98.312** **Complete traumatic amputation of** left **midfoot**   `CC` `HCC`

    √7th **S98.319** **Complete traumatic amputation of unspecified midfoot**   `CC` `HCC`

√6th **S98.32** **Partial** traumatic amputation of midfoot

    √7th **S98.321** **Partial traumatic amputation of** right **midfoot**   `CC` `HCC`

    √7th **S98.322** **Partial traumatic amputation of** left **midfoot**   `CC` `HCC`

    √7th **S98.329** **Partial traumatic amputation of unspecified midfoot**   `CC` `HCC`

√5th **S98.9** **Traumatic amputation of foot, level unspecified**

√6th **S98.91** **Complete** traumatic amputation of foot, level unspecified

    √7th **S98.911** **Complete traumatic amputation of** right **foot, level unspecified**   `CC` `HCC`

    √7th **S98.912** **Complete traumatic amputation of** left **foot, level unspecified**   `CC` `HCC`

    √7th **S98.919** **Complete traumatic amputation of unspecified foot, level unspecified**   `CC` `HCC`

√6th **S98.92** **Partial** traumatic amputation of foot, level unspecified

    √7th **S98.921** **Partial traumatic amputation of** right **foot, level unspecified**   `CC` `HCC`

    √7th **S98.922** **Partial traumatic amputation of** left **foot, level unspecified**   `CC` `HCC`

    √7th **S98.929** **Partial traumatic amputation of unspecified foot, level unspecified**   `CC` `HCC`

√4th **S99** **Other and unspecified injuries of ankle and foot**
AHA: 2018,2Q,12; 2018,1Q,3; 2016,4Q,68-69

√5th **S99.0** **Physeal fracture of** calcaneus

> The appropriate 7th character is to be added to each code from subcategory S99.0.
> A   initial encounter for closed fracture
> B   initial encounter for open fracture
> D   subsequent encounter for fracture with routine healing
> G   subsequent encounter for fracture with delayed healing
> K   subsequent encounter for fracture with nonunion
> P   subsequent encounter for fracture with malunion
> S   sequela

√6th **S99.00** **Unspecified physeal fracture of** calcaneus

    √7th **S99.001** **Unspecified physeal fracture of** right **calcaneus**

    √7th **S99.002** **Unspecified physeal fracture of** left **calcaneus**

    √7th **S99.009** **Unspecified physeal fracture of unspecified calcaneus**

√6th **S99.01** **Salter-Harris Type I physeal fracture of calcaneus**

    √7th **S99.011** **Salter-Harris Type I physeal fracture of** right **calcaneus**

    √7th **S99.012** **Salter-Harris Type I physeal fracture of** left **calcaneus**

    √7th **S99.019** **Salter-Harris Type I physeal fracture of unspecified calcaneus**

√6th **S99.02** **Salter-Harris Type II physeal fracture of calcaneus**

    √7th **S99.021** **Salter-Harris Type II physeal fracture of** right **calcaneus**

    √7th **S99.022** **Salter-Harris Type II physeal fracture of** left **calcaneus**

    √7th **S99.029** **Salter-Harris Type II physeal fracture of unspecified calcaneus**

√6th **S99.03** **Salter-Harris Type III physeal fracture of calcaneus**

    √7th **S99.031** **Salter-Harris Type III physeal fracture of** right **calcaneus**

    √7th **S99.032** **Salter-Harris Type III physeal fracture of** left **calcaneus**

    √7th **S99.039** **Salter-Harris Type III physeal fracture of unspecified calcaneus**

√6th **S99.04** **Salter-Harris Type IV physeal fracture of calcaneus**

    √7th **S99.041** **Salter-Harris Type IV physeal fracture of** right **calcaneus**

    √7th **S99.042** **Salter-Harris Type IV physeal fracture of** left **calcaneus**

    √7th **S99.049** **Salter-Harris Type IV physeal fracture of unspecified calcaneus**

- ✓6ᵗʰ **S99.09**   **Other physeal fracture of calcaneus**
  - ✓7ᵗʰ **S99.091** Other physeal fracture of right calcaneus
  - ✓7ᵗʰ **S99.092** Other physeal fracture of left calcaneus
  - ✓7ᵗʰ **S99.099** Other physeal fracture of unspecified calcaneus
- ✓5ᵗʰ **S99.1**   **Physeal fracture of metatarsal**

  > The appropriate 7th character is to be added to each code from subcategory S99.1
  > A   initial encounter for closed fracture
  > B   initial encounter for open fracture
  > D   subsequent encounter for fracture with routine healing
  > G   subsequent encounter for fracture with delayed healing
  > K   subsequent encounter for fracture with nonunion
  > P   subsequent encounter for fracture with malunion
  > S   sequela

  - ✓6ᵗʰ **S99.10**   **Unspecified physeal fracture of metatarsal**
    - ✓7ᵗʰ **S99.101** Unspecified physeal fracture of right metatarsal
    - ✓7ᵗʰ **S99.102** Unspecified physeal fracture of left metatarsal
    - ✓7ᵗʰ **S99.109** Unspecified physeal fracture of unspecified metatarsal
  - ✓6ᵗʰ **S99.11**   **Salter-Harris Type I physeal fracture of metatarsal**
    - ✓7ᵗʰ **S99.111** Salter-Harris Type I physeal fracture of right metatarsal
    - ✓7ᵗʰ **S99.112** Salter-Harris Type I physeal fracture of left metatarsal
    - ✓7ᵗʰ **S99.119** Salter-Harris Type I physeal fracture of unspecified metatarsal
  - ✓6ᵗʰ **S99.12**   **Salter-Harris Type II physeal fracture of metatarsal**
    - ✓7ᵗʰ **S99.121** Salter-Harris Type II physeal fracture of right metatarsal
    - ✓7ᵗʰ **S99.122** Salter-Harris Type II physeal fracture of left metatarsal
    - ✓7ᵗʰ **S99.129** Salter-Harris Type II physeal fracture of unspecified metatarsal
  - ✓6ᵗʰ **S99.13**   **Salter-Harris Type III physeal fracture of metatarsal**
    - ✓7ᵗʰ **S99.131** Salter-Harris Type III physeal fracture of right metatarsal
    - ✓7ᵗʰ **S99.132** Salter-Harris Type III physeal fracture of left metatarsal
    - ✓7ᵗʰ **S99.139** Salter-Harris Type III physeal fracture of unspecified metatarsal
  - ✓6ᵗʰ **S99.14**   **Salter-Harris Type IV physeal fracture of metatarsal**
    - ✓7ᵗʰ **S99.141** Salter-Harris Type IV physeal fracture of right metatarsal
    - ✓7ᵗʰ **S99.142** Salter-Harris Type IV physeal fracture of left metatarsal
    - ✓7ᵗʰ **S99.149** Salter-Harris Type IV physeal fracture of unspecified metatarsal
  - ✓6ᵗʰ **S99.19**   **Other physeal fracture of metatarsal**
    - ✓7ᵗʰ **S99.191** Other physeal fracture of right metatarsal
    - ✓7ᵗʰ **S99.192** Other physeal fracture of left metatarsal
    - ✓7ᵗʰ **S99.199** Other physeal fracture of unspecified metatarsal
- ✓5ᵗʰ **S99.2**   **Physeal fracture of phalanx of toe**

  > The appropriate 7th character is to be added to each code from subcategories S99.2.
  > A   initial encounter for closed fracture
  > B   initial encounter for open fracture
  > D   subsequent encounter for fracture with routine healing
  > G   subsequent encounter for fracture with delayed healing
  > K   subsequent encounter for fracture with nonunion
  > P   subsequent encounter for fracture with malunion
  > S   sequela

  - ✓6ᵗʰ **S99.20**   **Unspecified physeal fracture of phalanx of toe**
    - ✓7ᵗʰ **S99.201** Unspecified physeal fracture of phalanx of right toe
    - ✓7ᵗʰ **S99.202** Unspecified physeal fracture of phalanx of left toe
    - ✓7ᵗʰ **S99.209** Unspecified physeal fracture of phalanx of unspecified toe
  - ✓6ᵗʰ **S99.21**   **Salter-Harris Type I physeal fracture of phalanx of toe**
    - ✓7ᵗʰ **S99.211** Salter-Harris Type I physeal fracture of phalanx of right toe

---

  - ✓7ᵗʰ **S99.212** Salter-Harris Type I physeal fracture of phalanx of left toe
  - ✓7ᵗʰ **S99.219** Salter-Harris Type I physeal fracture of phalanx of unspecified toe
- ✓6ᵗʰ **S99.22**   **Salter-Harris Type II physeal fracture of phalanx of toe**
  - ✓7ᵗʰ **S99.221** Salter-Harris Type II physeal fracture of phalanx of right toe
  - ✓7ᵗʰ **S99.222** Salter-Harris Type II physeal fracture of phalanx of left toe
  - ✓7ᵗʰ **S99.229** Salter-Harris Type II physeal fracture of phalanx of unspecified toe
- ✓6ᵗʰ **S99.23**   **Salter-Harris Type III physeal fracture of phalanx of toe**
  - ✓7ᵗʰ **S99.231** Salter-Harris Type III physeal fracture of phalanx of right toe
  - ✓7ᵗʰ **S99.232** Salter-Harris Type III physeal fracture of phalanx of left toe
  - ✓7ᵗʰ **S99.239** Salter-Harris Type III physeal fracture of phalanx of unspecified toe
- ✓6ᵗʰ **S99.24**   **Salter-Harris Type IV physeal fracture of phalanx of toe**
  - ✓7ᵗʰ **S99.241** Salter-Harris Type IV physeal fracture of phalanx of right toe
  - ✓7ᵗʰ **S99.242** Salter-Harris Type IV physeal fracture of phalanx of left toe
  - ✓7ᵗʰ **S99.249** Salter-Harris Type IV physeal fracture of phalanx of unspecified toe
- ✓6ᵗʰ **S99.29**   **Other physeal fracture of phalanx of toe**
  - ✓7ᵗʰ **S99.291** Other physeal fracture of phalanx of right toe
  - ✓7ᵗʰ **S99.292** Other physeal fracture of phalanx of left toe
  - ✓7ᵗʰ **S99.299** Other physeal fracture of phalanx of unspecified toe
- ✓5ᵗʰ **S99.8**   **Other specified injuries of ankle and foot**

  > The appropriate 7th character is to be added to each code from subcategory S99.8.
  > A   initial encounter
  > D   subsequent encounter
  > S   sequela

  - ✓6ᵗʰ **S99.81**   **Other specified injuries of ankle**
    - ✓7ᵗʰ **S99.811** Other specified injuries of right ankle
    - ✓7ᵗʰ **S99.812** Other specified injuries of left ankle
    - ✓7ᵗʰ **S99.819** Other specified injuries of unspecified ankle
  - ✓6ᵗʰ **S99.82**   **Other specified injuries of foot**
    - ✓7ᵗʰ **S99.821** Other specified injuries of right foot
    - ✓7ᵗʰ **S99.822** Other specified injuries of left foot
    - ✓7ᵗʰ **S99.829** Other specified injuries of unspecified foot
- ✓5ᵗʰ **S99.9**   **Unspecified injury of ankle and foot**

  > The appropriate 7th character is to be added to each code from subcategory S99.9.
  > A   initial encounter
  > D   subsequent encounter
  > S   sequela

  - ✓6ᵗʰ **S99.91**   **Unspecified injury of ankle**
    - ✓7ᵗʰ **S99.911** Unspecified injury of right ankle
    - ✓7ᵗʰ **S99.912** Unspecified injury of left ankle
    - ✓7ᵗʰ **S99.919** Unspecified injury of unspecified ankle
  - ✓6ᵗʰ **S99.92**   **Unspecified injury of foot**
    - ✓7ᵗʰ **S99.921** Unspecified injury of right foot
    - ✓7ᵗʰ **S99.922** Unspecified injury of left foot
    - ✓7ᵗʰ **S99.929** Unspecified injury of unspecified foot

Ⓝ Newborn: 0   Ⓟ Pediatric: 0-17   Ⓜ Maternity: 9-64   Ⓐ Adult: 15-124   **MCC** Major Complication/Comorbidity   **CC** Complication/Comorbidity   **SW** Severe Wound Dx

1126   ICD-10-CM 2020

INJURY, POISONING AND CERTAIN OTHER CONSEQUENCES OF EXTERNAL CAUSES (T07-T88)

Injuries involving multiple body regions (T07)

EXCLUDES 1 burns and corrosions (T20-T32)
frostbite (T33-T34)
insect bite or sting, venomous (T63.4)
sunburn (L55.-)

✓x7ᵗʰ **T07 Unspecified multiple injuries**

   EXCLUDES 1 injury NOS (T14.90)

   AHA: 2017,4Q,26

   The appropriate 7th character is to be added to code T07.
   A   initial encounter
   D   subsequent encounter
   S   sequela

Injury of unspecified body region (T14)

✓4ᵗʰ **T14 Injury of unspecified body region**

   EXCLUDES 1 multiple unspecified injuries (T07)

   AHA: 2017,4Q,26

   The appropriate 7th character is to be added to each code from category T14.
   A   initial encounter
   D   subsequent encounter
   S   sequela

   ✓x7ᵗʰ **T14.8 Other injury of unspecified body region**
      Abrasion NOS
      Contusion NOS
      Crush injury NOS
      Fracture NOS
      Skin injury NOS
      Vascular injury NOS
      Wound NOS

   ✓5ᵗʰ **T14.9 Unspecified injury**
      ✓x7ᵗʰ **T14.90 Injury, unspecified**
         Injury NOS
      ✓x7ᵗʰ **T14.91 Suicide attempt**   HCC
         Attempted suicide NOS

Effects of foreign body entering through natural orifice (T15-T19)

EXCLUDES 2 foreign body accidentally left in operation wound (T81.5-)
foreign body in penetrating wound — see open wound by body region
residual foreign body in soft tissue (M79.5)
splinter, without open wound — see superficial injury by body region

✓4ᵗʰ **T15 Foreign body on external eye**

   EXCLUDES 2 foreign body in penetrating wound of orbit and eye ball (S05.4-, S05.5-)
   open wound of eyelid and periocular area (S01.1-)
   retained foreign body in eyelid (H02.8-)
   retained (old) foreign body in penetrating wound of orbit and eye ball (H05.5-, H44.6-, H44.7-)
   superficial foreign body of eyelid and periocular area (S00.25-)

   The appropriate 7th character is to be added to each code from category T15.
   A   initial encounter
   D   subsequent encounter
   S   sequela

   ✓5ᵗʰ **T15.0 Foreign body in cornea**
      ✓x7ᵗʰ **T15.00 Foreign body in cornea, unspecified eye**
      ✓x7ᵗʰ **T15.01 Foreign body in cornea, right eye**
      ✓x7ᵗʰ **T15.02 Foreign body in cornea, left eye**

   ✓5ᵗʰ **T15.1 Foreign body in conjunctival sac**
      ✓x7ᵗʰ **T15.10 Foreign body in conjunctival sac, unspecified eye**
      ✓x7ᵗʰ **T15.11 Foreign body in conjunctival sac, right eye**
      ✓x7ᵗʰ **T15.12 Foreign body in conjunctival sac, left eye**

   ✓5ᵗʰ **T15.8 Foreign body in other and multiple parts of external eye**
      Foreign body in lacrimal punctum
      ✓x7ᵗʰ **T15.80 Foreign body in other and multiple parts of external eye, unspecified eye**

   ✓x7ᵗʰ **T15.81 Foreign body in other and multiple parts of external eye, right eye**
   ✓x7ᵗʰ **T15.82 Foreign body in other and multiple parts of external eye, left eye**

   ✓5ᵗʰ **T15.9 Foreign body on external eye, part unspecified**
      ✓x7ᵗʰ **T15.90 Foreign body on external eye, part unspecified, unspecified eye**
      ✓x7ᵗʰ **T15.91 Foreign body on external eye, part unspecified, right eye**
      ✓x7ᵗʰ **T15.92 Foreign body on external eye, part unspecified, left eye**

✓4ᵗʰ **T16 Foreign body in ear**

   INCLUDES foreign body in auditory canal

   The appropriate 7th character is to be added to each code from category T16.
   A   initial encounter
   D   subsequent encounter
   S   sequela

   ✓x7ᵗʰ **T16.1 Foreign body in right ear**
   ✓x7ᵗʰ **T16.2 Foreign body in left ear**
   ✓x7ᵗʰ **T16.9 Foreign body in ear, unspecified ear**

✓4ᵗʰ **T17 Foreign body in respiratory tract**

   The appropriate 7th character is to be added to each code from category T17.
   A   initial encounter
   D   subsequent encounter
   S   sequela

   CC Excl: For CC codes in category T17, unless otherwise noted: PDX collection 1374

   ✓x7ᵗʰ **T17.0 Foreign body in nasal sinus**
   ✓x7ᵗʰ **T17.1 Foreign body in nostril**
      Foreign body in nose NOS

   ✓5ᵗʰ **T17.2 Foreign body in pharynx**
      Foreign body in nasopharynx
      Foreign body in throat NOS
      ✓6ᵗʰ **T17.20 Unspecified foreign body in pharynx**
         ✓7ᵗʰ **T17.200 Unspecified foreign body in pharynx causing asphyxiation**
         ✓7ᵗʰ **T17.208 Unspecified foreign body in pharynx causing other injury**
      ✓6ᵗʰ **T17.21 Gastric contents in pharynx**
         Aspiration of gastric contents into pharynx
         Vomitus in pharynx
         ✓7ᵗʰ **T17.210 Gastric contents in pharynx causing asphyxiation**
         ✓7ᵗʰ **T17.218 Gastric contents in pharynx causing other injury**
      ✓6ᵗʰ **T17.22 Food in pharynx**
         Bones in pharynx
         Seeds in pharynx
         ✓7ᵗʰ **T17.220 Food in pharynx causing asphyxiation**
         ✓7ᵗʰ **T17.228 Food in pharynx causing other injury**
      ✓6ᵗʰ **T17.29 Other foreign object in pharynx**
         ✓7ᵗʰ **T17.290 Other foreign object in pharynx causing asphyxiation**
         ✓7ᵗʰ **T17.298 Other foreign object in pharynx causing other injury**

   ✓5ᵗʰ **T17.3 Foreign body in larynx**
      ✓6ᵗʰ **T17.30 Unspecified foreign body in larynx**
         ✓7ᵗʰ **T17.300 Unspecified foreign body in larynx causing asphyxiation**
         ✓7ᵗʰ **T17.308 Unspecified foreign body in larynx causing other injury**
      ✓6ᵗʰ **T17.31 Gastric contents in larynx**
         Aspiration of gastric contents into larynx
         Vomitus in larynx
         ✓7ᵗʰ **T17.310 Gastric contents in larynx causing asphyxiation**
         ✓7ᵗʰ **T17.318 Gastric contents in larynx causing other injury**
      ✓6ᵗʰ **T17.32 Food in larynx**
         Bones in larynx
         Seeds in larynx
         ✓7ᵗʰ **T17.320 Food in larynx causing asphyxiation**

√7ᵗʰ **T17.328 Food in larynx** causing other injury

√6ᵗʰ **T17.39 Other foreign object in larynx**

√7ᵗʰ **T17.390 Other foreign object in larynx** causing asphyxiation

√7ᵗʰ **T17.398 Other foreign object in larynx** causing other injury

√5ᵗʰ **T17.4 Foreign body in trachea**

CC Excl: For CC codes in subcategory T17.4: PDX collection 1373

√6ᵗʰ **T17.40 Unspecified foreign body in trachea**

√7ᵗʰ **T17.400 Unspecified foreign body in trachea** causing asphyxiation ᴄᴄ

√7ᵗʰ **T17.408 Unspecified foreign body in trachea** causing other injury ᴄᴄ

√6ᵗʰ **T17.41 Gastric contents in trachea**

Aspiration of gastric contents into trachea
Vomitus in trachea

√7ᵗʰ **T17.410 Gastric contents in trachea** causing asphyxiation ᴄᴄ

√7ᵗʰ **T17.418 Gastric contents in trachea** causing other injury ᴄᴄ

√6ᵗʰ **T17.42 Food in trachea**

Bones in trachea
Seeds in trachea

√7ᵗʰ **T17.420 Food in trachea** causing asphyxiation ᴄᴄ

√7ᵗʰ **T17.428 Food in trachea** causing other injury ᴄᴄ

√6ᵗʰ **T17.49 Other foreign object in trachea**

√7ᵗʰ **T17.490 Other foreign object in trachea** causing asphyxiation ᴄᴄ

√7ᵗʰ **T17.498 Other foreign object in trachea** causing other injury ᴄᴄ

√5ᵗʰ **T17.5 Foreign body in bronchus**

√6ᵗʰ **T17.50 Unspecified foreign body in bronchus**

√7ᵗʰ **T17.500 Unspecified foreign body in bronchus** causing asphyxiation ᴄᴄ

√7ᵗʰ **T17.508 Unspecified foreign body in bronchus** causing other injury ᴄᴄ

√6ᵗʰ **T17.51 Gastric contents in bronchus**

Aspiration of gastric contents into bronchus
Vomitus in bronchus

√7ᵗʰ **T17.510 Gastric contents in bronchus** causing asphyxiation ᴄᴄ

√7ᵗʰ **T17.518 Gastric contents in bronchus** causing other injury ᴄᴄ

√6ᵗʰ **T17.52 Food in bronchus**

Bones in bronchus
Seeds in bronchus

√7ᵗʰ **T17.520 Food in bronchus** causing asphyxiation ᴄᴄ

√7ᵗʰ **T17.528 Food in bronchus** causing other injury ᴄᴄ

√6ᵗʰ **T17.59 Other foreign object in bronchus**

√7ᵗʰ **T17.590 Other foreign object in bronchus** causing asphyxiation ᴄᴄ

√7ᵗʰ **T17.598 Other foreign object in bronchus** causing other injury ᴄᴄ

√5ᵗʰ **T17.8 Foreign body in other parts of respiratory tract**

Foreign body in bronchioles
Foreign body in lung

√6ᵗʰ **T17.80 Unspecified foreign body in other parts of respiratory tract**

√7ᵗʰ **T17.800 Unspecified foreign body in other parts of respiratory tract** causing asphyxiation ᴄᴄ

√7ᵗʰ **T17.808 Unspecified foreign body in other parts of respiratory tract** causing other injury ᴄᴄ

√6ᵗʰ **T17.81 Gastric contents in other parts of respiratory tract**

Aspiration of gastric contents into other parts of respiratory tract
Vomitus in other parts of respiratory tract

√7ᵗʰ **T17.810 Gastric contents in other parts of respiratory tract** causing asphyxiation ᴄᴄ

√7ᵗʰ **T17.818 Gastric contents in other parts of respiratory tract** causing other injury ᴄᴄ

√6ᵗʰ **T17.82 Food in other parts of respiratory tract**

Bones in other parts of respiratory tract
Seeds in other parts of respiratory tract

√7ᵗʰ **T17.820 Food in other parts of respiratory tract** causing asphyxiation ᴄᴄ

√7ᵗʰ **T17.828 Food in other parts of respiratory tract** causing other injury ᴄᴄ

√6ᵗʰ **T17.89 Other foreign object in other parts of respiratory tract**

√7ᵗʰ **T17.890 Other foreign object in other parts of respiratory tract** causing asphyxiation ᴄᴄ

√7ᵗʰ **T17.898 Other foreign object in other parts of respiratory tract** causing other injury ᴄᴄ

√5ᵗʰ **T17.9 Foreign body in respiratory tract, part unspecified**

√6ᵗʰ **T17.90 Unspecified foreign body in respiratory tract, part unspecified**

√7ᵗʰ **T17.900 Unspecified foreign body in respiratory tract, part unspecified** causing asphyxiation ᴄᴄ

√7ᵗʰ **T17.908 Unspecified foreign body in respiratory tract, part unspecified** causing other injury ᴄᴄ

√6ᵗʰ **T17.91 Gastric contents in respiratory tract, part unspecified**

Aspiration of gastric contents into respiratory tract, part unspecified
Vomitus in trachea respiratory tract, part unspecified

√7ᵗʰ **T17.910 Gastric contents in respiratory tract, part unspecified** causing asphyxiation ᴄᴄ

√7ᵗʰ **T17.918 Gastric contents in respiratory tract, part unspecified** causing other injury ᴄᴄ

√6ᵗʰ **T17.92 Food in respiratory tract, part unspecified**

Bones in respiratory tract, part unspecified
Seeds in respiratory tract, part unspecified

√7ᵗʰ **T17.920 Food in respiratory tract, part unspecified** causing asphyxiation ᴄᴄ

√7ᵗʰ **T17.928 Food in respiratory tract, part unspecified** causing other injury ᴄᴄ

√6ᵗʰ **T17.99 Other foreign object in respiratory tract, part unspecified**

√7ᵗʰ **T17.990 Other foreign object in respiratory tract, part unspecified in** causing asphyxiation ᴄᴄ

√7ᵗʰ **T17.998 Other foreign object in respiratory tract, part unspecified** causing other injury ᴄᴄ

√4ᵗʰ **T18 Foreign body in alimentary tract**

ᴇxᴄʟᴜᴅᴇꜱ 2   foreign body in pharynx (T17.2-)

The appropriate 7th character is to be added to each code from category T18.
A   initial encounter
D   subsequent encounter
S   sequela

√x7ᵗʰ **T18.0 Foreign body in mouth**

ℕ Newborn: 0   ℙ Pediatric: 0-17   Ⓜ Maternity: 9-64   Ⓐ Adult: 15-124   ᴍᴄᴄ Major Complication/Comorbidity   ᴄᴄ Complication/Comorbidity   ꜱᴡ Severe Wound Dx

1128   ICD-10-CM 2020

√5ᵗʰ **T18.1** **Foreign body in esophagus**

> EXCLUDES 2   *foreign body in respiratory tract (T17.-)*

√6ᵗʰ **T18.10** **Unspecified foreign body in esophagus**

√7ᵗʰ **T18.100** **Unspecified foreign body in esophagus causing compression of trachea**
> Unspecified foreign body in esophagus causing obstruction of respiration

√7ᵗʰ **T18.108** **Unspecified foreign body in esophagus causing other injury**

√6ᵗʰ **T18.11** **Gastric contents in esophagus**
> Vomitus in esophagus

√7ᵗʰ **T18.110** **Gastric contents in esophagus causing compression of trachea**
> Gastric contents in esophagus causing obstruction of respiration

√7ᵗʰ **T18.118** **Gastric contents in esophagus causing other injury**

√6ᵗʰ **T18.12** **Food in esophagus**
> Bones in esophagus
> Seeds in esophagus

√7ᵗʰ **T18.120** **Food in esophagus causing compression of trachea**
> Food in esophagus causing obstruction of respiration

√7ᵗʰ **T18.128** **Food in esophagus causing other injury**

√6ᵗʰ **T18.19** **Other foreign object in esophagus**
> **AHA:** 2015,1Q,23

√7ᵗʰ **T18.190** **Other foreign object in esophagus causing compression of trachea**   CC
> Other foreign body in esophagus causing obstruction of respiration
> **TIP:** Any foreign object lodged in the esophagus requires immediate treatment and is considered an injury. Assign this code when there is respiratory compromise or compression.

√7ᵗʰ **T18.198** **Other foreign object in esophagus causing other injury**
> **TIP:** Any foreign object lodged in the esophagus requires immediate treatment and is considered an injury. Assign this code when there is no respiratory compromise or compression.

√x7ᵗʰ **T18.2** **Foreign body in stomach**   CC

√x7ᵗʰ **T18.3** **Foreign body in small intestine**

√x7ᵗʰ **T18.4** **Foreign body in colon**

√x7ᵗʰ **T18.5** **Foreign body in anus and rectum**
> Foreign body in rectosigmoid (junction)

√x7ᵗʰ **T18.8** **Foreign body in other parts of alimentary tract**

√x7ᵗʰ **T18.9** **Foreign body of alimentary tract, part unspecified**
> Foreign body in digestive system NOS
> Swallowed foreign body NOS

√4ᵗʰ **T19** **Foreign body in genitourinary tract**

> EXCLUDES 2   *complications due to implanted mesh (T83.7-)*
> *mechanical complications of contraceptive device (intrauterine) (vaginal) (T83.3-)*
> *presence of contraceptive device (intrauterine) (vaginal) (Z97.5)*

> The appropriate 7th character is to be added to each code from category T19.
> A   initial encounter
> D   subsequent encounter
> S   sequela

√x7ᵗʰ **T19.0** **Foreign body in urethra**

√x7ᵗʰ **T19.1** **Foreign body in bladder**

√x7ᵗʰ **T19.2** **Foreign body in vulva and vagina**   ♀

√x7ᵗʰ **T19.3** **Foreign body in uterus**   ♀

√x7ᵗʰ **T19.4** **Foreign body in penis**   ♂

√x7ᵗʰ **T19.8** **Foreign body in other parts of genitourinary tract**

√x7ᵗʰ **T19.9** **Foreign body in genitourinary tract, part unspecified**

BURNS AND CORROSIONS (T20-T32)

INCLUDES   burns (thermal) from electrical heating appliances
> burns (thermal) from electricity
> burns (thermal) from flame
> burns (thermal) from friction
> burns (thermal) from hot air and hot gases
> burns (thermal) from hot objects
> burns (thermal) from lightning
> burns (thermal) from radiation
> chemical burn [corrosion] (external) (internal)
> scalds

EXCLUDES 2   *erythema [dermatitis] ab igne (L59.0)*
> *radiation-related disorders of the skin and subcutaneous tissue (L55-L59)*
> *sunburn (L55.-)*

AHA: 2016,2Q,4

Burns and corrosions of external body surface, specified by site (T20-T25)

INCLUDES   burns and corrosions of first degree [erythema]
> burns and corrosions of second degree [blisters] [epidermal loss]
> burns and corrosions of third degree [deep necrosis of underlying tissue] [full-thickness skin loss]

Use additional code from category T31 or T32 to identify extent of body surface involved

√4ᵗʰ **T20** **Burn and corrosion of head, face, and neck**

> EXCLUDES 2   *burn and corrosion of ear drum (T28.41, T28.91)*
> *burn and corrosion of eye and adnexa (T26.-)*
> *burn and corrosion of mouth and pharynx (T28.0)*

AHA: 2015,1Q,18-19

> The appropriate 7th character is to be added to each code from category T20.
> A   initial encounter
> D   subsequent encounter
> S   sequela

√5ᵗʰ **T20.0** **Burn of unspecified degree of head, face, and neck**
> Use additional external cause code to identify the source, place and intent of the burn (X00-X19, X75-X77, X96-X98, Y92)

√x7ᵗʰ **T20.00** **Burn of unspecified degree of head, face, and neck, unspecified site**

√6ᵗʰ **T20.01** **Burn of unspecified degree of ear [any part, except ear drum]**
> EXCLUDES 2   *burn of ear drum (T28.41-)*

√7ᵗʰ **T20.011** **Burn of unspecified degree of right ear [any part, except ear drum]**

√7ᵗʰ **T20.012** **Burn of unspecified degree of left ear [any part, except ear drum]**

√7ᵗʰ **T20.019** **Burn of unspecified degree of unspecified ear [any part, except ear drum]**

√x7ᵗʰ **T20.02** **Burn of unspecified degree of lip(s)**

√x7ᵗʰ **T20.03** **Burn of unspecified degree of chin**

√x7ᵗʰ **T20.04** **Burn of unspecified degree of nose (septum)**

√x7ᵗʰ **T20.05** **Burn of unspecified degree of scalp [any part]**

√x7ᵗʰ **T20.06** **Burn of unspecified degree of forehead and cheek**

√x7ᵗʰ **T20.07** **Burn of unspecified degree of neck**

√x7ᵗʰ **T20.09** **Burn of unspecified degree of multiple sites of head, face, and neck**

√5ᵗʰ **T20.1** **Burn of first degree of head, face, and neck**
> Use additional external cause code to identify the source, place and intent of the burn (X00-X19, X75-X77, X96-X98, Y92)

√x7ᵗʰ **T20.10** **Burn of first degree of head, face, and neck, unspecified site**

√6ᵗʰ **T20.11** **Burn of first degree of ear [any part, except ear drum]**
> EXCLUDES 2   *burn of ear drum (T28.41-)*

√7ᵗʰ **T20.111** **Burn of first degree of right ear [any part, except ear drum]**

√7ᵗʰ **T20.112** **Burn of first degree of left ear [any part, except ear drum]**

√7ᵗʰ **T20.119** **Burn of first degree of unspecified ear [any part, except ear drum]**

√x7ᵗʰ **T20.12** **Burn of first degree of lip(s)**

√x7ᵗʰ **T20.13** **Burn of first degree of chin**

√x7ᵗʰ **T20.14** **Burn of first degree of nose (septum)**

√x7ᵗʰ **T20.15** **Burn of first degree of scalp [any part]**

√x7ᵗʰ **T20.16** **Burn of first degree of forehead and cheek**

✓x7th   **T20.17**   Burn of first degree of **neck**

✓x7th   **T20.19**   Burn of first degree of **multiple sites** of head, face, and neck

Degree of Burns

Epidermis
Dermis
Subcutaneous

Normal   First Degree Burn

Epidermis
Dermis
Subcutaneous

Second Degree Burn   Third Degree Burn

✓5th   **T20.2**   **Burn of second degree of head, face, and neck**

Use additional external cause code to identify the source, place and intent of the burn (X00-X19, X75-X77, X96-X98, Y92)

✓x7th   **T20.20**   **Burn of second degree of head, face, and neck, unspecified site**

✓6th   **T20.21**   **Burn of second degree of ear [any part, except ear drum]**

    EXCLUDES 2   burn of ear drum (T28.41-)

✓7th   **T20.211**   Burn of second degree of **right ear** [any part, except ear drum]

✓7th   **T20.212**   Burn of second degree of **left ear** [any part, except ear drum]

✓7th   **T20.219**   Burn of second degree of **unspecified ear** [any part, except ear drum]

✓x7th   **T20.22**   Burn of second degree of **lip(s)**

✓x7th   **T20.23**   Burn of second degree of **chin**

✓x7th   **T20.24**   Burn of second degree of **nose (septum)**

✓x7th   **T20.25**   Burn of second degree of **scalp [any part]**

✓x7th   **T20.26**   Burn of second degree of **forehead and cheek**

✓x7th   **T20.27**   Burn of second degree of **neck**

✓x7th   **T20.29**   Burn of second degree of **multiple sites** of head, face, and neck

✓5th   **T20.3**   **Burn of third degree of head, face, and neck**

Use additional external cause code to identify the source, place and intent of the burn (X00-X19, X75-X77, X96-X98, Y92)

✓x7th   **T20.30**   **Burn of third degree of head, face, and neck, unspecified site**   `CC` `H5` `SW`

    CC Excl: PDX collection 1375

✓6th   **T20.31**   **Burn of third degree of ear [any part, except ear drum]**

    EXCLUDES 2   burn of ear drum (T28.41-)

    AHA: 2015,1Q,18

    CC Excl: For CC codes in subcategory T20.31: PDX collection 1376

✓7th   **T20.311**   Burn of third degree of **right ear** [any part, except ear drum]   `CC` `H5` `SW`

✓7th   **T20.312**   Burn of third degree of **left ear** [any part, except ear drum]   `CC` `H5` `SW`

✓7th   **T20.319**   Burn of third degree of **unspecified ear** [any part, except ear drum]   `CC` `H5` `SW`

✓x7th   **T20.32**   Burn of third degree of **lip(s)**   `CC` `H5` `SW`

    CC Excl: PDX collection 1377

✓x7th   **T20.33**   Burn of third degree of **chin**   `CC` `H5` `SW`

    CC Excl: PDX collection 1378

✓x7th   **T20.34**   Burn of third degree of **nose (septum)**   `CC` `H5` `SW`

    CC Excl: PDX collection 1379

✓x7th   **T20.35**   Burn of third degree of **scalp [any part]**   `CC` `H5` `SW`

    CC Excl: PDX collection 1380

✓x7th   **T20.36**   Burn of third degree of **forehead and cheek**   `CC` `H5` `SW`

    CC Excl: PDX collection 1381

✓x7th   **T20.37**   Burn of third degree of **neck**   `CC` `H5` `SW`

    CC Excl: PDX collection 1382

✓x7th   **T20.39**   Burn of third degree of **multiple sites** of head, face, and neck   `CC` `H5` `SW`

    CC Excl: PDX collection 1383

✓5th   **T20.4**   **Corrosion of unspecified degree of head, face, and neck**

Code first (T51-T65) to identify chemical and intent

Use additional external cause code to identify place (Y92)

✓x7th   **T20.40**   **Corrosion of unspecified degree of head, face, and neck, unspecified site**

✓6th   **T20.41**   **Corrosion of unspecified degree of ear [any part, except ear drum]**

    EXCLUDES 2   corrosion of ear drum (T28.91-)

✓7th   **T20.411**   Corrosion of unspecified degree of **right ear** [any part, except ear drum]

✓7th   **T20.412**   Corrosion of unspecified degree of **left ear** [any part, except ear drum]

✓7th   **T20.419**   Corrosion of unspecified degree of **unspecified ear** [any part, except ear drum]

✓x7th   **T20.42**   Corrosion of unspecified degree of **lip(s)**

✓x7th   **T20.43**   Corrosion of unspecified degree of **chin**

✓x7th   **T20.44**   Corrosion of unspecified degree of **nose (septum)**

✓x7th   **T20.45**   Corrosion of unspecified degree of **scalp [any part]**

✓x7th   **T20.46**   Corrosion of unspecified degree of **forehead and cheek**

✓x7th   **T20.47**   Corrosion of unspecified degree of **neck**

✓x7th   **T20.49**   Corrosion of unspecified degree of **multiple sites** of head, face, and neck

✓5th   **T20.5**   **Corrosion of first degree of head, face, and neck**

Code first (T51-T65) to identify chemical and intent

Use additional external cause code to identify place (Y92)

✓x7th   **T20.50**   **Corrosion of first degree of head, face, and neck, unspecified site**

✓6th   **T20.51**   **Corrosion of first degree of ear [any part, except ear drum]**

    EXCLUDES 2   corrosion of ear drum (T28.91-)

✓7th   **T20.511**   Corrosion of first degree of **right ear** [any part, except ear drum]

✓7th   **T20.512**   Corrosion of first degree of **left ear** [any part, except ear drum]

✓7th   **T20.519**   Corrosion of first degree of **unspecified ear** [any part, except ear drum]

✓x7th   **T20.52**   Corrosion of first degree of **lip(s)**

✓x7th   **T20.53**   Corrosion of first degree of **chin**

✓x7th   **T20.54**   Corrosion of first degree of **nose (septum)**

✓x7th   **T20.55**   Corrosion of first degree of **scalp [any part]**

✓x7th   **T20.56**   Corrosion of first degree of **forehead and cheek**

✓x7th   **T20.57**   Corrosion of first degree of **neck**

✓x7th   **T20.59**   Corrosion of first degree of **multiple sites** of head, face, and neck

✓5th   **T20.6**   **Corrosion of second degree of head, face, and neck**

Code first (T51-T65) to identify chemical and intent

Use additional external cause code to identify place (Y92)

✓x7th   **T20.60**   **Corrosion of second degree of head, face, and neck, unspecified site**

✓6th   **T20.61**   **Corrosion of second degree of ear [any part, except ear drum]**

    EXCLUDES 2   corrosion of ear drum (T28.91-)

✓7th   **T20.611**   Corrosion of second degree of **right ear** [any part, except ear drum]

✓7th   **T20.612**   Corrosion of second degree of **left ear** [any part, except ear drum]

✓7th   **T20.619**   Corrosion of second degree of **unspecified ear** [any part, except ear drum]

✓x7th   **T20.62**   Corrosion of second degree of **lip(s)**

✓x7th   **T20.63**   Corrosion of second degree of **chin**

✓x7th   **T20.64**   Corrosion of second degree of **nose (septum)**

`N` Newborn: 0   `P` Pediatric: 0-17   `M` Maternity: 9-64   `A` Adult: 15-124   `MCC` Major Complication/Comorbidity   `CC` Complication/Comorbidity   `SW` Severe Wound Dx

1130   ICD-10-CM 2020

√x7ᵗʰ **T20.65** **Corrosion of second degree of** scalp [any part]

√x7ᵗʰ **T20.66** **Corrosion of second degree of** forehead and cheek

√x7ᵗʰ **T20.67** **Corrosion of second degree of** neck

√x7ᵗʰ **T20.69** **Corrosion of second degree of** multiple sites of head, face, and neck

√5ᵗʰ **T20.7** **Corrosion of** third degree **of head, face, and neck**

Code first (T51-T65) to identify chemical and intent
Use additional external cause code to identify place (Y92)

√x7ᵗʰ **T20.70** **Corrosion of third degree of head, face, and neck, unspecified site**   CC H5 SW
CC Excl: PDX collection 1375

√6ᵗʰ **T20.71** **Corrosion of third degree of ear [any part, except ear drum]**
EXCLUDES 2 *corrosion of ear drum (T28.91-)*
CC Excl: For CC codes in subcategory T20.71: PDX collection 1376

√7ᵗʰ **T20.711** **Corrosion of third degree of right ear [any part, except ear drum]**   CC H5 SW

√7ᵗʰ **T20.712** **Corrosion of third degree of left ear [any part, except ear drum]**   CC H5 SW

√7ᵗʰ **T20.719** **Corrosion of third degree of unspecified ear [any part, except ear drum]**   CC H5 SW

√x7ᵗʰ **T20.72** **Corrosion of third degree of** lip(s)   CC H5 SW
CC Excl: PDX collection 1377

√x7ᵗʰ **T20.73** **Corrosion of third degree of** chin   CC H5 SW
CC Excl: PDX collection 1378

√x7ᵗʰ **T20.74** **Corrosion of third degree of** nose (septum)   CC H5 SW
CC Excl: PDX collection 1379

√x7ᵗʰ **T20.75** **Corrosion of third degree of** scalp [any part]   CC H5 SW
CC Excl: PDX collection 1380

√x7ᵗʰ **T20.76** **Corrosion of third degree of** forehead and cheek   CC H5 SW
CC Excl: PDX collection 1381

√x7ᵗʰ **T20.77** **Corrosion of third degree of** neck   CC H5 SW
CC Excl: PDX collection 1382

√x7ᵗʰ **T20.79** **Corrosion of third degree of** multiple sites of head, face, and neck   CC H5 SW
CC Excl: PDX collection 1383

√4ᵗʰ **T21** **Burn and corrosion of trunk**

INCLUDES   burns and corrosion of hip region
EXCLUDES 2 *burns and corrosion of axilla (T22.- with fifth character 4)*
burns and corrosion of scapular region (T22.- with fifth character 6)
burns and corrosion of shoulder (T22.- with fifth character 5)

The appropriate 7th character is to be added to each code from category T21.
A   initial encounter
D   subsequent encounter
S   sequela

√5ᵗʰ **T21.0** **Burn of unspecified degree of trunk**

Use additional external cause code to identify the source, place and intent of the burn (X00-X19, X75-X77, X96-X98, Y92)

√x7ᵗʰ **T21.00** **Burn of unspecified degree of trunk, unspecified site**

√x7ᵗʰ **T21.01** **Burn of unspecified degree of** chest wall
Burn of unspecified degree of breast

√x7ᵗʰ **T21.02** **Burn of unspecified degree of** abdominal wall
Burn of unspecified degree of flank
Burn of unspecified degree of groin

√x7ᵗʰ **T21.03** **Burn of unspecified degree of** upper back
Burn of unspecified degree of interscapular region

√x7ᵗʰ **T21.04** **Burn of unspecified degree of** lower back

√x7ᵗʰ **T21.05** **Burn of unspecified degree of** buttock
Burn of unspecified degree of anus

√x7ᵗʰ **T21.06** **Burn of unspecified degree of** male genital region   ♂
Burn of unspecified degree of penis
Burn of unspecified degree of scrotum
Burn of unspecified degree of testis

√x7ᵗʰ **T21.07** **Burn of unspecified degree of** female genital region   ♀
Burn of unspecified degree of labium (majus) (minus)
Burn of unspecified degree of perineum
Burn of unspecified degree of vulva
EXCLUDES 2 *burn of vagina (T28.3)*

√x7ᵗʰ **T21.09** **Burn of unspecified degree of other site of trunk**

√5ᵗʰ **T21.1** **Burn of** first degree **of trunk**

Use additional external cause code to identify the source, place and intent of the burn (X00-X19, X75-X77, X96-X98, Y92)

√x7ᵗʰ **T21.10** **Burn of first degree of trunk, unspecified site**

√x7ᵗʰ **T21.11** **Burn of first degree of** chest wall
Burn of first degree of breast

√x7ᵗʰ **T21.12** **Burn of first degree of** abdominal wall
Burn of first degree of flank
Burn of first degree of groin

√x7ᵗʰ **T21.13** **Burn of first degree of** upper back
Burn of first degree of interscapular region

√x7ᵗʰ **T21.14** **Burn of first degree of** lower back

√x7ᵗʰ **T21.15** **Burn of first degree of** buttock
Burn of first degree of anus

√x7ᵗʰ **T21.16** **Burn of first degree of** male genital region   ♂
Burn of first degree of penis
Burn of first degree of scrotum
Burn of first degree of testis

√x7ᵗʰ **T21.17** **Burn of first degree of** female genital region   ♀
Burn of first degree of labium (majus) (minus)
Burn of first degree of perineum
Burn of first degree of vulva
EXCLUDES 2 *burn of vagina (T28.3)*

√x7ᵗʰ **T21.19** **Burn of first degree of other site of trunk**

√5ᵗʰ **T21.2** **Burn of** second degree **of trunk**

Use additional external cause code to identify the source, place and intent of the burn (X00-X19, X75-X77, X96-X98, Y92)

√x7ᵗʰ **T21.20** **Burn of second degree of trunk, unspecified site**

√x7ᵗʰ **T21.21** **Burn of second degree of** chest wall
Burn of second degree of breast

√x7ᵗʰ **T21.22** **Burn of second degree of** abdominal wall
Burn of second degree of flank
Burn of second degree of groin

√x7ᵗʰ **T21.23** **Burn of second degree of** upper back
Burn of second degree of interscapular region

√x7ᵗʰ **T21.24** **Burn of second degree of** lower back

√x7ᵗʰ **T21.25** **Burn of second degree of** buttock
Burn of second degree of anus

√x7ᵗʰ **T21.26** **Burn of second degree of** male genital region   ♂
Burn of second degree of penis
Burn of second degree of scrotum
Burn of second degree of testis

√x7ᵗʰ **T21.27** **Burn of second degree of** female genital region   ♀
Burn of second degree of labium (majus) (minus)
Burn of second degree of perineum
Burn of second degree of vulva
EXCLUDES 2 *burn of vagina (T28.3)*

√x7ᵗʰ **T21.29** **Burn of second degree of other site of trunk**

√5ᵗʰ **T21.3** **Burn of** third degree **of trunk**

Use additional external cause code to identify the source, place and intent of the burn (X00-X19, X75-X77, X96-X98, Y92)

√x7ᵗʰ **T21.30** **Burn of third degree of trunk, unspecified site**   CC H5 SW
CC Excl: PDX collection 1384

√x7ᵗʰ **T21.31** **Burn of third degree of** chest wall   CC H5 SW
Burn of third degree of breast
AHA: 2016,2Q,5
CC Excl: PDX collection 1385

√x7ᵗʰ **T21.32** **Burn of third degree of** abdominal wall   CC H5 SW
Burn of third degree of flank
Burn of third degree of groin
CC Excl: PDX collection 1386

√x7ᵗʰ **T21.33** **Burn of third degree of upper back** `CC` `H5` `SW`
Burn of third degree of interscapular region
CC Excl: PDX collection 1387

√x7ᵗʰ **T21.34** **Burn of third degree of lower back** `CC` `H5` `SW`
CC Excl: PDX collection 1387

√x7ᵗʰ **T21.35** **Burn of third degree of buttock** `CC` `H5` `SW`
Burn of third degree of anus
CC Excl: PDX collection 1387

√x7ᵗʰ **T21.36** **Burn of third degree of male genital region** `CC` `H5` `SW` ♂
Burn of third degree of penis
Burn of third degree of scrotum
Burn of third degree of testis
CC Excl: PDX collection 1388

√x7ᵗʰ **T21.37** **Burn of third degree of female genital region** `CC` `H5` `SW` ♀
Burn of third degree of labium (majus) (minus)
Burn of third degree of perineum
Burn of third degree of vulva
EXCLUDES 2   *burn of vagina (T28.3)*
CC Excl: PDX collection 1388

√x7ᵗʰ **T21.39** **Burn of third degree of other site of trunk** `CC` `H5` `SW`
CC Excl: PDX collection 1384

√5ᵗʰ **T21.4** **Corrosion of unspecified degree of trunk**
Code first (T51-T65) to identify chemical and intent
Use additional external cause code to identify place (Y92)

√x7ᵗʰ **T21.40** **Corrosion of unspecified degree of trunk, unspecified site**

√x7ᵗʰ **T21.41** **Corrosion of unspecified degree of chest wall**
Corrosion of unspecified degree of breast

√x7ᵗʰ **T21.42** **Corrosion of unspecified degree of abdominal wall**
Corrosion of unspecified degree of flank
Corrosion of unspecified degree of groin

√x7ᵗʰ **T21.43** **Corrosion of unspecified degree of upper back**
Corrosion of unspecified degree of interscapular region

√x7ᵗʰ **T21.44** **Corrosion of unspecified degree of lower back**

√x7ᵗʰ **T21.45** **Corrosion of unspecified degree of buttock**
Corrosion of unspecified degree of anus

√x7ᵗʰ **T21.46** **Corrosion of unspecified degree of male genital region** ♂
Corrosion of unspecified degree of penis
Corrosion of unspecified degree of scrotum
Corrosion of unspecified degree of testis

√x7ᵗʰ **T21.47** **Corrosion of unspecified degree of female genital region** ♀
Corrosion of unspecified degree of labium (majus) (minus)
Corrosion of unspecified degree of perineum
Corrosion of unspecified degree of vulva
EXCLUDES 2   *corrosion of vagina (T28.8)*

√x7ᵗʰ **T21.49** **Corrosion of unspecified degree of other site of trunk**

√5ᵗʰ **T21.5** **Corrosion of first degree of trunk**
Code first (T51-T65) to identify chemical and intent
Use additional external cause code to identify place (Y92)

√x7ᵗʰ **T21.50** **Corrosion of first degree of trunk, unspecified site**

√x7ᵗʰ **T21.51** **Corrosion of first degree of chest wall**
Corrosion of first degree of breast

√x7ᵗʰ **T21.52** **Corrosion of first degree of abdominal wall**
Corrosion of first degree of flank
Corrosion of first degree of groin

√x7ᵗʰ **T21.53** **Corrosion of first degree of upper back**
Corrosion of first degree of interscapular region

√x7ᵗʰ **T21.54** **Corrosion of first degree of lower back**

√x7ᵗʰ **T21.55** **Corrosion of first degree of buttock**
Corrosion of first degree of anus

√x7ᵗʰ **T21.56** **Corrosion of first degree of male genital region** ♂
Corrosion of first degree of penis
Corrosion of first degree of scrotum
Corrosion of first degree of testis

√x7ᵗʰ **T21.57** **Corrosion of first degree of female genital region** ♀
Corrosion of first degree of labium (majus) (minus)
Corrosion of first degree of perineum
Corrosion of first degree of vulva
EXCLUDES 2   *corrosion of vagina (T28.8)*

√x7ᵗʰ **T21.59** **Corrosion of first degree of other site of trunk**

√5ᵗʰ **T21.6** **Corrosion of second degree of trunk**
Code first (T51-T65) to identify chemical and intent
Use additional external cause code to identify place (Y92)

√x7ᵗʰ **T21.60** **Corrosion of second degree of trunk, unspecified site**

√x7ᵗʰ **T21.61** **Corrosion of second degree of chest wall**
Corrosion of second degree of breast

√x7ᵗʰ **T21.62** **Corrosion of second degree of abdominal wall**
Corrosion of second degree of flank
Corrosion of second degree of groin

√x7ᵗʰ **T21.63** **Corrosion of second degree of upper back**
Corrosion of second degree of interscapular region

√x7ᵗʰ **T21.64** **Corrosion of second degree of lower back**

√x7ᵗʰ **T21.65** **Corrosion of second degree of buttock**
Corrosion of second degree of anus

√x7ᵗʰ **T21.66** **Corrosion of second degree of male genital region** ♂
Corrosion of second degree of penis
Corrosion of second degree of scrotum
Corrosion of second degree of testis

√x7ᵗʰ **T21.67** **Corrosion of second degree of female genital region** ♀
Corrosion of second degree of labium (majus) (minus)
Corrosion of second degree of perineum
Corrosion of second degree of vulva
EXCLUDES 2   *corrosion of vagina (T28.8)*

√x7ᵗʰ **T21.69** **Corrosion of second degree of other site of trunk**

√5ᵗʰ **T21.7** **Corrosion of third degree of trunk**
Code first (T51-T65) to identify chemical and intent
Use additional external cause code to identify place (Y92)

√x7ᵗʰ **T21.70** **Corrosion of third degree of trunk, unspecified site** `CC` `H5` `SW`
CC Excl: PDX collection 1384

√x7ᵗʰ **T21.71** **Corrosion of third degree of chest wall** `CC` `H5` `SW`
Corrosion of third degree of breast
CC Excl: PDX collection 1385

√x7ᵗʰ **T21.72** **Corrosion of third degree of abdominal wall** `CC` `H5` `SW`
Corrosion of third degree of flank
Corrosion of third degree of groin
CC Excl: PDX collection 1386

√x7ᵗʰ **T21.73** **Corrosion of third degree of upper back** `CC` `H5` `SW`
Corrosion of third degree of interscapular region
CC Excl: PDX collection 1387

√x7ᵗʰ **T21.74** **Corrosion of third degree of lower back** `CC` `H5` `SW`
CC Excl: PDX collection 1387

√x7ᵗʰ **T21.75** **Corrosion of third degree of buttock** `CC` `H5` `SW`
Corrosion of third degree of anus
CC Excl: PDX collection 1387

√x7ᵗʰ **T21.76** **Corrosion of third degree of male genital region** `CC` `H5` `SW` ♂
Corrosion of third degree of penis
Corrosion of third degree of scrotum
Corrosion of third degree of testis
CC Excl: PDX collection 1388

√x7ᵗʰ **T21.77** **Corrosion of third degree of female genital region** `CC` `H5` `SW` ♀
Corrosion of third degree of labium (majus) (minus)
Corrosion of third degree of perineum
Corrosion of third degree of vulva
EXCLUDES 2   *corrosion of vagina (T28.8)*
CC Excl: PDX collection 1388

√x7ᵗʰ **T21.79** **Corrosion of third degree of other site of trunk** `CC` `H5` `SW`
CC Excl: PDX collection 1384

`N` Newborn: 0   `P` Pediatric: 0-17   `M` Maternity: 9-64   `A` Adult: 15-124   `MCC` Major Complication/Comorbidity   `CC` Complication/Comorbidity   `SW` Severe Wound Dx

1132   ICD-10-CM 2020

√4ᵗʰ **T22 Burn and corrosion of shoulder and upper limb, except wrist and hand**

> EXCLUDES 2   *burn and corrosion of interscapular region (T21.-)*
> *burn and corrosion of wrist and hand (T23.-)*

> The appropriate 7th character is to be added to each code from category T22.
> A   initial encounter
> D   subsequent encounter
> S   sequela

√5ᵗʰ **T22.0 Burn of unspecified degree of shoulder and upper limb, except wrist and hand**

> Use additional external cause code to identify the source, place and intent of the burn (X00-X19, X75-X77, X96-X98, Y92)

√ₓ7ᵗʰ **T22.00 Burn of unspecified degree of shoulder and upper limb, except wrist and hand, unspecified site**

√6ᵗʰ **T22.01 Burn of unspecified degree of forearm**

√7ᵗʰ **T22.011 Burn of unspecified degree of right forearm**

√7ᵗʰ **T22.012 Burn of unspecified degree of left forearm**

√7ᵗʰ **T22.019 Burn of unspecified degree of unspecified forearm**

√6ᵗʰ **T22.02 Burn of unspecified degree of elbow**

√7ᵗʰ **T22.021 Burn of unspecified degree of right elbow**

√7ᵗʰ **T22.022 Burn of unspecified degree of left elbow**

√7ᵗʰ **T22.029 Burn of unspecified degree of unspecified elbow**

√6ᵗʰ **T22.03 Burn of unspecified degree of upper arm**

√7ᵗʰ **T22.031 Burn of unspecified degree of right upper arm**

√7ᵗʰ **T22.032 Burn of unspecified degree of left upper arm**

√7ᵗʰ **T22.039 Burn of unspecified degree of unspecified upper arm**

√6ᵗʰ **T22.04 Burn of unspecified degree of axilla**

√7ᵗʰ **T22.041 Burn of unspecified degree of right axilla**

√7ᵗʰ **T22.042 Burn of unspecified degree of left axilla**

√7ᵗʰ **T22.049 Burn of unspecified degree of unspecified axilla**

√6ᵗʰ **T22.05 Burn of unspecified degree of shoulder**

√7ᵗʰ **T22.051 Burn of unspecified degree of right shoulder**

√7ᵗʰ **T22.052 Burn of unspecified degree of left shoulder**

√7ᵗʰ **T22.059 Burn of unspecified degree of unspecified shoulder**

√6ᵗʰ **T22.06 Burn of unspecified degree of scapular region**

√7ᵗʰ **T22.061 Burn of unspecified degree of right scapular region**

√7ᵗʰ **T22.062 Burn of unspecified degree of left scapular region**

√7ᵗʰ **T22.069 Burn of unspecified degree of unspecified scapular region**

√6ᵗʰ **T22.09 Burn of unspecified degree of multiple sites of shoulder and upper limb, except wrist and hand**

√7ᵗʰ **T22.091 Burn of unspecified degree of multiple sites of right shoulder and upper limb, except wrist and hand**

√7ᵗʰ **T22.092 Burn of unspecified degree of multiple sites of left shoulder and upper limb, except wrist and hand**

√7ᵗʰ **T22.099 Burn of unspecified degree of multiple sites of unspecified shoulder and upper limb, except wrist and hand**

√5ᵗʰ **T22.1 Burn of first degree of shoulder and upper limb, except wrist and hand**

> Use additional external cause code to identify the source, place and intent of the burn (X00-X19, X75-X77, X96-X98, Y92)

√ₓ7ᵗʰ **T22.10 Burn of first degree of shoulder and upper limb, except wrist and hand, unspecified site**

√6ᵗʰ **T22.11 Burn of first degree of forearm**

√7ᵗʰ **T22.111 Burn of first degree of right forearm**

√7ᵗʰ **T22.112 Burn of first degree of left forearm**

√7ᵗʰ **T22.119 Burn of first degree of unspecified forearm**

√6ᵗʰ **T22.12 Burn of first degree of elbow**

√7ᵗʰ **T22.121 Burn of first degree of right elbow**

√7ᵗʰ **T22.122 Burn of first degree of left elbow**

√7ᵗʰ **T22.129 Burn of first degree of unspecified elbow**

√6ᵗʰ **T22.13 Burn of first degree of upper arm**

√7ᵗʰ **T22.131 Burn of first degree of right upper arm**

√7ᵗʰ **T22.132 Burn of first degree of left upper arm**

√7ᵗʰ **T22.139 Burn of first degree of unspecified upper arm**

√6ᵗʰ **T22.14 Burn of first degree of axilla**

√7ᵗʰ **T22.141 Burn of first degree of right axilla**

√7ᵗʰ **T22.142 Burn of first degree of left axilla**

√7ᵗʰ **T22.149 Burn of first degree of unspecified axilla**

√6ᵗʰ **T22.15 Burn of first degree of shoulder**

√7ᵗʰ **T22.151 Burn of first degree of right shoulder**

√7ᵗʰ **T22.152 Burn of first degree of left shoulder**

√7ᵗʰ **T22.159 Burn of first degree of unspecified shoulder**

√6ᵗʰ **T22.16 Burn of first degree of scapular region**

√7ᵗʰ **T22.161 Burn of first degree of right scapular region**

√7ᵗʰ **T22.162 Burn of first degree of left scapular region**

√7ᵗʰ **T22.169 Burn of first degree of unspecified scapular region**

√6ᵗʰ **T22.19 Burn of first degree of multiple sites of shoulder and upper limb, except wrist and hand**

√7ᵗʰ **T22.191 Burn of first degree of multiple sites of right shoulder and upper limb, except wrist and hand**

√7ᵗʰ **T22.192 Burn of first degree of multiple sites of left shoulder and upper limb, except wrist and hand**

√7ᵗʰ **T22.199 Burn of first degree of multiple sites of unspecified shoulder and upper limb, except wrist and hand**

√5ᵗʰ **T22.2 Burn of second degree of shoulder and upper limb, except wrist and hand**

> Use additional external cause code to identify the source, place and intent of the burn (X00-X19, X75-X77, X96-X98, Y92)

√ₓ7ᵗʰ **T22.20 Burn of second degree of shoulder and upper limb, except wrist and hand, unspecified site**

√6ᵗʰ **T22.21 Burn of second degree of forearm**

√7ᵗʰ **T22.211 Burn of second degree of right forearm**

√7ᵗʰ **T22.212 Burn of second degree of left forearm**

√7ᵗʰ **T22.219 Burn of second degree of unspecified forearm**

√6ᵗʰ **T22.22 Burn of second degree of elbow**

√7ᵗʰ **T22.221 Burn of second degree of right elbow**

√7ᵗʰ **T22.222 Burn of second degree of left elbow**

√7ᵗʰ **T22.229 Burn of second degree of unspecified elbow**

√6ᵗʰ **T22.23 Burn of second degree of upper arm**

√7ᵗʰ **T22.231 Burn of second degree of right upper arm**

√7ᵗʰ **T22.232 Burn of second degree of left upper arm**

√7ᵗʰ **T22.239 Burn of second degree of unspecified upper arm**

√6ᵗʰ **T22.24 Burn of second degree of axilla**

√7ᵗʰ **T22.241 Burn of second degree of right axilla**

√7ᵗʰ **T22.242 Burn of second degree of left axilla**

√7ᵗʰ **T22.249 Burn of second degree of unspecified axilla**

√6ᵗʰ **T22.25 Burn of second degree of shoulder**

√7ᵗʰ **T22.251 Burn of second degree of right shoulder**

√7ᵗʰ **T22.252 Burn of second degree of left shoulder**

√7ᵗʰ **T22.259 Burn of second degree of unspecified shoulder**

√6ᵗʰ **T22.26 Burn of second degree of scapular region**

√7ᵗʰ **T22.261 Burn of second degree of right scapular region**

√7ᵗʰ **T22.262 Burn of second degree of left scapular region**

√7ᵗʰ **T22.269 Burn of second degree of unspecified scapular region**

√6ᵗʰ **T22.29 Burn of second degree of multiple sites of shoulder and upper limb, except wrist and hand**

√7ᵗʰ **T22.291 Burn of second degree of multiple sites of right shoulder and upper limb, except wrist and hand**

☑ Additional Character Required   √ₓ7ᵗʰ Placeholder   Unacceptable PDx   Questionable PDx   Manifestation   Unspecified Dx   H1-H14 HAC   HCC CMS-HCC Dx   HIV HIV Dx

ICD-10-CM 2020   1133

√7ᵗʰ **T22.292** Burn of second degree of multiple sites of left shoulder and upper limb, except wrist and hand

√7ᵗʰ **T22.299** Burn of second degree of multiple sites of unspecified shoulder and upper limb, except wrist and hand

√5ᵗʰ **T22.3** Burn of third degree of shoulder and upper limb, except wrist and hand

Use additional external cause code to identify the source, place and intent of the burn (X00-X19, X75-X77, X96-X98, Y92)

√x7ᵗʰ **T22.30** Burn of third degree of shoulder and upper limb, except wrist and hand, unspecified site   `CC` `H5` `SW`

CC Excl: PDX collection 1389

√6ᵗʰ **T22.31** Burn of third degree of forearm

CC Excl: For CC codes in subcategory T22.31: PDX collection 1390

√7ᵗʰ **T22.311** Burn of third degree of right forearm   `CC` `H5` `SW`

√7ᵗʰ **T22.312** Burn of third degree of left forearm   `CC` `H5` `SW`

√7ᵗʰ **T22.319** Burn of third degree of unspecified forearm   `CC` `H5` `SW`

√6ᵗʰ **T22.32** Burn of third degree of elbow

CC Excl: For CC codes in subcategory T22.32: PDX collection 1391

√7ᵗʰ **T22.321** Burn of third degree of right elbow   `CC` `H5` `SW`

√7ᵗʰ **T22.322** Burn of third degree of left elbow   `CC` `H5` `SW`

√7ᵗʰ **T22.329** Burn of third degree of unspecified elbow   `CC` `H5` `SW`

√6ᵗʰ **T22.33** Burn of third degree of upper arm

CC Excl: For CC codes in subcategory T22.32: PDX collection 1392

√7ᵗʰ **T22.331** Burn of third degree of right upper arm   `CC` `H5` `SW`

√7ᵗʰ **T22.332** Burn of third degree of left upper arm   `CC` `H5` `SW`

√7ᵗʰ **T22.339** Burn of third degree of unspecified upper arm   `CC` `H5` `SW`

√6ᵗʰ **T22.34** Burn of third degree of axilla

CC Excl: For CC codes in subcategory T22.34: PDX collection 1393

√7ᵗʰ **T22.341** Burn of third degree of right axilla   `CC` `H5` `SW`

√7ᵗʰ **T22.342** Burn of third degree of left axilla   `CC` `H5` `SW`

√7ᵗʰ **T22.349** Burn of third degree of unspecified axilla   `CC` `H5` `SW`

√6ᵗʰ **T22.35** Burn of third degree of shoulder

CC Excl: For CC codes in subcategory T22.35: PDX collection 1394

√7ᵗʰ **T22.351** Burn of third degree of right shoulder   `CC` `H5` `SW`

√7ᵗʰ **T22.352** Burn of third degree of left shoulder   `CC` `H5` `SW`

√7ᵗʰ **T22.359** Burn of third degree of unspecified shoulder   `CC` `H5` `SW`

√6ᵗʰ **T22.36** Burn of third degree of scapular region

CC Excl: For CC codes in subcategory T22.36: PDX collection 1395

√7ᵗʰ **T22.361** Burn of third degree of right scapular region   `CC` `H5` `SW`

√7ᵗʰ **T22.362** Burn of third degree of left scapular region   `CC` `H5` `SW`

√7ᵗʰ **T22.369** Burn of third degree of unspecified scapular region   `CC` `H5` `SW`

√6ᵗʰ **T22.39** Burn of third degree of multiple sites of shoulder and upper limb, except wrist and hand

CC Excl: For CC codes in subcategory T22.39: PDX collection 1389

√7ᵗʰ **T22.391** Burn of third degree of multiple sites of right shoulder and upper limb, except wrist and hand   `CC` `H5` `SW`

√7ᵗʰ **T22.392** Burn of third degree of multiple sites of left shoulder and upper limb, except wrist and hand   `CC` `H5` `SW`

√7ᵗʰ **T22.399** Burn of third degree of multiple sites of unspecified shoulder and upper limb, except wrist and hand   `CC` `H5` `SW`

√5ᵗʰ **T22.4** Corrosion of unspecified degree of shoulder and upper limb, except wrist and hand

Code first (T51-T65) to identify chemical and intent

Use additional external cause code to identify place (Y92)

√x7ᵗʰ **T22.40** Corrosion of unspecified degree of shoulder and upper limb, except wrist and hand, unspecified site

√6ᵗʰ **T22.41** Corrosion of unspecified degree of forearm

√7ᵗʰ **T22.411** Corrosion of unspecified degree of right forearm

√7ᵗʰ **T22.412** Corrosion of unspecified degree of left forearm

√7ᵗʰ **T22.419** Corrosion of unspecified degree of unspecified forearm

√6ᵗʰ **T22.42** Corrosion of unspecified degree of elbow

√7ᵗʰ **T22.421** Corrosion of unspecified degree of right elbow

√7ᵗʰ **T22.422** Corrosion of unspecified degree of left elbow

√7ᵗʰ **T22.429** Corrosion of unspecified degree of unspecified elbow

√6ᵗʰ **T22.43** Corrosion of unspecified degree of upper arm

√7ᵗʰ **T22.431** Corrosion of unspecified degree of right upper arm

√7ᵗʰ **T22.432** Corrosion of unspecified degree of left upper arm

√7ᵗʰ **T22.439** Corrosion of unspecified degree of unspecified upper arm

√6ᵗʰ **T22.44** Corrosion of unspecified degree of axilla

√7ᵗʰ **T22.441** Corrosion of unspecified degree of right axilla

√7ᵗʰ **T22.442** Corrosion of unspecified degree of left axilla

√7ᵗʰ **T22.449** Corrosion of unspecified degree of unspecified axilla

√6ᵗʰ **T22.45** Corrosion of unspecified degree of shoulder

√7ᵗʰ **T22.451** Corrosion of unspecified degree of right shoulder

√7ᵗʰ **T22.452** Corrosion of unspecified degree of left shoulder

√7ᵗʰ **T22.459** Corrosion of unspecified degree of unspecified shoulder

√6ᵗʰ **T22.46** Corrosion of unspecified degree of scapular region

√7ᵗʰ **T22.461** Corrosion of unspecified degree of right scapular region

√7ᵗʰ **T22.462** Corrosion of unspecified degree of left scapular region

√7ᵗʰ **T22.469** Corrosion of unspecified degree of unspecified scapular region

√6ᵗʰ **T22.49** Corrosion of unspecified degree of multiple sites of shoulder and upper limb, except wrist and hand

√7ᵗʰ **T22.491** Corrosion of unspecified degree of multiple sites of right shoulder and upper limb, except wrist and hand

√7ᵗʰ **T22.492** Corrosion of unspecified degree of multiple sites of left shoulder and upper limb, except wrist and hand

√7ᵗʰ **T22.499** Corrosion of unspecified degree of multiple sites of unspecified shoulder and upper limb, except wrist and hand

√5ᵗʰ **T22.5** Corrosion of first degree of shoulder and upper limb, except wrist and hand

Code first (T51-T65) to identify chemical and intent

Use additional external cause code to identify place (Y92)

√x7ᵗʰ **T22.50** Corrosion of first degree of shoulder and upper limb, except wrist and hand unspecified site

√6ᵗʰ **T22.51** Corrosion of first degree of forearm

√7ᵗʰ **T22.511** Corrosion of first degree of right forearm

√7ᵗʰ **T22.512** Corrosion of first degree of left forearm

√7ᵗʰ **T22.519** Corrosion of first degree of unspecified forearm

√6ᵗʰ **T22.52** Corrosion of first degree of elbow

√7ᵗʰ **T22.521** Corrosion of first degree of right elbow

√7ᵗʰ **T22.522** Corrosion of first degree of left elbow

√7ᵗʰ **T22.529** Corrosion of first degree of unspecified elbow

`N` Newborn: 0   `P` Pediatric: 0-17   `M` Maternity: 9-64   `A` Adult: 15-124   `MCC` Major Complication/Comorbidity   `CC` Complication/Comorbidity   `SW` Severe Wound Dx

1134   ICD-10-CM 2020

√6ᵗʰ **T22.53** Corrosion of first degree of upper arm
  √7ᵗʰ **T22.531** Corrosion of first degree of right upper arm
  √7ᵗʰ **T22.532** Corrosion of first degree of left upper arm
  √7ᵗʰ **T22.539** Corrosion of first degree of unspecified upper arm

√6ᵗʰ **T22.54** Corrosion of first degree of axilla
  √7ᵗʰ **T22.541** Corrosion of first degree of right axilla
  √7ᵗʰ **T22.542** Corrosion of first degree of left axilla
  √7ᵗʰ **T22.549** Corrosion of first degree of unspecified axilla

√6ᵗʰ **T22.55** Corrosion of first degree of shoulder
  √7ᵗʰ **T22.551** Corrosion of first degree of right shoulder
  √7ᵗʰ **T22.552** Corrosion of first degree of left shoulder
  √7ᵗʰ **T22.559** Corrosion of first degree of unspecified shoulder

√6ᵗʰ **T22.56** Corrosion of first degree of scapular region
  √7ᵗʰ **T22.561** Corrosion of first degree of right scapular region
  √7ᵗʰ **T22.562** Corrosion of first degree of left scapular region
  √7ᵗʰ **T22.569** Corrosion of first degree of unspecified scapular region

√6ᵗʰ **T22.59** Corrosion of first degree of multiple sites of shoulder and upper limb, except wrist and hand
  √7ᵗʰ **T22.591** Corrosion of first degree of multiple sites of right shoulder and upper limb, except wrist and hand
  √7ᵗʰ **T22.592** Corrosion of first degree of multiple sites of left shoulder and upper limb, except wrist and hand
  √7ᵗʰ **T22.599** Corrosion of first degree of multiple sites of unspecified shoulder and upper limb, except wrist and hand

√5ᵗʰ **T22.6** Corrosion of second degree of shoulder and upper limb, except wrist and hand
  Code first (T51-T65) to identify chemical and intent
  Use additional external cause code to identify place (Y92)
  √x7ᵗʰ **T22.60** Corrosion of second degree of shoulder and upper limb, except wrist and hand, unspecified site

√6ᵗʰ **T22.61** Corrosion of second degree of forearm
  √7ᵗʰ **T22.611** Corrosion of second degree of right forearm
  √7ᵗʰ **T22.612** Corrosion of second degree of left forearm
  √7ᵗʰ **T22.619** Corrosion of second degree of unspecified forearm

√6ᵗʰ **T22.62** Corrosion of second degree of elbow
  √7ᵗʰ **T22.621** Corrosion of second degree of right elbow
  √7ᵗʰ **T22.622** Corrosion of second degree of left elbow
  √7ᵗʰ **T22.629** Corrosion of second degree of unspecified elbow

√6ᵗʰ **T22.63** Corrosion of second degree of upper arm
  √7ᵗʰ **T22.631** Corrosion of second degree of right upper arm
  √7ᵗʰ **T22.632** Corrosion of second degree of left upper arm
  √7ᵗʰ **T22.639** Corrosion of second degree of unspecified upper arm

√6ᵗʰ **T22.64** Corrosion of second degree of axilla
  √7ᵗʰ **T22.641** Corrosion of second degree of right axilla
  √7ᵗʰ **T22.642** Corrosion of second degree of left axilla
  √7ᵗʰ **T22.649** Corrosion of second degree of unspecified axilla

√6ᵗʰ **T22.65** Corrosion of second degree of shoulder
  √7ᵗʰ **T22.651** Corrosion of second degree of right shoulder
  √7ᵗʰ **T22.652** Corrosion of second degree of left shoulder
  √7ᵗʰ **T22.659** Corrosion of second degree of unspecified shoulder

√6ᵗʰ **T22.66** Corrosion of second degree of scapular region
  √7ᵗʰ **T22.661** Corrosion of second degree of right scapular region
  √7ᵗʰ **T22.662** Corrosion of second degree of left scapular region
  √7ᵗʰ **T22.669** Corrosion of second degree of unspecified scapular region

√6ᵗʰ **T22.69** Corrosion of second degree of multiple sites of shoulder and upper limb, except wrist and hand
  √7ᵗʰ **T22.691** Corrosion of second degree of multiple sites of right shoulder and upper limb, except wrist and hand
  √7ᵗʰ **T22.692** Corrosion of second degree of multiple sites of left shoulder and upper limb, except wrist and hand
  √7ᵗʰ **T22.699** Corrosion of second degree of multiple sites of unspecified shoulder and upper limb, except wrist and hand

√5ᵗʰ **T22.7** Corrosion of third degree of shoulder and upper limb, except wrist and hand
  Code first (T51-T65) to identify chemical and intent
  Use additional external cause code to identify place (Y92)
  √x7ᵗʰ **T22.70** Corrosion of third degree of shoulder and upper limb, except wrist and hand, unspecified site   CC H5 SW
    CC Excl: PDX collection 1389

√6ᵗʰ **T22.71** Corrosion of third degree of forearm
    CC Excl: For CC codes in subcategory T22.71: PDX collection 1390
  √7ᵗʰ **T22.711** Corrosion of third degree of right forearm   CC H5 SW
  √7ᵗʰ **T22.712** Corrosion of third degree of left forearm   CC H5 SW
  √7ᵗʰ **T22.719** Corrosion of third degree of unspecified forearm   CC H5 SW

√6ᵗʰ **T22.72** Corrosion of third degree of elbow
    CC Excl: For CC codes in subcategory T22.72: PDX collection 1391
  √7ᵗʰ **T22.721** Corrosion of third degree of right elbow   CC H5 SW
  √7ᵗʰ **T22.722** Corrosion of third degree of left elbow   CC H5 SW
  √7ᵗʰ **T22.729** Corrosion of third degree of unspecified elbow   CC H5 SW

√6ᵗʰ **T22.73** Corrosion of third degree of upper arm
    CC Excl: For CC codes in subcategory T22.73: PDX collection 1392
  √7ᵗʰ **T22.731** Corrosion of third degree of right upper arm   CC H5 SW
  √7ᵗʰ **T22.732** Corrosion of third degree of left upper arm   CC H5 SW
  √7ᵗʰ **T22.739** Corrosion of third degree of unspecified upper arm   CC H5 SW

√6ᵗʰ **T22.74** Corrosion of third degree of axilla
    CC Excl: For CC codes in subcategory T22.74: PDX collection 1393
  √7ᵗʰ **T22.741** Corrosion of third degree of right axilla   CC H5 SW
  √7ᵗʰ **T22.742** Corrosion of third degree of left axilla   CC H5 SW
  √7ᵗʰ **T22.749** Corrosion of third degree of unspecified axilla   CC H5 SW

√6ᵗʰ **T22.75** Corrosion of third degree of shoulder
    CC Excl: For CC codes in subcategory T22.75: PDX collection 1394
  √7ᵗʰ **T22.751** Corrosion of third degree of right shoulder   CC H5 SW
  √7ᵗʰ **T22.752** Corrosion of third degree of left shoulder   CC H5 SW
  √7ᵗʰ **T22.759** Corrosion of third degree of unspecified shoulder   CC H5 SW

√6ᵗʰ **T22.76** Corrosion of third degree of scapular region
    CC Excl: For CC codes in subcategory T22.76: PDX collection 1395
  √7ᵗʰ **T22.761** Corrosion of third degree of right scapular region   CC H5 SW
  √7ᵗʰ **T22.762** Corrosion of third degree of left scapular region   CC H5 SW
  √7ᵗʰ **T22.769** Corrosion of third degree of unspecified scapular region   CC H5 SW

Chapter 19. Injury, Poisoning and Certain Other Consequences of External Causes

✓6ᵗʰ **T22.79**   Corrosion of third degree of multiple sites of shoulder and upper limb, except wrist and hand
     CC Excl: For CC codes in subcategory T22.79: PDX collection 1389

     ✓7ᵗʰ **T22.791**   Corrosion of third degree of multiple sites of right shoulder and upper limb, except wrist and hand   [CC] [H5] [SW]

     ✓7ᵗʰ **T22.792**   Corrosion of third degree of multiple sites of left shoulder and upper limb, except wrist and hand   [CC] [H5] [SW]

     ✓7ᵗʰ **T22.799**   Corrosion of third degree of multiple sites of unspecified shoulder and upper limb, except wrist and hand   [CC] [H5] [SW]

✓4ᵗʰ **T23**   **Burn and corrosion of wrist and hand**
     AHA: 2015,1Q,19

     The appropriate 7th character is to be added to each code from category T23.
     A   initial encounter
     D   subsequent encounter
     S   sequela

✓5ᵗʰ **T23.0**   **Burn of unspecified degree of wrist and hand**
     Use additional external cause code to identify the source, place and intent of the burn (X00-X19, X75-X77, X96-X98, Y92)

     ✓6ᵗʰ **T23.00**   Burn of unspecified degree of hand, unspecified site
         ✓7ᵗʰ **T23.001**   Burn of unspecified degree of right hand, unspecified site
         ✓7ᵗʰ **T23.002**   Burn of unspecified degree of left hand, unspecified site
         ✓7ᵗʰ **T23.009**   Burn of unspecified degree of unspecified hand, unspecified site

     ✓6ᵗʰ **T23.01**   Burn of unspecified degree of thumb (nail)
         ✓7ᵗʰ **T23.011**   Burn of unspecified degree of right thumb (nail)
         ✓7ᵗʰ **T23.012**   Burn of unspecified degree of left thumb (nail)
         ✓7ᵗʰ **T23.019**   Burn of unspecified degree of unspecified thumb (nail)

     ✓6ᵗʰ **T23.02**   Burn of unspecified degree of single finger (nail) except thumb
         ✓7ᵗʰ **T23.021**   Burn of unspecified degree of single right finger (nail) except thumb
         ✓7ᵗʰ **T23.022**   Burn of unspecified degree of single left finger (nail) except thumb
         ✓7ᵗʰ **T23.029**   Burn of unspecified degree of unspecified single finger (nail) except thumb

     ✓6ᵗʰ **T23.03**   Burn of unspecified degree of multiple fingers (nail), not including thumb
         ✓7ᵗʰ **T23.031**   Burn of unspecified degree of multiple right fingers (nail), not including thumb
         ✓7ᵗʰ **T23.032**   Burn of unspecified degree of multiple left fingers (nail), not including thumb
         ✓7ᵗʰ **T23.039**   Burn of unspecified degree of unspecified multiple fingers (nail), not including thumb

     ✓6ᵗʰ **T23.04**   Burn of unspecified degree of multiple fingers (nail), including thumb
         ✓7ᵗʰ **T23.041**   Burn of unspecified degree of multiple right fingers (nail), including thumb
         ✓7ᵗʰ **T23.042**   Burn of unspecified degree of multiple left fingers (nail), including thumb
         ✓7ᵗʰ **T23.049**   Burn of unspecified degree of unspecified multiple fingers (nail), including thumb

     ✓6ᵗʰ **T23.05**   Burn of unspecified degree of palm
         ✓7ᵗʰ **T23.051**   Burn of unspecified degree of right palm
         ✓7ᵗʰ **T23.052**   Burn of unspecified degree of left palm
         ✓7ᵗʰ **T23.059**   Burn of unspecified degree of unspecified palm

     ✓6ᵗʰ **T23.06**   Burn of unspecified degree of back of hand
         ✓7ᵗʰ **T23.061**   Burn of unspecified degree of back of right hand
         ✓7ᵗʰ **T23.062**   Burn of unspecified degree of back of left hand
         ✓7ᵗʰ **T23.069**   Burn of unspecified degree of back of unspecified hand

✓6ᵗʰ **T23.07**   Burn of unspecified degree of wrist
     ✓7ᵗʰ **T23.071**   Burn of unspecified degree of right wrist
     ✓7ᵗʰ **T23.072**   Burn of unspecified degree of left wrist
     ✓7ᵗʰ **T23.079**   Burn of unspecified degree of unspecified wrist

✓6ᵗʰ **T23.09**   Burn of unspecified degree of multiple sites of wrist and hand
     ✓7ᵗʰ **T23.091**   Burn of unspecified degree of multiple sites of right wrist and hand
     ✓7ᵗʰ **T23.092**   Burn of unspecified degree of multiple sites of left wrist and hand
     ✓7ᵗʰ **T23.099**   Burn of unspecified degree of multiple sites of unspecified wrist and hand

✓5ᵗʰ **T23.1**   **Burn of first degree of wrist and hand**
     Use additional external cause code to identify the source, place and intent of the burn (X00-X19, X75-X77, X96-X98, Y92)

     ✓6ᵗʰ **T23.10**   Burn of first degree of hand, unspecified site
         ✓7ᵗʰ **T23.101**   Burn of first degree of right hand, unspecified site
         ✓7ᵗʰ **T23.102**   Burn of first degree of left hand, unspecified site
         ✓7ᵗʰ **T23.109**   Burn of first degree of unspecified hand, unspecified site

     ✓6ᵗʰ **T23.11**   Burn of first degree of thumb (nail)
         ✓7ᵗʰ **T23.111**   Burn of first degree of right thumb (nail)
         ✓7ᵗʰ **T23.112**   Burn of first degree of left thumb (nail)
         ✓7ᵗʰ **T23.119**   Burn of first degree of unspecified thumb (nail)

     ✓6ᵗʰ **T23.12**   Burn of first degree of single finger (nail) except thumb
         ✓7ᵗʰ **T23.121**   Burn of first degree of single right finger (nail) except thumb
         ✓7ᵗʰ **T23.122**   Burn of first degree of single left finger (nail) except thumb
         ✓7ᵗʰ **T23.129**   Burn of first degree of unspecified single finger (nail) except thumb

     ✓6ᵗʰ **T23.13**   Burn of first degree of multiple fingers (nail), not including thumb
         ✓7ᵗʰ **T23.131**   Burn of first degree of multiple right fingers (nail), not including thumb
         ✓7ᵗʰ **T23.132**   Burn of first degree of multiple left fingers (nail), not including thumb
         ✓7ᵗʰ **T23.139**   Burn of first degree of unspecified multiple fingers (nail), not including thumb

     ✓6ᵗʰ **T23.14**   Burn of first degree of multiple fingers (nail), including thumb
         ✓7ᵗʰ **T23.141**   Burn of first degree of multiple right fingers (nail), including thumb
         ✓7ᵗʰ **T23.142**   Burn of first degree of multiple left fingers (nail), including thumb
         ✓7ᵗʰ **T23.149**   Burn of first degree of unspecified multiple fingers (nail), including thumb

     ✓6ᵗʰ **T23.15**   Burn of first degree of palm
         ✓7ᵗʰ **T23.151**   Burn of first degree of right palm
         ✓7ᵗʰ **T23.152**   Burn of first degree of left palm
         ✓7ᵗʰ **T23.159**   Burn of first degree of unspecified palm

     ✓6ᵗʰ **T23.16**   Burn of first degree of back of hand
         ✓7ᵗʰ **T23.161**   Burn of first degree of back of right hand
         ✓7ᵗʰ **T23.162**   Burn of first degree of back of left hand
         ✓7ᵗʰ **T23.169**   Burn of first degree of back of unspecified hand

     ✓6ᵗʰ **T23.17**   Burn of first degree of wrist
         ✓7ᵗʰ **T23.171**   Burn of first degree of right wrist
         ✓7ᵗʰ **T23.172**   Burn of first degree of left wrist
         ✓7ᵗʰ **T23.179**   Burn of first degree of unspecified wrist

     ✓6ᵗʰ **T23.19**   Burn of first degree of multiple sites of wrist and hand
         ✓7ᵗʰ **T23.191**   Burn of first degree of multiple sites of right wrist and hand
         ✓7ᵗʰ **T23.192**   Burn of first degree of multiple sites of left wrist and hand
         ✓7ᵗʰ **T23.199**   Burn of first degree of multiple sites of unspecified wrist and hand

N Newborn: 0   **P** Pediatric: 0-17   **M** Maternity: 9-64   **A** Adult: 15-124   **MCC** Major Complication/Comorbidity   **CC** Complication/Comorbidity   **SW** Severe Wound Dx

1136   ICD-10-CM 2020

✓5ᵗʰ **T23.2 Burn of second degree of wrist and hand**

Use additional external cause code to identify the source, place and intent of the burn (X00-X19, X75-X77, X96-X98, Y92)

✓6ᵗʰ **T23.20 Burn of second degree of hand, unspecified site**

    ✓7ᵗʰ **T23.201 Burn of second degree of right hand, unspecified site**

    ✓7ᵗʰ **T23.202 Burn of second degree of left hand, unspecified site**

    ✓7ᵗʰ **T23.209 Burn of second degree of unspecified hand, unspecified site**

✓6ᵗʰ **T23.21 Burn of second degree of thumb (nail)**

    ✓7ᵗʰ **T23.211 Burn of second degree of right thumb (nail)**

    ✓7ᵗʰ **T23.212 Burn of second degree of left thumb (nail)**

    ✓7ᵗʰ **T23.219 Burn of second degree of unspecified thumb (nail)**

✓6ᵗʰ **T23.22 Burn of second degree of single finger (nail) except thumb**

    ✓7ᵗʰ **T23.221 Burn of second degree of single right finger (nail) except thumb**

    ✓7ᵗʰ **T23.222 Burn of second degree of single left finger (nail) except thumb**

    ✓7ᵗʰ **T23.229 Burn of second degree of unspecified single finger (nail) except thumb**

✓6ᵗʰ **T23.23 Burn of second degree of multiple fingers (nail), not including thumb**

    ✓7ᵗʰ **T23.231 Burn of second degree of multiple right fingers (nail), not including thumb**

    ✓7ᵗʰ **T23.232 Burn of second degree of multiple left fingers (nail), not including thumb**

    ✓7ᵗʰ **T23.239 Burn of second degree of unspecified multiple fingers (nail), not including thumb**

✓6ᵗʰ **T23.24 Burn of second degree of multiple fingers (nail), including thumb**

    ✓7ᵗʰ **T23.241 Burn of second degree of multiple right fingers (nail), including thumb**

    ✓7ᵗʰ **T23.242 Burn of second degree of multiple left fingers (nail), including thumb**

    ✓7ᵗʰ **T23.249 Burn of second degree of unspecified multiple fingers (nail), including thumb**

✓6ᵗʰ **T23.25 Burn of second degree of palm**

    ✓7ᵗʰ **T23.251 Burn of second degree of right palm**

    ✓7ᵗʰ **T23.252 Burn of second degree of left palm**

    ✓7ᵗʰ **T23.259 Burn of second degree of unspecified palm**

✓6ᵗʰ **T23.26 Burn of second degree of back of hand**

    ✓7ᵗʰ **T23.261 Burn of second degree of back of right hand**

    ✓7ᵗʰ **T23.262 Burn of second degree of back of left hand**

    ✓7ᵗʰ **T23.269 Burn of second degree of back of unspecified hand**

✓6ᵗʰ **T23.27 Burn of second degree of wrist**

    ✓7ᵗʰ **T23.271 Burn of second degree of right wrist**

    ✓7ᵗʰ **T23.272 Burn of second degree of left wrist**

    ✓7ᵗʰ **T23.279 Burn of second degree of unspecified wrist**

✓6ᵗʰ **T23.29 Burn of second degree of multiple sites of wrist and hand**

    ✓7ᵗʰ **T23.291 Burn of second degree of multiple sites of right wrist and hand**

    ✓7ᵗʰ **T23.292 Burn of second degree of multiple sites of left wrist and hand**

    ✓7ᵗʰ **T23.299 Burn of second degree of multiple sites of unspecified wrist and hand**

✓5ᵗʰ **T23.3 Burn of third degree of wrist and hand**

Use additional external cause code to identify the source, place and intent of the burn (X00-X19, X75-X77, X96-X98, Y92)

✓6ᵗʰ **T23.30 Burn of third degree of hand, unspecified site**

AHA: 2016, 2Q, 5

CC Excl: For CC codes in subcategory T23.30: PDX collection 1396

    ✓7ᵗʰ **T23.301 Burn of third degree of right hand, unspecified site** `CC` `H5` `SW`

    ✓7ᵗʰ **T23.302 Burn of third degree of left hand, unspecified site** `CC` `H5` `SW`

    ✓7ᵗʰ **T23.309 Burn of third degree of unspecified hand, unspecified site** `CC` `H5` `SW`

✓6ᵗʰ **T23.31 Burn of third degree of thumb (nail)**

CC Excl: For CC codes in subcategory T23.31: PDX collection 1397

    ✓7ᵗʰ **T23.311 Burn of third degree of right thumb (nail)** `CC` `H5` `SW`

    ✓7ᵗʰ **T23.312 Burn of third degree of left thumb (nail)** `CC` `H5` `SW`

    ✓7ᵗʰ **T23.319 Burn of third degree of unspecified thumb (nail)** `CC` `H5` `SW`

✓6ᵗʰ **T23.32 Burn of third degree of single finger (nail) except thumb**

CC Excl: For CC codes in subcategory T23.32: PDX collection 1398

    ✓7ᵗʰ **T23.321 Burn of third degree of single right finger (nail) except thumb** `CC` `H5` `SW`

    ✓7ᵗʰ **T23.322 Burn of third degree of single left finger (nail) except thumb** `CC` `H5` `SW`

    ✓7ᵗʰ **T23.329 Burn of third degree of unspecified single finger (nail) except thumb** `CC` `H5` `SW`

✓6ᵗʰ **T23.33 Burn of third degree of multiple fingers (nail), not including thumb**

CC Excl: For CC codes in subcategory T23.33: PDX collection 1399

    ✓7ᵗʰ **T23.331 Burn of third degree of multiple right fingers (nail), not including thumb** `CC` `H5` `SW`

    ✓7ᵗʰ **T23.332 Burn of third degree of multiple left fingers (nail), not including thumb** `CC` `H5` `SW`

    ✓7ᵗʰ **T23.339 Burn of third degree of unspecified multiple fingers (nail), not including thumb** `CC` `H5` `SW`

✓6ᵗʰ **T23.34 Burn of third degree of multiple fingers (nail), including thumb**

CC Excl: For CC codes in subcategory T23.34: PDX collection 1400

    ✓7ᵗʰ **T23.341 Burn of third degree of multiple right fingers (nail), including thumb** `CC` `H5` `SW`

    ✓7ᵗʰ **T23.342 Burn of third degree of multiple left fingers (nail), including thumb** `CC` `H5` `SW`

    ✓7ᵗʰ **T23.349 Burn of third degree of unspecified multiple fingers (nail), including thumb** `CC` `H5` `SW`

✓6ᵗʰ **T23.35 Burn of third degree of palm**

CC Excl: For CC codes in subcategory T23.35: PDX collection 1401

    ✓7ᵗʰ **T23.351 Burn of third degree of right palm** `CC` `H5` `SW`

    ✓7ᵗʰ **T23.352 Burn of third degree of left palm** `CC` `H5` `SW`

    ✓7ᵗʰ **T23.359 Burn of third degree of unspecified palm** `CC` `H5` `SW`

✓6ᵗʰ **T23.36 Burn of third degree of back of hand**

CC Excl: For CC codes in subcategory T23.36: PDX collection 1402

    ✓7ᵗʰ **T23.361 Burn of third degree of back of right hand** `CC` `H5` `SW`

    ✓7ᵗʰ **T23.362 Burn of third degree of back of left hand** `CC` `H5` `SW`

    ✓7ᵗʰ **T23.369 Burn of third degree of back of unspecified hand** `CC` `H5` `SW`

✓6ᵗʰ **T23.37 Burn of third degree of wrist**

CC Excl: For CC codes in subcategory T23.37: PDX collection 1403

    ✓7ᵗʰ **T23.371 Burn of third degree of right wrist** `CC` `H5` `SW`

    ✓7ᵗʰ **T23.372 Burn of third degree of left wrist** `CC` `H5` `SW`

    ✓7ᵗʰ **T23.379 Burn of third degree of unspecified wrist** `CC` `H5` `SW`

☑ Additional Character Required   ✓x7ᵗʰ Placeholder   Unacceptable PDx   Questionable PDx   Manifestation   Unspecified Dx   H1-H14 HAC   HCC CMS-HCC Dx   HIV HIV Dx

ICD-10-CM 2020   **1137**

√6ᵗʰ **T23.39** Burn of third degree of multiple sites of wrist and hand

> **CC Excl: For CC codes in subcategory T23.39:** PDX collection 1396

√7ᵗʰ **T23.391** Burn of third degree of multiple sites of right wrist and hand `CC` `H5` `SW`

√7ᵗʰ **T23.392** Burn of third degree of multiple sites of left wrist and hand `CC` `H5` `SW`

√7ᵗʰ **T23.399** Burn of third degree of multiple sites of unspecified wrist and hand `CC` `H5` `SW`

√5ᵗʰ **T23.4** Corrosion of unspecified degree of wrist and hand

> Code first (T51-T65) to identify chemical and intent
> Use additional external cause code to identify place (Y92)

√6ᵗʰ **T23.40** Corrosion of unspecified degree of hand, unspecified site

√7ᵗʰ **T23.401** Corrosion of unspecified degree of right hand, unspecified site

√7ᵗʰ **T23.402** Corrosion of unspecified degree of left hand, unspecified site

√7ᵗʰ **T23.409** Corrosion of unspecified degree of unspecified hand, unspecified site

√6ᵗʰ **T23.41** Corrosion of unspecified degree of thumb (nail)

√7ᵗʰ **T23.411** Corrosion of unspecified degree of right thumb (nail)

√7ᵗʰ **T23.412** Corrosion of unspecified degree of left thumb (nail)

√7ᵗʰ **T23.419** Corrosion of unspecified degree of unspecified thumb (nail)

√6ᵗʰ **T23.42** Corrosion of unspecified degree of single finger (nail) except thumb

√7ᵗʰ **T23.421** Corrosion of unspecified degree of single right finger (nail) except thumb

√7ᵗʰ **T23.422** Corrosion of unspecified degree of single left finger (nail) except thumb

√7ᵗʰ **T23.429** Corrosion of unspecified degree of unspecified single finger (nail) except thumb

√6ᵗʰ **T23.43** Corrosion of unspecified degree of multiple fingers (nail), not including thumb

√7ᵗʰ **T23.431** Corrosion of unspecified degree of multiple right fingers (nail), not including thumb

√7ᵗʰ **T23.432** Corrosion of unspecified degree of multiple left fingers (nail), not including thumb

√7ᵗʰ **T23.439** Corrosion of unspecified degree of unspecified multiple fingers (nail), not including thumb

√6ᵗʰ **T23.44** Corrosion of unspecified degree of multiple fingers (nail), including thumb

√7ᵗʰ **T23.441** Corrosion of unspecified degree of multiple right fingers (nail), including thumb

√7ᵗʰ **T23.442** Corrosion of unspecified degree of multiple left fingers (nail), including thumb

√7ᵗʰ **T23.449** Corrosion of unspecified degree of unspecified multiple fingers (nail), including thumb

√6ᵗʰ **T23.45** Corrosion of unspecified degree of palm

√7ᵗʰ **T23.451** Corrosion of unspecified degree of right palm

√7ᵗʰ **T23.452** Corrosion of unspecified degree of left palm

√7ᵗʰ **T23.459** Corrosion of unspecified degree of unspecified palm

√6ᵗʰ **T23.46** Corrosion of unspecified degree of back of hand

√7ᵗʰ **T23.461** Corrosion of unspecified degree of back of right hand

√7ᵗʰ **T23.462** Corrosion of unspecified degree of back of left hand

√7ᵗʰ **T23.469** Corrosion of unspecified degree of back of unspecified hand

√6ᵗʰ **T23.47** Corrosion of unspecified degree of wrist

√7ᵗʰ **T23.471** Corrosion of unspecified degree of right wrist

√7ᵗʰ **T23.472** Corrosion of unspecified degree of left wrist

√7ᵗʰ **T23.479** Corrosion of unspecified degree of unspecified wrist

√6ᵗʰ **T23.49** Corrosion of unspecified degree of multiple sites of wrist and hand

√7ᵗʰ **T23.491** Corrosion of unspecified degree of multiple sites of right wrist and hand

√7ᵗʰ **T23.492** Corrosion of unspecified degree of multiple sites of left wrist and hand

√7ᵗʰ **T23.499** Corrosion of unspecified degree of multiple sites of unspecified wrist and hand

√5ᵗʰ **T23.5** Corrosion of first degree of wrist and hand

> Code first (T51-T65) to identify chemical and intent
> Use additional external cause code to identify place (Y92)

√6ᵗʰ **T23.50** Corrosion of first degree of hand, unspecified site

√7ᵗʰ **T23.501** Corrosion of first degree of right hand, unspecified site

√7ᵗʰ **T23.502** Corrosion of first degree of left hand, unspecified site

√7ᵗʰ **T23.509** Corrosion of first degree of unspecified hand, unspecified site

√6ᵗʰ **T23.51** Corrosion of first degree of thumb (nail)

√7ᵗʰ **T23.511** Corrosion of first degree of right thumb (nail)

√7ᵗʰ **T23.512** Corrosion of first degree of left thumb (nail)

√7ᵗʰ **T23.519** Corrosion of first degree of unspecified thumb (nail)

√6ᵗʰ **T23.52** Corrosion of first degree of single finger (nail) except thumb

√7ᵗʰ **T23.521** Corrosion of first degree of single right finger (nail) except thumb

√7ᵗʰ **T23.522** Corrosion of first degree of single left finger (nail) except thumb

√7ᵗʰ **T23.529** Corrosion of first degree of unspecified single finger (nail) except thumb

√6ᵗʰ **T23.53** Corrosion of first degree of multiple fingers (nail), not including thumb

√7ᵗʰ **T23.531** Corrosion of first degree of multiple right fingers (nail), not including thumb

√7ᵗʰ **T23.532** Corrosion of first degree of multiple left fingers (nail), not including thumb

√7ᵗʰ **T23.539** Corrosion of first degree of unspecified multiple fingers (nail), not including thumb

√6ᵗʰ **T23.54** Corrosion of first degree of multiple fingers (nail), including thumb

√7ᵗʰ **T23.541** Corrosion of first degree of multiple right fingers (nail), including thumb

√7ᵗʰ **T23.542** Corrosion of first degree of multiple left fingers (nail), including thumb

√7ᵗʰ **T23.549** Corrosion of first degree of unspecified multiple fingers (nail), including thumb

√6ᵗʰ **T23.55** Corrosion of first degree of palm

√7ᵗʰ **T23.551** Corrosion of first degree of right palm

√7ᵗʰ **T23.552** Corrosion of first degree of left palm

√7ᵗʰ **T23.559** Corrosion of first degree of unspecified palm

√6ᵗʰ **T23.56** Corrosion of first degree of back of hand

√7ᵗʰ **T23.561** Corrosion of first degree of back of right hand

√7ᵗʰ **T23.562** Corrosion of first degree of back of left hand

√7ᵗʰ **T23.569** Corrosion of first degree of back of unspecified hand

√6ᵗʰ **T23.57** Corrosion of first degree of wrist

√7ᵗʰ **T23.571** Corrosion of first degree of right wrist

√7ᵗʰ **T23.572** Corrosion of first degree of left wrist

√7ᵗʰ **T23.579** Corrosion of first degree of unspecified wrist

√6ᵗʰ **T23.59** Corrosion of first degree of multiple sites of wrist and hand

√7ᵗʰ **T23.591** Corrosion of first degree of multiple sites of right wrist and hand

√7ᵗʰ **T23.592** Corrosion of first degree of multiple sites of left wrist and hand

√7ᵗʰ **T23.599** Corrosion of first degree of multiple sites of unspecified wrist and hand

`N` Newborn: 0 `P` Pediatric: 0-17 `M` Maternity: 9-64 `A` Adult: 15-124 `MCC` Major Complication/Comorbidity `CC` Complication/Comorbidity `SW` Severe Wound Dx

1138

ICD-10-CM 2020

√5ᵗʰ **T23.6** **Corrosion of second degree of wrist and hand**

Code first (T51-T65) to identify chemical and intent

Use additional external cause code to identify place (Y92)

√6ᵗʰ **T23.60** **Corrosion of second degree of hand, unspecified site**

√7ᵗʰ **T23.601** **Corrosion of second degree of right hand, unspecified site**

√7ᵗʰ **T23.602** **Corrosion of second degree of left hand, unspecified site**

√7ᵗʰ **T23.609** **Corrosion of second degree of unspecified hand, unspecified site**

√6ᵗʰ **T23.61** **Corrosion of second degree of thumb (nail)**

√7ᵗʰ **T23.611** **Corrosion of second degree of right thumb (nail)**

√7ᵗʰ **T23.612** **Corrosion of second degree of left thumb (nail)**

√7ᵗʰ **T23.619** **Corrosion of second degree of unspecified thumb (nail)**

√6ᵗʰ **T23.62** **Corrosion of second degree of single finger (nail) except thumb**

√7ᵗʰ **T23.621** **Corrosion of second degree of single right finger (nail) except thumb.**

√7ᵗʰ **T23.622** **Corrosion of second degree of single left finger (nail) except thumb**

√7ᵗʰ **T23.629** **Corrosion of second degree of unspecified single finger (nail) except thumb**

√6ᵗʰ **T23.63** **Corrosion of second degree of multiple fingers (nail), not including thumb**

√7ᵗʰ **T23.631** **Corrosion of second degree of multiple right fingers (nail), not including thumb**

√7ᵗʰ **T23.632** **Corrosion of second degree of multiple left fingers (nail), not including thumb**

√7ᵗʰ **T23.639** **Corrosion of second degree of unspecified multiple fingers (nail), not including thumb**

√6ᵗʰ **T23.64** **Corrosion of second degree of multiple fingers (nail), including thumb**

√7ᵗʰ **T23.641** **Corrosion of second degree of multiple right fingers (nail), including thumb**

√7ᵗʰ **T23.642** **Corrosion of second degree of multiple left fingers (nail), including thumb**

√7ᵗʰ **T23.649** **Corrosion of second degree of unspecified multiple fingers (nail), including thumb**

√6ᵗʰ **T23.65** **Corrosion of second degree of palm**

√7ᵗʰ **T23.651** **Corrosion of second degree of right palm**

√7ᵗʰ **T23.652** **Corrosion of second degree of left palm**

√7ᵗʰ **T23.659** **Corrosion of second degree of unspecified palm**

√6ᵗʰ **T23.66** **Corrosion of second degree of back of hand**

√7ᵗʰ **T23.661** **Corrosion of second degree back of right hand**

√7ᵗʰ **T23.662** **Corrosion of second degree back of left hand**

√7ᵗʰ **T23.669** **Corrosion of second degree back of unspecified hand**

√6ᵗʰ **T23.67** **Corrosion of second degree of wrist**

√7ᵗʰ **T23.671** **Corrosion of second degree of right wrist**

√7ᵗʰ **T23.672** **Corrosion of second degree of left wrist**

√7ᵗʰ **T23.679** **Corrosion of second degree of unspecified wrist**

√6ᵗʰ **T23.69** **Corrosion of second degree of multiple sites of wrist and hand**

√7ᵗʰ **T23.691** **Corrosion of second degree of multiple sites of right wrist and hand**

√7ᵗʰ **T23.692** **Corrosion of second degree of multiple sites of left wrist and hand**

√7ᵗʰ **T23.699** **Corrosion of second degree of multiple sites of unspecified wrist and hand**

√5ᵗʰ **T23.7** **Corrosion of third degree of wrist and hand**

Code first (T51-T65) to identify chemical and intent

Use additional external cause code to identify place (Y92)

√6ᵗʰ **T23.70** **Corrosion of third degree of hand, unspecified site**

CC Excl: For CC codes in subcategory T23.70: PDX collection 1396

√7ᵗʰ **T23.701** **Corrosion of third degree of right hand, unspecified site**   CC H5 SW

√7ᵗʰ **T23.702** **Corrosion of third degree of left hand, unspecified site**   CC H5 SW

√7ᵗʰ **T23.709** **Corrosion of third degree of unspecified hand, unspecified site**   CC H5 SW

√6ᵗʰ **T23.71** **Corrosion of third degree of thumb (nail)**

CC Excl: For CC codes in subcategory T23.71: PDX collection 1397

√7ᵗʰ **T23.711** **Corrosion of third degree of right thumb (nail)**   CC H5 SW

√7ᵗʰ **T23.712** **Corrosion of third degree of left thumb (nail)**   CC H5 SW

√7ᵗʰ **T23.719** **Corrosion of third degree of unspecified thumb (nail)**   CC H5 SW

√6ᵗʰ **T23.72** **Corrosion of third degree of single finger (nail) except thumb**

CC Excl: For CC codes in subcategory T23.72: PDX collection 1398

√7ᵗʰ **T23.721** **Corrosion of third degree of single right finger (nail) except thumb**   CC H5 SW

√7ᵗʰ **T23.722** **Corrosion of third degree of single left finger (nail) except thumb**   CC H5 SW

√7ᵗʰ **T23.729** **Corrosion of third degree of unspecified single finger (nail) except thumb**   CC H5 SW

√6ᵗʰ **T23.73** **Corrosion of third degree of multiple fingers (nail), not including thumb**

CC Excl: For CC codes in subcategory T23.73: PDX collection 1399

√7ᵗʰ **T23.731** **Corrosion of third degree of multiple right fingers (nail), not including thumb**   CC H5 SW

√7ᵗʰ **T23.732** **Corrosion of third degree of multiple left fingers (nail), not including thumb**   CC H5 SW

√7ᵗʰ **T23.739** **Corrosion of third degree of unspecified multiple fingers (nail), not including thumb**   CC H5 SW

√6ᵗʰ **T23.74** **Corrosion of third degree of multiple fingers (nail), including thumb**

CC Excl: For CC codes in subcategory T23.74: PDX collection 1400

√7ᵗʰ **T23.741** **Corrosion of third degree of multiple right fingers (nail), including thumb**   CC H5 SW

√7ᵗʰ **T23.742** **Corrosion of third degree of multiple left fingers (nail), including thumb**   CC H5 SW

√7ᵗʰ **T23.749** **Corrosion of third degree of unspecified multiple fingers (nail), including thumb**   CC H5 SW

√6ᵗʰ **T23.75** **Corrosion of third degree of palm**

CC Excl: For CC codes in subcategory T23.75: PDX collection 1401

√7ᵗʰ **T23.751** **Corrosion of third degree of right palm**   CC H5 SW

√7ᵗʰ **T23.752** **Corrosion of third degree of left palm**   CC H5 SW

√7ᵗʰ **T23.759** **Corrosion of third degree of unspecified palm**   CC H5 SW

√6ᵗʰ **T23.76** **Corrosion of third degree of back of hand**

CC Excl: For CC codes in subcategory T23.76: PDX collection 1402

√7ᵗʰ **T23.761** **Corrosion of third degree of back of right hand**   CC H5 SW

√7ᵗʰ **T23.762** **Corrosion of third degree of back of left hand**   CC H5 SW

√7ᵗʰ **T23.769** **Corrosion of third degree back of unspecified hand**   CC H5 SW

√6ᵗʰ **T23.77** **Corrosion of third degree of wrist**

CC Excl: For CC codes in subcategory T23.77: PDX collection 1403

√7ᵗʰ **T23.771** **Corrosion of third degree of right wrist**   CC H5 SW

√7ᵗʰ **T23.772** **Corrosion of third degree of left wrist**   CC H5 SW

√7ᵗʰ **T23.779** **Corrosion of third degree of unspecified wrist**   CC H5 SW

☑ Additional Character Required   √x7ᵗʰ Placeholder   Unacceptable PDx   Questionable PDx   Manifestation   Unspecified Dx   H1-H14 HAC   HCC CMS-HCC Dx   HIV HIV Dx

ICD-10-CM 2020   **1139**

√6ᵗʰ **T23.79 Corrosion of third degree of multiple sites of wrist and hand**
CC Excl: For CC codes in subcategory T23.79: PDX collection 1396

√7ᵗʰ **T23.791 Corrosion of third degree of multiple sites of right wrist and hand** `CC` `H5` `SW`

√7ᵗʰ **T23.792 Corrosion of third degree of multiple sites of left wrist and hand** `CC` `H5` `SW`

√7ᵗʰ **T23.799 Corrosion of third degree of multiple sites of unspecified wrist and hand** `CC` `H5` `SW`

√4ᵗʰ **T24 Burn and corrosion of lower limb, except ankle and foot**

EXCLUDES 2 *burn and corrosion of ankle and foot (T25.-)*
burn and corrosion of hip region (T21.-)

The appropriate 7th character is to be added to each code from category T24.
A initial encounter
D subsequent encounter
S sequela

√5ᵗʰ **T24.0 Burn of unspecified degree of lower limb, except ankle and foot**
Use additional external cause code to identify the source, place and intent of the burn (X00-X19, X75-X77, X96-X98, Y92)

√6ᵗʰ **T24.00 Burn of unspecified degree of unspecified site of lower limb, except ankle and foot**

√7ᵗʰ **T24.001 Burn of unspecified degree of unspecified site of right lower limb, except ankle and foot**

√7ᵗʰ **T24.002 Burn of unspecified degree of unspecified site of left lower limb, except ankle and foot**

√7ᵗʰ **T24.009 Burn of unspecified degree of unspecified site of unspecified lower limb, except ankle and foot**

√6ᵗʰ **T24.01 Burn of unspecified degree of thigh**

√7ᵗʰ **T24.011 Burn of unspecified degree of right thigh**

√7ᵗʰ **T24.012 Burn of unspecified degree of left thigh**

√7ᵗʰ **T24.019 Burn of unspecified degree of unspecified thigh**

√6ᵗʰ **T24.02 Burn of unspecified degree of knee**

√7ᵗʰ **T24.021 Burn of unspecified degree of right knee**

√7ᵗʰ **T24.022 Burn of unspecified degree of left knee**

√7ᵗʰ **T24.029 Burn of unspecified degree of unspecified knee**

√6ᵗʰ **T24.03 Burn of unspecified degree of lower leg**

√7ᵗʰ **T24.031 Burn of unspecified degree of right lower leg**

√7ᵗʰ **T24.032 Burn of unspecified degree of left lower leg**

√7ᵗʰ **T24.039 Burn of unspecified degree of unspecified lower leg**

√6ᵗʰ **T24.09 Burn of unspecified degree of multiple sites of lower limb, except ankle and foot**

√7ᵗʰ **T24.091 Burn of unspecified degree of multiple sites of right lower limb, except ankle and foot**

√7ᵗʰ **T24.092 Burn of unspecified degree of multiple sites of left lower limb, except ankle and foot**

√7ᵗʰ **T24.099 Burn of unspecified degree of multiple sites of unspecified lower limb, except ankle and foot**

√5ᵗʰ **T24.1 Burn of first degree of lower limb, except ankle and foot**
Use additional external cause code to identify the source, place and intent of the burn (X00-X19, X75-X77, X96-X98, Y92)

√6ᵗʰ **T24.10 Burn of first degree of unspecified site of lower limb, except ankle and foot**

√7ᵗʰ **T24.101 Burn of first degree of unspecified site of right lower limb, except ankle and foot**

√7ᵗʰ **T24.102 Burn of first degree of unspecified site of left lower limb, except ankle and foot**

√7ᵗʰ **T24.109 Burn of first degree of unspecified site of unspecified lower limb, except ankle and foot**

√6ᵗʰ **T24.11 Burn of first degree of thigh**

√7ᵗʰ **T24.111 Burn of first degree of right thigh**

√7ᵗʰ **T24.112 Burn of first degree of left thigh**

√7ᵗʰ **T24.119 Burn of first degree of unspecified thigh**

√6ᵗʰ **T24.12 Burn of first degree of knee**

√7ᵗʰ **T24.121 Burn of first degree of right knee**

√7ᵗʰ **T24.122 Burn of first degree of left knee**

√7ᵗʰ **T24.129 Burn of first degree of unspecified knee**

√6ᵗʰ **T24.13 Burn of first degree of lower leg**

√7ᵗʰ **T24.131 Burn of first degree of right lower leg**

√7ᵗʰ **T24.132 Burn of first degree of left lower leg**

√7ᵗʰ **T24.139 Burn of first degree of unspecified lower leg**

√6ᵗʰ **T24.19 Burn of first degree of multiple sites of lower limb, except ankle and foot**

√7ᵗʰ **T24.191 Burn of first degree of multiple sites of right lower limb, except ankle and foot**

√7ᵗʰ **T24.192 Burn of first degree of multiple sites of left lower limb, except ankle and foot**

√7ᵗʰ **T24.199 Burn of first degree of multiple sites of unspecified lower limb, except ankle and foot**

√5ᵗʰ **T24.2 Burn of second degree of lower limb, except ankle and foot**
Use additional external cause code to identify the source, place and intent of the burn (X00-X19, X75-X77, X96-X98, Y92)

√6ᵗʰ **T24.20 Burn of second degree of unspecified site of lower limb, except ankle and foot**

√7ᵗʰ **T24.201 Burn of second degree of unspecified site of right lower limb, except ankle and foot**

√7ᵗʰ **T24.202 Burn of second degree of unspecified site of left lower limb, except ankle and foot**

√7ᵗʰ **T24.209 Burn of second degree of unspecified site of unspecified lower limb, except ankle and foot**

√6ᵗʰ **T24.21 Burn of second degree of thigh**

√7ᵗʰ **T24.211 Burn of second degree of right thigh**

√7ᵗʰ **T24.212 Burn of second degree of left thigh**

√7ᵗʰ **T24.219 Burn of second degree of unspecified thigh**

√6ᵗʰ **T24.22 Burn of second degree of knee**

√7ᵗʰ **T24.221 Burn of second degree of right knee**

√7ᵗʰ **T24.222 Burn of second degree of left knee**

√7ᵗʰ **T24.229 Burn of second degree of unspecified knee**

√6ᵗʰ **T24.23 Burn of second degree of lower leg**

√7ᵗʰ **T24.231 Burn of second degree of right lower leg**

√7ᵗʰ **T24.232 Burn of second degree of left lower leg**

√7ᵗʰ **T24.239 Burn of second degree of unspecified lower leg**

√6ᵗʰ **T24.29 Burn of second degree of multiple sites of lower limb, except ankle and foot**

√7ᵗʰ **T24.291 Burn of second degree of multiple sites of right lower limb, except ankle and foot**

√7ᵗʰ **T24.292 Burn of second degree of multiple sites of left lower limb, except ankle and foot**

√7ᵗʰ **T24.299 Burn of second degree of multiple sites of unspecified lower limb, except ankle and foot**

√5ᵗʰ **T24.3 Burn of third degree of lower limb, except ankle and foot**
Use additional external cause code to identify the source, place and intent of the burn (X00-X19, X75-X77, X96-X98, Y92)

√6ᵗʰ **T24.30 Burn of third degree of unspecified site of lower limb, except ankle and foot**
CC Excl: For CC codes in subcategory T24.30: PDX collection 1404

√7ᵗʰ **T24.301 Burn of third degree of unspecified site of right lower limb, except ankle and foot** `CC` `H5` `SW`

√7ᵗʰ **T24.302 Burn of third degree of unspecified site of left lower limb, except ankle and foot** `CC` `H5` `SW`

√7ᵗʰ **T24.309 Burn of third degree of unspecified site of unspecified lower limb, except ankle and foot** `CC` `H5` `SW`

✓6ᵗʰ **T24.31   Burn of third degree of** thigh

CC Excl: For CC codes in subcategory T24.31: PDX collection 1405

✓7ᵗʰ **T24.311   Burn of third degree of right thigh**   `CC` `H5` `SW`

✓7ᵗʰ **T24.312   Burn of third degree of** left **thigh**   `CC` `H5` `SW`

✓7ᵗʰ **T24.319   Burn of third degree of unspecified thigh**   `CC` `H5` `SW`

✓6ᵗʰ **T24.32   Burn of third degree of** knee

CC Excl: For CC codes in subcategory T24.32: PDX collection 1406

✓7ᵗʰ **T24.321   Burn of third degree of right knee**   `CC` `H5` `SW`

✓7ᵗʰ **T24.322   Burn of third degree of** left **knee**   `CC` `H5` `SW`

✓7ᵗʰ **T24.329   Burn of third degree of unspecified knee**   `CC` `H5` `SW`

✓6ᵗʰ **T24.33   Burn of third degree of** lower leg

CC Excl: For CC codes in subcategory T24.33: PDX collection 1407

✓7ᵗʰ **T24.331   Burn of third degree of right lower leg**   `CC` `H5` `SW`

✓7ᵗʰ **T24.332   Burn of third degree of** left **lower leg**   `CC` `H5` `SW`

✓7ᵗʰ **T24.339   Burn of third degree of unspecified lower leg**   `CC` `H5` `SW`

✓6ᵗʰ **T24.39   Burn of third degree of** multiple sites **of lower limb, except ankle and foot**

AHA: 2016,2Q,4

CC Excl: For CC codes in subcategory T24.39: PDX collection 1404

✓7ᵗʰ **T24.391   Burn of third degree of multiple sites of** right **lower limb, except ankle and foot**   `CC` `H5` `SW`

✓7ᵗʰ **T24.392   Burn of third degree of multiple sites of** left **lower limb, except ankle and foot**   `CC` `H5` `SW`

✓7ᵗʰ **T24.399   Burn of third degree of multiple sites of unspecified lower limb, except ankle and foot**   `CC` `H5` `SW`

✓5ᵗʰ **T24.4   Corrosion of unspecified degree of lower limb, except ankle and foot**

Code first (T51-T65) to identify chemical and intent

Use additional external cause code to identify place (Y92)

✓6ᵗʰ **T24.40   Corrosion of unspecified degree of unspecified site of lower limb, except ankle and foot**

✓7ᵗʰ **T24.401   Corrosion of unspecified degree of unspecified site of** right **lower limb, except ankle and foot**

✓7ᵗʰ **T24.402   Corrosion of unspecified degree of unspecified site of** left **lower limb, except ankle and foot**

✓7ᵗʰ **T24.409   Corrosion of unspecified degree of unspecified site of unspecified lower limb, except ankle and foot**

✓6ᵗʰ **T24.41   Corrosion of unspecified degree of** thigh

✓7ᵗʰ **T24.411   Corrosion of unspecified degree of** right **thigh**

✓7ᵗʰ **T24.412   Corrosion of unspecified degree of** left **thigh**

✓7ᵗʰ **T24.419   Corrosion of unspecified degree of unspecified thigh**

✓6ᵗʰ **T24.42   Corrosion of unspecified degree of** knee

✓7ᵗʰ **T24.421   Corrosion of unspecified degree of** right **knee**

✓7ᵗʰ **T24.422   Corrosion of unspecified degree of** left **knee**

✓7ᵗʰ **T24.429   Corrosion of unspecified degree of unspecified knee**

✓6ᵗʰ **T24.43   Corrosion of unspecified degree of** lower leg

✓7ᵗʰ **T24.431   Corrosion of unspecified degree of** right **lower leg**

✓7ᵗʰ **T24.432   Corrosion of unspecified degree of** left **lower leg**

✓7ᵗʰ **T24.439   Corrosion of unspecified degree of unspecified lower leg**

✓6ᵗʰ **T24.49   Corrosion of unspecified degree of** multiple sites **of lower limb, except ankle and foot**

✓7ᵗʰ **T24.491   Corrosion of unspecified degree of multiple sites of** right **lower limb, except ankle and foot**

✓7ᵗʰ **T24.492   Corrosion of unspecified degree of multiple sites of** left **lower limb, except ankle and foot**

✓7ᵗʰ **T24.499   Corrosion of unspecified degree of multiple sites of unspecified lower limb, except ankle and foot**

✓5ᵗʰ **T24.5   Corrosion of** first degree **of lower limb, except ankle and foot**

Code first (T51-T65) to identify chemical and intent

Use additional external cause code to identify place (Y92)

✓6ᵗʰ **T24.50   Corrosion of** first degree **of unspecified site of lower limb, except ankle and foot**

✓7ᵗʰ **T24.501   Corrosion of first degree of unspecified site of** right **lower limb, except ankle and foot**

✓7ᵗʰ **T24.502   Corrosion of first degree of unspecified site of** left **lower limb, except ankle and foot**

✓7ᵗʰ **T24.509   Corrosion of first degree of unspecified site of unspecified lower limb, except ankle and foot**

✓6ᵗʰ **T24.51   Corrosion of first degree of** thigh

✓7ᵗʰ **T24.511   Corrosion of first degree of** right **thigh**

✓7ᵗʰ **T24.512   Corrosion of first degree of** left **thigh**

✓7ᵗʰ **T24.519   Corrosion of first degree of unspecified thigh**

✓6ᵗʰ **T24.52   Corrosion of first degree of** knee

✓7ᵗʰ **T24.521   Corrosion of first degree of** right **knee**

✓7ᵗʰ **T24.522   Corrosion of first degree of** left **knee**

✓7ᵗʰ **T24.529   Corrosion of first degree of unspecified knee**

✓6ᵗʰ **T24.53   Corrosion of first degree of** lower leg

✓7ᵗʰ **T24.531   Corrosion of first degree of** right **lower leg**

✓7ᵗʰ **T24.532   Corrosion of first degree of** left **lower leg**

✓7ᵗʰ **T24.539   Corrosion of first degree of unspecified lower leg**

✓6ᵗʰ **T24.59   Corrosion of first degree of** multiple sites **of lower limb, except ankle and foot**

✓7ᵗʰ **T24.591   Corrosion of first degree of multiple sites of** right **lower limb, except ankle and foot**

✓7ᵗʰ **T24.592   Corrosion of first degree of multiple sites of** left **lower limb, except ankle and foot**

✓7ᵗʰ **T24.599   Corrosion of first degree of multiple sites of unspecified lower limb, except ankle and foot**

✓5ᵗʰ **T24.6   Corrosion of** second degree **of lower limb, except ankle and foot**

Code first (T51-T65) to identify chemical and intent

Use additional external cause code to identify place (Y92)

✓6ᵗʰ **T24.60   Corrosion of second degree of unspecified site of lower limb, except ankle and foot**

✓7ᵗʰ **T24.601   Corrosion of second degree of unspecified site of** right **lower limb, except ankle and foot**

✓7ᵗʰ **T24.602   Corrosion of second degree of unspecified site of** left **lower limb, except ankle and foot**

✓7ᵗʰ **T24.609   Corrosion of second degree of unspecified site of unspecified lower limb, except ankle and foot**

✓6ᵗʰ **T24.61   Corrosion of second degree of** thigh

✓7ᵗʰ **T24.611   Corrosion of second degree of** right **thigh**

✓7ᵗʰ **T24.612   Corrosion of second degree of** left **thigh**

✓7ᵗʰ **T24.619   Corrosion of second degree of unspecified thigh**

✓6ᵗʰ **T24.62   Corrosion of second degree of** knee

✓7ᵗʰ **T24.621   Corrosion of second degree of** right **knee**

✓7ᵗʰ **T24.622   Corrosion of second degree of** left **knee**

✓7ᵗʰ **T24.629   Corrosion of second degree of unspecified knee**

✓6ᵗʰ **T24.63   Corrosion of second degree of** lower leg

✓7ᵗʰ **T24.631   Corrosion of second degree of** right **lower leg**

✓ Additional Character Required   ✓ₓ7ᵗʰ Placeholder   Unacceptable PDx   Questionable PDx   Manifestation   Unspecified Dx   `H1`-`H14` HAC   `HCC` CMS-HCC Dx   `HIV` HIV Dx

ICD-10-CM 2020

1141

√7ᵗʰ **T24.632** Corrosion of second degree of left lower leg

√7ᵗʰ **T24.639** Corrosion of second degree of unspecified lower leg

√6ᵗʰ **T24.69** Corrosion of second degree of multiple sites of lower limb, except ankle and foot

√7ᵗʰ **T24.691** Corrosion of second degree of multiple sites of right lower limb, except ankle and foot

√7ᵗʰ **T24.692** Corrosion of second degree of multiple sites of left lower limb, except ankle and foot

√7ᵗʰ **T24.699** Corrosion of second degree of multiple sites of unspecified lower limb, except ankle and foot

√5ᵗʰ **T24.7** Corrosion of third degree of lower limb, except ankle and foot

Code first (T51-T65) to identify chemical and intent
Use additional external cause code to identify place (Y92)

√6ᵗʰ **T24.70** Corrosion of third degree of unspecified site of lower limb, except ankle and foot

CC Excl: For CC codes in subcategory T24.70: PDX collection 1404

√7ᵗʰ **T24.701** Corrosion of third degree of unspecified site of right lower limb, except ankle and foot `CC` `H5` `SW`

√7ᵗʰ **T24.702** Corrosion of third degree of unspecified site of left lower limb, except ankle and foot `CC` `H5` `SW`

√7ᵗʰ **T24.709** Corrosion of third degree of unspecified site of unspecified lower limb, except ankle and foot `CC` `H5` `SW`

√6ᵗʰ **T24.71** Corrosion of third degree of thigh

CC Excl: For CC codes in subcategory T24.71: PDX collection 1405

√7ᵗʰ **T24.711** Corrosion of third degree of right thigh `CC` `H5` `SW`

√7ᵗʰ **T24.712** Corrosion of third degree of left thigh `CC` `H5` `SW`

√7ᵗʰ **T24.719** Corrosion of third degree of unspecified thigh `CC` `H5` `SW`

√6ᵗʰ **T24.72** Corrosion of third degree of knee

CC Excl: For CC codes in subcategory T24.72: PDX collection 1406

√7ᵗʰ **T24.721** Corrosion of third degree of right knee `CC` `H5` `SW`

√7ᵗʰ **T24.722** Corrosion of third degree of left knee `CC` `H5` `SW`

√7ᵗʰ **T24.729** Corrosion of third degree of unspecified knee `CC` `H5` `SW`

√6ᵗʰ **T24.73** Corrosion of third degree of lower leg

CC Excl: For CC codes in subcategory T24.73: PDX collection 1407

√7ᵗʰ **T24.731** Corrosion of third degree of right lower leg `CC` `H5` `SW`

√7ᵗʰ **T24.732** Corrosion of third degree of left lower leg `CC` `H5` `SW`

√7ᵗʰ **T24.739** Corrosion of third degree of unspecified lower leg `CC` `H5` `SW`

√6ᵗʰ **T24.79** Corrosion of third degree of multiple sites of lower limb, except ankle and foot

CC Excl: For CC codes in subcategory T24.79: PDX collection 1404

√7ᵗʰ **T24.791** Corrosion of third degree of multiple sites of right lower limb, except ankle and foot `CC` `H5` `SW`

√7ᵗʰ **T24.792** Corrosion of third degree of multiple sites of left lower limb, except ankle and foot `CC` `H5` `SW`

√7ᵗʰ **T24.799** Corrosion of third degree of multiple sites of unspecified lower limb, except ankle and foot `CC` `H5` `SW`

√4ᵗʰ **T25** Burn and corrosion of ankle and foot

The appropriate 7th character is to be added to each code from category T25.
A initial encounter
D subsequent encounter
S sequela

√5ᵗʰ **T25.0** Burn of unspecified degree of ankle and foot

Use additional external cause code to identify the source, place and intent of the burn (X00-X19, X75-X77, X96-X98, Y92)

√6ᵗʰ **T25.01** Burn of unspecified degree of ankle

√7ᵗʰ **T25.011** Burn of unspecified degree of right ankle

√7ᵗʰ **T25.012** Burn of unspecified degree of left ankle

√7ᵗʰ **T25.019** Burn of unspecified degree of unspecified ankle

√6ᵗʰ **T25.02** Burn of unspecified degree of foot

EXCLUDES 2 burn of unspecified degree of toe(s) (nail) (T25.03-)

√7ᵗʰ **T25.021** Burn of unspecified degree of right foot

√7ᵗʰ **T25.022** Burn of unspecified degree of left foot

√7ᵗʰ **T25.029** Burn of unspecified degree of unspecified foot

√6ᵗʰ **T25.03** Burn of unspecified degree of toe(s) (nail)

√7ᵗʰ **T25.031** Burn of unspecified degree of right toe(s) (nail)

√7ᵗʰ **T25.032** Burn of unspecified degree of left toe(s) (nail)

√7ᵗʰ **T25.039** Burn of unspecified degree of unspecified toe(s) (nail)

√6ᵗʰ **T25.09** Burn of unspecified degree of multiple sites of ankle and foot

√7ᵗʰ **T25.091** Burn of unspecified degree of multiple sites of right ankle and foot

√7ᵗʰ **T25.092** Burn of unspecified degree of multiple sites of left ankle and foot

√7ᵗʰ **T25.099** Burn of unspecified degree of multiple sites of unspecified ankle and foot

√5ᵗʰ **T25.1** Burn of first degree of ankle and foot

Use additional external cause code to identify the source, place and intent of the burn (X00-X19, X75-X77, X96-X98, Y92)

√6ᵗʰ **T25.11** Burn of first degree of ankle

√7ᵗʰ **T25.111** Burn of first degree of right ankle

√7ᵗʰ **T25.112** Burn of first degree of left ankle

√7ᵗʰ **T25.119** Burn of first degree of unspecified ankle

√6ᵗʰ **T25.12** Burn of first degree of foot

EXCLUDES 2 burn of first degree of toe(s) (nail) (T25.13-)

√7ᵗʰ **T25.121** Burn of first degree of right foot

√7ᵗʰ **T25.122** Burn of first degree of left foot

√7ᵗʰ **T25.129** Burn of first degree of unspecified foot

√6ᵗʰ **T25.13** Burn of first degree of toe(s) (nail)

√7ᵗʰ **T25.131** Burn of first degree of right toe(s) (nail)

√7ᵗʰ **T25.132** Burn of first degree of left toe(s) (nail)

√7ᵗʰ **T25.139** Burn of first degree of unspecified toe(s) (nail)

√6ᵗʰ **T25.19** Burn of first degree of multiple sites of ankle and foot

√7ᵗʰ **T25.191** Burn of first degree of multiple sites of right ankle and foot

√7ᵗʰ **T25.192** Burn of first degree of multiple sites of left ankle and foot

√7ᵗʰ **T25.199** Burn of first degree of multiple sites of unspecified ankle and foot

√5ᵗʰ **T25.2** Burn of second degree of ankle and foot

Use additional external cause code to identify the source, place and intent of the burn (X00-X19, X75-X77, X96-X98, Y92)

√6ᵗʰ **T25.21** Burn of second degree of ankle

√7ᵗʰ **T25.211** Burn of second degree of right ankle

√7ᵗʰ **T25.212** Burn of second degree of left ankle

√7ᵗʰ **T25.219** Burn of second degree of unspecified ankle

√6ᵗʰ **T25.22** Burn of second degree of foot

EXCLUDES 2 burn of second degree of toe(s) (nail) (T25.23-)

√7ᵗʰ **T25.221** Burn of second degree of right foot

√7ᵗʰ **T25.222** Burn of second degree of left foot

N Newborn: 0 | P Pediatric: 0-17 | M Maternity: 9-64 | A Adult: 15-124 | MCC Major Complication/Comorbidity | CC Complication/Comorbidity | SW Severe Wound Dx

1142 | ICD-10-CM 2020

√7ᵗʰ **T25.229** Burn of second degree of unspecified foot

√6ᵗʰ **T25.23** Burn of second degree of toe(s) (nail)

√7ᵗʰ **T25.231** Burn of second degree of right toe(s) (nail)

√7ᵗʰ **T25.232** Burn of second degree of left toe(s) (nail)

√7ᵗʰ **T25.239** Burn of second degree of unspecified toe(s) (nail)

√6ᵗʰ **T25.29** Burn of second degree of multiple sites of ankle and foot

√7ᵗʰ **T25.291** Burn of second degree of multiple sites of right ankle and foot

√7ᵗʰ **T25.292** Burn of second degree of multiple sites of left ankle and foot

√7ᵗʰ **T25.299** Burn of second degree of multiple sites of unspecified ankle and foot

√5ᵗʰ **T25.3** Burn of third degree of ankle and foot

Use additional external cause code to identify the source, place and intent of the burn (X00-X19, X75-X77, X96-X98, Y92)

√6ᵗʰ **T25.31** Burn of third degree of ankle

CC Excl: For CC codes in subcategory T25.31: PDX collection 1408

√7ᵗʰ **T25.311** Burn of third degree of right ankle   `CC` `H5` `SW`

√7ᵗʰ **T25.312** Burn of third degree of left ankle   `CC` `H5` `SW`

√7ᵗʰ **T25.319** Burn of third degree of unspecified ankle   `CC` `H5` `SW`

√6ᵗʰ **T25.32** Burn of third degree of foot

EXCLUDES 2   burn of third degree of toe(s) (nail) (T25.33-)

CC Excl: For CC codes in subcategory T25.32: PDX collection 1409

√7ᵗʰ **T25.321** Burn of third degree of right foot   `CC` `H5` `SW`

√7ᵗʰ **T25.322** Burn of third degree of left foot   `CC` `H5` `SW`

√7ᵗʰ **T25.329** Burn of third degree of unspecified foot   `CC` `H5` `SW`

√6ᵗʰ **T25.33** Burn of third degree of toe(s) (nail)

CC Excl: For CC codes in subcategory T25.33: PDX collection 1410

√7ᵗʰ **T25.331** Burn of third degree of right toe(s) (nail)   `CC` `H5` `SW`

√7ᵗʰ **T25.332** Burn of third degree of left toe(s) (nail)   `CC` `H5` `SW`

√7ᵗʰ **T25.339** Burn of third degree of unspecified toe(s) (nail)   `CC` `H5` `SW`

√6ᵗʰ **T25.39** Burn of third degree of multiple sites of ankle and foot

CC Excl: For CC codes in subcategory T25.39: PDX collection 1404

√7ᵗʰ **T25.391** Burn of third degree of multiple sites of right ankle and foot   `CC` `H5` `SW`

√7ᵗʰ **T25.392** Burn of third degree of multiple sites of left ankle and foot   `CC` `H5` `SW`

√7ᵗʰ **T25.399** Burn of third degree of multiple sites of unspecified ankle and foot   `CC` `H5` `SW`

√5ᵗʰ **T25.4** Corrosion of unspecified degree of ankle and foot

Code first (T51-T65) to identify chemical and intent

Use additional external cause code to identify place (Y92)

√6ᵗʰ **T25.41** Corrosion of unspecified degree of ankle

√7ᵗʰ **T25.411** Corrosion of unspecified degree of right ankle

√7ᵗʰ **T25.412** Corrosion of unspecified degree of left ankle

√7ᵗʰ **T25.419** Corrosion of unspecified degree of unspecified ankle

√6ᵗʰ **T25.42** Corrosion of unspecified degree of foot

EXCLUDES 2   corrosion of unspecified degree of toe(s) (nail) (T25.43-)

√7ᵗʰ **T25.421** Corrosion of unspecified degree of right foot

√7ᵗʰ **T25.422** Corrosion of unspecified degree of left foot

√7ᵗʰ **T25.429** Corrosion of unspecified degree of unspecified foot

√7ᵗʰ **T25.43** Corrosion of unspecified degree of toe(s) (nail)

√7ᵗʰ **T25.431** Corrosion of unspecified degree of right toe(s) (nail)

√7ᵗʰ **T25.432** Corrosion of unspecified degree of left toe(s) (nail)

√7ᵗʰ **T25.439** Corrosion of unspecified degree of unspecified toe(s) (nail)

√6ᵗʰ **T25.49** Corrosion of unspecified degree of multiple sites of ankle and foot

√7ᵗʰ **T25.491** Corrosion of unspecified degree of multiple sites of right ankle and foot

√7ᵗʰ **T25.492** Corrosion of unspecified degree of multiple sites of left ankle and foot

√7ᵗʰ **T25.499** Corrosion of unspecified degree of multiple sites of unspecified ankle and foot

√5ᵗʰ **T25.5** Corrosion of first degree of ankle and foot

Code first (T51-T65) to identify chemical and intent

Use additional external cause code to identify place (Y92)

√6ᵗʰ **T25.51** Corrosion of first degree of ankle

√7ᵗʰ **T25.511** Corrosion of first degree of right ankle

√7ᵗʰ **T25.512** Corrosion of first degree of left ankle

√7ᵗʰ **T25.519** Corrosion of first degree of unspecified ankle

√6ᵗʰ **T25.52** Corrosion of first degree of foot

EXCLUDES 2   corrosion of first degree of toe(s) (nail) (T25.53-)

√7ᵗʰ **T25.521** Corrosion of first degree of right foot

√7ᵗʰ **T25.522** Corrosion of first degree of left foot

√7ᵗʰ **T25.529** Corrosion of first degree of unspecified foot

√6ᵗʰ **T25.53** Corrosion of first degree of toe(s) (nail)

√7ᵗʰ **T25.531** Corrosion of first degree of right toe(s) (nail)

√7ᵗʰ **T25.532** Corrosion of first degree of left toe(s) (nail)

√7ᵗʰ **T25.539** Corrosion of first degree of unspecified toe(s) (nail)

√6ᵗʰ **T25.59** Corrosion of first degree of multiple sites of ankle and foot

√7ᵗʰ **T25.591** Corrosion of first degree of multiple sites of right ankle and foot

√7ᵗʰ **T25.592** Corrosion of first degree of multiple sites of left ankle and foot

√7ᵗʰ **T25.599** Corrosion of first degree of multiple sites of unspecified ankle and foot

√5ᵗʰ **T25.6** Corrosion of second degree of ankle and foot

Code first (T51-T65) to identify chemical and intent

Use additional external cause code to identify place (Y92)

√6ᵗʰ **T25.61** Corrosion of second degree of ankle

√7ᵗʰ **T25.611** Corrosion of second degree of right ankle

√7ᵗʰ **T25.612** Corrosion of second degree of left ankle

√7ᵗʰ **T25.619** Corrosion of second degree of unspecified ankle

√6ᵗʰ **T25.62** Corrosion of second degree of foot

EXCLUDES 2   corrosion of second degree of toe(s) (nail) (T25.63-)

√7ᵗʰ **T25.621** Corrosion of second degree of right foot

√7ᵗʰ **T25.622** Corrosion of second degree of left foot

√7ᵗʰ **T25.629** Corrosion of second degree of unspecified foot

√6ᵗʰ **T25.63** Corrosion of second degree of toe(s) (nail)

√7ᵗʰ **T25.631** Corrosion of second degree of right toe(s) (nail)

√7ᵗʰ **T25.632** Corrosion of second degree of left toe(s) (nail)

√7ᵗʰ **T25.639** Corrosion of second degree of unspecified toe(s) (nail)

√6ᵗʰ **T25.69** Corrosion of second degree of multiple sites of ankle and foot

√7ᵗʰ **T25.691** Corrosion of second degree of right ankle and foot

√7ᵗʰ **T25.692** Corrosion of second degree of left ankle and foot

√7ᵗʰ **T25.699** Corrosion of second degree of unspecified ankle and foot

✓ Additional Character Required   √x7ᵗʰ Placeholder   Unacceptable PDx   Questionable PDx   Manifestation   Unspecified Dx   `H1`-`H14` HAC   `HCC` CMS-HCC Dx   `HIV` HIV Dx

ICD-10-CM 2020   1143

√5ᵗʰ **T25.7 Corrosion of third degree of ankle and foot**

Code first (T51-T65) to identify chemical and intent
Use additional external cause code to identify place (Y92)

√6ᵗʰ **T25.71 Corrosion of third degree of ankle**

CC Excl: For CC codes in subcategory T25.71: PDX collection 1408

√7ᵗʰ **T25.711 Corrosion of third degree of right ankle** `CC` `H5` `SW`

√7ᵗʰ **T25.712 Corrosion of third degree of left ankle** `CC` `H5` `SW`

√7ᵗʰ **T25.719 Corrosion of third degree of unspecified ankle** `CC` `H5` `SW`

√6ᵗʰ **T25.72 Corrosion of third degree of foot**

EXCLUDES 2 corrosion of third degree of toe(s) (nail) (T25.73-)

CC Excl: For CC codes in subcategory T25.72: PDX collection 1409

√7ᵗʰ **T25.721 Corrosion of third degree of right foot** `CC` `H5` `SW`

√7ᵗʰ **T25.722 Corrosion of third degree of left foot** `CC` `H5` `SW`

√7ᵗʰ **T25.729 Corrosion of third degree of unspecified foot** `CC` `H5` `SW`

√6ᵗʰ **T25.73 Corrosion of third degree of toe(s) (nail)**

CC Excl: For CC codes in subcategory T25.73: PDX collection 1410

√7ᵗʰ **T25.731 Corrosion of third degree of right toe(s) (nail)** `CC` `H5` `SW`

√7ᵗʰ **T25.732 Corrosion of third degree of left toe(s) (nail)** `CC` `H5` `SW`

√7ᵗʰ **T25.739 Corrosion of third degree of unspecified toe(s) (nail)** `CC` `H5` `SW`

√6ᵗʰ **T25.79 Corrosion of third degree of multiple sites of ankle and foot**

CC Excl: For CC codes in subcategory T25.79: PDX collection 1404

√7ᵗʰ **T25.791 Corrosion of third degree of multiple sites of right ankle and foot** `CC` `H5` `SW`

√7ᵗʰ **T25.792 Corrosion of third degree of multiple sites of left ankle and foot** `CC` `H5` `SW`

√7ᵗʰ **T25.799 Corrosion of third degree of multiple sites of unspecified ankle and foot** `CC` `H5` `SW`

Burns and corrosions confined to eye and internal organs (T26-T28)

√4ᵗʰ **T26 Burn and corrosion confined to eye and adnexa**

The appropriate 7th character is to be added to each code from category T26.
A initial encounter
D subsequent encounter
S sequela

√5ᵗʰ **T26.0 Burn of eyelid and periocular area**

Use additional external cause code to identify the source, place and intent of the burn (X00-X19, X75-X77, X96-X98, Y92)

√7ᵗʰ **T26.00 Burn of unspecified eyelid and periocular area**

√7ᵗʰ **T26.01 Burn of right eyelid and periocular area**

√7ᵗʰ **T26.02 Burn of left eyelid and periocular area**

√5ᵗʰ **T26.1 Burn of cornea and conjunctival sac**

Use additional external cause code to identify the source, place and intent of the burn (X00-X19, X75-X77, X96-X98, Y92)

√7ᵗʰ **T26.10 Burn of cornea and conjunctival sac, unspecified eye**

√7ᵗʰ **T26.11 Burn of cornea and conjunctival sac, right eye**

√7ᵗʰ **T26.12 Burn of cornea and conjunctival sac, left eye**

√5ᵗʰ **T26.2 Burn with resulting rupture and destruction of eyeball**

Use additional external cause code to identify the source, place and intent of the burn (X00-X19, X75-X77, X96-X98, Y92)

√7ᵗʰ **T26.20 Burn with resulting rupture and destruction of unspecified eyeball** `CC` `H5`
CC Excl: No Excl

√7ᵗʰ **T26.21 Burn with resulting rupture and destruction of right eyeball** `CC` `H5`
CC Excl: No Excl

√7ᵗʰ **T26.22 Burn with resulting rupture and destruction of left eyeball** `CC` `H5`
CC Excl: No Excl

√5ᵗʰ **T26.3 Burns of other specified parts of eye and adnexa**

Use additional external cause code to identify the source, place and intent of the burn (X00-X19, X75-X77, X96-X98, Y92)

√7ᵗʰ **T26.30 Burns of other specified parts of unspecified eye and adnexa**

√7ᵗʰ **T26.31 Burns of other specified parts of right eye and adnexa**

√7ᵗʰ **T26.32 Burns of other specified parts of left eye and adnexa**

√5ᵗʰ **T26.4 Burn of eye and adnexa, part unspecified**

Use additional external cause code to identify the source, place and intent of the burn (X00-X19, X75-X77, X96-X98, Y92)

√7ᵗʰ **T26.40 Burn of unspecified eye and adnexa, part unspecified**

√7ᵗʰ **T26.41 Burn of right eye and adnexa, part unspecified**

√7ᵗʰ **T26.42 Burn of left eye and adnexa, part unspecified**

√5ᵗʰ **T26.5 Corrosion of eyelid and periocular area**

Code first (T51-T65) to identify chemical and intent
Use additional external cause code to identify place (Y92)

√7ᵗʰ **T26.50 Corrosion of unspecified eyelid and periocular area**

√7ᵗʰ **T26.51 Corrosion of right eyelid and periocular area**

√7ᵗʰ **T26.52 Corrosion of left eyelid and periocular area**

√5ᵗʰ **T26.6 Corrosion of cornea and conjunctival sac**

Code first (T51-T65) to identify chemical and intent
Use additional external cause code to identify place (Y92)

√7ᵗʰ **T26.60 Corrosion of cornea and conjunctival sac, unspecified eye**

√7ᵗʰ **T26.61 Corrosion of cornea and conjunctival sac, right eye**

√7ᵗʰ **T26.62 Corrosion of cornea and conjunctival sac, left eye**

√5ᵗʰ **T26.7 Corrosion with resulting rupture and destruction of eyeball**

Code first (T51-T65) to identify chemical and intent
Use additional external cause code to identify place (Y92)

√7ᵗʰ **T26.70 Corrosion with resulting rupture and destruction of unspecified eyeball** `CC` `H5`
CC Excl: No Excl

√7ᵗʰ **T26.71 Corrosion with resulting rupture and destruction of right eyeball** `CC` `H5`
CC Excl: No Excl

√7ᵗʰ **T26.72 Corrosion with resulting rupture and destruction of left eyeball** `CC` `H5`
CC Excl: No Excl

√5ᵗʰ **T26.8 Corrosions of other specified parts of eye and adnexa**

Code first (T51-T65) to identify chemical and intent
Use additional external cause code to identify place (Y92)

√7ᵗʰ **T26.80 Corrosions of other specified parts of unspecified eye and adnexa**

√7ᵗʰ **T26.81 Corrosions of other specified parts of right eye and adnexa**

√7ᵗʰ **T26.82 Corrosions of other specified parts of left eye and adnexa**

√5ᵗʰ **T26.9 Corrosion of eye and adnexa, part unspecified**

Code first (T51-T65) to identify chemical and intent
Use additional external cause code to identify place (Y92)

√7ᵗʰ **T26.90 Corrosion of unspecified eye and adnexa, part unspecified**

√7ᵗʰ **T26.91 Corrosion of right eye and adnexa, part unspecified**

√7ᵗʰ **T26.92 Corrosion of left eye and adnexa, part unspecified**

√4ᵗʰ **T27 Burn and corrosion of respiratory tract**

Use additional external cause code to identify the source and intent of the burn (X00-X19, X75-X77, X96-X98)
Use additional external cause code to identify place (Y92)

The appropriate 7th character is to be added to each code from category T27.
A initial encounter
D subsequent encounter
S sequela

CC Excl: For CC codes in category T27: PDX collection 1411

√7ᵗʰ **T27.0 Burn of larynx and trachea** `CC` `H5`

√7ᵗʰ **T27.1 Burn involving larynx and trachea with lung** `CC` `H5`

√7ᵗʰ **T27.2 Burn of other parts of respiratory tract** `CC` `H5`

Burn of thoracic cavity

√7ᵗʰ **T27.3 Burn of respiratory tract, part unspecified** `CC` `H5`

N Newborn: 0 | P Pediatric: 0-17 | M Maternity: 9-64 | A Adult: 15-124 | **MCC** Major Complication/Comorbidity | **CC** Complication/Comorbidity | **SW** Severe Wound Dx

1144 | ICD-10-CM 2020

✓x7ᵗʰ **T27.4** **Corrosion of larynx and trachea**   CC H5
     Code first (T51-T65) to identify chemical and intent

✓x7ᵗʰ **T27.5** **Corrosion involving larynx and trachea with lung**   CC H5
     ▶Code first (T51-T65) to identify chemical and intent◀

✓x7ᵗʰ **T27.6** **Corrosion of other parts of respiratory tract**   CC H5
     Code first (T51-T65) to identify chemical and intent

✓x7ᵗʰ **T27.7** **Corrosion of respiratory tract, part unspecified**   CC H5
     Code first (T51-T65) to identify chemical and intent

✓4ᵗʰ **T28** **Burn and corrosion of other internal organs**
     Use additional external cause code to identify the source and intent of the burn (X00-X19, X75-X77, X96-X98)
     Use additional external cause code to identify place (Y92)

> The appropriate 7th character is to be added to each code from category T28.
> A   initial encounter
> D   subsequent encounter
> S   sequela

✓x7ᵗʰ **T28.0** **Burn of mouth and pharynx**

✓x7ᵗʰ **T28.1** **Burn of esophagus**   CC H5
     CC Excl: PDX collection 1412

✓x7ᵗʰ **T28.2** **Burn of other parts of alimentary tract**   CC H5
     CC Excl: PDX collection 1413

✓x7ᵗʰ **T28.3** **Burn of internal genitourinary organs**

✓5ᵗʰ **T28.4** **Burns of other and unspecified internal organs**
     ~~Code first (T51-T65) to identify chemical and intent~~

     ✓x7ᵗʰ **T28.40** **Burn of unspecified internal organ**

     ✓6ᵗʰ **T28.41** **Burn of ear drum**

         ✓7ᵗʰ **T28.411** **Burn of right ear drum**

         ✓7ᵗʰ **T28.412** **Burn of left ear drum**

         ✓7ᵗʰ **T28.419** **Burn of unspecified ear drum**

     ✓x7ᵗʰ **T28.49** **Burn of other internal organ**

✓x7ᵗʰ **T28.5** **Corrosion of mouth and pharynx**
     Code first (T51-T65) to identify chemical and intent

✓x7ᵗʰ **T28.6** **Corrosion of esophagus**   CC H5
     Code first (T51-T65) to identify chemical and intent
     CC Excl: PDX collection 1412

✓x7ᵗʰ **T28.7** **Corrosion of other parts of alimentary tract**   CC H5
     Code first (T51-T65) to identify chemical and intent
     CC Excl: PDX collection 1413

✓x7ᵗʰ **T28.8** **Corrosion of internal genitourinary organs**
     Code first (T51-T65) to identify chemical and intent

✓5ᵗʰ **T28.9** **Corrosions of other and unspecified internal organs**
     Code first (T51-T65) to identify chemical and intent

     ✓x7ᵗʰ **T28.90** **Corrosions of unspecified internal organs**

     ✓6ᵗʰ **T28.91** **Corrosions of ear drum**

         ✓7ᵗʰ **T28.911** **Corrosions of right ear drum**

         ✓7ᵗʰ **T28.912** **Corrosions of left ear drum**

         ✓7ᵗʰ **T28.919** **Corrosions of unspecified ear drum**

     ✓x7ᵗʰ **T28.99** **Corrosions of other internal organs**

Burns and corrosions of multiple and unspecified body regions (T30-T32)

CC Excl: For CC/MCC codes in categories T30-T32: PDX collection 1414

✓4ᵗʰ **T30** **Burn and corrosion, body region unspecified**

     T30.0 **Burn of unspecified body region, unspecified degree**
         This code is not for inpatient use. Code to specified site and degree of burns
         Burn NOS
         Multiple burns NOS

     T30.4 **Corrosion of unspecified body region, unspecified degree**
         This code is not for inpatient use. Code to specified site and degree of corrosion
         Corrosion NOS
         Multiple corrosion NOS

✓4ᵗʰ **T31** **Burns classified according to extent of body surface involved**

     NOTE   This category is to be used as the primary code only when the site of the burn is unspecified. It should be used as a supplementary code with categories T20-T25 when the site is specified.

     T31.0 **Burns involving less than 10% of body surface**

✓5ᵗʰ **T31.1** **Burns involving 10-19% of body surface**

     T31.10 **Burns involving 10-19% of body surface with 0% to 9% third degree burns**   CC H5
         Burns involving 10-19% of body surface NOS

     T31.11 **Burns involving 10-19% of body surface with 10-19% third degree burns**   CC H5 HCC

✓5ᵗʰ **T31.2** **Burns involving 20-29% of body surface**

     T31.20 **Burns involving 20-29% of body surface with 0% to 9% third degree burns**   CC H5
         Burns involving 20-29% of body surface NOS

     T31.21 **Burns involving 20-29% of body surface with 10-19% third degree burns**   MCC H5 HCC

     T31.22 **Burns involving 20-29% of body surface with 20-29% third degree burns**   MCC H5 HCC

✓5ᵗʰ **T31.3** **Burns involving 30-39% of body surface**

     T31.30 **Burns involving 30-39% of body surface with 0% to 9% third degree burns**   CC H5
         Burns involving 30-39% of body surface NOS

     T31.31 **Burns involving 30-39% of body surface with 10-19% third degree burns**   MCC H5 HCC

     T31.32 **Burns involving 30-39% of body surface with 20-29% third degree burns**   MCC H5 HCC

     T31.33 **Burns involving 30-39% of body surface with 30-39% third degree burns**   MCC H5 HCC

✓5ᵗʰ **T31.4** **Burns involving 40-49% of body surface**

     T31.40 **Burns involving 40-49% of body surface with 0% to 9% third degree burns**   CC H5
         Burns involving 40-49% of body surface NOS

     T31.41 **Burns involving 40-49% of body surface with 10-19% third degree burns**   MCC H5 HCC

     T31.42 **Burns involving 40-49% of body surface with 20-29% third degree burns**   MCC H5 HCC

     T31.43 **Burns involving 40-49% of body surface with 30-39% third degree burns**   MCC H5 HCC

     T31.44 **Burns involving 40-49% of body surface with 40-49% third degree burns**   MCC H5 HCC

✓5ᵗʰ **T31.5** **Burns involving 50-59% of body surface**

     T31.50 **Burns involving 50-59% of body surface with 0% to 9% third degree burns**   CC H5
         Burns involving 50-59% of body surface NOS

     T31.51 **Burns involving 50-59% of body surface with 10-19% third degree burns**   MCC H5 HCC

     T31.52 **Burns involving 50-59% of body surface with 20-29% third degree burns**   MCC H5 HCC

     T31.53 **Burns involving 50-59% of body surface with 30-39% third degree burns**   MCC H5 HCC

     T31.54 **Burns involving 50-59% of body surface with 40-49% third degree burns**   MCC H5 HCC

     T31.55 **Burns involving 50-59% of body surface with 50-59% third degree burns**   MCC H5 HCC

✓5th **T31.6** **Burns involving** 60-69% **of body surface**

T31.60 **Burns involving 60-69% of body surface with 0% to 9% third degree burns** `CC` `H5`
Burns involving 60-69% of body surface NOS

T31.61 **Burns involving 60-69% of body surface with 10-19% third degree burns** `MCC` `H5` `HCC`

T31.62 **Burns involving 60-69% of body surface with 20-29% third degree burns** `MCC` `H5` `HCC`

T31.63 **Burns involving 60-69% of body surface with 30-39% third degree burns** `MCC` `H5` `HCC`

T31.64 **Burns involving 60-69% of body surface with 40-49% third degree burns** `MCC` `H5` `HCC`

T31.65 **Burns involving 60-69% of body surface with 50-59% third degree burns** `MCC` `H5` `HCC`

T31.66 **Burns involving 60-69% of body surface with 60-69% third degree burns** `MCC` `H5` `HCC`

✓5th **T31.7** **Burns involving** 70-79% **of body surface**

T31.70 **Burns involving 70-79% of body surface with 0% to 9% third degree burns** `CC` `H5`
Burns involving 70-79% of body surface NOS

T31.71 **Burns involving 70-79% of body surface with 10-19% third degree burns** `MCC` `H5` `HCC`

T31.72 **Burns involving 70-79% of body surface with 20-29% third degree burns** `MCC` `H5` `HCC`

T31.73 **Burns involving 70-79% of body surface with 30-39% third degree burns** `MCC` `H5` `HCC`

T31.74 **Burns involving 70-79% of body surface with 40-49% third degree burns** `MCC` `H5` `HCC`

T31.75 **Burns involving 70-79% of body surface with 50-59% third degree burns** `MCC` `H5` `HCC`

T31.76 **Burns involving 70-79% of body surface with 60-69% third degree burns** `MCC` `H5` `HCC`

T31.77 **Burns involving 70-79% of body surface with 70-79% third degree burns** `MCC` `H5` `HCC`

✓5th **T31.8** **Burns involving** 80-89% **of body surface**

T31.80 **Burns involving 80-89% of body surface with 0% to 9% third degree burns** `CC` `H5`
Burns involving 80-89% of body surface NOS

T31.81 **Burns involving 80-89% of body surface with 10-19% third degree burns** `MCC` `H5` `HCC`

T31.82 **Burns involving 80-89% of body surface with 20-29% third degree burns** `MCC` `H5` `HCC`

T31.83 **Burns involving 80-89% of body surface with 30-39% third degree burns** `MCC` `H5` `HCC`

T31.84 **Burns involving 80-89% of body surface with 40-49% third degree burns** `MCC` `H5` `HCC`

T31.85 **Burns involving 80-89% of body surface with 50-59% third degree burns** `MCC` `H5` `HCC`

T31.86 **Burns involving 80-89% of body surface with 60-69% third degree burns** `MCC` `H5` `HCC`

T31.87 **Burns involving 80-89% of body surface with 70-79% third degree burns** `MCC` `H5` `HCC`

T31.88 **Burns involving 80-89% of body surface with 80-89% third degree burns** `MCC` `H5` `HCC`

✓5th **T31.9** **Burns involving** 90% or more **of body surface**

T31.90 **Burns involving 90% or more of body surface with 0% to 9% third degree burns** `CC` `H5`
Burns involving 90% or more of body surface NOS

T31.91 **Burns involving 90% or more of body surface with 10-19% third degree burns** `MCC` `H5` `HCC`

T31.92 **Burns involving 90% or more of body surface with 20-29% third degree burns** `MCC` `H5` `HCC`

T31.93 **Burns involving 90% or more of body surface with 30-39% third degree burns** `MCC` `H5` `HCC`

T31.94 **Burns involving 90% or more of body surface with 40-49% third degree burns** `MCC` `H5` `HCC`

T31.95 **Burns involving 90% or more of body surface with 50-59% third degree burns** `MCC` `H5` `HCC`

T31.96 **Burns involving 90% or more of body surface with 60-69% third degree burns** `MCC` `H5` `HCC`

T31.97 **Burns involving 90% or more of body surface with 70-79% third degree burns** `MCC` `H5` `HCC`

T31.98 **Burns involving 90% or more of body surface with 80-89% third degree burns** `MCC` `H5` `HCC`

T31.99 **Burns involving 90% or more of body surface with 90% or more third degree burns** `MCC` `H5` `HCC`

Rule of Nines Estimation of Total Body Surface Burned

Head and neck 9%
Each arm 9%
Anterior trunk 18%
Genitalia 1%
Anterior leg 9%
Posterior trunk 18%
Posterior leg 9%

✓4th **T32** **Corrosions classified according to extent of body surface involved**

`NOTE` This category is to be used as the primary code only when the site of the corrosion is unspecified. It may be used as a supplementary code with categories T20-T25 when the site is specified.

T32.0 **Corrosions involving** less than 10% **of body surface**

✓5th **T32.1** **Corrosions involving** 10-19% **of body surface**

T32.10 **Corrosions involving 10-19% of body surface with 0% to 9% third degree corrosion** `CC` `H5`
Corrosions involving 10-19% of body surface NOS

T32.11 **Corrosions involving 10-19% of body surface with 10-19% third degree corrosion** `CC` `H5` `HCC`

✓5th **T32.2** **Corrosions involving** 20-29% **of body surface**

T32.20 **Corrosions involving 20-29% of body surface with 0% to 9% third degree corrosion** `CC` `H5`

T32.21 **Corrosions involving 20-29% of body surface with 10-19% third degree corrosion** `MCC` `H5` `HCC`

T32.22 **Corrosions involving 20-29% of body surface with 20-29% third degree corrosion** `MCC` `H5` `HCC`

`N` Newborn: 0   `P` Pediatric: 0-17   `M` Maternity: 9-64   `A` Adult: 15-124   `MCC` Major Complication/Comorbidity   `CC` Complication/Comorbidity   `SW` Severe Wound Dx

1146   ICD-10-CM 2020

✓5ᵗʰ **T32.3** **Corrosions involving 30-39% of body surface**

T32.30 Corrosions involving 30-39% of body surface with 0% to 9% third degree corrosion   `CC` `H5`

T32.31 Corrosions involving 30-39% of body surface with 10-19% third degree corrosion   `MCC` `H5` `HCC`

T32.32 Corrosions involving 30-39% of body surface with 20-29% third degree corrosion   `MCC` `H5` `HCC`

T32.33 Corrosions involving 30-39% of body surface with 30-39% third degree corrosion   `MCC` `H5` `HCC`

✓5ᵗʰ **T32.4** **Corrosions involving 40-49% of body surface**

T32.40 Corrosions involving 40-49% of body surface with 0% to 9% third degree corrosion   `CC` `H5`

T32.41 Corrosions involving 40-49% of body surface with 10-19% third degree corrosion   `MCC` `H5` `HCC`

T32.42 Corrosions involving 40-49% of body surface with 20-29% third degree corrosion   `MCC` `H5` `HCC`

T32.43 Corrosions involving 40-49% of body surface with 30-39% third degree corrosion   `MCC` `H5` `HCC`

T32.44 Corrosions involving 40-49% of body surface with 40-49% third degree corrosion   `MCC` `H5` `HCC`

✓5ᵗʰ **T32.5** **Corrosions involving 50-59% of body surface**

T32.50 Corrosions involving 50-59% of body surface with 0% to 9% third degree corrosion   `CC` `H5`

T32.51 Corrosions involving 50-59% of body surface with 10-19% third degree corrosion   `MCC` `H5` `HCC`

T32.52 Corrosions involving 50-59% of body surface with 20-29% third degree corrosion   `MCC` `H5` `HCC`

T32.53 Corrosions involving 50-59% of body surface with 30-39% third degree corrosion   `MCC` `H5` `HCC`

T32.54 Corrosions involving 50-59% of body surface with 40-49% third degree corrosion   `MCC` `H5` `HCC`

T32.55 Corrosions involving 50-59% of body surface with 50-59% third degree corrosion   `MCC` `H5` `HCC`

✓5ᵗʰ **T32.6** **Corrosions involving 60-69% of body surface**

T32.60 Corrosions involving 60-69% of body surface with 0% to 9% third degree corrosion   `CC` `H5`

T32.61 Corrosions involving 60-69% of body surface with 10-19% third degree corrosion   `MCC` `H5` `HCC`

T32.62 Corrosions involving 60-69% of body surface with 20-29% third degree corrosion   `MCC` `H5` `HCC`

T32.63 Corrosions involving 60-69% of body surface with 30-39% third degree corrosion   `MCC` `H5` `HCC`

T32.64 Corrosions involving 60-69% of body surface with 40-49% third degree corrosion   `MCC` `H5` `HCC`

T32.65 Corrosions involving 60-69% of body surface with 50-59% third degree corrosion   `MCC` `H5` `HCC`

T32.66 Corrosions involving 60-69% of body surface with 60-69% third degree corrosion   `MCC` `H5` `HCC`

✓5ᵗʰ **T32.7** **Corrosions involving 70-79% of body surface**

T32.70 Corrosions involving 70-79% of body surface with 0% to 9% third degree corrosion   `CC` `H5`

T32.71 Corrosions involving 70-79% of body surface with 10-19% third degree corrosion   `MCC` `H5` `HCC`

T32.72 Corrosions involving 70-79% of body surface with 20-29% third degree corrosion   `MCC` `H5` `HCC`

T32.73 Corrosions involving 70-79% of body surface with 30-39% third degree corrosion   `MCC` `H5` `HCC`

T32.74 Corrosions involving 70-79% of body surface with 40-49% third degree corrosion   `MCC` `H5` `HCC`

T32.75 Corrosions involving 70-79% of body surface with 50-59% third degree corrosion   `MCC` `H5` `HCC`

T32.76 Corrosions involving 70-79% of body surface with 60-69% third degree corrosion   `MCC` `H5` `HCC`

T32.77 Corrosions involving 70-79% of body surface with 70-79% third degree corrosion   `MCC` `H5` `HCC`

✓5ᵗʰ **T32.8** **Corrosions involving 80-89% of body surface**

T32.80 Corrosions involving 80-89% of body surface with 0% to 9% third degree corrosion   `CC` `H5`

T32.81 Corrosions involving 80-89% of body surface with 10-19% third degree corrosion   `MCC` `H5` `HCC`

T32.82 Corrosions involving 80-89% of body surface with 20-29% third degree corrosion   `MCC` `H5` `HCC`

T32.83 Corrosions involving 80-89% of body surface with 30-39% third degree corrosion   `MCC` `H5` `HCC`

T32.84 Corrosions involving 80-89% of body surface with 40-49% third degree corrosion   `MCC` `H5` `HCC`

T32.85 Corrosions involving 80-89% of body surface with 50-59% third degree corrosion   `MCC` `H5` `HCC`

T32.86 Corrosions involving 80-89% of body surface with 60-69% third degree corrosion   `MCC` `H5` `HCC`

T32.87 Corrosions involving 80-89% of body surface with 70-79% third degree corrosion   `MCC` `H5` `HCC`

T32.88 Corrosions involving 80-89% of body surface with 80-89% third degree corrosion   `MCC` `H5` `HCC`

✓5ᵗʰ **T32.9** **Corrosions involving 90% or more of body surface**

T32.90 Corrosions involving 90% or more of body surface with 0% to 9% third degree corrosion   `CC` `H5`

T32.91 Corrosions involving 90% or more of body surface with 10-19% third degree corrosion   `MCC` `H5` `HCC`

T32.92 Corrosions involving 90% or more of body surface with 20-29% third degree corrosion   `MCC` `H5` `HCC`

T32.93 Corrosions involving 90% or more of body surface with 30-39% third degree corrosion   `MCC` `H5` `HCC`

T32.94 Corrosions involving 90% or more of body surface with 40-49% third degree corrosion   `MCC` `H5` `HCC`

T32.95 Corrosions involving 90% or more of body surface with 50-59% third degree corrosion   `MCC` `H5` `HCC`

T32.96 Corrosions involving 90% or more of body surface with 60-69% third degree corrosion   `MCC` `H5` `HCC`

T32.97 Corrosions involving 90% or more of body surface with 70-79% third degree corrosion   `MCC` `H5` `HCC`

T32.98 Corrosions involving 90% or more of body surface with 80-89% third degree corrosion   `MCC` `H5` `HCC`

T32.99 Corrosions involving 90% or more of body surface with 90% or more third degree corrosion   `MCC` `H5` `HCC`

Frostbite (T33-T34)

EXCLUDES 2 *hypothermia and other effects of reduced temperature (T68, T69.-)*

√4ᵗʰ **T33 Superficial frostbite**

> **INCLUDES** frostbite with partial thickness skin loss

> The appropriate 7th character is to be added to each code from category T33.
> A   initial encounter
> D   subsequent encounter
> S   sequela

> **CC Excl:** For CC codes in category T33, unless otherwise noted: PDX collection 1416

√5ᵗʰ **T33.0 Superficial frostbite of head**

> **CC Excl:** For CC codes in subcategory T33.0: PDX collection 1415

√6ᵗʰ **T33.01 Superficial frostbite of ear**

√7ᵗʰ **T33.011 Superficial frostbite of right ear** CC H5

√7ᵗʰ **T33.012 Superficial frostbite of left ear** CC H5

√7ᵗʰ **T33.019 Superficial frostbite of unspecified ear** CC H5

√x7ᵗʰ **T33.02 Superficial frostbite of nose** CC H5

√x7ᵗʰ **T33.09 Superficial frostbite of other part of head** CC H5

√x7ᵗʰ **T33.1 Superficial frostbite of neck** CC H5

> **CC Excl:** PDX collection 1415

√x7ᵗʰ **T33.2 Superficial frostbite of thorax** CC H5

√x7ᵗʰ **T33.3 Superficial frostbite of abdominal wall, lower back and pelvis** CC H5

√5ᵗʰ **T33.4 Superficial frostbite of arm**

> **EXCLUDES 2** *superficial frostbite of wrist and hand (T33.5-)*

√x7ᵗʰ **T33.40 Superficial frostbite of unspecified arm** CC H5

√x7ᵗʰ **T33.41 Superficial frostbite of right arm** CC H5

√x7ᵗʰ **T33.42 Superficial frostbite of left arm** CC H5

√5ᵗʰ **T33.5 Superficial frostbite of wrist, hand, and fingers**

> **CC Excl:** For CC codes in subcategory T33.5: PDX collection 1417

√6ᵗʰ **T33.51 Superficial frostbite of wrist**

√7ᵗʰ **T33.511 Superficial frostbite of right wrist** CC H5

√7ᵗʰ **T33.512 Superficial frostbite of left wrist** CC H5

√7ᵗʰ **T33.519 Superficial frostbite of unspecified wrist** CC H5

√6ᵗʰ **T33.52 Superficial frostbite of hand**

> **EXCLUDES 2** *superficial frostbite of fingers (T33.53-)*

√7ᵗʰ **T33.521 Superficial frostbite of right hand** CC H5

√7ᵗʰ **T33.522 Superficial frostbite of left hand** CC H5

√7ᵗʰ **T33.529 Superficial frostbite of unspecified hand** CC H5

√6ᵗʰ **T33.53 Superficial frostbite of finger(s)**

√7ᵗʰ **T33.531 Superficial frostbite of right finger(s)** CC H5

√7ᵗʰ **T33.532 Superficial frostbite of left finger(s)** CC H5

√7ᵗʰ **T33.539 Superficial frostbite of unspecified finger(s)** CC H5

√5ᵗʰ **T33.6 Superficial frostbite of hip and thigh**

√x7ᵗʰ **T33.60 Superficial frostbite of unspecified hip and thigh** CC H5

√x7ᵗʰ **T33.61 Superficial frostbite of right hip and thigh** CC H5

√x7ᵗʰ **T33.62 Superficial frostbite of left hip and thigh** CC H5

√5ᵗʰ **T33.7 Superficial frostbite of knee and lower leg**

> **EXCLUDES 2** *superficial frostbite of ankle and foot (T33.8-)*

√x7ᵗʰ **T33.70 Superficial frostbite of unspecified knee and lower leg** CC H5

√x7ᵗʰ **T33.71 Superficial frostbite of right knee and lower leg** CC H5

√x7ᵗʰ **T33.72 Superficial frostbite of left knee and lower leg** CC H5

√5ᵗʰ **T33.8 Superficial frostbite of ankle, foot, and toe(s)**

> **CC Excl:** For CC codes in subcategory T33.8: PDX collection 1418

√6ᵗʰ **T33.81 Superficial frostbite of ankle**

√7ᵗʰ **T33.811 Superficial frostbite of right ankle** CC H5

√7ᵗʰ **T33.812 Superficial frostbite of left ankle** CC H5

√7ᵗʰ **T33.819 Superficial frostbite of unspecified ankle** CC H5

√6ᵗʰ **T33.82 Superficial frostbite of foot**

√7ᵗʰ **T33.821 Superficial frostbite of right foot** CC H5

√7ᵗʰ **T33.822 Superficial frostbite of left foot** CC H5

√7ᵗʰ **T33.829 Superficial frostbite of unspecified foot** CC H5

√6ᵗʰ **T33.83 Superficial frostbite of toe(s)**

√7ᵗʰ **T33.831 Superficial frostbite of right toe(s)** CC H5

√7ᵗʰ **T33.832 Superficial frostbite of left toe(s)** CC H5

√7ᵗʰ **T33.839 Superficial frostbite of unspecified toe(s)** CC H5

√5ᵗʰ **T33.9 Superficial frostbite of other and unspecified sites**

√x7ᵗʰ **T33.90 Superficial frostbite of unspecified sites** CC H5

> Superficial frostbite NOS

√x7ᵗʰ **T33.99 Superficial frostbite of other sites** CC H5

> Superficial frostbite of leg NOS
> Superficial frostbite of trunk NOS

√4ᵗʰ **T34 Frostbite with tissue necrosis**

> The appropriate 7th character is to be added to each code from category T34.
> A   initial encounter
> D   subsequent encounter
> S   sequela

> **CC Excl:** For CC codes in category T34, unless otherwise noted: PDX collection 1416

√5ᵗʰ **T34.0 Frostbite with tissue necrosis of head**

> **CC Excl:** For CC codes in subcategory T34.0: PDX collection 1415

√6ᵗʰ **T34.01 Frostbite with tissue necrosis of ear**

√7ᵗʰ **T34.011 Frostbite with tissue necrosis of right ear** CC H5

√7ᵗʰ **T34.012 Frostbite with tissue necrosis of left ear** CC H5

√7ᵗʰ **T34.019 Frostbite with tissue necrosis of unspecified ear** CC H5

√x7ᵗʰ **T34.02 Frostbite with tissue necrosis of nose** CC H5

√x7ᵗʰ **T34.09 Frostbite with tissue necrosis of other part of head** CC H5

√x7ᵗʰ **T34.1 Frostbite with tissue necrosis of neck** CC H5

> **CC Excl:** PDX collection 1415

√x7ᵗʰ **T34.2 Frostbite with tissue necrosis of thorax** CC H5

√x7ᵗʰ **T34.3 Frostbite with tissue necrosis of abdominal wall, lower back and pelvis** CC H5

√5ᵗʰ **T34.4 Frostbite with tissue necrosis of arm**

> **EXCLUDES 2** *frostbite with tissue necrosis of wrist and hand (T34.5-)*

√x7ᵗʰ **T34.40 Frostbite with tissue necrosis of unspecified arm** CC H5

√x7ᵗʰ **T34.41 Frostbite with tissue necrosis of right arm** CC H5

√x7ᵗʰ **T34.42 Frostbite with tissue necrosis of left arm** CC H5

√5ᵗʰ **T34.5 Frostbite with tissue necrosis of wrist, hand, and finger(s)**

> **CC Excl:** For CC codes in subcategory T34.5: PDX collection 1417

√6ᵗʰ **T34.51 Frostbite with tissue necrosis of wrist**

√7ᵗʰ **T34.511 Frostbite with tissue necrosis of right wrist** CC H5

√7ᵗʰ **T34.512 Frostbite with tissue necrosis of left wrist** CC H5

√7ᵗʰ **T34.519 Frostbite with tissue necrosis of unspecified wrist** CC H5

N Newborn: 0   P Pediatric: 0-17   M Maternity: 9-64   A Adult: 15-124   MCC Major Complication/Comorbidity   CC Complication/Comorbidity   SW Severe Wound Dx

1148   ICD-10-CM 2020

√6ᵗʰ **T34.52 Frostbite with tissue necrosis of hand**

     EXCLUDES 2   *frostbite with tissue necrosis of finger(s)*
             (T34.53-)

     √7ᵗʰ **T34.521 Frostbite with tissue**   CC H5
                 necrosis of right hand

     √7ᵗʰ **T34.522 Frostbite with tissue**   CC H5
                 necrosis of left hand

     √7ᵗʰ **T34.529 Frostbite with tissue**   CC H5
                 necrosis of unspecified
                 hand

√6ᵗʰ **T34.53 Frostbite with tissue necrosis of finger(s)**

     √7ᵗʰ **T34.531 Frostbite with tissue**   CC H5
                 necrosis of right finger(s)

     √7ᵗʰ **T34.532 Frostbite with tissue**   CC H5
                 necrosis of left finger(s)

     √7ᵗʰ **T34.539 Frostbite with tissue**   CC H5
                 necrosis of unspecified
                 finger(s)

√5ᵗʰ **T34.6 Frostbite with tissue necrosis of hip and thigh**

     √x7ᵗʰ **T34.60 Frostbite with tissue necrosis of**   CC H5
              unspecified hip and thigh

     √7ᵗʰ **T34.61 Frostbite with tissue necrosis of**   CC H5
              right hip and thigh

     √x7ᵗʰ **T34.62 Frostbite with tissue necrosis of left**   CC H5
              hip and thigh

√5ᵗʰ **T34.7 Frostbite with tissue necrosis of knee and lower leg**

     EXCLUDES 2   *frostbite with tissue necrosis of ankle and foot*
             (T34.8-)

     √x7ᵗʰ **T34.70 Frostbite with tissue necrosis of**   CC H5
              unspecified knee and lower leg

     √x7ᵗʰ **T34.71 Frostbite with tissue necrosis of**   CC H5
              right knee and lower leg

     √x7ᵗʰ **T34.72 Frostbite with tissue necrosis of left**   CC H5
              knee and lower leg

√5ᵗʰ **T34.8 Frostbite with tissue necrosis of ankle, foot, and toe(s)**

     **CC Excl: For CC codes in subcategory T34.8: PDX collection
1418**

     √6ᵗʰ **T34.81 Frostbite with tissue necrosis of ankle**

         √7ᵗʰ **T34.811 Frostbite with tissue**   CC H5
                 necrosis of right ankle

         √7ᵗʰ **T34.812 Frostbite with tissue**   CC H5
                 necrosis of left ankle

         √7ᵗʰ **T34.819 Frostbite with tissue**   CC H5
                 necrosis of unspecified
                 ankle

     √6ᵗʰ **T34.82 Frostbite with tissue necrosis of foot**

         √7ᵗʰ **T34.821 Frostbite with tissue**   CC H5
                 necrosis of right foot

         √7ᵗʰ **T34.822 Frostbite with tissue**   CC H5
                 necrosis of left foot

         √7ᵗʰ **T34.829 Frostbite with tissue**   CC H5
                 necrosis of unspecified
                 foot

     √6ᵗʰ **T34.83 Frostbite with tissue necrosis of toe(s)**

         √7ᵗʰ **T34.831 Frostbite with tissue**   CC H5
                 necrosis of right toe(s)

         √7ᵗʰ **T34.832 Frostbite with tissue**   CC H5
                 necrosis of left toe(s)

         √7ᵗʰ **T34.839 Frostbite with tissue**   CC H5
                 necrosis of unspecified
                 toe(s)

√5ᵗʰ **T34.9 Frostbite with tissue necrosis of other and unspecified sites**

     √x7ᵗʰ **T34.90 Frostbite with tissue necrosis of**   CC H5
              unspecified sites

              Frostbite with tissue necrosis NOS

     √x7ᵗʰ **T34.99 Frostbite with tissue necrosis of**   CC H5
              other sites

              Frostbite with tissue necrosis of leg NOS
              Frostbite with tissue necrosis of trunk NOS

Poisoning by, adverse effects of and underdosing of drugs, medicaments and biological substances (T36-T50)

INCLUDES   adverse effect of correct substance properly administered
           poisoning by overdose of substance
           poisoning by wrong substance given or taken in error
           underdosing by (inadvertently) (deliberately) taking less substance
             than prescribed or instructed

Code first, for adverse effects, the nature of the adverse effect, such as:
   adverse effect NOS (T88.7)
   aspirin gastritis (K29.-)
   blood disorders (D56-D76)
   contact dermatitis (L23-L25)
   dermatitis due to substances taken internally (L27.-)
   nephropathy (N14.0-N14.2)

NOTE   The drug giving rise to the adverse effect should be identified by
           use of codes from categories T36-T50 with fifth or sixth character 5.

Use additional code(s) to specify:
   manifestations of poisoning
   underdosing or failure in dosage during medical and surgical care (Y63.6,
     Y63.8-Y63.9)
   underdosing of medication regimen (Z91.12-, Z91.13-)

EXCLUDES 1   *toxic reaction to local anesthesia in pregnancy (O29.3-)*
EXCLUDES 2   *abuse and dependence of psychoactive substances (F10-F19)*
             abuse of non-dependence-producing substances (F55.-)
             drug reaction and poisoning affecting newborn (P00-P96)
             pathological drug intoxication (inebriation) (F10-F19)

AHA: 2018,4Q,71; 2016,2Q,8; 2015,3Q,22

√4ᵗʰ **T36 Poisoning by, adverse effect of and underdosing of systemic antibiotics**

     EXCLUDES 1   *antineoplastic antibiotics (T45.1-)*
                 locally applied antibiotic NEC (T49.0)
                 topically used antibiotic for ear, nose and throat (T49.6)
                 topically used antibiotic for eye (T49.5)

     The appropriate 7th character is to be added to each code from
     category T36.
     A   initial encounter
     D   subsequent encounter
     S   sequela

√5ᵗʰ **T36.0 Poisoning by, adverse effect of and underdosing of penicillins**

     √6ᵗʰ **T36.0X Poisoning by, adverse effect of and underdosing
of penicillins**

         √7ᵗʰ **T36.0X1 Poisoning by penicillins, accidental
(unintentional)**

                 Poisoning by penicillins NOS

       7   √7ᵗʰ **T36.0X2 Poisoning by penicillins,**   HCC
                 intentional self-harm

         √7ᵗʰ **T36.0X3 Poisoning by penicillins, assault**

         √7ᵗʰ **T36.0X4 Poisoning by penicillins, undetermined**

         √7ᵗʰ **T36.0X5 Adverse effect of penicillins**

         √7ᵗʰ **T36.0X6 Underdosing of penicillins**

√5ᵗʰ **T36.1 Poisoning by, adverse effect of and underdosing of
cephalosporins and other beta-lactam antibiotics**

     √6ᵗʰ **T36.1X Poisoning by, adverse effect of and underdosing
of cephalosporins and other beta-lactam antibiotics**

         √7ᵗʰ **T36.1X1 Poisoning by cephalosporins and other
beta-lactam antibiotics, accidental
(unintentional)**

                 Poisoning by cephalosporins and other
                     beta-lactam antibiotics NOS

       7   √7ᵗʰ **T36.1X2 Poisoning by**   HCC
                 cephalosporins and other
                 beta-lactam antibiotics,
                 intentional self-harm

         √7ᵗʰ **T36.1X3 Poisoning by cephalosporins and other
beta-lactam antibiotics, assault**

         √7ᵗʰ **T36.1X4 Poisoning by cephalosporins and other
beta-lactam antibiotics, undetermined**

         √7ᵗʰ **T36.1X5 Adverse effect of cephalosporins and
other beta-lactam antibiotics**

         √7ᵗʰ **T36.1X6 Underdosing of cephalosporins and other
beta-lactam antibiotics**

√5ᵗʰ **T36.2 Poisoning by, adverse effect of and underdosing of
chloramphenicol group**

     √6ᵗʰ **T36.2X Poisoning by, adverse effect of and underdosing
of chloramphenicol group**

         √7ᵗʰ **T36.2X1 Poisoning by chloramphenicol group,
accidental (unintentional)**

                 Poisoning by chloramphenicol group NOS

☑ Additional Character Required   √x7ᵗʰ Placeholder   Unacceptable PDx   Questionable PDx   Manifestation   Unspecified Dx   H1 - H14 HAC   HCC CMS-HCC Dx   HIV HIV Dx

ICD-10-CM 2020

1149

7 √7ᵗʰ **T36.2X2 Poisoning by** HCC
chloramphenicol group,
intentional self-harm

√7ᵗʰ **T36.2X3 Poisoning by chloramphenicol group,**
assault

√7ᵗʰ **T36.2X4 Poisoning by chloramphenicol group,**
undetermined

√7ᵗʰ **T36.2X5 Adverse effect of chloramphenicol group**

√7ᵗʰ **T36.2X6 Underdosing of chloramphenicol group**

√5ᵗʰ **T36.3 Poisoning by, adverse effect of and underdosing of**
macrolides

√6ᵗʰ **T36.3X Poisoning by, adverse effect of and underdosing**
of macrolides

√7ᵗʰ **T36.3X1 Poisoning by macrolides, accidental**
(unintentional)
Poisoning by macrolides NOS

7 √7ᵗʰ **T36.3X2 Poisoning by macrolides,** HCC
intentional self-harm

√7ᵗʰ **T36.3X3 Poisoning by macrolides, assault**

√7ᵗʰ **T36.3X4 Poisoning by macrolides, undetermined**

√7ᵗʰ **T36.3X5 Adverse effect of macrolides**

√7ᵗʰ **T36.3X6 Underdosing of macrolides**

√5ᵗʰ **T36.4 Poisoning by, adverse effect of and underdosing of**
tetracyclines

√6ᵗʰ **T36.4X Poisoning by, adverse effect of and underdosing**
of tetracyclines

√7ᵗʰ **T36.4X1 Poisoning by tetracyclines, accidental**
(unintentional)
Poisoning by tetracyclines NOS

7 √7ᵗʰ **T36.4X2 Poisoning by** HCC
tetracyclines, intentional
self-harm

√7ᵗʰ **T36.4X3 Poisoning by tetracyclines, assault**

√7ᵗʰ **T36.4X4 Poisoning by tetracyclines, undetermined**

√7ᵗʰ **T36.4X5 Adverse effect of tetracyclines**

√7ᵗʰ **T36.4X6 Underdosing of tetracyclines**

√5ᵗʰ **T36.5 Poisoning by, adverse effect of and underdosing of**
aminoglycosides
Poisoning by, adverse effect of and underdosing of streptomycin

√6ᵗʰ **T36.5X Poisoning by, adverse effect of and underdosing**
of aminoglycosides

√7ᵗʰ **T36.5X1 Poisoning by aminoglycosides, accidental**
(unintentional)
Poisoning by aminoglycosides NOS

7 √7ᵗʰ **T36.5X2 Poisoning by** HCC
aminoglycosides,
intentional self-harm

√7ᵗʰ **T36.5X3 Poisoning by aminoglycosides, assault**

√7ᵗʰ **T36.5X4 Poisoning by aminoglycosides,**
undetermined

√7ᵗʰ **T36.5X5 Adverse effect of aminoglycosides**

√7ᵗʰ **T36.5X6 Underdosing of aminoglycosides**

√5ᵗʰ **T36.6 Poisoning by, adverse effect of and underdosing of**
rifampicins

√6ᵗʰ **T36.6X Poisoning by, adverse effect of and underdosing**
of rifampicins

√7ᵗʰ **T36.6X1 Poisoning by rifampicins, accidental**
(unintentional)
Poisoning by rifampicins NOS

7 √7ᵗʰ **T36.6X2 Poisoning by rifampicins,** HCC
intentional self-harm

√7ᵗʰ **T36.6X3 Poisoning by rifampicins, assault**

√7ᵗʰ **T36.6X4 Poisoning by rifampicins, undetermined**

√7ᵗʰ **T36.6X5 Adverse effect of rifampicins**

√7ᵗʰ **T36.6X6 Underdosing of rifampicins**

√5ᵗʰ **T36.7 Poisoning by, adverse effect of and underdosing of**
antifungal antibiotics, systemically used

√6ᵗʰ **T36.7X Poisoning by, adverse effect of and underdosing**
of antifungal antibiotics, systemically used

√7ᵗʰ **T36.7X1 Poisoning by antifungal antibiotics,**
systemically used, accidental
(unintentional)
Poisoning by antifungal antibiotics,
systemically used NOS

7 √7ᵗʰ **T36.7X2 Poisoning by antifungal** HCC
antibiotics, systemically
used, intentional
self-harm

√7ᵗʰ **T36.7X3 Poisoning by antifungal antibiotics,**
systemically used, assault

√7ᵗʰ **T36.7X4 Poisoning by antifungal antibiotics,**
systemically used, undetermined

√7ᵗʰ **T36.7X5 Adverse effect of antifungal antibiotics,**
systemically used

√7ᵗʰ **T36.7X6 Underdosing of antifungal antibiotics,**
systemically used

√5ᵗʰ **T36.8 Poisoning by, adverse effect of and underdosing of other**
systemic antibiotics

√6ᵗʰ **T36.8X Poisoning by, adverse effect of and underdosing**
of other systemic antibiotics
AHA: 2017,1Q,39

√7ᵗʰ **T36.8X1 Poisoning by other systemic antibiotics,**
accidental (unintentional)
Poisoning by other systemic antibiotics
NOS

7 √7ᵗʰ **T36.8X2 Poisoning by other** HCC
systemic antibiotics,
intentional self-harm

√7ᵗʰ **T36.8X3 Poisoning by other systemic antibiotics,**
assault

√7ᵗʰ **T36.8X4 Poisoning by other systemic antibiotics,**
undetermined

√7ᵗʰ **T36.8X5 Adverse effect of other systemic**
antibiotics

√7ᵗʰ **T36.8X6 Underdosing of other systemic antibiotics**

√5ᵗʰ **T36.9 Poisoning by, adverse effect of and underdosing of**
unspecified systemic antibiotic

√x7ᵗʰ **T36.91 Poisoning by unspecified systemic antibiotic,**
accidental (unintentional)
Poisoning by systemic antibiotic NOS

7 √x7ᵗʰ **T36.92 Poisoning by unspecified systemic** HCC
antibiotic, intentional self-harm

√x7ᵗʰ **T36.93 Poisoning by unspecified systemic antibiotic,**
assault

√x7ᵗʰ **T36.94 Poisoning by unspecified systemic antibiotic,**
undetermined

√x7ᵗʰ **T36.95 Adverse effect of unspecified systemic antibiotic**

√x7ᵗʰ **T36.96 Underdosing of unspecified systemic antibiotic**

√4ᵗʰ **T37 Poisoning by, adverse effect of and underdosing of other systemic**
anti-infectives and antiparasitics
EXCLUDES 1 anti-infectives topically used for ear, nose and throat (T49.6-)
anti-infectives topically used for eye (T49.5-)
locally applied anti-infectives NEC (T49.0-)

The appropriate 7th character is to be added to each code from
category T37.
A initial encounter
D subsequent encounter
S sequela

√5ᵗʰ **T37.0 Poisoning by, adverse effect of and underdosing of**
sulfonamides

√6ᵗʰ **T37.0X Poisoning by, adverse effect of and underdosing**
of sulfonamides

√7ᵗʰ **T37.0X1 Poisoning by sulfonamides, accidental**
(unintentional)
Poisoning by sulfonamides NOS

7 √7ᵗʰ **T37.0X2 Poisoning by** HCC
sulfonamides, intentional
self-harm

√7ᵗʰ **T37.0X3 Poisoning by sulfonamides, assault**

√7ᵗʰ **T37.0X4 Poisoning by sulfonamides,**
undetermined

√7ᵗʰ **T37.0X5 Adverse effect of sulfonamides**

√7ᵗʰ **T37.0X6 Underdosing of sulfonamides**

√5ᵗʰ **T37.1 Poisoning by, adverse effect of and underdosing of**
antimycobacterial drugs
EXCLUDES 1 rifampicins (T36.6-)
streptomycin (T36.5-)

√6ᵗʰ **T37.1X Poisoning by, adverse effect of and underdosing**
of antimycobacterial drugs

√7ᵗʰ **T37.1X1 Poisoning by antimycobacterial drugs,**
accidental (unintentional)
Poisoning by antimycobacterial drugs NOS

7 √7ᵗʰ **T37.1X2 Poisoning by** HCC
antimycobacterial drugs,
intentional self-harm

√7ᵗʰ **T37.1X3 Poisoning by antimycobacterial drugs,**
assault

✓7th **T37.1X4 Poisoning by antimycobacterial drugs, undetermined**

✓7th **T37.1X5** Adverse effect **of antimycobacterial drugs**

✓7th **T37.1X6** Underdosing **of antimycobacterial drugs**

✓5th **T37.2 Poisoning by, adverse effect of and underdosing of antimalarials and drugs acting on other blood protozoa**
> EXCLUDES 1   *hydroxyquinoline derivatives (T37.8-)*

  ✓6th **T37.2X Poisoning by, adverse effect of and underdosing of antimalarials and drugs acting on other blood protozoa**

    ✓7th **T37.2X1 Poisoning by antimalarials and drugs acting on other blood protozoa, accidental (unintentional)**
> Poisoning by antimalarials and drugs acting on other blood protozoa NOS

    7 ✓7th **T37.2X2 Poisoning by antimalarials and drugs acting on other blood protozoa, intentional self-harm** HCC

    ✓7th **T37.2X3 Poisoning by antimalarials and drugs acting on other blood protozoa, assault**

    ✓7th **T37.2X4 Poisoning by antimalarials and drugs acting on other blood protozoa, undetermined**

    ✓7th **T37.2X5** Adverse effect **of antimalarials and drugs acting on other blood protozoa**

    ✓7th **T37.2X6** Underdosing **of antimalarials and drugs acting on other blood protozoa**

✓5th **T37.3 Poisoning by, adverse effect of and underdosing of other antiprotozoal drugs**

  ✓6th **T37.3X Poisoning by, adverse effect of and underdosing of other antiprotozoal drugs**

    ✓7th **T37.3X1 Poisoning by other antiprotozoal drugs, accidental (unintentional)**
> Poisoning by other antiprotozoal drugs NOS

    7 ✓7th **T37.3X2 Poisoning by other antiprotozoal drugs, intentional self-harm** HCC

    ✓7th **T37.3X3 Poisoning by other antiprotozoal drugs, assault**

    ✓7th **T37.3X4 Poisoning by other antiprotozoal drugs, undetermined**

    ✓7th **T37.3X5** Adverse effect **of other antiprotozoal drugs**

    ✓7th **T37.3X6** Underdosing **of other antiprotozoal drugs**

✓5th **T37.4 Poisoning by, adverse effect of and underdosing of anthelminthics**

  ✓6th **T37.4X Poisoning by, adverse effect of and underdosing of anthelminthics**

    ✓7th **T37.4X1 Poisoning by anthelminthics, accidental (unintentional)**
> Poisoning by anthelminthics NOS

    7 ✓7th **T37.4X2 Poisoning by anthelminthics, intentional self-harm** HCC

    ✓7th **T37.4X3 Poisoning by anthelminthics, assault**

    ✓7th **T37.4X4 Poisoning by anthelminthics, undetermined**

    ✓7th **T37.4X5** Adverse effect **of anthelminthics**

    ✓7th **T37.4X6** Underdosing **of anthelminthics**

✓5th **T37.5 Poisoning by, adverse effect of and underdosing of antiviral drugs**
> EXCLUDES 1   *amantadine (T42.8-)*
> *cytarabine (T45.1-)*

  ✓6th **T37.5X Poisoning by, adverse effect of and underdosing of antiviral drugs**

    ✓7th **T37.5X1 Poisoning by antiviral drugs, accidental (unintentional)**
> Poisoning by antiviral drugs NOS

    7 ✓7th **T37.5X2 Poisoning by antiviral drugs, intentional self-harm** HCC

    ✓7th **T37.5X3 Poisoning by antiviral drugs, assault**

    ✓7th **T37.5X4 Poisoning by antiviral drugs, undetermined**

    ✓7th **T37.5X5** Adverse effect **of antiviral drugs**

    ✓7th **T37.5X6** Underdosing **of antiviral drugs**

✓5th **T37.8 Poisoning by, adverse effect of and underdosing of other specified systemic anti-infectives and antiparasitics**
> Poisoning by, adverse effect of and underdosing of hydroxyquinoline derivatives
> EXCLUDES 1   *antimalarial drugs (T37.2-)*

  ✓6th **T37.8X Poisoning by, adverse effect of and underdosing of other specified systemic anti-infectives and antiparasitics**

    ✓7th **T37.8X1 Poisoning by other specified systemic anti-infectives and antiparasitics, accidental (unintentional)**
> Poisoning by other specified systemic anti-infectives and antiparasitics NOS

    7 ✓7th **T37.8X2 Poisoning by other specified systemic anti-infectives and antiparasitics, intentional self-harm** HCC

    ✓7th **T37.8X3 Poisoning by other specified systemic anti-infectives and antiparasitics, assault**

    ✓7th **T37.8X4 Poisoning by other specified systemic anti-infectives and antiparasitics, undetermined**

    ✓7th **T37.8X5** Adverse effect **of other specified systemic anti-infectives and antiparasitics**

    ✓7th **T37.8X6** Underdosing **of other specified systemic anti-infectives and antiparasitics**

✓5th **T37.9 Poisoning by, adverse effect of and underdosing of unspecified systemic anti-infective and antiparasitics**

  ✓x7th **T37.91 Poisoning by unspecified systemic anti-infective and antiparasitics, accidental (unintentional)**
> Poisoning by, adverse effect of and underdosing of systemic anti-infective and antiparasitics NOS

  7 ✓x7th **T37.92 Poisoning by unspecified systemic anti-infective and antiparasitics, intentional self-harm** HCC

  ✓x7th **T37.93 Poisoning by unspecified systemic anti-infective and antiparasitics, assault**

  ✓x7th **T37.94 Poisoning by unspecified systemic anti-infective and antiparasitics, undetermined**

  ✓x7th **T37.95** Adverse effect **of unspecified systemic anti-infective and antiparasitic**

  ✓x7th **T37.96** Underdosing **of unspecified systemic anti-infectives and antiparasitics**

✓4th **T38 Poisoning by, adverse effect of and underdosing of hormones and their synthetic substitutes and antagonists, not elsewhere classified**
> EXCLUDES 1   *mineralocorticoids and their antagonists (T50.0-)*
> *oxytocic hormones (T48.0-)*
> *parathyroid hormones and derivatives (T50.9-)*

> The appropriate 7th character is to be added to each code from category T38.
> A   initial encounter
> D   subsequent encounter
> S   sequela

✓5th **T38.0 Poisoning by, adverse effect of and underdosing of glucocorticoids and synthetic analogues**
> EXCLUDES 1   *glucocorticoids, topically used (T49.-)*

  ✓6th **T38.0X Poisoning by, adverse effect of and underdosing of glucocorticoids and synthetic analogues**

    ✓7th **T38.0X1 Poisoning by glucocorticoids and synthetic analogues, accidental (unintentional)**
> Poisoning by glucocorticoids and synthetic analogues NOS

    7 ✓7th **T38.0X2 Poisoning by glucocorticoids and synthetic analogues, intentional self-harm** HCC

    ✓7th **T38.0X3 Poisoning by glucocorticoids and synthetic analogues, assault**

    ✓7th **T38.0X4 Poisoning by glucocorticoids and synthetic analogues, undetermined**

    ✓7th **T38.0X5** Adverse effect **of glucocorticoids and synthetic analogues**

    ✓7th **T38.0X6** Underdosing **of glucocorticoids and synthetic analogues**

Chapter 19. Injury, Poisoning and Certain Other Consequences of External Causes

T38.1–T38.801

✓5ᵗʰ **T38.1** **Poisoning by, adverse effect of and underdosing of thyroid hormones and substitutes**
- ✓6ᵗʰ **T38.1X** **Poisoning by, adverse effect of and underdosing of thyroid hormones and substitutes**
  - ✓7ᵗʰ **T38.1X1** **Poisoning by thyroid hormones and substitutes, accidental (unintentional)**
    Poisoning by thyroid hormones and substitutes NOS
  - 7 ✓7ᵗʰ **T38.1X2** **Poisoning by thyroid hormones and substitutes, intentional self-harm** `HCC`
  - ✓7ᵗʰ **T38.1X3** **Poisoning by thyroid hormones and substitutes, assault**
  - ✓7ᵗʰ **T38.1X4** **Poisoning by thyroid hormones and substitutes, undetermined**
  - ✓7ᵗʰ **T38.1X5** **Adverse effect of thyroid hormones and substitutes**
  - ✓7ᵗʰ **T38.1X6** **Underdosing of thyroid hormones and substitutes**

✓5ᵗʰ **T38.2** **Poisoning by, adverse effect of and underdosing of antithyroid drugs**
- ✓6ᵗʰ **T38.2X** **Poisoning by, adverse effect of and underdosing of antithyroid drugs**
  - ✓7ᵗʰ **T38.2X1** **Poisoning by antithyroid drugs, accidental (unintentional)**
    Poisoning by antithyroid drugs NOS
  - 7 ✓7ᵗʰ **T38.2X2** **Poisoning by antithyroid drugs, intentional self-harm** `HCC`
  - ✓7ᵗʰ **T38.2X3** **Poisoning by antithyroid drugs, assault**
  - ✓7ᵗʰ **T38.2X4** **Poisoning by antithyroid drugs, undetermined**
  - ✓7ᵗʰ **T38.2X5** **Adverse effect of antithyroid drugs**
  - ✓7ᵗʰ **T38.2X6** **Underdosing of antithyroid drugs**

✓5ᵗʰ **T38.3** **Poisoning by, adverse effect of and underdosing of insulin and oral hypoglycemic [antidiabetic] drugs**
- ✓6ᵗʰ **T38.3X** **Poisoning by, adverse effect of and underdosing of insulin and oral hypoglycemic [antidiabetic] drugs**
  - ✓7ᵗʰ **T38.3X1** **Poisoning by insulin and oral hypoglycemic [antidiabetic] drugs, accidental (unintentional)**
    Poisoning by insulin and oral hypoglycemic [antidiabetic] drugs NOS
  - 7 ✓7ᵗʰ **T38.3X2** **Poisoning by insulin and oral hypoglycemic [antidiabetic] drugs, intentional self-harm** `HCC`
  - ✓7ᵗʰ **T38.3X3** **Poisoning by insulin and oral hypoglycemic [antidiabetic] drugs, assault**
  - ✓7ᵗʰ **T38.3X4** **Poisoning by insulin and oral hypoglycemic [antidiabetic] drugs, undetermined**
  - ✓7ᵗʰ **T38.3X5** **Adverse effect of insulin and oral hypoglycemic [antidiabetic] drugs**
  - ✓7ᵗʰ **T38.3X6** **Underdosing of insulin and oral hypoglycemic [antidiabetic] drugs**

✓5ᵗʰ **T38.4** **Poisoning by, adverse effect of and underdosing of oral contraceptives**
  Poisoning by, adverse effect of and underdosing of multiple- and single-ingredient oral contraceptive preparations
- ✓6ᵗʰ **T38.4X** **Poisoning by, adverse effect of and underdosing of oral contraceptives**
  - ✓7ᵗʰ **T38.4X1** **Poisoning by oral contraceptives, accidental (unintentional)**
    Poisoning by oral contraceptives NOS
  - 7 ✓7ᵗʰ **T38.4X2** **Poisoning by oral contraceptives, intentional self-harm** `HCC`
  - ✓7ᵗʰ **T38.4X3** **Poisoning by oral contraceptives, assault**
  - ✓7ᵗʰ **T38.4X4** **Poisoning by oral contraceptives, undetermined**
  - ✓7ᵗʰ **T38.4X5** **Adverse effect of oral contraceptives**
  - ✓7ᵗʰ **T38.4X6** **Underdosing of oral contraceptives**

✓5ᵗʰ **T38.5** **Poisoning by, adverse effect of and underdosing of other estrogens and progestogens**
  Poisoning by, adverse effect of and underdosing of estrogens and progestogens mixtures and substitutes
- ✓6ᵗʰ **T38.5X** **Poisoning by, adverse effect of and underdosing of other estrogens and progestogens**
  - ✓7ᵗʰ **T38.5X1** **Poisoning by other estrogens and progestogens, accidental (unintentional)**
    Poisoning by other estrogens and progestogens NOS
  - 7 ✓7ᵗʰ **T38.5X2** **Poisoning by other estrogens and progestogens, intentional self-harm** `HCC`
  - ✓7ᵗʰ **T38.5X3** **Poisoning by other estrogens and progestogens, assault**
  - ✓7ᵗʰ **T38.5X4** **Poisoning by other estrogens and progestogens, undetermined**
  - ✓7ᵗʰ **T38.5X5** **Adverse effect of other estrogens and progestogens**
  - ✓7ᵗʰ **T38.5X6** **Underdosing of other estrogens and progestogens**

✓5ᵗʰ **T38.6** **Poisoning by, adverse effect of and underdosing of antigonadotrophins, antiestrogens, antiandrogens, not elsewhere classified**
  Poisoning by, adverse effect of and underdosing of tamoxifen
- ✓6ᵗʰ **T38.6X** **Poisoning by, adverse effect of and underdosing of antigonadotrophins, antiestrogens, antiandrogens, not elsewhere classified**
  - ✓7ᵗʰ **T38.6X1** **Poisoning by antigonadotrophins, antiestrogens, antiandrogens, not elsewhere classified, accidental (unintentional)**
    Poisoning by antigonadotrophins, antiestrogens, antiandrogens, not elsewhere classified NOS
  - 7 ✓7ᵗʰ **T38.6X2** **Poisoning by antigonadotrophins, antiestrogens, antiandrogens, not elsewhere classified, intentional self-harm** `HCC`
  - ✓7ᵗʰ **T38.6X3** **Poisoning by antigonadotrophins, antiestrogens, antiandrogens, not elsewhere classified, assault**
  - ✓7ᵗʰ **T38.6X4** **Poisoning by antigonadotrophins, antiestrogens, antiandrogens, not elsewhere classified, undetermined**
  - ✓7ᵗʰ **T38.6X5** **Adverse effect of antigonadotrophins, antiestrogens, antiandrogens, not elsewhere classified**
  - ✓7ᵗʰ **T38.6X6** **Underdosing of antigonadotrophins, antiestrogens, antiandrogens, not elsewhere classified**

✓5ᵗʰ **T38.7** **Poisoning by, adverse effect of and underdosing of androgens and anabolic congeners**
- ✓6ᵗʰ **T38.7X** **Poisoning by, adverse effect of and underdosing of androgens and anabolic congeners**
  - ✓7ᵗʰ **T38.7X1** **Poisoning by androgens and anabolic congeners, accidental (unintentional)**
    Poisoning by androgens and anabolic congeners NOS
  - 7 ✓7ᵗʰ **T38.7X2** **Poisoning by androgens and anabolic congeners, intentional self-harm** `HCC`
  - ✓7ᵗʰ **T38.7X3** **Poisoning by androgens and anabolic congeners, assault**
  - ✓7ᵗʰ **T38.7X4** **Poisoning by androgens and anabolic congeners, undetermined**
  - ✓7ᵗʰ **T38.7X5** **Adverse effect of androgens and anabolic congeners**
  - ✓7ᵗʰ **T38.7X6** **Underdosing of androgens and anabolic congeners**

✓5ᵗʰ **T38.8** **Poisoning by, adverse effect of and underdosing of other and unspecified hormones and synthetic substitutes**
- ✓6ᵗʰ **T38.80** **Poisoning by, adverse effect of and underdosing of unspecified hormones and synthetic substitutes**
  - ✓7ᵗʰ **T38.801** **Poisoning by unspecified hormones and synthetic substitutes, accidental (unintentional)**
    Poisoning by unspecified hormones and synthetic substitutes NOS

Ⓝ Newborn: 0   Ⓟ Pediatric: 0-17   Ⓜ Maternity: 9-64   Ⓐ Adult: 15-124   `MCC` Major Complication/Comorbidity   `CC` Complication/Comorbidity   `SW` Severe Wound Dx

1152   ICD-10-CM 2020

7 √7ᵗʰ **T38.802** **Poisoning by unspecified hormones and synthetic substitutes, intentional self-harm** `HCC`

√7ᵗʰ **T38.803** **Poisoning by unspecified hormones and synthetic substitutes, assault**

√7ᵗʰ **T38.804** **Poisoning by unspecified hormones and synthetic substitutes, undetermined**

√7ᵗʰ **T38.805** **Adverse effect of unspecified hormones and synthetic substitutes**

√7ᵗʰ **T38.806** **Underdosing of unspecified hormones and synthetic substitutes**

√6ᵗʰ **T38.81** **Poisoning by, adverse effect of and underdosing of anterior pituitary [adenohypophyseal] hormones**

√7ᵗʰ **T38.811** **Poisoning by anterior pituitary [adenohypophyseal] hormones, accidental (unintentional)**
Poisoning by anterior pituitary [adenohypophyseal] hormones NOS

7 √7ᵗʰ **T38.812** **Poisoning by anterior pituitary [adenohypophyseal] hormones, intentional self-harm** `HCC`

√7ᵗʰ **T38.813** **Poisoning by anterior pituitary [adenohypophyseal] hormones, assault**

√7ᵗʰ **T38.814** **Poisoning by anterior pituitary [adenohypophyseal] hormones, undetermined**

√7ᵗʰ **T38.815** **Adverse effect of anterior pituitary [adenohypophyseal] hormones**

√7ᵗʰ **T38.816** **Underdosing of anterior pituitary [adenohypophyseal] hormones**

√6ᵗʰ **T38.89** **Poisoning by, adverse effect of and underdosing of other hormones and synthetic substitutes**

√7ᵗʰ **T38.891** **Poisoning by other hormones and synthetic substitutes, accidental (unintentional)**
Poisoning by other hormones and synthetic substitutes NOS

7 √7ᵗʰ **T38.892** **Poisoning by other hormones and synthetic substitutes, intentional self-harm** `HCC`

√7ᵗʰ **T38.893** **Poisoning by other hormones and synthetic substitutes, assault**

√7ᵗʰ **T38.894** **Poisoning by other hormones and synthetic substitutes, undetermined**

√7ᵗʰ **T38.895** **Adverse effect of other hormones and synthetic substitutes**

√7ᵗʰ **T38.896** **Underdosing of other hormones and synthetic substitutes**

√5ᵗʰ **T38.9** **Poisoning by, adverse effect of and underdosing of other and unspecified hormone antagonists**

√6ᵗʰ **T38.90** **Poisoning by, adverse effect of and underdosing of unspecified hormone antagonists**

√7ᵗʰ **T38.901** **Poisoning by unspecified hormone antagonists, accidental (unintentional)**
Poisoning by unspecified hormone antagonists NOS

7 √7ᵗʰ **T38.902** **Poisoning by unspecified hormone antagonists, intentional self-harm** `HCC`

√7ᵗʰ **T38.903** **Poisoning by unspecified hormone antagonists, assault**

√7ᵗʰ **T38.904** **Poisoning by unspecified hormone antagonists, undetermined**

√7ᵗʰ **T38.905** **Adverse effect of unspecified hormone antagonists**

√7ᵗʰ **T38.906** **Underdosing of unspecified hormone antagonists**

√6ᵗʰ **T38.99** **Poisoning by, adverse effect of and underdosing of other hormone antagonists**

√7ᵗʰ **T38.991** **Poisoning by other hormone antagonists, accidental (unintentional)**
Poisoning by other hormone antagonists NOS

7 √7ᵗʰ **T38.992** **Poisoning by other hormone antagonists, intentional self-harm** `HCC`

√7ᵗʰ **T38.993** **Poisoning by other hormone antagonists, assault**

√7ᵗʰ **T38.994** **Poisoning by other hormone antagonists, undetermined**

√7ᵗʰ **T38.995** **Adverse effect of other hormone antagonists**

√7ᵗʰ **T38.996** **Underdosing of other hormone antagonists**

√4ᵗʰ **T39** **Poisoning by, adverse effect of and underdosing of nonopioid analgesics, antipyretics and antirheumatics**

The appropriate 7th character is to be added to each code from category T39.
A   initial encounter
D   subsequent encounter
S   sequela

√5ᵗʰ **T39.0** **Poisoning by, adverse effect of and underdosing of salicylates**

√6ᵗʰ **T39.01** **Poisoning by, adverse effect of and underdosing of aspirin**
Poisoning by, adverse effect of and underdosing of acetylsalicylic acid

√7ᵗʰ **T39.011** **Poisoning by aspirin, accidental (unintentional)**

7 √7ᵗʰ **T39.012** **Poisoning by aspirin, intentional self-harm** `HCC`

√7ᵗʰ **T39.013** **Poisoning by aspirin, assault**

√7ᵗʰ **T39.014** **Poisoning by aspirin, undetermined**

√7ᵗʰ **T39.015** **Adverse effect of aspirin**
AHA: 2016,1Q,15

√7ᵗʰ **T39.016** **Underdosing of aspirin**

√6ᵗʰ **T39.09** **Poisoning by, adverse effect of and underdosing of other salicylates**

√7ᵗʰ **T39.091** **Poisoning by salicylates, accidental (unintentional)**
Poisoning by salicylates NOS

7 √7ᵗʰ **T39.092** **Poisoning by salicylates, intentional self-harm** `HCC`

√7ᵗʰ **T39.093** **Poisoning by salicylates, assault**

√7ᵗʰ **T39.094** **Poisoning by salicylates, undetermined**

√7ᵗʰ **T39.095** **Adverse effect of salicylates**

√7ᵗʰ **T39.096** **Underdosing of salicylates**

√5ᵗʰ **T39.1** **Poisoning by, adverse effect of and underdosing of 4-Aminophenol derivatives**

√6ᵗʰ **T39.1X** **Poisoning by, adverse effect of and underdosing of 4-Aminophenol derivatives**

√7ᵗʰ **T39.1X1** **Poisoning by 4-Aminophenol derivatives, accidental (unintentional)**
Poisoning by 4-Aminophenol derivatives NOS

7 √7ᵗʰ **T39.1X2** **Poisoning by 4-Aminophenol derivatives, intentional self-harm** `HCC`

√7ᵗʰ **T39.1X3** **Poisoning by 4-Aminophenol derivatives, assault**

√7ᵗʰ **T39.1X4** **Poisoning by 4-Aminophenol derivatives, undetermined**

√7ᵗʰ **T39.1X5** **Adverse effect of 4-Aminophenol derivatives**

√7ᵗʰ **T39.1X6** **Underdosing of 4-Aminophenol derivatives**

√5ᵗʰ **T39.2** **Poisoning by, adverse effect of and underdosing of pyrazolone derivatives**

√6ᵗʰ **T39.2X** **Poisoning by, adverse effect of and underdosing of pyrazolone derivatives**

√7ᵗʰ **T39.2X1** **Poisoning by pyrazolone derivatives, accidental (unintentional)**
Poisoning by pyrazolone derivatives NOS

7 √7ᵗʰ **T39.2X2** **Poisoning by pyrazolone derivatives, intentional self-harm** `HCC`

√7ᵗʰ **T39.2X3** **Poisoning by pyrazolone derivatives, assault**

√7ᵗʰ **T39.2X4** **Poisoning by pyrazolone derivatives, undetermined**

√7ᵗʰ **T39.2X5** **Adverse effect of pyrazolone derivatives**

√7ᵗʰ **T39.2X6** **Underdosing of pyrazolone derivatives**

Chapter 19. Injury, Poisoning and Certain Other Consequences of External Causes

✓5th **T39.3** **Poisoning by, adverse effect of and underdosing of other nonsteroidal anti-inflammatory drugs [NSAID]**

    ✓6th **T39.31** **Poisoning by, adverse effect of and underdosing of propionic acid derivatives**

        Poisoning by, adverse effect of and underdosing of fenoprofen

        Poisoning by, adverse effect of and underdosing of flurbiprofen

        Poisoning by, adverse effect of and underdosing of ibuprofen

        Poisoning by, adverse effect of and underdosing of ketoprofen

        Poisoning by, adverse effect of and underdosing of naproxen

        Poisoning by, adverse effect of and underdosing of oxaprozin

        ✓7th **T39.311** **Poisoning by propionic acid derivatives, accidental (unintentional)**

        7 ✓7th **T39.312** **Poisoning by propionic acid derivatives, intentional self-harm** HCC

        ✓7th **T39.313** **Poisoning by propionic acid derivatives, assault**

        ✓7th **T39.314** **Poisoning by propionic acid derivatives, undetermined**

        ✓7th **T39.315** **Adverse effect of propionic acid derivatives**

        ✓7th **T39.316** **Underdosing of propionic acid derivatives**

    ✓6th **T39.39** **Poisoning by, adverse effect of and underdosing of other nonsteroidal anti-inflammatory drugs [NSAID]**

        ✓7th **T39.391** **Poisoning by other nonsteroidal anti-inflammatory drugs [NSAID], accidental (unintentional)**

            Poisoning by other nonsteroidal anti-inflammatory drugs NOS

        7 ✓7th **T39.392** **Poisoning by other nonsteroidal anti-inflammatory drugs [NSAID], intentional self-harm** HCC

        ✓7th **T39.393** **Poisoning by other nonsteroidal anti-inflammatory drugs [NSAID], assault**

        ✓7th **T39.394** **Poisoning by other nonsteroidal anti-inflammatory drugs [NSAID], undetermined**

        ✓7th **T39.395** **Adverse effect of other nonsteroidal anti-inflammatory drugs [NSAID]**

        ✓7th **T39.396** **Underdosing of other nonsteroidal anti-inflammatory drugs [NSAID]**

✓5th **T39.4** **Poisoning by, adverse effect of and underdosing of antirheumatics, not elsewhere classified**

    EXCLUDES 1   poisoning by, adverse effect of and underdosing of glucocorticoids (T38.0-)

             poisoning by, adverse effect of and underdosing of salicylates (T39.0-)

    ✓6th **T39.4X** **Poisoning by, adverse effect of and underdosing of antirheumatics, not elsewhere classified**

        ✓7th **T39.4X1** **Poisoning by antirheumatics, not elsewhere classified, accidental (unintentional)**

            Poisoning by antirheumatics, not elsewhere classified NOS

        7 ✓7th **T39.4X2** **Poisoning by antirheumatics, not elsewhere classified, intentional self-harm** HCC

        ✓7th **T39.4X3** **Poisoning by antirheumatics, not elsewhere classified, assault**

        ✓7th **T39.4X4** **Poisoning by antirheumatics, not elsewhere classified, undetermined**

        ✓7th **T39.4X5** **Adverse effect of antirheumatics, not elsewhere classified**

        ✓7th **T39.4X6** **Underdosing of antirheumatics, not elsewhere classified**

✓5th **T39.8** **Poisoning by, adverse effect of and underdosing of other nonopioid analgesics and antipyretics, not elsewhere classified**

    ✓6th **T39.8X** **Poisoning by, adverse effect of and underdosing of other nonopioid analgesics and antipyretics, not elsewhere classified**

        ✓7th **T39.8X1** **Poisoning by other nonopioid analgesics and antipyretics, not elsewhere classified, accidental (unintentional)**

            Poisoning by other nonopioid analgesics and antipyretics, not elsewhere classified NOS

        7 ✓7th **T39.8X2** **Poisoning by other nonopioid analgesics and antipyretics, not elsewhere classified, intentional self-harm** HCC

        ✓7th **T39.8X3** **Poisoning by other nonopioid analgesics and antipyretics, not elsewhere classified, assault**

        ✓7th **T39.8X4** **Poisoning by other nonopioid analgesics and antipyretics, not elsewhere classified, undetermined**

        ✓7th **T39.8X5** **Adverse effect of other nonopioid analgesics and antipyretics, not elsewhere classified**

        ✓7th **T39.8X6** **Underdosing of other nonopioid analgesics and antipyretics, not elsewhere classified**

✓5th **T39.9** **Poisoning by, adverse effect of and underdosing of unspecified nonopioid analgesic, antipyretic and antirheumatic**

    ✓x7th **T39.91** **Poisoning by unspecified nonopioid analgesic, antipyretic and antirheumatic, accidental (unintentional)**

        Poisoning by nonopioid analgesic, antipyretic and antirheumatic NOS

    7 ✓x7th **T39.92** **Poisoning by unspecified nonopioid analgesic, antipyretic and antirheumatic, intentional self-harm** HCC

    ✓x7th **T39.93** **Poisoning by unspecified nonopioid analgesic, antipyretic and antirheumatic, assault**

    ✓x7th **T39.94** **Poisoning by unspecified nonopioid analgesic, antipyretic and antirheumatic, undetermined**

    ✓x7th **T39.95** **Adverse effect of unspecified nonopioid analgesic, antipyretic and antirheumatic**

    ✓x7th **T39.96** **Underdosing of unspecified nonopioid analgesic, antipyretic and antirheumatic**

✓4th **T40** **Poisoning by, adverse effect of and underdosing of narcotics and psychodysleptics [hallucinogens]**

    EXCLUDES 2   drug dependence and related mental and behavioral disorders due to psychoactive substance use (F10.-F19.-)

    The appropriate 7th character is to be added to each code from category T40.

    A   initial encounter

    D   subsequent encounter

    S   sequela

✓5th **T40.0** **Poisoning by, adverse effect of and underdosing of opium**

    ✓6th **T40.0X** **Poisoning by, adverse effect of and underdosing of opium**

        6 ✓7th **T40.0X1** **Poisoning by opium, accidental (unintentional)** HCC

            Poisoning by opium NOS

        7 ✓7th **T40.0X2** **Poisoning by opium, intentional self-harm** HCC

        ✓7th **T40.0X3** **Poisoning by opium, assault**

        6 ✓7th **T40.0X4** **Poisoning by opium, undetermined** HCC

        ✓7th **T40.0X5** **Adverse effect of opium**

        ✓7th **T40.0X6** **Underdosing of opium**

✓5th **T40.1** **Poisoning by and adverse effect of heroin**

    ✓6th **T40.1X** **Poisoning by and adverse effect of heroin**

        6 ✓7th **T40.1X1** **Poisoning by heroin, accidental (unintentional)** HCC

            Poisoning by heroin NOS

        7 ✓7th **T40.1X2** **Poisoning by heroin, intentional self-harm** HCC

        ✓7th **T40.1X3** **Poisoning by heroin, assault**

        6 ✓7th **T40.1X4** **Poisoning by heroin, undetermined** HCC

N Newborn: 0   P Pediatric: 0-17   M Maternity: 9-64   A Adult: 15-124   MCC Major Complication/Comorbidity   CC Complication/Comorbidity   SW Severe Wound Dx

1154   ICD-10-CM 2020

√5th **T40.2** **Poisoning by, adverse effect of and underdosing of other opioids**

√6th **T40.2X** **Poisoning by, adverse effect of and underdosing of other opioids**

6 √7th **T40.2X1** **Poisoning by other opioids, accidental (unintentional)**   HCC
Poisoning by other opioids NOS

7 √7th **T40.2X2** **Poisoning by other opioids, intentional self-harm**   HCC

√7th **T40.2X3** **Poisoning by other opioids, assault**

6 √7th **T40.2X4** **Poisoning by other opioids, undetermined**   HCC

√7th **T40.2X5** Adverse effect of other opioids

√7th **T40.2X6** Underdosing of other opioids

√5th **T40.3** **Poisoning by, adverse effect of and underdosing of methadone**

√6th **T40.3X** **Poisoning by, adverse effect of and underdosing of methadone**

6 √7th **T40.3X1** **Poisoning by methadone, accidental (unintentional)**   HCC
Poisoning by methadone NOS

7 √7th **T40.3X2** **Poisoning by methadone, intentional self-harm**   HCC

√7th **T40.3X3** **Poisoning by methadone, assault**

6 √7th **T40.3X4** **Poisoning by methadone, undetermined**   HCC

√7th **T40.3X5** Adverse effect of methadone

√7th **T40.3X6** Underdosing of methadone

√5th **T40.4** **Poisoning by, adverse effect of and underdosing of other synthetic narcotics**

√6th **T40.4X** **Poisoning by, adverse effect of and underdosing of other synthetic narcotics**

6 √7th **T40.4X1** **Poisoning by other synthetic narcotics, accidental (unintentional)**   HCC
Poisoning by other synthetic narcotics NOS

7 √7th **T40.4X2** **Poisoning by other synthetic narcotics, intentional self-harm**   HCC

√7th **T40.4X3** **Poisoning by other synthetic narcotics, assault**

6 √7th **T40.4X4** **Poisoning by other synthetic narcotics, undetermined**   HCC

√7th **T40.4X5** Adverse effect of other synthetic narcotics

√7th **T40.4X6** Underdosing of other synthetic narcotics

√5th **T40.5** **Poisoning by, adverse effect of and underdosing of cocaine**

√6th **T40.5X** **Poisoning by, adverse effect of and underdosing of cocaine**

6 √7th **T40.5X1** **Poisoning by cocaine, accidental (unintentional)**   HCC
Poisoning by cocaine NOS
AHA: 2016,2Q,8

7 √7th **T40.5X2** **Poisoning by cocaine, intentional self-harm**   HCC

√7th **T40.5X3** **Poisoning by cocaine, assault**

6 √7th **T40.5X4** **Poisoning by cocaine, undetermined**   HCC

√7th **T40.5X5** Adverse effect of cocaine

√7th **T40.5X6** Underdosing of cocaine

√5th **T40.6** **Poisoning by, adverse effect of and underdosing of other and unspecified narcotics**

√6th **T40.60** **Poisoning by, adverse effect of and underdosing of unspecified narcotics**

6 √7th **T40.601** **Poisoning by unspecified narcotics, accidental (unintentional)**   HCC
Poisoning by narcotics NOS

7 √7th **T40.602** **Poisoning by unspecified narcotics, intentional self-harm**   HCC

√7th **T40.603** **Poisoning by unspecified narcotics, assault**

6 √7th **T40.604** **Poisoning by unspecified narcotics, undetermined**   HCC

√7th **T40.605** Adverse effect of unspecified narcotics

√7th **T40.606** Underdosing of unspecified narcotics

√6th **T40.69** **Poisoning by, adverse effect of and underdosing of other narcotics**

6 √7th **T40.691** **Poisoning by other narcotics, accidental (unintentional)**   HCC
Poisoning by other narcotics NOS

7 √7th **T40.692** **Poisoning by other narcotics, intentional self-harm**   HCC

√7th **T40.693** **Poisoning by other narcotics, assault**

6 √7th **T40.694** **Poisoning by other narcotics, undetermined**   HCC

√7th **T40.695** Adverse effect of other narcotics

√7th **T40.696** Underdosing of other narcotics

√5th **T40.7** **Poisoning by, adverse effect of and underdosing of cannabis (derivatives)**

√6th **T40.7X** **Poisoning by, adverse effect of and underdosing of cannabis (derivatives)**

√7th **T40.7X1** **Poisoning by cannabis (derivatives), accidental (unintentional)**
Poisoning by cannabis NOS

7 √7th **T40.7X2** **Poisoning by cannabis (derivatives), intentional self-harm**   HCC

√7th **T40.7X3** **Poisoning by cannabis (derivatives), assault**

√7th **T40.7X4** **Poisoning by cannabis (derivatives), undetermined**

√7th **T40.7X5** Adverse effect of cannabis (derivatives)

√7th **T40.7X6** Underdosing of cannabis (derivatives)

√5th **T40.8** **Poisoning by and adverse effect of lysergide [LSD]**

√6th **T40.8X** **Poisoning by and adverse effect of lysergide [LSD]**

6 √7th **T40.8X1** **Poisoning by lysergide [LSD], accidental (unintentional)**   HCC
Poisoning by lysergide [LSD] NOS

7 √7th **T40.8X2** **Poisoning by lysergide [LSD], intentional self-harm**   HCC

√7th **T40.8X3** **Poisoning by lysergide [LSD], assault**

6 √7th **T40.8X4** **Poisoning by lysergide [LSD], undetermined**   HCC

√5th **T40.9** **Poisoning by, adverse effect of and underdosing of other and unspecified psychodysleptics [hallucinogens]**

√6th **T40.90** **Poisoning by, adverse effect of and underdosing of unspecified psychodysleptics [hallucinogens]**

6 √7th **T40.901** **Poisoning by unspecified psychodysleptics [hallucinogens], accidental (unintentional)**   HCC

7 √7th **T40.902** **Poisoning by unspecified psychodysleptics [hallucinogens], intentional self-harm**   HCC

√7th **T40.903** **Poisoning by unspecified psychodysleptics [hallucinogens], assault**

6 √7th **T40.904** **Poisoning by unspecified psychodysleptics [hallucinogens], undetermined**   HCC

√7th **T40.905** Adverse effect of unspecified psychodysleptics [hallucinogens]

√7th **T40.906** Underdosing of unspecified psychodysleptics [hallucinogens]

√6th **T40.99** **Poisoning by, adverse effect of and underdosing of other psychodysleptics [hallucinogens]**

6 √7th **T40.991** **Poisoning by other psychodysleptics [hallucinogens], accidental (unintentional)**   HCC
Poisoning by other psychodysleptics [hallucinogens] NOS

7 √7th **T40.992** **Poisoning by other psychodysleptics [hallucinogens], intentional self-harm**   HCC

√7th **T40.993** **Poisoning by other psychodysleptics [hallucinogens], assault**

6 √7th **T40.994** **Poisoning by other psychodysleptics [hallucinogens], undetermined**   HCC

✔ Additional Character Required   √x7th Placeholder   Unacceptable PDx   Questionable PDx   Manifestation   Unspecified Dx   H1-H14 HAC   HCC CMS-HCC Dx   HIV HIV Dx

√7ᵗʰ **T40.995** Adverse effect of other psychodysleptics [hallucinogens]

√7ᵗʰ **T40.996** Underdosing of other psychodysleptics [hallucinogens]

√4ᵗʰ **T41** **Poisoning by, adverse effect of and underdosing of anesthetics and therapeutic gases**

> EXCLUDES 1   benzodiazepines (T42.4-)
> cocaine (T40.5-)
> complications of anesthesia during labor and delivery (O74.-)
> complications of anesthesia during pregnancy (O29.-)
> complications of anesthesia during the puerperium (O89.-)
> opioids (T40.0-T40.2-)

> The appropriate 7th character is to be added to each code from category T41.
> A   initial encounter
> D   subsequent encounter
> S   sequela

√5ᵗʰ **T41.0** **Poisoning by, adverse effect of and underdosing of inhaled anesthetics**

> EXCLUDES 1   oxygen (T41.5-)

√6ᵗʰ **T41.0X** **Poisoning by, adverse effect of and underdosing of inhaled anesthetics**

√7ᵗʰ **T41.0X1** Poisoning by inhaled anesthetics, accidental (unintentional)
Poisoning by inhaled anesthetics NOS

7 √7ᵗʰ **T41.0X2** Poisoning by inhaled anesthetics, intentional self-harm   HCC

√7ᵗʰ **T41.0X3** Poisoning by inhaled anesthetics, assault

√7ᵗʰ **T41.0X4** Poisoning by inhaled anesthetics, undetermined

√7ᵗʰ **T41.0X5** Adverse effect of inhaled anesthetics

√7ᵗʰ **T41.0X6** Underdosing of inhaled anesthetics

√5ᵗʰ **T41.1** **Poisoning by, adverse effect of and underdosing of intravenous anesthetics**
Poisoning by, adverse effect of and underdosing of thiobarbiturates

√6ᵗʰ **T41.1X** **Poisoning by, adverse effect of and underdosing of intravenous anesthetics**

√7ᵗʰ **T41.1X1** Poisoning by intravenous anesthetics, accidental (unintentional)
Poisoning by intravenous anesthetics NOS

7 √7ᵗʰ **T41.1X2** Poisoning by intravenous anesthetics, intentional self-harm   HCC

√7ᵗʰ **T41.1X3** Poisoning by intravenous anesthetics, assault

√7ᵗʰ **T41.1X4** Poisoning by intravenous anesthetics, undetermined

√7ᵗʰ **T41.1X5** Adverse effect of intravenous anesthetics

√7ᵗʰ **T41.1X6** Underdosing of intravenous anesthetics

√5ᵗʰ **T41.2** **Poisoning by, adverse effect of and underdosing of other and unspecified general anesthetics**

√6ᵗʰ **T41.20** **Poisoning by, adverse effect of and underdosing of unspecified general anesthetics**

√7ᵗʰ **T41.201** Poisoning by unspecified general anesthetics, accidental (unintentional)
Poisoning by general anesthetics NOS

7 √7ᵗʰ **T41.202** Poisoning by unspecified general anesthetics, intentional self-harm   HCC

√7ᵗʰ **T41.203** Poisoning by unspecified general anesthetics, assault

√7ᵗʰ **T41.204** Poisoning by unspecified general anesthetics, undetermined

√7ᵗʰ **T41.205** Adverse effect of unspecified general anesthetics
AHA: 2016,4Q,73

√7ᵗʰ **T41.206** Underdosing of unspecified general anesthetics

√6ᵗʰ **T41.29** **Poisoning by, adverse effect of and underdosing of other general anesthetics**

√7ᵗʰ **T41.291** Poisoning by other general anesthetics, accidental (unintentional)
Poisoning by other general anesthetics NOS

7 √7ᵗʰ **T41.292** Poisoning by other general anesthetics, intentional self-harm   HCC

√7ᵗʰ **T41.293** Poisoning by other general anesthetics, assault

√7ᵗʰ **T41.294** Poisoning by other general anesthetics, undetermined

√7ᵗʰ **T41.295** Adverse effect of other general anesthetics

√7ᵗʰ **T41.296** Underdosing of other general anesthetics

√5ᵗʰ **T41.3** **Poisoning by, adverse effect of and underdosing of local anesthetics**
Cocaine (topical)

> EXCLUDES 2   poisoning by cocaine used as a central nervous system stimulant (T40.5X1-T40.5X4)

√6ᵗʰ **T41.3X** **Poisoning by, adverse effect of and underdosing of local anesthetics**

√7ᵗʰ **T41.3X1** Poisoning by local anesthetics, accidental (unintentional)
Poisoning by local anesthetics NOS

7 √7ᵗʰ **T41.3X2** Poisoning by local anesthetics, intentional self-harm   HCC

√7ᵗʰ **T41.3X3** Poisoning by local anesthetics, assault

√7ᵗʰ **T41.3X4** Poisoning by local anesthetics, undetermined

√7ᵗʰ **T41.3X5** Adverse effect of local anesthetics

√7ᵗʰ **T41.3X6** Underdosing of local anesthetics

√5ᵗʰ **T41.4** **Poisoning by, adverse effect of and underdosing of unspecified anesthetic**

√x7ᵗʰ **T41.41** Poisoning by unspecified anesthetic, accidental (unintentional)
Poisoning by anesthetic NOS

7 √x7ᵗʰ **T41.42** Poisoning by unspecified anesthetic, intentional self-harm   HCC

√x7ᵗʰ **T41.43** Poisoning by unspecified anesthetic, assault

√x7ᵗʰ **T41.44** Poisoning by unspecified anesthetic, undetermined

√x7ᵗʰ **T41.45** Adverse effect of unspecified anesthetic

√x7ᵗʰ **T41.46** Underdosing of unspecified anesthetics

√5ᵗʰ **T41.5** **Poisoning by, adverse effect of and underdosing of therapeutic gases**

√6ᵗʰ **T41.5X** **Poisoning by, adverse effect of and underdosing of therapeutic gases**

√7ᵗʰ **T41.5X1** Poisoning by therapeutic gases, accidental (unintentional)
Poisoning by therapeutic gases NOS

7 √7ᵗʰ **T41.5X2** Poisoning by therapeutic gases, intentional self-harm   HCC

√7ᵗʰ **T41.5X3** Poisoning by therapeutic gases, assault

√7ᵗʰ **T41.5X4** Poisoning by therapeutic gases, undetermined

√7ᵗʰ **T41.5X5** Adverse effect of therapeutic gases

√7ᵗʰ **T41.5X6** Underdosing of therapeutic gases

√4ᵗʰ **T42** **Poisoning by, adverse effect of and underdosing of antiepileptic, sedative- hypnotic and antiparkinsonism drugs**

> EXCLUDES 2   drug dependence and related mental and behavioral disorders due to psychoactive substance use (F10.- – F19.-)

> The appropriate 7th character is to be added to each code from category T42.
> A   initial encounter
> D   subsequent encounter
> S   sequela

√5ᵗʰ **T42.0** **Poisoning by, adverse effect of and underdosing of hydantoin derivatives**

√6ᵗʰ **T42.0X** **Poisoning by, adverse effect of and underdosing of hydantoin derivatives**

√7ᵗʰ **T42.0X1** Poisoning by hydantoin derivatives, accidental (unintentional)
Poisoning by hydantoin derivatives NOS

7 √7ᵗʰ **T42.0X2** Poisoning by hydantoin derivatives, intentional self-harm   HCC

√7ᵗʰ **T42.0X3** Poisoning by hydantoin derivatives, assault

√7ᵗʰ **T42.0X4** Poisoning by hydantoin derivatives, undetermined

√7ᵗʰ **T42.0X5** Adverse effect of hydantoin derivatives

√7ᵗʰ **T42.0X6** Underdosing of hydantoin derivatives

✓5ᵗʰ **T42.1** **Poisoning by, adverse effect of and underdosing of iminostilbenes**

Poisoning by, adverse effect of and underdosing of carbamazepine

   ✓6ᵗʰ **T42.1X** **Poisoning by, adverse effect of and underdosing of iminostilbenes**

     ✓7ᵗʰ **T42.1X1** **Poisoning by iminostilbenes, accidental (unintentional)**

Poisoning by iminostilbenes NOS

     7 ✓7ᵗʰ **T42.1X2** **Poisoning by iminostilbenes, intentional self-harm** `HCC`

     ✓7ᵗʰ **T42.1X3** **Poisoning by iminostilbenes, assault**

     ✓7ᵗʰ **T42.1X4** **Poisoning by iminostilbenes, undetermined**

     ✓7ᵗʰ **T42.1X5** **Adverse effect of iminostilbenes**

     ✓7ᵗʰ **T42.1X6** **Underdosing of iminostilbenes**

✓5ᵗʰ **T42.2** **Poisoning by, adverse effect of and underdosing of succinimides and oxazolidinediones**

   ✓6ᵗʰ **T42.2X** **Poisoning by, adverse effect of and underdosing of succinimides and oxazolidinediones**

     ✓7ᵗʰ **T42.2X1** **Poisoning by succinimides and oxazolidinediones, accidental (unintentional)**

Poisoning by succinimides and oxazolidinediones NOS

     7 ✓7ᵗʰ **T42.2X2** **Poisoning by succinimides and oxazolidinediones, intentional self-harm** `HCC`

     ✓7ᵗʰ **T42.2X3** **Poisoning by succinimides and oxazolidinediones, assault**

     ✓7ᵗʰ **T42.2X4** **Poisoning by succinimides and oxazolidinediones, undetermined**

     ✓7ᵗʰ **T42.2X5** **Adverse effect of succinimides and oxazolidinediones**

     ✓7ᵗʰ **T42.2X6** **Underdosing of succinimides and oxazolidinediones**

✓5ᵗʰ **T42.3** **Poisoning by, adverse effect of and underdosing of barbiturates**

    EXCLUDES 1   *poisoning by, adverse effect of and underdosing of thiobarbiturates (T41.1-)*

   ✓6ᵗʰ **T42.3X** **Poisoning by, adverse effect of and underdosing of barbiturates**

     ✓7ᵗʰ **T42.3X1** **Poisoning by barbiturates, accidental (unintentional)**

Poisoning by barbiturates NOS

     7 ✓7ᵗʰ **T42.3X2** **Poisoning by barbiturates, intentional self-harm** `HCC`

     ✓7ᵗʰ **T42.3X3** **Poisoning by barbiturates, assault**

     ✓7ᵗʰ **T42.3X4** **Poisoning by barbiturates, undetermined**

     ✓7ᵗʰ **T42.3X5** **Adverse effect of barbiturates**

     ✓7ᵗʰ **T42.3X6** **Underdosing of barbiturates**

✓5ᵗʰ **T42.4** **Poisoning by, adverse effect of and underdosing of benzodiazepines**

   ✓6ᵗʰ **T42.4X** **Poisoning by, adverse effect of and underdosing of benzodiazepines**

     ✓7ᵗʰ **T42.4X1** **Poisoning by benzodiazepines, accidental (unintentional)**

Poisoning by benzodiazepines NOS

     7 ✓7ᵗʰ **T42.4X2** **Poisoning by benzodiazepines, intentional self-harm** `HCC`

     ✓7ᵗʰ **T42.4X3** **Poisoning by benzodiazepines, assault**

     ✓7ᵗʰ **T42.4X4** **Poisoning by benzodiazepines, undetermined**

     ✓7ᵗʰ **T42.4X5** **Adverse effect of benzodiazepines**

     ✓7ᵗʰ **T42.4X6** **Underdosing of benzodiazepines**

✓5ᵗʰ **T42.5** **Poisoning by, adverse effect of and underdosing of mixed antiepileptics**

   ✓6ᵗʰ **T42.5X** **Poisoning by, adverse effect of and underdosing of antiepileptics**

     ✓7ᵗʰ **T42.5X1** **Poisoning by mixed antiepileptics, accidental (unintentional)**

Poisoning by mixed antiepileptics NOS

     7 ✓7ᵗʰ **T42.5X2** **Poisoning by mixed antiepileptics, intentional self-harm** `HCC`

     ✓7ᵗʰ **T42.5X3** **Poisoning by mixed antiepileptics, assault**

     ✓7ᵗʰ **T42.5X4** **Poisoning by mixed antiepileptics, undetermined**

     ✓7ᵗʰ **T42.5X5** **Adverse effect of mixed antiepileptics**

     ✓7ᵗʰ **T42.5X6** **Underdosing of mixed antiepileptics**

✓5ᵗʰ **T42.6** **Poisoning by, adverse effect of and underdosing of other antiepileptic and sedative-hypnotic drugs**

Poisoning by, adverse effect of and underdosing of methaqualone

Poisoning by, adverse effect of and underdosing of valproic acid

    EXCLUDES 1   *poisoning by, adverse effect of and underdosing of carbamazepine (T42.1-)*

   ✓6ᵗʰ **T42.6X** **Poisoning by, adverse effect of and underdosing of other antiepileptic and sedative-hypnotic drugs**

     ✓7ᵗʰ **T42.6X1** **Poisoning by other antiepileptic and sedative-hypnotic drugs, accidental (unintentional)**

Poisoning by other antiepileptic and sedative-hypnotic drugs NOS

     7 ✓7ᵗʰ **T42.6X2** **Poisoning by other antiepileptic and sedative-hypnotic drugs, intentional self-harm** `HCC`

     ✓7ᵗʰ **T42.6X3** **Poisoning by other antiepileptic and sedative-hypnotic drugs, assault**

     ✓7ᵗʰ **T42.6X4** **Poisoning by other antiepileptic and sedative-hypnotic drugs, undetermined**

     ✓7ᵗʰ **T42.6X5** **Adverse effect of other antiepileptic and sedative-hypnotic drugs**

     ✓7ᵗʰ **T42.6X6** **Underdosing of other antiepileptic and sedative-hypnotic drugs**

✓5ᵗʰ **T42.7** **Poisoning by, adverse effect of and underdosing of unspecified antiepileptic and sedative-hypnotic drugs**

   ✓x7ᵗʰ **T42.71** **Poisoning by unspecified antiepileptic and sedative-hypnotic drugs, accidental (unintentional)**

Poisoning by antiepileptic and sedative-hypnotic drugs NOS

   7 ✓x7ᵗʰ **T42.72** **Poisoning by unspecified antiepileptic and sedative-hypnotic drugs, intentional self-harm** `HCC`

   ✓x7ᵗʰ **T42.73** **Poisoning by unspecified antiepileptic and sedative-hypnotic drugs, assault**

   ✓x7ᵗʰ **T42.74** **Poisoning by unspecified antiepileptic and sedative-hypnotic drugs, undetermined**

   ✓x7ᵗʰ **T42.75** **Adverse effect of unspecified antiepileptic and sedative-hypnotic drugs**

   ✓x7ᵗʰ **T42.76** **Underdosing of unspecified antiepileptic and sedative-hypnotic drugs**

✓5ᵗʰ **T42.8** **Poisoning by, adverse effect of and underdosing of antiparkinsonism drugs and other central muscle-tone depressants**

Poisoning by, adverse effect of and underdosing of amantadine

   ✓6ᵗʰ **T42.8X** **Poisoning by, adverse effect of and underdosing of antiparkinsonism drugs and other central muscle-tone depressants**

     ✓7ᵗʰ **T42.8X1** **Poisoning by antiparkinsonism drugs and other central muscle-tone depressants, accidental (unintentional)**

Poisoning by antiparkinsonism drugs and other central muscle-tone depressants NOS

     7 ✓7ᵗʰ **T42.8X2** **Poisoning by antiparkinsonism drugs and other central muscle-tone depressants, intentional self-harm** `HCC`

     ✓7ᵗʰ **T42.8X3** **Poisoning by antiparkinsonism drugs and other central muscle-tone depressants, assault**

     ✓7ᵗʰ **T42.8X4** **Poisoning by antiparkinsonism drugs and other central muscle-tone depressants, undetermined**

     ✓7ᵗʰ **T42.8X5** **Adverse effect of antiparkinsonism drugs and other central muscle-tone depressants**

     ✓7ᵗʰ **T42.8X6** **Underdosing of antiparkinsonism drugs and other central muscle-tone depressants**

✔ Additional Character Required   ✓x7ᵗʰ Placeholder   Unacceptable PDx   Questionable PDx   Manifestation   Unspecified Dx   H1-H4 HAC   HCC CMS-HCC Dx   HIV HIV Dx

ICD-10-CM 2020   1157

☑4ᵗʰ **T43** **Poisoning by, adverse effect of and underdosing of psychotropic drugs, not elsewhere classified**

> EXCLUDES 1   appetite depressants (T50.5-)
> barbiturates (T42.3-)
> benzodiazepines (T42.4-)
> methaqualone (T42.6-)
> psychodysleptics [hallucinogens] (T40.7-T40.9-)
> EXCLUDES 2   drug dependence and related mental and behavioral disorders due to psychoactive substance use (F10.- – F19.-)

> The appropriate 7th character is to be added to each code from category T43.
> A   initial encounter
> D   subsequent encounter
> S   sequela

☑5ᵗʰ **T43.0** **Poisoning by, adverse effect of and underdosing of tricyclic and tetracyclic antidepressants**

☑6ᵗʰ **T43.01** **Poisoning by, adverse effect of and underdosing of tricyclic antidepressants**

☑7ᵗʰ **T43.011** **Poisoning by tricyclic antidepressants, accidental (unintentional)**
Poisoning by tricyclic antidepressants NOS

7 ☑7ᵗʰ **T43.012** **Poisoning by tricyclic antidepressants, intentional self-harm**   HCC

☑7ᵗʰ **T43.013** **Poisoning by tricyclic antidepressants, assault**

☑7ᵗʰ **T43.014** **Poisoning by tricyclic antidepressants, undetermined**

☑7ᵗʰ **T43.015** **Adverse effect of tricyclic antidepressants**

☑7ᵗʰ **T43.016** **Underdosing of tricyclic antidepressants**

☑6ᵗʰ **T43.02** **Poisoning by, adverse effect of and underdosing of tetracyclic antidepressants**

☑7ᵗʰ **T43.021** **Poisoning by tetracyclic antidepressants, accidental (unintentional)**
Poisoning by tetracyclic antidepressants NOS

7 ☑7ᵗʰ **T43.022** **Poisoning by tetracyclic antidepressants, intentional self-harm**   HCC

☑7ᵗʰ **T43.023** **Poisoning by tetracyclic antidepressants, assault**

☑7ᵗʰ **T43.024** **Poisoning by tetracyclic antidepressants, undetermined**

☑7ᵗʰ **T43.025** **Adverse effect of tetracyclic antidepressants**

☑7ᵗʰ **T43.026** **Underdosing of tetracyclic antidepressants**

☑5ᵗʰ **T43.1** **Poisoning by, adverse effect of and underdosing of monoamine-oxidase-inhibitor antidepressants**

☑6ᵗʰ **T43.1X** **Poisoning by, adverse effect of and underdosing of monoamine-oxidase-inhibitor antidepressants**

☑7ᵗʰ **T43.1X1** **Poisoning by monoamine-oxidase-inhibitor antidepressants, accidental (unintentional)**
Poisoning by monoamine-oxidase-inhibitor antidepressants NOS

7 ☑7ᵗʰ **T43.1X2** **Poisoning by monoamine-oxidase-inhibitor antidepressants, intentional self-harm**   HCC

☑7ᵗʰ **T43.1X3** **Poisoning by monoamine-oxidase-inhibitor antidepressants, assault**

☑7ᵗʰ **T43.1X4** **Poisoning by monoamine-oxidase-inhibitor antidepressants, undetermined**

☑7ᵗʰ **T43.1X5** **Adverse effect of monoamine-oxidase-inhibitor antidepressants**

☑7ᵗʰ **T43.1X6** **Underdosing of monoamine-oxidase-inhibitor antidepressants**

☑5ᵗʰ **T43.2** **Poisoning by, adverse effect of and underdosing of other and unspecified antidepressants**

☑6ᵗʰ **T43.20** **Poisoning by, adverse effect of and underdosing of unspecified antidepressants**

☑7ᵗʰ **T43.201** **Poisoning by unspecified antidepressants, accidental (unintentional)**
Poisoning by antidepressants NOS

7 ☑7ᵗʰ **T43.202** **Poisoning by unspecified antidepressants, intentional self-harm**   HCC

☑7ᵗʰ **T43.203** **Poisoning by unspecified antidepressants, assault**

☑7ᵗʰ **T43.204** **Poisoning by unspecified antidepressants, undetermined**

☑7ᵗʰ **T43.205** **Adverse effect of unspecified antidepressants**
Antidepressant discontinuation syndrome

☑7ᵗʰ **T43.206** **Underdosing of unspecified antidepressants**

☑6ᵗʰ **T43.21** **Poisoning by, adverse effect of and underdosing of selective serotonin and norepinephrine reuptake inhibitors**
Poisoning by, adverse effect of and underdosing of SSNRI antidepressants

☑7ᵗʰ **T43.211** **Poisoning by selective serotonin and norepinephrine reuptake inhibitors, accidental (unintentional)**

7 ☑7ᵗʰ **T43.212** **Poisoning by selective serotonin and norepinephrine reuptake inhibitors, intentional self-harm**   HCC

☑7ᵗʰ **T43.213** **Poisoning by selective serotonin and norepinephrine reuptake inhibitors, assault**

☑7ᵗʰ **T43.214** **Poisoning by selective serotonin and norepinephrine reuptake inhibitors, undetermined**

☑7ᵗʰ **T43.215** **Adverse effect of selective serotonin and norepinephrine reuptake inhibitors**

☑7ᵗʰ **T43.216** **Underdosing of selective serotonin and norepinephrine reuptake inhibitors**

☑6ᵗʰ **T43.22** **Poisoning by, adverse effect of and underdosing of selective serotonin reuptake inhibitors**
Poisoning by, adverse effect of and underdosing of SSRI antidepressants

☑7ᵗʰ **T43.221** **Poisoning by selective serotonin reuptake inhibitors, accidental (unintentional)**

7 ☑7ᵗʰ **T43.222** **Poisoning by selective serotonin reuptake inhibitors, intentional self-harm**   HCC

☑7ᵗʰ **T43.223** **Poisoning by selective serotonin reuptake inhibitors, assault**

☑7ᵗʰ **T43.224** **Poisoning by selective serotonin reuptake inhibitors, undetermined**

☑7ᵗʰ **T43.225** **Adverse effect of selective serotonin reuptake inhibitors**

☑7ᵗʰ **T43.226** **Underdosing of selective serotonin reuptake inhibitors**

☑6ᵗʰ **T43.29** **Poisoning by, adverse effect of and underdosing of other antidepressants**

☑7ᵗʰ **T43.291** **Poisoning by other antidepressants, accidental (unintentional)**
Poisoning by other antidepressants NOS

7 ☑7ᵗʰ **T43.292** **Poisoning by other antidepressants, intentional self-harm**   HCC

☑7ᵗʰ **T43.293** **Poisoning by other antidepressants, assault**

☑7ᵗʰ **T43.294** **Poisoning by other antidepressants, undetermined**

☑7ᵗʰ **T43.295** **Adverse effect of other antidepressants**

☑7ᵗʰ **T43.296** **Underdosing of other antidepressants**

N Newborn: 0   P Pediatric: 0-17   M Maternity: 9-64   A Adult: 15-124   MCC Major Complication/Comorbidity   CC Complication/Comorbidity   SW Severe Wound Dx

1158   **ICD-10-CM 2020**

✓5ᵗʰ **T43.3 Poisoning by, adverse effect of and underdosing of phenothiazine antipsychotics and neuroleptics**

  ✓6ᵗʰ **T43.3X Poisoning by, adverse effect of and underdosing of phenothiazine antipsychotics and neuroleptics**

    ✓7ᵗʰ **T43.3X1 Poisoning by phenothiazine antipsychotics and neuroleptics, accidental (unintentional)**
      Poisoning by phenothiazine antipsychotics and neuroleptics NOS

    7 ✓7ᵗʰ **T43.3X2 Poisoning by phenothiazine antipsychotics and neuroleptics, intentional self-harm**   HCC

    ✓7ᵗʰ **T43.3X3 Poisoning by phenothiazine antipsychotics and neuroleptics, assault**

    ✓7ᵗʰ **T43.3X4 Poisoning by phenothiazine antipsychotics and neuroleptics, undetermined**

    ✓7ᵗʰ **T43.3X5 Adverse effect of phenothiazine antipsychotics and neuroleptics**

    ✓7ᵗʰ **T43.3X6 Underdosing of phenothiazine antipsychotics and neuroleptics**

✓5ᵗʰ **T43.4 Poisoning by, adverse effect of and underdosing of butyrophenone and thiothixene neuroleptics**

  ✓6ᵗʰ **T43.4X Poisoning by, adverse effect of and underdosing of butyrophenone and thiothixene neuroleptics**

    ✓7ᵗʰ **T43.4X1 Poisoning by butyrophenone and thiothixene neuroleptics, accidental (unintentional)**
      Poisoning by butyrophenone and thiothixene neuroleptics NOS

    7 ✓7ᵗʰ **T43.4X2 Poisoning by butyrophenone and thiothixene neuroleptics, intentional self-harm**   HCC

    ✓7ᵗʰ **T43.4X3 Poisoning by butyrophenone and thiothixene neuroleptics, assault**

    ✓7ᵗʰ **T43.4X4 Poisoning by butyrophenone and thiothixene neuroleptics, undetermined**

    ✓7ᵗʰ **T43.4X5 Adverse effect of butyrophenone and thiothixene neuroleptics**

    ✓7ᵗʰ **T43.4X6 Underdosing of butyrophenone and thiothixene neuroleptics**

✓5ᵗʰ **T43.5 Poisoning by, adverse effect of and underdosing of other and unspecified antipsychotics and neuroleptics**

    EXCLUDES 1   poisoning by, adverse effect of and underdosing of rauwolfia (T46.5-)

  ✓6ᵗʰ **T43.50 Poisoning by, adverse effect of and underdosing of unspecified antipsychotics and neuroleptics**

    ✓7ᵗʰ **T43.501 Poisoning by unspecified antipsychotics and neuroleptics, accidental (unintentional)**
      Poisoning by antipsychotics and neuroleptics NOS

    7 ✓7ᵗʰ **T43.502 Poisoning by unspecified antipsychotics and neuroleptics, intentional self-harm**   HCC

    ✓7ᵗʰ **T43.503 Poisoning by unspecified antipsychotics and neuroleptics, assault**

    ✓7ᵗʰ **T43.504 Poisoning by unspecified antipsychotics and neuroleptics, undetermined**

    ✓7ᵗʰ **T43.505 Adverse effect of unspecified antipsychotics and neuroleptics**

    ✓7ᵗʰ **T43.506 Underdosing of unspecified antipsychotics and neuroleptics**

  ✓6ᵗʰ **T43.59 Poisoning by, adverse effect of and underdosing of other antipsychotics and neuroleptics**
    AHA: 2017,1Q,40

    ✓7ᵗʰ **T43.591 Poisoning by other antipsychotics and neuroleptics, accidental (unintentional)**
      Poisoning by other antipsychotics and neuroleptics NOS

    7 ✓7ᵗʰ **T43.592 Poisoning by other antipsychotics and neuroleptics, intentional self-harm**   HCC

    ✓7ᵗʰ **T43.593 Poisoning by other antipsychotics and neuroleptics, assault**

    ✓7ᵗʰ **T43.594 Poisoning by other antipsychotics and neuroleptics, undetermined**

    ✓7ᵗʰ **T43.595 Adverse effect of other antipsychotics and neuroleptics**

    ✓7ᵗʰ **T43.596 Underdosing of other antipsychotics and neuroleptics**

✓5ᵗʰ **T43.6 Poisoning by, adverse effect of and underdosing of psychostimulants**

    EXCLUDES 1   poisoning by, adverse effect of and underdosing of cocaine (T40.5-)

  ✓6ᵗʰ **T43.60 Poisoning by, adverse effect of and underdosing of unspecified psychostimulant**

    6 ✓7ᵗʰ **T43.601 Poisoning by unspecified psychostimulants, accidental (unintentional)**   HCC
      Poisoning by psychostimulants NOS

    7 ✓7ᵗʰ **T43.602 Poisoning by unspecified psychostimulants, intentional self-harm**   HCC

    ✓7ᵗʰ **T43.603 Poisoning by unspecified psychostimulants, assault**

    6 ✓7ᵗʰ **T43.604 Poisoning by unspecified psychostimulants, undetermined**   HCC

    ✓7ᵗʰ **T43.605 Adverse effect of unspecified psychostimulants**

    ✓7ᵗʰ **T43.606 Underdosing of unspecified psychostimulants**

  ✓6ᵗʰ **T43.61 Poisoning by, adverse effect of and underdosing of caffeine**

    6 ✓7ᵗʰ **T43.611 Poisoning by caffeine, accidental (unintentional)**   HCC
      Poisoning by caffeine NOS

    7 ✓7ᵗʰ **T43.612 Poisoning by caffeine, intentional self-harm**   HCC

    ✓7ᵗʰ **T43.613 Poisoning by caffeine, assault**

    6 ✓7ᵗʰ **T43.614 Poisoning by caffeine, undetermined**   HCC

    ✓7ᵗʰ **T43.615 Adverse effect of caffeine**

    ✓7ᵗʰ **T43.616 Underdosing of caffeine**

  ✓6ᵗʰ **T43.62 Poisoning by, adverse effect of and underdosing of amphetamines**
    Poisoning by, adverse effect of and underdosing of methamphetamines

    6 ✓7ᵗʰ **T43.621 Poisoning by amphetamines, accidental (unintentional)**   HCC
      Poisoning by amphetamines NOS

    7 ✓7ᵗʰ **T43.622 Poisoning by amphetamines, intentional self-harm**   HCC

    ✓7ᵗʰ **T43.623 Poisoning by amphetamines, assault**

    6 ✓7ᵗʰ **T43.624 Poisoning by amphetamines, undetermined**   HCC

    ✓7ᵗʰ **T43.625 Adverse effect of amphetamines**

    ✓7ᵗʰ **T43.626 Underdosing of amphetamines**

  ✓6ᵗʰ **T43.63 Poisoning by, adverse effect of and underdosing of methylphenidate**

    6 ✓7ᵗʰ **T43.631 Poisoning by methylphenidate, accidental (unintentional)**   HCC
      Poisoning by methylphenidate NOS

    7 ✓7ᵗʰ **T43.632 Poisoning by methylphenidate, intentional self-harm**   HCC

    ✓7ᵗʰ **T43.633 Poisoning by methylphenidate, assault**

    6 ✓7ᵗʰ **T43.634 Poisoning by methylphenidate, undetermined**   HCC

    ✓7ᵗʰ **T43.635 Adverse effect of methylphenidate**

    ✓7ᵗʰ **T43.636 Underdosing of methylphenidate**

  ✓6ᵗʰ **T43.64 Poisoning by ecstasy**
    Poisoning by MDMA
    Poisoning by 3,4-methylenedioxymethamphetamine
    AHA: 2018,4Q,30-31

    6 ✓7ᵗʰ **T43.641 Poisoning by ecstasy, accidental (unintentional)**   HCC
      Poisoning by ecstasy NOS

    7 ✓7ᵗʰ **T43.642 Poisoning by ecstasy, intentional self-harm**   HCC

    ✓7ᵗʰ **T43.643 Poisoning by ecstasy, assault**

✓ Additional Character Required   ✓x7ᵗʰ Placeholder   Unacceptable PDx   Questionable PDx   Manifestation   Unspecified Dx   H1-H14 HAC   HCC CMS-HCC Dx   HIV HIV Dx

ICD-10-CM 2020   1159

Chapter 19. Injury, Poisoning and Certain Other Consequences of External Causes

T43.644–T44.3X6

6 ✓7ᵗʰ **T43.644 Poisoning by ecstasy, undetermined** [HCC]

✓6ᵗʰ **T43.69 Poisoning by, adverse effect of and underdosing of other psychostimulants**

  6 ✓7ᵗʰ **T43.691 Poisoning by other psychostimulants, accidental (unintentional)** [HCC]
    Poisoning by other psychostimulants NOS

  7 ✓7ᵗʰ **T43.692 Poisoning by other psychostimulants, intentional self-harm** [HCC]

  ✓7ᵗʰ **T43.693 Poisoning by other psychostimulants, assault**

  6 ✓7ᵗʰ **T43.694 Poisoning by other psychostimulants, undetermined** [HCC]

  ✓7ᵗʰ **T43.695 Adverse effect of other psychostimulants**

  ✓7ᵗʰ **T43.696 Underdosing of other psychostimulants**

✓5ᵗʰ **T43.8 Poisoning by, adverse effect of and underdosing of other psychotropic drugs**

✓6ᵗʰ **T43.8X Poisoning by, adverse effect of and underdosing of other psychotropic drugs**

  ✓7ᵗʰ **T43.8X1 Poisoning by other psychotropic drugs, accidental (unintentional)**
    Poisoning by other psychotropic drugs NOS

  7 ✓7ᵗʰ **T43.8X2 Poisoning by other psychotropic drugs, intentional self-harm** [HCC]

  ✓7ᵗʰ **T43.8X3 Poisoning by other psychotropic drugs, assault**

  ✓7ᵗʰ **T43.8X4 Poisoning by other psychotropic drugs, undetermined**

  ✓7ᵗʰ **T43.8X5 Adverse effect of other psychotropic drugs**

  ✓7ᵗʰ **T43.8X6 Underdosing of other psychotropic drugs**

✓5ᵗʰ **T43.9 Poisoning by, adverse effect of and underdosing of unspecified psychotropic drug**

  ✓x7ᵗʰ **T43.91 Poisoning by unspecified psychotropic drug, accidental (unintentional)**
    Poisoning by psychotropic drug NOS

  7 ✓x7ᵗʰ **T43.92 Poisoning by unspecified psychotropic drug, intentional self-harm** [HCC]

  ✓x7ᵗʰ **T43.93 Poisoning by unspecified psychotropic drug, assault**

  ✓x7ᵗʰ **T43.94 Poisoning by unspecified psychotropic drug, undetermined**

  ✓x7ᵗʰ **T43.95 Adverse effect of unspecified psychotropic drug**

  ✓x7ᵗʰ **T43.96 Underdosing of unspecified psychotropic drug**

✓4ᵗʰ **T44 Poisoning by, adverse effect of and underdosing of drugs primarily affecting the autonomic nervous system**

The appropriate 7th character is to be added to each code from category T44.
A   initial encounter
D   subsequent encounter
S   sequela

✓5ᵗʰ **T44.0 Poisoning by, adverse effect of and underdosing of anticholinesterase agents**

✓6ᵗʰ **T44.0X Poisoning by, adverse effect of and underdosing of anticholinesterase agents**

  ✓7ᵗʰ **T44.0X1 Poisoning by anticholinesterase agents, accidental (unintentional)**
    Poisoning by anticholinesterase agents NOS

  7 ✓7ᵗʰ **T44.0X2 Poisoning by anticholinesterase agents, intentional self-harm** [HCC]

  ✓7ᵗʰ **T44.0X3 Poisoning by anticholinesterase agents, assault**

  ✓7ᵗʰ **T44.0X4 Poisoning by anticholinesterase agents, undetermined**

  ✓7ᵗʰ **T44.0X5 Adverse effect of anticholinesterase agents**

  ✓7ᵗʰ **T44.0X6 Underdosing of anticholinesterase agents**

✓5ᵗʰ **T44.1 Poisoning by, adverse effect of and underdosing of other parasympathomimetics [cholinergics]**

✓6ᵗʰ **T44.1X Poisoning by, adverse effect of and underdosing of other parasympathomimetics [cholinergics]**

  ✓7ᵗʰ **T44.1X1 Poisoning by other parasympathomimetics [cholinergics], accidental (unintentional)**
    Poisoning by other parasympathomimetics [cholinergics] NOS

  7 ✓7ᵗʰ **T44.1X2 Poisoning by other parasympathomimetics [cholinergics], intentional self-harm** [HCC]

  ✓7ᵗʰ **T44.1X3 Poisoning by other parasympathomimetics [cholinergics], assault**

  ✓7ᵗʰ **T44.1X4 Poisoning by other parasympathomimetics [cholinergics], undetermined**

  ✓7ᵗʰ **T44.1X5 Adverse effect of other parasympathomimetics [cholinergics]**

  ✓7ᵗʰ **T44.1X6 Underdosing of other parasympathomimetics [cholinergics]**

✓5ᵗʰ **T44.2 Poisoning by, adverse effect of and underdosing of ganglionic blocking drugs**

✓6ᵗʰ **T44.2X Poisoning by, adverse effect of and underdosing of ganglionic blocking drugs**

  ✓7ᵗʰ **T44.2X1 Poisoning by ganglionic blocking drugs, accidental (unintentional)**
    Poisoning by ganglionic blocking drugs NOS

  7 ✓7ᵗʰ **T44.2X2 Poisoning by ganglionic blocking drugs, intentional self-harm** [HCC]

  ✓7ᵗʰ **T44.2X3 Poisoning by ganglionic blocking drugs, assault**

  ✓7ᵗʰ **T44.2X4 Poisoning by ganglionic blocking drugs, undetermined**

  ✓7ᵗʰ **T44.2X5 Adverse effect of ganglionic blocking drugs**

  ✓7ᵗʰ **T44.2X6 Underdosing of ganglionic blocking drugs**

✓5ᵗʰ **T44.3 Poisoning by, adverse effect of and underdosing of other parasympatholytics [anticholinergics and antimuscarinics] and spasmolytics**

Poisoning by, adverse effect of and underdosing of papaverine

✓6ᵗʰ **T44.3X Poisoning by, adverse effect of and underdosing of other parasympatholytics [anticholinergics and antimuscarinics] and spasmolytics**

  ✓7ᵗʰ **T44.3X1 Poisoning by other parasympatholytics [anticholinergics and antimuscarinics] and spasmolytics, accidental (unintentional)**
    Poisoning by other parasympatholytics [anticholinergics and antimuscarinics] and spasmolytics NOS

  7 ✓7ᵗʰ **T44.3X2 Poisoning by other parasympatholytics [anticholinergics and antimuscarinics] and spasmolytics, intentional self-harm** [HCC]

  ✓7ᵗʰ **T44.3X3 Poisoning by other parasympatholytics [anticholinergics and antimuscarinics] and spasmolytics, assault**

  ✓7ᵗʰ **T44.3X4 Poisoning by other parasympatholytics [anticholinergics and antimuscarinics] and spasmolytics, undetermined**

  ✓7ᵗʰ **T44.3X5 Adverse effect of other parasympatholytics [anticholinergics and antimuscarinics] and spasmolytics**

  ✓7ᵗʰ **T44.3X6 Underdosing of other parasympatholytics [anticholinergics and antimuscarinics] and spasmolytics**

Ⓝ Newborn: 0   Ⓟ Pediatric: 0-17   Ⓜ Maternity: 9-64   Ⓐ Adult: 15-124   MCC Major Complication/Comorbidity   CC Complication/Comorbidity   SW Severe Wound Dx

1160   ICD-10-CM 2020

√5ᵗʰ **T44.4** **Poisoning by, adverse effect of and underdosing of predominantly alpha-adrenoreceptor agonists**
Poisoning by, adverse effect of and underdosing of metaraminol

√6ᵗʰ **T44.4X** **Poisoning by, adverse effect of and underdosing of** predominantly alpha-adrenoreceptor agonists

√7ᵗʰ **T44.4X1** **Poisoning by predominantly alpha-adrenoreceptor agonists, accidental (unintentional)**
Poisoning by predominantly alpha-adrenoreceptor agonists NOS

7 √7ᵗʰ **T44.4X2** **Poisoning by predominantly alpha-adrenoreceptor agonists, intentional self-harm** 　HCC

√7ᵗʰ **T44.4X3** **Poisoning by predominantly alpha-adrenoreceptor agonists, assault**

√7ᵗʰ **T44.4X4** **Poisoning by predominantly alpha-adrenoreceptor agonists, undetermined**

√7ᵗʰ **T44.4X5** **Adverse effect of predominantly alpha-adrenoreceptor agonists**

√7ᵗʰ **T44.4X6** **Underdosing of predominantly alpha-adrenoreceptor agonists**

√5ᵗʰ **T44.5** **Poisoning by, adverse effect of and underdosing of predominantly beta-adrenoreceptor agonists**
EXCLUDES 1 poisoning by, adverse effect of and underdosing of beta-adrenoreceptor agonists used in asthma therapy (T48.6-)

√6ᵗʰ **T44.5X** **Poisoning by, adverse effect of and underdosing of** predominantly beta-adrenoreceptor agonists

√7ᵗʰ **T44.5X1** **Poisoning by predominantly beta-adrenoreceptor agonists, accidental (unintentional)**
Poisoning by predominantly beta-adrenoreceptor agonists NOS

7 √7ᵗʰ **T44.5X2** **Poisoning by predominantly beta-adrenoreceptor agonists, intentional self-harm** 　HCC

√7ᵗʰ **T44.5X3** **Poisoning by predominantly beta-adrenoreceptor agonists, assault**

√7ᵗʰ **T44.5X4** **Poisoning by predominantly beta-adrenoreceptor agonists, undetermined**

√7ᵗʰ **T44.5X5** **Adverse effect of predominantly beta-adrenoreceptor agonists**

√7ᵗʰ **T44.5X6** **Underdosing of predominantly beta-adrenoreceptor agonists**

√5ᵗʰ **T44.6** **Poisoning by, adverse effect of and underdosing of alpha-adrenoreceptor antagonists**
EXCLUDES 1 poisoning by, adverse effect of and underdosing of ergot alkaloids (T48.0)

√6ᵗʰ **T44.6X** **Poisoning by, adverse effect of and underdosing of** alpha-adrenoreceptor antagonists

√7ᵗʰ **T44.6X1** **Poisoning by alpha-adrenoreceptor antagonists, accidental (unintentional)**
Poisoning by alpha-adrenoreceptor antagonists NOS

7 √7ᵗʰ **T44.6X2** **Poisoning by alpha-adrenoreceptor antagonists, intentional self-harm** 　HCC

√7ᵗʰ **T44.6X3** **Poisoning by alpha-adrenoreceptor antagonists, assault**

√7ᵗʰ **T44.6X4** **Poisoning by alpha-adrenoreceptor antagonists, undetermined**

√7ᵗʰ **T44.6X5** **Adverse effect of alpha-adrenoreceptor antagonists**

√7ᵗʰ **T44.6X6** **Underdosing of alpha-adrenoreceptor antagonists**

√5ᵗʰ **T44.7** **Poisoning by, adverse effect of and underdosing of beta-adrenoreceptor antagonists**

√6ᵗʰ **T44.7X** **Poisoning by, adverse effect of and underdosing of** beta-adrenoreceptor antagonists

√7ᵗʰ **T44.7X1** **Poisoning by beta-adrenoreceptor antagonists, accidental (unintentional)**
Poisoning by beta-adrenoreceptor antagonists NOS

7 √7ᵗʰ **T44.7X2** **Poisoning by beta-adrenoreceptor antagonists, intentional self-harm** 　HCC

√7ᵗʰ **T44.7X3** **Poisoning by beta-adrenoreceptor antagonists, assault**

√7ᵗʰ **T44.7X4** **Poisoning by beta-adrenoreceptor antagonists, undetermined**

√7ᵗʰ **T44.7X5** **Adverse effect of beta-adrenoreceptor antagonists**

√7ᵗʰ **T44.7X6** **Underdosing of beta-adrenoreceptor antagonists**

√5ᵗʰ **T44.8** **Poisoning by, adverse effect of and underdosing of centrally-acting and adrenergic-neuron- blocking agents**
EXCLUDES 1 poisoning by, adverse effect of and underdosing of clonidine (T46.5)
poisoning by, adverse effect of and underdosing of guanethidine (T46.5)

√6ᵗʰ **T44.8X** **Poisoning by, adverse effect of and underdosing of** centrally-acting and adrenergic- neuron-blocking agents

√7ᵗʰ **T44.8X1** **Poisoning by centrally-acting and adrenergic-neuron-blocking agents, accidental (unintentional)**
Poisoning by centrally-acting and adrenergic-neuron-blocking agents NOS

7 √7ᵗʰ **T44.8X2** **Poisoning by centrally-acting and adrenergic-neuron-blocking agents, intentional self-harm** 　HCC

√7ᵗʰ **T44.8X3** **Poisoning by centrally-acting and adrenergic-neuron-blocking agents, assault**

√7ᵗʰ **T44.8X4** **Poisoning by centrally-acting and adrenergic-neuron-blocking agents, undetermined**

√7ᵗʰ **T44.8X5** **Adverse effect of centrally-acting and adrenergic-neuron-blocking agents**

√7ᵗʰ **T44.8X6** **Underdosing of centrally-acting and adrenergic-neuron-blocking agents**

√5ᵗʰ **T44.9** **Poisoning by, adverse effect of and underdosing of other and unspecified drugs primarily affecting the autonomic nervous system**
Poisoning by, adverse effect of and underdosing of drug stimulating both alpha and beta-adrenoreceptors

√6ᵗʰ **T44.90** **Poisoning by, adverse effect of and underdosing of unspecified drugs primarily affecting the autonomic nervous system**

√7ᵗʰ **T44.901** **Poisoning by unspecified drugs primarily affecting the autonomic nervous system, accidental (unintentional)**
Poisoning by unspecified drugs primarily affecting the autonomic nervous system NOS

7 √7ᵗʰ **T44.902** **Poisoning by unspecified drugs primarily affecting the autonomic nervous system, intentional self-harm** 　HCC

√7ᵗʰ **T44.903** **Poisoning by unspecified drugs primarily affecting the autonomic nervous system, assault**

√7ᵗʰ **T44.904** **Poisoning by unspecified drugs primarily affecting the autonomic nervous system, undetermined**

√7ᵗʰ **T44.905** **Adverse effect of unspecified drugs primarily affecting the autonomic nervous system**

√7ᵗʰ **T44.906** **Underdosing of unspecified drugs primarily affecting the autonomic nervous system**

√6ᵗʰ **T44.99** **Poisoning by, adverse effect of and underdosing of other drugs primarily affecting the autonomic nervous system**

√7ᵗʰ **T44.991** **Poisoning by other drug primarily affecting the autonomic nervous system, accidental (unintentional)**
Poisoning by other drugs primarily affecting the autonomic nervous system NOS

7 ✓7ᵗʰ **T44.992** **Poisoning by other drug primarily affecting the autonomic nervous system, intentional self-harm**   HCC

✓7ᵗʰ **T44.993** **Poisoning by other drug primarily affecting the autonomic nervous system, assault**

✓7ᵗʰ **T44.994** **Poisoning by other drug primarily affecting the autonomic nervous system, undetermined**

✓7ᵗʰ **T44.995** **Adverse effect of other drug primarily affecting the autonomic nervous system**

✓7ᵗʰ **T44.996** **Underdosing of other drug primarily affecting the autonomic nervous system**

✓4ᵗʰ **T45** **Poisoning by, adverse effect of and underdosing of primarily systemic and hematological agents, not elsewhere classified**

> The appropriate 7th character is to be added to each code from category T45.
> A   initial encounter
> D   subsequent encounter
> S   sequela

✓5ᵗʰ **T45.0** **Poisoning by, adverse effect of and underdosing of antiallergic and antiemetic drugs**

> EXCLUDES 1   poisoning by, adverse effect of and underdosing of phenothiazine-based neuroleptics (T43.3)

✓6ᵗʰ **T45.0X** **Poisoning by, adverse effect of and underdosing of antiallergic and antiemetic drugs**

✓7ᵗʰ **T45.0X1** **Poisoning by antiallergic and antiemetic drugs, accidental (unintentional)**
> Poisoning by antiallergic and antiemetic drugs NOS

7 ✓7ᵗʰ **T45.0X2** **Poisoning by antiallergic and antiemetic drugs, intentional self-harm**   HCC

✓7ᵗʰ **T45.0X3** **Poisoning by antiallergic and antiemetic drugs, assault**

✓7ᵗʰ **T45.0X4** **Poisoning by antiallergic and antiemetic drugs, undetermined**

✓7ᵗʰ **T45.0X5** **Adverse effect of antiallergic and antiemetic drugs**

✓7ᵗʰ **T45.0X6** **Underdosing of antiallergic and antiemetic drugs**

✓5ᵗʰ **T45.1** **Poisoning by, adverse effect of and underdosing of antineoplastic and immunosuppressive drugs**

> EXCLUDES 1   poisoning by, adverse effect of and underdosing of tamoxifen (T38.6)

> AHA: 2019,1Q,17,20; 2014,4Q,22

✓6ᵗʰ **T45.1X** **Poisoning by, adverse effect of and underdosing of antineoplastic and immunosuppressive drugs**

✓7ᵗʰ **T45.1X1** **Poisoning by antineoplastic and immunosuppressive drugs, accidental (unintentional)**
> Poisoning by antineoplastic and immunosuppressive drugs NOS

7 ✓7ᵗʰ **T45.1X2** **Poisoning by antineoplastic and immunosuppressive drugs, intentional self-harm**   HCC

✓7ᵗʰ **T45.1X3** **Poisoning by antineoplastic and immunosuppressive drugs, assault**

✓7ᵗʰ **T45.1X4** **Poisoning by antineoplastic and immunosuppressive drugs, undetermined**

✓7ᵗʰ **T45.1X5** **Adverse effect of antineoplastic and immunosuppressive drugs**
> AHA: 2019,2Q,24,28

✓7ᵗʰ **T45.1X6** **Underdosing of antineoplastic and immunosuppressive drugs**

Chemo correctly administered

✓5ᵗʰ **T45.2** **Poisoning by, adverse effect of and underdosing of vitamins**

> EXCLUDES 2   poisoning by, adverse effect of and underdosing of iron (T45.4)
> poisoning by, adverse effect of and underdosing of nicotinic acid (derivatives) (T46.7)
> poisoning by, adverse effect of and underdosing of vitamin K (T45.7)

✓6ᵗʰ **T45.2X** **Poisoning by, adverse effect of and underdosing of vitamins**

✓7ᵗʰ **T45.2X1** **Poisoning by vitamins, accidental (unintentional)**
> Poisoning by vitamins NOS

7 ✓7ᵗʰ **T45.2X2** **Poisoning by vitamins, intentional self-harm**   HCC

✓7ᵗʰ **T45.2X3** **Poisoning by vitamins, assault**

✓7ᵗʰ **T45.2X4** **Poisoning by vitamins, undetermined**

✓7ᵗʰ **T45.2X5** **Adverse effect of vitamins**

✓7ᵗʰ **T45.2X6** **Underdosing of vitamins**
> EXCLUDES 1   vitamin deficiencies (E50-E56)

✓5ᵗʰ **T45.3** **Poisoning by, adverse effect of and underdosing of enzymes**

✓6ᵗʰ **T45.3X** **Poisoning by, adverse effect of and underdosing of enzymes**

✓7ᵗʰ **T45.3X1** **Poisoning by enzymes, accidental (unintentional)**
> Poisoning by enzymes NOS

7 ✓7ᵗʰ **T45.3X2** **Poisoning by enzymes, intentional self-harm**   HCC

✓7ᵗʰ **T45.3X3** **Poisoning by enzymes, assault**

✓7ᵗʰ **T45.3X4** **Poisoning by enzymes, undetermined**

✓7ᵗʰ **T45.3X5** **Adverse effect of enzymes**

✓7ᵗʰ **T45.3X6** **Underdosing of enzymes**

✓5ᵗʰ **T45.4** **Poisoning by, adverse effect of and underdosing of iron and its compounds**

✓6ᵗʰ **T45.4X** **Poisoning by, adverse effect of and underdosing of iron and its compounds**

✓7ᵗʰ **T45.4X1** **Poisoning by iron and its compounds, accidental (unintentional)**
> Poisoning by iron and its compounds NOS

7 ✓7ᵗʰ **T45.4X2** **Poisoning by iron and its compounds, intentional self-harm**   HCC

✓7ᵗʰ **T45.4X3** **Poisoning by iron and its compounds, assault**

✓7ᵗʰ **T45.4X4** **Poisoning by iron and its compounds, undetermined**

✓7ᵗʰ **T45.4X5** **Adverse effect of iron and its compounds**

✓7ᵗʰ **T45.4X6** **Underdosing of iron and its compounds**
> EXCLUDES 1   iron deficiency (E61.1)

✓5ᵗʰ **T45.5** **Poisoning by, adverse effect of and underdosing of anticoagulants and antithrombotic drugs**

✓6ᵗʰ **T45.51** **Poisoning by, adverse effect of and underdosing of anticoagulants**

✓7ᵗʰ **T45.511** **Poisoning by anticoagulants, accidental (unintentional)**
> Poisoning by anticoagulants NOS

7 ✓7ᵗʰ **T45.512** **Poisoning by anticoagulants, intentional self-harm**   HCC

✓7ᵗʰ **T45.513** **Poisoning by anticoagulants, assault**

✓7ᵗʰ **T45.514** **Poisoning by anticoagulants, undetermined**

✓7ᵗʰ **T45.515** **Adverse effect of anticoagulants**
> AHA: 2016,1Q,14; 2013,2Q,34

✓7ᵗʰ **T45.516** **Underdosing of anticoagulants**

✓6ᵗʰ **T45.52** **Poisoning by, adverse effect of and underdosing of antithrombotic drugs**
> Poisoning by, adverse effect of and underdosing of antiplatelet drugs
> EXCLUDES 2   poisoning by, adverse effect of and underdosing of aspirin (T39.01-)
> poisoning by, adverse effect of and underdosing of acetylsalicylic acid (T39.01-)

✓7ᵗʰ **T45.521** **Poisoning by antithrombotic drugs, accidental (unintentional)**
> Poisoning by antithrombotic drug NOS

N Newborn: 0   P Pediatric: 0-17   M Maternity: 9-64   A Adult: 15-124   MCC Major Complication/Comorbidity   CC Complication/Comorbidity   SW Severe Wound Dx

1162   ICD-10-CM 2020

7 √7ᵗʰ **T45.522 Poisoning by**   HCC
antithrombotic drugs,
intentional self-harm

√7ᵗʰ **T45.523 Poisoning by antithrombotic drugs,**
assault

√7ᵗʰ **T45.524 Poisoning by antithrombotic drugs,**
undetermined

√7ᵗʰ **T45.525 Adverse effect of antithrombotic drugs**
AHA: 2016,1Q,15

√7ᵗʰ **T45.526 Underdosing of antithrombotic drugs**

√5ᵗʰ **T45.6 Poisoning by, adverse effect of and underdosing of**
fibrinolysis-affecting drugs

√6ᵗʰ **T45.60 Poisoning by, adverse effect of and underdosing**
of unspecified fibrinolysis-affecting drugs

√7ᵗʰ **T45.601 Poisoning by unspecified**
fibrinolysis-affecting drugs, accidental
(unintentional)
Poisoning by fibrinolysis-affecting drug
NOS

7 √7ᵗʰ **T45.602 Poisoning by unspecified**   HCC
fibrinolysis-affecting
drugs, intentional
self-harm

√7ᵗʰ **T45.603 Poisoning by unspecified**
fibrinolysis-affecting drugs, assault

√7ᵗʰ **T45.604 Poisoning by unspecified**
fibrinolysis-affecting drugs,
undetermined

√7ᵗʰ **T45.605 Adverse effect of unspecified**
fibrinolysis-affecting drugs

√7ᵗʰ **T45.606 Underdosing of unspecified**
fibrinolysis-affecting drugs

√6ᵗʰ **T45.61 Poisoning by, adverse effect of and underdosing**
of thrombolytic drugs

√7ᵗʰ **T45.611 Poisoning by thrombolytic drug,**
accidental (unintentional)
Poisoning by thrombolytic drug NOS

7 √7ᵗʰ **T45.612 Poisoning by thrombolytic**   HCC
drug, intentional
self-harm

√7ᵗʰ **T45.613 Poisoning by thrombolytic drug, assault**

√7ᵗʰ **T45.614 Poisoning by thrombolytic drug,**
undetermined

√7ᵗʰ **T45.615 Adverse effect of thrombolytic drugs**
AHA: 2017,2Q,9

√7ᵗʰ **T45.616 Underdosing of thrombolytic drugs**

√6ᵗʰ **T45.62 Poisoning by, adverse effect of and underdosing**
of hemostatic drugs

√7ᵗʰ **T45.621 Poisoning by hemostatic drug, accidental**
(unintentional)
Poisoning by hemostatic drug NOS

7 √7ᵗʰ **T45.622 Poisoning by hemostatic**   HCC
drug, intentional
self-harm

√7ᵗʰ **T45.623 Poisoning by hemostatic drug, assault**

√7ᵗʰ **T45.624 Poisoning by hemostatic drug,**
undetermined

√7ᵗʰ **T45.625 Adverse effect of hemostatic drug**

√7ᵗʰ **T45.626 Underdosing of hemostatic drugs**

√6ᵗʰ **T45.69 Poisoning by, adverse effect of and underdosing**
of other fibrinolysis-affecting drugs

√7ᵗʰ **T45.691 Poisoning by other fibrinolysis-affecting**
drugs, accidental (unintentional)
Poisoning by other fibrinolysis-affecting
drug NOS

7 √7ᵗʰ **T45.692 Poisoning by other**   HCC
fibrinolysis-affecting
drugs, intentional
self-harm

√7ᵗʰ **T45.693 Poisoning by other fibrinolysis-affecting**
drugs, assault

√7ᵗʰ **T45.694 Poisoning by other fibrinolysis-affecting**
drugs, undetermined

√7ᵗʰ **T45.695 Adverse effect of other**
fibrinolysis-affecting drugs

√7ᵗʰ **T45.696 Underdosing of other**
fibrinolysis-affecting drugs

√5ᵗʰ **T45.7 Poisoning by, adverse effect of and underdosing of**
anticoagulant antagonists, vitamin K and other coagulants

√6ᵗʰ **T45.7X Poisoning by, adverse effect of and underdosing**
of anticoagulant antagonists, vitamin K and other
coagulants

√7ᵗʰ **T45.7X1 Poisoning by anticoagulant antagonists,**
vitamin K and other coagulants,
accidental (unintentional)
Poisoning by anticoagulant antagonists,
vitamin K and other coagulants NOS

7 √7ᵗʰ **T45.7X2 Poisoning by**   HCC
anticoagulant
antagonists, vitamin K and
other coagulants,
intentional self-harm

√7ᵗʰ **T45.7X3 Poisoning by anticoagulant antagonists,**
vitamin K and other coagulants, assault

√7ᵗʰ **T45.7X4 Poisoning by anticoagulant antagonists,**
vitamin K and other coagulants,
undetermined

√7ᵗʰ **T45.7X5 Adverse effect of anticoagulant**
antagonists, vitamin K and other
coagulants

√7ᵗʰ **T45.7X6 Underdosing of anticoagulant**
antagonist, vitamin K and other
coagulants
EXCLUDES 1 *vitamin K deficiency (E56.1)*

√5ᵗʰ **T45.8 Poisoning by, adverse effect of and underdosing of other**
primarily systemic and hematological agents
Poisoning by, adverse effect of and underdosing of liver
preparations and other antianemic agents
Poisoning by, adverse effect of and underdosing of natural
blood and blood products
Poisoning by, adverse effect of and underdosing of plasma
substitute
EXCLUDES 2 *poisoning by, adverse effect of and underdosing of*
immunoglobulin (T50.Z1)
poisoning by, adverse effect of and underdosing of
iron (T45.4)
transfusion reactions (T80.-)

√6ᵗʰ **T45.8X Poisoning by, adverse effect of and underdosing**
of other primarily systemic and hematological
agents

√7ᵗʰ **T45.8X1 Poisoning by other primarily systemic**
and hematological agents, accidental
(unintentional)
Poisoning by other primarily systemic and
hematological agents NOS

7 √7ᵗʰ **T45.8X2 Poisoning by other**   HCC
primarily systemic and
hematological agents,
intentional self-harm

√7ᵗʰ **T45.8X3 Poisoning by other primarily systemic**
and hematological agents, assault

√7ᵗʰ **T45.8X4 Poisoning by other primarily systemic**
and hematological agents, undetermined

√7ᵗʰ **T45.8X5 Adverse effect of other primarily systemic**
and hematological agents
AHA: 2016,4Q,42

√7ᵗʰ **T45.8X6 Underdosing of other primarily systemic**
and hematological agents

√5ᵗʰ **T45.9 Poisoning by, adverse effect of and underdosing of**
unspecified primarily systemic and hematological agent

√x7ᵗʰ **T45.91 Poisoning by unspecified primarily systemic and**
hematological agent, accidental (unintentional)
Poisoning by primarily systemic and hematological
agent NOS

7 √x7ᵗʰ **T45.92 Poisoning by unspecified primarily**   HCC
systemic and hematological agent,
intentional self-harm

√x7ᵗʰ **T45.93 Poisoning by unspecified primarily systemic and**
hematological agent, assault

√x7ᵗʰ **T45.94 Poisoning by unspecified primarily systemic and**
hematological agent, undetermined

√x7ᵗʰ **T45.95 Adverse effect of unspecified primarily systemic**
and hematological agent

√x7ᵗʰ **T45.96 Underdosing of unspecified primarily systemic and**
hematological agent

✅ Additional Character Required   √x7ᵗʰ Placeholder   Unacceptable PDx   Questionable PDx   Manifestation   Unspecified Dx   H1-H14 HAC   HCC CMS-HCC Dx   HIV HIV Dx

ICD-10-CM 2020   1163

√4ᵗʰ **T46** **Poisoning by, adverse effect of and underdosing of agents primarily affecting the cardiovascular system**

> EXCLUDES 1 *poisoning by, adverse effect of and underdosing of metaraminol (T44.4)*

> The appropriate 7th character is to be added to each code from category T46.
> A initial encounter
> D subsequent encounter
> S sequela

√5ᵗʰ **T46.Ø** **Poisoning by, adverse effect of and underdosing of cardiac-stimulant glycosides and drugs of similar action**

√6ᵗʰ **T46.ØX** **Poisoning by, adverse effect of and underdosing of cardiac-stimulant glycosides and drugs of similar action**

√7ᵗʰ **T46.ØX1** **Poisoning by cardiac-stimulant glycosides and drugs of similar action, accidental (unintentional)**
Poisoning by cardiac-stimulant glycosides and drugs of similar action NOS

7 √7ᵗʰ **T46.ØX2** **Poisoning by cardiac-stimulant glycosides and drugs of similar action, intentional self-harm** HCC

√7ᵗʰ **T46.ØX3** **Poisoning by cardiac-stimulant glycosides and drugs of similar action, assault**

√7ᵗʰ **T46.ØX4** **Poisoning by cardiac-stimulant glycosides and drugs of similar action, undetermined**

√7ᵗʰ **T46.ØX5** **Adverse effect of cardiac-stimulant glycosides and drugs of similar action**

√7ᵗʰ **T46.ØX6** **Underdosing of cardiac-stimulant glycosides and drugs of similar action**

√5ᵗʰ **T46.1** **Poisoning by, adverse effect of and underdosing of calcium-channel blockers**

√6ᵗʰ **T46.1X** **Poisoning by, adverse effect of and underdosing of calcium-channel blockers**

√7ᵗʰ **T46.1X1** **Poisoning by calcium-channel blockers, accidental (unintentional)**
Poisoning by calcium-channel blockers NOS

7 √7ᵗʰ **T46.1X2** **Poisoning by calcium-channel blockers, intentional self-harm** HCC

√7ᵗʰ **T46.1X3** **Poisoning by calcium-channel blockers, assault**

√7ᵗʰ **T46.1X4** **Poisoning by calcium-channel blockers, undetermined**

√7ᵗʰ **T46.1X5** **Adverse effect of calcium-channel blockers**

√7ᵗʰ **T46.1X6** **Underdosing of calcium-channel blockers**

√5ᵗʰ **T46.2** **Poisoning by, adverse effect of and underdosing of other antidysrhythmic drugs, not elsewhere classified**

> EXCLUDES 1 *poisoning by, adverse effect of and underdosing of beta-adrenoreceptor antagonists (T44.7-)*

√6ᵗʰ **T46.2X** **Poisoning by, adverse effect of and underdosing of other antidysrhythmic drugs**

√7ᵗʰ **T46.2X1** **Poisoning by other antidysrhythmic drugs, accidental (unintentional)**
Poisoning by other antidysrhythmic drugs NOS

7 √7ᵗʰ **T46.2X2** **Poisoning by other antidysrhythmic drugs, intentional self-harm** HCC

√7ᵗʰ **T46.2X3** **Poisoning by other antidysrhythmic drugs, assault**

√7ᵗʰ **T46.2X4** **Poisoning by other antidysrhythmic drugs, undetermined**

√7ᵗʰ **T46.2X5** **Adverse effect of other antidysrhythmic drugs**

√7ᵗʰ **T46.2X6** **Underdosing of other antidysrhythmic drugs**

√5ᵗʰ **T46.3** **Poisoning by, adverse effect of and underdosing of coronary vasodilators**
Poisoning by, adverse effect of and underdosing of dipyridamole

> EXCLUDES 1 *poisoning by, adverse effect of and underdosing of calcium-channel blockers (T46.1)*

√6ᵗʰ **T46.3X** **Poisoning by, adverse effect of and underdosing of coronary vasodilators**

√7ᵗʰ **T46.3X1** **Poisoning by coronary vasodilators, accidental (unintentional)**
Poisoning by coronary vasodilators NOS

7 √7ᵗʰ **T46.3X2** **Poisoning by coronary vasodilators, intentional self-harm** HCC

√7ᵗʰ **T46.3X3** **Poisoning by coronary vasodilators, assault**

√7ᵗʰ **T46.3X4** **Poisoning by coronary vasodilators, undetermined**

√7ᵗʰ **T46.3X5** **Adverse effect of coronary vasodilators**

√7ᵗʰ **T46.3X6** **Underdosing of coronary vasodilators**

√5ᵗʰ **T46.4** **Poisoning by, adverse effect of and underdosing of angiotensin-converting-enzyme inhibitors**

√6ᵗʰ **T46.4X** **Poisoning by, adverse effect of and underdosing of angiotensin-converting-enzyme inhibitors**

√7ᵗʰ **T46.4X1** **Poisoning by angiotensin-converting-enzyme inhibitors, accidental (unintentional)**
Poisoning by angiotensin-converting-enzyme inhibitors NOS

7 √7ᵗʰ **T46.4X2** **Poisoning by angiotensin-converting-enzyme inhibitors, intentional self-harm** HCC

√7ᵗʰ **T46.4X3** **Poisoning by angiotensin-converting-enzyme inhibitors, assault**

√7ᵗʰ **T46.4X4** **Poisoning by angiotensin-converting-enzyme inhibitors, undetermined**

√7ᵗʰ **T46.4X5** **Adverse effect of angiotensin-converting-enzyme inhibitors**

√7ᵗʰ **T46.4X6** **Underdosing of angiotensin-converting-enzyme inhibitors**

√5ᵗʰ **T46.5** **Poisoning by, adverse effect of and underdosing of other antihypertensive drugs**

> EXCLUDES 2 *poisoning by, adverse effect of and underdosing of beta-adrenoreceptor antagonists (T44.7)*
> *poisoning by, adverse effect of and underdosing of calcium-channel blockers (T46.1)*
> *poisoning by, adverse effect of and underdosing of diuretics (T50.Ø-T50.2)*

√6ᵗʰ **T46.5X** **Poisoning by, adverse effect of and underdosing of other antihypertensive drugs**

√7ᵗʰ **T46.5X1** **Poisoning by other antihypertensive drugs, accidental (unintentional)**
Poisoning by other antihypertensive drugs NOS

7 √7ᵗʰ **T46.5X2** **Poisoning by other antihypertensive drugs, intentional self-harm** HCC

√7ᵗʰ **T46.5X3** **Poisoning by other antihypertensive drugs, assault**

√7ᵗʰ **T46.5X4** **Poisoning by other antihypertensive drugs, undetermined**

√7ᵗʰ **T46.5X5** **Adverse effect of other antihypertensive drugs**

√7ᵗʰ **T46.5X6** **Underdosing of other antihypertensive drugs**

√5ᵗʰ **T46.6** **Poisoning by, adverse effect of and underdosing of antihyperlipidemic and antiarteriosclerotic drugs**

√6ᵗʰ **T46.6X** **Poisoning by, adverse effect of and underdosing of antihyperlipidemic and antiarteriosclerotic drugs**

√7ᵗʰ **T46.6X1** **Poisoning by antihyperlipidemic and antiarteriosclerotic drugs, accidental (unintentional)**
Poisoning by antihyperlipidemic and antiarteriosclerotic drugs NOS

7 √7ᵗʰ **T46.6X2** Poisoning by antihyperlipidemic and antiarteriosclerotic drugs, intentional self-harm   `HCC`

√7ᵗʰ **T46.6X3** Poisoning by antihyperlipidemic and antiarteriosclerotic drugs, assault

√7ᵗʰ **T46.6X4** Poisoning by antihyperlipidemic and antiarteriosclerotic drugs, undetermined

√7ᵗʰ **T46.6X5** Adverse effect of antihyperlipidemic and antiarteriosclerotic drugs

√7ᵗʰ **T46.6X6** Underdosing of antihyperlipidemic and antiarteriosclerotic drugs

√5ᵗʰ **T46.7** Poisoning by, adverse effect of and underdosing of peripheral vasodilators

Poisoning by, adverse effect of and underdosing of nicotinic acid (derivatives)

EXCLUDES 1   *poisoning by, adverse effect of and underdosing of papaverine (T44.3)*

√6ᵗʰ **T46.7X** Poisoning by, adverse effect of and underdosing of peripheral vasodilators

√7ᵗʰ **T46.7X1** Poisoning by peripheral vasodilators, accidental (unintentional)

Poisoning by peripheral vasodilators NOS

7 √7ᵗʰ **T46.7X2** Poisoning by peripheral vasodilators, intentional self-harm   `HCC`

√7ᵗʰ **T46.7X3** Poisoning by peripheral vasodilators, assault

√7ᵗʰ **T46.7X4** Poisoning by peripheral vasodilators, undetermined

√7ᵗʰ **T46.7X5** Adverse effect of peripheral vasodilators

√7ᵗʰ **T46.7X6** Underdosing of peripheral vasodilators

√5ᵗʰ **T46.8** Poisoning by, adverse effect of and underdosing of antivaricose drugs, including sclerosing agents

√6ᵗʰ **T46.8X** Poisoning by, adverse effect of and underdosing of antivaricose drugs, including sclerosing agents

√7ᵗʰ **T46.8X1** Poisoning by antivaricose drugs, including sclerosing agents, accidental (unintentional)

Poisoning by antivaricose drugs, including sclerosing agents NOS

7 √7ᵗʰ **T46.8X2** Poisoning by antivaricose drugs, including sclerosing agents, intentional self-harm   `HCC`

√7ᵗʰ **T46.8X3** Poisoning by antivaricose drugs, including sclerosing agents, assault

√7ᵗʰ **T46.8X4** Poisoning by antivaricose drugs, including sclerosing agents, undetermined

√7ᵗʰ **T46.8X5** Adverse effect of antivaricose drugs, including sclerosing agents

√7ᵗʰ **T46.8X6** Underdosing of antivaricose drugs, including sclerosing agents

√5ᵗʰ **T46.9** Poisoning by, adverse effect of and underdosing of other and unspecified agents primarily affecting the cardiovascular system

√6ᵗʰ **T46.90** Poisoning by, adverse effect of and underdosing of unspecified agents primarily affecting the cardiovascular system

√7ᵗʰ **T46.901** Poisoning by unspecified agents primarily affecting the cardiovascular system, accidental (unintentional)

7 √7ᵗʰ **T46.902** Poisoning by unspecified agents primarily affecting the cardiovascular system, intentional self-harm   `HCC`

√7ᵗʰ **T46.903** Poisoning by unspecified agents primarily affecting the cardiovascular system, assault

√7ᵗʰ **T46.904** Poisoning by unspecified agents primarily affecting the cardiovascular system, undetermined

√7ᵗʰ **T46.905** Adverse effect of unspecified agents primarily affecting the cardiovascular system

√7ᵗʰ **T46.906** Underdosing of unspecified agents primarily affecting the cardiovascular system

√6ᵗʰ **T46.99** Poisoning by, adverse effect of and underdosing of other agents primarily affecting the cardiovascular system

√7ᵗʰ **T46.991** Poisoning by other agents primarily affecting the cardiovascular system, accidental (unintentional)

7 √7ᵗʰ **T46.992** Poisoning by other agents primarily affecting the cardiovascular system, intentional self-harm   `HCC`

√7ᵗʰ **T46.993** Poisoning by other agents primarily affecting the cardiovascular system, assault

√7ᵗʰ **T46.994** Poisoning by other agents primarily affecting the cardiovascular system, undetermined

√7ᵗʰ **T46.995** Adverse effect of other agents primarily affecting the cardiovascular system

√7ᵗʰ **T46.996** Underdosing of other agents primarily affecting the cardiovascular system

√4ᵗʰ **T47** Poisoning by, adverse effect of and underdosing of agents primarily affecting the gastrointestinal system

The appropriate 7th character is to be added to each code from category T47.
A   initial encounter
D   subsequent encounter
S   sequela

√5ᵗʰ **T47.0** Poisoning by, adverse effect of and underdosing of histamine H2-receptor blockers

√6ᵗʰ **T47.0X** Poisoning by, adverse effect of and underdosing of histamine H2-receptor blockers

√7ᵗʰ **T47.0X1** Poisoning by histamine H2-receptor blockers, accidental (unintentional)

Poisoning by histamine H2-receptor blockers NOS

7 √7ᵗʰ **T47.0X2** Poisoning by histamine H2-receptor blockers, intentional self-harm   `HCC`

√7ᵗʰ **T47.0X3** Poisoning by histamine H2-receptor blockers, assault

√7ᵗʰ **T47.0X4** Poisoning by histamine H2-receptor blockers, undetermined

√7ᵗʰ **T47.0X5** Adverse effect of histamine H2-receptor blockers

√7ᵗʰ **T47.0X6** Underdosing of histamine H2-receptor blockers

√5ᵗʰ **T47.1** Poisoning by, adverse effect of and underdosing of other antacids and anti-gastric-secretion drugs

√6ᵗʰ **T47.1X** Poisoning by, adverse effect of and underdosing of other antacids and anti-gastric-secretion drugs

√7ᵗʰ **T47.1X1** Poisoning by other antacids and anti-gastric-secretion drugs, accidental (unintentional)

Poisoning by other antacids and anti-gastric-secretion drugs NOS

7 √7ᵗʰ **T47.1X2** Poisoning by other antacids and anti-gastric-secretion drugs, intentional self-harm   `HCC`

√7ᵗʰ **T47.1X3** Poisoning by other antacids and anti-gastric-secretion drugs, assault

√7ᵗʰ **T47.1X4** Poisoning by other antacids and anti-gastric-secretion drugs, undetermined

√7ᵗʰ **T47.1X5** Adverse effect of other antacids and anti-gastric-secretion drugs

√7ᵗʰ **T47.1X6** Underdosing of other antacids and anti-gastric-secretion drugs

√5ᵗʰ **T47.2** Poisoning by, adverse effect of and underdosing of stimulant laxatives

√6ᵗʰ **T47.2X** Poisoning by, adverse effect of and underdosing of stimulant laxatives

√7ᵗʰ **T47.2X1** Poisoning by stimulant laxatives, accidental (unintentional)

Poisoning by stimulant laxatives NOS

7 √7ᵗʰ **T47.2X2** Poisoning by stimulant laxatives, intentional self-harm   `HCC`

√7ᵗʰ **T47.2X3** Poisoning by stimulant laxatives, assault

√7ᵗʰ **T47.2X4** Poisoning by stimulant laxatives, undetermined

✅ Additional Character Required   √x7ᵗʰ Placeholder   Unacceptable PDx   Questionable PDx   Manifestation   Unspecified Dx   `H1`-`H14` HAC   `HCC` CMS-HCC Dx   `HIV` HIV Dx

✓7ᵗʰ **T47.2X5** Adverse effect of stimulant laxatives

✓7ᵗʰ **T47.2X6** Underdosing of stimulant laxatives

✓5ᵗʰ **T47.3** Poisoning by, adverse effect of and underdosing of saline and osmotic laxatives

✓6ᵗʰ **T47.3X** Poisoning by and adverse effect of saline and osmotic laxatives

✓7ᵗʰ **T47.3X1** Poisoning by saline and osmotic laxatives, accidental (unintentional)

Poisoning by saline and osmotic laxatives NOS

7 ✓7ᵗʰ **T47.3X2** Poisoning by saline and osmotic laxatives, intentional self-harm HCC

✓7ᵗʰ **T47.3X3** Poisoning by saline and osmotic laxatives, assault

✓7ᵗʰ **T47.3X4** Poisoning by saline and osmotic laxatives, undetermined

✓7ᵗʰ **T47.3X5** Adverse effect of saline and osmotic laxatives

✓7ᵗʰ **T47.3X6** Underdosing of saline and osmotic laxatives

✓5ᵗʰ **T47.4** Poisoning by, adverse effect of and underdosing of other laxatives

✓6ᵗʰ **T47.4X** Poisoning by, adverse effect of and underdosing of other laxatives

✓7ᵗʰ **T47.4X1** Poisoning by other laxatives, accidental (unintentional)

Poisoning by other laxatives NOS

7 ✓7ᵗʰ **T47.4X2** Poisoning by other laxatives, intentional self-harm HCC

✓7ᵗʰ **T47.4X3** Poisoning by other laxatives, assault

✓7ᵗʰ **T47.4X4** Poisoning by other laxatives, undetermined

✓7ᵗʰ **T47.4X5** Adverse effect of other laxatives

✓7ᵗʰ **T47.4X6** Underdosing of other laxatives

✓5ᵗʰ **T47.5** Poisoning by, adverse effect of and underdosing of digestants

✓6ᵗʰ **T47.5X** Poisoning by, adverse effect of and underdosing of digestants

✓7ᵗʰ **T47.5X1** Poisoning by digestants, accidental (unintentional)

Poisoning by digestants NOS

7 ✓7ᵗʰ **T47.5X2** Poisoning by digestants, intentional self-harm HCC

✓7ᵗʰ **T47.5X3** Poisoning by digestants, assault

✓7ᵗʰ **T47.5X4** Poisoning by digestants, undetermined

✓7ᵗʰ **T47.5X5** Adverse effect of digestants

✓7ᵗʰ **T47.5X6** Underdosing of digestants

✓5ᵗʰ **T47.6** Poisoning by, adverse effect of and underdosing of antidiarrheal drugs

EXCLUDES 2 poisoning by, adverse effect of and underdosing of systemic antibiotics and other anti-infectives (T36-T37)

✓6ᵗʰ **T47.6X** Poisoning by, adverse effect of and underdosing of antidiarrheal drugs

✓7ᵗʰ **T47.6X1** Poisoning by antidiarrheal drugs, accidental (unintentional)

Poisoning by antidiarrheal drugs NOS

7 ✓7ᵗʰ **T47.6X2** Poisoning by antidiarrheal drugs, intentional self-harm HCC

✓7ᵗʰ **T47.6X3** Poisoning by antidiarrheal drugs, assault

✓7ᵗʰ **T47.6X4** Poisoning by antidiarrheal drugs, undetermined

✓7ᵗʰ **T47.6X5** Adverse effect of antidiarrheal drugs

✓7ᵗʰ **T47.6X6** Underdosing of antidiarrheal drugs

✓5ᵗʰ **T47.7** Poisoning by, adverse effect of and underdosing of emetics

✓6ᵗʰ **T47.7X** Poisoning by, adverse effect of and underdosing of emetics

✓7ᵗʰ **T47.7X1** Poisoning by emetics, accidental (unintentional)

Poisoning by emetics NOS

7 ✓7ᵗʰ **T47.7X2** Poisoning by emetics, intentional self-harm HCC

✓7ᵗʰ **T47.7X3** Poisoning by emetics, assault

✓7ᵗʰ **T47.7X4** Poisoning by emetics, undetermined

✓7ᵗʰ **T47.7X5** Adverse effect of emetics

✓7ᵗʰ **T47.7X6** Underdosing of emetics

✓5ᵗʰ **T47.8** Poisoning by, adverse effect of and underdosing of other agents primarily affecting gastrointestinal system

✓6ᵗʰ **T47.8X** Poisoning by, adverse effect of and underdosing of other agents primarily affecting gastrointestinal system

✓7ᵗʰ **T47.8X1** Poisoning by other agents primarily affecting gastrointestinal system, accidental (unintentional)

Poisoning by other agents primarily affecting gastrointestinal system NOS

7 ✓7ᵗʰ **T47.8X2** Poisoning by other agents primarily affecting gastrointestinal system, intentional self-harm HCC

✓7ᵗʰ **T47.8X3** Poisoning by other agents primarily affecting gastrointestinal system, assault

✓7ᵗʰ **T47.8X4** Poisoning by other agents primarily affecting gastrointestinal system, undetermined

✓7ᵗʰ **T47.8X5** Adverse effect of other agents primarily affecting gastrointestinal system

✓7ᵗʰ **T47.8X6** Underdosing of other agents primarily affecting gastrointestinal system

✓5ᵗʰ **T47.9** Poisoning by, adverse effect of and underdosing of unspecified agents primarily affecting the gastrointestinal system

✓x7ᵗʰ **T47.91** Poisoning by unspecified agents primarily affecting the gastrointestinal system, accidental (unintentional)

Poisoning by agents primarily affecting the gastrointestinal system NOS

7 ✓x7ᵗʰ **T47.92** Poisoning by unspecified agents primarily affecting the gastrointestinal system, intentional self-harm HCC

✓x7ᵗʰ **T47.93** Poisoning by unspecified agents primarily affecting the gastrointestinal system, assault

✓x7ᵗʰ **T47.94** Poisoning by unspecified agents primarily affecting the gastrointestinal system, undetermined

✓x7ᵗʰ **T47.95** Adverse effect of unspecified agents primarily affecting the gastrointestinal system

✓x7ᵗʰ **T47.96** Underdosing of unspecified agents primarily affecting the gastrointestinal system

✓4ᵗʰ **T48** Poisoning by, adverse effect of and underdosing of agents primarily acting on smooth and skeletal muscles and the respiratory system

The appropriate 7th character is to be added to each code from category T48.
A initial encounter
D subsequent encounter
S sequela

✓5ᵗʰ **T48.0** Poisoning by, adverse effect of and underdosing of oxytocic drugs

EXCLUDES 1 poisoning by, adverse effect of and underdosing of estrogens, progestogens and antagonists (T38.4-T38.6)

✓6ᵗʰ **T48.0X** Poisoning by, adverse effect of and underdosing of oxytocic drugs

✓7ᵗʰ **T48.0X1** Poisoning by oxytocic drugs, accidental (unintentional)

Poisoning by oxytocic drugs NOS

7 ✓7ᵗʰ **T48.0X2** Poisoning by oxytocic drugs, intentional self-harm HCC

✓7ᵗʰ **T48.0X3** Poisoning by oxytocic drugs, assault

✓7ᵗʰ **T48.0X4** Poisoning by oxytocic drugs, undetermined

✓7ᵗʰ **T48.0X5** Adverse effect of oxytocic drugs

✓7ᵗʰ **T48.0X6** Underdosing of oxytocic drugs

✓5ᵗʰ **T48.1** Poisoning by, adverse effect of and underdosing of skeletal muscle relaxants [neuromuscular blocking agents]

✓6ᵗʰ **T48.1X** Poisoning by, adverse effect of and underdosing of skeletal muscle relaxants [neuromuscular blocking agents]

✓7ᵗʰ **T48.1X1** Poisoning by skeletal muscle relaxants [neuromuscular blocking agents], accidental (unintentional)

Poisoning by skeletal muscle relaxants [neuromuscular blocking agents] NOS

7 √7th **T48.1X2 Poisoning by skeletal**   HCC
**muscle relaxants
[neuromuscular blocking
agents], intentional
self-harm**

√7th **T48.1X3 Poisoning by skeletal muscle relaxants
[neuromuscular blocking agents], assault**

√7th **T48.1X4 Poisoning by skeletal muscle relaxants
[neuromuscular blocking agents],
undetermined**

√7th **T48.1X5 Adverse effect of skeletal muscle
relaxants [neuromuscular blocking
agents]**

√7th **T48.1X6 Underdosing of skeletal muscle relaxants
[neuromuscular blocking agents]**

√5th **T48.2 Poisoning by, adverse effect of and underdosing of other
and unspecified drugs acting on muscles**

√6th **T48.20 Poisoning by, adverse effect of and underdosing
of unspecified drugs acting on muscles**

√7th **T48.201 Poisoning by unspecified drugs acting on
muscles, accidental (unintentional)**
Poisoning by unspecified drugs acting on
muscles NOS

7 √7th **T48.202 Poisoning by unspecified**   HCC
**drugs acting on muscles,
intentional self-harm**

√7th **T48.203 Poisoning by unspecified drugs acting on
muscles, assault**

√7th **T48.204 Poisoning by unspecified drugs acting on
muscles, undetermined**

√7th **T48.205 Adverse effect of unspecified drugs
acting on muscles**

√7th **T48.206 Underdosing of unspecified drugs acting
on muscles**

√6th **T48.29 Poisoning by, adverse effect of and underdosing
of other drugs acting on muscles**

√7th **T48.291 Poisoning by other drugs acting on
muscles, accidental (unintentional)**
Poisoning by other drugs acting on
muscles NOS

7 √7th **T48.292 Poisoning by other drugs**   HCC
**acting on muscles,
intentional self-harm**

√7th **T48.293 Poisoning by other drugs acting on
muscles, assault**

√7th **T48.294 Poisoning by other drugs acting on
muscles, undetermined**

√7th **T48.295 Adverse effect of other drugs acting on
muscles**

√7th **T48.296 Underdosing of other drugs acting on
muscles**

√5th **T48.3 Poisoning by, adverse effect of and underdosing of
antitussives**

√6th **T48.3X Poisoning by, adverse effect of and underdosing
of antitussives**

√7th **T48.3X1 Poisoning by antitussives, accidental
(unintentional)**
Poisoning by antitussives NOS

7 √7th **T48.3X2 Poisoning by antitussives,**   HCC
intentional self-harm

√7th **T48.3X3 Poisoning by antitussives, assault**

√7th **T48.3X4 Poisoning by antitussives, undetermined**

√7th **T48.3X5 Adverse effect of antitussives**

√7th **T48.3X6 Underdosing of antitussives**

√5th **T48.4 Poisoning by, adverse effect of and underdosing of
expectorants**

√6th **T48.4X Poisoning by, adverse effect of and underdosing
of expectorants**

√7th **T48.4X1 Poisoning by expectorants, accidental
(unintentional)**
Poisoning by expectorants NOS

7 √7th **T48.4X2 Poisoning by**   HCC
**expectorants, intentional
self-harm**

√7th **T48.4X3 Poisoning by expectorants, assault**

√7th **T48.4X4 Poisoning by expectorants,
undetermined**

√7th **T48.4X5 Adverse effect of expectorants**

√7th **T48.4X6 Underdosing of expectorants**

√5th **T48.5 Poisoning by, adverse effect of and underdosing of other
anti-common-cold drugs**
Poisoning by, adverse effect of and underdosing of
decongestants
EXCLUDES 2   *poisoning by, adverse effect of and underdosing of
antipyretics, NEC (T39.9-)*
*poisoning by, adverse effect of and underdosing of
non-steroidal antiinflammatory drugs (T39.3-)*
*poisoning by, adverse effect of and underdosing of
salicylates (T39.0-)*

√6th **T48.5X Poisoning by, adverse effect of and underdosing
of other anti-common-cold drugs**

√7th **T48.5X1 Poisoning by other anti-common-cold
drugs, accidental (unintentional)**
Poisoning by other anti-common-cold
drugs NOS

7 √7th **T48.5X2 Poisoning by other**   HCC
**anti-common-cold drugs,
intentional self-harm**

√7th **T48.5X3 Poisoning by other anti-common-cold
drugs, assault**

√7th **T48.5X4 Poisoning by other anti-common-cold
drugs, undetermined**

√7th **T48.5X5 Adverse effect of other anti-common-cold
drugs**

√7th **T48.5X6 Underdosing of other anti-common-cold
drugs**

√5th **T48.6 Poisoning by, adverse effect of and underdosing of
antiasthmatics, not elsewhere classified**
Poisoning by, adverse effect of and underdosing of
beta-adrenoreceptor agonists used in asthma therapy
EXCLUDES 1   *poisoning by, adverse effect of and underdosing of
anterior pituitary [adenohypophyseal]
hormones (T38.8)*
*poisoning by, adverse effect of and underdosing of
beta-adrenoreceptor agonists not used in
asthma therapy (T44.5)*

√6th **T48.6X Poisoning by, adverse effect of and underdosing
of antiasthmatics**

√7th **T48.6X1 Poisoning by antiasthmatics, accidental
(unintentional)**
Poisoning by antiasthmatics NOS

7 √7th **T48.6X2 Poisoning by**   HCC
**antiasthmatics,
intentional self-harm**

√7th **T48.6X3 Poisoning by antiasthmatics, assault**

√7th **T48.6X4 Poisoning by antiasthmatics,
undetermined**

√7th **T48.6X5 Adverse effect of antiasthmatics**

√7th **T48.6X6 Underdosing of antiasthmatics**

√5th **T48.9 Poisoning by, adverse effect of and underdosing of other
and unspecified agents primarily acting on the respiratory
system**

√6th **T48.90 Poisoning by, adverse effect of and underdosing
of unspecified agents primarily acting on the
respiratory system**

√7th **T48.901 Poisoning by unspecified agents
primarily acting on the respiratory
system, accidental (unintentional)**

7 √7th **T48.902 Poisoning by unspecified**   HCC
**agents primarily acting on
the respiratory system,
intentional self-harm**

√7th **T48.903 Poisoning by unspecified agents
primarily acting on the respiratory
system, assault**

√7th **T48.904 Poisoning by unspecified agents
primarily acting on the respiratory
system, undetermined**

√7th **T48.905 Adverse effect of unspecified agents
primarily acting on the respiratory system**

√7th **T48.906 Underdosing of unspecified agents
primarily acting on the respiratory system**

√6th **T48.99 Poisoning by, adverse effect of and underdosing
of other agents primarily acting on the respiratory
system**

√7th **T48.991 Poisoning by other agents primarily
acting on the respiratory system,
accidental (unintentional)**

Chapter 19. Injury, Poisoning and Certain Other Consequences of External Causes

T48.1X2–T48.991

Chapter 19. Injury, Poisoning and Certain Other Consequences of External Causes

7 √7ᵗʰ **T48.992** **Poisoning by other agents primarily acting on the respiratory system, intentional self-harm**   `HCC`

√7ᵗʰ **T48.993** **Poisoning by other agents primarily acting on the respiratory system,** assault

√7ᵗʰ **T48.994** **Poisoning by other agents primarily acting on the respiratory system, undetermined**

√7ᵗʰ **T48.995** Adverse effect **of other agents primarily acting on the respiratory system**

√7ᵗʰ **T48.996** Underdosing **of other agents primarily acting on the respiratory system**

√4ᵗʰ **T49** **Poisoning by, adverse effect of and underdosing of topical agents primarily affecting skin and mucous membrane and by ophthalmological, otorhinolaryngological and dental drugs**

> INCLUDES   poisoning by, adverse effect of and underdosing of glucocorticoids, topically used

> The appropriate 7th character is to be added to each code from category T49.
> A   initial encounter
> D   subsequent encounter
> S   sequela

√5ᵗʰ **T49.0** **Poisoning by, adverse effect of and underdosing of local antifungal, anti-infective and anti-inflammatory drugs**

√6ᵗʰ **T49.0X** **Poisoning by, adverse effect of and underdosing of** local antifungal, anti-infective and anti-inflammatory drugs

√7ᵗʰ **T49.0X1** **Poisoning by local antifungal, anti-infective and anti-inflammatory drugs,** accidental (unintentional)
Poisoning by local antifungal, anti-infective and anti-inflammatory drugs NOS

7 √7ᵗʰ **T49.0X2** **Poisoning by local antifungal, anti-infective and anti-inflammatory drugs,** intentional self-harm   `HCC`

√7ᵗʰ **T49.0X3** **Poisoning by local antifungal, anti-infective and anti-inflammatory drugs,** assault

√7ᵗʰ **T49.0X4** **Poisoning by local antifungal, anti-infective and anti-inflammatory drugs,** undetermined

√7ᵗʰ **T49.0X5** Adverse effect **of local antifungal, anti-infective and anti-inflammatory drugs**

√7ᵗʰ **T49.0X6** Underdosing **of local antifungal, anti-infective and anti-inflammatory drugs**

√5ᵗʰ **T49.1** **Poisoning by, adverse effect of and underdosing of antipruritics**

√6ᵗʰ **T49.1X** **Poisoning by, adverse effect of and underdosing of** antipruritics

√7ᵗʰ **T49.1X1** **Poisoning by antipruritics,** accidental (unintentional)
Poisoning by antipruritics NOS

7 √7ᵗʰ **T49.1X2** **Poisoning by antipruritics,** intentional self-harm   `HCC`

√7ᵗʰ **T49.1X3** **Poisoning by antipruritics,** assault

√7ᵗʰ **T49.1X4** **Poisoning by antipruritics,** undetermined

√7ᵗʰ **T49.1X5** Adverse effect **of antipruritics**

√7ᵗʰ **T49.1X6** Underdosing **of antipruritics**

√5ᵗʰ **T49.2** **Poisoning by, adverse effect of and underdosing of local astringents and local detergents**

√6ᵗʰ **T49.2X** **Poisoning by, adverse effect of and underdosing of** local astringents and local detergents

√7ᵗʰ **T49.2X1** **Poisoning by local astringents and local detergents,** accidental (unintentional)
Poisoning by local astringents and local detergents NOS

7 √7ᵗʰ **T49.2X2** **Poisoning by local astringents and local detergents,** intentional self-harm   `HCC`

√7ᵗʰ **T49.2X3** **Poisoning by local astringents and local detergents,** assault

√7ᵗʰ **T49.2X4** **Poisoning by local astringents and local detergents,** undetermined

√7ᵗʰ **T49.2X5** Adverse effect **of local astringents and local detergents**

√7ᵗʰ **T49.2X6** Underdosing **of local astringents and local detergents**

√5ᵗʰ **T49.3** **Poisoning by, adverse effect of and underdosing of emollients, demulcents and protectants**

√6ᵗʰ **T49.3X** **Poisoning by, adverse effect of and underdosing of** emollients, demulcents and protectants

√7ᵗʰ **T49.3X1** **Poisoning by emollients, demulcents and protectants,** accidental (unintentional)
Poisoning by emollients, demulcents and protectants NOS

7 √7ᵗʰ **T49.3X2** **Poisoning by emollients, demulcents and protectants,** intentional self-harm   `HCC`

√7ᵗʰ **T49.3X3** **Poisoning by emollients, demulcents and protectants,** assault

√7ᵗʰ **T49.3X4** **Poisoning by emollients, demulcents and protectants,** undetermined

√7ᵗʰ **T49.3X5** Adverse effect **of emollients, demulcents and protectants**

√7ᵗʰ **T49.3X6** Underdosing **of emollients, demulcents and protectants**

√5ᵗʰ **T49.4** **Poisoning by, adverse effect of and underdosing of keratolytics, keratoplastics, and other hair treatment drugs and preparations**

√6ᵗʰ **T49.4X** **Poisoning by, adverse effect of and underdosing of** keratolytics, keratoplastics, and other hair treatment drugs and preparations

√7ᵗʰ **T49.4X1** **Poisoning by keratolytics, keratoplastics, and other hair treatment drugs and preparations,** accidental (unintentional)
Poisoning by keratolytics, keratoplastics, and other hair treatment drugs and preparations NOS

7 √7ᵗʰ **T49.4X2** **Poisoning by keratolytics, keratoplastics, and other hair treatment drugs and preparations,** intentional self-harm   `HCC`

√7ᵗʰ **T49.4X3** **Poisoning by keratolytics, keratoplastics, and other hair treatment drugs and preparations,** assault

√7ᵗʰ **T49.4X4** **Poisoning by keratolytics, keratoplastics, and other hair treatment drugs and preparations,** undetermined

√7ᵗʰ **T49.4X5** Adverse effect **of keratolytics, keratoplastics, and other hair treatment drugs and preparations**

√7ᵗʰ **T49.4X6** Underdosing **of keratolytics, keratoplastics, and other hair treatment drugs and preparations**

√5ᵗʰ **T49.5** **Poisoning by, adverse effect of and underdosing of ophthalmological drugs and preparations**

√6ᵗʰ **T49.5X** **Poisoning by, adverse effect of and underdosing of** ophthalmological drugs and preparations

√7ᵗʰ **T49.5X1** **Poisoning by ophthalmological drugs and preparations,** accidental (unintentional)
Poisoning by ophthalmological drugs and preparations NOS

7 √7ᵗʰ **T49.5X2** **Poisoning by ophthalmological drugs and preparations,** intentional self-harm   `HCC`

√7ᵗʰ **T49.5X3** **Poisoning by ophthalmological drugs and preparations,** assault

√7ᵗʰ **T49.5X4** **Poisoning by ophthalmological drugs and preparations,** undetermined

√7ᵗʰ **T49.5X5** Adverse effect **of ophthalmological drugs and preparations**

√7ᵗʰ **T49.5X6** Underdosing **of ophthalmological drugs and preparations**

√5ᵗʰ **T49.6** **Poisoning by, adverse effect of and underdosing of otorhinolaryngological drugs and preparations**

√6ᵗʰ **T49.6X** **Poisoning by, adverse effect of and underdosing of** otorhinolaryngological drugs and preparations

√7ᵗʰ **T49.6X1** **Poisoning by otorhinolaryngological drugs and preparations,** accidental (unintentional)
Poisoning by otorhinolaryngological drugs and preparations NOS

7 √7ᵗʰ **T49.6X2** **Poisoning by otorhinolaryngological drugs and preparations,** intentional self-harm   `HCC`

√7ᵗʰ **T49.6X3** **Poisoning by otorhinolaryngological drugs and preparations, assault**

√7ᵗʰ **T49.6X4** **Poisoning by otorhinolaryngological drugs and preparations, undetermined**

√7ᵗʰ **T49.6X5** Adverse effect of otorhinolaryngological drugs and preparations

√7ᵗʰ **T49.6X6** Underdosing of otorhinolaryngological drugs and preparations

√5ᵗʰ **T49.7** **Poisoning by, adverse effect of and underdosing of dental drugs, topically applied**

√6ᵗʰ **T49.7X** **Poisoning by, adverse effect of and underdosing of dental drugs, topically applied**

√7ᵗʰ **T49.7X1** **Poisoning by dental drugs, topically applied, accidental (unintentional)**
Poisoning by dental drugs, topically applied NOS

7 √7ᵗʰ **T49.7X2** **Poisoning by dental drugs, topically applied, intentional self-harm** `HCC`

√7ᵗʰ **T49.7X3** **Poisoning by dental drugs, topically applied, assault**

√7ᵗʰ **T49.7X4** **Poisoning by dental drugs, topically applied, undetermined**

√7ᵗʰ **T49.7X5** Adverse effect of dental drugs, topically applied

√7ᵗʰ **T49.7X6** Underdosing of dental drugs, topically applied

√5ᵗʰ **T49.8** **Poisoning by, adverse effect of and underdosing of other topical agents**
Poisoning by, adverse effect of and underdosing of spermicides

√6ᵗʰ **T49.8X** **Poisoning by, adverse effect of and underdosing of other topical agents**

√7ᵗʰ **T49.8X1** **Poisoning by other topical agents, accidental (unintentional)**
Poisoning by other topical agents NOS

7 √7ᵗʰ **T49.8X2** **Poisoning by other topical agents, intentional self-harm** `HCC`

√7ᵗʰ **T49.8X3** **Poisoning by other topical agents, assault**

√7ᵗʰ **T49.8X4** **Poisoning by other topical agents, undetermined**

√7ᵗʰ **T49.8X5** Adverse effect of other topical agents

√7ᵗʰ **T49.8X6** Underdosing of other topical agents

√5ᵗʰ **T49.9** **Poisoning by, adverse effect of and underdosing of unspecified topical agent**

√x7ᵗʰ **T49.91** **Poisoning by unspecified topical agent, accidental (unintentional)**

7 √x7ᵗʰ **T49.92** **Poisoning by unspecified topical agent, intentional self-harm** `HCC`

√x7ᵗʰ **T49.93** **Poisoning by unspecified topical agent, assault**

√x7ᵗʰ **T49.94** **Poisoning by unspecified topical agent, undetermined**

√x7ᵗʰ **T49.95** Adverse effect of unspecified topical agent

√x7ᵗʰ **T49.96** Underdosing of unspecified topical agent

√4ᵗʰ **T50** **Poisoning by, adverse effect of and underdosing of diuretics and other and unspecified drugs, medicaments and biological substances**

The appropriate 7th character is to be added to each code from category T50.
A   initial encounter
D   subsequent encounter
S   sequela

√5ᵗʰ **T50.0** **Poisoning by, adverse effect of and underdosing of mineralocorticoids and their antagonists**

√6ᵗʰ **T50.0X** **Poisoning by, adverse effect of and underdosing of mineralocorticoids and their antagonists**

√7ᵗʰ **T50.0X1** **Poisoning by mineralocorticoids and their antagonists, accidental (unintentional)**
Poisoning by mineralocorticoids and their antagonists NOS

7 √7ᵗʰ **T50.0X2** **Poisoning by mineralocorticoids and their antagonists, intentional self-harm** `HCC`

√7ᵗʰ **T50.0X3** **Poisoning by mineralocorticoids and their antagonists, assault**

√7ᵗʰ **T50.0X4** **Poisoning by mineralocorticoids and their antagonists, undetermined**

√7ᵗʰ **T50.0X5** Adverse effect of mineralocorticoids and their antagonists

√7ᵗʰ **T50.0X6** Underdosing of mineralocorticoids and their antagonists

√5ᵗʰ **T50.1** **Poisoning by, adverse effect of and underdosing of loop [high-ceiling] diuretics**

√6ᵗʰ **T50.1X** **Poisoning by, adverse effect of and underdosing of loop [high-ceiling] diuretics**

√7ᵗʰ **T50.1X1** **Poisoning by loop [high-ceiling] diuretics, accidental (unintentional)**
Poisoning by loop [high-ceiling] diuretics NOS

7 √7ᵗʰ **T50.1X2** **Poisoning by loop [high-ceiling] diuretics, intentional self-harm** `HCC`

√7ᵗʰ **T50.1X3** **Poisoning by loop [high-ceiling] diuretics, assault**

√7ᵗʰ **T50.1X4** **Poisoning by loop [high-ceiling] diuretics, undetermined**

√7ᵗʰ **T50.1X5** Adverse effect of loop [high-ceiling] diuretics

√7ᵗʰ **T50.1X6** Underdosing of loop [high-ceiling] diuretics

√5ᵗʰ **T50.2** **Poisoning by, adverse effect of and underdosing of carbonic-anhydrase inhibitors, benzothiadiazides and other diuretics**
Poisoning by, adverse effect of and underdosing of acetazolamide

√6ᵗʰ **T50.2X** **Poisoning by, adverse effect of and underdosing of carbonic-anhydrase inhibitors, benzothiadiazides and other diuretics**

√7ᵗʰ **T50.2X1** **Poisoning by carbonic-anhydrase inhibitors, benzothiadiazides and other diuretics, accidental (unintentional)**
Poisoning by carbonic-anhydrase inhibitors, benzothiadiazides and other diuretics NOS

7 √7ᵗʰ **T50.2X2** **Poisoning by carbonic-anhydrase inhibitors, benzothiadiazides and other diuretics, intentional self-harm** `HCC`

√7ᵗʰ **T50.2X3** **Poisoning by carbonic-anhydrase inhibitors, benzothiadiazides and other diuretics, assault**

√7ᵗʰ **T50.2X4** **Poisoning by carbonic-anhydrase inhibitors, benzothiadiazides and other diuretics, undetermined**

√7ᵗʰ **T50.2X5** Adverse effect of carbonic-anhydrase inhibitors, benzothiadiazides and other diuretics

√7ᵗʰ **T50.2X6** Underdosing of carbonic-anhydrase inhibitors, benzothiadiazides and other diuretics

√5ᵗʰ **T50.3** **Poisoning by, adverse effect of and underdosing of electrolytic, caloric and water-balance agents**
Poisoning by, adverse effect of and underdosing of oral rehydration salts

√6ᵗʰ **T50.3X** **Poisoning by, adverse effect of and underdosing of electrolytic, caloric and water-balance agents**

√7ᵗʰ **T50.3X1** **Poisoning by electrolytic, caloric and water-balance agents, accidental (unintentional)**
Poisoning by electrolytic, caloric and water-balance agents NOS

7 √7ᵗʰ **T50.3X2** **Poisoning by electrolytic, caloric and water-balance agents, intentional self-harm** `HCC`

√7ᵗʰ **T50.3X3** **Poisoning by electrolytic, caloric and water-balance agents, assault**

√7ᵗʰ **T50.3X4** **Poisoning by electrolytic, caloric and water-balance agents, undetermined**

√7ᵗʰ **T50.3X5** Adverse effect of electrolytic, caloric and water-balance agents

√7ᵗʰ **T50.3X6** Underdosing of electrolytic, caloric and water-balance agents

Chapter 19. Injury, Poisoning and Certain Other Consequences of External Causes

T50.4–T50.B13

✓5ᵗʰ **T50.4** Poisoning by, adverse effect of and underdosing of drugs affecting uric acid metabolism

   ✓6ᵗʰ **T50.4X** Poisoning by, adverse effect of and underdosing of drugs affecting uric acid metabolism

     ✓7ᵗʰ **T50.4X1** Poisoning by drugs affecting uric acid metabolism, accidental (unintentional)

        Poisoning by drugs affecting uric acid metabolism NOS

     7 ✓7ᵗʰ **T50.4X2** Poisoning by drugs affecting uric acid metabolism, intentional self-harm   HCC

     ✓7ᵗʰ **T50.4X3** Poisoning by drugs affecting uric acid metabolism, assault

     ✓7ᵗʰ **T50.4X4** Poisoning by drugs affecting uric acid metabolism, undetermined

     ✓7ᵗʰ **T50.4X5** Adverse effect of drugs affecting uric acid metabolism

     ✓7ᵗʰ **T50.4X6** Underdosing of drugs affecting uric acid metabolism

✓5ᵗʰ **T50.5** Poisoning by, adverse effect of and underdosing of appetite depressants

   ✓6ᵗʰ **T50.5X** Poisoning by, adverse effect of and underdosing of appetite depressants

     ✓7ᵗʰ **T50.5X1** Poisoning by appetite depressants, accidental (unintentional)

        Poisoning by appetite depressants NOS

     7 ✓7ᵗʰ **T50.5X2** Poisoning by appetite depressants, intentional self-harm   HCC

     ✓7ᵗʰ **T50.5X3** Poisoning by appetite depressants, assault

     ✓7ᵗʰ **T50.5X4** Poisoning by appetite depressants, undetermined

     ✓7ᵗʰ **T50.5X5** Adverse effect of appetite depressants

     ✓7ᵗʰ **T50.5X6** Underdosing of appetite depressants

✓5ᵗʰ **T50.6** Poisoning by, adverse effect of and underdosing of antidotes and chelating agents

   Poisoning by, adverse effect of and underdosing of alcohol deterrents

   ✓6ᵗʰ **T50.6X** Poisoning by, adverse effect of and underdosing of antidotes and chelating agents

     ✓7ᵗʰ **T50.6X1** Poisoning by antidotes and chelating agents, accidental (unintentional)

        Poisoning by antidotes and chelating agents NOS

     7 ✓7ᵗʰ **T50.6X2** Poisoning by antidotes and chelating agents, intentional self-harm   HCC

     ✓7ᵗʰ **T50.6X3** Poisoning by antidotes and chelating agents, assault

     ✓7ᵗʰ **T50.6X4** Poisoning by antidotes and chelating agents, undetermined

     ✓7ᵗʰ **T50.6X5** Adverse effect of antidotes and chelating agents

     ✓7ᵗʰ **T50.6X6** Underdosing of antidotes and chelating agents

✓5ᵗʰ **T50.7** Poisoning by, adverse effect of and underdosing of analeptics and opioid receptor antagonists

   ✓6ᵗʰ **T50.7X** Poisoning by, adverse effect of and underdosing of analeptics and opioid receptor antagonists

     ✓7ᵗʰ **T50.7X1** Poisoning by analeptics and opioid receptor antagonists, accidental (unintentional)

        Poisoning by analeptics and opioid receptor antagonists NOS

     7 ✓7ᵗʰ **T50.7X2** Poisoning by analeptics and opioid receptor antagonists, intentional self-harm   HCC

     ✓7ᵗʰ **T50.7X3** Poisoning by analeptics and opioid receptor antagonists, assault

     ✓7ᵗʰ **T50.7X4** Poisoning by analeptics and opioid receptor antagonists, undetermined

     ✓7ᵗʰ **T50.7X5** Adverse effect of analeptics and opioid receptor antagonists

     ✓7ᵗʰ **T50.7X6** Underdosing of analeptics and opioid receptor antagonists

✓5ᵗʰ **T50.8** Poisoning by, adverse effect of and underdosing of diagnostic agents

   ✓6ᵗʰ **T50.8X** Poisoning by, adverse effect of and underdosing of diagnostic agents

     ✓7ᵗʰ **T50.8X1** Poisoning by diagnostic agents, accidental (unintentional)

        Poisoning by diagnostic agents NOS

     7 ✓7ᵗʰ **T50.8X2** Poisoning by diagnostic agents, intentional self-harm   HCC

     ✓7ᵗʰ **T50.8X3** Poisoning by diagnostic agents, assault

     ✓7ᵗʰ **T50.8X4** Poisoning by diagnostic agents, undetermined

     ✓7ᵗʰ **T50.8X5** Adverse effect of diagnostic agents

     ✓7ᵗʰ **T50.8X6** Underdosing of diagnostic agents

✓5ᵗʰ **T50.A** Poisoning by, adverse effect of and underdosing of bacterial vaccines

   ✓6ᵗʰ **T50.A1** Poisoning by, adverse effect of and underdosing of pertussis vaccine, including combinations with a pertussis component

     ✓7ᵗʰ **T50.A11** Poisoning by pertussis vaccine, including combinations with a pertussis component, accidental (unintentional)

     7 ✓7ᵗʰ **T50.A12** Poisoning by pertussis vaccine, including combinations with a pertussis component, intentional self-harm   HCC

     ✓7ᵗʰ **T50.A13** Poisoning by pertussis vaccine, including combinations with a pertussis component, assault

     ✓7ᵗʰ **T50.A14** Poisoning by pertussis vaccine, including combinations with a pertussis component, undetermined

     ✓7ᵗʰ **T50.A15** Adverse effect of pertussis vaccine, including combinations with a pertussis component

     ✓7ᵗʰ **T50.A16** Underdosing of pertussis vaccine, including combinations with a pertussis component

   ✓6ᵗʰ **T50.A2** Poisoning by, adverse effect of and underdosing of mixed bacterial vaccines without a pertussis component

     ✓7ᵗʰ **T50.A21** Poisoning by mixed bacterial vaccines without a pertussis component, accidental (unintentional)

     7 ✓7ᵗʰ **T50.A22** Poisoning by mixed bacterial vaccines without a pertussis component, intentional self-harm   HCC

     ✓7ᵗʰ **T50.A23** Poisoning by mixed bacterial vaccines without a pertussis component, assault

     ✓7ᵗʰ **T50.A24** Poisoning by mixed bacterial vaccines without a pertussis component, undetermined

     ✓7ᵗʰ **T50.A25** Adverse effect of mixed bacterial vaccines without a pertussis component

     ✓7ᵗʰ **T50.A26** Underdosing of mixed bacterial vaccines without a pertussis component

   ✓6ᵗʰ **T50.A9** Poisoning by, adverse effect of and underdosing of other bacterial vaccines

     ✓7ᵗʰ **T50.A91** Poisoning by other bacterial vaccines, accidental (unintentional)

     7 ✓7ᵗʰ **T50.A92** Poisoning by other bacterial vaccines, intentional self-harm   HCC

     ✓7ᵗʰ **T50.A93** Poisoning by other bacterial vaccines, assault

     ✓7ᵗʰ **T50.A94** Poisoning by other bacterial vaccines, undetermined

     ✓7ᵗʰ **T50.A95** Adverse effect of other bacterial vaccines

     ✓7ᵗʰ **T50.A96** Underdosing of other bacterial vaccines

✓5ᵗʰ **T50.B** Poisoning by, adverse effect of and underdosing of viral vaccines

   ✓6ᵗʰ **T50.B1** Poisoning by, adverse effect of and underdosing of smallpox vaccines

     ✓7ᵗʰ **T50.B11** Poisoning by smallpox vaccines, accidental (unintentional)

     7 ✓7ᵗʰ **T50.B12** Poisoning by smallpox vaccines, intentional self-harm   HCC

     ✓7ᵗʰ **T50.B13** Poisoning by smallpox vaccines, assault

---

N Newborn: 0   P Pediatric: 0-17   M Maternity: 9-64   A Adult: 15-124   MCC Major Complication/Comorbidity   CC Complication/Comorbidity   SW Severe Wound Dx

1170   ICD-10-CM 2020

√7ᵗʰ **T50.B14** Poisoning by smallpox vaccines, undetermined

√7ᵗʰ **T50.B15** Adverse effect of smallpox vaccines

√7ᵗʰ **T50.B16** Underdosing of smallpox vaccines

√6ᵗʰ **T50.B9** Poisoning by, adverse effect of and underdosing of other viral vaccines

√7ᵗʰ **T50.B91** Poisoning by other viral vaccines, accidental (unintentional)

7 √7ᵗʰ **T50.B92** Poisoning by other viral vaccines, intentional self-harm   HCC

√7ᵗʰ **T50.B93** Poisoning by other viral vaccines, assault

√7ᵗʰ **T50.B94** Poisoning by other viral vaccines, undetermined

√7ᵗʰ **T50.B95** Adverse effect of other viral vaccines

√7ᵗʰ **T50.B96** Underdosing of other viral vaccines

√5ᵗʰ **T50.Z** Poisoning by, adverse effect of and underdosing of other vaccines and biological substances

√6ᵗʰ **T50.Z1** Poisoning by, adverse effect of and underdosing of immunoglobulin

√7ᵗʰ **T50.Z11** Poisoning by immunoglobulin, accidental (unintentional)

7 √7ᵗʰ **T50.Z12** Poisoning by immunoglobulin, intentional self-harm   HCC

√7ᵗʰ **T50.Z13** Poisoning by immunoglobulin, assault

√7ᵗʰ **T50.Z14** Poisoning by immunoglobulin, undetermined

√7ᵗʰ **T50.Z15** Adverse effect of immunoglobulin

√7ᵗʰ **T50.Z16** Underdosing of immunoglobulin

√6ᵗʰ **T50.Z9** Poisoning by, adverse effect of and underdosing of other vaccines and biological substances

√7ᵗʰ **T50.Z91** Poisoning by other vaccines and biological substances, accidental (unintentional)

7 √7ᵗʰ **T50.Z92** Poisoning by other vaccines and biological substances, intentional self-harm   HCC

√7ᵗʰ **T50.Z93** Poisoning by other vaccines and biological substances, assault

√7ᵗʰ **T50.Z94** Poisoning by other vaccines and biological substances, undetermined

√7ᵗʰ **T50.Z95** Adverse effect of other vaccines and biological substances

√7ᵗʰ **T50.Z96** Underdosing of other vaccines and biological substances

√5ᵗʰ **T50.9** Poisoning by, adverse effect of and underdosing of other and unspecified drugs, medicaments and biological substances

AHA: 2016,1Q,38; 2015,1Q,21

√6ᵗʰ **T50.90** Poisoning by, adverse effect of and underdosing of unspecified drugs, medicaments and biological substances

√7ᵗʰ **T50.901** Poisoning by unspecified drugs, medicaments and biological substances, accidental (unintentional)

7 √7ᵗʰ **T50.902** Poisoning by unspecified drugs, medicaments and biological substances, intentional self-harm   HCC

√7ᵗʰ **T50.903** Poisoning by unspecified drugs, medicaments and biological substances, assault

√7ᵗʰ **T50.904** Poisoning by unspecified drugs, medicaments and biological substances, undetermined

√7ᵗʰ **T50.905** Adverse effect of unspecified drugs, medicaments and biological substances

√7ᵗʰ **T50.906** Underdosing of unspecified drugs, medicaments and biological substances

√6ᵗʰ **T50.91** Poisoning by, adverse effect of and underdosing of multiple unspecified drugs, medicaments and biological substances

Multiple drug ingestion NOS

Code also any specific drugs, medicaments and biological substances

√7ᵗʰ **T50.911** Poisoning by multiple unspecified drugs, medicaments and biological substances, accidental (unintentional)

√7ᵗʰ **T50.912** Poisoning by multiple unspecified drugs, medicaments and biological substances, intentional self-harm

√7ᵗʰ **T50.913** Poisoning by multiple unspecified drugs, medicaments and biological substances, assault

√7ᵗʰ **T50.914** Poisoning by multiple unspecified drugs, medicaments and biological substances, undetermined

√7ᵗʰ **T50.915** Adverse effect of multiple unspecified drugs, medicaments and biological substances

√7ᵗʰ **T50.916** Underdosing of multiple unspecified drugs, medicaments and biological substances

√6ᵗʰ **T50.99** Poisoning by, adverse effect of and underdosing of other drugs, medicaments and biological substances

√7ᵗʰ **T50.991** Poisoning by other drugs, medicaments and biological substances, accidental (unintentional)

7 √7ᵗʰ **T50.992** Poisoning by other drugs, medicaments and biological substances, intentional self-harm   HCC

√7ᵗʰ **T50.993** Poisoning by other drugs, medicaments and biological substances, assault

√7ᵗʰ **T50.994** Poisoning by other drugs, medicaments and biological substances, undetermined

√7ᵗʰ **T50.995** Adverse effect of other drugs, medicaments and biological substances

√7ᵗʰ **T50.996** Underdosing of other drugs, medicaments and biological substances

Toxic effects of substances chiefly nonmedicinal as to source (T51-T65)

NOTE When no intent is indicated code to accidental. Undetermined intent is only for use when there is specific documentation in the record that the intent of the toxic effect cannot be determined.

Use additional code(s) for all associated manifestations of toxic effect, such as:
personal history of foreign body fully removed (Z87.821)
respiratory conditions due to external agents (J60-J70)
to identify any retained foreign body, if applicable (Z18.-)

EXCLUDES 1 contact with and (suspected) exposure to toxic substances (Z77.-)

AHA: 2017,1Q,39-40

√4ᵗʰ **T51 Toxic effect of alcohol**

The appropriate 7th character is to be added to each code from category T51.
A initial encounter
D subsequent encounter
S sequela

√5ᵗʰ **T51.0 Toxic effect of ethanol**

Toxic effect of ethyl alcohol

EXCLUDES 2 acute alcohol intoxication or "hangover" effects (F10.129, F10.229, F10.929)
drunkenness (F10.129, F10.229, F10.929)
pathological alcohol intoxication (F10.129, F10.229, F10.929)

√6ᵗʰ **T51.0X Toxic effect of ethanol**

6 √7ᵗʰ **T51.0X1 Toxic effect of ethanol, accidental (unintentional)**   HCC
Toxic effect of ethanol NOS

7 √7ᵗʰ **T51.0X2 Toxic effect of ethanol, intentional self-harm**   HCC

√7ᵗʰ **T51.0X3 Toxic effect of ethanol, assault**

6 √7ᵗʰ **T51.0X4 Toxic effect of ethanol, undetermined**   HCC

√5ᵗʰ **T51.1 Toxic effect of methanol**

Toxic effect of methyl alcohol

√6ᵗʰ **T51.1X Toxic effect of methanol**

√7ᵗʰ **T51.1X1 Toxic effect of methanol, accidental (unintentional)**
Toxic effect of methanol NOS

7 √7ᵗʰ **T51.1X2 Toxic effect of methanol, intentional self-harm**   HCC

√7ᵗʰ **T51.1X3 Toxic effect of methanol, assault**

√7ᵗʰ **T51.1X4 Toxic effect of methanol, undetermined**

✓ Additional Character Required   √x7ᵗʰ Placeholder   Unacceptable PDx   Questionable PDx   Manifestation   Unspecified Dx   H1-H14 HAC   HCC CMS-HCC Dx   HIV HIV Dx

ICD-10-CM 2020   1171

Chapter 19. Injury, Poisoning and Certain Other Consequences of External Causes

T51.2–T53.0X4

√5th **T51.2** **Toxic effect of 2-Propanol**
　　Toxic effect of isopropyl alcohol
　　√6th **T51.2X** **Toxic effect of 2-Propanol**
　　　　√7th **T51.2X1** **Toxic effect of 2-Propanol, accidental (unintentional)**
　　　　　　Toxic effect of 2-Propanol NOS
　　　　7 √7th **T51.2X2** **Toxic effect of 2-Propanol, intentional self-harm** HCC
　　　　√7th **T51.2X3** **Toxic effect of 2-Propanol, assault**
　　　　√7th **T51.2X4** **Toxic effect of 2-Propanol, undetermined**

√5th **T51.3** **Toxic effect of fusel oil**
　　Toxic effect of amyl alcohol
　　Toxic effect of butyl [1-butanol] alcohol
　　Toxic effect of propyl [1-propanol] alcohol
　　√6th **T51.3X** **Toxic effect of fusel oil**
　　　　√7th **T51.3X1** **Toxic effect of fusel oil, accidental (unintentional)**
　　　　　　Toxic effect of fusel oil NOS
　　　　7 √7th **T51.3X2** **Toxic effect of fusel oil, intentional self-harm** HCC
　　　　√7th **T51.3X3** **Toxic effect of fusel oil, assault**
　　　　√7th **T51.3X4** **Toxic effect of fusel oil, undetermined**

√5th **T51.8** **Toxic effect of other alcohols**
　　√6th **T51.8X** **Toxic effect of other alcohols**
　　　　√7th **T51.8X1** **Toxic effect of other alcohols, accidental (unintentional)**
　　　　　　Toxic effect of other alcohols NOS
　　　　7 √7th **T51.8X2** **Toxic effect of other alcohols, intentional self-harm** HCC
　　　　√7th **T51.8X3** **Toxic effect of other alcohols, assault**
　　　　√7th **T51.8X4** **Toxic effect of other alcohols, undetermined**

√5th **T51.9** **Toxic effect of unspecified alcohol**
　　√x7th **T51.91** **Toxic effect of unspecified alcohol, accidental (unintentional)**
　　7 √x7th **T51.92** **Toxic effect of unspecified alcohol, intentional self-harm** HCC
　　√x7th **T51.93** **Toxic effect of unspecified alcohol, assault**
　　√x7th **T51.94** **Toxic effect of unspecified alcohol, undetermined**

√4th **T52** **Toxic effect of organic solvents**
　　EXCLUDES 1 　halogen derivatives of aliphatic and aromatic hydrocarbons (T53.-)

　　The appropriate 7th character is to be added to each code from category T52.
　　A　initial encounter
　　D　subsequent encounter
　　S　sequela

√5th **T52.0** **Toxic effects of petroleum products**
　　Toxic effects of ether petroleum
　　Toxic effects of gasoline [petrol]
　　Toxic effects of kerosene [paraffin oil]
　　Toxic effects of naphtha petroleum
　　Toxic effects of paraffin wax
　　Toxic effects of spirit petroleum
　　√6th **T52.0X** **Toxic effects of petroleum products**
　　　　√7th **T52.0X1** **Toxic effect of petroleum products, accidental (unintentional)**
　　　　　　Toxic effects of petroleum products NOS
　　　　7 √7th **T52.0X2** **Toxic effect of petroleum products, intentional self-harm** HCC
　　　　√7th **T52.0X3** **Toxic effect of petroleum products, assault**
　　　　√7th **T52.0X4** **Toxic effect of petroleum products, undetermined**

√5th **T52.1** **Toxic effects of benzene**
　　EXCLUDES 1 　homologues of benzene (T52.2)
　　　　　　nitroderivatives and aminoderivatives of benzene and its homologues (T65.3)
　　√6th **T52.1X** **Toxic effects of benzene**
　　　　√7th **T52.1X1** **Toxic effect of benzene, accidental (unintentional)**
　　　　　　Toxic effects of benzene NOS

7 √7th **T52.1X2** **Toxic effect of benzene, intentional self-harm** HCC
√7th **T52.1X3** **Toxic effect of benzene, assault**
√7th **T52.1X4** **Toxic effect of benzene, undetermined**

√5th **T52.2** **Toxic effects of homologues of benzene**
　　Toxic effects of toluene [methylbenzene]
　　Toxic effects of xylene [dimethylbenzene]
　　√6th **T52.2X** **Toxic effects of homologues of benzene**
　　　　√7th **T52.2X1** **Toxic effect of homologues of benzene, accidental (unintentional)**
　　　　　　Toxic effects of homologues of benzene NOS
　　　　7 √7th **T52.2X2** **Toxic effect of homologues of benzene, intentional self-harm** HCC
　　　　√7th **T52.2X3** **Toxic effect of homologues of benzene, assault**
　　　　√7th **T52.2X4** **Toxic effect of homologues of benzene, undetermined**

√5th **T52.3** **Toxic effects of glycols**
　　√6th **T52.3X** **Toxic effects of glycols**
　　　　√7th **T52.3X1** **Toxic effect of glycols, accidental (unintentional)**
　　　　　　Toxic effects of glycols NOS
　　　　7 √7th **T52.3X2** **Toxic effect of glycols, intentional self-harm** HCC
　　　　√7th **T52.3X3** **Toxic effect of glycols, assault**
　　　　√7th **T52.3X4** **Toxic effect of glycols, undetermined**

√5th **T52.4** **Toxic effects of ketones**
　　√6th **T52.4X** **Toxic effects of ketones**
　　　　√7th **T52.4X1** **Toxic effect of ketones, accidental (unintentional)**
　　　　　　Toxic effects of ketones NOS
　　　　7 √7th **T52.4X2** **Toxic effect of ketones, intentional self-harm** HCC
　　　　√7th **T52.4X3** **Toxic effect of ketones, assault**
　　　　√7th **T52.4X4** **Toxic effect of ketones, undetermined**

√5th **T52.8** **Toxic effects of other organic solvents**
　　√6th **T52.8X** **Toxic effects of other organic solvents**
　　　　√7th **T52.8X1** **Toxic effect of other organic solvents, accidental (unintentional)**
　　　　　　Toxic effects of other organic solvents NOS
　　　　7 √7th **T52.8X2** **Toxic effect of other organic solvents, intentional self-harm** HCC
　　　　√7th **T52.8X3** **Toxic effect of other organic solvents, assault**
　　　　√7th **T52.8X4** **Toxic effect of other organic solvents, undetermined**

√5th **T52.9** **Toxic effects of unspecified organic solvent**
　　√x7th **T52.91** **Toxic effect of unspecified organic solvent, accidental (unintentional)**
　　7 √x7th **T52.92** **Toxic effect of unspecified organic solvent, intentional self-harm** HCC
　　√x7th **T52.93** **Toxic effect of unspecified organic solvent, assault**
　　√x7th **T52.94** **Toxic effect of unspecified organic solvent, undetermined**

√4th **T53** **Toxic effect of halogen derivatives of aliphatic and aromatic hydrocarbons**

　　The appropriate 7th character is to be added to each code from category T53.
　　A　initial encounter
　　D　subsequent encounter
　　S　sequela

√5th **T53.0** **Toxic effects of carbon tetrachloride**
　　Toxic effects of tetrachloromethane
　　√6th **T53.0X** **Toxic effects of carbon tetrachloride**
　　　　√7th **T53.0X1** **Toxic effect of carbon tetrachloride, accidental (unintentional)**
　　　　　　Toxic effects of carbon tetrachloride NOS
　　　　7 √7th **T53.0X2** **Toxic effect of carbon tetrachloride, intentional self-harm** HCC
　　　　√7th **T53.0X3** **Toxic effect of carbon tetrachloride, assault**
　　　　√7th **T53.0X4** **Toxic effect of carbon tetrachloride, undetermined**

√5ᵗʰ **T53.1** **Toxic effects of chloroform**
Toxic effects of trichloromethane

√6ᵗʰ **T53.1X** **Toxic effects of** chloroform

√7ᵗʰ **T53.1X1** **Toxic effect of chloroform,** accidental (unintentional)
Toxic effects of chloroform NOS

7 √7ᵗʰ **T53.1X2** **Toxic effect of chloroform,** intentional self-harm   HCC

√7ᵗʰ **T53.1X3** **Toxic effect of chloroform,** assault

√7ᵗʰ **T53.1X4** **Toxic effect of chloroform,** undetermined

√5ᵗʰ **T53.2** **Toxic effects of trichloroethylene**
Toxic effects of trichloroethene

√6ᵗʰ **T53.2X** **Toxic effects of** trichloroethylene

√7ᵗʰ **T53.2X1** **Toxic effect of trichloroethylene,** accidental (unintentional)
Toxic effects of trichloroethylene NOS

7 √7ᵗʰ **T53.2X2** **Toxic effect of trichloroethylene,** intentional self-harm   HCC

√7ᵗʰ **T53.2X3** **Toxic effect of trichloroethylene,** assault

√7ᵗʰ **T53.2X4** **Toxic effect of trichloroethylene,** undetermined

√5ᵗʰ **T53.3** **Toxic effects of tetrachloroethylene**
Toxic effects of perchloroethylene
Toxic effect of tetrachloroethene

√6ᵗʰ **T53.3X** **Toxic effects of** tetrachloroethylene

√7ᵗʰ **T53.3X1** **Toxic effect of tetrachloroethylene,** accidental (unintentional)
Toxic effects of tetrachloroethylene NOS

7 √7ᵗʰ **T53.3X2** **Toxic effect of tetrachloroethylene,** intentional self-harm   HCC

√7ᵗʰ **T53.3X3** **Toxic effect of tetrachloroethylene,** assault

√7ᵗʰ **T53.3X4** **Toxic effect of tetrachloroethylene,** undetermined

√5ᵗʰ **T53.4** **Toxic effects of dichloromethane**
Toxic effects of methylene chloride

√6ᵗʰ **T53.4X** **Toxic effects of** dichloromethane

√7ᵗʰ **T53.4X1** **Toxic effect of dichloromethane,** accidental (unintentional)
Toxic effects of dichloromethane NOS

7 √7ᵗʰ **T53.4X2** **Toxic effect of dichloromethane,** intentional self-harm   HCC

√7ᵗʰ **T53.4X3** **Toxic effect of dichloromethane,** assault

√7ᵗʰ **T53.4X4** **Toxic effect of dichloromethane,** undetermined

√5ᵗʰ **T53.5** **Toxic effects of chlorofluorocarbons**

√6ᵗʰ **T53.5X** **Toxic effects of** chlorofluorocarbons

√7ᵗʰ **T53.5X1** **Toxic effect of chlorofluorocarbons,** accidental (unintentional)
Toxic effects of chlorofluorocarbons NOS

7 √7ᵗʰ **T53.5X2** **Toxic effect of chlorofluorocarbons,** intentional self-harm   HCC

√7ᵗʰ **T53.5X3** **Toxic effect of chlorofluorocarbons,** assault

√7ᵗʰ **T53.5X4** **Toxic effect of chlorofluorocarbons,** undetermined

√5ᵗʰ **T53.6** **Toxic effects of other halogen derivatives of aliphatic hydrocarbons**

√6ᵗʰ **T53.6X** **Toxic effects of** other halogen derivatives of aliphatic hydrocarbons

√7ᵗʰ **T53.6X1** **Toxic effect of other halogen derivatives of aliphatic hydrocarbons,** accidental (unintentional)
Toxic effects of other halogen derivatives of aliphatic hydrocarbons NOS

7 √7ᵗʰ **T53.6X2** **Toxic effect of other halogen derivatives of aliphatic hydrocarbons,** intentional self-harm   HCC

√7ᵗʰ **T53.6X3** **Toxic effect of other halogen derivatives of aliphatic hydrocarbons,** assault

√7ᵗʰ **T53.6X4** **Toxic effect of other halogen derivatives of aliphatic hydrocarbons,** undetermined

√5ᵗʰ **T53.7** **Toxic effects of other halogen derivatives of aromatic hydrocarbons**

√6ᵗʰ **T53.7X** **Toxic effects of** other halogen derivatives of aromatic hydrocarbons

√7ᵗʰ **T53.7X1** **Toxic effect of other halogen derivatives of aromatic hydrocarbons,** accidental (unintentional)
Toxic effects of other halogen derivatives of aromatic hydrocarbons NOS

7 √7ᵗʰ **T53.7X2** **Toxic effect of other halogen derivatives of aromatic hydrocarbons,** intentional self-harm   HCC

√7ᵗʰ **T53.7X3** **Toxic effect of other halogen derivatives of aromatic hydrocarbons,** assault

√7ᵗʰ **T53.7X4** **Toxic effect of other halogen derivatives of aromatic hydrocarbons,** undetermined

√5ᵗʰ **T53.9** **Toxic effects of unspecified halogen derivatives of aliphatic and aromatic hydrocarbons**

√x7ᵗʰ **T53.91** **Toxic effect of unspecified halogen derivatives of aliphatic and aromatic hydrocarbons,** accidental (unintentional)

7 √x7ᵗʰ **T53.92** **Toxic effect of unspecified halogen derivatives of aliphatic and aromatic hydrocarbons,** intentional self-harm   HCC

√x7ᵗʰ **T53.93** **Toxic effect of unspecified halogen derivatives of aliphatic and aromatic hydrocarbons,** assault

√x7ᵗʰ **T53.94** **Toxic effect of unspecified halogen derivatives of aliphatic and aromatic hydrocarbons,** undetermined

√4ᵗʰ **T54** **Toxic effect of corrosive substances**

The appropriate 7th character is to be added to each code from category T54.
A   initial encounter
D   subsequent encounter
S   sequela

√5ᵗʰ **T54.0** **Toxic effects of phenol and phenol homologues**

√6ᵗʰ **T54.0X** **Toxic effects of** phenol and phenol homologues

√7ᵗʰ **T54.0X1** **Toxic effect of phenol and phenol homologues,** accidental (unintentional)
Toxic effects of phenol and phenol homologues NOS

7 √7ᵗʰ **T54.0X2** **Toxic effect of phenol and phenol homologues,** intentional self-harm   HCC

√7ᵗʰ **T54.0X3** **Toxic effect of phenol and phenol homologues,** assault

√7ᵗʰ **T54.0X4** **Toxic effect of phenol and phenol homologues,** undetermined

√5ᵗʰ **T54.1** **Toxic effects of other corrosive organic compounds**

√6ᵗʰ **T54.1X** **Toxic effects of other corrosive organic compounds**

√7ᵗʰ **T54.1X1** **Toxic effect of other corrosive organic compounds,** accidental (unintentional)
Toxic effects of other corrosive organic compounds NOS

7 √7ᵗʰ **T54.1X2** **Toxic effect of other corrosive organic compounds,** intentional self-harm   HCC

√7ᵗʰ **T54.1X3** **Toxic effect of other corrosive organic compounds,** assault

√7ᵗʰ **T54.1X4** **Toxic effect of other corrosive organic compounds,** undetermined

√5ᵗʰ **T54.2** **Toxic effects of corrosive acids and acid-like substances**
Toxic effects of hydrochloric acid
Toxic effects of sulfuric acid

√6ᵗʰ **T54.2X** **Toxic effects of** corrosive acids and acid-like substances

√7ᵗʰ **T54.2X1** **Toxic effect of corrosive acids and acid-like substances,** accidental (unintentional)
Toxic effects of corrosive acids and acid-like substances NOS

7 √7ᵗʰ **T54.2X2** **Toxic effect of corrosive acids and acid-like substances,** intentional self-harm   HCC

√7ᵗʰ **T54.2X3** **Toxic effect of corrosive acids and acid-like substances,** assault

✓7ᵗʰ **T54.2X4** **Toxic effect of corrosive acids and acid-like substances, undetermined**

✓5ᵗʰ **T54.3** **Toxic effects of corrosive alkalis and alkali-like substances**

Toxic effects of potassium hydroxide
Toxic effects of sodium hydroxide

✓6ᵗʰ **T54.3X** **Toxic effects of corrosive alkalis and alkali-like substances**

✓7ᵗʰ **T54.3X1** **Toxic effect of corrosive alkalis and alkali-like substances, accidental (unintentional)**

Toxic effects of corrosive alkalis and alkali-like substances NOS

⁷ ✓7ᵗʰ **T54.3X2** **Toxic effect of corrosive alkalis and alkali-like substances, intentional self-harm** `HCC`

✓7ᵗʰ **T54.3X3** **Toxic effect of corrosive alkalis and alkali-like substances, assault**

✓7ᵗʰ **T54.3X4** **Toxic effect of corrosive alkalis and alkali-like substances, undetermined**

✓5ᵗʰ **T54.9** **Toxic effects of unspecified corrosive substance**

✓x7ᵗʰ **T54.91** **Toxic effect of unspecified corrosive substance, accidental (unintentional)**

⁷ ✓x7ᵗʰ **T54.92** **Toxic effect of unspecified corrosive substance, intentional self-harm** `HCC`

✓x7ᵗʰ **T54.93** **Toxic effect of unspecified corrosive substance, assault**

✓x7ᵗʰ **T54.94** **Toxic effect of unspecified corrosive substance, undetermined**

✓4ᵗʰ **T55** **Toxic effect of soaps and detergents**

The appropriate 7th character is to be added to each code from category T55.
A   initial encounter
D   subsequent encounter
S   sequela

✓5ᵗʰ **T55.0** **Toxic effect of soaps**

✓6ᵗʰ **T55.0X** **Toxic effect of soaps**

✓7ᵗʰ **T55.0X1** **Toxic effect of soaps, accidental (unintentional)**

Toxic effect of soaps NOS

⁷ ✓7ᵗʰ **T55.0X2** **Toxic effect of soaps, intentional self-harm** `HCC`

✓7ᵗʰ **T55.0X3** **Toxic effect of soaps, assault**

✓7ᵗʰ **T55.0X4** **Toxic effect of soaps, undetermined**

✓5ᵗʰ **T55.1** **Toxic effect of detergents**

✓6ᵗʰ **T55.1X** **Toxic effect of detergents**

✓7ᵗʰ **T55.1X1** **Toxic effect of detergents, accidental (unintentional)**

Toxic effect of detergents NOS

⁷ ✓7ᵗʰ **T55.1X2** **Toxic effect of detergents, intentional self-harm** `HCC`

✓7ᵗʰ **T55.1X3** **Toxic effect of detergents, assault**

✓7ᵗʰ **T55.1X4** **Toxic effect of detergents, undetermined**

✓4ᵗʰ **T56** **Toxic effect of metals**

`INCLUDES`   toxic effects of fumes and vapors of metals
toxic effects of metals from all sources, except medicinal substances

Use additional code to identify any retained metal foreign body, if applicable (Z18.0-, T18.1-)

`EXCLUDES 1`   *arsenic and its compounds (T57.0)*
manganese and its compounds (T57.2)

The appropriate 7th character is to be added to each code from category T56.
A   initial encounter
D   subsequent encounter
S   sequela

✓5ᵗʰ **T56.0** **Toxic effects of lead and its compounds**

✓6ᵗʰ **T56.0X** **Toxic effects of lead and its compounds**

✓7ᵗʰ **T56.0X1** **Toxic effect of lead and its compounds, accidental (unintentional)**

Toxic effects of lead and its compounds NOS

⁷ ✓7ᵗʰ **T56.0X2** **Toxic effect of lead and its compounds, intentional self-harm** `HCC`

✓7ᵗʰ **T56.0X3** **Toxic effect of lead and its compounds, assault**

✓7ᵗʰ **T56.0X4** **Toxic effect of lead and its compounds, undetermined**

✓5ᵗʰ **T56.1** **Toxic effects of mercury and its compounds**

✓6ᵗʰ **T56.1X** **Toxic effects of mercury and its compounds**

✓7ᵗʰ **T56.1X1** **Toxic effect of mercury and its compounds, accidental (unintentional)**

Toxic effects of mercury and its compounds NOS

⁷ ✓7ᵗʰ **T56.1X2** **Toxic effect of mercury and its compounds, intentional self-harm** `HCC`

✓7ᵗʰ **T56.1X3** **Toxic effect of mercury and its compounds, assault**

✓7ᵗʰ **T56.1X4** **Toxic effect of mercury and its compounds, undetermined**

✓5ᵗʰ **T56.2** **Toxic effects of chromium and its compounds**

✓6ᵗʰ **T56.2X** **Toxic effects of chromium and its compounds**

✓7ᵗʰ **T56.2X1** **Toxic effect of chromium and its compounds, accidental (unintentional)**

Toxic effects of chromium and its compounds NOS

⁷ ✓7ᵗʰ **T56.2X2** **Toxic effect of chromium and its compounds, intentional self-harm** `HCC`

✓7ᵗʰ **T56.2X3** **Toxic effect of chromium and its compounds, assault**

✓7ᵗʰ **T56.2X4** **Toxic effect of chromium and its compounds, undetermined**

✓5ᵗʰ **T56.3** **Toxic effects of cadmium and its compounds**

✓6ᵗʰ **T56.3X** **Toxic effects of cadmium and its compounds**

✓7ᵗʰ **T56.3X1** **Toxic effect of cadmium and its compounds, accidental (unintentional)**

Toxic effects of cadmium and its compounds NOS

⁷ ✓7ᵗʰ **T56.3X2** **Toxic effect of cadmium and its compounds, intentional self-harm** `HCC`

✓7ᵗʰ **T56.3X3** **Toxic effect of cadmium and its compounds, assault**

✓7ᵗʰ **T56.3X4** **Toxic effect of cadmium and its compounds, undetermined**

✓5ᵗʰ **T56.4** **Toxic effects of copper and its compounds**

✓6ᵗʰ **T56.4X** **Toxic effects of copper and its compounds**

✓7ᵗʰ **T56.4X1** **Toxic effect of copper and its compounds, accidental (unintentional)**

Toxic effects of copper and its compounds NOS

⁷ ✓7ᵗʰ **T56.4X2** **Toxic effect of copper and its compounds, intentional self-harm** `HCC`

✓7ᵗʰ **T56.4X3** **Toxic effect of copper and its compounds, assault**

✓7ᵗʰ **T56.4X4** **Toxic effect of copper and its compounds, undetermined**

✓5ᵗʰ **T56.5** **Toxic effects of zinc and its compounds**

✓6ᵗʰ **T56.5X** **Toxic effects of zinc and its compounds**

✓7ᵗʰ **T56.5X1** **Toxic effect of zinc and its compounds, accidental (unintentional)**

Toxic effects of zinc and its compounds NOS

⁷ ✓7ᵗʰ **T56.5X2** **Toxic effect of zinc and its compounds, intentional self-harm** `HCC`

✓7ᵗʰ **T56.5X3** **Toxic effect of zinc and its compounds, assault**

✓7ᵗʰ **T56.5X4** **Toxic effect of zinc and its compounds, undetermined**

✓5ᵗʰ **T56.6** **Toxic effects of tin and its compounds**

✓6ᵗʰ **T56.6X** **Toxic effects of tin and its compounds**

✓7ᵗʰ **T56.6X1** **Toxic effect of tin and its compounds, accidental (unintentional)**

Toxic effects of tin and its compounds NOS

⁷ ✓7ᵗʰ **T56.6X2** **Toxic effect of tin and its compounds, intentional self-harm** `HCC`

✓7ᵗʰ **T56.6X3** **Toxic effect of tin and its compounds, assault**

√7ᵗʰ **T56.6X4 Toxic effect of tin and its compounds, undetermined**

√5ᵗʰ **T56.7 Toxic effects of beryllium and its compounds**

√6ᵗʰ **T56.7X Toxic effects of beryllium and its compounds**

√7ᵗʰ **T56.7X1 Toxic effect of beryllium and its compounds, accidental (unintentional)**
Toxic effects of beryllium and its compounds NOS

7 √7ᵗʰ **T56.7X2 Toxic effect of beryllium and its compounds, intentional self-harm** HCC

√7ᵗʰ **T56.7X3 Toxic effect of beryllium and its compounds, assault**

√7ᵗʰ **T56.7X4 Toxic effect of beryllium and its compounds, undetermined**

√5ᵗʰ **T56.8 Toxic effects of other metals**

√6ᵗʰ **T56.81 Toxic effect of thallium**

√7ᵗʰ **T56.811 Toxic effect of thallium, accidental (unintentional)**
Toxic effect of thallium NOS

7 √7ᵗʰ **T56.812 Toxic effect of thallium, intentional self-harm** HCC

√7ᵗʰ **T56.813 Toxic effect of thallium, assault**

√7ᵗʰ **T56.814 Toxic effect of thallium, undetermined**

√6ᵗʰ **T56.89 Toxic effects of other metals**

√7ᵗʰ **T56.891 Toxic effect of other metals, accidental (unintentional)**
Toxic effects of other metals NOS

7 √7ᵗʰ **T56.892 Toxic effect of other metals, intentional self-harm** HCC

√7ᵗʰ **T56.893 Toxic effect of other metals, assault**

√7ᵗʰ **T56.894 Toxic effect of other metals, undetermined**

√5ᵗʰ **T56.9 Toxic effects of unspecified metal**

√x7ᵗʰ **T56.91 Toxic effect of unspecified metal, accidental (unintentional)**

7 √x7ᵗʰ **T56.92 Toxic effect of unspecified metal, intentional self-harm** HCC

√x7ᵗʰ **T56.93 Toxic effect of unspecified metal, assault**

√x7ᵗʰ **T56.94 Toxic effect of unspecified metal, undetermined**

√4ᵗʰ **T57 Toxic effect of other inorganic substances**

The appropriate 7th character is to be added to each code from category T57.
A initial encounter
D subsequent encounter
S sequela

√5ᵗʰ **T57.0 Toxic effect of arsenic and its compounds**

√6ᵗʰ **T57.0X Toxic effect of arsenic and its compounds**

√7ᵗʰ **T57.0X1 Toxic effect of arsenic and its compounds, accidental (unintentional)**
Toxic effect of arsenic and its compounds NOS

7 √7ᵗʰ **T57.0X2 Toxic effect of arsenic and its compounds, intentional self-harm** HCC

√7ᵗʰ **T57.0X3 Toxic effect of arsenic and its compounds, assault**

√7ᵗʰ **T57.0X4 Toxic effect of arsenic and its compounds, undetermined**

√5ᵗʰ **T57.1 Toxic effect of phosphorus and its compounds**

EXCLUDES 1 organophosphate insecticides (T60.0)

√6ᵗʰ **T57.1X Toxic effect of phosphorus and its compounds**

√7ᵗʰ **T57.1X1 Toxic effect of phosphorus and its compounds, accidental (unintentional)**
Toxic effect of phosphorus and its compounds NOS

7 √7ᵗʰ **T57.1X2 Toxic effect of phosphorus and its compounds, intentional self-harm** HCC

√7ᵗʰ **T57.1X3 Toxic effect of phosphorus and its compounds, assault**

√7ᵗʰ **T57.1X4 Toxic effect of phosphorus and its compounds, undetermined**

√5ᵗʰ **T57.2 Toxic effect of manganese and its compounds**

√6ᵗʰ **T57.2X Toxic effect of manganese and its compounds**

√7ᵗʰ **T57.2X1 Toxic effect of manganese and its compounds, accidental (unintentional)**
Toxic effect of manganese and its compounds NOS

7 √7ᵗʰ **T57.2X2 Toxic effect of manganese and its compounds, intentional self-harm** HCC

√7ᵗʰ **T57.2X3 Toxic effect of manganese and its compounds, assault**

√7ᵗʰ **T57.2X4 Toxic effect of manganese and its compounds, undetermined**

√5ᵗʰ **T57.3 Toxic effect of hydrogen cyanide**

√6ᵗʰ **T57.3X Toxic effect of hydrogen cyanide**

√7ᵗʰ **T57.3X1 Toxic effect of hydrogen cyanide, accidental (unintentional)**
Toxic effect of hydrogen cyanide NOS

7 √7ᵗʰ **T57.3X2 Toxic effect of hydrogen cyanide, intentional self-harm** HCC

√7ᵗʰ **T57.3X3 Toxic effect of hydrogen cyanide, assault**

√7ᵗʰ **T57.3X4 Toxic effect of hydrogen cyanide, undetermined**

√5ᵗʰ **T57.8 Toxic effect of other specified inorganic substances**

√6ᵗʰ **T57.8X Toxic effect of other specified inorganic substances**

√7ᵗʰ **T57.8X1 Toxic effect of other specified inorganic substances, accidental (unintentional)**
Toxic effect of other specified inorganic substances NOS

7 √7ᵗʰ **T57.8X2 Toxic effect of other specified inorganic substances, intentional self-harm** HCC

√7ᵗʰ **T57.8X3 Toxic effect of other specified inorganic substances, assault**

√7ᵗʰ **T57.8X4 Toxic effect of other specified inorganic substances, undetermined**

√5ᵗʰ **T57.9 Toxic effect of unspecified inorganic substance**

√x7ᵗʰ **T57.91 Toxic effect of unspecified inorganic substance, accidental (unintentional)**

7 √x7ᵗʰ **T57.92 Toxic effect of unspecified inorganic substance, intentional self-harm** HCC

√x7ᵗʰ **T57.93 Toxic effect of unspecified inorganic substance, assault**

√x7ᵗʰ **T57.94 Toxic effect of unspecified inorganic substance, undetermined**

√4ᵗʰ **T58 Toxic effect of carbon monoxide**

INCLUDES asphyxiation from carbon monoxide
toxic effect of carbon monoxide from all sources

The appropriate 7th character is to be added to each code from category T58.
A initial encounter
D subsequent encounter
S sequela

√5ᵗʰ **T58.0 Toxic effect of carbon monoxide from motor vehicle exhaust**
Toxic effect of exhaust gas from gas engine
Toxic effect of exhaust gas from motor pump

√x7ᵗʰ **T58.01 Toxic effect of carbon monoxide from motor vehicle exhaust, accidental (unintentional)**

7 √x7ᵗʰ **T58.02 Toxic effect of carbon monoxide from motor vehicle exhaust, intentional self-harm** HCC

√x7ᵗʰ **T58.03 Toxic effect of carbon monoxide from motor vehicle exhaust, assault**

√x7ᵗʰ **T58.04 Toxic effect of carbon monoxide from motor vehicle exhaust, undetermined**

√5ᵗʰ **T58.1 Toxic effect of carbon monoxide from utility gas**
Toxic effect of acetylene
Toxic effect of gas NOS used for lighting, heating, cooking
Toxic effect of water gas

√x7ᵗʰ **T58.11 Toxic effect of carbon monoxide from utility gas, accidental (unintentional)**

7 √x7ᵗʰ **T58.12 Toxic effect of carbon monoxide from utility gas, intentional self-harm** HCC

√x7ᵗʰ **T58.13 Toxic effect of carbon monoxide from utility gas, assault**

√x7ᵗʰ **T58.14** **Toxic effect of carbon monoxide from utility gas, undetermined**

√5ᵗʰ **T58.2** **Toxic effect of carbon monoxide from incomplete combustion of other domestic fuels**

Toxic effect of carbon monoxide from incomplete combustion of coal, coke, kerosene, wood

√6ᵗʰ **T58.2X** **Toxic effect of carbon monoxide from incomplete combustion of other domestic fuels**

√7ᵗʰ **T58.2X1** **Toxic effect of carbon monoxide from incomplete combustion of other domestic fuels, accidental (unintentional)**

7 √7ᵗʰ **T58.2X2** **Toxic effect of carbon monoxide from incomplete combustion of other domestic fuels, intentional self-harm** HCC

√7ᵗʰ **T58.2X3** **Toxic effect of carbon monoxide from incomplete combustion of other domestic fuels, assault**

√7ᵗʰ **T58.2X4** **Toxic effect of carbon monoxide from incomplete combustion of other domestic fuels, undetermined**

√5ᵗʰ **T58.8** **Toxic effect of carbon monoxide from other source**

Toxic effect of carbon monoxide from blast furnace gas
Toxic effect of carbon monoxide from fuels in industrial use
Toxic effect of carbon monoxide from kiln vapor

√6ᵗʰ **T58.8X** **Toxic effect of carbon monoxide from other source**

√7ᵗʰ **T58.8X1** **Toxic effect of carbon monoxide from other source, accidental (unintentional)**

7 √7ᵗʰ **T58.8X2** **Toxic effect of carbon monoxide from other source, intentional self-harm** HCC

√7ᵗʰ **T58.8X3** **Toxic effect of carbon monoxide from other source, assault**

√7ᵗʰ **T58.8X4** **Toxic effect of carbon monoxide from other source, undetermined**

√5ᵗʰ **T58.9** **Toxic effect of carbon monoxide from unspecified source**

√x7ᵗʰ **T58.91** **Toxic effect of carbon monoxide from unspecified source, accidental (unintentional)**

7 √x7ᵗʰ **T58.92** **Toxic effect of carbon monoxide from unspecified source, intentional self-harm** HCC

√x7ᵗʰ **T58.93** **Toxic effect of carbon monoxide from unspecified source, assault**

√x7ᵗʰ **T58.94** **Toxic effect of carbon monoxide from unspecified source, undetermined**

√4ᵗʰ **T59** **Toxic effect of other gases, fumes and vapors**

INCLUDES   aerosol propellants

EXCLUDES 1   *chlorofluorocarbons (T53.5)*

The appropriate 7th character is to be added to each code from category T59.
A   initial encounter
D   subsequent encounter
S   sequela

√5ᵗʰ **T59.0** **Toxic effect of nitrogen oxides**

√6ᵗʰ **T59.0X** **Toxic effect of nitrogen oxides**

√7ᵗʰ **T59.0X1** **Toxic effect of nitrogen oxides, accidental (unintentional)**
Toxic effect of nitrogen oxides NOS

7 √7ᵗʰ **T59.0X2** **Toxic effect of nitrogen oxides, intentional self-harm** HCC

√7ᵗʰ **T59.0X3** **Toxic effect of nitrogen oxides, assault**

√7ᵗʰ **T59.0X4** **Toxic effect of nitrogen oxides, undetermined**

√5ᵗʰ **T59.1** **Toxic effect of sulfur dioxide**

√6ᵗʰ **T59.1X** **Toxic effect of sulfur dioxide**

√7ᵗʰ **T59.1X1** **Toxic effect of sulfur dioxide, accidental (unintentional)**
Toxic effect of sulfur dioxide NOS

7 √7ᵗʰ **T59.1X2** **Toxic effect of sulfur dioxide, intentional self-harm** HCC

√7ᵗʰ **T59.1X3** **Toxic effect of sulfur dioxide, assault**

√7ᵗʰ **T59.1X4** **Toxic effect of sulfur dioxide, undetermined**

√5ᵗʰ **T59.2** **Toxic effect of formaldehyde**

√6ᵗʰ **T59.2X** **Toxic effect of formaldehyde**

√7ᵗʰ **T59.2X1** **Toxic effect of formaldehyde, accidental (unintentional)**
Toxic effect of formaldehyde NOS

7 √7ᵗʰ **T59.2X2** **Toxic effect of formaldehyde, intentional self-harm** HCC

√7ᵗʰ **T59.2X3** **Toxic effect of formaldehyde, assault**

√7ᵗʰ **T59.2X4** **Toxic effect of formaldehyde, undetermined**

√5ᵗʰ **T59.3** **Toxic effect of lacrimogenic gas**

Toxic effect of tear gas

√6ᵗʰ **T59.3X** **Toxic effect of lacrimogenic gas**

√7ᵗʰ **T59.3X1** **Toxic effect of lacrimogenic gas, accidental (unintentional)**
Toxic effect of lacrimogenic gas NOS

7 √7ᵗʰ **T59.3X2** **Toxic effect of lacrimogenic gas, intentional self-harm** HCC

√7ᵗʰ **T59.3X3** **Toxic effect of lacrimogenic gas, assault**

√7ᵗʰ **T59.3X4** **Toxic effect of lacrimogenic gas, undetermined**

√5ᵗʰ **T59.4** **Toxic effect of chlorine gas**

√6ᵗʰ **T59.4X** **Toxic effect of chlorine gas**

√7ᵗʰ **T59.4X1** **Toxic effect of chlorine gas, accidental (unintentional)**
Toxic effect of chlorine gas NOS

7 √7ᵗʰ **T59.4X2** **Toxic effect of chlorine gas, intentional self-harm** HCC

√7ᵗʰ **T59.4X3** **Toxic effect of chlorine gas, assault**

√7ᵗʰ **T59.4X4** **Toxic effect of chlorine gas, undetermined**

√5ᵗʰ **T59.5** **Toxic effect of fluorine gas and hydrogen fluoride**

√6ᵗʰ **T59.5X** **Toxic effect of fluorine gas and hydrogen fluoride**

√7ᵗʰ **T59.5X1** **Toxic effect of fluorine gas and hydrogen fluoride, accidental (unintentional)**
Toxic effect of fluorine gas and hydrogen fluoride NOS

7 √7ᵗʰ **T59.5X2** **Toxic effect of fluorine gas and hydrogen fluoride, intentional self-harm** HCC

√7ᵗʰ **T59.5X3** **Toxic effect of fluorine gas and hydrogen fluoride, assault**

√7ᵗʰ **T59.5X4** **Toxic effect of fluorine gas and hydrogen fluoride, undetermined**

√5ᵗʰ **T59.6** **Toxic effect of hydrogen sulfide**

√6ᵗʰ **T59.6X** **Toxic effect of hydrogen sulfide**

√7ᵗʰ **T59.6X1** **Toxic effect of hydrogen sulfide, accidental (unintentional)**
Toxic effect of hydrogen sulfide NOS

7 √7ᵗʰ **T59.6X2** **Toxic effect of hydrogen sulfide, intentional self-harm** HCC

√7ᵗʰ **T59.6X3** **Toxic effect of hydrogen sulfide, assault**

√7ᵗʰ **T59.6X4** **Toxic effect of hydrogen sulfide, undetermined**

√5ᵗʰ **T59.7** **Toxic effect of carbon dioxide**

√6ᵗʰ **T59.7X** **Toxic effect of carbon dioxide**

√7ᵗʰ **T59.7X1** **Toxic effect of carbon dioxide, accidental (unintentional)**
Toxic effect of carbon dioxide NOS

7 √7ᵗʰ **T59.7X2** **Toxic effect of carbon dioxide, intentional self-harm** HCC

√7ᵗʰ **T59.7X3** **Toxic effect of carbon dioxide, assault**

√7ᵗʰ **T59.7X4** **Toxic effect of carbon dioxide, undetermined**

N Newborn: 0   P Pediatric: 0-17   M Maternity: 9-64   A Adult: 15-124   MCC Major Complication/Comorbidity   CC Complication/Comorbidity   SW Severe Wound Dx

1176   ICD-10-CM 2020

√5ᵗʰ **T59.8** **Toxic effect of other specified gases, fumes and vapors**

     √6ᵗʰ **T59.81** **Toxic effect of** smoke

         Smoke inhalation

         EXCLUDES 2   *toxic effect of cigarette (tobacco) smoke (T65.22-)*

         √7ᵗʰ **T59.811** **Toxic effect of smoke, accidental (unintentional)**

             Toxic effect of smoke NOS

             AHA: 2013,4Q,121

         7 √7ᵗʰ **T59.812** **Toxic effect of smoke,**   HCC **intentional self-harm**

         √7ᵗʰ **T59.813** **Toxic effect of smoke, assault**

         √7ᵗʰ **T59.814** **Toxic effect of smoke, undetermined**

     √6ᵗʰ **T59.89** **Toxic effect of other specified gases, fumes and vapors**

         √7ᵗʰ **T59.891** **Toxic effect of other specified gases, fumes and vapors, accidental (unintentional)**

         7 √7ᵗʰ **T59.892** **Toxic effect of other**   HCC **specified gases, fumes and vapors, intentional self-harm**

         √7ᵗʰ **T59.893** **Toxic effect of other specified gases, fumes and vapors, assault**

         √7ᵗʰ **T59.894** **Toxic effect of other specified gases, fumes and vapors, undetermined**

√5ᵗʰ **T59.9** **Toxic effect of unspecified gases, fumes and vapors**

     √x7ᵗʰ **T59.91** **Toxic effect of unspecified gases, fumes and vapors, accidental (unintentional)**

     7 √x7ᵗʰ **T59.92** **Toxic effect of unspecified gases,**   HCC **fumes and vapors, intentional self-harm**

     √x7ᵗʰ **T59.93** **Toxic effect of unspecified gases, fumes and vapors, assault**

     √x7ᵗʰ **T59.94** **Toxic effect of unspecified gases, fumes and vapors, undetermined**

√4ᵗʰ **T60** **Toxic effect of pesticides**

     INCLUDES   toxic effect of wood preservatives

     The appropriate 7th character is to be added to each code from category T60.
     A   initial encounter
     D   subsequent encounter
     S   sequela

     √5ᵗʰ **T60.0** **Toxic effect of organophosphate and carbamate insecticides**

         √6ᵗʰ **T60.0X** **Toxic effect of** organophosphate and carbamate insecticides

             √7ᵗʰ **T60.0X1** **Toxic effect of organophosphate and carbamate insecticides, accidental (unintentional)**

                 Toxic effect of organophosphate and carbamate insecticides NOS

             7 √7ᵗʰ **T60.0X2** **Toxic effect of**   HCC **organophosphate and carbamate insecticides, intentional self-harm**

             √7ᵗʰ **T60.0X3** **Toxic effect of organophosphate and carbamate insecticides, assault**

             √7ᵗʰ **T60.0X4** **Toxic effect of organophosphate and carbamate insecticides, undetermined**

     √5ᵗʰ **T60.1** **Toxic effect of halogenated insecticides**

         EXCLUDES 1   *chlorinated hydrocarbon (T53.-)*

         √6ᵗʰ **T60.1X** **Toxic effect of** halogenated insecticides

             √7ᵗʰ **T60.1X1** **Toxic effect of halogenated insecticides, accidental (unintentional)**

                 Toxic effect of halogenated insecticides NOS

             7 √7ᵗʰ **T60.1X2** **Toxic effect of**   HCC **halogenated insecticides, intentional self-harm**

             √7ᵗʰ **T60.1X3** **Toxic effect of halogenated insecticides, assault**

             √7ᵗʰ **T60.1X4** **Toxic effect of halogenated insecticides, undetermined**

√5ᵗʰ **T60.2** **Toxic effect of other insecticides**

     √6ᵗʰ **T60.2X** **Toxic effect of** other insecticides

         √7ᵗʰ **T60.2X1** **Toxic effect of other insecticides, accidental (unintentional)**

             Toxic effect of other insecticides NOS

         7 √7ᵗʰ **T60.2X2** **Toxic effect of other**   HCC **insecticides, intentional self-harm**

         √7ᵗʰ **T60.2X3** **Toxic effect of other insecticides, assault**

         √7ᵗʰ **T60.2X4** **Toxic effect of other insecticides, undetermined**

√5ᵗʰ **T60.3** **Toxic effect of herbicides and fungicides**

     √6ᵗʰ **T60.3X** **Toxic effect of** herbicides and fungicides

         √7ᵗʰ **T60.3X1** **Toxic effect of herbicides and fungicides, accidental (unintentional)**

             Toxic effect of herbicides and fungicides NOS

         7 √7ᵗʰ **T60.3X2** **Toxic effect of herbicides**   HCC **and fungicides, intentional self-harm**

         √7ᵗʰ **T60.3X3** **Toxic effect of herbicides and fungicides, assault**

         √7ᵗʰ **T60.3X4** **Toxic effect of herbicides and fungicides, undetermined**

√5ᵗʰ **T60.4** **Toxic effect of rodenticides**

     EXCLUDES 1   *strychnine and its salts (T65.1)*

                     thallium (T56.81-)

     √6ᵗʰ **T60.4X** **Toxic effect of** rodenticides

         √7ᵗʰ **T60.4X1** **Toxic effect of rodenticides, accidental (unintentional)**

             Toxic effect of rodenticides NOS

         7 √7ᵗʰ **T60.4X2** **Toxic effect of**   HCC **rodenticides, intentional self-harm**

         √7ᵗʰ **T60.4X3** **Toxic effect of rodenticides, assault**

         √7ᵗʰ **T60.4X4** **Toxic effect of rodenticides, undetermined**

√5ᵗʰ **T60.8** **Toxic effect of other pesticides**

     √6ᵗʰ **T60.8X** **Toxic effect of other pesticides**

         √7ᵗʰ **T60.8X1** **Toxic effect of other pesticides, accidental (unintentional)**

             Toxic effect of other pesticides NOS

         7 √7ᵗʰ **T60.8X2** **Toxic effect of other**   HCC **pesticides, intentional self-harm**

         √7ᵗʰ **T60.8X3** **Toxic effect of other pesticides, assault**

         √7ᵗʰ **T60.8X4** **Toxic effect of other pesticides, undetermined**

√5ᵗʰ **T60.9** **Toxic effect of unspecified pesticide**

     √x7ᵗʰ **T60.91** **Toxic effect of unspecified pesticide, accidental (unintentional)**

     7 √x7ᵗʰ **T60.92** **Toxic effect of unspecified pesticide,**   HCC **intentional self-harm**

     √x7ᵗʰ **T60.93** **Toxic effect of unspecified pesticide, assault**

     √x7ᵗʰ **T60.94** **Toxic effect of unspecified pesticide, undetermined**

☑ Additional Character Required   √x7ᵗʰ Placeholder   Unacceptable PDx   Questionable PDx   Manifestation   Unspecified Dx   H1-H14 HAC   HCC CMS-HCC Dx   HIV HIV Dx

ICD-10-CM 2020   **1177**

Chapter 19. Injury, Poisoning and Certain Other Consequences of External Causes

✓4ᵗʰ T61 Toxic effect of noxious substances eaten as seafood

> **EXCLUDES 1**   *allergic reaction to food, such as:*
>   *anaphylactic reaction or shock due to adverse food reaction (T78.0-)*
>   *bacterial foodborne intoxications (A05.-)*
>   *dermatitis (L23.6, L25.4, L27.2)*
>   *food protein-induced enterocolitis syndrome (K52.21)*
>   *food protein-induced enteropathy (K52.22)*
>   *gastroenteritis (noninfective) (K52.29)*
>   *toxic effect of aflatoxin and other mycotoxins (T64)*
>   *toxic effect of cyanides (T65.0-)*
>   *toxic effect of harmful algae bloom (T65.82-)*
>   *toxic effect of hydrogen cyanide (T57.3-)*
>   *toxic effect of mercury (T56.1-)*
>   *toxic effect of red tide (T65.82-)*

> The appropriate 7th character is to be added to each code from category T61.
> A   initial encounter
> D   subsequent encounter
> S   sequela

✓5ᵗʰ T61.0 Ciguatera fish poisoning

   ✓x7ᵗʰ **T61.01 Ciguatera fish poisoning, accidental (unintentional)**

   7 ✓x7ᵗʰ **T61.02 Ciguatera fish poisoning, intentional self-harm**   HCC

   ✓x7ᵗʰ **T61.03 Ciguatera fish poisoning, assault**

   ✓x7ᵗʰ **T61.04 Ciguatera fish poisoning, undetermined**

✓5ᵗʰ T61.1 Scombroid fish poisoning

     Histamine-like syndrome

   ✓x7ᵗʰ **T61.11 Scombroid fish poisoning, accidental (unintentional)**

   7 ✓x7ᵗʰ **T61.12 Scombroid fish poisoning, intentional self-harm**   HCC

   ✓x7ᵗʰ **T61.13 Scombroid fish poisoning, assault**

   ✓x7ᵗʰ **T61.14 Scombroid fish poisoning, undetermined**

✓5ᵗʰ T61.7 Other fish and shellfish poisoning

   ✓6ᵗʰ **T61.77 Other fish poisoning**

     ✓7ᵗʰ **T61.771 Other fish poisoning, accidental (unintentional)**

     7 ✓7ᵗʰ **T61.772 Other fish poisoning, intentional self-harm**   HCC

     ✓7ᵗʰ **T61.773 Other fish poisoning, assault**

     ✓7ᵗʰ **T61.774 Other fish poisoning, undetermined**

   ✓6ᵗʰ **T61.78 Other shellfish poisoning**

     ✓7ᵗʰ **T61.781 Other shellfish poisoning, accidental (unintentional)**

     7 ✓7ᵗʰ **T61.782 Other shellfish poisoning, intentional self-harm**   HCC

     ✓7ᵗʰ **T61.783 Other shellfish poisoning, assault**

     ✓7ᵗʰ **T61.784 Other shellfish poisoning, undetermined**

✓5ᵗʰ T61.8 Toxic effect of other seafood

   ✓6ᵗʰ **T61.8X Toxic effect of other seafood**

     ✓7ᵗʰ **T61.8X1 Toxic effect of other seafood, accidental (unintentional)**

     7 ✓7ᵗʰ **T61.8X2 Toxic effect of other seafood, intentional self-harm**   HCC

     ✓7ᵗʰ **T61.8X3 Toxic effect of other seafood, assault**

     ✓7ᵗʰ **T61.8X4 Toxic effect of other seafood, undetermined**

✓5ᵗʰ T61.9 Toxic effect of unspecified seafood

   ✓x7ᵗʰ **T61.91 Toxic effect of unspecified seafood, accidental (unintentional)**

   7 ✓x7ᵗʰ **T61.92 Toxic effect of unspecified seafood, intentional self-harm**   HCC

   ✓x7ᵗʰ **T61.93 Toxic effect of unspecified seafood, assault**

   ✓x7ᵗʰ **T61.94 Toxic effect of unspecified seafood, undetermined**

✓4ᵗʰ T62 Toxic effect of other noxious substances eaten as food

> **EXCLUDES 1**   *allergic reaction to food, such as:*
>   *anaphylactic shock (reaction) due to adverse food reaction (T78.0-)*
>   *bacterial food borne intoxications (A05.-)*
>   *dermatitis (L23.6, L25.4, L27.2)*
>   *food protein-induced enterocolitis syndrome (K52.21)*
>   *food protein-induced enteropathy (K52.22)*
>   *gastroenteritis (noninfective) (K52.29)*
>   *toxic effect of aflatoxin and other mycotoxins (T64)*
>   *toxic effect of cyanides (T65.0-)*
>   *toxic effect of hydrogen cyanide (T57.3-)*
>   *toxic effect of mercury (T56.1-)*

> The appropriate 7th character is to be added to each code from category T62.
> A   initial encounter
> D   subsequent encounter
> S   sequela

✓5ᵗʰ T62.0 Toxic effect of ingested mushrooms

   ✓6ᵗʰ **T62.0X Toxic effect of ingested mushrooms**

     ✓7ᵗʰ **T62.0X1 Toxic effect of ingested mushrooms, accidental (unintentional)**
       Toxic effect of ingested mushrooms NOS

     7 ✓7ᵗʰ **T62.0X2 Toxic effect of ingested mushrooms, intentional self-harm**   HCC

     ✓7ᵗʰ **T62.0X3 Toxic effect of ingested mushrooms, assault**

     ✓7ᵗʰ **T62.0X4 Toxic effect of ingested mushrooms, undetermined**

✓5ᵗʰ T62.1 Toxic effect of ingested berries

   ✓6ᵗʰ **T62.1X Toxic effect of ingested berries**

     ✓7ᵗʰ **T62.1X1 Toxic effect of ingested berries, accidental (unintentional)**
       Toxic effect of ingested berries NOS

     7 ✓7ᵗʰ **T62.1X2 Toxic effect of ingested berries, intentional self-harm**   HCC

     ✓7ᵗʰ **T62.1X3 Toxic effect of ingested berries, assault**

     ✓7ᵗʰ **T62.1X4 Toxic effect of ingested berries, undetermined**

✓5ᵗʰ T62.2 Toxic effect of other ingested (parts of) plant(s)

   ✓6ᵗʰ **T62.2X Toxic effect of other ingested (parts of) plant(s)**

     ✓7ᵗʰ **T62.2X1 Toxic effect of other ingested (parts of) plant(s), accidental (unintentional)**
       Toxic effect of other ingested (parts of) plant(s) NOS

     7 ✓7ᵗʰ **T62.2X2 Toxic effect of other ingested (parts of) plant(s), intentional self-harm**   HCC

     ✓7ᵗʰ **T62.2X3 Toxic effect of other ingested (parts of) plant(s), assault**

     ✓7ᵗʰ **T62.2X4 Toxic effect of other ingested (parts of) plant(s), undetermined**

✓5ᵗʰ T62.8 Toxic effect of other specified noxious substances eaten as food

   ✓6ᵗʰ **T62.8X Toxic effect of other specified noxious substances eaten as food**

     ✓7ᵗʰ **T62.8X1 Toxic effect of other specified noxious substances eaten as food, accidental (unintentional)**
       Toxic effect of other specified noxious substances eaten as food NOS

     7 ✓7ᵗʰ **T62.8X2 Toxic effect of other specified noxious substances eaten as food, intentional self-harm**   HCC

     ✓7ᵗʰ **T62.8X3 Toxic effect of other specified noxious substances eaten as food, assault**

     ✓7ᵗʰ **T62.8X4 Toxic effect of other specified noxious substances eaten as food, undetermined**

✓5ᵗʰ T62.9 Toxic effect of unspecified noxious substance eaten as food

   ✓x7ᵗʰ **T62.91 Toxic effect of unspecified noxious substance eaten as food, accidental (unintentional)**
     Toxic effect of unspecified noxious substance eaten as food NOS

N Newborn: 0   P Pediatric: 0-17   M Maternity: 9-64   A Adult: 15-124   MCC Major Complication/Comorbidity   CC Complication/Comorbidity   SW Severe Wound Dx

1178   ICD-10-CM 2020

7 √x7ᵗʰ **T62.92** Toxic effect of unspecified noxious substance eaten as food, intentional self-harm   HCC

√x7ᵗʰ **T62.93** Toxic effect of unspecified noxious substance eaten as food, assault

√x7ᵗʰ **T62.94** Toxic effect of unspecified noxious substance eaten as food, undetermined

√4ᵗʰ **T63** Toxic effect of contact with venomous animals and plants

INCLUDES   bite or touch of venomous animal
pricked or stuck by thorn or leaf

EXCLUDES 2   ingestion of toxic animal or plant (T61.-, T62.-)

The appropriate 7th character is to be added to each code from category T63.
A   initial encounter
D   subsequent encounter
S   sequela

√5ᵗʰ **T63.0** Toxic effect of snake venom

√6ᵗʰ **T63.00** Toxic effect of unspecified snake venom

√7ᵗʰ **T63.001** Toxic effect of unspecified snake venom, accidental (unintentional)
Toxic effect of unspecified snake venom NOS

7 √7ᵗʰ **T63.002** Toxic effect of unspecified snake venom, intentional self-harm   HCC

√7ᵗʰ **T63.003** Toxic effect of unspecified snake venom, assault

√7ᵗʰ **T63.004** Toxic effect of unspecified snake venom, undetermined

√6ᵗʰ **T63.01** Toxic effect of rattlesnake venom

√7ᵗʰ **T63.011** Toxic effect of rattlesnake venom, accidental (unintentional)
Toxic effect of rattlesnake venom NOS

7 √7ᵗʰ **T63.012** Toxic effect of rattlesnake venom, intentional self-harm   HCC

√7ᵗʰ **T63.013** Toxic effect of rattlesnake venom, assault

√7ᵗʰ **T63.014** Toxic effect of rattlesnake venom, undetermined

√6ᵗʰ **T63.02** Toxic effect of coral snake venom

√7ᵗʰ **T63.021** Toxic effect of coral snake venom, accidental (unintentional)
Toxic effect of coral snake venom NOS

7 √7ᵗʰ **T63.022** Toxic effect of coral snake venom, intentional self-harm   HCC

√7ᵗʰ **T63.023** Toxic effect of coral snake venom, assault

√7ᵗʰ **T63.024** Toxic effect of coral snake venom, undetermined

√6ᵗʰ **T63.03** Toxic effect of taipan venom

√7ᵗʰ **T63.031** Toxic effect of taipan venom, accidental (unintentional)
Toxic effect of taipan venom NOS

7 √7ᵗʰ **T63.032** Toxic effect of taipan venom, intentional self-harm   HCC

√7ᵗʰ **T63.033** Toxic effect of taipan venom, assault

√7ᵗʰ **T63.034** Toxic effect of taipan venom, undetermined

√6ᵗʰ **T63.04** Toxic effect of cobra venom

√7ᵗʰ **T63.041** Toxic effect of cobra venom, accidental (unintentional)
Toxic effect of cobra venom NOS

7 √7ᵗʰ **T63.042** Toxic effect of cobra venom, intentional self-harm   HCC

√7ᵗʰ **T63.043** Toxic effect of cobra venom, assault

√7ᵗʰ **T63.044** Toxic effect of cobra venom, undetermined

√6ᵗʰ **T63.06** Toxic effect of venom of other North and South American snake

√7ᵗʰ **T63.061** Toxic effect of venom of other North and South American snake, accidental (unintentional)
Toxic effect of venom of other North and South American snake NOS

7 √7ᵗʰ **T63.062** Toxic effect of venom of other North and South American snake, intentional self-harm   HCC

√7ᵗʰ **T63.063** Toxic effect of venom of other North and South American snake, assault

√7ᵗʰ **T63.064** Toxic effect of venom of other North and South American snake, undetermined

√6ᵗʰ **T63.07** Toxic effect of venom of other Australian snake

√7ᵗʰ **T63.071** Toxic effect of venom of other Australian snake, accidental (unintentional)
Toxic effect of venom of other Australian snake NOS

7 √7ᵗʰ **T63.072** Toxic effect of venom of other Australian snake, intentional self-harm   HCC

√7ᵗʰ **T63.073** Toxic effect of venom of other Australian snake, assault

√7ᵗʰ **T63.074** Toxic effect of venom of other Australian snake, undetermined

√6ᵗʰ **T63.08** Toxic effect of venom of other African and Asian snake

√7ᵗʰ **T63.081** Toxic effect of venom of other African and Asian snake, accidental (unintentional)
Toxic effect of venom of other African and Asian snake NOS

7 √7ᵗʰ **T63.082** Toxic effect of venom of other African and Asian snake, intentional self-harm   HCC

√7ᵗʰ **T63.083** Toxic effect of venom of other African and Asian snake, assault

√7ᵗʰ **T63.084** Toxic effect of venom of other African and Asian snake, undetermined

√6ᵗʰ **T63.09** Toxic effect of venom of other snake

√7ᵗʰ **T63.091** Toxic effect of venom of other snake, accidental (unintentional)
Toxic effect of venom of other snake NOS

7 √7ᵗʰ **T63.092** Toxic effect of venom of other snake, intentional self-harm   HCC

√7ᵗʰ **T63.093** Toxic effect of venom of other snake, assault

√7ᵗʰ **T63.094** Toxic effect of venom of other snake, undetermined

√5ᵗʰ **T63.1** Toxic effect of venom of other reptiles

√6ᵗʰ **T63.11** Toxic effect of venom of gila monster

√7ᵗʰ **T63.111** Toxic effect of venom of gila monster, accidental (unintentional)
Toxic effect of venom of gila monster NOS

7 √7ᵗʰ **T63.112** Toxic effect of venom of gila monster, intentional self-harm   HCC

√7ᵗʰ **T63.113** Toxic effect of venom of gila monster, assault

√7ᵗʰ **T63.114** Toxic effect of venom of gila monster, undetermined

√6ᵗʰ **T63.12** Toxic effect of venom of other venomous lizard

√7ᵗʰ **T63.121** Toxic effect of venom of other venomous lizard, accidental (unintentional)
Toxic effect of venom of other venomous lizard NOS

7 √7ᵗʰ **T63.122** Toxic effect of venom of other venomous lizard, intentional self-harm   HCC

√7ᵗʰ **T63.123** Toxic effect of venom of other venomous lizard, assault

√7ᵗʰ **T63.124** Toxic effect of venom of other venomous lizard, undetermined

√6ᵗʰ **T63.19** Toxic effect of venom of other reptiles

√7ᵗʰ **T63.191** Toxic effect of venom of other reptiles, accidental (unintentional)
Toxic effect of venom of other reptiles NOS

7 √7ᵗʰ **T63.192** Toxic effect of venom of other reptiles, intentional self-harm   HCC

√7ᵗʰ **T63.193** Toxic effect of venom of other reptiles, assault

√7ᵗʰ **T63.194** Toxic effect of venom of other reptiles, undetermined

☑ Additional Character Required   √x7ᵗʰ Placeholder   Unacceptable PDx   Questionable PDx   Manifestation   Unspecified Dx   H1-H14 HAC   HCC CMS-HCC Dx   HIV HIV Dx

ICD-10-CM 2020   1179

✓5ᵗʰ **T63.2** Toxic effect of venom of scorpion

✓6ᵗʰ   **T63.2X**   Toxic effect of venom of scorpion

    ✓7ᵗʰ **T63.2X1** Toxic effect of venom of scorpion, accidental (unintentional)
         Toxic effect of venom of scorpion NOS

   7 ✓7ᵗʰ **T63.2X2** Toxic effect of venom of scorpion, intentional self-harm   HCC

    ✓7ᵗʰ **T63.2X3** Toxic effect of venom of scorpion, assault

    ✓7ᵗʰ **T63.2X4** Toxic effect of venom of scorpion, undetermined

✓5ᵗʰ **T63.3** Toxic effect of venom of spider

✓6ᵗʰ   **T63.30**   Toxic effect of unspecified spider venom

    ✓7ᵗʰ **T63.301** Toxic effect of unspecified spider venom, accidental (unintentional)

   7 ✓7ᵗʰ **T63.302** Toxic effect of unspecified spider venom, intentional self-harm   HCC

    ✓7ᵗʰ **T63.303** Toxic effect of unspecified spider venom, assault

    ✓7ᵗʰ **T63.304** Toxic effect of unspecified spider venom, undetermined

✓6ᵗʰ   **T63.31**   Toxic effect of venom of black widow spider

    ✓7ᵗʰ **T63.311** Toxic effect of venom of black widow spider, accidental (unintentional)

   7 ✓7ᵗʰ **T63.312** Toxic effect of venom of black widow spider, intentional self-harm   HCC

    ✓7ᵗʰ **T63.313** Toxic effect of venom of black widow spider, assault

    ✓7ᵗʰ **T63.314** Toxic effect of venom of black widow spider, undetermined

✓6ᵗʰ   **T63.32**   Toxic effect of venom of tarantula

    ✓7ᵗʰ **T63.321** Toxic effect of venom of tarantula, accidental (unintentional)

   7 ✓7ᵗʰ **T63.322** Toxic effect of venom of tarantula, intentional self-harm   HCC

    ✓7ᵗʰ **T63.323** Toxic effect of venom of tarantula, assault

    ✓7ᵗʰ **T63.324** Toxic effect of venom of tarantula, undetermined

✓6ᵗʰ   **T63.33**   Toxic effect of venom of brown recluse spider

    ✓7ᵗʰ **T63.331** Toxic effect of venom of brown recluse spider, accidental (unintentional)

   7 ✓7ᵗʰ **T63.332** Toxic effect of venom of brown recluse spider, intentional self-harm   HCC

    ✓7ᵗʰ **T63.333** Toxic effect of venom of brown recluse spider, assault

    ✓7ᵗʰ **T63.334** Toxic effect of venom of brown recluse spider, undetermined

✓6ᵗʰ   **T63.39**   Toxic effect of venom of other spider

    ✓7ᵗʰ **T63.391** Toxic effect of venom of other spider, accidental (unintentional)

   7 ✓7ᵗʰ **T63.392** Toxic effect of venom of other spider, intentional self-harm   HCC

    ✓7ᵗʰ **T63.393** Toxic effect of venom of other spider, assault

    ✓7ᵗʰ **T63.394** Toxic effect of venom of other spider, undetermined

✓5ᵗʰ **T63.4** Toxic effect of venom of other arthropods

✓6ᵗʰ   **T63.41**   Toxic effect of venom of centipedes and venomous millipedes

    ✓7ᵗʰ **T63.411** Toxic effect of venom of centipedes and venomous millipedes, accidental (unintentional)

   7 ✓7ᵗʰ **T63.412** Toxic effect of venom of centipedes and venomous millipedes, intentional self-harm   HCC

    ✓7ᵗʰ **T63.413** Toxic effect of venom of centipedes and venomous millipedes, assault

    ✓7ᵗʰ **T63.414** Toxic effect of venom of centipedes and venomous millipedes, undetermined

✓6ᵗʰ   **T63.42**   Toxic effect of venom of ants

    ✓7ᵗʰ **T63.421** Toxic effect of venom of ants, accidental (unintentional)

   7 ✓7ᵗʰ **T63.422** Toxic effect of venom of ants, intentional self-harm   HCC

    ✓7ᵗʰ **T63.423** Toxic effect of venom of ants, assault

    ✓7ᵗʰ **T63.424** Toxic effect of venom of ants, undetermined

✓6ᵗʰ   **T63.43**   Toxic effect of venom of caterpillars

    ✓7ᵗʰ **T63.431** Toxic effect of venom of caterpillars, accidental (unintentional)

   7 ✓7ᵗʰ **T63.432** Toxic effect of venom of caterpillars, intentional self-harm   HCC

    ✓7ᵗʰ **T63.433** Toxic effect of venom of caterpillars, assault

    ✓7ᵗʰ **T63.434** Toxic effect of venom of caterpillars, undetermined

✓6ᵗʰ   **T63.44**   Toxic effect of venom of bees

    ✓7ᵗʰ **T63.441** Toxic effect of venom of bees, accidental (unintentional)

   7 ✓7ᵗʰ **T63.442** Toxic effect of venom of bees, intentional self-harm   HCC

    ✓7ᵗʰ **T63.443** Toxic effect of venom of bees, assault

    ✓7ᵗʰ **T63.444** Toxic effect of venom of bees, undetermined

✓6ᵗʰ   **T63.45**   Toxic effect of venom of hornets

    ✓7ᵗʰ **T63.451** Toxic effect of venom of hornets, accidental (unintentional)

   7 ✓7ᵗʰ **T63.452** Toxic effect of venom of hornets, intentional self-harm   HCC

    ✓7ᵗʰ **T63.453** Toxic effect of venom of hornets, assault

    ✓7ᵗʰ **T63.454** Toxic effect of venom of hornets, undetermined

✓6ᵗʰ   **T63.46**   Toxic effect of venom of wasps
         Toxic effect of yellow jacket

    ✓7ᵗʰ **T63.461** Toxic effect of venom of wasps, accidental (unintentional)

   7 ✓7ᵗʰ **T63.462** Toxic effect of venom of wasps, intentional self-harm   HCC

    ✓7ᵗʰ **T63.463** Toxic effect of venom of wasps, assault

    ✓7ᵗʰ **T63.464** Toxic effect of venom of wasps, undetermined

✓6ᵗʰ   **T63.48**   Toxic effect of venom of other arthropod

    ✓7ᵗʰ **T63.481** Toxic effect of venom of other arthropod, accidental (unintentional)

   7 ✓7ᵗʰ **T63.482** Toxic effect of venom of other arthropod, intentional self-harm   HCC

    ✓7ᵗʰ **T63.483** Toxic effect of venom of other arthropod, assault

    ✓7ᵗʰ **T63.484** Toxic effect of venom of other arthropod, undetermined

✓5ᵗʰ **T63.5** Toxic effect of contact with venomous fish

    EXCLUDES 2   poisoning by ingestion of fish (T61.-)

✓6ᵗʰ   **T63.51**   Toxic effect of contact with stingray

    ✓7ᵗʰ **T63.511** Toxic effect of contact with stingray, accidental (unintentional)

   7 ✓7ᵗʰ **T63.512** Toxic effect of contact with stingray, intentional self-harm   HCC

    ✓7ᵗʰ **T63.513** Toxic effect of contact with stingray, assault

    ✓7ᵗʰ **T63.514** Toxic effect of contact with stingray, undetermined

✓6ᵗʰ   **T63.59**   Toxic effect of contact with other venomous fish

    ✓7ᵗʰ **T63.591** Toxic effect of contact with other venomous fish, accidental (unintentional)

   7 ✓7ᵗʰ **T63.592** Toxic effect of contact with other venomous fish, intentional self-harm   HCC

    ✓7ᵗʰ **T63.593** Toxic effect of contact with other venomous fish, assault

    ✓7ᵗʰ **T63.594** Toxic effect of contact with other venomous fish, undetermined

---

Ⓝ Newborn: 0   Ⓟ Pediatric: 0-17   Ⓜ Maternity: 9-64   Ⓐ Adult: 15-124   MCC Major Complication/Comorbidity   CC Complication/Comorbidity   SW Severe Wound Dx

√5ᵗʰ **T63.6** **Toxic effect of contact with other venomous marine animals**
    EXCLUDES 1   sea-snake venom (T63.09)
    EXCLUDES 2   poisoning by ingestion of shellfish (T61.78-)

   √6ᵗʰ **T63.61** **Toxic effect of contact with Portugese Man-o-war**
      Toxic effect of contact with bluebottle

      √7ᵗʰ **T63.611** **Toxic effect of contact with Portugese Man-o-war, accidental (unintentional)**

      7 √7ᵗʰ **T63.612** **Toxic effect of contact with Portugese Man-o-war, intentional self-harm**   HCC

      √7ᵗʰ **T63.613** **Toxic effect of contact with Portugese Man-o-war, assault**

      √7ᵗʰ **T63.614** **Toxic effect of contact with Portugese Man-o-war, undetermined**

   √6ᵗʰ **T63.62** **Toxic effect of contact with other jellyfish**

      √7ᵗʰ **T63.621** **Toxic effect of contact with other jellyfish, accidental (unintentional)**

      7 √7ᵗʰ **T63.622** **Toxic effect of contact with other jellyfish, intentional self-harm**   HCC

      √7ᵗʰ **T63.623** **Toxic effect of contact with other jellyfish, assault**

      √7ᵗʰ **T63.624** **Toxic effect of contact with other jellyfish, undetermined**

   √6ᵗʰ **T63.63** **Toxic effect of contact with sea anemone**

      √7ᵗʰ **T63.631** **Toxic effect of contact with sea anemone, accidental (unintentional)**

      7 √7ᵗʰ **T63.632** **Toxic effect of contact with sea anemone, intentional self-harm**   HCC

      √7ᵗʰ **T63.633** **Toxic effect of contact with sea anemone, assault**

      √7ᵗʰ **T63.634** **Toxic effect of contact with sea anemone, undetermined**

   √6ᵗʰ **T63.69** **Toxic effect of contact with other venomous marine animals**

      √7ᵗʰ **T63.691** **Toxic effect of contact with other venomous marine animals, accidental (unintentional)**

      7 √7ᵗʰ **T63.692** **Toxic effect of contact with other venomous marine animals, intentional self-harm**   HCC

      √7ᵗʰ **T63.693** **Toxic effect of contact with other venomous marine animals, assault**

      √7ᵗʰ **T63.694** **Toxic effect of contact with other venomous marine animals, undetermined**

√5ᵗʰ **T63.7** **Toxic effect of contact with venomous plant**

   √6ᵗʰ **T63.71** **Toxic effect of contact with venomous marine plant**

      √7ᵗʰ **T63.711** **Toxic effect of contact with venomous marine plant, accidental (unintentional)**

      7 √7ᵗʰ **T63.712** **Toxic effect of contact with venomous marine plant, intentional self-harm**   HCC

      √7ᵗʰ **T63.713** **Toxic effect of contact with venomous marine plant, assault**

      √7ᵗʰ **T63.714** **Toxic effect of contact with venomous marine plant, undetermined**

   √6ᵗʰ **T63.79** **Toxic effect of contact with other venomous plant**

      √7ᵗʰ **T63.791** **Toxic effect of contact with other venomous plant, accidental (unintentional)**

      7 √7ᵗʰ **T63.792** **Toxic effect of contact with other venomous plant, intentional self-harm**   HCC

      √7ᵗʰ **T63.793** **Toxic effect of contact with other venomous plant, assault**

      √7ᵗʰ **T63.794** **Toxic effect of contact with other venomous plant, undetermined**

√5ᵗʰ **T63.8** **Toxic effect of contact with other venomous animals**

   √6ᵗʰ **T63.81** **Toxic effect of contact with venomous frog**
      EXCLUDES 1   contact with nonvenomous frog (W62.0)

      √7ᵗʰ **T63.811** **Toxic effect of contact with venomous frog, accidental (unintentional)**

      7 √7ᵗʰ **T63.812** **Toxic effect of contact with venomous frog, intentional self-harm**   HCC

      √7ᵗʰ **T63.813** **Toxic effect of contact with venomous frog, assault**

      √7ᵗʰ **T63.814** **Toxic effect of contact with venomous frog, undetermined**

   √6ᵗʰ **T63.82** **Toxic effect of contact with venomous toad**
      EXCLUDES 1   contact with nonvenomous toad (W62.1)

      √7ᵗʰ **T63.821** **Toxic effect of contact with venomous toad, accidental (unintentional)**

      7 √7ᵗʰ **T63.822** **Toxic effect of contact with venomous toad, intentional self-harm**   HCC

      √7ᵗʰ **T63.823** **Toxic effect of contact with venomous toad, assault**

      √7ᵗʰ **T63.824** **Toxic effect of contact with venomous toad, undetermined**

   √6ᵗʰ **T63.83** **Toxic effect of contact with other venomous amphibian**
      EXCLUDES 1   contact with nonvenomous amphibian (W62.9)

      √7ᵗʰ **T63.831** **Toxic effect of contact with other venomous amphibian, accidental (unintentional)**

      7 √7ᵗʰ **T63.832** **Toxic effect of contact with other venomous amphibian, intentional self-harm**   HCC

      √7ᵗʰ **T63.833** **Toxic effect of contact with other venomous amphibian, assault**

      √7ᵗʰ **T63.834** **Toxic effect of contact with other venomous amphibian, undetermined**

   √6ᵗʰ **T63.89** **Toxic effect of contact with other venomous animals**

      √7ᵗʰ **T63.891** **Toxic effect of contact with other venomous animals, accidental (unintentional)**

      7 √7ᵗʰ **T63.892** **Toxic effect of contact with other venomous animals, intentional self-harm**   HCC

      √7ᵗʰ **T63.893** **Toxic effect of contact with other venomous animals, assault**

      √7ᵗʰ **T63.894** **Toxic effect of contact with other venomous animals, undetermined**

√5ᵗʰ **T63.9** **Toxic effect of contact with unspecified venomous animal**

   √x7ᵗʰ **T63.91** **Toxic effect of contact with unspecified venomous animal, accidental (unintentional)**

   7 √x7ᵗʰ **T63.92** **Toxic effect of contact with unspecified venomous animal, intentional self-harm**   HCC

   √x7ᵗʰ **T63.93** **Toxic effect of contact with unspecified venomous animal, assault**

   √x7ᵗʰ **T63.94** **Toxic effect of contact with unspecified venomous animal, undetermined**

√4ᵗʰ **T64** **Toxic effect of aflatoxin and other mycotoxin food contaminants**

> The appropriate 7th character is to be added to each code from category T64.
> A   initial encounter
> D   subsequent encounter
> S   sequela

√5ᵗʰ **T64.0** **Toxic effect of aflatoxin**

   √x7ᵗʰ **T64.01** **Toxic effect of aflatoxin, accidental (unintentional)**

   7 √x7ᵗʰ **T64.02** **Toxic effect of aflatoxin, intentional self-harm**   HCC

   √x7ᵗʰ **T64.03** **Toxic effect of aflatoxin, assault**

   √x7ᵗʰ **T64.04** **Toxic effect of aflatoxin, undetermined**

√5ᵗʰ **T64.8** **Toxic effect of other mycotoxin food contaminants**

   √x7ᵗʰ **T64.81** **Toxic effect of other mycotoxin food contaminants, accidental (unintentional)**

   7 √x7ᵗʰ **T64.82** **Toxic effect of other mycotoxin food contaminants, intentional self-harm**   HCC

   √x7ᵗʰ **T64.83** **Toxic effect of other mycotoxin food contaminants, assault**

   √x7ᵗʰ **T64.84** **Toxic effect of other mycotoxin food contaminants, undetermined**

✓4ᵗʰ **T65 Toxic effect of other and unspecified substances**

> The appropriate 7th character is to be added to each code from category T65.
> A initial encounter
> D subsequent encounter
> S sequela

✓5ᵗʰ **T65.0 Toxic effect of cyanides**

EXCLUDES 1 *hydrogen cyanide (T57.3-)*

✓6ᵗʰ **T65.0X Toxic effect of** cyanides

✓7ᵗʰ **T65.0X1 Toxic effect of cyanides, accidental (unintentional)**
Toxic effect of cyanides NOS

⁷ ✓7ᵗʰ **T65.0X2 Toxic effect of cyanides, intentional self-harm** HCC

✓7ᵗʰ **T65.0X3 Toxic effect of cyanides, assault**

✓7ᵗʰ **T65.0X4 Toxic effect of cyanides, undetermined**

✓5ᵗʰ **T65.1 Toxic effect of strychnine and its salts**

✓6ᵗʰ **T65.1X Toxic effect of** strychnine and its salts

✓7ᵗʰ **T65.1X1 Toxic effect of strychnine and its salts, accidental (unintentional)**
Toxic effect of strychnine and its salts NOS

⁷ ✓7ᵗʰ **T65.1X2 Toxic effect of strychnine and its salts, intentional self-harm** HCC

✓7ᵗʰ **T65.1X3 Toxic effect of strychnine and its salts, assault**

✓7ᵗʰ **T65.1X4 Toxic effect of strychnine and its salts, undetermined**

✓5ᵗʰ **T65.2 Toxic effect of tobacco and nicotine**

EXCLUDES 2 *nicotine dependence (F17.-)*

✓6ᵗʰ **T65.21 Toxic effect of** chewing tobacco

✓7ᵗʰ **T65.211 Toxic effect of chewing tobacco, accidental (unintentional)**
Toxic effect of chewing tobacco NOS

⁷ ✓7ᵗʰ **T65.212 Toxic effect of chewing tobacco, intentional self-harm** HCC

✓7ᵗʰ **T65.213 Toxic effect of chewing tobacco, assault**

✓7ᵗʰ **T65.214 Toxic effect of chewing tobacco, undetermined**

✓6ᵗʰ **T65.22 Toxic effect of** tobacco cigarettes
Toxic effect of tobacco smoke
Use additional code for exposure to second hand tobacco smoke (Z57.31, Z77.22)

✓7ᵗʰ **T65.221 Toxic effect of tobacco cigarettes, accidental (unintentional)**
Toxic effect of tobacco cigarettes NOS

⁷ ✓7ᵗʰ **T65.222 Toxic effect of tobacco cigarettes, intentional self-harm** HCC

✓7ᵗʰ **T65.223 Toxic effect of tobacco cigarettes, assault**

✓7ᵗʰ **T65.224 Toxic effect of tobacco cigarettes, undetermined**

✓6ᵗʰ **T65.29 Toxic effect of** other tobacco and nicotine

✓7ᵗʰ **T65.291 Toxic effect of other tobacco and nicotine, accidental (unintentional)**
Toxic effect of other tobacco and nicotine NOS

⁷ ✓7ᵗʰ **T65.292 Toxic effect of other tobacco and nicotine, intentional self-harm** HCC

✓7ᵗʰ **T65.293 Toxic effect of other tobacco and nicotine, assault**

✓7ᵗʰ **T65.294 Toxic effect of other tobacco and nicotine, undetermined**

✓5ᵗʰ **T65.3 Toxic effect of nitroderivatives and aminoderivatives of benzene and its homologues**
Toxic effect of anilin [benzenamine]
Toxic effect of nitrobenzene
Toxic effect of trinitrotoluene

✓6ᵗʰ **T65.3X Toxic effect of** nitroderivatives and aminoderivatives of benzene and its homologues

✓7ᵗʰ **T65.3X1 Toxic effect of nitroderivatives and aminoderivatives of benzene and its homologues, accidental (unintentional)**
Toxic effect of nitroderivatives and aminoderivatives of benzene and its homologues NOS

⁷ ✓7ᵗʰ **T65.3X2 Toxic effect of nitroderivatives and aminoderivatives of benzene and its homologues, intentional self-harm** HCC

✓7ᵗʰ **T65.3X3 Toxic effect of nitroderivatives and aminoderivatives of benzene and its homologues, assault**

✓7ᵗʰ **T65.3X4 Toxic effect of nitroderivatives and aminoderivatives of benzene and its homologues, undetermined**

✓5ᵗʰ **T65.4 Toxic effect of carbon disulfide**

✓6ᵗʰ **T65.4X Toxic effect of** carbon disulfide

✓7ᵗʰ **T65.4X1 Toxic effect of carbon disulfide, accidental (unintentional)**
Toxic effect of carbon disulfide NOS

⁷ ✓7ᵗʰ **T65.4X2 Toxic effect of carbon disulfide, intentional self-harm** HCC

✓7ᵗʰ **T65.4X3 Toxic effect of carbon disulfide, assault**

✓7ᵗʰ **T65.4X4 Toxic effect of carbon disulfide, undetermined**

✓5ᵗʰ **T65.5 Toxic effect of nitroglycerin and other nitric acids and esters**
Toxic effect of 1,2,3-Propanetriol trinitrate

✓6ᵗʰ **T65.5X Toxic effect of** nitroglycerin and other nitric acids and esters

✓7ᵗʰ **T65.5X1 Toxic effect of nitroglycerin and other nitric acids and esters, accidental (unintentional)**
Toxic effect of nitroglycerin and other nitric acids and esters NOS

⁷ ✓7ᵗʰ **T65.5X2 Toxic effect of nitroglycerin and other nitric acids and esters, intentional self-harm** HCC

✓7ᵗʰ **T65.5X3 Toxic effect of nitroglycerin and other nitric acids and esters, assault**

✓7ᵗʰ **T65.5X4 Toxic effect of nitroglycerin and other nitric acids and esters, undetermined**

✓5ᵗʰ **T65.6 Toxic effect of paints and dyes, not elsewhere classified**

✓6ᵗʰ **T65.6X Toxic effect of** paints and dyes, not elsewhere classified

✓7ᵗʰ **T65.6X1 Toxic effect of paints and dyes, not elsewhere classified, accidental (unintentional)**
Toxic effect of paints and dyes NOS

⁷ ✓7ᵗʰ **T65.6X2 Toxic effect of paints and dyes, not elsewhere classified, intentional self-harm** HCC

✓7ᵗʰ **T65.6X3 Toxic effect of paints and dyes, not elsewhere classified, assault**

✓7ᵗʰ **T65.6X4 Toxic effect of paints and dyes, not elsewhere classified, undetermined**

✓5ᵗʰ **T65.8 Toxic effect of other specified substances**

✓6ᵗʰ **T65.81 Toxic effect of** latex

✓7ᵗʰ **T65.811 Toxic effect of latex, accidental (unintentional)**
Toxic effect of latex NOS

⁷ ✓7ᵗʰ **T65.812 Toxic effect of latex, intentional self-harm** HCC

✓7ᵗʰ **T65.813 Toxic effect of latex, assault**

✓7ᵗʰ **T65.814 Toxic effect of latex, undetermined**

N Newborn: 0   P Pediatric: 0-17   M Maternity: 9-64   A Adult: 15-124   MCC Major Complication/Comorbidity   CC Complication/Comorbidity   SW Severe Wound Dx

√6ᵗʰ **T65.82** **Toxic effect of harmful algae and algae toxins**

Toxic effect of (harmful) algae bloom NOS
Toxic effect of blue-green algae bloom
Toxic effect of brown tide
Toxic effect of cyanobacteria bloom
Toxic effect of Florida red tide
Toxic effect of pfiesteria piscicida
Toxic effect of red tide

√7ᵗʰ **T65.821** **Toxic effect of harmful algae and algae toxins, accidental (unintentional)**

Toxic effect of harmful algae and algae toxins NOS

7 √7ᵗʰ **T65.822** **Toxic effect of harmful algae and algae toxins, intentional self-harm**   HCC

√7ᵗʰ **T65.823** **Toxic effect of harmful algae and algae toxins, assault**

√7ᵗʰ **T65.824** **Toxic effect of harmful algae and algae toxins, undetermined**

√6ᵗʰ **T65.83** **Toxic effect of fiberglass**

√7ᵗʰ **T65.831** **Toxic effect of fiberglass, accidental (unintentional)**

Toxic effect of fiberglass NOS

7 √7ᵗʰ **T65.832** **Toxic effect of fiberglass, intentional self-harm**   HCC

√7ᵗʰ **T65.833** **Toxic effect of fiberglass, assault**

√7ᵗʰ **T65.834** **Toxic effect of fiberglass, undetermined**

√6ᵗʰ **T65.89** **Toxic effect of other specified substances**

√7ᵗʰ **T65.891** **Toxic effect of other specified substances, accidental (unintentional)**

Toxic effect of other specified substances NOS

AHA: 2018,1Q,5

7 √7ᵗʰ **T65.892** **Toxic effect of other specified substances, intentional self-harm**   HCC

√7ᵗʰ **T65.893** **Toxic effect of other specified substances, assault**

√7ᵗʰ **T65.894** **Toxic effect of other specified substances, undetermined**

√5ᵗʰ **T65.9** **Toxic effect of unspecified substance**

√7ᵗʰ **T65.91** **Toxic effect of unspecified substance, accidental (unintentional)**

Poisoning NOS

7 √7ᵗʰ **T65.92** **Toxic effect of unspecified substance, intentional self-harm**   HCC

√7ᵗʰ **T65.93** **Toxic effect of unspecified substance, assault**

√7ᵗʰ **T65.94** **Toxic effect of unspecified substance, undetermined**

Other and unspecified effects of external causes (T66-T78)

√x7ᵗʰ **T66** **Radiation sickness, unspecified**

EXCLUDES 1   specified adverse effects of radiation, such as:
     burns (T20-T31)
     leukemia (C91-C95)
     radiation gastroenteritis and colitis (K52.0)
     radiation pneumonitis (J70.0)
     radiation related disorders of the skin and subcutaneous tissue (L55-L59)
     radiation sunburn (L55.-)

The appropriate 7th character is to be added to code T66.
A   initial encounter
D   subsequent encounter
S   sequela

√4ᵗʰ **T67** **Effects of heat and light**

EXCLUDES 1   erythema [dermatitis] ab igne (L59.0)
     malignant hyperpyrexia due to anesthesia (T88.3)
     radiation-related disorders of the skin and subcutaneous tissue (L55-L59)

EXCLUDES 2   burns (T20-T31)
     sunburn (L55.-)
     sweat disorder due to heat (L74-L75)

The appropriate 7th character is to be added to each code from category T67.
A   initial encounter
D   subsequent encounter
S   sequela

√5ᵗʰ **T67.0** **Heatstroke and sunstroke**

~~Heat apoplexy~~
~~Heat pyrexia~~
~~Siriasis~~
~~Thermoplegia~~

Use additional code(s) to identify any associated complications of heatstroke, such as:
     coma and stupor (R40.-)
     ►rhabdomyolysis (M62.82)◄
     systemic inflammatory response syndrome (R65.1-)

DEF: Headache, vertigo, cramps, and elevated body temperature due to prolonged exposure to high environmental temperatures that requires emergency intervention.

√x7ᵗʰ **T67.01** **Heatstroke and sunstroke**   CC

Heat apoplexy
Heat pyrexia
Siriasis
Thermoplegia

√x7ᵗʰ **T67.02** **Exertional heatstroke**   CC

√x7ᵗʰ **T67.09** **Other heatstroke and sunstroke**   CC

√x7ᵗʰ **T67.1** **Heat syncope**

Heat collapse

√x7ᵗʰ **T67.2** **Heat cramp**

√x7ᵗʰ **T67.3** **Heat exhaustion, anhydrotic**

Heat prostration due to water depletion

EXCLUDES 1   heat exhaustion due to salt depletion (T67.4)

√x7ᵗʰ **T67.4** **Heat exhaustion due to salt depletion**

Heat prostration due to salt (and water) depletion

√x7ᵗʰ **T67.5** **Heat exhaustion, unspecified**

Heat prostration NOS

√x7ᵗʰ **T67.6** **Heat fatigue, transient**

√x7ᵗʰ **T67.7** **Heat edema**

√x7ᵗʰ **T67.8** **Other effects of heat and light**

√x7ᵗʰ **T67.9** **Effect of heat and light, unspecified**

√x7ᵗʰ **T68** **Hypothermia**

Accidental hypothermia
Hypothermia NOS

Use additional code to identify source of exposure:
     exposure to excessive cold of man-made origin (W93)
     exposure to excessive cold of natural origin (X31)

EXCLUDES 1   hypothermia following anesthesia (T88.51)
     hypothermia not associated with low environmental temperature (R68.0)
     hypothermia of newborn (P80.-)

EXCLUDES 2   frostbite (T33-T34)

The appropriate 7th character is to be added to code T68.
A   initial encounter
D   subsequent encounter
S   sequela

Chapter 19. Injury, Poisoning and Certain Other Consequences of External Causes   T69–T71.144

√4ᵗʰ **T69   Other effects of reduced temperature**

Use additional code to identify source of exposure:
exposure to excessive cold of man-made origin (W93)
exposure to excessive cold of natural origin (X31)

EXCLUDES 2   frostbite (T33-T34)

The appropriate 7th character is to be added to each code from category T69.
A   initial encounter
D   subsequent encounter
S   sequela

√5ᵗʰ   **T69.0   Immersion hand and foot**

   √6ᵗʰ   **T69.01   Immersion hand**

     √7ᵗʰ   **T69.011   Immersion hand, right hand**

     √7ᵗʰ   **T69.012   Immersion hand, left hand**

     √7ᵗʰ   **T69.019   Immersion hand, unspecified hand**

   √6ᵗʰ   **T69.02   Immersion foot**

     Trench foot
     CC Excl: For CC codes in subcategory T69.02: PDX collection 1420

     √7ᵗʰ   **T69.021   Immersion foot, right foot**   CC H5

     √7ᵗʰ   **T69.022   Immersion foot, left foot**   CC H5

     √7ᵗʰ   **T69.029   Immersion foot, unspecified foot**   CC H5

√x7ᵗʰ   **T69.1   Chilblains**

DEF: Red, swollen, itchy skin primarily affecting the fingers and toes, nose and ears, and legs. Chilblains follows damp-cold exposure, and can also be associated with pruritus and a burning feeling.

√x7ᵗʰ   **T69.8   Other specified effects of reduced temperature**

√x7ᵗʰ   **T69.9   Effect of reduced temperature, unspecified**

√4ᵗʰ **T70   Effects of air pressure and water pressure**

The appropriate 7th character is to be added to each code from category T70.
A   initial encounter
D   subsequent encounter
S   sequela

√x7ᵗʰ   **T70.0   Otitic barotrauma**

Aero-otitis media
Effects of change in ambient atmospheric pressure or water pressure on ears

√x7ᵗʰ   **T70.1   Sinus barotrauma**

Aerosinusitis
Effects of change in ambient atmospheric pressure on sinuses

√5ᵗʰ   **T70.2   Other and unspecified effects of high altitude**

EXCLUDES 2   polycythemia due to high altitude (D75.1)

   √x7ᵗʰ   **T70.20   Unspecified effects of high altitude**

   √x7ᵗʰ   **T70.29   Other effects of high altitude**

     Alpine sickness
     Anoxia due to high altitude
     Barotrauma NOS
     Hypobaropathy
     Mountain sickness

√x7ᵗʰ   **T70.3   Caisson disease [decompression sickness]**   CC H5

Compressed-air disease
Diver's palsy or paralysis
DEF: Rapid reduction in air pressure while breathing compressed air. Symptoms include skin lesions, joint pains, and respiratory and neurological problems.
CC Excl: PDX collection 1421

√x7ᵗʰ   **T70.4   Effects of high-pressure fluids**

Hydraulic jet injection (industrial)
Pneumatic jet injection (industrial)
Traumatic jet injection (industrial)

√x7ᵗʰ   **T70.8   Other effects of air pressure and water pressure**

√x7ᵗʰ   **T70.9   Effect of air pressure and water pressure, unspecified**

√4ᵗʰ **T71   Asphyxiation**

Mechanical suffocation
Traumatic suffocation

EXCLUDES 1   acute respiratory distress (syndrome) (J80)
anoxia due to high altitude (T70.2)
asphyxia NOS (R09.01)
asphyxia from carbon monoxide (T58.-)
asphyxia from inhalation of food or foreign body (T17.-)
asphyxia from other gases, fumes and vapors (T59.-)
respiratory distress (syndrome) in newborn (P22.-)

The appropriate 7th character is to be added to each code from category T71.
A   initial encounter
D   subsequent encounter
S   sequela

CC Excl: For CC codes in category T71: PDX collection 1422

√5ᵗʰ   **T71.1   Asphyxiation due to mechanical threat to breathing**

Suffocation due to mechanical threat to breathing

   √6ᵗʰ   **T71.11   Asphyxiation due to smothering under pillow**

     √7ᵗʰ   **T71.111   Asphyxiation due to smothering under pillow, accidental**   CC H5

       Asphyxiation due to smothering under pillow NOS

     7 √7ᵗʰ   **T71.112   Asphyxiation due to smothering under pillow, intentional self-harm**   CC H5 HCC

     √7ᵗʰ   **T71.113   Asphyxiation due to smothering under pillow, assault**   CC H5

     √7ᵗʰ   **T71.114   Asphyxiation due to smothering under pillow, undetermined**   CC H5

   √6ᵗʰ   **T71.12   Asphyxiation due to plastic bag**

     √7ᵗʰ   **T71.121   Asphyxiation due to plastic bag, accidental**   CC H5

       Asphyxiation due to plastic bag NOS

     7 √7ᵗʰ   **T71.122   Asphyxiation due to plastic bag, intentional self-harm**   CC H5 HCC

     √7ᵗʰ   **T71.123   Asphyxiation due to plastic bag, assault**   CC H5

     √7ᵗʰ   **T71.124   Asphyxiation due to plastic bag, undetermined**   CC H5

   √6ᵗʰ   **T71.13   Asphyxiation due to being trapped in bed linens**

     √7ᵗʰ   **T71.131   Asphyxiation due to being trapped in bed linens, accidental**   CC H5

       Asphyxiation due to being trapped in bed linens NOS

     7 √7ᵗʰ   **T71.132   Asphyxiation due to being trapped in bed linens, intentional self-harm**   CC H5 HCC

     √7ᵗʰ   **T71.133   Asphyxiation due to being trapped in bed linens, assault**   CC H5

     √7ᵗʰ   **T71.134   Asphyxiation due to being trapped in bed linens, undetermined**   CC H5

   √6ᵗʰ   **T71.14   Asphyxiation due to smothering under another person's body (in bed)**

     √7ᵗʰ   **T71.141   Asphyxiation due to smothering under another person's body (in bed), accidental**   CC H5

       Asphyxiation due to smothering under another person's body (in bed) NOS

     √7ᵗʰ   **T71.143   Asphyxiation due to smothering under another person's body (in bed), assault**   CC H5

     √7ᵗʰ   **T71.144   Asphyxiation due to smothering under another person's body (in bed), undetermined**   CC H5

N Newborn: 0   P Pediatric: 0-17   M Maternity: 9-64   A Adult: 15-124   MCC Major Complication/Comorbidity   CC Complication/Comorbidity   SW Severe Wound Dx

1184   ICD-10-CM 2020

✓6ᵗʰ **T71.15** **Asphyxiation due to** smothering in furniture

    ✓7ᵗʰ **T71.151** **Asphyxiation due to**   CC H5
       smothering in furniture, **accidental**
       Asphyxiation due to smothering in furniture NOS

    7 ✓7ᵗʰ **T71.152** **Asphyxiation due to**   CC H5 HCC
       smothering in furniture, **intentional self-harm**

    ✓7ᵗʰ **T71.153** **Asphyxiation due to**   CC H5
       smothering in furniture, **assault**

    ✓7ᵗʰ **T71.154** **Asphyxiation due to**   CC H5
       smothering in furniture, **undetermined**

✓6ᵗʰ **T71.16** **Asphyxiation due to** hanging

    Hanging by window shade cord
    Use additional code for any associated injuries, such as:
    crushing injury of neck (S17.-)
    fracture of cervical vertebrae (S12.0-S12.2-)
    open wound of neck (S11.-)

    ✓7ᵗʰ **T71.161** **Asphyxiation due to**   CC H5
       hanging, accidental
       Asphyxiation due to hanging NOS
       Hanging NOS

    7 ✓7ᵗʰ **T71.162** **Asphyxiation due to**   CC H5 HCC
       hanging, intentional **self-harm**

    ✓7ᵗʰ **T71.163** **Asphyxiation due to**   CC H5
       hanging, assault

    ✓7ᵗʰ **T71.164** **Asphyxiation due to**   CC H5
       hanging, undetermined

✓6ᵗʰ **T71.19** **Asphyxiation due to mechanical threat to breathing** **due to other causes**

    ✓7ᵗʰ **T71.191** **Asphyxiation due to**   CC H5
       mechanical threat to **breathing due to other** **causes, accidental**
       Asphyxiation due to other causes NOS

    7 ✓7ᵗʰ **T71.192** **Asphyxiation due to**   CC H5 HCC
       mechanical threat to **breathing due to other** **causes, intentional** **self-harm**

    ✓7ᵗʰ **T71.193** **Asphyxiation due to**   CC H5
       mechanical threat to **breathing due to other** **causes, assault**

    ✓7ᵗʰ **T71.194** **Asphyxiation due to**   CC H5
       mechanical threat to **breathing due to other** **causes, undetermined**

✓5ᵗʰ **T71.2** **Asphyxiation due to** systemic oxygen deficiency due to low oxygen content in ambient air

    Suffocation due to systemic oxygen deficiency due to low oxygen content in ambient air

    ✓x7ᵗʰ **T71.20** **Asphyxiation due to systemic**   CC H5
       oxygen deficiency due to low oxygen **content in ambient air due to** **unspecified cause**

    ✓x7ᵗʰ **T71.21** **Asphyxiation due to cave-in or**   CC H5
       falling earth
       Use additional code for any associated cataclysm (X34-X38)

    ✓6ᵗʰ **T71.22** **Asphyxiation due to** being trapped in a car trunk

       ✓7ᵗʰ **T71.221** **Asphyxiation due to being**   CC
          trapped in a car trunk, **accidental**

       7 ✓7ᵗʰ **T71.222** **Asphyxiation due to being**   CC HCC
          trapped in a car trunk, **intentional self-harm**

       ✓7ᵗʰ **T71.223** **Asphyxiation due to being**   CC
          trapped in a car trunk, **assault**

       ✓7ᵗʰ **T71.224** **Asphyxiation due to being**   CC
          trapped in a car trunk, **undetermined**

    ✓6ᵗʰ **T71.23** **Asphyxiation due to being** trapped in a (discarded) refrigerator

       ✓7ᵗʰ **T71.231** **Asphyxiation due to being**   CC
          trapped in a (discarded) **refrigerator, accidental**

---

    7 ✓7ᵗʰ **T71.232** **Asphyxiation due to being**   CC HCC
       trapped in a (discarded) **refrigerator, intentional** **self-harm**

    ✓7ᵗʰ **T71.233** **Asphyxiation due to being**   CC
       trapped in a (discarded) **refrigerator, assault**

    ✓7ᵗʰ **T71.234** **Asphyxiation due to being**   CC
       trapped in a (discarded) **refrigerator,** **undetermined**

✓x7ᵗʰ **T71.29** **Asphyxiation due to being trapped**   CC H5
    in other low oxygen environment

✓x7ᵗʰ **T71.9** **Asphyxiation due to unspecified cause**   CC H5
    Suffocation (by strangulation) due to unspecified cause
    Suffocation NOS
    Systemic oxygen deficiency due to low oxygen content in ambient air due to unspecified cause
    Systemic oxygen deficiency due to mechanical threat to breathing due to unspecified cause
    Traumatic asphyxia NOS

✓4ᵗʰ **T73** **Effects of other deprivation**

    The appropriate 7th character is to be added to each code from category T73.
    A   initial encounter
    D   subsequent encounter
    S   sequela

✓x7ᵗʰ **T73.0** **Starvation**
    Deprivation of food

✓x7ᵗʰ **T73.1** **Deprivation of water**

✓x7ᵗʰ **T73.2** **Exhaustion due to exposure**

✓x7ᵗʰ **T73.3** **Exhaustion due to excessive exertion**
    Exhaustion due to overexertion

✓x7ᵗʰ **T73.8** **Other effects of deprivation**

✓x7ᵗʰ **T73.9** **Effect of deprivation, unspecified**

✓4ᵗʰ **T74** **Adult and child abuse, neglect and other maltreatment,** confirmed

    Use additional code, if applicable, to identify any associated current injury
    Use additional external cause code to identify perpetrator, if known (Y07.-)
    EXCLUDES 1   abuse and maltreatment in pregnancy (O9A.3-, O9A.4-, O9A.5-)
          adult and child maltreatment, suspected (T76.-)

    The appropriate 7th character is to be added to each code from category T74.
    A   initial encounter
    D   subsequent encounter
    S   sequela

    CC Excl: For CC codes in category T74, unless otherwise noted: PDX collection 2033

✓5ᵗʰ **T74.0** **Neglect or abandonment, confirmed**

    ✓x7ᵗʰ **T74.01** **Adult neglect or abandonment,**   CC A
       confirmed

    ✓x7ᵗʰ **T74.02** **Child neglect or abandonment,**   CC P
       confirmed

✓5ᵗʰ **T74.1** **Physical abuse, confirmed**
    EXCLUDES 2   sexual abuse (T74.2-)

    ✓x7ᵗʰ **T74.11** **Adult physical abuse, confirmed**   CC A

    ✓x7ᵗʰ **T74.12** **Child physical abuse, confirmed**   CC P
       EXCLUDES 2   shaken infant syndrome (T74.4)

✓5ᵗʰ **T74.2** **Sexual abuse, confirmed**
    Rape, confirmed
    Sexual assault, confirmed

    ✓x7ᵗʰ **T74.21** **Adult sexual abuse, confirmed**   CC A

    ✓x7ᵗʰ **T74.22** **Child sexual abuse, confirmed**   CC P

✓5ᵗʰ **T74.3** **Psychological abuse, confirmed**
    Bullying and intimidation, confirmed
    Intimidation through social media, confirmed

    ✓x7ᵗʰ **T74.31** **Adult psychological abuse,**   A
       confirmed

    ✓x7ᵗʰ **T74.32** **Child psychological abuse,**   CC P
       confirmed

✓x7ᵗʰ **T74.4** **Shaken infant syndrome**   CC P

√5ᵗʰ T74.5 Forced sexual exploitation, confirmed
> AHA: 2018,4Q,32-33,65

     √x7ᵗʰ T74.51 Adult forced sexual exploitation, `CC` `A`
         confirmed
         CC Excl: PDX collection 1423

     √x7ᵗʰ T74.52 Child sexual exploitation, confirmed `CC` `P`
         CC Excl: PDX collection 1423

√5ᵗʰ T74.6 Forced labor exploitation, confirmed
> AHA: 2018,4Q,32-33,65

     √x7ᵗʰ T74.61 Adult forced labor exploitation, `CC` `A`
         confirmed
         CC Excl: PDX collection 2029

     √x7ᵗʰ T74.62 Child forced labor exploitation, `CC` `P`
         confirmed
         CC Excl: PDX collection 2030

√5ᵗʰ T74.9 Unspecified maltreatment, confirmed

     √x7ᵗʰ T74.91 Unspecified adult maltreatment, `CC` `A`
         confirmed
         CC Excl: PDX collection 1424

     √x7ᵗʰ T74.92 Unspecified child maltreatment, `CC` `P`
         confirmed

√4ᵗʰ T75 Other and unspecified effects of other external causes
> EXCLUDES 1   adverse effects NEC (T78.-)
> EXCLUDES 2   burns (electric) (T20-T31)

> The appropriate 7th character is to be added to each code from category T75.
> A   initial encounter
> D   subsequent encounter
> S   sequela

√5ᵗʰ T75.0 Effects of lightning
> Struck by lightning

     √x7ᵗʰ T75.00 Unspecified effects of lightning
         Struck by lightning NOS

     √x7ᵗʰ T75.01 Shock due to being struck by lightning

     √x7ᵗʰ T75.09 Other effects of lightning
         Use additional code for other effects of lightning

√x7ᵗʰ T75.1 Unspecified effects of drowning and nonfatal `CC` `H5`
submersion
> Immersion
> EXCLUDES 1   specified effects of drowning — code to effects
> CC Excl: PDX collection 1425

√5ᵗʰ T75.2 Effects of vibration

     √x7ᵗʰ T75.20 Unspecified effects of vibration

     √x7ᵗʰ T75.21 Pneumatic hammer syndrome

     √x7ᵗʰ T75.22 Traumatic vasospastic syndrome

     √x7ᵗʰ T75.23 Vertigo from infrasound
         EXCLUDES 1   vertigo NOS (R42)

     √x7ᵗʰ T75.29 Other effects of vibration

√x7ᵗʰ T75.3 Motion sickness
> Airsickness
> Seasickness
> Travel sickness
> Use additional external cause code to identify vehicle or type of motion (Y92.81-, Y93.5-)

√x7ᵗʰ T75.4 Electrocution
> Shock from electric current
> Shock from electroshock gun (taser)

√5ᵗʰ T75.8 Other specified effects of external causes

     √x7ᵗʰ T75.81 Effects of abnormal gravitation [G] forces

     √x7ᵗʰ T75.82 Effects of weightlessness

     √x7ᵗʰ T75.89 Other specified effects of external causes

√4ᵗʰ T76 Adult and child abuse, neglect and other maltreatment, suspected
> Use additional code, if applicable, to identify any associated current injury
> EXCLUDES 1   adult and child maltreatment, confirmed (T74.-)
>   suspected abuse and maltreatment in pregnancy (O9A.3-, O9A.4-, O9A.5-)
>   suspected adult physical abuse, ruled out (Z04.71)
>   suspected adult sexual abuse, ruled out (Z04.41)
>   suspected child physical abuse, ruled out (Z04.72)
>   suspected child sexual abuse, ruled out (Z04.42)

> AHA: 2018,4Q,72

> The appropriate 7th character is to be added to each code from category T76.
> A   initial encounter
> D   subsequent encounter
> S   sequela

> CC Excl: For CC codes in category T76, unless otherwise noted: PDX collection 2033

√5ᵗʰ T76.0 Neglect or abandonment, suspected

     √x7ᵗʰ T76.01 Adult neglect or abandonment, `CC` `A`
         suspected

     √x7ᵗʰ T76.02 Child neglect or abandonment, `CC` `P`
         suspected

√5ᵗʰ T76.1 Physical abuse, suspected

     √x7ᵗʰ T76.11 Adult physical abuse, suspected `CC` `A`

     √x7ᵗʰ T76.12 Child physical abuse, suspected `CC` `P`
         AHA: 2019,2Q,12

√5ᵗʰ T76.2 Sexual abuse, suspected
> Rape, suspected
> EXCLUDES 1   alleged abuse, ruled out (Z04.7)

     √x7ᵗʰ T76.21 Adult sexual abuse, suspected `CC` `A`

     √x7ᵗʰ T76.22 Child sexual abuse, suspected `CC` `P`

√5ᵗʰ T76.3 Psychological abuse, suspected
> Bullying and intimidation, suspected
> Intimidation through social media, suspected

     √x7ᵗʰ T76.31 Adult psychological abuse, `A`
         suspected

     √x7ᵗʰ T76.32 Child psychological abuse, suspected `CC` `P`

√5ᵗʰ T76.5 Forced sexual exploitation, suspected
> AHA: 2018,4Q,32-33,65

     √x7ᵗʰ T76.51 Adult forced sexual exploitation, `CC` `A`
         suspected
         CC Excl: PDX collection 1423

     √x7ᵗʰ T76.52 Child sexual exploitation, suspected `CC` `P`
         CC Excl: PDX collection 1423

√5ᵗʰ T76.6 Forced labor exploitation, suspected
> AHA: 2018,4Q,32-33,65

     √x7ᵗʰ T76.61 Adult forced labor exploitation, `CC` `A`
         suspected
         CC Excl: PDX collection 2031

     √x7ᵗʰ T76.62 Child forced labor exploitation, `CC` `P`
         suspected
         CC Excl: PDX collection 2032

√5ᵗʰ T76.9 Unspecified maltreatment, suspected

     √x7ᵗʰ T76.91 Unspecified adult maltreatment, `CC` `A`
         suspected
         CC Excl: PDX collection 1424

     √x7ᵗʰ T76.92 Unspecified child maltreatment, `CC` `P`
         suspected

√4ᵗʰ T78 Adverse effects, not elsewhere classified
> EXCLUDES 2   complications of surgical and medical care NEC (T80-T88)

> The appropriate 7th character is to be added to each code from category T78.
> A   initial encounter
> D   subsequent encounter
> S   sequela

> CC Excl: For CC codes in category T78: PDX collection 1426

√5ᵗʰ T78.0 Anaphylactic reaction due to food
> Anaphylactic reaction due to adverse food reaction
> Anaphylactic shock or reaction due to nonpoisonous foods
> Anaphylactoid reaction due to food

     √x7ᵗʰ T78.00 Anaphylactic reaction due to `CC`
         unspecified food

`N` Newborn: 0   `P` Pediatric: 0-17   `M` Maternity: 9-64   `A` Adult: 15-124   `MCC` Major Complication/Comorbidity   `CC` Complication/Comorbidity   `SW` Severe Wound Dx

1186   ICD-10-CM 2020

√x7ᵗʰ **T78.Ø1** **Anaphylactic reaction due to** `CC`
peanuts

√x7ᵗʰ **T78.Ø2** **Anaphylactic reaction due to** `CC`
shellfish (crustaceans)

√x7ᵗʰ **T78.Ø3** **Anaphylactic reaction due to other** `CC`
fish

√x7ᵗʰ **T78.Ø4** **Anaphylactic reaction due to fruits** `CC`
and vegetables

√x7ᵗʰ **T78.Ø5** **Anaphylactic reaction due to tree** `CC`
nuts and seeds
EXCLUDES 2 *anaphylactic reaction due to peanuts*
(T78.Ø1)

√x7ᵗʰ **T78.Ø6** **Anaphylactic reaction due to food** `CC`
additives

√x7ᵗʰ **T78.Ø7** **Anaphylactic reaction due to milk** `CC`
and dairy products

√x7ᵗʰ **T78.Ø8** **Anaphylactic reaction due to eggs** `CC`

√x7ᵗʰ **T78.Ø9** **Anaphylactic reaction due to other** `CC`
food products

√x7ᵗʰ **T78.1** **Other adverse food reactions, not elsewhere classified**
Use additional code to identify the type of reaction, if applicable
EXCLUDES 1 *anaphylactic reaction or shock due to adverse food*
reaction (T78.Ø-)
anaphylactic reaction due to food (T78.Ø-)
bacterial food borne intoxications (AØ5.-)
EXCLUDES 2 *allergic and dietetic gastroenteritis and colitis*
(K52.29)
allergic rhinitis due to food (J3Ø.5)
dermatitis due to food in contact with skin (L23.6,
L24.6, L25.4)
dermatitis due to ingested food (L27.2)
food protein-induced enterocolitis syndrome (K52.21)
food protein-induced enteropathy (K52.22)

√x7ᵗʰ **T78.2** **Anaphylactic shock, unspecified** `CC`
Allergic shock
Anaphylactic reaction
Anaphylaxis
EXCLUDES 1 *anaphylactic reaction or shock due to adverse effect*
of correct medicinal substance properly
administered (T88.6)
anaphylactic reaction or shock due to adverse food
reaction (T78.Ø-)
anaphylactic reaction or shock due to serum (T8Ø.5-)

√x7ᵗʰ **T78.3** **Angioneurotic edema**
Allergic angioedema
Giant urticaria
Quincke's edema
EXCLUDES 1 *serum urticaria (T8Ø.6-)*
urticaria (L5Ø.-)

√5ᵗʰ **T78.4** **Other and unspecified allergy**
EXCLUDES 1 *specified types of allergic reaction such as:*
allergic diarrhea (K52.29)
allergic gastroenteritis and colitis (K52.29)
dermatitis (L23-L25, L27.-)
food protein-induced enterocolitis syndrome
(K52.21)
food protein-induced enteropathy (K52.22)
hay fever (J3Ø.1)

√x7ᵗʰ **T78.4Ø** **Allergy, unspecified**
Allergic reaction NOS
Hypersensitivity NOS

√x7ᵗʰ **T78.41** **Arthus phenomenon**
Arthus reaction

√x7ᵗʰ **T78.49** **Other allergy**

√x7ᵗʰ **T78.8** **Other adverse effects, not elsewhere classified**

Certain early complications of trauma (T79)

√4ᵗʰ **T79** **Certain early complications of trauma, not elsewhere classified**
EXCLUDES 2 *acute respiratory distress syndrome (J8Ø)*
complications occurring during or following medical
procedures (T8Ø-T88)
complications of surgical and medical care NEC (T8Ø-T88)
newborn respiratory distress syndrome (P22.Ø)

The appropriate 7th character is to be added to each code from
category T79.
A   initial encounter
D   subsequent encounter
S   sequela

6 √x7ᵗʰ **T79.Ø** **Air embolism (traumatic)** `MCC` `HCC`
EXCLUDES 1 *air embolism complicating abortion or ectopic or*
molar pregnancy (OØØ-OØ7, OØ8.2)
air embolism complicating pregnancy, childbirth and
the puerperium (O88.Ø)
air embolism following infusion, transfusion, and
therapeutic injection (T8Ø.Ø)
air embolism following procedure NEC (T81.7-)
DEF: Arterial or venous obstruction due to the introduction of air
bubbles into the blood vessels following surgery or trauma.
CC Excl: PDX collection 1427

6 √x7ᵗʰ **T79.1** **Fat embolism (traumatic)** `MCC` `HCC`
EXCLUDES 1 *fat embolism complicating:*
abortion or ectopic or molar pregnancy (OØØ-OØ7,
OØ8.2)
pregnancy, childbirth and the puerperium (O88.8)
DEF: Arterial blockage due to the entrance of fat into the
circulatory system after a fracture of the large bones or
administration of corticosteroids.
CC Excl: PDX collection 1428

6 √x7ᵗʰ **T79.2** **Traumatic secondary and recurrent** `CC` `HCC`
hemorrhage and seroma
CC Excl: PDX collection 1429

6 √x7ᵗʰ **T79.4** **Traumatic shock** `MCC` `HCC`
Shock (immediate) (delayed) following injury
EXCLUDES 1 *anaphylactic shock due to adverse food reaction*
(T78.Ø-)
anaphylactic shock due to correct medicinal
substance properly administered (T88.6)
anaphylactic shock due to serum (T8Ø.5-)
anaphylactic shock NOS (T78.2)
anesthetic shock (T88.2)
electric shock (T75.4)
nontraumatic shock NEC (R57.-)
obstetric shock (O75.1)
postprocedural shock (T81.1-)
septic shock (R65.21)
shock complicating abortion or ectopic or molar
pregnancy (OØØ-OØ7, OØ8.3)
shock due to lightning (T75.Ø1)
shock NOS (R57.9)
CC Excl: PDX collection 1430

6 √x7ᵗʰ **T79.5** **Traumatic anuria** `MCC` `HCC`
Crush syndrome
Renal failure following crushing
CC Excl: PDX collection 1431

6 √x7ᵗʰ **T79.6** **Traumatic ischemia of muscle** `HCC`
Traumatic rhabdomyolysis
Volkmann's ischemic contracture
EXCLUDES 2 *anterior tibial syndrome (M76.8)*
compartment syndrome (traumatic) (T79.A-)
nontraumatic ischemia of muscle (M62.2-)
AHA: 2019,2Q,12

6 √x7ᵗʰ **T79.7** **Traumatic subcutaneous emphysema** `CC` `HCC`
EXCLUDES 1 *emphysema NOS (J43)*
emphysema (subcutaneous) resulting from a
procedure (T81.82)
CC Excl: PDX collection 1432

Chapter 19. Injury, Poisoning and Certain Other Consequences of External Causes

√5ᵗʰ **T79.A Traumatic compartment syndrome**

EXCLUDES 1 fibromyalgia (M79.7)
nontraumatic compartment syndrome (M79.A-)
traumatic ischemic infarction of muscle (T79.6)

EXCLUDES 2 ▶traumatic ischemic infarction of muscle (T79.6)◀

DEF: Compression of nerves and blood vessels within an enclosed muscle space due to previous trauma, which leads to impaired blood flow and muscle and nerve damage.

6 √7ᵗʰ **T79.A0 Compartment syndrome, unspecified** CC HCC

Compartment syndrome NOS

CC Excl: PDX collection 896

√6ᵗʰ **T79.A1 Traumatic compartment syndrome of upper extremity**

Traumatic compartment syndrome of shoulder, arm, forearm, wrist, hand, and fingers

CC Excl: For CC codes in subcategory T79.A1: PDX collection 1433

6 √7ᵗʰ **T79.A11 Traumatic compartment syndrome of right upper extremity** CC HCC

6 √7ᵗʰ **T79.A12 Traumatic compartment syndrome of left upper extremity** CC HCC

6 √7ᵗʰ **T79.A19 Traumatic compartment syndrome of unspecified upper extremity** CC HCC

√6ᵗʰ **T79.A2 Traumatic compartment syndrome of lower extremity**

Traumatic compartment syndrome of hip, buttock, thigh, leg, foot, and toes

CC Excl: For CC codes in subcategory T79.A2: PDX collection 1433

6 √7ᵗʰ **T79.A21 Traumatic compartment syndrome of right lower extremity** CC HCC

6 √7ᵗʰ **T79.A22 Traumatic compartment syndrome of left lower extremity** CC HCC

6 √7ᵗʰ **T79.A29 Traumatic compartment syndrome of unspecified lower extremity** CC HCC

6 √7ᵗʰ **T79.A3 Traumatic compartment syndrome of abdomen** CC HCC

CC Excl: PDX collection 1434

6 √7ᵗʰ **T79.A9 Traumatic compartment syndrome of other sites** CC HCC

CC Excl: PDX collection 896

6 √7ᵗʰ **T79.8 Other early complications of trauma** HCC

6 √7ᵗʰ **T79.9 Unspecified early complication of trauma** HCC

Complications of surgical and medical care, not elsewhere classified (T80-T88)

Use additional code for adverse effect, if applicable, to identify drug (T36-T50 with fifth or sixth character 5)

Use additional code(s) to identify the specified condition resulting from the complication

Use additional code to identify devices involved and details of circumstances (Y62-Y82)

EXCLUDES 2 any encounters with medical care for postprocedural conditions in which no complications are present, such as:
artificial opening status (Z93.-)
closure of external stoma (Z43.-)
fitting and adjustment of external prosthetic device (Z44.-)
burns and corrosions from local applications and irradiation (T20-T32)
complications of surgical procedures during pregnancy, childbirth and the puerperium (O00-O9A)
mechanical complication of respirator [ventilator] (J95.850)
poisoning and toxic effects of drugs and chemicals (T36-T65 with fifth or sixth character 1-4 or 6)
postprocedural fever (R50.82)
specified complications classified elsewhere, such as:
cerebrospinal fluid leak from spinal puncture (G97.0)
colostomy malfunction (K94.0-)
disorders of fluid and electrolyte imbalance (E86-E87)
functional disturbances following cardiac surgery (I97.0-I97.1)
intraoperative and postprocedural complications of specified body systems (D78.-, E36.-, E89.-, G97.3-, G97.4, H59.3-, H59.-, H95.2-, H95.3, I97.4-, I97.5, J95.6-, J95.7, K91.6-, L76.-, M96.-, N99.-)
ostomy complications (J95.0-, K94.-, N99.5-)
postgastric surgery syndromes (K91.1)
postlaminectomy syndrome NEC (M96.1)
postmastectomy lymphedema syndrome (I97.2)
postsurgical blind-loop syndrome (K91.2)
ventilator associated pneumonia (J95.851)

AHA: 2015,1Q,15

√4ᵗʰ **T80 Complications following infusion, transfusion and therapeutic injection**

INCLUDES complications following perfusion

EXCLUDES 2 bone marrow transplant rejection (T86.01)
febrile nonhemolytic transfusion reaction (R50.84)
fluid overload due to transfusion (E87.71)
posttransfusion purpura (D69.51)
transfusion associated circulatory overload (TACO) (E87.71)
transfusion (red blood cell) associated hemochromatosis (E83.111)
transfusion related acute lung injury (TRALI) (J95.84)

The appropriate 7th character is to be added to each code from category T80.
A initial encounter
D subsequent encounter
S sequela

√7ᵗʰ **T80.0 Air embolism following infusion, transfusion and therapeutic injection** MCC H2

CC Excl: PDX collection 1435

√7ᵗʰ **T80.1 Vascular complications following infusion, transfusion and therapeutic injection** CC

Use additional code to identify the vascular complication

EXCLUDES 2 extravasation of vesicant agent (T80.81-)
infiltration of vesicant agent (T80.81-)
postprocedural vascular complications (T81.7-)
vascular complications specified as due to prosthetic devices, implants and grafts (T82.8-, T83.8-, T84.8-, T85.8-)

CC Excl: PDX collection 1436

N Newborn: 0 | P Pediatric: 0-17 | M Maternity: 9-64 | A Adult: 15-124 | MCC Major Complication/Comorbidity | CC Complication/Comorbidity | SW Severe Wound Dx

1188 ICD-10-CM 2020

√5ᵗʰ **T80.2** **Infections** following infusion, transfusion and therapeutic injection

Use additional code to identify the specific infection, such as: sepsis (A41.9)

Use additional code (R65.2-) to identify severe sepsis, if applicable

EXCLUDES 2   *infections specified as due to prosthetic devices, implants and grafts (T82.6-T82.7, T83.5-T83.6, T84.5-T84.7, T85.7)*

postprocedural infections (T81.4-)

AHA: 2018,4Q,62

CC Excl: For CC codes in subcategory T80.2: PDX collection 948

√6ᵗʰ **T80.21** **Infection** due to central venous catheter

Infection due to pulmonary artery catheter (Swan-Ganz catheter)

AHA: 2019,1Q,13-14

TIP: Only centrally placed catheters are captured with this subcategory. Infections resulting from catheters that are not central lines, including those used for hemodialysis, should be coded to T82.7-.

√7ᵗʰ **T80.211** **Bloodstream infection due to central venous catheter**   CC H7

Catheter-related bloodstream infection (CRBSI) NOS

Central line-associated bloodstream infection (CLABSI)

Bloodstream infection due to Hickman catheter

Bloodstream infection due to peripherally inserted central catheter (PICC)

Bloodstream infection due to portacath (port-a-cath)

Bloodstream infection due to pulmonary artery catheter

Bloodstream infection due to triple lumen catheter

Bloodstream infection due to umbilical venous catheter

AHA: 2019,1Q,13,14; 2018,4Q,89

√7ᵗʰ **T80.212** **Local infection** due to **central venous catheter**   CC H7

Exit or insertion site infection

Local infection due to Hickman catheter

Local infection due to peripherally inserted central catheter (PICC)

Local infection due to portacath (port-a-cath)

Local infection due to pulmonary artery catheter

Local infection due to triple lumen catheter

Local infection due to umbilical venous catheter

Port or reservoir infection

Tunnel infection

√7ᵗʰ **T80.218** **Other infection due to central venous catheter**   CC H7

Other central line-associated infection

Other infection due to Hickman catheter

Other infection due to peripherally inserted central catheter (PICC)

Other infection due to portacath (port-a-cath)

Other infection due to pulmonary artery catheter

Other infection due to triple lumen catheter

Other infection due to umbilical venous catheter

√7ᵗʰ **T80.219** **Unspecified infection due to central venous catheter**   CC H7

Central line-associated infection NOS

Unspecified infection due to Hickman catheter

Unspecified infection due to peripherally inserted central catheter (PICC)

Unspecified infection due to portacath (port-a-cath)

Unspecified infection due to pulmonary artery catheter

Unspecified infection due to triple lumen catheter

Unspecified infection due to umbilical venous catheter

√x7ᵗʰ **T80.22** **Acute infection following transfusion, infusion, or injection of blood and blood products**   CC

√x7ᵗʰ **T80.29** **Infection following other infusion, transfusion and therapeutic injection**   CC

√5ᵗʰ **T80.3** **ABO incompatibility reaction** due to transfusion of blood or blood products

EXCLUDES 1   *minor blood group antigens reactions (Duffy) (E) (K) (Kell) (Kidd) (Lewis) (M) (N) (P) (S) (T80.A-)*

CC Excl: For CC codes in subcategory T80.3: PDX collection 1437

√x7ᵗʰ **T80.30** **ABO incompatibility reaction due to transfusion of blood or blood products, unspecified**   CC H3

ABO incompatibility blood transfusion NOS

Reaction to ABO incompatibility from transfusion NOS

√6ᵗʰ **T80.31** **ABO incompatibility** with hemolytic transfusion reaction

√7ᵗʰ **T80.310** **ABO incompatibility with acute hemolytic transfusion reaction**   CC H3

ABO incompatibility with hemolytic transfusion reaction less than 24 hours after transfusion

Acute hemolytic transfusion reaction (AHTR) due to ABO incompatibility

√7ᵗʰ **T80.311** **ABO incompatibility with delayed hemolytic transfusion reaction**   CC H3

ABO incompatibility with hemolytic transfusion reaction 24 hours or more after transfusion

Delayed hemolytic transfusion reaction (DHTR) due to ABO incompatibility

√7ᵗʰ **T80.319** **ABO incompatibility with hemolytic transfusion reaction, unspecified**   CC H3

ABO incompatibility with hemolytic transfusion reaction at unspecified time after transfusion

Hemolytic transfusion reaction (HTR) due to ABO incompatibility NOS

√x7ᵗʰ **T80.39** **Other ABO incompatibility reaction due to transfusion of blood or blood products**   CC H3

Delayed serologic transfusion reaction (DSTR) from ABO incompatibility

Other ABO incompatible blood transfusion

Other reaction to ABO incompatible blood transfusion

√5ᵗʰ **T80.4** **Rh incompatibility reaction** due to transfusion of blood or blood products

Reaction due to incompatibility of Rh antigens (C) (c) (D) (E) (e)

CC Excl: For CC codes in subcategory T80.4, unless otherwise noted: PDX collection 1437

√x7ᵗʰ **T80.40** **Rh incompatibility reaction due to transfusion of blood or blood products, unspecified**   CC

Reaction due to Rh factor in transfusion NOS

Rh incompatible blood transfusion NOS

☑ Additional Character Required   √x7ᵗʰ Placeholder   Unacceptable PDx   Questionable PDx   Manifestation   Unspecified Dx   H1-H14 HAC   HCC CMS-HCC Dx   HIV HIV Dx

ICD-10-CM 2020   1189

✓6ᵗʰ **T80.41 Rh incompatibility with hemolytic transfusion reaction**

✓7ᵗʰ **T80.410 Rh incompatibility with acute hemolytic transfusion reaction** CC

Acute hemolytic transfusion reaction (AHTR) due to Rh incompatibility

Rh incompatibility with hemolytic transfusion reaction less than 24 hours after transfusion

✓7ᵗʰ **T80.411 Rh incompatibility with delayed hemolytic transfusion reaction** CC

Delayed hemolytic transfusion reaction (DHTR) due to Rh incompatibility

Rh incompatibility with hemolytic transfusion reaction 24 hours or more after transfusion

✓7ᵗʰ **T80.419 Rh incompatibility with hemolytic transfusion reaction, unspecified** CC

Rh incompatibility with hemolytic transfusion reaction at unspecified time after transfusion

Hemolytic transfusion reaction (HTR) due to Rh incompatibility NOS

✓x7ᵗʰ **T80.49 Other Rh incompatibility reaction due to transfusion of blood or blood products** CC

Delayed serologic transfusion reaction (DSTR) from Rh incompatibility

Other reaction to Rh incompatible blood transfusion

CC Excl: PDX collection 1438

✓5ᵗʰ **T80.A Non-ABO incompatibility reaction due to transfusion of blood or blood products**

Reaction due to incompatibility of minor antigens (Duffy) (Kell) (Kidd) (Lewis) (M) (N) (P) (S)

CC Excl: For CC codes in subcategory T80.A, unless otherwise noted: PDX collection 1438

✓7ᵗʰ **T80.A0 Non-ABO incompatibility reaction due to transfusion of blood or blood products, unspecified** CC

Non-ABO antigen incompatibility reaction from transfusion NOS

✓6ᵗʰ **T80.A1 Non-ABO incompatibility with hemolytic transfusion reaction**

✓7ᵗʰ **T80.A10 Non-ABO incompatibility with acute hemolytic transfusion reaction** CC

Acute hemolytic transfusion reaction (AHTR) due to non-ABO incompatibility

Non-ABO incompatibility with hemolytic transfusion reaction less than 24 hours after transfusion

✓7ᵗʰ **T80.A11 Non-ABO incompatibility with delayed hemolytic transfusion reaction** CC

Delayed hemolytic transfusion reaction (DHTR) due to non-ABO incompatibility

Non-ABO incompatibility with hemolytic transfusion reaction 24 or more hours after transfusion

✓7ᵗʰ **T80.A19 Non-ABO incompatibility with hemolytic transfusion reaction, unspecified** CC

Hemolytic transfusion reaction (HTR) due to non-ABO incompatibility NOS

Non-ABO incompatibility with hemolytic transfusion reaction at unspecified time after transfusion

✓x7ᵗʰ **T80.A9 Other non-ABO incompatibility reaction due to transfusion of blood or blood products** CC

Delayed serologic transfusion reaction (DSTR) from non-ABO incompatibility

Other reaction to non-ABO incompatible blood transfusion

CC Excl: PDX collection 1437

✓5ᵗʰ **T80.5 Anaphylactic reaction due to serum**

Allergic shock due to serum

Anaphylactic shock due to serum

Anaphylactoid reaction due to serum

Anaphylaxis due to serum

EXCLUDES 1 *ABO incompatibility reaction due to transfusion of blood or blood products (T80.3-)*

allergic reaction or shock NOS (T78.2)

anaphylactic reaction or shock NOS (T78.2)

anaphylactic reaction or shock due to adverse effect of correct medicinal substance properly administered (T88.6)

other serum reaction (T80.6-)

DEF: Life-threatening hypersensitivity to a foreign serum causing respiratory distress, vascular collapse, and shock.

CC Excl: For CC codes in subcategory T80.5: PDX collection 1439

✓x7ᵗʰ **T80.51 Anaphylactic reaction due to administration of blood and blood products** CC

✓x7ᵗʰ **T80.52 Anaphylactic reaction due to vaccination** CC

✓x7ᵗʰ **T80.59 Anaphylactic reaction due to other serum** CC

✓5ᵗʰ **T80.6 Other serum reactions**

Intoxiation by serum

Protein sickness

Serum rash

Serum sickness

Serum urticaria

EXCLUDES 2 *serum hepatitis (B16-B19)*

DEF: Serum sickness: Hypersensitivity to a foreign serum that causes fever, hives, swelling, and lymphadenopathy.

CC Excl: For CC codes in subcategory T80.6: PDX collection 1439

✓x7ᵗʰ **T80.61 Other serum reaction due to administration of blood and blood products** CC

✓x7ᵗʰ **T80.62 Other serum reaction due to vaccination** CC

✓x7ᵗʰ **T80.69 Other serum reaction due to other serum** CC

Code also, if applicable, arthropathy in hypersensitivity reactions classified elsewhere (M36.4)

CC Excl: PDX collection 1440

✓5ᵗʰ **T80.8 Other complications following infusion, transfusion and therapeutic injection**

✓6ᵗʰ **T80.81 Extravasation of vesicant agent**

Infiltration of vesicant agent

✓7ᵗʰ **T80.810 Extravasation of vesicant antineoplastic chemotherapy** CC

Infiltration of vesicant antineoplastic chemotherapy

CC Excl: PDX collection 1436

✓7ᵗʰ **T80.818 Extravasation of other vesicant agent** CC

Infiltration of other vesicant agent

CC Excl: PDX collection 1436

✓x7ᵗʰ **T80.89 Other complications following infusion, transfusion and therapeutic injection** CC

Delayed serologic transfusion reaction (DSTR), unspecified incompatibility

Use additional code to identify graft-versus-host reaction, if applicable, (D89.81-)

✓5ᵗʰ **T80.9 Unspecified complication following infusion, transfusion and therapeutic injection**

✓x7ᵗʰ **T80.90 Unspecified complication following infusion and therapeutic injection**

✓6ᵗʰ **T80.91** **Hemolytic transfusion reaction, unspecified incompatibility**

EXCLUDES 1   *ABO incompatibility with hemolytic transfusion reaction (T80.31-)*
non-ABO incompatibility with hemolytic transfusion reaction (T80.A1-)
Rh incompatibility with hemolytic transfusion reaction (T80.41-)

CC Excl: For CC codes in subcategory T80.91: PDX collection 1437

✓7ᵗʰ **T80.910** **Acute hemolytic transfusion reaction, unspecified incompatibility**   CC

✓7ᵗʰ **T80.911** **Delayed hemolytic transfusion reaction, unspecified incompatibility**   CC

✓7ᵗʰ **T80.919** **Hemolytic transfusion reaction, unspecified incompatibility, unspecified as acute or delayed**   CC

Hemolytic transfusion reaction NOS

✓7ᵗʰ **T80.92** **Unspecified transfusion reaction**

Transfusion reaction NOS

✓4ᵗʰ **T81** **Complications of procedures, not elsewhere classified**

Use additional code for adverse effect, if applicable, to identify drug (T36-T50 with fifth or sixth character 5)

EXCLUDES 2   *complications following immunization (T88.0-T88.1)*
complications following infusion, transfusion and therapeutic injection (T80.-)
complications of transplanted organs and tissue (T86.-)
specified complications classified elsewhere, such as:
complication of prosthetic devices, implants and grafts (T82-T85)
dermatitis due to drugs and medicaments (L23.3, L24.4, L25.1, L27.0-L27.1)
endosseous dental implant failure (M27.6-)
floppy iris syndrome (IFIS) (intraoperative) (H21.81)
intraoperative and postprocedural complications of specific body system (D78.-, E36.-, E89.-, G97.3-, G97.4, H59.3-, H59.-, H95.2-, H95.3, I97.4-, I97.5, J95, K91.-, L76.-, M96.-, N99.-)
ostomy complications (J95.0-, K94.-, N99.5-)
plateau iris syndrome (post-iridectomy) (postprocedural) H21.82
poisoning and toxic effects of drugs and chemicals (T36-T65 with fifth or sixth character 1-4 or 6)

AHA: 2019,2Q,21

The appropriate 7th character is to be added to each code from category T81.
A   initial encounter
D   subsequent encounter
S   sequela

✓5ᵗʰ **T81.1** **Postprocedural shock**

Shock during or resulting from a procedure, not elsewhere classified

EXCLUDES 1   *anaphylactic shock due to correct substance properly administered (T88.6)*
anaphylactic shock due to serum (T80.5-)
anaphylactic shock NOS (T78.2)
anesthetic shock (T88.2)
electric shock (T75.4)
obstetric shock (O75.1)
septic shock (R65.21)
shock following abortion or ectopic or molar pregnancy (O00-O07, O08.3)
traumatic shock (T79.4)

CC Excl: For CC/MCC codes in subcategory T81.1: PDX collection 1441

✓7ᵗʰ **T81.10** **Postprocedural shock unspecified**   CC

Collapse NOS during or resulting from a procedure, not elsewhere classified
Postprocedural failure of peripheral circulation
Postprocedural shock NOS

6 ✓7ᵗʰ **T81.11** **Postprocedural cardiogenic shock**   MCC HCC

6 ✓7ᵗʰ **T81.12** **Postprocedural septic shock**   MCC HCC

Postprocedural endotoxic shock resulting from a procedure, not elsewhere classified
Postprocedural gram-negative shock resulting from a procedure, not elsewhere classified
Code first underlying infection
Use additional code, to identify any associated acute organ dysfunction, if applicable

AHA: 2018,4Q,63

✓7ᵗʰ **T81.19** **Other postprocedural shock**   MCC

Postprocedural hypovolemic shock

✓5ᵗʰ **T81.3** **Disruption of wound, not elsewhere classified**

Disruption of any suture materials or other closure methods

EXCLUDES 1   *breakdown (mechanical) of permanent sutures (T85.612)*
displacement of permanent sutures (T85.622)
disruption of cesarean delivery wound (O90.0)
disruption of perineal obstetric wound (O90.1)
mechanical complication of permanent sutures NEC (T85.692)

AHA: 2014,1Q,23

CC Excl: For CC codes in subcategory T81.3: PDX collection 1442

✓7ᵗʰ **T81.30** **Disruption of wound, unspecified**   CC SW

Disruption of wound NOS

✓7ᵗʰ **T81.31** **Disruption of external operation (surgical) wound, not elsewhere classified**   CC SW

Dehiscence of operation wound NOS
Disruption of operation wound NOS
Disruption or dehiscence of closure of cornea
Disruption or dehiscence of closure of mucosa
Disruption or dehiscence of closure of skin and subcutaneous tissue
Full-thickness skin disruption or dehiscence
Superficial disruption or dehiscence of operation wound

EXCLUDES 1   *dehiscence of amputation stump (T87.81)*

✓7ᵗʰ **T81.32** **Disruption of internal operation (surgical) wound, not elsewhere classified**   CC SW

Deep disruption or dehiscence of operation wound NOS
Disruption or dehiscence of closure of internal organ or other internal tissue
Disruption or dehiscence of closure of muscle or muscle flap
Disruption or dehiscence of closure of ribs or rib cage
Disruption or dehiscence of closure of skull or craniotomy
Disruption or dehiscence of closure of sternum or sternotomy
Disruption or dehiscence of closure of tendon or ligament
Disruption or dehiscence of closure of superficial or muscular fascia

AHA: 2017,3Q,4

✓7ᵗʰ **T81.33** **Disruption of traumatic injury wound repair**   CC

Disruption or dehiscence of closure of traumatic laceration (external) (internal)

√5ᵗʰ **T81.4 Infection following a procedure**

Wound abscess following a procedure

Use additional code to identify infection

Use additional code (R65.2-) to identify severe sepsis, if applicable

EXCLUDES 2 bleb associated endophthalmitis (H59.4-)

infection due to infusion, transfusion and therapeutic injection (T80.2-)

infection due to prosthetic devices, implants and grafts (T82.6-T82.7, T83.5-T83.6, T84.5-T84.7, T85.7)

obstetric surgical wound infection (O86.0-)

postprocedural fever NOS (R50.82)

postprocedural retroperitoneal abscess (K68.11)

AHA: 2018,4Q,33-34,62; 2014,1Q,23

CC Excl: For CC codes in subcategory T81.4: PDX collection 805

√x7ᵗʰ **T81.40 Infection following a procedure, unspecified** CC H11 H12 H13

√x7ᵗʰ **T81.41 Infection following a procedure, superficial incisional surgical site** CC H11 H12 H13

Subcutaneous abscess following a procedure

Stitch abscess following a procedure

√x7ᵗʰ **T81.42 Infection following a procedure, deep incisional surgical site** CC H11 H12 H13

Intra-muscular abscess following a procedure

√x7ᵗʰ **T81.43 Infection following a procedure, organ and space surgical site** CC H11 H12 H13

Intra-abdominal abscess following a procedure

Subphrenic abscess following a procedure

6 √x7ᵗʰ **T81.44 Sepsis following a procedure** CC H11 H12 H13 HCC

Use additional code to identify the sepsis

√x7ᵗʰ **T81.49 Infection following a procedure, other surgical site** CC H11 H12 H13

√5ᵗʰ **T81.5 Complications of foreign body accidentally left in body following procedure**

AHA: 2014,4Q,24

CC Excl: For CC codes in subcategory T81.5: PDX collection 1443

√6ᵗʰ **T81.50 Unspecified complication of foreign body accidentally left in body following procedure**

√7ᵗʰ **T81.500 Unspecified complication of foreign body accidentally left in body following surgical operation** CC H1

√7ᵗʰ **T81.501 Unspecified complication of foreign body accidentally left in body following infusion or transfusion** CC H1

√7ᵗʰ **T81.502 Unspecified complication of foreign body accidentally left in body following kidney dialysis** CC H1 HCC

√7ᵗʰ **T81.503 Unspecified complication of foreign body accidentally left in body following injection or immunization** CC H1

√7ᵗʰ **T81.504 Unspecified complication of foreign body accidentally left in body following endoscopic examination** CC H1

√7ᵗʰ **T81.505 Unspecified complication of foreign body accidentally left in body following heart catheterization** CC H1

√7ᵗʰ **T81.506 Unspecified complication of foreign body accidentally left in body following aspiration, puncture or other catheterization** CC H1

√7ᵗʰ **T81.507 Unspecified complication of foreign body accidentally left in body following removal of catheter or packing** CC H1

√7ᵗʰ **T81.508 Unspecified complication of foreign body accidentally left in body following other procedure** CC H1

√7ᵗʰ **T81.509 Unspecified complication of foreign body accidentally left in body following unspecified procedure** CC H1

√6ᵗʰ **T81.51 Adhesions due to foreign body accidentally left in body following procedure**

√7ᵗʰ **T81.510 Adhesions due to foreign body accidentally left in body following surgical operation** CC H1

√7ᵗʰ **T81.511 Adhesions due to foreign body accidentally left in body following infusion or transfusion** CC H1

√7ᵗʰ **T81.512 Adhesions due to foreign body accidentally left in body following kidney dialysis** CC H1 HCC

√7ᵗʰ **T81.513 Adhesions due to foreign body accidentally left in body following injection or immunization** CC H1

√7ᵗʰ **T81.514 Adhesions due to foreign body accidentally left in body following endoscopic examination** CC H1

√7ᵗʰ **T81.515 Adhesions due to foreign body accidentally left in body following heart catheterization** CC H1

√7ᵗʰ **T81.516 Adhesions due to foreign body accidentally left in body following aspiration, puncture or other catheterization** CC H1

√7ᵗʰ **T81.517 Adhesions due to foreign body accidentally left in body following removal of catheter or packing** CC H1

√7ᵗʰ **T81.518 Adhesions due to foreign body accidentally left in body following other procedure** CC H1

√7ᵗʰ **T81.519 Adhesions due to foreign body accidentally left in body following unspecified procedure** CC H1

√6ᵗʰ **T81.52 Obstruction due to foreign body accidentally left in body following procedure**

√7ᵗʰ **T81.520 Obstruction due to foreign body accidentally left in body following surgical operation** CC H1

√7ᵗʰ **T81.521 Obstruction due to foreign body accidentally left in body following infusion or transfusion** CC H1

√7ᵗʰ **T81.522 Obstruction due to foreign body accidentally left in body following kidney dialysis** CC H1 HCC

√7ᵗʰ **T81.523 Obstruction due to foreign body accidentally left in body following injection or immunization** CC H1

√7ᵗʰ **T81.524 Obstruction due to foreign body accidentally left in body following endoscopic examination** CC H1

√7ᵗʰ **T81.525 Obstruction due to foreign body accidentally left in body following heart catheterization** CC H1

√7ᵗʰ **T81.526 Obstruction due to foreign body accidentally left in body following aspiration, puncture or other catheterization** CC H1

N Newborn: 0 | P Pediatric: 0-17 | M Maternity: 9-64 | A Adult: 15-124 | MCC Major Complication/Comorbidity | CC Complication/Comorbidity | SW Severe Wound Dx

1192 | ICD-10-CM 2020

√7ᵗʰ **T81.527 Obstruction due to foreign body accidentally left in body following removal of catheter or packing** `CC` `H1`

√7ᵗʰ **T81.528 Obstruction due to foreign body accidentally left in body following other procedure** `CC` `H1`

√7ᵗʰ **T81.529 Obstruction due to foreign body accidentally left in body following unspecified procedure** `CC` `H1`

√6ᵗʰ **T81.53 Perforation due to foreign body accidentally left in body following procedure**

√7ᵗʰ **T81.530 Perforation due to foreign body accidentally left in body following surgical operation** `CC` `H1`

√7ᵗʰ **T81.531 Perforation due to foreign body accidentally left in body following infusion or transfusion** `CC` `H1`

√7ᵗʰ **T81.532 Perforation due to foreign body accidentally left in body following kidney dialysis** `CC` `H1` `HCC`

√7ᵗʰ **T81.533 Perforation due to foreign body accidentally left in body following injection or immunization** `CC` `H1`

√7ᵗʰ **T81.534 Perforation due to foreign body accidentally left in body following endoscopic examination** `CC` `H1`

√7ᵗʰ **T81.535 Perforation due to foreign body accidentally left in body following heart catheterization** `CC` `H1`

√7ᵗʰ **T81.536 Perforation due to foreign body accidentally left in body following aspiration, puncture or other catheterization** `CC` `H1`

√7ᵗʰ **T81.537 Perforation due to foreign body accidentally left in body following removal of catheter or packing** `CC` `H1`

√7ᵗʰ **T81.538 Perforation due to foreign body accidentally left in body following other procedure** `CC` `H1`

√7ᵗʰ **T81.539 Perforation due to foreign body accidentally left in body following unspecified procedure** `CC` `H1`

√6ᵗʰ **T81.59 Other complications of foreign body accidentally left in body following procedure**

EXCLUDES 2   obstruction or perforation due to prosthetic devices and implants intentionally left in body (T82.0-T82.5, T83.0-T83.4, T83.7, T84.0-T84.4, T85.0-T85.6)

√7ᵗʰ **T81.590 Other complications of foreign body accidentally left in body following surgical operation** `CC` `H1`

√7ᵗʰ **T81.591 Other complications of foreign body accidentally left in body following infusion or transfusion** `CC` `H1`

√7ᵗʰ **T81.592 Other complications of foreign body accidentally left in body following kidney dialysis** `CC` `H1` `HCC`

√7ᵗʰ **T81.593 Other complications of foreign body accidentally left in body following injection or immunization** `CC` `H1`

√7ᵗʰ **T81.594 Other complications of foreign body accidentally left in body following endoscopic examination** `CC` `H1`

√7ᵗʰ **T81.595 Other complications of foreign body accidentally left in body following heart catheterization** `CC` `H1`

√7ᵗʰ **T81.596 Other complications of foreign body accidentally left in body following aspiration, puncture or other catheterization** `CC` `H1`

√7ᵗʰ **T81.597 Other complications of foreign body accidentally left in body following removal of catheter or packing** `CC` `H1`

√7ᵗʰ **T81.598 Other complications of foreign body accidentally left in body following other procedure** `CC` `H1`

√7ᵗʰ **T81.599 Other complications of foreign body accidentally left in body following unspecified procedure** `CC` `H1`

√5ᵗʰ **T81.6 Acute reaction to foreign substance accidentally left during a procedure**

EXCLUDES 2   complications of foreign body accidentally left in body cavity or operation wound following procedure (T81.5-)

CC Excl: For CC codes in subcategory T81.6: PDX collection 1444

√x7ᵗʰ **T81.60 Unspecified acute reaction to foreign substance accidentally left during a procedure** `CC` `H1`

√x7ᵗʰ **T81.61 Aseptic peritonitis due to foreign substance accidentally left during a procedure** `CC` `H1`

Chemical peritonitis

√x7ᵗʰ **T81.69 Other acute reaction to foreign substance accidentally left during a procedure** `CC` `H1`

√5ᵗʰ **T81.7 Vascular complications following a procedure, not elsewhere classified**

Air embolism following procedure NEC

Phlebitis or thrombophlebitis resulting from a procedure

EXCLUDES 1   embolism complicating abortion or ectopic or molar pregnancy (O00-O07, O08.2)

embolism complicating pregnancy, childbirth and the puerperium (O88.-)

traumatic embolism (T79.0)

EXCLUDES 2   embolism due to prosthetic devices, implants and grafts (T82.8-, T83.81, T84.8-, T85.81-)

embolism following infusion, transfusion and therapeutic injection (T80.0)

AHA: 2019,2Q,22

CC Excl: For CC codes in subcategory T81.7, unless otherwise stated: PDX collection 1446

√6ᵗʰ **T81.71 Complication of artery following a procedure, not elsewhere classified**

√7ᵗʰ **T81.710 Complication of mesenteric artery following a procedure, not elsewhere classified** `CC`

CC Excl: PDX collection 1445

√7ᵗʰ **T81.711 Complication of renal artery following a procedure, not elsewhere classified** `CC`

CC Excl: PDX collection 1445

√7ᵗʰ **T81.718 Complication of other artery following a procedure, not elsewhere classified** `CC`

AHA: 2019,2Q,21-22

√7ᵗʰ **T81.719 Complication of unspecified artery following a procedure, not elsewhere classified** `CC`

√x7ᵗʰ **T81.72 Complication of vein following a procedure, not elsewhere classified** `CC`

√5ᵗʰ **T81.8 Other complications of procedures, not elsewhere classified**

EXCLUDES 2   hypothermia following anesthesia (T88.51)

malignant hyperpyrexia due to anesthesia (T88.3)

√x7ᵗʰ **T81.81 Complication of inhalation therapy**

√x7ᵗʰ **T81.82 Emphysema (subcutaneous) resulting from a procedure**

☑ Additional Character Required   √x7ᵗʰ Placeholder   Unacceptable PDx   Questionable PDx   Manifestation   Unspecified Dx   `H1`-`H14` HAC   `HCC` CMS-HCC Dx   `HIV` HIV Dx

ICD-10-CM 2020

1193

Chapter 19. Injury, Poisoning and Certain Other Consequences of External Causes

√x7th **T81.83** **Persistent postprocedural fistula** `CC` `SW`
     AHA: 2017,3Q,3-4
     CC Excl: PDX collection 1447

√x7th **T81.89** **Other complications of procedures, not elsewhere classified** `SW`
     Use additional code to specify complication, such as: postprocedural delirium (F05)
     AHA: 2014,1Q,23

√x7th **T81.9** **Unspecified complication of procedure**

√4th **T82** **Complications of cardiac and vascular prosthetic devices, implants and grafts**
     EXCLUDES 2   *failure and rejection of transplanted organs and tissue (T86.-)*

The appropriate 7th character is to be added to each code from category T82.
A   initial encounter
D   subsequent encounter
S   sequela

√5th **T82.0** **Mechanical complication of heart valve prosthesis**
     Mechanical complication of artificial heart valve
     EXCLUDES 1   *mechanical complication of biological heart valve graft (T82.22-)*
     CC Excl: For CC codes in subcategory T82.0: PDX collection 1448

√x7th **T82.01** **Breakdown (mechanical) of heart valve prosthesis** `CC`

√x7th **T82.02** **Displacement of heart valve prosthesis** `CC`
     Malposition of heart valve prosthesis

√x7th **T82.03** **Leakage of heart valve prosthesis** `CC`

√x7th **T82.09** **Other mechanical complication of heart valve prosthesis** `CC`
     Obstruction (mechanical) of heart valve prosthesis
     Perforation of heart valve prosthesis
     Protrusion of heart valve prosthesis

√5th **T82.1** **Mechanical complication of cardiac electronic device**
     CC Excl: For CC codes in subcategory T82.1, unless otherwise noted: PDX collection 1449

√6th **T82.11** **Breakdown (mechanical) of cardiac electronic device**

√7th **T82.110** **Breakdown (mechanical) of cardiac electrode** `CC`

√7th **T82.111** **Breakdown (mechanical) of cardiac pulse generator (battery)** `CC`

√7th **T82.118** **Breakdown (mechanical) of other cardiac electronic device** `CC`
     CC Excl: PDX collection 1450

√7th **T82.119** **Breakdown (mechanical) of unspecified cardiac electronic device** `CC`
     CC Excl: No Excl

√6th **T82.12** **Displacement of cardiac electronic device**
     Malposition of cardiac electronic device

√7th **T82.120** **Displacement of cardiac electrode** `CC`

√7th **T82.121** **Displacement of cardiac pulse generator (battery)** `CC`

√7th **T82.128** **Displacement of other cardiac electronic device** `CC`
     CC Excl: PDX collection 1450

√7th **T82.129** **Displacement of unspecified cardiac electronic device** `CC`
     CC Excl: No Excl

√6th **T82.19** **Other mechanical complication of cardiac electronic device**
     Leakage of cardiac electronic device
     Obstruction of cardiac electronic device
     Perforation of cardiac electronic device
     Protrusion of cardiac electronic device

√7th **T82.190** **Other mechanical complication of cardiac electrode** `CC`

√7th **T82.191** **Other mechanical complication of cardiac pulse generator (battery)** `CC`

√7th **T82.198** **Other mechanical complication of other cardiac electronic device** `CC`
     CC Excl: PDX collection 1450

√7th **T82.199** **Other mechanical complication of unspecified cardiac device** `CC`
     CC Excl: No Excl

√5th **T82.2** **Mechanical complication of coronary artery bypass graft and biological heart valve graft**
     EXCLUDES 1   *mechanical complication of artificial heart valve prosthesis (T82.0-)*

√6th **T82.21** **Mechanical complication of coronary artery bypass graft**
     CC Excl: For CC codes in subcategory T82.21: PDX collection 1451

√7th **T82.211** **Breakdown (mechanical) of coronary artery bypass graft** `CC`

√7th **T82.212** **Displacement of coronary artery bypass graft** `CC`
     Malposition of coronary artery bypass graft

√7th **T82.213** **Leakage of coronary artery bypass graft** `CC`

√7th **T82.218** **Other mechanical complication of coronary artery bypass graft** `CC`
     Obstruction, mechanical of coronary artery bypass graft
     Perforation of coronary artery bypass graft
     Protrusion of coronary artery bypass graft

√6th **T82.22** **Mechanical complication of biological heart valve graft**
     CC Excl: For CC codes in subcategory T82.22: PDX collection 1450

√7th **T82.221** **Breakdown (mechanical) of biological heart valve graft** `CC`

√7th **T82.222** **Displacement of biological heart valve graft** `CC`
     Malposition of biological heart valve graft

√7th **T82.223** **Leakage of biological heart valve graft** `CC`

√7th **T82.228** **Other mechanical complication of biological heart valve graft** `CC`
     Obstruction of biological heart valve graft
     Perforation of biological heart valve graft
     Protrusion of biological heart valve graft

√5th **T82.3** **Mechanical complication of other vascular grafts**
     CC Excl: For CC codes in subcategory T82.3: PDX collection 1452

√6th **T82.31** **Breakdown (mechanical) of other vascular grafts**

6 √7th **T82.310** **Breakdown (mechanical) of aortic (bifurcation) graft (replacement)** `CC` `HCC`

6 √7th **T82.311** **Breakdown (mechanical) of carotid arterial graft (bypass)** `CC` `HCC`

6 √7th **T82.312** **Breakdown (mechanical) of femoral arterial graft (bypass)** `CC` `HCC`

6 √7th **T82.318** **Breakdown (mechanical) of other vascular grafts** `CC` `HCC`

6 √7th **T82.319** **Breakdown (mechanical) of unspecified vascular grafts** `CC` `HCC`

√6th **T82.32** **Displacement of other vascular grafts**
     Malposition of other vascular grafts

6 √7th **T82.320** **Displacement of aortic (bifurcation) graft (replacement)** `CC` `HCC`

6 √7th **T82.321** **Displacement of carotid arterial graft (bypass)** `CC` `HCC`

6 √7th **T82.322** **Displacement of femoral arterial graft (bypass)** `CC` `HCC`

6 √7th **T82.328** **Displacement of other vascular grafts** `CC` `HCC`

6 √7th **T82.329** **Displacement of unspecified vascular grafts** `CC` `HCC`

N Newborn: 0   P Pediatric: 0-17   M Maternity: 9-64   A Adult: 15-124   MCC Major Complication/Comorbidity   CC Complication/Comorbidity   SW Severe Wound Dx

1194   ICD-10-CM 2020

√6ᵗʰ **T82.33** **Leakage** of other vascular grafts

6 √7ᵗʰ **T82.330** **Leakage** of aortic (bifurcation) graft (replacement)   `CC` `HCC`

6 √7ᵗʰ **T82.331** **Leakage** of carotid arterial graft (bypass)   `CC` `HCC`

6 √7ᵗʰ **T82.332** **Leakage** of femoral arterial graft (bypass)   `CC` `HCC`

6 √7ᵗʰ **T82.338** **Leakage** of other vascular grafts   `CC` `HCC`

6 √7ᵗʰ **T82.339** **Leakage** of unspecified vascular graft   `CC` `HCC`

√6ᵗʰ **T82.39** **Other mechanical complication** of other vascular grafts

Obstruction (mechanical) of other vascular grafts
Perforation of other vascular grafts
Protrusion of other vascular grafts

6 √7ᵗʰ **T82.390** **Other mechanical complication** of aortic (bifurcation) graft (replacement)   `CC` `HCC`

6 √7ᵗʰ **T82.391** **Other mechanical complication** of carotid arterial graft (bypass)   `CC` `HCC`

6 √7ᵗʰ **T82.392** **Other mechanical complication** of femoral arterial graft (bypass)   `CC` `HCC`

6 √7ᵗʰ **T82.398** **Other mechanical complication** of other vascular grafts   `CC` `HCC`

6 √7ᵗʰ **T82.399** **Other mechanical complication** of unspecified vascular grafts   `CC` `HCC`

√5ᵗʰ **T82.4** **Mechanical complication** of vascular dialysis catheter

Mechanical complication of hemodialysis catheter

EXCLUDES 1   *mechanical complication of intraperitoneal dialysis catheter (T85.62)*

CC Excl: For CC codes in subcategory T82.4: PDX collection 1452

√x 7ᵗʰ **T82.41** **Breakdown (mechanical)** of vascular dialysis catheter   `CC` `HCC`

√x 7ᵗʰ **T82.42** **Displacement** of vascular dialysis catheter   `CC` `HCC`

Malposition of vascular dialysis catheter

√x 7ᵗʰ **T82.43** **Leakage** of vascular dialysis catheter   `CC` `HCC`

√x 7ᵗʰ **T82.49** **Other complication** of vascular dialysis catheter   `CC` `HCC`

Obstruction (mechanical) of vascular dialysis catheter
Perforation of vascular dialysis catheter
Protrusion of vascular dialysis catheter

√5ᵗʰ **T82.5** **Mechanical complication** of other cardiac and vascular devices and implants

EXCLUDES 2   *mechanical complication of epidural and subdural infusion catheter (T85.61)*

CC Excl: For CC codes in subcategory T82.5, unless otherwise noted: PDX collection 1452

√6ᵗʰ **T82.51** **Breakdown (mechanical)** of other cardiac and vascular devices and implants

6 √7ᵗʰ **T82.510** **Breakdown (mechanical)** of surgically created arteriovenous fistula   `CC` `HCC`

6 √7ᵗʰ **T82.511** **Breakdown (mechanical)** of surgically created arteriovenous shunt   `CC` `HCC`

√7ᵗʰ **T82.512** **Breakdown (mechanical)** of artificial heart   `CC`
CC Excl: PDX collection 1450

6 √7ᵗʰ **T82.513** **Breakdown (mechanical)** of balloon (counterpulsation) device   `CC` `HCC`

6 √7ᵗʰ **T82.514** **Breakdown (mechanical)** of infusion catheter   `CC` `HCC`

6 √7ᵗʰ **T82.515** **Breakdown (mechanical)** of umbrella device   `CC` `HCC`

6 √7ᵗʰ **T82.518** **Breakdown (mechanical)** of other cardiac and vascular devices and implants   `CC` `HCC`

√7ᵗʰ **T82.519** **Breakdown (mechanical)** of unspecified cardiac and vascular devices and implants   `CC`
CC Excl: PDX collection 1453

√6ᵗʰ **T82.52** **Displacement** of other cardiac and vascular devices and implants

Malposition of other cardiac and vascular devices and implants

6 √7ᵗʰ **T82.520** **Displacement** of surgically created arteriovenous fistula   `CC` `HCC`

6 √7ᵗʰ **T82.521** **Displacement** of surgically created arteriovenous shunt   `CC` `HCC`

√7ᵗʰ **T82.522** **Displacement** of artificial heart   `CC`
CC Excl: PDX collection 1450

6 √7ᵗʰ **T82.523** **Displacement** of balloon (counterpulsation) device   `CC` `HCC`

6 √7ᵗʰ **T82.524** **Displacement** of infusion catheter   `CC` `HCC`

6 √7ᵗʰ **T82.525** **Displacement** of umbrella device   `CC` `HCC`

6 √7ᵗʰ **T82.528** **Displacement** of other cardiac and vascular devices and implants   `CC` `HCC`

√7ᵗʰ **T82.529** **Displacement** of unspecified cardiac and vascular devices and implants   `CC`

√6ᵗʰ **T82.53** **Leakage** of other cardiac and vascular devices and implants

6 √7ᵗʰ **T82.530** **Leakage** of surgically created arteriovenous fistula   `CC` `HCC`

6 √7ᵗʰ **T82.531** **Leakage** of surgically created arteriovenous shunt   `CC` `HCC`

√7ᵗʰ **T82.532** **Leakage** of artificial heart   `CC`
CC Excl: PDX collection 1450

6 √7ᵗʰ **T82.533** **Leakage** of balloon (counterpulsation) device   `CC` `HCC`

6 √7ᵗʰ **T82.534** **Leakage** of infusion catheter   `CC` `HCC`

6 √7ᵗʰ **T82.535** **Leakage** of umbrella device   `CC` `HCC`

6 √7ᵗʰ **T82.538** **Leakage** of other cardiac and vascular devices and implants   `CC` `HCC`

√7ᵗʰ **T82.539** **Leakage** of unspecified cardiac and vascular devices and implants   `CC`
CC Excl: PDX collection 1453

√6ᵗʰ **T82.59** **Other mechanical complication** of other cardiac and vascular devices and implants

Obstruction (mechanical) of other cardiac and vascular devices and implants
Perforation of other cardiac and vascular devices and implants
Protrusion of other cardiac and vascular devices and implants

6 √7ᵗʰ **T82.590** **Other mechanical complication** of surgically created arteriovenous fistula   `CC` `HCC`

6 √7ᵗʰ **T82.591** **Other mechanical complication** of surgically created arteriovenous shunt   `CC` `HCC`

√7ᵗʰ **T82.592** **Other mechanical complication** of artificial heart   `CC`
CC Excl: PDX collection 1450

6 √7ᵗʰ **T82.593** **Other mechanical complication** of balloon (counterpulsation) device   `CC` `HCC`

6 √7ᵗʰ **T82.594** **Other mechanical complication** of infusion catheter   `CC` `HCC`
CC Excl: PDX collection 1450

6 √7ᵗʰ **T82.595** **Other mechanical complication** of umbrella device   `CC` `HCC`

✅ Additional Character Required   √x7ᵗʰ Placeholder   Unacceptable PDx   Questionable PDx   Manifestation   Unspecified Dx   H1-H14 HAC   HCC CMS-HCC Dx   HIV HIV Dx

ICD-10-CM 2020

1195

6 √7ᵗʰ **T82.598** **Other mechanical complication of other cardiac and vascular devices and implants** `CC` `HCC`
CC Excl: PDX collection 1450

√7ᵗʰ **T82.599** **Other mechanical complication of unspecified cardiac and vascular devices and implants** `CC`
CC Excl: PDX collection 1453

6 √x7ᵗʰ **T82.6** **Infection and inflammatory reaction due to cardiac valve prosthesis** `CC` `H13` `HCC`
Use additional code to identify infection
CC Excl: PDX collection 1454

6 √x7ᵗʰ **T82.7** **Infection and inflammatory reaction due to other cardiac and vascular devices, implants and grafts** `CC` `H13` `HCC`
Use additional code to identify infection
AHA: 2019,1Q,13-14
TIP: Assign this code for infections and/or cellulitis resulting from catheters that are not centrally placed (e.g., midline catheters).
CC Excl: PDX collection 1454

√5ᵗʰ **T82.8** **Other specified complications of cardiac and vascular prosthetic devices, implants and grafts**
AHA: 2016,4Q,70

√6ᵗʰ **T82.81** **Embolism due to cardiac and vascular prosthetic devices, implants and grafts**

√7ᵗʰ **T82.817** **Embolism due to cardiac prosthetic devices, implants and grafts** `CC`
CC Excl: PDX collection 1455

6 √7ᵗʰ **T82.818** **Embolism due to vascular prosthetic devices, implants and grafts** `CC` `HCC`
CC Excl: PDX collection 1454

√6ᵗʰ **T82.82** **Fibrosis due to cardiac and vascular prosthetic devices, implants and grafts**

√7ᵗʰ **T82.827** **Fibrosis due to cardiac prosthetic devices, implants and grafts** `CC`
CC Excl: PDX collection 1455

6 √7ᵗʰ **T82.828** **Fibrosis due vascular prosthetic devices, implants and grafts** `CC` `HCC`
CC Excl: PDX collection 1454

√6ᵗʰ **T82.83** **Hemorrhage due to cardiac and vascular prosthetic devices, implants and grafts**

√7ᵗʰ **T82.837** **Hemorrhage due to cardiac prosthetic devices, implants and grafts** `CC`
CC Excl: PDX collection 1455

6 √7ᵗʰ **T82.838** **Hemorrhage due to vascular prosthetic devices, implants and grafts** `CC` `HCC`
CC Excl: PDX collection 1454

√6ᵗʰ **T82.84** **Pain due to cardiac and vascular prosthetic devices, implants and grafts**

√7ᵗʰ **T82.847** **Pain due to cardiac prosthetic devices, implants and grafts** `CC`
CC Excl: PDX collection 1455

6 √7ᵗʰ **T82.848** **Pain due to vascular prosthetic devices, implants and grafts** `CC` `HCC`
CC Excl: PDX collection 1454

√6ᵗʰ **T82.85** **Stenosis due to cardiac and vascular prosthetic devices, implants and grafts**

√7ᵗʰ **T82.855** **Stenosis of coronary artery stent** `CC`
In-stent stenosis (restenosis) of coronary artery stent
Restenosis of coronary artery stent
CC Excl: PDX collection 1455

6 √7ᵗʰ **T82.856** **Stenosis of peripheral vascular stent** `CC` `HCC`
In-stent stenosis (restenosis) of peripheral vascular stent
Restenosis of peripheral vascular stent
CC Excl: PDX collection 1454

√7ᵗʰ **T82.857** **Stenosis of other cardiac prosthetic devices, implants and grafts** `CC`
CC Excl: PDX collection 1455

6 √7ᵗʰ **T82.858** **Stenosis of other vascular prosthetic devices, implants and grafts** `CC` `HCC`
CC Excl: PDX collection 1454

√6ᵗʰ **T82.86** **Thrombosis of cardiac and vascular prosthetic devices, implants and grafts**

√7ᵗʰ **T82.867** **Thrombosis due to cardiac prosthetic devices, implants and grafts** `CC`
CC Excl: PDX collection 1455

6 √7ᵗʰ **T82.868** **Thrombosis due to vascular prosthetic devices, implants and grafts** `CC` `HCC`
CC Excl: PDX collection 1454

√6ᵗʰ **T82.89** **Other specified complication of cardiac and vascular prosthetic devices, implants and grafts**

√7ᵗʰ **T82.897** **Other specified complication of cardiac prosthetic devices, implants and grafts** `CC`
AHA: 2019,2Q,33
CC Excl: PDX collection 1455

6 √7ᵗʰ **T82.898** **Other specified complication of vascular prosthetic devices, implants and grafts** `CC` `HCC`
CC Excl: PDX collection 1454

√x7ᵗʰ **T82.9** **Unspecified complication of cardiac and vascular prosthetic device, implant and graft** `CC`
CC Excl: PDX collection 1455

√4ᵗʰ **T83** **Complications of genitourinary prosthetic devices, implants and grafts**
EXCLUDES 2 failure and rejection of transplanted organs and tissue (T86.-)
AHA: 2016,4Q,70-71

The appropriate 7th character is to be added to each code from category T83.
A initial encounter
D subsequent encounter
S sequela

CC Excl: For CC codes in category T83, unless otherwise noted: PDX collection 1456

√5ᵗʰ **T83.0** **Mechanical complication of urinary catheter**
EXCLUDES 2 complications of stoma of urinary tract (N99.5-)

√6ᵗʰ **T83.01** **Breakdown (mechanical) of urinary catheter**

6 √7ᵗʰ **T83.010** **Breakdown (mechanical) of cystostomy catheter** `CC` `HCC`

6 √7ᵗʰ **T83.011** **Breakdown (mechanical) of indwelling urethral catheter** `HCC`

6 √7ᵗʰ **T83.012** **Breakdown (mechanical) of nephrostomy catheter** `HCC`

6 √7ᵗʰ **T83.018** **Breakdown (mechanical) of other urinary catheter** `HCC`
Breakdown (mechanical) of Hopkins catheter
Breakdown (mechanical) of ileostomy catheter
Breakdown (mechanical) urostomy catheter

√6ᵗʰ **T83.02** **Displacement of urinary catheter**
Malposition of urinary catheter

6 √7ᵗʰ **T83.020** **Displacement of cystostomy catheter** `CC` `HCC`

6 √7ᵗʰ **T83.021** **Displacement of indwelling urethral catheter** `HCC`

6 √7ᵗʰ **T83.022** **Displacement of nephrostomy catheter** `HCC`

6 √7ᵗʰ **T83.028** **Displacement of other urinary catheter** `HCC`
Displacement of Hopkins catheter
Displacement of ileostomy catheter
Displacement of urostomy catheter

√6ᵗʰ **T83.03** **Leakage of urinary catheter**

6 √7ᵗʰ **T83.030** **Leakage of cystostomy catheter** `CC` `HCC`

6 √7th **T83.031** **Leakage of** indwelling urethral **catheter** HCC

6 √7th **T83.032** **Leakage of** nephrostomy **catheter** HCC

6 √7th **T83.038** **Leakage of other urinary catheter** HCC

Leakage of Hopkins catheter
Leakage of ileostomy catheter
Leakage of urostomy catheter

√6th **T83.09** **Other mechanical complication of urinary catheter**

Obstruction (mechanical) of urinary catheter
Perforation of urinary catheter
Protrusion of urinary catheter

6 √7th **T83.090** **Other mechanical complication of** cystostomy **catheter** CC HCC

6 √7th **T83.091** **Other mechanical complication of** indwelling urethral **catheter** HCC

6 √7th **T83.092** **Other mechanical complication of** nephrostomy **catheter** HCC

6 √7th **T83.098** **Other mechanical complication of other urinary catheter** HCC

Other mechanical complication of Hopkins catheter
Other mechanical complication of ileostomy catheter
Other mechanical complication of urostomy catheter

√5th **T83.1** **Mechanical complication of other urinary devices and implants**

√6th **T83.11** **Breakdown (mechanical) of other urinary devices and implants**

6 √7th **T83.110** **Breakdown (mechanical) of urinary** electronic **stimulator device** CC HCC

EXCLUDES 2 breakdown (mechanical) of electrode (lead) for sacral nerve neurostimulator (T85.111)
breakdown (mechanical) of implanted electronic sacral neurostimulator, pulse generator or receiver (T85.113)

6 √7th **T83.111** **Breakdown (mechanical) of implanted urinary sphincter** CC HCC

6 √7th **T83.112** **Breakdown (mechanical) of indwelling ureteral stent** CC HCC

6 √7th **T83.113** **Breakdown (mechanical) of other urinary stents** CC HCC

Breakdown (mechanical) of ileal conduit stent
Breakdown (mechanical) of nephroureteral stent

6 √7th **T83.118** **Breakdown (mechanical) of other urinary devices and implants** CC HCC

√6th **T83.12** **Displacement of other urinary devices and implants**

Malposition of other urinary devices and implants

6 √7th **T83.120** **Displacement of urinary electronic stimulator device** CC HCC

EXCLUDES 2 displacement of electrode (lead) for sacral nerve neurostimulator (T85.121)
displacement of implanted electronic sacral neurostimulator, pulse generator or receiver (T85.123)

6 √7th **T83.121** **Displacement of implanted urinary sphincter** CC HCC

6 √7th **T83.122** **Displacement of indwelling ureteral stent** CC HCC

6 √7th **T83.123** **Displacement of other urinary stents** CC HCC

Displacement of ileal conduit stent
Displacement of nephroureteral stent

6 √7th **T83.128** **Displacement of other urinary devices and implants** CC HCC

√6th **T83.19** **Other mechanical complication of other urinary devices and implants**

Leakage of other urinary devices and implants
Obstruction (mechanical) of other urinary devices and implants
Perforation of other urinary devices and implants
Protrusion of other urinary devices and implants

6 √7th **T83.190** **Other mechanical complication of urinary electronic stimulator device** CC HCC

EXCLUDES 2 other mechanical complication of electrode (lead) for sacral nerve neurostimulator (T85.191)
other mechanical complication of implanted electronic sacral neurostimulator, pulse generator or receiver (T85.193)

6 √7th **T83.191** **Other mechanical complication of** implanted urinary sphincter CC HCC

6 √7th **T83.192** **Other mechanical complication of** indwelling ureteral stent CC HCC

6 √7th **T83.193** **Other mechanical complication of other urinary stent** CC HCC

Other mechanical complication of ileal conduit stent
Other mechanical complication of nephroureteral stent

6 √7th **T83.198** **Other mechanical complication of other urinary devices and implants** CC HCC

√5th **T83.2** **Mechanical complication of graft of urinary organ**

6 √x7th **T83.21** **Breakdown (mechanical) of graft of urinary organ** CC HCC

6 √x7th **T83.22** **Displacement of graft of urinary organ** CC HCC

Malposition of graft of urinary organ

6 √x7th **T83.23** **Leakage of graft of urinary organ** CC HCC

6 √x7th **T83.24** **Erosion of graft of urinary organ** CC HCC

6 √x7th **T83.25** **Exposure of graft of urinary organ** CC HCC

6 √x7th **T83.29** **Other mechanical complication of graft of urinary organ** CC HCC

Obstruction (mechanical) of graft of urinary organ
Perforation of graft of urinary organ
Protrusion of graft of urinary organ

√5th **T83.3** **Mechanical complication of intrauterine contraceptive device**

√x7th **T83.31** **Breakdown (mechanical) of intrauterine contraceptive device** ♀

√x7th **T83.32** **Displacement of intrauterine contraceptive device** ♀

Malposition of intrauterine contraceptive device
Missing string of intrauterine contraceptive device
AHA: 2018,1Q,5

√x7th **T83.39** **Other mechanical complication of intrauterine contraceptive device** ♀

Leakage of intrauterine contraceptive device
Obstruction (mechanical) of intrauterine contraceptive device
Perforation of intrauterine contraceptive device
Protrusion of intrauterine contraceptive device

√5th **T83.4** **Mechanical complication of other prosthetic devices, implants and grafts of genital tract**

√6th **T83.41** **Breakdown (mechanical) of other prosthetic devices, implants and grafts of genital tract**

6 √7th **T83.410** **Breakdown (mechanical) of implanted penile prosthesis** `CC` `HCC` ♂

     Breakdown (mechanical) of penile prosthesis cylinder

     Breakdown (mechanical) of penile prosthesis pump

     Breakdown (mechanical) of penile prosthesis reservoir

6 √7th **T83.411** **Breakdown (mechanical) of implanted testicular prosthesis** `CC` `HCC`

6 √7th **T83.418** **Breakdown (mechanical) of other prosthetic devices, implants and grafts of genital tract** `CC` `HCC`

√6th **T83.42** **Displacement of other prosthetic devices, implants and grafts of genital tract**

     Malposition of other prosthetic devices, implants and grafts of genital tract

6 √7th **T83.420** **Displacement of implanted penile prosthesis** `CC` `HCC` ♂

     Displacement of penile prosthesis cylinder

     Displacement of penile prosthesis pump

     Displacement of penile prosthesis reservoir

6 √7th **T83.421** **Displacement of implanted testicular prosthesis** `CC` `HCC`

6 √7th **T83.428** **Displacement of other prosthetic devices, implants and grafts of genital tract** `CC` `HCC`

     AHA: 2018,1Q,5

√6th **T83.49** **Other mechanical complication of other prosthetic devices, implants and grafts of genital tract**

     Leakage of other prosthetic devices, implants and grafts of genital tract

     Obstruction, mechanical of other prosthetic devices, implants and grafts of genital tract

     Perforation of other prosthetic devices, implants and grafts of genital tract

     Protrusion of other prosthetic devices, implants and grafts of genital tract

6 √7th **T83.490** **Other mechanical complication of implanted penile prosthesis** `CC` `HCC` ♂

     Other mechanical complication of penile prosthesis cylinder

     Other mechanical complication of penile prosthesis pump

     Other mechanical complication of penile prosthesis reservoir

6 √7th **T83.491** **Other mechanical complication of implanted testicular prosthesis** `CC` `HCC`

6 √7th **T83.498** **Other mechanical complication of other prosthetic devices, implants and grafts of genital tract** `CC` `HCC`

√5th **T83.5** **Infection and inflammatory reaction due to prosthetic device, implant and graft in urinary system**

     Use additional code to identify infection

     CC Excl: For CC codes in subcategory T83.5, unless otherwise noted: PDX collection 1458

√6th **T83.51** **Infection and inflammatory reaction due to urinary catheter**

     EXCLUDES 2   complications of stoma of urinary tract (N99.5-)

6 √7th **T83.510** **Infection and inflammatory reaction due to cystostomy catheter** `CC` `HCC`

6 √7th **T83.511** **Infection and inflammatory reaction due to indwelling urethral catheter** `CC` `H6` `HCC`

     CC Excl: PDX collection 1457

6 √7th **T83.512** **Infection and inflammatory reaction due to nephrostomy catheter** `CC` `HCC`

6 √7th **T83.518** **Infection and inflammatory reaction due to other urinary catheter** `CC` `H6` `HCC`

     Infection and inflammatory reaction due to Hopkins catheter

     Infection and inflammatory reaction due to ileostomy catheter

     Infection and inflammatory reaction due to urostomy catheter

√6th **T83.59** **Infection and inflammatory reaction due to prosthetic device, implant and graft in urinary system**

6 √7th **T83.590** **Infection and inflammatory reaction due to implanted urinary neurostimulation device** `CC` `HCC`

     EXCLUDES 2   *infection and inflammatory reaction due to electrode lead of sacral nerve neurostimulator (T85.732)*

     infection and inflammatory reaction due to pulse generator or receiver of sacral nerve neurostimulator (T85.734)

6 √7th **T83.591** **Infection and inflammatory reaction due to implanted urinary sphincter** `CC` `HCC`

6 √7th **T83.592** **Infection and inflammatory reaction due to indwelling ureteral stent** `CC` `HCC`

6 √7th **T83.593** **Infection and inflammatory reaction due to other urinary stents** `CC` `HCC`

     Infection and inflammatory reaction due to ileal conduit stents

     Infection and inflammatory reaction due to nephroureteral stent

6 √7th **T83.598** **Infection and inflammatory reaction due to other prosthetic device, implant and graft in urinary system** `CC` `HCC`

√5th **T83.6** **Infection and inflammatory reaction due to prosthetic device, implant and graft in genital tract**

     Use additional code to identify infection

     CC Excl: For CC codes in subcategory T83.6: PDX collection 1458

6 √x7th **T83.61** **Infection and inflammatory reaction due to implanted penile prosthesis** `CC` `HCC`

     Infection and inflammatory reaction due to penile prosthesis cylinder

     Infection and inflammatory reaction due to penile prosthesis pump

     Infection and inflammatory reaction due to penile prosthesis reservoir

6 √x7th **T83.62** **Infection and inflammatory reaction due to implanted testicular prosthesis** `CC` `HCC`

6 √x7th **T83.69** **Infection and inflammatory reaction due to other prosthetic device, implant and graft in genital tract** `CC` `HCC`

N Newborn: 0   P Pediatric: 0-17   M Maternity: 9-64   A Adult: 15-124   MCC Major Complication/Comorbidity   CC Complication/Comorbidity   SW Severe Wound Dx

1198   ICD-10-CM 2020

√5ᵗʰ **T83.7** **Complications due to implanted mesh and other prosthetic materials**

    √6ᵗʰ **T83.71** **Erosion of implanted mesh and other prosthetic materials**

        6 √7ᵗʰ **T83.711** **Erosion of implanted vaginal mesh to surrounding organ or tissue**   HCC ♀

            Erosion of implanted vaginal mesh into pelvic floor muscles

        6 √7ᵗʰ **T83.712** **Erosion of implanted urethral mesh to surrounding organ or tissue**   CC HCC

            Erosion of implanted female urethral sling

            Erosion of implanted male urethral sling

            Erosion of implanted urethral mesh into pelvic floor muscles

        6 √7ᵗʰ **T83.713** **Erosion of implanted urethral bulking agent to surrounding organ or tissue**   CC HCC

        6 √7ᵗʰ **T83.714** **Erosion of implanted ureteral bulking agent to surrounding organ or tissue**   CC HCC

        6 √7ᵗʰ **T83.718** **Erosion of other implanted mesh to organ or tissue**   CC HCC

        6 √7ᵗʰ **T83.719** **Erosion of other prosthetic materials to surrounding organ or tissue**   CC HCC

    √6ᵗʰ **T83.72** **Exposure of implanted mesh and other prosthetic materials into surrounding organ or tissue**

        Extrusion of implanted mesh

        6 √7ᵗʰ **T83.721** **Exposure of implanted vaginal mesh into vagina**   HCC ♀

            Exposure of implanted vaginal mesh through vaginal wall

        6 √7ᵗʰ **T83.722** **Exposure of implanted urethral mesh into urethra**   CC HCC

            Exposure of implanted female urethral sling

            Exposure of implanted male urethral sling

            Exposure of implanted urethral mesh through urethral wall

        6 √7ᵗʰ **T83.723** **Exposure of implanted urethral bulking agent into urethra**   CC HCC

        6 √7ᵗʰ **T83.724** **Exposure of implanted ureteral bulking agent into ureter**   CC HCC

        6 √7ᵗʰ **T83.728** **Exposure of other implanted mesh into organ or tissue**   CC HCC

        6 √7ᵗʰ **T83.729** **Exposure of other prosthetic materials into organ or tissue**   CC HCC

    6 √x7ᵗʰ **T83.79** **Other specified complications due to other genitourinary prosthetic materials**   CC HCC

        CC Excl: PDX collection 1458

√5ᵗʰ **T83.8** **Other specified complications of genitourinary prosthetic devices, implants and grafts**

    CC Excl: For CC codes in subcategory T83.8: PDX collection 1458

    6 √x7ᵗʰ **T83.81** **Embolism due to genitourinary prosthetic devices, implants and grafts**   CC HCC

    6 √x7ᵗʰ **T83.82** **Fibrosis due to genitourinary prosthetic devices, implants and grafts**   CC HCC

    6 √x7ᵗʰ **T83.83** **Hemorrhage due to genitourinary prosthetic devices, implants and grafts**   CC HCC

    6 √x7ᵗʰ **T83.84** **Pain due to genitourinary prosthetic devices, implants and grafts**   CC HCC

    6 √x7ᵗʰ **T83.85** **Stenosis due to genitourinary prosthetic devices, implants and grafts**   CC HCC

    6 √x7ᵗʰ **T83.86** **Thrombosis due to genitourinary prosthetic devices, implants and grafts**   CC HCC

6 √x7ᵗʰ **T83.89** **Other specified complication of genitourinary prosthetic devices, implants and grafts**   CC HCC

6 √x7ᵗʰ **T83.9** **Unspecified complication of genitourinary prosthetic device, implant and graft**   CC HCC

    CC Excl: PDX collection 1458

√4ᵗʰ **T84** **Complications of internal orthopedic prosthetic devices, implants and grafts**

    EXCLUDES 2   failure and rejection of transplanted organs and tissues (T86.-)

            fracture of bone following insertion of orthopedic implant, joint prosthesis or bone plate (M96.6)

    The appropriate 7th character is to be added to each code from category T84.

    A   initial encounter

    D   subsequent encounter

    S   sequela

    CC Excl: For CC codes in category T84, unless otherwise noted: PDX collection 911

√5ᵗʰ **T84.0** **Mechanical complication of internal joint prosthesis**

    √6ᵗʰ **T84.01** **Broken internal joint prosthesis**

        Breakage (fracture) of prosthetic joint

        Broken prosthetic joint implant

        EXCLUDES 1   periprosthetic joint implant fracture (M97-)

        AHA: 2016,4Q,42

        6 √7ᵗʰ **T84.010** **Broken internal right hip prosthesis**   CC HCC

        6 √7ᵗʰ **T84.011** **Broken internal left hip prosthesis**   CC HCC

        6 √7ᵗʰ **T84.012** **Broken internal right knee prosthesis**   CC HCC

        6 √7ᵗʰ **T84.013** **Broken internal left knee prosthesis**   CC HCC

        6 √7ᵗʰ **T84.018** **Broken internal joint prosthesis, other site**   CC HCC

            Use additional code to identify the joint (Z96.6-)

        6 √7ᵗʰ **T84.019** **Broken internal joint prosthesis, unspecified site**   CC HCC

    √6ᵗʰ **T84.02** **Dislocation of internal joint prosthesis**

        Instability of internal joint prosthesis

        Subluxation of internal joint prosthesis

        AHA: 2019,2Q,27

        6 √7ᵗʰ **T84.020** **Dislocation of internal right hip prosthesis**   CC HCC

        6 √7ᵗʰ **T84.021** **Dislocation of internal left hip prosthesis**   CC HCC

        6 √7ᵗʰ **T84.022** **Instability of internal right knee prosthesis**   CC HCC

        6 √7ᵗʰ **T84.023** **Instability of internal left knee prosthesis**   CC HCC

        6 √7ᵗʰ **T84.028** **Dislocation of other internal joint prosthesis**   CC HCC

            Use additional code to identify the joint (Z96.6-)

        6 √7ᵗʰ **T84.029** **Dislocation of unspecified internal joint prosthesis**   CC HCC

    √6ᵗʰ **T84.03** **Mechanical loosening of internal prosthetic joint**

        Aseptic loosening of prosthetic joint

        6 √7ᵗʰ **T84.030** **Mechanical loosening of internal right hip prosthetic joint**   CC HCC

        6 √7ᵗʰ **T84.031** **Mechanical loosening of internal left hip prosthetic joint**   CC HCC

        6 √7ᵗʰ **T84.032** **Mechanical loosening of internal right knee prosthetic joint**   CC HCC

        6 √7ᵗʰ **T84.033** **Mechanical loosening of internal left knee prosthetic joint**   CC HCC

        6 √7ᵗʰ **T84.038** **Mechanical loosening of other internal prosthetic joint**   CC HCC

            Use additional code to identify the joint (Z96.6-)

        6 √7ᵗʰ **T84.039** **Mechanical loosening of unspecified internal prosthetic joint**   CC HCC

☑ Additional Character Required   √x7ᵗʰ Placeholder   Unacceptable PDx   Questionable PDx   Manifestation   Unspecified Dx   H1-H14 HAC   HCC CMS-HCC Dx   HIV HIV Dx

ICD-10-CM 2020   1199

Chapter 19. Injury, Poisoning and Certain Other Consequences of External Causes

T84.05   **Periprosthetic osteolysis of internal prosthetic joint**

Use additional code to identify major osseous defect, if applicable (M89.7-)

6 ✓7ᵗʰ **T84.050**   **Periprosthetic osteolysis of internal prosthetic right hip joint**   CC HCC

6 ✓7ᵗʰ **T84.051**   **Periprosthetic osteolysis of internal prosthetic left hip joint**   CC HCC

6 ✓7ᵗʰ **T84.052**   **Periprosthetic osteolysis of internal prosthetic right knee joint**   CC HCC

6 ✓7ᵗʰ **T84.053**   **Periprosthetic osteolysis of internal prosthetic left knee joint**   CC HCC

6 ✓7ᵗʰ **T84.058**   **Periprosthetic osteolysis of other internal prosthetic joint**   CC HCC

Use additional code to identify the joint (Z96.6-)

6 ✓7ᵗʰ **T84.059**   **Periprosthetic osteolysis of unspecified internal prosthetic joint**   CC HCC

✓6ᵗʰ **T84.06**   **Wear of articular bearing surface of internal prosthetic joint**

6 ✓7ᵗʰ **T84.060**   **Wear of articular bearing surface of internal prosthetic right hip joint**   CC HCC

6 ✓7ᵗʰ **T84.061**   **Wear of articular bearing surface of internal prosthetic left hip joint**   CC HCC

6 ✓7ᵗʰ **T84.062**   **Wear of articular bearing surface of internal prosthetic right knee joint**   CC HCC

6 ✓7ᵗʰ **T84.063**   **Wear of articular bearing surface of internal prosthetic left knee joint**   CC HCC

6 ✓7ᵗʰ **T84.068**   **Wear of articular bearing surface of other internal prosthetic joint**   CC HCC

Use additional code to identify the joint (Z96.6-)

6 ✓7ᵗʰ **T84.069**   **Wear of articular bearing surface of unspecified internal prosthetic joint**   CC HCC

✓6ᵗʰ **T84.09**   **Other mechanical complication of internal joint prosthesis**

Prosthetic joint implant failure NOS

AHA: 2019,1Q,20

6 ✓7ᵗʰ **T84.090**   **Other mechanical complication of internal right hip prosthesis**   CC HCC

6 ✓7ᵗʰ **T84.091**   **Other mechanical complication of internal left hip prosthesis**   CC HCC

6 ✓7ᵗʰ **T84.092**   **Other mechanical complication of internal right knee prosthesis**   CC HCC

6 ✓7ᵗʰ **T84.093**   **Other mechanical complication of internal left knee prosthesis**   CC HCC

6 ✓7ᵗʰ **T84.098**   **Other mechanical complication of other internal joint prosthesis**   CC HCC

Use additional code to identify the joint (Z96.6-)

6 ✓7ᵗʰ **T84.099**   **Other mechanical complication of unspecified internal joint prosthesis**   CC HCC

✓5ᵗʰ **T84.1**   **Mechanical complication of internal fixation device of bones of limb**

EXCLUDES 2   mechanical complication of internal fixation device of bones of feet (T84.2-)

mechanical complication of internal fixation device of bones of fingers (T84.2-)

mechanical complication of internal fixation device of bones of hands (T84.2-)

mechanical complication of internal fixation device of bones of toes (T84.2-)

✓6ᵗʰ **T84.11**   **Breakdown (mechanical) of internal fixation device of bones of limb**

6 ✓7ᵗʰ **T84.110**   **Breakdown (mechanical) of internal fixation device of right humerus**   CC HCC

6 ✓7ᵗʰ **T84.111**   **Breakdown (mechanical) of internal fixation device of left humerus**   CC HCC

6 ✓7ᵗʰ **T84.112**   **Breakdown (mechanical) of internal fixation device of bone of right forearm**   CC HCC

6 ✓7ᵗʰ **T84.113**   **Breakdown (mechanical) of internal fixation device of bone of left forearm**   CC HCC

6 ✓7ᵗʰ **T84.114**   **Breakdown (mechanical) of internal fixation device of right femur**   CC HCC

6 ✓7ᵗʰ **T84.115**   **Breakdown (mechanical) of internal fixation device of left femur**   CC HCC

6 ✓7ᵗʰ **T84.116**   **Breakdown (mechanical) of internal fixation device of bone of right lower leg**   CC HCC

6 ✓7ᵗʰ **T84.117**   **Breakdown (mechanical) of internal fixation device of bone of left lower leg**   CC HCC

6 ✓7ᵗʰ **T84.119**   **Breakdown (mechanical) of internal fixation device of unspecified bone of limb**   CC HCC

✓6ᵗʰ **T84.12**   **Displacement of internal fixation device of bones of limb**

Malposition of internal fixation device of bones of limb

6 ✓7ᵗʰ **T84.120**   **Displacement of internal fixation device of right humerus**   CC HCC

6 ✓7ᵗʰ **T84.121**   **Displacement of internal fixation device of left humerus**   CC HCC

6 ✓7ᵗʰ **T84.122**   **Displacement of internal fixation device of bone of right forearm**   CC HCC

6 ✓7ᵗʰ **T84.123**   **Displacement of internal fixation device of bone of left forearm**   CC HCC

6 ✓7ᵗʰ **T84.124**   **Displacement of internal fixation device of right femur**   CC HCC

6 ✓7ᵗʰ **T84.125**   **Displacement of internal fixation device of left femur**   CC HCC

6 ✓7ᵗʰ **T84.126**   **Displacement of internal fixation device of bone of right lower leg**   CC HCC

6 ✓7ᵗʰ **T84.127**   **Displacement of internal fixation device of bone of left lower leg**   CC HCC

6 ✓7ᵗʰ **T84.129**   **Displacement of internal fixation device of unspecified bone of limb**   CC HCC

✓6ᵗʰ **T84.19**   **Other mechanical complication of internal fixation device of bones of limb**

Obstruction (mechanical) of internal fixation device of bones of limb

Perforation of internal fixation device of bones of limb

Protrusion of internal fixation device of bones of limb

6 ✓7ᵗʰ **T84.190**   **Other mechanical complication of internal fixation device of right humerus**   CC HCC

N Newborn: 0   P Pediatric: 0-17   M Maternity: 9-64   A Adult: 15-124   **MCC** Major Complication/Comorbidity   **CC** Complication/Comorbidity   **SW** Severe Wound Dx

1200   ICD-10-CM 2020

6 √7ᵗʰ **T84.191** Other mechanical complication of internal fixation device of left humerus   `CC` `HCC`

6 √7ᵗʰ **T84.192** Other mechanical complication of internal fixation device of bone of right forearm   `CC` `HCC`

6 √7ᵗʰ **T84.193** Other mechanical complication of internal fixation device of bone of left forearm   `CC` `HCC`

6 √7ᵗʰ **T84.194** Other mechanical complication of internal fixation device of right femur   `CC` `HCC`

6 √7ᵗʰ **T84.195** Other mechanical complication of internal fixation device of left femur   `CC` `HCC`

6 √7ᵗʰ **T84.196** Other mechanical complication of internal fixation device of bone of right lower leg   `CC` `HCC`

6 √7ᵗʰ **T84.197** Other mechanical complication of internal fixation device of bone of left lower leg   `CC` `HCC`

6 √7ᵗʰ **T84.199** Other mechanical complication of internal fixation device of unspecified bone of limb   `CC` `HCC`

√5ᵗʰ **T84.2** Mechanical complication of internal fixation device of other bones

   √6ᵗʰ **T84.21** Breakdown (mechanical) of internal fixation device of other bones

     6 √7ᵗʰ **T84.210** Breakdown (mechanical) of internal fixation device of bones of hand and fingers   `CC` `HCC`

     6 √7ᵗʰ **T84.213** Breakdown (mechanical) of internal fixation device of bones of foot and toes   `CC` `HCC`

     6 √7ᵗʰ **T84.216** Breakdown (mechanical) of internal fixation device of vertebrae   `CC` `HCC`

     6 √7ᵗʰ **T84.218** Breakdown (mechanical) of internal fixation device of other bones   `CC` `HCC`

   √6ᵗʰ **T84.22** Displacement of internal fixation device of other bones

     Malposition of internal fixation device of other bones

     6 √7ᵗʰ **T84.220** Displacement of internal fixation device of bones of hand and fingers   `CC` `HCC`

     6 √7ᵗʰ **T84.223** Displacement of internal fixation device of bones of foot and toes   `CC` `HCC`

     6 √7ᵗʰ **T84.226** Displacement of internal fixation device of vertebrae   `CC` `HCC`

     6 √7ᵗʰ **T84.228** Displacement of internal fixation device of other bones   `CC` `HCC`

   √6ᵗʰ **T84.29** Other mechanical complication of internal fixation device of other bones

     Obstruction (mechanical) of internal fixation device of other bones

     Perforation of internal fixation device of other bones

     Protrusion of internal fixation device of other bones

     6 √7ᵗʰ **T84.290** Other mechanical complication of internal fixation device of bones of hand and fingers   `CC` `HCC`

     6 √7ᵗʰ **T84.293** Other mechanical complication of internal fixation device of bones of foot and toes   `CC` `HCC`

     6 √7ᵗʰ **T84.296** Other mechanical complication of internal fixation device of vertebrae   `CC` `HCC`

6 √7ᵗʰ **T84.298** Other mechanical complication of internal fixation device of other bones   `CC` `HCC`

√5ᵗʰ **T84.3** Mechanical complication of other bone devices, implants and grafts

   EXCLUDES 2   other complications of bone graft (T86.83-)

   √6ᵗʰ **T84.31** Breakdown (mechanical) of other bone devices, implants and grafts

     6 √7ᵗʰ **T84.310** Breakdown (mechanical) of electronic bone stimulator   `CC` `HCC`

     6 √7ᵗʰ **T84.318** Breakdown (mechanical) of other bone devices, implants and grafts   `CC` `HCC`

   √6ᵗʰ **T84.32** Displacement of other bone devices, implants and grafts

     Malposition of other bone devices, implants and grafts

     6 √7ᵗʰ **T84.320** Displacement of electronic bone stimulator   `CC` `HCC`

     6 √7ᵗʰ **T84.328** Displacement of other bone devices, implants and grafts   `CC` `HCC`

      AHA: 2014,4Q,28

   √6ᵗʰ **T84.39** Other mechanical complication of other bone devices, implants and grafts

     Obstruction (mechanical) of other bone devices, implants and grafts

     Perforation of other bone devices, implants and grafts

     Protrusion of other bone devices, implants and grafts

     6 √7ᵗʰ **T84.390** Other mechanical complication of electronic bone stimulator   `CC` `HCC`

     6 √7ᵗʰ **T84.398** Other mechanical complication of other bone devices, implants and grafts   `CC` `HCC`

√5ᵗʰ **T84.4** Mechanical complication of other internal orthopedic devices, implants and grafts

   √6ᵗʰ **T84.41** Breakdown (mechanical) of other internal orthopedic devices, implants and grafts

     6 √7ᵗʰ **T84.410** Breakdown (mechanical) of muscle and tendon graft   `CC` `HCC`

     6 √7ᵗʰ **T84.418** Breakdown (mechanical) of other internal orthopedic devices, implants and grafts   `CC` `HCC`

   √6ᵗʰ **T84.42** Displacement of other internal orthopedic devices, implants and grafts

     Malposition of other internal orthopedic devices, implants and grafts

     6 √7ᵗʰ **T84.420** Displacement of muscle and tendon graft   `CC` `HCC`

     6 √7ᵗʰ **T84.428** Displacement of other internal orthopedic devices, implants and grafts   `CC` `HCC`

   √6ᵗʰ **T84.49** Other mechanical complication of other internal orthopedic devices, implants and grafts

     Mechanical complication of other internal orthopedic devices, implants and grafts NOS

     Obstruction (mechanical) of other internal orthopedic devices, implants and grafts

     Perforation of other internal orthopedic devices, implants and grafts

     Protrusion of other internal orthopedic devices, implants and grafts

     6 √7ᵗʰ **T84.490** Other mechanical complication of muscle and tendon graft   `CC` `HCC`

     6 √7ᵗʰ **T84.498** Other mechanical complication of other internal orthopedic devices, implants and grafts   `CC` `HCC`

☑ Additional Character Required   √x7ᵗʰ Placeholder   Unacceptable PDx   Questionable PDx   Manifestation   Unspecified Dx   `H1`-`H14` HAC   `HCC` CMS-HCC Dx   `HIV` HIV Dx

ICD-10-CM 2020   1201

Chapter 19. Injury, Poisoning and Certain Other Consequences of External Causes

T84.5–T85.09

√5ᵗʰ **T84.5** **Infection and inflammatory reaction due to internal joint prosthesis**
    Use additional code to identify infection
    AHA: 2015,1Q,16
    CC Excl: For CC codes in subcategory T84.5: PDX collection 1459

6 √x7ᵗʰ **T84.50** Infection and inflammatory reaction due to unspecified internal joint prosthesis   CC HCC

6 √x7ᵗʰ **T84.51** Infection and inflammatory reaction due to internal **right hip prosthesis**   CC HCC

6 √x7ᵗʰ **T84.52** Infection and inflammatory reaction due to internal **left hip prosthesis**   CC HCC

6 √x7ᵗʰ **T84.53** Infection and inflammatory reaction due to internal **right knee prosthesis**   CC HCC

6 √x7ᵗʰ **T84.54** Infection and inflammatory reaction due to internal **left knee prosthesis**   CC HCC

6 √x7ᵗʰ **T84.59** Infection and inflammatory reaction due to other internal joint prosthesis   CC HCC

√5ᵗʰ **T84.6** **Infection and inflammatory reaction due to internal fixation device**
    Use additional code to identify infection
    CC Excl: For CC codes in subcategory T84.6: PDX collection 1459

6 √x7ᵗʰ **T84.60** Infection and inflammatory reaction due to internal fixation device of unspecified site   CC H12 HCC

√6ᵗʰ **T84.61** Infection and inflammatory reaction due to internal fixation device of **arm**

    6 √7ᵗʰ **T84.610** Infection and inflammatory reaction due to internal fixation device of **right humerus**   CC H12 HCC

    6 √7ᵗʰ **T84.611** Infection and inflammatory reaction due to internal fixation device of **left humerus**   CC H12 HCC

    6 √7ᵗʰ **T84.612** Infection and inflammatory reaction due to internal fixation device of **right radius**   CC H12 HCC

    6 √7ᵗʰ **T84.613** Infection and inflammatory reaction due to internal fixation device of **left radius**   CC H12 HCC

    6 √7ᵗʰ **T84.614** Infection and inflammatory reaction due to internal fixation device of **right ulna**   CC H12 HCC

    6 √7ᵗʰ **T84.615** Infection and inflammatory reaction due to internal fixation device of **left ulna**   CC H12 HCC

    6 √7ᵗʰ **T84.619** Infection and inflammatory reaction due to internal fixation device of unspecified bone of arm   CC H12 HCC

√6ᵗʰ **T84.62** Infection and inflammatory reaction due to internal fixation device of **leg**

    6 √7ᵗʰ **T84.620** Infection and inflammatory reaction due to internal fixation device of **right femur**   CC HCC

    6 √7ᵗʰ **T84.621** Infection and inflammatory reaction due to internal fixation device of **left femur**   CC HCC

    6 √7ᵗʰ **T84.622** Infection and inflammatory reaction due to internal fixation device of **right tibia**   CC HCC

    6 √7ᵗʰ **T84.623** Infection and inflammatory reaction due to internal fixation device of **left tibia**   CC HCC

    6 √7ᵗʰ **T84.624** Infection and inflammatory reaction due to internal fixation device of **right fibula**   CC HCC

    6 √7ᵗʰ **T84.625** Infection and inflammatory reaction due to internal fixation device of **left fibula**   CC HCC

6 √7ᵗʰ **T84.629** Infection and inflammatory reaction due to internal fixation device of unspecified bone of leg   CC HCC

6 √x7ᵗʰ **T84.63** Infection and inflammatory reaction due to internal fixation device of **spine**   CC H12 HCC

6 √x7ᵗʰ **T84.69** Infection and inflammatory reaction due to internal fixation device of other site   CC H12 HCC

6 √x7ᵗʰ **T84.7** **Infection and inflammatory reaction due to other internal orthopedic prosthetic devices, implants and grafts**   CC H12 HCC
    Use additional code to identify infection
    CC Excl: PDX collection 1459

√5ᵗʰ **T84.8** **Other specified complications of internal orthopedic prosthetic devices, implants and grafts**
    CC Excl: For CC codes in subcategory T84.8: PDX collection 1459

6 √x7ᵗʰ **T84.81** **Embolism** due to internal orthopedic prosthetic devices, implants and grafts   CC HCC

6 √x7ᵗʰ **T84.82** **Fibrosis** due to internal orthopedic prosthetic devices, implants and grafts   CC HCC

6 √x7ᵗʰ **T84.83** **Hemorrhage** due to internal orthopedic prosthetic devices, implants and grafts   CC HCC

6 √x7ᵗʰ **T84.84** **Pain** due to internal orthopedic prosthetic devices, implants and grafts   CC HCC

6 √x7ᵗʰ **T84.85** **Stenosis** due to internal orthopedic prosthetic devices, implants and grafts   CC HCC

6 √x7ᵗʰ **T84.86** **Thrombosis** due to internal orthopedic prosthetic devices, implants and grafts   CC HCC

6 √x7ᵗʰ **T84.89** **Other specified complication** of internal orthopedic prosthetic devices, implants and grafts   CC HCC

6 √x7ᵗʰ **T84.9** **Unspecified complication of internal orthopedic prosthetic device, implant and graft**   CC HCC
    CC Excl: PDX collection 1459

√4ᵗʰ **T85** **Complications of other internal prosthetic devices, implants and grafts**
    EXCLUDES 2   failure and rejection of transplanted organs and tissue (T86.-)
    AHA: 2016,4Q,71-72

    The appropriate 7th character is to be added to each code from category T85.
    A   initial encounter
    D   subsequent encounter
    S   sequela

√5ᵗʰ **T85.0** **Mechanical complication of ventricular intracranial (communicating) shunt**
    CC Excl: For CC codes in subcategory T85.0: PDX collection 1460

6 √x7ᵗʰ **T85.01** **Breakdown (mechanical)** of ventricular intracranial (communicating) shunt   CC HCC

6 √x7ᵗʰ **T85.02** **Displacement** of ventricular intracranial (communicating) shunt   CC HCC
    Malposition of ventricular intracranial (communicating) shunt

6 √x7ᵗʰ **T85.03** **Leakage** of ventricular intracranial (communicating) shunt   CC HCC

6 √x7ᵗʰ **T85.09** **Other mechanical complication** of ventricular intracranial (communicating) shunt   CC HCC
    Obstruction (mechanical) of ventricular intracranial (communicating) shunt
    Perforation of ventricular intracranial (communicating) shunt
    Protrusion of ventricular intracranial (communicating) shunt

√5ᵗʰ **T85.1** **Mechanical complication of** implanted electronic stimulator of nervous system

CC Excl: For CC codes in subcategory T85.1: PDX collection 1460

√6ᵗʰ **T85.11** **Breakdown (mechanical) of implanted electronic stimulator of nervous system**

6 √7ᵗʰ **T85.110** **Breakdown (mechanical) of implanted electronic neurostimulator** of brain electrode (lead)   `CC` `HCC`

6 √7ᵗʰ **T85.111** **Breakdown (mechanical) of implanted electronic neurostimulator of** peripheral nerve electrode (lead)   `CC` `HCC`

Breakdown of electrode (lead) for cranial nerve neurostimulators

Breakdown of electrode (lead) for gastric neurostimulator

Breakdown of electrode (lead) for sacral nerve neurostimulator

Breakdown of electrode (lead) for vagal nerve neurostimulators

6 √7ᵗʰ **T85.112** **Breakdown (mechanical) of implanted electronic neurostimulator** of spinal cord electrode (lead)   `CC` `HCC`

6 √7ᵗʰ **T85.113** **Breakdown (mechanical) of implanted electronic neurostimulator, generator**   `CC` `HCC`

Breakdown (mechanical) of implanted electronic neurostimulator generator, brain, peripheral, gastric, spinal

Breakdown (mechanical) of implanted electronic sacral neurostimulator, pulse generator or receiver

6 √7ᵗʰ **T85.118** **Breakdown (mechanical) of other implanted electronic stimulator of nervous system**   `CC` `HCC`

√6ᵗʰ **T85.12** **Displacement of implanted electronic stimulator of nervous system**

Malposition of implanted electronic stimulator of nervous system

6 √7ᵗʰ **T85.120** **Displacement of implanted electronic neurostimulator** of brain electrode (lead)   `CC` `HCC`

6 √7ᵗʰ **T85.121** **Displacement of implanted electronic neurostimulator of** peripheral nerve electrode (lead)   `CC` `HCC`

Displacement of electrode (lead) for cranial nerve neurostimulators

Displacement of electrode (lead) for gastric neurostimulator

Displacement of electrode (lead) for sacral nerve neurostimulator

Displacement of electrode (lead) for vagal nerve neurostimulators

6 √7ᵗʰ **T85.122** **Displacement of implanted electronic neurostimulator** of spinal cord electrode (lead)   `CC` `HCC`

6 √7ᵗʰ **T85.123** **Displacement of implanted electronic neurostimulator, generator**   `CC` `HCC`

Displacement of implanted electronic neurostimulator generator, brain, peripheral, gastric, spinal

Displacement of implanted electronic sacral neurostimulator, pulse generator or receiver

6 √7ᵗʰ **T85.128** **Displacement of other implanted electronic stimulator of nervous system**   `CC` `HCC`

√6ᵗʰ **T85.19** **Other mechanical complication of implanted electronic stimulator of nervous system**

Leakage of implanted electronic stimulator of nervous system

Obstruction (mechanical) of implanted electronic stimulator of nervous system

Perforation of implanted electronic stimulator of nervous system

Protrusion of implanted electronic stimulator of nervous system

6 √7ᵗʰ **T85.190** **Other mechanical complication of implanted electronic neurostimulator of brain electrode (lead)**   `CC` `HCC`

6 √7ᵗʰ **T85.191** **Other mechanical complication of implanted electronic neurostimulator of peripheral nerve electrode (lead)**   `CC` `HCC`

Other mechanical complication of electrode (lead) for cranial nerve neurostimulators

Other mechanical complication of electrode (lead) for gastric neurostimulator

Other mechanical complication of electrode (lead) for sacral nerve neurostimulator

Other mechanical complication of electrode (lead) for vagal nerve neurostimulators

6 √7ᵗʰ **T85.192** **Other mechanical complication of implanted electronic neurostimulator of spinal cord electrode (lead)**   `CC` `HCC`

6 √7ᵗʰ **T85.193** **Other mechanical complication of implanted electronic neurostimulator, generator**   `CC` `HCC`

Other mechanical complication of implanted electronic neurostimulator generator, brain, peripheral, gastric, spinal

Other mechanical complication of implanted electronic sacral neurostimulator, pulse generator or receiver

6 √7ᵗʰ **T85.199** **Other mechanical complication of other implanted electronic stimulator of nervous system**   `CC` `HCC`

√5ᵗʰ **T85.2** **Mechanical complication of** intraocular lens

CC Excl: For CC codes in subcategory T85.2: PDX collection 1461

√x7ᵗʰ **T85.21** **Breakdown (mechanical) of intraocular lens**   `CC`

√x7ᵗʰ **T85.22** **Displacement of intraocular lens**   `CC`

Malposition of intraocular lens

√x7ᵗʰ **T85.29** **Other mechanical complication of intraocular lens**   `CC`

Obstruction (mechanical) of intraocular lens

Perforation of intraocular lens

Protrusion of intraocular lens

√5ᵗʰ **T85.3** **Mechanical complication of other ocular prosthetic devices, implants and grafts**

EXCLUDES 2   other complications of corneal graft (T86.84-)

CC Excl: For CC codes in subcategory T85.3: PDX collection 1462

√6ᵗʰ **T85.31** **Breakdown (mechanical) of other ocular prosthetic devices, implants and grafts**

√7ᵗʰ **T85.310** **Breakdown (mechanical) of prosthetic orbit of right eye**   `CC`

√7ᵗʰ **T85.311** **Breakdown (mechanical) of prosthetic orbit of left eye**   `CC`

√7ᵗʰ **T85.318** **Breakdown (mechanical) of other ocular prosthetic devices, implants and grafts**

✔ Additional Character Required   √x7ᵗʰ Placeholder   Unacceptable PDx   Questionable PDx   Manifestation   Unspecified Dx   `H1`-`H14` HAC   `HCC` CMS-HCC Dx   `HIV` HIV Dx

ICD-10-CM 2020   1203

√6ᵗʰ **T85.32 Displacement** of other ocular prosthetic devices, implants and grafts

Malposition of other ocular prosthetic devices, implants and grafts

√7ᵗʰ **T85.320 Displacement of prosthetic orbit of right eye**   CC

√7ᵗʰ **T85.321 Displacement of prosthetic orbit of left eye**   CC

√7ᵗʰ **T85.328 Displacement of other ocular prosthetic devices, implants and grafts**

√6ᵗʰ **T85.39 Other mechanical complication of other ocular prosthetic devices, implants and grafts**

Obstruction (mechanical) of other ocular prosthetic devices, implants and grafts

Perforation of other ocular prosthetic devices, implants and grafts

Protrusion of other ocular prosthetic devices, implants and grafts

√7ᵗʰ **T85.390 Other mechanical complication of prosthetic orbit of right eye**   CC

√7ᵗʰ **T85.391 Other mechanical complication of prosthetic orbit of left eye**   CC

√7ᵗʰ **T85.398 Other mechanical complication of other ocular prosthetic devices, implants and grafts**

√5ᵗʰ **T85.4 Mechanical complication of breast prosthesis and implant**

CC Excl: For CC codes in subcategory T85.4: PDX collection 1463

√x7ᵗʰ **T85.41 Breakdown (mechanical) of breast prosthesis and implant**   CC

√x7ᵗʰ **T85.42 Displacement of breast prosthesis and implant**   CC

Malposition of breast prosthesis and implant

√x7ᵗʰ **T85.43 Leakage of breast prosthesis and implant**   CC

√x7ᵗʰ **T85.44 Capsular contracture of breast implant**   CC

√x7ᵗʰ **T85.49 Other mechanical complication of breast prosthesis and implant**   CC

Obstruction (mechanical) of breast prosthesis and implant

Perforation of breast prosthesis and implant

Protrusion of breast prosthesis and implant

√5ᵗʰ **T85.5 Mechanical complication of gastrointestinal prosthetic devices, implants and grafts**

CC Excl: For CC codes in subcategory T85.5: PDX collection 1464

√6ᵗʰ **T85.51 Breakdown (mechanical) of gastrointestinal prosthetic devices, implants and grafts**

√7ᵗʰ **T85.510 Breakdown (mechanical) of bile duct prosthesis**   CC

√7ᵗʰ **T85.511 Breakdown (mechanical) of esophageal anti-reflux device**   CC

√7ᵗʰ **T85.518 Breakdown (mechanical) of other gastrointestinal prosthetic devices, implants and grafts**   CC

√6ᵗʰ **T85.52 Displacement of gastrointestinal prosthetic devices, implants and grafts**

Malposition of gastrointestinal prosthetic devices, implants and grafts

√7ᵗʰ **T85.520 Displacement of bile duct prosthesis**   CC

√7ᵗʰ **T85.521 Displacement of esophageal anti-reflux device**   CC

√7ᵗʰ **T85.528 Displacement of other gastrointestinal prosthetic devices, implants and grafts**   CC

√6ᵗʰ **T85.59 Other mechanical complication of gastrointestinal prosthetic devices, implants and**

Obstruction, mechanical of gastrointestinal prosthetic devices, implants and grafts

Perforation of gastrointestinal prosthetic devices, implants and grafts

Protrusion of gastrointestinal prosthetic devices, implants and grafts

√7ᵗʰ **T85.590 Other mechanical complication of bile duct prosthesis**   CC

√7ᵗʰ **T85.591 Other mechanical complication of esophageal anti-reflux device**   CC

√7ᵗʰ **T85.598 Other mechanical complication of other gastrointestinal prosthetic devices, implants and grafts**   CC

√5ᵗʰ **T85.6 Mechanical complication of other specified internal and external prosthetic devices, implants and grafts**

√6ᵗʰ **T85.61 Breakdown (mechanical) of other specified internal prosthetic devices, implants and grafts**

√7ᵗʰ **T85.610 Breakdown (mechanical) of cranial or spinal infusion catheter**   CC

Breakdown (mechanical) of epidural infusion catheter

Breakdown (mechanical) of intrathecal infusion catheter

Breakdown (mechanical) of subarachnoid infusion catheter

Breakdown (mechanical) of subdural infusion catheter

CC Excl: PDX collection 1465

√7ᵗʰ **T85.611 Breakdown (mechanical) of intraperitoneal dialysis catheter**   CC HCC

EXCLUDES 1   mechanical complication of vascular dialysis catheter (T82.4-)

CC Excl: PDX collection 1466

√7ᵗʰ **T85.612 Breakdown (mechanical) of permanent sutures**   CC

EXCLUDES 1   mechanical complication of permanent (wire) suture used in bone repair (T84.1-T84.2)

CC Excl: PDX collection 1467

√7ᵗʰ **T85.613 Breakdown (mechanical) of artificial skin graft and decellularized allodermis**   CC

Failure of artificial skin graft and decellularized allodermis

Non-adherence of artificial skin graft and decellularized allodermis

Poor incorporation of artificial skin graft and decellularized allodermis

Shearing of artificial skin graft and decellularized allodermis

CC Excl: PDX collection 1468

√7ᵗʰ **T85.614 Breakdown (mechanical) of insulin pump**   CC

CC Excl: PDX collection 1469

6 √7ᵗʰ **T85.615 Breakdown (mechanical) of other nervous system device, implant or graft**   CC HCC

Breakdown (mechanical) of intrathecal infusion pump

CC Excl: PDX collection 1467

√7ᵗʰ **T85.618 Breakdown (mechanical) of other specified internal prosthetic devices, implants and grafts**   CC

CC Excl: PDX collection 1467

N Newborn: 0   P Pediatric: 0-17   M Maternity: 9-64   A Adult: 15-124   MCC Major Complication/Comorbidity   CC Complication/Comorbidity   SW Severe Wound Dx

1204   ICD-10-CM 2020

✓6ᵗʰ T85.62   Displacement of other specified internal prosthetic devices, implants and grafts

Malposition of other specified internal prosthetic devices, implants and grafts

✓7ᵗʰ T85.620   Displacement of cranial or spinal infusion catheter   `CC`

Displacement of epidural infusion catheter

Displacement of intrathecal infusion catheter

Displacement of subarachnoid infusion catheter

Displacement of subdural infusion catheter

CC Excl: PDX collection 1465

✓7ᵗʰ T85.621   Displacement of intraperitoneal dialysis catheter   `CC` `HCC`

> *EXCLUDES 1*   mechanical complication of vascular dialysis catheter (T82.4-)

CC Excl: PDX collection 1466

✓7ᵗʰ T85.622   Displacement of permanent sutures   `CC`

> *EXCLUDES 1*   mechanical complication of permanent (wire) suture used in bone repair (T84.1-T84.2)

CC Excl: PDX collection 1467

✓7ᵗʰ T85.623   Displacement of artificial skin graft and decellularized allodermis   `CC`

Dislodgement of artificial skin graft and decellularized allodermis

CC Excl: PDX collection 1468

✓7ᵗʰ T85.624   Displacement of insulin pump   `CC`

CC Excl: PDX collection 1469

6 ✓7ᵗʰ T85.625   Displacement of other nervous system device, implant or graft   `CC` `HCC`

Displacement of intrathecal infusion pump

CC Excl: PDX collection 1467

✓7ᵗʰ T85.628   Displacement of other specified internal prosthetic devices, implants and grafts   `CC`

CC Excl: PDX collection 1467

✓6ᵗʰ T85.63   Leakage of other specified internal prosthetic devices, implants and grafts

✓7ᵗʰ T85.630   Leakage of cranial or spinal infusion catheter   `CC`

Leakage of epidural infusion catheter

Leakage of intrathecal infusion catheter infusion catheter

Leakage of subdural infusion catheter

Leakage of subarachnoid infusion catheter

CC Excl: PDX collection 1465

✓7ᵗʰ T85.631   Leakage of intraperitoneal dialysis catheter   `CC` `HCC`

> *EXCLUDES 1*   mechanical complication of vascular dialysis catheter (T82.4)

CC Excl: PDX collection 1466

✓7ᵗʰ T85.633   Leakage of insulin pump   `CC`

CC Excl: PDX collection 1469

6 ✓7ᵗʰ T85.635   Leakage of other nervous system device, implant or graft   `CC` `HCC`

Leakage of intrathecal infusion pump

CC Excl: PDX collection 1467

✓7ᵗʰ T85.638   Leakage of other specified internal prosthetic devices, implants and grafts   `CC`

CC Excl: PDX collection 1467

✓6ᵗʰ T85.69   Other mechanical complication of other specified internal prosthetic devices, implants and grafts

Obstruction, mechanical of other specified internal prosthetic devices, implants and grafts

Perforation of other specified internal prosthetic devices, implants and grafts

Protrusion of other specified internal prosthetic devices, implants and grafts

✓7ᵗʰ T85.690   Other mechanical complication of cranial or spinal infusion catheter   `CC`

Other mechanical complication of epidural infusion catheter

Other mechanical complication of intrathecal infusion catheter

Other mechanical complication of subarachnoid infusion catheter

Other mechanical complication of subdural infusion catheter

CC Excl: PDX collection 1465

✓7ᵗʰ T85.691   Other mechanical complication of intraperitoneal dialysis catheter   `CC` `HCC`

> *EXCLUDES 1*   mechanical complication of vascular dialysis catheter (T82.4)

CC Excl: PDX collection 1466

✓7ᵗʰ T85.692   Other mechanical complication of permanent sutures   `CC`

> *EXCLUDES 1*   mechanical complication of permanent (wire) suture used in bone repair (T84.1-T84.2)

CC Excl: PDX collection 1467

✓7ᵗʰ T85.693   Other mechanical complication of artificial skin graft and decellularized allodermis   `CC`

CC Excl: PDX collection 1468

✓7ᵗʰ T85.694   Other mechanical complication of insulin pump   `CC`

CC Excl: PDX collection 1469

6 ✓7ᵗʰ T85.695   Other mechanical complication of other nervous system device, implant or graft   `CC` `HCC`

Other mechanical complication of intrathecal infusion pump

CC Excl: PDX collection 1467

✓7ᵗʰ T85.698   Other mechanical complication of other specified internal prosthetic devices, implants and grafts   `CC`

Mechanical complication of nonabsorbable surgical material NOS

CC Excl: PDX collection 1467

✓5ᵗʰ T85.7   Infection and inflammatory reaction due to other internal prosthetic devices, implants and grafts

Use additional code to identify infection

CC Excl: For CC codes in subcategory T85.7, unless otherwise noted: PDX collection 1470

✓x7ᵗʰ T85.71   Infection and inflammatory reaction due to peritoneal dialysis catheter   `CC` `HCC`

CC Excl: PDX collection 1467

6 ✓x7ᵗʰ T85.72   Infection and inflammatory reaction due to insulin pump   `CC` `HCC`

✓6ᵗʰ T85.73   Infection and inflammatory reaction due to nervous system devices, implants and graft

6 ✓7ᵗʰ T85.730   Infection and inflammatory reaction due to ventricular intracranial (communicating) shunt   `CC` `HCC`

6 ✓7ᵗʰ T85.731   Infection and inflammatory reaction due to implanted electronic neurostimulator of brain, electrode (lead)   `CC` `HCC`

6 ✓7ᵗʰ **T85.732 Infection and** `CC` `HCC`
inflammatory reaction due to implanted electronic neurostimulator of peripheral nerve, electrode (lead)

Infection and inflammatory reaction due to electrode (lead) for cranial nerve neurostimulators

Infection and inflammatory reaction due to electrode (lead) for gastric neurostimulator

Infection and inflammatory reaction due to electrode (lead) for sacral nerve neurostimulator

Infection and inflammatory reaction due to electrode (lead) for vagal nerve neurostimulators

6 ✓7ᵗʰ **T85.733 Infection and** `CC` `HCC`
inflammatory reaction due to implanted electronic neurostimulator of spinal cord, electrode (lead)

6 ✓7ᵗʰ **T85.734 Infection and** `CC` `HCC`
inflammatory reaction due to implanted electronic neurostimulator, generator

Generator pocket infection

6 ✓7ᵗʰ **T85.735 Infection and** `CC` `HCC`
inflammatory reaction to cranial or spinal infusion catheter

Infection and inflammatory reaction due to epidural catheter

Infection and inflammatory reaction due to intrathecal infusion catheter

Infection and inflammatory reaction due to subarachnoid catheter

Infection and inflammatory reaction due to subdural catheter

6 ✓7ᵗʰ **T85.738 Infection and** `CC` `HCC`
inflammatory reaction due to other nervous system device, implant or graft

Infection and inflammatory reaction due to intrathecal infusion pump

6 ✓x7ᵗʰ **T85.79 Infection and inflammatory reaction** `CC` `HCC`
due to other internal prosthetic devices, implants and grafts

✓5ᵗʰ **T85.8 Other specified complications of internal prosthetic devices, implants and grafts, not elsewhere classified**

CC Excl: For codes in subcategory T85.8:
CC with 7th character A or D: PDX collection 1470

✓6ᵗʰ **T85.81 Embolism due to internal prosthetic devices, implants and grafts, not elsewhere classified**

5,6 ✓7ᵗʰ **T85.810 Embolism due to nervous** `CC` `HCC`
system prosthetic devices, implants and grafts

✓7ᵗʰ **T85.818 Embolism due to other internal prosthetic devices, implants and grafts**

✓6ᵗʰ **T85.82 Fibrosis due to internal prosthetic devices, implants and grafts, not elsewhere classified**

5,6 ✓7ᵗʰ **T85.820 Fibrosis due to nervous** `CC` `HCC`
system prosthetic devices, implants and grafts

✓7ᵗʰ **T85.828 Fibrosis due to other internal prosthetic devices, implants and grafts**

✓6ᵗʰ **T85.83 Hemorrhage due to internal prosthetic devices, implants and grafts, not elsewhere classified**

5,6 ✓7ᵗʰ **T85.830 Hemorrhage due to** `CC` `HCC`
nervous system prosthetic devices, implants and grafts

✓7ᵗʰ **T85.838 Hemorrhage due to other internal prosthetic devices, implants and grafts**

✓6ᵗʰ **T85.84 Pain due to internal prosthetic devices, implants and grafts, not elsewhere classified**

5,6 ✓7ᵗʰ **T85.840 Pain due to nervous** `CC` `HCC`
system prosthetic devices, implants and grafts

✓7ᵗʰ **T85.848 Pain due to other internal prosthetic devices, implants and grafts**

✓6ᵗʰ **T85.85 Stenosis due to internal prosthetic devices, implants and grafts, not elsewhere classified**

5,6 ✓7ᵗʰ **T85.850 Stenosis due to nervous** `CC` `HCC`
system prosthetic devices, implants and grafts

✓7ᵗʰ **T85.858 Stenosis due to other internal prosthetic devices, implants and grafts**

✓6ᵗʰ **T85.86 Thrombosis due to internal prosthetic devices, implants and grafts, not elsewhere classified**

5,6 ✓7ᵗʰ **T85.860 Thrombosis due to** `CC` `HCC`
nervous system prosthetic devices, implants and grafts

✓7ᵗʰ **T85.868 Thrombosis due to other internal prosthetic devices, implants and grafts**

✓6ᵗʰ **T85.89 Other specified complication of internal prosthetic devices, implants and grafts, not elsewhere classified**

Erosion or breakdown of subcutaneous device pocket

5,6 ✓7ᵗʰ **T85.890 Other specified** `CC` `HCC`
complication of nervous system prosthetic devices, implants and grafts

✓7ᵗʰ **T85.898 Other specified complication of other internal prosthetic devices, implants and grafts**

✓x7ᵗʰ **T85.9 Unspecified complication of internal prosthetic device, implant and graft**

Complication of internal prosthetic device, implant and graft NOS

✓4ᵗʰ **T86 Complications of transplanted organs and tissue**

Use additional code to identify other transplant complications, such as:
graft-versus-host disease (D89.81-)
malignancy associated with organ transplant (C80.2)
post-transplant lymphoproliferative disorders (PTLD) (D47.Z1)

✓5ᵗʰ **T86.0 Complications of bone marrow transplant**

CC Excl: For CC codes in subcategory T86.0: PDX collection 514

T86.00 Unspecified complication of bone `CC` `HCC`
marrow transplant

T86.01 Bone marrow transplant rejection `CC` `HCC`

T86.02 Bone marrow transplant failure `CC` `HCC`

T86.03 Bone marrow transplant infection `CC` `HCC`

T86.09 Other complications of bone marrow `CC` `HCC`
transplant

✓5ᵗʰ **T86.1 Complications of kidney transplant**

CC Excl: For CC codes in subcategory T86.1: PDX collection 1471

T86.10 Unspecified complication of kidney `CC`
transplant

T86.11 Kidney transplant rejection `CC`

T86.12 Kidney transplant failure `CC`

AHA: 2013,1Q,24

T86.13 Kidney transplant infection `CC`

Use additional code to specify infection

T86.19 Other complication of kidney `CC`
transplant

AHA: 2019,2Q,7

✓5ᵗʰ **T86.2 Complications of heart transplant**

EXCLUDES 1 complication of:
artificial heart device (T82.5)
heart-lung transplant (T86.3)

CC Excl: For CC codes in subcategory T86.2: PDX collection 1472

T86.20 Unspecified complication of heart `CC` `HCC`
transplant

T86.21 Heart transplant rejection `CC` `HCC`

T86.22 Heart transplant failure `CC` `HCC`

T86.23 Heart transplant infection `CC` `HCC`

Use additional code to specify infection

✓6ᵗʰ **T86.29 Other complications of heart transplant**

T86.290 Cardiac allograft `CC` `HCC`
vasculopathy

EXCLUDES 1 atherosclerosis of coronary arteries (I25.75-, I25.76-, I25.81-)

T86.298 Other complications of `CC` `HCC`
heart transplant

Ⓝ Newborn: 0   Ⓟ Pediatric: 0-17   Ⓜ Maternity: 9-64   Ⓐ Adult: 15-124   `MCC` Major Complication/Comorbidity   `CC` Complication/Comorbidity   `SW` Severe Wound Dx

1206

ICD-10-CM 2020

√5ᵗʰ **T86.3 Complications of heart-lung transplant**

CC Excl: For CC codes in subcategory T86.3: PDX collection 1472

     T86.30 Unspecified complication of heart-lung transplant `CC` `HCC`

     T86.31 Heart-lung transplant rejection `CC` `HCC`

     T86.32 Heart-lung transplant failure `CC` `HCC`

     T86.33 Heart-lung transplant infection `CC` `HCC`

         Use additional code to specify infection

     T86.39 Other complications of heart-lung transplant `CC` `HCC`

√5ᵗʰ **T86.4 Complications of liver transplant**

CC Excl: For CC codes in subcategory T86.4: PDX collection 1473

     T86.40 Unspecified complication of liver transplant `CC` `HCC`

     T86.41 Liver transplant rejection `CC` `HCC`

     T86.42 Liver transplant failure `CC` `HCC`

     T86.43 Liver transplant infection `CC` `HCC`

         Use additional code to identify infection, such as: cytomegalovirus (CMV) infection (B25.-)

     T86.49 Other complications of liver transplant `CC` `HCC`

T86.5 Complications of stem cell transplant `CC` `HCC`

   Complications from stem cells from peripheral blood

   Complications from stem cells from umbilical cord

   CC Excl: PDX collection 1474

√5ᵗʰ **T86.8 Complications of other transplanted organs and tissues**

   √6ᵗʰ **T86.81 Complications of lung transplant**

       EXCLUDES 1 complication of heart-lung transplant (T86.3-)

       CC Excl: For CC codes in subcategory T86.81: PDX collection 1475

     T86.810 Lung transplant rejection `CC` `HCC`

     T86.811 Lung transplant failure `CC` `HCC`

     T86.812 Lung transplant infection `CC` `HCC`

         Use additional code to specify infection

     T86.818 Other complications of lung transplant `CC` `HCC`

         AHA: 2019,2Q,6

     T86.819 Unspecified complication of lung transplant `CC` `HCC`

   √6ᵗʰ **T86.82 Complications of skin graft (allograft) (autograft)**

       EXCLUDES 2 complication of artificial skin graft (T85.693)

       CC Excl: For CC codes in subcategory T86.82: PDX collection 1476

     T86.820 Skin graft (allograft) rejection `CC`

     T86.821 Skin graft (allograft) (autograft) failure `CC`

     T86.822 Skin graft (allograft) (autograft) infection `CC`

         Use additional code to specify infection

     T86.828 Other complications of skin graft (allograft) (autograft) `CC`

     T86.829 Unspecified complication of skin graft (allograft) (autograft) `CC`

   √6ᵗʰ **T86.83 Complications of bone graft**

       EXCLUDES 2 mechanical complications of bone graft (T84.3-)

       CC Excl: For CC codes in subcategory T86.83: PDX collection 1477

     T86.830 Bone graft rejection `CC`

     T86.831 Bone graft failure `CC`

     T86.832 Bone graft infection `CC`

         Use additional code to specify infection

     T86.838 Other complications of bone graft `CC`

     T86.839 Unspecified complication of bone graft `CC`

√6ᵗʰ **T86.84 Complications of corneal transplant**

     EXCLUDES 2 mechanical complications of corneal graft (T85.3-)

     CC Excl: For CC codes in subcategory T86.84, unless otherwise noted: PDX collection 1479

     T86.840 Corneal transplant rejection `CC`

         CC Excl: PDX collection 1478

     T86.841 Corneal transplant failure `CC`

         CC Excl: PDX collection 1478

     T86.842 Corneal transplant infection `CC` `HCC`

         Use additional code to specify infection

     T86.848 Other complications of corneal transplant `CC`

     T86.849 Unspecified complication of corneal transplant `CC`

√6ᵗʰ **T86.85 Complication of intestine transplant**

     CC Excl: For CC codes in subcategory T86.85: PDX collection 495

     T86.850 Intestine transplant rejection `CC` `HCC`

     T86.851 Intestine transplant failure `CC` `HCC`

     T86.852 Intestine transplant infection `CC` `HCC`

         Use additional code to specify infection

     T86.858 Other complications of intestine transplant `CC` `HCC`

     T86.859 Unspecified complication of intestine transplant `CC` `HCC`

√6ᵗʰ **T86.89 Complications of other transplanted tissue**

     Transplant failure or rejection of pancreas

     CC Excl: For CC codes in subcategory T86.89: PDX collection 1480

     T86.890 Other transplanted tissue rejection `CC`

     T86.891 Other transplanted tissue failure `CC`

     T86.892 Other transplanted tissue infection `CC`

         Use additional code to specify infection

     T86.898 Other complications of other transplanted tissue `CC`

     T86.899 Unspecified complication of other transplanted tissue `CC`

√5ᵗʰ **T86.9 Complication of unspecified transplanted organ and tissue**

   CC Excl: For CC codes in subcategory T86.9: PDX collection 495

     T86.90 Unspecified complication of unspecified transplanted organ and tissue `CC`

     T86.91 Unspecified transplanted organ and tissue rejection `CC`

     T86.92 Unspecified transplanted organ and tissue failure `CC`

     T86.93 Unspecified transplanted organ and tissue infection `CC`

         Use additional code to specify infection

     T86.99 Other complications of unspecified transplanted organ and tissue `CC`

√4ᵗʰ **T87 Complications peculiar to reattachment and amputation**

   √5ᵗʰ **T87.0 Complications of reattached (part of) upper extremity**

     √6ᵗʰ **T87.0X Complications of reattached (part of) upper extremity**

       CC Excl: For CC codes in subcategory T87.0X: PDX collection 1481

     T87.0X1 Complications of reattached (part of) right upper extremity `CC` `HCC`

     T87.0X2 Complications of reattached (part of) left upper extremity `CC` `HCC`

     T87.0X9 Complications of reattached (part of) unspecified upper extremity `CC` `HCC`

☑ Additional Character Required   √x7ᵗʰ Placeholder   Unacceptable PDx   Questionable PDx   Manifestation   Unspecified Dx   H1–H14 HAC   HCC CMS-HCC Dx   HIV HIV Dx

✓5ᵗʰ **T87.1** **Complications of reattached (part of) lower extremity**

✓6ᵗʰ **T87.1X** **Complications of reattached (part of) lower extremity**

CC Excl: For CC codes in subcategory T87.1X: PDX collection 1482

T87.1X1 **Complications of reattached (part of) right lower extremity** CC HCC

T87.1X2 **Complications of reattached (part of) left lower extremity** CC HCC

T87.1X9 **Complications of reattached (part of) unspecified lower extremity** CC HCC

T87.2 **Complications of other reattached body part** CC HCC

CC Excl: PDX collection 1483

✓5ᵗʰ **T87.3** **Neuroma of amputation stump**

DEF: Non-neoplastic tumor generated at the proximal end of severed, partially transected, or injured nerve following amputation.

T87.30 **Neuroma of amputation stump, unspecified extremity** HCC

T87.31 **Neuroma of amputation stump, right upper extremity** HCC

T87.32 **Neuroma of amputation stump, left upper extremity** HCC

T87.33 **Neuroma of amputation stump, right lower extremity** HCC

T87.34 **Neuroma of amputation stump, left lower extremity** HCC

✓5ᵗʰ **T87.4** **Infection of amputation stump**

CC Excl: For CC codes in subcategory T87.4: PDX collection 1484

T87.40 **Infection of amputation stump, unspecified extremity** CC HCC

T87.41 **Infection of amputation stump, right upper extremity** CC HCC

T87.42 **Infection of amputation stump, left upper extremity** CC HCC

T87.43 **Infection of amputation stump, right lower extremity** CC HCC

T87.44 **Infection of amputation stump, left lower extremity** CC HCC

✓5ᵗʰ **T87.5** **Necrosis of amputation stump**

T87.50 **Necrosis of amputation stump, unspecified extremity** HCC

T87.51 **Necrosis of amputation stump, right upper extremity** HCC

T87.52 **Necrosis of amputation stump, left upper extremity** HCC

T87.53 **Necrosis of amputation stump, right lower extremity** HCC

T87.54 **Necrosis of amputation stump, left lower extremity** HCC

✓5ᵗʰ **T87.8** **Other complications of amputation stump**

T87.81 **Dehiscence of amputation stump** HCC

T87.89 **Other complications of amputation stump** HCC

Amputation stump contracture

Amputation stump contracture of next proximal joint

Amputation stump flexion

Amputation stump edema

Amputation stump hematoma

EXCLUDES 2 *phantom limb syndrome (G54.6-G54.7)*

T87.9 **Unspecified complications of amputation stump** HCC

✓4ᵗʰ **T88** **Other complications of surgical and medical care, not elsewhere classified**

EXCLUDES 2 *complication following infusion, transfusion and therapeutic injection (T80.-)*

complication following procedure NEC (T81.-)

complications of anesthesia in labor and delivery (O74.-)

complications of anesthesia in pregnancy (O29.-)

complications of anesthesia in puerperium (O89.-)

complications of devices, implants and grafts (T82-T85)

complications of obstetric surgery and procedure (O75.4)

dermatitis due to drugs and medicaments (L23.3, L24.4, L25.1, L27.0-L27.1)

poisoning and toxic effects of drugs and chemicals (T36-T65 with fifth or sixth character 1-4 or 6)

specified complications classified elsewhere

The appropriate 7th character is to be added to each code from category T88.

A initial encounter

D subsequent encounter

S sequela

✓x7ᵗʰ **T88.0** **Infection following immunization** CC

Sepsis following immunization

AHA: 2018,4Q,62-63

CC Excl: PDX collection 948

✓x7ᵗʰ **T88.1** **Other complications following immunization, not elsewhere classified** CC

Generalized vaccinia

Rash following immunization

EXCLUDES 1 *vaccinia not from vaccine (B08.011)*

EXCLUDES 2 *anaphylactic shock due to serum (T80.5-)*

other serum reactions (T80.6-)

postimmunization arthropathy (M02.2)

postimmunization encephalitis (G04.02)

postimmunization fever (R50.83)

CC Excl: PDX collection 1485

✓x7ᵗʰ **T88.2** **Shock due to anesthesia** CC

Use additional code for adverse effect, if applicable, to identify drug (T41.- with fifth or sixth character 5)

EXCLUDES 1 *complications of anesthesia (in):*

labor and delivery (O74.-)

postprocedural shock NOS (T81.1-)

pregnancy (O29.-)

puerperium (O89.-)

CC Excl: PDX collection 1441

✓x7ᵗʰ **T88.3** **Malignant hyperthermia due to anesthesia** CC

Use additional code for adverse effect, if applicable, to identify drug (T41.- with fifth or sixth character 5)

CC Excl: PDX collection 1486

✓x7ᵗʰ **T88.4** **Failed or difficult intubation**

✓5ᵗʰ **T88.5** **Other complications of anesthesia**

Use additional code for adverse effect, if applicable, to identify drug (T41.- with fifth or sixth character 5)

✓x7ᵗʰ **T88.51** **Hypothermia following anesthesia**

✓x7ᵗʰ **T88.52** **Failed moderate sedation during procedure**

Failed conscious sedation during procedure

EXCLUDES 2 *personal history of failed moderate sedation (Z92.83)*

✓x7ᵗʰ **T88.53** **Unintended awareness under general anesthesia during procedure**

EXCLUDES 2 *personal history of unintended awareness under general anesthesia (Z92.84)*

AHA: 2016,4Q,72-73

✓x7ᵗʰ **T88.59** **Other complications of anesthesia**

✓x7ᵗʰ **T88.6** **Anaphylactic reaction due to adverse effect of correct drug or medicament properly administered** CC

Anaphylactic shock due to adverse effect of correct drug or medicament properly administered

Anaphylactoid reaction NOS

Use additional code for adverse effect, if applicable, to identify drug (T36-T50 with fifth or sixth character 5)

EXCLUDES 1 *anaphylactic reaction due to serum (T80.5-)*

anaphylactic shock or reaction due to adverse food reaction (T78.0-)

CC Excl: PDX collection 1426

N Newborn: 0 P Pediatric: 0-17 M Maternity: 9-64 A Adult: 15-124 MCC Major Complication/Comorbidity CC Complication/Comorbidity SW Severe Wound Dx

1208 ICD-10-CM 2020

☑x7ᵗʰ **T88.7** **Unspecified adverse effect of drug or medicament**

Drug hypersensitivity NOS

Drug reaction NOS

Use additional code for adverse effect, if applicable, to identify drug (T36-T50 with fifth or sixth character 5)

> EXCLUDES 1   *specified adverse effects of drugs and medicaments (A00-R94 and T80-T88.6, T88.8)*

☑x7ᵗʰ **T88.8** **Other specified complications of surgical and medical care, not elsewhere classified**

Use additional code to identify the complication

☑x7ᵗʰ **T88.9** **Complication of surgical and medical care, unspecified**

☑ Additional Character Required   ☑x7ᵗʰ Placeholder   Unacceptable PDx   Questionable PDx   Manifestation   Unspecified Dx   H1-H14 HAC   HCC CMS-HCC Dx   HIV HIV Dx

ICD-10-CM 2020   **1209**

Chapter 20. External Causes of Morbidity (V00–Y99)

Chapter-specific Guidelines with Coding Examples

The chapter-specific guidelines from the ICD-10-CM Official Guidelines for Coding and Reporting have been provided below. Along with these guidelines are coding examples, contained in the shaded boxes, that have been developed to help illustrate the coding and/or sequencing guidance found in these guidelines.

The external causes of morbidity codes should never be sequenced as the first-listed or principal diagnosis.

External cause codes are intended to provide data for injury research and evaluation of injury prevention strategies. These codes capture how the injury or health condition happened (cause), the intent (unintentional or accidental; or intentional, such as suicide or assault), the place where the event occurred the activity of the patient at the time of the event, and the person's status (e.g., civilian, military).

There is no national requirement for mandatory ICD-10-CM external cause code reporting. Unless a provider is subject to a state-based external cause code reporting mandate or these codes are required by a particular payer, reporting of ICD-10-CM codes in Chapter 20, External Causes of Morbidity, is not required. In the absence of a mandatory reporting requirement, providers are encouraged to voluntarily report external cause codes, as they provide valuable data for injury research and evaluation of injury prevention strategies.

a. General external cause coding guidelines

1) Used with any code in the range of A00.0–T88.9, Z00–Z99

An external cause code may be used with any code in the range of A00.0–T88.9, Z00–Z99, classification that represents a health condition due to an external cause. Though they are most applicable to injuries, they are also valid for use with such things as infections or diseases due to an external source, and other health conditions, such as a heart attack that occurs during strenuous physical activity.

> Actinic reticuloid due to tanning bed use
>
> **L57.1**   **Actinic reticuloid**
>
> **W89.1XXA**   **Exposure to tanning bed, initial encounter**
>
> *Explanation:* An external cause code may be used with any code in the range of A00.0–T88.9, Z00–Z99, classifications that describe health conditions due to an external cause. Code W89.1 Exposure to tanning bed requires a seventh character of A to report this initial encounter, with a placeholder X for the fifth and sixth characters.

2) External cause code used for length of treatment

Assign the external cause code, with the appropriate 7th character (initial encounter, subsequent encounter or sequela) for each encounter for which the injury or condition is being treated.

Most categories in chapter 20 have a 7th character requirement for each applicable code. Most categories in this chapter have three 7th character values: A, initial encounter, D, subsequent encounter and S, sequela. While the patient may be seen by a new or different provider over the course of treatment for an injury or condition, assignment of the 7th character for external cause should match the 7th character of the code assigned for the associated injury or condition for the encounter.

3) Use the full range of external cause codes

Use the full range of external cause codes to completely describe the cause, the intent, the place of occurrence, and if applicable, the activity of the patient at the time of the event, and the patient's status, for all injuries, and other health conditions due to an external cause.

4) Assign as many external cause codes as necessary

Assign as many external cause codes as necessary to fully explain each cause. If only one external code can be recorded, assign the code most related to the principal diagnosis.

5) The selection of the appropriate external cause code

The selection of the appropriate external cause code is guided by the Alphabetic Index of External Causes and by Inclusion and Exclusion notes in the Tabular List.

6) External cause code can never be a principal diagnosis

An external cause code can never be a principal (first-listed) diagnosis.

7) Combination external cause codes

Certain of the external cause codes are combination codes that identify sequential events that result in an injury, such as a fall which results in striking against an object. The injury may be due to either event or both.

The combination external cause code used should correspond to the sequence of events regardless of which caused the most serious injury.

> Toddler tripped and fell while walking and struck his head on an end table, sustaining a scalp contusion
>
> **S00.03XA**   **Contusion of scalp, initial encounter**
>
> **W01.190A**   **Fall on same level from slipping, tripping and stumbling with subsequent striking against furniture, initial encounter**
>
> *Explanation:* Combination external cause codes identify sequential events that result in an injury, such as a fall resulting in striking against an object. The injury may be due to either or both events.

8) No external cause code needed in certain circumstances

No external cause code from Chapter 20 is needed if the external cause and intent are included in a code from another chapter (e.g. T36.0X1-Poisoning by penicillins, accidental (unintentional)).

b. Place of occurrence guideline

Codes from category Y92, Place of occurrence of the external cause, are secondary codes for use after other external cause codes to identify the location of the patient at the time of injury or other condition.

Generally, a place of occurrence code is assigned only once, at the initial encounter for treatment. However, in the rare instance that a new injury occurs during hospitalization, an additional place of occurrence code may be assigned. No 7th characters are used for Y92.

Do not use place of occurrence code Y92.9 if the place is not stated or is not applicable.

> A farmer was working in his barn and sustained a foot contusion when the horse stepped on his left foot
>
> **S90.32XA**   **Contusion of left foot, initial encounter**
>
> **W55.19XA**   **Other contact with horse, initial encounter**
>
> **Y92.71**   **Barn as the place of occurrence of the external cause**
>
> *Explanation:* A place-of-occurrence code from category Y92 is assigned at the initial encounter to identify the location of the patient at the time the injury occurred.

c. Activity code

Assign a code from category Y93, Activity code, to describe the activity of the patient at the time the injury or other health condition occurred.

An activity code is used only once, at the initial encounter for treatment. Only one code from Y93 should be recorded on a medical record.

The activity codes are not applicable to poisonings, adverse effects, misadventures or sequela.

Do not assign Y93.9, Unspecified activity, if the activity is not stated.

A code from category Y93 is appropriate for use with external cause and intent codes if identifying the activity provides additional information about the event.

> Ranch hand who was grooming a horse sustained a foot contusion when the horse stepped on his left foot
>
> **S90.32XA**   **Contusion of left foot, initial encounter**
>
> **W55.19XA**   **Other contact with horse, initial encounter**
>
> **Y93.K3**   **Activity, grooming and shearing an animal**
>
> *Explanation:* One activity code from category Y93 is assigned at the initial encounter only to describe the activity of the patient at the time the injury occurred.

d. Place of occurrence, activity, and status codes used with other external cause code

When applicable, place of occurrence, activity, and external cause status codes are sequenced after the main external cause code(s). Regardless of the number of external cause codes assigned, generally there should be only one place of occurrence code, one activity code, and one external cause status code assigned to an encounter. However, in the rare instance that a new injury occurs during hospitalization, an additional place of occurrence code may be assigned.

e. If the reporting format limits the number of external cause codes

If the reporting format limits the number of external cause codes that can be used in reporting clinical data, report the code for the cause/intent most related to the principal diagnosis. If the format permits capture of additional external cause codes, the cause/intent, including medical misadventures, of the additional events should be reported rather than the codes for place, activity, or external status.

f. Multiple external cause coding guidelines

More than one external cause code is required to fully describe the external cause of an illness or injury. The assignment of external cause codes should be sequenced in the following priority:

If two or more events cause separate injuries, an external cause code should be assigned for each cause. The first-listed external cause code will be selected in the following order:

External codes for child and adult abuse take priority over all other external cause codes.

See Section I.C.19., Child and Adult abuse guidelines.

External cause codes for terrorism events take priority over all other external cause codes except child and adult abuse.

External cause codes for cataclysmic events take priority over all other external cause codes except child and adult abuse and terrorism.

External cause codes for transport accidents take priority over all other external cause codes except cataclysmic events, child and adult abuse and terrorism.

Activity and external cause status codes are assigned following all causal (intent) external cause codes.

The first-listed external cause code should correspond to the cause of the most serious diagnosis due to an assault, accident, or self-harm, following the order of hierarchy listed above..

3Ø-year-old man accidentally discharged his hunting rifle, sustaining an open gunshot wound to the right thigh, which caused him to fall down the stairs, resulting in closed displaced comminuted fracture of his left radial shaft	
S71.131A	Puncture wound without foreign body, right thigh, initial encounter
W33.Ø2XA	Accidental discharge of hunting rifle, initial encounter
S52.352A	Displaced comminuted fracture of shaft of radius, left arm, initial encounter for closed fracture
W1Ø.9XXA	Fall (on) (from) unspecified stairs and steps, initial encounter

Explanation: If two or more events cause separate injuries, an external cause code should be assigned for each cause.

g. Child and adult abuse guideline

Adult and child abuse, neglect and maltreatment are classified as assault. Any of the assault codes may be used to indicate the external cause of any injury resulting from the confirmed abuse.

For confirmed cases of abuse, neglect and maltreatment, when the perpetrator is known, a code from YØ7, Perpetrator of maltreatment and neglect, should accompany any other assault codes.

See Section I.C.19. Adult and child abuse, neglect and other maltreatment

h. Unknown or undetermined intent guideline

If the intent (accident, self-harm, assault) of the cause of an injury or other condition is unknown or unspecified, code the intent as accidental intent. All transport accident categories assume accidental intent.

1) Use of undetermined intent

External cause codes for events of undetermined intent are only for use if the documentation in the record specifies that the intent cannot be determined.

i. Sequelae (late effects) of external cause guidelines

1) Sequelae external cause codes

Sequela are reported using the external cause code with the 7th character "S" for sequela. These codes should be used with any report of a late effect or sequela resulting from a previous injury.

See Section I.B.1Ø Sequela (Late Effects)

2) Sequela external cause code with a related current injury

A sequela external cause code should never be used with a related current nature of injury code.

3) Use of sequela external cause codes for subsequent visits

Use a late effect external cause code for subsequent visits when a late effect of the initial injury is being treated. Do not use a late effect external cause code for subsequent visits for follow-up care (e.g., to assess healing, to receive rehabilitative therapy) of the injury when no late effect of the injury has been documented.

j. Terrorism guidelines

1) Cause of injury identified by the Federal Government (FBI) as terrorism

When the cause of an injury is identified by the Federal Government (FBI) as terrorism, the first-listed external cause code should be a code from category Y38, Terrorism. The definition of terrorism employed by the FBI is found at the inclusion note at the beginning of category Y38. Use additional code for place of occurrence (Y92.-). More than one Y38 code may be assigned if the injury is the result of more than one mechanism of terrorism.

2) Cause of an injury is suspected to be the result of terrorism

When the cause of an injury is suspected to be the result of terrorism a code from category Y38 should not be assigned. Suspected cases should be classified as assault.

3) Code Y38.9, Terrorism, secondary effects

Assign code Y38.9, Terrorism, secondary effects, for conditions occurring subsequent to the terrorist event. This code should not be assigned for conditions that are due to the initial terrorist act.

It is acceptable to assign code Y38.9 with another code from Y38 if there is an injury due to the initial terrorist event and an injury that is a subsequent result of the terrorist event.

k. External cause status

A code from category Y99, External cause status, should be assigned whenever any other external cause code is assigned for an encounter, including an Activity code, except for the events noted below. Assign a code from category Y99, External cause status, to indicate the work status of the person at the time the event occurred. The status code indicates whether the event occurred during military activity, whether a non-military person was at work, whether an individual including a student or volunteer was involved in a non-work activity at the time of the causal event.

A code from Y99, External cause status, should be assigned, when applicable, with other external cause codes, such as transport accidents and falls. The external cause status codes are not applicable to poisonings, adverse effects, misadventures or late effects.

Do not assign a code from category Y99 if no other external cause codes (cause, activity) are applicable for the encounter.

An external cause status code is used only once, at the initial encounter for treatment. Only one code from Y99 should be recorded on a medical record.

Do not assign code Y99.9, Unspecified external cause status, if the status is not stated.

Chapter 20. External Causes of Morbidity (V00-Y99)

NOTE This chapter permits the classification of environmental events and circumstances as the cause of injury, and as other adverse effects. Where a code from this section is applicable, it is intended that it shall be used secondary to a code from another chapter of the Classification indicating the nature of the condition. Most often, the condition will be classifiable to Chapter 19, Injury, poisoning and certain other consequences of external causes (S00-T88). Other conditions that may be stated to be due to external causes are classified in Chapters I to XVIII. For these conditions, codes from Chapter 20 should be used to provide additional information as to the cause of the condition.

AHA: 2018,4Q,58-60

This chapter contains the following blocks:

V00-X58	Accidents
V00-V99	Transport accidents
V00-V09	Pedestrian injured in transport accident
V10-V19	Pedal cycle rider injured in transport accident
V20-V29	Motorcycle rider injured in transport accident
V30-V39	Occupant of three-wheeled motor vehicle injured in transport accident
V40-V49	Car occupant injured in transport accident
V50-V59	Occupant of pick-up truck or van injured in transport accident
V60-V69	Occupant of heavy transport vehicle injured in transport accident
V70-V79	Bus occupant injured in transport accident
V80-V89	Other land transport accidents
V90-V94	Water transport accidents
V95-V97	Air and space transport accidents
V98-V99	Other and unspecified transport accidents
W00-X58	Other external causes of accidental injury
W00-W19	Slipping, tripping, stumbling and falls
W20-W49	Exposure to inanimate mechanical forces
W50-W64	Exposure to animate mechanical forces
W65-W74	Accidental non-transport drowning and submersion
W85-W99	Exposure to electric current, radiation and extreme ambient air temperature and pressure
X00-X08	Exposure to smoke, fire and flames
X10-X19	Contact with heat and hot substances
X30-X39	Exposure to forces of nature
X50	Overexertion and strenuous or repetitive movements
X52-X58	Accidental exposure to other specified factors
X71-X83	Intentional self-harm
X92-Y09	Assault
Y21-Y33	Event of undetermined intent
Y35-Y38	Legal intervention, operations of war, military operations, and terrorism
Y62-Y84	Complications of medical and surgical care
Y62-Y69	Misadventures to patients during surgical and medical care
Y70-Y82	Medical devices associated with adverse incidents in diagnostic and therapeutic use
Y83-Y84	Surgical and other medical procedures as the cause of abnormal reaction of the patient, or of later complication, without mention of misadventure at the time of the procedure
Y90-Y99	Supplementary factors related to causes of morbidity classified elsewhere

ACCIDENTS (V00-X58)

AHA: 2018,2Q,7-8

Transport accidents (V00-V99)

NOTE This section is structured in 12 groups. Those relating to land transport accidents (V00-V89) reflect the victim's mode of transport and are subdivided to identify the victim's 'counterpart' or the type of event. The vehicle of which the injured person is an occupant is identified in the first two characters since it is seen as the most important factor to identify for prevention purposes. A transport accident is one in which the vehicle involved must be moving or running or in use for transport purposes at the time of the accident.

Use additional code to identify:
airbag injury (W22.1)
type of street or road (Y92.4-)
use of cellular telephone and other electronic equipment at the time of the transport accident (Y93.C-)

EXCLUDES 1 *agricultural vehicles in stationary use or maintenance (W31.-)*
assault by crashing of motor vehicle (Y03.-)
automobile or motor cycle in stationary use or maintenance — code to type of accident
crashing of motor vehicle, undetermined intent (Y32)
intentional self-harm by crashing of motor vehicle (X82)

EXCLUDES 2 *transport accidents due to cataclysm (X34-X38)*

NOTE Definitions related to transport accidents:

(a) A transport accident (V00-V99) is any accident involving a device designed primarily for, or used at the time primarily for, conveying persons or good from one place to another.

(b) A public highway [trafficway] or street is the entire width between property lines (or other boundary lines) of land open to the public as a matter of right or custom for purposes of moving persons or property from one place to another. A roadway is that part of the public highway designed, improved and customarily used for vehicular traffic.

(c) A traffic accident is any vehicle accident occurring on the public highway [i.e. originating on, terminating on, or involving a vehicle partially on the highway]. A vehicle accident is assumed to have occurred on the public highway unless another place is specified, except in the case of accidents involving only off-road motor vehicles, which are classified as nontraffic accidents unless the contrary is stated.

(d) A nontraffic accident is any vehicle accident that occurs entirely in any place other than a public highway.

(e) A pedestrian is any person involved in an accident who was not at the time of the accident riding in or on a motor vehicle, railway train, streetcar or animal-drawn or other vehicle, or on a pedal cycle or animal. This includes, a person changing a tire, working on a parked car, or a person on foot. It also includes the user of a pedestrian conveyance such as a baby stroller, ice-skates, skis, sled, roller skates, a skateboard, nonmotorized or motorized wheelchair, motorized mobility scooter, or nonmotorized scooter.

(f) A driver is an occupant of a transport vehicle who is operating or intending to operate it.

(g) A passenger is any occupant of a transport vehicle other than the driver, except a person traveling on the outside of the vehicle.

(h) A person on the outside of a vehicle is any person being transported by a vehicle but not occupying the space normally reserved for the driver or passengers, or the space intended for the transport of property. This includes a person travelling on the bodywork, bumper, fender, roof, running board or step of a vehicle, as well as, hanging on the outside of the vehicle.

(i) A pedal cycle is any land transport vehicle operated solely by nonmotorized pedals including a bicycle or tricycle.

(j) A pedal cyclist is any person riding a pedal cycle or in a sidecar or trailer attached to a pedal cycle.

(k) A motorcycle is a two-wheeled motor vehicle with one or two riding saddles and sometimes with a third wheel for the support of a sidecar. The sidecar is considered part of the motorcycle. This includes a moped, motor scooter, or motorized bicycle.

(l) A motorcycle rider is any person riding a motorcycle or in a sidecar or trailer attached to the motorcycle.

(m) A three-wheeled motor vehicle is a motorized tricycle designed primarily for on-road use. This includes a motor-driven tricycle, a motorized rickshaw, or a three-wheeled motor car.

(n) A car [automobile] is a four-wheeled motor vehicle designed primarily for carrying up to 7 persons. A trailer being towed by the car is considered part of the car. It does not include a van or minivan — see definition (o).

(o) A pick-up truck or van is a four or six-wheeled motor vehicle designed for carrying passengers as well as property or cargo weighing less than the local limit for classification as a heavy goods vehicle, and not requiring a special driver's license. This includes a minivan and a sport-utility vehicle (SUV).

(p) A heavy transport vehicle is a motor vehicle designed primarily for carrying property, meeting local criteria for classification as a heavy goods vehicle in terms of weight and requiring a special driver's license.

(q) A bus (coach) is a motor vehicle designed or adapted primarily for carrying more than 10 passengers, and requiring a special driver's license.

(r) A railway train or railway vehicle is any device, with or without freight or passenger cars couple to it, designed for traffic on a railway track. This includes subterranean (subways) or elevated trains.

(s) A streetcar, is a device designed and used primarily for transporting passengers within a municipality, running on rails, usually subject to normal traffic control signals, and operated principally on a right-of-way that forms part of the roadway. This includes a tram or trolley that runs on rails. A trailer being towed by a streetcar is considered part of the streetcar.

(t) A special vehicle mainly used on industrial premises is a motor vehicle designed primarily for use within the buildings and premises of industrial or commercial establishments. This includes battery-powered airport passenger vehicles or baggage/mail trucks, forklifts, coal-cars in a coal mine, logging cars and trucks used in mines or quarries.

(u) A special vehicle mainly used in agriculture is a motor vehicle designed specifically for use in farming and agriculture (horticulture), to work the land, tend and harvest crops and transport materials on the farm. This includes harvesters, farm machinery and tractor and trailers.

(v) A special construction vehicle is a motor vehicle designed specifically for use on construction and demolition sites. This includes bulldozers, diggers, earth levellers, dump trucks. backhoes, front-end loaders, pavers, and mechanical shovels.

(w) A special all-terrain vehicle is a motor vehicle of special design to enable it to negotiate over rough or soft terrain, snow or sand. Examples of special design are high construction, special wheels and tires, tracks, and support on a cushion of air. This includes snow mobiles, All-terrain vehicles (ATV), and dune buggies. It does not include passenger vehicle designated as Sport Utility Vehicles. (SUV)

(x) A watercraft is any device designed for transporting passengers or goods on water. This includes motor or sailboats, ships, and hovercraft.

(y) An aircraft is any device for transporting passengers or goods in the air. This includes hot-air balloons, gliders, helicopters and airplanes.

(z) A military vehicle is any motorized vehicle operating on a public roadway owned by the military and being operated by a member of the military.

Pedestrian injured in transport accident (V00-V09)

INCLUDES   person changing tire on transport vehicle
person examining engine of vehicle broken down in (on side of) road

EXCLUDES 1   *fall due to non-transport collision with other person (W03)*
pedestrian on foot falling (slipping) on ice and snow (W00.-)
struck or bumped by another person (W51)

The appropriate 7th character is to be added to each code from categories V00-V09.
A   initial encounter
D   subsequent encounter
S   sequela

√4ᵗʰ **V00 Pedestrian conveyance accident**

Use additional place of occurrence and activity external cause codes, if known (Y92.-, Y93.-)

EXCLUDES 1   *collision with another person without fall (W51)*
fall due to person on foot colliding with another person on foot (W03)
fall from non-moving wheelchair, nonmotorized scooter and motorized mobility scooter without collision (W05.-)
pedestrian (conveyance) collision with other land transport vehicle (V01-V09)
pedestrian on foot falling (slipping) on ice and snow (W00.-)

√5ᵗʰ **V00.0 Pedestrian on foot injured in collision with pedestrian conveyance**

√x7ᵗʰ   **V00.01 Pedestrian on foot injured in collision with roller-skater**

√x7ᵗʰ   **V00.02 Pedestrian on foot injured in collision with skateboarder**

√x7ᵗʰ   **V00.09 Pedestrian on foot injured in collision with other pedestrian conveyance**

√5ᵗʰ **V00.1 Rolling-type pedestrian conveyance accident**

EXCLUDES 1   *accident with baby stroller (V00.82-)*
accident with motorized mobility scooter (V00.83-)
accident with wheelchair (powered) (V00.81-)

√6ᵗʰ   **V00.11 In-line roller-skate accident**

√7ᵗʰ   **V00.111 Fall from in-line roller-skates**

√7ᵗʰ   **V00.112 In-line roller-skater colliding with stationary object**

√7ᵗʰ   **V00.118 Other in-line roller-skate accident**

EXCLUDES 1   *roller-skater collision with other land transport vehicle (V01-V09 with 5th character 1)*

√6ᵗʰ   **V00.12 Non-in-line roller-skate accident**

√7ᵗʰ   **V00.121 Fall from non-in-line roller-skates**

√7ᵗʰ   **V00.122 Non-in-line roller-skater colliding with stationary object**

√7ᵗʰ   **V00.128 Other non-in-line roller-skating accident**

EXCLUDES 1   *roller-skater collision with other land transport vehicle (V01-V09 with 5th character 1)*

√6ᵗʰ **V00.13 Skateboard accident**

√7ᵗʰ   **V00.131 Fall from skateboard**

√7ᵗʰ   **V00.132 Skateboarder colliding with stationary object**

√7ᵗʰ   **V00.138 Other skateboard accident**

EXCLUDES 1   *skateboarder collision with other land transport vehicle (V01-V09 with 5th character 2)*

√6ᵗʰ **V00.14 Scooter (nonmotorized) accident**

EXCLUDES 1   *motor scooter accident (V20-V29)*

√7ᵗʰ   **V00.141 Fall from scooter (nonmotorized)**

√7ᵗʰ   **V00.142 Scooter (nonmotorized) colliding with stationary object**

√7ᵗʰ   **V00.148 Other scooter (nonmotorized) accident**

EXCLUDES 1   *scooter (nonmotorized) collision with other land transport vehicle (V01-V09 with fifth character 9)*

√6ᵗʰ **V00.15 Heelies accident**

Rolling shoe
Wheeled shoe
Wheelies accident

√7ᵗʰ   **V00.151 Fall from heelies**

√7ᵗʰ   **V00.152 Heelies colliding with stationary object**

√7ᵗʰ   **V00.158 Other heelies accident**

√6ᵗʰ **V00.18 Accident on other rolling-type pedestrian conveyance**

√7ᵗʰ   **V00.181 Fall from other rolling-type pedestrian conveyance**

√7ᵗʰ   **V00.182 Pedestrian on other rolling-type pedestrian conveyance colliding with stationary object**

√7ᵗʰ   **V00.188 Other accident on other rolling-type pedestrian conveyance**

√5ᵗʰ **V00.2 Gliding-type pedestrian conveyance accident**

√6ᵗʰ   **V00.21 Ice-skates accident**

√7ᵗʰ   **V00.211 Fall from ice-skates**

√7ᵗʰ   **V00.212 Ice-skater colliding with stationary object**

√7ᵗʰ   **V00.218 Other ice-skates accident**

EXCLUDES 1   *ice-skater collision with other land transport vehicle (V01-V09 with 5th character 9)*

√6ᵗʰ   **V00.22 Sled accident**

√7ᵗʰ   **V00.221 Fall from sled**

√7ᵗʰ   **V00.222 Sledder colliding with stationary object**

√7ᵗʰ   **V00.228 Other sled accident**

EXCLUDES 1   *sled collision with other land transport vehicle (V01-V09 with 5th character 9)*

√6ᵗʰ   **V00.28 Other gliding-type pedestrian conveyance accident**

√7ᵗʰ   **V00.281 Fall from other gliding-type pedestrian conveyance**

√7ᵗʰ   **V00.282 Pedestrian on other gliding-type pedestrian conveyance colliding with stationary object**

√7ᵗʰ   **V00.288 Other accident on other gliding-type pedestrian conveyance**

EXCLUDES 1   *gliding-type pedestrian conveyance collision with other land transport vehicle (V01-V09 with 5th character 9)*

√5ᵗʰ **V00.3 Flat-bottomed pedestrian conveyance accident**

√6ᵗʰ   **V00.31 Snowboard accident**

√7ᵗʰ   **V00.311 Fall from snowboard**

√7ᵗʰ   **V00.312 Snowboarder colliding with stationary object**

N Newborn: 0   **P** Pediatric: 0-17   **M** Maternity: 9-64   **A** Adult: 15-124   **MCC** Major Complication/Comorbidity   **CC** Complication/Comorbidity   **SW** Severe Wound Dx

1214   ICD-10-CM 2020

√7ᵗʰ **V00.318 Other snowboard accident**

> EXCLUDES 1   *snowboarder collision with other land transport vehicle (V01-V09 with 5th character 9)*

√6ᵗʰ **V00.32 Snow-ski accident**

√7ᵗʰ **V00.321 Fall from snow-skis**

√7ᵗʰ **V00.322 Snow-skier colliding with stationary object**

√7ᵗʰ **V00.328 Other snow-ski accident**

> EXCLUDES 1   *snow-skier collision with other land transport vehicle (V01-V09 with 5th character 9)*

√6ᵗʰ **V00.38 Other flat-bottomed pedestrian conveyance accident**

√7ᵗʰ **V00.381 Fall from other flat-bottomed pedestrian conveyance**

√7ᵗʰ **V00.382 Pedestrian on other flat-bottomed pedestrian conveyance colliding with stationary object**

√7ᵗʰ **V00.388 Other accident on other flat-bottomed pedestrian conveyance**

√5ᵗʰ **V00.8 Accident on other pedestrian conveyance**

√6ᵗʰ **V00.81 Accident with wheelchair (powered)**

√7ᵗʰ **V00.811 Fall from moving wheelchair (powered)**

> EXCLUDES 1   *fall from non-moving wheelchair (W05.0)*

√7ᵗʰ **V00.812 Wheelchair (powered) colliding with stationary object**

√7ᵗʰ **V00.818 Other accident with wheelchair (powered)**

√6ᵗʰ **V00.82 Accident with baby stroller**

√7ᵗʰ **V00.821 Fall from baby stroller**

√7ᵗʰ **V00.822 Baby stroller colliding with stationary object**

√7ᵗʰ **V00.828 Other accident with baby stroller**

√6ᵗʰ **V00.83 Accident with motorized mobility scooter**

√7ᵗʰ **V00.831 Fall from motorized mobility scooter**

> EXCLUDES 1   *fall from non-moving motorized mobility scooter (W05.2)*

√7ᵗʰ **V00.832 Motorized mobility scooter colliding with stationary object**

√7ᵗʰ **V00.838 Other accident with motorized mobility scooter**

√6ᵗʰ **V00.89 Accident on other pedestrian conveyance**

√7ᵗʰ **V00.891 Fall from other pedestrian conveyance**

√7ᵗʰ **V00.892 Pedestrian on other pedestrian conveyance colliding with stationary object**

√7ᵗʰ **V00.898 Other accident on other pedestrian conveyance**

> EXCLUDES 1   *other pedestrian (conveyance) collision with other land transport vehicle (V01-V09 with 5th character 9)*

√4ᵗʰ **V01 Pedestrian injured in collision with pedal cycle**

√5ᵗʰ **V01.0 Pedestrian injured in collision with pedal cycle in nontraffic accident**

√x7ᵗʰ **V01.00 Pedestrian on foot injured in collision with pedal cycle in nontraffic accident**

> Pedestrian NOS injured in collision with pedal cycle in nontraffic accident

√x7ᵗʰ **V01.01 Pedestrian on roller-skates injured in collision with pedal cycle in nontraffic accident**

√x7ᵗʰ **V01.02 Pedestrian on skateboard injured in collision with pedal cycle in nontraffic accident**

√x7ᵗʰ **V01.09 Pedestrian with other conveyance injured in collision with pedal cycle in nontraffic accident**

> Pedestrian with baby stroller injured in collision with pedal cycle in nontraffic accident
> Pedestrian on ice-skates injured in collision with pedal cycle in nontraffic accident
> Pedestrian on nonmotorized scooter injured in collision with pedal cycle in nontraffic accident
> Pedestrian on sled injured in collision with pedal cycle in nontraffic accident
> Pedestrian on snowboard injured in collision with pedal cycle in nontraffic accident
> Pedestrian on snow-skis injured in collision with pedal cycle in nontraffic accident
> Pedestrian in wheelchair (powered) injured in collision with pedal cycle in nontraffic accident
> Pedestrian in motorized mobility scooter injured in collision with pedal cycle in nontraffic accident

√5ᵗʰ **V01.1 Pedestrian injured in collision with pedal cycle in traffic accident**

√x7ᵗʰ **V01.10 Pedestrian on foot injured in collision with pedal cycle in traffic accident**

> Pedestrian NOS injured in collision with pedal cycle in traffic accident

√x7ᵗʰ **V01.11 Pedestrian on roller-skates injured in collision with pedal cycle in traffic accident**

√x7ᵗʰ **V01.12 Pedestrian on skateboard injured in collision with pedal cycle in traffic accident**

√x7ᵗʰ **V01.19 Pedestrian with other conveyance injured in collision with pedal cycle in traffic accident**

> Pedestrian with baby stroller injured in collision with pedal cycle in traffic accident
> Pedestrian on ice-skates injured in collision with pedal cycle in traffic accident
> Pedestrian on nonmotorized scooter injured in collision with pedal cycle in traffic accident
> Pedestrian on sled injured in collision with pedal cycle in traffic accident
> Pedestrian on snowboard injured in collision with pedal cycle in traffic accident
> Pedestrian on snow-skis injured in collision with pedal cycle in traffic accident
> Pedestrian in wheelchair (powered) injured in collision with pedal cycle in traffic accident
> Pedestrian in motorized mobility scooter injured in collision with pedal cycle in traffic accident

√5ᵗʰ **V01.9 Pedestrian injured in collision with pedal cycle, unspecified whether traffic or nontraffic accident**

√x7ᵗʰ **V01.90 Pedestrian on foot injured in collision with pedal cycle, unspecified whether traffic or nontraffic accident**

> Pedestrian NOS injured in collision with pedal cycle, unspecified whether traffic or nontraffic accident

√x7ᵗʰ **V01.91 Pedestrian on roller-skates injured in collision with pedal cycle, unspecified whether traffic or nontraffic accident**

√x7ᵗʰ **V01.92 Pedestrian on skateboard injured in collision with pedal cycle, unspecified whether traffic or nontraffic accident**

✓x 7ᵗʰ **V01.99** **Pedestrian with other conveyance injured in collision with pedal cycle, unspecified whether traffic or nontraffic accident**
  Pedestrian with baby stroller injured in collision with pedal cycle, unspecified whether traffic or nontraffic accident
  Pedestrian on ice-skates injured in collision with pedal cycle unspecified, whether traffic or nontraffic accident
  Pedestrian on nonmotorized scooter injured in collision with pedal cycle, unspecified whether traffic or nontraffic accident
  Pedestrian on sled injured in collision with pedal cycle unspecified, whether traffic or nontraffic accident
  Pedestrian on snowboard injured in collision with pedal cycle, unspecified whether traffic or nontraffic accident
  Pedestrian on snow-skis injured in collision with pedal cycle, unspecified whether traffic or nontraffic accident
  Pedestrian in wheelchair (powered) injured in collision with pedal cycle, unspecified whether traffic or nontraffic accident
  Pedestrian in motorized mobility scooter injured in collision with pedal cycle, unspecified whether traffic or nontraffic accident

✓4ᵗʰ **V02** **Pedestrian injured in collision with two- or three-wheeled motor vehicle**
  ✓5ᵗʰ **V02.0** **Pedestrian injured in collision with two- or three-wheeled motor vehicle in nontraffic accident**
    ✓x 7ᵗʰ **V02.00** **Pedestrian on foot injured in collision with two- or three-wheeled motor vehicle in nontraffic accident**
      Pedestrian NOS injured in collision with two- or three-wheeled motor vehicle in nontraffic accident
    ✓x 7ᵗʰ **V02.01** **Pedestrian on roller-skates injured in collision with two- or three-wheeled motor vehicle in nontraffic accident**
    ✓x 7ᵗʰ **V02.02** **Pedestrian on skateboard injured in collision with two- or three-wheeled motor vehicle in nontraffic accident**
    ✓x 7ᵗʰ **V02.09** **Pedestrian with other conveyance injured in collision with two- or three-wheeled motor vehicle in nontraffic accident**
      Pedestrian with baby stroller injured in collision with two- or three-wheeled motor vehicle in nontraffic accident
      Pedestrian on ice-skates injured in collision with two- or three-wheeled motor vehicle in nontraffic accident
      Pedestrian on nonmotorized scooter injured in collision with two- or three-wheeled motor vehicle in nontraffic accident
      Pedestrian on sled injured in collision with two- or three-wheeled motor vehicle in nontraffic accident
      Pedestrian on snowboard injured in collision with two- or three-wheeled motor vehicle in nontraffic accident
      Pedestrian on snow-skis injured in collision with two- or three-wheeled motor vehicle in nontraffic accident
      Pedestrian in wheelchair (powered) injured in collision with two- or three-wheeled motor vehicle in nontraffic accident
      Pedestrian in motorized mobility scooter injured in collision with two- or three-wheeled motor vehicle in nontraffic accident
  ✓5ᵗʰ **V02.1** **Pedestrian injured in collision with two- or three-wheeled motor vehicle in traffic accident**
    ✓x 7ᵗʰ **V02.10** **Pedestrian on foot injured in collision with two- or three-wheeled motor vehicle in traffic accident**
      Pedestrian NOS injured in collision with two- or three-wheeled motor vehicle in traffic accident
    ✓x 7ᵗʰ **V02.11** **Pedestrian on roller-skates injured in collision with two- or three-wheeled motor vehicle in traffic accident**
    ✓x 7ᵗʰ **V02.12** **Pedestrian on skateboard injured in collision with two- or three-wheeled motor vehicle in traffic accident**

✓x 7ᵗʰ **V02.19** **Pedestrian with other conveyance injured in collision with two- or three-wheeled motor vehicle in traffic accident**
  Pedestrian with baby stroller injured in collision with two- or three-wheeled motor vehicle in traffic accident
  Pedestrian on ice-skates injured in collision with two- or three-wheeled motor vehicle in traffic accident
  Pedestrian on nonmotorized scooter injured in collision with two- or three-wheeled motor vehicle in traffic accident
  Pedestrian on sled injured in collision with two- or three-wheeled motor vehicle in traffic accident
  Pedestrian on snowboard injured in collision with two- or three-wheeled motor vehicle in traffic accident
  Pedestrian on snow-skis injured in collision with two- or three-wheeled motor vehicle in traffic accident
  Pedestrian in wheelchair (powered) injured in collision with two- or three-wheeled motor vehicle in traffic accident
  Pedestrian in motorized mobility scooter injued in collision with two- or three-wheeled motor vehicle in traffic accident

✓5ᵗʰ **V02.9** **Pedestrian injured in collision with two- or three-wheeled motor vehicle, unspecified whether traffic or nontraffic accident**
  ✓x 7ᵗʰ **V02.90** **Pedestrian on foot injured in collision with two- or three-wheeled motor vehicle, unspecified whether traffic or nontraffic accident**
    Pedestrian NOS injured in collision with two- or three-wheeled motor vehicle, unspecified whether traffic or nontraffic accident
  ✓x 7ᵗʰ **V02.91** **Pedestrian on roller-skates injured in collision with two- or three-wheeled motor vehicle, unspecified whether traffic or nontraffic accident**
  ✓x 7ᵗʰ **V02.92** **Pedestrian on skateboard injured in collision with two- or three-wheeled motor vehicle, unspecified whether traffic or nontraffic accident**
  ✓x 7ᵗʰ **V02.99** **Pedestrian with other conveyance injured in collision with two- or three-wheeled motor vehicle, unspecified whether traffic or nontraffic accident**
    Pedestrian with baby stroller injured in collision with two- or three-wheeled motor vehicle, unspecified whether traffic or nontraffic accident
    Pedestrian on ice-skates injured in collision with two- or three-wheeled motor vehicle, unspecified whether traffic or nontraffic accident
    Pedestrian on nonmotorized scooter injured in collision with two- or three-wheeled motor vehicle, unspecified whether traffic or nontraffic accident
    Pedestrian on sled injured in collision with two- or three-wheeled motor vehicle, unspecified whether traffic or nontraffic accident
    Pedestrian on snowboard injured in collision with two- or three-wheeled motor vehicle, unspecified whether traffic or nontraffic accident
    Pedestrian on snow-skis injured in collision with two- or three-wheeled motor vehicle, unspecified whether traffic or nontraffic accident
    Pedestrian in wheelchair (powered) injured in collision with two- or three-wheeled motor vehicle, unspecified whether traffic or nontraffic accident
    Pedestrian in motorized mobility scooter injured in collision with two- or three wheeled motor vehicle, unspecified whether traffic or nontraffic accident

✓4ᵗʰ **V03** **Pedestrian injured in collision with car, pick-up truck or van**
  ✓5ᵗʰ **V03.0** **Pedestrian injured in collision with car, pick-up truck or van in nontraffic accident**
    ✓x 7ᵗʰ **V03.00** **Pedestrian on foot injured in collision with car, pick-up truck or van in nontraffic accident**
      Pedestrian NOS injured in collision with car, pick-up truck or van in nontraffic accident
    ✓x 7ᵗʰ **V03.01** **Pedestrian on roller-skates injured in collision with car, pick-up truck or van in nontraffic accident**

✓x7ᵗʰ **V03.02** Pedestrian on skateboard injured in collision with car, pick-up truck or van in nontraffic accident

✓x7ᵗʰ **V03.09** Pedestrian with other conveyance injured in collision with car, pick-up truck or van in nontraffic accident

Pedestrian with baby stroller injured in collision with car, pick-up truck or van in nontraffic accident

Pedestrian on ice-skates injured in collision with car, pick-up truck or van in nontraffic accident

Pedestrian on nonmotorized scooter injured in collision with car, pick-up truck or van in nontraffic accident

Pedestrian on sled injured in collision with car, pick-up truck or van in nontraffic accident

Pedestrian on snowboard injured in collision with car, pick-up truck or van in nontraffic accident

Pedestrian on snow-skis injured in collision with car, pick-up truck or van in nontraffic accident

Pedestrian in wheelchair (powered) injured in collision with car, pick-up truck or van in nontraffic accident

Pedestrian in motorized mobility scooter injured in collision with car, pick-up truck or van in nontraffic accident

✓5ᵗʰ **V03.1 Pedestrian injured in collision with car, pick-up truck or van in traffic accident**

✓x7ᵗʰ **V03.10 Pedestrian on foot injured in collision with car, pick-up truck or van in traffic accident**

Pedestrian NOS injured in collision with car, pick-up truck or van in traffic accident

✓x7ᵗʰ **V03.11 Pedestrian on roller-skates injured in collision with car, pick-up truck or van in traffic accident**

✓x7ᵗʰ **V03.12 Pedestrian on skateboard injured in collision with car, pick-up truck or van in traffic accident**

✓x7ᵗʰ **V03.19 Pedestrian with other conveyance injured in collision with car, pick-up truck or van in traffic accident**

Pedestrian with baby stroller injured in collision with car, pick-up truck or van in traffic accident

Pedestrian on ice-skates injured in collision with car, pick-up truck or van in traffic accident

Pedestrian on nonmotorized scooter injured in collision with car, pick-up truck or van in nontraffic accident

Pedestrian on sled injured in collision with car, pick-up truck or van in traffic accident

Pedestrian on snowboard injured in collision with car, pick-up truck or van in traffic accident

Pedestrian on snow-skis injured in collision with car, pick-up truck or van in traffic accident

Pedestrian in wheelchair (powered) injured in collision with car, pick-up truck or van in traffic accident

Pedestrian in motorized mobility scooter injured in collision with car, pick-up truck or van in nontraffic accident

✓5ᵗʰ **V03.9 Pedestrian injured in collision with car, pick-up truck or van, unspecified whether traffic or nontraffic accident**

✓x7ᵗʰ **V03.90 Pedestrian on foot injured in collision with car, pick-up truck or van, unspecified whether traffic or nontraffic accident**

Pedestrian NOS injured in collision with car, pick-up truck or van, unspecified whether traffic or nontraffic accident

✓x7ᵗʰ **V03.91 Pedestrian on roller-skates injured in collision with car, pick-up truck or van, unspecified whether traffic or nontraffic accident**

✓x7ᵗʰ **V03.92 Pedestrian on skateboard injured in collision with car, pick-up truck or van, unspecified whether traffic or nontraffic accident**

✓x7ᵗʰ **V03.99 Pedestrian with other conveyance injured in collision with car, pick-up truck or van, unspecified whether traffic or nontraffic accident**

Pedestrian with baby stroller injured in collision with car, pick-up truck or van, unspecified whether traffic or nontraffic accident

Pedestrian on ice-skates injured in collision with car, pick-up truck or van, unspecified whether traffic or nontraffic accident

Pedestrian on nonmotorized scooter injured in collision with car, pick-up truck or van, unspecified whether traffic or nontraffic accident

Pedestrian on sled injured in collision with car, pick-up truck or van in traffic accident

Pedestrian on snowboard injured in collision with car, pick-up truck or van, unspecified whether traffic or nontraffic accident

Pedestrian on snow-skis injured in collision with car, pick-up truck or van, unspecified whether traffic or nontraffic accident

Pedestrian in wheelchair (powered) injured in collision with car, pick-up truck or van, unspecified whether traffic or nontraffic accident

Pedestrian in motorized mobility scooter injured in collision with car, pick-up truck or van, unspecified whether traffic or nontraffic accident

✓4ᵗʰ **V04 Pedestrian injured in collision with heavy transport vehicle or bus**

EXCLUDES 1   *pedestrian injured in collision with military vehicle (V09.01, V09.21)*

✓5ᵗʰ **V04.0 Pedestrian injured in collision with heavy transport vehicle or bus in nontraffic accident**

✓x7ᵗʰ **V04.00 Pedestrian on foot injured in collision with heavy transport vehicle or bus in nontraffic accident**

Pedestrian NOS injured in collision with heavy transport vehicle or bus in nontraffic accident

✓x7ᵗʰ **V04.01 Pedestrian on roller-skates injured in collision with heavy transport vehicle or bus in nontraffic accident**

✓x7ᵗʰ **V04.02 Pedestrian on skateboard injured in collision with heavy transport vehicle or bus in nontraffic accident**

✓x7ᵗʰ **V04.09 Pedestrian with other conveyance injured in collision with heavy transport vehicle or bus in nontraffic accident**

Pedestrian with baby stroller injured in collision with heavy transport vehicle or bus in nontraffic accident

Pedestrian on ice-skates injured in collision with heavy transport vehicle or bus in nontraffic accident

Pedestrian on nonmotorized scooter injured in collision with heavy transport vehicle or bus in nontraffic accident

Pedestrian on sled injured in collision with heavy transport vehicle or bus in nontraffic accident

Pedestrian on snowboard injured in collision with heavy transport vehicle or bus in nontraffic accident

Pedestrian on snow-skis injured in collision with heavy transport vehicle or bus in nontraffic accident

Pedestrian in wheelchair (powered) injured in collision with heavy transport vehicle or bus in nontraffic accident

Pedestrian in motorized mobility scooter injured in collision with heavy transport vehicle or bus in nontraffic accident

✓5ᵗʰ **V04.1 Pedestrian injured in collision with heavy transport vehicle or bus in traffic accident**

✓x7ᵗʰ **V04.10 Pedestrian on foot injured in collision with heavy transport vehicle or bus in traffic accident**

Pedestrian NOS injured in collision with heavy transport vehicle or bus in traffic accident

✓x7ᵗʰ **V04.11 Pedestrian on roller-skates injured in collision with heavy transport vehicle or bus in traffic accident**

✓x7ᵗʰ **V04.12 Pedestrian on skateboard injured in collision with heavy transport vehicle or bus in traffic accident**

✓ Additional Char Req   ✓x7ᵗʰ Placeholder   Unacceptable PDx   Questionable PDx   Wrong Procedure   Manifestation   Unspecified Dx   H1–H14 HAC   HCC CMS-HCC Dx   HIV HIV Dx

ICD-10-CM 2020

1217

V03.02–V04.12

Chapter 20. External Causes of Morbidity

√x7ᵗʰ **V04.19** **Pedestrian with other conveyance injured in collision with heavy transport vehicle or bus in traffic accident**

Pedestrian with baby stroller injured in collision with heavy transport vehicle or bus in traffic accident

Pedestrian on ice-skates injured in collision with heavy transport vehicle or bus in traffic accident

Pedestrian on nonmotorized scooter injured in collision with heavy transport vehicle or bus in traffic accident

Pedestrian on sled injured in collision with heavy transport vehicle or bus in traffic accident

Pedestrian on snowboard injured in collision with heavy transport vehicle or bus in traffic accident

Pedestrian on snow-skis injured in collision with heavy transport vehicle or bus in traffic accident

Pedestrian in wheelchair (powered) injured in collision with heavy transport vehicle or bus in traffic accident

Pedestrian in motorized mobility scooter injured in collision with heavy transport vehicle or bus in traffic accident

√5ᵗʰ **V04.9** **Pedestrian injured in collision with heavy transport vehicle or bus, unspecified whether traffic or nontraffic accident**

√x7ᵗʰ **V04.90** **Pedestrian on foot injured in collision with heavy transport vehicle or bus, unspecified whether traffic or nontraffic accident**

Pedestrian NOS injured in collision with heavy transport vehicle or bus, unspecified whether traffic or nontraffic accident

√x7ᵗʰ **V04.91** **Pedestrian on roller-skates injured in collision with heavy transport vehicle or bus, unspecified whether traffic or nontraffic accident**

√x7ᵗʰ **V04.92** **Pedestrian on skateboard injured in collision with heavy transport vehicle or bus, unspecified whether traffic or nontraffic accident**

√x7ᵗʰ **V04.99** **Pedestrian with other conveyance injured in collision with heavy transport vehicle or bus, unspecified whether traffic or nontraffic accident**

Pedestrian with baby stroller injured in collision with heavy transport vehicle or bus, unspecified whether traffic or nontraffic accident

Pedestrian on ice-skates injured in collision with heavy transport vehicle or bus, unspecified whether traffic or nontraffic accident

Pedestrian on nonmotorized scooter injured in collision with heavy transport vehicle or bus, unspecified whether traffic or nontraffic accident

Pedestrian on sled injured in collision with heavy transport vehicle or bus, unspecified whether traffic or nontraffic accident

Pedestrian on snowboard injured in collision with heavy transport vehicle or bus, unspecified whether traffic or nontraffic accident

Pedestrian on snow-skis injured in collision with heavy transport vehicle or bus, unspecified whether traffic or nontraffic accident

Pedestrian in wheelchair (powered) injured in collision with heavy transport vehicle or bus, unspecified whether traffic or nontraffic accident

Pedestrian in motorized mobility scooter injured in collision with heavy transport vehicle or bus, unspecified whether traffic or nontraffic accident

√4ᵗʰ **V05** **Pedestrian injured in collision with railway train or railway vehicle**

√5ᵗʰ **V05.0** **Pedestrian injured in collision with railway train or railway vehicle in nontraffic accident**

√x7ᵗʰ **V05.00** **Pedestrian on foot injured in collision with railway train or railway vehicle in nontraffic accident**

Pedestrian NOS injured in collision with railway train or railway vehicle in nontraffic accident

√x7ᵗʰ **V05.01** **Pedestrian on roller-skates injured in collision with railway train or railway vehicle in nontraffic accident**

√x7ᵗʰ **V05.02** **Pedestrian on skateboard injured in collision with railway train or railway vehicle in nontraffic accident**

√x7ᵗʰ **V05.09** **Pedestrian with other conveyance injured in collision with railway train or railway vehicle in nontraffic accident**

Pedestrian with baby stroller injured in collision with railway train or railway vehicle in nontraffic accident

Pedestrian on ice-skates injured in collision with railway train or railway vehicle in nontraffic accident

Pedestrian on nonmotorized scooter injured in collision with railway train or railway vehicle in nontraffic accident

Pedestrian on sled injured in collision with railway train or railway vehicle in nontraffic accident

Pedestrian on snowboard injured in collision with railway train or railway vehicle in nontraffic accident

Pedestrian on snow-skis injured in collision with railway train or railway vehicle in nontraffic accident

Pedestrian in wheelchair (powered) injured in collision with railway train or railway vehicle in nontraffic accident

Pedestrian in motorized mobility scooter injured in collision with railway train or railway vehicle in nontraffic accident

√5ᵗʰ **V05.1** **Pedestrian injured in collision with railway train or railway vehicle in traffic accident**

√x7ᵗʰ **V05.10** **Pedestrian on foot injured in collision with railway train or railway vehicle in traffic accident**

Pedestrian NOS injured in collision with railway train or railway vehicle in traffic accident

√x7ᵗʰ **V05.11** **Pedestrian on roller-skates injured in collision with railway train or railway vehicle in traffic accident**

√x7ᵗʰ **V05.12** **Pedestrian on skateboard injured in collision with railway train or railway vehicle in traffic accident**

√x7ᵗʰ **V05.19** **Pedestrian with other conveyance injured in collision with railway train or railway vehicle in traffic accident**

Pedestrian with baby stroller injured in collision with railway train or railway vehicle in traffic accident

Pedestrian on ice-skates injured in collision with railway train or railway vehicle in traffic accident

Pedestrian on nonmotorized scooter injured in collision with railway train or railway vehicle in traffic accident

Pedestrian on sled injured in collision with railway train or railway vehicle in traffic accident

Pedestrian on snowboard injured in collision with railway train or railway vehicle in traffic accident

Pedestrian on snow-skis injured in collision with railway train or railway vehicle in traffic accident

Pedestrian in wheelchair (powered) injured in collision with railway train or railway vehicle in traffic accident

Pedestrian in motorized mobility scooter injured in collision with railway train or railway vehicle in traffic accident

√5ᵗʰ **V05.9** **Pedestrian injured in collision with railway train or railway vehicle, unspecified whether traffic or nontraffic accident**

√x7ᵗʰ **V05.90** **Pedestrian on foot injured in collision with railway train or railway vehicle, unspecified whether traffic or nontraffic accident**

Pedestrian NOS injured in collision with railway train or railway vehicle, unspecified whether traffic or nontraffic accident

√x7ᵗʰ **V05.91** **Pedestrian on roller-skates injured in collision with railway train or railway vehicle, unspecified whether traffic or nontraffic accident**

√x7ᵗʰ **V05.92** **Pedestrian on skateboard injured in collision with railway train or railway vehicle, unspecified whether traffic or nontraffic accident**

Ⓝ Newborn: 0   Ⓟ Pediatric: 0-17   Ⓜ Maternity: 9-64   Ⓐ Adult: 15-124   **MCC** Major Complication/Comorbidity   **CC** Complication/Comorbidity   **SW** Severe Wound Dx

1218   ICD-10-CM 2020

√x7ᵗʰ **V05.99** **Pedestrian with other conveyance injured in collision with railway train or railway vehicle, unspecified whether traffic or nontraffic accident**

Pedestrian with baby stroller injured in collision with railway train or railway vehicle, unspecified whether traffic or nontraffic

Pedestrian on ice-skates injured in collision with railway train or railway vehicle, unspecified whether traffic or nontraffic

Pedestrian on nonmotorized scooter injured in collision with railway train or railway vehicle, unspecified whether traffic or nontraffic

Pedestrian on sled injured in collision with railway train or railway vehicle, unspecified whether traffic or nontraffic

Pedestrian on snowboard injured in collision with railway train or railway vehicle, unspecified whether traffic or nontraffic

Pedestrian on snow-skis injured in collision with railway train or railway vehicle, unspecified whether traffic or nontraffic

Pedestrian in wheelchair (powered) injured in collision with railway train or railway vehicle, unspecified whether traffic or nontraffic

Pedestrian in motorized mobility scooter injured in collision with railway train or railway vehicle, unspecified whether traffic or nontraffic

√4ᵗʰ **V06 Pedestrian injured in collision with other nonmotor vehicle**

INCLUDES   collision with animal-drawn vehicle, animal being ridden, nonpowered streetcar

EXCLUDES 1   *pedestrian injured in collision with pedestrian conveyance (V00.0-)*

√5ᵗʰ **V06.0 Pedestrian injured in collision with other nonmotor vehicle in nontraffic accident**

√x7ᵗʰ **V06.00 Pedestrian on foot injured in collision with other nonmotor vehicle in nontraffic accident**

Pedestrian NOS injured in collision with other nonmotor vehicle in nontraffic accident

√x7ᵗʰ **V06.01 Pedestrian on roller-skates injured in collision with other nonmotor vehicle in nontraffic accident**

√x7ᵗʰ **V06.02 Pedestrian on skateboard injured in collision with other nonmotor vehicle in nontraffic accident**

√x7ᵗʰ **V06.09 Pedestrian with other conveyance injured in collision with other nonmotor vehicle in nontraffic accident**

Pedestrian with baby stroller injured in collision with other nonmotor vehicle in nontraffic accident

Pedestrian on ice-skates injured in collision with other nonmotor vehicle in nontraffic accident

Pedestrian on nonmotorized scooter injured in collision with other nonmotor vehicle in nontraffic accident

Pedestrian on sled injured in collision with other nonmotor vehicle in nontraffic accident

Pedestrian on snowboard injured in collision with other nonmotor vehicle in nontraffic accident

Pedestrian on snow-skis injured in collision with other nonmotor vehicle in nontraffic accident

Pedestrian in wheelchair (powered) injured in collision with other nonmotor vehicle in nontraffic accident

Pedestrian in motorized mobility scooter injured in collision with other nonmotor vehicle in nontraffic accident

√5ᵗʰ **V06.1 Pedestrian injured in collision with other nonmotor vehicle in traffic accident**

√x7ᵗʰ **V06.10 Pedestrian on foot injured in collision with other nonmotor vehicle in traffic accident**

Pedestrian NOS injured in collision with other nonmotor vehicle in traffic accident

√x7ᵗʰ **V06.11 Pedestrian on roller-skates injured in collision with other nonmotor vehicle in traffic accident**

√x7ᵗʰ **V06.12 Pedestrian on skateboard injured in collision with other nonmotor vehicle in traffic accident**

√x7ᵗʰ **V06.19 Pedestrian with other conveyance injured in collision with other nonmotor vehicle in traffic accident**

Pedestrian with baby stroller injured in collision with other nonmotor vehicle in nontraffic accident

Pedestrian on ice-skates injured in collision with other nonmotor vehicle in traffic accident

Pedestrian on nonmotorized scooter injured in collision with other nonmotor vehicle in traffic accident

Pedestrian on sled injured in collision with other nonmotor vehicle in traffic accident

Pedestrian on snowboard injured in collision with other nonmotor vehicle in traffic accident

Pedestrian on snow-skis injured in collision with other nonmotor vehicle in traffic accident

Pedestrian in wheelchair (powered) injured in collision with other nonmotor vehicle in traffic accident

Pedestrian in motorized mobility scooter injured in collision with other nonmotor vehicle in traffic accident

√5ᵗʰ **V06.9 Pedestrian injured in collision with other nonmotor vehicle, unspecified whether traffic or nontraffic accident**

√x7ᵗʰ **V06.90 Pedestrian on foot injured in collision with other nonmotor vehicle, unspecified whether traffic or nontraffic accident**

Pedestrian NOS injured in collision with other nonmotor vehicle, unspecified whether traffic or nontraffic accident

√x7ᵗʰ **V06.91 Pedestrian on roller-skates injured in collision with other nonmotor vehicle, unspecified whether traffic or nontraffic accident**

√x7ᵗʰ **V06.92 Pedestrian on skateboard injured in collision with other nonmotor vehicle, unspecified whether traffic or nontraffic accident**

√x7ᵗʰ **V06.99 Pedestrian with other conveyance injured in collision with other nonmotor vehicle, unspecified whether traffic or nontraffic accident**

Pedestrian with baby stroller injured in collision with other nonmotor vehicle, unspecified whether traffic or nontraffic accident

Pedestrian on ice-skates injured in collision with other nonmotor vehicle, unspecified whether traffic or nontraffic accident

Pedestrian on nonmotorized scooter injured in collision with other nonmotor vehicle, unspecified whether traffic or nontraffic accident

Pedestrian on sled injured in collision with other nonmotor vehicle, unspecified whether traffic or nontraffic accident

Pedestrian on snowboard injured in collision with other nonmotor vehicle, unspecified whether traffic or nontraffic accident

Pedestrian on snow-skis injured in collision with other nonmotor vehicle, unspecified whether traffic or nontraffic accident

Pedestrian in wheelchair (powered) injured in collision with other nonmotor vehicle, unspecified whether traffic or nontraffic accident

Pedestrian in motorized mobility scooter injured in collision with other nonmotorized vehicle, unspecified whether traffic or nontraffic accident

√4ᵗʰ **V09 Pedestrian injured in other and unspecified transport accidents**

√5ᵗʰ **V09.0 Pedestrian injured in nontraffic accident involving other and unspecified motor vehicles**

√x7ᵗʰ **V09.00 Pedestrian injured in nontraffic accident involving unspecified motor vehicles**

√x7ᵗʰ **V09.01 Pedestrian injured in nontraffic accident involving military vehicle**

√x7ᵗʰ **V09.09 Pedestrian injured in nontraffic accident involving other motor vehicles**

Pedestrian injured in nontraffic accident by special vehicle

√x7ᵗʰ **V09.1 Pedestrian injured in unspecified nontraffic accident**

√5ᵗʰ **V09.2 Pedestrian injured in traffic accident involving other and unspecified motor vehicles**

√x7ᵗʰ **V09.20 Pedestrian injured in traffic accident involving unspecified motor vehicles**

√x7ᵗʰ **V09.21 Pedestrian injured in traffic accident involving military vehicle**

✔ Additional Char Req   √x7ᵗʰ Placeholder   Unacceptable PDx   Questionable PDx   Wrong Procedure   Manifestation   Unspecified Dx   H1-H14 HAC   HCC CMS-HCC Dx   HIV HIV Dx

ICD-10-CM 2020   1219

Chapter 20. External Causes of Morbidity

V09.29–V18.3

√x7ᵗʰ **V09.29** **Pedestrian injured in traffic accident involving other motor vehicles**

√x7ᵗʰ **V09.3** **Pedestrian injured in unspecified** traffic **accident**

√x7ᵗʰ **V09.9** **Pedestrian injured in unspecified** transport **accident**

Pedal cycle rider injured in transport accident (V10-V19)

INCLUDES   any non-motorized vehicle, excluding an animal-drawn vehicle, or a sidecar or trailer attached to the pedal cycle

EXCLUDES 2   rupture of pedal cycle tire (W37.0)

The appropriate 7th character is to be added to each code from categories V10-V19.
A   initial encounter
D   subsequent encounter
S   sequela

√4ᵗʰ **V10** **Pedal cycle rider injured in collision with pedestrian or animal**

EXCLUDES 1   pedal cycle rider collision with animal-drawn vehicle or animal being ridden (V16.-)

√x7ᵗʰ **V10.0** **Pedal cycle** driver **injured in collision with pedestrian or animal** in nontraffic accident

√x7ᵗʰ **V10.1** **Pedal cycle** passenger **injured in collision with pedestrian or** animal **in nontraffic accident**

√x7ᵗʰ **V10.2** **Unspecified pedal cyclist injured in collision with pedestrian or animal in nontraffic accident**

√x7ᵗʰ **V10.3** Person boarding or alighting **a pedal cycle injured in collision with pedestrian or animal**

√x7ᵗʰ **V10.4** **Pedal cycle** driver **injured in collision with pedestrian or animal in traffic accident**

√x7ᵗʰ **V10.5** **Pedal cycle** passenger **injured in collision with pedestrian or animal** in traffic accident

√x7ᵗʰ **V10.9** **Unspecified pedal cyclist injured in collision with pedestrian or animal** in traffic accident

√4ᵗʰ **V11** **Pedal cycle rider injured in collision with other pedal cycle**

√x7ᵗʰ **V11.0** **Pedal cycle** driver **injured in collision with other pedal cycle** in nontraffic accident

√x7ᵗʰ **V11.1** **Pedal cycle** passenger **injured in collision with other pedal cycle in nontraffic accident**

√x7ᵗʰ **V11.2** **Unspecified pedal cyclist injured in collision with other pedal cycle in nontraffic accident**

√x7ᵗʰ **V11.3** Person boarding or alighting **a pedal cycle injured in collision with other pedal cycle**

√x7ᵗʰ **V11.4** **Pedal cycle** driver **injured in collision with other pedal cycle in traffic accident**

√x7ᵗʰ **V11.5** **Pedal cycle** passenger **injured in collision with other pedal cycle in traffic accident**

√x7ᵗʰ **V11.9** **Unspecified pedal cyclist injured in collision with other pedal cycle in traffic accident**

√4ᵗʰ **V12** **Pedal cycle rider injured in collision with two- or three-wheeled motor vehicle**

√x7ᵗʰ **V12.0** **Pedal cycle** driver **injured in collision with two- or three-wheeled motor vehicle** in nontraffic accident

√x7ᵗʰ **V12.1** **Pedal cycle** passenger **injured in collision with two- or three-wheeled motor vehicle in nontraffic accident**

√x7ᵗʰ **V12.2** **Unspecified pedal cyclist injured in collision with two- or three-wheeled motor vehicle** in nontraffic accident

√x7ᵗʰ **V12.3** Person boarding or alighting **a pedal cycle injured in collision with two- or three-wheeled motor vehicle**

√x7ᵗʰ **V12.4** **Pedal cycle** driver **injured in collision with two- or three-wheeled motor vehicle** in traffic accident

√x7ᵗʰ **V12.5** **Pedal cycle** passenger **injured in collision with two- or three-wheeled motor vehicle** in traffic accident

√x7ᵗʰ **V12.9** **Unspecified pedal cyclist injured in collision with two- or three-wheeled motor vehicle** in traffic accident

√4ᵗʰ **V13** **Pedal cycle rider injured in collision with car, pick-up truck or van**

√x7ᵗʰ **V13.0** **Pedal cycle** driver **injured in collision with car, pick-up truck or van** in nontraffic accident

√x7ᵗʰ **V13.1** **Pedal cycle** passenger **injured in collision with car, pick-up truck or van in nontraffic accident**

√x7ᵗʰ **V13.2** **Unspecified pedal cyclist injured in collision with car, pick-up truck or van in nontraffic accident**

√x7ᵗʰ **V13.3** Person boarding or alighting **a pedal cycle injured in collision with car, pick-up truck or van**

√x7ᵗʰ **V13.4** **Pedal cycle** driver **injured in collision with car, pick-up truck or van** in traffic accident

√x7ᵗʰ **V13.5** **Pedal cycle** passenger **injured in collision with car, pick-up truck or van** in traffic accident

√x7ᵗʰ **V13.9** **Unspecified pedal cyclist injured in collision with car, pick-up truck or van** in traffic accident

√4ᵗʰ **V14** **Pedal cycle rider injured in collision with heavy transport vehicle or bus**

EXCLUDES 1   pedal cycle rider injured in collision with military vehicle (V19.81)

√x7ᵗʰ **V14.0** **Pedal cycle** driver **injured in collision with heavy transport vehicle or bus** in nontraffic accident

√x7ᵗʰ **V14.1** **Pedal cycle** passenger **injured in collision with heavy transport vehicle or bus** in nontraffic accident

√x7ᵗʰ **V14.2** **Unspecified pedal cyclist injured in collision with heavy transport vehicle or bus** in nontraffic accident

√x7ᵗʰ **V14.3** Person boarding or alighting **a pedal cycle injured in collision with heavy transport vehicle or bus**

√x7ᵗʰ **V14.4** **Pedal cycle** driver **injured in collision with heavy transport vehicle or bus** in traffic accident

√x7ᵗʰ **V14.5** **Pedal cycle** passenger **injured in collision with heavy transport vehicle or bus** in traffic accident

√x7ᵗʰ **V14.9** **Unspecified pedal cyclist injured in collision with heavy transport vehicle or bus** in traffic accident

√4ᵗʰ **V15** **Pedal cycle rider injured in collision with railway train or railway vehicle**

√x7ᵗʰ **V15.0** **Pedal cycle** driver **injured in collision with railway train or railway vehicle** in nontraffic accident

√x7ᵗʰ **V15.1** **Pedal cycle** passenger **injured in collision with railway train or railway vehicle** in nontraffic accident

√x7ᵗʰ **V15.2** **Unspecified pedal cyclist injured in collision with railway train or railway vehicle** in nontraffic accident

√x7ᵗʰ **V15.3** Person boarding or alighting **a pedal cycle injured in collision with railway train or railway vehicle**

√x7ᵗʰ **V15.4** **Pedal cycle** driver **injured in collision with railway train or railway vehicle** in traffic accident

√x7ᵗʰ **V15.5** **Pedal cycle** passenger **injured in collision with railway train or railway vehicle** in traffic accident

√x7ᵗʰ **V15.9** **Unspecified pedal cyclist injured in collision with railway train or railway vehicle** in traffic accident

√4ᵗʰ **V16** **Pedal cycle rider injured in collision with other nonmotor vehicle**

INCLUDES   collision with animal-drawn vehicle, animal being ridden, streetcar

√x7ᵗʰ **V16.0** **Pedal cycle** driver **injured in collision with other nonmotor vehicle** in nontraffic accident

√x7ᵗʰ **V16.1** **Pedal cycle** passenger **injured in collision with other nonmotor vehicle** in nontraffic accident

√x7ᵗʰ **V16.2** **Unspecified pedal cyclist injured in collision with other nonmotor vehicle** in nontraffic accident

√x7ᵗʰ **V16.3** Person boarding or alighting **a pedal cycle injured in collision with other nonmotor vehicle** in nontraffic accident

√x7ᵗʰ **V16.4** **Pedal cycle** driver **injured in collision with other nonmotor vehicle** in traffic accident

√x7ᵗʰ **V16.5** **Pedal cycle** passenger **injured in collision with other nonmotor vehicle** in traffic accident

√x7ᵗʰ **V16.9** **Unspecified pedal cyclist injured in collision with other nonmotor vehicle** in traffic accident

√4ᵗʰ **V17** **Pedal cycle rider injured in collision with fixed or stationary object**

√x7ᵗʰ **V17.0** **Pedal cycle** driver **injured in collision with fixed or stationary object** in nontraffic accident

√x7ᵗʰ **V17.1** **Pedal cycle** passenger **injured in collision with fixed or stationary object** in nontraffic accident

√x7ᵗʰ **V17.2** **Unspecified pedal cyclist injured in collision with fixed or stationary object** in nontraffic accident

√x7ᵗʰ **V17.3** Person boarding or alighting **a pedal cycle injured in collision with fixed or stationary object**

√x7ᵗʰ **V17.4** **Pedal cycle** driver **injured in collision with fixed or stationary object** in traffic accident

√x7ᵗʰ **V17.5** **Pedal cycle** passenger **injured in collision with fixed or stationary object** in traffic accident

√x7ᵗʰ **V17.9** **Unspecified pedal cyclist injured in collision with fixed or stationary object** in traffic accident

√4ᵗʰ **V18** **Pedal cycle rider injured in noncollision transport accident**

INCLUDES   fall or thrown from pedal cycle (without antecedent collision)
overturning pedal cycle NOS
overturning pedal cycle without collision

√x7ᵗʰ **V18.0** **Pedal cycle** driver **injured in noncollision transport accident** in nontraffic accident

√x7ᵗʰ **V18.1** **Pedal cycle** passenger **injured in noncollision transport accident** in nontraffic accident

√x7ᵗʰ **V18.2** **Unspecified pedal cyclist injured in noncollision transport accident** in nontraffic accident

√x7ᵗʰ **V18.3** Person boarding or alighting **a pedal cycle injured in noncollision transport accident**

N Newborn: 0   P Pediatric: 0-17   M Maternity: 9-64   A Adult: 15-124   MCC Major Complication/Comorbidity   CC Complication/Comorbidity   SW Severe Wound Dx

1220   ICD-10-CM 2020

√x7ᵗʰ **V18.4** Pedal cycle driver injured in noncollision transport accident in traffic accident

√x7ᵗʰ **V18.5** Pedal cycle passenger injured in noncollision transport accident in traffic accident

√x7ᵗʰ **V18.9** Unspecified pedal cyclist injured in noncollision transport accident in traffic accident

√4ᵗʰ **V19** Pedal cycle rider injured in other and unspecified transport accidents

√5ᵗʰ **V19.0** Pedal cycle driver injured in collision with other and unspecified motor vehicles in nontraffic accident

√x7ᵗʰ **V19.00** Pedal cycle driver injured in collision with unspecified motor vehicles in nontraffic accident

√x7ᵗʰ **V19.09** Pedal cycle driver injured in collision with other motor vehicles in nontraffic accident

√5ᵗʰ **V19.1** Pedal cycle passenger injured in collision with other and unspecified motor vehicles in nontraffic accident

√x7ᵗʰ **V19.10** Pedal cycle passenger injured in collision with unspecified motor vehicles in nontraffic accident

√x7ᵗʰ **V19.19** Pedal cycle passenger injured in collision with other motor vehicles in nontraffic accident

√5ᵗʰ **V19.2** Unspecified pedal cyclist injured in collision with other and unspecified motor vehicles in nontraffic accident

√x7ᵗʰ **V19.20** Unspecified pedal cyclist injured in collision with unspecified motor vehicles in nontraffic accident
Pedal cycle collision NOS, nontraffic

√x7ᵗʰ **V19.29** Unspecified pedal cyclist injured in collision with other motor vehicles in nontraffic accident

√x7ᵗʰ **V19.3** Pedal cyclist (driver) (passenger) injured in unspecified nontraffic accident
Pedal cycle accident NOS, nontraffic
Pedal cyclist injured in nontraffic accident NOS

√5ᵗʰ **V19.4** Pedal cycle driver injured in collision with other and unspecified motor vehicles in traffic accident

√x7ᵗʰ **V19.40** Pedal cycle driver injured in collision with unspecified motor vehicles in traffic accident

√x7ᵗʰ **V19.49** Pedal cycle driver injured in collision with other motor vehicles in traffic accident

√5ᵗʰ **V19.5** Pedal cycle passenger injured in collision with other and unspecified motor vehicles in traffic accident

√x7ᵗʰ **V19.50** Pedal cycle passenger injured in collision with unspecified motor vehicles in traffic accident

√x7ᵗʰ **V19.59** Pedal cycle passenger injured in collision with other motor vehicles in traffic accident

√5ᵗʰ **V19.6** Unspecified pedal cyclist injured in collision with other and unspecified motor vehicles in traffic accident

√x7ᵗʰ **V19.60** Unspecified pedal cyclist injured in collision with unspecified motor vehicles in traffic accident
Pedal cycle collision NOS (traffic)

√x7ᵗʰ **V19.69** Unspecified pedal cyclist injured in collision with other motor vehicles in traffic accident

√5ᵗʰ **V19.8** Pedal cyclist (driver) (passenger) injured in other specified transport accidents

√x7ᵗʰ **V19.81** Pedal cyclist (driver) (passenger) injured in transport accident with military vehicle

√x7ᵗʰ **V19.88** Pedal cyclist (driver) (passenger) injured in other specified transport accidents

√x7ᵗʰ **V19.9** Pedal cyclist (driver) (passenger) injured in unspecified traffic accident
Pedal cycle accident NOS

Motorcycle rider injured in transport accident (V20-V29)

INCLUDES   moped
motorcycle with sidecar
motorized bicycle
motor scooter

EXCLUDES 1   three-wheeled motor vehicle (V30-V39)

The appropriate 7th character is to be added to each code from categories V20-V29.
A   initial encounter
D   subsequent encounter
S   sequela

√4ᵗʰ **V20** Motorcycle rider injured in collision with pedestrian or animal

EXCLUDES 1   motorcycle rider collision with animal-drawn vehicle or animal being ridden (V26.-)

√x7ᵗʰ **V20.0** Motorcycle driver injured in collision with pedestrian or animal in nontraffic accident

√x7ᵗʰ **V20.1** Motorcycle passenger injured in collision with pedestrian or animal in nontraffic accident

√x7ᵗʰ **V20.2** Unspecified motorcycle rider injured in collision with pedestrian or animal in nontraffic accident

√x7ᵗʰ **V20.3** Person boarding or alighting a motorcycle injured in collision with pedestrian or animal

√x7ᵗʰ **V20.4** Motorcycle driver injured in collision with pedestrian or animal in traffic accident

√x7ᵗʰ **V20.5** Motorcycle passenger injured in collision with pedestrian or animal in traffic accident

√x7ᵗʰ **V20.9** Unspecified motorcycle rider injured in collision with pedestrian or animal in traffic accident

√4ᵗʰ **V21** Motorcycle rider injured in collision with pedal cycle

√x7ᵗʰ **V21.0** Motorcycle driver injured in collision with pedal cycle in nontraffic accident

√x7ᵗʰ **V21.1** Motorcycle passenger injured in collision with pedal cycle in nontraffic accident

√x7ᵗʰ **V21.2** Unspecified motorcycle rider injured in collision with pedal cycle in nontraffic accident

√x7ᵗʰ **V21.3** Person boarding or alighting a motorcycle injured in collision with pedal cycle

√x7ᵗʰ **V21.4** Motorcycle driver injured in collision with pedal cycle in traffic accident

√x7ᵗʰ **V21.5** Motorcycle passenger injured in collision with pedal cycle in traffic accident

√x7ᵗʰ **V21.9** Unspecified motorcycle rider injured in collision with pedal cycle in traffic accident

√4ᵗʰ **V22** Motorcycle rider injured in collision with two- or three-wheeled motor vehicle

√x7ᵗʰ **V22.0** Motorcycle driver injured in collision with two- or three-wheeled motor vehicle in nontraffic accident

√x7ᵗʰ **V22.1** Motorcycle passenger injured in collision with two- or three-wheeled motor vehicle in nontraffic accident

√x7ᵗʰ **V22.2** Unspecified motorcycle rider injured in collision with two- or three-wheeled motor vehicle in nontraffic accident

√x7ᵗʰ **V22.3** Person boarding or alighting a motorcycle injured in collision with two- or three-wheeled motor vehicle

√x7ᵗʰ **V22.4** Motorcycle driver injured in collision with two- or three-wheeled motor vehicle in traffic accident

√x7ᵗʰ **V22.5** Motorcycle passenger injured in collision with two- or three-wheeled motor vehicle in traffic accident

√x7ᵗʰ **V22.9** Unspecified motorcycle rider injured in collision with two- or three-wheeled motor vehicle in traffic accident

√4ᵗʰ **V23** Motorcycle rider injured in collision with car, pick-up truck or van

√x7ᵗʰ **V23.0** Motorcycle driver injured in collision with car, pick-up truck or van in nontraffic accident

√x7ᵗʰ **V23.1** Motorcycle passenger injured in collision with car, pick-up truck or van in nontraffic accident

√x7ᵗʰ **V23.2** Unspecified motorcycle rider injured in collision with car, pick-up truck or van in nontraffic accident

√x7ᵗʰ **V23.3** Person boarding or alighting a motorcycle injured in collision with car, pick-up truck or van

√x7ᵗʰ **V23.4** Motorcycle driver injured in collision with car, pick-up truck or van in traffic accident

√x7ᵗʰ **V23.5** Motorcycle passenger injured in collision with car, pick-up truck or van in traffic accident

√x7ᵗʰ **V23.9** Unspecified motorcycle rider injured in collision with car, pick-up truck or van in traffic accident

√4ᵗʰ **V24** Motorcycle rider injured in collision with heavy transport vehicle or bus

EXCLUDES 1   motorcycle rider injured in collision with military vehicle (V29.81)

√x7ᵗʰ **V24.0** Motorcycle driver injured in collision with heavy transport vehicle or bus in nontraffic accident

√x7ᵗʰ **V24.1** Motorcycle passenger injured in collision with heavy transport vehicle or bus in nontraffic accident

√x7ᵗʰ **V24.2** Unspecified motorcycle rider injured in collision with heavy transport vehicle or bus in nontraffic accident

√x7ᵗʰ **V24.3** Person boarding or alighting a motorcycle injured in collision with heavy transport vehicle or bus

√x7ᵗʰ **V24.4** Motorcycle driver injured in collision with heavy transport vehicle or bus in traffic accident

√x7ᵗʰ **V24.5** Motorcycle passenger injured in collision with heavy transport vehicle or bus in traffic accident

√x7ᵗʰ **V24.9** Unspecified motorcycle rider injured in collision with heavy transport vehicle or bus in traffic accident

√4ᵗʰ **V25** Motorcycle rider injured in collision with railway train or railway vehicle

√x7ᵗʰ **V25.0** Motorcycle driver injured in collision with railway train or railway vehicle in nontraffic accident

√x7ᵗʰ **V25.1** Motorcycle passenger injured in collision with railway train or railway vehicle in nontraffic accident

Chapter 20. External Causes of Morbidity

V25.2 Unspecified motorcycle rider injured in collision with railway train or railway vehicle in nontraffic accident

V25.3 Person boarding or alighting a motorcycle injured in collision with railway train or railway vehicle

V25.4 Motorcycle driver injured in collision with railway train or railway vehicle in traffic accident

V25.5 Motorcycle passenger injured in collision with railway train or railway vehicle in traffic accident

V25.9 Unspecified motorcycle rider injured in collision with railway train or railway vehicle in traffic accident

V26 Motorcycle rider injured in collision with other nonmotor vehicle

INCLUDES   collision with animal-drawn vehicle, animal being ridden, streetcar

V26.0 Motorcycle driver injured in collision with other nonmotor vehicle in nontraffic accident

V26.1 Motorcycle passenger injured in collision with other nonmotor vehicle in nontraffic accident

V26.2 Unspecified motorcycle rider injured in collision with other nonmotor vehicle in nontraffic accident

V26.3 Person boarding or alighting a motorcycle injured in collision with other nonmotor vehicle

V26.4 Motorcycle driver injured in collision with other nonmotor vehicle in traffic accident

V26.5 Motorcycle passenger injured in collision with other nonmotor vehicle in traffic accident

V26.9 Unspecified motorcycle rider injured in collision with other nonmotor vehicle in traffic accident

V27 Motorcycle rider injured in collision with fixed or stationary object

V27.0 Motorcycle driver injured in collision with fixed or stationary object in nontraffic accident

V27.1 Motorcycle passenger injured in collision with fixed or stationary object in nontraffic accident

V27.2 Unspecified motorcycle rider injured in collision with fixed or stationary object in nontraffic accident

V27.3 Person boarding or alighting a motorcycle injured in collision with fixed or stationary object

V27.4 Motorcycle driver injured in collision with fixed or stationary object in traffic accident

V27.5 Motorcycle passenger injured in collision with fixed or stationary object in traffic accident

V27.9 Unspecified motorcycle rider injured in collision with fixed or stationary object in traffic accident

V28 Motorcycle rider injured in noncollision transport accident

INCLUDES   fall or thrown from motorcycle (without antecedent collision)
overturning motorcycle NOS
overturning motorcycle without collision

V28.0 Motorcycle driver injured in noncollision transport accident in nontraffic accident

V28.1 Motorcycle passenger injured in noncollision transport accident in nontraffic accident

V28.2 Unspecified motorcycle rider injured in noncollision transport accident in nontraffic accident

V28.3 Person boarding or alighting a motorcycle injured in noncollision transport accident

V28.4 Motorcycle driver injured in noncollision transport accident in traffic accident

V28.5 Motorcycle passenger injured in noncollision transport accident in traffic accident

V28.9 Unspecified motorcycle rider injured in noncollision transport accident in traffic accident

V29 Motorcycle rider injured in other and unspecified transport accidents

V29.0 Motorcycle driver injured in collision with other and unspecified motor vehicles in nontraffic accident

V29.00 Motorcycle driver injured in collision with unspecified motor vehicles in nontraffic accident

V29.09 Motorcycle driver injured in collision with other motor vehicles in nontraffic accident

V29.1 Motorcycle passenger injured in collision with other and unspecified motor vehicles in nontraffic accident

V29.10 Motorcycle passenger injured in collision with unspecified motor vehicles in nontraffic accident

V29.19 Motorcycle passenger injured in collision with other motor vehicles in nontraffic accident

V29.2 Unspecified motorcycle rider injured in collision with other and unspecified motor vehicles in nontraffic accident

V29.20 Unspecified motorcycle rider injured in collision with unspecified motor vehicles in nontraffic accident

Motorcycle collision NOS, nontraffic

V29.29 Unspecified motorcycle rider injured in collision with other motor vehicles in nontraffic accident

V29.3 Motorcycle rider (driver) (passenger) injured in unspecified nontraffic accident

Motorcycle accident NOS, nontraffic
Motorcycle rider injured in nontraffic accident NOS

V29.4 Motorcycle driver injured in collision with other and unspecified motor vehicles in traffic accident

V29.40 Motorcycle driver injured in collision with unspecified motor vehicles in traffic accident

V29.49 Motorcycle driver injured in collision with other motor vehicles in traffic accident

V29.5 Motorcycle passenger injured in collision with other and unspecified motor vehicles in traffic accident

V29.50 Motorcycle passenger injured in collision with unspecified motor vehicles in traffic accident

V29.59 Motorcycle passenger injured in collision with other motor vehicles in traffic accident

V29.6 Unspecified motorcycle rider injured in collision with other and unspecified motor vehicles in traffic accident

V29.60 Unspecified motorcycle rider injured in collision with unspecified motor vehicles in traffic accident

Motorcycle collision NOS (traffic)

V29.69 Unspecified motorcycle rider injured in collision with other motor vehicles in traffic accident

V29.8 Motorcycle rider (driver) (passenger) injured in other specified transport accidents

V29.81 Motorcycle rider (driver) (passenger) injured in transport accident with military vehicle

V29.88 Motorcycle rider (driver) (passenger) injured in other specified transport accidents

V29.9 Motorcycle rider (driver) (passenger) injured in unspecified traffic accident

Motorcycle accident NOS

Occupant of three-wheeled motor vehicle injured in transport accident (V30-V39)

INCLUDES   motorized tricycle
motorized rickshaw
three-wheeled motor car

EXCLUDES 1   all-terrain vehicles (V86.-)
motorcycle with sidecar (V20-V29)
vehicle designed primarily for off-road use (V86.-)

The appropriate 7th character is to be added to each code from categories V30-V39.
A   initial encounter
D   subsequent encounter
S   sequela

V30 Occupant of three-wheeled motor vehicle injured in collision with pedestrian or animal

EXCLUDES 1   three-wheeled motor vehicle collision with animal-drawn vehicle or animal being ridden (V36.-)

V30.0 Driver of three-wheeled motor vehicle injured in collision with pedestrian or animal in nontraffic accident

V30.1 Passenger in three-wheeled motor vehicle injured in collision with pedestrian or animal in nontraffic accident

V30.2 Person on outside of three-wheeled motor vehicle injured in collision with pedestrian or animal in nontraffic accident

V30.3 Unspecified occupant of three-wheeled motor vehicle injured in collision with pedestrian or animal in nontraffic accident

V30.4 Person boarding or alighting a three-wheeled motor vehicle injured in collision with pedestrian or animal

V30.5 Driver of three-wheeled motor vehicle injured in collision with pedestrian or animal in traffic accident

V30.6 Passenger in three-wheeled motor vehicle injured in collision with pedestrian or animal in traffic accident

V30.7 Person on outside of three-wheeled motor vehicle injured in collision with pedestrian or animal in traffic accident

V30.9 Unspecified occupant of three-wheeled motor vehicle injured in collision with pedestrian or animal in traffic accident

V31 Occupant of three-wheeled motor vehicle injured in collision with pedal cycle

V31.0 Driver of three-wheeled motor vehicle injured in collision with pedal cycle in nontraffic accident

N Newborn: 0   P Pediatric: 0-17   M Maternity: 9-64   A Adult: 15-124   MCC Major Complication/Comorbidity   CC Complication/Comorbidity   SW Severe Wound Dx

1222   ICD-10-CM 2020

√x7ᵗʰ **V31.1** Passenger in three-wheeled motor vehicle injured in collision with pedal cycle in nontraffic accident

√x7ᵗʰ **V31.2** Person on outside of three-wheeled motor vehicle injured in collision with pedal cycle in nontraffic accident

√x7ᵗʰ **V31.3** Unspecified occupant of three-wheeled motor vehicle injured in collision with pedal cycle in nontraffic accident

√x7ᵗʰ **V31.4** Person boarding or alighting a three-wheeled motor vehicle injured in collision with pedal cycle

√x7ᵗʰ **V31.5** Driver of three-wheeled motor vehicle injured in collision with pedal cycle in traffic accident

√x7ᵗʰ **V31.6** Passenger in three-wheeled motor vehicle injured in collision with pedal cycle in traffic accident

√x7ᵗʰ **V31.7** Person on outside of three-wheeled motor vehicle injured in collision with pedal cycle in traffic accident

√x7ᵗʰ **V31.9** Unspecified occupant of three-wheeled motor vehicle injured in collision with pedal cycle in traffic accident

√4ᵗʰ **V32 Occupant of three-wheeled motor vehicle injured in collision with two- or three-wheeled motor vehicle**

√x7ᵗʰ **V32.0** Driver of three-wheeled motor vehicle injured in collision with two- or three-wheeled motor vehicle in nontraffic accident

√x7ᵗʰ **V32.1** Passenger in three-wheeled motor vehicle injured in collision with two- or three-wheeled motor vehicle in nontraffic accident

√x7ᵗʰ **V32.2** Person on outside of three-wheeled motor vehicle injured in collision with two- or three-wheeled motor vehicle in nontraffic accident

√x7ᵗʰ **V32.3** Unspecified occupant of three-wheeled motor vehicle injured in collision with two- or three-wheeled motor vehicle in nontraffic accident

√x7ᵗʰ **V32.4** Person boarding or alighting a three-wheeled motor vehicle injured in collision with two- or three-wheeled motor vehicle

√x7ᵗʰ **V32.5** Driver of three-wheeled motor vehicle injured in collision with two- or three-wheeled motor vehicle in traffic accident

√x7ᵗʰ **V32.6** Passenger in three-wheeled motor vehicle injured in collision with two- or three-wheeled motor vehicle in traffic accident

√x7ᵗʰ **V32.7** Person on outside of three-wheeled motor vehicle injured in collision with two- or three-wheeled motor vehicle in traffic accident

√x7ᵗʰ **V32.9** Unspecified occupant of three-wheeled motor vehicle injured in collision with two- or three-wheeled motor vehicle in traffic accident

√4ᵗʰ **V33 Occupant of three-wheeled motor vehicle injured in collision with car, pick-up truck or van**

√x7ᵗʰ **V33.0** Driver of three-wheeled motor vehicle injured in collision with car, pick-up truck or van in nontraffic accident

√x7ᵗʰ **V33.1** Passenger in three-wheeled motor vehicle injured in collision with car, pick-up truck or van in nontraffic accident

√x7ᵗʰ **V33.2** Person on outside of three-wheeled motor vehicle injured in collision with car, pick-up truck or van in nontraffic accident

√x7ᵗʰ **V33.3** Unspecified occupant of three-wheeled motor vehicle injured in collision with car, pick-up truck or van in nontraffic accident

√x7ᵗʰ **V33.4** Person boarding or alighting a three-wheeled motor vehicle injured in collision with car, pick-up truck or van

√x7ᵗʰ **V33.5** Driver of three-wheeled motor vehicle injured in collision with car, pick-up truck or van in traffic accident

√x7ᵗʰ **V33.6** Passenger in three-wheeled motor vehicle injured in collision with car, pick-up truck or van in traffic accident

√x7ᵗʰ **V33.7** Person on outside of three-wheeled motor vehicle injured in collision with car, pick-up truck or van in traffic accident

√x7ᵗʰ **V33.9** Unspecified occupant of three-wheeled motor vehicle injured in collision with car, pick-up truck or van in traffic accident

√4ᵗʰ **V34 Occupant of three-wheeled motor vehicle injured in collision with heavy transport vehicle or bus**

EXCLUDES 1 *occupant of three-wheeled motor vehicle injured in collision with military vehicle (V39.81)*

√x7ᵗʰ **V34.0** Driver of three-wheeled motor vehicle injured in collision with heavy transport vehicle or bus in nontraffic accident

√x7ᵗʰ **V34.1** Passenger in three-wheeled motor vehicle injured in collision with heavy transport vehicle or bus in nontraffic accident

√x7ᵗʰ **V34.2** Person on outside of three-wheeled motor vehicle injured in collision with heavy transport vehicle or bus in nontraffic accident

√x7ᵗʰ **V34.3** Unspecified occupant of three-wheeled motor vehicle injured in collision with heavy transport vehicle or bus in nontraffic accident

√x7ᵗʰ **V34.4** Person boarding or alighting a three-wheeled motor vehicle injured in collision with heavy transport vehicle or bus

√x7ᵗʰ **V34.5** Driver of three-wheeled motor vehicle injured in collision with heavy transport vehicle or bus in traffic accident

√x7ᵗʰ **V34.6** Passenger in three-wheeled motor vehicle injured in collision with heavy transport vehicle or bus in traffic accident

√x7ᵗʰ **V34.7** Person on outside of three-wheeled motor vehicle injured in collision with heavy transport vehicle or bus in traffic accident

√x7ᵗʰ **V34.9** Unspecified occupant of three-wheeled motor vehicle injured in collision with heavy transport vehicle or bus in traffic accident

√4ᵗʰ **V35 Occupant of three-wheeled motor vehicle injured in collision with railway train or railway vehicle**

√x7ᵗʰ **V35.0** Driver of three-wheeled motor vehicle injured in collision with railway train or railway vehicle in nontraffic accident

√x7ᵗʰ **V35.1** Passenger in three-wheeled motor vehicle injured in collision with railway train or railway vehicle in nontraffic accident

√x7ᵗʰ **V35.2** Person on outside of three-wheeled motor vehicle injured in collision with railway train or railway vehicle in nontraffic accident

√x7ᵗʰ **V35.3** Unspecified occupant of three-wheeled motor vehicle injured in collision with railway train or railway vehicle in nontraffic accident

√x7ᵗʰ **V35.4** Person boarding or alighting a three-wheeled motor vehicle injured in collision with railway train or railway vehicle

√x7ᵗʰ **V35.5** Driver of three-wheeled motor vehicle injured in collision with railway train or railway vehicle in traffic accident

√x7ᵗʰ **V35.6** Passenger in three-wheeled motor vehicle injured in collision with railway train or railway vehicle in traffic accident

√x7ᵗʰ **V35.7** Person on outside of three-wheeled motor vehicle injured in collision with railway train or railway vehicle in traffic accident

√x7ᵗʰ **V35.9** Unspecified occupant of three-wheeled motor vehicle injured in collision with railway train or railway vehicle in traffic accident

√4ᵗʰ **V36 Occupant of three-wheeled motor vehicle injured in collision with other nonmotor vehicle**

INCLUDES collision with animal-drawn vehicle, animal being ridden, streetcar

√x7ᵗʰ **V36.0** Driver of three-wheeled motor vehicle injured in collision with other nonmotor vehicle in nontraffic accident

√x7ᵗʰ **V36.1** Passenger in three-wheeled motor vehicle injured in collision with other nonmotor vehicle in nontraffic accident

√x7ᵗʰ **V36.2** Person on outside of three-wheeled motor vehicle injured in collision with other nonmotor vehicle in nontraffic accident

√x7ᵗʰ **V36.3** Unspecified occupant of three-wheeled motor vehicle injured in collision with other nonmotor vehicle in nontraffic accident

√x7ᵗʰ **V36.4** Person boarding or alighting a three-wheeled motor vehicle injured in collision with other nonmotor vehicle

√x7ᵗʰ **V36.5** Driver of three-wheeled motor vehicle injured in collision with other nonmotor vehicle in traffic accident

√x7ᵗʰ **V36.6** Passenger in three-wheeled motor vehicle injured in collision with other nonmotor vehicle in traffic accident

√x7ᵗʰ **V36.7** Person on outside of three-wheeled motor vehicle injured in collision with other nonmotor vehicle in traffic accident

√x7ᵗʰ **V36.9** Unspecified occupant of three-wheeled motor vehicle injured in collision with other nonmotor vehicle in traffic accident

√4ᵗʰ **V37 Occupant of three-wheeled motor vehicle injured in collision with fixed or stationary object**

√x7ᵗʰ **V37.0** Driver of three-wheeled motor vehicle injured in collision with fixed or stationary object in nontraffic accident

√x7ᵗʰ **V37.1** Passenger in three-wheeled motor vehicle injured in collision with fixed or stationary object in nontraffic accident

√x7ᵗʰ **V37.2** Person on outside of three-wheeled motor vehicle injured in collision with fixed or stationary object in nontraffic accident

√x7ᵗʰ **V37.3** Unspecified occupant of three-wheeled motor vehicle injured in collision with fixed or stationary object in nontraffic accident

√x7ᵗʰ **V37.4** Person boarding or alighting a three-wheeled motor vehicle injured in collision with fixed or stationary object

√x7ᵗʰ **V37.5** Driver of three-wheeled motor vehicle injured in collision with fixed or stationary object in traffic accident

√x7ᵗʰ **V37.6** Passenger in three-wheeled motor vehicle injured in collision with fixed or stationary object in traffic accident

√x7ᵗʰ **V37.7** Person on outside of three-wheeled motor vehicle injured in collision with fixed or stationary object in traffic accident

√x7ᵗʰ **V37.9** Unspecified occupant of three-wheeled motor vehicle injured in collision with fixed or stationary object in traffic accident

✔ Additional Char Req   √x7ᵗʰ Placeholder   Unacceptable PDx   Questionable PDx   Wrong Procedure   Manifestation   Unspecified Dx   H1 - H14 HAC   HCC CMS-HCC Dx   HIV HIV Dx

ICD-10-CM 2020   1223

Chapter 20. External Causes of Morbidity   V31.1–V37.9

☑4ᵗʰ **V38 Occupant of three-wheeled motor vehicle injured in noncollision transport accident**

    INCLUDES   fall or thrown from three-wheeled motor vehicle

           overturning of three-wheeled motor vehicle NOS

           overturning of three-wheeled motor vehicle without collision

☑x7ᵗʰ **V38.0 Driver** of three-wheeled motor vehicle injured in noncollision transport accident **in nontraffic accident**

☑x7ᵗʰ **V38.1 Passenger** in three-wheeled motor vehicle injured in noncollision transport accident **in nontraffic accident**

☑x7ᵗʰ **V38.2 Person on outside** of three-wheeled motor vehicle injured in noncollision transport accident **in nontraffic accident**

☑x7ᵗʰ **V38.3 Unspecified occupant** of three-wheeled motor vehicle injured in noncollision transport accident **in nontraffic accident**

☑x7ᵗʰ **V38.4 Person boarding or alighting** a three-wheeled motor vehicle injured in noncollision transport accident

☑x7ᵗʰ **V38.5 Driver** of three-wheeled motor vehicle injured in noncollision transport accident **in traffic accident**

☑x7ᵗʰ **V38.6 Passenger** in three-wheeled motor vehicle injured in noncollision transport accident **in traffic accident**

☑x7ᵗʰ **V38.7 Person on outside** of three-wheeled motor vehicle injured in noncollision transport accident **in traffic accident**

☑x7ᵗʰ **V38.9 Unspecified occupant** of three-wheeled motor vehicle injured in noncollision transport accident **in traffic accident**

☑4ᵗʰ **V39 Occupant of three-wheeled motor vehicle injured in other and unspecified transport accidents**

☑5ᵗʰ **V39.0 Driver** of three-wheeled motor vehicle injured in collision with other and unspecified motor vehicles **in nontraffic accident**

    ☑x7ᵗʰ **V39.00** Driver of three-wheeled motor vehicle injured in collision with unspecified motor vehicles in nontraffic accident

    ☑x7ᵗʰ **V39.09** Driver of three-wheeled motor vehicle injured in collision with other motor vehicles in nontraffic accident

☑5ᵗʰ **V39.1 Passenger** in three-wheeled motor vehicle injured in collision with other and unspecified motor vehicles **in nontraffic accident**

    ☑x7ᵗʰ **V39.10** Passenger in three-wheeled motor vehicle injured in collision with unspecified motor vehicles in nontraffic accident

    ☑x7ᵗʰ **V39.19** Passenger in three-wheeled motor vehicle injured in collision with other motor vehicles in nontraffic accident

☑5ᵗʰ **V39.2 Unspecified occupant** of three-wheeled motor vehicle injured in collision with other and unspecified motor vehicles **in nontraffic accident**

    ☑x7ᵗʰ **V39.20** Unspecified occupant of three-wheeled motor vehicle injured in collision with unspecified motor vehicles in nontraffic accident

           Collision NOS involving three-wheeled motor vehicle, nontraffic

    ☑x7ᵗʰ **V39.29** Unspecified occupant of three-wheeled motor vehicle injured in collision with other motor vehicles in nontraffic accident

☑x7ᵗʰ **V39.3 Occupant (driver) (passenger)** of three-wheeled motor vehicle injured in unspecified nontraffic accident

           Accident NOS involving three-wheeled motor vehicle, nontraffic

           Occupant of three-wheeled motor vehicle injured in nontraffic accident NOS

☑5ᵗʰ **V39.4 Driver** of three-wheeled motor vehicle injured in collision with other and unspecified motor vehicles **in traffic accident**

    ☑x7ᵗʰ **V39.40** Driver of three-wheeled motor vehicle injured in collision with unspecified motor vehicles in traffic accident

    ☑x7ᵗʰ **V39.49** Driver of three-wheeled motor vehicle injured in collision with other motor vehicles in traffic accident

☑5ᵗʰ **V39.5 Passenger** in three-wheeled motor vehicle injured in collision with other and unspecified motor vehicles **in traffic accident**

    ☑x7ᵗʰ **V39.50** Passenger in three-wheeled motor vehicle injured in collision with unspecified motor vehicles in traffic accident

    ☑x7ᵗʰ **V39.59** Passenger in three-wheeled motor vehicle injured in collision with other motor vehicles in traffic accident

☑5ᵗʰ **V39.6 Unspecified occupant** of three-wheeled motor vehicle injured in collision with other and unspecified motor vehicles **in traffic accident**

    ☑x7ᵗʰ **V39.60** Unspecified occupant of three-wheeled motor vehicle injured in collision with unspecified motor vehicles in traffic accident

           Collision NOS involving three-wheeled motor vehicle (traffic)

    ☑x7ᵗʰ **V39.69** Unspecified occupant of three-wheeled motor vehicle injured in collision with other motor vehicles in traffic accident

☑5ᵗʰ **V39.8 Occupant (driver) (passenger)** of three-wheeled motor vehicle injured in other specified transport accidents

    ☑x7ᵗʰ **V39.81** Occupant (driver) (passenger) of three-wheeled motor vehicle injured in transport accident with military vehicle

    ☑x7ᵗʰ **V39.89** Occupant (driver) (passenger) of three-wheeled motor vehicle injured in other specified transport accidents

☑x7ᵗʰ **V39.9 Occupant (driver) (passenger)** of three-wheeled motor vehicle injured in unspecified traffic accident

           Accident NOS involving three-wheeled motor vehicle

Car occupant injured in transport accident (V40–V49)

    INCLUDES   a four-wheeled motor vehicle designed primarily for carrying passengers

           automobile (pulling a trailer or camper)

    EXCLUDES 1   bus (V50-V59)

           minibus (V50-V59)

           minivan (V50-V59)

           motorcoach (V70-V79)

           pick-up truck (V50-V59)

           sport utility vehicle (SUV) (V50-V59)

The appropriate 7th character is to be added to each code from categories V40-V49.

A   initial encounter

D   subsequent encounter

S   sequela

☑4ᵗʰ **V40 Car occupant injured in collision with pedestrian or animal**

    EXCLUDES 1   car collision with animal-drawn vehicle or animal being ridden (V46.-)

☑x7ᵗʰ **V40.0 Car driver** injured in collision with pedestrian or animal **in nontraffic accident**

☑x7ᵗʰ **V40.1 Car passenger** injured in collision with pedestrian or animal **in nontraffic accident**

☑x7ᵗʰ **V40.2 Person on outside** of car injured in collision with pedestrian or animal **in nontraffic accident**

☑x7ᵗʰ **V40.3 Unspecified car occupant** injured in collision with pedestrian or animal **in nontraffic accident**

☑x7ᵗʰ **V40.4 Person boarding or alighting** a car injured in collision with pedestrian or animal

☑x7ᵗʰ **V40.5 Car driver** injured in collision with pedestrian or animal **in traffic accident**

☑x7ᵗʰ **V40.6 Car passenger** injured in collision with pedestrian or animal **in traffic accident**

☑x7ᵗʰ **V40.7 Person on outside** of car injured in collision with pedestrian or animal **in traffic accident**

☑x7ᵗʰ **V40.9 Unspecified car occupant** injured in collision with pedestrian or animal **in traffic accident**

☑4ᵗʰ **V41 Car occupant injured in collision with pedal cycle**

☑x7ᵗʰ **V41.0 Car driver** injured in collision with pedal cycle **in nontraffic accident**

☑x7ᵗʰ **V41.1 Car passenger** injured in collision with pedal cycle **in nontraffic accident**

☑x7ᵗʰ **V41.2 Person on outside** of car injured in collision with pedal cycle **in nontraffic accident**

☑x7ᵗʰ **V41.3 Unspecified car occupant** injured in collision with pedal cycle **in nontraffic accident**

☑x7ᵗʰ **V41.4 Person boarding or alighting** a car injured in collision with pedal cycle

☑x7ᵗʰ **V41.5 Car driver** injured in collision with pedal cycle **in traffic accident**

☑x7ᵗʰ **V41.6 Car passenger** injured in collision with pedal cycle **in traffic accident**

☑x7ᵗʰ **V41.7 Person on outside** of car injured in collision with pedal cycle **in traffic accident**

☑x7ᵗʰ **V41.9 Unspecified car occupant** injured in collision with pedal cycle **in traffic accident**

N Newborn: 0   P Pediatric: 0-17   M Maternity: 9-64   A Adult: 15-124   MCC Major Complication/Comorbidity   CC Complication/Comorbidity   SW Severe Wound Dx

1224   ICD-10-CM 2020

☑4ᵗʰ **V42** **Car occupant injured in collision with two- or three-wheeled motor vehicle**

☑x7ᵗʰ **V42.0** Car driver injured in collision with two- or three-wheeled motor vehicle in nontraffic accident

☑x7ᵗʰ **V42.1** Car passenger injured in collision with two- or three-wheeled motor vehicle in nontraffic accident

☑x7ᵗʰ **V42.2** Person on outside of car injured in collision with two- or three-wheeled motor vehicle in nontraffic accident

☑x7ᵗʰ **V42.3** Unspecified car occupant injured in collision with two- or three-wheeled motor vehicle in nontraffic accident

☑x7ᵗʰ **V42.4** Person boarding or alighting a car injured in collision with two- or three-wheeled motor vehicle

☑x7ᵗʰ **V42.5** Car driver injured in collision with two- or three-wheeled motor vehicle in traffic accident

☑x7ᵗʰ **V42.6** Car passenger injured in collision with two- or three-wheeled motor vehicle in traffic accident

☑x7ᵗʰ **V42.7** Person on outside of car injured in collision with two- or three-wheeled motor vehicle in traffic accident

☑x7ᵗʰ **V42.9** Unspecified car occupant injured in collision with two- or three-wheeled motor vehicle in traffic accident

☑4ᵗʰ **V43** **Car occupant injured in collision with car, pick-up truck or van**

☑5ᵗʰ **V43.0** Car driver injured in collision with car, pick-up truck or van in nontraffic accident

☑x7ᵗʰ **V43.01** Car driver injured in collision with sport utility vehicle in nontraffic accident

☑x7ᵗʰ **V43.02** Car driver injured in collision with other type car in nontraffic accident

☑x7ᵗʰ **V43.03** Car driver injured in collision with pick-up truck in nontraffic accident

☑x7ᵗʰ **V43.04** Car driver injured in collision with van in nontraffic accident

☑5ᵗʰ **V43.1** Car passenger injured in collision with car, pick-up truck or van in nontraffic accident

☑x7ᵗʰ **V43.11** Car passenger injured in collision with sport utility vehicle in nontraffic accident

☑x7ᵗʰ **V43.12** Car passenger injured in collision with other type car in nontraffic accident

☑x7ᵗʰ **V43.13** Car passenger injured in collision with pick-up truck in nontraffic accident

☑x7ᵗʰ **V43.14** Car passenger injured in collision with van in nontraffic accident

☑5ᵗʰ **V43.2** Person on outside of car injured in collision with car, pick-up truck or van in nontraffic accident

☑x7ᵗʰ **V43.21** Person on outside of car injured in collision with sport utility vehicle in nontraffic accident

☑x7ᵗʰ **V43.22** Person on outside of car injured in collision with other type car in nontraffic accident

☑x7ᵗʰ **V43.23** Person on outside of car injured in collision with pick-up truck in nontraffic accident

☑x7ᵗʰ **V43.24** Person on outside of car injured in collision with van in nontraffic accident

☑5ᵗʰ **V43.3** Unspecified car occupant injured in collision with car, pick-up truck or van in nontraffic accident

☑x7ᵗʰ **V43.31** Unspecified car occupant injured in collision with sport utility vehicle in nontraffic accident

☑x7ᵗʰ **V43.32** Unspecified car occupant injured in collision with other type car in nontraffic accident

☑x7ᵗʰ **V43.33** Unspecified car occupant injured in collision with pick-up truck in nontraffic accident

☑x7ᵗʰ **V43.34** Unspecified car occupant injured in collision with van in nontraffic accident

☑5ᵗʰ **V43.4** Person boarding or alighting a car injured in collision with car, pick-up truck or van

☑x7ᵗʰ **V43.41** Person boarding or alighting a car injured in collision with sport utility vehicle

☑x7ᵗʰ **V43.42** Person boarding or alighting a car injured in collision with other type car

☑x7ᵗʰ **V43.43** Person boarding or alighting a car injured in collision with pick-up truck

☑x7ᵗʰ **V43.44** Person boarding or alighting a car injured in collision with van

☑5ᵗʰ **V43.5** Car driver injured in collision with car, pick-up truck or van in traffic accident

☑x7ᵗʰ **V43.51** Car driver injured in collision with sport utility vehicle in traffic accident

☑x7ᵗʰ **V43.52** Car driver injured in collision with other type car in traffic accident

☑x7ᵗʰ **V43.53** Car driver injured in collision with pick-up truck in traffic accident

☑x7ᵗʰ **V43.54** Car driver injured in collision with van in traffic accident

☑5ᵗʰ **V43.6** Car passenger injured in collision with car, pick-up truck or van in traffic accident

☑x7ᵗʰ **V43.61** Car passenger injured in collision with sport utility vehicle in traffic accident

☑x7ᵗʰ **V43.62** Car passenger injured in collision with other type car in traffic accident

☑x7ᵗʰ **V43.63** Car passenger injured in collision with pick-up truck in traffic accident

☑x7ᵗʰ **V43.64** Car passenger injured in collision with van in traffic accident

☑5ᵗʰ **V43.7** Person on outside of car injured in collision with car, pick-up truck or van in traffic accident

☑x7ᵗʰ **V43.71** Person on outside of car injured in collision with sport utility vehicle in traffic accident

☑x7ᵗʰ **V43.72** Person on outside of car injured in collision with other type car in traffic accident

☑x7ᵗʰ **V43.73** Person on outside of car injured in collision with pick-up truck in traffic accident

☑x7ᵗʰ **V43.74** Person on outside of car injured in collision with van in traffic accident

☑5ᵗʰ **V43.9** Unspecified car occupant injured in collision with car, pick-up truck or van in traffic accident

☑x7ᵗʰ **V43.91** Unspecified car occupant injured in collision with sport utility vehicle in traffic accident

☑x7ᵗʰ **V43.92** Unspecified car occupant injured in collision with other type car in traffic accident

☑x7ᵗʰ **V43.93** Unspecified car occupant injured in collision with pick-up truck in traffic accident

☑x7ᵗʰ **V43.94** Unspecified car occupant injured in collision with van in traffic accident

☑4ᵗʰ **V44** **Car occupant injured in collision with heavy transport vehicle or bus**

> **EXCLUDES 1**   car occupant injured in collision with military vehicle (V49.81)

☑x7ᵗʰ **V44.0** Car driver injured in collision with heavy transport vehicle or bus in nontraffic accident

☑x7ᵗʰ **V44.1** Car passenger injured in collision with heavy transport vehicle or bus in nontraffic accident

☑x7ᵗʰ **V44.2** Person on outside of car injured in collision with heavy transport vehicle or bus in nontraffic accident

☑x7ᵗʰ **V44.3** Unspecified car occupant injured in collision with heavy transport vehicle or bus in nontraffic accident

☑x7ᵗʰ **V44.4** Person boarding or alighting a car injured in collision with heavy transport vehicle or bus

☑x7ᵗʰ **V44.5** Car driver injured in collision with heavy transport vehicle or bus in traffic accident

☑x7ᵗʰ **V44.6** Car passenger injured in collision with heavy transport vehicle or bus in traffic accident

☑x7ᵗʰ **V44.7** Person on outside of car injured in collision with heavy transport vehicle or bus in traffic accident

☑x7ᵗʰ **V44.9** Unspecified car occupant injured in collision with heavy transport vehicle or bus in traffic accident

☑4ᵗʰ **V45** **Car occupant injured in collision with railway train or railway vehicle**

☑x7ᵗʰ **V45.0** Car driver injured in collision with railway train or railway vehicle in nontraffic accident

☑x7ᵗʰ **V45.1** Car passenger injured in collision with railway train or railway vehicle in nontraffic accident

☑x7ᵗʰ **V45.2** Person on outside of car injured in collision with railway train or railway vehicle in nontraffic accident

☑x7ᵗʰ **V45.3** Unspecified car occupant injured in collision with railway train or railway vehicle in nontraffic accident

☑x7ᵗʰ **V45.4** Person boarding or alighting a car injured in collision with railway train or railway vehicle

☑x7ᵗʰ **V45.5** Car driver injured in collision with railway train or railway vehicle in traffic accident

☑x7ᵗʰ **V45.6** Car passenger injured in collision with railway train or railway vehicle in traffic accident

☑x7ᵗʰ **V45.7** Person on outside of car injured in collision with railway train or railway vehicle in traffic accident

☑x7ᵗʰ **V45.9** Unspecified car occupant injured in collision with railway train or railway vehicle in traffic accident

☑4ᵗʰ **V46** **Car occupant injured in collision with other nonmotor vehicle**

> **INCLUDES**   collision with animal-drawn vehicle, animal being ridden, streetcar

☑x7ᵗʰ **V46.0** Car driver injured in collision with other nonmotor vehicle in nontraffic accident

☑x7ᵗʰ **V46.1** Car passenger injured in collision with other nonmotor vehicle in nontraffic accident

☑x7ᵗʰ **V46.2** Person on outside of car injured in collision with other nonmotor vehicle in nontraffic accident

---

☑ Additional Char Req   ☑x7ᵗʰ Placeholder   Unacceptable PDx   Questionable PDx   Wrong Procedure   Manifestation   Unspecified Dx   H1-H14 HAC   HCC CMS-HCC Dx   HIV HIV Dx

ICD-10-CM 2020   1225

√x7ᵗʰ **V46.3** **Unspecified car occupant** injured in collision with other nonmotor vehicle in nontraffic accident

√x7ᵗʰ **V46.4** **Person boarding or alighting** a car injured in collision with other nonmotor vehicle

√x7ᵗʰ **V46.5** **Car driver** injured in collision with other nonmotor vehicle in traffic accident

√x7ᵗʰ **V46.6** **Car passenger** injured in collision with other nonmotor vehicle in traffic accident

√x7ᵗʰ **V46.7** **Person on outside** of car injured in collision with other nonmotor vehicle in traffic accident

√x7ᵗʰ **V46.9** **Unspecified car occupant** injured in collision with other nonmotor vehicle in traffic accident

√4ᵗʰ **V47** **Car occupant injured in collision with fixed or stationary object**

AHA: 2016,4Q,73

√x7ᵗʰ **V47.0** **Car driver** injured in collision with fixed or stationary object in nontraffic accident

√x7ᵗʰ **V47.1** **Car passenger** injured in collision with fixed or stationary object in nontraffic accident

√x7ᵗʰ **V47.2** **Person on outside** of car injured in collision with fixed or stationary object in nontraffic accident

√x7ᵗʰ **V47.3** **Unspecified car occupant** injured in collision with fixed or stationary object in nontraffic accident

√x7ᵗʰ **V47.4** **Person boarding or alighting** a car injured in collision with fixed or stationary object

√x7ᵗʰ **V47.5** **Car driver** injured in collision with fixed or stationary object in traffic accident

√x7ᵗʰ **V47.6** **Car passenger** injured in collision with fixed or stationary object in traffic accident

√x7ᵗʰ **V47.7** **Person on outside** of car injured in collision with fixed or stationary object in traffic accident

√x7ᵗʰ **V47.9** **Unspecified car occupant** injured in collision with fixed or stationary object in traffic accident

√4ᵗʰ **V48** **Car occupant injured in noncollision transport accident**

INCLUDES   overturning car NOS
            overturning car without collision

√x7ᵗʰ **V48.0** **Car driver** injured in noncollision transport accident in nontraffic accident

√x7ᵗʰ **V48.1** **Car passenger** injured in noncollision transport accident in nontraffic accident

√x7ᵗʰ **V48.2** **Person on outside** of car injured in noncollision transport accident in nontraffic accident

√x7ᵗʰ **V48.3** **Unspecified car occupant** injured in noncollision transport accident in nontraffic accident

√x7ᵗʰ **V48.4** **Person boarding or alighting** a car injured in noncollision transport accident

√x7ᵗʰ **V48.5** **Car driver** injured in noncollision transport accident in traffic accident

√x7ᵗʰ **V48.6** **Car passenger** injured in noncollision transport accident in traffic accident

√x7ᵗʰ **V48.7** **Person on outside** of car injured in noncollision transport accident in traffic accident

√x7ᵗʰ **V48.9** **Unspecified car occupant** injured in noncollision transport accident in traffic accident

√4ᵗʰ **V49** **Car occupant injured in other and unspecified transport accidents**

√5ᵗʰ **V49.0** **Driver** injured in collision with other and unspecified motor vehicles in nontraffic accident

√x7ᵗʰ **V49.00** **Driver** injured in collision with unspecified motor vehicles in nontraffic accident

√x7ᵗʰ **V49.09** **Driver** injured in collision with other motor vehicles in nontraffic accident

√5ᵗʰ **V49.1** **Passenger** injured in collision with other and unspecified motor vehicles in nontraffic accident

√x7ᵗʰ **V49.10** **Passenger** injured in collision with unspecified motor vehicles in nontraffic accident

√x7ᵗʰ **V49.19** **Passenger** injured in collision with other motor vehicles in nontraffic accident

√5ᵗʰ **V49.2** **Unspecified car occupant** injured in collision with other and unspecified motor vehicles in nontraffic accident

√x7ᵗʰ **V49.20** **Unspecified car occupant** injured in collision with unspecified motor vehicles in nontraffic accident
      Car collision NOS, nontraffic

√x7ᵗʰ **V49.29** **Unspecified car occupant** injured in collision with other motor vehicles in nontraffic accident

√x7ᵗʰ **V49.3** **Car occupant (driver) (passenger)** injured in unspecified nontraffic accident
      Car accident NOS, nontraffic
      Car occupant injured in nontraffic accident NOS

√5ᵗʰ **V49.4** **Driver** injured in collision with other and unspecified motor vehicles in traffic accident

√x7ᵗʰ **V49.40** **Driver** injured in collision with unspecified motor vehicles in traffic accident

√x7ᵗʰ **V49.49** **Driver** injured in collision with other motor vehicles in traffic accident

√5ᵗʰ **V49.5** **Passenger** injured in collision with other and unspecified motor vehicles in traffic accident

√x7ᵗʰ **V49.50** **Passenger** injured in collision with unspecified motor vehicles in traffic accident

√x7ᵗʰ **V49.59** **Passenger** injured in collision with other motor vehicles in traffic accident

√5ᵗʰ **V49.6** **Unspecified car occupant** injured in collision with other and unspecified motor vehicles in traffic accident

√x7ᵗʰ **V49.60** **Unspecified car occupant** injured in collision with unspecified motor vehicles in traffic accident
      Car collision NOS (traffic)

√x7ᵗʰ **V49.69** **Unspecified car occupant** injured in collision with other motor vehicles in traffic accident

√5ᵗʰ **V49.8** **Car occupant (driver) (passenger)** injured in other specified transport accidents

√x7ᵗʰ **V49.81** **Car occupant (driver) (passenger)** injured in transport accident with military vehicle

√x7ᵗʰ **V49.88** **Car occupant (driver) (passenger)** injured in other specified transport accidents

√x7ᵗʰ **V49.9** **Car occupant (driver) (passenger)** injured in unspecified traffic accident
      Car accident NOS

Occupant of pick-up truck or van injured in transport accident (V50-V59)

INCLUDES   a four or six wheel motor vehicle designed primarily for carrying passengers and property but weighing less than the local limit for classification as a heavy goods vehicle
           minibus
           minivan
           sport utility vehicle (SUV)
           truck
           van

EXCLUDES 1   *heavy transport vehicle (V60-V69)*

The appropriate 7th character is to be added to each code from categories V50-V59.
A   initial encounter
D   subsequent encounter
S   sequela

√4ᵗʰ **V50** **Occupant of pick-up truck or van injured in collision with pedestrian or animal**

EXCLUDES 1   *pick-up truck or van collision with animal-drawn vehicle or animal being ridden (V56.-)*

√x7ᵗʰ **V50.0** **Driver** of pick-up truck or van injured in collision with pedestrian or animal in nontraffic accident

√x7ᵗʰ **V50.1** **Passenger** in pick-up truck or van injured in collision with pedestrian or animal in nontraffic accident

√x7ᵗʰ **V50.2** **Person on outside** of pick-up truck or van injured in collision with pedestrian or animal in nontraffic accident

√x7ᵗʰ **V50.3** **Unspecified occupant** of pick-up truck or van injured in collision with pedestrian or animal in nontraffic accident

√x7ᵗʰ **V50.4** **Person boarding or alighting** a pick-up truck or van injured in collision with pedestrian or animal

√x7ᵗʰ **V50.5** **Driver** of pick-up truck or van injured in collision with pedestrian or animal in traffic accident

√x7ᵗʰ **V50.6** **Passenger** in pick-up truck or van injured in collision with pedestrian or animal in traffic accident

√x7ᵗʰ **V50.7** **Person on outside** of pick-up truck or van injured in collision with pedestrian or animal in traffic accident

√x7ᵗʰ **V50.9** **Unspecified occupant** of pick-up truck or van injured in collision with pedestrian or animal in traffic accident

√4ᵗʰ **V51** **Occupant of pick-up truck or van injured in collision with pedal cycle**

√x7ᵗʰ **V51.0** **Driver** of pick-up truck or van injured in collision with pedal cycle in nontraffic accident

√x7ᵗʰ **V51.1** **Passenger** in pick-up truck or van injured in collision with pedal cycle in nontraffic accident

√x7ᵗʰ **V51.2** **Person on outside** of pick-up truck or van injured in collision with pedal cycle in nontraffic accident

√x7ᵗʰ **V51.3** **Unspecified occupant** of pick-up truck or van injured in collision with pedal cycle in nontraffic accident

√x7ᵗʰ **V51.4** **Person boarding or alighting** a pick-up truck or van injured in collision with pedal cycle

√x7ᵗʰ **V51.5** **Driver** of pick-up truck or van injured in collision with pedal cycle in traffic accident

√x7ᵗʰ **V51.6** Passenger in pick-up truck or van injured in collision with pedal cycle in traffic accident

√x7ᵗʰ **V51.7** Person on outside of pick-up truck or van injured in collision with pedal cycle in traffic accident

√x7ᵗʰ **V51.9** Unspecified occupant of pick-up truck or van injured in collision with pedal cycle in traffic accident

√4ᵗʰ **V52** Occupant of pick-up truck or van injured in collision with two- or three-wheeled motor vehicle

√x7ᵗʰ **V52.0** Driver of pick-up truck or van injured in collision with two- or three-wheeled motor vehicle in nontraffic accident

√x7ᵗʰ **V52.1** Passenger in pick-up truck or van injured in collision with two- or three-wheeled motor vehicle in nontraffic accident

√x7ᵗʰ **V52.2** Person on outside of pick-up truck or van injured in collision with two- or three-wheeled motor vehicle in nontraffic accident

√x7ᵗʰ **V52.3** Unspecified occupant of pick-up truck or van injured in collision with two- or three-wheeled motor vehicle in nontraffic accident

√x7ᵗʰ **V52.4** Person boarding or alighting a pick-up truck or van injured in collision with two- or three-wheeled motor vehicle

√x7ᵗʰ **V52.5** Driver of pick-up truck or van injured in collision with two- or three-wheeled motor vehicle in traffic accident

√x7ᵗʰ **V52.6** Passenger in pick-up truck or van injured in collision with two- or three-wheeled motor vehicle in traffic accident

√x7ᵗʰ **V52.7** Person on outside of pick-up truck or van injured in collision with two- or three-wheeled motor vehicle in traffic accident

√x7ᵗʰ **V52.9** Unspecified occupant of pick-up truck or van injured in collision with two- or three-wheeled motor vehicle in traffic accident

√4ᵗʰ **V53** Occupant of pick-up truck or van injured in collision with car, pick-up truck or van

√x7ᵗʰ **V53.0** Driver of pick-up truck or van injured in collision with car, pick-up truck or van in nontraffic accident

√x7ᵗʰ **V53.1** Passenger in pick-up truck or van injured in collision with car, pick-up truck or van in nontraffic accident

√x7ᵗʰ **V53.2** Person on outside of pick-up truck or van injured in collision with car, pick-up truck or van in nontraffic accident

√x7ᵗʰ **V53.3** Unspecified occupant of pick-up truck or van injured in collision with car, pick-up truck or van in nontraffic accident

√x7ᵗʰ **V53.4** Person boarding or alighting a pick-up truck or van injured in collision with car, pick-up truck or van

√x7ᵗʰ **V53.5** Driver of pick-up truck or van injured in collision with car, pick-up truck or van in traffic accident

√x7ᵗʰ **V53.6** Passenger in pick-up truck or van injured in collision with car, pick-up truck or van in traffic accident

√x7ᵗʰ **V53.7** Person on outside of pick-up truck or van injured in collision with car, pick-up truck or van in traffic accident

√x7ᵗʰ **V53.9** Unspecified occupant of pick-up truck or van injured in collision with car, pick-up truck or van in traffic accident

√4ᵗʰ **V54** Occupant of pick-up truck or van injured in collision with heavy transport vehicle or bus

EXCLUDES 1 occupant of pick-up truck or van injured in collision with military vehicle (V59.81)

√x7ᵗʰ **V54.0** Driver of pick-up truck or van injured in collision with heavy transport vehicle or bus in nontraffic accident

√x7ᵗʰ **V54.1** Passenger in pick-up truck or van injured in collision with heavy transport vehicle or bus in nontraffic accident

√x7ᵗʰ **V54.2** Person on outside of pick-up truck or van injured in collision with heavy transport vehicle or bus in nontraffic accident

√x7ᵗʰ **V54.3** Unspecified occupant of pick-up truck or van injured in collision with heavy transport vehicle or bus in nontraffic accident

√x7ᵗʰ **V54.4** Person boarding or alighting a pick-up truck or van injured in collision with heavy transport vehicle or bus

√x7ᵗʰ **V54.5** Driver of pick-up truck or van injured in collision with heavy transport vehicle or bus in traffic accident

√x7ᵗʰ **V54.6** Passenger in pick-up truck or van injured in collision with heavy transport vehicle or bus in traffic accident

√x7ᵗʰ **V54.7** Person on outside of pick-up truck or van injured in collision with heavy transport vehicle or bus in traffic accident

√x7ᵗʰ **V54.9** Unspecified occupant of pick-up truck or van injured in collision with heavy transport vehicle or bus in traffic accident

√4ᵗʰ **V55** Occupant of pick-up truck or van injured in collision with railway train or railway vehicle

√x7ᵗʰ **V55.0** Driver of pick-up truck or van injured in collision with railway train or railway vehicle in nontraffic accident

√x7ᵗʰ **V55.1** Passenger in pick-up truck or van injured in collision with railway train or railway vehicle in nontraffic accident

√x7ᵗʰ **V55.2** Person on outside of pick-up truck or van injured in collision with railway train or railway vehicle in nontraffic accident

√x7ᵗʰ **V55.3** Unspecified occupant of pick-up truck or van injured in collision with railway train or railway vehicle in nontraffic accident

√x7ᵗʰ **V55.4** Person boarding or alighting a pick-up truck or van injured in collision with railway train or railway vehicle

√x7ᵗʰ **V55.5** Driver of pick-up truck or van injured in collision with railway train or railway vehicle in traffic accident

√x7ᵗʰ **V55.6** Passenger in pick-up truck or van injured in collision with railway train or railway vehicle in traffic accident

√x7ᵗʰ **V55.7** Person on outside of pick-up truck or van injured in collision with railway train or railway vehicle in traffic accident

√x7ᵗʰ **V55.9** Unspecified occupant of pick-up truck or van injured in collision with railway train or railway vehicle in traffic accident

√4ᵗʰ **V56** Occupant of pick-up truck or van injured in collision with other nonmotor vehicle

INCLUDES collision with animal-drawn vehicle, animal being ridden, streetcar

√x7ᵗʰ **V56.0** Driver of pick-up truck or van injured in collision with other nonmotor vehicle in nontraffic accident

√x7ᵗʰ **V56.1** Passenger in pick-up truck or van injured in collision with other nonmotor vehicle in nontraffic accident

√x7ᵗʰ **V56.2** Person on outside of pick-up truck or van injured in collision with other nonmotor vehicle in nontraffic accident

√x7ᵗʰ **V56.3** Unspecified occupant of pick-up truck or van injured in collision with other nonmotor vehicle in nontraffic accident

√x7ᵗʰ **V56.4** Person boarding or alighting a pick-up truck or van injured in collision with other nonmotor vehicle

√x7ᵗʰ **V56.5** Driver of pick-up truck or van injured in collision with other nonmotor vehicle in traffic accident

√x7ᵗʰ **V56.6** Passenger in pick-up truck or van injured in collision with other nonmotor vehicle in traffic accident

√x7ᵗʰ **V56.7** Person on outside of pick-up truck or van injured in collision with other nonmotor vehicle in traffic accident

√x7ᵗʰ **V56.9** Unspecified occupant of pick-up truck or van injured in collision with other nonmotor vehicle in traffic accident

√4ᵗʰ **V57** Occupant of pick-up truck or van injured in collision with fixed or stationary object

√x7ᵗʰ **V57.0** Driver of pick-up truck or van injured in collision with fixed or stationary object in nontraffic accident

√x7ᵗʰ **V57.1** Passenger in pick-up truck or van injured in collision with fixed or stationary object in nontraffic accident

√x7ᵗʰ **V57.2** Person on outside of pick-up truck or van injured in collision with fixed or stationary object in nontraffic accident

√x7ᵗʰ **V57.3** Unspecified occupant of pick-up truck or van injured in collision with fixed or stationary object in nontraffic accident

√x7ᵗʰ **V57.4** Person boarding or alighting a pick-up truck or van injured in collision with fixed or stationary object

√x7ᵗʰ **V57.5** Driver of pick-up truck or van injured in collision with fixed or stationary object in traffic accident

√x7ᵗʰ **V57.6** Passenger in pick-up truck or van injured in collision with fixed or stationary object in traffic accident

√x7ᵗʰ **V57.7** Person on outside of pick-up truck or van injured in collision with fixed or stationary object in traffic accident

√x7ᵗʰ **V57.9** Unspecified occupant of pick-up truck or van injured in collision with fixed or stationary object in traffic accident

√4ᵗʰ **V58** Occupant of pick-up truck or van injured in noncollision transport accident

INCLUDES overturning pick-up truck or van NOS
overturning pick-up truck or van without collision

√x7ᵗʰ **V58.0** Driver of pick-up truck or van injured in noncollision transport accident in nontraffic accident

√x7ᵗʰ **V58.1** Passenger in pick-up truck or van injured in noncollision transport accident in nontraffic accident

√x7ᵗʰ **V58.2** Person on outside of pick-up truck or van injured in noncollision transport accident in nontraffic accident

√x7ᵗʰ **V58.3** Unspecified occupant of pick-up truck or van injured in noncollision transport accident in nontraffic accident

√x7ᵗʰ **V58.4** Person boarding or alighting a pick-up truck or van injured in noncollision transport accident

√x7ᵗʰ **V58.5** Driver of pick-up truck or van injured in noncollision transport accident in traffic accident

√x7ᵗʰ **V58.6** Passenger in pick-up truck or van injured in noncollision transport accident in traffic accident

√x7ᵗʰ **V58.7** Person on outside of pick-up truck or van injured in noncollision transport accident in traffic accident

√x7ᵗʰ **V58.9** Unspecified occupant of pick-up truck or van injured in noncollision transport accident in traffic accident

Chapter 20. External Causes of Morbidity

V51.6–V58.9

Chapter 20. External Causes of Morbidity

V59–V62.9

✓4ᵗʰ **V59** **Occupant of pick-up truck or van injured in other and unspecified transport accidents**

  ✓5ᵗʰ **V59.0** Driver of pick-up truck or van injured in collision with other and unspecified motor vehicles in nontraffic accident

    ✓x7ᵗʰ **V59.00** Driver of pick-up truck or van injured in collision with unspecified motor vehicles in nontraffic accident

    ✓x7ᵗʰ **V59.09** Driver of pick-up truck or van injured in collision with other motor vehicles in nontraffic accident

  ✓5ᵗʰ **V59.1** Passenger in pick-up truck or van injured in collision with other and unspecified motor vehicles in nontraffic accident

    ✓x7ᵗʰ **V59.10** Passenger in pick-up truck or van injured in collision with unspecified motor vehicles in nontraffic accident

    ✓x7ᵗʰ **V59.19** Passenger in pick-up truck or van injured in collision with other motor vehicles in nontraffic accident

  ✓5ᵗʰ **V59.2** Unspecified occupant of pick-up truck or van injured in collision with other and unspecified motor vehicles in nontraffic accident

    ✓x7ᵗʰ **V59.20** Unspecified occupant of pick-up truck or van injured in collision with unspecified motor vehicles in nontraffic accident

      Collision NOS involving pick-up truck or van, nontraffic

    ✓x7ᵗʰ **V59.29** Unspecified occupant of pick-up truck or van injured in collision with other motor vehicles in nontraffic accident

  ✓x7ᵗʰ **V59.3** Occupant (driver) (passenger) of pick-up truck or van injured in unspecified nontraffic accident

      Accident NOS involving pick-up truck or van, nontraffic
      Occupant of pick-up truck or van injured in nontraffic accident NOS

  ✓5ᵗʰ **V59.4** Driver of pick-up truck or van injured in collision with other and unspecified motor vehicles in traffic accident

    ✓x7ᵗʰ **V59.40** Driver of pick-up truck or van injured in collision with unspecified motor vehicles in traffic accident

    ✓x7ᵗʰ **V59.49** Driver of pick-up truck or van injured in collision with other motor vehicles in traffic accident

  ✓5ᵗʰ **V59.5** Passenger in pick-up truck or van injured in collision with other and unspecified motor vehicles in traffic accident

    ✓x7ᵗʰ **V59.50** Passenger in pick-up truck or van injured in collision with unspecified motor vehicles in traffic accident

    ✓x7ᵗʰ **V59.59** Passenger in pick-up truck or van injured in collision with other motor vehicles in traffic accident

  ✓5ᵗʰ **V59.6** Unspecified occupant of pick-up truck or van injured in collision with other and unspecified motor vehicles in traffic accident

    ✓x7ᵗʰ **V59.60** Unspecified occupant of pick-up truck or van injured in collision with unspecified motor vehicles in traffic accident

      Collision NOS involving pick-up truck or van (traffic)

    ✓x7ᵗʰ **V59.69** Unspecified occupant of pick-up truck or van injured in collision with other motor vehicles in traffic accident

  ✓5ᵗʰ **V59.8** Occupant (driver) (passenger) of pick-up truck or van injured in other specified transport accidents

    ✓x7ᵗʰ **V59.81** Occupant (driver) (passenger) of pick-up truck or van injured in transport accident with military vehicle

    ✓x7ᵗʰ **V59.88** Occupant (driver) (passenger) of pick-up truck or van injured in other specified transport accidents

  ✓x7ᵗʰ **V59.9** Occupant (driver) (passenger) of pick-up truck or van injured in unspecified traffic accident

      Accident NOS involving pick-up truck or van

Occupant of heavy transport vehicle injured in transport accident (V60-V69)

INCLUDES   18 wheeler
      armored car
      panel truck
EXCLUDES 1   *bus*
      motorcoach

The appropriate 7th character is to be added to each code from categories V60-V69.
A   initial encounter
D   subsequent encounter
S   sequela

✓4ᵗʰ **V60** **Occupant of heavy transport vehicle injured in collision with pedestrian or animal**

  EXCLUDES 1   *heavy transport vehicle collision with animal-drawn vehicle or animal being ridden (V66.-)*

  ✓x7ᵗʰ **V60.0** Driver of heavy transport vehicle injured in collision with pedestrian or animal in nontraffic accident

  ✓x7ᵗʰ **V60.1** Passenger in heavy transport vehicle injured in collision with pedestrian or animal in nontraffic accident

  ✓x7ᵗʰ **V60.2** Person on outside of heavy transport vehicle injured in collision with pedestrian or animal in nontraffic accident

  ✓x7ᵗʰ **V60.3** Unspecified occupant of heavy transport vehicle injured in collision with pedestrian or animal in nontraffic accident

  ✓x7ᵗʰ **V60.4** Person boarding or alighting a heavy transport vehicle injured in collision with pedestrian or animal

  ✓x7ᵗʰ **V60.5** Driver of heavy transport vehicle injured in collision with pedestrian or animal in traffic accident

  ✓x7ᵗʰ **V60.6** Passenger in heavy transport vehicle injured in collision with pedestrian or animal in traffic accident

  ✓x7ᵗʰ **V60.7** Person on outside of heavy transport vehicle injured in collision with pedestrian or animal in traffic accident

  ✓x7ᵗʰ **V60.9** Unspecified occupant of heavy transport vehicle injured in collision with pedestrian or animal in traffic accident

✓4ᵗʰ **V61** **Occupant of heavy transport vehicle injured in collision with pedal cycle**

  ✓x7ᵗʰ **V61.0** Driver of heavy transport vehicle injured in collision with pedal cycle in nontraffic accident

  ✓x7ᵗʰ **V61.1** Passenger in heavy transport vehicle injured in collision with pedal cycle in nontraffic accident

  ✓x7ᵗʰ **V61.2** Person on outside of heavy transport vehicle injured in collision with pedal cycle in nontraffic accident

  ✓x7ᵗʰ **V61.3** Unspecified occupant of heavy transport vehicle injured in collision with pedal cycle in nontraffic accident

  ✓x7ᵗʰ **V61.4** Person boarding or alighting a heavy transport vehicle injured in collision with pedal cycle while boarding or alighting

  ✓x7ᵗʰ **V61.5** Driver of heavy transport vehicle injured in collision with pedal cycle in traffic accident

  ✓x7ᵗʰ **V61.6** Passenger in heavy transport vehicle injured in collision with pedal cycle in traffic accident

  ✓x7ᵗʰ **V61.7** Person on outside of heavy transport vehicle injured in collision with pedal cycle in traffic accident

  ✓x7ᵗʰ **V61.9** Unspecified occupant of heavy transport vehicle injured in collision with pedal cycle in traffic accident

✓4ᵗʰ **V62** **Occupant of heavy transport vehicle injured in collision with two- or three-wheeled motor vehicle**

  ✓x7ᵗʰ **V62.0** Driver of heavy transport vehicle injured in collision with two- or three-wheeled motor vehicle in nontraffic accident

  ✓x7ᵗʰ **V62.1** Passenger in heavy transport vehicle injured in collision with two- or three-wheeled motor vehicle in nontraffic accident

  ✓x7ᵗʰ **V62.2** Person on outside of heavy transport vehicle injured in collision with two- or three-wheeled motor vehicle in nontraffic accident

  ✓x7ᵗʰ **V62.3** Unspecified occupant of heavy transport vehicle injured in collision with two- or three-wheeled motor vehicle in nontraffic accident

  ✓x7ᵗʰ **V62.4** Person boarding or alighting a heavy transport vehicle injured in collision with two- or three-wheeled motor vehicle

  ✓x7ᵗʰ **V62.5** Driver of heavy transport vehicle injured in collision with two- or three-wheeled motor vehicle in traffic accident

  ✓x7ᵗʰ **V62.6** Passenger in heavy transport vehicle injured in collision with two- or three-wheeled motor vehicle in traffic accident

  ✓x7ᵗʰ **V62.7** Person on outside of heavy transport vehicle injured in collision with two- or three-wheeled motor vehicle in traffic accident

  ✓x7ᵗʰ **V62.9** Unspecified occupant of heavy transport vehicle injured in collision with two- or three-wheeled motor vehicle in traffic accident

N Newborn: 0   P Pediatric: 0-17   M Maternity: 9-64   A Adult: 15-124   MCC Major Complication/Comorbidity   CC Complication/Comorbidity   SW Severe Wound Dx

1228   ICD-10-CM 2020

☑4ᵗʰ **V63 Occupant of heavy transport vehicle injured in collision with car, pick-up truck or van**

☑x7ᵗʰ **V63.0** Driver of heavy transport vehicle injured in collision with car, pick-up truck or van in nontraffic accident

☑x7ᵗʰ **V63.1** Passenger in heavy transport vehicle injured in collision with car, pick-up truck or van in nontraffic accident

☑x7ᵗʰ **V63.2** Person on outside of heavy transport vehicle injured in collision with car, pick-up truck or van in nontraffic accident

☑x7ᵗʰ **V63.3** Unspecified occupant of heavy transport vehicle injured in collision with car, pick-up truck or van in nontraffic accident

☑x7ᵗʰ **V63.4** Person boarding or alighting a heavy transport vehicle injured in collision with car, pick-up truck or van

☑x7ᵗʰ **V63.5** Driver of heavy transport vehicle injured in collision with car, pick-up truck or van in traffic accident

☑x7ᵗʰ **V63.6** Passenger in heavy transport vehicle injured in collision with car, pick-up truck or van in traffic accident

☑x7ᵗʰ **V63.7** Person on outside of heavy transport vehicle injured in collision with car, pick-up truck or van in traffic accident

☑x7ᵗʰ **V63.9** Unspecified occupant of heavy transport vehicle injured in collision with car, pick-up truck or van in traffic accident

☑4ᵗʰ **V64 Occupant of heavy transport vehicle injured in collision with heavy transport vehicle or bus**

> **EXCLUDES 1**   occupant of heavy transport vehicle injured in collision with military vehicle (V69.81)

☑x7ᵗʰ **V64.0** Driver of heavy transport vehicle injured in collision with heavy transport vehicle or bus in nontraffic accident

☑x7ᵗʰ **V64.1** Passenger in heavy transport vehicle injured in collision with heavy transport vehicle or bus in nontraffic accident

☑x7ᵗʰ **V64.2** Person on outside of heavy transport vehicle injured in collision with heavy transport vehicle or bus in nontraffic accident

☑x7ᵗʰ **V64.3** Unspecified occupant of heavy transport vehicle injured in collision with heavy transport vehicle or bus in nontraffic accident

☑x7ᵗʰ **V64.4** Person boarding or alighting a heavy transport vehicle injured in collision with heavy transport vehicle or bus while boarding or alighting

☑x7ᵗʰ **V64.5** Driver of heavy transport vehicle injured in collision with heavy transport vehicle or bus in traffic accident

☑x7ᵗʰ **V64.6** Passenger in heavy transport vehicle injured in collision with heavy transport vehicle or bus in traffic accident

☑x7ᵗʰ **V64.7** Person on outside of heavy transport vehicle injured in collision with heavy transport vehicle or bus in traffic accident

☑x7ᵗʰ **V64.9** Unspecified occupant of heavy transport vehicle injured in collision with heavy transport vehicle or bus in traffic accident

☑4ᵗʰ **V65 Occupant of heavy transport vehicle injured in collision with railway train or railway vehicle**

☑x7ᵗʰ **V65.0** Driver of heavy transport vehicle injured in collision with railway train or railway vehicle in nontraffic accident

☑x7ᵗʰ **V65.1** Passenger in heavy transport vehicle injured in collision with railway train or railway vehicle in nontraffic accident

☑x7ᵗʰ **V65.2** Person on outside of heavy transport vehicle injured in collision with railway train or railway vehicle in nontraffic accident

☑x7ᵗʰ **V65.3** Unspecified occupant of heavy transport vehicle injured in collision with railway train or railway vehicle in nontraffic accident

☑x7ᵗʰ **V65.4** Person boarding or alighting a heavy transport vehicle injured in collision with railway train or railway vehicle

☑x7ᵗʰ **V65.5** Driver of heavy transport vehicle injured in collision with railway train or railway vehicle in traffic accident

☑x7ᵗʰ **V65.6** Passenger in heavy transport vehicle injured in collision with railway train or railway vehicle in traffic accident

☑x7ᵗʰ **V65.7** Person on outside of heavy transport vehicle injured in collision with railway train or railway vehicle in traffic accident

☑x7ᵗʰ **V65.9** Unspecified occupant of heavy transport vehicle injured in collision with railway train or railway vehicle in traffic accident

☑4ᵗʰ **V66 Occupant of heavy transport vehicle injured in collision with other nonmotor vehicle**

> **INCLUDES**   collision with animal-drawn vehicle, animal being ridden, streetcar

☑x7ᵗʰ **V66.0** Driver of heavy transport vehicle injured in collision with other nonmotor vehicle in nontraffic accident

☑x7ᵗʰ **V66.1** Passenger in heavy transport vehicle injured in collision with other nonmotor vehicle in nontraffic accident

☑x7ᵗʰ **V66.2** Person on outside of heavy transport vehicle injured in collision with other nonmotor vehicle in nontraffic accident

☑x7ᵗʰ **V66.3** Unspecified occupant of heavy transport vehicle injured in collision with other nonmotor vehicle in nontraffic accident

☑x7ᵗʰ **V66.4** Person boarding or alighting a heavy transport vehicle injured in collision with other nonmotor vehicle

☑x7ᵗʰ **V66.5** Driver of heavy transport vehicle injured in collision with other nonmotor vehicle in traffic accident

☑x7ᵗʰ **V66.6** Passenger in heavy transport vehicle injured in collision with other nonmotor vehicle in traffic accident

☑x7ᵗʰ **V66.7** Person on outside of heavy transport vehicle injured in collision with other nonmotor vehicle in traffic accident

☑x7ᵗʰ **V66.9** Unspecified occupant of heavy transport vehicle injured in collision with other nonmotor vehicle in traffic accident

☑4ᵗʰ **V67 Occupant of heavy transport vehicle injured in collision with fixed or stationary object**

☑x7ᵗʰ **V67.0** Driver of heavy transport vehicle injured in collision with fixed or stationary object in nontraffic accident

☑x7ᵗʰ **V67.1** Passenger in heavy transport vehicle injured in collision with fixed or stationary object in nontraffic accident

☑x7ᵗʰ **V67.2** Person on outside of heavy transport vehicle injured in collision with fixed or stationary object in nontraffic accident

☑x7ᵗʰ **V67.3** Unspecified occupant of heavy transport vehicle injured in collision with fixed or stationary object in nontraffic accident

☑x7ᵗʰ **V67.4** Person boarding or alighting a heavy transport vehicle injured in collision with fixed or stationary object

☑x7ᵗʰ **V67.5** Driver of heavy transport vehicle injured in collision with fixed or stationary object in traffic accident

☑x7ᵗʰ **V67.6** Passenger in heavy transport vehicle injured in collision with fixed or stationary object in traffic accident

☑x7ᵗʰ **V67.7** Person on outside of heavy transport vehicle injured in collision with fixed or stationary object in traffic accident

☑x7ᵗʰ **V67.9** Unspecified occupant of heavy transport vehicle injured in collision with fixed or stationary object in traffic accident

☑4ᵗʰ **V68 Occupant of heavy transport vehicle injured in noncollision transport accident**

> **INCLUDES**   overturning heavy transport vehicle NOS
> overturning heavy transport vehicle without collision

☑x7ᵗʰ **V68.0** Driver of heavy transport vehicle injured in noncollision transport accident in nontraffic accident

☑x7ᵗʰ **V68.1** Passenger in heavy transport vehicle injured in noncollision transport accident in nontraffic accident

☑x7ᵗʰ **V68.2** Person on outside of heavy transport vehicle injured in noncollision transport accident in nontraffic accident

☑x7ᵗʰ **V68.3** Unspecified occupant of heavy transport vehicle injured in noncollision transport accident in nontraffic accident

☑x7ᵗʰ **V68.4** Person boarding or alighting a heavy transport vehicle injured in noncollision transport accident

☑x7ᵗʰ **V68.5** Driver of heavy transport vehicle injured in noncollision transport accident in traffic accident

☑x7ᵗʰ **V68.6** Passenger in heavy transport vehicle injured in noncollision transport accident in traffic accident

☑x7ᵗʰ **V68.7** Person on outside of heavy transport vehicle injured in noncollision transport accident in traffic accident

☑x7ᵗʰ **V68.9** Unspecified occupant of heavy transport vehicle injured in noncollision transport accident in traffic accident

☑4ᵗʰ **V69 Occupant of heavy transport vehicle injured in other and unspecified transport accidents**

☑5ᵗʰ **V69.0** Driver of heavy transport vehicle injured in collision with other and unspecified motor vehicles in nontraffic accident

     ☑x7ᵗʰ **V69.00** Driver of heavy transport vehicle injured in collision with unspecified motor vehicles in nontraffic accident

     ☑x7ᵗʰ **V69.09** Driver of heavy transport vehicle injured in collision with other motor vehicles in nontraffic accident

☑5ᵗʰ **V69.1** Passenger in heavy transport vehicle injured in collision with other and unspecified motor vehicles in nontraffic accident

     ☑x7ᵗʰ **V69.10** Passenger in heavy transport vehicle injured in collision with unspecified motor vehicles in nontraffic accident

     ☑x7ᵗʰ **V69.19** Passenger in heavy transport vehicle injured in collision with other motor vehicles in nontraffic accident

☑5ᵗʰ **V69.2** Unspecified occupant of heavy transport vehicle injured in collision with other and unspecified motor vehicles in nontraffic accident

     ☑x7ᵗʰ **V69.20** Unspecified occupant of heavy transport vehicle injured in collision with unspecified motor vehicles in nontraffic accident

        Collision NOS involving heavy transport vehicle, nontraffic

☑ Additional Char Req   ☑x7ᵗʰ Placeholder   Unacceptable PDx   Questionable PDx   Wrong Procedure   Manifestation   Unspecified Dx   H1-H14 HAC   HCC CMS-HCC Dx   HIV HIV Dx

ICD-10-CM 2020   1229

√x7th **V69.29** Unspecified occupant of heavy transport vehicle injured in collision with other motor vehicles in nontraffic accident

√x7th **V69.3** Occupant (driver) (passenger) of heavy transport vehicle injured in unspecified nontraffic accident

Accident NOS involving heavy transport vehicle, nontraffic

Occupant of heavy transport vehicle injured in nontraffic accident NOS

√5th **V69.4** Driver of heavy transport vehicle injured in collision with other and unspecified motor vehicles in traffic accident

√x7th **V69.40** Driver of heavy transport vehicle injured in collision with unspecified motor vehicles in traffic accident

√x7th **V69.49** Driver of heavy transport vehicle injured in collision with other motor vehicles in traffic accident

√5th **V69.5** Passenger in heavy transport vehicle injured in collision with other and unspecified motor vehicles in traffic accident

√x7th **V69.50** Passenger in heavy transport vehicle injured in collision with unspecified motor vehicles in traffic accident

√x7th **V69.59** Passenger in heavy transport vehicle injured in collision with other motor vehicles in traffic accident

√5th **V69.6** Unspecified occupant of heavy transport vehicle injured in collision with other and unspecified motor vehicles in traffic accident

√x7th **V69.60** Unspecified occupant of heavy transport vehicle injured in collision with unspecified motor vehicles in traffic accident

Collision NOS involving heavy transport vehicle (traffic)

√x7th **V69.69** Unspecified occupant of heavy transport vehicle injured in collision with other motor vehicles in traffic accident

√5th **V69.8** Occupant (driver) (passenger) of heavy transport vehicle injured in other specified transport accidents

√x7th **V69.81** Occupant (driver) (passenger) of heavy transport vehicle injured in transport accidents with military vehicle

√x7th **V69.88** Occupant (driver) (passenger) of heavy transport vehicle injured in other specified transport accidents

√x7th **V69.9** Occupant (driver) (passenger) of heavy transport vehicle injured in unspecified traffic accident

Accident NOS involving heavy transport vehicle

Bus occupant injured in transport accident (V70-V79)

INCLUDES motorcoach
EXCLUDES 1 minibus (V50-V59)

The appropriate 7th character is to be added to each code from categories V70-V79.
A initial encounter
D subsequent encounter
S sequela

√4th **V70** Bus occupant injured in collision with pedestrian or animal

EXCLUDES 1 bus collision with animal-drawn vehicle or animal being ridden (V76.-)

√x7th **V70.0** Driver of bus injured in collision with pedestrian or animal in nontraffic accident

√x7th **V70.1** Passenger on bus injured in collision with pedestrian or animal in nontraffic accident

√x7th **V70.2** Person on outside of bus injured in collision with pedestrian or animal in nontraffic accident

√x7th **V70.3** Unspecified occupant of bus injured in collision with pedestrian or animal in nontraffic accident

√x7th **V70.4** Person boarding or alighting from bus injured in collision with pedestrian or animal

√x7th **V70.5** Driver of bus injured in collision with pedestrian or animal in traffic accident

√x7th **V70.6** Passenger on bus injured in collision with pedestrian or animal in traffic accident

√x7th **V70.7** Person on outside of bus injured in collision with pedestrian or animal in traffic accident

√x7th **V70.9** Unspecified occupant of bus injured in collision with pedestrian or animal in traffic accident

√4th **V71** Bus occupant injured in collision with pedal cycle

√x7th **V71.0** Driver of bus injured in collision with pedal cycle in nontraffic accident

√x7th **V71.1** Passenger on bus injured in collision with pedal cycle in nontraffic accident

√x7th **V71.2** Person on outside of bus injured in collision with pedal cycle in nontraffic accident

√x7th **V71.3** Unspecified occupant of bus injured in collision with pedal cycle in nontraffic accident

√x7th **V71.4** Person boarding or alighting from bus injured in collision with pedal cycle

√x7th **V71.5** Driver of bus injured in collision with pedal cycle in traffic accident

√x7th **V71.6** Passenger on bus injured in collision with pedal cycle in traffic accident

√x7th **V71.7** Person on outside of bus injured in collision with pedal cycle in traffic accident

√x7th **V71.9** Unspecified occupant of bus injured in collision with pedal cycle in traffic accident

√4th **V72** Bus occupant injured in collision with two- or three-wheeled motor vehicle

√x7th **V72.0** Driver of bus injured in collision with two- or three-wheeled motor vehicle in nontraffic accident

√x7th **V72.1** Passenger on bus injured in collision with two- or three-wheeled motor vehicle in nontraffic accident

√x7th **V72.2** Person on outside of bus injured in collision with two- or three-wheeled motor vehicle in nontraffic accident

√x7th **V72.3** Unspecified occupant of bus injured in collision with two- or three-wheeled motor vehicle in nontraffic accident

√x7th **V72.4** Person boarding or alighting from bus injured in collision with two- or three-wheeled motor vehicle

√x7th **V72.5** Driver of bus injured in collision with two- or three-wheeled motor vehicle in traffic accident

√x7th **V72.6** Passenger on bus injured in collision with two- or three-wheeled motor vehicle in traffic accident

√x7th **V72.7** Person on outside of bus injured in collision with two- or three-wheeled motor vehicle in traffic accident

√x7th **V72.9** Unspecified occupant of bus injured in collision with two- or three-wheeled motor vehicle in traffic accident

√4th **V73** Bus occupant injured in collision with car, pick-up truck or van

√x7th **V73.0** Driver of bus injured in collision with car, pick-up truck or van in nontraffic accident

√x7th **V73.1** Passenger on bus injured in collision with car, pick-up truck or van in nontraffic accident

√x7th **V73.2** Person on outside of bus injured in collision with car, pick-up truck or van in nontraffic accident

√x7th **V73.3** Unspecified occupant of bus injured in collision with car, pick-up truck or van in nontraffic accident

√x7th **V73.4** Person boarding or alighting from bus injured in collision with car, pick-up truck or van

√x7th **V73.5** Driver of bus injured in collision with car, pick-up truck or van in traffic accident

√x7th **V73.6** Passenger on bus injured in collision with car, pick-up truck or van in traffic accident

√x7th **V73.7** Person on outside of bus injured in collision with car, pick-up truck or van in traffic accident

√x7th **V73.9** Unspecified occupant of bus injured in collision with car, pick-up truck or van in traffic accident

√4th **V74** Bus occupant injured in collision with heavy transport vehicle or bus

EXCLUDES 1 bus occupant injured in collision with military vehicle (V79.81)

√x7th **V74.0** Driver of bus injured in collision with heavy transport vehicle or bus in nontraffic accident

√x7th **V74.1** Passenger on bus injured in collision with heavy transport vehicle or bus in nontraffic accident

√x7th **V74.2** Person on outside of bus injured in collision with heavy transport vehicle or bus in nontraffic accident

√x7th **V74.3** Unspecified occupant of bus injured in collision with heavy transport vehicle or bus in nontraffic accident

√x7th **V74.4** Person boarding or alighting from bus injured in collision with heavy transport vehicle or bus

√x7th **V74.5** Driver of bus injured in collision with heavy transport vehicle or bus in traffic accident

√x7th **V74.6** Passenger on bus injured in collision with heavy transport vehicle or bus in traffic accident

√x7th **V74.7** Person on outside of bus injured in collision with heavy transport vehicle or bus in traffic accident

√x7th **V74.9** Unspecified occupant of bus injured in collision with heavy transport vehicle or bus in traffic accident

√4th **V75** Bus occupant injured in collision with railway train or railway vehicle

√x7th **V75.0** Driver of bus injured in collision with railway train or railway vehicle in nontraffic accident

√x7th **V75.1** Passenger on bus injured in collision with railway train or railway vehicle in nontraffic accident

√x7th **V75.2** Person on outside of bus injured in collision with railway train or railway vehicle in nontraffic accident

N Newborn: 0　**P** Pediatric: 0-17　**M** Maternity: 9-64　**A** Adult: 15-124　**MCC** Major Complication/Comorbidity　**CC** Complication/Comorbidity　**SW** Severe Wound Dx

1230　　　　　　　ICD-10-CM 2020

✓x7th **V75.3** Unspecified occupant of bus injured in collision with railway train or railway vehicle in nontraffic accident

✓x7th **V75.4** Person boarding or alighting from bus injured in collision with railway train or railway vehicle

✓x7th **V75.5** Driver of bus injured in collision with railway train or railway vehicle in traffic accident

✓x7th **V75.6** Passenger on bus injured in collision with railway train or railway vehicle in traffic accident

✓x7th **V75.7** Person on outside of bus injured in collision with railway train or railway vehicle in traffic accident

✓x7th **V75.9** Unspecified occupant of bus injured in collision with railway train or railway vehicle in traffic accident

✓4th **V76** Bus occupant injured in collision with other nonmotor vehicle

> INCLUDES   collision with animal-drawn vehicle, animal being ridden, streetcar

✓x7th **V76.0** Driver of bus injured in collision with other nonmotor vehicle in nontraffic accident

✓x7th **V76.1** Passenger on bus injured in collision with other nonmotor vehicle in nontraffic accident

✓x7th **V76.2** Person on outside of bus injured in collision with other nonmotor vehicle in nontraffic accident

✓x7th **V76.3** Unspecified occupant of bus injured in collision with other nonmotor vehicle in nontraffic accident

✓x7th **V76.4** Person boarding or alighting from bus injured in collision with other nonmotor vehicle

✓x7th **V76.5** Driver of bus injured in collision with other nonmotor vehicle in traffic accident

✓x7th **V76.6** Passenger on bus injured in collision with other nonmotor vehicle in traffic accident

✓x7th **V76.7** Person on outside of bus injured in collision with other nonmotor vehicle in traffic accident

✓x7th **V76.9** Unspecified occupant of bus injured in collision with other nonmotor vehicle in traffic accident

✓4th **V77** Bus occupant injured in collision with fixed or stationary object

✓x7th **V77.0** Driver of bus injured in collision with fixed or stationary object in nontraffic accident

✓x7th **V77.1** Passenger on bus injured in collision with fixed or stationary object in nontraffic accident

✓x7th **V77.2** Person on outside of bus injured in collision with fixed or stationary object in nontraffic accident

✓x7th **V77.3** Unspecified occupant of bus injured in collision with fixed or stationary object in nontraffic accident

✓x7th **V77.4** Person boarding or alighting from bus injured in collision with fixed or stationary object

✓x7th **V77.5** Driver of bus injured in collision with fixed or stationary object in traffic accident

✓x7th **V77.6** Passenger on bus injured in collision with fixed or stationary object in traffic accident

✓x7th **V77.7** Person on outside of bus injured in collision with fixed or stationary object in traffic accident

✓x7th **V77.9** Unspecified occupant of bus injured in collision with fixed or stationary object in traffic accident

✓4th **V78** Bus occupant injured in noncollision transport accident

> INCLUDES   overturning bus NOS
> overturning bus without collision

✓x7th **V78.0** Driver of bus injured in noncollision transport accident in nontraffic accident

✓x7th **V78.1** Passenger on bus injured in noncollision transport accident in nontraffic accident

✓x7th **V78.2** Person on outside of bus injured in noncollision transport accident in nontraffic accident

✓x7th **V78.3** Unspecified occupant of bus injured in noncollision transport accident in nontraffic accident

✓x7th **V78.4** Person boarding or alighting from bus injured in noncollision transport accident

✓x7th **V78.5** Driver of bus injured in noncollision transport accident in traffic accident

✓x7th **V78.6** Passenger on bus injured in noncollision transport accident in traffic accident

✓x7th **V78.7** Person on outside of bus injured in noncollision transport accident in traffic accident

✓x7th **V78.9** Unspecified occupant of bus injured in noncollision transport accident in traffic accident

✓4th **V79** Bus occupant injured in other and unspecified transport accidents

✓5th **V79.0** Driver of bus injured in collision with other and unspecified motor vehicles in nontraffic accident

✓x7th **V79.00** Driver of bus injured in collision with unspecified motor vehicles in nontraffic accident

✓x7th **V79.09** Driver of bus injured in collision with other motor vehicles in nontraffic accident

✓5th **V79.1** Passenger on bus injured in collision with other and unspecified motor vehicles in nontraffic accident

✓x7th **V79.10** Passenger on bus injured in collision with unspecified motor vehicles in nontraffic accident

✓x7th **V79.19** Passenger on bus injured in collision with other motor vehicles in nontraffic accident

✓5th **V79.2** Unspecified bus occupant injured in collision with other and unspecified motor vehicles in nontraffic accident

✓x7th **V79.20** Unspecified bus occupant injured in collision with unspecified motor vehicles in nontraffic accident

> Bus collision NOS, nontraffic

✓x7th **V79.29** Unspecified bus occupant injured in collision with other motor vehicles in nontraffic accident

✓x7th **V79.3** Bus occupant (driver) (passenger) injured in unspecified nontraffic accident

> Bus accident NOS, nontraffic
> Bus occupant injured in nontraffic accident NOS

✓5th **V79.4** Driver of bus injured in collision with other and unspecified motor vehicles in traffic accident

✓x7th **V79.40** Driver of bus injured in collision with unspecified motor vehicles in traffic accident

✓x7th **V79.49** Driver of bus injured in collision with other motor vehicles in traffic accident

✓5th **V79.5** Passenger on bus injured in collision with other and unspecified motor vehicles in traffic accident

✓x7th **V79.50** Passenger on bus injured in collision with unspecified motor vehicles in traffic accident

✓x7th **V79.59** Passenger on bus injured in collision with other motor vehicles in traffic accident

✓5th **V79.6** Unspecified bus occupant injured in collision with other and unspecified motor vehicles in traffic accident

✓x7th **V79.60** Unspecified bus occupant injured in collision with unspecified motor vehicles in traffic accident

> Bus collision NOS (traffic)

✓x7th **V79.69** Unspecified bus occupant injured in collision with other motor vehicles in traffic accident

✓5th **V79.8** Bus occupant (driver) (passenger) injured in other specified transport accidents

✓x7th **V79.81** Bus occupant (driver) (passenger) injured in transport accidents with military vehicle

✓x7th **V79.88** Bus occupant (driver) (passenger) injured in other specified transport accidents

✓x7th **V79.9** Bus occupant (driver) (passenger) injured in unspecified traffic accident

> Bus accident NOS

Other land transport accidents (V80-V89)

The appropriate 7th character is to be added to each code from categories V80-V89.
A   initial encounter
D   subsequent encounter
S   sequela

✓4th **V80** Animal-rider or occupant of animal-drawn vehicle injured in transport accident

✓5th **V80.0** Animal-rider or occupant of animal drawn vehicle injured by fall from or being thrown from animal or animal-drawn vehicle in noncollision accident

✓6th **V80.01** Animal-rider injured by fall from or being thrown from animal in noncollision accident

✓7th **V80.010** Animal-rider injured by fall from or being thrown from horse in noncollision accident

✓7th **V80.018** Animal-rider injured by fall from or being thrown from other animal in noncollision accident

✓x7th **V80.02** Occupant of animal-drawn vehicle injured by fall from or being thrown from animal-drawn vehicle in noncollision accident

> Overturning animal-drawn vehicle NOS
> Overturning animal-drawn vehicle without collision

✓5th **V80.1** Animal-rider or occupant of animal-drawn vehicle injured in collision with pedestrian or animal

> EXCLUDES 1   animal-rider or animal-drawn vehicle collision with animal-drawn vehicle or animal being ridden (V80.7)

✓x7th **V80.11** Animal-rider injured in collision with pedestrian or animal

✓x7th **V80.12** Occupant of animal-drawn vehicle injured in collision with pedestrian or animal

✓ Additional Char Req   ✓x7th Placeholder   Unacceptable PDx   Questionable PDx   Wrong Procedure   Manifestation   Unspecified Dx   H1-H14 HAC   HCC CMS-HCC Dx   HIV HIV Dx

ICD-10-CM 2020   1231

Chapter 20. External Causes of Morbidity

V80.2–V82.4

✓5ᵗʰ **V80.2** **Animal-rider or occupant of animal-drawn vehicle injured in collision with** pedal cycle

     ✓x7ᵗʰ **V80.21** Animal-rider injured in collision with pedal cycle

     ✓x7ᵗʰ **V80.22** Occupant of animal-drawn vehicle injured in collision with pedal cycle

✓5ᵗʰ **V80.3** **Animal-rider or occupant of animal-drawn vehicle injured in collision with** two- or three-wheeled motor vehicle

     ✓x7ᵗʰ **V80.31** Animal-rider injured in collision with two- or three-wheeled motor vehicle

     ✓x7ᵗʰ **V80.32** Occupant of animal-drawn vehicle injured in collision with two- or three-wheeled motor vehicle

✓5ᵗʰ **V80.4** **Animal-rider or occupant of animal-drawn vehicle injured in collision with** car, pick-up truck, van, heavy transport vehicle or bus

     EXCLUDES 1   *animal-rider injured in collision with military vehicle (V80.910)*

                occupant of animal-drawn vehicle injured in collision with military vehicle (V80.920)

     ✓x7ᵗʰ **V80.41** Animal-rider injured in collision with car, pick-up truck, van, heavy transport vehicle or bus

     ✓x7ᵗʰ **V80.42** Occupant of animal-drawn vehicle injured in collision with car, pick-up truck, van, heavy transport vehicle or bus

✓5ᵗʰ **V80.5** **Animal-rider or occupant of animal-drawn vehicle injured in collision with other specified motor vehicle**

     ✓x7ᵗʰ **V80.51** Animal-rider injured in collision with other specified motor vehicle

     ✓x7ᵗʰ **V80.52** Occupant of animal-drawn vehicle injured in collision with other specified motor vehicle

✓5ᵗʰ **V80.6** **Animal-rider or occupant of animal-drawn vehicle injured in collision with railway train or railway vehicle**

     ✓x7ᵗʰ **V80.61** Animal-rider injured in collision with railway train or railway vehicle

     ✓x7ᵗʰ **V80.62** Occupant of animal-drawn vehicle injured in collision with railway train or railway vehicle

✓5ᵗʰ **V80.7** **Animal-rider or occupant of animal-drawn vehicle injured in collision with other nonmotor vehicles**

     ✓6ᵗʰ **V80.71** Animal-rider or occupant of animal-drawn vehicle injured in collision with animal being ridden

         ✓7ᵗʰ **V80.710** Animal-rider injured in collision with other animal being ridden

         ✓7ᵗʰ **V80.711** Occupant of animal-drawn vehicle injured in collision with animal being ridden

     ✓6ᵗʰ **V80.72** Animal-rider or occupant of animal-drawn vehicle injured in collision with other animal-drawn vehicle

         ✓7ᵗʰ **V80.720** Animal-rider injured in collision with animal-drawn vehicle

         ✓7ᵗʰ **V80.721** Occupant of animal-drawn vehicle injured in collision with other animal-drawn vehicle

     ✓6ᵗʰ **V80.73** Animal-rider or occupant of animal-drawn vehicle injured in collision with streetcar

         ✓7ᵗʰ **V80.730** Animal-rider injured in collision with streetcar

         ✓7ᵗʰ **V80.731** Occupant of animal-drawn vehicle injured in collision with streetcar

     ✓6ᵗʰ **V80.79** Animal-rider or occupant of animal-drawn vehicle injured in collision with other nonmotor vehicles

         ✓7ᵗʰ **V80.790** Animal-rider injured in collision with other nonmotor vehicles

         ✓7ᵗʰ **V80.791** Occupant of animal-drawn vehicle injured in collision with other nonmotor vehicles

✓5ᵗʰ **V80.8** **Animal-rider or occupant of animal-drawn vehicle injured in collision with** fixed or stationary object

     ✓x7ᵗʰ **V80.81** Animal-rider injured in collision with fixed or stationary object

     ✓x7ᵗʰ **V80.82** Occupant of animal-drawn vehicle injured in collision with fixed or stationary object

✓5ᵗʰ **V80.9** **Animal-rider or occupant of animal-drawn vehicle injured in other and unspecified transport accidents**

     ✓6ᵗʰ **V80.91** Animal-rider injured in other and unspecified transport accidents

         ✓7ᵗʰ **V80.910** Animal-rider injured in transport accident with military vehicle

         ✓7ᵗʰ **V80.918** Animal-rider injured in other transport accident

         ✓7ᵗʰ **V80.919** Animal-rider injured in unspecified transport accident

            Animal rider accident NOS

✓6ᵗʰ **V80.92** Occupant of animal-drawn vehicle injured in other and unspecified transport accidents

     ✓7ᵗʰ **V80.920** Occupant of animal-drawn vehicle injured in transport accident with military vehicle

     ✓7ᵗʰ **V80.928** Occupant of animal-drawn vehicle injured in other transport accident

     ✓7ᵗʰ **V80.929** Occupant of animal-drawn vehicle injured in unspecified transport accident

         Animal-drawn vehicle accident NOS

✓4ᵗʰ **V81** **Occupant of railway train or railway vehicle injured in transport accident**

     INCLUDES   derailment of railway train or railway vehicle

               person on outside of train

     EXCLUDES 1   *streetcar (V82.-)*

✓x7ᵗʰ **V81.0** **Occupant of railway train or railway vehicle injured in collision with motor vehicle** in nontraffic accident

     EXCLUDES 1   *occupant of railway train or railway vehicle injured due to collision with military vehicle (V81.83)*

✓x7ᵗʰ **V81.1** **Occupant of railway train or railway vehicle injured in collision with motor vehicle** in traffic accident

     EXCLUDES 1   *occupant of railway train or railway vehicle injured due to collision with military vehicle (V81.83)*

✓x7ᵗʰ **V81.2** **Occupant of railway train or railway vehicle injured in collision with or** hit by rolling stock

✓x7ᵗʰ **V81.3** **Occupant of railway train or railway vehicle injured in collision with other object**

     Railway collision NOS

✓x7ᵗʰ **V81.4** **Person injured** while boarding or alighting **from railway train or railway vehicle**

✓x7ᵗʰ **V81.5** **Occupant of railway train or railway vehicle injured by** fall in railway train **or railway vehicle**

✓x7ᵗʰ **V81.6** **Occupant of railway train or railway vehicle injured by** fall from railway train **or railway vehicle**

✓x7ᵗʰ **V81.7** **Occupant of railway train or railway vehicle injured in** derailment without antecedent collision

✓5ᵗʰ **V81.8** **Occupant of railway train or railway vehicle injured in other specified railway accidents**

     ✓x7ᵗʰ **V81.81** Occupant of railway train or railway vehicle injured due to explosion or fire on train

     ✓x7ᵗʰ **V81.82** Occupant of railway train or railway vehicle injured due to object falling onto train

         Occupant of railway train or railway vehicle injured due to falling earth onto train

         Occupant of railway train or railway vehicle injured due to falling rocks onto train

         Occupant of railway train or railway vehicle injured due to falling snow onto train

         Occupant of railway train or railway vehicle injured due to falling trees onto train

     ✓x7ᵗʰ **V81.83** Occupant of railway train or railway vehicle injured due to collision with military vehicle

     ✓x7ᵗʰ **V81.89** Occupant of railway train or railway vehicle injured due to other specified railway accident

✓x7ᵗʰ **V81.9** **Occupant of railway train or railway vehicle injured in unspecified railway accident**

     Railway accident NOS

✓4ᵗʰ **V82** **Occupant of powered streetcar injured in transport accident**

     INCLUDES   interurban electric car

               person on outside of streetcar

               tram (car)

               trolley (car)

     EXCLUDES 1   *bus (V70-V79)*

               motorcoach (V70-V79)

               nonpowered streetcar (V76.-)

               train (V81.-)

✓x7ᵗʰ **V82.0** **Occupant of streetcar injured in collision with motor vehicle in nontraffic accident**

✓x7ᵗʰ **V82.1** **Occupant of streetcar injured in collision with motor vehicle in traffic accident**

✓x7ᵗʰ **V82.2** **Occupant of streetcar injured in collision with or** hit by rolling stock

✓x7ᵗʰ **V82.3** **Occupant of streetcar injured in collision with other object**

     EXCLUDES 1   *collision with animal-drawn vehicle or animal being ridden (V82.8)*

✓x7ᵗʰ **V82.4** **Person injured** while boarding or alighting **from streetcar**

Ⓝ Newborn: 0   Ⓟ Pediatric: 0-17   Ⓜ Maternity: 9-64   Ⓐ Adult: 15-124   **MCC** Major Complication/Comorbidity   **CC** Complication/Comorbidity   **SW** Severe Wound Dx

1232   ICD-10-CM 2020

✓x7th V82.5 Occupant of streetcar injured by fall in streetcar

EXCLUDES 1   *fall in streetcar:*
     while boarding or alighting (V82.4)
     with antecedent collision (V82.0-V82.3)

✓x7th V82.6 Occupant of streetcar injured by fall from streetcar

EXCLUDES 1   *fall from streetcar:*
     while boarding or alighting (V82.4)
     with antecedent collision (V82.0-V82.3)

✓x7th V82.7 Occupant of streetcar injured in derailment without antecedent collision

EXCLUDES 1   *occupant of streetcar injured in derailment with antecedent collision (V82.0-V82.3)*

✓x7th V82.8 Occupant of streetcar injured in other specified transport accidents

Streetcar collision with military vehicle
Streetcar collision with train or nonmotor vehicles

✓x7th V82.9 Occupant of streetcar injured in unspecified traffic accident

Streetcar accident NOS

✓4th V83 Occupant of special vehicle mainly used on industrial premises injured in transport accident

INCLUDES   battery-powered airport passenger vehicle
     battery-powered truck (baggage) (mail)
     coal-car in mine
     forklift (truck)
     logging car
     self-propelled industrial truck
     station baggage truck (powered)
     tram, truck, or tub (powered) in mine or quarry

EXCLUDES 1   *special construction vehicles (V85.-)*
     special industrial vehicle in stationary use or maintenance (W31.-)

✓x7th V83.0 Driver of special industrial vehicle injured in traffic accident

✓x7th V83.1 Passenger of special industrial vehicle injured in traffic accident

✓x7th V83.2 Person on outside of special industrial vehicle injured in traffic accident

✓x7th V83.3 Unspecified occupant of special industrial vehicle injured in traffic accident

✓x7th V83.4 Person injured while boarding or alighting from special industrial vehicle

✓x7th V83.5 Driver of special industrial vehicle injured in nontraffic accident

✓x7th V83.6 Passenger of special industrial vehicle injured in nontraffic accident

✓x7th V83.7 Person on outside of special industrial vehicle injured in nontraffic accident

✓x7th V83.9 Unspecified occupant of special industrial vehicle injured in nontraffic accident

Special-industrial-vehicle accident NOS

✓4th V84 Occupant of special vehicle mainly used in agriculture injured in transport accident

INCLUDES   self-propelled farm machinery
     tractor (and trailer)

EXCLUDES 1   *animal-powered farm machinery accident (W30.8-)*
     contact with combine harvester (W30.0)
     special agricultural vehicle in stationary use or maintenance (W30.-)

✓x7th V84.0 Driver of special agricultural vehicle injured in traffic accident

✓x7th V84.1 Passenger of special agricultural vehicle injured in traffic accident

✓x7th V84.2 Person on outside of special agricultural vehicle injured in traffic accident

✓x7th V84.3 Unspecified occupant of special agricultural vehicle injured in traffic accident

✓x7th V84.4 Person injured while boarding or alighting from special agricultural vehicle

✓x7th V84.5 Driver of special agricultural vehicle injured in nontraffic accident

✓x7th V84.6 Passenger of special agricultural vehicle injured in nontraffic accident

✓x7th V84.7 Person on outside of special agricultural vehicle injured in nontraffic accident

✓x7th V84.9 Unspecified occupant of special agricultural vehicle injured in nontraffic accident

Special-agricultural vehicle accident NOS

✓4th V85 Occupant of special construction vehicle injured in transport accident

INCLUDES   bulldozer
     digger
     dump truck
     earth-leveller
     mechanical shovel
     road-roller

EXCLUDES 1   *special industrial vehicle (V83.-)*
     special construction vehicle in stationary use or maintenance (W31.-)

✓x7th V85.0 Driver of special construction vehicle injured in traffic accident

✓x7th V85.1 Passenger of special construction vehicle injured in traffic accident

✓x7th V85.2 Person on outside of special construction vehicle injured in traffic accident

✓x7th V85.3 Unspecified occupant of special construction vehicle injured in traffic accident

✓x7th V85.4 Person injured while boarding or alighting from special construction vehicle

✓x7th V85.5 Driver of special construction vehicle injured in nontraffic accident

✓x7th V85.6 Passenger of special construction vehicle injured in nontraffic accident

✓x7th V85.7 Person on outside of special construction vehicle injured in nontraffic accident

✓x7th V85.9 Unspecified occupant of special construction vehicle injured in nontraffic accident

Special-construction-vehicle accident NOS

✓4th V86 Occupant of special all-terrain or other off-road motor vehicle, injured in transport accident

EXCLUDES 1   *special all-terrain vehicle in stationary use or maintenance (W31.-)*
     sport-utility vehicle (V50-V59)
     three-wheeled motor vehicle designed for on-road use (V30-V39)

AHA: 2017,4Q,26

✓5th V86.0 Driver of special all-terrain or other off-road motor vehicle injured in traffic accident

✓x7th V86.01 Driver of ambulance or fire engine injured in traffic accident

✓x7th V86.02 Driver of snowmobile injured in traffic accident

✓x7th V86.03 Driver of dune buggy injured in traffic accident

✓x7th V86.04 Driver of military vehicle injured in traffic accident

✓x7th V86.05 Driver of 3- or 4- wheeled all-terrain vehicle (ATV) injured in traffic accident

✓x7th V86.06 Driver of dirt bike or motor/cross bike injured in traffic accident

✓x7th V86.09 Driver of other special all-terrain or other off-road motor vehicle injured in traffic accident

~~Driver of dirt bike injured in traffic accident~~
Driver of go cart injured in traffic accident
Driver of golf cart injured in traffic accident

✓5th V86.1 Passenger of special all-terrain or other off-road motor vehicle injured in traffic accident

✓x7th V86.11 Passenger of ambulance or fire engine injured in traffic accident

✓x7th V86.12 Passenger of snowmobile injured in traffic accident

✓x7th V86.13 Passenger of dune buggy injured in traffic accident

✓x7th V86.14 Passenger of military vehicle injured in traffic accident

✓x7th V86.15 Passenger of 3- or 4- wheeled all-terrain vehicle (ATV) injured in traffic accident

✓x7th V86.16 Passenger of dirt bike or motor/cross bike injured in traffic accident

✓x7th V86.19 Passenger of other special all-terrain or other off-road motor vehicle injured in traffic accident

~~Passenger of dirt bike injured in traffic accident~~
Passenger of go cart injured in traffic accident
Passenger of golf cart injured in traffic accident

✓5th V86.2 Person on outside of special all-terrain or other off-road motor vehicle injured in traffic accident

✓x7th V86.21 Person on outside of ambulance or fire engine injured in traffic accident

✓x7th V86.22 Person on outside of snowmobile injured in traffic accident

✓x7th V86.23 Person on outside of dune buggy injured in traffic accident

☑ Additional Char Req   ✓x7th Placeholder   Unacceptable PDx   Questionable PDx   Wrong Procedure   Manifestation   Unspecified Dx   H1-H14 HAC   HCC CMS-HCC Dx   HIV HIV Dx

ICD-10-CM 2020   1233

Chapter 20. External Causes of Morbidity

V86.24–V87.7

√x7th **V86.24** Person on outside of military vehicle injured in traffic accident

√x7th **V86.25** Person on outside of 3- or 4- wheeled all-terrain vehicle (ATV) injured in traffic accident

√x7th **V86.26** Person on outside of dirt bike or motor/cross bike injured in traffic accident

√x7th **V86.29** Person on outside of other special all-terrain or other off-road motor vehicle injured in traffic accident

~~Person on outside of dirt bike injured in traffic accident~~

Person on outside of go cart in traffic accident

Person on outside of golf cart injured in traffic accident

√5th **V86.3** Unspecified occupant of special all-terrain or other off-road motor vehicle injured in traffic accident

√x7th **V86.31** Unspecified occupant of ambulance or fire engine injured in traffic accident

√x7th **V86.32** Unspecified occupant of snowmobile injured in traffic accident

√x7th **V86.33** Unspecified occupant of dune buggy injured in traffic accident

√x7th **V86.34** Unspecified occupant of military vehicle injured in traffic accident

√x7th **V86.35** Unspecified occupant of 3- or 4-wheeled all-terrain vehicle (ATV) injured in traffic accident

√x7th **V86.36** Unspecified occupant of dirt bike or motor/cross bike injured in traffic accident

√x7th **V86.39** Unspecified occupant of other special all-terrain or other off-road motor vehicle injured in traffic accident

~~Unspecified occupant of dirt bike injured in traffic accident~~

Unspecified occupant of go cart injured in traffic accident

Unspecified occupant of golf cart injured in traffic accident

√5th **V86.4** Person injured while boarding or alighting from special all-terrain or other off-road motor vehicle

√x7th **V86.41** Person injured while boarding or alighting from ambulance or fire engine

√x7th **V86.42** Person injured while boarding or alighting from snowmobile

√x7th **V86.43** Person injured while boarding or alighting from dune buggy

√x7th **V86.44** Person injured while boarding or alighting from military vehicle

√x7th **V86.45** Person injured while boarding or alighting from a 3- or 4- wheeled all-terrain vehicle (ATV)

√x7th **V86.46** Person injured while boarding or alighting from a dirt bike or motor/cross bike

√x7th **V86.49** Person injured while boarding or alighting from other special all-terrain or other off-road motor vehicle

~~Person injured while boarding or alighting from dirt bike~~

Person injured while boarding or alighting from go cart

Person injured while boarding or alighting from golf cart

√5th **V86.5** Driver of special all-terrain or other off-road motor vehicle injured in nontraffic accident

√x7th **V86.51** Driver of ambulance or fire engine injured in nontraffic accident

√x7th **V86.52** Driver of snowmobile injured in nontraffic accident

√x7th **V86.53** Driver of dune buggy injured in nontraffic accident

√x7th **V86.54** Driver of military vehicle injured in nontraffic accident

√x7th **V86.55** Driver of 3- or 4- wheeled all-terrain vehicle (ATV) injured in nontraffic accident

√x7th **V86.56** Driver of dirt bike or motor/cross bike injured in nontraffic accident

√x7th **V86.59** Driver of other special all-terrain or other off-road motor vehicle injured in nontraffic accident

~~Driver of dirt bike injured in nontraffic accident~~

Driver of go cart injured in nontraffic accident

Driver of golf cart injured in nontraffic accident

√5th **V86.6** Passenger of special all-terrain or other off-road motor vehicle injured in nontraffic accident

√x7th **V86.61** Passenger of ambulance or fire engine injured in nontraffic accident

√x7th **V86.62** Passenger of snowmobile injured in nontraffic accident

√x7th **V86.63** Passenger of dune buggy injured in nontraffic accident

√x7th **V86.64** Passenger of military vehicle injured in nontraffic accident

√x7th **V86.65** Passenger of 3- or 4- wheeled all-terrain vehicle (ATV) injured in nontraffic accident

√x7th **V86.66** Passenger of dirt bike or motor/cross bike injured in nontraffic accident

√x7th **V86.69** Passenger of other special all-terrain or other off-road motor vehicle injured in nontraffic accident

~~Passenger of dirt bike injured in nontraffic accident~~

Passenger of go cart injured in nontraffic accident

Passenger of golf cart injured in nontraffic accident

√5th **V86.7** Person on outside of special all-terrain or other off-road motor vehicle injured in nontraffic accident

√x7th **V86.71** Person on outside of ambulance or fire engine injured in nontraffic accident

√x7th **V86.72** Person on outside of snowmobile injured in nontraffic accident

√x7th **V86.73** Person on outside of dune buggy injured in nontraffic accident

√x7th **V86.74** Person on outside of military vehicle injured in nontraffic accident

√x7th **V86.75** Person on outside of 3- or 4- wheeled all-terrain vehicle (ATV) injured in nontraffic accident

√x7th **V86.76** Person on outside of dirt bike or motor/cross bike injured in nontraffic accident

√x7th **V86.79** Person on outside of other special all-terrain or other off-road motor vehicles injured in nontraffic accident

~~Person on outside of dirt bike injured in nontraffic accident~~

Person on outside of go cart injured in nontraffic accident

Person on outside of golf cart injured in nontraffic accident

√5th **V86.9** Unspecified occupant of special all-terrain or other off-road motor vehicle injured in nontraffic accident

√x7th **V86.91** Unspecified occupant of ambulance or fire engine injured in nontraffic accident

√x7th **V86.92** Unspecified occupant of snowmobile injured in nontraffic accident

√x7th **V86.93** Unspecified occupant of dune buggy injured in nontraffic accident

√x7th **V86.94** Unspecified occupant of military vehicle injured in nontraffic accident

√x7th **V86.95** Unspecified occupant of 3- or 4- wheeled all-terrain vehicle (ATV) injured in nontraffic accident

√x7th **V86.96** Unspecified occupant of dirt bike or motor/cross bike injured in nontraffic accident

√x7th **V86.99** Unspecified occupant of other special all-terrain or other off-road motor vehicle injured in nontraffic accident

Off-road motor-vehicle accident NOS

Other motor-vehicle accident NOS

Unspecified occupant of go cart injured in nontraffic accident

Unspecified occupant of golf cart injured in nontraffic accident

√4th **V87** Traffic accident of specified type but victim's mode of transport unknown

EXCLUDES 1 collision involving:

pedal cycle (V10-V19)

pedestrian (V01-V09)

√x7th **V87.0** Person injured in collision between car and two- or three-wheeled powered vehicle (traffic)

√x7th **V87.1** Person injured in collision between other motor vehicle and two- or three-wheeled motor vehicle (traffic)

√x7th **V87.2** Person injured in collision between car and pick-up truck or van (traffic)

√x7th **V87.3** Person injured in collision between car and bus (traffic)

√x7th **V87.4** Person injured in collision between car and heavy transport vehicle (traffic)

√x7th **V87.5** Person injured in collision between heavy transport vehicle and bus (traffic)

√x7th **V87.6** Person injured in collision between railway train or railway vehicle and car (traffic)

√x7th **V87.7** Person injured in collision between other specified motor vehicles (traffic)

N Newborn: 0 P Pediatric: 0-17 M Maternity: 9-64 A Adult: 15-124 MCC Major Complication/Comorbidity CC Complication/Comorbidity SW Severe Wound Dx

1234 | ICD-10-CM 2020

☑x7ᵗʰ **V87.8** **Person injured in other specified** noncollision **transport accidents** involving motor vehicle **(traffic)**

☑x7ᵗʰ **V87.9** **Person injured in other specified (collision)(noncollision) transport accidents** involving nonmotor vehicle **(traffic)**

☑4ᵗʰ **V88** **Nontraffic accident of specified type but victim's mode of transport unknown**

> EXCLUDES 1   *collision involving:*
> > *pedal cycle (V10-V19)*
> > *pedestrian (V01-V09)*

☑x7ᵗʰ **V88.0** **Person injured in collision between** car and two- or three-wheeled motor vehicle, **nontraffic**

☑x7ᵗʰ **V88.1** **Person injured in collision between other** motor vehicle and two- or three-wheeled motor vehicle, **nontraffic**

☑x7ᵗʰ **V88.2** **Person injured in collision between** car and pick-up truck or van, **nontraffic**

☑x7ᵗʰ **V88.3** **Person injured in collision between** car and bus, **nontraffic**

☑x7ᵗʰ **V88.4** **Person injured in collision between** car and heavy transport vehicle, **nontraffic**

☑x7ᵗʰ **V88.5** **Person injured in collision between** heavy transport vehicle and bus, **nontraffic**

☑x7ᵗʰ **V88.6** **Person injured in collision between** railway train or railway vehicle and car, **nontraffic**

☑x7ᵗʰ **V88.7** **Person injured in collision between other specified** motor vehicle, **nontraffic**

☑x7ᵗʰ **V88.8** **Person injured in other specified** noncollision **transport accidents** involving motor vehicle, **nontraffic**

☑x7ᵗʰ **V88.9** **Person injured in other specified (collision)(noncollision) transport accidents** involving nonmotor vehicle, **nontraffic**

☑4ᵗʰ **V89** **Motor- or nonmotor-vehicle accident, type of vehicle unspecified**

☑x7ᵗʰ **V89.0** **Person injured in unspecified** motor-vehicle **accident, nontraffic**
> Motor-vehicle accident NOS, nontraffic

☑x7ᵗʰ **V89.1** **Person injured in unspecified** nonmotor-vehicle **accident, nontraffic**
> Nonmotor-vehicle accident NOS (nontraffic)

☑x7ᵗʰ **V89.2** **Person injured in unspecified** motor-vehicle **accident, traffic**
> Motor-vehicle accident [MVA] NOS
> Road (traffic) accident [RTA] NOS

☑x7ᵗʰ **V89.3** **Person injured in unspecified** nonmotor-vehicle **accident, traffic**
> Nonmotor-vehicle traffic accident NOS

☑x7ᵗʰ **V89.9** **Person injured in unspecified vehicle accident**
> Collision NOS

Water transport accidents (V90-V94)

> The appropriate 7th character is to be added to each code from categories V90-V94.
> A   initial encounter
> D   subsequent encounter
> S   sequela

☑4ᵗʰ **V90** **Drowning and submersion due to accident to watercraft**

> EXCLUDES 1   *civilian water transport accident involving military watercraft (V94.81-)*
> > *fall into water not from watercraft (W16.-)*
> > *military watercraft accident in military or war operations (Y36.0-, Y37.0-)*
> > *water-transport-related drowning or submersion without accident to watercraft (V92.-)*

☑5ᵗʰ **V90.0** **Drowning and submersion due to** watercraft overturning

☑x7ᵗʰ **V90.00** **Drowning and submersion due to** merchant ship **overturning**

☑x7ᵗʰ **V90.01** **Drowning and submersion due to** passenger ship **overturning**
> Drowning and submersion due to Ferry-boat overturning
> Drowning and submersion due to Liner overturning

☑x7ᵗʰ **V90.02** **Drowning and submersion due to** fishing boat **overturning**

☑x7ᵗʰ **V90.03** **Drowning and submersion due to other** powered **watercraft overturning**
> Drowning and submersion due to Hovercraft (on open water) overturning
> Drowning and submersion due to Jet ski overturning

☑x7ᵗʰ **V90.04** **Drowning and submersion due to** sailboat **overturning**

☑x7ᵗʰ **V90.05** **Drowning and submersion due to** canoe or kayak **overturning**

☑x7ᵗʰ **V90.06** **Drowning and submersion due to (nonpowered)** inflatable craft **overturning**

☑x7ᵗʰ **V90.08** **Drowning and submersion due to other** unpowered **watercraft overturning**
> Drowning and submersion due to windsurfer overturning

☑x7ᵗʰ **V90.09** **Drowning and submersion due to unspecified watercraft overturning**
> Drowning and submersion due to boat NOS overturning
> Drowning and submersion due to ship NOS overturning
> Drowning and submersion due to watercraft NOS overturning

☑5ᵗʰ **V90.1** **Drowning and submersion due to** watercraft sinking

☑x7ᵗʰ **V90.10** **Drowning and submersion due to** merchant ship **sinking**

☑x7ᵗʰ **V90.11** **Drowning and submersion due to** passenger ship **sinking**
> Drowning and submersion due to Ferry-boat sinking
> Drowning and submersion due to Liner sinking

☑x7ᵗʰ **V90.12** **Drowning and submersion due to** fishing boat **sinking**

☑x7ᵗʰ **V90.13** **Drowning and submersion due to other** powered **watercraft sinking**
> Drowning and submersion due to Hovercraft (on open water) sinking
> Drowning and submersion due to Jet ski sinking

☑x7ᵗʰ **V90.14** **Drowning and submersion due to** sailboat **sinking**

☑x7ᵗʰ **V90.15** **Drowning and submersion due to** canoe or kayak **sinking**

☑x7ᵗʰ **V90.16** **Drowning and submersion due to (nonpowered)** inflatable craft **sinking**

☑x7ᵗʰ **V90.18** **Drowning and submersion due to other** unpowered **watercraft sinking**

☑x7ᵗʰ **V90.19** **Drowning and submersion due to unspecified watercraft sinking**
> Drowning and submersion due to boat NOS sinking
> Drowning and submersion due to ship NOS sinking
> Drowning and submersion due to watercraft NOS sinking

☑5ᵗʰ **V90.2** **Drowning and submersion due to** falling or jumping from burning watercraft

☑x7ᵗʰ **V90.20** **Drowning and submersion due to falling or jumping from burning** merchant ship

☑x7ᵗʰ **V90.21** **Drowning and submersion due to falling or jumping from burning** passenger ship
> Drowning and submersion due to falling or jumping from burning Ferry-boat
> Drowning and submersion due to falling or jumping from burning Liner

☑x7ᵗʰ **V90.22** **Drowning and submersion due to falling or jumping from burning** fishing boat

☑x7ᵗʰ **V90.23** **Drowning and submersion due to falling or jumping from other burning** powered **watercraft**
> Drowning and submersion due to falling and jumping from burning Hovercraft (on open water)
> Drowning and submersion due to falling and jumping from burning Jet ski

☑x7ᵗʰ **V90.24** **Drowning and submersion due to falling or jumping from burning** sailboat

☑x7ᵗʰ **V90.25** **Drowning and submersion due to falling or jumping from burning** canoe or kayak

☑x7ᵗʰ **V90.26** **Drowning and submersion due to falling or jumping from burning (nonpowered)** inflatable craft

☑x7ᵗʰ **V90.27** **Drowning and submersion due to falling or jumping from burning** water-skis

☑x7ᵗʰ **V90.28** **Drowning and submersion due to falling or jumping from other burning** unpowered **watercraft**
> Drowning and submersion due to falling and jumping from burning surf-board
> Drowning and submersion due to falling and jumping from burning windsurfer

☑ Additional Char Req   ☑x7ᵗʰ Placeholder   Unacceptable PDx   Questionable PDx   Wrong Procedure   Manifestation   Unspecified Dx   H1-H14 HAC   HCC CMS-HCC Dx   HIV HIV Dx

Chapter 20. External Causes of Morbidity *(side margin)*

✓x7ᵗʰ V90.29 **Drowning and submersion due to falling or jumping from unspecified burning watercraft**
Drowning and submersion due to falling or jumping from burning boat NOS
Drowning and submersion due to falling or jumping from burning ship NOS
Drowning and submersion due to falling or jumping from burning watercraft NOS

✓5ᵗʰ V90.3 **Drowning and submersion due to falling or jumping from crushed watercraft**

✓x7ᵗʰ V90.30 **Drowning and submersion due to falling or jumping from crushed merchant ship**

✓x7ᵗʰ V90.31 **Drowning and submersion due to falling or jumping from crushed passenger ship**
Drowning and submersion due to falling and jumping from crushed Ferry boat
Drowning and submersion due to falling and jumping from crushed Liner

✓x7ᵗʰ V90.32 **Drowning and submersion due to falling or jumping from crushed fishing boat**

✓x7ᵗʰ V90.33 **Drowning and submersion due to falling or jumping from other crushed powered watercraft**
Drowning and submersion due to falling and jumping from crushed Hovercraft
Drowning and submersion due to falling and jumping from crushed Jet ski

✓x7ᵗʰ V90.34 **Drowning and submersion due to falling or jumping from crushed sailboat**

✓x7ᵗʰ V90.35 **Drowning and submersion due to falling or jumping from crushed canoe or kayak**

✓x7ᵗʰ V90.36 **Drowning and submersion due to falling or jumping from crushed (nonpowered) inflatable craft**

✓x7ᵗʰ V90.37 **Drowning and submersion due to falling or jumping from crushed water-skis**

✓x7ᵗʰ V90.38 **Drowning and submersion due to falling or jumping from other crushed unpowered watercraft**
Drowning and submersion due to falling and jumping from crushed surf-board
Drowning and submersion due to falling and jumping from crushed windsurfer

✓x7ᵗʰ V90.39 **Drowning and submersion due to falling or jumping from crushed unspecified watercraft**
Drowning and submersion due to falling and jumping from crushed boat NOS
Drowning and submersion due to falling and jumping from crushed ship NOS
Drowning and submersion due to falling and jumping from crushed watercraft NOS

✓5ᵗʰ V90.8 **Drowning and submersion due to other accident to watercraft**

✓x7ᵗʰ V90.80 **Drowning and submersion due to other accident to merchant ship**

✓x7ᵗʰ V90.81 **Drowning and submersion due to other accident to passenger ship**
Drowning and submersion due to other accident to Ferry-boat
Drowning and submersion due to other accident to Liner

✓x7ᵗʰ V90.82 **Drowning and submersion due to other accident to fishing boat**

✓x7ᵗʰ V90.83 **Drowning and submersion due to other accident to other powered watercraft**
Drowning and submersion due to other accident to Hovercraft (on open water)
Drowning and submersion due to other accident to Jet ski

✓x7ᵗʰ V90.84 **Drowning and submersion due to other accident to sailboat**

✓x7ᵗʰ V90.85 **Drowning and submersion due to other accident to canoe or kayak**

✓x7ᵗʰ V90.86 **Drowning and submersion due to other accident to (nonpowered) inflatable craft**

✓x7ᵗʰ V90.87 **Drowning and submersion due to other accident to water-skis**

✓x7ᵗʰ V90.88 **Drowning and submersion due to other accident to other unpowered watercraft**
Drowning and submersion due to other accident to surf-board
Drowning and submersion due to other accident to windsurfer

✓x7ᵗʰ V90.89 **Drowning and submersion due to other accident to unspecified watercraft**
Drowning and submersion due to other accident to boat NOS
Drowning and submersion due to other accident to ship NOS
Drowning and submersion due to other accident to watercraft NOS

✓4ᵗʰ V91 **Other injury due to accident to watercraft**
INCLUDES   any injury except drowning and submersion as a result of an accident to watercraft
EXCLUDES 1   *civilian water transport accident involving military watercraft (V94.81-)*
military watercraft accident in military or war operations (Y36, Y37.-)
EXCLUDES 2   *drowning and submersion due to accident to watercraft (V90.-)*

✓5ᵗʰ V91.0 **Burn due to watercraft on fire**
EXCLUDES 1   *burn from localized fire or explosion on board ship without accident to watercraft (V93.-)*

✓x7ᵗʰ V91.00 **Burn due to merchant ship on fire**

✓x7ᵗʰ V91.01 **Burn due to passenger ship on fire**
Burn due to Ferry-boat on fire
Burn due to Liner on fire

✓x7ᵗʰ V91.02 **Burn due to fishing boat on fire**

✓x7ᵗʰ V91.03 **Burn due to other powered watercraft on fire**
Burn due to Hovercraft (on open water) on fire
Burn due to Jet ski on fire

✓x7ᵗʰ V91.04 **Burn due to sailboat on fire**

✓x7ᵗʰ V91.05 **Burn due to canoe or kayak on fire**

✓x7ᵗʰ V91.06 **Burn due to (nonpowered) inflatable craft on fire**

✓x7ᵗʰ V91.07 **Burn due to water-skis on fire**

✓x7ᵗʰ V91.08 **Burn due to other unpowered watercraft on fire**

✓x7ᵗʰ V91.09 **Burn due to unspecified watercraft on fire**
Burn due to boat NOS on fire
Burn due to ship NOS on fire
Burn due to watercraft NOS on fire

✓5ᵗʰ V91.1 **Crushed between watercraft and other watercraft or other object due to collision**
Crushed by lifeboat after abandoning ship in a collision
NOTE   Select the specified type of watercraft that the victim was on at the time of the collision

✓x7ᵗʰ V91.10 **Crushed between merchant ship and other watercraft or other object due to collision**

✓x7ᵗʰ V91.11 **Crushed between passenger ship and other watercraft or other object due to collision**
Crushed between Ferry-boat and other watercraft or other object due to collision
Crushed between Liner and other watercraft or other object due to collision

✓x7ᵗʰ V91.12 **Crushed between fishing boat and other watercraft or other object due to collision**

✓x7ᵗʰ V91.13 **Crushed between other powered watercraft and other watercraft or other object due to collision**
Crushed between Hovercraft (on open water) and other watercraft or other object due to collision
Crushed between Jet ski and other watercraft or other object due to collision

✓x7ᵗʰ V91.14 **Crushed between sailboat and other watercraft or other object due to collision**

✓x7ᵗʰ V91.15 **Crushed between canoe or kayak and other watercraft or other object due to collision**

✓x7ᵗʰ V91.16 **Crushed between (nonpowered) inflatable craft and other watercraft or other object due to collision**

√x7ᵗʰ **V91.18 Crushed between other** unpowered **watercraft and other watercraft or other object due to collision**
Crushed between surfboard and other watercraft or other object due to collision
Crushed between windsurfer and other watercraft or other object due to collision

√x7ᵗʰ **V91.19 Crushed between unspecified watercraft and other watercraft or other object due to collision**
Crushed between boat NOS and other watercraft or other object due to collision
Crushed between ship NOS and other watercraft or other object due to collision
Crushed between watercraft NOS and other watercraft or other object due to collision

√5ᵗʰ **V91.2 Fall due to collision between watercraft and other watercraft or other object**
Fall while remaining on watercraft after collision

> **NOTE**   Select the specified type of watercraft that the victim was on at the time of the collision

> **EXCLUDES 1**   crushed between watercraft and other watercraft and other object due to collision (V91.1-)
> drowning and submersion due to falling from crushed watercraft (V90.3-)

√x7ᵗʰ **V91.20 Fall due to collision between** merchant ship **and other watercraft or other object**

√x7ᵗʰ **V91.21 Fall due to collision between** passenger ship **and other watercraft or other object**
Fall due to collision between Ferry-boat and other watercraft or other object
Fall due to collision between Liner and other watercraft or other object

√x7ᵗʰ **V91.22 Fall due to collision between** fishing boat **and other watercraft or other object**

√x7ᵗʰ **V91.23 Fall due to collision between other** powered **watercraft and other watercraft or other object**
Fall due to collision between Hovercraft (on open water) and other watercraft or other object
Fall due to collision between Jet ski and other watercraft or other object

√x7ᵗʰ **V91.24 Fall due to collision between** sailboat **and other watercraft or other object**

√x7ᵗʰ **V91.25 Fall due to collision between** canoe or kayak **and other watercraft or other object**

√x7ᵗʰ **V91.26 Fall due to collision between (nonpowered)** inflatable craft **and other watercraft or other object**

√x7ᵗʰ **V91.29 Fall due to collision between unspecified watercraft and other watercraft or other object**
Fall due to collision between boat NOS and other watercraft or other object
Fall due to collision between ship NOS and other watercraft or other object
Fall due to collision between watercraft NOS and other watercraft or other object

√5ᵗʰ **V91.3 Hit or struck by falling object due to accident to watercraft**
Hit or struck by falling object (part of damaged watercraft or other object) after falling or jumping from damaged watercraft

> **EXCLUDES 2**   drowning or submersion due to fall or jumping from damaged watercraft (V90.2-, V90.3-)

√x7ᵗʰ **V91.30 Hit or struck by falling object due to accident to** merchant ship

√x7ᵗʰ **V91.31 Hit or struck by falling object due to accident to** passenger ship
Hit or struck by falling object due to accident to Ferry-boat
Hit or struck by falling object due to accident to Liner

√x7ᵗʰ **V91.32 Hit or struck by falling object due to accident to** fishing boat

√x7ᵗʰ **V91.33 Hit or struck by falling object due to accident to other** powered **watercraft**
Hit or struck by falling object due to accident to Hovercraft (on open water)
Hit or struck by falling object due to accident to Jet ski

√x7ᵗʰ **V91.34 Hit or struck by falling object due to accident to** sailboat

√x7ᵗʰ **V91.35 Hit or struck by falling object due to accident to** canoe or kayak

√x7ᵗʰ **V91.36 Hit or struck by falling object due to accident to (nonpowered)** inflatable craft

√x7ᵗʰ **V91.37 Hit or struck by falling object due to accident to** water-skis
Hit by water-skis after jumping off of waterskis

√x7ᵗʰ **V91.38 Hit or struck by falling object due to accident to other** unpowered **watercraft**
Hit or struck by surf-board after falling off damaged surf-board
Hit or struck by object after falling off damaged windsurfer

√x7ᵗʰ **V91.39 Hit or struck by falling object due to accident to unspecified watercraft**
Hit or struck by falling object due to accident to boat NOS
Hit or struck by falling object due to accident to ship NOS
Hit or struck by falling object due to accident to watercraft NOS

√5ᵗʰ **V91.8 Other injury due to other accident to watercraft**

√x7ᵗʰ **V91.80 Other injury due to other accident to** merchant ship

√x7ᵗʰ **V91.81 Other injury due to other accident to** passenger ship
Other injury due to other accident to Ferry-boat
Other injury due to other accident to Liner

√x7ᵗʰ **V91.82 Other injury due to other accident to** fishing boat

√x7ᵗʰ **V91.83 Other injury due to other accident to other** powered **watercraft**
Other injury due to other accident to Hovercraft (on open water)
Other injury due to other accident to Jet ski

√x7ᵗʰ **V91.84 Other injury due to other accident to** sailboat

√x7ᵗʰ **V91.85 Other injury due to other accident to** canoe or kayak

√x7ᵗʰ **V91.86 Other injury due to other accident to (nonpowered)** inflatable craft

√x7ᵗʰ **V91.87 Other injury due to other accident to** water-skis

√x7ᵗʰ **V91.88 Other injury due to other accident to other** unpowered **watercraft**
Other injury due to other accident to surf-board
Other injury due to other accident to windsurfer

√x7ᵗʰ **V91.89 Other injury due to other accident to unspecified watercraft**
Other injury due to other accident to boat NOS
Other injury due to other accident to ship NOS
Other injury due to other accident to watercraft NOS

√4ᵗʰ **V92 Drowning and submersion due to accident on board watercraft, without accident to watercraft**

> **EXCLUDES 1**   civilian water transport accident involving military watercraft (V94.81-)
> drowning or submersion due to accident to watercraft (V90-V91)
> drowning or submersion of diver who voluntarily jumps from boat not involved in an accident (W16.711, W16.721)
> fall into water without watercraft (W16.-)
> military watercraft accident in military or war operations (Y36, Y37)

√5ᵗʰ **V92.0 Drowning and submersion due to** fall off **watercraft**
Drowning and submersion due to fall from gangplank of watercraft
Drowning and submersion due to fall overboard watercraft

> **EXCLUDES 2**   hitting head on object or bottom of body of water due to fall from watercraft (V94.0-)

√x7ᵗʰ **V92.00 Drowning and submersion due to fall off** merchant ship

√x7ᵗʰ **V92.01 Drowning and submersion due to fall off** passenger ship
Drowning and submersion due to fall off Ferry-boat
Drowning and submersion due to fall off Liner

√x7ᵗʰ **V92.02 Drowning and submersion due to fall off** fishing boat

√x7ᵗʰ **V92.03 Drowning and submersion due to fall off other** powered **watercraft**
Drowning and submersion due to fall off Hovercraft (on open water)
Drowning and submersion due to fall off Jet ski

√x7ᵗʰ **V92.04 Drowning and submersion due to fall off** sailboat

√x7ᵗʰ **V92.05 Drowning and submersion due to fall off** canoe or kayak

---

☑ Additional Char Req   √x7ᵗʰ Placeholder   Unacceptable PDx   Questionable PDx   Wrong Procedure   Manifestation   Unspecified Dx   **H1**-**H14** HAC   **HCC** CMS-HCC Dx   **HIV** HIV Dx

√x7ᵗʰ **V92.06** **Drowning and submersion due to fall off (nonpowered) inflatable craft**

√x7ᵗʰ **V92.07** **Drowning and submersion due to fall off water-skis**

> EXCLUDES 1   *drowning and submersion due to falling off burning water-skis (V90.27)*
>
> *drowning and submersion due to falling off crushed water-skis (V90.37)*
>
> *hit by boat while water-skiing NOS (V94.X)*

√x7ᵗʰ **V92.08** **Drowning and submersion due to fall off other unpowered watercraft**

Drowning and submersion due to fall off surf-board

Drowning and submersion due to fall off windsurfer

> EXCLUDES 1   *drowning and submersion due to fall off burning unpowered watercraft (V90.28)*
>
> *drowning and submersion due to fall off crushed unpowered watercraft (V90.38)*
>
> *drowning and submersion due to fall off damaged unpowered watercraft (V90.88)*
>
> *drowning and submersion due to rider of nonpowered watercraft being hit by other watercraft (V94.-)*
>
> *other injury due to rider of nonpowered watercraft being hit by other watercraft (V94.-)*

√x7ᵗʰ **V92.09** **Drowning and submersion due to fall off unspecified watercraft**

Drowning and submersion due to fall off boat NOS

Drowning and submersion due to fall off ship

Drowning and submersion due to fall off watercraft NOS

√5ᵗʰ **V92.1** **Drowning and submersion due to being thrown overboard by motion of watercraft**

> EXCLUDES 1   *drowning and submersion due to fall off surf-board (V92.08)*
>
> *drowning and submersion due to fall off water-skis (V92.07)*
>
> *drowning and submersion due to fall off windsurfer (V92.08)*

√x7ᵗʰ **V92.10** **Drowning and submersion due to being thrown overboard by motion of merchant ship**

√x7ᵗʰ **V92.11** **Drowning and submersion due to being thrown overboard by motion of passenger ship**

Drowning and submersion due to being thrown overboard by motion of Ferry-boat

Drowning and submersion due to being thrown overboard by motion of Liner

√x7ᵗʰ **V92.12** **Drowning and submersion due to being thrown overboard by motion of fishing boat**

√x7ᵗʰ **V92.13** **Drowning and submersion due to being thrown overboard by motion of other powered watercraft**

Drowning and submersion due to being thrown overboard by motion of Hovercraft

√x7ᵗʰ **V92.14** **Drowning and submersion due to being thrown overboard by motion of sailboat**

√x7ᵗʰ **V92.15** **Drowning and submersion due to being thrown overboard by motion of canoe or kayak**

√x7ᵗʰ **V92.16** **Drowning and submersion due to being thrown overboard by motion of (nonpowered) inflatable craft**

√x7ᵗʰ **V92.19** **Drowning and submersion due to being thrown overboard by motion of unspecified watercraft**

Drowning and submersion due to being thrown overboard by motion of boat NOS

Drowning and submersion due to being thrown overboard by motion of ship NOS

Drowning and submersion due to being thrown overboard by motion of watercraft NOS

√5ᵗʰ **V92.2** **Drowning and submersion due to being washed overboard from watercraft**

Code first any associated cataclysm (X37.0-)

√x7ᵗʰ **V92.20** **Drowning and submersion due to being washed overboard from merchant ship**

√x7ᵗʰ **V92.21** **Drowning and submersion due to being washed overboard from passenger ship**

Drowning and submersion due to being washed overboard from Ferry-boat

Drowning and submersion due to being washed overboard from Liner

√x7ᵗʰ **V92.22** **Drowning and submersion due to being washed overboard from fishing boat**

√x7ᵗʰ **V92.23** **Drowning and submersion due to being washed overboard from other powered watercraft**

Drowning and submersion due to being washed overboard from Hovercraft (on open water)

Drowning and submersion due to being washed overboard from Jet ski

√x7ᵗʰ **V92.24** **Drowning and submersion due to being washed overboard from sailboat**

√x7ᵗʰ **V92.25** **Drowning and submersion due to being washed overboard from canoe or kayak**

√x7ᵗʰ **V92.26** **Drowning and submersion due to being washed overboard from (nonpowered) inflatable craft**

√x7ᵗʰ **V92.27** **Drowning and submersion due to being washed overboard from water-skis**

> EXCLUDES 1   *drowning and submersion due to fall off water-skis (V92.07)*

√x7ᵗʰ **V92.28** **Drowning and submersion due to being washed overboard from other unpowered watercraft**

Drowning and submersion due to being washed overboard from surf-board

Drowning and submersion due to being washed overboard from windsurfer

√x7ᵗʰ **V92.29** **Drowning and submersion due to being washed overboard from unspecified watercraft**

Drowning and submersion due to being washed overboard from boat NOS

Drowning and submersion due to being washed overboard from ship NOS

Drowning and submersion due to being washed overboard from watercraft NOS

√4ᵗʰ **V93** **Other injury due to accident on board watercraft, without accident to watercraft**

> EXCLUDES 1   *civilian water transport accident involving military watercraft (V94.81-)*
>
> *other injury due to accident to watercraft (V91.-)*
>
> *military watercraft accident in military or war operations (Y36, Y37.-)*
>
> EXCLUDES 2   *drowning and submersion due to accident on board watercraft, without accident to watercraft (V92.-)*

√5ᵗʰ **V93.0** **Burn due to localized fire on board watercraft**

> EXCLUDES 1   *burn due to watercraft on fire (V91.0-)*

√x7ᵗʰ **V93.00** **Burn due to localized fire on board merchant vessel**

√x7ᵗʰ **V93.01** **Burn due to localized fire on board passenger vessel**

Burn due to localized fire on board Ferry-boat

Burn due to localized fire on board Liner

√x7ᵗʰ **V93.02** **Burn due to localized fire on board fishing boat**

√x7ᵗʰ **V93.03** **Burn due to localized fire on board other powered watercraft**

Burn due to localized fire on board Hovercraft

Burn due to localized fire on board Jet ski

√x7ᵗʰ **V93.04** **Burn due to localized fire on board sailboat**

√x7ᵗʰ **V93.09** **Burn due to localized fire on board unspecified watercraft**

Burn due to localized fire on board boat NOS

Burn due to localized fire on board ship NOS

Burn due to localized fire on board watercraft NOS

√5ᵗʰ **V93.1** **Other burn on board watercraft**

Burn due to source other than fire on board watercraft

> EXCLUDES 1   *burn due to watercraft on fire (V91.0-)*

√x7ᵗʰ **V93.10** **Other burn on board merchant vessel**

√x7ᵗʰ **V93.11** **Other burn on board passenger vessel**

Other burn on board Ferry-boat

Other burn on board Liner

√x7ᵗʰ **V93.12** **Other burn on board fishing boat**

√x7ᵗʰ **V93.13** **Other burn on board other powered watercraft**

Other burn on board Hovercraft

Other burn on board Jet ski

√x7ᵗʰ **V93.14** **Other burn on board sailboat**

Ⓝ Newborn: 0   Ⓟ Pediatric: 0-17   Ⓜ Maternity: 9-64   Ⓐ Adult: 15-124   MCC Major Complication/Comorbidity   CC Complication/Comorbidity   SW Severe Wound Dx

1238   ICD-10-CM 2020

√x7ᵗʰ **V93.19** **Other burn on board unspecified watercraft**

Other burn on board boat NOS
Other burn on board ship NOS
Other burn on board watercraft NOS

√5ᵗʰ **V93.2** **Heat exposure on board watercraft**

EXCLUDES 1   *exposure to man-made heat not aboard watercraft (W92)*
exposure to natural heat while on board watercraft (X30)
exposure to sunlight while or board watercraft (X32)
EXCLUDES 2   *burn due to fire on board watercraft (V93.0-)*

√x7ᵗʰ **V93.20** **Heat exposure on board merchant ship**

√x7ᵗʰ **V93.21** **Heat exposure on board passenger ship**

Heat exposure on board Ferry-boat
Heat exposure on board Liner

√x7ᵗʰ **V93.22** **Heat exposure on board fishing boat**

√x7ᵗʰ **V93.23** **Heat exposure on board other powered watercraft**

Heat exposure on board hovercraft

√x7ᵗʰ **V93.24** **Heat exposure on board sailboat**

√x7ᵗʰ **V93.29** **Heat exposure on board unspecified watercraft**

Heat exposure on board boat NOS
Heat exposure on board ship NOS
Heat exposure on board watercraft NOS

√5ᵗʰ **V93.3** **Fall on board watercraft**

EXCLUDES 1   *fall due to collision of watercraft (V91.2-)*

√x7ᵗʰ **V93.30** **Fall on board merchant ship**

√x7ᵗʰ **V93.31** **Fall on board passenger ship**

Fall on board Ferry-boat
Fall on board Liner

√x7ᵗʰ **V93.32** **Fall on board fishing boat**

√x7ᵗʰ **V93.33** **Fall on board other powered watercraft**

Fall on board Hovercraft (on open water)
Fall on board Jet ski

√x7ᵗʰ **V93.34** **Fall on board sailboat**

√x7ᵗʰ **V93.35** **Fall on board canoe or kayak**

√x7ᵗʰ **V93.36** **Fall on board (nonpowered) inflatable craft**

√x7ᵗʰ **V93.38** **Fall on board other unpowered watercraft**

√x7ᵗʰ **V93.39** **Fall on board unspecified watercraft**

Fall on board boat NOS
Fall on board ship NOS
Fall on board watercraft NOS

√5ᵗʰ **V93.4** **Struck by falling object on board watercraft**

Hit by falling object on board watercraft
EXCLUDES 1   *struck by falling object due to accident to watercraft (V91.3)*

√x7ᵗʰ **V93.40** **Struck by falling object on merchant ship**

√x7ᵗʰ **V93.41** **Struck by falling object on passenger ship**

Struck by falling object on Ferry-boat
Struck by falling object on Liner

√x7ᵗʰ **V93.42** **Struck by falling object on fishing boat**

√x7ᵗʰ **V93.43** **Struck by falling object on other powered watercraft**

Struck by falling object on Hovercraft

√x7ᵗʰ **V93.44** **Struck by falling object on sailboat**

√x7ᵗʰ **V93.48** **Struck by falling object on other unpowered watercraft**

√x7ᵗʰ **V93.49** **Struck by falling object on unspecified watercraft**

√5ᵗʰ **V93.5** **Explosion on board watercraft**

Boiler explosion on steamship
EXCLUDES 2   *fire on board watercraft (V93.0-)*

√x7ᵗʰ **V93.50** **Explosion on board merchant ship**

√x7ᵗʰ **V93.51** **Explosion on board passenger ship**

Explosion on board Ferry-boat
Explosion on board Liner

√x7ᵗʰ **V93.52** **Explosion on board fishing boat**

√x7ᵗʰ **V93.53** **Explosion on board other powered watercraft**

Explosion on board Hovercraft
Explosion on board Jet ski

√x7ᵗʰ **V93.54** **Explosion on board sailboat**

√x7ᵗʰ **V93.59** **Explosion on board unspecified watercraft**

Explosion on board boat NOS
Explosion on board ship NOS
Explosion on board watercraft NOS

√5ᵗʰ **V93.6** **Machinery accident on board watercraft**

EXCLUDES 1   *machinery explosion on board watercraft (V93.4-)*
machinery fire on board watercraft (V93.0-)

√x7ᵗʰ **V93.60** **Machinery accident on board merchant ship**

√x7ᵗʰ **V93.61** **Machinery accident on board passenger ship**

Machinery accident on board Ferry-boat
Machinery accident on board Liner

√x7ᵗʰ **V93.62** **Machinery accident on board fishing boat**

√x7ᵗʰ **V93.63** **Machinery accident on board other powered watercraft**

Machinery accident on board Hovercraft

√x7ᵗʰ **V93.64** **Machinery accident on board sailboat**

√x7ᵗʰ **V93.69** **Machinery accident on board unspecified watercraft**

Machinery accident on board boat NOS
Machinery accident on board ship NOS
Machinery accident on board watercraft NOS

√5ᵗʰ **V93.8** **Other injury due to other accident on board watercraft**

Accidental poisoning by gases or fumes on watercraft

√x7ᵗʰ **V93.80** **Other injury due to other accident on board merchant ship**

√x7ᵗʰ **V93.81** **Other injury due to other accident on board passenger ship**

Other injury due to other accident on board Ferry-boat
Other injury due to other accident on board Liner

√x7ᵗʰ **V93.82** **Other injury due to other accident on board fishing boat**

√x7ᵗʰ **V93.83** **Other injury due to other accident on board other powered watercraft**

Other injury due to other accident on board Hovercraft
Other injury due to other accident on board Jet ski

√x7ᵗʰ **V93.84** **Other injury due to other accident on board sailboat**

√x7ᵗʰ **V93.85** **Other injury due to other accident on board canoe or kayak**

√x7ᵗʰ **V93.86** **Other injury due to other accident on board (nonpowered) inflatable craft**

√x7ᵗʰ **V93.87** **Other injury due to other accident on board water-skis**

Hit or struck by object while waterskiing

√x7ᵗʰ **V93.88** **Other injury due to other accident on board other unpowered watercraft**

Hit or struck by object while surfing
Hit or struck by object while on board windsurfer

√x7ᵗʰ **V93.89** **Other injury due to other accident on board unspecified watercraft**

Other injury due to other accident on board boat NOS
Other injury due to other accident on board ship NOS
Other injury due to other accident on board watercraft NOS

√4ᵗʰ **V94** **Other and unspecified water transport accidents**

EXCLUDES 1   *military watercraft accidents in military or war operations (Y36, Y37)*

√x7ᵗʰ **V94.0** **Hitting object or bottom of body of water due to fall from watercraft**

EXCLUDES 2   *drowning and submersion due to fall from watercraft (V92.0-)*

√5ᵗʰ **V94.1** **Bather struck by watercraft**

Swimmer hit by watercraft

√x7ᵗʰ **V94.11** **Bather struck by powered watercraft**

√x7ᵗʰ **V94.12** **Bather struck by nonpowered watercraft**

√5ᵗʰ **V94.2** **Rider of nonpowered watercraft struck by other watercraft**

√x7ᵗʰ **V94.21** **Rider of nonpowered watercraft struck by other nonpowered watercraft**

Canoer hit by other nonpowered watercraft
Surfer hit by other nonpowered watercraft
Windsurfer hit by other nonpowered watercraft

√x7ᵗʰ **V94.22** **Rider of nonpowered watercraft struck by** powered **watercraft**
     Canoer hit by motorboat
     Surfer hit by motorboat
     Windsurfer hit by motorboat

√5ᵗʰ **V94.3** **Injury to rider of (inflatable) watercraft being pulled behind other watercraft**

√x7ᵗʰ **V94.31** **Injury to rider of (inflatable)** recreational **watercraft being pulled behind other watercraft**
     Injury to rider of inner-tube pulled behind motor boat

√x7ᵗʰ **V94.32** **Injury to rider of** non-recreational **watercraft being pulled behind other watercraft**
     Injury to occupant of dingy being pulled behind boat or ship
     Injury to occupant of life-raft being pulled behind boat or ship

√x7ᵗʰ **V94.4** **Injury to barefoot water-skier**
     Injury to person being pulled behind boat or ship

√5ᵗʰ **V94.8** **Other water transport accident**

√6ᵗʰ **V94.81** **Water transport accident involving military watercraft**

√7ᵗʰ **V94.810** **Civilian watercraft involved in water transport accident with military watercraft**
     Passenger on civilian watercraft injured due to accident with military watercraft

√7ᵗʰ **V94.811** **Civilian in water injured by military watercraft**

√7ᵗʰ **V94.818** **Other water transport accident involving military watercraft**

√x7ᵗʰ **V94.89** **Other water transport accident**

√x7ᵗʰ **V94.9** **Unspecified water transport accident**
     Water transport accident NOS

Air and space transport accidents (V95-V97)

EXCLUDES 1   *military aircraft accidents in military or war operations (Y36, Y37)*

The appropriate 7th character is to be added to each code from categories V95-V97.
A   initial encounter
D   subsequent encounter
S   sequela

√4ᵗʰ **V95** **Accident to powered aircraft causing injury to occupant**

√5ᵗʰ **V95.0** **Helicopter accident injuring occupant**

√x7ᵗʰ **V95.00** **Unspecified helicopter accident injuring occupant**

√x7ᵗʰ **V95.01** **Helicopter** crash **injuring occupant**

√x7ᵗʰ **V95.02** **Forced landing of helicopter injuring occupant**

√x7ᵗʰ **V95.03** **Helicopter** collision **injuring occupant**
     Helicopter collision with any object, fixed, movable or moving

√x7ᵗʰ **V95.04** **Helicopter** fire **injuring occupant**

√x7ᵗʰ **V95.05** **Helicopter** explosion **injuring occupant**

√x7ᵗʰ **V95.09** **Other helicopter accident injuring occupant**

√5ᵗʰ **V95.1** **Ultralight, microlight or powered-glider accident injuring occupant**

√x7ᵗʰ **V95.10** **Unspecified ultralight, microlight or powered-glider accident injuring occupant**

√x7ᵗʰ **V95.11** **Ultralight, microlight or powered-glider** crash **injuring occupant**

√x7ᵗʰ **V95.12** **Forced landing of ultralight, microlight or powered-glider injuring occupant**

√x7ᵗʰ **V95.13** **Ultralight, microlight or powered-glider** collision **injuring occupant**
     Ultralight, microlight or powered-glider collision with any object, fixed, movable or moving

√x7ᵗʰ **V95.14** **Ultralight, microlight or powered-glider** fire **injuring occupant**

√x7ᵗʰ **V95.15** **Ultralight, microlight or powered-glider** explosion **injuring occupant**

√x7ᵗʰ **V95.19** **Other ultralight, microlight or powered-glider accident injuring occupant**

√5ᵗʰ **V95.2** **Other private fixed-wing aircraft accident injuring occupant**

√x7ᵗʰ **V95.20** **Unspecified accident to other private fixed-wing aircraft, injuring occupant**

√x7ᵗʰ **V95.21** **Other private fixed-wing aircraft crash injuring occupant**

√x7ᵗʰ **V95.22** **Forced landing of other private fixed-wing aircraft injuring occupant**

√x7ᵗʰ **V95.23** **Other private fixed-wing aircraft** collision **injuring occupant**
     Other private fixed-wing aircraft collision with any object, fixed, movable or moving

√x7ᵗʰ **V95.24** **Other private fixed-wing aircraft** fire **injuring occupant**

√x7ᵗʰ **V95.25** **Other private fixed-wing aircraft** explosion **injuring occupant**

√x7ᵗʰ **V95.29** **Other accident to other private fixed-wing aircraft injuring occupant**

√5ᵗʰ **V95.3** **Commercial fixed-wing aircraft accident injuring occupant**

√x7ᵗʰ **V95.30** **Unspecified accident to commercial fixed-wing aircraft injuring occupant**

√x7ᵗʰ **V95.31** **Commercial fixed-wing aircraft** crash **injuring occupant**

√x7ᵗʰ **V95.32** **Forced landing of commercial fixed-wing aircraft injuring occupant**

√x7ᵗʰ **V95.33** **Commercial fixed-wing aircraft** collision **injuring occupant**
     Commercial fixed-wing aircraft collision with any object, fixed, movable or moving

√x7ᵗʰ **V95.34** **Commercial fixed-wing aircraft** fire **injuring occupant**

√x7ᵗʰ **V95.35** **Commercial fixed-wing aircraft** explosion **injuring occupant**

√x7ᵗʰ **V95.39** **Other accident to commercial fixed-wing aircraft injuring occupant**

√5ᵗʰ **V95.4** **Spacecraft accident injuring occupant**

√x7ᵗʰ **V95.40** **Unspecified spacecraft accident injuring occupant**

√x7ᵗʰ **V95.41** **Spacecraft** crash **injuring occupant**

√x7ᵗʰ **V95.42** **Forced landing of spacecraft injuring occupant**

√x7ᵗʰ **V95.43** **Spacecraft** collision **injuring occupant**
     Spacecraft collision with any object, fixed, moveable or moving

√x7ᵗʰ **V95.44** **Spacecraft** fire **injuring occupant**

√x7ᵗʰ **V95.45** **Spacecraft** explosion **injuring occupant**

√x7ᵗʰ **V95.49** **Other spacecraft accident injuring occupant**

√x7ᵗʰ **V95.8** **Other powered aircraft accidents injuring occupant**

√x7ᵗʰ **V95.9** **Unspecified aircraft accident injuring occupant**
     Aircraft accident NOS
     Air transport accident NOS

√4ᵗʰ **V96** **Accident to nonpowered aircraft causing injury to occupant**

√5ᵗʰ **V96.0** **Balloon accident injuring occupant**

√x7ᵗʰ **V96.00** **Unspecified balloon accident injuring occupant**

√x7ᵗʰ **V96.01** **Balloon** crash **injuring occupant**

√x7ᵗʰ **V96.02** **Forced landing of balloon injuring occupant**

√x7ᵗʰ **V96.03** **Balloon** collision **injuring occupant**
     Balloon collision with any object, fixed, moveable or moving

√x7ᵗʰ **V96.04** **Balloon** fire **injuring occupant**

√x7ᵗʰ **V96.05** **Balloon** explosion **injuring occupant**

√x7ᵗʰ **V96.09** **Other balloon accident injuring occupant**

√5ᵗʰ **V96.1** **Hang-glider accident injuring occupant**

√x7ᵗʰ **V96.10** **Unspecified hang-glider accident injuring occupant**

√x7ᵗʰ **V96.11** **Hang-glider** crash **injuring occupant**

√x7ᵗʰ **V96.12** **Forced landing of hang-glider injuring occupant**

√x7ᵗʰ **V96.13** **Hang-glider** collision **injuring occupant**
     Hang-glider collision with any object, fixed, moveable or moving

√x7ᵗʰ **V96.14** **Hang-glider** fire **injuring occupant**

√x7ᵗʰ **V96.15** **Hang-glider** explosion **injuring occupant**

√x7ᵗʰ **V96.19** **Other hang-glider accident injuring occupant**

√5ᵗʰ **V96.2** **Glider (nonpowered) accident injuring occupant**

√x7ᵗʰ **V96.20** **Unspecified glider (nonpowered) accident injuring occupant**

√x7ᵗʰ **V96.21** **Glider (nonpowered)** crash **injuring occupant**

√x7ᵗʰ **V96.22** **Forced landing of glider (nonpowered) injuring occupant**

√x7ᵗʰ **V96.23** **Glider (nonpowered) collision injuring occupant**

Glider (nonpowered) collision with any object, fixed, moveable or moving

√x7ᵗʰ **V96.24** **Glider (nonpowered) fire injuring occupant**

√x7ᵗʰ **V96.25** **Glider (nonpowered) explosion injuring occupant**

√x7ᵗʰ **V96.29** **Other glider (nonpowered) accident injuring occupant**

√x7ᵗʰ **V96.8** **Other nonpowered-aircraft accidents injuring occupant**

Kite carrying a person accident injuring occupant

√x7ᵗʰ **V96.9** **Unspecified nonpowered-aircraft accident injuring occupant**

Nonpowered-aircraft accident NOS

√4ᵗʰ **V97 Other specified air transport accidents**

√x7ᵗʰ **V97.0** **Occupant of aircraft injured in other specified air transport accidents**

Fall in, on or from aircraft in air transport accident

EXCLUDES 1   *accident while boarding or alighting aircraft (V97.1)*

√x7ᵗʰ **V97.1** **Person injured while boarding or alighting from aircraft**

√5ᵗʰ **V97.2** **Parachutist accident**

√x7ᵗʰ **V97.21** **Parachutist entangled in object**

Parachutist landing in tree

√x7ᵗʰ **V97.22** **Parachutist injured on landing**

√x7ᵗʰ **V97.29** **Other parachutist accident**

√5ᵗʰ **V97.3** **Person on ground injured in air transport accident**

√x7ᵗʰ **V97.31** **Hit by object falling from aircraft**

Hit by crashing aircraft
Injured by aircraft hitting house
Injured by aircraft hitting car

√x7ᵗʰ **V97.32** **Injured by rotating propeller**

√x7ᵗʰ **V97.33** **Sucked into jet engine**

√x7ᵗʰ **V97.39** **Other injury to person on ground due to air transport accident**

√5ᵗʰ **V97.8** **Other air transport accidents, not elsewhere classified**

EXCLUDES 1   *aircraft accident NOS (V95.9)*

exposure to changes in air pressure during ascent or descent (V94.-)

√6ᵗʰ **V97.81** **Air transport accident involving military aircraft**

√7ᵗʰ **V97.810** **Civilian aircraft involved in air transport accident with military aircraft**

Passenger in civilian aircraft injured due to accident with military aircraft

√7ᵗʰ **V97.811** **Civilian injured by military aircraft**

√7ᵗʰ **V97.818** **Other air transport accident involving military aircraft**

√x7ᵗʰ **V97.89** **Other air transport accidents, not elsewhere classified**

Injury from machinery on aircraft

Other and unspecified transport accidents (V98-V99)

EXCLUDES 1   *vehicle accident, type of vehicle unspecified (V89.-)*

The appropriate 7th character is to be added to each code from categories V98-V99.
A   initial encounter
D   subsequent encounter
S   sequela

√4ᵗʰ **V98 Other specified transport accidents**

√x7ᵗʰ **V98.0** **Accident to, on or involving cable-car, not on rails**

Caught or dragged by cable-car, not on rails
Fall or jump from cable-car, not on rails
Object thrown from or in cable-car, not on rails

√x7ᵗʰ **V98.1** **Accident to, on or involving land-yacht**

√x7ᵗʰ **V98.2** **Accident to, on or involving ice yacht**

√x7ᵗʰ **V98.3** **Accident to, on or involving ski lift**

Accident to, on or involving ski chair-lift
Accident to, on or involving ski-lift with gondola

√x7ᵗʰ **V98.8** **Other specified transport accidents**

√x7ᵗʰ **V99 Unspecified transport accident**

OTHER EXTERNAL CAUSES OF ACCIDENTAL INJURY (W00-X58)

Slipping, tripping, stumbling and falls (W00-W19)

EXCLUDES 1   *assault involving a fall (Y01-Y02)*
fall from animal (V80.-)
fall (in) (from) machinery (in operation) (W28-W31)
fall (in) (from) transport vehicle (V01-V99)
intentional self-harm involving a fall (X80-X81)

EXCLUDES 2   *at risk for fall (history of fall) Z91.81*
fall (in) (from) burning building (X00.-)
fall into fire (X00-X04, X08)

The appropriate 7th character is to be added to each code from categories W00-W19.
A   initial encounter
D   subsequent encounter
S   sequela

√4ᵗʰ **W00 Fall due to ice and snow**

INCLUDES   pedestrian on foot falling (slipping) on ice and snow

EXCLUDES 1   *fall on (from) ice and snow involving pedestrian conveyance (V00.-)*

fall from stairs and steps not due to ice and snow (W10.-)

AHA: 2016, 2Q, 4

√x7ᵗʰ **W00.0** **Fall on same level due to ice and snow**

√x7ᵗʰ **W00.1** **Fall from stairs and steps due to ice and snow**

√x7ᵗʰ **W00.2** **Other fall from one level to another due to ice and snow**

√x7ᵗʰ **W00.9** **Unspecified fall due to ice and snow**

√4ᵗʰ **W01 Fall on same level from slipping, tripping and stumbling**

INCLUDES   fall on moving sidewalk

EXCLUDES 1   *fall due to bumping (striking) against object (W18.0-)*
fall in shower or bathtub (W18.2-)
fall on same level NOS (W18.30)
fall on same level from slipping, tripping and stumbling due to ice or snow (W00.0)
fall off or from toilet (W18.1-)
slipping, tripping and stumbling NOS (W18.40)
slipping, tripping and stumbling without falling (W18.4-)

√x7ᵗʰ **W01.0** **Fall on same level from slipping, tripping and stumbling without subsequent striking against object**

Falling over animal

√5ᵗʰ **W01.1** **Fall on same level from slipping, tripping and stumbling with subsequent striking against object**

√x7ᵗʰ **W01.10** **Fall on same level from slipping, tripping and stumbling with subsequent striking against unspecified object**

√6ᵗʰ **W01.11** **Fall on same level from slipping, tripping and stumbling with subsequent striking against sharp object**

√7ᵗʰ **W01.110** **Fall on same level from slipping, tripping and stumbling with subsequent striking against sharp glass**

√7ᵗʰ **W01.111** **Fall on same level from slipping, tripping and stumbling with subsequent striking against power tool or machine**

√7ᵗʰ **W01.118** **Fall on same level from slipping, tripping and stumbling with subsequent striking against other sharp object**

√7ᵗʰ **W01.119** **Fall on same level from slipping, tripping and stumbling with subsequent striking against unspecified sharp object**

√6ᵗʰ **W01.19** **Fall on same level from slipping, tripping and stumbling with subsequent striking against other object**

√7ᵗʰ **W01.190** **Fall on same level from slipping, tripping and stumbling with subsequent striking against furniture**

√7ᵗʰ **W01.198** **Fall on same level from slipping, tripping and stumbling with subsequent striking against other object**

✓x7th **W03**   **Other fall on same level due to collision with another person**

Fall due to non-transport collision with other person

> EXCLUDES 1   *collision with another person without fall (W51)*
> *crushed or pushed by a crowd or human stampede (W52)*
> *fall involving pedestrian conveyance (V00-V09)*
> *fall due to ice or snow (W00)*
> *fall on same level NOS (W18.30)*

AHA: 2012,4Q,108

✓x7th **W04**   **Fall while being carried or supported by other persons**

Accidentally dropped while being carried

✓4th **W05**   **Fall from non-moving wheelchair, nonmotorized scooter and motorized mobility scooter**

> EXCLUDES 1   *fall from moving wheelchair (powered) (V00.811)*
> *fall from moving motorized mobility scooter (V00.831)*
> *fall from nonmotorized scooter (V00.141)*

✓x7th **W05.0**   **Fall from non-moving wheelchair**

AHA: 2019,2Q,27

✓x7th **W05.1**   **Fall from non-moving nonmotorized scooter**

✓x7th **W05.2**   **Fall from non-moving motorized mobility scooter**

✓x7th **W06**   **Fall from bed**

✓x7th **W07**   **Fall from chair**

✓x7th **W08**   **Fall from other furniture**

✓4th **W09**   **Fall on and from playground equipment**

> EXCLUDES 1   *fall involving recreational machinery (W31)*

✓x7th **W09.0**   **Fall on or from playground slide**

✓x7th **W09.1**   **Fall from playground swing**

✓x7th **W09.2**   **Fall on or from jungle gym**

✓x7th **W09.8**   **Fall on or from other playground equipment**

✓4th **W10**   **Fall on and from stairs and steps**

> EXCLUDES 1   *Fall from stairs and steps due to ice and snow (W00.1)*

✓x7th **W10.0**   **Fall (on)(from) escalator**

✓x7th **W10.1**   **Fall (on)(from) sidewalk curb**

✓x7th **W10.2**   **Fall (on)(from) incline**

Fall (on) (from) ramp

✓x7th **W10.8**   **Fall (on) (from) other stairs and steps**

✓x7th **W10.9**   **Fall (on) (from) unspecified stairs and steps**

✓x7th **W11**   **Fall on and from ladder**

✓x7th **W12**   **Fall on and from scaffolding**

✓4th **W13**   **Fall from, out of or through building or structure**

✓x7th **W13.0**   **Fall from, out of or through balcony**

Fall from, out of or through railing

✓x7th **W13.1**   **Fall from, out of or through bridge**

✓x7th **W13.2**   **Fall from, out of or through roof**

✓x7th **W13.3**   **Fall through floor**

✓x7th **W13.4**   **Fall from, out of or through window**

> EXCLUDES 2   *fall with subsequent striking against sharp glass (W01.110)*

✓x7th **W13.8**   **Fall from, out of or through other building or structure**

Fall from, out of or through viaduct

Fall from, out of or through wall

Fall from, out of or through flag-pole

✓x7th **W13.9**   **Fall from, out of or through building, not otherwise specified**

> EXCLUDES 1   *collapse of a building or structure (W20.-)*
> *fall or jump from burning building or structure (X00.-)*

✓x7th **W14**   **Fall from tree**

✓x7th **W15**   **Fall from cliff**

✓4th **W16**   **Fall, jump or diving into water**

> EXCLUDES 1   *accidental non-watercraft drowning and submersion not involving fall (W65-W74)*
> *effects of air pressure from diving (W94.-)*
> *fall into water from watercraft (V90-V94)*
> *hitting an object or against bottom when falling from watercraft (V94.0)*
>
> EXCLUDES 2   *striking or hitting diving board (W21.4)*

✓5th **W16.0**   **Fall into swimming pool**

Fall into swimming pool NOS

> EXCLUDES 1   *fall into empty swimming pool (W17.3)*

✓6th **W16.01**   **Fall into swimming pool striking water surface**

✓7th **W16.011**   **Fall into swimming pool striking water surface causing drowning and submersion**

> EXCLUDES 1   *drowning and submersion while in swimming pool without fall (W67)*

✓7th **W16.012**   **Fall into swimming pool striking water surface causing other injury**

✓6th **W16.02**   **Fall into swimming pool striking bottom**

✓7th **W16.021**   **Fall into swimming pool striking bottom causing drowning and submersion**

> EXCLUDES 1   *drowning and submersion while in swimming pool without fall (W67)*

✓7th **W16.022**   **Fall into swimming pool striking bottom causing other injury**

✓6th **W16.03**   **Fall into swimming pool striking wall**

✓7th **W16.031**   **Fall into swimming pool striking wall causing drowning and submersion**

> EXCLUDES 1   *drowning and submersion while in swimming pool without fall (W67)*

✓7th **W16.032**   **Fall into swimming pool striking wall causing other injury**

✓5th **W16.1**   **Fall into natural body of water**

Fall into lake

Fall into open sea

Fall into river

Fall into stream

✓6th **W16.11**   **Fall into natural body of water striking water surface**

✓7th **W16.111**   **Fall into natural body of water striking water surface causing drowning and submersion**

> EXCLUDES 1   *drowning and submersion while in natural body of water without fall (W69)*

✓7th **W16.112**   **Fall into natural body of water striking water surface causing other injury**

✓6th **W16.12**   **Fall into natural body of water striking bottom**

✓7th **W16.121**   **Fall into natural body of water striking bottom causing drowning and submersion**

> EXCLUDES 1   *drowning and submersion while in natural body of water without fall (W69)*

✓7th **W16.122**   **Fall into natural body of water striking bottom causing other injury**

✓6th **W16.13**   **Fall into natural body of water striking side**

✓7th **W16.131**   **Fall into natural body of water striking side causing drowning and submersion**

> EXCLUDES 1   *drowning and submersion while in natural body of water without fall (W69)*

✓7th **W16.132**   **Fall into natural body of water striking side causing other injury**

✓5th **W16.2**   **Fall in (into) filled bathtub or bucket of water**

✓6th **W16.21**   **Fall in (into) filled bathtub**

> EXCLUDES 1   *fall into empty bathtub (W18.2)*

✓7th **W16.211**   **Fall in (into) filled bathtub causing drowning and submersion**

> EXCLUDES 1   *drowning and submersion while in filled bathtub without fall (W65)*

✓7th **W16.212**   **Fall in (into) filled bathtub causing other injury**

N Newborn: 0   P Pediatric: 0-17   M Maternity: 9-64   A Adult: 15-124   MCC Major Complication/Comorbidity   CC Complication/Comorbidity   SW Severe Wound Dx

√6ᵗʰ **W16.22 Fall in (into)** bucket of water

   √7ᵗʰ **W16.221 Fall in (into) bucket of water causing** drowning and submersion

   √7ᵗʰ **W16.222 Fall in (into) bucket of water causing** other injury

√5ᵗʰ **W16.3 Fall into other water**

   Fall into fountain
   Fall into reservoir

  √6ᵗʰ **W16.31 Fall into other water** striking water surface

    √7ᵗʰ **W16.311 Fall into other water striking water surface causing** drowning and submersion

       EXCLUDES 1   *drowning and submersion while in other water without fall (W73)*

    √7ᵗʰ **W16.312 Fall into other water striking water surface causing** other injury

  √6ᵗʰ **W16.32 Fall into other water** striking bottom

    √7ᵗʰ **W16.321 Fall into other water striking bottom causing** drowning and submersion

       EXCLUDES 1   *drowning and submersion while in other water without fall (W73)*

    √7ᵗʰ **W16.322 Fall into other water striking bottom causing** other injury

  √6ᵗʰ **W16.33 Fall into other water** striking wall

    √7ᵗʰ **W16.331 Fall into other water striking wall causing** drowning and submersion

       EXCLUDES 1   *drowning and submersion while in other water without fall (W73)*

    √7ᵗʰ **W16.332 Fall into other water striking wall causing** other injury

√5ᵗʰ **W16.4 Fall into unspecified water**

  √x7ᵗʰ **W16.41 Fall into unspecified water causing** drowning and submersion

  √x7ᵗʰ **W16.42 Fall into unspecified water causing** other injury

√5ᵗʰ **W16.5 Jumping or diving into** swimming pool

  √6ᵗʰ **W16.51 Jumping or diving into swimming pool** striking water surface

    √7ᵗʰ **W16.511 Jumping or diving into swimming pool striking water surface causing** drowning and submersion

       EXCLUDES 1   *drowning and submersion while in swimming pool without jumping or diving (W67)*

    √7ᵗʰ **W16.512 Jumping or diving into swimming pool striking water surface causing** other injury

  √6ᵗʰ **W16.52 Jumping or diving into swimming pool** striking bottom

    √7ᵗʰ **W16.521 Jumping or diving into swimming pool striking bottom causing** drowning and submersion

       EXCLUDES 1   *drowning and submersion while in swimming pool without jumping or diving (W67)*

    √7ᵗʰ **W16.522 Jumping or diving into swimming pool striking bottom causing** other injury

  √6ᵗʰ **W16.53 Jumping or diving into swimming pool** striking wall

    √7ᵗʰ **W16.531 Jumping or diving into swimming pool striking wall causing** drowning and submersion

       EXCLUDES 1   *drowning and submersion while in swimming pool without jumping or diving (W67)*

    √7ᵗʰ **W16.532 Jumping or diving into swimming pool striking wall causing** other injury

√5ᵗʰ **W16.6 Jumping or diving into** natural body of water

   Jumping or diving into lake
   Jumping or diving into open sea
   Jumping or diving into river
   Jumping or diving into stream

  √6ᵗʰ **W16.61 Jumping or diving into natural body of water** striking water surface

    √7ᵗʰ **W16.611 Jumping or diving into natural body of water striking water surface causing** drowning and submersion

       EXCLUDES 1   *drowning and submersion while in natural body of water without jumping or diving (W69)*

    √7ᵗʰ **W16.612 Jumping or diving into natural body of water striking water surface causing** other injury

  √6ᵗʰ **W16.62 Jumping or diving into natural body of water** striking bottom

    √7ᵗʰ **W16.621 Jumping or diving into natural body of water striking bottom causing** drowning and submersion

       EXCLUDES 1   *drowning and submersion while in natural body of water without jumping or diving (W69)*

    √7ᵗʰ **W16.622 Jumping or diving into natural body of water striking bottom causing** other injury

√5ᵗʰ **W16.7 Jumping or diving** from boat

    EXCLUDES 1   *fall from boat into water — see watercraft accident (V90-V94)*

  √6ᵗʰ **W16.71 Jumping or diving from boat** striking water surface

    √7ᵗʰ **W16.711 Jumping or diving from boat striking water surface causing** drowning and submersion

    √7ᵗʰ **W16.712 Jumping or diving from boat striking water surface causing** other injury

  √6ᵗʰ **W16.72 Jumping or diving from boat** striking bottom

    √7ᵗʰ **W16.721 Jumping or diving from boat striking bottom causing** drowning and submersion

    √7ᵗʰ **W16.722 Jumping or diving from boat striking bottom causing** other injury

√5ᵗʰ **W16.8 Jumping or diving into other water**

   Jumping or diving into fountain
   Jumping or diving into reservoir

  √6ᵗʰ **W16.81 Jumping or diving into other water** striking water surface

    √7ᵗʰ **W16.811 Jumping or diving into other water striking water surface causing** drowning and submersion

       EXCLUDES 1   *drowning and submersion while in other water without jumping or diving (W73)*

    √7ᵗʰ **W16.812 Jumping or diving into other water striking water surface causing** other injury

  √6ᵗʰ **W16.82 Jumping or diving into other water** striking bottom

    √7ᵗʰ **W16.821 Jumping or diving into other water striking bottom causing** drowning and submersion

       EXCLUDES 1   *drowning and submersion while in other water without jumping or diving (W73)*

    √7ᵗʰ **W16.822 Jumping or diving into other water striking bottom causing** other injury

  √6ᵗʰ **W16.83 Jumping or diving into other water** striking wall

    √7ᵗʰ **W16.831 Jumping or diving into other water striking wall causing** drowning and submersion

       EXCLUDES 1   *drowning and submersion while in other water without jumping or diving (W73)*

    √7ᵗʰ **W16.832 Jumping or diving into other water striking wall causing** other injury

✓ Additional Char Req   √x7ᵗʰ Placeholder   Unacceptable PDx   Questionable PDx   Wrong Procedure   Manifestation   Unspecified Dx   H1-H14 HAC   HCC CMS-HCC Dx   HIV HIV Dx

ICD-10-CM 2020   1243

√5ᵗʰ **W16.9 Jumping or diving into unspecified water**

   √x7ᵗʰ **W16.91 Jumping or diving into unspecified water causing drowning and submersion**

   √x7ᵗʰ **W16.92 Jumping or diving into unspecified water causing other injury**

√4ᵗʰ **W17 Other fall from one level to another**

  √x7ᵗʰ **W17.0 Fall into well**

  √x7ᵗʰ **W17.1 Fall into storm drain or manhole**

  √x7ᵗʰ **W17.2 Fall into hole**

      Fall into pit

  √x7ᵗʰ **W17.3 Fall into empty swimming pool**

     EXCLUDES 1   *fall into filled swimming pool (W16.0-)*

  √x7ᵗʰ **W17.4 Fall from dock**

  √5ᵗʰ **W17.8 Other fall from one level to another**

    √x7ᵗʰ **W17.81 Fall down embankment (hill)**

    √x7ᵗʰ **W17.82 Fall from (out of) grocery cart**

        Fall due to grocery cart tipping over

    √x7ᵗʰ **W17.89 Other fall from one level to another**

        Fall from cherry picker

        Fall from lifting device

        Fall from mobile elevated work platform [MEWP]

        Fall from sky lift

        AHA: 2015,2Q,6

√4ᵗʰ **W18 Other slipping, tripping and stumbling and falls**

  √5ᵗʰ **W18.0 Fall due to bumping against object**

      Striking against object with subsequent fall

     EXCLUDES 1   *fall on same level due to slipping, tripping, or stumbling with subsequent striking against object (W01.1-)*

    √x7ᵗʰ **W18.00 Striking against unspecified object with subsequent fall**

    √x7ᵗʰ **W18.01 Striking against sports equipment with subsequent fall**

    √x7ᵗʰ **W18.02 Striking against glass with subsequent fall**

    √x7ᵗʰ **W18.09 Striking against other object with subsequent fall**

  √5ᵗʰ **W18.1 Fall from or off toilet**

    √x7ᵗʰ **W18.11 Fall from or off toilet without subsequent striking against object**

        Fall from (off) toilet NOS

    √x7ᵗʰ **W18.12 Fall from or off toilet with subsequent striking against object**

  √x7ᵗʰ **W18.2 Fall in (into) shower or empty bathtub**

     EXCLUDES 1   *fall in full bathtub causing drowning or submersion (W16.21-)*

  √5ᵗʰ **W18.3 Other and unspecified fall on same level**

    √x7ᵗʰ **W18.30 Fall on same level, unspecified**

    √x7ᵗʰ **W18.31 Fall on same level due to stepping on an object**

        Fall on same level due to stepping on an animal

     EXCLUDES 1   *slipping, tripping and stumbling without fall due to stepping on animal (W18.41)*

    √x7ᵗʰ **W18.39 Other fall on same level**

  √5ᵗʰ **W18.4 Slipping, tripping and stumbling without falling**

     EXCLUDES 1   *collision with another person without fall (W51)*

    √x7ᵗʰ **W18.40 Slipping, tripping and stumbling without falling, unspecified**

    √x7ᵗʰ **W18.41 Slipping, tripping and stumbling without falling due to stepping on object**

        Slipping, tripping and stumbling without falling due to stepping on animal

     EXCLUDES 1   *slipping, tripping and stumbling with fall due to stepping on animal (W18.31)*

    √x7ᵗʰ **W18.42 Slipping, tripping and stumbling without falling due to stepping into hole or opening**

    √x7ᵗʰ **W18.43 Slipping, tripping and stumbling without falling due to stepping from one level to another**

    √x7ᵗʰ **W18.49 Other slipping, tripping and stumbling without falling**

√x7ᵗʰ **W19 Unspecified fall**

    Accidental fall NOS

    AHA: 2012,4Q,95

Exposure to inanimate mechanical forces (W20-W49)

  EXCLUDES 1   *assault (X92-Y09)*

        contact or collision with animals or persons (W50-W64)

        exposure to inanimate mechanical forces involving military or war operations (Y36.-, Y37.-)

        intentional self-harm (X71-X83)

The appropriate 7th character is to be added to each code from categories W20-W49.
A   initial encounter
D   subsequent encounter
S   sequela

√4ᵗʰ **W20 Struck by thrown, projected or falling object**

    Code first any associated:

      cataclysm (X34-X39)

      lightning strike (T75.00)

     EXCLUDES 1   *falling object in machinery accident (W24, W28-W31)*

        falling object in transport accident (V01-V99)

        object set in motion by explosion (W35-W40)

        object set in motion by firearm (W32-W34)

        struck by thrown sports equipment (W21.-)

  √x7ᵗʰ **W20.0 Struck by falling object in cave-in**

     EXCLUDES 2   *asphyxiation due to cave-in (T71.21)*

  √x7ᵗʰ **W20.1 Struck by object due to collapse of building**

     EXCLUDES 1   *struck by object due to collapse of burning building (X00.2, X02.2)*

  √x7ᵗʰ **W20.8 Other cause of strike by thrown, projected or falling object**

     EXCLUDES 1   *struck by thrown sports equipment (W21.-)*

√4ᵗʰ **W21 Striking against or struck by sports equipment**

     EXCLUDES 1   *assault with sports equipment (Y08.0-)*

        striking against or struck by sports equipment with subsequent fall (W18.01)

  √5ᵗʰ **W21.0 Struck by hit or thrown ball**

    √x7ᵗʰ **W21.00 Struck by hit or thrown ball, unspecified type**

    √x7ᵗʰ **W21.01 Struck by football**

    √x7ᵗʰ **W21.02 Struck by soccer ball**

    √x7ᵗʰ **W21.03 Struck by baseball**

    √x7ᵗʰ **W21.04 Struck by golf ball**

    √x7ᵗʰ **W21.05 Struck by basketball**

    √x7ᵗʰ **W21.06 Struck by volleyball**

    √x7ᵗʰ **W21.07 Struck by softball**

    √x7ᵗʰ **W21.09 Struck by other hit or thrown ball**

  √5ᵗʰ **W21.1 Struck by bat, racquet or club**

    √x7ᵗʰ **W21.11 Struck by baseball bat**

    √x7ᵗʰ **W21.12 Struck by tennis racquet**

    √x7ᵗʰ **W21.13 Struck by golf club**

    √x7ᵗʰ **W21.19 Struck by other bat, racquet or club**

  √5ᵗʰ **W21.2 Struck by hockey stick or puck**

    √6ᵗʰ **W21.21 Struck by hockey stick**

      √7ᵗʰ **W21.210 Struck by ice hockey stick**

      √7ᵗʰ **W21.211 Struck by field hockey stick**

    √6ᵗʰ **W21.22 Struck by hockey puck**

      √7ᵗʰ **W21.220 Struck by ice hockey puck**

      √7ᵗʰ **W21.221 Struck by field hockey puck**

  √5ᵗʰ **W21.3 Struck by sports foot wear**

    √x7ᵗʰ **W21.31 Struck by shoe cleats**

        Stepped on by shoe cleats

    √x7ᵗʰ **W21.32 Struck by skate blades**

        Skated over by skate blades

    √x7ᵗʰ **W21.39 Struck by other sports foot wear**

  √x7ᵗʰ **W21.4 Striking against diving board**

      Use additional code for subsequent falling into water, if applicable (W16.-)

  √5ᵗʰ **W21.8 Striking against or struck by other sports equipment**

    √x7ᵗʰ **W21.81 Striking against or struck by football helmet**

    √x7ᵗʰ **W21.89 Striking against or struck by other sports equipment**

  √x7ᵗʰ **W21.9 Striking against or struck by unspecified sports equipment**

N Newborn: 0   P Pediatric: 0-17   M Maternity: 9-64   A Adult: 15-124   MCC Major Complication/Comorbidity   CC Complication/Comorbidity   SW Severe Wound Dx

1244   ICD-10-CM 2020

✓4ᵗʰ **W22 Striking against or struck by other objects**

     EXCLUDES 1   striking against or struck by object with subsequent fall (W18.09)

   ✓5ᵗʰ **W22.0 Striking against stationary object**

       EXCLUDES 1   striking against stationary sports equipment (W21.8)

     ✓7ᵗʰ **W22.01 Walked into wall**

     ✓7ᵗʰ **W22.02 Walked into lamppost**

     ✓7ᵗʰ **W22.03 Walked into furniture**

      ✓6ᵗʰ **W22.04 Striking against wall of swimming pool**

        ✓7ᵗʰ **W22.041 Striking against wall of swimming pool causing drowning and submersion**

          EXCLUDES 1   drowning and submersion while swimming without striking against wall (W67)

        ✓7ᵗʰ **W22.042 Striking against wall of swimming pool causing other injury**

     ✓7ᵗʰ **W22.09 Striking against other stationary object**

   ✓5ᵗʰ **W22.1 Striking against or struck by automobile airbag**

     ✓7ᵗʰ **W22.10 Striking against or struck by unspecified automobile airbag**

     ✓7ᵗʰ **W22.11 Striking against or struck by driver side automobile airbag**

     ✓7ᵗʰ **W22.12 Striking against or struck by front passenger side automobile airbag**

     ✓7ᵗʰ **W22.19 Striking against or struck by other automobile airbag**

   ✓7ᵗʰ **W22.8 Striking against or struck by other objects**

     Striking against or struck by object NOS

      EXCLUDES 1   struck by thrown, projected or falling object (W20.-)

✓4ᵗʰ **W23 Caught, crushed, jammed or pinched in or between objects**

     EXCLUDES 1   injury caused by cutting or piercing instruments (W25-W27)

           injury caused by firearms malfunction (W32.1, W33.1-, W34.1-)

           injury caused by lifting and transmission devices (W24.-)

           injury caused by machinery (W28-W31)

           injury caused by nonpowered hand tools (W27.-)

           injury caused by transport vehicle being used as a means of transportation (V01-V99)

           injury caused by struck by thrown, projected or falling object (W20.-)

   ✓7ᵗʰ **W23.0 Caught, crushed, jammed, or pinched between moving objects**

   ✓7ᵗʰ **W23.1 Caught, crushed, jammed, or pinched between stationary objects**

✓4ᵗʰ **W24 Contact with lifting and transmission devices, not elsewhere classified**

     EXCLUDES 1   transport accidents (V01-V99)

   ✓7ᵗʰ **W24.0 Contact with lifting devices, not elsewhere classified**

     Contact with chain hoist

     Contact with drive belt

     Contact with pulley (block)

   ✓7ᵗʰ **W24.1 Contact with transmission devices, not elsewhere classified**

     Contact with transmission belt or cable

✓7ᵗʰ **W25 Contact with sharp glass**

     Code first any associated:

     injury due to flying glass from explosion or firearm discharge (W32-W40)

     transport accident (V00-V99)

      EXCLUDES 1   fall on same level due to slipping, tripping and stumbling with subsequent striking against sharp glass ▶(W01.110)◀

           striking against sharp glass with subsequent fall (W18.02)

      EXCLUDES 2   glass embedded in skin (W45)

✓4ᵗʰ **W26 Contact with other sharp objects**

      EXCLUDES 2   sharp object(s) embedded in skin (W45)

     AHA: 2016,4Q,73

   ✓7ᵗʰ **W26.0 Contact with knife**

      EXCLUDES 1   contact with electric knife (W29.1)

   ✓7ᵗʰ **W26.1 Contact with sword or dagger**

   ✓7ᵗʰ **W26.2 Contact with edge of stiff paper**

     Paper cut

   ✓x7ᵗʰ **W26.8 Contact with other sharp object(s), not elsewhere classified**

     Contact with tin can lid

   ✓x7ᵗʰ **W26.9 Contact with unspecified sharp object(s)**

✓4ᵗʰ **W27 Contact with nonpowered hand tool**

   ✓x7ᵗʰ **W27.0 Contact with workbench tool**

     Contact with auger

     Contact with axe

     Contact with chisel

     Contact with handsaw

     Contact with screwdriver

   ✓x7ᵗʰ **W27.1 Contact with garden tool**

     Contact with hoe

     Contact with nonpowered lawn mower

     Contact with pitchfork

     Contact with rake

   ✓x7ᵗʰ **W27.2 Contact with scissors**

   ✓x7ᵗʰ **W27.3 Contact with needle (sewing)**

      EXCLUDES 1   contact with hypodermic needle (W46.-)

   ✓x7ᵗʰ **W27.4 Contact with kitchen utensil**

     Contact with fork

     Contact with ice-pick

     Contact with can-opener NOS

   ✓x7ᵗʰ **W27.5 Contact with paper-cutter**

   ✓x7ᵗʰ **W27.8 Contact with other nonpowered hand tool**

     Contact with nonpowered sewing machine

     Contact with shovel

✓x7ᵗʰ **W28 Contact with powered lawn mower**

     Powered lawn mower (commercial) (residential)

      EXCLUDES 1   contact with nonpowered lawn mower (W27.1)

      EXCLUDES 2   exposure to electric current (W86.-)

✓4ᵗʰ **W29 Contact with other powered hand tools and household machinery**

      EXCLUDES 1   contact with commercial machinery (W31.82)

           contact with hot household appliance (X15)

           contact with nonpowered hand tool (W27.-)

           exposure to electric current (W86)

   ✓x7ᵗʰ **W29.0 Contact with powered kitchen appliance**

     Contact with blender

     Contact with can-opener

     Contact with garbage disposal

     Contact with mixer

   ✓x7ᵗʰ **W29.1 Contact with electric knife**

   ✓x7ᵗʰ **W29.2 Contact with other powered household machinery**

     Contact with electric fan

     Contact with powered dryer (clothes) (powered) (spin)

     Contact with washing-machine

     Contact with sewing machine

   ✓x7ᵗʰ **W29.3 Contact with powered garden and outdoor hand tools and machinery**

     Contact with chainsaw

     Contact with edger

     Contact with garden cultivator (tiller)

     Contact with hedge trimmer

     Contact with other powered garden tool

      EXCLUDES 1   contact with powered lawn mower (W28)

   ✓x7ᵗʰ **W29.4 Contact with nail gun**

   ✓x7ᵗʰ **W29.8 Contact with other powered hand tools and household machinery**

     Contact with do-it-yourself tool NOS

✓4ᵗʰ **W30 Contact with agricultural machinery**

     INCLUDES   animal-powered farm machine

      EXCLUDES 1   agricultural transport vehicle accident (V01-V99)

           explosion of grain store (W40.8)

           exposure to electric current (W86.-)

   ✓x7ᵗʰ **W30.0 Contact with combine harvester**

     Contact with reaper

     Contact with thresher

   ✓x7ᵗʰ **W30.1 Contact with power take-off devices (PTO)**

   ✓x7ᵗʰ **W30.2 Contact with hay derrick**

   ✓x7ᵗʰ **W30.3 Contact with grain storage elevator**

      EXCLUDES 1   explosion of grain store (W40.8)

☑ Additional Char Req   ✓x7ᵗʰ Placeholder   Unacceptable PDx   Questionable PDx   Wrong Procedure   Manifestation   Unspecified Dx   H1-H14 HAC   HCC CMS-HCC Dx   HIV HIV Dx

√5ᵗʰ **W30.8** **Contact with other specified agricultural machinery**

√x7ᵗʰ **W30.81** **Contact with agricultural transport vehicle in stationary use**

Contact with agricultural transport vehicle under repair, not on public roadway

EXCLUDES 1 *agricultural transport vehicle accident (V01-V99)*

√x7ᵗʰ **W30.89** **Contact with other specified agricultural machinery**

√x7ᵗʰ **W30.9** **Contact with unspecified agricultural machinery**

Contact with farm machinery NOS

√4ᵗʰ **W31** **Contact with other and unspecified machinery**

EXCLUDES 1 *contact with agricultural machinery (W30.-)*

contact with machinery in transport under own power or being towed by a vehicle (V01-V99)

exposure to electric current (W86)

√x7ᵗʰ **W31.0** **Contact with mining and earth-drilling machinery**

Contact with bore or drill (land) (seabed)

Contact with shaft hoist

Contact with shaft lift

Contact with undercutter

√x7ᵗʰ **W31.1** **Contact with metalworking machines**

Contact with abrasive wheel

Contact with forging machine

Contact with lathe

Contact with mechanical shears

Contact with metal drilling machine

Contact with milling machine

Contact with power press

Contact with rolling-mill

Contact with metal sawing machine

√x7ᵗʰ **W31.2** **Contact with powered woodworking and forming machines**

Contact with band saw

Contact with bench saw

Contact with circular saw

Contact with molding machine

Contact with overhead plane

Contact with powered saw

Contact with radial saw

Contact with sander

EXCLUDES 1 *nonpowered woodworking tools (W27.0)*

√x7ᵗʰ **W31.3** **Contact with prime movers**

Contact with gas turbine

Contact with internal combustion engine

Contact with steam engine

Contact with water driven turbine

√5ᵗʰ **W31.8** **Contact with other specified machinery**

√x7ᵗʰ **W31.81** **Contact with recreational machinery**

Contact with roller coaster

√x7ᵗʰ **W31.82** **Contact with other commercial machinery**

Contact with commercial electric fan

Contact with commercial kitchen appliances

Contact with commercial powered dryer (clothes) (powered) (spin)

Contact with commercial washing-machine

Contact with commercial sewing machine

EXCLUDES 1 *contact with household machinery (W29.-)*

contact with powered lawn mower (W28)

√x7ᵗʰ **W31.83** **Contact with special construction vehicle in stationary use**

Contact with special construction vehicle under repair, not on public roadway

EXCLUDES 1 *special construction vehicle accident (V01-V99)*

√x7ᵗʰ **W31.89** **Contact with other specified machinery**

√x7ᵗʰ **W31.9** **Contact with unspecified machinery**

Contact with machinery NOS

√4ᵗʰ **W32** **Accidental handgun discharge and malfunction**

INCLUDES accidental discharge and malfunction of gun for single hand use

accidental discharge and malfunction of pistol

accidental discharge and malfunction of revolver

handgun discharge and malfunction NOS

EXCLUDES 1 *accidental airgun discharge and malfunction (W34.010, W34.110)*

accidental BB gun discharge and malfunction (W34.010, W34.110)

accidental pellet gun discharge and malfunction (W34.010, W34.110)

accidental shotgun discharge and malfunction (W33.01, W33.11)

assault by handgun discharge (X93)

handgun discharge involving legal intervention (Y35.0-)

handgun discharge involving military or war operations (Y36.4-)

intentional self-harm by handgun discharge (X72)

Very pistol discharge and malfunction (W34.09, W34.19)

√x7ᵗʰ **W32.0** **Accidental handgun discharge**

√x7ᵗʰ **W32.1** **Accidental handgun malfunction**

Injury due to explosion of handgun (parts)

Injury due to malfunction of mechanism or component of handgun

Injury due to recoil of handgun

Powder burn from handgun

√4ᵗʰ **W33** **Accidental rifle, shotgun and larger firearm discharge and malfunction**

INCLUDES rifle, shotgun and larger firearm discharge and malfunction NOS

EXCLUDES 1 *accidental airgun discharge and malfunction (W34.010, W34.110)*

accidental BB gun discharge and malfunction (W34.010, W34.110)

accidental handgun discharge and malfunction (W32.-)

accidental pellet gun discharge and malfunction (W34.010, W34.110)

assault by rifle, shotgun and larger firearm discharge (X94)

firearm discharge involving legal intervention (Y35.0-)

firearm discharge involving military or war operations (Y36.4-)

intentional self-harm by rifle, shotgun and larger firearm discharge (X73)

√5ᵗʰ **W33.0** **Accidental rifle, shotgun and larger firearm discharge**

√x7ᵗʰ **W33.00** **Accidental discharge of unspecified larger firearm**

Discharge of unspecified larger firearm NOS

√x7ᵗʰ **W33.01** **Accidental discharge of shotgun**

Discharge of shotgun NOS

√x7ᵗʰ **W33.02** **Accidental discharge of hunting rifle**

Discharge of hunting rifle NOS

√x7ᵗʰ **W33.03** **Accidental discharge of machine gun**

Discharge of machine gun NOS

√x7ᵗʰ **W33.09** **Accidental discharge of other larger firearm**

Discharge of other larger firearm NOS

√5ᵗʰ **W33.1** **Accidental rifle, shotgun and larger firearm malfunction**

Injury due to explosion of rifle, shotgun and larger firearm (parts)

Injury due to malfunction of mechanism or component of rifle, shotgun and larger firearm

Injury due to piercing, cutting, crushing or pinching due to (by) slide trigger mechanism, scope or other gun part

Injury due to recoil of rifle, shotgun and larger firearm

Powder burn from rifle, shotgun and larger firearm

√x7ᵗʰ **W33.10** **Accidental malfunction of unspecified larger firearm**

Malfunction of unspecified larger firearm NOS

√x7ᵗʰ **W33.11** **Accidental malfunction of shotgun**

Malfunction of shotgun NOS

√x7ᵗʰ **W33.12** **Accidental malfunction of hunting rifle**

Malfunction of hunting rifle NOS

√x7ᵗʰ **W33.13** **Accidental malfunction of machine gun**

Malfunction of machine gun NOS

N Newborn: 0   P Pediatric: 0-17   M Maternity: 9-64   A Adult: 15-124   MCC Major Complication/Comorbidity   CC Complication/Comorbidity   SW Severe Wound Dx

1246   ICD-10-CM 2020

☑x7ᵗʰ **W33.19**   **Accidental malfunction of other larger firearm**

Malfunction of other larger firearm NOS

☑4ᵗʰ **W34**   **Accidental discharge and malfunction from other and unspecified firearms and guns**

  ☑5ᵗʰ **W34.0**   **Accidental discharge from other and unspecified firearms and guns**

    ☑x7ᵗʰ **W34.00**   **Accidental discharge from unspecified firearms or gun**

Discharge from firearm NOS

Gunshot wound NOS

Shot NOS

    ☑6ᵗʰ **W34.01**   **Accidental discharge of gas, air or spring-operated guns**

      ☑7ᵗʰ **W34.010**   **Accidental discharge of airgun**

Accidental discharge of BB gun

Accidental discharge of pellet gun

      ☑7ᵗʰ **W34.011**   **Accidental discharge of paintball gun**

Accidental injury due to paintball discharge

      ☑7ᵗʰ **W34.018**   **Accidental discharge of other gas, air or spring-operated gun**

    ☑x7ᵗʰ **W34.09**   **Accidental discharge from other specified firearms**

Accidental discharge from Very pistol [flare]

  ☑5ᵗʰ **W34.1**   **Accidental malfunction from other and unspecified firearms and guns**

    ☑x7ᵗʰ **W34.10**   **Accidental malfunction from unspecified firearms or gun**

Firearm malfunction NOS

    ☑6ᵗʰ **W34.11**   **Accidental malfunction of gas, air or spring-operated guns**

      ☑7ᵗʰ **W34.110**   **Accidental malfunction of airgun**

Accidental malfunction of BB gun

Accidental malfunction of pellet gun

      ☑7ᵗʰ **W34.111**   **Accidental malfunction of paintball gun**

Accidental injury due to paintball gun malfunction

      ☑7ᵗʰ **W34.118**   **Accidental malfunction of other gas, air or spring-operated gun**

    ☑x7ᵗʰ **W34.19**   **Accidental malfunction from other specified firearms**

Accidental malfunction from Very pistol [flare]

☑x7ᵗʰ **W35**   **Explosion and rupture of boiler**

  EXCLUDES 1   *explosion and rupture of boiler on watercraft (V93.4)*

☑4ᵗʰ **W36**   **Explosion and rupture of gas cylinder**

  ☑x7ᵗʰ **W36.1**   **Explosion and rupture of aerosol can**

  ☑x7ᵗʰ **W36.2**   **Explosion and rupture of air tank**

  ☑x7ᵗʰ **W36.3**   **Explosion and rupture of pressurized-gas tank**

  ☑x7ᵗʰ **W36.8**   **Explosion and rupture of other gas cylinder**

  ☑x7ᵗʰ **W36.9**   **Explosion and rupture of unspecified gas cylinder**

☑4ᵗʰ **W37**   **Explosion and rupture of pressurized tire, pipe or hose**

  ☑x7ᵗʰ **W37.0**   **Explosion of bicycle tire**

  ☑x7ᵗʰ **W37.8**   **Explosion and rupture of other pressurized tire, pipe or hose**

☑x7ᵗʰ **W38**   **Explosion and rupture of other specified pressurized devices**

☑x7ᵗʰ **W39**   **Discharge of firework**

☑4ᵗʰ **W40**   **Explosion of other materials**

  EXCLUDES 1   *assault by explosive material (X96)*

    explosion involving legal intervention (Y35.1-)

    explosion involving military or war operations (Y36.0-, Y36.2-)

    intentional self-harm by explosive material (X75)

  ☑x7ᵗʰ **W40.0**   **Explosion of blasting material**

Explosion of blasting cap

Explosion of detonator

Explosion of dynamite

Explosion of explosive (any) used in blasting operations

  ☑x7ᵗʰ **W40.1**   **Explosion of explosive gases**

Explosion of acetylene

Explosion of butane

Explosion of coal gas

Explosion in mine NOS

Explosion of explosive gas

Explosion of fire damp

Explosion of gasoline fumes

Explosion of methane

Explosion of propane

  ☑x7ᵗʰ **W40.8**   **Explosion of other specified explosive materials**

Explosion in dump NOS

Explosion in factory NOS

Explosion in grain store

Explosion in munitions

    EXCLUDES 1   *explosion involving legal intervention (Y35.1-)*

      explosion involving military or war operations (Y36.0-, Y36.2-)

  ☑x7ᵗʰ **W40.9**   **Explosion of unspecified explosive materials**

Explosion NOS

☑4ᵗʰ **W42**   **Exposure to noise**

  ☑x7ᵗʰ **W42.0**   **Exposure to supersonic waves**

  ☑x7ᵗʰ **W42.9**   **Exposure to other noise**

Exposure to sound waves NOS

☑4ᵗʰ **W45**   **Foreign body or object entering through skin**

  INCLUDES   foreign body or object embedded in skin

    nail embedded in skin

  EXCLUDES 2   *contact with hand tools (nonpowered) (powered) (W27-W29)*

    contact with other sharp objects (W26.-)

    contact with sharp glass (W25.-)

    struck by objects (W20-W22)

  ☑x7ᵗʰ **W45.0**   **Nail entering through skin**

  ☑x7ᵗʰ **W45.8**   **Other foreign body or object entering through skin**

Splinter in skin NOS

☑4ᵗʰ **W46**   **Contact with hypodermic needle**

  ☑x7ᵗʰ **W46.0**   **Contact with hypodermic needle**

Hypodermic needle stick NOS

  ☑x7ᵗʰ **W46.1**   **Contact with contaminated hypodermic needle**

☑4ᵗʰ **W49**   **Exposure to other inanimate mechanical forces**

  INCLUDES   exposure to abnormal gravitational [G] forces

    exposure to inanimate mechanical forces NEC

  EXCLUDES 1   *exposure to inanimate mechanical forces involving military or war operations (Y36.-, Y37.-)*

  ☑5ᵗʰ **W49.0**   **Item causing external constriction**

    ☑x7ᵗʰ **W49.01**   **Hair causing external constriction**

    ☑x7ᵗʰ **W49.02**   **String or thread causing external constriction**

    ☑x7ᵗʰ **W49.03**   **Rubber band causing external constriction**

    ☑x7ᵗʰ **W49.04**   **Ring or other jewelry causing external constriction**

    ☑x7ᵗʰ **W49.09**   **Other specified item causing external constriction**

  ☑x7ᵗʰ **W49.9**   **Exposure to other inanimate mechanical forces**

Exposure to animate mechanical forces (W50-W64)

EXCLUDES 1   *toxic effect of contact with venomous animals and plants (T63.-)*

The appropriate 7th character is to be added to each code from categories W50-W64.

A   initial encounter

D   subsequent encounter

S   sequela

☑4ᵗʰ **W50**   **Accidental hit, strike, kick, twist, bite or scratch by another person**

  INCLUDES   hit, strike, kick, twist, bite, or scratch by another person NOS

  EXCLUDES 1   *assault by bodily force (Y04)*

    struck by objects (W20-W22)

  ☑x7ᵗʰ **W50.0**   **Accidental hit or strike by another person**

Hit or strike by another person NOS

  ☑x7ᵗʰ **W50.1**   **Accidental kick by another person**

Kick by another person NOS

  ☑x7ᵗʰ **W50.2**   **Accidental twist by another person**

Twist by another person NOS

☑ Additional Char Req   ☑x7ᵗʰ Placeholder   Unacceptable PDx   Questionable PDx   Wrong Procedure   Manifestation   Unspecified Dx   H1-H14 HAC   HCC CMS-HCC Dx   HIV HIV Dx

ICD-10-CM 2020   **1247**

√x7ᵗʰ **W50.3**   **Accidental bite by another person**
> Human bite
> Bite by another person NOS

√x7ᵗʰ **W50.4**   **Accidental scratch by another person**
> Scratch by another person NOS

√x7ᵗʰ **W51**   **Accidental striking against or bumped into by another person**
> EXCLUDES 1   *assault by striking against or bumping into by another person (Y04.2)*
> *fall due to collision with another person (W03)*

√x7ᵗʰ **W52**   **Crushed, pushed or stepped on by crowd or human stampede**
> Crushed, pushed or stepped on by crowd or human stampede with or without fall

√4ᵗʰ **W53**   **Contact with rodent**
> INCLUDES   contact with saliva, feces or urine of rodent

  √5ᵗʰ **W53.0**   **Contact with mouse**
    √x7ᵗʰ **W53.01**   **Bitten by mouse**
    √x7ᵗʰ **W53.09**   **Other contact with mouse**

  √5ᵗʰ **W53.1**   **Contact with rat**
    √x7ᵗʰ **W53.11**   **Bitten by rat**
    √x7ᵗʰ **W53.19**   **Other contact with rat**

  √5ᵗʰ **W53.2**   **Contact with squirrel**
    √x7ᵗʰ **W53.21**   **Bitten by squirrel**
    √x7ᵗʰ **W53.29**   **Other contact with squirrel**

  √5ᵗʰ **W53.8**   **Contact with other rodent**
    √x7ᵗʰ **W53.81**   **Bitten by other rodent**
    √x7ᵗʰ **W53.89**   **Other contact with other rodent**

√4ᵗʰ **W54**   **Contact with dog**
> INCLUDES   contact with saliva, feces or urine of dog

  √x7ᵗʰ **W54.0**   **Bitten by dog**

  √x7ᵗʰ **W54.1**   **Struck by dog**
> Knocked over by dog

  √x7ᵗʰ **W54.8**   **Other contact with dog**

√4ᵗʰ **W55**   **Contact with other mammals**
> INCLUDES   contact with saliva, feces or urine of mammal
> EXCLUDES 1   *animal being ridden — see transport accidents*
> *bitten or struck by dog (W54)*
> *bitten or struck by rodent (W53.-)*
> *contact with marine mammals (W56.-)*

  √5ᵗʰ **W55.0**   **Contact with cat**
    √x7ᵗʰ **W55.01**   **Bitten by cat**
    √x7ᵗʰ **W55.03**   **Scratched by cat**
    √x7ᵗʰ **W55.09**   **Other contact with cat**

  √5ᵗʰ **W55.1**   **Contact with horse**
    √x7ᵗʰ **W55.11**   **Bitten by horse**
    √x7ᵗʰ **W55.12**   **Struck by horse**
    √x7ᵗʰ **W55.19**   **Other contact with horse**

  √5ᵗʰ **W55.2**   **Contact with cow**
> Contact with bull
    √x7ᵗʰ **W55.21**   **Bitten by cow**
    √x7ᵗʰ **W55.22**   **Struck by cow**
>   Gored by bull
    √x7ᵗʰ **W55.29**   **Other contact with cow**

  √5ᵗʰ **W55.3**   **Contact with other hoof stock**
> Contact with goats
> Contact with sheep
    √x7ᵗʰ **W55.31**   **Bitten by other hoof stock**
    √x7ᵗʰ **W55.32**   **Struck by other hoof stock**
>   Gored by goat
>   Gored by ram
    √x7ᵗʰ **W55.39**   **Other contact with other hoof stock**

  √5ᵗʰ **W55.4**   **Contact with pig**
    √x7ᵗʰ **W55.41**   **Bitten by pig**
    √x7ᵗʰ **W55.42**   **Struck by pig**
    √x7ᵗʰ **W55.49**   **Other contact with pig**

  √5ᵗʰ **W55.5**   **Contact with raccoon**
    √x7ᵗʰ **W55.51**   **Bitten by raccoon**

    √x7ᵗʰ **W55.52**   **Struck by raccoon**
    √x7ᵗʰ **W55.59**   **Other contact with raccoon**

  √5ᵗʰ **W55.8**   **Contact with other mammals**
    √x7ᵗʰ **W55.81**   **Bitten by other mammals**
    √x7ᵗʰ **W55.82**   **Struck by other mammals**
    √x7ᵗʰ **W55.89**   **Other contact with other mammals**

√4ᵗʰ **W56**   **Contact with nonvenomous marine animal**
> EXCLUDES 1   *contact with venomous marine animal (T63.-)*

  √5ᵗʰ **W56.0**   **Contact with dolphin**
    √x7ᵗʰ **W56.01**   **Bitten by dolphin**
    √x7ᵗʰ **W56.02**   **Struck by dolphin**
    √x7ᵗʰ **W56.09**   **Other contact with dolphin**

  √5ᵗʰ **W56.1**   **Contact with sea lion**
    √x7ᵗʰ **W56.11**   **Bitten by sea lion**
    √x7ᵗʰ **W56.12**   **Struck by sea lion**
    √x7ᵗʰ **W56.19**   **Other contact with sea lion**

  √5ᵗʰ **W56.2**   **Contact with orca**
> Contact with killer whale
    √x7ᵗʰ **W56.21**   **Bitten by orca**
    √x7ᵗʰ **W56.22**   **Struck by orca**
    √x7ᵗʰ **W56.29**   **Other contact with orca**

  √5ᵗʰ **W56.3**   **Contact with other marine mammals**
    √x7ᵗʰ **W56.31**   **Bitten by other marine mammals**
    √x7ᵗʰ **W56.32**   **Struck by other marine mammals**
    √x7ᵗʰ **W56.39**   **Other contact with other marine mammals**

  √5ᵗʰ **W56.4**   **Contact with shark**
    √x7ᵗʰ **W56.41**   **Bitten by shark**
    √x7ᵗʰ **W56.42**   **Struck by shark**
    √x7ᵗʰ **W56.49**   **Other contact with shark**

  √5ᵗʰ **W56.5**   **Contact with other fish**
    √x7ᵗʰ **W56.51**   **Bitten by other fish**
    √x7ᵗʰ **W56.52**   **Struck by other fish**
    √x7ᵗʰ **W56.59**   **Other contact with other fish**

  √5ᵗʰ **W56.8**   **Contact with other nonvenomous marine animals**
    √x7ᵗʰ **W56.81**   **Bitten by other nonvenomous marine animals**
    √x7ᵗʰ **W56.82**   **Struck by other nonvenomous marine animals**
    √x7ᵗʰ **W56.89**   **Other contact with other nonvenomous marine animals**

√x7ᵗʰ **W57**   **Bitten or stung by nonvenomous insect and other nonvenomous arthropods**
> EXCLUDES 1   *contact with venomous insects and arthropods (T63.2-, T63.3-, T63.4-)*

√4ᵗʰ **W58**   **Contact with crocodile or alligator**

  √5ᵗʰ **W58.0**   **Contact with alligator**
    √x7ᵗʰ **W58.01**   **Bitten by alligator**
    √x7ᵗʰ **W58.02**   **Struck by alligator**
    √x7ᵗʰ **W58.03**   **Crushed by alligator**
    √x7ᵗʰ **W58.09**   **Other contact with alligator**

  √5ᵗʰ **W58.1**   **Contact with crocodile**
    √x7ᵗʰ **W58.11**   **Bitten by crocodile**
    √x7ᵗʰ **W58.12**   **Struck by crocodile**
    √x7ᵗʰ **W58.13**   **Crushed by crocodile**
    √x7ᵗʰ **W58.19**   **Other contact with crocodile**

√4ᵗʰ **W59**   **Contact with other nonvenomous reptiles**
> EXCLUDES 1   *contact with venomous reptile (T63.0-, T63.1-)*

  √5ᵗʰ **W59.0**   **Contact with nonvenomous lizards**
    √x7ᵗʰ **W59.01**   **Bitten by nonvenomous lizards**
    √x7ᵗʰ **W59.02**   **Struck by nonvenomous lizards**
    √x7ᵗʰ **W59.09**   **Other contact with nonvenomous lizards**
>   Exposure to nonvenomous lizards

  √5ᵗʰ **W59.1**   **Contact with nonvenomous snakes**
    √x7ᵗʰ **W59.11**   **Bitten by nonvenomous snake**
    √x7ᵗʰ **W59.12**   **Struck by nonvenomous snake**
    √x7ᵗʰ **W59.13**   **Crushed by nonvenomous snake**
    √x7ᵗʰ **W59.19**   **Other contact with nonvenomous snake**

√5ᵗʰ **W59.2** **Contact with** turtles
> EXCLUDES 1   contact with tortoises (W59.8-)

√x7ᵗʰ **W59.21** **Bitten by turtle**

√x7ᵗʰ **W59.22** **Struck by turtle**

√x7ᵗʰ **W59.29** **Other contact with turtle**
>   Exposure to turtles

√5ᵗʰ **W59.8** **Contact with other nonvenomous reptiles**

√x7ᵗʰ **W59.81** **Bitten by other nonvenomous reptiles**

√x7ᵗʰ **W59.82** **Struck by other nonvenomous reptiles**

√x7ᵗʰ **W59.83** **Crushed by other nonvenomous reptiles**

√x7ᵗʰ **W59.89** **Other contact with other nonvenomous reptiles**

√x7ᵗʰ **W60** **Contact with nonvenomous plant thorns and spines and sharp leaves**
> EXCLUDES 1   contact with venomous plants (T63.7-)

√4ᵗʰ **W61** **Contact with birds (domestic) (wild)**
> INCLUDES   contact with excreta of birds

√5ᵗʰ **W61.0** **Contact with** parrot

√x7ᵗʰ **W61.01** **Bitten by parrot**

√x7ᵗʰ **W61.02** **Struck by parrot**

√x7ᵗʰ **W61.09** **Other contact with parrot**
>   Exposure to parrots

√5ᵗʰ **W61.1** **Contact with** macaw

√x7ᵗʰ **W61.11** **Bitten by macaw**

√x7ᵗʰ **W61.12** **Struck by macaw**

√x7ᵗʰ **W61.19** **Other contact with macaw**
>   Exposure to macaws

√5ᵗʰ **W61.2** **Contact with other** psittacines

√x7ᵗʰ **W61.21** **Bitten by other psittacines**

√x7ᵗʰ **W61.22** **Struck by other psittacines**

√x7ᵗʰ **W61.29** **Other contact with other psittacines**
>   Exposure to other psittacines

√5ᵗʰ **W61.3** **Contact with** chicken

√x7ᵗʰ **W61.32** **Struck by chicken**

√x7ᵗʰ **W61.33** **Pecked by chicken**

√x7ᵗʰ **W61.39** **Other contact with chicken**
>   Exposure to chickens

√5ᵗʰ **W61.4** **Contact with** turkey

√x7ᵗʰ **W61.42** **Struck by turkey**

√x7ᵗʰ **W61.43** **Pecked by turkey**

√x7ᵗʰ **W61.49** **Other contact with turkey**

√5ᵗʰ **W61.5** **Contact with** goose

√x7ᵗʰ **W61.51** **Bitten by goose**

√x7ᵗʰ **W61.52** **Struck by goose**

√x7ᵗʰ **W61.59** **Other contact with goose**

√5ᵗʰ **W61.6** **Contact with** duck

√x7ᵗʰ **W61.61** **Bitten by duck**

√x7ᵗʰ **W61.62** **Struck by duck**

√x7ᵗʰ **W61.69** **Other contact with duck**

√5ᵗʰ **W61.9** **Contact with other birds**

√x7ᵗʰ **W61.91** **Bitten by other birds**

√x7ᵗʰ **W61.92** **Struck by other birds**

√x7ᵗʰ **W61.99** **Other contact with other birds**
>   Contact with bird NOS

√4ᵗʰ **W62** **Contact with nonvenomous amphibians**
> EXCLUDES 1   contact with venomous amphibians (T63.81-R63.83)

√x7ᵗʰ **W62.0** **Contact with nonvenomous** frogs

√x7ᵗʰ **W62.1** **Contact with nonvenomous** toads

√x7ᵗʰ **W62.9** **Contact with other nonvenomous amphibians**

√x7ᵗʰ **W64** **Exposure to other animate mechanical forces**
> INCLUDES   exposure to nonvenomous animal NOS
> EXCLUDES 1   contact with venomous animal (T63.-)

Accidental non-transport drowning and submersion (W65-W74)

> EXCLUDES 1   accidental drowning and submersion due to fall into water (W16.-)
>   accidental drowning and submersion due to water transport accident (V90.-, V92.-)
> EXCLUDES 2   accidental drowning and submersion due to cataclysm (X34-X39)

The appropriate 7th character is to be added to each code from categories W65-W74.
A   initial encounter
D   subsequent encounter
S   sequela

√x7ᵗʰ **W65** **Accidental drowning and submersion while in** bath-tub
> EXCLUDES 1   accidental drowning and submersion due to fall in (into) bathtub (W16.211)

√x7ᵗʰ **W67** **Accidental drowning and submersion while in** swimming-pool
> EXCLUDES 1   accidental drowning and submersion due to fall into swimming pool (W16.011, W16.021, W16.031)
>   accidental drowning and submersion due to striking into wall of swimming pool (W22.041)

√x7ᵗʰ **W69** **Accidental drowning and submersion while in** natural water
> Accidental drowning and submersion while in lake
> Accidental drowning and submersion while in open sea
> Accidental drowning and submersion while in river
> Accidental drowning and submersion while in stream
> EXCLUDES 1   accidental drowning and submersion due to fall into natural body of water (W16.111, W16.121, W16.131)

√x7ᵗʰ **W73** **Other specified cause of accidental non-transport drowning and submersion**
> Accidental drowning and submersion while in quenching tank
> Accidental drowning and submersion while in reservoir
> EXCLUDES 1   accidental drowning and submersion due to fall into other water (W16.311, W16.321, W16.331)

√x7ᵗʰ **W74** **Unspecified cause of accidental drowning and submersion**
> Drowning NOS

Exposure to electric current, radiation and extreme ambient air temperature and pressure (W85-W99)

> EXCLUDES 1   exposure to:
>   failure in dosage of radiation or temperature during surgical and medical care (Y63.2-Y63.5)
>   lightning (T75.0-)
>   natural cold (X31)
>   natural heat (X30)
>   natural radiation NOS (X39)
>   radiological procedure and radiotherapy (Y84.2)
>   sunlight (X32)

AHA: 2018,2Q,7-8

The appropriate 7th character is to be added to each code from categories W85-W99.
A   initial encounter
D   subsequent encounter
S   sequela

√x7ᵗʰ **W85** **Exposure to electric transmission lines**
> Broken power line

√4ᵗʰ **W86** **Exposure to other specified electric current**

√x7ᵗʰ **W86.0** **Exposure to domestic wiring and appliances**

√x7ᵗʰ **W86.1** **Exposure to industrial wiring, appliances and electrical machinery**
> Exposure to conductors
> Exposure to control apparatus
> Exposure to electrical equipment and machinery
> Exposure to transformers

√x7ᵗʰ **W86.8** **Exposure to other electric current**
> Exposure to wiring and appliances in or on farm (not farmhouse)
> Exposure to wiring and appliances outdoors
> Exposure to wiring and appliances in or on public building
> Exposure to wiring and appliances in or on residential institutions
> Exposure to wiring and appliances in or on schools

√4ᵗʰ **W88** **Exposure to ionizing radiation**
> EXCLUDES 1   exposure to sunlight (X32)

√x7ᵗʰ **W88.0** **Exposure to X-rays**

√x7ᵗʰ **W88.1** **Exposure to radioactive isotopes**

Chapter 20. External Causes of Morbidity

√x7ᵗʰ **W88.8**   **Exposure to other ionizing radiation**

√4ᵗʰ **W89**   **Exposure to man-made visible and ultraviolet light**
> INCLUDES   exposure to welding light (arc)
> EXCLUDES 1   *exposure to sunlight (X32)*

√x7ᵗʰ **W89.0**   **Exposure to welding light (arc)**

√x7ᵗʰ **W89.1**   **Exposure to tanning bed**

√x7ᵗʰ **W89.8**   **Exposure to other man-made visible and ultraviolet light**

√x7ᵗʰ **W89.9**   **Exposure to unspecified man-made visible and ultraviolet light**

√4ᵗʰ **W90**   **Exposure to other nonionizing radiation**
> EXCLUDES 1   *exposure to sunlight (X32)*
> AHA: 2019,1Q,21

√x7ᵗʰ **W90.0**   **Exposure to radiofrequency**

√x7ᵗʰ **W90.1**   **Exposure to infrared radiation**

√x7ᵗʰ **W90.2**   **Exposure to laser radiation**

√x7ᵗʰ **W90.8**   **Exposure to other nonionizing radiation**

√x7ᵗʰ **W92**   **Exposure to excessive heat of man-made origin**

√4ᵗʰ **W93**   **Exposure to excessive cold of man-made origin**

√5ᵗʰ **W93.0**   **Contact with or inhalation of dry ice**

√x7ᵗʰ **W93.01**   **Contact with dry ice**

√x7ᵗʰ **W93.02**   **Inhalation of dry ice**

√5ᵗʰ **W93.1**   **Contact with or inhalation of liquid air**

√x7ᵗʰ **W93.11**   **Contact with liquid air**
> Contact with liquid hydrogen
> Contact with liquid nitrogen

√x7ᵗʰ **W93.12**   **Inhalation of liquid air**
> Inhalation of liquid hydrogen
> Inhalation of liquid nitrogen

√x7ᵗʰ **W93.2**   **Prolonged exposure in deep freeze unit or refrigerator**

√x7ᵗʰ **W93.8**   **Exposure to other excessive cold of man-made origin**

√4ᵗʰ **W94**   **Exposure to high and low air pressure and changes in air pressure**

√x7ᵗʰ **W94.0**   **Exposure to prolonged high air pressure**

√5ᵗʰ **W94.1**   **Exposure to prolonged low air pressure**

√x7ᵗʰ **W94.11**   **Exposure to residence or prolonged visit at high altitude**

√x7ᵗʰ **W94.12**   **Exposure to other prolonged low air pressure**

√5ᵗʰ **W94.2**   **Exposure to rapid changes in air pressure during ascent**

√x7ᵗʰ **W94.21**   **Exposure to reduction in atmospheric pressure while surfacing from deep-water diving**

√x7ᵗʰ **W94.22**   **Exposure to reduction in atmospheric pressure while surfacing from underground**

√x7ᵗʰ **W94.23**   **Exposure to sudden change in air pressure in aircraft during ascent**

√x7ᵗʰ **W94.29**   **Exposure to other rapid changes in air pressure during ascent**

√5ᵗʰ **W94.3**   **Exposure to rapid changes in air pressure during descent**

√x7ᵗʰ **W94.31**   **Exposure to sudden change in air pressure in aircraft during descent**

√x7ᵗʰ **W94.32**   **Exposure to high air pressure from rapid descent in water**

√x7ᵗʰ **W94.39**   **Exposure to other rapid changes in air pressure during descent**

√x7ᵗʰ **W99**   **Exposure to other man-made environmental factors**

Exposure to smoke, fire and flames (X00-X08)

> EXCLUDES 1   *arson (X97)*
> EXCLUDES 2   *explosions (W35-W40)*
> *lightning (T75.0-)*
> *transport accident (V01-V99)*

AHA: 2018,2Q,7-8

The appropriate 7th character is to be added to each code from categories X00-X08.
A   initial encounter
D   subsequent encounter
S   sequela

√4ᵗʰ **X00**   **Exposure to uncontrolled fire in building or structure**
> INCLUDES   conflagration in building or structure
> Code first any associated cataclysm
> EXCLUDES 2   *exposure to ignition or melting of nightwear (X05)*
> *exposure to ignition or melting of other clothing and apparel (X06.-)*
> *exposure to other specified smoke, fire and flames (X08.-)*
> AHA: 2016,2Q,5

√x7ᵗʰ **X00.0**   **Exposure to flames in uncontrolled fire in building or structure**

√x7ᵗʰ **X00.1**   **Exposure to smoke in uncontrolled fire in building or structure**

√x7ᵗʰ **X00.2**   **Injury due to collapse of burning building or structure in uncontrolled fire**
> EXCLUDES 1   *injury due to collapse of building not on fire (W20.1)*

√x7ᵗʰ **X00.3**   **Fall from burning building or structure in uncontrolled fire**

√x7ᵗʰ **X00.4**   **Hit by object from burning building or structure in uncontrolled fire**
> AHA: 2016,2Q,4

√x7ᵗʰ **X00.5**   **Jump from burning building or structure in uncontrolled fire**

√x7ᵗʰ **X00.8**   **Other exposure to uncontrolled fire in building or structure**

√4ᵗʰ **X01**   **Exposure to uncontrolled fire, not in building or structure**
> INCLUDES   exposure to forest fire

√x7ᵗʰ **X01.0**   **Exposure to flames in uncontrolled fire, not in building or structure**

√x7ᵗʰ **X01.1**   **Exposure to smoke in uncontrolled fire, not in building or structure**

√x7ᵗʰ **X01.3**   **Fall due to uncontrolled fire, not in building or structure**

√x7ᵗʰ **X01.4**   **Hit by object due to uncontrolled fire, not in building or structure**

√x7ᵗʰ **X01.8**   **Other exposure to uncontrolled fire, not in building or structure**

√4ᵗʰ **X02**   **Exposure to controlled fire in building or structure**
> INCLUDES   exposure to fire in fireplace
> exposure to fire in stove

√x7ᵗʰ **X02.0**   **Exposure to flames in controlled fire in building or structure**

√x7ᵗʰ **X02.1**   **Exposure to smoke in controlled fire in building or structure**

√x7ᵗʰ **X02.2**   **Injury due to collapse of burning building or structure in controlled fire**
> EXCLUDES 1   *injury due to collapse of building not on fire (W20.1)*

√x7ᵗʰ **X02.3**   **Fall from burning building or structure in controlled fire**

√x7ᵗʰ **X02.4**   **Hit by object from burning building or structure in controlled fire**

√x7ᵗʰ **X02.5**   **Jump from burning building or structure in controlled fire**

√x7ᵗʰ **X02.8**   **Other exposure to controlled fire in building or structure**

√4ᵗʰ **X03**   **Exposure to controlled fire, not in building or structure**
> INCLUDES   exposure to bon fire
> exposure to camp-fire
> exposure to trash fire

√x7ᵗʰ **X03.0**   **Exposure to flames in controlled fire, not in building or structure**

√x7ᵗʰ **X03.1**   **Exposure to smoke in controlled fire, not in building or structure**

√x7ᵗʰ **X03.3**   **Fall due to controlled fire, not in building or structure**

√x7ᵗʰ **X03.4**   **Hit by object due to controlled fire, not in building or structure**

√x7ᵗʰ **X03.8**   **Other exposure to controlled fire, not in building or structure**

√x7ᵗʰ **X04 Exposure to ignition of highly flammable material**

Exposure to ignition of gasoline
Exposure to ignition of kerosene
Exposure to ignition of petrol
> EXCLUDES 2   *exposure to ignition or melting of nightwear (X05)*
> *exposure to ignition or melting of other clothing and apparel (X06)*

AHA: 2016,2Q,4

√x7ᵗʰ **X05 Exposure to ignition or melting of nightwear**

> EXCLUDES 2   *exposure to uncontrolled fire in building or structure (X00.-)*
> *exposure to uncontrolled fire, not in building or structure (X01.-)*
> *exposure to controlled fire in building or structure (X02.-)*
> *exposure to controlled fire, not in building or structure (X03.-)*
> *exposure to ignition of highly flammable materials (X04.-)*

√4ᵗʰ **X06 Exposure to ignition or melting of other clothing and apparel**

> EXCLUDES 2   *exposure to uncontrolled fire in building or structure (X00.-)*
> *exposure to uncontrolled fire, not in building or structure (X01.-)*
> *exposure to controlled fire in building or structure (X02.-)*
> *exposure to controlled fire, not in building or structure (X03.-)*
> *exposure to ignition of highly flammable materials (X04.-)*

√x7ᵗʰ **X06.0 Exposure to ignition of plastic jewelry**

√x7ᵗʰ **X06.1 Exposure to melting of plastic jewelry**

√x7ᵗʰ **X06.2 Exposure to ignition of other clothing and apparel**

√x7ᵗʰ **X06.3 Exposure to melting of other clothing and apparel**

√4ᵗʰ **X08 Exposure to other specified smoke, fire and flames**

√5ᵗʰ **X08.0 Exposure to bed fire**

Exposure to mattress fire

√x7ᵗʰ **X08.00 Exposure to bed fire due to unspecified burning material**

√x7ᵗʰ **X08.01 Exposure to bed fire due to burning cigarette**

√x7ᵗʰ **X08.09 Exposure to bed fire due to other burning material**

√5ᵗʰ **X08.1 Exposure to sofa fire**

√x7ᵗʰ **X08.10 Exposure to sofa fire due to unspecified burning material**

√x7ᵗʰ **X08.11 Exposure to sofa fire due to burning cigarette**

√x7ᵗʰ **X08.19 Exposure to sofa fire due to other burning material**

√5ᵗʰ **X08.2 Exposure to other furniture fire**

√x7ᵗʰ **X08.20 Exposure to other furniture fire due to unspecified burning material**

√x7ᵗʰ **X08.21 Exposure to other furniture fire due to burning cigarette**

√x7ᵗʰ **X08.29 Exposure to other furniture fire due to other burning material**

√x7ᵗʰ **X08.8 Exposure to other specified smoke, fire and flames**

Contact with heat and hot substances (X10-X19)

> EXCLUDES 1   *exposure to excessive natural heat (X30)*
> *exposure to fire and flames (X00-X08)*

AHA: 2018,2Q,7-8

The appropriate 7th character is to be added to each code from categories X10-X19.
A   initial encounter
D   subsequent encounter
S   sequela

√4ᵗʰ **X10 Contact with hot drinks, food, fats and cooking oils**

√x7ᵗʰ **X10.0 Contact with hot drinks**

√x7ᵗʰ **X10.1 Contact with hot food**

√x7ᵗʰ **X10.2 Contact with fats and cooking oils**

√4ᵗʰ **X11 Contact with hot tap-water**

> INCLUDES   contact with boiling tap-water
> contact with boiling water NOS
> EXCLUDES 1   *contact with water heated on stove (X12)*

√x7ᵗʰ **X11.0 Contact with hot water in bath or tub**

> EXCLUDES 1   *contact with running hot water in bath or tub (X11.1)*

√x7ᵗʰ **X11.1 Contact with running hot water**

Contact with hot water running out of hose
Contact with hot water running out of tap

√x7ᵗʰ **X11.8 Contact with other hot tap-water**

Contact with hot water in bucket
Contact with hot tap-water NOS

√x7ᵗʰ **X12 Contact with other hot fluids**

Contact with water heated on stove
> EXCLUDES 1   *hot (liquid) metals (X18)*

√4ᵗʰ **X13 Contact with steam and other hot vapors**

√x7ᵗʰ **X13.0 Inhalation of steam and other hot vapors**

√x7ᵗʰ **X13.1 Other contact with steam and other hot vapors**

√4ᵗʰ **X14 Contact with hot air and other hot gases**

√x7ᵗʰ **X14.0 Inhalation of hot air and gases**

√x7ᵗʰ **X14.1 Other contact with hot air and other hot gases**

√4ᵗʰ **X15 Contact with hot household appliances**

> EXCLUDES 1   *contact with heating appliances (X16)*
> *contact with powered household appliances (W29.-)*
> *exposure to controlled fire in building or structure due to household appliance (X02.8)*
> *exposure to household appliances electrical current (W86.0)*

√x7ᵗʰ **X15.0 Contact with hot stove (kitchen)**

√x7ᵗʰ **X15.1 Contact with hot toaster**

√x7ᵗʰ **X15.2 Contact with hotplate**

√x7ᵗʰ **X15.3 Contact with hot saucepan or skillet**

√x7ᵗʰ **X15.8 Contact with other hot household appliances**

Contact with cooker
Contact with kettle
Contact with light bulbs

√x7ᵗʰ **X16 Contact with hot heating appliances, radiators and pipes**

> EXCLUDES 1   *contact with powered appliances (W29.-)*
> *exposure to controlled fire in building or structure due to appliance (X02.8)*
> *exposure to industrial appliances electrical current (W86.1)*

√x7ᵗʰ **X17 Contact with hot engines, machinery and tools**

> EXCLUDES 1   *contact with hot heating appliances, radiators and pipes (X16)*
> *contact with hot household appliances (X15)*

√x7ᵗʰ **X18 Contact with other hot metals**

Contact with liquid metal

√x7ᵗʰ **X19 Contact with other heat and hot substances**

> EXCLUDES 1   *objects that are not normally hot, e.g., an object made hot by a house fire (X00-X08)*

Exposure to forces of nature (X30-X39)

AHA: 2018,2Q,7-8

The appropriate 7th character is to be added to each code from categories X30-X39.
A   initial encounter
D   subsequent encounter
S   sequela

√x7ᵗʰ **X30 Exposure to excessive natural heat**

Exposure to excessive heat as the cause of sunstroke
Exposure to heat NOS
> EXCLUDES 1   *excessive heat of man-made origin (W92)*
> *exposure to man-made radiation (W89)*
> *exposure to sunlight (X32)*
> *exposure to tanning bed (W89)*

√x7ᵗʰ **X31 Exposure to excessive natural cold**

Excessive cold as the cause of chilblains NOS
Excessive cold as the cause of immersion foot or hand
Exposure to cold NOS
Exposure to weather conditions
> EXCLUDES 1   *cold of man-made origin (W93.-)*
> *contact with or inhalation of dry ice (W93.-)*
> *contact with or inhalation of liquefied gas (W93.-)*

√x7ᵗʰ **X32 Exposure to sunlight**

> EXCLUDES 1   *man-made radiation (tanning bed) (W89)*
> EXCLUDES 2   *radiation-related disorders of the skin and subcutaneous tissue (L55-L59)*

☑ Additional Char Req   √x7ᵗʰ Placeholder   Unacceptable PDx   Questionable PDx   Wrong Procedure   Manifestation   Unspecified Dx   H1-H14 HAC   HCC CMS-HCC Dx   HIV HIV Dx

ICD-10-CM 2020   1251

√x7ᵗʰ **X34 Earthquake**

     EXCLUDES 2   *tidal wave (tsunami) due to earthquake (X37.41)*

√x7ᵗʰ **X35 Volcanic eruption**

     EXCLUDES 2   *tidal wave (tsunami) due to volcanic eruption (X37.41)*

√4ᵗʰ **X36 Avalanche, landslide and other earth movements**

     INCLUDES   victim of mudslide of cataclysmic nature

     EXCLUDES 1   *earthquake (X34)*

     EXCLUDES 2   *transport accident involving collision with avalanche or landslide not in motion (V01-V99)*

   √x7ᵗʰ **X36.0 Collapse of dam or man-made structure causing earth movement**

   √x7ᵗʰ **X36.1 Avalanche, landslide, or mudslide**

√4ᵗʰ **X37 Cataclysmic storm**

   √x7ᵗʰ **X37.0 Hurricane**

     Storm surge

     Typhoon

   √x7ᵗʰ **X37.1 Tornado**

     Cyclone

     Twister

   √x7ᵗʰ **X37.2 Blizzard (snow)(ice)**

   √x7ᵗʰ **X37.3 Dust storm**

   √5ᵗʰ **X37.4 Tidalwave**

     √x7ᵗʰ **X37.41 Tidal wave due to earthquake or volcanic eruption**

       Tidal wave NOS

       Tsunami

     √x7ᵗʰ **X37.42 Tidal wave due to storm**

     √x7ᵗʰ **X37.43 Tidal wave due to landslide**

   √x7ᵗʰ **X37.8 Other cataclysmic storms**

     Cloudburst

     Torrential rain

     EXCLUDES 2   *flood (X38)*

   √x7ᵗʰ **X37.9 Unspecified cataclysmic storm**

     Storm NOS

     EXCLUDES 1   *collapse of dam or man-made structure causing earth movement (X36.0)*

√x7ᵗʰ **X38 Flood**

     Flood arising from remote storm

     Flood of cataclysmic nature arising from melting snow

     Flood resulting directly from storm

     EXCLUDES 1   *collapse of dam or man-made structure causing earth movement (X36.0)*

               tidal wave NOS (X37.41)

               tidal wave caused by storm (X37.42)

√4ᵗʰ **X39 Exposure to other forces of nature**

   √5ᵗʰ **X39.0 Exposure to natural radiation**

     EXCLUDES 1   *contact with and (suspected) exposure to radon and other naturally occurring radiation (Z77.123)*

               exposure to man-made radiation (W88-W90)

               exposure to sunlight (X32)

     √x7ᵗʰ **X39.01 Exposure to radon**

     √x7ᵗʰ **X39.08 Exposure to other natural radiation**

   √x7ᵗʰ **X39.8 Other exposure to forces of nature**

Overexertion and strenuous or repetitive movements (X50)

√4ᵗʰ **X50 Overexertion and strenuous or repetitive movements**

     AHA: 2018,2Q,7-8; 2016,4Q,73-74

     The appropriate 7th character is to be added to each code from category X50.

     A   initial encounter

     D   subsequent encounter

     S   sequela

   √x7ᵗʰ **X50.0 Overexertion from strenuous movement or load**

     Lifting heavy objects

     Lifting weights

√x7ᵗʰ **X50.1 Overexertion from prolonged static or awkward postures**

     Prolonged bending

     Prolonged kneeling

     Prolonged reaching

     Prolonged sitting

     Prolonged standing

     Prolonged twisting

     Static bending

     Static kneeling

     Static reaching

     Static sitting

     Static standing

     Static twisting

√x7ᵗʰ **X50.3 Overexertion from repetitive movements**

     Use of hand as hammer

     EXCLUDES 2   *overuse from prolonged static or awkward postures (X50.1)*

√x7ᵗʰ **X50.9 Other and unspecified overexertion or strenuous movements or postures**

     Contact pressure

     Contact stress

Accidental exposure to other specified factors (X52-X58)

AHA: 2018,2Q,7-8

The appropriate 7th character is to be added to each code from categories X52-X58.

A   initial encounter

D   subsequent encounter

S   sequela

√x7ᵗʰ **X52 Prolonged stay in weightless environment**

     Weightlessness in spacecraft (simulator)

√x7ᵗʰ **X58 Exposure to other specified factors**

     Accident NOS

     Exposure NOS

Intentional self-harm (X71-X83)

Purposely self-inflicted injury

Suicide (attempted)

The appropriate 7th character is to be added to each code from categories X71-X83.

A   initial encounter

D   subsequent encounter

S   sequela

√4ᵗʰ **X71 Intentional self-harm by drowning and submersion**

   √x7ᵗʰ **X71.0 Intentional self-harm by drowning and submersion while in bathtub**   HCC

   √x7ᵗʰ **X71.1 Intentional self-harm by drowning and submersion while in swimming pool**   HCC

   √x7ᵗʰ **X71.2 Intentional self-harm by drowning and submersion after jump into swimming pool**   HCC

   √x7ᵗʰ **X71.3 Intentional self-harm by drowning and submersion in natural water**   HCC

   √x7ᵗʰ **X71.8 Other intentional self-harm by drowning and submersion**   HCC

   √x7ᵗʰ **X71.9 Intentional self-harm by drowning and submersion, unspecified**   HCC

√x7ᵗʰ **X72 Intentional self-harm by handgun discharge**   HCC

     Intentional self-harm by gun for single hand use

     Intentional self-harm by pistol

     Intentional self-harm by revolver

     EXCLUDES 1   *Very pistol (X74.8)*

√4ᵗʰ **X73 Intentional self-harm by rifle, shotgun and larger firearm discharge**

     EXCLUDES 1   *airgun (X74.01)*

   √x7ᵗʰ **X73.0 Intentional self-harm by shotgun discharge**   HCC

   √x7ᵗʰ **X73.1 Intentional self-harm by hunting rifle discharge**   HCC

   √x7ᵗʰ **X73.2 Intentional self-harm by machine gun discharge**   HCC

   √x7ᵗʰ **X73.8 Intentional self-harm by other larger firearm discharge**   HCC

   √x7ᵗʰ **X73.9 Intentional self-harm by unspecified larger firearm discharge**   HCC

N Newborn: 0   P Pediatric: 0-17   M Maternity: 9-64   A Adult: 15-124   MCC Major Complication/Comorbidity   CC Complication/Comorbidity   SW Severe Wound Dx

1252   ICD-10-CM 2020

☑4ᵗʰ X74 Intentional self-harm by other and unspecified firearm and gun discharge

    ☑5ᵗʰ X74.0 Intentional self-harm by gas, air or spring-operated guns

        ☑x7ᵗʰ X74.01 Intentional self-harm by airgun   HCC

            Intentional self-harm by BB gun discharge
            Intentional self-harm by pellet gun discharge

        ☑x7ᵗʰ X74.02 Intentional self-harm by paintball gun   HCC

        ☑x7ᵗʰ X74.09 Intentional self-harm by other gas, air or spring-operated gun   HCC

    ☑x7ᵗʰ X74.8 Intentional self-harm by other firearm discharge   HCC

        Intentional self-harm by Very pistol [flare] discharge

    ☑x7ᵗʰ X74.9 Intentional self-harm by unspecified firearm discharge   HCC

☑x7ᵗʰ X75 Intentional self-harm by explosive material   HCC

☑x7ᵗʰ X76 Intentional self-harm by smoke, fire and flames   HCC

☑4ᵗʰ X77 Intentional self-harm by steam, hot vapors and hot objects

    ☑x7ᵗʰ X77.0 Intentional self-harm by steam or hot vapors   HCC

    ☑x7ᵗʰ X77.1 Intentional self-harm by hot tap water   HCC

    ☑x7ᵗʰ X77.2 Intentional self-harm by other hot fluids   HCC

    ☑x7ᵗʰ X77.3 Intentional self-harm by hot household appliances   HCC

    ☑x7ᵗʰ X77.8 Intentional self-harm by other hot objects   HCC

    ☑x7ᵗʰ X77.9 Intentional self-harm by unspecified hot objects   HCC

☑4ᵗʰ X78 Intentional self-harm by sharp object

    ☑x7ᵗʰ X78.0 Intentional self-harm by sharp glass   HCC

    ☑x7ᵗʰ X78.1 Intentional self-harm by knife   HCC

    ☑x7ᵗʰ X78.2 Intentional self-harm by sword or dagger   HCC

    ☑x7ᵗʰ X78.8 Intentional self-harm by other sharp object   HCC

    ☑x7ᵗʰ X78.9 Intentional self-harm by unspecified sharp object   HCC

☑x7ᵗʰ X79 Intentional self-harm by blunt object   HCC

☑x7ᵗʰ X80 Intentional self-harm by jumping from a high place   HCC

    Intentional fall from one level to another

☑4ᵗʰ X81 Intentional self-harm by jumping or lying in front of moving object

    ☑x7ᵗʰ X81.0 Intentional self-harm by jumping or lying in front of motor vehicle   HCC

    ☑x7ᵗʰ X81.1 Intentional self-harm by jumping or lying in front of (subway) train   HCC

    ☑x7ᵗʰ X81.8 Intentional self-harm by jumping or lying in front of other moving object   HCC

☑4ᵗʰ X82 Intentional self-harm by crashing of motor vehicle

    ☑x7ᵗʰ X82.0 Intentional collision of motor vehicle with other motor vehicle   HCC

    ☑x7ᵗʰ X82.1 Intentional collision of motor vehicle with train   HCC

    ☑x7ᵗʰ X82.2 Intentional collision of motor vehicle with tree   HCC

    ☑x7ᵗʰ X82.8 Other intentional self-harm by crashing of motor vehicle   HCC

☑4ᵗʰ X83 Intentional self-harm by other specified means

    EXCLUDES 1   *intentional self-harm by poisoning or contact with toxic substance — see Table of Drugs and Chemicals*

    ☑x7ᵗʰ X83.0 Intentional self-harm by crashing of aircraft   HCC

    ☑x7ᵗʰ X83.1 Intentional self-harm by electrocution   HCC

    ☑x7ᵗʰ X83.2 Intentional self-harm by exposure to extremes of cold   HCC

    ☑x7ᵗʰ X83.8 Intentional self-harm by other specified means   HCC

Assault (X92-Y09)

INCLUDES   homicide
     injuries inflicted by another person with intent to injure or kill, by any means

EXCLUDES 1   *injuries due to legal intervention (Y35.-)*
     injuries due to operations of war (Y36.-)
     injuries due to terrorism (Y38.-)

> The appropriate 7th character is to be added to each code from categories X92-Y04 and Y08.
> A   initial encounter
> D   subsequent encounter
> S   sequela

☑4ᵗʰ X92 Assault by drowning and submersion

    ☑x7ᵗʰ X92.0 Assault by drowning and submersion while in bathtub

    ☑x7ᵗʰ X92.1 Assault by drowning and submersion while in swimming pool

    ☑x7ᵗʰ X92.2 Assault by drowning and submersion after push into swimming pool

    ☑x7ᵗʰ X92.3 Assault by drowning and submersion in natural water

    ☑x7ᵗʰ X92.8 Other assault by drowning and submersion

    ☑x7ᵗʰ X92.9 Assault by drowning and submersion, unspecified

☑x7ᵗʰ X93 Assault by handgun discharge

    Assault by discharge of gun for single hand use
    Assault by discharge of pistol
    Assault by discharge of revolver

    EXCLUDES 1   *Very pistol (X95.8)*

☑4ᵗʰ X94 Assault by rifle, shotgun and larger firearm discharge

    EXCLUDES 1   *airgun (X95.01)*

    ☑x7ᵗʰ X94.0 Assault by shotgun

    ☑x7ᵗʰ X94.1 Assault by hunting rifle

    ☑x7ᵗʰ X94.2 Assault by machine gun

    ☑x7ᵗʰ X94.8 Assault by other larger firearm discharge

    ☑x7ᵗʰ X94.9 Assault by unspecified larger firearm discharge

☑4ᵗʰ X95 Assault by other and unspecified firearm and gun discharge

    ☑5ᵗʰ X95.0 Assault by gas, air or spring-operated guns

        ☑x7ᵗʰ X95.01 Assault by airgun discharge

            Assault by BB gun discharge
            Assault by pellet gun discharge

        ☑x7ᵗʰ X95.02 Assault by paintball gun discharge

        ☑x7ᵗʰ X95.09 Assault by other gas, air or spring-operated gun

    ☑x7ᵗʰ X95.8 Assault by other firearm discharge

        Assault by Very pistol [flare] discharge

    ☑x7ᵗʰ X95.9 Assault by unspecified firearm discharge

☑4ᵗʰ X96 Assault by explosive material

    EXCLUDES 1   *incendiary device (X97)*
         terrorism involving explosive material (Y38.2-)

    ☑x7ᵗʰ X96.0 Assault by antipersonnel bomb

        EXCLUDES 1   *antipersonnel bomb use in military or war (Y36.2-)*

    ☑x7ᵗʰ X96.1 Assault by gasoline bomb

    ☑x7ᵗʰ X96.2 Assault by letter bomb

    ☑x7ᵗʰ X96.3 Assault by fertilizer bomb

    ☑x7ᵗʰ X96.4 Assault by pipe bomb

    ☑x7ᵗʰ X96.8 Assault by other specified explosive

    ☑x7ᵗʰ X96.9 Assault by unspecified explosive

☑x7ᵗʰ X97 Assault by smoke, fire and flames

    Assault by arson
    Assault by cigarettes
    Assault by incendiary device

☑4ᵗʰ X98 Assault by steam, hot vapors and hot objects

    ☑x7ᵗʰ X98.0 Assault by steam or hot vapors

    ☑x7ᵗʰ X98.1 Assault by hot tap water

    ☑x7ᵗʰ X98.2 Assault by hot fluids

    ☑x7ᵗʰ X98.3 Assault by hot household appliances

    ☑x7ᵗʰ X98.8 Assault by other hot objects

    ☑x7ᵗʰ X98.9 Assault by unspecified hot objects

☑ Additional Char Req   ☑x7ᵗʰ Placeholder   <u>Unacceptable PDx</u>   Questionable PDx   Wrong Procedure   Manifestation   Unspecified Dx   H1-H14 HAC   HCC CMS-HCC Dx   HIV HIV Dx

Chapter 20. External Causes of Morbidity

X99–Y08.89

√4ᵗʰ **X99** **Assault by sharp object**
> EXCLUDES 1   *assault by strike by sports equipment (Y08.0-)*

√x7ᵗʰ **X99.0** **Assault by sharp glass**

√x7ᵗʰ **X99.1** **Assault by knife**

√x7ᵗʰ **X99.2** **Assault by sword or dagger**

√x7ᵗʰ **X99.8** **Assault by other sharp object**

√x7ᵗʰ **X99.9** **Assault by unspecified sharp object**
> Assault by stabbing NOS

√x7ᵗʰ **Y00** **Assault by blunt object**
> EXCLUDES 1   *assault by strike by sports equipment (Y08.0-)*

√x7ᵗʰ **Y01** **Assault by pushing from high place**

√4ᵗʰ **Y02** **Assault by pushing or placing victim in front of moving object**

√x7ᵗʰ **Y02.0** **Assault by pushing or placing victim in front of motor vehicle**

√x7ᵗʰ **Y02.1** **Assault by pushing or placing victim in front of (subway) train**

√x7ᵗʰ **Y02.8** **Assault by pushing or placing victim in front of other moving object**

√4ᵗʰ **Y03** **Assault by crashing of motor vehicle**

√x7ᵗʰ **Y03.0** **Assault by being hit or run over by motor vehicle**

√x7ᵗʰ **Y03.8** **Other assault by crashing of motor vehicle**

√4ᵗʰ **Y04** **Assault by bodily force**
> EXCLUDES 1   *assault by:*
> *submersion (X92.-)*
> *use of weapon (X93-X95, X99, Y00)*

√x7ᵗʰ **Y04.0** **Assault by unarmed brawl or fight**

√x7ᵗʰ **Y04.1** **Assault by human bite**

√x7ᵗʰ **Y04.2** **Assault by strike against or bumped into by another person**

√x7ᵗʰ **Y04.8** **Assault by other bodily force**
> Assault by bodily force NOS

√4ᵗʰ **Y07** **Perpetrator of assault, maltreatment and neglect**
> **NOTE**   Codes from this category are for use only in cases of confirmed abuse (T74.-)
>
> Selection of the correct perpetrator code is based on the relationship between the perpetrator and the victim
>
> **INCLUDES**   perpetrator of abandonment
> perpetrator of emotional neglect
> perpetrator of mental cruelty
> perpetrator of physical abuse
> perpetrator of physical neglect
> perpetrator of sexual abuse
> perpetrator of torture

√5ᵗʰ **Y07.0** **Spouse or partner, perpetrator of maltreatment and neglect**
> Spouse or partner, perpetrator of maltreatment and neglect against spouse or partner

Y07.01 **Husband, perpetrator of maltreatment and neglect**

Y07.02 **Wife, perpetrator of maltreatment and neglect**

Y07.03 **Male partner, perpetrator of maltreatment and neglect**

Y07.04 **Female partner, perpetrator of maltreatment and neglect**

√5ᵗʰ **Y07.1** **Parent (adoptive) (biological), perpetrator of maltreatment and neglect**

Y07.11 **Biological father, perpetrator of maltreatment and neglect**

Y07.12 **Biological mother, perpetrator of maltreatment and neglect**

Y07.13 **Adoptive father, perpetrator of maltreatment and neglect**

Y07.14 **Adoptive mother, perpetrator of maltreatment and neglect**

√5ᵗʰ **Y07.4** **Other family member, perpetrator of maltreatment and neglect**

√6ᵗʰ **Y07.41** **Sibling, perpetrator of maltreatment and neglect**
> EXCLUDES 1   *stepsibling, perpetrator of maltreatment and neglect (Y07.435, Y07.436)*

Y07.410 **Brother, perpetrator of maltreatment and neglect**

Y07.411 **Sister, perpetrator of maltreatment and neglect**

√6ᵗʰ **Y07.42** **Foster parent, perpetrator of maltreatment and neglect**

Y07.420 **Foster father, perpetrator of maltreatment and neglect**

Y07.421 **Foster mother, perpetrator of maltreatment and neglect**

√6ᵗʰ **Y07.43** **Stepparent or stepsibling, perpetrator of maltreatment and neglect**

Y07.430 **Stepfather, perpetrator of maltreatment and neglect**

Y07.432 **Male friend of parent (co-residing in household), perpetrator of maltreatment and neglect**

Y07.433 **Stepmother, perpetrator of maltreatment and neglect**

Y07.434 **Female friend of parent (co-residing in household), perpetrator of maltreatment and neglect**

Y07.435 **Stepbrother, perpetrator or maltreatment and neglect**

Y07.436 **Stepsister, perpetrator of maltreatment and neglect**

√6ᵗʰ **Y07.49** **Other family member, perpetrator of maltreatment and neglect**

Y07.490 **Male cousin, perpetrator of maltreatment and neglect**

Y07.491 **Female cousin, perpetrator of maltreatment and neglect**

Y07.499 **Other family member, perpetrator of maltreatment and neglect**

√5ᵗʰ **Y07.5** **Non-family member, perpetrator of maltreatment and neglect**

Y07.50 **Unspecified non-family member, perpetrator of maltreatment and neglect**

√6ᵗʰ **Y07.51** **Daycare provider, perpetrator of maltreatment and neglect**

Y07.510 **At-home childcare provider, perpetrator of maltreatment and neglect**

Y07.511 **Daycare center childcare provider, perpetrator of maltreatment and neglect**

Y07.512 **At-home adultcare provider, perpetrator of maltreatment and neglect**

Y07.513 **Adultcare center provider, perpetrator of maltreatment and neglect**

Y07.519 **Unspecified daycare provider, perpetrator of maltreatment and neglect**

√6ᵗʰ **Y07.52** **Healthcare provider, perpetrator of maltreatment and neglect**

Y07.521 **Mental health provider, perpetrator of maltreatment and neglect**

Y07.528 **Other therapist or healthcare provider, perpetrator of maltreatment and neglect**
> Nurse perpetrator of maltreatment and neglect
> Occupational therapist perpetrator of maltreatment and neglect
> Physical therapist perpetrator of maltreatment and neglect
> Speech therapist perpetrator of maltreatment and neglect

Y07.529 **Unspecified healthcare provider, perpetrator of maltreatment and neglect**

Y07.53 **Teacher or instructor, perpetrator of maltreatment and neglect**
> Coach, perpetrator of maltreatment and neglect

Y07.59 **Other non-family member, perpetrator of maltreatment and neglect**

Y07.6 **Multiple perpetrators of maltreatment and neglect**
> AHA: 2018,4Q,32

Y07.9 **Unspecified perpetrator of maltreatment and neglect**

√4ᵗʰ **Y08** **Assault by other specified means**

√5ᵗʰ **Y08.0** **Assault by strike by sport equipment**

√x7ᵗʰ **Y08.01** **Assault by strike by hockey stick**

√x7ᵗʰ **Y08.02** **Assault by strike by baseball bat**

√x7ᵗʰ **Y08.09** **Assault by strike by other specified type of sport equipment**

√5ᵗʰ **Y08.8** **Assault by other specified means**

√x7ᵗʰ **Y08.81** **Assault by crashing of aircraft**

√x7ᵗʰ **Y08.89** **Assault by other specified means**

Y09 Assault by unspecified means

Assassination (attempted) NOS
Homicide (attempted) NOS
Manslaughter (attempted) NOS
Murder (attempted) NOS

Event of undetermined intent (Y21-Y33)

Undetermined intent is only for use when there is specific documentation in the record that the intent of the injury cannot be determined. If no such documentation is present, code to accidental (unintentional).

The appropriate 7th character is to be added to each code from categories Y21-Y33.
A   initial encounter
D   subsequent encounter
S   sequela

√4th **Y21 Drowning and submersion, undetermined intent**

√x7th **Y21.0 Drowning and submersion** while in bathtub, **undetermined intent**

√x7th **Y21.1 Drowning and submersion** after fall into bathtub, **undetermined intent**

√x7th **Y21.2 Drowning and submersion** while in swimming pool, **undetermined intent**

√x7th **Y21.3 Drowning and submersion** after fall into swimming pool, **undetermined intent**

√x7th **Y21.4 Drowning and submersion** in natural water, **undetermined intent**

√x7th **Y21.8 Other drowning and submersion, undetermined intent**

√x7th **Y21.9 Unspecified drowning and submersion, undetermined intent**

√x7th **Y22 Handgun discharge, undetermined intent**

Discharge of gun for single hand use, undetermined intent
Discharge of pistol, undetermined intent
Discharge of revolver, undetermined intent
EXCLUDES 2   Very pistol (Y24.8)

√4th **Y23 Rifle, shotgun and larger firearm discharge, undetermined intent**

EXCLUDES 2   airgun (Y24.0)

√x7th **Y23.0 Shotgun discharge, undetermined intent**

√x7th **Y23.1 Hunting rifle discharge, undetermined intent**

√x7th **Y23.2 Military firearm discharge, undetermined intent**

√x7th **Y23.3 Machine gun discharge, undetermined intent**

√x7th **Y23.8 Other larger firearm discharge, undetermined intent**

√x7th **Y23.9 Unspecified larger firearm discharge, undetermined intent**

√4th **Y24 Other and unspecified firearm discharge, undetermined intent**

√x7th **Y24.0 Airgun discharge, undetermined intent**

BB gun discharge, undetermined intent
Pellet gun discharge, undetermined intent

√x7th **Y24.8 Other firearm discharge, undetermined intent**

Paintball gun discharge, undetermined intent
Very pistol [flare] discharge, undetermined intent

√x7th **Y24.9 Unspecified firearm discharge, undetermined intent**

√x7th **Y25 Contact with explosive material, undetermined intent**

√x7th **Y26 Exposure to smoke, fire and flames, undetermined intent**

√4th **Y27 Contact with steam, hot vapors and hot objects, undetermined intent**

√x7th **Y27.0 Contact with steam and hot vapors, undetermined intent**

√x7th **Y27.1 Contact with hot tap water, undetermined intent**

√x7th **Y27.2 Contact with hot fluids, undetermined intent**

√x7th **Y27.3 Contact with hot household appliance, undetermined intent**

√x7th **Y27.8 Contact with other hot objects, undetermined intent**

√x7th **Y27.9 Contact with unspecified hot objects, undetermined intent**

√4th **Y28 Contact with sharp object, undetermined intent**

√x7th **Y28.0 Contact with sharp glass, undetermined intent**

√x7th **Y28.1 Contact with knife, undetermined intent**

√x7th **Y28.2 Contact with sword or dagger, undetermined intent**

√x7th **Y28.8 Contact with other sharp object, undetermined intent**

√x7th **Y28.9 Contact with unspecified sharp object, undetermined intent**

√x7th **Y29 Contact with blunt object, undetermined intent**

√x7th **Y30 Falling, jumping or pushed from a high place, undetermined intent**

Victim falling from one level to another, undetermined intent

√x7th **Y31 Falling, lying or running before or into moving object, undetermined intent**

√x7th **Y32 Crashing of motor vehicle, undetermined intent**

√x7th **Y33 Other specified events, undetermined intent**

Legal intervention, operations of war, military operations, and terrorism (Y35-Y38)

The appropriate 7th character is to be added to each code from categories Y35-Y38.
A   initial encounter
D   subsequent encounter
S   sequela

√4th **Y35 Legal intervention**

INCLUDES   any injury sustained as a result of an encounter with any law enforcement official, serving in any capacity at the time of the encounter, whether on-duty or off-duty. Includes injury to law enforcement official, suspect and bystander

√5th **Y35.0 Legal intervention involving firearm discharge**

√6th **Y35.00 Legal intervention involving unspecified firearm discharge**

Legal intervention involving gunshot wound
Legal intervention involving shot NOS

√7th **Y35.001 Legal intervention involving unspecified firearm discharge, law enforcement official injured**

√7th **Y35.002 Legal intervention involving unspecified firearm discharge, bystander injured**

√7th **Y35.003 Legal intervention involving unspecified firearm discharge, suspect injured**

√7th **Y35.009 Legal intervention involving unspecified firearm discharge, unspecified person injured**

√6th **Y35.01 Legal intervention involving injury by machine gun**

√7th **Y35.011 Legal intervention involving injury by machine gun, law enforcement official injured**

√7th **Y35.012 Legal intervention involving injury by machine gun, bystander injured**

√7th **Y35.013 Legal intervention involving injury by machine gun, suspect injured**

√7th **Y35.019 Legal intervention involving injury by machine gun, unspecified person injured**

√6th **Y35.02 Legal intervention involving injury by handgun**

√7th **Y35.021 Legal intervention involving injury by handgun, law enforcement official injured**

√7th **Y35.022 Legal intervention involving injury by handgun, bystander injured**

√7th **Y35.023 Legal intervention involving injury by handgun, suspect injured**

√7th **Y35.029 Legal intervention involving injury by handgun, unspecified person injured**

√6th **Y35.03 Legal intervention involving injury by rifle pellet**

√7th **Y35.031 Legal intervention involving injury by rifle pellet, law enforcement official injured**

√7th **Y35.032 Legal intervention involving injury by rifle pellet, bystander injured**

√7th **Y35.033 Legal intervention involving injury by rifle pellet, suspect injured**

√7th **Y35.039 Legal intervention involving injury by rifle pellet, unspecified person injured**

√6th **Y35.04 Legal intervention involving injury by rubber bullet**

√7th **Y35.041 Legal intervention involving injury by rubber bullet, law enforcement official injured**

√7th **Y35.042 Legal intervention involving injury by rubber bullet, bystander injured**

√7th **Y35.043 Legal intervention involving injury by rubber bullet, suspect injured**

√7th **Y35.049 Legal intervention involving injury by rubber bullet, unspecified person injured**

√6th **Y35.09 Legal intervention involving other firearm discharge**

√7th **Y35.091 Legal intervention involving other firearm discharge, law enforcement official injured**

√7th **Y35.092 Legal intervention involving other firearm discharge, bystander injured**

✔ Additional Char Req   √x7th Placeholder   Unacceptable PDx   Questionable PDx   Wrong Procedure   Manifestation   Unspecified Dx   H1 - H14 HAC   HCC CMS-HCC Dx   HIV HIV Dx

ICD-10-CM 2020   1255

Chapter 20. External Causes of Morbidity

Y35.093–Y35.831

    √7ᵗʰ **Y35.093** Legal intervention involving other firearm discharge, **suspect** injured

    √7ᵗʰ **Y35.099** Legal intervention involving other firearm discharge, unspecified person injured

√5ᵗʰ **Y35.1** Legal intervention involving **explosives**

  √6ᵗʰ **Y35.10** Legal intervention involving unspecified explosives

    √7ᵗʰ **Y35.101** Legal intervention involving unspecified explosives, **law enforcement official** injured

    √7ᵗʰ **Y35.102** Legal intervention involving unspecified explosives, **bystander** injured

    √7ᵗʰ **Y35.103** Legal intervention involving unspecified explosives, **suspect** injured

    √7ᵗʰ **Y35.109** Legal intervention involving unspecified explosives, unspecified person injured

  √6ᵗʰ **Y35.11** Legal intervention involving injury by **dynamite**

    √7ᵗʰ **Y35.111** Legal intervention involving injury by dynamite, **law enforcement official** injured

    √7ᵗʰ **Y35.112** Legal intervention involving injury by dynamite, **bystander** injured

    √7ᵗʰ **Y35.113** Legal intervention involving injury by dynamite, **suspect** injured

    √7ᵗʰ **Y35.119** Legal intervention involving injury by dynamite, unspecified person injured

  √6ᵗʰ **Y35.12** Legal intervention involving injury by **explosive shell**

    √7ᵗʰ **Y35.121** Legal intervention involving injury by explosive shell, **law enforcement official** injured

    √7ᵗʰ **Y35.122** Legal intervention involving injury by explosive shell, **bystander** injured

    √7ᵗʰ **Y35.123** Legal intervention involving injury by explosive shell, **suspect** injured

    √7ᵗʰ **Y35.129** Legal intervention involving injury by explosive shell, unspecified person injured

  √6ᵗʰ **Y35.19** Legal intervention involving other explosives

Legal intervention involving injury by grenade
Legal intervention involving injury by mortar bomb

    √7ᵗʰ **Y35.191** Legal intervention involving other explosives, **law enforcement official** injured

    √7ᵗʰ **Y35.192** Legal intervention involving other explosives, **bystander** injured

    √7ᵗʰ **Y35.193** Legal intervention involving other explosives, **suspect** injured

    √7ᵗʰ **Y35.199** Legal intervention involving other explosives, unspecified person injured

√5ᵗʰ **Y35.2** Legal intervention involving **gas**

Legal intervention involving asphyxiation by gas
Legal intervention involving poisoning by gas

  √6ᵗʰ **Y35.20** Legal intervention involving unspecified gas

    √7ᵗʰ **Y35.201** Legal intervention involving unspecified gas, **law enforcement official** injured

    √7ᵗʰ **Y35.202** Legal intervention involving unspecified gas, **bystander** injured

    √7ᵗʰ **Y35.203** Legal intervention involving unspecified gas, **suspect** injured

    √7ᵗʰ **Y35.209** Legal intervention involving unspecified gas, unspecified person injured

  √6ᵗʰ **Y35.21** Legal intervention involving injury by **tear gas**

    √7ᵗʰ **Y35.211** Legal intervention involving injury by tear gas, **law enforcement official** injured

    √7ᵗʰ **Y35.212** Legal intervention involving injury by tear gas, **bystander** injured

    √7ᵗʰ **Y35.213** Legal intervention involving injury by tear gas, **suspect** injured

    √7ᵗʰ **Y35.219** Legal intervention involving injury by tear gas, **unspecified person** injured

  √6ᵗʰ **Y35.29** Legal intervention involving other gas

    √7ᵗʰ **Y35.291** Legal intervention involving other gas, **law enforcement official** injured

    √7ᵗʰ **Y35.292** Legal intervention involving other gas, **bystander** injured

    √7ᵗʰ **Y35.293** Legal intervention involving other gas, **suspect** injured

    √7ᵗʰ **Y35.299** Legal intervention involving other gas, unspecified person injured

√5ᵗʰ **Y35.3** Legal intervention involving **blunt objects**

Legal intervention involving being hit or struck by blunt object

  √6ᵗʰ **Y35.30** Legal intervention involving unspecified blunt objects

    √7ᵗʰ **Y35.301** Legal intervention involving unspecified blunt objects, **law enforcement official** injured

    √7ᵗʰ **Y35.302** Legal intervention involving unspecified blunt objects, **bystander** injured

    √7ᵗʰ **Y35.303** Legal intervention involving unspecified blunt objects, **suspect** injured

    √7ᵗʰ **Y35.309** Legal intervention involving unspecified blunt objects, unspecified person injured

  √6ᵗʰ **Y35.31** Legal intervention involving **baton**

    √7ᵗʰ **Y35.311** Legal intervention involving baton, **law enforcement official** injured

    √7ᵗʰ **Y35.312** Legal intervention involving baton, **bystander** injured

    √7ᵗʰ **Y35.313** Legal intervention involving baton, **suspect** injured

    √7ᵗʰ **Y35.319** Legal intervention involving baton, unspecified person injured

  √6ᵗʰ **Y35.39** Legal intervention involving other blunt objects

    √7ᵗʰ **Y35.391** Legal intervention involving other blunt objects, **law enforcement official** injured

    √7ᵗʰ **Y35.392** Legal intervention involving other blunt objects, **bystander** injured

    √7ᵗʰ **Y35.393** Legal intervention involving other blunt objects, **suspect** injured

    √7ᵗʰ **Y35.399** Legal intervention involving other blunt objects, unspecified person injured

√5ᵗʰ **Y35.4** Legal intervention involving **sharp objects**

Legal intervention involving being cut by sharp objects
Legal intervention involving being stabbed by sharp objects

  √6ᵗʰ **Y35.40** Legal intervention involving unspecified sharp objects

    √7ᵗʰ **Y35.401** Legal intervention involving unspecified sharp objects, **law enforcement official** injured

    √7ᵗʰ **Y35.402** Legal intervention involving unspecified sharp objects, **bystander** injured

    √7ᵗʰ **Y35.403** Legal intervention involving unspecified sharp objects, **suspect** injured

    √7ᵗʰ **Y35.409** Legal intervention involving unspecified sharp objects, unspecified person injured

  √6ᵗʰ **Y35.41** Legal intervention involving **bayonet**

    √7ᵗʰ **Y35.411** Legal intervention involving bayonet, **law enforcement official** injured

    √7ᵗʰ **Y35.412** Legal intervention involving bayonet, **bystander** injured

    √7ᵗʰ **Y35.413** Legal intervention involving bayonet, **suspect** injured

    √7ᵗʰ **Y35.419** Legal intervention involving bayonet, unspecified person injured

  √6ᵗʰ **Y35.49** Legal intervention involving other sharp objects

    √7ᵗʰ **Y35.491** Legal intervention involving other sharp objects, **law enforcement official** injured

    √7ᵗʰ **Y35.492** Legal intervention involving other sharp objects, **bystander** injured

    √7ᵗʰ **Y35.493** Legal intervention involving other sharp objects, **suspect** injured

    √7ᵗʰ **Y35.499** Legal intervention involving other sharp objects, unspecified person injured

√5ᵗʰ **Y35.8** Legal intervention involving other specified means

  √6ᵗʰ **Y35.81** Legal intervention involving **manhandling**

    √7ᵗʰ **Y35.811** Legal intervention involving manhandling, **law enforcement official** injured

    √7ᵗʰ **Y35.812** Legal intervention involving manhandling, **bystander** injured

    √7ᵗʰ **Y35.813** Legal intervention involving manhandling, **suspect** injured

    √7ᵗʰ **Y35.819** Legal intervention involving manhandling, unspecified person injured

  √6ᵗʰ **Y35.83** Legal intervention involving a **conducted energy device**

Electroshock device (taser)
Stun gun

    √7ᵗʰ **Y35.831** Legal intervention involving a conducted energy device, **law enforcement official** injured

N Newborn: 0   P Pediatric: 0-17   M Maternity: 9-64   A Adult: 15-124   MCC Major Complication/Comorbidity   CC Complication/Comorbidity   SW Severe Wound Dx

1256   ICD-10-CM 2020

Chapter 20. External Causes of Morbidity

● ✓7ᵗʰ **Y35.832** **Legal intervention involving a conducted energy device, bystander injured**

● ✓7ᵗʰ **Y35.833** **Legal intervention involving a conducted energy device, suspect injured**

● ✓7ᵗʰ **Y35.839** **Legal intervention involving a conducted energy device, unspecified person injured**

✓6ᵗʰ **Y35.89** **Legal intervention involving other specified means**

✓7ᵗʰ **Y35.891** **Legal intervention involving other specified means, law enforcement official injured**

✓7ᵗʰ **Y35.892** **Legal intervention involving other specified means, bystander injured**

✓7ᵗʰ **Y35.893** **Legal intervention involving other specified means, suspect injured**

AHA: 2018,1Q,5

✓5ᵗʰ **Y35.9** **Legal intervention, means unspecified**

✓x7ᵗʰ **Y35.91** **Legal intervention, means unspecified, law enforcement official injured**

✓x7ᵗʰ **Y35.92** **Legal intervention, means unspecified, bystander injured**

✓x7ᵗʰ **Y35.93** **Legal intervention, means unspecified, suspect injured**

● ✓x7ᵗʰ **Y35.99** **Legal intervention, means unspecified, unspecified person injured**

✓4ᵗʰ **Y36** **Operations of war**

INCLUDES injuries to military personnel and civilians caused by war, civil insurrection, and peacekeeping missions

EXCLUDES 1 *injury to military personnel occurring during peacetime military operations (Y37.-)*

military vehicles involved in transport accidents with non-military vehicle during peacetime (V09.01, V09.21, V19.81, V29.81, V39.81, V49.81, V59.81, V69.81, V79.81)

AHA: 2014,3Q,4

✓5ᵗʰ **Y36.0** **War operations involving explosion of marine weapons**

✓6ᵗʰ **Y36.00** **War operations involving explosion of unspecified marine weapon**

War operations involving underwater blast NOS

✓7ᵗʰ **Y36.000** **War operations involving explosion of unspecified marine weapon, military personnel**

✓7ᵗʰ **Y36.001** **War operations involving explosion of unspecified marine weapon, civilian**

✓6ᵗʰ **Y36.01** **War operations involving explosion of depth-charge**

✓7ᵗʰ **Y36.010** **War operations involving explosion of depth-charge, military personnel**

✓7ᵗʰ **Y36.011** **War operations involving explosion of depth-charge, civilian**

✓6ᵗʰ **Y36.02** **War operations involving explosion of marine mine**

War operations involving explosion of marine mine, at sea or in harbor

✓7ᵗʰ **Y36.020** **War operations involving explosion of marine mine, military personnel**

✓7ᵗʰ **Y36.021** **War operations involving explosion of marine mine, civilian**

✓6ᵗʰ **Y36.03** **War operations involving explosion of sea-based artillery shell**

✓7ᵗʰ **Y36.030** **War operations involving explosion of sea-based artillery shell, military personnel**

✓7ᵗʰ **Y36.031** **War operations involving explosion of sea-based artillery shell, civilian**

✓6ᵗʰ **Y36.04** **War operations involving explosion of torpedo**

✓7ᵗʰ **Y36.040** **War operations involving explosion of torpedo, military personnel**

✓7ᵗʰ **Y36.041** **War operations involving explosion of torpedo, civilian**

✓6ᵗʰ **Y36.05** **War operations involving accidental detonation of onboard marine weapons**

✓7ᵗʰ **Y36.050** **War operations involving accidental detonation of onboard marine weapons, military personnel**

✓7ᵗʰ **Y36.051** **War operations involving accidental detonation of onboard marine weapons, civilian**

✓6ᵗʰ **Y36.09** **War operations involving explosion of other marine weapons**

✓7ᵗʰ **Y36.090** **War operations involving explosion of other marine weapons, military personnel**

✓7ᵗʰ **Y36.091** **War operations involving explosion of other marine weapons, civilian**

✓5ᵗʰ **Y36.1** **War operations involving destruction of aircraft**

✓6ᵗʰ **Y36.10** **War operations involving unspecified destruction of aircraft**

✓7ᵗʰ **Y36.100** **War operations involving unspecified destruction of aircraft, military personnel**

✓7ᵗʰ **Y36.101** **War operations involving unspecified destruction of aircraft, civilian**

✓6ᵗʰ **Y36.11** **War operations involving destruction of aircraft due to enemy fire or explosives**

War operations involving destruction of aircraft due to air to air missile

War operations involving destruction of aircraft due to explosive placed on aircraft

War operations involving destruction of aircraft due to rocket propelled grenade [RPG]

War operations involving destruction of aircraft due to small arms fire

War operations involving destruction of aircraft due to surface to air missile

✓7ᵗʰ **Y36.110** **War operations involving destruction of aircraft due to enemy fire or explosives, military personnel**

✓7ᵗʰ **Y36.111** **War operations involving destruction of aircraft due to enemy fire or explosives, civilian**

✓6ᵗʰ **Y36.12** **War operations involving destruction of aircraft due to collision with other aircraft**

✓7ᵗʰ **Y36.120** **War operations involving destruction of aircraft due to collision with other aircraft, military personnel**

✓7ᵗʰ **Y36.121** **War operations involving destruction of aircraft due to collision with other aircraft, civilian**

✓6ᵗʰ **Y36.13** **War operations involving destruction of aircraft due to onboard fire**

✓7ᵗʰ **Y36.130** **War operations involving destruction of aircraft due to onboard fire, military personnel**

✓7ᵗʰ **Y36.131** **War operations involving destruction of aircraft due to onboard fire, civilian**

✓6ᵗʰ **Y36.14** **War operations involving destruction of aircraft due to accidental detonation of onboard munitions and explosives**

✓7ᵗʰ **Y36.140** **War operations involving destruction of aircraft due to accidental detonation of onboard munitions and explosives, military personnel**

✓7ᵗʰ **Y36.141** **War operations involving destruction of aircraft due to accidental detonation of onboard munitions and explosives, civilian**

✓6ᵗʰ **Y36.19** **War operations involving other destruction of aircraft**

✓7ᵗʰ **Y36.190** **War operations involving other destruction of aircraft, military personnel**

✓7ᵗʰ **Y36.191** **War operations involving other destruction of aircraft, civilian**

✓5ᵗʰ **Y36.2** **War operations involving other explosions and fragments**

EXCLUDES 1 *war operations involving explosion of aircraft (Y36.1-)*

war operations involving explosion of marine weapons (Y36.0-)

war operations involving explosion of nuclear weapons (Y36.5-)

war operations involving explosion occurring after cessation of hostilities (Y36.8-)

✓6ᵗʰ **Y36.20** **War operations involving unspecified explosion and fragments**

War operations involving air blast NOS

War operations involving blast NOS

War operations involving blast fragments NOS

War operations involving blast wave NOS

War operations involving blast wind NOS

War operations involving explosion NOS

War operations involving explosion of bomb NOS

✓7ᵗʰ **Y36.200** **War operations involving unspecified explosion and fragments, military personnel**

✓7ᵗʰ **Y36.201** **War operations involving unspecified explosion and fragments, civilian**

☑ Additional Char Req   ✓x7ᵗʰ Placeholder   Unacceptable PDx   Questionable PDx   Wrong Procedure   Manifestation   Unspecified Dx   H1-H14 HAC   HCC CMS-HCC Dx   HIV HIV Dx

ICD-10-CM 2020   **1257**

Chapter 20. External Causes of Morbidity

✓6ᵗʰ **Y36.21** War operations involving explosion of aerial bomb

  ✓7ᵗʰ **Y36.210** War operations involving explosion of aerial bomb, military personnel

  ✓7ᵗʰ **Y36.211** War operations involving explosion of aerial bomb, civilian

✓6ᵗʰ **Y36.22** War operations involving explosion of guided missile

  ✓7ᵗʰ **Y36.220** War operations involving explosion of guided missile, military personnel

  ✓7ᵗʰ **Y36.221** War operations involving explosion of guided missile, civilian

✓6ᵗʰ **Y36.23** War operations involving explosion of improvised explosive device [IED]

  War operations involving explosion of person-borne improvised explosive device [IED]

  War operations involving explosion of vehicle-borne improvised explosive device [IED]

  War operations involving explosion of roadside improvised explosive device [IED]

  ✓7ᵗʰ **Y36.230** War operations involving explosion of improvised explosive device [IED], military personnel

  ✓7ᵗʰ **Y36.231** War operations involving explosion of improvised explosive device [IED], civilian

✓6ᵗʰ **Y36.24** War operations involving explosion due to accidental detonation and discharge of own munitions or munitions launch device

  ✓7ᵗʰ **Y36.240** War operations involving explosion due to accidental detonation and discharge of own munitions or munitions launch device, military personnel

  ✓7ᵗʰ **Y36.241** War operations involving explosion due to accidental detonation and discharge of own munitions or munitions launch device, civilian

✓6ᵗʰ **Y36.25** War operations involving fragments from munitions

  ✓7ᵗʰ **Y36.250** War operations involving fragments from munitions, military personnel

  ✓7ᵗʰ **Y36.251** War operations involving fragments from munitions, civilian

✓6ᵗʰ **Y36.26** War operations involving fragments of improvised explosive device [IED]

  War operations involving fragments of person-borne improvised explosive device [IED]

  War operations involving fragments of vehicle-borne improvised explosive device [IED]

  War operations involving fragments of roadside improvised explosive device [IED]

  ✓7ᵗʰ **Y36.260** War operations involving fragments of improvised explosive device [IED], military personnel

  ✓7ᵗʰ **Y36.261** War operations involving fragments of improvised explosive device [IED], civilian

✓6ᵗʰ **Y36.27** War operations involving fragments from weapons

  ✓7ᵗʰ **Y36.270** War operations involving fragments from weapons, military personnel

  ✓7ᵗʰ **Y36.271** War operations involving fragments from weapons, civilian

✓6ᵗʰ **Y36.29** War operations involving other explosions and fragments

  War operations involving explosion of grenade

  War operations involving explosions of land mine

  War operations involving shrapnel NOS

  ✓7ᵗʰ **Y36.290** War operations involving other explosions and fragments, military personnel

  ✓7ᵗʰ **Y36.291** War operations involving other explosions and fragments, civilian

✓5ᵗʰ **Y36.3** War operations involving fires, conflagrations and hot substances

War operations involving smoke, fumes, and heat from fires, conflagrations and hot substances

  EXCLUDES 1   war operations involving fires and conflagrations aboard military aircraft (Y36.1-)

     war operations involving fires and conflagrations aboard military watercraft (Y36.0-)

     war operations involving fires and conflagrations caused indirectly by conventional weapons (Y36.2-)

     war operations involving fires and thermal effects of nuclear weapons (Y36.53-)

✓6ᵗʰ **Y36.30** War operations involving unspecified fire, conflagration and hot substance

  ✓7ᵗʰ **Y36.300** War operations involving unspecified fire, conflagration and hot substance, military personnel

  ✓7ᵗʰ **Y36.301** War operations involving unspecified fire, conflagration and hot substance, civilian

✓6ᵗʰ **Y36.31** War operations involving gasoline bomb

  War operations involving incendiary bomb

  War operations involving petrol bomb

  ✓7ᵗʰ **Y36.310** War operations involving gasoline bomb, military personnel

  ✓7ᵗʰ **Y36.311** War operations involving gasoline bomb, civilian

✓6ᵗʰ **Y36.32** War operations involving incendiary bullet

  ✓7ᵗʰ **Y36.320** War operations involving incendiary bullet, military personnel

  ✓7ᵗʰ **Y36.321** War operations involving incendiary bullet, civilian

✓6ᵗʰ **Y36.33** War operations involving flamethrower

  ✓7ᵗʰ **Y36.330** War operations involving flamethrower, military personnel

  ✓7ᵗʰ **Y36.331** War operations involving flamethrower, civilian

✓6ᵗʰ **Y36.39** War operations involving other fires, conflagrations and hot substances

  ✓7ᵗʰ **Y36.390** War operations involving other fires, conflagrations and hot substances, military personnel

  ✓7ᵗʰ **Y36.391** War operations involving other fires, conflagrations and hot substances, civilian

✓5ᵗʰ **Y36.4** War operations involving firearm discharge and other forms of conventional warfare

✓6ᵗʰ **Y36.41** War operations involving rubber bullets

  ✓7ᵗʰ **Y36.410** War operations involving rubber bullets, military personnel

  ✓7ᵗʰ **Y36.411** War operations involving rubber bullets, civilian

✓6ᵗʰ **Y36.42** War operations involving firearms pellets

  ✓7ᵗʰ **Y36.420** War operations involving firearms pellets, military personnel

  ✓7ᵗʰ **Y36.421** War operations involving firearms pellets, civilian

✓6ᵗʰ **Y36.43** War operations involving other firearms discharge

  War operations involving bullets NOS

  EXCLUDES 1   war operations involving munitions fragments (Y36.25-)

     war operations involving incendiary bullets (Y36.32-)

  ✓7ᵗʰ **Y36.430** War operations involving other firearms discharge, military personnel

  ✓7ᵗʰ **Y36.431** War operations involving other firearms discharge, civilian

✓6ᵗʰ **Y36.44** War operations involving unarmed hand to hand combat

  EXCLUDES 1   war operations involving combat using blunt or piercing object (Y36.45-)

     war operations involving intentional restriction of air and airway (Y36.46-)

     war operations involving unintentional restriction of air and airway (Y36.47-)

  ✓7ᵗʰ **Y36.440** War operations involving unarmed hand to hand combat, military personnel

  ✓7ᵗʰ **Y36.441** War operations involving unarmed hand to hand combat, civilian

N Newborn: 0   P Pediatric: 0-17   M Maternity: 9-64   A Adult: 15-124   MCC Major Complication/Comorbidity   CC Complication/Comorbidity   SW Severe Wound Dx

1258   ICD-10-CM 2020

√6ᵗʰ **Y36.45** **War operations involving combat using** blunt or piercing object

    √7ᵗʰ **Y36.450** **War operations involving combat using blunt or piercing object,** military personnel

    √7ᵗʰ **Y36.451** **War operations involving combat using blunt or piercing object,** civilian

√6ᵗʰ **Y36.46** **War operations involving** intentional restriction of air and airway

    √7ᵗʰ **Y36.460** **War operations involving intentional restriction of air and airway,** military personnel

    √7ᵗʰ **Y36.461** **War operations involving intentional restriction of air and airway,** civilian

√6ᵗʰ **Y36.47** **War operations involving** unintentional restriction of air and airway

    √7ᵗʰ **Y36.470** **War operations involving unintentional restriction of air and airway,** military personnel

    √7ᵗʰ **Y36.471** **War operations involving unintentional restriction of air and airway,** civilian

√6ᵗʰ **Y36.49** **War operations involving other forms of conventional warfare**

    √7ᵗʰ **Y36.490** **War operations involving other forms of conventional warfare,** military personnel

    √7ᵗʰ **Y36.491** **War operations involving other forms of conventional warfare,** civilian

√5ᵗʰ **Y36.5** **War operations involving** nuclear weapons

War operations involving dirty bomb NOS

    √6ᵗʰ **Y36.50** **War operations involving unspecified effect of nuclear weapon**

        √7ᵗʰ **Y36.500** **War operations involving unspecified effect of nuclear weapon,** military personnel

        √7ᵗʰ **Y36.501** **War operations involving unspecified effect of nuclear weapon,** civilian

    √6ᵗʰ **Y36.51** **War operations involving** direct blast **effect of nuclear weapon**

War operations involving blast pressure of nuclear weapon

        √7ᵗʰ **Y36.510** **War operations involving direct blast effect of nuclear weapon,** military personnel

        √7ᵗʰ **Y36.511** **War operations involving direct blast effect of nuclear weapon,** civilian

    √6ᵗʰ **Y36.52** **War operations involving** indirect blast **effect of nuclear weapon**

War operations involving being thrown by blast of nuclear weapon

War operations involving being struck or crushed by blast debris of nuclear weapon

        √7ᵗʰ **Y36.520** **War operations involving indirect blast effect of nuclear weapon,** military personnel

        √7ᵗʰ **Y36.521** **War operations involving indirect blast effect of nuclear weapon,** civilian

    √6ᵗʰ **Y36.53** **War operations involving** thermal radiation **effect of nuclear weapon**

War operations involving direct heat from nuclear weapon

War operation involving fireball effects from nuclear weapon

        √7ᵗʰ **Y36.530** **War operations involving thermal radiation effect of nuclear weapon,** military personnel

        √7ᵗʰ **Y36.531** **War operations involving thermal radiation effect of nuclear weapon,** civilian

    √6ᵗʰ **Y36.54** **War operation involving** nuclear radiation **effects of nuclear weapon**

War operation involving acute radiation exposure from nuclear weapon

War operation involving exposure to immediate ionizing radiation from nuclear weapon

War operation involving fallout exposure from nuclear weapon

War operation involving secondary effects of nuclear weapons

        √7ᵗʰ **Y36.540** **War operation involving nuclear radiation effects of nuclear weapon,** military personnel

        √7ᵗʰ **Y36.541** **War operation involving nuclear radiation effects of nuclear weapon,** civilian

    √6ᵗʰ **Y36.59** **War operation involving other effects of nuclear weapons**

        √7ᵗʰ **Y36.590** **War operation involving other effects of nuclear weapons,** military personnel

        √7ᵗʰ **Y36.591** **War operation involving other effects of nuclear weapons,** civilian

√5ᵗʰ **Y36.6** **War operations involving biological weapons**

    √6ᵗʰ **Y36.6X** **War operations involving** biological weapons

        √7ᵗʰ **Y36.6X0** **War operations involving biological weapons,** military personnel

        √7ᵗʰ **Y36.6X1** **War operations involving biological weapons,** civilian

√5ᵗʰ **Y36.7** **War operations involving chemical weapons and other forms of unconventional warfare**

    EXCLUDES 1   *war operations involving incendiary devices (Y36.3-, Y36.5-)*

    √6ᵗʰ **Y36.7X** **War operations involving** chemical weapons and other forms of unconventional warfare

        √7ᵗʰ **Y36.7X0** **War operations involving chemical weapons and other forms of unconventional warfare,** military personnel

        √7ᵗʰ **Y36.7X1** **War operations involving chemical weapons and other forms of unconventional warfare,** civilian

√5ᵗʰ **Y36.8** **War operations occurring** after cessation of hostilities

War operations classifiable to categories Y36.0-Y36.8 but occurring after cessation of hostilities

    √6ᵗʰ **Y36.81** **Explosion of** mine **placed during war operations but exploding after cessation of hostilities**

        √7ᵗʰ **Y36.810** **Explosion of mine placed during war operations but exploding after cessation of hostilities,** military personnel

        √7ᵗʰ **Y36.811** **Explosion of mine placed during war operations but exploding after cessation of hostilities,** civilian

    √6ᵗʰ **Y36.82** **Explosion of** bomb **placed during war operations but exploding after cessation of hostilities**

        √7ᵗʰ **Y36.820** **Explosion of bomb placed during war operations but exploding after cessation of hostilities,** military personnel

        √7ᵗʰ **Y36.821** **Explosion of bomb placed during war operations but exploding after cessation of hostilities,** civilian

    √6ᵗʰ **Y36.88** **Other war operations occurring after cessation of hostilities**

        √7ᵗʰ **Y36.880** **Other war operations occurring after cessation of hostilities,** military personnel

        √7ᵗʰ **Y36.881** **Other war operations occurring after cessation of hostilities,** civilian

    √6ᵗʰ **Y36.89** **Unspecified war operations occurring after cessation of hostilities**

        √7ᵗʰ **Y36.890** **Unspecified war operations occurring after cessation of hostilities,** military personnel

        √7ᵗʰ **Y36.891** **Unspecified war operations occurring after cessation of hostilities,** civilian

√5ᵗʰ **Y36.9** **Other and unspecified war operations**

    √x7ᵗʰ **Y36.90** **War operations, unspecified**

    √x7ᵗʰ **Y36.91** **War operations involving unspecified** weapon of mass destruction [WMD]

    √x7ᵗʰ **Y36.92** **War operations involving** friendly fire

✓ Additional Char Req   √x7ᵗʰ Placeholder   Unacceptable PDx   Questionable PDx   Wrong Procedure   Manifestation   Unspecified Dx   H1-H14 HAC   HCC CMS-HCC Dx   HIV HIV Dx

ICD-10-CM 2020   1259

✓4ᵗʰ **Y37   Military operations**

> INCLUDES   injuries to military personnel and civilians occurring during peacetime on military property and during routine military exercises and operations
>
> EXCLUDES 1   military aircraft involved in aircraft accident with civilian aircraft (V97.81-)
>
> military vehicles involved in transport accident with civilian vehicle (V09.01, V09.21, V19.81, V29.81, V39.81, V49.81, V59.81, V69.81, V79.81)
>
> military watercraft involved in water transport accident with civilian watercraft (V94.81-)
>
> war operations (Y36.-)

✓5ᵗʰ **Y37.0   Military operations involving** explosion of marine weapons

   ✓6ᵗʰ **Y37.00   Military operations involving explosion of unspecified marine weapon**
> Military operations involving underwater blast NOS

     ✓7ᵗʰ **Y37.000   Military operations involving explosion of unspecified marine weapon, military personnel**

     ✓7ᵗʰ **Y37.001   Military operations involving explosion of unspecified marine weapon, civilian**

   ✓6ᵗʰ **Y37.01   Military operations involving explosion of depth-charge**

     ✓7ᵗʰ **Y37.010   Military operations involving explosion of depth-charge, military personnel**

     ✓7ᵗʰ **Y37.011   Military operations involving explosion of depth-charge, civilian**

   ✓6ᵗʰ **Y37.02   Military operations involving explosion of** marine mine
> Military operations involving explosion of marine mine, at sea or in harbor

     ✓7ᵗʰ **Y37.020   Military operations involving explosion of marine mine, military personnel**

     ✓7ᵗʰ **Y37.021   Military operations involving explosion of marine mine, civilian**

   ✓6ᵗʰ **Y37.03   Military operations involving explosion of** sea-based artillery shell

     ✓7ᵗʰ **Y37.030   Military operations involving explosion of sea-based artillery shell, military personnel**

     ✓7ᵗʰ **Y37.031   Military operations involving explosion of sea-based artillery shell, civilian**

   ✓6ᵗʰ **Y37.04   Military operations involving explosion of** torpedo

     ✓7ᵗʰ **Y37.040   Military operations involving explosion of torpedo, military personnel**

     ✓7ᵗʰ **Y37.041   Military operations involving explosion of torpedo, civilian**

   ✓6ᵗʰ **Y37.05   Military operations involving accidental detonation of onboard marine weapons**

     ✓7ᵗʰ **Y37.050   Military operations involving accidental detonation of onboard marine weapons, military personnel**

     ✓7ᵗʰ **Y37.051   Military operations involving accidental detonation of onboard marine weapons, civilian**

   ✓6ᵗʰ **Y37.09   Military operations involving explosion of other marine weapons**

     ✓7ᵗʰ **Y37.090   Military operations involving explosion of other marine weapons, military personnel**

     ✓7ᵗʰ **Y37.091   Military operations involving explosion of other marine weapons, civilian**

✓5ᵗʰ **Y37.1   Military operations involving** destruction of aircraft

   ✓6ᵗʰ **Y37.10   Military operations involving unspecified destruction of aircraft**

     ✓7ᵗʰ **Y37.100   Military operations involving unspecified destruction of aircraft, military personnel**

     ✓7ᵗʰ **Y37.101   Military operations involving unspecified destruction of aircraft, civilian**

✓6ᵗʰ **Y37.11   Military operations involving destruction of aircraft due to enemy fire or explosives**
> Military operations involving destruction of aircraft due to air to air missile
>
> Military operations involving destruction of aircraft due to explosive placed on aircraft
>
> Military operations involving destruction of aircraft due to rocket propelled grenade [RPG]
>
> Military operations involving destruction of aircraft due to small arms fire
>
> Military operations involving destruction of aircraft due to surface to air missile

   ✓7ᵗʰ **Y37.110   Military operations involving destruction of aircraft due to enemy fire or explosives, military personnel**

   ✓7ᵗʰ **Y37.111   Military operations involving destruction of aircraft due to enemy fire or explosives, civilian**

✓6ᵗʰ **Y37.12   Military operations involving destruction of aircraft due to collision with other aircraft**

   ✓7ᵗʰ **Y37.120   Military operations involving destruction of aircraft due to collision with other aircraft, military personnel**

   ✓7ᵗʰ **Y37.121   Military operations involving destruction of aircraft due to collision with other aircraft, civilian**

✓6ᵗʰ **Y37.13   Military operations involving destruction of aircraft due to onboard fire**

   ✓7ᵗʰ **Y37.130   Military operations involving destruction of aircraft due to onboard fire, military personnel**

   ✓7ᵗʰ **Y37.131   Military operations involving destruction of aircraft due to onboard fire, civilian**

✓6ᵗʰ **Y37.14   Military operations involving destruction of aircraft due to** accidental detonation of onboard munitions and explosives

   ✓7ᵗʰ **Y37.140   Military operations involving destruction of aircraft due to accidental detonation of onboard munitions and explosives, military personnel**

   ✓7ᵗʰ **Y37.141   Military operations involving destruction of aircraft due to accidental detonation of onboard munitions and explosives, civilian**

✓6ᵗʰ **Y37.19   Military operations involving other destruction of aircraft**

   ✓7ᵗʰ **Y37.190   Military operations involving other destruction of aircraft, military personnel**

   ✓7ᵗʰ **Y37.191   Military operations involving other destruction of aircraft, civilian**

✓5ᵗʰ **Y37.2   Military operations involving** other explosions and fragments

> EXCLUDES 1   military operations involving explosion of aircraft (Y37.1-)
>
> military operations involving explosion of marine weapons (Y37.0-)
>
> military operations involving explosion of nuclear weapons (Y37.5-)

✓6ᵗʰ **Y37.20   Military operations involving unspecified explosion and fragments**
> Military operations involving air blast NOS
>
> Military operations involving blast NOS
>
> Military operations involving blast fragments NOS
>
> Military operations involving blast wave NOS
>
> Military operations involving blast wind NOS
>
> Military operations involving explosion NOS
>
> Military operations involving explosion of bomb NOS

   ✓7ᵗʰ **Y37.200   Military operations involving unspecified explosion and fragments, military personnel**

   ✓7ᵗʰ **Y37.201   Military operations involving unspecified explosion and fragments, civilian**

✓6ᵗʰ **Y37.21   Military operations involving explosion of** aerial bomb

   ✓7ᵗʰ **Y37.210   Military operations involving explosion of aerial bomb, military personnel**

   ✓7ᵗʰ **Y37.211   Military operations involving explosion of aerial bomb, civilian**

✓6ᵗʰ **Y37.22   Military operations involving explosion of** guided missile

   ✓7ᵗʰ **Y37.220   Military operations involving explosion of guided missile, military personnel**

Ⓝ Newborn: 0   Ⓟ Pediatric: 0-17   Ⓜ Maternity: 9-64   Ⓐ Adult: 15-124   MCC Major Complication/Comorbidity   CC Complication/Comorbidity   SW Severe Wound Dx

1260   ICD-10-CM 2020

✓7ᵗʰ **Y37.221 Military operations involving explosion of guided missile, civilian**

✓6ᵗʰ **Y37.23 Military operations involving explosion of improvised explosive device [IED]**
Military operations involving explosion of person-borne improvised explosive device [IED]
Military operations involving explosion of vehicle-borne improvised explosive device [IED]
Military operations involving explosion of roadside improvised explosive device [IED]

✓7ᵗʰ **Y37.230 Military operations involving explosion of improvised explosive device [IED], military personnel**

✓7ᵗʰ **Y37.231 Military operations involving explosion of improvised explosive device [IED], civilian**

✓6ᵗʰ **Y37.24 Military operations involving explosion due to accidental detonation and discharge of own munitions or munitions launch device**

✓7ᵗʰ **Y37.240 Military operations involving explosion due to accidental detonation and discharge of own munitions or munitions launch device, military personnel**

✓7ᵗʰ **Y37.241 Military operations involving explosion due to accidental detonation and discharge of own munitions or munitions launch device, civilian**

✓6ᵗʰ **Y37.25 Military operations involving fragments from munitions**

✓7ᵗʰ **Y37.250 Military operations involving fragments from munitions, military personnel**

✓7ᵗʰ **Y37.251 Military operations involving fragments from munitions, civilian**

✓6ᵗʰ **Y37.26 Military operations involving fragments of improvised explosive device [IED]**
Military operations involving fragments of person-borne improvised explosive device [IED]
Military operations involving fragments of vehicle-borne improvised explosive device [IED]
Military operations involving fragments of roadside improvised explosive device [IED]

✓7ᵗʰ **Y37.260 Military operations involving fragments of improvised explosive device [IED], military personnel**

✓7ᵗʰ **Y37.261 Military operations involving fragments of improvised explosive device [IED], civilian**

✓6ᵗʰ **Y37.27 Military operations involving fragments from weapons**

✓7ᵗʰ **Y37.270 Military operations involving fragments from weapons, military personnel**

✓7ᵗʰ **Y37.271 Military operations involving fragments from weapons, civilian**

✓6ᵗʰ **Y37.29 Military operations involving other explosions and fragments**
Military operations involving explosion of grenade
Military operations involving explosions of land mine
Military operations involving shrapnel NOS

✓7ᵗʰ **Y37.290 Military operations involving other explosions and fragments, military personnel**

✓7ᵗʰ **Y37.291 Military operations involving other explosions and fragments, civilian**

✓5ᵗʰ **Y37.3 Military operations involving fires, conflagrations and hot substances**
Military operations involving smoke, fumes, and heat from fires, conflagrations and hot substances

EXCLUDES 1   *military operations involving fires and conflagrations aboard military aircraft (Y37.1-)*
military operations involving fires and conflagrations aboard military watercraft (Y37.0-)
military operations involving fires and conflagrations caused indirectly by conventional weapons (Y37.2-)
military operations involving fires and thermal effects of nuclear weapons (Y36.53-)

✓6ᵗʰ **Y37.30 Military operations involving unspecified fire, conflagration and hot substance**

✓7ᵗʰ **Y37.300 Military operations involving unspecified fire, conflagration and hot substance, military personnel**

✓7ᵗʰ **Y37.301 Military operations involving unspecified fire, conflagration and hot substance, civilian**

✓6ᵗʰ **Y37.31 Military operations involving gasoline bomb**
Military operations involving incendiary bomb
Military operations involving petrol bomb

✓7ᵗʰ **Y37.310 Military operations involving gasoline bomb, military personnel**

✓7ᵗʰ **Y37.311 Military operations involving gasoline bomb, civilian**

✓6ᵗʰ **Y37.32 Military operations involving incendiary bullet**

✓7ᵗʰ **Y37.320 Military operations involving incendiary bullet, military personnel**

✓7ᵗʰ **Y37.321 Military operations involving incendiary bullet, civilian**

✓6ᵗʰ **Y37.33 Military operations involving flamethrower**

✓7ᵗʰ **Y37.330 Military operations involving flamethrower, military personnel**

✓7ᵗʰ **Y37.331 Military operations involving flamethrower, civilian**

✓6ᵗʰ **Y37.39 Military operations involving other fires, conflagrations and hot substances**

✓7ᵗʰ **Y37.390 Military operations involving other fires, conflagrations and hot substances, military personnel**

✓7ᵗʰ **Y37.391 Military operations involving other fires, conflagrations and hot substances, civilian**

✓5ᵗʰ **Y37.4 Military operations involving firearm discharge and other forms of conventional warfare**

✓6ᵗʰ **Y37.41 Military operations involving rubber bullets**

✓7ᵗʰ **Y37.410 Military operations involving rubber bullets, military personnel**

✓7ᵗʰ **Y37.411 Military operations involving rubber bullets, civilian**

✓6ᵗʰ **Y37.42 Military operations involving firearms pellets**

✓7ᵗʰ **Y37.420 Military operations involving firearms pellets, military personnel**

✓7ᵗʰ **Y37.421 Military operations involving firearms pellets, civilian**

✓6ᵗʰ **Y37.43 Military operations involving other firearms discharge**
Military operations involving bullets NOS

EXCLUDES 1   *military operations involving munitions fragments (Y37.25-)*
military operations involving incendiary bullets (Y37.32-)

✓7ᵗʰ **Y37.430 Military operations involving other firearms discharge, military personnel**

✓7ᵗʰ **Y37.431 Military operations involving other firearms discharge, civilian**

✓6ᵗʰ **Y37.44 Military operations involving unarmed hand to hand combat**

EXCLUDES 1   *military operations involving combat using blunt or piercing object (Y37.45-)*
military operations involving intentional restriction of air and airway (Y37.46-)
military operations involving unintentional restriction of air and airway (Y37.47-)

✓7ᵗʰ **Y37.440 Military operations involving unarmed hand to hand combat, military personnel**

✓7ᵗʰ **Y37.441 Military operations involving unarmed hand to hand combat, civilian**

✓6ᵗʰ **Y37.45 Military operations involving combat using blunt or piercing object**

✓7ᵗʰ **Y37.450 Military operations involving combat using blunt or piercing object, military personnel**

✓7ᵗʰ **Y37.451 Military operations involving combat using blunt or piercing object, civilian**

✓6ᵗʰ **Y37.46 Military operations involving intentional restriction of air and airway**

✓7ᵗʰ **Y37.460 Military operations involving intentional restriction of air and airway, military personnel**

✓7ᵗʰ **Y37.461 Military operations involving intentional restriction of air and airway, civilian**

✓ Additional Char Req   ✓x7ᵗʰ Placeholder   Unacceptable PDx   Questionable PDx   Wrong Procedure   Manifestation   Unspecified Dx   H1-H14 HAC   HCC CMS-HCC Dx   HIV HIV Dx

ICD-10-CM 2020   1261

Chapter 20. External Causes of Morbidity

Y37.47–Y38.2X1

√6ᵗʰ **Y37.47** **Military operations involving** unintentional restriction of air and airway
- √7ᵗʰ **Y37.470** **Military operations involving** unintentional restriction of air and airway, **military personnel**
- √7ᵗʰ **Y37.471** **Military operations involving** unintentional restriction of air and airway, **civilian**

√6ᵗʰ **Y37.49** **Military operations involving other forms of conventional warfare**
- √7ᵗʰ **Y37.490** **Military operations involving other forms of conventional warfare, military personnel**
- √7ᵗʰ **Y37.491** **Military operations involving other forms of conventional warfare, civilian**

√5ᵗʰ **Y37.5** **Military operations involving** nuclear weapons

Military operation involving dirty bomb NOS

√6ᵗʰ **Y37.50** **Military operations involving unspecified effect of nuclear weapon**
- √7ᵗʰ **Y37.500** **Military operations involving unspecified effect of nuclear weapon, military personnel**
- √7ᵗʰ **Y37.501** **Military operations involving unspecified effect of nuclear weapon, civilian**

√6ᵗʰ **Y37.51** **Military operations involving** direct blast effect of nuclear weapon

Military operations involving blast pressure of nuclear weapon
- √7ᵗʰ **Y37.510** **Military operations involving direct blast effect of nuclear weapon, military personnel**
- √7ᵗʰ **Y37.511** **Military operations involving direct blast effect of nuclear weapon, civilian**

√6ᵗʰ **Y37.52** **Military operations involving** indirect blast effect of nuclear weapon

Military operations involving being thrown by blast of nuclear weapon

Military operations involving being struck or crushed by blast debris of nuclear weapon
- √7ᵗʰ **Y37.520** **Military operations involving indirect blast effect of nuclear weapon, military personnel**
- √7ᵗʰ **Y37.521** **Military operations involving indirect blast effect of nuclear weapon, civilian**

√6ᵗʰ **Y37.53** **Military operations involving** thermal radiation effect of nuclear weapon

Military operations involving direct heat from nuclear weapon

Military operation involving fireball effects from nuclear weapon
- √7ᵗʰ **Y37.530** **Military operations involving thermal radiation effect of nuclear weapon, military personnel**
- √7ᵗʰ **Y37.531** **Military operations involving thermal radiation effect of nuclear weapon, civilian**

√6ᵗʰ **Y37.54** **Military operation involving** nuclear radiation effects of nuclear weapon

Military operation involving acute radiation exposure from nuclear weapon

Military operation involving exposure to immediate ionizing radiation from nuclear weapon

Military operation involving fallout exposure from nuclear weapon

Military operation involving secondary effects of nuclear weapons
- √7ᵗʰ **Y37.540** **Military operation involving nuclear radiation effects of nuclear weapon, military personnel**
- √7ᵗʰ **Y37.541** **Military operation involving nuclear radiation effects of nuclear weapon, civilian**

√6ᵗʰ **Y37.59** **Military operation involving other effects of nuclear weapons**
- √7ᵗʰ **Y37.590** **Military operation involving other effects of nuclear weapons, military personnel**
- √7ᵗʰ **Y37.591** **Military operation involving other effects of nuclear weapons, civilian**

√5ᵗʰ **Y37.6** **Military operations involving** biological weapons
- √6ᵗʰ **Y37.6X** **Military operations involving biological weapons**
  - √7ᵗʰ **Y37.6X0** **Military operations involving biological weapons, military personnel**

√7ᵗʰ **Y37.6X1** **Military operations involving biological weapons, civilian**

√5ᵗʰ **Y37.7** **Military operations involving chemical weapons and other forms of unconventional warfare**

EXCLUDES 1   military operations involving incendiary devices (Y36.3-, Y36.5-)

√6ᵗʰ **Y37.7X** **Military operations involving** chemical weapons and other forms of unconventional warfare
- √7ᵗʰ **Y37.7X0** **Military operations involving chemical weapons and other forms of unconventional warfare, military personnel**
- √7ᵗʰ **Y37.7X1** **Military operations involving chemical weapons and other forms of unconventional warfare, civilian**

√5ᵗʰ **Y37.9** **Other and unspecified military operations**
- √x7ᵗʰ **Y37.90** **Military operations, unspecified**
- √x7ᵗʰ **Y37.91** **Military operations involving unspecified** weapon of mass destruction [WMD]
- √x7ᵗʰ **Y37.92** **Military operations involving** friendly fire

√4ᵗʰ **Y38 Terrorism**

NOTE   These codes are for use to identify injuries resulting from the unlawful use of force or violence against persons or property to intimidate or coerce a Government, the civilian population, or any segment thereof, in furtherance of political or social objective

Use additional code for place of occurrence (Y92.-)

√5ᵗʰ **Y38.0** **Terrorism involving explosion of marine weapons**

Terrorism involving depth-charge

Terrorism involving marine mine

Terrorism involving mine NOS, at sea or in harbor

Terrorism involving sea-based artillery shell

Terrorism involving torpedo

Terrorism involving underwater blast

√6ᵗʰ **Y38.0X** **Terrorism involving explosion of** marine weapons
- √7ᵗʰ **Y38.0X1** **Terrorism involving explosion of marine weapons, public safety official injured**
- √7ᵗʰ **Y38.0X2** **Terrorism involving explosion of marine weapons, civilian injured**
- √7ᵗʰ **Y38.0X3** **Terrorism involving explosion of marine weapons, terrorist injured**

√5ᵗʰ **Y38.1** **Terrorism involving destruction of aircraft**

Terrorism involving aircraft burned

Terrorism involving aircraft exploded

Terrorism involving aircraft being shot down

Terrorism involving aircraft used as a weapon

√6ᵗʰ **Y38.1X** **Terrorism involving** destruction of aircraft
- √7ᵗʰ **Y38.1X1** **Terrorism involving destruction of aircraft, public safety official injured**
- √7ᵗʰ **Y38.1X2** **Terrorism involving destruction of aircraft, civilian injured**
- √7ᵗʰ **Y38.1X3** **Terrorism involving destruction of aircraft, terrorist injured**

√5ᵗʰ **Y38.2** **Terrorism involving other explosions and fragments**

Terrorism involving antipersonnel (fragments) bomb

Terrorism involving blast NOS

Terrorism involving explosion NOS

Terrorism involving explosion of breech block

Terrorism involving explosion of cannon block

Terrorism involving explosion (fragments) of artillery shell

Terrorism involving explosion (fragments) of bomb

Terrorism involving explosion (fragments) of grenade

Terrorism involving explosion (fragments) of guided missile

Terrorism involving explosion (fragments) of land mine

Terrorism involving explosion of mortar bomb

Terrorism involving explosion of munitions

Terrorism involving explosion (fragments) of rocket

Terrorism involving explosion (fragments) of shell

Terrorism involving shrapnel

Terrorism involving mine NOS, on land

EXCLUDES 1   terrorism involving explosion of nuclear weapon (Y38.5)

terrorism involving suicide bomber (Y38.81)

√6ᵗʰ **Y38.2X** **Terrorism involving other explosions and fragments**
- √7ᵗʰ **Y38.2X1** **Terrorism involving other explosions and fragments, public safety official injured**

Ⓝ Newborn: 0   Ⓟ Pediatric: 0-17   Ⓜ Maternity: 9-64   Ⓐ Adult: 15-124   MCC Major Complication/Comorbidity   CC Complication/Comorbidity   SW Severe Wound Dx

1262   ICD-10-CM 2020

√7ᵗʰ **Y38.2X2** **Terrorism involving** other explosions and fragments, civilian **injured**

√7ᵗʰ **Y38.2X3** **Terrorism involving** other explosions and fragments, terrorist **injured**

√5ᵗʰ **Y38.3** **Terrorism involving fires, conflagration and hot substances**

Terrorism involving conflagration NOS

Terrorism involving fire NOS

Terrorism involving petrol bomb

EXCLUDES 1   *terrorism involving fire or heat of nuclear weapon (Y38.5)*

√6ᵗʰ **Y38.3X** **Terrorism involving fires, conflagration and hot substances**

√7ᵗʰ **Y38.3X1** **Terrorism involving fires, conflagration and hot substances, public safety official injured**

√7ᵗʰ **Y38.3X2** **Terrorism involving fires, conflagration and hot substances, civilian injured**

√7ᵗʰ **Y38.3X3** **Terrorism involving fires, conflagration and hot substances, terrorist injured**

√5ᵗʰ **Y38.4** **Terrorism involving firearms**

Terrorism involving carbine bullet

Terrorism involving machine gun bullet

Terrorism involving pellets (shotgun)

Terrorism involving pistol bullet

Terrorism involving rifle bullet

Terrorism involving rubber (rifle) bullet

√6ᵗʰ **Y38.4X** **Terrorism involving** firearms

√7ᵗʰ **Y38.4X1** **Terrorism involving firearms, public safety official injured**

√7ᵗʰ **Y38.4X2** **Terrorism involving firearms, civilian injured**

√7ᵗʰ **Y38.4X3** **Terrorism involving firearms, terrorist injured**

√5ᵗʰ **Y38.5** **Terrorism involving nuclear weapons**

Terrorism involving blast effects of nuclear weapon

Terrorism involving exposure to ionizing radiation from nuclear weapon

Terrorism involving fireball effect of nuclear weapon

Terrorism involving heat from nuclear weapon

√6ᵗʰ **Y38.5X** **Terrorism involving** nuclear weapons

√7ᵗʰ **Y38.5X1** **Terrorism involving nuclear weapons, public safety official injured**

√7ᵗʰ **Y38.5X2** **Terrorism involving nuclear weapons, civilian injured**

√7ᵗʰ **Y38.5X3** **Terrorism involving nuclear weapons, terrorist injured**

√5ᵗʰ **Y38.6** **Terrorism involving biological weapons**

Terrorism involving anthrax

Terrorism involving cholera

Terrorism involving smallpox

√6ᵗʰ **Y38.6X** **Terrorism involving** biological weapons

√7ᵗʰ **Y38.6X1** **Terrorism involving biological weapons, public safety official injured**

√7ᵗʰ **Y38.6X2** **Terrorism involving biological weapons, civilian injured**

√7ᵗʰ **Y38.6X3** **Terrorism involving biological weapons, terrorist injured**

√5ᵗʰ **Y38.7** **Terrorism involving chemical weapons**

Terrorism involving gases, fumes, chemicals

Terrorism involving hydrogen cyanide

Terrorism involving phosgene

Terrorism involving sarin

√6ᵗʰ **Y38.7X** **Terrorism involving** chemical weapons

√7ᵗʰ **Y38.7X1** **Terrorism involving chemical weapons, public safety official injured**

√7ᵗʰ **Y38.7X2** **Terrorism involving chemical weapons, civilian injured**

√7ᵗʰ **Y38.7X3** **Terrorism involving chemical weapons, terrorist injured**

√5ᵗʰ **Y38.8** **Terrorism involving other and unspecified means**

√x7ᵗʰ **Y38.80** **Terrorism involving unspecified means**

Terrorism NOS

√6ᵗʰ **Y38.81** **Terrorism involving** suicide bomber

√7ᵗʰ **Y38.811** **Terrorism involving suicide bomber, public safety official injured**

√7ᵗʰ **Y38.812** **Terrorism involving suicide bomber, civilian injured**

√6ᵗʰ **Y38.89** **Terrorism involving** other means

Terrorism involving drowning and submersion

Terrorism involving lasers

Terrorism involving piercing or stabbing instruments

√7ᵗʰ **Y38.891** **Terrorism involving other means, public safety official injured**

√7ᵗʰ **Y38.892** **Terrorism involving other means, civilian injured**

√7ᵗʰ **Y38.893** **Terrorism involving other means, terrorist injured**

√5ᵗʰ **Y38.9** **Terrorism, secondary effects**

NOTE   This code is for use to identify conditions occurring subsequent to a terrorist attack not those that are due to the initial terrorist attack

√6ᵗʰ **Y38.9X** **Terrorism,** secondary effects

√7ᵗʰ **Y38.9X1** **Terrorism, secondary effects, public safety official injured**

√7ᵗʰ **Y38.9X2** **Terrorism, secondary effects, civilian injured**

COMPLICATIONS OF MEDICAL AND SURGICAL CARE (Y62-Y84)

INCLUDES   complications of medical devices

surgical and medical procedures as the cause of abnormal reaction of the patient, or of later complication, without mention of misadventure at the time of the procedure

Misadventures to patients during surgical and medical care (Y62-Y69)

EXCLUDES 1   *surgical and medical procedures as the cause of abnormal reaction of the patient, without mention of misadventure at the time of the procedure (Y83-Y84)*

EXCLUDES 2   *breakdown or malfunctioning of medical device (during procedure) (after implantation) (ongoing use) (Y70-Y82)*

√4ᵗʰ **Y62** **Failure of** sterile precautions **during surgical and medical care**

Y62.0 **Failure of sterile precautions during** surgical operation

Y62.1 **Failure of sterile precautions during** infusion or transfusion

Y62.2 **Failure of sterile precautions during** kidney dialysis and other perfusion   **HCC**

Y62.3 **Failure of sterile precautions during** injection or immunization

Y62.4 **Failure of sterile precautions during** endoscopic examination

Y62.5 **Failure of sterile precautions during** heart catheterization

Y62.6 **Failure of sterile precautions during** aspiration, puncture and other catheterization

Y62.8 **Failure of sterile precautions during** other surgical and medical care

Y62.9 **Failure of sterile precautions during** unspecified surgical and medical care

√4ᵗʰ **Y63** **Failure in** dosage **during surgical and medical care**

EXCLUDES 2   *accidental overdose of drug or wrong drug given in error (T36-T50)*

Y63.0 **Excessive amount of blood or other fluid given during transfusion or infusion**

Y63.1 **Incorrect dilution of fluid used during infusion**

Y63.2 **Overdose of radiation given during therapy**

Y63.3 **Inadvertent exposure of patient to radiation during medical care**

Y63.4 **Failure in dosage in electroshock or insulin-shock therapy**

Y63.5 **Inappropriate temperature in local application and packing**

Y63.6 **Underdosing and nonadministration of necessary drug, medicament or biological substance**

AHA: 2018,4Q,72

Y63.8 **Failure in dosage during other surgical and medical care**

AHA: 2018,4Q,72

Y63.9 **Failure in dosage during unspecified surgical and medical care**

AHA: 2018,4Q,72

√4ᵗʰ **Y64** **Contaminated** medical or biological substances

Y64.0 **Contaminated medical or biological substance,** transfused or infused

Y64.1 **Contaminated medical or biological substance,** injected or used for immunization

Y64.8 **Contaminated medical or biological substance administered by other means**

✅ Additional Char Req   √x7ᵗʰ Placeholder   Unacceptable PDx   Questionable PDx   Wrong Procedure   Manifestation   Unspecified Dx   H1-H14 HAC   HCC CMS-HCC Dx   HIV HIV Dx

ICD-10-CM 2020   1263

Y64.9   **Contaminated medical or biological substance administered by unspecified means**
Administered contaminated medical or biological substance NOS

✓4ᵗʰ **Y65**   **Other misadventures during surgical and medical care**

    Y65.0   **Mismatched blood in transfusion**

    Y65.1   **Wrong fluid used in infusion**

    Y65.2   **Failure in suture or ligature during surgical operation**

    Y65.3   **Endotracheal tube wrongly placed during anesthetic procedure**

    Y65.4   **Failure to introduce or to remove other tube or instrument**

    ✓5ᵗʰ **Y65.5**   **Performance of** wrong procedure (operation)

       Y65.51   **Performance of wrong procedure (operation) on correct patient**
          Wrong device implanted into correct surgical site
          EXCLUDES 1   *performance of correct procedure (operation) on wrong side or body part (Y65.53)*

       Y65.52   **Performance of procedure (operation) on patient not scheduled for surgery**
          Performance of procedure (operation) intended for another patient
          Performance of procedure (operation) on wrong patient

       Y65.53   **Performance of correct procedure (operation) on wrong side or body part**
          Performance of correct procedure (operation) on wrong side
          Performance of correct procedure (operation) on wrong site

    Y65.8   **Other specified misadventures during surgical and medical care**
       AHA: 2019,2Q,23-24

Y66   **Nonadministration of surgical and medical care**
Premature cessation of surgical and medical care
    EXCLUDES 1   *DNR status (Z66)*
               palliative care (Z51.5)

Y69   **Unspecified misadventure during surgical and medical care**

Medical devices associated with adverse incidents in diagnostic and therapeutic use (Y70-Y82)

    INCLUDES   breakdown or malfunction of medical devices (during use) (after implantation) (ongoing use)
    EXCLUDES 2   *later complications following use of medical devices without breakdown or malfunctioning of device (Y83-Y84)*
          misadventure to patients during surgical and medical care, classifiable to (Y62-Y69)
          surgical and other medical procedures as the cause of abnormal reaction of the patient, or of later complication, without mention of misadventure at the time of the procedure (Y83-Y84)

✓4ᵗʰ **Y70**   **Anesthesiology devices associated with adverse incidents**

    Y70.0   **Diagnostic and monitoring anesthesiology devices associated with adverse incidents**

    Y70.1   **Therapeutic (nonsurgical) and rehabilitative anesthesiology devices associated with adverse incidents**

    Y70.2   **Prosthetic and other implants, materials and accessory anesthesiology devices associated with adverse incidents**

    Y70.3   **Surgical instruments, materials and anesthesiology devices (including sutures) associated with adverse incidents**

    Y70.8   **Miscellaneous anesthesiology devices associated with adverse incidents, not elsewhere classified**

✓4ᵗʰ **Y71**   **Cardiovascular devices associated with adverse incidents**

    Y71.0   **Diagnostic and monitoring cardiovascular devices associated with adverse incidents**

    Y71.1   **Therapeutic (nonsurgical) and rehabilitative cardiovascular devices associated with adverse incidents**

    Y71.2   **Prosthetic and other implants, materials and accessory cardiovascular devices associated with adverse incidents**

    Y71.3   **Surgical instruments, materials and cardiovascular devices (including sutures) associated with adverse incidents**

    Y71.8   **Miscellaneous cardiovascular devices associated with adverse incidents, not elsewhere classified**

✓4ᵗʰ **Y72**   **Otorhinolaryngological devices associated with adverse incidents**

    Y72.0   **Diagnostic and monitoring otorhinolaryngological devices associated with adverse incidents**

    Y72.1   **Therapeutic (nonsurgical) and rehabilitative otorhinolaryngological devices associated with adverse incidents**

    Y72.2   **Prosthetic and other implants, materials and accessory otorhinolaryngological devices associated with adverse incidents**

    Y72.3   **Surgical instruments, materials and otorhinolaryngological devices (including sutures) associated with adverse incidents**

    Y72.8   **Miscellaneous otorhinolaryngological devices associated with adverse incidents, not elsewhere classified**

✓4ᵗʰ **Y73**   **Gastroenterology and urology devices associated with adverse incidents**

    Y73.0   **Diagnostic and monitoring gastroenterology and urology devices associated with adverse incidents**

    Y73.1   **Therapeutic (nonsurgical) and rehabilitative gastroenterology and urology devices associated with adverse incidents**

    Y73.2   **Prosthetic and other implants, materials and accessory gastroenterology and urology devices associated with adverse incidents**

    Y73.3   **Surgical instruments, materials and gastroenterology and urology devices (including sutures) associated with adverse incidents**

    Y73.8   **Miscellaneous gastroenterology and urology devices associated with adverse incidents, not elsewhere classified**

✓4ᵗʰ **Y74**   **General hospital and personal-use devices associated with adverse incidents**

    Y74.0   **Diagnostic and monitoring general hospital and personal-use devices associated with adverse incidents**

    Y74.1   **Therapeutic (nonsurgical) and rehabilitative general hospital and personal-use devices associated with adverse incidents**

    Y74.2   **Prosthetic and other implants, materials and accessory general hospital and personal-use devices associated with adverse incidents**

    Y74.3   **Surgical instruments, materials and general hospital and personal-use devices (including sutures) associated with adverse incidents**

    Y74.8   **Miscellaneous general hospital and personal-use devices associated with adverse incidents, not elsewhere classified**

✓4ᵗʰ **Y75**   **Neurological devices associated with adverse incidents**

    Y75.0   **Diagnostic and monitoring neurological devices associated with adverse incidents**

    Y75.1   **Therapeutic (nonsurgical) and rehabilitative neurological devices associated with adverse incidents**

    Y75.2   **Prosthetic and other implants, materials and neurological devices associated with adverse incidents**

    Y75.3   **Surgical instruments, materials and neurological devices (including sutures) associated with adverse incidents**

    Y75.8   **Miscellaneous neurological devices associated with adverse incidents, not elsewhere classified**

✓4ᵗʰ **Y76**   **Obstetric and gynecological devices associated with adverse incidents**

    Y76.0   **Diagnostic and monitoring obstetric and gynecological devices associated with adverse incidents** ♀

    Y76.1   **Therapeutic (nonsurgical) and rehabilitative obstetric and gynecological devices associated with adverse incidents** ♀

    Y76.2   **Prosthetic and other implants, materials and accessory obstetric and gynecological devices associated with adverse incidents** ♀

    Y76.3   **Surgical instruments, materials and obstetric and gynecological devices (including sutures) associated with adverse incidents** ♀

    Y76.8   **Miscellaneous obstetric and gynecological devices associated with adverse incidents, not elsewhere classified** ♀

✓4ᵗʰ **Y77**   **Ophthalmic devices associated with adverse incidents**

    Y77.0   **Diagnostic and monitoring ophthalmic devices associated with adverse incidents**

    Y77.1   **Therapeutic (nonsurgical) and rehabilitative ophthalmic devices associated with adverse incidents**

    Y77.2   **Prosthetic and other implants, materials and accessory ophthalmic devices associated with adverse incidents**

    Y77.3   **Surgical instruments, materials and ophthalmic devices (including sutures) associated with adverse incidents**

    Y77.8   **Miscellaneous ophthalmic devices associated with adverse incidents, not elsewhere classified**

✓4ᵗʰ **Y78**   **Radiological devices associated with adverse incidents**

    Y78.0   **Diagnostic and monitoring radiological devices associated with adverse incidents**

    Y78.1   **Therapeutic (nonsurgical) and rehabilitative radiological devices associated with adverse incidents**

N Newborn: 0   **P** Pediatric: 0-17   **M** Maternity: 9-64   **A** Adult: 15-124   **MCC** Major Complication/Comorbidity   **CC** Complication/Comorbidity   **SW** Severe Wound Dx

1264   ICD-10-CM 2020

Y78.2   Prosthetic and other implants, materials and accessory radiological devices associated with adverse incidents

Y78.3   Surgical instruments, materials and radiological devices (including sutures) associated with adverse incidents

Y78.8   Miscellaneous radiological devices associated with adverse incidents, not elsewhere classified

✓4ᵗʰ **Y79**   **Orthopedic devices associated with adverse incidents**

Y79.Ø   Diagnostic and monitoring orthopedic devices associated with adverse incidents

Y79.1   Therapeutic (nonsurgical) and rehabilitative orthopedic devices associated with adverse incidents

Y79.2   Prosthetic and other implants, materials and accessory orthopedic devices associated with adverse incidents

Y79.3   Surgical instruments, materials and orthopedic devices (including sutures) associated with adverse incidents

Y79.8   Miscellaneous orthopedic devices associated with adverse incidents, not elsewhere classified

✓4ᵗʰ **Y8Ø**   **Physical medicine devices associated with adverse incidents**

Y8Ø.Ø   Diagnostic and monitoring physical medicine devices associated with adverse incidents

Y8Ø.1   Therapeutic (nonsurgical) and rehabilitative physical medicine devices associated with adverse incidents

Y8Ø.2   Prosthetic and other implants, materials and accessory physical medicine devices associated with adverse incidents

Y8Ø.3   Surgical instruments, materials and physical medicine devices (including sutures) associated with adverse incidents

Y8Ø.8   Miscellaneous physical medicine devices associated with adverse incidents, not elsewhere classified

✓4ᵗʰ **Y81**   **General- and plastic-surgery devices associated with adverse incidents**

Y81.Ø   Diagnostic and monitoring general- and plastic-surgery devices associated with adverse incidents

Y81.1   Therapeutic (nonsurgical) and rehabilitative general- and plastic-surgery devices associated with adverse incidents

Y81.2   Prosthetic and other implants, materials and accessory general- and plastic-surgery devices associated with adverse incidents

Y81.3   Surgical instruments, materials and general- and plastic-surgery devices (including sutures) associated with adverse incidents

Y81.8   Miscellaneous general- and plastic-surgery devices associated with adverse incidents, not elsewhere classified

✓4ᵗʰ **Y82**   **Other and unspecified medical devices associated with adverse incidents**

Y82.8   Other medical devices associated with adverse incidents

Y82.9   Unspecified medical devices associated with adverse incidents

Surgical and other medical procedures as the cause of abnormal reaction of the patient, or of later complication, without mention of misadventure at the time of the procedure (Y83-Y84)

EXCLUDES 1   misadventures to patients during surgical and medical care, classifiable to (Y62-Y69)

EXCLUDES 2   breakdown or malfunctioning of medical device (during procedure) (after implantation) (ongoing use) (Y7Ø-Y82)

✓4ᵗʰ **Y83**   **Surgical operation and other surgical procedures as the cause of abnormal reaction of the patient, or of later complication, without mention of misadventure at the time of the procedure**

Y83.Ø   Surgical operation with transplant of whole organ as the cause of abnormal reaction of the patient, or of later complication, without mention of misadventure at the time of the procedure

Y83.1   Surgical operation with implant of artificial internal device as the cause of abnormal reaction of the patient, or of later complication, without mention of misadventure at the time of the procedure

Y83.2   Surgical operation with anastomosis, bypass or graft as the cause of abnormal reaction of the patient, or of later complication, without mention of misadventure at the time of the procedure

Y83.3   Surgical operation with formation of external stoma as the cause of abnormal reaction of the patient, or of later complication, without mention of misadventure at the time of the procedure

Y83.4   Other reconstructive surgery as the cause of abnormal reaction of the patient, or of later complication, without mention of misadventure at the time of the procedure

Y83.5   Amputation of limb(s) as the cause of abnormal reaction of the patient, or of later complication, without mention of misadventure at the time of the procedure

Y83.6   Removal of other organ (partial) (total) as the cause of abnormal reaction of the patient, or of later complication, without mention of misadventure at the time of the procedure

Y83.8   Other surgical procedures as the cause of abnormal reaction of the patient, or of later complication, without mention of misadventure at the time of the procedure

Y83.9   Surgical procedure, unspecified as the cause of abnormal reaction of the patient, or of later complication, without mention of misadventure at the time of the procedure

✓4ᵗʰ **Y84**   **Other medical procedures as the cause of abnormal reaction of the patient, or of later complication, without mention of misadventure at the time of the procedure**

Y84.Ø   Cardiac catheterization as the cause of abnormal reaction of the patient, or of later complication, without mention of misadventure at the time of the procedure

Y84.1   Kidney dialysis as the cause of abnormal reaction of the patient, or of later complication, without mention of misadventure

Y84.2   Radiological procedure and radiotherapy as the cause of abnormal reaction of the patient, or of later complication, without mention of misadventure at the time of the procedure
     AHA: 2019,1Q,21; 2017,1Q,33

Y84.3   Shock therapy as the cause of abnormal reaction of the patient, or of later complication, without mention of misadventure at the time of the procedure

Y84.4   Aspiration of fluid as the cause of abnormal reaction of the patient, or of later complication, without mention of misadventure at the time of the procedure

Y84.5   Insertion of gastric or duodenal sound as the cause of abnormal reaction of the patient, or of later complication, without mention of misadventure at the time of the procedure

Y84.6   Urinary catheterization as the cause of abnormal reaction of the patient, or of later complication, without mention of misadventure at the time of the procedure

Y84.7   Blood-sampling as the cause of abnormal reaction of the patient, or of later complication, without mention of misadventure at the time of the procedure

Y84.8   Other medical procedures as the cause of abnormal reaction of the patient, or of later complication, without mention of misadventure at the time of the procedure
     AHA: 2014,4Q,24

Y84.9   Medical procedure, unspecified as the cause of abnormal reaction of the patient, or of later complication, without mention of misadventure at the time of the procedure

Supplementary factors related to causes of morbidity classified elsewhere (Y9Ø-Y99)

NOTE   These categories may be used to provide supplementary information concerning causes of morbidity. They are not to be used for single-condition coding.

✓4ᵗʰ **Y9Ø**   **Evidence of alcohol involvement determined by blood alcohol level**

Code first any associated alcohol related disorders (F1Ø)

Y9Ø.Ø   Blood alcohol level of less than 2Ø mg/1ØØ ml

Y9Ø.1   Blood alcohol level of 2Ø-39 mg/1ØØ ml

Y9Ø.2   Blood alcohol level of 4Ø-59 mg/1ØØ ml

Y9Ø.3   Blood alcohol level of 6Ø-79 mg/1ØØ ml

Y9Ø.4   Blood alcohol level of 8Ø-99 mg/1ØØ ml

Y9Ø.5   Blood alcohol level of 1ØØ-119 mg/1ØØ ml

Y9Ø.6   Blood alcohol level of 12Ø-199 mg/1ØØ ml

Y9Ø.7   Blood alcohol level of 2ØØ-239 mg/1ØØ ml

Y9Ø.8   Blood alcohol level of 24Ø mg/1ØØ ml or more

Y9Ø.9   Presence of alcohol in blood, level not specified

✓4ᵗʰ **Y92** **Place of occurrence of the external cause**

The following category is for use, when relevant, to identify the place of occurrence of the external cause. Use in conjunction with an activity code.

Place of occurrence should be recorded only at the initial encounter for treatment

✓5ᵗʰ **Y92.0** **Non-institutional (private) residence as the place of occurrence of the external cause**

EXCLUDES 1   *abandoned or derelict house (Y92.89)*

home under construction but not yet occupied (Y92.6-)

institutional place of residence (Y92.1-)

✓6ᵗʰ **Y92.00** **Unspecified non-institutional (private) residence as the place of occurrence of the external cause**

Y92.000 **Kitchen of unspecified non-institutional (private) residence as the place of occurrence of the external cause**

Y92.001 **Dining room of unspecified non-institutional (private) residence as the place of occurrence of the external cause**

Y92.002 **Bathroom of unspecified non-institutional (private) residence single-family (private) house as the place of occurrence of the external cause**

Y92.003 **Bedroom of unspecified non-institutional (private) residence as the place of occurrence of the external cause**

Y92.007 **Garden or yard of unspecified non-institutional (private) residence as the place of occurrence of the external cause**

Y92.008 **Other place in unspecified non-institutional (private) residence as the place of occurrence of the external cause**

Y92.009 **Unspecified place in unspecified non-institutional (private) residence as the place of occurrence of the external cause**

Home (NOS) as the place of occurrence of the external cause

✓6ᵗʰ **Y92.01** **Single-family non-institutional (private) house as the place of occurrence of the external cause**

Farmhouse as the place of occurrence of the external cause

EXCLUDES 1   *barn (Y92.71)*

chicken coop or hen house (Y92.72)

farm field (Y92.73)

orchard (Y92.74)

single family mobile home or trailer (Y92.02-)

slaughter house (Y92.86)

Y92.010 **Kitchen of single-family (private) house as the place of occurrence of the external cause**

Y92.011 **Dining room of single-family (private) house as the place of occurrence of the external cause**

Y92.012 **Bathroom of single-family (private) house as the place of occurrence of the external cause**

Y92.013 **Bedroom of single-family (private) house as the place of occurrence of the external cause**

Y92.014 **Private driveway to single-family (private) house as the place of occurrence of the external cause**

Y92.015 **Private garage of single-family (private) house as the place of occurrence of the external cause**

Y92.016 **Swimming-pool in single-family (private) house or garden as the place of occurrence of the external cause**

Y92.017 **Garden or yard in single-family (private) house as the place of occurrence of the external cause**

Y92.018 **Other place in single-family (private) house as the place of occurrence of the external cause**

Y92.019 **Unspecified place in single-family (private) house as the place of occurrence of the external cause**

✓6ᵗʰ **Y92.02** **Mobile home as the place of occurrence of the external cause**

Y92.020 **Kitchen in mobile home as the place of occurrence of the external cause**

Y92.021 **Dining room in mobile home as the place of occurrence of the external cause**

Y92.022 **Bathroom in mobile home as the place of occurrence of the external cause**

Y92.023 **Bedroom in mobile home as the place of occurrence of the external cause**

Y92.024 **Driveway of mobile home as the place of occurrence of the external cause**

Y92.025 **Garage of mobile home as the place of occurrence of the external cause**

Y92.026 **Swimming-pool of mobile home as the place of occurrence of the external cause**

Y92.027 **Garden or yard of mobile home as the place of occurrence of the external cause**

Y92.028 **Other place in mobile home as the place of occurrence of the external cause**

Y92.029 **Unspecified place in mobile home as the place of occurrence of the external cause**

✓6ᵗʰ **Y92.03** **Apartment as the place of occurrence of the external cause**

Condominium as the place of occurrence of the external cause

Co-op apartment as the place of occurrence of the external cause

Y92.030 **Kitchen in apartment as the place of occurrence of the external cause**

Y92.031 **Bathroom in apartment as the place of occurrence of the external cause**

Y92.032 **Bedroom in apartment as the place of occurrence of the external cause**

Y92.038 **Other place in apartment as the place of occurrence of the external cause**

Y92.039 **Unspecified place in apartment as the place of occurrence of the external cause**

✓6ᵗʰ **Y92.04** **Boarding-house as the place of occurrence of the external cause**

Y92.040 **Kitchen in boarding-house as the place of occurrence of the external cause**

Y92.041 **Bathroom in boarding-house as the place of occurrence of the external cause**

Y92.042 **Bedroom in boarding-house as the place of occurrence of the external cause**

Y92.043 **Driveway of boarding-house as the place of occurrence of the external cause**

Y92.044 **Garage of boarding-house as the place of occurrence of the external cause**

Y92.045 **Swimming-pool of boarding-house as the place of occurrence of the external cause**

Y92.046 **Garden or yard of boarding-house as the place of occurrence of the external cause**

Y92.048 **Other place in boarding-house as the place of occurrence of the external cause**

Y92.049 **Unspecified place in boarding-house as the place of occurrence of the external cause**

✓6ᵗʰ **Y92.09** **Other non-institutional residence as the place of occurrence of the external cause**

AHA: 2017,2Q,10

Y92.090 **Kitchen in other non-institutional residence as the place of occurrence of the external cause**

Y92.091 **Bathroom in other non-institutional residence as the place of occurrence of the external cause**

Y92.092 **Bedroom in other non-institutional residence as the place of occurrence of the external cause**

Y92.093 **Driveway of other non-institutional residence as the place of occurrence of the external cause**

Y92.094 **Garage of other non-institutional residence as the place of occurrence of the external cause**

Y92.095 **Swimming-pool of other non-institutional residence as the place of occurrence of the external cause**

Y92.096 **Garden or yard of other non-institutional residence as the place of occurrence of the external cause**

N Newborn: 0   P Pediatric: 0-17   M Maternity: 9-64   A Adult: 15-124   MCC Major Complication/Comorbidity   CC Complication/Comorbidity   SW Severe Wound Dx

1266   ICD-10-CM 2020

Y92.098 Other place in other non-institutional residence as the place of occurrence of the external cause

Y92.099 Unspecified place in other non-institutional residence as the place of occurrence of the external cause

✓5ᵗʰ **Y92.1** Institutional (nonprivate) residence as the place of occurrence of the external cause

Y92.10 Unspecified residential institution as the place of occurrence of the external cause

✓6ᵗʰ **Y92.11** Children's home and orphanage as the place of occurrence of the external cause

Y92.110 Kitchen in children's home and orphanage as the place of occurrence of the external cause

Y92.111 Bathroom in children's home and orphanage as the place of occurrence of the external cause

Y92.112 Bedroom in children's home and orphanage as the place of occurrence of the external cause

Y92.113 Driveway of children's home and orphanage as the place of occurrence of the external cause

Y92.114 Garage of children's home and orphanage as the place of occurrence of the external cause

Y92.115 Swimming-pool of children's home and orphanage as the place of occurrence of the external cause

Y92.116 Garden or yard of children's home and orphanage as the place of occurrence of the external cause

Y92.118 Other place in children's home and orphanage as the place of occurrence of the external cause

Y92.119 Unspecified place in children's home and orphanage as the place of occurrence of the external cause

✓6ᵗʰ **Y92.12** Nursing home as the place of occurrence of the external cause

Home for the sick as the place of occurrence of the external cause

Hospice as the place of occurrence of the external cause

AHA: 2017,2Q,10

Y92.120 Kitchen in nursing home as the place of occurrence of the external cause

Y92.121 Bathroom in nursing home as the place of occurrence of the external cause

Y92.122 Bedroom in nursing home as the place of occurrence of the external cause

Y92.123 Driveway of nursing home as the place of occurrence of the external cause

Y92.124 Garage of nursing home as the place of occurrence of the external cause

Y92.125 Swimming-pool of nursing home as the place of occurrence of the external cause

Y92.126 Garden or yard of nursing home as the place of occurrence of the external cause

Y92.128 Other place in nursing home as the place of occurrence of the external cause

Y92.129 Unspecified place in nursing home as the place of occurrence of the external cause

✓6ᵗʰ **Y92.13** Military base as the place of occurrence of the external cause

EXCLUDES 1   military training grounds (Y92.84)

Y92.130 Kitchen on military base as the place of occurrence of the external cause

Y92.131 Mess hall on military base as the place of occurrence of the external cause

Y92.133 Barracks on military base as the place of occurrence of the external cause

Y92.135 Garage on military base as the place of occurrence of the external cause

Y92.136 Swimming-pool on military base as the place of occurrence of the external cause

Y92.137 Garden or yard on military base as the place of occurrence of the external cause

Y92.138 Other place on military base as the place of occurrence of the external cause

Y92.139 Unspecified place military base as the place of occurrence of the external cause

✓6ᵗʰ **Y92.14** Prison as the place of occurrence of the external cause

Y92.140 Kitchen in prison as the place of occurrence of the external cause

Y92.141 Dining room in prison as the place of occurrence of the external cause

Y92.142 Bathroom in prison as the place of occurrence of the external cause

Y92.143 Cell of prison as the place of occurrence of the external cause

Y92.146 Swimming-pool of prison as the place of occurrence of the external cause

Y92.147 Courtyard of prison as the place of occurrence of the external cause

Y92.148 Other place in prison as the place of occurrence of the external cause

Y92.149 Unspecified place in prison as the place of occurrence of the external cause

✓6ᵗʰ **Y92.15** Reform school as the place of occurrence of the external cause

Y92.150 Kitchen in reform school as the place of occurrence of the external cause

Y92.151 Dining room in reform school as the place of occurrence of the external cause

Y92.152 Bathroom in reform school as the place of occurrence of the external cause

Y92.153 Bedroom in reform school as the place of occurrence of the external cause

Y92.154 Driveway of reform school as the place of occurrence of the external cause

Y92.155 Garage of reform school as the place of occurrence of the external cause

Y92.156 Swimming-pool of reform school as the place of occurrence of the external cause

Y92.157 Garden or yard of reform school as the place of occurrence of the external cause

Y92.158 Other place in reform school as the place of occurrence of the external cause

Y92.159 Unspecified place in reform school as the place of occurrence of the external cause

✓6ᵗʰ **Y92.16** School dormitory as the place of occurrence of the external cause

EXCLUDES 1   reform school as the place of occurrence of the external cause (Y92.15-)

school buildings and grounds as the place of occurrence of the external cause (Y92.2-)

school sports and athletic areas as the place of occurrence of the external cause (Y92.3-)

Y92.160 Kitchen in school dormitory as the place of occurrence of the external cause

Y92.161 Dining room in school dormitory as the place of occurrence of the external cause

Y92.162 Bathroom in school dormitory as the place of occurrence of the external cause

Y92.163 Bedroom in school dormitory as the place of occurrence of the external cause

Y92.168 Other place in school dormitory as the place of occurrence of the external cause

Y92.169 Unspecified place in school dormitory as the place of occurrence of the external cause

✓6ᵗʰ **Y92.19** Other specified residential institution as the place of occurrence of the external cause

AHA: 2017,2Q,10

Y92.190 Kitchen in other specified residential institution as the place of occurrence of the external cause

Y92.191 Dining room in other specified residential institution as the place of occurrence of the external cause

Y92.192 Bathroom in other specified residential institution as the place of occurrence of the external cause

Y92.193 Bedroom in other specified residential institution as the place of occurrence of the external cause

Y92.194 Driveway of other specified residential institution as the place of occurrence of the external cause

✓ Additional Char Req   ✓x7ᵗʰ Placeholder   Unacceptable PDx   Questionable PDx   Wrong Procedure   Manifestation   Unspecified Dx   H1–H14 HAC   HCC CMS-HCC Dx   HIV HIV Dx

ICD-10-CM 2020   1267

Y92.195 Garage of other specified residential institution as the place of occurrence of the external cause

Y92.196 Pool of other specified residential institution as the place of occurrence of the external cause

Y92.197 Garden or yard of other specified residential institution as the place of occurrence of the external cause

Y92.198 Other place in other specified residential institution as the place of occurrence of the external cause

Y92.199 Unspecified place in other specified residential institution as the place of occurrence of the external cause

✓5ᵗʰ **Y92.2** School, other institution and public administrative area as the place of occurrence of the external cause

Building and adjacent grounds used by the general public or by a particular group of the public

EXCLUDES 1　*building under construction as the place of occurrence of the external cause (Y92.6)*

residential institution as the place of occurrence of the external cause (Y92.1)

school dormitory as the place of occurrence of the external cause (Y92.16-)

sports and athletics area of schools as the place of occurrence of the external cause (Y92.3-)

✓6ᵗʰ **Y92.21** School (private) (public) (state) as the place of occurrence of the external cause

Y92.210 Daycare center as the place of occurrence of the external cause

Y92.211 Elementary school as the place of occurrence of the external cause

Kindergarten as the place of occurrence of the external cause

Y92.212 Middle school as the place of occurrence of the external cause

Y92.213 High school as the place of occurrence of the external cause

AHA: 2012,4Q,108

Y92.214 College as the place of occurrence of the external cause

University as the place of occurrence of the external cause

Y92.215 Trade school as the place of occurrence of the external cause

Y92.218 Other school as the place of occurrence of the external cause

Y92.219 Unspecified school as the place of occurrence of the external cause

Y92.22 Religious institution as the place of occurrence of the external cause

Church as the place of occurrence of the external cause

Mosque as the place of occurrence of the external cause

Synagogue as the place of occurrence of the external cause

✓6ᵗʰ **Y92.23** Hospital as the place of occurrence of the external cause

EXCLUDES 1　*ambulatory (outpatient) health services establishments (Y92.53-)*

home for the sick as the place of occurrence of the external cause (Y92.12-)

hospice as the place of occurrence of the external cause (Y92.12-)

nursing home as the place of occurrence of the external cause (Y92.12-)

Y92.230 Patient room in hospital as the place of occurrence of the external cause

Y92.231 Patient bathroom in hospital as the place of occurrence of the external cause

Y92.232 Corridor of hospital as the place of occurrence of the external cause

Y92.233 Cafeteria of hospital as the place of occurrence of the external cause

Y92.234 Operating room of hospital as the place of occurrence of the external cause

Y92.238 Other place in hospital as the place of occurrence of the external cause

Y92.239 Unspecified place in hospital as the place of occurrence of the external cause

✓6ᵗʰ **Y92.24** Public administrative building as the place of occurrence of the external cause

Y92.240 Courthouse as the place of occurrence of the external cause

Y92.241 Library as the place of occurrence of the external cause

Y92.242 Post office as the place of occurrence of the external cause

Y92.243 City hall as the place of occurrence of the external cause

Y92.248 Other public administrative building as the place of occurrence of the external cause

✓6ᵗʰ **Y92.25** Cultural building as the place of occurrence of the external cause

Y92.250 Art Gallery as the place of occurrence of the external cause

Y92.251 Museum as the place of occurrence of the external cause

Y92.252 Music hall as the place of occurrence of the external cause

Y92.253 Opera house as the place of occurrence of the external cause

Y92.254 Theater (live) as the place of occurrence of the external cause

Y92.258 Other cultural public building as the place of occurrence of the external cause

Y92.26 Movie house or cinema as the place of occurrence of the external cause

Y92.29 Other specified public building as the place of occurrence of the external cause

Assembly hall as the place of occurrence of the external cause

Clubhouse as the place of occurrence of the external cause

✓5ᵗʰ **Y92.3** Sports and athletics area as the place of occurrence of the external cause

✓6ᵗʰ **Y92.31** Athletic court as the place of occurrence of the external cause

EXCLUDES 1　*tennis court in private home or garden (Y92.09)*

Y92.310 Basketball court as the place of occurrence of the external cause

Y92.311 Squash court as the place of occurrence of the external cause

Y92.312 Tennis court as the place of occurrence of the external cause

Y92.318 Other athletic court as the place of occurrence of the external cause

✓6ᵗʰ **Y92.32** Athletic field as the place of occurrence of the external cause

Y92.320 Baseball field as the place of occurrence of the external cause

Y92.321 Football field as the place of occurrence of the external cause

Y92.322 Soccer field as the place of occurrence of the external cause

Y92.328 Other athletic field as the place of occurrence of the external cause

Cricket field as the place of occurrence of the external cause

Hockey field as the place of occurrence of the external cause

✓6ᵗʰ **Y92.33** Skating rink as the place of occurrence of the external cause

Y92.330 Ice skating rink (indoor) (outdoor) as the place of occurrence of the external cause

Y92.331 Roller skating rink as the place of occurrence of the external cause

Y92.34 Swimming pool (public) as the place of occurrence of the external cause

EXCLUDES 1　*swimming pool in private home or garden (Y92.016)*

Ⓝ Newborn: 0　Ⓟ Pediatric: 0-17　Ⓜ Maternity: 9-64　Ⓐ Adult: 15-124　MCC Major Complication/Comorbidity　CC Complication/Comorbidity　SW Severe Wound Dx

1268

ICD-10-CM 2020

Y92.39 **Other specified sports and athletic area as the place of occurrence of the external cause**

Golf-course as the place of occurrence of the external cause

Gymnasium as the place of occurrence of the external cause

Riding-school as the place of occurrence of the external cause

Stadium as the place of occurrence of the external cause

✓5ᵗʰ **Y92.4** **Street, highway and other paved roadways as the place of occurrence of the external cause**

EXCLUDES 1   private driveway of residence (Y92.014, Y92.024, Y92.043, Y92.093, Y92.113, Y92.123, Y92.154, Y92.194)

✓6ᵗʰ **Y92.41** **Street and highway as the place of occurrence of the external cause**

Y92.410 **Unspecified street and highway as the place of occurrence of the external cause**

Road NOS as the place of occurrence of the external cause

Y92.411 **Interstate highway as the place of occurrence of the external cause**

Freeway as the place of occurrence of the external cause

Motorway as the place of occurrence of the external cause

Y92.412 **Parkway as the place of occurrence of the external cause**

Y92.413 **State road as the place of occurrence of the external cause**

Y92.414 **Local residential or business street as the place of occurrence of the external cause**

Y92.415 **Exit ramp or entrance ramp of street or highway as the place of occurrence of the external cause**

✓6ᵗʰ **Y92.48** **Other paved roadways as the place of occurrence of the external cause**

Y92.480 **Sidewalk as the place of occurrence of the external cause**

Y92.481 **Parking lot as the place of occurrence of the external cause**

Y92.482 **Bike path as the place of occurrence of the external cause**

Y92.488 **Other paved roadways as the place of occurrence of the external cause**

✓5ᵗʰ **Y92.5** **Trade and service area as the place of occurrence of the external cause**

EXCLUDES 1   garage in private home (Y92.015)

schools and other public administration buildings (Y92.2-)

✓6ᵗʰ **Y92.51** **Private commercial establishments as the place of occurrence of the external cause**

Y92.510 **Bank as the place of occurrence of the external cause**

Y92.511 **Restaurant or café as the place of occurrence of the external cause**

Y92.512 **Supermarket, store or market as the place of occurrence of the external cause**

Y92.513 **Shop (commercial) as the place of occurrence of the external cause**

✓6ᵗʰ **Y92.52** **Service areas as the place of occurrence of the external cause**

Y92.520 **Airport as the place of occurrence of the external cause**

Y92.521 **Bus station as the place of occurrence of the external cause**

Y92.522 **Railway station as the place of occurrence of the external cause**

Y92.523 **Highway rest stop as the place of occurrence of the external cause**

Y92.524 **Gas station as the place of occurrence of the external cause**

Petroleum station as the place of occurrence of the external cause

Service station as the place of occurrence of the external cause

✓6ᵗʰ **Y92.53** **Ambulatory health services establishments as the place of occurrence of the external cause**

Y92.530 **Ambulatory surgery center as the place of occurrence of the external cause**

Outpatient surgery center, including that connected with a hospital as the place of occurrence of the external cause

Same day surgery center, including that connected with a hospital as the place of occurrence of the external cause

Y92.531 **Health care provider office as the place of occurrence of the external cause**

Physician office as the place of occurrence of the external cause

Y92.532 **Urgent care center as the place of occurrence of the external cause**

Y92.538 **Other ambulatory health services establishments as the place of occurrence of the external cause**

AHA: 2019,1Q,21

Y92.59 **Other trade areas as the place of occurrence of the external cause**

Office building as the place of occurrence of the external cause

Casino as the place of occurrence of the external cause

Garage (commercial) as the place of occurrence of the external cause

Hotel as the place of occurrence of the external cause

Radio or television station as the place of occurrence of the external cause

Shopping mall as the place of occurrence of the external cause

Warehouse as the place of occurrence of the external cause

✓5ᵗʰ **Y92.6** **Industrial and construction area as the place of occurrence of the external cause**

Y92.61 **Building [any] under construction as the place of occurrence of the external cause**

Y92.62 **Dock or shipyard as the place of occurrence of the external cause**

Dockyard as the place of occurrence of the external cause

Dry dock as the place of occurrence of the external cause

Shipyard as the place of occurrence of the external cause

Y92.63 **Factory as the place of occurrence of the external cause**

Factory building as the place of occurrence of the external cause

Factory premises as the place of occurrence of the external cause

Industrial yard as the place of occurrence of the external cause

Y92.64 **Mine or pit as the place of occurrence of the external cause**

Mine as the place of occurrence of the external cause

Y92.65 **Oil rig as the place of occurrence of the external cause**

Pit (coal) (gravel) (sand) as the place of occurrence of the external cause

Y92.69 **Other specified industrial and construction area as the place of occurrence of the external cause**

Gasworks as the place of occurrence of the external cause

Power-station (coal) (nuclear) (oil) as the place of occurrence of the external cause

Tunnel under construction as the place of occurrence of the external cause

Workshop as the place of occurrence of the external cause

✓5ᵗʰ **Y92.7** **Farm as the place of occurrence of the external cause**

Ranch as the place of occurrence of the external cause

EXCLUDES 1   farmhouse and home premises of farm (Y92.01-)

Y92.71 **Barn as the place of occurrence of the external cause**

Chapter 20. External Causes of Morbidity

Y92.72 **Chicken coop** as the place of occurrence of the external cause
> Hen house as the place of occurrence of the external cause

Y92.73 **Farm field** as the place of occurrence of the external cause

Y92.74 **Orchard** as the place of occurrence of the external cause

Y92.79 **Other farm location** as the place of occurrence of the external cause

✓5ᵗʰ **Y92.8** **Other places** as the place of occurrence of the external cause

   ✓6ᵗʰ **Y92.81** **Transport vehicle** as the place of occurrence of the external cause
> EXCLUDES 1   transport accidents (V00-V99)

        Y92.810 **Car** as the place of occurrence of the external cause

        Y92.811 **Bus** as the place of occurrence of the external cause

        Y92.812 **Truck** as the place of occurrence of the external cause

        Y92.813 **Airplane** as the place of occurrence of the external cause

        Y92.814 **Boat** as the place of occurrence of the external cause

        Y92.815 **Train** as the place of occurrence of the external cause

        Y92.816 **Subway car** as the place of occurrence of the external cause

        Y92.818 **Other transport vehicle** as the place of occurrence of the external cause

   ✓6ᵗʰ **Y92.82** **Wilderness area**

        Y92.820 **Desert** as the place of occurrence of the external cause

        Y92.821 **Forest** as the place of occurrence of the external cause

        Y92.828 **Other wilderness area** as the place of occurrence of the external cause
> Swamp as the place of occurrence of the external cause
> Mountain as the place of occurrence of the external cause
> Marsh as the place of occurrence of the external cause
> Prairie as the place of occurrence of the external cause

   ✓6ᵗʰ **Y92.83** **Recreation area** as the place of occurrence of the external cause

        Y92.830 **Public park** as the place of occurrence of the external cause

        Y92.831 **Amusement park** as the place of occurrence of the external cause

        Y92.832 **Beach** as the place of occurrence of the external cause
> Seashore as the place of occurrence of the external cause

        Y92.833 **Campsite** as the place of occurrence of the external cause

        Y92.834 **Zoological garden (Zoo)** as the place of occurrence of the external cause

        Y92.838 **Other recreation area** as the place of occurrence of the external cause

    Y92.84 **Military training ground** as the place of occurrence of the external cause

    Y92.85 **Railroad track** as the place of occurrence of the external cause

    Y92.86 **Slaughter house** as the place of occurrence of the external cause

    Y92.89 **Other specified places** as the place of occurrence of the external cause
> Derelict house as the place of occurrence of the external cause

Y92.9 **Unspecified place or not applicable**

✓4ᵗʰ **Y93** **Activity codes**

> **NOTE**   Category Y93 is provided for use to indicate the activity of the person seeking healthcare for an injury or health condition, such as a heart attack while shoveling snow, which resulted from, or was contributed to, by the activity. These codes are appropriate for use for both acute injuries, such as those from chapter 19, and conditions that are due to the long-term, cumulative effects of an activity, such as those from chapter 13. They are also appropriate for use with external cause codes for cause and intent if identifying the activity provides additional information on the event. These codes should be used in conjunction with codes for external cause status (Y99) and place of occurrence (Y92).

This section contains the following broad activity categories:

Y93.0	Activities involving walking and running
Y93.1	Activities involving water and water craft
Y93.2	Activities involving ice and snow
Y93.3	Activities involving climbing, rappelling, and jumping off
Y93.4	Activities involving dancing and other rhythmic movement
Y93.5	Activities involving other sports and athletics played individually
Y93.6	Activities involving other sports and athletics played as a team or group
Y93.7	Activities involving other specified sports and athletics
Y93.A	Activities involving other cardiorespiratory exercise
Y93.B	Activities involving other muscle strengthening exercises
Y93.C	Activities involving computer technology and electronic devices
Y93.D	Activities involving arts and handcrafts
Y93.E	Activities involving personal hygiene and interior property and clothing maintenance
Y93.F	Activities involving caregiving
Y93.G	Activities involving food preparation, cooking and grilling
Y93.H	Activities involving exterior property and land maintenance, building and construction
Y93.I	Activities involving roller coasters and other types of external motion
Y93.J	Activities involving playing musical instrument
Y93.K	Activities involving animal care
Y93.8	Activities, other specified
Y93.9	Activity, unspecified

✓5ᵗʰ **Y93.0** **Activities involving walking and running**
> EXCLUDES 1   activity, walking an animal (Y93.K1)
>   activity, walking or running on a treadmill (Y93.A1)

    Y93.01 **Activity,** walking, marching and hiking
> Activity, walking, marching and hiking on level or elevated terrain
> EXCLUDES 1   activity, mountain climbing (Y93.31)

    Y93.02 **Activity,** running

✓5ᵗʰ **Y93.1** **Activities involving water and water craft**
> EXCLUDES 1   activities involving ice (Y93.2-)

    Y93.11 **Activity,** swimming

    Y93.12 **Activity,** springboard and platform diving

    Y93.13 **Activity,** water polo

    Y93.14 **Activity,** water aerobics and water exercise

    Y93.15 **Activity,** underwater diving and snorkeling
> Activity, SCUBA diving

    Y93.16 **Activity,** rowing, canoeing, kayaking, rafting and tubing
> Activity, canoeing, kayaking, rafting and tubing in calm and turbulent water

    Y93.17 **Activity,** water skiing and wake boarding

    Y93.18 **Activity,** surfing, windsurfing and boogie boarding
> Activity, water sliding

    Y93.19 **Activity, other involving water and watercraft**
> Activity involving water NOS
> Activity, parasailing
> Activity, water survival training and testing

🅝 Newborn: 0   🅟 Pediatric: 0-17   🅜 Maternity: 9-64   🅐 Adult: 15-124   MCC Major Complication/Comorbidity   CC Complication/Comorbidity   SW Severe Wound Dx

1270   ICD-10-CM 2020

✓5ᵗʰ **Y93.2** **Activities involving ice and snow**
> *EXCLUDES 1*   *activity, shoveling ice and snow (Y93.H1)*

Y93.21 **Activity, ice skating**
Activity, figure skating (singles) (pairs)
Activity, ice dancing
> *EXCLUDES 1*   *activity, ice hockey (Y93.22)*

Y93.22 **Activity, ice hockey**

Y93.23 **Activity, snow (alpine) (downhill) skiing, snowboarding, sledding, tobogganing and snow tubing**
> *EXCLUDES 1*   *activity, cross country skiing (Y93.24)*

Y93.24 **Activity, cross country skiing**
Activity, nordic skiing

Y93.29 **Activity, other involving ice and snow**
Activity involving ice and snow NOS

✓5ᵗʰ **Y93.3** **Activities involving climbing, rappelling and jumping off**
> *EXCLUDES 1*   *activity, hiking on level or elevated terrain (Y93.01)*
> *activity, jumping rope (Y93.56)*
> *activity, trampoline jumping (Y93.44)*

Y93.31 **Activity, mountain climbing, rock climbing and wall climbing**

Y93.32 **Activity, rappelling**

Y93.33 **Activity, BASE jumping**
Activity, Building, Antenna, Span, Earth jumping

Y93.34 **Activity, bungee jumping**

Y93.35 **Activity, hang gliding**

Y93.39 **Activity, other involving climbing, rappelling and jumping off**

✓5ᵗʰ **Y93.4** **Activities involving dancing and other rhythmic movement**
> *EXCLUDES 1*   *activity, martial arts (Y93.75)*

Y93.41 **Activity, dancing**
AHA: 2012,4Q,108

Y93.42 **Activity, yoga**

Y93.43 **Activity, gymnastics**
Activity, rhythmic gymnastics
> *EXCLUDES 1*   *activity, trampolining (Y93.44)*

Y93.44 **Activity, trampolining**

Y93.45 **Activity, cheerleading**

Y93.49 **Activity, other involving dancing and other rhythmic movements**

✓5ᵗʰ **Y93.5** **Activities involving other sports and athletics played individually**
> *EXCLUDES 1*   *activity, dancing (Y93.41)*
> *activity, gymnastic (Y93.43)*
> *activity, trampolining (Y93.44)*
> *activity, yoga (Y93.42)*

Y93.51 **Activity, roller skating (inline) and skateboarding**

Y93.52 **Activity, horseback riding**

Y93.53 **Activity, golf**

Y93.54 **Activity, bowling**

Y93.55 **Activity, bike riding**

Y93.56 **Activity, jumping rope**

Y93.57 **Activity, non-running track and field events**
> *EXCLUDES 1*   *activity, running (any form) (Y93.02)*

Y93.59 **Activity, other involving other sports and athletics played individually**
> *EXCLUDES 1*   *activities involving climbing, rappelling, and jumping (Y93.3-)*
> *activities involving ice and snow (Y93.2-)*
> *activities involving walking and running (Y93.0-)*
> *activities involving water and watercraft (Y93.1-)*

✓5ᵗʰ **Y93.6** **Activities involving other sports and athletics played as a team or group**
> *EXCLUDES 1*   *activity, ice hockey (Y93.22)*
> *activity, water polo (Y93.13)*

Y93.61 **Activity, American tackle football**
Activity, football NOS

Y93.62 **Activity, American flag or touch football**

Y93.63 **Activity, rugby**

Y93.64 **Activity, baseball**
Activity, softball

Y93.65 **Activity, lacrosse and field hockey**

Y93.66 **Activity, soccer**

Y93.67 **Activity, basketball**

Y93.68 **Activity, volleyball (beach) (court)**

Y93.6A **Activity, physical games generally associated with school recess, summer camp and children**
Activity, capture the flag
Activity, dodge ball
Activity, four square
Activity, kickball

Y93.69 **Activity, other involving other sports and athletics played as a team or group**
Activity, cricket

✓5ᵗʰ **Y93.7** **Activities involving other specified sports and athletics**

Y93.71 **Activity, boxing**

Y93.72 **Activity, wrestling**

Y93.73 **Activity, racquet and hand sports**
Activity, handball
Activity, racquetball
Activity, squash
Activity, tennis

Y93.74 **Activity, frisbee**
Activity, ultimate frisbee

Y93.75 **Activity, martial arts**
Activity, combatives

Y93.79 **Activity, other specified sports and athletics**
> *EXCLUDES 1*   *sports and athletics activities specified in categories Y93.0-Y93.6*

✓5ᵗʰ **Y93.A** **Activities involving other cardiorespiratory exercise**
Activities involving physical training

Y93.A1 **Activity, exercise machines primarily for cardiorespiratory conditioning**
Activity, elliptical and stepper machines
Activity, stationary bike
Activity, treadmill

Y93.A2 **Activity, calisthenics**
Activity, jumping jacks
Activity, warm up and cool down

Y93.A3 **Activity, aerobic and step exercise**

Y93.A4 **Activity, circuit training**

Y93.A5 **Activity, obstacle course**
Activity, challenge course
Activity, confidence course

Y93.A6 **Activity, grass drills**
Activity, guerilla drills

Y93.A9 **Activity, other involving cardiorespiratory exercise**
> *EXCLUDES 1*   *activities involving cardiorespiratory exercise specified in categories Y93.0-Y93.7*

✓5ᵗʰ **Y93.B** **Activities involving other muscle strengthening exercises**

Y93.B1 **Activity, exercise machines primarily for muscle strengthening**

Y93.B2 **Activity, push-ups, pull-ups, sit-ups**

Y93.B3 **Activity, free weights**
Activity, barbells
Activity, dumbbells

Y93.B4 **Activity, pilates**

Y93.B9 **Activity, other involving muscle strengthening exercises**
> *EXCLUDES 1*   *activities involving muscle strengthening specified in categories Y93.0-Y93.A*

✓5ᵗʰ **Y93.C** **Activities involving computer technology and electronic devices**
> *EXCLUDES 1*   *activity, electronic musical keyboard or instruments (Y93.J-)*

Y93.C1 **Activity, computer keyboarding**
Activity, electronic game playing using keyboard or other stationary device

Y93.C2 **Activity, hand held interactive electronic device**
Activity, cellular telephone and communication device
Activity, electronic game playing using interactive device
> *EXCLUDES 1*   *activity, electronic game playing using keyboard or other stationary device (Y93.C1)*

Y93.C9 **Activity, other involving computer technology and electronic devices**

✓5ᵗʰ **Y93.D** **Activities involving arts and handcrafts**
> *EXCLUDES 1*   *activities involving playing musical instrument (Y93.J-)*

Y93.D1 **Activity, knitting and crocheting**

Chapter 20. External Causes of Morbidity

Y93.D2   **Activity, sewing**

Y93.D3   **Activity, furniture building and finishing**
     Activity, furniture repair

Y93.D9   **Activity, other involving arts and handcrafts**

✓5ᵗʰ **Y93.E**   **Activities involving personal hygiene and interior property and clothing maintenance**
     EXCLUDES 1   *activities involving cooking and grilling (Y93.G-)*
          activities involving exterior property and land maintenance, building and construction (Y93.H-)
          activities involving caregiving (Y93.F-)
          activity, dishwashing (Y93.G1)
          activity, food preparation (Y93.G1)
          activity, gardening (Y93.H2)

Y93.E1   **Activity, personal bathing and showering**

Y93.E2   **Activity, laundry**

Y93.E3   **Activity, vacuuming**

Y93.E4   **Activity, ironing**

Y93.E5   **Activity, floor mopping and cleaning**

Y93.E6   **Activity, residential relocation**
     Activity, packing up and unpacking involved in moving to a new residence

Y93.E8   **Activity, other personal hygiene**

Y93.E9   **Activity, other interior property and clothing maintenance**

✓5ᵗʰ **Y93.F**   **Activities involving caregiving**
     Activity involving the provider of caregiving

Y93.F1   **Activity, caregiving, bathing**

Y93.F2   **Activity, caregiving, lifting**

Y93.F9   **Activity, other caregiving**

✓5ᵗʰ **Y93.G**   **Activities involving food preparation, cooking and grilling**

Y93.G1   **Activity, food preparation and clean up**
     Activity, dishwashing

Y93.G2   **Activity, grilling and smoking food**

Y93.G3   **Activity, cooking and baking**
     Activity, use of stove, oven and microwave oven

Y93.G9   **Activity, other involving cooking and grilling**

✓5ᵗʰ **Y93.H**   **Activities involving exterior property and land maintenance, building and construction**

Y93.H1   **Activity, digging, shoveling and raking**
     Activity, dirt digging
     Activity, raking leaves
     Activity, snow shoveling

Y93.H2   **Activity, gardening and landscaping**
     Activity, pruning, trimming shrubs, weeding

Y93.H3   **Activity, building and construction**

Y93.H9   **Activity, other involving exterior property and land maintenance, building and construction**

✓5ᵗʰ **Y93.I**   **Activities involving roller coasters and other types of external motion**

Y93.I1   **Activity, rollercoaster riding**

Y93.I9   **Activity, other involving external motion**

✓5ᵗʰ **Y93.J**   **Activities involving playing musical instrument**
     Activity involving playing electric musical instrument

Y93.J1   **Activity, piano playing**
     Activity, musical keyboard (electronic) playing

Y93.J2   **Activity, drum and other percussion instrument playing**

Y93.J3   **Activity, string instrument playing**

Y93.J4   **Activity, winds and brass instrument playing**

✓5ᵗʰ **Y93.K**   **Activities involving animal care**
     EXCLUDES 1   *activity, horseback riding (Y93.52)*

Y93.K1   **Activity, walking an animal**

Y93.K2   **Activity, milking an animal**

Y93.K3   **Activity, grooming and shearing an animal**

Y93.K9   **Activity, other involving animal care**

✓5ᵗʰ **Y93.8**   **Activities, other specified**

Y93.81   **Activity, refereeing a sports activity**

Y93.82   **Activity, spectator at an event**

Y93.83   **Activity, rough housing and horseplay**

Y93.84   **Activity, sleeping**

Y93.85   **Activity, choking game**
     Activity, blackout game
     Activity, fainting game
     Activity, pass out game
     AHA: 2016,4Q,74-76

Y93.89   **Activity, other specified**

Y93.9   **Activity, unspecified**

Y95   **Nosocomial condition**
     AHA: 2013,4Q,119

✓4ᵗʰ **Y99**   **External cause status**
     NOTE   A single code from category Y99 should be used in conjunction with the external cause code(s) assigned to a record to indicate the status of the person at the time the event occurred.

Y99.0   **Civilian activity done for income or pay**
     Civilian activity done for financial or other compensation
     EXCLUDES 1   *military activity (Y99.1)*
          volunteer activity (Y99.2)

Y99.1   **Military activity**
     EXCLUDES 1   *activity of off duty military personnel (Y99.8)*

Y99.2   **Volunteer activity**
     EXCLUDES 1   *activity of child or other family member assisting in compensated work of other family member (Y99.8)*

Y99.8   **Other external cause status**
     Activity NEC
     Activity of child or other family member assisting in compensated work of other family member
     Hobby not done for income
     Leisure activity
     Off-duty activity of military personnel
     Recreation or sport not for income or while a student
     Student activity
     EXCLUDES 1   *civilian activity done for income or compensation (Y99.0)*
          military activity (Y99.1)
     AHA: 2012,4Q,108

Y99.9   **Unspecified external cause status**

Chapter 21. Factors Influencing Health Status and Contact with Health Services (Z00–Z99)

Chapter-specific Guidelines with Coding Examples

The chapter-specific guidelines from the ICD-10-CM Official Guidelines for Coding and Reporting have been provided below. Along with these guidelines are coding examples, contained in the shaded boxes, that have been developed to help illustrate the coding and/or sequencing guidance found in these guidelines.

Note: The chapter-specific guidelines provide additional information about the use of Z codes for specified encounters.

a. Use of Z Codes in any healthcare setting

Z codes are for use in any healthcare setting. Z codes may be used as either a first-listed (principal diagnosis code in the inpatient setting) or secondary code, depending on the circumstances of the encounter. Certain Z codes may only be used as first-listed or principal diagnosis.

Patient with middle lobe lung cancer admitted for initiation of chemotherapy

Z51.11   Encounter for antineoplastic chemotherapy

C34.2   Malignant neoplasm of middle lobe, bronchus or lung

Explanation: A Z code can be used as first-listed in this situation based on guidelines in this chapter as well as chapter 2, "Neoplasms."

b. Z Codes indicate a reason for an encounter

Z codes are not procedure codes. A corresponding procedure code must accompany a Z code to describe any procedure performed.

c. Categories of Z Codes

1) Contact/exposure

Category Z20 indicates contact with, and suspected exposure to, communicable diseases. These codes are for patients who do not show any sign or symptom of a disease but are suspected to have been exposed to it by close personal contact with an infected individual or are in an area where a disease is epidemic.

Category Z77, Other contact with and (suspected) exposures hazardous to health, indicates contact with and suspected exposures hazardous to health.

Contact/exposure codes may be used as a first-listed code to explain an encounter for testing, or, more commonly, as a secondary code to identify a potential risk.

2) Inoculations and vaccinations

Code Z23 is for encounters for inoculations and vaccinations. It indicates that a patient is being seen to receive a prophylactic inoculation against a disease. Procedure codes are required to identify the actual administration of the injection and the type(s) of immunizations given. Code Z23 may be used as a secondary code if the inoculation is given as a routine part of preventive health care, such as a well-baby visit.

3) Status

Status codes indicate that a patient is either a carrier of a disease or has the sequelae or residual of a past disease or condition. This includes such things as the presence of prosthetic or mechanical devices resulting from past treatment. A status code is informative, because the status may affect the course of treatment and its outcome. A status code is distinct from a history code. The history code indicates that the patient no longer has the condition.

A status code should not be used with a diagnosis code from one of the body system chapters, if the diagnosis code includes the information provided by the status code. For example, code Z94.1, Heart transplant status, should not be used with a code from subcategory T86.2, Complications of heart transplant. The status code does not provide additional information. The complication code indicates that the patient is a heart transplant patient.

For encounters for weaning from a mechanical ventilator, assign a code from subcategory J96.1, Chronic respiratory failure, followed by code Z99.11, Dependence on respirator [ventilator] status.

The status Z codes/categories are:

  Z14   Genetic carrier

          Genetic carrier status indicates that a person carries a gene, associated with a particular disease, which may be passed to offspring who may develop that disease. The person does not have the disease and is not at risk of developing the disease.

Z15   Genetic susceptibility to disease

        Genetic susceptibility indicates that a person has a gene that increases the risk of that person developing the disease.

        Codes from category Z15 should not be used as principal or first-listed codes. If the patient has the condition to which he/she is susceptible, and that condition is the reason for the encounter, the code for the current condition should be sequenced first. If the patient is being seen for follow-up after completed treatment for this condition, and the condition no longer exists, a follow-up code should be sequenced first, followed by the appropriate personal history and genetic susceptibility codes. If the purpose of the encounter is genetic counseling associated with procreative management, code Z31.5, Encounter for genetic counseling, should be assigned as the first-listed code, followed by a code from category Z15. Additional codes should be assigned for any applicable family or personal history.

Z16   Resistance to antimicrobial drugs

        This code indicates that a patient has a condition that is resistant to antimicrobial drug treatment. Sequence the infection code first.

Penicillin resistant streptococcus pneumoniae meningitis

G00.1   Pneumococcal meningitis

Z16.11   Resistance to penicillins

Explanation: The status Z code is used to describe the presence of a drug-resistant organism that most likely altered how the meningitis was treated.

Z17   Estrogen receptor status

Z18   Retained foreign body fragments

Z19   Hormone sensitivity malignancy status

Z21   Asymptomatic HIV infection status

        This code indicates that a patient has tested positive for HIV but has manifested no signs or symptoms of the disease.

Z22   Carrier of infectious disease

        Carrier status indicates that a person harbors the specific organisms of a disease without manifest symptoms and is capable of transmitting the infection.

Z28.3   Underimmunization status

Z33.1   Pregnant state, incidental

        This code is a secondary code only for use when the pregnancy is in no way complicating the reason for visit. Otherwise, a code from the obstetric chapter is required.

Z66   Do not resuscitate

        This code may be used when it is documented by the provider that a patient is on do not resuscitate status at any time during the stay.

Z67   Blood type

Z68   Body mass index (BMI)

        BMI codes should only be assigned when **there is an associated, reportable diagnosis (such as obesity).** Do not assign BMI codes during pregnancy.

        See Section I.B.14 for BMI documentation by clinicians other than the patient's provider.

Z74.01 Bed confinement status

Z76.82 Awaiting organ transplant status

Z78   Other specified health status

        Code Z78.1, Physical restraint status, may be used when it is documented by the provider that a patient has been put in restraints during the current encounter. Please note that this code should not be reported when it is documented by the provider that a patient is temporarily restrained during a procedure.

Z79 Long-term (current) drug therapy

Codes from this category indicate a patient's continuous use of a prescribed drug (including such things as aspirin therapy) for the long-term treatment of a condition or for prophylactic use. It is not for use for patients who have addictions to drugs. This subcategory is not for use of medications for detoxification or maintenance programs to prevent withdrawal symptoms in patients with drug dependence (e.g., methadone maintenance for opiate dependence). Assign the appropriate code for the drug dependence instead.

Assign a code from Z79 if the patient is receiving a medication for an extended period as a prophylactic measure (such as for the prevention of deep vein thrombosis) or as treatment of a chronic condition (such as arthritis) or a disease requiring a lengthy course of treatment (such as cancer). Do not assign a code from category Z79 for medication being administered for a brief period of time to treat an acute illness or injury (such as a course of antibiotics to treat acute bronchitis).

Z88 Allergy status to drugs, medicaments and biological substances

Except: Z88.9, Allergy status to unspecified drugs, medicaments and biological substances status

Z89 Acquired absence of limb

Z90 Acquired absence of organs, not elsewhere classified

Z91.0- Allergy status, other than to drugs and biological substances

Z92.82 Status post administration of tPA (rtPA) in a different facility within the last 24 hours prior to admission to a current facility

Assign code Z92.82, Status post administration of tPA (rtPA) in a different facility within the last 24 hours prior to admission to current facility, as a secondary diagnosis when a patient is received by transfer into a facility and documentation indicates they were administered tissue plasminogen activator (tPA) within the last 24 hours prior to admission to the current facility.

This guideline applies even if the patient is still receiving the tPA at the time they are received into the current facility.

The appropriate code for the condition for which the tPA was administered (such as cerebrovascular disease or myocardial infarction) should be assigned first.

Code Z92.82 is only applicable to the receiving facility record and not to the transferring facility record.

Z93 Artificial opening status

Z94 Transplanted organ and tissue status

Z95 Presence of cardiac and vascular implants and grafts

Z96 Presence of other functional implants

Z97 Presence of other devices

Z98 Other postprocedural states

Assign code Z98.85, Transplanted organ removal status, to indicate that a transplanted organ has been previously removed. This code should not be assigned for the encounter in which the transplanted organ is removed. The complication necessitating removal of the transplant organ should be assigned for that encounter.

See section I.C19. for information on the coding of organ transplant complications.

Z99 Dependence on enabling machines and devices, not elsewhere classified

Note: Categories Z89-Z90 and Z93-Z99 are for use only if there are no complications or malfunctions of the organ or tissue replaced, the amputation site or the equipment on which the patient is dependent.

4) **History (of)**

There are two types of history Z codes, personal and family. Personal history codes explain a patient's past medical condition that no longer exists and is not receiving any treatment, but that has the potential for recurrence, and therefore may require continued monitoring.

Family history codes are for use when a patient has a family member(s) who has had a particular disease that causes the patient to be at higher risk of also contracting the disease.

Personal history codes may be used in conjunction with follow-up codes and family history codes may be used in conjunction with screening codes to explain the need for a test or procedure. History codes are also acceptable on any medical record regardless of the reason for visit. A history of an illness, even if no longer present, is important information that may alter the type of treatment ordered.

The history Z code categories are:

Z80 Family history of primary malignant neoplasm

Z81 Family history of mental and behavioral disorders

Z82 Family history of certain disabilities and chronic diseases (leading to disablement)

Z83 Family history of other specific disorders

Z84 Family history of other conditions

Z85 Personal history of malignant neoplasm

Z86 Personal history of certain other diseases

Z87 Personal history of other diseases and conditions

Z91.4- Personal history of psychological trauma, not elsewhere classified

Z91.5 Personal history of self-harm

Z91.81 History of falling

Z91.82 Personal history of military deployment

Z92 Personal history of medical treatment

Except: Z92.0, Personal history of contraception

Except: Z92.82, Status post administration of tPA (rtPA) in a different facility within the last 24 hours prior to admission to a current facility

> Patient has chronic lymphocytic leukemia for which the patient had previous chemotherapy and is now in remission
>
> **C91.11** **Chronic lymphocytic leukemia of B-cell type in remission**
>
> **Z92.21** **Personal history of antineoplastic chemotherapy**
>
> *Explanation:* The personal history Z code is used to describe a secondary (supplementary) diagnosis to identify that this patient has had chemotherapy in the past.

5) **Screening**

Screening is the testing for disease or disease precursors in seemingly well individuals so that early detection and treatment can be provided for those who test positive for the disease (e.g., screening mammogram).

The testing of a person to rule out or confirm a suspected diagnosis because the patient has some sign or symptom is a diagnostic examination, not a screening. In these cases, the sign or symptom is used to explain the reason for the test.

A screening code may be a first-listed code if the reason for the visit is specifically the screening exam. It may also be used as an additional code if the screening is done during an office visit for other health problems. A screening code is not necessary if the screening is inherent to a routine examination, such as a pap smear done during a routine pelvic examination.

Should a condition be discovered during the screening then the code for the condition may be assigned as an additional diagnosis.

The Z code indicates that a screening exam is planned. A procedure code is required to confirm that the screening was performed.

The screening Z codes/categories:

Z11 Encounter for screening for infectious and parasitic diseases

Z12 Encounter for screening for malignant neoplasms

Z13 Encounter for screening for other diseases and disorders

Except: Z13.9, Encounter for screening, unspecified

Z36 Encounter for antenatal screening for mother

6) **Observation**

There are three observation Z code categories. They are for use in very limited circumstances when a person is being observed for a suspected condition that is ruled out. The observation codes are not for use if an injury or illness or any signs or symptoms related to the suspected condition are present. In such cases the diagnosis/symptom code is used with the corresponding external cause code.

The observation codes are to be used as principal diagnosis only. The only exception to this is when the principal diagnosis is required to be a code from category Z38, Liveborn infants according to place of birth and type of delivery. Then a code from category Z05, Encounter for observation and evaluation of newborn for suspected diseases and conditions ruled out, is sequenced after the Z38 code. Additional codes may be used in addition to the observation code but only if they are unrelated to the suspected condition being observed.

Codes from subcategory Z03.7, Encounter for suspected maternal and fetal conditions ruled out, may either be used as a first-listed or as an additional code assignment depending on the case. They are for use in very limited circumstances on a maternal record when an encounter is for a suspected maternal or fetal condition that is ruled out during that encounter (for example, a maternal or fetal condition may be suspected due to an abnormal test result). These codes should not be used when the condition is confirmed. In those cases, the confirmed condition should be coded. In addition, these codes are not for use if an illness or any signs or symptoms related to the suspected condition or problem are present. In such cases the diagnosis/symptom code is used.

Additional codes may be used in addition to the code from subcategory Z03.7, but only if they are unrelated to the suspected condition being evaluated.

Codes from subcategory Z03.7 may not be used for encounters for antenatal screening of mother. *See Section I.C.21. Screening.*

For encounters for suspected fetal condition that are inconclusive following testing and evaluation, assign the appropriate code from category O35, O36, O40 or O41.

The observation Z code categories:

Z03   Encounter for medical observation for suspected diseases and conditions ruled out

Z04   Encounter for examination and observation for other reasons
Except: Z04.9, Encounter for examination and observation for unspecified reason

Z05   Encounter for observation and evaluation of newborn for suspected diseases and conditions ruled out

> Upon initial examination, a heart murmur was heard in a newborn infant delivered vaginally in the hospital; however, after further observation, any serious cardiac conditions were ruled out.
>
> **Z38.00   Single liveborn infant, delivered vaginally**
>
> **Z05.0   Observation and evaluation of newborn for suspected cardiac condition ruled out**
>
> *Explanation:* Normally an observation code is used as the principal diagnosis except when the patient is a newborn. A code from category Z38 Liveborn infants according to place of birth and type of delivery code would be sequenced first, followed by the encounter for observation and evaluation of newborn for suspected diseases and conditions ruled out.

7) Aftercare

Aftercare visit codes cover situations when the initial treatment of a disease has been performed and the patient requires continued care during the healing or recovery phase, or for the long-term consequences of the disease. The aftercare Z code should not be used if treatment is directed at a current, acute disease. The diagnosis code is to be used in these cases. Exceptions to this rule are codes Z51.0, Encounter for antineoplastic radiation therapy, and codes from subcategory Z51.1, Encounter for antineoplastic chemotherapy and immunotherapy. These codes are to be first-listed, followed by the diagnosis code when a patient's encounter is solely to receive radiation therapy, chemotherapy, or immunotherapy for the treatment of a neoplasm. If the reason for the encounter is more than one type of antineoplastic therapy, code Z51.0 and a code from subcategory Z51.1 may be assigned together, in which case one of these codes would be reported as a secondary diagnosis.

The aftercare Z codes should also not be used for aftercare for injuries. For aftercare of an injury, assign the acute injury code with the appropriate 7th character (for subsequent encounter).

The aftercare codes are generally first-listed to explain the specific reason for the encounter. An aftercare code may be used as an additional code when some type of aftercare is provided in addition to the reason for admission and no diagnosis code is applicable. An example of this would be the closure of a colostomy during an encounter for treatment of another condition.

Aftercare codes should be used in conjunction with other aftercare codes or diagnosis codes to provide better detail on the specifics of an aftercare encounter visit, unless otherwise directed by the classification. The sequencing of multiple aftercare codes depends on the circumstances of the encounter.

Certain aftercare Z code categories need a secondary diagnosis code to describe the resolving condition or sequelae. For others, the condition is included in the code title.

Additional Z code aftercare category terms include fitting and adjustment, and attention to artificial openings.

Status Z codes may be used with aftercare Z codes to indicate the nature of the aftercare. For example code Z95.1, Presence of aortocoronary bypass graft, may be used with code Z48.812, Encounter for surgical aftercare following surgery on the circulatory system, to indicate the surgery for which the aftercare is being performed. A status code should not be used when the aftercare code indicates the type of status, such as using Z43.0, Encounter for attention to tracheostomy, with Z93.0, Tracheostomy status.

The aftercare Z category/codes:

Z42   Encounter for plastic and reconstructive surgery following medical procedure or healed injury

Z43   Encounter for attention to artificial openings

Z44   Encounter for fitting and adjustment of external prosthetic device

Z45   Encounter for adjustment and management of implanted device

Z46   Encounter for fitting and adjustment of other devices

Z47   Orthopedic aftercare

Z48   Encounter for other postprocedural aftercare

Z49   Encounter for care involving renal dialysis

Z51   Encounter for other aftercare and medical care

8) Follow-up

The follow-up codes are used to explain continuing surveillance following completed treatment of a disease, condition, or injury. They imply that the condition has been fully treated and no longer exists. They should not be confused with aftercare codes, or injury codes with a 7th character for subsequent encounter, that explain ongoing care of a healing condition or its sequelae. Follow-up codes may be used in conjunction with history codes to provide the full picture of the healed condition and its treatment. The follow-up code is sequenced first, followed by the history code.

A follow-up code may be used to explain multiple visits. Should a condition be found to have recurred on the follow-up visit, then the diagnosis code for the condition should be assigned in place of the follow-up code.

The follow-up Z code categories:

Z08   Encounter for follow-up examination after completed treatment for malignant neoplasm

Z09   Encounter for follow-up examination after completed treatment for conditions other than malignant neoplasm

Z39   Encounter for maternal postpartum care and examination

9) Donor

Codes in category Z52, Donors of organs and tissues, are used for living individuals who are donating blood or other body tissue. These codes are only for individuals donating for others, not for self-donations. They are not used to identify cadaveric donations.

10) Counseling

Counseling Z codes are used when a patient or family member receives assistance in the aftermath of an illness or injury, or when support is required in coping with family or social problems.

The counseling Z codes/categories:

Z30.0-   Encounter for general counseling and advice on contraception

Z31.5   Encounter for procreative genetic counseling

Z31.6-   Encounter for general counseling and advice on procreation

Z32.2   Encounter for childbirth instruction

Z32.3   Encounter for childcare instruction

Z69   Encounter for mental health services for victim and perpetrator of abuse

Z70   Counseling related to sexual attitude, behavior and orientation

Z71   Persons encountering health services for other counseling and medical advice, not elsewhere classified

Note: Code Z71.84, Encounter for health counseling related to travel, is to be used for health risk and safety counseling for future travel purposes.

Z76.81   Expectant mother prebirth pediatrician visit

11) Encounters for obstetrical and reproductive services

See Section I.C.15. Pregnancy, Childbirth, and the Puerperium, for further instruction on the use of these codes.

Z codes for pregnancy are for use in those circumstances when none of the problems or complications included in the codes from the Obstetrics chapter exist (a routine prenatal visit or postpartum care). Codes in category Z34, Encounter for supervision of normal pregnancy, are always first-listed and are not to be used with any other code from the OB chapter.

Codes in category Z3A, Weeks of gestation, may be assigned to provide additional information about the pregnancy. Category Z3A codes should not be assigned for pregnancies with abortive outcomes (categories O00-O08), elective termination of pregnancy (code Z33.2), nor for postpartum conditions, as category Z3A is not applicable to these conditions. The date of the admission should be used to determine weeks of gestation for inpatient admissions that encompass more than one gestational week.

The outcome of delivery, category Z37, should be included on all maternal delivery records. It is always a secondary code. Codes in category Z37 should not be used on the newborn record.

Z codes for family planning (contraceptive) or procreative management and counseling should be included on an obstetric record either during the pregnancy or the postpartum stage, if applicable.

Z codes/categories for obstetrical and reproductive services:

Z30	Encounter for contraceptive management
Z31	Encounter for procreative management
Z32.2	Encounter for childbirth instruction
Z32.3	Encounter for childcare instruction
Z33	Pregnant state
Z34	Encounter for supervision of normal pregnancy
Z36	Encounter for antenatal screening of mother
Z3A	Weeks of gestation
Z37	Outcome of delivery
Z39	Encounter for maternal postpartum care and examination
Z76.81	Expectant mother prebirth pediatrician visit

12) Newborns and infants

See Section I.C.16. Newborn (Perinatal) Guidelines, for further instruction on the use of these codes.

Newborn Z codes/categories:

Z76.1	Encounter for health supervision and care of foundling
Z00.1-	Encounter for routine child health examination
Z38	Liveborn infants according to place of birth and type of delivery

13) Routine and administrative examinations

The Z codes allow for the description of encounters for routine examinations, such as, a general check-up, or, examinations for administrative purposes, such as, a pre-employment physical. The codes are not to be used if the examination is for diagnosis of a suspected condition or for treatment purposes. In such cases the diagnosis code is used. During a routine exam, should a diagnosis or condition be discovered, it should be coded as an additional code. Pre-existing and chronic conditions and history codes may also be included as additional codes as long as the examination is for administrative purposes and not focused on any particular condition.

Some of the codes for routine health examinations distinguish between "with" and "without" abnormal findings. Code assignment depends on the information that is known at the time the encounter is being coded. For example, if no abnormal findings were found during the examination, but the encounter is being coded before test results are back, it is acceptable to assign the code for "without abnormal findings." When assigning a code for "with abnormal findings," additional code(s) should be assigned to identify the specific abnormal finding(s).

Pre-operative examination and pre-procedural laboratory examination Z codes are for use only in those situations when a patient is being cleared for a procedure or surgery and no treatment is given.

The Z codes/categories for routine and administrative examinations:

Z00	Encounter for general examination without complaint, suspected or reported diagnosis
Z01	Encounter for other special examination without complaint, suspected or reported diagnosis
Z02	Encounter for administrative examination
	Except: Z02.9, Encounter for administrative examinations, unspecified
Z32.0-	Encounter for pregnancy test

14) Miscellaneous Z codes

The miscellaneous Z codes capture a number of other health care encounters that do not fall into one of the other categories. Certain of these codes identify the reason for the encounter; others are for use as additional codes that provide useful information on circumstances that may affect a patient's care and treatment.

Prophylactic organ removal

For encounters specifically for prophylactic removal of an organ (such as prophylactic removal of breasts due to a genetic susceptibility to cancer or a family history of cancer), the principal or first-listed code should be a code from category Z40, Encounter for prophylactic surgery, followed by the appropriate codes to identify the associated risk factor (such as genetic susceptibility or family history).

If the patient has a malignancy of one site and is having prophylactic removal at another site to prevent either a new primary malignancy or metastatic disease, a code for the malignancy should also be assigned in addition to a code from subcategory Z40.0, Encounter for prophylactic surgery for risk factors related to malignant neoplasms. A Z40.0 code should not be assigned if the patient is having organ removal for treatment of a malignancy, such as the removal of the testes for the treatment of prostate cancer.

Female patient with cancer in lower inner quadrant of right breast and positive BRCA 1 noted on testing is admitted for mastectomy of right breast and prophylactic removal of left breast

C50.311	**Malignant neoplasm of lower-inner quadrant of right female breast**
Z40.01	**Encounter for prophylactic removal of breast**
Z15.01	**Genetic susceptibility to malignant neoplasm of breast**

Explanation: Removal of the current neoplastic disease in the right breast was the focus of treatment for this admission and is sequenced first. The removal of the left breast was not required to treat a current disease process but as a means of prevention. The two Z codes are informational; they capture the reason behind the removal of what is currently a healthy left breast.

Miscellaneous Z codes/categories:

Z28	Immunization not carried out
	Except: Z28.3, Underimmunization status
Z29	Encounter for other prophylactic measures
Z40	Encounter for prophylactic surgery
Z41	Encounter for procedures for purposes other than remedying health state
	Except: Z41.9, Encounter for procedure for purposes other than remedying health state, unspecified
Z53	Persons encountering health services for specific procedures and treatment, not carried out
Z55	Problems related to education and literacy
Z56	Problems related to employment and unemployment
Z57	Occupational exposure to risk factors
Z58	Problems related to physical environment
Z59	Problems related to housing and economic circumstances
Z60	Problems related to social environment
Z62	Problems related to upbringing
Z63	Other problems related to primary support group, including family circumstances
Z64	Problems related to certain psychosocial circumstances
Z65	Problems related to other psychosocial circumstances
Z72	Problems related to lifestyle
	Note: These codes should be assigned only when the documentation specifies that the patient has an associated problem
Z73	Problems related to life management difficulty
Z74	Problems related to care provider dependency
	Except: Z74.01, Bed confinement status
Z75	Problems related to medical facilities and other health care
Z76.0	Encounter for issue of repeat prescription
Z76.3	Healthy person accompanying sick person
Z76.4	Other boarder to healthcare facility
Z76.5	Malingerer [conscious simulation]
Z91.1-	Patient's noncompliance with medical treatment and regimen
Z91.83	Wandering in diseases classified elsewhere
Z91.84-	Oral health risk factors
Z91.89	Other specified personal risk factors, not elsewhere classified

See Section I.B.14 for Z55-Z65 Persons with potential health hazards related to socioeconomic and psychosocial circumstances, documentation by clinicians other than the patient's provider

15) Nonspecific Z codes

Certain Z codes are so non-specific, or potentially redundant with other codes in the classification, that there can be little justification for their use in the inpatient setting. Their use in the outpatient setting should be limited to those instances when there is no further documentation to permit more precise coding. Otherwise, any sign or symptom or any other reason for visit that is captured in another code should be used.

Nonspecific Z codes/categories:

Z02.9	Encounter for administrative examinations, unspecified
Z04.9	Encounter for examination and observation for unspecified reason
Z13.9	Encounter for screening, unspecified
Z41.9	Encounter for procedure for purposes other than remedying health state, unspecified
Z52.9	Donor of unspecified organ or tissue
Z86.59	Personal history of other mental and behavioral disorders
Z88.9	Allergy status to unspecified drugs, medicaments and biological substances status
Z92.0	Personal history of contraception

16) Z codes that may only be principal/first-listed diagnosis

The following Z codes/categories may only be reported as the principal/first-listed diagnosis, except when there are multiple encounters on the same day and the medical records for the encounters are combined:

Z00	Encounter for general examination without complaint, suspected or reported diagnosis
	Except: Z00.6
Z01	Encounter for other special examination without complaint, suspected or reported diagnosis
Z02	Encounter for administrative examination
Z03	Encounter for medical observation for suspected diseases and conditions ruled out
Z04	Encounter for examination and observation for other reasons
Z33.2	Encounter for elective termination of pregnancy
Z31.81	Encounter for male factor infertility in female patient
Z31.83	Encounter for assisted reproductive fertility procedure cycle
Z31.84	Encounter for fertility preservation procedure
Z34	Encounter for supervision of normal pregnancy
Z39	Encounter for maternal postpartum care and examination
Z38	Liveborn infants according to place of birth and type of delivery
Z40	Encounter for prophylactic surgery
Z42	Encounter for plastic and reconstructive surgery following medical procedure or healed injury
Z51.0	Encounter for antineoplastic radiation therapy
Z51.1-	Encounter for antineoplastic chemotherapy and immunotherapy
Z52	Donors of organs and tissues
	Except: Z52.9, Donor of unspecified organ or tissue
Z76.1	Encounter for health supervision and care of foundling
Z76.2	Encounter for health supervision and care of other healthy infant and child
Z99.12	Encounter for respirator [ventilator] dependence during power failure

Chapter 21. Factors Influencing Health Status and Contact With Health Services (Z00-Z99)

NOTE   Z codes represent reasons for encounters. A corresponding procedure code must accompany a Z code if a procedure is performed. Categories Z00-Z99 are provided for occasions when circumstances other than a disease, injury or external cause classifiable to categories A00-Y89 are recorded as "diagnoses" or "problems." This can arise in two main ways:

(a) When a person who may or may not be sick encounters the health services for some specific purpose, such as to receive limited care or service for a current condition, to donate an organ or tissue, to receive prophylactic vaccination (immunization), or to discuss a problem which is in itself not a disease or injury.

(b) When some circumstance or problem is present which influences the person's health status but is not in itself a current illness or injury.

AHA: 2018,4Q,60-61

This chapter contains the following blocks:

Z00-Z13   Persons encountering health services for examinations
Z14-Z15   Genetic carrier and genetic susceptibility to disease
Z16   Resistance to antimicrobial drugs
Z17   Estrogen receptor status
Z18   Retained foreign body fragments
Z19   Hormone sensitivity malignancy status
Z20-Z29   Persons with potential health hazards related to communicable diseases
Z30-Z39   Persons encountering health services in circumstances related to reproduction
Z40-Z53   Encounters for other specific health care
Z55-Z65   Persons with potential health hazards related to socioeconomic and psychosocial circumstances
Z66   Do not resuscitate status
Z67   Blood type
Z68   Body mass index (BMI)
Z69-Z76   Persons encountering health services in other circumstances
Z77-Z99   Persons with potential health hazards related to family and personal history and certain conditions influencing health status

Persons encountering health services for examinations (Z00-Z13)

NOTE   Nonspecific abnormal findings disclosed at the time of these examinations are classified to categories R70-R94.

EXCLUDES 1   *examinations related to pregnancy and reproduction (Z30-Z36, Z39.-)*

√4ᵗʰ **Z00**   **Encounter for general examination without complaint, suspected or reported diagnosis**

    EXCLUDES 1   *encounter for examination for administrative purposes (Z02.-)*
    EXCLUDES 2   *encounter for pre-procedural examinations (Z01.81-)*
            special screening examinations (Z11-Z13)

    AHA: 2017,4Q,95

√5ᵗʰ **Z00.0**   **Encounter for general adult medical examination**

      Encounter for adult periodic examination (annual) (physical) and any associated laboratory and radiologic examinations

      EXCLUDES 1   *encounter for examination of sign or symptom — code to sign or symptom*
               general health check-up of infant or child (Z00.12.-)

      Z00.00   **Encounter for general adult medical examination without abnormal findings**   [A]
           Encounter for adult health check-up NOS
           AHA: 2016,1Q,36

      Z00.01   **Encounter for general adult medical examination with abnormal findings**   [A]
           Use additional code to identify abnormal findings
           AHA: 2016,1Q,35-36

√5ᵗʰ **Z00.1**   **Encounter for newborn, infant and child health examinations**

    √6ᵗʰ **Z00.11**   **Newborn health examination**

        Health check for child under 29 days old
        Use additional code to identify any abnormal findings
        EXCLUDES 1   *health check for child over 28 days old (Z00.12.-)*

        Z00.110   **Health examination for newborn under 8 days old**   [N]
            Health check for newborn under 8 days old

        Z00.111   **Health examination for newborn 8 to 28 days old**   [N]
            Health check for newborn 8 to 28 days old
            Newborn weight check

√6ᵗʰ **Z00.12**   **Encounter for routine child health examination**

Health check (routine) for child over 28 days old
Immunizations appropriate for age
Routine developmental screening of infant or child
Routine vison and hearing testing

    EXCLUDES 1   *health check for child under 29 days old (Z00.11-)*
                health supervision of foundling or other healthy infant or child (Z76.1-Z76.2)
                newborn health examination (Z00.11-)

AHA: 2018,4Q,36

    Z00.121   **Encounter for routine child health examination with abnormal findings**   [P]
        Use additional code to identify abnormal findings
        AHA: 2016,1Q,34-35

    Z00.129   **Encounter for routine child health examination without abnormal findings**   [P]
        Encounter for routine child health examination NOS
        AHA: 2016,1Q,34

Z00.2   **Encounter for examination for period of rapid growth in childhood**   [P]

Z00.3   **Encounter for examination for adolescent development state**   [P]
    Encounter for puberty development state

Z00.5   **Encounter for examination of potential donor of organ and tissue**

Z00.6   **Encounter for examination for normal comparison and control in clinical research program**
    Examination of participant or control in clinical research program

√5ᵗʰ **Z00.7**   **Encounter for examination for period of delayed growth in childhood**

    Z00.70   **Encounter for examination for period of delayed growth in childhood without abnormal findings**   [P]

    Z00.71   **Encounter for examination for period of delayed growth in childhood with abnormal findings**   [P]
        Use additional code to identify abnormal findings

Z00.8   **Encounter for other general examination**
    Encounter for health examination in population surveys

√4ᵗʰ **Z01**   **Encounter for other special examination without complaint, suspected or reported diagnosis**

    INCLUDES   routine examination of specific system

    NOTE   Codes from category Z01 represent the reason for the encounter. A separate procedure code is required to identify any examinations or procedures performed

    EXCLUDES 1   *encounter for examination for administrative purposes (Z02.-)*
            encounter for examination for suspected conditions, proven not to exist (Z03.-)
            encounter for laboratory and radiologic examinations as a component of general medical examinations (Z00.0-)
            encounter for laboratory, radiologic and imaging examinations for sign(s) and symptom(s) — code to the sign(s) or symptom(s)

    EXCLUDES 2   *screening examinations (Z11-Z13)*

√5ᵗʰ **Z01.0**   **Encounter for examination of eyes and vision**

    EXCLUDES 1   *examination for driving license (Z02.4)*

    Z01.00   **Encounter for examination of eyes and vision without abnormal findings**
        Encounter for examination of eyes and vision NOS

    Z01.01   **Encounter for examination of eyes and vision with abnormal findings**
        Use additional code to identify abnormal findings
        AHA: 2016,4Q,21

Personal status - Z85-Z87 (handwritten)

✓6ᵗʰ Z01.02 Encounter for examination of eyes and vision following failed vision screening
> EXCLUDES 1   examination for examination of eyes and vision with abnormal findings (Z01.01)
> examination for examination of eyes and vision without abnormal findings (Z01.00)

● **Z01.020 Encounter for examination of eyes and vision following failed vision screening without abnormal findings**

● **Z01.021 Encounter for examination of eyes and vision following failed vision screening with abnormal findings**
> Use additional code to identify abnormal findings

✓5ᵗʰ Z01.1 Encounter for examination of ears and hearing

Z01.10 Encounter for examination of ears and hearing without abnormal findings
> Encounter for examination of ears and hearing NOS
> AHA: 2016,4Q,24

✓6ᵗʰ Z01.11 Encounter for examination of ears and hearing with abnormal findings
> AHA: 2016,3Q,17-18

Z01.110 Encounter for hearing examination following failed hearing screening

Z01.118 Encounter for examination of ears and hearing with other abnormal findings
> Use additional code to identify abnormal findings

Z01.12 Encounter for hearing conservation and treatment

✓5ᵗʰ Z01.2 Encounter for dental examination and cleaning

Z01.20 Encounter for dental examination and cleaning without abnormal findings
> Encounter for dental examination and cleaning NOS

Z01.21 Encounter for dental examination and cleaning with abnormal findings
> Use additional code to identify abnormal findings

✓5ᵗʰ Z01.3 Encounter for examination of blood pressure

Z01.30 Encounter for examination of blood pressure without abnormal findings
> Encounter for examination of blood pressure NOS

Z01.31 Encounter for examination of blood pressure with abnormal findings
> Use additional code to identify abnormal findings

✓5ᵗʰ Z01.4 Encounter for gynecological examination
> EXCLUDES 2   pregnancy examination or test (Z32.0-)
> routine examination for contraceptive maintenance (Z30.4-)

✓6ᵗʰ Z01.41 Encounter for routine gynecological examination
> Encounter for general gynecological examination with or without cervical smear
> Encounter for gynecological examination (general) (routine) NOS
> Encounter for pelvic examination (annual) (periodic)
> Use additional code:
>   for screening for human papillomavirus, if applicable, (Z11.51)
>   for screening vaginal pap smear, if applicable (Z12.72)
>   to identify acquired absence of uterus, if applicable (Z90.71-)
> EXCLUDES 1   gynecologic examination status-post hysterectomy for malignant condition (Z08)
> screening cervical pap smear not a part of a routine gynecological examination (Z12.4)

Z01.411 Encounter for gynecological examination (general) (routine) with abnormal findings   ♀
> Use additional code to identify abnormal findings

Z01.419 Encounter for gynecological examination (general) (routine) without abnormal findings   ♀

Z01.42 Encounter for cervical smear to confirm findings of recent normal smear following initial abnormal smear   ♀

✓5ᵗʰ Z01.8 Encounter for other specified special examinations

✓6ᵗʰ Z01.81 Encounter for preprocedural examinations
> Encounter for preoperative examinations
> Encounter for radiological and imaging examinations as part of preprocedural examination

Z01.810 Encounter for preprocedural cardiovascular examination

Z01.811 Encounter for preprocedural respiratory examination

Z01.812 Encounter for preprocedural laboratory examination
> Blood and urine tests prior to treatment or procedure

Z01.818 Encounter for other preprocedural examination
> Encounter for preprocedural examination NOS
> Encounter for examinations prior to antineoplastic chemotherapy

Z01.82 Encounter for allergy testing
> EXCLUDES 1   encounter for antibody response examination (Z01.84)

Z01.83 Encounter for blood typing
> Encounter for Rh typing

Z01.84 Encounter for antibody response examination
> Encounter for immunity status testing
> EXCLUDES 1   encounter for allergy testing (Z01.82)

Z01.89 Encounter for other specified special examinations

✓4ᵗʰ Z02 Encounter for administrative examination

Z02.0 Encounter for examination for admission to educational institution
> Encounter for examination for admission to preschool (education)
> Encounter for examination for re-admission to school following illness or medical treatment

Z02.1 Encounter for pre-employment examination

Z02.2 Encounter for examination for admission to residential institution
> EXCLUDES 1   examination for admission to prison (Z02.89)

Z02.3 Encounter for examination for recruitment to armed forces

Z02.4 Encounter for examination for driving license

Z02.5 Encounter for examination for participation in sport
> EXCLUDES 1   blood-alcohol and blood-drug test (Z02.83)

Z02.6 Encounter for examination for insurance purposes

✓5ᵗʰ Z02.7 Encounter for issue of medical certificate
> EXCLUDES 1   encounter for general medical examination (Z00-Z01, Z02.0-Z02.6, Z02.8-Z02.9)

Z02.71 Encounter for disability determination
> Encounter for issue of medical certificate of incapacity
> Encounter for issue of medical certificate of invalidity

Z02.79 Encounter for issue of other medical certificate

✓5ᵗʰ Z02.8 Encounter for other administrative examinations

Z02.81 Encounter for paternity testing

Z02.82 Encounter for adoption services

Z02.83 Encounter for blood-alcohol and blood-drug test
> Use additional code for findings of alcohol or drugs in blood (R78.-)

Z02.89 Encounter for other administrative examinations
> Encounter for examination for admission to prison
> Encounter for examination for admission to summer camp
> Encounter for immigration examination
> Encounter for naturalization examination
> Encounter for premarital examination
> EXCLUDES 1   health supervision of foundling or other healthy infant or child (Z76.1-Z76.2)

Z02.9 Encounter for administrative examinations, unspecified

✔ Additional Character Required   ✓x7ᵗʰ Placeholder   Unacceptable PDx   Questionable PDx   Manifestation   Unspecified Dx   H1 - H14 HAC   HCC CMS-HCC Dx   HIV HIV Dx

ICD-10-CM 2020   1279

✓4ᵗʰ Z03 Encounter for medical observation for suspected diseases and conditions ruled out

This category is to be used when a person without a diagnosis is suspected of having an abnormal condition, without signs or symptoms, which requires study, but after examination and observation, is ruled out. This category is also for use for administrative and legal observation status.

> **EXCLUDES 1**   *contact with and (suspected) exposures hazardous to health (Z77.-)*
> *encounter for observation and evaluation of newborn for suspected diseases and conditions ruled out (Z05.-)*
> *person with feared complaint in whom no diagnosis is made (Z71.1)*
> *signs or symptoms under study — code to signs or symptoms*

AHA: 2018,2Q,7-8; 2017,4Q,27

Z03.6 Encounter for observation for suspected toxic effect from ingested substance ruled out

Encounter for observation for suspected adverse effect from drug

Encounter for observation for suspected poisoning

✓5ᵗʰ Z03.7 Encounter for suspected maternal and fetal conditions ruled out

Encounter for suspected maternal and fetal conditions not found

> **EXCLUDES 1**   *known or suspected fetal anomalies affecting management of mother, not ruled out (O26.-, O35.-, O36.-, O40.-, O41.-)*

Z03.71 Encounter for suspected problem with amniotic cavity and membrane ruled out   M ♀

Encounter for suspected oligohydramnios ruled out

Encounter for suspected polyhydramnios ruled out

Z03.72 Encounter for suspected placental problem ruled out   M ♀

Z03.73 Encounter for suspected fetal anomaly ruled out   M ♀

Z03.74 Encounter for suspected problem with fetal growth ruled out   M ♀

Z03.75 Encounter for suspected cervical shortening ruled out   M ♀

Z03.79 Encounter for other suspected maternal and fetal conditions ruled out   M ♀

✓5ᵗʰ Z03.8 Encounter for observation for other suspected diseases and conditions ruled out

✓6ᵗʰ Z03.81 Encounter for observation for suspected exposure to biological agents ruled out

Z03.810 Encounter for observation for suspected exposure to anthrax ruled out

Z03.818 Encounter for observation for suspected exposure to other biological agents ruled out

Z03.89 Encounter for observation for other suspected diseases and conditions ruled out

✓4ᵗʰ Z04 Encounter for examination and observation for other reasons

> **INCLUDES**   encounter for examination for medicolegal reasons

This category is to be used when a person without a diagnosis is suspected of having an abnormal condition, without signs or symptoms, which requires study, but after examination and observation, is ruled-out. This category is also for use for administrative and legal observation status.

AHA: 2018,2Q,7-8

Z04.1 Encounter for examination and observation following transport accident

> **EXCLUDES 1**   *encounter for examination and observation following work accident (Z04.2)*

AHA: 2019,2Q,11; 2018,2Q,8

Z04.2 Encounter for examination and observation following work accident

Z04.3 Encounter for examination and observation following other accident

✓5ᵗʰ Z04.4 Encounter for examination and observation following alleged rape

Encounter for examination and observation of victim following alleged rape

Encounter for examination and observation of victim following alleged sexual abuse

Z04.41 Encounter for examination and observation following alleged adult rape   A

Suspected adult rape, ruled out

Suspected adult sexual abuse, ruled out

Z04.42 Encounter for examination and observation following alleged child rape   P

Suspected child rape, ruled out

Suspected child sexual abuse, ruled out

Z04.6 Encounter for general psychiatric examination, requested by authority

✓5ᵗʰ Z04.7 Encounter for examination and observation following alleged physical abuse

Z04.71 Encounter for examination and observation following alleged adult physical abuse   A

Suspected adult physical abuse, ruled out

> **EXCLUDES 1**   *confirmed case of adult physical abuse (T74.-)*
> *encounter for examination and observation following alleged adult sexual abuse (Z04.41)*
> *suspected case of adult physical abuse, not ruled out (T76.-)*

Z04.72 Encounter for examination and observation following alleged child physical abuse   P

Suspected child physical abuse, ruled out

> **EXCLUDES 1**   *confirmed case of child physical abuse (T74.-)*
> *encounter for examination and observation following alleged child sexual abuse (Z04.42)*
> *suspected case of child physical abuse, not ruled out (T76.-)*

✓5ᵗʰ Z04.8 Encounter for examination and observation for other specified reasons

Encounter for examination and observation for request for expert evidence

AHA: 2018,4Q,32,35,72

Z04.81 Encounter for examination and observation of victim following forced sexual exploitation

Z04.82 Encounter for examination and observation of victim following forced labor exploitation

Z04.89 Encounter for examination and observation for other specified reasons

Z04.9 Encounter for examination and observation for unspecified reason

Encounter for observation NOS

✓4ᵗʰ Z05 Encounter for observation and evaluation of newborn for suspected diseases and conditions ruled out

This category is to be used for newborns, within the neonatal period (the first 28 days of life), who are suspected of having an abnormal condition, but without signs or symptoms, and which, after examination and observation, is ruled out.

AHA: 2017,4Q,27; 2016,4Q,77

Z05.0 Observation and evaluation of newborn for suspected cardiac condition ruled out   N

Z05.1 Observation and evaluation of newborn for suspected infectious condition ruled out   N

AHA: 2019,2Q,10

Z05.2 Observation and evaluation of newborn for suspected neurological condition ruled out   N

Z05.3 Observation and evaluation of newborn for suspected respiratory condition ruled out   N

✓5ᵗʰ Z05.4 Observation and evaluation of newborn for suspected genetic, metabolic or immunologic condition ruled out

Z05.41 Observation and evaluation of newborn for suspected genetic condition ruled out   N

AHA: 2016,4Q,55

Z05.42 Observation and evaluation of newborn for suspected metabolic condition ruled out   N

N Newborn: 0   P Pediatric: 0-17   M Maternity: 9-64   A Adult: 15-124   **MCC** Major Complication/Comorbidity   **CC** Complication/Comorbidity   **SW** Severe Wound Dx

1280   ICD-10-CM 2020

Z05.43 Observation and evaluation of newborn for suspected immunologic condition ruled out N

Z05.5 Observation and evaluation of newborn for suspected gastrointestinal condition ruled out N

Z05.6 Observation and evaluation of newborn for suspected genitourinary condition ruled out N

√5ᵗʰ **Z05.7** Observation and evaluation of newborn for suspected skin, subcutaneous, musculoskeletal and connective tissue condition ruled out

  Z05.71 Observation and evaluation of newborn for suspected skin and subcutaneous tissue condition ruled out N

  Z05.72 Observation and evaluation of newborn for suspected musculoskeletal condition ruled out N

  Z05.73 Observation and evaluation of newborn for suspected connective tissue condition ruled out N

Z05.8 Observation and evaluation of newborn for other specified suspected condition ruled out N

Z05.9 Observation and evaluation of newborn for unspecified suspected condition ruled out N

Z08 Encounter for follow-up examination after completed treatment for malignant neoplasm

  Medical surveillance following completed treatment

  Use additional code to identify any acquired absence of organs (Z90.-)

  Use additional code to identify the personal history of malignant neoplasm (Z85.-)

  EXCLUDES 1   *aftercare following medical care (Z43-Z49, Z51)*

Z09 Encounter for follow-up examination after completed treatment for conditions other than malignant neoplasm

  Medical surveillance following completed treatment

  Use additional code to identify any applicable history of disease code (Z86.-. Z87.-)

  EXCLUDES 1   *aftercare following medical care (Z43-Z49, Z51)*

      surveillance of contraception (Z30.4-)

      surveillance of prosthetic and other medical devices (Z44-Z46)

  AHA: 2017,1Q,9; 2015,1Q,8

√4ᵗʰ **Z11** Encounter for screening for infectious and parasitic diseases

  Screening is the testing for disease or disease precursors in asymptomatic individuals so that early detection and treatment can be provided for those who test positive for the disease.

  EXCLUDES 1   *encounter for diagnostic examination — code to sign or symptom*

Z11.0 Encounter for screening for intestinal infectious diseases

Z11.1 Encounter for screening for respiratory tuberculosis

  ▶Encounter for screening for active tuberculosis disease◀

Z11.2 Encounter for screening for other bacterial diseases

Z11.3 Encounter for screening for infections with a predominantly sexual mode of transmission

  EXCLUDES 2   *encounter for screening for human immunodeficiency virus [HIV] (Z11.4)*

      encounter for screening for human papillomavirus (Z11.51)

Z11.4 Encounter for screening for human immunodeficiency virus [HIV]

√5ᵗʰ **Z11.5** Encounter for screening for other viral diseases

  EXCLUDES 2   *encounter for screening for viral intestinal disease (Z11.0)*

  Z11.51 Encounter for screening for human papillomavirus (HPV)

  Z11.59 Encounter for screening for other viral diseases

Z11.6 Encounter for screening for other protozoal diseases and helminthiases

  EXCLUDES 2   *encounter for screening for protozoal intestinal disease (Z11.0)*

Z11.7 Encounter for testing for latent tuberculosis infection

Z11.8 Encounter for screening for other infectious and parasitic diseases

  Encounter for screening for chlamydia

  Encounter for screening for rickettsial

  Encounter for screening for spirochetal

  Encounter for screening for mycoses

Z11.9 Encounter for screening for infectious and parasitic diseases, unspecified

√4ᵗʰ **Z12** Encounter for screening for malignant neoplasms

  Screening is the testing for disease or disease precursors in asymptomatic individuals so that early detection and treatment can be provided for those who test positive for the disease.

  Use additional code to identify any family history of malignant neoplasm (Z80.-)

  EXCLUDES 1   *encounter for diagnostic examination — code to sign or symptom*

Z12.0 Encounter for screening for malignant neoplasm of stomach

√5ᵗʰ **Z12.1** Encounter for screening for malignant neoplasm of intestinal tract

  AHA: 2017,1Q,8,9

  Z12.10 Encounter for screening for malignant neoplasm of intestinal tract, unspecified

  Z12.11 Encounter for screening for malignant neoplasm of colon

    Encounter for screening colonoscopy NOS

    AHA: 2019,1Q,32-33; 2018,1Q,6

  Z12.12 Encounter for screening for malignant neoplasm of rectum

    AHA: 2018,1Q,6

  Z12.13 Encounter for screening for malignant neoplasm of small intestine

Z12.2 Encounter for screening for malignant neoplasm of respiratory organs

√5ᵗʰ **Z12.3** Encounter for screening for malignant neoplasm of breast

  Z12.31 Encounter for screening mammogram for malignant neoplasm of breast

    EXCLUDES 1   *inconclusive mammogram (R92.2)*

    AHA: 2015,1Q,24

  Z12.39 Encounter for other screening for malignant neoplasm of breast

Z12.4 Encounter for screening for malignant neoplasm of cervix ♀

  Encounter for screening pap smear for malignant neoplasm of cervix

  EXCLUDES 1   *when screening is part of general gynecological examination (Z01.4-)*

  EXCLUDES 2   *encounter for screening for human papillomavirus (Z11.51)*

Z12.5 Encounter for screening for malignant neoplasm of prostate ♂

Z12.6 Encounter for screening for malignant neoplasm of bladder

√5ᵗʰ **Z12.7** Encounter for screening for malignant neoplasm of other genitourinary organs

  Z12.71 Encounter for screening for malignant neoplasm of testis ♂

  Z12.72 Encounter for screening for malignant neoplasm of vagina ♀

    Vaginal pap smear status-post hysterectomy for non-malignant condition

    Use additional code to identify acquired absence of uterus (Z90.71-)

    EXCLUDES 1   *vaginal pap smear status-post hysterectomy for malignant conditions (Z08)*

  Z12.73 Encounter for screening for malignant neoplasm of ovary ♀

  Z12.79 Encounter for screening for malignant neoplasm of other genitourinary organs

√5ᵗʰ **Z12.8** Encounter for screening for malignant neoplasm of other sites

  Z12.81 Encounter for screening for malignant neoplasm of oral cavity

  Z12.82 Encounter for screening for malignant neoplasm of nervous system

  Z12.83 Encounter for screening for malignant neoplasm of skin

  Z12.89 Encounter for screening for malignant neoplasm of other sites

Z12.9 Encounter for screening for malignant neoplasm, site unspecified

[handwritten annotations: "1st diagnosis" next to Z08; crossed-out X marks by Z08 and Z09; at bottom: "① screening 1st diagnosis w/ ② condition 2nd diagnosis"]

☑ Additional Character Required √x7ᵗʰ Placeholder Unacceptable PDx Questionable PDx Manifestation Unspecified Dx H1-H14 HAC HCC CMS-HCC Dx HIV HIV Dx

ICD-10-CM 2020   1281

Z05.43–Z12.9

✓4ᵗʰ **Z13 Encounter for screening for other diseases and disorders**

Screening is the testing for disease or disease precursors in asymptomatic individuals so that early detection and treatment can be provided for those who test positive for the disease.

> EXCLUDES 1 — encounter for diagnostic examination — code to sign or symptom

Z13.0 Encounter for screening for diseases of the blood and blood-forming organs and certain disorders involving the immune mechanism

Z13.1 Encounter for screening for diabetes mellitus

✓5ᵗʰ **Z13.2 Encounter for screening for nutritional, metabolic and other endocrine disorders**

Z13.21 Encounter for screening for nutritional disorder

✓6ᵗʰ **Z13.22 Encounter for screening for metabolic disorder**

Z13.220 Encounter for screening for lipoid disorders

Encounter for screening for cholesterol level

Encounter for screening for hypercholesterolemia

Encounter for screening for hyperlipidemia

Z13.228 Encounter for screening for other metabolic disorders

Z13.29 Encounter for screening for other suspected endocrine disorder

> EXCLUDES 1 — encounter for screening for diabetes mellitus (Z13.1)

✓5ᵗʰ **Z13.3 Encounter for screening examination for mental health and behavioral disorders**

AHA: 2018,4Q,35-36

Z13.30 Encounter for screening examination for mental health and behavioral disorders, unspecified

Z13.31 Encounter for screening for depression

Encounter for screening for depression, adult

Encounter for screening for depression for child or adolescent

Z13.32 Encounter for screening for maternal depression ♀

Encounter for screening for perinatal depression

Z13.39 Encounter for screening examination for other mental health and behavioral disorders

Encounter for screening for alcoholism

Encounter for screening for intellectual disabilities

✓5ᵗʰ **Z13.4 Encounter for screening for certain developmental disorders in childhood**

Encounter for development testing of infant or child

Encounter for screening for developmental handicaps in early childhood

> EXCLUDES 2 — encounter for routine child health examination (Z00.12-)

AHA: 2018,4Q,36

Z13.40 Encounter for screening for unspecified developmental delays

Z13.41 Encounter for autism screening

Z13.42 Encounter for screening for global developmental delays (milestones)

Encounter for screening for developmental handicaps in early childhood

Z13.49 Encounter for screening for other developmental delays

Z13.5 Encounter for screening for eye and ear disorders

> EXCLUDES 2 — encounter for general hearing examination (Z01.1-)
> encounter for general vision examination (Z01.0-)

AHA: 2016,3Q,17

Z13.6 Encounter for screening for cardiovascular disorders

✓5ᵗʰ **Z13.7 Encounter for screening for genetic and chromosomal anomalies**

> EXCLUDES 1 — genetic testing for procreative management (Z31.4-)

Z13.71 Encounter for nonprocreative screening for genetic disease carrier status

Z13.79 Encounter for other screening for genetic and chromosomal anomalies

✓5ᵗʰ **Z13.8 Encounter for screening for other specified diseases and disorders**

> EXCLUDES 2 — screening for malignant neoplasms (Z12.-)

✓6ᵗʰ **Z13.81 Encounter for screening for digestive system disorders**

Z13.810 Encounter for screening for upper gastrointestinal disorder

Z13.811 Encounter for screening for lower gastrointestinal disorder

> EXCLUDES 1 — encounter for screening for intestinal infectious disease (Z11.0)

Z13.818 Encounter for screening for other digestive system disorders

✓6ᵗʰ **Z13.82 Encounter for screening for musculoskeletal disorder**

Z13.820 Encounter for screening for osteoporosis

Z13.828 Encounter for screening for other musculoskeletal disorder

Z13.83 Encounter for screening for respiratory disorder NEC

> EXCLUDES 1 — encounter for screening for respiratory tuberculosis (Z11.1)

Z13.84 Encounter for screening for dental disorders

✓6ᵗʰ **Z13.85 Encounter for screening for nervous system disorders**

Z13.850 Encounter for screening for traumatic brain injury

Z13.858 Encounter for screening for other nervous system disorders

Z13.88 Encounter for screening for disorder due to exposure to contaminants

> EXCLUDES 1 — those exposed to contaminants without suspected disorders (Z57.-, Z77.-)

Z13.89 Encounter for screening for other disorder

Encounter for screening for genitourinary disorders

Z13.9 Encounter for screening, unspecified

Genetic carrier and genetic susceptibility to disease (Z14-Z15)

✓4ᵗʰ **Z14 Genetic carrier**

> DEF: Individuals carrying a gene mutation associated with a certain disease that typically do not develop the disease but are able to pass the mutated genes to offspring.

✓5ᵗʰ **Z14.0 Hemophilia A carrier**

Z14.01 Asymptomatic hemophilia A carrier

Z14.02 Symptomatic hemophilia A carrier

Z14.1 Cystic fibrosis carrier

Z14.8 Genetic carrier of other disease

✓4ᵗʰ **Z15 Genetic susceptibility to disease**

> INCLUDES — confirmed abnormal gene

Use additional code, if applicable, for any associated family history of the disease (Z80-Z84)

> EXCLUDES 1 — chromosomal anomalies (Q90-Q99)

✓5ᵗʰ **Z15.0 Genetic susceptibility to malignant neoplasm**

Code first, if applicable, any current malignant neoplasm (C00-C75, C81-C96)

Use additional code, if applicable, for any personal history of malignant neoplasm (Z85.-)

Z15.01 Genetic susceptibility to malignant neoplasm of breast

Z15.02 Genetic susceptibility to malignant neoplasm of ovary ♀

Z15.03 Genetic susceptibility to malignant neoplasm of prostate ♂

Z15.04 Genetic susceptibility to malignant neoplasm of endometrium ♀

Z15.09 Genetic susceptibility to other malignant neoplasm

✓5ᵗʰ **Z15.8 Genetic susceptibility to other disease**

Z15.81 Genetic susceptibility to multiple endocrine neoplasia [MEN]

> EXCLUDES 1 — multiple endocrine neoplasia [MEN] syndromes (E31.2-)

> DEF: Group of conditions in which several endocrine glands grow excessively (such as in adenomatous hyperplasia) and/or develop benign or malignant tumors. Tumors and hyperplasia associated with MEN often produce excess hormones, which impede normal physiology. There is no comprehensive cure known for MEN syndrome. Treatment is directed at the hyperplasia or tumors in each individual gland. Tumors are usually surgically removed and oral medications or hormonal injections are used to correct hormone imbalances.

Z15.89 Genetic susceptibility to other disease

genetic not 1st diagnosis

�N Newborn: 0 | P Pediatric: 0-17 | M Maternity: 9-64 | A Adult: 15-124 | MCC Major Complication/Comorbidity | CC Complication/Comorbidity | SW Severe Wound Dx

Resistance to antimicrobial drugs (Z16)

√4ᵗʰ **Z16 Resistance to antimicrobial drugs**

> **NOTE**   The codes in this category are provided for use as additional codes to identify the resistance and non-responsiveness of a condition to antimicrobial drugs.
>
> Code first the infection
>
> **EXCLUDES 1**   Methicillin resistant Staphylococcus aureus infection (A49.02)
> Methicillin resistant Staphylococcus aureus pneumonia (J15.212)
> sepsis due to Methicillin resistant Staphylococcus aureus (A41.02)

√5ᵗʰ **Z16.1 Resistance to beta lactam antibiotics**

     Z16.10 Resistance to unspecified beta lactam antibiotics

     Z16.11 Resistance to penicillins
       Resistance to amoxicillin
       Resistance to ampicillin

     Z16.12 Extended spectrum beta lactamase (ESBL) resistance   `CC`
       EXCLUDES 2   Methicillin resistant Staphylococcus aureus infection in diseases classified elsewhere (B95.62)

     Z16.19 Resistance to other specified beta lactam antibiotics
       Resistance to cephalosporins

√5ᵗʰ **Z16.2 Resistance to other antibiotics**

     Z16.20 Resistance to unspecified antibiotic
       Resistance to antibiotics NOS

     Z16.21 Resistance to vancomycin   `CC`

     Z16.22 Resistance to vancomycin related antibiotics

     Z16.23 Resistance to quinolones and fluoroquinolones

     Z16.24 Resistance to multiple antibiotics   `CC`

     Z16.29 Resistance to other single specified antibiotic
       Resistance to aminoglycosides
       Resistance to macrolides
       Resistance to sulfonamides
       Resistance to tetracyclines

√5ᵗʰ **Z16.3 Resistance to other antimicrobial drugs**
     EXCLUDES 1   resistance to antibiotics (Z16.1-, Z16.2-)

     Z16.30 Resistance to unspecified antimicrobial drugs
       Drug resistance NOS

     Z16.31 Resistance to antiparasitic drug(s)
       Resistance to quinine and related compounds

     Z16.32 Resistance to antifungal drug(s)

     Z16.33 Resistance to antiviral drug(s)

√6ᵗʰ   **Z16.34 Resistance to antimycobacterial drug(s)**
       Resistance to tuberculostatics

       Z16.341 Resistance to single antimycobacterial drug
         Resistance to antimycobacterial drug NOS

       Z16.342 Resistance to multiple antimycobacterial drugs

     Z16.35 Resistance to multiple antimicrobial drugs
       EXCLUDES 1   resistance to multiple antibiotics only (Z16.24)

     Z16.39 Resistance to other specified antimicrobial drug   `CC`

Estrogen receptor status (Z17)

√4ᵗʰ **Z17 Estrogen receptor status**

> Code first malignant neoplasm of breast (C50.-)
> **DEF:** Receptor status of breast cancer cells for the hormone estrogen that is used to help determine treatment and evaluate prognosis. ER+ breast cancer responds to hormone therapies while ER- breast cancer does not.

     Z17.0 Estrogen receptor positive status [ER+]

     Z17.1 Estrogen receptor negative status [ER-]

Retained foreign body fragments (Z18)

√4ᵗʰ **Z18 Retained foreign body fragments**

> **INCLUDES**   embedded fragment (status)
> embedded splinter (status)
> retained foreign body status
> **EXCLUDES 1**   artificial joint prosthesis status (Z96.6-)
> foreign body accidentally left during a procedure (T81.5-)
> foreign body entering through orifice (T15-T19)
> in situ cardiac device (Z95.-)
> organ or tissue replaced by means other than transplant (Z96.-, Z97.-)
> organ or tissue replaced by transplant (Z94.-)
> personal history of retained foreign body fully removed Z87.821
> superficial foreign body (non-embedded splinter) — code to superficial foreign body, by site
>
> **DEF:** Embedded or retained fragment, splinter, or foreign body, natural or synthetic that can cause infection.

√5ᵗʰ **Z18.0 Retained radioactive fragments**

     Z18.01 Retained depleted uranium fragments

     Z18.09 Other retained radioactive fragments
       Other retained depleted isotope fragments
       Retained nontherapeutic radioactive fragments

√5ᵗʰ **Z18.1 Retained metal fragments**

     EXCLUDES 1   retained radioactive metal fragments (Z18.01-Z18.09)

     Z18.10 Retained metal fragments, unspecified
       Retained metal fragment NOS

     Z18.11 Retained magnetic metal fragments

     Z18.12 Retained nonmagnetic metal fragments

     Z18.2 Retained plastic fragments
       Acrylics fragments
       Diethylhexyl phthalates fragments
       Isocyanate fragments

√5ᵗʰ **Z18.3 Retained organic fragments**

     Z18.31 Retained animal quills or spines

     Z18.32 Retained tooth

     Z18.33 Retained wood fragments

     Z18.39 Other retained organic fragments

√5ᵗʰ **Z18.8 Other specified retained foreign body**

     Z18.81 Retained glass fragments

     Z18.83 Retained stone or crystalline fragments
       Retained concrete or cement fragments

     Z18.89 Other specified retained foreign body fragments

     Z18.9 Retained foreign body fragments, unspecified material

Hormone sensitivity malignancy status (Z19)

√4ᵗʰ **Z19 Hormone sensitivity malignancy status**

> Code first malignant neoplasm — see Table of Neoplasms, by site, malignant
> **AHA:** 2016,4Q,76

     Z19.1 Hormone sensitive malignancy status

     Z19.2 Hormone resistant malignancy status
       Castrate resistant prostate malignancy status

Persons with potential health hazards related to communicable diseases (Z20-Z29)

√4ᵗʰ **Z20 Contact with and (suspected) exposure to communicable diseases**

> **EXCLUDES 1**   carrier of infectious disease (Z22.-)
> diagnosed current infectious or parasitic disease — see Alphabetic Index
> **EXCLUDES 2**   personal history of infectious and parasitic diseases (Z86.1-)

√5ᵗʰ   **Z20.0 Contact with and (suspected) exposure to intestinal infectious diseases**

     Z20.01 Contact with and (suspected) exposure to intestinal infectious diseases due to Escherichia coli (E. coli)

     Z20.09 Contact with and (suspected) exposure to other intestinal infectious diseases

     Z20.1 Contact with and (suspected) exposure to tuberculosis

     Z20.2 Contact with and (suspected) exposure to infections with a predominantly sexual mode of transmission

     Z20.3 Contact with and (suspected) exposure to rabies

     Z20.4 Contact with and (suspected) exposure to rubella

☑ Additional Character Required   √x7ᵗʰ Placeholder   Unacceptable PDx   Questionable PDx   Manifestation   Unspecified Dx   H1-H14 HAC   HCC CMS-HCC Dx   HIV HIV Dx

ICD-10-CM 2020   **1283**

Z20.5 Contact with and (suspected) exposure to **viral hepatitis**

Z20.6 Contact with and (suspected) exposure to **human immunodeficiency virus [HIV]**

> **EXCLUDES 1** asymptomatic human immunodeficiency virus [HIV] HIV infection status (Z21)

Z20.7 Contact with and (suspected) exposure to **pediculosis, acariasis and other infestations**

✓5th **Z20.8** Contact with and (suspected) exposure to other **communicable diseases**

  ✓6th **Z20.81** Contact with and (suspected) exposure to other **bacterial communicable diseases**

    Z20.810 Contact with and (suspected) exposure to **anthrax**

    Z20.811 Contact with and (suspected) exposure to **meningococcus**

    Z20.818 Contact with and (suspected) exposure to other bacterial communicable diseases

      AHA: 2019,2Q,10

  ✓6th **Z20.82** Contact with and (suspected) exposure to other **viral communicable diseases**

    Z20.820 Contact with and (suspected) exposure to **varicella**

    Z20.821 Contact with and (suspected) exposure to **Zika virus**

      AHA: 2018,4Q,35,64

    Z20.828 Contact with and (suspected) exposure to other viral communicable diseases

  Z20.89 Contact with and (suspected) exposure to other **communicable diseases**

Z20.9 Contact with and (suspected) exposure to unspecified **communicable disease**

Z21 Asymptomatic human immunodeficiency virus [HIV] infection status   HCC

  HIV positive NOS

  Code first human immunodeficiency virus [HIV] disease complicating pregnancy, childbirth and the puerperium, if applicable (O98.7-)

> **EXCLUDES 1** acquired immunodeficiency syndrome (B20)
> contact with human immunodeficiency virus [HIV] (Z20.6)
> exposure to human immunodeficiency virus [HIV] (Z20.6)
> human immunodeficiency virus [HIV] disease (B20)
> inconclusive laboratory evidence of human immunodeficiency virus [HIV] (R75)

  AHA: 2019,1Q,8-11

  DEF: Phase of human immunodeficiency virus (HIV) infection with no clinical symptoms. This phase may last for 10 years or more.

✓4th **Z22** Carrier of infectious disease

> **INCLUDES** colonization status
> suspected carrier
> **EXCLUDES 2** carrier of viral hepatitis (B18.-)

Z22.0 Carrier of **typhoid**

Z22.1 Carrier of other intestinal infectious diseases

Z22.2 Carrier of **diphtheria**

✓5th **Z22.3** Carrier of other specified bacterial diseases

  Z22.31 Carrier of bacterial disease due to **meningococci**

  ✓6th **Z22.32** Carrier of bacterial disease due to **staphylococci**

    Z22.321 Carrier or suspected carrier of **Methicillin susceptible** Staphylococcus aureus

      MSSA colonization

    Z22.322 Carrier or suspected carrier of **Methicillin resistant** Staphylococcus aureus

      MRSA colonization

      DEF: Carriers (colonization) of methicillin resistant Staphylococcus aureus (MRSA) have MRSA on their skin or in their body but do not exhibit signs of infection. These individuals are able to pass MRSA on to others who may develop an infection.

  ✓6th **Z22.33** Carrier of bacterial disease due to **streptococci**

    Z22.330 Carrier of **Group B** streptococcus

>   **EXCLUDES 1** carrier of streptococcus group B (GBS) complicating pregnancy, childbirth and the puerperium (O99.82-)

    Z22.338 Carrier of other streptococcus

  Z22.39 Carrier of other specified bacterial diseases

Z22.4 Carrier of **infections with a predominantly sexual mode of transmission**

Z22.6 Carrier of **human T-lymphotropic virus type-1 [HTLV-1] infection**

● **Z22.7** Latent tuberculosis

  Latent tuberculosis infection (LTBI)

> **EXCLUDES 1** nonspecific reaction to cell mediated immunity measurement of gamma interferon antigen response without active tuberculosis (R76.12)
> nonspecific reaction to tuberculin skin test without active tuberculosis (R76.11)

Z22.8 Carrier of other infectious diseases

Z22.9 Carrier of infectious disease, unspecified

Z23 Encounter for immunization

  Code first any routine childhood examination

> **NOTE** Procedure codes are required to identify the types of immunizations given

✓4th **Z28** Immunization not carried out and underimmunization status

> **INCLUDES** vaccination not carried out

✓5th **Z28.0** Immunization not carried out because of **contraindication**

  DEF: Contraindication: Situation where a drug, surgery, or other procedure may negatively affect or cause harm to a patient.

  Z28.01 Immunization not carried out because of **acute illness** of patient

  Z28.02 Immunization not carried out because of **chronic illness or condition** of patient

  Z28.03 Immunization not carried out because of **immune compromised state** of patient

  Z28.04 Immunization not carried out because of patient **allergy to vaccine or component**

  Z28.09 Immunization not carried out because of other contraindication

Z28.1 Immunization not carried out because of patient decision for **reasons of belief or group pressure**

  Immunization not carried out because of religious belief

✓5th **Z28.2** Immunization not carried out because of patient decision for **other and unspecified** reason

  Z28.20 Immunization not carried out because of patient decision for unspecified reason

  Z28.21 Immunization not carried out because of patient refusal

  Z28.29 Immunization not carried out because of patient decision for other reason

Z28.3 Underimmunization status

  Delinquent immunization status

  Lapsed immunization schedule status

✓5th **Z28.8** Immunization not carried out for other reason

  Z28.81 Immunization not carried out due to **patient having had the disease**

  Z28.82 Immunization not carried out because of **caregiver refusal**

    Immunization not carried out because of guardian refusal

    Immunization not carried out because of parent refusal

>   **EXCLUDES 1** immunization not carried out because of caregiver refusal because of religious belief (Z28.1)

  Z28.83 Immunization not carried out due to **unavailability of vaccine**

    Delay in delivery of vaccine

    Lack of availability of vaccine

    Manufacturer delay of vaccine

    AHA: 2018,4Q,36

  Z28.89 Immunization not carried out for other reason

Z28.9 Immunization not carried out for unspecified reason

✓4th **Z29** Encounter for other prophylactic measures

> **EXCLUDES 1** desensitization to allergens (Z51.6)
> prophylactic surgery (Z40.-)

  AHA: 2016,4Q,78-79

✓5th **Z29.1** Encounter for prophylactic immunotherapy

  Encounter for administration of immunoglobulin

  Z29.11 Encounter for prophylactic immunotherapy for respiratory syncytial virus (RSV)

  Z29.12 Encounter for prophylactic **antivenin**

  Z29.13 Encounter for prophylactic **Rho(D) immune globulin**

  Z29.14 Encounter for prophylactic **rabies immune globin**

Z29.3 Encounter for prophylactic **fluoride administration**

Z29.8 Encounter for other specified prophylactic measures

Z29.9 Encounter for prophylactic measures, unspecified

N Newborn: 0   P Pediatric: 0-17   M Maternity: 9-64   A Adult: 15-124   **MCC** Major Complication/Comorbidity   **CC** Complication/Comorbidity   **SW** Severe Wound Dx

Persons encountering health services in circumstances related to reproduction (Z30-Z39)

✓4ᵗʰ Z30 Encounter for contraceptive management

AHA: 2016,4Q,78

DEF: Contraceptive management to prevent pregnancy. Methods include oral medications, intrauterine devices, and surgical procedures for males and females (sterilization).

✓5ᵗʰ Z30.0 Encounter for general counseling and advice on contraception

  ✓6ᵗʰ Z30.01 Encounter for initial prescription of contraceptives

    EXCLUDES 1   *encounter for surveillance of contraceptives (Z30.4-)*

    Z30.011 Encounter for initial prescription of contraceptive pills ♀

    Z30.012 Encounter for prescription of emergency contraception ♀

      Encounter for postcoital contraception

    Z30.013 Encounter for initial prescription of injectable contraceptive ♀

    Z30.014 Encounter for initial prescription of intrauterine contraceptive device ♀

      EXCLUDES 1   *encounter for insertion of intrauterine contraceptive device (Z30.430, Z30.432)*

    Z30.015 Encounter for initial prescription of vaginal ring hormonal contraceptive ♀

    Z30.016 Encounter for initial prescription of transdermal patch hormonal contraceptive device

    Z30.017 Encounter for initial prescription of implantable subdermal contraceptive

    Z30.018 Encounter for initial prescription of other contraceptives ♀

      Encounter for initial prescription of barrier contraception

      Encounter for initial prescription of diaphragm

    Z30.019 Encounter for initial prescription of contraceptives, unspecified ♀

  Z30.02 Counseling and instruction in natural family planning to avoid pregnancy

  Z30.09 Encounter for other general counseling and advice on contraception

    Encounter for family planning advice NOS

Z30.2 Encounter for sterilization

✓5ᵗʰ Z30.4 Encounter for surveillance of contraceptives

  Z30.40 Encounter for surveillance of contraceptives, unspecified

  Z30.41 Encounter for surveillance of contraceptive pills ♀

    Encounter for repeat prescription for contraceptive pill

  Z30.42 Encounter for surveillance of injectable contraceptive ♀

  ✓6ᵗʰ Z30.43 Encounter for surveillance of intrauterine contraceptive device

    Z30.430 Encounter for insertion of intrauterine contraceptive device ♀

    Z30.431 Encounter for routine checking of intrauterine contraceptive device ♀

    Z30.432 Encounter for removal of intrauterine contraceptive device ♀

    Z30.433 Encounter for removal and reinsertion of intrauterine contraceptive device ♀

      Encounter for replacement of intrauterine contraceptive device

  Z30.44 Encounter for surveillance of vaginal ring hormonal contraceptive device ♀

  Z30.45 Encounter for surveillance of transdermal patch hormonal contraceptive device ♀

  Z30.46 Encounter for surveillance of implantable subdermal contraceptive ♀

    Encounter for checking, reinsertion or removal of implantable subdermal contraceptive

  Z30.49 Encounter for surveillance of other contraceptives ♀

    Encounter for surveillance of barrier contraception

    Encounter for surveillance of diaphragm

Z30.8 Encounter for other contraceptive management

  Encounter for postvasectomy sperm count

  Encounter for routine examination for contraceptive maintenance

  EXCLUDES 1   *sperm count following sterilization reversal (Z31.42)*

           sperm count for fertility testing (Z31.41)

Z30.9 Encounter for contraceptive management, unspecified

✓4ᵗʰ Z31 Encounter for procreative management

EXCLUDES 1   *complications associated with artificial fertilization (N98.-)*

           female infertility (N97.-)

           male infertility (N46.-)

Z31.0 Encounter for reversal of previous sterilization

✓5ᵗʰ Z31.4 Encounter for procreative investigation and testing

  EXCLUDES 1   *postvasectomy sperm count (Z30.8)*

  Z31.41 Encounter for fertility testing

    Encounter for fallopian tube patency testing

    Encounter for sperm count for fertility testing

  Z31.42 Aftercare following sterilization reversal

    Sperm count following sterilization reversal

  ✓6ᵗʰ Z31.43 Encounter for genetic testing of female for procreative management

    Use additional code for recurrent pregnancy loss, if applicable (N96, O26.2-)

    EXCLUDES 1   *nonprocreative genetic testing (Z13.7-)*

    Z31.430 Encounter of female for testing for genetic disease carrier status for procreative management ♀

    Z31.438 Encounter for other genetic testing of female for procreative management ♀

  ✓6ᵗʰ Z31.44 Encounter for genetic testing of male for procreative management

    EXCLUDES 1   *nonprocreative genetic testing (Z13.7-)*

    Z31.440 Encounter of male for testing for genetic disease carrier status for procreative management ♂

    Z31.441 Encounter for testing of male partner of patient with recurrent pregnancy loss A ♂

    Z31.448 Encounter for other genetic testing of male for procreative management A ♂

  Z31.49 Encounter for other procreative investigation and testing

Z31.5 Encounter for procreative genetic counseling

  AHA: 2017,4Q,27

✓5ᵗʰ Z31.6 Encounter for general counseling and advice on procreation

  Z31.61 Procreative counseling and advice using natural family planning

  Z31.62 Encounter for fertility preservation counseling

    Encounter for fertility preservation counseling prior to cancer therapy

    Encounter for fertility preservation counseling prior to surgical removal of gonads

  Z31.69 Encounter for other general counseling and advice on procreation

Z31.7 Encounter for procreative management and counseling for gestational carrier ♀

  EXCLUDES 1   *pregnant state, gestational carrier (Z33.3)*

  AHA: 2016,4Q,78

✓5ᵗʰ Z31.8 Encounter for other procreative management

  Z31.81 Encounter for male factor infertility in female patient ♀

  Z31.82 Encounter for Rh incompatibility status ♀

    AHA: 2015,3Q,40; 2014,4Q,17

✓ Additional Character Required   ✓x7ᵗʰ Placeholder   Unacceptable PDx   Questionable PDx   Manifestation   Unspecified Dx   H1-H14 HAC   HCC CMS-HCC Dx   HIV HIV Dx

ICD-10-CM 2020   1285

Chapter 21. Factors Influencing Health Status and Contact With Health Services

Z30–Z31.82

Z31.83   **Encounter for assisted reproductive fertility procedure cycle** ♀
Patient undergoing in vitro fertilization cycle
Use additional code to identify the type of infertility
EXCLUDES 1   *pre-cycle diagnosis and testing — code to reason for encounter*

Z31.84   **Encounter for fertility preservation procedure**
Encounter for fertility preservation procedure prior to cancer therapy
Encounter for fertility preservation procedure prior to surgical removal of gonads

Z31.89   **Encounter for other procreative management**

Z31.9   **Encounter for procreative management, unspecified**

✓4ᵗʰ **Z32**   **Encounter for pregnancy test and childbirth and childcare instruction**

  ✓5ᵗʰ **Z32.0**   **Encounter for pregnancy test**

    Z32.00   **Encounter for pregnancy test, result unknown** ♀
Encounter for pregnancy test NOS

    Z32.01   **Encounter for pregnancy test, result positive** M ♀

    Z32.02   **Encounter for pregnancy test, result negative** ♀

  Z32.2   **Encounter for childbirth instruction**

  Z32.3   **Encounter for childcare instruction**
Encounter for prenatal or postpartum childcare instruction

✓4ᵗʰ **Z33**   **Pregnant state**

  Z33.1   **Pregnant state, incidental** M ♀
Pregnant state NOS
EXCLUDES 1   *complications of pregnancy (O00–O9A)*
pregnant state, gestational carrier (Z33.3)

  Z33.2   **Encounter for elective termination of pregnancy** M ♀
EXCLUDES 1   *early fetal death with retention of dead fetus (O02.1)*
late fetal death (O36.4)
spontaneous abortion (O03)
TIP: Do not assign a code from category Z3A with this code.

  Z33.3   **Pregnant state, gestational carrier** M ♀
EXCLUDES 1   *encounter for procreative management and counseling for gestational carrier (Z31.7)*
AHA: 2016,4Q,78

✓4ᵗʰ **Z34**   **Encounter for supervision of normal pregnancy**
EXCLUDES 1   *any complication of pregnancy (O00–O9A)*
encounter for pregnancy test (Z32.0-)
encounter for supervision of high risk pregnancy (O09.-)
AHA: 2014,4Q,17

  ✓5ᵗʰ **Z34.0**   **Encounter for supervision of normal first pregnancy**

    Z34.00   **Encounter for supervision of normal first pregnancy, unspecified trimester** M ♀

    Z34.01   **Encounter for supervision of normal first pregnancy, first trimester** M ♀

    Z34.02   **Encounter for supervision of normal first pregnancy, second trimester** M ♀

    Z34.03   **Encounter for supervision of normal first pregnancy, third trimester** M ♀

  ✓5ᵗʰ **Z34.8**   **Encounter for supervision of other normal pregnancy**

    Z34.80   **Encounter for supervision of other normal pregnancy, unspecified trimester** M ♀

    Z34.81   **Encounter for supervision of other normal pregnancy, first trimester** M ♀

    Z34.82   **Encounter for supervision of other normal pregnancy, second trimester** M ♀

    Z34.83   **Encounter for supervision of other normal pregnancy, third trimester** M ♀

  ✓5ᵗʰ **Z34.9**   **Encounter for supervision of normal pregnancy, unspecified**

    Z34.90   **Encounter for supervision of normal pregnancy, unspecified, unspecified trimester** M ♀

    Z34.91   **Encounter for supervision of normal pregnancy, unspecified, first trimester** M ♀

    Z34.92   **Encounter for supervision of normal pregnancy, unspecified, second trimester** M ♀

    Z34.93   **Encounter for supervision of normal pregnancy, unspecified, third trimester** M ♀

✓4ᵗʰ **Z36**   **Encounter for antenatal screening of mother**
INCLUDES   encounter for placental sample (taken vaginally)
screening is the testing for disease or disease precursors in asymptomatic individuals so that early detection and treatment can be provided for those who test positive for the disease.
EXCLUDES 1   *diagnostic examination — code to sign or symptom*
encounter for suspected maternal and fetal conditions ruled out (Z03.7-)
suspected fetal condition affecting management of pregnancy — code to condition in Chapter 15
EXCLUDES 2   *abnormal findings on antenatal screening of mother (O28.-)*
genetic counseling and testing (Z31.43-, Z31.5)
routine prenatal care (Z34)
AHA: 2017,4Q,28

  Z36.0   **Encounter for antenatal screening for chromosomal anomalies** M ♀

  Z36.1   **Encounter for antenatal screening for raised alphafetoprotein level** M ♀
Encounter for antenatal screening for elevated maternal serum alphafetoprotein level
DEF: High levels of alpha-fetoprotein (AFP) that may indicate a possibility of spina bifida and other neural tube defects, anencephaly, or omphalocele in the fetus.

  Z36.2   **Encounter for other antenatal screening follow-up** M ♀
Non-visualized anatomy on a previous scan

  Z36.3   **Encounter for antenatal screening for malformations** M ♀
Screening for a suspected anomaly

  Z36.4   **Encounter for antenatal screening for fetal growth retardation** M ♀
Intrauterine growth restriction (IUGR)/small-for-dates

  Z36.5   **Encounter for antenatal screening for isoimmunization** M ♀

  ✓5ᵗʰ **Z36.8**   **Encounter for other antenatal screening**

    Z36.81   **Encounter for antenatal screening for hydrops fetalis** M ♀
DEF: Hydrops fetalis: Abnormal accumulation of fluid in two or more parts of the fetus, such as ascites, effusion of the pleural or pericardial tissues, or edema.

    Z36.82   **Encounter for antenatal screening for nuchal translucency** M ♀

    Z36.83   **Encounter for fetal screening for congenital cardiac abnormalities** M ♀

    Z36.84   **Encounter for antenatal screening for fetal lung maturity** M ♀

    Z36.85   **Encounter for antenatal screening for Streptococcus B** M ♀

    Z36.86   **Encounter for antenatal screening for cervical length** M ♀
Screening for risk of pre-term labor

    Z36.87   **Encounter for antenatal screening for uncertain dates** M ♀

    Z36.88   **Encounter for antenatal screening for fetal macrosomia** M ♀
Screening for large-for-dates

    Z36.89   **Encounter for other specified antenatal screening** M ♀

    Z36.8A   **Encounter for antenatal screening for other genetic defects** M ♀

  Z36.9   **Encounter for antenatal screening, unspecified** M ♀

✓4ᵗʰ **Z3A**   **Weeks of gestation**
NOTE   Codes from category Z3A are for use, only on the maternal record, to indicate the weeks of gestation of the pregnancy, if known.
Code first complications of pregnancy, childbirth and the puerperium (O09-O9A)
AHA: 2019,2Q,11; 2016,2Q,34; 2014,3Q,17; 2014,2Q,9; 2013,2Q,33
TIP: Do not assign a code from this category with codes from categories O00-O08 or code Z33.2.

  ✓5ᵗʰ **Z3A.0**   **Weeks of gestation of pregnancy, unspecified or less than 10 weeks**

    Z3A.00   **Weeks of gestation of pregnancy not specified** M ♀

    Z3A.01   **Less than 8 weeks gestation of pregnancy** M ♀

    Z3A.08   **8 weeks gestation of pregnancy** M ♀

    Z3A.09   **9 weeks gestation of pregnancy** M ♀

N Newborn: 0   P Pediatric: 0-17   M Maternity: 9-64   A Adult: 15-124   **MCC** Major Complication/Comorbidity   **CC** Complication/Comorbidity   **SW** Severe Wound Dx

1286   ICD-10-CM 2020

✓5ᵗʰ **Z3A.1 Weeks of gestation of pregnancy, weeks 1Ø-19**

Z3A.1Ø	**1Ø weeks** gestation of pregnancy	M ♀
Z3A.11	**11 weeks** gestation of pregnancy	M ♀
Z3A.12	**12 weeks** gestation of pregnancy	M ♀
Z3A.13	**13 weeks** gestation of pregnancy	M ♀
Z3A.14	**14 weeks** gestation of pregnancy	M ♀
Z3A.15	**15 weeks** gestation of pregnancy	M ♀
Z3A.16	**16 weeks** gestation of pregnancy	M ♀
Z3A.17	**17 weeks** gestation of pregnancy	M ♀
Z3A.18	**18 weeks** gestation of pregnancy	M ♀
Z3A.19	**19 weeks** gestation of pregnancy	M ♀

✓5ᵗʰ **Z3A.2 Weeks of gestation of pregnancy, weeks 2Ø-29**

Z3A.2Ø	**2Ø weeks** gestation of pregnancy	M ♀
Z3A.21	**21 weeks** gestation of pregnancy	M ♀
Z3A.22	**22 weeks** gestation of pregnancy	M ♀
Z3A.23	**23 weeks** gestation of pregnancy	M ♀
Z3A.24	**24 weeks** gestation of pregnancy	M ♀
Z3A.25	**25 weeks** gestation of pregnancy	M ♀
Z3A.26	**26 weeks** gestation of pregnancy	M ♀
Z3A.27	**27 weeks** gestation of pregnancy	M ♀
Z3A.28	**28 weeks** gestation of pregnancy	M ♀
Z3A.29	**29 weeks** gestation of pregnancy	M ♀

✓5ᵗʰ **Z3A.3 Weeks of gestation of pregnancy, weeks 3Ø-39**

Z3A.3Ø	**3Ø weeks** gestation of pregnancy	M ♀
Z3A.31	**31 weeks** gestation of pregnancy	M ♀
Z3A.32	**32 weeks** gestation of pregnancy	M ♀
Z3A.33	**33 weeks** gestation of pregnancy	M ♀
Z3A.34	**34 weeks** gestation of pregnancy	M ♀
Z3A.35	**35 weeks** gestation of pregnancy	M ♀
Z3A.36	**36 weeks** gestation of pregnancy	M ♀
Z3A.37	**37 weeks** gestation of pregnancy	M ♀
Z3A.38	**38 weeks** gestation of pregnancy	M ♀
Z3A.39	**39 weeks** gestation of pregnancy	M ♀

✓5ᵗʰ **Z3A.4 Weeks of gestation of pregnancy, weeks 4Ø or greater**

AHA: 2014,4Q,23

Z3A.4Ø	**4Ø weeks** gestation of pregnancy	M ♀
Z3A.41	**41 weeks** gestation of pregnancy	M ♀
Z3A.42	**42 weeks** gestation of pregnancy	M ♀
Z3A.49	**Greater than 42 weeks** gestation of pregnancy	M ♀

✓4ᵗʰ **Z37 Outcome of delivery**

This category is intended for use as an additional code to identify the outcome of delivery on the mother's record. It is not for use on the newborn record.

> **EXCLUDES 1**   *stillbirth (P95)*

Z37.0	**Single live birth**	M ♀

AHA: 2016,2Q,34; 2014,2Q,9

Z37.1	**Single stillbirth**	M ♀
Z37.2	**Twins, both liveborn**	M ♀
Z37.3	**Twins, one liveborn and one stillborn**	M ♀
Z37.4	**Twins, both stillborn**	M ♀

✓5ᵗʰ **Z37.5 Other multiple births, all liveborn**

Z37.5Ø	**Multiple births, unspecified, all liveborn**	M ♀
Z37.51	**Triplets, all liveborn**	M ♀
Z37.52	**Quadruplets, all liveborn**	M ♀
Z37.53	**Quintuplets, all liveborn**	M ♀
Z37.54	**Sextuplets, all liveborn**	M ♀
Z37.59	**Other multiple births, all liveborn**	M ♀

✓5ᵗʰ **Z37.6 Other multiple births, some liveborn**

Z37.6Ø	**Multiple births, unspecified, some liveborn**	M ♀
Z37.61	**Triplets, some liveborn**	M ♀
Z37.62	**Quadruplets, some liveborn**	M ♀
Z37.63	**Quintuplets, some liveborn**	M ♀
Z37.64	**Sextuplets, some liveborn**	M ♀

Z37.69	**Other multiple births, some liveborn**	M ♀
Z37.7	**Other multiple births, all stillborn**	M ♀
Z37.9	**Outcome of delivery, unspecified**	M ♀

Multiple birth NOS
Single birth NOS

✓4ᵗʰ **Z38 Liveborn infants according to place of birth and type of delivery**

This category is for use as the principal code on the initial record of a newborn baby. It is to be used for the initial birth record only. It is not to be used on the mother's record.

AHA: 2017,2Q,5-7; 2016,3Q,18; 2015,2Q,15

✓5ᵗʰ **Z38.0 Single liveborn infant, born in hospital**

Single liveborn infant, born in birthing center or other health care facility

Z38.00	**Single liveborn infant,** delivered vaginally	N
Z38.01	**Single liveborn infant,** delivered by cesarean	N
Z38.1	**Single liveborn infant, born outside hospital**	N
Z38.2	**Single liveborn infant, unspecified as to place of birth**	N

Single liveborn infant NOS

✓5ᵗʰ **Z38.3 Twin liveborn infant, born in hospital**

Z38.30	**Twin liveborn infant,** delivered vaginally	N
Z38.31	**Twin liveborn infant,** delivered by cesarean	N
Z38.4	**Twin liveborn infant, born outside hospital**	N
Z38.5	**Twin liveborn infant, unspecified as to place of birth**	N

✓5ᵗʰ **Z38.6 Other multiple liveborn infant, born in hospital**

Z38.61	**Triplet liveborn infant,** delivered vaginally	N
Z38.62	**Triplet liveborn infant,** delivered by cesarean	N
Z38.63	**Quadruplet liveborn infant,** delivered vaginally	N
Z38.64	**Quadruplet liveborn infant,** delivered by cesarean	N
Z38.65	**Quintuplet liveborn infant,** delivered vaginally	N
Z38.66	**Quintuplet liveborn infant,** delivered by cesarean	N
Z38.68	**Other multiple liveborn infant,** delivered vaginally	N
Z38.69	**Other multiple liveborn infant,** delivered by cesarean	N
Z38.7	**Other multiple liveborn infant, born outside hospital**	N
Z38.8	**Other multiple liveborn infant, unspecified as to place of birth**	N

✓4ᵗʰ **Z39 Encounter for maternal postpartum care and examination**

Z39.0	**Encounter for care and examination of mother immediately after delivery**	M ♀

1st Diagnoses

Care and observation in uncomplicated cases when the delivery occurs outside a healthcare facility

> **EXCLUDES 1**   *care for postpartum complication — see Alphabetic Index*

Z39.1	**Encounter for care and examination of lactating mother**	M ♀

Encounter for supervision of lactation

> **EXCLUDES 1**   *disorders of lactation (O92.-)*

Z39.2	**Encounter for routine postpartum follow-up**	M ♀

☑ Additional Character Required   ✓x7ᵗʰ Placeholder   Unacceptable PDx   Questionable PDx   Manifestation   Unspecified Dx   H1-H14 HAC   HCC CMS-HCC Dx   HIV HIV Dx

ICD-10-CM 2020   **1287**

Encounters for other specific health care (Z40-Z53)

Categories Z40-Z53 are intended for use to indicate a reason for care. They may be used for patients who have already been treated for a disease or injury, but who are receiving aftercare or prophylactic care, or care to consolidate the treatment, or to deal with a residual state

EXCLUDES 2   *follow-up examination for medical surveillance after treatment (Z08-Z09)*

✓4ᵗʰ Z40 Encounter for prophylactic surgery

    EXCLUDES 1   *organ donations (Z52.-)*

       therapeutic organ removal — code to condition

    DEF: Agent or treatment measure intended to prevent or ward off a disease condition.

    ✓5ᵗʰ Z40.0 Encounter for prophylactic surgery for risk factors related to malignant neoplasms

       Admission for prophylactic organ removal

       Use additional code to identify risk factor

       AHA: 2017,4Q,28-29

       Z40.00 Encounter for prophylactic removal of unspecified organ

       Z40.01 Encounter for prophylactic removal of breast

       Z40.02 Encounter for prophylactic removal of ovary(s) ♀

          Encounter for prophylactic removal of ovary(s) and fallopian tube(s)

       Z40.03 Encounter for prophylactic removal of fallopian tube(s) ♀

       Z40.09 Encounter for prophylactic removal of other organ

    Z40.8 Encounter for other prophylactic surgery

    Z40.9 Encounter for prophylactic surgery, unspecified

✓4ᵗʰ Z41 Encounter for procedures for purposes other than remedying health state

    Z41.1 Encounter for cosmetic surgery

       Encounter for cosmetic breast implant

       Encounter for cosmetic procedure

       EXCLUDES 1   *encounter for plastic and reconstructive surgery following medical procedure or healed injury (Z42.-)*

          encounter for post-mastectomy breast implantation (Z42.1)

    Z41.2 Encounter for routine and ritual male circumcision ♂

       AHA: 2018,3Q,15

       TIP: Do not report this code when circumcision is performed during the birth admission.

    Z41.3 Encounter for ear piercing

    Z41.8 Encounter for other procedures for purposes other than remedying health state

    Z41.9 Encounter for procedure for purposes other than remedying health state, unspecified

✓4ᵗʰ Z42 Encounter for plastic and reconstructive surgery following medical procedure or healed injury

    EXCLUDES 1   *encounter for cosmetic plastic surgery (Z41.1)*

       encounter for plastic surgery for treatment of current injury — code to relevent injury

    Z42.1 Encounter for breast reconstruction following mastectomy 🅰

       EXCLUDES 1   *deformity and disproportion of reconstructed breast (N65.1-)*

    Z42.8 Encounter for other plastic and reconstructive surgery following medical procedure or healed injury

       AHA: 2017,1Q,42

✓4ᵗʰ Z43 Encounter for attention to artificial openings

    INCLUDES   closure of artificial openings

       passage of sounds or bougies through artificial openings

       reforming artificial openings

       removal of catheter from artificial openings

       toilet or cleansing of artificial openings

    EXCLUDES 1   *complications of external stoma (J95.0-, K94.-, N99.5-)*

    EXCLUDES 2   *fitting and adjustment of prosthetic and other devices (Z44-Z46)*

    AHA: 2019,2Q,33

    Z43.0 Encounter for attention to tracheostomy HCC

    Z43.1 Encounter for attention to gastrostomy HCC

       EXCLUDES 2   *artificial opening status only, without need for care (Z93.-)*

    Z43.2 Encounter for attention to ileostomy HCC

    Z43.3 Encounter for attention to colostomy HCC

    Z43.4 Encounter for attention to other artificial openings of digestive tract HCC

    Z43.5 Encounter for attention to cystostomy HCC

    Z43.6 Encounter for attention to other artificial openings of urinary tract HCC

       Encounter for attention to nephrostomy

       Encounter for attention to ureterostomy

       Encounter for attention to urethrostomy

    Z43.7 Encounter for attention to artificial vagina

    Z43.8 Encounter for attention to other artificial openings HCC

    Z43.9 Encounter for attention to unspecified artificial opening HCC

✓4ᵗʰ Z44 Encounter for fitting and adjustment of external prosthetic device

    INCLUDES   removal or replacement of external prosthetic device

    EXCLUDES 1   *malfunction or other complications of device — see Alphabetical Index*

       presence of prosthetic device (Z97.-)

    ✓5ᵗʰ Z44.0 Encounter for fitting and adjustment of artificial arm

       ✓6ᵗʰ Z44.00 Encounter for fitting and adjustment of unspecified artificial arm

          Z44.001 Encounter for fitting and adjustment of unspecified right artificial arm

          Z44.002 Encounter for fitting and adjustment of unspecified left artificial arm

          Z44.009 Encounter for fitting and adjustment of unspecified artificial arm, unspecified arm

       ✓6ᵗʰ Z44.01 Encounter for fitting and adjustment of complete artificial arm

          Z44.011 Encounter for fitting and adjustment of complete right artificial arm

          Z44.012 Encounter for fitting and adjustment of complete left artificial arm

          Z44.019 Encounter for fitting and adjustment of complete artificial arm, unspecified arm

       ✓6ᵗʰ Z44.02 Encounter for fitting and adjustment of partial artificial arm

          Z44.021 Encounter for fitting and adjustment of partial artificial right arm

          Z44.022 Encounter for fitting and adjustment of partial artificial left arm

          Z44.029 Encounter for fitting and adjustment of partial artificial arm, unspecified arm

    ✓5ᵗʰ Z44.1 Encounter for fitting and adjustment of artificial leg

       ✓6ᵗʰ Z44.10 Encounter for fitting and adjustment of unspecified artificial leg

          Z44.101 Encounter for fitting and adjustment of unspecified right artificial leg HCC

          Z44.102 Encounter for fitting and adjustment of unspecified left artificial leg HCC

          Z44.109 Encounter for fitting and adjustment of unspecified artificial leg, unspecified leg HCC

       ✓6ᵗʰ Z44.11 Encounter for fitting and adjustment of complete artificial leg

          Z44.111 Encounter for fitting and adjustment of complete right artificial leg HCC

          Z44.112 Encounter for fitting and adjustment of complete left artificial leg HCC

          Z44.119 Encounter for fitting and adjustment of complete artificial leg, unspecified leg HCC

       ✓6ᵗʰ Z44.12 Encounter for fitting and adjustment of partial artificial leg

          Z44.121 Encounter for fitting and adjustment of partial artificial right leg HCC

          Z44.122 Encounter for fitting and adjustment of partial artificial left leg HCC

          Z44.129 Encounter for fitting and adjustment of partial artificial leg, unspecified leg HCC

— prosthetic device (handwritten note)

N Newborn: 0   **P** Pediatric: 0-17   **M** Maternity: 9-64   **A** Adult: 15-124   **MCC** Major Complication/Comorbidity   **CC** Complication/Comorbidity   **SW** Severe Wound Dx

1288   ICD-10-CM 2020

✓5ᵗʰ **Z44.2** **Encounter for fitting and adjustment of** artificial eye

    EXCLUDES 1　*mechanical complication of ocular prosthesis (T85.3)*

    Z44.20 **Encounter for fitting and adjustment of artificial eye, unspecified**

    Z44.21 **Encounter for fitting and adjustment of artificial right eye**

    Z44.22 **Encounter for fitting and adjustment of artificial left eye**

✓5ᵗʰ **Z44.3** **Encounter for fitting and adjustment of** external breast prosthesis

    EXCLUDES 1　*complications of breast implant (T85.4-)*

        encounter for adjustment or removal of breast implant (Z45.81-)

        encounter for initial breast implant insertion for cosmetic breast augmentation (Z41.1)

        encounter for breast reconstruction following mastectomy (Z42.1)

    Z44.30 **Encounter for fitting and adjustment of external breast prosthesis, unspecified breast**

    Z44.31 **Encounter for fitting and adjustment of external right breast prosthesis**

    Z44.32 **Encounter for fitting and adjustment of external left breast prosthesis**

Z44.8 **Encounter for fitting and adjustment of other external prosthetic devices**

Z44.9 **Encounter for fitting and adjustment of unspecified external prosthetic device**

✓4ᵗʰ **Z45** **Encounter for adjustment and management of implanted device**

    INCLUDES　removal or replacement of implanted device

    EXCLUDES 1　*malfunction or other complications of device — see Alphabetical Index*

    EXCLUDES 2　*encounter for fitting and adjustment of non-implanted device (Z46.-)*

✓5ᵗʰ **Z45.0** **Encounter for adjustment and management of** cardiac device

    ✓6ᵗʰ **Z45.01** **Encounter for adjustment and management of cardiac** pacemaker

        Encounter for adjustment and management of cardiac resynchronization therapy pacemaker (CRT-P)

        EXCLUDES 1　*encounter for adjustment and management of automatic implantable cardiac defibrillator with synchronous cardiac pacemaker (Z45.02)*

        Z45.010 **Encounter for checking and testing of cardiac pacemaker** pulse generator **[battery]**

            Encounter for replacing cardiac pacemaker pulse generator [battery]

        Z45.018 **Encounter for adjustment and management of other part of cardiac pacemaker**

            EXCLUDES 1　▶*presence of other part of cardiac pacemaker (Z95.0)*◀

            EXCLUDES 2　*presence of prosthetic and other devices ▶(Z95.1-Z95.5, Z95.811-Z97)◀*

    Z45.02 **Encounter for adjustment and management of** automatic implantable cardiac defibrillator

        Encounter for adjustment and management of automatic implantable cardiac defibrillator with synchronous cardiac pacemaker

        Encounter for adjustment and management of cardiac resynchronization therapy defibrillator (CRT-D)

    Z45.09 **Encounter for adjustment and management of other cardiac device**

Z45.1 **Encounter for adjustment and management of** infusion pump

Z45.2 **Encounter for adjustment and management of** vascular access device

    Encounter for adjustment and management of vascular catheters

    EXCLUDES 1　*encounter for adjustment and management of renal dialysis catheter (Z49.01)*

    AHA: 2018,3Q,20

✓5ᵗʰ **Z45.3** **Encounter for adjustment and management of implanted devices of the special senses**

    Z45.31 **Encounter for adjustment and management of implanted** visual **substitution device**

✓6ᵗʰ **Z45.32** **Encounter for adjustment and management of implanted** hearing **device**

    EXCLUDES 1　*encounter for fitting and adjustment of hearing aide (Z46.1)*

    Z45.320 **Encounter for adjustment and management of** bone conduction **device**

    Z45.321 **Encounter for adjustment and management of** cochlear **device**

    Z45.328 **Encounter for adjustment and management of other implanted hearing device**

✓5ᵗʰ **Z45.4** **Encounter for adjustment and management of implanted** nervous system device

    Z45.41 **Encounter for adjustment and management of** cerebrospinal fluid drainage **device**

        Encounter for adjustment and management of cerebral ventricular (communicating) shunt

    Z45.42 **Encounter for adjustment and management of** neurostimulator

        ▶Encounter for adjustment and management of brain neurostimulator◀

        ▶Encounter for adjustment and management of gastric neurostimulator◀

        ▶Encounter for adjustment and management of peripheral nerve neurostimulator◀

        ▶Encounter for adjustment and management of sacral nerve neurostimulator◀

        ▶Encounter for adjustment and management of spinal cord neurostimulator◀

        ▶Encounter for adjustment and management of vagus nerve neurostimulator◀

    Z45.49 **Encounter for adjustment and management of other implanted nervous system device**

        AHA: 2014,3Q,19

✓5ᵗʰ **Z45.8** **Encounter for adjustment and management of other implanted devices**

    ✓6ᵗʰ **Z45.81** **Encounter for adjustment or** removal of breast implant

        Encounter for elective implant exchange (different material) (different size)

        ▶Encounter removal of tissue expander with or without synchronous insertion of permanent implant◀

        EXCLUDES 1　*complications of breast implant (T85.4-)*

            encounter for initial breast implant insertion for cosmetic breast augmentation (Z41.1)

            encounter for breast reconstruction following mastectomy (Z42.1)

        Z45.811 **Encounter for adjustment or removal of** right breast implant

        Z45.812 **Encounter for adjustment or removal of** left breast implant

        Z45.819 **Encounter for adjustment or removal of unspecified breast implant**

    Z45.82 **Encounter for** adjustment or removal of myringotomy device **(stent) (tube)**

    Z45.89 **Encounter for adjustment and management of other implanted devices**

        AHA: 2014,4Q,26-28

Z45.9 **Encounter for adjustment and management of unspecified implanted device**

✓4ᵗʰ **Z46** **Encounter for fitting and adjustment of other devices**

    INCLUDES　removal or replacement of other device

    EXCLUDES 1　*malfunction or other complications of device — see Alphabetical Index*

    EXCLUDES 2　*encounter for fitting and management of implanted devices (Z45.-)*

        issue of repeat prescription only (Z76.0)

        presence of prosthetic and other devices (Z95-Z97)

Z46.0 **Encounter for fitting and adjustment of** spectacles and contact lenses

Z46.1 **Encounter for fitting and adjustment of** hearing aid

    EXCLUDES 1　*encounter for adjustment and management of implanted hearing device (Z45.32-)*

✔ Additional Character Required　✓x7ᵗʰ Placeholder　Unacceptable PDx　Questionable PDx　Manifestation　Unspecified Dx　H1-H14 HAC　HCC CMS-HCC Dx　HIV HIV Dx

ICD-10-CM 2020　　　1289

Z46.2   **Encounter for fitting and adjustment of other devices related to nervous system and special senses**
> *EXCLUDES 2*   *encounter for adjustment and management of implanted nervous system device (Z45.4-)*
> *encounter for adjustment and management of implanted visual substitution device (Z45.31)*

Z46.3   **Encounter for fitting and adjustment of dental prosthetic device**
> Encounter for fitting and adjustment of dentures

Z46.4   **Encounter for fitting and adjustment of orthodontic device**

√5ᵗʰ Z46.5   **Encounter for fitting and adjustment of other gastrointestinal appliance and device**
> *EXCLUDES 1*   *encounter for attention to artificial openings of digestive tract (Z43.1-Z43.4)*

    Z46.51   **Encounter for fitting and adjustment of gastric lap band**

    Z46.59   **Encounter for fitting and adjustment of other gastrointestinal appliance and device**

Z46.6   **Encounter for fitting and adjustment of urinary device**
> *EXCLUDES 2*   *attention to artificial openings of urinary tract (Z43.5, Z43.6)*

√5ᵗʰ Z46.8   **Encounter for fitting and adjustment of other specified devices**

    Z46.81   **Encounter for fitting and adjustment of insulin pump**
> Encounter for insulin pump instruction and training
> Encounter for insulin pump titration

    Z46.82   **Encounter for fitting and adjustment of non-vascular catheter**

    Z46.89   **Encounter for fitting and adjustment of other specified devices**
> Encounter for fitting and adjustment of wheelchair

Z46.9   **Encounter for fitting and adjustment of unspecified device**

√4ᵗʰ Z47   **Orthopedic aftercare**
> *EXCLUDES 1*   *aftercare for healing fracture — code to fracture with 7th character D*

Z47.1   **Aftercare following joint replacement surgery**
> Use additional code to identify the joint (Z96.6-)

Z47.2   **Encounter for removal of internal fixation device**
> *EXCLUDES 1*   *encounter for adjustment of internal fixation device for fracture treatment — code to fracture with appropriate 7th character*
> *encounter for removal of external fixation device — code to fracture with 7th character D*
> *infection or inflammatory reaction to internal fixation device (T84.6-)*
> *mechanical complication of internal fixation device (T84.1-)*

√5ᵗʰ Z47.3   **Aftercare following explantation of joint prosthesis**
> Aftercare following explantation of joint prosthesis, staged procedure
> Encounter for joint prosthesis insertion following prior explantation of joint prosthesis
> **AHA:** 2015,1Q,16

    Z47.31   **Aftercare following explantation of shoulder joint prosthesis**
> *EXCLUDES 1*   *acquired absence of shoulder joint following prior explantation of shoulder joint prosthesis (Z89.23-)*
> *shoulder joint prosthesis explantation status (Z89.23-)*

    Z47.32   **Aftercare following explantation of hip joint prosthesis**
> *EXCLUDES 1*   *acquired absence of hip joint following prior explantation of hip joint prosthesis (Z89.62-)*
> *hip joint prosthesis explantation status (Z89.62-)*

    Z47.33   **Aftercare following explantation of knee joint prosthesis**
> *EXCLUDES 1*   *acquired absence of knee joint following prior explantation of knee prosthesis (Z89.52-)*
> *knee joint prosthesis explantation status (Z89.52-)*

√5ᵗʰ Z47.8   **Encounter for other orthopedic aftercare**

    Z47.81   **Encounter for orthopedic aftercare following surgical amputation**
> Use additional code to identify the limb amputated (Z89.-)

    Z47.82   **Encounter for orthopedic aftercare following scoliosis surgery**

    Z47.89   **Encounter for other orthopedic aftercare**
> **AHA:** 2015,1Q,8

√4ᵗʰ Z48   **Encounter for other postprocedural aftercare**
> *EXCLUDES 1*   *encounter for aftercare following injury — code to Injury, by site, with appropriate 7th character for subsequent encounter*
> *encounter for follow-up examination after completed treatment (Z08-Z09)*
> *EXCLUDES 2*   *encounter for attention to artificial openings (Z43.-)*
> *encounter for fitting and adjustment of prosthetic and other devices (Z44-Z46)*
> **AHA:** 2015,4Q,38; 2015,1Q,6-7

√5ᵗʰ Z48.0   **Encounter for attention to dressings, sutures and drains**
> *EXCLUDES 1*   *encounter for planned postprocedural wound closure (Z48.1)*

    Z48.00   **Encounter for change or removal of nonsurgical wound dressing**
> Encounter for change or removal of wound dressing NOS

    Z48.01   **Encounter for change or removal of surgical wound dressing**
> **AHA:** 2019,2Q,33

    Z48.02   **Encounter for removal of sutures**
> Encounter for removal of staples

    Z48.03   **Encounter for change or removal of drains**
> **AHA:** 2019,2Q,33

Z48.1   **Encounter for planned postprocedural wound closure**
> *EXCLUDES 1*   *encounter for attention to dressings and sutures (Z48.0-)*

√5ᵗʰ Z48.2   **Encounter for aftercare following organ transplant**

    Z48.21   **Encounter for aftercare following heart transplant**   `CC` `HCC`
> **CC Excl:** PDX collection 1488

    Z48.22   **Encounter for aftercare following kidney transplant**   `CC`
> **CC Excl:** PDX collection 1489

    Z48.23   **Encounter for aftercare following liver transplant**   `CC` `HCC`
> **CC Excl:** PDX collection 1490

    Z48.24   **Encounter for aftercare following lung transplant**   `CC` `HCC`
> **CC Excl:** PDX collection 1491

    √6ᵗʰ Z48.28   **Encounter for aftercare following multiple organ transplant**

      Z48.280   **Encounter for aftercare following heart-lung transplant**   `CC` `HCC`
> **CC Excl:** PDX collection 1488

      Z48.288   **Encounter for aftercare following multiple organ transplant**

    √6ᵗʰ Z48.29   **Encounter for aftercare following other organ transplant**

      Z48.290   **Encounter for aftercare following bone marrow transplant**   `CC` `HCC`
> **CC Excl:** PDX collection 1492

      Z48.298   **Encounter for aftercare following other organ transplant**

    Z48.3   **Aftercare following surgery for neoplasm**
> Use additional code to identify the neoplasm

— dressings, sutures, drains, wounds

Ⓝ Newborn: 0   Ⓟ Pediatric: 0-17   Ⓜ Maternity: 9-64   Ⓐ Adult: 15-124   ᴹᶜᶜ Major Complication/Comorbidity   ᶜᶜ Complication/Comorbidity   ˢʷ Severe Wound Dx

1290   ICD-10-CM 2020

Z46.2–Z48.3

√5ᵗʰ **Z48.8 Encounter for other specified postprocedural aftercare**

√6ᵗʰ **Z48.81 Encounter for surgical aftercare following surgery on specified body systems**

These codes identify the body system requiring aftercare. They are for use in conjunction with other aftercare codes to fully explain the aftercare encounter. The condition treated should also be coded if still present.

EXCLUDES 1 *aftercare for injury — code the injury with 7th character D*
aftercare following surgery for neoplasm (Z48.3)

EXCLUDES 2 *aftercare following organ transplant (Z48.2-)*
orthopedic aftercare (Z47.-)

AHA: 2015,4Q,38

Z48.810 Encounter for surgical aftercare following surgery on the sense organs

Z48.811 Encounter for surgical aftercare following surgery on the nervous system

EXCLUDES 2 *encounter for surgical aftercare following surgery on the sense organs (Z48.810)*

Z48.812 Encounter for surgical aftercare following surgery on the circulatory system
AHA: 2012,4Q,96

Z48.813 Encounter for surgical aftercare following surgery on the respiratory system
AHA: 2019,2Q,33

Z48.814 Encounter for surgical aftercare following surgery on the teeth or oral cavity

Z48.815 Encounter for surgical aftercare following surgery on the digestive system

Z48.816 Encounter for surgical aftercare following surgery on the genitourinary system
EXCLUDES 1 *encounter for aftercare following sterilization reversal (Z31.42)*

Z48.817 Encounter for surgical aftercare following surgery on the skin and subcutaneous tissue

Z48.89 Encounter for other specified surgical aftercare

√4ᵗʰ **Z49 Encounter for care involving renal dialysis**

Code also associated end stage renal disease (N18.6)

√5ᵗʰ **Z49.0 Preparatory care for renal dialysis**

Encounter for dialysis instruction and training

Z49.01 Encounter for fitting and adjustment of extracorporeal dialysis catheter HCC
Removal or replacement of renal dialysis catheter
Toilet or cleansing of renal dialysis catheter

Z49.02 Encounter for fitting and adjustment of peritoneal dialysis catheter HCC

√5ᵗʰ **Z49.3 Encounter for adequacy testing for dialysis**

Z49.31 Encounter for adequacy testing for hemodialysis HCC

Z49.32 Encounter for adequacy testing for peritoneal dialysis HCC
Encounter for peritoneal equilibration test

√4ᵗʰ **Z51 Encounter for other aftercare and medical care**

Code also condition requiring care
EXCLUDES 1 *follow-up examination after treatment (Z08-Z09)*

Z51.0 Encounter for antineoplastic radiation therapy
AHA: 2017,4Q,103
TIP: Do not assign when admission is for insertion/implantation of radioactive elements. Assign a code for the malignancy instead. Any complications related to the radioactive elements should be assigned as secondary diagnoses.

√5ᵗʰ **Z51.1 Encounter for antineoplastic chemotherapy and immunotherapy**
EXCLUDES 2 *encounter for chemotherapy and immunotherapy for nonneoplastic condition — code to condition*

Z51.11 Encounter for antineoplastic chemotherapy
AHA: 2015,3Q,19

Z51.12 Encounter for antineoplastic immunotherapy

Z51.5 Encounter for palliative care
AHA: 2017,1Q,48

Hospice

Z51.6 Encounter for desensitization to allergens
AHA: 2016,4Q,77

√5ᵗʰ **Z51.8 Encounter for other specified aftercare**
EXCLUDES 1 *holiday relief care (Z75.5)*

Z51.81 Encounter for therapeutic drug level monitoring
Code also any long-term (current) drug therapy (Z79.-)
EXCLUDES 1 *encounter for blood-drug test for administrative or medicolegal reasons (Z02.83)*
DEF: Drug monitoring: Measurement of the level of a specific drug in the body or measurement of a specific function to assess effectiveness of a drug.

Z51.89 Encounter for other specified aftercare
AHA: 2012,4Q,95-97

√4ᵗʰ **Z52 Donors of organs and tissues**
INCLUDES autologous and other living donors
EXCLUDES 1 *cadaveric donor - omit code*
examination of potential donor (Z00.5)
AHA: 2012,4Q,99

√5ᵗʰ **Z52.0 Blood donor**

√6ᵗʰ **Z52.00 Unspecified blood donor**
Z52.000 Unspecified donor, whole blood
Z52.001 Unspecified donor, stem cells
Z52.008 Unspecified donor, other blood

√6ᵗʰ **Z52.01 Autologous blood donor**
Z52.010 Autologous donor, whole blood
Z52.011 Autologous donor, stem cells
Z52.018 Autologous donor, other blood

√6ᵗʰ **Z52.09 Other blood donor**
Volunteer donor
Z52.090 Other blood donor, whole blood
Z52.091 Other blood donor, stem cells
Z52.098 Other blood donor, other blood

√5ᵗʰ **Z52.1 Skin donor**
Z52.10 Skin donor, unspecified
Z52.11 Skin donor, autologous
Z52.19 Skin donor, other

√5ᵗʰ **Z52.2 Bone donor**
Z52.20 Bone donor, unspecified
Z52.21 Bone donor, autologous
Z52.29 Bone donor, other

Z52.3 Bone marrow donor
Z52.4 Kidney donor
Z52.5 Cornea donor
Z52.6 Liver donor

√5ᵗʰ **Z52.8 Donor of other specified organs or tissues**

√6ᵗʰ **Z52.81 Egg (Oocyte) donor**
Z52.810 Egg (Oocyte) donor under age 35, anonymous recipient ♀
Egg donor under age 35 NOS

Z52.811 Egg (Oocyte) donor under age 35, designated recipient ♀

Z52.812 Egg (Oocyte) donor age 35 and over, anonymous recipient ♀
Egg donor age 35 and over NOS

Z52.813 Egg (Oocyte) donor age 35 and over, designated recipient ♀

Z52.819 Egg (Oocyte) donor, unspecified ♀

Z52.89 Donor of other specified organs or tissues

Z52.9 Donor of unspecified organ or tissue
Donor NOS

√4ᵗʰ **Z53 Persons encountering health services for specific procedures and treatment, not carried out**

√5ᵗʰ **Z53.0 Procedure and treatment not carried out because of contraindication**
Z53.01 Procedure and treatment not carried out due to patient smoking
Z53.09 Procedure and treatment not carried out because of other contraindication

Z53.1 Procedure and treatment not carried out because of patient's decision for reasons of belief and group pressure

√5ᵗʰ **Z53.2 Procedure and treatment not carried out because of patient's decision for other and unspecified reasons**
Z53.20 Procedure and treatment not carried out because of patient's decision for unspecified reasons

---

Chapter 21. Factors Influencing Health Status and Contact With Health Services

Z53.21   **Procedure and treatment not carried out due to patient leaving prior to being seen by health care provider**

Z53.29   **Procedure and treatment not carried out because of patient's decision for other reasons**

√5ᵗʰ **Z53.3**   **Procedure converted to open procedure**
     AHA: 2016,4Q,79

     Z53.31   **Laparoscopic surgical procedure converted to open procedure**

     Z53.32   **Thoracoscopic surgical procedure converted to open procedure**

     Z53.33   **Arthroscopic surgical procedure converted to open procedure**

     Z53.39   **Other specified procedure converted to open procedure**

Z53.8   **Procedure and treatment not carried out for other reasons**

Z53.9   **Procedure and treatment not carried out, unspecified reason**

Persons with potential health hazards related to socioeconomic and psychosocial circumstances (Z55-Z65)

AHA: 2018,4Q,58,73; 2018,1Q,18
TIP: Codes from this code block can be assigned based on documentation from clinicians other than the diagnosing provider.

√4ᵗʰ **Z55**   **Problems related to education and literacy**
     EXCLUDES 1   *disorders of psychological development (F80-F89)*

     Z55.0   **Illiteracy and low-level literacy**
     Z55.1   **Schooling unavailable and unattainable**
     Z55.2   **Failed school examinations**
     Z55.3   **Underachievement in school**
     Z55.4   **Educational maladjustment and discord with teachers and classmates**
     Z55.8   **Other problems related to education and literacy**
         Problems related to inadequate teaching
     Z55.9   **Problems related to education and literacy, unspecified**
         Academic problems NOS

√4ᵗʰ **Z56**   **Problems related to employment and unemployment**
     EXCLUDES 2   *occupational exposure to risk factors (Z57.-)*
         problems related to housing and economic circumstances (Z59.-)

     Z56.0   **Unemployment, unspecified**
     Z56.1   **Change of job**   Ⓐ
     Z56.2   **Threat of job loss**
     Z56.3   **Stressful work schedule**
     Z56.4   **Discord with boss and workmates**
     Z56.5   **Uncongenial work environment**
         Difficult conditions at work
     Z56.6   **Other physical and mental strain related to work**
     √5ᵗʰ **Z56.8**   **Other problems related to employment**
         Z56.81   **Sexual harassment on the job**
         Z56.82   **Military deployment status**
             Individual (civilian or military) currently deployed in theater or in support of military war, peacekeeping and humanitarian operations
         Z56.89   **Other problems related to employment**
     Z56.9   **Unspecified problems related to employment**
         Occupational problems NOS

√4ᵗʰ **Z57**   **Occupational exposure to risk factors**
     Z57.0   **Occupational exposure to noise**
     Z57.1   **Occupational exposure to radiation**
     Z57.2   **Occupational exposure to dust**
     √5ᵗʰ **Z57.3**   **Occupational exposure to other air contaminants**
         Z57.31   **Occupational exposure to environmental tobacco smoke**
             EXCLUDES 2   *exposure to environmental tobacco smoke (Z77.22)*
         Z57.39   **Occupational exposure to other air contaminants**
     Z57.4   **Occupational exposure to toxic agents in agriculture**
         Occupational exposure to solids, liquids, gases or vapors in agriculture
     Z57.5   **Occupational exposure to toxic agents in other industries**
         Occupational exposure to solids, liquids, gases or vapors in other industries
     Z57.6   **Occupational exposure to extreme temperature**
     Z57.7   **Occupational exposure to vibration**
     Z57.8   **Occupational exposure to other risk factors**

Z57.9   **Occupational exposure to unspecified risk factor**

√4ᵗʰ **Z59**   **Problems related to housing and economic circumstances**
     EXCLUDES 2   *problems related to upbringing (Z62.-)*

     Z59.0   **Homelessness**   CC
     Z59.1   **Inadequate housing**
         Lack of heating
         Restriction of space
         Technical defects in home preventing adequate care
         Unsatisfactory surroundings
         EXCLUDES 1   *problems related to the natural and physical environment (Z77.1-)*
     Z59.2   **Discord with neighbors, lodgers and landlord**
     Z59.3   **Problems related to living in residential institution**
         Boarding-school resident
         EXCLUDES 1   *institutional upbringing (Z62.2)*
     Z59.4   **Lack of adequate food and safe drinking water**
         Inadequate drinking water supply
         EXCLUDES 1   *effects of hunger (T73.0)*
             inappropriate diet or eating habits (Z72.4)
             malnutrition (E40-E46)
     Z59.5   **Extreme poverty**
     Z59.6   **Low income**
     Z59.7   **Insufficient social insurance and welfare support**
     Z59.8   **Other problems related to housing and economic circumstances**
         Foreclosure on loan
         Isolated dwelling
         Problems with creditors
     Z59.9   **Problem related to housing and economic circumstances, unspecified**

√4ᵗʰ **Z60**   **Problems related to social environment**
     Z60.0   **Problems of adjustment to life-cycle transitions**
         Empty nest syndrome
         Phase of life problem
         Problem with adjustment to retirement [pension]
     Z60.2   **Problems related to living alone**
     Z60.3   **Acculturation difficulty**
         Problem with migration
         Problem with social transplantation
         DEF: Problem adapting to a different culture or environment not based on any coexisting mental disorder.
     Z60.4   **Social exclusion and rejection**
         Exclusion and rejection on the basis of personal characteristics, such as unusual physical appearance, illness or behavior.
         EXCLUDES 1   *target of adverse discrimination such as for racial or religious reasons (Z60.5)*
     Z60.5   **Target of (perceived) adverse discrimination and persecution**
         EXCLUDES 1   *social exclusion and rejection (Z60.4)*
     Z60.8   **Other problems related to social environment**
     Z60.9   **Problem related to social environment, unspecified**

√4ᵗʰ **Z62**   **Problems related to upbringing**
     INCLUDES   current and past negative life events in childhood
         current and past problems of a child related to upbringing
     EXCLUDES 2   *maltreatment syndrome (T74.-)*
         problems related to housing and economic circumstances (Z59.-)

     Z62.0   **Inadequate parental supervision and control**
     Z62.1   **Parental overprotection**
     √5ᵗʰ **Z62.2**   **Upbringing away from parents**
         EXCLUDES 1   *problems with boarding school (Z59.3)*
         Z62.21   **Child in welfare custody**   Ⓟ
             Child in care of non-parental family member
             Child in foster care
             EXCLUDES 2   *problem for parent due to child in welfare custody (Z63.5)*
         Z62.22   **Institutional upbringing**
             Child living in orphanage or group home
         Z62.29   **Other upbringing away from parents**
     Z62.3   **Hostility towards and scapegoating of child**   Ⓟ
     Z62.6   **Inappropriate (excessive) parental pressure**

Ⓝ Newborn: 0   Ⓟ Pediatric: 0-17   Ⓜ Maternity: 9-64   Ⓐ Adult: 15-124   MCC Major Complication/Comorbidity   CC Complication/Comorbidity   SW Severe Wound Dx

✓5ᵗʰ **Z62.8 Other specified problems related to upbringing**

  ✓6ᵗʰ **Z62.81 Personal history of abuse in childhood**

    Z62.810 Personal history of physical and sexual abuse in childhood
      EXCLUDES 1   current child physical abuse (T74.12, T76.12)
               current child sexual abuse (T74.22, T76.22)

    Z62.811 Personal history of psychological abuse in childhood
      EXCLUDES 1   current child psychological abuse (T74.32, T76.32)

    Z62.812 Personal history of neglect in childhood
      EXCLUDES 1   current child neglect (T74.02, T76.02)

    Z62.813 Personal history of forced labor or sexual exploitation in childhood
      AHA: 2018,4Q,32,35

    Z62.819 Personal history of unspecified abuse in childhood
      EXCLUDES 1   current child abuse NOS (T74.92, T76.92)

  ✓6ᵗʰ **Z62.82 Parent-child conflict**

    Z62.820 Parent-biological child conflict
      Parent-child problem NOS

    Z62.821 Parent-adopted child conflict

    Z62.822 Parent-foster child conflict

  ✓6ᵗʰ **Z62.89 Other specified problems related to upbringing**

    Z62.890 Parent-child estrangement NEC

    Z62.891 Sibling rivalry

    Z62.898 Other specified problems related to upbringing

Z62.9 Problem related to upbringing, unspecified

✓4ᵗʰ **Z63 Other problems related to primary support group, including family circumstances**

  EXCLUDES 2   maltreatment syndrome (T74.-, T76)
            parent-child problems (Z62.-)
            problems related to negative life events in childhood (Z62.-)
            problems related to upbringing (Z62.-)

Z63.0 Problems in relationship with spouse or partner
  Relationship distress with spouse or intimate partner
  EXCLUDES 1   counseling for spousal or partner abuse problems (Z69.1)
            counseling related to sexual attitude, behavior, and orientation (Z70.-)

Z63.1 Problems in relationship with in-laws

✓5ᵗʰ **Z63.3 Absence of family member**
  EXCLUDES 1   absence of family member due to disappearance and death (Z63.4)
            absence of family member due to separation and divorce (Z63.5)

  Z63.31 Absence of family member due to military deployment
    Individual or family affected by other family member being on military deployment
    EXCLUDES 1   family disruption due to return of family member from military deployment (Z63.71)

  Z63.32 Other absence of family member

Z63.4 Disappearance and death of family member
  Assumed death of family member
  Bereavement
  AHA: 2014,1Q,25

Z63.5 Disruption of family by separation and divorce
  Marital estrangement

Z63.6 Dependent relative needing care at home

✓5ᵗʰ **Z63.7 Other stressful life events affecting family and household**

  Z63.71 Stress on family due to return of family member from military deployment
    Individual or family affected by family member having returned from military deployment (current or past conflict)

  Z63.72 Alcoholism and drug addiction in family

  Z63.79 Other stressful life events affecting family and household
    Anxiety (normal) about sick person in family
    Health problems within family
    Ill or disturbed family member
    Isolated family

Z63.8 Other specified problems related to primary support group
  Family discord NOS
  Family estrangement NOS
  High expressed emotional level within family
  Inadequate family support NOS
  Inadequate or distorted communication within family

Z63.9 Problem related to primary support group, unspecified
  Relationship disorder NOS

✓4ᵗʰ **Z64 Problems related to certain psychosocial circumstances**

Z64.0 Problems related to unwanted pregnancy ♀

Z64.1 Problems related to multiparity ♀

Z64.4 Discord with counselors
  Discord with probation officer
  Discord with social worker

✓4ᵗʰ **Z65 Problems related to other psychosocial circumstances**

Z65.0 Conviction in civil and criminal proceedings without imprisonment

Z65.1 Imprisonment and other incarceration

Z65.2 Problems related to release from prison

Z65.3 Problems related to other legal circumstances
  Arrest
  Child custody or support proceedings
  Litigation
  Prosecution

Z65.4 Victim of crime and terrorism
  Victim of torture

Z65.5 Exposure to disaster, war and other hostilities
  EXCLUDES 1   target of perceived discrimination or persecution (Z60.5)

Z65.8 Other specified problems related to psychosocial circumstances
  Religious or spiritual problem

Z65.9 Problem related to unspecified psychosocial circumstances

Do not resuscitate status (Z66)

Z66 Do not resuscitate
  DNR status
  DEF: Medical order written by a physician that instructs others not to perform cardiopulmonary resuscitation (CPR), intubation, or advanced life support (ACLS). It prevents unnecessary invasive treatment to prolong life should breathing stop or cardiac arrest occur.

Blood type (Z67)

✓4ᵗʰ **Z67 Blood type**
     AHA: 2015,3Q,40

Blood Types

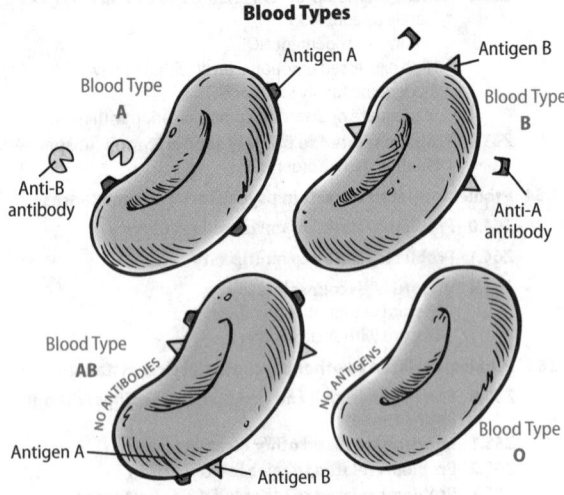

Antigen A • Antigen B

Blood Type **A** • Blood Type **B**

Anti-B antibody • Anti-A antibody

Blood Type **AB** • Blood Type **O**

NO ANTIBODIES • NO ANTIGENS

Antigen A • Antigen B

✓5ᵗʰ **Z67.1 Type A blood**
     Z67.1Ø Type A blood, Rh positive
     Z67.11 Type A blood, Rh negative

✓5ᵗʰ **Z67.2 Type B blood**
     Z67.2Ø Type B blood, Rh positive
     Z67.21 Type B blood, Rh negative

✓5ᵗʰ **Z67.3 Type AB blood**
     Z67.3Ø Type AB blood, Rh positive
     Z67.31 Type AB blood, Rh negative

✓5ᵗʰ **Z67.4 Type O blood**
     Z67.4Ø Type O blood, Rh positive
     Z67.41 Type O blood, Rh negative

✓5ᵗʰ **Z67.9 Unspecified blood type**
     Z67.9Ø Unspecified blood type, Rh positive
     Z67.91 Unspecified blood type, Rh negative

Body mass index [BMI] (Z68)

✓4ᵗʰ **Z68 Body mass index [BMI]**
     Kilograms per meters squared
     NOTE ▶BMI adult codes are for use for persons 2Ø years of age or older◀
         ▶BMI pediatric codes are for use for persons 2-19 years of age.◀
         ▶These percentiles are based on the growth charts published by the Centers for Disease Control and Prevention (CDC)◀
     AHA: 2018,4Q,73,77-83; 2017,1Q,39
     DEF: Index used to help determine whether an individual is underweight, a healthy weight, overweight, or obese.
     TIP: A BMI code may be assigned to support an associated condition based on medical record documentation from clinicians who are not the patient's provider.
     TIP: Do not assign when used in association with fluctuations in body fluid during an encounter, such as fluid overload or fluid retention.
     TIP: In order to assign a BMI code, the associated condition must meet the definition of a reportable diagnosis for nonoutpatient encounters, per section III of the *ICD-10-CM Official Guidelines for Coding and Reporting.*

     Z68.1 Body mass index [BMI] 19.9 or less, adult Ⓐ

✓5ᵗʰ **Z68.2 Body mass index [BMI] 2Ø-29, adult**
     Z68.2Ø Body mass index [BMI] 2Ø.Ø-2Ø.9, adult Ⓐ
     Z68.21 Body mass index [BMI] 21.Ø-21.9, adult Ⓐ
     Z68.22 Body mass index [BMI] 22.Ø-22.9, adult Ⓐ
     Z68.23 Body mass index [BMI] 23.Ø-23.9, adult Ⓐ
     Z68.24 Body mass index [BMI] 24.Ø-24.9, adult Ⓐ
     Z68.25 Body mass index [BMI] 25.Ø-25.9, adult Ⓐ
     Z68.26 Body mass index [BMI] 26.Ø-26.9, adult Ⓐ
     Z68.27 Body mass index [BMI] 27.Ø-27.9, adult Ⓐ

     Z68.28 Body mass index [BMI] 28.Ø-28.9, adult Ⓐ
     Z68.29 Body mass index [BMI] 29.Ø-29.9, adult Ⓐ

✓5ᵗʰ **Z68.3 Body mass index [BMI] 3Ø-39, adult**
     Z68.3Ø Body mass index [BMI] 3Ø.Ø-3Ø.9, adult Ⓐ
     Z68.31 Body mass index [BMI] 31.Ø-31.9, adult Ⓐ
     Z68.32 Body mass index [BMI] 32.Ø-32.9, adult Ⓐ
     Z68.33 Body mass index [BMI] 33.Ø-33.9, adult Ⓐ
     Z68.34 Body mass index [BMI] 34.Ø-34.9, adult Ⓐ
     Z68.35 Body mass index [BMI] 35.Ø-35.9, adult Ⓐ
     Z68.36 Body mass index [BMI] 36.Ø-36.9, adult Ⓐ
     Z68.37 Body mass index [BMI] 37.Ø-37.9, adult Ⓐ
     Z68.38 Body mass index [BMI] 38.Ø-38.9, adult Ⓐ
     Z68.39 Body mass index [BMI] 39.Ø-39.9, adult Ⓐ

✓5ᵗʰ **Z68.4 Body mass index [BMI] 4Ø or greater, adult**
     CC Excl: For CC codes in subcategory Z68.4: PDX collection 1494
     Z68.41 Body mass index [BMI] 4Ø.Ø-44.9, adult ᴴᶜᶜ Ⓐ
     Z68.42 Body mass index [BMI] 45.Ø-49.9, adult ᴴᶜᶜ Ⓐ
     Z68.43 Body mass index [BMI] 5Ø.Ø-59.9, adult ᶜᶜ ᴴᶜᶜ Ⓐ
     Z68.44 Body mass index [BMI] 6Ø.Ø-69.9, adult ᶜᶜ ᴴᶜᶜ Ⓐ
     Z68.45 Body mass index [BMI] 7Ø or greater, adult ᶜᶜ ᴴᶜᶜ Ⓐ

✓5ᵗʰ **Z68.5 Body mass index [BMI] pediatric**
     AHA: 2018,4Q,81-82
     Z68.51 Body mass index [BMI] pediatric, less than 5th percentile for age
     Z68.52 Body mass index [BMI] pediatric, 5th percentile to less than 85th percentile for age
     Z68.53 Body mass index [BMI] pediatric, 85th percentile to less than 95th percentile for age
     Z68.54 Body mass index [BMI] pediatric, greater than or equal to 95th percentile for age

Persons encountering health services in other circumstances (Z69-Z76)

✓4ᵗʰ **Z69 Encounter for mental health services for victim and perpetrator of abuse**
     INCLUDES counseling for victims and perpetrators of abuse

✓5ᵗʰ **Z69.Ø Encounter for mental health services for child abuse problems**

✓6ᵗʰ **Z69.Ø1 Encounter for mental health services for parental child abuse**

     Z69.Ø1Ø Encounter for mental health services for victim of parental child abuse ℙ
         Encounter for mental health services for victim of child abuse by parent
         Encounter for mental health services for victim of child neglect by parent
         Encounter for mental health services for victim of child psychological abuse by parent
         Encounter for mental health services for victim of child sexual abuse by parent

     Z69.Ø11 Encounter for mental health services for perpetrator of parental child abuse
         Encounter for mental health services for perpetrator of parental child neglect
         Encounter for mental health services for perpetrator of parental child psychological abuse
         Encounter for mental health services for perpetrator of parental child sexual abuse
         EXCLUDES 1 encounter for mental health services for non-parental child abuse (Z69.Ø2-)

√6ᵗʰ **Z69.02** **Encounter for mental health services for non-parental child abuse**

    Z69.020 **Encounter for mental health services for victim of non-parental child abuse**   P

        Encounter for mental health services for victim of non-parental child neglect

        Encounter for mental health services for victim of non-parental child psychological abuse

        Encounter for mental health services for victim of non-parental child sexual abuse

    Z69.021 **Encounter for mental health services for perpetrator of non-parental child abuse**

        Encounter for mental health services for perpetrator of non-parental child neglect

        Encounter for mental health services for perpetrator of non-parental child psychological abuse

        Encounter for mental health services for perpetrator of non-parental child sexual abuse

√5ᵗʰ **Z69.1** **Encounter for mental health services for spousal or partner abuse problems**

    Z69.11 **Encounter for mental health services for victim of spousal or partner abuse**

        Encounter for mental health services for victim of spouse or partner neglect

        Encounter for mental health services for victim of spouse or partner psychological abuse

        Encounter for mental health services for victim of spouse or partner violence, physical

    Z69.12 **Encounter for mental health services for perpetrator of spousal or partner abuse**

        Encounter for mental health services for perpetrator of spouse or partner neglect

        Encounter for mental health services for perpetrator of spouse or partner psychological abuse

        Encounter for mental health services for perpetrator of spouse or partner violence, physical

        Encounter for mental health services for perpetrator of spouse or partner violence, sexual

√5ᵗʰ **Z69.8** **Encounter for mental health services for victim or perpetrator of other abuse**

    Z69.81 **Encounter for mental health services for victim of other abuse**

        ~~Encounter for mental health services for perpetrator of non-spousal adult abuse~~

        Encounter for mental health services for victim of non-spousal adult abuse

        Encounter for mental health services for victim of spouse or partner violence, sexual

        Encounter for rape victim counseling

    Z69.82 **Encounter for mental health services for perpetrator of other abuse**

        ▶Encounter for mental health services for perpetrator of non-spousal adult abuse◀

√4ᵗʰ **Z70** **Counseling related to sexual attitude, behavior and orientation**

    INCLUDES   encounter for mental health services for sexual attitude, behavior and orientation

    EXCLUDES 2   *contraceptive or procreative counseling (Z30-Z31)*

Z70.0 **Counseling related to sexual attitude**

Z70.1 **Counseling related to patient's sexual behavior and orientation**

    Patient concerned regarding impotence

    Patient concerned regarding non-responsiveness

    Patient concerned regarding promiscuity

    Patient concerned regarding sexual orientation

Z70.2 **Counseling related to sexual behavior and orientation of third party**

    Advice sought regarding sexual behavior and orientation of child

    Advice sought regarding sexual behavior and orientation of partner

    Advice sought regarding sexual behavior and orientation of spouse

Z70.3 **Counseling related to combined concerns regarding sexual attitude, behavior and orientation**

Z70.8 **Other sex counseling**

    Encounter for sex education

Z70.9 **Sex counseling, unspecified**

√4ᵗʰ **Z71** **Persons encountering health services for other counseling and medical advice, not elsewhere classified**

    EXCLUDES 2   *contraceptive or procreation counseling (Z30-Z31)*

            sex counseling (Z70.-)

Z71.0 **Person encountering health services to consult on behalf of another person**

    Person encountering health services to seek advice or treatment for non-attending third party

    EXCLUDES 2   *anxiety (normal) about sick person in family (Z63.7)*

            expectant (adoptive) parent(s) pre-birth pediatrician visit (Z76.81)

Z71.1 **Person with feared health complaint in whom no diagnosis is made**

    Person encountering health services with feared condition which was not demonstrated

    Person encountering health services in which problem was normal state

    "Worried well"

    EXCLUDES 1   *medical observation for suspected diseases and conditions proven not to exist (Z03.-)*

Z71.2 **Person consulting for explanation of examination or test findings**

Z71.3 **Dietary counseling and surveillance**

    Use additional code for any associated underlying medical condition

    Use additional code to identify body mass index (BMI), if known (Z68.-)

√5ᵗʰ **Z71.4** **Alcohol abuse counseling and surveillance**

    Use additional code for alcohol abuse or dependence (F10.-)

    Z71.41 **Alcohol abuse counseling and surveillance of alcoholic**

    Z71.42 **Counseling for family member of alcoholic**

        Counseling for significant other, partner, or friend of alcoholic

√5ᵗʰ **Z71.5** **Drug abuse counseling and surveillance**

    Use additional code for drug abuse or dependence (F11-F16, F18-F19)

    Z71.51 **Drug abuse counseling and surveillance of drug abuser**

    Z71.52 **Counseling for family member of drug abuser**

        Counseling for significant other, partner, or friend of drug abuser

Z71.6 **Tobacco abuse counseling**

    Use additional code for nicotine dependence (F17.-)

Z71.7 **Human immunodeficiency virus [HIV] counseling**

√5ᵗʰ **Z71.8** **Other specified counseling**

    EXCLUDES 2   *counseling for contraception (Z30.0-)*

    AHA: 2017,4Q,27

    Z71.81 **Spiritual or religious counseling**

    Z71.82 **Exercise counseling**

    Z71.83 **Encounter for nonprocreative genetic counseling**

        EXCLUDES 1   *counseling for procreative genetics (Z31.5)*

             counseling for procreative management (Z31.6)

    Z71.84 **Encounter for health counseling related to travel**

        Encounter for health risk and safety counseling for (international) travel

        Code also, if applicable, encounter for immunization (Z23)

        EXCLUDES 2   *encounter for administrative examination (Z02.-)*

             encounter for other special examination without complaint, suspected or reported diagnosis (Z01.-)

    Z71.89 **Other specified counseling**

Z71.9 **Counseling, unspecified**

    Encounter for medical advice NOS

✔ Additional Character Required   √x7ᵗʰ Placeholder   Unacceptable PDx   Questionable PDx   Manifestation   Unspecified Dx   H1-H14 HAC   HCC CMS-HCC Dx   HIV HIV Dx

ICD-10-CM 2020   1295

✓4ᵗʰ **Z72 Problems related to lifestyle**

> *EXCLUDES 2*   problems related to life-management difficulty (Z73.-)
> problems related to socioeconomic and psychosocial circumstances (Z55-Z65)

Z72.0 Tobacco use
> Tobacco use NOS
> *EXCLUDES 1*   history of tobacco dependence (Z87.891)
> nicotine dependence (F17.2-)
> tobacco dependence (F17.2-)
> tobacco use during pregnancy (O99.33-)

Z72.3 Lack of physical exercise

Z72.4 Inappropriate diet and eating habits
> *EXCLUDES 1*   behavioral eating disorders of infancy or childhood (F98.2-F98.3)
> eating disorders (F50.-)
> lack of adequate food (Z59.4)
> malnutrition and other nutritional deficiencies (E40-E64)

✓5ᵗʰ **Z72.5 High risk sexual behavior**
> Promiscuity
> *EXCLUDES 1*   paraphilias (F65)

Z72.51 High risk heterosexual behavior

Z72.52 High risk homosexual behavior

Z72.53 High risk bisexual behavior

Z72.6 Gambling and betting
> *EXCLUDES 1*   compulsive or pathological gambling (F63.0)

✓5ᵗʰ **Z72.8 Other problems related to lifestyle**

✓6ᵗʰ **Z72.81 Antisocial behavior**
> *EXCLUDES 1*   conduct disorders (F91.-)

> **Z72.810 Child and adolescent antisocial behavior**   Ⓟ
> > Antisocial behavior (child) (adolescent) without manifest psychiatric disorder
> > Delinquency NOS
> > Group delinquency
> > Offenses in the context of gang membership
> > Stealing in company with others
> > Truancy from school

> **Z72.811 Adult antisocial behavior**   Ⓐ
> > Adult antisocial behavior without manifest psychiatric disorder

✓6ᵗʰ **Z72.82 Problems related to sleep**

> **Z72.820 Sleep deprivation**
> > Lack of adequate sleep
> > *EXCLUDES 1*   insomnia (G47.0-)

> **Z72.821 Inadequate sleep hygiene**
> > Bad sleep habits
> > Irregular sleep habits
> > Unhealthy sleep wake schedule
> > *EXCLUDES 1*   insomnia (F51.0-, G47.0-)

Z72.89 Other problems related to lifestyle
> Self-damaging behavior

Z72.9 Problem related to lifestyle, unspecified

✓4ᵗʰ **Z73 Problems related to life management difficulty**

> *EXCLUDES 2*   problems related to socioeconomic and psychosocial circumstances (Z55-Z65)

> **DEF:** State of emotional, mental, and physical exhaustion causing difficulties in managing personal, school, or work circumstances. It is usually due to prolonged stress or poor interpersonal relationship skills or parenting skills.

Z73.0 Burn-out

Z73.1 Type A behavior pattern

Z73.2 Lack of relaxation and leisure

Z73.3 Stress, not elsewhere classified
> Physical and mental strain NOS
> *EXCLUDES 1*   stress related to employment or unemployment (Z56.-)

Z73.4 Inadequate social skills, not elsewhere classified

Z73.5 Social role conflict, not elsewhere classified

Z73.6 Limitation of activities due to disability
> *EXCLUDES 1*   care-provider dependency (Z74.-)

✓5ᵗʰ **Z73.8 Other problems related to life management difficulty**

✓6ᵗʰ **Z73.81 Behavioral insomnia of childhood**
> **DEF:** Behaviors on the part of the child or caregivers that cause negative compliance with a child's sleep schedule resulting in lack of adequate sleep.

> **Z73.810 Behavioral insomnia of childhood, sleep-onset association type**   Ⓟ

> **Z73.811 Behavioral insomnia of childhood, limit setting type**   Ⓟ

> **Z73.812 Behavioral insomnia of childhood, combined type**   Ⓟ

> **Z73.819 Behavioral insomnia of childhood, unspecified type**   Ⓟ

Z73.82 Dual sensory impairment

Z73.89 Other problems related to life management difficulty

Z73.9 Problem related to life management difficulty, unspecified

✓4ᵗʰ **Z74 Problems related to care provider dependency**

> *EXCLUDES 2*   dependence on enabling machines or devices NEC (Z99.-)

✓5ᵗʰ **Z74.0 Reduced mobility**

> **Z74.01 Bed confinement status**
> > Bedridden

> **Z74.09 Other reduced mobility**
> > Chair ridden
> > Reduced mobility NOS
> > *EXCLUDES 2*   wheelchair dependence (Z99.3)

Z74.1 Need for assistance with personal care

Z74.2 Need for assistance at home and no other household member able to render care

Z74.3 Need for continuous supervision

Z74.8 Other problems related to care provider dependency

Z74.9 Problem related to care provider dependency, unspecified

✓4ᵗʰ **Z75 Problems related to medical facilities and other health care**

Z75.0 Medical services not available in home
> *EXCLUDES 1*   no other household member able to render care (Z74.2)

Z75.1 Person awaiting admission to adequate facility elsewhere

Z75.2 Other waiting period for investigation and treatment

Z75.3 Unavailability and inaccessibility of health-care facilities
> *EXCLUDES 1*   bed unavailable (Z75.1)

Z75.4 Unavailability and inaccessibility of other helping agencies

Z75.5 Holiday relief care

Z75.8 Other problems related to medical facilities and other health care

Z75.9 Unspecified problem related to medical facilities and other health care

✓4ᵗʰ **Z76 Persons encountering health services in other circumstances**

Z76.0 Encounter for issue of repeat prescription
> Encounter for issue of repeat prescription for appliance
> Encounter for issue of repeat prescription for medicaments
> Encounter for issue of repeat prescription for spectacles
> *EXCLUDES 2*   issue of medical certificate (Z02.7)
> repeat prescription for contraceptive (Z30.4-)

Z76.1 Encounter for health supervision and care of foundling

Z76.2 Encounter for health supervision and care of other healthy infant and child   Ⓟ
> Encounter for medical or nursing care or supervision of healthy infant under circumstances such as adverse socioeconomic conditions at home
> Encounter for medical or nursing care or supervision of healthy infant under circumstances such as awaiting foster or adoptive placement
> Encounter for medical or nursing care or supervision of healthy infant under circumstances such as maternal illness
> Encounter for medical or nursing care or supervision of healthy infant under circumstances such as number of children at home preventing or interfering with normal care

Z76.3 Healthy person accompanying sick person

Z76.4 Other boarder to healthcare facility
> *EXCLUDES 1*   homelessness (Z59.0)

Ⓝ Newborn: 0   Ⓟ Pediatric: 0-17   Ⓜ Maternity: 9-64   Ⓐ Adult: 15-124   **MCC** Major Complication/Comorbidity   **CC** Complication/Comorbidity   **SW** Severe Wound Dx

1296   ICD-10-CM 2020

Z76.5 Malingerer [conscious simulation]
Person feigning illness (with obvious motivation)
    EXCLUDES 1   factitious disorder (F68.1-, F68.A)
          peregrinating patient (F68.1-)
DEF: Act of intentionally exaggerating an illness or disability in order to receive personal gain or to avoid punishment or responsibility.

✓5th **Z76.8 Persons encountering health services in other specified circumstances**

Z76.81 Expectant parent(s) prebirth pediatrician visit
Pre-adoption pediatrician visit for adoptive parent(s)

Z76.82 Awaiting organ transplant status
Patient waiting for organ availability

Z76.89 Persons encountering health services in other specified circumstances
Persons encountering health services NOS
AHA: 2014,2Q,10

Persons with potential health hazards related to family and personal history and certain conditions influencing health status (Z77-Z99)

Code also any follow-up examination (Z08-Z09)

✓4th **Z77 Other contact with and (suspected) exposures hazardous to health**
    INCLUDES   contact with and (suspected) exposures to potential hazards to health
    EXCLUDES 2   contact with and (suspected) exposure to communicable diseases (Z20.-)
          exposure to (parental) (environmental) tobacco smoke in the perinatal period (P96.81)
          newborn affected by noxious substances transmitted via placenta or breast milk (P04.-)
          occupational exposure to risk factors (Z57.-)
          retained foreign body (Z18.-)
          retained foreign body fully removed (Z87.821)
          toxic effects of substances chiefly nonmedicinal as to source (T51-T65)

✓5th **Z77.0 Contact with and (suspected) exposure to hazardous, chiefly nonmedicinal, chemicals**

✓6th **Z77.01 Contact with and (suspected) exposure to hazardous metals**

Z77.010 Contact with and (suspected) exposure to arsenic

Z77.011 Contact with and (suspected) exposure to lead

Z77.012 Contact with and (suspected) exposure to uranium
    EXCLUDES 1   retained depleted uranium fragments (Z18.01)

Z77.018 Contact with and (suspected) exposure to other hazardous metals
Contact with and (suspected) exposure to chromium compounds
Contact with and (suspected) exposure to nickel dust

✓6th **Z77.02 Contact with and (suspected) exposure to hazardous aromatic compounds**

Z77.020 Contact with and (suspected) exposure to aromatic amines

Z77.021 Contact with and (suspected) exposure to benzene

Z77.028 Contact with and (suspected) exposure to other hazardous aromatic compounds
Aromatic dyes NOS
Polycyclic aromatic hydrocarbons

✓6th **Z77.09 Contact with and (suspected) exposure to other hazardous, chiefly nonmedicinal, chemicals**

Z77.090 Contact with and (suspected) exposure to asbestos

Z77.098 Contact with and (suspected) exposure to other hazardous, chiefly nonmedicinal, chemicals
Dyes NOS

✓5th **Z77.1 Contact with and (suspected) exposure to environmental pollution and hazards in the physical environment**

✓6th **Z77.11 Contact with and (suspected) exposure to environmental pollution**

Z77.110 Contact with and (suspected) exposure to air pollution

Z77.111 Contact with and (suspected) exposure to water pollution

Z77.112 Contact with and (suspected) exposure to soil pollution

Z77.118 Contact with and (suspected) exposure to other environmental pollution

✓6th **Z77.12 Contact with and (suspected) exposure to hazards in the physical environment**

Z77.120 Contact with and (suspected) exposure to mold (toxic)

Z77.121 Contact with and (suspected) exposure to harmful algae and algae toxins
Contact with and (suspected) exposure to (harmful) algae bloom NOS
Contact with and (suspected) exposure to blue-green algae bloom
Contact with and (suspected) exposure to brown tide
Contact with and (suspected) exposure to cyanobacteria bloom
Contact with and (suspected) exposure to Florida red tide
Contact with and (suspected) exposure to pfiesteria piscicida
Contact with and (suspected) exposure to red tide

Z77.122 Contact with and (suspected) exposure to noise

Z77.123 Contact with and (suspected) exposure to radon and other naturally occurring radiation
    EXCLUDES 2   radiation exposure as the cause of a confirmed condition (W88-W90, X39.0-)
          radiation sickness NOS (T66)

Z77.128 Contact with and (suspected) exposure to other hazards in the physical environment

✓5th **Z77.2 Contact with and (suspected) exposure to other hazardous substances**

Z77.21 Contact with and (suspected) exposure to potentially hazardous body fluids

Z77.22 Contact with and (suspected) exposure to environmental tobacco smoke (acute) (chronic)
Exposure to second hand tobacco smoke (acute) (chronic)
Passive smoking (acute) (chronic)
    EXCLUDES 1   nicotine dependence (F17.-)
          tobacco use (Z72.0)
    EXCLUDES 2   occupational exposure to environmental tobacco smoke (Z57.31)

Z77.29 Contact with and (suspected) exposure to other hazardous substances
AHA: 2016,2Q,33

Z77.9 Other contact with and (suspected) exposures hazardous to health

✓4th **Z78 Other specified health status**
    EXCLUDES 2   asymptomatic human immunodeficiency virus [HIV] infection status (Z21)
          postprocedural status (Z93-Z99)
          sex reassignment status (Z87.890)

Z78.0 Asymptomatic menopausal state   A ♀
Menopausal state NOS
Postmenopausal status NOS
    EXCLUDES 2   symptomatic menopausal state (N95.1)

Z78.1 Physical restraint status
    EXCLUDES 1   physical restraint due to a procedure — omit code
DEF: Application of mechanical restraining devices or manual restraints to limit physical mobility of a patient.

Z78.9 Other specified health status

☑4ᵗʰ Z79 Long term (current) drug therapy

INCLUDES long term (current) drug use for prophylactic purposes

Code also any therapeutic drug level monitoring (Z51.81)

EXCLUDES 2 *drug abuse and dependence (F11-F19)*

drug use complicating pregnancy, childbirth, and the puerperium (O99.32-)

long term (current) use of oral antidiabetic drugs (Z79.84)

long term (current) use of oral hypoglycemic drugs (Z79.84)

☑5ᵗʰ Z79.0 Long term (current) use of anticoagulants and antithrombotics/antiplatelets

EXCLUDES 2 *long term (current) use of aspirin (Z79.82)*

Z79.01 Long term (current) use of anticoagulants

Z79.02 Long term (current) use of antithrombotics/antiplatelets

Z79.1 Long term (current) use of non-steroidal anti-inflammatories (NSAID)

EXCLUDES 2 *long term (current) use of aspirin (Z79.82)*

Z79.2 Long term (current) use of antibiotics

Z79.3 Long term (current) use of hormonal contraceptives

Long term (current) use of birth control pill or patch

Z79.4 Long term (current) use of insulin ᴴᶜᶜ

TIP: When both long-term (current) insulin and long-term (current) oral hypoglycemic use is documented, assign only a code for the long-term insulin use.

☑5ᵗʰ Z79.5 Long term (current) use of steroids

Z79.51 Long term (current) use of inhaled steroids

Z79.52 Long term (current) use of systemic steroids

☑5ᵗʰ Z79.8 Other long term (current) drug therapy

☑6ᵗʰ Z79.81 Long term (current) use of agents affecting estrogen receptors and estrogen levels

Code first, if applicable:

malignant neoplasm of breast (C50.-)

malignant neoplasm of prostate (C61)

Use additional code, if applicable, to identify:

estrogen receptor positive status (Z17.0)

family history of breast cancer (Z80.3)

genetic susceptibility to malignant neoplasm (cancer) (Z15.0-)

personal history of breast cancer (Z85.3)

personal history of prostate cancer (Z85.46)

postmenopausal status (Z78.0)

EXCLUDES 1 *hormone replacement therapy (Z79.890)*

Z79.810 Long term (current) use of selective estrogen receptor modulators (SERMs)

Long term (current) use of raloxifene (Evista)

Long term (current) use of tamoxifen (Nolvadex)

Long term (current) use of toremifene (Fareston)

Z79.811 Long term (current) use of aromatase inhibitors

Long term (current) use of anastrozole (Arimidex)

Long term (current) use of exemestane (Aromasin)

Long term (current) use of letrozole (Femara)

Z79.818 Long term (current) use of other agents affecting estrogen receptors and estrogen levels

Long term (current) use of estrogen receptor downregulators

Long term (current) use of fulvestrant (Faslodex)

Long term (current) use of gonadotropin-releasing hormone (GnRH) agonist

Long term (current) use of goserelin acetate (Zoladex)

Long term (current) use of leuprolide acetate (leuprorelin) (Lupron)

Long term (current) use of megestrol acetate (Megace)

Z79.82 Long term (current) use of aspirin

Z79.83 Long term (current) use of bisphosphonates

AHA: 2016,4Q,42

Z79.84 Long term (current) use of oral hypoglycemic drugs

Long term (current) use of oral antidiabetic drugs

EXCLUDES 2 *long term (current) use of insulin (Z79.4)*

AHA: 2016,4Q,76

TIP: When both long-term (current) insulin and long-term (current) oral hypoglycemic use is documented, assign only code Z79.4 for the long-term insulin use.

☑6ᵗʰ Z79.89 Other long term (current) drug therapy

Z79.890 Hormone replacement therapy

Z79.891 Long term (current) use of opiate analgesic

Long term (current) use of methadone for pain management

EXCLUDES 1 *methadone use NOS (F11.9-)*

use of methodone for treatment of heroin addiction (F11.2-)

Z79.899 Other long term (current) drug therapy

AHA: 2015,4Q,34; 2015,3Q,21

☑4ᵗʰ Z80 Family history of primary malignant neoplasm

Z80.0 Family history of malignant neoplasm of digestive organs

Conditions classifiable to C15-C26

AHA: 2018,1Q,6

Z80.1 Family history of malignant neoplasm of trachea, bronchus and lung

Conditions classifiable to C33-C34

Z80.2 Family history of malignant neoplasm of other respiratory and intrathoracic organs

Conditions classifiable to C30-C32, C37-C39

Z80.3 Family history of malignant neoplasm of breast

Conditions classifiable to C50.-

☑5ᵗʰ Z80.4 Family history of malignant neoplasm of genital organs

Conditions classifiable to C51-C63

Z80.41 Family history of malignant neoplasm of ovary

Z80.42 Family history of malignant neoplasm of prostate

Z80.43 Family history of malignant neoplasm of testis

Z80.49 Family history of malignant neoplasm of other genital organs

☑5ᵗʰ Z80.5 Family history of malignant neoplasm of urinary tract

Conditions classifiable to C64-C68

Z80.51 Family history of malignant neoplasm of kidney

Z80.52 Family history of malignant neoplasm of bladder

Z80.59 Family history of malignant neoplasm of other urinary tract organ

Z80.6 Family history of leukemia

Conditions classifiable to C91-C95

Z80.7 Family history of other malignant neoplasms of lymphoid, hematopoietic and related tissues

Conditions classifiable to C81-C90, C96.-

Z80.8 Family history of malignant neoplasm of other organs or systems

Conditions classifiable to C00-C14, C40-C49, C69-C79

Z80.9 Family history of malignant neoplasm, unspecified

Conditions classifiable to C80.1

☑4ᵗʰ Z81 Family history of mental and behavioral disorders

Z81.0 Family history of intellectual disabilities

Conditions classifiable to F70-F79

Z81.1 Family history of alcohol abuse and dependence

Conditions classifiable to F10.-

Z81.2 Family history of tobacco abuse and dependence

Conditions classifiable to F17.-

Z81.3 Family history of other psychoactive substance abuse and dependence

Conditions classifiable to F11-F16, F18-F19

Z81.4 Family history of other substance abuse and dependence

Conditions classifiable to F55

Z81.8 Family history of other mental and behavioral disorders

Conditions classifiable elsewhere in F01-F99

☑4ᵗʰ Z82 Family history of certain disabilities and chronic diseases (leading to disablement)

Z82.0 Family history of epilepsy and other diseases of the nervous system

Conditions classifiable to G00-G99

Z82.1 Family history of blindness and visual loss

Conditions classifiable to H54.-

History

N Newborn: 0   **P** Pediatric: 0-17   **M** Maternity: 9-64   **A** Adult: 15-124   **MCC** Major Complication/Comorbidity   **CC** Complication/Comorbidity   **SW** Severe Wound Dx

1298   ICD-10-CM 2020

Z82.2   **Family history of deafness and hearing loss**
Conditions classifiable to H90-H91

Z82.3   **Family history of stroke**
Conditions classifiable to I60-I64

✓5ᵗʰ **Z82.4**   **Family history of ischemic heart disease and other diseases of the circulatory system**
Conditions classifiable to I00-I52, I65-I99

     Z82.41   **Family history of sudden cardiac death**

     Z82.49   **Family history of ischemic heart disease and other diseases of the circulatory system**

Z82.5   **Family history of asthma and other chronic lower respiratory diseases**
Conditions classifiable to J40-J47
     EXCLUDES 2   *family history of other diseases of the respiratory system (Z83.6)*

✓5ᵗʰ **Z82.6**   **Family history of arthritis and other diseases of the musculoskeletal system and connective tissue**
Conditions classifiable to M00-M99

     Z82.61   **Family history of arthritis**

     Z82.62   **Family history of osteoporosis**

     Z82.69   **Family history of other diseases of the musculoskeletal system and connective tissue**

✓5ᵗʰ **Z82.7**   **Family history of congenital malformations, deformations and chromosomal abnormalities**
Conditions classifiable to Q00-Q99

     Z82.71   **Family history of polycystic kidney**

     Z82.79   **Family history of other congenital malformations, deformations and chromosomal abnormalities**

Z82.8   **Family history of other disabilities and chronic diseases leading to disablement, not elsewhere classified**

✓4ᵗʰ **Z83**   **Family history of other specific disorders**
     EXCLUDES 2   *contact with and (suspected) exposure to communicable disease in the family (Z20.-)*

Z83.0   **Family history of human immunodeficiency virus [HIV] disease**
Conditions classifiable to B20

Z83.1   **Family history of other infectious and parasitic diseases**
Conditions classifiable to A00-B19, B25-B94, B99

Z83.2   **Family history of diseases of the blood and blood-forming organs and certain disorders involving the immune mechanism**
Conditions classifiable to D50-D89

Z83.3   **Family history of diabetes mellitus**
Conditions classifiable to E08-E13

✓5ᵗʰ **Z83.4**   **Family history of other endocrine, nutritional and metabolic diseases**
Conditions classifiable to E00-E07, E15-E88

     Z83.41   **Family history of multiple endocrine neoplasia [MEN] syndrome**

     Z83.42   **Family history of familial hypercholesterolemia**
     AHA: 2016,4Q,77

     ✓6ᵗʰ **Z83.43**   **Family history of other disorder of lipoprotein metabolism and other lipidemias**
     AHA: 2018,4Q,6,35

         Z83.430   **Family history of elevated lipoprotein(a)**
Family history of elevated Lp(a)

         Z83.438   **Family history of other disorder of lipoprotein metabolism and other lipidemia**
Family history of familial combined hyperlipidemia

     Z83.49   **Family history of other endocrine, nutritional and metabolic diseases**

✓5ᵗʰ **Z83.5**   **Family history of eye and ear disorders**

     ✓6ᵗʰ **Z83.51**   **Family history of eye disorders**
Conditions classifiable to H00-H53, H55-H59
     EXCLUDES 2   *family history of blindness and visual loss (Z82.1)*

         Z83.511   **Family history of glaucoma**

         Z83.518   **Family history of other specified eye disorder**

     Z83.52   **Family history of ear disorders**
Conditions classifiable to H60-H83, H92-H95
     EXCLUDES 2   *family history of deafness and hearing loss (Z82.2)*

Z83.6   **Family history of other diseases of the respiratory system**
Conditions classifiable to J00-J39, J60-J99
     EXCLUDES 2   *family history of asthma and other chronic lower respiratory diseases (Z82.5)*

✓5ᵗʰ **Z83.7**   **Family history of diseases of the digestive system**
Conditions classifiable to K00-K93

     Z83.71   **Family history of colonic polyps**
     EXCLUDES 2   *family history of malignant neoplasm of digestive organs (Z80.0)*

     Z83.79   **Family history of other diseases of the digestive system**

✓4ᵗʰ **Z84**   **Family history of other conditions**

Z84.0   **Family history of diseases of the skin and subcutaneous tissue**
Conditions classifiable to L00-L99

Z84.1   **Family history of disorders of kidney and ureter**
Conditions classifiable to N00-N29

Z84.2   **Family history of other diseases of the genitourinary system**
Conditions classifiable to N30-N99

Z84.3   **Family history of consanguinity**

✓5ᵗʰ **Z84.8**   **Family history of other specified conditions**

     Z84.81   **Family history of carrier of genetic disease**

     Z84.82   **Family history of sudden infant death syndrome**
Family history of SIDS
     AHA: 2016,4Q,77

     Z84.89   **Family history of other specified conditions**

✓4ᵗʰ **Z85**   **Personal history of malignant neoplasm**
Code first any follow-up examination after treatment of malignant neoplasm (Z08)
Use additional code to identify:
    alcohol use and dependence (F10.-)
    exposure to environmental tobacco smoke (Z77.22)
    history of tobacco dependence (Z87.891)
    occupational exposure to environmental tobacco smoke (Z57.31)
    tobacco dependence (F17.-)
    tobacco use (Z72.0)
     EXCLUDES 2   *personal history of benign neoplasm (Z86.01-)*
         personal history of carcinoma-in-situ (Z86.00-)
AHA: 2018,4Q,64

✓5ᵗʰ **Z85.0**   **Personal history of malignant neoplasm of digestive organs**
     AHA: 2017,1Q,9

     Z85.00   **Personal history of malignant neoplasm of unspecified digestive organ**

     Z85.01   **Personal history of malignant neoplasm of esophagus**
Conditions classifiable to C15

     ✓6ᵗʰ **Z85.02**   **Personal history of malignant neoplasm of stomach**

         Z85.020   **Personal history of malignant carcinoid tumor of stomach**
Conditions classifiable to C7A.092

         Z85.028   **Personal history of other malignant neoplasm of stomach**
Conditions classifiable to C16

     ✓6ᵗʰ **Z85.03**   **Personal history of malignant neoplasm of large intestine**

         Z85.030   **Personal history of malignant carcinoid tumor of large intestine**
Conditions classifiable to C7A.022-C7A.025, C7A.029

         Z85.038   **Personal history of other malignant neoplasm of large intestine**
Conditions classifiable to C18

     ✓6ᵗʰ **Z85.04**   **Personal history of malignant neoplasm of rectum, rectosigmoid junction, and anus**

         Z85.040   **Personal history of malignant carcinoid tumor of rectum**
Conditions classifiable to C7A.026

         Z85.048   **Personal history of other malignant neoplasm of rectum, rectosigmoid junction, and anus**
Conditions classifiable to C19-C21

     Z85.05   **Personal history of malignant neoplasm of liver**
Conditions classifiable to C22

✔ Additional Character Required   ✓x7ᵗʰ Placeholder   Unacceptable PDx   Questionable PDx   Manifestation   Unspecified Dx   H1-H14 HAC   HCC CMS-HCC Dx   HIV HIV Dx

ICD-10-CM 2020   1299

Chapter 21. Factors Influencing Health Status and Contact With Health Services

Z82.2–Z85.05

☑6ᵗʰ **Z85.06** **Personal history of malignant neoplasm of** small intestine

     Z85.060 **Personal history of malignant** carcinoid tumor **of small intestine**
         Conditions classifiable to C7A.01-

     Z85.068 **Personal history of other malignant neoplasm of small intestine**
         Conditions classifiable to C17

Z85.07 **Personal history of malignant neoplasm of** pancreas
     Conditions classifiable to C25

Z85.09 **Personal history of malignant neoplasm of other digestive organs**

☑5ᵗʰ **Z85.1** **Personal history of malignant neoplasm of** trachea, bronchus and lung

   ☑6ᵗʰ **Z85.11** **Personal history of malignant neoplasm of** bronchus and lung

     Z85.110 **Personal history of malignant** carcinoid tumor **of bronchus and lung**
         Conditions classifiable to C7A.090

     Z85.118 **Personal history of other malignant neoplasm of bronchus and lung**
         Conditions classifiable to C34

   Z85.12 **Personal history of malignant neoplasm of** trachea
     Conditions classifiable to C33

☑5ᵗʰ **Z85.2** **Personal history of malignant neoplasm of other** respiratory and intrathoracic organs

   Z85.20 **Personal history of malignant neoplasm of unspecified respiratory organ**

   Z85.21 **Personal history of malignant neoplasm of** larynx
     Conditions classifiable to C32

   Z85.22 **Personal history of malignant neoplasm of** nasal cavities, middle ear, and accessory sinuses
     Conditions classifiable to C30-C31

   ☑6ᵗʰ **Z85.23** **Personal history of malignant neoplasm of** thymus

     Z85.230 **Personal history of malignant** carcinoid tumor **of thymus**
         Conditions classifiable to C7A.091

     Z85.238 **Personal history of other malignant neoplasm of thymus**
         Conditions classifiable to C37

   Z85.29 **Personal history of malignant neoplasm of other respiratory and intrathoracic organs**

Z85.3 **Personal history of malignant neoplasm of** breast
     Conditions classifiable to C50.-

☑5ᵗʰ **Z85.4** **Personal history of malignant neoplasm of** genital organs
     Conditions classifiable to C51-C63

   Z85.40 **Personal history of malignant neoplasm of unspecified** female **genital organ** ♀

   Z85.41 **Personal history of malignant neoplasm of** cervix uteri ♀

   Z85.42 **Personal history of malignant neoplasm of other parts of uterus** ♀

   Z85.43 **Personal history of malignant neoplasm of ovary** ♀

   Z85.44 **Personal history of malignant neoplasm of other** female **genital organs** ♀

   Z85.45 **Personal history of malignant neoplasm of unspecified** male **genital organ** ♂

   Z85.46 **Personal history of malignant neoplasm of** prostate ♂

   Z85.47 **Personal history of malignant neoplasm of testis** ♂

   Z85.48 **Personal history of malignant neoplasm of** epididymis ♂

   Z85.49 **Personal history of malignant neoplasm of other** male **genital organs** ♂

☑5ᵗʰ **Z85.5** **Personal history of malignant neoplasm of** urinary tract
     Conditions classifiable to C64-C68

   Z85.50 **Personal history of malignant neoplasm of unspecified urinary tract organ**

   Z85.51 **Personal history of malignant neoplasm of** bladder

   ☑6ᵗʰ **Z85.52** **Personal history of malignant neoplasm of** kidney
     EXCLUDES 1   *personal history of malignant neoplasm of renal pelvis (Z85.53)*

     Z85.520 **Personal history of malignant** carcinoid tumor **of kidney**
         Conditions classifiable to C7A.093

     Z85.528 **Personal history of other malignant neoplasm of kidney**
         Conditions classifiable to C64

   Z85.53 **Personal history of malignant neoplasm of** renal pelvis

   Z85.54 **Personal history of malignant neoplasm of** ureter

   Z85.59 **Personal history of malignant neoplasm of other urinary tract organ**

Z85.6 **Personal history of** leukemia
     Conditions classifiable to C91-C95
     EXCLUDES 1   *leukemia in remission C91.0-C95.9 with 5th character 1*

☑5ᵗʰ **Z85.7** **Personal history of other malignant neoplasms of lymphoid, hematopoietic and related tissues**

   Z85.71 **Personal history of** Hodgkin lymphoma
     Conditions classifiable to C81

   Z85.72 **Personal history of** non-Hodgkin lymphomas
     Conditions classifiable to C82-C85

   Z85.79 **Personal history of other malignant neoplasms of lymphoid, hematopoietic and related tissues**
     Conditions classifiable to C88-C90, C96
     EXCLUDES 1   *multiple myeloma in remission (C90.01)*
         plasma cell leukemia in remission (C90.11)
         plasmacytoma in remission (C90.21)

☑5ᵗʰ **Z85.8** **Personal history of malignant neoplasms of other organs and systems**
     Conditions classifiable to C00-C14, C40-C49, C69-C75, C7A.098, C76-C79

   ☑6ᵗʰ **Z85.81** **Personal history of malignant neoplasm of** lip, oral cavity, and pharynx

     Z85.810 **Personal history of malignant neoplasm of** tongue

     Z85.818 **Personal history of malignant neoplasm of other sites of lip, oral cavity, and pharynx**

     Z85.819 **Personal history of malignant neoplasm of unspecified site of lip, oral cavity, and pharynx**

   ☑6ᵗʰ **Z85.82** **Personal history of malignant neoplasm of** skin

     Z85.820 **Personal history of malignant** melanoma **of skin**
         Conditions classifiable to C43

     Z85.821 **Personal history of** Merkel cell carcinoma
         Conditions classifiable to C4A

     Z85.828 **Personal history of other malignant neoplasm of skin**
         Conditions classifiable to C44

   ☑6ᵗʰ **Z85.83** **Personal history of malignant neoplasm of** bone and soft tissue

     Z85.830 **Personal history of malignant neoplasm of bone**

     Z85.831 **Personal history of malignant neoplasm of** soft tissue
         EXCLUDES 2   *personal history of malignant neoplasm of skin (Z85.82-)*

   ☑6ᵗʰ **Z85.84** **Personal history of malignant neoplasm of** eye and nervous tissue

     Z85.840 **Personal history of malignant neoplasm of eye**

     Z85.841 **Personal history of malignant neoplasm of brain**

     Z85.848 **Personal history of malignant neoplasm of other parts of nervous tissue**

   ☑6ᵗʰ **Z85.85** **Personal history of malignant neoplasm of endocrine glands**

     Z85.850 **Personal history of malignant neoplasm of** thyroid

     Z85.858 **Personal history of malignant neoplasm of other endocrine glands**

   Z85.89 **Personal history of malignant neoplasm of other organs and systems**

Z85.9 **Personal history of malignant neoplasm, unspecified**
     Conditions classifiable to C7A.00, C80.1

✓4ᵗʰ **Z86 Personal history of certain other diseases**

> Code first any follow-up examination after treatment (Z09)

✓5ᵗʰ **Z86.0 Personal history of in-situ and benign neoplasms and neoplasms of uncertain behavior**

> EXCLUDES 2 *personal history of malignant neoplasms (Z85.-)*
>
> AHA: 2017,1Q,9

✓6ᵗʰ **Z86.00 Personal history of in-situ neoplasm**

> Conditions classifiable to D00-D09

Z86.000 Personal history of in-situ neoplasm of breast

> ▶Conditions classifiable to D05◀

Z86.001 Personal history of in-situ neoplasm of cervix uteri ♀

> ▶Conditions classifiable to D06◀
>
> Personal history of cervical intraepithelial neoplasia III [CIN III]

Z86.002 Personal history of in-situ neoplasm of other and unspecified genital organs

> Conditions classifiable to D07
>
> Personal history of high-grade prostatic intraepithelial neoplasia III [HGPIN III]
>
> Personal history of vaginal intraepithelial neoplasia III [VAIN III]
>
> Personal history of vulvar intraepithelial neoplasia III [VIN III]

Z86.003 Personal history of in-situ neoplasm of oral cavity, esophagus and stomach

> Conditions classifiable to D00

Z86.004 Personal history of in-situ neoplasm of other and unspecified digestive organs

> Conditions classifiable to D01
>
> Personal history of anal intraepithelial neoplasia (AIN III)

Z86.005 Personal history of in-situ neoplasm of middle ear and respiratory system

> Conditions classifiable to D02

Z86.006 Personal history of melanoma in-situ

> Conditions classifiable to D03
>
> EXCLUDES 2 *sites other than skin — code to personal history of in-situ neoplasm of the site*

Z86.007 Personal history of in-situ neoplasm of skin

> Conditions classifiable to D04
>
> Personal history of carcinoma in situ of skin

Z86.008 Personal history of in-situ neoplasm of other site

> ▶Conditions classifiable to D09◀
>
> ~~Personal history of vaginal intraepithelial neoplasia III [VAIN III]~~
>
> ~~Personal history of vulvar intraepithelial neoplasia III [VIN III]~~

✓6ᵗʰ **Z86.01 Personal history of benign neoplasm**

Z86.010 Personal history of colonic polyps

> AHA: 2017,1Q,14

Z86.011 Personal history of benign neoplasm of the brain

Z86.012 Personal history of benign carcinoid tumor

Z86.018 Personal history of other benign neoplasm

> AHA: 2017,1Q,14

Z86.03 Personal history of neoplasm of uncertain behavior

✓5ᵗʰ **Z86.1 Personal history of infectious and parasitic diseases**

> Conditions classifiable to A00-B89, B99
>
> EXCLUDES 1 *personal history of infectious diseases specific to a body system*
>
> *sequelae of infectious and parasitic diseases (B90-B94)*

Z86.11 Personal history of tuberculosis

Z86.12 Personal history of poliomyelitis

Z86.13 Personal history of malaria

Z86.14 Personal history of Methicillin resistant Staphylococcus aureus infection

> Personal history of MRSA infection

Z86.15 Personal history of latent tuberculosis infection

Z86.19 Personal history of other infectious and parasitic diseases

Z86.2 Personal history of diseases of the blood and blood-forming organs and certain disorders involving the immune mechanism

> Conditions classifiable to D50-D89

✓5ᵗʰ **Z86.3 Personal history of endocrine, nutritional and metabolic diseases**

> Conditions classifiable to E00-E88

Z86.31 Personal history of diabetic foot ulcer

> EXCLUDES 2 *current diabetic foot ulcer (E08.621, E09.621, E10.621, E11.621, E13.621)*

Z86.32 Personal history of gestational diabetes ♀

> Personal history of conditions classifiable to O24.4-
>
> EXCLUDES 1 *gestational diabetes mellitus in current pregnancy (O24.4-)*

Z86.39 Personal history of other endocrine, nutritional and metabolic disease

✓5ᵗʰ **Z86.5 Personal history of mental and behavioral disorders**

> Conditions classifiable to F40-F59

Z86.51 Personal history of combat and operational stress reaction A

Z86.59 Personal history of other mental and behavioral disorders

✓5ᵗʰ **Z86.6 Personal history of diseases of the nervous system and sense organs**

> Conditions classifiable to G00-G99, H00-H95

Z86.61 Personal history of infections of the central nervous system

> Personal history of encephalitis
>
> Personal history of meningitis

Z86.69 Personal history of other diseases of the nervous system and sense organs

> AHA: 2016,4Q,24

✓5ᵗʰ **Z86.7 Personal history of diseases of the circulatory system**

> Conditions classifiable to I00-I99
>
> EXCLUDES 2 *old myocardial infarction (I25.2)*
>
> *personal history of anaphylactic shock (Z87.892)*
>
> *postmyocardial infarction syndrome (I24.1)*

✓6ᵗʰ **Z86.71 Personal history of venous thrombosis and embolism**

Z86.711 Personal history of pulmonary embolism

Z86.718 Personal history of other venous thrombosis and embolism

Z86.72 Personal history of thrombophlebitis

Z86.73 Personal history of transient ischemic attack (TIA), and cerebral infarction without residual deficits

> Personal history of prolonged reversible ischemic neurological deficit (PRIND)
>
> Personal history of stroke NOS without residual deficits
>
> EXCLUDES 1 *personal history of traumatic brain injury (Z87.820)*
>
> *sequelae of cerebrovascular disease (I69.-)*
>
> AHA: 2012,4Q,92

Z86.74 Personal history of sudden cardiac arrest

> Personal history of sudden cardiac death successfully resuscitated

Z86.79 Personal history of other diseases of the circulatory system

✓4ᵗʰ **Z87 Personal history of other diseases and conditions**

> Code first any follow-up examination after treatment (Z09)

✓5ᵗʰ **Z87.0 Personal history of diseases of the respiratory system**

> Conditions classifiable to J00-J99

Z87.01 Personal history of pneumonia (recurrent)

Z87.09 Personal history of other diseases of the respiratory system

✓5ᵗʰ **Z87.1 Personal history of diseases of the digestive system**

> Conditions classifiable to K00-K93

Z87.11 Personal history of peptic ulcer disease

Z87.19 Personal history of other diseases of the digestive system

> AHA: 2017,1Q,14

Z87.2 Personal history of diseases of the skin and subcutaneous tissue

> Conditions classifiable to L00-L99
>
> EXCLUDES 2 *personal history of diabetic foot ulcer (Z86.31)*

✔ Additional Character Required ✗7ᵗʰ Placeholder Unacceptable PDx Questionable PDx Manifestation Unspecified Dx H1-H14 HAC HCC CMS-HCC Dx HIV HIV Dx

ICD-10-CM 2020   1301

✓5ᵗʰ Z87.3　Personal history of diseases of the musculoskeletal system and connective tissue

Conditions classifiable to M00-M99

　EXCLUDES 2　personal history of (healed) traumatic fracture (Z87.81)

✓6ᵗʰ Z87.31　Personal history of (healed) nontraumatic fracture

Z87.310　Personal history of (healed) osteoporosis fracture

Personal history of (healed) fragility fracture

Personal history of (healed) collapsed vertebra due to osteoporosis

TIP: Assign for history of osteoporosis fractures that have resolved, even when a code from category M80 indicating current osteoporosis fracture is also reported.

Z87.311　Personal history of (healed) other pathological fracture

Personal history of (healed) collapsed vertebra NOS

　EXCLUDES 2　personal history of osteoporosis fracture (Z87.310)

Z87.312　Personal history of (healed) stress fracture

Personal history of (healed) fatigue fracture

Z87.39　Personal history of other diseases of the musculoskeletal system and connective tissue

✓5ᵗʰ Z87.4　Personal history of diseases of the genitourinary system

Conditions classifiable to N00-N99

✓6ᵗʰ Z87.41　Personal history of dysplasia of the female genital tract

　EXCLUDES 1　personal history of intraepithelial neoplasia III of female genital tract (Z86.001, Z86.008)

personal history of malignant neoplasm of female genital tract (Z85.40-Z85.44)

Z87.410　Personal history of cervical dysplasia　♀

Z87.411　Personal history of vaginal dysplasia　♀

Z87.412　Personal history of vulvar dysplasia　♀

Z87.42　Personal history of other diseases of the female genital tract　♀

✓6ᵗʰ Z87.43　Personal history of diseases of the male genital organs

Z87.430　Personal history of prostatic dysplasia　♂

　EXCLUDES 1　personal history of malignant neoplasm of prostate (Z85.46)

Z87.438　Personal history of other diseases of male genital organs　♂

✓6ᵗʰ Z87.44　Personal history of diseases of the urinary system

　EXCLUDES 1　personal history of malignant neoplasm of cervix uteri (Z85.41)

Z87.440　Personal history of urinary (tract) infections

Z87.441　Personal history of nephrotic syndrome

Z87.442　Personal history of urinary calculi

Personal history of kidney stones

Z87.448　Personal history of other diseases of urinary system

✓5ᵗʰ Z87.5　Personal history of complications of pregnancy, childbirth and the puerperium

Conditions classifiable to O00-O9A

　EXCLUDES 2　recurrent pregnancy loss (N96)

Z87.51　Personal history of pre-term labor　♀

　EXCLUDES 1　current pregnancy with history of pre-term labor (O09.21-)

Z87.59　Personal history of other complications of pregnancy, childbirth and the puerperium　♀

Personal history of trophoblastic disease

✓5ᵗʰ Z87.7　Personal history of (corrected) congenital malformations

Conditions classifiable to Q00-Q89 that have been repaired or corrected

　EXCLUDES 1　congenital malformations that have been partially corrected or repair but which still require medical treatment — code to condition

　EXCLUDES 2　other postprocedural states (Z98.-)

personal history of medical treatment (Z92.-)

presence of cardiac and vascular implants and grafts (Z95.-)

presence of other devices (Z97.-)

presence of other functional implants (Z96.-)

transplanted organ and tissue status (Z94.-)

✓6ᵗʰ Z87.71　Personal history of (corrected) congenital malformations of genitourinary system

Z87.710　Personal history of (corrected) hypospadias　♂

Z87.718　Personal history of other specified (corrected) congenital malformations of genitourinary system

✓6ᵗʰ Z87.72　Personal history of (corrected) congenital malformations of nervous system and sense organs

Z87.720　Personal history of (corrected) congenital malformations of eye

Z87.721　Personal history of (corrected) congenital malformations of ear

Z87.728　Personal history of other specified (corrected) congenital malformations of nervous system and sense organs

✓6ᵗʰ Z87.73　Personal history of (corrected) congenital malformations of digestive system

Z87.730　Personal history of (corrected) cleft lip and palate

Z87.738　Personal history of other specified (corrected) congenital malformations of digestive system

Z87.74　Personal history of (corrected) congenital malformations of heart and circulatory system

Z87.75　Personal history of (corrected) congenital malformations of respiratory system

Z87.76　Personal history of (corrected) congenital malformations of integument, limbs and musculoskeletal system

✓6ᵗʰ Z87.79　Personal history of other (corrected) congenital malformations

Z87.790　Personal history of (corrected) congenital malformations of face and neck

Z87.798　Personal history of other (corrected) congenital malformations

✓5ᵗʰ Z87.8　Personal history of other specified conditions

　EXCLUDES 2　personal history of self harm (Z91.5)

Z87.81　Personal history of (healed) traumatic fracture

　EXCLUDES 2　personal history of (healed) nontraumatic fracture (Z87.31-)

✓6ᵗʰ Z87.82　Personal history of other (healed) physical injury and trauma

Conditions classifiable to S00-T88, except traumatic fractures

Z87.820　Personal history of traumatic brain injury

　EXCLUDES 1　personal history of transient ischemic attack (TIA), and cerebral infarction without residual deficits (Z86.73)

Z87.821　Personal history of retained foreign body fully removed

Z87.828　Personal history of other (healed) physical injury and trauma

✓6ᵗʰ Z87.89　Personal history of other specified conditions

Z87.890　Personal history of sex reassignment

Z87.891　Personal history of nicotine dependence

　EXCLUDES 1　current nicotine dependence (F17.2-)

AHA: 2017,2Q,27

N Newborn: 0　　P Pediatric: 0-17　　M Maternity: 9-64　　A Adult: 15-124　　MCC Major Complication/Comorbidity　　CC Complication/Comorbidity　　SW Severe Wound Dx

1302　　　　　ICD-10-CM 2020

Z87.892 **Personal history of** anaphylaxis
Code also allergy status such as:
allergy status to drugs, medicaments and
biological substances (Z88.-)
allergy status, other than to drugs and
biological substances (Z91.0-)

Z87.898 **Personal history of other specified**
conditions
AHA: 2013,1Q,21

✓4ᵗʰ **Z88** **Allergy status to drugs, medicaments and biological substances**

EXCLUDES 2   *allergy status, other than to drugs and biological substances (Z91.0-)*

AHA: 2015,3Q,23

Z88.0 **Allergy status to** penicillin
Z88.1 **Allergy status to other antibiotic agents status**
Z88.2 **Allergy status to** sulfonamides **status**
Z88.3 **Allergy status to other anti-infective agents status**
Z88.4 **Allergy status to** anesthetic **agent status**
Z88.5 **Allergy status to** narcotic **agent status**
Z88.6 **Allergy status to** analgesic **agent status**
Z88.7 **Allergy status to** serum and vaccine **status**
Z88.8 **Allergy status to other drugs, medicaments and biological**
substances status
Z88.9 **Allergy status to unspecified drugs, medicaments and**
biological substances status

✓4ᵗʰ **Z89** **Acquired absence of limb**

INCLUDES   amputation status
postprocedural loss of limb
post-traumatic loss of limb

EXCLUDES 1   *acquired deformities of limbs (M20-M21)*
congenital absence of limbs (Q71-Q73)

✓5ᵗʰ **Z89.0** **Acquired absence of** thumb and other finger(s)

✓6ᵗʰ **Z89.01** **Acquired absence of** thumb
Z89.011 **Acquired absence of** right **thumb**
Z89.012 **Acquired absence of** left **thumb**
Z89.019 **Acquired absence of unspecified thumb**

✓6ᵗʰ **Z89.02** **Acquired absence of other** finger(s)
EXCLUDES 2   *acquired absence of thumb (Z89.01-)*
Z89.021 **Acquired absence of** right **finger(s)**
Z89.022 **Acquired absence of** left **finger(s)**
Z89.029 **Acquired absence of unspecified finger(s)**

✓5ᵗʰ **Z89.1** **Acquired absence of** hand and wrist

✓6ᵗʰ **Z89.11** **Acquired absence of** hand
Z89.111 **Acquired absence of** right **hand**
Z89.112 **Acquired absence of** left **hand**
Z89.119 **Acquired absence of unspecified hand**

✓6ᵗʰ **Z89.12** **Acquired absence of** wrist
Disarticulation at wrist
Z89.121 **Acquired absence of** right **wrist**
Z89.122 **Acquired absence of** left **wrist**
Z89.129 **Acquired absence of unspecified wrist**

✓5ᵗʰ **Z89.2** **Acquired absence of** upper limb above wrist

✓6ᵗʰ **Z89.20** **Acquired absence of upper limb, unspecified level**
Z89.201 **Acquired absence of** right **upper limb,**
unspecified level
Z89.202 **Acquired absence of** left **upper limb,**
unspecified level
Z89.209 **Acquired absence of unspecified upper**
limb, unspecified level
Acquired absence of arm NOS

✓6ᵗʰ **Z89.21** **Acquired absence of** upper limb below elbow
Z89.211 **Acquired absence of** right **upper limb**
below elbow
Z89.212 **Acquired absence of** left **upper limb**
below elbow
Z89.219 **Acquired absence of unspecified upper**
limb below elbow

✓6ᵗʰ **Z89.22** **Acquired absence of** upper limb above elbow
Disarticulation at elbow
Z89.221 **Acquired absence of** right **upper limb**
above elbow
Z89.222 **Acquired absence of** left **upper limb**
above elbow
Z89.229 **Acquired absence of unspecified upper**
limb above elbow

✓6ᵗʰ **Z89.23** **Acquired absence of** shoulder
Acquired absence of shoulder joint following
explantation of shoulder joint prosthesis, with
or without presence of antibiotic-impregnated
cement spacer
Z89.231 **Acquired absence of** right **shoulder**
Z89.232 **Acquired absence of** left **shoulder**
Z89.239 **Acquired absence of unspecified shoulder**

✓5ᵗʰ **Z89.4** **Acquired absence of** toe(s), foot, and ankle

✓6ᵗʰ **Z89.41** **Acquired absence of** great toe
Z89.411 **Acquired absence of** right **great toe**   HCC
Z89.412 **Acquired absence of** left **great toe**   HCC
Z89.419 **Acquired absence of unspecified great toe**   HCC

✓6ᵗʰ **Z89.42** **Acquired absence of other** toe(s)
EXCLUDES 2   *acquired absence of great toe (Z89.41-)*
Z89.421 **Acquired absence of other** right **toe(s)**   HCC
Z89.422 **Acquired absence of other** left **toe(s)**   HCC
Z89.429 **Acquired absence of other toe(s), unspecified side**   HCC

✓6ᵗʰ **Z89.43** **Acquired absence of** foot
Z89.431 **Acquired absence of** right **foot**   HCC
Z89.432 **Acquired absence of** left **foot**   HCC
Z89.439 **Acquired absence of unspecified foot**   HCC

✓6ᵗʰ **Z89.44** **Acquired absence of** ankle
Disarticulation of ankle
Z89.441 **Acquired absence of** right **ankle**   HCC
Z89.442 **Acquired absence of** left **ankle**   HCC
Z89.449 **Acquired absence of unspecified ankle**   HCC

✓5ᵗʰ **Z89.5** **Acquired absence of leg below knee**

✓6ᵗʰ **Z89.51** **Acquired absence of** leg below knee
Z89.511 **Acquired absence of** right **leg below knee**   HCC
Z89.512 **Acquired absence of** left **leg below knee**   HCC
Z89.519 **Acquired absence of unspecified leg below knee**   HCC

✓6ᵗʰ **Z89.52** **Acquired absence of** knee
Acquired absence of knee joint following explantation
of knee joint prosthesis, with or without presence
of antibiotic-impregnated cement spacer
Z89.521 **Acquired absence of** right **knee**
Z89.522 **Acquired absence of** left **knee**
Z89.529 **Acquired absence of unspecified knee**

✓5ᵗʰ **Z89.6** **Acquired absence of leg above knee**

✓6ᵗʰ **Z89.61** **Acquired absence of** leg above knee
Acquired absence of leg NOS
Disarticulation at knee
Z89.611 **Acquired absence of** right **leg above knee**   HCC
Z89.612 **Acquired absence of** left **leg above knee**   HCC
Z89.619 **Acquired absence of unspecified leg above knee**   HCC

✓6ᵗʰ **Z89.62** **Acquired absence of** hip
Acquired absence of hip joint following explantation
of hip joint prosthesis, with or without presence
of antibiotic-impregnated cement spacer
Disarticulation at hip
Z89.621 **Acquired absence of** right **hip joint**
Z89.622 **Acquired absence of** left **hip joint**
Z89.629 **Acquired absence of unspecified hip joint**

Z89.9 **Acquired absence of limb, unspecified**

✓4ᵗʰ **Z90** **Acquired absence of organs, not elsewhere classified**

INCLUDES   postprocedural or post-traumatic loss of body part NEC

EXCLUDES 1   *congenital absence — see Alphabetical Index*

EXCLUDES 2   *postprocedural absence of endocrine glands (E89.-)*

✓5ᵗʰ **Z90.0** **Acquired absence of part of** head and neck

Z90.01 **Acquired absence of** eye

✓ Additional Character Required   ✓x7ᵗʰ Placeholder   Unacceptable PDx   Questionable PDx   Manifestation   Unspecified Dx   H1-H14 HAC   HCC CMS-HCC Dx   HIV HIV Dx

ICD-10-CM 2020   **1303**

Z90.02   **Acquired absence of larynx**

Z90.09   **Acquired absence of other part of head and neck**
Acquired absence of nose
EXCLUDES 2   *teeth (K08.1)*

✓5ᵗʰ   **Z90.1**   **Acquired absence of breast and nipple**

Z90.10   **Acquired absence of unspecified breast and nipple**

Z90.11   **Acquired absence of right breast and nipple**

Z90.12   **Acquired absence of left breast and nipple**

Z90.13   **Acquired absence of bilateral breasts and nipples**

Z90.2   **Acquired absence of lung [part of]**

Z90.3   **Acquired absence of stomach [part of]**

✓5ᵗʰ   **Z90.4**   **Acquired absence of other specified parts of digestive tract**

✓6ᵗʰ   **Z90.41**   **Acquired absence of pancreas**
Code also exocrine pancreatic insufficiency (K86.81)
Use additional code to identify any associated:
diabetes mellitus, postpancreatectomy (E13.-)
insulin use (Z79.4)

Z90.410   **Acquired total absence of pancreas**
Acquired absence of pancreas NOS

Z90.411   **Acquired partial absence of pancreas**

Z90.49   **Acquired absence of other specified parts of digestive tract**

Z90.5   **Acquired absence of kidney**

Z90.6   **Acquired absence of other parts of urinary tract**
Acquired absence of bladder

✓5ᵗʰ   **Z90.7**   **Acquired absence of genital organ(s)**
EXCLUDES 1   *personal history of sex reassignment (Z87.890)*
EXCLUDES 2   *female genital mutilation status (N90.81-)*

✓6ᵗʰ   **Z90.71**   **Acquired absence of cervix and uterus**

Z90.710   **Acquired absence of both cervix and uterus**   ♀
Acquired absence of uterus NOS
Status post total hysterectomy

Z90.711   **Acquired absence of uterus with remaining cervical stump**   ♀
Status post partial hysterectomy with remaining cervical stump

Z90.712   **Acquired absence of cervix with remaining uterus**   ♀

✓6ᵗʰ   **Z90.72**   **Acquired absence of ovaries**

Z90.721   **Acquired absence of ovaries, unilateral**   ♀

Z90.722   **Acquired absence of ovaries, bilateral**   ♀

Z90.79   **Acquired absence of other genital organ(s)**

✓5ᵗʰ   **Z90.8**   **Acquired absence of other organs**

Z90.81   **Acquired absence of spleen**

Z90.89   **Acquired absence of other organs**

✓4ᵗʰ   **Z91**   **Personal risk factors, not elsewhere classified**
EXCLUDES 2   *contact with and (suspected) exposures hazardous to health (Z77.-)*
exposure to pollution and other problems related to physical environment (Z77.1-)
female genital mutilation status (N90.81-)
personal history of physical injury and trauma (Z87.81, Z87.82-)
occupational exposure to risk factors (Z57.-)

✓5ᵗʰ   **Z91.0**   **Allergy status, other than to drugs and biological substances**
EXCLUDES 2   *allergy status to drugs, medicaments, and biological substances (Z88.-)*

✓6ᵗʰ   **Z91.01**   **Food allergy status**
EXCLUDES 2   *food additives allergy status (Z91.02)*

Z91.010   **Allergy to peanuts**

Z91.011   **Allergy to milk products**
EXCLUDES 1   *lactose intolerance (E73.-)*

Z91.012   **Allergy to eggs**

Z91.013   **Allergy to seafood**
Allergy to shellfish
Allergy to octopus or squid ink

Z91.018   **Allergy to other foods**
Allergy to nuts other than peanuts

Z91.02   **Food additives allergy status**

✓6ᵗʰ   **Z91.03**   **Insect allergy status**

Z91.030   **Bee allergy status**

Z91.038   **Other insect allergy status**

✓6ᵗʰ   **Z91.04**   **Nonmedicinal substance allergy status**

Z91.040   **Latex allergy status**
Latex sensitivity status

Z91.041   **Radiographic dye allergy status**
Allergy status to contrast media used for diagnostic X-ray procedure

Z91.048   **Other nonmedicinal substance allergy status**

Z91.09   **Other allergy status, other than to drugs and biological substances**

✓5ᵗʰ   **Z91.1**   **Patient's noncompliance with medical treatment and regimen**

Z91.11   **Patient's noncompliance with dietary regimen**

✓6ᵗʰ   **Z91.12**   **Patient's intentional underdosing of medication regimen**
Code first underdosing of medication (T36-T50) with fifth or sixth character 6
EXCLUDES 1   *adverse effect of prescribed drug taken as directed — code to adverse effect*
poisoning (overdose) — code to poisoning
AHA: 2018,4Q,72

Z91.120   **Patient's intentional underdosing of medication regimen due to financial hardship**

Z91.128   **Patient's intentional underdosing of medication regimen for other reason**

✓6ᵗʰ   **Z91.13**   **Patient's unintentional underdosing of medication regimen**
Code first underdosing of medication (T36-T50) with fifth or sixth character 6
EXCLUDES 1   *adverse effect of prescribed drug taken as directed — code to adverse effect*
poisoning (overdose) — code to poisoning
AHA: 2018,4Q,72

Z91.130   **Patient's unintentional underdosing of medication regimen due to age-related debility**

Z91.138   **Patient's unintentional underdosing of medication regimen for other reason**

Z91.14   **Patient's other noncompliance with medication regimen**
Patient's underdosing of medication NOS
AHA: 2018,4Q,72

Z91.15   **Patient's noncompliance with renal dialysis**   HCC

Z91.19   **Patient's noncompliance with other medical treatment and regimen**
Nonadherence to medical treatment

✓5ᵗʰ   **Z91.4**   **Personal history of psychological trauma, not elsewhere classified**

✓6ᵗʰ   **Z91.41**   **Personal history of adult abuse**
EXCLUDES 2   *personal history of abuse in childhood (Z62.81-)*

Z91.410   **Personal history of adult physical and sexual abuse**   A
EXCLUDES 1   *current adult physical abuse (T74.11, T76.11)*
current adult sexual abuse (T74.21, T76.11)

Z91.411   **Personal history of adult psychological abuse**   A

Z91.412   **Personal history of adult neglect**   A
EXCLUDES 1   *current adult neglect (T74.01, T76.01)*

Z91.419   **Personal history of unspecified adult abuse**   A

Z91.42   **Personal history of forced labor or sexual exploitation**
AHA: 2018,4Q,32,35

Z91.49   **Other personal history of psychological trauma, not elsewhere classified**

Z91.5   **Personal history of self-harm**
Personal history of parasuicide
Personal history of self-poisoning
Personal history of suicide attempt

✓5ᵗʰ   **Z91.8**   **Other specified personal risk factors, not elsewhere classified**

Z91.81   **History of falling**
At risk for falling

N Newborn: 0   P Pediatric: 0-17   M Maternity: 9-64   A Adult: 15-124   MCC Major Complication/Comorbidity   CC Complication/Comorbidity   SW Severe Wound Dx

1304   ICD-10-CM 2020

Z91.82 **Personal history of military deployment** A

Individual (civilian or military) with past history of military war, peacekeeping and humanitarian deployment (current or past conflict)

Returned from military deployment

Z91.83 *Wandering in diseases classified elsewhere*

Code first underlying disorder such as:

Alzheimer's disease (G30.-)

autism or pervasive developmental disorder (F84.-)

intellectual disabilities (F70-F79)

unspecified dementia with behavioral disturbance (F03.9-)

√6ᵗʰ **Z91.84** **Oral health risk factors**

AHA: 2017,4Q,29

Z91.841 **Risk for dental caries, low**

Z91.842 **Risk for dental caries, moderate**

Z91.843 **Risk for dental caries, high**

Z91.849 **Unspecified risk for dental caries**

Z91.89 **Other specified personal risk factors, not elsewhere classified**

AHA: 2017,1Q,45

√4ᵗʰ **Z92** **Personal history of medical treatment**

EXCLUDES 2   *postprocedural states (Z98.-)*

Z92.0 **Personal history of contraception**

EXCLUDES 1   *counseling or management of current contraceptive practices (Z30.-)*

long term (current) use of contraception (Z79.3)

presence of (intrauterine) contraceptive device (Z97.5)

√5ᵗʰ **Z92.2** **Personal history of drug therapy**

EXCLUDES 2   *long term (current) drug therapy (Z79.-)*

Z92.21 **Personal history of antineoplastic chemotherapy**

Z92.22 **Personal history of monoclonal drug therapy**

Z92.23 **Personal history of estrogen therapy**

√6ᵗʰ **Z92.24** **Personal history of steroid therapy**

Z92.240 **Personal history of inhaled steroid therapy**

Z92.241 **Personal history of systemic steroid therapy**

Personal history of steroid therapy NOS

Z92.25 **Personal history of immunosupression therapy**

EXCLUDES 2   *personal history of steroid therapy (Z92.24)*

Z92.29 **Personal history of other drug therapy**

Z92.3 **Personal history of irradiation**

Personal history of exposure to therapeutic radiation

EXCLUDES 1   *exposure to radiation in the physical environment (Z77.12)*

occupational exposure to radiation (Z57.1)

√5ᵗʰ **Z92.8** **Personal history of other medical treatment**

Z92.81 **Personal history of extracorporeal membrane oxygenation (ECMO)**

Z92.82 **Status post administration of tPA (rtPA) in a different facility within the last 24 hours prior to admission to current facility**

Code first condition requiring tPA administration, such as:

acute cerebral infarction (I63.-)

acute myocardial infarction (I21.-, I22.-)

AHA: 2013,4Q,124

Z92.83 **Personal history of failed moderate sedation**

Personal history of failed conscious sedation

EXCLUDES 2   *failed moderate sedation during procedure (T88.52)*

Z92.84 **Personal history of unintended awareness under general anesthesia**

EXCLUDES 2   *unintended awareness under general anesthesia during procedure (T88.53)*

AHA: 2016,4Q,72-73,77

Z92.89 **Personal history of other medical treatment**

√4ᵗʰ **Z93** **Artificial opening status**

EXCLUDES 1   *artificial openings requiring attention or management (Z43.-)*

complications of external stoma (J95.0-, K94.-, N99.5-)

Z93.0 **Tracheostomy status** HCC

AHA: 2013,4Q,129

Z93.1 **Gastrostomy status** HCC

Z93.2 **Ileostomy status** HCC

Z93.3 **Colostomy status** HCC

Z93.4 **Other artificial openings of gastrointestinal tract status** HCC

√5ᵗʰ **Z93.5** **Cystostomy status**

Z93.50 **Unspecified cystostomy status** HCC

Z93.51 **Cutaneous-vesicostomy status** HCC

Z93.52 **Appendico-vesicostomy status** HCC

Z93.59 **Other cystostomy status** HCC

Z93.6 **Other artificial openings of urinary tract status**

Nephrostomy status

Ureterostomy status

Urethrostomy status

Z93.8 **Other artificial opening status** HCC

Z93.9 **Artificial opening status, unspecified** HCC

√4ᵗʰ **Z94** **Transplanted organ and tissue status**

INCLUDES   organ or tissue replaced by heterogenous or homogenous transplant

EXCLUDES 1   *complications of transplanted organ or tissue — see Alphabetical Index*

EXCLUDES 2   *presence of vascular grafts (Z95.-)*

✗ **Z94.0** **Kidney transplant status** — *not used w/ T86.11*

Z94.1 **Heart transplant status** HCC

EXCLUDES 1   *artificial heart status (Z95.812)*

heart-valve replacement status (Z95.2-Z95.4)

Z94.2 **Lung transplant status** HCC

Z94.3 **Heart and lungs transplant status** HCC

Z94.4 **Liver transplant status** HCC

Z94.5 **Skin transplant status**

Autogenous skin transplant status

Z94.6 **Bone transplant status**

Z94.7 **Corneal transplant status**

√5ᵗʰ **Z94.8** **Other transplanted organ and tissue status**

Z94.81 **Bone marrow transplant status** HCC

Z94.82 **Intestine transplant status** HCC

Z94.83 **Pancreas transplant status** HCC

Z94.84 **Stem cells transplant status** HCC

Z94.89 **Other transplanted organ and tissue status**

Z94.9 **Transplanted organ and tissue status, unspecified**

√4ᵗʰ **Z95** **Presence of cardiac and vascular implants and grafts**

EXCLUDES 2   *complications of cardiac and vascular devices, implants and grafts (T82.-)*

Z95.0 **Presence of cardiac pacemaker**

Presence of cardiac resynchronization therapy (CRT-P) pacemaker

EXCLUDES 1   *adjustment or management of cardiac device (Z45.0-)*

adjustment or management of cardiac pacemaker (Z45.0)

presence of automatic (implantable) cardiac defibrillator with synchronous cardiac pacemaker (Z95.810)

AHA: 2019,1Q,33

Z95.1 **Presence of aortocoronary bypass graft**

Presence of coronary artery bypass graft

Z95.2 **Presence of prosthetic heart valve**

Presence of heart valve NOS

Z95.3 **Presence of xenogenic heart valve**

Z95.4 **Presence of other heart-valve replacement**

Z95.5 **Presence of coronary angioplasty implant and graft**

EXCLUDES 1   *coronary angioplasty status without implant and graft (Z98.61)*

✓ Additional Character Required   ✗x7ᵗʰ Placeholder   Unacceptable PDx   Questionable PDx   Manifestation   Unspecified Dx   H1 - H14 HAC   HCC CMS-HCC Dx   HIV HIV Dx

ICD-10-CM 2020   1305

√5ᵗʰ **Z95.8** **Presence of other cardiac and vascular implants and grafts**

  √6ᵗʰ **Z95.81** **Presence of other cardiac implants and grafts**

    Z95.810 **Presence of automatic (implantable) cardiac defibrillator**

      Presence of automatic (implantable) cardiac defibrillator with synchronous cardiac pacemaker

      Presence of cardiac resynchronization therapy defibrillator (CRT-D)

      Presence of cardioverter-defibrillator (ICD)

    Z95.811 **Presence of heart assist device** `HCC`

    Z95.812 **Presence of fully implantable artificial heart** `HCC`

    Z95.818 **Presence of other cardiac implants and grafts**

  √6ᵗʰ **Z95.82** **Presence of other vascular implants and grafts**

    Z95.820 **Peripheral vascular angioplasty status with implants and grafts**

      EXCLUDES 1   peripheral vascular angioplasty without implant and graft (Z98.62)

    Z95.828 **Presence of other vascular implants and grafts**

      Presence of intravascular prosthesis NEC

Z95.9 **Presence of cardiac and vascular implant and graft, unspecified**

√4ᵗʰ **Z96** **Presence of other functional implants**

  EXCLUDES 2   complications of internal prosthetic devices, implants and grafts (T82-T85)

      fitting and adjustment of prosthetic and other devices (Z44-Z46)

Z96.0 **Presence of urogenital implants**

Z96.1 **Presence of intraocular lens**

  Presence of pseudophakia

√5ᵗʰ **Z96.2** **Presence of otological and audiological implants**

  Z96.20 **Presence of otological and audiological implant, unspecified**

  Z96.21 **Cochlear implant status**

  Z96.22 **Myringotomy tube(s) status**

  Z96.29 **Presence of other otological and audiological implants**

    Presence of bone-conduction hearing device

    Presence of eustachian tube stent

    Stapes replacement

Z96.3 **Presence of artificial larynx**

√5ᵗʰ **Z96.4** **Presence of endocrine implants**

  Z96.41 **Presence of insulin pump (external) (internal)**

  Z96.49 **Presence of other endocrine implants**

Z96.5 **Presence of tooth-root and mandibular implants**

√5ᵗʰ **Z96.6** **Presence of orthopedic joint implants**

  Z96.60 **Presence of unspecified orthopedic joint implant**

  √6ᵗʰ **Z96.61** **Presence of artificial shoulder joint**

    Z96.611 **Presence of right artificial shoulder joint**

    Z96.612 **Presence of left artificial shoulder joint**

    Z96.619 **Presence of unspecified artificial shoulder joint**

  √6ᵗʰ **Z96.62** **Presence of artificial elbow joint**

    Z96.621 **Presence of right artificial elbow joint**

    Z96.622 **Presence of left artificial elbow joint**

    Z96.629 **Presence of unspecified artificial elbow joint**

  √6ᵗʰ **Z96.63** **Presence of artificial wrist joint**

    Z96.631 **Presence of right artificial wrist joint**

    Z96.632 **Presence of left artificial wrist joint**

    Z96.639 **Presence of unspecified artificial wrist joint**

  √6ᵗʰ **Z96.64** **Presence of artificial hip joint**

    Hip-joint replacement (partial) (total)

    Z96.641 **Presence of right artificial hip joint**

    Z96.642 **Presence of left artificial hip joint**

    Z96.643 **Presence of artificial hip joint, bilateral**

    Z96.649 **Presence of unspecified artificial hip joint**

  √6ᵗʰ **Z96.65** **Presence of artificial knee joint**

    Z96.651 **Presence of right artificial knee joint**

    Z96.652 **Presence of left artificial knee joint**

    Z96.653 **Presence of artificial knee joint, bilateral**

    Z96.659 **Presence of unspecified artificial knee joint**

  √6ᵗʰ **Z96.66** **Presence of artificial ankle joint**

    Z96.661 **Presence of right artificial ankle joint**

    Z96.662 **Presence of left artificial ankle joint**

    Z96.669 **Presence of unspecified artificial ankle joint**

  √6ᵗʰ **Z96.69** **Presence of other orthopedic joint implants**

    Z96.691 **Finger-joint replacement of right hand**

    Z96.692 **Finger-joint replacement of left hand**

    Z96.693 **Finger-joint replacement, bilateral**

    Z96.698 **Presence of other orthopedic joint implants**

Z96.7 **Presence of other bone and tendon implants**

  Presence of skull plate

√5ᵗʰ **Z96.8** **Presence of other specified functional implants**

  Z96.81 **Presence of artificial skin**

  Z96.82 **Presence of neurostimulator**

    Presence of brain neurostimulator

    Presence of gastric neurostimulator

    Presence of peripheral nerve neurostimulator

    Presence of sacral nerve neurostimulator

    Presence of spinal cord neurostimulator

    Presence of vagus nerve neurostimulator

  Z96.89 **Presence of other specified functional implants**

Z96.9 **Presence of functional implant, unspecified**

√4ᵗʰ **Z97** **Presence of other devices**

  EXCLUDES 1   complications of internal prosthetic devices, implants and grafts (T82-T85)

      ~~fitting and adjustment of prosthetic and other devices (Z44-Z46)~~

  EXCLUDES 2   ▶fitting and adjustment of prosthetic and other devices (Z44-Z46)◀

      presence of cerebrospinal fluid drainage device (Z98.2)

Z97.0 **Presence of artificial eye**

√5ᵗʰ **Z97.1** **Presence of artificial limb (complete) (partial)**

  Z97.10 **Presence of artificial limb (complete) (partial), unspecified**

  Z97.11 **Presence of artificial right arm (complete) (partial)**

  Z97.12 **Presence of artificial left arm (complete) (partial)**

  Z97.13 **Presence of artificial right leg (complete) (partial)**

  Z97.14 **Presence of artificial left leg (complete) (partial)**

  Z97.15 **Presence of artificial arms, bilateral (complete) (partial)**

  Z97.16 **Presence of artificial legs, bilateral (complete) (partial)**

Z97.2 **Presence of dental prosthetic device (complete) (partial)**

  Presence of dentures (complete) (partial)

Z97.3 **Presence of spectacles and contact lenses**

Z97.4 **Presence of external hearing-aid**

Z97.5 **Presence of (intrauterine) contraceptive device** ♀

  EXCLUDES 1   checking, reinsertion or removal of implantable subdermal contraceptive (Z30.46)

      checking, reinsertion or removal of intrauterine contraceptive device (Z30.43-)

Z97.8 **Presence of other specified devices**

√4ᵗʰ **Z98** **Other postprocedural states**

  EXCLUDES 2   aftercare (Z43-Z49, Z51)

      follow-up medical care (Z08-Z09)

      postprocedural complication — see Alphabetical Index

Z98.0 **Intestinal bypass and anastomosis status**

  EXCLUDES 2   bariatric surgery status (Z98.84)

      gastric bypass status (Z98.84)

      obesity surgery status (Z98.84)

Z98.1 **Arthrodesis status**

Z98.2 **Presence of cerebrospinal fluid drainage device**

  Presence of CSF shunt

Z98.3 **Post therapeutic collapse of lung status**

  Code first underlying disease

√5ᵗʰ **Z98.4** **Cataract extraction status**

  Use additional code to identify intraocular lens implant status (Z96.1)

  EXCLUDES 1   aphakia (H27.0)

  Z98.41 **Cataract extraction status, right eye**

Ⓝ Newborn: 0   Ⓟ Pediatric: 0-17   Ⓜ Maternity: 9-64   Ⓐ Adult: 15-124   **MCC** Major Complication/Comorbidity   **CC** Complication/Comorbidity   **SW** Severe Wound Dx

1306   ICD-10-CM 2020

Z98.42   **Cataract extraction status, left eye**
Z98.49   **Cataract extraction status, unspecified eye**
✓5ᵗʰ   **Z98.5**   **Sterilization status**
    EXCLUDES 1   *female infertility (N97.-)*
               male infertility (N46.-)
   Z98.51   **Tubal ligation status**   ♀
   Z98.52   **Vasectomy status**   A ♂
✓5ᵗʰ   **Z98.6**   **Angioplasty status**
   Z98.61   **Coronary angioplasty status**
      EXCLUDES 1   *coronary angioplasty status with implant and graft (Z95.5)*
   Z98.62   **Peripheral vascular angioplasty status**
      EXCLUDES 1   *peripheral vascular angioplasty status with implant and graft (Z95.820)*
✓5ᵗʰ   **Z98.8**   **Other specified postprocedural states**
   ✓6ᵗʰ   **Z98.81**   **Dental procedure status**
      Z98.810   **Dental sealant status**
      Z98.811   **Dental restoration status**
           Dental crown status
           Dental fillings status
      Z98.818   **Other dental procedure status**
   Z98.82   **Breast implant status**
      EXCLUDES 1   *breast implant removal status (Z98.86)*
   Z98.83   **Filtering (vitreous) bleb after glaucoma surgery status**
      EXCLUDES 1   *inflammation (infection) of postprocedural bleb (H59.4-)*
   Z98.84   **Bariatric surgery status**
      Gastric banding status
      Gastric bypass status for obesity
      Obesity surgery status
      EXCLUDES 1   *bariatric surgery status complicating pregnancy, childbirth, or the puerperium (O99.84)*
      EXCLUDES 2   *intestinal bypass and anastomosis status (Z98.0)*
   Z98.85   **Transplanted organ removal status**
      Transplanted organ previously removed due to complication, failure, rejection or infection
      EXCLUDES 1   *encounter for removal of transplanted organ — code to complication of transplanted organ (T86.-)*
   Z98.86   **Personal history of breast implant removal**
   ✓6ᵗʰ   **Z98.87**   **Personal history of in utero procedure**
      Z98.870   **Personal history of in utero procedure during pregnancy**   ♀
         EXCLUDES 2   *complications from in utero procedure for current pregnancy (O35.7)*
                 supervision of current pregnancy with history of in utero procedure during previous pregnancy (O09.82-)
      Z98.871   **Personal history of in utero procedure while a fetus**
   ✓6ᵗʰ   **Z98.89**   **Other specified postprocedural states**
      Z98.890   **Other specified postprocedural states**
           Personal history of surgery, not elsewhere classified
      Z98.891   **History of uterine scar from previous surgery**   ♀
         EXCLUDES 1   *maternal care due to uterine scar from previous surgery (O34.2-)*
      AHA: 2016,4Q,51-52,76

✓4ᵗʰ   **Z99**   **Dependence on enabling machines and devices, not elsewhere classified**
     EXCLUDES 1   *cardiac pacemaker status (Z95.0)*
   Z99.0   **Dependence on aspirator**
   ✓5ᵗʰ   **Z99.1**   **Dependence on respirator**
      Dependence on ventilator
     Z99.11   **Dependence on respirator [ventilator] status**   HCC
         AHA: 2015,1Q,21

     Z99.12   **Encounter for respirator [ventilator] dependence during power failure**   HCC
         EXCLUDES 1   *mechanical complication of respirator [ventilator] (J95.850)*
   Z99.2   **Dependence on renal dialysis**   HCC
      Hemodialysis status
      Peritoneal dialysis status
      Presence of arteriovenous shunt for dialysis
      Renal dialysis status NOS
      EXCLUDES 1   *encounter for fitting and adjustment of dialysis catheter (Z49.0-)*
      EXCLUDES 2   *noncompliance with renal dialysis (Z91.15)*
      AHA: 2016,1Q,12; 2013,4Q,125
   Z99.3   **Dependence on wheelchair**
      Wheelchair confinement status
      Code first cause of dependence, such as:
        muscular dystrophy (G71.0-)
        obesity (E66.-)
   ✓5ᵗʰ   **Z99.8**   **Dependence on other enabling machines and devices**
     Z99.81   **Dependence on supplemental oxygen**
        Dependence on long-term oxygen
        AHA: 2013,4Q,129
     Z99.89   **Dependence on other enabling machines and devices**
        Dependence on machine or device NOS

A09	Infectious gastroenteritis and colitis, unspecified
A33	Tetanus neonatorum
A34	Obstetrical tetanus
A35	Other tetanus
A46	Erysipelas
A55	Chlamydial lymphogranuloma (venereum)
A57	Chancroid
A58	Granuloma inguinale
A64	Unspecified sexually transmitted disease
A65	Nonvenereal syphilis
A70	Chlamydia psittaci infections
A78	Q fever
A86	Unspecified viral encephalitis
A89	Unspecified viral infection of central nervous system
A90	Dengue fever [classical dengue]
A91	Dengue hemorrhagic fever
A94	Unspecified arthropod-borne viral fever
A99	Unspecified viral hemorrhagic fever
B03	Smallpox
B04	Monkeypox
B09	Unspecified viral infection characterized by skin and mucous membrane lesions
B20	Human immunodeficiency virus [HIV] disease
B49	Unspecified mycosis
B54	Unspecified malaria
B59	Pneumocystosis
B64	Unspecified protozoal disease
B72	Dracunculiasis
B75	Trichinellosis
B79	Trichuriasis
B80	Enterobiasis
B86	Scabies
B89	Unspecified parasitic disease
B91	Sequelae of poliomyelitis
B92	Sequelae of leprosy
C01	Malignant neoplasm of base of tongue
C07	Malignant neoplasm of parotid gland
C12	Malignant neoplasm of pyriform sinus
C19	Malignant neoplasm of rectosigmoid junction
C20	Malignant neoplasm of rectum
C23	Malignant neoplasm of gallbladder
C33	Malignant neoplasm of trachea
C37	Malignant neoplasm of thymus
C52	Malignant neoplasm of vagina
C55	Malignant neoplasm of uterus, part unspecified
C58	Malignant neoplasm of placenta
C61	Malignant neoplasm of prostate
C73	Malignant neoplasm of thyroid gland
D34	Benign neoplasm of thyroid gland
D45	Polycythemia vera
D62	Acute posthemorrhagic anemia
D65	Disseminated intravascular coagulation [defibrination A syndrome]
D66	Hereditary factor VIII deficiency
D67	Hereditary factor IX deficiency
D71	Functional disorders of polymorphonuclear neutrophils
D77	Other disorders of blood and blood-forming organs in diseases classified elsewhere
E02	Subclinical iodine-deficiency hypothyroidism
E15	Nondiabetic hypoglycemic coma
E35	Disorders of endocrine glands in diseases classified elsewhere
E40	Kwashiorkor
E41	Nutritional marasmus
E42	Marasmic kwashiorkor
E43	Unspecified severe protein-calorie malnutrition
E45	Retarded development following protein-calorie malnutrition

E46	Unspecified protein-calorie malnutrition
E52	Niacin deficiency [pellagra]
E54	Ascorbic acid deficiency
E58	Dietary calcium deficiency
E59	Dietary selenium deficiency
E60	Dietary zinc deficiency
E65	Localized adiposity
E68	Sequelae of hyperalimentation
F04	Amnestic disorder due to known physiological condition
F05	Delirium due to known physiological condition
F09	Unspecified mental disorder due to known physiological condition
F21	Schizotypal disorder
F22	Delusional disorders
F23	Brief psychotic disorder
F24	Shared psychotic disorder
F28	Other psychotic disorder not due to a substance or known physiological condition
F29	Unspecified psychosis not due to a substance or known physiological condition
F39	Unspecified mood [affective] disorder
F54	Psychological and behavioral factors associated with disorders or diseases classified elsewhere
F59	Unspecified behavioral syndromes associated with physiological disturbances and physical factors
F66	Other sexual disorders
F69	Unspecified disorder of adult personality and behavior
F70	Mild intellectual disabilities
F71	Moderate intellectual disabilities
F72	Severe intellectual disabilities
F73	Profound intellectual disabilities
F78	Other intellectual disabilities
F79	Unspecified intellectual disabilities
F82	Specific developmental disorder of motor function
F88	Other disorders of psychological development
F89	Unspecified disorder of psychological development
F99	Mental disorder, not otherwise specified
G01	Meningitis in bacterial diseases classified elsewhere
G02	Meningitis in other infectious and parasitic diseases classified elsewhere
G07	Intracranial and intraspinal abscess and granuloma in diseases classified elsewhere
G08	Intracranial and intraspinal phlebitis and thrombophlebitis
G09	Sequelae of inflammatory diseases of central nervous system
G10	Huntington's disease
G14	Postpolio syndrome
G20	Parkinson's disease
G26	Extrapyramidal and movement disorders in diseases classified elsewhere
G35	Multiple sclerosis
G53	Cranial nerve disorders in diseases classified elsewhere
G55	Nerve root and plexus compressions in diseases classified elsewhere
G59	Mononeuropathy in diseases classified elsewhere
G63	Polyneuropathy in diseases classified elsewhere
G64	Other disorders of peripheral nervous system
G92	Toxic encephalopathy
G94	Other disorders of brain in diseases classified elsewhere
H22	Disorders of iris and ciliary body in diseases classified elsewhere
H28	Cataract in diseases classified elsewhere
H32	Chorioretinal disorders in diseases classified elsewhere
H36	Retinal disorders in diseases classified elsewhere
H42	Glaucoma in diseases classified elsewhere
I00	Rheumatic fever without heart involvement
I10	Essential (primary) hypertension
I32	Pericarditis in diseases classified elsewhere
I38	Endocarditis, valve unspecified

I39	Endocarditis and heart valve disorders in diseases classified elsewhere
I41	Myocarditis in diseases classified elsewhere
I43	Cardiomyopathy in diseases classified elsewhere
I52	Other heart disorders in diseases classified elsewhere
I76	Septic arterial embolism
I81	Portal vein thrombosis
I96	Gangrene, not elsewhere classified
J00	Acute nasopharyngitis (common cold)
J13	Pneumonia due to Streptococcus pneumoniae
J14	Pneumonia due to Hemophilus influenzae
J17	Pneumonia in diseases classified elsewhere
J22	Unspecified acute lower respiratory infection
J36	Peritonsillar abscess
J40	Bronchitis, not specified as acute or chronic
J42	Unspecified chronic bronchitis
J60	Coalworker's pneumoconiosis
J61	Pneumoconiosis due to asbestos and other mineral fibers
J64	Unspecified pneumoconiosis
J65	Pneumoconiosis associated with tuberculosis
J80	Acute respiratory distress syndrome
J82	Pulmonary eosinophilia, not elsewhere classified
J90	Pleural effusion, not elsewhere classified
J99	Respiratory disorders in diseases classified elsewhere
K23	Disorders of esophagus in diseases classified elsewhere
K30	Functional dyspepsia
K36	Other appendicitis
K37	Unspecified appendicitis
K67	Disorders of peritoneum in infectious diseases classified elsewhere
K77	Liver disorders in diseases classified elsewhere
K87	Disorders of gallbladder, biliary tract and pancreas in diseases classified elsewhere
L00	Staphylococcal scalded skin syndrome
L14	Bullous disorders in diseases classified elsewhere
L22	Diaper dermatitis
L26	Exfoliative dermatitis
L42	Pityriasis rosea
L45	Papulosquamous disorders in diseases classified elsewhere
L52	Erythema nodosum
L54	Erythema in diseases classified elsewhere
L62	Nail disorders in diseases classified elsewhere
L80	Vitiligo
L83	Acanthosis nigricans
L84	Corns and callosities
L86	Keratoderma in diseases classified elsewhere
L88	Pyoderma gangrenosum
L99	Other disorders of skin and subcutaneous tissue in diseases classified elsewhere
N08	Glomerular disorders in diseases classified elsewhere
N10	Acute tubulo-interstitial nephritis
N12	Tubulo-interstitial nephritis, not specified as acute or chronic
N16	Renal tubulo-interstitial disorders in diseases classified elsewhere
N19	Unspecified kidney failure
N22	Calculus of urinary tract in diseases classified elsewhere
N23	Unspecified renal colic
N29	Other disorders of kidney and ureter in diseases classified elsewhere

N33	Bladder disorders in diseases classified elsewhere
N37	Urethral disorders in diseases classified elsewhere
N51	Disorders of male genital organs in diseases classified elsewhere
N62	Hypertrophy of breast
N72	Inflammatory disease of cervix uteri
N74	Female pelvic inflammatory disorders in diseases classified elsewhere
N86	Erosion and ectropion of cervix uteri
N96	Recurrent pregnancy loss
O68	Labor and delivery complicated by abnormality of fetal acid-base balance
O76	Abnormality in fetal heart rate and rhythm complicating labor and delivery
O80	Encounter for full-term uncomplicated delivery
O82	Encounter for cesarean delivery without indication
O85	Puerperal sepsis
O94	Sequelae of complication of pregnancy, childbirth, and the puerperium
P09	Abnormal findings on neonatal screening
P53	Hemorrhagic disease of newborn
P60	Disseminated intravascular coagulation of newborn
P84	Other problems with newborn
P90	Convulsions of newborn
P95	Stillbirth
Q02	Microcephaly
R05	Cough
R12	Heartburn
R17	Unspecified jaundice
R21	Rash and other nonspecific skin eruption
R32	Unspecified urinary incontinence
R34	Anuria and oliguria
R37	Sexual dysfunction, unspecified
R42	Dizziness and giddiness
R51	Headache
R52	Pain, unspecified
R54	Age-related physical debility
R55	Syncope and collapse
R58	Hemorrhage, not elsewhere classified
R61	Generalized hyperhidrosis
R64	Cachexia
R69	Illness, unspecified
R75	Inconclusive laboratory evidence of human immunodeficiency virus [HIV]
R81	Glycosuria
R99	Ill-defined and unknown cause of mortality
Y09	Assault by unspecified means
Y66	Nonadministration of surgical and medical care
Y69	Unspecified misadventure during surgical and medical care
Y95	Nosocomial condition
Z08	Encounter for follow-up examination after completed treatment for malignant neoplasm
Z09	Encounter for follow-up examination after completed treatment for conditions other than malignant neoplasm
Z21	Asymptomatic human immunodeficiency virus [HIV] infection status
Z23	Encounter for immunization
Z66	Do not resuscitate

Appendix B: Pharmacology List 2020

This section enables the coder to quickly review drugs, drug actions, and indications that are often associated with overlooked or undocumented diagnoses. The coder should review the patient's medication record and know what condition the physician is treating with the prescribed medication based on documentation in the medical record. When documentation is lacking, the coder can reference this section to locate the drug, determine the drug action, confirm drug indications, and when necessary query the physician. When applicable, some of the drugs provided in this resource have also been mapped to their appropriate Z code for long-term drug use.

Drug	Z Code	Drug Action/Classification	Indications
A-Methapred [methylprednisolone sodium succinate]	Z79.52	Corticosteroid	Severe inflammation
Abilify [aripiprazole]		Antipsychotic	Depression, bipolar disorder, schizophrenia, autism symptoms
Abstral [fentanyl citrate]	Z79.891	Analgesic, narcotic	Breakthrough cancer pain
Acarbose [acarbose]	Z79.84	Oral hypoglycemic	Diabetes mellitus
Accupril [quinapril hydrochloride]		ACE inhibitor	Congestive heart failure; hypertension
Acetaminophen with codeine [acetominophen/codeine phosphate]	Z79.891	Analgesic, narcotic	Pain, moderate to severe
Actemra [tocilizumab]		Antirheumatic	Rheumatoid arthritis
Actimmune [interferon gamma-1b]	Z79.899	Antineoplastic interferons; antiviral interferons	Chronic granulomatous disease; malignant osteopetrosis
Activella [estradiol/norethindrone acetate]	Z79.890	Estrogen therapy	Menopause symptoms; vaginal and vulvar atrophy; osteoporosis prevention
Actonel [risedronate sodium]	Z79.83	Biophosphonate	Decrease in bone loss in multiple myeloma patients; Paget's disease; hyperparathyroidism; osteoporosis
Actoplus Met [metformin hydrochloride/pioglitazone hydrochloride]	Z79.84	Oral hypoglycemic	Diabetes mellitus
Actos [pioglitazone hydrochloride]	Z79.84	Oral hypoglycemic	Diabetes mellitus
Aczone [dapsone]		Acne agent, topical	Acne vulgaris
Adalat CC [nifedipine]		Calcium channel blocker	Vasospastic angina; chronic stable angina; hypertension
Adderall XR [amphetamine aspartate and sulfate/dextroamphetamine saccharate and sulfate]		CNS stimulant	Attention deficit hyperactivity disorder (ADHD)
Admelog [insulin lispro]	Z79.4	Insulin	Diabetes mellitus
Advair [fluticasone propionate/salmeterol xinafoate]	Z79.51	Corticosteroid -inhaled; antiasthmatic	Prophylaxis and treatment of asthma and COPD
Advil [ibuprofen]	Z79.1	Nonsteroidal anti-inflammatory drug (NSAID)	Pain or fever relief
Aerospan HFA [flunisolide]	Z79.51	Corticosteroid -inhaled; antiasthmatic	Prophylaxis and treatment of asthma
Afrezza [human insulin recombinant]	Z79.4	Insulin -inhaled	Diabetes mellitus
Aggrastat [tirofiban hydrochloride]	Z79.02	Antiplatelet	Unstable angina; heart attacks
Aggrenox [aspirin/dipyridamole]	Z79.02	Antiplatelet	Lessening of the chance of heart attack or stroke
Aimovig [erenumab-aooe]		Antimigraine	Migraine headache
Airduo Respiclick [fluticasone propionate/salmeterol xinafoate]	Z79.51	Corticosteroid -- inhaled; antiasthmatic	Asthma
Aldactone [spironolactone]		Cardiovascular agent; antihypertensive agent; diuretic; electrolytic and renal agent	Severe heart failure; ascites associated with cirrhosis; hypokalemia
Aleve [naproxen sodium]	Z79.1	Nonsteroidal anti-inflammatory drug (NSAID)	Reduction of temporary aches and pains
Allegra allergy [fexofenadine hydrochloride]		Antihistamine	Seasonal allergic rhinitis
Allopurinol [allopurinol]		Antigout	Gouty arthritis, renal calculus, hyperuricemia, hyperuricemia secondary to leukemia, hyperuricemia secondary to lymphoma
Alora [estradiol]	Z79.890	Estrogen therapy	Menopause symptoms
Alphagan P [brimonidine tartrate]		Antiglaucoma agent (ophthalmic); antihypertensive, ocular	Open angle glaucoma or another condition in which pressure in the eye is too high (ocular hypertension)
Alprazolam [alprazolam]		Antianxiety; sedative/hypnotic	
Altabax [retapamulin]	Z79.2	Antibiotic, topical	Skin infections
Altace [ramipril]		ACE inhibitor	Congestive heart failure; hypertension
Altavera [ethinyl estradiol/levonorgestrel]	Z79.3	Contraceptive	Prevention of pregnancy
Alvesco [ciclesonide]	Z79.51	Corticosteroid -inhaled; antiasthmatic	Prophylaxis and treatment of asthma

Appendix B: Pharmacology List 2020

Drug	Z Code	Drug Action/Classification	Indications
Alyacen [ethinyl estradiol/norethindrone]	Z79.3	Contraceptive	Prevention of pregnancy
Amaryl [glimepiride]	Z79.84	Oral hypoglycemic	Diabetes mellitus
Ambien [zolpidem tartrate]		CNS depressant; anxiolytic/sedative/hypnotic	Insomnia
Amikacin [amikacin sulfate]	Z79.2	Antibiotic	Gram-negative bacterial infections such as Pseudomonas, Escherichia coli (E. coli), Proteus, Klebsiella-Enterobacter-Serratia
Amitriptyline HCl [amitriptyline hydrochloride]		Antidepressant	Depression
Amoxicillin [amoxicillin]	Z79.2	Antibiotic	Treatment of infections with a broad spectrum of bactericidal activity against many gram-positive and gram-negative micro-organisms; otitis media, gonorrhea, skin, respiratory, gastrointestinal, and genitourinary infections
Ampicillin [ampicillin sodium]	Z79.2	Antibiotic	Bacterial infections
Ampyra [dalfampridine]		Potassium channel blocker	Improvement in walking in patients with multiple sclerosis
Amrix [cyclobenzaprine hydrochloride]		Muscle relaxant	Adjunct to rest and physical therapy for muscle spasms
Anaprox DS [naproxen sodium]	Z79.1	Nonsteroidal anti-inflammatory drug (NSAID)	Pain, inflammation or fever relief
Anastrozole [anastrozole]	Z79.811	Aromatase inhibitor	Postmenopausal breast cancer
Ancef [cefazolin sodium]	Z79.2	Antibiotic	Respiratory tract infections due to Streptococcus pneumoniae, Klebsiella species, Haemophilus influenzae (H. influenzae), Staphylococcus aureus, and group A betahemolytic streptococci; urinary tract infections due to E. coli, Proteus mirabilis, Klebsiella species and some strains of Enterobacter and enterococci; skin and skin structure infections, biliary tract infections, bone and joint infections, genital infections, septicemia, and endocarditis
Androderm [testosterone]	Z79.890	Testosterone therapy -topical	Primary hypogonadism, hypogonadotropic hypogonadism
AndroGel [testosterone]	Z79.890	Testosterone therapy -topical	Primary hypogonadism, hypogonadotropic hypogonadism
Angeliq [drospirenone/estradiol]	Z79.890	Estrogen therapy	Menopause symptoms
Angiomax [bivalirudin]	Z79.01	Anticoagulant	Prevention of blood clots
Antabuse [disulfiram]		Alcohol treatment	Alcoholism
Antineoplastic/chemotherapy	Z79.899	Antineoplastic	Cancer
Apidra [insulin glulisine recombinant]	Z79.4	Insulin	Diabetes mellitus
Aranelle [ethinyl estradiol/norethindrone]	Z79.3	Contraceptive	Prevention of pregnancy; acne
Aranesp [darbepoetin alfa]		Erythropoiesis-stimulating agent (ESA)	Treatment of lower than normal blood cells (anemia) from disorders such as CKD and neoplasms
Argatroban [argatroban]	Z79.01	Anticoagulant	Prophylaxis and treatment of venous thrombosis in thrombocytopenia patients
Aricept [donepezil hydrochloride]		Acetylcholinesterase/cholinesterase inhibitors	Symptoms of mild to moderate Alzheimer's disease; can improve thinking ability in some patients
Arimidex [anastrozole]	Z79.811	Aromatase inhibitor	Postmenopausal breast cancer
Aristospan [triamcinolone hexacetonide]	Z79.52	Corticosteroid	Severe inflammation
Arixtra [fondaparinux sodium]	Z79.01	Anticoagulant	Venous thrombosis and pulmonary embolism
Armonair Respiclick [fluticasone propionate]	Z79.51	Corticosteroid -- inhaled; anitasthmatic	Asthma
Arnuity Ellipta [fluticasone furoate]	Z79.51	Corticosteroid -inhaled; antiasthmatic	Prophylaxis and treatment of asthma
Aromasin [exemestane]	Z79.811	Aromatase inhibitor	Postmenopausal breast cancer
Arthrotec [diclofenac sodium/misoprostol]	Z79.1	Non-steroidal anti-inflammatory drug (NSAID)-prostaglandin combo	Treatment of patients with arthritis who may develop stomach ulcers from taking nonsteroidal anti-inflammatory drugs (NSAIDs) alone; used to help relieve some symptoms of arthritis, such as inflammation, swelling, stiffness, and joint pain
Asacol HD [mesalamine]		Antiinflammatory	Ulcerative colitis
Ashlyna [ethinyl estradiol/levonorgestrel]	Z79.3	Contraceptive	Prevention of pregnancy
Asmanex [mometasone furoate]	Z79.51	Corticosteroid -inhaled; antiasthmatic	Prophylaxis and treatment of asthma
Astagraf XL [tacrolimus]	Z79.899	Immunosuppressant	Prophylaxis of organ transplant rejection
Atelvia [risedronate sodium]	Z79.83	Bisphosphonate	Prevention of thinning of the bones (osteoporosis)
Atenolol [atenolol]		Beta blocker	Angina pectoris; hypertension; acute myocardial infarction

Drug	Z Code	Drug Action/Classification	Indications
Ativan [lorazepam]		Antianxiety; sedative/hypnotic	Anxiety disorder associated with depressive symptoms; controls tension, agitation, irritability, and insomnia
Atripla [efavirenz/emtricitabine/tenofovir disoproxil fumarate]	Z79.899	Antiviral	HIV
Atrovent HFA [ipratropium bromide]		Antiasthmatic/bronchodilator	Chronic bronchitis, emphysema; bronchial asthma
Augmentin [amoxicillin/clavulanate potassium]	Z79.2	Antibiotic	Middle ear, lower respiratory, sinus, skin and skin structures, and urinary tract infections
Avandia [rosiglitazone maleate]	Z79.84	Oral hypoglycemic	Diabetes mellitus
Avapro [irbesartan]		Antihypertensive	Hypertension
Avelox [moxifloxacin hydrochloride]	Z79.2	Antibiotic	Bacterial infections, specifically pneumonia; skin; intra-abdominal; plague; acute sinusitis; acute chronic bronchitis
Aviane-28 [ethinyl estradiol/levonorgestrel]	Z79.3	Contraceptive	Prevention of pregnancy
Avonex [interferon beta-1a]	Z79.899	Antiviral	Treatment of relapsing multiple sclerosis
Axid AR [nizatidine]		Histamine H2-receptor antagonist	Acid/peptic disorder; gastroesophageal reflux; duodenal, gastric, and peptic ulcers
Azactam [aztreonam]	Z79.2	Antibiotic	Severe bacterial infections
Azithromycin [azithromycin]	Z79.2	Antibiotic	Bacterial infections
Bactrim [sulfamethoxazole/trimethoprim]	Z79.2	Antibiotic	Treatment of urinary tract infections, acute otitis media, acute exacerbation of chronic bronchitis, shigellosis, and pneumocystis carinii
Balziva-28 [ethinyl estradiol/norethindrone]	Z79.3	Contraceptive	Prevention of pregnancy
Basaglar [insulin glargine]	Z79.4	Insulin	Diabetes mellitus
Bayer [acetylsalicylic acid]	Z79.82	Aspirin	Prophylaxis and treatment of heart attacks, angina or strokes; reduction of fever, pain and inflammation
Beconase AQ [beclomethasone dipropionate monohydrate]		Corticosteroid -inhaled/nasal	Perennial and seasonal allergies; vasomotor rhinitis
Bekyree [desogestrel/ethinyl estradiol]	Z79.3	Contraceptive	Prevention of pregnancy
Betaseron [interferon beta-1b]	Z79.899	Antiviral	Treatment of relapsing multiple sclerosis
Betoptic [betaxolol hydrochloride]		Beta blocker; ophthalmic glaucoma agent	Lowering of intraocular pressure; also used for treatment of ocular hypertension and chronic open-angle glaucoma
Bevyxxa	Z79.01	Anticoagulant	Prophylaxis of venous thromboembolism
Beyaz [drospirenone/ethinyl estradiol/levomefolate calcium]	Z79.3	Contraceptive	Prevention of pregnancy; acne
Biaxin XL [clarithromycin]	Z79.2	Antibiotic	Acid/peptic disorder or ulcer, acute exacerbation chronic bronchitis, human immunodeficiency virus, lower and upper respiratory tract infection, sinus infection, prophylaxis mycobacterium avium complex, pharyngitis, pneumonia, tonsillitis
Bijuva [estradiol/progesterone]	Z79.890	Estrogen/progesterone therapy	Menopausal symptoms
Biltricide [praziquantel]		Antiparasitic	Infections from Schistosoma species and liver flukes
Binosto [alendronate sodium]	Z79.83	Bisphosphonate	Prevention of thinning of the bones (osteoporosis)
Boniva [ibandronate sodium]	Z79.83	Bisphosphonate	Prevention of thinning of the bones (osteoporosis)
Breo Ellipta [fluticasone furoate/vilanterol trifenatate]	Z79.51	Corticosteroid -- inhaled; anitasthmatic	Maintenance treatment of asthma and COPD
Brevicon 28-day [ethinyl estradiol/norethindrone]	Z79.3	Contraceptive	Prevention of pregnancy; acne
Briellyn [ethinyl estradiol/norethindrone]	Z79.3	Contraceptive	Prevention of pregnancy
Brilinta [ticagrelor]	Z79.02	Antiplatelet	Unstable angina; heart attacks; prevention of blood clots
Brisdelle [paroxetine]		Selective serotonin reuptake inhibitor (SSRI)	Vasomotor symptoms related to menopause
Buprenex [buprenorphine hydrochloride]	Z79.891	Analgesic, narcotic	Moderate to severe pain
Buprenorphine HCl and Naloxone HCl [buprenorphine hydrochloride/naloxone hydrochloride]	Z79.891	Analgesic, narcotic	Moderate to severe pain
Buspirone HCl [buspirone hydrochloride]		Antianxiety	Generalized anxiety disorder
Butorphanol tartrate [butorphanol tartrate]	Z79.891	Analgesic, narcotic	Moderate to severe postsurgical pain

Drug	Z Code	Drug Action/Classification	Indications
Butrans [buprenorphine]	Z79.891	Analgesic, narcotic	Chronic pain
Byetta [exenatide]		Antidiabetic — injectable	Diabetes mellitus
Calan [verapamil hydrochloride]		Calcium channel blocker	Angina pectoris at rest and chronic stable, arrhythmia, atrial fibrillation, atrial flutter, paroxysmal supraventricular tachycardia, ventricular arrhythmia, hypertension
Caldolor [ibuprofen]	Z79.1	Nonsteroidal anti-inflammatory drug (NSAID)	Pain or fever relief
Cambia [diclofenac potassium]	Z79.1	Nonsteroidal anti-inflammatory drug (NSAID)	Migraine headaches
Camila [norethindrone]	Z79.3	Contraceptive	Prevention of pregnancy; menstrual disorders
Cardizem CD [diltiazem hydrochloride]		Calcium channel blocker	Chronic stable angina, atrial fibrillation, atrial flutter, hypertension, paroxysmal supraventricular tachycardia
Cardura [doxazosin mesylate]		Antihypertensive	Benign prostatic hyperplasia; hypertension
Catapres [clonidine hydrochloride]		Antihypertensive	Hypertension
Cefprozil [cefprozil]	Z79.2	Antibiotic	Acute exacerbation and chronic bronchitis, lower respiratory tract infection, upper respiratory tract infection, pharyngitis, tonsillitis
Ceftriaxone [ceftriaxone sodium]	Z79.2	Antibiotic	Bacterial infections
Celebrex [celecoxib]	Z79.1	Nonsteroidal anti-inflammatory drug (NSAID)	Relief of some symptoms caused by arthritis, such as inflammation, swelling, stiffness, and joint pain
Celestone Soluspan [betamethasone acetate/betamethasone sodium phosphate]	Z79.52	Corticosteroid; antiasthmatic	Asthma; severe inflammation
Celexa [citalopram hydrobromide]		Antidepressant	Depression
Cellcept [mycophenolate mofetil]	Z79.899	Immunosuppressant	Prophylaxis of organ transplant rejection
Centany [mupirocin]	Z79.2	Antibiotic	Skin infections
Cephalexin [cephalexin]	Z79.2	Antibiotic	Bacterial infections
Chantix [varenicline tartrate]		Smoking cessation aid	Nicotine addiction, smoking
Cimduo [lamivudine/tenofovir disoproxil fumarate]	Z79.899	Antiviral	HIV
Cipro [ciprofloxacin hydrochloride]	Z79.2	Antibiotic	Cystitis, infectious diarrhea, gonorrhea, bone and joint infection, gastrointestinal tract infection, lower and upper respiratory tract infection, sinus infection, urinary tract infection, nosocomial pneumonia, chronic prostatitis
Ciprofloxacin [ciprofloxacin]	Z79.2	Antibiotic	Bacterial infections
Clarithromycin [clarithromycin]	Z79.2	Antibiotic	Skin and respiratory bacterial infections
Claritin [loratadine]		Antihistamine	Seasonal allergic rhinitis; chronic idiopathic urticaria
Cleocin [clindamycin phosphate]	Z79.2	Antibiotic	Bacterial infections
Climara [estradiol]	Z79.890	Estrogen therapy	Osteoporosis prevention and to treat menopausal symptoms; vaginal and vulvar atrophy; hypoestrogenism; ovarian failure
Clindamycin [clindamycin phosphate]	Z79.2	Antibiotic	Bacterial infections.
Clonazepam [clonazepam]		Anticonvulsant	Absence, akinetic and myoclonic epilepsy, Lennox-Gastaut syndrome
Clonidine HCl [clonidine hydrochloride]		Antihypertensive	Hypertension
Clopidogrel bisulfate [clopidogrel bisulfate]	Z79.02	Antiplatelet	Unstable angina; heart attacks; prevention of blood clots
Codeine [codeine sulfate]	Z79.891	Analgesic, narcotic	Mild to moderate pain
Cogentin [benztropine mesylate]		Antiparkinsonism	Parkinson's disease
Colace [docusate sodium]		Gastrointestinal agent; laxative, stool softener	Constipation
Colocort [hydrocortisone]	Z79.52	Corticosteroid	Inflammation of the colon
CombiPatch [ethinyl estradiol/norethindrone acetate]	Z79.890	Estrogen therapy	Menopause symptoms; vaginal and vulvar atrophy; osteoporosis prevention
Combivent respimat [ipratropium bromide/albuterol sulfate]		Antiasthmatic/bronchodilator	Chronic bronchitis, emphysema; bronchial asthma
Compro [prochlorperazine]		Antiemetic; antipsychotic	Nausea, vomiting, and manic phase of bipolar syndrome or schizophrenia
Copaxone [glatiramer acetate]		Immunostimulant	Treatment of relapsing multiple sclerosis
Coreg [carvedilol]		Beta blocker	Hypertension; chronic heart failure; left ventricular dysfunction following myocardial infarction

Drug	Z Code	Drug Action/Classification	Indications
Coreg CR [carvedilol phosphate]		Beta blocker	Hypertension; chronic heart failure; left ventricular dysfunction following myocardial infarction
Cortef [hydrocortisone]	Z79.52	Corticosteroid	Severe inflammation
Cortenema [hydrocortisone]	Z79.52	Corticosteroid	Inflammation of the colon
Cortifoam [hydrocortisone acetate]	Z79.52	Corticosteroid	Colon and rectum inflammation
Cortisone acetate [cortisone acetate]	Z79.52	Corticosteroid	Inflammation
Cortisporin [hydrocortisone acetate/neomycin sulfate/polymyxin B sulfate]		Topical anti-infective, topical steroid	Dermatosis
Cosentyx [secukinumab]	Z79.899	Immunosuppressant	Plaque psoriasis; psoriatic arthritis; ankylosing spondylitis
Coumadin [warfarin sodium]	Z79.Ø1	Anticoagulant	Prophylaxis and treatment of venous thrombosis, treatment of atrial fibrillation with embolization (pulmonary embolism), arrhythmias, myocardial infarction, and stroke prevention
Cozaar [losartan potassium]		Antihypertensive	Hypertension
Crestor [rosuvastatin calcium]		HMG-CoA reductase inhibitor (statin)	Hypercholesterolemia; hyperlipidemia; hyperproteinemia
Crixivan [indinavir sulfate]	Z79.899	Antiviral	HIV, asymptomatic HIV
Cryselle [ethinyl estradiol/norgestrel]	Z79.3	Contraceptive	Prevention of pregnancy
Cubicin [daptomycin]	Z79.2	Antibiotic	Bacterial skin infections; *Staphylococcus aureus* bloodstream infections
Cyclafem [ethinyl estradiol/norethindrone]	Z79.3	Contraceptive	Prevention of pregnancy
Cyclessa [desogestrel/ethinyl estradiol]	Z79.3	Contraceptive	Prevention of pregnancy
Cyclosporine [cyclosporine]	Z79.899	Immunosuppressant	Prophylaxis of organ transplant rejection
Cyltezo [adalimumab-abdm]	Z79.899	Antirheumatic	Rheumatoid arthritis; juvenile idiopathic arthritis; psoriatic arthritis; Crohn's disease; ulcerative colitis; plaque psoriasis
Cymbalta [duloxetine hydrochloride]		Antidepressant, serotonin and norepinephrine reuptake inhibitor (SNRI)	Major depressive disorder; general anxiety disorder; fibromyalgia; diabetic peripheral neuropathy; chronic musculoskeletal pain
Cytomel [liothyronine sodium]		Thyroid hormone	Hypothyroidism or prevention of euthyroid goiters
Daptomycin [daptomycin]	Z79.2	Antibiotic	Skin and underlying tissue bacterial infections
Dasetta [ethinyl estradiol/norethindrone]	Z79.3	Contraceptive	Prevention of pregnancy
Daypro [oxaprozin]	Z79.1	Nonsteroidal anti-inflammatory drug (NSAID)	Osteoarthritis and rheumatoid arthritis
Daysee [ethinyl estradiol/levonorgestrel]	Z79.3	Contraceptive	Prevention of pregnancy
Delestrogen [estradiol valerate]	Z79.89Ø	Estrogen therapy	Menopause symptoms
Demerol [meperidine hydrochloride]	Z79.891	Analgesic, narcotic	Moderate to severe pain
Depakote [divalproex sodium]		Anticonvulsant	Bipolar affective disorder; complex absence, complex partial and mixed pattern epilepsy; migraine headache
Depo-Medrol [methylprednisolone acetate]	Z79.52	Corticosteroid	Arthritis; joint disorders
Depo-Provera [medroxyprogesterone acetate]	Z79.3, Z79.89Ø	Antineoplastic; contraceptive; progestin	Amenorrhea; carcinoma, endometrium, adjunct; carcinoma, renal; Prevention of pregnancy; hemorrhage
Depo-SubQ Provera [medroxyprogesterone acetate]	Z79.3	Contraceptive	Prevention of pregnancy; menstrual disorder pain
Descovy [emtricitabine/tenofovir alafenamide]	Z79.899	Antiretroviral	HIV
Desogen [desogestrel/ethinyl estradiol]	Z79.3	Contraceptive	Prevention of pregnancy
Detrol [tolterodine tartrate]		Muscarinic receptor antagonist	Overactive bladders in patients with urinary frequency, urgency, or urge incontinence
Dexamethasone Intensol [dexamethasone]	Z79.52	Corticosteroid	Arthritis; allergic disorders; breathing disorders; lupus
Dexilant [dexlansoprazole]		Proton pump inhibitor	Healing of erosive esophagitis; relieve of heartburn; treatment of non-erosive gastroesophageal reflux disease
Diabinese [chlorpropamide]	Z79.84	Oral hypoglycemic	Diabetes mellitus
Diaβeta [glyburide]	Z79.84	Oral hypoglycemic	Diabetes mellitus
Diclegis [doxylamine succinate/pyridoxine hydrochloride]		Antiemetic	Nausea/vomiting in pregnancy
Didronel [etidronate disodium]	Z79.83	Bisphosphonate	Paget's disease and irregular bone growth
Dificid [fidaxomicin]	Z79.2	Antibiotic	Clostridium difficile

Drug	Z Code	Drug Action/Classification	Indications
Diflucan [fluconazole]		Antifungal	Oropharyngeal and esophageal candidiasis and cryptococcal meningitis in AIDS patients
Digoxin [digoxin]		Cardiotonic glycoside	Heart failure, atrial flutter, atrial fibrillation, and supraventricular tachycardia
Dilantin [phenytoin sodium]		Anticonvulsant	Grand mal and psychomotor seizures
Dilaudid [hydromorphone hydrochloride]	Z79.891	Analgesic, narcotic	Moderate to severe pain
Diovan [valsartan]		Angiotensin II receptor blocker	Hypertension
Diskets [methadone hydrochloride]		Opioid agonist	Treatment of opioid addiction
Divigel [estradiol]	Z79.890	Estrogen therapy -topical	Menopause symptoms
Dolophine HCl [methadone hydrochloride]	Z79.891	Analgesic, narcotic; opioid agonist	Pain; treatment of opioid addiction
Doxycycline [doxycycline]	Z79.2	Antibiotic	Bacterial infections; acne
Duavee [bazedoxifene acetate/conjugated estrogens]	Z79.890	Estrogen therapy	Menopause symptoms; osteoporosis prevention
Duetact [glimepiride/pioglitazone hydrochloride]	Z79.84	Oral hypoglycemic	Diabetes mellitus
Duexis [famotidine/ibuprofen]	Z79.1	Nonsteroidal anti-inflammatory drug (NSAID)	Symptomatic treatment of osteoarthritis and rheumatoid arthritis; reduce risk of ulcers
Dulera [formoterol fumarate/mometasone furoate]	Z79.51	Corticosteroid -inhaled; antiasthmatic	Prophylaxis and treatment of asthma
Duragesic [fentanyl]	Z79.891	Analgesic, narcotic	Chronic pain
Duramorph PF [morphine sulfate]	Z79.891	Analgesic, narcotic	Moderate to severe pain
Durlaza [aspirin]	Z79.82	Aspirin	Prevention of heart attack, stroke, angina
Dynacin [minocycline hydrochloride]	Z79.2	Antibiotic	Severe acne treatment
E.E.S. [erythromycin ethylsuccinate]	Z79.2	Antibiotic	Bacterial infections
Effexor XR [venlafaxine hydrochloride]		Antidepressant, serotonin and norepinephrine reuptake inhibitors (SNRIs)	Major depressive disorder; social anxiety disorder; panic disorder
Effient [prasugrel hydrochloride]	Z79.02	Antiplatelet	Lessening of the chance of heart attack or stroke
Elestrin [estradiol]	Z79.890	Estrogen therapy	Menopause symptoms
Eligard [leuprolide acetate]	Z79.818	Agents affecting estrogen receptors and estrogen levels	Palliative treatment of prostate cancer symptoms
Elinest [norgestrel/ethinyl estradiol]	Z79.3	Contraceptive	Prevention of pregnancy
Eliquis [apixaban]	Z79.01	Anticoagulant	Venous thrombosis
Embeda [morphine sulfate/naltrexone hydrochloride]	Z79.891	Analgesic, narcotic	Moderate to severe pain
Emoquette [ethinyl estradiol/desogestrel]	Z79.3	Contraceptive	Prevention of pregnancy
Emtriva [emtricitabine]	Z79.899	Antiretroviral	HIV
Enbrel [etanercept]	Z79.899	Antirheumatic	Rheumatoid arthritis; polyarticular juvenile idiopathic arthritis; psoriatic arthritis; ankylosing spondylitis, plaque psoriasis
Enpresse-28 [ethinyl estradiol/levonorgestrel]	Z79.3	Contraceptive	Prevention of pregnancy
Enskyce [desogestrel/ethinyl estradiol]	Z79.3	Contraceptive	Prevention of pregnancy
Entocort EC [budesonide]	Z79.52	Corticosteroid	Crohn's disease; ulcerative colitis
Entresto [sacubitril/valsartan]		Angiotensin II receptor blocker; neprilysin inhibitor	Chronic heart failure
Entyvio [vedolizumab]	Z79.899	Immunosuppressant	Ulcerative colitis; Crohn's disease
Envarsus XR [tacrolimus]	Z79.899	Immunosuppressant	Prophylaxis of organ transplant rejection
Epinephrine [epinephrine]		Bronchodilator, cardiotonic	Most commonly, relief of distress due to bronchospasm and restoration of cardiac rhythm in cardiac arrest
Epivir, Epivir-HBV [lamivudine]	Z79.899	Antiretroviral	HIV, hepatitis B (HBV), asymptomatic HIV
Erelzi [etanercept-szzs]	Z79.899	Antirheumatic	Rheumatoid arthritis; polyarticular juvenile idiopathic arthritis; psoriatic arthritis; ankylosing spondylitis, plaque psoriasis
Errin [norethindrone]	Z79.3	Contraceptive	Prevention of pregnancy
Ertapenem [ertapenem sodium]	Z79.2	Antibiotic	Stomach, urinary tract, pelvis, skin and lung infections
Ery-Tab [erythromycin]	Z79.2	Antibiotic	Bacterial infections
ERYC [erythromycin]	Z79.2	Antibiotic	Respiratory tract infections

Drug	Z Code	Drug Action/Classification	Indications
Erygel [erythromycin]	Z79.2	Antibiotic, topical	Bacterial skin infections
EryPed [erythromycin ethylsuccinate]	Z79.2	Antibiotic	Bacterial infections; rheumatic fever attacks
Erythrocin [erythromycin lactobionate]	Z79.2	Antibiotic	Bacterial infections
Erythromycin [erythromycin]	Z79.2	Antibiotic	Respiratory tract infections
Estarylla [ethinyl estradiol/norgestimate]	Z79.3	Contraceptive	Prevention of pregnancy
Estrace [estradiol]	Z79.890	Estrogen therapy	Vaginal cream for treatment of vaginal and vulvar atrophy
EstroGel [estradiol]	Z79.890	Estrogen therapy -topical	Menopause symptoms
Estrostep Fe [ethinyl estradiol/norethindrone acetate]	Z79.3	Contraceptive	Prevention of pregnancy
Evista [raloxifene hydrochloride]	Z79.810	Selective estrogen receptor modulator (SERM)	Prevention of thinning of the bones (osteoporosis) only in postmenopausal women
Exalgo [hydromorphone hydrochloride]	Z79.891	Analgesic, narcotic	Moderate to severe pain
Exemestane [exemestane]	Z79.811	Aromatase inhibitor	Postmenopausal breast cancer
Factive [gemifloxacin mesylate]	Z79.2	Antibiotic	Bacterial lung infections
Falmina [ethinyl estradiol/levonorgestrel]	Z79.3	Contraceptive	Prevention of pregnancy
Fareston [toremifene citrate]	Z79.810	Selective estrogen receptor modulator (SERM)	Treatment of metastatic breast cancer in postmenopausal women
Farxiga [dapagliflozin propanediol]	Z79.84	Oral hypoglycemic	Diabetes mellitus
Faslodex [fulvestrant]	Z79.818	Agents affecting estrogen receptors and estrogen levels	Hormone-related breast cancer; metastatic breast cancer
Feldene [piroxicam]	Z79.1	Nonsteroidal anti-inflammatory drug (NSAID)	Treatment of pain and inflammation due to arthritis
Femara [letrozole]	Z79.811	Aromatase inhibitor	Postmenopausal breast cancer
Femcon Fe [ethinyl estradiol/norethindrone]	Z79.3	Contraceptive	Prevention of pregnancy; acne
Femhrt [ethinyl estradiol/norethindrone acetate]	Z79.3, Z79.890	Contraceptive; estrogen therapy	Prevention of pregnancy; menopause symptoms; osteoporosis prevention
Femring [estradiol acetate]	Z79.890	Estrogen therapy	Osteoporosis prevention and to treat menopausal symptoms; hypoestrogenism; ovarian failure
Fentanyl citrate [fentanyl citrate]	Z79.891	Analgesic, narcotic	Postprocedural or chronic pain
Fentora [fentanyl citrate]	Z79.891	Analgesic, narcotic	Breakthrough cancer pain
Fiasp [insulin aspart]	Z79.4	Insulin	Diabetes mellitus
Fioricet with codeine [acetaminophen/butalbital/caffeine/codeine phosphate]	Z79.891	Analgesic, narcotic	Tension headaches
Firmagon [degarelix]	Z79.890	Hormone therapy	Prostate cancer
Flagyl [metronidazole]	Z79.2	Antibiotic	Bacterial infections
Flavoxate HCl [flavoxate hydrochloride]		Urinary tract spasmolytic	Relief of dysuria, urgency, nocturia, suprapubic pain, frequency, and incontinence associated with cystitis, prostatitis, urethritis, and urethrocystitis/urethrotrigonitis
Flomax [tamsulosin hydrochloride]		Antiadrenergic	Benign prostatic hyperplasia
Flonase allergy relief [fluticasone propionate]		Corticosteroid -inhaled/nasal	Perennial and seasonal allergic rhinitis
Flovent HFA [fluticasone propionate]	Z79.51	Corticosteroid -inhaled; antiasthmatic	Asthma
Fortamet [metformin hydrochloride]	Z79.84	Oral hypoglycemic	Diabetes mellitus
Fortaz [ceftazidime]	Z79.2	Antibiotic	Pneumonia and lower respiratory infections
Fosamax [alendronate sodium]	Z79.83	Biophosphonate	Osteoporosis; Paget's disease
Fosinopril sodium [fosinopril sodium]		ACE inhibitor	Hypertension
Fosrenol [lanthanum carbonate]		Phosphate binder	End-stage renal disease (ESRD)
Fragmin [dalteparin sodium]	Z79.01	Anticoagulant	Prophylaxis and treatment of blood clots
Gengraf [cyclosporine]	Z79.899	Immunosuppressant	Prophylaxis of organ transplant rejection
Gentamicin sulfate [gentamicin sulfate]	Z79.2	Antibiotic	Severe bacterial infections
Gildagia [ethinyl estradiol/norethindrone]	Z79.3	Contraceptive	Prevention of pregnancy
Gildess [ethinyl estradiol/norethindrone acetate]	Z79.3	Contraceptive	Prevention of pregnancy

Drug	Z Code	Drug Action/Classification	Indications
Glimepiride [glimepiride]	Z79.84	Oral hypoglycemic	Diabetes mellitus
Glucophage [metformin hydrochloride]	Z79.84	Oral hypoglycemic	Diabetes mellitus
Glucotrol [glipizide]	Z79.84	Oral hypoglycemic	Diabetes mellitus
Glucovance [glyburide/metformin hydrochloride]	Z79.84	Oral hypoglycemic	Diabetes mellitus
Glumetza [metformin hydrochloride]	Z79.84	Oral hypoglycemic	Diabetes mellitus
Glyburide (micronized) [glyburide]	Z79.84	Oral hypoglycemic	Diabetes mellitus
Glynase [glyburide]	Z79.84	Oral hypoglycemic	Diabetes mellitus
Glyset [miglitol]	Z79.84	Oral hypoglycemic	Diabetes mellitus
Harvoni [ledipasvir/sofosbuvir]	Z79.899	Antiviral	Chronic hepatitis C
Heparin sodium [heparin sodium]	Z79.01	Anticoagulant	Prophylaxis and treatment of venous thrombosis, pulmonary embolism; prevention of cerebral thrombosis, and treatment of consumptive coagulopathies
Humalog [insulin lispro recombinant]	Z79.4	Insulin	Diabetes mellitus
Humira [adalimumab]	Z79.899	Antirheumatic	Rheumatoid arthritis; juvenile idiopathic arthritis; psoriatic arthritis; Crohn's disease; ulcerative colitis; plaque psoriasis; hidradenitis suppurativa; uveitis
Humulin R [insulin recombinant]	Z79.4	Insulin	Diabetes mellitus
Hydrochlorothiazide [hydrochlorothiazide]		Diuretic; antihypertensive	Management of hypertension and in adjunctive therapy for edema associated with congestive heart failure; hepatic cirrhosis; corticosteroid, and estrogen therapy
Hydrocodone [acetaminophen/hydrocodone bitartrate]	Z79.891	Analgesic, narcotic	Moderate to severe pain
Hydrocodone bitartrate and acetaminophen [acetaminophen/hydrocodone bitartrate]	Z79.891	Analgesic, narcotic	Pain, moderate to severe
Hydrocortisone [hydrocortisone]	Z79.52	Corticosteroid	Addison's disease; arthritis; immune disorders; allergies; breathing problems
Hydromorphone HCl [hydromorphone hydrochloride]	Z79.891	Analgesic, narcotic	Moderate to severe pain
Hyrimoz [adalimumab-adaz]	Z79.899	Antirheumatic	Rheumatoid arthritis; juvenile idiopathic arthritis; psoriatic arthritis; Crohn's disease; ulcerative colitis; plaque psoriasis
Hyzaar [hydrochlorothiazide/ losartan potassium]		Antihypertensive	Hypertension
Ibuprofen [ibuprofen]	Z79.1	Nonsteroidal anti-inflammatory drug (NSAID)	Pain or fever relief
Imitrex [sumatriptan succinate]		Antimigraine	Migraine headache
Imuran [azathioprine]	Z79.899	Immunosuppressant	Rheumatoid arthritis
Inderal [propranolol hydrochloride]		Beta blocker	Angina pectoris; hypertension; cardiac arrhythmias
Indocin [indomethacin]	Z79.1	Nonsteroidal anti-inflammatory drug (NSAID)	Treatment of pain and inflammation
Integrilin [eptifibatide]	Z79.02	Antiplatelet	Unstable angina; heart attacks; prevention of blood clots
Intron A [interferon alfa 2-b]	Z79.899	Antineoplastic interferons; antiviral interferons	Cancer; hepatitis
Introvale [levonorgestrel/ethinyl estradiol]	Z79.3	Contraceptive	Prevention of pregnancy
Invanz [ertapeneum sodium]	Z79.2	Antibiotic	Stomach, urinary tract, pelvis, skin and lung infections
Invokamet [canagliflozin/metformin hydrochloride]	Z79.84	Oral hypoglycemic	Diabetes mellitus
Invokana [canagliflozin]	Z79.84	Oral hypoglycemic	Diabetes mellitus
Isoniazid [isoniazid]	Z79.2	Antibiotic	Tuberculosis
Isopto carpine [pilocarpine hydrochloride]		Cholinergic parasympathomimetic agent	Reduction of intraocular pressure in open-angle glaucoma or ocular hypertension; management of acute angle-closure glaucoma
Isordil [isosorbide dinitrate]		Smooth muscle relaxant	Acute anginal attacks
Isuprel [isoproterenol hydrochloride]		Adrenergic agent	Bronchodilator for asthma, chronic pulmonary emphysema, bronchitis, and other conditions accompanied by bronchospasm; can be used in cardiogenic shock cases

Drug	Z Code	Drug Action/Classification	Indications
Jantoven [warfarin sodium]	Z79.Ø1	Anticoagulant	Prophylaxis and treatment of venous thrombosis, pulmonary embolism; prevention of cerebral thrombosis, and treatment of consumptive coagulopathies
Janumet [metformin hydrochloride/sitagliptin phosphate]	Z79.84	Oral hypoglycemic	Diabetes mellitus
Januvia [sitagliptin phosphate]	Z79.84	Oral hypoglycemic	Diabetes mellitus
Jencycla [norethindrone]	Z79.3	Contraceptive	Prevention of pregnancy
Jentadueto [linagliptin/metformin hydrochloride]]	Z79.84	Oral hypoglycemic	Diabetes mellitus
Junel [ethinyl estradiol/norethindrone acetate]	Z79.3	Contraceptive	Prevention of pregnancy
K-Tab [potassium chloride]		Replaces potassium and maintains potassium level	Hypokalemia
Kadian [morphine sulfate]	Z79.891	Analgesic, narcotic	Moderate to severe pain
Kariva [desogestrel/ethinyl estradiol]	Z79.3	Contraceptive	Prevention of pregnancy
Kazano [alogliptin benzoate/metformin hydrochloride]	Z79.84	Oral hypoglycemic	Diabetes mellitus
Keflex [cephalexin]	Z79.2	Antibiotic	Bone, middle ear, skin and skin structures, upper respiratory tract and urinary tract infections; acute prostatitis
Kelnor [ethynodiol diacetate/ethinyl estradiol]	Z79.3	Contraceptive	Prevention of pregnancy
Kenalog-10; Kenalog-40 [triamcinolone acetonide]	Z79.52	Corticosteroid	Gouty arthritis; bursitis; tenosynovitis; epicondylitis; rheumatoid arthritis; synovitis; osteoarthritis
Keytruda [pembrolizumab]	Z79.899	Antineoplastic	Cancer
Kimidess [ethinyl estradiol/desogestrel]	Z79.3	Contraceptive	Prevention of pregnancy
Klaron [sulfacetamide sodium]	Z79.2	Antibiotic, topical	Acne vulgaris
Klonopin [clonazepam]		Anticonvulsant; CNS depressant	Epilepsy; seizures; panic disorder
Klor-Con [potassium chloride]		Replaces potassium and maintains potassium level	Hypokalemia
Kombiglyze [metformin hydrochloride/saxagliptin hydrochloride]	Z79.84	Oral hypoglycemic	Diabetes mellitus
Kurvelo [ethinyl estradiol/levonorgestrel]	Z79.3	Contraceptive	Prevention of pregnancy; menstrual disorders
Kyleena [levonorgestrel]	Z79.3	Contraceptive	Prevention of pregnancy
Lamisil [terbinafine hydrochloride]		Antifungal	Tinea cruris (jock itch), T. pedis (athlete's foot), T. corporis (ringworm)
Lanoxin [digoxin]		Cardiotonic glycoside	Congestive heart failure
Lantus [insulin glargine recombinant]	Z79.4	Insulin	Diabetes mellitus
Larin [ethinyl estradiol/norethindrone acetate]	Z79.3	Contraceptive	Prevention of pregnancy
Lasix [furosemide]		Antihypertensive; diuretic	Management of edema associated with congestive heart failure, renal disease, including nephrotic syndrome and hypertension
Lazanda [fentanyl citrate]	Z79.891	Analgesics, narcotic	Breakthrough cancer pain
Lescol XL [fluvastatin sodium]		HMG-CoA reductase inhibitor (statin)	Hypercholesterolemia; hyperlipidemia; hyperlipoproteinemia
Lessina-28 [ethinyl estradiol/levonorgestrel]	Z79.3	Contraceptive	Prevention of pregnancy
Letrozole [letrozole]	Z79.811	Aromatase inhibitor	Postmenopausal breast cancer
Levemir [insulin detemir recombinant]	Z79.4	Insulin	Diabetes mellitus
Levonest [levonorgestrel/ethinyl estradiol]	Z79.3	Contraceptive	Prevention of pregnancy; menstrual disorders; acne
Levora [levonorgestrel/ethinyl estradiol]	Z79.3	Contraceptive	Prevention of pregnancy
Levothroid [levothyroxine sodium]		Thyroid hormone	Hypothyroidism
Levoxyl [levothyroxine sodium]		Thyroid hormone	Euthyroid goiter; hypothyroidism
Lexapro [escitalopram oxalate]		Antidepressant, selective serotonin reuptake inhibitor (SSRI)	Depression; anxiety
Lialda [mesalamine]		Antiinflammatory	Ulcerative colitis
Librium [chlordiazepoxide hydrochloride]		Antianxiety	Acute withdrawal symptoms, especially from alcohol, or for other anxiety-producing conditions

Drug	Z Code	Drug Action/Classification	Indications
Lidocaine HCl [lidocaine hydrochloride]		Antiarrhythmic	Management of ventricular arrhythmias or during cardiac manipulation, such as cardiac surgery
Liletta [levonorgestrel]	Z79.3	Contraceptive	Intrauterine device for prevention of pregnancy
Lincocin [lincocin hydrochloride]	Z79.2	Antibiotic	Severe bacterial infections
Lipitor [atorvastatin calcium]		HMG-CoA reductase inhibitor (statin)	Hypercholesterolemia; hyperlipidemia; hyperproteinemia
Lithium carbonate [lithium carbonate]		Antimanic	Control of manic episodes in bipolar disorders
Lo Loestrin Fe [ethinyl estradiol/norethindrone acetate]	Z79.3	Contraceptive	Prevention of pregnancy
Locoid [hydrocotisone butyrate]	Z79.52	Corticosteroid -topical	Atopic dermatitis; other dermatoses
Loestrin [ethinyl estradiol/norethindrone acetate]	Z79.3	Contraceptive	Prevention of pregnancy
Lomotil [diphenoxylate hydrochloride/atropine sulfate]		Antidiarrheal	Symptoms of chronic and functional diarrhea
Lopid [gemfibrozil]		Lipid regulating agent	Hypercholesterolemia, hyperlipidemia, hyperlipoproteinemia, hypertriglyceridemia
Lopressor [metoprolol tartrate]		Beta blocker	Angina pectoris; hypertension; acute myocardial infarction
Lorazepam [lorazepam]		Antianxiety; sedative/hypnotic	Anxiety disorder associated with depressive symptoms; controls tension, agitation, irritability, and insomnia
Loryna [drospirenone/ethinyl estradiol]	Z79.3	Contraceptive	Prevention of pregnancy
LoSeasonique [ethinyl estradiol/levonorgestrel]	Z79.3	Contraceptive	Prevention of pregnancy
Lotensin [benazepril hydrochloride]		ACE inhibitor	Hypertension
Lotrel [amlodipine besylate/benazepril hydrochloride]		Antihypertensive	Hypertension
Lotrisone [clotrimazole/ betamethasone dipropionate]		Antifungal-corticosteroid	Relief of redness, swelling, itching, and other discomfort of fungus infections
Lovastatin [lovastatin]		HMG-CoA reductase inhibitor (statin)	Hypercholesterolemia; hyperlipidemia; hyperlipoproteinemia
Lovenox [enoxaparin sodium]	Z79.01	Anticoagulant	Prophylaxis and treatment of venous thrombosis and pulmonary embolism
Low-Ogestrel-28 [norgestrel/ethinyl estradiol]	Z79.3	Contraceptive	Prevention of pregnancy
Lupron [leuprolide acetate]	Z79.818	Agents affecting estrogen receptors and estrogen levels	Endometriosis symptoms; uterine fibroids
Macrobid [nitrofuantoin]	Z79.2	Antibiotic	Urinary tract infections
Macrodantin [nitrofurantoin]	Z79.2	Antibiotic	Urinary tract infections
Marlissa [ethinyl estradiol/levonorgestrel]	Z79.3	Contraceptive	Prevention of pregnancy
Maxipime [cefepime hydrochloride]	Z79.2	Antibiotic	Bacterial infections
Meclizine hydrochloride [meclizine hydrochloride]		Antihistamine	Nausea and vomiting, and dizziness associated with motion sickness
Medrol [methylprednisolone]	Z79.52	Corticosteroid	Endocrine, rheumatic, hematologic disorders; collagen, dermatological, ophthalmic, respiratory, neoplastic, gastrointestinal, nervous system disorders; allergic and edematous states
Mefoxin [cefoxitin sodium]	Z79.2	Antibiotic	Bacterial infections
Megace ES [megestrol acetate]	Z79.818	Agents affecting estrogen receptors and estrogen levels	Endometrial or advanced breast cancers; weight loss due to AIDS
Menest [esteriefied estrogens]	Z79.890	Estrogen therapy	Menopause symptoms; ovarian failure
Menostar [estradiol]	Z79.890	Estrogen therapy	Menopause symptoms; osteoporosis prevention
Mepron [atovaquone]	Z79.2	Antibiotic	Pneumonia due to penumocystis jiroveci
Merrem [meropenem]	Z79.2	Antibiotic	Bacterial infections of skin or stomach; bacterial meningitis
Metformin [metformin hydrochloride]	Z79.84	Oral hypoglycemic	Diabetes mellitus
Methadone HCl [methadone hydrochloride]	Z79.891	Analgesic, narcotic; opioid agonist	Pain; treatment of opioid addiction
Methadose [methadone hydrochloride]	Z79.891	Analgesic, narcotic	Acute and chronic pain
Methergine [methylergonovine maleate]		Oxytocic agent	Routine management of postpartum hemorrhage after delivery of placenta
Methylprednisolone [methylprednisolone]	Z79.52	Corticosteroid	Inflammatory disorders

Drug	Z Code	Drug Action/Classification	Indications
Metronidazole [metronidazole]	Z79.2	Antibiotic	Bacterial infections
Miacalcin [calcitonin salmon]		Calcitonin; a peptide hormone	Hypercalcemia, osteoporosis, postmenopausal symptoms, Paget's disease
Microgestin [ethinyl estradiol/norethindrone acetate]	Z79.3	Contraceptive	Prevention of pregnancy
Micronor [norethindrone]	Z79.3	Contraceptive	Prevention of pregnancy
Minastrin [ethinyl estradiol/norethindrone acetate]	Z79.3	Contraceptive	Prevention of pregnancy
Minivelle [estradiol]	Z79.890	Estrogen therapy	Menopause symptoms; osteoporosis prevention
Minocin [minocycline hydrochloride]	Z79.2	Antibiotic	Bacterial infections; acne
Mirena [levonorgestrel]	Z79.3	Contraceptive	Intrauterine device for prevention of pregnancy; menstrual disorders
Mobic [meloxicam]	Z79.1	Nonsteroidal anti-inflammatory drug (NSAID)	Treatment of pain and inflammation due to osteoarthritis and rheumatoid arthritis
Modicon 28 [ethinyl estradiol/norethindrone]	Z79.3	Contraceptive	Prevention of pregnancy
Mono-Linyah [norgestimate/ethinyl estradiol]	Z79.3	Contraceptive	Prevention of pregnancy; menstrual disorders; acne
Monoclonal antibodies	Z79.899	Monoclonal antibodies	Cancer; prophylaxis of organ transplant rejection
Monodox [doxycycline]	Z79.2	Antibiotic	Bacterial infections; acne
Monoket [isosorbide mononitrate]		Antianginal; coronary vasodilator, nitrate	Angina pectoris
Monurol [fosfomycin tromethamine]	Z79.2	Antibiotic	Bacterial bladder infections
Morphabond ER [morphine sulfate]	Z79.891	Analgesics, narcotic	Pain
Morphine sulfate [morphine sulfate]	Z79.891	Analgesic, narcotic	Moderate to severe pain
Motrin IB [ibuprofen]	Z79.1	Nonsteroidal anti-inflammatory drug (NSAID)	Pain or fever relief
MS Contin [morphine sulfate]	Z79.891	Analgesic, narcotic	Moderate to severe pain
Multaq [dronedarone hydrochloride]		Cardiac rhythm regulator	Treatment of patients with recent episodes of atrial fibrillation or atrial flutter
Mycobutin [rifabutin]	Z79.2	Antibiotic	Mycobacterium avium complex (MAC) prophylactic in HIV patients
Mytesi [crofelemer]		Antidiarrheal	Diarrhea occurring in HIV/AIDs patient's on anti-retroviral therapy
Myzilra [ethinyl estradiol/levonorgestrel]	Z79.3	Contraceptive	Prevention of pregnancy
Nabumetone [nabumetone]	Z79.1	Non-steroidal anti-inflammatory drug (NSAID)	Osteoarthritis and rheumatoid arthritis
Nalfon [fenoprofen calcium]	Z79.1	Nonsteroidal anti-inflammatory drug (NSAID)	Pain or inflammation relief
Namzaric [memantine/donepezil hydrochlroides]		Acetylcholinesterase/cholinesterase inhibitors	Dementia due to Alzheimer's
Naprelan [naproxen sodium]	Z79.1	Nonsteroidal anti-inflammatory drug (NSAID)	Pain or inflammation relief
Naprosyn [naproxen]	Z79.1	Nonsteroidal anti-inflammatory drug (NSAID)	Rheumatoid, gouty arthritis and osteoarthritis; ankylosing spondylitis; bursitis; dysmenorrhea; pain, mild to moderate; tendonitis
Natazia [estradiol valerate/dienogest]	Z79.3	Contraceptive	Prevention of pregnancy; menstrual disorders
Nebupent [pentamidine isethionate]	Z79.2	Antibiotic	Severe bacterial lung infection in high risk patients with HIV
Nefazodone HCl [nefazodone hydrochloride]		Antidepressant	Depression
Nembutal sodium [pentobarbital sodium]		Sedative/hypnotic	Adjunct medication in diagnostic procedures or for emergency use with convulsive disorders
NeoProfen [ibuprofen lysine]	Z79.1	Nonsteroidal anti-inflammatory drug (NSAID)	Pain or fever relief
Neoral [cyclosporine]	Z79.899	Immunosuppressant	Prophylaxis of organ transplant rejection
Neurontin [gabapentin]		Anticonvulsant	Epilepsy, partial
Nexium [esomeprazole magnesium]		Proton pump inhibitor	Gastroesophageal reflux disease (GERD), erosive esophagitis
Nexplanon [etonogestrel]	Z79.3	Contraceptive	Implantable device used for prevention of pregnancy
Nitrofurantoin [nitrofurantoin]	Z79.2	Antibiotic	Bacterial urinary tract infections
Nitropress [sodium nitroprusside]		Vasodilator	Potent, rapid action in reducing blood pressure in hypertensive crisis or for controlling bleeding during anesthesia by producing controlled hypotension

Appendix B: Pharmacology List 2020

Drug	Z Code	Drug Action/Classification	Indications
Nitrostat [nitroglycerin]		Muscle relaxant; antianginal; antihypertensive; coronary vasodilator	Prophylaxis and treatment of angina pectoris; heart failure associated with myocardial infarction; hypertension, perioperative; surgery, adjunct
Nor-QD [norethindrone]	Z79.3	Contraceptive	Prevention of pregnancy
Norco [acetaminophen/hydrocodone bitartrate]	Z79.891	Analgesic, narcotic	Moderate to severe pain
Norinyl [mestranol/norethisterone]	Z79.3	Contraceptive	Prevention of pregnancy
Norpace [disopyramide phosphate]		Antiarrhythmic	Coronary artery disease, for prevention, recurrence and control of unifocal, multifocal, and paired PVCs
Nortrel [ethinyl estradiol/norethindrone]	Z79.3	Contraceptive	Prevention of pregnancy
Norvasc [amlodipine besylate]		Calcium channel blocker	Hypertension, chronic stable angina, and vasospastic angina
Novolin [insulin recombinant]	Z79.4	Insulin	Diabetes mellitus
Novolog [insulin aspart recombinant]	Z79.4	Insulin	Diabetes mellitus
Nucynta [tapentadol hydrochloride]	Z79.891	Analgesic, narcotic	Moderate to severe pain
NuvaRing [etonogestrel/ethinyl estradiol]	Z79.3	Contraceptive	Vaginal ring for prevention of pregnancy
Ogestrel [norgestrel/ethinyl estradiol]	Z79.3	Contraceptive	Prevention of pregnancy
Onglyza [saxagliptin hydrochloride]	Z79.84	Oral hypoglycemic	Diabetes mellitus
Opana [oxymorphone hydrochloride]	Z79.891	Analgesic, narcotic	Moderate to severe pain
Oracea [doxycycline]	Z79.2	Antibiotic	Rosacea
Orapred ODT [prednisolone sodium phosphate]	Z79.52	Corticosteroid	Inflammatory disorders
Orbactiv [oritavancin diphosphate]	Z79.2	Antibiotic	Bacterial skin infections
Orencia [abatacept]	Z79.899	Antirheumatic	Rheumatoid arthritis; polyarticular juvenile idiopathic arthritis; psoriatic arthritis
Orilissa [elagolix]	Z79.890	Hormone therapy	Pain associated with endometriosis
Orphenadrine citrate [orphenadrine citrate]		Muscle relaxant	Acute spasms, tension, and post-trauma cases
Orsythia [ethinyl estradiol/levonorgestrel]	Z79.3	Contraceptive	Prevention of pregnancy
Ortho Cyclen-28 [ethinyl estradiol/norgestimate]	Z79.3	Contraceptive	Prevention of pregnancy
Ortho-Novum [norethindrone/ethinyl estradiol]	Z79.3	Contraceptive	Prevention of pregnancy
Ortho-Tri-Cyclen [ethinyl estradiol/norgestimate]	Z79.3	Contraceptive	Prevention of pregnancy
Oseni [alogliptin benzoate/pioglitazone hydrochloride]	Z79.84	Oral hypoglycemic	Diabetes mellitus
Osphena [ospemifene]	Z79.810, Z79.890	Selective estrogen receptor modulator (SERM)	Postmenopausal dyspareunia due to vaginal atrophy; osteoporosis prevention and treatment of menopausal symptoms
Otezla [apremilast]	Z79.899	Antirheumatic	Psoriatic arthritis; plaque psoriasis
Oxazepam [oxazepam]		Antianxiety	Anxiety, tension, and alcohol withdrawal
Oxycodone HCl [oxycodone hydrochloride]	Z79.891	Analgesic, narcotic	Moderate to severe pain
OxyContin [oxycodone hydrochloride]	Z79.891	Analgesic, narcotic	Moderate to severe pain
Ozempic [semaglutide]		Antidiabetic — injectable	Diabetes mellitus
Paxil [paroxetine hydrochloride]		Antidepressant	Anxiety with panic disorder and depression; obsessive-compulsive disorder
PediaPred [prednisolone sodium phosphate]	Z79.52	Corticosteroid	Inflammatory disorders
Pegintron [peginterferon alfa-2b]	Z79.899	Antiviral	Hepatitis C
Penicillin-VK [penicillin V potassium]	Z79.2	Antibiotic	Chorea, prevention; endocarditis, prevention, secondary to tooth extraction; erysipelas; infections of the skin and skin structures, upper respiratory tract; rheumatic fever, prophylaxis; scarlet fever; Vincent's gingivitis; Vincent's pharyngitis
Pentam [pentamidine isethionate]	Z79.2	Antibiotic	Severe bacterial lung infections
Pepcid [famotidine]		Histamine H2-receptor inhibitor	Acid/peptic disorder; adenoma, secretory; gastroesophageal reflux; duodenal and gastric ulcer; Zollinger-Ellison syndrome

Drug	Z Code	Drug Action/Classification	Indications
Percocet [oxycodone hydrochloride/acetaminophen]	Z79.891	Analgesic, narcotic	Pain, moderate to severe
Persantine [dipyridamole]	Z79.02	Antiplatelet	Therapy for chronic angina pectoris, preventing clots post heart valve surgery
Pfizerpen [penicillin g potassium]	Z79.2	Antibiotic	Severe bacterial infections
Phenobarbital [phenobarbital sodium]		Anticonvulsant	Grand mal epilepsy
Philith [ethinyl estradiol/norethindrone]	Z79.3	Contraceptive	Prevention of pregnancy
Pimtrea [desogestrel/ethinyl estradiol]	Z79.3	Contraceptive	Prevention of pregnancy
Pirmella [ethinyl estradiol/norethindrone]	Z79.3	Contraceptive	Prevention of pregnancy
Pitocin [oxytocin]		Uterotonic	Induction or stimulation of labor at term
Plan B One-Step [levonorgestrel]	Z79.3	Contraceptive	Prevention of pregnancy
Plavix [clopidogrel bisulfate]	Z79.02	Antiplatelet	Lessening of the chance of heart attack or stroke
Ponstel [mefenamic acid]	Z79.1	Nonsteroidal anti-inflammatory drug (NSAID)	Treatment of pain
Portia-28 [ethinyl estradiol/levonorgestrel]	Z79.3	Contraceptive	Prevention of pregnancy
Pradaxa [dabigatran etexilate mesylate]	Z79.01	Anticoagulant	Prophylaxis and treatment of blood clots in patients with atrial fibrillation
Prandimet [metformin hydrochloride/repaglinide]	Z79.84	Oral hypoglycemic	Diabetes mellitus
Prandin [repaglinide]	Z79.84	Oral hypoglycemic	Diabetes mellitus
Prasugrel [prasugrel hydrocloride]	Z79.02	Antiplatelet	Lessening the chance of heart attack or stroke
Pravachol [pravastatin sodium]		HMG-CoA reductase inhibitor (statin)	Hypercholesterolemia; hyperlipidemia; hyperlipoproteinemia
Precose [acarbose]	Z79.84	Oral hypoglycemic	Diabetes mellitus
Prednisolone [prednisolone]	Z79.52	Corticosteroid	Inflammatory disorders
Prednisone [prednisone]	Z79.52	Corticosteroid	Used for its immunosuppressant effects and for relief of inflammation; used in arthritis, polymyositis and other systemic diseases
Pregnyl [chorionic gonadotropin]		Gonadotropic hormone	Prepubertal cryptorchidism; hypogonadism; corpus luteum insufficiency and infertility
Prelone [prednisolone]	Z79.52	Corticosteroid	Inflammatory disorders
Prempro [conjugated estrogens/medroxyprogesterone acetate]	Z79.890	Estrogen/progesterone therapy	Menopause; osteoporosis; atrophic vaginitis
Prevacid [lansoprazole]		Proton pump inhibitor	Acid/peptic disorder, erosive esophagitis, duodenal ulcer, Zollinger-Ellison syndrome
Previfem [ethinyl estradiol/norgestimate]	Z79.3	Contraceptive	Prevention of pregnancy
Prezcobix [darunavir/cobicistat]	Z79.899	Antiviral	HIV
Prezista [darunavir ethanolate]	Z79.899	Antiviral	HIV
Priftin [rifapentine]	Z79.2	Antibiotic	Tuberculosis
Prilosec [omeprazole magnesium]		Proton pump inhibitor	Acid/peptic disorder; endocrine adenoma; erosive esophagitis; systemic mastocytosis; gastroesophageal reflux; duodenal, peptic and gastric ulcer; Zollinger-Ellison syndrome
Primaxin [cilastatin sodium/imipenem]	Z79.2	Antibiotic	Skin, stomach, female reproductive organs or lower respiratory tract infections
Prinivil [lisinopril]		ACE inhibitor	Congestive heart failure; hypertension
Pristiq [desvenlafaxine]		Antidepressant; serotonin and norepinephrine reuptake inhibitor (SNRI)	Major depressive disorder
Procardia [nifedipine]		Calcium channel blocker	Management of vasospastic angina and chronic stable angina, hypertension
Prograf [tacrolimus]	Z79.899	Immunosuppressant	Prophylaxis of organ transplant rejection
Prolia [denosumab]	Z79.899	Monoclonal antibody	Treatment and prevention of bone resorption and prevention of bone fracture
Promethazine hydrochloride [promethazine hydrochloride]		Anesthesia, adjunct to; antiemetic; antihistamine; antitussive/expectorant; sedative/hypnotic; vertigo/motion sickness/vomiting	Anesthesia; adjunct; angioedema; conjunctivitis; dermographism; hypersensitivity, motion sickness; pain; perennial, seasonal, and allergic rhinitis; sedation, obstetrical; urticaria

Drug	Z Code	Drug Action/Classification	Indications
Protonix [pantoprazole]		Proton pump inhibitor	Short-term treatment and maintenance therapy of erosive esophagitis associated with gastroesophageal reflux disease (GERD)
Protopic [tacrolimus]	Z79.899	Immunosuppressant	Atomic dermatitis (eczema)
Proventil-HFA [albuterol sulfate]		Antiasthmatic/bronchodilator	Asthma
Provera [medroxyprogesterone acetate]	Z79.3, Z79.890	Antineoplastic; contraceptive; progestin	Amenorrhea; carcinoma, endometrium, adjunct; carcinoma, renal; prevention of pregnancy; hemorrhage
Prozac [fluoxetine hydrochloride]		Selective serotonin reuptake inhibitor (SSRI)	Bulimia nervosa; depression; obsessive-compulsive disorder
Pulmicort [budesonide]	Z79.51	Corticosteroid -inhaled; antiasthmatic	Prophylaxis and treatment of asthma
Qnasl [beclomethasone dipropionate]		Corticosteroid -inhaled/nasal	Perennial and seasonal allergies; vasomotor rhinitis
Qtern [dapagliflozin propanediol/saxagliptin hydrochloride]	Z79.84	Oral hypoglycemic	Diabetes mellitus
Quartette [levonorgestrel/ethinyl estradiol]	Z79.3	Contraceptive	Prevention of pregnancy
Quasense [ethinyl estradiol/levonorgestrel]	Z79.3	Contraceptive	Prevention of pregnancy
Quinidine gluconate [quinidine gluconate]		Antiarrhythmic	Management of cardiac arrhythmias
Qvar [beclomethasone dipropionate]	Z79.51	Corticosteroid -inhaled; antiasthmatic	Prophylaxis and treatment of asthma
Raloxifene HCl [raloxifene hydrochloride]	Z79.810	Selective estrogen receptor modulator (SERM)	Prevention of thinning of the bones (osteoporosis) only in postmenopausal women
Rapaflo [silodosin]		Antiadrenergic	Benign prostatic hyperplasia
Rapamune [sirolimus]	Z79.899	Immunosuppressant	Prophylaxis of organ transplant rejection
Rayos [prednisone]	Z79.52	Corticosteroid; antiasthmatic	Arthritis; blood disorders; allergies; asthma
Rebetol [ribavirin]	Z79.899	Antiviral	Chronic hepatitis C
Rebif [interferon beta-1a]	Z79.899	Antiviral	Treatment of relapsing multiple sclerosis
Reclast [zoledronic acid]	Z79.83	Bisphosphonate	Prevention of thinning of the bones (osteoporosis); Paget's disease; bone cancer
Relenza [zanamivir]		Antiviral	Treat and prevent influenza A and B
Renvela [sevelamer carbonate]		Phosphate binder	Chronic kidney disease (CKD) on dialysis
Repaglinide [repaglinide]	Z79.84	Oral hypoglycemic	Diabetes mellitus
Reprexain [hydrocodone bitartrate/ibuprofen]	Z79.891	Analgesic, narcotic; nonsteroidal anti-inflammatory drug (NSAID)	Pain, inflammation or fever relief
Restasis [cyclosporine ophthalmic emulsion]		Antiinflammatory, ophthalmic	Ocular inflammation due to keratoconjunctivitis sicca
Restoril [temazepam]		Sedative/hypnotic	Insomnia
Retrovir [zidovudine]	Z79.899	Antiretroviral	Indicated in symptomatic HIV infection
Rifadin [rifampin]	Z79.2	Antibiotic	Tuberculosis
Rimactane [rifampin]	Z79.2	Antibiotic	Tuberculosis
Riomet [metformin hydrochloride]	Z79.84	Oral hypoglycemic	Diabetes mellitus
Risperdal [risperidone]		Antipsychotic/antimanic	Schizophrenia; bipolar I disorder
Ritalin [methylphenidate hydrochloride]		CNS stimulant	Depression; hyperkinetic activity in children
Roxicet [oxycodone hydrochloride/acetaminophen]	Z79.891	Analgesic, narcotic	Pain, moderate to severe
Roxicodone [oxycodone hydrochloride]	Z79.891	Analgesic, narcotic	Pain relief
Ryzodeg [insulin aspart/insulin degludec]	Z79.4	Insulin	Diabetes mellitus
Sabril [vigabatrin]		Anticonvulsant	Refractory complex partial seizures
Safyral [drospirenone/ethinyl estradiol/levomefolate calcium]	Z79.3	Contraceptive	Prevention of pregnancy
Sandimmune [cyclosporine]	Z79.899	Immunosuppressant	Prophylaxis of organ transplant rejection
Sarafem [fluoxetine hydrochloride]		Selective serotonin reuptake inhibitor (SSRI)	Premenstrual dysphoric disorder (PMDD)
Savaysa [edoxaban tosylate]	Z79.01	Anticoagulant	Prophylaxis and treatment of venous thrombosis, pulmonary embolism; prevention of blood clots due to atrial fibrillation
Seasonale [levonorgestrel/ethinyl estradiol]	Z79.3	Contraceptive	Prevention of pregnancy
Seasonique [ethinyl estradiol/levonorgestrel]	Z79.3	Contraceptive	Prevention of pregnancy

Drug	Z Code	Drug Action/Classification	Indications
Selfemra [fluoxetine hydrochloride]		Selective serotonin reuptake inhibitor (SSRI)	Premenstrual dysphoric disorder (PMDD)
Septra [sulfamethoxazole trimethoprim]	Z79.2	Antibiotic	Urinary tract infections, acute otitis media, acute exacerbations of chronic bronchitis, and shigellosis
Serevent [salmeterol xinafoate]		Bronchodilator	Asthma
Seromycin [cycloserine]	Z79.2	Antibiotic	Tuberculosis; urinary tract infections
Seroquel XR [quetiapine fumarate]		Antipsychotic	Schizophrenia; bipolar disorder; major depressive disorder
Setlakin [ethinyl estradiol/levonorgestrel]	Z79.3	Contraceptive	Prevention of pregnancy
Silvadene [silver sulfadiazine]	Z79.2	Antibiotic, topical	Wound sepsis due to second/third degree burns
Simulect [basiliximab]	Z79.899	Immunosuppressant	Prophylaxis of organ transplant rejection
Sinemet [carbidopa/levodopa]		Antiparkinsonism	Parkinson's disease
Singulair [montelukast sodium]		Antiasthmatic	Asthma; exercise-induced bronchoconstriction; perennial and seasonal allergic rhinitis
Sirolimus [sirolimus]	Z79.899	Immunosuppressant	Prophylaxis of organ transplant rejection
Sitagliptin [sitagliptin/metformin hydrochloride]	Z79.84	Oral hypoglycemic	Diabetes mellitus
Sivextro [tedizolid phosphate]	Z79.2	Antibiotic	Skin infections including MRSA
Skyla [levonorgestrel]	Z79.3	Contraceptive	Intrauterine device for prevention of pregnancy
Soliqua [insulin glargine/lixisenatide]	Z79.4	Insulin	Diabetes mellitus
Solodyn [minocycline hydrochloride]	Z79.2	Antibiotic	Bacterial infections
Soltamox [tamoxifen citrate]	Z79.810	Selective estrogen receptor modulator (SERM)	Breast cancer
Solu-Cortef [hydrocortisone sodium succinate]	Z79.52	Corticosteroid; antiasthmatic	Asthma; severe inflammation; allergic reactions
Solu-Medrol [methylprednisolone sodium succinate]	Z79.52	Corticosteroid	Anti-inflammatory and antiallergenic for shock and ulcerative colitis
Spiriva [tiotropium bromide]		Antiasthmatic/bronchodilator	Chronic obstructive pulmonary disease (COPD); asthma
Sprintec [norgestimate/ethinyl estradiol]	Z79.3	Contraceptive	Prevention of pregnancy
Starlix [nateglinide]	Z79.84	Oral hypoglycemic	Diabetes mellitus
Strattera [atomexetine hydrochloride]		CNS stimulant	Attention deficit hyperactivity disorder (ADHD)
Streptomycin sulfate [streptomycin sulfate]	Z79.2	Antibiotic	Severe bacterial infections
Sublimaze preservative free [fentanyl citrate]	Z79.891	Analgesic, narcotic	Pain relief
Supprelin LA [histrelin acetate]	Z79.818	Agents affecting estrogen receptors and estrogen levels	Precocious puberty
Suprax [cefixime]	Z79.2	Antibiotic	Bacterial infections
Sustiva [efavirenz]	Z79.899	Antiviral	HIV/AIDs
Syeda [drospirenone/ethinyl estradiol]	Z79.3	Contraceptive	Prevention of pregnancy
Sylatron [peginterferon alfa-2b]	Z79.899	Antineoplastic interferons; antiviral interferons	Prevention of recurrent malignant melanoma
Symbicort [budesonide/formoterol fumarate dihydrate]	Z79.51	Corticosteroid -inhaled; antiasthmatic	Prophylaxis and treatment of asthma and COPD
Symbyax [olanzapine/fluoxetine]		Antidepressant	Acute depressive episodes associated with bipolar I disorder; treatment resistant depression
Symtuza [darunavir/cobicistat/emtricitabine/tenofovir alafenamide]	Z79.899	Antiretroviral	HIV
Synarel [nafarelin acetate]	Z79.818	Agents affecting estrogen receptors and estrogen levels	Endometriosis symptoms; precocious puberty
Synercid [dalfopristin/quinupristin]	Z79.2	Antibiotic	Severe blood infections
Synjardy [empagliflozin/metformin hydrochloride]	Z79.84	Oral hypoglycemic	Diabetes mellitus
Synthroid [levothyroxine sodium]		Thyroid hormone	Hypothyroidism
Tacrolimus [tacrolimus]	Z79.899	Immunosuppressant	Prophylaxis of organ transplant rejection
Tamiflu [oseltamivir phosphate]		Antiviral	Treatment and prevention of influenza A and B
Tamoxifen citrate [tamoxifen citrate]	Z79.810	Selective estrogen receptor modulator (SERM)	Metastatic breast cancer in postmenopausal women

Appendix B: Pharmacology List 2020

Drug	Z Code	Drug Action/Classification	Indications
Tazicef [ceftazidime]	Z79.2	Antibiotic	Confirmed or suspected bacterial infections
Teflaro [ceftaroline fosamil]	Z79.2	Antibiotic	Bacterial skin infections; pneumonia
Tegretol [carbamazepine]		Anticonvulsant; analgesic	Epilepsy, especially with complex symptomatology; specific analgesic for trigeminal neuralgia
Tenormin [atenolol]		Beta blocker	Angina pectoris; hypertension; acute myocardial infarction
Terazosin HCl [terazosin hydrochloride]		Antiadrenergic	Benign prostatic hypertrophy; hypertension
Testim [testosterone]	Z79.890	Testosterone therapy -topical	Primary hypogonadism; hypogonadotropic hypogonadism
Tetracycline HCl [tetracycline hydrochloride]	Z79.2	Antibiotic	Bacterial infections
Tiazac [diltiazem hydrochloride]		Calcium channel blocker	Chronic stable angina, atrial fibrillation, atrial flutter, hypertension, paroxysmal supraventricular tachycardia
Tivorbex [indomethacin]	Z79.1	Nonsteroidal anti-inflammatory drug (NSAID)	Treatment of pain, inflammation and joint stiffness
Tobradex [tobramycin/dexamethasone]		Aminoglycoside ocular anti-infective; anti-inflammatory	Infectious conjunctivitis; dermatosis, corticosteroid-responsive with secondary infection; foreign body in eye; corneal inflammation; uveitis
Tobramycin [dexamethasone/tobramycin]	Z79.2	Antibiotic	Bacterial eye infections
Topamax [topiramate]		Anticonvulsant	Epilepsy; primary generalized tonic-clonic seizures; seizures associated with Lennox-Gastaut syndrome; migraine headache
Toprol-XL [metoprolol succinate]		Beta blocker	Angina pectoris; hypertension
Toremifene citrate [toremifene citrate]	Z79.810	Selective estrogen receptor modulator (SERM)	Metastatic breast cancer in postmenopausal women
Torisel [temsirolimus]	Z79.899	Antineoplastic	Renal cell carcinoma
Toujeo Solostar [insulin glargine recombinant]	Z79.4	Insulin	Diabetes mellitus
Tradjenta [linagliptin]	Z79.84	Oral hypoglycemic	Diabetes mellitus
Trazodone HCl [trazodone hydrochloride]		Antidepressant	Depression
Trelegy Ellipta [fluticasone furoate/umeclidinium bromide/vilanterol trifenatate]	Z79.51	Corticosteroid -- inhaled; anitasthmatic	COPD
Trelstar [triptorelin pamoate]	Z79.818	Agents affecting estrogen receptors and estrogen levels	Palliative treatment of prostate cancer symptoms
Tresiba [insulin degludec]	Z79.4	Insulin	Diabetes mellitus
Tri-Estarylla [ethinyl estradiol/norgestimate]	Z79.3	Contraceptive	Prevention of pregnancy; acne
Tri-Legest [ethinyl estradiol/norethindrone acetate]	Z79.3	Contraceptive	Prevention of pregnancy
Tri-Linyah [ethinyl estradiol/norgestimate]	Z79.3	Contraceptive	Prevention of pregnancy
Tri-Lo-Estarylla [ethinyl estradiol/norgestimate]	Z79.3	Contraceptive	Prevention of pregnancy
Tri-Lo-Sprintec [ethinyl estradiol/norgestimate]	Z79.3	Contraceptive	Prevention of pregnancy
Tri-Norinyl 28-day [ethinyl estradiol/norethindrone]	Z79.3	Contraceptive	Prevention of pregnancy
Tri-Previfem [ethinyl estradiol/norgestimate]	Z79.3	Contraceptive	Prevention of pregnancy
Tri-Sprintec [ethinyl estradiol/norgestimate]	Z79.3	Contraceptive	Prevention of pregnancy; acne
Triamterene and hydrochlorothiazide [triamterene/ hydrochlorothiazide]		Antihypertensive; diuretic	Edema; hypertension
Trimethoprim [trimethoprim]	Z79.2	Antibiotic	Acute exacerbation chronic bronchitis; travelers' diarrhea; infections of the middle, lower respiratory tract, and urinary tract; pneumonia, pneumocystis; shigellosis
Triptodur [triptorelin]	Z79.818	Agents affecting estrogen receptors and estrogen levels	Precocious puberty
Trivora-28 [ethinyl estradiol/ levonorgestrel]	Z79.3	Contraceptive	Prevention of pregnancy

Drug	Z Code	Drug Action/Classification	Indications
Trokendi XR [topiramate]		Anticonvulsant	Epilepsy; primary generalized tonic-clonic seizures; seizures associated with Lennox-Gastaut syndrome; migraine headache
Trulicity [dulaglutide]		Antidiabetic -injectable	Diabetes mellitus
Truvada [emtricitabine/ tenofovir disoproxil fumarate]	Z79.899	Antiviral	Treatment and prevention of HIV
Tygacil [tigecycline]	Z79.2	Antibiotic	Bacterial skin or digestive system infections; pneumonia
Tylenol with codeine [acetaminophen/codeine phosphate]	Z79.891	Analgesic, narcotic	Pain and cough
Ultram [tramadol hydrochloride]	Z79.891	Analgesic, non-narcotic (opiate, narcotic-like)	Moderate to severe pain
Unasyn [ampicillin sodium/sulbactam sodium]	Z79.2	Antibiotic	Bacterial infections
Vabomere [meropenem; vaborbactam]	Z79.2	Antibiotic	Complicated urinary tract infections; pyelonephritis
Vagifem [estradiol]	Z79.890	Estrogen therapy	Menopause symptoms
Valium [diazepam]		Antianxiety; muscle relaxant; anticonvulsant	Anxiety, tension, withdrawal from alcohol, muscle spasms and anticonvulsant therapy; epilepsy, generalized tonic-clonic; status epilepticus; stiff-man syndrome; tetanus
Vancocin HCl [vancomycin hydrochloride]	Z79.2	Antibiotic	Severe bacterial infections
Vancomycin HCl [vancomycin hydrochloride]	Z79.2	Antibiotic	Severe bacterial infections
Vantas [histrelin acetate]	Z79.818	Agents affecting estrogen receptors and estrogen levels	Palliative treatment of prostate cancer symptoms
Vasotec [enalaprilat maleate]		ACE inhibitor	Congestive heart failure; hypertension
Velivet [desogestrel/ethinyl estradiol]	Z79.3	Contraceptive	Prevention of pregnancy
Venlafaxine HCl [venlafaxine hydrochloride]		Antidepressant, serotonin and norepinephrine reuptake inhibitor (SNRI)	Major depressive disorder; social anxiety disorder; panic disorder
Ventolin HFA [albuterol sulfate]		Antiasthmatic/bronchodilator	Asthma
Verapamil HCL [verapamil hydrochloride]		Calcium channel blocker	Angina pectoris, chronic stable angina, atrial fibrillation, atrial flutter, paroxysmal supraventricular tachycardia, ventricular arrhythmia, hypertension
Viagra [sildenafil citrate]		Phosphodiesterase-5 (PDE5) inhibitor	Erectile dysfunction
Vibativ [telavancin hydrochloride]	Z79.2	Antibiotic	Pneumonia; severe bacterial skin infections
Vibramycin [doxycycline calcium]	Z79.2	Antibiotic	Bacterial infections
Victoza [liraglutide]		Antidiabetic -injectable	Diabetes mellitus
Vienva [ethinyl estradiol/levonorgestrel]	Z79.3	Contraceptive	Prevention of pregnancy
Viorele [desogestrel/ethinyl estradiol]	Z79.3	Contraceptive	Prevention of pregnancy
Virazole [ribavirin]	Z79.899	Antiviral	Respiratory syncytial virus (RSV)
Viread [tenofovir disoproxil fumarate]	Z79.899	Antiviral	HIV; chronic hepatitis B
Vistaril [hydroxyzine pamoate]		Antianxiety; antiemetic	Treatment of nausea and vomiting, for reducing narcotic requirement in surgery and as tranquilizer for tension, anxiety, or agitation states
Vivelle [estradiol]	Z79.890	Estrogen therapy	Menopause symptoms; osteoporosis prevention
Voltaren [diclofenac sodium]	Z79.1	Nonsteroidal anti-inflammatory drug (NSAID)	Treatment of pain, inflammation and joint stiffness due to arthritis
Vytorin [ezetimibe/simvastatin]		HMG-CoA reductase inhibitor (statin); cholesterol absorption inhibitor	Hyperlipidemia; hypercholesterolemia
Warfarin [warfarin sodium]	Z79.01	Anticoagulant	Prophylaxis and treatment of venous thrombosis, treatment of atrial fibrillation with embolization (pulmonary embolism), arrhythmias, myocardial infarction, and stroke prevention
Wellbutrin SR, Wellbutrin XL [bupropion hydrochloride]		Antidepressant	Depression
Wera [ethinyl estradiol/norethindrone]	Z79.3	Contraceptive	Prevention of pregnancy
Xalatan [latanoprost]		Prostaglandin F2α analogue	Glaucoma, open-angle; ocular hypertension
Xanax, Xanax XR [alprazolam]		Antianxiety; sedative/hypnotic	Anxiety disorders with panic disorder and depression
Xarelto [rivaraxaban]	Z79.01	Anticoagulant	Prophylaxis and treatment of venous thrombosis, pulmonary embolism; prevention of blood clots due to atrial fibrillation
Xeljanz [tofacitinib citrate]	Z79.899	Antirheumatic	Rheumatoid arthritis; psoriatic arthritis
Xgeva [denosumab]	Z79.899	Monoclonal antibody	Treatment and prevention of bone resorption and prevention of bone fracture

Drug	Z Code	Drug Action/Classification	Indications
Xifaxan [rifaximin]	Z79.2	Antibiotic	E. coli diarrhea
Xigduo [dapagliflozin propanediol/metformin hydrochloride]	Z79.84	Oral hypoglycemic	Diabetes mellitus
Xultophy [insulin degludec/liraglutide]	Z79.4	Insulin	Diabetes mellitus
Xyrem [sodium oxybate]		CNS depressant; anxiolytic/sedative/hypnotic	Cataplexy and/or excessive daytime sleepiness in narcolepsy
Xyzal [levocetirizine dihydrochloride]		Antihistamine	Perennial allergic rhinitis; chronic idiopathic urticaria
Yasmin [drospirenone/ethinyl estradiol]	Z79.3	Contraceptive	Prevention of pregnancy
Yaz [drospirenone/ethinyl estradiol]	Z79.3	Contraceptive	Prevention of pregnancy; menstrual disorders
Zantac [ranitidine hydrochloride]		Histamine H2-receptors inhibitor	Acid/peptic disorder, erosive esophagitis, gastrointestinal hypersecretion, mastocytosis, gastroesophageal reflux, peptic ulcer, Zollinger-Ellison syndrome
Zerbaxa [ceftolozane sulfate/tazobactam sodium]	Z79.2	Antibiotic	Complicated urinary tract and intra-abdominal infections
Zestoretic [lisinopril/hydrochlorothiazide]		ACE inhibitor	Congestive heart failure; hypertension
Zestril [lisinopril]		ACE inhibitor	Congestive heart failure; hypertension
Zetia [exetimibe]		Antihyperlipidemic	Hypercholesterolemia; sitosterolemia
Ziac [bisoprolol fumarate/ hydrochlorothiazide]		Antihypertensive	Hypertension
Zinacef [cefuroxime sodium]	Z79.2	Antibiotic	Bacterial infections
Zipsor [diclofenac potassium]	Z79.1	Nonsteroidal anti-inflammatory drug (NSAID)	Pain and inflammation relief
Zithromax [azithromycin]	Z79.2	Antibiotic	Infections of the cervix, lower respiratory tract, skin and skin structures, urethra, nongonococcal; mycobacterium avium complex; pharyngitis, streptococcal pneumonia; tonsillitis
Zocor [simvastatin]		HMG-CoA reductase inhibitor (statin)	Hypercholesterolemia; hyperlipidemia; hyperlipoproteinemia; hypertriglyceridemia
Zoladex [goserelin acetate]	Z79.818	Agents affecting estrogen receptors and estrogen levels	Palliative treatment of prostate cancer and breast cancer symptoms; endometriosis
Zoloft [sertraline hydrochloride]		Antidepressant	Anxiety with panic disorder and depression; obsessive-compulsive disorder
Zometa [zoledronic acid]	Z79.83	Bisphosphonate	Multiple myeloma; Paget's disease
Zorvolex [diclofenac]	Z79.1	Nonsteroidal anti-inflammatory drug (NSAID)	Pain, inflammation or fever relief
Zosyn [piperacillin sodium/tazobactam sodium]	Z79.2	Antibiotic	Bacterial infections
Zovia [ethynodiol diacetate/ethinyl estradiol]	Z79.3	Contraceptive	Prevention of pregnancy
Zovirax [acyclovir]		Antiviral	Genital herpes and herpes zoster infections
Zubsolv [buprenorphine/naloxone]		Opioid agonist	Treatment of opioid addiction
Zyban [bupropion hydrochloride]		Smoking cessation aid	Nicotine addiction, smoking
Zyflo [zileuton]		Antiasthmatic	Asthma
Zyloprim [allopurinol]		Antigout	Gouty arthritis, renal calculus, hyperuricemia, hyperuricemia secondary to leukemia, hyperuricemia secondary to lymphoma
Zyprexa [olanzapine]		Antipsychotic/antimanic	Psychotic disorders; schizophrenia
Zyrtec allergy [cetirizine hydrochloride]		Antihistamine	Perennial and seasonal allergic rhinitis; chronic urticaria
Zyvox [linezolid]	Z79.2	Antibiotic	Severe bacterial infections

Appendix C: Z Codes for Long-Term Drug Use with Associated Drugs

This resource correlates the Z codes that are used to identify current long-term drug use with a list of drugs that are typically categorized to that class of drug. These lists are not all-inclusive, providing only the more commonly used drugs.

Z79.Ø1 **Long term (current) use of anticoagulants**
Angiomax
Argatroban
Arixtra
Bevyxxa
Coumadin
Eliquis
Fragmin
Heparin
Jantoven
Lovenox
Pradaxa
Savaysa
Warfarin
Xarelto

Z79.Ø2 **Long term (current) use of antithrombotics/antiplatelets**
Aggrastat
Aggrenox
Brilinta
Clopidogrel bisulfate
Effient
Integrilin
Persantine
Plavix
Prasugrel

Z79.1 **Long term (current) use of non-steroidal anti-inflammatories (NSAID)**
Advil
Aleve
Anaprox DS
Arthrotec
Caldolor
Cambia
Celebrex
Daypro
Duexis
Feldene
Ibuprofen
Indocin
Mobic
Motrin IB
Nabumetone
Nalfon
Naprelan
Naprosyn
NeoProfen
Ponstel
Tivorbex
Voltaren
Zipsor
Zorvolex

Z79.2 **Long term (current) use of antibiotics**
Altabax
Amikacin
Amoxicillin
Ampicillin
Ancef
Augmentin
Avelox
Azactam
Azithromycin

Bactrim
Biaxin XL
Cefprozil
Ceftriaxone
Centany
Cephalexin
Cipro
Ciprofloxacin
Clarithromycin
Cleocin
Clindamycin
Cubicin
Daptomycin
Dificid
Doxycycline
Dynacin
E.E.S.
Ertapenem
ERYC
Erygel
EryPed
Ery-Tab
Erythrocin
Erythromycin
Factive
Flagyl
Fortaz
Gentamicin sulfate
Invanz
Isoniazid
Keflex
Klaron
Lincocin
Macrobid
Macrodantin
Maxipime
Mefoxin
Mepron
Merrem
Metronidazole
Minocin
Monodox
Monurol
Mycobutin
Nebupent
Nitrofurantoin
Oracea
Orbactiv
Penicillin-VK
Pentam
Pfizerpen
Priftin
Primaxin
Rifadin
Rimactane
Septra
Seromycin
Silvadene
Sivextro
Solodyn
Streptomycin sulfate
Suprax
Synercid
Tazicef

Teflaro
Tetracycline HCl
Tobramycin
Trimethoprim
Tygacil
Unasyn
Vabomere
Vancocin HCl
Vancomycin HCl
Vibativ
Vibramycin
Xifaxan
Zerbaxa
Zinacef
Zithromax
Zosyn
Zyvox

Z79.3 **Long term (current) use of hormonal contraceptives**
Altavera
Alyacen
Aranelle
Ashlyna
Aviane-28
Balziva-28
Bekyree
Beyaz
Brevicon 28-day
Briellyn
Camila
Cryselle
Cyclafem
Cyclessa
Dasetta
Daysee
Depo-Provera
Depo-SubQ Provera
Desogen
Elinest
Emoquette
Enpresse-28
Enskyce
Errin
Estarylla
Estrostep Fe
Falmina
Femcon Fe
Femhrt
Gildagia
Gildess
Introvale
Jencycla
Junel
Kariva
Kelnor
Kimidess
Kurvelo
Kyleena
Larin
Lessina-28
Levonest
Levora
Liletta
Lo Loestrin Fe

Loestrin
Loryna
LoSeasonique
Low-Ogestrel-28
Marlissa
Microgestin
Micronor
Minastrin
Mirena
Modicon 28
Mono-Linyah
Myzilra
Natazia
Nexplanon
Norinyl
Nor-QD
Nortrel
NuvaRing
Ogestrel
Orsythia
Ortho Cyclen-28
Ortho-Novum
Ortho-Tri-Cyclen
Philith
Pimtrea
Pirmella
Plan B One-Step
Portia-28
Previfem
Provera
Quartette
Quasense
Safyral
Seasonale
Seasonique
Setlakin
Skyla
Sprintec
Syeda
Tri-Estarylla
Tri-Legest
Tri-Linyah
Tri-Lo-Estarylla
Tri-Lo-Sprintec
Tri-Norinyl 28-day
Tri-Previfem
Tri-Sprintec
Trivora-28
Velivet
Vienva
Viorele
Wera
Yasmin
Yaz
Zovia

Z79.4   **Long term (current) use of insulin**
Admelog
Afrezza
Apidra
Basaglar
Fiasp
Humalog
Humulin R
Lantus
Levemir
Novolin
Novolog

Ryzodeg
Soliqua
Toujeo Solostar
Tresiba
Xultophy

Z79.51   **Long term (current) use of inhaled steroids**
Advair
Aerospan HFA
Alvesco
Airduo Respiclick
Armonair Respiclick
Arnuity Ellipta
Asmanex
Breo Ellipta
Dulera
Flovent
Pulmicort
Qvar
Symbicort
Trelegy Ellipta

Z79.52   **Long term (current) use of systemic steroids**
A-Methapred
Aristospan
Celestone Soluspan
Colocort
Cortef
Cortenema
Cortifoam
Cortisone acetate
Depo-Medrol
Dexamethasone Intensol
Entocort EC
Hydrocortisone
Kenalog-10
Kenalog-40
Locoid
Medrol
Methylprednisolone
Orapred ODT
PediaPred
Prednisolone
Prednisone
Prelone
Rayos
Solu-Cortef
Solu-Medrol

Z79.810   **Long term (current) use of selective estrogen receptor modulators (SERMs)**
Evista
Fareston
Osphena
Raloxifene HCl
Soltamox
Tamoxifen Citrate
Toremifene Citrate

Z79.811   **Long term (current) use of aromatase inhibitors**
Anastrozole
Arimidex
Aromasin
Exemestane
Femara
Letrozole

Z79.818   **Long term (current) use of other agents affecting estrogen receptors and estrogen levels**
Eligard
Faslodex
Lupron
Megace ES
Supprelin LA
Synarel
Trelstar
Triptodur
Vantas
Zoladex

Z79.82   **Long term (current) use of aspirin**
Bayer
Durlaza

Z79.83   **Long term (current) use of bisphosphonates**
Actonel
Atelvia
Binosto
Boniva
Didronel
Fosamax
Reclast
Zometa

Z79.84   **Long term (current) use of oral hypoglycemic drugs**
Acarbose
Actoplus Met
Actos
Amaryl
Avandia
Diabinese
DiaBeta
Duetact
Farxiga
Fortamet
Glimepiride
Glucophage
Glucotrol
Glucovance
Glumetza
Glyburide
Glynase
Glyset
Invokamet
Invokana
Janumet
Januvia
Jentadueto
Kazano
Kombiglyze
Metformin
Onglyza
Oseni
PrandiMet
Prandin
Precose
Qtern
Repaglinide
Riomet
Sitagliptin
Starlix
Synjardy
Tradjenta
Xigduo

Z79.890 Hormone replacement therapy
- Activella
- Alora
- Androderm
- AndroGel
- Angeliq
- Bijuva
- Climara
- CombiPatch
- Delestrogen
- Depo-Provera
- Divigel
- Duavee
- Elestrin
- Estrace
- EstroGel
- Femhrt
- Femring
- Firmagon
- Menest
- Menostar
- Minivelle
- Orlissa
- Osphena
- Prempro
- Provera
- Testim
- Vagifem
- Vivelle

Z79.891 Long term (current) use of opiate analgesic
- Abstral
- Acetaminophen with codeine
- Buprenex
- Buprenorphine HCl and Naloxone HCl
- Butorphanol tartrate
- Butrans
- Codeine
- Demerol
- Dilaudid
- Dolophine HCl
- Duragesic
- Duramorph PF

- Embeda
- Exalgo
- Fentanyl Citrate
- Fentora
- Fioricet with codeine
- Hydrocodone
- Hydrocodone bitartrate and acetaminophen
- Hydromorphone HCl
- Kadian
- Lazanda
- Methadone HCl
- Methadose
- Morphabond ER
- Morphine Sulfate
- MS Contin
- Norco
- Nucynta
- Opana
- Oxycodone HCl
- OxyContin
- Percocet
- Reprexain
- Roxicet
- Roxicodone
- Sublimaze Preservative Free
- Tylenol with codeine
- Ultram

Z79.899 Other long term (current) drug therapy
- Actimmune
- Antineoplastic/chemotherapy
- Astagraf XL
- Atripla
- Avonex
- Betaseron
- Cellcept
- Cimduo
- Cosentyx
- Crixivan
- Cyclosporine
- Cyltezo
- Descovy

- Emtriva
- Enbrel
- Entyvio
- Envarsus XR
- Epivir
- Erelzi
- Gengraf
- Harvoni
- Humira
- Hyrimoz
- Imuran
- Intron A
- Keytruda
- Monoclonal antibodies
- Neoral
- Orencia
- Otezla
- Pegintron
- Prezcobix
- Prezista
- Prograf
- Prolia
- Protopic
- Rapamune
- Rebetol
- Rebif
- Retrovir
- Sandimmune
- Simulect
- Sirolimus
- Sustiva
- Sylatron
- Symtuza
- Tacrolimus
- Torisel
- Truvada
- Virazole
- Viread
- Xeljanz
- Xgeva

Appendix D: Major Complication and Comorbidity (MCC) Code List

Note: The following list of MCCs are based on the *Federal Register,* volume 84, number 86, May 3, 2019 ("Hospital Inpatient Prospective Payment Systems for Acute Care Hospitals and the Long-Term Care Hospital Prospective Payment System and Proposed Policy Changes and Fiscal Year 2020 Rates; Proposed Rule"). The most current version, v37, of the ICD-10 MS-DRG Definitions Manual was not available at the time this book was printed. For the most current files related to IPPS please refer to the following:
https://www.cms.gov/Medicare/Medicare-Fee-for-Service-Payment/AcuteInpatientPPS/IPPS-Regulations-and-Notices.html.

Optum360 also provides the most current list (v37) of MCCs in an easily searchable data file that can be accessed at the following:
https://www.optum360coding.com/ProductUpdates/
Title: "2020 ICD-10-CM for Hospital IPPS Data File"
Password: OptumIPPS20

A02.1	A41.9	B37.81	E13.11	I26.02	I63.112	I63.529	J15.4	K27.2
A02.21	A42.7	B37.82	E13.641	I26.09	I63.113	I63.531	J15.5	K27.4
A02.22	A48.0	B38.4	E40	I26.90	I63.119	I63.532	J15.6	K27.5
A06.4	A48.1	B39.0	E41	I26.92	I63.12	I63.533	J15.7	K27.6
A06.5	A48.3	B39.1	E44.0	I26.93	I63.131	I63.539	J15.8	K28.0
A06.6	A50.41	B39.2	E51.2	I26.94	I63.132	I63.541	J15.9	K28.1
A17.0	A50.42	B44.0	E84.0	I26.99	I63.133	I63.542	J16.0	K28.2
A17.1	A51.41	B45.1	E84.11	I33.0	I63.139	I63.543	J16.8	K28.4
A17.81	A52.13	B46.0	E88.3	I33.9	I63.19	I63.549	J17	K28.5
A17.82	A52.14	B46.1	G00.0	I40.0	I63.20	I63.59	J18.0	K28.6
A17.83	A54.81	B46.2	G00.1	I40.1	I63.211	I63.6	J18.1	K29.01
A17.89	A54.86	B46.3	G00.2	I40.8	I63.212	I63.81	J18.8	K29.21
A18.31	A80.0	B46.4	G00.3	I40.9	I63.213	I63.89	J18.9	K29.31
A19.0	A80.1	B46.5	G00.8	I41	I63.219	I63.9	J45.51	K29.41
A19.1	A80.2	B46.8	G00.9	I50.21	I63.22	I67.0	J68.1	K29.51
A19.2	A80.30	B46.9	G01	I50.23	I63.231	I67.83	J69.0	K29.61
A19.8	A80.39	B50.9	G02	I50.31	I63.232	I71.01	J69.1	K29.71
A19.9	A83.0	B58.2	G03.0	I50.33	I63.233	I71.02	J69.8	K29.81
A20.0	A83.1	B58.3	G03.8	I50.41	I63.239	I71.03	J80	K29.91
A20.1	A83.2	B58.81	G03.9	I50.43	I63.29	I71.1	J81.0	K31.82
A20.2	A83.3	B59	G04.00	I60.00	I63.30	I71.3	J84.81	K40.10
A20.3	A83.4	B77.81	G04.01	I60.01	I63.311	I71.5	J84.83	K40.11
A20.7	A83.5	D57.212	G04.02	I60.02	I63.312	I71.8	J84.841	K40.40
A20.8	A83.6	D57.412	G04.2	I60.10	I63.313	I74.01	J84.842	K40.41
A20.9	A83.8	D59.3	G04.30	I60.11	I63.319	I77.70	J84.843	K41.10
A22.1	A83.9	D60.0	G04.31	I60.12	I63.321	I77.71	J84.848	K41.11
A22.7	A84.0	D60.1	G04.32	I60.2	I63.322	I77.72	J85.0	K41.40
A26.7	A84.1	D60.8	G04.39	I60.30	I63.323	I77.73	J85.1	K41.41
A27.81	A84.8	D60.9	G04.81	I60.31	I63.329	I77.74	J85.2	K42.1
A32.7	A84.9	D61.1	G04.89	I60.32	I63.331	I77.75	J85.3	K43.1
A33	A85.2	D61.2	G04.90	I60.4	I63.332	I77.76	J86.0	K43.4
A35	A92.30	D61.3	G04.91	I60.50	I63.333	I77.77	J86.9	K43.7
A37.01	A92.31	D61.89	G05.3	I60.51	I63.339	I77.79	J93.0	K44.1
A37.11	A92.32	D65	G05.4	I60.52	I63.341	I81	J95.2	K45.1
A37.81	A92.39	D66	G06.0	I60.6	I63.342	I82.0	J95.3	K46.1
A37.91	B00.3	D67	G06.1	I60.7	I63.343	I82.220	J95.822	K55.011
A39.0	B00.4	E03.5	G06.2	I60.8	I63.349	I82.221	J96.00	K55.012
A39.1	B00.7	E05.01	G07	I60.9	I63.39	I85.01	J96.01	K55.019
A39.2	B00.82	E05.11	G08	I61.0	I63.40	I85.11	J96.02	K55.021
A39.3	B01.11	E05.21	G21.0	I61.1	I63.411	J04.11	J96.20	K55.022
A39.4	B01.12	E05.31	G37.4	I61.2	I63.412	J04.31	J96.21	K55.029
A39.50	B01.2	E05.41	G40.301	I61.3	I63.413	J05.11	J96.22	K55.031
A39.51	B02.1	E05.81	G40.311	I61.4	I63.419	J09.X1	J96.90	K55.032
A39.52	B02.24	E05.91	G40.319	I61.5	I63.421	J10.00	J96.91	K55.039
A39.53	B05.0	E08.00	G70.01	I61.6	I63.422	J10.01	J96.92	K55.041
A39.81	B05.2	E08.01	G82.50	I61.8	I63.423	J10.08	J98.51	K55.042
A40.0	B06.01	E08.10	G82.51	I61.9	I63.429	J11.00	J98.59	K55.049
A40.1	B10.01	E08.11	G82.52	I62.00	I63.431	J11.08	K22.11	K55.051
A40.3	B10.09	E08.641	G82.54	I62.01	I63.432	J12.0	K22.3	K55.052
A40.8	B15.0	E09.00	G83.5	I62.02	I63.433	J12.1	K22.6	K55.059
A40.9	B16.0	E09.01	G92	I62.1	I63.439	J12.2	K25.0	K55.061
A41.01	B16.2	E09.10	G93.41	I63.00	I63.441	J12.3	K25.1	K55.062
A41.02	B17.11	E09.11	G93.6	I63.011	I63.442	J12.81	K25.2	K55.069
A41.1	B19.0	E09.641	G93.7	I63.012	I63.443	J12.89	K25.4	K55.21
A41.2	B19.11	E10.10	G95.11	I63.013	I63.449	J12.9	K25.5	K55.30
A41.3	B19.21	E10.11	I21.4	I63.019	I63.49	J13	K25.6	K55.31
A41.4	B25.0	E10.641	I21.9	I63.02	I63.50	J14	K26.0	K55.32
A41.50	B25.2	E11.01	I21.A1	I63.031	I63.511	J15.0	K26.1	K55.33
A41.51	B26.1	E11.10	I21.A9	I63.032	I63.512	J15.1	K26.2	K57.01
A41.52	B26.2	E11.11	I23.4	I63.033	I63.513	J15.20	K26.4	K57.11
A41.53	B37.1	E11.641	I23.5	I63.039	I63.519	J15.211	K26.5	K57.13
A41.59	B37.5	E13.00	I25.42	I63.09	I63.521	J15.212	K26.6	K57.21
A41.81	B37.6	E13.01	I26.01	I63.10	I63.522	J15.29	K27.0	K57.41
A41.89	B37.7	E13.10	I26.01	I63.111	I63.523	J15.3	K27.1	K57.51

Appendix D: Major Complication and Comorbidity (MCC) Code List

K57.53	O03.32	O41.1415	O60.14X9	P24.81	P91.5	R40.2323	S06.334A	S06.826A
K57.81	O03.81	O41.1419	O60.22X0	P25.0	P91.63	R40.2324	S06.335A	S06.827A
K57.91	O03.82	O41.1420	O60.22X1	P25.1	P92.01	R40.2340	S06.336A	S06.828A
K57.93	O04.7	O41.1421	O60.22X2	P25.2	Q00.0	R40.2341	S06.337A	S06.896A
K63.81	O04.81	O41.1422	O60.22X3	P25.3	Q00.1	R40.2342	S06.338A	S06.897A
K65.0	O04.82	O41.1423	O60.22X4	P25.8	Q00.2	R40.2343	S06.339A	S06.898A
K65.1	O07.2	O41.1424	O60.22X5	P26.0	Q04.0	R40.2344	S06.340A	S06.9X6A
K65.2	O07.31	O41.1425	O60.22X9	P26.1	Q04.1	R53.2	S06.341A	S06.9X7A
K65.3	O07.32	O41.1429	O60.23X0	P26.8	Q04.2	R57.0	S06.342A	S06.9X8A
K65.8	O08.2	O41.1430	O60.23X1	P26.9	Q04.3	R57.1	S06.343A	S11.011A
K65.9	O08.3	O41.1431	O60.23X2	P27.0	Q20.0	R57.8	S06.344A	S11.012A
K66.1	O08.4	O41.1432	O60.23X3	P27.1	Q20.1	R65.20	S06.345A	S11.013A
K67	O10.42	O41.1433	O60.23X4	P27.8	Q20.2	R65.21	S06.346A	S11.014A
K68.12	O11.1	O41.1434	O60.23X5	P27.9	Q20.3	R78.81	S06.347A	S11.015A
K68.19	O11.2	O41.1435	O60.23X9	P28.5	Q20.4	S02.0XXB	S06.348A	S11.019A
K68.9	O11.3	O41.1439	O67.0	P28.81	Q21.3	S02.101B	S06.349A	S11.021A
K70.41	O14.12	O44.11	O71.02	P29.30	Q22.0	S02.102B	S06.350A	S11.022A
K71.11	O14.13	O44.12	O71.03	P29.38	Q22.4	S02.109B	S06.351A	S11.023A
K72.00	O14.22	O44.13	O71.1	P29.81	Q22.5	S02.110B	S06.352A	S11.024A
K72.01	O14.23	O44.31	O75.1	P35.1	Q22.6	S02.111B	S06.353A	S11.025A
K72.11	O15.02	O44.32	O75.3	P35.2	Q22.8	S02.112B	S06.354A	S11.029A
K72.91	O15.03	O44.33	O85	P35.3	Q22.9	S02.113B	S06.355A	S11.031A
K75.0	O15.1	O44.51	O86.04	P35.4	Q23.4	S02.118B	S06.356A	S11.032A
K75.1	O15.2	O44.52	O86.81	P35.8	Q24.2	S02.119B	S06.357A	S11.033A
K76.2	O22.31	O44.53	O86.89	P35.9	Q24.4	S02.11AB	S06.358A	S11.034A
K76.3	O22.32	O45.001	O87.1	P36.0	Q24.6	S02.11BB	S06.359A	S11.035A
K76.7	O22.33	O45.002	O88.011	P36.10	Q25.5	S02.11CB	S06.360A	S11.039A
K83.1	O34.31	O45.003	O88.012	P36.19	Q25.6	S02.11DB	S06.361A	S12.000B
K83.2	O34.32	O45.011	O88.013	P36.2	Q25.71	S02.11EB	S06.362A	S12.001B
K85.00	O34.33	O45.012	O88.02	P36.30	Q25.72	S02.11FB	S06.363A	S12.01XB
K85.01	O41.1010	O45.013	O88.03	P36.39	Q25.79	S02.11GB	S06.364A	S12.02XB
K85.02	O41.1011	O45.021	O88.111	P36.4	Q28.2	S02.11HB	S06.365A	S12.030B
K85.10	O41.1012	O45.022	O88.112	P36.5	Q28.3	S02.121B	S06.366A	S12.031B
K85.11	O41.1013	O45.023	O88.113	P36.8	Q33.2	S02.122B	S06.367A	S12.040B
K85.12	O41.1014	O45.091	O88.12	P36.9	Q33.3	S02.129B	S06.368A	S12.041B
K85.20	O41.1015	O45.092	O88.13	P37.0	Q33.6	S02.19XB	S06.369A	S12.090B
K85.21	O41.1019	O45.093	O88.211	P37.1	Q39.0	S02.91XB	S06.370A	S12.091B
K85.22	O41.1020	O45.8X1	O88.212	P37.2	Q39.1	S06.1X0A	S06.376A	S12.100B
K85.30	O41.1021	O45.8X2	O88.213	P37.3	Q39.2	S06.1X1A	S06.377A	S12.101B
K85.31	O41.1022	O45.8X3	O88.22	P37.4	Q39.3	S06.1X2A	S06.378A	S12.110B
K85.32	O41.1023	O45.91	O88.23	P37.8	Q44.2	S06.1X3A	S06.380A	S12.111B
K85.80	O41.1024	O45.92	O88.311	P37.9	Q44.3	S06.1X4A	S06.386A	S12.112B
K85.81	O41.1025	O45.93	O88.312	P52.21	Q79.0	S06.1X5A	S06.387A	S12.120B
K85.82	O41.1029	O46.001	O88.313	P52.22	Q79.1	S06.1X6A	S06.388A	S12.121B
K85.90	O41.1030	O46.002	O88.32	P52.4	Q79.2	S06.1X7A	S06.4X0A	S12.130B
K85.91	O41.1031	O46.003	O88.33	P52.5	Q79.3	S06.1X8A	S06.4X1A	S12.131B
K85.92	O41.1032	O46.011	O88.811	P52.6	Q89.4	S06.1X9A	S06.4X2A	S12.14XB
K91.32	O41.1033	O46.012	O88.812	P52.8	R09.2	S06.2X6A	S06.4X3A	S12.150B
M31.1	O41.1034	O46.013	O88.813	P52.9	R40.20	S06.2X7A	S06.4X4A	S12.151B
M72.6	O41.1035	O46.021	O88.82	P54.1	R40.2110	S06.2X8A	S06.4X5A	S12.190B
N00.0	O41.1039	O46.022	O88.83	P54.2	R40.2111	S06.306A	S06.4X6A	S12.191B
N00.1	O41.1210	O46.023	O90.3	P54.3	R40.2112	S06.307A	S06.4X7A	S12.200B
N00.2	O41.1211	O46.091	O90.4	P56.0	R40.2113	S06.308A	S06.4X8A	S12.201B
N00.3	O41.1212	O46.092	O99.42	P56.90	R40.2114	S06.310A	S06.4X9A	S12.230B
N00.4	O41.1213	O46.093	P10.0	P56.99	R40.2120	S06.311A	S06.5X0A	S12.231B
N00.5	O41.1214	O60.02	P10.1	P57.0	R40.2121	S06.312A	S06.5X1A	S12.24XB
N00.6	O41.1215	O60.03	P10.3	P57.8	R40.2122	S06.313A	S06.5X2A	S12.250B
N00.7	O41.1219	O60.12X0	P10.4	P57.9	R40.2123	S06.314A	S06.5X3A	S12.251B
N00.8	O41.1220	O60.12X1	P10.8	P59.1	R40.2124	S06.315A	S06.5X4A	S12.290B
N00.9	O41.1221	O60.12X2	P10.9	P59.20	R40.2210	S06.316A	S06.5X5A	S12.291B
N01.0	O41.1222	O60.12X3	P11.0	P59.29	R40.2211	S06.317A	S06.5X6A	S12.300B
N01.1	O41.1223	O60.12X4	P11.2	P60	R40.2212	S06.318A	S06.5X7A	S12.301B
N01.2	O41.1224	O60.12X5	P11.9	P61.0	R40.2213	S06.319A	S06.5X8A	S12.330B
N01.3	O41.1225	O60.12X9	P22.0	P61.5	R40.2214	S06.320A	S06.5X9A	S12.331B
N01.4	O41.1229	O60.13X0	P23.0	P74.0	R40.2220	S06.321A	S06.6X0A	S12.34XB
N01.5	O41.1230	O60.13X1	P23.1	P77.1	R40.2221	S06.322A	S06.6X1A	S12.350B
N01.6	O41.1231	O60.13X2	P23.2	P77.2	R40.2222	S06.323A	S06.6X2A	S12.351B
N01.7	O41.1232	O60.13X3	P23.3	P77.3	R40.2223	S06.324A	S06.6X3A	S12.390B
N01.8	O41.1233	O60.13X4	P23.4	P77.9	R40.2224	S06.325A	S06.6X4A	S12.391B
N01.9	O41.1234	O60.13X5	P23.5	P78.0	R40.2310	S06.326A	S06.6X5A	S12.400B
N15.1	O41.1235	O60.13X9	P23.6	P83.2	R40.2311	S06.327A	S06.6X6A	S12.401B
N17.0	O41.1239	O60.14X0	P23.8	P90	R40.2312	S06.328A	S06.6X7A	S12.430B
N17.1	O41.1410	O60.14X1	P23.9	P91.0	R40.2313	S06.329A	S06.6X8A	S12.431B
N17.2	O41.1411	O60.14X2	P24.01	P91.1	R40.2314	S06.330A	S06.6X9A	S12.44XB
N73.3	O41.1412	O60.14X3	P24.11	P91.2	R40.2320	S06.331A	S06.816A	S12.450B
O03.2	O41.1413	O60.14X4	P24.21	P91.3	R40.2321	S06.332A	S06.817A	S12.451B
O03.31	O41.1414	O60.14X5	P24.31	P91.4	R40.2322	S06.333A	S06.818A	S12.490B

S12.491B	S21.329A	S22.23XB	S26.020A	S32.000B	S32.421B	S32.484A	S35.229A	S42.249B
S12.500B	S21.331A	S22.24XB	S26.021A	S32.001B	S32.422A	S32.484B	S35.231A	S42.251B
S12.501B	S21.332A	S22.31XB	S26.022A	S32.002B	S32.422B	S32.485A	S35.232A	S42.252B
S12.530B	S21.339A	S22.32XB	S26.12XA	S32.008B	S32.423A	S32.485B	S35.238A	S42.253B
S12.531B	S21.341A	S22.39XB	S26.92XA	S32.009B	S32.423B	S32.486A	S35.239A	S42.254B
S12.54XB	S21.342A	S22.41XB	S27.1XXA	S32.010B	S32.424A	S32.486B	S35.291A	S42.255B
S12.550B	S21.349A	S22.42XB	S27.2XXA	S32.011B	S32.424B	S32.491A	S35.292A	S42.256B
S12.551B	S21.351A	S22.43XB	S27.331A	S32.012B	S32.425A	S32.491B	S35.298A	S42.261B
S12.590B	S21.352A	S22.49XB	S27.332A	S32.018B	S32.425B	S32.492A	S35.299A	S42.262B
S12.591B	S21.359A	S22.5XXA	S27.339A	S32.019B	S32.426A	S32.492B	S35.311A	S42.263B
S12.600B	S21.401A	S22.5XXB	S27.401A	S32.020B	S32.426B	S32.499A	S35.318A	S42.264B
S12.601B	S21.402A	S22.9XXB	S27.402A	S32.021B	S32.431A	S32.499B	S35.319A	S42.265B
S12.630B	S21.409A	S24.0XXA	S27.409A	S32.022B	S32.431B	S32.501B	S35.321A	S42.266B
S12.631B	S21.411A	S24.101A	S27.411A	S32.028B	S32.432A	S32.502B	S35.328A	S42.291B
S12.64XB	S21.412A	S24.102A	S27.412A	S32.029B	S32.432B	S32.509B	S35.329A	S42.292B
S12.650B	S21.419A	S24.103A	S27.419A	S32.030B	S32.433A	S32.511B	S35.331A	S42.293B
S12.651B	S21.421A	S24.104A	S27.421A	S32.031B	S32.433B	S32.512B	S35.338A	S42.294B
S12.690B	S21.422A	S24.111A	S27.422A	S32.032B	S32.434A	S32.519B	S35.339A	S42.295B
S12.691B	S21.429A	S24.112A	S27.429A	S32.038B	S32.434B	S32.591B	S35.341A	S42.296B
S12.8XXA	S21.431A	S24.113A	S27.431A	S32.039B	S32.435A	S32.592B	S35.348A	S42.301B
S14.0XXA	S21.432A	S24.114A	S27.432A	S32.040B	S32.435B	S32.599B	S35.349A	S42.302B
S14.101A	S21.439A	S24.131A	S27.439A	S32.041B	S32.436A	S32.601B	S35.401A	S42.309B
S14.102A	S21.441A	S24.132A	S27.491A	S32.042B	S32.436B	S32.602B	S35.402A	S42.321B
S14.103A	S21.442A	S24.133A	S27.492A	S32.048B	S32.441A	S32.609B	S35.403A	S42.322B
S14.104A	S21.449A	S24.134A	S27.499A	S32.049B	S32.441B	S32.611B	S35.404A	S42.323B
S14.105A	S21.451A	S24.141A	S27.812A	S32.050B	S32.442A	S32.612B	S35.405A	S42.324B
S14.106A	S21.452A	S24.142A	S27.813A	S32.051B	S32.442B	S32.613B	S35.406A	S42.325B
S14.107A	S21.459A	S24.143A	S27.818A	S32.052B	S32.443A	S32.614B	S35.411A	S42.326B
S14.108A	S22.000B	S24.144A	S27.819A	S32.058B	S32.443B	S32.615B	S35.412A	S42.331B
S14.111A	S22.001B	S24.151A	S31.001A	S32.059B	S32.444A	S32.616B	S35.413A	S42.332B
S14.112A	S22.002B	S24.152A	S31.011A	S32.10XB	S32.444B	S32.691B	S35.414A	S42.333B
S14.113A	S22.008B	S24.153A	S31.021A	S32.110B	S32.445A	S32.692B	S35.415A	S42.334B
S14.114A	S22.009B	S24.154A	S31.031A	S32.111B	S32.445B	S32.699B	S35.416A	S42.335B
S14.115A	S22.010B	S25.00XA	S31.041A	S32.112B	S32.446A	S32.810B	S35.491A	S42.336B
S14.116A	S22.011B	S25.01XA	S31.051A	S32.119B	S32.446B	S32.811B	S35.492A	S42.341B
S14.117A	S22.012B	S25.02XA	S31.600A	S32.120B	S32.451A	S32.82XB	S35.493A	S42.342B
S14.118A	S22.018B	S25.09XA	S31.601A	S32.121B	S32.451B	S32.89XB	S35.494A	S42.343B
S14.121A	S22.019B	S25.101A	S31.602A	S32.122B	S32.452A	S32.9XXB	S35.495A	S42.344B
S14.122A	S22.020B	S25.102A	S31.603A	S32.129B	S32.452B	S34.01XA	S35.496A	S42.345B
S14.123A	S22.021B	S25.109A	S31.604A	S32.130B	S32.453A	S34.02XA	S35.50XA	S42.346B
S14.124A	S22.022B	S25.111A	S31.605A	S32.131B	S32.453B	S34.101A	S35.511A	S42.351B
S14.125A	S22.028B	S25.112A	S31.609A	S32.132B	S32.454A	S34.102A	S35.512A	S42.352B
S14.126A	S22.029B	S25.119A	S31.610A	S32.139B	S32.454B	S34.103A	S35.513A	S42.353B
S14.127A	S22.030B	S25.121A	S31.611A	S32.14XB	S32.455A	S34.104A	S35.514A	S42.354B
S14.128A	S22.031B	S25.122A	S31.612A	S32.15XB	S32.455B	S34.105A	S35.515A	S42.355B
S14.131A	S22.032B	S25.129A	S31.613A	S32.16XB	S32.456A	S34.109A	S35.516A	S42.356B
S14.132A	S22.038B	S25.191A	S31.614A	S32.17XB	S32.456B	S34.111A	S35.59XA	S42.361B
S14.133A	S22.039B	S25.192A	S31.615A	S32.19XB	S32.461A	S34.112A	S36.031A	S42.362B
S14.134A	S22.040B	S25.199A	S31.619A	S32.2XXB	S32.461B	S34.113A	S36.032A	S42.363B
S14.135A	S22.041B	S25.20XA	S31.620A	S32.301B	S32.462A	S34.114A	S36.115A	S42.364B
S14.136A	S22.042B	S25.21XA	S31.621A	S32.302B	S32.462B	S34.115A	S36.116A	S42.365B
S14.137A	S22.048B	S25.22XA	S31.622A	S32.309B	S32.463A	S34.119A	S37.061A	S42.366B
S14.138A	S22.049B	S25.29XA	S31.623A	S32.311B	S32.463B	S34.121A	S37.062A	S42.391B
S14.141A	S22.050B	S25.301A	S31.624A	S32.312B	S32.464A	S34.122A	S37.069A	S42.392B
S14.142A	S22.051B	S25.302A	S31.625A	S32.313B	S32.464B	S34.123A	S37.091A	S42.399B
S14.143A	S22.052B	S25.309A	S31.629A	S32.314B	S32.465A	S34.124A	S37.092A	S42.401B
S14.144A	S22.058B	S25.311A	S31.630A	S32.315B	S32.465B	S34.125A	S37.099A	S42.402B
S14.145A	S22.059B	S25.312A	S31.631A	S32.316B	S32.466A	S34.129A	S42.201B	S42.409B
S14.146A	S22.060B	S25.319A	S31.632A	S32.391B	S32.466B	S34.131A	S42.202B	S42.411B
S14.147A	S22.061B	S25.321A	S31.633A	S32.392B	S32.471A	S34.132A	S42.209B	S42.412B
S14.148A	S22.062B	S25.322A	S31.634A	S32.399B	S32.471B	S34.139A	S42.211B	S42.413B
S14.151A	S22.068B	S25.329A	S31.635A	S32.401B	S32.472A	S34.3XXA	S42.212B	S42.414B
S14.152A	S22.069B	S25.391A	S31.639A	S32.402B	S32.472B	S35.00XA	S42.213B	S42.415B
S14.153A	S22.070B	S25.392A	S31.640A	S32.409B	S32.473A	S35.01XA	S42.214B	S42.416B
S14.154A	S22.071B	S25.399A	S31.641A	S32.411A	S32.473B	S35.02XA	S42.215B	S42.421B
S14.155A	S22.072B	S25.401A	S31.642A	S32.411B	S32.474A	S35.09XA	S42.216B	S42.422B
S14.156A	S22.078B	S25.402A	S31.643A	S32.412A	S32.474B	S35.10XA	S42.221B	S42.423B
S14.157A	S22.079B	S25.409A	S31.644A	S32.412B	S32.475A	S35.11XA	S42.222B	S42.424B
S14.158A	S22.080B	S25.411A	S31.645A	S32.413A	S32.475B	S35.12XA	S42.223B	S42.425B
S21.301A	S22.081B	S25.412A	S31.649A	S32.413B	S32.476A	S35.19XA	S42.224B	S42.426B
S21.302A	S22.082B	S25.419A	S31.650A	S32.414A	S32.476B	S35.211A	S42.225B	S42.431B
S21.309A	S22.088B	S25.421A	S31.651A	S32.414B	S32.481A	S35.212A	S42.226B	S42.432B
S21.311A	S22.089B	S25.422A	S31.652A	S32.415A	S32.481B	S35.218A	S42.231B	S42.433B
S21.312A	S22.20XA	S25.429A	S31.653A	S32.415B	S32.482A	S35.219A	S42.232B	S42.434B
S21.319A	S22.20XB	S25.491A	S31.654A	S32.416A	S32.482B	S35.221A	S42.239B	S42.435B
S21.321A	S22.21XB	S25.492A	S31.655A	S32.416B	S32.483A	S35.222A	S42.241B	S42.436B
S21.322A	S22.22XB	S25.499A	S31.659A	S32.421A	S32.483B	S35.228A	S42.242B	S42.441B

S42.442B	S52.042C	S52.235B	S52.331C	S52.514B	S72.002C	S72.062B	S72.145C	S72.351C
S42.443B	S52.043B	S52.235C	S52.332B	S52.514C	S72.009A	S72.062C	S72.146B	S72.352A
S42.444B	S52.043C	S52.236B	S52.332C	S52.515B	S72.009B	S72.063A	S72.146C	S72.352B
S42.445B	S52.044B	S52.236C	S52.333B	S52.515C	S72.009C	S72.063B	S72.21XB	S72.352C
S42.446B	S52.044C	S52.241B	S52.333C	S52.516B	S72.011B	S72.063C	S72.21XC	S72.353A
S42.447B	S52.045B	S52.241C	S52.334B	S52.516C	S72.011C	S72.064A	S72.22XB	S72.353B
S42.448B	S52.045C	S52.242B	S52.334C	S52.531B	S72.012B	S72.064B	S72.22XC	S72.353C
S42.449B	S52.046B	S52.242C	S52.335B	S52.531C	S72.012C	S72.064C	S72.23XB	S72.354A
S42.451B	S52.046C	S52.243B	S52.335C	S52.532B	S72.019B	S72.065B	S72.23XC	S72.354B
S42.452B	S52.091B	S52.243C	S52.336B	S52.532C	S72.019C	S72.065C	S72.24XB	S72.354C
S42.453B	S52.091C	S52.244B	S52.336C	S52.539B	S72.021A	S72.066A	S72.24XC	S72.355A
S42.454B	S52.092B	S52.244C	S52.341B	S52.539C	S72.021B	S72.066B	S72.25XB	S72.355B
S42.455B	S52.092C	S52.245B	S52.341C	S52.541B	S72.021C	S72.066C	S72.25XC	S72.355C
S42.456B	S52.099B	S52.245C	S52.342B	S52.541C	S72.022A	S72.091A	S72.26XB	S72.356A
S42.461B	S52.099C	S52.246B	S52.342C	S52.542B	S72.022B	S72.091B	S72.26XC	S72.356B
S42.462B	S52.101B	S52.246C	S52.343B	S52.542C	S72.022C	S72.091C	S72.301B	S72.356C
S42.463B	S52.101C	S52.251B	S52.343C	S52.549B	S72.023A	S72.092A	S72.301C	S72.361A
S42.464B	S52.102B	S52.251C	S52.344B	S52.549C	S72.023B	S72.092B	S72.302B	S72.361B
S42.465B	S52.102C	S52.252B	S52.344C	S52.551B	S72.023C	S72.092C	S72.302C	S72.361C
S42.466B	S52.109B	S52.252C	S52.345B	S52.551C	S72.024A	S72.099A	S72.309B	S72.362A
S42.471B	S52.109C	S52.253B	S52.345C	S52.552B	S72.024B	S72.099B	S72.309C	S72.362B
S42.472B	S52.121B	S52.253C	S52.346B	S52.552C	S72.024C	S72.099C	S72.321A	S72.362C
S42.473B	S52.121C	S52.254B	S52.346C	S52.559B	S72.025A	S72.101A	S72.321B	S72.363A
S42.474B	S52.122B	S52.254C	S52.351B	S52.559C	S72.025B	S72.101B	S72.321C	S72.363B
S42.475B	S52.122C	S52.255B	S52.351C	S52.561B	S72.025C	S72.101C	S72.322A	S72.363C
S42.476B	S52.123B	S52.255C	S52.352B	S52.561C	S72.026A	S72.102A	S72.322B	S72.364A
S42.491B	S52.123C	S52.256B	S52.352C	S52.562B	S72.026B	S72.102B	S72.322C	S72.364B
S42.492B	S52.124B	S52.256C	S52.353B	S52.562C	S72.026C	S72.102C	S72.323A	S72.364C
S42.493B	S52.124C	S52.261B	S52.353C	S52.569B	S72.031A	S72.109A	S72.323B	S72.365A
S42.494B	S52.125B	S52.261C	S52.354B	S52.569C	S72.031B	S72.109B	S72.323C	S72.365B
S42.495B	S52.125C	S52.262B	S52.354C	S52.571B	S72.031C	S72.109C	S72.324A	S72.365C
S42.496B	S52.126B	S52.262C	S52.355B	S52.571C	S72.032A	S72.111B	S72.324B	S72.366A
S42.90XB	S52.126C	S52.263B	S52.355C	S52.572B	S72.032B	S72.111C	S72.324C	S72.366B
S42.91XB	S52.131B	S52.263C	S52.356B	S52.572C	S72.032C	S72.112B	S72.325A	S72.366C
S42.92XB	S52.131C	S52.264B	S52.356C	S52.579B	S72.033A	S72.112C	S72.325B	S72.391A
S45.001A	S52.132B	S52.264C	S52.361B	S52.579C	S72.033B	S72.113B	S72.325C	S72.391B
S45.002A	S52.132C	S52.265B	S52.361C	S52.591B	S72.033C	S72.113C	S72.326A	S72.391C
S45.009A	S52.133B	S52.265C	S52.362B	S52.591C	S72.034A	S72.114B	S72.326B	S72.392A
S45.011A	S52.133C	S52.266B	S52.362C	S52.592B	S72.034B	S72.114C	S72.326C	S72.392B
S45.012A	S52.134B	S52.266C	S52.363B	S52.592C	S72.034C	S72.115B	S72.331A	S72.392C
S45.019A	S52.134C	S52.271B	S52.363C	S52.599B	S72.035A	S72.115C	S72.331B	S72.399A
S45.091A	S52.135B	S52.271C	S52.364B	S52.599C	S72.035B	S72.116B	S72.331C	S72.399B
S45.092A	S52.135C	S52.272B	S52.364C	S52.601B	S72.035C	S72.116C	S72.332A	S72.399C
S45.099A	S52.136B	S52.272C	S52.365B	S52.601C	S72.036A	S72.121B	S72.332B	S72.401B
S52.001B	S52.136C	S52.279B	S52.365C	S52.602B	S72.036B	S72.121C	S72.332C	S72.401C
S52.001C	S52.181B	S52.279C	S52.366B	S52.602C	S72.036C	S72.122B	S72.333A	S72.402B
S52.002B	S52.181C	S52.281B	S52.366C	S52.609B	S72.041A	S72.122C	S72.333B	S72.402C
S52.002C	S52.182B	S52.281C	S52.371B	S52.609C	S72.041B	S72.123B	S72.333C	S72.409B
S52.009B	S52.182C	S52.282B	S52.371C	S52.611B	S72.041C	S72.123C	S72.334A	S72.409C
S52.009C	S52.189B	S52.282C	S52.372B	S52.611C	S72.042A	S72.124B	S72.334B	S72.411B
S52.021B	S52.189C	S52.283B	S52.372C	S52.612B	S72.042B	S72.124C	S72.334C	S72.411C
S52.021C	S52.201B	S52.283C	S52.379B	S52.612C	S72.042C	S72.125B	S72.335A	S72.412B
S52.022B	S52.201C	S52.291B	S52.379C	S52.613B	S72.043A	S72.125C	S72.335B	S72.412C
S52.022C	S52.202B	S52.291C	S52.381B	S52.613C	S72.043B	S72.126B	S72.335C	S72.413B
S52.023B	S52.202C	S52.292B	S52.381C	S52.614B	S72.043C	S72.126C	S72.336A	S72.413C
S52.023C	S52.209B	S52.292C	S52.382B	S52.614C	S72.044A	S72.131B	S72.336B	S72.414B
S52.024B	S52.209C	S52.299B	S52.382C	S52.615B	S72.044B	S72.131C	S72.336C	S72.414C
S52.024C	S52.221B	S52.299C	S52.389B	S52.615C	S72.044C	S72.132B	S72.341A	S72.415B
S52.025B	S52.221C	S52.301B	S52.389C	S52.616B	S72.045A	S72.132C	S72.341B	S72.415C
S52.025C	S52.222B	S52.301C	S52.391B	S52.616C	S72.045B	S72.133B	S72.341C	S72.416B
S52.026B	S52.222C	S52.302B	S52.391C	S52.691B	S72.045C	S72.133C	S72.342A	S72.416C
S52.026C	S52.223B	S52.302C	S52.392B	S52.691C	S72.046A	S72.134B	S72.342B	S72.421B
S52.031B	S52.223C	S52.309B	S52.392C	S52.692B	S72.046B	S72.134C	S72.342C	S72.421C
S52.031C	S52.224B	S52.309C	S52.399B	S52.692C	S72.046C	S72.135B	S72.343A	S72.422B
S52.032B	S52.224C	S52.321B	S52.399C	S52.699B	S72.051A	S72.135C	S72.343B	S72.422C
S52.032C	S52.225B	S52.321C	S52.501B	S52.699C	S72.051B	S72.136B	S72.343C	S72.423B
S52.033B	S52.225C	S52.322B	S52.501C	S52.90XB	S72.051C	S72.136C	S72.344A	S72.423C
S52.034B	S52.226B	S52.322C	S52.502B	S52.90XC	S72.052A	S72.141B	S72.344B	S72.424B
S52.034C	S52.226C	S52.323B	S52.502C	S52.91XB	S72.052B	S72.141C	S72.344C	S72.424C
S52.035B	S52.231B	S52.323C	S52.509B	S52.91XC	S72.052C	S72.142B	S72.345A	S72.425B
S52.035C	S52.231C	S52.324B	S52.509C	S52.92XB	S72.059A	S72.142C	S72.345B	S72.425C
S52.036B	S52.232B	S52.324C	S52.511B	S52.92XC	S72.059B	S72.143B	S72.345C	S72.426B
S52.036C	S52.232C	S52.325B	S52.511C	S72.001A	S72.059C	S72.143C	S72.346A	S72.426C
S52.041B	S52.233B	S52.325C	S52.512B	S72.001B	S72.061A	S72.144B	S72.346B	S72.431B
S52.041C	S52.233C	S52.326B	S52.512C	S72.001C	S72.061B	S72.144C	S72.346C	S72.431C
S52.042B	S52.234B	S52.326C	S52.513B	S72.002A	S72.061C	S72.145B	S72.351A	S72.432B
	S52.234C	S52.331B	S52.513C	S72.002B	S72.062A		S72.351B	S72.432C

Appendix D: Major Complication and Comorbidity (MCC) Code List

S72.433B	S72.8X1A	S79.099A	S82.144C	S82.235C	S82.409C	S82.461C	S85.591A	T32.32
S72.433C	S72.8X1B	S82.101B	S82.145B	S82.236B	S82.421B	S82.462B	S85.592A	T32.33
S72.434B	S72.8X1C	S82.101C	S82.145C	S82.236C	S82.421C	S82.462C	S85.599A	T32.41
S72.434C	S72.8X2A	S82.102B	S82.146B	S82.241B	S82.422B	S82.463B	T31.21	T32.42
S72.435B	S72.8X2B	S82.102C	S82.146C	S82.241C	S82.422C	S82.463C	T31.22	T32.43
S72.435C	S72.8X2C	S82.109B	S82.151B	S82.242B	S82.423B	S82.464B	T31.31	T32.44
S72.436B	S72.8X9A	S82.109C	S82.151C	S82.242C	S82.423C	S82.464C	T31.32	T32.51
S72.436C	S72.8X9B	S82.111B	S82.152B	S82.243B	S82.424B	S82.465B	T31.33	T32.52
S72.441B	S72.8X9C	S82.111C	S82.152C	S82.243C	S82.424C	S82.465C	T31.41	T32.53
S72.441C	S72.90XA	S82.112B	S82.153B	S82.244B	S82.425B	S82.466B	T31.42	T32.54
S72.442B	S72.90XB	S82.112C	S82.153C	S82.244C	S82.425C	S82.466C	T31.43	T32.55
S72.442C	S72.90XC	S82.113B	S82.154B	S82.245B	S82.426B	S82.491B	T31.44	T32.61
S72.443B	S72.91XA	S82.113C	S82.154C	S82.245C	S82.426C	S82.491C	T31.51	T32.62
S72.443C	S72.91XB	S82.114B	S82.155B	S82.246B	S82.431B	S82.492B	T31.52	T32.63
S72.444B	S72.91XC	S82.114C	S82.155C	S82.246C	S82.431C	S82.492C	T31.53	T32.64
S72.444C	S72.92XA	S82.115B	S82.156B	S82.251B	S82.432B	S82.499B	T31.54	T32.65
S72.445B	S72.92XB	S82.115C	S82.156C	S82.251C	S82.432C	S82.499C	T31.55	T32.66
S72.445C	S72.92XC	S82.116B	S82.191B	S82.252B	S82.433B	S82.831B	T31.61	T32.71
S72.446B	S75.001A	S82.116C	S82.191C	S82.252C	S82.433C	S82.831C	T31.62	T32.72
S72.446C	S75.002A	S82.121B	S82.192B	S82.253B	S82.434B	S82.832B	T31.63	T32.73
S72.451B	S75.009A	S82.121C	S82.192C	S82.253C	S82.434C	S82.832C	T31.64	T32.74
S72.451C	S75.011A	S82.122B	S82.199B	S82.254B	S82.435B	S82.839B	T31.65	T32.75
S72.452B	S75.012A	S82.122C	S82.199C	S82.254C	S82.435C	S82.839C	T31.66	T32.76
S72.452C	S75.019A	S82.123B	S82.201B	S82.255B	S82.436B	S82.861B	T31.71	T32.77
S72.453B	S75.021A	S82.123C	S82.201C	S82.255C	S82.436C	S82.861C	T31.72	T32.81
S72.453C	S75.022A	S82.124B	S82.202B	S82.256B	S82.441B	S82.862B	T31.73	T32.82
S72.454B	S75.029A	S82.124C	S82.202C	S82.256C	S82.441C	S82.862C	T31.74	T32.83
S72.454C	S75.091A	S82.125B	S82.209B	S82.261B	S82.442B	S82.863B	T31.75	T32.84
S72.455B	S75.092A	S82.125C	S82.209C	S82.261C	S82.442C	S82.863C	T31.76	T32.85
S72.455C	S75.099A	S82.126B	S82.221B	S82.262B	S82.443B	S82.864B	T31.77	T32.86
S72.456B	S75.101A	S82.126C	S82.221C	S82.262C	S82.443C	S82.864C	T31.81	T32.87
S72.456C	S75.102A	S82.131B	S82.222B	S82.263B	S82.444B	S82.865B	T31.82	T32.88
S72.461B	S75.109A	S82.131C	S82.222C	S82.263C	S82.444C	S82.865C	T31.83	T32.91
S72.461C	S75.111A	S82.132B	S82.223B	S82.264B	S82.445B	S82.866B	T31.84	T32.92
S72.462B	S75.112A	S82.132C	S82.223C	S82.264C	S82.445C	S82.866C	T31.85	T32.93
S72.462C	S75.119A	S82.133B	S82.224B	S82.265B	S82.446B	S85.001A	T31.86	T32.94
S72.463B	S75.121A	S82.133C	S82.224C	S82.265C	S82.446C	S85.002A	T31.87	T32.95
S72.463C	S75.122A	S82.134B	S82.225B	S82.266B	S82.451B	S85.009A	T31.88	T32.96
S72.464B	S75.129A	S82.134C	S82.225C	S82.266C	S82.451C	S85.011A	T31.91	T32.97
S72.464C	S75.191A	S82.135B	S82.226B	S82.291B	S82.452B	S85.012A	T31.92	T32.98
S72.465B	S75.192A	S82.135C	S82.226C	S82.291C	S82.452C	S85.019A	T31.93	T32.99
S72.465C	S75.199A	S82.136B	S82.231B	S82.292B	S82.453B	S85.091A	T31.94	T79.0XXA
S72.466B	S79.001A	S82.136C	S82.231C	S82.292C	S82.453C	S85.092A	T31.95	T79.1XXA
S72.466C	S79.002A	S82.141B	S82.232B	S82.299B	S82.454B	S85.099A	T31.96	T79.4XXA
S72.491B	S79.009A	S82.141C	S82.232C	S82.299C	S82.454C	S85.501A	T31.97	T79.5XXA
S72.491C	S79.011A	S82.142B	S82.233B	S82.401B	S82.455B	S85.502A	T31.98	T80.0XXA
S72.492B	S79.012A	S82.142C	S82.233C	S82.401C	S82.455C	S85.509A	T31.99	T81.11XA
S72.492C	S79.019A	S82.143B	S82.234B	S82.402B	S82.456B	S85.511A	T32.21	T81.12XA
S72.499B	S79.091A	S82.143C	S82.234C	S82.402C	S82.456C	S85.512A	T32.22	T81.19XA
S72.499C	S79.092A	S82.144B	S82.235B	S82.409B	S82.461B	S85.519A	T32.31	

Appendix E: Complication and Comorbidity (CC) Code List

Note: The following list of CCs are based on the *Federal Register*, volume 84, number 86, May 3, 2019 ("Hospital Inpatient Prospective Payment Systems for Acute Care Hospitals and the Long-Term Care Hospital Prospective Payment System and Proposed Policy Changes and Fiscal Year 2020 Rates; Proposed Rule"). The most current version, v37, of the ICD-10 MS-DRG Definitions Manual was not available at the time this book was printed. For the most current files related to IPPS please refer to the following:
https://www.cms.gov/Medicare/Medicare-Fee-for-Service-Payment/AcuteInpatientPPS/IPPS-Regulations-and-Notices.html.

Optum360 also provides the most current list (v37) of CCs in an easily searchable data file that can be accessed at the following:
https://www.optum360coding.com/ProductUpdates/
Title: "2020 ICD-10-CM for Hospital IPPS Data File"
Password: OptumIPPS20

A00.0	A15.7	A30.0	A50.02	A54.03	A82.1	B02.7	B40.0	B58.01
A00.1	A15.8	A30.1	A50.03	A54.09	A82.9	B02.8	B40.1	B58.09
A00.9	A15.9	A30.2	A50.04	A54.1	A85.0	B03	B40.2	B58.1
A01.00	A17.9	A30.3	A50.05	A54.21	A85.1	B04	B40.3	B58.82
A01.01	A18.01	A30.4	A50.06	A54.22	A85.8	B05.1	B40.7	B58.83
A01.02	A18.02	A30.5	A50.07	A54.23	A86	B05.4	B40.81	B58.89
A01.03	A18.03	A30.8	A50.08	A54.24	A87.0	B05.81	B40.89	B58.9
A01.04	A18.09	A30.9	A50.09	A54.29	A87.1	B05.89	B40.9	B60.0
A01.05	A18.10	A31.0	A50.2	A54.30	A87.2	B06.00	B41.0	B60.10
A01.09	A18.11	A31.1	A50.30	A54.31	A87.8	B06.02	B41.7	B60.19
A01.1	A18.12	A31.2	A50.31	A54.32	A87.9	B06.09	B41.8	B60.2
A01.2	A18.13	A31.8	A50.32	A54.33	A88.0	B06.81	B41.9	B65.0
A01.3	A18.14	A31.9	A50.39	A54.39	A88.8	B06.82	B44.1	B65.1
A01.4	A18.15	A32.0	A50.40	A54.40	A89	B06.89	B44.2	B65.2
A02.0	A18.16	A32.11	A50.43	A54.41	A90	B08.3	B44.7	B65.3
A02.23	A18.17	A32.12	A50.44	A54.42	A91	B08.71	B44.81	B65.8
A02.24	A18.18	A32.81	A50.45	A54.43	A92.0	B15.9	B44.89	B65.9
A02.25	A18.2	A32.82	A50.49	A54.49	A92.1	B16.1	B44.9	B66.0
A02.29	A18.32	A32.89	A50.51	A54.82	A92.2	B16.9	B45.0	B66.1
A02.8	A18.39	A32.9	A50.52	A54.83	A92.4	B17.0	B45.2	B66.2
A02.9	A18.4	A34	A50.53	A54.84	A92.5	B17.10	B45.3	B66.3
A03.0	A18.50	A36.0	A50.54	A54.85	A92.8	B17.2	B45.7	B66.4
A04.0	A18.51	A36.1	A50.55	A54.89	A92.9	B17.8	B45.8	B66.5
A04.1	A18.52	A36.2	A50.56	A54.9	A93.0	B17.9	B45.9	B66.8
A04.2	A18.53	A36.3	A50.57	A68.0	A93.1	B18.0	B47.0	B67.0
A04.3	A18.54	A36.81	A50.59	A68.1	A93.2	B18.1	B47.1	B67.1
A04.4	A18.59	A36.82	A51.31	A68.9	A93.8	B18.8	B47.9	B67.2
A04.5	A18.6	A36.83	A51.32	A69.1	A94	B18.9	B48.2	B67.31
A04.6	A18.7	A36.84	A51.39	A69.21	A95.0	B19.10	B48.3	B67.32
A04.71	A18.81	A36.85	A51.42	A69.22	A95.1	B19.9	B48.4	B67.39
A04.72	A18.82	A36.86	A51.43	A69.23	A95.9	B20	B48.8	B67.4
A04.8	A18.83	A36.89	A51.44	A69.29	A96.0	B25.1	B49	B67.5
A04.9	A18.84	A36.9	A51.45	A70	A96.1	B25.8	B50.0	B67.61
A05.0	A18.85	A37.00	A51.46	A75.0	A96.8	B25.9	B50.8	B67.69
A05.1	A18.89	A37.10	A51.49	A75.1	A96.9	B26.0	B51.0	B67.7
A05.2	A21.0	A37.80	A52.00	A75.2	A98.0	B26.3	B51.8	B67.8
A05.3	A21.1	A37.90	A52.01	A75.3	A98.1	B26.81	B51.9	B67.90
A05.4	A21.2	A38.0	A52.02	A75.9	A98.2	B26.82	B52.0	B67.99
A05.5	A21.3	A38.1	A52.03	A77.0	A98.5	B26.83	B52.8	B68.0
A05.8	A21.7	A38.8	A52.04	A77.1	A98.8	B26.84	B52.9	B68.1
A06.0	A21.8	A38.9	A52.05	A77.2	A99	B26.85	B53.0	B68.9
A06.1	A21.9	A39.82	A52.06	A77.3	B00.2	B26.89	B53.1	B69.0
A06.2	A22.0	A39.83	A52.09	A77.40	B00.50	B33.1	B53.8	B69.1
A06.3	A22.2	A39.84	A52.10	A77.41	B00.51	B33.20	B54	B69.81
A06.81	A22.8	A39.89	A52.11	A77.49	B00.52	B33.21	B55.0	B69.89
A06.82	A22.9	A39.9	A52.12	A77.8	B00.53	B33.22	B55.1	B69.9
A06.89	A23.8	A42.0	A52.15	A77.9	B00.59	B33.23	B55.2	B70.0
A07.1	A23.9	A42.1	A52.16	A78	B00.81	B33.4	B55.9	B70.1
A07.2	A24.0	A42.2	A52.17	A79.0	B00.89	B34.3	B56.0	B71.0
A07.3	A24.1	A42.81	A52.19	A79.1	B01.0	B37.0	B56.1	B71.1
A07.4	A24.2	A42.82	A52.2	A79.81	B01.81	B37.41	B56.9	B71.8
A07.8	A24.3	A42.89	A52.3	A79.89	B01.89	B37.49	B57.0	B72
A07.9	A24.9	A42.9	A52.71	A79.9	B01.9	B37.83	B57.1	B73.00
A08.0	A25.0	A43.0	A52.72	A81.00	B02.0	B37.84	B57.2	B73.01
A08.11	A25.1	A43.1	A52.73	A81.01	B02.21	B37.89	B57.30	B73.02
A08.19	A25.9	A43.8	A52.74	A81.09	B02.22	B38.0	B57.31	B73.09
A08.2	A27.0	A43.9	A52.75	A81.1	B02.23	B38.1	B57.32	B73.1
A08.31	A27.89	A44.0	A52.76	A81.2	B02.29	B38.2	B57.39	B74.0
A08.32	A27.9	A44.1	A52.77	A81.81	B02.30	B38.3	B57.40	B74.1
A08.39	A28.0	A44.8	A52.78	A81.82	B02.31	B38.7	B57.41	B74.2
A15.0	A28.1	A44.9	A52.79	A81.83	B02.32	B38.81	B57.42	B74.3
A15.4	A28.2	A48.51	A54.00	A81.89	B02.33	B38.89	B57.49	B74.4
A15.5	A28.8	A48.52	A54.01	A81.9	B02.34	B38.9	B57.5	B74.8
A15.6	A28.9	A50.01	A54.02	A82.0	B02.39	B39.3	B58.00	B74.9

B75	D78.81	E46	E72.23	E87.4	F12.951	F17.223	F32.1	G40.804
B76.0	D78.89	E51.11	E72.29	E88.02	F13.121	F17.293	F32.2	G40.811
B76.1	D80.0	E51.12	E72.3	E88.40	F13.150	F18.121	F32.3	G40.812
B76.8	D80.1	E51.8	E72.4	E88.41	F13.151	F18.150	F33.1	G40.813
B76.9	D80.2	E51.9	E72.50	E88.42	F13.20	F18.151	F33.2	G40.814
B77.0	D80.3	E53.0	E72.51	E88.49	F13.221	F18.17	F33.3	G40.821
B77.89	D80.4	E55.0	E72.52	E89.1	F13.230	F18.20	F33.40	G40.823
B77.9	D80.5	E64.0	E72.53	E89.6	F13.231	F18.221	F33.8	G40.824
B78.0	D80.6	E66.2	E72.59	E89.810	F13.232	F18.250	F33.9	G40.89
B78.7	D80.7	E70.0	E72.81	E89.811	F13.239	F18.251	F34.81	G40.911
B78.9	D80.8	E70.1	E72.89	E89.820	F13.250	F18.259	F34.89	G40.919
B79	D80.9	E70.20	E72.9	E89.821	F13.251	F18.27	F34.9	G40.A11
B80	D81.0	E70.21	E74.00	E89.822	F13.259	F18.280	F50.0	G40.A19
B81.0	D81.1	E70.29	E74.01	E89.823	F13.26	F18.288	F50.01	G40.B01
B81.1	D81.2	E70.30	E74.02	E89.89	F13.27	F18.921	F50.02	G40.B09
B81.2	D81.30	E70.310	E74.03	F01.51	F13.280	F18.950	F50.2	G40.B11
B81.3	D81.31	E70.311	E74.04	F02.81	F13.281	F18.951	F63.89	G40.B19
B81.4	D81.32	E70.318	E74.09	F03.91	F13.282	F18.97	F63.9	G43.601
B81.8	D81.39	E70.319	E74.20	F05	F13.288	F19.121	F68.10	G43.609
B82.0	D81.4	E70.320	E74.21	F06.0	F13.921	F19.150	F68.12	G43.611
B97.21	D81.5	E70.321	E74.29	F06.2	F13.930	F19.151	F68.A	G43.619
B97.33	D81.6	E70.328	E74.4	F06.30	F13.931	F19.17	F84.3	G45.8
B97.34	D81.7	E70.329	E74.8	F06.31	F13.932	F19.20	G03.1	G45.9
B97.35	D81.89	E70.330	E75.00	F06.4	F13.939	F19.221	G03.2	G46.0
C40.81	D81.9	E70.331	E75.01	F07.81	F13.950	F19.222	G04.1	G46.1
C68.1	D82.0	E70.338	E75.02	F09	F13.951	F19.230	G12.23	G46.2
C82.17	D82.1	E70.339	E75.09	F10.121	F13.97	F19.231	G12.24	G60.1
C83.00	D83.0	E70.39	E75.10	F10.14	F14.121	F19.232	G12.25	G61.0
C83.01	D83.1	E70.40	E75.11	F10.151	F14.150	F19.239	G21.11	G61.81
D59.4	D83.2	E70.41	E75.19	F10.159	F14.151	F19.250	G21.19	G62.81
D59.9	D83.8	E70.49	E75.23	F10.180	F14.221	F19.251	G21.2	G70.80
D61.01	D83.9	E70.5	E75.25	F10.181	F14.222	F19.259	G21.3	G70.81
D61.09	D84.8	E70.8	E75.26	F10.188	F14.229	F19.26	G21.8	G71.2
D61.810	D84.9	E70.9	E75.29	F10.221	F14.23	F19.27	G21.9	G72.0
D61.811	D89.810	E71.0	E75.4	F10.230	F14.250	F19.280	G23.0	G72.1
D61.818	D89.811	E71.110	E76.01	F10.231	F14.251	F19.281	G23.8	G72.2
D61.82	D89.812	E71.111	E76.02	F10.232	F14.259	F19.282	G23.9	G72.81
D68.0	D89.813	E71.118	E76.03	F10.239	F14.280	F19.288	G24.01	G73.1
D68.1	E06.0	E71.120	E76.1	F10.24	F14.281	F19.921	G24.02	G73.3
D68.2	E07.81	E71.121	E76.210	F10.251	F14.282	F19.930	G24.09	G80.0
D68.311	E08.52	E71.128	E76.211	F10.259	F14.288	F19.931	G24.2	G81.00
D68.312	E09.52	E71.19	E76.219	F10.27	F14.921	F19.932	G25.82	G81.01
D68.318	E09.65	E71.2	E76.22	F10.280	F14.950	F19.939	G25.9	G81.02
D68.32	E09.69	E71.310	E76.29	F10.281	F14.951	F19.950	G31.2	G81.03
D68.4	E09.8	E71.311	E76.3	F10.288	F15.121	F19.951	G31.81	G81.04
D68.8	E09.9	E71.312	E76.8	F10.29	F15.150	F19.97	G31.82	G81.10
D68.9	E10.52	E71.313	E76.9	F10.921	F15.151	F20.0	G32.0	G81.11
D69.0	E11.52	E71.314	E78.71	F10.94	F15.20	F20.1	G32.81	G81.12
D69.1	E13.52	E71.318	E78.72	F10.951	F15.221	F20.2	G36.0	G81.13
D69.3	E15	E71.32	E79.1	F10.959	F15.222	F20.5	G36.1	G81.14
D69.41	E22.1	E71.39	E79.2	F10.980	F15.23	F20.81	G36.8	G81.90
D69.42	E22.2	E71.50	E79.8	F10.981	F15.250	F20.89	G36.9	G81.91
D70.0	E22.8	E71.510	E79.9	F10.988	F15.251	F22	G37.0	G81.92
D70.1	E22.9	E71.511	E80.0	F11.121	F15.259	F23	G37.1	G81.93
D70.2	E23.2	E71.518	E80.1	F11.150	F15.280	F28	G37.2	G81.94
D70.3	E24.0	E71.520	E80.20	F11.151	F15.281	F29	G37.3	G82.20
D70.4	E24.2	E71.521	E80.21	F11.20	F15.282	F30.10	G37.5	G82.21
D70.8	E24.3	E71.522	E80.29	F11.221	F15.288	F30.11	G37.8	G82.22
D70.9	E24.4	E71.528	E80.3	F11.222	F15.921	F30.12	G37.9	G83.0
D71	E24.8	E71.529	E83.111	F11.23	F15.93	F30.13	G40.001	G83.4
D74.0	E24.9	E71.53	E83.39	F11.250	F15.950	F30.2	G40.009	G90.1
D74.8	E27.0	E71.540	E83.51	F11.251	F15.951	F30.9	G40.011	G90.3
D74.9	E27.1	E71.541	E84.19	F11.259	F16.121	F31.0	G40.019	G90.50
D75.81	E27.2	E71.542	E84.8	F11.281	F16.150	F31.10	G40.101	G90.511
D75.82	E27.3	E71.548	E84.9	F11.282	F16.151	F31.11	G40.109	G90.512
D76.1	E27.40	E72.00	E85.0	F11.288	F16.20	F31.12	G40.111	G90.513
D76.2	E27.49	E72.01	E85.1	F11.921	F16.221	F31.13	G40.119	G90.519
D76.3	E27.5	E72.02	E85.2	F11.93	F16.250	F31.2	G40.201	G90.521
D78.01	E32.1	E72.03	E85.3	F11.950	F16.251	F31.30	G40.209	G90.522
D78.02	E34.0	E72.04	E85.4	F11.951	F16.259	F31.31	G40.211	G90.523
D78.11	E36.01	E72.09	E85.81	F12.121	F16.280	F31.32	G40.219	G90.529
D78.12	E36.02	E72.10	E85.82	F12.150	F16.283	F31.4	G40.411	G90.59
D78.21	E36.11	E72.11	E85.89	F12.151	F16.288	F31.5	G40.419	G91.0
D78.22	E36.12	E72.12	E85.9	F12.221	F16.921	F31.60	G40.501	G91.1
D78.31	E42	E72.19	E87.0	F12.250	F16.950	F31.61	G40.509	G91.2
D78.32	E43	E72.20	E87.1	F12.251	F16.951	F31.62	G40.802	G91.3
D78.33	E44.1	E72.21	E87.2	F12.921	F17.203	F31.63	G40.803	G91.8
D78.34	E45	E72.22	E87.3	F12.950	F17.213	F31.64		

G91.9	H30.141	H35.82	H59.013	H95.51	I25.799	I69.154	I70.631	I80.232
G93.1	H30.142	H40.211	H59.019	H95.52	I25.810	I69.159	I70.632	I80.233
G93.40	H30.143	H40.212	H59.031	H95.53	I25.811	I69.251	I70.633	I80.239
G93.49	H30.149	H40.213	H59.032	H95.54	I25.812	I69.252	I70.634	I80.241
G93.5	H30.891	H40.219	H59.033	H95.811	I27.0	I69.253	I70.638	I80.242
G93.82	H30.892	H44.001	H59.039	H95.812	I27.1	I69.254	I70.639	I80.243
G95.0	H30.893	H44.002	H59.091	H95.813	I27.81	I69.259	I70.641	I80.249
G95.19	H30.899	H44.003	H59.092	H95.819	I27.82	I69.351	I70.642	I80.291
G95.20	H30.90	H44.009	H59.093	H95.88	I28.0	I69.352	I70.643	I80.292
G95.29	H30.91	H44.011	H59.099	H95.89	I28.1	I69.353	I70.644	I80.293
G95.81	H30.92	H44.012	H59.111	I01.0	I30.0	I69.354	I70.648	I80.299
G95.89	H30.93	H44.013	H59.112	I01.1	I30.1	I69.359	I70.649	I82.1
G95.9	H31.321	H44.019	H59.113	I01.2	I30.8	I69.851	I70.661	I82.210
G96.0	H31.322	H44.021	H59.119	I01.8	I30.9	I69.852	I70.662	I82.211
G96.11	H31.323	H44.022	H59.121	I01.9	I31.0	I69.853	I70.663	I82.290
G97.0	H31.329	H44.023	H59.122	I02.0	I31.1	I69.854	I70.668	I82.291
G97.2	H31.401	H44.029	H59.123	I02.9	I31.2	I69.859	I70.669	I82.3
G97.31	H31.402	H44.111	H59.129	I09.0	I31.3	I69.951	I70.731	I82.401
G97.32	H31.403	H44.112	H59.211	I09.2	I31.4	I69.952	I70.732	I82.402
G97.41	H31.409	H44.113	H59.212	I09.81	I31.8	I69.953	I70.733	I82.403
G97.48	H31.411	H44.119	H59.213	I12.0	I31.9	I69.954	I70.734	I82.409
G97.49	H31.412	H44.121	H59.219	I13.0	I32	I69.959	I70.738	I82.411
G97.51	H31.413	H44.122	H59.221	I13.11	I38	I70.261	I70.739	I82.412
G97.52	H31.419	H44.123	H59.222	I13.2	I39	I70.262	I70.741	I82.413
G97.61	H31.421	H44.129	H59.223	I16.1	I42.0	I70.263	I70.742	I82.419
G97.62	H31.422	H44.131	H59.229	I16.9	I42.6	I70.268	I70.743	I82.421
G97.63	H31.423	H44.132	H59.311	I20.0	I42.7	I70.269	I70.744	I82.422
G97.64	H31.429	H44.133	H59.312	I20.1	I42.8	I70.331	I70.748	I82.423
G97.81	H33.121	H44.139	H59.313	I21.01	I42.9	I70.332	I70.749	I82.429
G97.82	H33.122	H44.19	H59.319	I21.02	I43	I70.333	I70.761	I82.431
G99.0	H33.123	H46.00	H59.321	I21.09	I44.2	I70.334	I70.762	I82.432
G99.2	H33.129	H46.01	H59.322	I21.11	I45.2	I70.338	I70.763	I82.433
H05.011	H33.20	H46.02	H59.323	I21.19	I45.3	I70.339	I70.768	I82.439
H05.012	H33.21	H46.03	H59.329	I21.21	I47.0	I70.341	I70.769	I82.441
H05.013	H33.22	H46.10	H59.331	I21.29	I47.1	I70.342	I70.92	I82.442
H05.019	H33.23	H46.11	H59.332	I21.3	I47.2	I70.343	I71.00	I82.443
H05.021	H33.40	H46.12	H59.333	I22.0	I48.11	I70.344	I73.01	I82.449
H05.022	H33.41	H46.13	H59.339	I22.1	I48.19	I70.348	I74.09	I82.451
H05.023	H33.42	H46.8	H59.341	I22.2	I48.20	I70.349	I74.10	I82.452
H05.029	H33.43	H46.9	H59.342	I22.8	I48.21	I70.361	I74.11	I82.453
H05.031	H33.8	H47.10	H59.343	I22.9	I48.3	I70.362	I74.19	I82.459
H05.032	H34.00	H47.11	H59.349	I23.0	I48.4	I70.363	I74.2	I82.491
H05.033	H34.01	H47.41	H59.351	I23.1	I48.92	I70.368	I74.3	I82.492
H05.039	H34.02	H47.42	H59.352	I23.2	I49.01	I70.369	I74.4	I82.493
H20.00	H34.03	H47.43	H59.353	I23.3	I49.02	I70.431	I74.5	I82.499
H20.011	H34.10	H47.49	H59.359	I23.6	I49.2	I70.432	I74.8	I82.4Y1
H20.012	H34.11	H47.511	H59.361	I23.7	I50.1	I70.433	I74.9	I82.4Y2
H20.013	H34.12	H47.512	H59.362	I23.8	I50.20	I70.434	I75.011	I82.4Y3
H20.019	H34.13	H47.519	H59.363	I24.0	I50.30	I70.438	I75.012	I82.4Y9
H20.021	H34.211	H47.521	H59.369	I24.1	I50.40	I70.439	I75.013	I82.4Z1
H20.022	H34.212	H47.522	H59.811	I24.8	I51.0	I70.441	I75.019	I82.4Z2
H20.023	H34.213	H47.529	H59.812	I24.9	I51.1	I70.442	I75.021	I82.4Z3
H20.029	H34.219	H47.531	H59.813	I25.110	I51.2	I70.443	I75.022	I82.4Z9
H20.031	H34.231	H47.532	H59.819	I25.3	I51.3	I70.444	I75.023	I82.501
H20.032	H34.232	H47.539	H59.88	I25.700	I51.81	I70.448	I75.029	I82.502
H20.033	H34.233	H47.621	H59.89	I25.710	I62.03	I70.449	I75.81	I82.503
H20.039	H34.239	H47.622	H60.20	I25.711	I62.9	I70.461	I75.89	I82.509
H20.9	H34.8110	H47.629	H60.21	I25.718	I65.03	I70.462	I76	I82.511
H21.331	H34.8111	H47.631	H60.22	I25.719	I67.3	I70.463	I77.2	I82.512
H21.332	H34.8112	H47.632	H60.23	I25.720	I67.4	I70.468	I77.4	I82.513
H21.333	H34.8120	H47.639	H70.001	I25.721	I67.5	I70.469	I77.5	I82.519
H21.339	H34.8121	H47.641	H70.002	I25.728	I67.6	I70.531	I80.10	I82.521
H30.101	H34.8122	H47.642	H70.003	I25.729	I67.7	I70.532	I80.11	I82.522
H30.102	H34.8130	H47.649	H70.009	I25.730	I67.81	I70.533	I80.12	I82.523
H30.103	H34.8131	H49.811	H70.011	I25.731	I67.82	I70.534	I80.13	I82.529
H30.109	H34.8132	H49.812	H70.012	I25.738	I67.841	I70.538	I80.201	I82.531
H30.111	H34.8190	H49.813	H70.013	I25.739	I67.848	I70.539	I80.202	I82.532
H30.112	H34.8191	H49.819	H70.019	I25.750	I67.850	I70.541	I80.203	I82.533
H30.113	H34.8192	H53.121	H70.091	I25.751	I67.858	I70.542	I80.209	I82.539
H30.119	H35.70	H53.122	H70.092	I25.758	I68.2	I70.543	I80.211	I82.541
H30.121	H35.721	H53.123	H70.093	I25.759	I69.051	I70.544	I80.212	I82.542
H30.122	H35.722	H53.129	H70.099	I25.760	I69.052	I70.548	I80.213	I82.543
H30.123	H35.723	H53.131	H95.21	I25.761	I69.053	I70.549	I80.219	I82.549
H30.129	H35.729	H53.132	H95.22	I25.768	I69.054	I70.561	I80.221	I82.551
H30.131	H35.731	H53.133	H95.31	I25.769	I69.059	I70.562	I80.222	I82.552
H30.132	H35.732	H53.139	H95.32	I25.790	I69.151	I70.563	I80.223	I82.553
H30.133	H35.733	H59.011	H95.41	I25.791	I69.152	I70.568	I80.229	I82.559
H30.139	H35.739	H59.012	H95.42	I25.798	I69.153	I70.569	I80.231	I82.591

Appendix E: Complication and Comorbidity (CC) Code List

I82.592	I83.214	J44.0	K12.2	K63.0	K94.03	L10.4	L89.124	L89.504
I82.593	I83.215	J44.1	K22.10	K63.1	K94.09	L10.5	L89.126	L89.506
I82.599	I83.218	J45.21	K25.3	K63.2	K94.11	L10.81	L89.129	L89.509
I82.5Y1	I83.219	J45.22	K25.7	K63.3	K94.12	L10.89	L89.130	L89.510
I82.5Y2	I83.221	J45.31	K25.9	K65.4	K94.13	L10.9	L89.131	L89.511
I82.5Y3	I83.222	J45.32	K26.3	K68.11	K94.19	L12.0	L89.132	L89.512
I82.5Y9	I83.223	J45.41	K27.3	K76.1	K94.22	L12.30	L89.133	L89.513
I82.5Z1	I83.224	J45.42	K28.3	K76.6	K94.23	L12.31	L89.134	L89.514
I82.5Z2	I83.225	J45.52	K29.00	K77	K94.30	L12.35	L89.136	L89.516
I82.5Z3	I83.228	J45.901	K31.0	K80.01	K94.31	L12.8	L89.139	L89.519
I82.5Z9	I83.229	J45.902	K31.1	K80.11	K94.32	L12.9	L89.140	L89.520
I82.601	I85.00	J47.0	K31.5	K80.13	K94.33	L27.0	L89.141	L89.521
I82.602	I85.10	J47.1	K31.6	K80.19	K94.39	L27.1	L89.142	L89.522
I82.603	I87.011	J67.7	K31.7	K80.21	K95.01	L49.3	L89.143	L89.523
I82.609	I87.012	J67.8	K31.811	K80.30	K95.09	L49.4	L89.144	L89.524
I82.611	I87.013	J67.9	K35.80	K80.31	K95.81	L49.5	L89.146	L89.526
I82.612	I87.019	J68.0	K35.890	K80.32	K95.89	L49.6	L89.149	L89.529
I82.613	I87.031	J70.0	K35.891	K80.33	L02.211	L49.7	L89.150	L89.600
I82.619	I87.032	J70.1	K40.00	K80.34	L02.212	L49.8	L89.151	L89.601
I82.621	I87.033	J81.1	K40.01	K80.35	L02.213	L49.9	L89.152	L89.602
I82.622	I87.039	J82	K40.30	K80.36	L02.214	L51.1	L89.153	L89.603
I82.623	I87.1	J84.01	K40.31	K80.37	L02.215	L51.2	L89.154	L89.604
I82.629	I87.311	J84.02	K41.00	K80.40	L02.216	L51.3	L89.156	L89.606
I82.701	I87.312	J84.03	K41.01	K80.41	L02.31	L53.0	L89.159	L89.609
I82.702	I87.313	J84.09	K41.30	K80.42	L02.411	L53.1	L89.200	L89.610
I82.703	I87.319	J84.114	K41.31	K80.43	L02.412	L53.2	L89.201	L89.611
I82.709	I87.331	J84.116	K42.0	K80.44	L02.611	L53.3	L89.202	L89.612
I82.711	I87.332	J84.117	K43.0	K80.45	L02.612	L76.01	L89.203	L89.613
I82.712	I87.333	J84.2	K43.3	K80.46	L02.619	L76.02	L89.204	L89.614
I82.713	I87.339	J84.82	K43.6	K80.47	L03.111	L76.11	L89.206	L89.616
I82.719	I96	J90	K44.0	K80.50	L03.112	L76.12	L89.209	L89.619
I82.721	I97.110	J91.0	K45.0	K80.51	L03.113	L76.21	L89.210	L89.620
I82.722	I97.111	J91.8	K46.0	K80.60	L03.114	L76.22	L89.211	L89.621
I82.723	I97.120	J93.11	K51.212	K80.61	L03.115	L76.31	L89.212	L89.622
I82.729	I97.121	J93.12	K51.413	K80.62	L03.116	L76.32	L89.213	L89.623
I82.811	I97.130	J93.81	K51.811	K80.63	L03.119	L76.33	L89.214	L89.624
I82.812	I97.131	J93.82	K51.812	K80.64	L03.121	L76.34	L89.216	L89.626
I82.813	I97.190	J93.83	K51.813	K80.65	L03.122	L88	L89.219	L89.629
I82.819	I97.191	J93.9	K51.814	K80.66	L03.123	L89.000	L89.220	L89.810
I82.890	I97.410	J94.0	K51.818	K80.67	L03.124	L89.001	L89.221	L89.811
I82.891	I97.411	J94.2	K51.819	K80.70	L03.125	L89.002	L89.222	L89.812
I82.90	I97.418	J94.8	K51.911	K80.71	L03.126	L89.003	L89.223	L89.813
I82.91	I97.42	J95.00	K51.912	K80.81	L03.129	L89.004	L89.224	L89.814
I82.A11	I97.51	J95.01	K51.913	K81.0	L03.211	L89.006	L89.226	L89.816
I82.A12	I97.52	J95.02	K51.914	K81.2	L03.212	L89.009	L89.229	L89.819
I82.A13	I97.610	J95.03	K51.918	K82.0	L03.213	L89.010	L89.300	L89.890
I82.A19	I97.611	J95.04	K51.919	K82.2	L03.221	L89.011	L89.301	L89.891
I82.A21	I97.618	J95.09	K52.0	K82.3	L03.222	L89.012	L89.302	L89.892
I82.A22	I97.620	J95.1	K52.1	K82.A2	L03.311	L89.013	L89.303	L89.893
I82.A23	I97.621	J95.4	K56.0	K83.01	L03.312	L89.014	L89.304	L89.894
I82.A29	I97.622	J95.5	K56.1	K83.09	L03.313	L89.016	L89.306	L89.896
I82.B11	I97.630	J95.61	K56.2	K83.3	L03.314	L89.019	L89.309	L89.899
I82.B12	I97.631	J95.62	K56.3	K91.30	L03.315	L89.020	L89.310	L89.90
I82.B13	I97.638	J95.71	K56.41	K91.31	L03.316	L89.021	L89.311	L89.91
I82.B19	I97.640	J95.72	K56.49	K91.61	L03.317	L89.022	L89.312	L89.92
I82.B21	I97.641	J95.811	K56.50	K91.62	L03.319	L89.023	L89.313	L89.93
I82.B22	I97.648	J95.812	K56.51	K91.71	L03.321	L89.024	L89.314	L89.94
I82.B23	I97.710	J95.821	K56.52	K91.72	L03.322	L89.026	L89.316	L89.95
I82.B29	I97.711	J95.830	K56.600	K91.81	L03.323	L89.029	L89.319	L89.96
I82.C11	I97.790	J95.831	K56.601	K91.82	L03.324	L89.100	L89.320	L97.101
I82.C12	I97.791	J95.84	K56.609	K91.83	L03.325	L89.101	L89.321	L97.102
I82.C13	I97.810	J95.850	K56.690	K91.840	L03.326	L89.102	L89.322	L97.103
I82.C19	I97.811	J95.851	K56.691	K91.841	L03.327	L89.103	L89.323	L97.104
I82.C21	I97.820	J95.859	K56.699	K91.850	L03.329	L89.104	L89.324	L97.105
I82.C22	I97.821	J95.860	K56.7	K91.858	L03.811	L89.106	L89.326	L97.106
I82.C23	I97.88	J95.861	K57.00	K91.86	L03.818	L89.109	L89.329	L97.108
I82.C29	I97.89	J95.862	K57.20	K91.870	L03.891	L89.110	L89.40	L97.109
I83.201	J05.10	J95.863	K57.31	K91.871	L03.898	L89.111	L89.41	L97.111
I83.202	J10.1	J95.88	K57.32	K91.872	L03.90	L89.112	L89.42	L97.112
I83.203	J18.2	J95.89	K57.33	K91.873	L03.91	L89.113	L89.43	L97.113
I83.204	J21.0	J96.10	K57.40	K91.89	L05.01	L89.114	L89.44	L97.114
I83.205	J21.1	J96.11	K57.52	K92.0	L05.02	L89.116	L89.45	L97.115
I83.208	J21.8	J96.12	K57.80	K92.1	L08.1	L89.119	L89.46	L97.116
I83.209	J21.9	J98.01	K57.92	K92.2	L10.0	L89.120	L89.500	L97.118
I83.211	J36	J98.11	K59.2	K92.81	L10.1	L89.121	L89.501	L97.119
I83.212	J39.0	J98.19	K59.31	K94.01	L10.2	L89.122	L89.502	L97.121
I83.213	J39.1	K04.02	K59.39	K94.02	L10.3	L89.123	L89.503	L97.122

L97.123	L97.429	M00.039	M00.852	M33.02	M48.57XA	M80.021K	M80.831K	M84.343P
L97.124	L97.505	M00.041	M00.859	M33.03	M48.58XA	M80.021P	M80.831K	M84.344K
L97.125	L97.506	M00.042	M00.861	M33.09	M50.00	M80.022A	M80.831P	M84.344P
L97.126	L97.508	M00.049	M00.862	M33.10	M50.01	M80.022K	M80.832A	M84.345K
L97.128	L97.515	M00.051	M00.869	M33.11	M50.020	M80.022P	M80.832K	M84.345P
L97.129	L97.516	M00.052	M00.871	M33.12	M50.021	M80.029A	M80.832P	M84.346K
L97.201	L97.518	M00.059	M00.872	M33.13	M50.022	M80.029K	M80.839A	M84.346P
L97.202	L97.525	M00.061	M00.879	M33.19	M50.023	M80.029P	M80.839K	M84.350K
L97.203	L97.526	M00.062	M00.88	M33.20	M50.03	M80.031A	M80.839P	M84.350P
L97.204	L97.528	M00.069	M00.89	M33.21	M51.04	M80.031K	M80.841A	M84.351K
L97.205	L97.801	M00.071	M00.9	M33.22	M51.05	M80.031P	M80.841K	M84.351P
L97.206	L97.802	M00.072	M01.X0	M33.29	M51.06	M80.032A	M80.841P	M84.352K
L97.208	L97.803	M00.079	M01.X11	M33.90	M60.000	M80.032K	M80.842A	M84.352P
L97.209	L97.804	M00.08	M01.X12	M33.91	M60.001	M80.032P	M80.842K	M84.353K
L97.211	L97.805	M00.09	M01.X19	M33.92	M60.002	M80.039A	M80.842P	M84.353P
L97.212	L97.806	M00.10	M01.X21	M33.93	M60.003	M80.039K	M80.849A	M84.359K
L97.213	L97.808	M00.111	M01.X22	M33.99	M60.004	M80.039P	M80.849K	M84.359P
L97.214	L97.809	M00.112	M01.X29	M34.81	M60.005	M80.041A	M80.849P	M84.361K
L97.215	L97.811	M00.119	M01.X31	M34.82	M60.009	M80.041K	M80.851A	M84.361P
L97.216	L97.812	M00.121	M01.X32	M35.03	M60.011	M80.041P	M80.851K	M84.362K
L97.218	L97.813	M00.122	M01.X39	M35.1	M60.012	M80.042A	M80.851P	M84.362P
L97.219	L97.814	M00.129	M01.X41	M35.2	M60.019	M80.042K	M80.852A	M84.363K
L97.221	L97.815	M00.131	M01.X42	M35.5	M60.021	M80.042P	M80.852K	M84.363P
L97.222	L97.816	M00.132	M01.X49	M35.8	M60.022	M80.049A	M80.852P	M84.364K
L97.223	L97.818	M00.139	M01.X51	M36.0	M60.029	M80.049K	M80.859A	M84.364P
L97.224	L97.819	M00.141	M01.X52	M46.20	M60.031	M80.049P	M80.859K	M84.369K
L97.225	L97.821	M00.142	M01.X59	M46.21	M60.032	M80.051A	M80.859P	M84.369P
L97.226	L97.822	M00.149	M01.X61	M46.22	M60.039	M80.051K	M80.861A	M84.371K
L97.228	L97.823	M00.151	M01.X62	M46.23	M60.041	M80.051P	M80.861K	M84.371P
L97.229	L97.824	M00.152	M01.X69	M46.24	M60.042	M80.052A	M80.861P	M84.372K
L97.301	L97.825	M00.159	M01.X71	M46.25	M60.043	M80.052K	M80.862A	M84.372P
L97.302	L97.826	M00.161	M01.X72	M46.26	M60.044	M80.052P	M80.862K	M84.373K
L97.303	L97.828	M00.162	M01.X79	M46.27	M60.045	M80.059A	M80.862P	M84.373P
L97.304	L97.829	M00.169	M01.X8	M46.28	M60.046	M80.059K	M80.869A	M84.374K
L97.305	L97.901	M00.171	M01.X9	M46.30	M60.051	M80.059P	M80.869K	M84.374P
L97.306	L97.902	M00.172	M25.00	M46.31	M60.052	M80.061A	M80.869P	M84.375K
L97.308	L97.903	M00.179	M25.011	M46.32	M60.059	M80.061K	M80.871A	M84.375P
L97.309	L97.904	M00.18	M25.012	M46.33	M60.061	M80.061P	M80.871K	M84.376K
L97.311	L97.905	M00.19	M25.019	M46.34	M60.062	M80.062A	M80.871P	M84.376P
L97.312	L97.906	M00.20	M25.021	M46.35	M60.069	M80.062K	M80.872A	M84.377K
L97.313	L97.908	M00.211	M25.022	M46.36	M60.070	M80.062P	M80.872K	M84.377P
L97.314	L97.909	M00.212	M25.029	M46.37	M60.071	M80.069A	M80.872P	M84.378K
L97.315	L97.911	M00.219	M25.031	M46.38	M60.072	M80.069K	M80.879A	M84.378P
L97.316	L97.912	M00.221	M25.032	M46.39	M60.073	M80.069P	M80.879K	M84.379K
L97.318	L97.913	M00.222	M25.039	M47.011	M60.074	M80.071A	M80.879P	M84.379P
L97.319	L97.914	M00.229	M25.041	M47.012	M60.075	M80.071K	M80.88XA	M84.38XK
L97.321	L97.915	M00.231	M25.042	M47.013	M60.076	M80.071P	M80.88XK	M84.38XP
L97.322	L97.916	M00.232	M25.049	M47.014	M60.077	M80.072A	M80.88XP	M84.40XA
L97.323	L97.918	M00.239	M25.051	M47.015	M60.078	M80.072K	M84.30XK	M84.40XK
L97.324	L97.919	M00.241	M25.052	M47.016	M60.08	M80.072P	M84.30XP	M84.40XP
L97.325	L97.921	M00.242	M25.059	M47.019	M60.09	M80.079A	M84.311K	M84.411A
L97.326	L97.922	M00.249	M25.061	M47.021	M62.3	M80.079K	M84.311P	M84.411K
L97.328	L97.923	M00.251	M25.062	M47.022	M62.82	M80.079P	M84.312K	M84.411P
L97.329	L97.924	M00.252	M25.069	M47.029	M75.121	M80.08XA	M84.312P	M84.412A
L97.401	L97.925	M00.259	M25.071	M47.10	M75.122	M80.08XK	M84.319K	M84.412K
L97.402	L97.926	M00.261	M25.072	M47.11	M79.3	M80.08XP	M84.319P	M84.412P
L97.403	L97.928	M00.262	M25.073	M47.12	M79.A11	M80.80XA	M84.321K	M84.419A
L97.404	L97.929	M00.269	M25.074	M47.13	M79.A12	M80.80XK	M84.321P	M84.419K
L97.405	L98.3	M00.271	M25.075	M47.14	M79.A19	M80.80XP	M84.322K	M84.419P
L97.406	L98.415	M00.272	M25.076	M47.15	M79.A21	M80.811A	M84.322P	M84.421A
L97.408	L98.416	M00.279	M25.08	M47.16	M79.A22	M80.811K	M84.329K	M84.421K
L97.409	L98.418	M00.28	M30.0	M48.30	M79.A29	M80.811P	M84.329P	M84.421P
L97.411	L98.425	M00.29	M30.1	M48.31	M79.A3	M80.812A	M84.331K	M84.422A
L97.412	L98.426	M00.80	M30.2	M48.32	M79.A9	M80.812K	M84.331P	M84.422K
L97.413	L98.428	M00.811	M30.3	M48.33	M80.00XA	M80.812P	M84.332K	M84.422P
L97.414	L98.495	M00.812	M30.8	M48.34	M80.00XK	M80.819A	M84.332P	M84.429A
L97.415	L98.496	M00.819	M31.0	M48.35	M80.00XP	M80.819K	M84.333K	M84.429K
L97.416	L98.498	M00.821	M31.2	M48.36	M80.011A	M80.819P	M84.333P	M84.429P
L97.418	M00.00	M00.822	M31.31	M48.37	M80.011K	M80.821A	M84.334K	M84.431A
L97.419	M00.011	M00.829	M31.4	M48.38	M80.011P	M80.821K	M84.334P	M84.431K
L97.421	M00.012	M00.831	M31.7	M48.50XA	M80.012A	M80.821P	M84.339K	M84.431P
L97.422	M00.019	M00.832	M31.8	M48.51XA	M80.012K	M80.822A	M84.339P	M84.432A
L97.423	M00.021	M00.839	M31.9	M48.52XA	M80.012P	M80.822K	M84.341K	M84.432K
L97.424	M00.022	M00.841	M32.11	M48.53XA	M80.019A	M80.822P	M84.341P	M84.432P
L97.425	M00.029	M00.842	M32.12	M48.54XA	M80.019K	M80.829A	M84.342K	M84.433A
L97.426	M00.031	M00.849	M33.00	M48.55XA	M80.019P	M80.829K	M84.342P	M84.433K
L97.428	M00.032	M00.851	M33.01	M48.56XA	M80.021A	M80.829P	M84.343K	M84.433P

Appendix E: Complication and Comorbidity (CC) Code List

M84.434A	M84.478P	M84.564K	M84.652A	M86.012	M86.331	M86.649	M87.135	M87.311
M84.434K	M84.479A	M84.564P	M84.652K	M86.019	M86.332	M86.651	M87.136	M87.312
M84.434P	M84.479K	M84.569A	M84.652P	M86.021	M86.339	M86.652	M87.137	M87.319
M84.439A	M84.479P	M84.569K	M84.653A	M86.022	M86.341	M86.659	M87.138	M87.321
M84.439K	M84.48XA	M84.569P	M84.653K	M86.029	M86.342	M86.661	M87.139	M87.322
M84.439P	M84.48XK	M84.571A	M84.653P	M86.031	M86.349	M86.662	M87.141	M87.329
M84.441A	M84.48XP	M84.571K	M84.659A	M86.032	M86.351	M86.669	M87.142	M87.331
M84.441K	M84.50XA	M84.571P	M84.659K	M86.039	M86.352	M86.671	M87.143	M87.332
M84.441P	M84.50XK	M84.572A	M84.659P	M86.041	M86.359	M86.672	M87.144	M87.333
M84.442A	M84.50XP	M84.572K	M84.661A	M86.042	M86.361	M86.679	M87.145	M87.334
M84.442K	M84.511A	M84.572P	M84.661K	M86.049	M86.362	M86.68	M87.146	M87.335
M84.442P	M84.511K	M84.573A	M84.661P	M86.051	M86.369	M86.69	M87.150	M87.336
M84.443A	M84.511P	M84.573K	M84.662A	M86.052	M86.371	M86.8X0	M87.151	M87.337
M84.443K	M84.512A	M84.573P	M84.662K	M86.059	M86.372	M86.8X1	M87.152	M87.338
M84.443P	M84.512K	M84.574A	M84.662P	M86.061	M86.379	M86.8X2	M87.159	M87.339
M84.444A	M84.512P	M84.574K	M84.663A	M86.062	M86.38	M86.8X3	M87.161	M87.341
M84.444K	M84.519A	M84.574P	M84.663K	M86.069	M86.39	M86.8X4	M87.162	M87.342
M84.444P	M84.519K	M84.575A	M84.663P	M86.071	M86.40	M86.8X5	M87.163	M87.343
M84.445A	M84.519P	M84.575K	M84.664A	M86.072	M86.411	M86.8X6	M87.164	M87.344
M84.445K	M84.521A	M84.575P	M84.664K	M86.079	M86.412	M86.8X7	M87.165	M87.345
M84.445P	M84.521K	M84.576A	M84.664P	M86.08	M86.419	M86.8X8	M87.166	M87.346
M84.446A	M84.521P	M84.576K	M84.669A	M86.09	M86.421	M86.8X9	M87.171	M87.350
M84.446K	M84.522A	M84.576P	M84.669K	M86.10	M86.422	M86.9	M87.172	M87.351
M84.446P	M84.522K	M84.58XA	M84.669P	M86.111	M86.429	M87.00	M87.173	M87.352
M84.451A	M84.522P	M84.58XK	M84.671A	M86.112	M86.431	M87.011	M87.174	M87.353
M84.451K	M84.529A	M84.58XP	M84.671K	M86.119	M86.432	M87.012	M87.175	M87.361
M84.451P	M84.529K	M84.60XA	M84.671P	M86.121	M86.439	M87.019	M87.176	M87.362
M84.452A	M84.529P	M84.60XK	M84.672A	M86.122	M86.441	M87.021	M87.177	M87.363
M84.452K	M84.531A	M84.60XP	M84.672K	M86.129	M86.442	M87.022	M87.178	M87.364
M84.452P	M84.531K	M84.611A	M84.672P	M86.131	M86.449	M87.029	M87.179	M87.365
M84.453A	M84.532A	M84.611K	M84.673A	M86.132	M86.451	M87.031	M87.180	M87.366
M84.453K	M84.532K	M84.611P	M84.673K	M86.139	M86.452	M87.032	M87.188	M87.371
M84.453P	M84.532P	M84.612A	M84.673P	M86.141	M86.459	M87.033	M87.19	M87.372
M84.454A	M84.533A	M84.612K	M84.674A	M86.142	M86.461	M87.034	M87.20	M87.373
M84.454K	M84.533K	M84.612P	M84.674K	M86.149	M86.462	M87.035	M87.211	M87.374
M84.454P	M84.533P	M84.619A	M84.674P	M86.151	M86.469	M87.036	M87.212	M87.375
M84.459A	M84.534A	M84.619K	M84.675A	M86.152	M86.471	M87.037	M87.219	M87.376
M84.459K	M84.534K	M84.619P	M84.675K	M86.159	M86.472	M87.038	M87.221	M87.377
M84.459P	M84.534P	M84.621A	M84.675P	M86.161	M86.479	M87.039	M87.222	M87.378
M84.461A	M84.539A	M84.621K	M84.676A	M86.162	M86.48	M87.041	M87.229	M87.379
M84.461K	M84.539K	M84.621P	M84.676K	M86.169	M86.49	M87.042	M87.231	M87.38
M84.461P	M84.539P	M84.622A	M84.676P	M86.171	M86.50	M87.043	M87.232	M87.39
M84.462A	M84.541A	M84.622K	M84.68XA	M86.172	M86.511	M87.044	M87.233	M87.80
M84.462K	M84.541K	M84.622P	M84.68XK	M86.179	M86.512	M87.045	M87.234	M87.811
M84.462P	M84.541P	M84.629A	M84.68XP	M86.18	M86.519	M87.046	M87.235	M87.812
M84.463A	M84.542A	M84.629K	M84.750A	M86.19	M86.521	M87.050	M87.236	M87.819
M84.463K	M84.542K	M84.629P	M84.750K	M86.20	M86.522	M87.051	M87.237	M87.821
M84.463P	M84.542P	M84.631A	M84.750P	M86.211	M86.529	M87.052	M87.238	M87.822
M84.464A	M84.549A	M84.631K	M84.751A	M86.212	M86.531	M87.059	M87.239	M87.829
M84.464K	M84.549K	M84.631P	M84.751K	M86.219	M86.532	M87.061	M87.241	M87.831
M84.464P	M84.549P	M84.632A	M84.751P	M86.221	M86.539	M87.062	M87.242	M87.832
M84.469A	M84.550A	M84.632K	M84.752A	M86.222	M86.541	M87.063	M87.243	M87.833
M84.469K	M84.550K	M84.632P	M84.752K	M86.229	M86.542	M87.064	M87.244	M87.834
M84.469P	M84.550P	M84.633A	M84.752P	M86.231	M86.549	M87.065	M87.245	M87.835
M84.471A	M84.551A	M84.633K	M84.753A	M86.232	M86.551	M87.066	M87.246	M87.836
M84.471K	M84.551K	M84.633P	M84.753K	M86.239	M86.552	M87.071	M87.250	M87.837
M84.471P	M84.551P	M84.634A	M84.753P	M86.241	M86.559	M87.072	M87.251	M87.838
M84.472A	M84.552A	M84.634K	M84.754A	M86.242	M86.561	M87.073	M87.252	M87.839
M84.472K	M84.552K	M84.634P	M84.754K	M86.249	M86.562	M87.074	M87.256	M87.841
M84.472P	M84.552P	M84.639A	M84.754P	M86.251	M86.569	M87.075	M87.261	M87.842
M84.473A	M84.553A	M84.639K	M84.755A	M86.252	M86.571	M87.076	M87.262	M87.843
M84.473K	M84.553K	M84.639P	M84.755K	M86.259	M86.572	M87.077	M87.263	M87.844
M84.473P	M84.553P	M84.641A	M84.755P	M86.261	M86.579	M87.078	M87.264	M87.845
M84.474A	M84.559A	M84.641K	M84.756A	M86.262	M86.58	M87.079	M87.265	M87.849
M84.474K	M84.559K	M84.641P	M84.756K	M86.269	M86.59	M87.08	M87.266	M87.850
M84.474P	M84.559P	M84.642A	M84.756P	M86.271	M86.60	M87.09	M87.271	M87.851
M84.475A	M84.561A	M84.642K	M84.757A	M86.272	M86.611	M87.10	M87.272	M87.852
M84.475K	M84.561K	M84.642P	M84.757K	M86.279	M86.612	M87.111	M87.273	M87.859
M84.475P	M84.561P	M84.649A	M84.757P	M86.28	M86.619	M87.112	M87.274	M87.861
M84.476A	M84.562A	M84.649K	M84.758A	M86.29	M86.621	M87.119	M87.275	M87.862
M84.476K	M84.562K	M84.649P	M84.758K	M86.30	M86.622	M87.121	M87.276	M87.863
M84.476P	M84.562P	M84.650A	M84.758P	M86.311	M86.629	M87.122	M87.277	M87.864
M84.477A	M84.563A	M84.650K	M84.759A	M86.312	M86.631	M87.129	M87.278	M87.865
M84.477K	M84.563K	M84.650P	M84.759K	M86.319	M86.632	M87.131	M87.279	M87.869
M84.477P	M84.563P	M84.651A	M84.759P	M86.321	M86.639	M87.132	M87.28	M87.871
M84.478A	M84.564A	M84.651K	M86.00	M86.322	M86.641	M87.133	M87.29	M87.872
M84.478K		M84.651P	M86.011	M86.329	M86.642	M87.134	M87.30	M87.873

M87.874	N02.3	N48.30	O03.80	O22.8X1	O26.879	O36.0121	O60.10X1	O98.713
M87.875	N02.4	N48.31	O03.83	O22.8X2	O30.023	O36.0122	O60.10X2	O98.72
M87.876	N02.5	N48.32	O03.84	O22.8X3	O30.101	O36.0123	O60.10X3	O98.73
M87.877	N02.6	N48.33	O03.85	O22.8X9	O30.102	O36.0124	O60.10X4	O98.811
M87.878	N02.7	N48.39	O03.86	O22.90	O30.103	O36.0125	O60.10X5	O98.812
M87.879	N02.8	N70.01	O03.87	O23.01	O30.111	O36.0129	O60.10X9	O98.813
M87.88	N02.9	N70.02	O03.88	O23.02	O30.112	O36.0130	O60.20X0	O98.82
M87.89	N03.0	N70.03	O03.89	O23.03	O30.113	O36.0131	O60.20X1	O98.83
M87.9	N03.1	N71.0	O04.5	O23.11	O30.121	O36.0132	O60.20X2	O98.911
M90.50	N03.2	N73.0	O04.80	O23.12	O30.122	O36.0133	O60.20X3	O98.912
M90.511	N03.3	N73.4	O04.83	O23.13	O30.123	O36.0134	O60.20X4	O98.913
M90.512	N03.4	N75.1	O04.84	O23.21	O30.131	O36.0135	O60.20X5	O98.92
M90.519	N03.5	N76.81	O04.85	O23.22	O30.132	O36.0139	O60.20X9	O98.93
M90.521	N03.6	N82.0	O04.86	O23.23	O30.133	O36.0910	O63.9	O99.111
M90.522	N03.7	N82.1	O04.87	O23.31	O30.191	O36.0911	O68	O99.112
M90.529	N03.8	N82.2	O04.88	O23.32	O30.192	O36.0912	O70.20	O99.113
M90.531	N03.9	N82.3	O04.89	O23.33	O30.193	O36.0913	O70.21	O99.119
M90.532	N04.0	N82.4	O07.0	O23.41	O30.201	O36.0914	O70.22	O99.12
M90.539	N04.1	N82.5	O07.1	O23.42	O30.202	O36.0915	O70.23	O99.13
M90.541	N04.2	N82.8	O07.30	O23.43	O30.203	O36.0919	O70.3	O99.321
M90.542	N04.3	N82.9	O07.33	O23.511	O30.211	O36.0920	O70.4	O99.322
M90.549	N04.4	N83.511	O07.34	O23.512	O30.212	O36.0921	O71.2	O99.323
M90.551	N04.5	N83.512	O07.35	O23.513	O30.213	O36.0922	O71.3	O99.324
M90.552	N04.6	N83.519	O07.36	O23.521	O30.221	O36.0923	O71.4	O99.325
M90.559	N04.7	N83.521	O07.37	O23.522	O30.222	O36.0924	O71.5	O99.354
M90.561	N04.8	N83.522	O07.38	O23.523	O30.223	O36.0925	O71.6	O99.355
M90.562	N04.9	N83.529	O07.39	O23.591	O30.231	O36.0929	O71.7	O99.411
M90.569	N05.2	N83.53	O08.0	O23.592	O30.232	O36.0930	O72.0	O99.412
M90.571	N05.3	N98.0	O08.1	O23.593	O30.233	O36.0931	O72.1	O99.413
M90.572	N05.4	N98.1	O08.5	O23.91	O30.291	O36.0932	O72.2	O99.43
M90.579	N05.5	N98.2	O08.6	O23.92	O30.292	O36.0933	O75.2	O99.830
M90.58	N06.2	N98.3	O08.7	O23.93	O30.293	O36.0934	O76	O99.834
M90.59	N06.3	N98.8	O08.81	O24.011	O30.801	O36.0935	O86.11	O99.835
M96.0	N06.4	N98.9	O08.82	O24.012	O30.802	O36.0939	O86.12	P10.2
M96.621	N06.5	N99.510	O08.83	O24.013	O30.803	O36.1910	O86.13	P12.2
M96.622	N07.2	N99.511	O08.89	O24.019	O30.811	O36.1911	O86.19	P28.0
M96.629	N07.3	N99.512	O08.9	O24.02	O30.812	O36.4XX0	O86.20	P28.10
M96.631	N07.4	N99.518	O10.011	O24.03	O30.813	O36.4XX1	O86.21	P28.11
M96.632	N07.5	N99.61	O10.012	O24.111	O30.821	O36.4XX2	O86.22	P28.19
M96.639	N11.1	N99.62	O10.013	O24.112	O30.822	O36.4XX3	O86.29	P28.2
M96.65	N11.8	N99.71	O10.02	O24.113	O30.823	O36.4XX4	O86.4	P28.3
M96.661	N11.9	N99.72	O10.411	O24.119	O30.831	O36.4XX5	O87.0	P28.4
M96.662	N12	N99.820	O10.412	O24.12	O30.832	O36.4XX9	O87.2	P35.0
M96.669	N13.0	N99.821	O10.413	O24.13	O30.833	O41.01X0	O87.3	P38.1
M96.671	N13.1	N99.840	O10.43	O24.311	O30.891	O41.01X1	O87.8	P38.9
M96.672	N13.2	N99.841	O10.911	O24.312	O30.892	O41.01X2	O88.319	P39.0
M96.679	N13.30	N99.842	O10.912	O24.313	O30.893	O41.01X3	O98.011	P39.2
M96.69	N13.39	N99.843	O10.913	O24.319	O31.8X10	O41.01X4	O98.012	P39.3
M96.810	N13.4	O00.00	O10.92	O24.32	O31.8X11	O41.01X5	O98.013	P39.4
M96.811	N13.6	O00.01	O12.11	O24.33	O31.8X12	O41.01X9	O98.02	P39.8
M96.820	N13.8	O00.101	O12.12	O24.414	O31.8X13	O41.02X0	O98.03	P39.9
M96.821	N17.8	O00.102	O12.13	O24.415	O31.8X14	O41.02X1	O98.111	P52.0
M96.830	N17.9	O00.109	O12.21	O24.424	O31.8X15	O41.02X2	O98.112	P52.1
M96.831	N18.6	O00.111	O12.22	O24.425	O31.8X19	O41.02X3	O98.113	P52.3
M96.840	N20.1	O00.112	O12.23	O24.434	O31.8X20	O41.02X4	O98.12	P53
M96.841	N20.2	O00.119	O14.02	O24.435	O31.8X21	O41.02X5	O98.13	P54.4
M96.842	N25.1	O00.201	O14.03	O24.811	O31.8X22	O41.02X9	O98.211	P61.2
M96.843	N25.81	O00.202	O14.92	O24.812	O31.8X23	O41.03X0	O98.212	P61.3
M96.89	N28.0	O00.209	O14.93	O24.813	O31.8X24	O41.03X1	O98.213	P61.4
M97.01XA	N28.84	O00.211	O16.1	O24.819	O31.8X25	O41.03X2	O98.22	P61.6
M97.02XA	N28.85	O00.212	O16.2	O24.82	O31.8X29	O41.03X3	O98.23	P70.2
M97.11XA	N28.86	O00.219	O16.3	O24.83	O31.8X30	O41.03X4	O98.411	P70.8
M97.12XA	N30.40	O00.80	O20.0	O24.911	O31.8X31	O41.03X5	O98.412	P71.0
M97.21XA	N30.41	O00.81	O20.9	O24.912	O31.8X32	O41.03X9	O98.413	P71.1
M97.22XA	N32.1	O00.90	O22.20	O24.913	O31.8X33	O44.01	O98.42	P71.2
M97.31XA	N32.2	O00.91	O22.21	O24.919	O31.8X34	O44.02	O98.43	P71.3
M97.32XA	N34.0	O03.0	O22.22	O24.92	O31.8X35	O44.03	O98.511	P71.4
M97.41XA	N36.0	O03.30	O22.23	O24.93	O31.8X39	O44.21	O98.512	P71.8
M97.42XA	N39.0	O03.33	O22.30	O26.611	O33.0	O44.22	O98.513	P71.9
M97.8XXA	N41.2	O03.34	O22.40	O26.612	O36.0110	O44.23	O98.53	P72.0
M97.9XXA	N43.1	O03.35	O22.41	O26.613	O36.0111	O44.41	O98.611	P72.1
M99.10	N44.00	O03.36	O22.42	O26.62	O36.0112	O44.42	O98.612	P72.2
M99.11	N44.01	O03.37	O22.43	O26.831	O36.0113	O44.43	O98.613	P72.8
M99.18	N44.02	O03.38	O22.50	O26.832	O36.0114	O47.02	O98.62	P74.41
N02.0	N44.03	O03.39	O22.51	O26.833	O36.0115	O47.03	O98.63	P74.5
N02.1	N44.04	O03.5	O22.52	O26.872	O36.0119	O47.1	O98.711	P74.6
N02.2	N45.4	O03.7	O22.53	O26.873	O36.0120	O60.10X0	O98.712	P74.8

Appendix E: Complication and Comorbidity (CC) Code List

P76.1	Q33.4	Q85.9	S02.11AK	S02.601A	S02.82XK	S05.70XA	S11.10XA	S12.291K
P83.0	Q39.4	Q87.40	S02.11BA	S02.601B	S02.831A	S05.71XA	S11.11XA	S12.300A
P83.30	Q39.5	Q87.410	S02.11BK	S02.601K	S02.831B	S05.72XA	S11.12XA	S12.300K
P83.39	Q39.6	Q87.418	S02.11CA	S02.602A	S02.831K	S05.8X1A	S11.13XA	S12.301A
P91.60	Q39.8	Q87.42	S02.11CK	S02.602B	S02.832A	S05.8X2A	S11.14XA	S12.301K
P91.61	Q39.9	Q87.43	S02.11DA	S02.602K	S02.832B	S05.8X9A	S11.15XA	S12.330A
P91.62	Q41.0	Q87.5	S02.11DK	S02.609A	S02.832K	S05.91XA	S11.20XA	S12.330K
P93.0	Q41.1	Q93.51	S02.11EA	S02.609B	S02.839A	S05.92XA	S11.21XA	S12.331A
P93.8	Q41.2	Q93.59	S02.11EK	S02.609K	S02.839B	S06.0X0A	S11.22XA	S12.331K
P94.0	Q41.8	Q93.81	S02.11FA	S02.610A	S02.839K	S06.0X1A	S11.23XA	S12.34XA
P96.1	Q41.9	Q93.82	S02.11FK	S02.610B	S02.841A	S06.0X9A	S11.24XA	S12.34XK
P96.2	Q42.0	Q93.88	S02.11GA	S02.610K	S02.841B	S06.2X1A	S11.25XA	S12.350A
Q01.0	Q42.1	Q93.89	S02.11GK	S02.611A	S02.841K	S06.2X2A	S12.000A	S12.350K
Q01.1	Q42.2	Q93.9	S02.11HA	S02.611B	S02.842A	S06.2X3A	S12.000K	S12.351A
Q01.2	Q42.3	R04.0	S02.11HK	S02.611K	S02.842B	S06.2X4A	S12.001A	S12.351K
Q01.8	Q42.8	R04.1	S02.121A	S02.612A	S02.842K	S06.2X5A	S12.001K	S12.390A
Q01.9	Q42.9	R04.2	S02.121K	S02.612B	S02.849A	S06.2X9A	S12.01XA	S12.390K
Q04.4	Q43.1	R04.81	S02.122A	S02.612K	S02.849B	S06.301A	S12.01XK	S12.391A
Q04.5	Q43.2	R04.89	S02.122K	S02.620A	S02.849K	S06.302A	S12.02XA	S12.391K
Q04.6	Q43.3	R04.9	S02.129A	S02.620B	S02.85XA	S06.303A	S12.02XK	S12.400A
Q04.8	Q43.4	R06.3	S02.129K	S02.620K	S02.85XB	S06.304A	S12.030A	S12.400K
Q05.0	Q43.5	R09.01	S02.19XA	S02.621A	S02.85XK	S06.305A	S12.030K	S12.401A
Q05.1	Q43.6	R13.0	S02.19XK	S02.621B	S02.91XA	S06.309A	S12.031A	S12.401K
Q05.2	Q43.7	R17	S02.2XXB	S02.621K	S02.91XK	S06.371A	S12.031K	S12.430A
Q05.3	Q43.8	R18.0	S02.2XXK	S02.622A	S02.92XA	S06.372A	S12.040A	S12.430K
Q05.4	Q43.9	R18.8	S02.30XA	S02.622B	S02.92XB	S06.373A	S12.040K	S12.431A
Q07.02	Q44.0	R29.0	S02.30XB	S02.622K	S02.92XK	S06.374A	S12.041A	S12.431K
Q07.03	Q44.1	R29.1	S02.30XK	S02.630A	S04.011A	S06.375A	S12.041K	S12.44XA
Q20.5	Q44.4	R29.5	S02.31XA	S02.630B	S04.012A	S06.379A	S12.090A	S12.44XK
Q22.1	Q44.5	R39.0	S02.31XB	S02.630K	S04.019A	S06.381A	S12.090K	S12.450A
Q22.2	Q44.6	R40.3	S02.31XK	S02.631A	S04.02XA	S06.382A	S12.091A	S12.450K
Q22.3	Q44.7	R41.4	S02.32XA	S02.631B	S04.031A	S06.383A	S12.091K	S12.451A
Q24.0	Q45.0	R44.0	S02.32XB	S02.631K	S04.032A	S06.384A	S12.100A	S12.451K
Q24.1	Q45.1	R44.2	S02.32XK	S02.632A	S04.039A	S06.385A	S12.100K	S12.490A
Q24.3	Q45.2	R44.3	S02.400A	S02.632B	S04.041A	S06.389A	S12.101A	S12.490K
Q25.0	Q45.3	R45.851	S02.400B	S02.632K	S04.042A	S06.811A	S12.101K	S12.491A
Q25.1	Q61.8	R47.01	S02.400K	S02.640A	S04.049A	S06.812A	S12.110A	S12.491K
Q25.21	Q61.9	R50.2	S02.401A	S02.640B	S04.10XA	S06.813A	S12.110K	S12.500A
Q25.29	Q62.0	R50.82	S02.401B	S02.640K	S04.11XA	S06.814A	S12.111A	S12.500K
Q25.3	Q62.10	R56.00	S02.401K	S02.641A	S04.12XA	S06.815A	S12.111K	S12.501A
Q25.40	Q62.11	R56.01	S02.402A	S02.641B	S04.20XA	S06.819A	S12.112A	S12.501K
Q25.41	Q62.12	R56.1	S02.402B	S02.641K	S04.21XA	S06.821A	S12.112K	S12.530A
Q25.42	Q62.2	R57.9	S02.402K	S02.642A	S04.22XA	S06.822A	S12.120A	S12.530K
Q25.43	Q62.31	R58	S02.40AA	S02.642B	S04.30XA	S06.823A	S12.120K	S12.531A
Q25.44	Q62.32	R60.1	S02.40AB	S02.642K	S04.31XA	S06.824A	S12.121A	S12.531K
Q25.45	Q62.39	R62.7	S02.40AK	S02.650A	S04.32XA	S06.825A	S12.121K	S12.54XA
Q25.46	Q64.10	R63.3	S02.40BA	S02.650B	S04.40XA	S06.829A	S12.130A	S12.54XK
Q25.47	Q64.11	R64	S02.40BB	S02.650K	S04.41XA	S06.891A	S12.130K	S12.550A
Q25.48	Q64.12	R65.10	S02.40BK	S02.651A	S04.42XA	S06.892A	S12.131A	S12.550K
Q25.49	Q64.19	R65.11	S02.40CA	S02.651B	S04.50XA	S06.893A	S12.131K	S12.551A
Q25.8	Q64.2	R71.0	S02.40CB	S02.651K	S04.51XA	S06.894A	S12.14XA	S12.551K
Q25.9	Q64.31	R82.0	S02.40CK	S02.652A	S04.52XA	S06.895A	S12.14XK	S12.590A
Q26.0	Q64.32	R82.1	S02.40DA	S02.652B	S04.60XA	S06.899A	S12.150A	S12.590K
Q26.1	Q64.33	S01.101A	S02.40DB	S02.652K	S04.61XA	S06.9X1A	S12.150K	S12.591A
Q26.2	Q64.39	S01.102A	S02.40DK	S02.66XA	S04.62XA	S06.9X2A	S12.151A	S12.591K
Q26.3	Q67.5	S01.109A	S02.40EA	S02.66XB	S04.70XA	S06.9X3A	S12.151K	S12.600A
Q26.4	Q67.8	S02.0XXA	S02.40EB	S02.66XK	S04.71XA	S06.9X4A	S12.190A	S12.600K
Q26.8	Q68.1	S02.0XXK	S02.40EK	S02.670A	S04.72XA	S06.9X5A	S12.190K	S12.601A
Q26.9	Q74.3	S02.101A	S02.40FA	S02.670B	S04.811A	S06.9X9A	S12.191A	S12.601K
Q27.30	Q76.3	S02.101K	S02.40FB	S02.670K	S04.812A	S07.0XXA	S12.191K	S12.630A
Q27.4	Q76.425	S02.102A	S02.40FK	S02.671A	S04.819A	S07.1XXA	S12.200A	S12.630K
Q28.0	Q76.426	S02.102K	S02.411A	S02.671B	S04.891A	S07.8XXA	S12.200K	S12.631A
Q28.1	Q76.427	S02.109A	S02.411B	S02.671K	S04.892A	S07.9XXA	S12.201A	S12.631K
Q28.8	Q76.428	S02.109K	S02.411K	S02.672A	S04.899A	S09.0XXA	S12.201K	S12.64XA
Q28.9	Q76.429	S02.110A	S02.412A	S02.672B	S04.9XXA	S09.20XA	S12.230A	S12.64XK
Q31.1	Q76.6	S02.110K	S02.412B	S02.672K	S05.20XA	S09.21XA	S12.230K	S12.650A
Q31.2	Q76.7	S02.111A	S02.412K	S02.69XA	S05.21XA	S09.22XA	S12.231A	S12.650K
Q31.3	Q76.8	S02.111K	S02.413A	S02.69XB	S05.22XA	S09.301A	S12.231K	S12.651A
Q31.5	Q76.9	S02.112A	S02.413B	S02.69XK	S05.30XA	S09.302A	S12.24XA	S12.651K
Q31.8	Q77.2	S02.112K	S02.413K	S02.80XA	S05.31XA	S09.309A	S12.24XK	S12.690A
Q31.9	Q78.0	S02.113A	S02.42XA	S02.80XB	S05.32XA	S09.311A	S12.250A	S12.690K
Q32.0	Q78.2	S02.113K	S02.42XB	S02.80XK	S05.40XA	S09.312A	S12.250K	S12.691A
Q32.1	Q79.4	S02.118A	S02.42XK	S02.81XA	S05.41XA	S09.313A	S12.251A	S12.691K
Q32.2	Q79.51	S02.118K	S02.5XXK	S02.81XB	S05.42XA	S09.319A	S12.251K	S12.9XXA
Q32.3	Q79.59	S02.119A	S02.600A	S02.81XK	S05.50XA	S09.391A	S12.290A	S13.0XXA
Q32.4	Q85.1	S02.119K	S02.600B	S02.82XA	S05.51XA	S09.392A	S12.290K	S13.100A
Q33.0	Q85.8	S02.11AA	S02.600K	S02.82XB	S05.52XA	S09.399A	S12.291A	S13.101A

S13.110A	S21.121A	S22.059K	S25.99XA	S32.032A	S32.314K	S32.612K	S36.269A	S37.031A
S13.111A	S21.122A	S22.060A	S26.00XA	S32.032K	S32.315A	S32.613A	S36.290A	S37.032A
S13.120A	S21.129A	S22.060K	S26.01XA	S32.038A	S32.315K	S32.613K	S36.291A	S37.039A
S13.121A	S21.131A	S22.061A	S26.09XA	S32.038K	S32.316A	S32.614A	S36.292A	S37.041A
S13.130A	S21.132A	S22.061K	S26.10XA	S32.039A	S32.316K	S32.614K	S36.299A	S37.042A
S13.131A	S21.139A	S22.062A	S26.11XA	S32.039K	S32.391A	S32.615A	S36.30XA	S37.049A
S13.140A	S21.141A	S22.062K	S26.19XA	S32.040A	S32.391K	S32.615K	S36.32XA	S37.051A
S13.141A	S21.142A	S22.068A	S26.90XA	S32.040K	S32.392A	S32.616A	S36.33XA	S37.052A
S13.150A	S21.149A	S22.068K	S26.91XA	S32.041A	S32.392K	S32.616K	S36.39XA	S37.059A
S13.151A	S21.151A	S22.069A	S26.99XA	S32.041K	S32.399A	S32.691A	S36.400A	S37.10XA
S13.160A	S21.152A	S22.069K	S27.0XXA	S32.042A	S32.399K	S32.691K	S36.408A	S37.12XA
S13.161A	S21.159A	S22.070A	S27.301A	S32.042K	S32.401A	S32.692A	S36.409A	S37.13XA
S13.170A	S21.90XA	S22.070K	S27.302A	S32.048A	S32.401K	S32.692K	S36.410A	S37.19XA
S13.171A	S21.91XA	S22.071A	S27.309A	S32.048K	S32.402A	S32.699A	S36.418A	S37.20XA
S13.180A	S21.92XA	S22.071K	S27.311A	S32.049A	S32.402K	S32.699K	S36.419A	S37.22XA
S13.181A	S21.93XA	S22.072A	S27.312A	S32.049K	S32.409A	S32.810A	S36.420A	S37.23XA
S13.20XA	S21.94XA	S22.072K	S27.319A	S32.050A	S32.409K	S32.810K	S36.428A	S37.29XA
S13.29XA	S21.95XA	S22.078A	S27.321A	S32.050K	S32.411K	S32.811A	S36.429A	S37.30XA
S15.001A	S22.000A	S22.078K	S27.322A	S32.051A	S32.412K	S32.811K	S36.430A	S37.32XA
S15.002A	S22.000K	S22.079A	S27.329A	S32.051K	S32.413K	S32.82XA	S36.438A	S37.33XA
S15.009A	S22.001A	S22.079K	S27.391A	S32.052A	S32.414K	S32.82XK	S36.439A	S37.39XA
S15.011A	S22.001K	S22.080A	S27.392A	S32.052K	S32.415K	S32.89XA	S36.490A	S37.60XA
S15.012A	S22.002A	S22.080K	S27.399A	S32.058A	S32.416K	S32.89XK	S36.498A	S37.62XA
S15.019A	S22.002K	S22.081A	S27.50XA	S32.058K	S32.421K	S32.9XXA	S36.499A	S37.63XA
S15.021A	S22.008A	S22.081K	S27.51XA	S32.059A	S32.422K	S32.9XXK	S36.500A	S37.69XA
S15.022A	S22.008K	S22.082A	S27.52XA	S32.059K	S32.423K	S35.531A	S36.501A	S37.812A
S15.029A	S22.009A	S22.082K	S27.53XA	S32.10XA	S32.424K	S35.532A	S36.502A	S37.813A
S15.091A	S22.009K	S22.088A	S27.59XA	S32.10XK	S32.425K	S35.533A	S36.503A	S37.818A
S15.092A	S22.010A	S22.088K	S27.60XA	S32.110A	S32.426K	S35.534A	S36.508A	S37.819A
S15.099A	S22.010K	S22.089A	S27.63XA	S32.110K	S32.431K	S35.535A	S36.509A	S37.892A
S15.101A	S22.011A	S22.089K	S27.69XA	S32.111A	S32.432K	S35.536A	S36.510A	S37.893A
S15.102A	S22.011K	S22.20XK	S27.802A	S32.111K	S32.433K	S35.8X1A	S36.511A	S37.898A
S15.109A	S22.012A	S22.21XA	S27.803A	S32.112A	S32.434K	S35.8X8A	S36.512A	S37.899A
S15.111A	S22.012K	S22.21XK	S27.808A	S32.112K	S32.435K	S35.8X9A	S36.513A	S37.90XA
S15.112A	S22.018A	S22.22XA	S27.809A	S32.119A	S32.436K	S35.90XA	S36.518A	S37.92XA
S15.119A	S22.018K	S22.22XK	S27.892A	S32.119K	S32.441K	S35.91XA	S36.519A	S37.93XA
S15.121A	S22.019A	S22.23XA	S27.893A	S32.120A	S32.442K	S35.99XA	S36.520A	S37.99XA
S15.122A	S22.019K	S22.23XK	S27.898A	S32.120K	S32.443K	S36.00XA	S36.521A	S42.001B
S15.129A	S22.020A	S22.24XA	S27.899A	S32.121A	S32.444K	S36.020A	S36.522A	S42.001K
S15.191A	S22.020K	S22.24XK	S27.9XXA	S32.121K	S32.445K	S36.021A	S36.523A	S42.001P
S15.192A	S22.021A	S22.31XA	S28.1XXA	S32.122A	S32.446K	S36.029A	S36.528A	S42.002B
S15.199A	S22.021K	S22.31XK	S29.021A	S32.122K	S32.451K	S36.030A	S36.529A	S42.002K
S15.201A	S22.022A	S22.32XA	S29.029A	S32.129A	S32.452K	S36.039A	S36.530A	S42.002P
S15.202A	S22.022K	S22.32XK	S32.000A	S32.129K	S32.453K	S36.09XA	S36.531A	S42.009B
S15.209A	S22.028A	S22.39XA	S32.000K	S32.130A	S32.454K	S36.112A	S36.532A	S42.009K
S15.211A	S22.028K	S22.39XK	S32.001A	S32.130K	S32.455K	S36.113A	S36.533A	S42.009P
S15.212A	S22.029A	S22.41XA	S32.001K	S32.131A	S32.456K	S36.114A	S36.538A	S42.011B
S15.219A	S22.029K	S22.41XK	S32.002A	S32.131K	S32.461K	S36.118A	S36.539A	S42.011K
S15.221A	S22.030A	S22.42XA	S32.002K	S32.132A	S32.462K	S36.119A	S36.590A	S42.011P
S15.222A	S22.030K	S22.42XK	S32.008A	S32.132K	S32.463K	S36.122A	S36.591A	S42.012B
S15.229A	S22.031A	S22.43XA	S32.008K	S32.139A	S32.464K	S36.123A	S36.592A	S42.012K
S15.291A	S22.031K	S22.43XK	S32.009A	S32.139K	S32.465K	S36.128A	S36.593A	S42.012P
S15.292A	S22.032A	S22.49XA	S32.009K	S32.14XA	S32.466K	S36.129A	S36.598A	S42.013B
S15.299A	S22.032K	S22.49XK	S32.010A	S32.14XK	S32.471K	S36.13XA	S36.599A	S42.013K
S15.301A	S22.038A	S22.5XXK	S32.010K	S32.15XA	S32.472K	S36.200A	S36.60XA	S42.013P
S15.302A	S22.038K	S22.9XXA	S32.011A	S32.15XK	S32.473K	S36.201A	S36.61XA	S42.014B
S15.309A	S22.039A	S22.9XXK	S32.011K	S32.16XA	S32.474K	S36.202A	S36.62XA	S42.014K
S15.311A	S22.039K	S25.501A	S32.012A	S32.16XK	S32.475K	S36.209A	S36.63XA	S42.014P
S15.312A	S22.040A	S25.502A	S32.012K	S32.17XA	S32.476K	S36.220A	S36.69XA	S42.015B
S15.319A	S22.040K	S25.509A	S32.018A	S32.17XK	S32.481K	S36.221A	S36.81XA	S42.015K
S15.321A	S22.041A	S25.511A	S32.018K	S32.19XA	S32.482K	S36.222A	S36.892A	S42.015P
S15.322A	S22.041K	S25.512A	S32.019A	S32.19XK	S32.483K	S36.229A	S36.893A	S42.016B
S15.329A	S22.042A	S25.519A	S32.019K	S32.2XXA	S32.484K	S36.230A	S36.898A	S42.016K
S15.391A	S22.042K	S25.591A	S32.020A	S32.2XXK	S32.485K	S36.231A	S36.899A	S42.016P
S15.392A	S22.048A	S25.592A	S32.020K	S32.301A	S32.486K	S36.232A	S36.90XA	S42.017B
S15.399A	S22.048K	S25.599A	S32.021A	S32.301K	S32.491K	S36.239A	S36.92XA	S42.017K
S15.8XXA	S22.049A	S25.801A	S32.021K	S32.302A	S32.492K	S36.240A	S36.93XA	S42.017P
S15.9XXA	S22.049K	S25.802A	S32.022A	S32.302K	S32.499K	S36.241A	S36.99XA	S42.018B
S17.0XXA	S22.050A	S25.809A	S32.022K	S32.309A	S32.601A	S36.242A	S37.001A	S42.018K
S17.8XXA	S22.050K	S25.811A	S32.028A	S32.309K	S32.601K	S36.249A	S37.002A	S42.018P
S17.9XXA	S22.051A	S25.812A	S32.028K	S32.311A	S32.602A	S36.250A	S37.009A	S42.019B
S21.101A	S22.051K	S25.819A	S32.029A	S32.311K	S32.602K	S36.251A	S37.011A	S42.019K
S21.102A	S22.052A	S25.891A	S32.029K	S32.312A	S32.609A	S36.252A	S37.012A	S42.019P
S21.109A	S22.052K	S25.892A	S32.030A	S32.312K	S32.609K	S36.259A	S37.019A	S42.021B
S21.111A	S22.058A	S25.899A	S32.030K	S32.313A	S32.611A	S36.260A	S37.021A	S42.021K
S21.112A	S22.058K	S25.90XA	S32.031A	S32.313K	S32.611K	S36.261A	S37.022A	S42.021P
S21.119A	S22.059A	S25.91XA	S32.031K	S32.314A	S32.612A	S36.262A	S37.029A	S42.022B

Appendix E: Complication and Comorbidity (CC) Code List

S42.022K	S42.131B	S42.212P	S42.264K	S42.333A	S42.401P	S42.446K	S42.492A	S45.899A
S42.022P	S42.131K	S42.213A	S42.264P	S42.333K	S42.402A	S42.446P	S42.492K	S45.901A
S42.023B	S42.131P	S42.213K	S42.265K	S42.333P	S42.402K	S42.447A	S42.492P	S45.902A
S42.023K	S42.132B	S42.213P	S42.265P	S42.334A	S42.402P	S42.447K	S42.493A	S45.909A
S42.023P	S42.132K	S42.214A	S42.266A	S42.334K	S42.409A	S42.447P	S42.493K	S45.911A
S42.024B	S42.132P	S42.214K	S42.266K	S42.334P	S42.409K	S42.448A	S42.493P	S45.912A
S42.024K	S42.133B	S42.214P	S42.266P	S42.335A	S42.409P	S42.448K	S42.494A	S45.919A
S42.024P	S42.133K	S42.215A	S42.271A	S42.335K	S42.411A	S42.448P	S42.494K	S45.991A
S42.025B	S42.133P	S42.215K	S42.271K	S42.335P	S42.411K	S42.449A	S42.494P	S45.992A
S42.025K	S42.134B	S42.215P	S42.271P	S42.336A	S42.411P	S42.449K	S42.495A	S45.999A
S42.025P	S42.134K	S42.216A	S42.272A	S42.336K	S42.412A	S42.449P	S42.495K	S46.021A
S42.026B	S42.134P	S42.216K	S42.272K	S42.336P	S42.412K	S42.451A	S42.495P	S46.022A
S42.026K	S42.135B	S42.216P	S42.272P	S42.341A	S42.412P	S42.451K	S42.496A	S46.029A
S42.026P	S42.135K	S42.221A	S42.279A	S42.341K	S42.413A	S42.451P	S42.496K	S46.121A
S42.031B	S42.135P	S42.221K	S42.279K	S42.341P	S42.413K	S42.452A	S42.496P	S46.122A
S42.031K	S42.136B	S42.221P	S42.279P	S42.342A	S42.413P	S42.452K	S42.90XA	S46.129A
S42.031P	S42.136K	S42.222A	S42.291A	S42.342K	S42.414A	S42.452P	S42.90XK	S46.221A
S42.032B	S42.136P	S42.222K	S42.291K	S42.342P	S42.414K	S42.453A	S42.90XP	S46.222A
S42.032K	S42.141B	S42.222P	S42.291P	S42.343A	S42.414P	S42.453K	S42.91XA	S46.229A
S42.032P	S42.141K	S42.223A	S42.292A	S42.343K	S42.415A	S42.453P	S42.91XK	S46.321A
S42.033B	S42.141P	S42.223K	S42.292K	S42.343P	S42.415K	S42.454A	S42.91XP	S46.322A
S42.033K	S42.142B	S42.223P	S42.292P	S42.344A	S42.415P	S42.454K	S42.92XA	S46.329A
S42.033P	S42.142K	S42.224A	S42.293A	S42.344K	S42.416A	S42.454P	S42.92XK	S46.821A
S42.034B	S42.142P	S42.224K	S42.293K	S42.344P	S42.416K	S42.455A	S42.92XP	S46.822A
S42.034K	S42.143B	S42.224P	S42.293P	S42.345A	S42.416P	S42.455K	S43.201A	S46.829A
S42.034P	S42.143K	S42.225A	S42.294A	S42.345K	S42.421A	S42.455P	S43.202A	S46.921A
S42.035B	S42.143P	S42.225K	S42.294K	S42.345P	S42.421K	S42.456A	S43.203A	S46.922A
S42.035K	S42.144B	S42.225P	S42.294P	S42.346A	S42.421P	S42.456K	S43.204A	S46.929A
S42.035P	S42.144K	S42.226A	S42.295A	S42.346K	S42.422A	S42.456P	S43.205A	S48.011A
S42.036B	S42.144P	S42.226K	S42.295K	S42.346P	S42.422K	S42.461A	S43.206A	S48.012A
S42.036K	S42.145B	S42.226P	S42.295P	S42.351A	S42.422P	S42.461K	S43.211A	S48.019A
S42.036P	S42.145K	S42.231A	S42.296A	S42.351K	S42.423A	S42.461P	S43.212A	S48.021A
S42.101B	S42.145P	S42.231K	S42.296K	S42.351P	S42.423K	S42.462A	S43.213A	S48.022A
S42.101K	S42.146B	S42.231P	S42.296P	S42.352A	S42.423P	S42.462K	S43.214A	S48.029A
S42.101P	S42.146K	S42.232A	S42.301A	S42.352K	S42.424A	S42.462P	S43.215A	S48.111A
S42.102B	S42.146P	S42.232K	S42.301K	S42.352P	S42.424K	S42.463A	S43.216A	S48.112A
S42.102K	S42.151B	S42.232P	S42.301P	S42.353A	S42.424P	S42.463K	S43.221A	S48.119A
S42.102P	S42.151K	S42.239A	S42.302A	S42.353K	S42.425A	S42.463P	S43.222A	S48.121A
S42.109B	S42.151P	S42.239K	S42.302K	S42.353P	S42.425K	S42.464A	S43.223A	S48.122A
S42.109K	S42.152B	S42.239P	S42.302P	S42.354A	S42.425P	S42.464K	S43.224A	S48.129A
S42.109P	S42.152K	S42.241A	S42.309A	S42.354K	S42.426A	S42.464P	S43.225A	S48.911A
S42.111B	S42.152P	S42.241K	S42.309K	S42.354P	S42.426K	S42.465A	S43.226A	S48.912A
S42.111K	S42.153B	S42.241P	S42.309P	S42.355A	S42.426P	S42.465K	S45.101A	S48.919A
S42.111P	S42.153K	S42.242A	S42.311A	S42.355K	S42.431A	S42.465P	S45.102A	S48.921A
S42.112B	S42.153P	S42.242K	S42.311K	S42.355P	S42.431K	S42.466A	S45.109A	S48.922A
S42.112K	S42.154B	S42.242P	S42.311P	S42.356A	S42.431P	S42.466K	S45.111A	S48.929A
S42.112P	S42.154K	S42.249A	S42.312A	S42.356K	S42.432A	S42.466P	S45.112A	S49.001A
S42.113B	S42.154P	S42.249K	S42.312K	S42.356P	S42.432K	S42.471A	S45.119A	S49.001K
S42.113K	S42.155B	S42.249P	S42.312P	S42.361A	S42.432P	S42.471K	S45.191A	S49.001P
S42.113P	S42.155K	S42.251A	S42.319A	S42.361K	S42.433A	S42.471P	S45.192A	S49.002A
S42.114B	S42.155P	S42.251K	S42.319K	S42.361P	S42.433K	S42.472A	S45.199A	S49.002K
S42.114K	S42.156B	S42.251P	S42.319P	S42.362A	S42.433P	S42.472K	S45.201A	S49.002P
S42.114P	S42.156K	S42.252A	S42.321A	S42.362K	S42.434A	S42.472P	S45.202A	S49.009A
S42.115B	S42.156P	S42.252K	S42.321K	S42.362P	S42.434K	S42.473A	S45.209A	S49.009K
S42.115K	S42.191B	S42.252P	S42.321P	S42.363A	S42.434P	S42.473K	S45.211A	S49.009P
S42.115P	S42.191K	S42.253A	S42.322A	S42.363K	S42.435A	S42.473P	S45.212A	S49.011A
S42.116B	S42.191P	S42.253K	S42.322K	S42.363P	S42.435K	S42.474A	S45.219A	S49.011K
S42.116K	S42.192B	S42.253P	S42.322P	S42.364A	S42.435P	S42.474K	S45.291A	S49.011P
S42.116P	S42.192K	S42.254A	S42.323A	S42.364K	S42.436A	S42.474P	S45.292A	S49.012A
S42.121B	S42.192P	S42.254K	S42.323K	S42.364P	S42.436K	S42.475A	S45.299A	S49.012K
S42.121K	S42.199B	S42.254P	S42.323P	S42.365A	S42.436P	S42.475K	S45.301A	S49.012P
S42.121P	S42.199K	S42.255A	S42.324A	S42.365K	S42.441A	S42.475P	S45.302A	S49.019A
S42.122B	S42.199P	S42.255K	S42.324K	S42.365P	S42.441K	S42.476A	S45.309A	S49.019K
S42.122K	S42.201A	S42.255P	S42.324P	S42.366A	S42.441P	S42.476K	S45.311A	S49.019P
S42.122P	S42.201K	S42.256A	S42.325A	S42.366K	S42.442A	S42.476P	S45.312A	S49.021A
S42.123B	S42.201P	S42.256K	S42.325K	S42.366P	S42.442K	S42.481A	S45.319A	S49.021K
S42.123K	S42.202A	S42.256P	S42.325P	S42.391A	S42.442P	S42.481K	S45.391A	S49.021P
S42.123P	S42.202K	S42.261A	S42.326A	S42.391K	S42.443A	S42.481P	S45.392A	S49.022A
S42.124B	S42.202P	S42.261K	S42.326K	S42.391P	S42.443K	S42.482A	S45.399A	S49.022K
S42.124K	S42.209A	S42.261P	S42.326P	S42.392A	S42.443P	S42.482K	S45.801A	S49.022P
S42.124P	S42.209K	S42.262A	S42.331A	S42.392K	S42.444A	S42.482P	S45.802A	S49.029A
S42.125B	S42.209P	S42.262K	S42.331K	S42.392P	S42.444K	S42.489A	S45.809A	S49.029K
S42.125K	S42.211A	S42.262P	S42.331P	S42.399A	S42.444P	S42.489K	S45.811A	S49.029P
S42.125P	S42.211K	S42.263A	S42.332A	S42.399K	S42.445A	S42.489P	S45.812A	S49.031A
S42.126B	S42.211P	S42.263K	S42.332K	S42.399P	S42.445K	S42.491A	S45.819A	S49.031K
S42.126K	S42.212A	S42.263P	S42.332K	S42.401A	S42.445P	S42.491K	S45.891A	S49.031P
S42.126P	S42.212K	S42.264A	S42.332P	S42.401K	S42.446A	S42.491P	S45.892A	S49.032A

S49.032K	S52.001K	S52.033N	S52.101M	S52.133P	S52.222K	S52.241K	S52.256K	S52.282P
S49.032P	S52.001M	S52.033P	S52.101N	S52.133Q	S52.222M	S52.241M	S52.256M	S52.282Q
S49.039A	S52.001N	S52.033Q	S52.101P	S52.133R	S52.222N	S52.241N	S52.256N	S52.282R
S49.039K	S52.001P	S52.033R	S52.101Q	S52.134K	S52.222P	S52.241P	S52.256P	S52.283A
S49.039P	S52.001Q	S52.034K	S52.101R	S52.134M	S52.222Q	S52.241Q	S52.256Q	S52.283K
S49.041A	S52.001R	S52.034M	S52.102K	S52.134N	S52.222R	S52.241R	S52.256R	S52.283M
S49.041K	S52.002K	S52.034N	S52.102M	S52.134P	S52.223A	S52.242A	S52.261A	S52.283N
S49.041P	S52.002M	S52.034P	S52.102N	S52.134Q	S52.223K	S52.242K	S52.261K	S52.283P
S49.042A	S52.002N	S52.034Q	S52.102P	S52.134R	S52.223N	S52.242M	S52.261M	S52.283Q
S49.042K	S52.002P	S52.034R	S52.102Q	S52.135K	S52.223P	S52.242N	S52.261N	S52.283R
S49.042P	S52.002Q	S52.035K	S52.102R	S52.135M	S52.223Q	S52.242P	S52.261P	S52.291A
S49.049A	S52.002R	S52.035M	S52.109K	S52.135N	S52.223R	S52.242Q	S52.261Q	S52.291K
S49.049K	S52.009K	S52.035N	S52.109M	S52.135P	S52.224A	S52.242R	S52.261R	S52.291M
S49.049P	S52.009M	S52.035P	S52.109N	S52.135Q	S52.224K	S52.243A	S52.262A	S52.291N
S49.091A	S52.009N	S52.035Q	S52.109P	S52.135R	S52.224N	S52.243K	S52.262K	S52.291P
S49.091K	S52.009P	S52.035R	S52.109Q	S52.136K	S52.224P	S52.243M	S52.262M	S52.291Q
S49.091P	S52.009Q	S52.036K	S52.109R	S52.136M	S52.224Q	S52.243N	S52.262N	S52.291R
S49.092A	S52.009R	S52.036M	S52.111A	S52.136N	S52.224R	S52.243P	S52.262P	S52.292A
S49.092K	S52.011A	S52.036N	S52.111K	S52.136P	S52.225A	S52.243Q	S52.262Q	S52.292K
S49.092P	S52.011K	S52.036P	S52.111P	S52.136Q	S52.225K	S52.243R	S52.262R	S52.292M
S49.099A	S52.011P	S52.036Q	S52.112A	S52.136R	S52.225M	S52.244A	S52.263A	S52.292N
S49.099K	S52.012A	S52.036R	S52.112K	S52.181K	S52.225N	S52.244K	S52.263K	S52.292P
S49.099P	S52.012K	S52.041K	S52.112P	S52.181M	S52.225P	S52.244M	S52.263M	S52.292Q
S49.101A	S52.012P	S52.041M	S52.119A	S52.181N	S52.225Q	S52.244N	S52.263N	S52.292R
S49.101K	S52.019A	S52.041N	S52.119K	S52.181P	S52.225R	S52.244P	S52.263P	S52.299A
S49.101P	S52.019K	S52.041P	S52.119P	S52.181Q	S52.226A	S52.244Q	S52.263Q	S52.299K
S49.102A	S52.019P	S52.041Q	S52.121K	S52.181R	S52.226K	S52.244R	S52.263R	S52.299M
S49.102K	S52.021K	S52.041R	S52.121M	S52.182K	S52.226M	S52.245A	S52.264A	S52.299N
S49.102P	S52.021M	S52.042K	S52.121N	S52.182M	S52.226N	S52.245K	S52.264K	S52.299P
S49.109A	S52.021N	S52.042N	S52.121P	S52.182N	S52.226P	S52.245M	S52.264M	S52.299Q
S49.109K	S52.021P	S52.042P	S52.121R	S52.182P	S52.226Q	S52.245N	S52.264N	S52.299R
S49.109P	S52.021Q	S52.042Q	S52.122K	S52.182Q	S52.226R	S52.245P	S52.264P	S52.301A
S49.111A	S52.021R	S52.042R	S52.122M	S52.182R	S52.231A	S52.245Q	S52.264Q	S52.301K
S49.111K	S52.022K	S52.043K	S52.122N	S52.189K	S52.231K	S52.245R	S52.264R	S52.301M
S49.111P	S52.022M	S52.043M	S52.122P	S52.189M	S52.231M	S52.246A	S52.265A	S52.301N
S49.112A	S52.022N	S52.043N	S52.122Q	S52.189N	S52.231N	S52.246K	S52.265K	S52.301P
S49.112K	S52.022P	S52.043P	S52.122R	S52.189P	S52.231P	S52.246M	S52.265M	S52.301Q
S49.112P	S52.022Q	S52.043Q	S52.123K	S52.189Q	S52.231Q	S52.246P	S52.265P	S52.301R
S49.119A	S52.022R	S52.043R	S52.123M	S52.189R	S52.231R	S52.246Q	S52.265Q	S52.302A
S49.119K	S52.023K	S52.044K	S52.123N	S52.201A	S52.232A	S52.246R	S52.265R	S52.302K
S49.119P	S52.023M	S52.044M	S52.123P	S52.201K	S52.232K	S52.251A	S52.266A	S52.302M
S49.121A	S52.023N	S52.044N	S52.123Q	S52.201M	S52.232K	S52.251K	S52.266K	S52.302N
S49.121K	S52.023P	S52.044P	S52.123R	S52.201N	S52.232M	S52.251M	S52.266M	S52.302P
S49.121P	S52.023Q	S52.044Q	S52.124K	S52.201P	S52.232N	S52.251N	S52.266N	S52.302Q
S49.122A	S52.023R	S52.044R	S52.124M	S52.201Q	S52.232P	S52.251P	S52.266P	S52.302R
S49.122K	S52.024K	S52.045K	S52.124N	S52.201R	S52.232Q	S52.251Q	S52.266Q	S52.309A
S49.122P	S52.024M	S52.045M	S52.124P	S52.202A	S52.232R	S52.251R	S52.266R	S52.309K
S49.129A	S52.024N	S52.045N	S52.124Q	S52.202K	S52.233A	S52.252A	S52.271K	S52.309M
S49.129K	S52.024P	S52.045P	S52.124R	S52.202M	S52.233K	S52.252K	S52.271M	S52.309N
S49.129P	S52.024Q	S52.045Q	S52.125K	S52.202N	S52.233M	S52.252M	S52.271N	S52.309P
S49.131A	S52.024R	S52.045R	S52.125M	S52.202P	S52.233N	S52.252N	S52.271P	S52.309Q
S49.131K	S52.025K	S52.046K	S52.125N	S52.202Q	S52.233P	S52.252P	S52.271Q	S52.309R
S49.131P	S52.025M	S52.046M	S52.125P	S52.202R	S52.233Q	S52.252Q	S52.271R	S52.311A
S49.132A	S52.025N	S52.046N	S52.125Q	S52.209A	S52.233R	S52.252R	S52.272K	S52.311K
S49.132K	S52.025P	S52.046P	S52.125R	S52.209K	S52.234A	S52.253A	S52.272M	S52.311P
S49.132P	S52.025Q	S52.046Q	S52.126K	S52.209M	S52.234K	S52.253K	S52.272N	S52.312A
S49.139A	S52.025R	S52.046R	S52.126M	S52.209N	S52.234M	S52.253M	S52.272P	S52.312K
S49.139K	S52.026K	S52.091K	S52.126N	S52.209P	S52.234N	S52.253N	S52.272Q	S52.312P
S49.139P	S52.026M	S52.091M	S52.126P	S52.209Q	S52.234P	S52.253P	S52.272R	S52.319A
S49.141A	S52.026N	S52.091N	S52.126Q	S52.209R	S52.234Q	S52.253Q	S52.279K	S52.319K
S49.141K	S52.026P	S52.091P	S52.126R	S52.211A	S52.234R	S52.253R	S52.279M	S52.319P
S49.141P	S52.026Q	S52.091Q	S52.131K	S52.211K	S52.235A	S52.254A	S52.279N	S52.321A
S49.142A	S52.026R	S52.091R	S52.131M	S52.211P	S52.235K	S52.254K	S52.279P	S52.321K
S49.142K	S52.031K	S52.091R	S52.131N	S52.212A	S52.235M	S52.254M	S52.279Q	S52.321M
S49.142P	S52.031M	S52.092K	S52.131P	S52.212K	S52.235N	S52.254N	S52.279R	S52.321N
S49.149A	S52.031N	S52.092M	S52.131Q	S52.212P	S52.235P	S52.254P	S52.281A	S52.321Q
S49.149K	S52.031P	S52.092N	S52.131R	S52.219A	S52.235Q	S52.254Q	S52.281K	S52.321R
S49.149P	S52.031Q	S52.092P	S52.132K	S52.219K	S52.235R	S52.254R	S52.281M	S52.322A
S49.191A	S52.031R	S52.092Q	S52.132M	S52.219P	S52.236A	S52.255A	S52.281N	S52.322K
S49.191K	S52.032K	S52.092R	S52.132N	S52.221A	S52.236K	S52.255K	S52.281P	S52.322M
S49.191P	S52.032M	S52.099K	S52.132P	S52.221K	S52.236M	S52.255M	S52.281Q	S52.322N
S49.192A	S52.032N	S52.099N	S52.132Q	S52.221M	S52.236N	S52.255N	S52.281R	S52.322P
S49.192K	S52.032P	S52.099P	S52.132R	S52.221N	S52.236P	S52.255P	S52.282A	S52.322Q
S49.192P	S52.032Q	S52.099Q	S52.133K	S52.221P	S52.236Q	S52.255Q	S52.282K	S52.322R
S49.199A	S52.032R	S52.099R	S52.133M	S52.221Q	S52.236R	S52.255R	S52.282M	S52.323A
S49.199K	S52.033K	S52.101K	S52.133N	S52.221R	S52.241A	S52.256A	S52.282N	S52.323K
S49.199P	S52.033M							

S52.323M	S52.342M	S52.361M	S52.389M	S52.515M	S52.559A	S52.602A	S52.692Q	S56.029A
S52.323N	S52.342N	S52.361N	S52.389N	S52.515N	S52.559K	S52.602K	S52.692R	S56.121A
S52.323P	S52.342P	S52.361P	S52.389P	S52.515P	S52.559M	S52.602M	S52.699A	S56.122A
S52.323Q	S52.342Q	S52.361Q	S52.389Q	S52.515Q	S52.559N	S52.602N	S52.699K	S56.123A
S52.323R	S52.342R	S52.361R	S52.389R	S52.515R	S52.559P	S52.602P	S52.699M	S56.124A
S52.324A	S52.343A	S52.362A	S52.391A	S52.516A	S52.559Q	S52.602Q	S52.699N	S56.125A
S52.324K	S52.343K	S52.362K	S52.391K	S52.516K	S52.559R	S52.602R	S52.699P	S56.126A
S52.324M	S52.343M	S52.362M	S52.391M	S52.516M	S52.561A	S52.609A	S52.699Q	S56.127A
S52.324N	S52.343P	S52.362N	S52.391N	S52.516N	S52.561K	S52.609K	S52.699R	S56.128A
S52.324P	S52.343Q	S52.362P	S52.391P	S52.516P	S52.561M	S52.609M	S52.90XA	S56.129A
S52.324Q	S52.343R	S52.362Q	S52.391Q	S52.516Q	S52.561N	S52.609N	S52.90XK	S56.221A
S52.324R	S52.344A	S52.362R	S52.391R	S52.516R	S52.561P	S52.609P	S52.90XM	S56.222A
S52.325A	S52.344K	S52.363A	S52.392A	S52.521A	S52.561Q	S52.609Q	S52.90XN	S56.229A
S52.325K	S52.344M	S52.363K	S52.392K	S52.521K	S52.561R	S52.609R	S52.90XP	S56.321A
S52.325M	S52.344N	S52.363M	S52.392M	S52.521P	S52.562A	S52.611A	S52.90XQ	S56.322A
S52.325N	S52.344P	S52.363N	S52.392N	S52.522A	S52.562K	S52.611K	S52.90XR	S56.329A
S52.325P	S52.344Q	S52.363P	S52.392P	S52.522K	S52.562M	S52.611M	S52.91XA	S56.421A
S52.325Q	S52.344R	S52.363Q	S52.392Q	S52.522P	S52.562N	S52.611N	S52.91XK	S56.422A
S52.325R	S52.345A	S52.363R	S52.392R	S52.529A	S52.562P	S52.611P	S52.91XM	S56.423A
S52.326A	S52.345K	S52.364A	S52.399A	S52.529K	S52.562Q	S52.611Q	S52.91XN	S56.424A
S52.326K	S52.345M	S52.364K	S52.399K	S52.529P	S52.562R	S52.611R	S52.91XP	S56.425A
S52.326M	S52.345N	S52.364M	S52.399M	S52.531A	S52.569A	S52.612A	S52.91XQ	S56.426A
S52.326N	S52.345P	S52.364N	S52.399N	S52.531K	S52.569K	S52.612K	S52.91XR	S56.427A
S52.326P	S52.345Q	S52.364P	S52.399P	S52.531M	S52.569M	S52.612M	S52.92XA	S56.428A
S52.326Q	S52.345R	S52.364Q	S52.399Q	S52.531N	S52.569N	S52.612N	S52.92XK	S56.429A
S52.326R	S52.346A	S52.364R	S52.399R	S52.531P	S52.569P	S52.612P	S52.92XM	S56.521A
S52.331A	S52.346K	S52.365A	S52.501A	S52.531Q	S52.569Q	S52.612Q	S52.92XN	S56.522A
S52.331K	S52.346M	S52.365K	S52.501K	S52.531R	S52.569R	S52.612R	S52.92XP	S56.529A
S52.331M	S52.346N	S52.365M	S52.501M	S52.532A	S52.571A	S52.613A	S52.92XQ	S56.821A
S52.331N	S52.346P	S52.365N	S52.501N	S52.532K	S52.571K	S52.613K	S52.92XR	S56.822A
S52.331P	S52.346Q	S52.365P	S52.501P	S52.532M	S52.571M	S52.613M	S55.001A	S56.829A
S52.331Q	S52.346R	S52.365Q	S52.501Q	S52.532N	S52.571N	S52.613N	S55.002A	S56.921A
S52.331R	S52.351A	S52.365R	S52.501R	S52.532P	S52.571P	S52.613P	S55.009A	S56.922A
S52.332A	S52.351K	S52.366A	S52.502A	S52.532Q	S52.571Q	S52.613Q	S55.011A	S56.929A
S52.332K	S52.351M	S52.366K	S52.502K	S52.532R	S52.571R	S52.613R	S55.012A	S58.011A
S52.332M	S52.351N	S52.366M	S52.502M	S52.539A	S52.572A	S52.614A	S55.019A	S58.012A
S52.332N	S52.351P	S52.366N	S52.502N	S52.539K	S52.572K	S52.614K	S55.091A	S58.019A
S52.332P	S52.351Q	S52.366P	S52.502P	S52.539M	S52.572M	S52.614M	S55.092A	S58.021A
S52.332Q	S52.351R	S52.366Q	S52.502Q	S52.539N	S52.572N	S52.614N	S55.099A	S58.022A
S52.332R	S52.352A	S52.366R	S52.502R	S52.539P	S52.572P	S52.614P	S55.101A	S58.029A
S52.333A	S52.352K	S52.371A	S52.509A	S52.539Q	S52.572Q	S52.614Q	S55.102A	S58.111A
S52.333K	S52.352M	S52.371K	S52.509K	S52.539R	S52.572R	S52.614R	S55.109A	S58.112A
S52.333M	S52.352N	S52.371M	S52.509M	S52.541A	S52.579A	S52.615A	S55.111A	S58.119A
S52.333N	S52.352P	S52.371N	S52.509N	S52.541K	S52.579K	S52.615K	S55.112A	S58.121A
S52.333P	S52.352Q	S52.371P	S52.509P	S52.541M	S52.579M	S52.615M	S55.119A	S58.122A
S52.333Q	S52.352R	S52.371Q	S52.509Q	S52.541N	S52.579N	S52.615N	S55.191A	S58.129A
S52.333R	S52.353A	S52.371R	S52.509R	S52.541P	S52.579P	S52.615P	S55.192A	S58.911A
S52.334A	S52.353K	S52.372A	S52.511A	S52.541Q	S52.579Q	S52.615Q	S55.199A	S58.912A
S52.334K	S52.353M	S52.372K	S52.511K	S52.541R	S52.579R	S52.615R	S55.201A	S58.919A
S52.334M	S52.353N	S52.372M	S52.511M	S52.542A	S52.591A	S52.616A	S55.202A	S58.921A
S52.334N	S52.353P	S52.372N	S52.511N	S52.542K	S52.591K	S52.616K	S55.209A	S58.922A
S52.334P	S52.353Q	S52.372P	S52.511P	S52.542M	S52.591M	S52.616M	S55.211A	S58.929A
S52.334Q	S52.353R	S52.372Q	S52.511Q	S52.542N	S52.591N	S52.616N	S55.212A	S59.001A
S52.334R	S52.354A	S52.372R	S52.511R	S52.542P	S52.591P	S52.616P	S55.219A	S59.001K
S52.335A	S52.354K	S52.379A	S52.512A	S52.542Q	S52.591Q	S52.616Q	S55.291A	S59.001P
S52.335K	S52.354M	S52.379K	S52.512K	S52.542R	S52.591R	S52.616R	S55.292A	S59.002A
S52.335M	S52.354M	S52.379M	S52.512M	S52.549A	S52.592A	S52.621A	S55.299A	S59.002K
S52.335N	S52.354N	S52.379N	S52.512N	S52.549K	S52.592K	S52.621K	S55.801A	S59.002P
S52.335P	S52.354P	S52.379P	S52.512P	S52.549M	S52.592M	S52.621P	S55.802A	S59.009A
S52.335Q	S52.354Q	S52.379Q	S52.512Q	S52.549N	S52.592N	S52.622A	S55.809A	S59.009K
S52.335R	S52.354R	S52.379R	S52.512R	S52.549P	S52.592P	S52.622K	S55.811A	S59.009P
S52.336A	S52.355A	S52.381A	S52.513A	S52.549Q	S52.592Q	S52.622P	S55.812A	S59.011A
S52.336K	S52.355K	S52.381K	S52.513K	S52.549R	S52.592R	S52.629A	S55.819A	S59.011K
S52.336M	S52.355M	S52.381M	S52.513M	S52.551A	S52.599A	S52.629K	S55.891A	S59.011P
S52.336N	S52.355N	S52.381N	S52.513N	S52.551K	S52.599K	S52.629P	S55.892A	S59.012A
S52.336P	S52.355P	S52.381P	S52.513P	S52.551M	S52.599M	S52.691A	S55.899A	S59.012K
S52.336Q	S52.355Q	S52.381Q	S52.513Q	S52.551N	S52.599N	S52.691K	S55.901A	S59.012P
S52.336R	S52.355R	S52.381R	S52.513R	S52.551P	S52.599P	S52.691M	S55.902A	S59.019A
S52.341A	S52.356A	S52.382A	S52.514A	S52.551Q	S52.599Q	S52.691N	S55.909A	S59.019K
S52.341K	S52.356K	S52.382K	S52.514K	S52.551R	S52.599R	S52.691P	S55.911A	S59.019P
S52.341M	S52.356M	S52.382M	S52.514M	S52.552A	S52.601A	S52.691Q	S55.912A	S59.021A
S52.341N	S52.356N	S52.382N	S52.514N	S52.552K	S52.601K	S52.691R	S55.919A	S59.021K
S52.341P	S52.356P	S52.382P	S52.514P	S52.552M	S52.601M	S52.692A	S55.991A	S59.021P
S52.341Q	S52.356Q	S52.382Q	S52.514Q	S52.552N	S52.601N	S52.692K	S55.992A	S59.022A
S52.341R	S52.356R	S52.382R	S52.514R	S52.552P	S52.601P	S52.692M	S55.999A	S59.022K
S52.342A	S52.361A	S52.389A	S52.515A	S52.552Q	S52.601Q	S52.692N	S56.021A	S59.022P
S52.342K	S52.361K	S52.389K	S52.515K	S52.552R	S52.601R	S52.692P	S56.022A	S59.029A

S59.029K	S59.212A	S62.023P	S62.132K	S62.174B	S62.235P	S62.309K	S62.335B	S62.360P
S59.029P	S59.212K	S62.024B	S62.132P	S62.174K	S62.236B	S62.309P	S62.335K	S62.361B
S59.031A	S59.212P	S62.024K	S62.133B	S62.174P	S62.236K	S62.310B	S62.335P	S62.361K
S59.031K	S59.219A	S62.024P	S62.133P	S62.175B	S62.236P	S62.310K	S62.336B	S62.361P
S59.031P	S59.219K	S62.025B	S62.134B	S62.175K	S62.241B	S62.310P	S62.336K	S62.362B
S59.032A	S59.219P	S62.025K	S62.134K	S62.175P	S62.241K	S62.311B	S62.336P	S62.362K
S59.032K	S59.221A	S62.025P	S62.134P	S62.176B	S62.241P	S62.311K	S62.337B	S62.362P
S59.032P	S59.221K	S62.026B	S62.135B	S62.176K	S62.242B	S62.311P	S62.337K	S62.363B
S59.039A	S59.221P	S62.026K	S62.135K	S62.176P	S62.242K	S62.312B	S62.337P	S62.363K
S59.039K	S59.222A	S62.026P	S62.135P	S62.181B	S62.242P	S62.312K	S62.338B	S62.363P
S59.039P	S59.222K	S62 031B	S62.136B	S62.181K	S62.243B	S62.312P	S62.338K	S62.364B
S59.041A	S59.222P	S62.031K	S62.136K	S62.181P	S62.243K	S62.313B	S62.338P	S62.364K
S59.041K	S59.229A	S62.031P	S62.136P	S62.182B	S62.243P	S62.313K	S62.339B	S62.364P
S59.041P	S59.229K	S62.032B	S62.141B	S62.182K	S62.244B	S62.313P	S62.339K	S62.365B
S59.042A	S59.229P	S62.032K	S62.141K	S62.182P	S62.244K	S62.314B	S62.339P	S62.365K
S59.042K	S59.231A	S62.032P	S62.141P	S62.183B	S62.244P	S62.314K	S62.340B	S62.365P
S59.042P	S59.231K	S62.033B	S62.142B	S62.183K	S62.245B	S62.314P	S62.340K	S62.366B
S59.049A	S59.231P	S62.033K	S62.142K	S62.183P	S62.245K	S62.315B	S62.340P	S62.366K
S59.049K	S59.232A	S62.033P	S62.142P	S62.184B	S62.245P	S62.315K	S62.341B	S62.366P
S59.049P	S59.232K	S62.034B	S62.143B	S62.184K	S62.246B	S62.315P	S62.341K	S62.367B
S59.091A	S59.232P	S62.034K	S62.143K	S62.184P	S62.246K	S62.316B	S62.341P	S62.367K
S59.091K	S59.239A	S62.034P	S62.143P	S62.185B	S62.246P	S62.316K	S62.342B	S62.367P
S59.091P	S59.239K	S62.035B	S62.144B	S62.185K	S62.251B	S62.316P	S62.342K	S62.368B
S59.092A	S59.239P	S62.035K	S62.144K	S62.185P	S62.251K	S62.317B	S62.342P	S62.368K
S59.092K	S59.241A	S62.035P	S62.144P	S62.186B	S62.251P	S62.317K	S62.343B	S62.368P
S59.092P	S59.241K	S62.036B	S62.145B	S62.186K	S62.252B	S62.317P	S62.343K	S62.369B
S59.099A	S59.241P	S62.036K	S62.145K	S62.186P	S62.252K	S62.318B	S62.343P	S62.369K
S59.099K	S59.242A	S62.036P	S62.145P	S62.201B	S62.252P	S62.318K	S62.344B	S62.369P
S59.099P	S59.242K	S62.101B	S62.146B	S62.201K	S62.253B	S62.318P	S62.344K	S62.390B
S59.101K	S59.242P	S62.101K	S62.146K	S62.201P	S62.253K	S62.319B	S62.344P	S62.390K
S59.101P	S59.249A	S62.101P	S62.146P	S62.202B	S62.253P	S62.319K	S62.345B	S62.390P
S59.102K	S59.249K	S62.102B	S62.151B	S62.202K	S62.254B	S62.319P	S62.345K	S62.391B
S59.102P	S59.249P	S62.102K	S62.151K	S62.202P	S62.254K	S62.320B	S62.345P	S62.391K
S59.109K	S59.291A	S62.102P	S62.151P	S62.209B	S62.254P	S62.320K	S62.346B	S62.391P
S59.109P	S59.291K	S62.109B	S62.152B	S62.209K	S62.255B	S62.320P	S62.346K	S62.392B
S59.111K	S59.291P	S62.109K	S62.152K	S62.209P	S62.255K	S62.321B	S62.346P	S62.392K
S59.111P	S59.292A	S62.109P	S62.152P	S62.211B	S62.255P	S62.321K	S62.347B	S62.392P
S59.112K	S59.292K	S62.111B	S62.153B	S62.211K	S62.256B	S62.321P	S62.347K	S62.393B
S59.112P	S59.292P	S62.111K	S62.153K	S62.211P	S62.256K	S62.322B	S62.347P	S62.393K
S59.119K	S59.299A	S62.111P	S62.153P	S62.212B	S62.256P	S62.322K	S62.348B	S62.393P
S59.119P	S59.299K	S62.112B	S62.154B	S62.212K	S62.291B	S62.322P	S62.348K	S62.394B
S59.121K	S59.299P	S62.112K	S62.154K	S62.212P	S62.291K	S62.323B	S62.348P	S62.394K
S59.121P	S62.001B	S62.112P	S62.154P	S62.213B	S62.291P	S62.323K	S62.349B	S62.394P
S59.122K	S62.001K	S62.113B	S62.155B	S62.213K	S62.292B	S62.323P	S62.349K	S62.395B
S59.122P	S62.001P	S62.113K	S62.155K	S62.213P	S62.292K	S62.324B	S62.349P	S62.395K
S59.129K	S62.002B	S62.113P	S62.155P	S62.221B	S62.292P	S62.324K	S62.350B	S62.395P
S59.129P	S62.002K	S62.114B	S62.156B	S62.221K	S62.299B	S62.324P	S62.350K	S62.396B
S59.131K	S62.002P	S62.114K	S62.156K	S62.221P	S62.299K	S62.325B	S62.350P	S62.396K
S59.131P	S62.009B	S62.114P	S62.156P	S62.222B	S62.299P	S62.325K	S62.351B	S62.396P
S59.132K	S62.009K	S62.115B	S62.161B	S62.222K	S62.300B	S62.325P	S62.351K	S62.397B
S59.132P	S62.009P	S62.115K	S62.161K	S62.222P	S62.300K	S62.326B	S62.351P	S62.397K
S59.139K	S62.011B	S62.115P	S62.161P	S62.223B	S62.300P	S62.326K	S62.352B	S62.397P
S59.139P	S62.011K	S62.116B	S62.162B	S62.223K	S62.301B	S62.326P	S62.352K	S62.398B
S59.141K	S62.011P	S62.116K	S62.162K	S62.223P	S62.301K	S62.327B	S62.352P	S62.398K
S59.141P	S62.012B	S62.116P	S62.162P	S62.224B	S62.301P	S62.327K	S62.353B	S62.398P
S59.142K	S62.012K	S62.121B	S62.163B	S62.224K	S62.302B	S62.327P	S62.353K	S62.399B
S59.142P	S62.012P	S62.121K	S62.163K	S62.224P	S62.302K	S62.328B	S62.353P	S62.399K
S59.149K	S62.013B	S62.121P	S62.163P	S62.225B	S62.302P	S62.328K	S62.354B	S62.399P
S59.149P	S62.013K	S62.122B	S62.164B	S62.225K	S62.303B	S62.328P	S62.354K	S62.501B
S59.191K	S62.013P	S62.122K	S62.164K	S62.225P	S62.303K	S62.329B	S62.354P	S62.501K
S59.191P	S62.014B	S62.122P	S62.164P	S62.226B	S62.303P	S62.329K	S62.355B	S62.501P
S59.192K	S62.014K	S62.123B	S62.165B	S62.226K	S62.304B	S62.329P	S62.355K	S62.502B
S59.192P	S62.014P	S62.123K	S62.165K	S62.226P	S62.304K	S62.330B	S62.355P	S62.502K
S59.199K	S62.015B	S62.123P	S62.165P	S62.231B	S62.304P	S62.330K	S62.356B	S62.502P
S59.199P	S62.015K	S62.124B	S62.166B	S62.231K	S62.305B	S62.330P	S62.356K	S62.509B
S59.201A	S62.016B	S62.124K	S62.166K	S62.231P	S62.305K	S62.331B	S62.356P	S62.509K
S59.201K	S62.016K	S62.124P	S62.166P	S62.232B	S62.305P	S62.331K	S62.357B	S62.509P
S59.201P	S62.016P	S62.125B	S62.171B	S62.232K	S62.306B	S62.331P	S62.357K	S62.511B
S59.202A	S62.021B	S62.125K	S62.171K	S62.232P	S62.306K	S62.332B	S62.357P	S62.511K
S59.202K	S62.021K	S62.125P	S62.171P	S62.233B	S62.306P	S62.332K	S62.358B	S62.511P
S59.202P	S62.021P	S62.126B	S62.172B	S62.233K	S62.307B	S62.332P	S62.358K	S62.512B
S59.209A	S62.022B	S62.126K	S62.172K	S62.233P	S62.307K	S62.333B	S62.358P	S62.512K
S59.209K	S62.022K	S62.126P	S62.172P	S62.234B	S62.307P	S62.333K	S62.359B	S62.512P
S59.209P	S62.022P	S62.131B	S62.173B	S62.234K	S62.308B	S62.333P	S62.359K	S62.513B
S59.211A	S62.023B	S62.131K	S62.173K	S62.234P	S62.308K	S62.334B	S62.359P	S62.513K
S59.211K	S62.023K	S62.131P	S62.173P	S62.235B	S62.308P	S62.334K	S62.360B	S62.513P
S59.211P		S62.132B		S62.235K	S62.309B	S62.334P	S62.360K	S62.514B

S62.514K	S62.617B	S62.642P	S62.668K	S65.518A	S68.419A	S72.025Q	S72.046P	S72.101N
S62.514P	S62.617K	S62.643B	S62.668P	S65.519A	S68.421A	S72.025R	S72.046Q	S72.101P
S62.515B	S62.617P	S62.643K	S62.669B	S65.590A	S68.422A	S72.026K	S72.046R	S72.101Q
S62.515K	S62.618B	S62.643P	S62.669K	S65.591A	S68.429A	S72.026M	S72.051K	S72.101R
S62.515P	S62.618K	S62.644B	S62.669P	S65.592A	S68.711A	S72.026N	S72.051M	S72.102K
S62.516B	S62.618P	S62.644K	S62.90XB	S65.593A	S68.712A	S72.026P	S72.051N	S72.102M
S62.516K	S62.619B	S62.644P	S62.90XK	S65.594A	S68.719A	S72.026Q	S72.051P	S72.102N
S62.516P	S62.619K	S62.645B	S62.90XP	S65.595A	S68.721A	S72.026R	S72.051Q	S72.102P
S62.521B	S62.619P	S62.645K	S62.91XB	S65.596A	S68.722A	S72.031K	S72.051R	S72.102Q
S62.521K	S62.620B	S62.645P	S62.91XK	S65.597A	S68.729A	S72.031M	S72.052K	S72.102R
S62.521P	S62.620K	S62.646B	S62.91XP	S65.598A	S72.001K	S72.031N	S72.052M	S72.109K
S62.522B	S62.620P	S62.646K	S62.92XB	S65.599A	S72.001M	S72.031P	S72.052N	S72.109M
S62.522K	S62.621B	S62.646P	S62.92XK	S65.801A	S72.001N	S72.031Q	S72.052P	S72.109N
S62.522P	S62.621K	S62.647B	S62.92XP	S65.802A	S72.001P	S72.031R	S72.052Q	S72.109P
S62.523B	S62.621P	S62.647K	S65.001A	S65.809A	S72.001Q	S72.032K	S72.052R	S72.109Q
S62.523K	S62.622B	S62.647P	S65.002A	S65.811A	S72.001R	S72.032M	S72.059K	S72.109R
S62.523P	S62.622K	S62.648B	S65.009A	S65.812A	S72.002K	S72.032N	S72.059N	S72.111A
S62.524B	S62.622P	S62.648K	S65.011A	S65.819A	S72.002M	S72.032P	S72.059N	S72.111K
S62.524K	S62.623B	S62.648P	S65.012A	S65.891A	S72.002N	S72.032Q	S72.059P	S72.111M
S62.524P	S62.623K	S62.649B	S65.019A	S65.892A	S72.002P	S72.032R	S72.059Q	S72.111N
S62.525B	S62.623P	S62.649K	S65.091A	S65.899A	S72.002Q	S72.033K	S72.059R	S72.111P
S62.525K	S62.624B	S62.649P	S65.092A	S65.901A	S72.002R	S72.033M	S72.061K	S72.111Q
S62.525P	S62.624K	S62.650B	S65.099A	S65.902A	S72.009K	S72.033N	S72.061M	S72.111R
S62.526B	S62.624P	S62.650K	S65.101A	S65.909A	S72.009M	S72.033P	S72.061N	S72.112A
S62.526K	S62.625B	S62.650P	S65.102A	S65.911A	S72.009N	S72.033Q	S72.061P	S72.112K
S62.526P	S62.625K	S62.651B	S65.109A	S65.912A	S72.009P	S72.033R	S72.061Q	S72.112M
S62.600B	S62.625P	S62.651K	S65.111A	S65.919A	S72.009Q	S72.034K	S72.061R	S72.112N
S62.600K	S62.626B	S62.651P	S65.112A	S65.991A	S72.009R	S72.034M	S72.062K	S72.112P
S62.600P	S62.626K	S62.652B	S65.119A	S65.992A	S72.011A	S72.034N	S72.062M	S72.112Q
S62.601B	S62.626P	S62.652K	S65.191A	S65.999A	S72.011K	S72.034P	S72.062N	S72.112R
S62.601K	S62.627B	S62.652P	S65.192A	S66.021A	S72.011M	S72.034Q	S72.062P	S72.113A
S62.601P	S62.627K	S62.653B	S65.199A	S66.022A	S72.011N	S72.034R	S72.062Q	S72.113K
S62.602B	S62.627P	S62.653K	S65.201A	S66.029A	S72.011P	S72.035K	S72.062R	S72.113M
S62.602K	S62.628B	S62.653P	S65.202A	S66.120A	S72.011Q	S72.035M	S72.063K	S72.113N
S62.602P	S62.628K	S62.654B	S65.209A	S66.121A	S72.011R	S72.035N	S72.063M	S72.113P
S62.603B	S62.628P	S62.654K	S65.211A	S66.122A	S72.012A	S72.035P	S72.063N	S72.113Q
S62.603K	S62.629B	S62.654P	S65.212A	S66.123A	S72.012K	S72.035Q	S72.063P	S72.113R
S62.603P	S62.629K	S62.655B	S65.219A	S66.124A	S72.012N	S72.035R	S72.063Q	S72.114A
S62.604B	S62.629P	S62.655K	S65.291A	S66.125A	S72.012P	S72.036K	S72.063R	S72.114K
S62.604K	S62.630B	S62.655P	S65.292A	S66.126A	S72.012Q	S72.036M	S72.064K	S72.114M
S62.604P	S62.630K	S62.656B	S65.299A	S66.127A	S72.012R	S72.036N	S72.064M	S72.114N
S62.605B	S62.630P	S62.656K	S65.301A	S66.128A	S72.019A	S72.036P	S72.064N	S72.114P
S62.605K	S62.631B	S62.656P	S65.302A	S66.129A	S72.019K	S72.036Q	S72.064P	S72.114Q
S62.605P	S62.631K	S62.657B	S65.309A	S66.221A	S72.019M	S72.036R	S72.064Q	S72.114R
S62.606B	S62.631P	S62.657K	S65.311A	S66.222A	S72.019N	S72.041K	S72.064R	S72.115A
S62.606K	S62.632B	S62.657P	S65.312A	S66.229A	S72.019P	S72.041M	S72.065K	S72.115K
S62.607B	S62.632K	S62.658B	S65.319A	S66.320A	S72.019Q	S72.041N	S72.065M	S72.115M
S62.607K	S62.632P	S62.658K	S65.391A	S66.321A	S72.019R	S72.041P	S72.065N	S72.115N
S62.607P	S62.633B	S62.658P	S65.392A	S66.322A	S72.021K	S72.041Q	S72.065P	S72.115P
S62.608B	S62.633K	S62.659B	S65.399A	S66.323A	S72.021M	S72.041R	S72.065Q	S72.115Q
S62.608K	S62.633P	S62.659K	S65.401A	S66.324A	S72.021N	S72.042K	S72.065R	S72.115R
S62.608P	S62.634B	S62.659P	S65.402A	S66.325A	S72.021P	S72.042M	S72.066K	S72.116A
S62.609B	S62.634K	S62.660B	S65.409A	S66.326A	S72.021Q	S72.042N	S72.066M	S72.116K
S62.609K	S62.634P	S62.660K	S65.411A	S66.327A	S72.021R	S72.042P	S72.066N	S72.116M
S62.609P	S62.635B	S62.660P	S65.412A	S66.328A	S72.022K	S72.042Q	S72.066P	S72.116N
S62.610B	S62.635K	S62.661B	S65.419A	S66.329A	S72.022M	S72.042R	S72.066Q	S72.116P
S62.610K	S62.635P	S62.661K	S65.491A	S66.421A	S72.022N	S72.043K	S72.066R	S72.116Q
S62.610P	S62.636B	S62.661P	S65.492A	S66.422A	S72.022P	S72.043M	S72.091K	S72.116R
S62.611B	S62.636K	S62.662B	S65.499A	S66.429A	S72.022Q	S72.043N	S72.091M	S72.121A
S62.611K	S62.636P	S62.662K	S65.500A	S66.520A	S72.022R	S72.043P	S72.091N	S72.121K
S62.611P	S62.637B	S62.662P	S65.501A	S66.521A	S72.023K	S72.043Q	S72.091P	S72.121M
S62.612B	S62.637K	S62.663B	S65.502A	S66.522A	S72.023M	S72.043R	S72.091Q	S72.121N
S62.612K	S62.637P	S62.663K	S65.503A	S66.523A	S72.023N	S72.044K	S72.091R	S72.121P
S62.612P	S62.638B	S62.663P	S65.504A	S66.524A	S72.023P	S72.044M	S72.092K	S72.121Q
S62.613B	S62.638K	S62.664B	S65.505A	S66.525A	S72.023Q	S72.044N	S72.092M	S72.121R
S62.613K	S62.638P	S62.664K	S65.506A	S66.526A	S72.023R	S72.044P	S72.092N	S72.122A
S62.613P	S62.639B	S62.664P	S65.507A	S66.527A	S72.024K	S72.044Q	S72.092P	S72.122K
S62.614B	S62.639K	S62.665B	S65.508A	S66.528A	S72.024M	S72.044R	S72.092Q	S72.122M
S62.614K	S62.639P	S62.665K	S65.509A	S66.529A	S72.024N	S72.045K	S72.092R	S72.122N
S62.614P	S62.640B	S62.665P	S65.510A	S66.821A	S72.024P	S72.045M	S72.099K	S72.122P
S62.615B	S62.640K	S62.666B	S65.511A	S66.822A	S72.024Q	S72.045N	S72.099N	S72.122Q
S62.615K	S62.640P	S62.666K	S65.512A	S66.829A	S72.024R	S72.045P	S72.099N	S72.122R
S62.615P	S62.641B	S62.666P	S65.513A	S66.921A	S72.025K	S72.045Q	S72.099P	S72.123A
S62.616B	S62.641K	S62.667B	S65.514A	S66.922A	S72.025M	S72.045R	S72.099Q	S72.123K
S62.616K	S62.641P	S62.667K	S65.515A	S66.929A	S72.025N	S72.046K	S72.099R	S72.123M
S62.616P	S62.642B	S62.667P	S65.516A	S68.411A	S72.025P	S72.046M	S72.101K	S72.123N
	S62.642K	S62.668B	S65.517A	S68.412A			S72.101M	S72.123P

S72.123Q	S72.142Q	S72.301Q	S72.335M	S72.356K	S72.409N	S72.425N	S72.444N	S72.463N
S72.123R	S72.142R	S72.301R	S72.335N	S72.356M	S72.409P	S72.425P	S72.444P	S72.463P
S72.124A	S72.143A	S72.302A	S72.335P	S72.356N	S72.409Q	S72.425Q	S72.444Q	S72.463Q
S72.124K	S72.143K	S72.302K	S72.335Q	S72.356P	S72.409R	S72.425R	S72.444R	S72.463R
S72.124M	S72.143M	S72.302M	S72.335R	S72.356Q	S72.411A	S72.426A	S72.445A	S72.464A
S72.124N	S72.143N	S72.302N	S72.336K	S72.356R	S72.411K	S72.426K	S72.445K	S72.464K
S72.124P	S72.143P	S72.302P	S72.336M	S72.361K	S72.411M	S72.426M	S72.445M	S72.464M
S72.124Q	S72.143Q	S72.302Q	S72.336N	S72.361M	S72.411N	S72.426N	S72.445N	S72.464N
S72.124R	S72.143R	S72.302R	S72.336P	S72.361N	S72.411P	S72.426P	S72.445P	S72.464P
S72.125A	S72.144A	S72.309A	S72.336Q	S72.361P	S72.411Q	S72.426Q	S72.445Q	S72.464Q
S72.125K	S72.144K	S72.309K	S72.336R	S72.361Q	S72.411R	S72.426R	S72.445R	S72.464R
S72.125M	S72.144M	S72.309M	S72.341K	S72.361R	S72.412A	S72.431A	S72.446A	S72.465A
S72.125N	S72.144N	S72.309N	S72.341M	S72.362K	S72.412K	S72.431K	S72.446K	S72.465K
S72.125P	S72.144P	S72.309P	S72.341N	S72.362M	S72.412M	S72.431M	S72.446M	S72.465M
S72.125Q	S72.144Q	S72.309Q	S72.341P	S72.362N	S72.412N	S72.431N	S72.446N	S72.465N
S72.125R	S72.144R	S72.309R	S72.341Q	S72.362P	S72.412P	S72.431P	S72.446P	S72.465P
S72.126A	S72.145A	S72.321K	S72.341R	S72.362Q	S72.412Q	S72.431Q	S72.446Q	S72.465Q
S72.126K	S72.145K	S72.321M	S72.342K	S72.362R	S72.412R	S72.431R	S72.446R	S72.465R
S72.126M	S72.145M	S72.321N	S72.342M	S72.363K	S72.413A	S72.432A	S72.451A	S72.466A
S72.126N	S72.145N	S72.321P	S72.342N	S72.363M	S72.413K	S72.432K	S72.451K	S72.466K
S72.126P	S72.145P	S72.321Q	S72.342P	S72.363N	S72.413M	S72.432M	S72.451M	S72.466M
S72.126Q	S72.145Q	S72.321R	S72.342Q	S72.363P	S72.413N	S72.432N	S72.451N	S72.466N
S72.126R	S72.145R	S72.322K	S72.342R	S72.363Q	S72.413P	S72.432P	S72.451P	S72.466P
S72.131A	S72.146A	S72.322M	S72.343K	S72.363R	S72.413Q	S72.432Q	S72.451Q	S72.466Q
S72.131K	S72.146K	S72.322N	S72.343M	S72.364K	S72.413R	S72.432R	S72.451R	S72.466R
S72.131M	S72.146M	S72.322P	S72.343N	S72.364M	S72.414A	S72.433A	S72.452A	S72.471A
S72.131N	S72.146N	S72.322Q	S72.343P	S72.364N	S72.414K	S72.433K	S72.452K	S72.471K
S72.131P	S72.146P	S72.322R	S72.343Q	S72.364P	S72.414M	S72.433M	S72.452M	S72.471P
S72.131Q	S72.146Q	S72.323K	S72.343R	S72.364Q	S72.414N	S72.433N	S72.452N	S72.472A
S72.131R	S72.146R	S72.323M	S72.344K	S72.364R	S72.414P	S72.433P	S72.452P	S72.472K
S72.132A	S72.21XA	S72.323N	S72.344M	S72.365K	S72.414Q	S72.433Q	S72.452Q	S72.472P
S72.132K	S72.21XK	S72.323P	S72.344N	S72.365M	S72.414R	S72.433R	S72.452R	S72.479A
S72.132M	S72.21XM	S72.323Q	S72.344P	S72.365N	S72.415A	S72.434A	S72.453A	S72.479K
S72.132N	S72.21XN	S72.323R	S72.344Q	S72.365P	S72.415K	S72.434K	S72.453K	S72.479P
S72.132P	S72.21XP	S72.324K	S72.344R	S72.365Q	S72.415M	S72.434M	S72.453M	S72.491A
S72.132Q	S72.21XQ	S72.324M	S72.345K	S72.365R	S72.415N	S72.434N	S72.453N	S72.491K
S72.132R	S72.21XR	S72.324N	S72.345M	S72.366K	S72.415P	S72.434P	S72.453P	S72.491M
S72.133A	S72.22XA	S72.324P	S72.345N	S72.366M	S72.415Q	S72.434Q	S72.453Q	S72.491N
S72.133K	S72.22XK	S72.324Q	S72.345P	S72.366N	S72.415R	S72.434R	S72.453R	S72.491P
S72.133M	S72.22XM	S72.324R	S72.345Q	S72.366P	S72.416A	S72.435A	S72.454A	S72.491Q
S72.133N	S72.22XN	S72.325K	S72.345R	S72.366Q	S72.416K	S72.435K	S72.454K	S72.491R
S72.133P	S72.22XP	S72.325M	S72.346K	S72.366R	S72.416M	S72.435M	S72.454M	S72.492A
S72.133Q	S72.22XQ	S72.325N	S72.346M	S72.391K	S72.416N	S72.435N	S72.454N	S72.492K
S72.133R	S72.22XR	S72.325P	S72.346N	S72.391M	S72.416P	S72.435P	S72.454P	S72.492M
S72.134A	S72.23XA	S72.325Q	S72.346P	S72.391N	S72.416Q	S72.435Q	S72.454Q	S72.492N
S72.134K	S72.23XK	S72.325R	S72.346Q	S72.391P	S72.416R	S72.435R	S72.454R	S72.492P
S72.134M	S72.23XM	S72.326K	S72.346R	S72.391Q	S72.421A	S72.436A	S72.455A	S72.492Q
S72.134N	S72.23XN	S72.326M	S72.351K	S72.391R	S72.421K	S72.436K	S72.455K	S72.492R
S72.134P	S72.23XP	S72.326N	S72.351M	S72.392K	S72.421M	S72.436M	S72.455M	S72.499A
S72.134Q	S72.23XQ	S72.326P	S72.351N	S72.392M	S72.421N	S72.436N	S72.455N	S72.499K
S72.134R	S72.23XR	S72.326Q	S72.351P	S72.392N	S72.421P	S72.436P	S72.455P	S72.499M
S72.135A	S72.24XA	S72.326R	S72.351Q	S72.392P	S72.421Q	S72.436Q	S72.455Q	S72.499N
S72.135K	S72.24XK	S72.331K	S72.351R	S72.392Q	S72.421R	S72.436R	S72.455R	S72.499P
S72.135M	S72.24XM	S72.331M	S72.352K	S72.392R	S72.422A	S72.441A	S72.456A	S72.499Q
S72.135N	S72.24XN	S72.331N	S72.352M	S72.399K	S72.422K	S72.441K	S72.456K	S72.499R
S72.135P	S72.24XP	S72.331P	S72.352N	S72.399M	S72.422M	S72.441M	S72.456M	S72.8X1K
S72.135Q	S72.24XQ	S72.331Q	S72.352P	S72.399N	S72.422N	S72.441N	S72.456N	S72.8X1M
S72.135R	S72.24XR	S72.331R	S72.352Q	S72.399P	S72.422P	S72.441P	S72.456P	S72.8X1N
S72.136A	S72.25XA	S72.332K	S72.352R	S72.399Q	S72.422Q	S72.441Q	S72.456Q	S72.8X1P
S72.136K	S72.25XK	S72.332M	S72.353K	S72.399R	S72.422R	S72.441R	S72.456R	S72.8X1Q
S72.136M	S72.25XM	S72.332N	S72.353M	S72.401A	S72.423A	S72.442A	S72.461A	S72.8X1R
S72.136N	S72.25XN	S72.332P	S72.353N	S72.401K	S72.423K	S72.442K	S72.461K	S72.8X2K
S72.136P	S72.25XP	S72.332Q	S72.353P	S72.401M	S72.423M	S72.442M	S72.461M	S72.8X2M
S72.136Q	S72.25XQ	S72.332R	S72.353Q	S72.401N	S72.423N	S72.442N	S72.461N	S72.8X2N
S72.136R	S72.25XR	S72.333K	S72.353R	S72.401P	S72.423P	S72.442P	S72.461P	S72.8X2P
S72.141A	S72.26XA	S72.333M	S72.354K	S72.401Q	S72.423Q	S72.442Q	S72.461Q	S72.8X2Q
S72.141K	S72.26XK	S72.333N	S72.354M	S72.401R	S72.423R	S72.442R	S72.461R	S72.8X2R
S72.141M	S72.26XM	S72.333P	S72.354N	S72.402A	S72.424A	S72.443A	S72.462A	S72.8X9K
S72.141N	S72.26XN	S72.333Q	S72.354P	S72.402K	S72.424K	S72.443K	S72.462K	S72.8X9M
S72.141P	S72.26XP	S72.333R	S72.354Q	S72.402M	S72.424M	S72.443M	S72.462M	S72.8X9N
S72.141Q	S72.26XQ	S72.334K	S72.354R	S72.402N	S72.424N	S72.443N	S72.462N	S72.8X9P
S72.141R	S72.26XR	S72.334M	S72.355K	S72.402P	S72.424P	S72.443P	S72.462P	S72.8X9Q
S72.142A	S72.301A	S72.334N	S72.355M	S72.402Q	S72.424Q	S72.443Q	S72.462Q	S72.8X9R
S72.142K	S72.301K	S72.334P	S72.355N	S72.402R	S72.424R	S72.443R	S72.462R	S72.90XK
S72.142M	S72.301M	S72.334Q	S72.355P	S72.409A	S72.425A	S72.444A	S72.463A	S72.90XM
S72.142N	S72.301N	S72.334R	S72.355Q	S72.409K	S72.425K	S72.444K	S72.463K	S72.90XN
S72.142P	S72.301P	S72.335K	S72.355R	S72.409M	S72.425M	S72.444M	S72.463M	S72.90XP

Appendix E: Complication and Comorbidity (CC) Code List

S72.90XQ	S76.121A	S79.121P	S82.012Q	S82.025K	S82.041R	S82.101P	S82.123P	S82.142P
S72.90XR	S76.122A	S79.122A	S82.012R	S82.025M	S82.042A	S82.101Q	S82.123Q	S82.142Q
S72.91XK	S76.129A	S79.122K	S82.013A	S82.025N	S82.042B	S82.101R	S82.123R	S82.142R
S72.91XM	S76.221A	S79.122P	S82.013B	S82.025P	S82.042C	S82.102A	S82.124A	S82.143A
S72.91XN	S76.222A	S79.129A	S82.013C	S82.025Q	S82.042K	S82.102K	S82.124K	S82.143K
S72.91XP	S76.229A	S79.129K	S82.013K	S82.025R	S82.042M	S82.102M	S82.124M	S82.143M
S72.91XQ	S76.321A	S79.129P	S82.013M	S82.026A	S82.042N	S82.102N	S82.124N	S82.143N
S72.91XR	S76.322A	S79.131A	S82.013N	S82.026B	S82.042P	S82.102P	S82.124P	S82.143P
S72.92XK	S76.329A	S79.131K	S82.013P	S82.026C	S82.042Q	S82.102Q	S82.124Q	S82.143Q
S72.92XM	S76.821A	S79.131P	S82.013Q	S82.026K	S82.043A	S82.102R	S82.124R	S82.143R
S72.92XN	S76.822A	S79.132A	S82.013R	S82.026M	S82.043B	S82.109A	S82.125A	S82.144A
S72.92XP	S76.829A	S79.132K	S82.014A	S82.026N	S82.043C	S82.109K	S82.125K	S82.144K
S72.92XQ	S76.921A	S79.132P	S82.014B	S82.026P	S82.043K	S82.109M	S82.125M	S82.144M
S72.92XR	S76.922A	S79.139A	S82.014C	S82.026Q	S82.043M	S82.109N	S82.125N	S82.144N
S73.001A	S76.929A	S79.139K	S82.014K	S82.026R	S82.043N	S82.109P	S82.125P	S82.144P
S73.002A	S77.00XA	S79.139P	S82.014M	S82.031A	S82.043P	S82.109Q	S82.125Q	S82.144Q
S73.003A	S77.01XA	S79.141A	S82.014N	S82.031B	S82.043Q	S82.109R	S82.125R	S82.144R
S73.004A	S77.02XA	S79.141K	S82.014P	S82.031C	S82.043R	S82.111A	S82.126A	S82.145A
S73.005A	S77.10XA	S79.141P	S82.014Q	S82.031K	S82.044A	S82.111K	S82.126K	S82.145K
S73.006A	S77.11XA	S79.142A	S82.014R	S82.031M	S82.044B	S82.111M	S82.126M	S82.145M
S73.011A	S77.12XA	S79.142K	S82.015A	S82.031N	S82.044C	S82.111N	S82.126N	S82.145N
S73.012A	S78.011A	S79.142P	S82.015B	S82.031P	S82.044K	S82.111P	S82.126P	S82.145P
S73.013A	S78.012A	S79.149A	S82.015C	S82.031Q	S82.044M	S82.111Q	S82.126Q	S82.145Q
S73.014A	S78.019A	S79.149K	S82.015K	S82.031R	S82.044N	S82.111R	S82.126R	S82.145R
S73.015A	S78.021A	S79.149P	S82.015M	S82.032A	S82.044P	S82.112A	S82.131A	S82.146A
S73.016A	S78.022A	S79.191A	S82.015N	S82.032B	S82.044Q	S82.112K	S82.131K	S82.146K
S73.021A	S78.029A	S79.191K	S82.015P	S82.032C	S82.044R	S82.112M	S82.131M	S82.146M
S73.022A	S78.111A	S79.191P	S82.015Q	S82.032K	S82.045A	S82.112N	S82.131N	S82.146N
S73.023A	S78.112A	S79.192A	S82.015R	S82.032M	S82.045B	S82.112P	S82.131P	S82.146P
S73.024A	S78.119A	S79.192K	S82.016A	S82.032P	S82.045C	S82.112Q	S82.131Q	S82.146Q
S73.025A	S78.121A	S79.192P	S82.016B	S82.032Q	S82.045K	S82.112R	S82.131R	S82.146R
S73.026A	S78.122A	S79.199A	S82.016C	S82.032R	S82.045M	S82.113A	S82.132A	S82.151A
S73.031A	S78.129A	S79.199K	S82.016K	S82.033A	S82.045N	S82.113K	S82.132K	S82.151K
S73.032A	S78.911A	S79.199P	S82.016M	S82.033B	S82.045P	S82.113M	S82.132M	S82.151M
S73.033A	S78.912A	S82.001A	S82.016N	S82.033C	S82.045Q	S82.113N	S82.132N	S82.151N
S73.034A	S78.919A	S82.001B	S82.016P	S82.033K	S82.045R	S82.113P	S82.132P	S82.151P
S73.035A	S78.921A	S82.001C	S82.016Q	S82.033N	S82.046A	S82.113Q	S82.132Q	S82.151Q
S73.036A	S78.922A	S82.001K	S82.016R	S82.033P	S82.046B	S82.113R	S82.132R	S82.151R
S73.041A	S78.929A	S82.001M	S82.021A	S82.033Q	S82.046C	S82.114A	S82.133A	S82.152A
S73.042A	S79.001K	S82.001N	S82.021B	S82.033R	S82.046K	S82.114K	S82.133K	S82.152K
S73.043A	S79.001P	S82.001P	S82.021C	S82.034A	S82.046M	S82.114M	S82.133M	S82.152M
S73.044A	S79.002K	S82.001Q	S82.021K	S82.034B	S82.046N	S82.114N	S82.133N	S82.152N
S73.045A	S79.002P	S82.001R	S82.021M	S82.034C	S82.046P	S82.114P	S82.133P	S82.152P
S73.046A	S79.009K	S82.002A	S82.021N	S82.034K	S82.046Q	S82.114Q	S82.133Q	S82.152Q
S75.201A	S79.009P	S82.002B	S82.021P	S82.034M	S82.046R	S82.114R	S82.133R	S82.152R
S75.202A	S79.011K	S82.002C	S82.021Q	S82.034N	S82.091A	S82.115A	S82.134A	S82.153A
S75.209A	S79.011P	S82.002K	S82.021R	S82.034P	S82.091B	S82.115K	S82.134K	S82.153K
S75.211A	S79.012K	S82.002M	S82.022A	S82.034Q	S82.091C	S82.115M	S82.134M	S82.153M
S75.212A	S79.012P	S82.002N	S82.022B	S82.034R	S82.091K	S82.115N	S82.134N	S82.153N
S75.219A	S79.019K	S82.002P	S82.022C	S82.035A	S82.091M	S82.115P	S82.134P	S82.153P
S75.221A	S79.019P	S82.002Q	S82.022K	S82.035B	S82.091N	S82.115Q	S82.134Q	S82.153Q
S75.222A	S79.091K	S82.002R	S82.022M	S82.035C	S82.091P	S82.115R	S82.134R	S82.153R
S75.229A	S79.091P	S82.009B	S82.022N	S82.035K	S82.091Q	S82.116A	S82.135A	S82.154A
S75.291A	S79.092K	S82.009C	S82.022P	S82.035M	S82.091R	S82.116K	S82.135K	S82.154K
S75.292A	S79.092P	S82.009K	S82.022Q	S82.035N	S82.092A	S82.116M	S82.135M	S82.154M
S75.299A	S79.099K	S82.009M	S82.022R	S82.035P	S82.092B	S82.116N	S82.135N	S82.154N
S75.801A	S79.099P	S82.009N	S82.023A	S82.035Q	S82.092C	S82.116P	S82.135P	S82.154P
S75.802A	S79.101A	S82.009P	S82.023B	S82.035R	S82.092K	S82.116Q	S82.135Q	S82.154Q
S75.809A	S79.101K	S82.009P	S82.023C	S82.036A	S82.092M	S82.116R	S82.135R	S82.154R
S75.811A	S79.101P	S82.009Q	S82.023K	S82.036B	S82.092N	S82.121A	S82.136A	S82.155A
S75.812A	S79.102A	S82.009Q	S82.023M	S82.036C	S82.092P	S82.121K	S82.136K	S82.155K
S75.819A	S79.102K	S82.009R	S82.023N	S82.036K	S82.092Q	S82.121M	S82.136M	S82.155M
S75.891A	S79.102P	S82.011A	S82.023P	S82.036M	S82.092R	S82.121N	S82.136N	S82.155N
S75.892A	S79.109A	S82.011B	S82.023Q	S82.036N	S82.099A	S82.121P	S82.136P	S82.155P
S75.899A	S79.109K	S82.011C	S82.023R	S82.036P	S82.099B	S82.121Q	S82.136Q	S82.155Q
S75.901A	S79.109P	S82.011K	S82.024A	S82.036Q	S82.099C	S82.121R	S82.136R	S82.155R
S75.902A	S79.111A	S82.011M	S82.024B	S82.036R	S82.099K	S82.122A	S82.141A	S82.156A
S75.909A	S79.111K	S82.011N	S82.024C	S82.041A	S82.099M	S82.122K	S82.141K	S82.156K
S75.911A	S79.111P	S82.011P	S82.024K	S82.041B	S82.099N	S82.122M	S82.141M	S82.156M
S75.912A	S79.112A	S82.011Q	S82.024M	S82.041C	S82.099P	S82.122N	S82.141N	S82.156N
S75.919A	S79.112K	S82.011R	S82.024N	S82.041K	S82.099Q	S82.122P	S82.141P	S82.156P
S75.991A	S79.112P	S82.012A	S82.024P	S82.041M	S82.099R	S82.122Q	S82.141R	S82.156Q
S75.992A	S79.119A	S82.012B	S82.024Q	S82.041N	S82.101A	S82.122R	S82.142A	S82.156R
S75.999A	S79.119K	S82.012C	S82.024R	S82.041P	S82.101K	S82.123A	S82.142K	S82.161A
S76.021A	S79.119P	S82.012M	S82.025A	S82.041Q	S82.101M	S82.123K	S82.142M	S82.161K
S76.022A	S79.121A	S82.012N	S82.025B		S82.101N	S82.123M	S82.142N	S82.161P
S76.029A	S79.121K	S82.012P	S82.025C			S82.123N		S82.162A

S82.162K	S82.225M	S82.244M	S82.263M	S82.319A	S82.426N	S82.451M	S82.492K	S82.63XC
S82.162P	S82.225N	S82.244N	S82.263N	S82.319K	S82.426P	S82.451N	S82.492M	S82.63XK
S82.169A	S82.225P	S82.244P	S82.263Q	S82.319P	S82.426Q	S82.451Q	S82.492N	S82.63XM
S82.169K	S82.225Q	S82.244Q	S82.263R	S82.391B	S82.426R	S82.451R	S82.492P	S82.63XN
S82.169P	S82.225R	S82.244R	S82.264A	S82.391C	S82.431K	S82.452K	S82.492Q	S82.63XP
S82.191A	S82.226A	S82.245A	S82.264K	S82.391K	S82.431M	S82.452M	S82.492R	S82.63XQ
S82.191K	S82.226K	S82.245K	S82.264M	S82.391M	S82.431N	S82.452N	S82.499K	S82.63XR
S82.191M	S82.226M	S82.245M	S82.264N	S82.391N	S82.431P	S82.452P	S82.499M	S82.64XB
S82.191N	S82.226N	S82.245N	S82.264Q	S82.391P	S82.431Q	S82.452Q	S82.499N	S82.64XC
S82.191P	S82.226P	S82.245P	S82.264R	S82.391Q	S82.431R	S82.452R	S82.499P	S82.64XK
S82.191Q	S82.226Q	S82.245Q	S82.265A	S82.391R	S82.432K	S82.453K	S82.499Q	S82.64XM
S82.191R	S82.226R	S82.245R	S82.265K	S82.392B	S82.432M	S82.453M	S82.499R	S82.64XN
S82.192A	S82.231A	S82.246A	S82.265M	S82.392C	S82.432N	S82.453N	S82.51XB	S82.64XP
S82.192K	S82.231K	S82.246K	S82.265N	S82.392K	S82.432P	S82.453P	S82.51XC	S82.64XQ
S82.192M	S82.231M	S82.246M	S82.265Q	S82.392M	S82.432Q	S82.453Q	S82.51XK	S82.64XR
S82.192N	S82.231N	S82.246N	S82.265R	S82.392N	S82.432R	S82.453R	S82.51XM	S82.65XB
S82.192P	S82.231P	S82.246P	S82.266A	S82.392P	S82.433K	S82.454K	S82.51XN	S82.65XC
S82.192Q	S82.231Q	S82.246Q	S82.266K	S82.392Q	S82.433N	S82.454M	S82.51XP	S82.65XK
S82.192R	S82.231R	S82.246R	S82.266M	S82.392R	S82.433P	S82.454N	S82.51XQ	S82.65XM
S82.199A	S82.232A	S82.251A	S82.266N	S82.399B	S82.433Q	S82.454P	S82.51XR	S82.65XN
S82.199K	S82.232K	S82.251K	S82.266Q	S82.399C	S82.433R	S82.454Q	S82.52XB	S82.65XP
S82.199M	S82.232M	S82.251M	S82.266R	S82.399K	S82.434K	S82.454R	S82.52XC	S82.65XQ
S82.199N	S82.232N	S82.251N	S82.266P	S82.399M	S82.434M	S82.455M	S82.52XK	S82.65XR
S82.199P	S82.232P	S82.251P	S82.266P	S82.399N	S82.434N	S82.455N	S82.52XM	S82.66XB
S82.199Q	S82.232Q	S82.251Q	S82.266Q	S82.399P	S82.434P	S82.455P	S82.52XN	S82.66XC
S82.199R	S82.232R	S82.251R	S82.266R	S82.399Q	S82.434Q	S82.455Q	S82.52XP	S82.66XK
S82.201A	S82.233A	S82.252A	S82.291A	S82.399R	S82.434R	S82.455R	S82.52XQ	S82.66XM
S82.201K	S82.233K	S82.252K	S82.291K	S82.401K	S82.435K	S82.455R	S82.52XR	S82.66XN
S82.201M	S82.233M	S82.252M	S82.291M	S82.401M	S82.435M	S82.456K	S82.53XB	S82.66XP
S82.201N	S82.233N	S82.252N	S82.291N	S82.401N	S82.435N	S82.456M	S82.53XC	S82.66XQ
S82.201P	S82.233P	S82.252P	S82.291P	S82.401P	S82.435P	S82.456N	S82.53XM	S82.66XR
S82.201Q	S82.233Q	S82.252Q	S82.291Q	S82.401Q	S82.435Q	S82.456P	S82.53XN	S82.811K
S82.201R	S82.233R	S82.252R	S82.291R	S82.401R	S82.435R	S82.456Q	S82.53XP	S82.811P
S82.202A	S82.234A	S82.253A	S82.292A	S82.402K	S82.436K	S82.456R	S82.53XQ	S82.812K
S82.202K	S82.234K	S82.253K	S82.292K	S82.402M	S82.436M	S82.461K	S82.53XR	S82.812P
S82.202M	S82.234M	S82.253M	S82.292M	S82.402N	S82.436N	S82.461M	S82.54XB	S82.819K
S82.202N	S82.234N	S82.253N	S82.292N	S82.402P	S82.436P	S82.461N	S82.54XC	S82.819P
S82.202P	S82.234P	S82.253P	S82.292P	S82.402Q	S82.436Q	S82.461P	S82.54XK	S82.821K
S82.202Q	S82.234Q	S82.253Q	S82.292Q	S82.402R	S82.436R	S82.461Q	S82.54XM	S82.821P
S82.202R	S82.234R	S82.253R	S82.292R	S82.409K	S82.441K	S82.461R	S82.54XN	S82.822K
S82.209A	S82.235A	S82.254A	S82.299A	S82.409M	S82.441M	S82.462K	S82.54XP	S82.822P
S82.209K	S82.235K	S82.254K	S82.299K	S82.409N	S82.441N	S82.462M	S82.54XQ	S82.829K
S82.209M	S82.235M	S82.254M	S82.299M	S82.409P	S82.441P	S82.462N	S82.54XR	S82.829P
S82.209N	S82.235N	S82.254N	S82.299N	S82.409Q	S82.441Q	S82.462P	S82.55XB	S82.831K
S82.209P	S82.235P	S82.254P	S82.299P	S82.409R	S82.441R	S82.462Q	S82.55XC	S82.831M
S82.209Q	S82.235Q	S82.254Q	S82.299Q	S82.421K	S82.442K	S82.462R	S82.55XK	S82.831N
S82.209R	S82.235R	S82.254R	S82.299R	S82.421M	S82.442M	S82.463K	S82.55XM	S82.831P
S82.221A	S82.236A	S82.255A	S82.301B	S82.421N	S82.442N	S82.463M	S82.55XN	S82.831Q
S82.221K	S82.236K	S82.255K	S82.301C	S82.421P	S82.442P	S82.463N	S82.55XP	S82.831R
S82.221M	S82.236M	S82.255M	S82.301K	S82.421Q	S82.442Q	S82.463P	S82.55XQ	S82.832K
S82.221N	S82.236N	S82.255N	S82.301M	S82.421R	S82.442R	S82.463Q	S82.55XR	S82.832M
S82.221P	S82.236P	S82.255P	S82.301N	S82.422K	S82.443K	S82.463R	S82.56XB	S82.832N
S82.221Q	S82.236Q	S82.255Q	S82.301P	S82.422M	S82.443M	S82.464K	S82.56XC	S82.832P
S82.221R	S82.236R	S82.255R	S82.301Q	S82.422N	S82.443N	S82.464M	S82.56XK	S82.832Q
S82.222A	S82.241A	S82.256A	S82.301R	S82.422P	S82.443P	S82.464N	S82.56XM	S82.832R
S82.222K	S82.241K	S82.256K	S82.302B	S82.422Q	S82.443Q	S82.464P	S82.56XN	S82.839K
S82.222M	S82.241M	S82.256M	S82.302C	S82.422R	S82.443R	S82.464Q	S82.56XP	S82.839M
S82.222N	S82.241N	S82.256N	S82.302K	S82.423K	S82.444K	S82.464R	S82.56XQ	S82.839N
S82.222P	S82.241P	S82.256P	S82.302M	S82.423M	S82.444M	S82.465K	S82.56XR	S82.839P
S82.222Q	S82.241Q	S82.256Q	S82.302N	S82.423N	S82.444N	S82.465M	S82.61XB	S82.839Q
S82.222R	S82.241R	S82.256R	S82.302P	S82.423P	S82.444P	S82.465N	S82.61XC	S82.839R
S82.223A	S82.242A	S82.261A	S82.302Q	S82.423Q	S82.444Q	S82.465P	S82.61XK	S82.841B
S82.223K	S82.242K	S82.261K	S82.302R	S82.423R	S82.444R	S82.465Q	S82.61XM	S82.841C
S82.223M	S82.242M	S82.261M	S82.309B	S82.424K	S82.445K	S82.465R	S82.61XN	S82.841K
S82.223N	S82.242N	S82.261N	S82.309C	S82.424M	S82.445M	S82.466K	S82.61XP	S82.841M
S82.223P	S82.242P	S82.261P	S82.309K	S82.424N	S82.445N	S82.466M	S82.61XQ	S82.841N
S82.223Q	S82.242Q	S82.261Q	S82.309M	S82.424P	S82.445P	S82.466N	S82.61XR	S82.841P
S82.223R	S82.242R	S82.261R	S82.309N	S82.424Q	S82.445Q	S82.466P	S82.62XB	S82.841Q
S82.224A	S82.243A	S82.262A	S82.309P	S82.424R	S82.445R	S82.466Q	S82.62XC	S82.841R
S82.224K	S82.243K	S82.262K	S82.309Q	S82.425K	S82.446K	S82.466R	S82.62XK	S82.842B
S82.224M	S82.243M	S82.262M	S82.309R	S82.425M	S82.446M	S82.491K	S82.62XM	S82.842C
S82.224N	S82.243N	S82.262N	S82.311A	S82.425N	S82.446N	S82.491M	S82.62XN	S82.842K
S82.224P	S82.243P	S82.262P	S82.311K	S82.425P	S82.446P	S82.491N	S82.62XP	S82.842M
S82.224Q	S82.243Q	S82.262Q	S82.311P	S82.425Q	S82.446Q	S82.491P	S82.62XQ	S82.842N
S82.224R	S82.243R	S82.262R	S82.312A	S82.425R	S82.446R	S82.491Q	S82.62XR	S82.842Q
S82.225A	S82.244A	S82.263A	S82.312K	S82.426K	S82.451K	S82.491R	S82.63XB	S82.842R
S82.225K	S82.244K	S82.263K	S82.312P	S82.426M	S82.451K			

S82.843B	S82.856P	S82.875Q	S85.162A	S88.111A	S89.119P	S92.002K	S92.051B	S92.125P
S82.843C	S82.856Q	S82.875R	S85.169A	S88.112A	S89.121K	S92.002P	S92.051K	S92.126B
S82.843K	S82.856R	S82.876B	S85.171A	S88.119A	S89.121P	S92.009B	S92.051P	S92.126K
S82.843M	S82.861K	S82.876C	S85.172A	S88.121A	S89.122K	S92.009K	S92.052B	S92.126P
S82.843N	S82.861M	S82.876K	S85.179A	S88.122A	S89.122P	S92.009P	S92.052K	S92.131B
S82.843P	S82.861N	S82.876M	S85.181A	S88.129A	S89.129K	S92.011B	S92.052P	S92.131K
S82.843Q	S82.861P	S82.876N	S85.182A	S88.911A	S89.129P	S92.011K	S92.053B	S92.131P
S82.843R	S82.861Q	S82.876P	S85.189A	S88.912A	S89.131K	S92.011P	S92.053K	S92.132B
S82.844B	S82.861R	S82.876Q	S85.201A	S88.919A	S89.131P	S92.012B	S92.053P	S92.132K
S82.844C	S82.862K	S82.876R	S85.202A	S88.921A	S89.132K	S92.012K	S92.054B	S92.132P
S82.844K	S82.862M	S82.891B	S85.209A	S88.922A	S89.132P	S92.012P	S92.054K	S92.133B
S82.844M	S82.862N	S82.891C	S85.211A	S88.929A	S89.139K	S92.013B	S92.054P	S92.133K
S82.844N	S82.862P	S82.891K	S85.212A	S89.001A	S89.139P	S92.013K	S92.055B	S92.133P
S82.844P	S82.862Q	S82.891M	S85.219A	S89.001K	S89.141K	S92.013P	S92.055K	S92.134B
S82.844Q	S82.862R	S82.891N	S85.291A	S89.001P	S89.141P	S92.014B	S92.055P	S92.134K
S82.844R	S82.863K	S82.891P	S85.292A	S89.002A	S89.142K	S92.014K	S92.056B	S92.134P
S82.845B	S82.863M	S82.891Q	S85.299A	S89.002K	S89.142P	S92.014P	S92.056K	S92.135B
S82.845C	S82.863N	S82.891R	S85.301A	S89.002P	S89.149K	S92.015B	S92.056P	S92.135K
S82.845K	S82.863P	S82.892B	S85.302A	S89.009A	S89.149P	S92.015K	S92.061B	S92.135P
S82.845M	S82.863Q	S82.892C	S85.309A	S89.009K	S89.191K	S92.015P	S92.061K	S92.136B
S82.845N	S82.863R	S82.892K	S85.311A	S89.009P	S89.191P	S92.016B	S92.061P	S92.136K
S82.845P	S82.864K	S82.892M	S85.312A	S89.011A	S89.192K	S92.016K	S92.062B	S92.136P
S82.845Q	S82.864M	S82.892N	S85.319A	S89.011K	S89.192P	S92.016P	S92.062K	S92.141B
S82.845R	S82.864N	S82.892P	S85.391A	S89.011P	S89.199K	S92.021B	S92.062P	S92.141K
S82.846B	S82.864P	S82.892Q	S85.392A	S89.012A	S89.199P	S92.021K	S92.063B	S92.141P
S82.846C	S82.864Q	S82.892R	S85.399A	S89.012K	S89.201K	S92.021P	S92.063K	S92.142B
S82.846K	S82.864R	S82.899B	S85.401A	S89.012P	S89.201P	S92.022B	S92.063P	S92.142K
S82.846M	S82.865K	S82.899C	S85.402A	S89.019A	S89.202K	S92.022K	S92.064B	S92.142P
S82.846N	S82.865M	S82.899K	S85.409A	S89.019K	S89.202P	S92.022P	S92.064K	S92.143B
S82.846P	S82.865N	S82.899M	S85.411A	S89.019P	S89.209K	S92.023B	S92.064P	S92.143K
S82.846Q	S82.865P	S82.899N	S85.412A	S89.021A	S89.209P	S92.023K	S92.065B	S92.143P
S82.846R	S82.865Q	S82.899P	S85.419A	S89.021K	S89.211K	S92.023P	S92.065K	S92.144B
S82.851B	S82.865R	S82.899Q	S85.491A	S89.021P	S89.211P	S92.024B	S92.065P	S92.144K
S82.851C	S82.866K	S82.899R	S85.492A	S89.022A	S89.212K	S92.024K	S92.066B	S92.144P
S82.851K	S82.866M	S82.90XB	S85.499A	S89.022K	S89.212P	S92.024P	S92.066K	S92.145B
S82.851M	S82.866N	S82.90XC	S85.801A	S89.022P	S89.219K	S92.025B	S92.066P	S92.145K
S82.851N	S82.866P	S82.90XK	S85.802A	S89.029A	S89.219P	S92.025K	S92.101B	S92.145P
S82.851P	S82.866Q	S82.90XM	S85.809A	S89.029K	S89.221K	S92.025P	S92.101K	S92.146B
S82.851Q	S82.866R	S82.90XN	S85.811A	S89.029P	S89.221P	S92.026B	S92.101P	S92.146K
S82.851R	S82.871B	S82.90XP	S85.812A	S89.031A	S89.222K	S92.026K	S92.102B	S92.146P
S82.852B	S82.871C	S82.90XQ	S85.819A	S89.031K	S89.222P	S92.026P	S92.102K	S92.151B
S82.852C	S82.871K	S82.90XR	S85.891A	S89.031P	S89.229K	S92.031B	S92.102P	S92.151K
S82.852K	S82.871M	S82.91XB	S85.892A	S89.032A	S89.229P	S92.031K	S92.109B	S92.151P
S82.852M	S82.871N	S82.91XC	S85.899A	S89.032K	S89.291K	S92.031P	S92.109K	S92.152B
S82.852N	S82.871P	S82.91XK	S85.901A	S89.032P	S89.291P	S92.032B	S92.109P	S92.152K
S82.852P	S82.871Q	S82.91XM	S85.909A	S89.039A	S89.292K	S92.032K	S92.111B	S92.152P
S82.852Q	S82.871R	S82.91XN	S85.911A	S89.039K	S89.292P	S92.032P	S92.111K	S92.153B
S82.852R	S82.872B	S82.91XP	S85.912A	S89.039P	S89.299K	S92.033B	S92.111P	S92.153K
S82.853B	S82.872C	S82.91XQ	S85.919A	S89.041A	S89.299P	S92.033K	S92.112B	S92.153P
S82.853C	S82.872K	S82.91XR	S85.991A	S89.041K	S89.301K	S92.033P	S92.112K	S92.154B
S82.853K	S82.872M	S82.92XB	S85.992A	S89.041P	S89.301P	S92.034B	S92.112P	S92.154K
S82.853M	S82.872N	S82.92XC	S85.999A	S89.042A	S89.302K	S92.034K	S92.113B	S92.154P
S82.853P	S82.872P	S82.92XK	S86.021A	S89.042K	S89.302P	S92.034P	S92.113K	S92.155B
S82.853Q	S82.872Q	S82.92XM	S86.022A	S89.042P	S89.309K	S92.035B	S92.113P	S92.155K
S82.853R	S82.872R	S82.92XN	S86.029A	S89.049A	S89.309P	S92.035K	S92.114B	S92.155P
S82.854B	S82.873B	S82.92XP	S86.121A	S89.049K	S89.311K	S92.035P	S92.114K	S92.156B
S82.854C	S82.873C	S82.92XQ	S86.122A	S89.049P	S89.311P	S92.036B	S92.114P	S92.156K
S82.854K	S82.873K	S82.92XR	S86.129A	S89.091A	S89.312K	S92.036K	S92.115B	S92.156P
S82.854M	S82.873M	S85.101A	S86.221A	S89.091K	S89.312P	S92.036P	S92.115K	S92.191B
S82.854N	S82.873N	S85.102A	S86.222A	S89.091P	S89.319K	S92.041B	S92.115P	S92.191K
S82.854P	S82.873P	S85.109A	S86.229A	S89.092A	S89.319P	S92.041K	S92.116B	S92.191P
S82.854Q	S82.873Q	S85.111A	S86.321A	S89.092K	S89.321K	S92.041P	S92.116K	S92.192B
S82.854R	S82.873R	S85.112A	S86.322A	S89.092P	S89.321P	S92.042B	S92.116P	S92.192K
S82.855B	S82.874B	S85.119A	S86.329A	S89.099A	S89.322K	S92.042K	S92.121B	S92.192P
S82.855C	S82.874C	S85.121A	S86.821A	S89.099K	S89.322P	S92.042P	S92.121K	S92.199B
S82.855K	S82.874K	S85.122A	S86.822A	S89.099P	S89.329K	S92.043B	S92.121P	S92.199K
S82.855M	S82.874M	S85.129A	S86.829A	S89.101K	S89.329P	S92.043K	S92.122B	S92.199P
S82.855N	S82.874N	S85.131A	S86.921A	S89.101P	S89.391K	S92.043P	S92.122K	S92.201B
S82.855P	S82.874P	S85.132A	S86.922A	S89.102K	S89.391P	S92.044B	S92.122P	S92.201K
S82.855Q	S82.874Q	S85.139A	S86.929A	S89.102P	S89.392K	S92.044K	S92.123B	S92.201P
S82.855R	S82.874R	S85.141A	S88.011A	S89.109K	S89.392P	S92.044P	S92.123K	S92.202B
S82.856B	S82.875B	S85.142A	S88.012A	S89.109P	S89.399K	S92.045B	S92.123P	S92.202K
S82.856C	S82.875C	S85.149A	S88.019A	S89.111K	S89.399P	S92.045K	S92.124B	S92.202P
S82.856K	S82.875M	S85.152A	S88.021A	S89.112K	S92.001K	S92.046B	S92.124K	S92.209K
S82.856M	S82.875N	S85.159A	S88.022A	S89.112P	S92.001P	S92.046K	S92.124P	S92.209P
S82.856N	S82.875P	S85.161A	S88.029A	S89.119K	S92.002B	S92.046P	S92.125K	S92.211B

S92.211K	S92.253B	S92.341P	S92.501P	S95.001A	S98.929A	T22.329A	T23.741A	T27.2XXA
S92.211P	S92.253K	S92.342B	S92.502K	S95.002A	T17.400A	T22.331A	T23.742A	T27.3XXA
S92.212B	S92.253P	S92.342K	S92.502P	S95.009A	T17.408A	T22.332A	T23.749A	T27.4XXA
S92.212K	S92.254B	S92.342P	S92.503K	S95.011A	T17.410A	T22.339A	T23.751A	T27.5XXA
S92.212P	S92.254K	S92.343B	S92.503P	S95.012A	T17.418A	T22.341A	T23.752A	T27.6XXA
S92.213B	S92.254P	S92.343K	S92.504K	S95.019A	T17.420A	T22.342A	T23.759A	T27.7XXA
S92.213K	S92.255B	S92.343P	S92.504P	S95.091A	T17.428A	T22.349A	T23.761A	T28.1XXA
S92.213P	S92.255K	S92.344B	S92.505K	S95.092A	T17.490A	T22.351A	T23.762A	T28.2XXA
S92.214B	S92.255P	S92.344K	S92.505P	S95.099A	T17.498A	T22.352A	T23.769A	T28.6XXA
S92.214K	S92.256B	S92.344P	S92.506K	S95.101A	T17.500A	T22.359A	T23.771A	T28.7XXA
S92.214P	S92.256K	S92.345B	S92.506P	S95.102A	T17.508A	T22.361A	T23.772A	T31.10
S92.215B	S92.256P	S92.345K	S92.511K	S95.109A	T17.510A	T22.362A	T23.779A	T31.11
S92.215K	S92.301B	S92.345P	S92.511P	S95.111A	T17.518A	T22.369A	T23.791A	T31.20
S92.215P	S92.301K	S92.346B	S92.512K	S95.112A	T17.520A	T22.391A	T23.792A	T31.30
S92.216B	S92.301P	S92.346K	S92.512P	S95.119A	T17.528A	T22.392A	T23.799A	T31.40
S92.216K	S92.302B	S92.346P	S92.513K	S95.191A	T17.590A	T22.399A	T24.301A	T31.50
S92.216P	S92.302K	S92.351B	S92.513P	S95.192A	T17.598A	T22.70XA	T24.302A	T31.60
S92.221B	S92.302P	S92.351K	S92.514K	S95.199A	T17.800A	T22.711A	T24.309A	T31.70
S92.221K	S92.309B	S92.351P	S92.514P	S95.201A	T17.808A	T22.712A	T24.311A	T31.80
S92.221P	S92.309K	S92.352B	S92.515K	S95.202A	T17.810A	T22.719A	T24.312A	T31.90
S92.222B	S92.309P	S92.352K	S92.515P	S95.209A	T17.818A	T22.721A	T24.319A	T32.10
S92.222K	S92.311B	S92.352P	S92.516K	S95.211A	T17.820A	T22.722A	T24.321A	T32.11
S92.222P	S92.311K	S92.353B	S92.516P	S95.212A	T17.828A	T22.729A	T24.322A	T32.20
S92.223B	S92.311P	S92.353K	S92.521K	S95.219A	T17.890A	T22.731A	T24.329A	T32.30
S92.223K	S92.312B	S92.353P	S92.521P	S95.291A	T17.898A	T22.732A	T24.331A	T32.40
S92.223P	S92.312K	S92.354B	S92.522K	S95.292A	T17.900A	T22.739A	T24.332A	T32.50
S92.224B	S92.312P	S92.354K	S92.522P	S95.299A	T17.910A	T22.741A	T24.339A	T32.60
S92.224K	S92.313B	S92.354P	S92.523K	S95.801A	T17.920A	T22.742A	T24.391A	T32.70
S92.224P	S92.313K	S92.355B	S92.523P	S95.802A	T17.990A	T22.749A	T24.392A	T32.80
S92.225B	S92.313P	S92.355K	S92.524K	S95.809A	T18.190A	T22.751A	T24.399A	T32.90
S92.225K	S92.314B	S92.355P	S92.524P	S95.811A	T18.2XXA	T22.752A	T24.701A	T33.011A
S92.225P	S92.314K	S92.356B	S92.525K	S95.812A	T20.30XA	T22.759A	T24.702A	T33.012A
S92.226B	S92.314P	S92.356K	S92.525P	S95.819A	T20.311A	T22.761A	T24.709A	T33.019A
S92.226K	S92.315B	S92.356P	S92.526K	S95.891A	T20.312A	T22.762A	T24.711A	T33.02XA
S92.226P	S92.315K	S92.401K	S92.526P	S95.892A	T20.319A	T22.769A	T24.712A	T33.09XA
S92.231B	S92.315P	S92.401P	S92.531K	S95.899A	T20.32XA	T22.791A	T24.719A	T33.1XXA
S92.231K	S92.316B	S92.402K	S92.531P	S95.901A	T20.33XA	T22.792A	T24.721A	T33.2XXA
S92.231P	S92.316K	S92.402P	S92.532K	S95.902A	T20.34XA	T22.799A	T24.722A	T33.3XXA
S92.232B	S92.316P	S92.403K	S92.532P	S95.909A	T20.35XA	T23.301A	T24.729A	T33.40XA
S92.232K	S92.321B	S92.403P	S92.533K	S95.911A	T20.36XA	T23.302A	T24.731A	T33.41XA
S92.232P	S92.321K	S92.404K	S92.533P	S95.912A	T20.37XA	T23.309A	T24.732A	T33.42XA
S92.233B	S92.321P	S92.404P	S92.534K	S95.919A	T20.39XA	T23.311A	T24.739A	T33.511A
S92.233K	S92.322B	S92.405K	S92.534P	S95.991A	T20.70XA	T23.312A	T24.791A	T33.512A
S92.233P	S92.322K	S92.405P	S92.535K	S95.992A	T20.711A	T23.319A	T24.792A	T33.519A
S92.234B	S92.322P	S92.406K	S92.535P	S95.999A	T20.712A	T23.321A	T24.799A	T33.521A
S92.234K	S92.323B	S92.406P	S92.536K	S96.021A	T20.719A	T23.322A	T25.311A	T33.522A
S92.234P	S92.323K	S92.411K	S92.536P	S96.022A	T20.72XA	T23.329A	T25.312A	T33.529A
S92.235B	S92.323P	S92.411P	S92.591K	S96.029A	T20.73XA	T23.331A	T25.319A	T33.531A
S92.235K	S92.324B	S92.412K	S92.591P	S96.121A	T20.74XA	T23.332A	T25.321A	T33.532A
S92.235P	S92.324K	S92.412P	S92.592K	S96.122A	T20.75XA	T23.339A	T25.322A	T33.539A
S92.236B	S92.324P	S92.413K	S92.592P	S96.129A	T20.76XA	T23.341A	T25.329A	T33.60XA
S92.236K	S92.325B	S92.413P	S92.599K	S96.221A	T20.77XA	T23.342A	T25.331A	T33.61XA
S92.236P	S92.325K	S92.414K	S92.599P	S96.222A	T20.79XA	T23.349A	T25.332A	T33.62XA
S92.241B	S92.325P	S92.414P	S92.811B	S96.229A	T21.30XA	T23.351A	T25.339A	T33.70XA
S92.241K	S92.326B	S92.415K	S92.811K	S96.821A	T21.31XA	T23.352A	T25.391A	T33.71XA
S92.241P	S92.326K	S92.415P	S92.811P	S96.822A	T21.32XA	T23.359A	T25.392A	T33.72XA
S92.242B	S92.326P	S92.416K	S92.812B	S96.829A	T21.33XA	T23.361A	T25.399A	T33.811A
S92.242K	S92.331B	S92.416P	S92.812K	S96.921A	T21.34XA	T23.362A	T25.711A	T33.812A
S92.242P	S92.331K	S92.421K	S92.812P	S96.922A	T21.35XA	T23.369A	T25.712A	T33.819A
S92.243B	S92.331P	S92.421P	S92.819B	S96.929A	T21.36XA	T23.371A	T25.719A	T33.821A
S92.243K	S92.332B	S92.422K	S92.819K	S98.011A	T21.37XA	T23.372A	T25.721A	T33.822A
S92.243P	S92.332K	S92.422P	S92.819P	S98.012A	T21.39XA	T23.379A	T25.722A	T33.829A
S92.244B	S92.332P	S92.423K	S92.901B	S98.019A	T21.70XA	T23.391A	T25.729A	T33.831A
S92.244K	S92.333B	S92.423P	S92.901K	S98.021A	T21.71XA	T23.392A	T25.731A	T33.832A
S92.244P	S92.333K	S92.424K	S92.901P	S98.022A	T21.72XA	T23.399A	T25.732A	T33.839A
S92.245B	S92.333P	S92.424P	S92.902B	S98.029A	T21.73XA	T23.701A	T25.739A	T33.90XA
S92.245K	S92.334B	S92.425K	S92.902K	S98.311A	T21.74XA	T23.702A	T25.791A	T33.99XA
S92.245P	S92.334K	S92.425P	S92.902P	S98.312A	T21.75XA	T23.709A	T25.792A	T34.011A
S92.246B	S92.334P	S92.426K	S92.909B	S98.319A	T21.76XA	T23.711A	T25.799A	T34.012A
S92.246K	S92.335B	S92.426P	S92.909K	S98.321A	T21.77XA	T23.712A	T26.20XA	T34.019A
S92.246P	S92.335K	S92.491K	S92.909P	S98.322A	T21.79XA	T23.719A	T26.21XA	T34.02XA
S92.251B	S92.335P	S92.491P	S92.911K	S98.329A	T22.30XA	T23.721A	T26.22XA	T34.09XA
S92.251K	S92.336B	S92.492K	S92.911P	S98.911A	T22.311A	T23.722A	T26.70XA	T34.1XXA
S92.251P	S92.336K	S92.492P	S92.912K	S98.912A	T22.312A	T23.729A	T26.71XA	T34.2XXA
S92.252B	S92.336P	S92.499K	S92.912P	S98.919A	T22.319A	T23.731A	T26.72XA	T34.3XXA
S92.252K	S92.341B	S92.499P	S92.919K	S98.921A	T22.321A	T23.732A	T27.0XXA	T34.40XA
S92.252P	S92.341K	S92.501K	S92.919P	S98.922A	T22.322A	T23.739A	T27.1XXA	T34.41XA

Appendix E: Complication and Comorbidity (CC) Code List

T34.42XA	T74.22XA	T80.A9XA	T82.119A	T82.828A	T83.9XXA	T84.320A	T85.520A	T86.41
T34.511A	T74.32XA	T81.10XA	T82.120A	T82.837A	T84.010A	T84.328A	T85.521A	T86.42
T34.512A	T74.4XXA	T81.30XA	T82.121A	T82.838A	T84.011A	T84.390A	T85.528A	T86.43
T34.519A	T74.51XA	T81.31XA	T82.128A	T82.847A	T84.012A	T84.398A	T85.590A	T86.49
T34.521A	T74.52XA	T81.32XA	T82.129A	T82.848A	T84.013A	T84.410A	T85.591A	T86.5
T34.522A	T74.61XA	T81.33XA	T82.190A	T82.855A	T84.018A	T84.418A	T85.598A	T86.810
T34.529A	T74.62XA	T81.40XA	T82.191A	T82.856A	T84.019A	T84.420A	T85.610A	T86.811
T34.531A	T74.91XA	T81.41XA	T82.198A	T82.857A	T84.020A	T84.428A	T85.611A	T86.812
T34.532A	T74.92XA	T81.42XA	T82.199A	T82.858A	T84.021A	T84.490A	T85.612A	T86.818
T34.539A	T75.1XXA	T81.43XA	T82.211A	T82.867A	T84.022A	T84.498A	T85.613A	T86.819
T34.60XA	T76.01XA	T81.44XA	T82.212A	T82.868A	T84.023A	T84.50XA	T85.614A	T86.820
T34.61XA	T76.02XA	T81.49XA	T82.213A	T82.897A	T84.028A	T84.51XA	T85.615A	T86.821
T34.62XA	T76.11XA	T81.500A	T82.218A	T82.898A	T84.029A	T84.52XA	T85.618A	T86.822
T34.70XA	T76.12XA	T81.501A	T82.221A	T82.9XXA	T84.030A	T84.53XA	T85.620A	T86.828
T34.71XA	T76.21XA	T81.502A	T82.222A	T83.010A	T84.031A	T84.54XA	T85.621A	T86.829
T34.72XA	T76.22XA	T81.503A	T82.223A	T83.020A	T84.032A	T84.59XA	T85.622A	T86.830
T34.811A	T76.32XA	T81.504A	T82.228A	T83.030A	T84.033A	T84.60XA	T85.623A	T86.831
T34.812A	T76.51XA	T81.505A	T82.310A	T83.090A	T84.038A	T84.610A	T85.624A	T86.832
T34.819A	T76.52XA	T81.506A	T82.311A	T83.110A	T84.039A	T84.611A	T85.625A	T86.838
T34.821A	T76.61XA	T81.507A	T82.312A	T83.111A	T84.050A	T84.612A	T85.628A	T86.839
T34.822A	T76.62XA	T81.508A	T82.318A	T83.112A	T84.051A	T84.613A	T85.630A	T86.840
T34.829A	T76.91XA	T81.509A	T82.319A	T83.113A	T84.052A	T84.614A	T85.631A	T86.841
T34.831A	T76.92XA	T81.510A	T82.320A	T83.118A	T84.053A	T84.615A	T85.633A	T86.842
T34.832A	T78.00XA	T81.511A	T82.321A	T83.120A	T84.058A	T84.619A	T85.635A	T86.848
T34.839A	T78.01XA	T81.512A	T82.322A	T83.121A	T84.059A	T84.620A	T85.638A	T86.849
T34.90XA	T78.02XA	T81.513A	T82.328A	T83.122A	T84.060A	T84.621A	T85.690A	T86.850
T34.99XA	T78.03XA	T81.514A	T82.329A	T83.123A	T84.061A	T84.622A	T85.691A	T86.851
T67.01XA	T78.04XA	T81.515A	T82.330A	T83.128A	T84.062A	T84.623A	T85.692A	T86.852
T67.02XA	T78.05XA	T81.516A	T82.331A	T83.190A	T84.063A	T84.624A	T85.693A	T86.858
T67.09XA	T78.06XA	T81.517A	T82.332A	T83.191A	T84.068A	T84.625A	T85.694A	T86.859
T69.021A	T78.07XA	T81.518A	T82.338A	T83.192A	T84.069A	T84.629A	T85.695A	T86.890
T69.022A	T78.08XA	T81.519A	T82.339A	T83.193A	T84.090A	T84.63XA	T85.698A	T86.891
T69.029A	T78.09XA	T81.520A	T82.390A	T83.198A	T84.091A	T84.69XA	T85.71XA	T86.892
T70.3XXA	T78.2XXA	T81.521A	T82.391A	T83.21XA	T84.092A	T84.7XXA	T85.72XA	T86.898
T71.111A	T79.2XXA	T81.522A	T82.392A	T83.22XA	T84.093A	T84.81XA	T85.730A	T86.899
T71.112A	T79.7XXA	T81.523A	T82.398A	T83.23XA	T84.098A	T84.82XA	T85.731A	T86.90
T71.113A	T79.A0XA	T81.524A	T82.399A	T83.24XA	T84.099A	T84.83XA	T85.732A	T86.91
T71.114A	T79.A11A	T81.525A	T82.41XA	T83.25XA	T84.110A	T84.84XA	T85.733A	T86.92
T71.121A	T79.A12A	T81.526A	T82.42XA	T83.29XA	T84.111A	T84.85XA	T85.734A	T86.93
T71.122A	T79.A19A	T81.527A	T82.43XA	T83.410A	T84.112A	T84.86XA	T85.735A	T86.99
T71.123A	T79.A21A	T81.528A	T82.49XA	T83.411A	T84.113A	T84.89XA	T85.738A	T87.0X1
T71.124A	T79.A22A	T81.529A	T82.510A	T83.418A	T84.114A	T84.9XXA	T85.79XA	T87.0X2
T71.131A	T79.A29A	T81.530A	T82.511A	T83.420A	T84.115A	T85.01XA	T85.810A	T87.0X9
T71.132A	T79.A3XA	T81.531A	T82.512A	T83.421A	T84.116A	T85.02XA	T85.810D	T87.1X1
T71.133A	T79.A9XA	T81.532A	T82.513A	T83.428A	T84.117A	T85.03XA	T85.820A	T87.1X2
T71.134A	T80.1XXA	T81.533A	T82.514A	T83.490A	T84.119A	T85.09XA	T85.820D	T87.1X9
T71.141A	T80.211A	T81.534A	T82.515A	T83.491A	T84.120A	T85.110A	T85.830A	ICD87.2
T71.143A	T80.212A	T81.535A	T82.518A	T83.498A	T84.121A	T85.111A	T85.830D	T87.40
T71.144A	T80.218A	T81.536A	T82.519A	T83.510A	T84.122A	T85.112A	T85.840A	T87.41
T71.151A	T80.219A	T81.537A	T82.520A	T83.511A	T84.123A	T85.113A	T85.840D	T87.42
T71.152A	T80.22XA	T81.538A	T82.521A	T83.512A	T84.124A	T85.118A	T85.850A	T87.43
T71.153A	T80.29XA	T81.539A	T82.522A	T83.518A	T84.125A	T85.120A	T85.850D	T87.44
T71.154A	T80.30XA	T81.590A	T82.523A	T83.590A	T84.126A	T85.121A	T85.860A	T88.0XXA
T71.161A	T80.310A	T81.591A	T82.524A	T83.591A	T84.127A	T85.122A	T85.860D	T88.1XXA
T71.162A	T80.311A	T81.592A	T82.525A	T83.592A	T84.129A	T85.123A	T85.890A	T88.2XXA
T71.163A	T80.319A	T81.593A	T82.528A	T83.593A	T84.190A	T85.128A	T85.890D	T88.3XXA
T71.164A	T80.39XA	T81.594A	T82.529A	T83.598A	T84.191A	T85.190A	T86.00	T88.6XXA
T71.191A	T80.40XA	T81.595A	T82.530A	T83.61XA	T84.192A	T85.191A	T86.01	Z16.12
T71.192A	T80.410A	T81.596A	T82.531A	T83.62XA	T84.193A	T85.192A	T86.02	Z16.21
T71.193A	T80.411A	T81.597A	T82.532A	T83.69XA	T84.194A	T85.193A	T86.03	Z16.24
T71.194A	T80.419A	T81.598A	T82.533A	T83.712A	T84.195A	T85.199A	T86.09	Z16.39
T71.20XA	T80.49XA	T81.599A	T82.534A	T83.713A	T84.196A	T85.21XA	T86.10	Z48.21
T71.21XA	T80.51XA	T81.60XA	T82.535A	T83.714A	T84.197A	T85.22XA	T86.11	Z48.22
T71.221A	T80.60XA	T81.61XA	T82.538A	T83.718A	T84.199A	T85.29XA	T86.12	Z48.23
T71.222A	T80.52XA	T81.69XA	T82.539A	T83.719A	T84.210A	T85.310A	T86.13	Z48.24
T71.223A	T80.59XA	T81.710A	T82.590A	T83.722A	T84.213A	T85.311A	T86.19	Z48.280
T71.224A	T80.61XA	T81.711A	T82.591A	T83.723A	T84.216A	T85.320A	T86.20	Z48.290
T71.231A	T80.62XA	T81.718A	T82.592A	T83.724A	T84.218A	T85.321A	T86.21	Z59.0
T71.232A	T80.69XA	T81.719A	T82.593A	T83.728A	T84.220A	T85.390A	T86.22	Z68.43
T71.233A	T80.810A	T81.72XA	T82.594A	T83.729A	T84.223A	T85.391A	T86.23	Z68.44
T71.234A	T80.818A	T81.83XA	T82.595A	T83.79XA	T84.226A	T85.41XA	T86.290	Z68.45
T71.29XA	T80.89XA	T82.01XA	T82.598A	T83.81XA	T84.228A	T85.42XA	T86.298	
T71.9XXA	T80.910A	T82.02XA	T82.599A	T83.82XA	T84.290A	T85.43XA	T86.30	
T74.01XA	T80.911A	T82.03XA	T82.6XXA	T83.83XA	T84.293A	T85.44XA	T86.31	
T74.02XA	T80.919A	T82.09XA	T82.7XXA	T83.84XA	T84.296A	T85.49XA	T86.32	
T74.11XA	T80.A0XA	T82.110A	T82.817A	T83.85XA	T84.298A	T85.510A	T86.33	
T74.12XA	T80.A10A	T82.111A	T82.818A	T83.86XA	T84.310A	T85.511A	T86.39	
T74.21XA	T80.A11A	T82.118A	T82.827A	T83.89XA	T84.318A	T85.518A	T86.40	
	T80.A19A							

Present-on-admission (POA) indicators are required on all diagnoses and external cause-of-injury codes for all inpatient acute care hospital discharges, according to the requirement outlined in the Deficit Reduction Act of 2005, section 5001(c). The only exception is for a select group of codes that have been designated as exempt from the POA regulations. Certain facilities are also exempt from this reporting requirement and include the following:

- Critical access hospitals
- Long-term care hospitals
- Cancer hospitals
- Inpatient psychiatric hospitals
- Inpatient rehabilitation facilities
- Veterans Administration/Department of Defense Hospitals
- Children's inpatient facilities

The POA indicator guidelines are not intended to replace the official *ICD-10-CM Official Guidelines for Coding and Reporting*. Nor will the POA guidelines supersede the Uniform Hospital Discharge Data Set (UHDDS) definition of principal diagnosis, defined as the condition established after study to be chiefly responsible for occasioning the admission of the patient to the hospital. The definition of "additional diagnoses" also remains the same. Coders must report all conditions that coexist at the time of admission, develop subsequently, or that affect the treatment received and/or the length of stay. This significantly affects assignment of the POA indicators. Because the POA indicator should accurately reflect the patient's conditions upon admission, review of POA guidelines as well as the *ICD-10-CM Official Guidelines for Coding and Reporting* is required.

The following is a summary of the POA guidelines:

- A POA condition is defined not only as one that is clearly present at the time of admission, but also one that was clearly present but not diagnosed until after the time of admission.

- Present on admission is defined as present at the time the order for an inpatient admission is made, whether or not the patient's episode of care originated in the emergency department, ambulatory surgery area, or other outpatient area. Conditions that develop during an outpatient encounter are considered present on admission.

- A POA indicator is assigned to the principal diagnosis, secondary diagnoses, and the external cause-of-injury codes.

- The POA guidelines are not intended to replace any of the other *ICD-10-CM Official Guidelines for Coding and Reporting*.

- The intent of the POA guidelines is not to determine whether or not a condition should be coded, but rather how to apply the POA indicator.

The following reporting options, with definitions, should be used to indicate whether a condition was POA:

Y   *Yes: Present at the time of inpatient admission*
N   *No: Not present at the time of inpatient admission*
U   *Unknown: Documentation is insufficient to determine if condition is present at the time of inpatient admission*
W   *Clinically undetermined: Provider is unable to clinically determine whether condition was or was not present at the time of inpatient admission*

Unreported/not used—(exempt from POA reporting)—Most ICD-10-CM codes require the assignment of a POA indicator. However, there are some diagnoses that are considered exempt from the POA reporting. For these exempt conditions the POA field should be left blank.

Note: *A data file of all POA exempt codes can be accessed at the following: http://www.optum360coding.com/ProductUpdates/ Title: "2020 ICD-10-CM for Hospitals POA Exemption Data File" Password: OptumPOAExempt20*

Timeframe for POA identification and documentation

There is no timeframe during the encounter in which a condition must be diagnosed to be considered present on admission. In many cases, it is not clinically possible for the provider to determine a definitive diagnosis until well into the admission, after labs, imaging, and other tests have been performed and results examined. In these cases the condition is still considered to be present on admission, indicated with Y.

Examples

- A patient was admitted for diagnostic work-up for cachexia. The final diagnosis was malignant neoplasm of lung with metastasis.

  Assign Y in the POA field for the malignant neoplasm, which was clearly present on admission, although it was not diagnosed until after the admission occurred.

- A patient with severe cough and difficulty breathing was diagnosed during his hospitalization to have lung cancer.

  Assign Y in the POA field for the lung cancer. Even though the cancer was not diagnosed until after admission, it is a chronic condition that was clearly present before the patient's admission.

- A urine culture was obtained on admission. The provider documented urinary tract infection when the culture results became available a few days later.

  Assign Y to the urinary tract infection since the diagnosis is based on test results from a specimen obtained on admission. It may not be possible for a provider to make a definitive diagnosis for a period of time after admission. There is no required timeframe as to when a provider must identify or document a condition for it to be considered present on admission.

Condition is on the "Exempt from Reporting" list

The POA field is left blank for codes excluded from POA reporting.

Examples

- A patient was admitted for inpatient surgery on a burn contracture from scar tissue from a burn five years ago.

  Assign Y for the principal condition of the scar; however, the secondary code for the specifics of the burn injury with a seventh character for sequela is left blank since it is excluded from POA reporting.

- A patient was admitted to inpatient for a PEG tube insertion because of residual dysphagia due to a recent CVA.

  No POA indicator is assigned for the dysphagia following a CVA. Codes under I69.- are defined as sequela of cerebrovascular disease and are exempt from POA reporting.

- A patient was admitted to inpatient for corrective surgery for a malunion of a closed femur fracture.

  No POA indicator is assigned for the malunion of a closed fracture because the seventh character for malunion of fractures is considered a subsequent encounter and is exempt from POA reporting.

- A patient was admitted for breast reconstruction following mastectomy.

  The POA indicator field is left blank as this Z code is exempt from POA reporting.

- A patient was admitted for changing the battery in his AICD as it is at the end of its useful life.

  The POA indicator field is left blank as this Z code is exempt from POA reporting.

POA explicitly documented

If the provider explicitly documents a condition as being present on admission or not present on admission, assign the appropriate Y or N POA indicator based on that documentation. If there is conflicting documentation by different providers, query the attending physician.

Examples

- Even though sepsis is not diagnosed in the ED, the discharge summary states that the patient presented with sepsis at the time of admission.

  The provider explicitly stated that the sepsis was present on admission and therefore the Y POA indicator should be used.

- The patient was admitted with chills and cough and two days later diagnosed with pneumonia. The discharge summary documents that the pneumonia was not present on admission.

  Although the patient showed some symptoms of pneumonia on admission, the provider may have clinical evidence (e.g., chest x-rays, cultures) that indicates that pneumonia did not develop until after admission. Since this was explicitly stated in the discharge summary, the appropriate POA indicator is N.

- A consult note states that a patient came in with renal failure while the discharge summary states that the renal failure was not present on admission.

    When in doubt and there is conflicting documentation, query the attending physician.

Conditions diagnosed prior to inpatient admission

Conditions that were diagnosed prior to admission—for example, chronic conditions such as hypertension, diabetes, and asthma—are assigned the POA indicator of Y. A tip to help establish that a condition was POA is to check the patient's medication history for drugs that are routinely prescribed for these types of chronic conditions.

Examples

- The history and physical states that the patient has a history of hypertension and seizure disorder, and it is noted that the patient is currently on Atenolol and Dilantin.

    The hypertension and seizure disorder existed prior to admission; therefore, the appropriate POA indicator is Y. Verification that the patient is on long-term use of Atenolol and Dilantin can help solidify that these conditions are currently being treated.

- A 56-year-old male was admitted as an inpatient for multi-trauma wounds. Because the patient was unconscious on admission, his medical history was unknown. A progress note two days into the stay noted that the patient was on Metformin for history of type 2 diabetes.

    The timeframe of the diagnosis is irrelevant to POA. Even though it was not discovered until two days into the encounter that the patient had a history of DM2, the DM2 was still present prior to this admission and would be identified as such with the Y POA indicator.

- A patient was admitted to an inpatient facility from the ED. The admitting provider indicated that the patient had a current history of lung cancer and chronic kidney disease.

    Both of these conditions are indicated with Y, present on admission.

- During the course of an eight-day inpatient stay with surgery, a patient was diagnosed postoperatively with hypertension and discharged on Metoprolol.

    The hypertension was not diagnosed prior to admission and would be reported with an N POA indicator.

Conditions diagnosed during the admission but clearly present before admission

The POA indicator Y is assigned for conditions that clearly presented with applicable signs and symptoms but may have not been definitively diagnosed until later on, or even at the end of the encounter. Even if the presenting diagnosis was documented on admission as suspected, possible, or rule out, or written as a differential diagnosis and later confirmed, it is still considered present on admission.

Examples

- A patient was admitted with jaundice, fatigue, and mental confusion. Differential diagnosis on admission lists possible liver failure. The definitive diagnosis of liver failure is not made until two days after admission.

    Assign Y to the liver failure since the symptoms were present on admission and the differential diagnosis listed "possible" liver failure on admission even though the final diagnosis was two days later.

- An aid worker recently returned from Afghanistan presents to the ED with hematemesis, chest pain, and fever. Patient is put into inpatient isolation with suspected TB documented on the H & P. TB is confirmed the next day.

    The POA indicator Y is assigned because, even though the TB was only "suspected" on admission, it was confirmed the next day.

Condition develops during outpatient encounter prior to inpatient admission

Assign Y for any condition that develops during an outpatient encounter such as same-day surgery, observation, or extended recovery prior to a written order for inpatient admission. This also pertains to conditions that develop in

facilities such as transitional care units, skilled nursing homes, long-term care, hospice, or rehabilitation facilities with the patient transferring to inpatient hospital admission.

Examples

- A patient underwent outpatient surgery. During the recovery period, the patient developed atrial fibrillation and was subsequently admitted to the hospital as an inpatient.

    Assign Y on the POA field for the atrial fibrillation since it developed prior to a written order for inpatient admission.

- A patient was treated in observation and while in observation fell out of bed and broke a hip. The patient was subsequently admitted as an inpatient to treat the hip fracture.

    Assign Y on the POA field for the hip fracture since it developed prior to a written order for inpatient admission.

- An elderly patient underwent outpatient surgery with plans to go home after the surgery. In recovery, the patient developed shortness of breath, chest pain, and fever. A sputum sample was taken, and the surgeon decided to admit the patient to inpatient. The next day the patient was diagnosed with staphylococcal pneumonia based on sputum results and admitting chest x-ray.

    Assign Y to the staphylococcal pneumonia even though it was not diagnosed until the day following the admission. Even though the patient had undergone outpatient surgery, the sputum sample, signs, and symptoms were evident prior to the inpatient admission.

Documentation does not indicate whether condition was present on admission

If the documentation in the medical record is unclear as to the presence of a condition on admission, assign a U for unknown. This should be used sparingly and, if possible, the physician should be queried for further clarification.

Example

- A wheelchair-bound patient was admitted in respiratory failure from a long-term care facility to an inpatient hospital with severe aspiration pneumonia. A progress note three days into the admission listed a pressure ulcer stage 2 on the lower back.

    Assign U for the stage 2 pressure ulcer if unknown whether it was present on admission. Since the patient was wheelchair-bound and critically ill on admission, it is possible that the ulcer was present and not immediately addressed. The admitting physician can be queried to clarify, or a U is assigned if that is not possible.

Documentation states it cannot be determined whether the condition was or was not present on admission

A W is assigned when the documentation states that it cannot be clinically determined whether the condition was POA or not.

Examples

- An elderly patient was admitted with multi-trauma injuries from a motor vehicle accident. Two days into the admission, a urinary tract infection was diagnosed. No labs or urine cultures had been taken on admission as focus was stabilization from traumatic wounds. Documentation from the provider in a progress note stated that it was not clinically possible to determine whether the UTI was present on admission.

    Assign W for the UTI as it was specifically stated that it was not clinically possible to determine whether it was present on admission.

- A patient was admitted with high fever and pneumonia. The patient rapidly deteriorated and became septic. The discharge diagnosis listed sepsis and pneumonia. The documentation was unclear as to whether the sepsis was present on admission or developed shortly after admission.

    Query the physician as to whether the sepsis was present on admission, developed shortly after admission, or it cannot be clinically determined as to whether it was or was not present on admission.

Chronic condition with acute exacerbation during the admission

If a single code identifies only the chronic condition and not the acute exacerbation, assign Y. For instance, when there is no code for the acute exacerbation of a chronic condition as in acute exacerbation of chronic leukemia, the Y is assigned for the chronic leukemia.

For a single combination code that identifies both the chronic and acute exacerbation, see the combination code instructions.

Example

- Documentation on admission stated that the patient had chronic myelomonocytic leukemia. A progress note three days into the stay stated that the patient had, since admission, developed an acute exacerbation of his myelomonocytic leukemia.

  There is no code for an acute exacerbation of chronic myelomonocytic leukemia; therefore, assign Y since the chronic leukemia (either not specified as in remission, or in relapse) is represented by a single code and was present on admission.

Acute and chronic conditions

Assign Y to acute conditions present on admission and N to acute conditions not present at the time of admission.

Assign Y to conditions specified as chronic, even though they may not be diagnosed until after admission.

See the POA guideline "Codes that contain multiple clinical concepts" for a single code that identifies both the acute and chronic condition.

Examples

- A patient was admitted to the hospital for coronary artery bypass surgery. Postoperatively he developed a pulmonary embolism.

  Assign N in the POA field for the pulmonary embolism. This is an acute condition that was not present on admission.

- A patient admitted with sepsis due to pneumonia with acute respiratory failure, developed acute renal failure on day three.

  Assign Y for the sepsis, pneumonia, and acute respiratory failure, which were all acute conditions, present on admission. Assign N for the acute renal failure; even though it is an acute condition, it was not present until after the patient was admitted.

- A patient admitted with hypoglycemia, weakness, confusion, and slurred speech was diagnosed the next day with type 2 diabetes.

  Assign Y to the type 2 diabetes since it is a chronic condition that was present on admission, even though it was not diagnosed until the next day.

Codes that contain multiple clinical concepts

If at least one of the clinical concepts included in a code was not present on admission, assign N. If all the clinical concepts included in a code are present on admission, assign Y.

Examples

- Patient has history of gastrojejunal ulcer which started bleeding two days into the encounter.

  Assign a POA indicator of N to chronic gastrojejunal ulcer with bleeding; although the gastrojejunal ulcer is a chronic condition that was present at the time of admission, the bleeding did not occur until after the admission.

- A patient with chronic diastolic heart failure decompensated after admission.

  Assign N to the code for acute on chronic diastolic (congestive) heart failure. Although the heart failure was present on admission, the acute decompensation of the failure was not.

- A patient with viral hepatitis B progressed to hepatic coma after admission.

  Assign N for the viral hepatitis B with hepatic coma because a condition described by part of the code description did not develop until after admission.

- A patient with known systolic congestive heart failure was admitted to the hospital with decompensated systolic heart failure.

  Assign Y in the POA field for the acute on chronic systolic (congestive) heart failure as both the chronic and acute parts of the condition were present on admission.

Assign Y for infection codes that include the organism if the infection was present on admission even though the culture results are not available until after admission.

Example

- A patient was septic on admission with blood, sputum, and urine cultures taken. Two days later, *E. coli* was determined to be the causal organism.

  Assign Y even though the test results were not confirmed until after admission.

Conditions documented as possible, probable, suspected, or rule out at the time of discharge or conditions documented as impending or threatened at the time of discharge

If the final diagnosis contains language identifying a condition as possible, probable, suspected, or rule out, or as an impending or threatened diagnosis but the diagnosis is based on signs and symptoms that were present on admission, the POA indicator is Y. If those signs and symptoms were not present on admission, the appropriate POA indicator is N.

Examples

- A patient underwent inpatient surgery, after which the patient developed fever and was treated aggressively. The physician's final diagnosis documented "possible postoperative infection following surgery."

  Assign N on the POA field for the postoperative infection since final diagnoses that contain the terms "possible," "probable," "suspected," or "rule out" and that are based on symptoms or clinical findings that were not present on admission should be reported as N.

- A patient with prior cardiac intervention history was admitted with chest pain. After two days, the chest pain diminished with no underlying cause found. The discharge summary stated, "Suspected costochondritis or coronary artery spasm. Pain resolved. Follow up at regular cardiology office visit."

  Since the chest pain was present on admission, both suspected conditions of costochondritis and coronary artery spasm are represented by the POA indicator of Y.

- A patient was admitted with a known history of coronary atherosclerosis, status post myocardial infarction five years ago, and was then admitted for treatment of impending myocardial infarction. The patient was transferred to a larger facility with a cath lab. The final diagnosis was documented as "impending myocardial infarction."

  Assign Y to the impending myocardial infarction because the condition is present on admission.

Same diagnosis code for two or more conditions

When two or more separate conditions are classified to the same diagnosis code in the same encounter, assign Y if all conditions represented by the single code were present on admission and N if any of the conditions were not present on admission.

Examples

- A patient was admitted with diabetes type 2 with ketoacidosis.

  Assign Y since both the diabetes and ketoacidosis were present on admission.

- A patient involved in a car accident was admitted with hemorrhage to the abdomen secondary to the trauma; shortly after being admitted the patient also developed a seroma as a result of the trauma.

  The secondary traumatic hemorrhage was present on admission, and the traumatic seroma did not develop until after admission. Both of these conditions are classified to one code, but because both conditions were not present when the patient was admitted, a POA of N should be assigned.

Obstetrical conditions

The POA assignment for obstetrical conditions is not affected by whether the patient delivers during the encounter but rather by whether the pregnancy

Appendix F: Present on Admission (POA) Tutorial

complication was or was not present at the time of admission. If two or more conditions are classified to a single code, all conditions represented by that single code must be present on admission to correctly assign a Y. If all conditions are not present at the time of admission, the appropriate POA indicator is N. Several obstetrics codes are listed in the POA exclusion list; for obstetrics codes that are not on the exclusion list, all applicable POA guidelines apply.

Examples

- A female patient was admitted to the hospital and underwent a normal delivery.

  Leave the "present on admission" (POA) field blank. Code O80 Normal delivery, is on the "exempt from reporting" list.
- A patient was admitted in late pregnancy due to excessive vomiting and dehydration. During admission, the patient went into premature labor.

  Assign Y for the excessive vomiting and the dehydration. Assign N for the premature labor.
- A patient was admitted in active labor. During the stay, a breast abscess was noted when the mother attempted to breastfeed. The provider was unable to clinically determine whether the abscess was present on admission.

  Assign W for the breast abscess since the provider was unable to clinically determine whether the abscess was present on admission.
- A patient was admitted in active labor. After 12 hours of labor, it was noted that the infant was in fetal distress, and a cesarean section was performed.

  Assign N for the fetal distress even if it is used for the principal diagnosis, since it did not develop until later in the admission. In obstetrics cases, the principal diagnosis may have a POA indicator of N.

Perinatal and congenital conditions

Newborns are not considered admitted until after birth; therefore all conditions that develop in utero, occur during delivery, or are present at birth are represented by the POA indicator Y. Any conditions that develop after birth and admission are represented by N.

All congenital conditions and anomalies not found in chapter 17 should have a POA indicator of Y assigned. Chapter 17 codes in categories Q00–Q99 are exempt from POA reporting. All congenital conditions, regardless of the coding chapter to which they are assigned, are considered present on admission.

Examples

- A single liveborn infant was delivered in the hospital via cesarean section. The physician documented fetal bradycardia during labor as the final diagnosis in the newborn record.

  Assign Y because the bradycardia developed prior to the newborn admission (birth).
- A newborn developed diarrhea, which was believed to be due to the hospital baby formula.

  Assign N because the diarrhea developed after admission.
- A newborn was diagnosed with cephalhematoma due to birth injury.

  Assign Y because the injury occurred during delivery.
- A newborn was diagnosed with congenital pneumonia.

  Assign Y for the congenital pneumonia. Congenital conditions from chapter 16 are always considered present on admission and require the POA indicator.
- A newborn was diagnosed with congenital hydrocephalus.

  There should be no POA indicator assigned. This condition is coded in chapter 17 and is excluded from POA reporting.
- A 10-year-old boy was admitted for complications of spina bifida with hydrocephalus.

  No POA indicator is assigned. This condition is coded in chapter 17 and is excluded from POA reporting.

External cause and injury codes

If an injury or poisoning occurred prior to or at the time of admission and the seventh character indicates an initial encounter or active treatment, the code for the injury/poisoning is reported with POA indicator Y. Injury and poisoning codes S00–T88 with the seventh character indicating subsequent or sequela

are exempt from POA indicators since, in order to be a subsequent or sequela encounter, the condition must have occurred before the admission. Many of the external causes of morbidity codes from chapters V, W, and X are also exempt from POA reporting when the seventh character of S or D, representing subsequent or sequela encounters, are used.

Coders should be extremely careful in assigning the appropriate POA indicator if a patient suffers an injury while an inpatient. For example, if a patient falls from the hospital bed and fractures a hip, the codes representing that injury (along with the appropriate initial-encounter seventh character) should be assigned N for the corresponding POA indicator.

Examples

- A 12-year-old was admitted for treatment of fractured arm from falling out of a tree house.

  The injury itself and the cause of the injury are both assigned a Y POA indicator.

  Note: *The injury code and external cause code POA indicators should always match.*
- A patient admitted for pneumonia sustained a laceration of the right arm after falling and hitting his arm against a cart in the hospital room, requiring stitches.

  Assign N for the laceration for the right arm because it was not present on admission. The external cause code POA indicator should also be N.
- A patient was admitted for manipulation of a knee contracture due to a scar from a burn injury 10 years ago.

  Assign Y for the code for the scar, but leave blank the POA indicator for the burn injury with the seventh character of S for sequela. Sequela and subsequent-encounter codes in chapter 19 are exempt from POA reporting.

Appendix G: Hospital Acquired Conditions

Hospital-acquired conditions (HACs) are conditions considered reasonably preventable through the application of evidence-based guidelines. These conditions, in and of themselves, are either a complication or comorbidity (CC) or major complication or comorbidity (MCC) that as a secondary diagnosis will move the MS-DRG assignment from a lower-paying MS-DRG to a higher-paying MS-DRG. However, if these conditions are not present on admission (meaning they developed during the hospital stay), the CC or MCC designation is nullified and the case will not group to the higher-paying MS-DRG based solely upon the reporting of the HAC code.

HACs are grouped into 14 categories. ICD-10-CM codes in the tabular section of this book that are grouped to one of these HAC categories are identified by an icon specific to that category. As many of these HACs are conditional, this resource provides any additional stipulations that may be required before the code can be considered a HAC. For example, code I26.02 has an **H10** indicating it falls in the HAC 10 category for Deep Vein Thrombosis (DVT) or Pulmonary Embolism (PE) with Total Knee or Hip Replacement. However I26.02 is not, by itself, a HAC there must also be a specific ICD-10-PCS code, such as 0SR9019 Replacement of Right Hip Joint with Metal Synthetic Substitute, Cemented, Open Approach, applied in order for I26.02 to act as a HAC.

Note: The resource used to compile this list is the fiscal 2019 ICD-10 MS-DRG Definitions Manual Files v36. The most current version, v37, of ICD-10 MS-DRG Definitions Manual was not available at the time this book was printed. For the most current files related to IPPS please refer to the following: https://www.cms.gov/Medicare/Medicare-Fee-for-Service-Payment/AcuteInpatientPPS/IPPS-Regulations-and-Notices.html.

HAC 01: Foreign Object Retained After Surgery
Secondary diagnosis not POA:

T81.500A
T81.501A
T81.502A
T81.503A
T81.504A
T81.505A
T81.506A
T81.507A
T81.508A
T81.509A
T81.510A
T81.511A
T81.512A
T81.513A
T81.514A
T81.515A
T81.516A
T81.517A
T81.518A
T81.519A
T81.520A
T81.521A
T81.522A
T81.523A
T81.524A
T81.525A
T81.526A
T81.527A
T81.528A
T81.529A
T81.530A
T81.531A
T81.532A
T81.533A
T81.534A
T81.535A
T81.536A
T81.537A
T81.538A
T81.539A
T81.590A
T81.591A
T81.592A
T81.593A
T81.594A
T81.595A
T81.596A
T81.597A
T81.598A
T81.599A
T81.60XA
T81.61XA
T81.69XA

HAC 02: Air Embolism
Secondary diagnosis not POA:

T80.0XXA

HAC 03: Blood Incompatibility
Secondary diagnosis not POA:

T80.30XA
T80.310A
T80.311A
T80.319A
T80.39XA

HAC 04: Stage III and IV Pressure Ulcers
Secondary diagnosis not POA:

L89.003
L89.004
L89.013
L89.014
L89.023
L89.024
L89.103
L89.104
L89.113
L89.114
L89.123
L89.124
L89.133
L89.134
L89.143
L89.144
L89.153
L89.154
L89.203
L89.204
L89.213
L89.214
L89.223
L89.224
L89.303
L89.304
L89.313
L89.314
L89.323
L89.324
L89.43
L89.44
L89.503
L89.504
L89.513
L89.514
L89.523
L89.524

L89.603
L89.604
L89.613
L89.614
L89.623
L89.624
L89.813
L89.814
L89.893
L89.894
L89.93
L89.94

HAC 05: Falls and Trauma
Secondary diagnosis not POA:

M99.10
M99.11
M99.18
S02.0XXA
S02.0XXB
S02.101A
S02.101B
S02.102A
S02.102B
S02.109A
S02.109B
S02.110A
S02.110B
S02.111A
S02.111B
S02.112A
S02.112B
S02.113A
S02.113B
S02.118A
S02.118B
S02.119A
S02.119B
S02.11AA
S02.11AB
S02.11BA
S02.11BB
S02.11CA
S02.11CB
S02.11DA
S02.11DB
S02.11EA
S02.11EB
S02.11FA
S02.11FB
S02.11GA
S02.11GB
S02.11HA
S02.11HB
S02.19XA

S02.19XB
S02.2XXB
S02.30XA
S02.30XB
S02.31XA
S02.31XB
S02.32XA
S02.32XB
S02.400A
S02.400B
S02.401A
S02.401B
S02.402A
S02.402B
S02.40AA
S02.40AB
S02.40BA
S02.40BB
S02.40CA
S02.40CB
S02.40DA
S02.40DB
S02.40EA
S02.40EB
S02.40FA
S02.40FB
S02.411A
S02.411B
S02.412A
S02.412B
S02.413A
S02.413B
S02.42XA
S02.42XB
S02.600A
S02.600B
S02.601A
S02.601B
S02.602A
S02.602B
S02.609A
S02.609B
S02.610A
S02.610B
S02.611A
S02.611B
S02.612A
S02.612B
S02.620A
S02.620B
S02.621A
S02.621B
S02.622A
S02.622B
S02.630A
S02.630B
S02.631A

S02.631B
S02.632A
S02.632B
S02.640A
S02.640B
S02.641A
S02.641B
S02.642A
S02.642B
S02.650A
S02.650B
S02.651A
S02.651B
S02.652A
S02.652B
S02.66XA
S02.66XB
S02.670A
S02.670B
S02.671A
S02.671B
S02.672A
S02.672B
S02.69XA
S02.69XB
S02.80XA
S02.80XB
S02.81XA
S02.81XB
S02.82XA
S02.82XB
S02.91XA
S02.91XB
S02.92XA
S02.92XB
S06.0X1A
S06.0X9A
S06.1X1A
S06.1X2A
S06.1X3A
S06.1X4A
S06.1X5A
S06.1X6A
S06.1X7A
S06.1X8A
S06.1X9A
S06.2X1A
S06.2X2A
S06.2X3A
S06.2X4A
S06.2X5A
S06.2X6A
S06.2X7A
S06.2X8A
S06.2X9A
S06.301A
S06.302A

S06.303A
S06.304A
S06.305A
S06.306A
S06.307A
S06.308A
S06.309A
S06.310A
S06.311A
S06.312A
S06.313A
S06.314A
S06.315A
S06.316A
S06.317A
S06.318A
S06.319A
S06.320A
S06.321A
S06.322A
S06.323A
S06.324A
S06.325A
S06.326A
S06.327A
S06.328A
S06.329A
S06.330A
S06.331A
S06.332A
S06.333A
S06.334A
S06.335A
S06.336A
S06.337A
S06.338A
S06.339A
S06.340A
S06.341A
S06.342A
S06.343A
S06.344A
S06.345A
S06.346A
S06.347A
S06.348A
S06.349A
S06.350A
S06.351A
S06.352A
S06.353A
S06.354A
S06.355A
S06.356A
S06.357A
S06.358A

Appendix G: Hospital Acquired Conditions

HAC 05: Falls and Trauma (continued)

S06.359A	S06.826A	S12.201B	S12.64XA	S22.008A	S22.081B
S06.360A	S06.827A	S12.230A	S12.64XB	S22.008B	S22.082A
S06.361A	S06.828A	S12.230B	S12.650A	S22.009A	S22.082B
S06.362A	S06.829A	S12.231A	S12.650B	S22.009B	S22.088A
S06.363A	S06.891A	S12.231B	S12.651A	S22.010A	S22.088B
S06.364A	S06.892A	S12.24XA	S12.651B	S22.010B	S22.089A
S06.365A	S06.893A	S12.24XB	S12.690A	S22.011A	S22.089B
S06.366A	S06.894A	S12.250A	S12.690B	S22.011B	S22.20XA
S06.367A	S06.895A	S12.250B	S12.691A	S22.012A	S22.20XB
S06.368A	S06.896A	S12.251A	S12.691B	S22.012B	S22.21XA
S06.369A	S06.897A	S12.251B	S12.8XXA	S22.018A	S22.21XB
S06.370A	S06.898A	S12.290A	S12.9XXA	S22.018B	S22.22XA
S06.371A	S06.899A	S12.290B	S13.0XXA	S22.019A	S22.22XB
S06.372A	S06.9X1A	S12.291A	S13.100A	S22.019B	S22.23XA
S06.373A	S06.9X2A	S12.291B	S13.101A	S22.020A	S22.23XB
S06.374A	S06.9X3A	S12.300A	S13.110A	S22.020B	S22.24XA
S06.375A	S06.9X4A	S12.300B	S13.111A	S22.021A	S22.24XB
S06.376A	S06.9X5A	S12.301A	S13.120A	S22.021B	S22.31XA
S06.377A	S06.9X6A	S12.301B	S13.121A	S22.022A	S22.31XB
S06.378A	S06.9X7A	S12.330A	S13.130A	S22.022B	S22.32XA
S06.379A	S06.9X8A	S12.330B	S13.131A	S22.028A	S22.32XB
S06.380A	S06.9X9A	S12.331A	S13.140A	S22.028B	S22.39XA
S06.381A	S07.0XXA	S12.331B	S13.141A	S22.029A	S22.39XB
S06.382A	S07.1XXA	S12.34XA	S13.150A	S22.029B	S22.41XA
S06.383A	S07.8XXA	S12.34XB	S13.151A	S22.030A	S22.41XB
S06.384A	S07.9XXA	S12.350A	S13.160A	S22.030B	S22.42XA
S06.385A	S12.000A	S12.350B	S13.161A	S22.031A	S22.42XB
S06.386A	S12.000B	S12.351A	S13.170A	S22.031B	S22.43XA
S06.387A	S12.001A	S12.351B	S13.171A	S22.032A	S22.43XB
S06.388A	S12.001B	S12.390A	S13.180A	S22.032B	S22.49XA
S06.389A	S12.01XA	S12.390B	S13.181A	S22.038A	S22.49XB
S06.4X0A	S12.01XB	S12.391A	S13.20XA	S22.038B	S22.5XXA
S06.4X1A	S12.02XA	S12.391B	S13.29XA	S22.039A	S22.5XXB
S06.4X2A	S12.02XB	S12.400A	S14.101A	S22.039B	S22.9XXA
S06.4X3A	S12.030A	S12.400B	S14.102A	S22.040A	S22.9XXB
S06.4X4A	S12.030B	S12.401A	S14.103A	S22.040B	S24.101A
S06.4X5A	S12.031A	S12.401B	S14.104A	S22.041A	S24.102A
S06.4X6A	S12.031B	S12.430A	S14.105A	S22.041B	S24.103A
S06.4X7A	S12.040A	S12.430B	S14.106A	S22.042A	S24.104A
S06.4X8A	S12.040B	S12.431A	S14.107A	S22.042B	S24.111A
S06.4X9A	S12.041A	S12.431B	S14.111A	S22.048A	S24.112A
S06.5X0A	S12.041B	S12.44XA	S14.112A	S22.048B	S24.113A
S06.5X1A	S12.090A	S12.44XB	S14.113A	S22.049A	S24.114A
S06.5X2A	S12.090B	S12.450A	S14.114A	S22.049B	S24.131A
S06.5X3A	S12.091A	S12.450B	S14.115A	S22.050A	S24.132A
S06.5X4A	S12.091B	S12.451A	S14.116A	S22.050B	S24.133A
S06.5X5A	S12.100A	S12.451B	S14.117A	S22.051A	S24.134A
S06.5X6A	S12.100B	S12.490A	S14.121A	S22.051B	S24.151A
S06.5X7A	S12.101A	S12.490B	S14.122A	S22.052A	S24.152A
S06.5X8A	S12.101B	S12.491A	S14.123A	S22.052B	S24.153A
S06.5X9A	S12.110A	S12.491B	S14.124A	S22.058A	S24.154A
S06.6X0A	S12.110B	S12.500A	S14.125A	S22.058B	S32.000A
S06.6X1A	S12.111A	S12.500B	S14.126A	S22.059A	S32.000B
S06.6X2A	S12.111B	S12.501A	S14.127A	S22.059B	S32.001A
S06.6X3A	S12.112A	S12.501B	S14.131A	S22.060A	S32.001B
S06.6X4A	S12.112B	S12.530A	S14.132A	S22.060B	S32.002A
S06.6X5A	S12.120A	S12.530B	S14.133A	S22.061A	S32.002B
S06.6X6A	S12.120B	S12.531A	S14.134A	S22.061B	S32.008A
S06.6X7A	S12.121A	S12.531B	S14.135A	S22.062A	S32.008B
S06.6X8A	S12.121B	S12.54XA	S14.136A	S22.062B	S32.009A
S06.6X9A	S12.130A	S12.54XB	S14.137A	S22.068A	S32.009B
S06.811A	S12.130B	S12.550A	S14.151A	S22.068B	S32.010A
S06.812A	S12.131A	S12.550B	S14.152A	S22.069A	S32.010B
S06.813A	S12.131B	S12.551A	S14.153A	S22.069B	S32.011A
S06.814A	S12.14XA	S12.551B	S14.154A	S22.070A	S32.011B
S06.815A	S12.14XB	S12.590A	S14.155A	S22.070B	S32.012A
S06.816A	S12.150A	S12.590B	S14.156A	S22.071A	S32.012B
S06.817A	S12.150B	S12.591A	S14.157A	S22.071B	S32.018A
S06.818A	S12.151A	S12.591B	S17.0XXA	S22.072A	S32.018B
S06.819A	S12.151B	S12.600A	S17.8XXA	S22.072B	S32.019A
S06.821A	S12.190A	S12.600B	S17.9XXA	S22.078A	S32.019B
S06.822A	S12.190B	S12.601A	S22.000A	S22.078B	S32.020A
S06.823A	S12.191A	S12.601B	S22.000B	S22.079A	S32.020B
S06.824A	S12.191B	S12.630A	S22.001A	S22.079B	S32.021A
S06.825A	S12.200A	S12.630B	S22.001B	S22.080A	S32.021B
	S12.200B	S12.631A	S22.002A	S22.080B	S32.022A
	S12.201A	S12.631B	S22.002B	S22.081A	S32.022B

HAC 05: Falls and Trauma (continued)

S32.028A	S32.302B	S32.452A	S32.611B	S42.112B	S42.252B
S32.028B	S32.309A	S32.452B	S32.612A	S42.113B	S42.253A
S32.029A	S32.309B	S32.453A	S32.612B	S42.114B	S42.253B
S32.029B	S32.311A	S32.453B	S32.613A	S42.115B	S42.254A
S32.030A	S32.311B	S32.454A	S32.613B	S42.116B	S42.254B
S32.030B	S32.312A	S32.454B	S32.614A	S42.121B	S42.255A
S32.031A	S32.312B	S32.455A	S32.614B	S42.122B	S42.255B
S32.031B	S32.313A	S32.455B	S32.615A	S42.123B	S42.256A
S32.032A	S32.313B	S32.456A	S32.615B	S42.124B	S42.256B
S32.032B	S32.314A	S32.456B	S32.616A	S42.125B	S42.261A
S32.038A	S32.314B	S32.461A	S32.616B	S42.126B	S42.261B
S32.038B	S32.315A	S32.461B	S32.691A	S42.131B	S42.262A
S32.039A	S32.315B	S32.462A	S32.691B	S42.132B	S42.262B
S32.039B	S32.316A	S32.462B	S32.692A	S42.133B	S42.263A
S32.040A	S32.316B	S32.463A	S32.692B	S42.134B	S42.263B
S32.040B	S32.391A	S32.463B	S32.699A	S42.135B	S42.264A
S32.041A	S32.391B	S32.464A	S32.699B	S42.136B	S42.264B
S32.041B	S32.392A	S32.464B	S32.810A	S42.141B	S42.265A
S32.042A	S32.392B	S32.465A	S32.810B	S42.142B	S42.265B
S32.042B	S32.399A	S32.465B	S32.811A	S42.143B	S42.266A
S32.048A	S32.399B	S32.466A	S32.811B	S42.144B	S42.266B
S32.048B	S32.401A	S32.466B	S32.82XA	S42.145B	S42.271A
S32.049A	S32.401B	S32.471A	S32.82XB	S42.146B	S42.272A
S32.049B	S32.402A	S32.471B	S32.89XA	S42.151B	S42.279A
S32.050A	S32.402B	S32.472A	S32.89XB	S42.152B	S42.291A
S32.050B	S32.409A	S32.472B	S32.9XXA	S42.153B	S42.291B
S32.051A	S32.409B	S32.473A	S32.9XXB	S42.154B	S42.292A
S32.051B	S32.411A	S32.473B	S34.101A	S42.155B	S42.292B
S32.052A	S32.411B	S32.474A	S34.102A	S42.156B	S42.293A
S32.052B	S32.412A	S32.474B	S34.103A	S42.191B	S42.293B
S32.058A	S32.412B	S32.475A	S34.104A	S42.192B	S42.294A
S32.058B	S32.413A	S32.475B	S34.105A	S42.199B	S42.294B
S32.059A	S32.413B	S32.476A	S34.109A	S42.201A	S42.295A
S32.059B	S32.414A	S32.476B	S34.111A	S42.201B	S42.295B
S32.10XA	S32.414B	S32.481A	S34.112A	S42.202A	S42.296A
S32.10XB	S32.415A	S32.481B	S34.113A	S42.202B	S42.296B
S32.110A	S32.415B	S32.482A	S34.114A	S42.209A	S42.301A
S32.110B	S32.416A	S32.482B	S34.115A	S42.209B	S42.301B
S32.111A	S32.416B	S32.483A	S34.119A	S42.211A	S42.302A
S32.111B	S32.421A	S32.483B	S34.121A	S42.211B	S42.302B
S32.112A	S32.421B	S32.484A	S34.122A	S42.212A	S42.309A
S32.112B	S32.422A	S32.484B	S34.123A	S42.212B	S42.309B
S32.119A	S32.422B	S32.485A	S34.124A	S42.213A	S42.311A
S32.119B	S32.423A	S32.485B	S34.125A	S42.213B	S42.312A
S32.120A	S32.423B	S32.486A	S34.129A	S42.214A	S42.319A
S32.120B	S32.424A	S32.486B	S34.131A	S42.214B	S42.321A
S32.121A	S32.424B	S32.491A	S34.132A	S42.215A	S42.321B
S32.121B	S32.425A	S32.491B	S34.139A	S42.215B	S42.322A
S32.122A	S32.425B	S32.492A	S34.3XXA	S42.216A	S42.322B
S32.122B	S32.426A	S32.492B	S42.001B	S42.216B	S42.323A
S32.129A	S32.426B	S32.499A	S42.002B	S42.221A	S42.323B
S32.129B	S32.431A	S32.499B	S42.009B	S42.221B	S42.324A
S32.130A	S32.431B	S32.501A	S42.011B	S42.222A	S42.324B
S32.130B	S32.432A	S32.501B	S42.012B	S42.222B	S42.325A
S32.131A	S32.432B	S32.502A	S42.013B	S42.223A	S42.325B
S32.131B	S32.433A	S32.502B	S42.014B	S42.223B	S42.326A
S32.132A	S32.433B	S32.509A	S42.015B	S42.224A	S42.326B
S32.132B	S32.434A	S32.509B	S42.016B	S42.224B	S42.331A
S32.139A	S32.434B	S32.511A	S42.017B	S42.225A	S42.331B
S32.139B	S32.435A	S32.511B	S42.018B	S42.225B	S42.332A
S32.14XA	S32.435B	S32.512A	S42.019B	S42.226A	S42.332B
S32.14XB	S32.436A	S32.512B	S42.021B	S42.226B	S42.333A
S32.15XA	S32.436B	S32.519A	S42.022B	S42.231A	S42.333B
S32.15XB	S32.441A	S32.519B	S42.023B	S42.231B	S42.334A
S32.16XA	S32.441B	S32.591A	S42.024B	S42.232A	S42.334B
S32.16XB	S32.442A	S32.591B	S42.025B	S42.232B	S42.335A
S32.17XA	S32.442B	S32.592A	S42.026B	S42.239A	S42.335B
S32.17XB	S32.443A	S32.592B	S42.031B	S42.239B	S42.336A
S32.19XA	S32.443B	S32.599A	S42.032B	S42.241A	S42.336B
S32.19XB	S32.444A	S32.599B	S42.033B	S42.241B	S42.341A
S32.2XXA	S32.444B	S32.601A	S42.034B	S42.242A	S42.341B
S32.2XXB	S32.445A	S32.601B	S42.035B	S42.242B	S42.342A
S32.301A	S32.445B	S32.602A	S42.036B	S42.249A	S42.342B
ICD.301B	S32.446A	S32.602B	S42.101B	S42.249B	S42.343A
S32.302A	S32.446B	S32.609A	S42.102B	S42.251A	S42.343B
	S32.451A	S32.609B	S42.109B	S42.251B	S42.344A
	S32.451B	S32.611A	S42.111B	S42.252A	

HAC 05: Falls and Trauma (continued)

S42.344B	S42.436A	S43.201A	S52.032B	S52.212A	S52.262A
S42.345A	S42.436B	S43.202A	S52.032C	S52.219A	S52.262B
S42.345B	S42.441A	S43.203A	S52.033B	S52.221A	S52.262C
S42.346A	S42.441B	S43.204A	S52.033C	S52.221B	S52.263A
S42.346B	S42.442A	S43.205A	S52.034B	S52.221C	S52.263B
S42.351A	S42.442B	S43.206A	S52.034C	S52.222A	S52.263C
S42.351B	S42.443A	S43.211A	S52.035B	S52.222B	S52.264A
S42.352A	S42.443B	S43.212A	S52.035C	S52.222C	S52.264B
S42.352B	S42.444A	S43.213A	S52.036B	S52.223A	S52.264C
S42.353A	S42.444B	S43.214A	S52.036C	S52.223B	S52.265A
S42.353B	S42.445A	S43.215A	S52.041B	S52.223C	S52.265B
S42.354A	S42.445B	S43.216A	S52.041C	S52.224A	S52.265C
S42.354B	S42.446A	S43.221A	S52.042B	S52.224B	S52.266A
S42.355A	S42.446B	S43.222A	S52.042C	S52.224C	S52.266B
S42.355B	S42.447A	S43.223A	S52.043B	S52.225A	S52.266C
S42.356A	S42.447B	S43.224A	S52.043C	S52.225B	S52.271B
S42.356B	S42.448A	S43.225A	S52.044B	S52.225C	S52.271C
S42.361A	S42.448B	S43.226A	S52.044C	S52.226A	S52.272B
S42.361B	S42.449A	S49.001A	S52.045B	S52.226B	S52.272C
S42.362A	S42.449B	S49.002A	S52.045C	S52.226C	S52.279B
S42.362B	S42.451A	S49.009A	S52.046B	S52.231A	S52.279C
S42.363A	S42.451B	S49.011A	S52.046C	S52.231B	S52.281A
S42.363B	S42.452A	S49.012A	S52.091B	S52.231C	S52.281B
S42.364A	S42.452B	S49.019A	S52.091C	S52.232A	S52.281C
S42.364B	S42.453A	S49.021A	S52.092B	S52.232B	S52.282A
S42.365A	S42.453B	S49.022A	S52.092C	S52.232C	S52.282B
S42.365B	S42.454A	S49.029A	S52.099B	S52.233A	S52.282C
S42.366A	S42.454B	S49.031A	S52.099C	S52.233B	S52.283A
S42.366B	S42.455A	S49.032A	S52.101B	S52.233C	S52.283B
S42.391A	S42.455B	S49.039A	S52.101C	S52.234A	S52.283C
S42.391B	S42.456A	S49.041A	S52.102B	S52.234B	S52.291A
S42.392A	S42.456B	S49.042A	S52.102C	S52.234C	S52.291B
S42.392B	S42.461A	S49.049A	S52.109B	S52.235A	S52.291C
S42.399A	S42.461B	S49.091A	S52.109C	S52.235B	S52.292A
S42.399B	S42.462A	S49.092A	S52.111A	S52.235C	S52.292B
S42.401A	S42.462B	S49.099A	S52.112A	S52.236A	S52.292C
S42.401B	S42.463A	S49.101A	S52.119A	S52.236B	S52.299A
S42.402A	S42.463B	S49.102A	S52.121B	S52.236C	S52.299B
S42.402B	S42.464A	S49.109A	S52.121C	S52.241A	S52.299C
S42.409A	S42.464B	S49.111A	S52.122B	S52.241B	S52.301A
S42.409B	S42.465A	S49.112A	S52.122C	S52.241C	S52.301B
S42.411A	S42.465B	S49.119A	S52.123B	S52.242A	S52.301C
S42.411B	S42.466A	S49.121A	S52.123C	S52.242B	S52.302A
S42.412A	S42.466B	S49.122A	S52.124B	S52.242C	S52.302B
S42.412B	S42.471A	S49.129A	S52.124C	S52.243A	S52.302C
S42.413A	S42.471B	S49.131A	S52.125B	S52.243B	S52.309A
S42.413B	S42.472A	S49.132A	S52.125C	S52.243C	S52.309B
S42.414A	S42.472B	S49.139A	S52.126B	S52.244A	S52.309C
S42.414B	S42.473A	S49.141A	S52.126C	S52.244B	S52.311A
S42.415A	S42.473B	S49.142A	S52.131B	S52.244C	S52.312A
S42.415B	S42.474A	S49.149A	S52.131C	S52.245A	S52.319A
S42.416A	S42.474B	S49.191A	S52.132B	S52.245B	S52.321A
S42.416B	S42.475A	S49.192A	S52.132C	S52.245C	S52.321B
S42.421A	S42.475B	S49.199A	S52.133B	S52.246A	S52.321C
S42.421B	S42.476A	S52.001B	S52.133C	S52.246B	S52.322A
S42.422A	S42.476B	S52.001C	S52.134B	S52.246C	S52.322B
S42.422B	S42.481A	S52.002B	S52.134C	S52.251A	S52.322C
S42.423A	S42.482A	S52.002C	S52.135B	S52.251B	S52.323A
S42.423B	S42.489A	S52.009B	S52.135C	S52.251C	S52.323B
S42.424A	S42.491A	S52.009C	S52.136B	S52.252A	S52.323C
S42.424B	S42.491B	S52.011A	S52.136C	S52.252B	S52.324A
S42.425A	S42.492A	S52.012A	S52.181B	S52.252C	S52.324B
S42.425B	S42.492B	S52.019A	S52.181C	S52.253A	S52.325A
S42.426A	S42.493A	S52.021B	S52.182B	S52.253B	S52.325B
S42.426B	S42.493B	S52.021C	S52.182C	S52.253C	S52.325C
S42.431A	S42.494A	S52.022B	S52.189B	S52.254A	S52.326A
S42.431B	S42.494B	S52.022C	S52.189C	S52.254B	S52.326B
S42.432A	S42.495A	S52.023B	S52.201A	S52.254C	S52.326C
S42.432B	S42.495B	S52.023C	S52.201B	S52.255A	S52.331A
S42.433A	S42.496A	S52.024B	S52.201C	S52.255B	S52.331B
S42.433B	S42.496B	S52.024C	S52.202A	S52.255C	S52.331C
S42.434A	S42.90XA	S52.025B	S52.202B	S52.256A	S52.332A
S42.434B	S42.90XB	S52.025C	S52.202C	S52.256B	S52.332B
S42.435A	S42.91XA	S52.026B	S52.209A	S52.256C	S52.332C
S42.435B	S42.91XB	S52.026C	S52.209B	S52.261A	S52.333A
	S42.92XA	S52.031B	S52.209C	S52.261B	S52.333B
	S42.92XB	S52.031C	S52.211A	S52.261C	

HAC 05: Falls and Trauma (continued)					
S52.333C	S52.381C	S52.562B	S59.021A	S62.146B	S62.319B
S52.334A	S52.382A	S52.562C	S59.022A	S62.151B	S62.320B
S52.334B	S52.382B	S52.569A	S59.029A	S62.152B	S62.321B
S52.334C	S52.382C	S52.569B	S59.031A	S62.153B	S62.322B
S52.335A	S52.389A	S52.569C	S59.032A	S62.154B	S62.323B
S52.335B	S52.389B	S52.571A	S59.039A	S62.155B	S62.324B
S52.335C	S52.389C	S52.571B	S59.041A	S62.156B	S62.325B
S52.336A	S52.391A	S52.571C	S59.042A	S62.161B	S62.326B
S52.336B	S52.391B	S52.572A	S59.049A	S62.162B	S62.327B
S52.336C	S52.391C	S52.572B	S59.091A	S62.163B	S62.328B
S52.341A	S52.392A	S52.572C	S59.092A	S62.164B	S62.329B
S52.341B	S52.392B	S52.579A	S59.099A	S62.165B	S62.330B
S52.341C	S52.392C	S52.579B	S59.201A	S62.166B	S62.331B
S52.342A	S52.399A	S52.579C	S59.202A	S62.171B	S62.332B
S52.342B	S52.399B	S52.591A	S59.209A	S62.172B	S62.333B
S52.342C	S52.399C	S52.591B	S59.211A	S62.173B	S62.334B
S52.343A	S52.501A	S52.591C	S59.212A	S62.174B	S62.335B
S52.343B	S52.501B	S52.592A	S59.219A	S62.175B	S62.336B
S52.343C	S52.501C	S52.592B	S59.221A	S62.176B	S62.337B
S52.344A	S52.502A	S52.592C	S59.222A	S62.181B	S62.338B
S52.344B	S52.502B	S52.599A	S59.229A	S62.182B	S62.339B
S52.344C	S52.502C	S52.599B	S59.231A	S62.183B	S62.340B
S52.345A	S52.509A	S52.599C	S59.232A	S62.184B	S62.341B
S52.345B	S52.509B	S52.601A	S59.239A	S62.185B	S62.342B
S52.345C	S52.509C	S52.601B	S59.241A	S62.186B	S62.343B
S52.346A	S52.511A	S52.601C	S59.242A	S62.201B	S62.344B
S52.346B	S52.511B	S52.602A	S59.249A	S62.202B	S62.345B
S52.346C	S52.511C	S52.602B	S59.291A	S62.209B	S62.346B
S52.351A	S52.512A	S52.602C	S59.292A	S62.211B	S62.347B
S52.351B	S52.512B	S52.609A	S59.299A	S62.212B	S62.348B
S52.351C	S52.512C	S52.609B	S62.001B	S62.213B	S62.349B
S52.352A	S52.513A	S52.609C	S62.002B	S62.221B	S62.350B
S52.352B	S52.513B	S52.611A	S62.009B	S62.222B	S62.351B
S52.352C	S52.513C	S52.611B	S62.011B	S62.223B	S62.352B
S52.353A	S52.514A	S52.611C	S62.012B	S62.224B	S62.353B
S52.353B	S52.514B	S52.612A	S62.013B	S62.225B	S62.354B
S52.353C	S52.514C	S52.612B	S62.014B	S62.226B	S62.355B
S52.354A	S52.515A	S52.612C	S62.015B	S62.231B	S62.356B
S52.354B	S52.515B	S52.613A	S62.016B	S62.232B	S62.357B
S52.354C	S52.515C	S52.613B	S62.021B	S62.233B	S62.358B
S52.355A	S52.516A	S52.613C	S62.022B	S62.234B	S62.359B
S52.355B	S52.516B	S52.614A	S62.023B	S62.235B	S62.360B
S52.355C	S52.516C	S52.614B	S62.024B	S62.236B	S62.361B
S52.356A	S52.521A	S52.614C	S62.025B	S62.241B	S62.362B
S52.356B	S52.522A	S52.615A	S62.026B	S62.242B	S62.363B
S52.356C	S52.529A	S52.615B	S62.031B	S62.243B	S62.364B
S52.361A	S52.531A	S52.615C	S62.032B	S62.244B	S62.365B
S52.361B	S52.531B	S52.616A	S62.033B	S62.245B	S62.366B
S52.361C	S52.531C	S52.616B	S62.034B	S62.246B	S62.367B
S52.362A	S52.532A	S52.616C	S62.035B	S62.251B	S62.368B
S52.362B	S52.532B	S52.621A	S62.036B	S62.252B	S62.369B
S52.362C	S52.532C	S52.622A	S62.101B	S62.253B	S62.390B
S52.363A	S52.539A	S52.629A	S62.102B	S62.254B	S62.391B
S52.363B	S52.539B	S52.691A	S62.109B	S62.255B	S62.392B
S52.363C	S52.539C	S52.691B	S62.111B	S62.256B	S62.393B
S52.364A	S52.541A	S52.691C	S62.112B	S62.291B	S62.394B
S52.364B	S52.541B	S52.692A	S62.113B	S62.292B	S62.395B
S52.364C	S52.541C	S52.692B	S62.114B	S62.299B	S62.396B
S52.365A	S52.542A	S52.692C	S62.115B	S62.300B	S62.397B
S52.365B	S52.542B	S52.699A	S62.116B	S62.301B	S62.398B
S52.365C	S52.542C	S52.699B	S62.121B	S62.302B	S62.399B
S52.366A	S52.549A	S52.699C	S62.122B	S62.303B	S62.501B
S52.366B	S52.549B	S52.90XA	S62.123B	S62.304B	S62.502B
S52.366C	S52.549C	S52.90XB	S62.124B	S62.305B	S62.509B
S52.371A	S52.551A	S52.90XC	S62.125B	S62.306B	S62.511B
S52.371B	S52.551B	S52.91XA	S62.126B	S62.307B	S62.512B
S52.371C	S52.551C	S52.91XB	S62.131B	S62.308B	S62.513B
S52.372A	S52.552A	S52.91XC	S62.132B	S62.309B	S62.514B
S52.372B	S52.552B	S52.92XA	S62.133B	S62.310B	S62.515B
S52.372C	S52.552C	S52.92XB	S62.134B	S62.311B	S62.516B
S52.379A	S52.559A	S52.92XC	S62.135B	S62.312B	S62.521B
S52.379B	S52.559B	S59.001A	S62.136B	S62.313B	S62.522B
S52.379C	S52.559C	S59.002A	S62.141B	S62.314B	S62.523B
ICD52.381A	S52.561A	S59.009A	S62.142B	S62.315B	S62.524B
S52.381B	S52.561B	S59.011A	S62.143B	S62.316B	S62.525B
	S52.561C	S59.012A	S62.144B	S62.317B	S62.526B
	S52.562A	S59.019A	S62.145B	S62.318B	S62.600B

Appendix G: Hospital Acquired Conditions *(left margin)*

HAC 05: Falls and Trauma (continued)					
S62.601B	S72.002A	S72.059C	S72.132B	S72.331A	S72.392C
S62.602B	S72.002B	S72.061A	S72.132C	S72.331B	S72.399A
S62.603B	S72.002C	S72.061B	S72.133A	S72.331C	S72.399B
S62.604B	S72.009A	S72.061C	S72.133B	S72.332A	S72.399C
S62.605B	S72.009B	S72.062A	S72.133C	S72.332B	S72.401A
S62.606B	S72.009C	S72.062B	S72.134A	S72.332C	S72.401B
S62.607B	S72.011A	S72.062C	S72.134B	S72.333A	S72.401C
S62.608B	S72.011B	S72.063A	S72.134C	S72.333B	S72.402A
S62.609B	S72.011C	S72.063B	S72.135A	S72.333C	S72.402B
S62.610B	S72.012A	S72.063C	S72.135B	S72.334A	S72.402C
S62.611B	S72.012B	S72.064A	S72.135C	S72.334B	S72.409A
S62.612B	S72.012C	S72.064B	S72.136A	S72.334C	S72.409B
S62.613B	S72.019A	S72.064C	S72.136B	S72.335A	S72.409C
S62.614B	S72.019B	S72.065A	S72.136C	S72.335B	S72.411A
S62.615B	S72.019C	S72.065B	S72.141A	S72.335C	S72.411B
S62.616B	S72.021A	S72.065C	S72.141B	S72.336A	S72.411C
S62.617B	S72.021B	S72.066A	S72.141C	S72.336B	S72.412A
S62.618B	S72.021C	S72.066B	S72.142A	S72.336C	S72.412B
S62.619B	S72.022A	S72.066C	S72.142B	S72.341A	S72.412C
S62.620B	S72.022B	S72.091A	S72.142C	S72.341B	S72.413A
S62.621B	S72.022C	S72.091B	S72.143A	S72.341C	S72.413B
S62.622B	S72.023A	S72.091C	S72.143B	S72.342A	S72.413C
S62.623B	S72.023B	S72.092A	S72.143C	S72.342B	S72.414A
S62.624B	S72.023C	S72.092B	S72.144A	S72.342C	S72.414B
S62.625B	S72.024A	S72.092C	S72.144B	S72.343A	S72.414C
S62.626B	S72.024B	S72.099A	S72.144C	S72.343B	S72.415A
S62.627B	S72.024C	S72.099B	S72.145A	S72.343C	S72.415B
S62.628B	S72.025A	S72.099C	S72.145B	S72.344A	S72.415C
S62.629B	S72.025B	S72.101A	S72.145C	S72.344B	S72.416A
S62.630B	S72.025C	S72.101B	S72.146A	S72.344C	S72.416B
S62.631B	S72.026A	S72.101C	S72.146B	S72.345A	S72.416C
S62.632B	S72.026B	S72.102A	S72.146C	S72.345B	S72.421A
S62.633B	S72.026C	S72.102B	S72.21XA	S72.345C	S72.421B
S62.634B	S72.031A	S72.102C	S72.21XB	S72.346A	S72.421C
S62.635B	S72.031B	S72.109A	S72.21XC	S72.346B	S72.422A
S62.636B	S72.031C	S72.109B	S72.22XA	S72.346C	S72.422B
S62.637B	S72.032A	S72.109C	S72.22XB	S72.351A	S72.422C
S62.638B	S72.032B	S72.111A	S72.22XC	S72.351B	S72.423A
S62.639B	S72.032C	S72.111B	S72.23XA	S72.351C	S72.423B
S62.640B	S72.033A	S72.111C	S72.23XB	S72.352A	S72.423C
S62.641B	S72.033B	S72.112A	S72.23XC	S72.352B	S72.424A
S62.642B	S72.033C	S72.112B	S72.24XA	S72.352C	S72.424B
S62.643B	S72.034A	S72.112C	S72.24XB	S72.353A	S72.424C
S62.644B	S72.034B	S72.113A	S72.24XC	S72.353B	S72.425A
S62.645B	S72.034C	S72.113B	S72.25XA	S72.353C	S72.425B
S62.646B	S72.035A	S72.113C	S72.25XB	S72.354A	S72.425C
S62.647B	S72.035B	S72.114A	S72.25XC	S72.354B	S72.426A
S62.648B	S72.035C	S72.114B	S72.26XA	S72.354C	S72.426B
S62.649B	S72.036A	S72.114C	S72.26XB	S72.355A	S72.426C
S62.650B	S72.036B	S72.115A	S72.26XC	S72.355B	S72.431A
S62.651B	S72.036C	S72.115B	S72.301A	S72.355C	S72.431B
S62.652B	S72.041A	S72.115C	S72.301B	S72.356A	S72.431C
S62.653B	S72.041B	S72.116A	S72.301C	S72.356B	S72.432A
S62.654B	S72.041C	S72.116B	S72.302A	S72.356C	S72.432B
S62.655B	S72.042A	S72.116C	S72.302B	S72.361A	S72.432C
S62.656B	S72.042B	S72.121A	S72.302C	S72.361B	S72.433A
S62.657B	S72.042C	S72.121B	S72.309A	S72.361C	S72.433B
S62.658B	S72.043A	S72.121C	S72.309B	S72.362A	S72.433C
S62.659B	S72.043B	S72.122A	S72.309C	S72.362B	S72.434A
S62.660B	S72.043C	S72.122B	S72.321A	S72.362C	S72.434B
S62.661B	S72.044A	S72.122C	S72.321B	S72.363A	S72.434C
S62.662B	S72.044B	S72.123A	S72.321C	S72.363B	S72.435A
S62.663B	S72.044C	S72.123B	S72.322A	S72.363C	S72.435B
S62.664B	S72.045A	S72.123C	S72.322B	S72.364A	S72.435C
S62.665B	S72.045B	S72.124A	S72.322C	S72.364B	S72.436A
S62.666B	S72.045C	S72.124B	S72.323A	S72.364C	S72.436B
S62.667B	S72.046A	S72.124C	S72.323B	S72.365A	S72.436C
S62.668B	S72.046B	S72.125A	S72.323C	S72.365B	S72.441A
S62.669B	S72.046C	S72.125B	S72.324A	S72.365C	S72.441B
S62.90XB	S72.051A	S72.125C	S72.324B	S72.366A	S72.441C
S62.91XB	S72.051B	S72.126A	S72.324C	S72.366B	S72.442A
S62.92XB	S72.051C	S72.126B	S72.325A	S72.366C	S72.442B
S72.001A	S72.052A	S72.126C	S72.325B	S72.391A	S72.442C
S72.001B	S72.052B	S72.131A	S72.325C	S72.391B	S72.443A
S72.001C	S72.052C	S72.131B	S72.326A	S72.391C	S72.443B
	S72.059A	S72.131C	S72.326B	S72.392A	S72.443C
	S72.059B	S72.132A	S72.326C	S72.392B	S72.444A

HAC 05: Falls and Trauma (continued)

S72.444B	S73.002A	S82.013A	S82.101C	S82.146B	S82.241A
S72.444C	S73.003A	S82.013B	S82.102A	S82.146C	S82.241B
S72.445A	S73.004A	S82.013C	S82.102B	S82.151A	S82.241C
S72.445B	S73.005A	S82.014A	S82.102C	S82.151B	S82.242A
S72.445C	S73.006A	S82.014B	S82.109A	S82.151C	S82.242B
S72.446A	S73.011A	S82.014C	S82.109B	S82.152A	S82.242C
S72.446B	S73.012A	S82.015A	S82.109C	S82.152B	S82.243A
S72.446C	S73.013A	S82.015B	S82.111A	S82.152C	S82.243B
S72.451A	S73.014A	S82.015C	S82.111B	S82.153A	S82.243C
S72.451B	S73.015A	S82.016A	S82.111C	S82.153B	S82.244A
S72.451C	S73.016A	S82.016B	S82.112A	S82.153C	S82.244B
S72.452A	S73.021A	S82.016C	S82.112B	S82.154A	S82.244C
S72.452B	S73.022A	S82.021A	S82.112C	S82.154B	S82.245A
S72.452C	S73.023A	S82.021B	S82.113A	S82.154C	S82.245B
S72.453A	S73.024A	S82.021C	S82.113B	S82.155A	S82.245C
S72.453B	S73.025A	S82.022A	S82.113C	S82.155B	S82.246A
S72.453C	S73.026A	S82.022B	S82.114A	S82.155C	S82.246B
S72.454A	S73.031A	S82.022C	S82.114B	S82.156A	S82.246C
S72.454B	S73.032A	S82.023A	S82.114C	S82.156B	S82.251A
S72.454C	S73.033A	S82.023B	S82.115A	S82.156C	S82.251B
S72.455A	S73.034A	S82.023C	S82.115B	S82.161A	S82.251C
S72.455B	S73.035A	S82.024A	S82.115C	S82.162A	S82.252A
S72.455C	S73.036A	S82.024B	S82.116A	S82.169A	S82.252B
S72.456A	S73.041A	S82.024C	S82.116B	S82.191A	S82.252C
S72.456B	S73.042A	S82.025A	S82.116C	S82.191B	S82.253A
S72.456C	S73.043A	S82.025B	S82.121A	S82.191C	S82.253B
S72.461A	S73.044A	S82.025C	S82.121B	S82.192A	S82.253C
S72.461B	S73.045A	S82.026A	S82.121C	S82.192B	S82.254A
S72.461C	S73.046A	S82.026B	S82.122A	S82.192C	S82.254B
S72.462A	S77.00XA	S82.026C	S82.122B	S82.199A	S82.254C
S72.462B	S77.01XA	S82.031A	S82.122C	S82.199B	S82.255A
S72.462C	S77.02XA	S82.031B	S82.123A	S82.199C	S82.255B
S72.463A	S77.10XA	S82.031C	S82.123B	S82.201A	S82.255C
S72.463B	S77.11XA	S82.032A	S82.123C	S82.201B	S82.256A
S72.463C	S77.12XA	S82.032B	S82.124A	S82.201C	S82.256B
S72.464A	S79.001A	S82.032C	S82.124B	S82.202A	S82.256C
S72.464B	S79.002A	S82.033A	S82.124C	S82.202B	S82.261A
S72.464C	S79.009A	S82.033B	S82.125A	S82.202C	S82.261B
S72.465A	S79.011A	S82.033C	S82.125B	S82.209A	S82.261C
S72.465B	S79.012A	S82.034A	S82.125C	S82.209B	S82.262A
S72.465C	S79.019A	S82.034B	S82.126A	S82.209C	S82.262B
S72.466A	S79.091A	S82.034C	S82.126B	S82.221A	S82.262C
S72.466B	S79.092A	S82.035A	S82.126C	S82.221B	S82.263A
S72.466C	S79.099A	S82.035B	S82.131A	S82.221C	S82.263B
S72.471A	S79.101A	S82.035C	S82.131B	S82.222A	S82.263C
S72.472A	S79.102A	S82.036A	S82.131C	S82.222B	S82.264A
S72.479A	S79.109A	S82.036B	S82.132A	S82.222C	S82.264B
S72.491A	S79.111A	S82.036C	S82.132B	S82.223A	S82.264C
S72.491B	S79.112A	S82.041A	S82.132C	S82.223B	S82.265A
S72.491C	S79.119A	S82.041B	S82.133A	S82.223C	S82.265B
S72.492A	S79.121A	S82.041C	S82.133B	S82.224A	S82.265C
S72.492B	S79.122A	S82.042A	S82.133C	S82.224B	S82.266A
S72.492C	S79.129A	S82.042B	S82.134A	S82.224C	S82.266B
S72.499A	S79.131A	S82.042C	S82.134B	S82.225A	S82.266C
S72.499B	S79.132A	S82.043A	S82.134C	S82.225B	S82.291A
S72.499C	S79.139A	S82.043B	S82.135A	S82.225C	S82.291B
S72.8X1A	S79.141A	S82.043C	S82.135B	S82.226A	S82.291C
S72.8X1B	S79.142A	S82.044A	S82.135C	S82.226B	S82.292A
S72.8X1C	S79.149A	S82.044B	S82.136A	S82.226C	S82.292B
S72.8X2A	S79.191A	S82.044C	S82.136B	S82.231A	S82.292C
S72.8X2B	S79.192A	S82.045A	S82.136C	S82.231B	S82.299A
S72.8X2C	S79.199A	S82.045B	S82.141A	S82.231C	S82.299B
S72.8X9A	S82.001A	S82.045C	S82.141B	S82.232A	S82.299C
S72.8X9B	S82.001B	S82.046A	S82.141C	S82.232B	S82.301B
S72.8X9C	S82.001C	S82.046B	S82.142A	S82.232C	S82.301C
S72.90XA	S82.002A	S82.046C	S82.142B	S82.233A	S82.302B
S72.90XB	S82.002B	S82.091A	S82.142C	S82.233B	S82.302C
S72.90XC	S82.002C	S82.091B	S82.143A	S82.233C	S82.309B
S72.91XA	S82.009A	S82.091C	S82.143B	S82.234A	S82.309C
S72.91XB	S82.009B	S82.092A	S82.143C	S82.234B	S82.311A
S72.91XC	S82.009C	S82.092B	S82.144A	S82.234C	S82.312A
S72.92XA	S82.011A	S82.092C	S82.144B	S82.235A	S82.319A
S72.92XB	S82.011B	S82.099A	S82.144C	S82.235B	S82.391B
S72.92XC	S82.011C	S82.099B	S82.145A	S82.235C	S82.391C
S73.001A	S82.012A	S82.099C	S82.145B	S82.236A	S82.392B
	S82.012B	S82.101A	S82.145C	S82.236B	S82.392C
	S82.012C	S82.101B	S82.146A	S82.236C	S82.399B

HAC 05: Falls and Trauma (continued)	S82.52XB	S82.891C	S92.121B	S92.333B	T22.359A
S82.399C	S82.52XC	S82.892B	S92.122B	S92.334B	T22.361A
S82.401B	S82.53XB	S82.892C	S92.123B	S92.335B	T22.362A
S82.401C	S82.53XC	S82.899B	S92.124B	S92.336B	T22.369A
S82.402B	S82.54XB	S82.899C	S92.125B	S92.341B	T22.391A
S82.402C	S82.54XC	S82.90XB	S92.126B	S92.342B	T22.392A
S82.409B	S82.55XB	S82.90XC	S92.131B	S92.343B	T22.399A
S82.409C	S82.55XC	S82.91XB	S92.132B	S92.344B	T22.70XA
S82.421B	S82.56XB	S82.91XC	S92.133B	S92.345B	T22.711A
S82.421C	S82.56XC	S82.92XB	S92.134B	S92.346B	T22.712A
S82.422B	S82.61XB	S82.92XC	S92.135B	S92.351B	T22.719A
S82.422C	S82.61XC	S89.001A	S92.136B	S92.352B	T22.721A
S82.423B	S82.62XB	S89.002A	S92.141B	S92.353B	T22.722A
S82.423C	S82.62XC	S89.009A	S92.142B	S92.354B	T22.729A
S82.424B	S82.63XB	S89.011A	S92.143B	S92.355B	T22.731A
S82.424C	S82.63XC	S89.012A	S92.144B	S92.356B	T22.732A
S82.425B	S82.64XB	S89.019A	S92.145B	S92.811B	T22.739A
S82.425C	S82.64XC	S89.021A	S92.146B	S92.812B	T22.741A
S82.426B	S82.65XB	S89.022A	S92.151B	S92.819B	T22.742A
S82.426C	S82.65XC	S89.029A	S92.152B	S92.901B	T22.749A
S82.431B	S82.66XB	S89.031A	S92.153B	S92.902B	T22.751A
S82.431C	S82.66XC	S89.032A	S92.154B	S92.909B	T22.752A
S82.432B	S82.831B	S89.039A	S92.155B	T20.30XA	T22.759A
S82.432C	S82.831C	S89.041A	S92.156B	T20.311A	T22.761A
S82.433B	S82.832B	S89.042A	S92.191B	T20.312A	T22.762A
S82.433C	S82.832C	S89.049A	S92.192B	T20.319A	T22.769A
S82.434B	S82.839B	S89.091A	S92.199B	T20.32XA	T22.791A
S82.434C	S82.839C	S89.092A	S92.201B	T20.33XA	T22.792A
S82.435B	S82.841B	S89.099A	S92.202B	T20.34XA	T22.799A
S82.435C	S82.841C	S92.001B	S92.209B	T20.35XA	T23.301A
S82.436B	S82.842B	S92.002B	S92.211B	T20.36XA	T23.302A
S82.436C	S82.842C	S92.009B	S92.212B	T20.37XA	T23.309A
S82.441B	S82.843B	S92.011B	S92.213B	T20.39XA	T23.311A
S82.441C	S82.843C	S92.012B	S92.214B	T20.70XA	T23.312A
S82.442B	S82.844B	S92.013B	S92.215B	T20.711A	T23.319A
S82.442C	S82.844C	S92.014B	S92.216B	T20.712A	T23.321A
S82.443B	S82.845B	S92.015B	S92.221B	T20.719A	T23.322A
S82.443C	S82.845C	S92.016B	S92.222B	T20.72XA	T23.329A
S82.444B	S82.846B	S92.021B	S92.223B	T20.73XA	T23.331A
S82.444C	S82.846C	S92.022B	S92.224B	T20.74XA	T23.332A
S82.445B	S82.851B	S92.023B	S92.225B	T20.75XA	T23.339A
S82.445C	S82.851C	S92.024B	S92.226B	T20.76XA	T23.341A
S82.446B	S82.852B	S92.025B	S92.231B	T20.77XA	T23.342A
S82.446C	S82.852C	S92.026B	S92.232B	T20.79XA	T23.349A
S82.451B	S82.853B	S92.031B	S92.233B	T21.30XA	T23.351A
S82.451C	S82.853C	S92.032B	S92.234B	T21.31XA	T23.352A
S82.452B	S82.854B	S92.033B	S92.235B	T21.32XA	T23.359A
S82.452C	S82.854C	S92.034B	S92.236B	T21.33XA	T23.361A
S82.453B	S82.855B	S92.035B	S92.241B	T21.34XA	T23.362A
S82.453C	S82.855C	S92.036B	S92.242B	T21.35XA	T23.369A
S82.454B	S82.856B	S92.041B	S92.243B	T21.36XA	T23.371A
S82.454C	S82.856C	S92.042B	S92.244B	T21.37XA	T23.372A
S82.455B	S82.861B	S92.043B	S92.245B	T21.39XA	T23.379A
S82.455C	S82.861C	S92.044B	S92.246B	T21.70XA	T23.391A
S82.456B	S82.862B	S92.045B	S92.251B	T21.71XA	T23.392A
S82.456C	S82.862C	S92.046B	S92.252B	T21.72XA	T23.399A
S82.461B	S82.863B	S92.051B	S92.253B	T21.73XA	T23.701A
S82.461C	S82.863C	S92.052B	S92.254B	T21.74XA	T23.702A
S82.462B	S82.864B	S92.053B	S92.255B	T21.75XA	T23.709A
S82.462C	S82.864C	S92.054B	S92.256B	T21.76XA	T23.711A
S82.463B	S82.865B	S92.055B	S92.301B	T21.77XA	T23.712A
S82.463C	S82.865C	S92.056B	S92.302B	T21.79XA	T23.719A
S82.464B	S82.866B	S92.061B	S92.309B	T22.30XA	T23.721A
S82.464C	S82.866C	S92.062B	S92.311B	T22.311A	T23.722A
S82.465B	S82.871B	S92.063B	S92.312B	T22.312A	T23.729A
S82.465C	S82.871C	S92.064B	S92.313B	T22.319A	T23.731A
S82.466B	S82.872B	S92.065B	S92.314B	T22.321A	T23.732A
S82.466C	S82.872C	S92.066B	S92.315B	T22.322A	T23.739A
S82.491B	S82.873B	S92.101B	S92.316B	T22.329A	T23.741A
S82.491C	S82.873C	S92.102B	S92.321B	T22.331A	T23.742A
S82.492B	S82.874B	S92.109B	S92.322B	T22.332A	T23.749A
S82.492C	S82.874C	S92.111B	S92.323B	T22.339A	T23.751A
S82.499B	S82.875B	S92.112B	S92.324B	T22.341A	T23.752A
S82.499C	S82.875C	S92.113B	S92.325B	T22.342A	T23.759A
S82.51XB	S82.876B	S92.114B	S92.326B	T22.349A	T23.761A
S82.51XC	S82.876C	S92.115B	S92.331B	T22.351A	T23.762A
	S82.891B	S92.116B	S92.332B	T22.352A	T23.769A

HAC 05: Falls and Trauma (continued)					
T23.771A	T25.732A	T31.77	T32.82	T34.02XA	T71.161A
T23.772A	T25.739A	T31.80	T32.83	T34.09XA	T71.162A
T23.779A	T25.791A	T31.81	T32.84	T34.1XXA	T71.163A
T23.791A	T25.792A	T31.82	T32.85	T34.2XXA	T71.164A
T23.792A	T25.799A	T31.83	T32.86	T34.3XXA	T71.191A
T23.799A	T26.20XA	T31.84	T32.87	T34.40XA	T71.192A
T24.301A	T26.21XA	T31.85	T32.88	T34.41XA	T71.193A
T24.302A	T26.22XA	T31.86	T32.90	T34.42XA	T71.194A
T24.309A	T26.70XA	T31.87	T32.91	T34.511A	T71.20XA
T24.311A	T26.71XA	T31.88	T32.92	T34.512A	T71.21XA
T24.312A	T26.72XA	T31.90	T32.93	T34.519A	T71.29XA
T24.319A	T27.0XXA	T31.91	T32.94	T34.521A	T71.9XXA
T24.321A	T27.1XXA	T31.92	T32.95	T34.522A	T75.1XXA
T24.322A	T27.2XXA	T31.93	T32.96	T34.529A	
T24.329A	T27.3XXA	T31.94	T32.97	T34.531A	**HAC 06: Catheter**
T24.331A	T27.4XXA	T31.95	T32.98	T34.532A	**Associated Urinary**
T24.332A	T27.5XXA	T31.96	T32.99	T34.539A	**Tract Infection (UTI)**
T24.339A	T27.6XXA	T31.97	T33.011A	T34.60XA	Secondary diagnosis
T24.391A	T27.7XXA	T31.98	T33.012A	T34.61XA	not POA:
T24.392A	T28.1XXA	T31.99	T33.019A	T34.62XA	T83.511A
T24.399A	T28.2XXA	T32.10	T33.02XA	T34.70XA	T83.518A
T24.701A	T28.6XXA	T32.11	T33.09XA	T34.71XA	
T24.702A	T28.7XXA	T32.20	T33.1XXA	T34.72XA	**With or Without**
T24.709A	T31.10	T32.21	T33.2XXA	T34.811A	Secondary diagnosis
T24.711A	T31.11	T32.22	T33.3XXA	T34.812A	(also not POA) of:
T24.712A	T31.20	T32.30	T33.40XA	T34.819A	B37.41
T24.719A	T31.21	T32.31	T33.41XA	T34.821A	B37.49
T24.721A	T31.22	T32.32	T33.42XA	T34.822A	N10
T24.722A	T31.30	T32.33	T33.511A	T34.829A	N11.9
T24.729A	T31.31	T32.40	T33.512A	T34.831A	N12
T24.731A	T31.32	T32.41	T33.519A	T34.832A	N13.6
T24.732A	T31.33	T32.42	T33.521A	T34.839A	N15.1
T24.739A	T31.40	T32.43	T33.522A	T34.90XA	N28.84
T24.791A	T31.41	T32.44	T33.529A	T34.99XA	N28.85
T24.792A	T31.42	T32.50	T33.531A	T69.021A	N28.86
T24.799A	T31.43	T32.51	T33.532A	T69.022A	N30.00
T25.311A	T31.44	T32.52	T33.539A	T69.029A	N30.01
T25.312A	T31.50	T32.53	T33.60XA	T70.3XXA	N34.0
T25.319A	T31.51	T32.54	T33.61XA	T71.111A	N39.0
T25.321A	T31.52	T32.55	T33.62XA	T71.112A	
T25.322A	T31.53	T32.60	T33.70XA	T71.113A	**HAC 07: Vascular**
T25.329A	T31.54	T32.61	T33.71XA	T71.114A	**Catheter Associated**
T25.331A	T31.55	T32.62	T33.72XA	T71.121A	**Infection**
T25.332A	T31.60	T32.63	T33.811A	T71.122A	Secondary diagnosis
T25.339A	T31.61	T32.64	T33.812A	T71.123A	not POA:
T25.391A	T31.62	T32.65	T33.819A	T71.124A	T80.211A
T25.392A	T31.63	T32.66	T33.821A	T71.131A	T80.212A
T25.399A	T31.64	T32.70	T33.822A	T71.132A	T80.218A
T25.711A	T31.65	T32.71	T33.829A	T71.133A	T80.219A
T25.712A	T31.66	T32.72	T33.831A	T71.134A	
T25.719A	T31.70	T32.73	T33.832A	T71.141A	
T25.721A	T31.71	T32.74	T33.839A	T71.143A	
T25.722A	T31.72	T32.75	T33.90XA	T71.144A	
T25.729A	T31.73	T32.76	T33.99XA	T71.151A	
T25.731A	T31.74	T32.77	T34.011A	T71.152A	
	T31.75	T32.80	T34.012A	T71.153A	
	T31.76	T32.81	T34.019A	T71.154A	

Appendix G: Hospital Acquired Conditions

HAC 08: Surgical Site Infection of Mediastinitis after Coronary Bypass Graft (CABG)

Secondary diagnosis not POA:
- J98.51
- J98.59

AND

Any of the following procedures:

0210083   Bypass Coronary Artery, One Artery from Coronary Artery with Zooplastic Tissue, Open Approach

0210088   Bypass Coronary Artery, One Artery from Right Internal Mammary with Zooplastic Tissue, Open Approach

0210089   Bypass Coronary Artery, One Artery from Left Internal Mammary with Zooplastic Tissue, Open Approach

021008C   Bypass Coronary Artery, One Artery from Thoracic Artery with Zooplastic Tissue, Open Approach

021008F   Bypass Coronary Artery, One Artery from Abdominal Artery with Zooplastic Tissue, Open Approach

021008W   Bypass Coronary Artery, One Artery from Aorta with Zooplastic Tissue, Open Approach

0210093   Bypass Coronary Artery, One Artery from Coronary Artery with Autologous Venous Tissue, Open Approach

0210098   Bypass Coronary Artery, One Artery from Right Internal Mammary with Autologous Venous Tissue, Open Approach

0210099   Bypass Coronary Artery, One Artery from Left Internal Mammary with Autologous Venous Tissue, Open Approach

021009C   Bypass Coronary Artery, One Artery from Thoracic Artery with Autologous Venous Tissue, Open Approach

021009F   Bypass Coronary Artery, One Artery from Abdominal Artery with Autologous Venous Tissue, Open Approach

021009W   Bypass Coronary Artery, One Artery from Aorta with Autologous Venous Tissue, Open Approach

02100A3   Bypass Coronary Artery, One Artery from Coronary Artery with Autologous Arterial Tissue, Open Approach

02100A8   Bypass Coronary Artery, One Artery from Right Internal Mammary with Autologous Arterial Tissue, Open Approach

02100A9   Bypass Coronary Artery, One Artery from Left Internal Mammary with Autologous Arterial Tissue, Open Approach

02100AC   Bypass Coronary Artery, One Artery from Thoracic Artery with Autologous Arterial Tissue, Open Approach

02100AF   Bypass Coronary Artery, One Artery from Abdominal Artery with Autologous Arterial Tissue, Open Approach

02100AW   Bypass Coronary Artery, One Artery from Aorta with Autologous Arterial Tissue, Open Approach

02100J3   Bypass Coronary Artery, One Artery from Coronary Artery with Synthetic Substitute, Open Approach

02100J8   Bypass Coronary Artery, One Artery from Right Internal Mammary with Synthetic Substitute, Open Approach

02100J9   Bypass Coronary Artery, One Artery from Left Internal Mammary with Synthetic Substitute, Open Approach

02100JC   Bypass Coronary Artery, One Artery from Thoracic Artery with Synthetic Substitute, Open Approach

02100JF   Bypass Coronary Artery, One Artery from Abdominal Artery with Synthetic Substitute, Open Approach

02100JW   Bypass Coronary Artery, One Artery from Aorta with Synthetic Substitute, Open Approach

02100K3   Bypass Coronary Artery, One Artery from Coronary Artery with Nonautologous Tissue Substitute, Open Approach

02100K8   Bypass Coronary Artery, One Artery from Right Internal Mammary with Nonautologous Tissue Substitute, Open Approach

02100K9   Bypass Coronary Artery, One Artery from Left Internal Mammary with Nonautologous Tissue Substitute, Open Approach

02100KC   Bypass Coronary Artery, One Artery from Thoracic Artery with Nonautologous Tissue Substitute, Open Approach

02100KF   Bypass Coronary Artery, One Artery from Abdominal Artery with Nonautologous Tissue Substitute, Open Approach

02100KW   Bypass Coronary Artery, One Artery from Aorta with Nonautologous Tissue Substitute, Open Approach

02100Z3   Bypass Coronary Artery, One Artery from Coronary Artery, Open Approach

02100Z8   Bypass Coronary Artery, One Artery from Right Internal Mammary, Open Approach

02100Z9   Bypass Coronary Artery, One Artery from Left Internal Mammary, Open Approach

02100ZC   Bypass Coronary Artery, One Artery from Thoracic Artery, Open Approach

02100ZF   Bypass Coronary Artery, One Artery from Abdominal Artery, Open Approach

0210483   Bypass Coronary Artery, One Artery from Coronary Artery with Zooplastic Tissue, Percutaneous Endoscopic Approach

0210488   Bypass Coronary Artery, One Artery from Right Internal Mammary with Zooplastic Tissue, Percutaneous Endoscopic Approach

0210489   Bypass Coronary Artery, One Artery from Left Internal Mammary with Zooplastic Tissue, Percutaneous Endoscopic Approach

021048C   Bypass Coronary Artery, One Artery from Thoracic Artery with Zooplastic Tissue, Percutaneous Endoscopic Approach

021048F   Bypass Coronary Artery, One Artery from Abdominal Artery with Zooplastic Tissue, Percutaneous Endoscopic Approach

021048W   Bypass Coronary Artery, One Artery from Aorta with Zooplastic Tissue, Percutaneous Endoscopic Approach

0210493   Bypass Coronary Artery, One Artery from Coronary Artery with Autologous Venous Tissue, Percutaneous Endoscopic Approach

0210498   Bypass Coronary Artery, One Artery from Right Internal Mammary with Autologous Venous Tissue, Percutaneous Endoscopic Approach

0210499   Bypass Coronary Artery, One Artery from Left Internal Mammary with Autologous Venous Tissue, Percutaneous Endoscopic Approach

021049C   Bypass Coronary Artery, One Artery from Thoracic Artery with Autologous Venous Tissue, Percutaneous Endoscopic Approach

021049F   Bypass Coronary Artery, One Artery from Abdominal Artery with Autologous Venous Tissue, Percutaneous Endoscopic Approach

021049W   Bypass Coronary Artery, One Artery from Aorta with Autologous Venous Tissue, Percutaneous Endoscopic Approach

02104A3   Bypass Coronary Artery, One Artery from Coronary Artery with Autologous Arterial Tissue, Percutaneous Endoscopic Approach

02104A8   Bypass Coronary Artery, One Artery from Right Internal Mammary with Autologous Arterial Tissue, Percutaneous Endoscopic Approach

02104A9   Bypass Coronary Artery, One Artery from Left Internal Mammary with Autologous Arterial Tissue, Percutaneous Endoscopic Approach

02104AC   Bypass Coronary Artery, One Artery from Thoracic Artery with Autologous Arterial Tissue, Percutaneous Endoscopic Approach

02104AF   Bypass Coronary Artery, One Artery from Abdominal Artery with Autologous Arterial Tissue, Percutaneous Endoscopic Approach

02104AW   Bypass Coronary Artery, One Artery from Aorta with Autologous Arterial Tissue, Percutaneous Endoscopic Approach

02104J3   Bypass Coronary Artery, One Artery from Coronary Artery with Synthetic Substitute, Percutaneous Endoscopic Approach

02104J8   Bypass Coronary Artery, One Artery from Right Internal Mammary with Synthetic Substitute, Percutaneous Endoscopic Approach

02104J9   Bypass Coronary Artery, One Artery from Left Internal Mammary with Synthetic Substitute, Percutaneous Endoscopic Approach

02104JC   Bypass Coronary Artery, One Artery from Thoracic Artery with Synthetic Substitute, Percutaneous Endoscopic Approach

02104JF   Bypass Coronary Artery, One Artery from Abdominal Artery with Synthetic Substitute, Percutaneous Endoscopic Approach

02104JW   Bypass Coronary Artery, One Artery from Aorta with Synthetic Substitute, Percutaneous Endoscopic Approach

02104K3   Bypass Coronary Artery, One Artery from Coronary Artery with Nonautologous Tissue Substitute, Percutaneous Endoscopic Approach

02104K8   Bypass Coronary Artery, One Artery from Right Internal Mammary with Nonautologous Tissue Substitute, Percutaneous Endoscopic Approach

02104K9   Bypass Coronary Artery, One Artery from Left Internal Mammary with Nonautologous Tissue Substitute, Percutaneous Endoscopic Approach

02104KC   Bypass Coronary Artery, One Artery from Thoracic Artery with Nonautologous Tissue Substitute, Percutaneous Endoscopic Approach

02104KF   Bypass Coronary Artery, One Artery from Abdominal Artery with Nonautologous Tissue Substitute, Percutaneous Endoscopic Approach

02104KW   Bypass Coronary Artery, One Artery from Aorta with Nonautologous Tissue Substitute, Percutaneous Endoscopic Approach

02104Z3   Bypass Coronary Artery, One Artery from Coronary Artery, Percutaneous Endoscopic Approach

HAC 08: Surgical Artery Infection of Mediastinitis after Coronary Bypass Graft (CABG) (continued)

0210 4Z8 Bypass Coronary Artery, One Artery from Right Internal Mammary, Percutaneous Endoscopic Approach

0210 4Z9 Bypass Coronary Artery, One Artery from Left Internal Mammary, Percutaneous Endoscopic Approach

0210 4ZC Bypass Coronary Artery, One Artery from Thoracic Artery, Percutaneous Endoscopic Approach

0210 4ZF Bypass Coronary Artery, One Artery from Abdominal Artery, Percutaneous Endoscopic Approach

0211 083 Bypass Coronary Artery, Two Arteries from Coronary Artery with Zooplastic Tissue, Open Approach

0211 088 Bypass Coronary Artery, Two Arteries from Right Internal Mammary with Zooplastic Tissue, Open Approach

0211 089 Bypass Coronary Artery, Two Arteries from Left Internal Mammary with Zooplastic Tissue, Open Approach

0211 08C Bypass Coronary Artery, Two Arteries from Thoracic Artery with Zooplastic Tissue, Open Approach

0211 08F Bypass Coronary Artery, Two Arteries from Abdominal Artery with Zooplastic Tissue, Open Approach

0211 08W Bypass Coronary Artery, Two Arteries from Aorta with Zooplastic Tissue, Open Approach

0211 093 Bypass Coronary Artery, Two Arteries from Coronary Artery with Autologous Venous Tissue, Open Approach

0211 098 Bypass Coronary Artery, Two Arteries from Right Internal Mammary with Autologous Venous Tissue, Open Approach

0211 099 Bypass Coronary Artery, Two Arteries from Left Internal Mammary with Autologous Venous Tissue, Open Approach

0211 09C Bypass Coronary Artery, Two Arteries from Thoracic Artery with Autologous Venous Tissue, Open Approach

0211 09F Bypass Coronary Artery, Two Arteries from Abdominal Artery with Autologous Venous Tissue, Open Approach

0211 09W Bypass Coronary Artery, Two Arteries from Aorta with Autologous Venous Tissue, Open Approach

0211 0A3 Bypass Coronary Artery, Two Arteries from Coronary Artery with Autologous Arterial Tissue, Open Approach

0211 0A8 Bypass Coronary Artery, Two Arteries from Right Internal Mammary with Autologous Arterial Tissue, Open Approach

0211 0A9 Bypass Coronary Artery, Two Arteries from Left Internal Mammary with Autologous Arterial Tissue, Open Approach

0211 0AC Bypass Coronary Artery, Two Arteries from Thoracic Artery with Autologous Arterial Tissue, Open Approach

0211 0AF Bypass Coronary Artery, Two Arteries from Abdominal Artery with Autologous Arterial Tissue, Open Approach

0211 0AW Bypass Coronary Artery, Two Arteries from Aorta with Autologous Arterial Tissue, Open Approach

0211 0J3 Bypass Coronary Artery, Two Arteries from Coronary Artery with Synthetic Substitute, Open Approach

0211 0J8 Bypass Coronary Artery, Two Arteries from Right Internal Mammary with Synthetic Substitute, Open Approach

0211 0J9 Bypass Coronary Artery, Two Arteries from Left Internal Mammary with Synthetic Substitute, Open Approach

0211 0JC Bypass Coronary Artery, Two Arteries from Thoracic Artery with Synthetic Substitute, Open Approach

0211 0JF Bypass Coronary Artery, Two Arteries from Abdominal Artery with Synthetic Substitute, Open Approach

0211 0JW Bypass Coronary Artery, Two Arteries from Aorta with Synthetic Substitute, Open Approach

0211 0K3 Bypass Coronary Artery, Two Arteries from Coronary Artery with Nonautologous Tissue Substitute, Open Approach

0211 0K8 Bypass Coronary Artery, Two Arteries from Right Internal Mammary with Nonautologous Tissue Substitute, Open Approach

0211 0K9 Bypass Coronary Artery, Two Arteries from Left Internal Mammary with Nonautologous Tissue Substitute, Open Approach

0211 0KC Bypass Coronary Artery, Two Arteries from Thoracic Artery with Nonautologous Tissue Substitute, Open Approach

0211 0KF Bypass Coronary Artery, Two Arteries from Abdominal Artery with Nonautologous Tissue Substitute, Open Approach

0211 0KW Bypass Coronary Artery, Two Arteries from Aorta with Nonautologous Tissue Substitute, Open Approach

0211 0Z3 Bypass Coronary Artery, Two Arteries from Coronary Artery, Open Approach

0211 0Z8 Bypass Coronary Artery, Two Arteries from Right Internal Mammary, Open Approach

0211 0Z9 Bypass Coronary Artery, Two Arteries from Left Internal Mammary, Open Approach

0211 0ZC Bypass Coronary Artery, Two Arteries from Thoracic Artery, Open Approach

0211 0ZF Bypass Coronary Artery, Two Arteries from Abdominal Artery, Open Approach

0211 483 Bypass Coronary Artery, Two Arteries from Coronary Artery with Zooplastic Tissue, Percutaneous Endoscopic Approach

0211 488 Bypass Coronary Artery, Two Arteries from Right Internal Mammary with Zooplastic Tissue, Percutaneous Endoscopic Approach

0211 489 Bypass Coronary Artery, Two Arteries from Left Internal Mammary with Zooplastic Tissue, Percutaneous Endoscopic Approach

0211 48C Bypass Coronary Artery, Two Arteries from Thoracic Artery with Zooplastic Tissue, Percutaneous Endoscopic Approach

0211 48F Bypass Coronary Artery, Two Arteries from Abdominal Artery with Zooplastic Tissue, Percutaneous Endoscopic Approach

0211 48W Bypass Coronary Artery, Two Arteries from Aorta with Zooplastic Tissue, Percutaneous Endoscopic Approach

0211 493 Bypass Coronary Artery, Two Arteries from Coronary Artery with Autologous Venous Tissue, Percutaneous Endoscopic Approach

0211 498 Bypass Coronary Artery, Two Arteries from Right Internal Mammary with Autologous Venous Tissue, Percutaneous Endoscopic Approach

0211 499 Bypass Coronary Artery, Two Arteries from Left Internal Mammary with Autologous Venous Tissue, Percutaneous Endoscopic Approach

0211 49C Bypass Coronary Artery, Two Arteries from Thoracic Artery with Autologous Venous Tissue, Percutaneous Endoscopic Approach

0211 49F Bypass Coronary Artery, Two Arteries from Abdominal Artery with Autologous Venous Tissue, Percutaneous Endoscopic Approach

0211 49W Bypass Coronary Artery, Two Arteries from Aorta with Autologous Venous Tissue, Percutaneous Endoscopic Approach

0211 4A3 Bypass Coronary Artery, Two Arteries from Coronary Artery with Autologous Arterial Tissue, Percutaneous Endoscopic Approach

0211 4A8 Bypass Coronary Artery, Two Arteries from Right Internal Mammary with Autologous Arterial Tissue, Percutaneous Endoscopic Approach

0211 4A9 Bypass Coronary Artery, Two Arteries from Left Internal Mammary with Autologous Arterial Tissue, Percutaneous Endoscopic Approach

0211 4AC Bypass Coronary Artery, Two Arteries from Thoracic Artery with Autologous Arterial Tissue, Percutaneous Endoscopic Approach

0211 4AF Bypass Coronary Artery, Two Arteries from Abdominal Artery with Autologous Arterial Tissue, Percutaneous Endoscopic Approach

0211 4AW Bypass Coronary Artery, Two Arteries from Aorta with Autologous Arterial Tissue, Percutaneous Endoscopic Approach

0211 4J3 Bypass Coronary Artery, Two Arteries from Coronary Artery with Synthetic Substitute, Percutaneous Endoscopic Approach

0211 4J8 Bypass Coronary Artery, Two Arteries from Right Internal Mammary with Synthetic Substitute, Percutaneous Endoscopic Approach

0211 4J9 Bypass Coronary Artery, Two Arteries from Left Internal Mammary with Synthetic Substitute, Percutaneous Endoscopic Approach

0211 4JC Bypass Coronary Artery, Two Arteries from Thoracic Artery with Synthetic Substitute, Percutaneous Endoscopic Approach

0211 4JF Bypass Coronary Artery, Two Arteries from Abdominal Artery with Synthetic Substitute, Percutaneous Endoscopic Approach

0211 4JW Bypass Coronary Artery, Two Arteries from Aorta with Synthetic Substitute, Percutaneous Endoscopic Approach

0211 4K3 Bypass Coronary Artery, Two Arteries from Coronary Artery with Nonautologous Tissue Substitute, Percutaneous Endoscopic Approach

0211 4K8 Bypass Coronary Artery, Two Arteries from Right Internal Mammary with Nonautologous Tissue Substitute, Percutaneous Endoscopic Approach

HAC 08: Surgical Site Infection of Mediastinitis after Coronary Bypass Graft (CABG) (continued)

Ø2114K9   Bypass Coronary Artery, Two Arteries from Left Internal Mammary with Nonautologous Tissue Substitute, Percutaneous Endoscopic Approach

Ø2114KC   Bypass Coronary Artery, Two Arteries from Thoracic Artery with Nonautologous Tissue Substitute, Percutaneous Endoscopic Approach

Ø2114KF   Bypass Coronary Artery, Two Arteries from Abdominal Artery with Nonautologous Tissue Substitute, Percutaneous Endoscopic Approach

Ø2114KW   Bypass Coronary Artery, Two Arteries from Aorta with Nonautologous Tissue Substitute, Percutaneous Endoscopic Approach

Ø2114Z3   Bypass Coronary Artery, Two Arteries from Coronary Artery, Percutaneous Endoscopic Approach

Ø2114Z8   Bypass Coronary Artery, Two Arteries from Right Internal Mammary, Percutaneous Endoscopic Approach

Ø2114Z9   Bypass Coronary Artery, Two Arteries from Left Internal Mammary, Percutaneous Endoscopic Approach

Ø2114ZC   Bypass Coronary Artery, Two Arteries from Thoracic Artery, Percutaneous Endoscopic Approach

Ø2114ZF   Bypass Coronary Artery, Two Arteries from Abdominal Artery, Percutaneous Endoscopic Approach

Ø212Ø83   Bypass Coronary Artery, Three Arteries from Coronary Artery with Zooplastic Tissue, Open Approach

Ø212Ø88   Bypass Coronary Artery, Three Arteries from Right Internal Mammary with Zooplastic Tissue, Open Approach

Ø212Ø89   Bypass Coronary Artery, Three Arteries from Left Internal Mammary with Zooplastic Tissue, Open Approach

Ø212Ø8C   Bypass Coronary Artery, Three Arteries from Thoracic Artery with Zooplastic Tissue, Open Approach

Ø212Ø8F   Bypass Coronary Artery, Three Arteries from Abdominal Artery with Zooplastic Tissue, Open Approach

Ø212Ø8W   Bypass Coronary Artery, Three Arteries from Aorta with Zooplastic Tissue, Open Approach

Ø212Ø93   Bypass Coronary Artery, Three Arteries from Coronary Artery with Autologous Venous Tissue, Open Approach

Ø212Ø98   Bypass Coronary Artery, Three Arteries from Right Internal Mammary with Autologous Venous Tissue, Open Approach

Ø212Ø99   Bypass Coronary Artery, Three Arteries from Left Internal Mammary with Autologous Venous Tissue, Open Approach

Ø212Ø9C   Bypass Coronary Artery, Three Arteries from Thoracic Artery with Autologous Venous Tissue, Open Approach

Ø212Ø9F   Bypass Coronary Artery, Three Arteries from Abdominal Artery with Autologous Venous Tissue, Open Approach

Ø212Ø9W   Bypass Coronary Artery, Three Arteries from Aorta with Autologous Venous Tissue, Open Approach

Ø212ØA3   Bypass Coronary Artery, Three Arteries from Coronary Artery with Autologous Arterial Tissue, Open Approach

Ø212ØA8   Bypass Coronary Artery, Three Arteries from Right Internal Mammary with Autologous Arterial Tissue, Open Approach

Ø212ØA9   Bypass Coronary Artery, Three Arteries from Left Internal Mammary with Autologous Arterial Tissue, Open Approach

Ø212ØAC   Bypass Coronary Artery, Three Arteries from Thoracic Artery with Autologous Arterial Tissue, Open Approach

Ø212ØAF   Bypass Coronary Artery, Three Arteries from Abdominal Artery with Autologous Arterial Tissue, Open Approach

Ø212ØAW   Bypass Coronary Artery, Three Arteries from Aorta with Autologous Arterial Tissue, Open Approach

Ø212ØJ3   Bypass Coronary Artery, Three Arteries from Coronary Artery with Synthetic Substitute, Open Approach

Ø212ØJ8   Bypass Coronary Artery, Three Arteries from Right Internal Mammary with Synthetic Substitute, Open Approach

Ø212ØJ9   Bypass Coronary Artery, Three Arteries from Left Internal Mammary with Synthetic Substitute, Open Approach

Ø212ØJC   Bypass Coronary Artery, Three Arteries from Thoracic Artery with Synthetic Substitute, Open Approach

Ø212ØJF   Bypass Coronary Artery, Three Arteries from Abdominal Artery with Synthetic Substitute, Open Approach

Ø212ØJW   Bypass Coronary Artery, Three Arteries from Aorta with Synthetic Substitute, Open Approach

Ø212ØK3   Bypass Coronary Artery, Three Arteries from Coronary Artery with Nonautologous Tissue Substitute, Open Approach

Ø212ØK8   Bypass Coronary Artery, Three Arteries from Right Internal Mammary with Nonautologous Tissue Substitute, Open Approach

Ø212ØK9   Bypass Coronary Artery, Three Arteries from Left Internal Mammary with Nonautologous Tissue Substitute, Open Approach

Ø212ØKC   Bypass Coronary Artery, Three Arteries from Thoracic Artery with Nonautologous Tissue Substitute, Open Approach

Ø212ØKF   Bypass Coronary Artery, Three Arteries from Abdominal Artery with Nonautologous Tissue Substitute, Open Approach

Ø212ØKW   Bypass Coronary Artery, Three Arteries from Aorta with Nonautologous Tissue Substitute, Open Approach

Ø212ØZ3   Bypass Coronary Artery, Three Arteries from Coronary Artery, Open Approach

Ø212ØZ8   Bypass Coronary Artery, Three Arteries from Right Internal Mammary, Open Approach

Ø212ØZ9   Bypass Coronary Artery, Three Arteries from Left Internal Mammary, Open Approach

Ø212ØZC   Bypass Coronary Artery, Three Arteries from Thoracic Artery, Open Approach

Ø212ØZF   Bypass Coronary Artery, Three Arteries from Abdominal Artery, Open Approach

Ø212483   Bypass Coronary Artery, Three Arteries from Coronary Artery with Zooplastic Tissue, Percutaneous Endoscopic Approach

Ø212488   Bypass Coronary Artery, Three Arteries from Right Internal Mammary with Zooplastic Tissue, Percutaneous Endoscopic Approach

Ø212489   Bypass Coronary Artery, Three Arteries from Left Internal Mammary with Zooplastic Tissue, Percutaneous Endoscopic Approach

Ø21248C   Bypass Coronary Artery, Three Arteries from Thoracic Artery with Zooplastic Tissue, Percutaneous Endoscopic Approach

Ø21248F   Bypass Coronary Artery, Three Arteries from Abdominal Artery with Zooplastic Tissue, Percutaneous Endoscopic Approach

Ø21248W   Bypass Coronary Artery, Three Arteries from Aorta with Zooplastic Tissue, Percutaneous Endoscopic Approach

Ø212493   Bypass Coronary Artery, Three Arteries from Coronary Artery with Autologous Venous Tissue, Percutaneous Endoscopic Approach

Ø212498   Bypass Coronary Artery, Three Arteries from Right Internal Mammary with Autologous Venous Tissue, Percutaneous Endoscopic Approach

Ø212499   Bypass Coronary Artery, Three Arteries from Left Internal Mammary with Autologous Venous Tissue, Percutaneous Endoscopic Approach

Ø21249C   Bypass Coronary Artery, Three Arteries from Thoracic Artery with Autologous Venous Tissue, Percutaneous Endoscopic Approach

Ø21249F   Bypass Coronary Artery, Three Arteries from Abdominal Artery with Autologous Venous Tissue, Percutaneous Endoscopic Approach

Ø21249W   Bypass Coronary Artery, Three Arteries from Aorta with Autologous Venous Tissue, Percutaneous Endoscopic Approach

Ø2124A3   Bypass Coronary Artery, Three Arteries from Coronary Artery with Autologous Arterial Tissue, Percutaneous Endoscopic Approach

Ø2124A8   Bypass Coronary Artery, Three Arteries from Right Internal Mammary with Autologous Arterial Tissue, Percutaneous Endoscopic Approach

Ø2124A9   Bypass Coronary Artery, Three Arteries from Left Internal Mammary with Autologous Arterial Tissue, Percutaneous Endoscopic Approach

Ø2124AC   Bypass Coronary Artery, Three Arteries from Thoracic Artery with Autologous Arterial Tissue, Percutaneous Endoscopic Approach

Ø2124AF   Bypass Coronary Artery, Three Arteries from Abdominal Artery with Autologous Arterial Tissue, Percutaneous Endoscopic Approach

Ø2124AW   Bypass Coronary Artery, Three Arteries from Aorta with Autologous Arterial Tissue, Percutaneous Endoscopic Approach

Ø2124J3   Bypass Coronary Artery, Three Arteries from Coronary Artery with Synthetic Substitute, Percutaneous Endoscopic Approach

Ø2124J8   Bypass Coronary Artery, Three Arteries from Right Internal Mammary with Synthetic Substitute, Percutaneous Endoscopic Approach

HAC 08: Surgical Site Infection of Mediastinitis after Coronary Bypass Graft (CABG) (continued)

Ø2124J9 Bypass Coronary Artery, Three Arteries from Left Internal Mammary with Synthetic Substitute, Percutaneous Endoscopic Approach

Ø2124JC Bypass Coronary Artery, Three Arteries from Thoracic Artery with Synthetic Substitute, Percutaneous Endoscopic Approach

Ø2124JF Bypass Coronary Artery, Three Arteries from Abdominal Artery with Synthetic Substitute, Percutaneous Endoscopic Approach

Ø2124JW Bypass Coronary Artery, Three Arteries from Aorta with Synthetic Substitute, Percutaneous Endoscopic Approach

Ø2124K3 Bypass Coronary Artery, Three Arteries from Coronary Artery with Nonautologous Tissue Substitute, Percutaneous Endoscopic Approach

Ø2124K8 Bypass Coronary Artery, Three Arteries from Right Internal Mammary with Nonautologous Tissue Substitute, Percutaneous Endoscopic Approach

Ø2124K9 Bypass Coronary Artery, Three Arteries from Left Internal Mammary with Nonautologous Tissue Substitute, Percutaneous Endoscopic Approach

Ø2124KC Bypass Coronary Artery, Three Arteries from Thoracic Artery with Nonautologous Tissue Substitute, Percutaneous Endoscopic Approach

Ø2124KF Bypass Coronary Artery, Three Arteries from Abdominal Artery with Nonautologous Tissue Substitute, Percutaneous Endoscopic Approach

Ø2124KW Bypass Coronary Artery, Three Arteries from Aorta with Nonautologous Tissue Substitute, Percutaneous Endoscopic Approach

Ø2124Z3 Bypass Coronary Artery, Three Arteries from Coronary Artery, Percutaneous Endoscopic Approach

Ø2124Z8 Bypass Coronary Artery, Three Arteries from Right Internal Mammary, Percutaneous Endoscopic Approach

Ø2124Z9 Bypass Coronary Artery, Three Arteries from Left Internal Mammary, Percutaneous Endoscopic Approach

Ø2124ZC Bypass Coronary Artery, Three Arteries from Thoracic Artery, Percutaneous Endoscopic Approach

Ø2124ZF Bypass Coronary Artery, Three Arteries from Abdominal Artery, Percutaneous Endoscopic Approach

Ø213Ø83 Bypass Coronary Artery, Four or More Arteries from Coronary Artery with Zooplastic Tissue, Open Approach

Ø213Ø88 Bypass Coronary Artery, Four or More Arteries from Right Internal Mammary with Zooplastic Tissue, Open Approach

Ø213Ø89 Bypass Coronary Artery, Four or More Arteries from Left Internal Mammary with Zooplastic Tissue, Open Approach

Ø213Ø8C Bypass Coronary Artery, Four or More Arteries from Thoracic Artery with Zooplastic Tissue, Open Approach

Ø213Ø8F Bypass Coronary Artery, Four or More Arteries from Abdominal Artery with Zooplastic Tissue, Open Approach

Ø213Ø8W Bypass Coronary Artery, Four or More Arteries from Aorta with Zooplastic Tissue, Open Approach

Ø213Ø93 Bypass Coronary Artery, Four or More Arteries from Coronary Artery with Autologous Venous Tissue, Open Approach

Ø213Ø98 Bypass Coronary Artery, Four or More Arteries from Right Internal Mammary with Autologous Venous Tissue, Open Approach

Ø213Ø99 Bypass Coronary Artery, Four or More Arteries from Left Internal Mammary with Autologous Venous Tissue, Open Approach

Ø213Ø9C Bypass Coronary Artery, Four or More Arteries from Thoracic Artery with Autologous Venous Tissue, Open Approach

Ø213Ø9F Bypass Coronary Artery, Four or More Arteries from Abdominal Artery with Autologous Venous Tissue, Open Approach

Ø213Ø9W Bypass Coronary Artery, Four or More Arteries from Aorta with Autologous Venous Tissue, Open Approach

Ø213ØA3 Bypass Coronary Artery, Four or More Arteries from Coronary Artery with Autologous Arterial Tissue, Open Approach

Ø213ØA8 Bypass Coronary Artery, Four or More Arteries from Right Internal Mammary with Autologous Arterial Tissue, Open Approach

Ø213ØA9 Bypass Coronary Artery, Four or More Arteries from Left Internal Mammary with Autologous Arterial Tissue, Open Approach

Ø213ØAC Bypass Coronary Artery, Four or More Arteries from Thoracic Artery with Autologous Arterial Tissue, Open Approach

Ø213ØAF Bypass Coronary Artery, Four or More Arteries from Abdominal Artery with Autologous Arterial Tissue, Open Approach

Ø213ØAW Bypass Coronary Artery, Four or More Arteries from Aorta with Autologous Arterial Tissue, Open Approach

Ø213ØJ3 Bypass Coronary Artery, Four or More Arteries from Coronary Artery with Synthetic Substitute, Open Approach

Ø213ØJ8 Bypass Coronary Artery, Four or More Arteries from Right Internal Mammary with Synthetic Substitute, Open Approach

Ø213ØJ9 Bypass Coronary Artery, Four or More Arteries from Left Internal Mammary with Synthetic Substitute, Open Approach

Ø213ØJC Bypass Coronary Artery, Four or More Arteries from Thoracic Artery with Synthetic Substitute, Open Approach

Ø213ØJF Bypass Coronary Artery, Four or More Arteries from Abdominal Artery with Synthetic Substitute, Open Approach

Ø213ØJW Bypass Coronary Artery, Four or More Arteries from Aorta with Synthetic Substitute, Open Approach

Ø213ØK3 Bypass Coronary Artery, Four or More Arteries from Coronary Artery with Nonautologous Tissue Substitute, Open Approach

Ø213ØK8 Bypass Coronary Artery, Four or More Arteries from Right Internal Mammary with Nonautologous Tissue Substitute, Open Approach

Ø213ØK9 Bypass Coronary Artery, Four or More Arteries from Left Internal Mammary with Nonautologous Tissue Substitute, Open Approach

Ø213ØKC Bypass Coronary Artery, Four or More Arteries from Thoracic Artery with Nonautologous Tissue Substitute, Open Approach

Ø213ØKF Bypass Coronary Artery, Four or More Arteries from Abdominal Artery with Nonautologous Tissue Substitute, Open Approach

Ø213ØKW Bypass Coronary Artery, Four or More Arteries from Aorta with Nonautologous Tissue Substitute, Open Approach

Ø213ØZ3 Bypass Coronary Artery, Four or More Arteries from Coronary Artery, Open Approach

Ø213ØZ8 Bypass Coronary Artery, Four or More Arteries from Right Internal Mammary, Open Approach

Ø213ØZ9 Bypass Coronary Artery, Four or More Arteries from Left Internal Mammary, Open Approach

Ø213ØZC Bypass Coronary Artery, Four or More Arteries from Thoracic Artery, Open Approach

Ø213ØZF Bypass Coronary Artery, Four or More Arteries from Abdominal Artery, Open Approach

Ø213483 Bypass Coronary Artery, Four or More Arteries from Coronary Artery with Zooplastic Tissue, Percutaneous Endoscopic Approach

Ø213488 Bypass Coronary Artery, Four or More Arteries from Right Internal Mammary with Zooplastic Tissue, Percutaneous Endoscopic Approach

Ø213489 Bypass Coronary Artery, Four or More Arteries from Left Internal Mammary with Zooplastic Tissue, Percutaneous Endoscopic Approach

Ø21348C Bypass Coronary Artery, Four or More Arteries from Thoracic Artery with Zooplastic Tissue, Percutaneous Endoscopic Approach

Ø21348F Bypass Coronary Artery, Four or More Arteries from Abdominal Artery with Zooplastic Tissue, Percutaneous Endoscopic Approach

Ø21348W Bypass Coronary Artery, Four or More Arteries from Aorta with Zooplastic Tissue, Percutaneous Endoscopic Approach

Ø213493 Bypass Coronary Artery, Four or More Arteries from Coronary Artery with Autologous Venous Tissue, Percutaneous Endoscopic Approach

Ø213498 Bypass Coronary Artery, Four or More Arteries from Right Internal Mammary with Autologous Venous Tissue, Percutaneous Endoscopic Approach

Ø213499 Bypass Coronary Artery, Four or More Arteries from Left Internal Mammary with Autologous Venous Tissue, Percutaneous Endoscopic Approach

Ø21349C Bypass Coronary Artery, Four or More Arteries from Thoracic Artery with Autologous Venous Tissue, Percutaneous Endoscopic Approach

Ø21349F Bypass Coronary Artery, Four or More Arteries from Abdominal Artery with Autologous Venous Tissue, Percutaneous Endoscopic Approach

Ø21349W Bypass Coronary Artery, Four or More Arteries from Aorta with Autologous Venous Tissue, Percutaneous Endoscopic Approach

HAC 08: Surgical Site Infection of Mediastinitis after Coronary Bypass Graft (CABG) (continued)

02134A3 Bypass Coronary Artery, Four or More Arteries from Coronary Artery with Autologous Arterial Tissue, Percutaneous Endoscopic Approach

02134A8 Bypass Coronary Artery, Four or More Arteries from Right Internal Mammary with Autologous Arterial Tissue, Percutaneous Endoscopic Approach

02134A9 Bypass Coronary Artery, Four or More Arteries from Left Internal Mammary with Autologous Arterial Tissue, Percutaneous Endoscopic Approach

02134AC Bypass Coronary Artery, Four or More Arteries from Thoracic Artery with Autologous Arterial Tissue, Percutaneous Endoscopic Approach

02134AF Bypass Coronary Artery, Four or More Arteries from Abdominal Artery with Autologous Arterial Tissue, Percutaneous Endoscopic Approach

02134AW Bypass Coronary Artery, Four or More Arteries from Aorta with Autologous Arterial Tissue, Percutaneous Endoscopic Approach

02134J3 Bypass Coronary Artery, Four or More Arteries from Coronary Artery with Synthetic Substitute, Percutaneous Endoscopic Approach

02134J8 Bypass Coronary Artery, Four or More Arteries from Right Internal Mammary with Synthetic Substitute, Percutaneous Endoscopic Approach

02134J9 Bypass Coronary Artery, Four or More Arteries from Left Internal Mammary with Synthetic Substitute, Percutaneous Endoscopic Approach

02134JC Bypass Coronary Artery, Four or More Arteries from Thoracic Artery with Synthetic Substitute, Percutaneous Endoscopic Approach

02134JF Bypass Coronary Artery, Four or More Arteries from Abdominal Artery with Synthetic Substitute, Percutaneous Endoscopic Approach

02134JW Bypass Coronary Artery, Four or More Arteries from Aorta with Synthetic Substitute, Percutaneous Endoscopic Approach

02134K3 Bypass Coronary Artery, Four or More Arteries from Coronary Artery with Nonautologous Tissue Substitute, Percutaneous Endoscopic Approach

02134K8 Bypass Coronary Artery, Four or More Arteries from Right Internal Mammary with Nonautologous Tissue Substitute, Percutaneous Endoscopic Approach

02134K9 Bypass Coronary Artery, Four or More Arteries from Left Internal Mammary with Nonautologous Tissue Substitute, Percutaneous Endoscopic Approach

02134KC Bypass Coronary Artery, Four or More Arteries from Thoracic Artery with Nonautologous Tissue Substitute, Percutaneous Endoscopic Approach

02134KF Bypass Coronary Artery, Four or More Arteries from Abdominal Artery with Nonautologous Tissue Substitute, Percutaneous Endoscopic Approach

02134KW Bypass Coronary Artery, Four or More Arteries from Aorta with Nonautologous Tissue Substitute, Percutaneous Endoscopic Approach

02134Z3 Bypass Coronary Artery, Four or More Arteries from Coronary Artery, Percutaneous Endoscopic Approach

02134Z8 Bypass Coronary Artery, Four or More Arteries from Right Internal Mammary, Percutaneous Endoscopic Approach

02134Z9 Bypass Coronary Artery, Four or More Arteries from Left Internal Mammary, Percutaneous Endoscopic Approach

02134ZC Bypass Coronary Artery, Four or More Arteries from Thoracic Artery, Percutaneous Endoscopic Approach

02134ZF Bypass Coronary Artery, Four or More Arteries from Abdominal Artery, Percutaneous Endoscopic Approach

HAC 09: Manifestations of Poor Glycemic Control

Secondary diagnosis not POA:

E08.00
E08.01
E08.10
E09.00
E09.01
E09.10
E10.10
E11.00
E11.01
E13.00
E13.01
E13.10
E15

HAC 10: Deep Vein Thrombosis (DVT) or Pulmonary Embolism (PE) with Total Knee or Hip Replacement

Secondary diagnosis not POA:

I26.02
I26.09
I26.92
I26.99
I82.401
I82.402
I82.403
I82.409
I82.411
I82.412
I82.413
I82.419
I82.421
I82.422
I82.423
I82.429
I82.431
I82.432
I82.433
I82.439
I82.441
I82.442
I82.443
I82.449
I82.491
I82.492
I82.493
I82.499
I82.4Y1
I82.4Y2
I82.4Y3
I82.4Y9
I82.4Z1
I82.4Z2
I82.4Z3
I82.4Z9

AND

Any of the following procedures:

0SR9019 Replacement of Right Hip Joint with Metal Synthetic Substitute, Cemented, Open Approach

0SR901A Replacement of Right Hip Joint with Metal Synthetic Substitute, Uncemented, Open Approach

0SR901Z Replacement of Right Hip Joint with Metal Synthetic Substitute, Open Approach

0SR9029 Replacement of Right Hip Joint with Metal on Polyethylene Synthetic Substitute, Cemented, Open Approach

0SR902A Replacement of Right Hip Joint with Metal on Polyethylene Synthetic Substitute, Uncemented, Open Approach

0SR902Z Replacement of Right Hip Joint with Metal on Polyethylene Synthetic Substitute, Open Approach

0SR9039 Replacement of Right Hip Joint with Ceramic Synthetic Substitute, Cemented, Open Approach

0SR903A Replacement of Right Hip Joint with Ceramic Synthetic Substitute, Uncemented, Open Approach

0SR903Z Replacement of Right Hip Joint with Ceramic Synthetic Substitute, Open Approach

0SR9049 Replacement of Right Hip Joint with Ceramic on Polyethylene Synthetic Substitute, Cemented, Open Approach

0SR904A Replacement of Right Hip Joint with Ceramic on Polyethylene Synthetic Substitute, Uncemented, Open Approach

0SR904Z Replacement of Right Hip Joint with Ceramic on Polyethylene Synthetic Substitute, Open Approach

0SR9069 Replacement of Right Hip Joint with Oxidized Zirconium on Polyethylene Synthetic Substitute, Cemented, Open Approach

0SR906A Replacement of Right Hip Joint with Oxidized Zirconium on Polyethylene Synthetic Substitute, Uncemented, Open Approach

0SR906Z Replacement of Right Hip Joint with Oxidized Zirconium on Polyethylene Synthetic Substitute, Open Approach

0SR907Z Replacement of Right Hip Joint with Autologous Tissue Substitute, Open Approach

0SR90EZ Replacement of Right Hip Joint with Articulating Spacer, Open Approach

0SR90J9 Replacement of Right Hip Joint with Synthetic Substitute, Cemented, Open Approach

0SR90JA Replacement of Right Hip Joint with Synthetic Substitute, Uncemented, Open Approach

0SR90JZ Replacement of Right Hip Joint with Synthetic Substitute, Open Approach

0SR90KZ Replacement of Right Hip Joint with Nonautologous Tissue Substitute, Open Approach

0SRA009 Replacement of Right Hip Joint, Acetabular Surface with Polyethylene Synthetic Substitute, Cemented, Open Approach

0SRA00A Replacement of Right Hip Joint, Acetabular Surface with Polyethylene Synthetic Substitute, Uncemented, Open Approach

0SRA00Z Replacement of Right Hip Joint, Acetabular Surface with Polyethylene Synthetic Substitute, Open Approach

0SRA019 Replacement of Right Hip Joint, Acetabular Surface with Metal Synthetic Substitute, Cemented, Open Approach

0SRA01A Replacement of Right Hip Joint, Acetabular Surface with Metal Synthetic Substitute, Uncemented, Open Approach

HAC 10: Deep Vein Thrombosis (DVT) or Pulmonary Embolism (PE) with Total Knee or Hip Replacement (continued)

ØSRAØ1Z   Replacement of Right Hip Joint, Acetabular Surface with Metal Synthetic Substitute, Open Approach

ØSRAØ39   Replacement of Right Hip Joint, Acetabular Surface with Ceramic Synthetic Substitute, Cemented, Open Approach

ØSRAØ3A   Replacement of Right Hip Joint, Acetabular Surface with Ceramic Synthetic Substitute, Uncemented, Open Approach

ØSRAØ3Z   Replacement of Right Hip Joint, Acetabular Surface with Ceramic Synthetic Substitute, Open Approach

ØSRAØ7Z   Replacement of Right Hip Joint, Acetabular Surface with Autologous Tissue Substitute, Open Approach

ØSRAØJ9   Replacement of Right Hip Joint, Acetabular Surface with Synthetic Substitute, Cemented, Open Approach

ØSRAØJA   Replacement of Right Hip Joint, Acetabular Surface with Synthetic Substitute, Uncemented, Open Approach

ØSRAØJZ   Replacement of Right Hip Joint, Acetabular Surface with Synthetic Substitute, Open Approach

ØSRAØKZ   Replacement of Right Hip Joint, Acetabular Surface with Nonautologous Tissue Substitute, Open Approach

ØSRBØ19   Replacement of Left Hip Joint with Metal Synthetic Substitute, Cemented, Open Approach

ØSRBØ1A   Replacement of Left Hip Joint with Metal Synthetic Substitute, Uncemented, Open Approach

ØSRBØ1Z   Replacement of Left Hip Joint with Metal Synthetic Substitute, Open Approach

ØSRBØ29   Replacement of Left Hip Joint with Metal on Polyethylene Synthetic Substitute, Cemented, Open Approach

ØSRBØ2A   Replacement of Left Hip Joint with Metal on Polyethylene Synthetic Substitute, Uncemented, Open Approach

ØSRBØ2Z   Replacement of Left Hip Joint with Metal on Polyethylene Synthetic Substitute, Open Approach

ØSRBØ39   Replacement of Left Hip Joint with Ceramic Synthetic Substitute, Cemented, Open Approach

ØSRBØ3A   Replacement of Left Hip Joint with Ceramic Synthetic Substitute, Uncemented, Open Approach

ØSRBØ3Z   Replacement of Left Hip Joint with Ceramic Synthetic Substitute, Open Approach

ØSRBØ49   Replacement of Left Hip Joint with Ceramic on Polyethylene Synthetic Substitute, Cemented, Open Approach

ØSRBØ4A   Replacement of Left Hip Joint with Ceramic on Polyethylene Synthetic Substitute, Uncemented, Open Approach

ØSRBØ4Z   Replacement of Left Hip Joint with Ceramic on Polyethylene Synthetic Substitute, Open Approach

ØSRBØ69   Replacement of Left Hip Joint with Oxidized Zirconium on Polyethylene Synthetic Substitute, Cemented, Open Approach

ØSRBØ6A   Replacement of Left Hip Joint with Oxidized Zirconium on Polyethylene Synthetic Substitute, Uncemented, Open Approach

ØSRBØ6Z   Replacement of Left Hip Joint with Oxidized Zirconium on Polyethylene Synthetic Substitute, Open Approach

ØSRBØ7Z   Replacement of Left Hip Joint with Autologous Tissue Substitute, Open Approach

ØSRBØEZ   Replacement of Left Hip Joint with Articulating Spacer, Open Approach

ØSRBØJ9   Replacement of Left Hip Joint with Synthetic Substitute, Cemented, Open Approach

ØSRBØJA   Replacement of Left Hip Joint with Synthetic Substitute, Uncemented, Open Approach

ØSRBØJZ   Replacement of Left Hip Joint with Synthetic Substitute, Open Approach

ØSRBØKZ   Replacement of Left Hip Joint with Nonautologous Tissue Substitute, Open Approach

ØSRCØ69   Replacement of Right Knee Joint with Oxidized Zirconium on Polyethylene Synthetic Substitute, Cemented, Open Approach

ØSRCØ6A   Replacement of Right Knee Joint with Oxidized Zirconium on Polyethylene Synthetic Substitute, Uncemented, Open Approach

ØSRCØ6Z   Replacement of Right Knee Joint with Oxidized Zirconium on Polyethylene Synthetic Substitute, Open Approach

ØSRCØ7Z   Replacement of Right Knee Joint with Autologous Tissue Substitute, Open Approach

ØSRCØEZ   Replacement of Right Knee Joint with Articulating Spacer, Open Approach

ØSRCØJ9   Replacement of Right Knee Joint with Synthetic Substitute, Cemented, Open Approach

ØSRCØJA   Replacement of Right Knee Joint with Synthetic Substitute, Uncemented, Open Approach

ØSRCØJZ   Replacement of Right Knee Joint with Synthetic Substitute, Open Approach

ØSRCØKZ   Replacement of Right Knee Joint with Nonautologous Tissue Substitute, Open Approach

ØSRCØL9   Replacement of Right Knee Joint with Medial Unicondylar Synthetic Substitute, Cemented, Open Approach

ØSRCØLA   Replacement of Right Knee Joint with Medial Unicondylar Synthetic Substitute, Uncemented, Open Approach

ØSRCØLZ   Replacement of Right Knee Joint with Medial Unicondylar Synthetic Substitute, Open Approach

ØSRCØM9   Replacement of Right Knee Joint with Lateral Unicondylar Synthetic Substitute, Cemented, Open Approach

ØSRCØMA   Replacement of Right Knee Joint with Lateral Unicondylar Synthetic Substitute, Uncemented, Open Approach

ØSRCØMZ   Replacement of Right Knee Joint with Lateral Unicondylar Synthetic Substitute, Open Approach

ØSRCØN9   Replacement of Right Knee Joint with Patellofemoral Synthetic Substitute, Cemented, Open Approach

ØSRCØNA   Replacement of Right Knee Joint with Patellofemoral Synthetic Substitute, Uncemented, Open Approach

ØSRCØNZ   Replacement of Right Knee Joint with Patellofemoral Synthetic Substitute, Open Approach

ØSRDØ69   Replacement of Left Knee Joint with Oxidized Zirconium on Polyethylene Synthetic Substitute, Cemented, Open Approach

ØSRDØ6A   Replacement of Left Knee Joint with Oxidized Zirconium on Polyethylene Synthetic Substitute, Uncemented, Open Approach

ØSRDØ6Z   Replacement of Left Knee Joint with Oxidized Zirconium on Polyethylene Synthetic Substitute, Open Approach

ØSRDØ7Z   Replacement of Left Knee Joint with Autologous Tissue Substitute, Open Approach

ØSRDØEZ   Replacement of Left Knee Joint with Articulating Spacer, Open Approach

ØSRDØJ9   Replacement of Left Knee Joint with Synthetic Substitute, Cemented, Open Approach

ØSRDØJA   Replacement of Left Knee Joint with Synthetic Substitute, Uncemented, Open Approach

ØSRDØJZ   Replacement of Left Knee Joint with Synthetic Substitute, Open Approach

ØSRDØKZ   Replacement of Left Knee Joint with Nonautologous Tissue Substitute, Open Approach

ØSRDØL9   Replacement of Left Knee Joint with Medial Unicondylar Synthetic Substitute, Cemented, Open Approach

ØSRDØLA   Replacement of Left Knee Joint with Medial Unicondylar Synthetic Substitute, Uncemented, Open Approach

ØSRDØLZ   Replacement of Left Knee Joint with Medial Unicondylar Synthetic Substitute, Open Approach

ØSRDØM9   Replacement of Left Knee Joint with Lateral Unicondylar Synthetic Substitute, Cemented, Open Approach

ØSRDØMA   Replacement of Left Knee Joint with Lateral Unicondylar Synthetic Substitute, Uncemented, Open Approach

ØSRDØMZ   Replacement of Left Knee Joint with Lateral Unicondylar Synthetic Substitute, Open Approach

ØSRDØN9   Replacement of Left Knee Joint with Patellofemoral Synthetic Substitute, Cemented, Open Approach

ØSRDØNA   Replacement of Left Knee Joint with Patellofemoral Synthetic Substitute, Uncemented, Open Approach

ØSRDØNZ   Replacement of Left Knee Joint with Patellofemoral Synthetic Substitute, Open Approach

ØSREØ09   Replacement of Left Hip Joint, Acetabular Surface with Polyethylene Synthetic Substitute, Cemented, Open Approach

ØSREØØA   Replacement of Left Hip Joint, Acetabular Surface with Polyethylene Synthetic Substitute, Uncemented, Open Approach

ØSREØØZ   Replacement of Left Hip Joint, Acetabular Surface with Polyethylene Synthetic Substitute, Open Approach

ØSREØ19   Replacement of Left Hip Joint, Acetabular Surface with Metal Synthetic Substitute, Cemented, Open Approach

ØSREØ1A   Replacement of Left Hip Joint, Acetabular Surface with Metal Synthetic Substitute, Uncemented, Open Approach

ØSREØ1Z   Replacement of Left Hip Joint, Acetabular Surface with Metal Synthetic Substitute, Open Approach

ØSREØ39   Replacement of Left Hip Joint, Acetabular Surface with Ceramic Synthetic Substitute, Cemented, Open Approach

ØSREØ3A   Replacement of Left Hip Joint, Acetabular Surface with Ceramic Synthetic Substitute, Uncemented, Open Approach

ØSREØ3Z   Replacement of Left Hip Joint, Acetabular Surface with Ceramic Synthetic Substitute, Open Approach

HAC 10: Deep Vein Thrombosis (DVT) or Pulmonary Embolism (PE) with Total Knee or Hip Replacement (continued)

ØSRE07Z   Replacement of Left Hip Joint, Acetabular Surface with Autologous Tissue Substitute, Open Approach

ØSREØJ9   Replacement of Left Hip Joint, Acetabular Surface with Synthetic Substitute, Cemented, Open Approach

ØSREØJA   Replacement of Left Hip Joint, Acetabular Surface with Synthetic Substitute, Uncemented, Open Approach

ØSREØJZ   Replacement of Left Hip Joint, Acetabular Surface with Synthetic Substitute, Open Approach

ØSREØKZ   Replacement of Left Hip Joint, Acetabular Surface with Nonautologous Tissue Substitute, Open Approach

ØSRR019   Replacement of Right Hip Joint, Femoral Surface with Metal Synthetic Substitute, Cemented, Open Approach

ØSRR01A   Replacement of Right Hip Joint, Femoral Surface with Metal Synthetic Substitute, Uncemented, Open Approach

ØSRR01Z   Replacement of Right Hip Joint, Femoral Surface with Metal Synthetic Substitute, Open Approach

ØSRR039   Replacement of Right Hip Joint, Femoral Surface with Ceramic Synthetic Substitute, Cemented, Open Approach

ØSRR03A   Replacement of Right Hip Joint, Femoral Surface with Ceramic Synthetic Substitute, Uncemented, Open Approach

ØSRR03Z   Replacement of Right Hip Joint, Femoral Surface with Ceramic Synthetic Substitute, Open Approach

ØSRR07Z   Replacement of Right Hip Joint, Femoral Surface with Autologous Tissue Substitute, Open Approach

ØSRRØJ9   Replacement of Right Hip Joint, Femoral Surface with Synthetic Substitute, Cemented, Open Approach

ØSRRØJA   Replacement of Right Hip Joint, Femoral Surface with Synthetic Substitute, Uncemented, Open Approach

ØSRRØJZ   Replacement of Right Hip Joint, Femoral Surface with Synthetic Substitute, Open Approach

ØSRRØKZ   Replacement of Right Hip Joint, Femoral Surface with Nonautologous Tissue Substitute, Open Approach

ØSRS019   Replacement of Left Hip Joint, Femoral Surface with Metal Synthetic Substitute, Cemented, Open Approach

ØSRS01A   Replacement of Left Hip Joint, Femoral Surface with Metal Synthetic Substitute, Uncemented, Open Approach

ØSRS01Z   Replacement of Left Hip Joint, Femoral Surface with Metal Synthetic Substitute, Open Approach

ØSRS039   Replacement of Left Hip Joint, Femoral Surface with Ceramic Synthetic Substitute, Cemented, Open Approach

ØSRS03A   Replacement of Left Hip Joint, Femoral Surface with Ceramic Synthetic Substitute, Uncemented, Open Approach

ØSRS03Z   Replacement of Left Hip Joint, Femoral Surface with Ceramic Synthetic Substitute, Open Approach

ØSRS07Z   Replacement of Left Hip Joint, Femoral Surface with Autologous Tissue Substitute, Open Approach

ØSRSØJ9   Replacement of Left Hip Joint, Femoral Surface with Synthetic Substitute, Cemented, Open Approach

ØSRSØJA   Replacement of Left Hip Joint, Femoral Surface with Synthetic Substitute, Uncemented, Open Approach

ØSRSØJZ   Replacement of Left Hip Joint, Femoral Surface with Synthetic Substitute, Open Approach

ØSRSØKZ   Replacement of Left Hip Joint, Femoral Surface with Nonautologous Tissue Substitute, Open Approach

ØSRT07Z   Replacement of Right Knee Joint, Femoral Surface with Autologous Tissue Substitute, Open Approach

ØSRTØJ9   Replacement of Right Knee Joint, Femoral Surface with Synthetic Substitute, Cemented, Open Approach

ØSRTØJA   Replacement of Right Knee Joint, Femoral Surface with Synthetic Substitute, Uncemented, Open Approach

ØSRTØJZ   Replacement of Right Knee Joint, Femoral Surface with Synthetic Substitute, Open Approach

ØSRTØKZ   Replacement of Right Knee Joint, Femoral Surface with Nonautologous Tissue Substitute, Open Approach

ØSRU07Z   Replacement of Left Knee Joint, Femoral Surface with Autologous Tissue Substitute, Open Approach

ØSRUØJ9   Replacement of Left Knee Joint, Femoral Surface with Synthetic Substitute, Cemented, Open Approach

ØSRUØJA   Replacement of Left Knee Joint, Femoral Surface with Synthetic Substitute, Uncemented, Open Approach

ØSRUØJZ   Replacement of Left Knee Joint, Femoral Surface with Synthetic Substitute, Open Approach

ØSRUØKZ   Replacement of Left Knee Joint, Femoral Surface with Nonautologous Tissue Substitute, Open Approach

ØSRV07Z   Replacement of Right Knee Joint, Tibial Surface with Autologous Tissue Substitute, Open Approach

ØSRVØJ9   Replacement of Right Knee Joint, Tibial Surface with Synthetic Substitute, Cemented, Open Approach

ØSRVØJA   Replacement of Right Knee Joint, Tibial Surface with Synthetic Substitute, Uncemented, Open Approach

ØSRVØJZ   Replacement of Right Knee Joint, Tibial Surface with Synthetic Substitute, Open Approach

ØSRVØKZ   Replacement of Right Knee Joint, Tibial Surface with Nonautologous Tissue Substitute, Open Approach

ØSRW07Z   Replacement of Left Knee Joint, Tibial Surface with Autologous Tissue Substitute, Open Approach

ØSRWØJ9   Replacement of Left Knee Joint, Tibial Surface with Synthetic Substitute, Cemented, Open Approach

ØSRWØJA   Replacement of Left Knee Joint, Tibial Surface with Synthetic Substitute, Uncemented, Open Approach

ØSRWØJZ   Replacement of Left Knee Joint, Tibial Surface with Synthetic Substitute, Open Approach

ØSRWØKZ   Replacement of Left Knee Joint, Tibial Surface with Nonautologous Tissue Substitute, Open Approach

ØSU90BZ   Supplement Right Hip Joint with Resurfacing Device, Open Approach

ØSUAØBZ   Supplement Right Hip Joint, Acetabular Surface with Resurfacing Device, Open Approach

ØSUBØBZ   Supplement Left Hip Joint with Resurfacing Device, Open Approach

ØSUEØBZ   Supplement Left Hip Joint, Acetabular Surface with Resurfacing Device, Open Approach

ØSURØBZ   Supplement Right Hip Joint, Femoral Surface with Resurfacing Device, Open Approach

ØSUSØBZ   Supplement Left Hip Joint, Femoral Surface with Resurfacing Device, Open Approach

HAC 11: Surgical Site Infection—Bariatric Surgery

Principal diagnosis of:

E66.Ø1

AND

Secondary diagnosis not POA:

K68.11
K95.Ø1
K95.81
T81.40XA
T81.41XA
T81.42XA
T81.43XA
T81.44XA
T81.49XA

AND

Any of the following procedures:

ØD16079   Bypass Stomach to Duodenum with Autologous Tissue Substitute, Open Approach

ØD1607A   Bypass Stomach to Jejunum with Autologous Tissue Substitute, Open Approach

ØD1607B   Bypass Stomach to Ileum with Autologous Tissue Substitute, Open Approach

ØD1607L   Bypass Stomach to Transverse Colon with Autologous Tissue Substitute, Open Approach

ØD160J9   Bypass Stomach to Duodenum with Synthetic Substitute, Open Approach

ØD160JA   Bypass Stomach to Jejunum with Synthetic Substitute, Open Approach

ØD160JB   Bypass Stomach to Ileum with Synthetic Substitute, Open Approach

ØD160JL   Bypass Stomach to Transverse Colon with Synthetic Substitute, Open Approach

ØD160K9   Bypass Stomach to Duodenum with Nonautologous Tissue Substitute, Open Approach

ØD160KA   Bypass Stomach to Jejunum with Nonautologous Tissue Substitute, Open Approach

ØD160KB   Bypass Stomach to Ileum with Nonautologous Tissue Substitute, Open Approach

ØD160KL   Bypass Stomach to Transverse Colon with Nonautologous Tissue Substitute, Open Approach

ØD160Z9   Bypass Stomach to Duodenum, Open Approach

ØD160ZA   Bypass Stomach to Jejunum, Open Approach

ØD160ZB   Bypass Stomach to Ileum, Open Approach

ØD160ZL   Bypass Stomach to Transverse Colon, Open Approach

ØD16479   Bypass Stomach to Duodenum with Autologous Tissue Substitute, Percutaneous Endoscopic Approach

ØD1647A   Bypass Stomach to Jejunum with Autologous Tissue Substitute, Percutaneous Endoscopic Approach

ØD1647B   Bypass Stomach to Ileum with Autologous Tissue Substitute, Percutaneous Endoscopic Approach

HAC 11: Surgical Site Infection—Bariatric Surgery (continued)

ØD1647L   Bypass Stomach to Transverse Colon with Autologous Tissue Substitute, Percutaneous Endoscopic Approach

ØD164J9   Bypass Stomach to Duodenum with Synthetic Substitute, Percutaneous Endoscopic Approach

ØD164JA   Bypass Stomach to Jejunum with Synthetic Substitute, Percutaneous Endoscopic Approach

ØD164JB   Bypass Stomach to Ileum with Synthetic Substitute, Percutaneous Endoscopic Approach

ØD164JL   Bypass Stomach to Transverse Colon with Synthetic Substitute, Percutaneous Endoscopic Approach

ØD164K9   Bypass Stomach to Duodenum with Nonautologous Tissue Substitute, Percutaneous Endoscopic Approach

ØD164KA   Bypass Stomach to Jejunum with Nonautologous Tissue Substitute, Percutaneous Endoscopic Approach

ØD164KB   Bypass Stomach to Ileum with Nonautologous Tissue Substitute, Percutaneous Endoscopic Approach

ØD164KL   Bypass Stomach to Transverse Colon with Nonautologous Tissue Substitute, Percutaneous Endoscopic Approach

ØD164Z9   Bypass Stomach to Duodenum, Percutaneous Endoscopic Approach

ØD164ZA   Bypass Stomach to Jejunum, Percutaneous Endoscopic Approach

ØD164ZB   Bypass Stomach to Ileum, Percutaneous Endoscopic Approach

ØD164ZL   Bypass Stomach to Transverse Colon, Percutaneous Endoscopic Approach

ØD16879   Bypass Stomach to Duodenum with Autologous Tissue Substitute, Via Natural or Artificial Opening Endoscopic

ØD1687A   Bypass Stomach to Jejunum with Autologous Tissue Substitute, Via Natural or Artificial Opening Endoscopic

ØD1687B   Bypass Stomach to Ileum with Autologous Tissue Substitute, Via Natural or Artificial Opening Endoscopic

ØD1687L   Bypass Stomach to Transverse Colon with Autologous Tissue Substitute, Via Natural or Artificial Opening Endoscopic

ØD168J9   Bypass Stomach to Duodenum with Synthetic Substitute, Via Natural or Artificial Opening Endoscopic

ØD168JA   Bypass Stomach to Jejunum with Synthetic Substitute, Via Natural or Artificial Opening Endoscopic

ØD168JB   Bypass Stomach to Ileum with Synthetic Substitute, Via Natural or Artificial Opening Endoscopic

ØD168JL   Bypass Stomach to Transverse Colon with Synthetic Substitute, Via Natural or Artificial Opening Endoscopic

ØD168K9   Bypass Stomach to Duodenum with Nonautologous Tissue Substitute, Via Natural or Artificial Opening Endoscopic

ØD168KA   Bypass Stomach to Jejunum with Nonautologous Tissue Substitute, Via Natural or Artificial Opening Endoscopic

ØD168KB   Bypass Stomach to Ileum with Nonautologous Tissue Substitute, Via Natural or Artificial Opening Endoscopic

ØD168KL   Bypass Stomach to Transverse Colon with Nonautologous Tissue Substitute, Via Natural or Artificial Opening Endoscopic

ØD168Z9   Bypass Stomach to Duodenum, Via Natural or Artificial Opening Endoscopic

ØD168ZA   Bypass Stomach to Jejunum, Via Natural or Artificial Opening Endoscopic

ØD168ZB   Bypass Stomach to Ileum, Via Natural or Artificial Opening Endoscopic

ØD168ZL   Bypass Stomach to Transverse Colon, Via Natural or Artificial Opening Endoscopic

ØDV64CZ   Restriction of Stomach with Extraluminal Device, Percutaneous Endoscopic Approach

HAC 12: Surgical Site Infection—Certain Orthopedic Procedures of the Spine, Shoulder, and Elbow

Secondary diagnosis not POA:

K68.11
T81.40XA
T81.41XA
T81.42XA
T81.43XA
T81.44XA
T81.49XA
T84.60XA
T84.610A
T84.611A
T84.612A
T84.613A
T84.614A
T84.615A
T84.619A
T84.63XA
T84.69XA
T84.7XXA

AND

Any of the following procedures:

ØRG0070   Fusion of Occipital-cervical Joint with Autologous Tissue Substitute, Anterior Approach, Anterior Column, Open Approach

ØRG0071   Fusion of Occipital-cervical Joint with Autologous Tissue Substitute, Posterior Approach, Posterior Column, Open Approach

ØRG007J   Fusion of Occipital-cervical Joint with Autologous Tissue Substitute, Posterior Approach, Anterior Column, Open Approach

ØRG00A0   Fusion of Occipital-cervical Joint with Interbody Fusion Device, Anterior Approach, Anterior Column, Open Approach

ØRG00AJ   Fusion of Occipital-cervical Joint with Interbody Fusion Device, Posterior Approach, Anterior Column, Open Approach

ØRG00J0   Fusion of Occipital-cervical Joint with Synthetic Substitute, Anterior Approach, Anterior Column, Open Approach

ØRG00J1   Fusion of Occipital-cervical Joint with Synthetic Substitute, Posterior Approach, Posterior Column, Open Approach

ØRG00JJ   Fusion of Occipital-cervical Joint with Synthetic Substitute, Posterior Approach, Anterior Column, Open Approach

ØRG00K0   Fusion of Occipital-cervical Joint with Nonautologous Tissue Substitute, Anterior Approach, Anterior Column, Open Approach

ØRG00K1   Fusion of Occipital-cervical Joint with Nonautologous Tissue Substitute, Posterior Approach, Posterior Column, Open Approach

ØRG00KJ   Fusion of Occipital-cervical Joint with Nonautologous Tissue Substitute, Posterior Approach, Anterior Column, Open Approach

ØRG0370   Fusion of Occipital-cervical Joint with Autologous Tissue Substitute, Anterior Approach, Anterior Column, Percutaneous Approach

ØRG0371   Fusion of Occipital-cervical Joint with Autologous Tissue Substitute, Posterior Approach, Posterior Column, Percutaneous Approach

ØRG037J   Fusion of Occipital-cervical Joint with Autologous Tissue Substitute, Posterior Approach, Anterior Column, Percutaneous Approach

ØRG03A0   Fusion of Occipital-cervical Joint with Interbody Fusion Device, Anterior Approach, Anterior Column, Percutaneous Approach

ØRG03AJ   Fusion of Occipital-cervical Joint with Interbody Fusion Device, Posterior Approach, Anterior Column, Percutaneous Approach

ØRG03J0   Fusion of Occipital-cervical Joint with Synthetic Substitute, Anterior Approach, Anterior Column, Percutaneous Approach

ØRG03J1   Fusion of Occipital-cervical Joint with Synthetic Substitute, Posterior Approach, Posterior Column, Percutaneous Approach

ØRG03JJ   Fusion of Occipital-cervical Joint with Synthetic Substitute, Posterior Approach, Anterior Column, Percutaneous Approach

ØRG03K0   Fusion of Occipital-cervical Joint with Nonautologous Tissue Substitute, Anterior Approach, Anterior Column, Percutaneous Approach

ØRG03K1   Fusion of Occipital-cervical Joint with Nonautologous Tissue Substitute, Posterior Approach, Posterior Column, Percutaneous Approach

ØRG03KJ   Fusion of Occipital-cervical Joint with Nonautologous Tissue Substitute, Posterior Approach, Anterior Column, Percutaneous Approach

ØRG0470   Fusion of Occipital-cervical Joint with Autologous Tissue Substitute, Anterior Approach, Anterior Column, Percutaneous Endoscopic Approach

ØRG0471   Fusion of Occipital-cervical Joint with Autologous Tissue Substitute, Posterior Approach, Posterior Column, Percutaneous Endoscopic Approach

ØRG047J   Fusion of Occipital-cervical Joint with Autologous Tissue Substitute, Posterior Approach, Anterior Column, Percutaneous Endoscopic Approach

ØRG04A0   Fusion of Occipital-cervical Joint with Interbody Fusion Device, Anterior Approach, Anterior Column, Percutaneous Endoscopic Approach

ØRG04AJ   Fusion of Occipital-cervical Joint with Interbody Fusion Device, Posterior Approach, Anterior Column, Percutaneous Endoscopic Approach

ØRG04J0   Fusion of Occipital-cervical Joint with Synthetic Substitute, Anterior Approach, Anterior Column, Percutaneous Endoscopic Approach

ØRG04J1   Fusion of Occipital-cervical Joint with Synthetic Substitute, Posterior Approach, Posterior Column, Percutaneous Endoscopic Approach

ØRG04JJ   Fusion of Occipital-cervical Joint with Synthetic Substitute, Posterior Approach, Anterior Column, Percutaneous Endoscopic Approach

ØRG04K0   Fusion of Occipital-cervical Joint with Nonautologous Tissue Substitute, Anterior Approach, Anterior Column, Percutaneous Endoscopic Approach

HAC 12: Surgical Site Infection—Certain Orthopedic Procedures of the Spine, Shoulder, and Elbow (continued)

ØRGØ4K1   Fusion of Occipital-cervical Joint with Nonautologous Tissue Substitute, Posterior Approach, Posterior Column, Percutaneous Endoscopic Approach

ØRGØ4KJ   Fusion of Occipital-cervical Joint with Nonautologous Tissue Substitute, Posterior Approach, Anterior Column, Percutaneous Endoscopic Approach

ØRG1Ø7Ø   Fusion of Cervical Vertebral Joint with Autologous Tissue Substitute, Anterior Approach, Anterior Column, Open Approach

ØRG1Ø71   Fusion of Cervical Vertebral Joint with Autologous Tissue Substitute, Posterior Approach, Posterior Column, Open Approach

ØRG1Ø7J   Fusion of Cervical Vertebral Joint with Autologous Tissue Substitute, Posterior Approach, Anterior Column, Open Approach

ØRG1ØAØ   Fusion of Cervical Vertebral Joint with Interbody Fusion Device, Anterior Approach, Anterior Column, Open Approach

ØRG1ØAJ   Fusion of Cervical Vertebral Joint with Interbody Fusion Device, Posterior Approach, Anterior Column, Open Approach

ØRG1ØJØ   Fusion of Cervical Vertebral Joint with Synthetic Substitute, Anterior Approach, Anterior Column, Open Approach

ØRG1ØJ1   Fusion of Cervical Vertebral Joint with Synthetic Substitute, Posterior Approach, Posterior Column, Open Approach

ØRG1ØJJ   Fusion of Cervical Vertebral Joint with Synthetic Substitute, Posterior Approach, Anterior Column, Open Approach

ØRG1ØKØ   Fusion of Cervical Vertebral Joint with Nonautologous Tissue Substitute, Anterior Approach, Anterior Column, Open Approach

ØRG1ØK1   Fusion of Cervical Vertebral Joint with Nonautologous Tissue Substitute, Posterior Approach, Posterior Column, Open Approach

ØRG1ØKJ   Fusion of Cervical Vertebral Joint with Nonautologous Tissue Substitute, Posterior Approach, Anterior Column, Open Approach

ØRG137Ø   Fusion of Cervical Vertebral Joint with Autologous Tissue Substitute, Anterior Approach, Anterior Column, Percutaneous Approach

ØRG1371   Fusion of Cervical Vertebral Joint with Autologous Tissue Substitute, Posterior Approach, Posterior Column, Percutaneous Approach

ØRG137J   Fusion of Cervical Vertebral Joint with Autologous Tissue Substitute, Posterior Approach, Anterior Column, Percutaneous Approach

ØRG13AØ   Fusion of Cervical Vertebral Joint with Interbody Fusion Device, Anterior Approach, Anterior Column, Percutaneous Approach

ØRG13AJ   Fusion of Cervical Vertebral Joint with Interbody Fusion Device, Posterior Approach, Anterior Column, Percutaneous Approach

ØRG13JØ   Fusion of Cervical Vertebral Joint with Synthetic Substitute, Anterior Approach, Anterior Column, Percutaneous Approach

ØRG13J1   Fusion of Cervical Vertebral Joint with Synthetic Substitute, Posterior Approach, Posterior Column, Percutaneous Approach

ØRG13JJ   Fusion of Cervical Vertebral Joint with Synthetic Substitute, Posterior Approach, Anterior Column, Percutaneous Approach

ØRG13KØ   Fusion of Cervical Vertebral Joint with Nonautologous Tissue Substitute, Anterior Approach, Anterior Column, Percutaneous Approach

ØRG13K1   Fusion of Cervical Vertebral Joint with Nonautologous Tissue Substitute, Posterior Approach, Posterior Column, Percutaneous Approach

ØRG13KJ   Fusion of Cervical Vertebral Joint with Nonautologous Tissue Substitute, Posterior Approach, Anterior Column, Percutaneous Approach

ØRG147Ø   Fusion of Cervical Vertebral Joint with Autologous Tissue Substitute, Anterior Approach, Anterior Column, Percutaneous Endoscopic Approach

ØRG1471   Fusion of Cervical Vertebral Joint with Autologous Tissue Substitute, Posterior Approach, Posterior Column, Percutaneous Endoscopic Approach

ØRG147J   Fusion of Cervical Vertebral Joint with Autologous Tissue Substitute, Posterior Approach, Anterior Column, Percutaneous Endoscopic Approach

ØRG14AØ   Fusion of Cervical Vertebral Joint with Interbody Fusion Device, Anterior Approach, Anterior Column, Percutaneous Endoscopic Approach

ØRG14AJ   Fusion of Cervical Vertebral Joint with Interbody Fusion Device, Posterior Approach, Anterior Column, Percutaneous Endoscopic Approach

ØRG14JØ   Fusion of Cervical Vertebral Joint with Synthetic Substitute, Anterior Approach, Anterior Column, Percutaneous Endoscopic Approach

ØRG14J1   Fusion of Cervical Vertebral Joint with Synthetic Substitute, Posterior Approach, Posterior Column, Percutaneous Endoscopic Approach

ØRG14JJ   Fusion of Cervical Vertebral Joint with Synthetic Substitute, Posterior Approach, Anterior Column, Percutaneous Endoscopic Approach

ØRG14KØ   Fusion of Cervical Vertebral Joint with Nonautologous Tissue Substitute, Anterior Approach, Anterior Column, Percutaneous Endoscopic Approach

ØRG14K1   Fusion of Cervical Vertebral Joint with Nonautologous Tissue Substitute, Posterior Approach, Posterior Column, Percutaneous Endoscopic Approach

ØRG14KJ   Fusion of Cervical Vertebral Joint with Nonautologous Tissue Substitute, Posterior Approach, Anterior Column, Percutaneous Endoscopic Approach

ØRG2Ø7Ø   Fusion of 2 or more Cervical Vertebral Joints with Autologous Tissue Substitute, Anterior Approach, Anterior Column, Open Approach

ØRG2Ø71   Fusion of 2 or more Cervical Vertebral Joints with Autologous Tissue Substitute, Posterior Approach, Posterior Column, Open Approach

ØRG2Ø7J   Fusion of 2 or more Cervical Vertebral Joints with Autologous Tissue Substitute, Posterior Approach, Anterior Column, Open Approach

ØRG2ØAØ   Fusion of 2 or more Cervical Vertebral Joints with Interbody Fusion Device, Anterior Approach, Anterior Column, Open Approach

ØRG2ØAJ   Fusion of 2 or more Cervical Vertebral Joints with Interbody Fusion Device, Posterior Approach, Anterior Column, Open Approach

ØRG2ØJØ   Fusion of 2 or more Cervical Vertebral Joints with Synthetic Substitute, Anterior Approach, Anterior Column, Open Approach

ØRG2ØJ1   Fusion of 2 or more Cervical Vertebral Joints with Synthetic Substitute, Posterior Approach, Posterior Column, Open Approach

ØRG2ØJJ   Fusion of 2 or more Cervical Vertebral Joints with Synthetic Substitute, Posterior Approach, Anterior Column, Open Approach

ØRG2ØKØ   Fusion of 2 or more Cervical Vertebral Joints with Nonautologous Tissue Substitute, Anterior Approach, Anterior Column, Open Approach

ØRG2ØK1   Fusion of 2 or more Cervical Vertebral Joints with Nonautologous Tissue Substitute, Posterior Approach, Posterior Column, Open Approach

ØRG2ØKJ   Fusion of 2 or more Cervical Vertebral Joints with Nonautologous Tissue Substitute, Posterior Approach, Anterior Column, Open Approach

ØRG237Ø   Fusion of 2 or more Cervical Vertebral Joints with Autologous Tissue Substitute, Anterior Approach, Anterior Column, Percutaneous Approach

ØRG2371   Fusion of 2 or more Cervical Vertebral Joints with Autologous Tissue Substitute, Posterior Approach, Posterior Column, Percutaneous Approach

ØRG237J   Fusion of 2 or more Cervical Vertebral Joints with Autologous Tissue Substitute, Posterior Approach, Anterior Column, Percutaneous Approach

ØRG23AØ   Fusion of 2 or more Cervical Vertebral Joints with Interbody Fusion Device, Anterior Approach, Anterior Column, Percutaneous Approach

ØRG23AJ   Fusion of 2 or more Cervical Vertebral Joints with Interbody Fusion Device, Posterior Approach, Anterior Column, Percutaneous Approach

ØRG23JØ   Fusion of 2 or more Cervical Vertebral Joints with Synthetic Substitute, Anterior Approach, Anterior Column, Percutaneous Approach

ØRG23J1   Fusion of 2 or more Cervical Vertebral Joints with Synthetic Substitute, Posterior Approach, Posterior Column, Percutaneous Approach

ØRG23JJ   Fusion of 2 or more Cervical Vertebral Joints with Synthetic Substitute, Posterior Approach, Anterior Column, Percutaneous Approach

ØRG23KØ   Fusion of 2 or more Cervical Vertebral Joints with Nonautologous Tissue Substitute, Anterior Approach, Anterior Column, Percutaneous Approach

ØRG23K1   Fusion of 2 or more Cervical Vertebral Joints with Nonautologous Tissue Substitute, Posterior Approach, Posterior Column, Percutaneous Approach

ØRG23KJ   Fusion of 2 or more Cervical Vertebral Joints with Nonautologous Tissue Substitute, Posterior Approach, Anterior Column, Percutaneous Approach

HAC 12: Surgical Site Infection— Certain Orthopedic Procedures of the Spine, Shoulder, and Elbow (continued)

ØRG2470   Fusion of 2 or more Cervical Vertebral Joints with Autologous Tissue Substitute, Anterior Approach, Anterior Column, Percutaneous Endoscopic Approach

ØRG2471   Fusion of 2 or more Cervical Vertebral Joints with Autologous Tissue Substitute, Posterior Approach, Posterior Column, Percutaneous Endoscopic Approach

ØRG247J   Fusion of 2 or more Cervical Vertebral Joints with Autologous Tissue Substitute, Posterior Approach, Anterior Column, Percutaneous Endoscopic Approach

ØRG24AØ   Fusion of 2 or more Cervical Vertebral Joints with Interbody Fusion Device, Anterior Approach, Anterior Column, Percutaneous Endoscopic Approach

ØRG24AJ   Fusion of 2 or more Cervical Vertebral Joints with Interbody Fusion Device, Posterior Approach, Anterior Column, Percutaneous Endoscopic Approach

ØRG24JØ   Fusion of 2 or more Cervical Vertebral Joints with Synthetic Substitute, Anterior Approach, Anterior Column, Percutaneous Endoscopic Approach

ØRG24J1   Fusion of 2 or more Cervical Vertebral Joints with Synthetic Substitute, Posterior Approach, Posterior Column, Percutaneous Endoscopic Approach

ØRG24JJ   Fusion of 2 or more Cervical Vertebral Joints with Synthetic Substitute, Posterior Approach, Anterior Column, Percutaneous Endoscopic Approach

ØRG24KØ   Fusion of 2 or more Cervical Vertebral Joints with Nonautologous Tissue Substitute, Anterior Approach, Anterior Column, Percutaneous Endoscopic Approach

ØRG24K1   Fusion of 2 or more Cervical Vertebral Joints with Nonautologous Tissue Substitute, Posterior Approach, Posterior Column, Percutaneous Endoscopic Approach

ØRG24KJ   Fusion of 2 or more Cervical Vertebral Joints with Nonautologous Tissue Substitute, Posterior Approach, Anterior Column, Percutaneous Endoscopic Approach

ØRG4070   Fusion of Cervicothoracic Vertebral Joint with Autologous Tissue Substitute, Anterior Approach, Anterior Column, Open Approach

ØRG4071   Fusion of Cervicothoracic Vertebral Joint with Autologous Tissue Substitute, Posterior Approach, Posterior Column, Open Approach

ØRG407J   Fusion of Cervicothoracic Vertebral Joint with Autologous Tissue Substitute, Posterior Approach, Anterior Column, Open Approach

ØRG40AØ   Fusion of Cervicothoracic Vertebral Joint with Interbody Fusion Device, Anterior Approach, Anterior Column, Open Approach

ØRG40AJ   Fusion of Cervicothoracic Vertebral Joint with Interbody Fusion Device, Posterior Approach, Anterior Column, Open Approach

ØRG40JØ   Fusion of Cervicothoracic Vertebral Joint with Synthetic Substitute, Anterior Approach, Anterior Column, Open Approach

ØRG40J1   Fusion of Cervicothoracic Vertebral Joint with Synthetic Substitute, Posterior Approach, Posterior Column, Open Approach

ØRG40JJ   Fusion of Cervicothoracic Vertebral Joint with Synthetic Substitute, Posterior Approach, Anterior Column, Open Approach

ØRG40KØ   Fusion of Cervicothoracic Vertebral Joint with Nonautologous Tissue Substitute, Anterior Approach, Anterior Column, Open Approach

ØRG40K1   Fusion of Cervicothoracic Vertebral Joint with Nonautologous Tissue Substitute, Posterior Approach, Posterior Column, Open Approach

ØRG40KJ   Fusion of Cervicothoracic Vertebral Joint with Nonautologous Tissue Substitute, Posterior Approach, Anterior Column, Open Approach

ØRG4370   Fusion of Cervicothoracic Vertebral Joint with Autologous Tissue Substitute, Anterior Approach, Anterior Column, Percutaneous Approach

ØRG4371   Fusion of Cervicothoracic Vertebral Joint with Autologous Tissue Substitute, Posterior Approach, Posterior Column, Percutaneous Approach

ØRG437J   Fusion of Cervicothoracic Vertebral Joint with Autologous Tissue Substitute, Posterior Approach, Anterior Column, Percutaneous Approach

ØRG43AØ   Fusion of Cervicothoracic Vertebral Joint with Interbody Fusion Device, Anterior Approach, Anterior Column, Percutaneous Approach

ØRG43AJ   Fusion of Cervicothoracic Vertebral Joint with Interbody Fusion Device, Posterior Approach, Anterior Column, Percutaneous Approach

ØRG43JØ   Fusion of Cervicothoracic Vertebral Joint with Synthetic Substitute, Anterior Approach, Anterior Column, Percutaneous Approach

ØRG43J1   Fusion of Cervicothoracic Vertebral Joint with Synthetic Substitute, Posterior Approach, Posterior Column, Percutaneous Approach

ØRG43JJ   Fusion of Cervicothoracic Vertebral Joint with Synthetic Substitute, Posterior Approach, Anterior Column, Percutaneous Approach

ØRG43KØ   Fusion of Cervicothoracic Vertebral Joint with Nonautologous Tissue Substitute, Anterior Approach, Anterior Column, Percutaneous Approach

ØRG43K1   Fusion of Cervicothoracic Vertebral Joint with Nonautologous Tissue Substitute, Posterior Approach, Posterior Column, Percutaneous Approach

ØRG43KJ   Fusion of Cervicothoracic Vertebral Joint with Nonautologous Tissue Substitute, Posterior Approach, Anterior Column, Percutaneous Approach

ØRG4470   Fusion of Cervicothoracic Vertebral Joint with Autologous Tissue Substitute, Anterior Approach, Anterior Column, Percutaneous Endoscopic Approach

ØRG4471   Fusion of Cervicothoracic Vertebral Joint with Autologous Tissue Substitute, Posterior Approach, Posterior Column, Percutaneous Endoscopic Approach

ØRG447J   Fusion of Cervicothoracic Vertebral Joint with Autologous Tissue Substitute, Posterior Approach, Anterior Column, Percutaneous Endoscopic Approach

ØRG44AØ   Fusion of Cervicothoracic Vertebral Joint with Interbody Fusion Device, Anterior Approach, Anterior Column, Percutaneous Endoscopic Approach

ØRG44AJ   Fusion of Cervicothoracic Vertebral Joint with Interbody Fusion Device, Posterior Approach, Anterior Column, Percutaneous Endoscopic Approach

ØRG44JØ   Fusion of Cervicothoracic Vertebral Joint with Synthetic Substitute, Anterior Approach, Anterior Column, Percutaneous Endoscopic Approach

ØRG44J1   Fusion of Cervicothoracic Vertebral Joint with Synthetic Substitute, Posterior Approach, Posterior Column, Percutaneous Endoscopic Approach

ØRG44JJ   Fusion of Cervicothoracic Vertebral Joint with Synthetic Substitute, Posterior Approach, Anterior Column, Percutaneous Endoscopic Approach

ØRG44KØ   Fusion of Cervicothoracic Vertebral Joint with Nonautologous Tissue Substitute, Anterior Approach, Anterior Column, Percutaneous Endoscopic Approach

ØRG44K1   Fusion of Cervicothoracic Vertebral Joint with Nonautologous Tissue Substitute, Posterior Approach, Posterior Column, Percutaneous Endoscopic Approach

ØRG44KJ   Fusion of Cervicothoracic Vertebral Joint with Nonautologous Tissue Substitute, Posterior Approach, Anterior Column, Percutaneous Endoscopic Approach

ØRG6070   Fusion of Thoracic Vertebral Joint with Autologous Tissue Substitute, Anterior Approach, Anterior Column, Open Approach

ØRG6071   Fusion of Thoracic Vertebral Joint with Autologous Tissue Substitute, Posterior Approach, Posterior Column, Open Approach

ØRG607J   Fusion of Thoracic Vertebral Joint with Autologous Tissue Substitute, Posterior Approach, Anterior Column, Open Approach

ØRG60AØ   Fusion of Thoracic Vertebral Joint with Interbody Fusion Device, Anterior Approach, Anterior Column, Open Approach

ØRG60AJ   Fusion of Thoracic Vertebral Joint with Interbody Fusion Device, Posterior Approach, Anterior Column, Open Approach

ØRG60JØ   Fusion of Thoracic Vertebral Joint with Synthetic Substitute, Anterior Approach, Anterior Column, Open Approach

ØRG60J1   Fusion of Thoracic Vertebral Joint with Synthetic Substitute, Posterior Approach, Posterior Column, Open Approach

ØRG60JJ   Fusion of Thoracic Vertebral Joint with Synthetic Substitute, Posterior Approach, Anterior Column, Open Approach

ØRG60KØ   Fusion of Thoracic Vertebral Joint with Nonautologous Tissue Substitute, Anterior Approach, Anterior Column, Open Approach

ØRG60K1   Fusion of Thoracic Vertebral Joint with Nonautologous Tissue Substitute, Posterior Approach, Posterior Column, Open Approach

ØRG60KJ   Fusion of Thoracic Vertebral Joint with Nonautologous Tissue Substitute, Posterior Approach, Anterior Column, Open Approach

ØRG6370   Fusion of Thoracic Vertebral Joint with Autologous Tissue Substitute, Anterior Approach, Anterior Column, Percutaneous Approach

HAC 12: Surgical Site Infection—Certain Orthopedic Procedures of the Spine, Shoulder, and Elbow (continued)

ØRG6371 Fusion of Thoracic Vertebral Joint with Autologous Tissue Substitute, Posterior Approach, Posterior Column, Percutaneous Approach

ØRG637J Fusion of Thoracic Vertebral Joint with Autologous Tissue Substitute, Posterior Approach, Anterior Column, Percutaneous Approach

ØRG63AØ Fusion of Thoracic Vertebral Joint with Interbody Fusion Device, Anterior Approach, Anterior Column, Percutaneous Approach

ØRG63AJ Fusion of Thoracic Vertebral Joint with Interbody Fusion Device, Posterior Approach, Anterior Column, Percutaneous Approach

ØRG63JØ Fusion of Thoracic Vertebral Joint with Synthetic Substitute, Anterior Approach, Anterior Column, Percutaneous Approach

ØRG63J1 Fusion of Thoracic Vertebral Joint with Synthetic Substitute, Posterior Approach, Posterior Column, Percutaneous Approach

ØRG63JJ Fusion of Thoracic Vertebral Joint with Synthetic Substitute, Posterior Approach, Anterior Column, Percutaneous Approach

ØRG63KØ Fusion of Thoracic Vertebral Joint with Nonautologous Tissue Substitute, Anterior Approach, Anterior Column, Percutaneous Approach

ØRG63K1 Fusion of Thoracic Vertebral Joint with Nonautologous Tissue Substitute, Posterior Approach, Posterior Column, Percutaneous Approach

ØRG63KJ Fusion of Thoracic Vertebral Joint with Nonautologous Tissue Substitute, Posterior Approach, Anterior Column, Percutaneous Approach

ØRG647Ø Fusion of Thoracic Vertebral Joint with Autologous Tissue Substitute, Anterior Approach, Anterior Column, Percutaneous Endoscopic Approach

ØRG6471 Fusion of Thoracic Vertebral Joint with Autologous Tissue Substitute, Posterior Approach, Posterior Column, Percutaneous Endoscopic Approach

ØRG647J Fusion of Thoracic Vertebral Joint with Autologous Tissue Substitute, Posterior Approach, Anterior Column, Percutaneous Endoscopic Approach

ØRG64AØ Fusion of Thoracic Vertebral Joint with Interbody Fusion Device, Anterior Approach, Anterior Column, Percutaneous Endoscopic Approach

ØRG64AJ Fusion of Thoracic Vertebral Joint with Interbody Fusion Device, Posterior Approach, Anterior Column, Percutaneous Endoscopic Approach

ØRG64JØ Fusion of Thoracic Vertebral Joint with Synthetic Substitute, Anterior Approach, Anterior Column, Percutaneous Endoscopic Approach

ØRG64J1 Fusion of Thoracic Vertebral Joint with Synthetic Substitute, Posterior Approach, Posterior Column, Percutaneous Endoscopic Approach

ØRG64JJ Fusion of Thoracic Vertebral Joint with Synthetic Substitute, Posterior Approach, Anterior Column, Percutaneous Endoscopic Approach

ØRG64KØ Fusion of Thoracic Vertebral Joint with Nonautologous Tissue Substitute, Anterior Approach, Anterior Column, Percutaneous Endoscopic Approach

ØRG64K1 Fusion of Thoracic Vertebral Joint with Nonautologous Tissue Substitute, Posterior Approach, Posterior Column, Percutaneous Endoscopic Approach

ØRG64KJ Fusion of Thoracic Vertebral Joint with Nonautologous Tissue Substitute, Posterior Approach, Anterior Column, Percutaneous Endoscopic Approach

ØRG7Ø7Ø Fusion of 2 to 7 Thoracic Vertebral Joints with Autologous Tissue Substitute, Anterior Approach, Anterior Column, Open Approach

ØRG7Ø71 Fusion of 2 to 7 Thoracic Vertebral Joints with Autologous Tissue Substitute, Posterior Approach, Posterior Column, Open Approach

ØRG7Ø7J Fusion of 2 to 7 Thoracic Vertebral Joints with Autologous Tissue Substitute, Posterior Approach, Anterior Column, Open Approach

ØRG7ØAØ Fusion of 2 to 7 Thoracic Vertebral Joints with Interbody Fusion Device, Anterior Approach, Anterior Column, Open Approach

ØRG7ØAJ Fusion of 2 to 7 Thoracic Vertebral Joints with Interbody Fusion Device, Posterior Approach, Anterior Column, Open Approach

ØRG7ØJØ Fusion of 2 to 7 Thoracic Vertebral Joints with Synthetic Substitute, Anterior Approach, Anterior Column, Open Approach

ØRG7ØJ1 Fusion of 2 to 7 Thoracic Vertebral Joints with Synthetic Substitute, Posterior Approach, Posterior Column, Open Approach

ØRG7ØJJ Fusion of 2 to 7 Thoracic Vertebral Joints with Synthetic Substitute, Posterior Approach, Anterior Column, Open Approach

ØRG7ØKØ Fusion of 2 to 7 Thoracic Vertebral Joints with Nonautologous Tissue Substitute, Anterior Approach, Anterior Column, Open Approach

ØRG7ØK1 Fusion of 2 to 7 Thoracic Vertebral Joints with Nonautologous Tissue Substitute, Posterior Approach, Posterior Column, Open Approach

ØRG7ØKJ Fusion of 2 to 7 Thoracic Vertebral Joints with Nonautologous Tissue Substitute, Posterior Approach, Anterior Column, Open Approach

ØRG737Ø Fusion of 2 to 7 Thoracic Vertebral Joints with Autologous Tissue Substitute, Anterior Approach, Anterior Column, Percutaneous Approach

ØRG7371 Fusion of 2 to 7 Thoracic Vertebral Joints with Autologous Tissue Substitute, Posterior Approach, Posterior Column, Percutaneous Approach

ØRG737J Fusion of 2 to 7 Thoracic Vertebral Joints with Autologous Tissue Substitute, Posterior Approach, Anterior Column, Percutaneous Approach

ØRG73AØ Fusion of 2 to 7 Thoracic Vertebral Joints with Interbody Fusion Device, Anterior Approach, Anterior Column, Percutaneous Approach

ØRG73AJ Fusion of 2 to 7 Thoracic Vertebral Joints with Interbody Fusion Device, Posterior Approach, Anterior Column, Percutaneous Approach

ØRG73JØ Fusion of 2 to 7 Thoracic Vertebral Joints with Synthetic Substitute, Anterior Approach, Anterior Column, Percutaneous Approach

ØRG73J1 Fusion of 2 to 7 Thoracic Vertebral Joints with Synthetic Substitute, Posterior Approach, Posterior Column, Percutaneous Approach

ØRG73JJ Fusion of 2 to 7 Thoracic Vertebral Joints with Synthetic Substitute, Posterior Approach, Anterior Column, Percutaneous Approach

ØRG73KØ Fusion of 2 to 7 Thoracic Vertebral Joints with Nonautologous Tissue Substitute, Anterior Approach, Anterior Column, Percutaneous Approach

ØRG73K1 Fusion of 2 to 7 Thoracic Vertebral Joints with Nonautologous Tissue Substitute, Posterior Approach, Posterior Column, Percutaneous Approach

ØRG73KJ Fusion of 2 to 7 Thoracic Vertebral Joints with Nonautologous Tissue Substitute, Posterior Approach, Anterior Column, Percutaneous Approach

ØRG747Ø Fusion of 2 to 7 Thoracic Vertebral Joints with Autologous Tissue Substitute, Anterior Approach, Anterior Column, Percutaneous Endoscopic Approach

ØRG7471 Fusion of 2 to 7 Thoracic Vertebral Joints with Autologous Tissue Substitute, Posterior Approach, Posterior Column, Percutaneous Endoscopic Approach

ØRG747J Fusion of 2 to 7 Thoracic Vertebral Joints with Autologous Tissue Substitute, Posterior Approach, Anterior Column, Percutaneous Endoscopic Approach

ØRG74AØ Fusion of 2 to 7 Thoracic Vertebral Joints with Interbody Fusion Device, Anterior Approach, Anterior Column, Percutaneous Endoscopic Approach

ØRG74AJ Fusion of 2 to 7 Thoracic Vertebral Joints with Interbody Fusion Device, Posterior Approach, Anterior Column, Percutaneous Endoscopic Approach

ØRG74JØ Fusion of 2 to 7 Thoracic Vertebral Joints with Synthetic Substitute, Anterior Approach, Anterior Column, Percutaneous Endoscopic Approach

ØRG74J1 Fusion of 2 to 7 Thoracic Vertebral Joints with Synthetic Substitute, Posterior Approach, Posterior Column, Percutaneous Endoscopic Approach

ØRG74JJ Fusion of 2 to 7 Thoracic Vertebral Joints with Synthetic Substitute, Posterior Approach, Anterior Column, Percutaneous Endoscopic Approach

ØRG74KØ Fusion of 2 to 7 Thoracic Vertebral Joints with Nonautologous Tissue Substitute, Anterior Approach, Anterior Column, Percutaneous Endoscopic Approach

ØRG74K1 Fusion of 2 to 7 Thoracic Vertebral Joints with Nonautologous Tissue Substitute, Posterior Approach, Posterior Column, Percutaneous Endoscopic Approach

ØRG74KJ Fusion of 2 to 7 Thoracic Vertebral Joints with Nonautologous Tissue Substitute, Posterior Approach, Anterior Column, Percutaneous Endoscopic Approach

ØRG8Ø7Ø Fusion of 8 or More Thoracic Vertebral Joints with Autologous Tissue Substitute, Anterior Approach, Anterior Column, Open Approach

ØRG8Ø71 Fusion of 8 or More Thoracic Vertebral Joints with Autologous Tissue Substitute, Posterior Approach, Posterior Column, Open Approach

HAC 12: Surgical Site Infection—Certain Orthopedic Procedures of the Spine, Shoulder, and Elbow (continued)

ØRG8Ø7J Fusion of 8 or More Thoracic Vertebral Joints with Autologous Tissue Substitute, Posterior Approach, Anterior Column, Open Approach

ØRG8ØAØ Fusion of 8 or More Thoracic Vertebral Joints with Interbody Fusion Device, Anterior Approach, Anterior Column, Open Approach

ØRG8ØAJ Fusion of 8 or More Thoracic Vertebral Joints with Interbody Fusion Device, Posterior Approach, Anterior Column, Open Approach

ØRG8ØJØ Fusion of 8 or More Thoracic Vertebral Joints with Synthetic Substitute, Anterior Approach, Anterior Column, Open Approach

ØRG8ØJ1 Fusion of 8 or More Thoracic Vertebral Joints with Synthetic Substitute, Posterior Approach, Posterior Column, Open Approach

ØRG8ØJJ Fusion of 8 or More Thoracic Vertebral Joints with Synthetic Substitute, Posterior Approach, Anterior Column, Open Approach

ØRG8ØKØ Fusion of 8 or More Thoracic Vertebral Joints with Nonautologous Tissue Substitute, Anterior Approach, Anterior Column, Open Approach

ØRG8ØK1 Fusion of 8 or More Thoracic Vertebral Joints with Nonautologous Tissue Substitute, Posterior Approach, Posterior Column, Open Approach

ØRG8ØKJ Fusion of 8 or More Thoracic Vertebral Joints with Nonautologous Tissue Substitute, Posterior Approach, Anterior Column, Open Approach

ØRG837Ø Fusion of 8 or More Thoracic Vertebral Joints with Autologous Tissue Substitute, Anterior Approach, Anterior Column, Percutaneous Approach

ØRG8371 Fusion of 8 or More Thoracic Vertebral Joints with Autologous Tissue Substitute, Posterior Approach, Posterior Column, Percutaneous Approach

ØRG837J Fusion of 8 or More Thoracic Vertebral Joints with Autologous Tissue Substitute, Posterior Approach, Anterior Column, Percutaneous Approach

ØRG83AØ Fusion of 8 or More Thoracic Vertebral Joints with Interbody Fusion Device, Anterior Approach, Anterior Column, Percutaneous Approach

ØRG83AJ Fusion of 8 or More Thoracic Vertebral Joints with Interbody Fusion Device, Posterior Approach, Anterior Column, Percutaneous Approach

ØRG83JØ Fusion of 8 or More Thoracic Vertebral Joints with Synthetic Substitute, Anterior Approach, Anterior Column, Percutaneous Approach

ØRG83J1 Fusion of 8 or More Thoracic Vertebral Joints with Synthetic Substitute, Posterior Approach, Posterior Column, Percutaneous Approach

ØRG83JJ Fusion of 8 or More Thoracic Vertebral Joints with Synthetic Substitute, Posterior Approach, Anterior Column, Percutaneous Approach

ØRG83KØ Fusion of 8 or More Thoracic Vertebral Joints with Nonautologous Tissue Substitute, Anterior Approach, Anterior Column, Percutaneous Approach

ØRG83K1 Fusion of 8 or More Thoracic Vertebral Joints with Nonautologous Tissue Substitute, Posterior Approach, Posterior Column, Percutaneous Approach

ØRG83KJ Fusion of 8 or More Thoracic Vertebral Joints with Nonautologous Tissue Substitute, Posterior Approach, Anterior Column, Percutaneous Approach

ØRG847Ø Fusion of 8 or More Thoracic Vertebral Joints with Autologous Tissue Substitute, Anterior Approach, Anterior Column, Percutaneous Endoscopic Approach

ØRG8471 Fusion of 8 or More Thoracic Vertebral Joints with Autologous Tissue Substitute, Posterior Approach, Posterior Column, Percutaneous Endoscopic Approach

ØRG847J Fusion of 8 or More Thoracic Vertebral Joints with Autologous Tissue Substitute, Posterior Approach, Anterior Column, Percutaneous Endoscopic Approach

ØRG84AØ Fusion of 8 or More Thoracic Vertebral Joints with Interbody Fusion Device, Anterior Approach, Anterior Column, Percutaneous Endoscopic Approach

ØRG84AJ Fusion of 8 or More Thoracic Vertebral Joints with Interbody Fusion Device, Posterior Approach, Anterior Column, Percutaneous Endoscopic Approach

ØRG84JØ Fusion of 8 or More Thoracic Vertebral Joints with Synthetic Substitute, Anterior Approach, Anterior Column, Percutaneous Endoscopic Approach

ØRG84J1 Fusion of 8 or More Thoracic Vertebral Joints with Synthetic Substitute, Posterior Approach, Posterior Column, Percutaneous Endoscopic Approach

ØRG84JJ Fusion of 8 or More Thoracic Vertebral Joints with Synthetic Substitute, Posterior Approach, Anterior Column, Percutaneous Endoscopic Approach

ØRG84KØ Fusion of 8 or More Thoracic Vertebral Joints with Nonautologous Tissue Substitute, Anterior Approach, Anterior Column, Percutaneous Endoscopic Approach

ØRG84K1 Fusion of 8 or More Thoracic Vertebral Joints with Nonautologous Tissue Substitute, Posterior Approach, Posterior Column, Percutaneous Endoscopic Approach

ØRG84KJ Fusion of 8 or More Thoracic Vertebral Joints with Nonautologous Tissue Substitute, Posterior Approach, Anterior Column, Percutaneous Endoscopic Approach

ØRGAØ7Ø Fusion of Thoracolumbar Vertebral Joint with Autologous Tissue Substitute, Anterior Approach, Anterior Column, Open Approach

ØRGAØ71 Fusion of Thoracolumbar Vertebral Joint with Autologous Tissue Substitute, Posterior Approach, Posterior Column, Open Approach

ØRGAØ7J Fusion of Thoracolumbar Vertebral Joint with Autologous Tissue Substitute, Posterior Approach, Anterior Column, Open Approach

ØRGAØAØ Fusion of Thoracolumbar Vertebral Joint with Interbody Fusion Device, Anterior Approach, Anterior Column, Open Approach

ØRGAØAJ Fusion of Thoracolumbar Vertebral Joint with Interbody Fusion Device, Posterior Approach, Anterior Column, Open Approach

ØRGAØJØ Fusion of Thoracolumbar Vertebral Joint with Synthetic Substitute, Anterior Approach, Anterior Column, Open Approach

ØRGAØJ1 Fusion of Thoracolumbar Vertebral Joint with Synthetic Substitute, Posterior Approach, Posterior Column, Open Approach

ØRGAØJJ Fusion of Thoracolumbar Vertebral Joint with Synthetic Substitute, Posterior Approach, Anterior Column, Open Approach

ØRGAØKØ Fusion of Thoracolumbar Vertebral Joint with Nonautologous Tissue Substitute, Anterior Approach, Anterior Column, Open Approach

ØRGAØK1 Fusion of Thoracolumbar Vertebral Joint with Nonautologous Tissue Substitute, Posterior Approach, Posterior Column, Open Approach

ØRGAØKJ Fusion of Thoracolumbar Vertebral Joint with Nonautologous Tissue Substitute, Posterior Approach, Anterior Column, Open Approach

ØRGA37Ø Fusion of Thoracolumbar Vertebral Joint with Autologous Tissue Substitute, Anterior Approach, Anterior Column, Percutaneous Approach

ØRGA371 Fusion of Thoracolumbar Vertebral Joint with Autologous Tissue Substitute, Posterior Approach, Posterior Column, Percutaneous Approach

ØRGA37J Fusion of Thoracolumbar Vertebral Joint with Autologous Tissue Substitute, Posterior Approach, Anterior Column, Percutaneous Approach

ØRGA3AØ Fusion of Thoracolumbar Vertebral Joint with Interbody Fusion Device, Anterior Approach, Anterior Column, Percutaneous Approach

ØRGA3AJ Fusion of Thoracolumbar Vertebral Joint with Interbody Fusion Device, Posterior Approach, Anterior Column, Percutaneous Approach

ØRGA3JØ Fusion of Thoracolumbar Vertebral Joint with Synthetic Substitute, Anterior Approach, Anterior Column, Percutaneous Approach

ØRGA3J1 Fusion of Thoracolumbar Vertebral Joint with Synthetic Substitute, Posterior Approach, Posterior Column, Percutaneous Approach

ØRGA3JJ Fusion of Thoracolumbar Vertebral Joint with Synthetic Substitute, Posterior Approach, Anterior Column, Percutaneous Approach

ØRGA3KØ Fusion of Thoracolumbar Vertebral Joint with Nonautologous Tissue Substitute, Anterior Approach, Anterior Column, Percutaneous Approach

ØRGA3K1 Fusion of Thoracolumbar Vertebral Joint with Nonautologous Tissue Substitute, Posterior Approach, Posterior Column, Percutaneous Approach

ØRGA3KJ Fusion of Thoracolumbar Vertebral Joint with Nonautologous Tissue Substitute, Posterior Approach, Anterior Column, Percutaneous Approach

ØRGA47Ø Fusion of Thoracolumbar Vertebral Joint with Autologous Tissue Substitute, Anterior Approach, Anterior Column, Percutaneous Endoscopic Approach

ØRGA471 Fusion of Thoracolumbar Vertebral Joint with Autologous Tissue Substitute, Posterior Approach, Posterior Column, Percutaneous Endoscopic Approach

Appendix G: Hospital Acquired Conditions

HAC 12: Surgical Site Infection—Certain Orthopedic Procedures of the Spine, Shoulder, and Elbow (continued)

ØRGA47J Fusion of Thoracolumbar Vertebral Joint with Autologous Tissue Substitute, Posterior Approach, Anterior Column, Percutaneous Endoscopic Approach

ØRGA4AØ Fusion of Thoracolumbar Vertebral Joint with Interbody Fusion Device, Anterior Approach, Anterior Column, Percutaneous Endoscopic Approach

ØRGA4AJ Fusion of Thoracolumbar Vertebral Joint with Interbody Fusion Device, Posterior Approach, Anterior Column, Percutaneous Endoscopic Approach

ØRGA4JØ Fusion of Thoracolumbar Vertebral Joint with Synthetic Substitute, Anterior Approach, Anterior Column, Percutaneous Endoscopic Approach

ØRGA4J1 Fusion of Thoracolumbar Vertebral Joint with Synthetic Substitute, Posterior Approach, Posterior Column, Percutaneous Endoscopic Approach

ØRGA4JJ Fusion of Thoracolumbar Vertebral Joint with Synthetic Substitute, Posterior Approach, Anterior Column, Percutaneous Endoscopic Approach

ØRGA4KØ Fusion of Thoracolumbar Vertebral Joint with Nonautologous Tissue Substitute, Anterior Approach, Anterior Column, Percutaneous Endoscopic Approach

ØRGA4K1 Fusion of Thoracolumbar Vertebral Joint with Nonautologous Tissue Substitute, Posterior Approach, Posterior Column, Percutaneous Endoscopic Approach

ØRGA4KJ Fusion of Thoracolumbar Vertebral Joint with Nonautologous Tissue Substitute, Posterior Approach, Anterior Column, Percutaneous Endoscopic Approach

ØRGE04Z Fusion of Right Sternoclavicular Joint with Internal Fixation Device, Open Approach

ØRGE07Z Fusion of Right Sternoclavicular Joint with Autologous Tissue Substitute, Open Approach

ØRGE0JZ Fusion of Right Sternoclavicular Joint with Synthetic Substitute, Open Approach

ØRGE0KZ Fusion of Right Sternoclavicular Joint with Nonautologous Tissue Substitute, Open Approach

ØRGE34Z Fusion of Right Sternoclavicular Joint with Internal Fixation Device, Percutaneous Approach

ØRGE37Z Fusion of Right Sternoclavicular Joint with Autologous Tissue Substitute, Percutaneous Approach

ØRGE3JZ Fusion of Right Sternoclavicular Joint with Synthetic Substitute, Percutaneous Approach

ØRGE3KZ Fusion of Right Sternoclavicular Joint with Nonautologous Tissue Substitute, Percutaneous Approach

ØRGE44Z Fusion of Right Sternoclavicular Joint with Internal Fixation Device, Percutaneous Endoscopic Approach

ØRGE47Z Fusion of Right Sternoclavicular Joint with Autologous Tissue Substitute, Percutaneous Endoscopic Approach

ØRGE4JZ Fusion of Right Sternoclavicular Joint with Synthetic Substitute, Percutaneous Endoscopic Approach

ØRGE4KZ Fusion of Right Sternoclavicular Joint with Nonautologous Tissue Substitute, Percutaneous Endoscopic Approach

ØRGF04Z Fusion of Left Sternoclavicular Joint with Internal Fixation Device, Open Approach

ØRGF07Z Fusion of Left Sternoclavicular Joint with Autologous Tissue Substitute, Open Approach

ØRGF0JZ Fusion of Left Sternoclavicular Joint with Synthetic Substitute, Open Approach

ØRGF0KZ Fusion of Left Sternoclavicular Joint with Nonautologous Tissue Substitute, Open Approach

ØRGF34Z Fusion of Left Sternoclavicular Joint with Internal Fixation Device, Percutaneous Approach

ØRGF37Z Fusion of Left Sternoclavicular Joint with Autologous Tissue Substitute, Percutaneous Approach

ØRGF3JZ Fusion of Left Sternoclavicular Joint with Synthetic Substitute, Percutaneous Approach

ØRGF3KZ Fusion of Left Sternoclavicular Joint with Nonautologous Tissue Substitute, Percutaneous Approach

ØRGF44Z Fusion of Left Sternoclavicular Joint with Internal Fixation Device, Percutaneous Endoscopic Approach

ØRGF47Z Fusion of Left Sternoclavicular Joint with Autologous Tissue Substitute, Percutaneous Endoscopic Approach

ØRGF4JZ Fusion of Left Sternoclavicular Joint with Synthetic Substitute, Percutaneous Endoscopic Approach

ØRGF4KZ Fusion of Left Sternoclavicular Joint with Nonautologous Tissue Substitute, Percutaneous Endoscopic Approach

ØRGG04Z Fusion of Right Acromioclavicular Joint with Internal Fixation Device, Open Approach

ØRGG07Z Fusion of Right Acromioclavicular Joint with Autologous Tissue Substitute, Open Approach

ØRGG0JZ Fusion of Right Acromioclavicular Joint with Synthetic Substitute, Open Approach

ØRGG0KZ Fusion of Right Acromioclavicular Joint with Nonautologous Tissue Substitute, Open Approach

ØRGG34Z Fusion of Right Acromioclavicular Joint with Internal Fixation Device, Percutaneous Approach

ØRGG37Z Fusion of Right Acromioclavicular Joint with Autologous Tissue Substitute, Percutaneous Approach

ØRGG3JZ Fusion of Right Acromioclavicular Joint with Synthetic Substitute, Percutaneous Approach

ØRGG3KZ Fusion of Right Acromioclavicular Joint with Nonautologous Tissue Substitute, Percutaneous Approach

ØRGG44Z Fusion of Right Acromioclavicular Joint with Internal Fixation Device, Percutaneous Endoscopic Approach

ØRGG47Z Fusion of Right Acromioclavicular Joint with Autologous Tissue Substitute, Percutaneous Endoscopic Approach

ØRGG4JZ Fusion of Right Acromioclavicular Joint with Synthetic Substitute, Percutaneous Endoscopic Approach

ØRGG4KZ Fusion of Right Acromioclavicular Joint with Nonautologous Tissue Substitute, Percutaneous Endoscopic Approach

ØRGH04Z Fusion of Left Acromioclavicular Joint with Internal Fixation Device, Open Approach

ØRGH07Z Fusion of Left Acromioclavicular Joint with Autologous Tissue Substitute, Open Approach

ØRGH0JZ Fusion of Left Acromioclavicular Joint with Synthetic Substitute, Open Approach

ØRGH0KZ Fusion of Left Acromioclavicular Joint with Nonautologous Tissue Substitute, Open Approach

ØRGH34Z Fusion of Left Acromioclavicular Joint with Internal Fixation Device, Percutaneous Approach

ØRGH37Z Fusion of Left Acromioclavicular Joint with Autologous Tissue Substitute, Percutaneous Approach

ØRGH3JZ Fusion of Left Acromioclavicular Joint with Synthetic Substitute, Percutaneous Approach

ØRGH3KZ Fusion of Left Acromioclavicular Joint with Nonautologous Tissue Substitute, Percutaneous Approach

ØRGH44Z Fusion of Left Acromioclavicular Joint with Internal Fixation Device, Percutaneous Endoscopic Approach

ØRGH47Z Fusion of Left Acromioclavicular Joint with Autologous Tissue Substitute, Percutaneous Endoscopic Approach

ØRGH4JZ Fusion of Left Acromioclavicular Joint with Synthetic Substitute, Percutaneous Endoscopic Approach

ØRGH4KZ Fusion of Left Acromioclavicular Joint with Nonautologous Tissue Substitute, Percutaneous Endoscopic Approach

ØRGJ04Z Fusion of Right Shoulder Joint with Internal Fixation Device, Open Approach

ØRGJ07Z Fusion of Right Shoulder Joint with Autologous Tissue Substitute, Open Approach

ØRGJ0JZ Fusion of Right Shoulder Joint with Synthetic Substitute, Open Approach

ØRGJ0KZ Fusion of Right Shoulder Joint with Nonautologous Tissue Substitute, Open Approach

ØRGJ34Z Fusion of Right Shoulder Joint with Internal Fixation Device, Percutaneous Approach

ØRGJ37Z Fusion of Right Shoulder Joint with Autologous Tissue Substitute, Percutaneous Approach

ØRGJ3JZ Fusion of Right Shoulder Joint with Synthetic Substitute, Percutaneous Approach

ØRGJ3KZ Fusion of Right Shoulder Joint with Nonautologous Tissue Substitute, Percutaneous Approach

ØRGJ44Z Fusion of Right Shoulder Joint with Internal Fixation Device, Percutaneous Endoscopic Approach

ØRGJ47Z Fusion of Right Shoulder Joint with Autologous Tissue Substitute, Percutaneous Endoscopic Approach

ØRGJ4JZ Fusion of Right Shoulder Joint with Synthetic Substitute, Percutaneous Endoscopic Approach

ØRGJ4KZ Fusion of Right Shoulder Joint with Nonautologous Tissue Substitute, Percutaneous Endoscopic Approach

ØRGK04Z Fusion of Left Shoulder Joint with Internal Fixation Device, Open Approach

ØRGK07Z Fusion of Left Shoulder Joint with Autologous Tissue Substitute, Open Approach

ØRGK0JZ Fusion of Left Shoulder Joint with Synthetic Substitute, Open Approach

ØRGK0KZ Fusion of Left Shoulder Joint with Nonautologous Tissue Substitute, Open Approach

ØRGK34Z Fusion of Left Shoulder Joint with Internal Fixation Device, Percutaneous Approach

ØRGK37Z Fusion of Left Shoulder Joint with Autologous Tissue Substitute, Percutaneous Approach

HAC 12: Surgical Site Infection—Certain Orthopedic Procedures of the Spine, Shoulder, and Elbow (continued)

ØRGK3JZ Fusion of Left Shoulder Joint with Synthetic Substitute, Percutaneous Approach

ØRGK3KZ Fusion of Left Shoulder Joint with Nonautologous Tissue Substitute, Percutaneous Approach

ØRGK44Z Fusion of Left Shoulder Joint with Internal Fixation Device, Percutaneous Endoscopic Approach

ØRGK47Z Fusion of Left Shoulder Joint with Autologous Tissue Substitute, Percutaneous Endoscopic Approach

ØRGK4JZ Fusion of Left Shoulder Joint with Synthetic Substitute, Percutaneous Endoscopic Approach

ØRGK4KZ Fusion of Left Shoulder Joint with Nonautologous Tissue Substitute, Percutaneous Endoscopic Approach

ØRGLØ4Z Fusion of Right Elbow Joint with Internal Fixation Device, Open Approach

ØRGLØ5Z Fusion of Right Elbow Joint with External Fixation Device, Open Approach

ØRGLØ7Z Fusion of Right Elbow Joint with Autologous Tissue Substitute, Open Approach

ØRGLØJZ Fusion of Right Elbow Joint with Synthetic Substitute, Open Approach

ØRGLØKZ Fusion of Right Elbow Joint with Nonautologous Tissue Substitute, Open Approach

ØRGL34Z Fusion of Right Elbow Joint with Internal Fixation Device, Percutaneous Approach

ØRGL35Z Fusion of Right Elbow Joint with External Fixation Device, Percutaneous Approach

ØRGL37Z Fusion of Right Elbow Joint with Autologous Tissue Substitute, Percutaneous Approach

ØRGL3JZ Fusion of Right Elbow Joint with Synthetic Substitute, Percutaneous Approach

ØRGL3KZ Fusion of Right Elbow Joint with Nonautologous Tissue Substitute, Percutaneous Approach

ØRGL44Z Fusion of Right Elbow Joint with Internal Fixation Device, Percutaneous Endoscopic Approach

ØRGL45Z Fusion of Right Elbow Joint with External Fixation Device, Percutaneous Endoscopic Approach

ØRGL47Z Fusion of Right Elbow Joint with Autologous Tissue Substitute, Percutaneous Endoscopic Approach

ØRGL4JZ Fusion of Right Elbow Joint with Synthetic Substitute, Percutaneous Endoscopic Approach

ØRGL4KZ Fusion of Right Elbow Joint with Nonautologous Tissue Substitute, Percutaneous Endoscopic Approach

ØRGMØ4Z Fusion of Left Elbow Joint with Internal Fixation Device, Open Approach

ØRGMØ5Z Fusion of Left Elbow Joint with External Fixation Device, Open Approach

ØRGMØ7Z Fusion of Left Elbow Joint with Autologous Tissue Substitute, Open Approach

ØRGMØJZ Fusion of Left Elbow Joint with Synthetic Substitute, Open Approach

ØRGMØKZ Fusion of Left Elbow Joint with Nonautologous Tissue Substitute, Open Approach

ØRGM34Z Fusion of Left Elbow Joint with Internal Fixation Device, Percutaneous Approach

ØRGM35Z Fusion of Left Elbow Joint with External Fixation Device, Percutaneous Approach

ØRGM37Z Fusion of Left Elbow Joint with Autologous Tissue Substitute, Percutaneous Approach

ØRGM3JZ Fusion of Left Elbow Joint with Synthetic Substitute, Percutaneous Approach

ØRGM3KZ Fusion of Left Elbow Joint with Nonautologous Tissue Substitute, Percutaneous Approach

ØRGM44Z Fusion of Left Elbow Joint with Internal Fixation Device, Percutaneous Endoscopic Approach

ØRGM45Z Fusion of Left Elbow Joint with External Fixation Device, Percutaneous Endoscopic Approach

ØRGM47Z Fusion of Left Elbow Joint with Autologous Tissue Substitute, Percutaneous Endoscopic Approach

ØRGM4JZ Fusion of Left Elbow Joint with Synthetic Substitute, Percutaneous Endoscopic Approach

ØRGM4KZ Fusion of Left Elbow Joint with Nonautologous Tissue Substitute, Percutaneous Endoscopic Approach

ØRQEØZZ Repair Right Sternoclavicular Joint, Open Approach

ØRQE3ZZ Repair Right Sternoclavicular Joint, Percutaneous Approach

ØRQE4ZZ Repair Right Sternoclavicular Joint, Percutaneous Endoscopic Approach

ØRQEXZZ Repair Right Sternoclavicular Joint, External Approach

ØRQFØZZ Repair Left Sternoclavicular Joint, Open Approach

ØRQF3ZZ Repair Left Sternoclavicular Joint, Percutaneous Approach

ØRQF4ZZ Repair Left Sternoclavicular Joint, Percutaneous Endoscopic Approach

ØRQFXZZ Repair Left Sternoclavicular Joint, External Approach

ØRQGØZZ Repair Right Acromioclavicular Joint, Open Approach

ØRQG3ZZ Repair Right Acromioclavicular Joint, Percutaneous Approach

ØRQG4ZZ Repair Right Acromioclavicular Joint, Percutaneous Endoscopic Approach

ØRQGXZZ Repair Right Acromioclavicular Joint, External Approach

ØRQHØZZ Repair Left Acromioclavicular Joint, Open Approach

ØRQH3ZZ Repair Left Acromioclavicular Joint, Percutaneous Approach

ØRQH4ZZ Repair Left Acromioclavicular Joint, Percutaneous Endoscopic Approach

ØRQHXZZ Repair Left Acromioclavicular Joint, External Approach

ØRQJØZZ Repair Right Shoulder Joint, Open Approach

ØRQJ3ZZ Repair Right Shoulder Joint, Percutaneous Approach

ØRQJ4ZZ Repair Right Shoulder Joint, Percutaneous Endoscopic Approach

ØRQJXZZ Repair Right Shoulder Joint, External Approach

ØRQKØZZ Repair Left Shoulder Joint, Open Approach

ØRQK3ZZ Repair Left Shoulder Joint, Percutaneous Approach

ØRQK4ZZ Repair Left Shoulder Joint, Percutaneous Endoscopic Approach

ØRQKXZZ Repair Left Shoulder Joint, External Approach

ØRQLØZZ Repair Right Elbow Joint, Open Approach

ØRQL3ZZ Repair Right Elbow Joint, Percutaneous Approach

ØRQL4ZZ Repair Right Elbow Joint, Percutaneous Endoscopic Approach

ØRQLXZZ Repair Right Elbow Joint, External Approach

ØRQMØZZ Repair Left Elbow Joint, Open Approach

ØRQM3ZZ Repair Left Elbow Joint, Percutaneous Approach

ØRQM4ZZ Repair Left Elbow Joint, Percutaneous Endoscopic Approach

ØRQMXZZ Repair Left Elbow Joint, External Approach

ØRUEØ7Z Supplement Right Sternoclavicular Joint with Autologous Tissue Substitute, Open Approach

ØRUEØJZ Supplement Right Sternoclavicular Joint with Synthetic Substitute, Open Approach

ØRUEØKZ Supplement Right Sternoclavicular Joint with Nonautologous Tissue Substitute, Open Approach

ØRUE37Z Supplement Right Sternoclavicular Joint with Autologous Tissue Substitute, Percutaneous Approach

ØRUE3JZ Supplement Right Sternoclavicular Joint with Synthetic Substitute, Percutaneous Approach

ØRUE3KZ Supplement Right Sternoclavicular Joint with Nonautologous Tissue Substitute, Percutaneous Approach

ØRUE47Z Supplement Right Sternoclavicular Joint with Autologous Tissue Substitute, Percutaneous Endoscopic Approach

ØRUE4JZ Supplement Right Sternoclavicular Joint with Synthetic Substitute, Percutaneous Endoscopic Approach

ØRUE4KZ Supplement Right Sternoclavicular Joint with Nonautologous Tissue Substitute, Percutaneous Endoscopic Approach

ØRUFØ7Z Supplement Left Sternoclavicular Joint with Autologous Tissue Substitute, Open Approach

ØRUFØJZ Supplement Left Sternoclavicular Joint with Synthetic Substitute, Open Approach

ØRUFØKZ Supplement Left Sternoclavicular Joint with Nonautologous Tissue Substitute, Open Approach

ØRUF37Z Supplement Left Sternoclavicular Joint with Autologous Tissue Substitute, Percutaneous Approach

ØRUF3JZ Supplement Left Sternoclavicular Joint with Synthetic Substitute, Percutaneous Approach

ØRUF3KZ Supplement Left Sternoclavicular Joint with Nonautologous Tissue Substitute, Percutaneous Approach

ØRUF47Z Supplement Left Sternoclavicular Joint with Autologous Tissue Substitute, Percutaneous Endoscopic Approach

ØRUF4JZ Supplement Left Sternoclavicular Joint with Synthetic Substitute, Percutaneous Endoscopic Approach

ØRUF4KZ Supplement Left Sternoclavicular Joint with Nonautologous Tissue Substitute, Percutaneous Endoscopic Approach

ØRUGØ7Z Supplement Right Acromioclavicular Joint with Autologous Tissue Substitute, Open Approach

ØRUGØJZ Supplement Right Acromioclavicular Joint with Synthetic Substitute, Open Approach

ØRUGØKZ Supplement Right Acromioclavicular Joint with Nonautologous Tissue Substitute, Open Approach

ØRUG37Z Supplement Right Acromioclavicular Joint with Autologous Tissue Substitute, Percutaneous Approach

HAC 12: Surgical Site Infection—Certain Orthopedic Procedures of the Spine, Shoulder, and Elbow (continued)

ØRUG3JZ   Supplement Right Acromioclavicular Joint with Synthetic Substitute, Percutaneous Approach

ØRUG3KZ   Supplement Right Acromioclavicular Joint with Nonautologous Tissue Substitute, Percutaneous Approach

ØRUG47Z   Supplement Right Acromioclavicular Joint with Autologous Tissue Substitute, Percutaneous Endoscopic Approach

ØRUG4JZ   Supplement Right Acromioclavicular Joint with Synthetic Substitute, Percutaneous Endoscopic Approach

ØRUG4KZ   Supplement Right Acromioclavicular Joint with Nonautologous Tissue Substitute, Percutaneous Endoscopic Approach

ØRUH07Z   Supplement Left Acromioclavicular Joint with Autologous Tissue Substitute, Open Approach

ØRUH0JZ   Supplement Left Acromioclavicular Joint with Synthetic Substitute, Open Approach

ØRUH0KZ   Supplement Left Acromioclavicular Joint with Nonautologous Tissue Substitute, Open Approach

ØRUH37Z   Supplement Left Acromioclavicular Joint with Autologous Tissue Substitute, Percutaneous Approach

ØRUH3JZ   Supplement Left Acromioclavicular Joint with Synthetic Substitute, Percutaneous Approach

ØRUH3KZ   Supplement Left Acromioclavicular Joint with Nonautologous Tissue Substitute, Percutaneous Approach

ØRUH47Z   Supplement Left Acromioclavicular Joint with Autologous Tissue Substitute, Percutaneous Endoscopic Approach

ØRUH4JZ   Supplement Left Acromioclavicular Joint with Synthetic Substitute, Percutaneous Endoscopic Approach

ØRUH4KZ   Supplement Left Acromioclavicular Joint with Nonautologous Tissue Substitute, Percutaneous Endoscopic Approach

ØRUJ07Z   Supplement Right Shoulder Joint with Autologous Tissue Substitute, Open Approach

ØRUJ0JZ   Supplement Right Shoulder Joint with Synthetic Substitute, Open Approach

ØRUJ0KZ   Supplement Right Shoulder Joint with Nonautologous Tissue Substitute, Open Approach

ØRUJ37Z   Supplement Right Shoulder Joint with Autologous Tissue Substitute, Percutaneous Approach

ØRUJ3JZ   Supplement Right Shoulder Joint with Synthetic Substitute, Percutaneous Approach

ØRUJ3KZ   Supplement Right Shoulder Joint with Nonautologous Tissue Substitute, Percutaneous Approach

ØRUJ47Z   Supplement Right Shoulder Joint with Autologous Tissue Substitute, Percutaneous Endoscopic Approach

ØRUJ4JZ   Supplement Right Shoulder Joint with Synthetic Substitute, Percutaneous Endoscopic Approach

ØRUJ4KZ   Supplement Right Shoulder Joint with Nonautologous Tissue Substitute, Percutaneous Endoscopic Approach

ØRUK07Z   Supplement Left Shoulder Joint with Autologous Tissue Substitute, Open Approach

ØRUK0JZ   Supplement Left Shoulder Joint with Synthetic Substitute, Open Approach

ØRUK0KZ   Supplement Left Shoulder Joint with Nonautologous Tissue Substitute, Open Approach

ØRUK37Z   Supplement Left Shoulder Joint with Autologous Tissue Substitute, Percutaneous Approach

ØRUK3JZ   Supplement Left Shoulder Joint with Synthetic Substitute, Percutaneous Approach

ØRUK3KZ   Supplement Left Shoulder Joint with Nonautologous Tissue Substitute, Percutaneous Approach

ØRUK47Z   Supplement Left Shoulder Joint with Autologous Tissue Substitute, Percutaneous Endoscopic Approach

ØRUK4JZ   Supplement Left Shoulder Joint with Synthetic Substitute, Percutaneous Endoscopic Approach

ØRUK4KZ   Supplement Left Shoulder Joint with Nonautologous Tissue Substitute, Percutaneous Endoscopic Approach

ØRUL07Z   Supplement Right Elbow Joint with Autologous Tissue Substitute, Open Approach

ØRUL0JZ   Supplement Right Elbow Joint with Synthetic Substitute, Open Approach

ØRUL0KZ   Supplement Right Elbow Joint with Nonautologous Tissue Substitute, Open Approach

ØRUL37Z   Supplement Right Elbow Joint with Autologous Tissue Substitute, Percutaneous Approach

ØRUL3JZ   Supplement Right Elbow Joint with Synthetic Substitute, Percutaneous Approach

ØRUL3KZ   Supplement Right Elbow Joint with Nonautologous Tissue Substitute, Percutaneous Approach

ØRUL47Z   Supplement Right Elbow Joint with Autologous Tissue Substitute, Percutaneous Endoscopic Approach

ØRUL4JZ   Supplement Right Elbow Joint with Synthetic Substitute, Percutaneous Endoscopic Approach

ØRUL4KZ   Supplement Right Elbow Joint with Nonautologous Tissue Substitute, Percutaneous Endoscopic Approach

ØRUM07Z   Supplement Left Elbow Joint with Autologous Tissue Substitute, Open Approach

ØRUM0JZ   Supplement Left Elbow Joint with Synthetic Substitute, Open Approach

ØRUM0KZ   Supplement Left Elbow Joint with Nonautologous Tissue Substitute, Open Approach

ØRUM37Z   Supplement Left Elbow Joint with Autologous Tissue Substitute, Percutaneous Approach

ØRUM3JZ   Supplement Left Elbow Joint with Synthetic Substitute, Percutaneous Approach

ØRUM3KZ   Supplement Left Elbow Joint with Nonautologous Tissue Substitute, Percutaneous Approach

ØRUM47Z   Supplement Left Elbow Joint with Autologous Tissue Substitute, Percutaneous Endoscopic Approach

ØRUM4JZ   Supplement Left Elbow Joint with Synthetic Substitute, Percutaneous Endoscopic Approach

ØRUM4KZ   Supplement Left Elbow Joint with Nonautologous Tissue Substitute, Percutaneous Endoscopic Approach

ØSG0070   Fusion of Lumbar Vertebral Joint with Autologous Tissue Substitute, Anterior Approach, Anterior Column, Open Approach

ØSG0071   Fusion of Lumbar Vertebral Joint with Autologous Tissue Substitute, Posterior Approach, Posterior Column, Open Approach

ØSG007J   Fusion of Lumbar Vertebral Joint with Autologous Tissue Substitute, Posterior Approach, Anterior Column, Open Approach

ØSG00A0   Fusion of Lumbar Vertebral Joint with Interbody Fusion Device, Anterior Approach, Anterior Column, Open Approach

ØSG00AJ   Fusion of Lumbar Vertebral Joint with Interbody Fusion Device, Posterior Approach, Anterior Column, Open Approach

ØSG00J0   Fusion of Lumbar Vertebral Joint with Synthetic Substitute, Anterior Approach, Anterior Column, Open Approach

ØSG00J1   Fusion of Lumbar Vertebral Joint with Synthetic Substitute, Posterior Approach, Posterior Column, Open Approach

ØSG00JJ   Fusion of Lumbar Vertebral Joint with Synthetic Substitute, Posterior Approach, Anterior Column, Open Approach

ØSG00K0   Fusion of Lumbar Vertebral Joint with Nonautologous Tissue Substitute, Anterior Approach, Anterior Column, Open Approach

ØSG00K1   Fusion of Lumbar Vertebral Joint with Nonautologous Tissue Substitute, Posterior Approach, Posterior Column, Open Approach

ØSG00KJ   Fusion of Lumbar Vertebral Joint with Nonautologous Tissue Substitute, Posterior Approach, Anterior Column, Open Approach

ØSG0370   Fusion of Lumbar Vertebral Joint with Autologous Tissue Substitute, Anterior Approach, Anterior Column, Percutaneous Approach

ØSG0371   Fusion of Lumbar Vertebral Joint with Autologous Tissue Substitute, Posterior Approach, Posterior Column, Percutaneous Approach

ØSG037J   Fusion of Lumbar Vertebral Joint with Autologous Tissue Substitute, Posterior Approach, Anterior Column, Percutaneous Approach

ØSG03A0   Fusion of Lumbar Vertebral Joint with Interbody Fusion Device, Anterior Approach, Anterior Column, Percutaneous Approach

ØSG03AJ   Fusion of Lumbar Vertebral Joint with Interbody Fusion Device, Posterior Approach, Anterior Column, Percutaneous Approach

ØSG03J0   Fusion of Lumbar Vertebral Joint with Synthetic Substitute, Anterior Approach, Anterior Column, Percutaneous Approach

ØSG03J1   Fusion of Lumbar Vertebral Joint with Synthetic Substitute, Posterior Approach, Posterior Column, Percutaneous Approach

ØSG03JJ   Fusion of Lumbar Vertebral Joint with Synthetic Substitute, Posterior Approach, Anterior Column, Percutaneous Approach

ØSG03K0   Fusion of Lumbar Vertebral Joint with Nonautologous Tissue Substitute, Anterior Approach, Anterior Column, Percutaneous Approach

ØSG03K1   Fusion of Lumbar Vertebral Joint with Nonautologous Tissue Substitute, Posterior Approach, Posterior Column, Percutaneous Approach

HAC 12: Surgical Site Infection—Certain Orthopedic Procedures of the Spine, Shoulder, and Elbow (continued)

ØSG03KJ Fusion of Lumbar Vertebral Joint with Nonautologous Tissue Substitute, Posterior Approach, Anterior Column, Percutaneous Approach

ØSG0470 Fusion of Lumbar Vertebral Joint with Autologous Tissue Substitute, Anterior Approach, Anterior Column, Percutaneous Endoscopic Approach

ØSG0471 Fusion of Lumbar Vertebral Joint with Autologous Tissue Substitute, Posterior Approach, Posterior Column, Percutaneous Endoscopic Approach

ØSG047J Fusion of Lumbar Vertebral Joint with Autologous Tissue Substitute, Posterior Approach, Anterior Column, Percutaneous Endoscopic Approach

ØSG04AØ Fusion of Lumbar Vertebral Joint with Interbody Fusion Device, Anterior Approach, Anterior Column, Percutaneous Endoscopic Approach

ØSG04AJ Fusion of Lumbar Vertebral Joint with Interbody Fusion Device, Posterior Approach, Anterior Column, Percutaneous Endoscopic Approach

ØSG04JØ Fusion of Lumbar Vertebral Joint with Synthetic Substitute, Anterior Approach, Anterior Column, Percutaneous Endoscopic Approach

ØSG04J1 Fusion of Lumbar Vertebral Joint with Synthetic Substitute, Posterior Approach, Posterior Column, Percutaneous Endoscopic Approach

ØSG04JJ Fusion of Lumbar Vertebral Joint with Synthetic Substitute, Posterior Approach, Anterior Column, Percutaneous Endoscopic Approach

ØSG04KØ Fusion of Lumbar Vertebral Joint with Nonautologous Tissue Substitute, Anterior Approach, Anterior Column, Percutaneous Endoscopic Approach

ØSG04K1 Fusion of Lumbar Vertebral Joint with Nonautologous Tissue Substitute, Posterior Approach, Posterior Column, Percutaneous Endoscopic Approach

ØSG04KJ Fusion of Lumbar Vertebral Joint with Nonautologous Tissue Substitute, Posterior Approach, Anterior Column, Percutaneous Endoscopic Approach

ØSG1070 Fusion of 2 or More Lumbar Vertebral Joints with Autologous Tissue Substitute, Anterior Approach, Anterior Column, Open Approach

ØSG1071 Fusion of 2 or More Lumbar Vertebral Joints with Autologous Tissue Substitute, Posterior Approach, Posterior Column, Open Approach

ØSG107J Fusion of 2 or More Lumbar Vertebral Joints with Autologous Tissue Substitute, Posterior Approach, Anterior Column, Open Approach

ØSG10AØ Fusion of 2 or More Lumbar Vertebral Joints with Interbody Fusion Device, Anterior Approach, Anterior Column, Open Approach

ØSG10AJ Fusion of 2 or More Lumbar Vertebral Joints with Interbody Fusion Device, Posterior Approach, Anterior Column, Open Approach

ØSG10JØ Fusion of 2 or More Lumbar Vertebral Joints with Synthetic Substitute, Anterior Approach, Anterior Column, Open Approach

ØSG10J1 Fusion of 2 or More Lumbar Vertebral Joints with Synthetic Substitute, Posterior Approach, Posterior Column, Open Approach

ØSG10JJ Fusion of 2 or More Lumbar Vertebral Joints with Synthetic Substitute, Posterior Approach, Anterior Column, Open Approach

ØSG10KØ Fusion of 2 or More Lumbar Vertebral Joints with Nonautologous Tissue Substitute, Anterior Approach, Anterior Column, Open Approach

ØSG10K1 Fusion of 2 or More Lumbar Vertebral Joints with Nonautologous Tissue Substitute, Posterior Approach, Posterior Column, Open Approach

ØSG10KJ Fusion of 2 or More Lumbar Vertebral Joints with Nonautologous Tissue Substitute, Posterior Approach, Anterior Column, Open Approach

ØSG1370 Fusion of 2 or More Lumbar Vertebral Joints with Autologous Tissue Substitute, Anterior Approach, Anterior Column, Percutaneous Approach

ØSG1371 Fusion of 2 or More Lumbar Vertebral Joints with Autologous Tissue Substitute, Posterior Approach, Posterior Column, Percutaneous Approach

ØSG137J Fusion of 2 or More Lumbar Vertebral Joints with Autologous Tissue Substitute, Posterior Approach, Anterior Column, Percutaneous Approach

ØSG13AØ Fusion of 2 or More Lumbar Vertebral Joints with Interbody Fusion Device, Anterior Approach, Anterior Column, Percutaneous Approach

ØSG13AJ Fusion of 2 or More Lumbar Vertebral Joints with Interbody Fusion Device, Posterior Approach, Anterior Column, Percutaneous Approach

ØSG13JØ Fusion of 2 or More Lumbar Vertebral Joints with Synthetic Substitute, Anterior Approach, Anterior Column, Percutaneous Approach

ØSG13J1 Fusion of 2 or More Lumbar Vertebral Joints with Synthetic Substitute, Posterior Approach, Posterior Column, Percutaneous Approach

ØSG13JJ Fusion of 2 or More Lumbar Vertebral Joints with Synthetic Substitute, Posterior Approach, Anterior Column, Percutaneous Approach

ØSG13KØ Fusion of 2 or More Lumbar Vertebral Joints with Nonautologous Tissue Substitute, Anterior Approach, Anterior Column, Percutaneous Approach

ØSG13K1 Fusion of 2 or More Lumbar Vertebral Joints with Nonautologous Tissue Substitute, Posterior Approach, Posterior Column, Percutaneous Approach

ØSG13KJ Fusion of 2 or More Lumbar Vertebral Joints with Nonautologous Tissue Substitute, Posterior Approach, Anterior Column, Percutaneous Approach

ØSG1470 Fusion of 2 or More Lumbar Vertebral Joints with Autologous Tissue Substitute, Anterior Approach, Anterior Column, Percutaneous Endoscopic Approach

ØSG1471 Fusion of 2 or More Lumbar Vertebral Joints with Autologous Tissue Substitute, Posterior Approach, Posterior Column, Percutaneous Endoscopic Approach

ØSG147J Fusion of 2 or More Lumbar Vertebral Joints with Autologous Tissue Substitute, Posterior Approach, Anterior Column, Percutaneous Endoscopic Approach

ØSG14AØ Fusion of 2 or More Lumbar Vertebral Joints with Interbody Fusion Device, Anterior Approach, Anterior Column, Percutaneous Endoscopic Approach

ØSG14AJ Fusion of 2 or More Lumbar Vertebral Joints with Interbody Fusion Device, Posterior Approach, Anterior Column, Percutaneous Endoscopic Approach

ØSG14JØ Fusion of 2 or More Lumbar Vertebral Joints with Synthetic Substitute, Anterior Approach, Anterior Column, Percutaneous Endoscopic Approach

ØSG14J1 Fusion of 2 or More Lumbar Vertebral Joints with Synthetic Substitute, Posterior Approach, Posterior Column, Percutaneous Endoscopic Approach

ØSG14JJ Fusion of 2 or More Lumbar Vertebral Joints with Synthetic Substitute, Posterior Approach, Anterior Column, Percutaneous Endoscopic Approach

ØSG14KØ Fusion of 2 or More Lumbar Vertebral Joints with Nonautologous Tissue Substitute, Anterior Approach, Anterior Column, Percutaneous Endoscopic Approach

ØSG14K1 Fusion of 2 or More Lumbar Vertebral Joints with Nonautologous Tissue Substitute, Posterior Approach, Posterior Column, Percutaneous Endoscopic Approach

ØSG14KJ Fusion of 2 or More Lumbar Vertebral Joints with Nonautologous Tissue Substitute, Posterior Approach, Anterior Column, Percutaneous Endoscopic Approach

ØSG3070 Fusion of Lumbosacral Joint with Autologous Tissue Substitute, Anterior Approach, Anterior Column, Open Approach

ØSG3071 Fusion of Lumbosacral Joint with Autologous Tissue Substitute, Posterior Approach, Posterior Column, Open Approach

ØSG307J Fusion of Lumbosacral Joint with Autologous Tissue Substitute, Posterior Approach, Anterior Column, Open Approach

ØSG30AØ Fusion of Lumbosacral Joint with Interbody Fusion Device, Anterior Approach, Anterior Column, Open Approach

ØSG30AJ Fusion of Lumbosacral Joint with Interbody Fusion Device, Posterior Approach, Anterior Column, Open Approach

ØSG30JØ Fusion of Lumbosacral Joint with Synthetic Substitute, Anterior Approach, Anterior Column, Open Approach

ØSG30J1 Fusion of Lumbosacral Joint with Synthetic Substitute, Posterior Approach, Posterior Column, Open Approach

ØSG30JJ Fusion of Lumbosacral Joint with Synthetic Substitute, Posterior Approach, Anterior Column, Open Approach

ØSG30KØ Fusion of Lumbosacral Joint with Nonautologous Tissue Substitute, Anterior Approach, Anterior Column, Open Approach

ØSG30K1 Fusion of Lumbosacral Joint with Nonautologous Tissue Substitute, Posterior Approach, Posterior Column, Open Approach

ØSG30KJ Fusion of Lumbosacral Joint with Nonautologous Tissue Substitute, Posterior Approach, Anterior Column, Open Approach

Appendix G: Hospital Acquired Conditions

HAC 12: Surgical Site Infection—Certain Orthopedic Procedures of the Spine, Shoulder, and Elbow (continued)

ØSG337Ø Fusion of Lumbosacral Joint with Autologous Tissue Substitute, Anterior Approach, Anterior Column, Percutaneous Approach

ØSG3371 Fusion of Lumbosacral Joint with Autologous Tissue Substitute, Posterior Approach, Posterior Column, Percutaneous Approach

ØSG337J Fusion of Lumbosacral Joint with Autologous Tissue Substitute, Posterior Approach, Anterior Column, Percutaneous Approach

ØSG33AØ Fusion of Lumbosacral Joint with Interbody Fusion Device, Anterior Approach, Anterior Column, Percutaneous Approach

ØSG33AJ Fusion of Lumbosacral Joint with Interbody Fusion Device, Posterior Approach, Anterior Column, Percutaneous Approach

ØSG33JØ Fusion of Lumbosacral Joint with Synthetic Substitute, Anterior Approach, Anterior Column, Percutaneous Approach

ØSG33J1 Fusion of Lumbosacral Joint with Synthetic Substitute, Posterior Approach, Posterior Column, Percutaneous Approach

ØSG33JJ Fusion of Lumbosacral Joint with Synthetic Substitute, Posterior Approach, Anterior Column, Percutaneous Approach

ØSG33KØ Fusion of Lumbosacral Joint with Nonautologous Tissue Substitute, Anterior Approach, Anterior Column, Percutaneous Approach

ØSG33K1 Fusion of Lumbosacral Joint with Nonautologous Tissue Substitute, Posterior Approach, Posterior Column, Percutaneous Approach

ØSG33KJ Fusion of Lumbosacral Joint with Nonautologous Tissue Substitute, Posterior Approach, Anterior Column, Percutaneous Approach

ØSG347Ø Fusion of Lumbosacral Joint with Autologous Tissue Substitute, Anterior Approach, Anterior Column, Percutaneous Endoscopic Approach

ØSG3471 Fusion of Lumbosacral Joint with Autologous Tissue Substitute, Posterior Approach, Posterior Column, Percutaneous Endoscopic Approach

ØSG347J Fusion of Lumbosacral Joint with Autologous Tissue Substitute, Posterior Approach, Anterior Column, Percutaneous Endoscopic Approach

ØSG34AØ Fusion of Lumbosacral Joint with Interbody Fusion Device, Anterior Approach, Anterior Column, Percutaneous Endoscopic Approach

ØSG34AJ Fusion of Lumbosacral Joint with Interbody Fusion Device, Posterior Approach, Anterior Column, Percutaneous Endoscopic Approach

ØSG34JØ Fusion of Lumbosacral Joint with Synthetic Substitute, Anterior Approach, Anterior Column, Percutaneous Endoscopic Approach

ØSG34J1 Fusion of Lumbosacral Joint with Synthetic Substitute, Posterior Approach, Posterior Column, Percutaneous Endoscopic Approach

ØSG34JJ Fusion of Lumbosacral Joint with Synthetic Substitute, Posterior Approach, Anterior Column, Percutaneous Endoscopic Approach

ØSG34KØ Fusion of Lumbosacral Joint with Nonautologous Tissue Substitute, Anterior Approach, Anterior Column, Percutaneous Endoscopic Approach

ØSG34K1 Fusion of Lumbosacral Joint with Nonautologous Tissue Substitute, Posterior Approach, Posterior Column, Percutaneous Endoscopic Approach

ØSG34KJ Fusion of Lumbosacral Joint with Nonautologous Tissue Substitute, Posterior Approach, Anterior Column, Percutaneous Endoscopic Approach

ØSG704Z Fusion of Right Sacroiliac Joint with Internal Fixation Device, Open Approach

ØSG707Z Fusion of Right Sacroiliac Joint with Autologous Tissue Substitute, Open Approach

ØSG70JZ Fusion of Right Sacroiliac Joint with Synthetic Substitute, Open Approach

ØSG70KZ Fusion of Right Sacroiliac Joint with Nonautologous Tissue Substitute, Open Approach

ØSG734Z Fusion of Right Sacroiliac Joint with Internal Fixation Device, Percutaneous Approach

ØSG737Z Fusion of Right Sacroiliac Joint with Autologous Tissue Substitute, Percutaneous Approach

ØSG73JZ Fusion of Right Sacroiliac Joint with Synthetic Substitute, Percutaneous Approach

ØSG73KZ Fusion of Right Sacroiliac Joint with Nonautologous Tissue Substitute, Percutaneous Approach

ØSG744Z Fusion of Right Sacroiliac Joint with Internal Fixation Device, Percutaneous Endoscopic Approach

ØSG747Z Fusion of Right Sacroiliac Joint with Autologous Tissue Substitute, Percutaneous Endoscopic Approach

ØSG74JZ Fusion of Right Sacroiliac Joint with Synthetic Substitute, Percutaneous Endoscopic Approach

ØSG74KZ Fusion of Right Sacroiliac Joint with Nonautologous Tissue Substitute, Percutaneous Endoscopic Approach

ØSG804Z Fusion of Left Sacroiliac Joint with Internal Fixation Device, Open Approach

ØSG807Z Fusion of Left Sacroiliac Joint with Autologous Tissue Substitute, Open Approach

ØSG80JZ Fusion of Left Sacroiliac Joint with Synthetic Substitute, Open Approach

ØSG80KZ Fusion of Left Sacroiliac Joint with Nonautologous Tissue Substitute, Open Approach

ØSG834Z Fusion of Left Sacroiliac Joint with Internal Fixation Device, Percutaneous Approach

ØSG837Z Fusion of Left Sacroiliac Joint with Autologous Tissue Substitute, Percutaneous Approach

ØSG83JZ Fusion of Left Sacroiliac Joint with Synthetic Substitute, Percutaneous Approach

ØSG83KZ Fusion of Left Sacroiliac Joint with Nonautologous Tissue Substitute, Percutaneous Approach

ØSG844Z Fusion of Left Sacroiliac Joint with Internal Fixation Device, Percutaneous Endoscopic Approach

ØSG847Z Fusion of Left Sacroiliac Joint with Autologous Tissue Substitute, Percutaneous Endoscopic Approach

ØSG84JZ Fusion of Left Sacroiliac Joint with Synthetic Substitute, Percutaneous Endoscopic Approach

ØSG84KZ Fusion of Left Sacroiliac Joint with Nonautologous Tissue Substitute, Percutaneous Endoscopic Approach

XRG0092 Fusion of Occipital-cervical Joint using Nanotextured Surface Interbody Fusion Device, Open Approach, New Technology Group 2

XRG00F3 Fusion of Occipital-cervical Joint using Radiolucent Porous Interbody Fusion Device, Open Approach, New Technology Group 3

XRG1092 Fusion of Cervical Vertebral Joint using Nanotextured Surface Interbody Fusion Device, Open Approach, New Technology Group 2

XRG10F3 Fusion of Cervical Vertebral Joint using Radiolucent Porous Interbody Fusion Device, Open Approach, New Technology Group 3

XRG2092 Fusion of 2 or more Cervical Vertebral Joints using Nanotextured Surface Interbody Fusion Device, Open Approach, New Technology Group 2

XRG20F3 Fusion of 2 or more Cervical Vertebral Joints using Radiolucent Porous Interbody Fusion Device, Open Approach, New Technology Group 3

XRG4092 Fusion of Cervicothoracic Vertebral Joint using Nanotextured Surface Interbody Fusion Device, Open Approach, New Technology Group 2

XRG40F3 Fusion of Cervicothoracic Vertebral Joint using Radiolucent Porous Interbody Fusion Device, Open Approach, New Technology Group 3

XRG6092 Fusion of Thoracic Vertebral Joint using Nanotextured Surface Interbody Fusion Device, Open Approach, New Technology Group 2

XRG60F3 Fusion of Thoracic Vertebral Joint using Radiolucent Porous Interbody Fusion Device, Open Approach, New Technology Group 3

XRG7092 Fusion of 2 to 7 Thoracic Vertebral Joints using Nanotextured Surface Interbody Fusion Device, Open Approach, New Technology Group 2

XRG70F3 Fusion of 2 to 7 Thoracic Vertebral Joints using Radiolucent Porous Interbody Fusion Device, Open Approach, New Technology Group 3

XRG8092 Fusion of 8 or more Thoracic Vertebral Joints using Nanotextured Surface Interbody Fusion Device, Open Approach, New Technology Group 2

XRG80F3 Fusion of 8 or more Thoracic Vertebral Joints using Radiolucent Porous Interbody Fusion Device, Open Approach, New Technology Group 3

XRGA092 Fusion of Thoracolumbar Vertebral Joint using Nanotextured Surface Interbody Fusion Device, Open Approach, New Technology Group 2

XRGA0F3 Fusion of Thoracolumbar Vertebral Joint using Radiolucent Porous Interbody Fusion Device, Open Approach, New Technology Group 3

XRGB092 Fusion of Lumbar Vertebral Joint using Nanotextured Surface Interbody Fusion Device, Open Approach, New Technology Group 2

HAC 12: Surgical Site Infection—Certain Orthopedic Procedures of the Spine, Shoulder, and Elbow (continued)

XRGB0F3   Fusion of Lumbar Vertebral Joint using Radiolucent Porous Interbody Fusion Device, Open Approach, New Technology Group 3

XRGC092   Fusion of 2 or more Lumbar Vertebral Joints using Nanotextured Surface Interbody Fusion Device, Open Approach, New Technology Group 2

XRGC0F3   Fusion of 2 or more Lumbar Vertebral Joints using Radiolucent Porous Interbody Fusion Device, Open Approach, New Technology Group 3

XRGD092   Fusion of Lumbosacral Joint using Nanotextured Surface Interbody Fusion Device, Open Approach, New Technology Group 2

XRGD0F3   Fusion of Lumbosacral Joint using Radiolucent Porous Interbody Fusion Device, Open Approach, New Technology Group 3

HAC 13: Surgical Site Infection (SSI) Following Cardiac Implantable Electronic Device (CIED) Procedures

Secondary diagnosis not POA:

K68.11
T81.40XA
T81.41XA
T81.42XA
T81.43XA
T81.44XA
T81.49XA
T82.6XXA
T82.7XXA

AND

Any of the following procedures:

02H43JZ   Insertion of Pacemaker Lead into Coronary Vein, Percutaneous Approach

02H43KZ   Insertion of Defibrillator Lead into Coronary Vein, Percutaneous Approach

02H43MZ   Insertion of Cardiac Lead into Coronary Vein, Percutaneous Approach

02H63JZ   Insertion of Pacemaker Lead into Right Atrium, Percutaneous Approach

02H63MZ   Insertion of Cardiac Lead into Right Atrium, Percutaneous Approach

02H73JZ   Insertion of Pacemaker Lead into Left Atrium, Percutaneous Approach

02H73MZ   Insertion of Cardiac Lead into Left Atrium, Percutaneous Approach

02HK3JZ   Insertion of Pacemaker Lead into Right Ventricle, Percutaneous Approach

02HL3JZ   Insertion of Pacemaker Lead into Left Ventricle, Percutaneous Approach

02HN0JZ   Insertion of Pacemaker Lead into Pericardium, Open Approach

02HN0MZ   Insertion of Cardiac Lead into Pericardium, Open Approach

02HN3JZ   Insertion of Pacemaker Lead into Pericardium, Percutaneous Approach

02HN3MZ   Insertion of Cardiac Lead into Pericardium, Percutaneous Approach

02HN4JZ   Insertion of Pacemaker Lead into Pericardium, Percutaneous Endoscopic Approach

02HN4MZ   Insertion of Cardiac Lead into Pericardium, Percutaneous Endoscopic Approach

02PA0MZ   Removal of Cardiac Lead from Heart, Open Approach

02PA3MZ   Removal of Cardiac Lead from Heart, Percutaneous Approach

02PA4MZ   Removal of Cardiac Lead from Heart, Percutaneous Endoscopic Approach

02PAXMZ   Removal of Cardiac Lead from Heart, External Approach

02WA0MZ   Revision of Cardiac Lead in Heart, Open Approach

02WA3MZ   Revision of Cardiac Lead in Heart, Percutaneous Approach

02WA4MZ   Revision of Cardiac Lead in Heart, Percutaneous Endoscopic Approach

0JH604Z   Insertion of Pacemaker, Single Chamber into Chest Subcutaneous Tissue and Fascia, Open Approach

0JH605Z   Insertion of Pacemaker, Single Chamber Rate Responsive into Chest Subcutaneous Tissue and Fascia, Open Approach

0JH606Z   Insertion of Pacemaker, Dual Chamber into Chest Subcutaneous Tissue and Fascia, Open Approach

0JH607Z   Insertion of Cardiac Resynchronization Pacemaker Pulse Generator into Chest Subcutaneous Tissue and Fascia, Open Approach

0JH608Z   Insertion of Defibrillator Generator into Chest Subcutaneous Tissue and Fascia, Open Approach

0JH609Z   Insertion of Cardiac Resynchronization Defibrillator Pulse Generator into Chest Subcutaneous Tissue and Fascia, Open Approach

0JH60PZ   Insertion of Cardiac Rhythm Related Device into Chest Subcutaneous Tissue and Fascia, Open Approach

0JH634Z   Insertion of Pacemaker, Single Chamber into Chest Subcutaneous Tissue and Fascia, Percutaneous Approach

0JH635Z   Insertion of Pacemaker, Single Chamber Rate Responsive into Chest Subcutaneous Tissue and Fascia, Percutaneous Approach

0JH636Z   Insertion of Pacemaker, Dual Chamber into Chest Subcutaneous Tissue and Fascia, Percutaneous Approach

0JH637Z   Insertion of Cardiac Resynchronization Pacemaker Pulse Generator into Chest Subcutaneous Tissue and Fascia, Percutaneous Approach

0JH638Z   Insertion of Defibrillator Generator into Chest Subcutaneous Tissue and Fascia, Percutaneous Approach

0JH639Z   Insertion of Cardiac Resynchronization Defibrillator Pulse Generator into Chest Subcutaneous Tissue and Fascia, Percutaneous Approach

0JH63PZ   Insertion of Cardiac Rhythm Related Device into Chest Subcutaneous Tissue and Fascia, Percutaneous Approach

0JH804Z   Insertion of Pacemaker, Single Chamber into Abdomen Subcutaneous Tissue and Fascia, Open Approach

0JH805Z   Insertion of Pacemaker, Single Chamber Rate Responsive into Abdomen Subcutaneous Tissue and Fascia, Open Approach

0JH806Z   Insertion of Pacemaker, Dual Chamber into Abdomen Subcutaneous Tissue and Fascia, Open Approach

0JH807Z   Insertion of Cardiac Resynchronization Pacemaker Pulse Generator into Abdomen Subcutaneous Tissue and Fascia, Open Approach

0JH808Z   Insertion of Defibrillator Generator into Abdomen Subcutaneous Tissue and Fascia, Open Approach

0JH809Z   Insertion of Cardiac Resynchronization Defibrillator Pulse Generator into Abdomen Subcutaneous Tissue and Fascia, Open Approach

0JH80PZ   Insertion of Cardiac Rhythm Related Device into Abdomen Subcutaneous Tissue and Fascia, Open Approach

0JH834Z   Insertion of Pacemaker, Single Chamber into Abdomen Subcutaneous Tissue and Fascia, Percutaneous Approach

0JH835Z   Insertion of Pacemaker, Single Chamber Rate Responsive into Abdomen Subcutaneous Tissue and Fascia, Percutaneous Approach

0JH836Z   Insertion of Pacemaker, Dual Chamber into Abdomen Subcutaneous Tissue and Fascia, Percutaneous Approach

0JH837Z   Insertion of Cardiac Resynchronization Pacemaker Pulse Generator into Abdomen Subcutaneous Tissue and Fascia, Percutaneous Approach

0JH838Z   Insertion of Defibrillator Generator into Abdomen Subcutaneous Tissue and Fascia, Percutaneous Approach

0JH839Z   Insertion of Cardiac Resynchronization Defibrillator Pulse Generator into Abdomen Subcutaneous Tissue and Fascia, Percutaneous Approach

0JH83PZ   Insertion of Cardiac Rhythm Related Device into Abdomen Subcutaneous Tissue and Fascia, Percutaneous Approach

0JPT0PZ   Removal of Cardiac Rhythm Related Device from Trunk Subcutaneous Tissue and Fascia, Open Approach

0JPT3PZ   Removal of Cardiac Rhythm Related Device from Trunk Subcutaneous Tissue and Fascia, Percutaneous Approach

0JWT0PZ   Revision of Cardiac Rhythm Related Device in Trunk Subcutaneous Tissue and Fascia, Open Approach

0JWT3PZ   Revision of Cardiac Rhythm Related Device in Trunk Subcutaneous Tissue and Fascia, Percutaneous Approach

HAC 14: Iatrogenic Pneumothorax with Venous Catheterization

Secondary diagnosis not POA:

J95.811

AND

Any of the following procedures:

02H633Z   Insertion of Infusion Device into Right Atrium, Percutaneous Approach

02HK33Z   Insertion of Infusion Device into Right Ventricle, Percutaneous Approach

02HS33Z   Insertion of Infusion Device into Right Pulmonary Vein, Percutaneous Approach

02HS43Z   Insertion of Infusion Device into Right Pulmonary Vein, Percutaneous Endoscopic Approach

02HT33Z   Insertion of Infusion Device into Left Pulmonary Vein, Percutaneous Approach

02HT43Z   Insertion of Infusion Device into Left Pulmonary Vein, Percutaneous Endoscopic Approach

02HV33Z   Insertion of Infusion Device into Superior Vena Cava, Percutaneous Approach

02HV43Z   Insertion of Infusion Device into Superior Vena Cava, Percutaneous Endoscopic Approach

05H033Z   Insertion of Infusion Device into Azygos Vein, Percutaneous Approach

05H043Z   Insertion of Infusion Device into Azygos Vein, Percutaneous Endoscopic Approach

05H133Z   Insertion of Infusion Device into Hemiazygos Vein, Percutaneous Approach

05H143Z   Insertion of Infusion Device into Hemiazygos Vein, Percutaneous Endoscopic Approach

HAC 14: Iatrogenic Pneumothorax with Venous Catheterization (continued)

Ø5H333Z　Insertion of Infusion Device into Right Innominate Vein, Percutaneous Approach

Ø5H343Z　Insertion of Infusion Device into Right Innominate Vein, Percutaneous Endoscopic Approach

Ø5H433Z　Insertion of Infusion Device into Left Innominate Vein, Percutaneous Approach

Ø5H443Z　Insertion of Infusion Device into Left Innominate Vein, Percutaneous Endoscopic Approach

Ø5H533Z　Insertion of Infusion Device into Right Subclavian Vein, Percutaneous Approach

Ø5H543Z　Insertion of Infusion Device into Right Subclavian Vein, Percutaneous Endoscopic Approach

Ø5H633Z　Insertion of Infusion Device into Left Subclavian Vein, Percutaneous Approach

Ø5H643Z　Insertion of Infusion Device into Left Subclavian Vein, Percutaneous Endoscopic Approach

Ø5HM33Z　Insertion of Infusion Device into Right Internal Jugular Vein, Percutaneous Approach

Ø5HN33Z　Insertion of Infusion Device into Left Internal Jugular Vein, Percutaneous Approach

Ø5HP33Z　Insertion of Infusion Device into Right External Jugular Vein, Percutaneous Approach

Ø5HQ33Z　Insertion of Infusion Device into Left External Jugular Vein, Percutaneous Approach

ØJH63XZ　Insertion of Vascular Access Device into Chest Subcutaneous Tissue and Fascia, Percutaneous Approach

Appendix H: Centers for Medicare & Medicaid Services Hierarchical Condition Categories (CMS-HCC)

In the 1970s, Medicare began demonstration projects that contracted with health maintenance organizations (HMOs) to provide care for Medicare beneficiaries in exchange for prospective payments. In 1985, this project changed from demonstration status to a regular part of the Medicare program, Medicare Part C. The Balanced Budget Act (BBA) of 1997 named Medicare's Part C managed care program Medicare+Choice, and the Medicare Modernization Act (MMA) of 2003 again renamed it to Medicare Advantage (MA).

Medicare is one of the world's largest health insurance programs, and about one-third of the beneficiaries on Medicare are enrolled in a MA private health care plan. Due to the great variance in the health status of Medicare beneficiaries, risk adjustment provides a means of adequately compensating those plans with large numbers of seriously ill patients while not overburdening other plans that have healthier individuals. Medicare Advantage (MA) plans have been using the Hierarchical Condition Category (HCC) risk adjustment model since 2004.

The Risk Adjustment Model

The primary purpose of a risk adjustment model is to predict (on average) the future health care costs for specific consortiums enrolled in Medicare Advantage (MA) health plans. CMS is then able to provide capitation payments to these private health plans. Capitation payments are an incentive for health plans to enroll not only healthier individuals but those with chronic conditions or who are more seriously ill by removing some of the financial burden.

The MA risk adjustment model uses HCCs to assess the disease burden of its enrollees. HCC diagnostic groupings were created after examining claims data so that enrollees with similar disease processes, and consequently similar health care expenditures, could be pooled into a larger data set in which an average expenditure rate could be determined. The medical conditions included in HCC categories are those that were determined to most predictably affect the health status and health care costs of any individual. Several important principles to the risk adjustment model and the development of the HCC categories include but are not limited to:

1. The HCC diagnostic categories should be clinically meaningful.

   • Diagnostic categories are well-defined.

   • Clinically specific diseases or medical conditions are grouped to each category.

2. The HCC diagnostic categories should predict medical expenditures.

   • The diagnoses grouped to a specific category should have as close to the same cost burden not only in the current year but also in the future.

3. The HCC diagnostic categories should have adequate sample sizes and discretionary categories excluded to be as accurate and stable in their estimate of costs as possible.

   • A diagnostic category that groups extremely rare diseases or conditions would not be reliably effective in determining current or future costs.

   • Codes that are not credible as cost predictors or may be subject to coding variation should be excluded, when possible.

4. The HCC diagnostic categories should be both hierarchical and additive.

   • Hierarchical measurement is used within a specific disease process.

   • Disease processes that are unrelated to each other are measured additively.

5. The diagnostic classification should encourage specificity and should not reward coding proliferation.

   • More diagnosis codes and vague diagnosis codes do not equal greater disease burden.

More than 10,000 ICD-10-CM diagnosis codes map to 86 HCCs in the current risk adjustment model. Diagnoses are excluded from mapping when they do not predict future cost or are vague or variable in diagnosis, coding, or treatment, such as symptoms or osteoarthritis. Also excluded are diagnosis codes from laboratories, radiology, and home health claims.

Risk Adjustment Factors

The CMS-HCC risk adjustment model uses "risk adjustment factors" to calculate a risk score for each member. This score summarizes that particular patient's expected cost of care relative to other members'. Each member's risk score is based on demographic and health status information and is calculated as the sum of these demographic and health factors weighted by their estimated marginal contributions to total risk. The model also takes into account where the patient resides (community or institutional), Medicaid eligibility (full or partial benefits), the patient's Medicare enrollment status (new or established), age, disability status, whether the patient is frail or has end-stage renal disease (ESRD), and even prescription drug use.

No procedure codes, ICD-10-PCS or CPT, are included in the MA risk adjustment model. The model relies solely on diagnostic and demographic data. Not all ICD-10-CM diagnoses map to an HCC, and there is no specific code sequencing involved. The CMS-HCC model is additive as well as hierarchical. The additive functionality allows a patient to have more than one HCC category assigned, providing a more complete clinical picture and prediction of resource consumption. The hierarchical aspect of the model provides a means of ranking diagnoses that are similar in disease process, by severity. The hierarchy of the condition categories ensures the patient's conditions are classified to the most severe condition within the related group. Less severe conditions within a particular hierarchy are superseded by more severe diagnoses within the same group. The hierarchy and additive relationship permits this model to characterize the person's illness level within each disease process, while still allowing the effects of unrelated disease processes to be counted in the patient's overall score.

Certain combinations of coexisting diagnoses for an individual can increase medical costs. The CMS-HCC model adjusts for these higher costs by the addition of "disease interaction" factors. For each patient, multiple HCCs assigned, along with demographic and disease interaction factors, are used to calculate a single, combined risk adjustment factor (RAF). The RAF score for an individual member represents all of the HCCs that have been submitted from all sources for that member to CMS during the course of an entire calendar year.

There are separate CMS-HCC models for new enrollees and continuing enrollees. The new enrollee model uses demographic factors only, such as age, sex, and disability status, and is used when the enrollee has less than 12 months of medical history. The community model accounts for age, sex, original reason for Medicare entitlement (age or disability), Medicaid eligibility, and clinical conditions as measured by HCCs. In the second step, expected costs are adjusted for outliers based on the member's risk score and whether the patient has ESRD.

Demographic data (age, sex, eligibility) as well as health status (diagnoses codes submitted on claims to CMS) of an MA population are used to determine the reimbursement to the health plan to care for their members.

CMS considers a RAF score of 1.0 as the benchmark to indicate the score of the average healthy patient with the same demographic and diagnostic factors. These patients are expected to use average or lower-than-average resources. When the RAF score is higher than 1.0, CMS considers the patient to be sicker than the average patient with the same criteria and expects greater-than-average resource utilization.

A low RAF score may accurately indicate a healthier patient, but it may also falsely indicate a healthier patient due to incomplete or inaccurate coding, incomplete or insufficient record documentation, or patients who fail to complete an annual assessment.

A high RAF score may accurately indicate a sicker patient, or it may be falsely inflated from overcoding due to diagnoses that are reported but not documented, or from copying and pasting from previous encounters or problem lists of resolved conditions.

Documentation Requirements

Payment is made per HCC category (not per diagnosis code). No matter how many times in the year the diagnosis codes are reported, a single payment is made to the MA plan each year. Each year the list of HCCs and the RAF for each patient is "reset." This means the annual health assessment is extremely important, and adequate documentation is critical. Accurate risk adjustment payment relies on complete medical record documentation and diagnosis coding. CMS requires that all applicable diagnosis codes be reported and that all diagnoses be reported to the highest level of specificity and that these be substantiated by the medical record.

CMS's Guiding Principle:

The risk adjustment diagnosis must be based on clinical medical record documentation from a face-to-face encounter, coded according to the *ICD-10-CM Guidelines for Coding and Reporting*; assigned based on dates of service within the data collection period, submitted to the MA organization from an appropriate risk adjustment provider type and an appropriate risk adjustment physician data source.

A "face-to-face" health service encounter between a patient and healthcare provider describes an encounter between the patient and the provider (MD, DO), including qualified nonphysician practitioners (NPP) (e.g. nurse practitioner or physician's assistant), which is face-to-face with the patient. CMS provides a current listing of acceptable physician specialty types for risk adjustment data submission within the 2012 Regional Technical Assistance Participant Guide. The only exception to the face-to-face encounter requirement is pathology services (professional component only). Currently, CMS does not provide a listing of all services that are considered face-to-face visits for risk adjustment data, but does provide guidance on what types of services are not acceptable for risk adjustment in the Participant Guide. For example, diagnostic radiology does not qualify because diagnostic radiologists typically do not document confirmed diagnoses. Other examples of services that are not acceptable include diagnostic reports that have not been interpreted, such as laboratory reports.

It is essential that the medical record documentation show evidence by provider authentication that the direct face-to-face service was personally furnished by the physician or qualified NPP. Examples of these services include office visits, hospital visits, preoperative anesthesia assessment, and surgical and invasive procedures.

Risk adjustment relies on annual health information. Each enrollee is assigned an individual risk score based on the health status information obtained from the diagnosis codes on the claims. The CMS-HCC model relies on ICD-10-CM coding specificity for accurate risk adjustment by using the most specific code available that is substantiated by the documentation in the medical record. Providers should fully document and accurately code the evaluation and management of all severe and chronic conditions to ensure a full, complete, and accurate clinical record of the patient's condition and reflect the work involved in caring for the patient, particularly those with complex and challenging health issues. All conditions affecting the treatment or management of the patient's health should be documented at least once a year, as applicable to care provided, to accurately describe the true complexity and severity of the patient's health. If the diagnosis coding on the claim is not accurate or complete, the claim may indicate that the provider did much less medical decision-making, evaluation, and management than was actually performed.

Documentation to support or validate risk adjustment conditions may be found anywhere in the note for the face-to-face encounter. It is important to ensure that the note accurately reflects all chronic conditions that affect the health and care of the patient. Each encounter must be unique and reflect only that visit as it occurred. Insufficient documentation influences the assignment of diagnosis codes and directly affects the patient's risk score.

Documentation should properly validate all reported conditions. Each page of progress notes should be properly authenticated and include the patient's name and the date.

Providers should document each clinical diagnosis to the highest degree of specificity per encounter, including all complications and/or manifestations, including clear links to causal conditions. Only confirmed conditions should be documented—no rule-out conditions or abnormal findings without clinical significance. All known conditions, including chronic conditions, that affect the care and treatment of the patient at least once per year should be noted.

Providers should specifically document the condition and clinical significance, and any pertinent changes, using terminology such as decreased, increased, worsening, improving, or unchanged, or abnormal findings.

Documentation Tips
- Document all cause-and-effect relationships.
- Report the most specific diagnosis code available that is supported by the documentation.
- Include all current diagnoses as part of the current medical decision-making, and document for every visit.
- Identify diagnoses that are current or chronic problems rather than a past medical history or previous resolved condition.
- Document history of heart attack, status codes, etc., that affect the patient's care as "history of" or "PMH" when they no longer exist or are not current conditions.
- Ensure each progress note has the date, signature, and credentials/specialty.
- Document the thought processes used to assess each condition.
- Know high revenue HCCs that are often undiagnosed or undercoded.
- Avoid "unspecified" codes.

- Ensure the codes reported are accurate.
- Ensure each encounter is billed.
- Review rejection reports, and audit reports to assess risks.

Audits
Because reimbursement is by patient, rather than based on an average of the entire population, and is based upon documentation, there is the potential for upcoding. Audits are conducted by the MA plan and CMS recovery auditors.

Initial Validation Audit (IVA)
CMS requires that the MA plan validate HCCs. This is usually performed by an independent auditor working with the plan or a contracted vendor to validate the MA plan's data submitted to CMS.

The MA plan submits the one best medical record that supports each HCC identified for the beneficiary.

Risk Adjustment Data Validation Audit
Risk adjustment data validation (RADV) audits were introduced in 2011 and updated for 2015. They are performed by CMS to validate the integrity and accuracy of risk-adjusted payments by verifying that the diagnosis codes the MA plans submit are supported by the medical record documentation for a member.

MA plans can be selected by CMS for RADV audits annually and if chosen are required to submit their members' medical records to CMS. Providers are required to assist the MA plan by providing the medical record documentation included in the audit. Even though each diagnosis needs to be reported only once in a calendar year, during a RADV audit up to five dates of service may be submitted to support any one HCC.

To be validated, medical record documentation must meet certain criteria and standards. Even if the diagnosis is documented and coded correctly, any deficiency in the documentation can make the encounter and the HCC invalid. Diagnoses that cannot be validated are considered payment errors. The results of the audit are communicated to the MA plan, which then communicates these results to the provider. Under- and overpayments are subject to payment adjustment. The results of RADV audits can be extrapolated over the MA plan population to calculate potential payment errors and overpayments/recoupments. Regulations include a RADV appeal process, a document dispute process, and a procedure for obtaining physician-signature attestations.

The following items are reviewed during the validation process:
- The record is for the correct enrollee.
- The record is from the correct calendar year for the payment year being audited.
- The record is legible.
- The date of service is present on the records and is for a face-to-face visit.
- The record is from a valid provider type.
- Valid credentials and/or a valid physician specialty are documented on the record.
- The record contains a signature from an acceptable type of physician.
- There is a diagnosis on the record.
- The diagnosis supports an HCC.
- The diagnosis supports the submitted HCC.

Mitigate audit risk by coding each reportable diagnosis each time it meets reporting guidelines. Audit regularly to assess areas of risk and in need of improvement and to capture conditions documented but not coded. Check for additional qualifying HCCs. Ensure claims are submitted and that corrected claims are submitted when indicated. There are three claims submission deadlines: January, March, and September. CMS adjusts each member's risk score twice a year, with the final reconciliation in August of the year after the plan year.

If providers emphasize correct coding and documentation and perform internal audits to determine where the risks are and prepare for audits, incorrect payment is less likely.

For additional information on risk adjustment coding, see Optum360's *Risk Adjustment Coding and HCC Guide*.

Appendix I: Long-term Care Hospital Prospective Payment System Overview

Information in this appendix is based on the Centers for Medicare and Medicaid Services (CMS) FY 2019 long-term care hospital prospective payment system (LTCH PPS) final rule published in the *Federal Register*, volume 83, number 160, August 17, 2018 ("Hospital Inpatient Prospective Payment Systems for Acute Care Hospitals and the Long-Term Care Hospital Prospective Payment System and Policy Changes and Fiscal Year 2019 Rates").

Classification As a Long-term Care Hospital

Under the regulations at § 412.23(e)(1), to qualify to be paid under the long-term care hospital prospective payment system (LTCH PPS), a hospital must have a provider agreement with Medicare. Furthermore, § 412.23(e)(2)(i), which implements section 1886(d)(1)(B)(iv) of the Social Security Act, requires that a hospital have an average Medicare inpatient length of stay of greater than 25 days to be paid under the LTCH PPS. In accordance with section 1206(a)(3) of the Pathway for SGR Reform Act of 2013 (Pub. L. 113–67), as amended by section 15007 of Public Law 114–255, CMS amended the regulations to specify that Medicare Advantage plans' and site-neutral payment rate discharges are excluded from the calculation of the average length of stay for all LTCHs, for discharges occurring in cost reporting period beginning on or after October 1, 2015.

The following hospitals are paid under special payment provisions, as described in § 412.22(c) and, therefore, are not subject to the LTCH PPS rules:

- Veterans Administration hospitals
- Hospitals that are reimbursed under state cost control systems approved under 42 CFR part 403
- Hospitals that are reimbursed in accordance with demonstration projects authorized under section 402(a) of the Social Security Amendments of 1967 (Pub. L. 90-248) (42 U.S.C. 1395b-1), section 222(a) of the Social Security Amendments of 1972 (Pub. L. 92-603) (42 U.S.C. 1395b-1 (note)) (statewide all-payer systems, subject to the rate-of-increase test at section 1814(b) of the Act), or section 3201 of the Patient Protection and Affordable Care Act (Pub. L. 111-148 (42 U.S.C. 1315a))
- Nonparticipating hospitals furnishing emergency services to Medicare beneficiaries

Medicare Severity Long-Term Care Diagnosis-Related Groups

The LTCH PPS uses Medicare severity long-term care diagnosis-related groups (MS-LTC-DRG) as a patient classification system. The MS-LTC-DRGs are the same Medicare severity DRGs (MS-DRGs) CMS uses under the inpatient prospective payment system (IPPS), weighted to reflect the different resources LTCHs use. Each patient stay is grouped into an MS-LTC-DRG based on:

- Diagnoses (including secondary diagnoses)
- Procedures performed
- Age
- Gender
- Discharge status

Each MS-LTC-DRG has a predetermined average length of stay (ALOS), which is the typical LOS for a patient classified to the MS-LTC-DRG. CMS updates the ALOS annually based on the latest available LTCH discharge data. Under the LTCH PPS, if the discharge is excluded from the site-neutral payment rate, the LTCH is paid for each Medicare patient based on the MS-LTC-DRG to which that patient's stay is grouped. This reflects the typical resources used for treating such a patient. Medicare pays cases assigned to an MS-LTC-DRG based on the federal payment rate, including any payment and policy adjustments.

Methodology for Determining FY 2019 Relative Weights for MS-LTC-DRGs

When the LTCH PPS was implemented for cost-reporting periods beginning on or after October 1, 2002, CMS adopted the same DRG patient classification system used at that time under the IPPS. Since this patient classification system is a component of the LTCH PPS, CMS referred to it as the "long-term care diagnosis-related groups (LTC-DRGs)." Although the patient classification system used under both the LTCH PPS and the IPPS are the same, the relative weights are different. The established relative weight methodology and data used under the LTCH PPS result in relative weights under the LTCH PPS that reflect the differences in patient resource use of LTCH patients, consistent with section

123(a)(1) of the Balanced Budget Refinement Act of 1999 (BBRA) (Pub. L. 106-113).

As part of CMS's efforts to better recognize severity of illness among patients, in the FY 2008 IPPS final rule with comment period (72 FR 47130), the MS-DRGs and the MS-LTC-DRGs were adopted under the IPPS and the LTCH PPS, respectively, effective beginning October 1, 2007 (FY 2008). (CMS notes that, in that same final rule, it revised the regulations at § 412.503 to specify that for LTCH discharges occurring on or after October 1, 2007, when applying the provisions of 42 CFR part 412, subpart O, applicable to LTCHs for policy descriptions and payment calculations, all references to LTC-DRGs would be considered a reference to MS-LTC-DRGs. For the remainder of this section, the discussion is presented in terms of the current MS-LTC-DRG patient classification system unless specifically referring to the previous LTC-DRG patient classification system that was in effect before October 1, 2007.)

The MS-DRG classifications are updated annually. For FY 2019, there were 761 MS-DRG groupings. Consistent with section 123 of the BBRA, as amended by section 307(b)(1) of the Benefits Improvement and Protection Act of 2000 (BIPA) and § 412.515 of the regulations, CMS used information derived from LTCH PPS patient records to classify LTCH discharges into distinct MS-LTC-DRGs based on clinical characteristics and estimated resource needs. An appropriate weight is then assigned to the MS-LTC-DRGs to account for the difference in patients' resource use, exhibiting the case complexity and multiple medical problems characteristic of LTCHs.

As CMS proposed, the final rule for FY 2019 states that CMS will continue to use the existing methodology to determine the MS-LTC-DRG relative weights. As previously established when CMS implemented the dual rate LTCH PPS payment structure codified under § 412.522, which began in FY 2016, the annual recalibration of the MS-LTC-DRG relative weights are determined: (1) using only data from available LTCH PPS claims that would have qualified for payment under the new LTCH PPS standard federal payment rate if that rate had been in effect at the time of discharge when claims data from time periods before the dual rate LTCH PPS payment structure applies are used to calculate the relative weights; and (2) using only data from available LTCH PPS claims that qualify for payment under the new LTCH PPS standard federal payment rate when claims data from time periods after the dual rate LTCH PPS payment structure applies are used to calculate the relative weights (80 FR 49624). That is, under the current methodology, MS-LTC-DRG relative weight calculations do not use data from cases paid at the site-neutral payment rate under § 412.522(c)(1) or data from cases that would have been paid at the site-neutral payment rate if the dual rate LTCH PPS payment structure had been in effect at the time of that discharge. For the remainder of this discussion, the phrase "applicable LTCH cases" or "applicable LTCH data" is used when referring to the resulting claims data set used to calculate the relative weights. In addition, in the FY 2019 IPPS/LTCH PPS final rule, CMS is continuing to exclude the data from all-inclusive rate providers and LTCHs paid in accordance with demonstration projects, as well as any Medicare Advantage claims from the MS-LTC-DRG relative weight calculations.

Furthermore, for FY 2019, in using data from applicable LTCH cases to establish MS-LTC-DRG relative weights, CMS will continue to establish low-volume MS-LTC-DRGs (that is, MS-LTC-DRGs with less than 25 cases) using existing quintile methodology in determining the MS-LTC-DRG relative weights because LTCHs do not typically treat the full range of diagnoses as do acute care hospitals. Therefore, for purposes of determining the relative weights for the large number of low-volume MS-LTC-DRGs, CMS groups all of the low-volume MS-LTC-DRGs into five quintiles based on average charges per discharge. Then, under the existing methodology, adjustments made to LTCH PPS standard federal payments for short-stay outlier (SSO) cases are accounted for (that is, cases where the covered length of stay at the LTCH is less than or equal to five-sixths of the geometric average length of stay for the MS-LTC-DRG), and adjustments are made to account for nonmonotonically increasing weights, when necessary. The methodology is premised on more severe cases under the MS-LTC-DRG system requiring greater expenditure of medical care resources and higher average charges such that, in the severity levels within a base MS-LTC-DRG, the relative weights should increase monotonically with severity from the lowest to highest severity level.

Changes to the MS-LTC-DRGs for FY2019

As specified by § 412.517(a), which requires that the MS-LTC-DRG classifications and relative weights be updated annually, and consistent with historical practice of using the same patient classification system under the LTCH PPS as is used under the IPPS, in the FY 2019 IPPS/LTCH PPS final rule, CMS updated the MS-LTC-DRG classifications effective October 1, 2018, through September 30,

2019 (FY 2019), consistent with the changes specific to the MS-DRG classifications.

Accordingly, the MS-LTC-DRGs for FY 2019 presented in the final rule are the same as the MS-DRGs that are being used under the IPPS for FY 2019. In addition, because the MS-LTC-DRGs for FY 2019 are the same as the MS-DRGs for FY 2019, the other changes that affect MS-DRG (and by extension MS-LTC-DRG) assignments under Grouper version 36, including the changes to the MCE software and the ICD-10-CM/PCS coding system, are also applicable under the LTCH PPS for FY 2019.

For FY 2019, consistent with historical relative weight methodology and as proposed, CMS is establishing a relative weight of 0.0000 for the following transplant MS-LTC-DRGs: Heart Transplant or Implant of Heart Assist System with MCC (MS-LTC-DRG 001); Heart Transplant or Implant of Heart Assist System without MCC (MS-LTC-DRG 002); Liver Transplant with MCC or Intestinal Transplant (MS-LTC-DRG 005); Liver Transplant without MCC (MS-LTC-DRG 006); Lung Transplant (MS-LTC-DRG 007); Simultaneous Pancreas/Kidney Transplant (MS-LTC-DRG 008); Pancreas Transplant (MS-LTC-DRG 010); and Kidney Transplant (MS-LTC-DRG 652). This is because Medicare covers these procedures only if they are performed at a hospital that Medicare has certified for the specific procedures and presently no LTCH has been so certified. Currently, CMS includes these eight transplant MS-LTC-DRGs in the Grouper program for administrative purposes only. Because CMS uses the same Grouper program for LTCHs as is used under the IPPS, removing these MS-LTC-DRGs would be administratively burdensome.

In addition, consistent with historical policy and as proposed, CMS is establishing a relative weight of 0.0000 for the 2 "error" MS-LTC-DRGs (that is, MS-LTC-DRG 998 [Principal Diagnosis Invalid as Discharge Diagnosis] and MS-LTC-DRG 999 [Ungroupable]) because applicable LTCH cases grouped to these MS-LTC-DRGs cannot be properly assigned to an MS-LTC-DRG according to the grouping logic.

In the final rule, consistent with CMS practice in FYs 2016 through 2018 and as proposed, CMS is establishing a relative weight for FY 2019 equal to the respective FY 2015 relative weight of the MS-LTC-DRGs for the following psychiatric or rehabilitation MS-LTC-DRGs: MS-LTC-DRG 876 (O.R. Procedure with Principal Diagnoses of Mental Illness); MS-LTC-DRG 880 (Acute Adjustment Reaction & Psychosocial Dysfunction); MS-LTC-DRG 881 (Depressive Neuroses); MS-LTC-DRG 882 (Neuroses Except Depressive); MS-LTC-DRG 883 (Disorders of Personality & Impulse Control); MS-LTC-DRG 884 (Organic Disturbances & Mental Retardation); MS-LTC-DRG 885 (Psychoses); MS-LTC-DRG 886 (Behavioral & Developmental Disorders); MS-LTC-DRG 887 (Other Mental Disorder Diagnoses); MS-LTC-DRG 894 (Alcohol/Drug Abuse or Dependence, Left AMA); MS-LTC-DRG 895 (Alcohol/Drug Abuse or Dependence, with Rehabilitation Therapy); MS-LTC-DRG 896 (Alcohol/Drug Abuse or Dependence, without Rehabilitation Therapy with MCC); MS-LTC-DRG 897 (Alcohol/Drug Abuse or Dependence, without Rehabilitation Therapy without MCC); MS-LTC-DRG 945 (Rehabilitation with CC/MCC); and MS-LTC-DRG 946 (Rehabilitation without CC/MCC). When CMS implemented the dual-rate LTCH PPS payment structure, LTCH discharges that are grouped to these 15 psychiatric and rehabilitation MS-LTC-DRGs did not meet the criteria for exclusion from the site-neutral payment rate.

Therefore, under the criterion for a principal diagnosis relating to a psychiatric diagnosis or to rehabilitation, there are no applicable LTCH cases to use in calculating a relative weight for the psychiatric and rehabilitation MS-LTC-DRGs. In other words, any LTCH PPS discharges grouped to any of the 15 psychiatric and rehabilitation MS-LTC-DRGs would always be paid at the site-neutral payment rate, and, therefore, those MS-LTC-DRGs would never include any LTCH cases that meet the criteria for exclusion from the site-neutral payment rate. However, section 1886(m)(6)(B) of the Social Security Act establishes a transitional payment method for cases that would be paid at the site-neutral payment rate for LTCH discharges occurring in cost reporting periods beginning during FY 2016 or FY 2017, which was extended to include FYs 2018 and 2019 under Public Law 115–123. Under the transitional payment method for site-neutral payment rate cases, for LTCH discharges occurring in cost reporting periods beginning on or after October 1, 2018, and on or before September 30, 2019, site-neutral payment rate cases are paid a blended payment rate, calculated as 50 percent of the applicable site-neutral payment rate amount for the discharge and 50 percent of the applicable LTCH PPS standard federal payment rate. Because the LTCH PPS standard Federal payment rate is based on the relative weight of the MS-LTC-DRG, in order to determine the transitional blended payment for site-neutral payment rate cases grouped to one of the "psychiatric or rehabilitation" MS-LTC-DRGs in FY 2019, CMS assigned a relative weight to these MS-LTC-DRGs for FY 2019 that is the same as the FY 2018 relative weight (which is also the same as the FYs 2016 and 2017 relative weight). CMS believes that using the respective FY 2015 relative weight for each of the "psychiatric or rehabilitation" MS-LTC-DRGs results in appropriate payments for LTCH cases that are paid at the site-neutral payment rate under the transition policy provided by the statute because there are no clinically similar MS-LTC-DRGs for which CMS was able to determine relative weights based on applicable LTCH cases in the

March 2018 update of the FY 2017 MedPAR file data using the steps described above. Furthermore, CMS believes that it would be administratively burdensome and introduce unnecessary complexity to the MS-LTC-DRG relative weight calculation to use the LTCH discharges in the MedPAR file data to calculate a relative weight for those 15 "psychiatric and rehabilitation" MS-LTC-DRGs to be used for the sole purposes of determining half of the transitional blended payment for site-neutral payment rate cases during the transition period (80 FR 49631 through 49632) or payment for discharges from spinal cord specialty hospitals under § 412.522(b)(4).

In summary, for FY 2019, CMS is establishing a relative weight (and average length of stay thresholds) equal to the respective FY 2015 relative weight of the MS-LTC-DRGs for the 15 "psychiatric or rehabilitation" MS-LTC-DRGs listed previously (that is, MS-LTC-DRGs 876, 880, 881, 882, 883, 884, 885, 886, 887, 894, 895, 896, 897, 945, and 946).

Site-Neutral Payment Rate

For cost reporting periods beginning on or after October 1, 2015, LTCH discharges that do not meet specific criteria will be paid at a new site-neutral payment rate, which is generally the lower of:

- The IPPS comparable per diem amount (as calculated under CMS's short-stay outlier [SSO] policy)
- The estimated costs of the case (calculated by multiplying the allowable charges by the LTCH's Cost-to-Charge Ratio [CCR])

For a discharge to be excluded from the site-neutral payment rate and paid based on the standard federal payment rate:

- The discharge must not have a principal diagnosis in the LTCH of a psychiatric diagnosis or rehabilitation as indicated by the grouping of the discharge into one of 15 psychiatric and rehabilitation MS-LTC-DRGs (MS-LTC-DRGs 876, 880, 881, 882, 883, 884, 885, 886, 887, 894, 895, 896, 897, 945, and 946).
- The discharge must have been immediately preceded by a subsection (d) hospital discharge. "Immediately preceded" means that the LTCH admission occurred within one day of the subsection (d) hospital discharge based on the admission date on the LTCH claim and the discharge date on the subsection (d) hospital claim.
- The patient discharged from the LTCH must have either:
  - Spent at least three days in an intensive care unit during the immediately preceding subsection (d) hospital stay. Discharges that meet this criterion are identified by the use of revenue center codes 020x and 021x on the subsection (d) hospital discharge claim.
  - Received at least 96 hours of respiratory ventilation services during the LTCH stay that are generally identified by using ICD-10-PCS code 5A1955Z on the LTCH claim.
- The patient was treated for a severe wound and discharged from a grandfathered LTCH hospital-within-hospital (HwH) located in a rural area or treated as being located in a rural area. To find the list of severe wounds by category identified by ICD-10 code, visit CMS.gov/Medicare/Medicare-Fee-for-Service-Payment/LongTermCareHospitalPPS/download.html. Discharges that meet the definition of infected wound and wounds with morbid obesity are identified by using payer-only condition codes.
- Discharges fall into a grandfathered LTCH HwH for a severe wound grouped into MS-LTC-DRG 602, 603, 539, or 540. To find the list of severe wounds by category identified by ICD-10 code, visit CMS.gov/Medicare/Medicare-Fee-for-Service-Payment/LongTermCare HospitalPPS/download.html.
- All discharges from spinal cord specialty hospitals in their FY 2018 and 2019 cost reporting periods.

Payment Policy Adjustments

This section discusses the short-stay outlier (SSO), high cost outlier (HCO), fixed-loss amounts, and interrupted stay payment policy adjustments (unless otherwise noted, these policies apply to both site-neutral and standard federal payment rate discharges).

Short-Stay Outlier

The SSO, which helps prevent inappropriate payment for cases that do not have a full episode of care, is an adjustment to the federal payment rate for LTCH stays that are generally much shorter than the ALOS for an MS-LTC-DRG. An SSO payment adjustment to the standard Federal payment rate may apply when a patient:

- Experiences an acute condition that requires urgent treatment or requires more intensive rehabilitation, and the LTCH facility then discharges the patient to another facility

- Does not require the level of care provided in an LTCH, which then discharges the patient to another facility

- Discharges to his or her home

- Dies within the first several days of admission to an LTCH or

- Exhausts benefits during the LTCH stay (see the section "SSO Payments When the Patient's Benefits Are Exhausted During an LTCH Stay" for more information about exhausted benefits)

An adjustment applies when the LOS ranges from one day through 5/6 of the ALOS for the MS-LTC-DRG to which the case is grouped, and the MS-LTC-DRG payment is subject to SSO adjustment. An adjustment is not applied when the LOS is more than 5/6 of the ALOS for the MS-LTC-DRG to which the case is grouped, and the LTCH facility receives the full MS-LTC-DRG payment. This policy does not apply to site-neutral discharges.

Note: If the ALOS for a particular MS-LTC-DRG is 30 days, the SSO policy applies to stays that are 25 days or less in length (5/6 of 30 days = 25 days).

Prior to October 1, 2017, Medicare paid an SSO case using the least of one of these case-level adjustment calculation methods:

1. The full payment for the MS-LTC-DRG assigned to the case.

2. An amount that is 120 percent of the MS-LTC-DRG per diem. To calculate the per diem, divide the full MS-LTC-DRG payment by the ALOS for the MS-LTC-DRG and multiply by the actual LOS of the case.

3. An amount that is 100 percent of the estimated cost of the case, which is calculated using the provider-specific CCR.

4. For SSO discharge dates:

   – On or before December 28, 2012—A blend of an amount comparable to what Medicare would otherwise pay under the IPPS, calculated as a per diem and capped at the full IPPS comparable amount, and 120 percent of the MS-LTC-DRG per diem amount

   – On or after December 29, 2012—One of these amounts:

     – When the LOS is greater than the IPPS-comparable threshold, which is one standard deviation from the geometric average LOS for the same MS-DRG under the IPPS, for the MS-LTC-DRG assigned to the case—A blend of an amount comparable to what Medicare would otherwise pay under the IPPS, calculated as a per diem and capped at the full IPPS comparable amount, and 120 percent of the MS-LTC-DRG per diem amount

     – When the LOS is equal to or less than the IPPS comparable threshold for the MS-LTC-DRG assigned to the case—An IPPS comparable amount, calculated on a per diem basis, capped at an amount comparable to but not exceeding what would have been a full payment under the IPPS.

   – On or after October 1, 2017—A blend of an amount comparable to what Medicare would otherwise pay under the IPPS, calculated as a per diem and capped at the full IPPS comparable amount and the MS-LTC-DRG per diem amount.

SSO Payments When the Patient's Benefits Are Exhausted During an LTCH Stay

Medicare pays for covered benefit days only until the LOS triggers a full MS-LTC-DRG payment. In other words, a patient's remaining amount of benefit days and the length of a hospital stay can affect LTCH payment, resulting in an SSO payment adjustment. These tables provide examples of SSO payments for patients whose benefits have been exhausted.

When Benefits Are Exhausted and LOS Is Below the MS-LTC-DRG Threshold		
If …	Then …	Example
The patient uses all regular benefit days for an episode during an LOS that does not reach the SSO threshold for an MS-LTC-DRG.	The patient is liable for any noncovered days. The LTCH will receive an SSO payment for the patient's covered hospital stay.	The MS-LTC-DRG SSO threshold is 25 days, and the patient's LOS is 20 days. The LTCH will receive an SSO payment. Patient benefit days end on day 15. The LTCH will be paid only the 15 covered days under the short-stay policy. The patient is liable for days 16 through 20 of the stay.
The patient uses all benefit days for an episode during an LOS that exceeds the SSO threshold for an MS-LTC-DRG.	The patient is not liable for any noncovered days. The LTCH will receive the full MS-LTC-DRG payment.	The MS-LTC-DRG SSO threshold is 25 days, and the patient's benefit days end on day 30. The patient's LOS is 35 days. He or she is not liable for days 31 through 35 (the short-stay policy does not apply). Because the LTCH will receive the full MS-LTC-DRG payment, the patient is not liable until the first day the stay qualifies as an HCO.

Note: Medicare provides 90 covered benefit days for an episode of care under the inpatient hospital benefit. Each patient has an additional 60 lifetime reserve days. The patient may use these lifetime reserve days to cover additional noncovered days of an episode of care that exceeds 90 days.

Any changes to an SSO outlier payment made as a result of reconciliation of SSO payments do not retroactively affect a patient's lifetime reserve days or coverage status, benefits, and payments under Medigap or Medicaid.

High-Cost Outlier

The high-cost outlier (HCO) is an adjustment to the applicable LTCH PPS payment rate (either the site-neutral rate or the standard federal rate) for LTCH stays with unusually high costs that exceed the typical cost for cases with a similar case mix. It equals 80 percent of the difference between the estimated cost of the case and the outlier threshold, and it is made in addition to the applicable LTCH PPS payment rate. In the case of a standard federal payment rate, it is made in addition to the full MS-LTC-DRG payment or the adjusted SSO amount for the case. To qualify for the HCO payment, the estimated costs to treat the case must exceed the outlier threshold. Note that site-neutral cases paid based on costs cannot qualify for the HCO adjustment. The applicable outlier threshold is calculated as the applicable LTCH PPS payment for the case plus the applicable fixed-loss amount. Beginning in FY 2016, CMS sets two fixed-loss amounts: one for the site-neutral payment rate and one for the standard federal rate.

The HCO adjustment:

- Strongly improves the accuracy of the LTCH PPS in determining patient and hospital resource costs

- Reduces financial losses that could result from treating patients who require more costly care

- Limits the loss to the fixed-loss amount and the percentage of costs above the marginal cost factor

- Reduces the incentive to underserve high-cost patients

Upon receipt of a claim, the Medicare administrative contractor (MAC) determines HCO payments using Pricer software and based on whether there are enough benefit days for each medically necessary day in the outlier period. If the patient has enough benefit days, the claim is processed as usual, and no further action is necessary. If the patient does not have enough benefit days, the claim is returned for correction, with the appropriate HCO threshold amount indicated.

For SSO cases, the MAC determines the outlier threshold by adding the fixed-loss amount to the adjusted SSO payment for the MS-LTC-DRG (not the full

MS-LTC-DRG payment). If the estimated cost of the SSO case exceeds the HCO threshold, it also qualifies as an HCO case.

HCO Payments When the Patient's Benefits Are Exhausted During an LTCH Stay

The HCO payment is made only for:

- Days that the patient has Medicare coverage (regular, coinsurance, or lifetime reserve days) for the portion of the stay beyond the HCO threshold
- Covered costs associated with medically necessary days for which the patient has a benefit day available

Note: Medicare provides 90 covered benefit days for an episode of care under the inpatient hospital benefit. Each patient has an additional 60 lifetime reserve days. The patient may use these lifetime reserve days to cover additional noncovered days of an episode of care that exceeds 90 days.

Fixed-Loss Amounts

Beginning October 1, 2015, under the new dual-rate LTCH PPS payment structure, CMS set two fixed-loss amounts: one for standard federal rate payments and one for site-neutral rate payments. The fixed-loss amount for cases paid based on the federal rate is set at an amount that allows the projected total HCO payments in a given year to equal 8 percent of the total LTCH PPS standard federal rate payments estimated for that year (the full MS-LTC-DRG payments or the adjusted SSO amount plus HCO payments). For FY 2019, CMS established that the applicable HCO threshold for site-neutral payment rate cases is the sum of the site-neutral payment rate for the case and the IPPS fixed-loss amount. That is, a fixed-loss amount was established for site-neutral payment rate cases of $25,769, which is the same FY 2019 IPPS fixed-loss amount.

The cost of each case is estimated using CCRs from the Provider Specific File (PSF). For those LTCHs for which CCRs in the PSF are unavailable, the applicable statewide average CCR is used. The MAC estimates the cost of a case by multiplying Medicare-covered charges for the case by the LTCH's overall CCR, which is calculated from the most recently settled or tentatively settled cost report. These CCR revisions or determinations may also apply:

- MACs may use an alternate CCR, as directed by CMS, which more accurately reflects recent substantial increases or decreases in a hospital's charges.
- Upon approval by the respective CMS regional office (RO), LTCHs may request, based on substantial evidence, that MACs use a higher or lower CCR.
- On an annual basis, MACs assign the statewide average CCR to LTCHs with CCRs above the maximum ceiling.
- MACs do not assign the statewide average CCR for LTCHs with CCRs below the minimum floor; rather, the LTCH's actual CCR is used.
- MACs may use the statewide average CCR when the LTCH CCR is undetermined (such as when a new LTCH has not submitted its first Medicare cost report or when data are not available to calculate an CCR due to being missing or faulty).

The LTCH PPS outlier policy allows for reconciliation of HCO (and SSO) payments at cost report settlement and accounts for differences between the estimated CCR and the actual CCR for the period during which the discharge occurs.

Interrupted Stay

An interrupted stay occurs when a patient is discharged from an LTCH and, after a specific number of days, is readmitted to the same LTCH for further medical treatment. For example, an LTCH patient may be discharged for treatment and services that are not available in the LTCH. Each stay is evaluated separately to make certain that it meets the interrupted stay criteria. A case may have multiple interrupted stays. A case with interrupted stays may be eligible for other case-level adjustments (such as the HCO payment).

The two types of interrupted stays are three-day or less interruption of stay and greater than three-day interruption of stay.

Three-day or less interruption of stay—For discharges and readmissions to the same LTCH within three days, the patient may:

- Receive outpatient or inpatient tests, treatment, or care at an inpatient acute care hospital, inpatient rehabilitation facility (IRF), or skilled nursing facility (SNF)/swing bed
- Have an intervening patient stay at home for up to three days without the delivery of additional tests, treatment, or care

Any test, procedure, or care provided to an LTCH patient on an outpatient basis and any inpatient treatment during the interruption is the responsibility of the

LTCH under arrangements, which means that such care (including inpatient surgical care at an inpatient acute care hospital) is part of that single episode of LTCH care and bundled into the payment. The LTCH facility must pay any other providers without additional Medicare program payment liability. If the patient receives any tests or procedures any time during the three-day interruption and the LTCH pays the intervening provider under arrangements, the total day count for the patient includes all days of the interruption. If the patient does not receive any care during the three-day interruption, the total day count for the patient stay does not include the days away from the LTCH.

If a patient discharges to home and returns to the LTCH within three days without getting additional medical treatment, the days away from the LTCH are not included in the total LOS; however, if he or she receives treatment on any of the 3 days (for which the LTCH is responsible for under arrangements), the days must be counted in the total LOS.

Greater than three-day interruption of stay—If a patient is discharged to an inpatient acute care hospital, IRF, or SNF/swing bed and then readmitted after three days, these fixed-day periods apply:

- Inpatient acute care hospital—between four and nine days
- IRF—between four and 27 days
- SNF/swing bed—between four and 45 days

To meet the full definition of a greater than three-day interruption of stay, the patient must also be discharged:

- Directly from the LTCH and admitted directly to an inpatient acute care hospital, IRF, or SNF/swing bed
- Back to the original LTCH after an LOS that falls within the applicable fixed-day period

The interrupted stay day count begins on the day of discharge from the LTCH and continues until the ninth, 27th, or 45th day after discharge (depending on the facility type). Although the greater than three-day interruption of stay policy governs from the fourth day forward, the day count of the interruption begins on the first day the patient is away from the LTCH. For example, if a patient leaves the LTCH on Monday and returns during the same week on Wednesday, Wednesday is considered day three.

If the applicable interrupted stay criteria are met, the days prior to the original discharge from the LTCH are added to the number of days following the readmission at the receiving facility. The days before and after an interrupted stay determine the total LOS for the episode of care.

If the patient is discharged to home, the greater than three-day interruption of stay adjustment will not apply. If, however, the patient is discharged to home for three days or less, the three-day or less interruption of stay adjustment applies as described above. If the patient's stay at an inpatient acute care hospital, IRF, or SNF/swing bed falls respectively within the fixed-day period, when the patient is readmitted to the LTCH, the entire stay is considered an interrupted stay. The LTCH receives one payment (either a full MS-LTC-DRG payment or an adjusted SSO payment, as applicable) based on the initial admission. (The payment for an interrupted stay is eligible for a high-cost outlier payment, as applicable.) The inpatient acute care hospital, IRF, or SNF/swing bed receives a separate payment if the greater than three-day interruption of stay policy governs the patient stay. If the interruption in the LTCH stay exceeds the fixed-day period, the readmission to the LTCH is treated as a separate LTCH stay, and the LTCH facility is paid an additional payment when the patient is discharged.

If the applicable interrupted stay criteria are met, the principal diagnosis should not be changed when the patient returns to the LTCH from the receiving facility. If other medical conditions are apparent on the patient's return, additional diagnosis codes should be noted on the claim.

FY 2019 LTCH PPS Payment Changes

Annual Update to the LTCH PPS Standard Federal Payment Rate for FY 2019

Under § 412.523(c)(3) of the regulations, for LTCH PPS FYs 2012 through 2017, CMS updated the standard Federal payment rate by the most recent estimate of the LTCH PPS market basket at that time, including additional statutory adjustments required by sections 1886(m)(3)(A)(i) (citing sections 1886(b)(3)(B)(xi)(II), 1886(m)(3)(A)(ii), and 1886(m)(4) of the Act as set forth in the regulations at §412.523(c)(3)(viii) through (c)(3)(xiii)). (For a summary of the payment rate development prior to FY 2012, see the FY 2018 IPPS/LTCH PPS final rule (82 FR 38310 through 38312).)

Sections 1886(m)(3)(A) and 1886(m)(3)(C) of the Act specify that, for rate year 2010 and each subsequent rate year, except FY 2018, any annual update to the standard Federal payment rate shall be reduced:

- For rate year 2010 through 2019, by the "other adjustment" specified in section 1886(m)(3)(A)(ii) and (m)(4) of the Act; and

- For rate year 2012 and each subsequent year, by the productivity adjustment described in section 1886(b)(3)(B)(xi)(II) of the Act (referred to as "the multifactor productivity (MFP) adjustment").

This section of the Act further provides that the application of section 1886(m)(3)(B) of the Act may result in the annual update being less than zero for a rate year, and may result in payment rates for a rate year being less than such payment rates for the preceding rate year. (CMS has adopted the term "fiscal year" (FY) rather than "rate year" (RY) under the LTCH PPS beginning October 1, 2010. Therefore, for purposes of clarity, when discussing the annual update for the LTCH PPS, including the provisions of the Affordable Care Act, the term "fiscal year" rather than "rate year" is used for 2011 and subsequent years.)

For LTCHs that fail to submit the required quality reporting data in accordance with the LTCH QRP, the annual update is reduced by 2.0 percentage points as required by section 1886(m)(5) of the Act.

In the FY 2019 IPPS/LTCH PPS final rule, CMS is establishing an annual update to the LTCH PPS standard Federal payment rate of 1.35 percent. Accordingly, under § 412.523(c)(3)(xv), a factor of 1.0135 was applied to the FY 2018 LTCH PPS standard Federal payment rate of $41,415.11 to determine the FY 2019 LTCH PPS standard Federal payment rate. Also, under § 412.523(c)(3)(xv), applied in conjunction with the provisions of § 412.523(c)(4), CMS is establishing an annual update to the LTCH PPS standard Federal payment rate of -0.65 percent (that is, an update factor of 0.9935) for FY 2019 for LTCHs that fail to submit the required quality reporting data for FY 2019 as required under the LTCH QRP. Consistent with § 412.523(d)(4), an area wage level budget neutrality factor was applied to the FY 2019 LTCH PPS standard Federal payment rate of 0.999713 based on the best available data at the time, to ensure that any changes to the area wage level adjustment (that is, the annual update of the wage index values and labor-related share) would not result in any change (increase or decrease) in estimated aggregate LTCH PPS standard Federal payment rate. Finally, CMS applied temporary budget neutrality adjustment factor of 0.990884 to LTCH PPS standard Federal payment rate cases only for the cost of the elimination of the 25-percent threshold policy for FY 2019. Accordingly, an LTCH PPS standard Federal payment rate was established of $41,579.65 (calculated as $41,415.11 × 1.0135 × 0.999713 × 0.990884) for FY 2019 (calculations performed on rounded numbers). For LTCHs that fail to submit quality reporting data for FY 2019, in accordance with the requirements of the LTCH QRP under section 1866(m)(5) of the Act, CMS established an LTCH PPS standard Federal payment rate of $40,759.12 (calculated as $41,415.11 × 0.9935 × 0.999713 × 0.990884) (calculations performed on rounded numbers) for FY 2019.

Elimination of the "25-Percent Threshold Policy" Adjustment

The "25-percent threshold policy" is a per discharge payment adjustment in the LTCH PPS that is applied to payments for Medicare patient discharges from an LTCH when the number of such patients originating from any single referring hospital is in excess of the applicable threshold for a given cost reporting period (such threshold is generally set at 25 percent, with exceptions for rural and urban single or MSA-dominant hospitals). If an LTCH exceeds the applicable threshold during a cost reporting period, payment for the discharge that puts the LTCH over its threshold and all discharges subsequent to that discharge in the cost reporting period from the referring hospital are adjusted at cost report settlement (discharges not in excess of the threshold are unaffected by the 25-percent threshold policy). The 25-percent threshold policy was originally established in the FY 2005 IPPS final rule for LTCH HwHs and satellites (69 FR 49191 through 49214). CMS later expanded the 25-percent threshold policy in the RY 2008 LTCH PPS final rule to include all LTCHs and LTCH satellite facilities (72 FR 26919 through 26944). Several laws have mandated delayed implementation of the 25-percent threshold policy. For more details on the various laws that delayed the full implementation of the 25-percent threshold policy, CMS refers readers to the FY 2018 IPPS/LTCH PPS final rule (82 FR 38318 through 38319).

In light of the further statutory delays and continued consideration of public comments received in response to the proposal to consolidate and streamline the 25-percent threshold policy in the FY 2017 IPPS/LTCH PPS proposed rule, in the FY 2018 IPPS/ LTCH PPS final rule (82 FR 38320), CMS adopted a 1-year regulatory moratorium on the implementation of the 25-percent threshold policy; that is, CMS imposed a regulatory moratorium on the implementation of the provisions of § 412.538 until October 1, 2018.

In the proposed rule, CMS indicated the goal of eliminating the 25-percent threshold policy would be to reduce unnecessary regulatory burden. Independent of this goal, CMS continues to believe aggregate LTCH PPS payments are sufficient. Therefore, CMS does not believe that it would be appropriate to change the aggregate amount of LTCH PPS payments on a permanent basis. As described earlier, the 25-percent threshold policy would have reduced the LTCH PPS payments for certain discharges, and that eliminating the 25-percent threshold policy would result in an increase in aggregate LTCH PPS payments. As a result, CMS also stated in the proposed rule that they believe this proposal should be accomplished in a budget neutral manner.

To do this, CMS proposed to remove the provisions of § 412.538, reserving this section, and add a new paragraph (d)(6) to § 412.523 to provide for a one-time permanent budget neutrality factor adjustment to the LTCH PPS standard Federal payment rate to ensure that removal of the 25-percent threshold policy at existing § 412.538 is budget neutral. In addition, it was proposed to make conforming technical changes to remove paragraph (c)(2)(v) of § 412.522 and paragraph (d)(6) of § 412.525.

CMS has determined the following budget neutrality adjustment factors for the costs of the elimination of the 25-percent threshold policy:

- For FY 2019, a temporary, one-time factor of 0.990884

- For FY 2020, a temporary, one-time factor of 0.990741

- For FY 2021 and subsequent years, a permanent, one-time factor of 0.991249

This budget neutrality adjustment will only be applied to the LTCH PPS standard federal payment rate (or such portion of a transitional blended payment) because payments made under the site-neutral payment rate are unaffected by the 25-percent threshold policy.

Appendix J: Long-Term Care Hospital Quality Reporting Program

Information in this appendix is based on the Centers for Medicare and Medicaid Services (CMS) FY 2019 long-term care hospital prospective payment system (LTCH PPS) final rule published in the *Federal Register*, volume 83, number 160, August 17, 2018 ("Hospital Inpatient Prospective Payment Systems for Acute Care Hospitals and the Long-Term Care Hospital Prospective Payment System and Policy Changes and Fiscal Year 2019 Rates").

Background

The LTCH QRP is authorized by section 1886(m)(5) of the Act and applies to all hospitals certified by Medicare as long-term care hospitals (LTCHs). Under the LTCH QRP, the Secretary reduces by 2 percentage points the annual update to the LTCH PPS standard Federal rate for discharges for an LTCH during a fiscal year if the LTCH fails to submit data in accordance with the LTCH QRP requirements specified for that fiscal year. As part of agency-wide efforts under the Meaningful Measures Initiative to use a parsimonious set of the most meaningful measures for patients and clinicians in the quality programs and the Patients Over Paperwork Initiative to reduce cost and burden and program complexity, CMS is removing three measures from the LTCH QRP, adopting a new measure removal factor, and codifying the measure removal factors in CMS regulations. In addition, regulations are updated to expand the methods by which an LTCH is notified of noncompliance with the requirements of the LTCH QRP for a program year and how CMS will notify an LTCH of a reconsideration decision.

For more detailed information on the requirements CMS has adopted for the LTCH QRP, the reader is referred to the FY 2012 IPPS/LTCH PPS final rule (76 FR 51743 through 51744), the FY 2013 IPPS/LTCH PPS final rule (77 FR 53614), the FY 2014 IPPS/LTCH PPS final rule (78 FR 50853), the FY 2015 IPPS/LTCH PPS final rule (79 FR 50286), the FY 2016 IPPS/LTCH PPS final rule (80 FR 49723 through 49725), the FY 2017 IPPS/LTCH PPS final rule (81 FR 57193), and the FY 2018 IPPS/LTCH PPS final rule (82 FR 38425 through 38426).

Although CMS has historically used the preamble to the IPPS/LTCH PPS proposed and final rules each year as a reminder of all previously finalized program requirements, repeating the same discussion each year is not felt necessary for every requirement, especially if the requirements have been codified into the regulations. Accordingly, the following is limited as much as possible to policies being finalizing for future years of the LTCH QRP, and represents the approach CMS intends to use in their rulemakings for this program going forward.

General Considerations Used for Selection of Quality Measures for the LTCH QRP

For a detailed discussion of the considerations historically used for the selection of LTCH QRP quality, resource use, and other measures, readers are referred to the FY 2016 IPPS/LTCH PPS final rule (80 FR 49728).

Accounting for Social Risk Factors in the LTCH QRP

In the FY 2018 IPPS/LTCH PPS final rule (82 FR 38428 through 38429), CMS discussed the importance of improving beneficiary outcomes including reducing health disparities. Also discussed was the commitment by CMS to ensuring that medically complex patients, as well as those with social risk factors, receive excellent care. CMS discussed how studies show that social risk factors, such as being near or below the poverty level as determined by HHS, belonging to a racial or ethnic minority group, or living with a disability, can be associated with poor health outcomes and how some of this disparity is related to the quality of health care. Among the core objectives, CMS aims to improve health outcomes, attain health equity for all beneficiaries, and ensure that complex patients as well as those with social risk factors receive excellent care. Within this context, reports by the Office of the Assistant Secretary for Planning and Evaluation (ASPE) and the National Academy of Medicine have examined the influence of social risk factors in the value-based purchasing programs. As noted in the FY 2018 IPPS/LTCH PPS final rule (82 FR 38404), ASPE's report to Congress, which was required by the IMPACT Act, found that, in the context of value-based purchasing programs, dual eligibility was the most powerful predictor of poor health care outcomes among those social risk factors that they examined and tested. ASPE is continuing to examine this issue in its second report required by the IMPACT Act, which was due to Congress in the fall of 2019. In addition, as noted in the FY 2018 IPPS/LTCH PPS final rule (82 FR 38428), the National Quality Forum (NQF) undertook a 2-year trial period in which certain new measures and measures undergoing maintenance review have been assessed to determine if risk adjustment for social risk factors is appropriate for these measures. The trial period ended in April 2017 and a final report is available at: http://www.qualityforum.org/SES_Trial_Period.aspx. The trial concluded that "measures with a conceptual basis for adjustment generally did not demonstrate an empirical relationship" between social risk factors and the outcomes measured. This discrepancy may be explained in part by the methods used for adjustment and the limited availability of robust data on social risk factors. NQF has extended the socioeconomic status (SES) trial, allowing further examination of social risk factors in outcome measures.

New Measure Removal Factor for Previously Adopted LTCH QRP Measures

As a part of the Meaningful Measures Initiative, CMS strives to put patients first, ensuring that they, along with their clinicians, are empowered to make decisions about their own healthcare using data-driven information that is increasingly aligned with a parsimonious set of meaningful quality measures. CMS began reviewing the LTCH QRP's measures in accordance with the Meaningful Measures Initiative, and is working to identify how to move the LTCH QRP forward in the least burdensome manner possible, while continuing to incentivize improvement in the quality of care provided to patients.

Specifically, CMS believes the goals of the LTCH QRP and the measures used in the program cover most of the Meaningful Measures Initiative priorities, including making care safer, strengthening person and family engagement, promoting coordination of care, promoting effective prevention and treatment, and making care affordable.

CMS also evaluated the appropriateness and completeness of the LTCH QRP's current measure removal factors, and had previously finalized that a notice and comment rulemaking would be used to remove measures from the LTCH QRP based on the following factors:

- Factor 1. Measure performance among LTCHs is so high and unvarying that meaningful distinctions in improvements in performance can no longer be made.

- Factor 2. Performance or improvement on a measure does not result in better patient outcomes.

- Factor 3. A measure does not align with current clinical guidelines or practice.

- Factor 4. A more broadly applicable measure (across settings, populations, or conditions) for the particular topic is available.

- Factor 5. A measure that is more proximal in time to desired patient outcomes for the particular topic is available.

- Factor 6. A measure that is more strongly associated with desired patient outcomes for the particular topic is available.

- Factor 7. Collection or public reporting of a measure leads to negative unintended consequences other than patient harm.

CMS continues to believe that these measure removal factors are appropriate for use in the LTCH QRP. However, even if one or more of the measure removal factors applies, the measure may be retained for certain specified reasons. Examples of such instances could include occasions in which a particular measure addresses a gap in quality that is so significant that removing the measure could, in turn, result in poor quality, or in the event that a given measure is statutorily required. CMS notes further that, consistent with other quality reporting programs, these factors are applied on a case-by-case basis.

In the FY 2019 IPPS/LTCH PPS final rule, an additional factor was adopted to consider when evaluating potential measures for removal from the LTCH QRP measure set: Factor 8, the costs associated with a measure outweigh the benefit of its continued use in the program. CMS believes the new measure removal factor adds a new criterion that is not captured in the other seven factors and will help advance the goals of the Meaningful Measures Initiative, which aims to improve outcomes for patients, their families, and health care providers while reducing burden and costs for clinicians and providers.

Quality Measures Currently Adopted for the FY 2020 LTCH QRP

The LTCH QRP currently has 19 measures for the FY 2020 program year, which are outlined in the following table:

Quality Measures Currently Adopted for the FY 2020 LTCH QRP	
Short Name	Measure Name & Data Source
LTCH CARE Data Set	
Pressure Ulcer	Percent of Residents or Patients with Pressure Ulcers That Are New or Worsened (Short Stay) (NQF #0678)*

Quality Measures Currently Adopted for the FY 2020 LTCH QRP	
Short Name	**Measure Name & Data Source**
Pressure Ulcer/Injury	Changes in Skin Integrity Post-Acute Care: Pressure Ulcer/Injury
Patient Influenza Vaccine	Percent of Residents or Patients Who Were Assessed and Appropriately Given the Seasonal Influenza Vaccine (Short Stay) (NQF #0680)
Application of Falls	Application of Percent of Residents Experiencing One or More Falls with Major Injury (Long Stay) (NQF #0674)
Functional Assessment	Percent of Long-Term Care Hospital (LTCH) Patients with an Admission and Discharge Functional Assessment and a Care Plan That Addresses Function (NQF #2631)
Application of Functional Assessment	Application of Percent of Long-Term Care Hospital (LTCH) Patients with an Admission and Discharge Functional Assessment and a Care Plan That Addresses Function (NQF #2631)
Change in Mobility	Functional Outcome Measure: Change in Mobility Among Long-Term Care Hospital (LTCH) Patients Requiring Ventilator Support (NQF #2632)
DRR	Drug Regimen Review Conducted With Follow-Up for Identified Issues—Post Acute Care (PAC) Long-Term Care Hospital (LTCH) Quality Reporting Program (QRP)
Compliance with SBT	Compliance with Spontaneous Breathing Trial (SBT) by Day 2 of the LTCH Stay
Ventilator Liberation	Ventilator Liberation Rate
NHSN	
CAUTI	National Healthcare Safety Network (NHSN) Catheter-Associated Urinary Tract Infection (CAUTI) Outcome Measure (NQF #0138)
CLABSI	National Healthcare Safety Network (NHSN) Central Line-Associated Bloodstream Infection (CLABSI) Outcome Measure (NQF #0139)
MRSA	National Healthcare Safety Network (NHSN) Facility-wide Inpatient Hospital-onset Methicillin-resistant *Staphylococcus aureus* (MRSA) Bacteremia Outcome Measure (NQF #1716)
CDI	National Healthcare Safety Network (NHSN) Facility-wide Inpatient Hospital-onset *Clostridium difficile* Infection (CDI) Outcome Measure (NQF #1717)
HCP Influenza Vaccine	Influenza Vaccination Coverage among Healthcare Personnel (NQF #0431)
VAE	National Healthcare Safety Network (NHSN) Ventilator-Associated Event (VAE) Outcome Measure
Claims-based	
MSPB LTCH	Medicare Spending Per Beneficiary (MSPB)—Post Acute Care (PAC) Long-Term Care Hospital (LTCH) Quality Reporting Program (QRP)
DTC	Discharge to Community—Post Acute Care (PAC) Long-Term Care Hospital (LTCH) Quality Reporting Program (QRP)
PPR	Potentially Preventable 30-Day Post-Discharge Readmission Measure for Long-Term Care Hospital (LTCH) Quality Reporting Program (QRP)

* The measure was replaced with the Changes in Skin Integrity Post-Acute Care: Pressure Ulcer/Injury measure, effective July 1, 2018.

Removal of Three LTCH QRP Measures

In the FY 2019 IPPS/LTCH PPS proposed rule (83 FR 20513 through 20515), CMS proposed to remove three measures from the LTCH QRP measure set.

Beginning with the FY 2020 LTCH QRP, CMS proposed to remove two measures: (1) National Healthcare Safety Network (NHSN) Facility-wide Inpatient Hospital-onset Methicillin-resistant *Staphylococcus aureus* (MRSA) Bacteremia Outcome Measure (NQF #1716); and (2) National Healthcare Safety Network (NHSN) Ventilator-Associated Event (VAE) Outcome Measure. Additionally, CMS proposed to remove one measure beginning with the FY 2021 LTCH QRP: Percent of Residents or Patients Who Were Assessed and Appropriately Given the Seasonal Influenza Vaccine (Short Stay) (NQF #0680).

Removal of the National Healthcare Safety Network (NHSN) Facility-Wide Inpatient Hospital-Onset Methicillin-Resistant *Staphylococcus aureus* (MRSA) Bacteremia Outcome Measure (NQF #1716)

One of the main goals of the Meaningful Measures Initiative is to apply a parsimonious set of the most meaningful measures available to track patient outcomes and impact. CMS currently collects data on two measures of healthcare-associated bacteremia infections in the LTCH QRP: (1) NHSN Central line-associated Bloodstream Infection (CLABSI) Outcome Measure (NQF #0139); and (2) NHSN Facility-wide Inpatient Hospital-onset Methicillin-resistant *Staphylococcus aureus* (MRSA) Bacteremia Outcome Measure (NQF #1716).

In reviewing these measures used in the LTCH QRP, CMS believes that it is appropriate to remove the NHSN Facility-wide Inpatient Hospital-onset Methicillin-resistant *Staphylococcus aureus* (MRSA) Bacteremia Outcome Measure (NQF #1716) based on: (1) Factor 6, a measure that is more strongly associated with desired patient outcomes for the particular topic is available; and (2) Factor 8, the costs associated with a measure outweigh the benefit of its continued use in the program.

CMS believes that the NHSN CLABSI Outcome Measure (NQF #0139) is more strongly associated with the desired patient outcome for bloodstream infections than the NHSN Facility-wide Inpatient Hospital-Onset MRSA Bacteremia Outcome Measure (NQF #1716). Bloodstream infections are serious infections typically causing a prolongation of hospital stay and increased cost and risk of mortality. The NHSN CLABSI Outcome Measure (NQF #0139) assesses the results of the quality of care provided to patients, and it is risk-adjusted to compare the infection rate for a particular location or locations in a hospital with an expected infection rate for those locations (which is calculated using national NHSN data for those locations in a predictive model). The NHSN CLABSI Outcome Measure (NQF #0139) is more strongly associated with the desired patient outcome of better results in the quality of care provided to patients because it covers a wide range of bloodstream infections, while the NHSN Facility-wide Inpatient Hospital-Onset MRSA Bacteremia Outcome Measure (NQF #1716) only covers observed hospital-onset unique blood source MRSA laboratory-identified events. The NHSN CLABSI Outcome Measure (NQF #0139) also captures the MRSA bloodstream events, creating potential duplicative collection and reporting.

CMS also believes that the costs associated with the NHSN Facility-wide Inpatient Hospital-Onset MRSA Bacteremia Outcome Measure (NQF #1716) outweigh the benefit of its continued use in the LTCH QRP. The NHSN Facility-wide Inpatient Hospital-Onset MRSA Bacteremia Outcome Measure (NQF #1716) was adopted to assess MRSA infections caused by a strain of MRSA bacteremia that has become resistant to antibiotics commonly used to treat MRSA infections. The NHSN Facility-wide Inpatient Hospital-Onset MRSA Bacteremia Outcome Measure (NQF #1716) and NHSN CLABSI Outcome Measure (NQF #0139) capture the same type of MRSA infection. This overlap results in the data submission on two measures that cover the same quality issue. CMS believes that this results in redundant efforts on the part of LTCHs that are costly and burdensome. In addition, the maintenance of these two measures in the LTCH QRP is costly for CMS. Lastly, CMS believes that the removal of the NHSN Facility-wide Inpatient Hospital-Onset MRSA Bacteremia Outcome Measure (NQF #1716) would benefit the public by eliminating the potential confusion of seeing two different measure rates on LTCH Compare that capture MRSA bacteremia. Beginning with October 1, 2018 admissions and discharges, LTCHs are no longer required to submit data on this measure for the purposes of the LTCH QRP.

Removal of the National Healthcare Safety Network (NHSN) Ventilator-Associated Event (VAE) Outcome Measure

CMS finalized the National Healthcare Safety Network (NHSN) Ventilator-Associated Event (VAE) Outcome Measure in the FY 2015 IPPS/LTCH PPS final rule (79 FR 50301 through 50305) to assess whether LTCHs monitor ventilator use and identify improvements in preventing complications associated with mechanical ventilation. CMS also adopted for the LTCH QRP three other assessment-based quality measures on the topic of ventilator support: (1) Functional Outcome Measure: Change in Mobility among Long-Term Care Hospital Patients Requiring Ventilator Support (NQF #2632) (79 FR 50298 through 50301); (2) Compliance with Spontaneous Breathing Trials (SBT) by Day 2 of the LTCH Stay (82 FR 38439 through 38443); and (3) Ventilator Liberation Rate (82 FR 38443 through 38446).

CMS believes that these three other assessment-based quality measures are more strongly associated with desired patient outcomes than the National Healthcare Safety Network (NHSN) Ventilator-Associated Event (VAE) Outcome Measure. The three assessment-based measures assess activities that reduce the potential for serious complications and other adverse events as a result of mechanical ventilation. Specifically, the Functional Outcome Measure: Change in Mobility among Long-Term Care Hospital Patients Requiring Ventilator Support (NQF #2632) focuses on improvement in functional mobility for patients requiring mechanical ventilation. The Compliance with SBT by Day 2 of the LTCH Stay measure focuses on successfully liberating patients from mechanical ventilation as soon as possible, which reduces the risk associated with events as a result of prolonged ventilator support. The Ventilator Liberation Rate measure assesses whether the patient was fully liberated from mechanical ventilation at discharge. Together, these three ventilator-related assessment-based quality measures assess positive outcomes and track patient goals of avoiding adverse outcomes associated with mechanical ventilation and successful ventilator weaning.

The inclusion in the LTCH QRP measure set of these three ventilator-related assessment-based measures, which focus on quality of care through promotion of positive outcomes, have reduced poor outcomes associated with the complications of ventilator care, which is the same focus of the National Healthcare Safety Network (NHSN) Ventilator-Associated Event (VAE) Outcome Measure (for example, worsening oxygenation, infection or inflammation, ventilator-associated pneumonia, or even death). As a result, CMS does not believe that it is necessary to retain all four of these measures in the LTCH QRP. By retaining the three ventilator-related assessment-based measures but removing the National Healthcare Safety Network (NHSN) Ventilator-Associated Event (VAE) Outcome Measure, it is believed that the focus can be on the topic of mechanical ventilation measures that promote positive outcomes while indirectly promoting a reduction in ventilator support complications.

For these reasons, CMS will remove the National Healthcare Safety Network (NHSN) Ventilator-Associated Event (VAE) Outcome Measure from the LTCH QRP beginning with the FY 2020 LTCH QRP under Factor 6, the measure that is more strongly associated with desired patient outcomes for the particular topic is available. Beginning with October 1, 2018 admissions and discharges, LTCHs are no longer required to submit data on this measure for the purposes of the LTCH QRP.

Removal of the Percent of Residents or Patients Who Were Assessed and Appropriately Given the Seasonal Influenza Vaccine (Short Stay) (NQF #0680) Measure

This process measure reports the percentage of stays in which a patient was assessed and appropriately given the influenza vaccine for the most recent influenza vaccination season and was adopted in the FY 2013 IPPS/LTCH PPS final rule (77 FR 53624 through 53627) to assess vaccination rates among older adults with the goal of reducing the incidence of influenza in this population. Specifically, adoption of the measure in the LTCH QRP was intended to act as a safeguard for patients who did not receive vaccinations prior to admission to an LTCH, since many patients receiving care in the LTCH setting are older adults (those 65 years and older) and are considered to be the target population for the influenza vaccination.

In the CMS evaluation of the LTCH QRP measure set, analysis of this particular measure revealed that for the 2016–2017 influenza season, nearly every patient was assessed by the LTCH upon admission and that less than 0.04 percent of patients were not assessed for the vaccination. Of those assessed, the data show that most patients who could receive the vaccine had already received the vaccine outside of the LTCH facility, prior to admission.

In addition, CMS believes that removing this measure would reduce provider costs and burden by eliminating duplicative patient assessments across healthcare settings, minimizing data collection and reporting, and avoiding potentially confusing public reporting of other influenza-related quality measures, such as the Influenza Vaccination Coverage Among Healthcare Personnel (NQF #0431) measure.

Therefore, CMS will remove this measure from the LTCH QRP beginning with the FY 2021 LTCH QRP under measure removal factor 8, the costs associated with a measure outweigh the benefit of its continued use in the program. LTCHs will no longer be required to report the data elements necessary to calculate this measure beginning with October 1, 2018 admissions and discharges.

IMPACT Act Implementation Update

In the FY 2018 IPPS/LTCH PPS final rule (82 FR 38449), CMS stated their intention to specify two measures that would satisfy the domain of accurately communicating the existence and provision of the transfer of health information and care preferences under section 1899B(c)(1)(E) of the Act no later than October 1, 2018, and intended to propose to adopt them for the FY 2021 LTCH QRP with data collection beginning on or about April 1, 2019.

In the FY 2019 IPPS/LTCH PPS proposed rule (83 FR 20515), CMS stated that as a result of the input provided during a public comment period between November 10, 2016 and December 11, 2016, input provided by a technical expert panel (TEP), and pilot measure testing conducted in 2017, the decision had been made to engage in continued development work on these two measures, including supplementary measure testing and providing the public with an opportunity for comment in 2018. A TEP reconvened in April 2018. CMS stated their intention to specify the measures under section 1899B(c)(1)(E) of the Act no later than October 1, 2019 and intend to propose to adopt the measures for the FY 2022 LTCH QRP, with data collection beginning with April 1, 2020 admissions and discharges. For more information on the pilot testing, readers are referred to: https://www.cms.gov/Medicare/Quality-Initiatives-Patient-Assessment-Instruments/Post-Acute-Care-Quality-Initiatives/IMPACT-Act-of-2014/IMPACT-Act-Downloads-and-Videos.html.

Form, Manner, and Timing of Data Submission Under the LTCH QRP

Under the current CMS policy, LTCHs report data on LTCH QRP assessment-based measures and standardized patient assessment data by reporting the designated data elements for each applicable patient on the LTCH CARE Data Set patient assessment instrument and then submitting the completed instruments to CMS using the Quality Improvement and Evaluation System (QIES) Assessment and Submission Processing (ASAP) system. Data on LTCH QRP measures that are also collected by the CDC for other purposes are reported by LTCHs to the CDC through the NHSN, and the CDC then transmits the relevant data to CMS. Readers are referred to the FY 2018 IPPS/LTCH PPS final rule (82 FR 38454 through 38456) for the data collection and submission timeframes that were finalized for the LTCH QRP.

In the FY 2019 IPPS/LTCH PPS proposed rule (83 FR 20515), CMS sought input on whether the implementation date of any new version of the LTCH CARE Data Set should be moved from the usual release date of April to October in the future. CMS would like to clarify that in proposing any updates to the LTCH CARE Data Set, the implementation date of the new version of the LTCH CARE Data Set would not occur until the following year at the earliest. For example, with the proposal of this change in April 2019, the implementation of the new version of the LTCH CARE Data Set would not occur until October 1, 2020 at the earliest, as opposed to April 1, 2020. This would give LTCHs an additional six months (April-October) to update their systems so that they can comply with new reporting requirements.

Changes to the LTCH QRP Reconsideration Requirements

Section 412.560(d)(1) of the regulations states that CMS will send an LTCH written notification of a decision of noncompliance with the measures data and standardized patient assessment data reporting requirements for a particular fiscal year. It also states that CMS will use the QIES ASAP system to provide notification of noncompliance to the LTCH.

In the FY 2019 final rule, CMS is revising § 412.560(d)(1) of the regulations to state that LTCHs will be notified of noncompliance with the LTCH QRP via a notification sent through at least one of the following methods: the QIES ASAP system, the United States Postal Service, or via an email from the MAC. CMS also finalized the proposal to revise § 412.560(d)(3) of the regulations to clarify that LTCHs would be notified, in writing, of the final decision by CMS regarding any reconsideration request using the same notification process. This policy was effective October 1, 2018.

Appendix K: Severe Wound Diagnosis Codes by Category

The following lists the ICD-10-CM codes describing severe wound diagnoses. CMS allows for a temporary exception for certain wound care discharges from the site-neutral payment rate for certain long-term care hospitals (LTCHs). This exception applies to discharges occurring during FY2018 (that is, for cost reporting period beginning on or after October 1, 2017, and on or before September 30, 2018) from LTCHs that are grandfathered hospitals-within-hospitals (HwHs) (that is, hospitals that are described under § 412.23(e)(2)(i) that meet the criteria of § 412.22(f)) when the individual discharged "has a severe wound." Based upon the FY 2018 IPPS/LTCH final rule classification, the definition of "severe wound" has been refined to include only five categories (stage 3 wound, stage 4 wound, unstageable wound, nonhealing surgical wound, and fistula) and exclusions are limited to discharges that both meet the definition of a severe wound and are additionally grouped to certain specified MS-LTC-DRGs.

Note: An updated ICD-10-CM list was not available at the time this publication was printed and therefore does not reflect any FY 2020 code changes. An updated list of severe wound codes, effective October 1, 2019, can be found at: https://www.cms.gov/Medicare/Medicare-Fee-for-Service-Payment/LongTermCareHospitalPPS/download.html.

Stage 3 Wound

L89.003	L89.123	L89.213	L89.43	L89.613	L97.112	L97.124	L97.922
L89.013	L89.133	L89.223	L89.503	L89.623	L97.113	L97.912	L97.923
L89.023	L89.143	L89.303	L89.513	L89.813	L97.114	L97.913	L97.924
L89.103	L89.153	L89.313	L89.523	L89.893	L97.122	L97.914	
L89.113	L89.203	L89.323	L89.603	L89.93	L97.123	L97.921	

Stage 4 Wound

L89.004	L89.104	L89.134	L89.204	L89.304	L89.44	L89.524	L89.624	L89.94
L89.014	L89.114	L89.144	L89.214	L89.314	L89.504	L89.604	L89.814	
L89.024	L89.124	L89.154	L89.224	L89.324	L89.514	L89.614	L89.894	

Unstageable Wound

L89.000	T20.319D	T20.72XA	T21.34XS	T21.77XD	T22.341A	T22.399S	T22.742D	T23.302A
L89.010	T20.319S	T20.72XD	T21.35XA	T21.77XS	T22.341D	T22.70XA	T22.742S	T23.302D
L89.020	T20.32XA	T20.72XS	T21.35XD	T21.79XA	T22.341S	T22.70XD	T22.749A	T23.302S
L89.100	T20.32XD	T20.73XA	T21.35XS	T21.79XD	T22.342A	T22.70XS	T22.749D	T23.309A
L89.110	T20.32XS	T20.73XD	T21.36XA	T21.79XS	T22.342D	T22.711A	T22.749S	T23.309D
L89.120	T20.33XA	T20.73XS	T21.36XD	T22.30XA	T22.342S	T22.711D	T22.751A	T23.309S
L89.130	T20.33XD	T20.74XA	T21.36XS	T22.30XD	T22.349A	T22.711S	T22.751D	T23.311A
L89.140	T20.33XS	T20.74XD	T21.37XA	T22.30XS	T22.349D	T22.712A	T22.751S	T23.311D
L89.150	T20.34XA	T20.74XS	T21.37XD	T22.311A	T22.349S	T22.712D	T22.752A	T23.311S
L89.200	T20.34XD	T20.75XA	T21.37XS	T22.311D	T22.351A	T22.712S	T22.752D	T23.312A
L89.210	T20.34XS	T20.75XD	T21.39XA	T22.311S	T22.351D	T22.719A	T22.752S	T23.312D
L89.220	T20.35XA	T20.75XS	T21.39XD	T22.312A	T22.351S	T22.719D	T22.759A	T23.312S
L89.300	T20.35XD	T20.76XA	T21.39XS	T22.312D	T22.352A	T22.719S	T22.759D	T23.319A
L89.310	T20.35XS	T20.76XD	T21.70XA	T22.312S	T22.352D	T22.721A	T22.759S	T23.319D
L89.320	T20.36XA	T20.76XS	T21.70XD	T22.319A	T22.352S	T22.721D	T22.761A	T23.319S
L89.45	T20.36XD	T20.77XA	T21.70XS	T22.319D	T22.359A	T22.721S	T22.761D	T23.321A
L89.500	T20.36XS	T20.77XD	T21.71XA	T22.319S	T22.359D	T22.722A	T22.761S	T23.321D
L89.510	T20.37XA	T20.77XS	T21.71XD	T22.321A	T22.359S	T22.722D	T22.762A	T23.321S
L89.520	T20.37XD	T20.79XA	T21.71XS	T22.321D	T22.361A	T22.722S	T22.762D	T23.322A
L89.600	T20.37XS	T20.79XD	T21.72XA	T22.321S	T22.361D	T22.729A	T22.762S	T23.322D
L89.610	T20.39XA	T20.79XS	T21.72XD	T22.322A	T22.361S	T22.729D	T22.769A	T23.322S
L89.620	T20.39XD	T21.30XA	T21.72XS	T22.322D	T22.362A	T22.729S	T22.769D	T23.329A
L89.810	T20.39XS	T21.30XD	T21.73XA	T22.322S	T22.362D	T22.731A	T22.769S	T23.329D
L89.890	T20.70XA	T21.30XS	T21.73XD	T22.329A	T22.362S	T22.731D	T22.791A	T23.329S
L89.95	T20.70XD	T21.31XA	T21.73XS	T22.329D	T22.369A	T22.731S	T22.791D	T23.331A
T20.30XA	T20.70XS	T21.31XD	T21.74XA	T22.329S	T22.369D	T22.732A	T22.791S	T23.331D
T20.30XD	T20.711A	T21.31XS	T21.74XD	T22.331A	T22.369S	T22.732D	T22.792A	T23.331S
T20.30XS	T20.711D	T21.32XA	T21.74XS	T22.331D	T22.391A	T22.732S	T22.792D	T23.332A
T20.311A	T20.711S	T21.32XD	T21.75XA	T22.331S	T22.391D	T22.739A	T22.792S	T23.332D
T20.311D	T20.712A	T21.32XS	T21.75XD	T22.332A	T22.391S	T22.739D	T22.799A	T23.332S
T20.311S	T20.712D	T21.33XA	T21.75XS	T22.332D	T22.392A	T22.739S	T22.799D	T23.339A
T20.312A	T20.712S	T21.33XD	T21.76XA	T22.332S	T22.392D	T22.741A	T22.799S	T23.339D
T20.312D	T20.719A	T21.33XS	T21.76XD	T22.339A	T22.392S	T22.741D	T23.301A	T23.339S
T20.312S	T20.719D	T21.34XA	T21.76XS	T22.339D	T22.399A	T22.741S	T23.301D	T23.341A
T20.319A	T20.719S	T21.34XD	T21.77XA	T22.339S	T22.399D	T22.742A	T23.301S	T23.341D

Appendix K: Severe Wound Diagnosis Codes by Category

Unstageable Wound (continued)

T23.341S	T23.379D	T23.722A	T23.759S	T24.302D	T24.391A	T24.729A	T25.321S	T25.719D
T23.342A	T23.379S	T23.722D	T23.761A	T24.302S	T24.391D	T24.729D	T25.322A	T25.719S
T23.342D	T23.391A	T23.722S	T23.761D	T24.309A	T24.391S	T24.729S	T25.322D	T25.721A
T23.342S	T23.391D	T23.729A	T23.761S	T24.309D	T24.392A	T24.731A	T25.322S	T25.721D
T23.349A	T23.391S	T23.729D	T23.762A	T24.309S	T24.392D	T24.731D	T25.329A	T25.721S
T23.349D	T23.392A	T23.729S	T23.762D	T24.311A	T24.392S	T24.731S	T25.329D	T25.722A
T23.349S	T23.392D	T23.731A	T23.762S	T24.311D	T24.399A	T24.732A	T25.329S	T25.722D
T23.351A	T23.392S	T23.731D	T23.769A	T24.311S	T24.399D	T24.732D	T25.331A	T25.722S
T23.351D	T23.399A	T23.731S	T23.769D	T24.312A	T24.701A	T24.732S	T25.331D	T25.729A
T23.351S	T23.399D	T23.732A	T23.769S	T24.312D	T24.701D	T24.739A	T25.331S	T25.729D
T23.352A	T23.399S	T23.732D	T23.771A	T24.312S	T24.701S	T24.739D	T25.332A	T25.729S
T23.352D	T23.701A	T23.732S	T23.771D	T24.319A	T24.702A	T24.739S	T25.332D	T25.731A
T23.352S	T23.701D	T23.739A	T23.771S	T24.319D	T24.702D	T24.791A	T25.332S	T25.731D
T23.359A	T23.701S	T23.739D	T23.772A	T24.319S	T24.702S	T24.791D	T25.339A	T25.731S
T23.359D	T23.702A	T23.739S	T23.772D	T24.321A	T24.709A	T24.791S	T25.339D	T25.732A
T23.359S	T23.702D	T23.741A	T23.772S	T24.321D	T24.709D	T24.792A	T25.339S	T25.732D
T23.361A	T23.702S	T23.741D	T23.779A	T24.321S	T24.709S	T24.792D	T25.391A	T25.732S
T23.361D	T23.709A	T23.741S	T23.779D	T24.322A	T24.711A	T24.792S	T25.391D	T25.739A
T23.361S	T23.709D	T23.742A	T23.779S	T24.322D	T24.711D	T24.799A	T25.391S	T25.739D
T23.362A	T23.709S	T23.742D	T23.791A	T24.322S	T24.711S	T24.799D	T25.392A	T25.739S
T23.362D	T23.711A	T23.742S	T23.791D	T24.329A	T24.712A	T24.799S	T25.392D	T25.791A
T23.362S	T23.711D	T23.749A	T23.791S	T24.329D	T24.712D	T25.311A	T25.392S	T25.791D
T23.369A	T23.711S	T23.749D	T23.792A	T24.329S	T24.712S	T25.311D	T25.399A	T25.791S
T23.369D	T23.712A	T23.749S	T23.792D	T24.331A	T24.719A	T25.311S	T25.399D	T25.792A
T23.369S	T23.712D	T23.751A	T23.792S	T24.331D	T24.719D	T25.312A	T25.399S	T25.792D
T23.371A	T23.712S	T23.751D	T23.799A	T24.331S	T24.719S	T25.312D	T25.711A	T25.792S
T23.371D	T23.719A	T23.751S	T23.799D	T24.332A	T24.721A	T25.312S	T25.711D	T25.799A
T23.371S	T23.719D	T23.752A	T23.799S	T24.332D	T24.721D	T25.319A	T25.711S	T25.799D
T23.372A	T23.719S	T23.752D	T24.301A	T24.332S	T24.721S	T25.319D	T25.712A	T25.799S
T23.372D	T23.721A	T23.752S	T24.301D	T24.339A	T24.722A	T25.319S	T25.712D	
T23.372S	T23.721D	T23.759A	T24.301S	T24.339D	T24.722D	T25.321A	T25.712S	
T23.379A	T23.721S	T23.759D	T24.302A	T24.339S	T24.722S	T25.321D	T25.719A	

Non-Healing Surgical Wound

L97.102	L97.214	L97.313	L97.412	L97.504	L97.803	L97.902	L98.424	T81.32XA
L97.103	L97.222	L97.314	L97.413	L97.512	L97.804	L97.903	L98.492	T81.32XD
L97.104	L97.223	L97.322	L97.414	L97.513	L97.812	L97.904	L98.493	T81.89XA
L97.202	L97.224	L97.323	L97.422	L97.514	L97.813	L98.412	L98.494	T81.89XD
L97.203	L97.302	L97.324	L97.423	L97.522	L97.814	L98.413	T81.30XA	
L97.204	L97.303	L97.402	L97.424	L97.523	L97.822	L98.414	T81.30XD	
L97.212	L97.304	L97.403	L97.502	L97.524	L97.823	L98.422	T81.31XA	
L97.213	L97.312	L97.404	L97.503	L97.802	L97.824	L98.423	T81.31XD	

Fistula* (which includes osteomyelitis)

H04.611	H83.12	K50.113	K51.813	L05.92	M25.131	M25.159	M25.175	Q18.1
H04.612	H83.13	K50.813	K51.913	M25.10	M25.132	M25.161	M25.176	T81.83XA
H04.613	H83.19	K50.913	K60.3	M25.111	M25.139	M25.162	M25.18	T81.83XD
H04.619	J86.0	K51.013	K60.4	M25.112	M25.141	M25.169	N82.0	T81.83XS
H70.811	K04.6	K51.213	K60.5	M25.119	M25.142	M25.171	N82.2	
H70.812	K11.4	K51.313	K63.2	M25.121	M25.149	M25.172	N82.3	
H70.813	K31.6	K51.413	L05.01	M25.122	M25.151	M25.173	N82.4	
H70.819	K50.013	K51.513	L05.02	M25.129	M25.152	M25.174	N82.5	

Chapter 3. Diseases of the Blood and Blood-forming Organs and Certain Disorders Involving the Immune Mechanism (D50–D89)

Red Blood Cells

White Blood Cell

Platelet

Coagulation

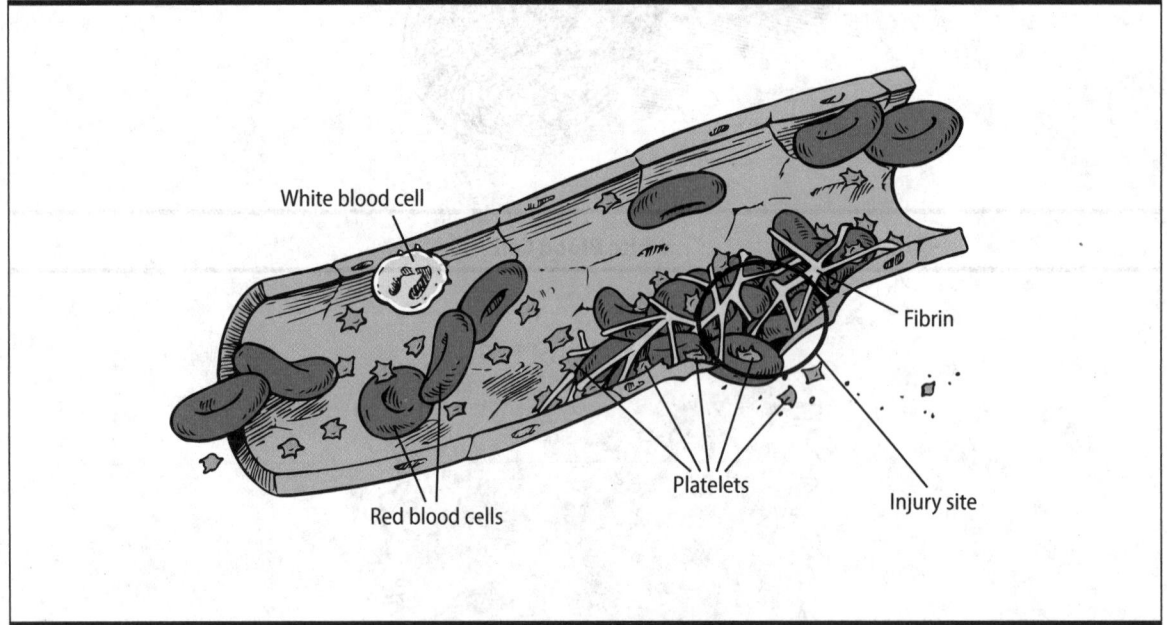

Spleen Anatomical Location and External Structures

Spleen Interior Structures

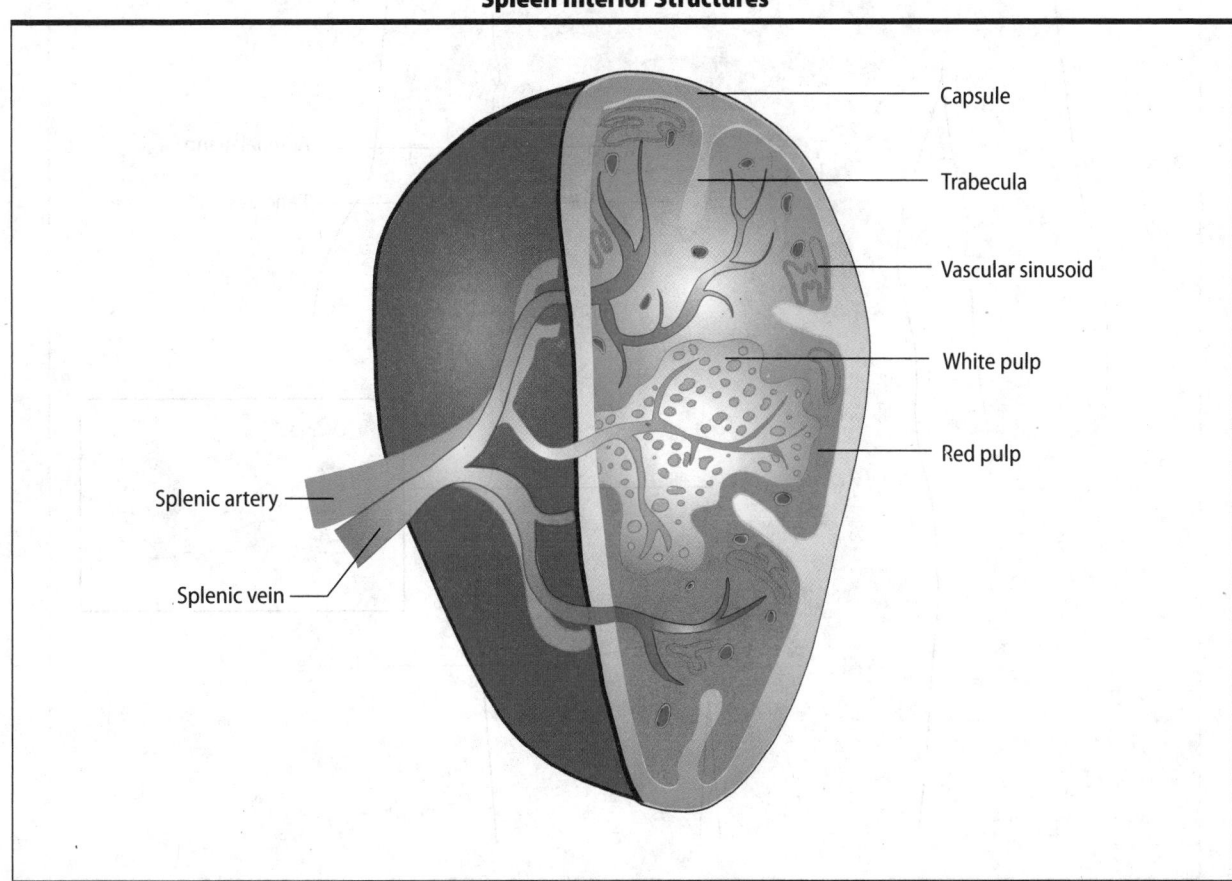

Chapter 4. Endocrine, Nutritional and Metabolic Diseases (E00–E89)

Endocrine System

Thyroid

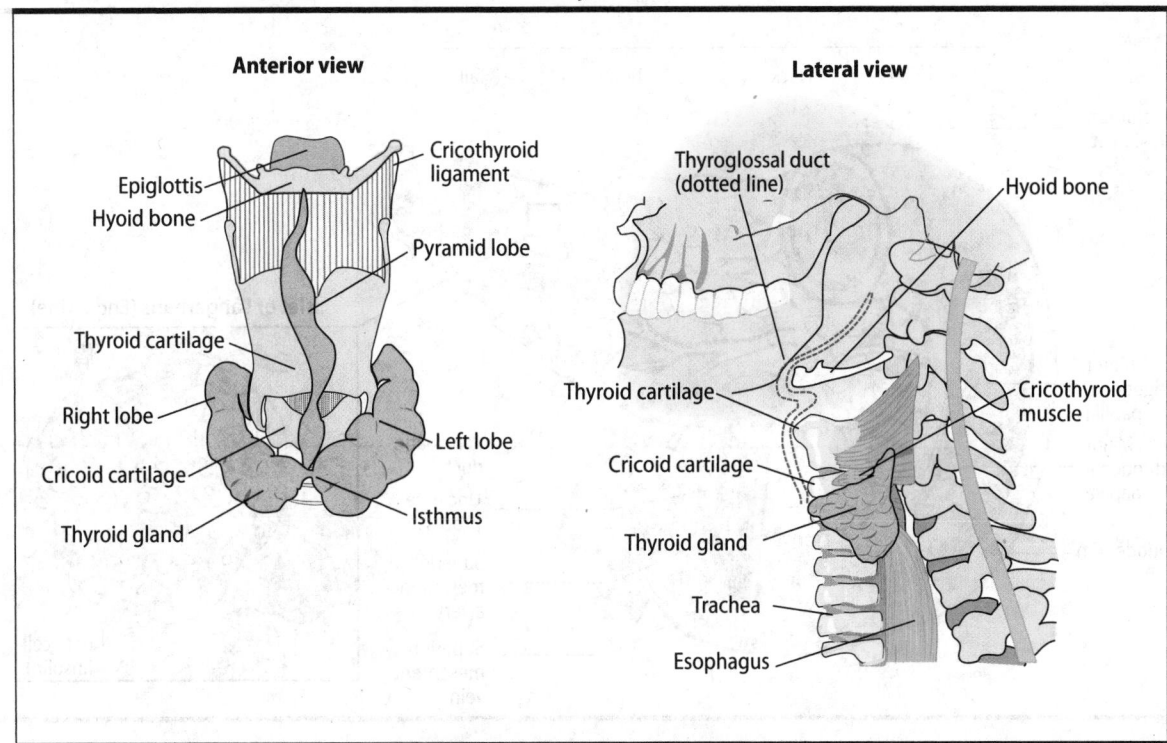

Thyroid and Parathyroid Glands

Pancreas

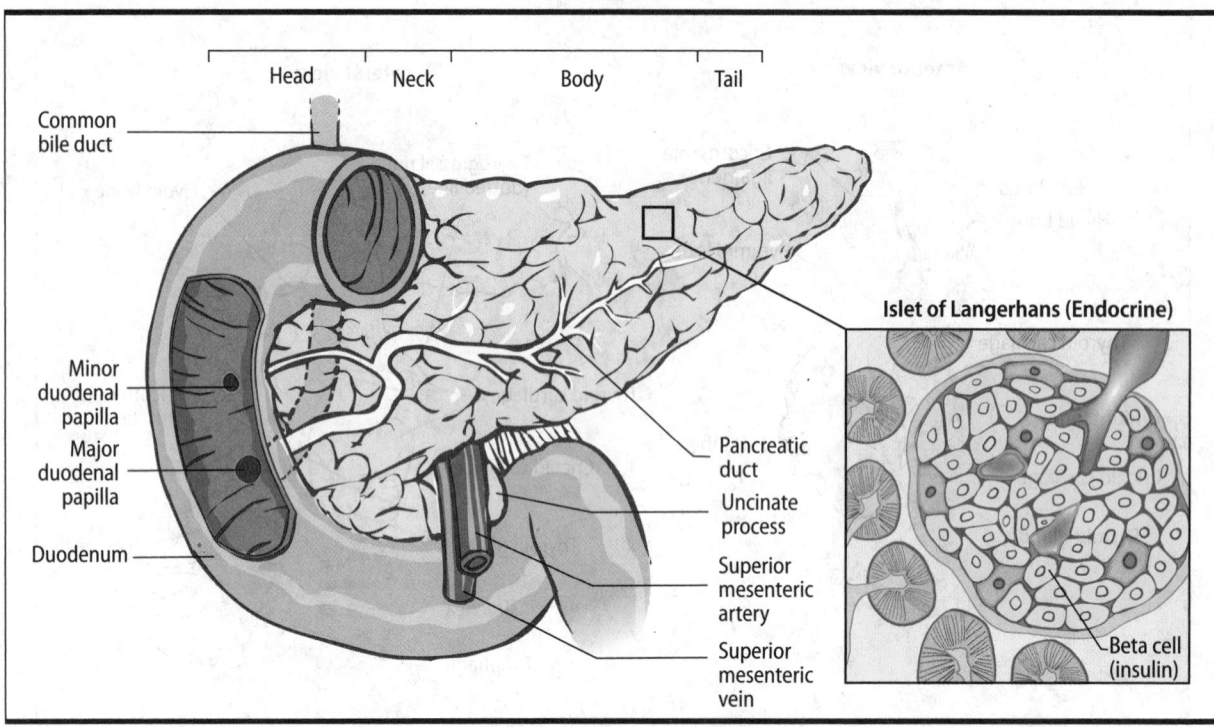

Islet of Langerhans (Endocrine)

Anatomy of the Adrenal Gland

Structure of an Ovary

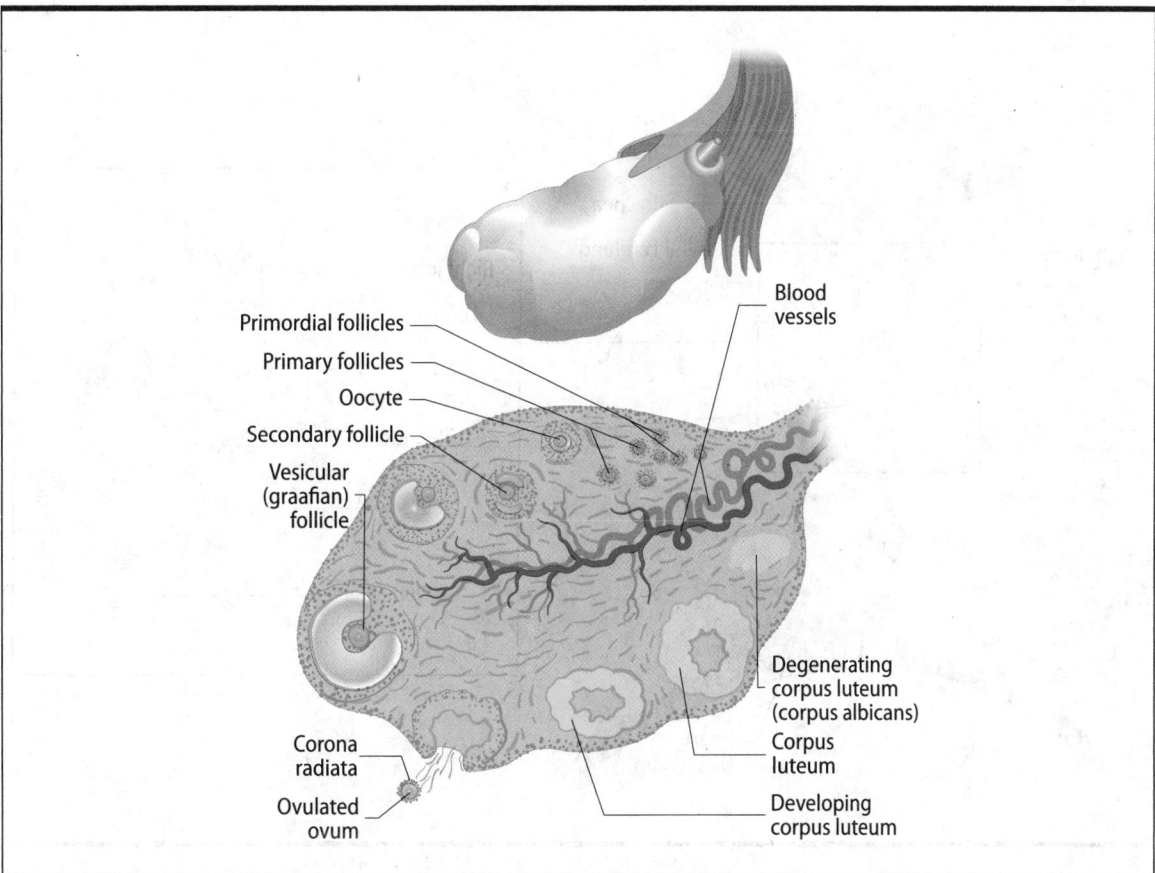

Testis and Associated Structures

Thymus

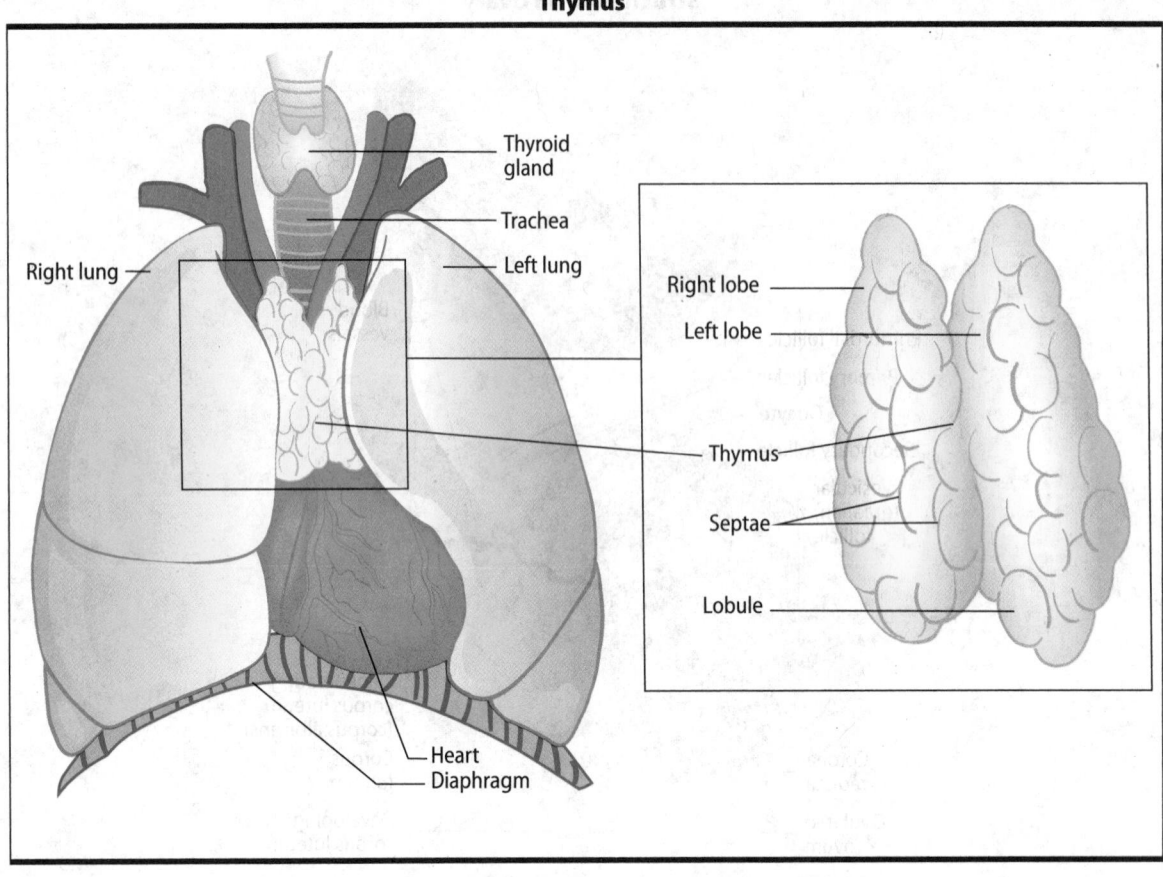

Chapter 6. Diseases of the Nervous System (G00–G99)

Brain

Cranial Nerves

Peripheral Nervous System

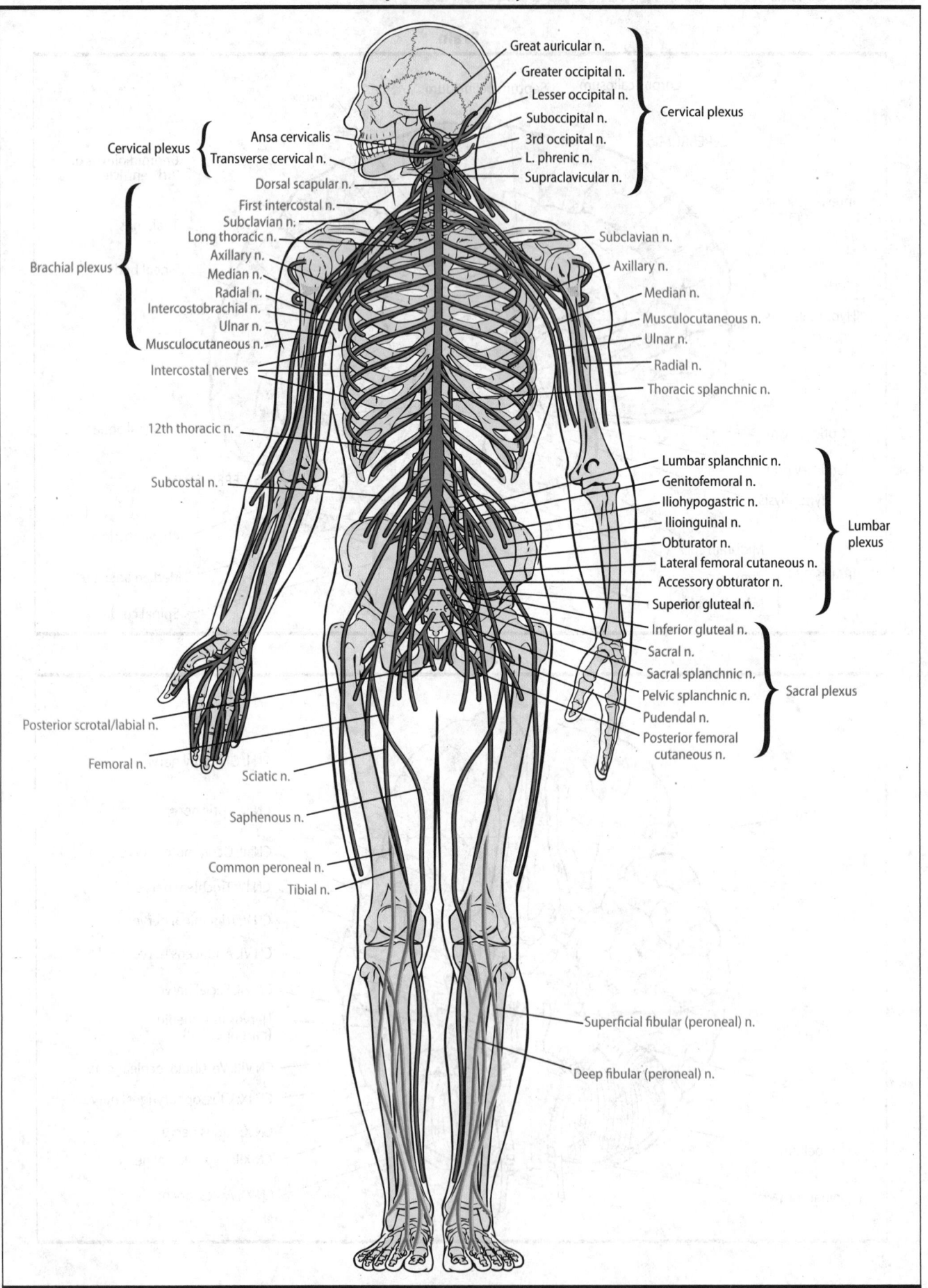

Great auricular n.
Greater occipital n.
Lesser occipital n.
Suboccipital n.
3rd occipital n.
L. phrenic n.
Supraclavicular n.

Cervical plexus

Ansa cervicalis
Transverse cervical n.

Cervical plexus

Dorsal scapular n.
First intercostal n.
Subclavian n.
Long thoracic n.
Axillary n.
Median n.
Radial n.
Intercostobrachial n.
Ulnar n.
Musculocutaneous n.

Brachial plexus

Intercostal nerves

12th thoracic n.

Subcostal n.

Subclavian n.
Axillary n.
Median n.
Musculocutaneous n.
Ulnar n.
Radial n.
Thoracic splanchnic n.

Lumbar splanchnic n.
Genitofemoral n.
Iliohypogastric n.
Ilioinguinal n.
Obturator n.
Lateral femoral cutaneous n.
Accessory obturator n.
Superior gluteal n.

Lumbar plexus

Inferior gluteal n.
Sacral n.
Sacral splanchnic n.
Pelvic splanchnic n.
Pudendal n.
Posterior femoral cutaneous n.

Sacral plexus

Posterior scrotal/labial n.

Femoral n.

Sciatic n.

Saphenous n.

Common peroneal n.
Tibial n.

Superficial fibular (peroneal) n.

Deep fibular (peroneal) n.

Peripheral Nervous System

Spinal Cord and Spinal Nerves

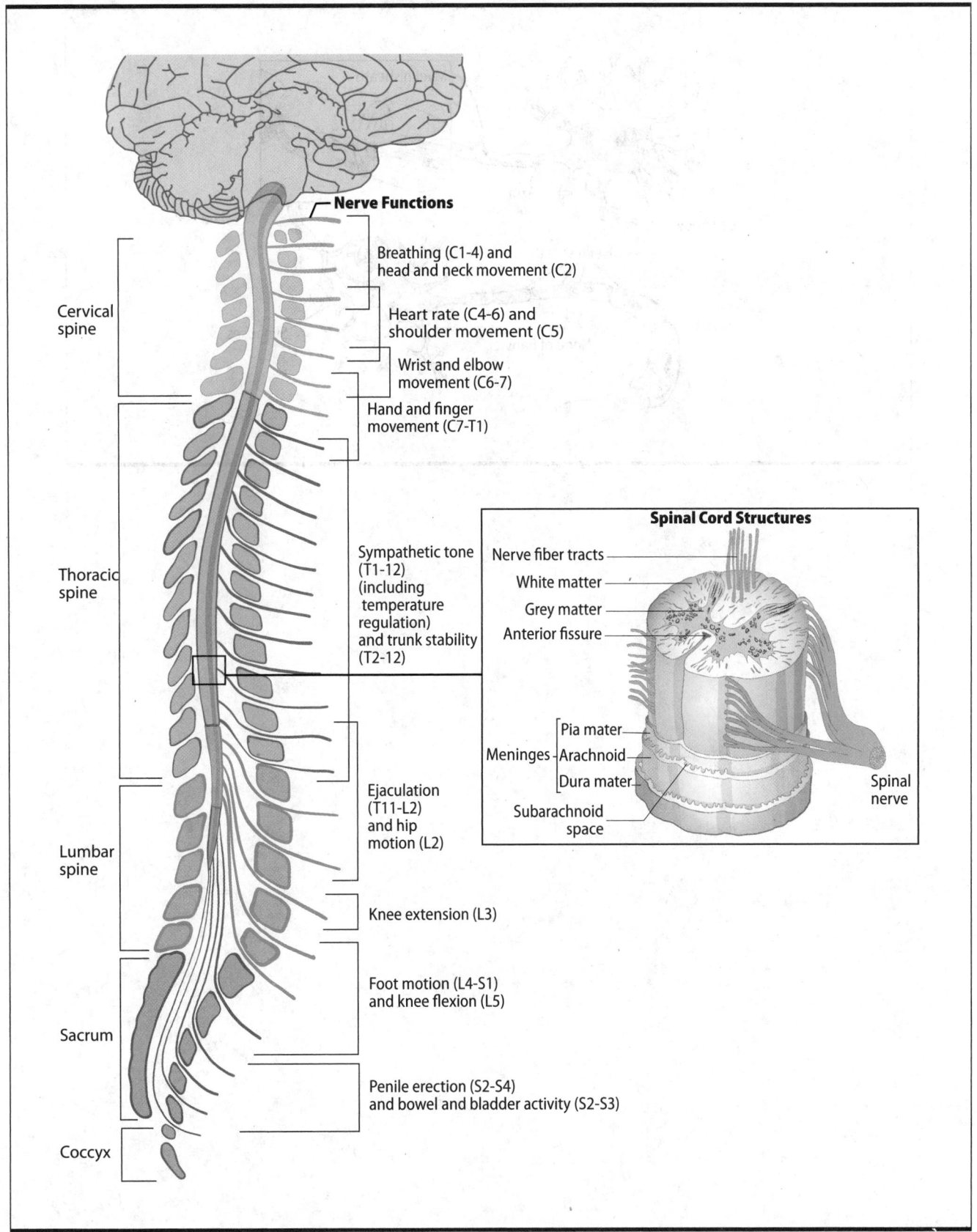

Nerve Functions

Breathing (C1-4) and head and neck movement (C2)

Heart rate (C4-6) and shoulder movement (C5)

Wrist and elbow movement (C6-7)

Hand and finger movement (C7-T1)

Cervical spine

Thoracic spine

Sympathetic tone (T1-12) (including temperature regulation) and trunk stability (T2-12)

Ejaculation (T11-L2) and hip motion (L2)

Lumbar spine

Knee extension (L3)

Foot motion (L4-S1) and knee flexion (L5)

Sacrum

Penile erection (S2-S4) and bowel and bladder activity (S2-S3)

Coccyx

Spinal Cord Structures

Nerve fiber tracts

White matter

Grey matter

Anterior fissure

Meninges — Pia mater / Arachnoid / Dura mater

Subarachnoid space

Spinal nerve

Nerve Cell

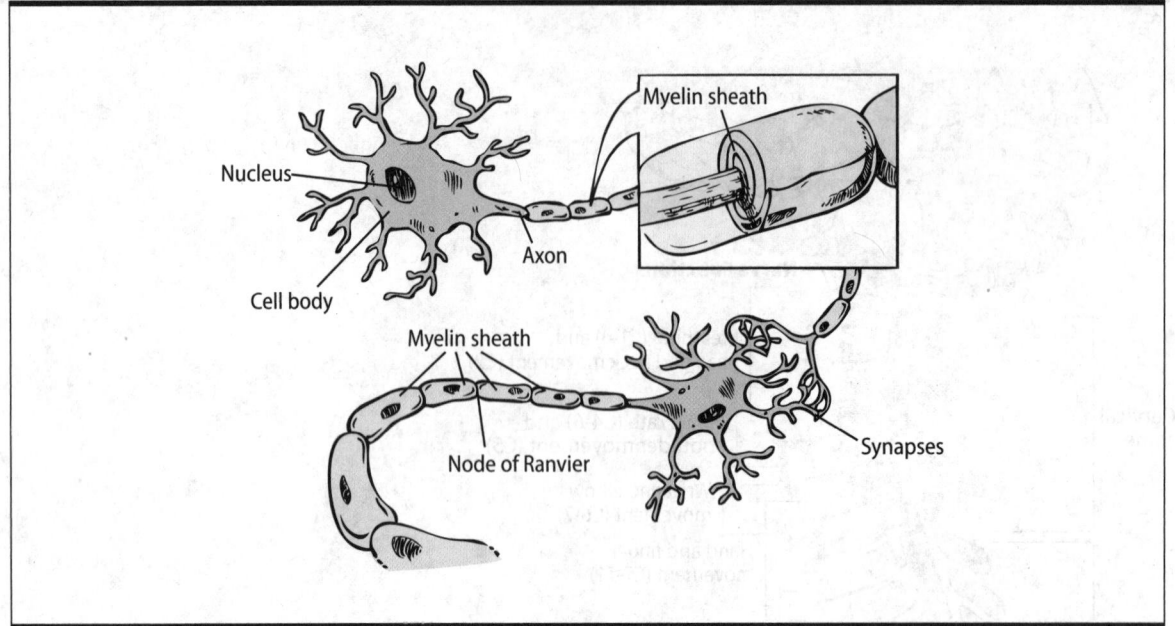

Chapter 7. Diseases of the Eye and Adnexa (HØØ–H59)

Eye

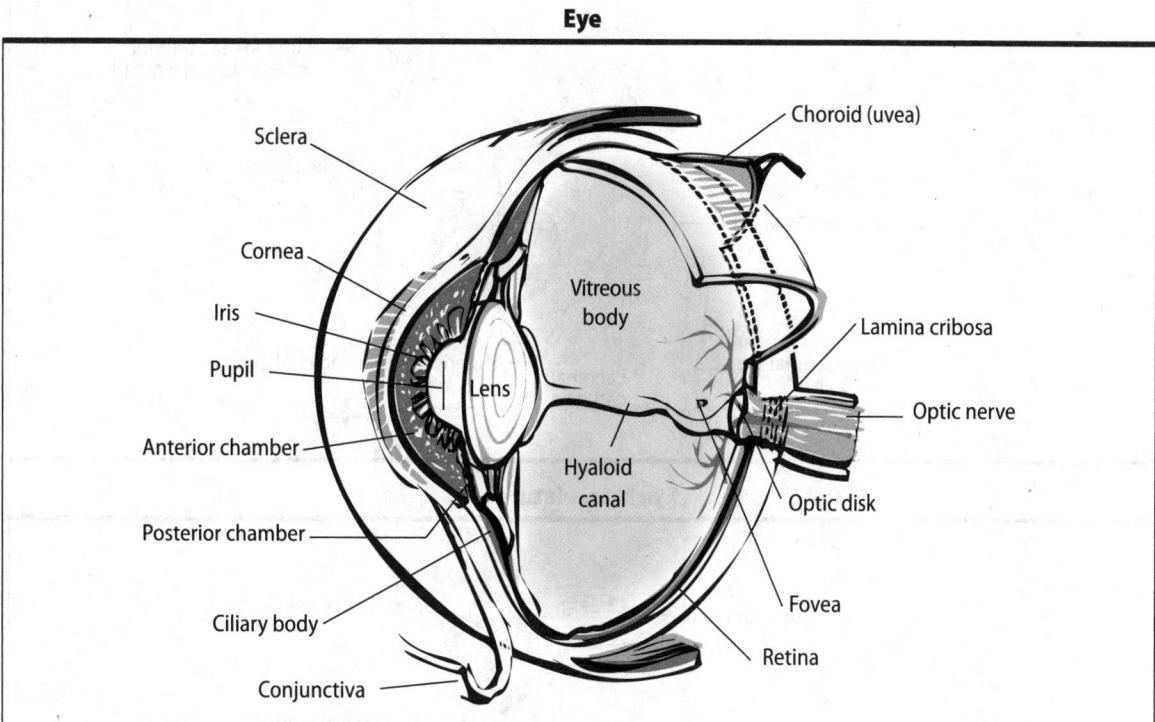

Posterior Pole of Globe/Flow of Aqueous Humor

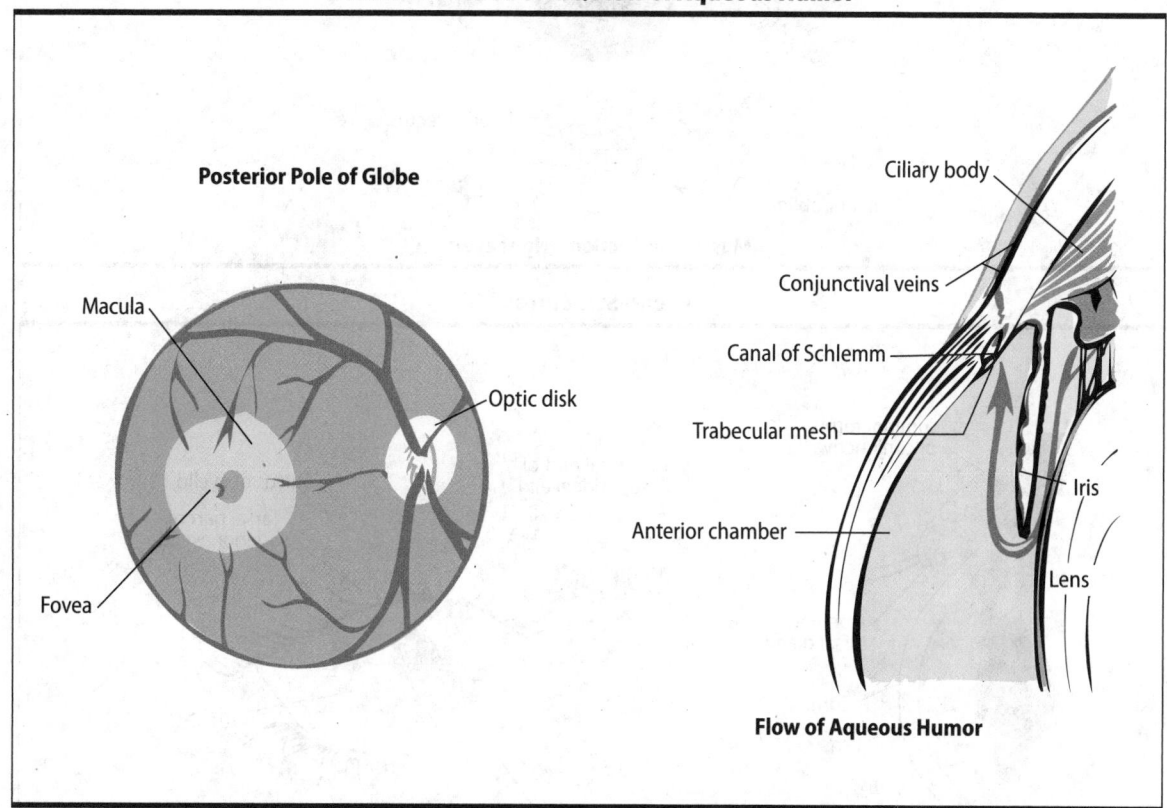

Posterior Pole of Globe

Flow of Aqueous Humor

Lacrimal System

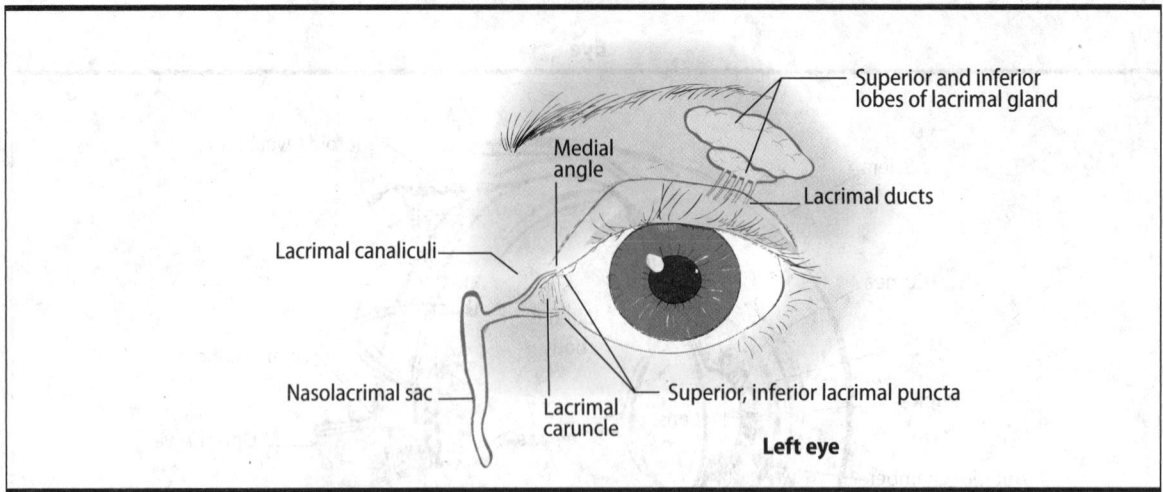

Left eye

Eye Musculature

Muscles and actions (right eye)

Eyelid Structures

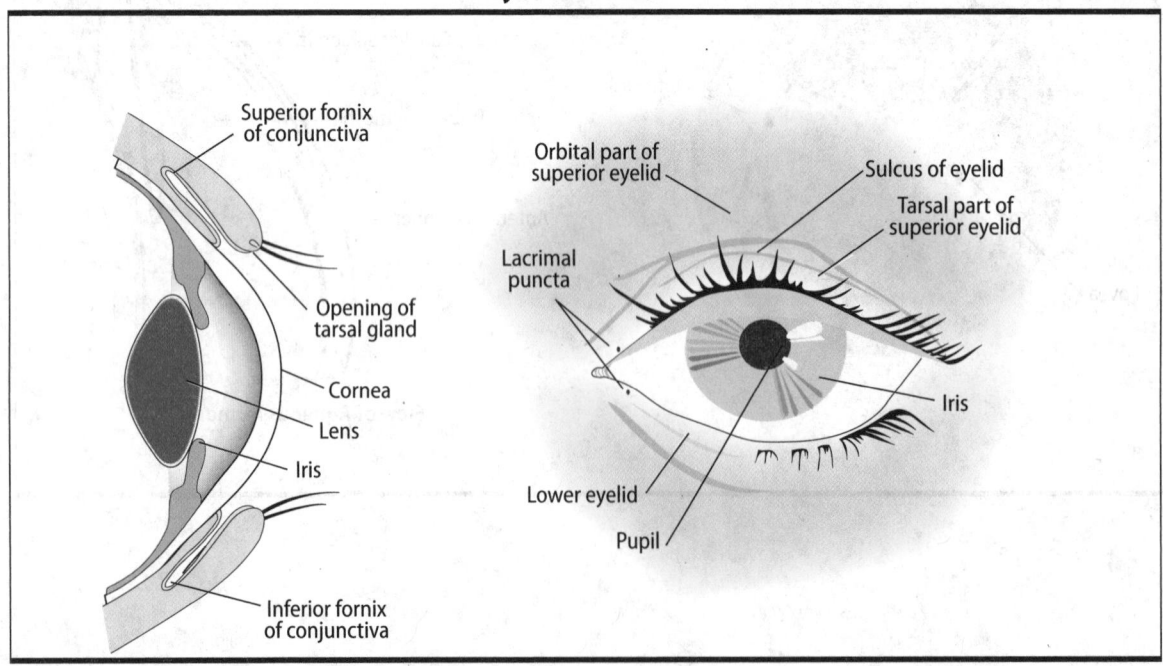

Chapter 8. Diseases of the Ear and Mastoid Process (H60–H95)

Ear Anatomy

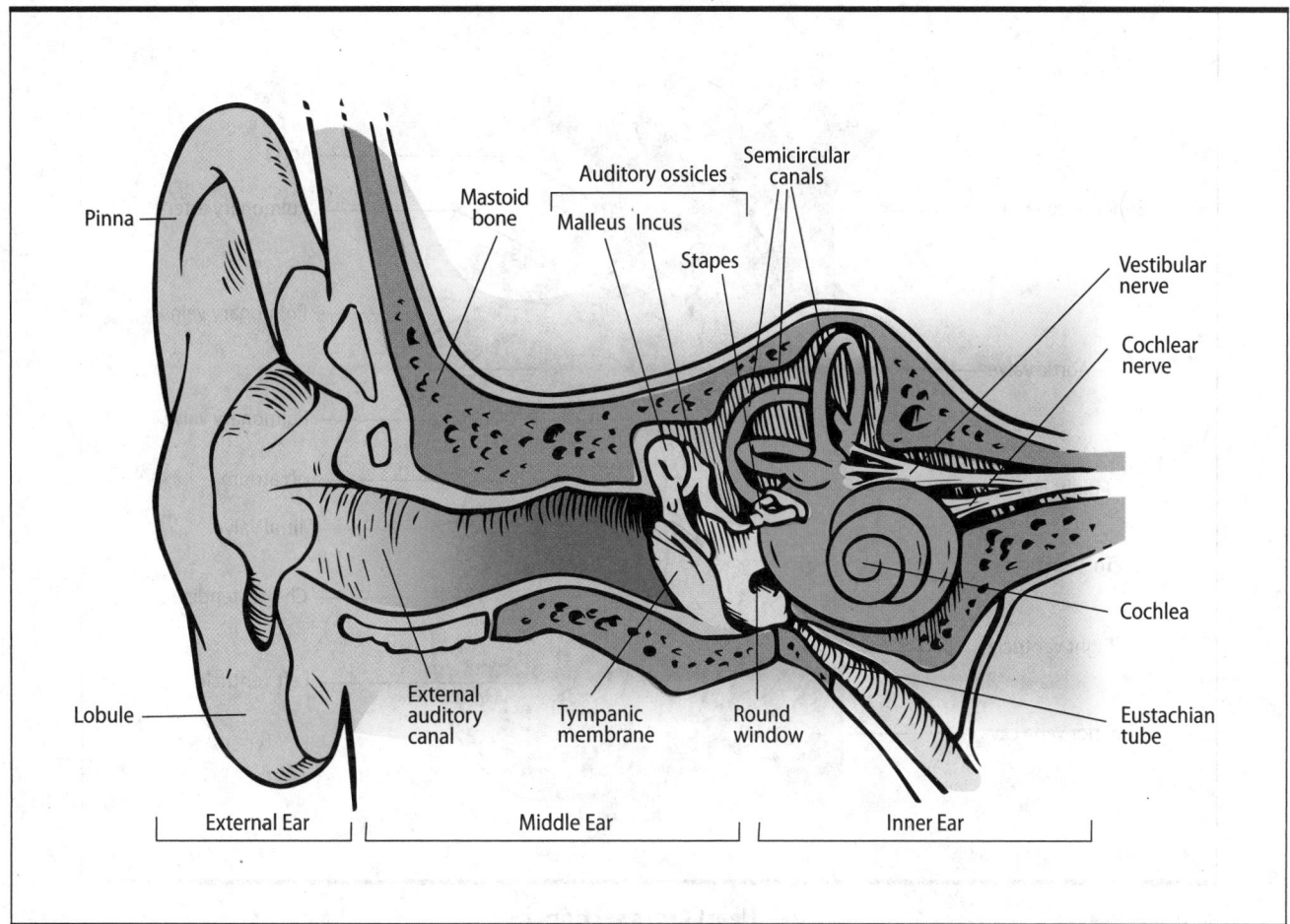

Chapter 9. Diseases of the Circulatory System (I00–I99)

Anatomy of the Heart

Heart Cross Section

Heart Valves

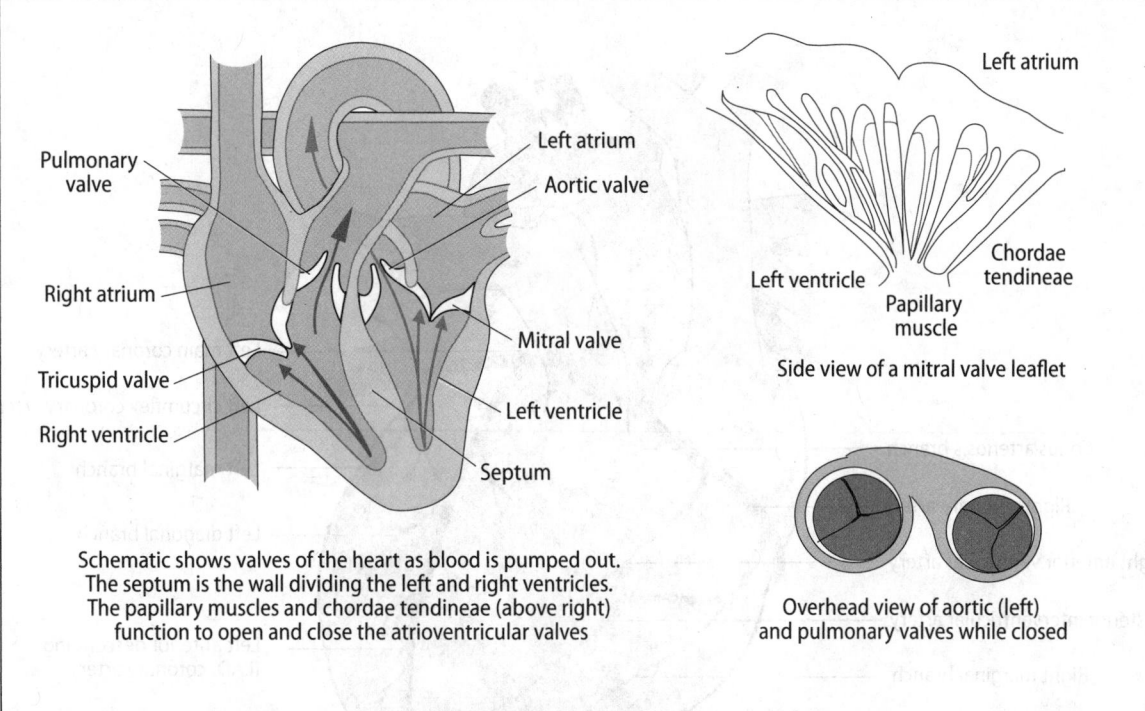

Schematic shows valves of the heart as blood is pumped out.
The septum is the wall dividing the left and right ventricles.
The papillary muscles and chordae tendineae (above right)
function to open and close the atrioventricular valves

Side view of a mitral valve leaflet

Overhead view of aortic (left)
and pulmonary valves while closed

Heart Conduction System

Coronary Arteries

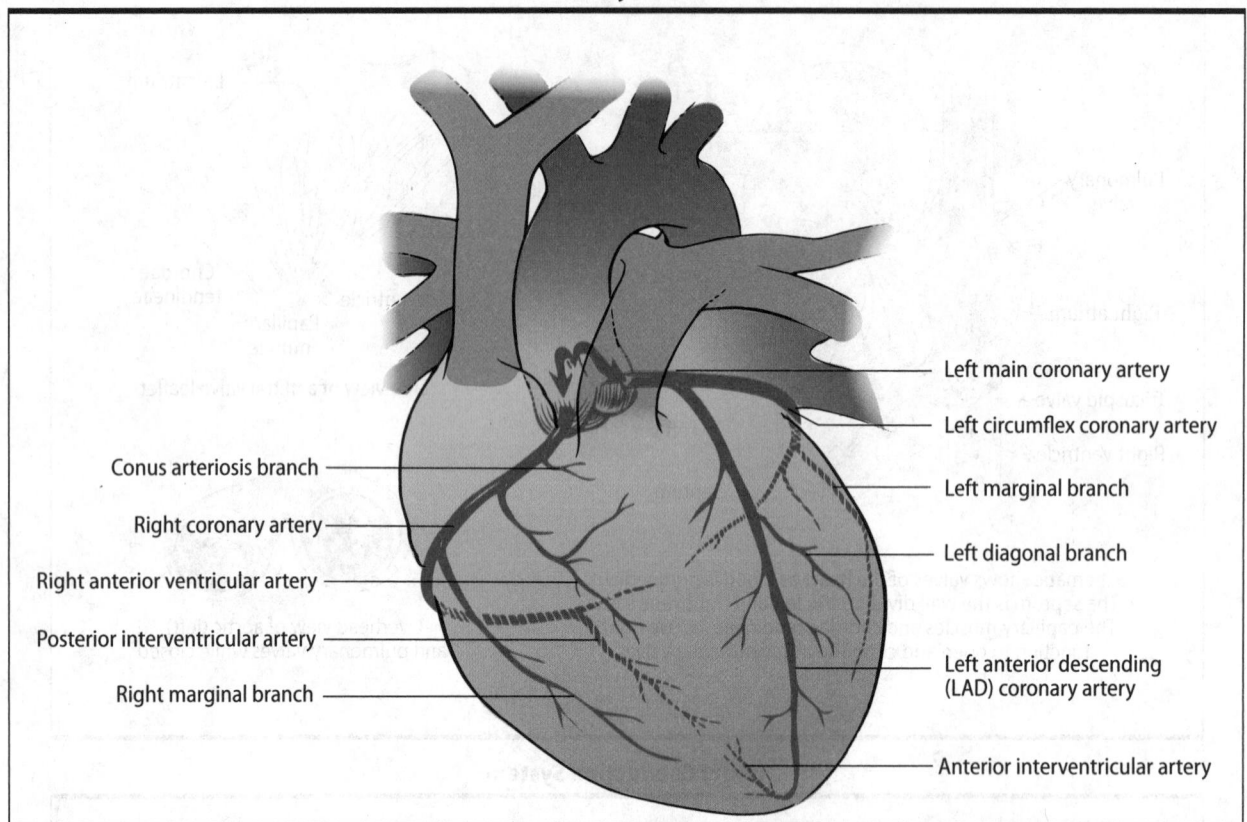

Left main coronary artery

Left circumflex coronary artery

Conus arteriosis branch

Left marginal branch

Right coronary artery

Left diagonal branch

Right anterior ventricular artery

Posterior interventricular artery

Left anterior descending (LAD) coronary artery

Right marginal branch

Anterior interventricular artery

Arteries

Veins

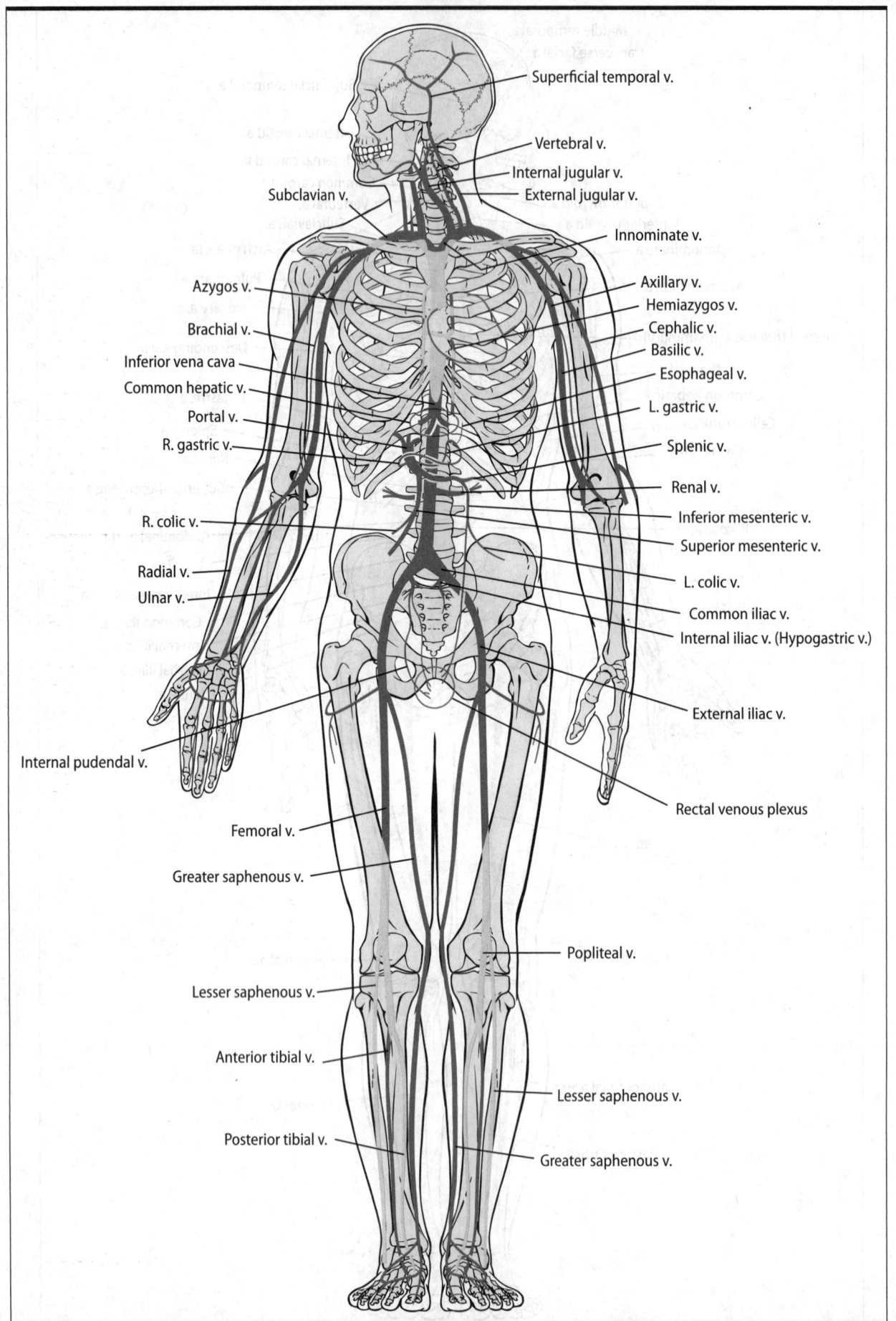

- Superficial temporal v.
- Vertebral v.
- Internal jugular v.
- External jugular v.
- Subclavian v.
- Innominate v.
- Azygos v.
- Axillary v.
- Hemiazygos v.
- Brachial v.
- Cephalic v.
- Inferior vena cava
- Basilic v.
- Common hepatic v.
- Esophageal v.
- Portal v.
- L. gastric v.
- R. gastric v.
- Splenic v.
- Renal v.
- R. colic v.
- Inferior mesenteric v.
- Superior mesenteric v.
- Radial v.
- L. colic v.
- Ulnar v.
- Common iliac v.
- Internal iliac v. (Hypogastric v.)
- External iliac v.
- Internal pudendal v.
- Rectal venous plexus
- Femoral v.
- Greater saphenous v.
- Popliteal v.
- Lesser saphenous v.
- Anterior tibial v.
- Lesser saphenous v.
- Posterior tibial v.
- Greater saphenous v.

Internal Carotid and Vertebral Arteries and Branches

Side View

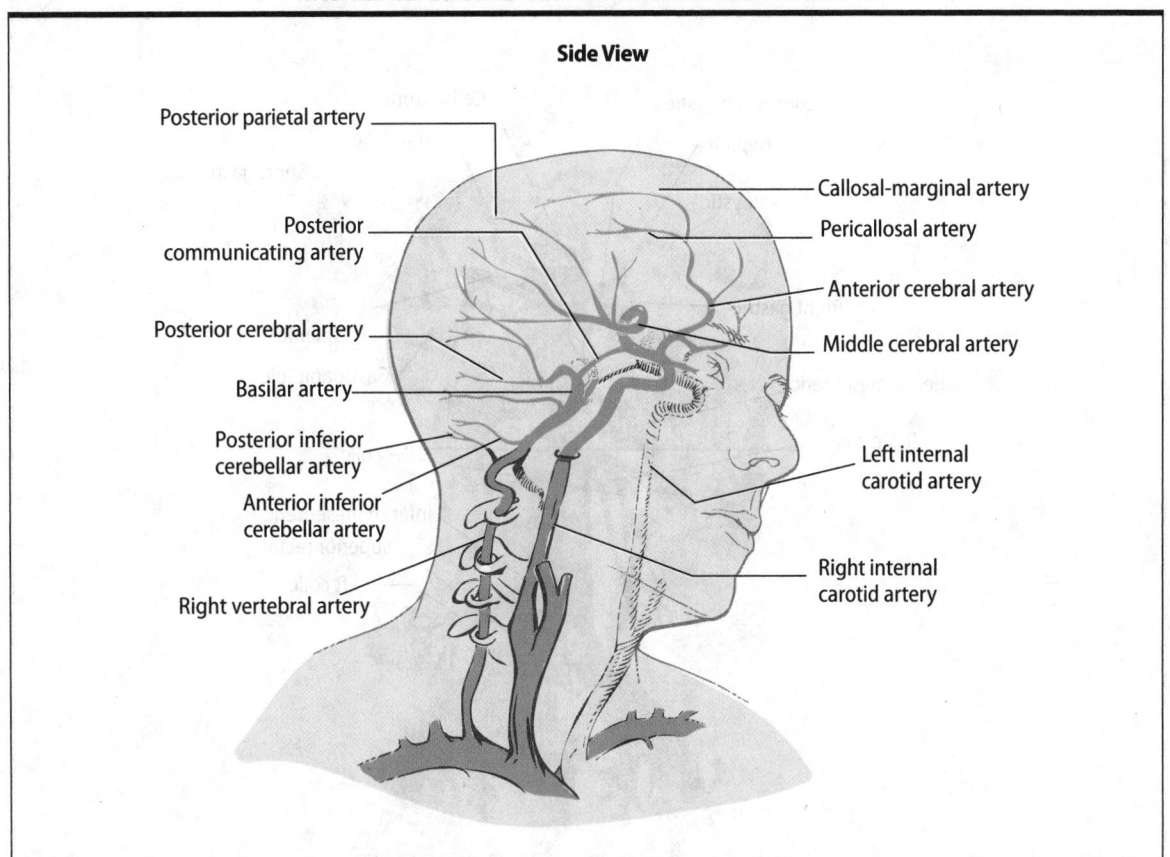

External Carotid Artery and Branches

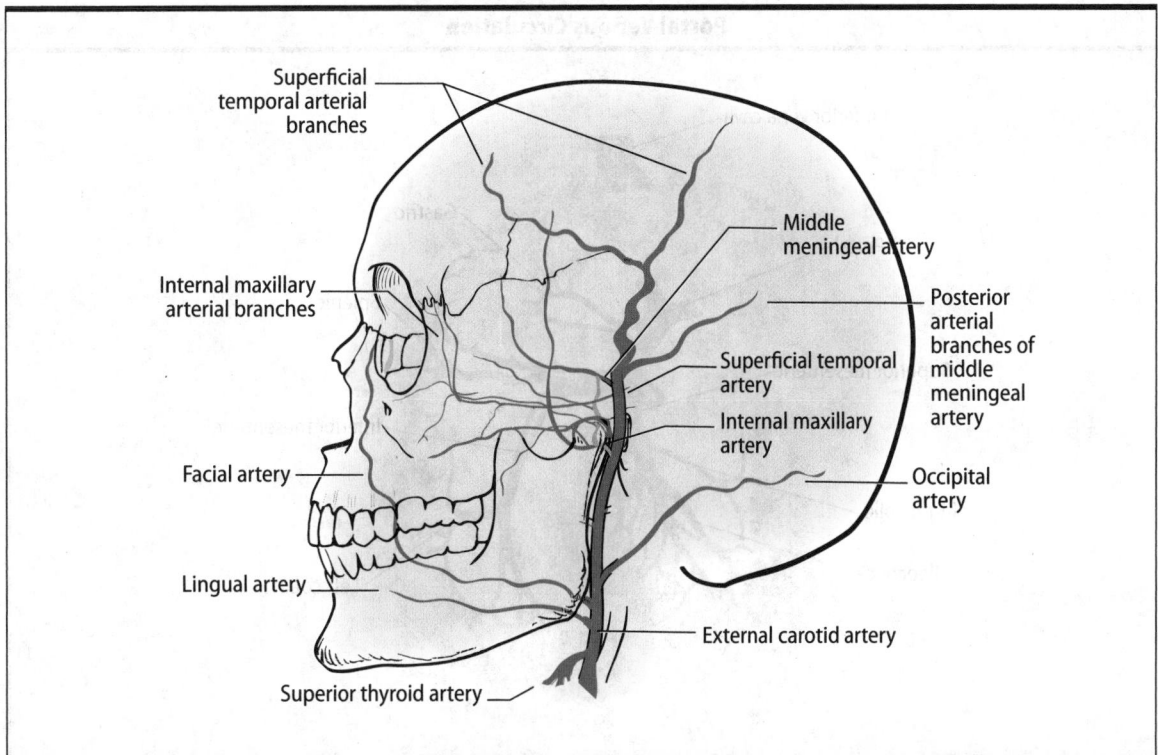

Branches of Abdominal Aorta

Portal Venous Circulation

Lymphatic System

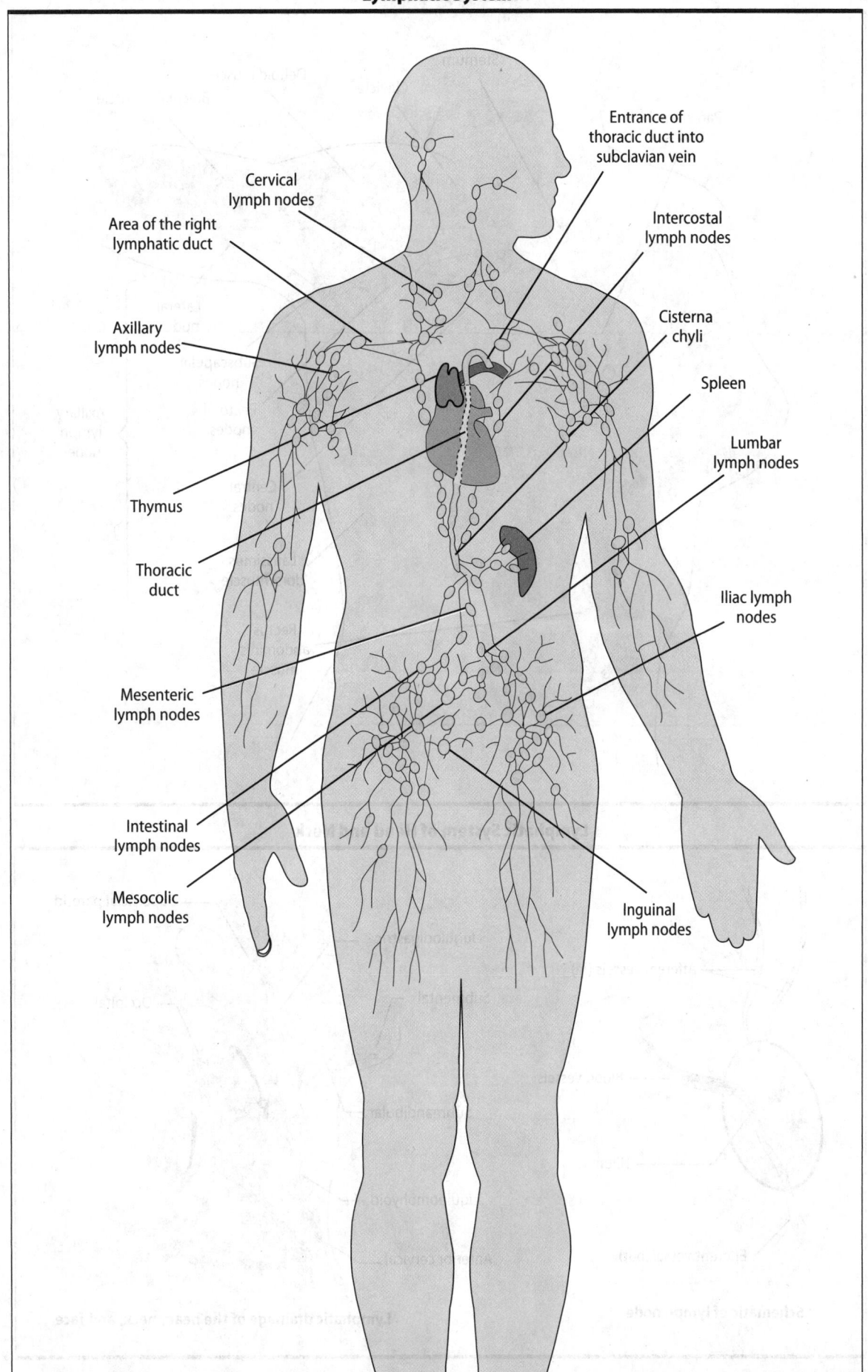

Axillary Lymph Nodes

Parasternal nodes

Sternum

Clavicle

Deltoid muscle

Brachialis muscle

Lateral nodes

Subscapular nodes

Pectoral nodes

Axillary lymph nodes

Central nodes

Latissimus dorsi muscle

Rectus abdominis muscle

Lymphatic System of Head and Neck

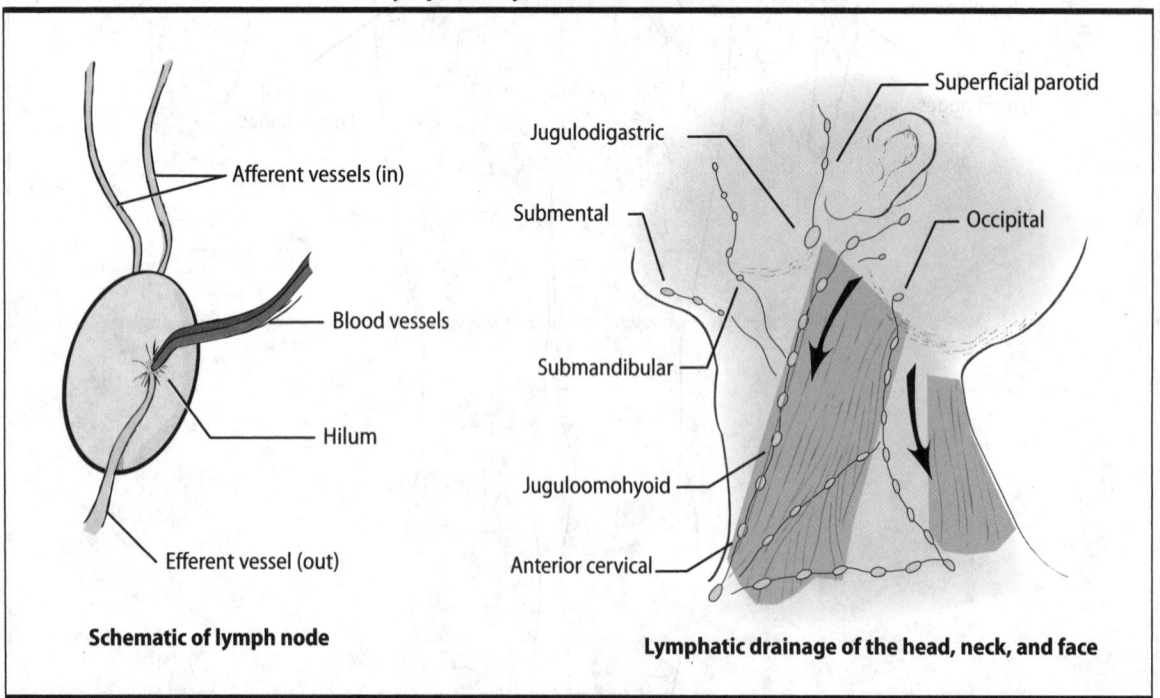

Afferent vessels (in)

Blood vessels

Hilum

Efferent vessel (out)

Jugulodigastric

Superficial parotid

Submental

Occipital

Submandibular

Juguloomohyoid

Anterior cervical

Schematic of lymph node

Lymphatic drainage of the head, neck, and face

Lymphatic Capillaries

Schematic of lymphatic capillaries

Valves

Tissue cells

Endothelial cells

Fluids and particles can enter the capillary through overlapping valves

Lymphatic Drainage

Lymphatic drainage of the colon follows blood supply

Middle colic nodes

Paracolic nodes

Left colic nodes

Ascending colon

Cecum

Rectum

Chapter 10. Diseases of the Respiratory System (J00–J99)

Respiratory System

Upper Respiratory System

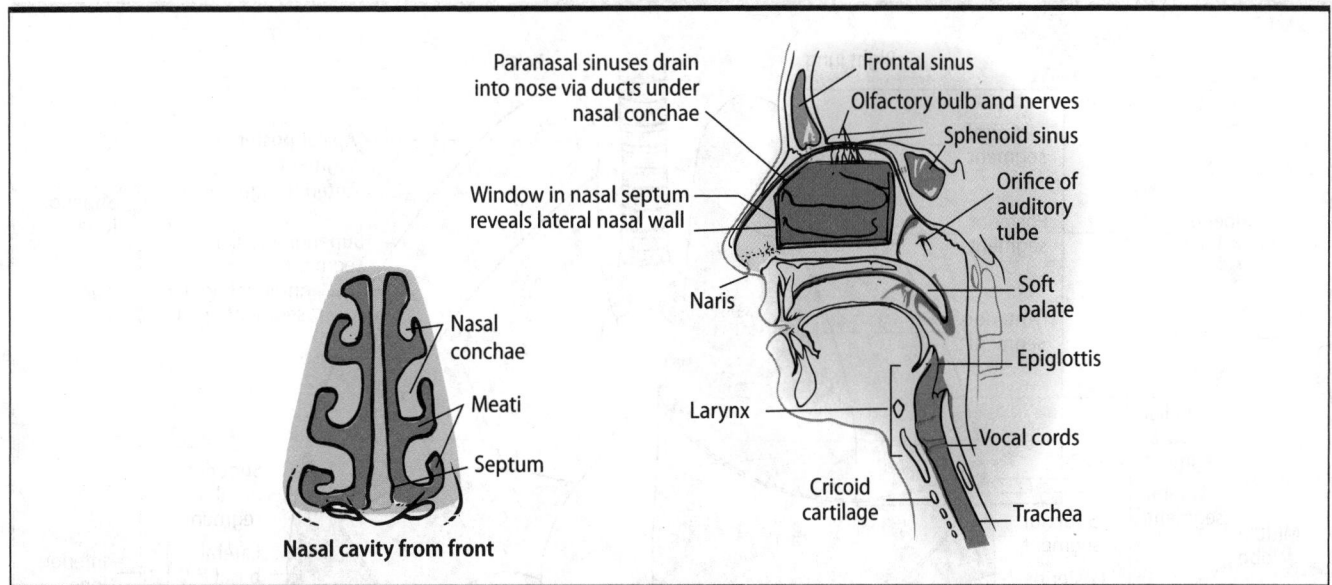

Paranasal sinuses drain into nose via ducts under nasal conchae

Window in nasal septum reveals lateral nasal wall

Frontal sinus

Olfactory bulb and nerves

Sphenoid sinus

Orifice of auditory tube

Naris

Soft palate

Nasal conchae

Meati

Septum

Larynx

Epiglottis

Vocal cords

Cricoid cartilage

Trachea

Nasal cavity from front

Lower Respiratory System

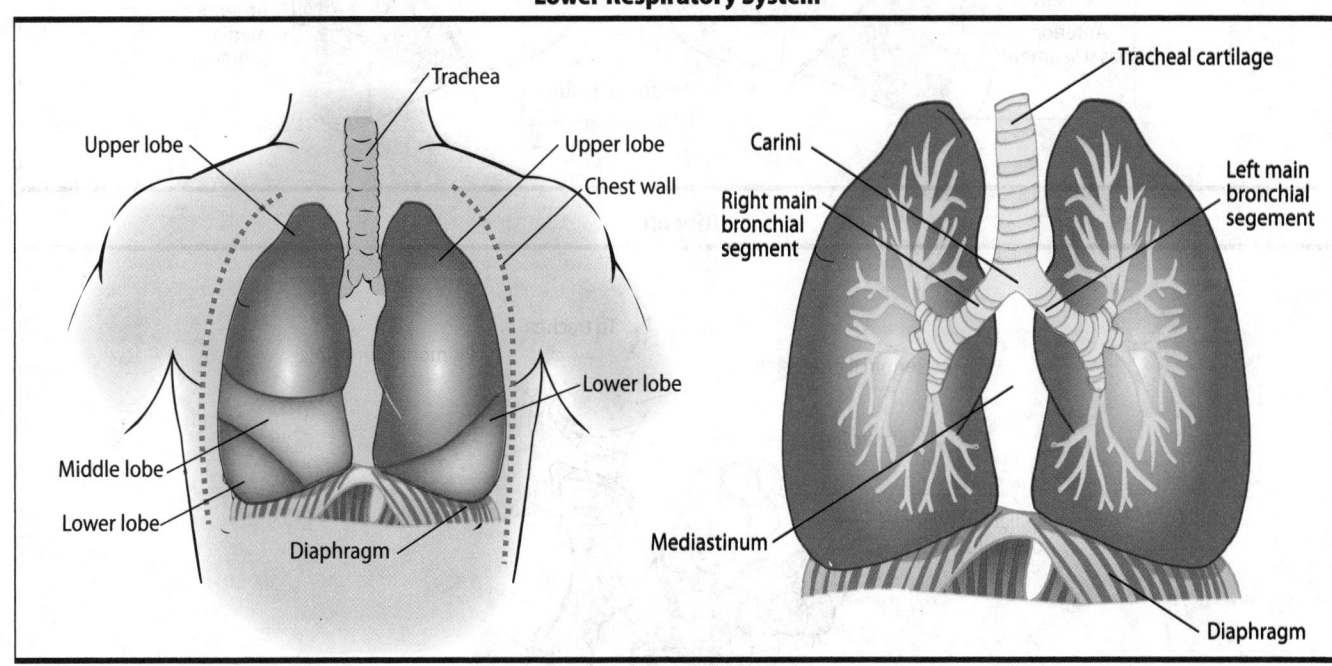

Trachea

Upper lobe

Upper lobe

Chest wall

Lower lobe

Middle lobe

Lower lobe

Diaphragm

Tracheal cartilage

Carini

Right main bronchial segment

Left main bronchial segment

Mediastinum

Diaphragm

Paranasal Sinuses

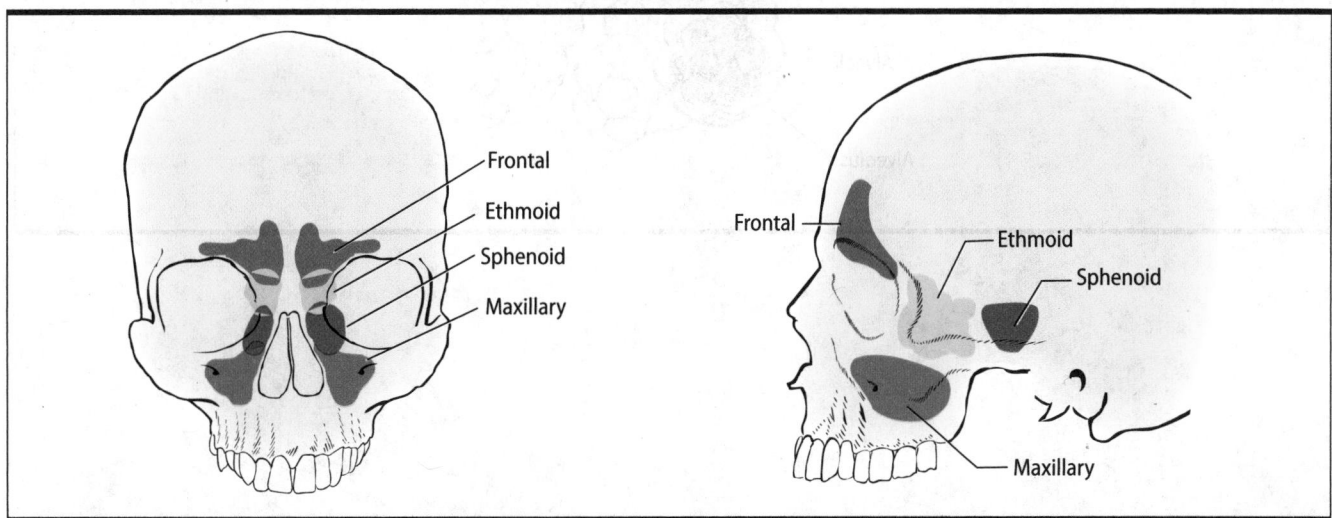

Frontal

Ethmoid

Sphenoid

Maxillary

Frontal

Ethmoid

Sphenoid

Maxillary

Lung Segments

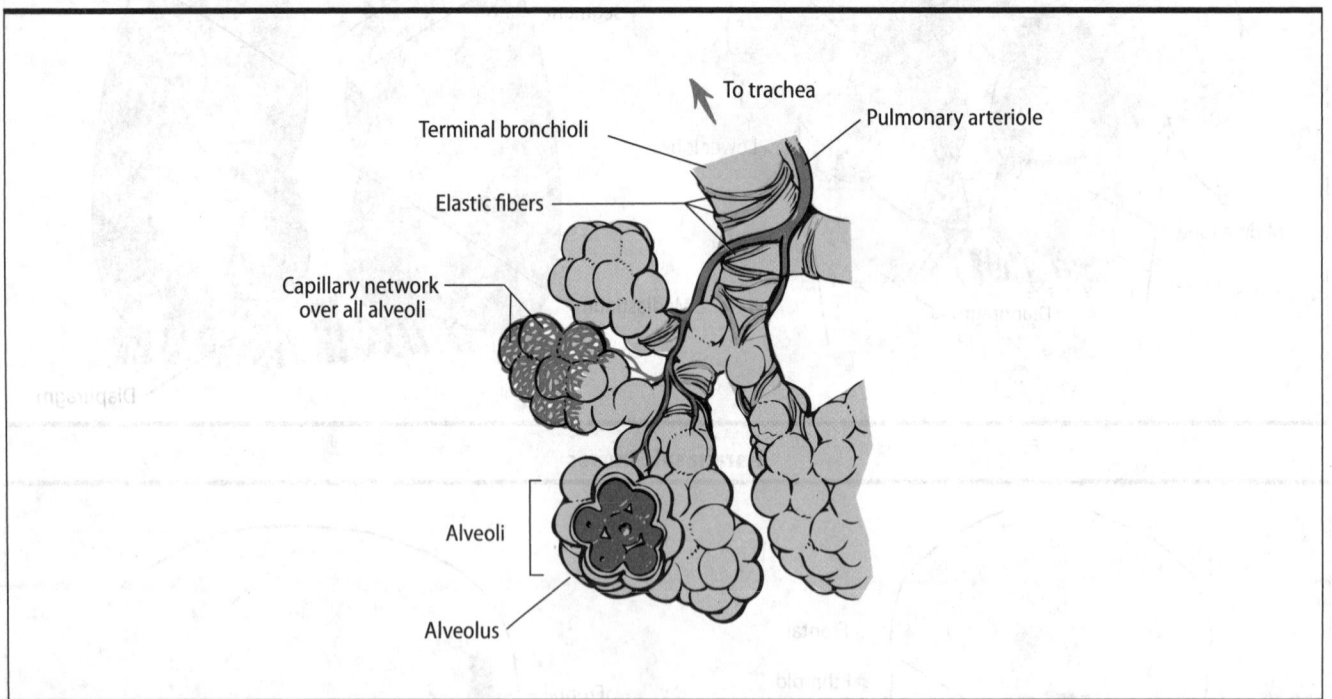

Right lung

Left lung

Apical segment

Apical-posterior segment

Anterior segment

Superior lobe

Posterior segment

Superior lingular segment

Inferior lingular segment

Anterior segment

Superior lobe

Medial basal segment

Superior basal segment

Lateral segment

Lateral basal segment

Middle lobe

Superior segment

Inferior lobe

Inferior lobe

Posterior basal segment

Anterior medial segment

Anterior basal segment

Horizontal fissure

Oblique fissures

Alveoli

To trachea

Terminal bronchioli

Pulmonary arteriole

Elastic fibers

Capillary network over all alveoli

Alveoli

Alveolus

Chapter 11. Diseases of the Digestive System (KØØ–K95)

Digestive System

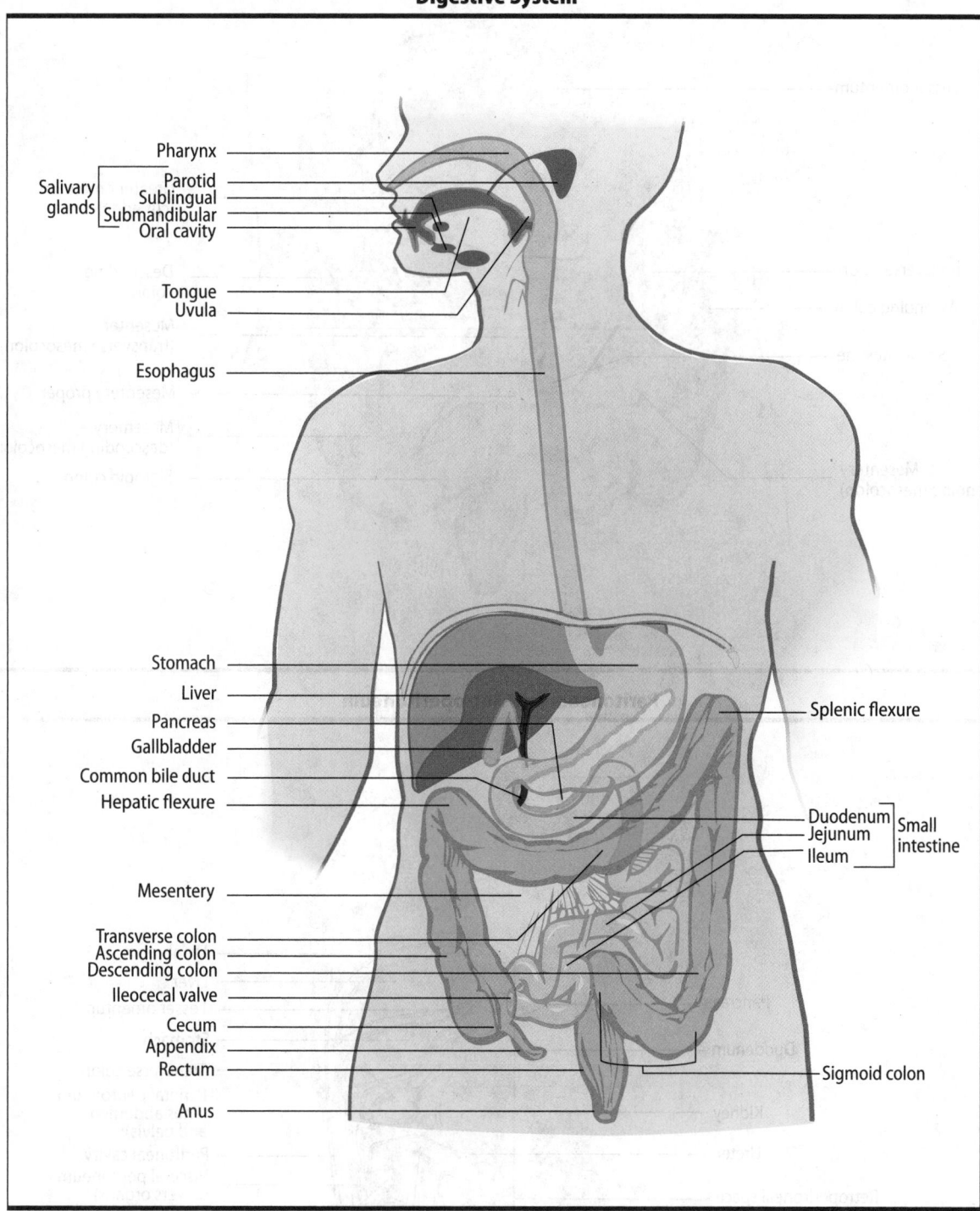

Omentum and Mesentery

Lesser omentum

Transverse colon

Ascending colon

Small intestine

Mesentery
(ascending mesocolon)

Greater omentum
(cut edge)

Descending
colon

Mesentery
(transverse mesocolon)

Mesentery proper

Mesentery
(descending mesocolon)

Sigmoid colon

Peritoneum and Retroperitoneum

Pancreas

Duodenum

Kidney

Ureter

Retroperitoneal space

Sigmoid colon

Bladder

Rectum

Diaphragm

Liver

Lesser omentum

Stomach

Transverse colon

Parietal peritoneum
(lines abdomen
and pelvis)

Peritoneal cavity

Visceral peritoneum
(covers organs)

Small intestine

Mesentery

Greater omentum

Chapter 12. Diseases of the Skin and Subcutaneous Tissue (LØØ–L99)

Nail Anatomy

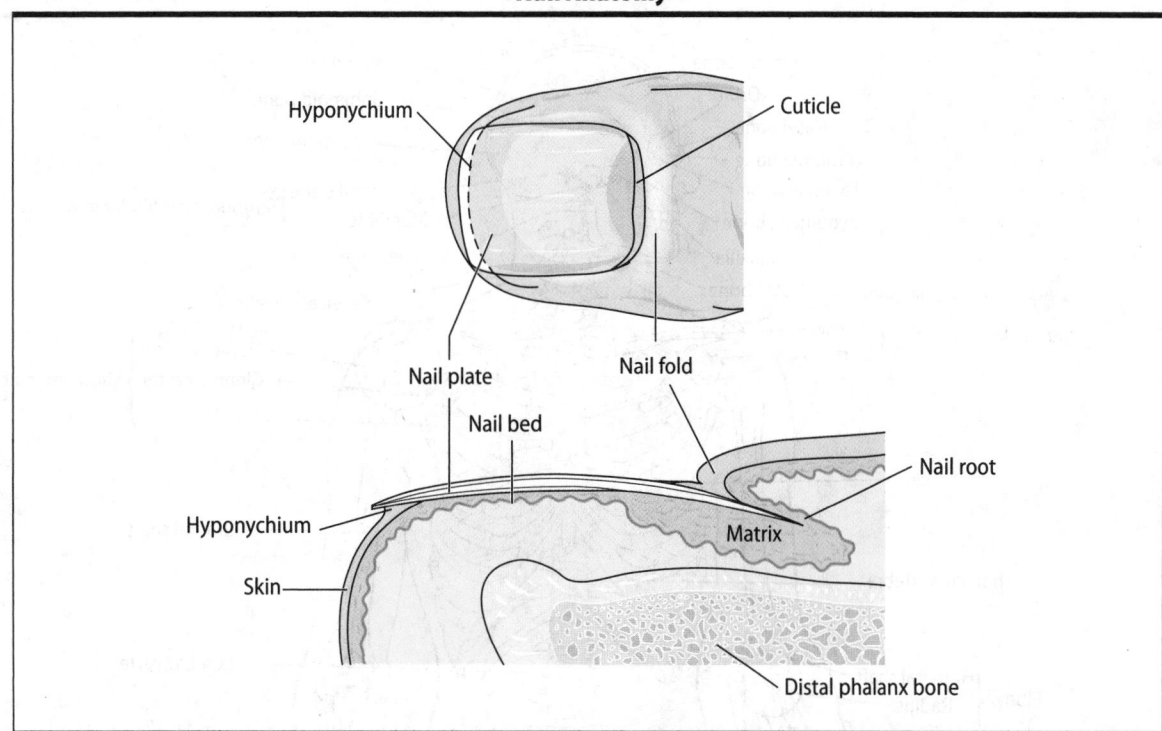

Skin and Subcutaneous Tissue

Chapter 13. Diseases of the Musculoskeletal System and Connective Tissue (MØØ–M99)

Bones and Joints

Shoulder Anterior View

Shoulder Posterior View

Elbow Anterior View

Elbow Posterior View

Hand

Hip Anterior View

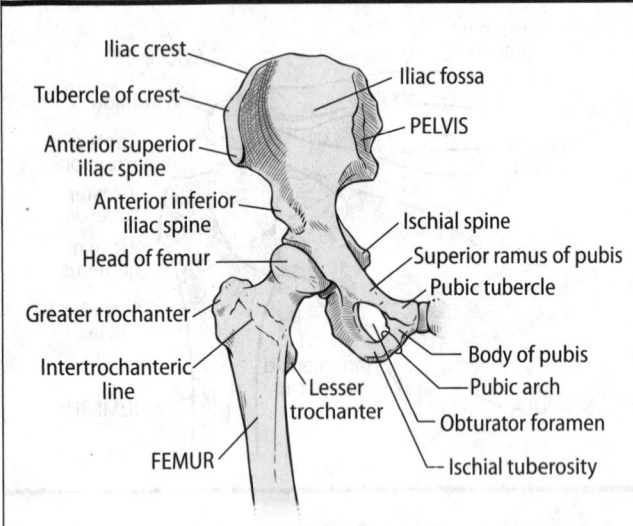

Iliac crest
Tubercle of crest
Anterior superior iliac spine
Anterior inferior iliac spine
Head of femur
Greater trochanter
Intertrochanteric line
FEMUR
Lesser trochanter

Iliac fossa
PELVIS
Ischial spine
Superior ramus of pubis
Pubic tubercle
Body of pubis
Pubic arch
Obturator foramen
Ischial tuberosity

Hip Posterior View

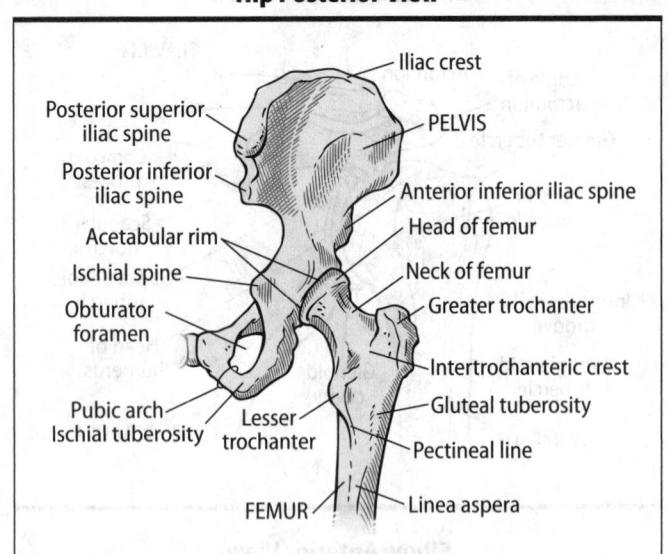

Posterior superior iliac spine
Posterior inferior iliac spine
Acetabular rim
Ischial spine
Obturator foramen
Pubic arch
Ischial tuberosity
Lesser trochanter
FEMUR

Iliac crest
PELVIS
Anterior inferior iliac spine
Head of femur
Neck of femur
Greater trochanter
Intertrochanteric crest
Gluteal tuberosity
Pectineal line
Linea aspera

Knee Anterior View

Lateral epicondyle
Lateral femoral condyle
Lateral tibial condyle
Head of fibula
Neck of fibula
Lateral surface
FIBULA

FEMUR
PATELLA
Adductor tubercle
Medial epicondyle
Medial tibial condyle
Tibial tuberosity
Medial surface
Anterior border
TIBIA

Knee Posterior View

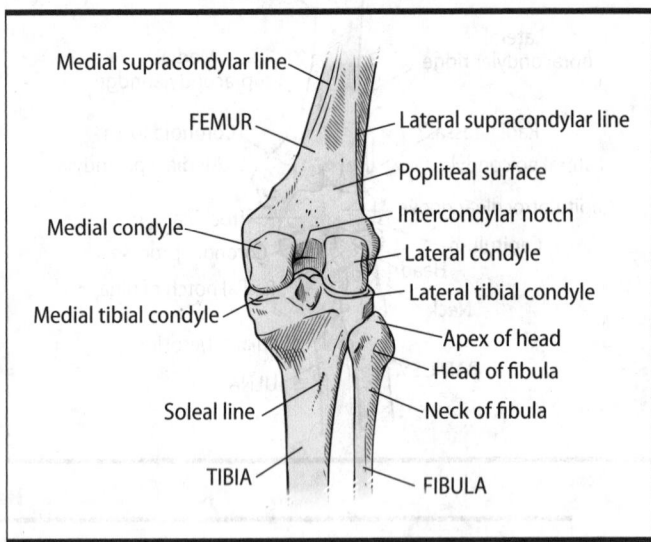

Medial supracondylar line
FEMUR
Medial condyle
Medial tibial condyle
Soleal line
TIBIA

Lateral supracondylar line
Popliteal surface
Intercondylar notch
Lateral condyle
Lateral tibial condyle
Apex of head
Head of fibula
Neck of fibula
FIBULA

Foot

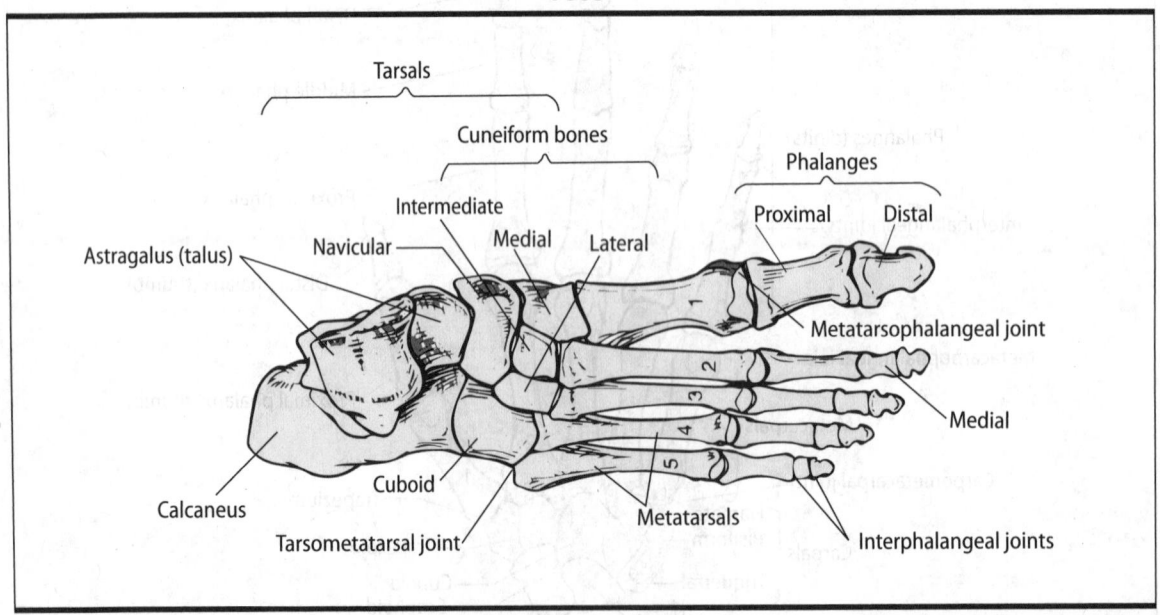

Tarsals
Cuneiform bones
Phalanges
Intermediate
Medial
Lateral
Proximal
Distal
Astragalus (talus)
Navicular
Metatarsophalangeal joint
Calcaneus
Cuboid
Medial
Tarsometatarsal joint
Metatarsals
Interphalangeal joints

Muscles

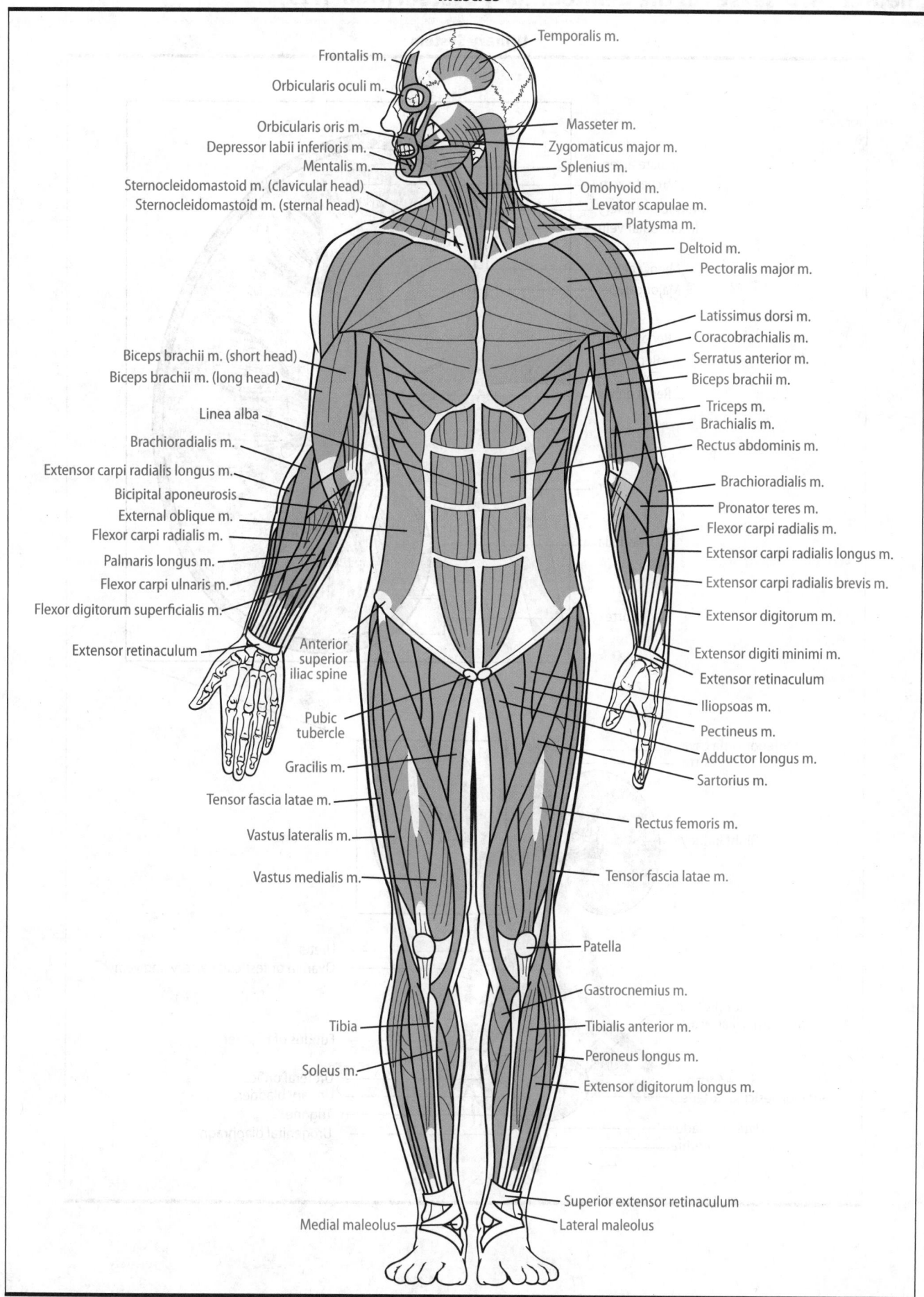

Chapter 14. Diseases of the Genitourinary System (N00–N99)

Urinary System

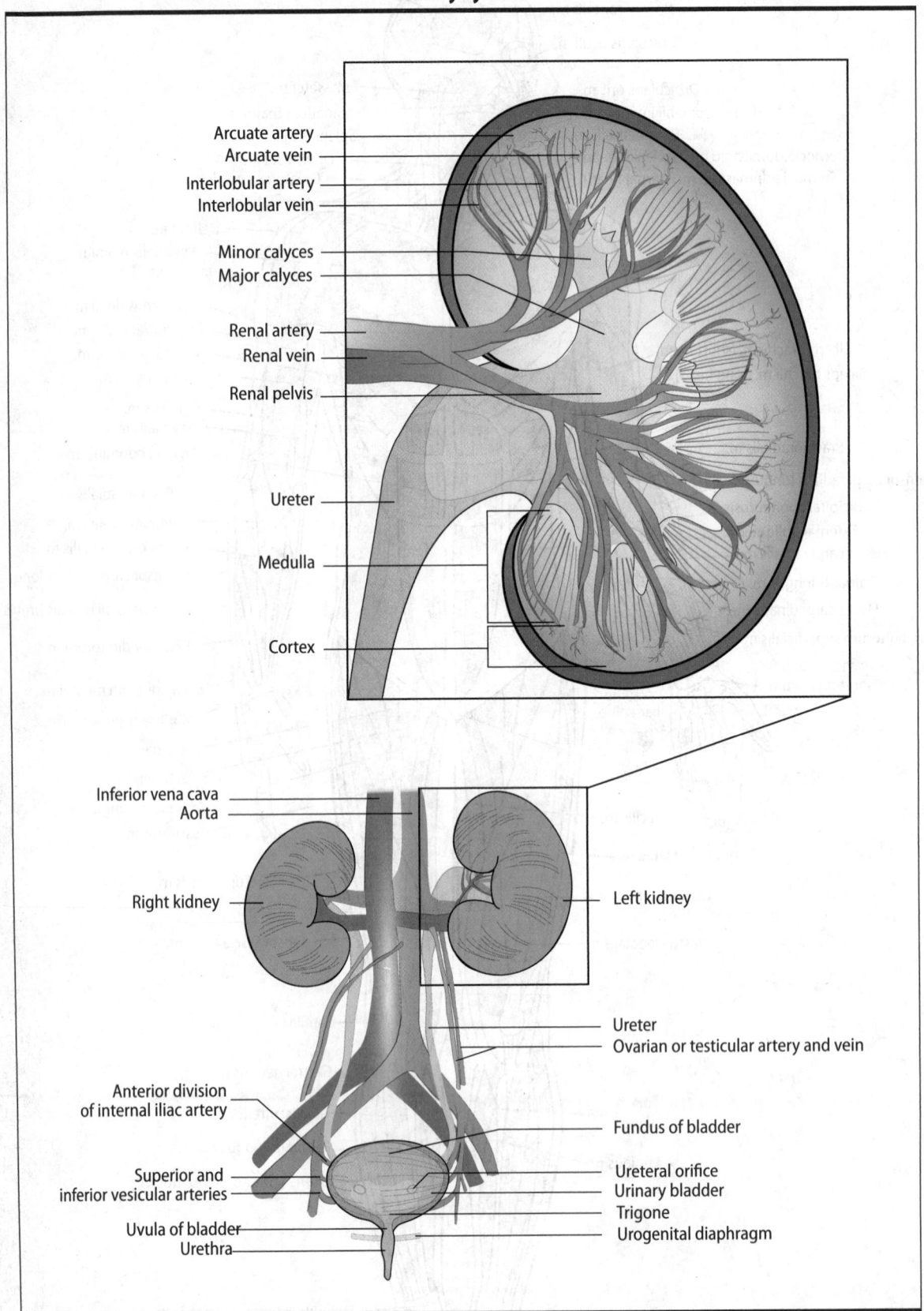

Arcuate artery
Arcuate vein
Interlobular artery
Interlobular vein
Minor calyces
Major calyces
Renal artery
Renal vein
Renal pelvis
Ureter
Medulla
Cortex

Inferior vena cava
Aorta
Right kidney
Left kidney
Ureter
Ovarian or testicular artery and vein
Anterior division
of internal iliac artery
Fundus of bladder
Superior and
inferior vesicular arteries
Ureteral orifice
Urinary bladder
Trigone
Uvula of bladder
Urethra
Urogenital diaphragm

Male Genitourinary System

Female Internal Genitalia

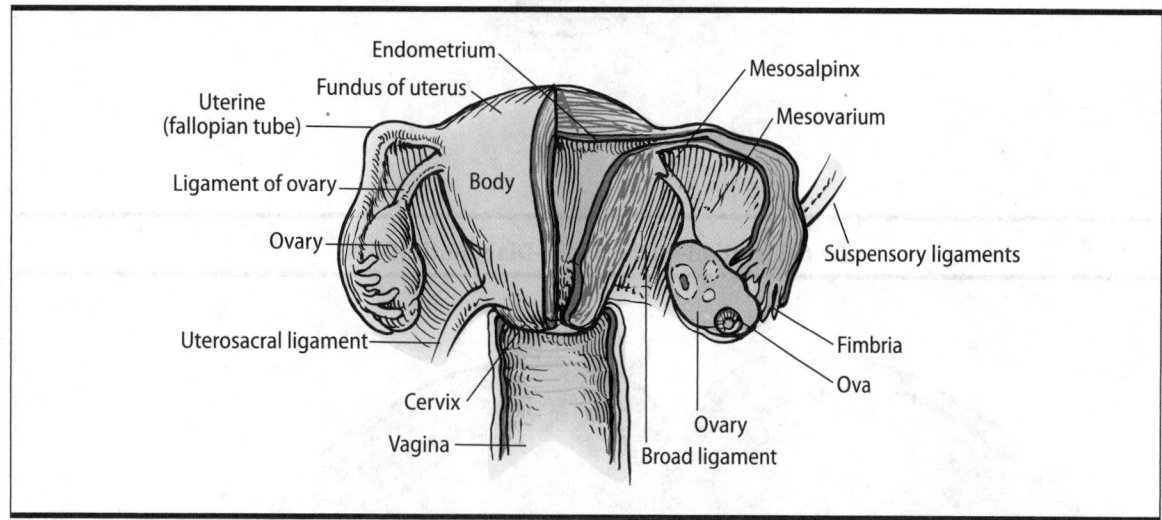

Female Genitourinary Tract Lateral View

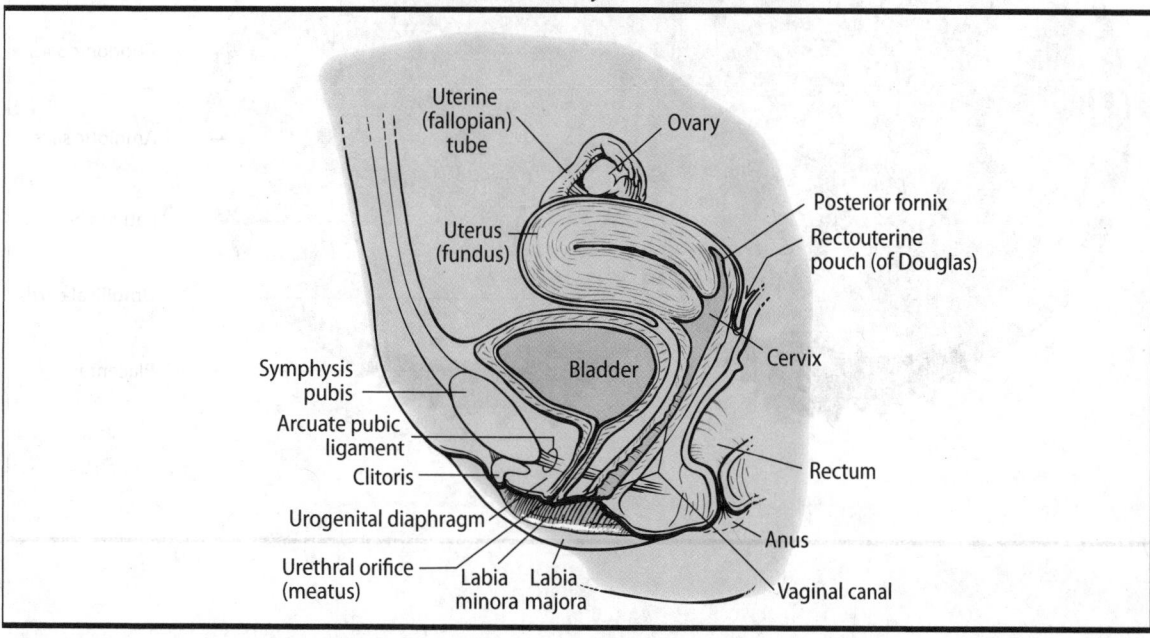

Chapter 15. Pregnancy, Childbirth and the Puerperium (O00–O9A)

Term Pregnancy – Single Gestation

Twin Gestation–Dichorionic–Diamniotic (DI-DI)

Twin Gestation–Monochorionic–Diamniotic (MO-DI)

1 Chorionic sac

2 Amniotic sacs

2 Fetuses

2 Umbilical cords

1 Placenta

Twin Gestation–Monochorionic–Monoamniotic (MO-MO)

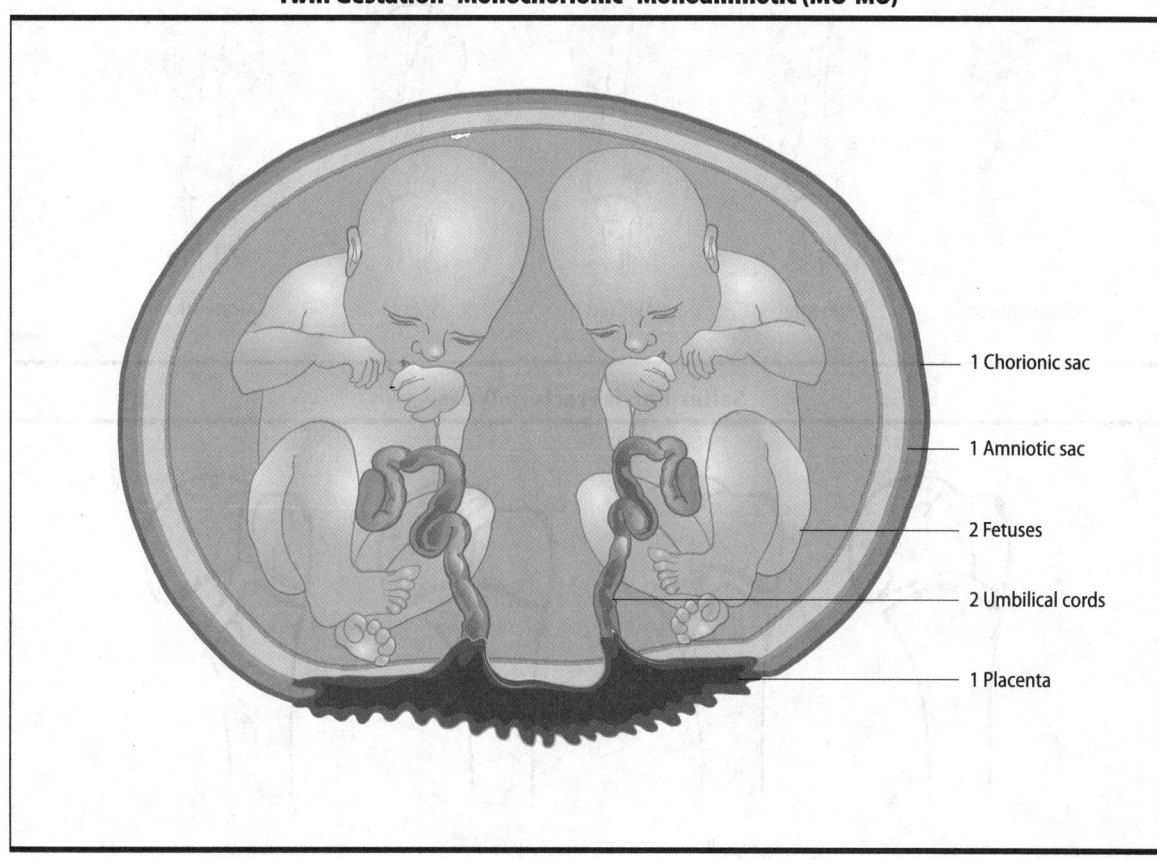

1 Chorionic sac

1 Amniotic sac

2 Fetuses

2 Umbilical cords

1 Placenta

Chapter 19. Injury, Poisoning and Certain Other Consequences of External Causes (SØØ–T88)

Types of Fractures

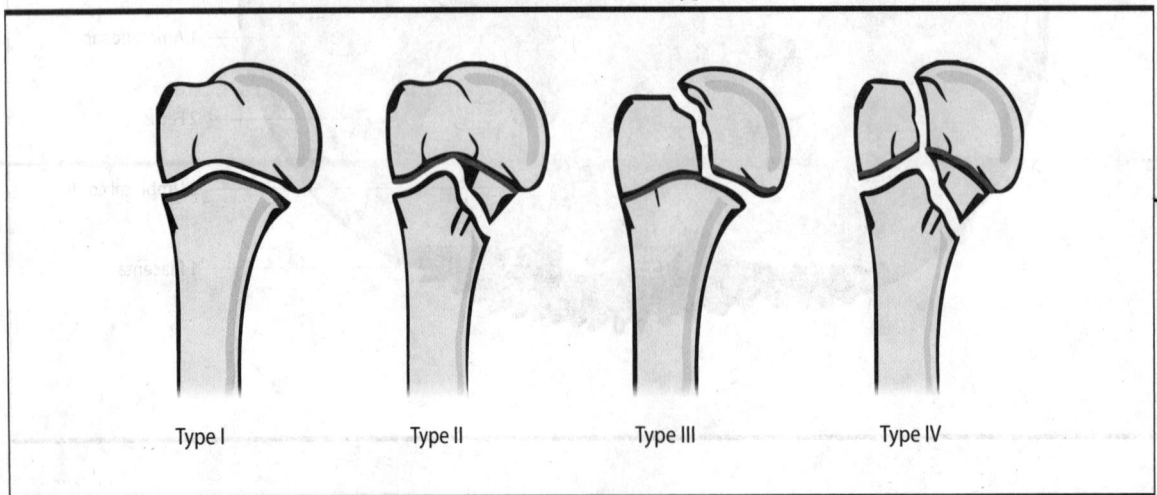

| Normal | Transverse | Open/Compound | Oblique | Oblique displaced |

| Comminuted | Segmental | Avulsed | Spiral | Greenstick |

Salter-Harris Fracture Types

| Type I | Type II | Type III | Type IV |